TABLE 295-3   CAGE Questionnaire

C: Have you ever felt that you should *cut* down on your drinking?
A: Have people ever *annoyed* you by criticizing your drinking?
G: Have you ever felt bad or *guilty* about your drinking?
E: Have you ever had a drink first thing in the morning to steady your nerves or get rid of a hangover (*eye opener*)?

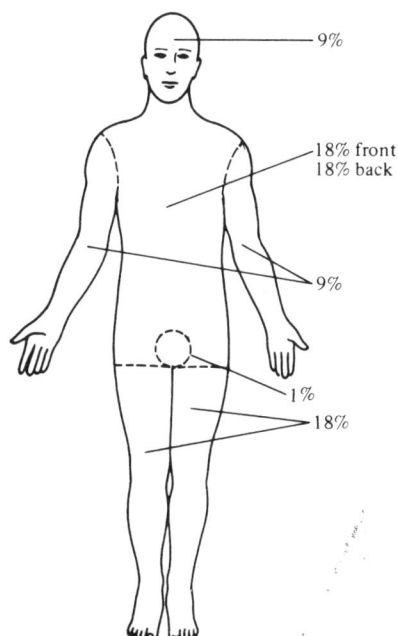

FIG. 199-1. Rule of Nines.

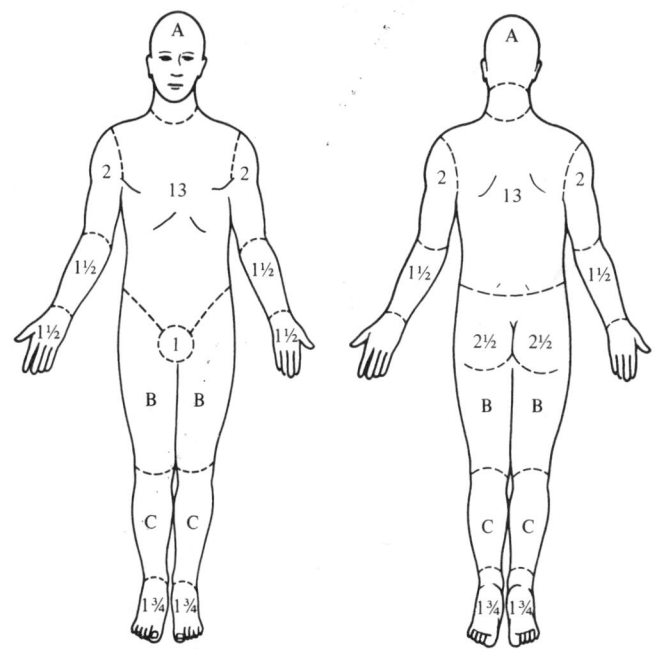

Relative Percentages of Areas Affected by Growth (Age in Years)

	0	1	5	10	15	Adult
A: half of head	9½	8½	6½	5½	4½	3½
B: half of thigh	2¾	3¼	4	4¼	4½	4¾
C: half of leg	2½	2½	2¾	3	3¼	3½

Second-degree _____ and

Third-degree _____ =

Total percent burned _____

FIG. 199-2. Lund and Browder diagram to estimate percentage of pediatric burn.

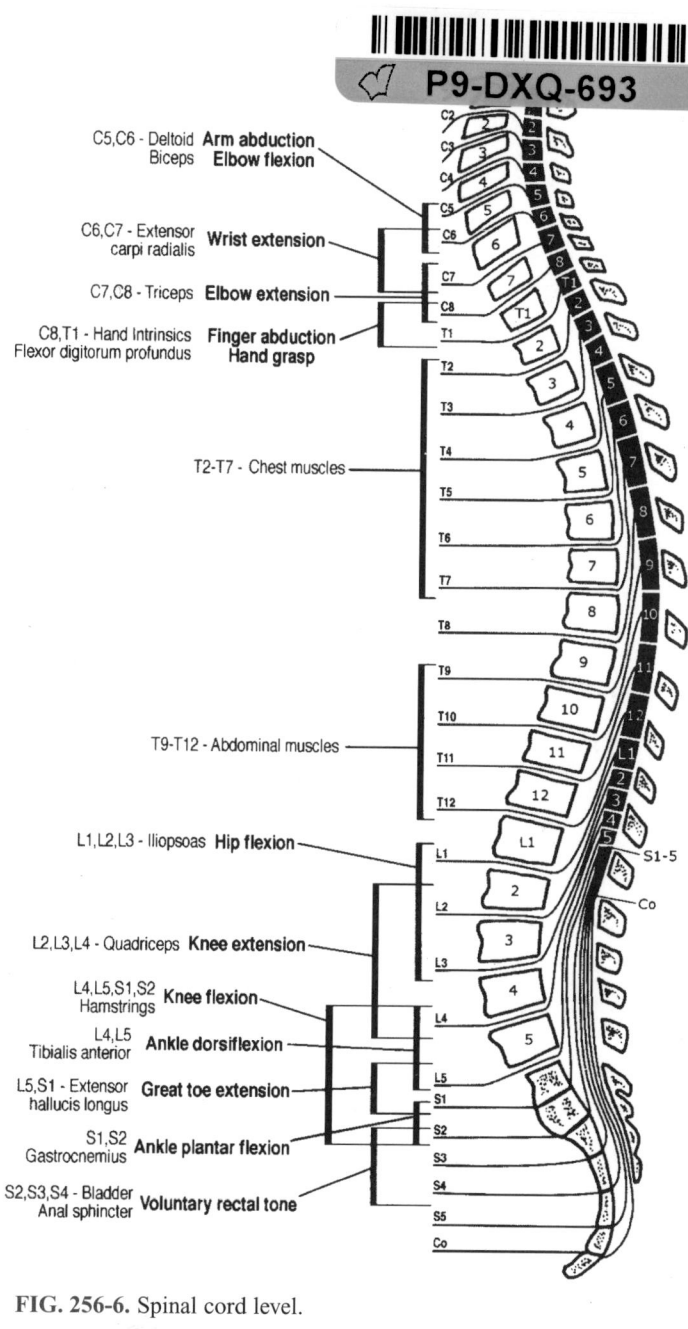

FIG. 256-6. Spinal cord level.

TABLE 199-2   Parkland Formula

Adults
LR 4 mL × weight (kg) × % BSA* over initial 24 h
Half over the first 8 h from the time of burn
Other half over the subsequent 16 h
Example: 70-kg adult with 40% second- and third-degree burns
4 mL × 70 kg × 40 = 11,200 mL over 24 h

Children
LR 3 mL × weight (kg) × % BSA* over initial 24 h plus maintenance
Half over the first 8 h from the time of burn
Other half over the subsequent 16 h

*Second- and third-degree burns only.

EMERGENCY MEDICINE

A COMPREHENSIVE STUDY GUIDE

sixth edition

EMERGENCY MEDICINE

A COMPREHENSIVE STUDY GUIDE

Editor-in-Chief

Judith E. Tintinalli, MD, MS

Professor and Chair
Department of Emergency Medicine
Adjunct Professor
Department of Health Policy and Administration
University of North Carolina at Chapel Hill
Chapel Hill, North Carolina

Co-Editors

Gabor D. Kelen, MD

Professor and Chair
Department of Emergency Medicine
Johns Hopkins University
Baltimore, Maryland

J. Stephan Stapczynski, MD

Professor and Former Chair
Department of Emergency Medicine
University of Kentucky College of Medicine
Lexington, Kentucky

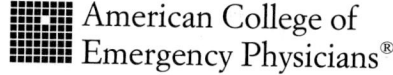 American College of
Emergency Physicians®

McGraw-Hill

Medical Publishing Division

New York   Chicago   San Francisco   Lisbon   London   Madrid   Mexico City   Milan   New Delhi
San Juan   Seoul   Singapore   Sydney   Toronto

EMERGENCY MEDICINE: A Comprehensive Study Guide

5 6 7 8 9 0   DOW/DOW   0 9 8 7

ISBN: 0-07-138875-3

This book was set in Times New Roman by ATLIS Graphics, Inc.
The editors were Andrea Seils, Nicky Fernando, and Michelle Watt.
The production supervisor was Catherine H. Saggese.
The cover designer was Aimee Nordin.
The index was prepared by Jerry Ralya.
RR Donnelley was the printer and binder.
This book is printed on acid-free paper.

LIBRARY OF CONGRESS CATALOGING-IN-PUBLICATION DATA
Emergency medicine : a comprehensive study guide / [edited by] Judith E. Tintinalli,
Gabor D. Kelen, J. Stephan Stapczynski.—6th ed.
        p. ; cm.
    Includes bibliographical references and index.
    ISBN: 0-07-138875-3
        1. Emergency medicine.   I. Tintinalli, Judith E. II. Kelen, Gabor D.
III. Stapczynski, J. Stephan.
        [DNLM: 1. Emergency Medicine. 2. Emergencies. WB 105 E552 2004]
    RC86.7 .E57828 2004
    616.02'5—dc21

To students and practitioners of Emergency Medicine around the world.
JET

To Laurie, Ardie and Mikey, whose love and support sustained me through this endeavor.
GDK

To those who have taught me, my gratitude for their patience and wisdom; to those I have taught, my encouragement for life-long learning.
JSS

CONTENTS

Section One Prehospital Care 1

Section Two Disaster Preparedness 27

Section Three Resuscitative Problems and Techniques 61

Section Four Shock 219

Section Five Analgesia, Anesthesia, and Sedation 257

Section Six Emergency Wound Management 287

Section Seven Cardiovascular Disease 333

Section Eight Pulmonary Emergencies 437

Section Nine Gastrointestinal Emergencies 487

Section Ten Renal and Genitourinary Disorders 593

Section Eleven Gynecology and Obstetrics 647

Section Twelve Pediatrics 727

Section Thirteen Infectious Diseases 909

Section Fourteen Toxicology and Pharmacology 1015

Section Fifteen Environmental Injuries 1175

Section Sixteen Emergency Medicine in Unique Environments 1251

Section Seventeen Endocrine Emergencies 1283

Section Eighteen Hematologic and Oncologic Emergencies 1319

Section Nineteen Neurology 1369

Section Twenty Eye, Ear, Nose, Throat, and Oral Surgery 1449

Section Twenty-One Disorders of the Skin 1507

Section Twenty-Two Trauma 1537

Section Twenty-Three Injuries to the Bones, Joints, and Soft Tissue 1651

Section Twenty-Four Nontraumatic Musculoskeletal Disorders 1769

Section Twenty-Five Psychosocial Disorders 1807

Section Twenty-Six Abuse and Assault 1847

Section Twenty-Seven Principles of Imaging 1865

Section Twenty-Eight Special Situations 1891

Color plates fall between pages 1542 and 1543.

CONTRIBUTORS*

STEPHANIE B. ABBUHL, MD [304]
Associate Professor and Medical Director
Department of Emergency Medicine
Hospital of the University of PA
University of PA School of Medicine
Philadelphia, Pennsylvania

RIYAD B. ABU-LABAN, MD, MHSc [87]
Assistant Professor and Research Director
Division of Emergency Medicine
University of British Columbia
Department of Emergency Medicine
Vancouver General Hospital
Vancouver, British Columbia, Canada

WILLIAM AHRENS, MD [132]
Director of Pediatric Emergency Medicine
University of Illinois
Chicago, Illinois

MICHAEL F. ALTIERI, MD [140]
Associate Clinical Professor of Emergency Medicine
George Washington University
Washington, DC
Inova-Fairfax Hospital for Children
Department of Pediatrics
Falls Church, Virginia

ERIC ANDERSON, MD, MBA [64]
Associate Director of Operations
Department of Emergency Medicine
The Cleveland Clinic Foundation
Assistant Professor of Emergency Medicine
The Ohio State University
Cleveland, Ohio

WILLIAM T. ANDERSON, MD [150]
Chief, Department of Emergency Medicine
William Beaumont Hospital
Troy, Michigan

THOMAS P. AUFDERHEIDE, MD [85]
Professor of Emergency Medicine and Research Director
Medical College of Wisconsin
Department of Emergency Medicine
Milwaukee, Wisconsin

CHENICHERI BALAKRISHNAN, MD [199]
Associate Professor of Surgery
Department of Emergency Medicine
Wayne State University
Detroit Receiving Hospital
Detroit, Michigan

JEFFREY D. BAND, MD [148]
Director, Infectious Diseases and International Medicine
William Beaumont Hospital
Royal Oak, Michigan
Clinical Professor of Medicine
Wayne State University School of Medicine
Detroit, Michigan

JOSEPH A. BARBERA, MD [7]
Associate Professor of Engineering Management
Clinical Associate Professor of Emergency Medicine
Co-Director, Institute for Crisis, Disaster, and Risk Management
The George Washington University
Washington, DC

ROBERT A. BARISH, MD [76]
Associate Dean for Clinical Affairs
Professor of Emergency Medicine and Surgery
University of Maryland School of Medicine
Baltimore, Maryland

BONNY J. BARON, MD [256, 258]
Associate Professor
Department of Emergency Medicine
State University of New York Downstate Medical Center
Director of Trauma, Emergency Department
Kings County Hospital Center
Brooklyn, New York

CHRISTOPHER W. BARTON, MD [24]
Clinical Professor of Medicine
University of California San Francisco
Medical Director, Emergency Services
San Francisco General Hospital
San Francisco, California

DANIEL G. BATTON, MD [118]
Director, Neonatal Intensive Care Unit
William Beaumont Hospital
Royal Oak, Michigan

BRIGITTE M. BAUMANN, MD, DTM&H [306]
Head, Division of Clinical Research
Department of Emergency Medicine
UMDNJ-Robert Wood Johnson Medical School
Cooper Health System
Camden, New Jersey

NORMAN J. BEAUCHAMP, JR., MD [237]
Professor and Chair
University of Washington
Department of Radiology
Seattle, Washington

RONALD W. BEAUDREAU, DMD, MD [242]
Doctor's Hospital
Department of Emergency Medicine
Augusta, Georgia
Medical Evacuation Services
SOS International
Shanghai, China

MARY HARKINS BECKER, MD [80]
Department of Emergency Medicine
Maine Medical Center
Assistant Clinical Professor
Department of Surgery
University of Vermont
Portland, Maine

*The numbers in brackets following the contributors' names indicate the chapter(s) written or cowritten by that contributor.

MARY P. BEDARD, MD [13]
Clinical Director, Neonatal Intensive Care Unit
Medical Director, Transport Program
Children's Hospital of Michigan
Associate Professor of Pediatrics
Wayne State University
Detroit, Michigan

AMY J. BEHRMAN, MD [109]
Associate Professor
Department of Emergency Medicine
Director, Occupational Medicine
Hospital of the University of Pennsylvania
Philadelphia, Pennsylvania

WILLIAM A. BERK, MD [21, 166, 295]
Associate Professor
Department of Emergency Medicine
Wayne State University
Vice-Chief, Emergency Department
Detroit Receiving Hospital
Detroit, Michigan

CAROL D. BERKOWITZ, MD [115, 119, 297]
Executive Vice Chair and Professor
Department of Pediatrics
Harbor-UCLA Medical Center
David Geffen School of Medicine at UCLA
Torrance, California

EDWARD BERNSTEIN, MD [295]
Professor and Vice Chair for Academic Affairs
Department of Emergency Medicine
Boston University School of Medicine
Professor of Social and Behavioral Sciences
Boston University School of Public Health
Boston, Massachusetts

JUDITH BERNSTEIN, RNC, PhD [295]
Associate Professor
Department of Maternal and Child Health
Boston University School of Public Health
Director, MCH Certificate Program
Boston University School of Medicine
Department of Emergency Medicine
Boston, Massachusetts

HOWARD A. BESSEN, MD [192]
Professor of Medicine
UCLA School of Medicine
Los Angeles, California
Director, Emergency Medicine Residency Program
Department of Emergency Medicine
Harbor-UCLA Medical Center
Torrance, California

EDWARD S. BESSMAN, MD [22]
Assistant Professor
Department of Emergency Medicine
The Johns Hopkins University
Baltimore, Maryland
Clinical Director
Department of Emergency Medicine
Johns Hopkins Bayview Medical Center
Baltimore, Maryland

MICHAEL B. BEUHLER, MD [180]
Medical Director
Carolinas Poison Center
Charlotte, North Carolina
Adjunct Instructor of Emergency Medicine
University of North Carolina at Chapel Hill
Chapel Hill, North Carolina

JESSICA L. BIENSTOCK, MD [105]
Residency Program Director
Assistant Professor
Johns Hopkins Hospital
Baltimore, Maryland

PAUL BLACKBURN, DO [225]
Residency Program Director
Department of Emergency Medicine
Maricopa Medical Center
Phoenix, Arizona

BARBARA K. BLOK, MD [52]
Assistant Professor
Department of Emergency Medicine
Johns Hopkins Hospital
Baltimore, Maryland

DAVID A. BLUEMKE, MD, PhD [61]
Associate Professor, Radiology
Clinical Director, MRI
Johns Hopkins University and Hospital
Department of Radiology
Baltimore, Maryland

ANDY BOGGUST, MD [2]
Department of Emergency Medicine
Mayo Clinic School of Medicine
Rochester, Minnesota

MARK P. BOGNER, MD [94, 97]
Assistant Clinical Professor
Department of Emergency Medicine
University of Wisconsin Medical School
Madison, Wisconsin

EDMUND BOLTON, MD [28]
EM Healthcare Physicians
Westmont, Illinois

MICHAEL J. BONO, MD [91]
Associate Professor
Associate Residency Program Director
Department of Emergency Medicine
Eastern Virginia Medical School
Norfolk, Virginia

ASHLEY E. BOOTH, MD [142]
University of Florida Health Sciences Center-Jacksonville
Department of Emergency Medicine
Jacksonville, Florida

CARL BOSE, MD [4]
Chief, Division of Neonatal-Perinatal Medicine
Professor of Pediatrics
University of North Carolina
Chapel Hill, North Carolina

GEORGE M. BOSSE, MD [164]
Associate Professor of Emergency Medicine
Department of Emergency Medicine
University of Louisville
Medical Director-Kentucky Regional Poison Center
Louisville, Kentucky

SHARON A. BOSWELL, RN, BSN, CRNP [260]
Clinical Nurse Practitioner
R. Adams Cowley Shock Trauma Center
Baltimore, Maryland

JAMES K. BOUZOUKIS, MD [82]
Department of Emergency Medicine
Medical Center of Delaware
Wilmington, Delaware

WILLIAM M. BOWLING, MD [259]
Department of Surgery
Washington University School of Medicine
St. Louis, Missouri

WILLIAM J. BRADY, MD [85, 161, 210, 245, 246]
Associate Professor
Vice Chair and Program Director of Emergency Medicine
Department of Emergency Medicine
University of Virginia School of Medicine
Charlottesville, Virginia
Medical Director
Charlottesville-Albemarle Rescue Squad
Charlottesville, Virginia

G. RICHARD BRAEN, MD [186]
Professor and Chairman
Department of Emergency Medicine
State University of New York at Buffalo
Buffalo, New York

ANNE F. BRAYER, MD [204]
Assistant Professor of Emergency Medicine and Pediatrics
University of Rochester School of Medicine
Department of Emergency Medicine
Rochester, New York

JASON H. BREDENKAMP, MD [270]
Rockford Memorial Hospital
Department of Emergency Medicine
Rockford, Illinois

JANE H. BRICE, MD, MPH [153]
Assistant Professor
Department of Emergency Medicine
Medical Director, Orange County Emergency Medical Services
University of North Carolina
Chapel Hill, North Carolina

JOSHUA S. BRODER, MD [86]
Assistant Professor
Coordinator, International Programs
Department of Emergency Medicine
University of North Carolina at Chapel Hill
Chapel Hill, North Carolina

TONIA J. BROUSSEAU, DO [117]
Department of Emergency Medicine
Division of Pediatric Emergency Medicine
The University of Florida Health Science Center
Jacksonville, Florida

JAMES BROWN, MD [294]
Assistant Professor and Residency Program Director
Wright State University
Department of Emergency Medicine
Dayton, Ohio

KATHLEEN BROWN, MD [123]
State University of New York—Upstate
Department of Emergency Medicine
Syracuse, New York

ROBERT A. BROWNSTEIN, MD [143]
Department of Emergency Medicine
Rex Hospital
Raleigh, North Carolina

G. RICHARD BRUNO, MD [172, 181, 187]
Director of Emergency Services
University Hospital Brooklyn
Assistant Professor of Emergency Medicine
Vice Chairman for Clinical Services
Department of Emergency Medicine
SUNY Downstate Medical Center
State University of New York
Brooklyn, New York

TIMOTHY G. BUCHMAN, PhD., MD [259]
Edison Professor of Surgery
Professor of Anesthesiology and Medicine
Department of Surgery
Washington University in St. Louis
St. Louis, Missouri

BRIAN E. BURGESS, MD [82]
Clinical Assistant Professor of Emergency Medicine
Jefferson Medical College
Attending Physician, Christiana Care Health System
Newark, Delaware
Clinical Assistant Professor
Physician Assistant Program
Drexel University School of Nursing
Hockessin, Delaware

JOHN H. BURTON, MD [286]
Research Director
Department of Emergency Medicine
Maine Medical Center
Portland, Maine

DAVID G. CALDICOTT, MD [196]
Emergency and Trauma Registrar
Royal Adelaide Hospital
Adelaide, South Australia
Australia

MARY CAMARCA, MD [140]
Division of Pediatric Emergency Medicine
Inova Fairfax Hospital for Children
Falls Church, Virginia

DONNA L. CARDEN, MD [146]
Professor of Emergency and Internal Medicine
Louisiana State University Health Sciences Center
Departments of Internal & Emergency Medicine
   and Molecular & Cellular Physiology
Shreveport, Lousiana

TERESA M. CARLIN, MD [175]
St. Christopher's Hospital for Children
Division of Pediatric Emergency Medicine
Philadelphia, Pennsylvania
Instructor, Department of Emergency Medicine
Johns Hopkins University School of Medicine
Baltimore, Maryland

STUART CARR, MD [34]
Assistant Clinical Professor
Stollery Children's Hospital
Department of Pediatrics
Edmonton, Alberta
Canada

WALLACE A. CARTER, MD [41, 44, 172, 181, 187]
Emergency Medicine Residency Director
New York Presbyterian Hospital
Associate Professor of Emergency Medicine
Weill Medical College of Cornell University
Associate Professor of Medicine
College of Physicians & Surgeons of Columbia University
New York, New York

CHRISTINA L. CATLETT, MD [10, 232]
Assistant Professor
Johns Hopkins Hospital
Department of Emergency Medicine
Baltimore, Maryland

ALAN L. CAUSEY, MD [198]
Clinical Assistant Professor of Pediatrics and Medicine
University of South Florida College of Medicine
Tampa, Florida
Attending Physician, Pediatric Emergency Medicine
Tampa General Hospital
Tampa, Florida
Attending Physician
All Children's Hospital
St. Petersburg, Florida

EUGENE E. CEPEDA, MD [13]
Director, Newborn Nursery
Hutzel Hospital
Assistant Professor of Pediatrics
Wayne State University
Detroit, Michigan

RICHARD C. CHANDLER, MD [284]
Associate Program Director
Emergency Medicine Residency
Maine Medical Center
Department of Emergency Medicine
Portland, Maine

ARJUN CHANMUGAM, MD, MBA [57, 177]
Assistant Professor and Residency Director
The Johns Hopkins University School of Medicine
Department of Emergency Medicine
Baltimore, Maryland

MICHAEL E. CHANSKY, MD [211]
Chair, Department of Emergency Medicine
Associate Professor of Emergency Medicine and Internal Medicine
Robert Wood Johnson Medical School/Camden
The Cooper Health System
Camden, New Jersey

BENNETT CHIN, MD [61]
Assistant Professor
Department of Radiology
Johns Hopkins University and Hospital
Baltimore, Maryland

ANIL CHOPRA, MD [59]
Assistant Professor
Department of Medicine
University Health Network
University of Toronto
Toronto, Ontario
Canada

RICHARD A. CHRISTOPH, MD [136]
Front Royal Pediatrics
Front Royal, Virginia

PATTY CHU, MD [222]
Department of Emergency Medicine
Methodist Willowbrook Hospital
Houston, Texas

RICHARD F. CLARK, MD [194]
Professor of Medicine
Director, UCSD Division of Medical Toxicology
Medical Director, San Diego Division
California Poison Control System
UCSD Medical Center
San Diego, California

ELIZABETH A. CLEMENTS, PharmD [29]
Clinical Specialist Emergency Medicine
Adjunct Assistant Professor
Department of Pharmacy Practice
Spectrum Health Butterworth Campus
Grand Rapids, Michigan
Assistant Professor
Department of Emergency Medicine
Wayne State University
Detroit, Michigan

DAVID M. CLINE, MD [39, 54]
Associate Professor and Research Director
Wake Forest University
Baptist Medical Center
Department of Emergency Medicine
Winston-Salem, North Carolina

REB CLOSE, MD [102]
Department of Emergency Medicine
Hospital of the Monterey Peninsula
Monterey, California

WENDY C. COATES, MD [43]
Director Emergency Medicine Education
Harbor-UCLA Medical Center
Associate Professor of Medicine
Vice-Chair, Acute Care College
David Geffen School of Medicine at UCLA
Torrance, California

DANIEL J. COBAUGH, PharmD [162]
Finger Lakes Regional Poison and Drug Information Center
Assistant Professor
Department of Emergency Medicine
University of Rochester Medical Center
Rochester, New York

IRENE COLETSOS, MS [295]
University of Massachusetts School of Medicine
Worcester, Massachusetts

STEPHEN A. COLUCCIELLO, MD [257]
Assistant Chair
Director of Clinical Services and Trauma Coordinator
Department of Emergency Medicine
Carolinas Medical Center
Charlotte, North Carolina
Assistant Clinical Professor
Department of Emergency Medicine
University of North Carolina at Chapel Hill
Chapel Hill, North Carolina

ALASDAIR K. T. CONN, MD [261]
Chief of Emergency Services
Massachusetts General Hospital
Assistant Professor of Surgery
Harvard Medical School
Boston, Massachusetts

MARCO COPPOLA, DO [282]
Professor of Emergency Medicine
Texas A&M University System Health Science Center
Temple, Texas

RANDOLPH CORDLE, MD [129, 133]
Department of Pediatric Emergency Medicine
Boise, Idaho

EDWARD E. CORNWELL, III, MD [251]
Associate Professor Surgery, Anesthesiology and Critical Care Medicine
Johns Hopkins Hospital
Department of Surgery
Baltimore, Maryland

C. JAMES CORRALL, MD, MPH [120]
Clinical Associate Professor of Emergency Medicine and Pediatrics
Adjunct Associate Professor of Clinical Pharmacology
Department of Emergency Medicine
Emergency Medicine and Trauma Center
Methodist Hospital of Indiana
Indiana University School of Medicine
Indianapolis, Indiana

FRANCIS L. COUNSELMAN, MD [279]
EVMS Distinguished Professor of Emergency Medicine
Chairman and Program Director
Department of Emergency Medicine
Eastern Virginia Medical School and
    Emergency Physicians of Tidewater
Norfolk, Virginia

PAT CROSKERRY, MD, PhD [312]
Associate Professor
Dalhousie University
Halifax, Nova Scotia
Canada
Dartmouth General Hospital
Department of Emergency Medicine
Dartmouth, Nova Scotia
Canada

NATALIE CULLEN, MD [130]
Department of Emergency Medicine
Wright State University
Dayton, Ohio

RITA K. CYDULKA, MD, MS [68, 69]
Associate Professor
Department of Emergency Medicine
Case Western Reserve University School of Medicine
Department of Emergency Medicine
MetroHealth Medical Center
Cleveland, Ohio

FRANK F. S. DALY, MD, MBBS [195]
Rocky Mountain Poison and Drug Center
University of Colorado Health Sciences Center
Denver, Colorado

DANIEL F. DANZL, MD [19]
Professor and Chair
Department of Emergency Medicine
University of Louisville School of Medicine
Louisville, Kentucky

RICHARD C. DART, MD, PhD [195]
Director, Rocky Mountain Poison and Drug Center
Denver Health Authority
Professor, University of Colorado Health Sciences Center
Denver, Colorado

ELIZABETH M. DATNER, MD [16]
Assistant Professor of Emergency Medicine
University of Pennsylvania School of Medicine
Department of Emergency Medicine
Philadelphia, Pennsylvania

MOHAK DAVE, MD [69]
Department of Emergency Medicine
Case Western Reserve University/MetroHealth Medical Center
Cleveland, Ohio

DANIEL J. DEBEHNKE, MD [246]
Associate Professor of Emergency Medicine
Director of Clinical Operations and Vice Chair
Department of Emergency Medicine
Medical College of Wisconsin
Milwaukee, Wisconsin

KATHLEEN A. DELANEY, MD [188]
Professor of Emergency Medicine
University of Texas Southwestern Medical Center
Dallas, Texas

GEORGE DELGADO, JR., PharmD [157]
Clinical Pharmacy Specialist
Emergency Medicine, Coordinator
Emergency Medicine Specialty Residency
Adjunct Assistant Professor
Pharmacy Practice, Wayne State University
Detroit Receiving Hospital & University Health Center
Department of Pharmacy Services
Detroit, Michigan

DAVID DELLA-GIUSTINA, MD [282, 283]
Chairman and Program Director
Emergency Medicine Residency
Madigan Army Medical Center
Department of Emergency Medicine
Tacoma, Washington

CHRISTOPHER J. DENNY, MD [227]
Division of Emergency Medicine
Faculty of Medicine
University of Toronto
Toronto, Ontario
Canada
Sunnybrook and Women's Hospital
Institute for Clinical Evaluative Sciences
Toronto, Ontario
Canada

CHAYAN C. DEY, MD, MPH [206]
Assistant Professor
Director, International Emergency Medicine Fellowship Program
Department of Emergency Medicine
Johns Hopkins University
Baltimore, Maryland

DEBORAH B. DIERCKS, MD [51]
Assistant Professor of Internal Medicine and Emergency Medicine
University of California
Davis Medical Center
Sacramento, California

GAIL D'ONOFRIO, MD [295]
Associate Professor
Yale University School of Medicine
Director of Research
Section of Emergency Medicine
Yale New Haven Hospital
New Haven, Connecticut

SUZANNE DOYON, MD [167]
Medical Director
Maryland Poison Center
Baltimore, Maryland

WILLIAM DRIBBEN, MD [174]
Assistant Professor
Division of Emergency Medicine
Washington University School of Medicine
St. Louis, Missouri

OLLY DUCKETT, MD [139]
Assistant Director, Pediatric Emergency Medicine
Wake Medical Center
Raleigh, North Carolina
Adjunct Instructor
Department of Emergency Medicine
University of North Carolina at Chapel Hill

COL. EDWARD M. EITZEN, JR., MD, MPH [8, 185]
Chief
Division of Operational Medicine
USAMRIID
Ft. Detrick, Maryland
Associate Clinical Professor
Uniformed Services
University of the Health Sciences
Bethesda, Maryland

STEFANIE R. ELLISON, MD [273]
Assistant Professor
Department of Emergency Medicine
Truman Medical Center and University of Missouri-Kansas City
Kansas City, Missouri

CHARLES L. EMERMAN, MD [63, 173]
Professor and Chairman
Department of Emergency Medicine
MetroHealth Medical Center
Cleveland, Ohio

JOHN ENG, MD [302]
Assistant Professor of Radiology
Department of Radiology and Radiological Science
Johns Hopkins University
Baltimore, Maryland

RAKESH ENGINEER, MD [96]
Cleveland Clinic Foundation
Department of Emergency Medicine
Cleveland, Ohio

MERT EROGUL, MD [99]
Assistant Professor
State University of New York
Downstate Medical Center
Department of Emergency Medicine
Brooklyn, New York

ROBERT H. ESCARZA, MD [269]
Clinical Assistant Professor of Surgery
Department of Surgery
University of Illinois College of Medicine at Rockford
Rockford Memorial Hospital
Rockford, Illinois

BRIAN EUERLE, MD [35]
Assistant Professor
University of Maryland School of Medicine
Department of Emergency Medicine
Baltimore, Maryland

RAWDEN EVANS, MD, PhD [86]
Assistant Professor
Department of Emergency Medicine
University of Michigan Medical Center
Ann Arbor, Michigan

MARTIN L. FACKLER, MD [264]
President
International Wound Ballistics Association
Hawthorne, Florida

KIM M. FELDHAUS, MD [298]
Associate Professor
Division of Emergency Medicine
Denver Health Medical Center
University of Colorado Health Sciences Center
Denver, Colorado

RAYMOND M. FISH, MD, PhD [201, 202]
Adjunct Professor in Bioengineering
Electrical and Computer Engineering
University of Illinois, Urbana-Champaign
Clinical Assistant Professor of Emergency Medicine
The Medical School at the University of Illinois
Urbana, Illinois

DENIS J. FITZGERALD, MD [78]
Assistant Professor of Military and Emergency Medicine
Uniformed Services University of the Health Sciences
Adjunct Assistant Professor of Emergency Medicine
University of Cincinnati
Cincinnati, Ohio

STEVEN G. FOLSTAD, MD, [152]
Mid-Atlantic Emergency Medical Associates
Charlotte, North Carolina

KIMBERLEY B. FORTNER, MD [107]
Division of Emergency Medicine
University of Toronto
Sunnybrook and Women's College Health Sciences Center
Toronto, Ontario, Canada

MARK W. FOURRE, MD [285]
Program Director
Emergency Medicine Residency
Maine Medical Center
Portland, Maine
Associate Professor of Surgery
University of Vermont School of Medicine
Burlington, Vermont

DAVID R. FOWLER, MD [265]
Chief Medical Examiner State of Maryland
Maryland Forensic Medicine Center
Office of the Chief Medical Examiner
Baltimore, Maryland

HAROLD E. FOX, MD, MS [105]
Professor and Chair
Residency Program Director
Obstetrician/Gynecologist-in-Chief
Department of OB/GYN
Johns Hopkins University School of Medicine
Johns Hopkins Hospital
Baltimore, Maryland

WILLIAM J. FROHNA, MD [281]
Chair, Department of Emergency Medicine
Franklin Square Hospital Center
Baltimore, Maryland
Attending Physician
Department of Emergency Medicine
Washington Hospital Center and Children's National Medical Center
Washington, DC

SUSAN FUCHS, MD [121]
Associate Professor of Pediatrics
Feinberg School of Medicine
Northwestern University
Associate Director
Division of Pediatric Emergency Medicine
Children's Memorial Hospital
Chicago, Illinois

WADE R. GAASCH, MD [76]
Assistant Professor of Surgery
Division of Emergency Medicine
University of Maryland School of Medicine
Baltimore, Maryland

E. JOHN GALLAGHER, MD [72]
Professor and University Chair
Department of Emergency Medicine
Albert Einstein College of Medicine
Bronx, New York

FIONA E. GALLAHUE, MD [44]
Associate Residency Director
New York Methodist Hospital
Department of Emergency Medicine
Brooklyn, New York

DAVID R. GENS, MD [20]
Associate Professor of Surgery
R. Adams Cowley Shock Trauma Center
Program in Trauma at the University of Maryland School of Medicine
Baltimore, Maryland

WILLIE GILFORD, JR., MD [123]
Assistant Professor of Emergency Medicine
University of Alabama at Birmingham
Department of Emergency Medicine
Birmingham, Alabama

JEFFREY N. GLASPY, MD [274]
Assistant Professor of Emergency Medicine
Associate Residency Program Director
UMKC-Truman Medical Center
Department of Emergency Medicine
Kansas City, Missouri

LEWIS R. GOLDFRANK, MD [310]
Professor and Chair
Department of Emergency Medicine
New York University Medical Center
Bellevue Hospital Center
New York, New York

BRIAN GOLDMAN, MD [231]
Staff Emergency Physician
Mount Sinai Hospital
Toronto, Canada
Assistant Professor
Department of Family and Community Medicine
University of Toronto
Toronto, Ontario
Canada

PHILLIP V. GORDON, MD, PhD [4]
Assistant Professor of Pediatrics
Division of Neonatology
University of Virginia Health Science Center
Department of Pediatrics
Charlottesville, Virginia

SUSAN J. GOTTLIEB, PhD [291]
Department of Psychiatry
William Beaumont Hospital
Royal Oak, Michigan

CHARLES S. GRAFFEO, MD [214]
Associate Professor
Eastern Virginia Medical School
Department of Emergency Medicine
Norfolk, Virginia

MATTHEW C. GRATTON, MD [77]
Associate Professor
Department of Emergency Medicine
Truman Medical Center
University of Missouri at Kansas City School of Medicine
Kansas City, Missouri
EMS Medical Director
Missouri EMS System
Kansas City, Missouri

GARY B. GREEN, MD, MPH [49]
Associate Professor of Emergency Medicine and Pathology
Johns Hopkins University School of Medicine
Department of Emergency Medicine
Baltimore, Maryland

KELLY L. GROGAN, MD [26]
Johns Hopkins Hospital
Department of Anesthesiology and Critical Care Medicine
Baltimore, Maryland

JASON B. HACK, MD [156]
Assistant Professor
Department of Emergency Medicine
Brody School of Medicine
East Carolina University
Greenville, North Carolina

THERESA A. HACKELING, MD [244]
Wake Medical Center
Department of Emergency Medicine
Raleigh, North Carolina

PETER H. HACKETT, MD [207]
Clinical Associate Professor
Division of Emergency Medicine
University of Colorado School of Medicine
Denver, Colorado
President, International Society for Mountain Medicine
Ridgeway, Colorado

ROBERT HADDON, MD, MS [240]
The Cleveland Clinic Foundation
Department of Emergency Medicine
Cleveland, Ohio

BRUCE L. HALL, MD, PhD, MBA [259]
Assistant Professor of Surgery
School of Medicine
Adjunct Professor of Business Administration
Olin School of Business Administration
Washington University in Saint Louis
St. Louis, Missouri

PAUL R. HALLER, MD [275, 278]
Assistant Professor
Department of Emergency Medicine
University of Minnesota
Minneapolis, Minnesota

GLENN HAMILTON, MD, MSM [294]
Professor and Chair
Wright State University
Department of Emergency Medicine
Kettering, Ohio

DARCIE HAMMER, MD [27]
Department of Emergency Medicine
The Johns Hopkins Hospital
Baltimore, Maryland

DANIEL G. HANKINS, MD [2]
Department of Emergency Medicine
Co-Medical Director, Mayo Medical Transport
Mayo Clinic
Rochester, Minnesota

KAREN N. HANSEN, MD [169]
Assistant Professor
University of Maryland School of Medicine
Baltimore, Maryland

CHRISTINA E. HANTSCH, MD [104]
Middle Tennessee Poison Center
Center for Clinical Toxicology
Vanderbilt University Medical Center
Nashville, Tennessee

FRED P. HARCHELROAD, JR., MD [200]
Allegheny General Hospital
Department of Emergency Medicine
Pittsburgh, Pennsylvania

KAREN M. HARDART, MD [112]
Attending Physician
Anne Arundel Medical Center
Annapolis, Maryland

RICHARD A. HARRIGAN, MD [161, 210]
Associate Professor of Emergency Medicine
Temple University Hospital and School of Medicine
Department of Emergency Medicine
Philadelphia, Pennsylvania

BENJAMIN HARRISON, MD [283]
Residency Director
Madigan Army Medical Center
Department of Emergency Medicine
Tacoma, Washington

NAEL HASAN, MD [257]
Lynchburg General Hospital
Department of Emergency Medicine
Lynchburg, Virginia

WILLIAM E. HAUDA II, MD [14, 131, 252]
Assistant Clinical Professor of Emergency Medicine
George Washington University School of Medicine
Washington, DC
Inova Fairfax Hospital
Department of Emergency Medicine
Falls Church, Virginia
Adult Services Medical Director
Falls Church, Virginia

KENNON HEARD, MD [176]
Assistant Professor, Division of Emergency Medicine
Rocky Mountain Poison and Drug Center
University of Colorado Health Sciences Center
Denver, Colorado

MICHAEL B. HELLER, MD [303]
Clinical Professor, Emergency Medicine
Temple University School of Medicine
Program Director, Emergency Medicine Residency
St. Lukes Hospital
Bethlehem, Pennsylvania

ROBIN R. HEMPHILL, MD [218, 219, 220, 221, 222]
Assistant Professor of Emergency Medicine
Associate Residency Program Director
Vanderbilt University School of Medicine
Department of Emergency Medicine
Nashville, Tennessee

WILMA V. HENDERSON, MD [166]
Assistant Professor, Department of Emergency Medicine
Wayne State University
Detroit Receiving Hospital
Detroit, Michigan

JENNIFER J. HESS, MD [83]
Department of Emergency Medicine
Mayo Clinic
Rochester, Minnesota

ARMANDO HEVIA, MD [312]
Assistant Professor
Department of Emergency Medicine
Louisiana State University
New Orleans, Louisiana

ERIC HIGGINBOTHAM, MD [37]
Department of Emergency Medicine
University of North Carolina at Chapel Hill
Assistant Consulting Professor
Division of Emergency Medicine
Duke University
Durham, North Carolina

PETER M. HILL, MD, MSc [49]
Assistant Chief of Service
Johns Hopkins Bayview Medical Center
Instructor, Department of Emergency Medicine
Johns Hopkins University
Baltimore, Maryland

JON MARK HIRSHON, MD, MPH [12]
Assistant Professor
University of Maryland School of Medicine
Division of Emergency Medicine
Departments of Surgery, Epidemiology and
    Preventative Medicine
Baltimore, Maryland

CHERRI HOBGOOD, MD [312]
Assistant Professor
Department of Emergency Medicine
University of North Carolina at Chapel Hill
Chapel Hill, North Carolina

ROBERT S. HOFFMAN, MD [156, 168]
Associate Professor of Emergency Medicine
New York University School of Medicine
Attending Physician, Bellevue Hospital Center
Director, New York City Poison Control Center
New York, New York

DAVID E. HOGAN, DO [193]
Oklahoma State University
Integris Southwest Medical Center
Division of Emergency Medicine
Oklahoma City, Oklahoma

JUDD E. HOLLANDER, MD, [40, 42, 48, 50, 51]
Professor and Clinical Research Director
Hospital of the University of Pennsylvania
Department of Emergency Medicine
Philadelphia, Pennsylvania

JEREMY J. HOLLERMAN, MD [264]
Department of Radiology
Hennepin County Medical Center and
    University of Minnesota
Minneapolis, Minnesota

CHRISTOPHER M. HOLMES, MD [126]
Department of Emergency Medicine
Swedish Medical Center
Englewood, Colorado
Senior Clinical Instructor
University of Colorado Health Sciences Center
Denver, Colorado

EDMOND A. HOOKER, MD [88, 89]
Associate Professor and Research Director
Department of Emergency Medicine
University of Louisville
Louisville, Kentucky

COURTNEY HOPKINS-MANN, MD [136]
Department of Pediatric Emergency Medicine
Wake Medical Center
Raleigh, North Carolina
Adjunct Instructor
Department of Emergency Medicine
University of North Carolina at Chapel Hill
Chapel Hill, North Carolina

MARK A. HOSTETLER, MD, MPH [205]
Assistant Professor
Section of Emergency Medicine
Department of Pediatrics
The University of Chicago
Medical Director
Pediatric Emergency Department
University of Chicago Children's Hospital
Chicago, Illinois

DEBRA E. HOURY, MD, MPH [266]
Assistant Professor
Department of Emergency Medicine
Associate Director, Center for Injury Control
Emory University School of Medicine
Atlanta, Georgia

DAVID S. HOWES, MD [94, 97]
Program Director
University of Chicago Emergency Medicine Residency
Associate Professor of Medicine
University of Chicago Pritzker School of Medicine
Chicago, Illinois

J. STEPHEN HUFF, MD [226, 229, 230]
Associate Professor of Emergency Medicine and Neurology
Departments of Emergency Medicine and Neurology
University of Virginia Health System
Charlottesville, Virginia

ROGER L. HUMPHRIES, MD [66]
Assistant Professor and Residency Director
University of Kentucky College of Medicine
Department of Emergency Medicine
Lexington, Kentucky

OLIVER L. HUNG, MD [171]
Assistant Professor of Clinical Surgery and
    Emergency Medicine
Department of Emergency Medicine
Bellevue Hospital Center and New York
    University Medical Center
New York, New York

D. MONTE HUNTER, MD [283]
Division of Sports Medicine
Department of Orthopedics
UCLA Medical Center
Los Angeles, California

JEFFERY C. HUTZLER, MD [289]
Department of Psychiatry
Ohio State University
Columbus, Ohio

GEOFFREY K. ISBISTER, BSc, MBBS [196]
Clinical Toxicologist and Emergency Physician
Newcastle Mater Hospital
Lecturer, Discipline of Clinical Pharmacology
University of Newcastle
Newcastle, Australia

KENNETH C. JACKIMCZYK, MD [293]
Associate Chairman
Maricopa Medical Center
Emergency Department
Phoenix, Arizona

DAVID M. JAFFE, MD [121]
Dana Brown Professor of Pediatrics
Washington University School of Medicine
Director of Emergency Services
St. Louis Children's Hospital
Department of Emergency Pediatrics
St. Louis, Missouri

F. MICHAEL JAGGI, MD [224]
Clinical Assistant Professor
Department of Emergency Medicine
University of Michigan Medical Center
Ann Arbor, Michigan
Chief of Emergency Medicine
Hurley Medical Center
Flint, Michigan

DAVID M. JANICKE, MD, PhD [103]
Associate Research Director
State University of New York at Buffalo
Department of Emergency Medicine
Buffalo, New York

DIETRICH V.K. JEHLE, MD [113]
Director of Emergency Services
Erie County Medical Center
Associate Professor and Vice Chaiman
Department of Emergency Medicine,
    SUNY at Buffalo School of Medicine
Buffalo, New York

MICHAEL N. JOHNSTON, MD [134]
Assistant Professor of Clinical Pediatrics
Division of Pediatric Emergency Medicine
Louisiana State University Health Sciences Center
New Orleans, Lousiana

GARY A. JOHNSON, MD [58]
Associate Professor
SUNY Upstate Medical University
Department of Emergency Medicine
Syracuse, New York

CARROLL P. JONES, MD [280]
Department of Orthopaedics
University of North Carolina School of Medicine
Chapel Hill, North Carolina

ELAINE B. JOSEPHSON, MD [98]
Assistant Clinical Professor of Medicine
Columbia University College of Physicians and Surgeons
Department of Emergency Medicine
St. Lukes-Roosevelt Hospital Center
New York, New York

JONATHAN JUI, MD, MPH [32]
Professor
Oregon Health Sciences University
Department of Emergency Medicine
Portland, Oregon

LAURENCE M. KATZ, MD [24]
Associate Professor
Department of Emergency Medicine
University of North Carolina
Chapel Hill, North Carolina

GABOR D. KELEN, MD [25, 27, 144, 259, 262]
Professor and Chair
Department of Emergency Medicine
Johns Hopkins University
Baltimore, Maryland

ARTHUR L. KELLERMAN, MD, MPH [266]
Professor and Chair
Department of Emergency Medicine
Director, Center for Injury Control
Emory University School of Medicine
Atlanta, Georgia

SCOTT S. KELLEY, MD [280]
Clinical Professor
Duke University Department of Surgery
Division of Orthopaedics
Durham, North Carolina

MARK A. KIRK, MD [174]
Medical Toxicology Fellowship Director
Division of Medical Toxicology
Department of Emergency Medicine
University of Virginia
Blue Ridge Poison Center
Charlottesville, Virginia

THOMAS D. KIRSCH, MD, MPH [255]
Maricopa Medical Center
Phoenix, Arizona
Medical Director
Department of Emergency Medicine
Chandler Regional Hospital
Chandler, Arizona

NIRANJAN KISSOON, MD [117]
Professor of Pediatrics and Emergency Medicine
Chief, Division of Critical Care Medicine
University of Florida Health Sciences Center-Jacksonville
Department of Pediatrics
Jacksonville, Florida

KELLY R. KLEIN, MD [8, 185]
Regional Poison Control Center
Children's Hospital of Michigan
Detroit, Michigan

JEFFREY A. KLINE, MD [56, 176]
Director of Research
Carolinas Medical Center
Department of Emergency Medicine
Charlotte, North Carolina
Adjunct Associate Professor
Department of Emergency Medicine
University of North Carolina at Chapel Hill

SANFORD H. KOLTONOW, MD, Psy.S. [296]
Department of Emergency Medicine and
    Director of Physician Wellness Programs
William Beaumont Hospital
Royal Oak, Michigan
Assistant Clinical Professor
Department of Emergency Medicine
Wayne State University
Detroit, Michigan

MAYBELLE KOU, MD [124, 137]
Department of Emergency Medicine
Pediatric Emergency Medicine Fellowship Director
Inova Fairfax Hospital
Falls Church, Virginia
Assistant Professor of Pediatrics
Georgetown University School of Medicine and
    George Washington University School of Medicine
Washington, DC

GARY S. KRAUSE, MD, MS [23]
Edward S. Thomas Distinguished Professor
Department of Emergency Medicine
    and the Center for Molecular Medicine and Genetics
Wayne State University School of Medicine
Detroit, Michigan

RICHARD S. KRAUSE, MD [103]
Residency Director
State University of New York at Buffalo
Department of Emergency Medicine
Buffalo, New York

JOEL KRAVITZ, MD [141]
Assistant Residency Director
Department of Emergency Medicine
Albert Einstein Medical Center
Philadelphia, Pennsylvania

STEVEN KRONICK, MD, PhD [90]
Clinical Assistant Professor
University of Michigan
Department of Emergency Medicine
Ann Arbor, Michigan

BRYAN R. KUHN, PharmD [29]
Department of Emergency Medicine
Specialty Pharmacy Services
Detroit Receiving Hospital and University Health Center
Department of Pharmacy Services
Detroit, Michigan

GLORIA J. KUHN, DO, PhD [106, 108]
Associate Professor and Vice-Chair
Department of Emergency Medicine
Wayne State University
Detroit Receiving Hospital
Detroit, Michigan

ALAN M. KUMAR, MD [263]
Lutheran General Hospital
Department of Emergency Medicine
Park Ridge, Illinois

JAY LADDE, MD [236]
Assistant Professor
Valencia Community College
Department of Emergency Medical Services
Orlando Regional Medical Center
Orlando, Florida

RICHARD L. LAMMERS, MD [46]
Associate Professor of Emergency Medicine
Michigan State University/Kalamazoo Center for Medical Studies
Department of Emergency Medicine
Kalamazoo, Michigan

JAMES L. LARSON, JR., MD [272]
Assistant Professor
Assistant Residency Director
Clinical Director, Department of Emergency Medicine
University of North Carolina at Chapel Hill
Chapel Hill, North Carolina

FRANK W. LAVOIE, MD [80]
Chief, Department of Emergency Medicine
Southern Maine Medical Center
Biddeford, Maine
Clinical Associate Professor
University of Vermont
College of Medicine
Burlington, Vermont
and
University of New England
College of Osteopathic Medicine
Biddeford, Maine

DAVID LEADER, DO [136]
Department of Emergency Medicine
Wake Medical Center
Raleigh, North Carolina
Adjunct Assistant Professor
Department of Emergency Medicine
University of North Carolina at Chapel Hill

FREDERICK LEVY, MD [262]
Assistant Professor
Department of Emergency Medicine
Johns Hopkins University
Baltimore, Maryland

HORACE K. LIANG, MD, MA [215, 216]
Assistant Professor
Department of Emergency Medicine
Johns Hopkins Hospital
Baltimore, Maryland

ERICA L. LIEBELT, MD [134]
Director
Medical Toxicology Services
Division of Pediatric Emergency Medicine
Children's Hospital
Birmingham, Alabama

G. PATRICK LILJA, MD [1]
Clinical Professor, Emergency Medicine
University of Minnesota Medical School
Medical Director,
    Emergency and Trauma Services
North Memorial Medical Center
Minneapolis, Minnesota

JOAO A.C. LIMA, MD [61]
Assistant Professor, Cardiology
Clinical Director, Echocardiology Lab
Johns Hopkins University and Hospital
Department of Cardiology
Baltimore, Maryland

CHRISTOPHER A. LIPINSKI, MD [255]
Assistant Professor of Clinical Surgery
    and Director of Emergency Medicine Research
University of Arizona College of Medicine
Phoenix Programs
Maricopa Medical Center
Phoenix, Arizona

MICHAEL LONDNER, MD, MPH, MBA [27, 111]
Assistant Professor
Clinical Director
Johns Hopkins Hospital
Department of Emergency Medicine
Baltimore, Maryland

HEATHER LONG, MD [184]
Department of Emergency Medicine
North Shore University Hospital
Manhasset, New York

KEITH E. LORING, MD, MPH [235]
Medical Director and Chief
Department of Emergency Medicine
St. Mary's Medical Center
San Francisco, California
Assistant Clinical Professor of Surgery
Department of Surgery
Division of Emergency Services
University of California
San Francisco General Hospital
San Francisco, California

CARY L. LUBKIN, MD [211]
Assitant Director
Assistant Professor of Emergency Medicine
Department of Emergency Medicine
UMDNJ-Robert Wood Johnson
    Medical School at Camden
The Cooper Health System
Camden, New Jersey

MICHAEL LUCCHESI, MD [239]
Associate Professor and Chairman
Downstate Medical Center
State University of New York
Department of Emergency Medicine
Brooklyn, New York

DESMOND J. LUGG, MD [208]
Chief, Medicine of Extreme Environments
Office of the Chief Health and Medical Officer
NASA Headquarters, Code AM,
Washington, DC
Distinguished Research Professor
George Mason University
Fairfax, Virginia
Head
Polar Medicine Australian Antarctic Division
Kingston, Tasmania
Australia

O. JOHN MA, MD [253]
Vice Chair
Department of Emergency Medicine
Truman Medical Center
Associate Professor of Emergency Medicine
University of Missouri-Kansas City School of Medicine
Kansas City, Missouri

ANTHONY G. MACINTYRE, MD [7]
Associate Professor of Emergency Medicine
George Washington University
Department of Emergency Medicine
Washington, DC

RICHARD MALLEY, MD [122]
Assistant Professor in Pediatrics
Harvard Medical School
Children's Hospital
Divisions of Emergency Medicine and
    Infectious Diseases
Boston, Massachusetts

ANN E. MALONEY, MD [292]
Department of Psychiatry
University of North Carolina
Chapel Hill, North Carolina

JAMES E. MANNING, MD [24, 31]
Associate Professor and Vice Chair
University of North Carolina School of Medicine
Department of Emergency Medicine
Chapel Hill, North Carolina

CATHERINE A. MARCO, MD [17, 144, 145]
Associate Professor, Medical College of Ohio
Acute Care Services, St. Vincent Mercy Medical Center
Toledo, Ohio

HEATHER MARSHALL, DO [173]
Department of Emergency Medicine
Case Western Reserve University
Cleveland, Ohio

MARCUS L. MARTIN, MD [245]
Professor and Chair
University of Virginia School of Medicine
Department of Emergency Medicine
Charlottesville, Virginia

MARIA G. MATHEUS, MD [237]
Visiting Professor, Neuroradiology
Department of Radiology
Chapel Hill, North Carolina

LISA MAY, MD [247, 248, 249, 250]
Biltmore Dermatology Associates
Ashville, North Carolina

THOM MAYER, MD [124, 128, 131, 137, 140]
President, Emergency Physicians of Northern Virginia, Ltd.
Professor of Emergency Medicine and Pediatrics
Georgetown University & George Washington
   University Schools of Medicine
Inova-Fairfax Hospital
Department of Emergency Medicine
Falls Church, Virginia

MARSHALL C. McCOY, MD [301]
Associate Professor
Medical Director, UNC AirCare
University of North Carolina
Department of Emergency Medicine
Chapel Hill, North Carolina

ROBERT McNAMARA, MD [73]
Professor and Chair
Department of Emergency Medicine
Temple University School of Medicine
Philadelphia, Pennsylvania

WILLIAM J. MEGGS, MD, PhD [182]
Professor and Chief of Division of Toxicology
Brody School of Medicine at
   East Carolina University
Department of Emergency Medicine
Greenville, North Carolina

HAGOP S. MEKHJIAN, MD [81]
Professor, Division of Gastroenterology
Department of Internal Medicine
The Ohio State University College of Medicine and
   Public Health
Columbus, Ohio

SCOTT W. MELANSON, MD [303]
Associate Director
Emergency Medicine Residency
St. Luke's Hospital
Bethlehem, Pennsylvania
Assistant Clinical Professor
Temple University School of Medicine
Philadelphia, Pennsylvania

STEPHEN W. MELDON, MD [253]
Associate Professor of Emergency Medicine
Case Western Reserve University
Cleveland, Ohio
MetroHealth Medical Center
Department of Emergency Medicine
Cleveland, Ohio

FRANTZ R. MELIO, MD, FACEP [287]
Executive Director ED Operations
St Vincent Hospital
Santa Fe, New Mexico
President
Northern New Mexico Emergency Medical Services

PETER MELLIS, MD [114, 116]
Associate Clinical Professor of Pediatrics
Virginia Commonwealth University Health System
Director, Pediatric Emergency Services
Chippenham Medical Center
Midlothian, Virginia

MOSS H. MENDELSON, MD [75]
Associate Professor
Eastern Virginia School of Medicine
Department of Emergency Medicine
Norfolk, Virginia

JEFFREY S. MENKES, MD [267]
Hartford Medical Group
Hartford Hospital
Hartford, Connecticut
Clinical Instructor of Emergency Medicine
University of Connecticut School of Medicine
Farmington, Connecticut

JOHN T. MEREDITH, MD, [151]
Clinical Associate Professor of
   Emergency Medicine
Brody School of Medicine at
   East Carolina University
Department of Emergency Medicine
Greenville, North Carolina

DANIELA MESHKAT, MD [111]
Department of Obstetrics and Gynecology
The Howard County General Hospital
Baltimore, Maryland

JOHN A. MICHAEL, MD [276, 277]
Department of Emergency Medicine
The Northshore Medical Center
Salem, Massachusetts

MICHAEL R. MILL, MD [60]
Professor and Chief
Cardiothoracic Surgery
University of North Carolina School of Medicine
Director, Transplantation Services,
   University of North Carolina Hospitals
University of North Carolina at Chapel Hill
Chapel Hill, North Carolina

MICHELLE S. MILL, RN, BSN, CCTC [60]
Heart Transplant Coordinator
University of North Carolina at Chapel Hill
Chapel Hill, North Carolina

KIRK C. MILLS, MD [158, 159, 160]
Clinical Assistant Professor
Wayne State University
Detroit, Michigan

JOHN D. MITCHELL, MD [238]
Senior Attending Surgeon
Washington National Eye Center/
   Washington Hospital Center
Washington, DC

DONALD A. MOFFA, JR., MD [63]
Department of Emergency Medicine
Case Western Reserve University
MetroHealth Emergency Medicine
Cleveland Clinic Foundation
Cleveland, Ohio

GREGORY P. MOORE, MD, JD [293]
Department of Emergency Medicine
Kaiser Sacramento/Roseville
Sacramento, California
Volunteer Clinical Faculty
University of California at Davis
Department of Emergency Medicine

DONNA MORO-SUTHERLAND, MD [136, 138]
Department of Pediatric Emergency Medicine
Wake Medical Center
Raleigh, North Carolina
Adjunct Assistant Professor
Departments of Emergency Medicine and Pediatrics
University of North Carolina at Chapel Hill
Chapel Hill, North Carolina

DEAN MORRELL, MD [247, 248, 249, 250]
Assistant Professor
Director of Pediatric and Adolescent Dermatology
University of North Carolina
Department of Dermatology
Chapel Hill, North Carolina

LAURIE J. MORRISON, MSc, MD [101]
Associate Professor, Division of Emergency Medicine
University of Toronto
Sunnybrook and Women's College
   Health Sciences Center
Toronto, Ontario

ROBERT L. MUELLEMAN, MD [268]
Professor and Chief
University of Nebraska Medical Center
Department of Emergency Medicine
Omaha, Nebraska

J. BRENT MYERS, MD, MPH [153]
Assistant Professor
Department of Emergency Medicine
Director, Wake County Emergency Medical Services
University of North Carolina
Chapel Hill, North Carolina

LEWIS S. NELSON, MD [171, 179, 184, 189, 190]
Assistant Clinical Professor of Emergency Medicine
New York University School of Medicine
Director, Medical Toxicology Fellowship
New York City Poison Center
New York, New York

TOM NEUMAN, MD [197]
Professor of Medicine and Surgery
Department of Emergency Medicine
Director, Hyperbaric Medicine Center
University of California, San Diego Medical Center
San Diego, California

TINA M. NEWMAN, MD [52]
Piedmont Emergency Medicine Associates
Charlotte, North Carolina

H. BRYANT NGUYEN, MD, MS [30]
Instructor
Loma Linda University School of Medicine
Department of Emergency Medicine
Loma Linda, California

LINDA M. NICHOLAS, MD, MS [292]
Associate Professor
University of North Carolina School of Medicine
Department of Psychiatry
Chapel Hill, North Carolina

MARK A. NICHTER, MD [198]
Affiliate Associate Professor of Pediatrics
University of South Florida School of Medicine
Chief, Division of Pediatric Critical Care Medicine
All Children's Hospital
St. Petersburg, Florida

DAVID D. NICOLAOU, MD [25, 38]
Assistant Professor
Department of Emergency Medicine and
   Division of Health Sciences Informatics
Johns Hopkins University School of Medicine
Johns Hopkins Hospital
Baltimore, Maryland

JAMES T. NIEMANN, MD [55]
Professor of Medicine
Harbor-University of California at Los Angeles Medical Center
Department of Emergency Medicine
Torrance, California

MICHAEL A. NIGRO, DO [125]
Professor of Pediatrics and Neurology
Wayne State University School of Medicine
Detroit, Michigan
Michigan Institute for Neurological Disorders
Farmington Hills, Michigan

RICHARD A. NOCKOWITZ, MD [290]
Department of Psychiatry
The Ohio State University School of Medicine
Columbus, Ohio

THOMAS P. NOELLER, MD [70]
EPS/TeamHealth
St. John Westshore Hospital
Westlake, Ohio
Southwest General Health Center
Middleberg Heights, Ohio

ERIC K. NOJI, MD, MPH [6]
Special Assistant to the US Surgeon General for
   Homeland Security and Disaster Medicine
US Public Health Service
Washington, DC

JOHN N. OH, MD [308]
Assistant Professor
University of North Carolina at Chapel Hill
Department of Physical Medicine & Rehabilitation
Chapel Hill, North Carolina

JOSEPH P. ORNATO, MD [11]
Professor and Chairman
Virginia Commonwealth University Health System
Department of Emergency Medicine
Richmond, Virginia

HAROLD H. OSBORN, MD [149, 178]
Bronx Lebanon Hospital
Emergency Department
Bronx, New York

ERIC W. OSSMANN, MD [5]
Assistant Professor
Emory University School of Medicine
Department of Emergency Medicine
Atlanta, Georgia

RONNY M. OTERO, MD [30]
Assistant Professor
Division of Emergency Medicine
Duke University
Durham, North Carlonia

DAVID T. OVERTON, MD [74]
Professor and Chairman
Department of Emergency Medicine
Emergency Medicine Program Director
Michigan State University College of
    Human Medicine
Michigan State Kalmazoo Center for Medical Studies
Kalamazoo, Michigan

JOSEPH PAGANE, MD [236]
Clinical Assistant Professor
University of Florida
Department of Emergency Medicine
Orlando, Florida

PETER J. PAGANUSSI [137]
Department of Pediatric Emergency Medicine
Inova-Fairfax Hospital
Falls Church, Virginia

ARTHUR M. PANCIOLI, MD, FACEP [78]
Associate Professor and Vice Chairman
University of Cincinnati College of Medicine
Department of Emergency Medicine
Cincinnatti, Ohio

PETER R. PEACOCK, JR., MD [92]
Assistant Professor
State University of New York-Downstate
Kings County Hospital Center
Department of Emergency Medicine
Brooklyn, New York

W. FRANKLIN PEACOCK IV, MD [33, 53, 96, 240, 241]
Associate Professor
The Ohio State University
Emergency Department Clinical Operations Director
Medical Director, Event Medicine
The Cleveland Clinic Foundation
Department of Emergency Medicine
Cleveland, Ohio

DEBRA G. PERINA [213]
Associate Professor
Department of Emergency Medicine
University of Virginia School of Medicine
Charlottesville, Virginia

ANDREW D. PERRON, MD [226, 245, 246]
Department of Emergency Medicine
Maine Medical Center
Portland, Maine

JEANMARIE PERRONE, MD [168]
Co-Director
Division of Toxicology
Assistant Professor
Department of Emergency Medicine
University of Pennsylvania School of Medicine
Attending Physician
Emergency Department
Hospital of the University of Pennsylvania
Philadelphia, Pennsylvania

SHAWNA J. PERRY, MD [142]
Assistant Professor and Assistant Chair
University of Florida Health Sciences Center-Jacksonville
Department of Emergency Medicine
Jacksonville, Florida

PAMELA L. PIGGOTT, MD [10]
Department of Emergency Medicine
Pitt County Memorial Hospital
East Carolina University School of Medicine
Greenville, North Carolina

JAMIE PILAROWSKI, PharmD [157]
Clinical Pharmacist
Detroit Receiving Hospital/Detroit Medical Center
Department of Pharmacy Services
Detroit, Michigan

FREDERICK PLACE, MD [128]
Department of Pediatric Emergency Medicine
Emergency Physicians of Northern Virginia
Inova Fairfax Hospital
Falls Church, Virginia

CHARLES V. POLLACK, JR., MD [224]
Associate Professor
Department of Emergency Medicine
University of Pennsylvania Medical Center
Philadelphia, Pennsylvania

NANCY POOK, MD [130]
Clinical Assistant Professor of Emergency Medicine
Department of Emergency Medicine and Pediatrics
Wright State University
Dayton, Ohio

JANET M. POPONICK, MD [65, 71]
MetroHealth Medical Center
Department of Emergency Medicine
Cleveland, Ohio

ROBERT D. POWERS, MD, MPH [47]
Professor of Emergency Medicine
Chief of Emergency Medicine
University of Connecticut School of Medicine
Hartford Hospital
Department of Emergency Medicine
Hartford, Connecticut

TIMOTHY G. PRICE, MD [79]
Assistant Professor
Department of Emergency Medicine
University of Louisville
Louisville, Kentucky

LOUISE A. PRINCE, MD [58]
Assistant Professor
State University of New York-Upstate
Department of Emergency Medicine
Syracuse, New York

SUSAN B. PROMES, MD [16, 141]
Associate Clinical Professor of Surgery
Residency Director
Division of Emergency Medicine
Duke University Medical Center
Chapel Hill, North Carolina

PETER PRONOVOST, MD, PhD [26]
Associate Professor
Departments of Anesthesiology & Critical
  Care, Surgery, & Health Policy
Management Medical Director
Center for Innovations in Quality Patient Care
The Johns Hopkins University School of Medicine
Johns Hopkins Hospital
Baltimore, Maryland

ARTHUR F. PROUST, MD [270]
Associate Director Emergency Medicine
Department of Emergency Medicine
Rockford Memorial Hospital
Clinical Assistant Professor
Department of Surgery
University of Illinois
  College of Medicine Rockford
Rockford, Illinois

KATHERINE M. PRYBYS, DO [169]
Assistant Professor of Emergency Medicine
University of Maryland School of Medicine
Baltimore, Maryland

KIMBERLY S. QUAYLE, MD [121]
Assistant Professor of Pediatrics
Washington University School of Medicine
St. Louis Children's Hospital
Division of Pediatric Emergency Medicine
St. Louis, Missouri

RALPH H. RAASCH, PharmD [155]
Associate Professor of Pharmacy
Clinical Associate Professor of Medicine
University of North Carolina at Chapel Hill
School of Pharmacy
Chapel Hill, North Carolina

MARK B. RABOLD, MD [191]
Medical Director
Emergency Department
St. Peter's Hospital
Helena, Montana

KATHLEEN A. RAFTERY, MD [311]
Department of Emergency Medicine
Brigham & Women's Hospital
Boston, Massachusetts

RAMA B. RAO, MD [310]
Assistant Clinical Professor
Bellevue Hospital Center
New York University Medical Center
Department of Emergency Medicine
New York, New York

ROBERT F. REARDON, MD [113]
Assistant Professor of Clinical Emergency Medicine
University of Minnesota
Department of Emergency Medicine
Hennepin County Medical Center
Minneapolis, Minnesota

SEAN M. REES, MD [189]
Department of Emergency Medicine
Bethesda and Good Samaritan Hospitals
Cincinnati, Ohio

EARL J. REISDORFF, MD [45]
Director of Medical Education
Ingham Regional Medical Center
Associate Professor of Emergency Medicine
Michigan State University
Lansing, Michigan

JOSEPH G. RELLA, MD [179, 190]
Assistant Professor of Emergency Medicine
University School of Medicine and Dentistry of New Jersey
Consultant, New Jersey Poison and Information Education System
Newark, New Jersey

KATHY J. RINNERT, MD, MPH [154]
Assistant Professor of Emergency Medicine
University of Texas-Southwestern Medical Center
Division of Emergency Medicine
Department of Surgery
Dallas, Texas

EMANUEL P. RIVERS, MD, MPH [30]
Associate Professor and Senior Staff Attending Physician
Departments of Emergency Medicine and Surgery
Director of Research
Case Western Reserve University
Cleveland, Ohio
Henry Ford Hospital
Department of Emergency Medicine
Detroit, Michigan

WALTER C. ROBEY III, MD [182]
Clinical Associate Professor of Emergency Medicine
Brody School of Medicine at East Carolina University
Department of Emergency Medicine
Greenville, North Carolina

A. MICHAEL ROMAN, MD [18]
Department of Emergency Medicine
University of Arkansas
Little Rock, Arkansas

ALEXANDER M. ROSENAU, DO [135]
Department of Emergency Medicine
Lehigh Valley Hospital
Allentown, Pennsylvania

RICHARD E. ROTHMAN, MD, PhD [144, 145]
Assistant Professor
Department of Emergency Medicine
The Johns Hopkins University
Baltimore, Maryland

DAVID M. ROTTINGHAUS, MD [200]
Fellow, Medical Toxicology
Department of Emergency Medicine
Allegheny General Hospital
Pittsburgh, Pennsylvania

BRIAN H. ROWE, MD, MSc [34]
Canada Research Chair in Emergency Airway Diseases
Research Director, Division of Emergency Medicine
Professor, University of Alberta
University of Alberta Hospital
Edmonton, Alberta
Canada

MARCIE RUBIN, MD [15]
Department of Emergency Medicine
Beth Israel Deaconess Hospital
Boston, Massachusetts

JOHN P. RUDZINSKI, MD [271]
Department of Emergency Medicine
Rockford Memorial Hospital
Rockford, Illinois

DOUGLAS A. RUND, MD [81, 288, 289, 290]
Professor and Chairman
Ohio State University
Department of Emergency Medicine
Columbus, Ohio

MICHAEL D. RUSH, MD [212]
Assistant Professor
University of Missouri-Kansas City
Truman Medical Center
Department of Emergency Medicine
Kansas City, Missouri

WILLIAM A. RUTALA, PhD, MPH [147]
University of North Carolina at Chapel Hill
Division of Infectious Diseases
Chapel Hill, North Carolina

SAMY SAAD, MD [139]
Department of Pediatric Emergency Medicine
Wake Medical Center
Raleigh, North Carolina
Adjunct Assistant Professor
Department of Emergency Medicine
University of North Carolina at Chapel Hill

ALEXANDER H. SACKEYFIO, MD [291]
Coordinator-Eating Disorders Program
William Beaumont Hospital
Royal Oak, Michigan
Associate Professor of Psychiatry
Michigan State University
East Lansing, Michigan

ANNIE T. SADOSTY, MD [83]
Assistant Professor of Emergency Medicine
Mayo Clinic
Department of Emergency Medicine
Rochester, Minnesota

NICHOLAS SADOVNIKOFF, MD [15]
Department of Anesthesiology
Critical Care Medicine
Brigham & Women's Hospital
Boston, Massachusetts

PATRICIA R. SALBER, MD, MBA [299]
Senior Medical Director
Center for Health Improvement
Blue Shield of California
San Francisco, California

ARTHUR B. SANDERS, MD [307]
Professor of Emergency Medicine
Department of Emergency Medicine
University of Arizona College of Medicine
Tucson, Arizona

SALLY A. SANTEN, MD [223]
Assistant Professor
Vanderbilt University School of Medicine
Assistant Program Director
Vanderbilt University
    Emergency Medicine Residency
Department of Emergency Medicine
Nashville, Tennessee

THOMAS M. SCALEA, MD [35, 256, 260]
Physician-in-Chief
R. Adams Cowley Shock Trauma Center
Francis X Kelly Professor of Trauma Surgery
University of Maryland School of Medicine
Baltimore, Maryland

ROBERT W. SCHAFERMEYER, MD [127]
Associate Chair
Department of Emergency Medicine
Carolinas Medical Center
Charlotte, North Carolina
Clinical Professor Emergency Medicine and
    Pediatrics
University of North Carolina School of Medicine
Chapel Hill, North Carolina

RAQUEL M. SCHEARS, MD, MPH [163, 165]
Assistant Professor in Emergency Medicine
Mayo Clinic, St. Mary's Hospital
Department of Emergency Medicine
Rochester, Minnesota

ROBERT E. SCHNEIDER, MD [95]
Department of Emergency Medicine
Carolinas Medical Center
Charlotte, North Carolina
Clinical Assistant Professor
Department of Emergency Medicine
University of North Carolina at Chapel Hill

SANDRA M. SCHNEIDER, MD [162, 204, 205]
Professor and Chair
Department of Emergency Medicine
University of Rochester School of Medicine and Dentistry
Rochester, New York

AARON B. SCHNEIR, MD [194]
Assistant Clinical Professor of Medicine
University of California at San Diego Medical Center
Department of Emergency Medicine
Division of Medical Toxicolgy
San Diego, California

CHARLES N. SCHOENFELD, MD [217]
Assistant Professor
John Hopkins School of Medicine
Department of Emergency Medicine
Baltimore, Maryland

MICHAEL J. SCHULL, MD, MSc [227]
Assistant Professor
Department of Medicine, Division of Emergency Medicine
University of Toronto
Emergency Department
Sunnybrook and Women's College Health Sciences Center
Toronto, Ontario
Canada

ROBERT A. SCHWAB, MD [47]
Professor and Chair
University of Missouri-Kansas City School of Medicine
Truman Medical Center
Department of Emergency Medicine
Kansas City, Missouri

LAWRENCE R. SCHWARTZ, MD [199]
Assistant Professor
Department of Emergency Medicine
Wayne State University School of Medicine
Detroit Receiving Hospital
Detroit, Michigan

PHILLIP A. SCOTT, MD [228]
Assistant Professor
University of Michigan
Department of Emergency Medicine
Ann Arbor, Michigan

DONNA L. SEGER, MD [104]
Assistant Professor of Medicine and Emergency Medicine
Vanderbilt University School of Medicine
Medical Director
Middle Tennessee Poison Center
Nashville, Tennessee

EMILY H. SHEFFER, MD [100]
St. Luke's-Roosevelt Hospital
Department of Emergency Medicine
New York, New York

SUZANNE M. SHEPHERD, MD, MS [109, 306]
Associate Professor, Emergency Medicine
Director of Education & Research
Hospital of the University of Pennsylvania
Department of Emergency Medicine
Philadelphia, Pennsylvania

RICHARD O. SHIELDS, JR., MD [84]
Chairman, Department of Emergency Medicine
Candler Hospital
Savannah, Georgia

WILLIAM H. SHOFF, MD [109]
Associate Professor, Emergency Medicine
Director, PENN Travel Medicine
Hospital of the University of Pennsylvania
Department of Emergency Medicine
Philadelphia, Pennsylvania

CAROL G. SHORES, MD, PhD [243, 244]
Assistant Professor
University of North Carolina School of Medicine
Department of Otolaryngology/Head and Neck Surgery
Chapel Hill, North Carolina

SUSAN L. SIEGFREID, MD [292]
Kansas City VA Medical Center
Kansas City, Missouri
Clinical Assistant Professor
University of Kansas Medical Center
Kansas City, Kansas

LINMARIE SIKICH, MD [309]
Medical Director
Adolescent Inpatient Unit
Assistant Professor of Psychiatry
University of North Carolina at Chapel Hill
Division of Child Psychiatry
Chapel Hill, North Carolina

MICHAEL A. SILVERMAN, MD [112]
Associate Director
Department of Emergency Medicine
St. Agnes Healthcare
Baltimore, Maryland
Instructor of Emergency Medicine
The Johns Hopkins University School of Medicine
Baltimore, Maryland

RICHARD SINERT, DO [92, 93, 99]
Associate Professor
State University of New York
Downstate Medical Center
Department of Emergency Medicine
Brooklyn, New York

JONATHAN I. SINGER, MD [130]
Professor of Emergency Medicine and Pediatrics
Wright State University School of Medicine
Vice Chairman of Emergency Medicine
Associate Emergency Medicine Residency Program Director
Wright State University
Department of Emergency Medicine
Dayton, Ohio

ADAM J. SINGER, MD [40, 42, 48]
Associate Professor
Director of Clinical Research
Stony Brook University
Department of Emergency Medicine
Stony Brook, New York

JATINDER SINGH, MD [98]
St. Luke's-Roosevelt Hospital Center
Department of Emergency Medicine
New York, New York

EDWARD P. SLOAN, MD, MPH [234]
Associate Professor and Research Development Director
Department of Emergency Medicine
University of Illinois College of Medicine
Attending Physician, Emergency Services
University of Illinois Hospital
University of Illinois-Chicago
Chicago, Illinois

JOHN E. SMIALEK, MD [265]*
Head, Forensic Pathology
Associate Professor
Department of Pathology
University of Maryland
Baltimore, Maryland

SUMMER A. SMITH, MD [126]
Departments of Emergency Medicine and Pediatrics
Swedish Hospital
Englewood, Colorado

BRIAN SNYDER, MD [197]
Assistant Clinical Professor of Medicine
Hyperbaric Medicine Center
University of California, San Diego Medical Center
Department of Emergency Medicine
San Diego, California

MARK SPEKTOR, DO [93]
Assistant Professor
Assistant Residency Director
State University of New York
Downstate Medical Center
Kings County Hospital Center
Department of Emergency Medicine
Brooklyn, New York

JULIE M. SPENCE, MD [101]
Assistant Professor
St. Michael's Hospital
Division of Emergency Medicine
Toronto, Ontario
Canada

J. STEPHAN STAPCZYNSKI, MD [62]
Professor and Former Chair
Department of Emergency Medicine
University of Kentucky College of Medicine
Lexington, Kentucky

MICHAEL STAVA, MD [67]
Voluntary Professor
Department of Emergency Medicine
University of Kentucky College of Medicine
Lexington, Kentucky

MARK T. STEELE, MD [273, 274]
Professor and Associate Dean
University of Missouri-Kansas City School of Medicine
Chief Medical Officer
Truman Medical Center
Department of Emergency Medicine
Kansas City, Missouri

IAN G. STIELL, MD, MSc [276, 277]
Professor and Head
Department of Emergency Medicine
University of Ottawa
Chair of Emergency Medicine Research
Ottawa Health Research Institute
Senior Scientist, Clinical Epidemiology Unit
Distinguished Investigator, Canadian Institutes of Health Research
Ottawa Hospital Civic Campus
Clinical Epidemiology Unit
Ottawa, Ontario
Canada

C. KEITH STONE, MD [3]
Chairman
Department of Emergency Medicine
Texas A&M University Health Science Center
Scott and White Memorial Hospital
Temple, Texas

SUSAN STONE, MD, MPH [41]
Associate Residency Director
Assistant Professor
University of Southern California School of Medicine
Department of Emergency Medicine
Los Angeles, California

BHARAT SUTARIYA, MD [21]
Clinical Assistant Professor
Department of Emergency Medicine
Wayne State University
Attending Physician, Emergency Medicine
Detroit Receiving and Huron Valley-Sinai Hospitals
Detroit, Michigan

ELLEN H. TALIAFERRO, MD [300]
Professor of Surgery
Division of Emergency Medicine
San Francisco General Hospital
San Francisco, California

NELSON TANG, MD [254]
Assistant Professor
Department of Emergency Medicine
The Johns Hopkins University
Director, Division of Special Operations
The Johns Hopkins Medical Institutions
Baltimore, Maryland

PAUL J.W. TAWNEY, MD [308]
Associate Professor
University of North Carolina at Chapel Hill
Department of Physical Medicine & Rehabilitation
Chapel Hill, North Carolina

MALEK TEBACHE, MD [61]
Department of Radiology
Johns Hopkins Hospital
Baltimore, Maryland

STEPHEN H. THOMAS, MD, MPH [3]
Assistant in Emergency Services
Massachusetts General Hospital
Assistant Professor of Surgery
Harvard Medical School
Associate Medical Director, Boston MedFlight
Boston, Massachusetts

KEITH THOMASSET, MD [177]
Department of Emergency Medicine
Johns Hopkins University School of Medicine
Baltimore, Maryland

CAROLINE A. TIMMERMAN, MD [228]
Department of Emergency Medicine
University of Michigan
Detroit, Michigan

ANNE TINTINALLI, MD [239]
Clinical Instructor
Department of Emergency Medicine
Wayne State University
Detroit Receiving Hospital
Detroit, Michigan

JUDITH E. TINTINALLI, MD, MS [85]
Professor and Chair
Department of Emergency Medicine
Adjunct Professor
Department of Health Policy and Administration
University of North Carolina at Chapel Hill
Chapel Hill, North Carolina

RUDOLPH J. TRIANA JR., MD [244]
MidWest Ear Nose & Throat
Evansville, Indiana

DOUGLAS R. TROSCINSKI, MD [138]
Assistant Emergency Medicine Residency Director
Wake Medical Center
Raleigh, North Carolina
Assistant Professor
Department of Emergency Medicine
University of North Carolina at Chapel Hill

DENNIS T. UEHARA, MD [269, 270, 271]
Chairman, Department of Emergency Medicine
Rockford Memorial Hospital
Clinical Professor of Surgery, Department of Surgery
University of Illinois College of Medicine Rockford
Rockford, Illinois

KEITH W. VAN METER, MD [203]
Clinical Professor of Medicine
Louisiana State University School of Medicine
Louisiana State University Section Head of
   Emergency Medicine
Charity Hospital of Louisiana-LSU
New Orleans, Louisiana

MICHAEL J. VANROOYEN, MD, MPH [107, 206]
Associate Professor and Vice Chair
Director, Center for International Emergency, Disaster and
   Refugee Studies
Johns Hopkins University
Department of Emergency Medicine
Baltimore, Maryland

LARISSA I. VELEZ, MD [188]
Assistant Professor of Emergency Medicine
University of Texas-Southwestern Medical Center
Division of Emergency Medicine
Dallas, Texas

RAGHU VENUGOPAL, MD [206]
Center for International Emergency,
   Disaster and Refugee Studies
Johns Hopkins University
Department of Emergency Medicine
Baltimore, Maryland

SALVATOR J. VICARIO, MD [79]
Associate Professor of Emergency Medicine
University of Louisville School of Medicine
Department of Emergency Medicine
Louisville, Kentucky

ROBERT J. VISSERS, MD [19, 37, 87, 311]
Residency Director and Assistant Professor
University of North Carolina
Department of Emergency Medicine
Chapel Hill, North Carolina

MICHAEL C. WADMAN, MD [268]
Assistant Professor
Section of Emergency Medicine
University of Nebraska College of Medicine
Omaha, Nebraska

JAMES S. WALKER, DO [193]
Department of Emergency Medicine
Oklahoma Heart Hospital
Oklahoma City, Oklahoma
Clinical Professor of Surgery
University of Oklahoma Health Sciences Center
Oklahoma City, Oklahoma

MICHAEL M. WANG, MD, PhD [233]
Assistant Professor
Departments of Neurology and Anesthesiology/Critical Care Medicine
Johns Hopkins University
Johns Hopkins Hospital
Baltimore, Maryland

MARY CHESTER MORGAN WASKO, MD [284]
Department of Medicine
Division of Rheumatology and Clinical Immunology
University of Pittsburgh
Pittsburgh, Pennsylvania

THOMAS A. WATERS, MD [241]
Clinical Instructor
Case Western Reserve University
Director of Education
Department of Emergency Medicine
The Cleveland Clinic Foundation
Cleveland, Ohio

PAUL M. WAX, MD [180, 183]
Fellowship Director, Medical Toxicology
Banner Samaritan Medical Center
Professor of Clinical Emergency Medicine
University of Arizona School of Medicine
Phoenix, Arizona

BARRY A. WAYNE, MD, CDR, MC, USN [9]
Assistant Professor and Director, Education Division
Department of Military and Emergency Medicine
Uniformed Services University of the Health Sciences
Bethesda, Maryland

ROBERT L. WEARS, MD, MS [312]
Professor
Department of Emergency Medicine
University of Florida Health Sciences Center-Jacksonville
Jacksonville, Florida

DAVID J. WEBER, MD, MPH [147]
Professor of Medicine, Pediatrics, and Epidemiology
University of North Carolina at Chapel Hill
Director of Hospital Epidemiology
Medical Director of Occupational Health Services
UNC Heathcare Systems
Chapel Hill, North Carolina

JIM EDWARD WEBER, DO [33, 224]
Assistant Professor
University of Michigan Medical School
Department of Emergency Medicine
Ann Arbor, Michigan

MICHAEL S. WEINSTOCK, MD [135]
Lehigh Valley Hospital
Department of Emergency Medicine
Allentown, Pennsylvania

IRWIN D. WEISMAN, MD, PhD [305]
Consulting Radiologists, Ltd.
Minneapolis, Minnesota
Clinical Assistant Professor of Radiology
University of Minnesota
Cambridge Medical Center
Cambridge, Minnesota

HOWARD A. WERMAN, MD [81]
Professor of Clinical Emergency Medicine
Medical Director, MedFlight
The Ohio State University College of
  Medicine and Public Health
Department of Emergency Medicine
Columbus, Ohio

BLAINE C. WHITE, MD [23]
Professor and Associate Chair
Department of Emergency Medicine
Professor
Department of Physiology, and the Center for
  Molecular Medicine and Genetics
Wayne State University School of Medicine
Detroit, Michigan

DREW WHITE, MD [254]
Instructor
Department of Emergency Medicine
The Johns Hopkins University
Assistant Chief of Service
The Johns Hopkins Medical Institutions
Johns Hopkins Hospital
Baltimore, Maryland

SUZANNE R. WHITE, MD [8, 185]
Assistant Professor of Emergency Medicine and Pediatrics
Medical Director
Resgional Poison Control Center
Children's Hospital of Michigan
Detroit, Michigan

DANIEL E. WIENER, MD [100]
Chairman, Department of Emergency Medicine
Assistant Professor of Clinical Medicine
Columbia College of Physicians and Surgeons
St. Luke's-Roosevelt Hospital
Department of Emergency Medicine
New York, New York

JOHN M. WIGHTMAN, MD [9]
Associate Professor
Department of Emergency Medicine
Wright State University School of Medicine
Dayton, Ohio

DAVID WILLIAMS, MD, PhD [209]
Director
Space and Life Sciences Directorate
NASA Johnson Space Center
Astronaut Office
Houston, Texas

SONIA WINSLETT, MD [212]
Senior Staff Physician
Emergency Medicine
Henry Ford Hospital System
Detroit, Michigan

KIMERLEY DAWN WISDOM, MD [212]
Surgeon General
State of Michigan
Attending Emergency Physician
Henry Ford Hospital System
Detroit, Michigan

MARY A. WITTLER, MD [219]
Vanderbilt University School of Medicine
Department of Emergency Medicine
Nashville, Tennessee

DAVID A. WOHL, MD [147]
University of North Carolina at Chapel Hill
Division of Infectious Diseases
Chapel Hill, North Carolina

DEAN WOLANYNK, MD [269]
Clinical Associate Professor of Surgery and Medicine
University of Illinois College of Medicine at Rockford
Director, Department of Emergency Medicine
Harvard Memorial Hospital
Harvard, Illinois

WILLIAM A. WOODS, MD [213]
Injury Prevention Program Director
University of Virginia
Department of Emergency Medicine
Charlottesville, Virginia

MELISSA M. WU, MD, MBA [57]
Assistant Professor
Director, Urgent Care Center
Johns Hopkins University School of Medicine
Department of Emergency Medicine
Baltimore, Maryland

ARTHUR H. YANCEY II, MD, MPH [5]
Assistant Professor
Emory University School of Medicine
Department of Emergency Medicine
Atlanta, Georgia

SAMUEL YANG, MD [145]
Instructor of Emergency Medicine
Department of Emergency Medicine
The Johns Hopkins University
Baltimore, Maryland

LUKE YIP, MD [170]
Attending Physician
Rocky Mountain Poison and Drug Center
Denver Health Medical Center
Denver, Colorado
Clinical Assistant Professor, School of Pharmacy
Department of Pharmaceutical Sciences
University of Colorado Health Sciences Center

WILLIAM FRANKLIN YOUNG, JR., MD [66, 67]
Assistant Professor
University of Kentucky College of Medicine
Department of Emergency Medicine
Lexington, Kentucky

JANET SIMMONS YOUNG, MD [110]
Assistant Professor
University of North Carolina at Chapel Hill
Department of Emergency Medicine
Chapel Hill, North Carolina

RICHARD D. ZANE, MD [263]
Brigham and Women's Hospital
Harvard Medical School
Department of Emergency Medicine
Boston, Massachusetts

GARY D. ZIMMER, MD [36]
Assistant Chief of Service
Johns Hopkins Hospital
Department of Emergency Medicine
Baltimore, Maryland

*Deceased.

This is the seventh *Study Guide* since 1979, when the first edition was published by the American College of Emergency Physicians. The first McGraw-Hill edition was published in 1985.

The maturation of the *Study Guide* matches the development and maturation of the specialty of Emergency Medicine. As a matter of fact, the phrase 'study guide' was coined in 1979 because the scope of practice of emergency medicine was felt to be so large that no one text could possibly cover all of the conditions encountered in a busy emergency medicine practice.

Each successive edition has expanded in scope and depth. We three editors are active teachers and practitioners of emergency medicine.

We have tried to make sure that the likely, and unlikely, conditions encountered during a busy practice have been reflected in this text.

This book would not be possible without the contributions of more than 400 authors. They have incorporated evidence-based medicine into the text wherever possible. We editors have cross-checked references, and double checked drugs against standard pharmacological references.

We thank our readers who have corresponded with us to point out inconsistencies or omissions. And we thank the practitioners of emergency medicine around the world who have motivated us, and charged us with the responsibility of establishing high clinical standards for emergency medicine practice.

JET
Chapel Hill, North Carolina
October 2003

The authors wish to acknowledge Cinnamon Larson for her fine illustrations; David Nielsen, MD, Elizabeth Mejia-Millan, PharmD, and Kelly Summers, PharmD for helping us to review the accuracy of the manuscript; and Amy Ahlquist for her excellent administrative support.

EMERGENCY MEDICINE

A COMPREHENSIVE STUDY GUIDE

EMERGENCY MEDICAL SERVICES
G. Patrick Lilja

Emergency medical services (EMS) constitute the extension of emergency medical care into the community. Strong emergency physician leadership is essential to a safe and effective EMS system.

The current EMS system in the United States started with the 1966 National Highway Safety Act, which authorized the U.S. Department of Transportation (DOT) to fund ambulances, communications, and training programs for prehospital medical services. Coincidentally, in 1967, J. F. Pantridge began using a mobile coronary care unit in Belfast, Northern Ireland, to extend coronary care into the prehospital setting.

In 1973, Public Law 93-154 defined a goal of improving emergency medical care and EMS on a national scale. Although much has changed in EMS since passage of that initial act, the original definition of an EMS system is useful for understanding its functions. This law identified 15 elements of an EMS system: (1) personnel, (2) training, (3) communications, (4) transportation, (5) facilities, (6) critical care units, (7) public safety agencies, (8) consumer participation, (9) access to care, (10) transfer of care, (11) standardization of patients' records, (12) public information and education, (13) indepen-dent review and evaluation, (14) disaster linkage, and (15) mutual aid agreements. Thus an EMS system is the entire system in place to provide care to emergency patients from the initial call to definitive care.

In the United States, individual state EMS laws and regulations typically define levels of ambulance service capability, training requirements, equipment requirements, and requirements for physician leadership and accountability. In addition, the state health department may be the lead agency in promoting and funding EMS activity.

LOCAL ROLE IN EMERGENCY MEDICAL SERVICES

To be effective, an EMS system should be planned, organized, and operated at the local level. Local communities identify the needs and allocate resources to meet the demands for emergency care. The 15 elements of an EMS system defined by Public Law 93-154 can provide guidance in this process.

Personnel

In most urban areas, paid public safety and ambulance personnel provide prehospital medical care, but in rural or wilderness areas, citizen volunteers, park rangers, or ski patrols are commonly employed.

Training

Training begins with education of the private citizen in EMS system access, CPR, and other forms of first aid. Communications media can be used to reach large populations with the information necessary to educate citizens to respond to medical emergencies.

Currently, there are four DOT EMS training curriculum levels. These are first responder (FR), Emergency Medical Technician (EMT) basic (EMT-B), EMT intermediate (EMT-I), and EMT paramedic (EMT-P). The DOT FR course is designed primarily for individuals who may be the first to arrive at a medical emergency; typically police officers, firefighters, first aid teams, and/or other community EMS responders. This course provides instruction in CPR, spinal immobilization, bleeding control, and other basic emergency care procedures. The FR course is not designed for personnel working primarily on ambulances.

The three DOT EMT levels are designed for individuals who will function as members of an ambulance crew. Some states have additional EMT levels other than the three recognized by the DOT. The EMT-Bs have the necessary first aid skills to take care of immediately life-threatening prehospital emergency conditions. These skills include CPR, use of an automated external defibrillator (AED), and safe extrication, immobilization, and transportation of emergency victims. EMT-Bs are now being trained to assist patients in using their own nitroglycerin, epinephrine, and inhalers. There is an optional module in the DOT EMT-B curriculum on advanced airway techniques: endotracheal intubation or an advanced airway adjunct, such as a pharyngeal-tracheal lumen airway or laryngeal-mask airway. The decision to teach the optional airway module generally is made by the state EMS agency. EMT-I training includes additional skills in patient assessment but also adds such skills as intravenous therapy, defibrillation, basic electrocardiogram (ECG) interpretation, and the ability to give some cardiac medications. The EMT-I curriculum was changed recently to add medications. There are, however, some states that are still using the previous EMT-I curriculum that did not include delivery of medications. The highest level of EMT training, that of EMT-P, adds additional skills in patient assessment as well as additional background in basic medical physiology. Besides the skills of the EMT-I, the paramedics are trained in the ability to give additional medications and to have a better understanding of the pathophysiology and pharmacology needed for interventions in various medical conditions. Clearly, physicians need to be deeply involved in EMT training to ensure that knowledge and skills are being taught appropriately.

Communications

The universal emergency telephone number (e.g., 911 in the United States and Canada, 000 in Australia, 999 in the United Kingdom, and 112 in the European Union member countries) has greatly facilitated citizens' access to emergency medical care. In many systems, the answering centers have enhanced equipment (e.g., E-911) that provides automatic number and location identification as well as additional information to assist the responding personnel. However, the advent of cellular telephones has complicated this process. In some urban areas, up to 25 percent of all emergency calls are made from cellular phones. Technology is being developed to address this issue.

The emergency call is the essential front door of the EMS system; those answering the calls should have the knowledge and training to obtain initial medical information properly, dispatch appropriate personnel, and offer first aid information to the caller when appropriate. The training level for individuals answering emergency medical calls in dispatching ambulances is a curriculum called the Emergency Medical Dispatch (EMD) course. EMDs are trained to collect information in a structured manner in order to direct the most appropriate EMS response. This process is called *priority dispatch*. Information obtained by the EMD allows for the provision of basic instructions to help care for the patient prior to the arrival of EMS personnel. This process is called *prearrival instruction*.

Ambulance personnel should be able directly or indirectly to communicate with the hospital of destination. Most EMTs operate in the field under *offline* medical control, according to standing orders and patient care protocols developed by physicians. However, there are times when EMS personnel may require *online* medical control, in which they talk directly with a physician for specific direction or orders. The EMS communications system should function to provide public access, prompt dispatch of the appropriate vehicles and personnel, timely hospital notification, and online medical control. The public should be encouraged to use the universal emergency telephone number rather than call a hospital or physician when life-threatening symptoms (e.g., acute chest pain, dyspnea, loss of consciousness, or focal weakness) occur.

Transportation

Ground ambulances have evolved from transport vehicles into sophisticated and efficient mobile patient care areas where lifesaving maneuvers can be performed. The most important aspect of ambulance design is that the attendants must be able to provide airway and ventilatory support while transporting the patient safely. Basic life support (BLS) ambulances carry equipment appropriate for attendants trained at the EMT-B level. Advanced life support (ALS) ambulances are equipped for EMT-Ps or other health care personnel capable of providing drug therapy and performing other advanced medical procedures. Ground transportation is appropriate for the majority of ill or injured patients, especially in urban and suburban areas. Air transport should be considered if the time elapsed before definitive care is important and air transport would shorten that interval.

Facilities

In general, emergency patients should be transported to the closest appropriate hospital or, if there are multiple hospitals within the same transport time, to the hospital of the patient's choice. However, if the EMS system has identified a specific hospital with better resources to treat seriously ill or injured patients (e.g., trauma center, cardiac center), the patient should be transported to that institution, bypassing closer hospitals. Several systems of categorizing hospitals exist, and this process should precede or coincide with the development of the EMS system. In a number of regions, the state has the statutory authority to designate certain specialty hospitals to receive a subset of patients (most commonly trauma patients) based on an objective review of the hospitals' capabilities. Some states and the American College of Surgeons also have developed a process to provide external verification of trauma centers. This process requires a review of hospital facilities, treatment processes, and patient outcomes to confirm that quality trauma care is in place. EMS systems are now also identifying hospitals as specialized receiving facilities that can provide emergency angioplasty for patients with acute myocardial infarction (AMI) or that have special expertise with thrombolytic therapy for acute stroke patients.

Decisions to divert patients to specialty centers have substantial health care and monetary implications. These decisions should be made in a collaborative manner for the EMS region based on clearly defined criteria.

Critical Care Units

Tertiary care facilities should be identified by every EMS system to provide specialty care that is not available in typical community hospitals. These facilities may be either within the EMS service area or, more commonly, outside the area. Usually, patients are transported initially to a local hospital for assessment and treatment and then transferred to a tertiary center. In some EMS regions, it may be possible to develop criteria for the transport of patients requiring tertiary specialty care directly from the scene to these centers. The most common reasons for tertiary care emergency transfer are trauma, neonatal intensive care, high-risk obstetrics, burns, spinal cord injury, and neurosurgical and cardiac care. It is not cost-effective or feasible for every community to support all these specialty services.

Public Safety Agencies

The EMS system should have strong ties with police and fire departments. Public safety agencies provide first-response services because their personnel are often the first on the scene of an emergency, and they are vital links in the delivery of emergency care. For example, police in some municipalities have begun carrying automatic defibrillators in order to improve outcomes for patients suffering cardiac arrest.[1] Conversely, EMS personnel often require support from police and fire departments to provide medical care in hazardous circumstances.

Consumer Participation

Laypersons should be represented on EMS councils. Public support, both political and financial, is necessary for a good EMS system. Two important components of a successful EMS system are lay public first aid training and the implementation of a universal telephone number system.

Access to Care

A successful EMS system ensures that all individuals have access to emergency care regardless of their ability to pay or type of insurance coverage. Often the EMS system is a patient's only point of entry into the health care system. In an effort to control health care costs, patients may be discouraged from accessing the EMS system for perceived emergencies. An important principle of EMS is that all individuals deserve timely access to the system when necessary.

A more difficult problem exists when population densities or terrain dictate longer response times for some citizens than others. EMS councils should address such inequities by providing accurate information and advice to local political entities responsible for EMS service.

Transfer of Care

Patients sometimes are transferred from one medical care facility to another either within or outside of the EMS service area. Safe transfer is an important concept, and many problems can be avoided if both the transferring and receiving medical facilities develop transfer agreements in advance. For example, the prospective agreement to accept a trauma patient decreases the time spent arranging for transfer of a critical patient. The receiving physician should be assured of receiving all relevant information about the patient on arrival. Having appropriate medical personnel accompany the patient ensures medical support during transfer.

Standardization of Patients' Records

Patient care often depends on good medical records, and prehospital records are no exception. It is desirable that all ambulance services within a specific region use a similar reporting form that can be interpreted quickly and easily by receiving nurses and physicians. It is more difficult to standardize emergency department records. However, flow sheets that are easily interpretable by receiving physicians and nurses can be used. Uniform data elements for EMS care have been developed by the NHTSA and are coming into common use.[2] Uniform data elements for emergency department care also have been developed by a cooperative effort among the NHTSA, the Centers for Disease Control and Prevention (CDC), and many emergency medical organizations. It is wise to design record systems that facilitate data extraction for trauma registries, severity scoring, and cardiac arrest outcome studies.

Public Information and Education

In designing a public information program, the local EMS council should consider that the public (1) understands how the community stands to benefit from an excellent EMS system, (2) is prepared to render first aid care, (3) knows how to quickly access the EMS system, and (4) understands that patients may not be delivered to the hospital of their choice under life-threatening conditions.

Independent Review and Evaluation

Governing agencies should be assured that there is ongoing review of the EMS system. Monitoring of radio communications, review of response times, and review of patient care records are relatively mechanical methods of quality control that are implemented easily. Outcome studies of such entities as cardiac arrest and multiple trauma require considerable physician input and cooperation. The system medical director should require that mechanisms be in place to ensure and improve the quality of EMS care. EMS system access to hospital charts should be a requirement for participating hospitals, with proper controls to ensure patient confidentiality.

Disaster Linkage

The EMS system is an integral part of disaster preparedness and should be involved in planning and practice drills along with public safety agencies and others. Public safety agencies should keep the EMS system informed of potential disaster situations or hazards that may be present temporarily. Also, hospitals should be prepared to keep the EMS system informed of their capacity to receive certain kinds of patients under disaster conditions.

Mutual Aid Agreements

EMS services should develop mutual aid agreements with neighboring jurisdictions so that uninterrupted emergency care is available when local agencies are overwhelmed or unable to provide services.

Research

While not one of the original 15 elements of an EMS system, research is needed to determine which therapeutic interventions are beneficial and which are not. Unfortunately, much of what has been done in prehospital emergency care has been based on assumptions, many of which have not been subjected to scientific investigation. An investment in research is the key to improved EMS practice.[3]

MEDICAL CONTROL

A safe and effective EMS system requires considerable physician input and surveillance.[4] Medical control can be either online (immediate and direct) or offline (indirect).

Online medical control is the provision of direct medical communication to personnel in the field either in person or by radio or phone communication. The EMS medical director may delegate this authority to other physicians who understand the protocols under which EMTs administer care. Also, the medical director may allow ambulance personnel to carry out certain standing orders when timely contact with the controlling physician is not feasible.

Offline medical control is the responsibility of the ambulance service medical director. Three main components of offline medical control are (1) development of protocols, (2) development of medical accountability (quality assurance), and (3) development of ongoing education. Protocol development determines treatment procedures that prehospital personnel may perform under the medical license of the medical director. Protocols not only should address medical treatment but also should specify the use of medical devices and equipment. It is the medical director's responsibility to approve the medical devices used by EMS personnel. EMS medical protocols should be reviewed and revised to keep pace with current medical knowledge. Quality assurance requires ongoing surveillance and study of the system. Enlisting other physicians to review existing protocols and suggest improvement is recommended. Finally, the medical director is responsible for the ongoing educational needs of the prehospital care providers under his or her direction. The medical director is responsible for the quality and content of that training.

MEDICAL BASIS FOR EMERGENCY MEDICAL SERVICES

While a relatively small number of emergency physicians are involved in the direction and control of an EMS system, virtually every emergency physician deals with prehospital care in day-to-day clinical practice.

Emergency Cardiac Care

The impetus for starting paramedic ambulance programs in the United States grew out of the recognition that sudden cardiac death was the leading cause of out-of-hospital deaths in the United States. At the same time, J. F. Pantridge in Belfast, Ireland, investigated bringing the hospital to the patient's side in the form of a mobile coronary care unit to treat life-threatening cardiac arrhythmias and improve patient survival. Subsequently, it was recognized that rather than sending physicians and nurses to the patient's side, that ambulance technicians could be trained to appropriately recognize and treat many cardiac rhythm disturbances, particularly ventricular fibrillation (VF). This resulted in communities having over 20 percent of patients resuscitated successfully from an out-of-hospital cardiac arrest. Over time it became apparent that the most effective treatment for cardiac arrest was rapid electrical defibrillation for patients in VF.[5] This observation led to the development of automated external defibrillators (AEDs) that could be used by individuals with as little as 2 to 4 h of training. Currently, the American Heart Association (AHA) recommends that AEDs be available for all individuals who may respond to cardiac emergencies and, in addition, has proposed that they be distributed widely in communities in a program known as Public Access Defibrillation. Observations from casinos and airports found that bystanders or trained security personnel could use a publicly accessible AED to obtain a survival rate of over 50 percent for victims of sudden cardiac arrest.[6,7]

With the advent of reperfusion therapy for AMI, EMS systems have attempted to identify patients in the field who may benefit from this intervention. Some systems perform 12-lead ECGs in the field and notify hospitals if the patient has ECG evidence of an AMI so that the hospital may prepare to intervene promptly on patient arrival, reducing the time needed to initiate reperfusion therapy.[8] In addition, thrombolytic agents also may be given by paramedics; a meta-analysis of six studies indicated that prehospital thrombolytic administration decreases time to drug administration and in-hospital mortality.[9] For patients with angina and unstable angina, there is evidence that prehospital drug therapy (nitroglycerin and aspirin) improves the patient's symptoms and reduces hospital use.[10]

Trauma Care

While the care of trauma patients is more controversial than cardiac care for EMS systems, there is widespread agreement that delivery of critically injured trauma patients to trauma centers saves lives.[11]

Trauma triage protocols are designed to bypass certain hospitals under predetermined protocols based on the mechanism of injury or the patient's physiologic status.

There is less agreement on what therapy should be given by EMS providers to trauma victims in the field and en route.[12] While the value of providing a secure airway is unarguable, the value of prehospital intravenous fluid administration has been challenged. A study from the Houston EMS system found that for hypotensive victims of penetrating truncal trauma who required surgical repair, withholding fluid and blood in both the prehospital and emergency department phases until arrival in the operating room improved survival rates, reduced the amount of blood loss, and shortened the overall hospital stay compared with patients who received fluid and blood in the field and emergency department.[13] A case-control study from Pennsylvania for hypotensive blunt trauma victims found that prehospital fluid administration had no effect on survival or length of hospital stay.[14] Thus, questions concerning the value of prehospital fluid therapy for trauma victims remain.[15] Until further studies are done, emphasis remains on rapid transport and airway support of trauma victims, with intravenous fluid administration an unproven but commonly performed treatment.

Adult Medical Care

While much of initial EMS care centered on cardiac and traumatic emergencies, interest has evolved in the management of other emergencies by EMS providers as they have broadened their scope of practice.[10] The management of airway obstruction and respiratory arrest is an important function of the EMS system. Paramedics can achieve airway control by endotracheal and nasotracheal intubation with a high success rate and an acceptable complication rate. Early advanced airway measures for upper airway obstruction from burns, trauma, foreign bodies, or allergic causes may be lifesaving. Neuromuscular paralytic agents, such as succinylcholine, may be used safely by paramedics in the field with appropriate instruction and close medical oversight.[16]

Respiratory distress in patients with chronic obstructive pulmonary disease (COPD) and asthma is a common clinical entity treated in EMS systems. Beta-2 agonists and ipratropium have been shown to be safe and effective bronchodilators for field use. Pulse oximetric studies for the evaluation of occult hypoxemia have become widely used. Devices capable of delivering continuous positive airway pressure (CPAP) have become available for use on ambulances.[17] There are initial observations indicating that this treatment may add benefit to the care of patients with acute exacerbations of COPD and perhaps also for other disorders such as asthma.

Paramedics are commonly called to evaluate patients with altered mental status. Glucose is given routinely to hypoglycemic patients and naloxone to patients with suspected opioid overdose. Similarly, control of seizures with diazepam or lorazepam and airway support for status epilepticus are important EMS functions.[18]

Pediatric Care

With the development of pediatric emergency care as an area of interest, experts and organizations have started to review the care of children in EMS systems.[19] It is estimated that 5 to 10 percent of an EMS system's volume consists of pediatric cases, and the most common pediatric emergencies are trauma, respiratory emergencies, and seizures. Cardiac arrest in children is rare (approximately 1 per 10,000 children per year in the United States), usually with a dismal outcome. The ability of paramedics to perform procedures to treat pediatric cardiac arrest, respiratory emergencies, and trauma is extremely variable and age-dependent. For most age groups, endotracheal intubation success rates are comparable with those for adults. As would be expected, endotracheal intubation and intravenous access have poorer success in infants and small children. Conversely, the benefit of these procedures in the field for pediatric patients remains unproven. For example, a study of pediatric prehospital intubation in Los Angeles County found no increase in patient survival compared with bag-mask ventilation.[20]

RURAL EMERGENCY MEDICAL SERVICES

Most EMS literature has been developed by urban and suburban systems, with little emphasis on rural EMS care. The rural environment provides a number of unique challenges to providers of emergency care. Long distances over which to reach and transport patients are the central issue. Specialized search and rescue capabilities may be needed for off-road and wilderness emergencies. Because of the low population density of rural areas, there is a decreased likelihood that an emergency will be witnessed and emergency aid summoned. Compared with urban and suburban populations, the population in rural areas tends to be less affluent, older, and less likely to request emergency aid unless it is truly needed.

Implementation of a universal emergency telephone number has not occurred in some rural communities. Enhanced emergency telephone service, which provides automatic location identifiers, may not be as useful in rural locations because there may not be addresses to guide emergency providers. The infrastructure for basic radio communications may not be as well developed or supported. The contraction of the health care system in the United States has caused the closure of a number of hospitals, most of them in rural areas. If an emergency facility exists, it may not have specialty or critical care services. Therefore, access to air or ground interfacility transport services is important.

Rural EMS systems face particular challenges in maintaining a cadre of EMS personnel. The volume of EMS responses in most rural communities is too low to allow for the employment of full-time EMS providers; thus rural EMS services often use volunteers or on-call part-time personnel who are paid only when called out. Volunteer and part-time personnel have limited time for initial training and continuing education and limited experience necessary for skill maintenance. Most, but not all, rural EMS services are provided at the EMT-B level. The DOT EMT-B curriculum now allows for an increased level of service by EMT-Bs that may be useful in rural areas. Some states have adopted rules allowing EMT-Bs to use certain medications such as nitroglycerin for chest pain, epinephrine for anaphylaxis, and β_2 agonists for asthma. These modifications allow a higher level of basic EMT service without having to commit rural providers to the much longer time required to obtain a higher level of certification. Innovative approaches to continuing education are also needed, particularly in isolated areas. Distance learning approaches, often in collaboration with local schools, are invaluable. Videotape conferences, satellite transmissions of lectures, and computer- and Internet-based education programs are all valuable adjuncts to rural EMS continuing education.

The provision of lifesaving services on a volunteer basis entails particular obstacles. Daytime coverage for service is a challenge because most volunteers or part-time personnel have other full-time employment. As a result, many services hire a cadre of full-time providers to respond during business hours. Dispatching volunteers from home or work directly to the scene may be one method of providing daytime coverage and reducing response times. Recruitment and retention of providers is an ongoing problem; incentives such as retirement benefits, death benefits, and scholarships for volunteers and their children are useful. Undoubtedly, the most powerful incentive for EMS volunteers is the fellowship bonds that develop within volunteer EMS agencies.

Medical leadership of any EMS system is crucial. Identification of a physician who is knowledgeable and experienced in emergency care and willing to take time away from his or her family and practice is a difficult problem for rural systems. Many systems depend on non-emergency physicians, such as family physicians with an interest in community health or general surgeons with an interest in acute surgical care, to provide medical leadership.

REFERENCES

1. Mossesso VN, Newman MM, Ornato JP, et al: Law enforcement agency defibrillation (LEA-D): Proceedings of the National Center for Early Defibrillation Police AED issues forum. *Prehosp Emerg Care* 6:273, 2002.
2. Spaite D, Benoit R, Brown D, et al: Uniform prehospital data elements and definitions: A report from the uniform prehospital emergency medical services data conference. *Ann Emerg Med* 25:525, 1995.
3. Sayre MR, White LJ, Brown LH, et al: National EMS research agenda. *Prehosp Emerg Care* 6(3 suppl):S1, 2002.
4. Alonso-Serra H, Blanton D, O'Connor RE: Physician medical direction in EMS. *Prehosp Emerg Care* 2:153, 1998.
5. Eisenberg MS, Pantridge JF, Cobb LA, Geddes JS: The revolution and evolution of prehospital cardiac care. *Arch Intern Med* 156:1611, 1996.
6. Valenzuela TD, Roe DJ, Nichol G, et al: Outcome of rapid defibrillation by security officers after cardiac arrest in casinos. *New Engl J Med* 343:1206, 2000.
7. Caffrey SL, Willoughby PJ, Pepe PE, Becker LB: Public use of automated external defibrillators. *New Engl J Med* 347:1242, 2002.
8. Patel RJ, Vilke GM, Chan TC: The prehospital electrocardiogram. *J Emerg Med* 21:35, 2001.
9. Morrison LJ, Verbeek PR, McDonald AC, et al: Mortality and prehospital thrombolysis for acute myocardial infarction: A meta-analysis. *JAMA* 283:2686, 2000.
10. Ferrazzi S, Waltner-Toews D, Abernathy T, et al: The effects of prehospital advanced life support drug treatment on patient improvement and in-hospital utilization. *Prehosp Emerg Care* 5:252, 2001.
11. Mann NC, Mullins RJ, MacKenzie EJ, et al: Systematic review of published evidence regarding trauma system effectiveness. *J Trauma* 47(3 suppl):S25, 1999.
12. Pepe PE, Eckstein M: Reappraising the prehospital care of the patient with major trauma. *Emerg Med Clin North Am* 16:1, 1998.
13. Bickell WH, Wall MJ, Pepe PE, et al: Immediate vs. delayed fluid resuscitation for hypotensive patients with penetrating torso injuries. *New Engl J Med* 331:1105, 1994.
14. Dula DJ, Wood GC, Rejmer AR, et al: Use of prehospital fluids in hypotensive blunt trauma patients. *Prehosp Emerg Care* 6:417, 2002.
15. Pepe PE, Mosesso VN, Falk JL: Prehospital fluid resuscitation of the patient with major trauma. *Prehosp Emerg Care* 6:81, 2002.
16. Wayne MA, Friedland E: Prehospital use of succinylcholine: A 20 year review. *Prehosp Emerg Care* 3:107, 1999.
17. Kosowsky JM, Stephanides SL, Branson RD, Sayre MR: Prehospital use of continuous positive airway pressure (CPAP) for presumed pulmonary edema: A preliminary case series. *Prehosp Emerg Care* 5:190, 2001.
18. Alldredge BK, Gelb AM, Isaacs SM, et al: A comparison of lorazepam, diazepam, and placebo for the treatment of out-of-hospital status epilepticus. *New Engl J Med* 345:631, 2001.
19. Gausche M, Henderson DP, Brownstein D, Foltin GL: The education of out-of-hospital emergency medical personnel in pediatrics: Report of a national task force. *Prehosp Emerg Care* 2:56, 1998.
20. Gausche M, Lewis RJ, Stratton SJ, et al: A prospective, randomized study of the effect of out-of-hospital pediatric intubation on patient outcome. *JAMA* 283:783, 2000.

PREHOSPITAL EQUIPMENT AND ADJUNCTS

Daniel G. Hankins

Andy Boggust

To a large extent, early emergency medical service (EMS) equipment began as hospital equipment that was extrapolated to the field; it was assumed that if something worked in the hospital, then it would work in the field. It soon became apparent that this hospital equipment did not always perform under the more rigorous conditions of out-of-hospital care. Over the last 30 years, equipment has evolved specifically for EMS that is better adapted to field use in terms of size, weight, and durability. This equipment is directed at resuscitating and packaging the patient for transport to the hospital and for maintenance of stability during emergency or interfacility transport. As the science of EMS continues to mature, more and more equipment will be scrutinized for effectiveness.[1] The four basic questions regarding EMS equipment are: (1) Does it do the job? (2) Is it safe? (3) Does it do the job and is it safe in the field environment? and (4) Does it do the job and is it safe in the field environment in the hands of field personnel?

The nature of EMS equipment is changing due to expanded scope of practice by paramedics and the blurring of care levels between basic and advanced life support (BLS versus ALS) personnel. Equipment once considered only for ALS care is now being carried routinely on BLS ambulances (e.g., defibrillators and airway adjuncts).

VEHICLES

The equipment used in out-of-hospital care includes the vehicles and everything on them. The vehicles may be ground ambulances, helicopters, fixed-wing aircraft, or even first-response vehicles of every sort (fire engines, police cruisers, or pickup rescue vehicles). The most common vehicle used is the ground ambulance, categorized into three common varieties: (1) type I, a standard truck (e.g., pickup) chassis with a separate modular box to carry personnel, patient, and equipment; (2) type II, an enlarged van-type vehicle, and (3) type III, a van chassis with an integrated modular box on the back for medical care and equipment. In types II and III, there is physical access between the driver's and patient care compartments, as opposed to type I, where these spaces are separate.

Ground vehicles typically have warning devices (lights and siren) as part of their equipment. Unwarranted use of red lights and sirens is dangerous for the EMS crew, the patient onboard (if present), and the general public on the streets. Protocols or guidelines to limit the use of these devices only to times when they are medically indicated is important.

COMMUNICATIONS

The two-way radio is an important piece of equipment carried by prehospital providers. As the arena of wireless communication changes, EMS systems will need to adapt their communications system to best fit their needs. The spectrum of frequencies available for emergency services is limited and is shared with other industries that require wireless communications. In the United States, EMS services may use specific frequencies (*channels*) in the very high frequency (VHF, around 170 MHz), ultra high frequency (UHF, around 460 MHz), and public safety (around 800 MHz) bands. In an attempt to create more channels for users, the Federal Communications Commission (FCC) has decreased channel spacing from 25 to 12.5 kHz, and there is an FCC mandate to continue spacing down to 6.25 kHz. Although newer radio equipment can be reprogrammed to allow for the change in channel spacing, older equipment may not function correctly with this spacing.

EMS systems in rural or suburban settings may have no difficulties with local communications; however, as they transport patients into urban settings and attempt to communicate with urban providers, the problem of compatible frequencies and channel congestion may develop. Urban systems may use *trunking,* where communications pathways are managed by a central processor between end users, allowing large numbers of users to share a relatively small number of communications frequencies. Trunked systems may be analog, VHF/UHF digital radio, or 800-MHz digital radio. An 800-MHz digital trunked system is popular because of the advantages of shared equipment between different providers (EMS, police, and fire), enhanced radio coverage, shared or lowered cost, and wide-area communications. The main disadvantage with all trunked systems is the cost necessary to upgrade the current system.

Many urban and suburban EMS providers are choosing cellular/personal communication systems (PCS) as a means of communications. These systems are abundant in urban settings because they are often inexpensive and easier to use. However, at times these PCS systems are congested, and there are still dead spots even in urban areas.

ELECTRONIC PATIENT RECORD

Although many vendors provide software to generate electronic medical records on different platforms (desktops, laptops, or handheld devices), there are no prospective or retrospective studies that support the use of any of these products on any given platform. This may be a catch-22 of EMS. It is difficult to do research in EMS because there are limited good data. However, platforms employing such software, which may help generate these data, are not used because there is no evidence to support their use.

Large systems with enough resources often have their own software specifically written for that system. However, smaller EMS systems often use off-the-shelf alternatives. Using one of these products may require either modification of a vendor's product (often costly) or modification of the EMS system to make the software fully functional.

Many states are in the process of or have already generated a common data set and are collecting statewide data. As noted before, these data are essential for prehospital research. Local EMS systems should have the ability to query their databases to provide the state with patient information for this common data set.

UNIVERSAL PRECAUTIONS

Every EMS provider must be protected against exposure to blood and other body fluids from patients. This includes masks, goggles, and gloves for routine use. On occasion, more protection may be needed, such as gowns or perhaps heavier gloves. This equipment should be carried on every EMS vehicle.

PERSONAL PROTECTIVE EQUIPMENT (PPE)

The equipment needed for universal precautions may not provide the protection necessary when personnel are exposed to hazardous material or biologic or chemical weapons of mass destruction. Minimum PPE for such exposure should include a filtered (HEPA, M95, N95, or chemical-specific) mask, goggles, gloves, and protective clothing. Protective clothing should be nonabsorbent and puncture-resistant (Figure 2-1).

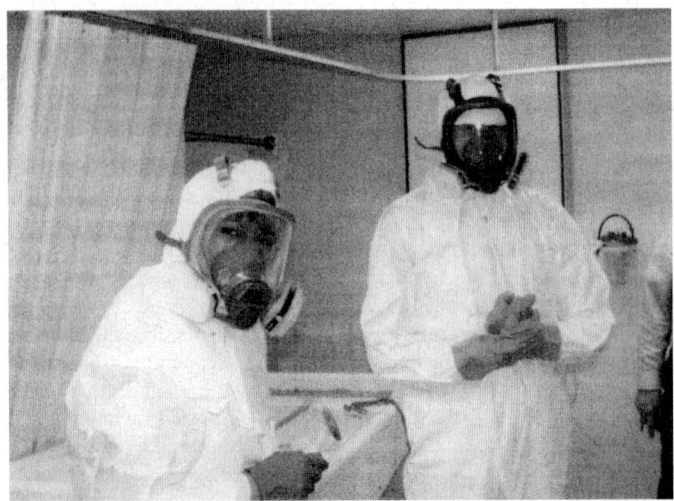

FIG. 2-1. Personal protective equipment: filtered (HEPA, M95, N95, or chemical-specific) mask, goggles, gloves, and protective clothing.

A growing number of urban EMS providers wear soft body armor as a standard part of the uniform. Suburban and rural providers can be placed in situations that necessitate similar protection. With advances in soft-armor technology, there are now a variety of styles and levels of protection from which to choose. Although each service must consider such variables as comfort, heat, weight, and cost, for EMS providers, a combination of ballistic/stab protection is optimal.

RESUSCITATION EQUIPMENT AND THERAPEUTIC MODALITIES

Defibrillators

Defibrillators have been an essential part of prehospital care since Pantridge showed that defibrillation could be done in the field on the streets of Belfast in 1965. Early defibrillation is the most important factor in survival from a cardiac arrest. Because of this, defibrillators have gotten smaller and less costly in order to expand their use. Paramedic-staffed ALS services typically carry manual monitor/defibrillators, often with additional functions (e.g., 12-lead electrocardiogram, external cardiac pacing, and synchronized cardioversion). An increasing percentage of BLS services carry automated external defibrillators (AEDs). These devices are *shock advisory defibrillators;* AEDs analyze the patient's rhythm by computer algorithm, determines if the rhythm meets defibrillation criteria, informs the operator that a shock is advised, charges the capacitor, and delivers a defibrillation when the operator pushes the appropriate button. AEDs are designed only to shock ventricular fibrillation and very fast ventricular or supraventricular tachycardias (usually over 180 beats/min). AEDs have become so easy to use and are so effective that many health and medical organizations are promoting these devices for first-responder public safety personnel and for public-access defibrillation by laypersons.[2–4]

As mentioned earlier, AEDs are simple and relatively inexpensive. They often do not have monitor screens that display the patient's rhythm. This actually may be better because a rhythm on the screen may only serve to distract a non-ALS operator. The device should have recording capabilities in order that the cardiac arrest can later be reviewed for medical oversight and quality assurance reasons. The medical director should be involved in choosing such devices, training in their use, establishing protocols for their use, and reviewing their use afterwards for quality assurance reasons.

A defibrillator used by ALS personnel is typically a different, more sophisticated device, usually with additional functions. Defibrillation is facilitated using hands-off combination monitoring/defibrillation adhesive pads rather than with handheld paddles. These pads give better contact with the skin and decreased resistance of the skin to allow for a higher success rate of rhythm conversion. It is also safer for the operator who does not have direct contact with the patient when the shock is delivered. The ALS defibrillator has a screen for interpreting rhythms and so is also used for ongoing monitoring of patients' rhythms and may be used for countershocking rhythms other than lethal ones or pacing brady-asystolic rhythms. Additional critical-care patient monitoring can be incorporated into an ALS defibrillator: noninvasive blood pressure, pulse oximetry, end-tidal Pco_2 in intubated patients, as well as other physiologic parameters. ALS personnel can use these machines for closely monitoring very ill patients during emergent calls or interfacility transfers.

The most recent development in defibrillator technology is the development of biphasic waveforms for shock delivery (as opposed to the traditional monophasic waveform). It appears from preliminary data that these biphasic defibrillators may be more successful at lower energy levels for both defibrillation and cardioversion, but papers have been few as of yet.[5] Every manufacturer is developing its own biphasic waveform for the defibrillatory shock. The debate and data may become moot in the sense that soon only biphasic models may be available.

Airway and Ventilation Adjuncts

In a patient with acute respiratory failure or arrest, these devices maintain a patent airway that otherwise would have to be maintained by the paramedic. In addition, some airway adjuncts aid in preventing complications of airway management such as gastric distention or aspiration (Figure 2-2).

The simplest devices for airway management after manual airway maneuvers are the oropharyngeal and nasopharyngeal airways. These basic airway adjuncts usually are paired in the field with a simple bag-valve mask device for ventilation and will work quite well together. Ventilation with the bag-valve mask is deceptively complex and difficult for a single person to both attain a good seal with the mask and to compress the bag to produce an adequate tidal volume for the patient. It is probably more effective (especially for first-responder and ambulance personnel who do not perform the skill often) to make this a two-person task (one to maintain the seal and one to compress the bag to maintain tidal volume). Along with these adjuncts, effective portable suction devices are available to be carried to the patient's side to help clear the airway.

More advanced airway devices are used if the patient appears to need more prolonged airway management or is at greater risk for aspiration. At the BLS ambulance level, these more invasive airways include the pharyngeal tracheal lumen (PTL) airway, the esophagotracheal Combitube (or simply Combitube), and the laryngeal mask airway (LMA). Each of these is used in conjunction with a bag-valve mask for ventilation. These devices are great improvements over the old esophageal obturator airway (EOA) and esophageal gastric tube airway (EGTA), which both had unacceptably high complication rates and are no longer recommended for use. Both the PTL airway and the Combitube are for adult patients in full cardiac arrest. They improve the airway seal to promote better ventilation than the bag-valve mask with the oral airway and seal the esophagus off with a balloon to prevent aspiration. If either device goes into the trachea, which happens a small percentage of the time, it can function equivalently to an endotracheal tube. There is some evidence that the Combitube is a more reliable device than the PTL airway because the large PTL mouth balloon is more easily broken than the more robust Combitube balloon and the Combitube may be easier for basic EMTs to ventilate with.[6]

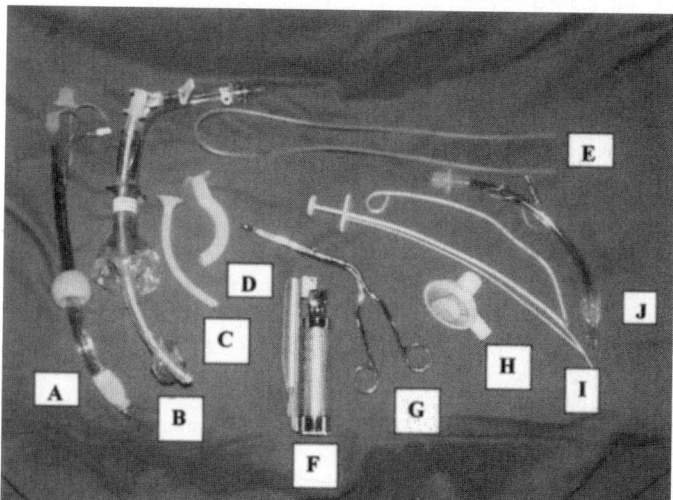

FIG. 2-2. Airway devices and adjuncts. **A.** Combitube. **B.** Pharyngeal tracheal lumen airway. **C.** Nasopharyngeal airway. **D.** Oropharyngeal airway. **E.** Tube exchanger. **F.** Laryngoscope. **G.** Magill forceps. **H.** Qualitative expiratory CO_2 detector. **I.** Stylets for endotracheal intubation. **J.** Endotracheal tube.

There are few data on use of the LMA for out-of-hospital care. It provides a seal for ventilation but may not prevent aspiration. One possible advantage of the LMA is that it is cheaper than the Combitube or the PTL airway. The PTL airway or Combitube are mostly used by BLS ambulance personnel but may be used by ALS personnel (or even by hospital personnel) as a fallback rescue device for a patient who has a difficult airway and cannot be intubated with an endotracheal tube.

The disadvantages of the PTL airway, Combitube, or LMA is that they cannot be used in small adults, children, or patients who are somewhat responsive with a gag reflex. Endotracheal intubation is the "gold standard" for airway management in all patients and is especially useful in patients in whom the other airways cannot be used. The majority of ALS systems use endotracheal intubation as the airway of choice for patients in respiratory failure or with an unprotected airway. Different-sized endotracheal tubes, laryngoscope blades with handles, stylets, lubricant, and Magill forceps should be carried in the airway kit to handle the variety of patients encountered. Tube-exchanger catheters or gum bougies also can aid in placing a difficult endotracheal tube.

The basic EMT curriculum has an optional module for endotracheal intubation training. Therefore, intubation equipment may be found on some BLS ambulances around the country. Increasing the number of ambulance personnel in need of endotracheal intubation training in an EMS system may cause logistic problems for the medical director. It is sometimes difficult to obtain adequate live intubation opportunities for the personnel in an EMS system in order to maintain skills. Some studies have shown that basic EMTs do not maintain endotracheal intubation skills and have low rates of successful completion.[7,8] This would suggest that intubation remain an ALS skill.

Another intubation-related modality that has bearing on the equipment carried on an ambulance is rapid-sequence intubation (RSI). Critical-care transport services have been doing RSI for more than a decade, but now this is being done in some ALS systems as well with good success. RSI raises the level of training, judgment, and psychomotor skills needed by the paramedic but has the advantage of being able to secure more difficult airways. In addition to the usual equipment required for intubation, RSI requires these ALS services to carry the drugs needed for sedation and paralysis.[11] RSI increases the need for oversight and vigilance by the medical director if this treatment modality is added to the ambulance providers' armamentarium.[9]

Vascular Access Equipment

The equipment used to establish intravenous access is the same as at the hospital: tourniquets, cleaning agent, intravenous (IV) catheters, IV fluid bags, and IV tubing. ALS ambulances use this treatment modality for fluid resuscitation and for administration of drugs. In general, vascular access for drug administration is completed as soon as possible after the patient is assessed and it is determined that pharmacologic intervention is needed. For fluid resuscitation, usually in trauma patients, vascular access usually is started en route to the hospital after the patient is immobilized, unless there is prolonged scene time due to extrication. This is to avoid prolonged scene times that may be detrimental to a trauma patient who may need intervention in the operating room. In any event, the amount of fluid that can be administered during transport is modest and may not be physiologically significant. There is also evidence that aggressive fluid resuscitation of hypovolemic trauma patients is detrimental in that it may increase morbidity and mortality by enhancing exsanguination from vascular or organ injury requiring operative intervention. The difference between hospital and EMS usage of IVs is that the medical director must provide guidelines for when and how to institute vascular access to allow appropriate interventions at the appropriate time. Use of vascular access should be examined in the quality assurance process in an ongoing manner. Sternal interosseous devices for establishing vascular access in patients with no other sites have been developed recently; it is too early yet to determine how useful these devices will be in out-of-hospital care.

Vascular access is also used by some U.S. BLS services for fluid resuscitation. Since BLS services are usually more rural and have longer transport times, fluid resuscitation may be more beneficial in these rural hypovolemic trauma patients who tend to have blunt rather than penetrating trauma.

Military Antishock Trousers (MASTs)

The MAST garment is a one-piece layered device made of polyvinyl fabric that encircles the legs and lower abdomen and can be inflated to apply external pressure to the enclosed body parts. The legs and lower abdomen are each enclosed separately, allowing access to the perineal area. The three compartments are fastened with Velcro. Some versions of the garment allow separate inflation and deflation of each compartment. The MAST is usually inflated with a foot pump, and some are equipped with an interposed inflation pressure monitoring gauge. Internal pressures of the suit are limited by a pressure-relief valve (set at 104 mm Hg) and the ability of the Velcro fastener to withstand stress. Pulmonary edema is an absolute contraindication to use of the MAST garment. Relative contraindications for MAST use are pregnancy, impaled objects, evisceration of the abdominal contents, and thoracic and diaphragmatic injuries.

The MAST garment has fallen into considerable disfavor because there is little evidence that it improves survival in hemorrhagic shock after trauma, and it may even be detrimental in penetrating thoracic trauma with short transport times. It is not clear whether MASTs may be useful in other situations or in disease entities other than trauma. For instance, they may be useful in blunt trauma patients with long transport times, in ruptured abdominal aortic aneurysms (AAA), and in pelvic fractures. A position paper from the National Association of EMS Physicians (NAEMSP) categorizes possible indications for MAST use into class I (useful and effective), class IIA (weight of evidence favors usefulness and efficacy), class IIB (may be helpful, probably not harmful), and class III (not indicated); the only class I intervention for MASTs was hypotension due to ruptured AAA.[10] It may be reasonable to keep the MAST garment on ambulances for now, especially on rural services, with medical oversight on its use.

SPINAL IMMOBILIZATION

Preservation of the integrity of the spinal column and spinal cord is of paramount importance in the field. The first person to assess the patient should immobilize the cervical spine immediately and simultaneously perform a modified jaw thrust to open the airway, if necessary. Manual stabilization of the neck is not released until the patient has been transferred and securely strapped to a board. Short or long boards, either alone or in combination, are used to immobilize the spine depending on the initial position in which the patient is found by the EMT or first responder.

Carrying boarded patients takes a heavy toll on the backs of EMTs and paramedics. Evaluation of the boarded patient is more expensive and time-consuming in the emergency department because of the need to clear the cervical spine. A reasonable approach is to set criteria down in protocols/guidelines written by the medical director to clinically clear the spine in the field. A patient with no neck pain or tenderness (neck pain must be defined liberally and include stiffness or "feels funny"), not in the extremes of age (below age 10 or above age 65), no altered sensorium (no drugs or alcohol present, no head injury), and no distracting injuries (long bone fracture, abdominal or chest injury) may be cleared in the field because there is an extraordinarily low probability of neck injury.[11]

Spinal Boards and Cervical Collars

Spinal boards, either short or long, are made from plastic or wood to provide a rigid surface on which to bind the patient to ensure that no movement occurs in the cervical, thoracic, or lumbar spine. Straps are used to secure the patient for transport. Some boards are provided with firm rubber blocks on either side of the head and straps to go across these blocks to keep the head steady between them. Blanket rolls secured to the board with tape are also effective head blocks. A popular and effective variation of the short board is the Kendrick extrication device (KED board), which consists of slats of rigid material bound together by heavy cloth. This board immobilizes the cervical spine, wraps partly around the patient, and is then strapped the rest of the way around the thorax and around the thighs for secure immobilization. The patient can be lifted by the KED straps, allowing for easier and safer extrication from a vehicle upward, if this is the appropriate way to remove the patient.

Rigid cervical collars are more accurately called *cervical extrication devices*. Multiple types are used in the field, such as the Philadelphia collar, the Stiffneck, and the Neck-Loc. The collars come in two asymmetric pieces, which are used and marked for back and front, or as a single piece that is folded into the correct shape. By themselves, collars are not adequate for cervical immobilization but require additional lateral support to avoid movement in that direction. For adequate immobilization, the patient needs to be strapped on the back board and secured with head blocks and head straps. Once the patient is well secured to the board, the collar does not add a significant amount of stabilization and actually can be removed without compromise of the spine; however, it is often left in place for added protection. Patients with mandible or soft tissue neck injuries probably should not have a collar applied because of the potential for airway compromise, which could be masked by the collar. Newer collars have openings in the front to allow observation of the trachea and jugular veins, but this may not be adequate for observing other neck areas. Soft cervical collars are not adequate or appropriate for out-of-hospital care.

Sequence of Spinal Immobilization

Prehospital personnel are taught to have a high index of suspicion for spine trauma. If the patient is sitting in a car after an accident and is stable from respiratory and circulatory standpoints, the short spine board and rigid cervical collar or KED are first used to get the patient out of the vehicle safely and onto a long spine board. If the situation at hand is a critical one because of the patient's condition or the threat of hazards such as chemicals, fire, or water, the patient can be extricated more rapidly using only the cervical collar without the short board or KED. After applying the cervical collar, the patient is carefully rotated out and slid onto the waiting long board.

At a non-critical scene, when the patient is still sitting in the vehicle, one EMT secures the neck with his or her hands and applies the necessary airway maneuvers, while the second EMT applies the rigid cervical collar. The short board is then slid in behind the patient, and the patient is strapped to the short spine board. (Short boards are not used if the patient is not seated in a vehicle.) The first EMT maintains manual stabilization of the neck until the patient is secured to the short board. The patient's head and truck can then be rotated around as one unit and slid directly on to the long board positioned on the car seat or on the ambulance cot. The MAST garment, if needed, is often already placed on the long board underneath the patient. The patient is then strapped to the long board and then to the cot. A properly boarded patient can be turned on the board or even stood on end if necessary to move the patient to the ambulance. If the patient vomits, for instance, the board can be partly log-rolled up to prevent aspiration.

Because of the difference in relative size and positions of head and body, adults and children need slightly different positioning on a backboard. An adult needs more padding under the head, whereas a child needs more padding under the body to maintain neutral neck position.

If a patient is walking at the scene when the paramedical personnel arrive but complains of neck pain, the patient can be boarded from a standing position. If the patient is lying on the ground when the EMTs arrive, the patient can be carefully log-rolled by several attendants onto a long backboard.

Immobilization on a rigid board produces midline cervical pain and tenderness, so examination and radiographs should be done promptly on arrival.[12] Radiographs can be done without difficulty through short and long boards. In general, patients should not be removed from immobilization until the spine has been cleared clinically and roentgenographically. Transfer from the hard out-of-hospital board to a padded board at the hospital is desirable if the patient may spend prolonged time immobilized.

Football Helmet Removal

The National Athletic Trainer's Association (NATA, www.nata.org) and the Inter-Association Task Force for the Appropriate Care of the Spine-Injured Athlete have developed guidelines for the prehospital care of athletes with potential spine injury. These guidelines recommend that the face mask of a football helmet should be removed at the earliest opportunity, before transportation and regardless of respiratory status. However, because a properly fitted football helmet with shoulder pads holds the head in position of neutral spinal alignment, field removal of these devices is not recommended. It is recommended that the helmet and shoulder pads remain on as the athlete is immobilized and transported on a rigid backboard. Simultaneous removal of the helmet and shoulder pads should be done after clinical assessment and radiographs at the hospital, although radiographs may have to be repeated after equipment removal.[13]

Removal of football shoulder pads and helmet requires at least four individuals to maintain spinal alignment.[14] One individual stands at the head of the bed to stabilize the patient's head, neck, and helmet. All straps and laces that secure the pads to the torso and arms are cut, not unbuckled or unsnapped. The laces or straps over the sternum are cut, allowing the right and left anterior portions to be spread open exposing the chest. The posterior portion of the shoulder pads are kept in place to maintain spinal alignment with the helmet. Another individual cuts the chin strap from below while standing beside the patient's chest. Accessible internal padding should be removed from inside the helmet and any air bladders deflated. The individual standing alongside the patient's chest then reaches up into the helmet to stabilize the head by placing a hand with fingers and thumbs spread alongside the jaw, mastoid region, and occiput.

Two additional individuals stand alongside the patient's chest and place their hands directly on the skin in the thoracic region. On command, the patient is lifted slightly, with all four individuals maintaining spinal alignment. The individual standing at the head of the bed can remove the helmet by a slight forward rotation to slide it off the occiput. Slight traction or anteroposterior motion may be necessary, but care should be taken not to move the head and neck unit. Attempting to assist removal by pulling on the ear holes tightens the helmet in the forehead and occipital regions and does not help. The posterior portion of the shoulder pads is removed, and the patient is lowered. A rigid cervical collar can then be placed.

Other Athletic Helmets

Studies with standard lacrosse and ice hockey helmets also support the principle of maintaining spinal immobilization by leaving the helmet on and securing the patient to a rigid spine board for transport from the field to the hospital. Because of variations in helmet design, this principle cannot be extrapolated to other circumstances.[15]

Motorcycle Helmets

Because motorcycle helmets do hot fit snugly on the head and are not worn with shoulder pads, they do not maintain a neutral spine position when the patient lays down on a flat surface. Therefore, motorcycle helmets should be removed in the field. The two-person technique, one above to remove the helmet and one below to reach up inside to stabilize the mandible and occiput similar to football helmet removal is recommended.

EXTREMITY IMMOBILIZATION

Most fractures encountered in the field are splinted for patient comfort and ease of transport. Air splints or circumferential bladders that are inflated by mouth are adequate for most distal fractures of the upper and lower extremities. In hot weather, air splints can be difficult to remove because they stick to the skin. It is better to use an air splint with a zipper and powder the inside for easy removal. The MAST garment can function as an air splint for one or both lower extremities. Other splinting possibilities include simple sling and swathe, tying the legs together with cravats to splint one injured leg with the other normal one, or using a pillow wrapped around an extremity and secured with tape. A pillow splint is comfortable and secure for the patient either out of hospital or in the emergency department. Other splints are available on the market, such as vacuum splints, but they add cost with perhaps no clearcut advantages over older, cheaper splinting methods.

Traction Splints

Pelvic fractures and fractures of the femoral shaft are potentially life- and limb-threatening. Field or emergency department stabilization of pelvic fractures is difficult; the only effective method is the MAST garment with all compartments inflated. Radiographs can be performed through the MAST garment.

Fractures of the femur can damage vessels and nerves when bony fragments move. Stabilization in the field is imperative to minimize blood loss and soft tissue damage. While MAST garments are used often to stabilize femur fractures, they do limit patient assessment and cannot reduce the fracture. The femoral traction splint is the preferred device for femur fractures.

Several leg traction splint variations are available for use. The two most commonly used types are the Hare (Dyna Med) splint and the Sager (Minto Research and Development, Inc.) splint. Other traction splints (Thomas Ring, Donway, and Klippel) are used less commonly. The underlying mechanism is the application of traction by a hitch on the ankle against resistance when the splint impinges proximally on the pelvis. The padded proximal end of the Hare splint abuts the ischial tuberosity (Figure 2-3). The proximal end of the Sager splint (Figure 2-4) rests against the pubic symphysis. These splints cannot be used if a pelvic fracture is suspected because the pressure on the pelvis may further displace a fracture and cause more bleeding. Another contraindication to traction splint use is the presence of a hip dislocation.

Leg traction splints also may be used for tibial shaft fractures. Traction splints should not be used for fractures near the knee because longitudinal traction may damage neurovascular structures in the

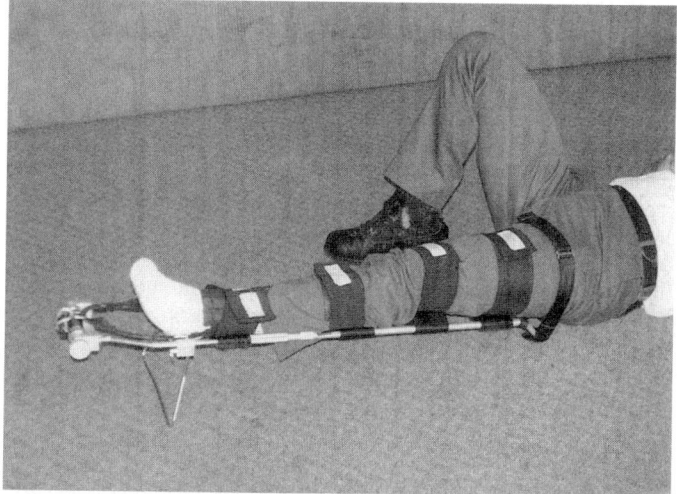

FIG. 2-3. Hare traction splint.

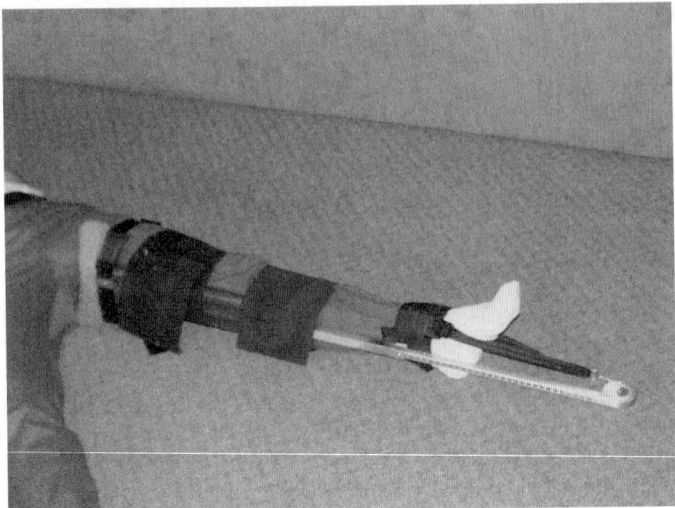

FIG. 2-4. Sager traction splint.

popliteal region. Traction splints for the tibia should be reserved for angulated or displaced fractures; otherwise, an air splint, a pillow splint, or a MAST garment would suffice.

At the scene, clothing is removed, and the extremity is assessed for injury and distal neurovascular function. If the Hare is used, the proximal half ring is placed in the crease of the buttocks against the ischial tuberosity. Traction is placed on the ankle with the padded ankle strap by one rescuer while the splint is strapped to the leg. The ankle strap is then attached to a ratcheting mechanism, and traction is tightened (see Figure 2-3). If a Sager splint (see Figure 2-4) is used, the splint is placed on the medial side of the limb up against the groin. The padded ankle hitch is applied, and traction is applied until malalignment is reduced and pain is relieved. Elastic straps are then applied to hold the splint to the leg.

The Hare splint can be longer than an ambulance cot when fully extended, and care needs to be taken when closing the rear door of the ambulance. The Sager splint is shorter than the Hare splint, and one Sager splint can be used to splint both legs simultaneously. The Sager splint is less bulky and therefore takes up less room in an ambulance or a helicopter, which can be very important in the latter.

PHARMACEUTICAL EQUIPMENT

Another area where practice is becoming blurred between BLS and ALS is in the realm of medications. The new basic EMT curriculum has modules on certain classes of pharmaceuticals to prepare basic EMTs for helping patients administer their medication in a limited fashion. These include such things as nitroglycerin for chest pain, inhaled beta agonists for bronchospasm, glucagon for hypoglycemia, and epinephrine-preloaded injections for anaphylaxis. These scenarios occur when the patient already has the medication and the EMT is simply assisting; the drugs are not carried on the ambulance. Some states have gone beyond this and allow limited carrying of medications on the BLS ambulance. The drugs carried by ALS services are more extensive, but it must be emphasized here that out-of-hospital pharmaceutical interventions are limited to a few that will make a real difference before the patient gets to the hospital. The drugs that can make a real difference when administered by a paramedic include oxygen for hypoxia; glucose for hypoglycemia; nitroglycerin for chest pain and to decrease afterload on the heart; inhaled beta agonists for bronchospasm; naloxone for suspected narcotic overdose; morphine for pain; benzodiazepines for seizures, extreme agitation, or intubation; furosemide for fluid overload; epinephrine for cardiac arrests and anaphylaxis; and lidocaine, magnesium, and amiodarone for cardiac arrest. Adenosine and diltiazem are useful for rate control of the various

tachycardias. Calcium and sodium bicarbonate are helpful for suspected or known hyperkalemia. In some systems, paralytic drugs (succinylcholine, vecuronium) are used for RSI along with sedating agents.

THE FUTURE OF EMS THERAPEUTIC MODALITIES

Small portable laboratories are already being used during critical-care transports. Most ALS services already use glucometers, but the portable laboratory or similar device would allow for other determinations in the field: low hemoglobins, high potassiums, high calciums, and high Pco_2 readings. Several companies are working on bloodless analyzers for glucose, electrolytes, and hemoglobin. While it is clear that these devices can be used in the field, it is not yet clear if the laboratory value obtained has any impact on out-of-hospital care or patient outcomes.

If proved safe and effective, oxygen-carrying resuscitation fluids (blood substitutes) may be used eventually in the out-of-hospital care arena. The roles of EMTs and paramedics are changing. Perhaps paramedics will be giving immunizations or suturing in the field. Different roles will require different equipment on the vehicle. The vehicle of the future may not look much like its current counterpart. Perhaps the paramedics will respond in a nontransporting vehicle such as a smaller truck, and the transporting vehicle will come to the scene only if asked to respond after the paramedics evaluate the situation. Digital video cameras can be used to send live visual information back to the medical control physician in those unusual complicated circumstances where the paramedics need acute advice. All these options for treatments, devices, and expanded scope of practice will need to be evaluated carefully, with physician participation, to determine their indications, usefulness, and mode of implementation.

REFERENCES

1. Callaham M: Quantifying the scanty science of prehospital emergency care. *Ann Emerg Med* 30:785, 1997.
2. Mosesso VN, Newman MM, Ornato JP, et al: Law enforcement agency defibrillation (LEA-D): Proceedings of the National Center for Early Defibrillation Police AED issues forum. *Prehosp Emerg Care* 6:273, 2002.
3. Valenzuela TD, Roe DJ, Nichol G, et al: Outcome of rapid defibrillation by security officers after cardiac arrest in casinos. *New Engl J Med* 343:1206, 2000.
4. Caffrey SL, Willoughby PJ, Pepe PE, Becker LB: Public use of automated external defibrillators. *New Engl J Med* 347:1242, 2002.
5. Higgins SL, Herre JM, Epstein AE, et al: A comparison of biphasic and monophasic shocks for external defibrillation. *Prehosp Emerg Care* 4:305, 2000.
6. Rumball CJ, MacDonald D: The PTL, Combitube, laryngeal mask, and oral airway: A randomized prehospital comparative study of ventilatory device effectiveness and cost-effectiveness in 470 cases of cardiorespiratory arrest. *Prehosp Emerg Care* 1:1, 1997.
7. Bradley JS, Billows GL, Olinger ML, et al.: Prehospital oral endotracheal intubation by rural basic emergency medical technicians. *Ann Emerg Med* 32:26, 1998.
8. Sayre MR, Sakles JC, Mistler AF, et al: Field trial of endotracheal intubation by basic EMTs. *Ann Emerg Med* 31:228, 1998.
9. Wang HE, O'Connor RE, Domeier RM: Prehospital rapid-sequence intubation. *Prehosp Emerg Care* 5:40, 2001.
10. Domeier RM, O'Connor RE, Delbridge TR, Hunt RC: Use of pneumatic anti-shock garment (PASG). *Prehosp Emerg Care* 1:32, 1997.
11. Hankins DG, Rivera-Rivera EJ, Ornato JP, et al: Spinal immobilization in the field: Clinical clearance criteria and implementation. *Prehosp Emerg Care* 5:88, 2001.
12. March JA, Ausband SC, Brown LH: Changes in physical examination caused by use of spinal immobilization. *Prehosp Emerg Care* 6:421, 2002.
13. Davidson RM, Burton JH, Snowise M, Owens WB: Football protective gear and cervical spine imaging. *Ann Emerg Med* 38:26, 2001.
14. Peries MD, Donaldson WF, Towers J, et al: Helmet and shoulder pad removal in suspected cervical spine injury: Human control model. *Spine* 27:995, 2002.

15. Waninger KN, Richards JG, Pan WT, et al: An evaluation of head movement in backboard-immobilized helmeted football, lacrosse, and ice hockey players. *Clin J Sport Med* 11:82, 2002.

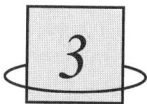

AIR MEDICAL TRANSPORT
C. Keith Stone
Stephen H. Thomas

Air medical transport consists of helicopter (or rotor-wing) and airplane (or fixed-wing) transport serving as an important component of emergency medical service (EMS) systems for prehospital care and interfacility transport. Rotor-wing and fixed-wing aircraft have different capabilities and advantage/disadvantage profiles. These specialized vehicles offer fast speeds, ranging from 100 to 200 miles per h for helicopters to over 500 miles per h for airplanes, but planning for appropriate vehicle use involves many other logistic factors as well as speed. While many ill and injured patients can be transported safely by ground, air medical transport provides added medical assessment and care capabilities beyond those of the paramedic-staffed ground ambulance. Guidelines for the use of air medical transport exist, but field EMS personnel and physicians involved in transfer decision making should be able to consider situational circumstances to determine the appropriate transportation mode.

With the occasionally important exception of ground transport legs (e.g., from a landing zone to the patient or from an airport to the hospital), air transport modalities are not limited by traffic or road quality. Weather can be an operational limitation, particularly for helicopters. Service radii differ among various helicopters and between helicopters and fixed-wing craft, but as a general rule, fixed-wing transport is considered when weather is bad or when transport distances exceed 150 to 200 miles.

The complexity of air transport far exceeds the simple act of loading a patient onto an airborne vehicle. National organizations such as the Air Medical Physician Association (AMPA), the Committee on Accreditation of Medical Transport Systems (CAMTS), and the National Association of EMS Physicians (NAEMSP) have published texts, position statements, and guidelines covering aspects of air medical transport. The AMPA *(www.ampa.org) Air Medical Physician Handbook* is a particularly helpful resource for medical issues. The CAMTS *(www.camts.org)* accreditation standards address medical, aviation, organizational, and operational issues. NAEMSP *(www.naemsp.org)* has created detailed position statements and guidelines addressing helicopter EMS (HEMS) trauma and nontrauma triage criteria as well as training of physicians involved as air medical crew or medical directors.

The effectiveness of air medical services is enabled by attention to myriad factors that come into play before, during, and after actual patient transport. The transport service should disseminate protocols guiding appropriate triage, and the program's communications personnel (as well as its physician consultants) should be versed and available for rapid decision making as to appropriate vehicle use. Ongoing training of referring agencies should occur to ensure safe and efficient operations during air transport service arrival (e.g., securing of landing zones) and transition of patient care to the flight crew (e.g., loading of patients onto the aircraft). Rigorous training programs, covering both cognitive and procedural skills, enable flight crews to provide a high level of intratransport care. In-flight communications capabilities should include the ability of the air medical crew to speak with medical control physicians, as well as arrange for any change of plan (e.g., direct transport to the operating suite) necessitated by patient condition. Some posttransport issues include utilization review, continuous quality improvement, and flight crew participation in continuing medical education conferences in which their patients are discussed. In terms of the "big picture," the air transport program should be integrated into the EMS system plans for both primary (i.e., scene response) and secondary (i.e., interfacility) missions. Because of their role in disaster operations, air medical services should be integrated into regional disaster plans.

HELICOPTER TRANSPORT

History and Aviation Issues

The first use of rotor-wing aircraft for evacuation of wounded occurred in Burma during World War II, but large-scale use of helicopters commenced with the transport of 20,000 soldiers during the Korean War. The experience in Korea led to further development of rotor-wing evacuation techniques in Vietnam, with hundreds of thousands of soldiers airlifted to medical care. Inevitably, the success of military helicopter evacuation translated into enthusiasm for development of civilian HEMS programs with the founding of the first program in the United States in Denver in 1972. HEMS grew rapidly thereafter, with approximately 200 programs in the United States and over 500 programs worldwide by 2002.

Individual hospitals or hospital consortia run most U.S. civilian air transport programs. Since helicopters are expensive (ranging from $750,000 to over $5 million) and other aviation needs (e.g., maintenance, pilot training) are also resource-intensive, most programs lease their helicopters from vendors. The air medical program typically provides and equips communications and medical personnel, whereas the aircraft vendor supplies the helicopters, pilots, and maintenance personnel. Though costs vary depending on geographic region, patient case mix, equipment and aircraft used, and even the methods used for their calculation, annual operating costs for a rotor-wing service typically exceed $2 million.

Safety is an overriding consideration for air transport. Optimization of safety begins well before an actual air transport, with training of the flight crew and of those who interact with them at scenes and hospitals. Training is especially important for scene responses, in which the helicopter may be landing in an unknown area with more nearby obstacles (e.g., wires, trees) than the hospital helipad. Scene setup (depending on the aircraft, an area of up to 100 × 100 ft is required) and demarcation, as well as safety of nearby personnel, must be taught to ground EMS services and others who call for HEMS transport. Some relevant rules include the following: (1) The aircraft always should be approached from the front, where the pilot can see approaching personnel and can then acknowledge their presence and motion them into the helicopter, (2) when rotors are turning, non-flight team personnel should approach the aircraft only with escort from a flight team member, (3) a rotor-wing aircraft should never be approached from the rear because the turning tail rotor is virtually invisible, and (4) since landings and takeoffs are the most likely times for adverse incidents to occur, ground personnel need to be well clear during these operations.

In addition to providing training for referring agencies, HEMS pilots and medical crew should undergo both initial and recurrent safety training. For added protection, most HEMS programs have followed the lessons of the military experience and adopted injury-prevention maneuvers such as the use of helmets and fire-resistant clothing. As another safety issue, the pilot should be "blinded" to the nature of the call during mission planning; this eliminates introduction of acuity-related subjectivity as the pilot considers whether the mission should be accepted. During a mission, the pilot has chief responsibility for safety, but the medical crew also should participate by maintaining a sterile cockpit (e.g., no nonaviation dialogue) at appropriate times and by pointing out obstacles or other aircraft.

Safety is partially behind the transition of HEMS programs from single-engine helicopters with visual flight rules (VFR) capability to twin-engine helicopters that can fly under instrument flight rules (IFR) conditions. The latter aircraft have greater lifting capacity, range, and speed and usually can execute controlled landings in the event of failure of one engine. A VFR aircraft can fly only during good visibility, whereas IFR aircraft operate safely in poorer conditions; both comply with visibility limitations imposed by the Federal Aviation Administration (FAA), but the IFR helicopter has fewer restrictions. If the pilot unexpectedly encounters bad weather during a flight, an IFR helicopter (as compared with a VFR aircraft) has a better chance of completing the mission successfully and safely. Due to the complexity of IFR operations, some programs (especially those with frequent bad weather periods) have elected to use two-pilot IFR.

Air medical programs operate under rules established by the national aviation authority—in the United States, the FAA. Additionally, the industry itself has set forth stringent standards under the auspices of CAMTS. On request, CAMTS performs site visits of air medical programs to certify that they comply with strict safety and operational (as well as clinical) standards. As of 2002, nearly 100 U.S. transport programs (including both rotary- and fixed-wing services) were accredited by CAMTS.

The Air Medical Crew

The primary considerations with regard to medical members of the flight crew are background (i.e., crew configuration) and training. While there are few absolutes with regard to optimal configuration, it is clear that initial and recurrent training are at least as important as the credentials of the flight team members.

The air medical team can have multiple compositions: nurse-paramedic, nurse-nurse, nurse-physician, or nurse-respiratory therapist. Further subdivisions also can be made. For example, should transport nurse hiring focus on those experienced in emergency department care, intensive care unit practice, or both? Even within the physician crew category, there would appear to be a wide difference—without casting aspersion on either party—between the capabilities and expertise of an anesthesiologist on a German HEMS unit as compared with those of a junior emergency medicine resident in a U.S. service. These differences may be one reason that the literature has failed to answer definitively the seemingly simple question of whether a physician should be on board the helicopter. Though there are a few studies that suggest outcome improvement associated with physician staffing of HEMS programs, most experts (at least in the United States) agree that physicians are not a necessary component to HEMS crews, and individual program staffing configurations generally have remained stable during the ongoing debate on optimal team makeup.[1–3]

For a number of reasons, it is unlikely that further efforts to define the optimal crew configuration will result in a consensus. The capabilities of most U.S. nonphysician crews represent an *extended scope of practice*. For instance, flight paramedics and/or nurses frequently are credentialed to perform such procedures as neuromuscular blockade-assisted endotracheal intubation and cricothyrotomy. This example of extended practice scope is important, given the importance of prehospital airway considerations and the fact that flight crews represent a highly trained group with particular expertise in this area. This level of achievement is reflected in part by the 98 percent success rate for airway establishment by the nonphysician personnel for one air medical program during a 6-year period.[4] This ability of nonphysicians to perform advanced procedures—and to perform them well—blurs the procedural skills demarcation between physician and nonphysician crew. Thus crew configuration-based outcome analyses often emphasize assessment of a more subjective (e.g., cognitive) physician contribution; these contributions are inherently difficult to quantify or associate with patient survival.[1,2]

At this time, the best recommendation with regard to crew configuration is for programs to continue to do what works for them; the relevant literature is not of sufficient strength to prompt undertaking major changes toward any single model. With this in mind, some crew configuration guidelines have relatively widespread applicability. As a good starting place, the mission profile of the HEMS program should be a consideration in determining optimal staffing. The staffing needs of a program performing primarily interfacility cardiac transports differ from the needs of a program transporting mostly trauma scene patients. Most U.S. programs perform a variety of scene and interfacility missions for trauma and nontrauma indications, so the nurse-paramedic configuration, combining the complementary skills of prehospital and hospital-based practitioners, is most popular in this country. Some transport population heterogeneity can be addressed by the accommodation of extra crew members (e.g., neonatal nurses, intraaortic balloon pump technicians) when logistics allow.

Regardless of the background of the air medical crew, initial and recurrent training in both cognitive and procedural skills is necessary to ensure an optimal level of care. Organizations such as CAMTS and NAEMSP have promulgated education and training guidelines for medical crew, as well as medical directors, of air transport programs. In addition to the considerations (e.g., airway management) applicable to acute-care provision in any setting, education of the air medical crew must address issues specific to transport in the helicopter (or fixed-wing) setting.

Environmental Factors of Air Transport

Patient care in any transport vehicle (including a ground ambulance) differs from that provided while the patient is on a hospital stretcher. Vehicle vibrations, bumpy rides, noise, physiologic stress, ergonomic constraints, and motion sickness are among the factors that can affect care. The higher acuity of air-transported patients, with the attendant need for more monitoring and interventions, is probably behind the increased focus on vehicle-related patient care limitations of air (as opposed to ground) vehicles. However, many of the same constraints probably apply to both types of transport, and even absent speed issues, there are some vehicle considerations in which helicopters may be preferable to ground ambulances (e.g., smoothness of the ride for a patient with a spinal column injury).

The impact of most vehicle-related issues in HEMS can be eliminated or at least reduced. Some solutions are easy (i.e., visual rather than aural alarms on ventilators), but flight crew must learn to "work around" other limitations (e.g., perform preflight intubation on patients who appear likely to deteriorate). Some problems will be specific to a service's particular aircraft, mission profile, or crew background; individual program patient care protocols thus should take into account the service's equipment and personnel-related capabilities and limitations.

One transport-related issue that cannot be avoided is the question of altitude and its potential effects on the patient and the crew. In the absence of unusual circumstances (i.e., ground transport over a mountain pass), these considerations are not problematic for ground transport. In fact, altitude considerations vary with location—a Denver-based program has concerns that are different from those of a Miami service. Environmental conditions also have an impact on altitude considerations, since aircraft operating under IFR frequently fly at higher altitudes than those operating under VFR. Of course, fixed-wing transports have more pronounced altitude considerations.

Helicopter (or fixed-wing) altitude and environment are known to have potential effects on patient pathology as well as the crew's ability to monitor and care for the patient. Helicopters generally transport patients at about 1000 to 3500 ft above ground level (not necessarily sea level), although sometimes these altitudes are increased for IFR flights or for clearing of obstacles or terrain. Therefore, the altitude-related problems tend to be mild, as is the case for hypoxemia, and/or relatively easily overcome, as are the cases with dehydration and cold temperatures. As noted previously, however, geographic differences are important; some western U.S. programs fly with supplemental oxygen for the medical crews.

Pressure-related problems related to Boyle's law may represent the most important consideration for helicopter-transported patients. For example, even the relatively low transport altitude range for HEMS may affect patients with certain diagnoses (e.g., decompression sickness, cerebral arterial gas embolism) or instrumentation (e.g., tamponading devices for esophageal variceal hemorrhage). In some cases, understanding of altitude issues is important for provision of prophylactic care. To minimize aspiration risk, gastric intubation should be performed for unconscious patients transported by air. Alternatively, understanding of the relevant science can be employed to prevent overreaction to potential barometric risks. The best example of this is the fact that not all patients with small pneumothoraces (i.e., who do not otherwise require tube thoracostomy) require pretransport chest decompression simply because they are to be transported by air.

CLINICAL USE OF HELICOPTERS

The roots of HEMS are clearly in the trauma arena, and trauma transports still constitute a major portion of helicopter transports for most programs. However, with more diagnoses becoming time-critical and in part due to medical care regionalization, helicopters are being used increasingly for noninjured patients. There are many logical schemes (e.g., adult/pediatric age group, scene/interfacility mission type) for categorization of HEMS transports, but an attempt to incorporate evidence-based information is perhaps best aided by parsing HEMS use into trauma and nontrauma diagnostic categories. Some issues, primarily logistic in nature, can be applied (at least in part) to both patient groups, and therefore, these are considered first.

Logistics and HEMS Utilization

Some general logistic factors have been mentioned already, but this type of detail is a prime example of information often best considered on a case-by-case basis. For example, if a mildly ill or injured patient requiring evacuation is miles away from road access, then HEMS is likely the best transport choice. This accessibility issue can be broadened to complications (e.g., traffic conditions) other than topography.

Time and distance factors, discussed earlier in relation to triage to rotary- or fixed-wing aircraft, come into play in determining whether air transport is indicated at all. A severe trauma or medical situation in an urban area, close to a major hospital, does not present the same vehicle triage implications as would the same situation occurring in a rural area—either at a small hospital or at a trauma scene—many miles from a major hospital.

A general logistic indication for helicopter use is whether delays involved in ground transport are likely to affect the patient adversely. Some logistic prompts for helicopter consideration, used primarily for scene trauma but also for other selected circumstances, include (1) lengthy transport time for ground ambulances to reach the tertiary center, (2) ground vehicle transport time to the local hospital exceeds the time required for helicopter transport to the tertiary center, and (3) for entrapped trauma patients, extrication time is expected to exceed 20 min. In some cases, HEMS is used because local ground EMS personnel lack the expertise requisite to providing the indicated level of intratransport care. Another important consideration is whether a region's ground EMS system can provide transport to the receiving tertiary center while still maintaining the ability to cover their base area with appropriate ALS care.

HEMS Use in Trauma Patients

There is no easy solution to the problem of designing helicopter trauma response guidelines that are sufficiently sensitive that nearly all appropriate patients are responded to, yet do not result in over-

triage. Various anatomic, physiologic, and mechanism criteria have been tested without agreement on any detailed protocol. National organizations have used the extant triage literature to generate consensus guidelines intended to aid localities in designing HEMS triage criteria optimally suited to their needs and resources. Reasonably appropriate triage is achievable when local ground EMS providers use such guidelines in addition to clinical judgment.[5] Critical to the process, especially for trauma scene response, is retrospective utilization review, whereby ongoing educational efforts strive to maximize appropriate HEMS use while minimizing overtriage.

There is one group of trauma patients—those in traumatic cardiac arrest—for whom air medical scene response has shown a very low rate of resuscitation and essentially zero survival.[6] Most HEMS programs have their crews accompany traumatic arrest patients by ground to the nearest facility. Outside sporadic clinical situations (e.g., hypothermic cold-water drowning in a child), there is no benefit to loading an asystolic trauma patient onto the aircraft.

After the initial triage response decision, the larger issue is whether HEMS actually improves outcome for *any* injured patients. Disagreement over this question is evidenced in the medical literature.

One tool commonly used to compare air and ground transport is the TRISS method. This methodology incorporates physiologic (Trauma Score), anatomic (Injury Severity Score, or ISS), and age (55 years as cutoff) as independent variables to predict mortality using the multivariate logistic regression model (with β coefficients derived from a large trauma database) that then can be compared with actual mortality. Studies assessing HEMS patients' survival versus that predicted by TRISS can incorporate a ground control group by simultaneously evaluating whether ground-transported patients' survival was equivalent to that predicted by TRISS.

TRISS methods have provided argument for blunt trauma mortality benefit associated with HEMS use, but there have also been nobenefit studies. The most commonly cited study that failed to identify a benefit associated with HEMS transport was conducted in London, England.[7] The authors analyzed scene transports to either a specialized trauma center or one of 19 regional nontrauma centers and concluded that there was little, if any, HEMS-associated benefit. However, further study in the same transport service during the same era but assessing only patients transported to specialized trauma center care reached an opposite conclusion: 4.2 additional lives were saved per 100 HEMS transports.[8] This difference in results likely was due to improved methodology and the use of a *W* statistic that was standardized to account for the fact that the London case mix was different from that on which TRISS methodology was based.

There have been at least seven other TRISS studies examining adult and pediatric patients transported from scenes and community hospitals that have found mortality benefit to air transport.[9] A pediatric trauma study of scene and interfacility transports concluded that for every 1000 patients flown (as compared with a control group transported by ground), 11 lives were saved.[10] Two TRISS methodology papers focused on crew configuration but also suggested an HEMS-associated mortality benefit: a 30 to 45 percent reduction in patient deaths compared with TRISS-predicted mortality.[1,2]

Two large-scale multivariate logistic regression design studies have found a reduction in blunt trauma mortality with HEMS use. HEMS transport produced improved survival for patients with moderate injury severity (ISS between 16 and 60).[11] HEMS was associated with a 24 percent reduction in mortality compared with ground transport in a large-sample study ($n = 16,699$ air and ground patients) using logistic regression analysis to control for demographic factors, ISS, mission type (i.e., scene or interfacility), and prehospital level of care (i.e., BLS or ALS).[9]

The small role of penetrating trauma in the HEMS outcomes literature is likely a reflection of the fact that most civilian HEMS programs transport few patients with this injury mechanism. Another shortcoming of the literature is that studies generally address only the hard end point of mortality, with little emphasis on either mechanisms for survival improvement or on nonmortality end points. Regardless of these shortcomings, however, the primary issue for trauma HEMS is not whether some patients benefit, but rather how well those patients most likely to benefit from helicopter use can be identified by ongoing work on improved triage criteria.

HEMS Use in Nontrauma Patients

The reason that HEMS trauma literature is (relatively) abundant is that there are ready means for controlling for the differing acuities of air- and ground-transported patients. Unfortunately, there is no such easy methodology for patients with nontrauma diagnoses, and acuity scales for nontrauma patients generally have not been accepted for use in assessing association between transport mode and outcome.

As is the case with use of HEMS for trauma, some general guidelines are applicable, and the logistic considerations noted previously apply to nontrauma flights. Rural areas have more potential use for nontrauma scene flights (or modified scene flights, in which ground ambulances transporting deteriorating patients are intercepted by a helicopter). Also, patients who are in cardiac arrest generally are transported to the nearest hospital rather than loaded onto the aircraft. Conversely, cardiac arrest patients who have been resuscitated at community hospitals may benefit from interfacility HEMS transport.[12]

NAEMSP has developed criteria for use of HEMS in nontrauma diagnoses based on a literature that suggests that time savings and the high level of HEMS care are beneficial, especially in the critically ill. The relevant studies suggest utility of HEMS for a myriad of patients ranging from premature neonates to elderly stroke victims.[13]

In most HEMS programs, the largest single nontrauma diagnostic category is cardiac. Transport for primary or rescue coronary intervention is a frequent indication for helicopter use.[14] Cardiac patients, including those with pacemakers or those who have received thrombolytics, can be transported safely and effectively by HEMS.[15]

Obstetrics transports are a special consideration for air transport because many high-risk patients are best delivered at tertiary care centers. The question for this population is primarily one of safety during transport; in-flight deliveries of such patients would doubtless represent a major resuscitation problem for both mother and infant. Experience has provided some reassurance that the use of HEMS to transport high-risk obstetric patients did not result in deliveries in the back of the helicopter, and neonatal outcomes are not adversely impacted by transport. HEMS transport of obstetric patients in an urban area is a viable solution to the problem of traffic congestion, and helicopters reduce response times for patient transport. An important aspect is the pretransport screening for the appropriateness of HEMS use.

COST AND REIMBURSEMENT

Using only direct comparison of costs to perform a single transport, which can exceed $4000 for a U.S. HEMS service, helicopters are clearly more expensive than ground ambulances. The fees charged by almost all U.S. programs include a base fee for liftoff plus a fee for loaded (one-way) mileage. Depending on staffing and local considerations, some programs charge for professional services and drugs or medical supplies used in flight.

Reimbursement by medical insurance companies for HEMS transport varies among companies and over time. Since helicopter transport services must respond when called, there is no prospective screening of ability to pay. Insurance reimbursement guidelines require adjustment to keep up with increasing calls on helicopter services to transport patients (e.g., with ischemic stroke) who historically have not warranted HEMS. Some states have regulatory guidelines for HEMS utilization and appropriateness, and there are ongoing efforts to revise the reimbursement adjudication process.

Fixed-wing transport reimbursement is less problematic than that for rotor-wing service. One reason is that fixed-wing transports are more likely to be nonemergent. Time, regulatory, and ethical considerations dictate that HEMS must respond when called, without reference to ability of the transported party to pay. These considerations less commonly come into play for airplane transports. As a result, fixed-wing transport services often can ensure reimbursement before dispatching aircraft. There are important exceptions to this rule. For example, fixed-wing services may provide emergency evacuation in regions with considerable interhospital distances or in areas where weather situations such as fog sometimes preclude helicopter operations and surface transport is not an option.

Closely related to the issue of reimbursement is demonstration of favorable cost-benefit ratios associated with HEMS use. As noted, HEMS outcomes literature limitations (e.g., lack of nonmortality end points) preclude a definitive cost-benefit analysis. However, economic analysis of HEMS for trauma patients concluded that helicopter transport is at least as cost-beneficial as many other medical interventions commonly performed in the United States.[16]

The studies just mentioned do not completely account for all aspects pertinent to true analysis of cost-benefit analysis of helicopter as compared with ground transport. The costs of helicopter transport are compared with transport by a single ambulance unit only at the peril of neglecting important systems costs. Economic analyses and expert commentary suggest that there would be little (if any) savings if helicopter coverage in a specific geographic area were replaced with ground critical-care ambulances characterized by similar response times.[17,18]

FIXED-WING AIR MEDICAL TRANSPORT

Fixed-wing aircraft can serve a wide variety of missions, from urgent to routine, over great distances. Since airplanes land only at airports, they cannot make scene flights, and they need ground ambulance connections at both ends of the flight to transport the patient between the hospital and airport. Because of these factors, fixed-wing flights generally take longer to arrange and are uncommonly used for truly emergent patients.

Unlike the situation with helicopters, which are virtually always dedicated as air medical transport vehicles when used by U.S. HEMS services, airplanes used for medical transport may have other roles. When such fixed-wing aircraft are to be used for air medical transport, their cabins must be reconfigured in a sometimes time-consuming step that may result in a transport vehicle not optimally suited for medical care. To aid with this potential problem and to ensure the presence of adequate medical equipment, vendors have developed removable medical equipment modules that can be placed relatively quickly in the aircraft cabin.

On a per-mile basis, fixed-wing transports are less expensive than HEMS transports. Excluding weather considerations, fixed-wing transfer generally becomes preferred when distances exceed 150 to 200 miles. However, the optimal transport radius for fixed-wing triage varies with regional and patient-specific considerations.

Airplanes vary in size and speed. Turboprop aircraft typically cruise at 200 to 300 miles per h; jets are twice as fast. The appropriate aircraft to use for any one mission depends on many factors: distance, the nature of the airport at the patient's pickup point, the condition of the patient, the amount of equipment, and the crew required in transport. The more critically ill the patient, the more equipment and crew may be needed and the larger the aircraft required. The choice of aircraft also must take into account the comfort of the crew and the patient for a trip of that distance (e.g., bathroom facilities for a plane making a 6 h cross-country trip). The cabins of fixed-wing aircraft are larger than those of rotor-wing craft, although the cabin's cylindrical build can be more of a constraint than its absolute volume. A larger plane that can be pressurized can fly above 3000 m (10,000 ft), which means that the aircraft can travel faster, farther, and more comfortably. At these higher altitudes, flight crews must have a deeper understanding of altitude physiology issues. Cabin pressure (i.e., indicated altitude above sea level) should be recorded on medical records because of the importance of pressure issues to physiology, and crew safety training should include measures to take in case of inadvertent cabin depressurization.

All fixed-wing services must comply with civil aviation authority rules for airplanes. As is the case with helicopters used for medical transport, CAMTS has developed standards for air medical fixed-wing transport. These standards, which are also a useful primer for more detailed information about fixed-wing air medical transport, deal with aircraft configuration, medical equipment requirements, medical crew configuration and training, and medical director qualifications.

MEDICAL DIRECTION OF AIR MEDICAL SERVICES

Medical direction may be even more important with rotor- and fixed-wing services than with ground services; it is certainly more complicated because it involves most aspects of ground EMS in addition to vehicle-specific and altitude- and acuity-related issues. The medical director should be familiar with the physiology and stress of flight on patients and should oversee the teaching of these and other applicable principles to the air medical crew. Overall, a flight crew requires more initial and ongoing training than do most ground EMS personnel due to the higher patient acuity and extended practice scope. Because flight crews are often far from their base of operations and may be out of voice contact, they must be sufficiently trained that they can act independently when necessary. For nonphysician crew, standing orders or protocols (especially for advanced procedures such as cricothyrotomy) are needed. Periodic review and updating of these protocols, as well as close inspection of every transport record, are among the many responsibilities of the medical director. Information on the responsibilities and function of the air medical program physician director have been published by AMPA and NAEMSP.

REFERENCES

1. Baxt W, Moody PG: The impact of a physician as part of the aeromedical prehospital team in patients with blunt trauma. *JAMA* 257:3246, 1987.
2. Hamman BL, Cue JI, Miller FB, et al: Helicopter transport of trauma victims: Does a physician make a difference? *J Trauma* 31:490, 1991.
3. Gisvold SE: Helicopter emergency medical service with specially trained physicians: Does it make a difference? *Acta Anaesthesiol Scand* 46:757, 2002.
4. Thomas SH, Harrison T, Wedel SK: Flight crew airway management in four settings: A six-year review. *Prehosp Emerg Care* 3:310, 1999.
5. Emerman CL, Shade B, Kubincanek J: A comparison of EMT judgment and prehospital trauma triage instruments. *J Trauma* 31:1369, 1991.
6. Wright SW, Dronen SC, Combs TJ, Storer D: Aeromedical transport of patients with posttraumatic cardiac arrest. *Ann Emerg Med* 18:721, 1989.
7. Nicholl JP, Brazier JE, Snooks HA: Effects of London helicopter EMS on survival after trauma. *Br Med J* 311:217, 1995.
8. Younge PA, Coats TJ, Gurney K, Kirk CJC: Interpretation of the *Ws* statistic: Application to an integrated trauma system. *J Trauma* 43:511, 1997.
9. Thomas SH, Harrison TH, Buras WR, et al: Helicopter transport and blunt trauma outcome. *J Trauma* 52:136, 2002.
10. Moront ML, Gotschall CS, Eichelberger MR: Helicopter transport of injured children: System effectiveness and triage criteria. *J Pediatr Surg* 31:1183, 1996.
11. Brathwaite CEM, Rosko M, McDowell R, et al: A critical analysis of on-scene helicopter transport on survival in a statewide trauma system. *J Trauma* 45:140, 1998.
12. Werman HA, Falcone RA, Shaner S, et al: Helicopter transport of patients to tertiary care centers after cardiac arrest. *Am J Emerg Med* 17:130, 1999.
13. Thomas SH, Cheema F, Cumming M, et al: Nontrauma helicopter EMS transport: Annotated review of selected outcomes-related literature. *Prehosp Emerg Care* 6:242, 2002.
14. Straumann E, Yoon S, Naegeli B, et al: Hospital transfer for primary coronary angioplasty in high-risk patients with acute myocardial infarction. *Heart* 82:415, 1999.
15. Berns KS, Hankins DG, Zietlow SP: Comparison of air and ground transport of cardiac patients. *Air Med J* 20:33, 2001.
16. Gearhart PA, Wuerz RW, Localio AR: Cost-effectiveness analysis of helicopter EMS for trauma patients. *Ann Emerg Med* 30:500, 1997.
17. Bruhn JD, Williams KA, Aghababian R: True costs of air medical vs. ground ambulance systems. *Air Med J* 12:262, 1993.
18. Mackenzie JR: Are scene flights for penetrating trauma justified? (Commentary). *J Trauma* 43:83, 1997.

4

NEONATAL AND PEDIATRIC TRANSPORT

Phillip V. Gordon
Carl Bose

Regionalized intensive care is a concept that has gained wide acceptance in neonatology and pediatric care.[1] This concept mandates that expensive, high-technology, labor-intensive therapies be limited to a few regional centers. Because patients in need of these services may initially present to other hospitals, interfacility transport has developed as a complement to regionalized intensive care.[2]

Either the referring hospital or, more commonly, the regional center may assume the responsibility for transport of a patient to a regional center. Because community emergency medical services (EMS) systems often are not equipped to transport critically ill children, the interfacility transport of pediatric patients frequently is conducted by specialized transport services.[2] Under these circumstances, the referring hospital and its medical care staff still have important responsibilities related to transport; emergency department personnel most often assume these responsibilities because the emergency department is the site of initial care.

THE TRANSPORT ENVIRONMENT

Moving critically ill patients between hospitals invariably adds to the risks of the illness or injury because of the hazards associated with the transport environment, particularly during the transport of neonatal and pediatric patients.[3] An understanding of the transport environment is important for individuals who participate in the preparation of a patient for transport, as well as for those who conduct the transport.

Features

The features of transport that distinguish this environment from the inpatient setting and the effects of these features on patients and caretakers include the following:

1. *Excessive noise.* The acute effects of excessive noise on older pediatric and adult patients probably are minimal. By contrast, persistent sound in excess of 80 dB significantly increases the frequency of arterial oxygen desaturation in premature infants. In addition, excessive noise makes it virtually impossible to use the sense of hearing to evaluate patients during transport.
2. *Vibration.* The effects of vibration on patients are uncertain but probably are not of great significance. However, vibration may limit the reliability of transport equipment. Monitor artifact must be recognized, and alternative techniques for monitoring should be employed as needed.
3. *Inadequate lighting.* Inadequate lighting is rarely a problem during the transport of adult patients because EMS vehicles generally have lighting designed for adult patients on stretchers. However, task lighting for illuminating small areas and small patients is usually not available.
4. *Variable ambient temperature.* Although the range of ambient temperatures encountered during transport rarely influences the body temperature of adult patients, environmental conditions can markedly influence the body temperature of neonates and small children.

5. *Changes in barometric pressure.* Changes in barometric pressure during ascent in nonpressurized aircraft cause expansion of gases in closed spaces (e.g., with endotracheal tube cuffs or pulmonary interstitial emphysema) and a fall in the partial pressure of oxygen. These changes are rarely of sufficient magnitude to influence physiologic characteristics unless the change in altitude is greater than 1500 m (5000 ft).

6. *Confined space.* The confined space in transport vehicles is an obvious handicap because it limits the number of caretakers and the amount of support equipment.

7. *Limited support services and personnel.* Similarly, the extent and precision of care are limited during transport by the lack of support services (e.g., radiographic and laboratory services) and specialty personnel.

8. *Equipment failure.* Equipment failure during transport is common and is particularly problematic because replacement equipment is less likely to be available in the vehicle than in an inpatient setting. A common problem is the unexpected exhaustion of an oxygen tank.

9. *Motion-induced illness.* Many medical personnel develop motion-induced illnesses during transport. Symptoms often are categorized into one of two syndromes: the Sopite syndrome, which is characterized by drowsiness and inability to concentrate, and the nausea syndrome. Either syndrome may impair the ability of personnel to provide skilled care.

Precautions

Suggested guidelines to minimize the impact of the handicaps inherent in a transport environment are

1. *Stabilize the patient carefully prior to transport.* Unless the immediate needs of the patient can only be met in the receiving hospital (e.g., severe trauma), ample time should be devoted to stabilizing the patient in the referring hospital.

2. *Anticipate deterioration.* Preparation of the patient should include not only care for the identified problems but also anticipation of problems that may arise during transport.

3. *Monitor as many physiologic parameters as possible electronically.* Because physical examination is nearly impossible during transport, and because pediatric patients often are transported during dynamic changes in their physiologic condition, electronic monitoring is essential. The following monitors are commonly used during transport:

   a. *Heart rate and respiratory monitor.* All transported patients should be monitored with impedance electrocardiogram (ECG) and respiratory monitoring. The selection of a monitor should be based on its size, weight, battery life, and resistance to motion artifact. The monitor should include a screen with a graphic display of ECG and respiratory tracings. Ideally, the monitor should display pressure waveforms and digital readings of systolic, diastolic, and mean blood pressures from transduced intravascular catheters. It is not essential that the monitoring system include the capability of electrical cardioversion or pacing; the need for such a device in the care of pediatric patients is extremely rare. However, this capability should be available during the transport of patients with known arrhythmias or patients at risk for such problems (e.g., tricyclic antidepressant poisoning or complex heart disease).

   b. *Pulse oximetry.* Continuous pulse oximetry is essential in patients with cardiorespiratory illness. Devices that display a plethysmographic waveform are ideal because they assist in identifying motion artifact.

   c. *Body temperature monitor.* Continuous temperature monitoring is helpful in neonates and small infants because of their predisposition to hypothermia.

   d. *Carbon dioxide monitor.* Continuous estimation of Pa_{CO_2} is helpful in patients with respiratory failure. Capnography, using continuous in-line infrared analysis to measure end-tidal carbon dioxide, is becoming increasingly popular as an alternative to transcutaneous carbon dioxide monitoring or arterial blood analysis. Colorimetric CO_2 detectors to confirm endotracheal tube placement in the airway are readily available and are especially helpful during transport when there is emergent concern of inadvertent extubation.

   e. *Blood pressure monitor.* Noninvasive blood pressure monitoring is advisable in children without indwelling arterial catheters. The cuff should cycle frequently enough to provide meaningful information about changes in hemodynamics. Arterial pressure can be monitored directly in patients with indwelling arterial catheters. Direct monitoring is preferable because it is more accurate and provides an alarm system in the event that arterial pressure suddenly falls (e.g., if the line becomes disconnected and the neonate suddenly has unimpeded arterial hemorrhage). Noninvasive blood pressure monitoring also may be useful in patients with direct monitoring to differentiate abnormal findings from technical artifacts.

   f. *Portable blood analyzer.* Small battery-powered devices are now available for the performance of blood gas analysis and measurement of selected blood chemistries (e.g., electrolytes and blood glucose). These devices are valuable for monitoring patients with dynamic diseases, particularly when the transit time between hospitals is long, and such devices are rapidly becoming the standard of care for neonatal transport teams.

4. *Prepare the transport vehicle.* If repeated transport of pediatric patients is anticipated, one or more vehicles should be prepared to meet the special needs of these patients (e.g., accessory lighting and a more precisely controlled thermal environment).

PREPARATION OF A PATIENT FOR TRANSPORT

Decision to Transport

A pediatric patient should be transferred to a regional center if the current or anticipated medical care needs of the patient exceed the resources of the local hospital. Arranging transfer to the regional center can occur simultaneously with assessment, resuscitation, and stabilization at the local hospital.

Basic Preparation

Extensive preparation and planning are required for transfer of a critically ill child from one institution to another. This preparation should be completed by the referring hospital personnel to the limits of their abilities and resources, regardless of whether they or a receiving hospital will perform the transport. Two of the most important aspects of care are airway management and vascular access.

AIRWAY MANAGEMENT Intubation and mechanical ventilation in a pediatric patient usually are done to (1) protect the airway from obstruction, (2) provide adequate oxygenation, or (3) ensure adequate ventilation. This principle applies to both inpatients and those being prepared for transport. However, the threshold for intervention is lowered for patients requiring transport.[4] For example, an infant with a Pa_{CO_2} of 50 mm Hg might be observed without ventilatory support in the inpatient setting but probably should be intubated and ventilated in preparation for transport. In addition, children without respiratory failure but in whom deterioration is anticipated should be intubated in preparation for transport. This more aggressive approach to airway management is justified because the ability to identify respiratory failure and to intubate often is impaired during transport.

Emergency departments should be supplied with equipment to intubate and ventilate patients of all sizes (Table 4-1). A weight- and

TABLE 4-1 Intubation Guide for Neonatal and Pediatric Patients

Age/ Weight	Laryngoscope Blade	Tube Size (mm)*	Insertion Distance (cm)†
<1 kg	Straight 0	2.5	6.0–7.0
1–2 kg	Straight 0	3.0	7.0–8.0
2–3 kg	Straight 0 or 1	3.0–3.5	8.0–9.0
3–4 kg	Straight 1	3.5–4.0	9.0–9.5
0.5–3 years	Straight 1	4.0–4.5	‡
3–5 years	Straight or curved 2	4.5–5.5	‡
5–8 years	Straight or curved 2	5.5–6.5	‡
>8 years	Straight or curved 2 or 3	6.5–7.5	‡

* Cuffed endotracheal tubes should not be used in children <7 years of age.
† Insertion distance is the distance from the tip of the tube to the lip.
‡ See Chap. 15 for more details.

size-appropriate endotracheal (ET) tube should be used. In an observational study of pediatric air medical transports, about 15 percent of intubated patients had an inappropriate ET tube size, almost always too small.[5] All nonneonatal patients should be medicated prior to intubation unless they are unconscious or in extreme distress. Neonatal patients should be premedicated only if they are alert and vigorous. An opiate analgesic (morphine or fentanyl) should be administered intravenously to patients less than approximately 3 months of age. Older children should be intubated following rapid-sequence anesthesia and paralysis.

Neonatal intubation may be challenging for personnel not experienced in airway management within this population. Attention to the following problems may increase the likelihood of success:

1. A common mistake made during neonatal intubation is to insert the blade into the esophagus and then fail to withdraw it far enough to visualize the glottis.
2. The glottis is in a more ventral position in infants than in older children; therefore, it is more difficult to visualize. This problem can be minimized by avoiding overextension of the neck and by applying gentle pressure to the cricoid. Too much pressure should be avoided because it can occlude the airway and prevent intubation.
3. Premature infants have very small mouths and upper airways, making insertion of an ET tube difficult. Gentle traction on the infant's mouth, pulled in a fishhook fashion on the right side by an assistant, often can augment the opening, allowing insertion of the ET tube just to the right of the blade. This maneuver also helps preserve the intubator's field of view.
4. Because the skin of newborns is usually moist, extra care must be taken during taping of the ET tube.

Because the distance between the thoracic inlet and the carina is extremely short in small children, the position of the tip of the ET tube should be confirmed with a chest radiograph as soon after insertion as possible. A radiograph should be obtained even when reassuring signs of a successful intubation are present (condensation on the wall of the tube, symmetric chest rise and breath sounds, and positive CO_2 detection). In the previously mentioned pediatric air medical transport study, 55 percent of intubated patients did not have the ET tube inserted to the recommended depth; almost always it was inserted too deep.[5] Right mainstem intubation is common in neonates. Prolonged right mainstem intubation increases the likelihood of pneumothorax and is particularly hazardous in premature infants. Soon after the initiation of mechanical ventilation, arterial blood gas analysis should be performed to ensure appropriate ventilator settings. Overventilation is a common error that may have serious consequences in the preterm neonate.

VASCULAR ACCESS All patients should have intravascular access during transport. Critically ill children should have at least two lines in case one becomes dislodged or several drugs must be administered simultaneously. Access should be through a device that includes a nonmetallic intravascular component. The metal butterfly needles previously used in pediatric inpatient units are not satisfactory during transport because they frequently perforate the vessel as a result of vibration and movement. Intraosseous cannulation is an alternative technique for fluid and drug administration when intravascular lines cannot be placed and the severity of illness demands immediate access.

In small children, intravenous lines should be infused with the use of pumps. Open "drips" should not be used, even with volumetric drip chambers, because of the risk of fluid intoxication from inadvertent administration of large boluses. The amount of fluid administered should be monitored and recorded carefully.

CONDUCT OF A TRANSPORT

The transport of a critically ill child from the emergency department in a community hospital to a regional center is facilitated by preestablished transfer protocols. These protocols should provide information about each regional center to which a patient might be referred, including (1) special services available, (2) criteria for referral, (3) telephone numbers for consultation, referral, and transport, (4) distance and usual response time, (5) type of transport personnel and their capabilities, (6) type of transport vehicles, and (7) protocols for preparation of patients. It is also advisable to establish formal agreements with regional centers that outline the circumstances under which patients can be transported without prior administrative approval.

Once the decision has been made to transport a child, the referring hospital has certain obligations in addition to medical care.[6] In the United States, federal law specifies some of these responsibilities; the referring physician must obtain acceptance from a receiving physician, the patient must be stabilized to the best of the transferring hospital's ability prior to transport, and the patient must be transported using a medically appropriate transport vehicle.

In preparation for transport, the referring hospital should assemble all available information pertinent to the current illness. This generally includes a copy of the emergency department record, laboratory data, radiographs, and old medical records, if available. The referring physician should inform the parents of the need for transfer and discuss the mechanism by which the child will be transferred. Consent to transport should be obtained from a parent or other responsible individual.

Receiving physicians often make recommendations regarding stabilization of the patient, sometimes at the request of the referring doctor. However, referring physicians are not obligated to follow these recommendations if they are considered to be medically inappropriate or beyond the capabilities of the referring hospital. Under these circumstances, it is advisable for the referring and receiving physicians to develop an alternative plan.[6]

For most critically ill pediatric patients, ideal care is provided when the emergency department of the referring hospital devotes its energy to providing emergent short-term care and the responsibility for transport is left to the regional center. This is particularly true for neonatal patients because of the special equipment and expertise required for transport. It is rarely in the best interest of critically ill neonates to "pick them up and run." When transport services are not provided by the regional center or when time is critical, it may be appropriate for the referring hospital to provide transport. In these circumstances, it is the referring hospital's responsibility to ensure the adequacy of care during transport.

In many areas, physicians have a choice between air and ground transportation. Again, this decision should be made collaboratively.[7] Air transport should be reserved for situations in which reduction of a critical period of time during transport is likely to reduce morbidity or mortality. In some emergencies, the critical period ends with arrival of the receiving hospital's transport team because the team is able to administer a definitive intervention for most medical emergencies. Under these circumstances, the advantage of air compared with ground transport is related directly to the reduction in time between the referral and the arrival of the team at the referring hospital. Air transport may offer the greatest advantage when definitive therapy is available only in the receiving hospital (e.g., a surgical procedure) because the patient benefits from the reduction in transit time between the receiving and referring hospitals.

When the transport team arrives, the referring physician should be present to coordinate the transition of care. Under most circumstances, a transport team originating from a hospital other than the referring hospital does not receive a detailed history of the patient's illness prior to arrival. It is essential that the referring physician be available to provide this history and a brief review of recent events. In addition to the referring physician, one or two support personnel also should be available to aid the transport team with further stabilization.

SPECIAL PROBLEMS OF THE NEONATE

The stabilization and transport of critically ill neonates are complicated by their dependence on extrinsic factors to maintain homeostasis. This is particularly true when birth occurs prior to term. In fact, the complexity of care often is inversely related to birth weight and gestational age. Neonatal conditions and aspects of clinical care that deserve special consideration when preparing for a transport include the following:

Hypothermia

Humans conserve body temperature by several mechanisms: (1) shunting blood from the skin and periphery to the core, (2) increasing basal metabolic rate, (3) voluntary muscle activity, (4) shivering, and (5) nonshivering thermogenesis. With the exception of nonshivering thermogenesis, all these mechanisms are less effective in the neonate. Although older children and adults can maintain normal core body temperature when subjected to a wide range of environmental conditions, neonates, particularly premature infants, are very limited in this regard. In addition, even under conditions in which a neonate can maintain normal body temperature, this is often accomplished at the expense of increased oxygen consumption and carbon dioxide production. These consequences are particularly onerous in infants with respiratory failure.

Neonates should be cared for in a neutral thermal environment in which core temperature remains normal and oxygen consumption is minimized. Such an environment is best provided by treating a neonate on or within a thermo-controlled bed specially designed for neonates. Thermo-controlled beds come in two varieties: an open platform heated with an overhead radiant heat source and a closed plastic incubator heated with a convection heater. Although not satisfactory for transport, open incubators with radiant heaters are ideal for the care of critically ill neonates in the emergency department because they permit access by several caretakers. An alternative is the use of a portable overhead heat lamp and a standard crib. These devices should be used with extreme caution because they do not usually include a servo-control mechanism. The patient's body temperature should be monitored frequently to avoid hyperthermia. The neutral thermal environment is presumed when the infant's body temperature is normal and there is a minimal gradient between the core and the skin temperature.

Neonates, especially preterm infants, are particularly susceptible to heat loss because they have a relatively large surface-to-body-mass ratio when compared with older patients. Also, their skin is more permeable to water vapor, and they may have a paucity of subcutaneous tissue. In addition to providing a heat source, attempts to create a neutral thermal environment should include provisions to minimize heat loss.

1. Infants should be thoroughly dried to avoid evaporative heat loss. This is critical after an emergent delivery; drying should not be delayed under any circumstances. If emergent procedures are necessary, such as intubation, another caretaker should simultaneously dry the infant.
2. Whenever possible, infants should be placed on a prewarmed surface to avoid conductive heat loss. The temperature of these surfaces or auxiliary heat sources (e.g., hot water bottles) should not exceed 40°C (104°F) because of the risk of thermal injury.
3. When treating an infant in an open crib or platform warmer, the room temperature should be increased to avoid convective heat loss. The infant should be located away from drafts (e.g., heat and/or air-conditioning vents).
4. An infant should be clothed to the extent that it does not interfere with patient care and should not be placed near cold surfaces (e.g., exterior windows) to avoid radiant heat loss. At a minimum, a covering or hat should be placed on the infant's head.

Hypoxemia

Newborn infants delivered in an emergency department or those brought to the emergency department soon after delivery outside the hospital are most often healthy. However, some may have respiratory failure with severe hypoxemia. The disease that most often causes severe hypoxemia in newborns is respiratory distress syndrome (RDS). Persistent pulmonary hypertension of the newborn (PPHN) and cyanotic congenital heart disease (CHD) also may cause severe hypoxemia in this population. It is critical that the cause of hypoxemia be identified with accuracy so that specific therapies (e.g., surfactant therapy) can be initiated promptly and/or referral to centers with appropriate subspecialty support (e.g., pediatric cardiology) can be made.

RESPIRATORY DISTRESS SYNDROME (RDS) Premature infants with RDS present with progressively worsening retractions, tachypnea, and oxygen requirements because their lungs are too immature to synthesize surfactant (a lipid-protein complex that reduces the surface tension of the alveoli). This disease has a characteristic pattern on x-ray that includes "ground glass" opacity in the lung parenchyma and prominent air bronchograms (Figure 4-1). Two postnatal strategies are employed to minimize further lung damage and rescue the patient. First, the stenting of airways with continuous positive airway pressure (CPAP) reduces the collapse of the alveoli and thereby limits further damage. CPAP can be administered through specially designed nasal cannula-type devices (with a continuous pressure of 4 to 6 cmH$_2$O) in the nonintubated patient with mild respiratory distress. A similar strategy should be used as an adjunct therapy in the intubated patient by adjusting the ventilator to provide a positive end-expiratory pressure (PEEP) of 4 or 5 cmH$_2$O such that there is never a period of negative pressure during passive exhalation. The second intervention is administration of surfactant through the ET tube. This procedure can result in rapid changes in pulmonary compliance, can cause transient airways obstruction, and sometimes is associated with pulmonary hemorrhage. For these reasons, only experienced personnel should administer surfactant. When an infant needs surfactant but the referring institution is unable to administer it, transport always should be performed by the receiving hospital. This allows the transport clinicians to administer surfactant as soon as they arrive on site, thereby minimizing further treatment delay.

During transport, most neonates are ventilated with time-cycled, pressure-limited ventilators using intermittent mandatory ventilation. As with volume ventilation, the clinician determines the fraction of inspired oxygen (Fio$_2$) and the ventilator rate. In contrast to volume ventilation, the tidal volume is not set and, in fact, is not known with many infant ventilators. The volume of each breath is determined by setting a peak inspiratory pressure (PIP), a positive end-expiratory pressure (PEEP), and an inspiratory time (T$_i$) with suggested initial ventilator

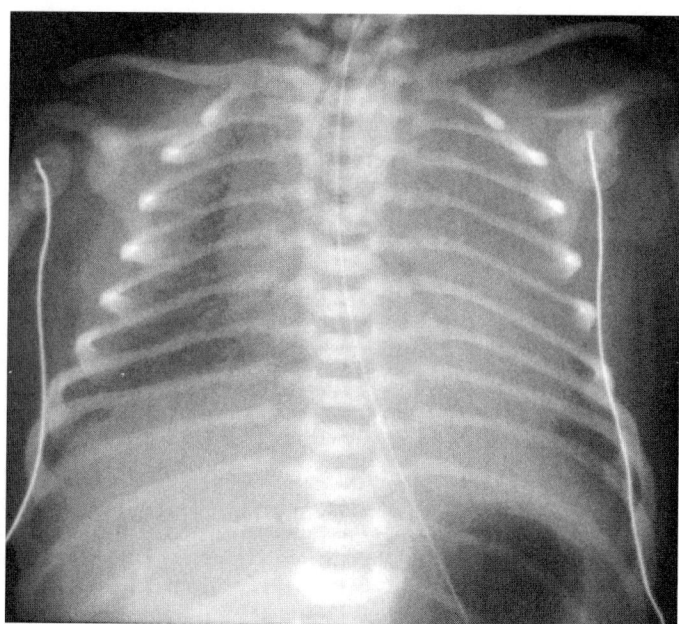

FIG. 4-1. Chest x-ray of an intubated infant illustrating classic findings of respiratory distress syndrome (RDS). Note the granular or "ground glass" appearance of the lung parenchyma, the poor inflation, the lack of focal opacities (typically seen with pneumonia), and the prominent air bronchograms. These findings correlate clinically with moderate to severe retractions and oxygen dependence in premature infants with RDS.

settings for infants that vary according to the severity of lung disease (Table 4-2).

The adequacy of oxygenation and ventilation should be assessed immediately after initiation of ventilation by observing the degree of chest expansion, skin color, and oxygen saturation. Arterial blood gases are the best means to fine-tune ventilator settings, but capillary or venous blood is acceptable for measurement of the P_{CO_2} and pH in the absence of access to arterial blood. The target ranges for oxygenation and ventilation of neonates differ according to the disease process and gestational age (Table 4-3). The blending of oxygen and air to deliver the minimum F_{IO_2} required to achieve adequate oxygenation is highly desirable, particularly in premature infants, in whom hyperoxia may lead to retinopathy.

PERSISTENT PULMONARY HYPERTENSION (PPHN)   Pulmonary circulation is attenuated in the fetus due to high intrinsic vascular resistance in the pulmonary arterioles and bypass shunting around the lungs via the ductus arteriosus. The rapid transition from fetal to newborn circulation includes a precipitous drop in pulmonary vascular resistance concomitant with lung expansion, followed by increased pulmonary blood flow in the first minutes of life and then a gradual closing of the ductus arteriosus over the next 48 h. Unfortunately, there

TABLE 4-2   Suggested Initial Ventilator Settings for Neonates

Severity of Respiratory Disease	Mild	Moderate	Severe
PIP (cmH$_2$O)	18	24	28
PEEP (cmH$_2$O)	4	4	5
T_i, s	0.5	0.4	0.4
Rate, breaths/min	20	24	30

Note: The appropriateness of initial ventilator settings should always be tested by blood gas analysis.

TABLE 4-3   Target Ranges for Oxygenation and Ventilation of Neonates

Oxygenation	Arterial Blood Gas	Pulse Oximetry
Premature infant with RDS	Pa$_{O_2}$ 50–70 mm Hg	Sa$_{O_2}$ 93–98%
Term infant (no lung disease)	Pa$_{O_2}$ 60–100 mm Hg	Sa$_{O_2}$ 96–100%
Infant with PPHN	Pa$_{O_2}$ >100 mm Hg	Sa$_{O_2}$ 100%
Infant with CHD	Pa$_{O_2}$ 35–50 mm Hg	Sa$_{O_2}$ 75–95%
Ventilation		
Premature infant with RDS	Pa$_{CO_2}$ 45–55 mm Hg	
Term infant (no lung disease)	Pa$_{CO_2}$ 35–50 mm Hg	
Infant with PPHN	Pa$_{CO_2}$ 30–35 mm Hg	
Infant with CHD	Pa$_{CO_2}$ 35–50 mm Hg	

Abbreviations: CHD = cyanotic heart disease; PPHN = persistent pulmonary hypertension; RDS = respiratory distress syndrome; Sa$_{O_2}$ = arterial oxygen saturation.

are several common conditions that can disrupt this progression, including infection, meconium aspiration, and asphyxiation. Infants with PPHN can be quite ill and require significant experience and expertise on the part of the caregivers to manage in the long term. Fortunately, the stabilization algorithm for PPHN is reasonably concise. The challenge comes in diagnosing PPHN early enough to prevent patient morbidity.

Infants with PPHN demonstrate labile oxygenation despite adequate ventilation due to right-to-left shunting of blood through the ductus arteriosus (Figure 4-2). This usually can be detected by placing a pulse oximetry probe on the right hand (preductal) and a second probe on a foot (postductal). If the preductal oximeter exceeds the post-ductal oximeter by more than 5 percent in a newborn, right-to-left

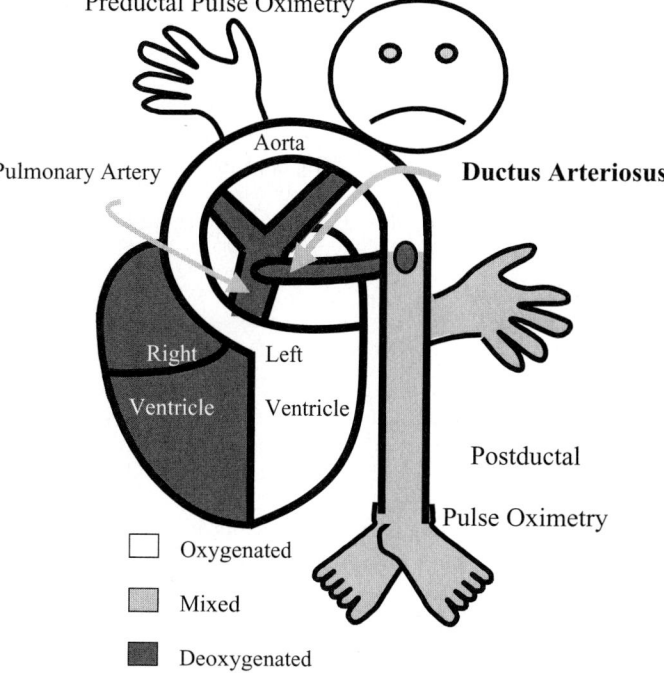

FIG. 4-2. Homunculus illustrating right-to-left shunting through the ductus arteriosus due to persistent pulmonary hypertension.

shunting is present. This finding, in combination with labile oxygenation, indicates a diagnosis of PPHN until proven otherwise with echocardiography.

Initial management of severe PPHN includes a variety of interventions designed to optimize pulmonary blood flow. These include intubation, administration of 100% oxygen (a pulmonary vasodilator), optimization of ventilation to promote lung expansion (see Table 4-3), maintenance of high-normal blood pressures to slow ductal shunting (with saline boluses and pressors if necessary), and sedation with paralysis (to minimize intrathoracic pressure). These therapies may transiently stabilize critically ill infants with PPHN but are damaging in the long term. Nitric oxide (NO) is a potent pulmonary vasodilator that has revolutionized the management of PPHN, and many neonatal transport teams now have portable NO tanks. When possible, transport of a neonate with PPHN should be performed by a team that can administer NO, thus minimizing the time to treatment. Infants that do not respond adequately to the preceding interventions are likely to require extracorporal membrane oxygenation (ECMO) for survival. For this reason, infants with PPHN should be transported preferentially to ECMO centers.

CYANOTIC HEART DISEASE (CHD) Because fetal oxygenation occurs through the placenta, cyanotic heart lesions usually are asymptomatic in the fetus. Likewise, a large number of cyanotic heart lesions become dependent on the ductus arteriosus for pulmonary blood flow at birth but remain clinically silent until the time of ductal closure. This sequence of events can result in delayed diagnosis of CHD and a subsequent need for emergency management.

The classic emergency maneuver for confirming the suspected diagnosis of CHD in a newborn is to draw an arterial blood gas while the patient is on 100% oxygen. A PaO_2 of less than 100 mm Hg indicates the presence of right-to-left shunting. However, distinguishing CHD from PPHN requires additional assessments.[8] Whenever possible, the diagnosis of CHD should be confirmed with an echocardiogram.

Emergent management of CHD relies on two strategies: (1) supportive interim management and (2) reopening and maintaining ductus arteriosus patency with a prostaglandin E_1 infusion (PGE_1). Supportive interim management may include administration of oxygen, mechanical ventilation, correction of acidosis, augmentation of cardiac contractility with pressors, and sedation. PGE_1 typically is started at 0.05 μg/kg per min and titrated according to oxygen saturation up to 0.1 μg/kg per min when trying to reopen the ductus in a severely ill patient. Mild hyperthermia and profound apnea are two side effects that are seen more commonly with the higher dosage.

Once stabilized, the primary issue for transport is typically retaining intravenous access and ensuring a continuous, steady flow of PGE_1. Patients with previously undiagnosed cyanotic heart lesions should be transferred to a tertiary facility that can perform pediatric cardiovascular surgery (preferably to a service that does at least 100 pediatric cases annually).

Hypoglycemia

During fetal life, the placenta and the maternal circulation closely regulate metabolic homeostasis. In healthy full-term neonates, homeostasis is maintained by the infant's autoregulatory mechanisms. Unfortunately, these mechanisms often fail during acute illness or after preterm birth.

The most common metabolic abnormality in newborns is hypoglycemia. At birth, blood glucose in the neonate is approximately 60 to 70 percent of the maternal level. Within 1 to 2 h, the level falls to approximately 40 mg/dL. This decline may be accentuated in premature infants, acutely ill infants of any gestational age, and certain other high-risk infants (e.g., infants of diabetic mothers).

Because of the risk of hypoglycemia, all neonates should receive glucose-containing fluids in preparation for and during transport. Thus D10 infused at a rate of 80 mL/kg per d should be used in infants with birth weights greater than 1000 g. In infants smaller than 1000 g in weight, D5 infused at a rate of approximately 100 mL/kg per d should be used because of the risk of hyperglycemia using the more concentrated solution and the relatively larger fluid requirements of the smaller neonate. In all infants at risk for hypoglycemia, measurement of blood sugar should be repeated at frequent intervals, at least every 2 h.

Vascular Access

Peripheral venous access in the neonate may be technically challenging and usually is performed successfully only by caretakers skilled in this technique. Femoral line placement is difficult in neonates and should be considered rarely. Intravascular lines placed through the umbilicus are a simple and desirable alternative for both arterial and venous access in infants less than 1 week of age. The most rapid way to obtain vascular access is to temporarily place an umbilical venous catheter (UVC) 2 to 3 cm below the level of the skin. A UVC located in this position can be used to administer fluids and medications in emergency situations, but it is not a sufficiently stable form of access during transport. By contrast, UVCs with the tip located near the junction of the inferior vena cava and the right atrium are ideal for all infusions during both stabilization and transport. The position of the tip of the catheter should be determined radiographically prior to use to ensure that medications are not being infused into the liver. An umbilical artery catheter is desirable when frequent blood gas analysis is anticipated or central blood pressure monitoring is crucial. However, umbilical artery catheters generally should not be used for the administration of pressors.

Infection

Signs and symptoms of infection in a neonate are often nonspecific and may be indistinguishable from those associated with other diseases. Therefore, infection should be presumed as a cause of illness in any sick neonate. Broad-spectrum antibiotics should be administered unless the signs and symptoms can be attributed with reasonable certainty to a cause other than infection. Antibiotics also should be administered to premature infants because uterine and placental infection is a common cause of preterm labor. Antibiotics should be administered as soon as possible because early treatment decreases mortality and morbidity rates. It is preferable to collect a blood culture prior to the initiation of antibiotic therapy, but therapy should not be withheld because of difficulties in collecting a blood culture.

Viability

Delivery of premature infants who are at the limits of viability is not an uncommon occurrence in the emergency department. Under these circumstances, the first priority of the physician caring for the infant is to determine whether resuscitation is justified. In the United States, an infant born at a gestational age of less than 23 weeks, weighing less than 400 g, with gelatinous/translucent skin and fused eyes generally should not be resuscitated or transported. By contrast, infants born at 24 weeks or older are capable of relatively good outcomes and should be supported aggressively after birth. The decision to initiate support must be made immediately because any significant delay can worsen the child's prognosis dramatically. If the decision is not clear, proceed immediately with a full resuscitation. There is never a reason to do a "slow" code in a newborn.

The death of an infant judged to be nonviable often does not occur rapidly, even in the absence of spontaneous respiration. After a decision has been made to withhold interventional care, it is important that the staff remain supportive and available to the parents. If the parents desire, the child can be held in a quiet place with a physician checking periodically to determine the time of death. This period, around the time of death, may be emotionally difficult for the staff as well as for the family. However, families often recall these irreplaceable moments (and the facility in which they occurred) with tenderness and gratitude. Futile efforts at resuscitation or interfacility transport should not be a substitute for compassionate support without medical intervention.

SPECIAL PROBLEMS ASSOCIATED WITH PEDIATRIC PATIENTS

Consent for Transport

In most of the United States, the legal age of majority is 18 years. However, mothers of younger ages have consenting authority for medical therapies for their offspring unless specifically prohibited by court order. Likewise, in many states, medical care to minors can be given without parental consent when it involves reproductive health (e.g., a teenager with a tubal pregnancy). Thus the definition of the age of majority is situational and must be addressed on an individual basis within the confines of both federal and state law.

In situations where transport of a minor patient is advisable and a parent or guardian is not available (such as is often the case with pediatric traumas in intercity areas), the minor patient can be transported under the philosophical auspices of beneficence. In these cases, legal authorization for interhospital transport requires documented consent from the referring physician explicitly stating that failure to transport would endanger the patient's well-being.

Stranger Anxiety

Young children often exhibit anxiety during contact with strangers. This behavior becomes especially significant when a child's condition is compromised by an unstable airway. In particular, patients with croup, epiglottitis, and inhaled foreign bodies can become acutely unstable when agitated. Sedation, which may reduce anxiety, may incur the risk of compromising respiratory drive and/or causing paradoxical agitation. Often the best adjunct to management of an anxious child with airway obstruction is to allow a parent to hold the child while treatment is administered (e.g., nebulized bronchodilators).

Respiratory Fatigue

Infants and small children have remarkable respiratory reserve. Infants in particular can maintain respiratory rates above 100 breaths per min for days without significant fatigue. Unfortunately, when infants or small children do experience respiratory fatigue, little time may elapse before they become apneic and unconscious. Therefore, caretakers need to be prepared for sudden respiratory failure. A laryngoscope, an appropriately sized ET tube, oxygen, and a bag-mask device should be readily available during the care of children in whom respiratory fatigue is a possibility. When respiratory fatigue appears imminent, a controlled rapid-sequence intubation is recommended prior to transport.

Transport Decisions in Children with Terminal Diseases

In the past decade, the deaths of children with terminal diseases have occurred more frequently in the home.[9] In some regions, the role of hospice and physician-directed end-of-life care provides these patients with a desirable alternative to death in the hospital. These patients may have highly evolved plans and specific limitations on end-of-life care. To be valid, these documents must be signed by both the patient's legal decision maker and his or her primary physician. These documents typically are kept at the bedside or on the refrigerator door. Despite these measures, EMS personnel sometimes are requested because the

patient is experiencing intolerable discomfort or because caregivers become uncomfortable with the dying process. Under these circumstances, EMS personnel generally are obligated to take patients to the closest appropriate medical facility, placing them at risk for having to experience the very fate that the end-of-life directive was designed to avoid. In these instances, it is of paramount importance that the patient's end-of-life directives be honored.

REFERENCES

1. American Academy of Pediatrics/American College of Critical Care Medicine: Consensus report for regionalization of services for critically ill or injured children. *Pediatrics* 105:152, 2000.
2. Woodward GA, Insoft RM, Pearson-Shaver AL, et al: The state of pediatric interfacility transport: Consensus of the second national pediatric and neonatal interfacility transport medicine leadership conference. *Pediatr Emerg Care* 18:38, 2002.
3. AAP Section on Transport Medicine: *Guidelines for Air and Ground Transport of Neonatal and Pediatric Patients,* 2d ed. Elk Grove, IL, American Academy of Pediatrics, 1999.
4. Nieman CT, Merlino JI, Kovach B, et al: Intubated pediatric patients requiring transport: A review of patients, indication, and standards. *Air Med* 21:22, 2002.
5. Orf J, Thomas SH, Ahmed W, et al: Appropriateness of endotracheal tube size and insertion depth in children undergoing air medical transport. *Pediatr Emerg Care* 16:321, 2000.
6. Bolte R: Responsibilities of the referring physician and hospital, in McCloskey KAL, Orr RA (eds): *Pediatric Transport Medicine.* St. Louis, Mosby, 1995, pp. 33.
7. Jaimovich DG, Vidyasagar D (eds): *Handbook of Pediatric and Neonatal Transport Medicine,* 2d ed. Philadelphia, Lippincott Williams & Wilkins, 2002.
8. Gordon PV: Cyanotic heart disease in the newborn (a focus on rapid diagnosis and basic management in the transport environment). *Air Med* 5:10, 1999.
9. Feudtner C, Silveira MJ, Christakis DA. Where do children with complex chronic conditions die? Patterns in Washington State, 1980–1998. *Pediatrics* 109:656, 2002.

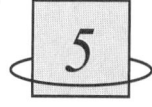

MASS GATHERINGS
Eric W. Ossmann
Arthur H. Yancey II

Mass gatherings have been defined as any voluntary and temporary collection of greater than 1000 people at one site or location for a common purpose.[1] Gatherings can be short-term (for a few hours as in a sporting contest) or longer (for several days to weeks as in the Olympic games). The event can be held on one location (e.g., a stadium) or spread over different sites. While mass gatherings imply a sports or entertainment event, smaller gatherings have many similar characteristics for medical care. These smaller gatherings include commercial airliners, passenger trains, and offshore transportation modes, such as ferries or hydrofoils, that create a situation where varying numbers of people are crowded into a limited area.

A major sporting event in an outdoor stadium will typically involve 60 to 80,000 spectators, although some university stadiums can accommodate more than 100,000 fans. Indoor arenas for basketball, ice hockey, and concerts can seat up to 20 to 25,000 people. Outdoor music festivals or motor racing can have more than 300,000 people in attendance. Not included in these figures are the thousands who attend events as diverse as high school athletics, local and state fairs, air shows, parades, and religious, political, or professional gatherings. A common feature of all these gatherings is that the injury and illness rates of those present are greater than the average non-gathered population.[2]

Several features of mass gatherings create unique medical treatment and transportation challenges not found in the general population.

Densely clustered crowds and physical barriers prevent access to, on-scene care of, and timely safe evacuation of patients. Exposure to the climatic elements and intentional injury can result in mass casualty incidents, quickly overwhelming dedicated, on-site resources. Distances within the site or between different venues, as well as interaction with public resource managers, require reliance on wireless communications. Medical care for mass gatherings represents an intersection of emergency medicine with public health and public safety, requiring working talents in business, logistics, disaster preparedness, telecommunications, and public relations.

The American College of Emergency Physicians (www.acep.org) and the National Association of Emergency Medical Service Physicians (www.naesmp.org) have developed recommendations for the provision of medical care at mass gatherings; relevant documents can be accessed through their websites. However, as noted in the NAESMP Position on Mass Gathering Medical Care, there is little scientific evidence to substantiate many of the recommendations stated in these documents.

EPIDEMIOLOGY

The modern era of mass gathering medical care began in 1965, when two spectators collapsed and died in the University of Nebraska Football Stadium. Staff or equipment to provide CPR was not available. To address this problem, personnel and equipment were placed within the stadium to provide emergency medical care. In the 8 years that followed, 18 spectators developed a cardiac or pulmonary emergency; 9 experienced cardiac arrest, 8 of whom were successfully resuscitated and discharged from the hospital.[3] Since then, reported specific experiences on mass gathering medical care include professional and collegiate football, summer and winter Olympic Games; World's Fair Expositions; motor racing; and rock concert festivals.

Statistics generated from sporting events have shown the incidence of medical problems ranging from 0.12 to 17 per 1000 spectators and cardiac arrests ranging from 0.3 to 4.0 per 1,000,000 spectators.[4,5] Statistics from major rock concerts demonstrate a 3 to 10 times higher incidence for spectator medical care than at sporting events. For events with a large number of participants engaged in physical activity (e.g., biking, running, and walking marathons) the demand for medical care (24 per 1000) can far exceed that from events at which spectators are the majority of the event population. These numbers reflect the unique medical setting for which a medical care plan and program is indicated.

MEDICAL DIRECTION

The event medical director is ultimately responsible for the conduct of medical care provided at the event. The goal should be the provision of medical care to at least the standard of that in the surrounding community. To accomplish this goal, the directorship position should be integrated into the overall event administrative structure, with clear lines of responsibility and authority to event management and medical care providers. In addition to the requisite state licensure, the medical director must be knowledgeable and experienced in the care of acutely ill and injured patients. Further, the medical director should have education and experience in out-of-hospital [i.e., emergency medical services (EMS)] medical care. Emergency medicine is an ideal background for the medical director.

On-site medical direction has several advantages over off-site medical direction. Critical medical issues requiring the expertise of a physician can be addressed in the most appropriate and timely manner, including the perspective of both in-transit care level and destination facility capability. The quality of decisions about nontransport and triage is improved by on-scene evaluations. The credibility of care and disposition decisions is enhanced in circumstances where a physician

spectator intercedes in event emergency care. Ultimately, the medical director's presence symbolizes organized medicine's commitment to the highest level of care possible at the event, an attribute likely to be appreciated by event management, as well as by patients. However, because of potential conflict with oversight duties, the medical director should avoid all but brief direct patient care responsibilities. When on-site, the medical director should be easily and readily identifiable by uniform or vest. In spite of these perceived benefits by those with mass gathering medical experience, physicians do not need to be on-site for events of low acuity, small to moderate size, with on-site patient times of less than 30 min.[6]

MEDICAL DIRECTOR AND EVENT MANAGER NEGOTIATIONS

The medical director should meet with the event managers during the planning phase to discuss the issues relevant to medical coverage. The medical director should inspect each event venue and anticipate medical demand based on either past experience or research of the literature. These findings should be discussed with the event managers. A final meeting should result in an agreement upon which the medical care plan is based. Elements to be addressed by the medical care plan include personnel issues covering medicolegal liability, credentialing, scope of practice, compensation, labor laws (uniformed medics); logistical support covering potable water, meals, sanitation facilities, parking, lodging, work-cycle assignments; communications system design for physician supervision of all event medical personnel and liaison to event managers responsible for functions impacting medical care; facility supplies, medical equipment, and pharmaceuticals. The agreement should be documented and contractual because of the risk management and medicolegal implications of the anticipated duties.

EVENT RECONNAISSANCE

The Physical Setting

Preparation should begin with repeated reconnaissance of the event setting with respect to the event type and expected population. Will the participants be seated at a sports event in a stadium or a political rally at a convention center or arena? Or will they be ambulatory at a golf or racecourse, aviation exhibit, cross-country running, biking, or equestrian event? The extent of spectator mobility has important implications for the population density and expected morbidity. At events where spectators are predominantly ambulatory, especially on irregular terrain, lower extremity trauma should be anticipated. Reports from both the 1984 Los Angeles and 1996 Atlanta Summer Olympics revealed the highest medical care use in venues where spectators moved about during the events.[7,8]

Internally, the medical director must investigate the total geographic area of medical responsibility, as well as the physical barriers to accessing potential patients. These factors can affect the ability to discover, locate, and extricate victims from a crowd as well as transport them to the most appropriate treatment site. Are on-site treatment facilities needed, or will on-scene stabilization and immediate patient evacuation off-site, or some combination of both be instituted? Externally, are dedicated public safety ingress and egress routes adequate to handle anticipated medical needs? What is the estimated transport time to the nearest hospital for noncritical patients and the nearest appropriate facility for critical patients? These factors hold profound implications for both the number and expertise of event medical care providers needed as well as their mode(s) of transportation within the venue.

For indoor events, adequate ventilation and access to exits are important issues, usually determined by jurisdictional fire codes. For outdoor events with climatic exposure, access to shelter and protection from indigenous species must be anticipated. In both settings, access to potable water, adequate numbers and distribution of restrooms, and public address system geographic range must be investigated. The history of severe weather conditions during the time of the event should be researched in anticipation of resultant illness/injury such as heat syndromes or hypothermia-frostbite.

Expected Populations and Hazardous Exposures

The event attendance bears some relationship to the expected patient volume with implications for the numbers and type of medical staff needed. However, retrospective research has not yielded any universally acceptable mathematical relationship, and the event's hazardous exposures bear a much greater relationship to patient volume than to crowd size. In studying Syracuse University's rock concert, basketball, and football events for 7 years, De Lorenzo found a correlation of crowd size with patient volume only for the concerts.[1] Event duration also correlates with patient volume through time of exposure to event and population health risk factors; the 1982 U.S. Rock Music Festival experienced a significant increase in daily patient volume on the second day of the 3-day event.

Therefore, investigating expected population characteristics and hazardous exposures is crucial to planning for their medical care. The expected density and range of ambulatory movement within a venue may foretell the risk of heat exhaustion. Will this event attract an older population at risk for sudden cerebrovascular and cardiovascular events or one in which a younger population will likely be exposed to the attendant morbidity of street drugs? Children presenting the danger of separation from responsible adults can be tagged with identification upon entry to the event. Will alcohol be allowed and/or served, and if so, what is the history of its effect on participants' behavior and health at previous and similar events? Will food be offered at the event, and if so, what public health official(s) has responsibility for monitoring and enforcing its sanitation and disposal? Is the access to toilet facilities and potable water adequate, especially at outdoor and rural sites? What is the public address system range? Will VIPs (very important persons such as politicians, heads of state, diplomats, media personalities, and corporate heads) participate, and if so, what special health and medical care measures are planned? Who are the officials responsible for these measures?

INTERACTIONS

Plans for medical care should proceed simultaneously along interdisciplinary and intradisciplinary lines. Coordination with fire/rescue/hazardous material (HAZMAT), public health, and law enforcement/security is essential. What law enforcement agency and official(s) are responsible for precautions against terrorism and the coordinated response to it? What agency and official(s) are responsible for the jurisdictional disaster/multicasualty incident (MCI) plan? What is the communications path to officials responsible for initiating execution of the plan and what intra-venue officials are in the decision tree to trigger the request?

What EMS service is responsible for responding to emergency calls within the jurisdiction surrounding the venue? The patient transport capacity of that service should be determined. If the transport service becomes saturated, when is the MCI plan activated? The extra patient transport capacity afforded by any existing mutual aid agreements with other services should be examined. What potential patient capacities do the surrounding hospitals possess? Limited external medical facilities (i.e., rural setting) may force more advanced care to be performed on site, requiring more medical staff at a higher level of expertise, more supplies, and intravenue facilities. Both the medical and administrative directors of potentially affected EMS and hospital emergency services should be repeatedly updated on medical care plans for the event and their suggestions actively solicited.

RESPONSIBILITY FOR COVERAGE

The owner or promoter of any mass gathering has an obligation to provide for the safety and security of its participants, spectators, and workers. Very few venues have enough events on a regular basis to provide for permanent, in-house medical care without outside assistance. On-site emergency medical care is typically secured through an affiliation or contractual arrangement with an EMS system and/or a health care provider, such as a hospital. The goal of any venue should be to provide the same quality of health care and security one could reasonably expect as a normal citizen outside of the venue. Failure to provide this level of service could result in a significant liability for the venue owner or event promoter. Inappropriate and/or inadequate resources or care is also a liability to the medical director, EMS system, or hospital that is assisting with the medical services.

The medical director plays a key role in the planning of any on-site medical facility and the care it is to provide during a mass gathering. The medical director should be involved in the plan, setup, and maintenance of any medical facility; and the selection, training, and function of the medical team. This requires involvement not only in the event planning, but, if possible, during the design and construction of the facility.

Licensing and credentialing all medical personnel is important. Typical good samaritan laws provide only limited protection to health care workers who provide emergency care on a voluntary basis and are not designed to cover medical personnel assigned specific responsibilities at a scheduled event. The relevant statues and law should be investigated prior to the event.[9] Health care providers should be licensed to perform their function during the event.

Liability insurance is also important for the medical director as well as the health care providers. The owner or promoter of the event may be able to obtain coverage for the medical care, or coverage may extend from the health care provider or their employer.

Several legal issues should be addressed in a contract between the medical director and event organizer/manager. A contract should give the medical director the authority to obtain whatever supplies or resources are appropriate prior to and during the event. The contract should specify financial responsibility for equipment, resources, and personnel. At a minimum, the contract should include start and end dates, fee structures, health department and medical license structures, equipment and personnel requirements, minimum medical care requirements, medical direction authority level, and emergency provisions for disaster or mass casualty situations. As much detail as possible should be listed with respect to the medical treatment facility size, location, and physical construction; the transportation of patients and personnel; the personnel's lodging, parking, food, and hygiene issues; and the communications system and devices.

ANATOMY OF A MEDICAL CARE SYSTEM

Planning

The first step in designing a mass gathering medical care system is to determine the sophistication of medical care that is needed or desired. On-site levels of care may be basic life support (BLS), on-site treatment with jurisdictional EMS transportation, advanced life support (ALS), or some combination thereof. The patient population for which medical direction is responsible should also be established; this may be participants or performers, spectators or employees. The goal is to provide the maximum care possible with the resources available. For events involving significant risk of injury to performers, separate medical personnel and resources should exist for both spectators and participants; so that care to one sector does not interrupt coverage to the other. This requires that the system be cooperative, adjustable, organized, intelligent, and prepared.

If possible, the design of a medical care system should be based on interventions that can positively affect patient outcome. For instance, a response time of 3 to 5 min can positively influence the ability to successfully resuscitate a cardiac arrest victim. Rapid (optimally, bystander) CPR is the cornerstone of BLS care, as is airway management and early defibrillation for ALS care. Therefore, responders who are trained at least to a BLS level should be stationed within 3 min of anyone in the venue.

Medical personnel and supplies should be allocated based on the anticipated number of patients and the seriousness of the anticipated medical problems. The medical problems encountered at mass gatherings are often similar. The volume and complaints can depend to a large degree on the variables previously discussed. If possible, it is helpful to obtain pre-event medical intelligence from the records of previous and/or similar events or law enforcement agencies that have had experience with the particular event. This may give insight to the potential for violence, and alcohol and drug use.

Patient Care Path

The medical care plan should address the flow of patient care from the occurrence and possible scenes of the medical events to their definitive care. Ushers, volunteers, and security personnel should be equipped with adequate communications devices and trained to relay information concerning any individual in need of medical care. Those without communication devices should be informed of the location of the nearest security officer or device for contacting the command center. Training should include the ability to communicate the appropriate information in a clear, concise format. These individuals must also act as first responders in providing a path to the patient and when necessary, providing bystander CPR.

The command center or dispatch center is responsible for coordinating the response to a medical incident. Provision of a clear, concise chief complaint to the center is vital to coordinating an appropriate response. The command center should provide all the necessary medical and security resources for response. Command staff should include managers of facility maintenance to address plumbing and electrical mishaps, parking, public relations, security and ushers. The command center is also responsible for the flexibility of personnel duties and the positioning of the response teams within the facility to provide the best response time.

Once dispatched, the response team should locate the victim and initiate care. This is best accomplished by the rapid extrication of the patient from the crowd to the nearest space (tunnel, open entryway) isolated by security personnel. At this point, stabilization/treatment can be initiated by protocol or with on-line medical direction. The amount of treatment provided at this point depends on the medical condition of the patient and the layout of the facility. Transport to a designated on-site treatment facility or ambulance should occur as soon as possible so that a specialist can provide care at the highest level appropriate to definitive treatment.

Transportation from the event should be by the most efficient mode possible considering all factors. If no access roads are available, helicopter transport may be the most appropriate option. A medical care plan should integrate the local EMS system to allow for increased transport capabilities to external hospitals if needed. This can be done by dispatching units in service within the jurisdictional system to sites of medical occurrences at the event or to a site previously occupied by a unit transporting a patient.

MEDICAL CARE RESOURCES

Personnel

Often events are staffed by a combination of paid personnel and volunteers. The number of personnel is based on the layout of the facility, the size and characteristics of the crowd, the adequacy of EMS cover-

age, and the proximity to adequate off-site (hospital) facilities. These factors determine the level of intravenue care needed. Response teams should be located throughout the facility to keep response times within a 3- to 5-min time period needed to successfully resuscitate cardiac arrest victims. It is often very beneficial to couple security officers with medical personnel in order to provide a safer environment and a quicker response. In special situations, it may be necessary to add others to the response team, such as fire fighters or water rescuers. Each response team should be efficiently staffed and equipped to easily transport a nonambulatory patient.

Treatment facilities should be staffed with definitive emergency care-level personnel; usually a mixture of nurses, physician assistants, emergency medical technicians, paramedics, and physicians. It is the function of the medical director to determine how to best meet the demands of patient care in the context of the event budget dedicated to medical care. The appropriate expertise of nonphysician personnel varies greatly. Their availability can have a direct impact on the number of physicians required. The number of physicians recommended for on-site care ranges from 1 for every 5000 to 1 for every 50,000 people. These staffing requirements should be part of a formal contract with the facility management.

Equipment

It is the responsibility of the medical director to determine the supply level and type of equipment to be used within the facility, and to incorporate these specifications into both the contract and medical care plan.[10] Often this is dictated by the local EMS system, which provides equipment for the event. Response teams should be equipped with basic airway and first aid equipment. The teams must also have adequate extrication and intravenue transportation modes (e.g., motorized carts) based on the layout and terrain of the facility. In the event of a cardiac arrest, a defibrillator should be available to be sent to the location of the patient along with ALS personnel with advanced airway equipment. This may not be necessary if an intravenue treatment facility is within a 3- to 5-min transport time under actual event conditions. The medical care system should have enough defibrillators to allow any location in the facility to have access to one in 5 min or less.

Equipment within the on-site treatment facilities should be based on the level of care provided, the number of patients anticipated, and the length of time each patient would be required to stay at the site awaiting disposition or transportation. Transportation, if not on-site, should be established in the plan to have the capabilities of transporting the patient to a hospital within 30 min of the request.

Communications

Audio communications represent the glue that joins not only the myriad of medical care and surveillance components into an efficiently functioning system, but also the venue health care system to the other systems vital to managing a mass gathering.

The spectator level presents the greatest challenge. The first "first responders" are always fellow performers or spectators. Upon entry to an event, they should be educated in how to link knowledge of an illness/injury occurrence to the venue's medical care system so that rapid assistance can be rendered. In preparation for the 1996 Olympics, health promotion brochures were mailed with ticket information. Concise information on ticket stubs accompanied by periodic public service announcements can serve the same purpose.

At the medical care system personnel level, every event official, from ushers, volunteers, security, and public relations personnel to the top rung of management, must be educated in and updated on the most expedient manner in which to obtain medical assistance. Because radios are expensive, for the most numerous event workers, usually ushers, alternatives such as flag systems have been organized. At the U.S. Open Tennis Tournament, Forrest Hills, New York, a flare system has been organized. All event personnel should know the venue location of the nearest official who has a radio.

Among those officials with radios, frequencies and/or "talk groups" (e.g., 800 MHz trunking) can be organized to minimize interruptions and maximize effective radio traffic from incident discovery through responders to definitive caregivers. At the most highly evolved events, discovery of a victim(s) by the system usually proceeds from bystanders, ushers, or vendors to on-site security to a central communications or command center where the event medical director is based. Venue surveillance cameras can augment verbal reports on victim location as well as examine the scope of the incident. The medical director can then select and radio-dispatch the nearest most appropriate responders with adequate security and/or public relations assistance. Responding event field providers, dedicated event ambulance crews, on-site medical facilities, the medical director, and the medical command center should be able to communicate with each other. Additionally, medical command should have voice access to all area hospital emergency facilities.

RELATIONSHIP OF FUNCTIONAL AREAS

Optimally, a central location should be designated for stationing the directors of the following functions: medical emergencies, event management, logistics, facility maintenance, public relations, and security/law enforcement, ushers and event performers/athletes. If not within this immediate area, fire/rescue, public health, and public transportation and parking directors must be easily and reliably accessible by telephone and/or radio. From the medical care perspective, the leadership's close physical proximity is especially important if on-site care is provided, as it will allow for efficient information exchange and problem solving among the directors whose functional areas are integral to medical care delivery. A less-reliable alternative involves intra-venue radio links among the directors of these functional areas.

Internally, event management has to mediate issues at the interface of one functional area with another. Event management is the contact for accessing outside resources, a vital function in the management of multicasualty incidents. Whenever depletion of operational resources is threatened, logistics personnel should immediately access and deliver additional equipment and supplies as patient demand dictates. The medical director and logistics supervisor should prospectively determine a threshold level of each essential supply item, below which resupply is undertaken. Facility maintenance has a major public health role in providing and maintaining an adequate potable water supply, sanitary facilities, and the venue electrical system vital to operating the public address system, air conditioning/ventilation, and lighting. Public relations plays a crucial role in directing crowd control and informing the event population of preventive public health measures as well as the location of medical care. Security/law enforcement personnel serve the entire spectrum of illness/injury prevention. Their primary prevention role includes pedestrian safety in regulating the interface of vehicular and pedestrian traffic, clearance of emergency vehicle access routes and venue pedestrian entrances/exits, and surveillance for and investigation of terrorist threats. Their discovery of the ill/injured by direct sight or television surveillance, subsequent dispatch of medical care providers, then clearance of the path through crowds to gain access to patients represents their secondary prevention role. Similarly, ushers play a crucial role in the direct-sight discovery of victims and must know how to relay medical event information to the predesignated personnel responsible for dispatching medical response teams. Like security/law enforcement, their ubiquitous positioning make them invaluable in the delivery of response time-sensitive CPR.

Event participants or performers, be they athletes, politicians, musicians, or animals, represent a separate and distinct population requiring medical care specifically geared to their talent(s) and/or position in society; their care is best provided by a cadre of personnel most familiar with their specific health care needs. When affordable, a separate medical care system and resources should be provided to ensure that care for performers and spectators do not interfere with each other.

QUALITY MANAGEMENT

Documentation

A medical record should be generated for each medical encounter, the type based on the severity of the complaint. An officially sanctioned event form should be used to record the encounter date and time, patient's name, sex, age, race, medical complaint, drug allergies, relevant medical history, and examination findings. The tentative diagnosis and treatment plan should be documented, complete with discharge instructions. Because most all patients provided ALS care will be transported to a hospital, the transporting EMS patient care report form can conveniently document the continuum of care provided at the scene and in transit.

Event Training

Event training represents prospective quality management. Optimally, all of the personnel functions described in the preceding relationship of the functional areas should be represented at event training sessions held on-site. Ironically, especially with regard to public safety, health, and medical care personnel, the major obstacle to their training participation in one place at the same time is their regularly scheduled duties, the skills from which will translate into their event duties. Possible alternatives to address this problem include videoconferencing and virtual-reality applications. However, both of these modes preclude a realistic grasp of time-space relationships (i.e., patient access obstacles) that are facilitated by drills at the venue.

A central goal of event orientation should include instruction in the following venue locations: the command center, medical care facilities, ambulance, radio-equipped security postings, and emergency ingress and egress routes. All personnel must know their geographic postings and coverage areas, receive instruction in communications equipment use, and practice the appropriate communications pathways to be used for medical care. Instruction in filling out a standardized medical care report form should be provided. Practice scenarios should include a mock MCI requiring designation of ambulance staging and contingent triage zones, and a request for outside intervention. Contingency plans for critical incident stress debriefing should be made and explained. Difficult access extrication, hyper- and/or hypothermia prevention and treatment, cardiac arrest, event player/performer(s) injury, and dignitary/VIP care should be rehearsed. Within each of these scenarios, communication (radio, cell phone) and physical routes to optimal care (ambulance evacuation, on-site facility care) should be tested.

Retrospective quality management can be done through instruments that document the quality of care (patient care report forms), measures of the public image of care rendered at the event (patient-targeted surveys), and management's degree of satisfaction with the results. The medical director should review all medical records. If the patient volume has been large or included a multicasualty incident, an audit and review committee should perform the review.

SPECIAL CONSIDERATIONS

Cardiac Arrests

As discussed, the incidence of cardiac arrests in mass gatherings is higher than in the normal population. It has been postulated that because of the natural excitement generated by competitive sports, individuals who have cardiac disease are more likely to become symptomatic. However, medical systems at mass gatherings have demonstrated much higher success rates than even the most advanced EMS systems. This is primarily a result of the ability to provide early bystander CPR, airway control, defibrillation, and ALS care. Survival rates for hospital discharge have varied from 20 to 100 percent survival from documented cardiac arrest. This evidence would also support the use of automatic external defibrillators (AEDs) in mass gatherings where ALS support is not available in less than 5 min.

Positioning of emergency care providers with AEDs requires careful attention during the planning stages for any mass gathering. Optimally, BLS and AED should be available to all event participants within 3 min of collapse. Factors such as event layout, slope and crowd density all need to be evaluated when positioning AED-equipped first responders.

Commercial Airline In-flight Emergencies

The population density, temporary isolation, and common purpose on commercial airliners is one situation where many of the principles of mass gathering medical care applies.[11] Since 1986, U.S. airlines have been required to carry mandated emergency medical kits. In April 2001, the rule was changed to require all U.S. airlines to carry an enhanced emergency medical kit (accessible to the flight crew but to be used only by medical professionals) and an AED, plus providing the flight crew with appropriate AED and CPR training.

Medical problems encountered on board commercial airliners resemble those seen at ground-level mass gatherings. A survey of 5 U.S. domestic airlines between 1996 and 1997 found 1132 in-flight medical incidents with use of the medical kit in 47 percent of these events.[12,13] A major airline can expect approximately three in-flight medical emergencies per day and one life-threatening (asthma, choking, cardiac arrest, heart attack, loss of consciousness, stroke) emergency every 2 to 3 days. The most frequent (in decreasing order) complaints were neurologic, syncopal, cardiac, psychiatric, and respiratory. Intentional injury of crews by unruly passengers has increased, with 174 incidents reported in 1995.

The airplane environment presents several unique aspects of medical emergencies and their treatment. Following discovery of a medical incident, the response time to on board care is minimal. Caregivers' access to victims is compromised by their seated position in a setting similar to that in a crowded stadium. The victim's safe, timely extraction to a secured space allowing the supine (left lateral decubitus for pregnant patients) position is a foremost priority but a formidable challenge in such a confined environment not dedicated to even provisional medical care. Oxygen sources are plentiful but their location is not configured for optimal patient care. At cruising altitude, despite cabin pressurization, ambient air oxygen availability is below that at sea level [Po_2 (partial pressure of oxygen) is typically 118 mm Hg while in-flight versus 159 mm Hg at sea level] and has the potential to cause respiratory problems in the marginally compensated patient.

Flight attendants receive basic first aid training to a degree that varies among airlines. A 2-year monitoring period following institution of the Federal Aviation Administration (FAA)-mandated basic medical kit in 1986, found that physicians responded in 85 percent of the 2322 cases when it was used. A review of the kit contents supports the inclusion of bronchodilator inhalers, oral antihistamines and non-opioid analgesics.[12] The demonstrated efficacy of AEDs on commercial aircraft has prompted the FAA to require them on U.S. carriers.[13] Recent reports document a survival-to-discharge rate of up to 40 percent for witnessed arrests in-flight when an AED is available.

When addressing in-flight medical emergencies, the issue of plane diversion arises. Diversion is considered when the patient is in immediate need of care and the expertise needed to provide that care is not available on board. The decision to divert a commercial aircraft rests ultimately with the pilot. However, in 2321 cases from U.S. domestic air carriers between 1990 and 1993, the crews complied with a physician's recommendation to divert 97 percent of the time. In addition to the time sensitivity of the patient's condition, diversion involves issues of proximity to an airport suitable for the aircraft versus the original destination port, availability of adequate EMS resources (ALS versus BLS) to meet the diverted craft, and proximity of appropriate hospital resources to the diversion airport. Many of the U.S. air carriers contract with in-flight medical consultation companies to assist crews and on-board medical personnel in making an appropriate diversion decision. Emergency physicians, by virtue of their expertise, have collaborated with the airlines to improve in-flight medical care.

REFERENCES

1. DeLorenzo RA: Mass gathering medicine: A review. *Prehospital Disaster Med* 12:68, 1997.
2. Flabouris A, Bridgewater F: An analysis of demand for first-aid care at a major public event. *Prehospital Disaster Med* 11:48, 1996.
3. Carveth SW: Eight-year experience with a stadium-based mobile coronary-care unit. *Heart Lung* 3:770, 1974.
4. Michael JA, Barbera JA: Mass gathering medical care: A twenty-five year review. *Prehospital Disaster Med* 12:305, 1997
5. Arbon P, Bridgewater FH, Smith C: Mass gathering medicine: A predictive model for patient presentation and transport rates. *Prehospital Disaster Med* 16:150, 2001.
6. McDonald CC, Koenigsberg MD, Ward S: Medical control of mass gatherings: Can paramedics perform without physicians on-site? *Prehospital Disaster Med* 8:327, 1993.
7. Baker WM, Simone BM, Niemann JT, et al: Special event medical care: The 1984 Los Angeles Summer Olympics experience. *Ann Emerg Med* 15:185, 1986.
8. Wetterhall SF, Coulombier DM, Herndon JM, et al: Medical care delivery at the 1996 Olympic Games. *JAMA* 279:1463, 1998.
9. Jaslow D, Drake M, Lewis J: Characteristics of state legislation governing medical care at mass gatherings. *Prehosp Emerg Care* 3:316, 1999.
10. Sullivan FM, Kleinman G, Suner S, St Jean J: Development of an equipment and supply list for emergency medical services delivery at an annual air show. *Prehospital Disaster Med* 14:100, 1999.
11. DeHart RL: Health issues of air travel. *Annu Rev Public Health* 24:08.1, 2003.
12. DeJohn CA, Wolbrink AM, Veronneau SJ, et al: An evaluation of in-flight medical care in the U.S. *Aviat Space Environ Med* 73:580, 2002.
13. DeJohn CA, Veronneau SJ, Wolbrink AM, et al: An evaluation of the U.S. in-flight medical kit. *Aviat Space Environ Med* 73:496, 2002.
14. Groeneveld PW, Kwong JL, Liu Y, et al: Cost-effectiveness of automated external defibrillators on airlines. *JAMA* 286:1482, 2001.

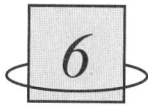

DISASTER MEDICAL SERVICES
Eric K. Noji
Gabor D. Kelen

Natural disasters such as earthquakes, tornadoes, floods, and hurricanes have claimed approximately 3.5 million lives worldwide during the past 25 years, adversely affecting the lives of at least 1 billion more people, and have resulted in property damages exceeding $50 billion. While past disasters have produced their share of mass casualty situations, the future appears to be even more bleak. Increasing population density in flood plains and seismic and hurricane-prone areas, the development and transportation of thousands of toxic and hazardous materials on the nations' roads, the potential risks that can occur from incidents at fixed-site industrial facilities, and the catastrophic possibilities from nuclear, explosive, biological, and chemical terrorism, all point to the probability of major emergencies in the future. Recent significant disasters have included Hurricane Mitch (1998); a series of devastating tornadoes in Oklahoma; record flooding in eastern Texas; a number of major earthquakes in India, Turkey, El Salvador, Taiwan, and southern Italy; the terrorist passenger plane attacks on the World Trade Center, followed by intentional anthrax releases up and down the East Coast; and, most recently, the deadly terrorist bombing of a crowded tourist venue on the island of Bali and the nightclub fire in Rhode Island.

The emergency physician has extensive responsibilities for community disaster preparedness and other disaster medical services. Since 1976, the American College of Emergency Physicians (ACEP) has taken the position that emergency medicine should assume a primary role in the medical aspects of disaster planning, management, and patient care. Despite efficient field management of disaster victims, a rapid flow of victims from a disaster scene can quickly overwhelm a hospital emergency department. The point at which the emergency department becomes overwhelmed often varies according to the time of day, the nature of the injuries, and the amount of preparation time prior to the arrival of victims.[1] When it appears that normal procedures will be overwhelmed, emergency departments must have a specific set of protocols that direct the mobilization of personnel and equipment outside of the emergency department and permit rapid assessment, stabilization, and triage to definitive care of victims of a mass casualty incident.[2]

DEFINITION OF DISASTER

A multivehicle crash involving four or five seriously injured persons, or a family presenting with carbon monoxide poisoning that would overwhelm the resources of a small rural community hospital may be a rather routine event at a large university teaching medical center. On the other hand, greater than 25 patients at one time will overwhelm even the best staffed trauma center. According to the World Health Organization, a disaster can be defined as a sudden ecologic phenomenon of sufficient magnitude to require external assistance. From the perspective of the emergency department, however, a disaster exists when the number of patients presenting in a given space of time are such that the emergency department cannot offer even minimal care for them without external assistance. Disasters that are characterized by the production of large numbers of deaths and injuries are also referred to as "mass casualty incidents."[3] Note that disasters are not defined simply by a given number of victims. A single case of smallpox may paralyze an entire hospital let alone the ED. The arrival of one important political person or celebrity with severe injuries (e.g., the president of the United States, the Pope, a rock star) will completely disrupt normal operations of even the most efficient emergency department. Thus, the definition of disaster incorporates the concept of "massive disruptive impact."

The hospital and, more specifically, the emergency department should have a preestablished protocol for effectively dealing with such an extraordinary situation. These protocols (e.g., for intentionally infected, chemically contaminated patients or for the mobilization of appropriate outside assistance) should be instituted rapidly in order to prevent death or severe complications.

In many hospitals in the United States, disasters are often divided further into external or internal events. *External disasters* are events that occur physically outside the hospital (e.g., transportation accidents, industrial explosions, terrorist actions). Patients are brought to the hospital from the outside, usually to the emergency department. Unlike patients contaminated from a chemical, nuclear, or biologic contagion incident, the hospital and its staff, patients, and visitors are in no immediate physical danger from victims of explosives, blast, or other simple but devastating traumas.

Internal disasters are events that occur within the physical plant of the hospital itself (e.g., fire, laboratory accident involving radioactive material, power failure, contaminated water) that severely compromise the ability of the hospital to function.[4] A disaster may be both internal and external; for example, an earthquake or explosion that severely damages the hospital.

CHARACTER OF MASS CASUALTY EVENTS INVOLVING EMERGENCY DEPARTMENTS

Extensive social and organizational research, conducted on the management of mass casualty events prior to September 11, 2001 (9/11), has shown that emergency departments experience great difficulty coping with even moderate numbers of patients following a disaster. The reasons for this difficulty include confusion, lack of planning, lack of training in principles of disaster management, and lack of practice drills. Hospitals are often not well integrated into the surrounding community's disaster planning efforts. Shortcomings of hospital disaster plans include:

Delayed or improper notification
Poor delineation of command structure
Overloaded or broken communications networks
Improper or incomplete identification
Lack of supplies
Lack of public relations

The World Trade Center and Pentagon attacks have forced virtually all public hospitals to focus on these issues.

In mass casualty events, the emergency medical services (EMS) protocols that call for transport of patients in equitable distribution to appropriate centers is easily foiled because of confusion, route obstacles, and difficulty in communications. This was quite evident in New York City on 9/11. As a result, the highly injured and ill are often transported to the nearest hospital ED, which often does not have appropriate facilities and expertise to best care for the seriously injured and ill. Unfortunately, the problem is compounded by the fact the "walking wounded" and "worried well," that is, those who need the least medical attention, also arrive at the nearby hospital(s); often in overwhelming numbers. In an urban setting, patients can be expected at the nearest hospital(s) within minutes, and peak volumes can be expected within 2 to 3 h.[5] More than half of all patients likely to require or seek medical care within 48 h will be seen within 7 h of the event.[5] During the World Trade Center disaster, 18 percent of the 790 injured survivors were admitted.[5] The vast majority of patients are not transported by the EMS system. Announcements of numbers of patients to be brought to the ED by the local emergency communications center or by the on-site command will invariably underestimate the total number of patients who actually arrive.

Those with minor injuries travel by alternate means of transport (private automobiles, police vehicles, buses, cabs, and on foot),[6] and are likely to arrive in great numbers, even before many of the seriously ill are transported via EMS. The more severely injured, who often need extrication (e.g., from collapsed buildings following earthquakes and explosive devices), arrive at a later stage. Thus, without careful planning, less-severely injured patients often tend to be treated before the more seriously injured.

Other factors that may hinder effective ED disaster management include:

- Poor communications with the scene and within the facility (often considered the greatest problem)
- Incident Command System not followed
- Convergence of rescuers, emergency medical technicians, and the media in the ED
- Convergence in the ED of other hospital physicians and nurses, who are unfamiliar with their roles and have little experience caring for traumatized or nuclear, chemical, or biologic agent-exposed patients.
- Convergence of friends and family searching for loved ones

It does not take a mass casualty event to essentially paralyze an ED. In the early phase of the anthrax release, even one case of possible exposure could paralyze an ED. In at least one major academic ED, local law enforcement, the FBI, hospital infection control, hospital corporate security, hospital safety officials, and city and state health departments all converged in various ways in the ED as part of the investigation (G. D. Kelen, personal communication, Nov. 21, 2002), illustrating clearly that a disaster is not defined by numbers, but by impact.

DISASTER PLANNING

Overview

Roles, responsibilities, and working relationships between those responsible for disaster operations should be clarified in the planning process to lessen the confusion that invariably occurs during a disaster event.[7] Selected protocols should require personnel to perform functions that are relatively similar to their day-to-day activities.

The disaster planning process should begin by answering the following questions:

- What types of disasters are most likely to occur in the community (e.g., hazard analysis)?
- What are the disaster planning requirements of the Joint Commission on Accreditation of Healthcare Organizations (JCAHO),[2] as well as other accreditation bodies (e.g., local and state health agencies)?
- What are the capabilities and responsibilities of the hospital?

Hazard Analysis

Hospital disaster planners should plan for those disasters most likely to occur in their community. For example, hospitals in Hawaii and along the Gulf and Atlantic Coasts of the United States should plan for hurricanes, those in California should plan for earthquakes,[8,9] and those near chemical industries should have facilities for decontamination. Regarding the latter, hospitals located near facilities using large amounts of hazardous materials are required by Title III of the Super-

fund Amendments and Reauthorization Act (SARA III) to participate in local emergency planning committees (LEPCs).[10] Factors such as the presence of nearby transportation facilities (e.g., airports, harbors), festivals, stadiums, and amusement parks should be included within the risk assessment. Because different disasters are characterized by very different morbidity and mortality patterns, anticipation of health care requirements can be specific.[11] For example, earthquakes cause many deaths and severe injuries.[12,13] Hurricanes cause mostly property damage; however, deaths are usually low and injuries minor.[14] Pulmonary irritation may result from fires or hazardous chemicals, requiring large supplies of oxygen, as the 1984 Bhopal industrial accident demonstrated,[15] or a specific antidote (atropine), as occurred following the Tokyo sarin chemical weapon attack in 1995.[16]

JCAHO Requirements for Hospital Disaster Planning

There are other motivations for hospitals to plan for potential disasters. The JCAHO requires that member hospitals have a written plan for the timely care of casualties arising from both external and internal disasters, and the hospital must document the rehearsal of these plans.[2]

Hospital-Community Cooperation in Disaster Planning

The Medical and Health Incident Management (MaHIM) System was recently developed as a model for planning a regional response that allows customizable organization of available assets for mass casualty response[17] (more than 500 casualties). The health system and its component hospitals play a vital role. Every hospital should integrate its own disaster plan with those of community disaster management agencies. This is especially important regarding disaster notification and communications, transportation of casualties and provisions for dispatch of hospital medical teams to a disaster site. Strong relationships with community agencies (e.g., the fire department, the regional EMS system, local emergency management or civil defense agency) are important to ensure a coordinated disaster response. The number of community agencies that have some responsibility for disaster planning and response can be bewildering. Table 6-1 lists just a few.

TABLE 6-1 Key Agencies that May Play a Role in Health-Related Disasters

Community Agency	Responsibilities
FBI	Initial incident command if a federal crime may be involved
FEMA	Incident command in public health disaster
State governor	Authority to declare health emergency; requests federal assistance (e.g., from FEMA); responsible for public safety
State health department	Authorized by governor to coordinate disaster response
State emergency management association	State-level equivalent to FEMA
City/county health department	May have jurisdiction for local disasters
EMS service	Patient triage in the field, stabilization, and transfer to definitive care facility
Fire service	Overall scene command; victim rescue and hazard control
Police service	Traffic management and scene security
Public works	Support equipment and personnel; structural safety expertise

Abbreviations: EMS = emergency medical services; FBI = Federal Bureau of Investigation; FEMA = Federal Emergency Management Agency.

Other organizations that a hospital may interact with during the disaster planning process may include the military, local chapters of the American Red Cross, LEPCs, Citizens' Corps Councils, and other volunteer agencies, along with state and federal agencies [e.g., National Disaster Medical System, Metropolitan Medical Response System, Centers for Disease Control and Prevention (CDC)]. The CDC in and of itself is advisory and has no official jurisdiction.

Medical planning for disasters in the community is usually the responsibility of local EMS councils, health departments, or boards of health.

Each hospital should have mutual aid agreements or memoranda of understanding with hospitals outside the immediate area should hospital capacities be exceeded.

Hospital disaster planners should anticipate that information about specific hazards (e.g., chemicals, radiation), expert personnel (e.g., poison control), and special supplies (e.g., antidotes) not readily available may be needed in a particular disaster situation. Plans should consider how to rapidly access these resources. Plans for obtaining additional shelter, food, and water should also be considered.

INTEGRATION WITH OTHER RESPONSE ASSETS   Some of the federal response resources with which the emergency clinician should have familiarity are listed below. They all are subsidiary agencies to the Department of Health and Human Services (DHHS), with the exception of the Federal Bureau of Investigation (FBI). During a response, these agencies may play pivotal roles and may interface and coordinate with hospitals and emergency medicine clinicians.

United States Public Health Service/Office of Emergency Response [formerly Office of Emergency Preparedness (USPHS/OER)]   This agency is an office within the DHHS dedicated to the management and coordination of federal health and medical activities related to preparation, response, and recovery from major emergencies and Presidentially declared disasters. One of the most significant programs developed by the Office of Emergency Preparedness (OEP) is the Metropolitan Medical Response System (MMRS) (www.mmrs.hhs.gov). Initiated in 1996, MMRS was originally a program with a team-oriented approach to responding to weapons of mass destruction events including bioterrorism. Teams were hosted by local jurisdictions and then provided funding, equipment, and supplies by OEP to make them operational. The concept was developed on the basis that local responders would be more rapidly able to respond to incidents in an individual jurisdiction. Since then, the MMRS program has evolved to include a more primary focus of enhancing local emergency preparedness systems as opposed to developing stand-alone teams. The MMRS program promotes coordination between various types of local responders [police, fire, hazardous material (HAZMAT), EMS, hospital, law enforcement, and others] to affect an adequate community response system. This is accomplished through contractual requirements that prompt participating jurisdiction to meet in developing specific elements of their weapons of mass destruction response plans. By the end of 2002, it is expected that 120 U.S. cities will have funding in place for an MMRS.

OEP also manages and participates in other programs which could potentially play a role in a bioterrorist event. OEP is the principal coordinator of the National Disaster Medical System (NDMS). NDMS is an asset-sharing program between DHHS, the Federal Emergency Management Agency (FEMA), Department of Defense (DoD), Veteran's Health Administration (VA), and public/private organizations. Originally developed to provide surge capacity for injured victims of catastrophic natural disasters and for wartime military casualties, the system also has utility in a large-scale bioterrorist event. Key components of NDMS are the Disaster Medical Assistance Teams (DMATs), patient transport systems, and agreements with definitive care facilities across the United States to care for casualties. DMATs are teams comprised of physicians, nurses, medics, pharmacists, and logisticians that deploy in response to federally declared disasters and emergencies

to support a local jurisdiction's response. Several specialty teams, based on the DMAT concept, have been developed to respond to chemical, biological, and radiologic events (National Medical Response Teams or NMRTs). OEP has additional assets such as the Commissioned Corps Readiness Force (CCRF), which draws on volunteers from within the U.S. Public Health Service (USPHS) commissioned officers corp. Disaster Mortuary Operations Response Teams (DMORTs) are designed to handle the increased demands of processing the deceased after a disaster and could potentially be utilized as well.

Centers for Disease Control and Prevention   The CDC is the lead federal agency in developing and applying disease prevention and control and also sits within the DHHS. Though responsible for diseases of all types, the traditional focus has been on infectious diseases, making the CDC a natural resource for bioterrorism response. Many programs managed by the CDC are related to bioterrorism response, and some of them are described below.[18]

Rapid Response Teams: These include CDC epidemiologists on standby to assist with local efforts in investigating potential outbreaks, confirmation of cases and exposures, and environmental clean-up. This, most likely, is the program with which emergency clinicians will have direct contact.

Laboratory Response Network (LRN): The CDC has developed a program designed to link state and local public health laboratories to advanced-capacity labs including military, clinical, veterinarian, agricultural, water, and food testing labs.

Rapid Response and Advanced Technologies lab (RRAT): The CDC has laboratory capability to provide diagnostic, confirmatory, and reference support to terrorism response teams.

National Electronic Disease Surveillance System (NEDSS): Using the development of standards to advance efficient and integrated surveillance systems, the CDC promotes a national surveillance system for health departments.

Health Alert Network (HAN): Health departments and others are connected via internet communications that allows for early warning broadcast alerts for potential emerging infectious diseases.

National Pharmaceutical Stockpile (NPS): The NPS is a two-part system designed to supply local jurisdictions with medications, vaccines, and equipment during response to a chemical or biological event. The first part of the system relies on prepackaged caches that can be delivered within 12 h in the United States. The second part relies on the vendor-managed inventory, which takes 36 h to arrive.

Federal Bureau of Investigation   The FBI is designated as the lead federal agency for crisis management and, as such, has the authority to conduct law enforcement investigations into acts of terrorism. Clinicians may be approached by these persons during investigations.

THE HOSPITAL DISASTER PLAN

The Hospital Emergency Incident Command System (HEICS) was developed to mitigate confusion and chaos that can paralyze hospitals' response during a disaster. HEICS employs a clear management structure with defined responsibilities and mechanisms of reporting using a uniform nomenclature that allows clear communication and understanding between hospitals and with other emergency responders. HEICS has become the standard, and all hospitals should use this system. It includes the following components[19]:

Common language
Defined and predictable chain of management
Flexible response
Prioritized response
Accountability of position function
Documentation guidelines for accountability and cost recovery

Basic Requirements of Hospital Planning

Hospital disaster planning is the responsibility of administration, nursing, and the entire medical staff. It should provide for an organized response of the hospital for the management of casualties transported to the hospital from the disaster site. In addition, it should plan for disasters arising within or near the hospital that require hospital evacuation.[20]

Disaster research has demonstrated that staff who perform most efficiently are those who are performing relatively familiar tasks. The disaster plan should take this into account by relying on standard operating procedures as much as possible.

The hospital plan should describe several key functions, including:

Activation of the plan
Assessment of the hospital's capacity
Establishment of a disaster command
Communications
Supplies
Hospital disaster administrative and treatment areas
Training and drills
Security and crowd control

Activation of the Disaster Plan

The plan should designate a (set of) individual(s) who can put the hospital's disaster plan into effect. This is not the equivalent of taking incident command. Situations that warrant activation of the plan should also be defined. Disaster protocols should define how it is determined to what degree to mobilize ED staff and staff from other departments.

Following activation of the plan, there should be immediate mobilization of all disaster resources likely to be needed. These include personnel, supplies, equipment, communications, and transportation.

Assessment of the Hospital's Capacity

Before the hospital can receive casualties, it must be determined if the hospital itself has sustained any structural damage or loss of utility as a result of a disaster. These include blocked passageways or inoperable elevators; potential for fire, explosion, or building collapse; failure of any utility; loss of equipment and/or supplies including oxygen; contamination of water; and outside access problems. This damage assessment is usually the responsibility of the plant safety officer or hospital engineer. If the hospital's structural integrity has been compromised, it may be necessary to evacuate staff and patients.

Once it is determined that the hospital itself is safe, the hospital should determine how many casualties from the disaster site it can safely manage. This may be limited by available personnel, beds, operating room and intensive care unit (ICU) capacity, and supplies, as well as by the type of disaster and the availability of other community resources. At the time of disaster notification, it is necessary to know the status of many of the hospital's capabilities: how many beds are available; how much critical supplies and medications (including blood) are available; how many personnel are on duty; what damage has been done; how many operating rooms are in use; which doctors are present in the hospital; and so forth. Ideally, a mechanism to collect these data in short order is delineated in the plan.

Establishment of Disaster Command

A command site within the hospital should be established, preferably in a predesignated area (e.g., disaster control center). This center should be able to communicate with the patient-receiving area (triage site), patient care areas, and with regional EMS, police, fire, and government authorities. Provisions for multiple (redundant) modes of communication (cellular telephones, two-way radios, runners, etc.) should be made. The command personnel should include at least a physician, a nurse, and an administrator. The command structure itself should be clear.

Communication

Establishment of good communications is critical in any disaster or mass casualty situation. Without a clear method of communication, the best disaster plans fail. Unfortunately, experience shows that this essential function is difficult to achieve for a variety of reasons. Many communication modes become inoperative during a disaster. A major goal should be full use of all possible communication resources, including citizens' band groups, cellular phones, blackboards, e-mail, intercoms, closed-circuit television, shortwave radio, and radio-equipped individuals of all kinds, even messenger and courier services.

Interhospital and intrahospital communication needs should be considered. It may be necessary because of shortages of life-saving supplies such as blood, antibiotics, and intravenous fluids; certain equipment, such as incubators and surgical instruments; or personnel, such as nurses, x-ray technicians, respiratory therapists, and physicians. Unfortunately, most hospitals in the United States today have limited "surge capacity" regarding both staff and stores of supplies and medications. An overloaded hospital may also wish to transfer patients to a prearranged receiving hospital. (Interestingly, during the World Trade Center disaster, ICU capacity was not stressed.[21]) Unfortunately, interhospital communications may present a weak link in the community's disaster response.

Supplies

During a disaster, necessary supplies and equipment must be ready for immediate distribution to appropriate locations in the hospital (e.g., stretchers and wheelchairs to the receiving area). Each hospital will need to estimate the amount of supplies that will be needed in stock over and above their regular hospital supply. Unfortunately, whereas 10 years ago many medical centers kept a month's supply of many items in stock, most now keep only 2 to 3 days' worth of consumable supplies and medications such as antibiotics. The CDC has arranged a series of medication push-packs throughout the United States that can be delivered to any area of disaster within 12 h. Unfortunately, it is up to each jurisdiction or state to determine how the contents will be distributed.

Hospital Disaster Administrative and Treatment Areas

As part of disaster planning, it is essential that certain areas of the hospital be designated for specific functions such as reception of casualties, treatment, and discharge of patients. The plan should be quite specific as to the function of these areas, staffing requirements, and basic supplies to be used. The areas to be incorporated in each plan are discussed below.

DISASTER CONTROL CENTER   A disaster control center should be established remote from the ED. Apart from establishing a hospital-based incident command, the center coordinates hospital activities with those at the disaster site. Good communication is absolutely essential. Other responsibilities include opening up additional hospital wards or clinics, obtaining outside assistance, evacuation of endangered patients, assignment of staff to treatment areas, and revision of original job assignments.

TRIAGE   To maximize efficiency, entry of all patients should be restricted to only one location, the triage area. The primary functions of a disaster triage area are rapid assessment of all incoming casualties or ill patients, the assignment of priorities for management, and classification of dispositions (i.e., distribution of patients to various other patient care areas in the hospital). Without a triage area to manage the patient flow, the major treatment area may become overwhelmed.

PATIENT CARE STATIONS   One suggested method of organizing patient care stations includes major trauma and medicine and minor trauma–primary care.

Major Trauma and Medicine From the triage location, most, if not all, of the seriously injured patients will be sent to the major trauma–medicine area (e.g., trauma and cardiac resuscitation, treatment of hypovolemic or septic shock, severe respiratory distress). This is usually physically located in the emergency department.

Minor Trauma–Primary Care In most disaster situations, the majority of patients are not very seriously injured. A great percentage of these will be classified as the "walking wounded" or the "worried well." These low-priority patients can be sent to an "urgent care" area, often designated as the minor trauma–primary care area, for definitive care including splinting of fractures, primary closure of lacerations, and tetanus prophylaxis. This minor trauma–primary care area can be established in the hospital's outpatient clinics.

ADMISSION PRESURGICAL HOLDING Most trauma patients stabilized in the major trauma area (emergency department) will be sent to the admission presurgical holding area.

SURGERY The number of operating rooms that can be staffed is the main limiting factor in the provision of definitive care for a large number of severely injured casualties. The most experienced (not necessarily most senior) surgeon available should take the responsibility to prioritize cases and to assign surgeons to these cases as rapidly as possible.

MORGUE Many disasters can result in a large number of fatalities. This may require that present morgue capacities be expanded possibly to outside facilities such as a church, school auditorium, or stadium.[22] Because the vast majority of patients reaching a hospital are salvageable, this is historically usually not an immediate concern for a given hospital.

DECONTAMINATION JCAHO requires hospitals to have provisions for emergency treatment and decontamination of individuals who are radioactively or chemically contaminated.[2] Some basic requirements for hospitals are:

A safe area for decontamination
A means of washing external contamination from the patients
A method of containment of contaminated materials
Adequate protection for persons handling the patient, and other hospital personnel
Disposable/cleanable medical equipment

The goals are to reduce external contamination, contain the contamination that remains, and prevent further spread of potentially dangerous substances. The decontamination area should have the ability to provide major resuscitative efforts which are never subservient to decontamination itself.

PSYCHIATRY In the event of a disaster involving mass casualties, and even property damage with loss of possessions, it is common for patients to present with episodes of anxiety and depression, as well as psychotic episodes. Hysterical persons, whether patients, visitors, or staff, can be extremely disruptive to hospital disaster operations. A separate isolated area should be predesignated to receive individuals in need of psychological intervention. The issue of stress and the need for ongoing debriefing among all who provide assistance in a disaster (including hospital staff) is becoming increasingly recognized.

FAMILY WAITING AND DISCHARGE AREA As past experience in disasters has shown, families and friends will converge en masse to the hospital seeking information about victims. This convergence can seriously interfere with efforts of the hospital to respond effectively to the situation. For this reason, a separate area should be predesignated for family members seeking information. This area may also be utilized to discharge in-hospital patients and victims of the disaster.

VOLUNTEER PROGRAM In major disasters, the potential of large numbers of volunteers, including those wishing to donate blood, should be anticipated. While some of these may have appropriate clinical skills, they are unlikely to be familiar with the hospital functions and could be more hindrance than help.[21] A separate place should be identified to handle these volunteers and if appropriate credential and decide how they may best be used.

Training and Drills

Regular training and drills help to familiarize staff with their disaster roles and responsibilities. They also serve to point out weaknesses or omissions in the plan that require additions or revisions. Drills can range from full-scale community-wide simulations with moulage victims, to tabletop triage scenarios, to mini-drills that test only certain components of the disaster plan, such as call-up of personnel, and test of communications. The JCAHO requires two drills a year; the scenarios should reflect incidents that are likely to occur in the community.[2]

CATASTROPHIC CASUALTY MANAGEMENT: DISASTER OPERATIONS

Field Medical Care

In the field, rescue personnel often use a simple triage and rapid treatment (START) technique that depends on a quick assessment of respirations, perfusion, and mental status (RPM).[23] Subsequently, determining how much and what type of care to administer at the disaster site depends on several factors. If the number of patients is small and there are sufficient prehospital personnel and transportation resources available, on-site medical care can proceed in a fairly normal manner, with rapid stabilization and transportation to nearby hospitals. When extrication will be prolonged, it is important that potentially life-saving interventions be instituted in the field, such as intravenous fluids for hypovolemic shock. On the other hand, early, rapid transportation with a minimum of treatment should be practiced when there is danger to rescuers and casualties from fire, explosion, falling buildings, hazardous materials, and extreme weather conditions.

When there is an overwhelming number of casualties that exceed transportation capacities, advanced field medical and surgical treatment may be beneficial because it may be hours before seriously injured patients can be evacuated. This may necessitate the establishment of field hospitals with operating theater capabilities. Such a field hospital may be set up in a large building such as a school gymnasium or church. Casualties are brought here from the disaster site for further assessment and initial treatment of their injuries. After a period of observation and stabilization, they are either sent home or transported to a hospital.

When local hospitals are likely to be, or are, overwhelmed prior to transporting victims, it may be better to treat victims in the field. To address these considerations, the "secondary assessment of victim endpoint" (SAVE) system of triage was proposed.[24] The SAVE triage system is designed to identify patients who are most likely to benefit from the care available under austere field conditions. When combined with the START protocol, the SAVE triage is useful for any scenario wherein multiple patients experience a prolonged delay in accessing definitive care. The SAVE triage methodology divides patients into three categories: (1) those who will die regardless of how much care they receive; (2) those who will survive whether or not they receive care; and (3) those who will benefit significantly from austere field interventions.

Incident Command System

The incident command system (ICS) is a standard emergency management system used throughout the country to provide a flexible command and control structure upon which to organize a response.[25] The ICS is generally used when there is an identifiable single scene for a disaster event such as the site of a plane crash. By standardizing an organizational structure and using common terminology, the ICS provides a management system that is adaptable to incidents involving a multiagency or multijurisdictional response. At the most basic level there are five main components to the organizational structure: (1) incident command; (2) operations; (3) planning; (4) logistics; and (5) finance. With this type of organizational infrastructure and the flexibility to expand and collapse as needed, an orderly and efficient response to any incident can theoretically be implemented.

Communication from Disaster Site to Hospital

The local emergency communications or disaster operations center should alert hospitals in the affected area of a possible mass or multiple casualty situation. Ideally, this report should include number of injured, specifically the number of seriously injured (who may need ICU capability) and number for whom ambulatory treatment is sufficient. Hospitals should report to the local emergency communications center the following information: bed availability, number of casualties received thus far, number of additional casualties that the hospital is prepared to accept, and specific items in short supply.

Distribution of Casualties to Receiving Hospitals

Victims of a mass casualty incident usually are distributed unequally as described above. However, to decrease the possibility of this occurring, good communications should be maintained between hospitals and on-site EMS command. The on-scene incident commander should be alerted immediately by a potentially overloaded hospital. In this situation, the less injured and more stable can be sent a further distance to outlying hospitals. Secondary triage from one hospital to another may also be necessary if the hospital's capability to handle victims has been exceeded.

Casualties with special problems, such as major burns, carbon monoxide poisoning, spinal cord injuries, or victims of chemical or biological terrorism may need to be transferred directly to specialized units, although it may not be possible for these units to accept a large number of ill or injured.

On-Site Disaster Medical Teams from Hospitals

On-site disaster medical teams dispatched from local hospitals may be of value in situations where victims require prolonged extrication; transportation routes are blocked, preventing easy evacuation to hospitals; or the number of casualties are of such magnitude that they exceed transportation capacities. Such a team should be dispatched with great caution. Most physicians and nurses function well in an in-hospital setting; few, however, are prepared to work under austere field conditions either by training, inclination, or experience. Such hospital-based teams should probably not come from the emergency department staff until backup staff has arrived to care for patients arriving from the disaster site or who are already present. How such personnel are placed in action should be explicitly described in the hospital disaster plan and should be coordinated with state and local agencies through memoranda of understanding.

The resources for such field response teams should be carefully planned on a regional basis. The capability to send hospital teams to a disaster site can be developed in a number of ways. For example, an on-site triage team of physicians and nurses can come from teaching hospitals or be created from a pool of volunteer medical staff in office practice. Ideally, at least one institution from each region should maintain such a capability. The designated hospital should store disaster triage kits containing essential resuscitation and stabilization equipment in the emergency department for such circumstances.

THE EMERGENCY DEPARTMENT

The emergency department is the most critical part of the hospital's initial response to virtually any type of external disaster. It is often the hospital department that usually receives first notification that a disaster has occurred, and it is usually the entry point for incoming victims.

Initial Response

When a call is made to the hospital informing them of a disaster or potential mass-casualty-producing event, the receiver of the call must have a procedure to follow for verification of the incident. A disaster notification form is usually used by some facilities to remind the staff of the questions they are to ask the caller.

The appropriate hospital official or administrator on duty is then given this information. When the emergency department is notified by hospital administration (now disaster control) that the external disaster plan is in effect, it sets in motion a series of activities. The information obtained from the call is given to the charge nurse; the nursing and medical personnel in the department are notified of the impending arrival of casualties; and the emergency department's plan for calling additional staff is activated. Many hospital plans call for specific action by other doctors and allied personnel that is department-specific (e.g., surgeons, ICU staff, respiratory therapy, operating room staff).

An initial needs assessment is conducted by the nurse and physician in charge, given the information available. They should evaluate the current status of the patients in the department and make the appropriate decisions concerning their care and disposition. The ED physician becomes the on-site incident commander until the plan-designated disaster control physician arrives on the scene. Among the decisions to be made are those related to the admission, discharge, or transfer of patients, and decisions about the priority of patient care. All nonemergency patients should be discharged from the emergency department with responsible individuals (e.g., friends and relatives).

Based on the initial assessment, the number of patients that the department can receive is determined and communicated to the prehospital disaster communications center. The nurse and the physician in charge then determine whether more physician and nursing coverage is required in the emergency department and assign staff to those areas in the department to be used during the disaster.

As predetermined by the plan, a designated waiting area for family members should be located away from the emergency department.

Personnel Notification

The director of the emergency department or the director's designee should have a phone list of appropriate personnel to be called in to work during a disaster. Lists of addresses and phone numbers of these individuals should be distributed to all key personnel should it be impossible to locate the director or his or her assistant. Every position, address, and telephone number listed should be updated at least quarterly.

If hospital telephone communications have been completely disrupted, ED personnel may have to be reached by radio, cellular phone, e-mail, or television announcement (if power lines are down). Alternatively, a calling station remote from the hospital, such as an administrator's, physician's, or nurse's residence, may be able to handle this extensive calling job without taxing the hospital's phone system.

Security and Traffic Control

Hospital security play a key role in the emergency department by diverting nonessential vehicles and ensuring a smooth, one-way flow of traffic to the ambulance entrance. Once patients, family, and media arrive, security is also responsible for protecting the treatment areas.

Reception of Patients

Many seeking help will arrive independent of the official or formal EMS system. They will be brought by neighbors or friends or even hitchhike. Plans should include appropriate triage of these patients so that they do not overwhelm the ED prior to the arrival of the more severely injured, who arrive at a later stage.

All available litters and wheelchairs should be taken to the ambulance ramp immediately on announcement of the disaster status. Patients from the disaster site are met at the receiving area by hospital escorts who assist the EMTs in transferring patients to wheelchairs or stretchers.

Essential equipment such as endotracheal tubes, intravenous solutions, cervical collars, splints, and bandages should be placed near to the ambulance entrance to permit convenient restocking of the ambulance and rapid return to the disaster site.

THERAPEUTIC MANAGEMENT DURING DISASTER SITUATIONS

Triage

PURPOSES   In general, triage can be defined as the prioritization of patient care based on severity of injury/illness, prognosis, and availability of resources. For those responsible for the triage of patients arriving in the emergency department, the purpose of triage is to determine to which predesignated patient care area the patient should be sent. The location to which patients are "triaged" establishes priorities for care. For example, some patients may need immediate decontamination as they arrive, regardless of their severity of injury. Those needing immediate care (e.g., respiratory failure, shock) are taken to resuscitation areas ("crash" rooms), while the dead are moved directly to the morgue. The severely but less critically injured are taken to the major trauma–medical area described earlier, where they are further assessed and initial treatment commenced. The walking injured are directed to the minor surgery–primary care treatment area, often located in outpatient clinic areas.

PERSONNEL   A team consisting of a physician (preferably an emergency physician or a surgeon), an emergency department nurse, and a medical records or admitting clerk should receive every patient. In extraordinary situations, several triage teams may be required to handle the casualty load. The physician performing hospital triage should be acknowledged as being in command of the triage area, should be clearly identified by a specially colored vest or other garment, and must understand all triage options.

If a physician is not available, an emergency nurse with training in the concepts of casualty triage and disaster patient assessment can be designated as the triage officer.

RESPONSIBILITIES   Although likely triaged at the scene, patients should undergo a second process of triage upon arrival at the hospital, preferably at the ambulance entrance to the emergency department. Responsibilities of members of the triage team include:

1. Assigning disaster patients to appropriate treatment areas (e.g., resuscitation room, major surgical, minor surgical) according to the assessment of their immediate needs and the availability of resources.
2. Instituting the most basic of life-support measures, such as inserting oral airways, cardiopulmonary resuscitation, and the external control of hemorrhage.

Assessment of severity of injury should be accomplished by conducting a rapid primary survey supplemented by obtaining prehospital information from the patient or prehospital personnel. The triage team

communicates information on number of casualties, severity of injuries, and the need for additional resources to both the emergency department and the hospital disaster control center. If phones are tied up, this notification can be accomplished by using runners, cellular phones, or portable radios. Likewise, triage personnel need to be informed about the capability of the various treatment areas (e.g., major and minor surgery) to handle additional casualties or special problems such as eye injuries or burns. They also need to know about the establishment and location of patient overflow areas.

The triage physician should also be aware of the location of a family waiting and public relations area within the institution, because family, friends, and the media will otherwise attempt to enter the triage area.

The admitting clerk's role as part of the triage team is to complete tags, attach them to victims, and retrieve valuables and clothing for bagging. The admitting clerk then tags the bag and completes the triage area casualty log.

Principles of Triage

The approach to patient evaluation and treatment is quite different under disaster situations resulting in large numbers of casualties.[26] In mass casualty situations, one no longer has the luxury of concentrating all resources on the management of a single critical patient. To accomplish the most good for the most number of patients, the triage team should evaluate all patients arriving at the ED doors and classify their conditions with regard to severity of injury and need for treatment. Some principles of medical care must be altered to achieve the best overall result. There clearly is no role for resuscitation or definitive care at this stage. Care should be limited to manually opening airways, and controlling external hemorrhage.

The most common triage classification in the United States still involves assigning patients to one of four color-coded categories (red, yellow, green, or black), depending on injury severity and prognosis (Table 6-2). In addition to the nature and urgency of the patient's systemic condition, triage decisions should be sensitive to factors affecting prognosis, such as age, general health, and prior physical condition of the patient, and the qualifications of the responders and availability of key supplies and equipment.

TABLE 6-2   Triage Categories

Red
First priority
Most urgent
Life-threatening shock or hypoxia is present or imminent, but the patient can likely be stabilized and, if given immediate care, will probably survive

Yellow
Second priority
Urgent
The injuries have systemic implications or effects, but patients are not yet in life-threatening shock or hypoxia; although systemic decline may ensue, given appropriate care, can likely withstand a 45- to 60-min wait without immediate risk

Green
Third priority
Nonurgent
Injuries are localized without immediate systemic implications; with a minimum of care, these patients generally are unlikely to deteriorate for several hours, if at all

Black
Dead
No distinction can be made between clinical and biologic death in a mass casualty incident, and any unresponsive patient who has no spontaneous ventilation or circulation is classified as dead. Some place catastrophically injured patients who have a poor chance for survival regardless of care in this triage category

Catastrophically injured patients who have a minimal chance for survival despite optimal medical care should be classified as "expectant" (i.e., "black": e.g., burns involving 95 percent body surface area, patients in full cardiac arrest, anthrax-infected patients in septic shock). Spending time on patients who are not likely to live leaves other patients who are truly salvageable awaiting care. If too much time intercedes, these patients also may become nonsalvageable. The goal with these "expectant" patients should be adequate pain control and the opportunity to be with friends and family.

PATIENT CARE IN THE EMERGENCY DEPARTMENT

Mass casualty care cannot be covered appropriately here, but some concepts of care are not within emergency routine. For example, wound infections may occur in virtually all types of disasters. Infected wounds and gangrene were major problems following the earthquakes in Armenia (1988) and Turkey (1999) and tornadoes in Illinois (1991) and Oklahoma (2000). In hurricanes or tornadoes, persons may be cut by flying glass and other potentially highly contaminated material. Because of this, all wounds should be copiously flushed with saline. Primary closure of heavily contaminated wounds may result in major complications, as was the case following the Armero volcanic eruption in Colombia in 1985. If lacerations are old (more than 6 to 12 h) or appear contaminated, they should be treated by débridement and left open for primary delayed closure in a 3-day period. This will allow one an opportunity to observe the wound for the development of infection. Tetanus prophylaxis and tetanus immunoglobulin (TIG) should be administered as indicated.

Patients with blunt trauma, for example, victims of earthquakes who have been trapped by rubble for several hours or days, should be watched very closely for signs and symptoms of crush syndrome such as cardiac arrhythmias, hyperkalemia, and renal failure.[27] Fulminant pulmonary edema or pneumonia from dust inhalation may also be a delayed cause of mortality for victims of building collapse as with patients injured by blast waves from explosions ("white butterfly sign").[28]

Radiographic and Laboratory Studies

Radiographic and laboratory studies should be used sparingly, if at all, in a mass casualty situation, and only if the results of such tests will change therapeutic intervention. For example, x-rays of closed, nonangulated potential fractures can be safely delayed for 24 to 48 h, during which time effective splinting, elevation, and ice can be used. A chest film may be appropriate in those patients complaining of chest pain, dyspnea, or abnormal chest wall motion, or who were potentially exposed to blast waves secondary to bombs. The abdominal film in most cases of trauma does not provide much useful information. Cervical spine films and pelvic and femur x-rays may be indicated, considering the potential seriousness of injuries thus detected (e.g., permanent neurologic impairment, potential blood loss from internal injuries). Ultrasonography for FAST examination and detection of pneumothorax can be both timesaving and cost-effective.

There are few indications for laboratory testing in disaster medicine (exception: patients suspected of exposure to biologic weapons). For example, in cases of hemorrhagic shock, obtain a baseline hematocrit in addition to type- and cross-matching for blood. Urine test strip for blood may be useful to detect kidney or urinary tract injuries. In patients who are short of breath, or who demonstrate ventilatory impairment, it may be useful to have baseline arterial blood gases. All other laboratory studies should be considered accessory and only ordered in specific circumstances (e.g., carboxyhemoglobin in cases of smoke inhalation).

Blood Bank

In a disaster situation involving many casualties, it is recommended that the blood bank have as many as 50 units of blood available. It is also important that the blood bank have ready access to a source of volunteer donors who can be rapidly mobilized. Other potential sources of blood include friends and family members of patients, as well as the "walking wounded."

Patient Identification and Record Keeping

In past disasters ED records of disaster victims have usually been poor to nonexistent. The general absence of detailed and systematic record keeping in disasters, except for serious cases admitted to hospitals for surgery or to intensive care units, has many implications ranging from problems of cost of care, billings, reimbursement, and insurance collection to the difficulty of making any evaluations of the quality of medical care given and the possible efficacy of treatment procedures.[29]

Documentation of the patient's hospital course starts in the triage area. Proper tagging with a hospital disaster tag is essential for proper identification, documentation of medical care rendered, and for supplying information for relatives and the news media.

One member of the triage team (admitting or medical records clerk) should be assigned the job of recording the victim's name on the disaster tag along with the triaged destination within the hospital. If identification of the patient is not available, ethnicity, gender, and approximate age should be noted on the tag. An initial diagnostic impression should also be registered on the tag. This information is entered into a department log and is also placed in a triage logbook.

Media Relations

In a disaster, the hospital may become inundated by more members of the media than by actual disaster victims. Witness the recent intense media coverage of anthrax cases in the autumn of 2001 and during the sniper attacks in metropolitan Washington, DC, in the fall of 2002. The unauthorized presence of the press in patient care areas can definitely impair the performance of an already stressed hospital staff. Members of the media should be directed to a room or office of the hospital away from the emergency department and closely supervised by a hospital administrator or public relations specialist. This person should be in direct contact with the disaster control center. Hospital staff should leave all communications with the press to this person and should direct any member of the media to the public relations area so as to have consistent information given out by the hospital.

Handling of Family Members

Similarly, a separate area should be predesignated for family members seeking information. Family members should not be allowed into patient care areas, unless to see patients who are critically ill or who have died. The hospital operator will also be inundated with calls of inquiry regarding the presence and status of individual patients from concerned family members. These calls should be directed to a single predesignated desk or office for handling them.

AFTERMATH OF DISASTER

As soon as possible, efforts should be directed toward returning the hospital to normal operations. Besides restocking and cleaning, consideration should be given to the emotional stress experienced by both prehospital EMS and hospital staff. Short- and long-term emotional problems, particularly among rescuers, have been reported on numerous occasions including posttraumatic stress disorder. All those involved should be encouraged to talk with one another and with counselors as needed. In an attempt to reduce the psychologic impact of these events on medical responders, a technique known as critical incident stress debriefing (CISD) was introduced in 1993.[30]

The CISD is an important part of the overall disaster response. Implementation of this stress management strategy offers immediate emotional support to health care workers. Data from previous experiences suggest that such intervention can assist providers in maintaining job performance and satisfaction, resulting in improved patient care.[31]

Deficiencies in a hospital's disaster plan that are revealed during a disaster should be carefully recorded, reviewed, and criticized. Immediate steps should then be taken to correct these flaws in the plan.

REFERENCES

1. Hogan DE, Lillibridge SR, Waeckerle J, et al: Emergency department impact of the Oklahoma City terrorist bombing. *Ann Emerg Med* 34:160, 1999.
2. Joint Commission on Accreditation of Healthcare Organizations (JCAHO): *Emergency Management Standard.* Oak Brook Terrace, IL, JCAHO, 2001.
3. Koenig KL, Dinerman N, Kuehl AE: Disaster nomenclature: A functional impact approach. *Acad Emerg Med* 3:723, 1996.
4. Aghababian R, Lewis CP, Gans L, et al: Disasters within hospitals. *Ann Emerg Med* 23:771, 1994.
5. Centers for Disease Control: Rapid assessment of injuries among survivors of the terrorist attack on the World Trade Center—New York City, September 2001. *MMWR* 51:1, 2002.
6. Orr M, Robinson A: The Hyatt Regency skywalk collapse: An EMS-based disaster response. *Ann Emerg Med* 12:601, 1983.
7. Waeckerle JF: Disaster planning and response. *New Engl J Med* 324:815, 1991.
8. Schultz CH, Koenig KL, Noji EK: A medical disaster response to reduce immediate mortality after an earthquake. *New Engl J Med* 334:438, 1996.
9. Palafox J, Pointer JE, Martchenke J, et al: The 1989 Loma Prieta earthquake: Issues in medical control. *Prehosp Disaster Med* 8:291, 1993.
10. Leonard RB, Calabro JJ, Noji EK, Leviton RH: SARA (Superfund Amendments and Reauthorization Act): Implications for emergency medicine. *Ann Emerg Med* 18:1212, 1989.
11. Noji EK, Sivertson KT: Injury prevention in natural disasters: A theoretical framework. *Disasters* 11:290, 1987.
12. Noji EK, Kelen GD, Armenian HK, et al: The 1988 earthquake in Soviet Armenia: A case study. *Ann Emerg Med* 19:891, 1990.
13. Durkin ME, Thiel CC, Schneider JE, et al: Injuries and emergency medical response in the Loma Prieta earthquake. *Bull Seismological Soc Am* 81:2143, 1991.
14. Sincell M: Natural disasters. Texas Medical Center staggered by deadly tropical storm. *Science* 292(5525):2226, 2001.
15. Dhara RV: Health effects of the Bhopal gas leak: A review. *Arch Environ Health* 47:385, 1992.
16. Okumura T, Takasu N, Ishimatsu S, et al: Report on 640 victims of the Tokyo subway sarin attack. *Ann Emerg Med* 28:129, 1996.
17. Barbera JA, Macintyre AG: Medical and Health Incident Management (MaHIM) System. A comprehensive functional system description for Mass Casualty Medical and Health Incident Management. Institute for Crisis, Disaster, and Risk Management, The George Washington University. Washington D.C., October 2002.
18. Centers for Disease Control and Prevention: *Public Health Emergency Preparedness and Response: Bioterrorism. What has the CDC Accomplished?* Available from: URL http://www.bt.cdc.gov/Documents/BTInitiative.asp, accessed Aug 1, 2002.
19. Hospital Emergency Incident Command System Update Project, available at www.emsa.cahwnet.gov/dms2/heics3.htm, last accessed July 23, 2003.
20. Landesman LY: *Emergency Preparedness in Health Care Organizations.* Oak Brook Terrace, IL, JCAHO, 1996.
21. Kratan V: The World Trade Center attack. Is critical care prepared for terrorism? *Crit Care* 5:321, 2001.
22. Hooft PJ, Noji EK, Van de Voorde HP: Fatality management in mass-casualty incidents. *Forensic Sci Int* 40:3, 1989.
23. Super G, Groth S, Hook R, et al: *START: Simple Triage and Rapid Treatment Plan.* Newport Beach, CA, Hoag Memorial Hospital Presbyterian, 1994.
24. Benson M, Koenig KL, Schultz CH: Disaster triage: START, then SAVE—A new method of dynamic triage for victims of a catastrophic earthquake. *Prehosp Disaster Med* 11:117, 1996.
25. Koenig KL, Schultz CH: Disaster medicine: Advances in local catastrophic disaster response. *Acad Emerg Med* 1:133, 1994.
26. Garner A, Lee A, Harrison K, Schultz CH: Comparative analysis of multiple-casualty incident triage algorithms. *Ann Emerg Med* 38:541, 2001.
27. Oda Y, Shindoh M, Yukioka H, et al: Crush syndrome sustained in the 1995 Kobe, Japan, earthquake: Treatment and outcome. *Ann Emerg Med* 30:507, 1997.
28. Feliciano DV, Anderson GV, Rozycki GS, et al: Management of casualties from the bombing at the centennial Olympics. *Am J Surg* 176:538, 1998.
29. American College of Emergency Physicians (ACEP): Disaster data collection, in: *ACEP Policy Compendium*, 2001 ed. Dallas, TX, ACEP, 2001, p. 12.
30. Mitchell J, Everly GS: *Critical Incident Stress Debriefing: An Operations Manual for the Prevention of Traumatic Stress among Emergency and Disaster Workers.* Ellicott City, MD, Chevron Publishing, 1993.
31. Gerrity ET: Critical incident stress debriefing (CISD): Value and limitations in disaster response. *Nat Ctr PTSD Clin Quart* 4:17, 1994.

BIOTERRORISM RESPONSE: IMPLICATIONS FOR THE EMERGENCY CLINICIAN

Anthony G. MacIntyre
Joseph A. Barbera

Of all the issues facing the modern emergency physician, the potential threat of bioterrorism is one of the most challenging. An adequate response to a bioterrorist event of any magnitude requires the effective coordination of many disparate health and medical entities beyond the emergency department. Although the emergency physician plays a critical role in these types of events, many other essential functions must be addressed by individuals and organizations representing public health, mental health, law enforcement, emergency management, and others. Emergency physicians may find themselves working closely with organizations that are not traditionally encountered in everyday emergency medical practice.

A bioterrorist event involves the release of a biological agent among a civilian population for the purpose of creating fear, illness, and death. In extreme instances, disruption of the social and economic infrastructure may result. Biological agents are classified into two groups: infectious agents and biologically produced toxins. In most circumstances, biological toxins act as chemical agents in their human impact. The response requirements for these are very similar to those for chemical terrorism incidents and therefore are not discussed in this chapter. Infectious agents may be subdivided into two categories: contagious (propagating person to person) and noncontagious.

The use of infectious agents has been an increasing concern of the U.S. federal government since the mid 1990s (after waning at the end of the Cold War). This concern has been due in part to the biological weapons development programs in existence in certain countries and the capabilities of transnational terrorism. Throughout history, biological agents have been investigated as potential weapons for military campaigns, but current realities raise the specter of attacks that primarily target noncombatants. A bioterrorist event in the civilian setting often has been described as a low probability, high impact event.

Until the fall of 2001, only two small events had occurred in recent U.S. history involving a biological agent deployed against civilians.[1,2] These events might be more appropriately described as criminal rather than terrorist in nature, because there was no associated terror message aimed at a larger audience. Concern for bioterrorism grew more acute after the events of September 11, 2001. Public trepidation was validated by the subsequent anthrax dissemination incident, in which the U.S. Postal Service was used to deliver letters containing spores of *Bacillus anthracis*. Although the environmental contamination was widespread, only 22 diagnosed cases of anthrax infection occurred: 11 cases of inhalational and 11 cases of cutaneous anthrax. Five patients died as a direct result of the anthrax exposure.[3] The limited numbers of actual diagnosed cases belies the fact that multiple communities on the eastern seaboard of the United States were severely affected, with thousands receiving prophylaxis for anthrax.[4] The fear then spread across the entire nation as concern increased for a wider delivery of anthrax in mid-western and western locales. Much of this national concern may have been exacerbated by the perception of an inadequate public health response capability, with the deficiencies demonstrating a critical need to integrate acute care medicine and the public health response.

It is difficult to comprehensively cover the complex topic of bioterrorism in this limited format. General event characteristics are presented with focused information on specific biological agents of concern. References for more comprehensive information on specific agents are identified. Response to bioterrorism is a rapidly evolving discipline, with the U.S. response systems and the understanding of individual agents in constant transition.

AGENTS OF CONCERN

Many infectious biologic organisms have the potential to be used as bioterrorism agents. Certain characteristics, however, make individual organisms particularly attractive as weapons for generating widespread fear, illness, and death among civilian populations. In an effort to risk stratify agents of concern, the Centers for Disease Control and Prevention (CDC) convened a multidisciplinary working group to designate select organisms and the diseases they cause as the priority for focused preparation.[5] Agent selection was based on four general criteria:

1. Potential for public health impact
2. Delivery potential (an estimation of the ease for development and dissemination, including the potential for person-to-person transmission of infection)
3. Public perception (fear) of the agent
4. Special requirements for public health preparedness (diagnostic, logistical, etc.)

The selected agents were then ranked in three categories, based on their overall potential for adverse public health impact (Table 7-1). Class A agents have the most severe potential and include viruses and bacteria such as *Variola major* (smallpox), *Bacillus anthracis* (anthrax), and *Yersinia pestis* (plague). Class B agents are considered to have less potential for causing widespread illness and death, and class C agents are those that, as technology improves, could emerge as future threats. It is important to recognize that many other, more common pathogens could be used to cause intentional injury, and the intentional etiology of the infections may be apparent only through epidemiologic cohort evaluation.

RECOGNITION OF A BIOTERRORIST EVENT

Unlike the more common scenario from terrorist bombings, a biological agent attack may not be immediately recognizable. Unless the release of an agent is openly announced or the terrorist is caught in the process of delivering the agent, initial indications of attack may be subtle. Recognition that a biological attack has caused a disease outbreak is complicated further by the fact that initial symptoms of most agents of concern are not readily distinguished from more common, less threatening illnesses. Fever, body aches, and malaise could be the initial presenting symptoms of a victim of bioterrorism (anthrax and others) or of influenza, parainfluenza, or many common illnesses. This is more than a theoretical risk, as demonstrated when some agents of concern have been documented to occur in the non-bioterrorism setting. For example, cases of human plague in the Southwest United States (where plague is endemic) initially were diagnosed as nonspecific viral illnesses and dismissed as benign. Only later, when symptoms became more severe, was bubonic plague diagnosed.[6] During the anthrax dissemination event of 2001, several anthrax-infected postal workers were evaluated by physicians early in their illness, but their relatively nonspecific symptoms were attributed to other causes, and

they were discharged home without antibiotic therapy.[7] Two postal workers in this cohort died from inhalational anthrax.

The actual recognition of any future, surreptitious biologic attack could occur through several pathways:

1. A patient presents with signs, symptoms, or immediately available diagnostic results that obviously indicate a suspect disease process.
2. A patient presents with protean symptoms, but an astute clinician establishes enough criteria (suspicious historical information, signs, symptoms, short turn-around laboratory results, public health corroborative information, etc.) to designate the patient as a presumptive case until diagnostic confirmation can be accomplished.
3. Patient presents, is evaluated and admitted or released, but not suspected as being a victim of bioterrorism. Diagnostic test results (blood cultures, immunoassays, etc.) subsequently establish a diagnosis, potentially even postmortem.
4. Multiple patients present over a defined period with similar symptoms or historical characteristics, raising the suspicions of a practitioner and causing that individual to report the concern. Further investigation with diagnostic testing and/or public health epidemiological investigation of the cohort establishes the cause.
5. Public health surveillance systems establish unusual patterns of signs, symptoms, or disease in the community and correlate with further investigation to establish the etiology.

Currently, the first three scenarios appear to be the most likely ways in which a bioterrorist event will be detected. Scenario 3 is how inhalational anthrax was initially diagnosed in Florida during the fall of 2001.[8] The initial inhalational anthrax infection in a postal worker was recognized as in scenario 2. Thus, the emergency clinician, perhaps more than any other medical specialist, should have an operational knowledge of the biological agents of concern. This knowledge should include basic pathologic principles for each agent, modes of dissemination and transmission, disease signs and symptoms, recommended diagnostic testing, recommended therapy (medicines, immunizations, or prophylaxis), and infection control practices. For example, every emergency clinician should be capable of listing the distinguishing characteristics of the rash caused by smallpox and how to differentiate it from chickenpox or other pox viruses. Another example of diagnostically important knowledge was noted during the anthrax dissemination event of 2001. All symptomatic patients presenting with inhalational anthrax had abnormal chest x-rays and/or thoracic computed tomographic scans at presentation (most with a widened mediastinum), providing an important diagnostic indicator in suspicious cases.[7]

Enhanced knowledge among practitioners is currently the best method for improving the capability to detect a bioterrorist event. Some formalized education efforts are underway to address this,[9] and changes to the curricula of emergency medicine residencies have been proposed.[10] In addition, access to references for specific clinical information, such as distinguishing signs and symptoms for agents of concern, can be very useful in identifying suspect patients. Pictorial resources made widely available during the anthrax dissemination incident, for distinguishing between cutaneous anthrax and other cutaneous lesions, were exceptionally reassuring for clinicians in the national capital area.[11]

Unfortunately, currently available technology for virtually all emergency clinicians does not provide real-time diagnostic studies to reliably confirm or exclude the presence of most potential agents of concern (which actually do not differ from most common infectious processes). Confirmatory tests, however, may not even be available at the individual hospital or even in the community, and may require specialized studies through state or federal laboratories. The clinician therefore should command sufficient knowledge of agent diagnosis to confidently order appropriate tests and provide appropriate medical interventions when *suspicious* of a patient's clinical presentation.

The emergency clinician also should be prepared to appropriately respond to notification of potential disease by another health or med-

TABLE 7-1   Agents of Concern as Defined by the Centers for Disease Control and Prevention

Biological Agent	Disease Caused	Incubation Period	Signs and Symptoms
Class A agents			
Variola major	Smallpox	12–14 d	Initially fever, severe myalgias, prostration; followed within 2 d by papular rash on the face spreading to extremities (affecting palms and soles) and then to trunk (lesser extent than chickenpox); lesions progress at same rate, becoming vesicular and then pustular with subsequent scab formation
Bacillus anthracis	Cutaneous anthrax	Usually <1 d, up to 2 wk reported	Macule or papule enlarging into eschar with surrounding vesicles and edema; sepsis possible, less common
	GI anthrax	Usually 1–7 d	Abdominal pain, vomiting, GI bleeding progressing to sepsis; mesenteric adenopathy on CT
	Oropharyngeal anthrax	Usually 1–7 d	Sore throat, ulcers on base of tongue, marked unilateral neck swelling
	Inhalational anthrax	Usually <1 wk, 43 d reported at Sverdlovsk*	First stage is nonspecific (fever, dyspnea, cough, headache, vomiting, abdominal pain, chest pain); second stage (dyspnea, diaphoresis, shock); hemorrhagic mediastinitis with widened mediastinum on x-ray
Yersinia pestis	Bubonic plague	2–8 d	Initially fever, chills, painful swollen lymph node(s); node progresses to bubo (sometimes suppurative)
	Pneumonic plague	2–3 d	Fever chills, cough, dyspnea, nausea, vomiting, abdominal pain; clinical condition consistent with gram-negative sepsis
	Primary septicemic plague	2–8 d	After bubo formation, the clinical condition is consistent with gram-negative sepsis, DIC
Clostridium botulinum	Food-borne botulism	1–5 d	GI symptoms followed by symmetric cranial neuropathies, blurred vision, progressing to descending paralysis
	Inhalational botulism†	12–72 h	Symmetric cranial nerve palsies followed by descending paralysis
Francisella tularensis	Tularemia	2–5 d	Abrupt nonspecific febrile illness progressing to pleuropneumonitis; may have mucocutaneous lesions
Filoviruses and arenaviruses (e.g., *Ebola virus*)	Viral hemorrhagic fevers	2 d–3 wk depending on virus	Initial nonspecific febrile illness, sometimes with rash; progresses to bloody vomiting, diarrhea, shock.
Class B agents			
Coxiella burnetii	Q fever	2–3 wk	Fever, myalgias, headache, 30% develop pneumonia, rarely lethal (2%)
Brucella spp.	Brucellosis	2–4 wk	Fever, myalgias, back pain; CNS infections and endocarditis possible
Burkholderia mallei	Glanders	10–14 d	Local infection: ulcers, suppurative; pneumonia, pulmonic abscesses, sepsis possible
Burkholderia pseudomallei	Melioidosis	2 d to years reported	Local infection: nodule; pneumonia, pulmonic abscesses, sepsis
Alphaviruses (VEE, EEE, WEE)	Encephalitis	Variable	Fever, headache, aseptic meningitis, encephalitis, focal paralysis, seizures
Rickettsia prowazekii	Typhus fever	7–14 d	Fever, headache, rash
Toxins (e.g., Ricin, *Staphylococcus,* Enterotoxin B)	Toxic syndromes		
Chlamydia psittaci	Psittacosis	6–19 d	Fever, headache, dry cough, pneumonia, endocarditis
Food safety threats (e.g., *Salmonella* spp., *Eschericia coli* O157:H7)			
Water safety threats (e.g., *Vibrio cholera, Cryptosporidium parvum*)			
Class C threats			
Emerging threat agents (e.g., *Nipah virus,* hantavirus)			

*Data from Meselson M, Guillemin J, Hugh-Jones M, et al: The Sverdlovsk anthrax outbreak of 1979. *Science* 266:1202, 1994.
†Inhalational botulism may not be preceded by GI symptoms. Inhalational and food-borne botulisms are caused by botulinum toxin, not the bacteria itself.
Abbreviations: CNS = central nervous system; CT = computed tomography; DIC = disseminated intravascular coagulation; EEE = Eastern equine encephalitis; GI = gastrointestinal; VEE = Venezuelan equine encephalitis; WEE = Western equine encephalitis.

ical professional (laboratory technician, radiologist, pathologist, or medical examiner). Carefully querying the source for pertinent specific information, including methodology of the testing that produced the concern (specimen collection technique and the sensitivity and specificity of the test procedure), and time until confirmatory test re-sults become available are important factors in considering further actions, such as those delineated below.

Situations that pose great challenge to emergency department operations are those in which patients present after having been exposed to an unidentified substance (e.g., white powder), with circumstances that have raised suspicion for terrorism (threatening letter, high profile location, a "very important person," etc.). The source substance may not have been properly evaluated or secured, and any recommended treatment necessarily will involve coordination with outside agencies (public health and law enforcement). If no testing was performed, one may attempt to obtain confirmatory studies (through the local public health authorities) if the substance remains available. Otherwise, the difficult task of stratifying patient exposure risk is necessary, using arguably nonspecific factors such as patient demographics and the specific characteristics of the event (e.g., white powder found in a local business vs. a high-level federal official's office). The public health authorities with jurisdiction over the involved communities should be consulted early in this process, ideally by using preplanned notification processes and decision support tools (see Chap. 6). When testing has been performed by others, the emergency clinician should request specific information on the testing methodology and judge the reliability of the test procedure. For instance, anthrax environmental testing may be performed with a wide range of procedures, including immune-based assays, assays based on polymerase chain reaction, and confirmatory culture testing.[12] Numerous instances of false positive environmental tests, when reported in the press, have created serious public concern. Several widely used field tests for anthrax, long recognized as unreliable, have now been officially discredited.[13]

Currently, much effort in the United States is focused on developing broad-based public health surveillance systems for detection of disease. The surveillance systems currently in use or under development are based on collecting and analyzing public health information and/or patient diagnostic information in specific communities. Information is sought from many disparate sources, including hospitals, clinics, nursing homes, pharmacies, emergency medical service systems, independent laboratories, medical examiners, and general businesses (e.g., absenteeism rates). Information collected from emergency departments often is based on symptom complexes (syndromic surveillance). Proposed methods for detection of a biologic event include the recognition of unusual epidemiologic phenomena such as a high incidence of nonspecific illness, clusters or large numbers of rapidly fatal cases, and steep infection curves.[14] The City of New York's Department of Health has operated this type of surveillance system since the late 1990s.[15]

Even though modeling suggests earlier detection and recognition, it has not yet been proven that currently proposed syndromic surveillance systems are sensitive and specific enough to detect an anomaly at a sufficiently early stage and to recognize the anomaly as a bioterrorism event to allow the earliest possible response. Most new infectious events (e.g., hantavirus and West Nile virus) were noted first by astute practitioners evaluating the initial cases. However, public health surveillance systems may have an important role during an actual event, if they also can assist with defining the size and scope of the event, the at-risk population, the effects of response interventions, and other epidemiologic characteristics. Critical data likely will be generated from patients in emergency departments, so emergency physicians should participate in surveillance systems. Emergency medicine should, however, be involved in the design and implementation of their community surveillance systems to assure that the resulting system meets the following criteria that the author's propose:

1. Clinical duties are minimally affected (does not consume valuable clinician or support staff time and attention)
2. Financial investment is not carried by the hospital or professional staff (especially in the current fiscal environment)
3. Patient privacy and hospital proprietary issues are appropriately addressed
4. Participation in the system provides direct benefit to the acute care medical community (i.e., all pertinent epidemiologic information is disseminated in real time to the practitioners)

Past attempts at surveillance system development and implementation have occurred without adequately addressing these principles (e.g.,

temporary surveillance for a presidential inauguration).[16] The resulting hospital and emergency department participation was limited.

INITIAL RESPONSE TO A POTENTIAL BIOTERRORIST THREAT

Every receiving facility and emergency department should have plans and policies to manage a bioterrorism threat. The initial response to a suspected or confirmed bioterrorist event should involve many different hospital departments and agencies outside the hospital. Initial actions taken by the emergency physician can be pivotal in the success of the hospital efforts and the overall community response.

If the emergency clinician has diagnosed a confirmed or probable victim of bioterrorism, a critical action is adequate initial notification and plan activation. Infection control procedures should be used as appropriate (see below). Within the hospital, administration should be notified, as should other departments such as infection control, infectious diseases, and laboratory services (if not already involved in the case). If contaminating bioagent is an issue, as may be the case with anthrax, security and environmental services should be notified. The plan should address efficient methods of information flow to all departments of the hospital regarding the suspected agent, its characteristics including potential for person-to-person transmission, and efforts to protect the staff. Consideration should be given to activating a facility's full emergency operations plan (EOP). Implementation of the EOP should provide a preplanned surge capacity configuration. Nonmedical departments that require special attention include security (to aid in protection of the facility and staff) and media relations. Media personnel for the hospital ideally should coordinate any information released in briefings with the department of public health to prevent the presentation of conflicting information. Ideally, the hospital EOP fully integrates the hospital into the community response, which is critical in any bioterrorist event.[17]

Depending on the details of the plan or the circumstances of the incident, the emergency clinician also may have the responsibility for notifying the respective jurisdictional public health department. This necessitates that a reliable 24-h contact method be established and regularly tested. The information should be provided to public health as soon as a presumptive diagnosis is made to aid in the community response. Information that should be conveyed includes:

1. Diagnosed or suspected agent of concern
2. Whether it is a presumed or definitive diagnosis (and how any "definitive" diagnosis was made)
3. Patient demographics (including occupation)
4. Recent history of travel or participation in special events (mass gatherings, high-profile events, or at-risk gatherings)
5. Patient condition
6. Initial testing performed and further diagnostic testing being conducted
7. Treatment being provided
8. Public health assistance required (including testing)
9. Preferred method of contacting hospital or treating physicians for follow-up

The local department of health then has the responsibility to notify regional or state public health departments (as applicable) and the CDC. With some agents, the CDC would notify the World Health Organization, because the potential impact could be global (e.g., smallpox). Public health (city or state) also would have the responsibility of notifying local law enforcement and the Federal Bureau of Investigation.

Another critical initial action for the emergency clinician is to establish the appropriate infection control guidelines respective to the diagnosed or suspected agent. This is essential in protecting the clinician, hospital staff, and other patients present in the hospital. It is also critical in maintaining the ability of the hospital to continue its regular medical commitment to the community. In 1999, the Association for

Professionals in Infection Control and Epidemiology published guidelines for hospital infection control in response to a bioterrorist event.[18] Fortunately, most agents of concern require only standard precautions (gloves, mucous membrane protection when potential for splashing exists, and gown when potential exists for soiling). The more troubling agents are those that are capable of airborne transmission. A case of pneumonic plague will require droplet protection and patient isolation, very similar to current procedures for active tuberculosis cases. Smallpox would require airborne and contact precautions and therefore full patient isolation. Appropriately fitting face masks should be protective against these agents. Adequately providing these types of protection can pose one of the greater challenges to hospitals when multiple patients are involved.

Aside from actual medical treatment of the individual patient, another important initial consideration is whether patient decontamination is indicated. Decontamination should be a consideration only if a patient presents shortly after acute exposure to a substance suspected or confirmed as a biologic weapon, in contrast to the presentation of the patient who has already developed symptoms of an infectious disease. Public health authorities consider the risk of secondarily cross contaminating hospital staff from resuspension of an agent on this type of patient as unlikely.[19] If a realistic concern exists, simple disrobing of the patient and showering with soap and warm water should be adequate decontamination. Clothing and personal belongings may need to be secured to assist with the public health and law enforcement investigations. Decontaminants, such as diluted bleach, should be avoided, due to their potential for harm and the lack of any demonstrated clinical efficacy (hypochlorite requires prolonged contact time for its agent-cidal action and can in itself cause skin injury).

INTEGRATION WITH LOCAL DEPARTMENT OF HEALTH

In any suspected or confirmed case of bioterrorism, the emergency physician can expect to interface with multiple diverse agencies, the most critical of which is the local public health department. In most communities, public health epidemiologists are assigned the task of defining the size and scope of an incident, the at-risk population, and other incident parameters. This type of information becomes critical to acute care clinicians, other medical care providers, and hospitals in the evaluation and treatment of patients and in the anticipation of surge capacity requirements. Challenges, such as the evaluation of minimally symptomatic individuals or the evaluation of large volumes of patients, can be facilitated by the provision of clear and concise information from the public health department.

The most important assistance public health can provide to all clinicians is in the development of a communitywide patient evaluation and treatment protocol. Evaluation and treatment protocols provide a clear delineation of epidemiologic criteria that establish a patient's individual risk for exposure and, hence, how to further evaluate and treat the individual. This kind of tool is essential for the practitioner once an event has been recognized, because confirmatory testing will rarely be immediately available. It therefore assists the practitioner in risk stratifying a patient or groups of patients. The protocol also should include the recommended testing, treatment methodologies, and patient and public education. During the response to the anthrax event in the fall of 2001, initial epidemiologic investigations using nasal swabs were misunderstood by some practitioners and the public as having individual diagnostic utility. It was merely an epidemiologic surveillance tool. Anxiety and confusion, however, resulted when individuals received nasal swabbing at some health care locations and were told it was not useful for diagnosis at other locations.

During the initial stages of a biologic event, the screening criteria for potential exposure may be necessarily broad. As the epidemiologic investigation ensues, these criteria should rapidly become more conclusive. Information coordination between health care providers and public health epidemiologists is necessary to rapidly accomplish an epidemiologic profile of the incident. Evaluation protocols may evolve during this epidemiologic investigation and will require reliable dissemination of the recommendations with regularly scheduled updates. Ideally, the medical community should receive incident updates and changes in recommendations before general release to the public. This allows clinicians time to respond to changes and to provide further explanation and reassurance to anxious inquiring patients.

An important advantage of a single evaluation and treatment protocol is that it provides a uniform method across a community to evaluate patients presenting with possible exposure. This is important not only for individual practitioners but also for the public. During the response to the anthrax dissemination event in the Washington-Baltimore corridor, no early standardized protocol was developed; instead, hospitals implemented their own protocols to limit variation of practice between clinicians at individual hospitals. The variability between each institution's approach caused great consternation for patients and, hence, for providers. The protocols used at George Washington University Hospital were modified daily, based upon updated information. The operationalization of the public health approach can be quite complex.

Critical information that the public health system should provide is a clear and concise case definition for the particular agent in question. A case definition provides clinical and diagnostic criteria for an individual patient to be considered as a definitive victim of the infectious agent in question. Within the case definition, criteria also should be supplied that define "suspicious" cases for patients awaiting confirmatory testing. This kind of tool is simple and allows practitioners to officially designate victims as confirmed or suspicious for infection. A similar "exposure" definition would be helpful for defining the criteria for confirmed or suspected exposure. In many cases, the epidemiologic investigation that can initially define and later refine these definitions requires close information sharing and collaboration between clinicians seeing cases and the public health authorities.

Other critical information for the clinician includes reporting requirements (surveillance) for suspected or diagnosed cases. Specific points as to what information should be reported and the method in which it should be conveyed are essential (phone, fax, or Internet). Contact methods should be provided that allow for 24-h access and for technical advice. Ideal reporting systems affect the clinician minimally (as described above) and provide confirmation of receipt of transmitted information. The reporting format should promote rapid processing of the communitywide data, with dissemination of composite information to the reporting sources. This demonstration of the value of the system will promote clinician participation and provide clear value in participating in a coordinated, overall incident management system.

Integration with Other Response Assets   Requests for assistance or for assets not available within an individual hospital should be coordinated through hospital administration to the local department of health and/or the local emergency managment agency. From there, requests may be transmitted to the regional, state, or federal level. Other response assets are discussed in Chap. 6

TREATMENT, PROPHYLAXIS, AND IMMUNIZATION

General treatment principles for victims of bioterrorism should be understood by the practitioner. Specific therapies for individual class A agents are listed in Table 7-2. Limitations of morbidity and mortality are based on preventing exposure, providing prophylaxis and immunization (when available for the specific pathogen), and providing treatment to those infected. Treatment may involve specific pharmaceuticals or general supportive care. Depending on the agent involved, prophylaxis or immunization of the hospital staff may be warranted (e.g., smallpox). It is important to recognize that therapeutics may be

TABLE 7-2   Category A Agents: Treatment, Prophylaxis, and Vaccination

Biological Agent	Vaccination	Prophylaxis	Treatment
Class A agents			
Variola major	Vaccinia vaccination: currently not recommended for general public use because of its association with limited numbers of deaths and complications in immunocompromised individuals and those with eczema; useful in preventing disease if given within 4 d of exposure	Vaccinia immune globulin: best given within 2–3 d of exposure; limited supplies are available; consider giving to those exposed who have contraindications to vaccine	Mainly supportive; Cidovir has demonstrated some efficacy in monkey models
Bacillus anthracis	Anthrax vaccination: 6-part series vaccination at 0, 2, and 4 wk and then at 6, 12, and 18 mo; annual boosters required; currently not available to the public; efficacy in preventing inhalational anthrax demonstrated in animal models	Ciprofloxacin or doxycycline for 60 d (amoxicillin if strain not resistant); 60-d term established by using latency period for last infection occurring at Sverdlovsk*; consideration for concurrent vaccination	Ciprofloxacin or doxycycline (amoxicillin if strain not resistant) *in combination* with two others including clindamycin, rifampin, imipenem, aminoglycoside, chloramphenicol, vancomycin, streptomycin, and some macrolides
Yersinia pestis	Killed whole bacilli vaccine no longer available by producers; vaccine had efficacy in preventing bubonic disease but not the pneumonic form	Ciprofloxacin or doxycycline; alternative: chloramphenicol; prophylaxis for 7 d	Streptomycin or gentamicin preferred choices; alternatives: doxycycline, ciprofloxacin, chloramphenicol
Clostridium botulinum	Vaccine not available to the public: pentavalent toxoid of C botulinum toxin types A–E; 3-part series with yearly booster	Not applicable	Antitoxin: requires procurement through local public health agency (state or the CDC); antitoxin may preserve remaining neurologic function but does not reverse paralysis; may require prolonged, assisted mechanical ventilation and supportive care
Francisella tularensis	Live attenuated vaccine under investigation by FDA	Ciprofloxacin or doxycycline for 14 d	Streptomycin or gentamicin preferred choices; alternatives: doxycycline, ciprofloxacin, chloramphenicol
Filoviruses and arenaviruses (e.g., *Ebola virus*)	Not applicable	Not applicable	Supportive therapy; ribavirin may have applicability in arenaviruses

*Data from Meselson M, Guillemin J, Hugh-Jones M, et al: The Sverdlovsk anthrax outbreak of 1979. *Science* 266:1202, 1994.
Abbreviations: CDC = Centers for Disease Control and Prevention; FDA = Food and Drug Administration.

indicated even without obvious signs of disease or definitive information about exposure. This makes the practitioner heavily reliant on the public health sector to stratify patient risk as to their exposure and to provide science-based prophylaxis and treatment recommendations.

One of the critical issues in providing treatment to victims of bioterrorism is the development of an adequate surge capacity. This issue is complicated by the current health care industry practice of minimizing staff and maintaining just-in-time inventory. For the individual practitioner, ideal surge capacity is provided by first maximizing health care facility response assets and coordinating with regional resources. State and federal assistance should be included in planning, but not relied on, for the initial stages of an event (up to at least 48 h).

General Emergency Operations Plans

Patients will self-refer to hospitals and emergency departments, even if instructed to do otherwise (as occurred in the anthrax dissemination event). All emergency department and hospital surge capacity should be based on a sound and well-practiced hospital EOP that can manage a large surge in general patient volume.

Specialty Requirements

Specialty needs also should be addressed for patients with unusual medical conditions and those who present contagion or contamination risks to staff and other patients. Separate treatment areas may need to be established within the health care facility to allow normal emergency department operations to continue. This also may be necessary if the potential agent is capable of person-to-person transmission.

Disease Containment

Isolation of large numbers of infectious patients may be necessary (e.g., smallpox). Adequate plans for this procedure should be investigated before an incident. Current hospital configurations often prohibit large-scale containment of patients in official isolation rooms, but entire wings could be adapted (using doors and ventilation re-routing) to serve as isolation wards. Plans to provide adequate separation from other, noninfected patients, to designate specific staff to care for these patients, and to furnish proper personal protective equipment should be accomplished.

Management of Personnel

Large numbers of patients require additional staff to manage them. Staff recruitment may be complicated by reluctance of staff to care for potentially infectious patients. Lack of training of temporary personnel from staffing agencies makes this more difficult and is addressed only through regionwide training efforts.

Logistics

Just-in-time inventory may limit the amount of pharmaceuticals and supplies available for treating patients. Further, vendors for emergency backup supplies and equipment are commonly shared by multiple institutions, each counting the backup cache as their own. Having a communitywide mutual aid system between all the hospitals promotes sharing of critical supplies, equipment, and staff during an emergency. If prescriptions are being written for antibiotics, consideration must be given to the supply local pharmacies have on hand (an issue during the anthrax incident in 2001). Integration of National Pharmaceutical Stockpile (NPS) supplies into a medical community has specific requirements that are available for review through the CDC, and that require specific planning by the community emergency management and public health agencies.

Patient Management

Addressing the requirements of each patient encounter can facilitate the overall processing of victims. For those patients who are potentially exposed but not physically ill, the patient interaction may require sophisticated explanations as to why the individual is or is not receiving a particular therapy. Preprinted instructions (indicating category of risk stratification and why the patient was placed in that category) can be helpful for patients being treated and released. These instructions should clearly indicate how the disease is transmitted, measures that prevent spread, and early signs and symptoms of disease, with appropriate steps if they should occur. Appropriate follow-up should be established (in a large-scale event, this may not be with a primary care physician but through public health avenues). It is important to note any change in the epidemiology of the event (e.g., new site tests positive for an agent) or if new information becomes available on the etiological agent (antibiotic resistance patterns, etc.), and patients may need to be contacted to change their therapy. Proper record keeping and organization of charts based on assigned risk category can assist with this process. Entering all patients into a reliable long-term surveillance data base should be a task for the public health agency, but hospitals and emergency departments could facilitate this process.

For agents of concern that have a vaccine (e.g., anthrax and smallpox), recommendations at the time of this writing are that they not be given in a pre-event setting to the general public. Anthrax vaccination requires a series of six injections followed by yearly updates. Smallpox vaccine has not been given to the general public for nearly three decades. Even those who received vaccine in the past are expected to have a waning immunity to the virus. At the time of writing of this chapter, recommendations are under review to re-introduce this vaccine. The risk of potential life-threatening side effects, such as generalized vaccinia, complicate the recommendations of smallpox vaccination in the absence of known disease.

Recommended therapies for some bioterrorism agents normally are not approved for children or pregnant or lactating women. In many instances, these recommendations have been relaxed where the risk of infection and its consequences exceeds the risks of the medications or vaccines. Examples include using ciprofloxacin in children for anthrax exposure. Preparation to explain this concept to patients is imperative.

Fatality Management

Large numbers of deceased patients can pose a burden on a health care facility, especially when death is caused by a contagious disease. In intentional events, the forensic requirements add complications, because the bodies are considered evidence and must be processed through an official medical examiner or coroner.

SOURCES OF EXPERT INFORMATION

There are many sources of expert information available on the World Wide Web that present specific knowledge on individual agents of concern. Some of these are listed below:

1. The Journal of the American Medical Association has published a series of articles on individual agents. These are available online at http://jama.ama-assn.org
2. The CDC provides individual agent information at: http://www.bt.cdc.gov

3. The Department of Defense has a military textbook available online that discusses biological and chemical agents. It is available at: http://chemdef.apgea.army.mil/textbook/contents.asp
4. The Association for Professionals in Infection Control and Epidemiology has infection control guidelines available at: http://www.apic.org

Information is also available through telephone resources. An individual practitioner should start by contacting the local department of public health for quick information reference. Certain poison control centers are now updating their databases to include information on biological agent and patient management. The CDC also may be contacted directly as a backup resource for information (after first contacting local public health). The CDC's emergency response center telephone number is 1-770-488-7100.

REFERENCES

1. Torok T, Tauxe R, Wise R, et al: A large community outbreak of salmonellosis caused by intentional contamination of restaurant salad bars. *JAMA* 278:389, 1997.
2. Kolavic S, Kimura A, Simons S, et al: An outbreak of shigella dysenteriae type 2 among laboratory workers due to intentional food contamination. *JAMA* 278:396, 1997.
3. Inglesby T, O'Toole T, Henderson D, et al: Anthrax as a biological weapon, 2002 updated recommendations for management. *JAMA* 287:2236, 2002.
4. Update: Investigation of bioterrorism-related anthrax and adverse events from antimicrobial prophylaxis. *MMWR* 50:973, 2001.
5. Rotz L, Khan A, Lillibridge S, et al: Public health assessment of potential biological terrorism agents. *Emerg Infect Dis* 8:225, 2002. Available at: http://www.cdc.gov/ncidod/eid/vol8no2/01-0164.htm. Accessed August 1, 2002.
6. Fatal human plague—Arizona and Colorado, 1996. *MMWR* 46:617, 1997.
7. Jernigan J, Stephens D, Ashford D, et al: Bioterrorism-related inhalational anthrax: The first 10 cases reported in the United States. *Emerg Infect Dis* 7:993, 2001. Available at: http://www.cdc.gov/ncidod/eid/vol7no6/jernigan.htm. Accessed August 1, 2002.
8. Bush L, Abrams B, Beall A, et al: Index case of anthrax due to bioterrorism in the United States. *New Eng J Med* 345:1607, 2001.
9. Domestic Preparedness Program, Defense Against Weapons of Mass Destruction: *Technician-Hospital Provider Course Manual.* Aberdeen, MD, US Army SBCCOM, Domestic Preparedness Office, 1997.
10. Waeckerle J, Seamans S, Whiteside M, et al: Task Force of Health Care and Emergency Services Professionals on preparedness for nuclear, biological, and chemical incidents, executive summary: Developing objectives, content, and competencies for the training of emergency medical technicians, emergency physicians, and emergency nurses to care for casualties resulting from nuclear, biological, or chemical incidents. *Ann Emerg Med* 37:587, 2001.
11. *Clinical Clues to the Diagnosis of Cutaneous Anthrax. The Gorgas Course in Clinical Tropical Medicine.* Santiago, Universidad Peruana Cayetano Heredia. Available at: http://info.dom.uab.edu/gorgas/anthrax.html. Accessed August 20, 2002.
12. Notice to readers: Use of onsite technologies for rapidly assessing environmental *Bacillus anthracis* contamination on surfaces of buildings. *MMWR* 50:1087, 2001.
13. Hauer J: *Handheld Systems for Detection of Anthrax and Other Biologic Agents. Personal Communication from the Acting Assistant Secretary for Public Health and Emergency Preparedness to State and Local Health Officials.* Washington, DC, Department of Health and Human Services, July 26, 2002.
14. Pavlin J: Epidemiology of bioterrorism. *Emerg Infect Dis* 5:528, 2001. Available at: http://www.cdc.gov/ncidod/EID/vol5no4/pavlin.htm. Accessed August 1, 2002.
15. Connolly C: In New York, on alert for bioterrorism: City's tracking system is viewed as model. *Washington Post,* November 24, 2001, A1.
16. *Defense Advanced Research Projects Agency Epidemiology Software Used During Presidential Inauguration* [press release]. March 9, 2001. Available at: http://www.darpa.mil/dso/success/encompass.html. Accessed October 17, 2002.

17. Joint Commission on Accreditation of Healthcare Organizations: Using JCAHO standards as a starting point to prepare for an emergency. *Perspectives* 21:4, 2001.

18. Association for Professionals in Infection Control and Epidemiology Bioterrorism Task Force and Centers for Disease Control and Prevention Bioterrorism Working Group: *Bioterrorism Readiness Plan: A Template for Healthcare Facilities.* April 13, 1999. Available at: http://www.apic.org/educ/readinow.cfm. Accessed October 17, 2002.

19. Keim M, Kaufmann A: Principles for emergency response to bioterrorism. *Ann Emerg Med* 34:177, 1999.

DISASTER MANAGEMENT FOR CHEMICAL AGENTS OF MASS DESTRUCTION

Suzanne R. White

Kelly R. Klein

Col. Edward M. Eitzen, Jr.

". . . [T]he effect of chemical and biological weapons is so deadly to the unprepared that we can never afford to neglect the question."

General Pershing

INTRODUCTION

Chemical warfare is the intentional use of weapons (agents) designed to kill, injure, or incapacitate on the basis of toxic or noxious chemical properties. The battlefield use of chemical agents was first documented in 1000 B.C. in the form of Chinese arsenical smokes. Other notable military deployments included picric acid use during the 1899 Boer War, and the large-scale use of multiple agents such as chlorine, phosgene, cyanogen chloride, hydrogen cyanide, and, most significantly, the sulfur mustards during WWI. While both the U.S. and Germany had stockpiled nerve agents during World War II, the only chemical incident documented was the nautical release of mustard from an allied ship bombed in Bari, Italy. In the 1980s, Iraq allegedly used multiple agents against the Kurdish nationals and Iranians, resulting in thousands of fatalities. Following Desert Storm in the early 1990s, defectors ultimately disclosed the extent of the Iraqi arsenal and thousands of tons of chemical agents loaded into bombs were then located and destroyed. Current intelligence suggests that despite chemical weapons treaties, offensive programs are proliferating in at least 17 countries hostile to the U.S., many of whom are signatories to these agreements.

Recent terrorist events highlight the potential for chemical agent use extending beyond the war theatre. Specifically, chemical releases could be sponsored by parastate, paramilitary, militia, or extremist groups or by deranged individuals, for the furtherance of political or social objectives. For example, Aum Shinrikyo, a cult of educated, wealthy multinationals twice carried out the release of the nerve agent sarin. The first attack occurred in Matsumoto, Japan, in 1994, killing 7 and injuring more than 600 people. A larger scale release into the Tokyo subway system 1 year later caused 5510 people to seek medical attention. During this incident, 640 chemically contaminated patients arrived by private conveyance within the first few hours to a single health care facility. Twenty-three percent of the ED staff at that hospital became secondarily poisoned as the nerve agent was essentially transported via contaminated victims from the scene to the hospital.[1,2] Other chemical events around the same period included the aversion of a large-scale plot to release chlorine gas at Disneyland and the discovery that cyanide had been involved in the 1993 World Trade Center bombing in New York. As a recent example of nonbattlefield use,

the Russian military ended a hostage crisis in Moscow, in 2002, by deploying a potent "gas." More than 100 fatalities and more than 400 hospitalizations resulted. Definitive identification of the chemical is pending at this time, but based on clinical features that included a response to naloxone, an opioid derivative is suspected.

Chemical weapon disasters from terrorism are low-probability, high-impact events. Casualties are not only poisoned but may be contaminated. They may also have serious concomitant injuries, such as trauma, burns, or smoke inhalation. Those victims able to flee the scene are likely to seek their own transportation to the hospital, which then potentially becomes a crime scene and a secondary "hot zone." Other problems include communication breakdown and chaos among medical personnel who may be unfamiliar with the agents involved, unaware of available resources, or themselves secondarily contaminated. In addition, widespread or prolonged psychological impact may occur. As seen both in drill and in real-life scenarios, chemical disasters quickly overwhelm prehospital and hospital medical resources. The need for emergency medical planning and preparedness to mitigate the consequences of such events has become a priority for emergency physicians.

PLANNING AND PREPAREDNESS

Every hospital emergency department should be prepared to receive and treat contaminated victims who arrive unannounced. Survival of victims will largely be determined by awareness training and preeducation of emergency staff, the practice of contingency plans, and effective communication at the time of the incident. The following are planning priorities:

Recognition that chemical terrorism has occurred;

Rapid identification of the agent(s) involved;

Information retrieval on the toxicity and secondary contamination potential of the agent;

Proper protection of self, hospital personnel, already-hospitalized patients and the facility itself from secondary contamination or loss of serviceability to other patients;

Decontamination and triage of victims;

Stabilization and medical treatment of victims; and

Protection of the community-at-large from secondary contamination.

A critical step in planning is the identification of those chemical agents that pose the greatest threat. Along these lines, the Centers for Disease Control (CDC) has established a list of agents of most concern for chemical terrorism (Table 8-1).[3] The inclusive nature of this list illustrates the difficulty in performing a chemical-threat assessment. In reality, the specific agent used is limited only by the determination and creativity of the terrorist, with common industrial chemicals potentially representing a greater hazard than military agents. To this end, close integration of hospital planning committees with public agencies is essential. In the wake of the largest chemical disaster ever, in which 2500 fatalities resulted from the release of methylisocyanate in Bhopal, India, the Emergency Planning and Community Right-to-Know Act of 1986, also known as the Superfund Amendments and Reauthorization Act (SARA Title III) emerged. This law requires the establishment of State Emergency Response Commissions to oversee the activities of local emergency planning committees (LEPCs). LEPCs, in turn, are responsible for the development of comprehensive emergency response plans for community hazardous materials incidents. Active emergency physician participation in LEPC activities promotes medical community awareness of the major chemical hazards that exist at industrial and worksites nearby. Once community response plans are established, drills concentrating on the types of hazards likely to be encountered locally should be practiced annually. Finally, a formal critique of each drill, as well as each "live" incident, should be carried out with the involved medical personnel to allow for plan revision. Refer to Chap. 185 for a toxicologic review of important chemical agents.

TABLE 8-1 Chemical Agents

Chemical agents that might be used by terrorists range from warfare agents to toxic chemicals commonly used in industry. Criteria for determining priority chemical agents include:

Chemical agents already known to be used as weaponry;
Availability of chemical agents to potential terrorists;
Chemical agents likely to cause major morbidity or mortality;
Potential of agents for causing public panic and social disruption; and
Agents that require special action for public health preparedness (Box 4).

Categories of chemical agents include:

Nerve agents
tabun (ethyl N,N-dimethylphosphoramidocyanidate)
sarin (isopropyl methylphosphanofluoridate)
soman (pinacolyl methyl phosphonofluoridate)
GF (cyclohexylmethylphosphonofluoridate)
VX (o-ethyl-[S]-[2-diisopropylaminoethyl]-methylphosphonothioate)

Blood agents
hydrogen cyanide
cyanogen chloride

Blister agents
lewisite (an aliphatic arsenic compound, 2-chlorovinyldichloroarsine)
nitrogen and sulfur mustards
phosgene oxime

Heavy metals
arsenic
lead
mercury

Volatile toxins
benzene
chloroform
trihalomethanes

Pulmonary agents
phosgene
chlorine
vinyl chloride

Incapacitating agents
BZ (3-quinuclidinyl benzilate)

Pesticides, persistent and nonpersistent

Dioxins, furans, and polychlorinated biphenyls (PCBs)

Explosive nitro compounds and oxidizers
ammonium nitrate combined with fuel oil

Flammable industrial gases and liquids
gasoline
propane

Poison industrial gases, liquids, and solids
cyanides
nitriles
and

Corrosive industrial acids and bases
nitric acid
sulfuric acid

*www.cdc.gov/mmwr/preview/mmwrhtml/rr4904@1.htm.

A standard operating procedure for mass casualty decontamination should be developed as part of the hospital disaster plan. It should include a plan for outdoor hospital decontamination of patients, types and location of protective and decontamination equipment, designation of personnel responsibilities, medical treatment guidelines for expected toxic agents, and reference lists of information resources (Table 8-2). One excellent resource for designing such procedures is the Agency for Toxic Substances and Disease Registry's *ATSDR Medical Management Guidelines for Acute Chemical Exposures.*[4] At the time of this writing, most hospitals in the United States are not adequately prepared to treat contaminated patients, many assuming that other local facilities or agencies will handle such events or that patients will undergo prehospital decontamination. It is true that Hazardous Materials Response (HAZMAT) Teams and some fire departments are trained and equipped to provide on-scene chemical decontamination; however, response times and availability of such resources vary widely. In reality, typically less than 20 percent of contaminated victims receive decontamination and treatment at the scene. Furthermore, most victims of a chemical disaster, especially the "walking wounded," will flee the scene and seek out the closest hospital for their medical care regardless of that institution's capabilities.

In a chemical disaster situation, it is possible that first responders will not initially recognize a hazardous material situation and will transport contaminated victims to the ED, potentially contaminating the ED as well as themselves. Accidents occurring at industrial sites, on farms, or on freeways or railways are always suspect for a chemical involvement. Other clues are the presence of multiple victims, vapor clouds, fires or explosions, or patients with burns, unusual odors, colors, or patterns of skin irritation.[5] The emergency physician's interface with a large cross-section of the community confers unique perspective and opportunity toward the early detection of illness from chemical hazards.

ACTIVATION OF THE RESPONSE PLAN

If prenotification allows, several steps should be taken to prepare for patient arrival. Communication with prehospital providers is desirable to ascertain the type of the incident, number of victims, signs and symptoms exhibited, nature of injuries, identification of chemical(s), presence of radioactive materials, prior decontamination, and estimated time of arrival. At this point, consideration should be given to the potential for a specific method of decontamination. Is there an antidote or distinct method of treatment for this exposure, and if so, what is its availability at the receiving and or surrounding institution(s)? Do hospital entrances need to be secured? A determination should be made as to whether the hospital's disaster plan should be activated and which community facilities in the area are prepared to assist with overflow of large numbers of victims. Examples of individuals to be prenotified include the medical toxicologist, poison control center, industrial hygienist or occupational physician, safety officer, radiation safety officer, security, hospital administrator, and media relations representative.

ADVANCE INFORMATION RETRIEVAL

Detailed information about the chemical(s) involved is most helpful if received prior to patient arrival. Regional poison control centers (PCCs) are often already integrated into the emergency medical, hazardous materials, and Metropolitan Medical Response Systems (MMRS) and provide 24-h availability.[6] Another information resource is the Material Safety Data Sheet (MSDS), a document that identifies health and safety information for any product containing hazardous chemicals.[7] MSDSs may be obtained by facsimile from the work-site employer or safety officer, regional PCCs, Chemtrec, NRC, the Internet, and computer databases such as Dolphin. Included are chemical and physical hazard data as well as information regarding safe use, handling, and storage. Basic first aid procedures are outlined, but advanced medical information usually is not included. While the merit of MSDSs has been questioned,[8] at the least they will assist with correct identification and spelling of the chemical agent(s) involved. Limitations of MSDS use are that they may not exist for all toxic substances, they are not always comprehensive with regard to ingredients listing or toxicity data, they may not be up to date, ingredients listed as inert may be toxic, and "trade secret" ingredients may be deleted (although trade secret toxicity data must be listed, and the treating physician is entitled to immediate identity on request). Other resources that may assist with hazard identification and determination of toxicity are listed in Table 8-2.

Ascertain the reason for the incident (explosion, spill, act of terrorism), the presence and status of other victims, the route of exposure, whether exposure was within a confined space, and the duration of exposure.

DECONTAMINATION ZONES

Patient decontamination ideally should occur outside the hospital. Hot, warm, and cold zones should be established and cordoned off with brightly colored tape. The *hot zone* is the area of the spill or chemical release (at the scene) or the hospital area where arriving patients with no prior decontamination are held. Therefore, only people who are trained and properly attired may enter. Only the most immediate life threats are addressed in the hot zone (opening of the airway, cervical spine immobilization, brushing off of gross contaminants, and application of pressure to stop arterial bleeding). The *warm zone* is an area where thorough decontamination and further medical stabilization occur. Theoretically, this area poses no risk of primary contamination (direct exposure to the toxin), but secondary contamination (transfer of the toxic material from the victim to personnel or equipment) may still occur. Access, therefore, is also restricted, and the use of protective clothing is required. The *cold zone* is the area to which fully decontaminated patients are transferred. There is no personnel flow between hot/warm or warm/cold areas.

PERSONAL PROTECTION

The various levels of personal protection are levels A through D. *Level A* attire [fully encapsulating chemical-resistant suit and self-contained breathing apparatus (SCBA)] is recommended when the highest level of eye, mucous membrane, skin, and respiratory protection is needed. Lower levels of protection include level B (splash protection with chemical-resistant clothing and an SCBA) and level C (splash protection with chemical-resistant clothing and a full-faced, air-purifying canister-equipped respirator). Level D protection is a standard work uniform and includes firefighter bunker gear. Military mission-oriented protective posture (MOPP) level IV gear, comprised of an air-purifying respirator, protective mask, hood, charcoal-impregnated suit, and butyl rubber gloves and boots, affords effective protection against the biochemical weapons of mass destruction.

While level A protection is recommended by the National Institute of Occupational Safety and Health (NIOSH) and the Environmental Protection Agency (EPA) in situations where the concentration or identity of toxins involved is unknown (i.e., most hazardous materials incidents), there is no consensus regarding the level of protection needed for health care workers decontaminating patients at the hospital.[8] Only limited patient care can be rendered while wearing level A or level B gear, and air availability restricts its use to only short periods of time. Furthermore, specialized protective gear is only recommended for those with prior training and fitting, given the added level of physical and heat stress and false sense of security that its use may render. Despite these limitations, if level A or B protection is to be used by the emergency staff, it is recommended that the hospital coordinate equipment acquisition with the local fire departments or hazardous materials teams so that regulator fittings (replacement air bottles) are interchangeable. Practically speaking, most hospitals have only level C protection available to employees. Powered air-purifying respirators (PAPRs) allow for increased mobility and may be used for longer periods of time in oxygen-sufficient environments, such as most emergency departments. Ideally, persons responsible for selecting the personal protective equipment and decontamination process should be trained to the first-responder operations level under the Occupational Safety and Health Act (OSHA 29 CFR 1910.120).

TRIAGE

The first wave of minimally exposed victims arrives within 30 min of the incident and has the potential to overwhelm the emergency department and impede the care of sicker patients who arrive later.[9] Emergency department triage must be efficient and should occur outdoors. **First and foremost, the contaminated patient should not be allowed to enter the ED.** Second, personnel who are not in an appro-

priate level of protective gear must not be allowed in the triage/decontamination area. The incoming ambulance or ambulatory patients should be met by a triage officer, an individual in appropriate level of personal protective gear, to determine whether decontamination has been performed and, if so, its adequacy. The most difficult situations involve victims who are seriously injured and who have bypassed the field decontamination procedure. A management dilemma is created between immediate medical treatment and decontamination. While the appropriate response varies depending on the chemical(s) involved, many situations involve unknown chemicals and therefore unknown risk to personnel. **It is always prudent to err on the side of decontamination before treatment in unknown situations.** Examples of substances with little or no risk of secondary contamination include gases, vapors, and substances with no serious toxicity or skin absorption. Patients exposed to gases or vapors only, with no symptoms other than respiratory irritation and no signs of condensation of vapor on the clothing, do not require decontamination beyond clothing removal. This may not hold true, however, for large numbers of victims exposed to nerve agent vapor or for those exposed in confined spaces. Substances with high risk of secondary contamination include highly toxic substances that are readily absorbed dermally, radioactive agents, and certain biologic agents. Patient triage is covered in more detail in Chap. 6. Table 8-2 lists aids in chemical identification and hazard determination.

TABLE 8-2   Aids in Chemical Identification and Hazard Determination

Department of Transportation (DOT) placards (used with DOT ERG*)
   Diamond-shaped placards on tank truck or rail cars
United Nations Classification numbering system on vehicles:
   At bottoms of placards or on shipping papers, defines hazard
Bill of lading (cargo manifest in cab of truck)
Waybill (with train conductor)
Shipping papers
National Fire Protection Association (NFPA) 704 marking system labels on containers (at fixed facilities)
Material safety data sheet (MSDS)
Company records or company safety officer
CAS number: unique number assigned to specific chemical or mixture (http://chemfinder.cambridgesoft.com/)
On-scene chemical analysis (by fire department or HazMat Team)
Regional poison control center: 1-800-222-1222
Chemtrec: 24-h assistance to emergency responders regarding chemicals spills: 1-800-424-9300 or www.chemtrec.org/Chemtrec/chemtrec.nsf/NavERFS
REAC/TS: 24-h emergency consultative assistance for radiation accidents: 423-576-3131; after business hours: 423-481-1000
Motherisk program: teratology information service: 416-813-6780; after business hours: 416-813-5900
ATSDR Emergency Response 24-h Hotline: 404-639-0615
EPA Environmental Response Hotline: 201-321-6660
National Response Center: 800-424-8802
Local emergency planning committee (LEPC): _____
Local FBI representative (suspected terrorist incident): _____
Local health department (suspected terrorist incident): _____
Other local government agencies
U.S. Army Medical Research Institute of Infectious Diseases (USAMRIID), Fort Detrick, Maryland: 888-872-7443
Centers for Disease Control and Prevention (CDC): 404-639-3311
National Pesticide Telecommunication Network: 800-858-7378
Computer databases: Poisindex, Dolphin, Tomes Plus, ToxNet, others
Other references:
   ATSDR Managing Hazardous Materials Incidents: Obtain by calling 404-639-6360 or online at www.atsdr.cdc.gov/mhmi.html

*DOT *Emergency Response Guidebook 2000* (obtain by calling 1-800-327-6868 or online at www.tc.gc.ca/canutec/erg_gmu/erg2000_menu.htm).
Source: Reproduced from Sullivan JB, Krieger GR (eds): *Hazardous Materials Toxicology: Clinical Principles of Environmental Health.* Baltimore, Lippincott, Williams & Wilkins, 2001.

PATIENT DECONTAMINATION

Outside portable decontamination systems include portable showers, large inflatable heated tents, or a series of kiddy pools with privacy screens. Attempts to contain effluent should not delay patient decontamination. Disposable equipment should be used wherever feasible. Suggested equipment for outdoor hospital decontamination is listed in Table 8-3. Decontamination inside the hospital should only be done in a designated room with a separate entrance, separate ventilation, and ideally, a separate water drainage system.

The goal of decontamination is to decrease the absorbed dose for the victim and prevent secondary contamination of health care providers. Clothing should be removed quickly because this is thought to accomplish 80 percent of the decontamination. Particulate or radioactive matter should removed by careful roll-down of clothing. Further particulate matter should be brushed away prior to showering because interaction of some dry chemicals with water may produce heat. All clothing should be double bagged and treated as toxic waste. All patient belongings and waste must be accounted for by a tracking log. Jewelry and valuables should be bagged separately from clothing, which may require disposal.

The critically ill, nonambulatory contaminated patient should have a patent airway ensured, the cervical spine immobilized, oxygen administered, ventilation assisted, and pressure maintained on arterial bleeding. Further medical care, such as intubation or intravenous line insertion, is delayed until gross decontamination has been completed and the patient has been transferred to the cold zone. Ocular exposures take precedence and should be treated first with immediate eye irrigation. Ideally, this should have begun in the prehospital phase. Wounds are the next decontamination priority and should be irrigated, debrided of gross contaminants, and then covered with a water-occlusive dressing to prevent recontamination during subsequent showering. Whole-body decontamination should begin with the head and proceed downward. Along with the hands, the face and head generally are the most heavily contaminated areas and should be washed or shampooed in the head-back position to avoid runoff onto other body parts and incorporation of toxic material. This may be best accomplished initially in the sitting position, prior to showering. Most agents are readily removed with copious amounts of water. A mild soap, shampoo, or detergent may be necessary for nonpolar, water-insoluble substances. Tincture of green soap has been recommended by some based on its small concentration of ethanol that enhances dissolution of certain agents such as hydrocarbons. Typically, 3 to 5 min of showering is recommended, although 15 min may be required for concentrated, strongly alkaline

materials or oily, adherent substances. The use of abrasives, such as corn meal or scrub brushes, generally is not advised because abrading the skin may increase toxin absorption. New amphoteric decontamination solutions, such as Diphoterine or Hexafluorine, for specific acid, base, solvent, oxidizer, and reducing-agent exposures are under investigation. Water temperature should be tepid because heat potentially will increase dermal absorption of some toxins.

Certain agents may be removed more effectively with the use of specific decontamination solutions. Dilute household bleach solutions (9 parts water to 1 part bleach) will inactivate nerve agents and most biologic agents, but its use on patients is controversial. The use of neutralizing solutions for acid or alkaline exposures generally is not recommended. Other agents requiring targeted decontamination solutions include phenol and hydrofluoric acid and are discussed below. One should not delay decontamination if such solutions are not readily available but rather begin washing with deluge volumes of water in an attempt to prevent toxin absorption through massive dilution.

Certain metals such as sodium, lithium, and potassium react violently with water, releasing heat, hydroxide ion, and hydrogen gas and potentially causing thermal burns. Proper treatment of alkali metal burns involves clothing removal, covering the affected area with mineral or cooking oil, followed by removal of any remaining metal with dry forceps. Only then can wounds be copiously irrigated with water. Burning fragments should be extinguished by smothering or with a class D fire extinguisher. Again, in the absence of proper solutions, decontamination with deluge volumes of water may be considered. Other water-reactive chemicals are listed in Table 8-4. In contrast to water-reactive chemicals, white phosphorus ignites spontaneously on exposure to air. Burns from this agent must be kept continuously moist with water or saline dressings until adequate debridement is accomplished. Each phosphorus particle must be removed. The application of copper sulfate solution blackens the phosphorus to aid in visualization and provides neutralization. Alternatively, a Wood's lamp may be used. Some adherent toxins are extremely difficult to remove from the skin. Epoxy resins and cyanoacrylates (glues) may be removed by swabbing with acetone. Use of vegetable or mineral oil or saline-soaked gauze pads for the eyes and mucous membranes is safe. Hot tar, typically inflicting burns to the face and upper extremities, should be allowed to cool prior to removal. Effective tar removal has then been reported using Neosporin cream, Tween 80, plain Vaseline, Shur Clens, Desolv-It, or mayonnaise. No attempt should be made to remove tar by mechanical means because this may increase tissue destruction and result in hair follicle loss.

Nausea and vomiting are common following chemical exposures. These symptoms may indicate toxin ingestion with gastrointestinal irritation or, more commonly, systemic toxin effect or hysteria. Regardless of the cause, secondary contamination by toxic vomitus may occur, and the need for its containment should be anticipated. Furthermore, some materials may react with stomach acid to produce toxic gas (sodium azide → hydrazoic acid, cyanide salts → hydrogen cyanide gas). Suction with outdoor venting should be available to prevent secondary poisoning of personnel. If spontaneous emesis has not occurred already, gastric emptying or the administration of charcoal may be considered for certain large chemical ingestions. Induction of vomiting is not recommended. If an alkaline corrosive material is

TABLE 8-3 Suggested Equipment for Outdoor Hospital Decontamination

Biohazard/radiation hazard tape
Decontamination stretcher (alternative fiberglass backboard with sawhorses)
Hose with warm water and soft-stream shower head
Disposable butyl rubber, nitrile rubber, and neoprene rubber gloves in various sizes
Disposable chemical-resistant jump suits (Tyvek or Saranex) with hoods and boots
Rubber aprons
Mild soap/shampoo
Splash protective goggles
Plastic bags for clothing and waste container liners
Multiple wading pools for ambulatory patients (to contain runoff)
Adsorbent materials (for diking of waste water)
Oxygen tanks with delivery supplies
Disposable towels and gauze
Blankets and sheets for patient privacy
Portable privacy barriers

Source: Modified from ATSDR: *Managing Hazardous Materials Incidents: Medical Guidelines for Acute Chemical Exposures.* Washington, US Department of Health and Human Services, Agency for Toxic Substances and Disease Registry, 2001.

TABLE 8-4 Water-Reactive Substances

Acetic anhydride, acetyl chloride
Alkali metals: lithium, sodium, potassium (also form caustic sodium and potassium hydroxides) calcium
Chlorosulfonic acid
Concentrated sulfuric acid (oleum), concentrated muriatic acid
Dry lime (calcium oxide), calcium carbide
Hydrides: boranes, silanes
Inorganic chlorides (some): titanium tetrachloride peroxides
Organometallics: alkylaluminums, zinc phosphide

ingested, 4 to 8 oz of water may be administered if the patient is conscious. Other decisions regarding gastrointestinal tract decontamination may be guided by the regional PCC.

Following decontamination, zipping patients into body bags or placing them into hooded Tyvek suits prior to transport to the support zone is no longer recommended. This technique is not effective in minimizing the transfer of toxin to hospital staff and poses the risk of increased toxin absorption by the patient. The patient simply should be wrapped in clean blankets or sheets prior to transfer to the cold zone.

Complete medical assessment and specific medical treatment can be carried out in the support zone (cold zone). **Emergency department personnel in this area should maintain protective gear (chemical-resistant gowns, latex gloves, eye protection) until the chemical has been definitively identified and the risk of secondary contamination is known.**

REFERENCES

1. Okumura T, Takasu N, Ishimatsu S: Report on 640 victims of the Tokyo subway sarin attack. *Ann Emerg Med* 28:129, 1996.
2. Okumura T, Suzuki K, Fukada A, et al: The Tokyo subway sarin attack: Disaster management, part 2: Hospital response. *Acad Emerg Med* 5:618, 1998.
3. Kahn AS, Age MJ: Biological and chemical terrorism: Strategic plan for preparedness and response. *MMWR* 49(RR04): 1, 2000.
4. *ATSDR Managing Hazardous Materials Incidents, Medical Guidelines for Acute Chemical Exposures.* Washington, DC, US Department of Health and Human Services. Agency for Toxic Substances and Disease Registry, 2001. www.atsdr.cdc.gov/mhmi.html.
5. Sidell FR, Urbanetti JS, Smith WJ et al, in Sidell FR, Takafuji ET, Franz DR (eds): *Medical Aspects of Chemical and Biological Warfare.* Washington, DC, Office of the Surgeon General, TMM Publications, 1997, p. 179.
6. Burgess JL, Keifer MC, Barnhart S, et al: Hazardous materials exposure information service: Development, analysis, and medical implications. *Ann Emerg Med* 29:248, 1997.
7. Greenberg MI, Cone DC, Roberts JR: Material Safety Data Sheet: A useful resource for the emergency physician. *Ann Emerg Med* 27:347, 1996.
8. Burgess JL, Kirk M, Borron SW et al: Emergency Department Hazardous Materials Protocol for Contaminated Patients. *Ann Emerg Med* 34:205, 1999.
9. Waeckerle JF: Disaster planning and response. *New Engl J Med* 324:815, 1991.

BLAST AND CRUSH INJURIES
John M. Wightman
Barry A. Wayne

Sudden force and rapid acceleration of body surfaces to high peak velocities, but relatively small amounts of actual displacement, characterize the interaction of blast waves with victims caught near explosions. Slower application of force, weaker acceleration, and lower peak velocity, but relatively greater surface displacement, are typical of crushing injuries.[1] Both can create internal tissue damage and pathophysiologic derangement, which may be clinically occult to providers managing patients soon after the time of injury. Stress waves are created by the brief acceleration of a surface, and are transmitted deep into the body through the fluid of the tissues akin to the sonic pressure wave produced by a high-velocity bullet. Damage occurs when the stress wave encounters tissues of different densities, thus creating differential pressure forces, motion, stretching, and eventual tearing. Shear waves are created by body deformation, which stretches tissues tangentially to the displaced surface. Primary blast injury (PBI) of the ears, lungs, and bowel are mostly caused by stress waves. Damage from blunt trauma and crushing injuries is mostly due to shear waves.

BLAST INJURIES

Intentional detonation of high explosives or accidental ignition of many explosive substances lead to virtually instantaneous release of large amounts of energy in the form of expanding gasses.[2] These gases compress and superheat the surrounding air or water so rapidly that a shock wave is created. This wave (also called a blast wave) delivers high overpressures to surfaces it contacts. Solid surfaces such as concrete and glass are poorly compliant and tend to shatter. Body surfaces, accelerated through the force created by differentials in air or water pressure between the blast wave, ambient medium, and body surface, "spring back" to their original shape because they are more compliant. Unlike other internal organs, bone tends to shatter like other solids. Although applied for only milliseconds due to the supersonic speed of the shock wave passing a human body, extreme accelerations on the order of hundreds of km/s^2 can induce stress and shear waves, which can tear tissues by exceeding their tensile strengths.[3]

Pathophysiology

Stress waves propagated through solid organs of relatively homogenous liquid densities generally do not cause significant effects until overpressures are high enough to cause multiple obvious external injuries. However, stress waves in hollow organs constantly encounter different densities at air-tissue interfaces, which result in macroscopic and microscopic distortions leading to tissue tearing. Bleeding and air escape are the two principal manifestations of PBI (i.e., damage caused by the blast wave itself).

EAR   Bleeding of the tympanic membrane (TM) can be seen as petechiae or hemotympanum. More likely, however, the TM will rupture from even relatively low pressure differentials between the external canal and middle ear. Occasionally, the ossicles may be fractured or dislocated. Forces transmitted to the inner ear may cause temporary or permanent hearing loss.

SINUSES   Sinus bleeding has been described, but unless their bony supports yield to the pressure differentials, there will not be significant injury at these air-tissue interfaces.

LUNGS   Tearing of pulmonary tissue can result in blood or air escaping their normal confines into the parenchyma or pleural cavity or being exchanged between the respiratory tree and the pulmonary vascular circuit. A pulmonary laceration can cause hemo- or pneumothorax. Large tears of the bronchi or lungs may create bronchopleural fistulae with unilateral or bilateral tension pneumothoraces.[4] Extreme tension pneumothorax can lead to tension pneumoperitoneum.[5] Parenchymal hemorrhage results in pulmonary contusion, which may be localized, patchy, or diffuse. Blood in tissues and small airways impairs gas exchange between alveoli and pulmonary capillaries. Air escape into pulmonary tissues will result in pseudocyst formation called a pneumatocele. Blood entry into the larger bronchi may compromise airway patency and prevent oxygen from reaching many alveoli. Air entry into the pulmonary venous circuit can lead to systemic arterial air embolism (AAE) with impaction in any organ and subsequent distal ischemia.[6] Two conditions that, alone or in combination, make AAE more likely are high airway pressures and low venous pressures.[2]

BOWEL   Bleeding from the walls of the gastrointestinal tract can leak into the lumen, the bowel wall, the intraperitoneal cavity, or other extraperitoneal space. In addition to blood loss, transmural tears of the stomach, small bowel, or colon can result in peritonitis following spillage of intraluminal contents. Stretching of the bowel wall or intraparenchymal hemorrhage can result in ischemia with delayed perforation.[7]

OTHER   Most of the injuries seen in survivors of explosions are from missiles, generally causing penetrating trauma to exposed body regions, particularly the eyes. Blunt trauma can also result from flying objects. The blast wind created by differentials in pressure between the shock wave and ambient air can be hundreds of mph, which is sufficient to throw or tumble people along the ground or into objects, also creating blunt and penetrating trauma. Miscellaneous injuries include burns, toxic inhalations, and traumatic amputations, as well as crushing injuries if victims are caught within a structural collapse.

Detection and Intervention

With the exception of ruptured TMs, the management of various PBIs may not be well known because they are not commonly encountered. Additionally, standard emergency interventions, useful for most trauma victims, may have to be altered in the presence of pulmonary PBI in order not to cause iatrogenic harm as discussed below.

AIRWAY COMPROMISE   Selective bronchial intubation may be used for massive hemoptysis when there is more blood coming from one side than the other.[2,8] Otherwise, airway patency is at risk from all of the usual mechanisms such as depressed level of consciousness, facial or neck trauma, and inhalational injury.

VENTILATORY INSUFFICIENCY   High-flow oxygen should be administered to all victims with any period of dyspnea, evidence of hemorrhage, or obviously serious injuries. Continuous positive airway pressure (CPAP) has been used successfully. Positive-pressure ventilation (PPV) may be required for persistent hypoxemia or inability to exchange gasses. **However, PPV can increase the risk of AAE, so spontaneous (negative-pressure) respirations in victims with blast injuries are desirable whenever adequate.** In severe cases with marked lung stiffness, permissive hypercapnia[9] or other ventilation strategies used for the acute respiratory distress syndrome (ARDS)[2] may be necessary.

EXTERNAL HEMORRHAGE   Bleeding from external wounds is likely to be the most commonly encountered life-threatening finding based on military experience. Whether venous or arterial, blood loss from multiple wounds may have a cumulative effect (or be combined with internal hemorrhage) sufficient to cause hypovolemic shock. All external bleeding must be quickly controlled with direct pressure. Tourniquets should be considered for extremity hemorrhage whenever blood loss cannot be controlled with direct pressure or the resources required to maintain direct pressure are insufficient during either treatment or transportation.

TENSION PNEUMOTHORAX   Asymmetrical breath sounds and any evidence of shock should mandate immediate performance of a needle thoracostomy on the side of decreased or absent breath sounds to relieve any potential tension pneumothorax. If there is no improvement in the patient's hemodynamic status, a tube thoracostomy should quickly follow. If a large-bore chest tube connected to an underwater seal and 20 cm H_2O of suction still does not evacuate sufficient air from the pleural space, the presence of a bronchopleural fistula should be assumed.[2] At this stage, either more chest tubes must be placed or air should be prevented from entering the affected lung by selectively intubating the opposite mainstem bronchus.[2,8]

SHOCK   Shock, which persists after external hemorrhage, tension pneumothorax, and hypoxia have been addressed, could be due to internal blood loss; traumatic deep venous thrombosis (DVT) with pulmonary embolism following blunt trauma; crush syndrome; sepsis, if rescue and care were delayed; or AAE, causing brainstem stroke, myo-

cardial infarction, or injury to the spinal cord. Plain chest and pelvis radiography and focused abdominal sonography for trauma (FAST) or diagnostic peritoneal tap and lavage (DPTL) are the most rapid studies used to exclude immediately life-threatening internal hemorrhage. There are no studies commonly available in the ED that are sufficiently sensitive to rule out the other possibilities rapidly, so clinical suspicion and judgment must be used to determine their likelihood and priority for additional diagnostic testing. Perfusion of vital organs should be restored with small, repeated boluses of crystalloid fluids or blood products to avoid secondary injury of contused lungs or edematous brain.

ARTERIAL AIR EMBOLISM   Although blunt trauma can cause many of the same manifestations, **AAE should be considered for any evidence of localized ischemia of the skin or mucous membranes, or such findings as altered mental status, seizures, focal neurologic deficits, chest pain, dysrhythmia, pulmonary edema, abdominal pain, or hematuria.**[2] AAE should also be considered when there is a sudden deterioration after an intervention such as intubation or change in altitude. Other clues may be an acute myocardial infarction in a young victim without evident chest trauma, paraplegia in absence of spinal cord injury, or focal neurologic deficits without head trauma. Pulmonary venous pressure must be maintained by correcting hypovolemia and PPV should be avoided whenever possible.[6] Specific treatment involves hyperbaric oxygen (HBO) therapy. Since most centers do not have a hyperbaric chamber, risks related to transportation to the nearest accepting center would have to be considered.

Additional Evaluation

Classic descriptions of blast injuries are divided into primary, secondary, tertiary, and miscellanous.[2] Secondary blast injuries are caused by flying objects, whereas tertiary blast injuries result from the victim's body being placed in motion by the blast wind associated with the high pressures of the blast wave. These clinical entities do not differ in their clinical presentation from those caused by different mechanisms, and most of these are obvious or easily detected during the normal evaluation of trauma victims. However, manifestations of pulmonary and gastrointestinal PBI are commonly occult.

PULMONARY PBI   Symptoms of pulmonary PBI include dyspnea and chest pain. Pharyngeal petechiae or hemoptysis may be clinical predictors of possible pulmonary PBI,[2] but TM rupture probably is not.[10] Plain chest radiography is the mainstay of the ED diagnosis of pulmonary injury. Hemo- and pneumothoraces, interstitial infiltrates representing pulmonary contusion, pneumatoceles, and manifestations of blunt and penetrating trauma can all be identified. Additionally, arterial blood gas analysis may be helpful as a predictor of which patients may require ventilatory assistance using the Pao_2/Fio_2 ratio (PFR).[4] Table 9-1 shows how this ratio correlates with early requirements for standard and nonstandard PPV.[2] Computed tomography (CT) of the chest can identify smaller degrees of pneumothorax and pulmonary contusion, but is unlikely to be as helpful early in the course of ED care.

GASTROINTESTINAL PBI   Symptoms of abdominal injury include abdominal or testicular pain, nausea or vomiting, and an urge to defecate. Hemtochezia is a clinical sign predictive of gastrointestinal PBI. The evaluation for intra- and extraperitoneal injury should proceed as for blunt abdominopelvic trauma. However, each ED will have to assess how to best employ individual or combined tests such as physical examination, FAST, DPTL, and CT, given that the likelihood of injury to hollow organs is increased.[2]

Management Caveats

Although the approach to patients with blast injuries is the same as for other victims of trauma, there are specific issues that require awareness: (1) External hemorrhage is much more likely than airway compromise,

TABLE 9-1 Severity Categories for Primary Blast Injury of the Lung

	Mild	Moderate	Severe
Radiographic infiltrates	Unilateral	Asymmetrical	Diffuse
PFR (mm Hg)	>200	60–200	<60
Bronchopleural fistula	No		Yes
PPV requirement	Unlikely for respiratory problem	Highly likely but conventional methods usually	Universal and unconventional methods common
PEEP requirement (cm H_2O)	<5 if PPV needed	5–10 usually needed	>10 commonly needed

Abbreviation: PFR = Pao_2/Fio_2.
Source: From Wightman.[2]

and thus requires primary attention. (2) Trauma victims usually receive vigorous ventilatory assistance as per standard practice. However, risk of pneumothorax and air embolism is very high, and needs to be considered. In fact, air embolism from positive-pressure ventilation is the most common cause of early death among immediate survivors. (3) Ideal positioning of the patient may not be supine. The risk of AAE may be lower with the patient placed on the left side slightly forward prone. (4) Rapid infusion of crystalloid fluids as may occur in typical trauma patients may be harmful due to the high risk of pulmonary contusion. Small boluses with frequent assessment would be a better approach. (5) Casualties may attempt to assist rescue efforts in the field, but this should be prevented if possible. Exertion may worsen clinically occult blast lung injury.

Disposition

Patients with no chest or abdominal complaints, normal plain chest radiography, normal arterial blood gases, and no other indications for admission 4 h after injury may be candidates for discharge. Detailed instructions should be provided for follow-up care, as delayed manifestations of pulmonary contusion or bowel perforation would be the most likely late PBI complications in those discharged. All other victims should be admitted for management or observation in a facility with capabilities for surgery, pulmonology, and critical care.

CRUSH INJURIES

Blunt or compressive trauma may result from a great variety of mechanisms: industrial machinery accidents, building collapse following explosion or earthquake, combat injuries, drug overdose, mining accidents, torture,[11] and transportation and construction accidents. Apart from isolated limb entrapment, these mechanisms frequently result in multiple trauma and/or multiple victims. The term "crush injury" is imprecisely used in the literature, at times referring to the mechanism, and at others referring to the sequelae, such as "crush syndrome" or "compartment syndrome." The term *acute traumatic ischemia* (ATI) is preferable in the majority of these cases, particularly because it focuses attention on the underlying problem that is common to these injuries.

Pathophysiology

The basic cause of ATI is a disruption of adequate perfusion of the affected tissues by oxygenated blood. The underlying mechanisms fall into two broad categories (Figure 9-1). One is direct macroscopic muscular and vascular trauma, typically resulting from energy applied to the tissue in a brief but intense pulse. The other is microvascular trauma, which may result from a less intense though prolonged application of compressive force, or from hypoperfusion or hypoxia alone. Hemorrhage, associated with either the specific injury or with other internal or external injuries, may also lead to hypoperfusion due to the anemia it produces. Hemorrhage into an intact compartment may lead to a compartment syndrome (see Chap. 278) and an ongoing cycle of increased pressure and decreased perfusion. Hypoperfusion may also be the result of tearing or compressive vascular trauma despite the presence of adequate total-body vascular volume. Microvascular trauma may lead to extracellular edema, and if this occurs in an intact compartment, a compartment syndrome as well. If neurologic structures are involved as they are in many myofascial compartments, the result may also be a Volkmann's contracture.[12]

The net result of hemorrhage, edema, and hypoperfusion is tissue hypoxia and ischemia. Capillary blood flow in muscular compartments is compromised at pressures exceeding 20 mm Hg and hypoxic injury results from tissue oxygen tensions below 30 mm Hg.[12] At the cellular level, this lack of substrate and oxygen translates into a decrease in available ATP and cellular acidosis. An inadequate level of energy results in decreased membrane sodium-potassium-ATPase pump activity and eventual bidirectional sarcolemma leakage. The derangement of intracellular organelles that results leads to an ever-increasing cycle toward cellular death and rhabdomyolysis.[13,14] Upon cellular lysis, there is a release of mediators of inflammation that promotes vasoconstriction, platelet aggregation, and vascular permeability, which causes further edema and decreased tissue perfusion. Cellular death also results in the release of potassium, phosphate, and myoglobin—aspects of acute traumatic rhabdomyolysis that are responsible for the creation of a crush syndrome (see Chap. 279).

Clinical Approach

The standard approach to any trauma victim should be followed (see Chap. 251). Apart from those cases that result in clinically apparent compartment syndromes, or those that result in crush syndrome, there remains the significant clinical entity of ATI. While ATI may initially not cause compartment syndromes or systemically profound rhabdomyolysis, it does require appropriate intervention to prevent their development. Unfortunately, a history of a crushing mechanism or the time elapsed from the moment of injury may not be obtainable in many cases due to an obtunded patient or lack of witnesses. A disruption in the medical infrastructure or a large number of casualties may also delay care. Clues to the presence of ATI include: mechanisms of injury, prolonged immobilization following the injury, a history consistent with the possibility of a crush mechanism, and, in cases of a conscious patient, pain out of proportion to the apparent extent of the injury.

Although any tissue can be affected, nerve and muscle within myofascial compartments are at particular risk. The affected limb may not appear to be diffusely swollen or particularly painful until the onset of an actual compartment syndrome, though a tensely swollen limb with shiny overlying skin is an indication that a compartment syndrome has probably already developed. These relatively unyielding compartments may contain increased pressure without a marked change in the external appearance. It is essential that the skin be cleansed of dirt, soot, and debris in order to determine if there are any changes or asymmetries in skin color. Areas that are blanched, as well as areas of erythema, should prompt concern and an expanded evaluation. Palpation of the entire body should be done to determine if there are areas of crepitus, swelling, or tenderness. Although the utility of capillary refill has been called into question, it may provide a useful screening tool for detecting asymmetry and for serial checks.

Following a thorough neurologic examination, and removal of any clothing or jewelry, which may be potentially constrictive, any affected limbs should be immobilized with padded splints in a position that will enhance local circulation. Frequent neurologic and vascular checks are essential to detect developing processes that may have been occult to the examiner initially.

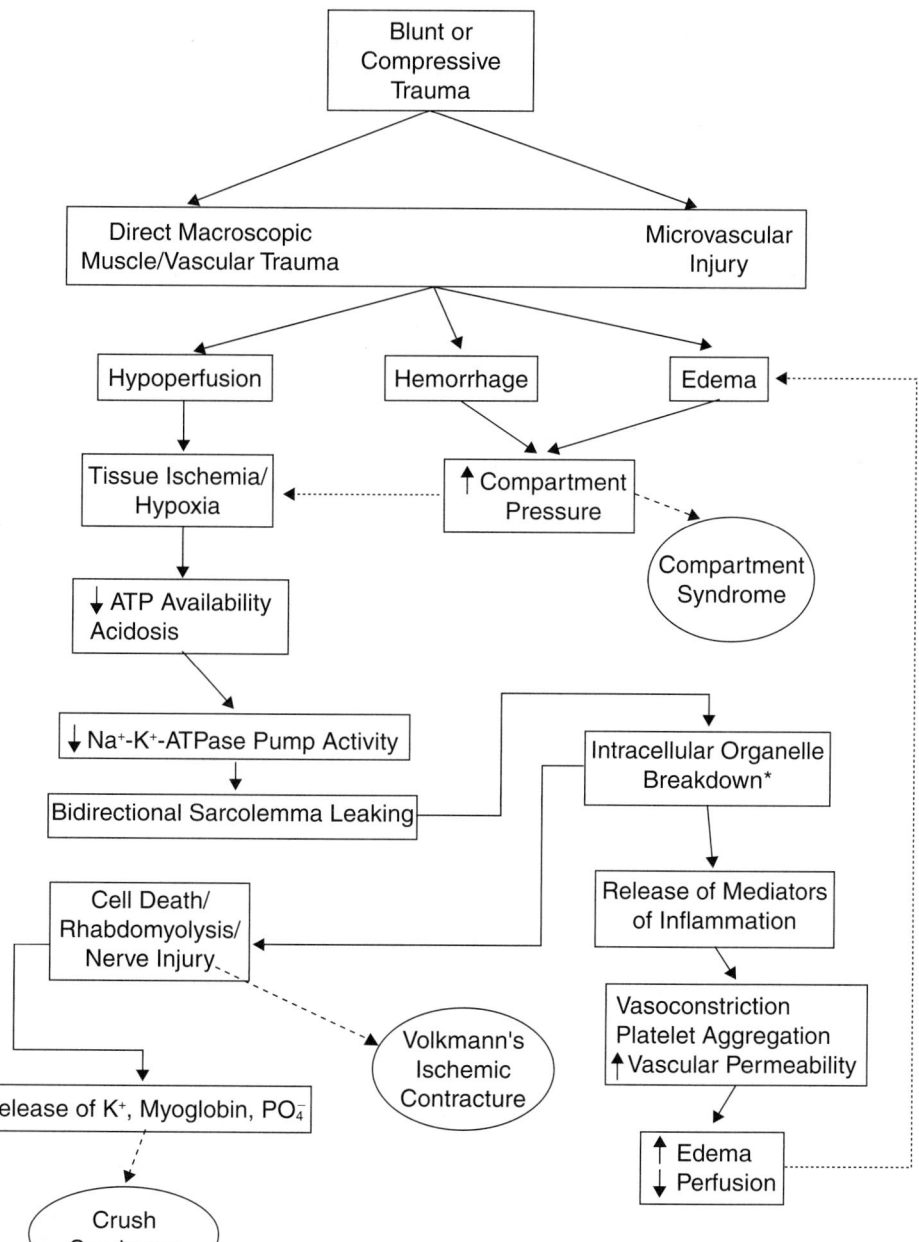

FIG. 9-1. Pathophysiologic cascade of acute traumatic ischemia (ATI). *The intracellular derangement includes swelling of the mitochondria, a breakdown in the endoplasmic reticulum, and gradual breakdown of the cell membrane, all leading to increased intracellular calcium, lysosome breakdown, and the release of multiple enzymes. These enzymes (lipase, protease, etc) further accelerate the autocatabolism and result in cell death.

Apart from any laboratory tests needed for concomitant injuries, blood should be drawn for CBC, BUN, creatinine, electrolytes, phosphorus, calcium, and creatine kinase (CK) activity. Urine should be sent for urinalysis and urine myoglobin concentration. Samples should be collected from freshly produced urine, not the pretrauma specimen that the bladder initially contains. Prior to results being returned, the presence of myoglobin can be assumed when a urine test strip is positive for blood but microscopic examination reveals no red blood cells. Serial laboratory examinations of serum potassium and CK, as well as urine myoglobin, should likewise be obtained, particularly if the initial results are normal in a clinical context that strongly suggests the possibility of ATI.

Management

Standard trauma protocols should be followed. Supplemental oxygen should be provided to keep the hemoglobin saturation greater than 95 percent, and blood transfused to keep the hemoglobin concentration greater than 10 g/dL. Continuous cardiac monitoring and pulse oxime-

try should be performed. Initial fluid resuscitation should be done with 250-mL aliquots of NS every 15 min until urine is produced at a rate of 2 mL/kg per h. Large fluid boluses should be avoided. The goal is a resuscitated mean arterial pressure greater than 80 mm Hg. The use of furosemide and mannitol is controversial. Furosemide 40 to 120 mg IV may be given. Furosemide causes renal vasodilation, decreased oxygen demands by the kidney, and increased renal intratubular flow.[14]

It should be realized that, particularly in the case of mass casualty incidents or disasters, that amputation of a nonviable limb may be a life-saving procedure in terms of preventing the sequelae found in crush syndrome.

Disposition

All patients with suspected ATI require admission for intravenous hydration; serial monitoring of potassium, CK, and myoglobin; and close monitoring for the onset of compartment syndromes by performing frequent neurologic and vascular examinations. The treatment of hyperkalemia, hypercalcemia, hypophosphatemia, and myoglobinuria associated with rhabdomyolysis is discussed in Chap. 279. HBO therapy has recently been demonstrated in a double-blind trial to be effective in extremity ATI,[15] and could also be considered.

REFERENCES

1. Viano DC, Lau IV: A viscous tolerance criterion for soft tissue injury assessment. *J Biomech* 21:387, 1988.
2. Wightman JM, Gladish SL: Explosions and blast injuries. *Ann Emerg Med* 37:664, 2001.
3. Stuhmiller JH, Phillips YY, Richmond DR: The physics and mechanisms of primary blast injury, in Bellamy RF, Zajtchuk R (eds): *Conventional Warfare: Ballistic, Blast, and Burn Injuries.* Washington: Office of the Surgeon General of the United States Army, 1991, pp. 241.
4. Pizov R, Oppenheim-Eden A, Matot I, et al: Blast lung injury from an explosion on a civilian bus. *Chest* 115:165, 1999.
5. Oppenheim A, Pizov R, Pikarsky A, et al: Tension pneumoperitoneum after blast injury: Dramatic improvement in ventilatory and hemodynamic parameters after surgical decompression. *J Trauma* 44:915, 1998.
6. Ho AM-H, Ling E: Systemic air embolism after lung trauma. *Anesthesiology* 90:564, 1999.
7. Paran H, Neufeld D, Shwartz I, et al: Perforation of the terminal ileum induced by blast injury: Delayed diagnosis or delayed perforation? *J Trauma* 40:472, 1996.
8. Ost D, Corbridge T: Independent lung ventilation. *Clin Chest Med* 17:591, 1996.
9. Sorkine P, Szold O, Kluger Y, et al: Permissive hypercapnia ventilation in patients with severe pulmonary blast injury. *J Trauma* 45:35, 1998.
10. Leibovici D, Gofrit ON, Shapira SC: Eardrum perforation in explosion survivors: Is it a marker of pulmonary blast injury? *Ann Emerg Med* 34:168, 1999.
11. Bloom AI, Gideon Z, Muggia M, et al: Torture rhabdomyorhexis—a pseudo-crush syndrome. *J Trauma* 38:252, 1995.
12. von Schroeder HP, Botte MJ: Crush syndrome of the upper extremity. *Hand Clin* 14:451, 1998.
13. Hofmeister EP, Shin AY: The role of prophylactic fasciotomy and medical treatment in limb ischemia and revascularization. *Hand Clin* 14:457, 1998.
14. Better OS: Rescue and salvage of casualties suffering from the crush syndrome after mass disasters. *Mil Med* 164:366, 1999.
15. Bouachour G, Cronier P, Couello JP, et al: Hyperbaric oxygen therapy in the management of crush injuries: A randomized double-blind, placebo controlled, clinical trial. *J Trauma* 41:333, 1996.

RADIATION INJURIES
Christina L. Catlett
Pamela L. Piggott

INTRODUCTION

In the last 40 years, the public's concern with radiation injuries centered around nuclear power plant accidents and the threat of use of a nuclear weapon in a war setting. However, with today's widespread use of radiation technology in medicine, research, industry, power production, and national defense, there is a growing potential for radiation injuries. Of further concern is the potential for large numbers of casualties from a terrorist attack employing a nuclear weapon or radioactive material. As a front-line responder, the emergency physician must be prepared to recognize and treat injuries sustained in a radiation event.

RADIATION EVENT SCENARIOS

Radiation events may be accidental or intentional. Accidents may occur at any facility utilizing a radioactive source, or during transport of radioactive materials. Accidents can also occur in the medical setting, involving erroneous dosing of radiotherapy.

Nonmalevolent theft of radioactive sources for financial gain can result in accidental exposure to radiation. Sealed medical and industrial sources, such as cobalt-60, cesium-137, and iridium-192, could be targets for thieves. These sources can also be abandoned, lost, misplaced, or embezzled, thereby ending up in the wrong or unsuspecting hands.

Recently, the threat of a radiation event as a result of terrorist activity has arisen. A "dirty bomb" is one in which conventional explosives are linked to a radioactive source with the intention of dispersing radioactive particles over a large area. While this may not be likely to cause many radiation injuries, the ensuing panic and psychological distress would be devastating. Terrorists may also attempt to attack a nuclear installation (such as a power plant or waste repository) in an effort to disperse radioactive material. In the worst-case scenario, terrorists may manage to obtain a nuclear weapon for detonation.

Radiation injury can also occur if an individual has contact with a radiation source without being aware of its hazardous nature. Four major cases of this occurred in Thailand (2000), Egypt (2000), Estonia (1994), and Brazil (1987), in which unsuspecting villagers gained possession of lost or abandoned radioactive sources (scavenging scrap metal in two of the incidents) and were exposed to radiation. The average time from first exposure to diagnosis for these four events was 22 days.[1] The ability to recognize signs and symptoms of radiation injury will enable the physician to deliver more prompt and effective treatment to these types of patients.

INCIDENCE OF RADIATION EVENTS

The most recognized and comprehensive record of radiation accidents is the registry maintained by an asset of the U.S. Department of Energy, the Radiation Emergency Assistance Center/Training Site (REACTS). Since the inception of the registry in 1944, 426 radiation accidents have been recorded worldwide with a total of 133,811 victims; 3063 had significant exposure and there were 134 fatalities. The 1986 Chernobyl accident accounted for 116,500 individuals and 28 acute fatalities. The most frequent radiation accident is one of high-dose local exposure, usually to the hands, from a radiation device. The majority of these accidents have occurred in the industrial setting with inadvertent exposure from radiation devices used in radiography to verify integrity of metals such as pipe welds.[2]

FUNDAMENTALS OF RADIATION PHYSICS

An understanding of basic radiation physics and pathogenesis of injury will aid the emergency physician in the triage and initial management of radiation injuries.

Nonionizing and Ionizing Radiation

The electromagnetic radiation spectrum includes long-wavelength, low-frequency, low-energy forms of nonionizing radiation and progresses to short-wavelength, high-frequency, high-energy forms of ionizing radiation. *Ionizing* refers to the ability of high-energy radiation to displace electrons from atoms and cause matter through which it passes to become electrically charged. Alpha and beta particles, neutrons, x-rays, and gamma waves are ionizing forms of radiation. Nonionizing forms include ultraviolet rays, visible light rays, infrared rays, microwaves, and radio waves. Lasers, ultrasound, and nuclear magnetic resonance systems are other examples of devices that use nonionizing radiation in the medical field.

Types of Ionizing Radiation

Radiation is emitted as either particles or waves. Particulate radiation includes alpha, beta, and neutrons, whereas gamma and x-rays are electromagnetic waves (Table 10-1).

TABLE 10-1   Types of Radiation

Type (Symbol)	Mass*	Charge	Penetration	Shield	Hazard	Source
Alpha (α)	4	+2	Few cm in air	Paper, keratin layer of skin	Internal contamination only	Transuranic elements, i.e., plutonium found in nuclear weapons and isotope production facilities
Beta (β)	1/200	−1	~8 mm into skin	Clothing	Skin and internal contamination	Most radioisotopes decay by β followed by γ emission
Neutron (N)	1	0	Variable	Material with high hydrogen content	Whole-body irradiation	Nuclear power plants, particle accelerators, weapons assembly plants
Gamma (γ) and x-rays	0	0	Several cm in tissue	Concrete Lead	Whole-body irradiation	Most radioisotopes emit γ following β decay

*Approximate measurement in atomic mass units (AMU).

ALPHA PARTICLES   Alpha radiation is a heavy, highly charged particle composed of two protons and two neutrons. Because of its large mass and charge, alpha particles travel at a low velocity and interact readily with matter. This form of radiation deposits a large amount of energy in a small volume of tissue; however, the energy dissipates quickly. Therefore, alpha radiation possesses a significant biological hazard only when internalized. Alpha radiation is easily shielded and cannot penetrate paper or the keratin layer of skin. Heavy radioisotopes with an atomic number above 82, such as uranium and plutonium, are sources of alpha particle emission. Specialized devices are required to detect alpha particles.

BETA PARTICLES   Beta particles have a smaller mass and charge and generally have a greater velocity than alpha particles. Beta radiation can travel several meters in air and penetrates approximately 8 mm into exposed skin and can cause serious burns. Like alpha, beta is also a hazard if internally deposited, but to a lesser extent. Most radioisotopes decay by beta radiation followed by gamma emission.

NEUTRONS   Neutrons are electrically neutral particles with a wide range of energy, velocity, and penetration power. Exposure to neutrons is unique. Unlike irradiation by other forms, high-level neutron exposure can induce radioactivity. That is, neutron irradiation can cause previously stable atoms of the absorbing material to become radioactive. In human tissue, the induced radioactive isotope is primarily Na-24, which can be detected in blood and urine specimens. In peacetime, neutron exposure is unlikely and sources of neutrons are limited primarily to nuclear power plants, particle accelerators, and weapon assembly sites.

GAMMA AND X-RAYS   Gamma and x-rays are electromagnetic waves with no mass and no charge that travel at the speed of light. X-rays have longer wavelengths, lower frequency, and lower energy than gamma rays. Gamma rays are the most penetrating type of ionizing radiation and travel several meters in air and many centimeters into tissue; therefore dense materials are required to shield from gamma radiation. Exposure to an external source of gamma or high-energy x-rays presents a significant whole-body radiation hazard and high doses may result in acute radiation syndrome.

Units of Measure

Radiation can be measured as activity, exposure, or dose (Table 10-2). Conventional units include the curie, roentgen, rad, and rem. The International System (SI) is now more widely used and includes the becquerel, gray, and sievert.

The curie (Ci) and becquerel (Bq) are units of activity and describe the amount of radioactivity present, which is a function of the radioisotope's rate of decay or number of disintegrations per second. The roentgen (R) is a unit of exposure and measures the amount of x-ray or gamma radiation that produces a given number of ionizations in air. Many radiation survey instruments record exposure rate per h of x-ray or gamma radiation. The SI equivalent of roentgen is coulomb per kilogram (coul/kg). The rad (r) and gray (Gy) are units of absorbed dose and reflect the amount of energy that the radiation imparts to matter through which it passes.

Because the different types of radiation have different magnitudes of biological effect on humans, units of dose-equivalent are used to provide a common scale of measurement for the different types of radiation. The

TABLE 10-2   Radiation Units of Measure

Description	Conventional Units	SI Unit	Conversion
Activity Units of activity describe the amount of radioactivity present.	Curie (Ci)	Becquerel (Bq)	1 Bq ~2.7 × 10⁻¹¹ Ci 1 Ci ~3.7 × 10¹⁰ Bq
Exposure Units of exposure measure the amount of x-ray or gamma radiation that produces a given number of ionizations in air.	Roentgen (R)	Coulombs per kg (coul/kg)	1 R = 2.58 × 10⁻⁴ coul/kg
Absorbed Dose Units of absorbed dose can be applied to any type of radiation and reflects the energy imparted to matter.	Rad (r)	Gray (Gy)	1 rad = 0.01 Gy 1 Gy = 100 rad
Dose Equivalent Units that provide a common scale of measure for the different types of radiation.	Rem	Sievert (Sv)	1 rem = 0.01 Sv 1 Sv = 100 rem
Internalized Radiation Term that reflects the amount of radiation that will be delivered to the body from internally deposited radioisotopes.	Body burden	N/A	

rem and sievert (Sv) are units of dose-equivalent and are obtained by multiplying the absorbed dose by modifying factors. Differentiation between units of absorbed dose and dose equivalent is most important with high-energy transfer radiation, particularly alpha radiation. Because of the large amount of energy that alpha particles deposit in a concentrated area, the potential of alpha particles to cause biological damage is greater. The dose equivalent of alpha radiation is approximately 20 times the absorbed dose. In other words, one rad (or gray) of alpha radiation is approximately equivalent to 20 rem (or sievert).

For beta, x-ray, and gamma radiation, the dose equivalent is essentially equal to the absorbed dose. In simplified terms, a rad (or gray) of beta, x-ray, or gamma radiation is roughly equivalent to a rem (or sievert). For these types of low-energy-transfer radiation, units of absorbed dose and dose-equivalent are often used interchangeably.

Body burden is used in reference to internally deposited radioactive material. Different radionuclides will deliver varying amounts of radiation to the body when internalized. The amount of radioactivity that may be present in the body for a working lifetime and pose no reasonable expectation of health risk is referred to as the maximum permissible body burden (MPBB). The amount of internally deposited radioactive material is quantified as a percentage of the MPBB that has been established for the particular radionuclide. The MPBB is based on continuous exposure in a working lifetime, thus the MPBB must be interpreted with caution in an accident setting involving acute exposure. Annual limit of intake (ALI) is a newer term that is also used to quantify internally deposited radioactive material.

Biologic Effect of Ionizing Radiation

The biologic effect of ionizing radiation occurs at the cellular level. DNA and other macromolecules of the cell may be directly ionized by radiation or indirectly damaged by highly reactive free radicals created by ionization of cellular water. High levels of radiation exposure may directly cause cell death. More commonly, lower levels of radiation interrupt the cell's reproductive process by damaging its mitotic capability, making it unable to divide. Injury occurs at the time of exposure, but the onset of clinical manifestations of radiation injury varies among cell types. Short-lived cells, such as blood cells, are quickly depleted and injury may become evident before new cells are generated. Longer-lived cells, such as in the lens of the eye, regenerate slowly and thus injury may not become apparent for years after the exposure.

Radiosensitivity is the response of cells to acute manifestations of radiation injury. In general, poorly differentiated cells and cells with a short lifespan and high turnover rate are most vulnerable to the detrimental effects of radiation. Rapidly proliferating cells, such as those of the hematopoietic, gastrointestinal, and reproductive systems, are more radiosensitive than the more slowly dividing cells of the nervous and musculoskeletal systems.

Radiation Monitoring Equipment

Common radiation monitoring equipment includes dosimeters and survey meters (Table 10-3). Dosimeters are small devices that are typically worn on the upper torso to record the cumulative amount of radiation an individual receives while wearing the device. Survey instruments are rate meters that record the amount of radiation detected in an area per unit of time. Both of these monitoring devices should be available to the emergency department for use during a radiologic emergency. Survey meters should be used to monitor contamination of victims and staff, and personal dosimeters should be worn by personnel working in the radiation emergency area (see below).

PERSONAL DOSIMETERS   A thermoluminescent dosimeter (TLD), or film badge, is used to provide permanent records of cumulative dose received. Most of these devices measure beta, x-ray, and gamma radiation. The dose is recorded in rem or sievert. Dose measurements are not immediately available to the wearer because these devices require processing. Self-reading pocket dosimeters may be used in addition to TLDs. These devices provide immediate estimates of cumulative exposure of x-ray and gamma radiation. Most pocket dosimeters can be directly read when held up to a light source. Estimates are typically recorded in milliroentgen (mR).

RADIATION SURVEY METERS   Ion chambers are common types of survey meters for recording exposure rates of x-ray and gamma radiation. Some types of ion chambers are also equipped to detect beta radiation with a Mylar window beneath a removable shield. These instruments are usually calibrated in mR/h. Geiger-Müeller (GM) instruments are commonly used to perform surveys for external contamination. These instruments detect lower exposure rates of x-ray and gamma radiation, as well as beta radiation. With special instrument probes, alpha radiation can also be detected. The units recorded are typically counts per minute (cpm). For comparison, 2500 cpm is approximately equal to 1 mR per h.

Lethal Dose of Radiation

The LD50/60 from exposure to ionizing radiation is defined as the dose of penetrating ionizing radiation that will result in the deaths of 50 percent of the exposed population within 60 days. Three values are commonly cited regarding human survival. The most commonly cited value is LD50/60 of approximately 4.5 Gy (450 rad). This value assumes intensive medical therapy is provided, including antibiotics, blood products, and reverse isolation. With only minimal treatment, such as basic first aid, the LD50/60 falls to approximately 3.4 Gy (340 rad). Victims of the Chernobyl nuclear accident have demonstrated that humans can survive radiation doses greater than anticipated. Intensive medical support for Chernobyl victims allowed a high survival rate in individuals receiving less than 6 Gy (600 rad). With newer advances in medical treatment, such as stem cell transplantation and hematopoietic growth factor administration, it may be possible to raise the LD50/60 to 11 Gy (1100 rad).[3]

RADIATION EVENT MANAGEMENT

Advance Planning

Every EMS system should have a prehospital plan for the evacuation of victims from a radiation disaster. HazMat is often the responsible entity. In addition, every hospital is required by the Joint Commission

TABLE 10-3   Radiation Monitoring Equipment

Equipment Type	Device	Common Type of Measurement	Units Commonly Recorded
Dosimeter	Thermoluminescent dosimeter or film badge	Cumulative dose of beta, x-ray, and gamma	Rem or Sievert
Dosimeter	Pocket dosimeter	Cumulative exposure to x-ray and gamma	mR
Survey meter	Geiger-Müeller tube	Low exposure rates of x-ray, gamma, and beta†	cpm*
Survey meter	Ion chamber	Higher exposure rates of x-ray and gamma	mR per h

*2500 counts per minute (cpm) equal approximately 1 mR per h.
†With special instrument probes, alpha radiation can also be detected.

on Accreditation of Healthcare Organizations (JCAHO) to have a written protocol detailing instructions for receiving and treating radiation event victims. The initial medical evaluation and treatment of the victims often falls under the purview of the emergency department; therefore the emergency physician should take an active role in the development of the hospital's radiation event plan.[4,5] Further, the hospital should stage regular disaster drills and train personnel in decontamination procedures, use of personal protective equipment, and radiologic monitoring.

Prehospital Emergency Medical Management

Emergency responders rapidly establish incident command in a situation involving radioactive materials. Responders secure the scene and attempt to identify the hazard. Personal protective equipment, respiratory protection, and turnout gear are used per protocols. Radiation dosimeters or survey meters are utilized, if available. Victims are extricated, and life-saving medical interventions are administered. Care and transportation of seriously injured victims should not be delayed, even if the patient is contaminated. In medically stable patients, radiation control measures will be undertaken at the scene, such as radiation monitoring, removal of the patient's clothing, covering of wounds, and transfer of the patient to a clean stretcher and ambulance if possible. First responders must communicate with hospitals prior to arrival to allow adequate preparation.

Emergency Department Notification and Preparation

When receiving notification of a radiation event, the emergency department should request information that will facilitate the necessary preparation, including:

1. Circumstances of the accident or event
2. Number of victims
3. Medical condition and physical injuries of the victims
4. Type and extent of radiologic insult: irradiated, externally contaminated, or internally contaminated
5. Identification of the radioactive material, if known
6. If victims were able to be surveyed in the field
7. Exposure to other hazardous material that may be chemically toxic or corrosive

If contamination of the victim is unknown, the patient should be assumed to be contaminated and undergo decontamination measures (see below).

Notification alone should serve to activate the radiation event protocol. Elements of the protocol include: clear identification of the members of the radiation emergency response team, individual responsibilities, location and type of radiation emergency supplies, specific details for physical preparation of the emergency department, and procedures to ensure ED staff and patient safety (Table 10-4).

Initial activation of the protocol should instruct ED personnel how to contact predetermined local radiation specialists, and ideally, health physics professionals. Radiation specialists may assist by monitoring radiation doses of personnel, surveying personnel and areas for contamination, directing contamination control and decontamination efforts, and disposing of contaminated wastes.

Triage and Treatment Philosophies

When there are multiple casualties, triage should be based on the patient's acute medical condition and not specifically on radiation exposure. Radioactive contamination (external or internal) is never immediately life-threatening. Therefore radiologic surveying or decontamination should never supercede life-saving medical interventions.

If all patients are medically stable, then the suggested priority of providing treatment is:

1. Externally contaminated patients (to prevent spread of contamination and internal contamination)

TABLE 10-4   Emergency Department Preparation

Establish the radiation emergency area (REA)
Locate away from usual traffic or patient flow
Establish "buffer zone"
Adequate size for anticipated number of victims
Police or security strictly control access
Boundaries identified with rope or signs
Cover floors with plastic or paper secured with heavy tape
Pregnant women, nonessential personnel not allowed
Obtain preassembled emergency kits
Supplies for REA set-up and decontamination
Personal dosimeters
Radiation survey meters
Specimen collection containers
Resuscitation equipment (intubation equipment, IV supplies and fluids, drugs, etc.) and trauma supplies (chest tubes, dressings, etc.)
Portable ultrasound
Don protective gear
Water-repellent coveralls or aprons and shoe covers
Surgical gown, mask, eye protection, cap
Double pair of latex gloves, with inner glove taped in place, outer pair changed after contact with contamination
Fasten dosimeter on torso, on outermost clothing layer
Meet the patient(s)
At the ambulance if the ED has the capability to decontaminate patients prior to entry into the hospital
At the entrance to the REA if the patient must be decontaminated within the ED

---

2. Internally contaminated patients
3. Externally irradiated patients

Additional precautions are required when managing radiation events, because unlike incidents involving hazardous material of other types, incidents that involve radiation and radioactive material can only be detected by monitoring devices. Contamination control is necessary in order to protect the safety of patients, health care providers, and the environment. The goal of treatment is to limit exposure of the patients and staff to the hazardous substance, thereby minimizing morbidity and mortality, and to contain the spread of the hazardous material.

TYPES OF RADIATION EXPOSURE

A radiation accident or event can expose a victim through several different means. *External contamination* occurs when radioactive materials are deposited on the skin. These patients require decontamination to prevent further exposure to the patient and hospital staff.

External irradiation occurs when all or part of the body is exposed to a penetrating radiation source. The irradiation may occur locally (i.e., to the hands) or diffusely, resulting in acute radiation syndrome. Localized injuries, which rarely cause systemic illness, are the most common type of radiation exposure.

Internal contamination can occur through an accidental or intentional ingestion of a radioactive source, or via absorption of radioactive materials through wounds or the lungs. Internal contamination can result in *incorporation,* or uptake of the radioactive material into cells, tissues, and organs such as bone, thyroid, liver, or kidneys.

CLINICAL PRESENTATION AND MANAGEMENT

The presentation, emergency management, and long-term care of a radiation victim varies based on the mechanism of exposure to radiation. For ease of discussion, the following four exposure scenarios will be addressed: externally contaminated patients; localized radiation injuries; whole-body irradiation; and internally contaminated patients. For each scenario, patient presentation, decontamination, emergency department treatment, and inpatient treatment shall be discussed. For a summary of recommendations for the medical treatment of radiation victims, please refer to Table 10-5.

Externally Contaminated Patients

A patient is externally contaminated when radioactive materials are physically deposited onto the patient's skin or clothing. All victims of radiation events should be handled as if contaminated until known otherwise.

Upon arrival at the hospital, all patients should be surveyed for contamination. If radiation monitoring devices are not available, patients should be routinely decontaminated and then surveyed for contamination when monitoring equipment is obtained.

The dose from external contamination to either the patient or the medical staff is rarely significant. Spreading the contamination in the environment and the potential of internalization are the main hazards with external contamination. Thus special precautions are required for receiving and treating these patients. Specific contamination control principles, physical decontamination techniques, and personal protective equipment are required for the care of these patients (see Tables 10-4 and 10-6).

It is not immediately crucial to know the identity of the radionuclide; however, it is important to determine whether the nuclide emits beta-gamma radiation and/or alpha radiation. Commonly used radiation survey meters easily detect beta and gamma radiation. Detection of alpha radiation requires special instrument probes and careful monitoring techniques. Alpha radiation is shielded by any moisture, including perspiration and blood. Therefore only trained individuals should perform surveys for alpha-emitting contamination.

Local Radiation Injury

The majority of radiation accidents in the United States result in local radiation injury from partial-body exposure. In contrast to whole-body irradiation, partial-body irradiation rarely causes systemic manifestations. A rare exception is the development of acute radiation syndrome (see below) following partial-body irradiation that affects a significant amount of the bone marrow. Most commonly, a portion of the extremities is affected and the clinical picture consists of cutaneous changes.

The extent and course of cutaneous involvement is dose dependent. Generally, within the first week following localized radiation exposure, the patient may be asymptomatic or experience some transient erythema, hyperesthesia, and itching. In the second week, true erythema develops along with progressive epilation. In week 3, the skin becomes warm, painful, swollen, and pruritic. By the fourth week, dry or wet desquamation and/or ulceration ensues, depending on the radiation dose received (Table 10-7).[6]

These skin manifestations may appear similar to thermal burns. However, unlike thermal burns, cutaneous radiation injury may be associated with waves of transient erythema described above, as well as with a delayed onset of pain, followed by a more prolonged and severe pain. Another important distinction of radiation injury is that the clinical changes evolve over a more prolonged time period. The exception is very high doses on the order of 50 Gy (5000 rad), that result in prompt transdermal injury resembling a thermal third-degree burn. The pain is immediate and excruciating. Surgical resection and grafting may be required.

Emergency department care of cutaneous radiation injury is limited to analgesics, routine burn care, and if indicated, surgical referral. Inpatient treatment may not be required. However, close follow-up is essential. Physical therapy and splinting may be useful for preventing contractures and preserving joint range of motion. These patients should be carefully monitored for hemorrhage, infection, and necrosis. In addition, prolonged close follow-up is needed for later neoplastic changes of the skin.

Whole-Body Irradiation/Acute Radiation Syndrome

Characteristic and relatively predictable signs and symptoms develop when a significant portion of the body is exposed to a high level of penetrating radiation over a short period of time, typically less that 24 h. These signs and symptoms are collectively referred to as *acute radiation syndrome* (ARS) (Table 10-8). A whole-body gamma dose in excess of 2 Gy (200 rad) is the primary cause of acute radiation syndrome. Alpha and low-energy beta radiation lack sufficient energy to penetrate the skin and deliver a whole-body radiation dose. Neutron exposure is rare, but high-level neutron irradiation is also capable of producing ARS. Additionally, there are a few reports of ARS following significant amounts of internal radioactive contamination.

Four distinct phases are seen in the unfolding of ARS. The *prodromal phase* is a transient period of self-limiting symptoms that may occur within minutes, hours, or days after exposure. The acuity of onset and the duration of this phase are directly related to the dose received. The prodromal phase is an autonomic nervous system response that initiates gastrointestinal symptoms such as anorexia, nausea, vomiting, and with high doses, diarrhea. In addition, neuromuscular symptoms often accompany the autonomic response and may include hy-

TABLE 10-5 Medical Management of Radiation Event Victims

Radiologic Insult	Key Actions
External Contamination	Initiate contamination control practices and decontamination techniques described in Tables 10–4 and 10–6.
Localized Radiation Injury	Provide adequate analgesics. Routine burn care. Surgical referral as indicated.
Internal Contamination	After swabs have been obtained, irrigate wounds with normal saline. Begin collection of body excreta (sputum, urine, feces, emesis) for bioassay to identify and quantify radioisotopes. Continue collection of urine and feces for 4 days to monitor excretion rate. If ingestion is suspected, begin gut decontamination methods. If high levels of internal contamination are suspected, particularly radioiodine or alpha-emitting radiation, obtain expert consultation for assistance with decorporation procedures.
Whole-Body Irradiation	Obtain blood specimens for dose estimation and for cell and HLA typing. Document time of onset of all symptoms, i.e., anorexia, nausea, vomiting. Symptomatic treatment, i.e., antiemetics, pain management, anxiolytics. Supportive treatment, i.e., IV fluids, blood products, total parenteral nutrition. Consider prophylactic measures, i.e., reverse isolation, prophylactic antibiotics, and antifungals. If severe bone marrow suppression is anticipated, consider administration of hematopoietic growth factors. If neutron irradiation is a concern, obtain blood and urine specimens and monitor for induced radioactivity of Na-24. Monitor all metals on the patient's body for induced radioactivity.

TABLE 10-6   Key Decontamination Techniques

Remove the patient's clothing. This may remove as much as 90% of external contamination. Ideally, this is done at the accident scene prior to transport, or prior to entrance into the ED. Potentially contaminated items are placed in plastic bags and labeled for further management by the Radiation Safety Officer.
Survey the patient for radiation. Document the location and level of contamination.
Decontaminate the patient:

1. If the hospital has permanent showers or prefabricated (temporary) decontamination tents, the patient should be decontaminated prior to entrance into the hospital. Resuscitation and stabilization supplies should be available in the decontamination area. Management of decontamination run-off should be discussed with the state's Environmental Protection Agency (EPA) office prior to an actual event. If a patient still surveys positive for radiation following general decontamination, he or she should be brought into the REA for further decontamination.
2. If the hospital has an approved decontamination room(s) with water containment capability, this may be used.
3. If neither is available, the patient may be decontaminated in the REA (see Table 10-4). If contamination is localized, the area is irrigated and the washings are collected in a container. If contamination is generalized, the patient is cleansed with washcloths, warm water, and a mild soap. Washcloths should be placed in a plastic bag.

Wounds and body orifces are the first priority of decontamination because of the potential for systemic absorption. Intact skin with the highest level of surface contamination follows, progressing to the area of lowest contamination. Attention should be paid to skin folds, where contamination may collect.
Resurvey the patient after each decontamination attempt. Remaining contamination may be removed with mild soap and gentle scrubbing. Vigorous decontamination may damage the skin and thus facilitate absorption. Surgical debridement or excision may be necessary if contamination is embedded in a wound. Emergency procedures that must be performed immediately (e.g., intubation, relief of tension pneumothorax) may need to occur in the REA.
Swab samples should be obtained (time and location noted) for contamined areas of skin, wounds, nares and assessed by Geiger counter.
If radioactivity persists, suspect skin folds or internal contamination (absorption, inhalation, or ingestion). Nasogastric suction may be appropriate of ingestions.
If significant uptake is suspected, request assistance from expert consultants for management of internal contamination. All excreta should be collected, bagged, labeled by site and time, and sent to the appropriate laboratory (per the Radiation Safety Officer or Health Physicist) for isotope analysis.
Following decontamination (accomplished when the reading on the radiation monitor is at or below twice background level), a clean stretcher is rolled over plastic to the patient, and the patient is transferred to the clean stretcher for transfer out of the REA.
Any patient, staff, supplies, and/or equipment leaving the REA are assessed for contamination by the Radiation Safety Officer or Health Physics personnel to prevent spread of contamination into the ED.
Life-saving surgical procedures should not be delayed for decontamination. If necessary, the patient may be covered with clean sheets and transferred to the operating room. The operating room will require decontamination prior to further use.

Source: Mettler FA: Emergency room management of radiation accidents, in, Gusev IA, Guskova AK, Mettler FA (eds): *Medical Management of Radiation Accidents,* 2d ed, CRC Press, NY, 2001, p 437.

potension, pyrexia, diaphoresis, cephalgia, and fatigue. The *latent phase* is a symptom-free interval that follows the resolution of the prodromal phase. Shorter latent phases correspond to higher levels of dose received. The latent period may last 1 to 3 weeks with a dose of less than 4 Gy (400 rad), but may last only a few hours when a dose above 15 Gy (1500 rads) is received.

The *manifest illness phase* is often divided into three dose-dependent subsyndromes. In ascending order of severity, these syndromes are clinically related to injury of the hematopoietic, gastrointestinal, and cardiovascular and central nervous systems. The toxic effects to these organ systems are not discrete. There is considerable overlap as well as additive detrimental effects among these syndromes.

HEMATOPOIETIC SYNDROME   The hematopoietic system is the first organ system to manifest injury and symptoms are seen from doses above 1.5 to 2 Gy (150 to 200 rad). Self-limiting prodromal symptoms begin within several hours or days and typically resolve within 48 h. An asymptomatic latent period follows and typically lasts for 1 to 3 weeks. Radiation destroys circulating lymphocytes and damages stem cells in the bone marrow and lymphatic system. The rapid

TABLE 10-7   Deterministic Thresholds for Local Radiation Injury

Dosage	Cutaneous Manifestation	Time From Exposure
3 gy	Epilation	2–3 weeks
6 gy	Erythema	First day Recurs in 2–3 weeks
10–15 gy	Dry desquamation	2–3 weeks
20–50 gy	Wet desquamation	2–3 weeks
>50 gy	Overt radionecrosis and ulceration	1–2 weeks

Source: From Goans.[1]

decline in lymphocytes is a hallmark of the hematopoietic syndrome and is one of the best early indicators of the extent of radiation injury. Granulocytes, and to a lesser extent, platelet counts display an initial rise followed by an accelerated decrease, reaching a nadir at about 30 days. The red blood cell population also decreases in concentration with resultant mild anemia, but to a lesser extent than other blood cell lines (Figure 10-1). This syndrome results in pancytopenia and immunosuppression with subsequent hemorrhage and infection as the principal causes of morbidity and mortality. Survival is possible with extensive medical intervention.

GASTROINTESTINAL SYNDROME   Gastrointestinal syndrome is the second subsyndrome of the manifest illness phase of ARS and may occur after doses above 6 to 7 Gy (600 to 700 rad) are received. This syndrome is distinguished from the hematopoietic syndrome by the onset of nausea, vomiting, and often diarrhea within hours after exposure. These prodromal symptoms are followed by a short latent period of 1 week or less. Reappearance of gastrointestinal symptoms then occurs with severe nausea, vomiting, diarrhea, and abdominal pain. There is damage of the intestinal mucosal barrier with massive fluid losses resulting in profound volume loss and electrolyte disturbances. The denuded gastrointestinal mucosa allows enteric flora to disseminate into the bloodstream. Declines in blood cell populations are similar to that which occurs with the hematopoietic syndrome, but abnormalities occur sooner and with greater magnitude. With the concurrent immunocompromised state, a fulminating enterocolitis follows. There are few documented cases of gastrointestinal syndrome in humans, all of which resulted in fatalities.

CARDIOVASCULAR AND CENTRAL NERVOUS SYSTEM SYNDROME   The cardiovascular and central nervous system syndrome is the third subsyndrome of the manifest illness phase of ARS that occurs after doses above 20 to 30 Gy (2000 to 3000 rad) are received. This syndrome presents with immediate prostration, nausea, vomiting, and explosive bloody diarrhea as well as hypotension. Alterations in

TABLE 10-8   Acute Radiation Syndrome

Approximate Dose	Onset of Prodrome	Duration of Latent Phase	Manifest Illness
>2 gy (200 rad)	Within 2 days	1–3 weeks	Hematopoietic syndrome with pancytopenia, infection, and hemorrhage; survival possible
>6 gy (600 rad)	Within hours	<1 week	GI syndrome with dehydration, electrolyte abnormalities, GI bleeding, and fulminant enterocolitis; uniformly fatal
>30 gy (3000 rad)	Within minutes	None	Cardiovascular/CNS syndrome with refractory hypotension and circulatory collapse; fatal within 24–72 h

consciousness including lethargy, disorientation, ataxia, tremors, and convulsions occur within hours after exposure. Hypotension is persistent and refractory to treatment. The lymphocyte count promptly falls to near-zero levels. This syndrome is universally fatal with death occurring within 24 to 72 h, predominately due to circulatory collapse.

In addition to these organ system injuries of the manifest illness syndromes, radiation doses above 8 to 9 Gy (800 to 900 rad) may damage the pulmonary system with resulting pneumonitis, fibrosis, and interstitial edema.[7]

TREATMENT OF WHOLE-BODY IRRADIATION   The patient who has been exposed only to an external source of penetrating radiation is not radioactive or contaminated and therefore requires no special precautions for handling or treating. A rare exception is exposure to high-level neutron irradiation, which can induce radioactivity. In the unlikely event of a nuclear plant accident, neutron exposure becomes a concern. Patient specimens of blood and urine should be collected and assayed for induced radioactivity in the body, predominately Na-24. In addition, all metal objects on the patient's body or clothing should be monitored for potential radioactivity, including jewelry, coins, dental fillings, wristwatches, and buttons.

Treatment of the irradiated patient in the emergency department is directed toward alleviating the symptoms of the prodromal phase. Although metoclopramide has been used to prevent nausea and vomiting with some success, studies show that 5-HT3 receptor antagonists (e.g., ondansetron 10 mg IV q4 to 6 h, or 8 mg PO tid) are a more effective way to control nausea and vomiting.[8] Anxiolytics or pain management may be required. Medical treatment has been unsuccessful in the few documented cases of high radiation doses that cause major damage to the GI or CV and CNS systems, but comfort care should be provided. Survival is possible for individuals with lower radiation doses resulting in the hematopoietic form of ARS.

The absence or time of onset of nausea and vomiting are useful for assessing the injury severity. Diarrhea is a less useful symptom unless

there is prompt, explosive, bloody diarrhea, which indicates a likely fatal outcome. Individuals who have received doses less than 1 Gy (100 rad) seldom experience nausea or vomiting. Less than 1 Gy is a reliable dose estimate for individuals who remain asymptomatic 24 h postexposure; further hospitalization of these individuals is generally unnecessary.[9]

Serial blood specimens should be obtained for hematologic and cytogenetic dose assessment. The earliest laboratory indicator of biological damage from radiation is a marked decrease in peripheral lymphocytes, often within 8 h postexposure. The more precipitous the decline in lymphocytes, the greater the dose received (Figure 10-2). The lymphocyte count 24 h postexposure is useful in predicting the patient's clinical course. If the lymphocyte count is maintained above 1200/μL, no clinical support is required. If the count falls below 500/μL, a severe clinical course can be anticipated. If the entire lymphocyte count is depleted within 6 h, a fatal outcome is likely.

Cytogenetic analysis of circulating lymphocytes is another method of dose estimation. Radiation induces some characteristic chromosome aberrations, particularly rings and dicentrics, in a dose-dependent manner. The frequency of these abnormalities can be scored in cytogenetic laboratories to obtain estimates of radiation dose received. This process is technically challenging, time consuming, and expensive, but is the most sensitive biologic measurement for quantifying dose from whole-body irradiation.[10]

Obtaining data and specimens for dose estimation is a crucial aspect of planning inpatient therapy and predicting the patient's clinical course. The time of onset of all clinical symptoms should be carefully observed and documented.

The ultimate long-term treatment goal is to provide support during the period of deficient defenses against infection and hemorrhage until marrow recovery occurs. Supportive treatment may include intravenous fluids, blood products, and total parenteral nutrition, as well as reverse isolation, prophylactic antibiotics, and antifungal medications.

Anemia, granulocytopenia and thrombocytopenia can be expected within a month following significant radiation exposure (see Figure

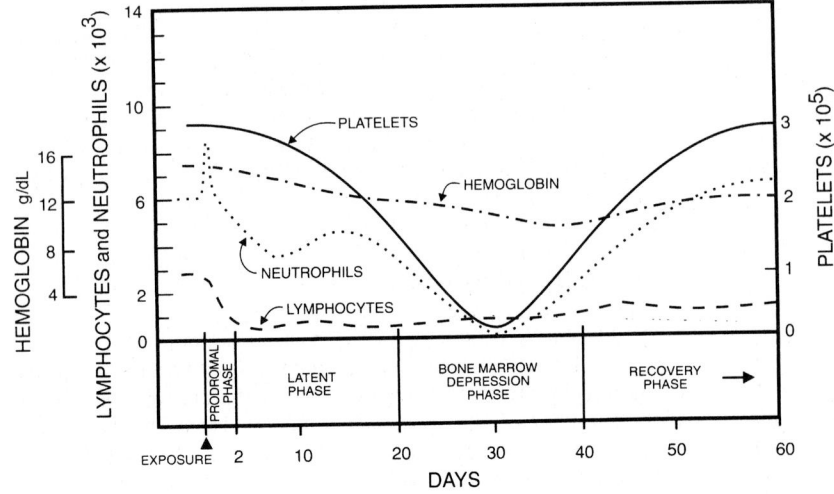

FIG. 10-1. Typical hematologic course and clinical stages after sublethal (~300 rad) exposure to total body irradiation. [Reprinted with permission from *Radiobiological Factors in Manned Space Flight,* © 1965 by the National Academy of Sciences. Washington: National Academy Press, 1965.]

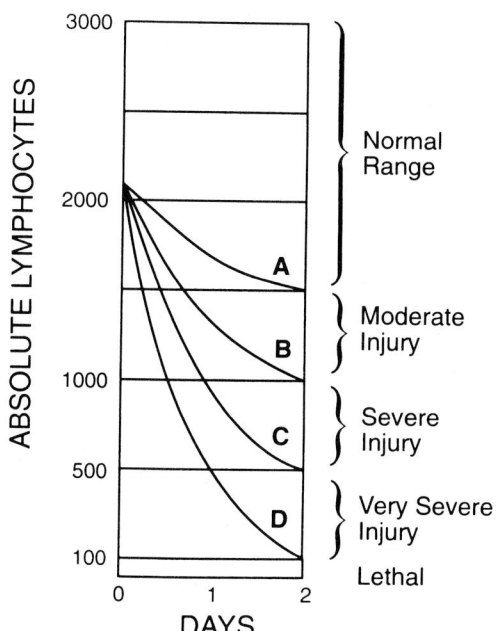

FIG. 10-2. Estimated radiation dose and degree of injury from early changes in lymphocyte counts. Approximate whole-body dose: Curve A–3.1 Gy (310 rad); Curve B–4.4 Gy (440 rad); Curve C–5.6 Gy (560 rad); Curve D–7.1 Gy (710 rad). [Reproduced from *Health Physics* 72:514, 1997 with permission from the Health Physics Society. Figure has been modified from its original version.]

10-1). Therefore the patient, as well as family members who may be potential blood donors, should undergo HLA typing in preparation for white cell and platelet transfusions if marrow suppression becomes severe. The most severe marrow depression occurs at 2 to 3 weeks after exposure. Spontaneous recovery of granulocytes and platelets is quite rapid after the fifth week.

Two approaches have been used to combat bone marrow suppression in victims of radiation injury. Hematopoietic growth factors are cytokines such as erythropoietin, interleukins, and colony-stimulating factors, that have been shown to stimulate the proliferation and differentiation of the surviving stem cells and thus accelerate reconstitution of the bone marrow.[11] Hematopoietic stem cell transplants are also being studied to improve survival.[12]

If significant radiation dose was received, the patient should have long-term periodic follow-up for potential delayed effects of radiation damage such as cataracts, infertility, thyroid dysfunction, leukemia, or other neoplasms.

Internally Contaminated Patients

Radioactive material gains entry into the body by three principal routes: inhalation, ingestion, or absorption from contaminated mucous membranes or abraded skin. Misadministration of a radiopharmaceutical is a potential source of internal contamination that can occur in the hospital setting. Internal contamination becomes a major concern if large amounts of radioactive material are released into the atmosphere as a result of nuclear weapon detonation, large-scale nuclear power plant accident, or even a volcanic eruption. Such events may result in inhalation of airborne radioactive material or ingestion of radioactive material deposited onto agricultural land with subsequent transfer into the food chain.

Internally deposited radioactive material will continue to irradiate tissues until it decays to a stable isotope or is biologically eliminated. The biochemical nature of the radionuclide determines if it is disseminated throughout the body or concentrated in a specific organ. The term *critical organ* is used to describe the organ that receives the highest dose of radiation or is the site of the most significant biologic damage.

In contrast to external contamination, identification of the specific radionuclides that become internalized is important for determining the method of treatment. When the substance is not known, laboratory identification is possible. Internally deposited radionuclides are identified by radioanalysis of swabs from the nares, oropharynx, and wounds, as well as sputum, urine, and fecal specimens. All body excreta from internally contaminated patients should be collected for several days because repeated measurements are used to monitor the elimination rates of the radionuclide.

Radioactivity within the body can also be measured in vivo by a device called a whole-body counter. These detectors predominately measure gamma-emitting radiation and some high-energy beta radiation. Internalized alpha and lower-energy beta-emitting radiation do not escape from the body and are not detected by these devices. Whole-body counters are very sensitive and give false measurements if external contamination is present on the body. For this reason and because these detectors are not readily accessible, whole-body counters are generally not practical in the acute setting of a radiation event.

TREATMENT OF INTERNAL CONTAMINATION   When the contaminating radionuclide is not known, radiochemical laboratory identification of radioisotopes may take several days. Prior to obtaining identification, methods can be initiated for removal of the most commonly encountered radionuclides that are suspected for the particular radiation event. Treatment is aimed at reducing absorption or hastening elimination. After all swabs have been obtained, wounds should be irrigated with physiologic saline.

Pulmonary clearance of inhaled radioactive particles is not effectively enhanced by medications. If large quantities of insoluble radioactive material have been inhaled, bronchopulmonary lavage may be considered. This treatment carries the associated risk of general anesthesia and is performed more commonly in Britain than in this country.

In the emergency department, reduction in gastrointestinal absorption may be accomplished with gastric lavage, emetics, and purgatives. Additionally, antacids containing aluminum cause many metals to precipitate as insoluble hydroxides. Cathartics can then be administered to decrease the transit time of these precipitants.

Decorporation Treatment: Once the radioactive material crosses into the extracellular fluid, incorporation has occurred and elimination is more difficult. Methods of decorporation include blocking agents, isotopic dilution, displacement, mobilizing agents, and chelation.

Frequently treated causes of internal contamination are radioactive forms of iodine, plutonium, cesium, and hydrogen (Table 10-9). Of particular importance and effectiveness are the treatments discussed below for radioiodine and alpha-emitting contamination such as plutonium.

Radioiodine: Inhalation or ingestion of radioiodine is particularly hazardous to the thyroid with a potential risk of causing hypothyroidism or thyroid cancer. I-131 is the predominant internal contaminate resulting from incidents that involve the release of nuclear fission products such as a nuclear reactor accident or nuclear weapons test. Studies on the health effects of the Chernobyl accident have shown that populations in heavily contaminated areas have an increase in thyroid cancer. The number of thyroid cancers reported in these areas continues to increase, with the highest prevalence in individuals who were under the age of 10 years at the time of the accident.[13]

Rapid detection of radioiodine uptake is essential because treatment is most beneficial when administered within 12 h. Radioiodine is a soluble nuclide that is detected in the urine immediately after exposure, allowing early identification of radioiodine uptake. A more rapid, but less sensitive, method is direct measurement with a survey meter held over the thyroid gland.

TABLE 10-9   Commonly Treated Forms of Internal Contamination

Radionuclide	Primary Route of Intake	Principal Hazard	Treatment Mechanism	Agent	Usual Administration*
I-131	Inhalation Ingestion Percutaneous absorption	Thyroid	Block thyroid uptake	KI	130 mg PO for adults ages 18–40 y, and pregnant or lactating women, dosed daily until significant risk of exposure to radioiodine no longer exists 65 mg a day for school-age children 32 mg a day 1 mo to 3 y 16 mg a day for 0 to 1 mo Adults >40 y need KI only when a large internal radiation dose ≥5 gy is predicted
Pu-239	Inhalation Ingestion Absorption through wounds	Bone Liver Lung	Chelation Increase excretion	Ca-DTPA or Zn-DTPA†	1 g/d for 5 d, IV or aerosol IV: 1 g in 250 mL NS or D5W over 30 min Aerosol: 1 g in nebulizer; inhale over 15 to 20 min
H-3	Inhalation Ingestion Percutaneous absorption	Whole-body dose	Isotopic dilution Increase excretion	Water	Oral: 3–4 liters a day for 2 wks
Cs-137	Inhalation Ingestion	Whole-body dose	Mobilization Decrease GI uptake	Ferric Ferrocyanide (Prussian blue)	Oral: 1 g in 100–200 mL water tid for several days

*Duration of therapy is based on dose estimations from radiochemical measurements of urine and fecal samples.
†Calcium and zinc salts of diethylenetriamine pentaacetic acid.
Abbreviation: KI = potassium iodide.

Early administration of stable potassium iodine (KI) is recommended for high levels of radioiodine exposure. Realizing that it may be difficult to assess the risk or level of radioiodine exposure to the public, the FDA has recommended that the administration of KI should begin before or immediately coincident with the passage of a radioactive cloud. Oral administration of KI (see Table 10-9 for dosing) within 1 h of exposure is approximately 90 percent effective at blocking the thyroid uptake of radioiodine. KI administered 6 h after exposure reduces thyroid uptake by approximately 50 percent. Little protective effect is seen when KI is given after 12 h of exposure.[14] KI should be continued daily until significant risk of exposure to radioiodine no longer exists. Administration of antithyroid medications, such as propylthiouracil or methimazole, may be considered if the time since exposure is more than 12 h.[15] In the event of widespread release of radioiodine, the FDA has approved the use of nonprescription KI. State and local officials are responsible for the procurement and distribution of KI to the general public.

Alpha Contamination: Early treatment is recommended for contamination with alpha-emitting radionuclides such as Pu-239. Alpha radiation has potential for significant damage when internally deposited. This internal contamination hazard is a result of alpha's emission of large amounts of energy for a short range, thus causing intense ionization in a concentrated area. This potential damage is made worse by the fact that many of the radioisotopes that emit alpha radiation have very long half-lives.

Chelating agents such as calcium and zinc salts of diethylenetriamine pentaacetic acid (Ca-DTPA and Zn-DTPA, respectively) are effective treatments for contamination with heavy metals and rare earths that emit alpha radiation. If alpha-emitting contamination is detected in wounds or in the nares or oropharynx, treatment with DTPA should be initiated promptly, ideally within 1 to 2 h after contamination has occurred. Potential contraindications for the use of DTPA are severe renal dysfunction, thrombocytopenia, or leukopenia. DTPA is administered systemically by slow intravenous push or by aerosol administration. Ca-DTPA has been shown to be more effective in animal studies and is the preferred form of drug for the initial 1 to 2 d of treatment. Zn-DTPA is less toxic and recommended for treatments of longer duration and of pregnant females. For aerosol administration, Ca-DTPA is preferred because of the metallic taste associated with Zn-DTPA. Of note, most DTPA solutions in nuclear medicine departments are too dilute a concentration for effective decorporation. The success of decorporation techniques depends on early administration. The risks associated with therapy must be weighed against the risk of untreated internal radiation exposure. Assistance from expert consultants should be requested prior to beginning decorporation therapy.

Prenatal Exposures

When a pregnant female is exposed to ionizing radiation, special consideration must be given to the radiosensitive unborn child.[16,17] Fetal cells are largely undifferentiated and highly proliferative and thus have increased radiosensitivity depending on the phase of gestation. At 0 to 2 weeks postconception, there is an all-or-none phenomenon. Irradiation during this time usually results in death with resorption of the conceptus or no observable damage. This phenomenon is a result of the pluripotential of the early blastomeres that allows injured cells to be replaced by remaining cells when the damage is not extensive. After 2 weeks' gestation, organogenesis begins and the embryo is at risk of congenital malformations. The risk of injury is greatest for the particular organ system that is under development at the time of radiation exposure. After 7 weeks, major organogenesis is complete, with the exception of the CNS. The CNS has continued susceptibility to radiation injury during the early fetal period.[17]

Data derived from Japanese atomic bomb survivors suggest the most common in utero injuries are related to the CNS, particularly microcephaly and mental retardation. Other malformations, such as growth restriction and ocular defects, have been reported less frequently.[17]

If a fetal dose is above 500 millirem (5 milliSv), particularly during the vulnerable period of 8 to 15 weeks' gestation, risks such as CNS damage or growth defects must be considered. In such a case, a physician with expertise in radiation injury should be consulted to provide counseling to the expecting parents.

SOURCES OF ASSISTANCE

Emergency department personnel should be familiar with authorities that can provide advice and assistance when radiation accidents occur. Radiation emergency call lists may be prepared in advance and include the following contacts:

1. Local facilities which staff medical and health physics professionals trained in radiation accidents
2. Local civil defense or disaster offices
3. State radiologic health office (title may vary by state)
4. Federal Emergency Management Agency (FEMA)

In addition, there are two organizations that provide current medical advice for the treatment of radiation casualties. The first is the Radiation Emergency Assistance Center/Training Site (REACTS), sponsored by the Department of Energy and managed by the Oak Ridge Institute for Science and Education. REACTS provides training programs, consultation assistance, and treatment capabilities. It has the capability to dispatch an emergency response team of health professionals to assist at an accident site. After initial treatment and decontamination actions are complete, REACTS may also accept severely contaminated or irradiated patients for transfer to its facilities for more definitive care. REACTS contact information is:

Radiation Emergency Assistance Center/Training Site
Oak Ridge Institute for Science and Education
P.O. Box 117, MS 39, Oak Ridge, TN 37831-0117
(865) 576-3131 (daytime phone)
(865) 576-1005 (24-h emergency number)

The second organization available for medical consultation is the Medical Radiobiology Advisory Team, sponsored by the Department of Defense and managed by the Armed Forces Radiobiology Research Institute. The contact information is:

Medical Radiobiology Advisory Team (MRAT)
Armed Forces Radiobiology Research Institute
National Naval Medical Center
8901 Wisconsin Avenue, Building 42
Bethesda, MD 20889-5603
(301) 295-0316

REFERENCES

1. Goans RE: Clinical care of the radiation-accident patient: Patient presentation, assessment, and initial diagnosis, in Ricks R, Berger M, O'Hara FM (eds): *The Medical Basis for Radiation-Accident Preparedness*. New York, The Parthenon Publishing Group, 2002, p. 12.
2. Barabanova AV: Local radiation injury, in Gusev IA, Guskova AK, Mettler FA (eds): *Medical Management of Radiation Accidents, 2d ed*. Boca Raton, FL, CRC Press, 2001, p. 224.
3. Gale RP: Immediate medical consequences of nuclear accidents. Lessons from Chernobyl. *JAMA* 285:627, 1987.
4. Armed Forces Radiobiology Research Laboratory: *Medical Management of Radiological Casualties Handbook*. Bethesda, MD, Armed Forces Radiobiology Research Laboratory, 1999.
5. National Council on Radiation Protection and Measurements: Management of Terrorist Events Involving Radioactive Material (NCRP Report No. 138). Bethesda, MD, National Council on Radiation Protection and Measurements, 2001.
6. Goans RE: Clinical care of the radiation-accident patient: Patient presentation, assessment, and initial diagnosis, in Ricks R, Berger M, O'Hara FM (eds): *The Medical Basis for Radiation-Accident Preparedness*. New York, The Parthenon Publishing Group, 2002, p. 14.
7. Wald N: Acute radiation injury and their medical management, in Mossman KL, Mills WA (eds): *The Biological Basis of Radiation Protection Practice*. Baltimore, Health Physics Society, Williams & Wilkins, 1992, p. 188.
8. Fasano A: Pathophysiology and management of radiation injury of the gastrointestinal tract, in Ricks R, Berger M, O'Hara FM (eds): *The Medical Basis for Radiation-Accident Preparedness*. New York, The Parthenon Publishing Group, 2002, p. 154.
9. Mettler FA, Guskova AK: Treatment of acute radiation sickness, in Gusev IA, Guskova AK, Mettler FA (eds): *Medical Management of Radiation Accidents, 2d ed*. Boca Raton, FL, CRC Press, 2001, p. 56.
10. Kastengerg WE: Principal issues and future projects of nuclear energy, in Champlin RE (ed): Radiation Accidents and Nuclear Energy: Medical Consequences and Therapy. *Ann Intern Med* 109:739, 1998.
11. MacVittie TJ, Farese AM: Cytokine-based treatment for acute radiation-induced myelosuppression: Preclinical and clinical perspective, in Ricks R, Berger M, O'Hara FM (eds): *The Medical Basis for Radiation-Accident Preparedness*. New York, The Parthenon Publishing Group, 2002, p. 53.
12. Georges GE, Storb RF: Experimental and clinical experience with hematopoietic stem cell transplants, in Ricks R, Berger M, O'Hara FM (eds): *The Medical Basis for Radiation-Accident Preparedness*. New York, The Parthenon Publishing Group, 2002, p. 73.
13. McCarthy PL Jr: A perspective on clinical disorders of radiation accident victims. *Stem Cells* 15(Suppl 2):122, 1997.
14. Voelz GL, Bushberg JT: Medical management of internal contamination accidents, in Raabe O (ed): Internal Radiation Dosimetry. Madison, WI, Proceedings of the Health Physics Society, Medical Physics Publishers, 1994, p. 602.
15. Voelz GL: Assessment and treatment of internal contamination: General principles, in Gusev IA, Guskova AK, Mettler FA (eds): *Medical Management of Radiation Accidents, 2d ed*. Boca Raton, FL, CRC Press, 2001, p. 332.
16. Streffer C, Lake JV, Bock GR, Cardew G (eds): Biological effects of prenatal irradiation, in Lake JV, Bock GR, Cardew G (eds): *Health Impacts of Large Releases of Radionuclides*. Ciba Foundation Symposium 203. New York, John Wiley, 1997, p. 155.
17. Mettler FA Jr, Upton AC (eds): Radiation exposure in utero, in Mettler FA Jr, Upton AC (eds): *Medical Effects of Ionizing Radiation*, 2d ed. Philadelphia, WB Saunders, 1995, p. 322.

RESUSCITATIVE PROBLEMS AND TECHNIQUES

SUDDEN CARDIAC DEATH
Joseph P. Ornato

Sudden cardiac death (SCD) as a consequence of unexpected cardiac arrest claims the lives of more than 460,000 adult Americans each year and accounts for approximately 63 percent of all deaths from cardiovascular causes.[1] Despite advances in resuscitation and emergency medical services (EMS), only approximately 3 to 8 percent of all cardiac arrest victims survive to leave the hospital neurologically intact. However, there is substantial variability in the odds for survival among various geographic locations, with published survival to hospital discharge for patients with all initial rhythms ranging from 1 percent to 25 percent.[2–4] This chapter reviews the epidemiology and pathophysiology of SCD in adults, and the strategies to prevent and treat the problem. Sudden infant death syndrome and cardiac arrest in children are discussed in Chaps. 13 and 14, respectively.

EPIDEMIOLOGY

Most episodes of unexpected SCD in adults occur in the home.[5] The most common victim is a male who is 50 to 75 years of age. The majority of SCD victims have underlying structural heart disease, usually in the form of coronary atherosclerosis and/or cardiomegaly.[6] A recent review surmised that structural coronary artery abnormalities and their consequences (e.g., myocardial ischemia and infarction) are associated with 80 percent of fatal arrhythmias.[7] Dilated and hypertrophic cardiomyopathies are the next most common cardiac abnormalities causing SCD. Other cardiovascular disorders, including valvular or congenital heart disease, acquired infiltrative disorders, primary electrophysiologic abnormalities (e.g., hereditary prolonged Q-T interval syndromes), genetically determined ion-channel abnormalities (e.g., Brugada syndrome), account for only a small proportion of SCD cases.

Epidemiologic studies have identified both a circadian and a seasonal pattern of SCD and acute myocardial infarction (AMI), suggesting the presence of underlying biologic triggers of the onset of both disease processes.[8] Both SCD and AMI are most likely to occur within the first few hours after awakening from sleep, at a time when there is increased sympathetic stimulation. β-blockade appears to protect against SCD, particularly in patients with known coronary artery disease who have had an AMI and have a low ejection fraction. In addition, both SCD and AMI are much more likely to occur during climatic winter rather than summer.[8,9] These and other epidemiologic and experimental findings suggest that neurophysiologic factors, such as autonomic tone, may alter the heart's propensity to develop and sustain a serious ventricular dysrhythmia. An alternative possibility is that there are factors external to the atherosclerotic plaque, such as triggers of plaque rupture or thrombus formation, which may affect the onset of ischemic cardiac events.

PATHOPHYSIOLOGY

Ventricular Tachyarrhythmias

Sudden cardiac death is usually caused by chance arrhythmic events that are triggered by an interaction between structural heart abnormalities and transient, functional electrophysiologic disturbances. In the majority of cases, the initiating event is a ventricular tachyarrhythmia, either pulseless ventricular tachycardia (VT) that degenerates rapidly to ventricular fibrillation (VF) or "primary" VF.[10,11] From a public health standpoint, strategies for preventing and treating SCD in the community can be targeted primarily at VT and VF because these rhythms are not only the most frequent, but also the most potentially treatable, currently identified initiating event.

The mechanisms responsible for triggering fatal ventricular dysrhythmias are only partially understood. Frequent ventricular ectopy alone, in the absence of significant underlying structural heart disease, does not generally result in cardiac arrest. However, ventricular extrasystoles in the presence of transient myocardial ischemia, left ventricular dysfunction, and/or cardiomegaly may trigger runs of VT that may degenerate into pulseless VT or VF.

Many types of structural heart disease can predispose to SCD. One common denominator is dispersion of ventricular depolarization and/or repolarization, allowing "islands" of ventricular tissue to depolarize and repolarize at different rates. This lack of homogeneity in electrical activation and recovery fosters the development of circus movement reentry, which can initiate and sustain ventricular tachyarrhythmias. Myocardial ischemia and/or infarction can also diminish transiently the homogeneity of left ventricular depolarization and repolarization.

Left ventricular hypertrophy (often a result of hypertension and/or valvular heart disease) or conduction disturbances (left or right bundle-branch block or a nonspecific intraventricular conduction disturbance) can create similar functional disturbances on a more chronic basis. Preexcitation, such as the Wolf-Parkinson-White (WPW) syndrome, can trigger SCD if atrial fibrillation occurs and is conducted into the ventricles at a rate rapid enough to initiate VF. Other electrophysiologic mechanisms, such as Brugada syndrome [syncope with or without SCD caused by polymorphic ventricular tachycardia and associated with a distinctive electrocardiogram (ECG) pattern], can also cause SCD. Brugada syndrome is caused by an autosomal dominant, genetic defect resulting in total loss of function of the sodium channel or in acceleration of recovery from sodium channel activation.[12] It most commonly affects men and can be recognized by its pathognomonic ECG pattern (downsloping ST-segment elevation in leads V_{1-3}, often associated with a RBBB pattern) (Figure 11-1). It can be distinguished from benign early repolarization because Brugada syndrome causes right precordial ST-segment elevation that is downsloping and followed by a negative T wave, whereas early repolarization usually has ST elevation in V_{2-6} with an upward concavity, a notched J point, and a positive T wave. Although its prevalence in the United States is unknown, Brugada syndrome accounts for 40 to 50 percent of idiopathic ventricular fibrillation cases in some countries in Southeast Asia. Current treatment includes implantation of a cardioverter-defibrillator.

The long QT syndrome, in which the corrected QT interval (QT_c) is prolonged pathologically, is also associated with SCD.[12] Prolongation of the QT_c probably represents dispersion in ventricular repolarization and can be congenital (with or without nerve deafness) or acquired (caused by hypokalemia, hypomagnesemia, hypocalcemia, anorexia, ischemia, central nervous system pathology, terfenadine-ketoconazole combinations, or certain antipsychotic or antiarrhythmic drugs). The "QT_c" can be calculated by Bazett's equation:

$$QT_c = \frac{QT_m}{\sqrt{R - R}}$$

where QT_c is the corrected QT interval in seconds, QT_m is the measured QT interval in seconds, and $R - R$ is the interval between any two consecutive R waves on the ECG in seconds. Because the QT interval

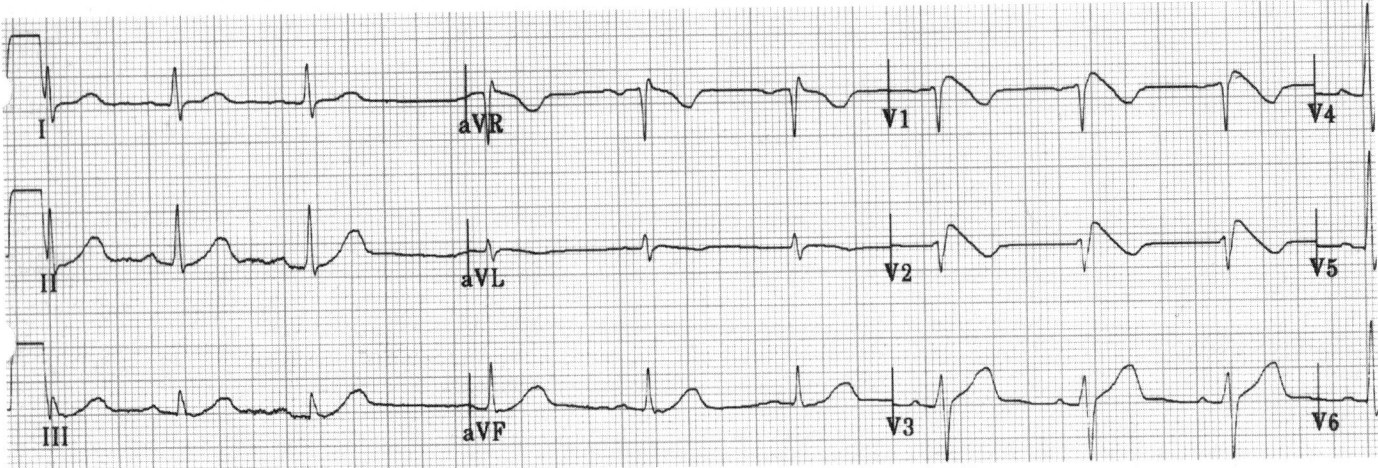

FIG. 11-1. Twelve-lead ECG typical of Brugada syndrome shows characteristic downsloping ST-segment elevation in leads V_1 and V_2 and QRS morphology resembling a right bundle-branch block. (Reproduced with permission from *Ann Emerg Med* 36:157, 2000.)

is heart-rate dependent, the formula "corrects" the measured QT interval to a heart rate of 60 beats/min (at which the R−R interval is 1.0 s). Because the square root of $1 = 1$, the QT_c equals the QT_m at a heart rate of 60 beats/min (at which the normal QT interval limits are 0.35 to 0.44 s).

Most SCD victims have cardiac abnormalities on postmortem examination. The most common autopsy findings in SCD victims are evidence of coronary atherosclerosis and its complications, cardiomegaly with left ventricular hypertrophy and contraction band necrosis. The latter appears to be a marker for catecholamine stimulation and occurs with high frequency regardless of whether CPR was performed.[13]

Factors affecting survival from out-of-hospital VF include witnessed collapse, prompt initiation of CPR, early defibrillation, younger age, and arrest occurring away from home.[14] Comorbid illnesses, such as a history of congestive heart failure, contribute to hospital mortality following successful resuscitation but only account for one-fourth of the variation in survival from SCD. Cardiac arrest during AMI is associated with a significantly *improved* outcome compared to cases not occurring in the setting of AMI.[15] Although the reason for improved long-term survival of AMI patients is not fully known, it probably occurs because such patients have *transient* electrical instability, unlike patients with chronic cardiomyopathy in whom there is a persistent vulnerability to VT or VF.

The outcome of resuscitation is influenced strongly by the patient's initial cardiac rhythm. The likelihood of survival is relatively high (up to 60 percent) if the initial rhythm is VT or VF (particularly if the VF is "coarse," the arrest is witnessed, and prompt CPR and defibrillation are provided). If the initial rhythm is not VT or VF, survival is typically less than 5 percent in most reported series. Asystolic patients whose cardiac arrest is unwitnessed rarely survive neurologically intact to hospital discharge. The only common exceptions are witnessed cardiac arrest patients whose initial asystole is a result of increased vagal tone or other relatively easily correctible factors, such as hypoxia of brief duration.

Bradyasystole

Although this chapter emphasizes VT and VF, an important minority of SCD events begin with a bradyarrhythmia[16] or an organized rhythm without a pulse [e.g., pulseless electrical activity (PEA)]. Bradyasystole refers to a cardiac rhythm that has a ventricular rate below 60 beats/min in adults and/or periods of absent heart rhythm (asystole). Bradyasystolic states are clinical situations during which bradyasystole is the dominant heart rhythm.

Bradyasystolic rhythms other than asystole can either be accompanied by a pulse or there can be no discernible pulse with each QRS (PEA). Bradyasystole with a pulse is often accompanied by a significant decrease in cardiac output, leading to hypotension and/or syncope. Bradycardia with or without a pulse occurs frequently during cardiac arrest, either as the initial rhythm, during the course of resuscitation, or following electrical defibrillation. Obviously, asystole occurs eventually in all dying patients.

To ensure that VF is not masquerading as asystole, the American Heart Association recommends confirmation of asystole by switching to another lead whenever a "flat line" is recorded on the ECG during resuscitation. Although there are anecdotal case reports in the literature suggesting that this phenomenon can occur in humans, "masquerading" VF probably occurs rarely during clinical resuscitation and is not responsible for the misdiagnosis of large numbers of cases of asystole.[17]

Primary bradyasystole occurs when the heart's electrical system intrinsically fails to generate and/or propagate an adequate number of ventricular depolarizations per minute to sustain consciousness and other vital functions. Secondary bradyasystole is present when factors external to the heart's electrical system cause it to fail (e.g., hypoxia). It is unclear why conventional treatment of bradyasystolic cardiac arrest with atropine, epinephrine, or electrical pacemakers rarely results in survival to hospital discharge.

Cellular metabolic functions must be intact for normal electrical impulse generation and propagation to occur. Severe ischemia of the sinoatrial (SA) node can disable cellular metabolism, preventing pacemaker cells from actively transporting the ions necessary to control the transmembrane action potential. Proximal occlusion of the right coronary artery (RCA) can cause ischemia and/or infarction of both the SA and atrioventricular (AV) nodes, because in humans, the SA node is supplied by a branch from the proximal RCA in 55 percent, and the AV node receives its nourishment from a branch of the distal RCA 90 percent of the time. Ischemia or infarction of the AV node can disrupt normal conduction, causing bradycardia as a consequence of AV block. Because the bundle branches receive their blood supply from multiple coronary arteries, bradyasystole caused by ischemic bilateral bundle-branch block is rare and generally only occurs when there is extensive myocardial infarction caused by severe, multivessel coronary artery disease.

The spectrum of disorders affecting the heart's primary pacemaker, known as the *sick sinus syndrome*, can cause intermittent lightheadedness, syncope, or SCD. The disorder affects both men and women. Although it is more common with advancing age, primary electrical failure of the heart can occur in infants and children. The precise cause of sick sinus syndrome is unknown. Pathologic studies usually reveal histologic degeneration of the SA node. In addition, the disorder often involves the AV node and the conduction tissue between the SA and AV nodes. Thus, sick sinus syndrome should be thought of as a diffuse degenerative disease of the heart's electrical generation and conduction system. Idiopathic sclerodegeneration of the AV node and the bundle branches (Lenègre disease) or invasion of the conduction system by fibrosis or calcification spreading from adjacent cardiac structures (Lev disease) can lead to bradyasystolic heart block with or without cardiac arrest. In rare cases, a clinical presentation resembling the sick sinus syndrome can occur when the heart's electrical system is affected by systemic disease, vascular compromise, or tumor (e.g., melanoma metastatic to the AV node).

Atropine, transcutaneous pacing, dopamine, or epinephrine can be used to treat acute, symptomatic bradyasystole (including cardiac arrest) that is caused by the sick sinus syndrome. Permanent ventricular or AV sequential pacing is usually necessary for patients with persistent symptomatic bradycardia. Patients who manifest the tachycardia-bradycardia variant (periods of supraventricular tachycardia followed by prolonged sinus arrest or bradycardia) may also require antiarrhythmic therapy or radiofrequency ablation.

Pacemaker cells and conducting tissue can be affected by a variety of endogenous chemical, hormonal, pharmacologic, toxicologic, and neurogenic influences. Hypoxia and hypercarbia, because of respiratory arrest, frequently cause bradyasystole as a consequence of both a direct depressant effect on cardiac pacemaker cells and increased parasympathetic discharge. Common clinical conditions that often cause bradyasystole include suffocation, near drowning, stroke, and opiate overdose. β-Adrenergic blocking agents, calcium channel blockers, digitalis glycosides, parasympathomimetic agents (e.g., edrophonium), hypoxia, hypercarbia, adenosine, and adenosine triphosphate can also cause bradyasystole.

Endogenous adenosine that is released when there is myocardial hypoxia and ischemia relaxes vascular smooth muscle, decreases atrial and ventricular contractility, depresses pacemaker automaticity, and impairs AV conduction. During normal aerobic metabolism, adenosine is formed primarily by intracellular degradation of S-adenosyl-L-homocysteine (SAH), catalyzed by the enzyme SAH hydrolase (SAH pathway). During myocardial ischemia, adenosine is formed primarily by dephosphorylation of adenosine monophosphate (AMP), catalyzed by the enzyme 5' nucleotidase [adenosine triphosphate (ATP) pathway].

The cellular electrophysiologic effects of adenosine can be antagonized competitively by methylxanthines but not by atropine. A specific adenosine antagonist (BW-A1433U) reverses and prevents postdefibrillation bradyasystole and hemodynamic depression in a domestic pig model. In small pilot studies, aminophylline, a competitive nonspecific adenosine antagonist, restored cardiac electrical activity within 30 s in more than half of the bradyasystolic cardiac arrest patients who were refractory to atropine and epinephrine.[18,19]

Myocardial ischemia excites cardiac vagal and sympathetic afferents, leading to vagally mediated depressor reflexes and/or sympathetic reflex cardioexcitation. In addition, myocardial infarction can interrupt afferent and efferent neural transmission, potentially triggering dysrhythmias. Autonomic disturbances have been documented in the majority of AMI patients, especially during the first 30 to 60 min after coronary artery occlusion. Stimulation of afferent vagal cardiac receptors, particularly those located in the posterior left ventricle, during ischemia or infarction can trigger sympathetic inhibition producing vasodilation, bradycardia, and hypotension (the Bezold-Jarisch reflex). Activation of this reflex may explain the higher incidence of nausea and vomiting in patients with inferior (69 percent) compared to anterior (29 percent) infarction. Bradyasystole triggered by the Bezold-Jarisch reflex is usually short-lived and often responds to atropine.

One of the most baffling mysteries of bradyasystolic cardiac arrest relates to myocardial mechanics. Bradyasystole, unlike ventricular fibrillation, is accompanied by very little myocardial oxygen consumption in animal models. Because of this, myocardial high-energy phosphate stores should decay relatively slowly during bradyasystole. This should theoretically result in a high incidence of return of spontaneous circulation following restoration of a more normal rhythm (e.g., with the early use of electrical pacing). However, return of spontaneous circulation is infrequent, and long-term neurologically intact survival is rare in bradyasystolic cardiac arrest.

These findings strongly suggest that other factors must play a determining role in the pathophysiology and subsequent outcome of bradyasystolic cardiac arrest. Bradyasystolic arrest is not just a disorder of rhythm generation or propagation; it is a perplexing syndrome characterized by such rhythm disturbances accompanied, in many cases, by profound depression of myocardial and vascular function. The causes of the latter derangements have yet to be elucidated. Suspected causes include endogenous myocardial depressants (including downregulation of catecholamine receptors and/or toxic influences of intense sympathetic stimulation), neurogenic influences, postischemic myocardial stunning, and/or free radical injury.

Pulseless Electrical Activity

Pulseless electrical activity can be caused by a variety of pathophysiologic conditions. The sine qua non of this syndrome is the presence of an organized rhythm without the presence of a detectable pulse in an individual who is clinically in cardiac arrest. The latter is important to differentiate conditions in which the rescuer is unable to detect a pulse, but there is unmistakable evidence that there is adequate blood pressure and cardiac output to maintain vital organ perfusion (e.g., a conscious patient with profound vasoconstriction caused by hypothermia, or "pseudo-PEA"). There is evidence that PEA encompasses a spectrum of pathophysiologic effects ranging from good left ventricular (LV) function with an empty ventricle or widely dilated arterial bed, to a stiff ventricle.

The underlying physiologic cause of PEA is a marked reduction in cardiac output that is a result of either profound myocardial depression or mechanical factors that reduce venous return or impede the flow of blood through the cardiovascular system. Common conditions that can cause PEA are shown in Table 11-1. In one recent analysis, PEA was present initially during resuscitation in 22 percent of cardiac arrest cases.[20] Compared to other patients, individuals with PEA were more likely to be women whose cardiac arrest was unwitnessed, at night, and without bystander-initiated CPR. Only 2 percent of these patients

TABLE 11-1   Common Causes of PEA

Hypovolemia
Tension pneumothorax
Pericardial tamponade
Pulmonary embolism
Massive myocardial dysfunction
  Infarction or ischemia
  Myocarditis
  Toxic myocardial depression
Profound shock of any cause
Hypoxia
Acidosis
Severe hypercarbia
Auto-PEEP
Cardiotoxins
  Tricyclic antidepressants
  β-blockers
  Calcium channel blockers
Hypothermia
Hyperkalemia
Pseudo-PEA
Post defibrillation pulselessness

Abbreviations: PEA = Pulseless electrical activity; PEEP = Positive expiratory pressure.

survived to hospital discharge. The management of patients with PEA is directed at identifying and treating the underlying cause or causes.

SCD PREVENTION

Prediction of SCD

It is necessary to accurately predict who is at risk for SCD for any prevention strategy to be of value. Unfortunately, the majority of future SCD victims cannot be identified in advance. Prodromal symptoms in the days to weeks preceding cardiac arrest are common but usually too nonspecific to be of important predictive value. In one of the largest series in which survivors of SCD were questioned about events preceding their collapse, Goldstein et al[21] found that 71 percent of SCD survivors reported no prodromal symptoms or symptoms of 1 h or less in duration. Prodromal symptoms were present for more than 1 h in only 29 percent of patients. The most common symptoms reported by SCD survivors or family members of SCD victims are chest pain, dyspnea, and palpitations.

Even aggressive attempts to predict SCD in high-risk patients, such as those who have suffered a prior AMI or those with a chronic cardiomyopathy, have been of limited value (Table 11-2). Various diagnostic techniques have been used to try to "risk stratify" these patients, including invasive and noninvasive assessment of left ventricular ejection fraction; coronary angiography; ambulatory ECG (Holter) monitoring; exercise testing; detection of ventricular late potentials by using signal averaging; programmed ventricular stimulation of the heart to test the inducibility of ventricular tachydysrhythmias; assessment of heart rate variability; and T-wave alternans (alternating T-wave amplitude from beat to beat on the ECG, which is only visible with special recording equipment).[6,22] None of these tests, alone or in combination, has sufficient sensitivity and specificity to identify more than a small fraction of those who will develop SCD. For example, only 15 to 30 percent of even "high-risk" post-AMI patients identified by a variety of these screening tests will experience a sustained ventricular tachydysrhythmia over the next several years of follow-up.[23] Despite this reality, it is critically important for emergency physicians to recognize signs and symptoms of the syndromes that place a patient at higher SCD risk and to admit or refer such patients for proper evaluation and preventive intervention promptly.

Antidysrhythmic Drug Therapy

Results of large randomized, controlled, clinical trials of antidysrhythmic agents for primary and secondary prevention of VT and VF are changing traditional beliefs regarding the actions, efficacy, and risk of these agents. The Cardiac Arrhythmia Suppression Trial (CAST) showed that potent class I sodium channel-blocking antidysrhythmic drugs (encainide, flecainide, and moricizine) are proarrhythmic and paradoxically increase the odds of developing SCD, as compared to placebo, in patients at relatively low risk for death.[24] Conversely, Class III agents (amiodarone, sotalol) and/or β-blockers may be of some protective value in patients at high SCD risk.

TABLE 11-2 Common Risk Factors for SCD in Adults Older than 35 Years of Age

Age
Male gender
Coronary artery disease (i.e., prior or acute myocardial infarction or unstable angina)
Cardiomegaly with left ventricular hypertrophy
Impaired left ventricular function (i.e., ejection fraction <30% and/or congestive heart failure)
Prolonged QT$_c$ interval
Ventricular arrhythmias, particularly sustained, inducible ventricular tachycardia

Implantable Cardioverter-Defibrillator Therapy

The benefits of β-blockade, sotalol, and amiodarone in decreasing mortality from SCD pale in comparison to the protective effects of the implantable cardioverter-defibrillator (ICD) on high-risk patients.[25] Treatment with an ICD is more effective than antidysrhythmic agents at reducing mortality in patients at high risk for SCD, as defined by a reduced left ventricular ejection fraction, documented nonsustained VT, and/or inducibility of sustained VT during programmed electrical stimulation.[26,27] Although these devices are expensive to insert, their effectiveness over conventional therapy results in a cost of less than $30,000 per year of life saved, which is highly cost-effective.[28] At present, these devices are indicated for preventing SCD in high-risk patients, particularly those with clinically significant coronary artery disease, depressed left ventricular function, and spontaneous life-threatening and/or inducible ventricular dysrhythmias. However, in some patients with advanced coronary atherosclerosis and a low ejection fraction who are candidates for mechanical revascularization, effective revascularization may obviate the need for ICD therapy. Prophylactic ICD insertion does not appear to provide additional survival benefit beyond that achieved with effective coronary revascularization.

Further research is ongoing to determine the value of ICD therapy in patients with nonischemic cardiomyopathy accompanied by reduced left ventricular function.

RESCUE FROM SCD

Emergency medical services and in-hospital resuscitation (also known as code blue or code 99) systems are the most effective means currently known to rescue patients from SCD. Survival from pulseless VT or VF is inversely related to the time interval between its onset and its termination. Each minute that a patient remains in VF, the odds of survival decrease by 7 to 10 percent. Survival is optimal when both CPR and advanced cardiac life support (ACLS), including defibrillation and drug therapy, are provided early.

The American Heart Association has introduced the "chain-of-survival" concept to represent a sequence of events that ideally should occur to maximize the odds of successful resuscitation from cardiac arrest.[11] The links in the chain include early access (recognition of the problem and activation of the EMS system by a bystander), early CPR, early defibrillation for patients who need it, and early advanced cardiac life support.

Early Access and Early CPR

Bystanders who witness the event can improve a victim's chances for survival significantly by alerting the emergency response system promptly. Although the value of bystander CPR was once debatable, virtually all recent studies show that early initiation of CPR by a bystander improves survival from cardiac arrest significantly, and it also results in improved neurologic outcome of survivors.[11] The presumed mechanism by which CPR by a bystander improves outcome is the preservation of flow to the heart, brain, and other vital organs, providing a "holding action" until other therapies (e.g., defibrillation) can result in restoration of spontaneous circulation.

Public CPR education can improve the behavior of bystanders significantly when a cardiac emergency occurs in the community. However, there are a number of problems associated with training the public to perform CPR. The typical cardiac arrest victim is male, age 50 to 75 years, and usually arrests at home, often in the presence of a spouse of similar age. Most citizens who have taken CPR training are younger than 30 years of age; typically, fewer than 10 percent live with family members known to have heart disease. Most citizens who have received CPR training never actually witness or participate in managing a cardiac arrest; conversely, bystanders who witness a cardiac arrest usually do not know how to perform CPR. Many laypersons who attempt to perform CPR out of hospital are actually employed or volunteer their services as health professionals. The best solution to the problem is to target CPR training to "high-risk" individuals, such as middle-aged persons, senior center residents and staff, and family members (particularly the spouse) of patients who are survivors of AMI or cardiac arrest or who have other risk factors for SCD.

Skill retention is also a problem because CPR is a psychomotor technique that deteriorates rapidly over time unless practiced or used. In Belgium, 46 percent of bystanders who performed CPR forgot to perform mouth-to-mouth breathing; chest compressions were not done 17 percent of the time.[29] As important as it is to receive at least annual reinforcement, only about 20 percent of trainees return for annual training in the United States. Fear of communicable disease, particularly infection with the human immunodeficiency virus (HIV), that is disproportionate to the known minimal risk of disease transmission may decrease the likelihood that trained rescuers will actually perform mouth-to-mouth ventilation on strangers.[30]

Early Defibrillation

The rationale for the use of early defibrillation stems from four observations: (1) ventricular tachydysrhythmias are the most common cause of SCD in adults; (2) defibrillation is the most effective treatment for VT and VF; (3) the effectiveness of defibrillation diminishes rapidly over time; and (4) unless treated promptly, VF becomes less coarse and eventually converts to the less treatable rhythm of fine VF or asystole.

Pulseless VT and VF in adults occur regularly in the electrophysiology laboratories. Prompt defibrillation (typically within 20 to 30 s of dysrhythmia onset) results in virtually 100 percent survival. Defibrillation, which can be performed within the first minute or two in cardiac rehabilitation programs, results in as many as 90 percent of patients resuscitated, with return to their prearrest neurologic status. Survival from out-of-hospital VT and VF treated by police officers equipped with automatic external defibrillators (AEDs) in Rochester, Minnesota, has averaged 50 percent resuscitation, with a median time from collapse to defibrillation of about 5 min. Outcomes in many locations with EMS systems that cannot provide defibrillation until 10 min or more after a patient's collapse typically yield survival rates of less than 10 percent.[11]

The best survival is attained in EMS systems that can provide early defibrillation to a large percentage of patients. In most cases, this is most cost-effectively accomplished by a tiered response system, in which large numbers of rapid first-response firefighters or emergency medical technicians (EMTs) are trained and equipped to provide first aid, CPR, and early defibrillation using an AED. Unfortunately, not all communities in the United States have yet implemented a comprehensive, tiered EMS system. Many systems, particularly in suburban or rural areas, have EMTs who are neither trained nor equipped to defibrillate. For such areas, adding rapid defibrillation capability offers a cost-effective alternative that can significantly improve survival from out-of-hospital VF or pulseless VT.

The American Heart Association advocates the widespread implementation of rapid defibrillation programs throughout the nation, including the training of all emergency personnel (volunteer or professional) whose activities require response or competence in managing cardiac arrest. All emergency ambulances and other emergency vehicles that respond to or transport cardiac patients should be equipped with a defibrillator.[31]

More novel strategies have also been tried to increase the availability of rapid defibrillation in the community. There are many densely populated public areas in which conventional EMS systems *cannot* respond within an acceptable response time interval. The most innovative idea is termed *public access defibrillation* (PAD), so named because the intent is to have citizens from outside the health care fields perform early defibrillation using AEDs.

There are three "levels" of PAD based on the type of potential first responder expected to use the AED. There has been considerable experience demonstrating benefit with minimal risk for level 1 nontraditional responders (e.g., police, firefighters, security personnel, sports marshals, ski patrol members, ferryboat crews, flight attendants, airport personnel) who have a duty to respond as part of their everyday responsibilities.

Level 2 refers to targeted, trained "citizen responders" who may be employed by a worksite with a PAD program but who do not have an explicit duty to respond. There has been good experience with level 2 AED workplace use in British rail stations, oil platforms in the North Sea, electricity plants, passenger cruise ships, gambling casinos, and merchant marine vessels.[11] Level 3 responders are trained family members and/or friends living with or visiting a person at high risk for SCD. There has been little experience thus far with level 3 AED use, and the few studies that have been reported have been somewhat disappointing. For example, Eisenberg et al. trained family members of 59 patients who had survived out-of-hospital cardiac arrest in King County, Washington.[32] Only 6 of 10 cardiac arrests that occurred in these patients were defibrillated successfully, and only 1 patient survived for a few months with sustained new neurologic impairment. Further study is needed to determine the risks and benefits of AED use by the general public, and also to identify optimal locations for AED placement.

Early ACLS

Physicians provide prehospital ACLS by staffing specially equipped ambulances in many countries (e.g., Western Europe, Scandinavia, Czech Republic, and Canada). In the United States, "intermediate"-level EMTs or paramedics provide most prehospital ACLS intervention (e.g., defibrillation or synchronized cardioversion, endotracheal intubation, intravenous fluid therapy, or drug administration). Intermediate EMTs (often called cardiac technicians) typically receive several hundred hours of training; paramedics usually receive 1000 or more hours. Adding field ACLS capability appears to affect survival from out-of-hospital cardiac arrest favorably, although the degree of benefit is relatively minimal compared to the powerful effect of early defibrillation.[11]

REFERENCES

1. Centers for Disease Control and Prevention: State-specific mortality from sudden cardiac death-United States, 1999. *MMWR* 51:123–126, 2002.
2. Lombardi G, Gallagher J, Gennis P: Outcome of out of hospital cardiac arrest in New York City: The Pre-Hospital Arrest Survival Evaluation (PHASE) study. *JAMA* 271:678, 1994.
3. Becker LB, Ostrander MP, Barrett J, et al: Outcome of CPR in a large metropolitan area: Where are the survivors? *Ann Emerg Med* 20:355, 1991.
4. Eisenberg MS Howard BT, Cummins RO, et al: Cardiac arrest and resuscitation: A tale of 29 cities. *Ann Emerg Med* 19:179, 1990.
5. Becker L, Eisenberg M, Fahrenbruck C, Cobb L: Public locations of cardiac arrest: Implications for public access defibrillation. *Circulation* 97:2106, 1998.
6. Huikuri HV, Castellanos A, Myerburg RJ. Sudden death due to cardiac arrhythmias. *New Engl J Med* 345:1473, 2001.
7. Myerburg RJ, Interian A Jr, Mitrani RM, et al: Frequency of sudden cardiac death and profiles of risk. *Am J Cardiol* 80:10F, 1997.
8. Ornato JP, Peberdy MA, Chondra NC, Bush DE: Seasonal pattern of acute myocardial infarction in the National Registry of Myocardial Infarction. *J Am Coll Cardiol* 28:1684, 1996.
9. Hohnloser SH, Klingenheben T: Insights into the pathogenesis of sudden cardiac death from analysis of circadian fluctuations of potential triggering factors. *Pacing Clin Electrophysiol* 17:428, 1994.
10. Bayes de Luna A, Coumel P, Leclercq JF: Ambulatory sudden cardiac death: Mechanisms of production of fatal arrhythmia on the basis of data from 157 cases. *Am Heart J* 117:151, 1989.
11. Cummins RO, Ornato JP, Thies WH, Pepe PE: Improving survival from sudden cardiac arrest: the "chain of survival" concept: A statement for health professionals from the Advanced Cardiac Life Support Subcommittee and the Emergency Cardiac Care Committee, American Heart Association. *Circulation* 83:1832, 1991.

12. Brugada P, Geelen P: Some electrocardiographic patterns predicting sudden cardiac death that every doctor should recognize. *Acta Cardiol* 52:473, 1997.

13. Davies MJ: Anatomic features in victims of sudden coronary death: Coronary artery pathology. *Circulation* 85(suppl 1):119, 1992.

14. Hallstrom AP, Cobb LA, Ben Hui Y: Influence of comorbidity on the outcome of patients treated for out-of-hospital ventricular fibrillation. *Circulation* 93:2019, 1996.

15. Beuret P, Feihl F, Vogt P, et al: Cardiac arrest: Prognostic factors and outcome at one year. *Resuscitation* 25:171, 1993.

16. Ornato JP, Peberdy MA: The mystery of bradyasystole during cardiac arrest. *Ann Emerg Med* 27:576, 1996.

17. Cummins RO, Austin D Jr: The frequency of "occult" ventricular fibrillation masquerading as a flat line in prehospital cardiac arrest. *Ann Emerg Med* 17:813, 1988.

18. Viskin S, Belhassen B, Roth A, et al: Aminophylline for bradyasystolic cardiac arrest refractory to atropine and epinephrine. *Ann Intern Med* 118:279, 1993.

19. Mader TJ, Gibson P: Adenosine receptor antagonism in refractory asystolic cardiac arrest: Results of a human pilot study. *Resuscitation* 35:3, 1997.

20. Herlitz J, Estrom L, Wennerblom B, et al: Survival among patients with out-of-hospital cardiac arrest found in electromechanical dissociation. *Resuscitation* 29:97, 1995.

21. Goldstein S, Mendendorp SV, Landis JR, et al: Analysis of cardiac symptoms preceding cardiac arrest. *Am J Cardiol* 58:1195, 1986.

22. Breithardt G, Borggrefe M, Fetsch T, et al: Prognosis and risk stratification after myocardial infarction. *Eur Heart J* 16(suppl G):10, 1995.

23. Gilman JK, Jalal S, Naccarelli GV: Predicting and preventing sudden death from cardiac causes. *Circulation* 90:1083, 1994.

24. Pratt CM, Moye LA: The Cardiac Arrhythmia Suppression Trial: Background, interim results and implications. *Am J Cardiol* 65:20B, 1990.

25. Haverkamp W, Eckardt L, Borggrefe M, Breithardt G: Drugs versus devices in controlling ventricular tachycardia, ventricular fibrillation, and recurrent cardiac arrest. *Am J Cardiol* 80:67G, 1997.

26. Moss AJ, Hall WJ, Cannom DS, et al: Improved survival with an implanted defibrillator in patients with coronary disease at high risk for ventricular arrhythmia. *New Engl J Med* 335:1933, 1996.

27. Buxton AE, Lee KL, Fisher JD, et al: A randomized study of the prevention of sudden death in patients with coronary artery disease. *New Engl J Med* 341:1882, 1999.

28. Mushlin AI, Hall WJ, Zwanziger J, et al: The cost-effectiveness of automatic implantable cardiac defibrillators: Results from MADIT (Multicenter Automatic Defibrillator Implantation Trial). *Circulation* 97:2129, 1998.

29. Bossaert L, Van Hoeyweghen R: Cerebral Resuscitation Study Group: Evaluation of cardiopulmonary resuscitation (CPR) techniques. *Resuscitation* 17:S99, 1989.

30. Ornato JP, Hallagan LF, McMahan SB, et al: Attitudes of BCLS instructors about mouth-to-mouth resuscitation during the AIDS epidemic. *Ann Emerg Med* 19:151, 1990.

31. Kerber RE: Statement on early defibrillation from the Emergency Cardiac Care Committee, American Heart Association. *Circulation* 83:2233, 1991.

32. Eisenberg MS, Moore J, Cummins RO, et al: Use of the automatic external defibrillator in homes of survivors of out-of-hospital ventricular fibrillation. *Am J Cardiol* 63:443, 1989.

BASIC CARDIOPULMONARY RESUSCITATION IN ADULTS
Jon Mark Hirshon

CPR is a key part of emergency medical care designed to resuscitate individuals in cardiac arrest. The purpose of cardiopulmonary resuscitation is to temporarily provide effective oxygenation of vital organs, especially the brain and heart, through artificial circulation of oxygenated blood until the restoration of normal cardiac and respiratory activity occurs. The intended effect is to stop the degenerative processes of ischemia and anoxia caused by inadequate circulation and inadequate oxygenation. Quick initiation of cardiopulmonary resuscitation is critical to improve the likelihood of recovery; ideally, it should be started within 4 min of arrest, and advanced cardiac life support should be initiated within 8 min of arrest. While basic life support alone may be lifesaving in some instances, in most cases advanced interventions such as the delivery of electric current for defibrillation and the addition of various pharmacologic therapies are required to maximize the likelihood of patient recovery. Without rhythm-specific interventions, recovery from cardiac arrest is highly unlikely.[1]

This chapter reviews basic CPR for adults (≥8 years), including approach to an unresponsive patient, basic airway opening procedures including initial management of an obstructed airway, and the physiology and mechanics of closed-chest compression techniques.

Overview

As with all aspects of emergency medicine, it is important to approach basic CPR systematically. When someone is found unresponsive, the following should be performed rapidly and in sequence:

1. Assess responsiveness. If unresponsive, then
2. Obtain assistance and activate the local emergency medical service system, called "phone first" in American Heart Association Guidelines.[1]
3. Call for a defibrillator (if available).
4. Position the patient and open the airway (maintain cervical spine immobilization if trauma is potentially involved).
5. Assess breathing. If no breathing is noted, then
6. Give two slow breaths.
7. Assess circulation. If no pulse noted, then
8. Begin closed-chest compressions and continue ventilations. Use the defibrillator if available and indicated.

Initial Actions

Upon discovery of a collapsed individual, the first medical action should be to assess the victim and determine whether the person is unresponsive. However, prior to approaching a collapsed individual, the scene needs to be fully assessed for dangers to health care providers. Potential risks, whether from hazardous materials, an unstable physical environment, or personal violence should be considered. Once the patient is reached, the level of responsiveness to noxious stimuli can be determined quickly. If the individual is not responding, obtain help prior to starting ventilations and chest compressions. In a hospital, this may mean calling for the arrest team and requesting the arrest cart; outside the hospital, this is likely to involve activation of the local emergency medical services system or asking a bystander to do so. Additionally, efforts should be made to obtain a defibrillator. Rapid administration of rhythm-specific therapy, especially defibrillation for unstable ventricular tachycardia or ventricular fibrillation, is critical for the recovery of patients.

Open the Airway

The next step is to assess the upper airway of the victim. This usually requires positioning the individual supine on a flat, firm surface with arms along the sides of the body, followed by opening the person's airway. Unless trauma can be definitely excluded, any movement of the victim should take into account the potential of a spine injury; as the patient is placed supine, stabilize the cervical spine by maintaining the head, neck, and trunk in a straight line. If the neck is not already straight, then it should be moved the least possible that allows the establishment of an airway. If for some reason the patient cannot be placed supine, consider using the jaw-thrust maneuver (see below) from a lateral position to open the airway. Properly opening the airway is a critical and potentially lifesaving step. Common causes for airway obstruction in an unconscious patient are occlusion of the oropharynx by the tongue and laxity of the epiglottis. With loss of muscle tone, the tongue or the epiglottis can be forced back into the oropharynx upon inspiration. This can create the effect of a one-way valve at the entrance to the trachea, leading to airway obstruction manifesting as inspiratory stridor. After positioning the patient, the mouth and oropharynx should be inspected for secretions or foreign objects, including loose dentures. If secretions are present, they can be removed with the use of oropharyngeal suction if available; a foreign body may be dislodged by use of a finger sweep and then manually removed (see below).

Once the oropharynx has been cleared, two basic maneuvers for opening the airway may be tried to relieve upper airway obstruction. These are the head tilt–chin lift and the jaw thrust. These maneuvers help to open the airway by mechanically displacing the mandible and the attached tongue out of the oropharynx.

HEAD TILT–CHIN LIFT MANEUVER

The head tilt–chin lift is usually the first maneuver attempted if there is no concern for cervical spine injury. The head tilt is performed by gently extending the neck. This is done by placing one hand under the patient's neck and the other on the forehead and extending the head in relation to the neck. This should place the patient's head in the sniffing position with the nose pointing up. In conjunction with the head tilt, the chin lift is performed. This is done by carefully placing the hand which had been supporting the neck for the head tilt under the symphysis of the mandible, taking care not to compress the soft tissues of the submental triangle and the base of the tongue. The mandible is then lifted forward and up until the teeth barely touch. This supports the jaw and helps tilt the head back.

JAW-THRUST MANEUVER

The jaw thrust is the safest method for opening the airway if there is the possibility of cervical spine injury. It helps to maintain the cervical spine in a neutral position during resuscitation. The rescuer, who is positioned at the head of the patient, places the hands at the sides of the victim's face, grasps the mandible at its angle, and lifts the mandible forward (Figure 12-1). This lifts the jaw and opens the airway with minimal head movement.

Assess Breathing and Initiate Ventilation

Once the airway has been opened, assessment of respiratory effort and air movement should occur. The care provider should look for chest expansions and listen and feel for airflow. The simple act of opening the airway may be adequate for the return of spontaneous respirations. However, if the victim remains without adequate respiratory effort, then further intervention is required. If rescuers are reluctant to perform mouth-to-mouth ventilation, and the patient is in cardiac arrest, chest compressions alone can be effective (see Techniques of Closed-Chest Compressions below).

Two slow breaths over 2 s each should be given. At this point, if a foreign body obstruction is noted, as indicated by a lack of chest rise or airflow on ventilation, the obstruction requires removal (Figure 12-2). Agonal respirations in an individual who has just suffered a cardiac arrest are not considered adequate. Intermittent positive-pressure ventilation, if possible with oxygen-enriched air, should be initiated.

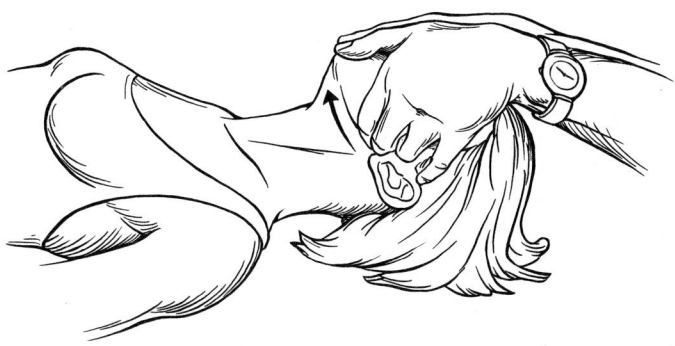

FIG. 12-1. Jaw-thrust maneuver.

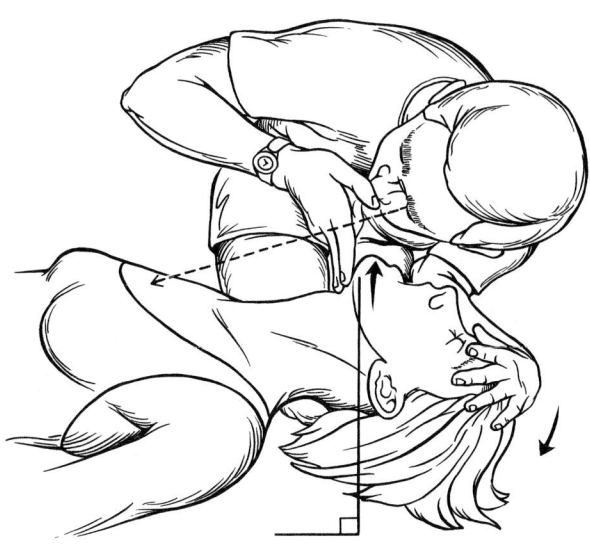

FIG. 12-2. Determine breathlessness.

VENTILATION TECHNIQUES

Ventilation
    Without Supplemental Oxygen
        Rate: 10 to 12 per min
        Amount: 10 mL/kg (700 to 1000 mL)

    With Supplemental Oxygen ($\geq$40 percent)
        Rate: 10 to 12 per min
        Amount: 6 to 7 mL/kg (400 to 600 mL)

There are a number of techniques for ventilating an individual, including mouth to mouth, mouth to nose, mouth to stoma, and mouth to mask. Rescue breaths with an inspiratory time of over 2 s each should be given at a rate of 10 to 12 per min, with a volume adequate to make the chest rise visibly (10 mL/kg; 700 to 1000 mL in adults). Expired air has a F_{IO_2} of 16 to 17 percent. Supplemental oxygen should be delivered as soon as possible. If supplemental oxygen ($\geq$40 percent) is available, a smaller tidal volume of 6 to 7 mL/kg (400 to 600 mL for adults) may be used.[1]

Too large a volume or too rapid an inspiratory flow rate will likely cause gastric distention, which can lead to regurgitation and aspiration. If an additional trained rescuer is available, cricoid pressure may be applied in an attempt to limit gastric inflation and distention. This is done by applying a moderate amount of firm pressure on the cricoid cartilage, located directly below the thyroid cartilage.

Mouth to Mouth With the airway open, the patient's nose should be gently pinched shut with the rescuer's thumb and index finger (Figure 12-3). This prevents air escape. After taking a deep breath, the rescuer places his or her lips around the patient's mouth, forming an airtight seal. The rescuer slowly exhales. Release the seal and allow adequate time for passive exhalation by the victim, and then repeat the procedure. Protective devices such as face shields are commonly available to decrease the risks to the provider of contracting an infectious disease, and can be purchased from most medical equipment stores.

Mouth to Nose In some cases, as with severe maxillofacial trauma, mouth-to-nose ventilation may be more effective. With the airway open, the rescuer lifts the patient's jaw, closing the mouth. After a deep breath, the rescuer places his or her lips around the patient's nose, forming an airtight seal. The rescuer slowly exhales.

Mouth to Stoma or Tracheostomy After laryngectomy or tracheotomy, the stoma or tracheostomy becomes the patient's airway. As with the other techniques, a seal is made around the stoma or tracheostomy tube, and the rescuer slowly exhales.

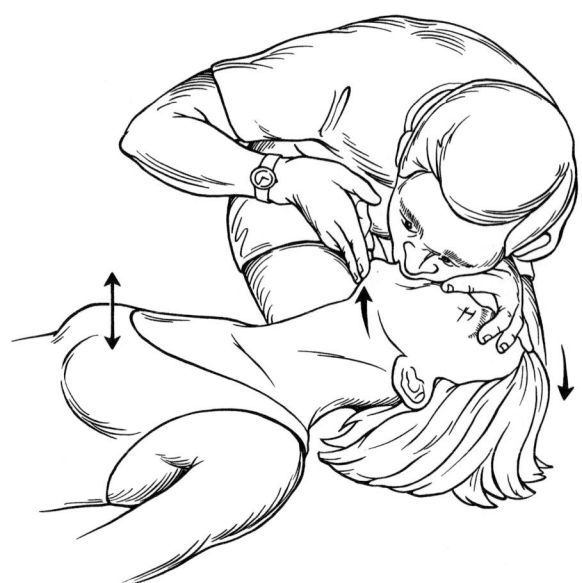

FIG. 12-3. Mouth-to-mouth rescue breathing.

Mouth to Mask   Placement of the mask properly and securely on a victim's face is important when using a mask for ventilation, either with a bag or via mouth to mask. The mask should be placed over the bridge of the patient's nose and around the mouth. The rescuer places the thumb on the part of the mask that is sitting on the patient's nose and places the index finger of the same hand on the part of the mask sitting on the patient's chin (Figure 12-4). The three other fingers of the same hand are then placed along the bony margin of the jaw. The mask can then be firmly sealed to the patient's face. Two hands may be used for this technique if a second rescuer is available. Ventilations are then performed through the mask; some masks also allow for supplemental oxygenation.

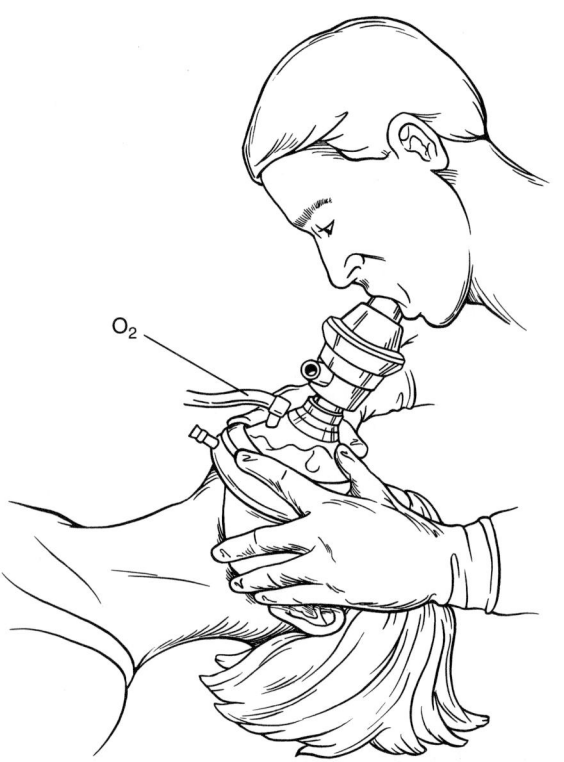

FIG. 12-4. Mouth-to-mask rescue breathing with proper mask placement.

Foreign Body Obstruction

It is important to recognize and be able to assist someone with an airway obstruction due to a foreign body. The National Safety Council reported that approximately 3200 deaths (1.2 per 100,000) were caused by foreign body airway obstruction in 1998.[2] An individual in distress from a compromised airway is likely to use the universal sign for an airway obstruction, which is for the individual to grab his or her neck with both hands. Foreign bodies can cause partial or complete obstruction. With a partial airway obstruction, air exchange may be adequate or inadequate. If the victim is able to speak, cough, and exchange air, then he or she should be encouraged to continue spontaneous efforts. Assistance, such as activation of the local emergency medical services system, should be obtained. No interference should be made with the patient's attempts to cough or expel the foreign body. If air exchange becomes inadequate, as indicated by an inability to speak, increased difficulty breathing, weak and ineffective cough, worsening inspiratory stridor, or cyanosis, immediate medical intervention should be performed. Inadequate air exchange from a severe partial or a complete airway obstruction should be managed the same way. In an unconscious person, the presence of airway obstruction may be ascertained by noting inadequate airflow and poor chest rise with efforts to ventilate.

OBSTRUCTION-RELIEVING MANEUVERS   Maneuvers used to relieve foreign body obstructions include the Heimlich maneuver (subdiaphragmatic abdominal thrusts), chest thrusts, and the finger sweep. In a conscious individual, the Heimlich maneuver is the recommended maneuver in most adults for relieving airway obstruction due to a solid object. It is not useful for liquids. In an unconscious individual suspected of having an aspirated foreign body, the recommended first step is the finger sweep. Otherwise, in an unconscious patient the recommended sequence is to perform the Heimlich maneuver up to five times, open the mouth and perform a finger sweep, and then attempt to ventilate. This sequence may be repeated as often as needed until the patient recovers or additional assistance arrives.

HEIMLICH MANEUVERS   Described by Dr. Heimlich in 1975, this maneuver creates an artificial cough by forcefully elevating the diaphragm and forcing air from the lungs.[3] It may be repeated multiple times; each individual thrust should be performed with the intention of removing the obstruction. It can be performed with the victim standing, sitting, or lying down, or it can be self-administered (Figure 12-5). To perform the maneuver with the patient standing or sitting, the rescuer stands behind the patient and places the thumb side of a fist against the victim's abdomen midline just above the navel and well below the xiphoid process (Figure 12-5). Grasping the fist with the other hand, the rescuer presses the fist into the victim's abdomen with a quick upward thrust. This is repeated until the item is dislodged or the patient becomes unconscious. For an unconscious patient, the individual is placed supine on a firm surface with the rescuer sitting astride the victim's thighs (Figure 12-6). The heel of a hand is positioned midline just above the patient's umbilicus, and the second hand is placed directly on top of the first. The rescuer then delivers quick upward thrusts. To self-administer thrusts, the individual can either use his or her own fist to deliver the thrusts or lean forcibly against a firm object, such as a porch rail or the back of a chair. Potential complications of the Heimlich maneuver include injury or rupture of abdominal or thoracic viscera and regurgitation of stomach contents.

CHEST THRUSTS   This maneuver is used primarily if someone is morbidly obese or in the late stages of pregnancy and the rescuer cannot reach around the patient's abdomen to perform abdominal thrusts (Figure 12-7). To perform chest thrusts with the patient standing or sitting, the rescuer stands behind the patient and places the thumb side of

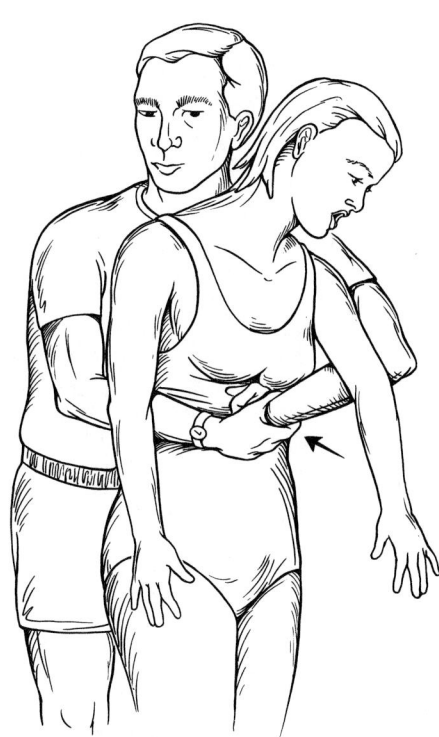

FIG. 12-5. Standing Heimlich maneuver administered to conscious victim of foreign body airway obstruction.

a fist against the victim's sternum, avoiding the costal margins and the xiphoid process. Grasping the fist with the other hand, the rescuer presses the fist into the victim's chest with a quick backward thrust. This is repeated until the item is dislodged or the patient becomes unconscious. For an unconscious patient, the individual is placed supine on a firm surface with the rescuer kneeling close to the victim's side. The hands are placed in the same position as for chest compression (i.e., the lower sternum), and quick thrusts are delivered.

FINGER SWEEP This maneuver is used only in unconscious patients (Figure 12-8). Using the thumb and fingers of one hand, the rescuer grasps both the tongue and the mandible and lifts. This may partially relieve the obstruction by lifting the tongue away from the back of the throat. With the other hand, the rescuer then inserts his or her

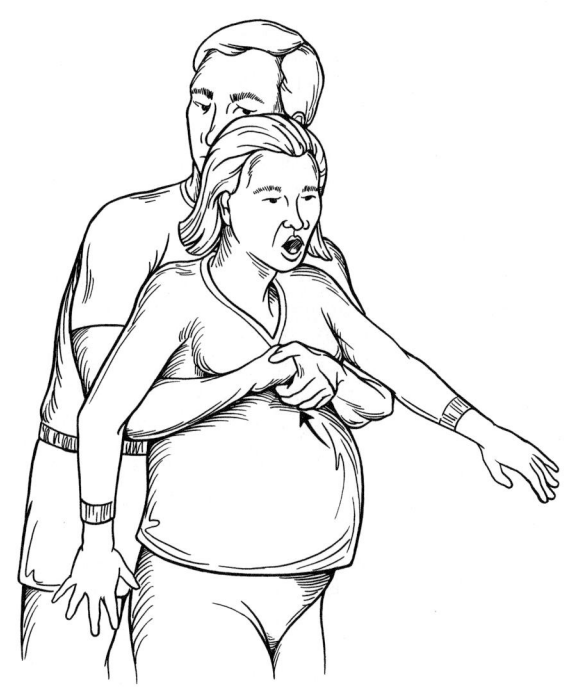

FIG. 12-7. Standing chest-thrust maneuver administered to conscious victim of foreign body airway obstruction.

index finger into the back of the throat and uses a hooking action in an attempt to dislodge the foreign body to move it into the mouth for manual removal. Care must be used so as to not push the foreign object deeper into the throat.

Assess Circulation and Initiate Compressions

The carotid artery is generally the most reliable and accessible location to palpate a pulse. The artery can be located by placing two fingers on the trachea and then sliding them down to the groove between

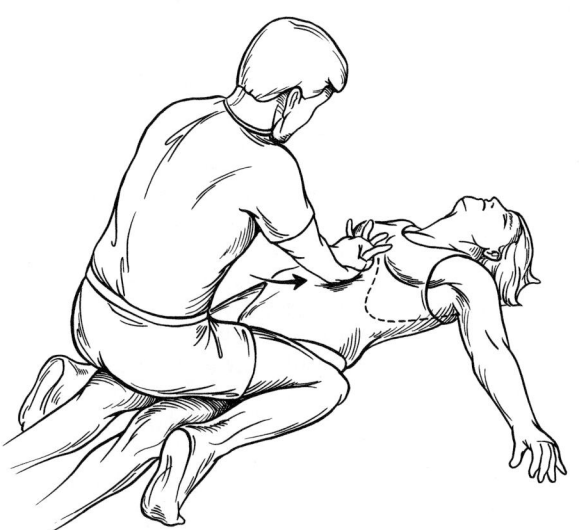

FIG. 12-6. Prone Heimlich maneuver administered to unconscious victim of foreign body airway obstruction.

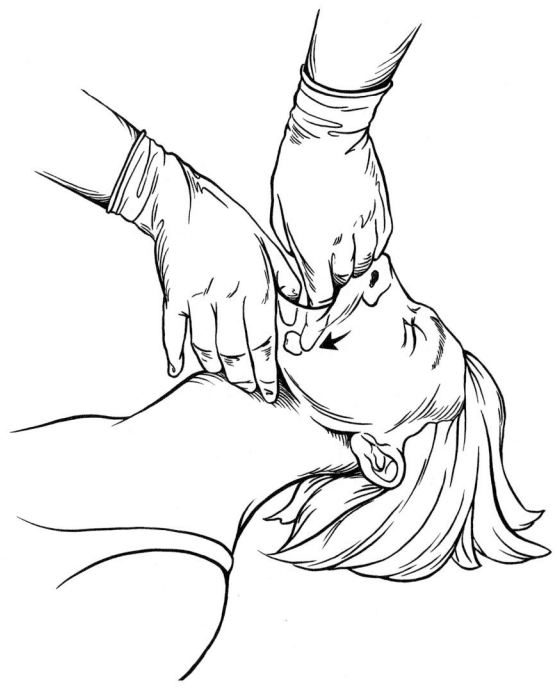

FIG. 12-8. Finger-sweep maneuver administered to unconscious victim of foreign body airway obstruction.

the trachea and the sternocleidomastoid muscle. Simultaneous palpation of both carotid arteries should not be performed because in low-pressure states this could obstruct cerebral blood flow and may interfere with the ability to detect a pulse. The femoral artery may be used as an alternative site to palpate a pulse. This can be found just below the inguinal ligament approximately halfway between the anterosuperior iliac spine and the pubic tubercle. If no pulse is felt after 5 to 10 s, chest compressions should begin.

PHYSIOLOGY OF CLOSED-CHEST COMPRESSIONS Since the technique of closed-chest compressions was put forth initially by Kouwenhoven and colleagues in the 1960s, there has been an active debate as to the exact mechanism that causes blood flow.[4,5] In a closed system, liquid flows when pressure gradients develop. There are three basic theories for how pressure gradients and flow are produced during closed-chest cardiac massage.[6,7] The conventional theory of blood flow during compressions is called the *cardiac pump theory*. This postulates that direct compression of the heart between the spine and the sternum leads to increased pressure in the ventricles. This causes closure of the mitral and tricuspid valves, leading to blood flow into the aorta and the pulmonary arteries. The *thoracic pump theory* postulates that compressions lead to an increase in pressure throughout the thoracic cavity, leading to a pressure gradient from intrathoracic to extrathoracic arteries. The third mechanism described is the *abdominal pump theory*, which has both an arterial and a venous component. The arterial component postulates blood flow into the peripheral arterial system from increased arterial pressure caused by abdominal compressions that forces blood from the abdominal aorta against the closed aortic valve. The venous component leads to blood return via the inferior vena cava from abdominal pressure. However, regardless of the mechanism, conventional chest compressions generate one-fourth to one-third of physiologic cardiac output. Lower ratios can be expected with delays in initiating compressions.

TECHNIQUES OF CLOSED-CHEST COMPRESSIONS
Closed-Chest Compressions:

1. Depth: $1\frac{1}{2}$ - 2 in (3.8 to 5.1 cm)
2. Rate: Approximately 100 per min

Ventilations:

1. Single rescuer or two rescuer non-intubated patient: 2 ventilations after every 15 compressions
2. Two rescuer, intubated patient: 1 ventilation after every fifth compression

Upon confirmation that an individual is without a pulse, serial rhythmic closed-chest compressions should be initiated. The victim is placed supine on a firm surface with the rescuer at the side. The care provider places the heel of one hand midline on the lower half of the sternum, approximately 2 in. (5 cm) cephalad of the xiphoid process (Figure 12-9). The heel of the hand should be parallel with the long axis of the patient's body. The second hand is then placed on top of the first hand so the hands are parallel with each other. The fingers of the two hands may be interlaced if desired, but they should not be touching the chest. The arms should be straight and the elbows preferably locked. The vector of the compression force should start from the rescuer's shoulders and be directed downward; lateral forces will decrease efficiency of the compressions and increase the likelihood of complications. The sternum should be depressed $1\frac{1}{2}$ to 2 in. (3.8 to 5.1 cm) in an adult at a rate of approximately 100 compressions per min. Rates lower than this are inadequate. The compression-release phases should be roughly equal in length. With a single rescuer or with two rescuers if the patient is not intubated, 2 ventilations should be given after every 15 compressions. With two rescuers assisting an intubated patient, a ventilation should be given after every fifth compression. Of

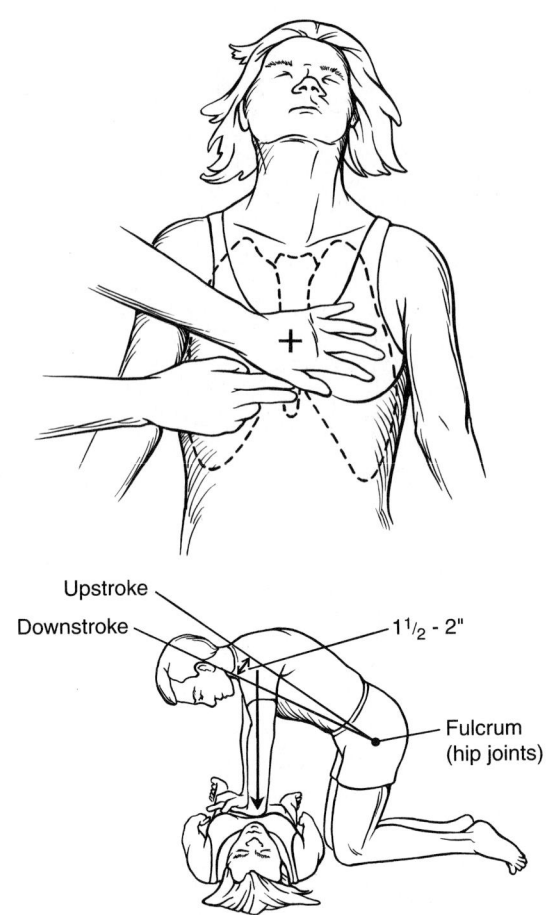

FIG. 12-9. Proper hand and rescuer positioning for chest compression.

note, while assisting ventilation is important, not everyone is willing to perform mouth-to-mouth breathing due to concerns over infectious disease transmission. Chest compressions alone can be effective and should be provided even if rescue breathing is not being performed.[8]

There are currently several experimental techniques for improving the effectiveness of closed-chest cardiac massage. In one method, circumferential chest compressions are performed by a pneumatic vest to more effectively increase intrathoracic pressure during chest compressions.[9] In interposed abdominal compression CPR, abdominal compression occurs during the relaxation phase of chest compression, causing increased aortic diastolic pressure and leading to improved blood flow to organs above the diaphragm.[10] In active compression-decompression CPR, a hand-held suction device is used to decrease intrathoracic pressure during the relaxation phase of chest compression and to improve ventricular filling.[11] Additionally, self-initiated cardiopulmonary resuscitation can be performed by forceful coughing. This increases intrathoracic pressure, leading to blood flow to the brain for as long as the patient remains conscious and able to cough.[12] Increased understanding of the physiology of cardiopulmonary resuscitation is leading to improved circulatory adjuncts, such as interposed abdominal compression CPR and active compression-decompression CPR, and may lead to improved CPR by experienced practitioners.[13,14] Currently, however, availability of these adjuncts should not delay the initiation of closed-chest cardiac massage.

Open-chest cardiac massage is an additional alternative to standard CPR, and has been shown to improve blood flow in animal models. While there are no data showing improved clinical outcome with the use of open-chest cardiac massage versus closed-chest cardiac massage, this technique may be considered in a number of situations, including (1) after penetrating chest trauma; (2) the perioperative period before or after cardiothoracic surgery; (3) cardiac arrest caused by hypothermia, pulmonary embolism, pericardial tamponade, or abdominal hemorrhage; (4) cases of chest deformity in which closed-chest CPR is ineffective; (5) penetrating abdominal trauma with deterioration and cardiac arrest; and (6) blunt trauma with cardiac arrest.[14] However, the use of this technique requires a well-coordinated multidisciplinary team (see Chap. 259).

Complications of Cardiopulmonary Resuscitation

Ventilations can cause insufflation of the stomach, leading to regurgitation and aspiration and possibly to gastric rupture. Closed-chest compressions can lead to fractures of the sternum or the ribs, separation of the ribs from the sternum, pulmonary contusion, pneumothorax, myocardial contusion, hemorrhagic pericardial effusions, splenic laceration, or liver laceration. Proper techniques can minimize these complications but cannot totally prevent them. Late complications include pulmonary edema, gastrointestinal hemorrhage, pneumonia, and recurrent cardiopulmonary arrest. Anoxic brain injury can occur in a resuscitated individual subjected to prolonged hypoxia; it is the most common cause of death in resuscitated patients.

Terminating Resuscitation

Efforts at resuscitation should be continued until the patient recovers spontaneous respirations and cardiac output, the rescuer becomes exhausted, or the patient is pronounced dead. An atraumatic individual who recovers spontaneous respirations and circulation should be placed on their side—the *recovery position*. Recovery from cardiac arrest depends on time to CPR and rhythm-specific intervention. Resuscitation and long-term outcome in normothermic patients with arrest times of 20 min or more are very poor.

Ethical Considerations in Resuscitation (also see Chap. 17)

While resuscitation attempts are initiated, efforts should be made to discover whether or not the victim has advance directives that prohibit CPR,[15] and these should be honored when possible. In addition, family members may wish to be present during resuscitation attempts.[15] This often requires support from social services and clergy. However, whenever possible family members should be given this option.

REFERENCES

1. The American Heart Association in collaboration with the International Liaison Committee on Resuscitation: Guidelines 2000 for Cardiopulmonary Resuscitation and Emergency Cardiovascular Care. Part 3: Adult basic life support. *Circulation* 102(8 Suppl):I22, 2000.
2. The National Safety Council: Injury Facts (formerly Accident Facts). Itasca, IL, 1999.
3. Heimlich HJ: A life-saving maneuver to prevent food-choking. *JAMA* 234:398, 1975.
4. Kouwenhoven WB, Jude JR, Knickerbocker GG: Closed-chest cardiac massage. *JAMA* 173:1064, 1960.
5. Jude JR, Kouwenhoven WB, Knickerbocker GG: Cardiac arrest: Report of application of external cardiac massage on 118 patients. *JAMA* 178:1063, 1961.
6. Halperin HR: Mechanisms of forward flow during CPR, in Paradis N, Nowak R, Halperin H (eds): *Cardiac Arrest: The Science and Practice of Resuscitation Medicine,* Baltimore, Williams & Wilkins, 1996.
7. Babbs CF: Circulatory adjunct: Newer methods of cardiopulmonary resuscitation. *Cardiol Clin* 20:37, 2002.
8. Hallstrom A, Cobb L, Johnson E, et al: Cardiopulmonary resuscitation by chest compression alone or with mouth-to-mouth ventilation *New Engl J Med* 342:1546, 2000.
9. Halperin HR, Tsitlik JE, Gelfand M, et al: A preliminary study of cardiopulmonary resuscitation by circumferential compression of the chest with use of a pneumatic vest. *New Engl J Med* 329:762, 1993.
10. Sack JB, Kasselbremmer MB, Bregman D, et al: Survival from in-hospital cardiac arrest with interposed abdominal counter pulsation during cardiopulmonary resuscitation. *JAMA* 267:379, 1992.
11. Cohen TJ, Goldner BG, Maccaro PC, et al: A comparison of active compression-decompression cardiopulmonary resuscitation with standard cardiopulmonary resuscitation for cardiac arrests occurring in the hospital. *New Engl J Med* 329:1918, 1993.
12. Criley JM, Blaufuss AH, Kissel GL: Cough-induced cardiac compression: Self-administered form of cardiopulmonary resuscitation. *JAMA* 236:1246, 1976.
13. Gazmuri RJ, Becker J: Cardiac resuscitation: The search for hemodynamically more effective methods. *Chest* 111:712, 1997.
14. Kern KB, Morley PT, Babbs CF, et al: Use of adjunctive devices in cardiopulmonary resuscitation. *Ann Emerg Med* 2001;37, S68.
15. Cummins RO, Hazinski MF: The most important changes in the international ECC and CPR guidelines 2000. *Circulation* 102(8 Suppl):I371, 2000.

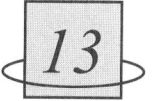

13
NEONATAL RESUSCITATION AND EMERGENCIES
Eugene E. Cepeda
Mary P. Bedard

NEONATAL RESUSCITATION

Approximately 6 percent of all newborns require life support in the delivery room or nursery, and in those neonates whose birthweights are less than 1500 g, the need for resuscitation rises to 60 percent. Personnel skilled in neonatal resuscitation should be available at every delivery.[1]

There are no guidelines available to assist in making the decision to resuscitate extremely premature infants in the emergency department. When in doubt, resuscitate. At the present time, survival at 22 weeks of gestation or younger is rare. However, an 11 to 30 percent survival rate is reported at 23 weeks' gestation, although often with severe resultant morbidity. About 30 to 50 percent of surviving children with birthweights less than 750 g or whose gestational age was younger than 25 weeks had moderate to severe disability including blindness, deafness, and cerebral palsy.[2]

The single most frequent reason for resuscitation of a newborn is prematurity. Factors associated with an increased risk for neonatal resuscitation are shown in Table 13-1. The following conditions should alert nursery personnel to the possibility that apnea may develop: previous need for resuscitation, prematurity, sepsis and/or meningitis, congenital abnormalities, respiratory distress, or seizures.

Normal newborns are equipped with physiologic, pharmacologic, and metabolic responses to enable them to survive the hypoxia that develops as a consequence of asphyxia. In general, brain injury occurs only when the asphyxia is severe enough to impair cerebral blood flow. Initially the injury is reversible, and only prolonged periods of ischemia lead to permanent damage. The pattern of injury is strongly influenced by the distribution of blood flow. During asphyxia, blood flow is redirected to the heart, brain, and adrenals at the expense of other organs, such as the kidneys and the gastrointestinal tract. Within the brain, flow is directed to the brain stem at the expense of the high cerebral structures, such as the cortex. In the preterm neonate, the periventricular white matter is susceptible to injury. In the full-term or post-term neonate, the gray matter regions, such as the overlying parasagittal "watershed" cortex, are more vulnerable to ischemic injury. When the asphyxial insult is severe or prolonged, hypoxic multiorgan dysfunction occurs, because of the redistribution of organ blood flow, and results in cardiopulmonary distress, renal failure, impaired

TABLE 13-1 Factors Potentiating the Need for Neonatal Resuscitation

Maternal factors
Inadequate prenatal care
Age <16 and >35 y
History of previous perinatal morbidity or mortality
Toxemia or hypertension
Diabetes
Chronic renal disease
Anemia
Drug therapy (e.g., reserpine, lithium, magnesium, adrenergic-blocking agents)
Substance abuse
Blood type or group isoimmunization
Oligohydramnios
Intrapartum factors
Abnormal presentation
Caesarean section
Prolonged labor or precipitous delivery
Prolonged rupture of membranes, chorioamnionitis
Cephalopelvic disproportion
Forceps delivery other than outlet or vacuum extraction
Prolapsed cord
Cord compression
Maternal hypotension, shock
Analgesic or sedative drugs given within 2 h of delivery
Fetal factors
Prematurity
Postmaturity
Intrauterine growth failure
Multiple gestation
Acidosis on fetal scalp capillary monitoring
Abnormal fetal heart rate per monitor
Thick meconium in amniotic fluid
Congenital infection
Fetal malformation or edema diagnosed by ultrasound

hepatic function, seizures and encephalopathy, gastrointestinal dysfunction, and coagulopathies.

PRINCIPLES OF RESUSCITATION

The Apgar score (Table 13-2) is assessed at 1 and 5 min of age for every newly delivered infant. Although the scoring system has been useful in evaluating the condition of the newborn, 1 min is too long to wait to make the decision to initiate resuscitation. If the 5-min score is less than 7, additional scores are obtained every 5 min for a total of 20 min.

Perinatal asphyxia is currently defined as the presence of umbilical artery acidemia (pH <7.00), 5-min Apgar score of 0 to 3, neonatal neurologic sequelae, and multiorgan dysfunction. Certain conditions require specific measures during resuscitation in addition to those outlined below. These conditions are discussed after the general principles.

TABLE 13-2 Apgar Score

Sign	0	1	2
Heart rate	Absent	<100/min	>100/min
Respiratory effort	Absent	Weak cry	Strong cry
Muscle tone	Limp	Some flexion	Good flexion
Reflex irritability (when feet stimulated)	No response	Some motion	Cry
Color	Blue, pale	Body pink, extremities blue	Pink

Infants who are successfully resuscitated at birth should have continuous monitoring of vital signs, blood gases, hematocrit, glucose levels, blood pressure, fluid status, and clinical condition. Complications associated with severe asphyxia are hypoxic-ischemic encephalopathy, seizures, intracranial hemorrhage, syndrome of inappropriate secretion of antidiuretic hormone, hypocalcemia, persistent pulmonary hypertension, ischemic cardiomyopathy, hypovolemia or shock, necrotizing enterocolitis, renal failure, and coagulopathy.

Equipment

Equipment necessary for resuscitation is listed in Table 13-3.

Resuscitation Steps

MAINTAIN BODY TEMPERATURE   The infant should be maintained below the level of the placenta before clamping the cord. When the cord is clamped, the infant is blotted dry with a sterile towel and placed under a preheated radiant warmer on a sterile table. Neonates should be placed on the back or the left side, somewhat in the Trendelenburg position, with the neck in a neutral position.

CLEAR THE AIRWAY   The nose and mouth are suctioned gently with a bulb syringe or mechanical suction apparatus with an 8-French suction catheter. A 5- to 10-s examination should be performed to determine the need for resuscitation. This examination should include an assessment of heart rate, respiratory effort, color, and muscular tone. If the infant has a lusty cry, is pink, has spontaneous respirations, and has a heart rate faster than 120 beats/min (Apgar >8), no further therapy is needed.

INITIATE BREATHING   If the infant is apneic or the heart rate is slow and irregular (<100 beats/min) and the color is cyanotic (Apgar 4 to 7), positive pressure ventilation is administered with the mask over the infant's face with 100 percent oxygen. The respiratory rate should be maintained at 40 to 60 breaths/min, with enough pressure applied to gently move the chest wall. In an infant who has not yet taken a breath, pressure over 30 cm H_2O may be necessary to expand the lungs. In mildly depressed infants, this amount will produce a prompt increase in heart rate and the onset of regular spontaneous respirations. If no improvement is noted in 15 to 30 s or the condition deteriorates (Apgar ≤4), the trachea should be intubated and assisted ventilation continued.

MECONIUM STAINING   Meconium staining of the amniotic fluid occurs in up to 20 percent of all births. Meconium aspiration syndrome is a cause of severe respiratory disease and often is associated

TABLE 13-3 Neonatal Resuscitation Equipment

Bag and mask with manometer attached, connected to a source of 100% oxygen (oxygen should be heated and humidified; bag should be a rubber anesthesia bag, a rebreathing bag of 500-mL capacity, or a self-inflating bag designed for newborns)
Rubber face masks of different sizes, 1, 2, 3, and 4
Wall suction, sterile catheters, and bulb syringes
DeLee suction catheter with mucus trap
Laryngoscope with 0 and 1 blades
Oral endotracheal tubes with stylet, sizes 2.5, 3.0, 3.5, and 4.0 mm
Radiant heater with servomechanism
Sterile umbilical vessel catheterization tray
Glucose blood test strips
Heart rate monitor with easily applicable leads
Intravenous infusion equipment
Pulse oximeter
Appropriate light
Infant stethoscope
Nasogastric tubes, 5 and 8 French
Clock with sweep second hand

with persistent pulmonary hypertension of the newborn. With proper obstetric and pediatric management, the incidence and severity of the disease can be significantly decreased. When meconium staining of the amniotic fluid is present, the infant's nose, mouth, and pharynx should be thoroughly suctioned after delivery of the head and before delivery of the shoulders. If the infant is vigorous after delivery, the oropharynx should be suctioned again with a bulb syringe or large-bore catheter. No further intervention is necessary.

If the infant is depressed at birth, direct suctioning of the trachea should be performed. Free-flow oxygen should be given throughout the procedure. The infant's trachea is visualized with a laryngoscope, and the mouth and pharynx are cleared with a 12- or 14-French suction catheter. An endotracheal tube is inserted into the trachea and attached to a suction device. Suction is applied as the endotracheal tube is slowly removed. This procedure should be repeated until little additional meconium is recovered.[3] If the heart rate remains slower than 100 beats/min, positive pressure ventilation and chest compressions should be initiated. If no suction device is available to attach to the endotracheal tube, a large-bore suction catheter can be inserted in the trachea and suction applied to remove meconium from the trachea. If the heart rate is remains slower than 100 beats/min after suctioning, bag-and-mask ventilation should be done. If the heart rate does not respond, the infant should be intubated and given positive pressure ventilation. Chest compressions and epinephrine should be given, as outlined below, if bradycardia persists.

Endotracheal intubation of the neonate is not particularly different from other young pediatric patients. Details of this technique are discussed in Chap. 15.

CARDIAC MASSAGE   If the heart rate is slower than 60 beats/min with assisted ventilation, cardiac massage should be initiated by placing both hands around the infant's chest with two thumbs over the midsternum, one finger's width below the intermammary line. The sternum is depressed one third of the distance to the vertebral column at 120 compressions per min. Chest compressions should be coordinated with ventilation at one breath for every three compressions. Cardiac massage may be stopped periodically to assess improvement. The chest should expand, bilateral breath sounds should be heard in the axilla, and heart rate should increase if the resuscitation is effective and the endotracheal tube is in good position. *In most instances* it is possible to obtain an adequate response with the use of external cardiac massage and assisted ventilation. If there is no response to these measures after 30 s, drug therapy should be considered. Any route of access to the circulatory system is acceptable, including a peripheral vein, the umbilical vein, or the endotracheal tube.

UMBILICAL VEIN CATHETERIZATION   The most expedient procedure for obtaining vascular access is to insert the venous catheter through the umbilicus via the umbilical vein and the ductus venosus into the inferior vena cava (Figure 13-1). The venous catheter should be inserted 10 to 12 cm and anchored to the abdominal wall. Radiographs of chest and abdomen should be obtained to rule out other abnormalities and evaluate the position of the catheters.

UMBILICAL ARTERY CATHETERIZATION   Umbilical artery catheterization is indicated for continuous monitoring of blood pressure and closer monitoring of arterial blood gases (Table 13-4). If the umbilical artery cannot be cannulated for a blood gas determination, the radial artery or warmed (arterialized) finger stick for capillary blood are alternatives.

Patency of the umbilical arterial line can be maintained by a continuous infusion of fluid. The catheter should be removed when the need for arterial blood gas monitoring is no longer necessary or complications occur.

Possible complications of umbilical artery catheterization are infection, thrombosis and vasospasm, and hemorrhage. Renal hypertension is a delayed complication.

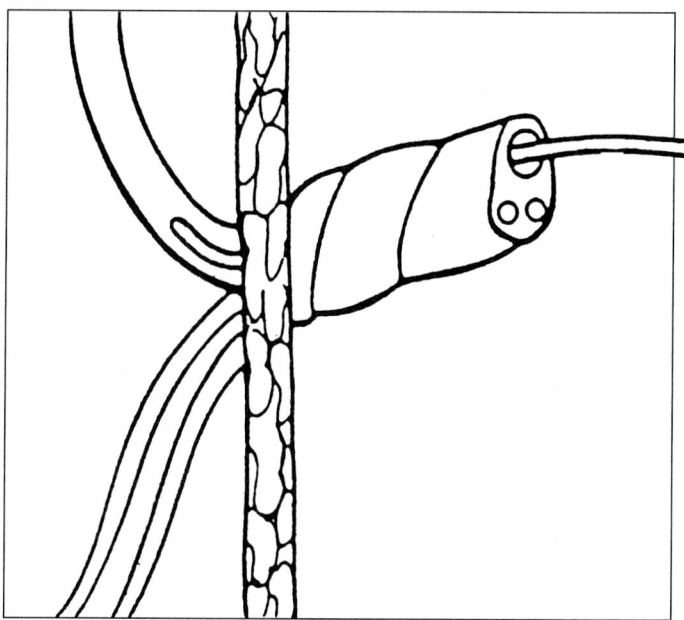

FIG. 13-1. Umbilical vein catheterization. The large vessel is the umbilical vein. The two smaller vessels are the umbilical arteries.

DRUG THERAPY IN RESUSCITATION

There is a minor role for drug therapy in resuscitation. Most resuscitative efforts in the delivery room respond to adequate support of ventilation and circulation without drug therapy (Table 13-5).

DEXTROSE   To provide metabolic substrate and expansion of plasma volume, D10W in water at 100 mL/kg a day or 6 to 8 mg/kg per min (0.06 to 0.08 mL/kg per min) should be infused. If the blood glucose is below 45 mg/dL, 2 mL/kg of D10W or D15W solution should be infused at a rate of 2 mL per min; 25 percent dextrose infusions should be avoided because of the risk of rebound hypoglycemia.

EPINEPHRINE   To stimulate heart rate if it is slower than 60 beats/min, 0.1 to 0.3 mL/kg of a 1:10,000 solution may be given IV. Epinephrine may be administered down the endotracheal tube at a dose that is 2 to 2.5 times larger than the IV dose. Cardiac massage should continue after epinephrine administration.

VOLUME EXPANSION   Infants who appear pale with weak pulses or who fail to respond to the above resuscitative measures may be hypovolemic and require volume expansion. The fluid of choice is an isotonic crystalloid solution, such as NS or LR. After intravenous access is established, administer 10 mL/kg of fluid by slow intravenous push over 5 to 10 min. If there is minimal response to the first dose, a second 10 mL/kg dose can be given. If acute blood loss is suspected, transfusion with 10 mL/kg of O-negative blood can be given.

BICARBONATE   The use of sodium bicarbonate during neonatal resuscitation remains controversial. If possible, a blood gas should be obtained to check adequacy of ventilation before sodium bicarbonate is given. During a prolonged arrest, it can be given once adequate ventilation and circulation have been established. Sodium bicarbonate is caustic and should be given intravenously, not by the endotracheal route. The dose is 1 to 2 mEq/kg of a 4.2 percent (0.5 mEq/mL) solution or 2 to 4 mL/kg. Blood gases should be obtained, and further treatment should be reassessed.

NALOXONE HYDROCHLORIDE   Naloxone hydrochloride is used to reverse narcotic respiratory depression and should not be given until adequate ventilation has been established. The dose is 0.1 mg/kg of

TABLE 13-4   Umbilical Artery Catheterization

Equipment:
Five 2 × 2 in. sponges
Curved hemostat
Two medicine glasses
Scalpel blade, no. 11
Two iris forceps, curved, serrated end, no teeth
Lacrimal probe
Needle holder
Debriding scissors
Umbilical tape, 6 in.
Knife handle
4-0 silk suture with needle
Three-way stopcock
Two 10-mL syringes
Povidone-iodine solution
3.5-French catheter for infant <1200 g
5.0-French catheter for infant >1200 g

Method:
1. Immobilize the patient. Measure the distance between the umbilicus and the right shoulder.
2. Clean the umbilical stump and surrounding area with povidone-iodine solution. Drape the umbilical area, but leave the infant's head and feet uncovered.
3. Tie the base of the cord with the umbilical tape, using a single throw, and apply traction to minimize blood loss.
4. Cut the cord cleanly across its length to 1 cm with the scalpel. The arteries are small and have pinpoint openings. The vein is larger and has thinner walls and a larger opening.
5. Grasp the edge of the cord with the forceps. Using the iris forceps, enlarge the opening of the umbilical artery first with the tip of one arm of the forceps.
6. Insert both arms of the forceps to dilate the artery so that it will accept the catheter.
7. The length of the catheter inserted for the low position is two thirds the distance from the umbilicus to the right shoulder, and the length for the high position is the full measurement from the right shoulder to the umbilicus.
8. Attach the three-way stopcock and aspirate blood with a syringe. Clear the catheter with normal saline.
9. Anchor the catheter with silk suture to the umbilical stump. The umbilical tape also can be used to secure the catheter.
10. Check the position of the catheter tip with an x-ray. It should be at the level of L4 for the low position or between T6 and T9, which is above the diaphragm, for the high position.

0.4 mg/mL solution. It may be administered intravenously or through the endotracheal tube. Intramuscular or subcutaneous administration is associated with a delayed onset of action. Naloxone hydrochloride may precipitate withdrawal in infants whose mothers are addicted to opiates.

DISCONTINUATION OF RESUSCITATION

If no heart rate is established after 15 min, it is appropriate to discontinue resuscitative efforts. Current data indicate that resuscitation after 10 min of asystole is very unlikely to result in survival without severe disability.

TRANSFERS

Once an infant has been successfully resuscitated, it should be transferred as soon as possible to an intensive care unit with equipment and trained personnel for the management of newborns.

EMERGENCIES IMMEDIATELY AFTER BIRTH

This section discusses selected emergencies that can develop immediately after birth. Chaps. 117, 118, and 120 discuss other aspects of neonatal problems in detail.

Apnea

Apnea is the absence of respirations for a period of 20 s or for shorter durations when associated with a heart rate slower than 80 beats/min and/or cyanosis or pallor. Apnea is categorized as *central apnea* when it originates from the central nervous system (CNS). There are no respiratory efforts and no gas flow in central apnea. In *obstructive apnea,* there is impaired gas flow in the presence of respiratory effort. In *mixed apnea,* there are components of central and obstructive apnea. *Periodic breathing* is apnea of a few seconds' duration in a 20-s span of otherwise normal breathing. In term infants, apnea is never physiologic and is usually secondary to a serious disorder. Pathologic conditions associated with neonatal apnea are listed in Table 13-6. Detailed discussion of apnea is provided in Chap. 119.

Neonatal Shock

The risk factors for shock and hypotension in newborn infants are low birthweight, perinatal sepsis, prolapsed cord, and acute blood loss. Clinical signs of hypovolemia are pallor, tachycardia, grunting respirations without pulmonary disease, mottling of skin, poor capillary filling, thready pulse and hypotension (systolic <40 mm Hg in a 1000-g premature neonate or <55 mm Hg in a term infant), and persistent metabolic acidosis. A hematocrit should be obtained, and, if anemia (hematocrit <35 vol%) or hypotension is diagnosed, immediate plasma expansion in the form of packed red blood cells, 10 to 15 mL/kg, or whole blood, fresh-frozen plasma, or 5 percent albumin, 10 mL/kg, should be given IV over 10 min.

Neonatal Seizures

Seizures in neonates are common, with an incidence of 1 in 200 live births, and may represent primary CNS disease or a systemic or metabolic disorder. Hypoxic-ischemic encephalopathy is the most common cause of neonatal seizures. The seizures usually occur between 6 and 18 h of life but may be seen as early as age 1 h. In full-term neonates, the hypoxic injury may result in a cerebral hemorrhage, watershed infarct, posterior fossa hematoma, or subarachnoid or subdural hemorrhage. In premature infants, hypoxic injury often results in periventricular-intraventricular hemorrhage. This type of seizure has a poor prognosis. Recent data suggest that seizure activity itself may adversely affect the growing brain. It is important to distinguish seizures from tremors or jitteriness, which may be seen in infants who have hypocalcemia, hypoglycemia, drug withdrawal, or no identifiable disease. Tremors are uniform, fine movements that respond to sensory stimuli, stop with manual stabilization, and do not occur spontaneously. They are not accompanied by eye, oral, or lingual movements. The types of neonatal seizures include subtle seizures, tonic seizures, multifocal clonic seizures, focal clonic seizures, and myoclonic seizures.

Subtle seizures occur in preterm and term neonates. These seizures consist of ocular, facial, oral, or lingual movements and respiratory manifestations, such as apnea or stertorous breathing.

Tonic seizures are characteristic of premature infants. The seizures appear as decerebrate or decorticate posturing. There are sustained deviation of the eyes and asymmetric posturing of the limbs and trunk.

Multifocal clonic seizures are seen in term infants. These are initially noted in one limb and migrate to another part of the body. There are rhythmic and slow movements at one to six times per second.

Focal clonic seizures are well localized and accompanied by specific sharp activity on the electroencephalogram (EEG). These seizures occur more commonly in full-term infants.

Myoclonic seizures are expressed as single or multiple jerks of flexion of the upper or lower extremities. They are rare and occur in premature and full-term infants.

TABLE 13-5   Neonatal Resuscitation Drug Chart

Drug, Concentration, and Indication	Syringe Size (mL)	Dose by Weight	PATIENT DOSE			Administration
			Weight (kg)	VOLUME (mL) IV	ET	
Epinephrine 1:10,000 (0.1 mg/mL) for bradycardia	1	0.01–0.03 mg/kg	1	0.2	0.5	IV push or ET followed by 1 mL NS solution. Repeat q5 min as needed. *Do not mix with sodium bicarbonate. Never inject into an artery.*
			2	0.4	1	
			3	0.6	1.5	
			4	0.8	2	
Sodium bicarbonate 4.2% (0.5 mEq/mL) for metabolic acidosis	6, 10, or 12	2 mEq/kg	1	4		IV over at least 2 min. **Do not mix with epinephrine.** Ensure adequate ventilation.
			2	8		
			3	12		
			4	16		
Whole blood, albumin 5%, NS, or LR for volume expansion	20 or 35	10 mL/kg	1	10		IV over at least 10 min.
			2	20		
			3	30		
			4	40		
Naloxone 0.4 mg/mL for opiate-induced respiratory depression	1	0.1 mg/kg	1	0.25	0.25	IV push or ET May repeat 2 to 3 times. *Use cautiously if maternal narcotic addiction is suspected.*
			2	0.50	0.50	
			3	0.75	0.75	
			4	1	1	

Abbreviation: ET = endotracheally.
Source: Adapted from Bloom RS, Cropley C: *Textbook of Neonatal Resuscitation.* Chicago, American Heart Association, 1994.

CLINICAL FEATURES   The metabolic disturbances associated with neonatal seizures include hypoglycemia, hypocalcemia, hypomagnesemia, hyperammonemia, hypernatremia, and hyponatremia. Hypoglycemia, hypocalcemia, and hypomagnesemia are often found in premature infants with perinatal asphyxia. Hypernatremia occurs in neonates with volume depletion secondary to excessive fluid losses or treatment with large doses of sodium bicarbonate. Hyponatremia may be seen secondary to inappropriate antidiuretic hormone secretion or acute volume overload. Inborn errors of amino acid metabolism also may present as seizures.

TABLE 13-6   Conditions Associated with Apnea

Central nervous system
  Asphyxia
  Cerebral infarction
  Hydrocephalus
  Intracranial hemorrhage
  Meningitis
  Seizures
Cardiovascular
  Congestive heart failure
  Patent ductus arteriosus
Respiratory
  Chronic lung disease
  Hypoxia
  Pneumonia
  Obstruction
Digestive
  Necrotizing enterocolitis
  Overfeeding
  Vagal response to a nasogastric tube
Other causes
  Anemia
  Polycythemia
  Sepsis
  Temperature instability
  Hyponatremia
  Hyperkalemia
  Hypocalcemia
  Hypermagnesemia
  High serum levels of phenobarbital, diazepam, opiates, and chloral hydrate

Seizures can result from bacterial meningitis, encephalitis associated with the TORCH complex (toxoplasmosis, rubella, cytomegalovirus infection, and herpes simplex infection), or enteroviral encephalitis. Developmental abnormalities, including congenital hydrocephalus, microcephaly, and other congenital brain anomalies, can cause seizures. Drug withdrawal from maternal use of methadone, barbiturates, alcohol, pentazocine (Talwin), and tripelennamine (Pyribenzamine) rarely presents as seizures. Pyridoxine dependence occurs rarely but should be considered in neonatal seizures unresponsive to standard therapy. A rare cause of neonatal seizures is inadvertent fetal scalp injection of maternal local anesthetic agents. Neonatal stroke diagnosed by computed tomography recently has been described in term infants with focal motor seizures. Neonatal stroke may occur in the setting of diverse cerebrovascular disorders, such as hypoxic-ischemic encephalopathy, polycythemia, acute severe hypertension, and cocaine use.

A careful history, including intrapartum monitoring data and physical examination, is essential when considering drug withdrawal, birth asphyxia, or metabolic disorders as a cause of the seizures. A lumbar puncture with analysis of cell count, culture, Gram stain, and blood specimens for culture and determinations of glucose, calcium, magnesium, and blood urea nitrogen levels should be obtained. The echoencephalogram and EEG can be obtained after the seizures have been controlled. In a full-term infant, computed tomography or magnetic resonance imaging of the head to look for ischemic injury may be necessary, because an echoencephalogram may not provide adequate visualization of the subarachnoid space or posterior fossa. Recently, positron emission tomography of the head has been used to evaluate the effects of asphyxia and seizures on cerebral blood flow.

TREATMENT   Repeated seizures in neonates may be accompanied by hypoventilation and apnea, resulting in hypercapnia and hypoxemia. Increases in cerebral blood flow and arterial hypertension occur with neonatal seizures. Treatment of seizures should be initiated while awaiting results of laboratory data. An intravenous access route should be established immediately, and the airway should be maintained; assisted ventilation should be initiated if apnea is present. Hypoglycemia is treated with 2 mL/kg of a D10W solution given IV at 2 mL per min, followed by a maintenance infusion of D10W at 80 mL/kg a day.

Hypocalcemia is total calcium less than 7 mg/dL and should be treated with 10 percent calcium gluconate, 2 mL/kg, given IV at a maximal rate of 3 mL per min. If the heart rate decreases, the infusion should be slowed or stopped. Hypomagnesemia, less than 1.6 mg/dL, is often associated with hypo-calcemia and should be treated IV or IM with 0.1 to 0.2 mL/kg of 50 percent magnesium sulfate solution. Blood glucose, calcium, and magnesium should be determined before treatment of seizures from low levels of these three substances.

The anticonvulsant drugs used most frequently include phenobarbital and phenytoin. The loading dose of phenobarbital is 20 mg/kg IV given slowly over 10 min, and the maintenance dose is 5 mg/kg a day IM or PO in two divided doses. If the initial 20 mg/kg dose of phenobarbital is not effective in controlling the seizures, additional doses of 5 mg/kg may be administered every 5 min until the seizures have ceased or the total dose of 40 mg/kg has been reached. In unresponsive cases, phenytoin may be administered with a similar loading dose followed by a maintenance dose of 3 to 5 mg/kg a day by the IV route in only two divided doses 20 min apart to avoid disturbance of cardiac function. Lorazepam is recommended for status epilepticus as long as ventilation and blood pressure are supported. The dose of lorazepam is 0.05 to 0.1 mg/kg administered IV. Infants with pyridoxine dependence respond immediately to an intravenous injection of pyridoxine, 50 to 100 mg. For further discussion, see Chap. 125.

Diaphragmatic Hernia

A failure of development of the posterolateral parts of the diaphragm at the Bochdalek foramen or retrosternally at the Morgagni foramen allows herniation of the gut into the chest cavity. Associated anomalies with diaphragmatic hernias include congenital heart diseases, genitourinary anomalies, and gastrointestinal anomalies. Frequently the lungs are hypoplastic bilaterally and have abnormal pulmonary vasculature, thus predisposing the infant to pulmonary hypertension.

Fifty percent of fetuses with diaphragmatic hernia have difficulty swallowing, and the condition may be associated with polyhydramnios. The diagnosis often can be made by prenatal ultrasonography.

CLINICAL FEATURES The clinical findings are localized to the respiratory and digestive tracts. The chest is large, and the abdomen is scaphoid. Bowel sounds may be heard in the left chest, and the heart is displaced to the right. Dyspnea, cyanosis, retractions, and vomiting are proportional to the amount of abdominal viscera herniated into the thorax. Radiologic study shows air-filled loops of bowel in the chest cavity and an absent diaphragmatic margin. The lungs are hypoplastic and have abnormal vasculature.

TREATMENT The neonate should be stabilized as much as possible before surgery. The infant should be intubated immediately, and little or no attempt should be made to ventilate with a mask. Rapid ventilatory rates and low peak inspiratory pressures are used to ventilate the infant and prevent reactive respiratory acidosis and hypercarbia, which are potentially conducive to the development of pulmonary hypertension. A large-caliber 10-French tube should be placed in the stomach, with low continuous suction applied. An umbilical artery catheter is useful to monitor blood gases. Any acidemia should be corrected, and the pH should be maintained in the normal range, if possible. Intravenous fluids should be given, and the patient should be kept warm.

The outcome of an infant with diaphragmatic hernia depends on the degree of pulmonary hypoplasia and vascular abnormalities leading to persistent pulmonary hypertension. The morbidity is higher when the symptoms present at birth and when the diaphragmatic hernia is detected prenatally. Common complications include pneumothorax, persistent pulmonary hypertension, and chylothorax. The introduction of extracorporeal membrane oxygenation (ECMO) for in-

fants with persistent pulmonary hypertension has had minimal effect on outcome.

Tracheoesophageal Fistula

A defect in the separation of the trachea from the esophagus results in a persistent channel connecting the trachea and the esophagus. There are five types of tracheoesophageal fistulas: (1) esophageal atresia with a distal fistula between the trachea and the esophagus, the most common presentation (85 percent); (2) isolated esophageal atresia; (3) H-type fistula; (4) esophageal atresia with a proximal fistula; and (5) esophageal atresia with proximal and distal fistulas. The potential exists for respiratory distress in the first hours after birth in neonates with a proximal fistula. A proximal fistula can lead to massive aspiration at the first feed. Other types of esophageal atresia can lead to respiratory distress from inability to handle oral secretions, aspiration, and choking.

Congenital heart malformation, vertebral anomalies, imperforate anus, and radial aplasia are associated anomalies.

The inability to pass a catheter from the nose or mouth to the stomach is the hallmark of esophageal atresia. A radiograph may show the air-filled proximal pouch, and the catheter, if left in place, may coil in the proximal esophagus. Recurrent pneumonias occur in infants with an H-type fistula.

It is important to provide respiratory support by assisted ventilation, if needed, to correct acidosis before any surgical repair can be undertaken. A plastic sump catheter should be left in the pouch and connected to constant, low-pressure suction. The patient should be maintained in the reverse Trendelenburg or semi-Fowler position to prevent further reflux of gastric secretions through the fistula into the trachea. Intravenous fluids and antibiotics are indicated. Consultation with a neonatologist is advised.

Most (80 percent) infants with tracheoesophageal fistula survive. Operative mortality is low.[4]

Pneumothorax

Pulmonary air leaks may present as pneumothorax, pulmonary interstitial emphysema, pneumomediastinum, pneumopericardium, or pneumoperitoneum. Spontaneous pneumothorax can occur in term and post-term infants after intrapartum asphyxia and aspiration syndromes. The incidence of pneumothorax is higher in infants who require positive airway pressure, mechanical ventilation, and cardiopulmonary resuscitation. Uneven ventilation caused by aspirated blood, mucus, meconium, and amniotic fluid debris also can result in an air leak. Atelectasis, poor ventilation, and air trapping are common predisposing factors. Premature, low-birthweight infants with surfactant deficiency have a high incidence of air leaks (30 percent), as do newborns with meconium aspiration syndrome (10 percent).

CLINICAL FEATURES The signs and symptoms of an air leak (pneumothorax) are those of respiratory distress and often present as an acute clinical deterioration. Grunting respirations and intercostal, sternal, and subcostal retractions may be seen. Cyanosis, elevated respiratory rate, and elevated heart rate are common. Auscultation of the chest reveals decreased breath sounds on the affected side of a pneumothorax, distant heart sounds, and a shift of the mediastinum. Transillumination of the chest with a high-intensity lamp may aid in the diagnosis. A chest radiograph is diagnostic. The accuracy can be improved with a cross-table lateral film of the chest, in addition to anteroposterior and lateral views.

TREATMENT An asymptomatic pneumothorax that is less than 20 percent of the volume of the affected side may be followed clinically with no therapy and with serial radiographic studies every 4 h. Any pneumothorax with severe respiratory distress and clinical deterioration needs emergency treatment. When there are mediastinal shift and cardiovascular collapse, rapid decompression at the fourth intercostal space with a 21-gauge needle alone or attached to a three-way stopcock and a large syringe can be lifesaving.

Indications for thoracostomy tube placement are post-decompression of a tension pneumothorax or relief of respiratory compromise for simple pneumothorax, hemopneumothorax, or pleural fluid. The same equipment used for adults is required. A 10-French chest tube is used for infants weighing less than 1500 g, whereas a 12-French chest tube is appropriate for infants weighing more 1500 g. The procedure is similar to that in adults and is described in Chap. 259. Placement of the tube can be at the second or third intercostal space in the midclavicular line or at the fifth or sixth intercostal space in the anterior axillary line. The same precaution regarding avoidance of injury to the intercostal nerve, artery, and vein, which run on the lower edge of the rib, is required. The skin wound is similarly closed, and the chest tube is severed. The position of the chest tube is verified with a chest x-ray. The lung should re-expand promptly after evacuation of the air in the pleural space.

Gastroschisis and Omphalocele

An omphalocele is a defect in the umbilical ring that allows the intestines to protrude out of the abdominal cavity in a sac. A gastroschisis is a defect in the abdominal wall that allows the antenatal evisceration of abdominal structures without a sac being present.

The emergency management of the two conditions is not different, especially when the sac in an omphalocele is ruptured. The eviscerated bowel should be wrapped in saline-soaked gauze and placed in a plastic bag to protect it from hypothermia and evaporative losses. A nasogastric tube should be inserted to decompress the intestines. Rapid infusion of LR 20 mL/kg, may be necessary to restore vital signs, after which the infusion should be adjusted to maintain a urine output of at least 2 mL/kg per h. Intravenous antibiotics should be administered.

Primary fascial closure is the treatment of choice and often is accomplished within hours after birth. The mortality of omphalocele is 25 to 30 percent, largely as a result of concomitant congenital heart disease and sepsis, whereas death in patients with gastroschisis is associated with intestinal atresia.

Cyanotic Newborns

Cyanosis in neonates may be central or peripheral. Central cyanosis is defined as cyanosis of the tongue, mucous membranes, and peripheral skin and indicates the presence of reduced hemoglobin. Peripheral cyanosis is defined as blue discoloration confined to the skin of the extremities; the arterial saturation is greater than 94 percent. Peripheral cyanosis is common in neonates and may persist for 2 to 3 days. It is usually due to vasomotor instability secondary to a cold environment.

Normal newborn infants have a partial pressure of oxygen above 50 mm Hg by 5 to 10 min of age; hence, it is pathologic for central cyanosis to persist beyond 20 min after birth. Diagnostic considerations in central cyanosis are presented in Table 13-7.

DIAGNOSTIC APPROACH TO CENTRAL CYANOSIS Neonates with cyanosis secondary to congenital heart disease rarely have respiratory symptoms other than tachypnea. A murmur may be present. Neonates with lung disease producing cyanosis have respiratory distress, grunting, tachypnea, and retractions. Cyanotic infants with CNS disturbances or sepsis have apnea, bradycardia, lethargy, and seizures. Neonates with methemoglobinemia have minimal distress despite their cyanotic appearance.

TABLE 13-7 Differential Diagnosis of Central Cyanosis in the Neonate

Congenital heart disease with intracardiac right-to-left shunt
    Transposition of the great vessels
    Tricuspid atresia
    Truncus arteriosus
    Tetralogy of Fallot
    Total anomalous pulmonary venous return with obstruction
    Pulmonary atresia
    Preductal coarctation
Pulmonary disorders
    Hyaline membrane disease
    Pneumonia
    Meconium aspiration syndrome
    Persistent pulmonary hypertension
    Pneumothorax
    Diaphragmatic hernia
    Lobar emphysema
    Mucous plugs
Other causes
    Central nervous system disorders (e.g., intracranial hemorrhage)
    Polycythemia
    Shock
    Sepsis

The "hyperoxia test" (arterial partial pressure of oxygen [PaO_2] in response to breathing 100 percent oxygen) may be of use in distinguishing heart disease from other causes of cyanosis. Neonates with cyanotic heart disease do not demonstrate an increase in PaO_2 over 20 mm Hg, because of the right-to-left shunting of the circulation. Most neonates with lung disease, however, demonstrate an increase in PaO_2 after breathing 100 percent oxygen for 20 min. The neonate with CNS disorders, polycythemia, sepsis, and shock also demonstrates an increase in PaO_2. Infants with persistent pulmonary hypertension may or may not demonstrate a significant rise in partial pressure of oxygen. There is no response elicited in the neonate with methemoglobinemia. When a blood specimen is exposed to air, it turns pink in all the conditions described above except in methemoglobinemia, where the blood remains chocolate colored.

The chest radiograph may demonstrate pulmonary oligemia with normal heart size in the tetralogy of Fallot and pulmonary or tricuspid atresia, and pulmonary vascularity is increased in transposition of great vessels, truncus arteriosus, anomalous pulmonary venous return, and hypoplastic left heart. Neonates with lung disease have radiographs characteristic of the underlying disease. The electrocardiogram and echocardiogram are useful in diagnosing congenital heart disease. Right ventricular hypertrophy may be seen in lung disease, with associated pulmonary hypertension.

TREATMENT Infants with cardiac causes of cyanosis that have decreased pulmonary blood flow or left heart obstruction are dependent on the postnatal patency of the ductus arteriosus for maintenance of adequate pulmonary blood flow and systemic oxygenation. Prostaglandin E1 infusion at 0.05 to 0.1 μg/kg per min in these infants has allowed stabilization before surgery. Oxygen and ventilation are indicated for other causes.

Congestive Cardiac Failure

Causes of congestive heart failure in newborn infants are listed in Table 13-8. For detailed discussion see Chap. 120.

Neonates with severe heart failure from left-to-right shunts with cardiogenic shock and bradycardia may require inotropic support. Dobutamine and/or dopamine at 5 to 15 μg/kg per min can be used. Isoproterenol infused at 0.01 to 0.04 μg/kg per min may be helpful if

TABLE 13-8   Etiologies of Newborn Congestive Heart Failure

Structural heart disease
Heart disease without structural abnormalities (myocarditis, cardiac
  dysrhythmias, glycogen storage disease, and endocardial fibroelastosis)
Respiratory disease with patent ductus arteriosus with left-to-right shunt
Anemia (hemoglobin <3.5 g/dL)
Polycythemia
Cerebral or other arteriovenous malformation
Sepsis
Systemic hypertension

the heart rate is slower than 140 beats/min. Careful monitoring of blood pressure and heart rate is required.

Neonatal Transfers

Many facilities will not be able to care for neonates after emergency department resuscitation. Providers should be aware of the nearest hospital able to accommodate transfers. A specially trained team is likely to do the transportation, whether by ground or by air (see Chap. 4).

REFERENCES

1. Kattwinkel J (ed): *Textbook of Neonatal Resuscitation,* 4th ed. Elk Grove Village, IL, American Academy of Pediatrics and American Heart Association, 2000.
2. MacDonald H, and the Committee on Fetus and Newborn: Perinatal care at the threshold of viability. *Pediatrics* 110:1024, 2002.
3. Wiswell TE: Handling the meconium-stained infant. *Semin Neonatol* 6:225, 2001.
4. Deurloo JA, Ekelkamp S, Schoorl M, et al: Esophageal atresia: Historical evolution of management and results in 371 patients. *Ann Thorac Surg* 73: 267, 2002.

14   PEDIATRIC CARDIOPULMONARY RESUSCITATION
William E. Hauda II

This chapter reviews CPR in children and pertinent differences from adults. One major difference between adult and pediatric cardiopulmonary arrest is etiology. The most common cause of primary cardiac arrest in adults is coronary artery disease. Children usually develop cardiac arrest secondary to respiratory arrest and shock syndromes.

Children have very poor survival rates from cardiac arrest, because it is often associated with prolonged hypoxia or shock.[1,2] After a cardiac arrest, the survival rate without devastating neurologic sequelae in children is only 2 percent.[3] The best chance for a good outcome is to recognize impending respiratory failure or shock and intervene to prevent the development of cardiopulmonary arrest.

Age-related differences are important within the pediatric population.[4] An appropriate drug dose for a 6 month old may be excessive for a 1 month old but inadequate for a 5 year old. Other aspects of resuscitation, such as endotracheal tube size, tidal volumes, cardiac compression rates, and respiratory rates, vary with a child's age.

The priorities of resuscitation are airway, oxygenation, ventilation, and shock management. Cardiopulmonary arrest may be prevented with prompt recognition of and intervention for compromised physiology.[4] International consensus guidelines for basic life support procedures[5] are listed in Table 14-1.

AIRWAY

Anatomy

A child's airway is much smaller than an adult's, and the size varies by age. The anatomic and functional differences are more pronounced in infants and young children. The airway is higher and more anterior in a child's than in an adult's neck. The tongue and epiglottis are relatively larger and thus more likely to be an obstructing element in a child's airway. Infants younger than 6 months are primarily nasal breathers. Thus, keeping the nasal passages clear is vital in a young, spontaneously breathing infant. When a child is supine, the prominent occiput causes flexion of the neck on the chest, thereby occluding the airway. The occlusion can be corrected by mild extension of the neck to the sniffing position. Overextension or hyperextension, acceptable for adults, causes obstruction and may kink the trachea, because the cartilaginous support is poor.

Positioning

The sniffing position can be maintained by placing a towel or other object beneath the shoulders. Despite good head position, a child's hypotonic mandibular tissues may still allow the relatively large tongue to occlude the airway posteriorly. This condition can be relieved by a chin lift or jaw thrust that elevates the mandible anteriorly and separates the tongue from the posterior pharyngeal wall. The jaw-thrust technique is preferred in a child with a possible cervical spine injury, because it minimizes the movement of the neck and allows maintenance of a neutral position of the cervical spine. If these maneuvers are unsuccessful, an oral airway or endotracheal tube should be considered.

TABLE 14-1   Guidelines for Pediatric Basic Life Support

Maneuver	Newborn	Infant <1 Year	Child 1–8 Years	Adult >8 Years
Airway	Head tilt/chin lift	Head tilt/chin lift	Head tilt/chin lift	Head tilt/chin lift
If trauma	Jaw thrust	Jaw thrust	Jaw thrust	Jaw thrust
If foreign body	Suction	Back blows and chest thrusts	Abdominal thrusts	Abdominal thrusts
Breathing rate	30–60/min (every 1–2 s)	20/min (every 3 s)	20/min (every 3 s)	12/min (every 5 s)
Circulation				
Pulse check	Umbilical	Brachial	Carotid	Carotid
Compression				
Location	1 finger below intramammary line	1 finger below intramammary line	Lower half of sternum	Lower half of sternum
Method	2 fingers or 2 thumbs	2 fingers	Heel of 1 hand	2 hands
Depth	$\frac{1}{3}$ of chest	$\frac{1}{3}$ of chest	$\frac{1}{3}$ of chest	$\frac{1}{3}$ of chest
Rate	120/min	100/min	100/min	100/min
Ventilation ratio	3:1	5:1	5:1	5:1 (15:2 for 1 rescuer)

Source: Circulation 95:2185, 1997.

NASOPHARYNGEAL AIRWAY Nasopharyngeal airways tend to be less useful in children, because of the small nasal passages and the presence of hypertrophic adenoid tissue in the posterior nasopharynx, which is easily traumatized when inserting a nasopharyngeal airway.

ORAL AIRWAY Oral airways, which should be used only in unconscious children, are most useful in patients who require a continuous jaw thrust or chin lift to maintain airway patency. Oral airways are inserted with a tongue depressor to push the tongue down into the mandible so that the airway can be inserted under direct vision.

Intubation

Endotracheal intubation of infants and children is felt by many to be easier than the same procedure in adults. There are, however, some differences related to a child's anatomy and proper sizing of equipment. Pediatric airway management is discussed in detail in Chap. 15. A brief overview is provided here for perspective.

POSITIONING Hyperextension of the neck must be avoided by placing the child in the sniffing position before intubation. Also, the stretcher should be raised so that the child's head is at least at the level of the intubator's waist. All equipment should be located within easy reach of the team, including the bag-valve mask, oxygen source, monitoring equipment, and, perhaps most importantly, the suction device.

LARYNGOSCOPE BLADES For two reasons, the curved (MacIntosh) blade is rarely used in children younger than 4 years. First, the relatively large and flaccid epiglottis is not effectively displaced by pulling on it indirectly from the vallecular space. Second, an exact-size blade must be used to fit the curvature of the tongue. For these reasons, a straight (Miller) blade is preferred. The straight blade is inserted in the midline with the tip underneath the epiglottis, such that the epiglottis is directly lifted up to allow tracheal visualization.

ENDOTRACHEAL TUBE Tracheal tube sizes vary with a patient's age. An often quoted rule is that the correct internal diameter tube size is approximately the same size as the end of the patient's little finger. However, this tenet has been disproved.[6,7] The age-based formula, (age + 16)/4, remains a better predictor of correct endotracheal tube size for children. **Uncuffed tubes are used for children up to 7 or 8 years old** (tube size, 2.5 to 5.5 mm), because in children (unlike adults) the subglottic trachea is the narrowest spot of the trachea and forms an adequate seal around the endotracheal tube in this age group. In patients older than 8 years, the vocal cords become the narrowest part to the airway, and a cuff is needed to provide an adequate seal for positive pressure ventilation. One can almost always intubate with a laryngoscope blade that is too large and with a tube that is too small, but not vice-versa.

SECURING THE AIRWAY Once a child has been intubated, one person should be assigned to hold the endotracheal tube in place until it is securely fastened. Confirmation of endotracheal intubation is similar to that in adults: adequate chest rise, symmetric breath sounds, capnographic or capnometric readings,[8] improved oxygenation, and clinical improvement.[4] Because a young child has a small chest, listening to breath sounds in each axilla and over the stomach will minimize the chance of hearing sounds transmitted from the other lung.[4] The tube should be taped to the upper lip and jaw, ideally from both sides of the face. Especially in small infants, small movements can easily displace the tube from the trachea into the esophagus. Tape or ties should not be wrapped around the head of a young child, because these can slide off the occiput and easily allow displacement of the tube. Mechanical ventilation is discussed in the section on Breathing, which follows.

Foreign-Body Management

There is controversy concerning the safest and most effective emergency maneuvers to use with a choking child. The American Heart Association specifically discourages two common maneuvers used with adult patients: (1) the Heimlich maneuver for patients younger than 1 year, because of the potential for injury to abdominal organs, and (2) blind finger sweeps, because of the possibility of pushing the foreign body farther into the airway.[4] Serious differences of opinion exist, but current recommendations rely on the back blow and chest thrust to clear an infant's airway.

CONSCIOUS CHILDREN A child who is choking but is able to maintain some ventilation or vocalization should be allowed to clear the airway by coughing. Once a child cannot cough, vocalize, or breathe, a sequence of steps must be instituted immediately. Choking infants are treated with an alternating sequence of five back blows and five chest thrusts. With the infant's torso positioned prone and head down along the rescuer's arm, or the older child draped prone and head down across the rescuer's knees, five blows are delivered to the interscapular area. The infant is then repositioned supinely along the rescuer's arm, or the larger infant can be placed on the floor, as for external cardiac compression, and five chest thrusts (cardiac compressions) are delivered. This sequence is continued until the child's airway obstruction is relieved or the child becomes unconscious. In older children, the Heimlich maneuver is used, with the rescuer kneeling or standing behind the child. The clenched fist is placed at the level of the umbilicus, and firm upward thrusts are continued until the obstruction is cleared or the child becomes unconscious.

UNCONSCIOUS CHILDREN In all cases in which a child becomes unconscious with the rescuer present, the rescuer should first attempt ventilation, because the object may have become dislodged. If an obstruction is still present, then airway clearance maneuvers must be continued. For infants, the same sequence is used, but between each cycle of back blows and chest thrusts (the same technique as for CPR), an attempt at ventilation should be made. Before attempting a ventilation, the airway should be inspected to see whether an object is present. Only a visible object is removed; blind finger sweeps should be avoided. If the obstruction persists, the sequence is repeated. For children older than 1 year, chest compressions are performed with the child lying on its back. Future investigation may well lead to revised recommendations.

The foregoing recommendations are directed primarily at a first responder who has neither access to nor the skills to use airway management equipment. For unconscious children in emergency departments, direct laryngoscopy, visualization, and removal of the foreign body with McGill forceps should be attempted rapidly. Until this equipment is ready, basic life support techniques should be used.

BREATHING

Mouth to Mouth

Whether to use mouth-to-mouth or mouth-to-mouth-and-nose ventilation depends on the size of the patient. The rate of ventilation is shown in Table 14-1. Ventilations are done slowly to avoid the generation of high airway pressures, which can overcome esophageal resistance and result in gastric distention.

Bag-Valve Mask

The self-inflating bag-valve mask system is most commonly used for ventilation. Ventilation bags used for infants and children should have a minimum volume of 450 mL. There is a common misconception that children are more susceptible to pneumothoraces at high inspiratory pressures. In fact, pediatric lung compliance is very good, and children can tolerate relatively high pressures. Pneumothoraces more commonly result from the administration of excessive tidal volume. The tidal volume necessary to ventilate children is the same as that for adults: 10 to 15 mL/kg. Because it is impractical to calculate the tidal volume in emergency situations, ventilation is started with the smallest volume that causes adequate chest rise. Careful monitoring of the rate of ventilation is crucial to avoid excessive hyperventilation, a very common mistake.

Mechanical Ventilation

If an endotracheal tube is placed, then mechanical ventilation should be instituted promptly. Determining appropriate initial settings for the mechanical ventilation of children can be difficult. For children weighing less than 10 kg, time-flow or pressure preset ventilators should be used. For time-flow ventilators, inspiratory and expiratory times are needed. Typical inspiratory times are 0.5 to 1 s, depending on ventilation frequency. For pressure ventilators, inflating pressures are determined by using pressures necessary to inflate the lungs and cause the chest to rise. Pressures usually range from 15 to 40 mm Hg. Excess pressures can cause barotrauma. For older children, volume ventilators can be used, starting with a tidal volume of 10 mL/kg, as for adults. If the lungs have normal compliance and the child does not require hyperventilation, then the respiratory rate should be started at half the normal rate for age (20 breaths/min for infants, 15 breaths/min for young children, and 10 breaths/min for older children and adolescents). Children should be adequately sedated and paralyzed during mechanical ventilation, until definitive care is started in a pediatric intensive care unit.

CIRCULATION

External Cardiac Compression

The brachial pulse is recommended for monitoring purposes for infants younger than 1 year. For older children, the femoral pulse is most easily accessible, but most guidelines recommend assessment of the carotid pulse by laypersons. Absence of pulse or poor perfusion, with a heart rate of 60 beats/min or slower, mandates external cardiac compression. Current standards advocate compressions over the lower sternum as opposed to the midsternum.[5] The depth of compressions should be approximately one third the anteroposterior diameter of the chest to be effective. Patients should be placed on a hard surface to improve the effectiveness of compressions. To assess the adequacy of the compression depth and rate, the femoral or carotid artery should be palpated during compressions.

INFANTS   The two-thumb technique is the recommended technique when two health care providers are present. Compressions should be at a rate of at least 100 per min. There should be a brief pause after five compressions to administer one ventilation. This ratio of 5:1 should be used whether there are one or two health care providers. If the patient is intubated, then compressions and ventilations may be performed without synchronization, but the rate of compressions should be maintained at 100 per min.

CHILDREN 1 TO 8 YEARS OLD   The heel of one hand should be used to compress the lower half of the sternum. If unable to adequately depress the sternum with one hand, then the two-hand technique should be used. At least 100 compressions per min must be achieved. Compressions should be performed in a series of 5:1 with interposed ventilation, whether there are one or two health care providers. If the patient is intubated, then compressions and ventilations may be per-

formed without synchronization, but the rate of compressions should be maintained at 100 per min.

CHILDREN OLDER THAN 8 YEARS   A significant change in the recent emergency care guidelines was the recommendation that children older than 8 years be treated similarly to adults with respect to basic life support. The two-hand technique of chest compressions should be performed. Compressions should be performed in sets of 15, with two interposed ventilations. If the patient is intubated, then compressions and ventilations may be performed without synchronization, but the rate of compressions should be maintained at 100 per min.

VASCULAR ACCESS

Difficulty in obtaining rapid IV access is certainly one of the major differences between adult and pediatric resuscitation (see Chap. 21). Two important facts should be kept in mind. First, a significant portion of children respond to airway management alone, because most cardiac arrests in children are secondary to hypoxia from respiratory arrest. Time spent securing vascular access at the expense of adequate airway management is a common mistake in dealing with children. Second, once a patient has been intubated, the tracheal route may be used to administer drugs, such as lidocaine, epinephrine, atropine, and naloxone (mnemonic: LEAN). The dose of endotracheal epinephrine for symptomatic bradycardia or pulseless cardiac arrest is 0.1 mg/kg, 1:1000 concentration, every 3 to 5 min. Although the ideal endotracheal doses for drugs other than epinephrine have never been studied in children, current recommendations support the use of two to three times the respective IV dose.[4]

Although central access would be ideal for administration of drugs during CPR, many emergency medicine practitioners are not highly skilled in placing central lines in children. Therefore, the most frequently used sites are peripheral: scalp, arm, hand, or antecubital veins; the external jugular vein; femoral vein; or distal saphenous vein via cutdown. Intraosseous infusion and fluid administration are quick, safe routes for resuscitation drugs (see Chap. 21). The general order of attempts during a resuscitation should be antecubital, hand or foot, and then intraosseous.

FLUIDS

In the face of hypotension due to volume depletion, isotonic fluid boluses of 20 mL/kg should be given as rapidly as possible and repeated, depending on response.[4] A syringe attached to a three-way stopcock and extension tubing can be used to deliver aliquots of fluid rapidly, until the entire bolus is administered. Gravity or pressure bags should not be relied upon. The bolus should be delivered in a maximum of 20 min, and then the child's condition should be reassessed. If volume depletion has been corrected (at most, three to four boluses) and hypotension persists, a pressor agent should be strongly considered, preferably with the aid of a central venous catheter. In normotensive patients or when the IV line is being used for drug administration only, it should be maintained at the minimum rate that will keep the vein open. Fine fluid and electrolyte calculations and adjustments can be made af-

TABLE 14-2   Body Weight Estimation Guidelines

Age		Weight (kg)
Term infant	3.5	Birthweight
6 Months	7	$2 \times$ birthweight
1 Year	10	$3 \times$ birthweight
4 Years	16	$\frac{1}{4}$ Adult weight of 70 kg
10 Years	35	$\frac{1}{2}$ Adult weight

ter the emergency treatment has been completed. Overhydration, even when IV lines are set to keep the vein open, is common when adult equipment is used in pediatric resuscitations. To enable easy monitoring of the total volume given and prevent accidental overhydration, a pediatric microdrip should always be used when resuscitating children.

PHARMACOLOGIC AGENTS

The indications for the use of specific drugs are essentially the same for children as for adults. Particular to pediatrics, however, is the problem of drug dosage. Proper dosage in children requires knowledge of the patient's weight (Table 14-2), knowledge of the dose (usually given in milligrams per kilogram), and error-free calculation and delivery. Problems may arise in remembering the correct dose, performing calculations in the crisis situation (a common error involves the misplacement of a decimal point and results in 10 times or one tenth the

correct dosage), and delivery of the correct dosage (because of an error in drawing up the correctly calculated amount). Use of a chart with precalculated drug doses can help reduce dosage errors (Tables 14-3 and 14-4). However, estimating a child's weight accurately so that the proper dosage can be determined from the table is not easy, especially in a crisis situation. Choosing the proper-size equipment for pediatric patients is similarly difficult. Valuable time can be lost in weight estimation, dosage calculations, and equipment selection.

Systems based on a direct measurement of a patient's length recently have been developed for estimating dosages and selecting equipment in pediatric emergencies (Table 14-5).[9] In children, length has a direct correlation with weight. Length also has been shown to be one of the most accurate predictors of correct equipment sizes for pediatric patients, especially endotracheal tube sizes. The use of a length-based system is currently included in the American Heart Association's Pediatric Advanced Life Support Course. These systems use a

TABLE 14-3   Drugs Commonly Used in Pediatric Resuscitation

Drug	Pediatric Dosage	Remarks
Adenosine	IV: 0.1–0.2 mg/kg, followed by 2–5 mL NS bolus Double dose and repeat × 1 if needed	Maximum single dose: 12 mg
Amiodarone	IV: 5 mg/kg over 20–60 min; then 5–15 μg/kg per min infusion	Maximum bolus repetition to 15 mg/kg per d. Use lowest effective dose. Bolus may be given more rapidly in shock states.
Atropine	IV: 0.02 mg/kg of 1:10,000 (0.1 mg/mL), repeat in 5 min (minimum single dose is 0.1 mg) ET: double IV dose and dilute with NS to 3–5 mL	Maximum single dose: 0.5 mg (child) and 1.0 mg (adolescent) Maximum cumulative dose: 1.0 mg (child) and 2.0 mg (adolescent)
Bretylium	IV: 5 mg/kg, may be increased to 10 mg/kg	Rapid IV. Dosage in pediatric patients not well defined
Calcium chloride (10%)	20 mg/kg	Slow push

Dopamine infusion	IV: 2.0–20 μg/kg per min titrate to desired effect
	Renal dose (dopaminergic effects):
	  IV: 2–5 μg/kg per min infusion
	Cardiac dose (β₁ effects)
	  IV: 5–10 μg/kg per min infusion
	Vasopressor dose (α effects):
	  IV: 10–20 μg/kg per min infusion
		6 × weight in kg = mg of drug to add to a diluent to make a final volume of 100 mL. 1 mL/h = 1 μg/kg per min

Dobutamine infusion	IV: 2.0–20 μg/kg per min, titrate to desired effect	6 × weight in kg = mg of drug to add to a diluent to make a final volume of 100 mL. 1 mL/h = 1 μg/kg per min

Epinephrine	Bradycardia:
	  IV/IO: 0.01 mg/kg (0.1 mL/kg of 1:10,000)
	  ET: 0.1 mg/kg (0.1 mL/kg of 1:1000)
	Pulseless arrest:
	  First dose:
	    IV/IO: 0.01 mg/kg (0.1 mL/kg of 1:10,000)
	    ET: 0.1 mg/kg (0.1 mL/kg of 1:1000)
	  Second dose:
	    IV/IO/ET: 0.1 mg/kg (0.1 mL/kg of 1:1000) q3 min
		Unlike other agents, epinephrine per ET tube is 10 times the IV dose. Follow ET dose with several positive pressure ventilations.

Epinephrine infusion	IV: 0.1–1.0 μg/kg per min	0.6 × weight in kg = mg of drug to add to a diluent to make a final volume of 100 mL. 1.0 mL/h = 0.1 μg/kg per min
Lidocaine	IV: 1.0 mg/kg bolus ET: double IV dose and dilute with NS to 3–5 mL	
Lidocaine infusion	IV: 20–50 μg/kg per min	60 × weight in kg = mg of drug to add to a diluent to make a final volume of 100 mL. 1 mL/h = 10 μg/kg per min
Naloxone	If <5 y or ≤20 kg: 0.1 mg/kg If >5 y and >20 kg: 2.0 mg	Titrate to desired effect
Nitroprusside infusion	IV/IO: 1–8 μg/kg per min	6 × weight in kg = mg of drug to add to a diluent to make a final volume of 100 mL. 1 mL/h = 1 μg/kg per min
Norepinephrine infusion	IV/IO: 0.1–2 μg/kg per min	0.6 × weight in kg = mg of drug to add to a diluent to make a final volume of 100 mL. 1 mL/h = 0.1 μg/kg per min
Sodium bicarbonate	IV/IO: 1 mEq/kg (1 mEq/mL)	Infuse slowly and use only if ventilation is adequate.

Abbreviations: ET = endotracheally; IO = intraosseously; NS = normal saline.
Source: Chameides L, Hazinski MF (eds): *Textbook of Pediatric Advanced Life Support.* Dallas: American Heart Association, 1997.

TABLE 14-4 Calculation for Dosage of Medications Delivered by Constant Infusion Using the Rule of 6

Drug	Continuous Infusion Dose	Conversion Factor	Delivery
Epinephrine dose	0.1–1.0 µg/kg per min	0.6 mg × wt (kg)	1 mL/h = 0.1 µg/kg per min
Dobutamine dose	5–20 µg/kg per min	6 mg × wt (kg)	1 mL/h = 1.0 µg/kg per min
Dopamine	5–20 µg/kg per min	6 mg × wt (kg)	1 mL/h = 1.0 µg/kg per min
Isoproterenol	0.1–1.0 µg/kg per min	0.6 mg × wt (kg)	1 mL/h = 0.1 µg/kg per min
Lidocaine	20–50 µg/kg per min	60 mg × wt (kg)	1 mL/h = 10 µg/kg per min

Dosage of medications delivered by constant infusions is calculated in terms of micrograms per kilogram per minute. Actual calculation can be confusing and a source of lethal decimal errors. The *rule of 6* can be used for *dopamine* and *dobutamine* to simplify dosage calculation:

$$6 \text{ mg} \times \text{wt (kg)}, \textit{fill to } 100 \text{ mL with D5W}$$

The medication is mixed in an intravenous set with a measured chamber and a microdrip (1 drop/min = 1 mL/h). Rate of administration is best set by an electric pump.

Example: For a 10-kg infant requiring dopamine:

$$6 \text{ mg} \times 10 = 60 \text{ mg dopamine}$$

In a measured chamber *fill* to 100 mL with D5W. Weight is now factored in so that

$$1 \text{ mL/h} = 1 \text{ µg/kg per min}$$
$$5 \text{ mL/h} = 5 \text{ µg/kg per min}$$
$$10 \text{ mL/h} = 10 \text{ µg/kg per min}$$

For *epinephrine* and *isoproterenol,* the rule of 6 is:

$$0.6 \text{ mg} \times \text{wt (kg)}, \textit{fill to } 100 \text{ mL with D5W}$$
$$1 \text{ mL/h} = 0.1 \text{ µg/kg per min}$$
$$5 \text{ mL/h} = 0.5 \text{ µg/kg per min}$$

Abbreviation: D5W = 5% dextrose in water.

tape to assist in making appropriate selections. Most tapes are two sided and display emergency resuscitation drug dosage and equipment selection based on length (Figures 14-1 to 14-3). Fluid volumes for resuscitation and appropriate basic life support techniques are often also displayed. To make optimal use of these systems, emergency personnel must be able to find the proper equipment rapidly. Equipment can be stored on shelves or in drawers labeled by age and weight, or a system of color codes can be used in which color-coded shelves, carts, or equipment organizers correspond to specific length categories.

The pharmacology of resuscitation drugs has been well described in other chapters (see Chap. 29), but a few peculiarities pertain to pediatric resuscitation drug use.

TABLE 14-5 Length-Based Equipment Chart (Length, cm)*

Item	54–70	70–85	85–95	95–107	107–124	124–138	138–155
Endotracheal tube size (mm)	3.5	4.0	4.5	5.0	5.5	6.0	6.5
Lip–tip length (mm)	10.5	12.0	13.5	15.0	16.5	18.0	19.5
Laryngoscope	1 Straight	1 Straight	2 Straight	2 Straight or curved	2 Straight or curved	2–3 Straight or curved	3 Straight or curved
Suction catheter	8F	8–10F	10F	10F	10F	10F	12F
Stylet	6F	6F	6F	6F	14F	14F	14F
Oral airway	Infant/small child	Small child	Child	Child	Child/small adult	Child/adult	Medium adult
Big-valve mask	Infant	Child	Child	Child	Child	Child/adult	Adult
Oxygen mask	Newborn	Pediatric	Pediatric	Pediatric	Pediatric	Adult	Adult
Vascular access (gauge)							
Catheter	22–24	20–22	18–22	18–22	18–20	18–20	16–20
Butterfly	23–25	23–25	21–23	21–23	21–23	21–22	18–21
Nasogastric tube	5–8F	8–10F	10F	10–12F	12–14F	14–18F	18F
Urinary catheter	5–8F	8–10F	10F	10–12F	10–12F	12F	12F
Chest tube	10–12F	16–20F	20–24F	20–24F	24–32F	28–32F	32–40F
Blood pressure cuff	Newborn/infant	Infant/child	Child	Child	Child	Child/adult	Adult

*Directions for use: (1) measure patient length with centimeter tape; (2) using measured length in centimeters, access appropriate equipment column.
Source: Luten RC, Wears RL, Broselow J, et al: Length-based endotracheal tube sizing and emergency equipment for pediatric resuscitation. *Ann Emerg Med* 21:900, 1992.

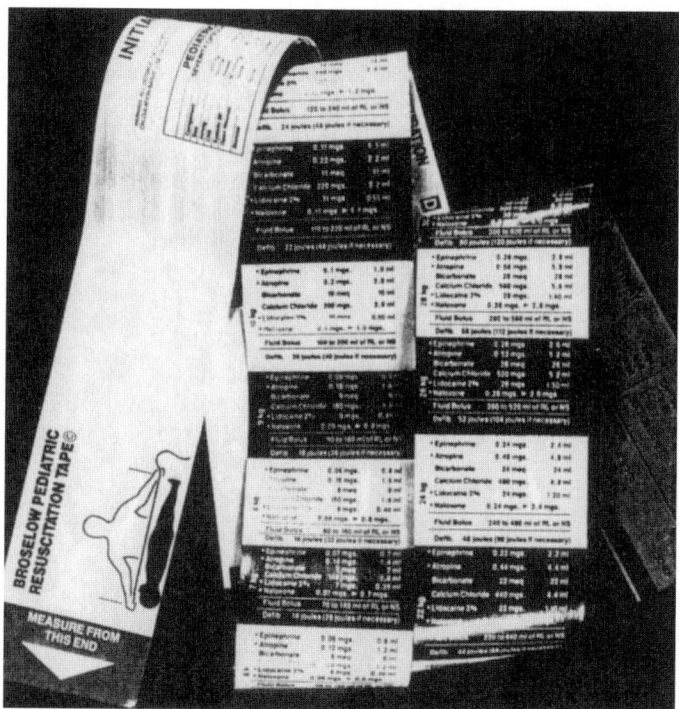

FIG. 14-1. The Broselow resuscitation tape.

Epinephrine

Epinephrine is the one drug proven beneficial in cases of cardiac arrest. It is specifically indicated for hypoxia- or ischemia-induced slow rates that fail to respond to adequate oxygenation and ventilation and for pulseless arrest situations (i.e., asystole, pulseless electrical activity, and ventricular fibrillation). If the initial dose of epinephrine is not effective, subsequent doses should be given at the same dose, although larger doses can be considered. The use of high-dose epinephrine 0.1 mg/kg of the 1:1000 concentration) for resuscitation in infants and children has not been associated with increased survival rate in any controlled prospective studies. The American Heart Association currently recommends that subsequent doses of epinephrine be at the standard dose.[4] High-dose epinephrine may be useful in catecholamine-resistant states, such as anaphylaxis, α- or β-blocker overdose, or severe sepsis. Adverse effects associated with the use of high-dose epinephrine in the clinical setting include intracranial hypertension, myocardial hemorrhage, and myocardial necrosis.[5]

Epinephrine, rather than dopamine, is the vasopressor infusion of choice in children (see Table 14-4), because dopamine requires release of endogenous norepinephrine. In children with cardiac arrest, norepinephrine stores may be low.

Amiodarone

Amiodarone has been added to the most recent guidelines for pediatric cardiopulmonary resuscitation to treat atrial and ventricular arrhythmias. The pharmacology of amiodarone is complex; the inhibition of a variety of receptor and ion channels explains the utility of amiodarone in a range of arrhythmias. Dosage for pediatric patients is 5 mg/kg over 20 to 60 min and may be repeated to a maximum of 15 mg/kg per d. Amiodarone is a potent vasodilator and a potential pro-arrhythmic agent. However, in shock-resistant ventricular tachycardia or ventricular fibrillation, the dose should be given rapidly.

Atropine

Although primary cardiac causes of slow rates are rare in the pediatric population, atropine is recommended for pharmacologic treatment of slow rates after adequate oxygenation and ventilation. The recommended dose of atropine is 0.02 mg/kg IV. The minimum dose is 0.1 mg, with maximum single doses of 0.5 mg for children and 1.0 mg for adolescents. The dose may be repeated once, with maximum total doses of 1.0 mg for children and 2.0 mg for adolescents. There is no particular proscription against additional doses, but the maximum dose is considered fully vagolytic. If no response to atropine is seen, then dosing beyond the vagolytic amount is unlikely to be effective. If an effect is seen but not maintained, additional doses should be considered.

Sodium Bicarbonate

Sodium bicarbonate is a recommended drug in only limited situations, because it worsens acidosis when administered in the presence of inadequate ventilation and perfusion. Because other resuscitation drugs are less effective in the face of severe acidosis, sodium bicarbonate may be a useful agent in prolonged resuscitations. An initial dose of 1 mEq/kg IV is given only after the airway has been secured, the patient is adequately ventilated, and CPR is initiated. In neonates or premature infants, sodium bicarbonate should be diluted 1:1 with sterile water, not with saline. Indications for bicarbonate include hyperkalemia, sodium channel blocker toxicity, and severe metabolic acidosis with adequate ventilation.

Calcium

Because of lack of proven efficacy and because of possible deleterious effects, routine calcium administration is not recommended during resuscitation. Calcium should be used for documented and symptomatic hyperkalemia, hypocalcemia, and calcium channel blocker overdose. Calcium may be given as calcium chloride 20 mg/kg (0.2 mL/kg of a 10 percent solution), or calcium gluconate 60 to 100 mg/kg (0.6 to 1.0 mL/kg of a 10 percent solution) via the IV or intraosseous route.

FIG. 14-2. Equipment side of the Broselow resuscitation tape. One of seven color equipment zones.

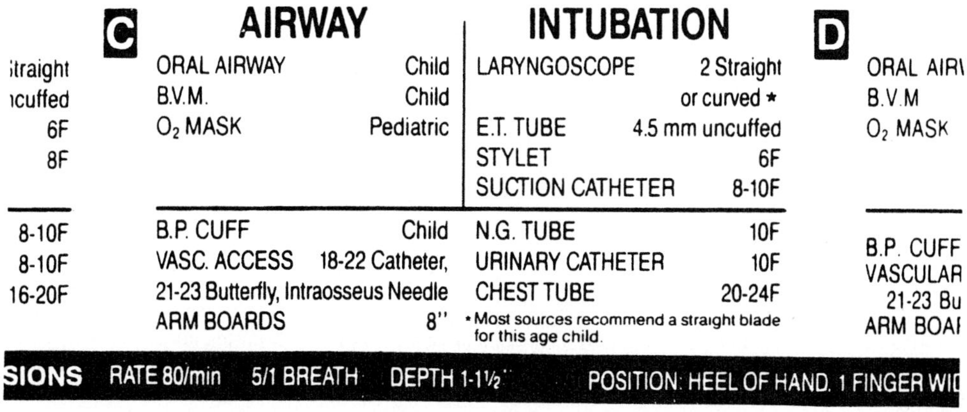

	C AIRWAY		INTUBATION		**D**
itraight	ORAL AIRWAY	Child	LARYNGOSCOPE	2 Straight	ORAL AIR\
icuffed	B.V.M.	Child		or curved ★	B.V.M
6F	O₂ MASK	Pediatric	E.T. TUBE	4.5 mm uncuffed	O₂ MASK
8F			STYLET	6F	
			SUCTION CATHETER	8-10F	
8-10F	B.P. CUFF	Child	N.G. TUBE	10F	
8-10F	VASC. ACCESS	18-22 Catheter,	URINARY CATHETER	10F	B.P. CUFF
16-20F	21-23 Butterfly, Intraosseus Needle		CHEST TUBE	20-24F	VASCULAR
	ARM BOARDS	8"	* Most sources recommend a straight blade		21-23 Bu
			for this age child.		ARM BOAI

| SIONS | RATE 80/min | 5/1 BREATH | DEPTH 1-1½" | POSITION: HEEL OF HAND. 1 FINGER WID |

* **Epinephrine**	**0.1 mgs.**	**1.0 ml**
* **Atropine**	**0.2 mgs.**	**2.0 ml**
Bicarbonate	**10 meq**	**10 ml**
Calcium Chloride	**200 mgs.**	**2.0 ml**
* **Lidocaine 2%**	**10 mgs.**	**0.50 ml**
* **Naloxone**	**0.1 mgs.** ▶	**1.0 mgs.**

10 kg

Fluid Bolus	**100 to 200 ml of RL or NS**

Defib.	**20 joules (40 joules if necessary)**

FIG. 14-3. Drug side of the Broselow resuscitation tape. One of 25 precalculated weight zones for resuscitation drugs.

The Rule of 6

Often there is great confusion when attempting to calculate the dose of a medication to be delivered by constant infusion. The *rule of 6* can be used to avoid mistakes (see Table 14-4), although there are limitations to using this technique in the older child. Length-based resuscitation aids or other resuscitation references should be used to assist with calculating infusion rates.

DYSRHYTHMIAS

Dysrhythmia management plays only a small role in the resuscitation of children. Because rhythm disturbances are usually secondary to hypoxia and not primary cardiac events, careful attention must be given to the correction of hypoxia, acidosis, and fluid balance. Ventilation and oxygenation must be accomplished first. Pulse oximetry, or arterial blood gas analysis, should be performed to assess oxygen and blood gas status. An IV of NS or LR solution should be established, and the child should be placed on a cardiac monitor.

A patient with an abnormal cardiac rhythm or rate, coupled with evidence of poor end-organ perfusion (cyanosis, mottled skin, lethargy, etc.), has an unstable cardiac rhythm and requires immediate intervention. The parameters of clinical assessment and expression of instability vary with a child's age. In neonates, blood pressure measurement is difficult, and a heart rate of 80 beats/min or slower, coupled with evidence of poor end-organ perfusion, requires immediate intervention. In infants and children, variations in heart rate may be well tolerated clinically, and a blood pressure of 70 plus (age in years) divided by 2 mm Hg or less, coupled with evidence of poor end-organ perfusion, is used to define instability. Figures 14-4, 14-5, and 14-6 summarize electrical and drug therapies of unstable cardiac rhythms in children.

The most common rhythms seen in pediatric arrest are the bradycardias, which lead to asystole if untreated. Treatment consists of maximizing oxygenation and ventilation. Chest compression should be started in children with a heart rate slower than 60 beats/min and signs of poor perfusion.

Paroxysmal atrial tachycardia (supraventricular tachycardia, or SVT) is seen most commonly in infants and most often presents as a narrow complex tachycardia with rates usually between 250 and 350 beats/min. Treatment of unstable patients consists of rapid synchronized cardioversion. Treatment of stable patients varies. Adenosine, vagal maneuvers, or cardioversion are used to treat stable SVT. Adenosine (0.1 mg/kg) is the current recommended drug for SVT in children. This dose can be doubled if the first dose is unsuccessful.

Differentiating a rapid secondary sinus tachycardia from a rapid primary cardiac tachycardia can be difficult. Although heart rates of 150 to 200 beats/min in adults are usually cardiac in origin, young children not uncommonly have compensatory sinus tachycardias as fast as 200 to 220 beats/min, especially small infants. Children can tolerate rapid primary cardiac heart rates for long periods before congestive heart failure or lethal dysrhythmias develop. Differentiating primary from secondary tachycardia is critical to patient management. However, an electrocardiogram may not be very helpful, because, at very fast rates, in sinus tachycardia or SVT, identifiable P waves may not be readily apparent. Historical features pointing to volume loss likely suggest sinus tachycardia. Evidence of congestive heart failure more likely is associated with a pathologic rhythm than a compensatory sinus tachycardia.

CARDIOVERSION, DEFIBRILLATION, AND PACING

Electric conversion is used on an emergency basis to treat ventricular fibrillation (defibrillation) and symptomatic tachydysrhythmia (cardioversion). Ventricular fibrillation as a cause of cardiac arrest is rare in children and even more rare in infants.

Paddle Size

Paddle size is usually 4.5 cm for infants (who weigh less than 10 kg) and 8 cm for children. The paddle should be in contact with the chest wall over its entire surface area. The larger 8-cm paddles can be used for infants in the anteroposterior position.

Interface

Electrode cream, electrode paste, and saline-soaked gauze pads are acceptable. Alcohol pads are to be discouraged, because serious burns may be produced. Care must be taken so that the interface substance from one paddle does not come in contact with the substance from the other paddle. This creates a short circuit, and insufficient energy may be delivered to the heart.

Electrode Position

One paddle is placed on the right of the sternum at the second intercostal space. The other is placed on the left midclavicular line at the level of the xiphoid. The anteroposterior approach also can be used.[4]

Defibrillation

Initially, 2 J/kg should be used. If that is unsuccessful, the amount should be doubled and performed twice at the higher energy level, if necessary. If the three attempts are unsuccessful, epinephrine should be given at the standard dose. The oxygenation and ventilation of the child should be maximized for 1 to 2 min before repeating a defibrillation attempt at the higher setting.

Cardioversion

Tachydysrhythmias are generally very sensitive to electric conversion. The initial dose is 0.5 J/kg. The energy level is doubled if the first attempt is unsuccessful. If the device has only a few energy settings available, the one closest to the desired energy setting is chosen. All tachydysrhythmias should be treated with synchronized cardioversion. If synchronization in not possible (i.e., if the device cannot identify the QRS), then the defibrillator is used in the unsynchronized mode.

Transcutaneous Pacing

Children with a severe bradycardia or asystole may respond to pacing. Because transvenous pacing requires central venous access with large tubing and proficient skill in placing the pacing electrodes, most emergency practitioners and prehospital providers should attempt only transcutaneous pacing. Adult patches should be used in children who

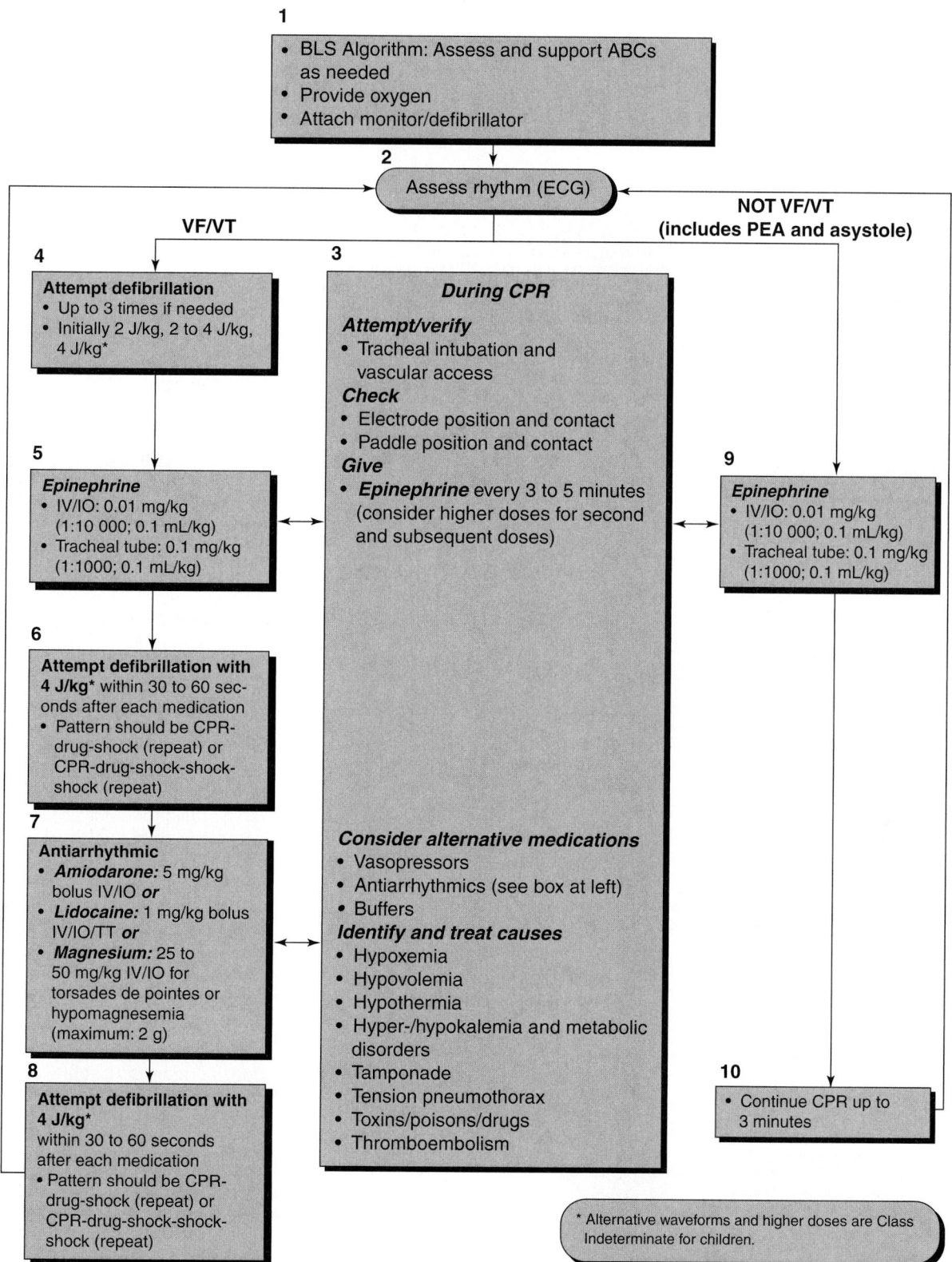

FIG. 14-4. Pediatric pulseless arrest decision tree. ET = endotracheal; IO = intraosseous; IV = intravenous. (Reproduced with permission from *Pediatric Advanced Life Support Instructors Manual.* American Heart Association, 2001.)

weigh more than 15 kg.[10] The negative electrode patch should be placed on the anterior chest at V3, and the positive electrode patch is placed on the posterior chest between the shoulder blades at the T4 vertebral level. Ventricular capture is determined by the palpation of a pulse or the appearance of an arterial waveform, if an arterial pressure catheter is present. Maximal energy output is used first. If ventricular capture occurs, then the energy setting is decreased progressively until the lowest setting is found that allows ventricular capture. The pacing rate should be set at a rate slightly higher than the normal rate for age. Transcutaneous pacing has not been associated with greatly

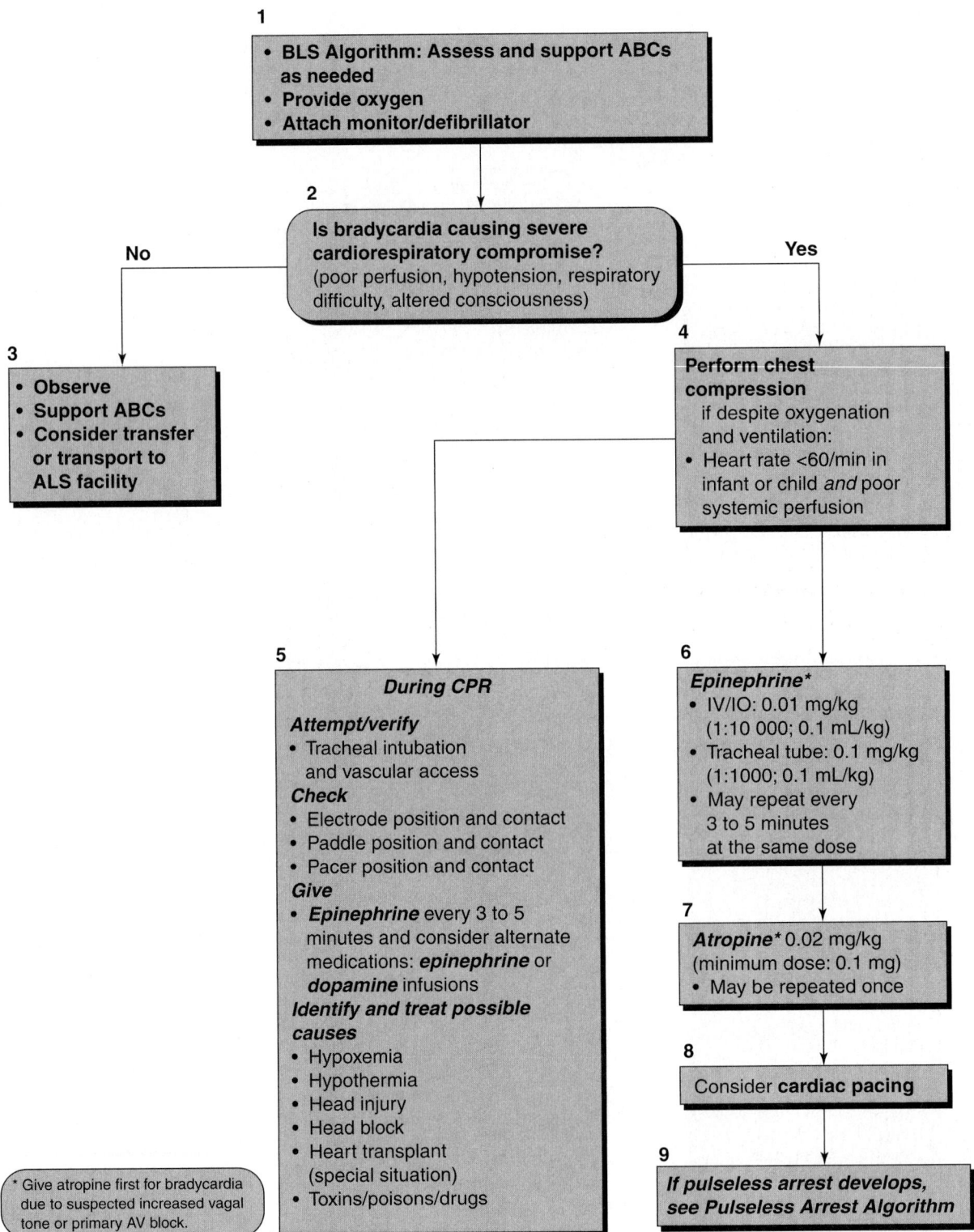

FIG. 14-5. Pediatric bradycardia decision tree. ET = endotracheal; IO = intraosseous; IV = intravenous. (Reproduced with permission from *Pediatric Advanced Life Support Instructors Manual.* American Heart Association, 2001.)

improved survival rates, but it can be lifesaving if applied quickly in a child with sudden asystole or bradycardia.

Automated External Defibrillators

A recent change to the American Heart Association guidelines includes the use of an automated external defibrillator (AED) in pedi-

atric patients. Because children 8 years and older may have life-threatening arrhythmias similar to adults and because their body weights approach those of adults, an AED may be used successfully in a pediatric resuscitation. Few AEDs allow changing the cardioversion energy levels, so infants and young children may receive a dose that is too high. A child older than 8 years and weighing more than 25 kg who suffers a sudden collapse should have an AED applied as soon as pos-

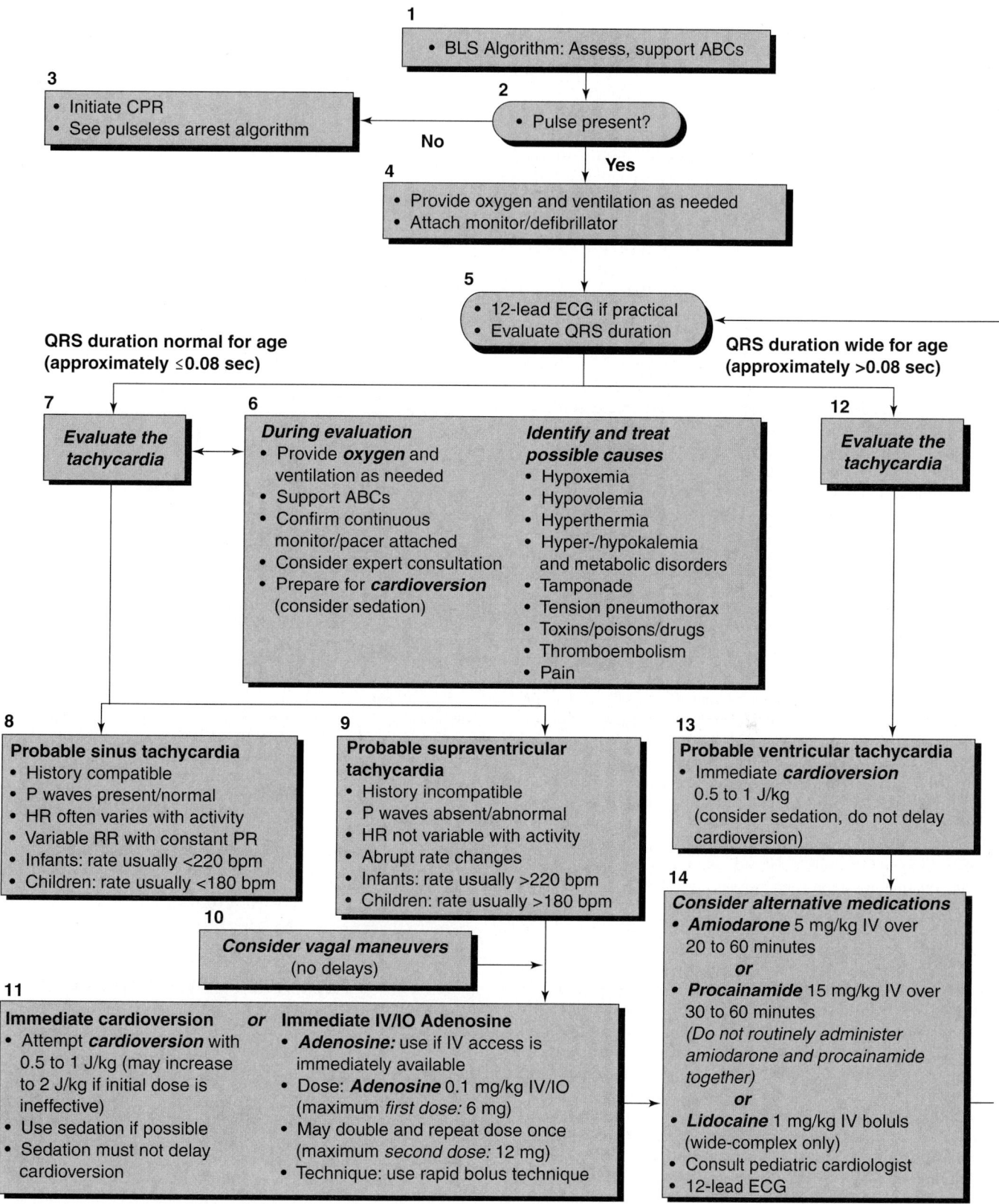

FIG. 14-6. Pediatric tachycardia decision tree for infants and children with rapid rhythm and poor perfusion. ET = endotracheal; IO = intraosseous; IV = intravenous. (Reproduced with permission from *Pediatric Advanced Life Support Instructors Manual.* American Heart Association, 2001.)

sible (class IIb recommendation). Should the AED not recommend defibrillation, then CPR should be initiated. The AED should remain applied until other means of cardiac monitoring become available to the health care provider.

TERMINATION OF EFFORTS

Pediatric cardiopulmonary arrest longer than 20 min or with no response to two doses of epinephrine has been associated with a dismal outcome.[1] **Resuscitation should be continued until a core temperature of 30°C is reached, if cardiac electrical activity is present in a child with hypothermia.**

COPING WITH THE DEATH OF A CHILD

Family members and member of the resuscitation team will mourn the death of a child. Little attention has been focused on this issue for the family or the ED staff. Several *tasks of mourning* have been described that must occur for successful resolution of grieving (Table 14-6).[11] Whether a child dies in the emergency department or after several days of hospitalization does not seem to affect the grieving process.[12] Pathologic grief reactions are often the result of fear that the child will be forgotten. Excessive focus of time, energy, and effort is spent on remembering the child without resolving the grief. Sharing feelings and memories about the child is crucial; persons who do not allow parents to express their feelings may mar the grieving process.[12]

Physicians and other health care providers can shape the way families remember the death of a child. Guidelines for communicating with parents are listed in Table 14-7.[12] Parents remember how compassionately the bad news is given, but most families still want the "bottom line" when they are first told of their child's death. They are waiting for it. Saying "I am very sorry, we did everything we could, but Sally died" is compassionate and direct. Most families do not want all the technical details about the resuscitation efforts. After delivering the bad news, have a chaplain or social worker stay with the family to allow the family time to deal initially with the shocking news. The physician should remain quietly in the room or return after a few minutes (or later, if other duties require) to answer questions. This is also the time to ask whether the family would like to see the child and to prepare them for what they will see. This is also the time to inquire about organ or tissue donation, if a regional transplant consortium does not provide this service already. Although parents do not regret organ donation, donation is not associated with a higher likelihood of successful grieving.[12]

Many hospitals have policies requiring that family wait outside the area where resuscitation efforts are being conducted, but family presence during resuscitation efforts is increasing in popularity. Positive and negative family responses can occur during resuscitation.[13] Family presence during the resuscitative effort may enable family members to begin appropriate grieving earlier. No studies have shown beneficial long-term effects on family grieving by allowing family presence during the resuscitation, however. Some family members may become distressed or exceedingly emotional while care is being given to a loved one. Worries by emergency department staff members about the family's critiques of the resuscitation or the family's unwillingness to terminate efforts contribute to the desire not to have the family present during resuscitation. However, the desire to have family members present during a resuscitation is a holistic approach to patient care, with the family's and the patient's needs addressed simultaneously. In general, the resistance of emergency department staff members to the

TABLE 14-6   Tasks of Family Mourning a Lost Child

Accept the reality of the loss
Work through painful grieving
Adjust to the life without the child
Emotional resolution and return to normal activities

TABLE 14-7   Giving Bad News Effectively

Use support staff such as chaplains and social workers
Early in your delivery of the news, let the family know the child has died
Use simple, direct, understandable language
Speak with compassion and caring
Answer questions from any family members honestly

presence of family members during a resuscitation has been diminishing. Policies are being created to train emergency department staff on how to assist family members and what to expect when families are present during a resuscitation.

REFERENCES

1. Schindler MB, Bohn D, Cox PN, et al: Outcome of out-of-hospital cardiac and respiratory arrest in children. *New Engl J Med* 335:1473, 1996.
2. Teach SJ, Moore PE, Fleisher GR: Death and resuscitation in the pediatric emergency department. *Ann Emerg Med* 25:799, 1995.
3. Ronco R, King W, Donley DK, et al: Outcome and cost at a children's hospital following resuscitation for out-of-hospital cardiopulmonary arrest. *Arch Pediatr Adolesc Med* 149:210, 1995.
4. *Textbook of Pediatric Advanced Life Support.* Dallas, American Heart Association, 2002.
5. Nadkarni V, Hazinski MF, Zideman D, et al: Pediatric resuscitation: An advisory statement from the Pediatric Working Group of the International Liaison Committee on Resuscitation. *Circulation* 95:2185, 1997.
6. King BR, Baker MD, Braitman LE, et al: Endotracheal tube selection in children: A comparison of four methods. *Ann Emerg Med* 22:530, 1993.
7. Van den Berg AA, Mphanza T: Choice of tracheal tube size for children: Finger size or age-related formula. *Anaesthesia* 52:695, 1997.
8. Bhende MS, Thompson AE: Evaluation of an end-tidal CO_2 detector during pediatric cardiopulmonary resuscitation. *Pediatrics* 95:395, 1995.
9. Luten RC, Wears RL, Broselow J, et al: Length-based endotracheal tube sizing and emergency equipment for pediatric resuscitation. *Ann Emerg Med* 21:900, 1992.
10. Beland MJ, Hesslein PS, Finlay CD, et al: Non-invasive transcutaneous cardiac pacing in children. *PACE* 10:1262, 1987.
11. Worden JW: Attachment, loss, and the tasks of mourning, in *Grief Counselling and Grief Therapy: A Handbook for the Mental Health Practitioner,* 2nd ed. New York, Springer-Verlag, 1991.
12. Oliver RC, Fallat ME: Traumatic childhood death: How well do parents cope? *J Trauma* 39:303, 1995.
13. Boudreaux ED, et al: Family presence during invasive procedures and resuscitations in the emergency department. *Ann Emerg Med* 40:193, 2002.

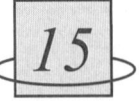

PEDIATRIC AIRWAY MANAGEMENT
Marcie Rubin
Nicholas Sadovnikoff

NORMAL PEDIATRIC AIRWAY ANATOMY

The normal airway of a pediatric patient has important anatomic differences from that of the adult. These differences are most apparent in infants and become relatively insignificant by age 8 years. Differences include the size of the occiput and the tongue in the infant, the high position of the larynx, the configuration of the larynx, and the position of the vocal cords.

The infant has a large occiput. Positioning of the head to obtain the optimum orientation for laryngoscopy, or the "sniffing position," is accomplished simply by rotating the head so that it rests on the occiput. Elevating the head with padding can lead to excessive flexion of the neck and may contribute to upper airway obstruction and difficulty during intubation. The infant's tongue is also relatively large, and this can impair laryngoscopy and contribute to upper airway obstruction. An infant's larynx is higher in the neck, located at the C3 level, than that of an adult, which is found at the C4 to C5 level. The larynx also has a funnel shape in infants, with the narrowest portion at the subglottic area, rather than at the level of the vocal cords, as in an adult. Hence, in infants and small children, an endotracheal tube that passes easily through the vocal cords may encounter resistance more distally. In addition, infants' vocal cords are slanted anteriorly rather than being perpendicular to the trachea, as in an adult, and this characteristic, too, can result in more difficult visualization and intubation in the pediatric population.[1]

ABNORMAL PEDIATRIC AIRWAYS

Congenital

Numerous airway anomalies may be present at birth or develop over the first several months of life. Although they rarely lead to the need for emergent airway control, their presence will complicate management of other emergencies requiring intubation.

Choanal atresia is the most common congenital anomaly of the nose. It may be unilateral or bilateral. Infants with this condition may not have difficulty breathing at birth if they can breathe PO, but they often present several months after birth when there is a concurrent problem, such as an upper respiratory infection. Maintaining an oral or tracheal airway overcomes the obstruction. ED treatment is placement of oral airway, tube feedings, and admission for surgical repair.

Cystic hygroma is a benign congenital tumor of lymphatic origin. About 60 percent appear within the first year of life, and 80 to 90 percent occur before the second year. Cystic hygroma usually occurs in the neck or tongue but may also be found in the mediastinum. Progressive growth can lead to compromise of the structures of the pharynx and trachea, leading to airway obstruction and impairing or preventing laryngoscopy. The treatment is surgical resection.[2]

There are five types of tracheoesophageal fistulas, the most common defect consisting of a blind upper esophageal pouch and a fistula between the lower esophagus and the trachea. The diagnosis is usually made soon after birth, when an infant becomes cyanotic and starts coughing after feeding or when a catheter cannot be passed into the stomach. Although most patients present soon after birth, a few with tracheoesophageal fistula with esophageal atresia present some time after discharge with pneumonia and cyanosis with feeding. Placement of the endotracheal tube in patients with tracheoesophageal fistula is crucial to avoid gastric insufflation and resultant aspiration. The tube should be above the carina but below the fistula. This is often achieved by intubation of the right mainstem bronchus and then pulling back until breath sounds are heard bilaterally.

The common congenital syndrome of trisomy 21 (Down syndrome) may present significant difficulties in airway management. Characteristic of these patients is a short neck, small mouth, narrow nasopharynx, and large tongue; moreover, approximately 20 percent have asymptomatic dislocation of the atlas on the axis.[3] All potential difficulties must be considered before initiating intubation. Many congenital syndromes include airway abnormalities (Table 15-1). In controlled settings, management is preceded by careful evaluation and planning. Unfortunately, in the ED, this is rarely possible, and thus the approach to airway management must be mastered in all facets by those whose practice, even infrequently, involves pediatrics.

Acquired

Acquired abnormalities in pediatric airways can be subdivided into acute and chronic. Acute obstruction can result from foreign-body aspiration, infection such as laryngotracheobronchitis or epiglottitis, subglottic edema secondary to previous intubation or allergy, or internal or external airway trauma. Chronic obstruction can result from subglottic stenosis (posttraumatic or postsurgical), tumor, or abscess formation.

TABLE 15-1 Pediatric Syndromes and Associated Airway Abnormalities

Prominent Airway Abnormality	Syndromes
Mandibular hypoplasia	Hallermann-Steiff-François Pierre-Robin Goldenhaber Nager Treacher Collins
Maxillary hypoplasia	Apert Pfeiffer Crouzon
Macroglossia	Trisomy 21 Beckwith-Wiedemann Hurler
Tracheomalacia	Apert Crouzon

Note: If patient has history of significant airway obstruction or apnea, premedication is best avoided or used with extreme caution.

The management of an infant or child with airway obstruction depends on the use of a safe, calculated approach to securing the airway. Such an approach requires a systematic evaluation of the pediatric airway, familiarity with pediatric airway equipment and pharmacologic agents, and recognition of a difficult airway and its appropriate management.

EVALUATION OF A PEDIATRIC AIRWAY

The first step in evaluating a pediatric airway is a directed history and physical examination. The time course of the present episode should be determined, as should a history of any recent fever, cough, or sore throat. Any history of previous airway problems should be elicited. If time permits, the history should include a review of the antenatal and perinatal periods, with an emphasis on feeding or sleeping difficulties. Any history of snoring or noisy breathing, recurrent croup or upper respiratory infections, or cyanosis or coughing during feedings should alert the clinician to the possibility of an abnormal airway.

The physical examination of a pediatric patient may be hindered by lack of cooperation, and care should be taken not to frighten the child. Visual signs of possible airway compromise include tachypnea, cyanosis, drooling, nasal flaring, and intercostal retractions. The child may assume a "tripod" position to enhance the use of accessory respiratory muscles. Auscultation may reveal stridor, wheezing, or grunting. Any change in the child's mental status, including agitation or somnolence, may further indicate airway difficulties. As in adults, features suggesting potentially difficult intubation include a small or recessed mandible, a prominent tongue, prominent upper incisors, and impairment of neck mobility.

Pediatric patients often have a period of compensated respiratory compromise before an arrest.[4] Pulse oximetric measurements should be monitored continuously, but adequate oxygen saturation should not be considered assurance of respiratory stability, because this measurement may not reflect declining ventilatory performance. All patients with potential airway compromise require attentive observation and frequent examination.

PEDIATRIC AIRWAY EQUIPMENT

Oropharyngeal and Nasopharyngeal Airways

Oropharyngeal airways are easy to use and available for pediatric patients of all ages. An oral airway should extend from the corner of the mouth to just cephalad to the angle of the mandible. To estimate the correct size, the airway can be placed next to the face. The oral airway should not be used in a conscious child, because it may induce vomiting. The nasopharyngeal airway can be used in awake or semicomatose patients. The proper length is estimated by measuring the distance from the tip of the nose to the tragus of the ear. Complications include damage to adenoid tissue, epistaxis, and laryngospasm. Because the diameters of the nasal airways are so small in the pediatric population, they easily may become obstructed with blood, mucus, or vomitus and thus require frequent suctioning.

Bag-Valve-Mask Devices

The ideal pediatric mask should provide an airtight seal between the mask and the patient's face. A poor mask fit results in gas leaks, inability to maintain positive pressure, and potential compromise to ventilation and oxygenation. Child-size and adult-size self-inflating bags (Ambu, Inc., Linthicum, MD) may be used for the entire range of infants and children. Maximum oxygen delivery occurs at an oxygen flow of 15 L/min.[1]

Laryngoscope Blades

Two types of blades are most commonly available in emergency departments for pediatric intubation: curved (Macintosh) and straight (Miller). The tip of the Macintosh blade is inserted into the vallecula anterior to the epiglottis, and, as the blade is lifted, the epiglottis is elevated passively beneath the blade tip to expose the glottic opening. The tip of the Miller blade is placed beneath the epiglottis, which is directly elevated as the blade is lifted. A straight blade is superior to a curved blade in children younger than 2 years. Table 15-2 presents a guide for laryngoscope selection in pediatric patients.

Endotracheal Tubes

There are numerous methods for selecting the correct endotracheal tube size for a given pediatric patient, including age, height, weight, and diameter of the fifth digit. Endotracheal tube size for premature and full-term infants usually is selected by weight, because, given the rapid growth during this period, age formulas become invalid. The rule usually employed is a 2.5-mm tube below 1.5 kg of body weight, a 3.0-mm tube between 1.5 and 2.5 kg, and a 3.5-mm tube above 2.5 kg. The most commonly used formula for age determination of endotracheal tube size in children older than 1 year is: tube size (in millimeters) = 4 + age (in years)/4.[5] However, single-formula methods based on age have been shown to lead frequently to inappropriate tube selection.[6] Resuscitation measuring tapes have been found to be more accurate than age-based formulas, which in turn are superior to the diameter of the fifth digit.[7,8]

The tube should fit sufficiently snugly to prevent any leakage at pressures up to 10 cm H_2O but should leak at a pressure lower than 30 cm H_2O. An insufficiently snug fit will result in difficulty ventilating, compromised airway protection, and leakage of inhalational agents if the patient undergoes anesthesia. An overly tight-fitting tube risks endotracheal injury, with the potential for development of subglottic stenosis due to the anatomic reasons noted above. For the same reason, **cuffed tubes are generally avoided in patients 8 years and younger.** Clearly, in the care of an unstable patient in the emergency department, a suboptimal tube that provides adequate ventilation is preferable to no airway at all, and exchange for a more appropriate tube can be deferred until the patient has been stabilized.

The ideal depth of placement is midway between the glottis and the carina. Because of substantial variability in tracheal length, especially before the age of 1 year, formulas predicting the distance to the lips are unreliable. Because most pediatric tubes have a series of marks at the distal end, one technique is to simply advance the tube so that the second mark is just past the vocal cords. This results in a conservatively high tube that will not risk bronchial intubation. However, inadvertent dislodgement of the tube with head and neck manipulation may occur. A second technique is to initially and deliberately perform a bronchial intubation by advancing the tube until breath sounds are heard only unilaterally and then to back the tube up to a point 1 cm above where the breath sounds are again heard bilaterally. This method results in a conservatively low tube, but with little risk of inadvertent displacement out of the airway.

Laryngeal Mask Airway

The laryngeal mask airway (LMA) has been used widely in the pediatric population.[9] It has been found to be extremely useful in the management of difficult airways. It consists of a large-bore tube terminating in an ovoid, fenestrated cup with an inflatable rim that, when properly placed, forms a seal over the laryngeal orifice (see Figure 18-6). The result is an airway that is superior to a face mask in that it prevents supraglottic obstruction and greatly reduces the likelihood of gastric insufflation, but it is less reliable at preventing aspiration than an endotracheal tube. Because it is placed blindly, it avoids the complications of endotracheal intubation that arise from the need to visualize and penetrate the glottic opening. It provides a useful rescue device in the event of a failed endotracheal intubation. Once in place, it can be used as a conduit for fiberoptically guided endotracheal intubation. Its applications and experience with its use continue to expand, and emergency physicians should be familiar with its insertion. Laryngeal mask airways can be sized from neonates to adults. Table 15-3 presents a guideline of sizes according to weight.

RAPID SEQUENCE INTUBATION OF THE PEDIATRIC PATIENT

Rapid sequence intubation (RSI) is the nearly simultaneous administration of a potent intravenous anesthetic agent and a neuromuscular blocking agent to facilitate endotracheal intubation. The process involves

TABLE 15-2 Laryngoscope Blade Selection for Pediatric Patients

Age	SIZE	
	Miller	Macintosh
Premature	0	
Neonate	0 or 1	
1 month to 2 years	1	
2–6 years	*	2
6–12 years	2	2 or 3
12 or older	2 or 3	3

*If a straight blade is desired in this age group, a Wis-Hipple 1.5 may be used.

TABLE 15-3 Laryngeal Mask Airway Size Selection

Weight, kg	LMA Size
<5	1
5–10	1.5
10–20	2
20–30	2.5
30–50	3
50–70	4
>70	5

preparation, preoxygenation, application of cricoid pressure (Sellick maneuver), induction of anesthesia, neuromuscular blockade, and intubation without attempting mask ventilation. Although some remain advocates of other airway management methods, this technique provides unsurpassed airway access and minimizes complications. Its use in critically ill children is well described, and it is regarded as the first choice in the absence of contraindications (see below).[10,11]

Preparation

Before undertaking an RSI, all necessary tools and materials should be prepared. A well-functioning intravenous line must be in place, and all drugs to be used for the RSI should be predrawn in syringes and labeled. Laryngoscopes with blades of the appropriate sizes, with lights checked and working, should be within reach, as should suction equipment and a bag-mask-ventilation apparatus connected to oxygen. Any materials for rescue maneuvers after failed intubation, such as LMAs, jet ventilation devices, and cricothyrotomy trays, should be immediately available. An endotracheal tube of the estimated size should be styletted, with tubes a size larger and a size smaller present. At least one additional experienced provider should be present to apply cricoid pressure and provide assistance as needed. **Continuous pulse oximetric monitoring and an exhaled CO_2 detection device are strongly recommended.**

Preoxygenation

Due to their relatively high oxygen consumption, smaller children, and especially infants, undergo rapid desaturation with cessation of ventilation, even with normal lungs. Once drugs have been administered in RSI, patients rapidly become apneic. Positive pressure mask ventilation is not performed at this point due to the risk of gastric insufflation and resultant regurgitation. Therefore, it is important to maximize the length of time that adequate saturation is maintained by maximizing the reservoir of oxygen in the lungs. The lung volume remaining at end-expiration, or functional residual capacity, contains less than 20 percent oxygen in a patient breathing room air, with nearly 80 percent occupied by nitrogen. Preoxygenation is effectively denitrogenation of functional residual capacity, and it increases by roughly fivefold the oxygen reservoir in the lungs once apnea occurs. Effective denitrogenation is ideally accomplished by having a patient breathe 100 percent oxygen from a tight-fitting mask for 2 min or for four vital capacity breaths. Often this is not possible with a critically ill pediatric patient, but as long a period of preoxygenation as circumstances permit should be provided before RSI.

Premedication

Atropine should be available and given preemptively when succinylcholine is being considered. Some authorities suggest the use of atropine (0.015 to 0.20 mg/kg IV push) for all RSI to prevent bradycardia associated with posterior pharynx stimulation. In patients in whom increased intracranial pressure is a consideration, premedication with lidocaine (1.5 mg/kg IV) 1 to 5 min prior to intubation is recommended. Lidocaine is believed to decrease the adrenergic response to laryngoscopy, sedatives, and neuromuscular blocking agents,[12] although of 25 studies reviewed by Lev and Rosen, only 60 percent claimed some cardiovascular benefit.[13] Lidocaine has also been shown to attenuate cough[14] and increases in intracranial[15] and intraocular pressure. The review by Lev and Rosen showed no adverse effects of premedication with lidocaine,[13] thus it appears appropriate to consider its use routinely in pediatric RSI.

Cricoid Pressure

Application of cricoid pressure entails the manual application of firm pressure at the level of the cricoid cartilage anteroposteriorly to oc-

clude the esophagus and minimize the risk of aspiration. It should not be applied over the thyroid cartilage or over the entire larynx. It should be initiated immediately before the administration of the RSI drugs and not released until correct endotracheal tube position is confirmed. The amount of pressure should be graded according to the size of the patient. In smaller patients, the person applying cricoid pressure may wish to use the other hand under the neck to avoid altering the neck position.

Induction of Anesthesia

Laryngoscopy and endotracheal intubations are extremely stimulating events that are powerfully resisted by the unanesthetized patient. The goal of RSI is to overcome this resistance while preserving hemodynamic stability. The term *induction of anesthesia* is used rather than *sedation,* because, although the distinction between the two is somewhat indistinct, performance of laryngoscopy and intubation without causing major hemodynamic perturbations requires a deep state of anesthesia, for which the term *sedation* is inappropriate. The drugs commonly used for induction of anesthesia and their pediatric doses are listed in Table 15-4. **Note the absence of opioid agents for induction, because they do not reliably induce rapid hypnosis.** These doses are appropriate for healthy, well-hydrated patients. The dose for critically ill patients and for those who have received other agents, such as opioid analgesics, should be adjusted downward accordingly. All of these drugs are appropriate for this indication; however, the profiles and side effects of each differ somewhat, as discussed below.

SODIUM THIOPENTAL Sodium thiopental is the most commonly employed drug for induction of anesthesia and has been in use for some five decades. It is very inexpensive and provides reliable induction of anesthesia within 1 min. It causes significant venodilation and moderate direct myocardial suppression, which result in decreases in blood pressure and cardiac output despite an increase in heart rate mediated by a minimally suppressed baroreceptor reflex. It lowers intracranial and intraocular pressures and has long been the drug of choice when elevations of these pressures are a concern. Only barbiturates, of all the pharmacologic interventions studied, have been shown to provide cerebroprotection in acute brain injury, leading to the preference for this drug in the setting of intracranial mass lesions or head trauma. Its side effects include histamine release, which may manifest as flushing, exaggerated hypotension, and wheezing in patients with reactive airways. Neuroexcitatory effects during induction, such as twitching, cough, and hiccups, are relatively common. It can cause extensive tissue necrosis if extravasated.

PROPOFOL Since its release in the United States in 1989, this drug has enjoyed increasing popularity, particularly in elective settings. Its onset of action is similar to that of thiopental, and it produces comparable decreases in blood pressure and cardiac output. Unlike thiopental, there is no reflex increase in heart rate. Propofol appears to be superior to thiopental at suppressing pharyngeal and laryngeal reflexes and for this reason is usually chosen for insertion of an LMA without paralysis. Like thiopental, it lowers intracranial and intraocular pressures, and although experience with propofol is less extensive, it is probably as good a choice as thiopental in similar settings. It does not cause histamine release or stimulate bronchospasm, and extravasation has not been reported to cause significant tissue injury. It is notorious for causing pain on injection, which may be markedly attenuated by preadministration of a small dose of lidocaine. It is significantly more expensive than thiopental, and, given the overall similarity of their profiles, propofol has not been widely adopted for use in RSI due to this factor. Because it is prepared as an emulsion that readily supports bacterial growth, propofol must be administered or discarded within 6 h of opening its container.

TABLE 15-4   Drugs for Pediatric Intubation

Drug	Dose	Duration	Comments
Neuromuscular blockade			
Vecuronium	0.15–0.20 mg/kg	to 60 min	Atropine 0.02 mg/kg
Rocuronium	0.9–1.2 mg/kg	to 60 min	Atropine 0.02 mg/kg
Succinylcholine	1–2 mg/kg	3–5 min	Atropine 0.02 mg/kg
Anesthetic agents			
Etomidate	0.3 mg/kg	5–10 min	Cardiostable; not an analgesic
Midazolam	0.1–0.2 mg/kg	30–45 min	Cardiostable; reversible
Ketamine	2 mg/kg	20–60 min	Cardiostable; use atropine
Thiopental	4 mg/kg	5–10 min	Hypotension, histamine release
Propofol	2.5–3.5 mg/kg	4–8 min	Hypotension

KETAMINE   Unlike any of the other induction agents, ketamine tends to increase heart rate, blood pressure, and cardiac output. These effects appear to be mediated through central sympathetic stimulation, because ketamine appears to be a weak myocardial depressant in isolated heart preparations. Such effects enhance its attractiveness in settings such as trauma with hypovolemia. It is also a bronchodilator with no suppression of ventilatory drive, making it an excellent choice for patients with known reactive airway disease. In addition, it has significant analgesic and amnestic properties. It can be given intramuscularly in a dose of 4 to 6 mg/kg, with onset of anesthesia within 5 min. This may be desirable in the combative patient in whom intravenous access has not been secured. Unfortunately, it also carries a number of undesirable side effects. Despite the bronchodilatation, there are marked increases in upper airway secretions, which can occur briskly and complicate airway management. It increases cerebral blood flow, intracranial pressure, and intraocular pressure and should not be used in patients in whom these effects are a concern. Moreover, it is associated with a significant incidence of emergence hallucinations, particularly in patients with a known history of psychosis, although this reaction is less common in children than in adults. This response can be attenuated by coadministration of benzodiazepines.

MIDAZOLAM   Of the benzodiazepines, midazolam is the most popular for induction of anesthesia due to its rapid onset time and lack of venous irritation. The doses required for induction are much larger than those used for sedation. The onset of action is still somewhat slower than with the other induction agents discussed in this section. As a consequence of the large dose, the time to recovery is prolonged compared with that for the other induction agents. Unlike the other induction agents, midazolam can be reversed by the benzodiazepine antagonist flumazenil, although this should be avoided due to the risk of seizures. Remarkably little hemodynamic perturbation occurs with an induction dose, although significant hypotension may occur in a hypovolemic or critically ill patient. Apnea is common, and coadministration of opioids markedly potentiates respiratory suppression. Amnesia is accomplished most reliably with this induction agent. Although expensive when compared with thiopental, it is commonly used in the emergency department due to its stable hemodynamic profile.

ETOMIDATE   Etomidate has a stable hemodynamic profile. An induction dose results in almost no change in heart rate, blood pressure, or cardiac output, because it appears to affect neither vascular tone nor baroreceptor reflex. It has little effect on ventilatory drive and none on airway smooth muscle. It lowers cerebral blood flow, intracranial pressure, and intraocular pressure much to the same degree as do thiopental and propofol. It completely lacks any analgesic properties and may require a low (2 to 4 μg/kg) dose of fentanyl to fully suppress the response to intubation. Side effects include pain on injection, myoclonic movements on induction, and a high incidence of subsequent nausea and vomiting. Reports suggesting adrenal suppression occurring with only an induction dose of the drug decreased its popularity, but evidence of the clinical significance of this observation has not been reported.

CHOICE OF AGENTS   The choice of agent should be dictated by the specifics of the patient's physiologic status and by the experience of the emergency physician. Factors such as cost and convenience of storage and administration affect a department's choice of options. Specific scenarios for which pharmacologic management may be tailored are discussed below.

Neuromuscular Blockade

The goal of neuromuscular blockade in RSI is to obtain the optimal conditions for laryngoscopy as quickly as possible. The neuromuscular-blocking drug (NMB) is thus injected immediately after the injection of the induction agent. Complete neuromuscular blockade enables maximal laryngoscopic displacement of the tongue and mandible to optimize the view of the glottic aperture. In most children without anatomic deformities, glottic visualization is relatively simple once neuromuscular blockade is accomplished. Neuromuscular blockade also ensures that the vocal cords will be open, thus facilitating atraumatic passage of the endotracheal tube. There are many NMBs available, but only those with the most rapid times of onset can be recommended for RSI. These include the depolarizing NMB, succinylcholine, and two nondepolarizing NMBs, vecuronium and rocuronium.

Although many practitioners may be more familiar with pancuronium, which is inexpensive and has a long history of use in the emergency department, its long time of onset and very long duration of action make it a suboptimal choice for RSI.

SUCCINYLCHOLINE   Succinylcholine, the only depolarizing NMB available in the United States, remains the drug of choice for RSI. Although the U.S. Food and Drug Administration has issued an advisory against its elective use in children, it continues to be approved for emergency airway management. The reason for the limitation of its use is that it has been associated with hyperkalemic arrest in children subsequently found to have underlying but undiagnosed myopathies (see below).

The advantages of succinylcholine include its extremely reliable and rapid time to onset of action; intubating conditions are obtained generally within 45 s. As noted, children become hypoxemic with apnea more rapidly than do adults, and even a 15-s advantage can be meaningful. Unlike nondepolarizing NMBs, duration of action is short. Spontaneous ventilation usually returns within 3 to 5 min. This is particularly important when ongoing neurologic assessment is desired, or when a difficult airway is anticipated or encountered, as options are preserved in the case of a failed intubation.

Unfortunately, the potential disadvantages of the drug are relatively numerous and include hyperkalemia; malignant hyperthermia; elevations in intracranial, intraocular, and intragastric pressures; prolonged blockade; and fasciculations. These are described in detail in Chapter 19. Fasciculations are not inherently dangerous as long as the patient is protected from involuntary physical injury. As in adults, they can be prevented by preadministration of a small "defasciculating" dose (10 percent of an intubating dose) of a nondepolarizing NMB 2 min before succinylcholine is given.

Bradycardia occurs unpredictably in some patients receiving succinylcholine and is more common after a second dose. When it does occur, hypoxia, rather than drug effect, should be the first consideration. This is of particular concern in small children and neonates, whose cardiac output is directly dependent on heart rate. **Premedication with atropine 0.015 to 0.20 mg/kg is advisable in children younger than 5 years or in any child with a heart rate slower than 120 beats/min.**

Prolonged blockade is not inherently dangerous in and of itself. The implication is that occasionally a patient has a prolonged apparent absence of neurologic function that could be mistaken for central nervous system injury. Train-of-four monitoring, the elicitation of muscular response after a standardized series of four electrical pulses stimulating a particular nerve, is used primarily in the operating room and intensive care unit settings. Absence of any twitch response to train-of-four muscular stimulation 10 min after a dose of succinylcholine reflects prolonged neuromuscular blockade.

A small subset of patients develops masseter spasm on receiving succinylcholine, making intubation more difficult. These patients are at increased risk of developing myoglobinuria and have a greater propensity for developing malignant hyperthermia. Fewer than 1 percent of patients manifest this complication.

In the event that succinylcholine is contraindicated, a fast-acting nondepolarizing NMB may be chosen with the knowledge that the onset will be slightly slower and the duration of action substantially longer.

VECURONIUM Vecuronium was the first nondepolarizing NMB to be recommended for use in RSI. To obtain intubating conditions in 60 to 90 s, a dose of 0.3 to 0.4 mg/kg is given. This results in a duration of action of 90 to 150 min. Alternatively, if time permits, a "priming" dose of 0.01 mg/kg should be given 2 to 3 min before an intubating dose of 0.15 to 0.2 mg/kg. The priming technique entails no clinically significant issues, but it speeds the onset of intubating conditions after the intubating dose and shortens the duration of action to 60 to 75 min. Vecuronium is essentially devoid of hemodynamic effects and does not cause histamine release. It is stored as a powder that is easily diluted for use.

ROCURONIUM Rocuronium is similar to vecuronium in its lack of hemodynamic effects. It is somewhat less potent, giving it a more rapid time to onset of intubating conditions, sufficiently so that priming is not considered necessary. Doses of 0.9 and 1.2 mg/kg have been shown in adults to result in times to intubating conditions of 75 and 55 s, respectively, approaching the 45 s typical of succinylcholine.[16] The duration of action is comparable to that of vecuronium 0.1 mg/kg, at the 0.9-mg/kg dose and somewhat longer at the 1.2-mg/kg dose. Rocuronium is supplied as a solution that requires refrigeration, making it slightly less convenient to stock and store than vecuronium.

Contraindications to RSI

There are few contraindications to RSI. A known difficult airway requires an alternative approach. A variety of other approaches may be considered in a patient known to have experienced failed laryngoscopic intubation in the past or whose anatomy or injuries preclude direct laryngoscopy. These approaches include blind techniques, fiberoptically assisted techniques, and techniques employing an LMA. (These are detailed in Chap. 19.) Invasive emergency airway management approaches are discussed below. Patients who are judged to be too ill to receive anesthetic drugs, such as those who are comatose, profoundly hypotensive, or without circulation, may be intubated without pharmacologic assistance. Cricoid pressure nonetheless should be applied, because regurgitation and aspiration may still occur in these patients.

INVASIVE AIRWAY TECHNIQUES

Needle Cricothyroidotomy

Emergency surgical airways are often difficult to establish in children and have high complication rates. Hence, needle cricothyroidotomy has been advocated as the preferred airway access technique in the pediatric population. Needle cricothyroidotomy is performed by first identifying the cricothyroid membrane. A large-bore (14-gauge) intravenous catheter is passed through the membrane into the airway at a 45-degree caudad angle. The needle is removed, and an adapter is placed on the catheter so a standard bag-valve-mask can be connected for oxygenation. This system has been shown to provide adequate oxygenation for prolonged periods. It cannot, however, provide adequate ventilation.[17]

Transtracheal jet ventilation (TTJV) allows ventilation and oxygenation through a catheter. Ventilation is provided with short, intermittent bursts of oxygen. This requires high-pressure (50 psi) oxygen-delivery systems. The system of choice is a jet injector regulated by a flow meter attached to a wall or tank unit. The less optimal choice is an unregulated wall or tank system. A 1-s jet of oxygen followed by a 4-s expiratory phase achieves satisfactory ventilation.[18]

Complications of needle cricothyroidotomy include bleeding, infection, esophageal perforation, breakage or bending of the needle, subcutaneous emphysema, pneumothorax, pneumomediastinum, and pneumopericardium.

Surgical Cricothyroidotomy and Tracheostomy

Emergency surgical cricothyroidotomy and tracheostomy in pediatric patients is much more difficult than in adults due to the smaller dimensions of the structures and the relatively higher position of the larynx in the neck. Cricothyroidotomy should be avoided in children under 10 years due to technical difficulties and TTJV is preferred. Few emergency physicians are experienced in emergency tracheostomy, and again TTJV or LMA should be considered. Sufficient literature documenting the true complication rates of these procedures in the pediatric population is not available.

SPECIAL CONSIDERATIONS

Head Trauma or Intracranial Mass Lesion

Securing the airway in a pediatric patient with head trauma or an intracranial mass lesion plays an important role by correcting or preventing hypercarbia and hypoxemia, factors that can increase intracranial pressure. Because endotracheal intubation itself is inherently stimulating to intracranial pressure, all possible precautions should be taken to suppress this response. In addition, in the setting of head trauma, RSI should be undertaken with strict head and neck immobilization due to the potential for concomitant cervical spine injuries.

Rapid sequence intubation is the preferred method of intubation in pediatric patients with suspected or known intracranial hypertension. In addition to the agents previously discussed, lidocaine at a dose of 1.5 mg/kg IV should be given before laryngoscopy.[19] This intervention blocks the rise in intracranial pressure that commonly accompanies endotracheal intubation. It is important to remember that in pediatric patients, as in adults, head injuries can also be associated with intra-oral and intratracheal injuries. When managing the airway of a head-injured patient, one must always be prepared for invasive airway management.

Epiglottitis and Croup

For a detailed discussion of pediatric upper airway obstruction, see Chap. 133. Optimal airway management for pediatric patients with epiglottitis is in the operating room. If the patient is stable, he or she should be transported to the operating room accompanied by a skilled airway manager and the proper equipment. A patient with complete airway obstruction often can be ventilated until an airway can be established. If this is unsuccessful, emergent orotracheal intubation should be attempted. If this fails, invasive airway techniques should be used.

Uncommonly, a child with croup may be unresponsive to medical management and may require an artificial airway. An endotracheal tube is optimally placed in the operating room, allowing for inhalation induction of anesthesia. Intubation, however, may have to be performed in the emergency department if the patient is in extremis.

Airway Foreign Bodies

Management of an unstable patient with acute airway obstruction requires immediate attention to the airway. In the prehospital setting, the American Heart Association recommends a series of five back blows and five chest thrusts in a child younger than 1 year (see Chap. 14). The child should have the oropharynx examined between each series. In a child older than 1 year, the recommendation is a series of abdominal thrusts in the upright or the supine position.

In the emergency department, the child with a partially obstructed airway should be rapidly assessed. If the child will tolerate it, a visual inspection of the hypopharyngeal and laryngeal areas should be attempted. Commonly, a child will tolerate this procedure poorly and thus should be taken to the operating room for general anesthesia and removal of the foreign body. In an unstable or completely obstructed patient, orotracheal intubation may dislodge the foreign body, and this should be attempted before needle cricothyroidotomy.

REFERENCES

1. Todres D: Pediatric airway control and ventilation. *Ann Emerg Med* 22:440, 1993.
2. Sie KC: Hemangiomas and vascular malformations of the airway. *Otolaryngol Clin North Am* 33:209, 2000.
3. Williams JP, Somerville GM, Miner ME, Reilly D: Atlanto-axial subluxation and trisomy 21: Another perioperative complication. *Anesthesiology* 67:253, 1987.
4. Emergency Cardiac Care Committee and Subcommittees, American Heart Association: Guidelines for cardiopulmonary resuscitation and emergency cardiac care. Part VI. Pediatric advanced life support. *JAMA* 268:2262, 1992.
5. Ferrari LR, Cunningham MJ: Determination of endotracheal tube size in pediatric patients. *Arch Otolaryngol Head Neck Surg* 118:448, 1992.
6. Mostafa SM: Variation in subglottic size in children. *Proc R Soc Med* 29:494, 1976.
7. Luten RC, Wears RL, Broselow J, et al: Length-based endotracheal tube and emergency equipment in pediatrics. *Ann Emerg Med* 21:900, 1992.
8. King BR, Baker MD, Braitman LE: Endotracheal tube selection in children: A comparison of four methods. *Ann Emerg Med* 22:530, 1993.
9. Lopez-Gil M, Brimacombe J, Alvarez M: Safety and efficacy of the laryngeal mask airway: A prospective survey of 1400 paediatric patients. *Anesthesia* 51:969, 1996.
10. Gerardi MJ, Sacchetti AD, Cantor RM, et al: Rapid-sequence intubation of the pediatric patient. Pediatric Emergency Medicine Committee of the American College of Emergency Physicians. *Ann Emerg Med* 28:55, 1996.
11. Walls RM: Rapid-sequence intubation comes of age. *Ann Emerg Med* 28:79, 1996.
12. Lee BS, Gausche-Hill M: Advances in pediatric resuscitation. *Clin Pediat Emerg Med* 2:91, 2001.
13. Lev R, Rosen P: Prophylactic lidocaine use preintubation: A review *J Emerg Med* 12:499, 1994.
14. Wilson IG, Meiklejohn BH, Smith G: Intravenous lignocaine and sympathoadrenal responses to laryngoscopy and intubation. *Anaesthesia* 46:177, 1991.
15. Brucia JJ, Owen DC, Rudy EB: The effects of lidocaine on intracranial hypertension. *J Neurosci Nursing* 24:205, 1992.
16. Magorian T, Flannery KB, Miller RD: Comparison of rocuronium, succinylcholine and vecuronium for rapid-sequence induction of anesthesia in adult patients. *Anesthesiology* 79:913, 1993.
17. Cote CJ, Eavey RD, Todres ID, et al: Crycoid membrane puncture: Oxygenation and ventilation in a dog model using an intravenous catheter. *Crit Care Med* 16:615, 1988.
18. Benumof JC, Scheller MS: The importance of transtracheal jet ventilation in the management of the difficult airway. *Anesthesiology* 71:769, 1989.
19. Walls RM: Rapid-sequence intubation in head trauma. *Ann Emerg Med* 22:1008, 1993.

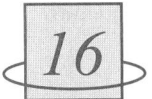

16

RESUSCITATION ISSUES IN PREGNANCY

Elizabeth M. Datner
Susan B. Promes

ETIOLOGY OF MATERNAL DEATH

Although cardiac arrest in pregnant patients is rare (it is estimated to occur once in every 30,000 deliveries), the incidence of maternal death has been increasing recently. In 1999, there were 11.8 deaths per 100,000 live births. However, the National Health Promotion and Disease Prevention Objectives of Healthy People 2010 identified a rate of no more than 3.3 maternal deaths per 100,000 live births as a national goal. Some of the factors associated with a higher risk of pregnancy-related death include advancing maternal age, race, increasing live birth order, lack of prenatal care, and unwed mothers.[1]

The leading causes of maternal death are pulmonary embolism, hemorrhage, pregnancy-induced hypertension, and infection[1] (Table 16-1). Although pulmonary embolism is considered the most common *medical* cause of death in pregnant women, several studies have indicated that maternal death from homicide is the most common form of fatal injury.[2,3] Domestic violence and its relation to pregnancy and homicide is poorly understood, but domestic violence indicators should be examined in all pregnant patients as a preventive measure.

MATERNAL AND FETAL PHYSIOLOGIC CHANGES THAT AFFECT CARDIAC ARREST

Uteroplacental blood flow is directly related to maternal blood volume and arterial pressure. Support of maternal blood volume and oxygenation is the best way to prevent fetal hypoxia. With this principle in mind, a detailed understanding of cardiac arrest physiology is important. A full discussion of fetomaternal physiology can be found in Chap. 104, but several points are discussed and put in perspective here.

The maternal cardiovascular system undergoes dramatic changes. Cardiac output increases to 30 to 45 percent above baseline levels by the twentieth week of gestation and remains at that level until delivery. In addition, the mean arterial blood pressure gradually falls throughout the first two trimesters of pregnancy and returns to baseline levels by term. This change is a result of decreased resistance in the pulmonary and uteroplacental circulations. The uteroplacental mass increases and requires 10 percent of systemic blood volume by term, compared with a baseline of 2 percent. By the second half of pregnancy, the uteroplacental vascular bed functions as a passive low-resistance system, with flow determined by maternal perfusion pressure. Thus, in a state of cardiac compromise, uterine blood flow is greatly diminished. The addition of vasopressors with α- and β-adrenergic effects can cause significant vasoconstriction, thereby decreasing uterine blood flow even further.

By the twentieth week of pregnancy, the enlarged uterus mechanically compresses the great vessels in the pelvis, particularly when the patient is in the supine position. As a result of decreased venous return from compression of the inferior vena cava, cardiac output is reduced 10 to 30 percent during spontaneous circulation (Figure 16-1). Administration of medications through intravenous sites in the infradiaphragmatic vessels, such as the femoral or saphenous vein, is also compromised because of poor venous flow. These vascular sites therefore are not recommended for intravenous access in the resuscitation of a pregnant patient with greater than 20 weeks gestation. Aortal compression also occurs, causing diminished distal blood flow. The untoward effects of great vessel compression are worsened in the setting of maternal hypotension and uterine contractions, leading to an even more pronounced decrease in uteroplacental blood flow.

Pregnancy also alters the respiratory system. A state of chronic respiratory alkalosis develops during the first trimester of pregnancy due

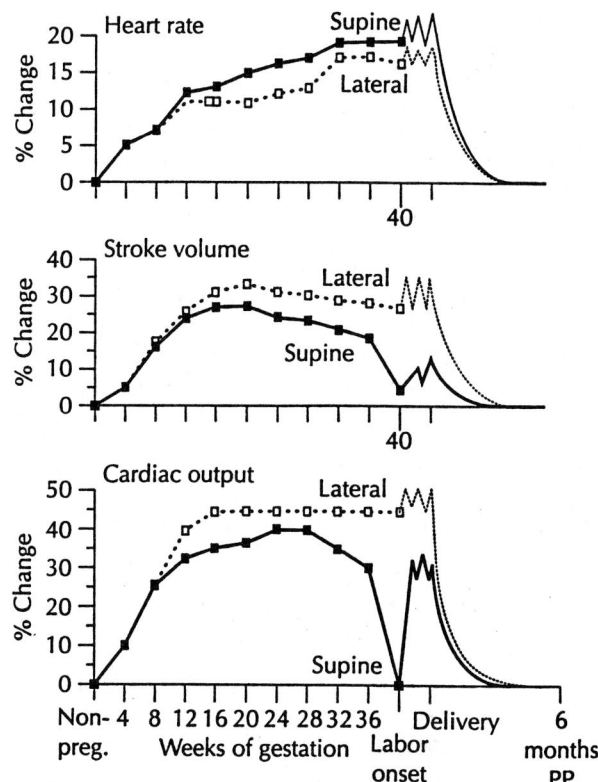

FIG. 16-1. Changes in maternal heart rate, stroke volume, and cardiac output during pregnancy, with the gravida in the supine and lateral positions. [Reproduced with permission from Barclay ML, Critical physiologic alterations in pregnancy, in Pearlman MD, Tintinalli JE (eds): *Emergency Care of the Woman.* New York, McGraw-Hill, 1998, p. 9.]

TABLE 16-1   Pregnancy-Related Etiologies of Maternal Cardiopulmonary Arrest

Obstetric complications
  Hemorrhage (17.2%)
    Uterine atony
    Placental abruption
    Placenta previa, accreta, increta, or percreta
    Disseminated intravascular coagulopathy
  Severe pregnancy-induced hypertension (15.7%)
  Amniotic fluid embolism
  Idiopathic peripartum cardiomyopathy (8.3%)
Iatrogenic events
  Failed intubation
  Pulmonary aspiration
  Intravascular local anesthetic overdose (1.6%)
  Drug error, overdose, or allergy
  Hypermagnesemia
Pulmonary embolism (19.6%)
  Thrombus
  Air
  Fat
Stroke (5%)
Trauma
  Homicide
  Suicide
  Motor vehicle accident
Infection or sepsis (12.6%)
Other (19.2%) (cardiovascular, pulmonary & neurologic comorbidities)

Sources: Adapted with permission from Johnson MD, Luppi CJ, Over D: Cardiopulmonary resuscitation in pregnancy, in Gambling DR, Douglas MJ (eds): *Obstetric Anesthesia and Uncommon Disorders.* Philadelphia, WB Saunders, 1997; Doan-Wiggins L: Cardiopulmonary resuscitation during pregnancy, in Benrubi GI (ed): *Obstetric and Gynecologic Emergencies.* Philadelphia, Lippincott, 1994, p. 77; and Pregnancy-related mortality surveillance United States—1991–1999, *MMWR* 52:SS-2, Feb 21, 2003.

to increased minute ventilation secondary to increased tidal volume and mild progesterone-stimulated hyperventilation. The resulting compensatory decrease in serum bicarbonate levels due to decreased partial pressure of carbon dioxide (Pco_2) makes the woman less able to buffer a state of acidosis from hypotension or cardiac arrest. In addition, the decreased functional residual capacity (FRC) and increased maternal oxygen consumption and basal metabolic rate during pregnancy results in more rapid onset of anoxia with respiratory arrest. Arterial oxygen content drops more quickly in pregnant than in nonpregnant patients. Rapid resumption of respiration, whether mechanical or spontaneous, is essential to minimize hypoxic damage. Progesterone also increases gastric emptying time and decreases lower esophageal sphincter tone, making the gravid patient prone to aspiration. This is another reason to initiate endotracheal intubation early.

Fetal physiology appears to be protective of severe hypoxia. There are several reports of fetal survival when delivery occurred more than 20 min after maternal cardiac arrest in patients receiving CPR. However, the trauma literature indicates that absence of maternal vital signs for longer than 20 min renders emergency cesarean section futile. It is unclear whether CPR plays a role in potential fetal survival beyond 20 min. The fetal oxyhemoglobin dissociation curve is shifted to the left relative to the maternal oxyhemoglobin dissociation curve, because of the greater affinity of hemoglobin F for oxygen. Thus, at any partial pressure of oxygen (Po_2), fetal hemoglobin will bind oxygen more strongly, resulting in greater saturation. Fetal Po_2 does not fall significantly unless maternal Po_2 falls below 60 mm Hg.[4] Below this level, only slight decreases in maternal Po_2 will result in significant decreases in fetal Po_2. In addition, there is a higher concentration of fetal hemoglobin in fetal erythrocytes than maternal hemoglobin in maternal erythrocytes, and the fetus exists in a physiologically acidemic state relative to the mother, which allows preferential oxygen transfer at the fetal tissue level. Acidemia favors a rightward shift of the oxyhemoglobin dissociation curve. Thus, a greater amount of oxygen is supplied to fetal tissues.

Fetal cardiac output protects against hypoxia with increases in umbilical blood flow and placental gas exchange. Fetal blood flow is then preferentially redistributed to vital tissues. As a result, fetuses exposed to short periods of maternal hypoxia may not suffer neurologic damage.

Resuscitation of a pregnant patient can become a chaotic event. Particularly in major centers, there may be other specialists involved, including pediatricians, neonatologists, anesthesiologists, obstetricians, and possibly others. These specialists have unique skills and experience that will help in the resuscitation. However, many of the specialists are poorly versed in emergency medicine and advanced cardiac life support (ACLS) protocols. It is particularly important that the team leader of the resuscitation take strict control of the events and the order in which they occur. The other specialists involved should not be allowed to deviate from the proper process. The team leader for such resuscitations may be decided by hospital policy. If such a policy does not exist, then typically the emergency physician should be the director of the resuscitation and take firm control.

AIRWAY ISSUES

The airway presents special concerns in obstetric patients. Attention to a few details, particularly in the setting of maternal cardiac arrest, may reduce morbidity and mortality. Airway management and its associated problems, most commonly failed intubation and aspiration of gastric contents, represent the greatest risk factors for anesthetic-related maternal deaths, most of which occur in the setting of an emergent cesarean section. Maternal death related to anesthesia most commonly results from aspiration of gastric contents or failure to intubate the trachea, resulting in hypoxia, which ultimately can result in cardiac arrest. Mask ventilation can be difficult and ineffectual in obstetric patients, because of low FRC, elevated diaphragms, and raised intra-abdominal pressure. Due to the risk of aspiration, mask ventilation should be avoided unless hypoxia is present. According to Hawthorne and colleagues, the incidence of failed intubation in the obstetric population is 0.4 percent.[5] Complicating the fact that pregnant patients develop hypoxia more quickly and are less tolerant of apneic periods, the airway poses more difficulties than in the general population. The potential factors accounting for these difficulties should be assessed before attempting an intubation.

Parturients in general are in an edematous state, which affects the tongue and supraglottic soft tissues.[6] The edema may compromise the airway lumen, making mask ventilation, laryngoscopy, and endotracheal intubation more challenging. The incidence of Mallampati class III airway increases as pregnancy progresses.[7] Smaller endotracheal tubes may be needed to achieve a successful intubation and should be readily available. Mucosal engorgement and increased friability make the airway more likely to bleed and swell. This in itself can cause rapid deterioration. Increased gastric emptying time and diminished lower esophageal sphincter tone allow for increased gastric insufflation and result in a greater risk of aspiration during intubation. The most experienced physician should undertake the intubation. Blind nasotracheal intubation is relatively contraindicated, and nasogastric tubes generally should be avoided, given the engorgement and friability of the mucosa in pregnant patients. Orogastric tubes may be used with caution in pregnant patients in cardiac arrest.

Several other physical conditions should be considered before intubating a parturient. Pregnant patients are likely to have full and intact dentition, and there may be little interdental distance in which to maneuver a laryngoscope. Obesity is relatively common in pregnant patients, causing relative neck extension when patients are supine, which results in greater anterior placement of the larynx. The neck is foreshortened, and there are often redundant pharyngeal and palatal folds in the airways of obese gravid women. In addition, enlarged and engorged breasts may obstruct placement of the laryngoscope in the mouth and the hand of an assistant attempting to maintain cricoid pressure.

The technique for intubating pregnant patients may require several modifications. As in any intubation, adjunctive equipment, including small endotracheal tubes, short laryngoscope handles, and stylets, should be readily available and familiar to the physician managing the airway. In addition, special airway devices, including the fiberoptic bronchoscope and the laryngeal mask airway, may be helpful in managing a difficult airway. The patient should be placed in the supine position, with the right hip elevated 10 to 12 cm to minimize aortocaval compression. The head and shoulders can be elevated with a pillow or folded sheets to achieve the sniffing position. This maneuver is particularly important in obese patients.

Use of rapid sequence induction with cricoid pressure has become the standard of care for intubating pregnant women, in particular unstable patients with airway compromise. Administration of an induction agent, such as thiopental or etomidate, is followed by administration of succinylcholine, the muscle relaxant of choice, unless there is a contraindication to its use. Standard doses are used (see Chap. 19). It is helpful to allow a sufficient period for muscle relaxants to take effect and for adequate preoxygenation before attempting laryngoscopy, given its potential hazards in pregnant patients. Preoxygenation, rather than mask ventilation with its associated risk of aspiration, before intubation is important because of the parturient's decreased FRC. However, hyperventilation may lead to respiratory alkalosis, which, in addition to shifting the oxyhemoglobin dissociation curve to the left, causes decreased uterine blood flow. Cricoid pressure must be applied carefully throughout the intubation procedure. In the case of failed intubation and inability to maintain oxygenation and ventilation with alternative airway devices (i.e., laryngeal mask airway, Combitube), more invasive maneuvers, such as percutaneous transtracheal jet ventilation or cricothyrotomy, may need to be performed to maintain oxygenation and prevent hypercarbia. Ventilator settings for pregnant patients are similar to those for nonpregnant patients, with minor modifications. Minute ventilation should aim to maintain a P_{CO_2} of approximately 30 mm Hg. Normal antepartum arterial blood gas values should be sought at term: pH, 7.43 ± 0.027; P_{CO_2} (mm Hg), 30.4 ± 2.7; and P_{O_2} (mm Hg), 102 ± 5, indicating a chronic respiratory alkalosis.[8] Significant respiratory alkalosis must be avoided to prevent decreased uterine blood flow.

MODIFICATIONS OF CARDIOPULMONARY RESUSCITATION

All common underlying conditions can be influential, and the etiology of cardiac arrest in pregnant patients is different from that in nonpregnant patients (see Table 16-1) and includes pulmonary embolism, amniotic fluid embolism, eclampsia, drug toxicity (e.g., magnesium sulfate or epidural anesthetics), cardiomyopathy, aortic dissection, trauma, and hemorrhage. As always, one should address the potential underlying etiology and the cardiovascular collapse.

Cardiopulmonary arrest in a pregnant patient must be considered under two scenarios: before fetal viability and after fetal viability. The accepted age of fetal viability may vary among institutions, but 24 to 26 weeks is generally considered the age of viability. The uterine fundus is palpable at the umbilicus at 20 weeks. After 20 weeks, the gestational age of the fetus can be estimated by measuring the fundus from the pubic symphysis to the top of the fundus. The fundal height in centimeters corresponds roughly to the gestational age in weeks. **Before 24 weeks' gestation, all efforts should focus on the mother, with no modifications to CPR.** However, early intubation and resumption of respirations and circulation are essential in all gravid arrests for the reasons mentioned earlier. Beyond 20 weeks or if the gravid uterus can be palpated above the umbilicus, several modifica-

TABLE 16-2 Algorithm for Cardiopulmonary Resuscitation in Pregnant Patients

Early intubation, protect vulnerable airway, supply oxygen
Tilt the patient, limit aortocaval compression
Obtain rapid intravenous access, avoid the femoral and saphenous veins
Follow current ACLS recommendations
Perimortem cesarean section within 5 min of maternal arrest if fetus >20 wks
Consider open chest CPR within 15 min of maternal arrest
Explore differential diagnosis, include iatrogenic causes, e.g., spinal analgesia
Consider cardiopulmonary bypass, if indicated

Abbreviation: ACLS = advanced cardiac life support.

tions of CPR should be instituted: (1) the patient should be positioned to minimize aortocaval compression, and (2) an emergency cesarean section should be considered and appropriate preparations made for its potential performance and for care of a viable fetus.

Aortocaval compression must be limited in all patients beyond the twentieth week of gestation. This can be achieved by (1) having someone manually displace the uterus to the left, (2) tilting the patient 15 to 30 degrees on a tiltable table, or (3) placement of a roll or a Cardiff wedge, if available, under the patient's right hip and flank. The Cardiff wedge provides a tilt of 27 percent, allowing 80 percent of the compressive force, compared with CPR in the supine position.[9] Even this is minimal blood flow, considering that correctly performed CPR maintains 30 percent or less of normal cardiac output in nonpregnant adults.[10,11] The "human wedge" has been advocated for bystander CPR. In this technique, the patient lies across the thighs of the rescuer, who is in a kneeling position. Despite relatively clear current recommendations regarding resuscitation in pregnancy, summarized in Table 16-2, there remains a paucity of research in this area.

Five factors have been suggested as important to improving the chance of fetal survival when the mother suffers cardiac arrest: gestational age older than 28 weeks or fetal weight greater than 1 kg, short interval between maternal death and delivery, a cause of maternal death not related to chronic hypoxia, fetal status before maternal death, availability of neonatal intensive care facilities, and quality of maternal resuscitation.[12]

The role of open chest CPR remains unclear. There is some evidence that early thoracotomy and open chest cardiac massage may improve maternal and fetal outcomes. If, after several minutes of external CPR (15 min has been suggested), a pregnant woman has failed to achieve return of spontaneous circulation, open chest CPR should be considered.

DEFIBRILLATION AND MEDICATIONS

Pregnant patients in cardiac arrest should be treated according to current ACLS guidelines. Defibrillation has never been found to have adverse effects on the fetus and thus is not contraindicated. The patient should be placed in the left lateral tilt position, if possible, before defibrillation or cardioversion. Large-bore intravenous lines should be placed, preferably above the diaphragm, and LR or NS solution infused. Supplemental oxygen should be given. Apgar scores and fetal outcome are positively affected by greater fetal oxygen reserves. In limited published reports, the standard medications used in ACLS have not been demonstrated to have adverse effects on the fetus and thus are recommended in the setting of cardiac arrest.[13] Table 16-3 presents details regarding ACLS medications. Vasopressors, such as epinephrine and dopamine, may be detrimental in the setting of maternal hypotension because they cause uteroplacental vasoconstriction, but should be used as needed during cardiac arrest. In the setting of hypotension alone without cardiac arrest, ephedrine, in standard doses (5 mg IV every 5 min until a response is seen), is the preferred pressor

TABLE 16-3 Medications Used During Cardiopulmonary Resuscitation—Considerations in Pregnancy

Drug	Indications	Considerations in Pregnancy
Epinephrine	Potentially beneficial in all forms of cardiac arrest	Category C. Has been shown to be teratogenic in animals in large doses; may induce uteroplacental vasoconstriction.
Lidocaine	Ventricular ectopy, tachycardia, and fibrillation	Category C. Use during pregnancy is not well studied; crosses the placenta but in therapeutic doses has no teratogenic effect on the fetus; may cause fetal bradycardia.
Bretylium	Ventricular fibrillation and tachycardia unresponsive to other therapy	Category C. No longer recommended as a first-line drug for resuscitation, because of potential risk of reduced uterine blood flow and fetal hypoxia (bradycardia); appropriate when benefits outweigh risks.
Atropine	Symptomatic bradycardia, asystole	Category B. Crosses placenta but results in no fetal abnormalities; can cause fetal tachycardia.
Sodium bicarbonate	Cardiac arrest unresponsive to other measures; documented preexisting metabolic acidosis	Category C. Studies to define risk of hypertonic sodium bicarbonate therapy in pregnancy have not been done.
Dopamine	Hemodynamically significant hypotension in the absence of hypovolemia	Category C. No teratogenic effects have been observed in laboratory animals, but sufficient studies in humans are lacking; use only when clearly indicated.
Dobutamine	Short-term inotropic support of patients with depressed myocardial contractility	Category C. Not found to be teratogenic in animal studies, but its effects in pregnant humans are unknown; use only if clearly indicated
Amiodarone	Ventricular fibrillation, tachycardia, and supraventricular tachycardia	Category D. Should not be used in pregnancy; serious fetal adverse effects have been observed.
Adenosine	Supraventricular tachycardia	Class C. Multiple case reports have described the safe use of adenosine to treat maternal and fetal supraventricular tachycardia.
Magnesium sulfate	Acute myocardial infarction and torsades de pointes	Class B. This drug is commonly used in pregnancy for toxemia and tocolysis with no reports of congenital defects; neonatal neurologic depression may occur with respiratory depression, muscle weakness, and loss of reflexes.

Sources: Tamari I, Eldar M, Rabinowitz B, Neufeld HN: Medical treatment of cardiovascular disorders during pregnancy. *Am Heart J* 104:1357, 1982; Gibler WB: Antiarrhythmics, in Barsan WG, Jastremski MS, Syverud SA (eds): *Emergency Drug Therapy.* Philadelphia, WB Saunders, 1991, p 147; Saunders CF: Vasoactive agents, in Barsan WG, Jastremski MS, Syverud SA (eds): *Emergency Drug Therapy.* Philadelphia, WB Saunders, 1991, p 281; Singal B: Acidifying and alkalizing agents, in Barsan WG, Jastremski MS, Syverud SA (eds): *Emergency Drug Therapy.* Philadelphia, WB Saunders, 1991, p 281; Briggs GG, Freeman RK, Yaffe SJ: *A Reference Guide to Fetal and Neonatal Risk—Drugs in Pregnancy and Lactation.* Philadelphia, Lippincott Williams & Wilkins, 2000.

when fluids fail to restore adequate blood pressure. The use of sodium bicarbonate is not well studied. Sodium bicarbonate crosses the placenta slowly and can be problematic for the fetus for the following reason. Rapid correction of maternal acidosis may decrease maternal respiratory drive and lead to a further rise in, or pseudonormalization of, maternal P_{CO_2}. As maternal P_{CO_2} increases, the concomitant rise in fetal P_{CO_2} occurs at a faster rate than does the rise in HCO_3^-, causing the fetus to become more acidemic.

COMPLICATIONS FROM CARDIOPULMONARY RESUSCITATION

Complications may occur from standard resuscitation. Maternal problems secondary to CPR include liver lacerations, uterine rupture, hemothorax, and hemopericardium. Potential fetal complications include cardiac dysrhythmias from maternal defibrillation and ACLS drugs, central nervous system toxicity from ACLS drugs, and altered uteroplacental blood flow from maternal hypoxia, acidosis, and vasoconstriction. Despite all of the aforementioned problems, standard ACLS protocols, with the addition of a pelvic tilt, are still the standard of care in resuscitating pregnant patients. The ultimate goal is to oxygenate the mother, and in turn the fetus, and achieve return of spontaneous circulation as soon as possible.

PERIMORTEM CESAREAN SECTION

Perimortem cesarean section must be considered as part of any resuscitation in the case of maternal cardiac arrest and a viable fetus. Prognosis for intact survival of the infant is excellent if delivery occurs within 5 min of maternal arrest and initiation of CPR. If the 5-min time frame has been exceeded, it is still recommended to perform a perimortem cesarean section. One case has been reported of a perimortem cesarean section performed 22 min after maternal cardiac arrest that resulted in a normal living infant.[14] No cases have been reported of live births by perimortem cesarean section beyond 25 min after maternal arrest. Ideally, an obstetrician and a pediatrician or neonatologist are present at the time of a perimortem cesarean section. In the absence of these specialists, the emergency physician must be prepared to perform the procedure. **It is not necessary and only delays a potentially lifesaving procedure to evaluate fetal viability before initiation of the cesarean section.** For the same reasons, the patient should not be moved to an operating suite, because this only wastes time. The decision to perform a perimortem cesarean section should be made by 4 min after cardiac arrest, with delivery of the fetus by 5 min post-arrest.

Maternal CPR should be continued throughout the procedure and for a brief time afterward, because a few cases of successful resuscitation after such a procedure have been reported. Necessary equipment is listed in Table 16-4. The goal of this procedure is to remove and resuscitate the fetus.

Abdominal preparation and insertion of a Foley catheter to decompress the bladder may be performed before initial incision, if time allows, but should not delay the procedure. No anesthesia is required, because the mother is in cardiac arrest. A vertical midline (classic) incision is made from 4 to 5 cm below the xiphoid process to the pubic symphysis through the abdominal wall. The rectus muscles may be separated with blunt dissection, and the peritoneum is entered with a midline incision that is continued superiorly and inferiorly to allow visualization of the uterus. A vertical uterine incision is made from the fundus to the point at which the opaque bladder is adherent to the uterus. An initial small inferior incision may be made until amniotic fluid is obtained and then extended with scissors by using the free hand to elevate the uterus, thereby avoiding injury to the fetus. An anterior placenta should be incised to reach the fetus. The fetus is then delivered and resuscitated. The placenta is then manually removed from the uterus, and the uterus is wiped clean of membranes with a sponge or towel. The uterus is closed with one or two layers with a locked running stitch using number 0 or number 1 semipermanent (e.g., chromic) suture and a large needle. The fascia and peritoneum may be closed with a permanent or semipermanent number 0 or number 1 suture with a running stitch. Finally, the skin is closed. Closure of the abdomen may be delayed until maternal pulse and blood pressure are restored, to allow direct observation of the uterus for ongoing bleeding. Uterine atony after perimortem cesarean section is common and may lead to significant blood loss when the uterus fails to contract after delivery. Because maternal blood circulation may not be sufficient to deliver intravenously administered medication, dilute oxytocin (10 U in 9 mL of NS solution) may be injected directly into the myometrium in divided doses until contraction occurs. Other possible therapeutic medications include ergometrine (intravenous or intramuscular) or prostaglandin $F_{2\alpha}$ injected into the uterus.

Informed consent for perimortem cesarean section is not necessary. The procedure needs to be performed expediently and should be considered part of the resuscitation. Perimortem cesarean section during cardiac arrest fulfills criteria for absence of malfeasance and beneficence for the mother and the fetus. Maternal and/or fetal death, and deciding to perform a perimortem cesarean section, impose a highly emotional impact on all parties involved in the resuscitation. Debriefing and counseling services should be provided to all participants in such cases.[15] The question of when emergent cesarean section should be performed in critically ill, prearrest patients has not been adequately addressed in the literature. In addition, the recommendations for perimortem cesarean section are based on multiple case reports. No experimental studies have evaluated this procedure.

CARDIAC ISCHEMIA

Pregnant women with acute cardiac ischemia are treated the same as nonpregnant patients, with the exception of thrombolytic therapy. Pregnancy is considered a relative contraindication to thrombolytic therapy by the American College of Cardiology and the American Heart Association.[16] No controlled trials using thrombolytic agents, such as streptokinase, urokinase, or tissue plasminogen activator, have been performed on pregnant women or are currently feasible. Patients with suspected myocardial infarction should be evaluated for emergent percutaneous interventional therapy or medical management.

PULMONARY EMBOLISM

Thromboembolic disease is increased in pregnancy. Anticoagulation with heparin is currently the treatment of choice for a pulmonary embolism, in addition to ensuring adequate oxygenation and treating hypotension. Either unfractionated or low-molecular-weight heparin are acceptable treatment regimens. When pulmonary embolism is suspected, empiric treatment with heparin should be started immediately, especially if the patient is hypoxic or hemodynamically unstable. Once treatment has begun, a CT scan or ventilation-perfusion scan should be obtained to confirm the diagnosis. Traditionally, thrombolytic ther-

TABLE 16-4 Equipment Required for Emergency Cesarean Section

Scalpel
Mayo scissors
Bandage scissors
Toothed forceps
Needle holders
No. 0 or 1 chromic sutures on a CT 1 needle
Richardson retractors
10 U/mL oxytocin vials
10-mL NS solution vials
10-mL syringe with intramuscular needle

apy for pulmonary embolism has been considered relatively contraindicated in pregnant patients. However, there are multiple case reports of pregnant women who have been treated successfully with thrombolytics for thromboembolic disease, with no untoward complications.[17] The use of thrombolytics should be reserved for patients in extremis for whom the potential benefit outweighs the potential risks.

AMNIOTIC FLUID EMBOLISM

The classic presentation of amniotic fluid embolism is the development of dyspnea and hypotension in association with labor or an abortion. Milder forms can present with sudden onset of shortness of breath and air hunger and a decreased oxygen saturation that resolves spontaneously. Amniotic fluid embolism can be difficult to distinguish from pulmonary embolism. Patients can develop cardiac arrest within minutes, and, if they survive, they will go on to develop disseminated intravascular coagulation and potentially multiorgan failure.[18] Treatment is primarily supportive care in addition to invasive cardiac monitoring and correction of the coagulopathy. The use of cardiopulmonary bypass and open pulmonary artery thromboembolectomy has been used with success in a moribund patient with amniotic fluid embolism.[19]

DISPOSITION

The presence of experienced obstetricians, anesthesiologists, and pediatricians or neonatologists will facilitate the care of pregnant patients with cardiac arrest. However, none of the required care and procedures should be delayed if these specialists are not available; further, many of these specialists are not well versed in orchestrating resuscitation or resuscitative techniques. When trained staff are available to perform external fetal tococardiography without diverting care from the mother, it should be provided for pregnancies beyond 20 weeks' gestation. If this technology is not available or personnel are limited, the often-quoted maxim, "maternal resuscitation is the best fetal resuscitation," should be kept in mind. The closest center providing neonatal services should be contacted as soon as possible to facilitate rapid transport of the newly delivered infant.

REFERENCES

1. Chang J, Elam-Evans LD, Berg CJ, et al: Pregnancy-related mortality surveillance—United States, 1991–1999. *MMWR Surveill Summ* 52:1, Feb. 21, 2003.
2. Harper M, Parsons L: Maternal deaths due to homicide and other injuries in North Carolina: 1992-1994. *Obstet Gynecol* 90:920, 1997.
3. Dannenberg AL, Carter DM, Lawson HW, et al: Homicide and other injuries as causes of maternal death in New York City, 1987 through 1991. *Am J Obstet Gynecol* 172:1557, 1995.
4. Sobrevilla LA, Cassinelli MT, Carcelen A, et al: Human fetal and maternal oxygen tension and acid-base status during delivery at high altitude. *Am J Obstet Gynecol* 111:1111, 1971.
5. Hawthorne L, Wilson R, Lyons G, et al: Failed intubation revisited: 17-Year experience in a teaching maternity unit. *Br J Anaesth* 76:680, 1996.
6. Cheek TG, Gutsche BB: Maternal physiologic alterations during pregnancy, in Shnider SM, Levinson G (eds): *Anesthesia for Obstetrics,* 3rd ed. Baltimore, Williams & Wilkins, 1993.
7. Campbell LA, Klocke RA: Update in nonpulmonary critical care-implications for the pregnant patient. *Am J Respir Crit Care Med* 163:1051, 2001.
8. Templeton A, Kellman GR: Maternal blood-gases, (Pa_{O_2}-Pa_{O_2}), physiological shunt and Vd/Vt in normal pregnancy. *Br J Anaesth* 48:1001, 1976.
9. Rees GA, Willis BA: Resuscitation in late pregnancy. *Anaesthesia* 43:347, 1988.
10. Ornato JP, Paradis N, Bircher N, et al: Future directions for resuscitation research: III. External cardiopulmonary resuscitation advanced life support. *Resuscitation* 32:139, 1996.
11. Chandra NC, et al: *Textbook of Basic Life Support for Healthcare Providers.* New York, American Heart Association, 1994.
12. Strong TH, Lowe RV: Perimortem cesarean section. *J Emerg Med* 7:489, 1989.
13. Selden BS, Burke TJ: Complete maternal and fetal recovery after prolonged cardiac arrest. *Ann Emerg Med* 17:346, 1988.
14. Oates S, Williams GL, Rees GGAD: Cardiopulmonary resuscitation in late pregnancy. *BMJ* 297:404, 1988.
15. Tang G, Nada W, Gyaneshwar R, et al: Perimortem caesarean section: Two case reports and a management protocol. *Aust N Z J Obstet Gynaecol* 40:405, 2000.
16. Ryan TJ, Antman EM, Brooks NH, et al: 1999 Update: ACC/AHA guidelines for the management of patients with acute myocardial infarction. *J AM Coll Cardiol* 34:890, 1999.
17. Turrentine MA, Braems G, Ramirez MM: Use of thrombolytics for the treatment of thromboembolic disease during pregnancy. *Obstet Gynecol Surv* 50:534, 1995.
18. Gei A, Hankins GDV: Amniotic fluid embolism: An update. *Contemp Obstet Gynecol* 45:53, 2000.
19. Esposito RA, Grossi EA, Coppa G, et al: Successful treatment of postpartum shock caused by amniotic fluid embolism with cardiopulmonary bypass and pulmonary artery thromboembolectomy. *Am J Obstet Gynecol* 163:572, 1990.

17 ETHICAL ISSUES OF RESUSCITATION
Catherine A. Marco

GENERAL PRINCIPLES OF MEDICAL ETHICS

The study of ethics has been defined as the way of *understanding and examining the moral life*[1] and as the discipline dealing with moral duty and obligation.[2] The Hippocratic Oath has been revered as one of the oldest codes of medical ethics. More recently, the American Medical Association (AMA) Code of Ethics (earliest version in 1847) and the American College of Emergency Physicians (ACEP) Code of Ethics (1997) have provided guidance to emergency physicians in application of ethical principles to clinical practice. Most ethical codes address common features, such as *beneficence* (doing good), *nonmaleficence* (*primum non nocere,* or "do no harm"), respect for patient *autonomy, confidentiality, honesty, distributive justice,* and *respect for the law.* Ethical dilemmas may arise when there is a potential conflict between two principles or values. Ethical dilemmas may be resolved by various means, including individual physician judgment, additional information gathering, and meetings with health care professionals, patients, and families. In some circumstances, the involvement of the institutional ethics committee or the judicial system may be sought.

CARDIAC RESUSCITATION AND OUTCOMES

There are 460,000 sudden deaths in the United States annually.[3] The outcome of resuscitative efforts for victims of cardiac arrest is uniformly poor but varies depending on a variety of factors. The most important factor determining outcome is the time elapsed since arrest *(down time).* Studies over several decades have demonstrated improved survival rates for patients who received early advanced cardiac life support (ACLS).[4,5] Another important prognostic factor is the presenting rhythm. Previous studies have demonstrated improved survival rates for patients with presenting rhythms of ventricular fibrillation or ventricular tachycardia and reduced survival rates for patients with asystole or pulseless electrical activity. The underlying medical condition of the patient is another important factor affecting outcome.

A potentially poor response to resuscitation can be expected for patients with metastatic disease, acute cerebrovascular accident, sepsis, renal failure, or pneumonia. Failure to respond to prehospital advanced life support (ALS) protocols leads to a survival rate of less than 2 percent. The age of the patient also affects predicted survival rate, with a nearly 0 percent survival rate for unwitnessed arrests of elderly patients[6] and for long-term care patients.[7] Overall, survival of victims of cardiac arrests to hospital discharge has been estimated in many studies to be between 0 and 10 percent.

Based on such data, several authors have suggested proposed criteria for withholding resuscitative efforts for patients in certain clinical settings with a low likelihood of successful resuscitation [e.g., apneic, pulseless for longer than 10 min prior to emergency medical service (EMS) arrival, no response to ACLS, and preexisting terminal disease].[8,9] Knowledge of data regarding resuscitation outcomes in various clinical settings is crucial when making evidence-based decisions regarding the risks and benefits of attempting CPR and the duration of the resuscitation attempt.

RISKS AND BENEFITS OF RESUSCITATIVE EFFORTS

When considering offering or withholding resuscitative efforts, risks and benefits of resuscitative efforts should be considered carefully. The goal of resuscitative efforts is to restore circulation and life to the patient. Other less tangible benefits may include such entities as resolution of guilt of the survivors and the additional time for acceptance of bad news for survivors.

However, often resuscitative measures are undertaken in clinical situations in which physiologic survival is very unlikely, if not all but impossible. In some situations, there is a substantial risk that if circulation is restored, significant anoxic brain injury will result, resulting in significant impairment of quality of life (dementia, persistent vegetative state, or other cognitive impairments).

Additionally, substantial resources (supply costs as well as personnel) are often invested in this clinical setting of low likelihood of benefit, while the care of many other patients is delayed (distributive justice). Another consideration for limiting resuscitative efforts is the potentially large investment of human resources that otherwise might be used for family counseling and communication.

FUTILITY AND NONBENEFICIAL INTERVENTIONS

The term *futility* is fraught with difficulties in definition and interpretation. Health care professionals may interpret futile interventions as those which carry an absolute impossibility of successful outcome, a low likelihood of success, a low likelihood of survival to discharge from the hospital, or a low likelihood of restoration of meaningful quality of life. Schneiderman and colleagues defined *futility* as "any effort to achieve a result that is possible but that reasoning or experience suggests is highly improbable and that cannot be systematically produced."[10] Several authors have demonstrated that there is no consensus among physicians about the meaning of futility. Because of these difficulties, it is probably more accurate to use the appropriate terminology, such as *nonbeneficial, ineffectual,* or *low likelihood of success.*

The withholding or limitation of medical interventions that have a predicted low likelihood of producing a successful outcome can be a difficult and far-reaching decision. Many emergency physicians continue to attempt resuscitation on patients in cardiac arrest in situations considered nonbeneficial, often because of fears of litigation or criticism.[11]

Many ethicists agree that physicians are under no obligation to render treatments that they deem of little or no benefit to the patient. There have been numerous ethical opinions supportive of the position of offering only those treatments judged to be of likely medical benefit. The AMA Council on Ethical and Judicial Affairs wrote that CPR may be withheld, even if requested by the patient, "when efforts to resuscitate a patient are judged by the treating physician to be futile."[12] Numerous other ethicists and authors support withholding of interventions deemed unlikely to benefit patients.[13]

Dilemmas regarding nonbeneficial interventions often arise due to inadequate or ineffective communication between physician, patient, and family. This is of particular concern in emergency medicine, where previous relationships with patients and family rarely exist and time is often inadequate to establish effective relationships. In fact, verification of family status is often impossible. Thus, when a difference of opinion exists, initial efforts should be made to improve communication, education, and joint decision making.

There exist several policies that may be of guidance in decision making regarding nonbeneficial interventions. The ACEP approved a policy statement on futile treatment in 1998. This policy asserts ACEP's belief that "physicians are under no ethical obligation to render treatments that they judge have no realistic likelihood of medical benefit to the patient." The policy goes on to state that emergency physicians' judgments should be unbiased, based on available scientific evidence and societal and professional standards, and sensitive to differences of opinion regarding the value of medical intervention in various situations.[14]

The AMA Council on Ethical and Judicial Affairs recommends a process-based approach to the determination of futility[15] to include such actions as

1. deliberation and resolution;
2. joint decision making with physician and patient or proxy;
3. assistance of a consultant or patient representative; and
4. use of an institutional committee (i.e., ethics committee).

Ultimately, the decision regarding CPR and its likelihood of benefit to the patient and decisions to provide, limit, or withhold resuscitative efforts are to be made by the emergency physician in the context of well-accepted research results, patient and family wishes, and professional judgment. Individual bias regarding quality of life or other related issues should be avoided. There are many cases where dying should be accepted as a natural process, even in an emergency setting.

ADVANCE DIRECTIVES

An *advance directive* refers to any proactive document stating the patient's wishes in various situations, should he or she be unable to state his or her wishes. The *living will,* which was adopted by many states in 1990, is a document suitable for terminally ill individuals, and the treating physician accepts the provisions in advance. Many state that no life support be used in cases where meaningful recovery will not occur. *Durable power of attorney* specifies a surrogate decision maker in the event that the patient no longer has the capacity to make medical decisions. In 1991, the Federal Patient Self-Determination Act mandated the opportunity to sign an advance directive for all patients admitted to a hospital. In many cases, the existence of an advance directive can facilitate the implementation of the patient's specific wishes.

Despite widespread advocacy and legal mandates (such as the 1991 Federal Patient Self-Determination Act) for the increased use of advance directives, only a minority of patients have completed an advance directive, and an even smaller minority presents to the emergency department with the necessary documentation.[16] Although some health care providers are reluctant to discuss issues such as end-of-life care and advance directives, many patients welcome the opportunity to discuss their wishes. Most patients have definite opinions regarding resuscitation preferences, despite the lack of completion of legal advance directives.[17] Without advance directives, surrogate decision makers and physicians often make erroneous assumptions regarding the preferences of patients.

Although studies conducted in other settings have demonstrated variable compliance with advance directives by medical personnel, recent studies have indicated that emergency medical personnel may comply with advance directives more often than previously believed. Most emergency physicians (78 percent) withhold resuscitation attempts for patients with a legal advance directive, indicating a willingness to honor patients' wishes regarding their own medical care.[11]

Additionally, most prehospital providers (89 percent) withhold resuscitation attempts for patients with a legal advance directive.[18] These results suggest that advance directives may be especially significant in medical decision making to emergency health care providers.

PUBLIC EDUCATION ABOUT RESUSCITATION AND ALTERNATIVES

Numerous studies have demonstrated that accurate knowledge regarding probability of survival influences patient preferences.[19] Improved knowledge base regarding resuscitation may be achieved through a variety of venues, including television, radio, online education, physicians' offices, and many others, and may contribute to improved knowledge and, in turn, action regarding communication of personal preferences regarding CPR, including advance directives.

FAMILY PRESENCE DURING RESUSCITATION

Although, traditionally, family members have not been allowed to witness resuscitation attempts, several recent reports have demonstrated positive results of this practice.[20,21] Although most research to date has addressed medical arrests, the practice also should be considered for traumatic procedures and arrests. Family presence may serve to relieve guilt or disappointment and may be a helpful part of the grieving process. Many families simply wish to have the option of being present. If family members are allowed to be present, a chaperone is recommended to assist with communication and education about procedures and other medical issues.

PROCEDURES ON RECENTLY DECEASED PATIENTS

The practices of teaching and performing procedures on recently deceased patients are controversial. The most important benefit of these practices is the fulfillment of the recognized need for hands-on practice for students and house staff, as well as experienced physicians.[22] The setting of the recently deceased patient provides a unique clinical setting with literally *no* tangible risk to the patient. Following this rationale, physicians so inclined forward the unsubstantiated assertion that such practice allows the performance of these procedures competently on future, living patients, resulting in overall benefit to society. However, this assertion has not been demonstrated. Further, informed consent is rarely obtained or available in these settings. Some consider performing procedures without informed consent to be disrespectful, deceptive, or unethical.[23]

In the absence of formal policy set by the local institution, and until formal policies are developed by governing organizations in emergency medicine, emergency physicians must make the choice most appropriate in the specific clinical situation encountered. Factors to be considered when making such decisions include availability of the family and feasibility of informed consent, teaching benefit to the student and his or her future patients, the overall benefit to society, invasiveness and disfigurement produced by the procedure(s), interference with forensic assessment, potential distress to the family, other potential avenues for teaching procedures, and any institutional policies on this issue.

RESUSCITATION RESEARCH

Research on resuscitation techniques and pharmaceuticals has been problematic due to the frequent inability to obtain informed consent and the constraints of the decision-making process. Ordinarily, the process of obtaining informed consent for human subject research is designed to ensure protection and autonomy of the subject. However, the process of obtaining informed consent is time-consuming and requires competence of the subject. Because of these difficulties, the Food and Drug Administration (FDA) recently issued guidelines under

which resuscitation research may be performed with a waiver of informed consent under certain conditions.[24] When designing such research protocols, factors to be considered include the patient's wishes (if known), expected safety of the study protocol, expected benefit of the therapeutic intervention, overall expected benefit to society by improved knowledge regarding resuscitation, related animal data, feasibility of surrogate consent, local institutional review board (IRB) opinion, and local general public opinion, if available. Waiver of consent is obtained by application with the FDA with local IRB approval.

COMMUNICATION AND COUNSELING FOR SURVIVORS

In many cases, the communication, care, and counseling provided for survivors (family, friends, and the like) of victims of cardiac arrest will have more impact than the actual resuscitative efforts. Optimal care should be provided for families and friends of victims of cardiac arrest, regardless of the level of treatment rendered and outcome. See Chap. 294 for detailed discussion on communication.

REFERENCES

1. Beauchamp TL, Childress JF: *Principles of Biomedical Ethics,* 5th ed. New York, Oxford University Press, 2003.
2. *Merriam-Webster's Collegiate Dictionary.* www.m-w.com; accessed August 27, 2002.
3. Centers for Disease Control and Prevention: State-specific mortality from sudden cardiac death—United States, 1999. *MMWR* 51:123, 2002.
4. Eisenberg MS, Bergner L, Hallstrom A: Cardiac resuscitation in the community: Importance of rapid provision and implications for program planning. *JAMA* 241:1905, 1979.
5. Kuisma M, Maatta T, Repo J: Cardiac arrests witnessed by EMS personnel in a multitiered system: Epidemiology and outcome. *Am J Emerg Med* 16:12, 1998.
6. Murphy DJ, Murray AM, Robinson BE, et al: Outcomes of cardiopulmonary resuscitation in the elderly. *Ann Intern Med* 111:199, 1989.
7. Awoke S, Mouton CP, Parrott M: Outcomes of skilled cardiopulmonary resuscitation in a long-term-care facility: Futile therapy? *J Am Geriatr Soc* 40:593, 1992.
8. Bonnin MJ, Pepe PE, Kimball KT, et al: Distinct criteria for termination of resuscitation in the out-of-hospital setting. *JAMA* 270:1457, 1993.
9. Kellerman AL, Hackman BB, Somes G: Predicting the outcome of unsuccessful prehospital advanced cardiac life support. *JAMA* 270:1433, 1993.
10. Schneiderman LJ, Jecker NS, Jonsen AR: Medical futility: Its meaning and ethical implications. *Ann Intern Med* 112:949, 1990.
11. Marco CA, Bessman ES, Schoenfeld CN, et al: Ethical issues of cardiopulmonary resuscitation: Current practice among emergency physicians. *Acad Emerg Med* 4:898, 1997.
12. AMA, Council on Ethical and Judicial Affairs: Guidelines for the Appropriate Use of Do-Not-Resusitate Orders. *JAMA* 265:1868, 1991.
13. Marco CA, Larkin GL, Moskop JC, Derse AR: The determination of "futility" in emergency medicine. *Ann Emerg Med* 35:604, 2000.
14. ACEP Policy Statement: Nonbeneficial ("futile") emergency medical interventions. American College of Emergency Physicians, Dallas, Texas, 1998.
15. AMA, Council on Ethical and Judicial Affairs: Medical futility in end-of-life care. *JAMA* 281:937, 1999
16. The SUPPORT Principle Investigators: A controlled trial to improve care for seriously ill hospitalized patients. *JAMA* 274:1591, 1995.
17. Schonwetter RS, Walker RM, Solomon M, et al: Life values, resuscitation preferences, and the applicability of living wills in an older population. *J Am Geriatr Soc* 44:954, 1996.
18. Marco CA, Schears RM: Prehospital resuscitation practices: A survey of prehospital providers. *J Emerg Med* 24:101, 2003.
19. de Vos R, Koster RW, de Haan RJ: Impact of survival probability, life expectancy, quality of life and patient preferences on do-not-attempt resuscitation orders in a hospital. *Resuscitation* 39:15, 1998.
20. Boyd R: Witnessed resuscitation by relatives. *Resuscitation* 43:171, 2000.
21. Boudreaux ED, et al: Family presence during invasive procedures and resuscitations in the emergency department. *Ann Emeg Med* 40:193, 2002.

22. Iserson KV: Law versus life: The ethical imperative to practice and teach using the newly dead emergency department patient. *Ann Emerg Med* 25:91, 1995.

23. Goldblatt AD: Don't ask, don't tell: Practicing minimally invasive resuscitative techniques on the newly dead. *Ann Emerg Med* 25:86, 1995.

24. Department of Health and Human Services, Food and Drug Administration: Protection of human subjects; informed consent and waiver of informed consent requirements in certain emergency research: Final rules. *Fed Reg* 96-24968, September 26, 1996.

18 NONINVASIVE AIRWAY MANAGEMENT
A. Michael Roman

ANATOMY AND PATHOPHYSIOLOGY

Prior to airway management procedures, when there is sufficient time, the physician should:

1. Inspect the patient's mouth for size of teeth and for size and mobility of the jaw.
2. Open the patient's mouth and observe the palate, tongue, and oropharynx.
3. Flex the stable neck (in the absence of trauma), assess mobility, and place in the sniffing position.
4. Examine the size and alignment of the neck.
5. Inspect the nasal openings for patency.
6. Listen for abnormal airway sounds such as stridor, hoarseness, or gurgling.
7. Ask the patient's history, if possible.
8. Be sure to have suction available at all times, especially during any procedures.

The anatomic airway (Figure 18-1) begins at the oral/nasal cavities and continues posteriorly to the tongue/turbinates, the tonsils/adenoids; past the palate; through the oropharynx; across the epiglottis, which protects the glottis (the narrowest portion of the airway); past the false and true vocal cords; and into the larynx. Surrounding the larynx is the thyroid cartilage, cricoid cartilage, and thyroid gland. The upper airway ends here. The lower airway then continues to the trachea and into the lungs. Potential obstruction may develop anywhere along this route. In infants and small children, the anatomy is somewhat different than in the adult. The tongue is relatively larger in relation to the mandible. The glottis is higher and more anterior and the vocal cords are angled more anteriorly and inferiorly. The epiglottis is large and floppy and may lie against the posterior wall of the pharynx.

AIRWAY OBSTRUCTION

Table 18-1 lists potential causes of upper airway obstruction. Basic management of the obstructed airway is discussed in Chap. 12. Most of these entities cause soft tissue swelling or themselves are soft tissue masses that compromise the upper airway, but a few need mentioning. Certain medical diseases, such as respiratory syncytial virus (RSV) and cystic fibrosis, produce copious secretions in the upper airway that can lead to partial or complete occlusion. Angioedema may present with soft tissue swelling sufficient to preclude an oral airway, requiring a nasal pharyngeal airway, nasotracheal intubation, or surgical intervention to reestablish patency. Laryngospasm, the feared complication of any invasive airway technique, needs to be considered in any patient with a compromised airway, especially in children. It is defined as closure of the glottis by the constriction of intrinsic/extrinsic laryngeal muscles, which can completely restrict ventilation. This pathophysiologic state often persists long after the stimulus has ceased. Laryngospasm may occur secondary to contact with the upper airway receptors on the tongue, palate, and oropharynx. Light touch to the upper airway, traction on the pelvic/abdominal viscera, chemical irritation, secretions, blood, water, and vomitus may all cause laryngospasm. Hypoxia and hypercapnia depress the activity of laryngeal adductor neurons, so laryngospasm is somewhat self-limited. Laryngospasm and bronchospasm occur more frequently in children and particularly following a recent respiratory tract infection.

FIG. 18-1. The anatomic airway.

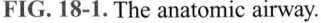

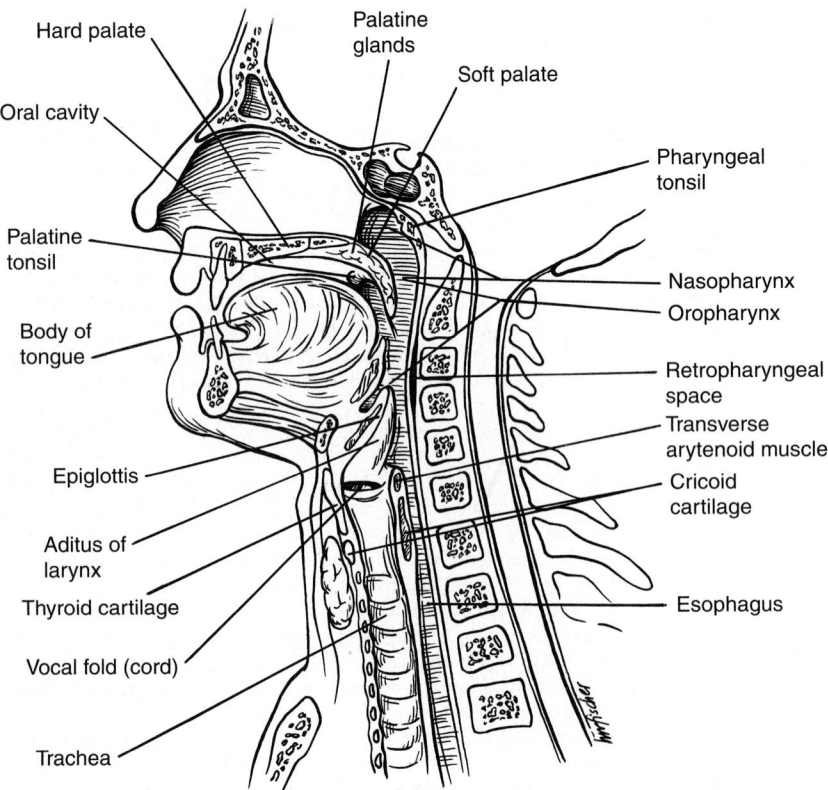

Hard palate
Palatine glands
Soft palate
Oral cavity
Pharyngeal tonsil
Palatine tonsil
Nasopharynx
Oropharynx
Body of tongue
Retropharyngeal space
Transverse arytenoid muscle
Epiglottis
Cricoid cartilage
Aditus of larynx
Thyroid cartilage
Esophagus
Vocal fold (cord)
Trachea

TABLE 18-1   Causes of Upper Airway Obstruction

Congenital/ Genetic	Infectious	Medical	Trauma/Tumor
Large tonsils	Tonsillitis	Cystic fibrosis	Laryngeal trauma
Macroglossia	Peritonsilar abscess	Angioedema	Hematoma/masses
Micrognathia	Retropharyngeal abscess	Laryngospasm	Smoke inhalation
Neck masses	Pretracheal abscess	Airway muscle relaxation	Thermal injuries
Large adenoids	Epiglottitis	Inflammatory	Foreign body
	Laryngitis/RSV*	Asthma	
	Ludwig angina		

*Respiratory syncytial virus.

Altered mental status, somnolence, or even sleep can depress the intrinsic and extrinsic muscle tone of the airway and produce obstruction. Some authors question the long-standing belief that the tongue falling back and occluding the lower pharynx is the major cause of airway obstruction in the somnolent or comatose patient. Recently, it was shown that during anesthesia in the supine patient, the tongue does, in fact, displace posteriorly, but it does not appear to occlude the pharynx. Upper airway obstruction in the unconscious patient occurs primarily because the epiglottis occludes the laryngeal inlet because of intrinsic muscle relaxation, which can be relieved simply by extending the neck. Extension of the neck and anterior displacement of the mandible moves the hyoid bone anteriorly and, in turn, lifts the epiglottis away from the laryngeal inlet. In a supine individual, the degree of extension of the head required to open the airway depends on elevation of the occiput above the horizontal plane. Relative to the neck, the more the occiput is elevated (to a degree), the less extension is required to open the airway, which explains why patients with airway compromise need to have their heads in the "sniffing" position. One can place a folded towel (not rolled) or foam rubber device underneath the patient's occiput (not neck) to create this position. Flexion of the neck has a marked effect of closing the airway, specifically the oropharynx. Recent magnetic resonance imaging (MRI) studies show that the soft palate also relaxes significantly during sedation, partially occluding the nasopharynx and causing complete obstruction when the patient is fully anesthetized. Moreover, extension of the anterior tongue does not appear to relieve this obstruction.[1]

Esophageal foreign bodies can also obstruct the airway. They can impinge upon the larynx or trachea, causing either acute or subacute obstruction. Some foreign bodies, such as large fruit pits, may have been present for some time; thus, there may not be a history of swallowing or choking on an object.

ORAL/NASAL AIRWAYS

The oral airway (Figure 18-2) is an "S"-shaped, rigid instrument that is used to prevent the base of the tongue from occluding the hypopharynx. It should be used to maintain the airway only in a patient with an absent gag reflex. The operator places the oral airway over the tongue, being careful not to push it further into the hypopharynx. A tongue blade can be used to aid insertion. The concave portion is placed cephalad, rotated 180 degrees, or aimed toward the ear and rotated 90 degrees inferiorly to hold the tongue away from the pharyngeal wall. It can also be used as a bite block during orotracheal intubation.

A nasal airway (nasopharyngeal tube) (Figure 18-3) is made of a pliable material that allows it to be placed into the nostril of a somnolent patient with an intact gag reflex. The nasal airway is a wonderful

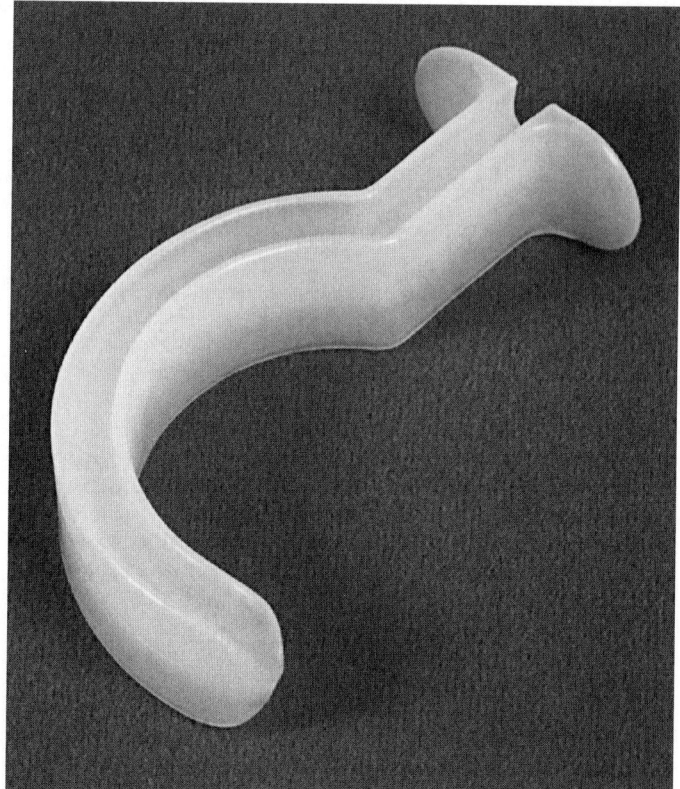

FIG. 18-2. An oral airway.

tool that can be quickly placed in a sonorous patient who may have decreased pharyngeal muscle tone and an obstructing soft palate and tongue. It allows air to bypass such obstructions, and if topical anesthesia is used as a lubricant, may ease subsequent passage of a nasogastric tube. The nasopharyngeal tube should be inserted into the most patent nostril (with the tip lubricated, ideally with a topical anesthetic such as lidocaine jelly) horizontal to the palate, and advanced until

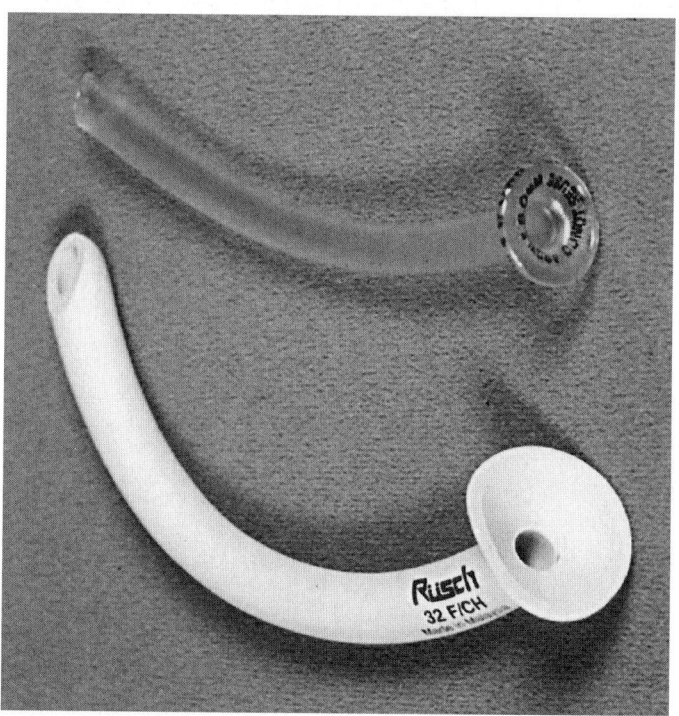

FIG. 18-3. Nasal airways.

maximal airflow is heard. It is important to use the correct size tube and to avoid inserting it far enough to stimulate the gag reflex.

THE BAG-VALVE-MASK UNIT

The bag-valve-mask (BVM) unit (Figure 18-4) is a self-inflating bag with a nonrebreathing valve that can be attached to a face mask. This design allows room air or oxygenated air to be manually delivered into the victim's lungs after any obstruction has been eliminated. This apparatus can be used initially while preparing for definitive airway maintenance. After the mask is placed, the handler clamps it snugly to the face. The thumb and index finger grasp the mask while the other fingers grasp the chin and pull it forward to hyperextend the stable neck. The other hand compresses the bag, expelling air into the patient's respiratory tree. This procedure can be used to manage respiratory failure temporarily, to assist poor inspiratory effort, or to temporize respiratory fatigue. The most common problem with a one-person operation is air leaks around the mask. A two-person operation employs two hands to hold the mask flush and has been shown to result in more effective ventilation.[2] Placement of an oral or nasal airway further facilitates airflow. The BVM unit may also be used prior to rapid-sequence intubation (RSI) to quickly assess the ease of BVM ventilation in cases where oral intubation fails. After an intubation, the BVM unit can be attached to the proximal end of the endotracheal tube.

To deliver 100 percent oxygen, there must be a reservoir with the same volume as the bag and an oxygen flow rate equal to the respiratory minute volume of the patient. By using a 2.5-L reservoir bag with an oxygen flow of 15 L per min, 100 percent oxygen can theoretically be delivered, although most nonrebreathers deliver about 75 percent oxygen. Similarly, a demand valve attached to the reservoir port of the ventilation bag will deliver a high concentration of oxygen.

ESOPHAGEAL AIRWAYS

Esophageal obturator airways (EOAs) (Figure 18-5)—the pharyngotracheal lumen airway and the esophageal tracheal Combitube—are all devices used in the prehospital setting when oral endotracheal intubation is not a viable option. These devices are designed to be placed in apneic, unconscious adults only.

Esophageal Obturator Airway/Esophageal Gastric Tube Airway

EOAs/esophageal gastric tube airways (EGTAs) are mentioned here only for historic reasons. They are rarely used now. The original primary benefit, placement without direct laryngeal visualization, has been supplanted by other more efficacious devices. The EGTA is a modification of the EOA and has an open distal tube containing a valve that allows passage of a nasogastric tube. Compared with the endotracheal tube (ETT), ventilation and oxygenation studies reveal varying results but suggest that the EOAs are adequate during cardiac

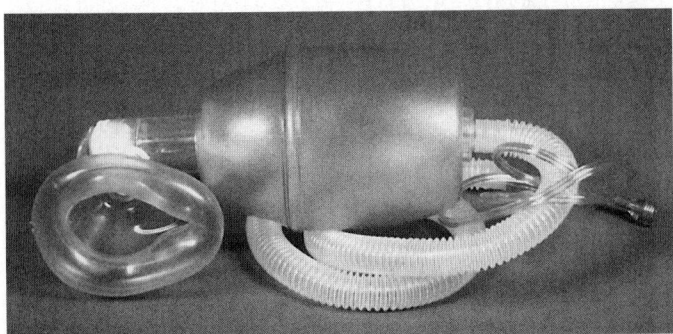

FIG. 18-4. Bag-valve-mask unit.

arrest.[2] One study showed that some physicians had never seen an EOA, and unfamiliarity is reason enough to avoid using this tool.

Pharyngotracheal Lumen Airway

The pharyngotracheal lumen airway (PTLA) (Figure 18-5A) is another two-tubed, cuffed airway that seals the oropharynx proximally and occludes the esophagus distally, allowing for ventilation through the short tube. There is no need for a face-to-mask seal. If the trachea is intubated by the long tube, ventilation can occur through the lumen, similar to an ETT.

Esophageal Tracheal Combitube

The esophageal tracheal Combitube (ETC) (Sheridan Catheter Corp.) (Figure 18-5B) is a plastic twin-lumen tube with a proximal low-pressure cuff that seals the pharyngeal area and a distal cuff that seals the esophagus, allowing ventilation between the cuffs. The proximal seal also removes the need for a facemask and, as compared with the PTLA, minimizes dental damage to the cuff. The distal cuff is similar to an ETT and serves to seal either the esophagus or the trachea when inflated. If the distal tube enters the esophagus, perforations in the esophageal lumen serve to ventilate the patient. If the trachea is intubated, the patient is ventilated directly, as with the cuffed ETT.

Tracheoesophageal Airway

The tracheoesophageal airway (TEA) (Figure 18-5C) is a standard ETT attached to a ventilation mask with two ports, one for the ETT and the other for oropharyngeal mask ventilation. It is designed to function equally well if inserted into the trachea or the esophagus. Tracheal intubation is facilitated by using cricoid pressure and extending the neck. While the tube is in the trachea, the cuff is inflated and the patient is ventilated normally. While the tube is in the esophagus, the patient is ventilated through the mask and the ETT allows for gastric venting or decompression.

Laryngeal Mask Airway

The laryngeal mask airway (LMA) (Intavent, Ltd.) (Figure 18-6) was developed by Brain, in 1983, as another artificial airway that can be placed blindly yet can provide a positive-pressure airway. The LMA consists of a tubular oropharyngeal airway similar to the ETT, but it is shorter and has a distal silicone laryngeal mask (balloon-type bulb) that inflates and provides a seal around the larynx. The LMA, when placed, is similar to other esophageal airways in that it can be inserted without manipulation of the patient's head. Because of its large diameter and short length, intubation of the bronchi or esophagus is circumvented. The hypopharynx, which is adapted to the passage of food, is less sensitive to a foreign body than the larynx and vocal cords, which have sensitive, protective reflexes.

Many published cases show the LMA to be an effective alternative when the ETT fails because of nonvisualization of the cords secondary to ETT difficulty, airway masses, or cervical pathology.[3] One study of LMA use by nonphysician emergency personnel in fasting patients found it easier to place than the ETT. In this study, there was no failure in LMA placement, whereas 21 percent of ETT placement attempts failed. Furthermore, the LMA required only half as many attempts and one-fifth the time to perform, and was rated equal to the ETT as an airway by anesthesiologists.[4] Complications of the LMA include partial or complete respiratory obstruction (approximately 3 percent) and general failure to protect against aspiration of gastric contents. The LMA is also inadequate in severe chronic obstructive pulmonary disease (COPD) because of the high pressure requirement.[5] Applying cricoid pressure in the acute setting almost always impedes insertion of the LMA and therefore reduces the chance of

FIG. 18-5. **A.** Pharyngotracheal lumen airway. **B.** Esophageal tracheal Combitube. **C.** Tracheo-esophageal airway (used with permission).

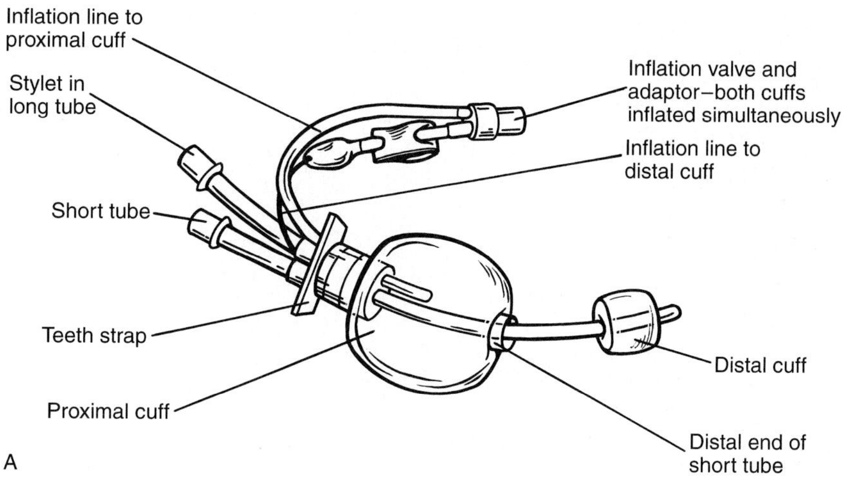

Inflation line to proximal cuff

Inflation valve and adaptor—both cuffs inflated simultaneously

Stylet in long tube

Inflation line to distal cuff

Short tube

Teeth strap

Distal cuff

Proximal cuff

Distal end of short tube

A

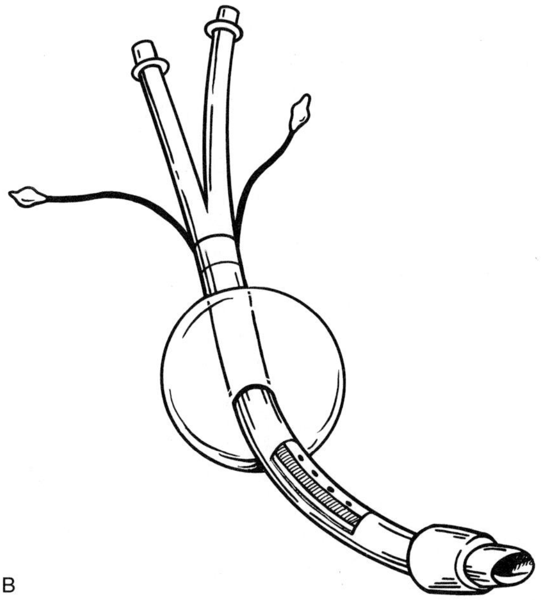

B

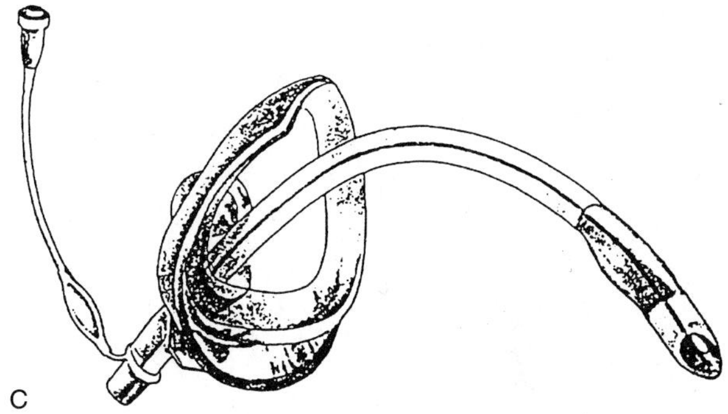

C

successful ventilation of the patient.[6] Therefore the LMA seems an effective alternative to the ETT when endotracheal intubation fails or when cervical pathology exists.

NONINVASIVE POSITIVE-PRESSURE VENTILATION

The widespread use of noninvasive positive-pressure ventilation (NIPPV) for chronic sleep apnea in the 1980s has prompted investigators to look at NIPPV in the acute setting today. NIPPV can be described as an application of a preset volume/pressure of inspiratory air through a face or nasal mask.

Inspiratory muscle fatigue is the final phase of ventilatory failure in patients with severe reactive airway disease, COPD, and end-state pulmonary edema/pneumonia. The airway resistance overcomes the patient's muscular ability to ventilate. An effective alternative to the traditional ETT, with its potential complications, is noninvasive, mechanically assisted ventilation with continuous positive airway pressure (CPAP) or bilevel positive airway pressure (BiPAP).

Continuous Positive Airway Pressure

CPAP is one method of NIPPV where positive pressure is held constant throughout the respiratory cycle and applied through a face or nasal mask. It recently received renewed application in the treatment of patients with *acute* hypoxemic respiratory failure.[7] CPAP improves

pulmonary function by reducing the work of breathing, maintaining inflation of atelectatic alveoli, and improving pulmonary compliance. CPAP also improves hemodynamics by reducing preload and afterload, therefore improving patient's cardiac output in left ventricular failure.

NIPPV has been used to support patients with acute respiratory failure but has been primarily studied in the intensive care setting. Only in the last decade have patient diagnostic categories individually been studied in the emergency department (ED) using CPAP. Those diseases include COPD, status asthmaticus, adult respiratory distress syndrome (ARDS), acute cardiogenic pulmonary edema (ACPE), pneumonia, or traumatic respiratory insufficiency. CPAP can be adjusted according to the patient's clinical response. Pressures of 5 to 10 cm of H_2O are most commonly used, and pressures above 15 are rare.

In early published and unpublished studies, CPAP at 10 cm of H_2O used in the hospital and prehospital settings showed more rapid improvement of vital signs (heart rate, respiratory rate, blood pressure) and oxygen saturation versus standard medical therapy alone in ACPE patients.[8] In other studies, using CPAP up to 10 to 12.5 cm H_2O, there was a significant improvement in Pao_2, stroke volume index, lower rate-pressure product, intrapulmonary shunt fraction, alveolar-arterial oxygen gradient, and, more importantly, lower rate of tracheal intubation.[9] After meta-analysis on the above studies, there was found a statistically significant reduction in the need for tracheal intubation and possibly a decrease in mortality.[10]

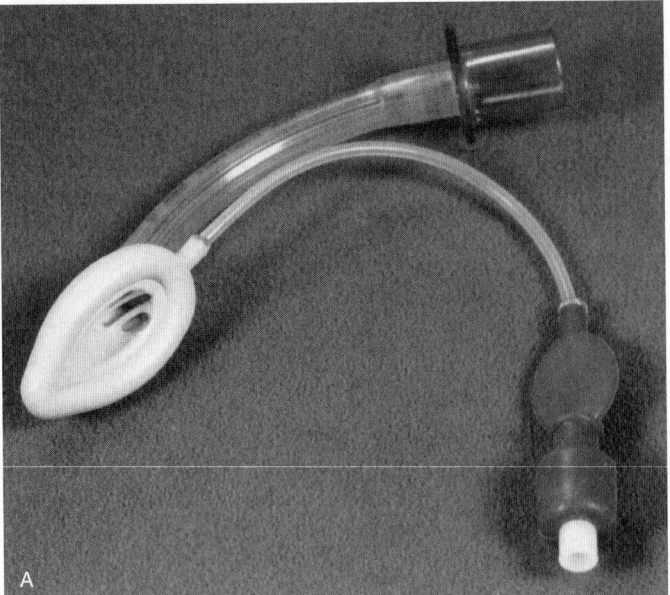

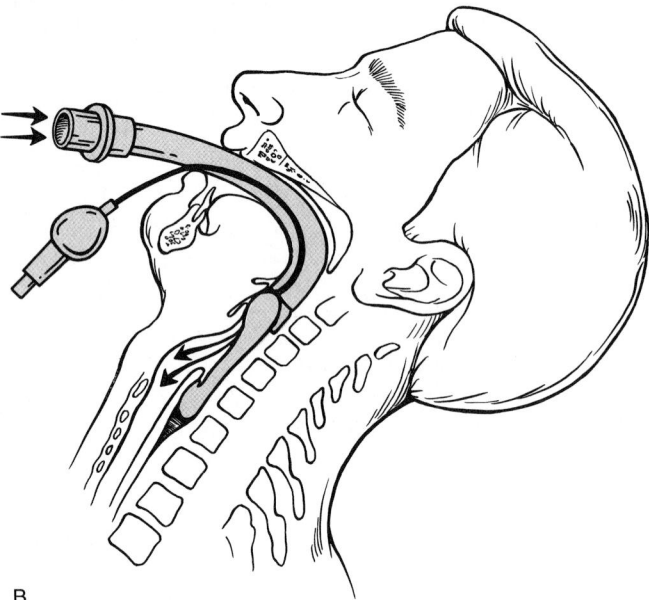

FIG. 18-6. **A.** Laryngeal mask airway (LMA). **B.** LMA diagram showing placement at the larynx (used with permission).

Bilevel Positive Airway Pressure

BiPAP is a method of NIPPV where positive airway pressure is used to assist the patient's spontaneous ventilation at a "bilevel." The positive airway pressure increases during inspiration and a positive expiratory pressure provides the physiological positive end-expiratory pressure known as PEEP. BiPAP machines respond to the patient's respiratory cycle by alternating between a higher flow rate during the inhalation phase of respiration and a lower flow rate during the exhalation phase.

The use of face-mask positive-pressure ventilation with acute exacerbation of COPD avoids intubation up to 76 percent of the time.[11] The benefits of BiPAP have been proven most effectively in the setting of severe COPD and is now being evaluated for ACPE. With the positive inspiratory pressure decreasing the work of breathing, and the positive expiratory pressure providing the physiologic CPAP, BiPAP has a theoretical advantage over CPAP alone. BiPAP has shown to reduce respiratory rate, dyspnea, and allow a more rapid improvement in both oxygenation and ventilation versus CPAP. Most recent studies us-

ing BiPAP with ACPE has shown to be an effective treatment in acute respiratory failure when compared to conventional oxygen therapy alone.[12–14]

NIPPV has been shown to decrease need for endotracheal intubation (ETI), thus decreasing the risks of ETI in the immunocompromised patient.[15] A major goal in the management of respiratory failure in the immunocompromised patient is avoiding ETI. These patients are at high risk of pneumonia, bronchitis, sinusitis, and ETI increases the risk of acquiring these diseases. In patients with pulmonary infiltrates, fever, and acute respiratory failure, early NIPPV has shown to decrease rates of ETI and the serious associated complications. Early NIPPV improves the likelihood of survival to hospital discharge.[15] One intensive care unit study showed that irrespective of the severity of the patient's illness, the use of NIPPV reduced the risk of ventilation-associated pneumonia and nosocomial infections.[16]

NIPPV decreases the requirement for mechanical support and lowers the average stay in the intensive care unit, among hemodynamically stable patients with impending respiratory failure.[17] Studies also demonstrate arterial blood gas improvement, intubation avoidance, and decreased respiratory rates with low complication risk.[7,18]

In the elderly, where the decision to intubate is more complex (because of age, illness, or cancer), nasal-mask ventilation yielded improvements in Pa_{O_2} similar to those of other studies (60 percent), but hypercarbia improved more slowly.[19] NIPPV should be considered for any patient where invasive respiratory support presents significant risk of sequelae.

In the pediatric patient population, BiPAP appears to improve respiratory rate, heart rate, Pa_{CO_2}, and O_2 saturation. It also decreases the need for intubation in obstructive apnea.

Trauma patients frequently have a significant loss of functional residual capacity (FRC) that often leads to mild to moderate respiratory insufficiency. In such instances, CPAP has been used to improve respiratory function and reduce hypoxemia.[20] CPAP is helpful in decreasing the work of breathing and improving FRC, thus preventing hypoxemia, hypocarbia, and tachypnea. Criteria for NIPPV have included spontaneous respirations, absence of respiratory acidemia/hypercarbia, intact mental status, a Pa_{O_2} above 65 mm Hg, presence of a functioning nasogastric tube, and absence of severe maxillofacial injury. Improvement may be seen starting at 5 cm H_2O. Studies show that a mean CPAP of 8.6 cm H_2O meets therapeutic goals. Duration of therapy may range from a few hours to 2 days. Trauma conditions that have been studied include pulmonary contusion, flail chest, pneumothorax, hemopneumothorax, and multiple chest and abdominal gunshot/stab wounds. In this setting, a functioning nasogastric tube and respective chest tube placement, when indicated, are extremely important. Patients suffering high esophageal or tracheal injuries should not be supported with a NIPPV. Maxillofacial and basilar skull fractures are also contraindications to NIPPV by face mask. Because many traumatized patients exhibit a remarkable capacity to breathe spontaneously and improvements in hemodynamics are one of the benefits of using spontaneous ventilation versus mechanical ventilation, CPAP/BiPAP is an appropriate adjunct for managing the airway in the trauma patient assuming non-airway related indications for ETI do not exist.

Technique

Nasal-mask or facial-mask ventilation employs a tight-fitting mask that allows for a CPAP or BiPAP support system. The patient with impending respiratory failure receives either continuous pressure or inspiratory/expiratory (bilevel) support, thus allowing a decrease in inspiratory effort, rest for respiratory and accessory muscles, improvement of gas exchange, avoidance of intubation, and improved comfort.[11,21] A nasal-mask protocol with BiPAP appears to be the most advanced protocol and appears to allow more sensitive changes during the course of treatment (Figure 18-7). The nasal mask allows the pa-

FIG. 18-7. A patient with severe COPD on nasal BiPAP (used with permission).

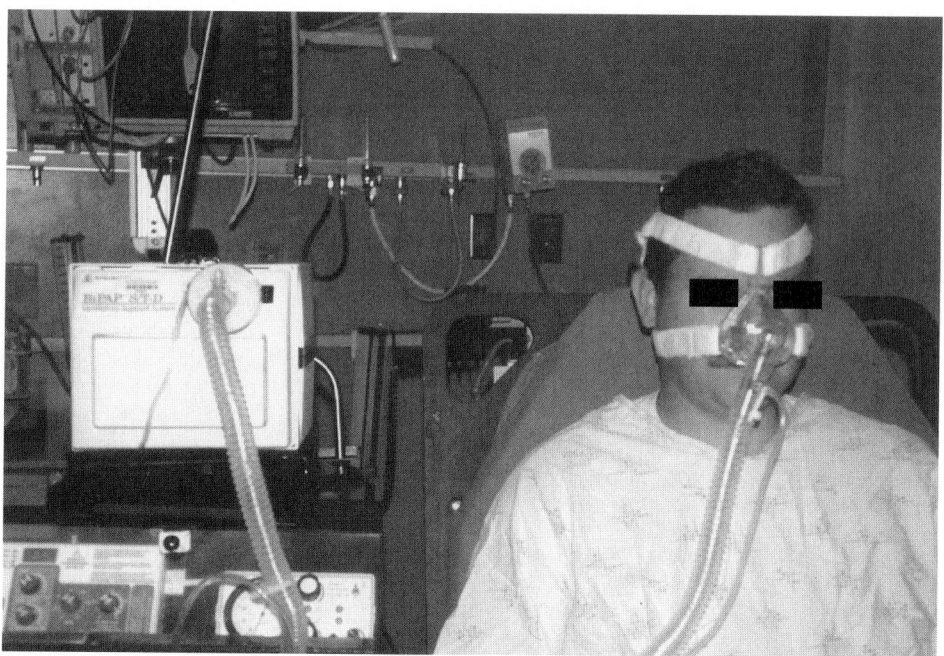

tient to eat, drink, and converse with the emergency staff. However, the nasal positive-pressure ventilation (NPPV) (distinct from NIPPV) does allow for air leaks through the mouth.

The ideal BiPAP ventilator is small, relatively inexpensive, very mobile, and tolerates some leaks. It is possible to set the inspiratory positive airway pressure (IPAP) and the expiratory positive airway pressure (EPAP/PEEP) independently. Three modes of ventilatory triggering are available: spontaneous, combined spontaneous/timed, and timed. The proper-size mask should be chosen (allowing no mouth coverage) and tight enough to allow a good, comfortable seal. Settings should include spontaneous mode, IPAP set at 10, EPAP set at 3 cm H_2O initially and increasing IPAP in 3-cm increments and EPAP slowly. Continuing hypercarbic failure is treated by increasing IPAP alone in 3-cm increments.[22] Caution must be applied when using NIPPV at pressures approaching 15 cm H_2O. There is evidence of increased risk of acute myocardial infarction with higher NIPPV pressures. BiPAP, CPAP, and NIPPV at high pressures (15 cm H_2O), may produce a greater fall in blood pressure because of a higher intrathoracic pressure reducing myocardial perfusion.[13,14]

Complications

Known complications include difficulty with mask seal requiring multiple readjustments, gastric distention, aspiration (rare), intolerance of the positive pressure, and facial skin breakdown (with long-term use). These complications appear to occur infrequently, but the most common intolerance is excessive respiratory secretions, which, in fact, may be a relative contraindication to NPPV along with life-threatening epistaxis, or pre-existing bullous lung disease. Other contraindications to NPPV are severe maxillofacial trauma and potential basilar skull fracture where pneumocephalus may occur, pneumothorax, pneumomediastinum, or hypotension due to or associated with intravascular volume depletion. Another problem with *mask* ventilation is that using a conventional ventilator can be difficult or even counterproductive because of the inadvertent triggering of alarms in systems in masks not designed for this use. The BiPAP ventilatory system, which is designed for NIPPV use, has been used with success, but may not be readily available in the ED, and respiratory services may have to be contacted for this setup.

Application of NPPV provides ventilatory support for impending respiratory failure and has been shown to decrease the workload of the respiratory muscles. Oxygen saturation, Pao_2, and pH remain stable or improve as compared with unassisted ventilation. Therefore this technique may prove useful in respiratory failure when complication of intubation is high.

This modality may decrease long-term hospital admissions, prevent unwanted intubations in the elderly or severely ill, and circumvent borderline respiratory failure intubations. Each patient must be closely monitored for tolerance of upper airway positive pressure and for instability.

Patients who receive NIPPV need to be cooperative and should not have life-threatening cardiac ischemia, dysrhythmias, or hypotension. NIPPV is inappropriate in patients who have absent or agonal respiratory effort, or who produce excessive airway secretions. Airway management and apparatus associated with NIPPV can be distracting. However, medical treatment, such as in-line nebulized updrafts, anticholinergics, steroids, and respiratory hygiene should proceed as appropriate.

REFERENCES

1. Nandi PR, Charlesworth CH, Taylor SJ, et al: Effects of general anesthesia on the pharynx. *Br J Anesth* 66:157, 1990.
2. Hammargren Y, Clinton JE, Ruiz E: A standard comparison of esophageal obturator airway and endotracheal tube ventilation in cardiac arrest. *Ann Emerg Med* 14:953, 1985.
3. Calder I, Ordman AJ, Jackowski A, Crockard HA: The Brain laryngeal mask airway-An alternative to emergency tracheal intubation. *Anaesthesia* 45:137, 1990.
4. Reinhart DJ, Simmons G: Comparison of placement of laryngeal mask airway with endotracheal tube by paramedics and respiratory therapists. *Ann Emerg Med* 24:260, 1994.
5. Maltby JR, Loken RG, Watson NC: The laryngeal mask airway: Clinical appraisal in 250 patients. *Can J Anesth* 37:509, 1990.
6. Gabbott DA, Sasada MP: Laryngeal mask airway insertion using cricoid pressure and manual in-line neck stabilization. *Anaesthesia* 50:674, 1995.
7. Meduri GU, Abou-Shala N, Fox RC: Noninvasive face mask mechanical ventilation in patients with acute hypercapnic respiratory failure. *Chest* 100:445, 1991.
8. Vaisanen IT, Rassanen J: Continuous positive airway pressure and supplemental oxygen in the treatment of cardiogenic pulmonary edema. *Chest* 92:481, 1987.
9. Lin M, Yang YF, Chiang HT, et al: Reappraisal of continuous positive airway pressure therapy in acute cardiogenic pulmonary edema. Short-term results and long-term follow up. *Chest* 107:1379, 1995.

10. Keenan SP, Kernerman PD, Cook DJ: The effect of noninvasive positive pressure ventilation on mortality in patients admitted with acute respiratory failure: A meta-analysis. *Crit Care Med* 25:1685, 1997.

11. Brochard L, Isabey D, Piquet J, et al: Reversal of acute exacerbations of chronic obstructive lung disease by inspiratory assistance with a facemask. *N Engl J Med* 323:1523, 1990.

12. Sacchetti AD, Harris RH, Paston C, et al: Bi-level positive airway pressure support system use in acute congestive heart failure: Preliminary case series. *Acad Emerg Med* 2:714, 1995.

13. Kosowsky JM, Storrow AB, Carleton SC: Continuous and bilevel positive airway pressure in the treatment of acute cardiogenic pulmonary edema [review]. *Am J Emerg Med* 18:91, 2000.

14. Mehta S, Jay GD, Woolard RH, et al: Randomized, prospective trial of bilevel vs continuous positive airway pressure in acute pulmonary edema. *Crit Care Med* 25:620, 1997.

15. Hilbert G, Gruson D, Vargas F, et al: Noninvasive ventilation in immunosuppressed patients with pulmonary infiltrates, fever, and acute respiratory failure. *N Engl J Med* 344(7):481, 2001.

16. Hill NS: Noninvasive ventilation for immunocompromised patients. *N Engl J Med* 344(7):522, 2001.

17. Bersten AD, Holt AW, Vedig AE, et al: Treatment of severe cardiogenic pulmonary edema with continuous positive airway pressure delivered by face mask. *N Engl J Med* 325:1825, 1991.

18. Pennock BE, Kaplan PD, Carlin BW, et al: Pressure support ventilation with a simplified ventilatory support system administered with a nasal mask in patients with respiratory failure. *Chest* 100:1371, 1991.

19. Benhamou D, Girault C, Raure C, et al: Nasal mark ventilation in acute respiratory failure. *Chest* 102:912, 1992.

20. Hurst JM, DeHaven CB, Branson RD: Use of CPAP mask as the sole mode of ventilatory support in trauma patients with mild to moderate respiratory insufficiency. *J Trauma* 25:1065, 1985.

21. Carrey Z, Stewart BG, Levy RD: Ventilatory muscle support in respiratory failure with nasal positive pressure ventilation. *Chest* 97:150, 1990.

22. Pennock BE, Crawshaw L, Kaplan PD: Noninvasive nasal mark ventilation for acute respiratory failure. *Chest* 105:441, 1994.

19

TRACHEAL INTUBATION AND MECHANICAL VENTILATION
Daniel F. Danzl
Robert J. Vissers

Airway integrity, assurance of oxygenation, ventilation, and prevention of aspiration are the mainstays of emergency airway management. The indications for tracheal intubation in the emergency setting most commonly include correction of hypoxia or hypercarbia, prevention of impending hypoventilation, and ensuring maintenance of a patent airway. Secondary indications include provision of a route for resuscitative medication administration and to permit temporizing paralysis during diagnostic testing.

OROTRACHEAL INTUBATION

The most reliable way to ensure a patent airway, provide oxygenation and ventilation, and prevent aspiration is endotracheal intubation. Many unconscious and even conscious patients may be unable to spontaneously clear the airway of secretions, may require mechanical ventilation, may have aspirated, or lack protective airway reflexes.[1]

Preparation

The clinical assessment of oxygenation and ventilation may be unreliable in a chaotic emergency department (ED). Continuous, noninvasive bedside monitoring of arterial oxygen saturation is helpful. Isolated oximetry does not assess the status of alveolar ventilation, whereas *capnography* does allow estimation of the partial pressure of carbon dioxide (Pa_{CO_2}) based on the waveform display of the end-tidal

partial pressure of carbon dioxide. *Capnometry* refers to the numerical display. In combination, these noninvasive modalities affect decisions regarding tracheal intubation.

Checking the necessary equipment should be standard procedure for ED clinicians at the beginning of their clinical duties. The following items should be available: oral and nasal airways, different-size orotracheal tubes, an O_2 setup that is appropriately connected, a self-inflating ventilation bag, different-size masks, and various sizes of Miller and Macintosh blades with the light checked and the suction attached and tested. When intubation is required, the appropriate-size tube and an additional tube (0.5 to 1 mm in diameter smaller) should be selected, and the cuffs should be checked for air leaks with a 10-mL syringe. Selecting a tube of the proper diameter is essential. The approximate sizes for endotracheal tubes are 8.0 to 8.5 mm inner diameter for an adult male and 7.5 to 8.0 mm inner diameter for an adult female. The second hole at the end of the tube above the bevel is called *Murphy eye*. This hole permits some uninterrupted airflow if the tip is occluded.

Endotracheal tubes (ETTs) with high-volume, low-pressure cuffs are the best design for adults. When properly inflated, thin-walled cuffs prevent aspiration better than medium-walled cuffs. The operator should test the light on the laryngoscope and then pick an appropriate-size blade. The straight Miller blade is used to physically lift the epiglottis. The curved Macintosh blade is placed in the vallecula above the epiglottis and is used to indirectly lift the epiglottis off the larynx owing to the traction on the frenulum.

The development of expertise with both blade types is desirable, because they offer different advantages. The curved blade may cause less trauma and be less likely to stimulate an airway reflex, because, when used properly, it does not directly touch the larynx. It also allows more room for adequate visualization during tube placement and is helpful in the obese patient. The straight blade is mechanically easier to insert in many patients who do not have large central incisors. Selecting the proper-size blade greatly facilitates intubation. In adults, the curved Macintosh no. 3 is the most popular, and no. 4 is more useful in large patients. The straight Miller no. 2 or 3 is popular for the same purposes.

The patient should be thoroughly preoxygenated before intubation, ideally for several minutes. Hypoxia develops more quickly in children, pregnant women, and patients in other hyperdynamic states. Flexion of the lower neck with extension at the atlantooccipital joint (sniffing position) aligns the oropharyngeal-laryngeal axis, allowing a direct view of the larynx (Figure 19-1). The inexperienced laryngoscopist's most common reasons for failure, inadequate equipment preparation and poor patient positioning, arise before using the laryngoscope.

Technique

The laryngoscope is held in the left hand, and an ETT or suction apparatus is held in the right. After dentures and any obscuring blood, secretions, or vomitus have been removed, the suction is exchanged for the ETT and inserted during the same laryngoscopy.

The blade is inserted into the right corner of the patient's mouth. If a curved Macintosh blade is used, the flange will push the tongue toward the left side of the oropharynx. If the blade is inserted directly down the middle, the tongue can force the line of sight posteriorly, which is a common reason for the putative "anterior larynx." After visualization of the arytenoids, the epiglottis is lifted directly with the straight blade or indirectly with the curved blade. The larynx is exposed by pulling the handle in the direction that it points, i.e., 90 degrees to the blade. Cocking the handle back, especially with the straight blade, risks fracturing central incisors and is ineffective at revealing the cords.

There are a variety of other straight and curved blades available. For example, the Guedel blade is a straight blade with an acute, 72-degree angle to the handle. The Schapira straight blade has a side concavity that helps cradle the large tongue and push it toward the left

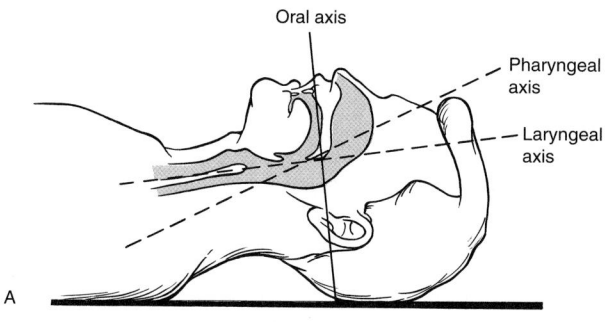

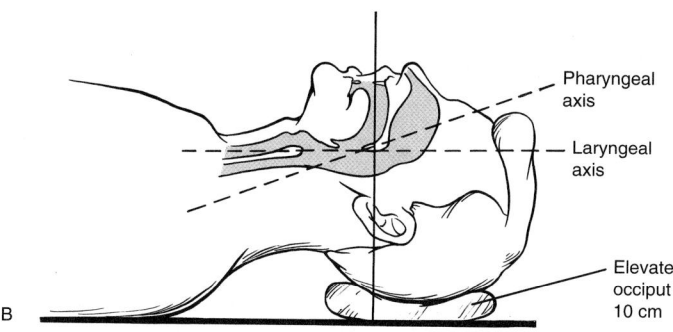

FIG. 19-1. A. Oral, pharyngeal, and laryngeal axes. **B.** Sniffing position.

side of the mouth. The CLM curved laryngoscope blade has a hinged tip, which permits elevation of the epiglottis with minimal force, as the fulcrum is repositioned down within the pharynx.

One technique that avoids the most common error, i.e., overly deep insertion of the blade, is to look for the arytenoid cartilages. If only the posterior commissure is visible, an assistant should apply more pressure on the cricoid (Sellick maneuver) or perform the laryngeal lift. Another option is the "burp" technique. The larynx is manually displaced posteriorly (backward) against the cervical vertebrae, superiorly (upward), and laterally to the right (rightward pressure). To avoid error, the cuff must be seen passing completely through the cords. "Last ditch" attempts at blind passage invite anoxia. The intubator should never be reluctant to abort the attempt if visualization of the larynx is not successful. Whenever feasible, an assistant should apply steady cricoid pressure with the thumb and index finger during the intubation to help prevent aspiration.

With proper technique and practice, semirigid, malleable, blunt-tipped metal, or plastic stylets are not usually necessary for most patients. Nevertheless, a selection of proper-size stylets should be available. The tip of the stylet should not extend beyond the end of the ETT or exit Murphy eye.

One aid to intubation with direct vision is the use of a thin, flexible intubation stylet. This type of stylet can be inserted blindly around the epiglottis into the trachea. The ETT is then threaded over it into the trachea, and the stylet is removed. The Eschmann tracheal tube introducer or stylet, also known as the "gum elastic bougie," is a valuable aid for difficult oral intubations. Another option is to use the tip on the laryngeal tracheal anesthesia kit. With either stylet, orient the tube so that Murphy eye is at the 12-o'clock position.

The tube should never be forced through the vocal cords, which can result in avulsion of the arytenoid cartilages or laceration of the vocal cords. Usually, any difficulty in passing the tube is a result of the tube being too large or too soft and flexible. Directed transoral or translaryngeal anesthesia with lidocaine can help relax the cords. If anesthesia fails, aligning the bevel with the glottic opening may be successful.

The tube should be advanced until the cuff disappears below the cords. Because head motion may move the tip of the tube 1 to 2 cm,

correct tube placement is a minimum of about 2 cm above the carina. From the corner of the mouth, this location is approximately 23 cm in men and 21 cm in women. The base of the pilot tube (a tube with the adapter to inflate the cuff) is usually at the level of the teeth. To avoid ischemia of the tracheal mucosa, cuff pressure should be kept below 40 cm H_2O. The minimal intracuff pressure to prevent aspiration is 25 cm H_2O.[2] The operator should secure the tube, being careful not to impede cervical venous return with the umbilical tape or fixator. The use of a modified clove-hitch knot or a commercial fixator is ideal and helps to avoid kinking the pilot tube.

CONFIRMATION OF INTUBATION   Endobronchial or esophageal intubation will result in hypoxia or hypercarbia. There is no clinically reliable substitute for direct visualization of the tube passing through the vocal cords. Hence the adage, "when in doubt, take it out." Nevertheless, there are a number of options to help confirm intratracheal tube positioning. Clinical assessments, including chest and epigastric auscultation, tube condensation, and symmetrical chest wall expansion, are not infallible in the ED. "Breath sounds" from the stomach can be transmitted through the chest after gastric insufflation.

The two basic categories of confirmatory adjuncts are end-tidal CO_2 (ETCO$_2$) detectors or monitors and esophageal detection devices. Both have advantages provided that the operator remains cognizant of the sources of interpretation error. Capnometers measure CO_2 in the expired air. The most commonly used capnometric devices in the ED are colorimetric, with a pH-sensitive purple filter paper. When in contact with CO_2, hydrogen ions are formed, resulting in color changes according to the concentration of CO_2. For example, with the Nellcor Easy Cap II, the paper turns yellow after exposure to 2 to 5 percent ETCO$_2$, which is equivalent to 15 to 38 mm Hg P_{CO_2}. There is no color change, the filter paper remains purple, with an ETCO$_2$ of less than 0.5 percent, equivalent to less than 4 mm Hg P_{CO_2}. Colorimetric capnometers are useful for general readings, as in assessing proper ETT placement, but are not accurate enough when precise determinations are necessary. Capnography displays real-time characteristic CO_2 waveforms.

The use of ETCO$_2$ pressure (P_{ETCO_2}) monitoring can help confirm endotracheal intubation.[2] Colorimetric or infrared detection of P_{ETCO_2}, however, may not occur even with proper ETT placement, during states of low pulmonary perfusion such as cardiac arrest, inadequate chest compressions during cardiopulmonary resuscitation, or massive pulmonary embolism. Another cause of false-negative interpretations is massive obesity. Severe pulmonary edema may obstruct the ETCO$_2$ or P_{ETCO_2} monitor with secretions. Alternatively, there may be an initial false-positive detection of CO_2 after esophageal intubation if carbonated beverages have been ingested by the patient or for a few minutes after bolus sodium bicarbonate administration. Another cause is gastric distention resulting from bag-valve-mask (BVM) ventilation. A heated humidifier or nebulizer or epinephrine instilled through the ETT also can cause false-positive interpretations.

After intubation and cuff inflation, the capnometer is attached to the ETT. Then a BVM unit is attached to the detector, and the patient is given about six ventilations to wash out residual CO_2. The P_{ETCO_2} monitor is then checked for color changes. If capnography is available, a persistent positive capnograph formation after clear and direct visualization of tube placement approaches certainty. On rare occasion, misplacement of the hypopharyngeal glottic tube tip may result in misleadingly normal oximetry and capnography. This error can be recognized by the inadequate depth of tube insertion or inadequate ventilatory volumes or on chest x-ray.

Esophageal detection devices also offer the potential to accurately determine tube location. The various designs depend on their proper function as inline aspirators of the ETT. The device adaptors fit over the 15-mm ETT connector. One advantage of the esophageal detection devices is that accuracy does not depend on adequate cardiac output and pulmonary perfusion. Rather, proper functioning is predicated on the anatomic differences between the esophagus and the trachea. When the ETT is in the esophagus, the soft, non-cartilaginous walls will collapse, and air cannot be aspirated easily.

To perform the syringe aspiration technique, the device should be attached after intubation but before ventilation. The syringe plunger should then be retracted. Resistance to aspiration reflects occlusion from esophageal collapse. If there is no resistance during aspiration, then the tube is assumed to be in the trachea. If a self-inflating bulb is used, the bulb should be compressed and then attached to the ETT. One advantage of the bulb is that it requires one hand.

COMPLICATIONS The emergency physician should never assume that continued airway patency is assured after ETT insertion.[3] Repeated suctioning is necessary to prevent thrombotic or inspissated secretions from obstructing the tube. Endobronchial ball-valve obstruction also can be caused by a clot. The clot can impair ventilation and produce hyperinflation of individual lobes. Cuff displacement or overinflation can result in ball-valve obstruction of the airway. Cuffs inflated in the field during frigid conditions will expand with warming. If tracheal ball-valve obstruction is suspected, the cuff should be deflated. If the tube is blocked, deflation will allow exhalation.

There are many other correctable intubation complications that should be kept in mind. If the ETT cuff leaks after the intubation, the inflation valve should be checked, because it may be defective. One simple remedy is to attach a three-way stopcock to the valve, re-inflate the cuff, and turn off the stopcock. A cuff that seems to be leaking slowly might be sealable. One type of sealant involves instilling an aspirable mixture of normal saline and 2 percent lidocaine jelly, at a 3:1 ratio, into the cuff.

If the ETT needs to be replaced, a tube changer might be considered. There are many commercially available, semirigid catheters that include 15-mm adaptors or connectors to permit ventilation during the tube exchange. These devices have quick-connect adapters that incorporate through-lumen designs to ensure adequate airflow during the procedure.

Although uncommon, morbidity related to emergent endotracheal intubation does occur and may be quite debilitating. Arytenoid cartilage avulsion or displacement, usually on the right, prevents the patient from phonating properly. Intubation of the pyriform sinus and pharyngeal-esophageal perforation has been reported. Chordal synechiae may develop anteriorly, or commissural stenosis can develop posteriorly.

Subglottic stenosis is the most disastrous sequela. The physician should avoid cuff overinflation and attempt to minimize tube motion in the larynx and trachea. Subglottic stenosis usually occurs in patients with poorly secured tubes who are combative or on ventilators.

ALTERNATIVE AIRWAY MANAGEMENT TECHNIQUES

Nasotracheal Intubation

Nasotracheal intubation (NTI) is an essential psychomotor skill that may be useful in many difficult situations. Operators adept at rapid sequence intubation (RSI) and NTI are in the best position to assess and act on the following prime considerations: What are the potential risks and benefits to having spontaneous respirations preserved rather than ablated? Is there a safe alternative in this patient that may avoid precipitating the need for a potentially unnecessary surgical airway?

Nasal intubation is helpful in situations where laryngoscopy or cricothyrotomy may be difficult and neuromuscular blockade hazardous.[4] Severely dyspneic patients with congestive heart failure, chronic obstructive pulmonary disease, or asthma and who are awake often cannot remain supine but can tolerate NTI in the sitting position. It may be impossible to align the oropharyngeal-laryngeal axis in patients with arthritis, masseter spasm, temporomandibular dislocation,

or recent oral surgical procedures. Patients with a peculiar body habitus may be difficult to intubate orally. Other considerations for NTI include persistent trismus from seizures, facial trauma, infection, tetanus, or decorticate-decerebrate rigidity. Patients with certain neuromuscular disorders or dystrophies or significant electrolyte abnormalities are not ideal candidates for oral intubation.

To minimize epistaxis, both nares should be sprayed with a topical vasoconstrictor anesthetic. During the brief period for the anesthetic to take effect, a cuffed ETT 0.5 to 1 mm smaller than optimal for oral intubation should be selected. The integrity of the cuff should be verified, and the tube adapter should be checked to ensure a snug fit. Because secretions and blood may be expelled into the air and onto the intubator's face, universal precautions should be observed. An option in addition to a face shield is the use of a protective filtering adapter, such as the Humid-Vent 1, which can be attached to the proximal end of the ETT (Gibeck Respiration, Stockholm, Sweden).

The tube, lubricated with a water-soluble (2 percent lidocaine or K-Y) jelly, is advanced along the nasal floor on the more patent side. Abrasions of the Kiesselbach plexus can be minimized by having the bevel face the septum. Steady, gentle pressure or slow rotation of the tube usually bypasses small obstructions. Passage of the tube is straight back toward the occiput (not upward). If the right side is not passable, the tube should be advanced along the other side before resorting to a smaller tube.

In patients with intact protective airway reflexes, directed transoral or translaryngeal anesthesia often facilitates intubation. Translaryngeal anesthesia, although not widely used in the ED, should be considered when the initial intubation attempt is unsuccessful. After palpating the superior border of the cricoid cartilage in the midline, the cricothyroid membrane is punctured with a 22- to 25-gauge 0.5- to 1-in. needle (Figure 19-2). The needle should be perpendicular to the membrane in the midline, with the point of injection just cephalad to the cricoid cartilage. Aspirate air, swiftly inject 1.5 to 2.0 mL of 4 percent lidocaine (sterile for injection), and press the site firmly with one finger for a few seconds. This technique prevents small degrees of subcutaneous emphysema that would erroneously suggest a laryngeal injury. Translaryngeal anesthesia is contraindicated if the landmarks are obscured by thyroid or tumor impingement on the cricothyroid membrane and in obese or combative patients.

An assistant should immobilize the patient's head and initially maintain it in a neutral or slightly extended position ("sniffing position"). The physician should stand beside the patient, with one hand on the tube and with the thumb and index finger of the other hand straddling the larynx. The tube is then advanced while rotating it medially 15 to 30 degrees until maximal airflow is heard through the tube. Then the tube is gently but somewhat swiftly advanced. The best time for advancement is at the initiation of inspiration. Entrance into the larynx may initiate a cough, and most expired air should exit through the tube even though the cuff is uninflated. **The presence of any vocal sounds indicates a failed attempt.**

The advancement of the tube toward the carina can be observed externally. The normal distance from the external nares to the carina is 32 cm in the adult male and 27 to 28 cm in the adult female. Therefore, before obtaining a chest x-ray, the optimal initial depth of tube placement for NTI in adults, measured at the nares, is 28 cm in men and 26 cm in women. Standard tube confirmation techniques should be performed. Secretions or blood in the tube should be removed before initiating positive-pressure ventilation.

If intubation is unsuccessful, the neck is carefully inspected to determine malposition of the tube. Most commonly, the tube is in the pyriform fossa on the same side as the nostril used. A bulge will be seen and can be palpated laterally. The tube is withdrawn into the retropharynx until breath sounds are heard. The tube is then redirected while the larynx is manually displaced toward the bulge. If there is no contraindication, flexion and rotation of the neck to the ipsilateral side while the tube is rotated medially often is effective.

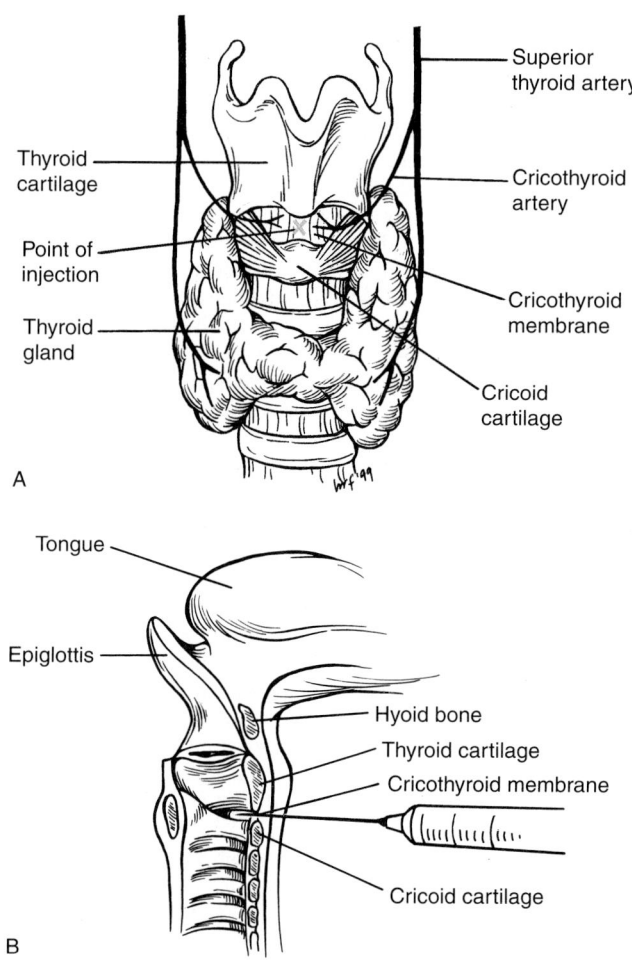

Thyroid cartilage

Point of injection

Thyroid gland

A

Superior thyroid artery

Cricothyroid artery

Cricothyroid membrane

Cricoid cartilage

Tongue

Epiglottis

Hyoid bone

Thyroid cartilage

Cricothyroid membrane

Cricoid cartilage

B

FIG. 19-2. Translaryngeal anesthesia via cricothyroid puncture. **A.** Anatomy, anterior view. **B.** Anatomy, cross-sectional view. Same landmarks as those for translaryngeal ventilation.

technique in the setting of obvious massive head trauma would be required for such an outcome. Severe traumatic nasal or pharyngeal hemorrhage may necessitate orotracheal intubation or cricothyrotomy. Contamination of the spinal fluid is a hazard with some basilar skull fractures.

Serious complications of NTI are rare. In a number of large series, there was no permanent laryngeal damage. Epistaxis will occur with inadequate topical vasoconstriction, excessive tube size, poor technique, or anatomic defects. Excessive force can damage the nasal septum or turbinates.

Frequent suctioning, especially if epistaxis or other upper airway hemorrhage is present, will help to prevent thrombotic occlusion of the tube or a mainstem bronchus. Retropharyngeal lacerations, abscesses, and nasal necrosis have been reported.

Paranasal sinusitis, especially occurring with prolonged NTI or severe cranial trauma, can be an unrecognized source of sepsis. The risk of postintubation sinusitis correlates with the duration of intubation, which often reflects the neurologic insult. In the setting of craniofacial trauma, any subsequent computed tomographic scans should include views of the paranasal sinuses. Other factors causing sinusitis include the presence of a nasogastric tube, sinus hemorrhage or fracture, and administration of glucocorticoids.

Digital Intubation

Digital intubation is an underused, noninvasive technique for ETT insertion. The performance of this maneuver requires tactile recognition of the epiglottis. Visual landmarks may be impossible to identify with a laryngoscope, because of patient positioning, anatomic disruption, or significant hemorrhage. Tactile digital intubation can avert cricothyrotomy when direct laryngoscopy after neuromuscular blockade has failed. Patients with micrognathia or temporomandibular immobility are poor candidates for this technique.

The patient must be deeply comatose, in cardiac arrest, or in a state of adequate neuromuscular blockade. Before insertion, the well-lubricated ETT should be shaped with a stylet into a J configuration. Then, unless the operator is quite confident, a bite block should be inserted in the opposite side of the mouth. The tongue should be lifted and the mandible pulled forward with the gloved dominant hand. The lubricated middle and index fingers of the gloved nondominant hand are inserted down the middle of the tongue and the cartilaginous epiglottis is palpated with the middle finger.

While the epiglottis is being palpated, the well-lubricated, J-shaped ETT and stylet are inserted and slid along the middle finger. The path from the corner of the mouth opposite the bite block to the epiglottis is the shortest distance. The index finger can help guide the tube from behind. As the larynx is entered, resistance will be encountered. At this point, it is essential to partly withdraw the stylet. Otherwise, the tube will lodge against the anterior wall of the trachea and become difficult to advance.

Transillumination

Transillumination with a lighted stylet can facilitate oral or nasal intubation and help to confirm ETT placement and positioning. This technique is particularly useful when direct laryngoscopy is anatomically impossible. Oral intubation is easiest with a semirigid stylet. Before insertion, the patient's cheek is transilluminated. This serves as a check of the ambient light and will predict the laryngeal light intensity. It may be necessary to dim or shield bright ambient light from the neck. Obese patients who do not transilluminate buccally may not do so laryngeally.

For oral insertion, the lubricated ETT and lighted stylet are inserted after pulling the tongue forward with a 4 × 4 in. gauze pad. The tube initially should be directed into the ipsilateral pyriform fossa to establish the depth of the epiglottis. Then the tube is slightly withdrawn, and

The other most common tube misplacement is posteriorly in the esophagus. There are no breath sounds through the tube, and the trachea is slightly elevated. The intubator should attempt redirection after extending the patient's head and performing Sellick maneuver. When cervical spine pathology is suspected, a directional tip-control tube (Endotrol) or a fiberoptic laryngoscope should be considered. Endotrol tubes smaller than 7.5 mm (inner diameter) tend to soften and obstruct and can be difficult to suction. However, the use of these directional-tip tubes often improves the success rate of the first attempt at NTI.

When the tube hangs up on the vocal cords, shrill, turbulent air noises will be heard. The tube can be rotated slightly to realign the bevel with the cords. Alternatively, 2 mL of 4 percent lidocaine (80 mg) can be administered down through the tube onto the cords if transoral or translaryngeal anesthesia was omitted.

Nasal intubation with a fiberoptic laryngoscope may be required when neoplastic lesions, lymphoid tissue, Ludwig angina, peritonsillar abscess, or epiglottitis obstructs the pharynx. The presence of facial trauma does not appear to be a contraindication to NTI.[5] Complex nasal and massive midfacial fractures and bleeding disorders are relative contraindications to NTI.

Conversely, oral intubation can impede prompt reduction and stabilization of some maxillary fractures. Because a LeFort I fracture does not extend to the cribriform plate, it is not a contraindication. Fiberoptic guidance or RSI is preferable for LeFort II and III fractures.

The risk of inadvertent intracranial passage of a nasotracheal tube is extremely low, unlike that with nasogastric tube insertion. Very poor

the tip is directed toward the midline. The intubator must discriminate between the light emanating from the larynx and the much dimmer light transmitted from the esophagus. Usually the "jack-o-lantern" glow arising from the larynx or trachea is not appreciated when the light source is misplaced in the esophagus. For nasal intubation, the flexible stylet or wand instrument is inserted into a directional-tip ETT (e.g., Endotrol). After positioning the tube in the retropharynx, very gentle traction is applied to the ring to achieve slight flexion of the tip of the ETT.

Intubating Laryngeal Mask Airway

The laryngeal mask airway (LMA) is a ventilatory device that looks like an ETT with an inflatable silicone mask on the distal end. The LMA is placed blindly, and the mask is inflated over the larynx to provide a supraglottic seal. The technique is quickly mastered, and in most cases the LMA is placed rapidly. LMA's inability to protect against aspiration has limited its role in the ED to a temporizing rescue device.

The intubating LMA (ILMA) addresses this deficiency by providing a conduit to facilitate endotracheal intubation.[6] This device also is inserted blindly and uses a rigid handle for insertion, making it an excellent rescue device. Ventilation is achieved in almost all patients, even those with difficult airways or distorted anatomy. Blind intubation through the ILMA with an ETT is over 90 percent successful and improves to almost 100 percent when a lighted stylet or fiberoptic bronchoscope is used to assist.[7]

The ILMA can be used successfully in cervical spine injuries. Its primary role is as a rescue device, although it has been used as an intubation technique in awake patients with known difficult airways. Aspiration of gastric contents is the most common complication with ILMA and continues to be a risk until successful placement of the ETT.

Fiberoptic Assistance

The flexible fiberoptic laryngoscope can be a valuable adjunct when there are anatomic or traumatic limitations that prevent visualization of the vocal cords. Clinical examples include conditions that prevent opening or movement of the mandible, massive tongue swelling (hemorrhage or angioedema), congenital anatomic abnormalities, and cervical spine immobility. These instruments allow visualization of laryngeal structures and can enable difficult intubations, including those around expanding hematomas (Figure 19-3). Patients in need of an immediate airway or those with ongoing hemorrhage or copious secretions are poor candidates.

Directed transoral or transnasal and translaryngeal topical anesthesia is essential. The nasal mucosa should be sprayed with a vasoconstrictor. Dual suctioning capability is needed; a suction port should be attached to a suction apparatus for oral blood and secretions. Tongue extrusion and anterior mandibular displacement are helpful if the oral route is chosen. Fragile equipment is more frequently damaged transorally. The nasal route is also preferred, because the optic tip can enter the glottis at a less acute angle.

For this procedure, the eyepiece is focused, and the flexible shaft is lubricated. The lens at the tip of the laryngoscope is then immersed in warm water to prevent fogging. The intubator should continuously monitor pulse oximetry and ensure that the gag reflex is not present. After attachment of oxygen tubing to the suction port, intermittent insufflation of oxygen at 10 to 15 L per min to keep the optic tip clear should be considered. Insufflation is usually superior to suction for clearing secretions.

The adapter initially is removed from an ETT that is at least 7.0 mm in inner diameter. To prevent barotrauma when high-flow oxygen is insufflated, an ETT of at least 7.5 mm in inner diameter is used. Then the lubricated ETT is slipped over the shaft up to the handle. The distal end of the fiberoptic laryngoscope must extend beyond the end of the ETT. The laryngoscope is held with the left hand, and tip deflection is controlled while advancing it through the cords. The laryngoscope will function as a stylet for the tube. After the laryngoscope is in the trachea, the ETT is advanced and the laryngoscope is removed.

Another option is to insert a nasotracheal tube blindly into the posterior pharynx and stop about 1 to 2 cm proximal to the epiglottis. The scope is then inserted through this hollow conduit, and the fiberoptic tip can be directed into the glottis. The lubricated scope should not pass through Murphy eye. If this occurs, it will be impossible to advance the ETT.

The fiberoptic scope cannot be used as a stylet to guide the ETT into the trachea. The stiffer ETT often will deflect the thin scope tip posteriorly into the esophagus. In addition, the concavity of the ETT is kept anterior toward the 12 o'clock position and places the tube tip and Murphy eye at 3 o'clock (90 degrees to the right). The tip then often hits the right arytenoid cartilage. Rotating the tube 90 degrees

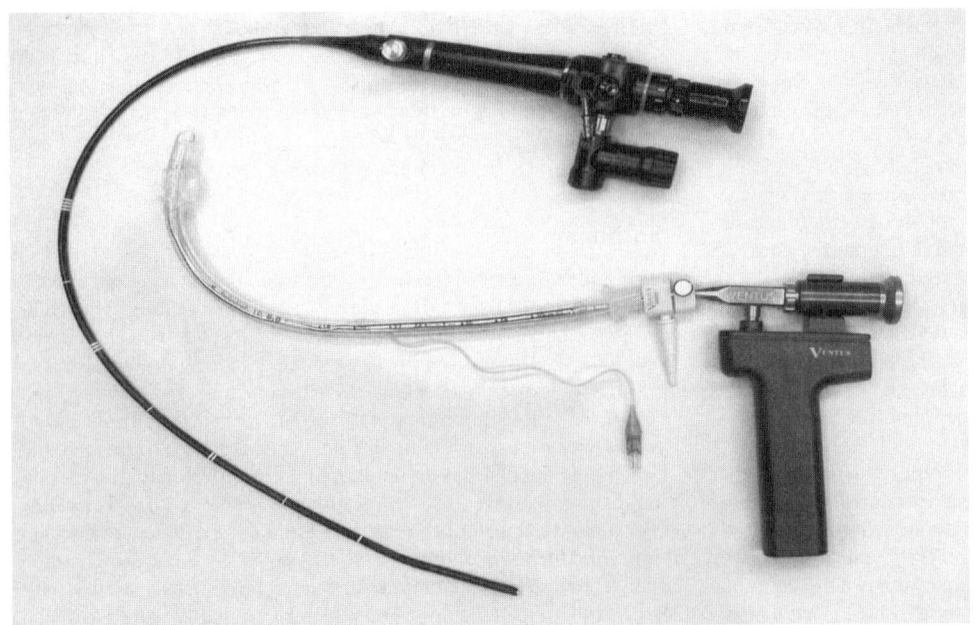

FIG. 19-3. A fiberoptic laryngoscope and a Shikani endoscope.

counterclockwise aligns the tip with the upper triangular entrance into the trachea.

Indirect Fiberoptic Laryngoscopes

There are many devices that incorporate fiberoptics into a laryngoscope, allowing for indirect visualization of the cords in potentially difficult airways. They are particularly useful when direct visualization of the larynx is impossible due to neck immobility, reduced oral opening, or an anterior larynx. They do not replace the diagnostic capabilities of a flexible fiberoptic scope and have the same visualization restrictions when blood and excessive secretions are present. The Bullard laryngoscope (Circon, ACMI, Stamford, CT), the Upsher-Scope (Mercury Medical, Clearwater, FL), and the WuScope (Pentax, Fremont, CA) are available. These devices are best used for the anticipated difficult airway as opposed to an emergent rescue device. Only the Bullard model has pediatric sizes.

The Shikani scope (Clarus Medical, Minneapolis, MN) is a device that incorporates the fiberoptics into a malleable stylet.[8] Similar to the other devices, the light source is in a portable handle. Setup only requires mounting the ETT. Pediatric sizes are available. The ability to manipulate the angle of the stylet and its brightness allows the use of a blind technique similar to that with the lighted stylet.

Fiberoptic ETTs also are commercially available. Direct line of sight can improve visualization in many difficult intubations. The advantages of direct vision include verification of tube positioning, identification of the right- or left-sided source of pulmonary hemorrhage, and inspection of tracheal injury.

Retrograde Tracheal Intubation

Retrograde tracheal intubation is another option when conventional airway approaches fail. The landmarks are the same as those for cricothyroid puncture (see Figure 19-2). Cervical or mandibular ankylosis and upper airway masses are some of the potential conditions in which retrograde tracheal intubation may help.

The insertion of a retrograde translaryngeal catheter is a less invasive option than cricothyrotomy. **This technique can be time consuming and will not be quick enough for apneic patients.** The initial angle of the needle should be 30 to 45 degrees cephalad, and a 70- to 75-cm flexible-tip guidewire is advanced through the needle. The wire is then grasped in the oropharynx or nares with Magill forceps. A J wire, which can be slowly twisted once it arrives at the oropharynx, can be easier to locate than a straight guidewire.

The next step is to clasp the guidewire securely with a hemostat at the neck. Then the proximal end of the guidewire is threaded through the Murphy eye on the ETT. This allows more of the ETT to enter the trachea before the guidewire is removed. With both hands, the wire is tightened, like a tightrope, and the tube is advanced. When the ETT will pass no farther, guidewire or catheter is cut flush with the cricothyroid membrane to minimize soft tissue contamination.

Rapid Sequence Intubation

The term *induction* refers to the production of a deep level of unconsciousness. *Rapid sequence induction* is the classic anesthesia term pertaining to the induction of anesthesia. In emergency medicine parlance, RSI most commonly involves the combined administration of a sedative and a neuromuscular blocking agent to facilitate tracheal intubation after preoxygenation (Table 19-1).[9,10] Tracheal intubation follows laryngoscopy, and cricoid pressure is maintained to prevent aspiration. Sellick maneuver is performed, beginning with the administration of the first RSI agent, and maintained until the cuff is passed through the cords and inflated. The principal contraindication to RSI is any condition preventing mask ventilation or intubation, because this may be the only way to ventilate a patient once the patient is paralyzed.[11]

TABLE 19-1   Rapid Sequence Intubation

1. Set up intravenous ×2; cardiac monitor, oximetry, and capnography
2. Prepare equipment, suction, difficult-airway cart
3. Explain procedure: document neurologic status
4. Preoxygenate (100%, fraction of inspired oxygen), ideally, for several minutes; no positive pressure ventilation
5. Consider sedation, analgesia, adjunctive lidocaine, and/or atropine
6. Defasciculation agent, if necessary
7. Induce with sedative agent
8. Perform Sellick maneuver
9. Give neuromuscular blocking agent
10. Intubate trachea and release Sellick maneuver
11. Confirm placement

Patient care is optimized if emergency physicians are adept with all methods for managing standard and difficult airways in nonfasting patients. Otherwise, the incidence of cricothyrotomy will exceed the current 1 to 2 percent of patients when RSI is selected and fails.[12] The prime goal is to avoid placing the breathing patient in the "can't ventilate, can't intubate" predicament.

PRETREATMENT AGENTS   Pretreatment agents attenuate the pathophysiologic responses to laryngoscopy and intubation that may be harmful in certain clinical circumstances (Table 19-2).[13] The reflex sympathetic response causes increases in heart rate and blood pressure, which may be harmful in patients with intracranial hemorrhage, myocardial ischemia, and aortic dissection. In children, the vagal response predominates and can result in significant bradycardia, even in the absence of succinylcholine. Patients without cerebral autoregulation can experience a centrally mediated rise in intracranial pressure (ICP). Laryngeal stimulation also can have respiratory effects, including laryngospasm, cough, and bronchospasm.

To be effective, pretreatment agents are usually given 3 to 5 min before initiation of RSI. Although there is evidence that the adverse effects listed above may be mitigated by use of these agents, it is unclear whether their use improves outcome. Constraints on time or resources may preclude their use in some circumstances, although every effort should be made to use atropine before intubation of children.

INDUCTION AGENTS   There is no single initial agent of choice for achieving hypnosis and sedation during RSI in the ED. All the commonly used agents offer distinct advantages in specific clinical conditions. Each agent also has significant potential side effects and specific contraindications (Table 19-3).

Barbiturates   Thiopental is a short-acting barbiturate sedative. An intravenous dose of 3.0 to 5.0 mg/kg will induce unconsciousness in 30 to 60 s and last 10 to 30 min. Hypotension is commonly observed because of myocardial depression and venous dilatation. An ultra-short-acting barbiturate option is methohexital. It is twice as potent as thiopental, with onset of action in 60 s and a duration of action of 5 to 7 min. These cerebroprotective agents should be avoided if systemic hypotension is a problem, as may be the case in the multiple trauma patient. Thiopental and methohexital should be avoided in the setting of left ventricular dysfunction, asthma, or porphyria. Methohexital also can cause laryngospasm. A very rare complication is trismus, or masseter muscle spasm, which also has been reported with fentanyl and propofol, often with rapid bolus administration. Methohexital can reduce the seizure threshold.

Ketamine   Ketamine, a phencyclidine derivative, is a potent bronchodilator to be considered particularly in difficult hypotensive or bronchospastic patients. This agent is indicated for refractory status asthmaticus. Because ketamine increases blood pressure, it is an appropriate choice in hypovolemic patients. It also can increase ICP and

TABLE 19-2   Pretreatment Agents Used in Rapid Sequence Intubation

Agent	Dose	Indications	Precautions
Lidocaine	1.5 mg/kg IV/topically	Elevated ICP Bronchospasm	May be ineffective Does not attenuate sympathetic response
Fentanyl	3 μg/kg IV	Elevated ICP Cardiac ischemia Aortic dissection	Respiratory depression Hypotension Chest wall rigidity
Atropine	0.02 mg/kg IV 0.01 mg/kg IV	Children <5 y Children <10 y receiving succinylcholine Bradycardia from repeat succinylcholine in adults	Minimal dose 0.10 mg
Defasciculating agents	10% of normal paralyzing dose	Elevated ICP	Weakness Occasional apnea
Haloperidol	5 mg aliquots	Combative Extreme agitation	Dystonia Rare hypotension
Midazolam	0.1 mg/kg IV	Sedation Reversible Amnesia	Wide therapeutic index No analgesia Apnea

Abbreviation: ICP = intracranial pressure.

thus should be avoided in patients with head injuries. Due to its inotropic and chronotropic cardiac effects, caution is indicated in the elderly. As consciousness returns, the patient may experience "emergence phenomenon" in the form of nightmares, visual hallucinations, and dissociative sensations, although benzodiazepines may attenuate this phenomenon. The dose of ketamine for induction is 1 to 2 mg/kg IV.

Etomidate   Etomidate is a non-barbiturate, non-receptor hypnotic. The advantages of etomidate include protection from myocardial and cerebral ischemia, minimal histamine release, a stable hemodynamic profile, and short duration of action.[14] This agent should be considered if patients are hypovolemic or have closed head injury. Myoclonus, nausea, and vomiting do occur, and seizure foci may be stimulated. The incidence of severe etomidate-induced myoclonus can be decreased by pretreatment with diazepam or fentanyl (see Table 19-2). Etomidate lacks analgesic efficacy and does not blunt the sympathetic response to intubation. With one administration as an induction agent, inhibition of adrenocortical function is not a major concern. The dose of etomidate is 0.3 mg/kg IV.

Propofol   Another option is propofol, a highly lipophilic, rapid-acting sedative. During RSI, this agent provides effective hypnosis. Propofol has a more rapid onset of action than does etomidate and a shorter duration of action. Some of the pharmacologic advantages include its anticonvulsant and antiemetic properties and its ability to lower intracranial pressure. A fluid challenge before propofol administration may minimize hypotension. The dose is .5 to 1.5 mg/kg IV.

Opioids   Although not first-line selections, opioids are potent reversible induction agents. Fentanyl has an onset of action of shorter than 2 min. The ideal dose is highly variable (3 to 8 μg/kg IV). Fentanyl is popular because of its sedative and analgesic properties. This agent provides a very neutral hemodynamic profile during RSI. Rapid injection of high doses may cause chest wall rigidity. Related compounds, alfentanil (3 to 8 μg/kg IV) and remifentanil (1 μg/kg IV over 30 to 60 s), are more potent and have a more immediate onset of action.

PARALYTIC AGENTS   Depolarizing and nondepolarizing neuromuscular blocking agents facilitate airway management of selected pa-

TABLE 19-3   Sedative Induction Agents

Agent	Dose	Induction	Duration	Benefits	Caveats
Thiopental	3–5 mg/kg IV	30–60 s	10–30 min	↓ ICP	↓ BP
Methohexital	1 mg/kg IV	<1 min	5–7 min	↓ ICP Short duration	↓ BP Seizures Laryngospasm
Ketamine	1–2 mg/kg IV	1 min	5 min	Bronchodilator "Dissociative" amnesia	↑ Secretions ↑ ICP Emergence phenomenon
Etomidate	0.3 mg/kg IV	<1 min	10–20 min	↓ ICP ↓ IOP Neutral BP	Myoclonic excitation Vomiting No analgesia
Propofol	0.5–1.5 mg/kg IV	20–40 s	8–15 min	Antiemetic Anticonvulsant ↓ ICP	Apnea ↓ BP No analgesia
Fentanyl	3–8 μg/kg IV	1–2 min	20–30 min	Reversible analgesia Neutral BP	Highly variable dose ICP: variable effects Chest wall rigidity

Abbreviations: ICP = intracranial pressure; IOP = intraocular pressure.

TABLE 19-4   Succinylcholine

Adult dose	1.0–1.5 mg/kg
Onset	45–60 s
Duration	5–9 min
Benefits	Rapid onset, short duration
Complications	Bradyarrhythmias Masseter spasm Increased intragastric, intraocular, and possibly intracranial pressure Malignant hyperthermia Hyperkalemia Prolonged apnea with pseudocholinesterase deficiency Fasciculation-induced musculoskeletal trauma Histamine release Cardiac arrest

tients in the ED. Depolarizing neuromuscular blocking agents have high affinity for cholinergic receptors of the motor end plate and are resistant to acetylcholinesterase. Initially they produce transient muscle fasciculations, followed by paralysis. This type of blockade is not antagonized, and may be enhanced, by anticholinesterase agents. Succinylcholine, a depolarizing agent, inhibits neuromuscular transmission as long as an adequate concentration remains at one receptor site. However, succinylcholine is rapidly hydrolyzed by plasma cholinesterase. Potential adverse effects are listed in Table 19-4. In contrast, nondepolarizing neuromuscular blocking agents compete with acetylcholine for the cholinergic receptors and usually can be antagonized by anticholinesterase agents. Vecuronium, doxacurium, atracurium, and rocuronium are commonly used nondepolarizing agents (Table 19-5).

In the ED, neuromuscular blockade can facilitate tracheal intubation, improve mechanical ventilation, and help control intracranial hypertension. Paralysis improves oxygenation and decreases peak airway pressures in a variety of disorders, including refractory pulmonary edema and the respiratory distress syndrome. Patients with refractory status asthmaticus, status epilepticus, or tetanic spasms resulting from clostridial infections or a variety of toxins, including strychnine, may improve with blockade. In addition, extremely violent, agitated patients who jeopardize air medical personnel or their own airway security, spinal cord integrity, or fracture stability may require the ultimate pharmacologic restraint (i.e., paralysis).

After documentation of the neurologic examination, including pupil size, pre-sedation with an induction agent is advised unless there are other mitigating circumstances, such as significant head injury or overdose. Neuromuscular blockers (NMBs) are neither anxiolytics nor analgesics. **Omission of sedation is a common error in patients who remain aware of their paralysis.** The resultant increased sympathetic tone can exacerbate dysrhythmias.

Succinylcholine   When the indication for neuromuscular blockade is tracheal intubation, succinylcholine is the most commonly used agent. It has a more rapid onset (45 to 60 s) and shorter duration of action (average, 5 to 9 min) than do the nondepolarizing agents. After a brief fasciculation, complete relaxation occurs at 60 s, with maximal paralysis at 2 to 3 min. Effective respirations resume in 9 to 12 min.

The dosage of succinylcholine is 1.0 to 1.5 mg/kg IV for adults. Succinylcholine can result in excellent intubation conditions. Succinylcholine is generally preferable to nondepolarizing agents for RSI in the ED. In the event of a failed airway, the duration of BVM ventilation is generally only 10 to 12 min. Giving an induction agent before succinylcholine should be considered to avoid the cognition scenario of the "sentient being in an unresponsive body."

Before injection of succinylcholine, atropine, 0.01 mg/kg IV, may attenuate muscarinic vagal effects, especially in vagotonic adults and adolescents. In infants and small children, atropine pretreatment is essential to avoid bradyarrhythmias and asystole. An additional pretreatment to consider is a subparalytic dose of vecuronium, 0.01 mg/kg, or another nondepolarizing agent of similar duration to prevent the initial muscle fasciculations, which may cause long bone fractures to become displaced. Such fasciculations are most pronounced in muscular adolescents.

Succinylcholine increases intraocular pressure. In addition, the increased intragastric pressure predisposes to aspiration, thus emphasizing the importance of cricoid pressure. Another concern with succinylcholine is its potential to increase ICP. There are no data establishing the clinical relevance of the transient intracranial pressor response to intubation, so it is not contraindicated in patients with head trauma.

Serum potassium will transiently rise an average of 0.5 mEq/L with succinylcholine. Hyperkalemia may be pronounced hours to days after muscle trauma or burns. A clinically significant hyperkalemic response should not be a factor in the immediate aftermath of such injury. Nevertheless, it may be advisable to avoid depolarizing agents in patients with burns, muscle trauma, crush injuries, myopathies, rhabdomyolysis, narrow-angle glaucoma, renal failure, or neurologic disorders. Any patient with "denervated musculature" (e.g., Guillain-Barré syndrome or spinal cord injury) is particularly at risk.

Genetically susceptible individuals may develop acute malignant hyperthermia. Dantrolene sodium should always be available. Patients with an atypical pseudocholinesterase will require prolonged ventilatory support, as will those with burns, cirrhosis, or carcinomas who have low plasma pseudocholinesterase levels. Also, patients recently abusing amphetamines or cocaine may have a prolonged duration of neuromuscular blockade, because cocaine is metabolized by plasma cholinesterase, which reduces the amount of enzyme available for succinylcholine metabolism.[15]

For the conditions described above, nondepolarizing agents are preferable to succinylcholine. Although the onset of action is delayed, nondepolarizing agents produce fewer adverse cardiovascular and histaminic effects and a longer duration of paralysis.

TABLE 19-5   Nondepolarizing Neuromuscular Relaxants

Agent	Adult Intubating IV Dose	Onset	Duration	Complications
Vecuronium (intermediate/long)	0.08–0.15 mg/kg 0.15–0.28 mg/kg (high-dose protocol)	2–4 min	25–40 min 60–120 min	Prolonged recovery time in obese or elderly, or if there is hepatorenal dysfunction
Rocuronium (intermediate/long)	0.6 mg/kg	1–3 min	30–45 min	Tachycardia
Doxacurium	0.05–0.08 mg/kg	3.5 min	80–100 min	Prolonged block
Atracurium (intermediate)	0.4–0.5 mg/kg	2–3 min	25–45 min	Hypotension Histamine release Bronchospasm

Nondepolarizing Agents Pancuronium and d-tubo curare have been largely supplanted by agents with more rapid onset, shorter durations of action, and more favorable hemodynamic profiles. *Vecuronium bromide* is an intermediate- to long-acting nondepolarizing agent. The usual dose of vecuronium is 0.08 to 0.15 mg/kg IV. Maximal paralysis occurs within 2 to 4 min, with full blockade lasting for 25 to 40 min. One advantage of vecuronium is the lack of hemodynamic alterations. Hypersensitivity reactions are rare, doses are only minimally cumulative, and excretion is biliary. Despite the lack of histamine release, hypotension may occur through two other mechanisms. Blockage of sympathetic ganglia occurs, and venous return is decreased from absent muscle tone and the positive-pressure ventilation.

Rocuronium is an intermediate-duration nondepolarizing agent that is an option for RSI when successful visualization of the trachea is a certainty. The onset of action is more rapid than that with vecuronium. By increasing the dose of rocuronium to 0.9 to 1.2 mg/kg, the onset approximates that of succinylcholine, but also prolongs its duration of action. There are fewer side effects and contraindications with rocuronium than with vecuronium.

Doxacurium chloride is a long-acting nondepolarizing NMB used to facilitate prolonged mechanical ventilation after tracheal intubation. It provides skeletal muscle relaxation, with no dose-related cardiovascular effects.

Atracurium is an agent well suited for patients with hepatic or renal failure. Elimination occurs by ester hydrolysis and Hoffman degradation, a non-enzymatic process. This nondepolarizing agent's elimination half-life is approximately 20 min, as opposed to 65 to 75 min for vecuronium. Recovery time is consistent and unaffected by anticonvulsants. This agent is suitable for intubated patients requiring brief diagnostic or therapeutic procedures. Atracurium also offers advantages when continuous infusion is essential to maintain a precise, required level of neuromuscular blockade. A disadvantage is that histamine release can cause bronchospasm and hypotension. The risk with prolonged infusion is accumulation of laudanosine, a neuroexcitatory metabolic byproduct.

Other nondepolarizing options include *cisatracurium* and *mivacurium*. Cisatracurium is an intermediate-duration NMB agent. None of the metabolites have NMB activity, and excretion is independent of hepatorenal function. Mivacurium is the nondepolarizing agent with the shortest duration of action. Histamine release can be minimized by slow infusion.

The reversal of nondepolarizing muscle relaxants is rarely necessary in the ED. Reversal should not be attempted before some sign of motion or spontaneous recovery, because these enzyme inhibitors will have no effect until at least 40 percent of spontaneous recovery has occurred. Reversal is not innocuous and requires atropine 0.01 mg/kg IV, to prevent muscarinic side effects, followed by edrophonium 0.5 to 1.0 mg/kg IV. Edrophonium is an acetylcholinesterase inhibitor with a faster onset of cholinergic and fewer muscarinic side effects than the longer-acting neostigmine. The onset of action is 30 to 60 s, with a duration of 10 to 30 min. This reversal may be shorter than the duration of the muscle relaxant.

The normal sequence in RSI is to induce sedation before administration of the depolarizing NMB agent. If a nondepolarizing agent has been selected, some physicians reverse the sequence of administration by giving the nondepolarizing agent first because of its longer onset of action. Giving a rapid-acting hypnotic agent seconds later results in both medications having a synchronized peak effect.

DIFFICULT AIRWAY

The management of the difficult airway in the ED is, in many ways, more challenging than in the controlled setting of the operating room. The patient generally has not been fasting and is not premedicated. There is rarely time for a leisurely evaluation of the "airway history" and "airway physical examination." The difficult airway constitutes the clinical scenario in which mask ventilation or tracheal intubation is challenging. Approximately 2 to 3 percent of tracheal intubations prove impossible with standard techniques. *Difficult mask ventilation* is defined as the inability to maintain O_2 saturation above 90 percent. Intubation is considered as difficult if more than three attempts are necessary or if conventional laryngoscopy requires more than 10 min. Many emergency physicians prefer to ensure the availability of the appropriate airway equipment by customizing the contents of a portable airway kit (Table 19-6).

The identification of a potentially difficult airway is perhaps more important than the subsequent management and may obviate a rescue airway in the "cannot-intubate, cannot-ventilate" scenario. Before any attempt at airway management, an assessment of potential difficulties with BVM ventilation and intubation must be performed. Once the potential for difficulty is identified, the management will vary with not only the type of airway difficulty but also the operator's experience and availability of alternative devices.[16]

Potential impediments of BVM ventilation should be considered before proceeding with RSI. The presence of two of the following five factors is predictive of difficult BVM: facial hair, obesity, edentulous patient, advanced age, and snoring. An inability to adequately ventilate with a BVM is usually solved by better positioning, jaw thrust, a tighter seal with two-person bagging, and the use of oral and nasal airways to improve patency. A poor seal due to a beard may be improved with a lubricant. Dentures facilitate BVM ventilation.

Multiple external features are also associated with difficult intubation. These features include facial hair, obesity, a short neck, small or large chin, buckteeth, high arched palate, and any airway deformity due to trauma, tumor, or inflammation. Most studies of airway difficulty use the grade of laryngoscopic view, which is impractical in the ED setting. A simple, systematic, and rapid evaluation of the airway is needed to predict a potentially poor laryngoscopic view before the initiation of neuromuscular blockade.

Clinical examination of the airway anatomy can identify more subtle predictors. The mandibular opening in an adult should be at least 4 cm, or two to three fingerbreadths. The ability of the mandible to accommodate the tongue can be estimated by the distance between the mentum and the hyoid bone, which should be three to four fingerbreadths. A small mandible is more likely to have a tongue that obstructs visualization during laryngoscopy. An unusually large mandible also may impair visualization by elongating the oral axis, referred to above. A high, anterior larynx is possible if the space between the mandible and top of the thyroid cartilage is narrower than two fingerbreadths. The degree to which the tongue obstructs the visualization of the posterior pharynx on mouth opening has some correlation with the visualization of the glottis. This correlation can be assessed with Mallampati's criteria, with classes III and IV being associated with poor visualization and higher failure rates (up to 5 and 20 percent, respectively) (Figure 19-4).[17] Neck immobility also interferes

TABLE 19-6 Difficult-Airway Kit

Endotracheal tubes: assorted sizes, designs, tip control, fiberoptic
Laryngoscope blades: alternate sizes and designs, fiberoptic (extra bulbs)
Laryngoscope handles: extra batteries
Stylets: Eschmann bougie, semirigid, hollow, light wand
Syringes, fixators, and Magill forceps
4% lidocaine and laryngotracheal anesthesia kit
1% phenylephrine (Neo-Synephrine), lidocaine jelly
Suction catheters
Emergency ventilation options
    Laryngeal mask airway and intubating laryngeal mask airway
    Translaryngeal ventilation equipment
    Esophageal tracheal Combitube
Retrograde tracheal intubation equipment
Cricothyrotomy equipment: dilators, no. 4 Shiley
Fiberoptic options

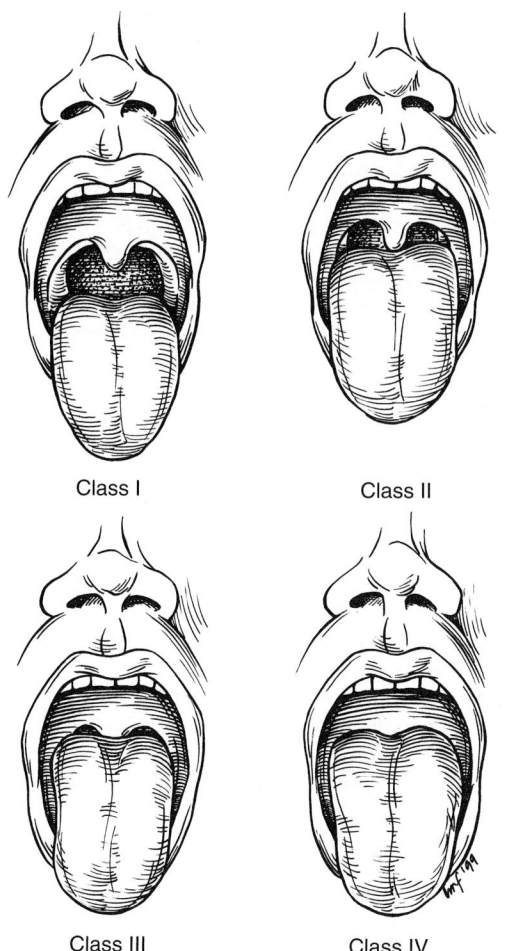

Class I   Class II

Class III   Class IV

FIG. 19-4. Classification of tongue size relative to the size of the oral cavity as described by Mallampati and colleagues.[17] Class I: Faucial pillars, soft palate, and uvula can be visualized. Class II: Faucial pillars and soft palate can be visualized, but the uvula is masked by the base of the tongue. Class III: Only the base of the uvula can be visualized. Class IV: None of the three structures can be visualized.

with the ability to align the visual axes by preventing the desired "sniffing position." Neck immobility may be imposed by the presence of a cervical collar. If there is no suspicion of cervical injury, atlanto-occipital extension should be assessed, even in the uncooperative patient.

Airway obstruction presents a particular difficulty in airway management. If evidence of obstruction is present, three aspects must be considered: the location of the obstruction, whether it is fixed (e.g., tumor) or mobile (e.g., epiglottis), and how rapidly it is progressing. The location may determine which approach or rescue device can be used. Oral airway obstruction from angioedema of the tongue may limit the physician to nasal techniques or surgical airways that use the cricothyroid membrane. The BVM method is more likely to be successful in mobile as opposed to fixed obstruction. The speed of progression determines whether the management can await transport to another facility, management in the operating room, or immediate management in the ED.

STRATEGIES FOR SPECIFIC CLINICAL SCENARIOS

Cerebral Perfusion Issues

Patients with suspected acute intracranial hypertension require aggressive airway management. Direct laryngoscopy can elevate the

ICP. Before oral or nasal intubation, pretreatment with intravenous lidocaine may help blunt this deleterious cardiovascular response. Fentanyl also will blunt the hemodynamic changes.

In certain situations, succinylcholine may increase ICP, so the intubator should consider prior use of a defasiculating dose of a nondepolarizing NMB agent. If one is selected, the use of a priming dose will shorten the onset of action. However, a significantly prolonged duration of action may be the result, thereby extending the risks if a difficult airway is encountered. Another consideration is the use of a short-acting sedative induction agent. Several of these drugs, including thiopental, fentanyl, and etomidate, directly decrease ICP.

Effective oxygenation and ventilation during cerebral resuscitation often require prolonged neuromuscular blockade. Autoregulation of cerebral blood flow (CBF) over a range of perfusion pressures may be impaired. As a result, CBF becomes pressure dependent: CBF = CPP/CVR, where CPP is cerebral perfusion pressure and CVR is cerebral vascular resistance. Autoregulation is usually intact when the CPP ranges between 50 and 150 mm Hg. The CPP equals the mean arterial pressure minus the ICP.

In traumatic brain injury, the goal therefore is to maintain the mean arterial pressure above 90 mm Hg throughout the patient's course; doing so usually will maintain the CPP above 70 mm Hg. Other treatment modalities, such as mannitol administration and hyperventilation, can exacerbate intracranial ischemia. Of note, when cerebral autoregulation is lost, the ability to vasoconstrict with hyperventilation may be maintained. Therefore, prophylactic hyperventilation therapy (Paco$_2$ <35 mm Hg) should be avoided during the first 24 h after injury.

Conversely, brief hyperventilation therapy should be initiated rapidly in the ED in patients with definite acute signs of intracranial hypertension. If the intracranial hypertension does not respond to adjunctive osmotic diuretics, sedation, neuromuscular blockade, and neurosurgical drainage of CSF, protracted hyperventilation may be necessary.

After blockade, the fraction of inspired oxygen (Fio$_2$) sufficient to maintain a Pao$_2$ of 100 mm Hg is selected. Significant hypoxia can increase reactive oxygen species and contribute to oxidative brain injury. Positive end-expiratory pressure (PEEP) of up to 5 cm H$_2$O may help prevent atelectasis. Higher levels will impair cerebral venous drainage, because of the elevated intrathoracic pressure. Excessively tight ETT straps, tight cervical collars, or Trendelenburg positioning potentiate increased ICP and should be avoided.

Cardiopulmonary Disease

Tracheal intubation and mechanical ventilation can have other significant physiologic consequences. Any conditions that result in the cardiovascular system's reliance on preload to maintain perfusion will predispose to hypotension and cardiac decompensation. Particular caution is needed when intubating previously hypotensive patients who require vasopressor support. In addition, patients with hypercarbia and chronic obstructive pulmonary disease require special consideration. Mechanical ventilation increases the positive intrathoracic pressure, which decreases the preload by decreasing venous return. Hypotension may be anticipated. Additional physiologic considerations include the decreased left ventricular compliance and the fact that most medications useful in RSI decrease the sympathetic tone.

Trauma Airway Management

Airway management of patients with the potential to have an unstable injury of the cervical spine challenges clinical judgment. There is no single best algorithm. Cervical spine radiography without a thorough and reliable neurologic examination does not "clear the neck." From 20 to 30 percent of cervical spine injuries are not appreciated on one cross-table lateral view. In addition, patients with blunt major trauma requiring tracheal intubation have associated unstable cervical spine injuries that range from 1 to 12 percent. Spinal cord injury without radiographic abnormality (SCIWORA) is an important consideration, especially in adolescents and children.

The initial decision is to determine whether immediate airway intervention is really needed. Patients not in urgent need of an airway should be neurologically and radiographically evaluated as thoroughly as is practical given their condition. The need for inline cervical stabilization should not be considered a license for axial inline traction. For example, attempting to visualize C7 radiographically by countertraction of the head and shoulders of the near-hanging patient can cause further distraction injury.

There is a large selection of airway options to consider while attempting to maintain cervical spine immobilization. The selection is far less critical than the timing. Rapid sequence intubation, NTI, transillumination, and fiberoptic laryngoscopy are commonly selected options. Oral intubation appears safe when achieved without hyperdistraction, flexion, or extension of the neck. Maintenance of cervical spine immobilization is the paramount objective, not the approach to secure the airway. Careful endotracheal intubation causes less cervical spine motion than does BVM ventilation.

Visualization of the larynx before cervical spine clearance is difficult, because alignment of the oropharyngeal-laryngeal axis is not possible. One method to move the tip of the tube anteriorly is to use a slightly flexed directional-tip tube (Endotrol) coupled with Sellick maneuver. Another is to use a flexible stylet, such as the Flexiguide, which passes through the tube and has a trigger similar to that of the Endotrol. Another option is to aim the tip of the tube anteriorly with Magill forceps while an assistant advances the tube.

There are several commercially available laryngoscope blade designs that allow vocal cord visualization without manipulation of the neck. Most designs have fiberoptic attachments to the blade, which allow elevation of the tongue to avoid the blood or secretions. Technically, these blades may prove simpler to use than conventional fiberoptic laryngoscopes.

Victims of trauma may be hypotensive due to hemorrhagic shock or maintain a "normal" blood pressure in compensated shock. Many agents used in RSI may cause myocardial depression and vasodilation, potentially worsening hypotension or precipitating decompensation. Barbiturates and benzodiazepines should be avoided in this scenario. Etomidate has a better hemodynamic profile and is the preferred induction agent. Although ketamine will maintain blood pressure, it should be avoided in patients with intracranial injury. If hypotension is due to a clinically suspected tension pneumothorax, a chest tube thoracostomy should be performed before, or simultaneously with airway management.

SUCTIONING

Many conditions render patients unable to clear their own secretions. Aspiration usually occurs when the tone of the lower esophageal sphincter is insufficient to deal with the increased intragastric pressure and the protective laryngeal airway reflexes are depressed. The common iatrogenic causes include BVM ventilation, the presence of nasogastric tubes, and pharmacologic neuromuscular paralysis. Some common predisposing conditions include trauma, bowel obstruction, obesity, overdose, pregnancy, hiatus hernia, and seizures.

Aspiration after urgent ETT intubation occurs infrequently in ED patients if there is attention to technique. The intubator should consider using large-diameter suction systems or tubing for the removal of particulate matter or clots that are larger than the standard Yankauer tip can handle. The rigid-tip plastic tonsil suction catheter can remove large quantities of oropharyngeal secretions.

When necessary, the patient is placed in a left lateral Trendelenburg position. This position helps get the tongue out of the laryngoscopist's way and facilitates immediate endotracheal suctioning. To suction the nasopharynx and tracheobronchial tree, a well-lubricated, soft, curved-tip catheter is used. Straight catheters usually will pass into the right mainstem bronchus. If a curved-tip catheter is available, turning the head to the right and rotating the catheter often will facilitate passage into the left bronchus. A suction catheter no larger than half the diameter of the tube to be suctioned should be selected to prevent pulmonic collapse from insufficient ventilation during suctioning. The patient should be oxygenated before and after suctioning to avoid transient desaturation. The catheter should be inserted without suctioning and then slowly removed while suctioning with rotation over 10 to 15 s.

Some complications of suctioning include hypoxia, cardiac dysrhythmias, hypotension, pulmonic collapse, and direct mucosal injury. The magnitude of the ICP increase during endotracheal suctioning may be related to the increase in intrathoracic pressure with coughing if lidocaine has been omitted.

MECHANICAL VENTILATORY SUPPORT

The knowledge of the pathophysiology of acute respiratory failure and the changes in lung physiology during positive-pressure ventilation will aid in the selection of an appropriate ventilatory modality and of the initial settings. Ventilators are pressure or volume cycled. Volume-cycled ventilators are used routinely in EDs. Other decisions with regard to mechanical ventilatory support in the ED include the rate, mode, F_{IO_2}, minute ventilation, use of PEEP, continuous positive airway pressure (CPAP), or bilevel pressure ventilation (BiPAP).

There are three common ventilator methods for providing the tidal volume: controlled mechanical ventilation, assist-control (A/C), and intermittent mandatory ventilation (IMV). The control mode is used for apneic patients. The A/C mode allows the patient to trigger a cycle by inhaling and lowering the air pressure, which can be adjusted by the ventilator's trigger "sensitivity" (1 to 3 cm H_2O). The ventilator will provide an untriggered "controlled" breath unless one is triggered during the selected time cycle. A predetermined number of ventilator-generated tidal volumes can be ensured either unsynchronized (IMV) or, more commonly, synchronized to patient effort (SIMV). In the ED, A/C or SIMV is the preferred initial mode, except as noted with an apneic patient.

The initial F_{IO_2} should be guided by the oximetry. Initially, the tidal volume is set at 10 mL/kg ideal body weight, and the rate is adjusted accordingly. Sufficient time should be allowed for expiration. The peak airway pressure is maintained below 35 to 45 cm H_2O to prevent barotrauma. The peak airway pressure appears to be related to barotrauma more than to the level of CPAP.

To reclaim lung volumes, PEEP or CPAP should be considered if the decreased pulmonary compliance prevents delivery of an adequate tidal volume or if hypoxemia persists despite 100 percent F_{IO_2}. Even low levels (3 to 5 cm H_2O) of PEEP/CPAP usually render ventilator "sighs" (1.5 × tidal volume) unnecessary. If hypotension develops, the respiratory rate and PEEP should be adjusted to lower the *mean* airway pressure.

Selected patients with acute respiratory failure will benefit from noninvasive BiPAP (see Chap. 19).[18] Nasal mask or full-face mask BiPAP can decrease length of stay and improve survival. Although pretrial arterial blood gas (ABG) levels do not predict success, a BiPAP trial for stable patients with acute respiratory failure can be followed by intubation and mechanical ventilation if there is inadequate improvement within 30 min.

EXTUBATION

Inherently more relaxing than intubation, extubation nevertheless can be hazardous. This maneuver is rarely indicated in the ED but may be required in some systems that have an observation center. Patients recovering their protective airway reflexes may "fight" the tube yet need to remain intubated. Instillation of 1 to 2 mL of 4 percent lidocaine (sterile for injection) down the ETT will decrease "bucking." The absorption of lidocaine through the airway yields a maximum serum level that is only slightly lower than that from an equivalent intravenous dose.

Before extubation, the physician should consider the impact of metabolic or circulatory abnormalities. The patient should be checked for respiratory insufficiency, and nasogastric decompression is advised. On command, the patient should have an inspiratory capacity of at least 15 mL/kg. Ideally, there should be no intercostal or suprasternal reactions, and the patient's grip should be firm.

After suctioning secretions, the physician should ensure adequate oxygenation and explain the procedure to the patient. Positive-pressure ventilation with a mask will help to exsufflate secretions while the cuff is deflated. At the end of a deep inspiration, the tube should be removed and oxygenation continued by mask to prevent secretory reaccumulation.`

The patient should be observed closely for stridor. Postextubation laryngospasm is treated initially with oxygen by positive pressure. If necessary, nebulized racemic epinephrine (0.5 mL of 2.25 percent epinephrine in 4 mL saline) is often helpful.

REFERENCES

1. Walls RM, Barton ED, McAfee AT: 2392 Emergency department intubations; first report of the ongoing National Emergency Airway Registry study (Near97). *Ann Emerg Med* 34(4):S14, 1999.
2. Barnhard WN, Cattrell JE, Sirakumarana C, et al: Adjustment of intracuff pressure to prevent aspiration. *Anesthesiology* 50:313, 1979.
3. Li J, Murphy-Lavoie H, Bugas C, et al: Complications of emergency intubation with or without paralysis. *Am J Emerg Med* 17:141, 1999.
4. Roppolo LP, Vilke GM, Chan TC, et al: Nasotracheal intubation in the emergency department, revisited. *J Emerg Med* 17:791, 1999.
5. Rosen CL, Wolfe RE, Chew SE, et al: Blind nasotracheal intubation in the presence of facial trauma. *J Emerg Med* 15:141, 1997.
6. Levitan RM, Ochroch EA, Stuart S, et al: Use of intubating laryngeal mask airway by medical and non medical personnel. *Am J Emerg Med* 18:12, 2000.
7. Ferson DZ, Rosenblatt WH, Johansen MJ, et al: Use of the intubating LMA-Fastrach in 254 patients with difficult-to-manage airways. *Anesthesiology* 95:1175, 2001.
8. Agro F, Cataldo R, Carassiti M, et al: The seeing stylet: A new device for tracheal intubation. *Resuscitation* 44:177, 2000.
9. Vissers RJ, Barton ED, Sagarin MJ, et al: Success and complication rates of rapid-sequence vs non rapid sequence intubation in 1200 emergency intubations. *Acad Emerg Med* 5:4, 1998.
10. Dronen S: Rapid-sequence intubation: A safe but ill-defined procedure. *Acad Emerg Med* 6:1, 1999.
11. Tayal VS, Riggs RW, Marx JA, et al: Rapid sequence intubation at an emergency medicine residency: Success rate and adverse events during a two-year period. *Acad Emerg Med* 6:31, 1999.
12. Sakles JC, Laurin EG, Rantapaa AA, et al: Airway management in the emergency department: A one year study of 610 tracheal intubations. *Ann Emerg Med* 31:325, 1998.
13. Sivilotti ML, Ducharme J: Randomized, double-blind study on sedatives and hemodynamics during rapid sequence intubation in the emergency department: The SHRED study. *Ann Emerg Med* 31:313, 1998.
14. Smith DC, Bergen JM, Smithline H, et al: A trial of etomidate for rapid sequence intubation in the emergency department. *J Emerg Med* 18:13, 2000.
15. Stibolt O, Wachowick-Anderson G: Altered response to IV thiopental and succinylcholine in acute amphetamine abuse. *Acta Anaesthesiol Scand* 46:609, 2002.
16. Caplan RA, Benumof JL, Berry FA, et al: Practice guidelines for management of difficult airway: A report by American Society of Anesthesiologists Task Force on Management of the Difficult Airway. *Anesthesiology* 78:597, 1993.
17. Mallampati SR, Gatt SP, Gugino LD, et al: A clinical sign to predict difficult tracheal intubation: A prospective study. *Can Anesth Soc J* 32:429, 1985.
18. Poponick JM, Renston JP, Bennett RP, et al: Use of a ventilatory support system (BiPAP) for acute respiratory failure in the emergency department. *Chest* 116:166, 1999.

SURGICAL AIRWAY MANAGEMENT
David R. Gens

The rate of failed ED intubations and subsequent surgical airway placement is below 0.6 percent.[1] About 3 percent of intubation attempts are in difficult airways where a surgical airway should be anticipated.[1]

The term *cricothyroidotomy* technically means "vertically incising (splitting) the cricoid and thyroid cartilages," and *coniotomy* means "incising the cricothyroid (conic) ligament," which runs from the cricoid to the thyroid cartilage. Although *coniotomy* is the correct term for incising between these two cartilages, the term *cricothyroidotomy* is now commonly used to denote this procedure.

CLINICAL FEATURES

The indications for an emergency surgical airway are several; however, most are due to an inability to establish an orotracheal or nasotracheal airway. This may be due to anatomy (short, obese neck), a disease state (epiglottitis, laryngeal edema, paralyzed vocal cords, or retropharyngeal abscess), trauma from distortion of the neck by hematoma (cervical fracture or major vessel injury), aspiration of blood (facial trauma), or loss of supporting structures (mandibular fractures). Clinical manifestations of acute airway obstruction are stridor (in a patient who is still able to breathe) or cyanosis. Clinical signs and symptoms are listed in Table 20-1.

SPECIFIC ISSUES THAT AFFECT EVALUATION AND TREATMENT

Age

Needle cricothyroidotomy is the preferred emergency surgical airway in children younger than approximately 10–12 years who cannot be intubated orotracheally or nasotracheally. A 12- or 14-gauge catheter over a needle will support ventilation and oxygenation in a child until a tracheostomy can be performed in the operating room by a surgeon familiar with the anatomy of a child's neck. The larynx is easily damaged by surgical cricothyroidotomy, and younger individuals have a higher incidence of late airway complications.[2]

Associated Injuries

The standard indications for an airway in emergency patients are mentioned below; however, some specific types of trauma usually have a

TABLE 20-1 Clinical Manifestations Associated with Acute Airway Obstruction

Etiology	Manifestation
Vascular	Hematoma External hemorrhage Hypotension Hemoptysis
Laryngotracheal	Stridor Subcutaneous air (massive) Hoarseness Dysphonia Hemoptysis
Pharyngeal and/or hypopharyngeal	Subcutaneous air Hematemesis Dysphagia Sucking wound

greater need for a surgical airway. Penetrating trauma to the neck (gunshot or stab wound) that injures a major artery (carotid, vertebral, or thyroid) and demonstrates an expanding hematoma around the injured artery may cause obstruction of the airway by pressure. The need for a surgical airway should be anticipated. Infrequently, free blood from concomitant vascular and pharyngeal or tracheal injuries spills into the oro- or hypopharynx and causes severe aspiration of blood; in such cases, a cuffed tube (surgical cricothyroidotomy, not needle cricothyroidotomy) is needed. Difficulty in establishing an airway occurs in approximately 10 percent of penetrating cervical trauma cases.[3]

Blunt trauma to the neck or face may cause hemorrhage of the soft tissues or injury to the trachea or larynx itself. The trachea may become detached from the larynx at the level of the first tracheal ring, and the larynx or the trachea may become ruptured. In either of these rare circumstances, an emergency tracheostomy is required. This procedure should be performed by someone with experience in surgery of the neck. It is difficult to perform an emergency tracheostomy, especially with an awake patient who is becoming hypoxic and combative. Severe edema of the larynx or, rarely, fracture of the cartilages of the larynx may obstruct the airway.

In blunt facial trauma, the principal cause of death is obstruction of the airway. This occurs for several reasons. In patients with mandibular fractures, the loss of supporting structure for the tongue allows the base of the tongue to fall back into the hypopharynx and obstruct the airway. Also, these patients, placed supine and with major facial bleeding, will often continuously aspirate blood.

Type of Emergency Airway and Tube Selection

Surgical cricothyroidotomy is always preferred over needle cricothyroidotomy (except for children younger than 10–12 years, as noted above), simply because of the larger diameter of the 6-mm (internal diameter) endotracheal or tracheostomy tube compared with the needle cricothyroidotomy catheter. Adequate ventilation is crucial in the early prevention of cerebral edema after brain injury. Ventilation is practically impossible through a 14- or 12-gauge catheter. Emergency tracheostomy is rarely indicated and extremely difficult to perform. This procedure should be performed only by physicians who are familiar with surgical anatomy and skilled in the procedure.

A tracheostomy tube is preferred to an endotracheal tube for several reasons. A tracheostomy tube has an obturator, which makes entry through the narrow cricothyroid membrane easier. The tracheostomy tube is shorter and therefore easier to suction. Most important, it has flanges on each side that allow it to be sutured to the neck and secured with a cloth ribbon around the neck (Figure 20-1). The endotracheal tube (when used for cricothyroidotomy) is very difficult to affix to the neck and moves easily no matter how well it has been secured with adhesive tape. Unfortunately, many EDs are not stocked with tracheostomy tubes, because of their infrequent need, or, when they are stocked, they may not be readily available. Therefore, an endotracheal tube is most commonly used and is readily available. When a tracheostomy tube becomes available, a tube change can be made by using Seldinger technique; a suction catheter with the suction vent cut off at one end is readily available and easy to use.

The diameter of the tube inserted is crucial. **A 6-mm tracheostomy or 6-mm endotracheal tube is preferred (never larger than 7 mm in either case).** Tubes with internal diameters larger than 7 mm are difficult to insert in the narrow space between the cricoid and thyroid cartilages. If airway pressures are high with the small-diameter tube, the cricothyroidotomy tube may be changed to a tracheostomy or endotracheal tube with a larger diameter at a later, convenient time.

Availability of Equipment and Staff Education

The success rates with either type of surgical airway depend largely on the preparedness of the ED and the training of the staff. Two recent

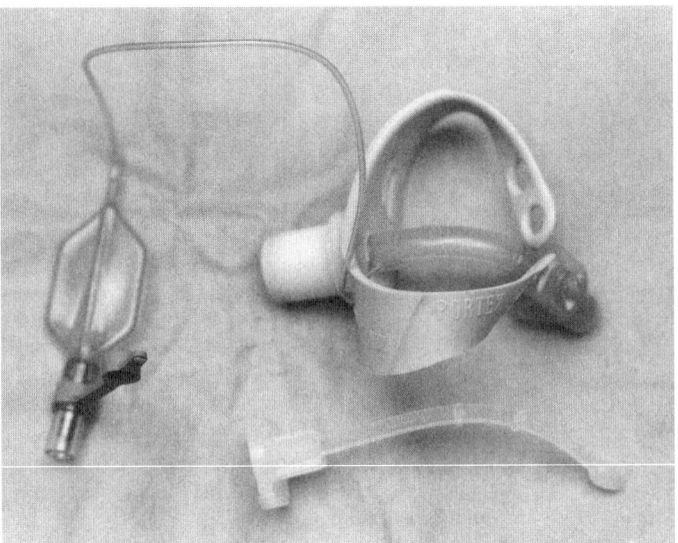

FIG. 20-1. Tracheostomy tube with obturator.

European studies have shown that EDs are rarely prepared for performing an emergency surgical airway. A recent study in Great Britain found that only 47 percent of EDs had made provisions for the immediate use of a needle cricothyroidotomy and only 45 percent of the physicians were conversant in its use.[4] In an Austrian study of intensive care staff, only 70 and 60 percent of the staff were able to successfully perform a surgical cricothyroidotomy and a needle cricothyroidotomy, respectively.[5] All ED staff should be trained in the performance of an emergency surgical airway (through advanced trauma life support), and all EDs should be properly equipped.

Conversion from Cricothyroidotomy to Tracheostomy

The question frequently arises as to how long to leave a cricothyroidotomy tube in place in the larynx. A tube left in the narrow space between the cricoid and thyroid cartilages can erode both cartilages, and a bacterial chondritis may occur. The cartilages will be destroyed and eventually scar, leading to stenosis and loss of the function of the larynx. Because cricothyroidotomy has a higher incidence of airway stenosis, a cricothyroidotomy should be converted to a tracheostomy.[6] As a rule of thumb, **if the airway will be needed for more than 2 to 3 days, the cricothyroidotomy should be changed to a tracheostomy.** Otherwise, the cricothyroid tube may stay in place.

PROCEDURE

Surgical Cricothyroidotomy

ANATOMY The cricothyroid membrane is located between the thyroid and cricoid cartilages (Figure 20-2A). Both structures are easily palpated. The cricothyroid membrane can be found approximately one third the distance from the manubrium to the chin in the midline in patients with normal habitus (see Figure 20-2B). In a patient with a short, obese neck, the membrane may be hidden at the level of the manubrium; in a patient with a thin, long neck, it may be midway between the chin and the manubrium. The thyroid gland overlies the trachea; both structures are difficult to palpate.

The only vascular structure that may be injured during the course of a properly performed cricothyroidotomy is the thyroid ima artery, a branch of the aorta that runs up to the thyroid gland in the midline and infrequently reaches the level of the cricothyroid membrane. When injured, it needs to be surgically ligated to control the hemorrhage.

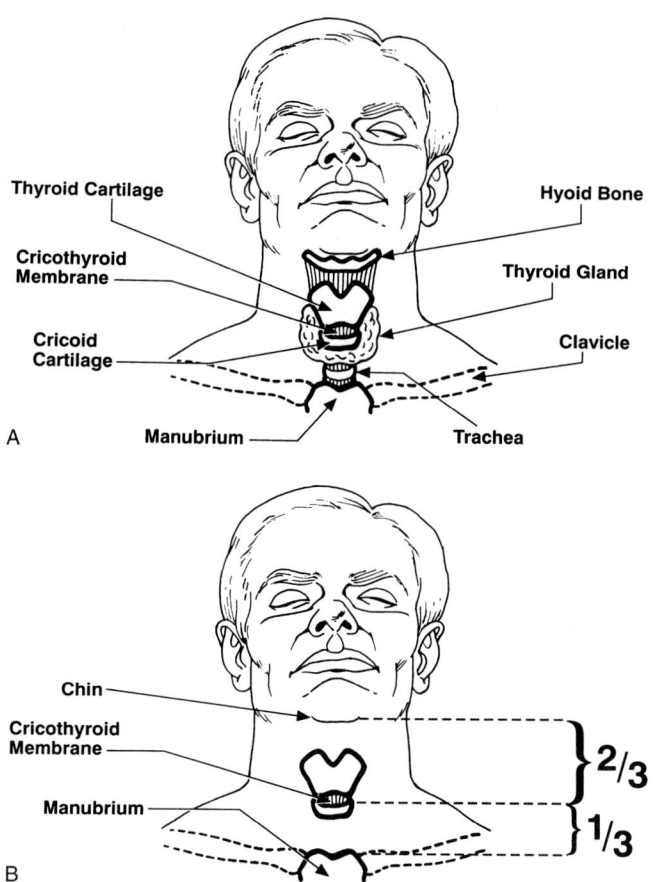

FIG. 20-2. **A.** Anatomy of the neck. **B.** Location of the cricothyroid membrane.

INDICATIONS AND CONTRAINDICATIONS

Inability to orotracheally intubate an emergency patient is the prime indication for surgical or needle cricothyroidotomy. Orotracheal (or nasotracheal) intubation should be attempted first. Inline cervical stabilization must be maintained in trauma patients. If orotracheal intubation is unsuccessful, then cricothyroidotomy should be considered.

Surgical cricothyroidotomy is reserved for patients older than 12 years and is contraindicated in patients younger than 12 years. Needle cricothyroidotomy is the procedure of choice in those younger than 12 years.

COMPLICATIONS

Acute complications after emergency cricothyroidotomy occur in up to approximately 10 percent of cases.[7]

Bleeding from the Insertion Site Venous bleeding almost always occurs from small veins and usually stops spontaneously (using a vertical neck incision decreases the chance of bleeding). Arterial bleeding can be from the thyroid ima artery or from a small artery at the base of the cricothyroid membrane. Gentle pressure is applied to stop the bleeding. If bleeding persists, surgical control may be necessary in the operating room.

Misplacement of the Tube In an obese neck, it is possible to place the tube anterior to the larynx and trachea into the mediastinum. Ventilation is not possible. Manifestations of an incorrectly positioned tube are high airway pressures, absent breath sounds, and massive subcutaneous emphysema. The tube should be removed and a second attempt should be made.

Laceration of the Structures of the Neck Laceration of the trachea, esophagus, or recurrent laryngeal nerves is extremely rare and is due to inadequate knowledge of the anatomy of the neck.

Pneumothorax This complication is probably secondary to barotrauma caused by ventilation initiated immediately after tube placement.

Late airway complications may occur in up to 52 percent of cases. These complications include voice changes and laryngeal and/or tracheal stenosis.[8–10]

EQUIPMENT NEEDED

1. Personal protective equipment
2. Scalpel with a no. 10 (preferable because of its greater width) or no. 11 blade
3. A 6-mm endotracheal tube or tracheostomy tube (preferred); tubes larger than 6 mm are difficult to place through the cricothyroid membrane.
4. Tape to secure the endotracheal tube in place; cloth ribbon and sutures to secure tracheostomy tube in place
5. Bag-valve-mask device and oxygen source

PATIENT PREPARATION AND POSITIONING

The patient should be placed supine, with the neck positioned in the midline. Povidone iodine solution should be quickly applied to the skin, if time permits. If the patient still has a patent airway (albeit minimal), oxygen should be administered by mask.

STEPS OF PROCEDURE

1. Stand to one side of the patient at the level of the neck. A right-handed practitioner should stand on the right side, and a left-handed practitioner should stand on the left side.
2. Locate the cricoid ring. Place the index finger at the sternal notch and palpate cephalad until the first rigid structure is felt (cricoid ring). Roll the index finger one finger breadth above to locate the "hollow" between the cricoid and thyroid cartilages. This is the cricothyroid membrane.
3. Using the thumb and middle finger of the nondominant hand, stabilize the two cartilages (Figure 20-3).
4. Use the scalpel to make a vertical incision in the midline between the two cartilages. The incision should go through the skin and subcutaneous tissues. The structures are superficial, and care should be taken not to incise deeper, because this may result in damage to the cricoid or thyroid cartilage or vascular structures (Figure 20-4).
5. With the scalpel blade positioned horizontally, perforate the cricothyroid membrane so that the blade goes in approximately half its length (Figure 20-5).

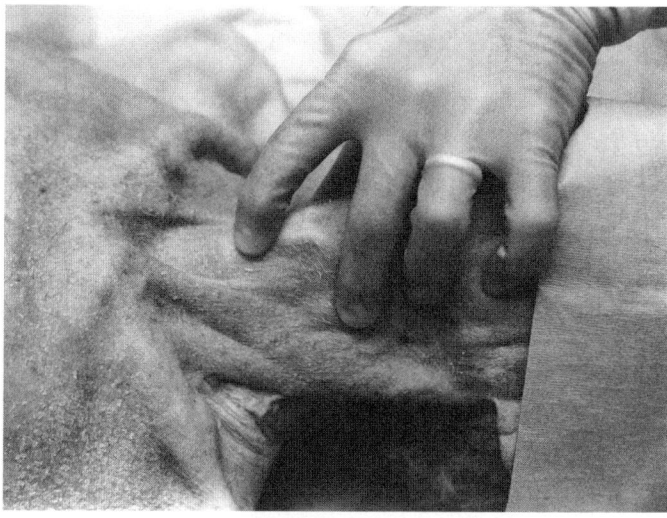

FIG. 20-3. Surgical cricothyroidotomy. Palpating the cricothyroid membrane and stabilizing the laryngeal cartilages.

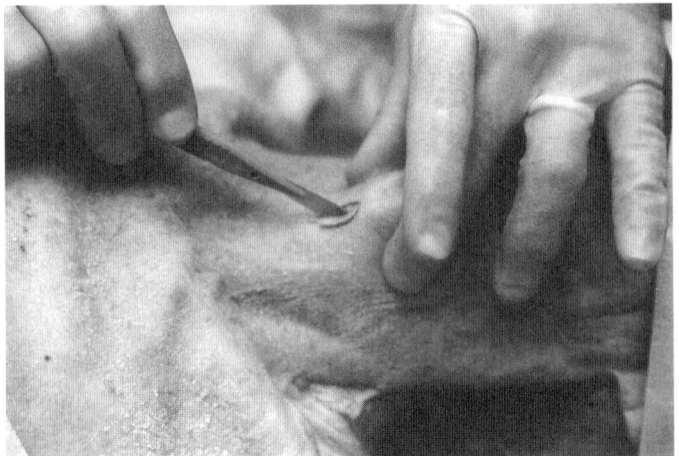

FIG. 20-4. Surgical cricothyroidotomy. Incision between the cricoid and thyroid cartilages.

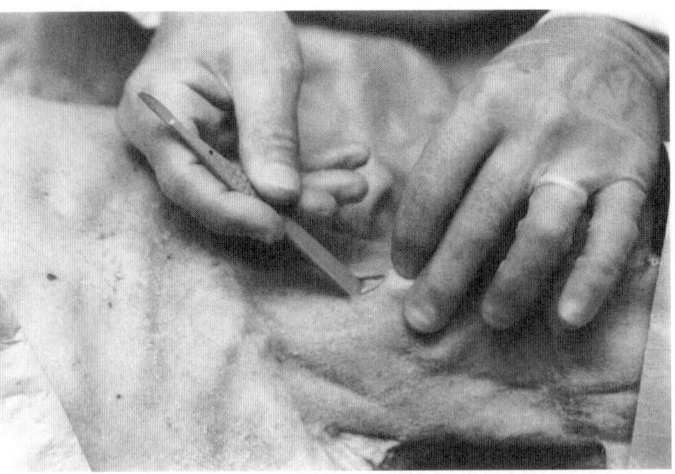

FIG. 20-6. Surgical cricothyroidotomy. Placing the scalpel handle to widen the hole in the cricothyroid membrane.

6. Place the back end of the scalpel handle into the incision in the cricothyroid membrane to widen the opening (Figure 20-6).
7. Place the endotracheal tube (or tracheostomy tube) in the opening (Figure 20-7).
8. Secure the tube carefully with a ribbon and/or adhesive tape. If using an endotracheal tube, take special care that the tube is inserted no more than 2 to 3 cm; otherwise, the tube will slip down the right main-stem bronchus with even minimal movement.
9. Connect to a bag-valve-mask device for ventilation. Check for breath sounds with ventilation. If no ventilation is heard bilaterally, then pull the tube out and reinsert it. Constantly recheck for breath sounds to ensure that the endotracheal tube is correctly positioned. If breath sounds are absent only on the left side, then the tube has been inserted down the right main-stem bronchus and needs to be pulled back a few centimeters. This usually occurs with the use of an endotracheal tube.

DRESSING AND STABILIZATION   If a tracheostomy tube has been used, a simple dressing may be fashioned by cutting a slit halfway down the middle of a 4 × 4 cm dressing and placing it under the tracheostomy tube. This tube may be secured with a ribbon placed through the flanges of the tracheostomy tube. For added security, 2-0 nylon sutures may be used to fix the tube to the skin. Endotracheal tubes are extremely difficult to secure properly to the neck and should be changed to tracheostomy tubes whenever possible.

DEVICE REMOVAL   The cricothyroidotomy tube may be removed once the patient has a patent airway or has been changed to a tracheostomy tube, as mentioned above. Patency may be evaluated by deflating the cuff of the tube and assessing airflow by breathing or by speech.

Needle Cricothyroidotomy

Needle cricothyroidotomy entails insertion of a catheter (generally an intravenous catheter) through the cricothyroid membrane. Although this procedure is easier to perform than surgical cricothyroidotomy, it is greatly inferior in providing adequate ventilation. The diameter of the catheter used is the limiting factor for airflow.

ANATOMY   See the discussion under "Surgical Cricothyroidotomy."

INDICATIONS AND CONTRAINDICATIONS   The general indications are listed under "Surgical Cricothyroidotomy." However, needle cricothyroidotomy is usually deemed the only type of emergency surgical airway that is indicated in children younger than 10–12 years. Although, in general, there are no contraindications to needle cricothyroidotomy, adult patients can be ventilated for only approximately 15 to 20 min and should have an alternative airway secured immediately (by surgical cricothyroidotomy, endotracheal intubation, or tracheostomy).

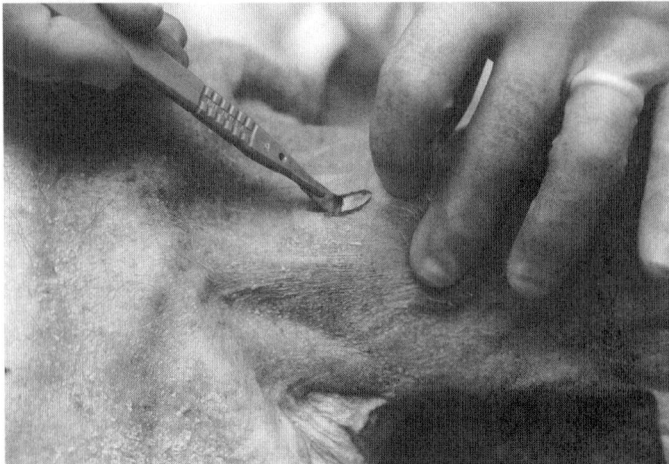

FIG. 20-5. Surgical cricothyroidotomy. Puncturing the cricothyroid membrane with a scalpel blade.

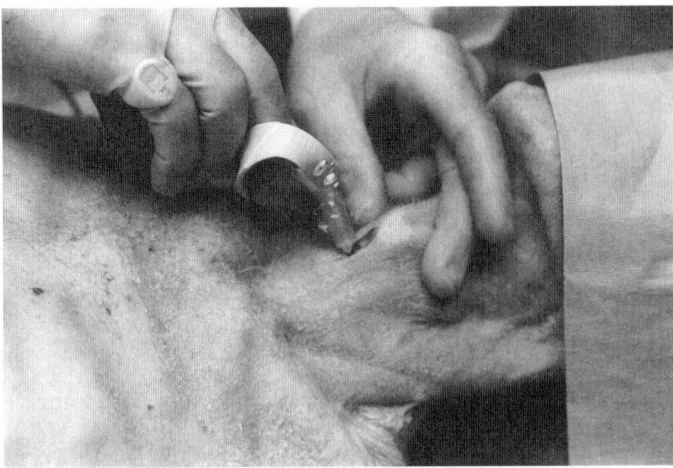

FIG. 20-7. Surgical cricothyroidotomy. Placement of tracheostomy tube with obturator.

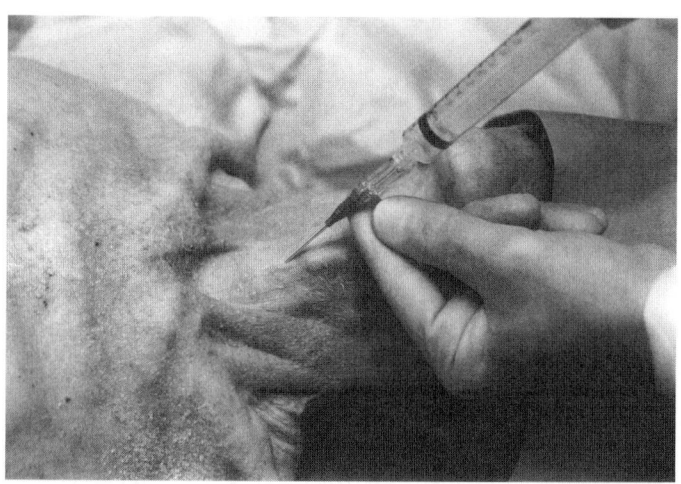

FIG. 20-8. Needle cricothyroidotomy. Puncturing the skin with needle and catheter.

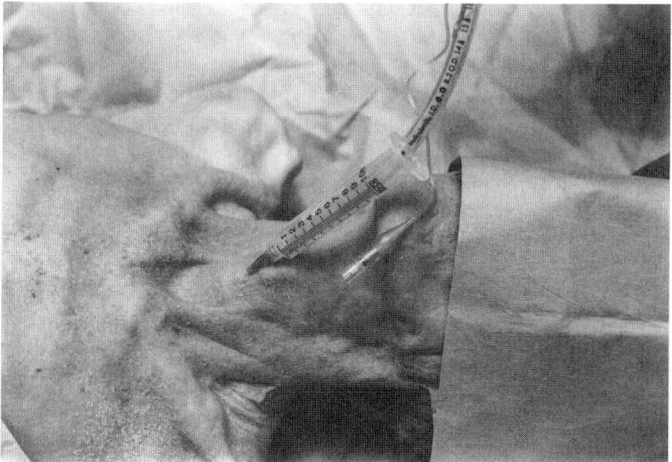

FIG. 20-10. Needle cricothyroidotomy. Endotracheal setup with tube, syringe, and catheter.

COMPLICATIONS Complications after needle cricothyroidotomy are less frequent than after surgical cricothyroidotomy. Bleeding at the puncture site and infection may occur. Inadvertent perforation of the esophagus or back wall of the trachea or larynx is infrequent. Massive subcutaneous emphysema will develop during ventilation. The catheter also may be misplaced in the soft tissues of the neck.

EQUIPMENT NEEDED

1. Personal protective equipment
2. A 14- or 12-gauge sheathed needle catheter
3. A 3-mL syringe
4. Adapter from the end of a 7-mm endotracheal tube
5. Wall oxygen source at 15 L/min (40 to 50 psi) connected by tubing with a Y connector or fashioned with a side hole (a bag-valve-mask device can be substituted but is not optimal)

PATIENT PREPARATION AND POSITIONING See the discussion under "Surgical Cricothyroidotomy."

STEPS OF PROCEDURE

1. The operator should be positioned above the head of the patient.
2. Locate the cricoid ring. Place the index finger at the sternal notch and palpate cephalad until the first rigid structure is felt (cricoid ring). Roll the finger one finger breadth above to locate the "hol-

low" between the cricoid and thyroid cartilages. This is the cricothyroid membrane (see Figure 20-3).
3. Attach a 3-mL syringe to the catheter (12 or 14 gauge).
4. Introduce the catheter into the subcutaneous tissue at a 90-degree angle to the skin. Aspirate gently while advancing the catheter over the needle. When air suddenly returns (indicating entry into the airway), change the angle to 45 degrees and advance the catheter over the needle into the larynx. Withdraw the needle and syringe (Figure 20-8).
5. Disconnect the 3-mL syringe from the bare needle.
6. Withdraw the plunger from the syringe and attach the plungerless 3-mL syringe barrel to the catheter in the neck.
7. Attach the adapter (from the end of a 7-mm endotracheal tube) to the open end of the 3-mL syringe (Figure 20-9), or place a 7-mm endotracheal tube into the empty syringe barrel and inflate the balloon (Figure 20-10).
8. Attach the oxygen source to the adapter and start ventilation with 100 percent oxygen. Intermittent jet insufflation (50 psi) can be achieved by occluding the Y connector or side hole in the connecting tubing. Insufflate for 1 s and then release the occlusion for 4 s. To achieve the required high pressures, it is best to use a jet injector regulated by a flowmeter attached to a wall unit on a tank. An unregulated wall unit or tank is a less optimal choice.
9. The operator must hold the catheter securely as it can become displaced with minimal movement. The inspiration-to-expiration ratio may need to be 1:10 to 1:15 to allow for expiration. Needle cricothyroidotomy does not provide for adequate ventilation and this technique is only a temporizing measure until definitive airway establishment.

DRESSING AND STABILIZATION Stabilization is maintained by the operator until another choice of airway is established, either tracheostomy or oro- or nasotracheal intubation (if possible). Dressings are not necessary.

DEVICE REMOVAL A needle cricothyroidotomy catheter should be removed as expediently as possible. The catheter almost always becomes inadvertently dislodged from the airway, and the ability to ventilate is poor.

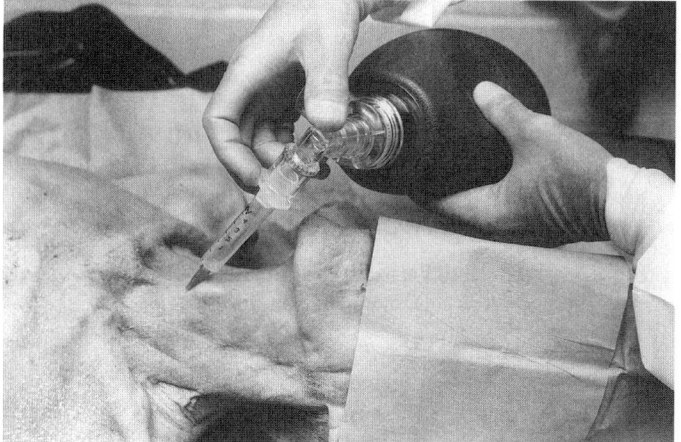

FIG. 20-9. Needle cricothyroidotomy. Catheter in place with adapter and syringe.

REFERENCES

1. Bair AE, Filbin MR, Kulkarnio RG et al: The failed intubation attempt in the emergency department: Analysis of prevalence, rescue techniques, and personnel. *J Emerg Med* 23:131, 2002.

2. Sise MJ, Shackford SR, Cruickshank JC, et al: Cricothyroidotomy for long-term tracheal access. A prospective analysis of morbidity and mortality in 76 patients. *Am Surg* 200:13, 1984.

3. Grewal H, Rao PM, Mukerji S, Ivantury RR: Management of laryngotracheal injuries. *Head Neck* 17:494, 1995.

4. Davies P: A stab in the dark! Are you ready to perform needle cricothyroidotomy? *Injury* 30:659, 1999.

5. Eisenburger P: Comparison of conventional surgical versus Seldinger technique emergency cricothyrotomy performed by inexperienced clinicians. *Anesthesiology* 92:687, 2000.

6. Esses BA, Jafek BW: Cricothyroidotomy: A decade of experience in Denver. *Ann Otol Rhinol Laryngol* 96:519, 1987.

7. Isaacs JH Jr, Pedersen AD: Emergency cricothyroidotomy. *Am Surg* 63:346, 1997.

8. Gleeson MJ, Pearson RC, Armistead S, Yates AK: Voice changes following cricothyroidotomy. *J Laryngol Otol* 98:1015, 1984.

9. Kuriloff DB, Setzen M, Portnoy W, Gadaleta D: Laryngotracheal injury following cricothyroidotomy. *Laryngoscope* 99:125, 1989.

10. Holst M, Hertegard S, Persson A: Vocal dysfunction following cricothyroidotomy: A prospective study. *Laryngoscope* 100:749, 1990.

21

VASCULAR ACCESS
William A. Berk
Bharat Sutariya

Obtaining access to the venous and arterial circulation enables the administration of drug, crystalloid, and blood products and measurement of central venous and arterial pressures. About one-third—or more than 33 million ED patients each year—require vascular access.

During resuscitation, venous access should be obtained at the site of the largest vein that is accessible without disrupting resuscitation. When peripheral sites are not available, central veins should be accessed for monitoring of central venous pressure or the administration of drugs directly into the central circulation.

ENDOTRACHEAL TUBE SUBSTITUTION FOR VASCULAR ACCESS

A number of medications may be administered by endotracheal tube in the critical minutes of resuscitation before intravenous access is obtained. These include atropine, diazepam, epinephrine, isoproterenol, lidocaine, and naloxone but *not* sodium bicarbonate or calcium chloride. Epinephrine as a preparation of 1 mg/mL (1:1000) should be given in a dosage of 0.1 mg/kg (standard dosage). The American Heart Association Advanced Cardiac Life Support (ACLS) and Pediatric Advanced Life Support (PALS) guidelines recommend increasing the intravenous dosages of other resuscitation medications by a factor of 2 to 3 and diluting with 3 to 5 mL of NS before administration via endotracheal tube. Drug administration is followed by several positive-pressure ventilations using a bag-to-tube device.

ISSUES OF FLOW DYNAMICS

Infusion rate is crucial in resuscitation for severe hypovolemia or hemorrhage. Fluid in a medical catheter behaves for practical purposes according to the Poiseuille law:

$$\text{Rate of flow} = \frac{\pi \times (\text{catheter radius})^4 \times \text{pressure gradient}}{8 \times \text{dynamic fluid viscosity}}$$

The fact that flow is a function of the fourth power of the radius of the tube lumen means that the internal catheter diameter is a major limiting factor.[1] A fluid delivery system is only as effective as its slowest component, whether this is intravenous tubing, in-line filters, or the catheter itself. Flow rates may also be affected by temperature, pressure, and viscosity, the latter being an especially important consideration in relation to red blood cell transfusion.[1] Rate of infusion is also directly proportional to catheter length, which is why a long central catheter will have a slower infusion rate than a shorter catheter of the same caliber in a peripheral vein.[2]

Placement of two large-bore 16-gauge or greater catheters is indicated in stable adult trauma patients whose injuries could cause potentially life-threatening hemorrhage or for initial therapy of medical patients with hypovolemic shock. In the management of exsanguination, an 8.5-F catheter with a manually operated pressure bag or a wall-mounted external pneumatic device delivers crystalloid at the rate of almost 0.5 L per min. A second catheter may be needed for drug infusion. Rapid infusion of larger volumes of fluid should be accompanied by careful monitoring for volume overload, especially in older patients or those with cardiovascular disease.

Volume repletion and measurement of central venous pressure can be accomplished by a Y-arm catheter sheath passed percutaneously into the femoral vein. An 8.5-F catheter can then be used for volume repletion, while a smaller catheter can simultaneously be inserted through the other arm of the Y and directed into the right atrium for the measurement of central venous pressure. Femoral catheters should generally be left in place no longer than 48 h, since iliofemoral thrombophlebitis can result. However, with sterile technique and the use of Silastic catheters, the deep femoral system may safely be employed for a longer duration.

Pressure infusion increases crystalloid flow two to three times above that achieved by gravity alone and is superior to the use of on-line hand-pumped bulbs. Pressure devices are also available for the administration of packed red blood cells. Use of a standard Y irrigation set augments flow rates by reducing resistance in the tubing leading to the catheter site. For maximum infusion rates of either blood or crystalloid, use of blood administration tubing eliminates on-line micropore filters, stopcocks, and one-way valves, all of which increase resistance. Addition of NS to packed red blood cell infusions decreases viscosity, increasing the speed of transfusion.[1]

Warming of crystalloid and blood before infusion is essential when volume resuscitation is massive. Crystalloid may be stored in a heating bath or oven, safely microwaved, or warmed with a heating coil or heat packs. Blood warming coils that allow transfusion rates of up to 500 mL per min are now available. Alternatively, cold-packed red blood cells may be warmed by diluting them with an equal amount of warmed saline (up to 60°C); this will also decrease viscosity and thus enhance flow.[1] An in-line microwave blood warmer may be used to heat blood safely to 49°C without any significant increase in hemolysis.[1,3]

VENOUS ACCESS SITES

Peripheral venous catheterization is a routine component of emergency medical practice. The normal human anatomy offers many potential sites for catheterization (Figures 21-1 and 21-2). The cephalic vein, in both the forearm and the upper arm, is large, constant, and straight; easily catheterized, it is the time-honored choice for peripheral access in both adults and children. The superficial radial vein at the wrist is well developed in adults, though it is difficult to locate in a small child. Veins of the hand are usually accessible even in obese persons but are short, tortuous, and difficult to stabilize. Veins in the antecubital fossa are excellent in emergency situations, but an armboard is necessary to prevent catheter kinking or dislodgement with movement, and the resulting elbow extension is a relatively uncomfortable position for patients if required for more than a few hours. The large basilic vein in the upper arm is usually not visible, but with practice it can be catheterized by palpating the brachial artery and searching blindly for the medially placed vein. Puncture of the brachial artery is common but rarely of clinical significance if care is taken to prevent hemorrhage or hematoma formation. Transitory paresthesias may also occur.

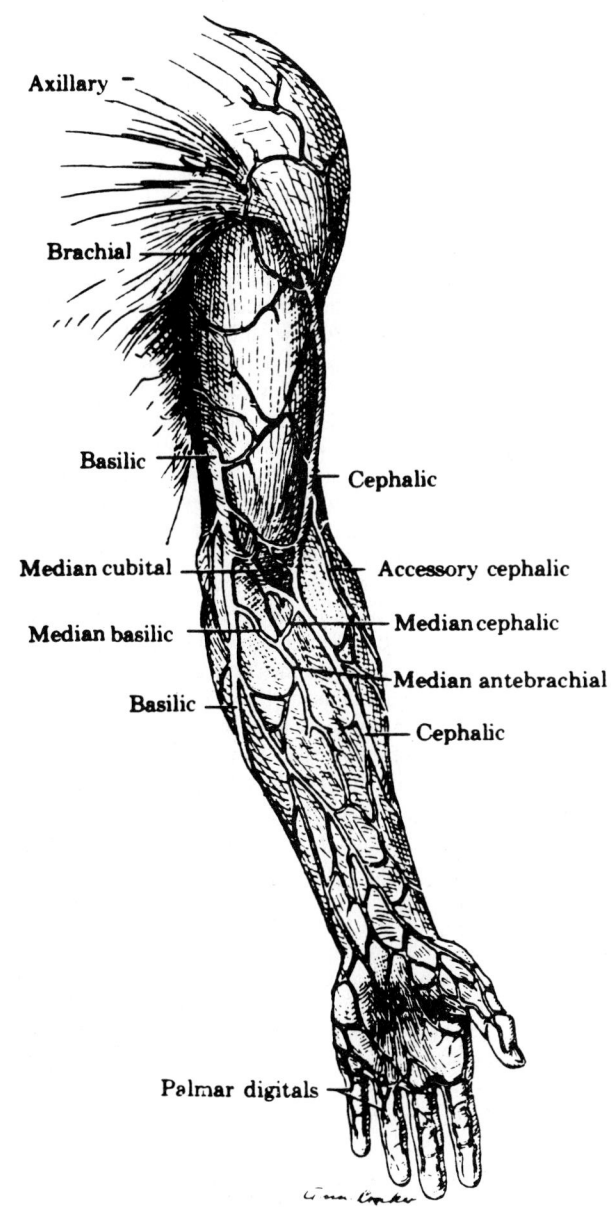

FIG. 21-1. Veins of the upper extremity.

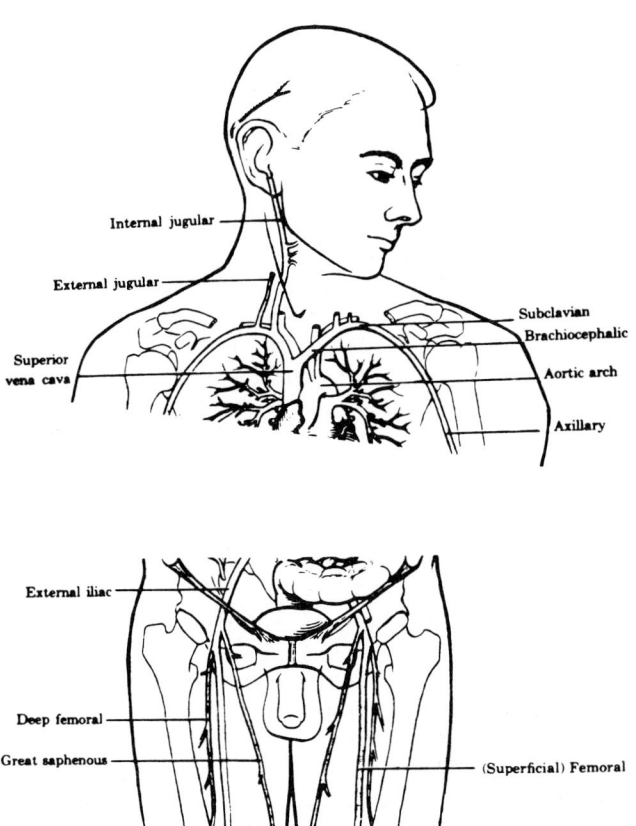

FIG. 21-2. Veins of the torso and lower extremities.

Internal jugular, subclavian, or femoral vein catheterization is performed when peripheral access is impossible or when the measurement of central venous pressure is desired. The relative risk for a catheter-related bloodstream infection is significantly higher with central than peripheral venous catheters.[4] The external jugular vein can provide reliable access in both adults and children. Although this vein is readily distended by the Valsalva or Trendelenburg maneuvers, scant subcutaneous support can make it difficult to catheterize. However, access to central veins without the risk that attends direct internal jugular and subclavian puncture is a major advantage. In young children, intraosseous infusion provides rapid and reliable access in emergencies (see Chap. 14).

TECHNIQUE FOR PERIPHERAL VENOUS ACCESS

Insertion of peripheral venous catheters should be preceded by wiping with an antiseptic solution and followed routinely by placement of a sterile transparent or gauze dressing. Although a 2 percent chlorhexidine-based preparation is preferred, tincture of iodine, an iodophor, or 70 percent alcohol may be used.[5] If peripheral veins are small, size and visibility can be enhanced by application of hot, moist compresses for 5 min, by tapping gently on the vein before attempting puncture, or by application of nitroglycerin ointment (0.4 percent for children less than 1 year old; 2 percent for others) over an area 1 in. in diameter for 2 min and then wiping it off. Once access has been obtained, gentle circumferential occlusive taping may be necessary if stability of the site is tenuous, with the intravenous line looped and secondarily secured to prevent traction at the point at which the line penetrates the skin. The size of the catheter can usually be determined by the color of the hub; otherwise, it should be written on the tape dressing. When venous access is required primarily for drug administration, consideration should be given to placing a saline or heparin lock.

Obtaining intravenous access in young children can be a challenge. Children tend to be more anxious and thus uncooperative. Generous

Veins in the legs often require cutdown for catheter placement. The superficial saphenous vein at the ankle is large, constant, and easy to isolate and cannulate. The proximal great saphenous vein in the thigh may be found reliably 5 cm below the inguinal ligament at the junction of the medial and middle third of the thigh (between the pubis symphysis and superior iliac spine) in the supine patient. The deep femoral vein is accessible percutaneously, just medial to the femoral artery which is found approximately midway between the superior iliac spine and the pubic symphysis below the inguinal ligament (see Figure 21-2). In the pulseless patient, the landmark is the junction of the medial and middle third of the inguinal ligament. From the great saphenous and deep femoral veins, advancement of catheters into the right atrium for the measurement of central venous pressure is possible.

Peripheral venous catheterization should not be attempted in an extremity distal to cellulitis, burns, or serious injury, or when potential for vascular disruption due to injury is anatomically proximate.

Catheterization of arms in the presence of an indwelling fistula or serious ipsilateral neck trauma should also be avoided. Hyperosmolar fluids and agents known to cause chemical phlebitis or sclerosis of peripheral veins should not be infused through such veins.

subcutaneous fat may prevent vessel palpation and direct visualization. Finally, a child's vessels are smaller, and children readily lose body heat, which promotes vasoconstriction. It is helpful to have an experienced assistant who can help in holding and distracting the child. When possible prior application of a topical anesthetic can reduce the pain of needle puncture (see Chap. 37).

Complications

Complications from placement of peripheral intravenous lines include hematoma formation, phlebitis, and cellulitis. Phlebitis may occur in up to 75 percent of hospitalized patients. There is general agreement that peripheral venous catheters should not be left in place for longer than 3 days before replacement. Nerve and tendon damage, deep venous thrombosis, suppurative thrombophlebitis, and septicemia are rare. The unusual event of extravasation of irritative, vasoconstricting, or tissue-toxic substances such as 50 percent dextrose, epinephrine, phenytoin, and some drugs used for chemotherapy of malignancies may cause problems ranging from minor pain and inflammation to full-thickness sloughing of skin, necessitating skin grafting. In rare situations, reactive arterial vasospasm has led to ischemia and ultimately tissue necrosis in extremities with very distally placed intravenous lines that have infiltrated. Catheter-over-needle assemblies are now in common use and provide more stable, reliable access than the steel needles they replaced. Microparticulate matter in intravenous solutions is removed by in-line micropore filters.

CENTRAL VENOUS PRESSURE CATHETERIZATION AND MONITORING

Central venous catheterization should be performed:

1. When access to the central circulation is necessary for procedures such as pulmonary artery catheter or pacemaker placement;
2. For access when peripheral veins cannot be cannulated; or
3. When measurement of central venous pressure is desired.

Hypovolemic shock by itself is not, however, an indication for central venous catheterization. Many patients who require large-volume infusions or transfusion with multiple units of blood can be managed with large-bore peripheral intravenous lines. Determination of central venous pressure is indicated when:

1. Massive volume repletion is administered to elderly patients or those with heart disease,
2. Fluid administration is being monitored in patients with visceral trauma and severe head injuries; or
3. Pericardial tamponade is suspected.

A variety of sites and techniques are available to access the central circulation. Most commonly, a catheter is placed in the superior vena cava via the internal jugular or subclavian vein; the external jugular vein is less commonly employed. The femoral vein may also be used, but it requires subsequent immobilization of the leg, and the procedure is accompanied by a higher risk of infection and thrombosis. Emergency physicians should become skilled in at least two approaches for central venous catheterization, using one as the primary while reserving the other as a backup.

Use of peripheral veins to access the central circulation and measure central venous pressure has the advantage of avoiding the risk associated with direct puncture of the subclavian and internal jugular veins. However, low flow is inevitable due to the long course of the catheter from the extremity to the superior vena cava. Peripheral sites also fail frequently due to catheter malposition and kinking. In the arm the brachial-basilic system must be used, since catheters in the cephalic system often become kinked in the plexus of veins at the shoulder. Smooth passage and correct tip positioning are more likely if the patient is sitting with his or her head angulated sharply toward

the catheterized arm, the arm is held abducted, and the catheter is wire-guided. In emergency situations, however, this time-consuming approach to the central circulation is often impractical.

Anatomy

A brief review of anatomy is warranted (Figures 21-1 and 21-3). The major veins of the upper thorax are deeply and centrally placed and well protected by the clavicles, sternum, and strap muscles. The internal jugular veins join the subclavian veins to form the brachiocephalics (innominates), which in turn join to become the superior vena cava. The sternocleidomastoid muscle attaches separately by two heads to the sternum and clavicle; the triangle formed by these two heads and the clavicle is just above the internal jugular vein. The right internal jugular has a straight path into the superior vena cava, whereas all the other major tributaries curve. Both external jugular veins enter the subclavian veins at close to right angles. The subclavian veins lie immediately posterior to the junction of the medial and middle thirds of the clavicle and are anterior and inferior to the artery; the pleura are immediately posterior and inferior to the subclavian vessels (Figure 21-4). The internal jugular vein usually lies anterolateral to the carotid. The basilic and brachial veins join to form the axillary vein. The cephalic vein joins the axillary vein more superiorly, just before it becomes the subclavian vein. The axillary vein continues the distal subclavian vein and runs medial to the axillary artery from the distal arm. The femoral vein is medial to the femoral artery. The relative locations of components of the neurovascular-lymphatic bundle in the groin from lateral to medial can be recalled by the mnemonic NAVEL (nerve, artery, vein, empty space, lymphatic).

Equipment and General Technique for Central Venous Catheterization

All equipment should be at the bedside, including a central venous (CV) pressure manometer if CV pressure monitoring is desired. Catheter-through-needle devices, whose large 14-gauge insertion needles are prone to complications and whose 16-gauge catheters allow maximum gravity-assisted flow of 100 to 150 mL per min, have been largely supplanted by wire-guided (Seldinger) catheters.[6] Their use allows use of a small needle to place any size catheter into a vessel.

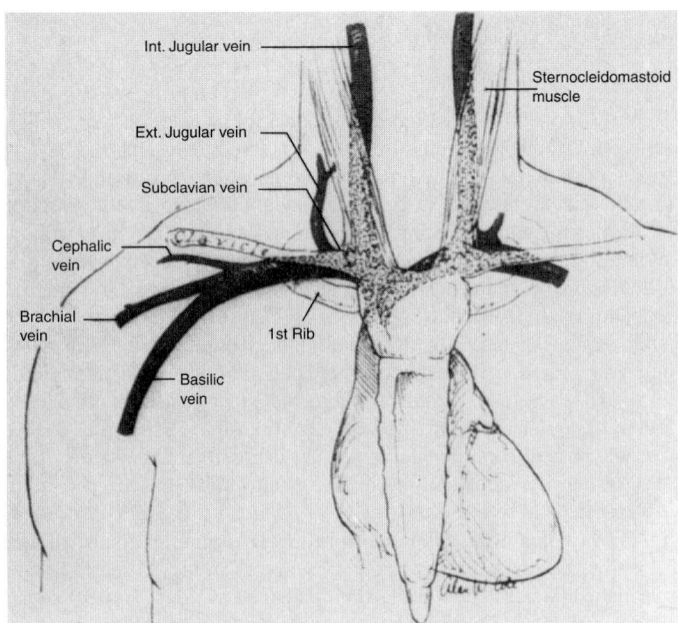

FIG. 21-3. Relationship of major torso veins to other anatomy.

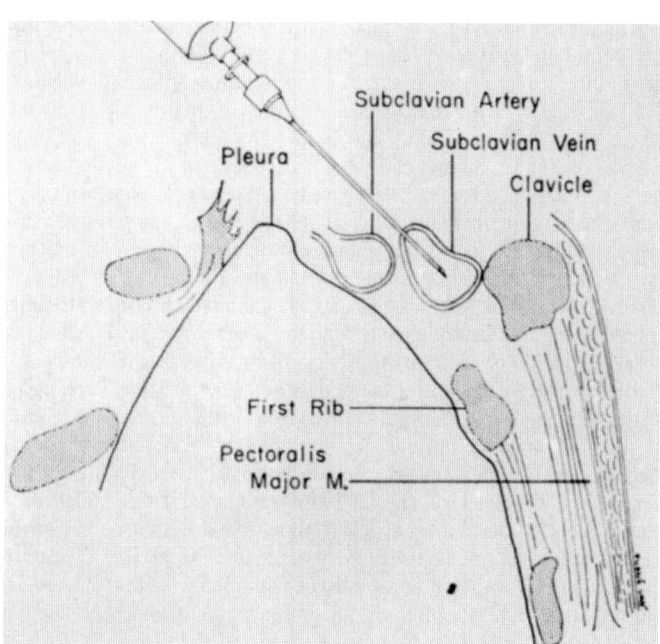

FIG. 21-4. Coronal section through the midclavicle.

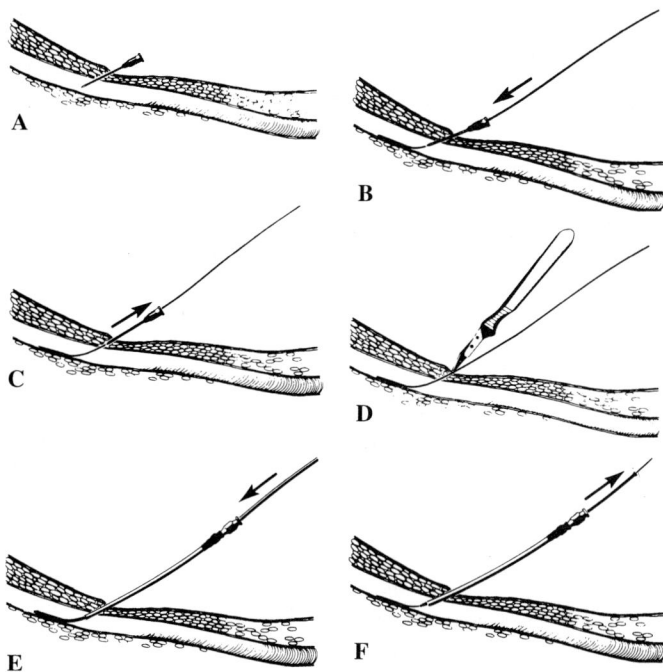

FIG. 21-5. Seldinger technique of catheter insertion (wire-guided). (Reproduced with permission from Conahan TJ III, Schwartz AJ, Geer RT: Percutaneous catheter introduction: The Seldinger technique. *JAMA* 237:446, 1977.)

The patient should be placed in a neutral to maximum of 30 degrees head rotation and 15 degrees Trendelenburg position, and the entire route of the neck should be prepped so that all three approaches are possible in case the primary approach fails. The right side is preferred over the left, since (1) the lung apex is slightly lower, (2) there is a straight relationship between the right internal jugular vein and the superior vena cava, and (3) the left-sided thoracic duct cannot be injured. With unilateral chest trauma in the absence of suspected vessel injury, the attempt should be on the injured side in order to protect the uninjured hemithorax in the event of complications from the procedure.

When the procedure is performed electively, preceding the approach for catheter placement with a 22-gauge needle attached to a 5- or 10-mL syringe filled with lidocaine facilitates local anesthesia and allows the operator to locate the vein. After landmarks are identified, an 18-gauge needle is then inserted into the vein (Figure 21-5A). Gentle, continuous negative pressure on the syringe should be maintained until free flow of blood is obtained. The syringe is removed and a fingertip is used to occlude the hub before wire insertion (Figure 21-5B). This often forgotten or ignored maneuver is important to prevent aspiration of air, particularly in internal jugular or subclavian vein catheterizations. The needle is then removed (Figure 21-5C), leaving just the wire in the vein. A small skin incision (1 to 2 mm) is often made over the wire (Figure 21-5D) to facilitate smooth entry of the catheter, which is threaded over the wire and into the vein with a twisting motion (Figure 21-5E). The wire is then removed, leaving only the catheter in place (Figure 21-5F). If a large-bore catheter is necessary, the apparatus is used with a venodilator. In this situation, the veno-dilator is removed with the wire, leaving the large-bore 8.5-F catheter sheath in place.

The principal advantages of wire-guided catheters are:

1. Use of a small (and thus safer) needle for insertion
2. The step-up capability with a venodilator, allowing for the higher flow rates often required in trauma resuscitation
3. The flexibility of exchanging standard intravenous catheters, central venous catheters, and pulmonary artery catheters without repeated stabs, and
4. The use of J wires to access the central circulation from the external jugular vein

Ultrasound visualization of the central vein while puncture is attempted reduces the number of punctures necessary for cannulation to establish central access, while also reducing the incidence of complications. The technique is particularly helpful when the traditional landmark-based techniques fail or are impractical due to vascular anomalies or body habitus, or when patients with a coagulopathy require central venous access.[7,8]

Complications

The three most common serious complications of central venous catheterization are mechanical problems (pneumothorax, arterial puncture, and malpositioning), catheter-related infection, and thrombosis (Table 21-1). A large body of reported experience suggests that for internal jugular access there are more arterial punctures but fewer catheter malpositions than with subclavian access. There is, however, no evidence of a difference in the incidence of hemo- or pneumothorax or vessel occlusion. Femoral venous catheterization is associated with greater risk of infection and thrombotic complications than subclavian catheterization.[9] In children, the success rate for subclavian catheterization is higher and the complication rate is lower (3.2 percent) than for internal jugular venous access. Other, less common complications include hydrothorax, chylothorax (left side), hydromediastinum, air or catheter embolism, vessel thrombosis, dysrhythmia, nerve injuries, osteomyelitis of the clavicle, catheter tip perforation of

TABLE 21-1 Central Venous Access Complication Rate

	Subclavian	Internal Jugular	Femoral
Infection	4–5%	8–9%	15–19%
Thrombosis	1–2%	1%	12–21%
Pneumothorax	1.5%	1.3%	0%
Arterial puncture	<1%	3%	8%
Malposition	9%	5%	<1%

Note: Data is compiled from a number of studies.

the superior vena cava (causing hydromediastinum or hydrothorax) or right atrium (causing hydropericardium), knotting with other catheters, and puncture of endotracheal tube cuffs.[10] Care in executing the procedure and in the selection of patients who will benefit from central venous catheterization will minimize the occurrence of complications.

Technique of Commonly Used Approaches

EXTERNAL JUGULAR VEIN   The external jugular vein is a superficial, readily accessible vessel that lies in the subcutaneous tissue over the sternocleidomastoid muscle. The vein courses inferior and joins the subclavian vein under the clavicle (see Figure 21-3). Central venous access via this route has an increased success rate if a J-wire-guided catheter assembly is used. Success is enhanced by introducing the wire through a 16-gauge catheter rather than through a needle, using a J tip with no more than a 3-mm radius, exaggerating head tilt with marked traction on the skin of the neck. The latter technique in particular should be tried before making a second attempt. Wire-through-needle techniques may be met with resistance at the level of the clavicle that can be overcome by twisting the tip of the J wire 180 degrees. It is also recommended that a small syringe (insulin or TB syringe) be attached to the introducing needle-catheter assembly for both stabilization and to maintain negative pressure. The external jugular vein is very pliable and collapses easily during initial skin puncture. Gently withdrawing the needle back while maintaining suction improves chances of successful catheterization.

The main disadvantage of external jugular catheterization is difficulty in securing the catheter in the neck. Other potential problems are:

1. The venous valves within its course may impede catheter placement
2. Patient movement makes most external jugular lines short-lived, and
3. Neck rotation impedes flow of the infusion, making the line unreliable for fluid or medications unless it is constantly watched

INTERNAL JUGULAR VEIN   There are three traditional approaches to catheterization of the internal jugular vein. In the central approach (Figure 21-6B), after the patient is placed in Trendelenburg position, the needle should puncture the skin 1 cm below the apex of a triangle at the midpoint formed by the tendinous and muscular heads of the stern-ocleidomastoid muscle. The palpation and definition of the margin of the carotid artery is not as important as in the anterior approach, but is helpful in locating the vein and to avoid puncture of the artery. Held at a 60 degree angle with the plane of the skin, the needle is directed slightly lateral to the axis of the body (lateral to the pulsation of the carotid artery). Common helpful landmarks for needle direction include the ipsilateral nipple and a plane parallel to the medial border of the lateral head of the sternocleidomastoid muscle. Blood return should be obtained within 3 cm, since the vein is very superficial here. If the attempt appears to fail, the needle should be withdrawn slowly, as success is often evident only on slight withdrawal. If the attempt has clearly failed, the needle should be withdrawn completely before the next attempt.

In the lateral or posterior approach, the head is turned slightly away from the selected side; after the patient is placed in Trendelenburg position, the needle is inserted at the posterior margin and deep to the sternocleidomastoid muscle two to three fingerbreadths above the clavicle and directed toward the suprasternal notch (Figure 21-6A). Frequently, the external jugular vein crosses the lateral wall of the sterno-cleidomastoid muscle at this point. If it does, the needle should be inserted at the junction of the crossing at a 90 degree angle to the external jugular vein. Blood should be aspirated within 4 to 5 cm. The carotid artery is just behind this path, albeit slightly posterior, and may be at increased risk for puncture.

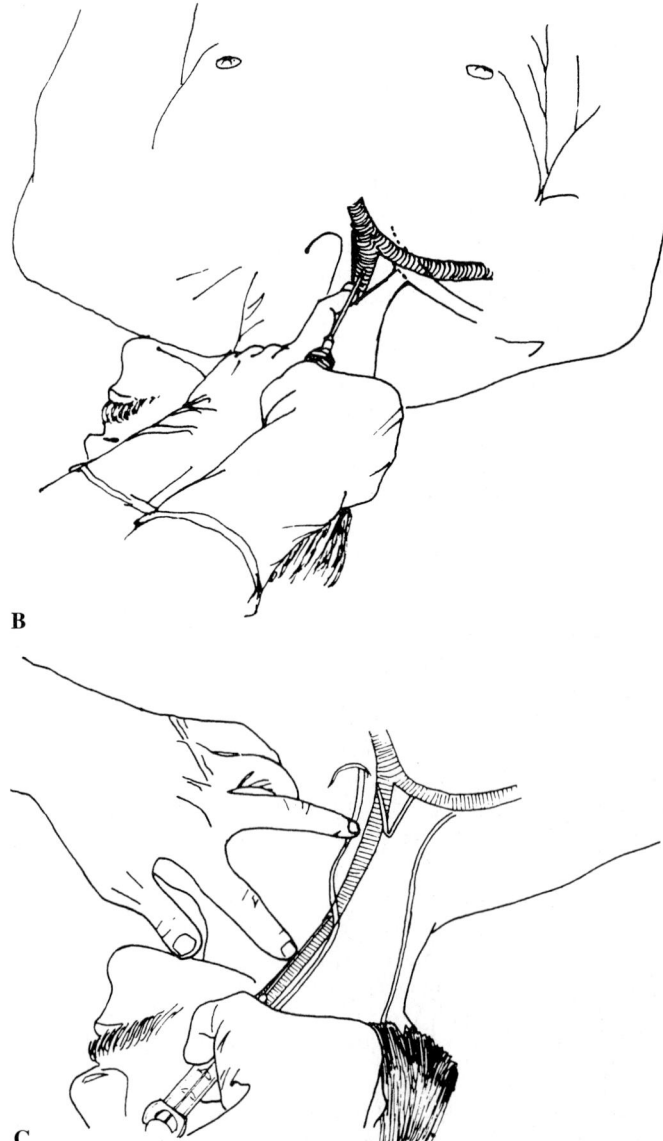

B

C

FIG. 21-6. A. Posterior approach for internal jugular venipuncture. **B.** Central approach. **C.** Anterior approach. (Reproduced with permission from *Textbook of Advanced Life Support,* 2d ed. Dallas: American Heart Association, 1990, pp. 149-150.)

A

The anterior approach (Figure 21-6C) and its variants may well be the most technically difficult. After the carotid is identified, the needle is entered at the midpart of the medial border of the sternocleidomastoid. With the fingers over the carotid, the needle is directed 30 to 45 degrees from the midline plane toward the ipsilateral nipple. This approach has the greatest likelihood of carotid puncture and appears to be the least favored of the intravenous cannulation approaches.

SUBCLAVIAN VEIN   The subclavian vein is still the most commonly used site for central venous access. The right side is preferred because the pleural dome is lower on that side. The fact that the point of insertion is in a broad, flat area of the chest makes it ideal for use when central venous access will be required for a prolonged period. The patient is placed in the Trendelenburg position. If the patient is a child, a towel is placed under the thoracic spine. This may also be helpful in some adults.

The *infraclavicular* subclavian approach is the most commonly taught technique. There is no universal agreement on exactly where the needle should enter. The bisection of the middle and medial thirds of the clavicle is an appropriate landmark. Another is a point just lateral and inferior to the junction of the clavicle and first rib. Using the former landmark (Figure 21-7), the skin is penetrated about 1 cm inferior to the clavicle and directed inferomedially. With the index or middle finger of the other hand in the suprasternal notch, the needle is aimed at the superior and most posterior portion of the ipsilateral clavicular head. Inferomedial orientation of the needle bevel facilitates entry of the wire or catheter into the vein. Vessel entry occurs at a depth of 3 to 4 cm.

For the *supraclavicular* subclavian approach, the patient's head is turned slightly away from the selected side. The needle enters just above the clavicle, 1 cm lateral to the insertion of the clavicular head of the sternocleidomastoid muscle and 1 cm posterior to the clavicle. It is then directed to bisect the angle formed between the sternocleidomastoid and the clavicle, at an angle of 10 degrees above the horizontal, with the tip pointing just caudad to the contralateral nipple. Keeping the bevel up prevents trapping of the wire or catheter against the inferior wall of the vessel. Vessel puncture occurs at a depth of 2 to 3 cm.

FEMORAL VEIN   Femoral vein catheterization is used when the vessels of the upper body are not suitable, and when access is required

above and below an injury. Although femoral vein catheterization is somewhat easier than subclavian or internal jugular catheterization, the insertion site is difficult to sterilize and keep clean, and patient movement may make it difficult to keep the line secured.

The patient should be supine with the ipsilateral hip in a neutral to slightly externally rotated position. The approximate position of the femoral vein can be determined by dividing the distance between the anterior superior iliac spine and the pubic tubercle into three equal segments (see Figure 21-2). In most patients, the femoral artery usually lies at the midpoint. If the femoral pulse is palpable, the needle puncture site should be 1.5 cm medial and 1.5 cm inferior to the inguinal ligament. Once venous blood is obtained, the guidewire is inserted though the needle, the needle is removed, and the catheter is inserted over the wire.

This access can be used for the measurement of central venous pressure, for intravenous pacing, for pulmonary artery catheterization, and to administer large volumes of fluids rapidly. The increased risk of infection and thrombosis make it less than ideal as a route for hyperalimentation. It is not an ideal central access site for administration of ACLS medications.

AXILLARY VEIN   The axillary vein (see Figure 21-2) is used for central venous access when the femoral, subclavian, and jugular veins are unavailable. This useful technique is unfortunately rarely used by emergency physicians. With practice, the success rate for central access via the axillary vein is similar to that for puncture of the internal jugular or subclavian vein. There is no risk of pneumothorax and the method has the advantage that if arterial puncture should occur, direct pressure can be applied.

Patients are placed supine with head-down tilt and the arm abducted to 45 degrees. In this position the axillary vein follows a straight course from the arm to the subclavian vein. An insertion point is chosen approximately 2.5 cm inferior to the axillary pulse and lateral to the midclavicular line. The introducer needle is then inserted along a line formed by the insertion point and suprasternal notch, at an angle of 30 degrees to the skin, and directed parallel to the course of the artery toward the chest wall. In children and thin adults, the artery is easily palpable.

VENOUS CUTDOWN

The basilic vein in the antecubital fossa and the saphenous vein in the leg are the most commonly utilized vessels for cutdowns. The basilic vein is located two fingerbreadths above and two fingerbreadths medial to the olecranon. The saphenous vein is just anterior to the medial malleolus at the ankle (Figure 21-8A) and is also accessible in the proximal thigh three fingerbreadths below the midpoint of the inguinal ligament (see Figure 21-2). Although experienced operators may be able to complete the procedure in less than a minute, for most operators 5 or 6 min will be required. In many situations, this implies that cutdown should be resorted to only when percutaneous access has failed or is deemed likely to be unsuccessful.

The operator begins by disinfecting and anesthetizing the skin (Figure 21-8). A transverse skin incision is made, and by blunt dissection the subcutaneous tissue is separated until the vein is exposed. Any accompanying artery is identified by slipping a forceps or hemostat under the vessels and applying pressure; pulsatile flow will be evident in the artery. (However, with patients who are in shock, this maneuver may be unsuccessful.) After freeing the vein from the surrounding tissues, two separate sutures are passed beneath the vein, one proximally and one distally. The proximal sutures are left untied, while the distal suture is tied to occlude the vein. The ends of the sutures are kept long so that they can be used for applying traction to the vein. A small incision is made in the vein between the proximal and the distal sutures (it should not be cut through and through). While applying traction on the vein, the operator inserts the catheter into the vein. Some cutdown

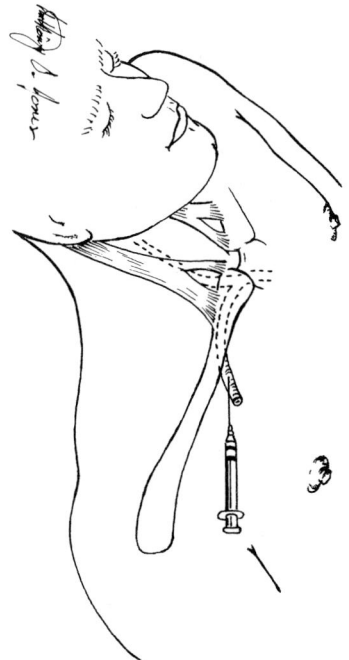

FIG. 21-7. Infraclavicular subclavian venipuncture.

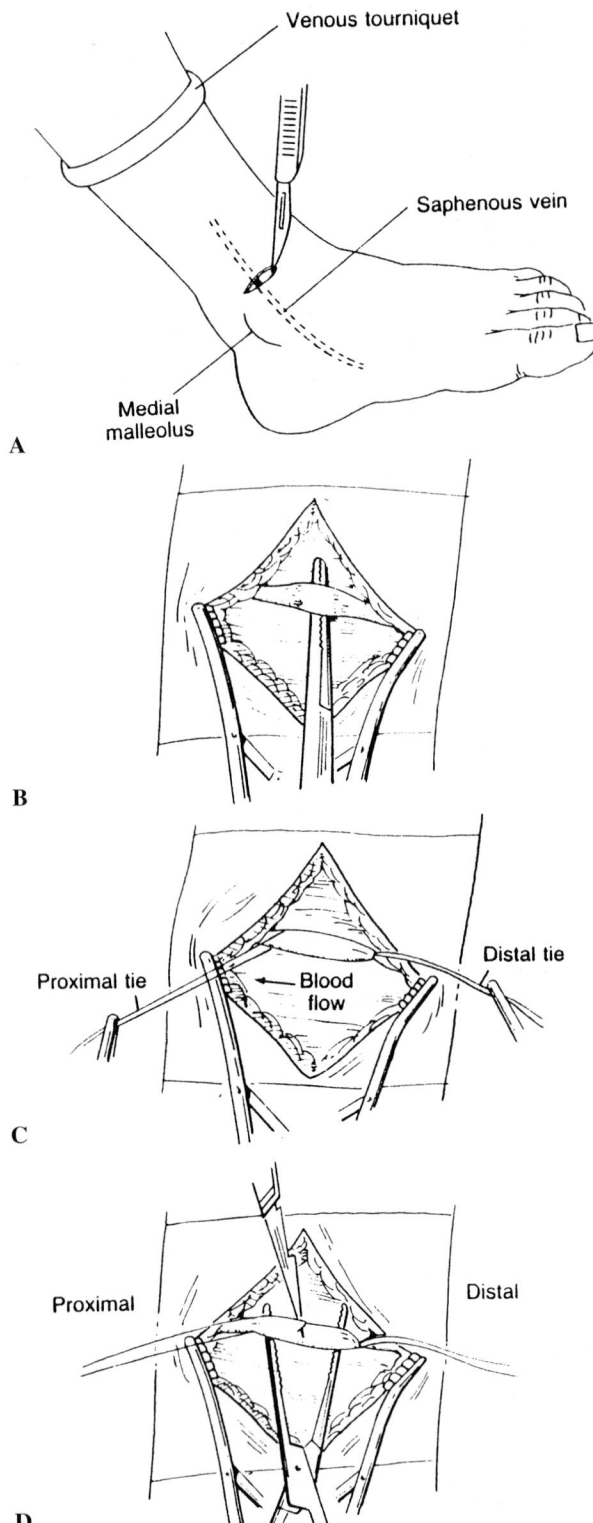

FIG. 21-8. Venous cutdown. **A.** A skin incision is made perpendicular to the course of the vein. **B.** Skin retracted and vein exposed. **C.** Proximal and distal ties are passed under the vein. If the vein is to be sacrificed, the distal suture is tied to prevent bleeding, and the ends are left long to help stabilize the vein during cannulation. The proximal tie is not tied at this point, but traction on it will control back bleeding. **D.** The vein is stretched flat and incised at a 45 degree angle. Approximately one-third of the lumen must be exposed. (Reproduced with permission from Roberts JR, Hedges JR: *Clinical Procedures in Emergency Medicine,* 2d ed. Philadelphia: Saunders, 1991, p. 321. Parts B and C first appeared in Vander Salm TJ, et al: *Atlas of Bedside Procedures.* Boston: Little, Brown, 1979.)

kits contain a vein "holder," which may help to prepare the vein to accept a catheter. The proximal suture is tied to secure the catheter in the vein and the skin is closed. Care must be exercised throughout the procedure, since poor technique can result in injury to a tendon or nerve or extensive hemorrhage from soft tissue.

An alternate method of cannulating the vessel is to perform a "mini-cutdown" (Figure 21-9). In this technique, the vein is fully exposed and an over-the-needle catheter is inserted into the vein under direct visualization. Great care must be taken to avoid through-and-through puncture. The advantage of this technique is that it is easier to perform, especially in young children, and the vessel does not have to be sacrificed. Extensive tissue dissection and complete isolation of the vein are avoided, there is no need to place proximal and distal suture ties, and the catheter can be discontinued with simple pressure at the site.

The potential complications of venous cutdown include infection, phlebitis, and laceration of a nerve or artery.

INTRAOSSEOUS VASCULAR ACCESS

When vascular access cannot be obtained through other sites, intraosseous infusion may be life- or limb-saving. This method of vascular access, usually considered for children, may be used in adults as well. After 5 years of age, however, red marrow is steadily replaced by yellow marrow in the limbs, making infusion more difficult, and decreasing the potential infusion rate.

Arterial supply to bones is by a nutrient artery that pierces the cortex and bifurcates into ascending and descending branches; these further divide into arterioles that pierce the endosteal surface to become capillaries. The capillaries drain into medullary venous sinusoids within the medullary space; these then drain into a central venous channel. Catheter placement in the sinusoids provides ready access to the venous circulation.

For pediatric patients up to 5 years of age, the tibia is the preferred site (Figure 21-10). In adults, the most commonly used site is the medial malleolus. Although the sternum offers higher infusion rates for adults, this approach is attended by the potentially disastrous complication of puncture into the thoracic cavity. The tibial approach is technically more difficult in adults than in children because the adult bone is thicker and the needle tends to slip off the bone. Other potential insertion sites include the distal femur, clavicle, humerus, and ileum.

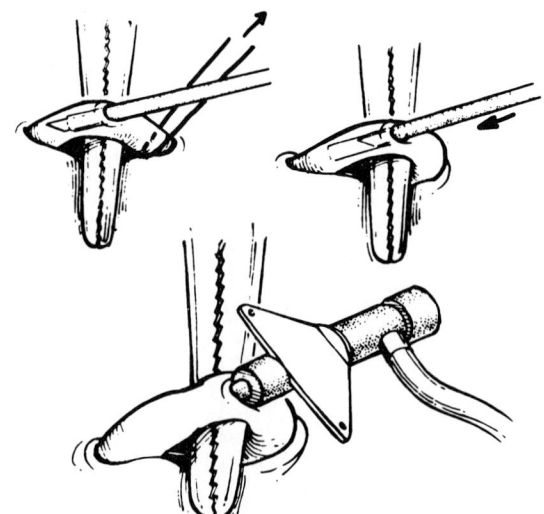

FIG. 21-9. A "mini-cutdown." The vessel is elevated with a hemostat and occluded with gentle traction from a distal tie. The needle is inserted and the sheath is advanced into the vessel. The vessel should not be tied off with this technique.

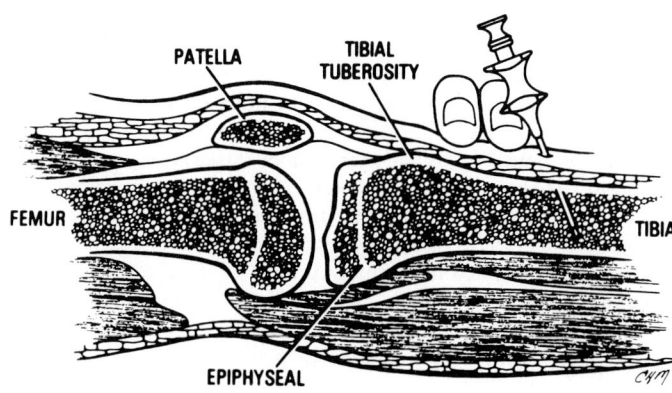

FIG. 21-10. The needle is inserted 2 cm distal to the tibial tuberosity on the medial aspect of the tibia. It is inserted in a caudal direction, away from the joint space.

Technique

Either standard bone marrow aspiration needles or specialized intraosseous infusion needles must be used because standard intravenous stylets and spinal needles are likely to bend during the procedure. For the proximal tibia, the puncture site is 1 to 2 cm distal to the midpoint between the tibial tuberosity and the medial aspect of the tibia; for the distal tibia, it is the medial surface of the ankle just proximal to the medial malleolus; and for the distal femur, it is the dorsal surface at the point where the condyles join the shaft of the bone. After disinfecting skin and anesthetizing skin and periosteum, the operator inserts the needle with the point directed away from the joint space (distally if the site is the proximal tibia, proximally at the other two sites). The needle is grasped in the palm of the hand and directed into the bone using a twisting motion to break through the cortex. Once this has occurred, resistance decreases and crepitus is encountered as the needle enters the marrow cavity. The stylet is then removed and aspiration with a syringe is performed to obtain blood and marrow for confirmation of positioning. If shock is present, aspiration may be unsuccessful; if this is the case, cautious infusion of several milliliters of NS should be attempted with careful observation for extravasation. If there is none, then the needle may be assumed to be positioned in the marrow cavity. A postprocedure x-ray should be performed to rule out the complication of iatrogenic fracture.

Complications

The incidence of infection, including both cellulitis and osteomyelitis, is less than 1 percent, similar to that for other techniques. The potential for infection can be minimized by limiting the duration of intraosseous infusion and avoiding hypertonic solutions. Fractures of the tibia have been reported. Fat embolism is rare and has been reported only in adult patients. Injury to the growth plate has also been mentioned as a potential complication, but there are no reports of serious morbidity arising from an injury to developing bone.

VASCULAR ACCESS IN CHILDREN

Scalp Vein Access

Scalp veins are easily accessible in children less than 1 year of age and provide a good route for maintenance fluid and drug administration (Figure 21-11). The superficial temporal, posterior auricular, and supratrochlear veins are the most easily catheterized scalp veins. In all cases, the vein must be differentiated from its respective artery. Arteries are generally more tortuous; they pulsate, and they fill from below, whereas veins fill from above.

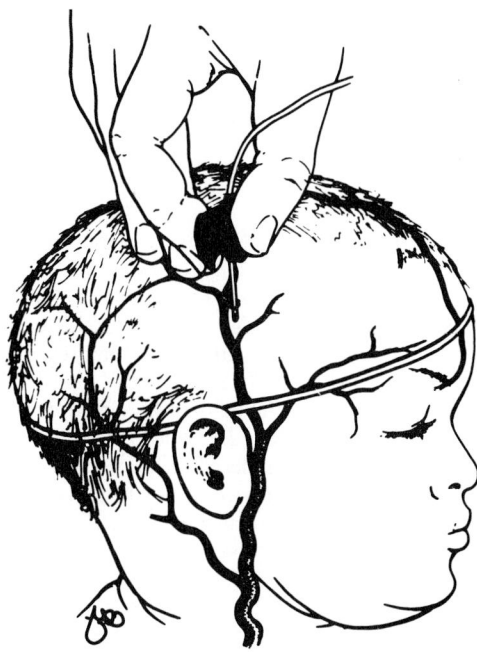

FIG. 21-11. A tourniquet is placed around the infant's head and the needle inserted 0.5 cm from the intended puncture site in the direction of blood flow.

The operator begins by shaving and disinfecting an area large enough to secure butterfly needle wings. A rubber-band tourniquet is placed around the head proximal to the venipuncture site and a butterfly needle—usually 23 to 27 gauge—is advanced into the vein. The needle is then taped at the skin entry point and at the butterfly is taped with cotton support under the wings. A cover (medicine cup) may be used to protect the area. Complications from this procedure include infection, bleeding, extravasation of fluid or medications, and inadvertent arterial puncture.

Umbilical Vein Access

In the first 1 to 2 weeks after birth, the umbilical vessels offer easy central venous access. Even a severely dehydrated umbilical stump may yield good vessels with adequate preparation. In a normal infant, there are two small umbilical arteries and a single larger vein. The arteries arise from the internal iliac artery while the vein is continuous with the portal vein.

The operator begins by cleansing the cord with an antiseptic. Avoid tincture of iodine because of the potential effect on the neonatal thyroid.[5] A transverse cut is made 1 cm above the junction of skin and cord, at which point a purse-string suture is placed. The single large vein and two smaller arteries are identified. A 3.5- to 5.0-F catheter is inserted into the vein and advanced to 4 to 5 cm in a term infant; further advancement may cause liver damage. The catheter should be filled with NS solution and flushed properly prior to placement to ensure an air-free system.

The most common complications relate to vascular insufficiency induced by the catheter. Evidence of ischemia—such as necrotizing enterocolitis, liver necrosis, poor peripheral circulation, or abdominal distention—is an indication for immediate removal of the catheter. The potential for infectious complications is equivalent to that for other indwelling catheters.

ARTERIAL ACCESS

Arterial access is predominantly concerned with arterial pressure monitoring or repeated arterial blood sampling. This is described in detail in Chap. 22, on invasive monitoring techniques.

SPECIAL PROBLEMS RELATED TO VENOUS ACCESS

Complications of Total Parenteral Nutrition

Central venous catheter placement for total parenteral nutrition (TPN) may be done short-term as a part of hospital care or long-term at home or in extended-care facilities. TPN is usually administered through a catheter placed into either the subclavian or jugular vein. The incidence of mechanical and septic complications depends on the skill, experience, and commitment of both the patient and the nutrition support team.[11] Suspicion of line sepsis demands immediate consultation. Most patients should be admitted, although the catheter may not need to be removed in selected cases.

Catheter occlusions occur in approximately 5 percent of patients receiving long-term TPN. If the first-line remedy of flushing the catheter with NS or heparin solution fails, thrombolytic agents, such as alteplase and reteplase may be used to lyse clots that obstruct the lumen of the catheter without obstructing the vessel. These agents are as effective as urokinase,[12,13] which was commonly used prior to its removal from the market in 1998. The recommended dose of alteplase is 1 to 2 mg, depending on the type of intravascular device and its filling volume. Alteplase is available in a small-dose 2 mg/2 mL vial (Cathflo). An appropriate volume of alteplase is instilled into the catheter, which is then clamped for 30 min. If no blood return is achieved, then one should wait another 120 min. If there is still no return, then a second attempt may be made with the same dosage and dwell times. Failure to clear the catheter after two dosages suggests either organized thrombus or anatomic abnormality; further diagnostic study such as angiography and ultrasound-Doppler duplex scanning may be indicated. Some authors have reported high success rates infusing ethanol (up to 3 mL of 70 percent solution) for presumed lipid occlusions, or hydrochloric acid (HCl 0.1N, up to 3 mL) to clear presumed mineral oil or other precipitates.

Catheter-related sepsis in patients receiving TPN is usually a result of catheter contamination by organisms colonizing the skin. Gram-negative bacteremia, sepsis syndrome, and fungemia are treated by removal of the catheter in association with appropriate antimicrobial therapy. Gram-positive infections can often be managed with the catheter left in place while antibiotic therapy is administered. The delivery of TPN through peripherally inserted central catheters (PICCs) is associated with slightly lower infection rates but a higher rate of mechanical failure. Because there is a considerably increased risk of both infection and thrombosis when femoral lines are used for TPN, this mode of access is less than optimal for patients requiring parenteral nutrition. Other reported complications include pulmonary embolism, line fracture, embolized catheter fragment, mediastinitis, superior vena cava syndrome, pneumothorax, air embolism, and lymphatic duct injury.

Accessing Indwelling Catheters

It is increasingly common for patients to present to EDs with specialized devices, such as Hickman catheters, which have been placed to provide long-term intravenous access. Such devices facilitate outpatient treatment in an era of increasing cost-consciousness. Emergency physicians can access these devices to obtain specimens for laboratory study as well as to administer intravenous fluids and medications.

When indwelling catheters are accessed, meticulous care should be taken to maintain sterility at the site. Depending on the type of device (implanted versus externalized), specialized equipment may be required to obtain access. Five milliliters of either NS or heparin flush (100 U/mL) is injected and then withdrawn gently to ensure catheter patency. Blood for laboratory study is collected only after a dead-space volume (5 to 10 mL) has been collected and discarded. Since these devices are heparinized, coagulation studies performed on such samples are unreliable; blood for these studies should be obtained from other sites. After access has been terminated, implanted devices should be flushed with heparin solution of 1000 U/mL strength. Other externalized devices should be flushed using a solution of 100 U/mL strength.

Arteriovenous fistulas and shunts should be used only for access in the most extreme of emergency situations, since complications, including loss of the access site, are common. The smallest needle appropriate to the task at hand should be inserted. Afterward, local pressure should be applied for 5 min or more, and these arterialized sites should be carefully monitored for hemorrhage for 12 h.

REFERENCES

1. Floccore DJ, Kelen GD, Altman NJ, et al: Rapid infusion of additive red blood cells: Alternative techniques for massive hemorrhage. *Ann Emerg Med* 19:129, 1990.
2. Dutky PA, Stevens SL, Maull KI: Factors affecting rapid fluid resuscitation with large bore intravenous catheters. *J Trauma* 29:856, 1989.
3. Herron DM, Grabowy R, Connolly R, et al: The limits of bloodwarming: Maximally heating blood with an inline microwave bloodwarmer. *J Trauma* 43:219, 1997.
4. Mermel LA: New technologies to prevent intravascular catheter-related bloodsteam infections. *Emerg Infect Dis* 7:197, 2001.
5. Centers for Disease Control and Prevention: Guidelines for the prevention of intravascular catheter-related infections. *MMWR* 51:(No. RR-10), 2002.
6. Conahan TJ, Schwartz AJ, Geer RT: Percutaneous catheter introduction: The Seldinger technique. *JAMA* 237:446, 1977.
7. Keenan SP: Use of ultrasound to place central lines. *J Crit Care* 17:126, 2002.
8. Slama M, Novara A, Safavian A, et al: Improvement of internal jugular vein cannulation using an ultrasound-guided technique. *Intensive Care Med* 23:916, 1997.
9. Merrer J, DeJonghe B, Golliot F, et al: Complications of femoral and subclavian venous catheterization in critically ill patients: A randomized controlled trial. *JAMA* 286:700, 2001.
10. Ruesch S, Walder B, Tramer MR: Complications of central venous catheters: Internal jugular versus subclavian access-a systematic review, *Crit Care Med* 30:454, 2002.
11. Savage AP, Picard M, Hopkins CC, et al: Complications and survival of multilumen central venous catheters used for total parenteral nutrition. *Br J Surg* 80:1287, 1993.
12. Castner D: The efficacy of reteplase in the treatment of thrombosed hemodialysis venous catheters. *Nephrol Nurs J* 28:403, 2001.
13. Walton T, Eyrich H: Tissue plasminogen activator use in maintaining patency in hemodialysis access catheters. *Am J Kidney Dis* 37:453, 2001.

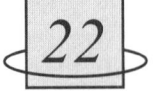

22

INVASIVE MONITORING, PACING TECHNIQUES, AND AUTOMATIC AND IMPLANTABLE DEFIBRILLATORS
Edward S. Bessman

INVASIVE MONITORING TECHNIQUES

General Considerations

Invasive pressure monitoring should never be the initial step in resuscitation. When clinically indicated, arterial line or pulmonary artery catheter (PAC) placement may be considered after initial stabilization is completed. If possible, these procedures should be deferred until the patient reaches the more controlled environment of the intensive care unit, unless there will be a significant delay.

The two essential components of any pressure monitoring system are a properly placed and secured catheter and a functioning pressure transducer-monitor. Ideally, the transducer and line for pressure monitoring should be set up and ready for use prior to the patient's arrival in the ED.

Arterial Cannulation

Arterial lines offer several advantages over monitoring blood pressure with an arm cuff. The arterial line provides continuous measurement of blood pressure and can be used for easy sequential sampling of blood gases. In the setting of marked vasoconstriction or hypotension, the arterial line usually gives more accurate pressure readings than a blood pressure cuff. The American College of Cardiology/American Heart Association practice guidelines for patients with acute myocardial infarction recommend intraarterial pressure monitoring for patients with severe hypotension or cardiogenic shock or who are receiving potent vasoactive infusions.[1] Other appropriate scenarios include hypertensive crisis, hypothermic cardiac arrest, and prolonged ED resuscitation.

Although the radial artery is the most frequently employed site, extensive experience using the brachial, femoral, and dorsalis pedis arteries has shown them to be equally satisfactory. In infants and neonates, the temporal or umbilical and dorsalis pedis arteries are most often accessed, although radial artery cannulation is also acceptable. While many operators are most familiar with the radial artery site, use of the femoral artery leaves the arm clear for other procedures and, in the presence of shock, the femoral artery is less difficult to cannulate percutaneously. Cutdown on the radial artery is an alternative in such patients.

Assessment

Although catheterization of the radial artery is associated with up to a 20 percent incidence of temporary flow obstruction by Doppler study, permanent ischemic complications requiring surgical reanastomosis or amputation are quite rare. Confirmation of collateral flow through a patent ulnar artery can be obtained by performing the Allen test: while the patient clenches the wrist for 1 min, the examiner compresses the radial and ulnar vessels with thumb and forefinger.[2] On release of ulnar compression, the patient partially extends the fingers, which are observed for accentuated rubor in comparison to the untested side. Patent ulnar circulation is indicated by return of rubor within 7 s; an equivocal result is 7 to 14 s. Greater than 14 s is considered definitely abnormal. If ulnar cannulation is contemplated, patency of the radial artery can be tested by the same test, with release of that vessel following compression. If the test result is positive, another site should be considered, but if that is not practical, then the clinician may have to proceed with radial artery cannulation in any case.[3]

Technique

Landmarks for radial and femoral artery cannulation are shown in Figure 22-1. The catheter (usually 20-gauge, 2 in. long for radial cannulation, and 18-gauge, 4 in. long for femoral cannulation) can be introduced by direct puncture threaded over the needle or by Seldinger technique threaded over a guidewire. Freely flowing, pulsatile, bright-red blood indicates proper placement. With marked hypotension or hypoxia, arterial blood flow may be mistaken for venous (nonpulsatile, dark blood returned). In all cases, connection to the transducer should reveal an arterial waveform if the catheter is in the proper position. Failure to visualize a waveform can be due to venous placement, air in the line, a closed stopcock, or a malfunction in the transducer or monitor.

Percutaneous cannulation of the brachial or femoral arteries may be possible when the radial pulse is absent in a hypotensive patient. The technique is similar to radial artery cannulation, although a careful groin preparation, preceded by removal of hair at that site to minimize the risk of infection, is necessary.

With profound hypotension, cutdown to the radial artery may be required to cannulate the artery. This is performed through a transverse incision similar to a venous cutdown (see Chap. 21). When 1 cm of artery is visible, the vessel is isolated by passing two lengths of silk suture beneath it using a hemostat. A catheter-through-needle device is passed through the skin distal to the area of exposure and advanced into the site. The artery may then be punctured and the catheter advanced. The suture, which is used only to control the artery, may then be removed and the skin incision closed.

Complications

Serious complications, such as infection and occlusion, are most closely related to duration of cannulation and are much more common among critically ill patients than among those undergoing adjunct monitoring. In the past, incidence of local infection in an ICU setting could approach 20 percent. Recent data indicates infection rates of less than 1 percent with no site differentiation (radial, brachial, femoral). Other complications that may be apparent in an ED include hematoma formation and hemorrhage. Both can usually be controlled with a pressure

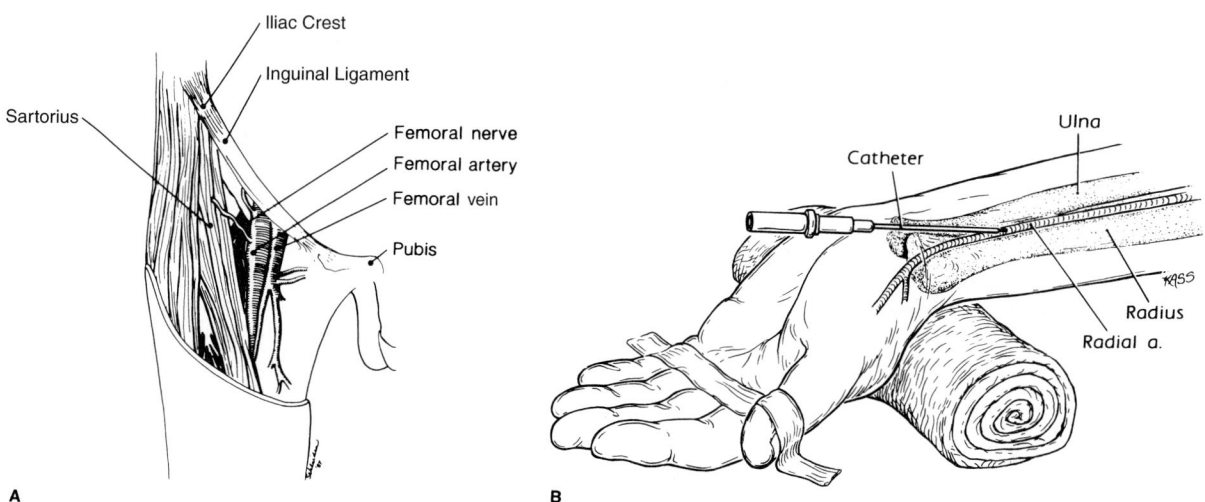

FIG. 22-1. Anatomic landmarks for arterial line placement. **A.** Fem-oral triangle. Note that the femoral artery lies lateral to the vein and midway between the pubis and the iliac crest. **B.** Radial aspect of the wrist. Note that mild extension of the wrist aids in successful placement. [Reproduced with permission from Beal JM (ed): *Critical Care for Surgical Patients.* New York: Macmillan, 1982.]

dressing. Arterial occlusion, thrombosis, or embolization with distal ischemia may occur. They are associated with placement in smaller vessels or in atherosclerotic vessels, with prolonged catheterization, and with use of end arteries that supply areas with poor collateral circulation. Permanent ischemic injury is very rare. Sepsis may result from local infection at the insertion site. Using the femoral or radial site can minimize these complications, along with proper attention to sterile technique and removal of the line as soon as feasible after the patient is stabilized.[1]

Pulmonary Artery Cannulation

A PAC is helpful in the measurement of critically ill patients with hemodynamic instability, particularly in the setting of acute myocardial infarction. Most important, the PAC can help to differentiate between shock due to intravascular volume depletion and that due to extensive left ventricular (LV) dysfunction. When the balloon tip of a PAC is properly inflated in a branch of the pulmonary artery, the pressure sensed by the catheter corresponds approximately to that in the left atrium. Left atrial pressure (which equals LV filling pressure) is an excellent indication of the adequacy of fluid resuscitation. If this pressure is low (<12 mm Hg), additional fluid resuscitation is indicated. If this pressure is high (>20 mm Hg), additional fluids are unlikely to improve cardiac performance; instead diuresis, afterload reduction, inotropic support, or vasopressors should be considered. Although the PAC can yield useful diagnostic information (Table 22-1), the distinction between the need for more fluids and the need for more LV support is its most useful application during resuscitation.[1] Volume assessment by central venous pressure monitoring is less reliable than PAC, especially in the presence of valvular or pulmonary disease.

A standard PAC is shown in Figure 22-2. The catheter has two fluid paths, one that terminates at the tip (the distal port) and a second that opens 10 to 15 cm from the tip (the proximal port). A third lumen connects to a 1.5-mL balloon located at the tip of the catheter. The balloon is ordinarily deflated except during insertion and when taking occlusion pressure measurements. When inflated during insertion, the balloon surrounds the tip of the PAC to prevent it from causing injury to the heart or great vessels as well as to help float the catheter through the heart as it is advanced. A temperature sensor is located about 5 cm proximal to the catheter tip and can be used to measure cardiac output via the thermodilution technique.

The procedure for insertion is described in detail elsewhere[4] but briefly is as follows. After central venous access is secured (see Chap. 21), the PAC, which has already been attached to a monitor and a pressure transducer, is slowly advanced through the introducer sheath. Once the tip of the catheter enters the vein, the balloon is inflated. By observing the pressure waveform transmitted via the distal port, the operator can follow the progress of the catheter through the heart, and ultimately into a branch of the pulmonary artery (Figure 22-3). Fluoroscopy is helpful to ensure quick and proper placement, but rarely is available in the ED.

With the PAC in position, the clinician can occlude the branch pulmonary artery by inflating the balloon. This gives the pulmonary artery occlusion pressure, or as it is more commonly known, the pulmonary capillary wedge pressure, which best reflects the pressure in the pulmonary capillary bed and the left atrium. The clinician can also rapidly measure pulmonary artery pressure, cardiac output, and central venous pressure. These measurements, when combined with arterial pressure measurement, enable the clinician to calculate systemic vascular resistance (see Chap. 30). These parameters are useful in the diagnosis and treatment of various shock states and in guiding therapy in acute myocardial infarction (see Table 50-8).

As with arterial cannulation, therapeutic procedures or definitive care should not be delayed solely to allow PAC placement. Complications include all the complications of central venous line placement (see Chap. 21). In addition, cardiac dysrhythmias and right bundle-branch block may occur as the catheter traverses the heart. Other potential complications include pulmonary embolism or infarction, knotting of the catheter, infection, and rupture of a small branch of the pulmonary artery.

The safety of PACs in the critical care environment has been questioned because of an association between its use and increased mortality rates.[5] Current consensus favors the continued use of PACs,[1] but underscores the need for definitive investigation. Benefits of PAC insertion in the ED have not been investigated. The advent of newer techniques, such as transesophageal echocardiography,[6] transthoracic impedance cardiography,[7] and magnetic resonance velocimetry[8] may further reduce the role of PACs in the ED. Recent studies have demonstrated the utility of these noninvasive hemodynamic monitoring techniques in the ED for both trauma and nontrauma patients.[9]

EMERGENCY PACING TECHNIQUES

General Considerations

Cardiac pacing serves to maintain or restore myocardial depolarization and thus ensure adequate cardiac output. In the ED, pacing may be performed therapeutically to correct an ongoing rhythm disturbance, or prophylactically in anticipation of possible conduction problems. Common situations that may respond to emergency pacing include bradyarrhythmias, asystole, and overdrive pacing of tachyarrhythmias. Detailed guidelines regarding the indications for emergency cardiac pacing may be found in Chap. 28. The techniques are described below.

Transcutaneous Pacing

Transcutaneous pacing has become the emergency technique of choice because of its easy application. It uses externally applied electrodes to deliver an electric impulse directly across the intact chest wall to stimulate the myocardium. Transcutaneous pacers differ from standard pulse generators in several important ways. The pulse duration of the stimulating impulse is longer and the current output higher than for internal pacing. Muscle contraction (usually the chest wall or diaphragm) is notable during pacing, especially at higher outputs. This results in a twitching or bucking activity that can make assessment of cardiac output by palpation of the radial, carotid, or femoral pulse unreliable during transcutaneous pacing. The higher current outputs used make cardiac monitoring with standard electrocardiogram (ECG) monitors problematic due to interference from the large-amplitude pacing spike. Most transcutaneous pacing units come equipped with a monitor that automatically filters the pacing spike so that simultaneous monitoring is possible.

The external pacing electrodes are quickly and easily applied to the chest and back. If separate defibrillator pads or paddles are used, they should be placed at least 2 to 3 cm away from the pacing pads. There is little risk of electrical injury to health care providers during transcutaneous pacing. **The electrodes are insulated, and chest compressions CPR can be administered directly over them** while pacing,

TABLE 22-1 Hemodynamic Diagnosis of Shock States

Type of Shock	CO	PCWP	SVR
Cardiogenic	↓	↑	↑
Hypovolemic	↓	↓	↑
Septic	↓ or ↑	↓	↓
Neurogenic	↑	↓	↓
Anaphylactic	↓	↓	↓

Abbreviations: CO = cardiac output; PCWP = pulmonary capillary wedge pressure; SVR = systemic vascular resistance; ↑ = increased; ↓ = decreased.

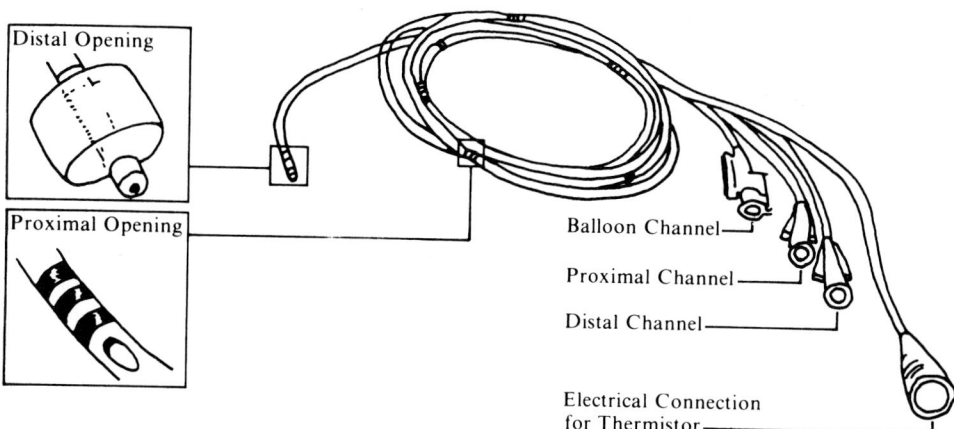

FIG. 22-2. Pulmonary artery thermodilution catheter. [Reproduced with permission from Beal JM (ed): *Critical Care for Surgical Patients.* New York: Macmillan, 1982.]

Distal Opening

Proximal Opening

Balloon Channel

Proximal Channel

Distal Channel

Electrical Connection for Thermistor

although it is recommended that pacing be discontinued during CPR to minimize inappropriate stimulation of the patient due to electrical artifacts. Inadvertent contact with the active pacing surface results only in a mild shock. In the setting of bradyasystolic arrest, it is reasonable to turn the stimulating current to maximum output and then decrease the output if capture is achieved. In a patient with a hemodynamically compromising bradycardia (but not in cardiac arrest), the operator should slowly increase the output from the minimum setting until capture is achieved; usually between 50–100 mA. Capture is assessed by following the ECG on the filtered monitor of the pacing unit and palpation of peripheral pulses. Bedside ultrasound may also be useful for determining external pacer capture.[10] The hemodynamic response to pacing must also be assessed, either by blood pressure cuff or arterial catheter. Ideally, pacing should be continued at 1.25 times the threshold of initial electrical capture.

As with other pacing systems, transcutaneous pacing may be fixed rate (asynchronous) or demand (synchronous). Asynchronous pacing delivers an electrical impulse at a regular interval without regard to intrinsic cardiac pacemaker activity. This creates the risk of precipitating

dysrhythmias if a pacing stimulus is given during the vulnerable period of ventricular repolarization. Synchronous pacing is therefore safer, since the pacing impulse is delivered only if an intrinsic electrical complex is not sensed within a preset interval. An increasing number of defibrillators include a built-in transcutaneous pacemaker. These units are equipped with multifunctional electrodes that allow defibrillation, pacing, and ECG monitoring through one set of pads. This development ensures that pacing will be available as soon as the defibrillator reaches the patient in cardiac arrest.

Failure to capture with transcutaneous pacing may be related to electrode placement or the patient's size. Patients who are conscious or who regain consciousness during transcutaneous pacing may experience discomfort due to muscle contraction. Analgesia with incremental doses of morphine or sedation with a benzodiazepine makes this discomfort tolerable. There is no evidence of clinically significant myocardial damage from properly performed transcutaneous pacing.[11] Nonetheless, transcutaneous pacing should be used for temporary stabilization only and should always be followed as soon as feasible by an internal pacing technique if there is a prolonged need for pacing.

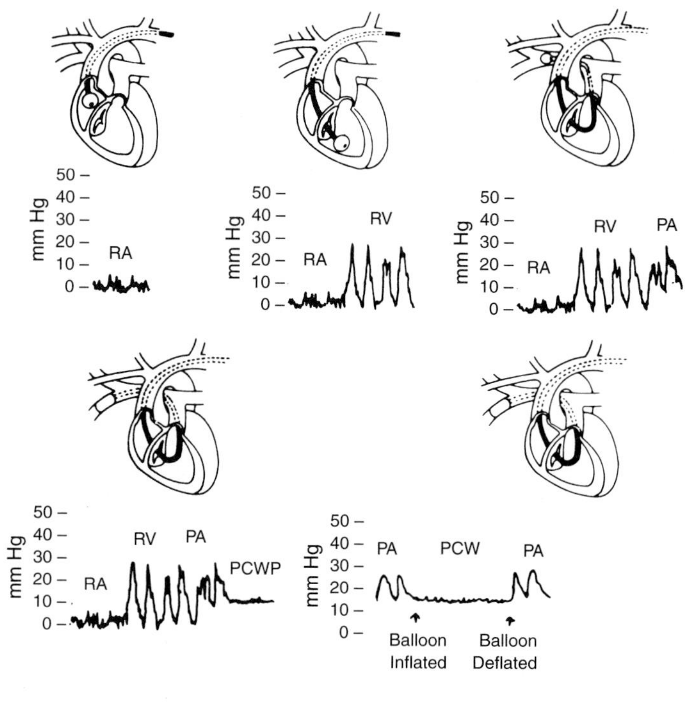

Transvenous Pacing

Transvenous pacing consists of endocardial stimulation of the right ventricle by an electrode introduced into a central vein. The most commonly encountered difficulties with transvenous pacing are securing venous access and obtaining proper placement of the stimulating electrode, both of which can be time-consuming. Venous access can be by any route. Transvenous pacing catheters can be inserted through a variety of venous introducers. A soft, flexible, semifloating bipolar catheter is preferred. This type of pacer is safest to use and takes advantage of any forward blood flow that may be present.

Placement of the catheter tip into the apex of the right ventricle is the key to successful transvenous pacing. Several techniques can aid successful placement. Fluoroscopic guidance is the surest method of right ventricular placement but is rarely available in the ED. Electrocardiographic guidance is useful in patients with narrow complexes and/or P waves when fluoroscopy is unavailable. There are some promising reports on the use of bedside ultrasound to guide transvenous pacemaker placement in the ED.[12,13] The safety and availability of ultrasound make this technique potentially very attractive. Balloon-tipped floating catheters may aid placement when used in conjunction with ECG and fluoroscopic guidance or when used alone. The balloon is inflated after catheter insertion into a central vein. Forward blood flow then directs the catheter tip toward the ventricle as the operator slowly advances the catheter. As with all balloon-tipped catheters, the balloon should always be deflated prior to withdrawal.

When patients have decreased or no forward blood flow (including many circumstances in which transvenous pacing would be used in the ED), positioning of the pacer tip within the right ventricle is difficult.

FIG. 22-3. Hemodynamic aspects of balloon catheter insertion into the pulmonary artery. [Reproduced with permission from Gottlieb AJ (ed): *The Whole Internist Catalog.* Philadelphia: Saunders, 1980.]

Balloon-tipped catheters are not much of an aid in placement during low- or no-flow states. In a true emergency, the pacemaker electrodes are connected to the power source and the catheter advanced blindly in hopes that the tip will encounter the endocardium of the right ventricle and that capture will result. In this setting a right internal jugular venous access route should be used. From this approach, the catheter traverses a straight line into the right ventricle and rarely curls in the atrium or deflects into the inferior vena cava.

Pacer settings vary with the clinical situation. An initial rate of 80 to 100 impulses/min is appropriate for most patients. Asynchronous mode (sensitivity off) is used initially in patients requiring emergency pacing for hemodynamically unstable bradycardias. The ECG should be followed to determine the presence or absence of capture (Figure 22-4). Output should initially be set at maximum (usually 20 mA) and then decreased after capture is achieved. With optimal tip position, capture should occur at less than 2 mA. Pacing should be continued at 1.5 to 2 times the threshold output required for capture. Subsequent rate and sensitivity settings should be adjusted as clinically indicated by the patient's hemodynamic status and underlying rhythm disturbance.

Chest radiographs should be obtained after the patient is stabilized to ensure proper tip placement and to evaluate the possibility of pneumothorax from the preceding central venous line placement. Finally, care should be taken to firmly affix the pacing catheter to the insertion site prior to transferring the patient. Transvenous pacing is best used in urgent rather than emergent situations, particularly when there is adequate time to utilize fluoroscopy. In the setting of cardiac arrest, transcutaneous pacing is preferred.

Transthoracic pacing is mentioned here largely for historic reasons, since external pacing techniques have largely replaced its use. However, whenever transvenous pacing is tried but unsuccessful, transthoracic pacing may still be attempted. When the latter technique is performed blindly, the likelihood of successful placement is low, with risk of liver, pulmonary artery, diaphragm, lung, or coronary artery puncture.[14] Although it has not been studied, use of ultrasound-guided placement may improve results.

AUTOMATIC AND IMPLANTABLE DEFIBRILLATORS

In 1933, William Kouwenhoven observed in dogs that closed-chest electrical shocks delivered within 30 s of inducing ventricular fibrillation (VF) were 98 percent effective in terminating the dysrhythmia. After 2 min of VF, the rate of resuscitation fell to 27 percent. He reported similar results in human subjects.[15] Modern research indicates that the likelihood for successful resuscitation decreases roughly 10 percent/min after the onset of VF. Thus the goal of emergency cardiac care is to deliver defibrillation as quickly as possible.

Two recent technologic developments have led to the more rapid application of defibrillation. Automatic external defibrillators allow first responders to rapidly institute defibrillation. Even laypersons, such as family members or bystanders, can learn to use these devices.

In addition, implanted defibrillators allow patients with frequent malignant ventricular dysrhythmias to carry their own defibrillators with them at all times. Emergency physicians need to be familiar with these devices and the special considerations associated with their use.

Automatic External Defibrillators

Automatic external defibrillators (AEDs) have relatively simple controls and can be used by minimally trained providers to initiate defibrillation. The operator places electrode pads at the patient's right sternal border and cardiac apex. Pads are used both for monitoring and defibrillating. Once applied, the AED must be turned on. The AED analyzes the cardiac rhythm and initiates its treatment algorithm. A fully automatic device will deliver a countershock once ventricular tachycardia or VF has been sensed. The AED gives an audible announcement that defibrillation will commence, and the only way the operator can prevent discharge is to turn off the device. A semiautomatic AED analyzes the rhythm and then advises whether a shock is indicated. The operator must press the control button in order to initiate defibrillation.

AEDs shock patients in VF several times sequentially until an organized cardiac rhythm results or until the maximum number of shocks allowed by the programmed algorithm is reached. Many devices also provide a record of rhythms and events during their use, which allows the emergency physician to subsequently reconstruct the sequence of events during resuscitation.

An AED may be placed on an unstable patient in anticipation of subsequent deterioration, but the device should not be activated until or unless the patient is pulseless. Since motion artifacts may confuse the rhythm-analysis circuitry, the **AED should not be in the sensing mode during CPR, during transport, or if the patient has a seizure.** Unlike transcutaneous pacemakers, AEDs can deliver a debilitating shock to the operator or other personnel, and the same precautions regarding contact with the patient during defibrillation should be followed with AEDs as with standard defibrillators. The failure of an AED to restore a perfusing rhythm is a poor prognostic sign often associated with long arrest times or arrest rhythms other than VF. When an AED fails to resuscitate a patient in arrest, advanced cardiac life support (ACLS) guidelines should be followed.

AEDs are most effective in tiered emergency medical services systems where AED-equipped first responders reach the patient rapidly and are backed up by the later arrival of paramedics with full advanced life-support capabilities. There is ongoing interest in making AEDs available for widespread use by nonmedical personnel and the lay public,[16-18] although this initiative is controversial.[19]

Implantable Cardioverter-Defibrillators

The first human placement of an implantable cardioverter-defibrillator (ICD) took place in 1980 at the Johns Hopkins Hospital. Since that

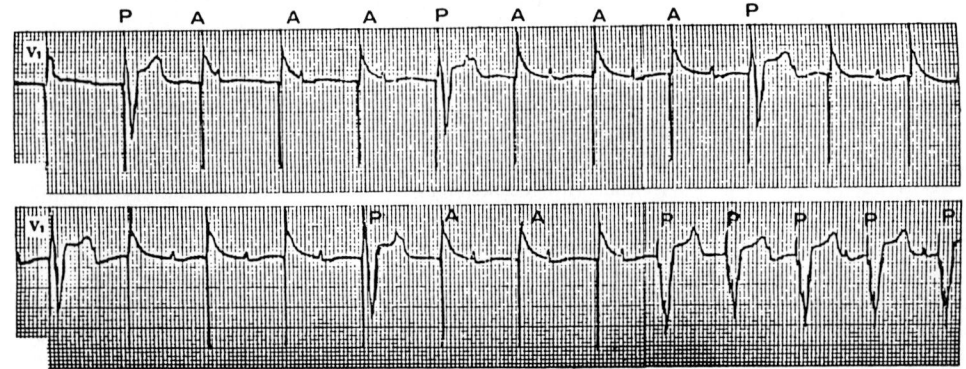

FIG. 22-4. Pacing with intermittent capture. "P" indicates paced beats and "A," pacer artifact without capture.

time it has become the treatment of choice for sudden cardiac death, reducing mortality from about 30 to 45 percent/year to less than 2 percent/year. This remarkable efficacy, coupled with the failure (and potentially proarrhythmic effects) of pharmacologic therapy and the increasing sophistication and miniaturization of the devices, has led to an explosion in ICD use. Through 1994 there had been roughly 50,000 ICDs implanted worldwide; in 1995 there were more than 20,000 implantations in the United States alone. Expanding indications for ICD implantation make it likely that emergency physicians will regularly see patients with these devices.[20]

An ICD consists of a pulse generator, a lead system with both sensing and shocking electrodes, circuitry to analyze the cardiac rhythm and trigger defibrillation, and a power supply. There are currently three generations of ICDs. In each successive generation, the devices have become smaller, more sophisticated, more reliable, and easier to implant. Second-generation ICDs are still quite common. These devices generally were placed by thoracotomy or sternotomy, and defibrillation occurred through electrodes positioned inside or outside the pericardium. Rate-sensing electrodes were placed epicardially or transvenously. The sensing algorithms for second-generation ICDs were relatively unsophisticated; they reliably detected ventricular tachycardia and VF, but would cause the devices to inappropriately shock supraventricular rhythms as well. Roughly one-third of patients with second-generation ICDs receive at least one shock triggered by a supraventricular tachycardia during the working life of the device.

Third-generation ICDs have a volume of about 60 mL, or roughly one-quarter that of second-generation devices. The sensing-pacing-defibrillation electrodes are placed transvenously, and the device itself is generally implanted subcutaneously in the subpectoral region or in an abdominal pocket. A subcutaneous patch electrode may be used to help lower the defibrillation threshold. On a chest radiograph, at first glance these devices can easily be mistaken for conventional pacemakers. Careful examination of the electrodes will reveal their true nature (Figure 22-5). Newer ICDs are better at discriminating supraventricular tachycardia and are capable of a variety of responses to ventricular tachycardia and VF. Most are programmed to follow a tiered approach to ventricular dysrhythmias: antitachycardia pacing, low-energy cardioversion, and finally defibrillation. Depending on the frequency of discharge and whether the pacemaker function is used, the latest ICDs have a projected life span of about 8 years.

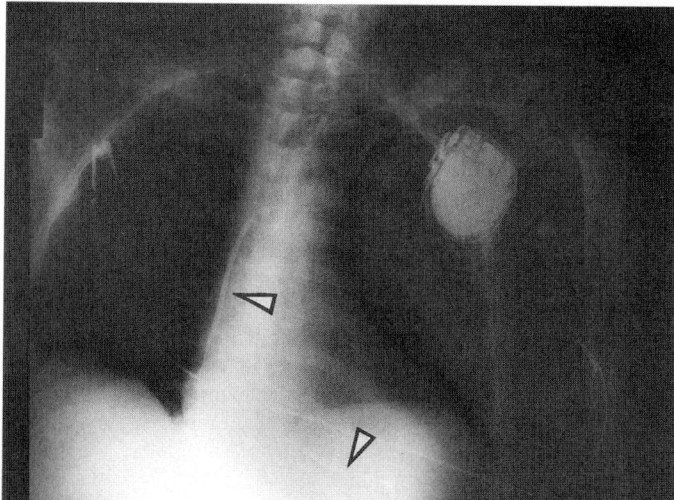

FIG. 22-5. Chest radiograph of a patient with a nonthoracotomy implanted third-generation defibrillator. The ICD is in the left subpectoral area. The electrodes *(arrows)* have been placed transvenously. The proximal spring electrode is positioned at the junction of the superior vena cava and the right atrium. The distal electrode is in the right ventricle.

EMERGENCY DEPARTMENT EVALUATION AND THERAPY

ICDs are remarkably effective in preventing sudden cardiac death. The most common cause of death in patients with ICDs is congestive heart failure, which should be managed in standard fashion in the ED. However, the most common reason an ICD patient comes to the ED is to be evaluated for the appropriateness of a previously delivered shock. Causes of inappropriate shock delivery are summarized in Table 22-2. It is important to determine the number of shocks delivered, the activity of the patient at the time, and any prodromal symptoms or postshock trauma. Recent changes in antiarrhythmic drug dosage should be noted. The physical examination should focus on the vital signs, the cardiovascular status, the generator pocket, and evidence of incidental trauma. The patient should be monitored during the evaluation. An ECG should be obtained and interpreted with the knowledge that ST-segment elevations or depressions due exclusively to the shock will resolve within 15 min. A chest radiograph may reveal electrode migration, displacement, or fracture. Drug levels of antiarrhythmics should be determined and electrolyte disturbances explored.

Admission criteria depends on the reason for shock delivery. The patient's cardiologist should be consulted and the ICD can be interrogated by external telemetry devices that are manufacturer and model specific. General admission recommendations include unstable patients, two or more shocks in a 1-week period, correctable causes of dysrhythmia, and any sign of infection or mechanical disruption of the ICD or lead system. The ICD can be interrogated by external telemetry devices that are specific to the individual ICD manufacturers and models.

For an ICD patient in cardiac arrest, normal basic and advanced resuscitation measures are followed. **If defibrillation is necessary, the operator should avoid placing either paddle directly over the ICD.** The presence of epicardial patch electrodes may shield the myocardium from the countershock and may therefore necessitate repositioning of the paddles. CPR may be performed in the usual fashion. If the ICD should discharge during CPR, the provider may perceive a small electrical shock, but it is neither uncomfortable nor dangerous.

Occasionally it may become necessary to temporarily deactivate the ICD, as in the case of inappropriate shock for a stable rhythm. Second-generation devices may be deactivated by placing a donut-shaped magnet over the right upper quadrant (Figure 22-6) of the pulse generator for 30 s until the intermittent beeping ceases and a solid tone is heard. The magnet is then removed. If this does not succeed, then deactivation is attempted by placing the magnet over the opposite corner of the pulse generator (some are surgically positioned upside down). The response of third-generation devices to a magnet can be complex, but generally defibrillation is deactivated only when the magnet is present. This requires taping the magnet to the skin overlying the ICD. Defibrillation can be reenabled by removing the magnet. Some third-generation devices are programmed so that they cannot be deactivated by a magnetic field. All ICDs should be evaluated by a cardiologist after exposure to a magnet.[21]

TABLE 22-2   Potential Causes of Inappropriate ICD Shock Delivery

False sensing
Supraventricular tachycardia with rapid ventricular response
Muscular activity (shivering, diaphragmatic contraction)
Extraneous source (tapping of chest wall, vibrations, pacer spikes)
Sensing T waves as QRS complex (double counting)
Sensing lead fracture or migration
Unsustained tachyarrhythmia
ICD-pacemaker interactions
Component failure

Source: Adapted from Munter WM, DeLacey WA: Automatic implantable cardioverter defibrillators. *Emerg Med Clin North Am* 12:579, 1994. Used with permission.

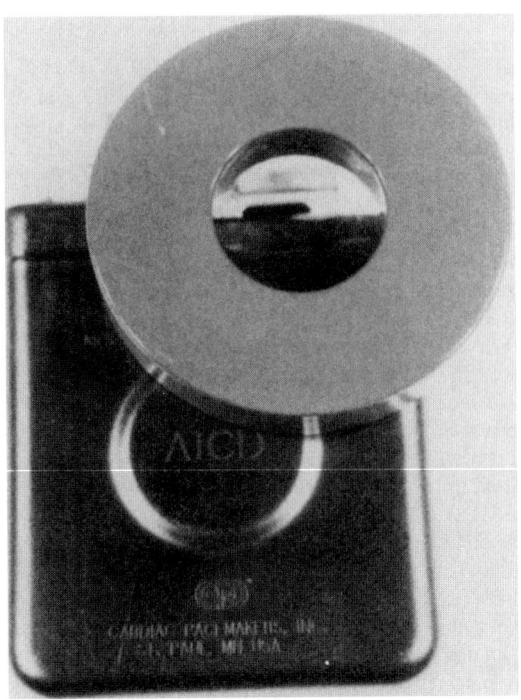

FIG. 22-6. Correct magnet placement to deactivate second-generation ICD. (Reproduced with permission from Chapman PD, Veseth-Rogers JL, Duquette SE: The implantable defibrillator and the emergency physician. *Ann Emerg Med* 18:579, 1989.)

REFERENCES

1. Ryan TJ, Anderson JL, Antman EM, et al: ACC/AHA guidelines for the management of patients with acute myocardial infarction: A report of the American College of Cardiology/American Heart Association Task Force on Practice Guidelines (Committee on Management of Acute Myocardial Infarction). *J Am Coll Cardiol* 28:1328, 1996.
2. Allen EV: Thromboangiitis obliterans: Methods of diagnosis of chronic occlusive arterial lesions distal to the wrist with illustrative cases. *Am J Med Sci* 178:237, 1929.
3. Slogoff S, Keats AS, Arlund C: On the safety of radial artery cannulation. *Anesthesiology* 59:42, 1983.
4. Kong R, Singer M: Insertion of a pulmonary artery flotation catheter: How to do it. *Br J Hosp Med* 57:432, 1997.
5. Connors AF, Speroff T, Dawson NV, et al: The effectiveness of right heart catheterization in the initial care of critically ill patients. *JAMA* 276:889, 1996.
6. Laupland KB, Bands CJ: Utility of esophageal Doppler as a minimally invasive hemodynamic monitor: A review. *Can J Anaesth* 49:393, 2002.
7. Woltjer HH, Bogaard HJ, Bronzwaer JG, et al: Prediction of pulmonary capillary wedge pressure and assessment of stroke volume by noninvasive impedance cardiography. *Am Heart J* 134:450, 1997.
8. Mohiaddin RH, Gatehouse PD, Henien M, et al: Cine MR fourier velocimetry of blood flow through cardiac valves: Comparison with Doppler echocardiography. *J Magn Reson Imaging* 7:657, 1997.
9. Shoemaker WC, Belzberg H, Wo CC, et al: Multicenter study of noninvasive monitoring systems as alternatives to invasive monitoring of acutely ill emergency patients. *Chest* 114:1643, 1998.
10. Ettin D, Cook T: Using ultrasound to determine external pacer capture. *J Emerg Med* 17:1007, 1999.
11. Hedges JR, Syverud S, Dalsey WC, et al: Threshold, enzymatic, and pathologic changes associated with prolonged transcutaneous pacing in a chronic heart block model. *J Emerg Med* 7:1, 1989.
12. Macedo W Jr, Sturman K, Kim JM, et al: Ultrasonic guidance of transvenous pacemaker insertion in the emergency department: A report of three cases. *J Emerg Med* 17:491, 1999.
13. Aguilera PA, Durham BA, Riley DA: Emergency transvenous cardiac pacing placement using ultrasound guidance. *Ann Emerg Med* 36:224, 2000.
14. Brown CG: Injuries associated with percutaneous placement of transthoracic pacemakers. *Ann Emerg Med* 14:223, 1985.
15. Kouwenhoven WB: Closed chest defibrillation of the heart. *Surgery* 42:550, 1952.
16. Kerber RE, Becker LB, Bourland JD, et al: Automatic external defibrillators for public access defibrillation: Recommendations for specifying and reporting arrhythmia analysis algorithm performance, incorporating new waveforms, and enhancing safety. A statement for health professionals from the American Heart Association Task Force on Automatic External Defibrillation, Subcommittee on AED Safety and Efficacy. *Circulation* 95:1677, 1997.
17. Myerburg RJ, Fenster J, Velez M, et al: Impact of community-wide police car deployment of automated external defibrillators on survival from out-of-hospital cardiac arrest. *Circulation* 106:1058, 2002.
18. Capucci A, Aschieri D, Piepoli MF, et al: Tripling survival from sudden cardiac arrest via early defibrillation without traditional education in cardiopulmonary resuscitation. *Circulation* 106:1065, 2002.
19. Pell JP, Sirel JM, Marsden AK, et al: Potential impact of public access defibrillators on survival after out of hospital cardiopulmonary arrest: Retrospective cohort study. *BMJ* 325:515, 2002.
20. Bigger JT: Expanding indications for implantable cardiac defibrillators. *New Engl J Med* 346:931, 2002.
21. Rasmussen MJ, Friedman PA, Hammill SC, et al: Unintentional deactivation of implantable cardioverter-defibrillators in health care settings. *Mayo Clin Proc* 77:855, 2002.

23 CEREBRAL RESUSCITATION
Gary S. Krause
Blaine C. White

Cerebral ischemia continues to affect a substantial portion of the population of the United States. Data from the ARIC (Atherosclerotic Risk in Communities), CHS (Cardiovascular Health Study), and the NHLBI (National Heart, Lung, and Blood Institute) show that about 600,000 people suffer a new or recurrent stroke each year. Furthermore, stroke is the leading cause of serious, long-term disability in the United States. Three million Americans are currently permanently disabled because of stroke, and 31 percent of stroke survivors need help caring for themselves, 20 percent need help walking, 71 percent have an impaired vocational capacity when examined an average of 7 years later, and 16 percent have to be institutionalized. The direct and indirect cost of stroke in 1998 was estimated at over $40 billion. In addition, cardiopulmonary resuscitation for victims of cardiac arrest, both within and outside of the hospital, succeeds in restoring spontaneous circulation in about 70,000 patients a year in the United States. At least 60 percent of these patients subsequently die in the hospital as a result of extensive brain damage; only 3 to 10 percent of resuscitated patients are finally able to resume their former lifestyles. Clearly, the development of effective interventions to prevent these sequelae of brain ischemia and reperfusion would enormously enhance the value of the investment already made and would return thousands of these impaired patients to renewed vigorous and productive time with their families and in our society.

There are two important issues involved in the ongoing effort to reduce this neurologic morbidity. One is discovery of the mechanisms involved in tissue injury and repair, and the other is the identification of clinically effective therapy. Clinical trials conducted more than a decade ago utilizing postresuscitation treatment with barbiturates or calcium antagonists were disappointing. More recently, clinical treatment of stroke with a radical scavenger (tirilazad), intercellular adhesion molecule-1 antagonist (enlimomab), glutamate receptor antagonist (aptiganel, gavestinel), glutamate release inhibitor (lubeluzole), ganglioside administration (GM1), calcium channel blockade, or upregulation of the GABA receptor (clomethiazole) were all found ineffective. This suggests that our understanding of the mechanisms involved in damage and repair of neurons remains incomplete.

Four major observations have provided the foundation for investigation of brain injury by ischemia and reperfusion:[1] (1) rapid loss of high-energy phosphate compounds during ischemia followed by their recovery within the first 15 min of reperfusion, (2) morphologic evidence that most structural damage occurs during reperfusion, especially in selectively vulnerable zones, (3) progressive brain hypoperfusion during postischemic reperfusion, and (4) prolonged suppression of protein synthesis in selectively vulnerable neurons. Cardiac arrest resulting in ischemic-anoxic brain injury is characterized by three phases: ischemia, early reperfusion, and late reperfusion. We have published extensive reviews of our theoretical model of the causal interactions of neuronal injury and repair mechanisms during ischemia and reperfusion.[1,2] Briefly, primary injury mechanisms include, at a minimum, activation of phospholipases and proteolytic enzymes (calpain) during ischemia and generation of radicals accompanied by lipid peroxidation and caspase activation during reperfusion. This chapter outlines the crucial role of calcium and iron in these injury mechanisms and suggests possible therapies to ameliorate brain injury following an ischemic insult.

ISCHEMIC PHASE

Morphologic studies have shown that the extent of tissue injury observed following ischemia largely reflects damage incurred during reperfusion and have identified specific populations of brain neurons that are exceptionally susceptible to damage and death. These selectively vulnerable neurons include the pyramidal neurons in layers 3 and 5 of the cortex and those found in the CA1 and hilum of the hippocampus. Minimal ultrastructural injury is seen in the brain during complete ischemia. Some margination and clumping of nuclear chromatin is seen by 10 to 15 min of complete ischemia. Mitochondria may be slightly swollen, but their structure does not show major degenerative alterations for up to 30 min of complete ischemia. Similarly, some swelling of the endoplasmic reticulum (ER) may be seen during ischemia, but the polyribosomes remain appropriately associated with the ER, and disaggregation of polyribosomes does not occur during complete ischemia. Nuclear and plasma membranes show a normal, well-defined bilaminar structure without evidence of holes or general structural disintegration.

In contrast to the paucity of morphologic findings, there are severe biochemical alterations. With the onset of cardiac arrest there is precipitous decline in brain oxygen content, which approaches zero within 6 to 12 s. Neurons have very limited reserves of glucose, glycogen, or phosphocreatine; therefore oxygen depletion leads to a sharp decline in tissue adenosine triphosphate (ATP) levels, which approach zero within 4 min. Anaerobic glycolysis and ATP depletion lead to lactic acidosis and hypoxanthine accumulation, respectively, during the ischemic phase. Since about 80 percent of the brain's ATP is used to maintain transmembrane ionic gradients for potassium, sodium, and calcium, these ionic gradients also decay rapidly. During complete ischemic anoxia, these ions equilibrate between the extra- and intracellular fluid within 5 to 10 min of the insult.

The high cytosolic calcium level, thought to be a major initiating event leading to cell death,[3] causes several key events: the activation of membrane phospholipase A_2, proteolytic cleavage of xanthine dehydrogenase, activation of the proteolytic enzyme calpain, activation of nitric oxide synthase (NOS), and release of excitatory neurotransmitters such as glutamate. Phospholipase A_2 cleaves a fatty acid, primarily arachidonate, from the cell membrane lipids, yielding a free fatty acid and in the process damaging the membrane's structure. The proteolysis of xanthine dehydrogenase in brain endothelial cells produces xanthine oxidase, which will react with hypoxanthine to produce the superoxide radical ($O_2^{\cdot-}$) upon reperfusion. Proteins that are degraded by calpain during either ischemia or reperfusion include microtubule-associated protein kinase-2, tubulin, neurofilament protein, spectrin, protein kinase C, calcium/calmodulin kinase II, and the translation initiation factors eIF4E and eIF4G (see below).

EARLY REPERFUSION

During early reperfusion, ATP levels and total adenylate charge recover rapidly. If the ischemic insult has been less than 20 min, the membrane ionic gradients also recover quickly. After much longer insults of 1 to 3 h, total tissue calcium loads actually increase during reperfusion. It is felt that this reflects extensive and irreversible cell membrane injury during these very prolonged periods of ischemia.

Arachidonate is rapidly oxidized by both cyclooxygenase and lipoxygenase, and returns to preischemic levels within 30 min of reperfusion. Several vasoactive substances are produced by the metabolism of arachidonate. The prostaglandins are the products of cyclooxygenase, and the leukotrienes are the products of lipoxygenase. The production of the vasodilatory prostaglandin prostacyclin is severely inhibited during early reperfusion. Thus vasospastic compounds predominate in the leukotriene and prostaglandin products. While the free arachidonic acid levels rapidly return to baseline during reperfusion, leukotrienes remain markedly elevated for at least 24 h. The time course of leukotriene elevation may explain the alterations in blood flow seen in the postischemic brain (the "no-reflow" phenomenon). Restoration of normal or mildly hypertensive systemic arterial pressure produces an initial brain hyperperfusion. However, within 1 h, global brain perfusion has dropped to levels of 20 to 40 percent of normal, where it remains for up to 1 to 2 days. This phenomenon occurs without a change in intracranial pressure and was originally thought to lead to failure of high-energy metabolism and neuronal death during reperfusion. However, therapy that inhibited postischemic brain hypoperfusion had little effect on neurologic outcome.

Membrane lipids are extensively peroxidized by iron-dependent radical reactions during reperfusion. Within the first 30 s of reperfusion, there is a brief burst of oxygen-based free radical production, although the precise identity of the radical species remains unknown. Xanthine oxidase and cyclooxygenase, whose substrates are hypoxanthine and arachidonate respectively, produce $O_2^{\cdot-}$ as a side product. In addition, $O_2^{\cdot-}$ reacts with nitric oxide produced by NOS to form peroxynitrite which may also initiate lipid peroxidation. Availability of a transition metal, such as iron, is required for reaction of oxygen radicals with tissue macromolecules, including lipids (lipid peroxidation). The brain glia have abundant stores of oxidized (ferric) iron, mostly in ferritin and transferrin, forms in which the iron is unable to act as a catalyst for oxygen radical reactions. However, $O_2^{\cdot-}$, which is present in excessive amounts during early reperfusion, promotes reduction of ferric iron and release of ferrous iron from ferritin, and lipid peroxidation in the reperfused brain has been demonstrated by many laboratories and maps to selectively vulnerable neurons. These reactions also appear to be involved in the genesis of the postischemic hypoperfusion phenomenon, which is inhibited by superoxide dismutase and deferoxamine or U74006F, a lipid peroxidation chain terminator.

Excitatory amino acid neurotransmitters appear to play a role in the injury produced by focal brain ischemia such as stroke; it is unclear whether the same holds true in global brain ischemia. However, excitatory neurotransmitter uptake is inhibited by arachidonate and products of lipid peroxidation, and thus continued stimulation of receptors may contribute to neuronal damage by as yet unidentified mechanisms.

Suppression of protein production has long been known to occur in the brain following ischemia and reperfusion and is likely to be an important contributing factor in neuronal death. The brain has a substantial requirement for protein synthesis just to maintain cerebral function. It expresses the largest percentage of its DNA of any organ, and its protein turnover is approximately equal to 100 percent of its protein content every 48 h. Additionally, as a result of ischemia and reperfusion, there is a significant need for replacement of proteins damaged by calpain-mediated proteolysis and membrane lipid peroxidation (neuronal membranes are ~50 percent protein). Because proteins have such fundamental roles in the cell, including enzymatic reactions governing intermediary metabolism, transport, and storage, as well as intracellular signaling and cellular structure, significant changes in the neurons' ability to produce and maintain proteins would be expected to have considerable effect on the cells' capacity to survive. Indeed, inhibition of protein synthesis may itself trigger apoptosis.

Protein synthesis is suppressed during ischemia by lack of ATP.[4] However, even with the rapid restoration of ATP levels that accompanies reperfusion, there is a severe suppression of protein synthesis that varies with duration of ischemia, brain region, and individual proteins. Whereas most regions of the brain recover their ability to synthesize protein following a short ischemic period, protein synthesis in the selectively vulnerable regions is depressed by about 90 percent early in reperfusion and does not recover significantly. Failure of protein synthesis is due to a disruption in the formation of new ribosomal translation complexes. Initiation, the rate-limiting step in translation, requires the coordinated assembly of the ribosomal subunits, the mRNA to be translated, and the amino-acyl tRNA for the first amino acid (always methionine in eukaryotes). This process is orchestrated by a family of proteins named *eukaryotic initiation factors* (eIFs). The eIF4 and eIF2 complexes are the major regulatory points for translation initiation. Cellular mRNAs vary greatly in their binding efficiency to eIF4E, and under normal physiologic situations, message selection for translation initiation is modulated by altering the phosphorylation of Ser^{209} on eIF4E. However, under conditions of cellular stress (e.g., heat shock, viral infection, or starvation), rates of global protein synthesis are downregulated by phosphorylating Ser^{51} on the α-subunit of eIF2 [eIF2α(P)].

Studies have now identified important changes in eIFs that occur during brain ischemia and reperfusion: (1) there is a modest degree of proteolytic degradation of eIF4E during ischemia, but without change in its phosphorylation state during either ischemia or reperfusion;[5,6] (2) there is substantial proteolytic degradation of eIF4G mediated by calpain during both ischemia and reperfusion;[7,8] and (3) probably most important, there is an approximately twentyfold increase in eIF2α(P) during early reperfusion. In nonischemic tissue, phosphorylated eIF2α is found exclusively in astrocytes.[9] After only 10 min postischemic reperfusion, there is prominent eIF2α(P) immunostaining in the cytoplasm of neurons in both the hippocampus and cortex. After 1 h of reperfusion, eIF2α(P) is prominent in both the nuclei and cytoplasm of selectively vulnerable neurons in both the hippocampus and cortex; nuclear eIF2α(P) is never seen in ischemia-resistant neurons. By 4 h reperfusion, the pattern of nuclear eIF2α(P) immunostaining in vulnerable neurons suggests nuclear condensation consistent with the early stages of apoptosis. These results provide a mechanism for the inhibition of protein synthesis in vulnerable neurons during reperfusion and, together with other evidence suggesting a role for eIF2α(P) in causing apoptosis, may represent a fundamental phenomenon in the causal pathway leading to the death of vulnerable neurons. It is interesting to note that animals treated with 20 units/kg insulin at resuscitation are able to dephosphorylate eIF2α(P) and recover protein synthesis in vulnerable hippocampal neurons by 90 min reperfusion. The activation of the eIF2α kinase PERK, which phosphorylates eIF2α during reperfusion, and the salutary effects of high-dose insulin imply that cell signaling pathways, in particular the unfolded protein response (UPR) and the PI-3 kinase/Akt pathway respectively, play a role in neuronal injury/survival mechanisms. Thus, growth factors, including fibroblast growth factor, nerve growth factor, insulin-like growth factor 1, and insulin, all of which have been shown to improve neuronal survival in the laboratory, may have a role in limiting and repairing neuronal damage.[10]

LATE EVENTS DURING REPERFUSION

After 15-min transient global ischemia, caspases have been proteolytically activated in the hippocampal CA1 neurons at 8 to 72 h of reperfusion, resulting in deoxyribonuclease activity, PKR activation and

eIF2α phosphorylation, cleavage of eIF4E-binding protein 1, which inhibits cap-dependent translation, and cleavage of eIF2α, eIF4B, and eIF4G. Studies will be needed to examine alterations in message translation and in intracellular signaling that occur following an ischemic insult.[11,12] Brain tissue ionic concentrations are indistinguishable from normal after 4 h of reperfusion following a 15-min cardiac arrest. The tissue iron has been recovered into high-molecular-weight species by 8 h of reperfusion. However, after 8 h large shifts of the concentrations of calcium, potassium, and sodium are observed. These shifts most likely reflect equilibration between the cytosol and the interstitial fluid for these ions. Electron microscopic examination of brains fixed in situ after 8 h reperfusion reveals an obvious general degradation of membrane structure with large holes in the plasmalemma in the vulnerable neurons. Nuclear chromatin is densely clumped, with grossly abnormal nuclear architecture. Mitochondrial architecture is well preserved. The ER is dilated and ragged, and normally arranged polyribosomes are virtually nonexistent. Histochemical evidence of lipid peroxidation can be seen by as early as 90 min following a 10-min arrest and involves approximately 30 percent of the neurons in the cortex and most neurons in CA1 and the hilum. Membrane injury by lipid peroxidation produces degradation of membrane structure to the point that the membrane becomes freely permeable to ions and the cell is irreversibly injured.

THERAPY

Clearly, the first priority in the treatment of cerebral ischemia is the reestablishment of blood flow. Methods of restoring spontaneous circulation in cardiac arrest are described in Chaps. 12, 14, and 24. Trials of thrombolytics have shown tissue plasminogen activator to be of some benefit in select subgroups of stroke patients, but it must be administered within a 3-h window.[13] Although neurons at the core of the ischemic area die within a few minutes of the onset of ischemia, animal studies indicate that there is an approximately 3- to 4-h therapeutic window when neuroprotective drugs may be beneficial before infarction occurs in the ischemic penumbra.

Because the ultimate extent of injury observed following ischemia largely reflects damage incurred during reperfusion (reperfusion injury), effective therapy must not only limit ongoing mechanisms of damage, but also facilitate repair of the damage that has already occurred. The optimal therapy for preventing continuing injury and salvaging viable brain tissue is unknown.[14] In addition to those agents mentioned above, several other therapies including pentobarbital coma, calcium antagonists, and glucocorticoids have been advocated, but human studies have failed to show efficacy.[15,16] However, a few general principles can be stated. Perfusion should be maintained at normal levels. It does not appear that intracranial pressure is increased in the postresuscitation period, and therefore therapies directed at increased intracranial pressure (hyperventilation and osmotic agents[17]) are unnecessary. Hypotension should be avoided for obvious reasons. Oxygenation should be maintained at or near normal levels. Hyperoxia should be avoided, because it is toxic to the lungs and may increase brain damage.[18] Pre- and post-arrest hyperglycemia is associated with poor neurologic outcome and must be avoided.[19,20]

Ischemic injury of the brain is complex, and this complexity indicates that single-drug therapeutic approaches will continue to fail. The pattern of ATP and ionic recovery and DNA transcription during reperfusion shows that several cellular systems are intact following prolonged ischemia and reperfusion. Future investigation of therapeutic approaches may combine calpain/caspase antagonists, iron chelators, lipid peroxidation chain reaction terminators, and growth factors to forestall further lipid peroxidation and to stimulate repair mechanisms. Phase I trials are underway in which clonal neuronal grafts are implanted into stroke victims. Effective therapeutic protocols will be identified only by continued studies.

REFERENCES

1. O'Neil BJ, Krause GS, Grossman LI, et al: Global brain ischemia and reperfusion by cardiac arrest and resuscitation: Mechanisms leading to death of vulnerable neurons and a fundamental basis for therapeutic approaches, in Paradis NA, Halperin HR, Nowak RM (eds): *Cardiac Arrest: The Science and Practice of Resuscitation Medicine.* Baltimore, Williams & Wilkins, 1996, pp. 84.
2. White BC, Sullivan JM, DeGracia DJ, et al: Brain ischemia and reperfusion: Molecular mechanisms of neuronal injury. *J Neurol Sci* 179:1, 2000.
3. Siesjo BK, Bengtsson F, Grampp W, et al: Calcium, excitotoxins, and neuronal death in the brain. *Ann NY Acad Sci* 568:234, 1989.
4. Krause GS, Tiffany BR: Protein synthesis in the reperfused brain. *Stroke* 24:747, 1993.
5. Krause GS, DeGracia DJ, Neumar RW, et al: eIF4E degradation during brain ischemia. *J Neurochem* 63:1391, 1995.
6. Neumar RW, DeGracia DJ, Konkoly LL, et al: Calpain I mediates eukaryotic initiation factor 4G degradation during global brain ischemia. *J Cereb Blood Flow Metab* 18:876, 1998.
7. DeGracia DJ, Neumar RW, White BC, Krause GS: Global brain ischemia and reperfusion: Modifications in eukaryotic initiation factors are associated with inhibition of translation initiation. *J Neurochem* 67:2005, 1996.
8. Neumar RW, Hagle SM, DeGracia DJ, et al: Brain calpain autolysis during global cerebral ischemia. *J Neurochem* 66:421, 1996.
9. DeGracia DJ, Sullivan JM, Neumar RW, et al: Effect of brain ischemia and reperfusion on the localization of phosphorylated eukaryotic initiation factor 2α. *J Cereb Blood Flow Metab* 17:1291, 1997.
10. White B, Grossman L, Krause G: Membrane damage and repair in brain injury by ischemia and reperfusion. *Neurology* 43:1656, 1993.
11. Folli F, Ghidella S, Bonfanti L, et al: The early intracellular signaling pathway for the insulin/insulin-like growth factor receptor family in the mammalian central nervous system. *Mol Neurobiol* 13:155, 1996.
12. DeGracia DJ, Kumar R, Owen CR, et al: Molecular pathways of protein synthesis inhibition during brain reperfusion: Implications for neuronal survival or death. *J Cereb Blood Flow Metab* 22:127, 2002.
13. National Institute of Neurological Disorders and Stroke rt-PA Stroke Study Group: Tissue plasminogen activator for acute ischemic stroke. *New Engl J Med* 333:1581, 1995.
14. del Zoppo GJ, Wagner S, Tagaya M: Trends and future developments in the pharmacological treatment of acute ischemic stroke. *Drugs* 54:9, 1997.
15. Grafton ST, Longstreth WT Jr: Steroids after cardiac arrest: A retrospective study with concurrent, nonrandomized controls. *Neurology* 38:1315, 1988.
16. Jastremski M, Sutton-Tyrrell K, Vaagenes P, et al: Glucocorticoid treatment does not improve neurological recovery following cardiac arrest: Brain Resuscitation Clinical Trial I Study Group. *JAMA* 262:3427, 1989.
17. Bereczki D, Liu M, do Prado GF, et al: Mannitol for acute stroke. *Cochrane Database Syst Rev* 1:CD001153, 2001.
18. Ronning OM, Guldvog B: Should stroke victims routinely receive supplemental oxygen? A quasi-randomized controlled study. *Stroke* 30:2033, 1999.
19. Kagansky N, Levy S, Knobler H: The role of hyperglycemia in acute stroke. *Arch Neurol* 58:1209, 2001.
20. Wass CT, Lanier WL: Glucose modulation of ischemic brain injury: Review and clinical recommendations. *Mayo Clin Proc* 71:801, 1996.

NEWER RESUSCITATIVE TECHNIQUES

James E. Manning

Christopher W. Barton

Laurence M. Katz

Despite advances in the science of cardiopulmonary and cerebral resuscitation, the prospects for long-term survival with good neurologic recovery remain exceedingly poor. A major limitation of present therapy is the marginal blood flow generated by closed chest CPR. Cardiac output has been reported to be 25 to 33 percent of normal at best and decreases with time delays to initiation of CPR. With increasing duration of arrest and progressive loss of peripheral arterial resistance, even optimally performed closed chest CPR is unlikely to result in return of spontaneous circulation (ROSC).

Successful resuscitation of the patient in cardiac arrest requires at least some minimal amount of blood flow to the heart. Myocardial perfusion during closed chest CPR is directly related to the pressure gradient across the coronary vasculature. This gradient is equal to the aortic pressure minus the right atrial pressure and is termed the *coronary perfusion pressure* (CPP). Aortic pressure largely determines the CPP gradient and depends on the level of residual peripheral arterial vasomotor tone. Research has shown that the CPP gradient is greatest during the relaxation phase of CPR chest compressions (CPR diastole). Laboratory and clinical data have indicated that a CPP of at least 15 mm Hg is almost always required to achieve ROSC. In contrast, human studies have indicated that CPP gradients attained with standard CPR are usually in the ineffective range of 1 to 8 mm Hg.

Much of the research into CPR has focused on methods to improve artificial perfusion during cardiac arrest. In addition to the originally described "conventional" CPR technique, several alternative methods of performing closed chest CPR have been investigated (Table 24-1). Vasoconstrictor agents have long been used as the pharmacologic adjunct to improve vital organ perfusion by increasing aortic pressure and CPP. Although epinephrine has been the principal drug, vasopressin has been added to the 2000 American Heart Association guidelines for advanced cardiac life support as an acceptable alternative to epinephrine for treating ventricular fibrillation (VF) and pulseless ventricular tachycardia.[1] A recent conference on the "Post-Resuscitative and Initial Utility in Life Saving Efforts," focused on strategies and priorities for future resuscitation research, with an emphasis on interventions that promote functional neurologic recovery.[2]

Noninvasive and invasive monitoring techniques have been examined to identify clinically useful and reliable parameters to guide resuscitative efforts (Table 24-2). Invasive perfusion techniques capable of providing near-normal artificial vital organ perfusion also have been described (Table 24-3). Direct mechanical ventricular assistance (or actuation) and cardiopulmonary bypass have been reported in laboratory models and a few clinical reports. Methods of artificial perfusion using aortic balloon catheters recently have been described in laboratory investigations. These newer invasive techniques have attempted to address the issue of clinical feasibility during sudden cardiac death.

TABLE 24-1 Alternative Methods of Closed Chest Cardiopulmonary Resuscitation

Mechanical piston cardiopulmonary resuscitation
Simultaneous compression and ventilation cardiopulmonary resuscitation
Interposed abdominal compression cardiopulmonary resuscitation
Cardiopulmonary resuscitation with abdominal binding
Cardiopulmonary resuscitation with Military Anti-Shock Trousers (MAST)
High-impulse cardiopulmonary resuscitation
Circumferential thoracic vest cardiopulmonary resuscitation
Active compression and decompression cardiopulmonary resuscitation
Phased chest and abdominal compression and decompression (Lifestick)

TABLE 24-2 Monitoring Techniques for Assessing Effectiveness of Cardiopulmonary Resuscitation

Noninvasive
  Ventricular fibrillation amplitude
  End-tidal carbon dioxide
  Median frequency of ventricular fibrillation
Invasive
  Arterial pressure
  Coronary perfusion pressure
  Central venous oxygen saturation

TABLE 24-3   Invasive Perfusion Techniques

Open chest manual cardiac compression
Minimally invasive direct cardiac massage
Direct mechanical ventricular assistance
Cardiopulmonary bypass
Hemopump
Aortic catheter perfusion techniques
   Intra-aortic balloon pump
   Selective aortic arch perfusion/selective aortic perfusion and oxygenation
   Intermittent ascending aortic occlusion
Suspended animation

Reperfusion-induced injury is a major focus of research in many fields of medicine and for numerous ischemic diseases states, including cardiac arrest, and is discussed in detail elsewhere (see Chap. 23). Cerebral resuscitation with favorable neurologic outcome after prolonged global ischemia will be the ultimate obstacle to overcome in cardiac arrest therapy. Brain-oriented therapies, such as hypothermia, may substantially improve post-resuscitation neuronal survival and functional neurologic recovery. Pharmacologic agents capable of limiting ischemia-induced cellular damage and reperfusion-induced injury from reactive oxygen species likely will be an important form of therapy for cardiac arrest patients in the resuscitation and post-resuscitation phases.

ALTERNATIVE METHODS OF CLOSED CHEST CPR

The rationale for most alternative methods of closed chest CPR that have been described are based on one of two proposed mechanisms of blood flow during CPR chest compression. The *cardiac pump theory* proposes that compression of the heart between the sternum and the spine squeezes blood out of the ventricles in a forward flow direction in a manner generally similar to normal myocardial contraction. The *thoracic pump theory* proposes that pressurization of the entire thorax, not just the heart, is responsible for blood flow and that the heart serves only as a passive or partially compressed conduit for blood flow. Net forward blood flow occurs due to competent closure of venous valves during diastole at the thoracic inlet during chest compression. The evidence for and against each theory is beyond the scope of this chapter, but it is accurate to state that the precise mechanism of blood flow during closed chest CPR remains controversial and may vary based on individual anatomic features. Alternative methods of performing closed chest CPR have been based largely on efforts to exploit one or both of the proposed mechanisms.

High-Impulse CPR

In 1984, Maier and colleagues reported a laboratory study comparing compression rates of 100 and 150 per min with the conventional rate of 60 per min advocated before 1986.[3] They observed increases in cardiac output that were roughly linear to the increase in compression rate, whereas stroke volume remained relatively constant. The compression force and velocity of impact used with these rapid CPR compression rates led to the term *high-impulse* CPR. This work was partly responsible for the increase in the recommended CPR compression rate from 60 per min to 80 to 100 per min.

Interposed Abdominal Compression CPR (IAC CPR)

Compression of the abdomen during cardiac arrest generates aortic pressures similar to those of chest compressions. The hypothesis that CPR diastolic aortic pressure and venous return from the abdomen might be augmented by abdominal compressions led to the idea of IAC CPR. One person performs the chest compressions of standard CPR, and another person applies a similar compression over the central abdomen during the relaxation phase of chest compression. The hemodynamic effects of IAC CPR in laboratory investigations have not been consistent, but most have shown increases in CPR diastolic aortic pressure, CPP, and cardiac output. Results of clinical studies of IAC CPR have been highly variable. Some studies have shown no evidence of improved resuscitation outcome, whereas others have demonstrated significant improvements in ROSC and survival to hospital discharge.[4] Differences in study populations and the technical performance of IAC CPR may be the reasons for the variable results obtained. At present, the data supporting the use of IAC CPR are not sufficient to recommend its routine application. It could also be argued that IAC CPR is physiologically very similar to high-impulse CPR with the compressions performed by two persons rather than one. However, if perfusion with standard CPR is judged to be inadequate, attempting IAC CPR is a reasonable alternative intervention.

Active Compression and Decompression CPR (ACD CPR)

Standard CPR involves a forceful, or "active," chest compression phase with elastic recoil of the chest wall during the relaxation phase ("passive" decompression). The ACD CPR device consists of a circular suction cup connected to a handle with a force gauge (Figure 24-1). With the suction cup securely attached at the midsternal chest, CPR is performed with force applied downward (active compression) and upward (active decompression) during CPR.[5] One advantage of the ACD CPR device is that it tends to decrease the venous system pressure to a greater extent than the arterial pressures during the active decompression phase. This may increase venous return and increase the CPP gradient during CPR diastole. Although initial clinical reports have indicated some improvement in ROSC and survival, a large randomized clinical trial in in-hospital cardiac arrest (773 patients) and out-of-hospital cardiac arrest (1011 patients) showed no improvement in survival for the ACD CPR device as compared with

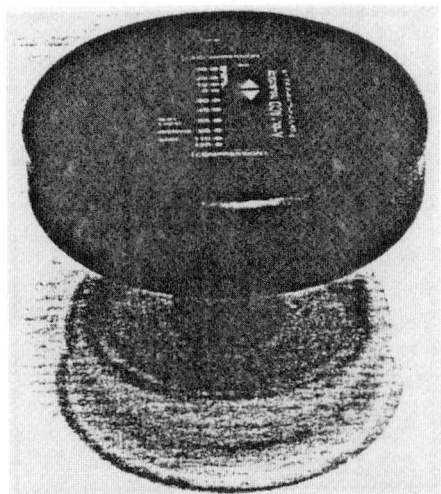

FIG. 24-1. The Ambu CardioPump (Ambu International Inc., Copenhagen, Denmark) is used for active compression and decompression cardiopulmonary resuscitation (CPR). The silicone rubber suction cup is positioned midchest at the level of the nipples. Using the circular plastic handle, the device is pushed downward during the compression phase, followed by active withdrawal during the decompression phase. Force of compression and decompression is measured by the gauge located within the handle and is easily viewed by the operator during CPR. (Reproduced with permission from Lurie KG, Shultz JJ, Callaham ML, et al: Evaluation of active compression-decompression CPR in victims of out-of-hospital cardiac arrest. *JAMA* 271:1405, 1994.)

standard CPR.[5] There is presently insufficient evidence to support the routine use of ACD CPR. However, as noted for other alternative CPR techniques, if standard CPR is judged to be ineffective, ACD CPR is another option. Unlike some of the other alternative techniques, ACD CPR requires a special device, and this limits its applicability.

Phased Chest and Abdominal Compression and Decompression

Tang and associates described the use of a device that combines the concepts of IAC CPR and ACD.[6] This technique involves the use of a device called the Lifestick resuscitator. This device has chest and abdominal pads connected to an adjustable rigid frame with a handle at each end (Figure 24-2). The pads are attached to the sternum and the upper abdomen by an adhesive. Using a seesaw motion, the chest and abdomen are compressed in an alternating pattern. The preliminary report of this technique by Tang and colleagues in a survival model of swine cardiac arrest showed improved CPP, ROSC, and 48-h survival. At present, there have been no reports of the use of this device in human cardiac arrests.

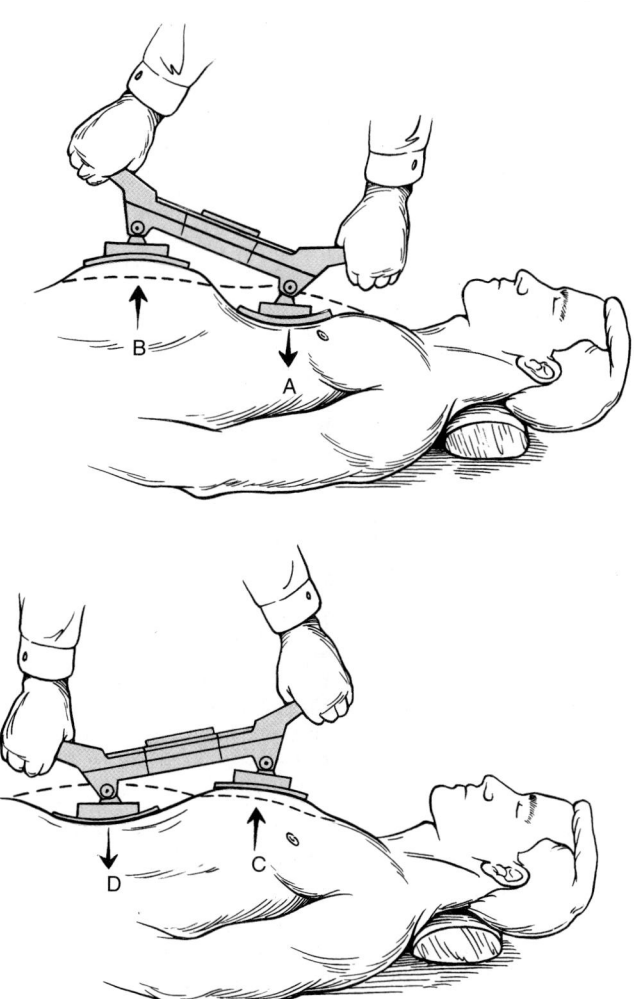

FIG. 24-2. Sequencing compression and decompression with the Lifestick resuscitator. The subject's head is on the right. Chest compression (**A**) is coincident with abdominal decompression (**B**). This is followed by chest decompression (**C**) and abdominal compression (**D**). (Reproduced with permission from Tang W, Weil MH, Schock RB, et al: Phased chest and abdominal compression-decompression: A new option for cardiopulmonary resuscitation. *Circulation* 95:1335, 1997.)

Circumferential Thoracic Vest CPR

The thoracic pump theory proposes that cyclic fluctuations in intrathoracic pressure created by CPR chest compressions are responsible for blood flow. Thus, efforts to maximize the intrathoracic pressure generated and limit trauma to the chest would be advantageous. This led to the conception of the circumferential thoracic vest CPR device. This method involves the placement of a vest around the thorax and pressurizing the thorax from all directions as opposed to localized pressure over the lower sternum (Figure 24-3). Halperin and colleagues reported their preliminary experience in humans with a refined circumferential vest CPR device and found significant improvements in CPP and initial ROSC.[7] In patients failing prolonged resuscitative efforts, peak CPR systolic aortic pressure increased from an average of 78 mm Hg with manual CPR to an average of 138 mm Hg with vest CPR. In 34 patients randomized to receive manual versus vest CPR, after an average of 11 min of unsuccessful manual CPR, 8 of 17 vest CPR patients had ROSC compared with only 3 of 17 manual CPR patients. Although this appears to be a promising alternative method of CPR, a substantial amount of clinical investigation is still needed to clarify its potential benefit.

Inspiratory Impedance Threshold Valve During CPR

Improving venous return to the thorax and heart during the relaxation phase of CPR should have a beneficial effect on the blood flow generated during the compression phase. To enhance this venous return, an inspiratory impedance threshold valve for the ventilation circuit was developed to augment the negative intrathoracic pressure that occurs during the relaxation phase of CPR. Laboratory study has demonstrated substantial increases in CPP and vital organ perfusion during standard CPR. The magnitude of effect has been shown to be even greater when combined with ACD CPR. Clinical experience with the inspiratory impedance threshold valve has been limited, but early reports have shown increased early survival.[8]

PHARMACOLOGIC INTERVENTIONS

Adrenergic Therapy

Adrenergic drugs have been the primary agents studied and used in all types of cardiac arrest. Epinephrine is the predominant adrenergic drug and remains the recommended agent. The mechanism of action of adrenergic therapy in cardiac resuscitation has been convincingly shown to be primarily α-adrenergic receptor-mediated vasoconstriction in the peripheral arterial system, resulting in increased aortic pressure and thus increased CPP. In addition to epinephrine, several other pure α-adrenergic or mixed α- and β-adrenergic agents have been studied. However, none of these agents has been shown to increase ROSC or long-term survival as compared with epinephrine.

The appropriate dosage of adrenergic drugs during cardiac arrest is the subject of ongoing controversy. Although based on early animal studies and on very limited anecdotal clinical evidence, an epinephrine dose of 1 mg was the standard recommendation for many years. Laboratory investigations and clinical reports in the 1980s suggested that substantially higher doses are required for optimal beneficial effect. These studies led to large, randomized, controlled clinical trials in the early 1990s that showed variable effects on the rate of ROSC but failed to show improvement in survival to hospital discharge or neurologic outcome.[1] Although no benefit was demonstrated, no adverse results were identified with the use of higher doses of epinephrine. Nonetheless, there have been anecdotal complaints from intensivists that the temporary ROSC achieved unnecessarily diverts intensive care resources for futile situations. The 2000 AHA ACLS guidelines largely discourage the use of higher doses of epinephrine but leave this open to the clinician's discretion if standard doses of epinephrine have been unsuccessful.[1]

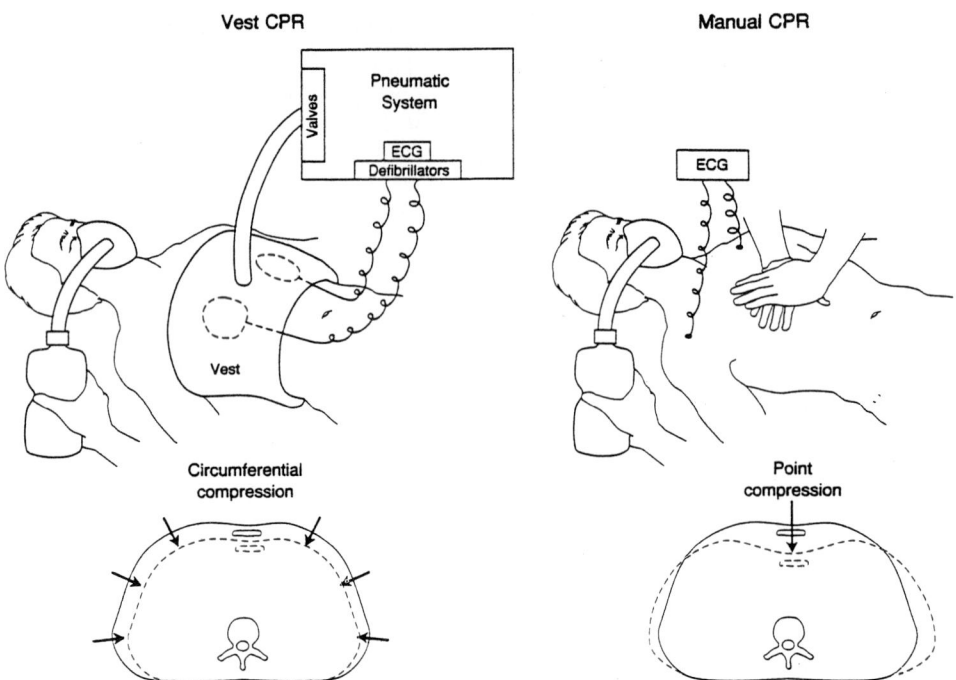

FIG. 24-3. A comparison of the thoracic vest system for cardiopulmonary resuscitation (vest CPR) with the standard manual CPR. The vest contains a bladder that is inflated and deflated by the pneumatic system. Defibrillation can be accomplished during chest compression through the flat defibrillator electrodes *(dashed circles)* under the vest. The electrocardiogram can be recorded through the same electrodes. The lower panels show schematic representations of transverse sections of the midthorax during vest CPR and manual CPR. The thoracic size during chest relaxation is shown by the *solid lines*. The *arrows* indicate force applied to the thorax during chest compression. With vest inflation, there is a relatively uniform decrease in the dimensions of the thorax. With manual CPR, the sternum is displaced during compression *(arrow),* and the lateral thorax can bulge, thereby increasing thoracic volume and reducing the intrathoracic pressure generated during compression. (Reproduced with permission from Halperin HR, Tsitlik JE, Gefand M, et al: A preliminary study of cardiopulmonary resuscitation by circumferential compression of the chest with use of a pneumatic vest. *New Engl J Med* 329:762, 1993.)

Nonadrenergic Vasoconstriction (Vasopressin)

The 40-year reign of epinephrine as the sole recommended vasoconstrictor during cardiac arrest has come to an end. Vasopressin, a nonadrenergic vasoconstrictor, now shares the podium with epinephrine in the 2000 AHA ACLS guidelines. Although vasopressin has undergone extensive laboratory investigation, the clinical evidence supporting the use of vasopressin over epinephrine remains limited. However, vasopressin appears to be at least as effective as epinephrine. The principal advantage of vasopressin may be its greater duration of action, which allows for more sustained increases in CPP during CPR than that seen with epinephrine due to its shorter duration of action. Linder and associates reported a small randomized clinical study comparing intravenous vasopressin (40 units) with intravenous epinephrine (1 mg) and showed a significant increase in initial ROSC, hospital admission, and 24-h survival.[9] There was also a trend toward improved survival to hospital discharge. Another nonadrenergic agent that has undergone only limited laboratory investigation is angiotensin II. **The use of vasopressin is now accepted for routine management of VF cardiac arrest.** The use of vasopressin or other nonadrenergic vasoconstrictor in conjunction with adrenergic vasoconstrictor agents may prove to be more effective than either alone.

Thrombolytic Therapy

Coronary thrombosis and pulmonary thromboembolism are known pathologic entities that can cause cardiac arrest, and both disorders are treatable with thrombolytic therapy. The estimated incidence of these disorders in cardiac arrest is variable, but estimates as high as 50 to 70 percent have been reported. Concern about bleeding complications in the setting of thoracic trauma associated with CPR chest compressions has discouraged its use in cardiac resuscitation. However, there has been growing interest in thrombolysis during cardiac arrest when initial standard resuscitative measures have failed. In addition to the obvious benefit of restoring blood flow to through an occluded vessel, thrombolytic therapy might improve microcirculatory reperfusion, most importantly cerebral perfusion, by reversing microcirculatory sludging. Several clinical anecdotes and case series have suggested that thrombolysis improves resuscitation success rates and early survival.[10] However, long-term survival benefit has not been clearly demonstrated. Prospective, randomized, controlled clinical studies are needed to determine whether these expensive agents are justified in the routine treatment of cardiac arrest. It seems reasonable to consider the use of thrombolytic agents in cardiac arrest victims with high suspicion for coronary thrombosis or massive pulmonary embolism.

Adenosine Antagonism

Release and accumulation of adenosine in ischemic tissues and adenosine's role as a depressant of cardiac pacemaker automaticity have been defined more clearly in recent years. There is limited clinical evidence to suggest that aminophylline can reverse these effects (by acting as an adenosine antagonist) and may be useful in the treatment of bradydysrhythmia associated with myocardial ischemia. Clinical studies have shown favorable initial response to aminophylline bolus, but long-term survival does not appear to be affected.[11] Laboratory studies have shown no apparent benefit of aminophylline in cardiac arrest. Thus, adenosine antagonism remains an unproven therapy. However, given the dismal prospects for survival associated with bradyasystolic arrest, use of aminophylline is not unreasonable and is unlikely to be harmful.

Amiodarone

Amiodarone is an antiarrhythmic agent with a complex electropharmacologic profile that has been used for long-term control of a variety of atrial and ventricular dysrhythmias. Despite its reportedly limited effect on ventricular effective refractory period after acute intravenous administration, it has been shown to be effective in the treatment of acute unstable ventricular dysrhythmias refractory to lidocaine and procainamide. In a recent randomized, double-blind, clinical trial, amiodarone was compared with lidocaine in victims of out-of-hospital cardiac arrest, with the primary end point being survival to hospital admission. Patients receiving amiodarone had a significantly greater survival to admission rate than patients receiving lidocaine (22.8 vs. 12 percent, respectively).[12] However, long-term survival benefit has not been clearly demonstrated. Nonetheless, based on the early benefit observed, **the 2000 AHA ACLS guidelines recommend amiodarone as an acceptable alternative to lidocaine in the treatment of VF and pulseless ventricular tachycardia.**

Magnesium

Clinical studies have shown improved survival with magnesium supplementation in the setting of acute myocardial infarction. The cardioprotective effects of magnesium are thought to be related to suppression of automaticity, coronary vasodilation, platelet inhibition, and inhibition of calcium influx. Although an association between hypomagnesemia and cardiac dysrhythmias has been recognized, the value of magnesium in the treatment of acute, life-threatening ventricular dysrhythmias has not been established. Thel and associates reported a randomized, double-blind, placebo-controlled clinical trial of magnesium administration in 156 in-hospital cardiac arrest patients (MAGIC trial).[13] Administration of magnesium (initial 2 g bolus during cardiac arrest followed by an infusion of 8 g over 24 h) showed no difference from placebo in ROSC, survival to 24 h, survival to hospital discharge, or Glasgow Coma Scale score on discharge. However, among survivors to hospital discharge (21 percent in each group), quality of life assessed by Karnofsky's performance status was better in the magnesium group, and no adverse effects of magnesium administration were noted. **Thus, the use of magnesium in cardiac arrest remains incompletely defined.** Magnesium administration during cardiac arrest seems acceptable based on clinical judgment, especially in cases of suspected hypomagnesemia or refractory cardiac arrest.

Sodium-Hydrogen Exchanger Inhibition

Studies in models of ischemic myocardium have shown that sodium-hydrogen exchanger inhibitors have a protective effect on the myocardium by limiting intracellular accumulation of calcium. One inhibitor, cariporide, has recently been studied in laboratory rat models of VF to determine its effect on subsequent defibrillation success. The remarkable finding in the early reports of administering cariporide during VF has been the predominant occurrence of spontaneous defibrillation without the need for electrical shock.[14] This finding of "pharmacologic defibrillation" has exciting prospects for the treatment of VF cardiac arrest. However, this has been demonstrated only in rat models at present, and further testing in larger animal models of VF will be necessary. Even if spontaneous defibrillation does not occur in larger animal models or, ultimately, in humans, sodium-hydrogen exchanger inhibitors may be a useful therapy if they enhance the VF energy profile and promote successful electrical defibrillation.

Routes for Medication Delivery

Recommended routes for the administration of resuscitation drugs include intravenous, endotracheal, and intraosseous. Intravenous administration is considered optimal, **with central venous delivery preferred over peripheral venous delivery,** provided there is no delay in gaining central venous access. Intracardiac drug injection has largely been discouraged. Central arterial administration of medications has received little attention but may be a useful alternative, especially for delivery of vasoconstrictor agents, which have their effector sites in the peripheral arterial system.

Catheterization to measure arterial pressure during cardiac arrest is becoming a more accepted intervention to help guide resuscitative efforts. Thoracic aortic catheterization via a femoral artery approach allows for pressure monitoring and homogeneous arterial drug administration. When aortic arch and central venous routes of epinephrine administration were compared in a laboratory model, aortic arch delivery resulted in a more rapid increase in CPR diastolic aortic pressure, a greater magnitude of aortic pressure increase, and a maximal response consistently seen within 30 to 50 s of injection.[15] The rapidity of initial and maximal aortic pressure responses suggests that adrenergic therapy could be rapidly adjusted based on a parameter reflecting vital organ perfusion. Thus, thoracic aortic catheterization allows for rapid delivery of vasoconstrictor agents to effector sites and rapid assessment of therapeutic effect, such that therapy can be rapidly titrated on an individual basis. The major limitation of this route is the need to establish central arterial access.

TECHNIQUES FOR ASSESSMENT OF RESUSCITATIVE EFFORTS

The lack of an accurate and readily measurable parameter to guide resuscitative efforts has long frustrated clinicians and clinical investigators. Pulse quality, pupillary reactivity, serial blood gases, and the coarseness of VF were the only parameters available until relatively recently. None of these was sufficiently accurate to allow for therapeutic adjustments on an individual basis. Fortunately, recent technologic advances have led to monitoring techniques that allow for much more accurate assessment and guidance of therapy.

Capnometry or End-Tidal Carbon Dioxide

Capnometry (the measurement of exhaled end-tidal carbon dioxide levels) has become a valuable and standard monitoring tool in the ED. Although used primarily to assess endotracheal tube placement and monitor ventilation, end-tidal carbon dioxide ($ETCO_2$) can be used to assess blood flow. End-tidal carbone dioxide is proportional to pulmonary perfusion, which in turn reflects systemic perfusion. It is this principle that makes $ETCO_2$ monitoring of value in the assessment of perfusion during CPR.

The use of quantitative or semiquantitative $ETCO_2$ as an indicator of the effectiveness of artificial perfusion has received considerable attention over the past decade or so. Laboratory models or cardiac arrest have demonstrated a statistically significant correlation between $ETCO_2$ and CPP. In one clinical study, the initial $ETCO_2$ served to predict which patients would regain a pulse during the resuscitation. Those patients with an $ETCO_2$ of at least 15 mm Hg on arrival in the ED had a greater than 90 percent probability of regaining a pulse, whereas those patients with an $ETCO_2$ of less than 15 mm Hg almost never regained a pulse.[16] In many of these patients, a sudden, dramatic increase in the $ETCO_2$ was noticed well before a pulse could be detected. Unfortunately, $ETCO_2$ does not always correlate precisely with CPP, and the relation between the two can be affected by therapeutic interventions such as adrenergic therapy. Although these studies cannot be used as an endorsement for deciding when to quit or continue CPR, they do lend support to the validity of $ETCO_2$ as a reflection of cardiac output. **End-tidal carbon dioxide is the most accurate noninvasive method of monitoring CPR effectiveness** currently available, and its use is encouraged. The most appropriate way to use $ETCO_2$ is to maintain minute ventilation relatively constant while adjusting the mechanics of CPR chest compression and titrating adrenergic therapy in an effort to maximize the $ETCO_2$.

Ventricular Fibrillation Waveform Analysis

It has long been recognized that the coarseness of the VF waveform has a rough correlation with the duration of cardiac arrest and the prospects for successful defibrillation with ROSC. With the onset of VF, there is a gradually progressive decrease in the peak-to-trough amplitude of the VF waveform in the absence of resuscitative interventions. The recorded amplitude of the VF waveform, however, is subject to such factors as body habitus, electrode location and contact, and instrumentation. By using mathematical formulas (the fast Fourier transform) and high-speed computers, a digital characterization of the VF waveform can be derived. This method provides a discrete digital number with which to describe the distribution of frequencies present in the waveform. One measure, the median or centroid frequency, has been found to correlate with defibrillation success and to predict the duration of VF. As VF continues without resuscitation, the median frequency gradually deteriorates over time. When effective resuscitation measures are instituted, the median frequency promptly increases.[17] Such interventions as invasive perfusion support or pharmacologic therapy with epinephrine or vasopressin have successfully raised the median frequency of VF and have been associated with enhanced resuscitation success in animal models. The median frequency (or other measures derived from the fast Fourier transform) may eventually find their way to the bedside in the form of a monitor used by the clinician to guide therapy during resuscitation attempts.

Invasive Hemodynamic Pressure Monitoring

Laboratory and clinical studies have demonstrated that aortic pressure and CPP correlate strongly with coronary blood flow and ROSC. Although placement of arterial pressure catheters is a common occurrence in critical care medicine, arterial catheterization is not routinely performed in cardiac arrest patients, in part because of the technical difficulties associated with performing this during CPR. However, arterial pressure monitoring provides a very useful parameter to guide resuscitative efforts. The CPR diastolic arterial pressure is the major predictor of the actual CPP. Thus, adjusting therapeutic interventions to maximize CPR diastolic arterial pressure will result in greater CPP and improved chances of survival.

Central venous catheterization in addition to arterial and aortic catheterization allows for the accurate measurement of the aortic-to-right atrial pressure gradient or CPP. Although clearly one of the most useful measurable parameters in human resuscitation, it has been studied by only a few investigators and only as an in-hospital procedure. Thus, out-of-hospital cardiac arrest patients undergoing CPP monitoring have generally been in arrest for an extended period. Paradis and colleagues reported that ROSC in the ED correlates with achieving a CPP greater than 15 mm Hg among patients with prolonged cardiac arrest.[18] None of the patients with ROSC survived, suggesting that CPP monitoring after prolonged cardiac arrest is likely to be of limited benefit. Thus, efforts to perform invasive monitoring more rapidly upon hospital arrival or even in the prehospital setting should be pursued. The feasibility of performing prehospital invasive hemodynamic monitoring has been demonstrated with the use of a commercially available, lightweight, and portable monitoring system that can be easily transported to the scene of out-of-hospital cardiac arrest.

Central Venous Oxygen Saturation Monitoring

Rivers and associates reported the use of central venous oximetry in the evaluation of cardiac arrest patients.[19] Central venous oxygen saturation provided important information about tissue oxygen delivery and consumption balance and was predictive of ROSC. A central venous oxygen saturation of less than 30 percent resulted in a 0 percent ROSC rate, whereas a value greater than 72 percent resulted in a 100 percent ROSC rate. Impending ROSC was foreshadowed by an abrupt or gradual increase in central venous oxygen saturation. Interestingly, a supranormal central venous oxygen saturation, termed *venous hyperoxia,* was seen frequently during the early phase of ROSC, followed by a return to normal levels.

INVASIVE PERFUSION TECHNIQUES

Direct Mechanical Ventricular Assistance

Direct mechanical ventricular assistance (DMVA) was first described by Anstadt and colleagues in 1965, and several laboratory studies have investigated this technique in cardiac arrest models. Direct mechanical ventricular assistance uses a cup-shaped device that fits around the ventricles and is held in place by a vacuum at the apex of the heart (Figure 24-4). Cyclic positive and negative pressures are transmitted to a flexible diaphragm on the inner surface of the cup, resulting in compression and re-expansion of the ventricles, respectively. The clinical utility of this technique in the treatment of cardiac arrest has not been established. The major advantage of DMVA is that it can be sustained for an extended period. The major limitation of DMVA is the requirement of a thoracotomy, which largely precludes its use within an effective time frame for most victims of out-of-hospital cardiac arrest.

Cardiopulmonary Bypass

Cardiopulmonary bypass (CPB; Figure 24-5) is an effective means of providing sustained global perfusion and has been advocated in the treatment of cardiac arrest. Several laboratory studies have demonstrated improved ROSC and neurologic recovery with CPB compared with standard ACLS interventions. There are also several case series describing the successful use of femorofemoral CPB in the treatment of cardiac arrest. The major advantages of CPB are that it can be performed with only a femoral vessel cutdown, artificial perfusion can be sustained for an extended period, and perfusion support can be gradually withdrawn. The major disadvantages are the equipment, skill, and time required to perform CPB. A recent report of 10 cardiac arrest victims in whom CPB was initiated in the ED showed that ROSC was achieved in all 10, but there were no long-term survivors.[20] The average time from onset of arrest to onset of CPB support was 32 min. To achieve long-term survival, the time interval to CPB support must be much shorter. Unless the technique can be extended to the prehospital setting, it will be of very limited value in the treatment of victims of out-of-hospital cardiac arrest. However, technologic advances offer the

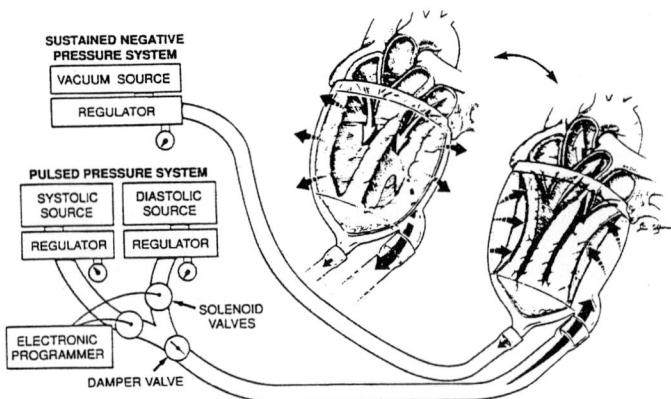

FIG. 24-4. Direct mechanical ventricular assistance (DMVA). Schematic diagram of DMVA drive system and cup. The device actuates the ventricular myocardium into systolic *(right)* and diastolic *(left)* configurations. (Reproduced with permission from Anstad MP, Anstad GL, Lowe JE: Direct mechanical ventricular actuation: A review. *Resuscitation* 21:7, 1991.)

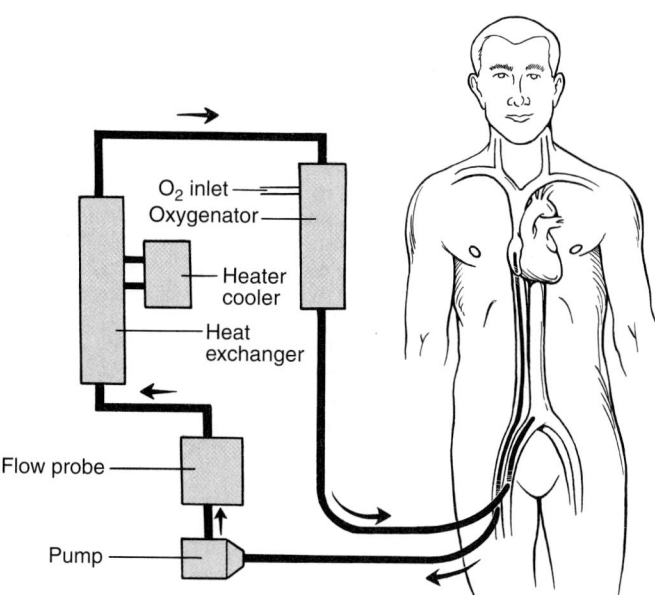

FIG. 24-5. Schematic diagram of a cardiopulmonary bypass system.

prospect of developing CPB devices that can be used in the prehospital setting.

Hemopump

The Hemopump is a catheter-based, temporary ventricular assist device consisting of an axial flow pump component at the distal end of the catheter powered by an external motor via a flexible drive cable that runs the length of the catheter. The distal tip of the axial flow pump component is advanced from a femoral artery into the left ventricle (Figure 24-6). When it is in operation, forward blood flow is generated by blood entering the axial flow pump component in the left ventricle and exiting in the aortic arch. Laboratory investigation in a cardiac arrest model has demonstrated sustained mean arterial pressures of approximately 60 mm Hg and cardiac output averaging 2.3 L per min.[21] The major drawback with the use of this device in the setting of cardiac arrest is that one must be able to insert the catheter from a femoral artery into the left ventricle.

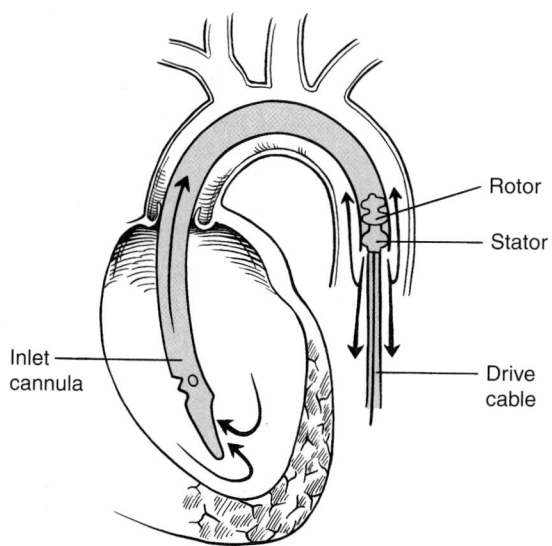

FIG. 24-6. Schematic diagram of the Hemopump positioned in the left ventricle.

Aortic Catheter Perfusion Techniques

During the past decade, there has been interest in the use of aortic balloon occlusion catheters to enhance vital organ perfusion during cardiac arrest. The use of standard intra-aortic balloon pumping has been shown to increase CPP during closed chest CPR, but the effect is not dramatic. However, the use of aortic balloon catheters for the infusion of resuscitation solutions during cardiac arrest holds greater promise for improving resuscitation outcome.

Selective aortic arch perfusion (SAAP), as described by Manning and associates,[22] or selective aortic perfusion and oxygenation, as described by Paradis and colleagues,[23] uses a large-lumen balloon occlusion catheter positioned in the descending aortic arch to provide selective perfusion of the heart and brain during cardiac arrest (Figure 24-7). The catheter is inserted into a femoral artery (percutaneously or via a cutdown) and blindly advanced into the thoracic aorta. With the balloon inflated and pressure cuffs applied to the upper arms, the coronary and cerebral circulations are relatively isolated for brief perfusion. The resuscitation solution infused consists of an oxygenated blood substitute, such as a perfluorocarbon emulsion or polymerized hemoglobin solution, that might contain various agents to enhance restoration of spontaneous cardiac contraction, maintain neuronal viability, and limit myocardial and neuronal reperfusion injuries. One major advantage of SAAP is the ability to administer agents to combat reperfusion injury at the moment of or just before reperfusion. In addition, the temperature of the infused resuscitation solution can be adjusted to rapidly induce protective hypothermia. Once ROSC is achieved, SAAP can be used to provide partial perfusion support dur-

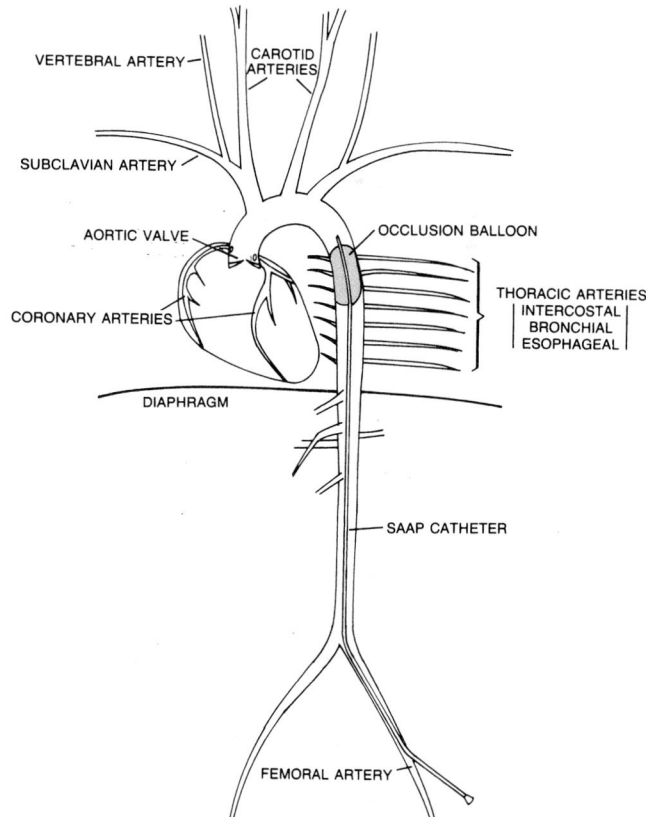

FIG. 24-7. Selective aortic arch perfusion (SAAP). Positioning of the SAAP balloon occlusion catheter at the end of the descending aortic arch through a femoral artery. Placement of the balloon at this level restricts flow to aortic arch vessels including coronary arteries. (Reproduced with permission from Manning JE, Murphy CA, Hertz CM, et al: Selective aortic arch perfusion during cardiac arrest: A new resuscitation technique. *Ann Emerg Med* 21:1058, 1992.)

ing the early post-resuscitation phase. The concept of SAAP was created primarily with a focus on the prehospital environment, but it also can be used in-hospital. The intravascular volume loading associated with SAAP therapy makes it particularly attractive for the treatment of hemorrhage-induced hypovolemic cardiac arrest. Although laboratory results in VF and exsanguination cardiac arrest models have been very favorable, the efficacy of this invasive perfusion technique in human cardiac arrest has not been studied.

Safar and colleagues recently described using a descending aortic arch balloon occlusion catheter for the purpose of infusing very cold fluid (4°C) to rapidly induce protective brain and heart hypothermia while in a persistent cardiac arrest.[24] The rationale for this "suspended animation" state is to protect the vital organs from further ischemic damage or reperfusion injury until the patient can be transported to a facility with CPB capability. Thereafter, CPB would be used for controlled reperfusion, leading to stable restoration of spontaneous circulation. This approach might minimize ischemic and reperfusion cellular injuries sufficiently to promote normal functional neurologic recovery. This approach has been shown to be effective in laboratory models of primary cardiac arrest and hemorrhage-induced cardiac arrest.

Tang and colleagues described the use of a balloon occlusion catheter positioned in the ascending aortic arch.[25] Laboratory investigations of this technique have shown marked increases in coronary perfusion with intermittent balloon occlusion. Infusion of fluid through the catheter results in isolated coronary artery perfusion. The technical feasibility of rapidly and reliably positioning the tip of this catheter in the ascending aortic arch may prove to be a significant challenge in the clinical setting.

Minimally Invasive Direct Cardiac Massage

In 1995, Buckman and colleagues reported the use of a relatively simple device for the rapid initiation of internal cardiac compression through a small thoracic incision.[26] The technique, called *minimally invasive direct cardiac massage,* uses a rectangular, curved, padded plate connected to a handle to compress the heart through an intercostal incision at the anterolateral left chest at the level of the lower sternum (Figure 24-8). In a swine cardiac arrest model, the device generated CPP and cardiac output similar to that produced by manual open chest cardiac massage. It has been suggested that a modified device could be inserted via a smaller (2 to 3 cm) intercostal incision.

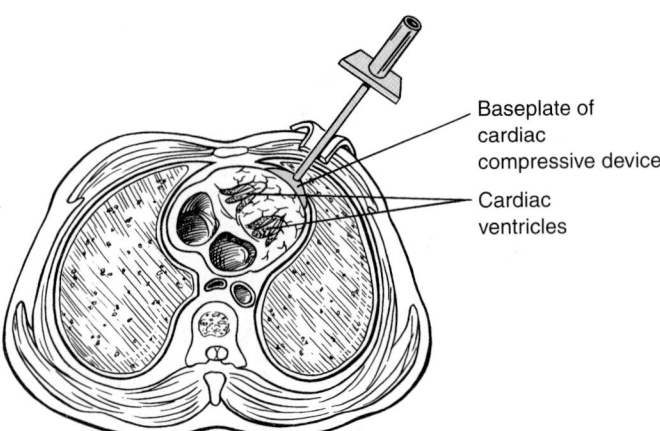

Baseplate of cardiac compressive device

Cardiac ventricles

FIG. 24-8. The heart-contacting baseplate and a portion of the stem of the cardiac compressive device are inserted into the thorax through a small, parasternal incision. The manually operated handle remains outside the chest. The base plate is positioned directly on the cardiac ventricles, lying within an intact pericardium. Manual depression of the device compresses the heart and produces an artificial systole.

REFERENCES

1. Guidelines 2000 for Cardiopulmonary Resuscitation and Emergency Cardiovascular Care. *Circulation* 102:1, 2000.
2. Becker LB, Weisfeldt ML, Weil MH, et al: The PULSE initiative: Scientific priorities and strategic planning for resuscitation research and life saving therapies. *Circulation* 105:2562, 2002.
3. Maier GW, Tyson GS, Olsen CO, et al: The physiology of external cardiac massage: High-impulse cardiopulmonary resuscitation. *Circulation* 70:86, 1984.
4. Sack JB, Kesselbrenner MB: Hemodynamics, survival benefits, and complications of interposed abdominal compression during cardiopulmonary resuscitation. *Acad Emerg Med* 1:490, 1994.
5. Stiell IG, Hebert PC, Wells GA, et al: The Ontario trial of active compression-decompression cardiopulmonary resuscitation for in-hospital and prehospital cardiac arrest. *JAMA* 267:2916, 1992.
6. Tang W, Weil MH, Schock RB, et al: Phased chest and abdominal compression-decompression: A new option for cardiopulmonary resuscitation. *Circulation* 95:1335, 1997.
7. Halperin HR, Tsitlik JE, Gefand M, et al: A preliminary study of cardiopulmonary resuscitation by circumferential compression of the chest with use of a pneumatic vest. *New Engl J Med* 329:762, 1993.
8. Lurie KG, Zielinski T, Voelckel W, et al: Augmentation of ventricular preload during treatment of cardiovascular collapse and cardiac arrest. *Crit Care Med* 30(suppl):S162, 2002.
9. Wenzel V, Lindner KH: Arginine vasopressin during cardiopulmonary resuscitation: Laboratory evidence, clinical experience and recommendations, and a view to the future. *Crit Care Med* 30(suppl):S157, 2002.
10. Bottiger BW, Bode C, Kern S, et al: Efficacy and safety of thrombolytic therapy after initially unsuccessful cardiopulmonary resuscitation: A prospective clinical trial. *Lancet* 357:1583, 2001.
11. Viskin S, Belhassen B, Roth A, et al: Aminophylline for bradyasystolic cardiac arrest refractory to atropine and epinephrine. *Ann Intern Med* 118:279, 1993.
12. Dorian DP, Cass D, Schwartz B, et al: Amiodarone as compared with lidocaine for shock-resistant ventricular fibrillation. *New Eng J Med* 346:884, 2002.
13. Thel MC, Armstrong AL, McNulty SE, et al: Randomised trial of magnesium in in-hospital cardiac arrest. *Lancet* 350:1272, 1997.
14. Gazmuri RJ, Ayoub IM, Kolarova JD, et al: Myocardial protection during ventricular fibrillation by inhibition of the sodium-hydrogen exchanger isoform-1. *Crit Care Med* 30(suppl):S166, 2002.
15. Manning JE, Murphy CA, Batson DN, et al: Aortic arch versus central venous epinephrine during CPR. *Ann Emerg Med* 22:703, 1993.
16. Callaham ML, Barton CW: Prediction of outcome of cardiopulmonary resuscitation from end-tidal carbon dioxide concentration. *Crit Care Med* 18:358, 1990.
17. Brown CG, Dzwonczyk R: Signal analysis of the human electrocardiogram during ventricular fibrillation: Frequency and amplitude parameters as predictors of successful countershock. *Ann Emerg Med* 27:184, 1996.
18. Paradis NA, Martin GB, Rivers EP, et al: Coronary perfusion pressure and the return of spontaneous circulation in human cardiopulmonary resuscitation. *JAMA* 263:1106, 1990.
19. Rivers EP, Martin GB, Smithline H, et al: The clinical implications of continuous central venous oxygen saturation during human CPR. *Ann Emerg Med* 21:1094, 1992.
20. Martin GB, Rivers EP, Paradis NA, et al: Emergency department cardiopulmonary bypass in the treatment of human cardiac arrest. *Chest* 113:743, 1998.
21. Schroder T, Hering JP, Uhlig P, et al: Efficiency of the left ventricle assist device Hemopump in cardiac fibrillation. *Br J Anaesth* 68:536, 1992.
22. Manning JE, Murphy CA, Hertz CM, et al: Selective aortic arch perfusion during cardiac arrest: A new resuscitation technique. *Ann Emerg Med* 21:1058, 1992.
23. Paradis NA, Rose MI, Gawryl MS: Selective aortic perfusion and oxygenation: An effective adjunct to external chest compression-based cardiopulmonary resuscitation. *J Am Coll Cardiol* 23:497, 1994.
24. Safar P, Tisherman SA, Behringer W, et al: Suspended animation for delayed resuscitation from prolonged cardiac arrest that is unresuscitable by standard cardiopulmonary-cerebral resuscitation. *Crit Care Med* 28:N214, 2000.
25. Tang W, Weil MH, Noc M, et al: Augmented efficacy of external CPR by intermittent occlusion of the ascending aorta. *Circulation* 88:1916, 1993.

26. Buckman RF Jr, Badellino MM, Mauro LH, et al: Direct cardiac massage without major thoracotomy: Feasibility and systemic blood flow. *Resuscitation* 29:237, 1995.

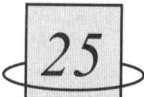

ACID-BASE DISORDERS
David D. Nicolaou
Gabor D. Kelen

Many diseases, including those presenting an imminent life threat, produce acid and base (acid-base) disturbances that provide important clues concerning the nature of the underlying illness and suggest immediate therapeutic interventions. This chapter describes a practical approach to the clinical evaluation of acid-base disorders.

MEASUREMENT OF PLASMA ACIDITY

Plasma hydrogen ion concentration ($[H^+]$) is normally 40 nmol/L, corresponding to a pH of 7.4. Because pH is a logarithmic transformation of $[H^+]$, the relation of $[H^+]$ to pH is not linear for all pH values (Table 25-1). However, for pH values from 7.20 to 7.50, the relation between $[H^+]$ and pH is nearly linear; pH changes of 0.01 correspond to approximately 1 nmol/L change in $[H^+]$. This linear relation allows very rapid bedside interpretation of blood gas and electrolyte results.

Plasma Acid Homeostasis

Plasma $[H^+]$ is influenced by the rate of endogenous production, the rate of excretion, and buffering capacity of the body. Buffers mitigate the impact of large changes in available hydrogen ion on plasma pH.

Buffer systems that are effective at physiologic pH include hemoglobin, phosphate, proteins, and bicarbonate (Figure 25-1).[1] One can consider the $[H^+]$ to be the result of all physiologic buffers acting on the common pool of hydrogen ions.

The familiar Henderson-Hasselbalch equation, shown in Eq. (1),

$$pH = pK + \log \frac{[HCO_3^-]}{[H_2CO_3]} \qquad (1)$$

demonstrates the interrelationship between carbonic acid, bicarbonate, and pH; any two of these determine the third.

However, the clinical utility of the Henderson-Hasselbalch equation is limited.

Nevertheless, if all constants are inserted into the Henderson-Hasselbalch equation and the anti-log of all its terms is taken, the resulting simplified Kaissirer-Bleich equation, shown in Eq. (2), is of great clinical utility.[2]

$$[H^+] = 24 \times \frac{P_{CO_2}}{[HCO_3^-]} \qquad (2)$$

The Kassirer-Bleich equation may be used to calculate the concentration of any component of the bicarbonate buffer system provided the concentrations of the other two components are known. It therefore allows clinicians to determine, for example, what the pH *must be* when the partial pressure of carbon dioxide (P_{CO_2}) and $[HCO_3^-]$ are known.* Performing such a calculation with values reported by the laboratory permits the clinician to check the internal consistency of the reported data. (In fact, in most hospital laboratories, the $[HCO_3^-]$

---

*The "bicarbonate concentration" measured by the clinical laboratory is actually the total CO_2, a figure that is the sum of bicarbonate and dissolved CO_2 plus H_2CO_3. The latter term is the P_{CO_2} multiplied by the solubility coefficient of CO_2 in blood (α), 0.03. Thus, total $CO_2 = [HCO_3^-] + (0.03)(P_{CO_2})$. Most clinicians simply neglect the second term when the P_{CO_2} is normal; when hypercapnia is present, however, the second term contributes significantly to total CO_2.[1]

TABLE 25-1   pH and Hydrogen Ion Concentrations

pH	$[H^+]$ nmol/L
6.8	158
6.9	126
7.0	100
7.1	79
7.2	63
7.3	50
7.4	40
7.5	32
7.6	25
7.7	20

Source: Narins RG, Emmett M: Simple and mixed acid–base disorders: A practical approach. *Medicine* 59:161, 1980.

reported as part of a blood gas analysis is not measured, but rather calculated from pH and P_{CO_2} measurements.)

PHYSIOLOGY OF ACID PRODUCTION AND EXCRETION

The quantity of $[HCO_3^-]$ in relation to carbonic acid buffer in the system is not fixed but varies according to physiologic need. This flexibility is largely provided by pulmonary excretion of P_{CO_2}, which can vary significantly and rapidly according to the exigencies of the acid-base milieu. The kidney regulates $[HCO_3^-]$ excretion and the formation of new $[HCO_3^-]$ and can change the rate of these processes when demanded by the acid-base milieu. However, renal response to pulmonary acid-base disturbances requires hours to days to reach equilibrium.

Hepatic Influence on Acid-Base Balance

Increasing attention is being given to the role of the liver in acid-base homeostasis. Approximately 1 mol each of $[HCO_3^-]$ and ammonium is generated every day by protein catabolism. The irreversible synthesis of urea by the liver results in consumption of virtually all of this $[HCO_3^-]$. The rate of this reaction is closely tied to extracellular pH and $[HCO_3^-]$. This control, mediated by glutaminase and carbonic anhydrase, can result in significant retention and neutralization of bicarbonate during acidosis. The fixation of ammonium ions into urea

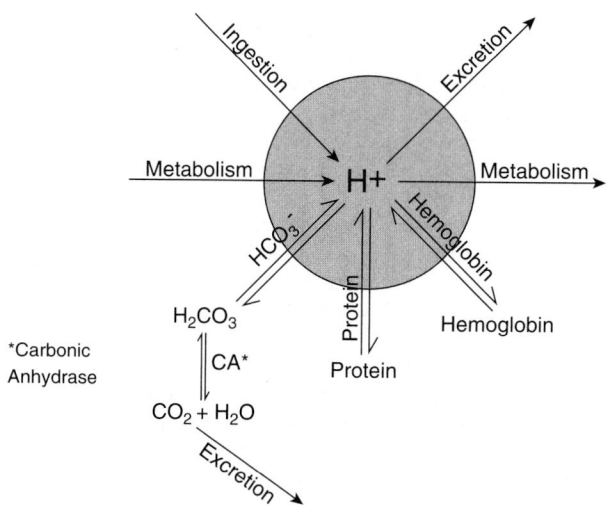

FIG. 25-1. Schematic representation of hydrogen ion homeostasis.

slows, but the kidney increases ammonia synthesis and excretion. This process not only prevents ammonia accumulation but also allows hydrogen ion trapping in the distal tubule. Further, hepatic cells without the cellular apparatus to fix ammonia into urea avidly use excess ammonia to synthesize glutamine.[3] Thus, the liver is the *"third organ"* of acid-base balance.

Renal Influence on Acid-Base Balance

Bicarbonate homeostasis requires the reclamation of filtered HCO_3^-, 85 percent of which occurs in the proximal convoluted tubule. Sodium is extruded from the tubular cell into the plasma in exchange for K^+ (via the Na^+/K^+-ATPase pump). To maintain equilibrium, cellular Na^+ is absorbed from the filtrate into the cell as H^+ is secreted into the lumen. This H^+ combines with the filtered HCO_3^- to produce carbonic acid (H_2CO_3), which carbonic anhydrase in turn converts to CO_2 and H_2O. To maintain equilibrium, CO_2 diffuses back into the cell, where cytoplasmic carbonic anhydrase regenerates H_2CO_3, which in turn completes the cycle by dissociating into $[HCO_3^-]$ and H^+ (thereby providing a supply of H^+ for extrusion). If tubular disease (such as occurs in renal tubular acidosis) inhibits H^+ extrusion, serum $[HCO_3^-]$ decreases to a steady-state level where reclaimed HCO_3^- effectively equals H^+ extrusion.

The balance (15 percent) of HCO_3^- reclamation occurs in the distal tubule. Via a *sodium-independent* process, cytoplasmic carbonic anhydrase generates H_2CO_3, which dissociates. HCO_3^- diffuses into plasma, and H^+ is secreted into the lumen by an H^+-ATPase pump, thereby maintaining cellular electrical neutrality. H^+ is trapped in the lumen by inorganic phosphate or ammonia $[NH_4^+]$. Failure of $[H^+]$ secretion is the underlying mechanism of distal renal tubular acidosis (RTA). A *sodium-dependent* process allows the generation of HCO_3^- in the distal tubule. Intracellular glutamine generates HCO_3^- and ammonia $[NH_4^+]$. The Na^+/K^+ pump moves $[Na^+]$ into the lumen, but $[Na^+]$ diffuses back across the cell membrane, and $[NH_4^+]$ is secreted into the lumen in exchange. Thus, the $[HCO_3^-]$ generated simply stays in the cell. Formation of $[HCO_3^-]$ by this process may require 4 to 5 days to reach equilibrium when acidosis so demands. Drugs that alter uptake or delivery of $[Na^+]$ to the distal tubule can significantly interfere. The process of acid secretion allows the regeneration of $[HCO_3^-]$ in proportion to the daily production of acid. Urine, especially under conditions of acidosis, can be made almost entirely free of $[HCO_3^-]$.

FUNDAMENTAL ACID-BASE DISORDERS

Any condition that disturbs acid-base balance by increasing $[H^+]$—whether through endogenous production, decreased buffering capacity, decreased excretion, or exogenous addition—is termed *acidosis*. Similarly, any condition that decreases $[H^+]$ is termed *alkalosis*. The terms *acidemia* and *alkalemia* refer to the net imbalance of $[H^+]$ in the blood. The difference between acidosis and acidemia is not merely semantic but of great clinical importance. For example, a patient with acidosis and alkalosis of equal magnitude will have a normal pH. Thus a patient with these disturbances has neither acidemia nor alkalemia but has two simultaneously occurring primary disturbances, acidosis and alkalosis. It is therefore important to appreciate that, although acidemia is diagnostic of acidosis and alkalemia of alkalosis, a normal or high pH does not exclude acidosis and a normal or low pH does not exclude alkalosis.

Acid-base disturbances are further classified as respiratory or metabolic. Respiratory acid-base disorders are due to primary changes in Pco_2, and metabolic disorders reflect primary changes in $[HCO_3^-]$. If there were no compensatory mechanism, the Kassirer-Bleich equation states that the magnitude of change in Pco_2 or $[HCO_3^-]$ would directly determine the magnitude of change in the pH. However, physiologic mechanisms tend to mitigate pH changes by effecting offsetting changes in bicarbonate and CO_2 levels. For example, the Pco_2 is elevated in respiratory acidosis, but the corresponding decrease in pH is attenuated over time by renal retention of bicarbonate.

Compensatory mechanisms are, by definition, not "disorders," but rather constitute normal physiologic responses to acid-base derangements. Terms such as *compensatory respiratory alkalosis* therefore are not only confusing but also misleading. The clinician is concerned with the adequacy of compensation, however, because failure of adequate compensation implies the presence of another primary acid-base disturbance. For example, a patient with metabolic acidosis who does not exhibit adequate respiratory compensation has a superimposed respiratory acidosis. Normal compensatory responses to each primary acid-base disturbance have been established through careful study and are presented later in this chapter.

It is important to note that compensatory mechanisms return the pH toward, but not completely to, normal.* The fact that compensatory mechanisms cannot become complete is evident when one considers that complete compensation would necessarily remove the (physiologic) stimulus driving the compensation.[1]

The "normal" values of pH, Pco_2, and $[HCO_3^-]$ for a given laboratory are ranges, intended to include 95 percent of patients without an acid-base disorder. The normal pH range is 7.35 to 7.45, the "normal" Pco_2 range is 35 to 45 mm Hg, and the "normal" $[HCO_3^-]$ is usually 21 to 28 mEq/L. However, a patient may have no value outside the "normal range" and still have significant acid-base disturbances. As detailed further below, a patient with a wide anion gap (AG) acidosis and a concomitant metabolic alkalosis of nearly equal magnitude will have a perfectly "normal" pH, Pco_2, and $[HCO_3^-]$. In contrast, abnormal-appearing values may, in fact, be appropriate for a given simple acid-base disturbance. For example, in the presence of a metabolic acidosis ($[HCO_3^-] = 15$; pH = 7.3), an appropriate respiratory compensation should result in a Pco_2 of about 30 mm Hg. The Pco_2 is below the "normal" range but at the expected level for the degree of (metabolic) acidosis. In this example, the finding of Pco_2 in the normal (35 to 45) range actually implies the presence of a respiratory acidosis, because the expected physiologic respiratory response is inadequate.

The Anion Gap

The principle of electrical neutrality requires that plasma have no net charge. The charge of the predominant plasma cation, sodium, therefore must be "balanced" by the charge of plasma anions. Although $[HCO_3^-]$ and $[Cl^-]$ constitute a significant fraction of plasma anions, the sum of their concentrations does not equal that of sodium. Therefore, there must be other anions present in the serum that preserve electrical neutrality. These anions are mostly serum proteins, phosphate, sulfate, and organic anions, such as lactate, and the conjugate bases of ketoacids. Because these substances are not commonly measured, they are termed *unmeasured anions* (UA). Unmeasured cations (UC) also exist, largely in the form of $[Ca^{2+}]$ and $[Mg^{2+}]$. Because all cations, measured and unmeasured, must equal all anions (measured and unmeasured),

$$MC + UC = MA + UA \qquad (3)$$

it follows that

$$MC - MA = UA - UC = AG \qquad (4)$$

Thus, substituting measured ions produces

$$[Na^+] - ([HCO_3^-] + [Cl^-]) = AG \qquad (5)$$

The difference between the serum $[Na^+]$ (the contribution of $[K^+]$, largely an intracellular ion, is usually neglected) and the sum of serum $[Cl^-]$ and $[HCO_3^-]$ equals the concentration of the unmeasured anions. For the purposes of AG determination, correction of serum $[Na^+]$ in the face of hyperglycemia is unnecessary, because this condition similarly dilutes $[Cl^-]$.[4]

---

*The sole exception is in chronic respiratory alkalosis, where bicarbonate levels may decline to a level that nearly normalizes the pH such that differentiating the actual pH from normal falls within the range of laboratory error.

The unmeasured anion concentration is commonly called the *anion gap,* and its normal value had been considered to be 12 ± 4 mEq/L. Recent reports have suggested that a normal AG value of 7 ± 4 mEq/L may be more appropriate to electrolyte measurements made with ion-specific electrodes.[5] However, the value used by the clinician should reflect institutional practice.[6] As with other acid-base concepts, the accepted "normal" range for the AG is less important than whether it has changed in relation to the patient's steady-state (baseline) value. Thus, a relative change in AG is more important than the actual value. However, virtually all values above 15 mEq/L can be considered abnormal, even when there are no previous comparison values available.

The AG may change even in the absence of acid-base disturbances. It may rise when (unmeasured) cations are decreased, as in severe states of hypomagnesemia, hypokalemia, and hypocalcemia. A reduced (narrow) or even negative anion gap may result from an increase in unmeasured *cations,* such as lithium, and unmeasured positively charged proteins resulting from myeloma and polyclonal gammopathies or from a decrease in unmeasured anions, such as albumin and γ globulin. A narrow or negative AG also may be the result of confounders of chloride measurement. Bromide is measured as chloride on an equimolar basis by chloride-specific electrodes. Other techniques of chloride measurement may produce even more inaccurate results in the presence of bromide.[7] Triglyceride levels greater than 600 mg/dL produce overestimation of chloride levels measured by colorimetric techniques and may result in underestimation of serum sodium, resulting in an apparently narrow or even negative AG.[4]

Although increases in the AG are traditionally considered in the context of metabolic acidosis, elevation of the AG may be seen with many acid-base disturbance. Metabolic and respiratory alkalosis, for example, may elevate the AG by 2 to 3 mEq/L, because of elevations in lactate produced by enhancement of glycolysis. Penicillin and carbenicillin, as anions, produce elevations in the AG. Their charges must be balanced by sodium, which is retained by renal tubules at the cost of enhancing secretion of potassium and hydrogen ions. This effect is enhanced by the presence of the poorly reabsorbed penicillin and carbenicillin ions in the tubule lumen, the negative charges of which serve as an electrical gradient for hydrogen and potassium ion secretions. The result is an elevated AG with a hypokalemic alkalosis, illustrating the principle that anions principally cleared by the kidney may elevate the AG, particularly when aldosterone activity is high.

However, elevation of the AG is most commonly associated with metabolic acidosis (Table 25-2). Traditional mnemonics for the differential diagnosis of an elevated AG acidosis unfortunately suggest that iron, theophylline, cyanide, biguanides, and other compounds *are* unmeasured anions. These substances actually elevate the AG by producing lactic acidosis, discussed later in this chapter. The result of using traditional mnemonics in evaluating elevated AG acidosis may result in a satisfaction-of-search error, where the discovery of lactic acidosis provides a ready explanation for the elevated AG and thereby inhibits consideration of the full differential diagnosis of lactic acidosis. We suggest that the differential diagnosis of metabolic acidosis with an elevated AG should emphasize distinctions between endogenous and exogenous unmeasured anion sources and avoid mixing the etiology of lactic acidosis with that of other increased unmeasured anions.

Clinical use of the AG requires an appreciation of its limitations. Although an AG greater than 30 mEq/L is usually caused by lactic acidosis or ketoacidosis, these conditions may exist even when the AG is normal. An AG value less than 25 mEq/L has been found to be an insensitive indicator of elevated lactate levels in critically ill patients[8]; in trauma patients, the post-resuscitation AG does not predict lactate levels.[9] Thus, a "normal" AG does not exclude the presence of increased concentrations of unmeasured anions. An AG increased from baseline but still within the "normal" range may be a clue. Direct measurements of lactate, formate, ketoacids, methanol (parent of formic acid), ethylene glycol (parent of oxalic acid and numerous other organic acids), and salicylate should be ordered when the presence of any of these substances is suspected but the AG is "normal" (particularly when the value is in the upper range of normal).

A common clinical problem is the diagnosis of mixed acid-base disturbances in the presence of an elevated AG. Simple acid-base disturbances that produce elevated AGs are referred to as *wide-AG metabolic acidoses.* If a wide-AG metabolic acidosis is the only disturbance, then the change (elevation from baseline) in value of the AG (sometimes referred to as the *delta gap*)[10] should exactly equal the change (decrease) in the $[HCO_3^-]$. This is a one-to-one relationship. This concept is represented mathematically in Eq. (6).

$$\Delta \uparrow AG = \Delta \downarrow [HCO_3^-] \qquad (6)$$

This simple relationship can be used to great advantage in determining the presence of other metabolic acid-base disturbances. If the $[HCO_3^-]$ is even lower than predicted by the delta AG, then there must be a concomitant hyperchloremic (i.e., non-AG type) metabolic acidosis (Figure 25-2A). Similarly, if the decrease in $[HCO_3^-]$ is less than expected based on the delta AG, there must be a concomitant metabolic alkalosis present. Note that acute respiratory conditions (respiratory acidosis or alkalosis) do not affect these determinations. Potential acid-base disturbances related to respiratory status must be further determined, as discussed below (Figure 25-2A to 25-2C).

Parameters Required for Clinical Acid-Base Evaluation

When taking a medical history, one should emphasize events that may result in the gain or loss of acid or base, such as vomiting, diarrhea, medications, or ingestions, and seek evidence of dysfunction of the organs of acid-base homeostasis: the liver, kidneys, and lungs.

Laboratory evaluation requires blood samples for determination of electrolyte concentrations ($[Na^+]$, $[K^+]$, $[Cl^-]$, $[HCO_3^-]$) and blood gases (pH, P_{CO_2}, and $[HCO_3^-]$). Most clinical laboratories measure

TABLE 25-2 Unmeasured Anions Associated with an Elevated Anion Gap and Metabolic Acidosis

Diagnostic Category	Species	Origin	Diagnostic Adjuncts
Renal failure (uremia)	$[PO_4^{2-}]$, $[SO_4^{2-}]$	Protein metabolism	BUN/Creatinine

Ketoacidosis
  Diabetic
  Alcoholic
  Starvation
	Ketoacids
	β-hydroxybutyrate
	Acetoacetate
		Fatty acid metabolism	Serum/urine ketones

Lactic acidosis	Lactate	Metabolism	Lactate level

Exogenous poisoning
  Methanol
  Ethylene glycol (EG)
 	
  Salicylate
	
	Formate
	Oxylate and organic anions
	
	Salicylate
		
		Methanol metabolism
		EG metabolism, also results in high NAD/NADH
		  ratio, favoring pyruvate conversion to lactate
		Salicylate, lactate, ketoacids
			
			Osmolal gap
			Osmolal gap
			Oxylate crystals (urine)
			Concomitant respiratory alkalosis
			  and metabolic alkalosis

Abbreviations: BUN = serum urea nitrogen; NAD = nicotinamide adenine dinucleotide.

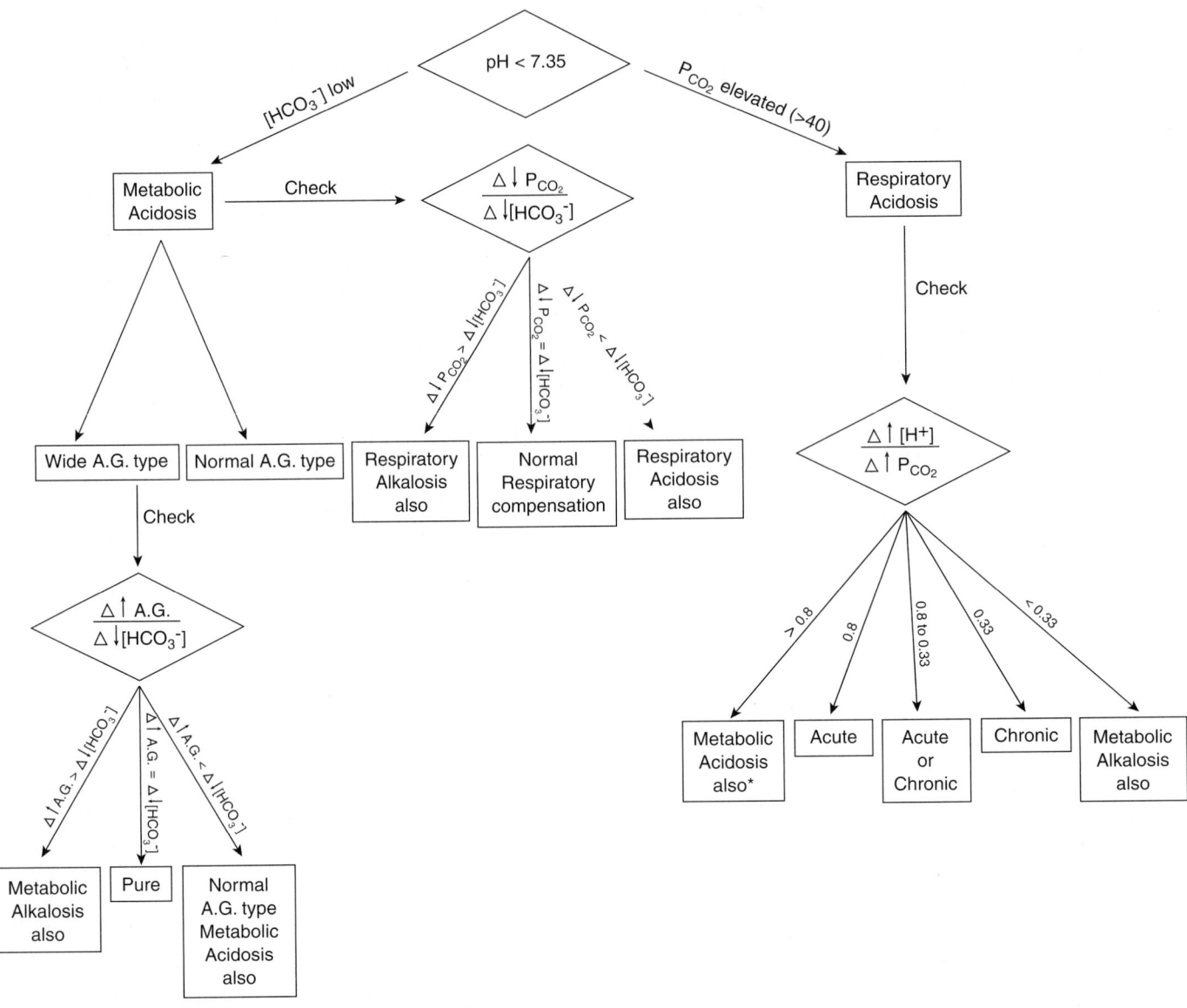

Key: *It is likely that [HCO₃⁻] is < 25 in this scenario and the tree could have been started on the left.
A.G., anion gap.

FIG. 25-2. A. Algorithm for determination of type of acidosis and mixed acid-base disturbances when pH indicates acidemia.

two of the parameters reported in blood gas results (most commonly the pH and P_{CO_2}) and use the Henderson-Hasselbalch equation to calculate the third ([HCO₃⁻]).

Blood samples for acid-base evaluation are traditionally obtained by arterial puncture, but there is some evidence that venous blood may be used instead. Arterial and capillary values of pH and CO_2 content in normal patients and those with diabetic ketoacidosis correlate well (correlation coefficients of 0.9 and 0.98, respectively). Recent work has demonstrated high correlations between arterial and venous pH ($r = 0.9689$) and between arterial and venous bicarbonate concentrations ($r = 0.9543$) in ED patients with diabetic ketoacidosis.[11] The correlation between venous and arterial blood gas values in patients with severe shock remains uncertain, but in other circumstances the use of venous values seems reasonable. Inexperienced clinicians frequently resort to arterial blood gas (ABG) determination as a means to "know" the pH. However, the pH per se is often the least important value for diagnosis and management. When respiratory status is not compromised, the pH can be calculated with the aid of the Kassirer-

Bleich equation [see Eq. (2)] from knowing the venous [HCO₃⁻] alone, as described below.

METABOLIC ACIDOSIS

Metabolic acidosis may result from [HCO₃⁻] loss per se, administration of acid, or endogenous production and accumulation of acid. Loss of [HCO₃⁻] occurs in externalization of intestinal contents (e.g., vomiting, enterocutaneous fistulae) and renal wasting of bicarbonate (e.g., renal tubular acidosis, carbonic anhydrase inhibitor therapy). Administration of acid (unlikely to be seen in the ED) occurs primarily in total parenteral nutrition, where patients receive hydrochloric salts of basic amino acids. Endogenous acids accumulate in renal tubular acidosis, ketoacidosis, and lactic acidosis.

Unopposed metabolic acidosis results in a decreased serum [HCO₃⁻] and an increase in serum [H⁺]. The increased [H⁺] stimulates the respiratory center, resulting in increased alveolar ventilation. The physiologically based "respiratory compensation" is an attempt to lower the [H⁺]

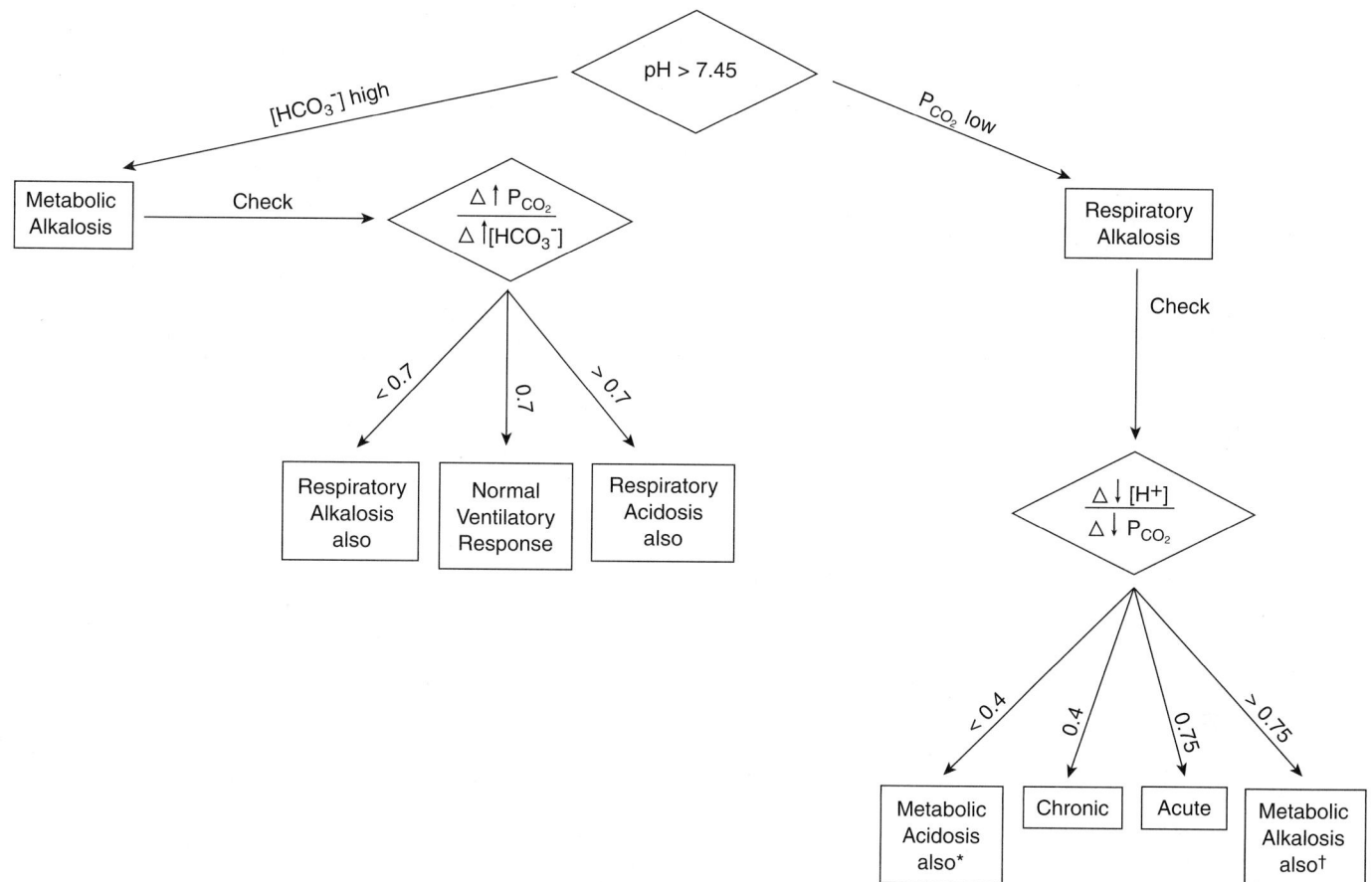

Key : *Implies that the △ in [H⁺] is not low, but elevated, and thus the pH would be < 7.40. Therefore, this algorithm would not be selected but rather Fig. 21-2A.
†It is likely that the HCO₃⁻ will be > 25 in this scenario and then the tree could have started on the left.
A.G., anion gap.

FIG. 25-2. B. Algorithm for determination of type of alkalosis and mixed acid-base disturbances when pH indicates alkalemia.

by a reduction in P_{CO_2}. The steady-state relationship between the P_{CO_2} and the $[HCO_3^-]$, determined from a study of 60 patients who had only metabolic acidosis of more than 24-h duration, is shown in Eq. (7).[12]*

$$P_{CO_2} = (1.5 \times [HCO_3^-] + 8) \pm 2 \qquad (7)$$

Equation (7) was derived from patients with more than 24 h of metabolic acidosis, although the respiratory response is almost immediate. When $[HCO_3^-]$ is greater than about 8 mEq/L, the relation between P_{CO_2} and $[HCO_3^-]$ is simpler: With normal respiratory compensation, P_{CO_2} *falls by 1 mm Hg for every 1-mEq/L fall in $[HCO_3^-]$.* Use of these relationships allows the clinician to calculate the expected P_{CO_2} (when respiratory compensation is normal) from the measured $[HCO_3^-]$. If the expected P_{CO_2} value differs from the measured value in uncomplicated steady-state metabolic acidosis, a primary respiratory disorder also exists. For example, if the $[HCO_3^-]$ is 15 mEq/L, the expected P_{CO_2} is about 30 mm Hg. If it is higher than this value (say 35 mm Hg), then by definition there is also a concomitant respiratory acidosis (see Figure 25-2A). If the value is lower than expected (say 25 mm Hg), then there is a concomitant respiratory alkalosis. This latter case is not an "overcompensation" but rather a second primary disturbance occurring simultaneously. These are important concepts. The body cannot tolerate metabolic and respiratory mechanisms for acidosis simultaneously, because one cannot buffer or compensate for the other.

*The constants in this equation ($P_{CO_2} = 1.54 \times [HCO_3^-] + 8.36 \pm 2$) have been rounded for ease of use.

Unfortunately, the ED patient's illness can rarely be assumed to be in steady state. Pierce and colleagues, in physiologic studies of otherwise healthy persons with acute metabolic acidosis caused by diarrhea, found that the completeness of the respiratory response to metabolic acidosis depends on the duration of the acidosis, the time course of its development, and its severity.[13] If acidosis develops quickly, the P_{CO_2} is often higher than that observed in steady state; the more rapid and severe the acidosis, the larger the difference between the observed P_{CO_2} and the predicted steady-state P_{CO_2}. When $[HCO_3^-]$ is then held constant, steady-state P_{CO_2} is reached in 11 to 24 h. When acidosis develops or is corrected more slowly, there is no lag in respiratory compensation.

There are limits to the adequacy of respiratory compensation during metabolic acidosis. In a study of diabetic ketoacidosis, Kety and colleagues found that respiratory minute volume actually declines when pH decreases below 7.10.[14] This finding led Albert and associates[12] and Pierce and colleagues[13] to initiate bicarbonate therapy when their subjects' pH fell below 7.10. These studies appear to have established 7.10 as the definition of "severe" metabolic acidosis. It is particularly important to appreciate any contribution to the acidosis from inadequate respiratory response. Simply initiating bicarbonate therapy when a pH of less than 7.1 is encountered may miss the respiratory insufficiency, which, if addressed, may obviate the use of solutions containing $[HCO_3^-]$. Further, administration of $[HCO_3^-]$ in the face of inadequate ventilatory response may actually exacerbate the respiratory acidosis, because the $[HCO_3^-]$ is converted to CO_2 and H_2O. The development of metabolic acidosis in which the pH is below 7.10 probably is associated with a very high risk of

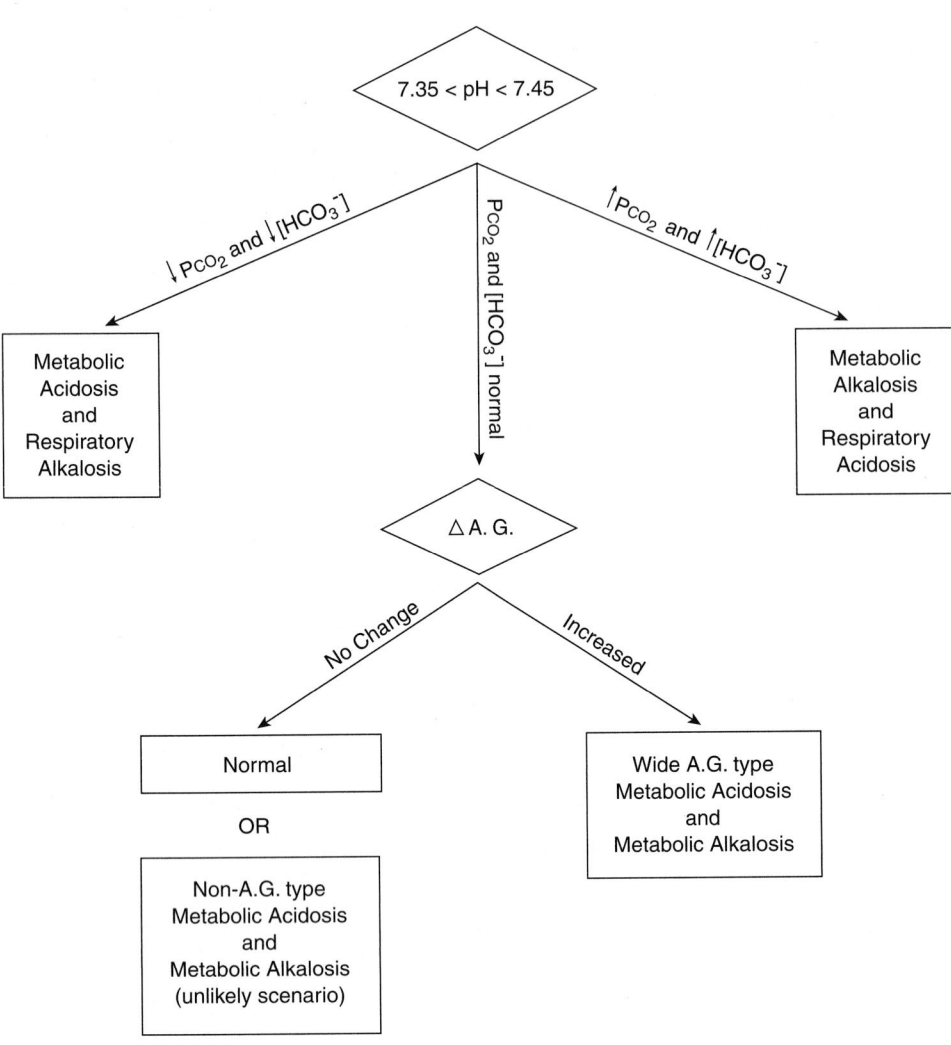

FIG. 25-2. C. Algorithm to check for acid-base disturbances when pH is within in the "normal" range.

Key : A.G., anion gap.

ventilatory insufficiency, because there is a limit to respiratory compensation. The lowest P_{CO_2} level achievable is about 12 mm Hg. The restriction of air movement and the CO_2 generated by the exertion required for rapid ventilation limits the attainable nadir for P_{CO_2}. The superimposition of respiratory acidosis on a patient in such straits will result in a rapid decline of pH to levels at which organ function and pharmacotherapy will fail. Mechanical ventilation usually should be instituted in such situations.

The serum $[K^+]$ level is affected by metabolic acidosis. The movement of H^+ into cells is associated with extrusion of K^+. Changes in $[K^+]$ are more substantial in inorganic acidosis, although elevated serum $[K^+]$ are typically seen in diabetic ketoacidosis (DKA). In general, for each 0.10 change in the pH, serum $[K^+]$ will increase by approximately 0.5 mEq/L. Whatever the mechanism of the acidosis, it is important to remember that normal in addition to low serum $[K^+]$ likely reflects severe intracellular K^+ depletion. The reversal of the acidosis in such circumstances may result in severe hypokalemia, with attendant cardiovascular effects.

Causes of Metabolic Acidosis

The causes of elevated-AG metabolic acidosis are listed in Table 25-2. We re-emphasize that the AG may be within the normal range, even when a metabolic acidosis associated with increased concentrations of unmeasured anions is present. A comparison with the patient's steady-state AG should occur whenever possible. Measurement or detection of specific anions may be indicated. However, caution is necessary when serum ketone testing is performed, because the chemical reac-

tion used to measure serum ketones has an important limitation: the nitroprusside reaction for ketones is positive only for species whose carbonyl moiety has an α-methyl group. The major ketone present in the sera of patients with untreated diabetic or alcoholic ketoacidosis may be β-hydroxybutyrate, which has no α-methyl group and is not detected by the nitroprusside reaction. The result may be a paradox: initial serum ketone assays in a patient with clinically severe diabetic ketoacidosis are only weakly positive yet rise despite clear clinical improvement. This occurs because appropriate treatment alters the hepatic ratio of nicotinamide adenine dinucleotide (NAD) to $NADH_2$, and the restoration of NAD concentrations allows oxidation of β-hydroxybutyrate to acetoacetate. The addition of several drops of hydrogen peroxide to serum also will oxidize β-hydroxybutyrate to acetoacetate in cases in which this distinction is clinically important. See Chap. 211 for a detailed discussion.

Lactic acidosis occurs whenever lactate production exceeds lactate use or metabolism and is classically of two types. The first, in which tissue hypoxia is present and lactate production is elevated, is referred to as *type A*. Normal tissue oxygenation and impairment of lactate use define the second, called *type B*. Type B lactic acidosis is further subdivided. Type B_1 lactic acidosis is associated with systemic disorders, such as diabetes, renal insufficiency, sepsis, and leukemia; type B_2 is associated with various substances, especially biguanides (phenformin, metformin), salicylates, methanol, iron, and isoniazid; and type B_3 is associated with hereditary metabolic diseases.

The pyruvate produced by glycolysis may be transported across mitochondrial membranes and metabolized in the Krebs cycle under aerobic conditions. However, under anaerobic conditions, it is oxidized to lactate by lactate dehydrogenase. This reaction is reversible, but the conversion of lactate to pyruvate in the liver requires NAD. Thus, it is not surprising that many patients with type B lactic acidosis have underlying liver disease. For example, an alcoholic may develop lactic acidosis after giving up heavy drinking, because impaired gluconeogenesis prevents pyruvate fixation into glucose, and the metabolism of ethanol has left little NAD available to convert lactate to pyruvate. The distinction between type A and type B lactic acidosis is useful in conceptualizing the therapeutic approach. However, there is some impairment of lactate use in both types, usually because of impaired hepatic oxygenation or perfusion, in the case of type A, and because of underlying liver disease, in the case of type B.

Differential Diagnoses of Wide-AG Acidosis

An ABG is completely immaterial in determining whether a wide-AG metabolic acidosis exists. The determination is made with simple venous electrolytes. The differential diagnosis falls into four broad categories: renal failure (uremia), lactic acidosis, ketoacidosis [DKA, alcoholic ketoacidosis (AKA), starvation ketoacidosis (SKA)], and ingestions (methanol, ethylene glycol, salicylates).

Renal failure should be evident from the serum chemistries. Positive serum ketones point to one of the ketoacidoses. In known insulin-dependent diabetes mellitus, DKA is likely, although there is usually a small component of lactic acidosis for reasons just described. In alcoholics who have recently stopped binge drinking, AKA should be considered. Starvation ketosis will be found in patients with inadequate recent oral intake (fasting, dieting, or protracted vomiting), although the magnitude of acid-base disturbance in starvation ketosis should be small.

Determination of the osmolal gap will help differentiate two of the ingestants from other etiologies. Elevated osmolal gaps are seen in methanol and ethylene glycol poisoning. Although methanol is measured in most hospital laboratories, determination of ethylene glycol levels is performed off-site in many institutions. A widened osmolal gap without evidence of methanol ingestion may determine the diagnosis long before confirmatory laboratory evidence is available. Calculation adjustments to the osmolal gap may need to be made if ethanol is a coingestant (see Chap. 27 for detailed discussion).

When the diagnosis remains in doubt or poor tissue perfusion is a diagnostic possibility, lactate levels should be specifically sent. It should be noted that several poisonings may result in lactic acidosis, including isoniazid, iron, carbon monoxide, methemoglobin, and cyanide. This is but one reason investigators shun the overtaught mnemonic of *MUDPILES*. For example, this mnemonic does not clearly reflect the fact that isoniazid and iron exert their effects on the AG through lactic acidosis. Also, ethanol is frequently cited as a cause of wide-AG acidosis. However, **ethanol should never be considered the etiologic source of any significant metabolic acidosis.** Although ethyl alcohol metabolism may lead indirectly to very mild lactic acidosis, usually due to AKA, neither the alcohol nor its metabolites directly contribute to the acidosis.

Severe acidosis that is resistant to treatment is seen in various type B_1 lactic acidoses and ingestions. AKA and SKA tend to be mild. Acidosis seen in initial stages of renal failure may be severe but tends to be stable ([HCO_3^-] about 15 mEq/L) in chronic renal failure. Concomitant acid-base disturbance may further assist in determining the etiology. The triple acid-base disturbance of wide-AG metabolic acidosis, metabolic alkalosis, and respiratory alkalosis is seen with sepsis (lactic acidosis) and salicylate poisoning. The latter also may be associated with a mild temperature elevation.

The relation of [HCO_3^-] to the AG and the [HCO_3^-] to the expected P_{CO_2} compensation must be examined in every patient with wide-AG acidosis to determine whether other (respiratory) acid-base disturbances exist (see Figure 25-2A).

Differential Diagnosis of Unchanged (Normal) AG Acidosis

The non-AG type of acidosis is often referred to as "normal" AG acidosis. Issues related to the AG are relative, so the term *unchanged* or

non-AG type is preferred. Some texts refer to this as *hyperchloremic metabolic acidosis.*

Non-AG acidosis results from loss of [HCO_3^-], failure to excrete [H^+], or administration of H^+. Bicarbonate may be lost from the urine or gastrointestinal tract and is usually accompanied by K^+ loss. However, potassium-sparing diuretics, hypoaldosteronism, urinary tract obstruction, and type IV renal tubular acidosis result in loss of [HCO_3^-] with retention of [K^+] (Table 25-3).

One should be wary of the traditional classification based on K^+, because serum [K^+] itself is dependent on the actual pH. Thus, in severe acidosis, a normal range [K^+] may be deceiving unless the clinician corrects for the degree of acidosis.

Because all diuretics have a tendency to result in mild contraction alkalosis, the metabolic acidosis that occurs simultaneously with potassium-sparing diuretics may not be evident, as the two distinct physiologic processes may simply cancel each other out (see Figure 25-2C). Because the AG is unchanged, there is no clue that two opposed processes may be occurring.

Acetazolamide exerts its effect through carbonic anhydrase inhibition, inducing a functional RTA.

Physiologic Consequences of Acidosis

Acidemia has numerous negative physiologic consequences that impair the function of many different organs through mechanisms not yet well understood. Cardiac contractile function is reduced, probably due to impaired oxidative phosphorylation, intracellular acidosis, and alterations in intracellular calcium concentration. The threshold for ventricular fibrillation falls, whereas the defibrillation threshold rises. Hepatic and renal perfusion and systemic blood pressure decline, whereas pulmonary vascular resistance increases. The physiologic effects of catecholamines are attenuated, and, when acidosis is sufficiently severe, vascular collapse may result. A catabolic state develops, including a generalized increase in metabolism, resistance to insulin, and inhibition of anaerobic glycolysis. The effect of hypoxia on all organs is aggravated.[15]

Treatment

The treatment of acidosis reflects that of the underlying disorder but particularly emphasizes restoration of normal tissue perfusion and oxygenation. The most important step is to determine whether there is a respiratory component to the acidosis (i.e., a primary respiratory acidosis), because the treatment approach differs. If there is inadequate respiratory compensation, the most appropriate treatment will be to first correct the respiratory problem.

Buffer Therapy in Acidosis

The adverse effects of acidemia make the concept of buffer therapy teleologically appealing, but the role of buffer therapy in cardiac arrest

TABLE 25-3 Causes of Normal Anion Gap Metabolic Acidosis

With a tendency to hyperkalemia	With a tendency to hypokalemia
Subsiding diabetic ketoacidosis	Renal tubular acidosis, type I (classical distal acidosis)
Early uremic acidosis	
Early obstructive uropathy	Renal tubular acidosis, type II (proximal acidosis)
Renal tubular acidosis, type IV	
Hypoaldosteronism (Addison disease)	Acetazolamide
	Acute diarrhea with losses of [HCO_3^-] and [K^+]
Infusion or ingestion of HCl, NH$_4$Cl, lysine-HCl, or arginine-HCl	Ureterosigmoidostomy with increased resorption of [H^+] and [Cl^-] and losses of [HCO_3^-] and [K^+]
Potassium-sparing diuretics	
	Obstruction of artificial ileal bladder
	Dilution acidosis

and severe metabolic acidosis is uncertain. The traditional therapeutic buffer, sodium bicarbonate, may have negative effects in the treatment of acidosis. Bicarbonate therapy results in the generation of significant quantities of CO_2, which diffuses readily into cells, in particular those of the central nervous system, and therefore may cause paradoxical worsening of intracellular acidosis. An abrupt CO_2 load also may exceed the ventilatory capacity of a maximally ventilating patient, thereby producing abrupt or worsening respiratory failure. After successful treatment with bicarbonate, "overshoot" alkalosis may result. Bicarbonate therapy imposes an osmotic and sodium load (1000 mEq/L of typical 1N solution). These concerns suggest that bicarbonate therapy should not be used in the ED treatment of mild to moderate metabolic acidosis.

Kraut and Kurtz recently reviewed the literature concerning buffer therapy in cardiac arrest, diabetic ketoacidosis, and lactic acidosis.[16] Several studies of HCO_3^- use (adult and pediatric, including patients with severe acidosis) failed to show any improvement in speed of recovery or complication rates with buffer therapy. However, it remains unclear whether certain subgroups of patients, for example, those with cardiac or other disease, may benefit from bicarbonate therapy in DKA.

Similarly, a review of studies of HCO_3^- use suggested that patients with mild lactic acidosis derive no mortality benefit from bicarbonate therapy, and such patients who also have severe cardiac disease may actually suffer deleterious effects. However, patients with severe acidosis demonstrated a mortality benefit when treated with "large" doses of bicarbonate and concomitant dialysis. The goal of high-dose bicarbonate and dialysis therapy in lactic acidosis may be to "bridge" the patient physiologically to definitive treatment of the etiology of the acidosis. Bicarbonate therapy seems reasonable, therefore, in situations in which the effects of lactic acidosis are so severe that they preclude or jeopardize therapy for the underlying disease (Table 25-4).

When $[HCO_3^-]$ is used, Adrogue and Madias[15] recommended administering $[HCO_3^-]$, 0.5 mEq/kg, for each milliequivalent per liter desired rise in $[HCO_3^-]$. The goal is to restore adequate buffer capacity ($[HCO_3^-] > 8$ mEq/L) or achieve clinical improvement in shock or dysrhythmias. Bicarbonate should be given as slowly as the clinical situation permits; 75 mL of 8.4 percent sodium bicarbonate in 500 mL of D5W produces a nearly isotonic solution for infusion. Adequate time should be allowed for the desired effect to be achieved, and close monitoring of acid-base balance, especially in patients with organic acidosis, is critical.

Newer buffers appear to show promise in the treatment of metabolic acidosis. Carbicarb, an equimolar solution of sodium bicarbonate and sodium carbonate $[CO_3^{2-}]$, produces significantly less CO_2 than an equimolar dose of bicarbonate. The carbonate ion, a strong base, combines avidly with protons to form bicarbonate, resulting in increased pH, an increased $[HCO_3^-]$, and limited CO_2 production. Clinical studies of Carbicarb use in lactic acidosis models have shown improvements in pH with little or no change in P_{CO_2}.[17,18] Trials of Carbicarb therapy in cardiac arrest have yielded equivocal results. Thus, Carbicarb, although a promising agent for buffer therapy, remains experimental. Tris-hydroxymethyl amino-methane (THAM), an inert amino acid, has been studied as a buffer; its promise resides in its pK_a (at 7.8, THAM should be a more effective buffer than HCO_3^-) and its ability to penetrate cells (in reducing intracellular P_{CO_2}). Limited studies, generally not in humans, have suggested that THAM provides salutary pH and P_{CO_2} changes when given in metabolic acidosis. However, information about its effects in humans and its role in treatment is still developing, and THAM is at present an experimental agent.

METABOLIC ALKALOSIS

Metabolic alkalosis is typically classified as chloride-sensitive and chloride-insensitive, thus indicating the treatment approach. Metabolic alkalosis results from gain of bicarbonate or loss of acid. The relation of metabolic alkalosis to chloride balance defines pathophysiologic features of the disease and its therapy. Bicarbonate and chloride represent the major serum anions whose concentrations may be readily altered, and their homeostasis is therefore closely intertwined.

Conditions that produce chloride loss, such as vomiting (which also produces acid loss), diarrhea, diuretic therapy, and chloride-wasting diseases (e.g., cystic fibrosis and chloride-wasting enteropathy) tend to reduce serum chloride concentration and extracellular volume. The reduction in extracellular volume increases mineralocorticoid activity, which enhances sodium reabsorption and potassium and hydrogen ion secretion in the distal tubule, which in turn enhance bicarbonate generation. The resulting increase in serum $[HCO_3^-]$ eventually exceeds the tubule's maximum ability to reabsorb filtered bicarbonate. The resulting alkaline urine, because its anionic content is mostly bicarbonate, is largely free of chloride (<10 mEq/L), although the urine chloride may be normal after diuretics have been administered. The result is hypokalemic, hypochloremic alkalosis that responds to normal saline (chloride-responsive alkalosis).

Other diseases that cause metabolic alkalosis are usually associated with normovolemia or hypervolemia and often hypertension. These diseases usually cause excess mineralocorticoid activity, resulting in the same pathophysiologic cascade described above. However, the excess mineralocorticoid activity is not associated with hypovolemia, so the urine chloride is generally normal or elevated (>10 mEq/L) and the alkalosis cannot be reversed with normal saline. Diseases producing "chloride-unresponsive alkalosis" and hypertension include renal artery stenosis, renin-secreting tumors, adrenal hyperplasia, hyperaldosteronism, Cushing syndrome, Liddle syndrome, and exogenous mineralocorticoids (e.g., licorice, fludrocortisone). Chloride-unresponsive alkalosis caused by Bartter and Gitelman syndromes usually is associated with normotension.

The compensation for metabolic alkalosis involves reduction in alveolar ventilation, but the exact relation between P_{CO_2} and $[H^+]$ is not well established. Most studies to date have been conducted in dialysis patients or patients with conditions that predispose to alveolar hyperventilation (e.g., sepsis, pneumonia). As a guideline, P_{CO_2} in patients with significant metabolic alkalosis should rise 0.7 mm Hg for each milliequivalent increase in $[HCO_3^-]$. The P_{CO_2} also rarely rises above 55 mm Hg in compensation for metabolic alkalosis.

Consequences of Alkalosis

The physiologic effects of alkalemia are substantial. Neurologic abnormalities, especially tetany, neuromuscular instability, and seizures, are common. Reduction in $[H^+]$ results in reductions in ionized calcium, potassium, magnesium, and phosphate levels. Constriction of arterioles occurs, resulting in reduced coronary and cerebral blood flow. Refractory dysrhythmias may develop.[15] Alkalemia may be of

TABLE 25-4   Indications for Bicarbonate Therapy in Metabolic Acidosis

Indication	Rationale
Severe hypobicarbonatemia (<4 mEq/L)	Insufficient buffer concentrations may lead to extreme increases in acidemia with small increases in acidosis
Severe acidemia (pH <7.20) with signs of shock or myocardial irritability that is not rapidly responsive to supportive measures	Therapy for the underlying cause of acidosis depends upon adequate organ perfusion
Severe hyperchloremic acidemia*	Lost bicarbonate must be regenerated by kidneys and liver, which may require days

*No specific threshold indication by pH exists. The presence of serious hemodynamic insufficiency despite supportive care should guide the use of bicarbonate therapy for this indication.

particular concern in patients with chronic obstructive pulmonary disease (COPD), because of the shift of the oxygen hemoglobin to the left, making O_2 less available to the tissues. Many such patients are taking diuretics, which lead to a contraction alkalosis. Also, the alkalemic environment tends to depress ventilatory drive further.

Treatment

Therapy of alkalemia, as with all acid-base disorders, emphasizes treatment of the underlying cause and careful supportive care. Acetazolamide produces significant bicarbonaturia and is effective in the treatment of metabolic alkalosis, but its use requires very careful monitoring of potassium, magnesium, and phosphate concentrations. If alkalosis is severe ($[HCO_3^-] > 45$ mmol/L) and associated with serious signs or symptoms not responsive to supportive care, the use of intravenous hydrochloric acid should be considered. A 0.1 normal solution (100 mmol/L), infused at no more than 0.2 mmol/kg per h through a central venous catheter is used; higher concentrations may degrade the catheter material.[19] The dose is calculated as shown in Eq. (8), with the result in millimoles of bicarbonate.

$$\text{Dose} = (\Delta[HCO_3^-])(\text{weight, in kg})(0.5) \qquad (8)$$

RESPIRATORY ACIDOSIS

Respiratory acidosis is defined by alveolar hypoventilation and is diagnosed when the P_{CO_2} is greater then the expected value. Acute respiratory acidosis may have origins in other conditions, such as increased CO_2 production (high-glucose diet) and abnormal gas exchange (e.g., pneumonia). However, the final common path is inadequate ventilation.

Inadequate minute ventilation is most frequently due to head trauma, chest trauma, lung disease or excess sedation. The chronic hypoventilation seen in extremely obese patients is often referred to as the *pickwickian syndrome,* after an obese character in Charles Dickens' *Pickwick Papers.* Patients with severe COPD have increased dead space and frequently also have a decreased minute ventilation.

In general, a rise in the P_{CO_2} stimulates the respiratory center to increase respiratory rate and minute ventilation. However, if the arterial P_{CO_2} chronically exceeds 60 to 70 mm Hg, as may occur in 5 to 10 percent of patients with severe emphysema, the respiratory acidosis may depress the respiratory center. Under such circumstances, the stimulus for ventilation is provided primarily by hypoxemia acting on chemoreceptors in the carotid and aortic bodies. Giving oxygen could remove the main stimulus to breathe, causing the P_{CO_2} to rise abruptly to extremely dangerous levels. Consequently, one should not administer oxygen to patients with COPD without carefully watching for the development of apnea or hypoventilation.

Evaluation of ventilation requires attention to several important clinical issues. First, the ventilation that would be expected based on assessment of the respiratory rate and depth should be compared with the actual ventilation of the patient (i.e., P_{CO_2}). A "normal" P_{CO_2} of 40 mm Hg in a tachypneic, dyspneic patient likely reflects significant ventilatory insufficiency. Second, the impact of respiratory acidosis on partial pressure of oxygen in the alveoli (P_{AO_2}) in such a patient may be considerable. The alveolar gas equation suggests that, if inspired oxygen concentration and respiratory quotient do not change, increases in P_{CO_2} will result in reductions in P_{AO_2}.

The relation of P_{CO_2} to hydrogen ion concentration in acute respiratory acidosis is suggested by the Kassirer-Bleich equation shown in Eq. (9):

$$\Delta[H^+] = 0.8(\Delta P_{CO_2}) \qquad (9)$$

Each 1-mm Hg increase in P_{CO_2} results in a 1-mmol increase in $[H^+]$. Across the linear portion of the pH-hydrogen ion concentration relationship, each 1-mmHg increase in P_{CO_2} should theoretically produce a 0.01 decrease in pH. The actual relation between changes in P_{CO_2} (up to values of 90 mm Hg) and changes in $[H^+]$ determined in normal humans is about 8 to 10, as shown in Eq. (9). Thus, a 10-mm Hg increment in P_{CO_2} produces an 8-mmol increase in $[H^+]$, with little change in bicarbonate concentration (usually 1 mEq/L) or urinary acid excretion.[20] If the $[H^+]$ is higher or lower than that suggested by the change in the P_{CO_2}, a mixed disorder is present.

The adaptation to chronic respiratory acidosis is complex. Over time, chronic elevation of P_{CO_2} reduces carotid sinus sensitivity to hypercapnia; ventilatory drive is then controlled by P_{AO_2}. The acidosis results in significant increases in renal HCO_3^- generation and avid reclamation of filtered HCO_3^-. The relation between $[H^+]$ and $[HCO_3^-]$ in chronic respiratory acidosis at steady state, derived from studies in humans, is shown in Eq. (10).

$$\Delta[H^+] = 0.3(\Delta P_{CO_2}) \qquad (10)$$

It is rarely certain during a given clinical encounter whether a patient has an acute respiratory acidosis, a chronic respiratory acidosis, or a mixed disorder. Evaluation of the acid-base status in such circumstances does not require "baseline" ABG values. Instead, the change in $[H^+]$ is compared with the change in P_{CO_2}. If this ratio is 0.3, the patient has a chronic respiratory acidosis; if it is 0.8, the patient has an acute respiratory acidosis. States resulting in other ratios suggest a mixed acid-base disturbance, as shown in Table 25-5.

Treatment of respiratory acidosis is designed primarily to improve alveolar ventilation. In general, if the minute ventilation is doubled, the P_{CO_2} will be reduced by 50 percent. In patients with COPD, bronchodilators such as β-agonists, anticholinergics, or systemic sympathomimetic agents, with careful administration of small amounts of oxygen, may substantially improve ventilation. However, ventilatory assistance (intubation or noninvasive ventilatory support) may be required in some patients who do not respond adequately to lesser measures, particularly if the pH falls below 7.25.

In patients with a chronic respiratory acidosis, reduction of the P_{CO_2} should generally proceed slowly. The minute ventilation for a 70-kg person is normally about 6 L/min; in COPD patients, it may be

---

TABLE 25-5 Evaluation of Acid–Base Status in Respiratory Acidosis

| | | RATIO = $\Delta[H^+]/\Delta P_{CO_2}$ | | |
Ratio < 0.3	Ratio = 0.3	0.3 < Ratio < 0.8	Ratio = 0.8	Ratio > 0.8
Change in hydrogen ion concentration is less than accounted for by chronic change in P_{CO_2}. Metabolic alkalosis is also present.	Change in hydrogen ion concentration matches chronic change in P_{CO_2}. Chronic respiratory acidosis is present.	Change in hydrogen ion concentration is larger than accounted for by chronic change in P_{CO_2}. Chronic respiratory acidosis plus either acute respiratory alkalosis or metabolic acidosis is present; examine pH.	Change in hydrogen ion concentration matches acute change in P_{CO_2}. Acute respiratory acidosis is present.	Change in hydrogen ion concentration is larger than accounted for by acute or chronic change in P_{CO_2}. Metabolic acidosis is also present.

Abbreviation: P_{CO_2} = partial pressure of carbon dioxide.

less than 4 L/min. It is beyond the scope of this chapter to discuss in detail the approach to management of a patient with COPD and severe hypercarbia. If treatment is indicated in the ED, it may be wise to start with a minute ventilation of about 5 L/min and then gradually increase it according to the clinical response and changes in P_{CO_2}.

In patients with a chronic respiratory acidosis, the arterial P_{CO_2} should not be reduced by more than 5.0 mm Hg/h. Rapid correction of a chronic respiratory acidosis can cause sudden development of a severe combined metabolic and respiratory alkalosis with resulting dysrhythmias. A rapid rise in pH can cause an abrupt fall in ionized calcium and in hypokalemia. Both may cause dangerous dysrhythmias or seizures.

RESPIRATORY ALKALOSIS

Respiratory alkalosis is defined by alveolar hyperventilation and exists when P_{CO_2} is less then expected. It is caused by conditions that stimulate respiratory centers, including central nervous system tumors or stroke, infections, pregnancy, hypoxia, and toxins (e.g., salicylates). Anxiety, pain, and iatrogenic overventilation of patients on mechanical ventilators also cause respiratory alkalosis.

Whatever the etiology, the clinical symptoms of acute respiratory alkalosis are predictable from its physiologic effects. Acute reduction in P_{CO_2} produces a reduction in [H⁺], resulting in an increase in negative charge on anionic buffers. The now relatively negatively charged proteins instead bind calcium, and, if sufficient, the reduction in ionized calcium produces carpopedal spasm and paresthesias.[15] Hypocapnia also produces substantial reductions in cerebral blood flow and results in reduced tissue oxygen delivery due to a leftward shift in the oxygen-hemoglobin dissociation curve (i.e., increased hemoglobin oxygen binding).

The theoretical relationship of [H⁺] and P_{CO_2} predicted by the Kassirer-Bleich equation is that a 1-mmol decrease in [H⁺] results from each 1-mm Hg reduction in P_{CO_2}. The actual observed relationship is very close to that predicted by the Kassirer-Bleich equation.[21] Each millimeter of mercury reduction in P_{CO_2} results in a 0.75-mmol reduction in [H⁺] (Eq. 11).[21]

$$\Delta[H^+] = 0.75(\Delta P_{CO_2}) \qquad (11)$$

Chronic respiratory alkalosis is unique among the acid-base disorders in that its compensation may be complete. Compensatory events include bicarbonaturia and a reduction in acid excretion, requiring 6 to 72 h to develop fully and at least 1 week to normalize pH. The steady-state relationship between [H⁺] and P_{CO_2} in chronic respiratory alkalosis observed in normal human subjects at high altitude is shown in Eq. (12).[22]

$$\Delta[H^+] = 0.4(\Delta P_{CO_2}) \qquad (12)$$

Therapy for acute respiratory alkalosis emphasizes identification and treatment of the underlying cause. The use of paper-bag rebreathing in the treatment of respiratory alkalosis should be avoided. Callaham evaluated paper-bag rebreathing in voluntarily hyperventilating volunteers and found that, although the inspired P_{CO_2} increased by 20 mm Hg in 30 s, it never increased above 40 mm Hg. However, inspired oxygen concentration decreased by an average of 27 mm Hg in 180 s, and in 5 percent of subjects the decrease was greater than or equal to 42 mm Hg.[23] If the cause of hyperventilation is actually cellular hypoxia, such a decrease could be catastrophic.[24] Further, there is evidence that expectation of efficacy and suggestion, rather than elevations, of inspired CO_2 tension are responsible for relief of symptoms in hyperventilation.[25] An oxygen mask might provide benefits similar to those of paper-bag rebreathing with less risk of hypoxia.

Chronic respiratory alkalosis is seen at high altitudes, in particular among mountaineers climbing over 3700 m (12,000 ft) (where the partial pressure of O_2 is significantly diminished). Acetazolamide is frequently prescribed to counter the physiologic respiratory effects of such ascents.

CLINICAL APPROACH TO ACID-BASE PROBLEMS AND MIXED ACID-BASE DISTURBANCES

The evaluation of an acid-base problem begins with a history and physical examination, with particular attention to sources of acid or alkali gain or loss and to diseases that affect renal, hepatic, or pulmonary function. Blood should be obtained for gas analysis and electrolyte determination, and the AG should be calculated. Blood gas results should be checked for internal consistency with the Henderson-Hasselbalch or Kassirer-Bleich equation [Eq. (1) or (2)].

In metabolic acidosis, where the respiratory response appears clinically appropriate, the P_{CO_2} and pH can be predicted. Thus, one ABG to prove there is no abnormal respiratory component may be sufficient, and further evaluation can be determined from serum (venous) [HCO₃⁻] alone. For example, when the [HCO₃⁻] is 15, the expected physiologic respiratory compensatory response is expected to be a decline in P_{CO_2} equal to the decline in [HCO₃⁻], i.e., in this scenario, 30 mm Hg. The values for known [HCO₃⁻] and predicted P_{CO_2} can then be inserted in the Kassirer-Bleich equation shown in Eq. (2) to determine the [H⁺], which in this case is calculated to be about 48. The [H⁺] can then be related to the corresponding pH, which is close to linear for values from 22 to 55 nmol/L, in this case, about 7.32.

Methodical interpretation of laboratory results followed by correlation with the clinical scenario are necessary to prevent erroneous acid-base evaluation. Although we suggest one method that has worked well for us, the particular method used matters less than the consistency of its application. However, **reliance on "acid-base disturbance maps" is discouraged.** First, they may be misleading, particularly when there is more than one primary disturbance. Second, they offer no understanding of the processes. Without an understanding of the complex but not difficult to master concepts of interrelationships in acid-base balance, the clinician misses diagnoses and has little understanding of the appropriate approach to therapy. As long as the method selected reflects the acid-base relationships presented in this chapter, the result should be the same. One suggested method follows:

1. Look at the pH. If it is decreased, the primary or predominant disturbance is acidosis. If the pH is increased, the predominant disturbance is alkalosis.
2. If the pH indicates acidosis, the primary (or predominant) mechanism can be ascertained by examining the [HCO₃⁻] and P_{CO_2} (see Figure 25-2A).
   a. If the [HCO₃⁻] is low (implying a primary metabolic acidosis), then the AG should be examined and, if possible, compared with a known steady-state value.
      i. If the AG is increased compared with the known previous value or is greater than 15, then by definition a wide-AG metabolic acidosis is present, and the absolute change in the AG should be compared with the absolute change in the [HCO₃⁻] from normal.
      ii. If the AG is unchanged, then the disturbance is (non-widened) *unchanged AG* or *hyperchloremic* metabolic acidosis.
      iii. If the change in the AG is equal to the change in the [HCO₃⁻], then the wide AG-acidosis is termed *pure*. If the AG has risen more than the [HCO₃⁻] has decreased, then there is also likely to be a concomitant metabolic alkalosis. If the change in the AG is less than the change in the [HCO₃⁻], then a non-AG acidosis is also present. (This is a difficult concept, but two separate physiologic mechanisms resulting in increased [H⁺] can occur simultaneously.) Next examine whether the ventilatory response is appropriate.
      (1) If the decrease in the P_{CO_2} equals the decrease in the [HCO₃⁻], there is appropriate respiratory compensation. Note that the pH will not return to normal.
      (2) If the decrease in the P_{CO_2} is greater than the decrease in the [HCO₃⁻], there is a concomitant respiratory alkalosis. (Although there are other formulas for this comparison, this is the simplest, as explained earlier in the text.)

(3) If the decrease in the P_{CO_2} is less than the decrease in $[HCO_3^-]$, there is also a concomitant respiratory acidosis.

b. If the P_{CO_2} is elevated (rather than the $[HCO_3^-]$ being decreased), the primary disturbance is respiratory acidosis (see Figure 25-2A). The next step is to determine which type it is by examining the ratio of (i.e., the change in) $[H^+]$ to (the upward change in) the P_{CO_2}.

   i. If the ratio is 0.8, it is considered acute.

   ii. If the ratio is 0.33, it is considered chronic.

   iii. If the ratio is between 0.8 and 0.33, it is probably an acute exacerbation of the chronic condition.

   iv. If the ratio is greater than 0.8, there must be a metabolic explanation for the excess $[H^+]$.

   v. If the ratio is less than 0.33, a metabolic alkalosis must also be present.

3. If the pH is greater than 7.45, the primary or predominant disturbance is alkalosis (see Figure 25-2B).

a. It is best to look at the $[HCO_3^-]$ first. If it is elevated, there is a primary metabolic alkalosis. There is an expected ventilatory response, although it is quite varied. The ratio of the change upward in P_{CO_2} to the change upward in $[HCO_3^-]$ can be examined. If the ratio is much less than 0.7, there is also a respiratory alkalosis (in addition to the metabolic alkalosis). If the ratio is more or less 0.7, this is likely to be a compensatory ventilatory response. If the ratio is well above 0.7, respiratory acidosis is concomitantly present.

b. If the P_{CO_2} is low, there is a primary respiratory alkalosis, and the ratio of the change in $[H^+]$ to the change in P_{CO_2} should be examined. Acute respiratory alkalosis has a ratio of about 0.75. If the ratio is well above 0.75, there is probably also a concomitant metabolic alkalosis to explain the greater than expected decline in $[H^+]$. If the ratio is smaller, the condition is chronic or there may also be a metabolic acidosis component.

4. Every ABG that shows no or minimal pH derangement should still call for examination of the P_{CO_2}, $[HCO_3^-]$, and the AG, because there may well be a mixed acid-base disturbance (see Figure 25-2C). It is quite possible for the pH, $[HCO_3^-]$, and P_{CO_2} to be normal and yet have significant acid-base disturbances. The only evident abnormality may be the AG. Take the example of an $[Na^+]$ of 145, $[Cl^-]$ of 97, $[K^+]$ of 4.5, and $[HCO_3^-]$ of 25 and a normal ABG. All the numbers look reasonably normal. However, the AG is 23, so by definition there must be a wide-AG metabolic acidosis. The only explanation for the normal numbers is a concomitant metabolic alkalosis.

REFERENCES

1. Narins RG, Emmett M: Simple and mixed acid-base disorders: A practical approach. *Medicine* 59:161, 1980.
2. Kassirer JP, Bleich HL: Rapid estimation of plasma carbon dioxide from pH and total carbon dioxide content. *New Engl J Med* 272:1067, 1965.
3. Häussinger D: Liver and kidney in acid-base regulation. *Nephrol Dial Transplant* 10:1536, 1995.
4. Graber ML, Quigg RJ, Stempsey WE, Weis S: Spurious hyperchloremia and decreased anion gap in hyperlipidemia. *Ann Intern Med* 98(pt 1):607, 1983.
5. Winter SD, Pearson JR, Gabow PA, et al: The fall of the serum anion gap. *Arch Intern Med* 150:311, 1990.
6. Roberts W, Johnson R: The serum anion gap: Has the reference interval really fallen? *Arch Pathol Lab Med* 121:568, 1997.
7. Elin R, Robertson E, Johnson E: Bromide interferes with determination of chloride by each of four methods. *Clin Chem* 27:778, 1981.
8. Levraut J, Bounatirou T, Ichai C, et al: Reliability of anion gap as an indicator of blood lactate in critically ill patients. *Intens Care Med* 23:417, 1997.
9. Mikulaschek A, Henry SM, Donovan R, Scalea TM: Serum lactate is not predicted by anion gap or base excess after trauma resuscitation. *J Trauma* 40:218, 1996.
10. Wrenn K: The delta (Δ) gap: An approach to mixed acid-base disorders. *Ann Emerg Med* 19:1310, 1990.
11. Brandenburg MA, Dire DJ: Comparison of arterial and venous blood gas values in the initial emergency department evaluation of patients with diabetic ketoacidosis. *Ann Emerg Med* 31:459, 1998.
12. Albert MS, Dell RB, Winters RW: Quantitative displacement of acid-base equilibrium in metabolic acidosis. *Ann Intern Med* 66:312, 1967.
13. Pierce NF, Fedson DS, Brigham KL, et al: The ventilatory response to acute base deficit in humans: Time course during development and correction of metabolic acidosis. *Ann Intern Med* 72:633, 1970.
14. Kety SS, Polis BD, Nadler CS, Schmidt CF: The blood flow and the oxygen consumption of the human brain in diabetic acidosis and coma. *J Clin Invest* 27:500, 1948.
15. Adrogue HJ, Madias NE: Management of life-threatening acid-base disorders: Second of two parts. *New Engl J Med* 338:107, 1998.
16. Kraut JA, Kurtz I: Use of base in the treatment of severe acidemic states. *Am J Kidney Dis* 38:703, 2001.
17. Kucera RR, Shapiro JI, Whalen MA, et al: Brain pH effects of $NaHCO_3$ and Carbicarb in lactic acidosis. *Crit Care Med* 17:1320, 1989.
18. Bersin RM, Arieff AI: Improved hemodynamic function during hypoxia with Carbicarb, a new agent for the management of acidosis. *Circulation* 77:227, 1988.
19. Kopel RF, Durbin CG Jr: Pulmonary artery catheter deterioration during hydrochloric acid infusion for the treatment of metabolic alkalosis. *Crit Care Med* 17:688, 1989.
20. Brackett NC, Cohen JJ, Schwartz WB: Carbon dioxide titration curve of normal man: Effect of increasing degrees of acute hypercapnia on acid-base equilibrium. *New Engl J Med* 272:6, 1965.
21. Arbus GS, Herbert LA, Levesque PR, et al: Characterization and clinical application of the "significance band" for acute respiratory alkalosis. *N Engl J Med* 280:117, 1969.
22. Krapf R, Beeler I, Hertner D, Hulter HN: Chronic respiratory alkalosis: The effect of sustained hyperventilation on renal regulation of acid-base equilibrium. *New Engl J Med* 324:1394, 1991.
23. Callaham M: Hypoxic hazards of traditional paper bag rebreathing in hyperventilating patients. *Ann Emerg Med* 18:622, 1989.
24. Callaham M: Panic disorders, hyperventilation, and the dreaded brown paper bag. *Ann Emerg Med* 30:838, 1997.
25. van der Hout MA, Boek C, van der Molen GM, et al: Rebreathing to cope with hyperventilation: Experimental tests of the paper bag method. *J Behav Med* 11:303, 1989.

BLOOD GASES: PATHOPHYSIOLOGY AND INTERPRETATION

Kelly L. Grogan
Peter Pronovost

Human lungs serve two distinct functions: ventilation and oxygenation. Ventilation, which determines the clearance of carbon dioxide from the body, is a function of the rate and depth of breathing. Oxygenation is the diffusion of oxygen from the lungs to the bloodstream for subsequent delivery to the tissues. The separation between oxygenation and ventilation is dramatically demonstrated by the apnea test for determining brain death. During this test, 100 percent oxygen is insufflated via a thin catheter placed near the carina in an apneic, unventilated patient. The peripheral oxygen saturation is 90 to 100 percent despite no clearance of carbon dioxide with severe respiratory acidosis. This distinction should be considered when managing patients who are receiving mechanical ventilation.

VENTILATION

Minute Ventilation

Minute ventilation (V_M), the total amount of new air moved in and out of the airways and lungs each minute, is equal to the tidal volume (V_T) multiplied by the respiratory rate (f).

$$V_M = V_T \times f \qquad (1)$$

The normal V_T is about 7 mL/kg, or 500 mL in an adult, and the normal f is 12 breaths per minute. Therefore, the normal minute ventilatory volume required to maintain a partial pressure of carbon dioxide (P_{CO_2}) of 40 mm Hg averages about 6 L/min. However, the V_M required to maintain a normal P_{CO_2} depends on the amount of CO_2 being produced and the amount of dead space in the lung. People who are exercising or patients who are febrile or hypermetabolic have increased CO_2 production and thus an increased V_M that can be greater than 20 L/min, while patients who are severely hypothermic may have decreased CO_2 production and thus a decreased V_M. A V_M less than 2 L/min, even in a hypothermic patient, leads to respiratory acidosis. The f occasionally rises to as high as 40 to 50 breaths per minute, and the V_T can become almost as great as the forced vital capacity, which is about 4500 to 5000 mL, or 65 to 70 mL/kg in a young adult male. However, a person usually cannot sustain a V_T greater than 40 percent of the vital capacity for more than a few hours.

Dead Space

Approximately 30 percent of the air that a person breathes does not participate in alveolar gas exchange and is thus called dead space ventilation (V_{DS}). Dead space ventilation is made up of anatomic dead space and alveolar dead space. Anatomic dead space is the volume of air that fills the conducting airways (trachea, bronchi, and bronchioles). Alveolar dead space, or high ventilation–perfusion ($\dot{V}/\dot{Q}$) mismatch, occurs when ventilation of an alveolar-capillary unit is normal but perfusion of the alveolar capillary is absent. The combination of alveolar and anatomic dead space is called the physiologic dead space, which is about 30 percent of the V_T or 150 mL (about 2 mL/kg) in a young male adult with a V_T of 500 mL. The normal ratio between dead (V_{DS}) space ventilation and tidal volume (V_T), V_{DS}/V_T, is 0.3.

When the physiologic dead space is increased, some of the work of ventilation is wasted because a greater fraction of ventilated air never reaches the functional alveolar-capillary units to exchange gas. Certain disease states, such as acute respiratory distress syndrome (ARDS) and chronic obstructive pulmonary disease (COPD), may have an increase in the physiologic dead space that can exceed 60 percent of the V_T. The increased dead space requires a tremendous increase in the V_M (usually by an increase in f) to prevent the development of respiratory acidosis. A patient with a dead space ratio greater than 0.6 generally requires mechanical ventilation to maintain a normal Pa_{CO_2}.

Alveolar Ventilation

The main function of the pulmonary ventilatory system is to continually renew the air in the alveoli, where it is brought into close proximity to the pulmonary capillary blood. The rate at which new air reaches these areas is called alveolar ventilation (V_A):

$$(V_A) = V_M - V_{DS} \qquad (2)$$

Consider a patient with myasthenia gravis who is developing progressive respiratory failure. The patient's baseline V_A is V_M (500 × 12 = 6 L/min) − V_{DS} (150 × 12 = 1.8 L/min) = V_A (4.2 L/min). If the patient's V_T is decreased to 250 due to weakness, the patient cannot simply double f, but must increase it almost four times, to 42 breaths per minute [(250 × 42 = 10.5 L/min) − (150 × 42 = 6.3 L/min) = 4.2 L/min], to maintain the same alveolar ventilation. An increased f increases the patient's work of breathing, which in and of itself generates increased CO_2 and may lead to respiratory failure.

DIFFUSION OF GASES

Factors Affecting the Rate of Gas Diffusion

Rate of gas diffusion in a fluid is directly related to (1) the partial pressure of the gas, (2) the solubility of the gas in the fluid, (3) the surface area available for diffusion, and inversely related to (4) the distance through which the gas must diffuse, and (5) the molecular weight of the gas. All these factors can be expressed in a single formula:

$$D = \frac{PAS}{d\sqrt{MW}} \qquad (3)$$

Where D = diffusion rate
  P = pressure difference between the two ends of the diffusion pathway
  A = cross-section area of the pathway
  S = solubility of the gas
  d = distance of diffusion
  MW = molecular weight of the gas

The solubility coefficient at body temperature for oxygen is 0.024; for carbon dioxide, 0.57; for carbon monoxide, 0.018; and for nitrogen, 0.012. Thus carbon dioxide is more than 20 times as soluble as oxygen, and oxygen is twice as soluble as nitrogen. The solubility helps to determine the quantity of gas dissolved in the fluids of the body, which is a major factor in determining the rate at which the gas can diffuse through tissues.

The characteristics of a gas determine its solubility and molecular weight, which determine the diffusion coefficient of the gas. The diffusion coefficient, which equals $S\sqrt{MW}$, determines the relative rates at which different gases at the same pressure will diffuse. If the diffusion coefficient of oxygen is 1.0, the relative diffusion coefficients of other gases of respiratory importance are carbon dioxide, 20.3; carbon monoxide, 0.81; nitrogen, 0.53; and helium, 0.95.

Oxygen, carbon dioxide, and nitrogen are all highly soluble in lipids and consequently are also highly soluble in cell membranes. The major limitation to the movement of these gases in tissues is the rate at which the gases can diffuse through the tissue water, an important consideration in pulmonary edema.

For oxygen (or any other gas) to move from the alveolus into the pulmonary capillary bed, it must pass through four separate layers, referred to collectively as the alveolar-capillary, or respiratory, membrane. These layers include (1) a layer of fluid, called alveolar fluid, lining the alveolus and containing surfactant that reduces its surface tension; (2) the alveolar epithelium, composed of very thin epithelial cells and a basement membrane; (3) a very thin interstitial space between the alveolar epithelium and the capillary membrane; and (4) the capillary endothelial membrane and its basement membrane, which fuses with the alveolar basement membrane in many places.

The average diameter of the pulmonary capillaries is less than 0.8 microns, which means that red blood cells must actually squeeze through them. Therefore at least part of the red blood cell membrane touches the capillary wall. Where this occurs, oxygen does not have to pass through significant amounts of plasma as it diffuses from the alveolus to the red blood cell. This reduces the diffusion distance and thus increases the rapidity of diffusion of gases between the alveolus and the hemoglobin molecules.

Diffusion Through the Respiratory Membrane

The total diffusing surface area of the lung is enormous (160 m^2) and very thin (averaging 0.63 mm). These characteristics, combined with the solubility of CO_2 and O_2, make the lungs very efficient for maximizing gas exchange. The factors that determine how rapidly a gas passes through the respiratory membrane are (1) the thickness of the membrane, (2) the surface area of the membrane, (3) the diffusion coefficient of the gas in the water of the membrane, and (4) the pressure difference between the two sides of the membrane.

Thickness of the membrane is rarely a significant impediment to the transfer of CO_2, but O_2, being 20 times less soluble than CO_2, can be affected by processes that increase the diffusion distance. Two common clinical entities that increase the diffusion distance are pulmonary edema and pulmonary fibrosis, which explains the common finding of hypoxemia (but not always hypercarbia) in patients with congestive heart failure. Another example of how the factors that determine gas diffusion can be applied clinically is the treatment of carbon monoxide poisoning with 100 percent oxygen, or hyperbaric oxygen. These therapies increase the pressure difference between the two sides of the alveolar capillary membrane and thus facilitate oxygen loading.

The surface area of the respiratory membrane may be greatly decreased by a variety of conditions, such as atelectasis, resection of lung tissue, or emphysema. When the total surface area of the lung is decreased to approximately one-third to one-fourth normal as may be seen with emphysema, exchange of gases through the membrane is impeded significantly. During strenuous exercise, even the slightest increase in dead space in patients with severe emphysema can seriously interfere with gas exchange.

The pressure difference across the respiratory membrane is the difference between the partial pressure of the gas in the alveoli and the partial pressure of the gas in the blood. In room air, the normal difference between the partial pressure of alveolar oxygen (PAO_2) and the partial pressure of arterial oxygen (PaO_2), ($PAO_2 - PaO_2$), or [$P(A - a)O_2$], is 2 to 10 mm Hg. The normal difference between the partial pressure of alveolar carbon dioxide ($PACO_2$) and the partial pressure of arterial carbon dioxide ($PaCO_2$), ($PACO_2 - PaCO_2$), or [$P(A - a)CO_2$], is zero. An increase in the $P(A - a)CO_2$ is due to an increase in dead space. The dead space air does not participate in gas exchange and thus dilutes the alveolar CO_2.

ALVEOLAR GASES

Inspired Gases

Air at sea level has an average barometric pressure of 760 mm Hg and contains approximately 21 percent oxygen and 0.04 percent carbon dioxide, with nitrogen making up most of the remainder. Thus the partial pressures of oxygen and carbon dioxide in the air at sea level are 159 and 0.3 mm Hg, respectively (Table 26-1).

Alveolar air does not have the same concentration of gases as atmospheric air. The reasons for the difference include the following: (1) dry atmospheric air that enters the respiratory passages is humidified before it reaches the alveoli; (2) alveolar air is only partially replaced by atmospheric air with each breath; (3) oxygen is constantly being absorbed from the alveolar air; and (4) carbon dioxide is constantly diffusing from the pulmonary blood into the alveoli.

Humidification of Inspired Air

When air enters the respiratory passageways, water immediately evaporates from the surfaces of these passages and humidifies the inhaled air. At 37°C (98.6°F), water has a vapor pressure of 47 mm Hg (regardless of barometric pressure). This partial pressure is designated PH_2O and must be subtracted from atmospheric pressure (760 mm Hg) prior to calculation of the partial pressures of the dry gases in the alve-

olus (760 − 47 = 713). The remaining gases are predominantly nitrogen (79 percent, or 563 mm Hg), oxygen (21 percent, or 149 mm Hg), and CO_2 (0.04 percent, or 0.3 mm Hg) (Table 26-1). If the patient is breathing 60 percent oxygen, the inspired oxygen pressure (PIO_2) in the trachea or bronchi is determined by the fraction of inspired oxygen (FIO_2) as follows:

$$PIO_2 = (PB - PH_2O)\, FIO_2 \tag{4}$$
$$= 427.8 \text{ mm Hg}$$

where PB is barometric pressure (assumed to be 760 mm Hg at sea level).

Rate at Which Alveolar Air Is Renewed by Atmospheric Air

The functional residual capacity of the lungs, which is the amount of air remaining in the lungs at the end of normal expiration, is approximately 2500 to 3000 mL (35 to 45 mL/kg). Only 350 mL of new air is brought into the alveoli with each new VT and the same amount of old alveolar air is expired.

The slow replacement of alveolar air helps prevent sudden changes in gas concentrations in the blood. This helps to prevent excessive changes in tissue oxygenation, tissue carbon dioxide concentration, and tissue pH when ventilation is temporarily interrupted. This is also the basis for preoxygenation of patients prior to elective intubation, which could be more accurately described as denitrogenation, or replacing the alveolar nitrogen with oxygen.

Oxygen Concentration and Partial Pressure in the Alveoli

Oxygen is continually being absorbed into the blood in the alveolar capillaries, and new oxygen is continually entering the alveoli from the atmosphere. The more rapidly oxygen is absorbed, the lower its concentration in the alveoli. The more rapidly new oxygen is brought into the alveoli from the atmosphere, the higher its concentration becomes. Therefore, oxygen concentration in the alveoli is controlled by the rate of absorption of oxygen into the blood and the rate of entry of new oxygen into the lung.

Carbon Dioxide Concentration in the Alveoli

Carbon dioxide is continually formed and discharged into the alveoli and continually removed from the alveoli by ventilation. Therefore, the two factors that determine the $PACO_2$ are (1) the rate of diffusion of carbon dioxide from the blood into the alveoli and (2) the rate at which carbon dioxide is removed from the alveoli by VA.

At a normal rate of VA of 4.2 L/min, the $PACO_2$ is usually 40 mm Hg. If VA is doubled, the $PACO_2$ is reduced to 20 mm Hg. If VA is decreased by half to 2.1 L/min, the $PACO_2$ rises to 80 mm Hg. These estimations change with metabolic activity, nutritional state, temperature, and so on.

Alveolar Gas Equation

Inspired gas in the trachea has a partial pressure of oxygen (PO_2) of about 149 mm Hg and a PCO_2 of about 0.3 mm Hg. As the warm, water-saturated air enters the alveoli, oxygen diffuses through the alveolar capillary membranes into the plasma and carbon dioxide diffuses from the blood into the alveoli. The mixed venous blood brought to the pulmonary capillaries normally has a PO_2 of about 40 mm Hg and a PCO_2 of 46 mm Hg. On the average, for each milliliter of oxygen that leaves the alveolus, 0.8 to 1.0 mL of carbon dioxide enters it. This relationship is defined as the respiratory quotient (RQ), which can be expressed as

$$RQ = \frac{\text{rate of } CO_2 \text{ production}}{\text{rate of } O_2 \text{ consumption}} \tag{5}$$

TABLE 26-1 Partial Pressure of Gases while Breathing Room Air, mm Hg

Value	Air	Inspired Air in Trachea	Average Alveolar Gas	Average Expired Gas
PO_2	159.0	149.3	104.0	120.0
PCO_2	0.3	0.3	40.0	28.0
PN_2	597.0	563.4	569.0	565.0
PH_2O	3.7	47.0	47.0	47.0
Total	760.0	760.0	760.0	760.0

To determine how well the lungs are functioning at oxygenation, the difference between P_{AO_2} and Pa_{O_2} is often estimated. To estimate P_{AO_2} from the P_{IO_2} and Pa_{CO_2}, one needs a correction factor to determine how much oxygen is consumed for each 1.0 mm Hg of Pa_{CO_2} resulting from carbon dioxide that enters the alveoli. Thus for the usual circumstances, in which the RQ is 0.8, the alveolar gas equation is

$$P_{AO_2} = (PB - P_{H_2O})(FiO_2) - (Pa_{CO_2}/RQ) \qquad (6)$$

In room air ($FiO_2 = 0.21$) at sea level with a Pa_{CO_2} of 40 mm Hg, the P_{AO_2} is expected to be

$$P_{AO_2} = (760 - 47)(0.21) - (40/0.8) = 150 - 50 = 100$$

The normal difference between P_{AO_2} and Pa_{O_2} is 2 to 10 mm Hg.

Expired Gases

Expired air is a combination of dead space air and alveolar air, and its overall composition is determined by the proportion of each in expired air. At the end of normal exhalation nothing but alveolar air is expired. Therefore, to collect alveolar air for study, one simply collects end-tidal gas. Determination of end-tidal carbon dioxide ($ETCO_2$) levels is a useful measure of the adequacy of ventilation. In patients with normal lungs, $ETCO_2$ is approximately 3 mm Hg lower than Pa_{CO_2}, but in patients with obstructive airways disease, typically asthma, there can be a large difference between $ETCO_2$ and Pa_{CO_2}, since dead space air is never fully exhaled and thus neither is pure alveolar air. In the ED, the use of $ETCO_2$ monitors helped to reduce undetected esophageal intubations.

ARTERIAL BLOOD GASES

Partial Pressure of Arterial Carbon Dioxide

ALVEOLAR VENTILATION   Carbon dioxide diffuses so rapidly that the Pa_{CO_2} usually provides an excellent index of the adequacy of ventilation. If the Pa_{CO_2} is greater than expected based on the HCO_3^-, one can assume that V_A is inadequate since by definition a respiratory acidosis exists. The patient may have a low respiratory rate or tidal volume or may also have increased dead space due to emphysema, pulmonary emboli, or increased carbon dioxide production as in thyroid storm or sepsis. An elevated Pa_{CO_2} in the presence of metabolic alkalosis usually reflects compensatory physiologic effects to restore arterial pH toward (but never all the way to) normal. An increased Pa_{CO_2} in a patient with metabolic acidosis is ominous and generally indicates impending respiratory failure.

TRANSPORT OF CARBON DIOXIDE IN THE BLOOD   Under resting conditions, each 100 mL of blood transports an average of 4 mL of carbon dioxide from the tissues to the lungs. Transport of carbon dioxide is not as great a problem as is transport of oxygen because, even under the most abnormal conditions, carbon dioxide can usually be transported in far greater quantities than can oxygen. However, carbon dioxide in the blood does affect acid-base balance.

The carbon dioxide formed in cells diffuses out in the form of carbon dioxide rather than bicarbonate because the cell membrane is almost impermeable to bicarbonate ions. As the carbon dioxide enters the capillary, it initiates a number of almost instantaneous reactions essential for carbon dioxide transport. Carbon dioxide is transported in the blood in three forms: as dissolved carbon dioxide, as bicarbonate, and in combination with proteins as carbamino compounds.

Dissolved   A small portion of the carbon dioxide is transported to the lungs dissolved in plasma. The dissolved portion is approximately 0.36 mL of carbon dioxide in each 100 mL of blood. This is about 9 percent of all carbon dioxide transported.

Bicarbonate   Much of the carbon dioxide in the blood reacts with water to form carbonic acid and subsequently to bicarbonate. The first reaction is very slow in plasma, but carbonic anhydrase inside the red blood cells speeds up the reaction about 500-fold. The reaction occurs so rapidly that it reaches almost complete equilibrium within a fraction of a second. This allows tremendous amounts of carbon dioxide to react with red blood cell water even before the blood leaves the tissue capillaries.

In another fraction of a second, the carbonic acid formed in the red blood cells dissociates into hydrogen and bicarbonate ions.

Some of the hydrogen ions liberated are bound to hemoglobin (Hb). Reduced Hb is less acidic than the oxygenated form, and is therefore a better proton acceptor. The presence of reduced Hb in the peripheral blood helps with the loading of CO_2, while the oxygenation that occurs in the pulmonary capillary assists in the unloading. Deoxygenation of the blood that increases its ability to carry CO_2 is known as the *Haldane effect*, and is quantitatively far more important in promoting CO_2 transport than the Bohr effect is in promoting O_2 transport (see "Oxyhemoglobin Saturation").

The reversible combination of carbon dioxide with water in the red blood cells, under the influence of carbonic anhydrase, accounts for at least 60 to 70 percent of all the carbon dioxide transported from the tissues. Indeed, when a carbonic anhydrase inhibitor (acetazolamide) is administered to block the action of carbonic anhydrase in the red blood cells, carbon dioxide transport from the tissues becomes very poor and the tissue P_{CO_2} rises abruptly.

Carbaminohemoglobin and Carbaminoproteins   Carbamino compounds are formed by the combination of CO_2 with terminal amine groups in blood proteins. The most important protein is the globin of hemoglobin to form carbaminohemoglobin ($HbCO_2$). Since this reversible reaction occurs with a very loose bond, the carbon dioxide is easily released into the alveoli, where the P_{CO_2} is lower than that in the tissue capillaries. Thus, again the unloading of O_2 in peripheral capillaries facilitates the loading of CO_2, while oxygenation has the opposite effect. A small amount of carbon dioxide (usually equivalent to about 0.5 to 1.0 mEq/L of bicarbonate) also reacts in this way with the plasma proteins, forming carbaminoproteins. This reaction is much less significant because the quantity of these proteins is only about one-fourth to one-half the quantity of hemoglobin.

The theoretical quantity of carbon dioxide that can be carried to the lungs in combination with hemoglobin and plasma proteins is approximately 20 to 30 percent of the total quantity transported—that is, about 1.5 mL of carbon dioxide in each 100 mL of blood. However, this reaction is much slower than the reaction of carbon dioxide with water, and it is doubtful that more than 15 to 25 percent of the total quantity of carbon dioxide is transported via hemoglobin and plasma proteins.

CHANGE IN BLOOD ACIDITY DURING CARBON DIOXIDE TRANSPORT   The transport of CO_2 has a profound effect on the acid-base status of the blood. The lung excretes over 10,000 mEq of carbonic anhydrase per day compared with less than 100 mEq of fixed acids by the kidney. Therefore, by altering alveolar ventilation and the elimination of CO_2, the body has great control over the acid-base balance.

The carbonic acid formed when carbon dioxide enters the blood in the tissue capillaries decreases the pH. However, the buffers of the blood prevent the hydrogen ion concentration from rising greatly. Ordinarily, arterial blood has a pH of approximately 7.40, and as the blood acquires carbon dioxide in the tissue capillaries, the pH falls to approximately 7.35. The reverse occurs when carbon dioxide is released from the blood in the lungs. Under conditions of high metabolic activity or when blood flow through the tissues is extremely sluggish, the decrease in pH in the blood as it leaves the tissues can be 0.50 or more.

Partial Pressure of Arterial Oxygen

The Pa_{O_2} in normal, healthy young adults breathing room air at sea level is considered to be 90 to 100 mm Hg. The Pa_{O_2} is extremely important because it not only reflects the functional capabilities of the lungs but also determines the rate at which oxygen enters the tissue cells.

FACTORS AFFECTING Pa_{O_2} Factors that affect the Pa_{O_2} include the V_A, the $F_{I_{O_2}}$, altitude, age, and the oxyhemoglobin dissociation curve (discussed later).

Alveolar Ventilation   If the patient hyperventilates, the Pa_{CO_2} tends to fall and the Pa_{O_2} tends to rise. In accordance with the law of additive properties, if the Pa_{CO_2} falls by 1 mm Hg, the Pa_{O_2} rises by about 1.0 to 1.2 mm Hg. The lungs can make up for some pulmonary dysfunction by hyperventilating. This is seen in pregnant patients who have normal arterial blood gas values at term showing normal pH, a Pa_{CO_2} of 30 to 32, a Pa_{O_2} of 110 to 115, and a serum bicarbonate level of 20 to 22 mEq/L. This is due to an increase in V_M (predominantly due to increased V_T), with resultant respiratory alkalosis with increased urinary excretion of bicarbonate to compensate.

Fraction of Inspired Oxygen   Unfortunately, the $F_{I_{O_2}}$ is often not considered adequately in evaluating the Pa_{O_2}. If a patient is receiving oxygen by nasal cannula, the actual delivered $F_{I_{O_2}}$ is usually only 25 to 30 percent. With a properly fitting face mask, the inhaled $F_{I_{O_2}}$ is usually less than half that delivered to the mask. The approximate Pa_{O_2} values that might be expected in normal persons who are inhaling various concentrations of oxygen are listed in Table 26-2.

The expected Pa_{O_2} when the patient is given oxygen can be estimated by multiplying the actual delivered percentage of oxygen by 6. Thus a patient getting 60 percent oxygen would be expected to have a Pa_{O_2} of about 60 × 6, or 360 mm Hg.

Altitude   The Pa_{O_2} expected when a patient is breathing room air varies with height above sea level. The greater the altitude, the lower the P_{O_2} in the air and the greater the tendency for the patient to hyperventilate (Table 26-3).

The Pa_{O_2} drops about 3 to 4 mm Hg for each 1000-foot rise above sea level. When a person breathes air at 30,000 ft, where the barometric pressure is about 226 mm Hg, the Pa_{O_2} is only 21 mm Hg. At this height above sea level, almost three-fourths of the alveolar air is nitrogen. However, if the person breathes pure oxygen instead of air, most of the space in the alveoli formerly occupied by nitrogen becomes occupied by oxygen. Nevertheless, even if the person is breathing 100 percent oxygen at 30,000 ft, the Pa_{O_2} is only 139 mm Hg (Table 26-4).

Age   Even in healthy individuals, pulmonary changes that cause a fall in the Pa_{O_2} occur with advancing age. On the average, the Pa_{O_2} falls about 3 to 4 mm Hg per decade after the patient reaches 20 to 30 years of age. Thus an otherwise normal 20-year-old patient with a Pa_{O_2} of about 90 to 100 mm Hg (breathing room air at sea level) might be expected to have a Pa_{O_2} of only about 75 to 80 mm Hg at 80 years of age.

TABLE 26-2   Expected Pa_{O_2} in Patients Inhaling Various Concentrations of Oxygen, mm Hg

$F_{I_{O_2}}$	0.21 (room air)	0.4	0.6	0.8	1.0
Pa_{O_2}*	100	227	370	512	655

*Assuming a Pa_{O_2} − Pa_{O_2} of 10 mm Hg and a P_{CO_2} of 40 mm Hg.
Note: Concentrations of inspired O_2 greater than 60% are not achievable by face mask regardless of flow rate.

TABLE 26-3   Changes in P_{O_2} at Various Altitudes

Altitude Above Sea Level, ft	Barometric Pressure, mm Hg	P_{O_2} in Air, mm Hg	Pa_{O_2}, mm Hg	Pa_{O_2}, mm Hg*
0	760	159	105	100
2000	707	148	97	92
4000	656	137	90	85
6000	609	127	84	79
8000	564	118	79	74
10,000	523	109	74	69
20,000	349	73	40	35
30,000	226	47	21	19

*Assuming ideal circumstances with a Pa_{O_2} − Pa_{O_2} of 5 mm Hg or less.

Alveolar-Arterial Oxygen Differences

One method of determining the degree to which lung function is impaired is to determine the alveolar-arterial oxygen gradient $[P(A - a)O_2]$. The Pa_{O_2} can be determined from arterial blood samples and the Pa_{O_2} can be determined using the alveolar air equation previously discussed (Equation 6). The $P(A - a)O_2$ is essentially:

$$Pa_{O_2} - Pa_{O_2} \qquad (7)$$

Generally speaking the $P(A - a)O_2$ should be about 10 plus one tenth the patient's age. A $P(A - a)O_2$ of 20 to 30 mm Hg on room air usually indicates mild pulmonary dysfunction, and a $P(A - a)O_2$ greater than 50 mm Hg on room air usually indicates severe pulmonary dysfunction. The causes of an increased A-a gradient include intrapulmonary shunt (relatively less ventilation than perfusion, or a low $\dot{V}/\dot{Q}$ ratio), intracardiac shunt, and diffusion abnormalities.

Physiologic Shunting in the Lung (Venous-Arterial Admixture)

Although abnormal gas diffusion or distribution in the lungs can cause abnormal blood gas values, the most important cause is usually $\dot{V}/\dot{Q}$ mismatching. When considering ventilation and perfusion, there can be four types of alveolar capillary units: (1) if ventilation and perfusion are normal, the unit is normal; (2) if there is ventilation without perfusion, the unit is considered to be dead space (or high $\dot{V}/\dot{Q}$); (3) if there is perfusion without ventilation, the unit is considered to be a (right-to-left) shunt (or low $\dot{V}/\dot{Q}$); and (4) if there is neither ventilation nor perfusion, the unit is silent.

TABLE 26-4   Effects of Acute Exposure to Low Atmospheric Pressure on Alveolar Gas Concentrations and on Sa_{O_2}

Altitude Above Sea Level, ft	Barometric Pressure, mm Hg	WHILE BREATHING AIR		WHILE BREATHING 100% O_2	
		Pa_{O_2}, mm Hg	Pa_{CO_2}, mm Hg	Pa_{O_2}, mm Hg	Oxygen Saturation, %
0	760	159	40	673	100
10,000	523	110	40	436	100
20,000	349	73	40	262	100
30,000	226	47	40	139	99
40,000	141	29	36	58	87
50,000	87	18	24	16	22

The amount of physiologic shunting in the lung, or venous-arterial admixture (QS/QT), is probably the most sensitive guide to the onset and progression of acute respiratory failure. The shunt is that fraction of blood passing through the lungs without being oxygenated. Normally, the amount for venous-arterial admixture is about 3 to 5 percent of the cardiac output. This small amount of shunting is largely due to the drainage of deoxygenated blood in bronchial veins into oxygenated blood in pulmonary veins.

Physiologic shunting is harder to determine than alveolar-arterial oxygen differences because it requires drawing both arterial and mixed venous (pulmonary artery) blood samples and determining their oxygen contents. Mixed venous samples from the pulmonary artery are preferable to those obtained from central venous pressure catheters. However, central venous blood does give a reasonable estimate of the amount of shunting present if cardiac output is relatively normal.

Although a F_{IO_2} of 1.0 was generally used in the past to determine the amount of physiologic shunting in the lung, the high F_{IO_2} in itself may cause increased shunting. The shunt with a F_{IO_2} of 0.4 is considered to be a better indicator of lung function.

Oxygen Availability

Oxygen availability is determined by the amount of oxygen brought to the capillaries, or oxygen delivery (D_{O_2}), and the dissociation of oxygen from hemoglobin at the tissues. Oxygen delivery is dependent upon oxygen content and cardiac output. Generally, a healthy heart that can increase cardiac output appropriately can make up for diseased lungs and a low hemoglobin level. The reverse is also true. However, a combination of poor oxygenation, low hemoglobin level, and low cardiac output may be rapidly fatal.

OXYGEN DELIVERY

Oxygen Content   Oxygen is carried in the blood either dissolved or in combination with hemoglobin. Primarily the hemoglobin level and the oxyhemoglobin saturation determine the oxygen content of blood. When fully saturated, each gram of hemoglobin measured clinically can carry 1.34 mL of oxygen. Thus a patient with a hemoglobin concentration of 15.0 g/dL can carry about 20.1 mL of oxygen per 100 mL in the red blood cells when the hemoglobin is fully saturated. Although the Pa_{O_2} determines the rate at which oxygen enters the tissues, it contributes very little to the total oxygen content of blood. Each millimeter of mercury of Pa_{O_2} represents only 0.003 mL of oxygen in 100 mL of blood. Thus a patient with a normal Pa_{O_2} of 100 mm Hg has only 0.3 mL of oxygen dissolved in the plasma.

The oxygen content of arterial blood (Ca_{O_2}) can be calculated from the following formula:

$$Ca_{O_2} = [Hb](1.34)(Sa_{O_2}/100) + (Pa_{O_2})(0.003)$$

Thus in a patient with a hemoglobin concentration of 15.0 g/dL, an Sa_{O_2} (arterial saturation of oxygen) of 98 percent, and a Pa_{O_2} of 100 mm Hg,

$$Ca_{O_2} = (15)(1.34)(98/100) + (100)(0.003)$$
$$= 20.0 \text{ mL O}_2 \text{ per deciliter of blood}$$

If the hemoglobin concentration falls to 10.0 g/dL, even if Sa_{O_2} and Pa_{O_2} remain the same, Ca_{O_2} falls by about a third. For example,

$$Ca_{O_2} = (10)(1.34)(98/100) + (100)(0.003)$$
$$= 13.132 + 0.30$$
$$= 13.4 \text{ mL O}_2 \text{ per deciliter of blood}$$

Even with only 10 g of hemoglobin, the red blood cells are carrying over 40 times as much oxygen as is the plasma. While the formula for Ca_{O_2} is complex, the only variables that can be affected through intervention are Hb (with transfusions of red blood cells) and oxygen saturation (with oxygen administration).

Cardiac Output   Oxygen content (in milliliters per liter of blood) multiplied by cardiac output (in liters per minute) is equal to D_{O_2}. Thus, the D_{O_2} in a patient with 15.0 g of 98 percent saturated hemoglobin, a Pa_{O_2} of 100 mm Hg, and a cardiac output (CO) of 5 L/min is

$$D_{O_2} = (Ca_{O_2})(10)(CO)$$
$$= [\text{hemoglobin}](1.34)(Sa_{O_2}/100) + (Pa_{O_2})(0.003)(10)(CO)$$
$$= (15)(1.34)(98/100) + (100)(0.003)(10)(5)$$
$$= 1000 \text{ mL/min}$$

The factor 10 is used to convert oxygen content from milliliters per 100 mL of blood to milliliters per liter of blood.

Since the normal oxygen consumption of an average resting adult male is about 250 to 300 mL/min or approximately 3 mL/kg per min, the tissue on average takes up about 25 percent of the oxygen brought to it, although the percent of oxygen extracted varies by organ. Thus, the Sa_{O_2} falls from about 98 percent in arterial blood to about 73 percent in mixed venous blood. If there is no change in oxygen consumption but cardiac output doubles to 10 L/min, the amount of oxygen removed from each liter of blood is halved, and the venous oxyhemoglobin saturation will be about 85 percent. On the other hand, if cardiac output falls to 2.5 L/min, venous oxyhemoglobin saturation will fall to about 48 percent.

OXYHEMOGLOBIN SATURATION

Normal Relationships   When arterial blood gas study results are obtained, Pa_{O_2} levels in the 60- to 90-mm Hg range often concern clinicians. A Pa_{O_2} of 60 mm Hg correlates to an Sa_{O_2} of 90 percent. Furthermore, if the hemoglobin level is 15.0 g/dL and the tissue removes 5.0 mL of oxygen from each 100 mL of blood, the P_{O_2} of the venous blood falls to about 36 mm Hg, which is only 4 mm Hg below the arterial value. Thus, the tissue P_{O_2} often changes minimally despite a marked fall in Pa_{O_2}.

On the other hand, if the Pa_{O_2} rises far above the upper limit of normal (90 to 100 mm Hg), the oxygen saturation of hemoglobin cannot rise above 100 percent. Therefore, even if the Pa_{O_2} rose to 600 mm Hg or more, the saturation of hemoglobin would increase only 1 to 2 percent because at Pa_{O_2} of 100 mm Hg the Sa_{O_2} is only 98 to 99 percent. This, combined with some evidence (predominantly in animals) that an F_{IO_2} greater than 50 can be associated with pulmonary toxicity, should guide the clinician to supply only the amount of oxygen required to produce a Pa_{O_2} between 70 and 100 mm Hg.

Under circumstances of normal body temperature [37°C (98.6°F)] and blood pH 7.40, certain standard relationships exist between the oxyhemoglobin saturation and the plasma P_{O_2} (Table 26-5 and Figure 26-1). The curved shape of the O_2 dissociation curve has several physiologic advantages. The flat portion means that even if the P_{O_2} in alveolar gas falls somewhat, loading of O_2 will be affected little. The steep lower part of the dissociation curve means that the peripheral tissue can withdraw large amounts of O_2 for only a small drop in capillary P_{O_2}. This maintenance of blood P_{O_2} assists the diffusion of O_2 in the tissue cells. Thus, the relationship between Sa_{O_2} and plasma P_{O_2} is almost linear when the Sa_{O_2} is 60 to 90 percent. However, as the Sa_{O_2} rises above 90 percent, the P_{O_2} begins to rise much faster than the saturation. A simplification to remember for clinical practice is that a Pa_{O_2} of 30, 40, 50, and 60 correspond approximately to an Sa_{O_2} of 60, 70, 80, and 90 percent, respectively.

Factors Affecting Oxyhemoglobin Dissociation   The best known of the factors affecting the oxyhemoglobin dissociation curve are pH,

TABLE 26-5   Relation Between Oxyhemoglobin Saturation and Plasma P_{O_2}

Oxygen saturation, %	100.0	98.4	95	90	80	73	60	50	40	35	30
P_{O_2}, mm Hg	677	100	80	59	48	40	30	26	23	21	18

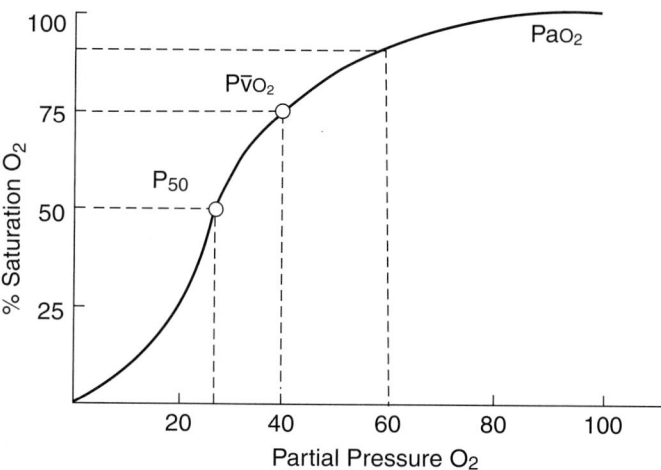

FIG. 26-1. The hemoglobin dissociation curve. This curve demonstrates the relationship of plasma oxygen partial pressure to the degree to which potential oxygen-carrying hemoglobin sites have oxygen attached. The P_{50} is the Po_2 at which hemoglobin is 50 percent saturated and correlates with Po_2 of 27 mm Hg normally. Normal mixed venous blood has an oxygen partial pressure (Pvo_2) of 40 mm Hg and an oxyhemoglobin saturation of 75 percent. A Po_2 of 60 percent normally results in approximately 90 percent saturation of hemoglobin. (Reprinted with permission from Civetti JM, Taylor RW, Kirby RR (eds): *Critical Care,* 3d ed. Baltimore, Lippincott Williams, & Wilkins, 1997.)

temperature, and the amount of 2,3-diphosphoglycerate (2,3-DPG) in the red blood cells. Other related factors include Pco_2 and exercise (Table 26-6).

pH   The more acidic the blood, the more readily hemoglobin gives up its oxygen and the higher the Pao_2 (the partial pressure of oxygen dissolved in blood) for a particular oxyhemoglobin saturation. In contrast, alkalosis makes hemoglobin hold on to its oxygen more tightly, lowering the Pao_2 present at a particular oxyhemoglobin saturation. In general, a rise or fall in pH of 0.10 causes a fall or rise (i.e., an opposite change) in the Pao_2 of about 10 percent (Table 26-7).

PARTIAL PRESSURE OF CARBON DIOXIDE   A shift of the oxyhemoglobin dissociation curve, as a result of changes in the blood levels of carbon dioxide (Haldane effect) and hydrogen ions (Bohr effect), enhances oxygenation of the blood in the lungs and promotes release of oxygen from the blood in the tissues. As the blood passes through the lungs, carbon dioxide diffuses from the blood into the alveoli. This reduces the blood Pco_2 and decreases the hydrogen ion concentration be-

TABLE 26-6   Factors Affecting Oxyhemoglobin Dissociation

Left Shift

    Alkalosis
    Hypothermia
    Abnormal and fetal hemoglobin
    Carboxyhemoglobin
    Methemoglobin
    Carbon monoxide
    Decreased 2,3-DPG

Right Shift

    Acidosis
    Increased Pco_2
    Hyperthermia
    Increased 2,3-DPG

Abbreviation: 2,3-DPG = 2,3-diphosphoglycerate.

TABLE 26-7   Changes in Pao_2 Related to pH

pH	7.60	7.50	7.40	7.30	7.20	7.10	7.00
Pao_2, mm Hg*	80	90	100	111	122	134	148

*Assuming a temperature of 37°C (98.6°F) and a hemoglobin saturation of 98.4%.

cause of the resulting decrease in the blood carbonic acid level. Both changes shift the oxyhemoglobin dissociation curve to the left. With a shift to the left, the quantity of oxygen binding to hemoglobin at any given Pao_2 is increased, allowing greater oxygen transport to the tissues. Then, when the blood reaches the tissue capillaries, the opposite effect occurs. Carbon dioxide entering the blood from the tissues shifts the curve to the right. This displaces oxygen from the hemoglobin and delivers oxygen to the tissues at a higher Po_2 than would otherwise occur.

TEMPERATURE   As blood temperature increases, hemoglobin gives up oxygen more readily, raising the Po_2 in the plasma. The opposite occurs during cooling. For each 1°C rise in temperature, the Pao_2 rises about 5 percent (Table 26-8). With hypothermia, the Pco_2 falls by about the same amount.

EXERCISE   During strenuous exercise, several factors can shift the oxyhemoglobin dissociation curve to the right. Exercising muscles release large quantities of carbon dioxide and other acids, increasing the hydrogen ion concentration in muscle capillary blood. In addition, the temperature of the muscle often rises as much as 3 to 4°C, and phosphate compounds are also released. All these factors acting together shift the oxyhemoglobin dissociation curve of the blood in the muscle capillaries considerably to the right. This allows oxygen to be released to the muscle at a Po_2 as high as 40 mm Hg even though as much as 75 percent of the oxygen has been removed from the hemoglobin. In the lungs, the shift occurs in the opposite direction, allowing pickup of extra amounts of oxygen from the alveoli.

2,3-DIPHOSPHOGLYCERATE   Except for hemoglobin, the compound present in greatest quantity in red blood cells is 2,3-DPG. A normal concentration of 2,3-DPG in a red blood cell keeps the oxyhemoglobin dissociation curve shifted slightly to the right all the time. In addition, under hypoxic conditions lasting longer than a few hours, the quantity of 2,3-DPG increases considerably, shifting the oxyhemoglobin dissociation curve even farther to the right. This can cause the Po_2 in the plasma to be as much as 10 mm Hg higher than it would have been otherwise. However, the presence of increased 2,3-DPG makes it more difficult for the hemoglobin to combine with oxygen in the lungs.

If the concentration of 2,3-DPG falls, as it does in stored blood or during sepsis, the hemoglobin holds on to its oxygen more tightly and the Pao_2 tends to fall. This is an important consideration during large-volume resuscitations with banked blood.

CARBON MONOXIDE   Carbon monoxide combines with hemoglobin at the same point on the hemoglobin molecule that oxygen does. Its presence shifts the oxyhemoglobin dissociation curve to the left. Its physiology is discussed in detail in Chap. 203.

Oxygen Reserve   The ability of blood to give up more oxygen (increasing the arteriovenous oxygen difference) as cardiac output falls and thus maintain oxygen delivery is an important defense mechanism sometimes referred to as oxygen reserve. Unfortunately, there is a

TABLE 26-8   Changes in Pao_2 Related to Temperature

Temperature, °F	104.0	102.2	100.4	98.6	95.0	89.6
Temperature, °C	40	39	38	37	35	32
Pao_2, mm Hg*	117	111	105	100	90	76

*Assuming a pH of 7.40 and a hemoglobin saturation of 98.4%.

limit to this "reserve" because the Po_2 in most tissues seldom falls below 26 mm Hg, which is the P_{50} for hemoglobin (Po_2 at which hemoglobin is 50 percent saturated).

The lowest value to which the Po_2 in capillaries can fall is about 18 to 20 mm Hg because this is the usual capillary-mitochondrial gradient for oxygen. The saturation at a Po_2 of 20 mm Hg is referred to as the S_{20}, and this is normally about 33 percent. The only places where the Po_2 in venous blood is normally as low as 20 mm Hg are the coronary sinus, renal medulla, and perhaps the jugular venous bulb at the base of the brain. A relatively mild degree of alkalosis can raise the S_{20} by 4 to 5 percent, thereby greatly reducing oxygen availability to the myocardium. Thus alkalosis (e.g., when metabolic acidosis is treated with bicarbonate) in low-flow states can be deleterious.

OTHER METHODS OF EVALUATING BLOOD GASES

Pao_2/Fio_2 RATIO   A quick way to estimate the impairment of oxygenation is to calculate the Pao_2/Fio_2 ratio. Normally, the ratio is about 500 to 600, which usually correlates to a pulmonary shunt (QS/QT) of about 3 to 5 percent. However, if a patient has a Pao_2 of 80 mm Hg on 40 percent oxygen, the Pao_2/Fio_2 ratio is 80/0.4, or 200. A Pao_2/Fio_2 ratio of less than 200 corresponds with a QS/QT of about 20 percent. The usual relationship between Pao_2/Fio_2 ratios and the QS/QT in patients with a normal cardiac output is shown in Table 26-9. Pao_2/Fio_2 ratios are also used as criteria for the diagnosis of ARDS/acute lung injury (ALI). In a patient with alveolar infiltrates in at least 3 of 4 quadrants on chest x-ray, a normal pulmonary capillary wedge pressure, and a mechanism known to cause ARDS/ALI, a Pao_2/Fio_2 of less than 300 indicates at least ALI, while a ratio less than 200 indicates ARDS. However, some researchers no longer distinguish between ARDS and ALI and classify all patients with a Pao_2/Fio_2 ratio less than 300 as having ARDS.

PULMONARY ARTERY CATHETERS   A number of pulmonary artery catheters have been developed to continuously monitor mixed venous oxygen saturation ($Smvo_2$). The normal $Smvo_2$ is about 70 to 75 percent. A change in Do_2 could serve as an early warning of inadequacy of perfusion and oxygenation. A rise in $Smvo_2$ can signal an increase in cardiac output and Do_2 beyond that required for metabolism, shunting of blood from tissues (sepsis), or an inability of the peripheral tissues to extract and utilize O_2 (cyanide poisoning). It can also be simply a reflection of the location of the catheter tip in a persistently wedged position so that pulmonary capillary (oxygenated) blood is being analyzed. A fall in $Smvo_2$ below 50 to 60 percent is usually due to a significant decrease in cardiac output or lung function and requires urgent investigation. It is important to remember that, while a change in $Smvo_2$ may indicate important physiologic change, there can be major changes in the patient's condition without corresponding changes in the $Smvo_2$. A major criticism of the use of $Smvo_2$ to guide therapy is that it is a measure of all of the blood returning to the lungs and gives little information about the adequacy of perfusion of individual organ systems, such as the kidneys, brain, heart, or liver.

CLINICAL EXAMINATION   A patient who is awake, alert, comfortable, and cooperative and has normal vital signs is generally oxygenating and ventilating adequately. However, if a patient is tachypneic and/or tachycardic and appears to be anxious and/or confused, hypercarbia or hypoxemia should be considered early. In comatose patients, it is sometimes very difficult to judge how well the patient is oxygenating or ventilating without serial blood gas determinations.

Because reduced Hb is purple, a low arterial O_2 saturation causes cyanosis. Since it is the amount of reduced Hb that is important, cyanosis as a sign of inadequate oxygenation is almost worthless when the hemoglobin is less than 10 g/dL. Under such circumstances, the arterial oxygen saturation (Sao_2) must be less than 65 percent, corresponding to a Pao_2 of about 30 to 35 mm Hg, before the patient looks cyanotic. It must be remembered that oxygenation and ventilation are two separate systems. **A common clinical misconception is that a patient with an adequate Sao_2 must be ventilating adequately. This assumption is incorrect and dangerous,** particularly with patients who are receiving supplemental oxygen. This is discussed further below.

PULSE OXIMETRY   The use of pulse oximetry for monitoring Sao_2 and pulse amplitude in the fingers, nose, or toes can provide early warning of pulmonary or cardiovascular deterioration before it is clinically apparent. This technique employs a microprocessor that continuously measures pulse rate and oxyhemoglobin saturation. The photosensor is not heated and does not require calibration. Oxyhemoglobin is red and reduced hemoglobin is blue, and each has a different absorption of light at their given wavelengths. Because the ratio of transmittance at each of the two wavelengths (660 nm for red and 940 nm for infrared) varies according to the percentage of oxyhemoglobin, pulse oximeters can be programmed to calculate and display the percentage of oxyhemoglobin saturation at each pulse.

There is a predictable correlation between noninvasive Sao_2 monitoring and measured arterial oxygen saturation from arterial blood gas over a wide range of values. Pulse oximetry has only a minimal error, of 1 to 2 percent, above 60 percent saturation. However, a number of factors can limit the effectiveness and accuracy of pulse oximetry, including impaired local perfusion (e.g., in patients who are hypothermic or on vasopressors); ambient light, particularly fluorescent (easily eliminated by placing a towel over the pulse oximeter); nail polish (particularly blue, which absorbs near 660 nm); abnormal hemoglobin; and very high Po_2.

Carboxyhemoglobin falsely raises oxyhemoglobin saturation readings because bedside pulse oximeters read carboxyhemoglobin as oxyhemoglobin, in contrast to methemoglobin, which lowers them (at high levels of methemoglobin the pulse oximeter will read 85 percent regardless of the actual blood oxygenation, as may be seen after the treatment of cyanide poisoning). Fetal hemoglobin has nearly the same absorption spectrum as hemoglobin A and thus has little effect on the readings.

It is important to remember that a pulse oximeter does not provide a good measure of the adequacy of ventilation of patients on supplemental oxygen. A quick calculation using the alveolar gas equation (see Equation 6) shows that a person on 50 percent oxygen would be able to increase the $Paco_2$ to greater than 230 mm Hg before the saturation would drop below 90 [$Pao_2 = (713)(0.5) - 230/0.8 = 356 - 287 = 69$].

CAPNOGRAPHY   By providing a real-time estimate of $Paco_2$, capnography is a useful and accurate means of assessing ventilation, respiratory gas exchange, and carbon dioxide production, and it can give some indication of cardiovascular status (primarily cardiac output).[1] The capnogram during expiration is normally divided into three phases (Figure 26-2)[2]: phase I represents the low CO_2 tension in gas expelled from the anatomic dead space; phase II represents the increasing CO_2 tension as the exhaled gas becomes composed of increasingly more alveolar gas; and phase III represents the CO_2 plateau

TABLE 26-9   Interpretation of Pao_2/Fio_2 Ratio

Pao_2, mm Hg	Fio_2, mm Hg	Ratio	QS/QT, %	Impairment of Oxygenation
240	0.4	600	5	None
120	0.4	300	10	Minimal
100	0.4	250	15	Mild
80	0.4	200	20	Moderate
60	0.4	150	30	Severe*
40	0.4	100	40	Very severe*

*In trauma or septic patients, ventilatory assistance and PEEP to reduce the QS/QT (pulmonary shunt) to 15 percent should be considered. The higher the QS/QT, the greater the need for ventilatory assistance and PEEP.

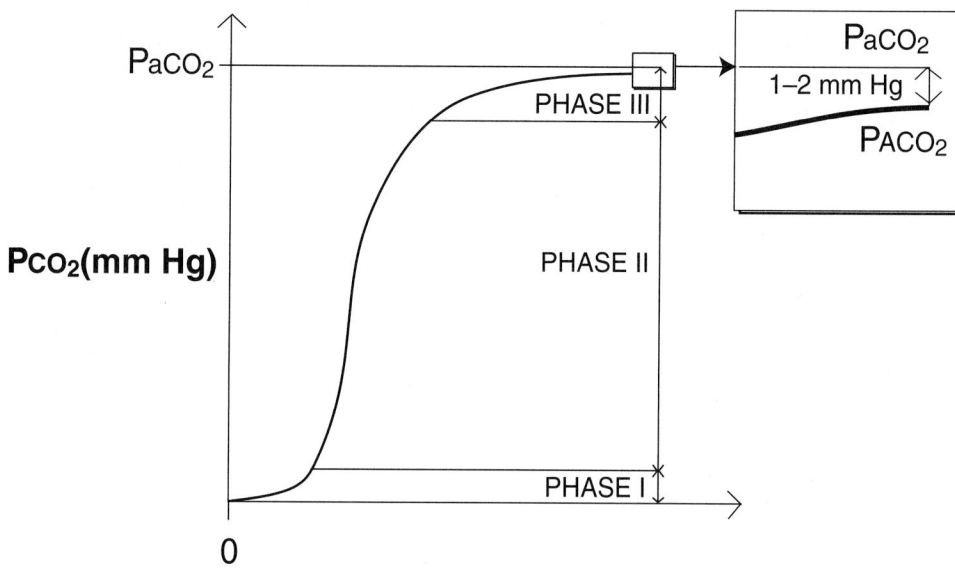

FIG. 26-2. A normal exhaled CO_2 curve. Phase I represents dead space. Phase II represents the increasing CO_2 tension as the exhaled gas becomes composed of increasingly more alveolar gas. Phase III represents the CO_2 plateau, where the exhaled gas is composed primarily of gas from the alveoli. The inset shows the normal disparity between Pa_{CO_2} and the carbon dioxide tension of end-exhalation (end-tidal) gas, which is less than 3 mm Hg. An increase in this disparity probably reflects increases in alveolar dead space ventilation. (Reprinted with permission from Civetti JM, Taylor RW, Kirby RR (eds): *Critical Care,* 3d ed. Baltimore, Lippincott Williams, & Wilkins, 1997.)

reached when the exhaled gas is composed primarily of gas from the alveoli. When inspiration starts, the CO_2 level drops sharply and there is a rapid downstroke of the curve to zero. The point at which the plateau ends just before inspiration is the pulmonary end-tidal CO_2 concentration (Pet_{CO_2}). Pet_{CO_2} is commonly used to estimate Pa_{CO_2} quantitatively; however, even in healthy people the Pet_{CO_2} is usually 3 mm Hg less than Pa_{CO_2}. This gradient is higher in situations that increase the physiologic dead space, cause $\dot{V}/\dot{Q}$ mismatch, or increase shunting. Pet_{CO_2} can be used reliably to estimate the Pa_{CO_2} as long as airway resistance and the V_{DS}/V_T ratio are unchanging. Table 26-10 describes the different clinical conditions that may affect Pet_{CO_2}.

Mainstream and sidestream infrared capnometers are commercially available. A mainstream capnometer connects directly to the endotracheal tube, thus providing real-time breath-by-breath analysis. The major disadvantages of this system are its size and bulk and that it cannot be used in nonintubated patients. Sidestream capnometers aspirate gas at the sample site. The principal advantages of this system are that it reduces mechanical dead space and can be used in nonintubated patients; however, many mechanical factors related to gas sampling require much expert attention and time, and can affect the results.

There are several clinical applications for capnography and $ETCO_2$. A frequent use of $ETCO_2$ is to evaluate the adequacy of alveolar ventilation in relatively healthy patients undergoing general anesthesia. Capnography has been shown to be useful during intubations to ensure tracheal, rather than esophageal, intubation. CO_2 may initially be detected with esophageal intubation from exhaled gas in the stomach; however, this is usually very low (3 to 5 mm Hg) and decreases to zero rapidly, within 3 to 5 breaths. Accidental tracheal extubation, endotracheal tube obstruction, or disconnect from a ventilation system can also be readily detected. These monitors can reduce the number of ar-

terial blood gas determinations obtained and can be very useful in weaning patients from mechanical ventilatory support.

Finally, they can also be useful in determining the adequacy of circulation during cardiopulmonary resuscitation.[3,4] The decrease in cardiac output and pulmonary blood flow during cardiac arrest results in decreased elimination of CO_2 by the lungs and therefore a low Pet_{CO_2}. Successful resuscitation results in an increase in cardiac output that will in turn lead to an increase in Pet_{CO_2}. Capnographic monitoring is a useful guide to the adequacy of closed cardiac compressions during CPR.

Pulse oximetry, and to some extent capnography, have become standard monitors in most locations that provide for the acute care of unstable patients. While understanding that they have limitations, the clinician can use them for second-to-second indications of the adequacy of ventilation and oxygenation.

REFERENCES

1. Soubani A: Noninvasive monitoring of oxygen and carbon dioxide. *Am J Emerg Med* 19:141, 2001.
2. Shapiro B, Peruzzi W: Blood gas analysis, in Civetti JM, Taylor RW, Kirby, RR (eds): *Critical Care.* Philadelphia, Lippincott Williams & Wilkins, 1997, p. 921.
3. Garnett A, Omato J, Gonzalez E, et al: End-tidal carbon dioxide monitoring during cardiopulmonary resuscitation. *JAMA* 257:512, 1986.
4. Falk J, Rackow E, Well M: End-tidal carbon dioxide concentration during cardiopulmonary resuscitation. *New Engl J Med* 318:607, 1988.

TABLE 26-10   Conditions That Affect Pet_{CO_2}

Increase in Pet_{CO_2}	Decrease in Pet_{CO_2}
Increased cardiac output	Decreased cardiac output
Hypoventilation	Hyperventilation
Hyperthermia	Hypothermia
Bicarbonate administration	Cardiac arrest
Insufflation of CO_2	Pulmonary embolism
(e.g., laparoscopic surgery)	Fat or air embolism
	Disruption of ventilation system (e.g., disconnect, circuit leak)
	Accidental extubation
	Endotracheal tube obstruction

FLUID AND ELECTROLYTE PROBLEMS

Michael Londner
Darcie Hammer
Gabor D. Kelen

FLUIDS

Compartments

The total body water (TBW) can be divided into intracellular and extracellular fluids (ICF and ECF, respectively). In addition, the ECF can be divided into interstitial and intravascular. Body fluid compartment sizes for an adult are diagrammed in Figure 27-1. The concentrations

As a function of	TBW	ICF	ECF	IF	IVF
Total Weight	60%	40%	20%	15%	5%
TBW		67%	33%	25%	8%
ECF compartment				75%	25%

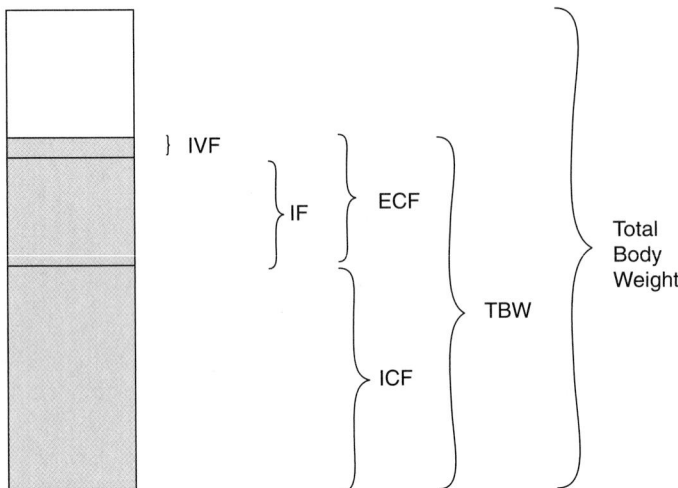

FIG. 27-1. Relation of fluid compartment to body weight and each other. ECF = extracellular fluid; ICF = intracellular fluid; IF = interstitial fluid; IVF = intravascular fluid; TBW = total body water.

of the most abundant anions and cations of the fluid compartments and the constituents of commonly used intravenous fluids are listed in Table 27-1.

Solutes

Concentrations are often expressed in moles, equivalents, or osmoles per liter. A *mole* (abbreviation: mol) of any compound contains 6.02×10^{23} molecules of that compound. The *molecular weight* of a substance is the weight, in grams, of a mole of that substance.

An *equivalent* of a substance is the mass (in grams) of a mole of that substance (molecular weight) divided by its charge. Therefore, 1 eq of Na^+ is equal to 23 g/1, or 23 g, whereas 1 eq of Ca^{2+} is equal to 40 g/2, or 20 g.

An osmole is the amount of a substance (in moles) that dissociates to form 1 mol of osmotically active particles. For example, 1 mol of NaCl dissolves to produce 1 mol of Na^+ and 1 mol of Cl^-, for a total of 2 mol of osmotically active particles. Therefore, 1 osmol of NaCl is 0.5 mol of NaCl.

Osmolarity is the number of osmoles per liter of solution, whereas *osmolality* is the number of osmoles per kilogram of solvent.

TABLE 27-1   Electrolyte Concentration of Body Fluids (mEq/L)

Solution	Plasma	Interstitial	Intracellular	NS	LR
Cations					
Sodium	142	144	10	154	130
Potassium	4	4.5	150		4
Magnesium	2	1	40		
Calcium	5	2.5			3
Total cations	153	152	200	154	137
Anions					
Chloride	104	113		154	109
Lactate					28
Phosphates	2	2	120		
Sulfates	1	1	30		
Bicarbonate	27	30	10		
Protein	13	1	40		
Organic acids	6	5			
Total anions	153	152	200	154	137

Abbreviations: LR = lactated Ringer; NS = normal saline.

The serum osmolality can be measured directly by determining the freezing point of the serum, because 1 mol of solute will lower the freezing point of 1 kg of water by 1.86°C. Osmolarity can be estimated by adding the measured $[Na^+]$, $[Cl^-]$, and bicarbonate to the glucose and blood nitrogen blood (BUN) divided by their respective molecular weights divided by 10 (to convert from dL to L):

$$\text{osmolarity (mosmol/L)} = 2 \times [Na^+] + \frac{\text{glucose}}{18} + \frac{\text{blood urea nitrogen}}{2.8}$$

Because the sum of the measured $[Cl^-]$ and bicarbonate approximates the measured $[Na^+]$, twice the measured $[Na^+]$ is generally used in this calculation. Because the density of water is 1 kg/L, the osmolarity (in osmol/L) is roughly equivalent to the osmolality (in osmol/kg) in water-based systems with limited temperature variation, such as the human body; thus, the terms are frequently interchanged in medical texts.

The normal serum osmolarity ranges from 275 to 295 mosmol/L. The presence of additional osmotically active agents should be suspected when the measured osmolality (measure via freezing point) differs from the calculated osmolality by more than 10. This is termed an *osmolar gap*. If an osmolar gap is encountered, the following possibilities should be considered:

1. Laboratory analytic error
2. Decreased serum water content: hyperlipidemia and hyperproteinemia
3. Additional low-molecular-weight substances in the serum, such as ethanol, methanol, isopropyl alcohol, ethylene glycol, acetone, ethyl ether, paraldehyde, lactate, or mannitol

If the substance ingested is known to be ethanol, the osmolar gap can be used to estimate the blood alcohol level, because osmolarity increases 22 mg/dL for every 100 mg/dL of ethanol. Other substances can be similarly estimated (see Table 166-1 in Chap. 166).

$$\text{blood alcohol level in mg/dL (estimated)} = \text{osmolar gap} \times (100/22) = \text{osmolar gap} \times 4.6$$

Homeostasis

To maintain fluid balance, an average normal adult requires approximately 2000 to 3000 mL of water per day. This accounts for the volume of water lost in a day due to insensible and urinary losses. The insensible losses include the respiratory tract (500 to 700 mL per d), the skin (250 to 350 mL per d), and the feces (100 mL per d). This insensible loss can accelerate dramatically in the setting of fever (500 mL/d per 1°C fever), sweating (up to 1500 mL), and gastrointestinal losses.

ELECTROLYTES

Each electrolyte disorder can be assessed with the same general approach. In general, increased concentration of an electrolyte (hyper-) is a result of (1) excess total body amount, (2) shift between compartments, and (3) a relative fluid loss. Similarly, decreased concentrations (hypo-) are a result of (1) depleted total body amount, (2) shift among compartments, and (3) relative fluid gain. It is usually the rate of change of an electrolyte rather than the absolute value that determines the severity of symptoms. Correction of electrolyte disturbance should follow a time frame similar to the development of the abnormality.

SODIUM (NA$^+$)

The total body Na$^+$ content is between 40 and 50 mEq/kg, which is approximately 2800 mEq in a normal 70-kg man. It is found predominantly in the ECF space (98 percent), with a concentration of approximately 140 mEq/L. The intracellular concentration is usually less than 10 to 12 mEq/L. Sodium passively moves into cells along its concentration gradient and is actively extruded via an adenosine triphosphatase (ATPase) dependent system.

Hyponatremia

Hyponatremia is strictly defined as a measured serum [Na$^+$] less than 135 mEq/L. This can result from primary water gain and/or Na$^+$ loss greater than that of water, alteration in the distribution of body water, or aberrant laboratory measurement. The development of symptoms is related more to the rate of change of the serum [Na$^+$] than to the absolute value. Values less than 120 mEq/L are more likely to lead to symptoms, even when slowly developing. Common presenting symptoms include, but are not limited to, confusion, lethargy, nausea, vomiting, anorexia, muscle cramps, and hypothermia and culminate ultimately in seizures and coma. Seizures are quite likely at [Na$^+$] of 113 mEq/L or less.

PATHOPHYSIOLOGY

Central Nervous System As serum [Na$^+$] decreases, the osmotic gradient that develops across the blood-brain barrier causes water to move into the brain, causing apathy, agitation, headache, altered consciousness, seizures, and even coma. The severity of symptoms is dependent on not only the rapidity but also the magnitude of the decrease in the serum [Na$^+$]. Acute hyponatremia occurring in 24 h or less and resulting in a serum [Na$^+$] of less than 120 mEq/L, or declining at a rate of 0.5 mEq/L or more per hour, can cause muscular twitching, seizures, and coma. The mortality rate with acute severe hyponatremia and central nervous system (CNS) changes has been reported to be as high as 50 percent in adults. Patients are usually less symptomatic when [Na$^+$] decreases gradually, but even patients with chronic hyponatremia may experience focal weakness, hemiparesis, ataxia, and a positive Babinski sign.

The brain has two mechanisms to protect against fluid shifts secondary to hyponatremia:(1) The increase in the hydrostatic pressure causes movement of interstitial fluid into the cerebrospinal fluid and via the arachnoid villi; and (2) The loss of cellular K$^+$/Na$^+$ and organic osmolytes decreases the osmotic gradients.

The adaptive changes that protect the brain from excessive swelling also render it susceptible to volume depletion during correction of the fluid and electrolyte problem. There is often more risk of brain damage during treatment than from the hyponatremia itself. The rate of rise of brain intracellular potassium and organic osmolytes during correction of the hyponatremia is much slower than the rate of loss of these substances during the development of the problem. If correction of hyponatremia occurs more rapidly than the brain can recover solute, the higher plasma osmolality may result in a fluid shift out of cells and injury to the brain. This is referred to as the *osmotic demyelination syndrome,* or *central pontine myelinolysis* (CPM). (See Complications of Therapy.)

Cardiovascular System In volume-depleted patients, hyponatremia can cause a further decrease in the intravascular volume by allowing movement of water out of the ECF compartment into the ICF space. Accordingly, shock occurs at lesser degrees of TBW depletion in hyponatremia than similar fluid deficits when the plasma is hypertonic or isotonic.

Antidiuretic hormone (ADH) release occurs in almost all hyponatremic conditions. The function of ADH in this setting initially may seem paradoxical, because it potentiates the hyponatremic state by increasing water reabsorption by the renal tubules. Antidiuretic hormone is also a potent vasoconstrictor, and, even at the low ADH concentrations that are characteristic of clinical hyponatremia, it increases peripheral vascular resistance, thereby increasing blood flow to the liver and kidneys at the expense of the skin and muscle.

Musculoskeletal System Most patients with hyponatremia have normal muscle tone and function. However, muscle cramps and weakness can occur during strenuous exercise, especially if excess sweating is replaced with water. These symptoms usually resolve rapidly when the serum [Na$^+$] is corrected back toward normal.

Renal System The usual renal response to hyponatremia is the production of dilute urine; however, this process is abrogated to some extent by the presence of increased concentrations of ADH. The amount of ADH present depends on the primary disease process and the effective arterial blood volume.

A urine [Na$^+$] less than 10 mEq/L usually indicates that the renal handling of Na$^+$ is intact and that the effective arterial blood volume is contracted. In contrast, a urine [Na$^+$] greater than 20 mEq/L often indicates intrinsic renal tubular damage or a natriuretic response to hypervolemia. The urine [Na$^+$] also will vary somewhat according to the ongoing gains and losses of salt and water. Urine [Na$^+$] will tend to increase if the underlying disease significantly impairs renal function.

DIAGNOSIS The actual [Na$^+$] does not confer information regarding volume status. Therefore, the first step in the evaluation of a patient with a low measured [Na$^+$] should include a clinical evaluation of ECF volume status and measured and calculated plasma osmolalities. This provides a means for the first tier in categorizing hyponatremic disorders. In *true* hyponatremia, the plasma osmolality is reduced; in *factitious* hyponatremic states, the plasma osmolality is normal or increased.

HYPERTONIC HYPONATREMIA (P$_{OSM}$ >295) Hyponatremia with an increase in osmotically active solutes occurs when there is an accumulation of large quantities of solutes restricted primarily to the ECF space. In this setting, there is a net movement of water from the ICF to the ECF, thereby effectively diluting the ECF [Na$^+$]. The most common cause of this is hyperglycemia. Each 100 mg/dL increase in plasma glucose decreases the serum [Na$^+$] by 1.6 to 1.8 mEq/L. The differential diagnosis of hypertonic hyponatremia is shown in Table 27-2. Treatment of hyponatremia in this class includes reduction of the ECF hypertonicity by correction of the underlying disorder with close observation. Unless detected during the very acute phase or in the face of renal failure, an osmotic diuresis is likely, resulting in total body Na$^+$ deficit. Volume depletion is often associated, so volume repletion with Na$^+$-containing fluids is required.

ISOTONIC HYPONATREMIA (P$_{OSM}$ 275 TO 295) Hyponatremia associated with normal plasma osmolality is often termed *pseudohy-*

TABLE 27-2   Etiology of Hyponatremia

Hypertonic hyponatremia (P_{osm} >295)
   Hyperglycemia
   Mannitol excess
   Glycerol therapy
Isotonic (pseudo)hyponatremia (P_{osm} 275–295)
   Hyperlipidemia
   Hyperproteinemia (e.g., multiple myeloma, Waldenström
      macroglobulinemia)
Hypotonic hyponatremia (P_{osm} <275)
   Hypovolemic (usually associated with volume replacement with
      hypotonic fluids)
      Renal
         Diuretic use
         Salt-wasting nephropathy (renal tubular acidosis, chronic renal
            failure, interstitial nephritis)
         Osmotic diuresis (glucose, urea, mannitol, hyperproteinemia)
         Mineralocorticoid (aldosterone) deficiency
      Extrarenal
         Volume replacement with hypotonic fluids
         Gastrointestinal loss (vomiting, diarrhea, fistula, tube suction)
         Third-space loss (e.g., burns, hemorrhagic pancreatitis, peritonitis)
         Sweating (e.g., cystic fibrosis)
   Hypervolemic
      Urinary [Na^+] >20 mEq/L
         Renal failure (inability to excrete free water)
      Urinary [Na^+] <20 mEq/L
         Congestive heart failure (perceived as low-flow state by kidneys,
            stimulates ADH)
         Nephrotic syndrome (low serum protein secondary to urinary loss)
         Cirrhosis (low intravascular oncotic pressure secondary to decreased
            protein production)
   Euvolemic (urine [Na^+] usually >20 mEq/L)
      SIADH (see Table 27-3)
      Hypothyroidism (possible increased ADH or deceased GFR)
      Pain, stress, nausea, psychosis (stimulates ADH)
      Drugs: ADH, nicotine, sulfonylureas, morphine, barbiturates, NSAIDs,
         acetaminophen, carbamazepine, phenothiazines, TCAs,
         colchicine, clofibrate, cyclophosphamide, isoproterenol,
         tolbutamide, vincristine, MAOI
      Water intoxication (psychogenic polydipsia, lesion in thirst center)
      Glucocorticoid deficiency (glucocorticoids required to suppress ADH)
      Positive-pressure ventilation
      Porphyria
      Essential (reset osmostat or sick cell syndrome—usually in the elderly)

Abbreviations: ADH = antidiuretic hormone; GFR = glomerular filtration rate; MAOI = monoamine oxidase inhibitor; NSAIDs = nonsteroidal antiinflammatory drugs; SIADH = syndrome of inappropriate secretion of antidiuretic hormone; TCAs = tricyclic antidepressants.

ponatremia. High levels of plasma proteins and lipids increase the non-aqueous, non-Na^+-containing fraction of plasma. Because traditional methods of Na^+ measurement use a "mass per volume" of serum method (such as flame emission spectrophotometry), the laboratory analysis reports a factitious lower value of [Na^+] than the serum truly contains. The true [Na^+] and osmolality of plasma water are normal. The differential diagnosis of isotonic hyponatremia is shown in Table 27-2. Treatment of hyponatremia in this class is not required.

HYPOTONIC HYPONATREMIA (P_{OSM} <275)   This category of hyponatremia results in intracellular volume expansion with consequent derangement of cellular functions. This category can be further subdivided into classifications based on functional ECF volume and urinary [Na^+] (accounting for possible recent use of diuretics). The assessment of ECF should focus on predisposing factors once volume status is ascertained. In addition to the electrolytes and plasma osmolality, urine electrolytes and osmolality should be obtained. This will help facilitate classification into hypovolemic, hypervolemic, and euvolemic categories.

Hypovolemic hyponatremia is associated with a loss of Na^+ and water, often with disproportionate water replacement through oral intake or the administration of hypotonic fluids. Losses of Na^+ may be renal or extrarenal.

Patients with extrarenal losses of Na^+ and water will demonstrate a urinary [Na^+] of less than 20 mEq/L. The unequal balance of electrolyte and water loss produces a contracted ECF and hyponatremia. This is maintained by the physiologic effect of volume depletion on the kidneys inhibiting the excretion of free water. The impairment of water excretion to defend ECF volume at the expense of tonicity is accomplished by four mechanisms:

1. Decreased glomerular filtration
2. Increased proximal tubular reabsorption of solute and water
3. Decreased delivery of fluid to the diluting segment of the nephron
4. Antidiuretic hormone released by nonosmotic stimuli

The differential diagnosis of hypovolemic hyponatremia from extrarenal losses is shown in Table 27-2.

The decreased ECF volume also may be due to renal losses. In this setting, the urinary [Na^+] will be greater than 20 mEq/L. The clinical manifestations are usually due to the volume deficit rather than to the hyponatremia. Treatment of hypovolemic hyponatremia includes reexpansion of the ECF volume with isotonic saline and appropriate correction of any underlying disorder.

Euvolemic hyponatremia is described as having a combination of normal volume status and hyponatremia. Although ECF volume may be slightly increased, patients are not clinically edematous and have nearly normal total body Na+ content despite the presence of hyponatremia. When symptoms are present, they usually relate to CNS hypotonicity. Urinary [Na^+] is usually greater than 20 mEq/L and may be much higher in instances of ADH excess. The most notable cause of euvolemic hyponatremia is the syndrome of inappropriate ADH secretion. This is characterized by six criteria:

1. Hypotonic hyponatremia
2. Inappropriately elevated urinary osmolality (usually >200 mosmol/kg)
3. Elevated urinary [Na^+] (typically >20 mEq/L)
4. Clinical euvolemia
5. Normal adrenal, renal, cardiac, hepatic, and thyroid functions
6. Correctable with water restriction

The diagnosis of syndrome of inappropriate ADH is made primarily by exclusion (Table 27-3). The other causes of euvolemic hyponatremia are listed in Table 27-2. Some of these may stimulate ADH secretion. Treatment for patients with euvolemic hyponatremia requires fluid restriction and appropriate diagnosis and management of the underlying disorder. Admission is usually warranted.

Hypervolemic hyponatremia is described as TBW in great excess. Patients have manifestations of volume overload, such as peripheral and/or pulmonary edema. They usually have impaired ability to excrete a water load. This allows for water retention in excess of Na^+ re-

TABLE 27-3   Etiology of Syndrome of Inappropriate Antidiuretic Hormone

Central Nervous System Disease	Pulmonary Disease	Carcinoma
Tumor	Tumor	Lung
Trauma	Pneumonia	Pancreas
Infection	Chronic obstructive pulmonary disease	Thymoma
Cerebral vascular accident, subarachnoid hemorrhage	Lung abscess	Ovary
Guillain-Barré syndrome	Tuberculosis	Lymphoma
Delerium tremens	Cystic fibrosis	
Multiple sclerosis		

tention. These patients can be further categorized into two groups (see Table 27-2). The first of these is generalized edematous states without advanced renal insufficiency. These patients have urinary [Na$^+$] of less than 20 mEq/L. They include patients with cirrhosis and/or ascites, congestive heart failure, and nephrotic syndrome. The second category is advanced acute or chronic renal insufficiency. These patients have urinary [Na$^+$] in excess of 20 mEq/L.

Management of patients with hypervolemic hyponatremia includes optimizing treatment for the underlying disorder coupled with judicious salt and water restriction. Often diuretics are required to aid in management. Dialysis may be necessary.

EMERGENCY TREATMENT OF SEVERE HYPONATREMIA   Although specific or general treatment of hyponatremia for the condition discussed may be initiated in the ED, there is little urgency to address the hyponatremia immediately when [Na$^+$] is above 120 mEq/L. In cases in which hyponatremia is severe (less than 115 mEq/L or when the patient is symptomatic), treatment should be initiated.

EVALUATION AND TREATMENT   Urine electrolytes are useful only before beginning treatment and therefore should be collected in the ED.

Situations that warrant consideration of emergent treatment are hypovolemic patients and patients in extremis, e.g., mental status changes or coma. In hypovolemic patients, the Na$^+$ deficit should be calculated and replaced with normal saline solution. The formula is:

$$\text{total body Na}^+ \text{ deficit (mEq/L)}$$
$$= (\text{desired plasma [Na}^+] - \text{actual plasma [Na}^+]) \times \text{TBW}$$

In cases in which hyponatremia is severe (<120 mEq/L), develops rapidly (>0.5-mEq/L decrease in serum [Na$^+$] per h), and is associated with a patient in extremis (i.e., coma or seizures), administration of 3 percent saline solution (513 mEq/L) should be considered. This can be administered at 25 to 100 mL/h, with careful observation for fluid overload and the rise in serum [Na$^+$] levels. **The rise in [Na$^+$] should be no greater than 0.5 to 1.0 mEq/L per h. In the face of seizures, this can be increased to 1 to 2 mEq/L per h.** It is sometimes necessary to administer concomitant furosemide to reduce the amount of water present in the body, thereby allowing more rapid correction of plasma [Na$^+$].

COMPLICATIONS OF THERAPY   Complications with the treatment of acute hyponatremia, especially when there is no underlying CNS, hepatic, or renal disorder, are uncommon and occur in fewer than 2 percent of patients. Patients with chronic hyponatremia appear to be at greater risk for CPM brain injury during the correction process. The injury reportedly occurs after hyponatremia has been corrected, and progresses in a predictable manner. These neurologic changes are believed to be due to correction of the serum [Na$^+$] at a rate faster than the brain can adapt to the higher osmolality. In patients with chronic hyponatremia, other factors contributing to CPM may include alcoholism, malnutrition, toxins, and metabolic imbalance. In patients with chronic severe hyponatremia, the threshold for the production of CPM is a rate of correction of [Na$^+$] levels faster than 0.5 mEq/L per h (12 mEq/L per d).

In typical cases, the neurologic findings include fluctuating levels of consciousness, behavioral disturbances, dysarthria, dysphagia, or convulsions progressing to pseudobulbar palsy and quadriparesis. Improvement may occur after several weeks of severe debilitation, but some patients are permanently impaired.

Hypernatremia

PATHOPHYSIOLOGY   Hypernatremia is defined as serum [Na$^+$] greater than 150 mEq/L and can be classified as a decrease in TBW (the most common cause) or, less likely, from increased sodium (from increased intake or decreased excretion; Table 27-4).

TABLE 27-4   Etiologic Classification of Hypernatremia

Inadequate water intake*
  Inability to obtain or swallow water
  Impaired thirst drive; examples include
      hypothalamic lesion
  Increased insensible loss
Excessive sodium
  Iatrogenic sodium administration
    Sodium bicarbonate
    Hypertonic saline
  Accidental/deliberate ingestion of large quantities of sodium
    Substitution of salt for sugar in infant formula or tube feedings
  Seawater ingestion or drowning
  Mineralocorticoid or glucocorticoid excess*
    Primary aldosteronism
    Cushing syndrome
    Ectopic adrenocorticotropic hormone production
  Peritoneal dialysis
Loss of water in excess of sodium (without simultaneous water intake)
  Gastrointestinal*
    Vomiting, diarrhea, intestinal fistula
  Renal loss
    Central diabetes insipidus
    Impaired renal concentrating ability
      Osmotic diuresis (multiple causes)*
      Hypercalcemia
      Decreased protein intake
      Prolonged, excessive water intake
      Sickle cell disease
      Multiple myeloma
      Amyloidosis
      Sarcoidosis
      Sjögren syndrome
      Nephrogenic diabetes insipidus
      Congenital
  Drugs, including
    Alcohol, lithium, phenytoin, propoxyphene, sulfonylurea
      hypoglycemic agents, amphotericin B, colchicine
  Skin loss
    Burns, sweating
Essential hypernatremia

*Likely or important emergency department diagnostic consideration.

The main defense against hypernatremia is thirst. A 2 percent increase in plasma osmolality should stimulate thirst to increase free water intake. The problem arises when patients, such as those in a coma or those who are bedridden, are unable to obtain adequate fluid.

Virtually all hypernatremia encountered in the ED is related to volume loss, usually severe. In otherwise healthy hypovolemic patients, conservation of free water by the kidneys results in low urine output (<20 mL per h) that has a high osmolality (usually >1000 mosmol/kg water). Although the urine is concentrated, it is of such low volume as to limit the excretion of sodium.

Diabetes Insipidus

In diabetes insipidus (DI), there is failure of central or peripheral ADH response. Urine osmolality is low (200 to 300 mosmol/kg, with urinary [Na$^+$] of 60 to 100 mEq/kg), resulting in excessive loss of hypotonic urine. Diabetes insipidus may be central (due to a failure of secretion of ADH) or nephrogenic (due to renal unresponsiveness to ADH) in origin. Specific causes are listed in Table 27-5. Diagnosis of central and nephrogenic DI is best achieved by noting the response of serum and urine osmolarity to water deprivation (trying to reach a serum osmolarity >295 mosmol/L) and the response to 5 units of subcutaneous aqueous vasopressin. A lack of response to fluid loss is diagnostic of DI. Patients with central DI respond well to vasopressin (urine osmolarity >800 mosmol/L), whereas patients with nephrogenic DI show little or no response to vasopressin.

TABLE 27-5   Causes of Diabetes Insipidus

Central	Nephrogenic
Neoplasms	Familial
Pituitary surgery	Hypercalcemia
Trauma	Hypokalemia
Granulomas	Renal disease
Idiopathic	Drug induced
	Hematologic disorders
	Malnutrition

SYMPTOMS   Acute symptomatology is seen in many patients once serum [Na$^+$] exceeds 158 mEq/L, although the rate of change of [Na$^+$] is an important factor. Neurologic symptoms predominate. Patients tend to become irritable. One may see increased muscle tone or even coma with eventual seizures. Fever can be a contributing cause and a result of hypernatremic dehydration.

The serum osmolality at which signs and symptoms occur can be found in Table 27-6. If the plasma osmolality exceeds 350 mosmol/kg, the incidence of severe morbidity or mortality may exceed 50 percent.

Hypocalcemia, which is frequently seen in patients with hypernatremia, may contribute to the CNS symptomatology. However, the mechanism of the hypocalcemia is unclear.

Massive brain hemorrhage or multiple small hemorrhages and thromboses may occur when hypernatremia causes enough cellular fluid loss and resultant brain shrinkage to cause tearing of cerebral blood vessels.

If the hypernatremia persists for more than a few days, brain water content may return to normal or near-normal levels due to accumulation in the brain cells of amino acids known as *idiogenic osmoles,* in particular taurine. The formation of these idiogenic osmoles increases intracellular osmolality, attracts water back into the brain cells, and restores their cellular volume. If the hypertonicity develops gradually, this protective mechanism tends to prevent severe brain cell shrinkage.

TREATMENT   The cornerstone of treatment is volume repletion. Volume should be replaced first with NS or LR. Either will have, by definition, a lower [Na$^+$] than the patient's serum. Some practitioners inappropriately fear using NS solution from concern that an [Na$^+$] of 154 mEq/L is higher than normal serum [Na$^+$]. However, in most hypernatremic states, there is a total body Na$^+$ deficit, and the use of NS allows a more gradual decrease in serum [Na$^+$]. Plasma-expanding fluids should continue until tissue perfusion is restored. Once perfusion has been established, the solution should be converted to 0.45 percent saline or other hypotonic solution. This should continue until the urine output is at least 0.5 mL/kg per h. The reduction in [Na$^+$] should not exceed 10 to 15 mEq/L per d. A calculation to estimate free water deficit is:

$$\text{water deficit } (L) = \text{TBW} \times \left[\left(\frac{\text{measured [Na}^+]}{\text{normal [Na}^+]} \right) - 1 \right]$$

As a general rule, each liter of water deficit results in serum [Na$^+$] rise of 3 to 5 mEq/L.

TABLE 27-6   Clinical Manifestations of Hypernatremic States Related to Serum Osmolality

Osmolality (mosmol/kg)	Manifestations
350–375	Restlessness, irritability
375–400	Tremulousness, ataxia
400–430	Hyperreflexia, twitching, spasticity
>430	Seizures and death

Unless the hypernatremia is of short duration, idiogenic osmoles are presumably present in brain cells. Consequently, too rapid rehydration and lowering of serum [Na$^+$] can cause brain cells to swell, resulting in cerebral edema and an increased likelihood of seizures, permanent neurologic sequelae, or even death. **In acute hypernatremia, serum [Na$^+$] levels can be corrected rather rapidly** with little fear of cerebral edema, because idiogenic osmoles will not yet be present in brain cells.

POTASSIUM (K$^+$)

Elemental K$^+$ is the major intracellular cation of the body. The normal intracellular concentration is 100 to 150 mEq/L, and the normal extracellular concentration is 3.5 to 5.0 mEq/L. The total body K$^+$ store ranges from 35 to 55 mEq/kg or 3500 mEq in a healthy 70-kg man. Approximately 70 to 75 percent of total body K$^+$ is found in muscle tissue; therefore, in patients with severe muscle wasting, total body stores may be as low as 20 to 30 mEq/kg. Daily intake of K$^+$ ranges from 50 to 150 mEq. Foods high in K$^+$ include oranges, grapefruit, tomatoes, bananas, avocados, and raisins. K$^+$ is excreted predominantly by the kidneys (90 percent), with some loss in the stool and by sweating. K$^+$ is filtered freely through the glomerulus and then reabsorbed in the proximal and ascending tubules. It is secreted in the distal tubule in exchange for Na$^+$. In healthy individuals, the kidneys are able to excrete up to 6 mEq/kg per d.

In the absence of an acid-base disturbance, measuring extracellular [K$^+$] is a reasonably accurate way to assess total body K$^+$ in relatively healthy patients. A decrease in measured serum [K$^+$] from 4 to 3 mEq/L (with pH remaining steady) represents a total body deficit of approximately 200 to 400 mEq. An increase in measured serum [K$^+$] from 4 to 5 mEq/L represents a total body K$^+$ increase of approximately 100 to 200 mEq. Extracellular K$^+$ represents about 2 percent of total body K$^+$, or 70 mEq, and is influenced by two important variables: total body K$^+$ stores and distribution between the ICF and ECF spaces. Significant and rapid intracellular to extracellular shifting occurs in response to severe injury (i.e., surgical stress, trauma, or burns), acid-base imbalance, catabolic states, increased extracellular osmolality, or insulin deficiency. These shifts are important when viewed in light of the role of K$^+$ in maintaining the resting membrane potential. The normally balanced intracellular to extracellular gradient facilitates propagation of electrical impulses. This is particularly important in the functioning of the heart.

Hypokalemia

PATHOPHYSIOLOGY   Hypokalemia is defined as a serum [K$^+$] of less than 3.5 mEq/L. The most frequent causes of hypokalemia are intracellular shifts and increased losses (Table 27-7). K$^+$ will shift into cells as the pH of the ECF rises in exchange for hydrogen ions. A rise in the pH of 0.10 generally causes a 0.5 mEq/L decrease in serum [K$^+$] levels. This relation applies to metabolic acid-base derangements. Although the reasons are unclear, respiratory alkalosis and acidosis have minimum effect on K$^+$ shift.

The clinical manifestations of hypokalemia usually start when serum concentrations reach 2.5 mEq/L, although they may appear sooner with rapid decreases in concentration (Table 27-8). The symptoms result from abnormalities in membrane polarization and affect almost every system.

TREATMENT   The treatment of hypokalemia is replacement of K$^+$. This can be done orally in stable patients who are able to tolerate oral intake. Foods rich in K$^+$, salt substitutes, or K$^+$ supplements will work. **The oral dose is 20 mEq K$^+$ every 60 min until the anticipated result is achieved.** Intravenous replacement is appropriate for patients with severe hypokalemia. To prevent sudden or excessive

TABLE 27-7 Etiology of Hypokalemia

Extracellular to intracellular potassium shifts
  Alkalosis*
  Increased plasma insulin (treatment of diabetic ketoacidosis)
  β-Adrenergics
  Hypokalemic periodic paralysis
Decreased intake
  Poor dietary intake, geophagia
Gastrointestinal loss*
  Vomiting, nasogastric suction, diarrhea (laxative, enema abuse),
    malabsorption, ureterosigmoidostomy, enteric fistula, villous adenoma
Renal loss
  Diuretic therapy*
  Primary aldosteronism
  Secondary aldosteronism
  Licorice ingestion
  Excessive use of chewing tobacco
  Renal tubular acidosis
  Postobstructive diuresis
  Osmotic diuresis
Drugs and toxins
  Carbenicillin, penicillin, amphotericin B, L-dopa, lithium, thalium,
    theophylline, dopamine
Sweat loss
  Heavy exercise, heatstroke, febrile illness
Other
  Hypomagnesemia, acute leukemia, state of rapid cellular synthesis,
    intravenous hyperalimentation, recovery from megaloblastic anemia

*Frequently encountered etiologies in the emergency department.

elevations in $[K^+]$, intravenous KCl should be administered in 10 mEq increments over 30 to 60 min, via a well running peripheral IV line. A cumulative dose of 20 mEq will raise serum $[K^+]$ by about 0.25 mEq/L. **No more than 40 mEq should be added to each L of IV fluid and infusion rates should be no greater than 40 mEq per h. Cardiac monitoring is recommended for infusion rates greater than 20 mEq per h.**

Hyperkalemia

PATHOPHYSIOLOGY Hyperkalemia is defined as measured serum $[K^+]$ of greater than 5.5 mEq/L. The most common cause is hemolysis during phlebotomy. Other causes are listed in Table 27-9.

TABLE 27-8 Symptoms and Signs of Hypokalema

Cardiovascular
  Hypertension
  Orthostatic hypotension
  Potentiation of digitalis toxicity
  Dysrhythmias (usually tachydysrhythmias)
  T-wave flattening, U waves, ST depression
Neuromuscular
  Malaise, weakness, fatigue
  Hyporeflexia
  Cramps
  Paresthesias
  Paralysis
  Rhabdomylosis
Gastrointestinal
  Ileus
Renal
  Increased ammonia production
  Urinary concentrating defects
  Metabolic alkalosis, paradoxical aciduria
  Nephrogenic diabetes insipidus
Endocrine
  Glucose intolerance

Clinical manifestations of hyperkalemia usually result from derangement in membrane polarization. Cardiac manifestations are the most serious. The following ECG changes are associated with hyperkalemia:

$[K^+]$ 6.5 to 7.5 mEq/L: tall peaked T waves, short QT interval, and prolonged PR interval
$[K^+]$ 7.5 to 8.0 mEq/L: QRS widening and flattening of the P wave
$[K^+]$ 10 to 12 mEq/L: the QRS complex may degrade into a "sine wave" pattern

In chronic or slowly developing hyperkalemia, ECG changes will occur at higher $[K^+]$ levels.

Ventricular fibrillation, complete heart block, and asystole may occur. Death from hyperkalemia is usually the result of diastolic arrest or ventricular fibrillation. Other symptoms include neuromuscular dysfunctional weakness, paresthesias, areflexia, ascending paralysis, and gastrointestinal (nausea, vomiting, and diarrhea).

TREATMENT If there are no cardiac derangements, the initial step in the treatment of hyperkalemia is to confirm the presence of "true" hyperkalemia by a repeat sample. Immediate cessation of further K^+ administration and clinical determination of severity will drive management. Asymptomatic patients with relatively small elevation of K^+ (5.0 to 6.0 mEq/L) require determination and treatment of the underlying cause. Emergent treatment for symptomatic patients is divided into three phases:

1. Membrane stabilization (especially cardiac tissue)
2. Shift of K^+ into cells
3. Removal of K^+ from the body

Therapies used to treat hyperkalemia are outlined in Table 27-10. **If calcium is to be given to a patient on digitalis, great caution must be exercised, because hypercalcemia potentiates the toxic cardiac effects of digitalis.** In severe hyperkalemia, however, the risk-to-benefit ratio may be such that giving Ca^{2+} is warranted.

CALCIUM (Ca^{2+})

Ca^{2+} is the most abundant mineral in the body. The total body Ca^{2+} is 15 g/kg of body weight, or about 1 kg in an average-sized adult. Ca^{2+} is 99 percent bound in bone as phosphate and carbonate (mineral apatite), with the remainder in the ECF compartment. The normal daily intake of Ca^{2+} is 800 to 3000 mg, one third of which is absorbed primarily in the small bowel by active (vitamin D dependent) and passive (concentration dependent) absorption. Excretion of Ca^{2+} is primarily via the stool.

The measured serum $[Ca^{2+}]$ ranges from 8.5 to 10.5 mg/dL and is maintained by the function of parathyroid hormone, vitamin D metabolites (1,25-dihydroxyvitamin D3, or calcitriol), and calcitonin.

Parathormone (parathyroid hormone, or PTH) is secreted by the parathyroid gland in response to low ionized Ca^{2+} levels. It raises $[Ca^{2+}]$ primarily by stimulating osteoclasts to increase bone resorption. It secondarily increases $[Ca^{2+}]$ by indirect action in the kidney (increases Ca^{2+} resorption and phosphorus excretion) and in conjunction with calcitriol to increase intestinal absorption. Calcitonin is influenced by elevations in $[Ca^{2+}]$, epinephrine, glucagon, and gastrin. Its primary effect is to inhibit the activity of osteoclasts, with a limited secondary effect to potentiate Ca^{2+} loss through the kidney.

The intravascular Ca^{2+} exists as 50 percent bound to plasma proteins, i.e., albumin, 45 percent free active ions, and 5 percent nonionized (bound to other substances in plasma and interstitial fluids). A laboratory value reported in milliequivalents per liter is equal to half the amount in milligrams per deciliter; e.g., a value of 4.2 mg/dL is equal to 2.1 mEq/L (or 1.05 mosmol/L).

Changes in $[H^+]$ result in changes of the ionized $[Ca^{2+}]$, because Ca^{2+} and protons competitively bind to proteins. For example, hyperventilation leads to respiratory alkalosis and an attendant decrease in $[H^+]$. The decreased $[H^+]$ causes an increase in protein-bound Ca^{2+}

TABLE 27-9　Etiology of Hyperkalemia

Pseudohyperkalemia	Intra- to Extracellular Potassium Shift	Potassium Load	Decreased Potassium Excretion
Tourniquet use	Acidosis*	Potassium supplements	Renal failure*
Hemolysis (in vitro)*	Heavy exercise	Potassium-rich foods	Drugs 　Potassium-sparing diuretics,* β blockade, NSAIDs, ACE inhibitors
Leukocytosis	β Blockade	Intravenous potassium	Aldosterone deficiency*
Thrombocytosis	Insulin deficiency Digitalis intoxication Hyperkalemic periodic paralysis	Potassium-containing drugs Transfusion of aged blood Hemolysis (in vivo) Gastrointestinal bleeding Cell destruction after chemotherapy Rhabdomyolysis/crush injury* Extensive tissue necrosis	Selective defect in renal potassium excretion 　Pseudohypoaldosteronism, SLE, sickle cell disease, obstructive uropathy, renal transplantation, Type IV renal tubular acidosis

*Frequent or important ED diagnostic consideratons.
Abbreviations: ACE = angiotensin-converting enzyme; NSAIDs = nonsteroidal anti-inflammatory drugs; SLE = systemic lupus erythematosus.

and a decrease in serum ionized Ca^{2+}. It is the ionized fraction that is physiologically activity.

Various factors affect $[Ca^{2+}]$ protein binding:

1. Serum protein, of which albumin is the major component. On average, 0.8 mg of Ca^{2+} binds to 1 g of protein. Therefore, total serum $[Ca^{2+}]$ is equal to ionized $[Ca^{2+}]$ plus the product of 0.8 and total protein. A 1 g decrease in albumin results in a 0.8 mg/dL decrease in total calcium, with no change in ionized fraction.
2. Alkalosis produces a decrease in ionized fraction with no change in the total serum $[Ca^{2+}]$. Each 0.1 rise in pH lowers ionized $[Ca^{2+}]$ by about 3 to 8 percent.
3. Acidosis produces an increase in ionized fraction with no change in the total serum $[Ca^{2+}]$.

Hypocalcemia

PATHOPHYSIOLOGY　Hypocalcemia is defined by an ionized $[Ca^{2+}]$ level of below 2.0 mEq/L. Normal ionized $[Ca^{2+}]$ is 2.1 to 2.6 mEq/L (1.05 to 1.3 mmol/L). Some common causes of hypocalcemia are shock, sepsis, renal failure, and pancreatitis. It is quite uncommon in ambulatory patients, except those with hypoparathyroidism (secondary to surgery) or chronic renal disease (Table 27-11).

Cellular Dysfunction　Any process that interferes with cell metabolism, such as shock or sepsis, will tend to reduce ionized $[Ca^{2+}]$ by al-

lowing increased net movement of Ca^{2+} across the cell membrane into the cytoplasm of the poorly functioning cells. After trauma, serum $[Ca^{2+}]$ may be low, especially with the fat embolism syndrome, not only because of cell dysfunction and binding of calcium to free fatty acids but also because of fatty inhibition of cell membrane calcium pumps.

Pancreatitis　Acute pancreatitis is an important cause of hypocalcemia. Pancreatic lipase breaks down fat into fatty acids and glycerol. The fatty acids combine with Ca^{2+} to form insoluble Ca^{2+} soaps and reduce serum $[Ca^{2+}]$. The combination of necrotic fat cells plus Ca^{2+} soaps makes up much of what is recognized as the fat necrosis of pancreatitis.

Drugs　Many drugs can cause hypocalcemia (Table 27-12).

Postoperative Hypocalcemia　Currently, more than 10 percent of post-parathyroidectomy patients may have hypoparathyroidism as defined by a fasting $[Ca^{2+}]$ of less than 8.5 mg/dL and a simultaneous inorganic phosphorus level of greater than 4.5 mg/dL. Postoperative hypocalcemia can be due to hypoparathyroidism from the permanent surgical removal of parathyroid tissue, from transient ischemia of the parathyroid glands in patients who have extensive bilateral neck surgery, or because of long-term hypercalcemic suppression of the nonadenomatous parathyroid glands.

TABLE 27-10　Emergency Therapy of Hyperkalemia

Therapy	Mechanism	Dose and Route	Onset of Action	Duration of Effect
Albuterol (nebulized)	Upregulates cAMP, shifts K^+ into cell	2.5 mg in 4 mL NS nebulized over 20 min	15–30 min	2–4 h
$CaCl_2$ (10%)*	Membrane stabilization	5–10 mL IV	1–3 min	30–50 min
Ca gluconate (10%)*	Membrane stabilization	10–20 mL IV	1–3 min	30–50 min
$NaHCO_3$	Shifts K^+ into cell	50–100 mEq IV	5–10 min	1–2 h
Insulin and glucose	Shifts K^+ into cell	10 units regular insulin 50 g glucose	30 min	4–6 h
Furosemide	Renal K^+ excretion	40 mg IV	Varies	Varies
Sodium polystyrene	GI K^+ excretion	25–50 g PO or PR	1–2 h	4–6 h
Hemodialysis	Removes K^+		Minutes	Varies

*Calcium chloride is 3 times as potent as calcium gluconate. 10% calcium chloride = 27.2 mg Ca^{++}/mL; 10% calcium gluconate = 9 mg Ca^{++}/mL.
Abbreviation: cAMP = cyclic adenosine monophosphate.

TABLE 27-11 Some Causes of Hypocalcemia

Decreased calcium absorption
    Vitamin D deficiency
    Malabsorption syndromes
Increased calcium excretion
    Alcoholism
    Chronic renal insufficiency
    Diuretics
Endocrine disorders
    Hypoparathyroidism
    Pseudohypoparathyroidism
Drugs (see Table 27-12)
Miscellaneous
    Sepsis
    Acute pancreatitis
    Massive transfusions
    Hypomagnesemia
    Rhabdomyolysis

TABLE 27-13 Symptoms and Signs of Hypocalcemia

General	Muscular
Weakness, fatigue	Spasms, cramps
Neurologic	Weakness
Tetany	Skeletal
Chvostek sign, Trousseau sign	Osteodystrophy
Circumoral and digital paresthesias	Rickets
Impaired memory, confusion	Osteomalacia
Hallucinations, dementia, seizures	Miscellaneous
Extrapyramidal disorders	Dental hypoplasia
Dermatologic	Cataracts
Hyperpigmentation	Decreased insulin secretion
Coarse, brittle hair	
Dry, scaly skin	
Cardiovascular	
Heart failure	
Vasoconstriction	

Renal Failure Hypocalcemia is a frequent finding in renal failure. This may be due in part to the resulting hyperphosphatemia, but there is also decreased production of 1,25-$(OH)_2$-vitamin D in the kidney, which in turn decreases intestinal absorption of calcium.

Phosphate Overload Phosphate overload from nonrenal causes also may lead to hypocalcemia. This is the presumed mechanism in the acute rhabdomyolysis of hyperpyrexia and major trauma. Hypomagnesemia in association with hypocalcemia may be seen in alcoholism, diuretic use, epilepsy, and renal failure.

Etiologies less likely to be encountered are listed in Table 27-11.

SYMPTOMS Serious physiologic changes do not usually occur until ionized levels in serum are less than 1.4 to 1.6 mEq/L (0.7 to 0.8 mmol/L; Table 27-13).

The severity of signs and symptoms depends greatly on the rapidity of the decrease in Ca^{2+}. As serum $[Ca^{2+}]$ fall, neuronal membranes become increasingly more permeable to sodium, thereby enhancing excitation.

Decreased ionized $[Ca^{2+}]$ reduces the strength of myocardial contraction primarily by inhibiting relaxation. Hypocalcemia decreases the sensitivity of the heart to digitalis.

The most characteristic initial symptom of hypocalcemia after thyroid or parathyroid surgery is paresthesias around the mouth or in the fingertips. Hypocalcemia should be suspected in any patient who is irritable and has hyperactive deep tendon reflexes after neck surgery. It also should be suspected in patients who have seizures, particularly if they have ever had thyroid surgery, even if many years previously.

A positive Chvostek or Trousseau sign is generally considered to be good clinical evidence of hypocalcemia. A positive Chvostek sign is a twitch at the corner of the mouth when the examiner taps over the

TABLE 27-12 Drugs That Can Cause Hypocalcemia

Phosphates (e.g., enemas, laxatives)
Phenytoin, phenobarbital
Gentamicin, tobramycin, actinomycin
Cisplatin
Heparin
Theophylline
Protamine
Glucagon
Norepinephrine
Citrate
Loop diuretics
Glucocorticoids
Magnesium sulfate
Sodium nitroprusside

facial nerve just in front of the ear. However, it is present in about 10 to 30 percent of normal individuals. Nevertheless, eyelid muscle contraction with the Chvostek maneuver is said to be almost diagnostic of hypocalcemia.

The Trousseau sign, which is generally a more reliable indicator of hypocalcemia, is positive if carpal spasm is produced when the examiner applies a blood pressure cuff to the upper arm and maintains a pressure above systolic for 3 min. The fingers are spastically extended at the interphalangeal joints and flexed at the metacarpophalangeal joints. The wrist is flexed and the forearm is pronated.

Decreased plasma levels of ionized Ca^{2+} are diagnostic, but one also should suspect hypocalcemia if a patient has decreased levels of total Ca^{2+} in the presence of normal plasma proteins.

Electrocardiography The most characteristic ECG finding in hypocalcemia is a prolonged QT interval. However, the T wave is of normal width, and it is the ST segment that is really prolonged. This finding is usually seen with total serum calcium levels below 6.0 mg/dL.

TREATMENT Treatment of hypocalcemia is tailored to the individual and directed toward the underlying cause. If a patient is asymptomatic, oral Ca^{2+} therapy with or without vitamin D may be sufficient. Ca^{2+} lactate, glubionate, ascorbate, carbonate, and gluconate are available in oral preparations. Milk, because of the large amount of phosphate present, is not really a very good source of Ca^{2+}, except in normal growing children who also need the phosphate.

If the patient is not symptomatic or if the hypocalcemia is not severe and prolonged for more than 10 to 14 days, treatment with Ca^{2+} may not be required. Symptomatic patients after thyroid or parathyroid surgery are often treated with parenteral Ca^{2+}. With severe acute hypocalcemia, 10 mL of 10 percent $CaCl_2$ (or 10 to 30 mL of 10 percent Ca^{2+} gluconate) may be given IV over 10 to 20 min followed by a continuous IV infusion of 10 percent $CaCl_2$ at 0.02 to 0.08 mL/kg per h (1.4 to 5.6 mL/h in a 70-kg patient). The serum $[Ca^{2+}]$ should be rechecked at that point before continuing parenteral Ca^{2+}. Intravenous calcium is recommended only in cases of symptomatic or severe hypocalcemia (ionized $[Ca^{2+}]$ <1.3 mEq/L or <0.65 mmol/L), because intravenous Ca^{2+} administration causes vasoconstriction and possible ischemia, especially in patients with low cardiac output who already have significant peripheral vasoconstriction. In addition, intravenous Ca^{2+} should be used with extreme caution in patients taking digitalis, because hypercalcemia can potentiate digitalis toxicity.

During massive transfusions, if the blood is being given faster than 1 unit every 5 min, 10 mL of 10 percent $CaCl_2$ can be given after every 4 to 6 units of blood if a patient is in shock or has heart failure despite adequate volume replacement therapy.

Similar to hypokalemia, hypocalcemia is difficult to correct in the setting of hypomagnesemia. Hypomagnesemic states reduce parathormone and Ca^{2+} releases from bone. Therefore, magnesium should be replaced before, or in conjunction with, Ca^{2+} replacement.

Hypercalcemia

PATHOPHYSIOLOGY   Hypercalcemia is a relatively common entity. It is defined as a total $[Ca^{2+}]$ exceeding 10.5 mg/dL or an ionized calcium level exceeding 2.7 mEq/L. More than 90 percent of occurrences are associated with hyperparathyroidism or malignancy, the latter being the most likely underlying presentation in the ED. A list of potential etiologies for hypercalcemia can be found in Table 27-14.

The effects of hypercalcemia can be neuromuscular, cardiovascular, gastrointestinal, renal, and skeletal. Neuromuscular changes include decreased sensitivity, responsiveness, and strength of muscular contraction and nerve conduction.

In mild hypercalcemic states, the heart's conduction is slowed and automaticity is decreased with a shortening of the refractory period. There is also increased sensitivity to digitalis preparations.

Loss of renal concentrating ability is the most frequent renal effect of hypercalcemia. This is a reversible tubular defect, which results in polyuria and volume depletion despite polydipsia. Potassium wasting results in hypokalemia in up to one third of patients. Nephrocalcinosis and nephrolithiasis are caused by the hypercalcemia and aggravated by volume depletion. As the hypercalcemia persists, increasing microscopic Ca^{2+} deposits in the kidney may result in progressive renal insufficiency.

SYMPTOMS   Hypercalcemic patients with plasma total $[Ca^{2+}]$ below 12.0 mg/dL are usually asymptomatic, but higher levels can cause a wide variety of symptoms and signs (Table 27-15).

Patients with total $[Ca^{2+}]$ above 14 to 16 mg/dL are usually very weak, lethargic, and confused. Polyuria and polydipsia are due to impaired renal tubular reabsorption of water and result in volume depletion. Total $[Ca^{2+}]$ above 15.0 mg/dL may cause somnolence, stupor, and even coma.

A mnemonic sometimes used for the signs and symptoms of hypercalcemia is *stones* (renal calculi), *bones* (osteolysis), *moans* (psychiatric disorders), and *groans* (peptic ulcer disease, pancreatitis, and constipation).

Hypercalcemia should be suspected in patients with extensive metastatic bone disease, particularly if the primary site involves the breast, lungs, or kidneys, and in individuals with combinations of clinical problems, such as renal calculi, pancreatitis, or ulcer disease.

TABLE 27-14   Causes of Hypercalcemia

Malignancy*	Granulomatous disease*
Lung (squamous cell cancer)	Sarcoidoses
Breast	Tuberculosis
Kidney	Histoplasmosis
Myeloma	Coccidioidomycosis
Leukemia	Immobilization
Endocrinopathies	Miscellaneous
Primary hyperparathyroidism	Paget's disease of bone
Hyperthyroidism	Postrenal transplantation
Pheochromocytoma	Recovery from acute renal failure
Adrenal insufficiency	Phosphate depletion syndrome
Acromegaly	
Drugs	
Hypervitaminosis D and A	
Thiazides	
Lithium*	
Hormonal therapy for breast cancer	

*More likely to be encountered in the ED.

TABLE 27-15   Symptoms and Signs of Hypercalcemia

General	Cardiovascular
Malaise, weakness	Hypertension
Polydipsia, dehydration	Dysrhythmias
Neurologic	Vascular calcifications
Confusion	ECG abnormalities
Apathy, depression, stupor	QT shortening
Decreased memory	Coving of ST–T wave
Irritability	Widening of T wave
Hallucinations	Digitalis sensitivity
Headache	Gastrointestinal
Ataxia	Anorexia, weight loss
Hyporeflexia, hypotonia	Nausea, vomiting
Mental retardation (infants)	Constipation
Metastatic calcification	Abdominal pain
Band keratopathy	Peptic ulcer disease
Conjunctivitis	Pancreatitis
Pruritus	Urologic
Skeletal	Polyuria, nocturia
Fractures	Renal insufficiency
Bone pain	Nephrolithiasis
Deformities	

Abbreviation: ECG = electrocardiogram.

On ECG, hypercalcemia may be associated with depressed ST segments, widened T waves, and shortened ST segments and QT intervals. Bradyarrhythmias may occur, and bundle branch patterns may progress to second-degree block and then to complete heart block. Levels above 20 mg/dL may cause cardiac arrest.

TREATMENT   Treatment for hypercalcemia should be initiated in any symptomatic patient, or if $[Ca^{2+}]$ is above 14 mg/dL. Treatment consists of volume repletion (with NS), increasing renal Ca^{2+} elimination, decreasing Ca^{2+} mobilization from bone, and correction of the underlying disorder. Up to one third of patients with hypercalcemia have hypokalemia. Hypomagnesemia also is common.

Renal elimination of Ca^{2+} can be increased with furosemide (40 to 100 mg IV every 2 to 4 h) or other loop diuretic. Care must be taken, because diuresis can worsen the volume depleted state, hypokalemia, and hypomagnesemia.

Decreased mobilization of Ca^{2+} from bone through reduction of osteoclast activity can be accomplished with several medications. Recommendations for initiating the following medications in the ED are generally lacking, but consideration should be given to using them if the patient is symptomatic or the $[Ca^{2+}]$ is greater than 14 mg/dL. Mithramycin (25 μg/kg IV) is particularly useful in patients with metastatic bone disease, but calcitonin (4 IU/kg SC or IM every 12 h) is less toxic. Glucocorticoids (hydrocortisone, 3 mg/kg per d in divided doses) are useful in patients with sarcoidosis, vitamin A or D intoxication, multiple myeloma, leukemia, or breast cancer. They work by inhibiting bone resorption and gastrointestinal absorption of Ca^{2+}. It is also postulated that they cause Ca^{2+} to shift inside cells, where it may become bound to mitochondria. Gallium nitrate has been approved for use in the United States. It acts by decreasing the solubility of base crystals. It potentiates nephropathy, and its use should be avoided in renal disease. Intravenous phosphates are no longer used.

MAGNESIUM (Mg^{2+})

The total body content of Mg^{2+} is 24 g, or 2000 mEq, 50 to 70 percent of which is fixed in bone and only slowly exchangeable. Most of the remaining Mg^{2+} is found in the ICF space, with a concentration of approximately 40 mEq/L. The distribution of Mg^{2+} is similar to that of K^+, with the major portion being intracellular. It is the second most abundant intracellular cation. Normal serum $[Mg^{2+}]$ ranges between 1.5 and 2.5 mEq/L. Mg^{2+} present in blood is 25 to 35 percent protein bound, 10 to 15 percent complexed, and 50 to 60 percent ionized. The normal dietary intake of Mg^{2+} is approximately 20 to 28 mEq per d, or 240 to 336 mg per d, and is found in vegetables such as dry beans and leafy greens, meat, and cereals. Sixty percent of excreted Mg^{2+} is via the stool, with the remainder via the urine. Mg^{2+} promotes enzyme reactions within the cell during metabolism, helps in the production of ATP, participates in protein synthesis, and plays a role in coagulation, platelet aggregation, and neuromuscular activity.

Hypomagnesemia

PATHOPHYSIOLOGY   A wide variety of problems can cause hypomagnesemia (Table 27-16). In adults, magnesium deficiencies are seen most frequently in alcoholics, in malnourished patients, and in patients with cirrhosis, pancreatitis, or excessive gastrointestinal fluid losses. Diarrhea produces greater Mg^{2+} losses ($[Mg^{2+}]$ of 10 to 14 mEq/L) than does upper gastrointestinal loss (1 to 2 mEq/L).

Intravenous hyperalimentation or treatment of diabetic ketoacidosis without providing adequate Mg^{2+}, especially in a previously malnourished patient, can cause an abrupt fall in plasma magnesium levels. Renal wasting of Mg^{2+} can be seen with loop diuretics, hypophosphatemia, ketoacidosis, aminoglycosides, and nephrotoxic chemotherapeutic agents.

Magnesium is essential to a large number of vital enzymes, including membrane-bound ATPase. Consequently, hypomagnesemia may result in a wide variety of neuromuscular, gastrointestinal, and cardiovascular changes (Table 27-17).

SYMPTOMS   The diagnosis of hypomagnesemia in the presence of normal serum calcium levels is suggested by increased neuromuscular irritability (hyperreflexia, positive Chvostek or Trousseau sign, tremor, tetany, or even convulsions). Hypomagnesemia should be suspected in alcoholics, cirrhotics, and patients on intravenous fluids for prolonged periods. Hypomagnesemia also may develop rapidly during intravenous hyperalimentation, especially when anabolism begins.

The ECG changes seen with magnesium deficiencies include prolonged PR and QT intervals, widened QRS complexes, depression of ST segments, and inversion of T waves, especially in the precordial leads. The changes may be somewhat similar to those caused by hypokalemia and/or hypocalcemia, and many of these changes may be related to Mg^{2+} deficiency altering cardiac intracellular potassium content.

TREATMENT   Hypokalemia, hypocalcemia, and hypophosphatemia are often present with severe hypomagnesemia and must be monitored carefully. Hypocalcemia does not develop until $[Mg^{2+}]$ falls below 1.2 mg/dL.

Patients with Mg^{2+} deficiency may require more than 50 mEq of oral Mg^{2+} (6 g of $MgSO_4$) per day. In chronic alcoholics with delirium tremens and in patients with severe proven hypomagnesemia, up to 8 to 12 g of $MgSO_4$ may be given IM or IV the first day. The first 10 to 15 mEq (1.5 to 2.0 g) of intravenous $MgSO_4$ can be given over 1 to 2 h. This may be followed by up to 4 to 6 g per d thereafter. Approximately half of the administered Mg^{2+} will be lost in the urine.

Hypermagnesemia

PATHOPHYSIOLOGY   Hypermagnesemia is rarely encountered in emergency practice. A small elevation in serum concentration has little clinical significance. The most common etiology for hypermagnesemia can be found in patients with renal insufficiency or renal failure who ingest Mg^{2+}-containing drugs. Hypermagnesemia may be seen in the perinatal setting in a mother and her neonate secondary to the treatment of preeclampsia or eclampsia. Other etiologies of hypermagnesemia include lithium ingestion, volume depletion, or familial hypocalciuric hypercalcemia (Table 27-18).

SYMPTOMS   Hypermagnesemia only rarely produces symptoms. Mg^{2+} decreases the transmission of neuromuscular messages and thus acts as a CNS depressant and decreases neuromuscular activity. Approximate $[Mg^{2+}]$ causing signs and symptoms can be found in Table 27-19.

EVALUATION AND TREATMENT   Serum $[Mg^{2+}]$ are usually diagnostic. The possibility of hypermagnesemia should be considered in patients with hyperkalemia or hypercalcemia. Hypermagnesemia also should be suspected in patients with renal failure, particularly in those who are taking magnesium-containing antacids (see Table 27-18).

The primary treatment available is the immediate cessation of Mg^{2+} administration. If renal failure is not evident, dilution by intravenous fluids followed by furosemide (40 to 80 mg IV) may be helpful. Calcium directly antagonizes the effects of magnesium; severe

TABLE 27-16   Causes of Hypomagnesemia

Redistribution	Extrarenal Loss	Decreased Intake	Increased Renal Loss

Postparathyroidectomy
Correction of diabetic ketoacidosis
	Nasogastric suction (infrequent)
	Lactation
		Alcoholism (cirrhosis)
		Malnutrition, poor intake
			Ketoacidosis
			Drugs: loop diuretics
			    Aminoglycosides
			    Amphotericin B
			    Vitamin D intoxication
			    Alcohol
			    Cisplatin

Intravenous glucose	Profuse sweating, burns, sepsis	Small bowel resection	SIADH
Intravenous hyperalimentation	Intestinal or biliary fistula	Malabsorption	Hyperthyroidism
Refeeding after starvation	Diarrhea		Hyperparathyroidism
Acute pancreatitis			Hypercalcemic states Primary or secondary aldosteronism Tubulointerstitial renal disease Postobstructive or postacute renal failure diuresis Saline or osmotic diuresis Potassium depletion Familial hypophosphatemia

Abbreviation: SIADH = syndrome of inappropriate antidiuretic hormone.

TABLE 27-17   Symptoms and Signs of Hypomagnesemia

Neuromuscular	Gastrointestinal
Tetany	Dysphagia
Muscle weakness	Anorexia, nausea
Cerebellar (ataxia, nystagmus, vertigo)	Cardiovascular
Confusion, obtundation, coma	Heart failure
Seizures	Dysrhythmias
Apathy, depression	Hypotension
Irritability	Miscellaneous
Paresthesias	Hypokalemia
	Hypocalcemia
	Anemia

TABLE 27-19   Symptoms and Signs of Hypermagnesemia

Level (mEq/L)	Symptom
2.0–3.0	Nausea
3.0–4.0	Somnolence
4.0–8.0	Loss of DTRs
8.0–12.0	Respiratory depression
12.0–15.0	Hypotension, heart block, cardiac arrest

Abbreviation: DTRs = deep tendon reflexes.

symptomatic hypermagnesemia can be treated with 5 mL 10 percent $CaCl_2$ IV over 5 min. Patients with renal failure may benefit from dialysis using a decreased Mg^{2+} bath that lowers serum $[Mg^{2+}]$.

CHLORIDE (Cl^-)

Alteration in serum chloride is seldom a primary disturbance. Chloride is a major extracellular anion that has the power of increasing or decreasing in concentration whenever changes occur in the concentration of other anions. For example, in non-anion gap metabolic acidosis, the decrease in serum $[HCO_3^-]$ is replaced by Cl^-. Cl^- plays a major role in the maintenance of urinary output, ECF, acid and base, and potassium balance. $[Cl^-]$ should be between 95 and 105 mEq/L. Cl^- is easily absorbed in the intestine by active and passive transport. Ninety percent of Cl^- is excreted through the kidney, with the remainder secreted in sweat and stool.

Hypochloremia

PATHOPHYSIOLOGY   Hypochloremia usually manifests when levels are below 95 mEq/L. It is usually caused by excessive diuresis, vomiting, or nasogastric tube drainage. Volume loss results in alkalosis. When Cl^- is lost via the urine or gastrointestinal fluids, there is an increase in Na^+ and HCO_3^- resorption secondary to the volume contraction. Na^+ may be resorbed in the kidney with Cl^- or HCO_3^-.

SYMPTOMS   There are no signs or symptoms specific for hypochloremia. The clinical approach is based on the findings of the secondary effects. It is important to determine the urinary $[Cl^-]$, because low urinary $[Cl^-]$ (<10 mEq/L) in the setting of metabolic alkalosis implies chloride-responsive alkalosis (see Chap. 25). If the urinary Cl^- levels are higher (>40 mEq/L), the hypochloremia may be secondary to volume overload or dilution. Increased urinary Cl^- also may result from increased mineralocorticoid activity, which leads to the retention of HCO_3^- and Na^+ at the expense of H^+, K^+, and Cl^-.

TABLE 27-18   Causes of Hypermagnesemia

Renal failure (acute or chronic)
Increased magnesium load
Magnesium-containing laxatives, antacids, or enemas*
Treatment of preeclampsia/eclampsia (mothers and neonates)
Diabetic ketoacidosis (untreated)*
Tumor lysis
Rhabdomyolysis*
Increased renal magnesium absorption
Hyperparathyroidism
Familial hypocalciuric hypercalcemia
Hypothyroidism
Mineralocorticoid deficiency, adrenal insufficiency

*Most likely presentation relevant to the ED.

TREATMENT   Generally speaking, emergency practice concerns itself with addressing the acute issues associated with the underlying condition. The treatment of chloride-responsive metabolic alkalosis (urinary $[Cl^-]$ = 10 mEq/L) is intravenous NS administration.

Hyperchloremia

PATHOPHYSIOLOGY   Excessive concentration of Cl^- is usually the result of administration of NaCl, volume depletion, or entities causing metabolic acidosis without a widened anion gap (see Chap. 25).

TREATMENT   Treatment is aimed at the underlying issues (see Chap. 25).

PHOSPHORUS

Phosphorus is an essential mineral that exists mainly as hydroxyapatite (85 percent) or as an intracellular constituent (10 to 15 percent). Only about 1 percent is in the ECF, so serum measurements may not accurately reflect total body stores. Serum phosphate levels decrease with age from a high of 4.0 to 7.0 mg/dL in newborns to 2.5 to 5.0 mg/dL in adults. The total body phosphorus in a normal man is approximately 700 g (10 to 15 g/kg). This amount is predominantly in bone (80 percent), where phosphorus plays a major role in structural integrity. Serum Ca^{2+} and phosphate are inversely proportional, and the product of their concentrations is maintained at approximately 30 to 40 mg/dL. Intracellular phosphorus is bound to protein or exists as organic esters.

Serum phosphorus, unlike the other elements, is 85 percent free and only 15 percent bound to proteins. Phosphate (PO_4^{3-}) may be present in different forms such as $H_2PO_4^-$ or HPO_4^{2-}. Plasma phosphorus levels, unlike Ca^{2+} or Mg^{2+}, demonstrate diurnal variation with a morning nadir and are affected by age, hormones (insulin and growth hormone), and the amount of carbohydrate ingestion. Therefore, fasting levels are the most useful, because glucose infusion and carbohydrate and phosphorus ingestion lower serum levels.

Normal daily intake is between 10 and 12 mmol. Phosphorus absorption is proportional to dietary intake. Approximately 70 percent is absorbed via passive transport, with the remainder via active transport, which is dependent on 1,25-$(OH)_2$-vitamin D. Excretion is predominantly in the urine by the glomerulus, with the majority resorbed in the proximal tubules. This is regulated by PTH, which acts to lower serum phosphate by increasing renal excretion. Proximal tubule absorption increases when serum PO_4^{3-} levels drop, and with hypoparathyroidism, volume depletion, hypocalcemia, or the presence of growth hormone. Excretion increases in the presence of volume expansion, hypercalcemia, acidosis, hypomagnesemia, hypokalemia, glucocorticoids, diuretics, calcitonin, or PTH. Phosphate is essential to a wide variety of biochemical reactions, especially energy metabolism in the form of high-energy phosphate and phosphocreatine.

Hypophosphatemia

PATHOPHYSIOLOGY   Because phosphorus is abundant in many foods and readily absorbed, hypophosphatemia is relatively unusual. Mechanisms leading to hypophosphatemia include movement of phosphate into cells, increased renal excretion, and decreased gastrointestinal absorption. Significant hypophosphatemia is unlikely to be encountered in the ED, because it is associated most often with hyperalimentation. There may be a shift into cells seen with alkalosis (respiratory or metabolic). Other conditions that may on occasion present to the ED with complications related to phosphate depletion include hyperparathyroidism, malignancy with hypercalcemia (phosphaturia), renal tubular defects, and use of phosphate-binding antacids. Conditions unlikely to be seen in ED practice but associated with hypophosphatemia include rapid healing, prolonged anabolic states, recovery from starvation or severe burns, and partial hepatectomy.

Redistribution phenomena also can occur with glucose infusion. Phosphorus is consumed during phosphorylation as glucose moves into cells. This is one of the theoretical reasons potassium phosphate is advocated as part of K^+ replacement regimens in the treatment for diabetic ketoacidosis. **However, it should not be the initial form of K^+ replacement in the ED, because significant hypophosphatemia is unlikely to occur for 12 to 24 h, and parenteral administration may cause precipitous falls in serum $[Ca^{2+}]$.** (Also see Chap. 211).

SYMPTOMS   Symptoms of hypophosphatemia are unlikely to appear until levels are quite low, usually below 1 mg/dL. Hypophosphatemia should be particularly sought as a potential complication 12 to 24 h after initiating treatment for diabetic ketoacidosis and 24 to 96 h after treatment for alcoholic ketoacidosis. Detecting total body depletion cannot reliably be ascertained from blood phosphorus levels, because the ratio of intracellular to extracellular phosphorus is approximately 100:1. Specific findings of hypophosphatemia are presented in Table 27-20.

TREATMENT   Fortunately, PO_4^{3-} deficiency is easily reversible by correcting the underlying disorder and replacing phosphorus. Milk is an excellent source of phosphorus and contains 1000 mg/L. Tablets come in the form of sodium or potassium phosphate. If symptoms are severe enough, intravenous PO_4^- may be necessary.

The oral replacement dosage for uncomplicated, mild hypophosphatemia (>2 mg/dL) is 1200 to 1500 mg daily, given in divided doses. Intravenous replacement for severe (<1 mg/dL) hypophosphatemia, concomitant cardiac, or respiratory compromise is 2.5 to 5 mg/kg (0.08 to 0.16 mmol/kg) over 6h. Electrolytes should be

TABLE 27-20   Symptoms and Signs of Hypophosphatemia

Hematologic
    Reduced survival of platelets and red and white blood cells
    Impaired platelet function
    Spherocytosis
    Tissue hypoxia secondary to decreased 2,3-DPG
    Impaired macrophage function
Neuromuscular
    Weakness
    Tremors
    Circumoral and fingertip paresthesias
    Decreased DTRs
    Decreased mental status
    Anorexia
    Hyperventilation
Cardiac
    Impaired myocardial function

Abbreviations: 2,3-DPG = 2,3-diphosphoglycerate; DTRs = deep tendon reflexes.

rechecked after 6 h before further replacement. Slower rates are required in patients with renal insufficiency, and less total replacement is given in patients with hypercalcemia to avoid metastatic calcifications.

Hyperphosphatemia

PATHOPHYSIOLOGY   Hyperphosphatemia may be due to reduced renal excretion, increased PO_4^{3-} movement out of cells into the ECF, or increased phosphorus or vitamin D intake. Hyperphosphatemia is most apt to be seen with renal dysfunction. It also may be seen with hypoparathyroidism or any problem associated with hypocalcemia or hypomagnesemia.

SYMPTOMS   Problems due to hyperphosphatemia are usually those due to associated renal failure, hypocalcemia, or the hypomagnesemia that is usually present.

TREATMENT   Therapy is aimed at treating the underlying cause and restricting calcium phosphate intake to less than 200 mg per d. With normal renal function, PO_4^{3-} excretion can be increased with saline (1 to 2 L every 4 to 6 h) and acetazolamide (500 mg every 6 h). Phosphorus absorption from the gastrointestinal tract can be decreased with oral phosphate binders (i.e., aluminum carbonate or hydroxide 30 to 45 mL daily). These binders also absorb PO_4^{3-} secreted into the gut lumen and are of benefit even if no oral phosphorus is given. In severe cases, hemodialysis may be required.

BIBLIOGRAPHY

Arthur C, Guyton J, Hall E (eds): *Textbook of Medical Physiology.* Philadelphia, WB Saunders, 2000.

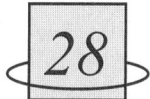

28   DISTURBANCES OF CARDIAC RHYTHM AND CONDUCTION
Edmund Bolton

THE NORMAL CARDIAC CONDUCTING SYSTEM

The heart consists of variations of three types of specialized tissue: (1) pacemaker cells that undergo spontaneous depolarization and can initiate an electric impulse (this property is called *automaticity*); (2) cells that conduct electrical waves more rapidly than other cardiac cells, causing a very rapid propagation of the electric impulse throughout the heart; and (3) contractile cells, which contract when electrically depolarized.

The sinus [sinoatrial (SA)] node is normally the dominant cardiac pacemaker unless disease or drugs depress its activity. The SA node is near the junction of the superior vena cava and right atrium. Blood supply is from the sinus node artery, which arises from the proximal few centimeters of the right coronary artery (in about 55 percent of individuals) or from the proximal few millimeters of the left circumflex artery (in the other 45 percent). Sympathetic and parasympathetic nerves, which are the primary controls of the heart rate, innervate the SA node. The normal sinus discharge rate is 60 to 100 beats/min.

The electric impulse generated by the SA node spreads in waves through the cardiac muscles of the atria, thus activating atrial contraction. In addition, specialized atrial conduction tracts (anterior, middle, and posterior internodal tracts) serve to propagate the electric impulse through the atria and between the sinus node and the atrioventricular (AV) node.

The atria and ventricles are insulated electrically from each other by the fibrous connective tissue of the AV ring (annulus fibrosus).

Normally, electrical impulses from the atria can reach the ventricles only by passing through the AV node and infranodal conducting system.

The AV node is under the surface of the right atrial endocardium and directly above the insertion of the septal leaflet of the tricuspid valve. The AV node receives its blood supply from the right coronary artery as it turns to form the posterior descending artery in 90 percent of individuals or as it comes off the left circumflex artery in the other 10 percent. This accounts for the common occurrence of AV conduction disturbances with acute inferior myocardial infarctions (MIs). The AV node is innervated by sympathetic and parasympathetic fibers. It has two important electrophysiologic characteristics: a slow conduction velocity and a long refractory period. The slow conduction velocity through the AV node allows time for atrial contraction to give an extra 10 percent ventricular filling, which increases stroke volume according to the Frank-Starling principle. This "atrial kick" is most important for patients with ventricular failure. The long refractory period of the AV node protects the ventricles from excessively rapid stimulation; very rapid heart rates decrease the diastolic filling period and thereby reduce cardiac output, which may cause deterioration into ventricular fibrillation or cardiac failure. Cells near the AV node have automaticity and will escape from the control of the SA node if its rate becomes too slow, normally slower than 60 beats/min.

Electrical impulses leave the inferior pole of the AV node along the bundle of His, which travels downward along the posterior margin of the membranous portion of the intraventricular septum to reach the top of the muscular portion. The bundle of His consists of Purkinje cells, which are the most rapidly conducting cells of the heart. The common bundle is only 1 to 2 cm in length before it divides at the crest of the muscular intraventricular septum into the right and left bundle branches (RBB and LBB, respectively). The RBB is a compact group of fibers that travels down to the apex of the right ventricle before separating into smaller branches. The LBB travels 2 to 3 cm before fanning out into a virtual sheet of fibers to cover the left ventricle. There are two relatively distinct pathways to the base of the papillary muscles, the left anterior superior fascicle (LASF) and the left posterior inferior fascicle (LPIF). These fascicles are distinguished more readily by electrical means than by anatomy in humans, but they can be seen clearly in animals.

The blood supply to the RBB and LASF is from the same sources: about half the time from the AV nodal artery and branches from the left anterior descending coronary artery and the other half from the left anterior descending artery alone. The LPIF is supplied about half the time from the AV nodal artery and the other half by the AV nodal artery and left anterior descending artery. Infarction in the region supplied by the left anterior descending artery can affect the RBB and LASF but very rarely the LPIF.

Accessory tracts are embryologic remnants of myocardium found in the AV annulus that can transmit electrical impulses between the atria and the ventricles and thus bypass all or part of the AV node and infranodal system. These bypass tracts conduct at different rates and are the anatomic basis for the preexcitation syndrome.

THE NORMAL ELECTROCARDIOGRAM

The clinical surface electrocardiogram (ECG) records the potential (voltage) differences between "neutral" ground and recording electrodes. The ECG is generated by the electrical activity of the heart and depicts the net sum of this activity recorded over time. By convention, a potential difference that points toward a recording electrode is assigned a positive deflection on the ECG, and a potential that points away from the recording electrode is assigned a negative deflection. Also by convention, routine ECG recordings are obtained with paper speed of 25 mm/s (2.5 cm/s) and signal calibration of 1.0 mV/10 mm (1.0 cm).

In Figure 28-1, depolarization starts on the left side of the ventricular septum and initially proceeds to the right; this action is recorded as a small negative deflection in the recording electrode. Subsequent

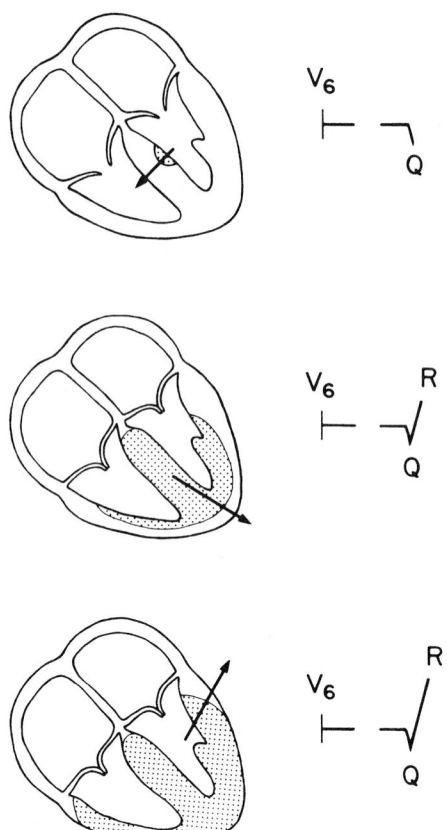

FIG. 28-1. Ventricular depolarization recorded in lead V_6.

depolarization involves the free walls of both ventricles; further, because the left side has a much larger mass, the net sum of electrical activity is directed toward the recording electrode, and a tall, positive deflection is recorded.

The P-QRS-T complex of the normal ECG represents electrical activity over one cardiac cycle (Figure 28-2). The P wave is caused by atrial depolarization. The QRS complex usually obscures atrial repolarization. The normal P-wave duration is shorter than 0.10 s (2.5 mm), and normal amplitude is less than 0.3 mV (3 mm). A P wave originating from the SA node is directed inferiorly and to the left on the frontal plane. The P-R interval is the time between the onset of depolarization in the atria and the onset of depolarization in the ventricles. It is commonly used as an estimation of AV nodal conduction time, because the AV node is the most likely site for delay in conduction. For adults in sinus rhythm, the P-R interval is 0.12 to 0.20 s (3 to 5 mm at 25 mm/s).

The QRS complex indicates ventricular depolarization. In general, depolarization starts on the endocardium and spreads outward to the epicardium. Despite the large amount of myocardium that must be depolarized, the specialized conducting system makes this a rapid process, and the normal QRS duration is 0.06 to 0.10 s (1.5 to 2.5 mm). Any delay in intraventricular conduction results in a wide QRS. Ectopic impulses that originate below the bundle of His or that arrive before repolarization of the bundle branches also result in a widened QRS, because they do not use the Purkinje network.

Although small negative initial deflections (Q waves) are normal, large Q waves can be due to an electrically nonexcitable area just under the recording electrode. **An abnormal Q wave has a width of 0.04 s or greater and a height one third that of the QRS complex.**

The ST segment represents the plateau phase of ventricular depolarization. Although the ST segment is usually isoelectric, a small deviation, less than 0.1 mV (1 mm), may be normal.

The T wave is caused by ventricular repolarization. Depolarization is a rapid, nearly simultaneous release of stored energy (like the re-

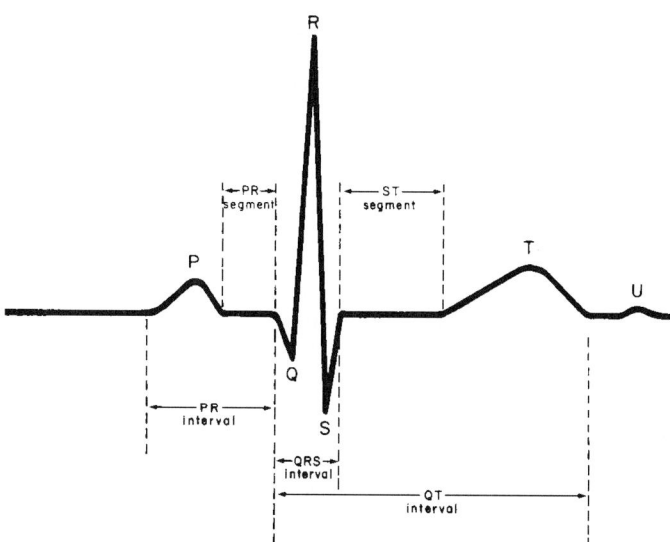

FIG. 28-2. Normal P-QRS-T electrocardiographic pattern.

lease of a compressed spring); repolarization is a slow, asynchronous event in which the metabolic machinery of each cell restores the transmembrane potential. Therefore, the T-wave duration is much longer and the amplitude much lower than those of the QRS complex. In general, repolarization starts on the epicardium and spreads to the endocardium. Many factors can influence this normal repolarization sequence: (1) metabolic factors (hypoxia, fever, drugs), (2) autonomic stimuli (abdominal pain, hyperventilation), (3) myocardial hypertrophy, (4) myocardial ischemia or inflammation, and (5) abnormal depolarization (bundle-branch block).

The QT interval represents ventricular depolarization and repolarization. QT duration is commonly between 0.33 and 0.42 s, but it does vary inversely with heart rate. The corrected interval is obtained by dividing the measured QT interval (in seconds) by the square root of the R-R interval (in seconds; i.e., $QT_c = QT/\sqrt{R\text{-}R}$). The normal corrected QT interval is shorter than 0.47 s. This corrected QT should be checked before giving drugs such as ibutilide, and other drugs that can prolong the QT interval and may cause torsade de pointes (TdP). The potential association of droperidol to prolongation of the QT interval has been recently questioned.[1]

The U wave may be seen as a normal component of the surface ECG. It is best seen in leads V_1 and V_2. There is still some dispute as to the origin of the U wave. The classic explanation is that the U wave represents the delayed repolarization of the Purkinje network. More recent research has shown that the U wave can be seen at the same time as early afterdepolarizations in patients with a prolonged QT interval and TdP.[1,2]

CARDIAC DYSRHYTHMIAS

There are many protocols for the classification of dysrhythmias and conduction disturbances. Dysrhythmias are basically classified in relation to the rate and site of abnormality. Conduction disturbances are usually classified as to the site and degree of block.

Cardiac dysrhythmias may decrease cardiac output if the ventricular rate is too fast or slow. In an adult without cardiac disease, heart rates between 40 and 160 beats/min are usually well tolerated, because physiologic adaptations can maintain adequate cardiac output and blood pressure. In adults with significant heart disease, rates slower than 50 or faster than 120 beats/min may decrease cardiac output based on a poorly functioning ventricle, because of basic myocardial cell damage, ischemic cells, valvular disease, or a combination of these.

Mechanisms of Tachydysrhythmia

There are three accepted mechanisms for tachydysrhythmias: (1) increased automaticity in a normal or ectopic site, (2) reentry in a normal or accessory pathway, and (3) afterdepolarizations causing triggered rhythms. Although treatment is best directed by an understanding of the underlying process, uncertainty still exists over the precise mechanism of many dysrhythmias, and therapy is often empiric.

An ectopic focus is an area of the heart, away from the normal sinus node pacemaker, that acquires independent pacemaker activity and usurps the pacemaking role. The result can be one extrasystole or multiple extra depolarizations. These ectopic pacemakers can be the result of (1) enhanced automaticity of subsidiary pacemaker cells (i.e., in the AV node or infranodal conducting system) or (2) abnormal automaticity of myocardial cells, which seldom possess pacemaking activity (i.e., Purkinje cells). Dysrhythmias due to an ectopic focus usually have a gradual onset ("warmup period"). The termination is also gradual, as opposed to the abrupt onset and termination seen with reentry or triggered mechanisms.

Reentry requires a temporary or permanent unidirectional block in one limb of a circuit and slower-than-normal conduction around the entire circuit. These conditions are secondary to disease, drugs, accessory pathways, or when tissue is stimulated during the partial refractory period (before full repolarization), as with premature depolarizations.

As indicated in Figure 28-3, the inciting impulse traveling in the normal downward direction encounters the two limbs, finds limb *a* blocked, and travels down limb *b*. Upon reaching the bottom portion of the circuit where the two limbs rejoin, the impulse can then travel retrograde up limb *a* and reach the upper connection of the circuit. Normally, conduction is so rapid that the impulse would encounter limb *b* still refractory to stimulation, and no further propagation would occur. However, if conduction around the circuit were slow enough, limb *b* would be able to conduct the impulse again in the antegrade direction. With the right size circuit and conduction velocity, an electrical impulse can continue traveling around the circuit in a cyclic manner. Each time the impulse passes the upper and lower limb connections, a depolarization occurs.

Reentry can occur around anatomically defined circuits, resulting in a regular rapid rhythm, such as paroxysmal supraventricular tachycardia (SVT). Conversely, reentry can occur in a disorganized and chaotic fashion through a syncytium of myocardial tissue as seen, for example, in atrial or ventricular fibrillation.

Triggered dysrhythmias are due to the oscillations of the transmembrane potential during or after repolarization (afterpotentials). Under ideal conditions of rate, afterpotentials reach threshold and trigger a complete depolarization (afterdepolarization). Once triggered, this process may be self-sustaining. Triggered dysrhythmias associated

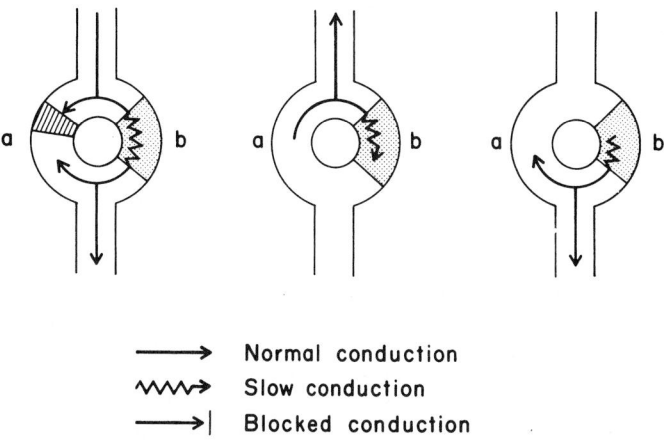

→ **Normal conduction**
〜〜→ **Slow conduction**
→| **Blocked conduction**

FIG. 28-3. Reentry circuit.

with early afterpotentials are enhanced by slow heart rates and usually treated by accelerating the ventricular rate with positive chronotropic drugs or electrical pacing. Triggered dysrhythmias associated with delayed afterpotentials are enhanced by fast heart rates. Treatment with agents that have a negative chronotropic action is usually effective.

The urgency with which tachydysrhythmias require treatment is guided by two considerations: (1) evidence of hypoperfusion (shock, altered mental status, anginal chest pain, or pulmonary edema) and (2) the potential to degenerate into a more serious dysrhythmia or cardiac arrest. The two treatment methods most commonly used are intravenous drugs for the clinically stable patient and synchronized cardioversion or defibrillation for the unstable patient. Some tachydysrhythmias are amenable to overdrive electrical pacing but frequently require rates faster than 200 beats/min to capture the ventricle.

Mechanisms of Bradydysrhythmia

Bradydysrhythmias can be caused by two mechanisms: depression of sinus nodal activity or conduction system blocks. In both situations, subsidiary pacemakers take over and pace the heart; provided the pacemaker is above the bifurcation of the bundle of His, the rate is generally adequate to maintain cardiac output.

The need for emergent treatment of bradycardias is guided by two considerations: (1) evidence of hypoperfusion and (2) the potential to degenerate into a more profound bradycardia or ventricular asystole. In general, emergent treatment is not required, unless (1) the heart rate is slower than 50 beats/min and there is clinical evidence of hypoperfusion or (2) the bradycardia is due to structural disease of the infranodal conducting system (transient or permanent) that has a risk of progressing to complete AV block. The first group of patients requires immediate treatment during assessment of the etiology of the bradycardia and consideration of whether internal pacing will be required. The second group of patients does not always require immediate treatment but should be monitored closely, with therapy readily available, while arrangements are made for further evaluation and possible internal cardiac pacing.

Three methods are currently available for emergent treatment of bradycardias: atropine, isoproterenol, and transcutaneous cardiac pacing.

Atropine should be the initial agent, at doses of 0.5 mg intravenously every 5 min until the desired response is achieved or a total vagolytic dose (about 0.05 mg/kg in humans) is given. Usually, if no response is seen after a cumulative dose of 2.0 mg, further doses are not effective. The vast majority of bradycardias due to problems of the sinus or AV node respond to atropine. Even some patients with infranodal blocks may respond, so atropine deserves consideration in most bradycardias when emergent treatment is desired. Atropine can increase rate and myocardial oxygen consumption; therefore, it has no place in an otherwise stable patient with bradycardia.

Isoproterenol can be used for refractory symptomatic bradycardia (when atropine is ineffective), generally as a result of disease of the infranodal conducting system. Isoproterenol is given as a constant infusion, starting at a rate of 0.5 to 2.0 μg/min and increasing to 10 μg/min, as required, to maintain a heart rate of 60 beats/min. Isoproterenol increases myocardial oxygen demand, stimulates ventricular ectopy, and produces peripheral vasodilation, making it a significantly less attractive agent than atropine. The reported response to isoproterenol is weaker than that observed with atropine, although isoproterenol is usually used only in patients who fail while receiving atropine. It is difficult to say how effective isoproterenol would be if used initially, but there is no recommendation for its use as a front-line agent.

External cardiac pacing represents a reemergence of an old concept with new electronics that make the technique more sensitive and likely to capture rhythm. This device should be available in every emergency facility. The emergency physician must become familiar with the technique of applying the transcutaneous pacemaker so that it will sense and pace appropriately.

Internal pacing is the definitive treatment for progressive or persistent bradycardias. Emergent internal pacing is possible with the use of balloon-tipped or semi-flexible flotation catheters, although, without fluoroscopic guidance, it is often technically difficult to achieve stable placement in a patient with low cardiac output.

Supraventricular Dysrhythmias

SINUS DYSRHYTHMIA   Some variation in the sinus node discharge rate is common, but **if the variation exceeds 0.12 s between the longest and shortest intervals, sinus dysrhythmia is present.** The ECG characteristics of sinus dysrhythmia are (1) normal sinus P waves and P-R intervals, (2) 1:1 AV conduction, and (3) variation of at least 0.12 s between the shortest and longest P-P interval (Figure 28-4).

Clinical Significance   Sinus dysrhythmia is frequently a normal finding in children and young adults; it tends to disappear with advancing age. Sinus dysrhythmia is most commonly a phasic (respiratory variation) variety and less commonly a nonphasic variety. In the phasic variety, the sinus node rate accelerates during inspiration and decelerates during expiration, because of changes in vagal tone occurring with respiration (Bainbridge reflex). The irregularity in the phasic or nonphasic varieties can be exaggerated by conditions that increase vagal tone. During long intervals of sinus dysrhythmia, junctional escape beats may occur.

Treatment   None is required.

SINUS BRADYCARDIA   Sinus bradycardia occurs when the sinus node rate falls below 60 beats/min. The ECG characteristics of sinus bradycardia are (1) normal sinus P waves and P-R intervals, (2) 1:1 AV conduction, and (3) atrial rate below 60 beats/min.

Clinical Significance   Sinus bradycardia represents a suppression of the sinus node discharge rate. Sinus bradycardia can be (1) physiologic (in well-conditioned athletes, during sleep, or with vagal stimulation), (2) pharmacologic (digoxin, opioids, reserpine, β-adrenergic antagonists, calcium channel blockers, quinidine), or (3) pathologic (acute inferior MI, increased intracranial pressure, carotid sinus hypersensitivity, hypothyroidism).

Treatment

1. Sinus bradycardia usually does not require specific treatment unless the heart rate is slower than 50 beats/min and there is evidence of hypoperfusion.
2. Therapy should begin with atropine as previously described. Most patients will respond to one or two doses.
3. Isoproterenol can be used if atropine is ineffective.
4. External cardiac pacing can be used in the patient refractory to atropine or isoproterenol.
5. Internal pacing is required in the patient with symptomatic recurrent or persistent sinus bradycardia.

SINUS TACHYCARDIA   Sinus tachycardia originates from acceleration of the sinus node discharge rate. The ECG characteristics of sinus tachycardia are (1) normal sinus P waves and P-R intervals, (2) 1:1 AV conduction, and (3) an atrial rate usually between 100 and 160 beats/min.

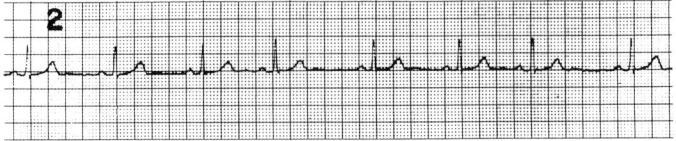

FIG. 28-4. Sinus dysrhythmia.

Clinical Significance Sinus tachycardia represents an acceleration of the sinus node discharge rate, usually in response to three categories of stimuli: (1) physiologic (infants and children, exertion, anxiety, emotions), (2) pharmacologic (atropine, epinephrine and other sympathomimetics, alcohol, nicotine, caffeine), or (3) pathologic (fever, hypoxia, anemia, hypovolemia, pulmonary embolism). In many of these conditions, the increased heart rate is due to an effort to increase cardiac output to match increased circulatory needs.

Treatment

1. No specific treatment is usually required, but any underlying conditions should be investigated and treated.
2. Some patients with acute MI have an "inappropriate" tachycardia and benefit from slowing heart rate with β-adrenergic antagonists.

PREMATURE ATRIAL CONTRACTIONS Premature atrial contractions (PACs) originate from ectopic pacemakers anywhere in the atrium other than the sinus node. The ECG characteristics of PACs are (1) an ectopic P′ wave that appears sooner (prematurely) than the next expected sinus beat, (2) an ectopic P′ wave that has a different shape and axis, and (3) the ectopic P′ wave may or may not be conducted through the AV node (Figure 28-5). A PAC is not conducted through the AV node if it reaches the AV node during the absolute refractory period and is conducted with a delay (longer P′R interval) during the relative refractory period. Most PACs are conducted with typical QRS complexes, but some may be conducted aberrantly through the infranodal system, if they reach a bundle branch during the refractory period. The sinus node is often depolarized and "reset," so that, although the interval after the PAC is often slightly longer than the previous cycle length, the pause is less than fully compensatory.

Clinical Significance Premature atrial contractions are common at all ages and often without heart disease. It is generally assumed, although it remains unproven, that stress, fatigue, alcohol, tobacco, and coffee may precipitate PACs. Frequent PACs may also be seen in chronic lung disease, ischemic heart disease, or digitalis toxicity. Premature atrial contractions may precipitate sustained atrial tachycardia, flutter, or fibrillation under certain circumstances.

Treatment

1. Any precipitating drugs or toxins should be discontinued.
2. Underlying disorders should be treated.

3. Premature atrial contractions that produce symptoms or initiate sustained tachycardias can be suppressed with calcium channel blockers, β-adrenergic antagonists, quinidine, or procainamide.

MULTIFOCAL ATRIAL TACHYCARDIA Multifocal atrial tachycardia (MFAT; also known as "chaotic atrial rhythm" or "wandering atrial pacemaker") is an irregular rhythm caused by at least three different sites of atrial ectopy. The ECG characteristics of MFAT are (1) three or more differently shaped P waves; (2) changing P-P, P-R, and R-R intervals; and (3) atrial rhythm usually between 100 and 180 beats/min (Figure 28-6). Multifocal atrial tachycardia is frequently confused with atrial flutter (AF) or fibrillation.

Clinical Significance Multifocal atrial tachycardia is found most often in elderly patients with decompensated chronic lung disease, but it may also complicate congestive heart failure (CHF) or sepsis or be caused by methylxanthine toxicity. Digoxin toxicity is an unlikely cause of MFAT.

Treatment

1. Treatment is directed toward the underlying disorder. With decompensated lung disease, oxygen and bronchodilators improve pulmonary function and arterial oxygenation and decrease atrial ectopy. Theophylline agents have been associated with the production or exacerbation of this dysrhythmia.
2. Specific antiarrhythmic treatment is rarely indicated. Standard antiarrhythmics appear to be ineffective in suppressing these multiple sites of atrial ectopy, and toxic side effects from these agents have been reported. Likewise, attempts to slow the ventricular rate by depressing AV nodal conduction with digoxin is difficult without producing toxic side effects. Recently, three modes of therapy have been described that may be helpful in some patients. Magnesium sulfate 2 g intravenously over 60 s, followed by a constant infusion of 1 to 2 g/h, has been shown to reduce atrial ectopy in these patients and is sometimes associated with conversion to sinus rhythm. The full antiarrhythmic effect of magnesium requires supplemental potassium to maintain serum potassium levels above 4 mEq/L. Intravenous verapamil (5 to 10 mg) slows the ventricular response in most patients, decreases atrial ectopy in some patients, and is associated with conversion to sinus rhythm in many patients. The β-adrenergic antagonists esmolol, acebutolol, and metoprolol decrease the ventricular rate in MFAT. However, theoretically, β-blocker therapy may worsen bronchospasm. The value of such specific antiarrhythmic treatment in MFAT is unproven.
3. Cardioversion has no effect on these multiple sites of atrial ectopy.

FIG. 28-5. Premature atrial contractions. *(Top)* Ectopic P′ waves *(arrows).* *(Bottom)* Atrial bigeminy.

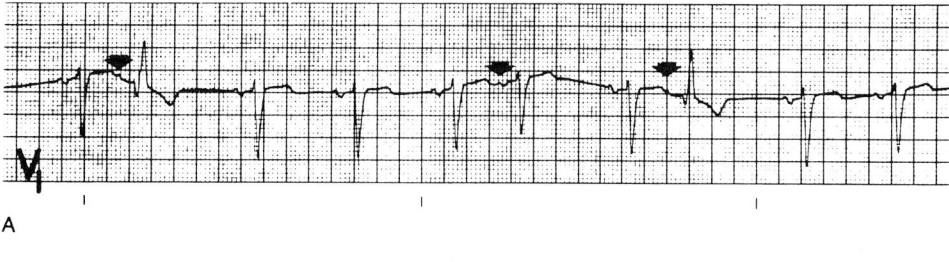

A

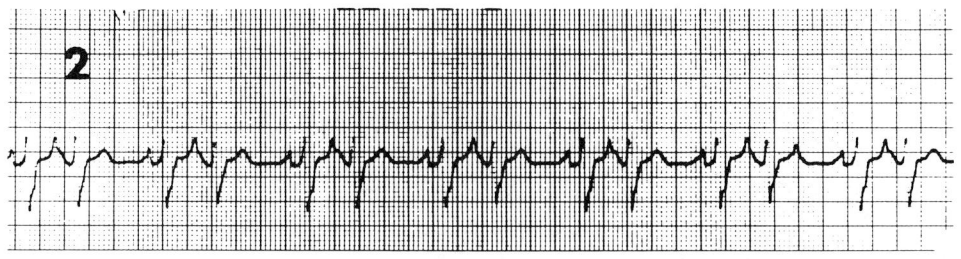

B

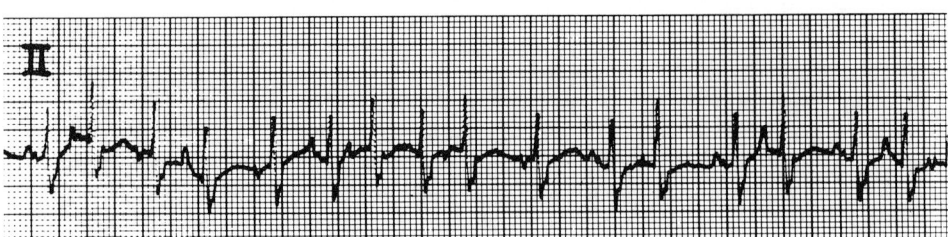

FIG. 28-6. Multifocal atrial tachycardia.

ATRIAL FLUTTER   Atrial flutter usually originates from a localized area within the atria. The exact mechanism (reentry, automatic focus, or triggered dysrhythmia) is not known. Intracardiac studies have demonstrated electrical activity usually originating in the inferior right atrium and propagating upward and to the left. The ECG characteristics of AF are (1) regular atrial rate between 250 and 350 beats/min (most commonly 280 and 320 beats/min); (2) sawtooth flutter waves directed superiorly and most visible in leads II, III, and aVF; and (3) AV block, usually at 2:1, but occasionally greater, causing a ventricular rate between 125–175 beats/min (Figure 28-7). One-to-one AV conduction may occur in the presence of bypass tracts or if drugs are used to slow the atrial rate to the level that the AV node can conduct one-to-one. A ventricular rate faster than 300 beats/min definitely should be investigated with electrophysiology (EP) studies. Carotid sinus massage is a useful technique to slow the ventricular response, increase the AV block, and unmask flutter waves.

Clinical Significance   Atrial flutter is usually associated with heart disease. It is found most commonly in patients with ischemic heart disease or acute MI. Less common causes include congestive cardiomyopathy, pulmonary embolus, myocarditis, blunt chest trauma, and, rarely, digoxin toxicity. Atrial flutter may be a transitional dysrhythmia between sinus rhythm and atrial fibrillation.

Treatment

1. Low-energy cardioversion (25 to 50 J) is very successful in converting more than 90 percent of cases of AF into sinus rhythm. Energies weaker than 10 J should be avoided, because they are more likely to convert AF into atrial fibrillation than into sinus rhythm.
2. If cardioversion is contraindicated, control of ventricular rate can be achieved with digoxin, verapamil, diltiazem, esmolol, or propranolol (see Chap. 29 for dosage). If there is 1:1 conduction and the rate is 300 beats/min and faster, preexcitation should be considered, and procainamide may be the drug of first choice.
3. Quinidine or procainamide can be used after ventricular rate control is achieved to chemically slow or convert AF or prevent recurrence of the dysrhythmia.
4. Intravenous esmolol will convert up to 60 percent of patients with new-onset AF to sinus rhythm.
5. Intravenous verapamil or diltiazem occasionally will convert AF into sinus rhythm.[3]
6. Some of the newer antiarrhythmics may have a role in the chemical conversion of AF. Ibutilide (0.01 mg/kg IV over 10 min) can convert AF and fibrillation to normal sinus rhythm. This drug should be used in new-onset AF, because of the chance of emboli if used in long-term AF. Ibutilide is very effective in the conversion of AF or atrial fibrillation; however, there is a significant possibility of initiating TdP. To reduce the chance of TdP, it is suggested that the $[K^+]$ and the corrected QT interval be checked before administration of the agent. This agent should not be given in the presence of hypokalemia, prolonged corrected QT interval, or history of CHF. The chance of TdP can extend 4 to 6 h after the drug is given.

ATRIAL FIBRILLATION   Atrial fibrillation occurs when there are multiple, small areas of atrial myocardium continuously discharging and contracting. There is no uniform atrial depolarization and contraction, but rather, only a quivering of the atrial wall. Although the atrial rate is usually faster than 400 beats/min, the ventricular rate is limited by the refractory period of the AV node or an accessory pathway. The ECG characteristics of atrial fibrillation are (1) fibrillatory waves of atrial activity, best seen in leads V_1, V_2, V_3, and aVF; and (2) irregular ventricular response, usually around 170 to 180 beats/min in patients with a healthy AV node (Figure 28-8). Disease or drugs (especially digoxin) may reduce AV node conduction and markedly slow ventricular response. A more rapid ventricular response may be seen in patients with bypass tracts, and the rate in these patients has been suggested as a way of estimating the refractory period of the accessory path. Ventricular rates faster than 300 beats/min are possible and dangerous. In this case, because ventricular activation occurs by way of the bypass tract, the QRS complex is usually wide. The configuration of the aberrancy may differ with the site of the accessory pathway.

Clinical Significance   Atrial fibrillation can occur in a paroxysmal or a sustained manner. Predisposing factors for atrial fibrillation are increased atrial size and mass, increased vagal tone, and variation in refractory periods between different parts of the atrial myocardium. Atrial fibrillation is usually found in association with four disorders: rheumatic heart disease, hypertension, ischemic heart disease, and thyrotoxicosis. Less common causes are chronic lung disease, pericarditis, acute alcoholic intoxication, pulmonary embolus, and atrial septal defect.

In patients with left ventricular failure, left atrial contraction contributes significantly to cardiac output. The loss of effective atrial contraction, as in atrial fibrillation, may produce heart failure in these patients. Atrial fibrillation also predisposes to peripheral venous and atrial emboli, with the risk of pulmonary and systemic arterial embolism. Up to 15 percent of patients in chronic atrial fibrillation have at least one embolic episode each year. Conversion from chronic atrial fibrillation to sinus rhythm also carries a 1 to 2 percent risk of arte-

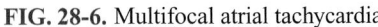

FIG. 28-7. Atrial flutter.

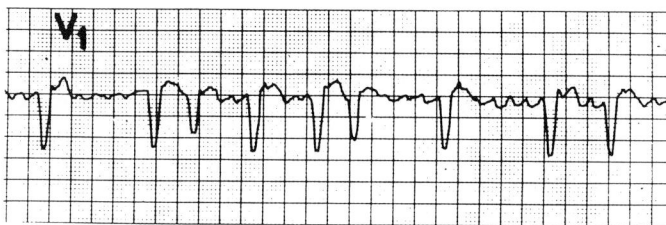

FIG. 28-8. Atrial fibrillation.

rial embolism. Patients with chronic atrial fibrillation are frequently anticoagulated.

Treatment

1. Atrial fibrillation with a rapid ventricular response and acute hemodynamic deterioration should be treated with synchronized cardioversion. More than 60 percent of patients can be converted with 100 J, and more than 80 percent can be converted with 200 J. Conversion to and retention in sinus rhythm are more likely when atrial fibrillation is of short duration and the atria are not greatly dilated. If initial cardioversion is unsuccessful, procainamide should be given intravenously to facilitate further cardioversion attempts. Oral quinidine or low-dose amiodarone can enhance maintenance of sinus rhythm. Meta-analysis and decision analysis of postconversion antiarrhythmic treatment have found that the benefits of maintaining sinus rhythm with antiarrhythmics are partly offset by an increase in sudden death, presumably due to the proarrhythmic properties of these drugs. In the ED setting, all other causes of hypotension, such as acute blood loss, should be ruled out before concluding that the rate is causing the hemodynamic deterioration.

2. In the more stable patient, the first priority is to achieve ventricular rate control. Diltiazem, 20 mg (0.25 mg/kg) given IV over 2 min, is extremely effective in achieving ventricular rate control, with the peak response seen in 2 to 7 min. An infusion of 5 mg/h is usually started after the initial dose to maintain control, and a second dose of 25 mg (0.35 mg/kg) can be given after 15 min if rate control is not achieved. Verapamil 5 to 10 mg IV is effective in slowing the ventricular response in 60 to 70 percent of patients with atrial fibrillation and converts 10 to 15 percent into sinus rhythm. Intravenous β-adrenergic blockers (e.g., esmolol and propranolol) are effective, especially in patients with thyrotoxicosis or rheumatic mitral stenosis, but the depressive effects on myocardial contractility make them poor agents to use in patients with ventricular failure. Intravenous digoxin is an effective agent for this purpose, although the onset of action is slow, with a mean time longer than 11 h to achieve ventricular rate control. With a rapid digitalization protocol, an effect may be seen within 3 to 6 h.

3. Once ventricular rate control has been achieved, chemical conversion can be considered with procainamide, quinidine, or verapamil. Intravenous procainamide has been used as a single agent to chemically convert atrial fibrillation of short duration into sinus rhythm; however, ibutilide is being touted as a better agent. Amiodarone (300 mg IV 1h; 20 mg/kg over the next 24 h) has recently been shown to be a safe and highly effective first-choice drug for restoring sinus rhythm in patients with atrial fibrillation who present to an ED.[4] Because of the risk of intraatrial thrombi and arterial embolization, patients with atrial fibrillation of more than 2 days' duration should be anticoagulated systemically for 1 to 3 weeks before attempts at chemical or electrical conversion. More recent work has indicated that there may be some increased risk of embolism even with AF of less than 2 days' duration. An alternative to prolonged preanticoagulation is to exclude atrial thrombi by transesophageal echocardiography. **Those without visible thrombi can be safely cardioverted following a loading dose of heparin and oral warfarin for one month.**[5]

4. Patients with a slow ventricular response not due to digitalis have AV node disease and probably a more generalized disorder of cardiac conduction (second- or third-degree AV block is seen in these patients when in sinus rhythm). These patients are at increased risk for profound bradycardias or asystole after cardioversion or antiarrhythmic drug therapy.

5. In some patients with a rapid ventricular response, conversion will reveal a very slow rate (tachybrady syndrome) because of underlying disease of the pacemaker tissue (sick sinus syndrome).

SUPRAVENTRICULAR TACHYCARDIA Supraventricular tachycardia is a regular, rapid rhythm that arises from reentry or an ectopic pacemaker in areas above the bifurcation of the bundle of His. The reentrant variety is clinically the most common. These patients often present with acute, symptomatic episodes termed *paroxysmal supraventricular tachycardia.*

Ectopic SVT usually originates in the atria, with an atrial rate of 100 to 250 beats/min (most commonly 140 to 200 beats/min; Figure 28-9). The regular P waves can be mistaken for AF or, if there is a 2:1 AV block, sinus rhythm.

Reentrant SVT is seen in most patients with SVT: about 60 percent of these patients have reentry within the AV node, and 20 percent have reentry involving a bypass tract. The remainder have reentry in other sites. In the normal heart, reentrant SVT at the typical rates of 160 to 200 beats/min is often tolerated for hours or days. However, cardiac output is usually depressed, regardless of the blood pressure, and rapid rates may produce heart failure depending on the health of the myocardium.

Reentrant SVT within the AV node usually is initiated when an ectopic atrial impulse encounters the AV node during the partial refractory period (Figure 28-10). There are two functionally different parallel conducting limbs within the AV node that are connected above, at the atrial end, and below, at the ventricular end of the node. This circuit is capable of sustained reentry when properly stimulated. In AV nodal reentry, the P wave is usually buried in the QRS complex and not visible, there is 1:1 conduction, and the QRS complex is normal.

Patients with bypass tracts have two parallel limbs of the reentry circuit, the AV node and the bypass tract, with connections at the atrial and ventricular ends by myocardial cells. Although reentry can occur in either direction, it usually occurs in a direction that is antegrade through the AV node and retrograde through the bypass tract, thus producing a narrow QRS complex (orthodromic conduction). In the Wolff-Parkinson-White (WPW) syndrome, about 85 percent of the reentrant SVTs have narrow QRS complexes. If the conduction is antegrade through the accessory bundle and retrograde through the AV node (antidromic conduction), the complexes are wide and difficult to differentiate from ventricular tachycardia.

Clinical Significance Ectopic SVT may be seen in patients with acute MI, chronic lung disease, pneumonia, alcohol intoxication, and digoxin toxicity (where it is often associated with AV block and termed *paroxysmal atrial tachycardia with block*). It is commonly held that a high percentage of SVT with block, as much as 75 percent, is due to digoxin toxicity. However, not all studies have found this to be the case.

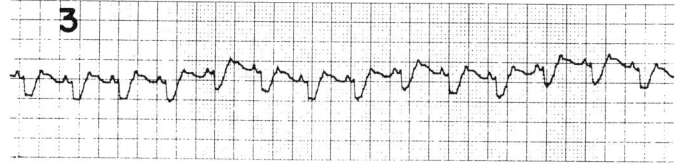

FIG. 28-9. Ectopic supraventricular tachycardia with 2:1 atrioventricular conduction.

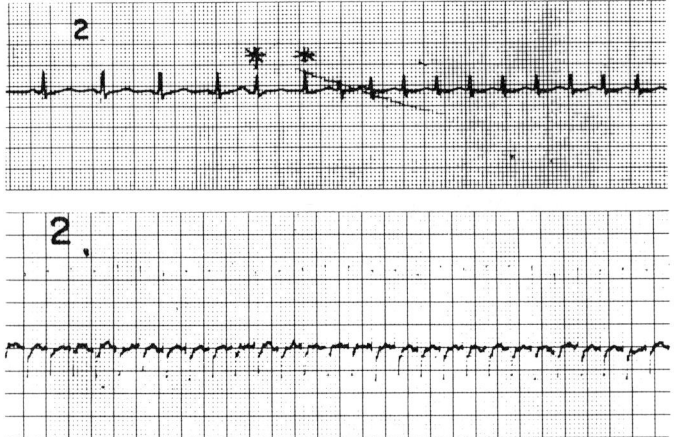

FIG. 28-10. Reentrant supraventricular tachycardia (SVT). *(Top)* initiates run of paroxysmal atrial tachycardia. *(Bottom)* SVT, rate of 286 beats/min.

Reentrant SVT can occur in a normal heart or in association with rheumatic heart disease, acute pericarditis, MI, mitral valve prolapse, or one of the preexcitation syndromes.

Supraventricular tachycardia often causes a sensation of palpitations and lightheadedness. In patients with coronary artery disease, anginal chest pain and dyspnea may occur from the rapid heart rate. Frank heart failure and pulmonary edema may occur in patients with poor left ventricular function. The decrease in diastolic filling period and subsequent decrease in cardiac output cannot be tolerated in the patient with left ventricular failure.

Treatment   Reentrant SVT can be converted by impeding conduction through one limb of the reentry circuit; sustained reentry is then impossible and extinguishes, allowing sinus rhythm to resume ventricular pacing. Because it is usually clinically impossible to differentiate ectopic from reentrant SVT, treatment is initially the same.

1. Maneuvers that increase vagal tone have been shown to slow conduction and prolong the refractory period in the AV node. These maneuvers can be done by themselves or after administration of drugs.
    a. Carotid sinus massage exerts pressure on the carotid sinus and baroreceptors against the transverse process of C6. Bruits should be discovered before the procedure. Massage should be done for 10 s at a time, first on the side of the nondominant cerebral hemisphere, and should never be done simultaneously on both sides. Prolonged AV block during carotid massage may occur in patients with AV node disease or who are taking digoxin. Patients with carotid artery stenosis may develop cerebral ischemia or infarction from overly vigorous carotid massage.
    b. Facial immersion in cold water is done for 6 to 7 s with the nostrils held closed ("diving reflex"). This maneuver is particularly effective in infants. The patient's parents may develop greater vagal tone than the infant, so this must be approached carefully.
    c. The Valsalva maneuver performed in the supine position appears to be the most effective vagal maneuver for the conversion of reentrant SVT. For maximal effectiveness, the strain phase must be adequate (usually at least 10 s), with slowing or conversion seen during the release phase.
2. Adenosine, an ultra-short-acting (20 s) agent, produces AV block and has been observed to convert over 90 percent of reentrant SVT.[6] The initial dose is a 6-mg rapid intravenous bolus. This **must be given in a large vein,** preferably in the antecubital space. If no effect is seen within 2 min, a second dose of 12 mg can be given. There is no proven benefit to repeated doses or administration of more than 20 mg. At least 50 percent of patients experience

distressing, albeit transient, side effects of facial flushing or chest pain. Obviously this should be discussed with the patient, when possible. Because adenosine possesses no sustained antiarrhythmic effect, subsequent ectopic beats can reinitiate the dysrhythmia, and early recurrences of SVT are seen in up to 25 percent of patients. The major advantage of adenosine is its ultrashort effect[7] and its lack of hypotensive or myocardial depressive activity. Adenosine is also safe and effective in unstable patients (chest pain and/or hypotension) with reentrant SVT. It is safe in pregnancy. In addition, it is not contraindicated in the presence of WPW syndrome.

3. Verapamil 0.075 to 0.15 mg/kg (3 to 10 mg) IV over 15 to 60 s, with a repeat dose in 30 min, can be used, if necessary. Studies have found that more than 90 percent of adults with reentrant SVT will respond within 1 to 2 min to verapamil. In patients with a normal blood pressure, intravenous verapamil is almost always associated with a decrease in blood pressure, even after successful conversion of SVT. The falls in systolic and mean arterial pressures are approximately 20 and 10 mm Hg, respectively. The drop in blood pressure due to verapamil can be prevented and/or treated with intravenous calcium without reducing the antiarrhythmic action of verapamil. Although the use of different calcium doses and salts has been reported, elemental calcium, 90 mg given IV over 3 to 6 min, appears safe and effective (90 mg elemental calcium = 10 mL calcium gluconate 10% solution = 3.3 mL calcium chloride 10% solution). Whenever verapamil is used IV, calcium should be readily available. Intravenous verapamil is generally considered to be contraindicated in the hypotensive patient. Many would consider cardioversion a better approach to the hypotensive patient with SVT.
4. Diltiazem 20 mg (0.25 mg/kg) IV over 2 min is reported to be 75 to 100 percent effective in converting reentrant SVT.
5. Vagal tone can be enhanced by pharmacologically elevating blood pressure with a pure peripheral vasoconstrictor; agents without β-adrenergic activity should be used. This method should be combined with carotid sinus massage. Blood pressure should be monitored frequently, and diastolic pressure should not be allowed to exceed 130 mm Hg. This method should not be used if hypertension is already present.
    a. Metaraminol 200 mg/500 mL D5W or norepinephrine 4 mg/ 500 mL D5W can be infused at rates of 1 to 2 mL/min and titrated until the rhythm converts.
    b. Methoxamine or phenylephrine, 0.5 to 1.0 mg IV over 2 to 3 min, can be administered, with repeat doses, as required.
6. Esmolol is an intravenous β-adrenergic blocker with an ultrashort duration of activity that can be titrated to effect. This agent can be used to control the ventricular rate in most tachycardias of supraventricular origin and is capable of converting about half of reentrant SVT. Esmolol is given as a bolus dose of 300 μg/kg over 60 s, followed by an infusion starting at 50 μg/kg per min. If there is an inadequate response after 2 to 5 min, a repeat bolus of 300 μg/kg should be given, and increases in the infusion rate in increments of 50 μg/kg per min should be made. The maximal recommended infusion rate is 300 μg/kg per min, although most patients respond to rates of 200 μg/kg or less per min. With aggressive dosing regimens, hypotension occurs in approximately 50 percent of patients but can be quickly reversed by halting the infusion.
7. Propranolol 0.5 to 1.0 mg IV, slowly over 60 s, can be repeated every 5 min, until the rhythm converts or the total dose reaches 0.1 mg/kg. Overall, propranolol has a nearly 50 percent success rate in converting reentrant SVT: about 80 percent with AV nodal reentry and 15 to 20 percent with accessory tract retrograde reentry.
8. Digoxin 0.5 mg IV, with repeat doses of 0.25 mg in 30 to 60 min, can be used until a response occurs or the total dose reaches 0.02 mg/kg. The chief drawback of digoxin has been its long onset of action and potential hazard in patients with accessory (bypass) tracts who develop atrial fibrillation or AF.

9. External noninvasive pacing has been used in a limited number of patients to terminate reentrant SVT. Asynchronous pacing with 2 to 10 external pulses at a rate 240 to 280 beats/min (typically 40 beats/min faster than the SVT rate) with an impulse amplitude of 120 mA is effective in young, hemodynamically stable adults. Most pacing units in the ED do not pace at 240 to 280 beats/min. Some automatic internal cardiac defibrillators have overdrive-pacing capability.

10. Synchronized cardioversion should be done in any unstable patient with hypotension, pulmonary edema, or severe chest pain. The dose required is usually small, less than 50 J.

Ectopic SVT due to digoxin toxicity is treated as follows:

1. Discontinuation of the digoxin.
2. As long as there is not a high-grade AV block, correction of any existing hypokalemia to bring serum potassium into the high-normal range in an effort to reduce atrial ectopy is indicated.
3. Digoxin-specific antibody fragments should be considered for patients with hemodynamic deterioration or serious ventricular dysrhythmias due to digoxin toxicity.
4. Phenytoin, lidocaine, or magnesium given intravenously can reduce atrial ectopy. Published reports are not methodologically adequate for determination of the response rate, risks, and benefits of each agent, so the choice is guided by personal preference. Historically, phenytoin has been the most commonly used drug, but its response rate has not been impressive and toxic side effects are common with full loading doses (15 to 18 mg/kg IV). Lidocaine has not been considered a useful agent for this dysrhythmia, but case reports have indicated some benefit. Recent studies have indicated that magnesium sulfate 1 g IV impressively reduces atrial ectopy due to digoxin toxicity, and perhaps this agent has a greater effect than phenytoin or lidocaine.
5. **Cardioversion is not effective and is potentially hazardous in digoxin-induced dysrhythmias.**

Junctional Dysrhythmias

Traditionally, a junctional impulse is considered to arise from the AV node or bundle of His above the bifurcation. Pacemaker tissue cannot be found in the AV node of experimental animals. The question is not settled in humans. From its source, probably in the junction, the impulse spreads retrogradely toward the atria and antegradely toward the ventricles. Depending on the site of origin, conduction velocity, and refractory periods, the atria may be activated before, during, or after ventricular depolarization. Atrial depolarization may not be visible if retrograde conduction is blocked or atrial activation occurs simultaneously with ventricular activation and the QRS complex obscures the P waves. Atrioventricular dissociation may occur if the rate of discharge from the junctional pacemaker is faster than the sinus node rate and the junctional impulse is blocked from retrograde conduction toward the atria.

JUNCTIONAL PREMATURE CONTRACTIONS   Junctional premature contractions (JPCs) are due to an ectopic pacemaker within the AV node or common AV bundle. The ECG characteristics of JPCs are as follows:

1. The ectopic QRS complex is premature.
2. The ectopic P′ wave has a different shape and direction (usually inverted in leads II, III, and aV_F).
3. The ectopic P′ wave may occur before or after the QRS complex.
4. The P-R interval of the ectopic beat is shorter than normal.
5. The QRS complex is usually of normal shape unless there is aberrant conduction.
6. The sinus node is usually affected, and the postectopic pause is not fully compensatory (Figure 28-11). Some JPCs do not conduct retrogradely; therefore, a compensatory pause may be seen.

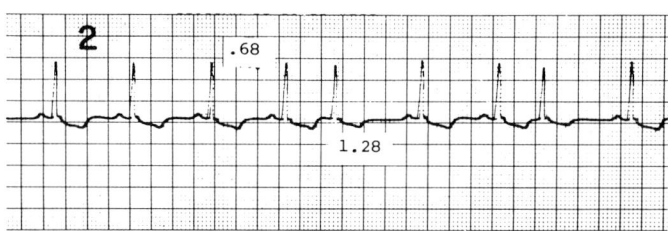

FIG. 28-11. Junctional premature contractions.

Junctional premature contractions may be isolated, multiple (as in bigeminy or trigeminy), or multifocal.

Clinical Significance   Junctional premature contractions are uncommon in healthy hearts. They occur in CHF, digoxin toxicity, ischemic heart disease, and acute MI (especially of the inferior wall).

Treatment

1. No specific treatment is usually required.
2. Treat the underlying disorder.
3. Antiarrhythmic therapy with quinidine or procainamide may be useful if JPCs are frequent, symptomatic, or initiate more serious dysrhythmias.

JUNCTIONAL RHYTHMS   Under normal circumstances, the sinus node discharges at a faster rate than the AV junction, so the pacemaker function of the AV junction and all other slower pacemakers is suppressed (overdrive suppression). If sinus node discharges slow or fail to reach the AV junction, then junctional escape beats may occur, usually at a rate between 40 and 60 beats/min, depending on the level of the pacemaker. In general, junctional escape beats do not conduct retrograde into the atria, so a QRS complex without a P′ wave is usually seen (Figure 28-12).

Under other circumstances, enhanced junctional automaticity may override the sinus node and produce an accelerated junctional rhythm (rate 60 to 100 beats/min) or junctional tachycardia (rate ≥100 beats/min). Usually, the enhanced junctional pacemaker (Figure 28-13) captures the atria and ventricles.

Clinical Significance   Junctional escape beats may occur whenever there is a long enough pause in the impulses reaching the AV junction: sinus bradycardia, slow phase of sinus dysrhythmia, AV block, or during the pause after premature beats. Sustained junctional escape rhythms may be seen with CHF, myocarditis, hypokalemia, or digoxin toxicity. If the ventricular rate is too slow, myocardial or cerebral ischemia may develop.

Accelerated junctional rhythm and junctional tachycardia may occur from digoxin toxicity, acute rheumatic fever, or inferior MI. With digoxin toxicity, the rate is usually between 70 and 130 beats/min. If this rhythm develops in a patient being treated with digoxin for atrial fibrillation, the ECG is characterized by regular QRS complexes superimposed on atrial fibrillatory waves. Regulation of ventricular response during digoxin therapy in a patient with atrial fibrillation should raise the suspicion of digoxin toxicity.

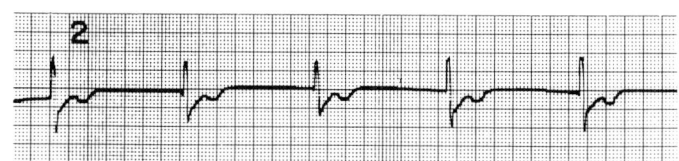

FIG. 28-12. Junctional escape rhythm, with a rate of 42 beats/min.

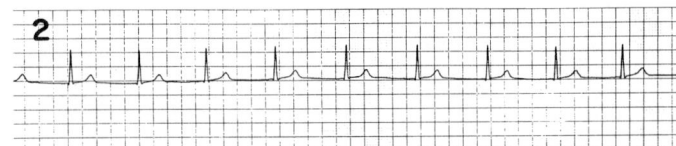

FIG. 28-13. Accelerated junctional rhythm, with a rate of 61 beats/ min.

Treatment

1. Isolated, infrequent junctional escape beats usually do not require specific treatment.
2. If sustained junctional escape rhythms are producing symptoms, the underlying cause should be treated. Atropine can be used to accelerate the sinus node discharge rate temporarily and enhance AV nodal conduction.
3. Accelerated junctional rhythm and junctional tachycardia usually do not produce significant symptoms. If the cause is digoxin toxicity, the drug should be discontinued. If the rate is fast and producing symptoms, giving supplemental potassium to increase the serum level into the high-normal range may decrease it.

Ventricular Dysrhythmias

PREMATURE VENTRICULAR CONTRACTIONS   Premature ventricular contractions (PVCs) are due to impulses originating from single or multiple areas in the ventricles. The ECG characteristics of PVCs are as follows:

1. There is a premature and wide QRS complex (Figure 28-14).
2. There is no preceding P wave.
3. The ST segment and T wave of the PVC are directed opposite the major QRS deflection.
4. Most PVCs do not affect the sinus node, so there is usually a fully compensatory postectopic pause or the PVC may be interpolated between two sinus beats (Figure 28-14).
5. Many PVCs have a fixed coupling interval (within 0.04 s) from the preceding sinus beat.
6. Some PVCs are conducted into the atria, producing a retrograde P wave.

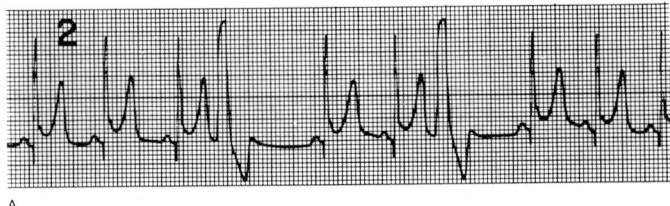

A

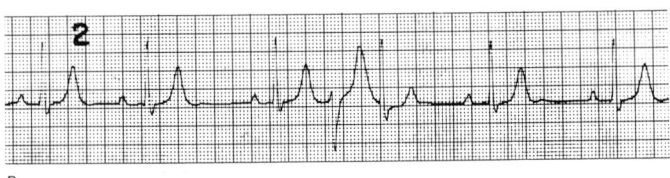

B

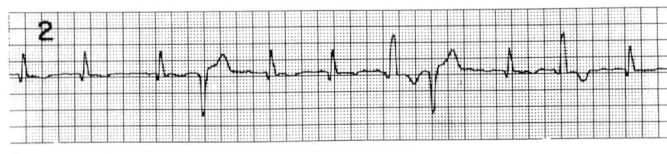

C

FIG. 28-14. Premature ventricular contractions: unifocal *(top),* interpolated *(center),* and multifocal *(bottom).*

Occasionally, a *ventricular fusion beat* occurs when supraventricular and ventricular impulses depolarize the ventricles almost simultaneously. The QRS configuration of a fusion beat contains features of the individual components.

A PVC may be confused with an aberrantly conducted supraventricular beat. Several clinical and ECG criteria can be used to help distinguish aberrantly conducted supraventricular beats from PVCs; this is discussed later in this section.

Clinical Significance   Premature ventricular contractions are very common, even in patients without evidence of heart disease. They occur in most patients with ischemic heart disease and are universally found in patients with acute MI. Other common causes of PVCs include digoxin toxicity, CHF, hypokalemia, alkalosis, hypoxia, and sympathomimetic drugs.

Although there is a correlation between the severity of underlying coronary artery disease and the degree of ventricular ectopy, there is disagreement as to whether ventricular ectopy itself is an independent risk factor for future morbidity or mortality. Most studies have indicated that repetitive PVCs (two or more in a row) do have some associated independent risk in patients with coronary artery disease, but the evidence for other forms of ventricular ectopy is less convincing. Lown has made an attempt with his classification to quantitate the risks associated with chronic ventricular ectopy, but his classification is not universally accepted (Table 28-1). It must be remembered that his classification was developed from patients with recent acute MIs.

In the setting of an acute MI, PVCs indicate the underlying electrical instability of the heart. The patients are at increased risk for the development of primary ventricular fibrillation. Current work indicates that various degrees of PVCs ("warning dysrhythmias") are not reliable predictors of subsequent ventricular fibrillation.

Although it is experimentally established that electrical impulses, such as PVCs, that occur during or soon after repolarization (the so-called vulnerable period) can initiate ventricular tachycardia or fibrillation, clinical studies have found that late-coupled PVCs initiate more paroxysms of ventricular tachycardia than early-coupled PVCs (R-on-T phenomenon).

Treatment

1. Most patients with acute myocardial disease and PVCs will respond to intravenous lidocaine, although some patients may require procainamide. In the setting of acute myocardial ischemia (unstable angina or acute MI), many physicians would treat frequent or multiform PVCs with the goal of reducing deaths due to sudden ventricular tachycardia or fibrillation. Although single studies have suggested benefit, **pooled data and meta-analyses have found no reduction in mortality from suppressive or prophylactic treatment of PVCs.**[8] The use of β-blockers may be a better choice, and at least metoprolol has been associated with better mortality reduction in post-MI patients.
2. In patients with chronic PVCs, there is no evidence that oral antiarrhythmics enhance survival. To the contrary, large, randomized studies of postinfarction patients found that treatment with en-

TABLE 28-1   Lown Grading System for Ventricular Ectopy

Grade	ECG Characteristics
1	Uniform PVCs < 30/h
2	Uniform PVCs > 30/h
3	Multiform PVCs
4A	Couplets (2 consecutive PVCs)
4B	Triplets (3 or more consecutive PVCs)
5	R-on-T PVCs

Abbreviations: ECG = electrocardiogram; PVC = premature ventricular contraction.

cainide, flecainide, or moricizine increased the incidence of cardiac arrest or arrhythmic death, probably related to their pro-arrhythmic effects.[9] Before treating chronic PVCs, the physician should consider several factors:

a. Underlying heart disease
b. The nature of the ectopy
c. The presence or absence of symptoms
d. The potential side effects of oral antiarrhythmic therapy
e. Which technique will be used to judge efficacy of therapy (continuous monitoring vs. EP studies)? Oral antiarrhythmic therapy requires careful monitoring. In some patients at risk of sudden cardiac death, automatic internal cardiac defibrillators are used in conjunction with antiarrhythmics.

VENTRICULAR PARASYSTOLE   Parasystole occurs when an independent ectopic pacemaker is protected from the influence of outside impulses (entrance block) and competes with the dominant pacemaker to produce myocardial depolarizations. A parasystolic pacemaker can arise anywhere in the heart but is most often in the ventricles, where it produces a rhythm that operates in competition with the sinus node. This ectopic pacemaker has an innate rate; however, not all beats depolarize the ventricle (exit block).

The ECG characteristics of ventricular parasystole are (1) variation in the coupling interval between the preceding sinus beat and the ectopic beat, (2) common relation between the interectopic beat intervals, and (3) occurrence of fusion beats (Figure 28-15). Usually, long rhythm strips are necessary to establish that the interectopic intervals are multiples of a common parasystolic pacemaker. Because of the difference in response to antiarrhythmics, it is important to recognize and differentiate parasystolic beats from PVCs.

Clinical Significance   Ventricular parasystole most often is associated with severe ischemic heart disease, acute MI, hypertensive heart disease, or electrolyte imbalance. Parasystole is often self-limited and benign but infrequently may lead to ventricular tachycardia or fibrillation.

Treatment

1. The underlying disease should be treated.
2. Antiarrhythmics are indicated in patients with symptomatic episodes or beats that initiate ventricular tachycardia.

ACCELERATED IDIOVENTRICULAR RHYTHM   Accelerated idioventricular rhythm (AIVR) is an ectopic rhythm of ventricular origin occurring at a rate of 40 to 100 beats/min. Even though AIVR is not a tachycardia, terms such as *idioventricular tachycardia, nonparoxysmal ventricular tachycardia,* or *slow ventricular tachycardia* are sometimes used to describe this rhythm.

The ECG characteristics of AIVR are (1) wide and regular QRS complexes, (2) a rate between 40 and 100 beats/min that is often close to the preceding sinus rate, (3) usually runs of short duration (3 to 30 beats/min), and (4) often beginning with a fusion beat (Figure 28-16).

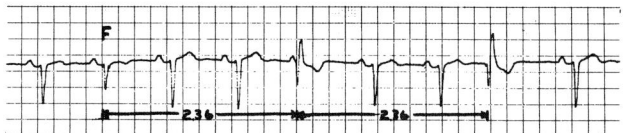

FIG. 28-15. The fifth and eighth ventricular complexes are premature and of similar morphology but have different coupling intervals. The second complex (*F*) represents a fusion beat. The interectopic interval is 2.36 s. (Reproduced with permission from Heger JW, Niemann JT, Boman KG, et al: *Cardiology for the House Officer.* Baltimore, Williams & Wilkins, 1982.)

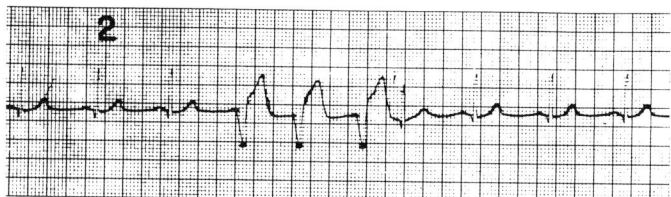

FIG. 28-16. Accelerated idioventricular rhythms.

Clinical Significance   This condition is found most commonly in the setting of an acute MI. Reports have indicated that AIVR sometimes appears during successful thrombolysis of an occluded coronary artery. Accelerated idioventricular rhythm and other ventricular dysrhythmias seen during this time are termed *reperfusion dysrhythmias.* Accelerated idioventricular rhythm may be seen infrequently in patients without organic heart disease. Although there is some variable association with ventricular tachycardia, there is no apparent association with ventricular fibrillation. Accelerated idioventricular rhythm usually produces no symptoms itself. Sometimes the loss of atrial contraction and subsequent fall in cardiac output may produce hemodynamic deterioration.

Treatment

1. Treatment is not necessary. On occasion, AIVR may be the only functioning pacemaker, and suppression with lidocaine can lead to cardiac asystole.
2. If sustained AIVR produces symptoms secondary to a decrease in cardiac output, treatment with atrial pacing may be required.

VENTRICULAR TACHYCARDIA   Ventricular tachycardia is the occurrence of three or more depolarizations from a ventricular ectopic pacemaker at a rate faster than 100 beats/min. The ECG characteristics of ventricular tachycardia are (1) wide QRS complexes; (2) rate faster than 100 beats/min (most commonly 150 to 200 beats/min); (3) rhythm usually regular, although there may be some beat-to-beat variation; and (4) QRS axis usually constant (Figure 28-17). Uncommonly (about 5 percent of episodes), ventricular tachycardia may have a narrow (<120 ms) QRS complex. In these cases, ECG criteria usually suggest a ventricular origin (see "Aberrant versus Ventricular Tachyarrhythmias," below). Ventricular tachycardia can occur in a nonsustained manner—usually short episodes, lasting seconds, with spontaneous termination—or in a sustained fashion—longer episodes that typically require treatment.

There are several variants of ventricular tachycardia. *Ventricular flutter* is the phrase used for a regular zigzag pattern without distinguishable QRS complexes or T waves. In *bidirectional ventricular tachycardia,* the QRS complexes alternate polarity as recorded in a single lead. In *alternating ventricular tachycardia,* the QRS complexes alternate in height (but not polarity) in a single lead. (Bidirectional and alternating ventricular tachycardias indicate serious myocardial disease and often are due to digitalis toxicity.)

In *polymorphic ventricular tachycardia,* the QRS complexes have many different shapes in one lead. This pattern has been recently described in Brugada syndrome, which consists of syncope, sudden death, unusual J-point elevation in V_1 and V_3, and RBB block.[10] It was initially described in 1991 and was not well known until late 1990s (Figure 28-18). **Brugada syndrome should be considered a potential cause of syncope**

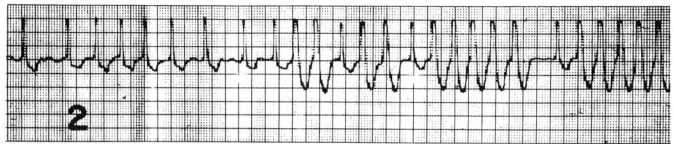

FIG. 28-17. Ventricular tachycardia.

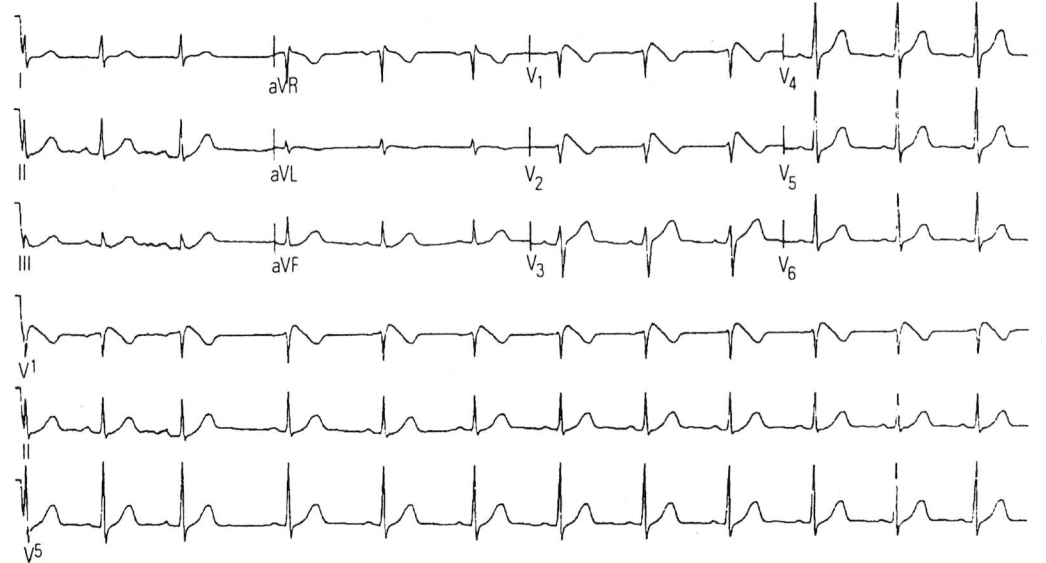

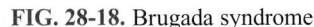
FIG. 28-18. Brugada syndrome.

in ED patients and a family history of sudden death. Further referral should be considered for provocative tests even with a normal ECG. The disease is genetically determined, with a very high incidence of sudden death. The only treatment available is an automatic implanted cardiac cardioverter-defibrillator. The ECG can be normal but frequently may be unmasked by procainamide, flecainide, or ajmaline. The abnormality is in the gene *SCN5A* on chromosome 3, and the electrophysiologic mechanism is theorized to concern the transient currents (Ito) at a myocardial cellular level.

Atypical ventricular tachycardia (TdP, or "twisting of the points") is where the QRS axis swings from a positive to a negative direction in a single lead (Figure 28-19). This rhythm results from a triggered arrhythmic mechanism. Torsade de pointes usually occurs in short runs of 5 to 15 s at a rate of 200 to 240 beats/min. This form of ventricular tachycardia generally occurs in patients with serious myocardial disease who have a prolonged and uneven ventricular repolarization (prolonged QT interval; Table 28-2).

Drugs that further prolong repolarization, such as quinidine, disopyramide, procainamide, phenothiazine, and tricyclic antidepressants, exacerbate this dysrhythmia. Conventional treatment with lidocaine often is ineffective. To date, treatment for TdP consisted of accelerating the heart rate (thereby shortening ventricular repolarization) with isoproterenol (2 to 8 µg/min) while making arrangements for a ventricular pacemaker to overdrive the heart at rates of 90 to 120 beats/min. Temporary pacing is the most effective and safest method to treat TdP and prevent its recurrence in the emergency setting. Recent reports have found that magnesium sulfate 1 to 2 g IV over 60 to 90 s, followed by an infusion of 1 to 2 g/h, is effective in abolishing these runs of TdP, although recurrences are seen despite continued infusion. A wide variety of other agents and antiarrhythmics have been reported anecdotal successes, but overall efficacy has been inconsistent.

Clinical Significance Ventricular tachycardia is very rare in patients without underlying heart disease. The most common causes of ventricular tachycardia are ischemic heart disease and acute MI. Less common causes include hypertrophic cardiomyopathy, mitral valve prolapse, and toxicity from many drugs (digoxin, quinidine, procainamide, and sympathomimetics). Hypoxia, alkalosis, and electrolyte abnormalities exacerbate the tendency toward ventricular ectopy and tachycardia.

It is a common misconception that patients with ventricular tachycardia appear clinically unstable; this is the basis for the mistaken assumption that patients who appear stable with a wide complex tachy-

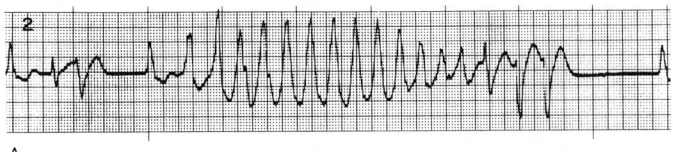

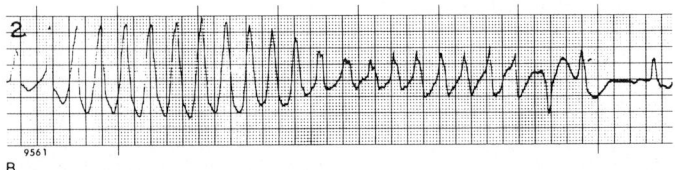

FIG. 28-19. Two examples of short runs of atypical ventricular tachycardia showing sinusoidal variation in amplitude and direction of the QRS complexes, i.e., torsade de pointes (twisting of the points). The top run was initiated by a late-occurring premature ventricular contraction (lead II).

TABLE 28-2   Etiologies and Associated Conditions in Torsade de Pointes

Familial
    Jervell and Lange-Nielsen syndrome (congenital deafness)
    Romano-Ward syndrome (without deafness)
Toxins and drugs
    Antiarrhythmics: most common with classes IA, IC, and III
    Psychotropics: tricyclic antidepressants, some phenothiazines (thioridazine), tetracyclics (maprotiline)
    Organophosphate insecticides
    Liquid protein diets
Cerebrovascular disease
    Cerebrovascular accidents, intracranial hemorrhage, carotid endarterectomy
Electrolyte disorders
    Hypokalemia, hypomagnesemia, hypocalcemia
Endocrine disorders
    Hypothyroidism
Cardiac disease
    Acute rheumatic carditis, mitral valve prolapse syndrome, inflammatory myocarditis
Coronary artery disease
    Myocardial ischemia or infarction, left ventricular failure
Pacemaker malfunction
Postoperative complication

cardia (WCT) have SVT with aberrancy rather than ventricular tachycardia. **Ventricular tachycardia cannot be differentiated from SVT with aberrancy on the basis of clinical symptoms, blood pressure, or heart rate.** Patients who are unstable should be cardioverted; this is effective for both dysrhythmias. In patients who are stable, a 12-lead ECG should be obtained first and examined for evidence favoring one dysrhythmia over another; but even then, it is often difficult to decide. Therefore, in general, it is best to treat all WCTs as ventricular tachycardia with lidocaine or procainamide. These drugs are obviously effective in ventricular tachycardia and often surprisingly effective in SVT with aberrancy, and they carry little risk of harming the patient. Conversely, verapamil is harmful in most patients with ventricular tachycardia, because it accelerates the heart rate and decreases blood pressure without converting the rhythm. Adenosine appears to do little harm in patients with ventricular tachycardia and has potential merit for the treatment for wide QRS complex tachycardias.

Treatment

1. Unstable patients or those in cardiac arrest should be treated with synchronized cardioversion. Symptomatic ventricular tachycardia with a pulse should be treated with synchronized cardioversion, beginning at 100 J. For pulseless ventricular tachycardia, unsynchronized cardioversion should begin with 200 J.
2. Clinically stable patients may be treated with intravenous antiarrhythmics.
   a. Lidocaine 75 mg (1.0 to 1.5 mg/kg) IV over 60 to 90 s can be used, followed by a constant infusion at 1 to 4 mg/min (10 to 40 μg/kg per min). A repeat bolus dose of 50 mg may be required during the first 20 min to avoid a subtherapeutic dip in serum level due to the early distribution phase.
   b. Amiodarone, 150 mg over the first 10 min, may be repeated every 10 min up to a total dose of 2 g. Or a maintenance dose of 0.5 mg/min over 18 h can be administered.
   c. Procainamide can be given at a rate slower than 50 mg/min IV until the dysrhythmia converts, the total dose reaches 15 to 17 mg/kg in normal patients (12 mg/kg in patients with CHF), or early signs of toxicity develop with hypotension or QRS prolongation. The loading dose should be followed by a maintenance infusion of 2.8 mg/kg per h in normal subjects (1.4 mg/kg per h in patients with renal insufficiency).
   d. A variety of other antiarrhythmics have been studied for the treatment of ventricular tachycardia. Most class I and III agents are effective for the acute termination of ventricular tachycardia when given IV. Recommendations concerning their routine use will have to await further studies.

VENTRICULAR FIBRILLATION   Ventricular fibrillation is the totally disorganized depolarization and contraction of small areas of ventricular myocardium: there is no effective ventricular pumping activity. The ECG of ventricular fibrillation shows a fine to coarse zigzag pattern without discernible P waves or QRS complexes (Figure 28-20).

A pulse or blood pressure never accompanies ventricular fibrillation. In patients who are awake and responsive, the ECG pattern of ventricular fibrillation is caused by a loose lead artifact or electrical interference.

Clinical Significance   Ventricular fibrillation is seen most commonly in patients with severe ischemic heart disease, with or without

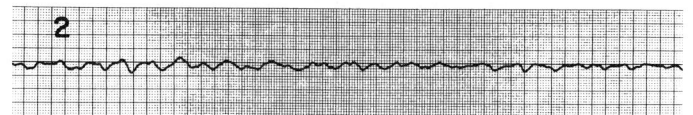

FIG. 28-20. Ventricular fibrillation.

an acute MI. Primary ventricular fibrillation occurs suddenly, without preceding hemodynamic deterioration, whereas secondary ventricular fibrillation occurs after a prolonged period of left ventricular failure and/or circulatory shock. Ventricular fibrillation also may occur from digoxin toxicity, quinidine toxicity, hypothermia, blunt chest trauma, severe electrolyte abnormality, or myocardial irritation caused by an intracardiac catheter or pacemaker electrode.

Treatment

1. Current Advanced Cardiac Life Support (ACLS) guidelines recommend immediate electrical defibrillation with 200 J. If ventricular fibrillation persists, defibrillation should be repeated immediately with 200 to 300 J for the second attempt and increased to 360 J for the third attempt.[11]
2. If the initial three attempts at defibrillation are unsuccessful, cardiopulmonary resuscitation should be initiated, and according to ACLS guidelines, further electrical defibrillations should be done after the administration of various intravenous drugs.

ABERRANT VERSUS VENTRICULAR TACHYDYSRHYTHMIAS   Differentiation between ectopic beats of ventricular origin and those of supraventricular origin but conducted aberrantly can be difficult, especially in sustained tachycardias with wide QRS complexes (WCT). In general, most **patients with WCT have ventricular tachycardia and should be approached as having ventricular tachycardia until proven otherwise.** Several guidelines might help in the distinction.

1. A preceding ectopic P′ wave is good evidence favoring aberrancy, although coincidental atrial and ventricular ectopic beats or retrograde conduction can occur. During a sustained run of tachycardia, AV dissociation greatly favors a ventricular origin of the dysrhythmia.
2. A postectopic, i.e., fully compensatory, pause is more likely after a ventricular beat, but exceptions do occur.
3. Fusion beats are good evidence for ventricular origin, but exceptions do occur.
4. A varying bundle branch block pattern suggests aberrancy.
5. Coupling intervals are usually constant with ventricular ectopic beats unless parasystole is present. Varying coupling intervals suggest aberrancy.
6. Response to carotid sinus massage or other vagal maneuvers will slow conduction through the AV node and may abolish reentrant SVT and slow the ventricular response in other SVTs. These maneuvers have essentially no effect on ventricular dysrhythmias.
7. A QRS duration longer than 0.14 s usually is found only in ventricular ectopy or tachycardia.
8. With regard to QRS morphology, Wellens and colleagues studied patients with ventricular tachycardia and SVT with aberrancy using His bundle electrocardiography.[12] Several morphologic ECG criteria were found useful in differentiating between the two (Table 28-3). In the ED, these morphologic criteria are less useful.
9. Historical criteria have been found to be useful: age older than 35 years and/or history of MI, CHF, or coronary artery bypass graft strongly suggest ventricular tachycardia in patients with WCT.

CONDUCTION DISTURBANCES

Sinoatrial Block

The sinus node discharge must be conducted into the atria to pace the heart during sinus rhythm. If sinus node discharges are delayed or blocked in their outward propagation (exit block), then SA block is present. Sinoatrial block is divided into first-, second-, and third-degree varieties.

In *first-degree SA block,* the impulse is delayed in its conduction out of the sinus node into the atria, a condition that cannot be recognized on the clinical ECG.

TABLE 28-3 Aberrancy versus Ventricular Ectopy

QRS Pattern in V_1	Favors	QRS Pattern in V_6	Favors
rSR′(RBBB pattern)	Aberrancy	qRS	Aberrancy
rR′			
R		rS	
qR		S	
RS	Ventricular	qR or QR	Ventricular
Slurred downslope R		R	
		qQ′	
Slurred upstroke R	Either	RS	Either
		Slurred R	

Abbreviation: RBBB = right bundle branch block.
Source: Wellens HJ, Bar FW, Lie KI: The value of the electrocardiogram in the differential diagnosis of tachycardia with a widened QRS complex. *Am J Med* 64:27, 1978.

In *second-degree SA block,* some impulses get through and some are blocked. Second-degree SA block can be suspected whenever an expected P wave and the corresponding QRS complex are absent. In the variable (Wenckebach) type of second-degree SA block, the missing P wave appears after a period of progressive prolongation of the conduction time from the sinus node to the atrium, something undetectable on the clinical ECG. However, another ECG finding common to the Wenckebach phenomenon can be seen: progressive shortening of the P-P intervals before the missing P wave (Figure 28-21). In the constant type of second-degree SA block, the SA conduction time remains constant before and after the blocked impulses. In this situation, the interval encompassing the missing beat is an exact or nearly exact multiple of the cycle length (Figure 28-22).

Third-degree SA block occurs when the sinus node discharge is completely blocked, and no P wave originating from the sinus is seen. There are three other causes of absent sinus P waves in addition to third-degree SA block: (1) sinus node failure, (2) a sinus node stimulus inadequate to activate the atria, and (3) atrial unresponsiveness.

Clinical Significance Sinoatrial block usually arises from myocardial disease (acute rheumatic fever, acute inferior MI, or other causes of myocarditis) or drug toxicity (digoxin, quinidine, salicylates, β-adrenergic blockers, or calcium channel blockers). In rare individuals, vagal stimulation can produce SA block.

Treatment

1. Treatment depends on the underlying cause, associated dysrhythmias, and whether symptoms of hypoperfusion are present.
2. Sinus node discharge rate and SA conduction can be facilitated by atropine or isoproterenol, when clinically required; however, ischemia may result from a rhythm that is accelerated.
3. Cardiac pacing is indicated for recurrent or persistent symptomatic bradycardia.

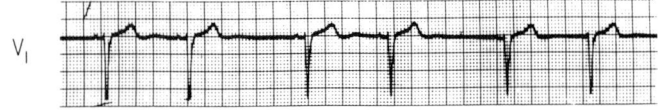

FIG. 28-21. Second-degree sinoatrial block type I (Wenckebach). (Reproduced with permission from Braunwald E: *Heart Disease. A Textbook of Cardiovascular Medicine.* Philadelphia, WB Saunders, 1980.)

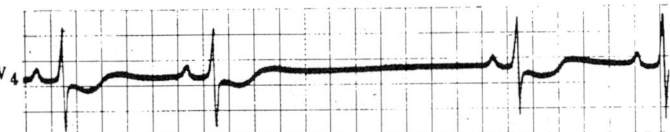

FIG. 28-22. Second-degree constant sinoatrial block type II (lead V_4).

Sinus Arrest (Pause)

Sinus pause is a failure of impulse formation within the sinus node. In sinus arrest, the P-P interval has no mathematical relation to the basic sinus node discharge rate (Figure 28-23).

Clinical Significance The same conditions that produce SA block can produce sinus arrest, especially digoxin toxicity and aging disease of the SA node, as in sick sinus syndrome, discussed below. **The combination of digoxin and carotid sinus massage is well known to be able to produce prolonged sinus arrest.** Brief periods of sinus arrest may occur in healthy individuals due to increased vagal tone. If sinus arrest is prolonged, AV junctional escape beats often occur.

Treatment

1. Treatment depends on the underlying cause, associated dysrhythmias, and whether symptoms of hypoperfusion are present.
2. If sinus arrest is symptomatic, atropine usually will increase the sinus node discharge rate.
3. Cardiac pacing is indicated for recurrent or persistent symptomatic bradycardia.

Atrioventricular Dissociation

Atrioventricular dissociation is a condition in which separate and independent pacemakers drive the atria and ventricles. It is not a primary rhythm disturbance but is secondary to another conduction or rhythm abnormality. There are two varieties of AV dissociation: passive (default or "escape") and active (usurpation).

Passive AV dissociation occurs when an impulse fails to reach the AV node because of sinus node failure or block. Usually an escape rhythm takes over and paces the ventricles. When the sinus node recovers, atrial activity resumes, but there may be a period during which the ventricles are still driven by the escape pacemaker and the P waves and QRS complexes occur independently of each other (Figure 28-24).

Active AV dissociation occurs when a slower pacemaker accelerates to usurp the sinus node and captures the ventricles but the atria are still paced as before (Figure 28-25).

In both varieties of AV dissociation, fusion beats are common. It is also common for the two pacemakers to operate with nearly identical rates, possibly as a result of mechanical or electrical influences that tend to keep them in phase with each other, a condition termed *isorhythmic dissociation.*

Clinical Significance Passive AV dissociation occurs when the sinus node discharge rate is slowed by sinus bradycardia, sinus dysrhythmia, SA block, or sinus pause. Common causes include (1) ischemic heart disease (especially acute inferior MI), (2) myocarditis (especially acute rheumatic fever), (3) drug toxicity (especially digoxin), and (4) vagal reflexes. It also may be seen in well-conditioned athletes.

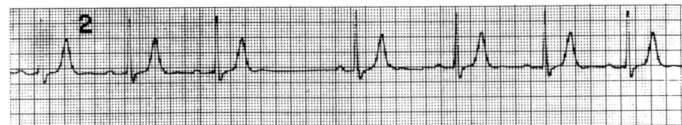

FIG. 28-23. Sinus pause.

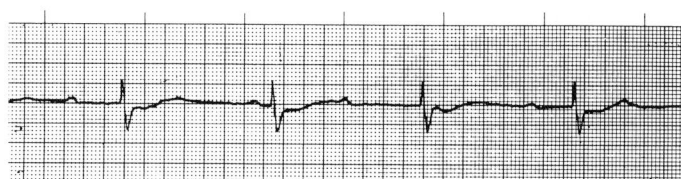

FIG. 28-24. Passive atrioventricular (AV) dissociation, secondary to third-degree AV block.

Active AV dissociation occurs when the automaticity of lower pacemakers is enhanced. Common causes include myocardial ischemia and drug toxicity (especially digoxin). This form of AV dissociation is seen only when the lower tachycardiac rhythm is not conducted to the sinus node with capture of the SA node. Ventricular tachycardia is the classic example of an active AV dissociation.

Treatment

1. Most occurrences of AV dissociation have an acceptable heart rate and are well tolerated.
2. Therapy, if any, is directed toward the underlying cause.

Atrioventricular Block

Clinical classification of AV block occurred before the sites and mechanisms involved in impairing conduction between the atria and ventricles were understood. As a matter of fact, Wenckebach described his block before the development of ECGs by looking at the A and V waves in the jugular veins. Mobitz described his classification after the invention of the ECG but before His bundle recordings. This classification is too simple to categorize all the problems that may occur with AV conduction. However, this system is used almost universally in respect to their observations.

First-degree AV block is characterized by a delay in AV conduction manifest by a prolonged P-R interval. Second-degree AV block is characterized by intermittent AV conduction: some atrial impulses reach the ventricles and others are blocked. Third-degree AV block is characterized by the complete interruption of AV conduction.

Precise localization of AV conduction blocks can be made with His bundle electrocardiography. Although this method is not available for use in the ED, correlations can be made between the clinical ECG, approximate location of the block, and risk of future progression.

Atrioventricular blocks also can be divided into nodal and infranodal blocks. This is an important distinction, because the clinical significance and prognosis differ with the site. Atrioventricular nodal blocks (block at the AH area) are usually due to reversible depression of conduction, are often self-limited, and generally have a stable infranodal escape pacemaker pacing the ventricles. Therefore, AV nodal

blocks usually do not have a serious prognosis. Infranodal blocks (block at the HV area) usually are due to organic disease of the His bundle or bundle branches; often the damage is irreversible. They generally have a slow and unstable ventricular escape rhythm pacing the ventricles, and they may have a serious prognosis, depending on the clinical circumstance.

FIRST-DEGREE AV BLOCK   In first-degree AV block, each atrial impulse is conducted into the ventricles, but more slowly than normal. This is recognized by a P-R interval longer than 0.20 s (Figure 28-26). The AV node is usually the site of conduction delay, although this block may occur at any infranodal level.

Clinical Significance   First-degree AV block occasionally is found in normal hearts. Other common causes include increased vagal tone (any cause), digoxin toxicity, acute inferior MI, and myocarditis. Patients with first-degree AV block without evidence of organic heart disease appear to have no significant difference in mortality compared with matched controls.

Treatment

1. None is usually required.
2. Prophylactic pacing in acute MI is not indicated unless more serious infranodal conduction disturbances are present.

Second-Degree Mobitz I (Wenckebach) AV Block

In this block there is progressive prolongation of AV conduction (and the P-R interval) until an atrial impulse is completely blocked (Figure 28-27). This property of a gradually increasing block until it is complete is a normal property of cardiac tissue. In the face of disease, this property occurs at a much slower rate. In the EP laboratory, a Wenckebach type of block is frequently seen when atrial pacing occurs at fast rates to uncover an accessory pathway. Conduction ratios are used to indicate the ratio of atrial to ventricular depolarizations: 3:2 indicates that two of three atrial impulses are conducted into the ventricles. Usually, one atrial impulse is blocked. After the dropped beat, the AV conduction returns to normal, and the cycle usually repeats itself with the same conduction ratio (fixed ratio) or a different conduction ratio (variable ratio). This type of block almost always occurs at the level of the AV node and is often due to reversible depression of AV nodal conduction.

The Wenckebach phenomenon involves a seeming paradox. Even though the P-R intervals progressively lengthen before the dropped beat, the increments by which they lengthen decrease with successive beats; this produces a progressive shortening of the R-R interval before the dropped beat (see Figure 28-27). This sign can be used to indicate that a Wenckebach phenomenon is occurring even when the conduction delay cannot be seen, as in Wenckebach SA block.

Wenckebach block is believed to occur because each successive depolarization produces prolongation of the refractory period of the AV node. When the next atrial impulse comes upon the node, it is earlier in the relative refractory period, and conduction occurs more slowly relative to the previous stimulus. This process is progressive until an atrial impulse reaches the AV node during the absolute refractory

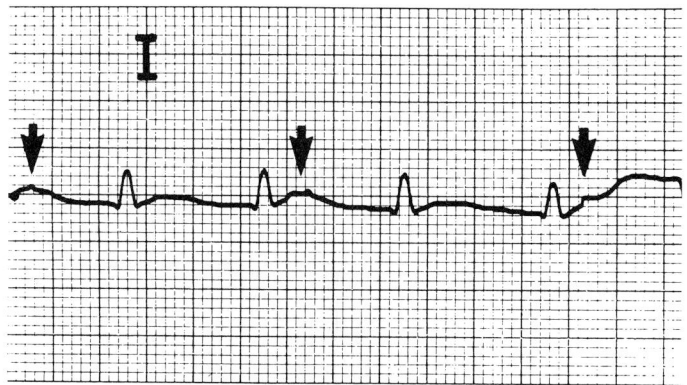

FIG. 28-25. Active atrioventricular dissociation (*arrows* = P waves).

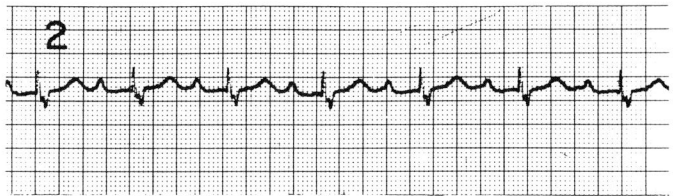

FIG. 28-26. First-degree atrioventricular block (P-R interval = 0.3 s).

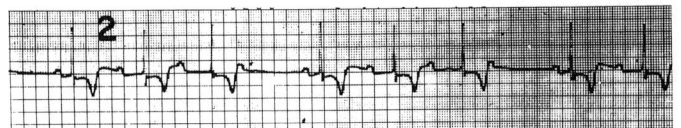

FIG. 28-27. Second-degree Mobitz I (Wenckebach) atrioventricular (AV) block with 4:3 AV conduction.

period, and conduction is blocked altogether. The pause allows the AV node to recover, and the process can resume.

Clinical Significance   This block is often transient and usually associated with an acute inferior MI, digoxin toxicity, or myocarditis, or it is seen after cardiac surgery. Wenckebach block may occur when a normal AV node is exposed to very rapid atrial rates.

Treatment

1. Specific treatment is not necessary unless slow ventricular rates produce signs of hypoperfusion.
2. Atropine 0.5 mg IV is the initial treatment of choice, repeated every 5 min as necessary, titrated to the desired effect, or until the total dose reaches 2.0 mg. Almost all patients will respond to atropine. The need for an increased rate and, one hopes, increased perfusion must be consistently balanced with the increased myocardial O_2 consumption in the ischemic patient.
3. Isoproterenol is hazardous in the setting of acute MI or digoxin toxicity, and its use should be avoided.
4. Transcutaneous or transvenous ventricular demand pacing should be initiated if atropine is unsuccessful. It must be confirmed that the hypoperfusion is due to the rate and not to decreased preload, as in some patients with inferior MI.

Second-Degree Mobitz II AV Block

In this block, the P-R interval remains constant before and after the nonconducted atrial beats (Figure 28-28). One or more beats may be nonconducted at one time.

Mobitz II blocks usually occur in the infranodal conducting system, often with coexistent fascicular or bundle branch blocks, and the QRS complexes therefore are usually wide. Even if the QRS complexes are narrow, the block is generally in the infranodal system.

When second-degree AV block occurs with a fixed conduction ratio of 2:1, it is not possible to differentiate between a Mobitz type I (Wenckebach) or Mobitz type II block (see Figure 28-28). If the QRS complex is narrow, then the block is in the AV node or infranodal system with about equal incidence. If the QRS complex is wide, the block is more likely to be in the infranodal system.

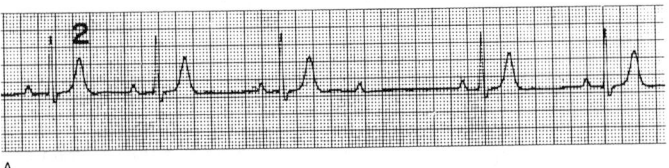

A

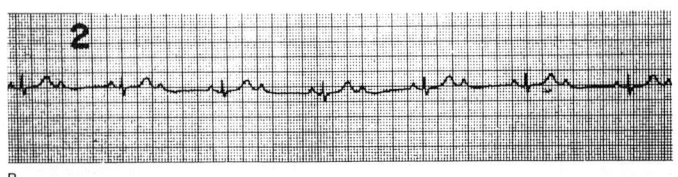

B

FIG. 28-28. *Top:* Second-degree Mobitz II atrioventricular (AV) block. *Bottom:* Second-degree AV block with 2:1 AV conduction.

Clinical Significance   Type II blocks imply structural damage to the infranodal conducting system, are usually permanent, and may progress suddenly to complete heart block, especially in the setting of an acute MI.

Treatment

1. Emergent treatment is required when slow ventricular rates produce symptoms of hypoperfusion. Atropine should be the first drug used, and up to 60 percent of patients will respond. Isoproterenol is effective in up to 50 percent of cases but is potentially hazardous in the setting of acute MI or digoxin toxicity, and its use should be avoided. Transcutaneous cardiac pacing is a useful modality in patients unresponsive to atropine.
2. Most patients, especially in the setting of acute MI, will require transvenous cardiac pacing.

Third-Degree (Complete) AV Block

In third-degree AV block, there is no AV conduction. An escape pacemaker at a rate slower than the atrial rate (Figure 28-29) paces the ventricles. Third-degree AV block can occur at nodal or infranodal levels.

When third-degree AV block occurs at the AV node, a junctional escape pacemaker takes over with a ventricular rate of 40 to 60 beats/min, and because the rhythm originates above the bifurcation of the bundle of His, the QRS complexes are narrow.

When third-degree AV block occurs at the infranodal level, the ventricles are driven by a ventricular escape rhythm at a rate slower than 40 beats/min. In third-degree AV block at the His bundle level, the escape rhythm has narrow QRS complexes about half of the time. Presumably in these cases, the escape pacemaker resides above the bifurcation of the conducting system into the separate bundle branches. Third-degree AV blocks in the bundle branch or elsewhere in the Purkinje system invariably have escape rhythms with wide QRS complexes.

Clinical Significance   Nodal third-degree AV block may develop in up to 8 percent of acute inferior MIs, where it is usually transient, although it may last for several days.

Infranodal third-degree AV blocks indicate structural damage to the infranodal conducting system, as seen with an extensive acute anterior MI. The ventricular escape pacemaker is usually inadequate to maintain cardiac output and is unstable, with periods of ventricular asystole. When third-degree block is seen in acute MI; mortality is increased even when rhythm is controlled with pacing.

Treatment

1. Nodal third-degree AV blocks should be treated like second-degree Mobitz I AV blocks with atropine or ventricular demand pacemaker, as required.
2. Infranodal third-degree AV blocks require a ventricular demand pacemaker. When other measures fail, isoproterenol can be used temporarily to accelerate the ventricular escape rhythm, or external cardiac pacing can be performed before transvenous pacemaker placement.

FASCICULAR BLOCKS

Unifascicular Block

Unifascicular block is a conduction block that affects one of the three major infranodal conduction pathways: RBB, LASF, or LPIF. A wide

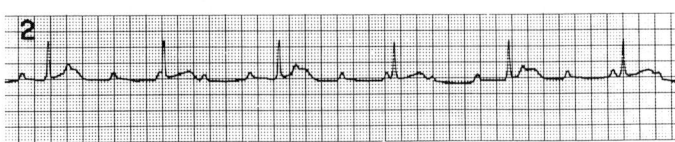

FIG. 28-29. Third-degree atrioventricular block.

FIG. 28-30. Left anterior superior fascicular block.

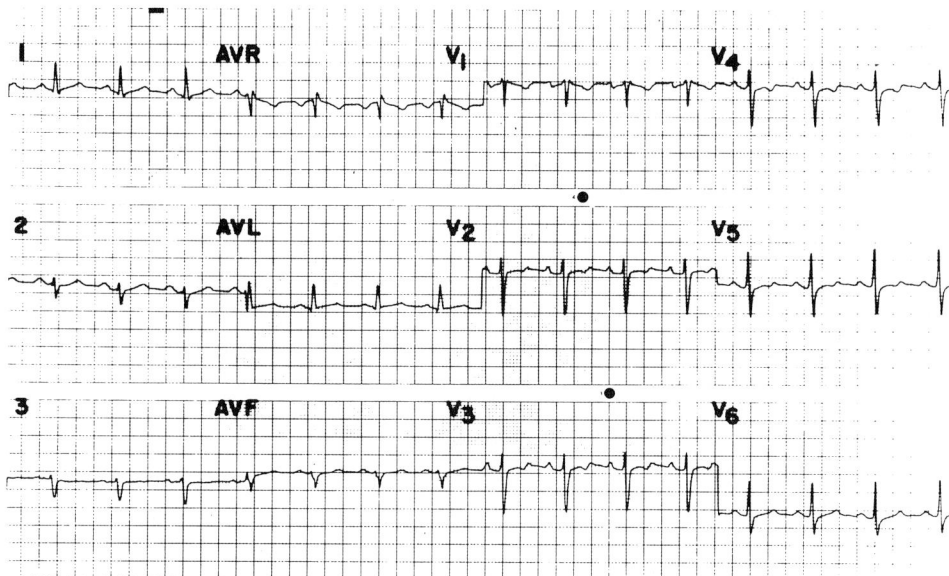

variety of disease processes can produce conduction block in the fascicles: ischemia, cardiomyopathies, valvular (especially aortic), myocarditis, cardiac surgery, congenital conditions, and degenerative processes affecting the conduction tissue (Lenègre or Lev diseases). The RBB and the LASF are relatively small and easily affected parts of the conduction system. The LPIF is very broad and is caused by disease affecting a large area of myocardium.

In LASF block, left ventricular activation is by way of the LPIF and proceeds in an inferior-to-superior and right-to-left direction. The ECG characteristics of LASF block are (1) normal QRS duration, (2) frontal plane mean QRS axis between −30 and −90 degrees, (3) R wave in lead I greater than the R waves in lead II or III, (4) a qR complex in lead aV_L, and (5) deep S wave in leads II, III, and aV_F (Figure 28-30). The LASF is small and easily affected by focal lesions. Other causes of left axis deviation should be excluded: inferior MI, hyperkalemia, preexcitation syndromes, or body habitus. Left ventricular hypertrophy can cause left axis deviation as seen with LASF block; however, the axis is infrequently less than −30 degrees.

In the LPIF block, left ventricular activation is by way of the LASF and proceeds in a superior-to-inferior and left-to-right direction. The ECG characteristics of LPIF block are (1) normal QRS duration, (2) frontal plane mean QRS axis between 110 and 180 degrees, (3) small r and deep S waves in lead I, (4) an R wave in lead III larger than the

R wave in lead II, and (5) a qR complex in lead III (Figure 28-31). The LPIF is broad and not affected by focal lesions; its presence indicates widespread organic heart disease. Other causes of right axis deviation are chronic cor pulmonale, right ventricular hypertrophy, and lateral MI.

In RBB block (RBBB), ventricular activation is by way of the LBB, proceeding from the left to the right ventricle. The ECG characteristics of RBB block are (1) prolonged QRS duration (≥0.12 s); (2) triphasic QRS complexes (RSR′) in lead V_1; (3) wide S waves in the lateral leads I, V_5, and V_6; and (4) normal onset of ventricular activation in lead V_6 (Figure 28-32). The frontal plane mean QRS axis is usually not deviated to the right, unless there is associated right ventricular hypertrophy or LPIF block.

Bifascicular Block

The term *bifascicular block* refers to conduction blocks over two fascicles: (1) RBB and LASF, (2) RBB and LPIF, or (3) LBB block (LBBB).

In LBBB, ventricular activation is by way of the RBB and proceeds from right to left and inferior to superior. The ECG characteristics of LBBB are (1) prolonged QRS duration (≥0.12 s); (2) large and wide R waves in leads I, aV_L, V_5, and V_6; (3) small r wave followed by deep S wave in leads II, III, aV_F, and V_1 to V_3; and (4) no q waves in leads I, V_5, and V_6 (Figure 28-33).

FIG. 28-31. Left posterior inferior fascicular block.

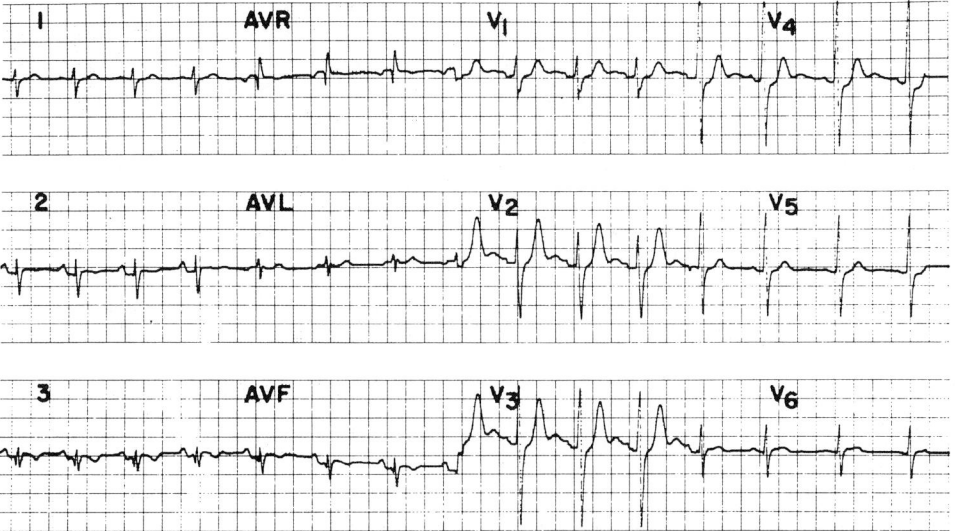

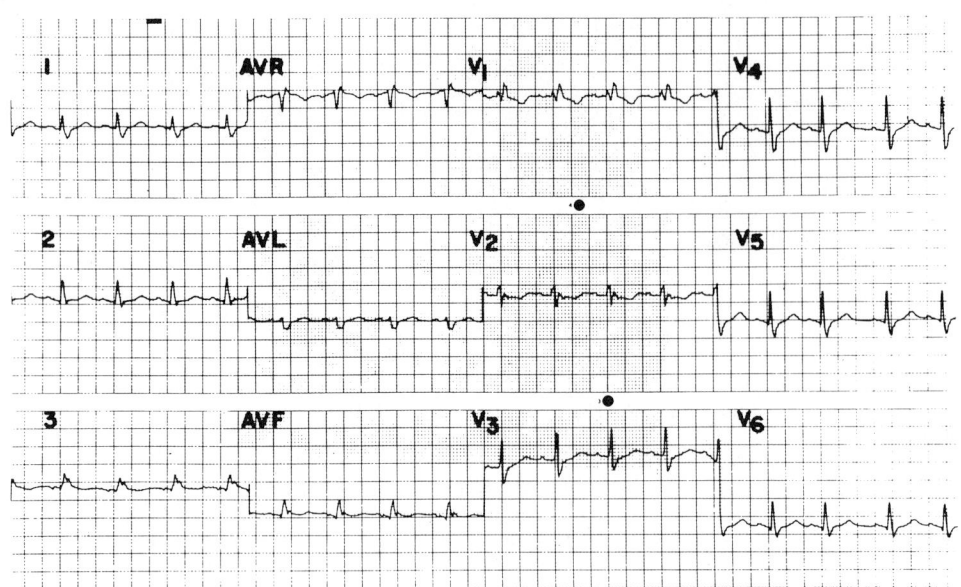

FIG. 28-32. Right bundle branch block.

Trifascicular Block

The term *trifascicular block* refers to a combination of conduction blocks in all three fascicles, either permanent or transient: (1) RBB and LASF with first-degree AV block, (2) RBB and LPIF with first-degree AV block, (3) LBB with first-degree AV block, or (4) alternating RBBB and LBBB.

Although bi- and trifascicular conduction blocks indicate advanced organic heart disease, long-term follow-up studies of ambulatory patients have indicated that the risk of sudden progression to complete heart block and sudden death due to ventricular asystole is not great. Placement of a ventricular demand pacemaker is indicated only for symptoms due to documented bradyarrhythmias.

In the face of an acute MI, the risks of complete heart block are much greater when new or preexisting bi- or trifascicular conduction blocks are present. In this setting, prophylactic placement of a ventricular demand pacemaker is indicated.

PRETERMINAL RHYTHMS

Several dysrhythmias may be seen during cardiac resuscitation. Ventricular tachycardia and fibrillation potentially are treatable, and re-suscitation may result in a functional survivor. The four other dysrhythmias included here have a low rate of successful resuscitation and are much less likely to result in a functional survivor.

Pulseless Electrical Activity

Pulseless electrical activity (PEA) is the presence of electrical complexes without accompanying mechanical contraction of the heart. In the setting of a cardiac arrest, PEA is due to a profound metabolic abnormality of the myocardium that renders it noncontractile. At this time, there is no clearly beneficial therapy; the best that can be recommended currently is continued cardiopulmonary resuscitation and α-adrenergic agents. Although calcium has been advocated traditionally, most studies have found no consistent benefit, and there are serious biophysiologic reasons to question the use of calcium in the setting of cardiac arrest. Electrical pacing is not effective.

Other conditions associated with PEA are (1) severe hypovolemia, (2) cardiac tamponade, (3) tension pneumothorax, (4) massive pulmonary embolus, and (5) rupture of the ventricular wall. The first three conditions are potentially treatable if recognized early.

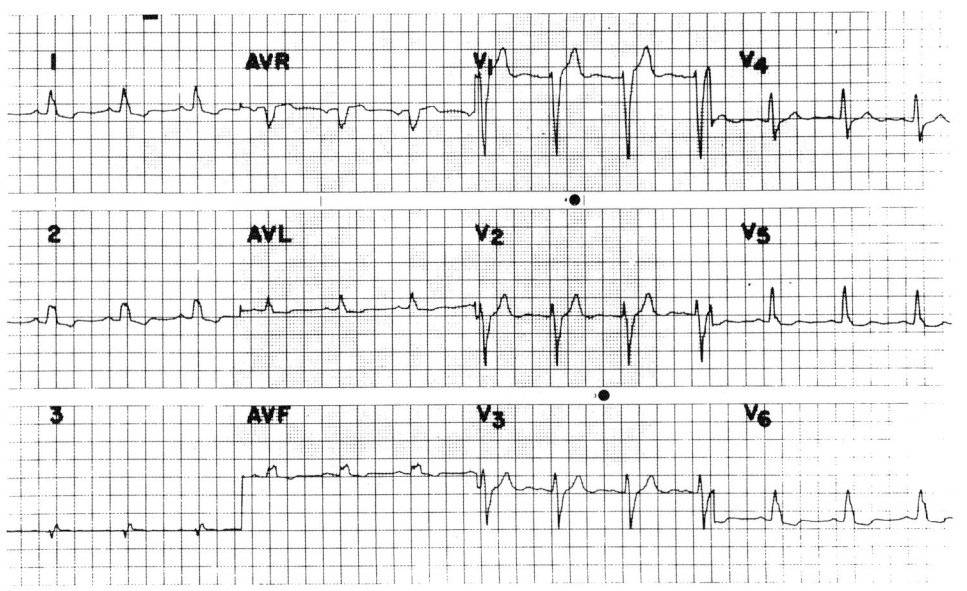

FIG. 28-33. Left bundle branch block.

Idioventricular Rhythm

An idioventricular rhythm is an escape rhythm of ventricular origin with very wide QRS complexes ($\geq$0.16 s) and a rate slower than 40 beats/min (Figure 28-34). Effective cardiac contractions and pulses may or may not be present. Idioventricular rhythm may occur as the result of complete infranodal AV block, acute MI, cardiac tamponade, or exsanguinating hemorrhage. Treatment consists of accelerating the heart rate and enhancing mechanical contractility by using cardiopulmonary resuscitation and α-adrenergic agents. There is no proven benefit to the use of atropine or isoproterenol to treat idioventricular rhythm during cardiac resuscitation.

Agonal Ventricular Rhythm

Agonal rhythm is the occurrence of very broad and irregular ventricular complexes at a slow rate, usually without associated ventricular contractions (Figure 28-35).

Cardiac Asystole (Cardiac Standstill)

Asystole is the complete absence of cardiac electrical activity. Treatment consists of stimulating electrical activity and mechanical contractions with continued cardiopulmonary resuscitation and α-adrenergic agents. Transthoracic or transvenous ventricular pacing occasionally may produce electrical capture but rarely yields effective pumping action if prior agents were unsuccessful.

TACHYCARDIA-BRADYCARDIA SYNDROME (SICK SINUS SYNDROME)

Sick sinus syndrome (SSS) is a heterogeneous disorder consisting of abnormalities of supraventricular impulse generation and conduction that produce a wide variety of intermittent supraventricular tachy- and bradydysrhythmias. The tachydysrhythmias are usually atrial fibrillation, junctional tachycardia, reentrant SVT, and AF. The bradydysrhythmias are marked sinus bradycardia, prolonged sinus arrest, and SA block, usually associated with AV nodal conduction abnormalities and inadequate AV junctional escape rhythms.

Clinical Significance   Symptoms of SSS are due to the effects of fast or slow heart rate. Common symptoms include syncope or near syncope, palpitations, dyspnea, chest pain, and cerebrovascular accidents.

A wide variety of cardiac diseases can affect the sinus and AV nodes and produce the dysrhythmias of SSS: ischemic and rheumatic disorders, myocarditis and pericarditis, rheumatologic disease, metastatic tumors, surgical damage, or cardiomyopathies.

Conditions such as abdominal pain, increased intracranial pressure, thyrotoxicosis, and hyperkalemia, which increase vagal tone, may exacerbate the abnormalities of SSS and increase symptoms. Drugs such as digoxin, quinidine, procainamide, disopyramide, nicotine, β-adrenergic antagonists, or calcium channel blockers also can increase symptoms.

Ambulatory ECG monitoring or EP studies are usually necessary for the diagnosis of SSS, because a routine ECG will not normally

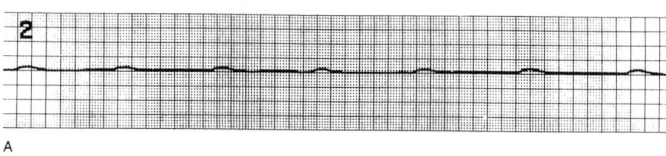

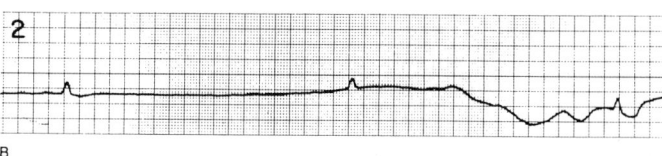

FIG. 28-35. Agonal ventricular rhythms: regular *(top)* and irregular *(bottom).*

demonstrate the intermittent dysrhythmias common in this syndrome. The demonstration of increased sensitivity of the sinus node to carotid sinus massage, the Valsalva maneuver, or atropine suggests sinus node dysfunction but is not conclusive proof for the diagnosis of SSS.

Treatment

1. Sick sinus syndrome is the most common indication for a permanent pacemaker. This disease of the SA and AV nodes accounts for 48 percent of primary pacemaker implants. Retrospective analysis indicates that a reduction in mortality and in the incidence of CHF, AF, and thromboembolism occurs in patients with atrial pacing (AAI or DDD) as opposed to ventricular pacing (VVI) (see Pacing, below).
2. Treatment of atrial tachyarrhythmias with digoxin, quinidine, disopyramide, procainamide, propranolol, or verapamil carries the risk of aggravating preexisting AV block or sinus arrest. Therefore, most patients should have pacemaker implantation before drug therapy is begun.

PREEXCITATION SYNDROMES

Preexcitation occurs when the ventricles are activated by an impulse from the atria sooner than would be expected if the impulse were transmitted down the normal conducting pathway (the AV node). Several different forms of preexcitation have been described, based on anatomic, clinical, ECG, and EP abnormalities. All forms of preexcitation are felt to be due to accessory tracts that bypass all or part of the normal conducting system. These bypass tracts have specific names (Figure 28-36).

James fibers (atriohisian connection) are a continuation of the posterior internodal tract and connect the atrium and proximal His bundles.

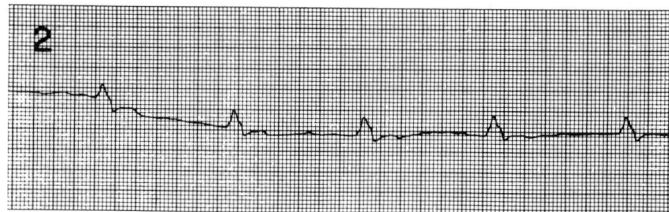

FIG. 28-34. Idioventricular rhythm.

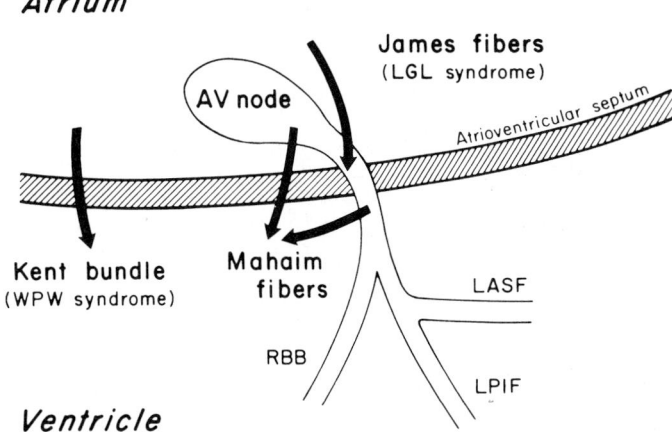

FIG. 28-36. Anatomic sites of bypass tracts.

Atrial impulses can therefore completely bypass the AV node to activate the ventricles. On ECG, this appears as (1) a short P-R interval because the usual delay in the AV node is bypassed and (2) a normal QRS because James fibers insert directly into the infranodal conducting system and the ventricles are activated normally. When this is associated with reentrant SVT, the clinical condition is termed *Lown-Ganong-Levine syndrome.*

Mahaim bundles are composed of myogenic tissue; they originate from the AV node, His bundle, or bundle branches and insert into the ventricles in the septal region. Atrial impulses pass through the AV node but then bypass all or part of the infranodal conducting system to activate the ventricles. Ventricular activation then occurs from two sources, the bypass tract and the normal conducting system, and the QRS complex represents a fusion of the two. The initial depolarization starts at the ventricular insertion of the bypass tract and is spread slowly by cell-to-cell transmission of the impulse. Subsequent depolarization by way of the faster normal conducting system then overtakes the initial depolarization and activates the bulk of ventricular myocardium. The QRS complex is basically normal, with a slurred and distorted initial portion termed a *delta wave.* On ECG, this wave appears as a normal P-R interval and an initial distortion of ventricular depolarization (delta wave).

Kent bundles are composed of myogenic tissue and directly link the atria to the ventricles, completely bypassing the AV node and infranodal system. This is the most common form of preexcitation and is the anatomic basis for the WPW syndrome. On ECG, this appears as a shortened P-R interval with an initial distortion of ventricular activation (delta wave). Sometimes the bypass tract does not conduct an atrial impulse in the antegrade direction and the QRS complex is entirely normal. However, these concealed bypass tracts may conduct retrogradely and be able to sustain reentrant SVT.

The WPW syndrome has been divided into types, depending on the direction of the initial delta wave on the surface ECG. This in turn is determined by where the bypass tract (bundle of Kent) inserts into the ventricles and which portion of the ventricles is activated first. In reality, accessory tracts can insert anywhere around the AV annulus; the three types are just the most common locations.

In type A WPW syndrome, ventricular activation first occurs in the inferior-posterior region of the left ventricle and the delta wave is directed anteriorly. A positive initial deflection with a dominant R wave is seen in lead V_1. Q waves in leads II, III, and aV_F are common (Figure 28-37).

In type B WPW syndrome, ventricular activation first occurs in the inferior-posterior region of the right ventricle and the delta wave is directed posteriorly and to the left. A negative initial deflection and RS or QS pattern are seen in lead V_1 (Figure 28-38).

In type C WPW syndrome, ventricular activation first occurs in the posterior-lateral region of the left ventricle and the delta wave is directed to the right, superiorly, and anteriorly. A positive delta wave is seen in lead V_1, with a negative or isoelectric delta wave in leads V_5 and V_6.

Because there is altered depolarization, repolarization is often abnormal, with changes in the ST segments and T waves. The ECG changes of WPW syndrome may mimic changes seen with myocardial ischemia, infarction, or ventricular hypertrophy. Type A WPW syndrome may imitate as a posterior MI, and type B WPW syndrome may imitate an inferior MI.

Clinical Significance   There is a high incidence of tachyarrhythmias in patients with WPW syndrome. Atrial flutter occurs in about 5 percent, atrial fibrillation in 10 to 20 percent, and paroxysmal reentrant SVT in 40 to 80 percent.

Reentrant SVT occurs when an impulse is sustained around a loop composed of the bypass tract and the AV conducting system, with the impulse traveling down one and up the other. Whether the QRS complex is wide or narrow depends on which limb of the circuit is used as the downward pathway to activate the ventricles. About 80 to 95 percent of the time, reentrant SVT occurs with the impulse being conducted down the normal AV conducting system and up the bypass tract (*orthodromic* AV reciprocating tachycardia). In this situation, ventricular activation occurs entirely over the normal system, the QRS complex is normal, and no delta wave is seen. Because the entire heart is used as the reentrant pathway, these arrhythmias are easily converted. Conversely, 5 to 10 percent of the time, the impulse is conducted down the bypass tract and retrogradely up the AV node (*antidromic* AV reciprocating tachycardia). In this case, the QRS complex is wide, and in the ED setting, this arrhythmia is treated as ventricular tachycardia. Reentry usually is initiated by a premature atrial contraction that encounters a bypass tract that is still refractory from the previous sinus beat, but the AV node has partly recovered and conducts the impulse more slowly than normal (Figure 28-39). In some patients, the bypass tract does not conduct antegradely during sinus rhythm, so no delta wave is seen, but it does conduct retrogradely, so reentrant SVT occurs. Patients with concealed bypass tracts account for about 20 percent of all patients with reentrant SVT.

If patients with WPW syndrome develop AF or atrial fibrillation, impulses can reach the ventricles via the accessory tract, the normal

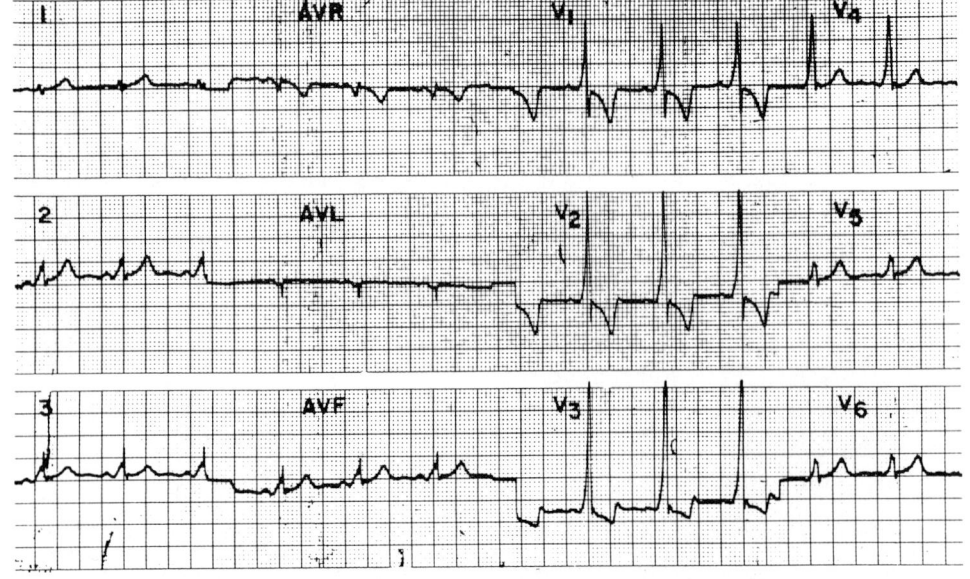

FIG. 28-37. Type A Wolff-Parkinson-White syndrome.

FIG. 28-38. Type B Wolff-Parkinson-White syndrome.

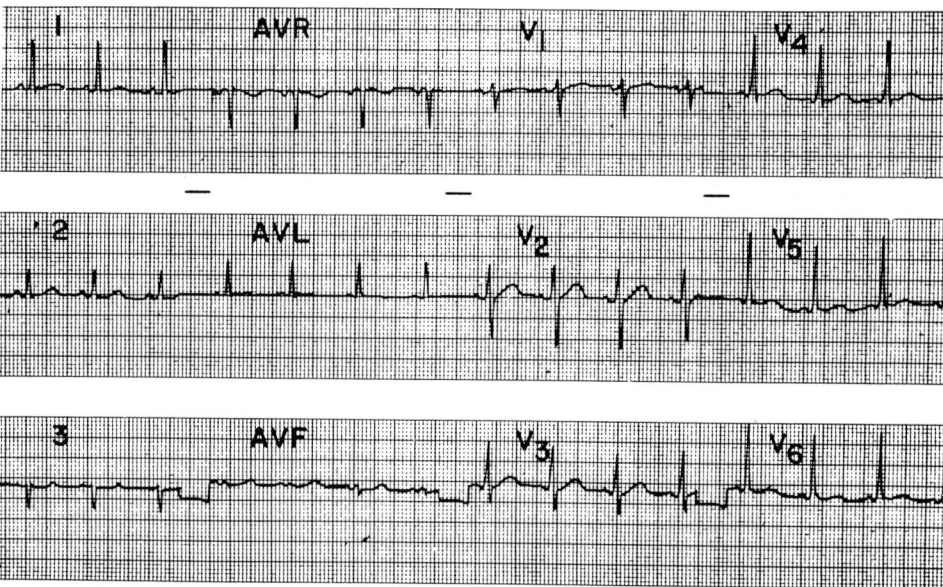

conducting system, or both. Which pathway is used depends on the refractory period of each. Most patients with WPW syndrome have longer refractory periods in their accessory tracts than in the AV node, but a minority has the opposite. In patients with short refractory periods in their accessory tracts, more atrial impulses can be conducted through the accessory tract than through the AV node, so most of the QRS complexes will be wide. In AF, 1:1 AV conduction is possible with ventricular rates of 300 beats/min (Figure 28-40). In atrial fibrillation, very rapid and irregular ventricular rates are possible. These rapid rhythms may resemble ventricular tachycardia, and excessive stimulation of the ventricles may precipitate ventricular fibrillation.

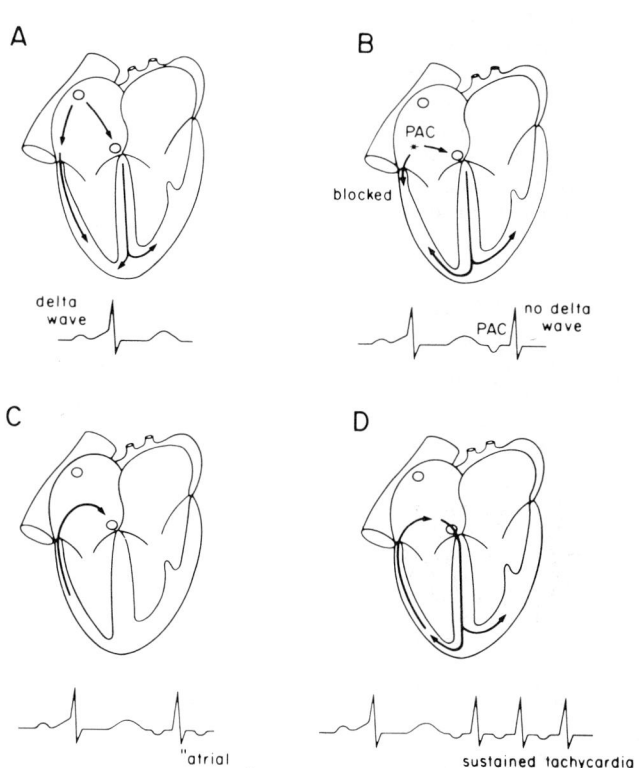

FIG. 28-39. Onset of reentrant supraventricular tachycardia in Wolff-Parkinson-White syndrome.

Any patient with a ventricular rate faster than 300 beats/min should raise the suspicion of preexcitation syndrome.

Treatment

1. Reentrant SVT (orthodromic AV reciprocating tachycardia, narrow QRS complex) in the WPW syndrome can be treated like other cases of reentrant SVT. Because the AV node is involved in the reentry circuit, any maneuver or drug that slows conduction through the AV node is usually effective. Verapamil in the patient who is not hypotensive or in CHF is by some accounts the optimal drug. Adenosine is very successful at terminating this dysrhythmia in patients with WPW; however, there is some proclivity to increase atrial vulnerability to AF and to ectopic atrial activity, which may reinitiate the dysrhythmia.

2. Antidromic tachycardia (antidromic AV reciprocating tachycardia, wide QRS complex) is usually associated with a short refractory period in the bypass tract, and such patients are at risk for rapid ventricular rates and degeneration into ventricular fibrillation. Stable patients should be treated with intravenous procainamide, and unstable patients should be cardioverted. **β-Blocking agents, adenosine, and calcium channel blockers should be avoided.**

3. Atrial flutter or fibrillation with a rapid ventricular response is best treated with cardioversion. As an alternative, agents that prolong the refractory period of the accessory tract, such as intravenous procainamide, can be used. Experimental studies with intravenous flecainide have shown promise. In general, phenytoin, esmolol, propranolol, or verapamil should not be used, because of their variable effects on accessory conduction. Digoxin is contraindicated, because it may shorten the refractory period and enhance conduction over the bypass tract.

DEFIBRILLATION AND SYNCHRONIZED CARDIOVERSION

Defibrillation and cardioversion is the technique of passing a short burst (about 5 ms) of direct electric current across the thorax to terminate tachyarrhythmias. The electric current simultaneously depolarizes all excitable cardiac tissue and terminates any areas of reentry by halting further propagation of the impulse around the reentry loop. This places all cardiac cells in the same depolarized state, and a dominant pacemaker (usually the sinus node) paces the heart in a regular manner.

Defibrillation or cardioversion uses the same type of equipment. A device stores a known quantity of electrical energy in a storage capacitor

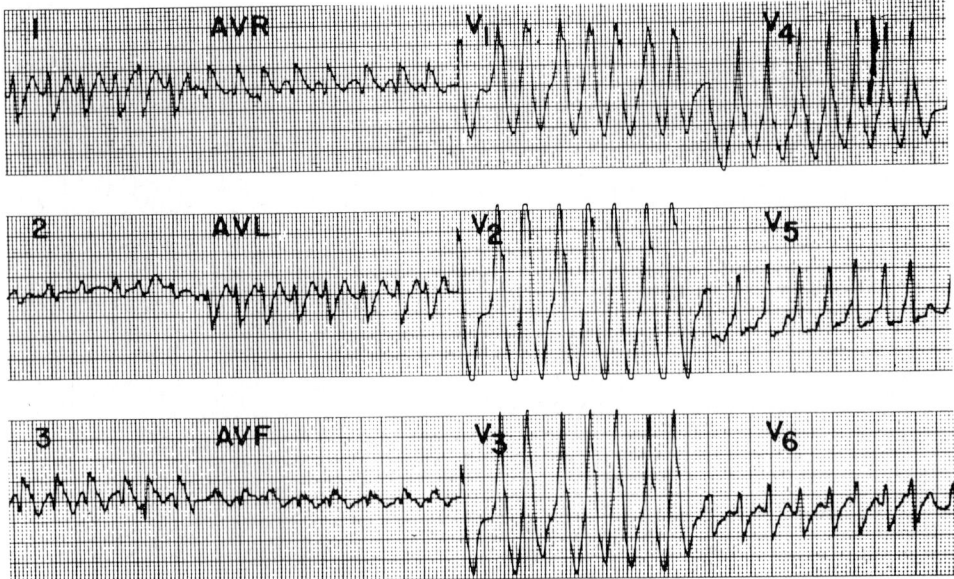

FIG. 28-40. Atrial fibrillation in Wolff-Parkinson-White syndrome.

and, on command, discharges it through two electrodes placed on the chest wall. Usually, a rhythm monitor and a synchronizer circuit are built into the device. Electrode placement can be anterior and posterior or apex and right parasternal. Whereas some investigators have used a lower energy requirement for conversion using anterior and posterior electrodes, others have not. For emergencies, electrode placement probably does not matter.

To reduce transthorax electrical impedance and increase the amount of current passing through the heart, certain techniques are important at the electrode-chest wall interface. Electrode paste, gel, or saline pads are applied to the surface of the electrodes. Firm pressure of 10 to 12.5 kg/cm^2 (20 to 25 lb/in.^{2}) is used to achieve good electrical contact. Larger electrodes or defibrillator pads, within reason, have a reduced impedance, but this does not appear to significantly influence the energy required for conversion.

Older devices had significant internal energy losses and delivered as little as 40 percent of the stored energy to the patient. This is not a problem with modern defibrillators, because they deliver very close to the stored amount.

Defibrillation should be done as soon as ventricular fibrillation is diagnosed. The longer ventricular fibrillation persists, the less likely it is that resuscitation will be successful. Current ACLS guidelines recommend 200 J for the first attempt, 200 to 300 J for the second attempt, and 360 J for subsequent defibrillations.[11] Several studies have found that most patients can be defibrillated with 160 to 200 J. Recommendations for children are 2 J/kg (1 J/lb) in the initial attempt and 4 J/kg in subsequent attempts.

Synchronized cardioversion applies the electric current at a time during the cardiac cycle well away from the vulnerable period when there is little chance of inducing ventricular fibrillation, usually about 10 ms after the peak of the R wave. On most machines, the synchronizer circuit must be turned on each time an impulse is desired. Many devices also display on the monitor screen or by a flashing light that the synchronizer circuit is properly detecting the QRS complex. Cable leads, rather than the paddles, should be used to monitor the cardiac rhythm to avoid any movement artifact that could be misinterpreted by the synchronizer circuit as the QRS complex.

Complications of defibrillation or cardioversion include the following:

1. Direct myocardial damage is unusual unless there are repeated shocks at high energy (≥325 J).
2. Incidence of ventricular fibrillation is less than 5 percent with a synchronized discharge but probably greater in the presence of digoxin or quinidine toxicity, hypokalemia, or acute MI. However,

patients on maintenance digoxin therapy can be safely cardioverted using low energies (≤50 J).
3. Systemic emboli occur in about 1.2 to 1.5 percent in patients with chronic atrial fibrillation.
4. ST-segment changes (transient elevations or depressions) usually resolving within 5 min.
5. Bradycardias are more common in patients with inferior MIs and those requiring multiple defibrillations and cardioversions. Bradycardias are usually evident during the first 5 s after shock and occasionally may persist for longer than 20 s and require external or internal pacing.
6. Tachycardias (usually sinus tachycardia, occasionally AF or fibrillation) usually resolving spontaneously within 5 min.
7. Atrial, junctional, or ventricular ectopy is usually transient and benign.
8. Pulmonary edema is uncommon but may occur in patients with mitral or aortic valvular disease or left ventricular failure.
9. Hypotension is rare, inexplicable, and may last for several hours before spontaneously resolving.
10. Muscle damage: elevated levels of creatine phosphokinase and lactate dehydrogenase are common, but other more specific indicators (CK-MB and troponin) are rarely abnormal.

Automated internal defibrillators are discussed in Chap. 22.

CARDIAC PACEMAKERS

Artificial cardiac pacemakers have two components: a power source (battery with pulse generator) and an electrode that delivers current to the heart (transvenous, epicardial, transthoracic, and transcutaneous). In permanent pacemaker placement, the power source is implanted subcutaneously, and the electrodes are run through the veins to inside the heart or through the subcutaneous tissue to the epicardial surface. In temporary pacemaker placement, the power source is external to the body, and electrodes are placed in one of two ways: transvenously to an intracardiac location or transcutaneously with electrodes placed on the thoracic skin. The pulse generator can be designated to operate in a fixed-rate mode (asynchronous or competitive) or a demand mode (synchronous or noncompetitive). In the fixed-rate mode, the pulse generator produces an electrical signal at the preset rate regardless of the patient's own intrinsic cardiac rhythm. Serious dysrhythmias or ventricular fibrillation may occur if the pacemaker discharges during the vulnerable period (T wave); for this reason, fixed-rate pacing is rarely done.

In the demand mode, the pulse generator has a sensing circuit that detects spontaneous cardiac activity and will discharge only if no cardiac depolarization is detected for a preset interval. Demand pacemakers may have two response modes, inhibited and triggered. Pacemakers set to be inhibited have a pulse generator that is inhibited by the sensed cardiac activity and do not generate an impulse. In the triggered-response mode, the pacemaker detects the patient's intrinsic cardiac activity and then discharges during the absolute refractory period. On ECG, this discharge appears as pacing spikes after each intrinsic QRS complex.

The most recent five-letter code system is shown in Table 28-4. This coding system has added antitachyarrhythmic and shocking capabilities of the latest pacemakers. Many patients carry cards indicating the type of pacemaker they have. The simplest type of pacemaker used, the ventricular-demand inhibited-response pacemaker, would be designated as VVI.

The modern permanent pacemaker is powered by a lithium battery that has an approximate lifetime of 8 to 12 years. Most units are preset for rates near 70 beats/min, with a pacing interval of 0.84 s. The demand pacemaker has a built-in refractory period (0.2 to 0.4 s) during which it will not sense. This prevents it from being inhibited by its own stimulus. Most demand pacemakers have a magnetic switch, which temporarily converts the pulse generator from the demand mode to the fixed-rate mode when a magnet is held over the unit. In this way, the pacing rate can be quickly determined, but the magnet should be applied for only short periods to avoid initiating tachyarrhythmias. The rate and stimulus strength can be reset by noninvasive means in programmable pacemakers. Some of the more sophisticated pacemakers can be interrogated to indicate events such as tachyarrhythmias and conversions. Because pacemaker complexity varies, the manufacturer supplies an identification card with each unit that patients should carry.

Temporary pacemakers are powered by 9-V radio-type batteries. On these pacemakers, there are settings for the mode (fixed or demand), rate (40 to 140 beats/min), and stimulus strength (0.2 to 20 mA). During emergency pacing, initial settings should be in the demand mode with a rate near 70 beats/min and stimulus strength near 3.0 mA. The negative terminal should be connected to the distal electrode.

The transvenous intracardiac electrode may be unipolar or bipolar. The unipolar setup has the negative electrode within the heart and the positive electrode in the chest wall. Permanent pacemakers using the unipolar setup have the positive electrode in the surface covering. Temporary pacemakers using the unipolar setup have their positive electrode connected to a needle implanted in the skin of the anterior thorax. With the bipolar setup, both electrodes are within a few millimeters of each other and both lie within the heart. Transvenous electrodes are placed most commonly into the apex of the right ventricle.

This causes an LBBB pattern when pacing. Different catheters are used depending on the clinical situation. Semirigid catheters (6 or 7 French) are inserted through a venous puncture or cutdown. They usually require fluoroscopy for correct placement. Semifloating (3 or 4 French) or flexible balloon-tipped catheters (3 or 5 French) can be introduced and directed into the right ventricle without fluoroscopy by using blood flow. Flexible catheters can become dislodged by patient or cardiac movement and are usually replaced with semirigid catheters within 24 h.

Transthoracic cardiac pacing has been largely replaced by transcutaneous pacing. Transthoracic pacing is fraught with many complications, including coronary artery laceration and cardiac tamponade in addition to pneumothorax.

Transcutaneous electrodes are self-adhesive pads that are usually placed with the negative electrode over the left anterior precordium and the positive electrode over the left infrascapular area. Transcutaneous pacing is then initiated by using the lowest current setting, which is increased until electrical capture is achieved. Most patients can be paced with 100 mA, but some may require up to 200 mA. The newer pacemakers cause much less discomfort, can be applied faster, and combine defibrillator and pacing functions from the same pads.

Indications for Emergency Pacing

Emergency cardiac pacing is indicated therapeutically (for symptomatic bradyarrhythmias) or prophylactically (for conduction defects that pose a high risk of sudden complete heart block or asystole).

Symptomatic bradyarrhythmias should be treated with atropine and/or isoproterenol as a temporary measure to support cardiac rhythm before pacemaker placement. Some patients may respond adequately to atropine alone and do not require pacemaker insertion.

Most investigators recommend prophylactic placement of a pacemaker in any patient with acute MI who has a new or age-indeterminate bi- or trifascicular block. In addition, second-degree Mobitz II and third-degree AV blocks are indications for pacemaker insertion or transcutaneous pacer pad placement. Despite successful pacing, many patients with acute MI and these serious conduction blocks have extensive left ventricular damage and a high mortality from pump failure.

Pacemaker Malfunction

Malfunction of a permanent pacemaker can be categorized as (1) failure to sense, (2) failure to pace, (3) oversensing, or (4) combinations of the first three. With current lithium batteries and reliable circuitry, most pacemaker malfunctions are due to problems with the electrodes and not the result of battery exhaustion or pulse-generator failure.

TABLE 28-4   NASPE/BPEG Generic Pacemaker Code

Letter Position	I	II	III	IV	V
Category	Chamber(s) Paced	Chamber(s) Sensed	Response to Sensing	Programmability, Rate	Antitachyarrhythmic Function(s)
	O, none	O, none	O, none	O, none	O, none
	A, atrium	A, atrium	T, triggered	P, simple programmable	P, pacing
	V, ventricle	V, ventricle	I, inhibited	M, multiprogrammable	S, shock
	D, dual (A + V)*	D, dual (A + V)*	D, dual (D + I)†	C, Communicating (telemetry)	D, dual (P + S)‡
	S, single chamber	S, single chamber		R, rate modulation	

Abbreviation: NASPE/BPEG, North American Society for Pacing and Electrophysiology/British Pacing and Electrophysiology Group.
*Atrial and ventricular.
†Dual (atrial and ventricular) and inhibited.
‡Pacing and shock.

Failure to sense may occur when the voltages of the patient's own intrinsic QRS complex is too low to be detected by the sensing circuit of the pacemaker. Changing from a bipolar to a unipolar setup (if possible) may help the pacemaker sense the intrinsic cardiac activity. Failure to sense may cause the pacemaker to become a fixed-rate pacemaker, discharge during the T wave, and trigger serious dysrhythmias.

Failure to pace may occur when tissue reaction around the electrode makes the myocardium insensitive to the electric discharge that is generated by the pacemaker. It is common for the pacing threshold to increase during the first few weeks after insertion, but further rises are infrequent.

Failure to sense and pace may be due to battery exhaustion, fracture of the wires in the catheter, or displacement of the electrodes. Battery exhaustion is indicated when the pacing rate slowly decreases. With lithium batteries, such decreases usually occur years before actual battery exhaustion. Greater than a 10 percent change from the initial rate is an urgent indication for replacement. Catheter wire fracture may cause sustained or intermittent interruption in electrical conductivity. Sudden onset of symptoms and/or bradyarrhythmias suggest catheter fracture. Catheter fractures are rarely seen on routine chest radiographs. The transvenous electrode is usually positioned in the right ventricular apex, with a characteristic appearance on the chest radiograph and ECG. Displacement can be suggested when changes on radiographs or ECG occur.

Oversensing is used to describe the situation in which the pacemaker senses electrical activity not associated with atrial or ventricular depolarizations; it is thus inhibited, and generation of the pacemaker impulse is suppressed. Causes of oversensing include physiologic electrical activity (T waves, muscle potentials), external electromagnetic interference, and signals generated by the interaction of different portions of the pacing system. Unipolar electrodes are more sensitive to physiologic electrical activity and electromagnetic interference than to bipolar electrodes.

Under certain conditions, pacemakers may initiate tachyarrhythmias despite functioning as designed; this usually results from an intrinsic depolarization occurring during the pacemaker refractory period, the depolarization not being sensed, and the pacemaker firing soon thereafter and initiating a reentrant tachycardia. In this setting, maintenance of the dysrhythmia does not require further participation of the pacemaker. Dual-chamber pacemakers also can induce and sustain dysrhythmias. In this situation, emergent treatment requires reprogramming the pacemaker, if possible, or converting to asynchronous mode by placing a magnet over the pulse generator.

EVALUATION OF PALPITATIONS

Palpitations are common symptoms that may be due to a dysrhythmia.[13] Frequently, palpitations are no longer present when the patient presents to the ED. The term is nonspecific, but certain descriptions may be helpful in pointing toward certain types of rhythm disturbances. Premature atrial or ventricular contractions followed by a compensatory pause are often described as a flip-flopping in the chest. Atrial or ventricular dysrhythmias can cause a fluttering feeling. Pounding in the neck can be felt when atrial and ventricular contractions are dissociated, as in supraventricular or junctional tachycardias. Inappropriate sinus tachycardia is also in the differential diagnosis.

History taking should include questions regarding prescribed medications, including herbals; recreational drugs; and use of caffeine-containing beverages. History suggestive of endocrine disorders such as hyperthyroidism should be sought. If the clinical presentation suggests potassium abnormality, electrolytes can be checked.

Palpitations associated with dizziness, syncope, or presyncope should be assumed to be associated with ventricular tachycardia until proven otherwise. Although panic attack is often assumed to be associated with palpitations, this diagnosis cannot be established in the ED.

The ECG should be examined for evidence of dysrhythmia, bypass tracts, and QT-interval prolongation. Patients with a family history of sudden death, syncope, or dysrhythmia; those with any evidence of organic heart disease; and those with presyncope, syncope, or dizziness can be admitted or placed in an observation unit for monitoring and EP testing. Patients felt to be at lower risk can be discharged, and ambulatory monitoring can be arranged by the continuing-care physician.

REFERENCES

1. Kao LW, Kirk MA, Evers SJ, Rosenfeld SH: Droperidol, QT prolongation, and sudden death: What is the evidence? *Ann Emerg Med* 41:546, 2003.
2. Anderson ME, Al-Khatib SM, Roden DM, Califf RM: Cardiac repolarization: Current knowledge, critical gaps, and new approaches to drug development and patient management. *Am Heart J* 144:769, 2002.
3. Phillips BG, Gandhi AJ, Sanoski CA, et al: Comparison of intravenous diltiazem and verapamil for the acute treatment of atrial fibrillation and atrial flutter. *Pharmacotherapy* 17:1238, 1997.
4. Vardas PE, Kochiadakis GE, Igoumenidis NE, et al: Amiodarone as a first-choice drug for restoring sinus rhythm in patients with atrial fibrillation: A randomized controlled study. *Chest* 117:1529, 2000.
5. Weigner MJ, Thomas LR, Patel U, et al: Early cardioversion of atrial fibrillation facilitated by transesophageal echocardiography: Short-term safety and impact on maintenance of sinus rhythm at 1 year. *Am J Med* 110:694, 2001.
6. Rankin AC, Brooks R, Ruskin JN, et al: Adenosine and the treatment of supraventricular tachycardia. *Am J Med* 92:655, 1992.
7. Marco CA, Cardinale JF: Adenosine for the treatment of supraventricular tachycardia in the ED. *Am J Emerg Med* 12:485, 1994.
8. Teo KK, Yusuf S, Furberg CD: Effects of prophylactic antiarrhythmic drug therapy in acute myocardial infarction. An overview of results from randomized controlled trials. *JAMA* 270:1589, 1993.
9. Epstein AE, Hallstrom AP, Rogers WJ, et al: Mortality following ventricular dysrhythmia suppression by encainide, flecainide, and moricizine after myocardial infarction: The original design concept of the Cardiac Dysrhythmia Suppression Trial (CAST). *JAMA* 270:2451, 1993.
10. Brugada P, Brugada J, Mont L, et al: A new approach to the differential diagnosis of regular tachycardia with a wide QRS complex. *Circulation* 83:1649, 1991.
11. American Heart Association: Guidelines 2000 for cardiopulmonary resuscitation and emergency cardiovascular care. *Circulation* 102(suppl):11, 2000.
12. Wellens HJ, Bar RW, Lie KI: The value of the electrocardiogram in the differential diagnosis of tachycardia with a widened QRS complex. *Am J Med* 64:27, 1978.
13. Zimetbaum P, Josephson ME: Evaluation of patients with palpitations. *New Engl J Med* 338:1369, 1998.

29 PHARMACOLOGY OF ANTIDYSRHYTHMIC AND VASOACTIVE MEDICATIONS
Elizabeth A. Clements
Bryan R. Kuhn

This chapter discusses the actions, indications, pharmacokinetics, dosing, and adverse effect profiles of antidysrhythmic and vasoactive drugs that are pertinent to emergency medicine practice. Specific antidysrhythmics and vasoactive medications also are discussed. Vasodilating agents, such as phentolamine, hydralazine, and clonidine, and other drugs used in hypertension management are discussed in Chap. 57.

ANTIDYSRHYTHMIC AGENTS

Optimal therapy of dysrhythmias requires knowledge of the mechanism of action, pharmacokinetics, indications, appropriate dosing and administration, and types of adverse effects that may occur with each medication. Antidysrhythmic drugs are divided into four classes based on their electrophysiologic properties (Table 29-1). Class I drugs are further subdivided into three subgroups.

TABLE 29-1 Electrophysiologic Actions of Antidysrhythmic Agents

Class	Subclass	Generic Name	Trade Name	Electrophysiologic Actions
I Fast sodium channel blockers	Ia	Quinidine Disopyramide Procainamide	— Norpace Pronestyl	↓↓ conduction velocity ↑ action potential duration 0/↓ automaticity (↓↓ automacticity in higher doses) ↑↑ effective refractory period 0/↑ PR, QRS, and QT intervals (drug- and dose-related)
	Ib	Lidocaine Phenytoin Mexiletine Tocainide	Xylocaine Dilantin Mexitil Tonocard	↓↓ phase 0 of action potential ↓ automaticity ↓↓ effective refractory period (in ischemic tissue) ↑ fibrillatory threshold ↓ repolarization period 0/↓ PR and QT intervals 0/↑ in AV nodal conduction
	Ic	Encainide Flecainide Propafenone Indecainide Moricizine*	Enkaid Tambocor Rhythmol Decabid Ethmozine	↓↓ phase 0 of action potential ↓ automaticity ↓↓ conduction velocity ↑ action potential duration ↑ effective refractory period ↑ PR and QRS intervals (drug- and dose-related) 0/↑ QT intervals
II β-blockers		Propranolol	Inderal	↓ conduction velocity ↑ automaticity ↑ effective refractory period ↓↓ AV nodal conduction 0/↑ PR interval 0/↓ QT interval
III		Bretylium	Bretylol	↑↑ effective refractory period 0/↑ in automaticity 0/↑ in AV conduction
		Amiodarone	Cordarone	↑ fibrillatory threshold ↑ action potential duration
		Sotalol	Betapace	0/↑ PR, QRS, and QT intervals (amiodarone)
IV Calcium channel blockers		Verapamil Diltiazem (also see text)	Isoptin Calan Cardizem	0/↓ automaticity ↓/↓↓ AV nodal conduction ↑ AV node effective refractory period ↑ PR interval
Unclassified		Digoxin Adenosine Magnesium sulfate	Lanoxin Adenocard —	0/↓ automaticity; ↑ automaticity in high levels ↓ AV nodal ↑ AV nodal refractory period ↓ refractory period in ventricle ↑ PR interval ↓ QT interval

*Very minimal negative inotropic effects.

Class I Antidysrhythmics

LIDOCAINE

Actions Lidocaine (Xylocaine), a class Ib antidysrhythmic drug, controls ventricular dysrhythmias by binding to fast sodium channels in their inactive state, thereby inhibiting recovery after repolarization in a time- and voltage-dependent manner. Lidocaine suppresses automaticity in the His-Purkinje system and spontaneous depolarization of the ventricles during diastole. Lidocaine appears to act preferentially on ischemic myocardial tissue, causing little or no effect on atrioventricular (AV) nodal or His-Purkinje conduction velocity in normal heart tissue. Lidocaine has local anesthetic effects that stabilize membranes, elevate ventricular fibrillation threshold, and suppress ventricular ectopy in tissues during myocardial ischemia. Unlike quinidine and procainamide, lidocaine has little effect on peripheral vascular tone, myocardial contractility, or cardiac output in normal doses. It does, however, possess central nervous system (CNS) depression activity and can produce sedative, analgesic, and anticonvulsant effects.[1]

Pharmacokinetics The onset of action after IV administration is 45 to 90 s, with a duration of action of 10 to 20 min. Subsequent bolus doses are generally required to maintain therapeutic plasma levels early in treatment; maintenance infusions started without an initial bolus will not attain therapeutic levels for up to 30 min to several hours. Lidocaine has apparent volumes of distribution (Vd) of 1.3 L/kg in normal patients and 0.9 L/kg in patients with liver disease, congestive heart failure (CHF), or hypotension. Lidocaine is only available for parenteral administration, because of poor gastrointestinal (GI) absorption and extensive first-pass metabolism.

Lidocaine has an initial distribution half-life of 7 to 30 min. The elimination half-life in healthy patients ranges from 80 to 108 min but may be up to 7 h in patients with CHF or liver disease, and is greatly prolonged in cardiac arrest. In healthy patients, the elimination half-lives of lidocaine's two active metabolites (MEGX and GX) are 2 and 10 h, respectively. Therapeutic serum levels range from 1.5 to 6 μg/mL; CNS effects can be seen with serum levels above 5 μg/mL.

Indications Lidocaine is used in the treatment of ventricular dysrhythmias and ectopy. In the most recent advanced cardiac life support (ACLS) guidelines, the use of lidocaine as the first-line agent in the treatment of pulseless ventricular tachycardia (VT) and ventricular fibrillation (VF) has been challenged.[2] Lidocaine may be used to maintain normal sinus rhythm after successful conversion of pulseless VT/VF by defibrillation and is a second-line agent (after procainamide and amiodarone) for hemodynamically stable VT.[3,4]

Dosing and Administration The loading dose is 1 to 1.5 mg/kg, with an additional bolus of 1 to 1.5 mg/kg to a maximum of 3 mg/kg, or 1 to 4 mg/min by continuous infusion. **The dose should be reduced by 50 percent in patients with CHF or liver disease and in those older than 70 years.** Toxicity is likely with infusions longer than 24 h, and in patients with hepatic or renal insufficiency.

The loading dose must be followed immediately by a maintenance infusion, usually starting at 2 mg/min, provided there is spontaneous circulation. With prolonged administration, serum levels should be obtained, and infusions should be adjusted accordingly. Lidocaine toxicity can result from prolonged infusions (>24 h) and in patients with renal dysfunction due to accumulation of active metabolites. Those patients who are successfully converted to normal sinus rhythm (NSR) with lidocaine and require long-term therapy should be converted to an oral antidysrhythmic within the first 24 h.

Adverse Effect Profile Adverse effects from lidocaine usually occur when excessive doses are administered or when a drug interaction potentiates toxicity. Symptoms of lidocaine toxicity that correlate with levels above 5 μg/mL include slurred speech, drowsiness, confusion, nausea, vertigo, ataxia, tinnitus, paresthesias, and muscle twitching. An abrupt change in mental status is indicative of lidocaine toxicity and may indicate that an excessive dose was administered. Serious symptoms occurring at plasma levels above 9 μg/mL may include psychosis, seizures, and respiratory depression. Lidocaine is contraindicated in patients with known sensitivities to amide-type anesthetics and those with high degrees of sinoatrial (SA) or AV block.

PROCAINAMIDE

Actions Procainamide (Pronestyl), a class Ia antidysrhythmic agent, shares the same mechanism of action as the other class Ia agents, disopyramide (Norpace) and quinidine (various). Class Ia antiarrhythmic agents suppress automaticity by binding with fast sodium channels in their inactive state and thereby inhibit recovery after repolarization in a time- and voltage-dependent manner. Procainamide prolongs the action potential duration and reduces the speed of impulse conduction, which directly depresses myocardial conduction, suppresses fibrillatory activity in the atria and ventricles, and prevents ectopic or reentrant dysrhythmias. In therapeutic plasma concentrations, procainamide causes prolongation of the PR and QT intervals, and the QRS complex.

Procainamide also has anticholinergic properties. Large doses can exaggerate the anticholinergic activity and may even increase automaticity (i.e., a pro-dysrhythmic effect). Class Ia antidysrhythmic agents may decrease the force of myocardial contraction by inhibition of calcium transport across the cell membrane. The negative inotropic effect is more pronounced in ischemic myocardial tissue. At high plasma concentrations, procainamide may result in hypotension

caused by vasodilation of the peripheral vasculature. This hypotension can produce a sinus tachycardia as a result of a reflexive sympathetic response to hypotension.

Pharmacokinetics The onset of action of procainamide is 5 to 10 min after IV administration and 10 to 30 min after IM injection. Procainamide has an initial half-life of 4 to 5 min and a terminal half-life of 2.5 to 4.7 h in patients with normal renal function. The apparent Vd is 2 L/kg. However, in patients with CHF and renal dysfunction, the elimination half-life may increase and the Vd decreases, thus requiring a smaller dose. Procainamide is metabolized via acetylation in the liver to an active metabolite, N-acetyl procainamide (NAPA). This metabolite has antidysrhythmic activity and may represent more than 50 percent of the total drug in plasma. N-acetyl procainamide has an average half-life of 7 h in patients with normal renal function. Acetylation is related to genetic phenotype, with rapid acetylators converting greater amounts of procainamide to NAPA than slow acetylators. Plasma procainamide levels of 4 to 8 μg/mL are usually required to suppress ventricular dysrhythmias. Refractory dysrhythmias may require levels up to 20 μg/mL (usually 10 to 15 μg/mL). However, adverse events are associated with plasma levels above 12 μg/mL.

Indications Procainamide is used to treat and prevent recurrence of ventricular dysrhythmias, specifically stable VT and wide complex tachycardia of unknown type in patients with preserved left ventricular (LV) function and unresponsive pulseless VT/VF. Procainamide also may be used for converting supraventricular tachycardias (SVT), including atrial flutter and fibrillation, even if associated with Wolff-Parkinson-White (WPW) syndrome and paroxysmal supraventricular tachycardia (PSVT). It is infrequently used in VF or pulseless VT, because the dosing requires prolonged administration times. Contraindications include complete AV heart block, second- or third-degree heart block (without an electrical pacemaker present), bundle-branch block or severe cardiac glycoside intoxication, prolonged QT interval, and torsades de pointes. Procainamide should be used with caution in patients with systemic lupus erythematosus (SLE), CHF, bone marrow suppression or cytopenia of any type, and hepatic or renal disease and those with allergies to procaine or ester-type local anesthetics.

Dosing and Administration Previous recommendations for IV loading of procainamide called for a bolus injection. However, a continuous infusion rate has been shown to be safer (fewer adverse effects). Typically, a loading dose starts at 20 mg/min (in urgent situations, 30 mg/min) and is instituted until any of the following occur: a maximum dose of 17 mg/kg is reached, termination of the dysrhythmia, prolongation of the QRS interval by greater than 50 percent of baseline, or hypotension. If procainamide loading suppresses the dysrhythmia, a continuous infusion of 1 to 4 mg/min is used to maintain the suppression. Alternatively, oral therapy may be started after IV loading with an immediate-release preparation (50 mg/kg daily given in divided doses every 3 h) or a sustained-release preparation (500 to 1000 mg PO every 6 to 8 h). Normal procainamide and NAPA levels are 4 to 12 μg/mL and 10 to 30 μg/mL, respectively. Lower doses may be required for patients with hypotension, CHF, and renal or hepatic dysfunction. Daily procainamide or NAPA levels should be followed in patients with risk factors for impaired clearance.

Adverse Effect Profile The most serious adverse effects of procainamide are from myocardial depression. Electrocardiographic changes may include QRS and QT interval prolongations, VT, VF, frequent premature ventricular contractions (PVCs), complete AV block, and torsades de pointes. Procainamide should be discontinued if any of these ECG changes appear. High doses or rapid infusion rates are associated with significant hypotension. The pro-dysrhythmic effects may be more pronounced in patients with extensive myocardial injury. Procainamide and NAPA levels should be monitored in the following patients: those receiving procainamide longer than 24 h, those on a maintenance infusion of 3 mg/min or higher, and those with acute CHF or renal failure.

Antinuclear antibodies are found in at least 50 percent of individuals receiving long-term therapy with procainamide (usually within 2 to 18 months) that can increase the risk of developing SLE. Hypersensitivity reactions may occur as a result of sensitization by the parent compound (an ester-type structure). Serious hematologic effect also can occur, including agranulocytosis, leukopenia, bone marrow suppression, hypoplastic anemia, and thrombocytopenia. **Procainamide is contraindicated in patients with myasthenia gravis,** because it may increase weakness.

OTHER CLASS I AGENTS   Propafenone and flecainide are class Ic antiarrhythmics that are available. Encainide is also a class Ic antiarrhythmic but was voluntarily withdrawn by the manufacturer in 1991. Flecainide use has been limited by significant adverse effects, although it can be used in the treatment of atrial fibrillation/flutter of recent-onset (<48 h) to convert rhythm to sinus in patients with preserved LV function. The dose of flecainide is 2 mg/kg at 10 mg/min IV (the IV preparation is not available in the United States).

Propafenone, interestingly, has recently been used in the treatment of recent-onset atrial fibrillation in the ED in Europe (namely Italy and Spain). In each of the two studies, patients with recent onset atrial fibrillation (<72 h) were randomized to propafenone, 450 to 750 mg PO as a single dose (Azpitarte) or 2 mg/kg IV for 10 min (Ganau), or placebo. Although both studies found significantly more patients receiving propafenone who converted to sinus rhythm early, the oral load study found no difference at 24 h when compared with placebo. Hypotension was the most common adverse effect in the propafenone-treated patients. This is known to occur especially in patients with LV dysfunction. In the acute setting, there is more evidence supporting the use of agents, such as ibutilide, amiodarone, or procainamide, all of which are available in intravenous form in the United States.[5,6]

Class II Antidysrhythmics: Beta Blockers

GENERAL INFORMATION

Actions and Pharmacokinetics   There are many β-blockers from which a clinician can choose to treat various disease states. Although these drugs share the principal characteristic of blocking catecholamine effects on β-receptors, they differ with respect to cardioselectivity, intrinsic sympathomimetic activity (ISA), α-adrenergic blocking activity, membrane-stabilizing effect, and pharmacokinetic properties.

Cardioselective β-blocking (specific for β_1-receptors) drugs include acebutolol, atenolol, esmolol, and metoprolol. They may be better choices for use in patients with a history of asthma, chronic obstructive pulmonary disease, or diabetes, because the blockade of β_2 receptors may result in adverse effects. At high doses, these drugs lose their cardioselectivity. Unfortunately, the dose at which this occurs has not been clearly established.

β-Blockers with ISA, such as acebutolol, carteolol, penbutolol, and pindolol, occupy the β receptor and produce a low level of stimulation. Despite this stimulation, the receptor is functionally blocked to high sympathetic tone. Theoretically, these drugs would be safer because of their intrinsic ability to stimulate the heart. This ability may prevent acute drug-induced heart failure, but this has not been proven in clinical trials.

β-Blockers with α-blocking activity are covered later in this chapter (see Labetalol).

Membrane-stabilizing effect is a characteristic of propranolol, acebutolol, pindolol, and alprenolol, which results in a reduction of membrane permeability to the fast inward current of sodium ions. This is otherwise known as a quinidine-like effect. Although the clinical relevance of this effect is unknown, the membrane-stabilizing effect is usually seen at supra-therapeutic doses and may precipitate a prolongation of the QRS complex.

Indications   With the exception of esmolol and sotalol, all β-blockers are indicated for the treatment of hypertension. Cardio-selective beta blockers are used in patients with asthma or insulin-dependent diabetes, but drugs with ISA may be better tolerated by some patients (e.g., CHF patients, although there are no clinical data to support this). Some β-blockers have been shown to decrease morbidity and mortality in patients with acute myocardial infarction (e.g., metoprolol and atenolol) and CHF (metoprolol and carvedilol). Beta-blockers should be administered within 12 h of an acute myocardial infarction[7] if no contraindications exist. β-Blockers in the acutely decompensated CHF patient may further aggravate the heart failure. β-Blockers, if desirable, are typically instituted in the stable CHF patient at doses lower than those used to treat hypertension.

Adverse Effect Profile   Adverse effects are remarkably similar across this class of agents and include nausea, vomiting, lightheadedness, mental depression, bradycardia, hypotension, bronchospasm, hyperglycemia, and pulmonary edema. Cardioselective drugs cause less bronchospasm and hyperglycemia than do nonselective drugs, but they can mask the symptoms of hypoglycemia (e.g., blocking tachycardia and blood pressure changes, but not sweating). These drugs are generally contraindicated in patients with heart block other than first-degree or cardiogenic shock.

ESMOLOL

Actions   Esmolol (Brevibloc) is a short-acting drug selectively blocking β_1-receptors in the myocardium, with minimal effect on β_2-receptors of bronchial and vascular smooth muscle. As with other β-blocking drugs, esmolol exhibits negative inotropic and chronotropic effects. Esmolol prevents excessive adrenergic stimulation of the myocardium by blocking the β_1-receptors, thus producing an increase in sinus cycle length, prolongation of SA nodal recovery time, and a decrease in conduction through the AV node. At higher doses (e.g., >300 µg/kg per min), the β_1 selectivity usually diminishes, and the drug will competitively inhibit β_1 and β_2-receptors. Esmolol is effective in treating SVT and elevated blood pressure. Antihypertensive effects may be due to its ability to decrease cardiac output, sympathetic outflow, and renin release from the kidneys.

Pharmacokinetics   Esmolol is available only in a parenteral formulation with an onset of action of 1 to 4 min. Compared with other β-blockers, esmolol has the shortest duration of action. The elimination half-life is approximately 9 min, and complete reversal of drug effects are seen within 30 min after discontinuation of IV administration. This short duration of action makes esmolol an attractive drug for the management of acute unstable SVT. Although 90 percent of esmolol is eliminated in urine as metabolites, the metabolites possess minimal, if any, β-blocking activity. Therefore, dosing adjustments are not required in renal or hepatic insufficiency.

Indications   Esmolol is an ultra-short-acting, cardioselective β-blocker that is effective in the treatment of supraventricular dysrhythmias, including atrial fibrillation/flutter and sinus tachycardia in acute myocardial ischemia.

Dosing and Administration   The loading dose is a 500 µg/kg bolus over 1 min, followed by an infusion at 50 µg/kg per min for 4 min. If there is no response, another 500 µg/kg bolus should be given and the infusion increased to 100 µg/kg per min. Thereafter, the bolus should be repeated and the infusion increased to 200 µg/kg per min. Hypotension is the most common adverse effect and depends on dose.

Infusion rates greater than 200 μg/kg per min have not been studied for safety.

Adverse Effect Profile   The most common adverse effect is hypotension. Other cardiovascular adverse effects include bradycardia, syncope, and heart block. Abrupt discontinuation may cause rebound hypertension or angina. Other adverse effects may include bronchospasm or pulmonary edema producing wheezing, dyspnea, rhonchi, and rales.

LABETALOL

Actions   Labetalol (Normodyne, Trandate) is a non-cardioselective β-adrenergic blocking agent and a selective α_1-adrenergic blocking agent. The β-blocking effects of labetalol are greater than the α_1-blocking effects, in ratios of 3:1 in the oral formulation and 7:1 in the parenteral formulation. The mechanisms by which labetalol elicits its antihypertensive effects may include any or all of the following: (1) synergistic effects resulting in hypotension when α_1 and β_1-receptors are blocked, (2) β_2-receptor stimulation, and (3) direct vasodilatory action. Labetalol decreases heart rate, contractility, cardiac output, cardiac work, and total peripheral resistance.

Pharmacokinetics   The onsets of action of labetalol are 2 to 5 min after IV administration and 20 min to 2 h after oral administration. The durations of action are 2 to 4 h after IV administration and 8 to 24 h after oral administration. Labetalol is eliminated primarily by the liver and undergoes extensive first-pass metabolism, with approximately 25 percent of an oral dose reaching the circulation. First-pass metabolism may be reduced in the elderly and those with hepatic dysfunction. Labetalol has an apparent Vd of 3.2 to 15.7 L/kg. The elimination half-life is approximately 2.5 to 8 h.

Indications   Labetalol is used principally for its antihypertensive effects. Intravenous labetalol rapidly and effectively reduces elevated blood pressures, causing only minimal alterations in heart rate and cardiac output. It is a good choice for treating hypertension in patients with myocardial ischemia. It has little effect on cerebral perfusion pressure or intracranial pressure and can be used in patients with acute neurologic emergencies. Oral labetalol may be substituted once control of blood pressure has been established. It has also been used safely during pregnancy.

Dosing and Administration   Labetalol can be administered intravenously by multiple boluses or as a continuous infusion. The initial dose for an IV bolus is 20 mg followed by repeat doses of 40 to 80 mg every 10 min until the desired effect is reached or a maximum cumulative dose of 300 mg is attained. It is best to double the previous dose when using multiple boluses to provide a gradual increase in dose. A smaller alternative dose would be 10 to 15 mg every 15 min. Alternatively, labetalol can be administered as a continuous IV infusion at a rate of 0.5 to 2 mg/min until the desired effect is reached. There are reports of labetalol being used as a continuous infusion for longer than 24 h in severe and refractory cases. **Patients receiving labetalol as a continuous infusion should be placed in a supine position** and remain so approximately 3 h after receiving any IV doses, because symptomatic orthostatic hypotension may occur. Acute dosing of IV labetalol can lead to a "cumulative effect," because each dose will persist for 2 to 4 h. These patients must be diligently observed to avoid hypotensive episodes. After stabilization, a patient can be converted to oral labetalol (up to 2400 mg per d in two to four divided doses).

Adverse Effect Profile   Labetalol has the same adverse effect profile as other β- and α-blocking agents. The most frequent adverse effect is symptomatic orthostatic hypotension, which can occur in up to 5 and 60 percent of patients after oral and IV administration, respectively. Symptomatic heart failure also may occur. Adverse CNS effects may include lightheadedness, drowsiness, dizziness, fatigue, lethargy, and vivid nightmares. However, these effects may be obviated by the slow, upward titration of the dosage over 4 to 12 weeks. Labetalol also may cause reversible increases in the hepatic enzymes or, rarely, jaundice and hepatitis.

PROPRANOLOL

Actions   In therapeutic doses, the major effect of propranolol (Inderal) is its β-adrenergic blocking activity. The drug competitively blocks the effects of β-adrenergic stimuli on receptors within the myocardium and bronchial and vascular smooth muscles. Propranolol is a non-cardioselective β-blocker without ISA. Inhibition of myocardial β-receptors decreases chronotropic, inotropic, and vasodilator responses to β-adrenergic stimuli. Propranolol slows the sinus rate, depresses AV conduction, decreases cardiac output, prevents exercise-induced increases in blood pressure, and reduces supine and standing blood pressures. Propranolol also decreases myocardial oxygen consumption.

Pharmacokinetics   The onset of action of propranolol is 1 to 2 h after an oral dose and within 1 min after IV administration. The half-life shows great variability. Short-term treatment has an elimination half-life of 2 to 3 h, whereas long-term treatment has an elimination half-life of 3.4 to 6 h. Propranolol is widely distributed throughout body tissue, undergoes extensive first-pass metabolism after oral administration, and is significantly bound to sites within the liver. For these reasons, propranolol has a low bioavailability when taken PO as opposed to IV administration, making the IV dose approximately one tenth of the oral dose. The Vd of propranolol is 6 L/kg, but varies widely in proportion to the fraction of unbound drug in whole blood. At least eight metabolites have been identified and are principally excreted in the urine. No dose adjustments are required for patients with renal insufficiency.

Indications   Propranolol is indicated for a wide variety of supraventricular dysrhythmias. These include multifocal atrial tachycardia (MFAT), in particular those dysrhythmias induced by digoxin or catecholamines; rate control of atrial flutter or fibrillation with preserved LV function excluding those associated with WPW; persistent atrial extrasystoles that do not respond to conventional therapy; and tachydysrhythmia associated with thyrotoxicosis. Propranolol is less effective for ventricular than for supraventricular dysrhythmias, but it can be used for ventricular tachycardias or ectopy due to digoxin or catecholamine toxicity and polymorphic ventricular tachycardia.

Other indications for propranolol include the management of angina, because it decreases myocardial oxygen demand; management of all chronic types of hypertension alone or in combination with other antihypertensive agents (propranolol is not indicated for hypertensive emergencies); the treatment of hypertrophic cardiomyopathy; prophylaxis for common migraine headaches; management of familial or hereditary essential tremor; and as an adjunctive drug after administration of an α-adrenergic blocker in controlling tachycardia due to pheochromocytoma. Propranolol has been used to reduce the autonomic symptoms associated with anxiety disorders (mild tremor, tachycardia, and sweating).

Dosing and Administration   The loading dose is 0.5 to 1 mg IV at a rate not to exceed 1 mg per min. The dose may be repeated after 2 min. Esmolol is as effective as propranolol in decreasing heart rate and is titrated more easily.

Because significant myocardial depression can occur with doses larger than 3 mg, caution should be used if additional doses are required.

Adverse Effect Profile   The adverse effect profile for propranolol is similar to that for the non-cardioselective β-blockers. The drug is generally not given to patients with asthma or allergic rhinitis and is contraindicated in those with sinus bradycardia or advanced SA or AV block and intermittent claudication. Propranolol also should not be used in CHF or cardiogenic shock, unless these conditions are due to tachydysrhythmia.

SOTALOL

Actions   Sotalol (Betapace) is a unique non-cardioselective β-blocker without ISA or membrane-stabilizing activity. The mechanism of action is similar to that of other non-cardioselective β-blockers by inhibiting the response of adrenergic stimuli in the myocardium and bronchial and vascular smooth muscles. Sotalol also exhibits electrophysiologic characteristics of class III antiarrhythmics (i.e., prolongs repolarization and refractoriness without affecting conduction). Sotalol is available only in an oral formulation in the United States, which contains a racemic mixture of the two optical isomers, although only the *l*-isomer exhibits β-blocking activity.

Pharmacokinetics   The onset of action after oral administration is 2 to 3 h, with duration of action of approximately 24 h after one dose. The elimination half-life is 7 to 18 h in the normal patient and depends on renal function. Patients with a creatinine clearance (CrCl) of 10 to 30 mL/min have an elimination half-life of 22 to 24 h and up to 97 h in patients with a CrCl of less than 10 mL/min. No metabolites are formed, and the drug is principally eliminated unchanged in the urine.

Indications   Sotalol has been shown to be an effective agent for the suppression of life-threatening ventricular dysrhythmias refractory to other antidysrhythmic drugs. Clinical trials have shown sotalol to be effective in patients who have been refractory to other conventional antidysrhythmic drugs. Although not approved for this indication by the U.S. Food and Drug Administration, double-blind trials have shown that sotalol can suppress SVT and atrial fibrillation.[2]

Dosing and Administration   The usual initial oral dose is 80 mg twice daily, which can be titrated every 3 days between dosing increments to allow for attainment of steady-state plasma concentrations and to monitor for changes in the QT interval. The usual maintenance dose is 160 to 320 mg per d. The dosing intervals should be increased to every 24 h when CrCl is 30 to 59 mL/min and to 36 to 48 h when CrCl is 10 to 29 mL/min. The dosing interval should be individualized when CrCl is less than 10 mL/min. The maximum dose is 480 to 640 mg per d and should be used only when the potential benefits outweigh the increased risk of adverse effects (e.g., pro-dysrhythmic activity).

Adverse Effect Profile   Sotalol is generally well tolerated, and the adverse effects are dose related; the most common are related to that of non-cardioselective β-blockade (e.g., bradycardia, hypotension, and hypo- or hyperglycemia). Sotalol also can have pro-dysrhythmic effects, particularly in patients with torsade de pointes, prolonged QTc intervals, hypokalemia, or those taking high doses of the drug.

Class III Antidysrhythmic Drugs

AMIODARONE

Actions   Although the exact mechanism of action has not been conclusively determined, amiodarone (Cordarone) is classified as a class III antidysrhythmic. The primary effect of the drug on cardiac tissue is to delay repolarization by prolonging the action potential duration and effective refractory period, especially when administered for a long period. Amiodarone slows the heart by impairing SA nodal function, depressing AV nodal conduction, modifying the automaticity of spontaneously firing fibers in the Purkinje system, and prolonging the refractory period in an accessory pathway (e.g., WPW syndrome). The drug also produces an inhibition of sodium channels and β-adrenergic activity, further contributing to the antidysrhythmic effects.

Pharmacokinetics   Most of the pharmacokinetic information in the literature is for the oral formulation. Due to a rapid redistribution phase, the concentration of amiodarone declines to 10 percent of peak values within 30 to 45 min after the end of IV infusion. Amiodarone is approximately 96 percent bound to plasma proteins. The apparent Vd of the major metabolite averages to 65.8 L/kg (range, 18.3 to 147.7 L/kg) after IV administration. Amiodarone is metabolized in the liver and eliminated by biliary excretion. The terminal half-life is 25 days after IV therapy. However, after chronic oral therapy, the terminal half-life increases to 40 to 55 days, with maximal antidysrhythmic effects usually seen within 1 to 5 months.

Indications   Oral amiodarone appears to be effective in the management of a wide variety of ventricular and supraventricular dysrhythmias. However, due to its potentially life-threatening adverse effect profile, chronic amiodarone therapy is used only to suppress and prevent the recurrence of life-threatening ventricular dysrhythmias that do not respond to documented adequate dosages of other currently available antidysrhythmic drugs or when these drugs cannot be tolerated. Amiodarone has been used effectively in the suppression and prevention of recurrent ventricular fibrillation and tachycardia, atrial fibrillation and flutter, and junctional and wide-complex tachycardias. It has recently been added to the ACLS pathway to treat patients with pulseless VT/VF and atrial dysrhythmias with a significant decrease in ejection fraction (i.e., ≤40 percent).

Dosing and Administration   For VF/pulseless VT, the loading dose is a 300-mg IV bolus that may be repeated with a 150-mg bolus. For other dysrhythmias, the dose is 150 mg IV in 100 mL D5W over 10 min. The loading dose is followed by an infusion at 1 mg/min for 6 h, and then 0.5 mg/min thereafter. Oral maintenance doses typically are 200 to 600 mg per d.

Amiodarone is available in oral and IV formulations. Either formulation is as effective as loading and maintenance doses in stable patients.

Alternatively, oral daily loading doses of 800 to 1600 mg per d are generally required for 1 to 3 weeks until an initial therapeutic response occurs. When adequate control of the dysrhythmia is achieved or adverse effects become apparent, the dosage should be reduced to 200 to 600 mg as a single oral dose. Short-term IV therapy is associated with bradycardia and hypotension. Long-term oral therapy is associated with thyroid disorders, pulmonary fibrosis, skin discoloration, hepatic dysfunction, and other conditions.Before long-term treatment, patients should undergo baseline ophthalmologic and pulmonary function tests.

Adverse Effect Profile   After IV administration, adverse effects are typically limited to hypotension and bradycardia, although asystole, cardiac arrest, and shock have been reported. However, after chronic oral therapy, amiodarone exhibits several serious and potentially fatal toxicities, including pulmonary fibrosis, pro-dysrhythmic activity, and hepatotoxicity. In patients receiving more than 400 mg per d, some adverse effects are present in up to 75 percent of those patients and will be responsible for discontinuance in up to 20 percent of patients. The most common adverse reactions requiring discontinuance of the drug are pulmonary infiltrates or fibrosis, paroxysmal ventricular tachycardia, CHF, and elevations in the serum hepatic enzyme concentrations. The likelihood of most adverse effects appears to increase after the first 6 months of therapy and remains relatively constant beyond 1 year of therapy. Corneal microdeposits are reported in all patients after chronic administration. Additional adverse effects include rash, skin discoloration, constipation and other GI symptoms, and falsely elevating or decreasing thyroid function tests. Amiodarone contains iodine, 37.3 percent by weight and, as such, is contraindicated in patients with an iodine or shellfish allergy.

Amiodarone is also responsible for several clinically significant drug interactions. Initiation of amiodarone therapy after warfarin therapy is stabilized can result in a 50 percent decrease in warfarin metabolism and subsequent increase risk of bleeding. Amiodarone increases serum concentrations of many drugs, including digoxin, procainamide, quinidine, theophylline, and others. Concurrent use of amiodarone with calcium channel or β-blockers may potentiate sinus bradycardia, sinus arrest, and AV block.

DOFETILIDE

Actions Dofetilide (Tikosyn) is a class III antidysrhythmic agent that prolongs repolarization without affecting the conduction velocity. Dofetilide is a pure class III antidysrhythmic, because it selectively blocks the cardiac delayed rectifier potassium current. Other class III antiarrhythmics, such as amiodarone or sotalol, possess class I or II antiarrhythmic properties in addition to class III properties. The cardiac delayed rectifier potassium current is responsible for termination of the action potential plateau. Dofetilide prolongs the action potential duration, atrial and ventricular effective refractory periods, and the effective refractory period of the accessory pathway. This results in prolongation of the QT and QTc intervals without change in the QRS interval. This result allows dofetilide to suppress dysrhythmias dependent on a reentry mechanism. Dofetilide produces a dose-dependent negative chronotropic effect but lacks negative inotropic effects. Given IV, it is effective for the conversion of atrial fibrillation to NSR.[8] However, only the oral formulation is available in the United States.

Pharmacokinetics The onset of action of dofetilide is 2 h, and the duration of action is 4 h after oral administration. The time to peak response occurs in 1 to 3 h after oral administration. Dofetilide is well absorbed from the GI tract, with a bioavailability of 96 to 100 percent and is not affected by food or antacids. The apparent Vd is 3 to 4 L/kg. Approximately 50 percent of a dose is metabolized by the liver (cytochrome $3A_4$) to inactive metabolites, with about 80 percent of the drug and metabolites eliminated in the urine. The elimination half-life is 7.5 to 10 h after oral administration and is increased in patients with renal insufficiency.

Indications Dofetilide is indicated for the conversion to, and maintenance of, NSR in patients with atrial fibrillation or flutter. However, because dofetilide has a significant pro-dysrhythmic effect, it should be reserved for patients in whom atrial fibrillation or flutter is highly symptomatic.

Dosing and Administration The loading dose is based on QTc interval and CrCl. If the baseline QTc interval is longer than 440 ms, dofetilide is contraindicated. The doses are 500 μg PO twice a day when the CrCl is greater than 60 mL/min, 250 μg PO twice a day when the CrCl is 40 to 60 mL/min, and 125 μg PO twice a day when the CrCl is 20 to 39 mL/min. Dofetilide is contraindicated if the CrCl is less than 20 mL/min, the baseline QTc interval is longer than 440 ms, or the QTc interval exceeds 500 ms while on therapy. The ECG is repeated 2 to 3 h after the dose. If the QTc interval is less than 15 percent from baseline, the current dose is continued; if it is greater than 15 percent from baseline, the dose is decreased.

Patients should be admitted for a minimum of 3 days to a facility that can provide CrCl calculations, continuous ECG monitoring, and cardiac resuscitation. Prescribing is restricted to physicians with evidence of having received educational information of dofetilide dosing and administration.

Adverse Effect Profile The most serious adverse effect of dofetilide is QTc interval prolongation, which can result in torsade de pointes. The risk of developing torsade de pointes is associated with larger dofetilide doses, occurring during the first few days of therapy, and in patients with electrolyte imbalances. Ventricular tachycardia is another adverse effect associated with dofetilide. The most common adverse effects reported in clinical trials are headache, dizziness, and chest pain. Dofetilide is contraindicated in patients with a CrCl of less than 20 mL/min or a QTc interval longer than 440 ms before initiating therapy or 500 ms at any time after initiating therapy.

IBUTILIDE

Actions Ibutilide (Corvert) is a class III antidysrhythmic agent that prolongs the action potential duration and effective refractory period in atrial and ventricular cardiac tissues. This action is caused by activation of a slow inward sodium current, as opposed to inhibition of outward potassium currents. However, data suggest that blockade of the delayed rectifier potassium current, which slows repolarization, may contribute, in a minor way, to its clinical effects.

Pharmacokinetics The onset of action of ibutilide is 20 to 30 min, with a duration of action of 24 h after one IV dose. The apparent Vd is 9 to 13 L/kg. Ibutilide is metabolized in the liver via oxidation to several metabolites, of which at least one has significant activity. Approximately 80 percent of an IV dose is eliminated in urine within 24 h, with the remaining 20 percent being excreted in feces over a period of 1 week. The elimination half-life of the parent compound is 2 to 12 h (average, 6 h) after IV administration.

Indications Ibutilide is indicated for the rapid conversion of recent-onset (<30 days) atrial fibrillation or flutter to NSR. Atrial dysrhythmias that are not of recent onset may be less likely to respond to ibutilide. Ibutilide may be used as an alternative to electrical cardioversion, which is one of the most rapid and frequently used methods of converting atrial fibrillation and atrial flutter of less than 48 h duration.

Dosing and Administration Ibutilide is administered only as an IV infusion. The loading dose is 1 mg IV in 50 mL D5W over 10 min (patient weight >60 kg) or 0.01 mg/kg IV in 50 mL D5W over 10 min (patient weight <60 kg). The dose may be repeated 10 min after completion of the first dose. Electrocardiographic monitoring is continued for at least 4 h or until the QTc interval returns to baseline, or longer if dysrhythmias are observed.

Adverse Effect Profile Cardiovascular adverse effects include hypotension, hypertension, bradycardia, sinus arrest, syncope, prolongation of the QTc interval, and CHF. Ibutilide is capable of inducing or exacerbating dysrhythmias, such as sustained polymorphic ventricular tachycardia including torsade de pointes, supraventricular and ventricular extrasystoles, and monomorphic ventricular tachycardia. Patients should be observed with continuous ECG monitoring for at least 4 h after infusion or until the QTc interval has returned to baseline. Longer monitoring is required if any dysrhythmic activity is noted.

Class IV Antidysrhythmic Drugs: Calcium Channel Antagonists

DILTIAZEM

Actions Diltiazem (Cardizem) is a non-dihydropyridine calcium channel antagonist that interferes with the influx of extracellular calcium through "slow" channels in the cardiac smooth muscle. At doses slightly higher than those used clinically, diltiazem also inhibits the influx of sodium through "fast" channels. The net result is a slowing of AV nodal conduction (although less than with equivalent doses of verapamil) and a prolongation of AV nodal refractoriness. Diltiazem produces minimal systemic vasodilation and preferentially dilates the coronary vasculature, allowing for a decrease in oxygen consumption, improved oxygen delivery, and an overall improvement in oxygen balance in those with chronic stable angina. Although diltiazem has no effect on sinus node recovery or the SA conduction time in patients without SA nodal dysfunction, patients with sick sinus syndrome experience a decrease in SA node automaticity.

Pharmacokinetics   The onset of action of diltiazem is 2 to 3 min after IV administration and 15 to 60 min after oral administration, with peak responses in 2 to 7 min and 1.5 to 4 h after IV and oral administrations, respectively. The duration of action is 1 to 3 h after single IV administration but can be prolonged up to 10 h after multiple IV doses. The bioavailability of oral diltiazem is 35 to 40 percent due to first-pass metabolism. The elimination half-life is 3.1 to 6.6 h. However, the extended- and controlled-release formulations have a longer time-to-peak response and longer elimination half-life: 3 to 6 h and 4.5 to 10 h, respectively. This results in once-daily dosing of the controlled-release formulations and twice-daily dosing of the extended-release formulations. The apparent Vd is 5.3 L/kg. Diltiazem undergoes extensive hepatic metabolism to active and inactive metabolites.

Indications   Intravenous diltiazem is effective for rapid conversion of PSVT to NSR and to slow ventricular response in atrial fibrillation or atrial flutter. It should not be used in patients with a wide-complex tachydysrhythmia suggesting an accessory bypass tract (e.g., WPW syndrome). Oral diltiazem is indicated for the treatment of vasospastic and chronic stable angina and is considered one of the drugs of choice for vasospastic angina. The extended-release formulations are indicated for the treatment of hypertension alone or in combination with other antihypertensives.

Dosing and Administration   The loading dose is 0.25 mg/kg (maximum, 20 mg) IV push over 2 min. The dose is repeated in 15 min with 0.35 mg/kg (maximum, 25 mg) IV push over 2 min, if the patient is not responsive.

The recommended initial infusion rate is 5 mg per h, (which can be increased to 15 mg per h if required). Once the heart rate is controlled, the patient can be converted from IV to oral diltiazem. The IV infusion should be continued for 1 h after the first oral dose to allow for adequate peak oral response.

The approximate oral dosage (in mg per d) can be calculated as follows: (infusion rate [mg/hr] $\times$ 3 + 3) $\times$ 10. This daily dose can be given as the short-acting formulation (in four divided doses) for the first 24 h and then converted to a long-acting formulation thereafter.

The maximal antihypertensive effect is usually observed within 14 days. Dose adjustments should be made accordingly. Dosages may need to be decreased in patients with hepatic or renal insufficiency.

Adverse Effect Profile   The cardiovascular side effects associated with diltiazem may include angina, bradycardia, asystole, CHF, AV block, bundle branch block, flushing, hypotension, palpitations, and peripheral edema. Noncardiac adverse effects may include headache, dizziness, nausea, constipation, rash, vomiting, diarrhea, dry mouth, pruritus, nervousness, somnolence, insomnia, tinnitus, depression, sexual dysfunction, hyperglycemia, and photosensitivity. Diltiazem also may cause transient increases in liver function test enzymes, which may resolve despite continued therapy with diltiazem. Cimetidine increases serum diltiazem through inhibition of its metabolism.

VERAPAMIL

Actions   Verapamil (Verelan, Isoptin, Calan, and Tarka), a non-dihydropyridine calcium channel antagonist, is a class IV antidysrhyth-

mic agent. Like other calcium channel antagonists, the principal action is to inhibit the transmembrane influx of extracellular calcium ions across the membrane of myocardial cells and vascular smooth muscle. However, unlike dihydropyridine calcium channel antagonists, verapamil has substantial inhibitory effects on the cardiac conduction system. It slows conduction and prolongs refractoriness in the AV node and, rarely, may reduce the resting heart rate and produce sinus arrest or SA block in patients with SA node dysfunction (e.g., sick sinus syndrome). In patients with PSVT, verapamil's effects at the AV node result in an interruption of the reentrant pathway and restoration of NSR. Verapamil also decreases the ventricular response in patients with atrial fibrillation/flutter. It has minimal or no effects on antegrade or retrograde conduction of the accessory pathways.

Pharmacokinetics   The onset of action of verapamil is within 5 min, a peak response of 10 to 20 min, and a duration of action of 30 to 60 min after IV administration. The onset, peak response, and duration after oral administration are 1 to 2 h, 4 to 11 h (depending on oral formulation), and 6 to 12 h, respectively. The apparent Vd is 12 L/kg. Verapamil is metabolized extensively in the liver to at least 12 metabolites, at least one of which is active (approximately 20 percent activity of the parent compound). Approximately 70 and 16 percent of oral and IV doses, respectively, are eliminated in the urine and feces as metabolites within 5 days. The elimination half-life after one oral dose or IV infusion is 2 to 8 h. After 1 to 2 days of therapy, the half-life increases to 4.5 to 12 h, presumably due to saturation of hepatic enzymes. Plasma half-life can be prolonged to 14 to 16 h in patients with hepatic insufficiency.

Indications   Verapamil is as effective as adenosine and diltiazem in terminating narrow-complex PSVT and for controlling the ventricular response in atrial fibrillation/flutter. Oral verapamil can be used for the management of vasospastic, chronic stable, and unstable angina and may be used for the prophylaxis of PSVT. It is also used for essential hypertension. Verapamil should not be used for the management of atrial fibrillation/flutter in patients with an accessory bypass tract (e.g., WPW or Lown-Ganong-Levine syndrome), because life-threatening adverse effects (e.g., ventricular fibrillation and/or cardiac arrest) may occur due to accelerated accessory bypass tract conduction.

Dosing and Administration   For the treatment of PSVT, the initial dose is 5 to 10 mg IV push over 2 min, although some experts recommend an initial dose of 2.5 to 5 mg IV push over 2 min to minimize adverse effects, particularly in elderly patients and those with hepatic dysfunction. Blood pressure should be checked immediately before and after verapamil administration. Pretreatment with calcium chloride or gluconate (500 to 1000 mg) can be given before or after verapamil administration to prevent or manage verapamil-induced hypotension, although calcium use is largely anecdotal. For the prevention of recurrent PSVT, oral administration of 240 to 480 mg per d should be given. Maximum antidysrhythmic effects are generally seen within 48 h after initiating verapamil therapy. For the treatment of vasospastic, unstable, or chronic stable angina, oral doses of 240 to 480 mg per d in three to four divided doses can be given, although efficacy with doses larger than 360 mg per d have not been proven. Conversion to an extended-release formulation should be done as soon as dose titration is completed with a satisfactory clinical response. The dose of the extended-release formulation is the total daily dose of the immediate-release formulation. The initial dose for the treatment of hypertension is 240 mg every morning, with titration upward by 120-mg increments in the evening. Antihypertensive effects are evident within the first week of therapy.

Adverse Effect Profile   Most adverse effects are related to its pharmacologic properties. The incidence of adverse effects is increased in patients with severe heart failure, cardiomyopathy, or conduction disturbances. Hypotension, bradycardia, AV block, bundle branch block, and pulmonary edema are possible cardiac adverse effects. Noncardiac adverse effects include constipation, dizziness, headache, and nausea. Verapamil should be given with caution to patients who are concurrently receiving β-blockers, other antihypertensives, and other antidysrhythmics, because their effects may be additive. Concurrent administration of digoxin and verapamil may result in increased digoxin serum concentrations.

Other Antidysrhythmic Drugs

ADENOSINE

Actions   Adenosine (Adenocard) is an endogenous nucleoside produced by the degradation of adenosine triphosphate (ATP). Adenosine and ATP have been shown to exert transient negative inotropic, dromotropic, and chronotropic effects on SA and AV nodal tissues. Adenosine produces a transient AV nodal block, which breaks the re-entrant circuit of atrial tachydysrhythmia involving the AV node. Re-entrant SVTs not involving the AV node are not terminated by adenosine. It has no effect on anterograde conduction over accessory pathways in patients with WPW syndrome. When administered as a rapid IV bolus, adenosine slows cardiac conduction and restores sinus rhythm. However, when administered as a continuous infusion, it is a potent vasodilator. Adenosine is rapidly metabolized by circulating adenosine deaminase to an inert compound, giving the drug a very short half-life (<10 s).

Pharmacokinetics   The onset of action of adenosine is 20 to 30 s, with a duration of action lasting approximately 60 to 90 s. The drug is rapidly metabolized by circulating adenosine deaminase to inosine, an inactive metabolite. Adenosine is also rapidly taken up by most types of cells, where deamination to the inactive metabolite occurs. This contributes to the less than 10-s half-life of adenosine. Other pharmacokinetic parameters such as Vd, therapeutic plasma concentrations, and clearance are difficult to assess due to the very short half-life of the drug.

Indications   Adenosine is used for the emergency treatment of SVT. Although adenosine is effective in the initial conversion of re-entrant PSVT, recurrence of the dysrhythmia may occur within minutes after conversion. Although repeat doses of adenosine may be used, consideration of a longer-acting antidysrhythmic agent often may be necessary. Adenosine may be a preferable agent for the treatment of PSVT in infants, children, and pregnant women. Adenosine shortens the action potential duration and slows the heart rate; it is contraindicated in second- or third-degree AV heart block or sick sinus syndrome if no pacemaker (implanted or external) is present. Adenosine is not effective in converting atrial fibrillation or flutter to NSR; rather, it can be used to distinguish these rhythms from other tachydysrhythmias.

Dosing and Administration   The initial dose for the treatment of PSVT is 6 mg given as a rapid IV bolus over 1 to 2 s directly into the vein or in the most proximal port of the IV tubing. The dose may be repeated with 12 mg IV push two times if dysrhythmia persists every 1 to 2 min. The bolus dose should be followed immediately by a 10- to 20-mL fluid flush, and the arm should be elevated to maximize distribution of the drug before its metabolism and inactivation. It is important to administer adenosine as fast as possible; if infused too slowly, it can cause systemic vasodilation and a reflexive tachycardia.

Adverse Effect Profile   The adverse effects of adenosine are typically minor and well tolerated, because they last less than 1 min due to the short half-life. The most common adverse effects include dyspnea, cough, syncope, vertigo, paresthesias, numbness, nausea, and metallic taste. Cardiovascular adverse effects include facial flushing, headache, palpitations, retrosternal chest pain, sinus bradydysrhythmia (i.e., bradycardia, sinus arrest, AV block), PVCs, and hypotension. These adverse effects rarely require specific management. Occasionally, patients will have feelings of impending doom and should be reassured. Dipyridamole and carbamazepine have been shown to enhance the negative chronotropic and dromotropic effects of adenosine and may increase the degree of adverse effects. In contrast, methylxanthines and caffeine compete for adenosine receptors. Therefore, patients receiving these drugs may require a higher dose of adenosine to achieve a therapeutic effect. Adenosine should be used with caution in asthmatics, because it may induce bronchoconstriction.

DIGOXIN

Actions   Digoxin has three basic actions: it increases the force, strength, and velocity of cardiac contractions (positive inotropic effect); it slows the heart rate (negative chronotropic effect); and it slows conduction velocity through the AV node (negative dromotropic effect). Digoxin inhibits $Na^+K^+ATPase$ enzyme pump system, which is responsible for maintaining a high intracellular potassium concentration and high extracellular sodium concentration in the normal resting myocyte. Inhibition of $Na^+K^+ATPase$ leads to a net loss of potassium and a net gain of sodium in the intracellular fluid, which activates a Na^+-Ca^{2+} channel that pumps sodium out and calcium into the cell. The increase in intracellular calcium improves the efficiency of excitation and contraction coupling of myocytes, resulting in increased myocardial contractility. There is an inverse relation between the extent of the positive inotropic effect and the initial condition of the myocardium. Thus greater improvements in contractility will be greater in a myocardium with decreased contractility.

Digoxin increases the refractory period and decreases the conduction velocity of the SA and AV nodes but shortens the refractory period and increases conduction velocity in atrial tissue, including atrial bypass tracts as present in WPW syndrome. Therefore, digoxin generally should *not* be used in the management of WPW syndrome, because it may enhance conduction via the accessory pathway and, in the presence of atrial fibrillation/flutter, result in extremely rapid ventricular rates and even VF. The primary effect on SA and AV nodal conduction is secondary to indirect vagal stimulation.

Slowing of the heart results in a prolonged diastolic period, allowing improved coronary blood flow and myocardial perfusion. A decrease in oxygen demand also may occur secondary to the decrease in heart rate.

Pharmacokinetics   The onsets of action of digoxin are approximately 5 to 30 min after IV administration and 30 to 120 min after oral administration, and peak effects are 1.5 to 4 h and 2 to 6 h for IV and oral administrations, respectively. The apparent Vd is 5.6 L/kg and is proportional to lean body mass, with muscular individuals having larger Vds than obese individuals based on body weight. As a result of a large Vd, hemo- and peritoneal dialyses are ineffective in removing significant amounts of digoxin.

The bioavailability varies with the tablet, elixir, and capsule formulations, being 70, 80, and 90 percent, respectively. Digoxin is eliminated primarily through the kidneys unchanged, with approximately 20 to 40 percent of the dose metabolized in the liver to two active metabolites and excreted in bile and feces. The half-life of digoxin in patients with normal renal function is 1.5 to 1.8 days and can be extended up to 4 to 6 days in patients with renal insufficiency.

Indications   Digoxin is indicated to improve cardiac output in CHF and to control the ventricular response in atrial fibrillation, atrial flutter, and PSVT. Digoxin can be used in CHF in conjunction with β-blockers, diuretics, and angiotensin-converting enzyme inhibitors to control symptoms of CHF. Unlike these medications, which have a demonstrated benefit on mortality, digoxin has been shown to reduce hospitalizations, not mortality. It is not recommended in patients with New York Heart Association class I failure. Digoxin is generally most effective in low-output failure secondary to hypertensive, atherosclerotic heart disease, primary myocardial disease, nonobstructive cardiomyopathies, and valvular heart disease. It is less effective in high-output heart failure caused by bronchopulmonary insufficiency, infection, hyperthyroidism, anemia, fever, or arteriovenous fistulas.

Dosing and Administration   Digoxin can be administered by the oral or IV route. The IV route is preferred when a more rapid onset of action and peak effect is desired. Due to increased bioavailability, the IV dose is 20 to 30 percent less than the oral dose. The IV dose is 10 to 15 μg/kg, or 0.75 to 1.5 mg given as a series of three injections: the first is half the total dose, and the second and third are one fourth the total dose each. The three doses should be separated by 4 to 8 h to allow for distribution and minimize toxicity. Administering digoxin by the IM route is not recommended, because it offers no advantages over oral or IV administration and can cause severe pain at the injection site. Therapy with oral digoxin should replace IV administration as soon as is feasible. The oral dose is 0.125 to 0.5 mg per d. The therapeutic serum digoxin level is 0.8 to 2 ng/mL. Oral and IV doses should be decreased in elderly patients and those with renal insufficiency. The dose to provide symptomatic relief in patients with CHF is lower (8 to 12 μg/kg) than that for treating SVT but is administered in the same manner. The loading dose should be calculated by using the patient's lean body weight, because this method generally provides therapeutic effects with minimal risk of toxicity. Intravenous digoxin should be administered slowly over 5 min or longer. Serum levels should not be obtained any sooner than 6 to 8 h after loading to allow for distribution of the drug. Reductions in maintenance doses are required in patients with renal insufficiency, dehydration, hypokalemia, hypocalcemia, hypomagnesemia, and hypothyroidism. Several drug interactions can increase serum digoxin levels, including amiodarone, verapamil, nifedipine, diltiazem, flecainide, quinidine, erythromycin, and tetracycline. In contrast, cholestyramine, metoclopramide, kaolin-pectin, penicillamine, and dietary fiber may result in decreased serum digoxin levels.

Adverse Effect Profile   Adverse effects of digoxin are generally GI in nature, including abdominal pain, diarrhea, nausea, and vomiting. Other adverse effects may include gynecomastia, skin rash, eosinophilia, and thrombocytopenia. Digoxin also can result in cardiac dysrhythmias, such as sinus bradycardia, AV or SA nodal block, and ventricular dysrhythmias. The clinician must be vigilant in recognizing the signs and symptoms associated with digoxin toxicity, which can be fatal if not properly treated. If digoxin toxicity is suspected, the drug should be discontinued and a serum level obtained.

Symptoms of digoxin toxicity include mental status changes, confusion, headache, drowsiness, anorexia, nausea, vomiting, weakness, visual disturbances, delirium, and seizures. Almost any type of dysrhythmia can manifest as a result of digoxin toxicity. The most common dysrhythmias include an increased number of unifocal or multifocal PVCs, VT, junctional tachycardia, high-degree AV block, SVT with block, and sinus arrest. Atrial fibrillation, bradycardia, bidirectional VT, and VF also may occur.

Although hypokalemia increases the risk of digoxin toxicity, significant digoxin toxicity itself may produce hyperkalemia. When digoxin toxicity is associated with hyperkalemia, a corresponding intracellular deficiency of potassium exists, which may be the causative factor of subsequent dysrhythmias. Lidocaine and phenytoin are antidysrhythmic drugs that have classically been used in digoxin toxicity, but their efficacy has not been proven. Atropine and transcutaneous pacing also have been used. Hemo- and peritoneal dialyses are ineffective in significantly reducing serum digoxin levels due to the large

Vd of digoxin. Charcoal hemoperfusion has been used with limited success for the same reasons. Digoxin antibody fragments (Digibind) is an antidote for digoxin toxicity and is indicated for life-threatening tachydysrhythmia, sinus bradydysrhythmia, severe AV blocks, and/or serum potassium greater than 5 mEq/L resulting from overdose or accidental ingestion of digoxin or other cardiac glycosides. Once digoxin antibody fragments has been administered, subsequent serum digoxin levels are of no use.

MAGNESIUM

Actions   Magnesium increases skeletal and smooth muscle contractility, vasomotor tone, and neuronal transmission by directly activating the Na$^+$K$^+$ATPase pump and indirectly by calcium channel blockade. It increases membrane potential, prolongs AV conduction, and increases the absolute refractory period. Hypomagnesemia can precipitate life-threatening dysrhythmias, symptoms of cardiac insufficiency, and sudden cardiac death after myocardial infarction. Supplementation with magnesium helps to replenish intracellular potassium in hypomagnesemic, hypokalemic patients; blocks calcium to cause vasodilation; and reduces platelet aggregation.

Pharmacokinetics   The onset of action of magnesium sulfate is immediate, with a duration of action of approximately 30 min after IV administration. The onset after IM administration increases to 1 h and a duration of 3 to 4 h. Magnesium is minimally eliminated via the urine at a rate that is directly proportional to the plasma concentration and glomerular filtration rate. A high percentage of magnesium is reabsorbed in the proximal tubule.

Indications   Magnesium is indicated for torsade de pointes and refractory VT/VF, regardless of pre-arrest serum magnesium levels. It has shown efficacy in treating MFAT, SVT, and ventricular dysrhythmias associated with cardiac arrest and/or digoxin toxicity in patients who are, or are likely to be, hypomagnesemic. Other uses for magnesium include seizures associated with toxemia/eclampsia/nephritis, hypomagnesemia (mild to severe), acute asthma exacerbations, and hyperalimentation.

Dosing and Administration   The loading dose is 1 to 4 g in 50 to 100 mL D5W over 20 to 60 min in patients with spontaneous circulation or 1 to 2 g in 10 mL D5W over 1 to 2 min in patients in cardiac arrest. The rate should be reduced or the infusion stopped temporarily if hypotension develops.

Adverse Effect Profile   Hypotension is the predominant adverse effect but is surprisingly uncommon, even when a 1- to 2-g IV push dose is given over 1 to 2 min. Other signs of hypermagnesemia, which may begin at serum concentrations of 4 mEq/L, include flushing, sweating, nausea, vomiting, CNS depression, depression of deep tendon reflexes, flaccid paralysis, depression of cardiac function, circulatory collapse, and respiratory depression.

VASOACTIVE DRUGS

ATROPINE

Actions   Atropine sulfate, a naturally occurring antimuscarinic drug, competitively antagonizes the effects of acetylcholine and other muscarinic agents. Its effect on the heart is to increase sinus node automaticity and AV conduction by blocking vagal activity. It thus has been termed a *parasympatholytic* drug.

Pharmacokinetics   The onset of action of atropine after IM, IV, and endotracheal (ET) administration is rapid, with peak increases in heart rate occurring within 2 to 4 min and a duration of action of up to 5 h.

The half-lives of atropine are 4 h in adults and 6.5 h in children but can be longer. Atropine elimination occurs at two rates: an initial fast rate of about 2 h and a slow rate ranging from 12.5 to 38 h. It is well absorbed and distributed throughout the body, metabolized in the liver, and excreted in the urine.

Indications Atropine sulfate reverses cholinergic-mediated decreases in heart rate. Atropine is useful in treating symptomatic sinus bradycardia (e.g., decreased heart rate with hypotension, altered mental status, "escape beats," or chest pain). Atropine is generally effective for AV block at the nodal level and ineffective when the block is infranodal. Atropine is rarely effective for pulseless electrical activity (PEA) with bradycardia and asystole.

Dosing and Administration For bradycardia, the loading dose is 0.5 mg rapid IV push every 3 to 5 min (maximum, 0.04 mg/kg). For PEA or asystole, the dose is 1 mg rapid IV push every 3 to 5 min (maximum, 0.04 mg/kg).

Atropine can be administered by several routes, including IV, IM, ET, SC, and intraosseous. When atropine is administered by ET tube, the dose should be increased 2 to 2.5 times the IV dose (the ET dose is diluted to 10 mL of the compatible solution). No dilution is required when administering the preloaded syringe (1 mg/10 mL), but dilution with 10 mL of NS is recommended when the 1 mg/mL ampules are used for ET administration. A total dose of 0.04 mg/kg produces complete vagal blockade.

Adverse Effect Profile Atropine is not indicated to correct bradycardia in the hemodynamically stable patient. If administered, marked increases in heart rate can increase myocardial oxygen consumption, possibly inducing ischemia and precipitating ventricular tachydysrhythmia. Doses smaller than 0.4 mg and therapeutic doses administered slowly can cause a paradoxical bradycardia that may be due in part to a central reflex stimulation of the vagus nerve. Other adverse effects may include other anticholinergic symptoms (e.g., blurred vision, dry mouth, CNS stimulation, hallucinations, mydriasis, and tachycardia).

DOBUTAMINE

Actions Dobutamine (Dobutrex) is a synthetic sympathomimetic drug that exerts potent inotropic and mild chronotropic activities. Dobutamine is formulated as a racemic mixture with β_1- and β_2-adrenergic and α-adrenergic agonist activities that are offset by α-adrenergic antagonist activity (Table 29-2). The net result is an increase in myocardial contractility and systemic vasodilation, with minimal changes in heart rate. Doses of up to 20 μg/kg per min will increase cardiac output, decrease peripheral vascular resistance, and decrease pulmonary occlusive pressures. Conversely, doses larger than 20 μg/kg per min will increase the heart rate and induce dysrhythmias.

TABLE 29-2 Ability of Commonly Used Sympathomimetic Agents to Stimulate Adrenergic Receptors

	Receptor Type			
	α	β_1	β_2	Dopamine
Phenylephrine	++/+++	−	−	
Norepinephrine	++++	++++	−	
Epinephrine	+++	++++	+++	
Dopamine	++/+++	++++	++	++++
Dobutamine	+	++++	++	
Isoproterenol	−	++++	++++	

Pharmacokinetics The onset of action of dobutamine is 1 to 2 min, and the peak response occurs within 10 min after IV administration. The apparent Vd is 0.2 L/kg, and the drug is metabolized primarily in tissue and the liver to inactive metabolites. The elimination half-life is 1 to 2 min, with the majority of the drug being eliminated within 48 h in the urine as inactive metabolites.

Indications Dobutamine is indicated for short-term positive inotropic support for the treatment of cardiovascular decompensation secondary to ventricular dysfunction or low-output heart failure. It is also usually the preferred agent in the management of cardiogenic shock.[9] Dobutamine increases cardiac output and renal and mesenteric blood flow without direct stimulation of the heart rate and decreases systemic vascular resistance.

Dosing and Administration Dobutamine is administered only as a continuous IV infusion. The dosage range is 2 to 20 μg/kg per min; however, most patients can be maintained on 10 μg/kg per min. Doses larger than 20 μg/kg per min are associated with increased risk of tachydysrhythmia. To assess effectiveness of the dose administered, patients should be monitored with a central venous pressure or pulmonary artery catheter.

Adverse Effects Profile The primary adverse effects of dobutamine are modest increases in heart rate (increases greater than 5 to 15 beats/min are uncommon), blood pressure (increases greater than 10 to 20 mm Hg are uncommon), and ectopic dysrhythmias (escape beats, unifocal and multifocal ventricular ectopic beats, and ventricular bigeminy). Less common adverse effects include headache, paresthesias, tremors, nausea, angina, and dyspnea. Heart rate increases greater than 10 percent may induce or exacerbate myocardial ischemia.

DOPAMINE

Actions Dopamine (Intropin) is an endogenous catecholamine and a precursor of norepinephrine and other endogenous catecholamines. It acts on dopaminergic, β_1- and α-adrenergic receptors. In low doses, dopamine causes vasodilation in the renal, mesenteric, coronary, and intracerebral vasculatures via stimulation of the dopaminergic receptors. This stimulation results in an increase in renal blood flow, glomerular filtration rate, sodium excretion, and urine output. Recently, however, the ability of dopamine to significantly increase urine output has been questioned.[10] At intermediate doses, dopamine stimulates β_1-adrenergic receptors, thereby improving myocardial contractility and cardiac output and increasing SA nodal conduction. At high doses, dopamine stimulates α-adrenergic receptors, causing peripheral vasoconstriction and increasing blood pressure. At very high doses, the α-adrenergic effects dominate, causing peripheral vasoconstriction and vasoconstriction of the mesenteric and renal vascular beds.

Pharmacokinetics The onset of action of dopamine is 5 min, with a duration of action of 10 min after IV administration. Dopamine is used only as a continuous IV infusion. The apparent Vd is 1.8 to 2.5 L/kg. Dopamine is 75 percent metabolized by monoamine oxidase and catechol-*O*-methyltransferase (COMT) in the liver, kidneys, and plasma to an inactive metabolite. The remaining 25 percent is metabolized to norepinephrine in the adrenergic nerve terminals. The elimination half-life is 2 min and is 80 percent eliminated by the kidneys as the inactive metabolite and norepinephrine. The elimination half-life may be prolonged in patients with hepatic or renal insufficiency and in pediatric patients.

Indications Dopamine is indicated for reversing hemodynamically significant hypotension caused by myocardial infarction, trauma, sepsis, heart failure, and renal failure when fluid resuscitation is unsuccessful or not appropriate. Dopamine is used to increase cardiac output, blood pressure, urine output, and peripheral perfusion.

Dosing and Administration The lowest dose of dopamine should be used to maintain a desired blood pressure based on the clinical presentation. Most patients can be maintained on doses between 0.5 and 20 μg/kg per min (continuous infusion). It is important to note that tachyphylaxis may occur with larger doses because the actions of dopamine are dependent on endogenous stores of norepinephrine and other catecholamines. As with all vasoactive drugs, dopamine should be discontinued by tapering the dose.

Adverse Effect Profile Dopamine produces dose-dependent adverse effects, including hypotension at low doses, hypertension at higher doses, ectopic beats, headache, nausea, vomiting, angina, palpitations, and tachycardia. Necrosis can develop if extravasation occurs. Gangrene of the extremities has been reported in patients with occlusive vascular disease or diabetes and in those who have received prolonged high-dose infusions. Monoamine oxidase inhibitors, halogenated anesthetics, sympathomimetics, and phosphodiesterase inhibitors will prolong and intensify the effects of dopamine. It is contraindicated in patients with pheochromocytoma or tachydysrhythmia. As with epinephrine, dopamine should not be infused in the same IV line with alkaline infusions.

EPINEPHRINE

Actions Epinephrine is an endogenous catecholamine and a nonselective α- and β-adrenergic agonist that is used in anaphylactic shock, a bronchodilator in acute asthma, and a myocardial stimulant in cardiac arrest. It increases heart rate, ventricular contractility, and peripheral vascular resistance. This effect causes vasoconstriction of arterioles in the skin mucosa and mesenteric vasculature by redistributing blood to the heart and brain. This leads to improved cardiac and cerebral perfusion during resuscitation. Epinephrine also causes bronchodilation and antagonizes the effects of histamine.

Pharmacokinetics The onset of action is 1 to 2 min, with a duration of action of 2 to 10 min after IV administration. The drug quickly becomes fixed in the tissues and is rapidly inactivated via oxidation by monoamine oxidase and methylation by COMT. The drug is eliminated via the kidneys predominantly as inactive metabolites.

Indications Epinephrine is indicated for the treatment of anaphylactic reactions and acute asthma exacerbations. It is considered a first-line agent in the treatment of cardiac arrest (i.e., pulseless VT/VF, asystole, and PEA). Epinephrine is also used as a vasopressor to increase blood pressure and to reverse bronchospasm due to anaphylactic and hypersensitivity reactions. Epinephrine infusions are used to increase heart rate in refractory symptomatic bradycardia.

Dosing and Administration For bradycardia, the dose is 2 to 10 μg/min IV. For asthma, the dose is 0.3 to 0.5 mL of a 1:1000 concentration SC every 20 to 30 min, for a maximum of three doses.

Epinephrine remains the adrenergic drug of choice in the ACLS guidelines. Although there have been various administration methods of epinephrine described in the past (e.g., escalating and high dose), the current guidelines recommend the administration of 1 mg IV every 3 to 5 min. In fact, the guidelines stress that doses larger than 1 mg are not recommended and may be harmful. However, if IV access is unavailable during a cardiac arrest situation, 2 to 2.5 mL of a 1:1000 solution, diluted with 10 to 20 mL of saline, can be administered via the ET tube, followed by several rapid mechanical ventilations to disperse the drug throughout the airways for maximal absorption.

Adverse Effect Profile Adverse effects are of minimal importance in the setting of cardiac arrest. Epinephrine significantly increases myocardial oxygen consumption and thus can exacerbate ventricular irritability in the setting of myocardial ischemia. Adverse effects are extensions of the drug's action and include hypertension, tachycardia, palpitations, and dysrhythmias. Epinephrine is not compatible in the same IV line with alkaline solutions.

INAMRINONE

Actions Inamrinone (Inocor) contains the same chemical formula as the previously available product, amrinone. The name was changed to prevent potential confusion with similarly sounding drugs. Inamrinone produces inotropic effects by inhibition of the phosphodiesterase enzyme, which is responsible for the degradation of intracellular cyclic adenosine monophosphate (cAMP). The increased intracellular concentration of cAMP results in an increase in intracellular calcium and thus increases myocardial contractility and the force of contractions. In addition to positive inotropic effects, inamrinone has vasodilatory properties. It appears to have a direct action on vascular smooth muscle but may also cause vasodilation secondary to a decrease in sympathetic tone resulting from improved myocardial contractility. The net affect is an increase in myocardial contractility and stroke volume, with a reduction in preload and afterload.

Pharmacokinetics The onset of action of inamrinone is 2 to 5 min, with peak affects seen within 10 min and a duration of action of 0.5 to 2 h after IV administration. The duration of action is dose dependent. The apparent Vd is 1.2 L/kg, and the terminal half-life is 3.6 h. The terminal half-life may be prolonged up to 8.3 h in patients with CHF. Inamrinone is metabolized by the liver to several metabolites, which are eliminated principally in the urine.

Indications Inamrinone is indicated for the short-term management of decompensated CHF. Because of the potential for serious adverse effects, inamrinone should be reserved for CHF refractory to or intolerant of conventional therapy (e.g., cardiac glycosides, diuretics, and/or vasodilators). Inamrinone has been used in clinical studies for up to 48 h, and prolonged use has not been found to be safe and effective.

Dosing and Administration The loading dose is a bolus of 0.75 mg/kg IV over 2 to 3 min, followed by a maintenance infusion of 5 to 15 μg/kg per min. A second bolus of 0.75 mg/kg may be given 30 min the after initial bolus dose.

Inamrinone is available only for IV administration. The total daily dose should not exceed 10 mg/kg. Inamrinone should be diluted in 0.45 or 0.9 percent saline solutions. Dextrose-containing solutions may eliminate the drug's activity. Adjustments in the maintenance dose should be titrated to clinical response.

Adverse Effect Profile The most common adverse effects are thrombocytopenia, ventricular and supraventricular dysrhythmias, hypotension, and nausea. Other adverse effects, which occur in fewer than 1 percent of patients, include vomiting, anorexia, fever, chest pain, and burning at the injection site. Hepatotoxicity has been reported, although rarely.

ISOPROTERENOL

Actions Isoproterenol (Isuprel) is a synthetic sympathomimetic agonist with β1- and β2-adrenergic receptor affinity only. The β1-receptor interaction results in increased chronotropic and inotropic activities in the myocardium and vasodilation by β2-receptor-mediated relaxation of smooth muscle.

Pharmacokinetics The onset of action of isoproterenol is 1 to 5 min and the duration of action is 1 to 2 h. Fifty percent of the dose is eliminated unchanged in the urine, and COMT is responsible for metabolizing 25 to 35 percent in the liver, lung, and other body tissues. The elimination half-life is 3 to 7 h.

Indications   Isoproterenol use is limited to refractory torsade de pointes and temporary control of refractory symptomatic bradycardia. Due to significant increases in myocardial oxygen demand with the use of isoproterenol, its use has been restricted to refractory arrhythmias.

Dosing and Administration   The dose is 2 to 10 μg/min IV by continuous infusion. Larger doses are considered harmful.

Adverse Effect Profile   The significant increases in heart rate seen with isoproterenol therapy causes dramatic increases in myocardial oxygen demand that can result in ischemic complications and tachy-dysrhythmia. The lowest possible effective dose should be used to prevent VT.

NESIRITIDE

Actions   Nesiritide (Natrecor) is a recombinant B-type natriuretic peptide that is endogenously produced in the human heart under conditions of increased pressure load or ventricular stretch, usually in association with increased intravascular volume. When B-type natriuretic peptide is produced and released from ventricular myocytes in response to increased pressure, it binds to and stimulates guanylate cyclase-linked GC-A receptors. This causes an increase in intracellular cyclic guanosine monophosphate, which results in its natriuretic, diuretic, vasodilatory, and smooth muscle relaxant activity. GC-A receptors are located primarily in the adrenal gland, lungs, kidneys, and endothelial and smooth muscle vasculatures. Nesiritide also inhibits renin-aldosterone release.

Pharmacokinetics   The onset of action of nesiritide is 15 to 30 min, with a peak response seen in approximately 60 min and a duration of action of 30 to 120 min after continuous IV administration. The apparent Vd is 0.19 L/kg. Metabolism occurs in the kidneys via proteolysis of nesiritide, although no dosage reduction is recommended in patients with renal insufficiency. The elimination half-life is 18 to 23 min.

Indications   Nesiritide is indicated for the treatment of acutely decompensated heart failure. It reduces pulmonary capillary wedge pressure and improves dyspnea. Nesiritide also can result in symptomatic hypotension comparable to nitroglycerin. However, when compared with dobutamine, ventricular dysrhythmias and cardiac arrest occur less frequently with nesiritide. Nesiritide is contraindicated in patients with a systolic blood pressure of less than 90 mm Hg.

Dosing and Administration   The loading dose is a 2 μg/kg IV bolus over 1 min followed by continuous infusion of 0.01 μg/kg per min. The infusion is titrated by 0.005 μg/kg per min every 3 h as needed, up to a maximal rate of 0.03 μg/kg per min.

Nesiritide is available only for continuous IV infusion. Hypotension is a dose-limiting effect and may necessitate a decrease in the infusion rate or discontinuation of the drug.

Adverse Effects Profile   Hypotension (11 percent) is the most common adverse effect of nesiritide and may require a reduction in dosage or discontinuation of the drug. Headache is also a common adverse effect. In at least 1 percent of patients who received nesiritide during clinical trials, bradycardia, ventricular dysrhythmias, and atrial fibrillation were reported. Less common adverse effects include confusion, paresthesias, somnolence, tremor, and lightheadedness.

NICARDIPINE

Actions   Nicardipine (Cardene) is a dihydropyridine calcium channel antagonist that is structurally similar to nifedipine. It inhibits the slow inward current of calcium into normal cardiac cells, resulting in coronary and peripheral vasodilation. Nicardipine will significantly increase cardiac index and output in a dose-related fashion, with reduction of systemic vascular resistance. Similar to other dihydropyridine calcium channel antagonists, nicardipine has little to no effect on SA and AV nodal conduction and, hence, is not associated with any negative inotropic or antidysrhythmic effects.

Pharmacokinetics   The onset of action of nicardipine is 1 min, with a duration of action of 3 h after IV administration. The apparent Vd is 0.64 L/kg. Metabolism occurs almost exclusively in the liver to an inactive metabolite, 65 percent of which is eliminated in the urine and 35 percent is excreted in feces. The elimination half-life is 44 to 107 min.

Indications   Nicardipine is available in oral and IV formulations. The IV formulation is indicated for the short-term management of hypertensive crises or essential hypertension when oral therapy is not feasible or desired.

Dosing and Administration   The loading dose is 5 mg/h by continuous infusion. The dose is titrated in increments of 2.5 mg per h every 15 min, to a maximum of 15 mg per h.

Adverse Effects Profile   Adverse effects associated with the IV formulation are usually dose dependent. Most common cardiovascular adverse effects include hypotension and tachycardia. Other adverse effects include headache, flushing, nausea, vomiting, and dizziness.

NIFEDIPINE

Actions   Nifedipine (Procardia and Adalat) is a dihydropyridine calcium channel antagonist with actions similar to other drugs in this class. Calcium channel inhibition in smooth muscle and cardiac cells results in a decrease in total peripheral resistance, a decrease in systemic blood pressure, a decrease in the afterload of the heart, a small reflex increase in the heart rate, and an increase in the cardiac index. Coronary artery vasodilation results in improved oxygen delivery, benefiting patients with vasospastic angina. Systemic artery vasodilation results in decreased afterload, leading to decreased oxygen consumption in patients with chronic stable angina. A reflexive increase in heart rate and cardiac output is seen with nifedipine use. Unlike verapamil or diltiazem, nifedipine has little effect on SA and AV nodal conduction. Nifedipine may, however, result in a decrease in left ventricular end diastolic pressure or left ventricular end diastolic volume in patients with moderately to severely impaired LV function, thereby worsening their condition.

Pharmacokinetics   The onset of action of nifedipine is 20 min, a peak response of 20 to 30 min and a duration of 6 h after oral immediate-release administration. The onset and duration of action after oral extended-release administration are 30 min and 12 h, respectively. Regardless of formulation, nifedipine has 45 to 70 percent bioavailability due to first-pass hepatic metabolism. Liver metabolism results in inactive metabolites, which are 90 percent eliminated in urine. The elimination half-life is 2 to 5 h and may be increased up to 7 h in patients with hepatic dysfunction. Nifedipine is 90 to 96 percent protein bound and should be taken on an empty stomach. Concurrent administration with grapefruit juice may increase serum concentration through inhibition of intestinal metabolism.

Indications   Previous recommendations for the sublingual use of the oral immediate-release formulation called for its use in the treatment of hypertensive emergencies. However, recent data have shown that a precipitous drop in blood pressure may worsen outcomes in these patients by the development of ischemic complications. Grossman and associates called for the abandonment of nifedipine in the routine treatment of hypertensive crisis based on reports of serious adverse effects, despite its effectiveness in reducing blood pressure.[11] Both oral formulations are indicated for the treatment of vasospastic and chronic stable angina. Nifedipine sustained-release, alone or in combination with other anti-hypertensive drugs, is indicated in the management of essential hypertension.

Dosing and Administration   For hypertension or angina, the dose is 30 to 60 mg per d of an extended-release formulation (maximum, 120 mg per d). For angina, the dose is 10 mg of immediate-release formulation (swallowed whole) three times daily (maximum, 180 mg per d). Sublingual or chewing the immediate-release formulation can cause a precipitous drop in blood pressure and has been implicated in ischemic events.

Adverse Effect Profile   Most adverse effects of nifedipine are related to its vasodilatory activity on the smooth muscle and include lightheadedness, flushing, headache, and hypotension. The most serious adverse effects reported with the sublingual use of the immediate-release formulation include cerebrovascular ischemia, stroke, severe hypotension, and acute myocardial infarction. Other, less severe, cardiovascular adverse effects include a peripheral edema, CHF, reflex tachycardia, and pulmonary edema. Noncardiac adverse effects include nervousness, sleep disturbances, blurred vision, nausea, somnolence, insomnia, and diarrhea. Concomitant administration with other antihypertensive drugs may enhance the hypotensive effects. Nifedipine should be used with caution in patients with CHF, aortic stenosis, and concomitant β-blocker therapy.

NIMODIPINE

Actions   Nimodipine (Nimotop) is a dihydropyridine calcium channel antagonist with actions similar to those of other calcium channel antagonists. Nimodipine has a relative selectivity for vascular smooth muscle when compared with the myocardium and therefore has minimal effects on conduction and inotropism of the myocardium. Because it dilates cerebral vessels to a greater extent than peripheral or coronary vessels, nimodipine's primary indication is in the treatment of subarachnoid hemorrhage (SAH). Nimodipine use results in an increase in cerebral blood flow and may shunt blood to ischemic areas. Although it is believed that prevention of vasospasm after a SAH may lead to improved outcomes, improved collateral blood flow and prevention of large calcium influxes in to neurons (causing cell destruction) may be of greater benefit.

Pharmacokinetics   The peak response seen after oral administration is 60 min. It is 95 percent protein bound and readily crosses the blood-brain barrier. Metabolism occurs extensively in the liver to numerous inactive metabolites that are eliminated almost entirely in the urine or feces. The elimination half-life is 8 to 9 h.

Indications   Nimodipine is indicated for the treatment of recent (within 96 h) SAH from ruptured congenital intracranial aneurysm.

Dosing and Administration   The loading dose is 60 mg PO every 4 h for 21 days. The dose may be changed to 30 mg PO every 2 h if hypotension develops. If oral administration is not feasible, the capsule can be punctured, with the contents administered through a nasogastric tube and flushed with 30 mL of saline.

Adverse Effect Profile   The most common adverse effect is hypotension, which is often dose related. In addition, edema and headache have been reported in patients with SAH. Other, less frequent, dose-related adverse effects include tachycardia, bradycardia, palpitations, flushing, hypertension, rebound vasospasm, CHF, and pulmonary edema.

NITROGLYCERIN

Action   Nitroglycerin (various trade names) is an organic nitrate that readily enters vascular smooth muscle, where it undergoes conversion to nitric oxide. Nitric oxide is a direct vasodilator that primarily produces systemic venodilatation by reducing preload as measured by pulmonary capillary wedge pressure and left ventricular end-diastolic volume and pressure. Venodilatation is typically seen at doses smaller than 100 μg per min, whereas arteriolar vasodilation is seen at doses larger than 200 μg per min.

Pharmacokinetics   Table 29-3 lists the onset and duration of action of various nitroglycerin formulations. Nitroglycerin has a half-life of 2 to 33 min and is metabolized by the liver to inactive metabolites. The apparent Vd is 3 L/kg. Oral nitroglycerin formulations undergo extensive first-pass metabolism.

Indications   Nitroglycerin, in its various formulations, is indicated for the prophylaxis and management of angina pectoris. Intravenous nitroglycerin may be preferable to sodium nitroprusside for decreasing preload in acute decompensated heart failure, due to its more favorable effects on regional ischemia and pulmonary artery pressure. Intravenous nitroglycerin is also used in the treatment of hypertensive crisis and for the management of perioperative hypertension, especially hypertension associated with cardiovascular procedures.

Dosing and Administration   Nitroglycerin can be administered sublingually, lingually, intrabuccally, PO, topically, or by IV infusion. See Table 29-3 for specific dosing regimens. The sublingual and intrabuccal formulations should not be swallowed, and the extended-release formulations should not be chewed. Patients should be in a sitting or supine position immediately after sublingual, lingual, or intrabuccal

TABLE 29-3   Nitroglycerin Chart

Sublingual: 0.3, 0.4, and 0.6 tablets
   Dissolve 1 tablet under tongue q5 min until pain relief or hypotension
      occurs
   Onset: 1–3 min
   DOA: 30–60 min
Translingual spray: 0.4 mg/spray
   1–2 metered-dose sprays into oral mucosa q3–5 min
   Onset: 2 min
   DOA: 30–60 min
Topical ointment: 2% nitroglycerin ointment
   Apply 1 to 2 in. to chest wall q4–8 h
   Onset: 20–60 min
   DOA: 2–12 h
Intravenous infusion
   Give 5–10 μg per min, titrate in increments of 5–10 μg per min q3–5 min
      until desired results (standard dose, 50–200 μg per min)
   Onset: 1–2 min
   DOA: 5–10 min
Sustained-release pill
   Starting dose is 2.5 mg PO TID
   Onset: 20–45 min
   DOA: 4–8 h
Transmucosal tablets
   Place 1-mg pill between lip and gum above incisors or between cheek
      and gum q3–5h while awake
   Onset: 1–2 min
   DOA: 3–5 h
Transdermal patch
   Apply to hair-free area and rotate sites. 2.5–15-mg patches are available;
      start with low dose and titrate upward
   Onset: 30–60 min
   DOA: up to 24 h

Abbreviation: DOA = duration of action.

administration. Intravenous nitroglycerin should be administered by an infusion pump. Patients may exhibit tolerance to nitroglycerin infusions of 24 h or longer and thus may need increasing infusion rates over time although tolerance may be seen with any formulation when dosed continuously for longer than 24 h. To minimize tolerance to nitroglycerin, IV infusion should be maintained at the lowest effective dose for the shortest duration possible. A "drug-free period" of 6 to 12 h is recommended for the oral, topical, and transdermal formulations. Intravenous nitroglycerin should not be discontinued abruptly. Rather, it should be titrated down slowly to minimize any rebound effects (e.g., angina or myocardial infarction).

Adverse Effect Profile   Most adverse effects are related to the cardiovascular actions caused by nitroglycerin. These effects include headache, dizziness, weakness, syncope, flushing, hypotension, reflex tachycardia, and, occasionally, bradycardia. Caution is advised when using nitroglycerin in patients who are hemodynamically unstable (including those who are volume depleted) or who have increased intracranial pressure or severe anemia. Nitroglycerin also should be used with caution in cases of constrictive pericarditis, pericardial tamponade, and hypertrophic cardiomyopathy. Extended-release formulations should be avoided in patients with GI hypermotility or malabsorption syndromes. Transdermal patches and topical ointment should be removed before defibrillation or synchronized cardioversion. Topical nitroglycerin formulations alter electrical conductivity and enhance the potential for electrical arcing to occur. Concurrent use with sildenafil (Viagra) has been reported to cause excessive hypotension and should be avoided.

NOREPINEPHRINE

Actions   Norepinephrine bitartrate (Levophed) is identical to the endogenous catecholamine synthesized in the adrenal medulla and sympathetic nervous tissue. Norepinephrine stimulates α and β_1-receptors. The net results are increases in arterial and venous vascular tone and increases in inotropic and chronotropic activity of the heart. Paradoxical decreases in heart rate may result from reflex increase in parasympathetic tone. Norepinephrine differs from epinephrine in that it has no effect on β_2-receptors.

Pharmacokinetics   The onset of action of norepinephrine is 1 to 2 min and the duration of action is 5 to 10 min after IV administration. Metabolism of norepinephrine occurs in the liver and other tissues, mainly by COMT. Elimination occurs via uptake by adrenergic neurons, with a small percentage being eliminated via the kidneys.

Indications   Norepinephrine is a direct-acting sympathomimetic and is used to produce vasoconstriction and cardiac stimulation as an adjunct to correct hemodynamic imbalances in the treatment of shock that persists after adequate fluid volume replacement. Norepinephrine may be particularly useful when endogenous stores of norepinephrine are low. This scenario may arise in patients who have been on prolonged infusions of dopamine. Other specific uses for norepinephrine include controlling hypotensive states during poliomyelitis, drug overdoses (various phenothiazines, and tricyclic antidepressants), spinal anesthesia, pheochromocytoma, and sympathectomy.

Dosing and Administration   The initial dose is 2 μg per min by constant infusion. The rate should be adjusted in increments of 1–2 μg per min every 3 to 5 min as needed. The maximal recommended dose is 12 μg per min.

Norepinephrine is available for continuous IV infusion only. As with any vasopressor, adequate fluid or blood replacement should be corrected before starting norepinephrine. Norepinephrine infusions should not be discontinued abruptly. Rather, a slow titration down should be instituted to avoid rebound hypotension.

Adverse Effect Profile   High doses of norepinephrine may result in ventricular irritability, cardiac depression, decreased renal blood flow, and a reflex bradycardia. Acute hypertension may occur in patients on monoamine oxidase inhibitors or tricyclic antidepressants. Care should be taken to avoid extravasation. To prevent necrosis and sloughing if extravasation occurs, the area should be infiltrated as soon as possible with 5 to 10 mg of phentolamine (Regitine). Norepinephrine is contraindicated in patients with hypotension resulting from cyclosporine or halogenated hydrocarbon anesthesia, uncorrected blood deficits, or in mesenteric or peripheral vascular thrombosis.

VASOPRESSIN

Actions   Vasopressin (Pitressin) is identical to endogenous vasopressin (antidiuretic hormone). The primary physiologic role of vasopressin is to maintain serum osmolality. It produces relatively concentrated urine by increasing reabsorption of water by the renal tubules. Maintenance of osmolality is mediated by renal vasopressin V_2 receptors, which are coupled to adenyl cyclase activity and cAMP formation. In doses larger than those required for antidiuretic effects, vasopressin directly stimulates contraction of smooth muscle V_1 receptors. Vascular V_1 receptors are coupled to phospholipase C, resulting in release of calcium from sarcoplasmic reticulum in smooth muscle cells, leading to vasoconstriction. Vasoconstriction, which occurs particularly in the capillaries and small arterioles, results in decreased blood flow to the splanchnic, coronary, GI, pancreatic, skin, and muscular systems. Endogenous vasopressin concentrations in patients undergoing cardiopulmonary resuscitation are higher in those who have a return of spontaneous circulation (ROSC) than in those who do not. This finding suggested that exogenous vasopressin might be beneficial during cardiac arrest.

Pharmacokinetics   The onset of action on vasopressin is immediate, with a duration of action of 10 to 30 min. Vasopressin has a half-life of approximately 10 to 20 min and is rapidly metabolized in the liver and kidneys.

Indications   Vasopressin is indicated for the prevention and treatment of diabetes insipidus, treatment of GI hemorrhage, and, more recently, as an alternative to epinephrine for its vasopressor effects as a nonadrenergic peripheral vasoconstrictor during cardiopulmonary resuscitation. Vasopressin is indicated only in the treatment of pulseless VT/VF. Preliminary clinical evidence shows that vasopressin may be effective in enhancing the probability of ROSC in patients with out-of-hospital VF. Low-dose vasopressin infusions have been shown to be an effective alternative to traditional high-dose catecholamine therapy in septic patients with refractory hypotension.

Dosing and Administration   The initial dose in cardiac arrest is 40 units IV push. If there is no ROSC in 10 min, epinephrine 1 mg every 3 to 5 min can be used. Vasopressin can be used in place of, but not concurrent with, the initial dose of epinephrine. There are no data to support the use of a second dose of vasopressin during cardiac arrest.

Adverse Effect Profile   In the dose recommended in cardiac arrest, vasopressin may produce increased blood pressure, bradycardia, dysrhythmias, premature atrial contractions, heart block, peripheral vascular constriction or collapse, coronary insufficiency, decreased cardiac output, myocardial ischemia, and mesenteric thrombosis.

ACKNOWLEDGMENT

The author acknowledges that parts of this chapter are based on previous work by David Levy, PharmD.

REFERENCES

1. Anderson WL, Slovis CM: Lidocaine in the treatment of status epilepticus. *Acad Emerg Med* 4:918, 1997.
2. ECC Guidelines: Guidelines 2000 for cardiopulmonary resuscitation and emergency cardiovascular care, international consensus on science. *Circulation* 102(suppl I):I1, 2000.
3. Gorgels AP, van den Dool A, Hofs A, et al: Comparison of procainamide and lidocaine in terminating sustained monomorphic ventricular tachycardia [see comments]. *Am J Cardiol* 78:43, 1996.
4. Akhtar M, Gilbert CJ, Shenasa M: Effect of lidocaine on atrioventricular response via the accessory pathway in patients with Wolff-Parkinson-White syndrome. *Circulation* 63:435, 1981.
5. Ganau G, Lenzi T. Intravenous propafenone for converting recent onset atrial fibrillation in emergency departments: A randomized placebo-controlled multicenter trial. FAPS Investigators Study Group. *J Emerg Med* 16:383, 1998.
6. Azpitarte J, Alvarez M, Baun O, et al: Value of single oral loading dose of propafenone in converting recent-onset atrial fibrillation. Results of a randomized, double-blind, controlled study. *Eur Heart J* 18:1649, 1997.
7. Ryan TJ, Antman EM, Brooks NH, et al: 1999 Update: ACC/AHA guidelines for the management of patients with acute myocardial infarction: Executive summary and recommendations: A report of the American College of Cardiology/American Heart Association Task Force on Practice Guidelines (Committee on Management of Acute Myocardial Infarction). *Circulation* 100:1016, 1999.
8. Krahn AD, Klein GJ, Yee R: A randomized, double-blind, placebo-controlled evaluation of the efficacy and safety of intravenously administered dofetilide in patients with Wolff-Parkinson-White syndrome. *Pacing Clin Electrophysiol* 24(8 pt 1):1258, 2001.
9. Hutchinson TA, Shahan DR (eds): *Drugdex® System,* 112th ed. Greenwood Village, CO, Micromedex, 2002.
10. Kellum JA, Decker J: Use of dopamine in acute renal failure: A meta-analysis. *Crit Care Med* 29:1638, 2001.
11. Grossman E, Messerli FH, Grodzicki T, Kowey P: Should a moratorium be placed on sublingual nifedipine capsules for hypertensive emergencies and pseudoemergencies? *JAMA* 276:1328, 1996.

BIBLIOGRAPHY

American Hospital Formulary Service Drug Information 2002. Bethesda, MD, American Society of Health-System Pharmacists, 2002.
Drug Facts and Comparisons. St. Louis, Lippincott, 2002.
Schreiner GF, Protter AA: B-type natriuretic peptide for the treatment of congestive heart failure. *Curr Opin Pharmacol* 2:142, 2002.
Silver MA, Horton DP, Ghali JK, Elkayam U: Effect of nesiritide versus dobutamine on short-term outcomes in the treatment of patients with acutely decompensated heart failure. *J Am Coll Cardiol* 39:798, 2002.

APPROACH TO THE PATIENT IN SHOCK

Emanuel P. Rivers

Ronny M. Otero

H. Bryant Nguyen

EPIDEMIOLOGY

More than 1 million cases of shock are estimated to present to U.S. hospital EDs each year.[1] The presentation may be cryptic, as in the patient with compensated heart failure, or obvious as in the ultimate shock state of cardiac arrest. Despite aggressive treatment, mortality from shock remains high. Approximately 30 to 45 percent of patients in septic shock, and 60 to 90 percent for those with cardiogenic shock, die within 1 month of presentation.[2,3] The definition and treatment of shock continues to evolve. With a contemporary understanding of the disease and new evolving technology, the emergency physician can recognize shock at an earlier stage and initiate expert, timely intervention. The general approach to a patient in the initial stages of shock follows similar principles regardless of the inciting factors or etiology.

PATHOPHYSIOLOGY

Shock is defined as circulatory insufficiency that creates an imbalance between tissue oxygen supply and oxygen demand. The result of shock is global tissue hypoperfusion and is associated with a decreased venous oxygen content and metabolic acidosis (lactic acidosis). Shock is classified into four categories by etiology: (1) hypovolemic (caused by inadequate circulating volume), (2) cardiogenic (caused by inadequate cardiac pump function), (3) distributive (caused by peripheral vasodilatation and maldistribution of blood flow), and (4) obstructive (caused by extra cardiac obstruction to blood flow). Clinically, shock may have a predominant cause, but as the shock state persists or progresses to irreversible end organ damage, other pathophysiologic mechanisms become operative.

Knowledge of the principles of oxygen delivery and consumption is important to the understanding of shock. A maximum of four molecules of oxygen is loaded onto each molecule of hemoglobin as it passes through the lungs. If all available oxygen sites are occupied (four per molecule of hemoglobin), arterial oxygen saturation (SaO_2) is 100 percent (Table 30-1). Arterial oxygen content (CaO_2) is the amount of oxygen bound to hemoglobin plus the amount dissolved in plasma (Table 30-2). Oxygen is delivered to the tissues by the pumping function (cardiac output) of the heart.

Systemic oxygen delivery (DO_2) is the product of the CaO_2 and cardiac output (CO). Systemic oxygen consumption (VO_2) comprises a sensitive balance between supply and demand. Normally, the tissues consume approximately 25 percent of the oxygen carried on hemoglobin, and venous blood returning to the right heart is approximately 75 percent saturated [mixed venous oxygen saturation (pulmonary artery) ($SmvO_2$)]. When oxygen supply is insufficient to meet demand, the first compensatory mechanism is an increase in CO. If the increase in CO is inadequate, the amount of oxygen extracted from hemoglobin by the tissues increases, which decreases $SmvO_2$.

When compensatory mechanisms fail to correct the imbalance between tissue supply and demand, anaerobic metabolism occurs, resulting in the formation of lactic acid. Lactic acid is rapidly buffered, resulting in the formation of measured lactate; normally between 0.5 and

1.5 mM/L. An elevated lactate level is associated with an $SmvO_2 < 50$ percent. Most cases of lactic acidosis are a result of inadequate oxygen delivery, but lactic acidosis occasionally can develop from an excessively high oxygen demand, for example, in status epilepticus. In other cases, lactic acidosis occurs because of an impairment in tissue oxygen utilization, as in septic shock and postresuscitation from cardiac arrest; a normal $SmvO_2$ with an elevated lactate indicates such an impairment. Elevated lactate is a marker of impaired oxygen delivery and/or utilization and correlates with short-term prognosis of critically ill patients in the ED.

$SmvO_2$ can also be used as a measure of the balance between tissue oxygen supply and demand. $SmvO_2$ is obtained from the pulmonary artery catheter, but similar information can be obtained by central venous blood cannulation ($ScvO_2$). $ScvO_2$ correlates well with $SmvO_2$ and can be more easily obtained in the ED setting.[4]

Shock is usually, but not always, associated with systemic arterial hypotension; i.e., systolic blood pressure less than 90 mm Hg. Pressure is the product of flow and resistance [mean arterial pressure (MAP) = CO × systemic vascular resistance (SVR)]. Blood pressure may not fall if there is increase in peripheral vascular resistance in the presence of decreased cardiac output, resulting in inadequate flow to the tissue or global tissue hypoperfusion. The insensitivity of blood pressure to detect global tissue hypoperfusion has been repeatedly confirmed. Thus, shock may occur with a normal blood pressure, and hypotension may occur without shock.

The onset of shock provokes a myriad of autonomic responses, many of which serve to maintain perfusion pressure to vital organs. Stimulation of the carotid baroreceptor stretch reflex activates the sympathetic nervous system leading to (1) arteriolar vasoconstriction, resulting in redistribution of blood flow from the skin, skeletal muscle, kidneys, and splanchnic viscera; (2) an increase in heart rate and contractility that increases cardiac output; (3) constriction of venous capacitance vessels, which augments venous return; (4) release of the vasoactive hormones epinephrine, norepinephrine, dopamine, and cortisol to increase arteriolar and venous tone; and (5) release of antidiuretic hormone and activation of the renin-angiotensin axis to enhance water and sodium conservation to maintain intravascular volume. These compensatory mechanisms attempt to maintain DO_2 to the most critical organs—the coronary and cerebral circulation. During this process, blood flow to other organs such as the kidneys and gastrointestinal tract may be compromised.

The cellular response to decreased DO_2 is adenosine triphosphate depletion leading to ion-pump dysfunction, influx of sodium, efflux of potassium, and reduction in membrane resting potential. Cellular edema occurs secondary to increased intracellular sodium, while cellular membrane receptors become poorly responsive to the stress hormones insulin, glucagon, cortisol, and catecholamines. As shock progresses, lysosomal enzymes are released into the cells with subsequent hydrolysis of membranes, deoxyribonucleic acid, ribonucleic acid, and phosphate esters. As the cascade of shock continues, the loss of cellular integrity and the breakdown in cellular homeostasis result in cellular death. These pathologic events give rise to the metabolic features of hemoconcentration, hyperkalemia, hyponatremia, prerenal azotemia, hyper- or hypoglycemia, and lactic acidosis.

In the early phases of septic shock, these physiologic changes produce a clinical syndrome called the systemic inflammatory response syndrome or SIRS, defined as the presence of two or more of the following features: (1) temperature greater than 38°C (100.4°F) or less than 36°C (96.8°F); (2) heart rate faster than 90 beats/min; (3) respiratory rate faster than 20 breaths/min; and (4) white blood cell count

TABLE 30-1 Definitions of Abbreviations

$(a-v)CO_2$	Arterial-central venous carbon dioxide difference
Cao_2	Arterial oxygen content
$Cmvo_2$	Mixed venous oxygen content
CI	Cardiac index (cardiac output/body surface area)
CO	Cardiac output
CPP	Coronary perfusion pressure
CVP	Central venous pressure
Do_2	Systemic oxygen delivery
DBP	Diastolic blood pressure
Hb	Hemoglobin
MAP	Mean arterial pressure
MODS	Multiorgan dysfunction syndrome
OER	Oxygen extraction ratio
$Paco_2$	Arterial carbon dioxide pressure
Pao_2	Arterial oxygen pressure
PAOP	Pulmonary artery occlusion (wedge) pressure
Sao_2	Arterial oxygen saturation
$Scvo_2$	Central venous oxygen saturation
$Smvo_2$	Mixed venous oxygen saturation (pulmonary artery)
$Srvo_2$	Retinal venous oxygen saturation
SIRS	Systemic inflammatory response syndrome
SVR	Systemic vascular resistance
Vo_2	Systemic oxygen consumption

greater than $12.0 \times 10^9/L$, less than $4.0 \times 10^9/L$, or with greater than 10 percent immature forms or bands.[5] As SIRS progresses, shock ensues, followed by multiorgan dysfunction syndrome (MODS) manifested by myocardial depression, adult respiratory distress syndrome, disseminated intravascular coagulation, hepatic failure, or renal failure. The fulminate progression from SIRS to MODS is determined by the balance of anti-inflammatory and proinflammatory mediators or cytokines that are released from endothelial cell disruption (Figure 30-1).

Global tissue hypoperfusion alone can independently activate the inflammatory response and serve as a comorbid variable in the pathogenesis of all forms of shock.[6] The failure to diagnose and treat global tissue hypoperfusion in a timely manner leads to an accumulation of an oxygen debt, the magnitude of which correlates with increased mortality.

CLINICAL FEATURES

History

Often, the presence of shock will be instantly apparent along with the underlying cause, such as acute myocardial infarction, anaphylaxis, or hemorrhage. Some patients may be in shock with few symptoms other than generalized weakness, lethargy, or altered mental status. Symptoms that suggest volume depletion include bleeding, vomiting, diarrhea, excessive urination, insensible losses because of fever, or orthostatic light-headedness. A history of cardiovascular disease is important, particularly episodes of chest pain or symptoms of congestive heart failure. Prior neurologic diseases can render patients more susceptible to complications from hypovolemia. Medication use, both prescribed and nonprescribed, is important. Some medication will cause volume depletion (e.g., diuretics) whereas others depress myocardial contractility (e.g., β-blockers and calcium channel blockers). The possibility of an anaphylactic reaction to a new medication, or cardiovascular depression as a consequence of drug toxicity should be considered.

Physical Examination

The clinical presentation of shock can be dramatic, as in profound hypotension caused by hemorrhage from a gunshot wound. On the other hand, shock can be subtle, as in heart failure, or, paradoxically, with hypertension. No single vital sign or value is diagnostic of shock as vital signs are insensitive in detecting and assessing the severity of tissue hypoperfusion. Measurement of blood pressure can be particularly difficult because of peripheral vascular disease, tachycardia with a small pulse pressure, and arrhythmias such as atrial fibrillation. Although not specific, physical findings taken as a composite may be useful in the assessment of patients in shock (Table 30-3).

DIAGNOSIS

Ancillary Studies

The clinical presentation and the presumptive etiology of shock will dictate the use of ancillary studies. A battery of standard hematologic,

TABLE 30-2 Oxygen Transport and Utilization Components

Arterial oxygen content	$Cao_2 = 0.0031 \times Pao_2 + 1.38 \times Hb \times Sao_2$

Cao_2 is the amount of O_2 within 100 mL blood. Oxygen is contained within blood in two forms: dissolved in plasma and chemically combined with hemoglobin. Assuming 15 g hemoglobin per 100 mL blood and an oxygen saturation of 97%, the representative normal value of Cao_2 is 20.1 mL/100 mL blood (vol%).

Central venous/mixed venous oxygen saturation	$Scvo_2$ or $Smvo_2$

$Smvo_2$ reflects physiologic efforts to meet tissue O_2 demands. Normal $Smvo_2$ is 65 to 75%. When the $Smvo_2$ falls below 50%, the body's limits to compensate have been reached and O_2 availability for tissue metabolism will be compromised, leading to lactic acidosis.

Central venous/mixed venous oxygen content	$Cmvo_2 = 0.0031 \times Pmvo_2 + 1.38 \times Hb \times Smvo_2$

$Cmvo_2$ is the amount of oxygen content returning to the heart. Normal $Cmvo_2$ is 15 mL/100 mL blood (vol%).

Systemic oxygen extraction ratio (OER)	$OER = C(a - v)O_2/Cao_2$

The amount of O_2 taken out of the blood by the tissues is the systemic OER. It is described as a percentage. Normal OER is about 25%. Lactic acid production, an indicator of anaerobic metabolism, usually accompanies an OER of greater than 50%.

Oxygen delivery	$Do_2 = CO \times Cao_2 \times 10$

Do_2 is the amount of O_2 delivered to the tissues per minute. Assuming a normal cardiac output of 5 L per min and a Cao_2 of 20.1 vol%; a normal value for O_2 delivery would be 1000 mL O_2 per min.

Oxygen consumption	$Vo_2 = CO \times Hb \times 1.38 \times (Sao_2 - Smvo_2) \times 10$

The amount of O_2 consumed by tissues each minute and is equal to the difference in O_2 delivered to tissues and the O_2 returning from tissues. The normal value is about 250 mL O_2 per min. Note that this formula ignores the small contribution from dissolved oxygen.

Oxygen affinity

Shifts in the oxyhemoglobin dissociation curve affect the release of O_2 in the peripheral circulation. Increased pH, decreased temperature, decreased carbon dioxide concentration (Pco_2) and decreases in 2,3-DPG levels all result in a shift of the oxyhemoglobin curve to the left. Thus, for any particular value of Pao_2, the O_2 saturation will be higher. This increased affinity of hemoglobin for O_2 makes O_2 loading easier, but release of O_2 in the peripheral tissues is impaired. The reverse is true with a decreased pH, increased temperature, increased Pco_2, and increased 2,3-DPG: there is a shift of the oxyhemoglobin dissociation curve to the right resulting in a decreased affinity of hemoglobin for O_2.

Note: See Table 30-1 for abbreviation definitions.

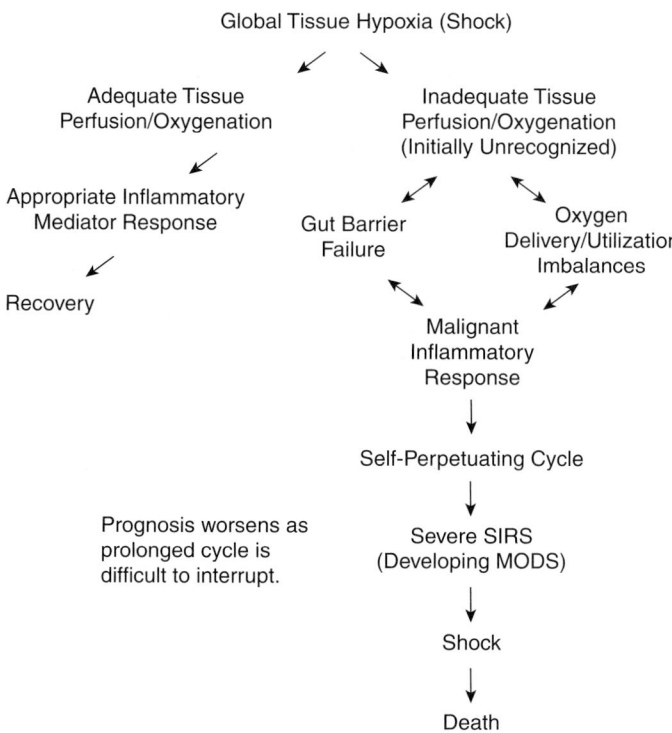

Global Tissue Hypoxia (Shock)

Adequate Tissue Perfusion/Oxygenation

Inadequate Tissue Perfusion/Oxygenation (Initially Unrecognized)

Appropriate Inflammatory Mediator Response

Gut Barrier Failure

Oxygen Delivery/Utilization Imbalances

Recovery

Malignant Inflammatory Response

Self-Perpetuating Cycle

Prognosis worsens as prolonged cycle is difficult to interrupt.

Severe SIRS (Developing MODS)

Shock

Death

FIG. 30-1. The pathophysiology of shock, SIRS, and MODS.

Hemodynamic monitoring is important in the assessment of patients in shock and evaluation of response to treatment. Monitoring capabilities will vary from institution to institution, but should include pulse oximetry, electrocardiographic monitoring, continuous noninvasive but preferably intraarterial blood pressure monitoring, end-tidal CO_2 monitoring, and central venous pressure (CVP) monitoring.[7] Because hemodynamic measurements are physiologic values, they should be used to answer specific physiologic questions rather than to serve as therapeutic end points.

TREATMENT

The Rationale for Early Intervention

The tenet of trauma resuscitation is to initiate care within the "golden hour" of disease presentation. A similar principle applies to patients with nonsurgical causes of shock. Current national increases in ED patient acuity and overcrowding have resulted in extending the golden hour into *hours* and even *days*, consequently requiring the provision of critical care in the ED. The benefit of timely ED intervention in nontraumatic critical illness is significant; standard ED care can significantly decrease the predicted mortality of critically ill patients in as little as 6 h of treatment.[8] Application of an algorithmic approach to optimize hemodynamic endpoints with early goal-directed therapy in the ED reduces mortality by 16 percent in patients with severe sepsis or septic shock.[9] The *ABCDE* tenets of shock resuscitation are establishing *A*irway, controlling the work of *B*reathing, optimizing the *C*irculation, assuring adequate oxygen *D*elivery, and achieving *E*nd points of resuscitation.

Establishing Airway

Airway control is best obtained through endotracheal intubation for airway protection, positive pressure ventilation (oxygenation), and pulmonary toilet. Sedatives, which are frequently used to facilitate intubation, can exacerbate hypotension through arterial vasodilatation,

coagulation, and biochemical tests usually provides an assessment of the patient's general physiologic condition and occasionally detects an abnormality that requires specific treatment (Table 30-4). A wide range of laboratory abnormalities may be encountered in shock, but most abnormal values merely point to the particular organ system that is either contributing to or being affected by the shock state. No single laboratory value is sensitive or specific for shock.

TABLE 30-3 Physical Examination

Temperature	Hyperthermia or hypothermia may be present. It is important to distinguish endogenous hypothermia (hypometabolic shock) from exogenous hypothermia secondary to environmental exposure. The treatment is obviously aggressive resuscitation in the former and exogenous heat application in the latter.
Heart rate	Usually elevated. However, paradoxical bradycardia can be seen in shock states such as hemorrhagic shock (up to 30%), hypoglycemia, β-blocker use, and preexisting cardiac disease.
Systolic blood pressure	May actually increase slightly when cardiac contractility increases in early shock and then fall as shock advances.
Diastolic blood pressure	Correlates with arteriolar vasoconstriction and may rise early in shock and then fall when cardiovascular compensation fails.
Pulse pressure	Systolic minus diastolic pressure and related to stroke volume and rigidity of the aorta. Increases early in shock and decreases before systolic pressure.
Pulsus paradoxus	The change in systolic blood pressure with respiration. The rise and fall in intrathoracic pressure affects cardiac output. This can be seen in asthma, cardiac tamponade, and severe cardiac decompensation.
Mean arterial blood pressure	Diastolic blood pressure + [pulse pressure/3]. The relationship between cardiac output and vascular resistance determines can be seen in asthma, cardiac tamponade, and severe cardiac decompensation.
Shock index	Shock index = heart rate/systolic blood pressure. Normal = 0.5 to 0.7. The shock index is related to left ventricular stroke work in acute circulatory failure. A persistent elevation of the shock index (>1.0) indicates an impaired left ventricular function (as a result of blood loss and/or cardiac depression) and carries a high mortality rate.[15]
Central nervous system	Acute delirium or brain failure; restlessness, disorientation, confusion, and coma secondary to decrease in cerebral perfusion pressure (mean arterial pressure − intracranial pressure). Patients with chronic hypertension may be symptomatic at normal blood pressures.
Skin	Pallor, pale, dusky, clammy, cyanosis, sweating, altered temperature, and decreased capillary refill.
Cardiovascular	Neck vein distention or flattening, tachycardia, and arrhythmias. An S3 may result from high-output states. Decreased coronary perfusion pressures can lead to ischemia, decreased ventricular compliance, increased left ventricular diastolic pressure, and pulmonary edema.
Respiratory	Tachypnea, increased minute ventilation, increased dead space, bronchospasm, hypocapnia with progression to respiratory failure, and adult respiratory distress syndrome.
Splanchnic organs	Ileus, gastrointestinal bleeding, pancreatitis, acalculous cholecystitis, and mesenteric ischemia can occur from low flow states.
Renal	Reduced glomerular filtration rate, renal blood flow redistributes from the renal cortex toward the renal medulla leading to oliguria. Paradoxical polyuria can occur in sepsis, which may be confused with adequate hydration status.
Metabolic	Respiratory alkalosis is the first acid–base abnormality, as shock progresses metabolic acidosis occurs. Hyperglycemia, hypoglycemia, and hyperkalemia.

TABLE 30-4   Ancillary Studies

Basic evaluation
  Hemogram: white blood cell count and differential, hemoglobin and
    hematocrit, platelet count
  Electrolytes, glucose, calcium, magnesium, phosphorus
  Blood urea nitrogen, creatinine
  Prothrombin time, partial thromboplastin time
  Urinalysis
  Chest radiograph
  Electrocardiogram
Moderate physiologic assessment
  Arterial blood gas (measured oxygen saturation)
  Serum lactate
  Fibrinogen, fibrin split products, d-dimer
  Hepatic function panel
Noninvasive hemodynamic assessment
  End-tidal carbon dioxide
  Noninvasive cardiac output measurement
  Echocardiogram
Invasive hemodynamic assessment
  Filling pressures: CVP or PAOP
  Cardiac output
  Central venous oxygen saturation: $Smvo_2$
  Calculation of hemodynamic values: SVR, CO, Do_2, Vo_2
As clinically indicated to define etiology or detect complications
  Blood, sputum, urine, and pelvic cultures
  CT of head and sinuses
  Lumbar puncture
  Culture suspicious wounds
  Cortisol level
  Pregnancy test
  Acute abdominal series
  Abdominal or pelvic ultrasound
  Abdominal or pelvic CT

Note: See Table 30-1 for abbreviation definitions.

venodilation, and myocardial suppression. Furthermore, positive pressure ventilation reduces preload and cardiac output. The combination of these interventions can lead to hemodynamic collapse. Volume resuscitation or application of vasoactive agents may be required prior to intubation and positive pressure ventilation.

Controlling the Work of Breathing

Control of breathing is required when tachypnea accompanies shock. Respiratory muscles are significant consumers of oxygen during shock and contribute to lactate production. Mechanical ventilation and sedation decrease the work of breathing and have been shown to improve survival. Sao_2 should be restored to greater than 93 percent and ventilation controlled to maintain a $Paco_2$ 35 to 40 mm Hg. Attempts to normalize pH above 7.3 by hyperventilation are not beneficial. Mechanical ventilation not only provides oxygenation and corrects hypercapnia but assists, controls, and synchronizes ventilation, which ultimately decreases the work of breathing. Neuromuscular blocking agents are used as adjuncts to further decrease respiratory muscle, oxygen consumption and preserve Do_2 to vital organs.

Optimizing the Circulation

Circulatory or hemodynamic stabilization begins with intravascular access through large-bore peripheral venous lines. Trendelenburg positioning, historically considered necessary for maintaining perfusion in the hypotensive patient, does not improve cardiopulmonary performance compared with the supine position. It may worsen pulmonary gas exchange and predispose to aspiration. If a volume challenge is urgently required, rather than using the Trendelenburg position, an alternative is to raise the patient's legs above the level of the heart with the patient supine. Central venous access will aid in assessing volume status (preload) and monitoring $Scvo_2$. It is the preferred route for the long-term administration of vasopressor therapy, and provides rapid access to the heart if pacemaker placement is required.

Fluid resuscitation begins with isotonic crystalloid; the amount and rate are determined by an estimate of the hemodynamic abnormality. Most patients in shock have either an absolute or relative volume deficit, except the patient in cardiogenic shock with pulmonary edema. Fluid is given rapidly, in set quantities (e.g., 500 or 1000 mL), with reassessment of the patient after each amount. Patients with modest degree of hypovolemia usually require an initial 20 mL/kg of isotonic crystalloid. More fluids may be necessary with profound volume deficits.

The colloid-versus-crystalloid resuscitation controversy remains despite evidence that there is a slight increase in mortality when colloids are used for volume replacement in critically ill patients.[10] Some studies have found a lower incidence of pulmonary edema, and possibly greater benefit, in elderly patients with colloid resuscitation, although survival is not statistically improved. In the acute situation with severe shock, colloids may be considered to achieve rapid plasma expansion using less volume compared to crystalloids.

Without invasive hemodynamic monitoring, noncardiogenic pulmonary edema may be difficult to differentiate from cardiogenic pulmonary edema in the ED. Even though the former may respond to fluids, fluids should be minimized in a patient with clinical or radiographic evidence of pulmonary edema until appropriate monitoring is established.

Vasopressor agents are used when there has been an inadequate response to volume resuscitation or when a patient has contraindications to volume infusion.[11] They are most effective when the vascular space is "full" and least effective when the vascular space is depleted. However, vasopressors may be necessary early in the treatment of shock, before volume resuscitation is complete, in order to prevent potentially lethal consequences of prolonged systemic arterial hypotension. This is especially important in elderly patients with significant coronary and cerebrovascular disease. Rapidly restoring the MAP to 60 mm Hg or systolic pressure to 90 mm Hg may avoid the coronary and cerebral complications of decreased blood flow. Vasopressor agents are based on the catecholamine molecule and have variable effects on the α-adrenergic, β-adrenergic, and dopaminergic receptors (Table 30-5).[11,12]

The use of vasopressors is accompanied with potential pitfalls. While improving perfusion pressure in the large vessels, they may decrease capillary blood flow in certain tissue beds, especially the bowel. Vasopressors also may alter the relationship between volume and pressure measurements through their effect on the pulmonary and peripheral vascular beds. In other words, vasopressors will falsely elevate intracardiac filling pressures (i.e., CVP). They should be used judiciously, generally only after volume resuscitation. When multiple vasopressors are used, they should be simplified as soon as the best therapeutic agent is identified.

Assuring Adequate Oxygen Delivery

Once blood pressure is stabilized through optimization of preload and afterload, Do_2 can be assessed and further manipulated. Arterial oxygen saturation should be returned to physiologic levels (93 to 95 percent) and hemoglobin maintained above 10 g/dL.[13] If cardiac output can be assessed, it should be increased by using volume infusion and inotropic agents in incremental amounts until venous oxygen saturation ($Smvo_2$ or $Scvo_2$) and lactate are normalized.

The control of Vo_2 is important in restoring the balance of oxygen supply and demand to tissues. A hyperadrenergic state results from the compensatory response to shock, physiologic stress, pain, and anxiety. Shivering frequently results when a patient is unclothed for examination and then left inadequately covered in a cold resuscitation room.

TABLE 30-5 Commonly Used Vasoactive Agents

Drug	Dose/Mixture*	Action	Cardiac Stimulation	Vasoconstriction	Vasodilation	Cardiac Output	Side Effects and Comments
Dopamine	0.5–25 μg/kg per min 400 mg/250 mL	α, β, and dopaminergic	++ at 2–10 μg/kg per min	++ at 7 μg/kg per min	+ at 0.5–5.0 μg/kg per min	Usually increases	Tachydysrhythmias, increases myocardial O_2 consumption, a cerebral, mesenteric, coronary and renal vasodilator at low doses
Norepinephrine	0.01–0.5 μg/kg per min 4 mg/250 mL	Primarily α_1, some β_1	++	++++	0	Slight decrease	Dose related, reflex bradycardia; useful when loss of venous tone predominates, spares the coronary circulation
Phenylephrine	0.15–0.75 μg/kg per min 10 mg/250 mL	Pure α	0	++++	0	Decrease	Reflex bradycardia, headache, restlessness, excitability, rarely arrhythmias; ideal for patients in shock with tachycardia or supraventricular arrhythmias
Ephedrine	5–25 mg	α and β	+++	++	+	Increases	Causes palpitations, hypertension, cardiac arrhythmias, an indirect-acting CNS stimulant; limited long-term value as therapy for shock.
Vasopressin	0.01–0.04 units per min 200 units/250 mL	α		++++			Primarily vasoconstriction, outcome data from its use is lacking; infusions of >0.04 units per min may lead to adverse, vasoconstriction-mediated events
Epinephrine	0.01–0.75 μg/kg per min 1 mg/250 mL	α and β	+++ at 0.03–0.15 μg/kg per min	++++ at 0.15–0.30 μg/kg per min	+++	Increases	Causes tachydysrhythmia, leukocytosis, increases myocardial oxygen consumption
Dobutamine	2.0–20 μg/kg per min 250 mg/250 mL	β_1, some β_2 and α_1 in large dosages	++++	+	++	Increase	Causes tachydysrhythmia, occasional GI distress, increases myocardial oxygen consumption, hypotension in volume depleted patient; has less peripheral vasoconstriction than dopamine, can cause fewer arrhythmias than isoproterenol
Isoproterenol	0.01–0.05 μg/kg per min 1 mg/250 mL	β_1 and some β_2	++++	0	++++	Increases	Causes tachydysrhythmia, facial flushing, hypotension in hypovolemic patients; increases myocardial oxygen consumption; never use alone in shock.

Note: 0 = no effect, + = mild effect, ++ = moderate effect, +++ = marked effect, ++++ = very marked effect.

Abbreviations: CNS = central nervous system; GI = gastrointestinal.

*Individual drugs may be diluted in D5W or NS, and may be diluted in larger volumes or concentrated into smaller volumes according to the fluid needs of the individual patient.

The combination of these variables increases systemic oxygen consumption. Pain further suppresses myocardial function, thus impairing Do_2 and Vo_2. Providing analgesia, muscle relaxation, warm covering, anxiolytics, and even paralytic agents, when appropriate, decreases this inappropriate Vo_2.

Tissue oxygen extraction assesses adequacy of the resuscitation in meeting the oxygen needs of the tissues. Sequential examination of lactate and $Smvo_2$ or $Scvo_2$ is a method to assess adequacy of tissue oxygen extraction. Continuous measurement of $Smvo_2$ or $Scvo_2$ through fiberoptic technology can be used in the ED.[4] A variety of other technologies have potential to assess tissue perfusion during resuscitation (Table 30-6).[14–17]

Achieving End Points of Resuscitation

Traditional end points have been normalization of blood pressure, heart rate, and urine output. Because these underestimate the degree of remaining hypoperfusion and oxygen debt, more physiologic end points have been investigated (Tables 30-7 and 30-8).[18] No therapeutic end point is universally effective, and only a few have been tested in prospective trials, with mixed results.[18] The goal of resuscitation is to maximize survival and minimize morbidity using objective hemodynamic and physiologic values to guide therapy. A goal-directed approach at achieving urine output >0.5 mL/kg per h, CVP 8 to 12 mm Hg, MAP 65 to 90 mm Hg, and $Scvo_2$ >70 percent during ED resuscitation of septic shock significantly decreases mortality.[9]

Troubleshooting a Persistently Hypotensive Patient

Treatment of a persistently hypotensive patient after maximal therapy can be a harrowing experience. Similar principles apply to both the trauma patient with ongoing hemorrhage and the persistently hypotensive medical patient. Issues to keep in mind include the following: (1) Is the patient appropriately monitored?[7] (2) Is there malfunction-ing arterial blood pressure monitoring, such as dampening of the arterial line or disconnection from the transducer? (3) Is the patient adequately volume resuscitated? (4) Does the early use of vasopressor falsely elevate CVP and disguise hypovolemia? (5) Is the intravenous tubing into which the vasopressors are running connected appropriately? (6) Are the vasopressor infusion pumps working? (7) Are the vasopressors mixed adequately? (8) Does the patient have a pneumothorax after placement of central venous access? (9) Has the patient been adequately assessed for an occult penetrating injury (a bullet hole or stab wound)? (10) Is there hidden bleeding from a ruptured spleen or ectopic pregnancy? (11) Does the patient have adrenal insufficiency? The incidence of adrenal dysfunction can be as high as 30 percent in this subset of patients.[19] (12) Is the patient allergic to the medication just given (e.g., penicillin) or taken before arrival? (13) Is there cardiac tamponade in the chronic renal failure patient on dialysis or cancer patient?

Bicarbonate Use in Shock

The primary treatment of acidosis in shock is to reverse the underlying cause. Because this goal is not rapidly attainable, intravenous bicarbonate is often administered. The rationale for giving bicarbonate is that it will diminish myocardial depression and counteract the insensitivity to endogenous catecholamines attributed to acidosis, but experimental data indicate that exogenous bicarbonate can actually worsen intracellular acidosis, and prospective studies have not shown benefit. Bicarbonate also shifts the oxygen-hemoglobin dissociation curve to the left and impairs tissue unloading of hemoglobin-bound oxygen. However, many clinicians remain uncomfortable withholding bicarbonate, which has created disparate opinions in the medical literature. A compromise is to partially correct the metabolic acidosis over time. The bicarbonate deficit is determined, which is equal to (normal HCO_3 minus the patient's HCO_3) $\times$ 0.5 $\times$ body weight (kilograms). One-half of this amount is infused slowly and the remainder over 6 to

TABLE 30-6   Adjuncts in Assessing Tissue Perfusion

Base deficit	Base deficit is an indicator of metabolic acidosis and is an index of hemodynamic and tissue perfusion changes in shock. Predicts illness severity in intra-abdominal hemorrhage and blunt trauma.
Invasive blood pressure monitoring	Intensive vasoconstriction caused by sympathetic activity or vasopressors given will cause the cuff pressure to underestimate true blood pressure. A Doppler may be used in conjunction with a sphygmomanometer may enable more accurate measure of systolic blood pressure once Korotkoff sound are no longer audible. Intra-arterial pressure measurement is preferable because vasoactive drugs may cause rapid swings in blood pressure and multiple blood samplings will typically be required.
Central venous pressure (CVP)	Aids in assessing volume status. Preferred for the long-term administration of vasopressor therapy and provides rapid access to the heart if pacemaker placement is required. May not reliably reflect the left ventricular filling pressure in clinical states such as pulmonary embolus, obstructive airway disease, right ventricular infarction, and pericardial effusion. Common iliac venous pressure can approximate CVP.
Central venous oximetry ($Scvo_2$)	$Scvo_2$ closely approximates mixed venous O_2 saturation ($Smvo_2$) and can be monitored continuously using infrared oximetry. This technology enables the clinician to detect clinically unrecognized tissue global tissue hypoperfusion in the treatment of myocardial infarction, general medical shock, trauma, hemorrhage, septic, hypovolemic, end-stage heart failure, and cardiogenic shock during and after cardiopulmonary arrest.
Arterial-central venous CO_2 difference	Increased arterial-mixed venous carbon dioxide gradients or $(a-v)CO_2$ are seen in acute circulatory failure, and inversely correlate with the cardiac index (CI).
Pulmonary artery catheterization	The standard of care for assessing cardiac status. Valuable in determining left-sided heart filling, pulmonary artery pressure, and assessing the cause of pulmonary edema. Can obtain cardiac output and mixed venous oxygen saturation. Will be able to calculate hemodynamic (i.e., SVR) and oxygen transport variables (VO_2 and DO_2). The effectiveness of this monitoring technique on improving outcome is challenged.
Noninvasive cardiac output	Cardiac output can be measured by transesophageal Doppler, cutaneous bioimpedance, and lithium dilution.
Gastric tonometry and sublingual capnography	Serial measurements of gastric and sublingual mucosal blood flow are based on hydrogen ion diffusion and carbon dioxide elimination. Inadequate visceral perfusion as evidenced by persistently low intramucosal pH or increased sublingual carbon dioxide concentration after resuscitation is associated with subsequent organ dysfunction and death.
Retinal venous O_2 saturation	Retinal venous O_2 saturation ($Srvo_2$) correlates with blood volume, central venous O_2 saturation and arterial O_2 saturation.
Metabolic cart	Directly measured VO_2 without a pulmonary artery catheter. A reduction in VO_2 (after acute myocardial infarction) predicts cardiogenic shock and mortality after human cardiac arrest.

TABLE 30-7   End Points of Resuscitation

Traditional: normalization of blood pressure, pulse, and urine output
Restoration of circulating volume
Restoration of all fluid compartments
Vascular space is "full"
Hemodynamic parameters are "normalized"
Tissue oxygen delivery is maximized
Restoration of aerobic metabolism, elimination of tissue acidosis, and
    repayment of oxygen debt

8 h. Additional bicarbonate should be withheld once arterial pH is 7.25 or greater.

DISPOSITION AND TRANSITION TO THE INTENSIVE CARE UNIT

Documentation and communication are important. Resuscitation in the ED is commonly performed in "ordered chaos." Even though resuscitation is systematic and thoughtful, miscommunication with the intensivist or subspecialist accepting the patient can undo the benefits of initial treatment. A system-oriented problem list with an assessment and plan, including all procedures and complications, should be verbally communicated and written or dictated prior to transfer. For prolonged ED stays, notations regarding patient status, diagnostic and therapeutic intervention, and sentinel events should be provided frequently.

PROGNOSIS

Outcome prediction at ED disposition has not been fully studied; however, some clinical variables are associated with poor outcome, such as severity of shock, temporal duration, underlying cause, preexisting vital organ dysfunction and reversibility. Direct noninvasive measurement of Vo_2 is predictive of outcome in patients who developed cardiogenic shock secondary to myocardial infarction and after cardiac arrest.[8] Persistent elevated lactate levels are prognostic in trauma, septic shock, and after cardiac arrest.[8] Base deficit is also correlated with the development of multisystem organ failure in trauma.[20] Elevated sublingual partial pressure of carbon dioxide (Pco_2) is associated with increased mortality.[14] Outcome predictions using physiologic scoring systems in the ED are also being studied.[8]

TABLE 30-8   Hemodynamic Resuscitation End Points

	Modality	Goals
Preload	CVP	10–12 mm Hg
	PAOP	12–18 mm Hg
Afterload	MAP	90–100 mm Hg
	SVR = (MAP − CVP/CO)(80)	800–1400 dyne · s/cm^5
Contractility	CO	5.0 L/min
	CI	2.5–4.5 L per min · m^2
	SV = CO/heart rate	50–60 mL per min
Heart rate	60–100 bpm	Avoid >100 bpm; this will decrease SV and increase myocardial oxygen consumption
Coronary perfusion pressure	CPP = DBP − CVP (or PAOP)	>60 mm Hg
Tissue oxygenation	Scvo$_2$ or Smvo$_2$	>70%
	Serum lactate	<2 mM/L

Note: See Table 30-1 for abbreviation definitions.
Abbreviation: bpm = beats per min.

REFERENCES

 1. McCaig LF, Ly N: National hospital ambulatory medical care survey: 2000 emergency department summary. Advance Data from Vital and Health Statistics; No. 326. Hyattsville, MD, National Center for Health Statistics, April 22, 2002.
 2. Moscucci M, Bates ER: Cardiogenic shock. *Cardiol Clin* 13:391, 1995.
 3. Angus DC, Linde-Zwirble WT, Lidicker J, et al: Epidemiology of severe sepsis in the United States: Analysis of incidence, outcome, and associated costs of care. *Crit Care Med* 29:1303, 2001.
 4. Rivers EP, Ander DS, Powell D: Central venous oxygen saturation monitoring in the critically ill patient. *Curr Opin Crit Care* 7:204, 2001.
 5. American College of Chest Physicians/Society of Critical Care Medicine consensus conference: Definitions for sepsis and organ failure and guidelines for the use of innovative therapies in sepsis. *Crit Care Med* 20:864, 1992.
 6. Karimova A, Pinsky DJ: The endothelial response to oxygen deprivation: Biology and clinical implications. *Intensive Care Med* 27:19, 2001.
 7. Boldt J: Clinical review: Hemodynamic monitoring in the intensive care unit. *Crit Care* 6:52, 2002.
 8. Nguyen HB, Rivers EP, Havstad S, et al: Critical care in the emergency department: A physiologic assessment and outcome evaluation. *Acad Emerg Med* 7:1354, 2000.
 9. Rivers E, Nguyen B, Havstad S, et al: Early goal-directed therapy in the treatment of severe sepsis and septic shock. *New Engl J Med* 345:1368, 2001.
10. Webb AR: The appropriate role of colloids in managing fluid imbalance: A critical review of recent meta-analytic findings. *Crit Care* 4(suppl 2):S26, 2000.
11. Reinhart K, Sakka SG, Meier-Hellmann A: Haemodynamic management of a patient with septic shock. *Eur J Anaesthesiol* 17:6, 2000.
12. Forrest P: Vasopressin and shock. *Anaesth Intensive Care* 29:463, 2001.
13. Hebert PC, Wells G, Tweeddale M, et al: Does transfusion practice affect mortality in critically ill patients? Transfusion Requirements in Critical Care (TRICC) Investigators and the Canadian Critical Care Trials Group. *Am J Respir Crit Care Med* 155:1618, 1997.
14. Rackow EC, O'Neil P, Astiz ME, Carpati CM: Sublingual capnometry and indexes of tissue perfusion in patients with circulatory failure. *Chest* 120:1633, 2001.
15. Rady MY, Rivers EP, Nowak RM: Resuscitation of the critically ill in the ED: Responses of blood pressure, heart rate, shock index, central venous oxygen saturation and lactate. *Ann Emerg Med* 14:218, 1996.
16. Lind L: Veno-arterial carbon dioxide and pH gradients and survival in critical illness. *Eur J Clin Invest* 25:201, 1995.
17. Denninghoff KR, Smith MH, Hillman LW, et al: Retinal venous oxygen saturation correlates with blood volume. *Acad Emerg Med* 5:577, 1998.
18. Porter JM, Ivatury RR: In search of the optimal end points of resuscitation in trauma patients: A review. *J Trauma* 44:908, 1998.
19. Rivers EP, Blake HC, Dereczyk B, et al: Adrenal dysfunction in hemodynamically unstable patients in the emergency department. *Acad Emerg Med* 6:626, 1999.
20. Rutherford EJ, Morris JA Jr, Reed GW, Hall KS: Base deficit stratifies mortality and determines therapy. *J Trauma* 33:417, 1992.

FLUID AND BLOOD RESUSCITATION
James E. Manning

Fluid resuscitation is the initial therapy for disorders causing intravascular volume depletion with resulting tissue hypoperfusion and organ dysfunction. In addition, other causes of shock may have a relative hypovolemia and benefit from fluid administration. Fluid and blood resuscitation serve as the bridge to maintain survival and limit morbidity until the underlying cause can be corrected. Acute hemorrhage is the predominant cause of acute intravascular volume loss requiring aggressive fluid resuscitation (Table 31-1). Other processes that cause loss of plasma fluid and electrolytes (e.g., dehydration, burns) may require aggressive fluid therapy, but blood replacement is usually not an

TABLE 31-1 Causes of Intravascular Volume Loss

Hemorrhagic hypovolemia
  Thorax
    Pulmonary parenchymal trauma
    Pulmonary vascular injury
    Intercostal vascular injury
    Aortic disruption
    Massive hemoptysis
  Abdomen/pelvis/retroperitoneum
    Solid organ injuries (liver, spleen, kidney)
    Vascular (trauma, aneurysmal rupture)
    Gastrointestinal hemorrhage (esophageal varices, ulcers, vascular
      anomalies, etc.)
    Gynecologic disorders (ruptured ectopic pregnancy, peripartum
      hemorrhage, abnormal uterine bleeding, ovarian cyst rupture, etc.)
  Orthopedic
    Pelvic fracture
    Large bone fractures
    Multiple fractures
  Extremity and skin surface
    Major vascular injuries
    Large soft tissue injuries
Nonhemorrhagic hypovolemia
    Gastrointestinal disorders: vomiting, diarrhea, ascites
    Burns
    Environmental exposure or neglect
    Renal salt wasting

issue. This chapter focuses on the issues related to fluid resuscitation in acute hemorrhagic shock.

Until recently, the widely accepted goal of fluid resuscitation was to restore a state of normovolemia (i.e., "to fill the tank"). However, laboratory studies and limited clinical reports have raised controversy about the presumed benefit of restoring normal intravascular volume in the setting of ongoing hemorrhage. Limited-volume "hypotensive" resuscitation and even "no fluid" resuscitation approaches have been proposed. Questions about the optimal initial resuscitation fluid to use and the extent of volume to administer remain.

The principal objective of fluid resuscitation is to restore sufficient intravascular volume and oxygen-carrying capacity to maintain cellular delivery of metabolic substrates (principally oxygen) in order to sustain cellular viability. Achieving this goal requires attentive responses by the clinician to the dynamic changes that occur during hemorrhage and the ability to accurately monitor, as best as possible, the physiological state of the patient.

PATHOPHYSIOLOGY

Injuries to major vascular structures, solid organs, and large bones are the major causes of severe traumatic hemorrhage. Common nontraumatic causes of hemorrhage include gastrointestinal bleeding, vascular aneurysm rupture, and ruptured ectopic pregnancy. The acute loss of intravascular volume triggers a wide range of physiological regulatory responses aimed at compensating for the blood loss and maintaining perfusion to the most important vascular beds. These compensatory mechanisms include cardiovascular, autonomic nervous system, endocrine, renal, coagulation system, and respiratory responses. Depending upon the severity of the hemorrhage and the ability of the body to compensate, variable regional or global hypoperfusion may result. Although transient, moderate hypoperfusion may be well tolerated, prolonged or severe hypoperfusion leads to shock physiology with progressive cellular and organ dysfunction.

At the cellular level, hemorrhagic shock can be defined as a state of impaired oxidative metabolism and homeostasis due to inadequate oxygen delivery and inadequate cellular waste removal resulting from hypoperfusion. The compensatory physiologic responses to acute hemorrhage seek to maintain adequate tissue oxygen delivery and sus-

tain cellular homeostasis. Loss of circulating blood volume leads to decreases in arterial blood pressure, venous return, and ventricular stroke volume. Cardiac stretch receptors and aortic baroreceptors are stimulated along with the sympathetic nervous system resulting in increased heart rate, arterial and venous vasoconstriction, increased ventricular contractility, and extravascular to intravascular fluid shift. Conversely, vagal tone is decreased. The kidneys, through stimulation of the renin-angiotensin-aldosterone system and antidiuretic hormone release, retain sodium and water to further support intravascular volume. Angiotensin II and vasopressin promote vasoconstriction. Activation of the coagulation system leads to platelet deposition and release of local mediators (thromboxane, platelet aggregating factor), local vasoconstriction at bleeding sites, platelet plug formation and fibrin deposition to seal vascular injury sites. Together these responses serve to increase intravascular volume, limit further blood loss, optimize cardiac output, and preserve vital organ perfusion.

Despite the activation of these physiologic responses, severe hemorrhage causes decreased cardiac output, and vital organ perfusion can only be maintained at the expense of nonvital organs. Progressive vasoconstriction in the splanchnic, musculoskeletal, and cutaneous vascular beds allows for sustained critical perfusion to the heart, brain, and kidneys. Renal perfusion is also sacrificed in severe states. This redistribution of blood flow is not without potential adverse effects since prolonged or severe splanchnic hypoperfusion could potentially trigger responses leading to subsequent multiple organ failure.[1] Renal hypoperfusion can lead to acute renal failure.

Progressive failure of oxidative metabolism with lactate production in hypoperfused areas leads to worsening systemic metabolic acidosis that will eventually overcome compensatory mechanisms. If hypoperfusion is not reversed or progresses beyond the capacity of the cardiovascular system, hemodynamic decompensation will occur as depression of myocardial contractility develops and local tissue acidosis and hypoxia result in loss of peripheral vasoconstriction. Death rapidly ensues. Even if the patient is resuscitated, release of inflammatory mediators and activation of cellular apoptotic pathways may be so advanced that survival is jeopardized. The goal of fluid resuscitation is to assist the body in its efforts to compensate and, above all, to avoid reaching the critical point of hemodynamic decompensation.

CLINICAL FEATURES

The clinical presentation of the patient with acute hemorrhage depends upon the cause, rate, volume, and duration of bleeding, the presence of other acute pathological processes, and the patient's baseline physiologic status. Nontraumatic causes will often have signs that indicate the source of bleeding and have symptoms specific to the disease process in addition to signs of hypovolemia. However, many causes of nontraumatic hemorrhage can have initially occult presentations. Traumatic injuries usually show some evidence of the source of bleeding, but the search must not end with the obvious since victims of major trauma can have multiple sites of significant bleeding. The presence of associated central nervous system trauma, alcohol and drug abuse, airway compromise, pulmonary injury, and other acute processes can significantly affect response to hemorrhage. Chronic underlying disease processes and medications that affect cardiovascular responsiveness can also affect response to hemorrhage.

The hemodynamic profile in response to significant acute hemorrhage-induced hypovolemia commonly includes tachycardia, hypotension, and signs of poor peripheral perfusion (cool, pale, clammy extremities with weak peripheral pulses and prolonged capillary refill). Arterial and venous vasoconstriction leads to a narrowing of the pulse pressure. Cerebral hypoperfusion causes alterations in mental status that range from subtle hypo-alertness (e.g., unusually quiet for the situation) to confusion and, ultimately, severe lethargy. Associated head injury or recreational substance intoxication can make it impossible to distinguish cerebral hypoperfusion, but this possibility should be kept in mind and evidence of systemic hypoperfusion should be sought.

With increasing blood loss, signs and symptoms of acute hemorrhage become more pronounced. The normal total circulating volume of an adult is approximately 7 percent of ideal body weight or about 5 L for an average 70-kg adult patient divided into about 3 L of plasma and 2 L of red blood cell (RBC) volume (Table 31-2). The American College of Surgeons classification of hemorrhage from their Advanced Trauma Life Support course is a useful guide for estimating blood loss and judging fluid resuscitation needs.[2] In general, loss of up to 15 percent (about 750 mL) of circulating blood volume (class I hemorrhage) is tolerated well in healthy patients. There is minimal or no tachycardic response, and changes in blood pressure usually do not occur. Without further bleeding, fluid replacement therapy is usually not needed. Blood loss of 15 to 30 percent (about 750 to 1500 mL) of total blood volume (class II hemorrhage) generally results in tachycardia and narrowed pulse pressure. The blood pressure response ranges from minimal to moderate hypotension as blood loss progresses. Compensatory peripheral vasoconstriction results in skin and pulse changes of decreased perfusion. There may be mild mental status changes. Provided the patient had a normal RBC volume before hemorrhage, this degree of blood loss is tolerated without RBC replacement provided circulating volume is restored. As blood loss increases beyond 30 percent (>1500 mL) (class III hemorrhage) there is worsening hypotension, tachycardia, peripheral hypoperfusion, and decline in mental status. At greater than 40 percent (>2 L) blood loss (class IV hemorrhage) the ability of the body to compensate has reached its limits and hemodynamic decompensation is imminent without effective resuscitation. Although this classification is helpful in estimating severity of hemorrhage, it must be remembered that there can be substantial individual variation related to baseline health status, intoxicants, and other factors.

Patients with excellent baseline physiologic status (e.g., young athletes) may have such a robust compensatory response to hemorrhage that they do not manifest tachycardia or hypotension in response to even significant hemorrhage. Such patients can appear deceptively stable for the severity of hemorrhage. Signs of peripheral hypoperfusion and subtle mental status alterations may be the only clues that the severity of hemorrhage is greater than predicted based on hemodynamic parameters. Elderly patients may not develop a tachycardic response to blood loss because of underlying heart disease or medications (e.g., β-adrenergic blocking agents). Bradycardia or lack of tachycardia may occur in approximately 30 percent of patients with intra-abdominal hemorrhage from increased vagal tone because of the hemoperitoneum. In a pregnant trauma patient, compression of the inferior vena cava by the gravid uterus can decrease central venous return, thereby worsening hypotension and tachycardia in the setting of less-severe hemorrhage.

Systemic hypoperfusion usually results in decreased urine output because of renal hypoperfusion and compensatory fluid reabsorption. Urine output is not helpful in the initial assessment of the patient with acute hemorrhage but is valuable over time in assessing response to therapy.

It must be remembered that hypotension in the setting of trauma does not always indicate hemorrhage. Other etiologies, such as primary myocardial dysfunction, airway compromise, hypoxemia as a result of lung injury, pericardial tamponade, tension pneumothorax, spinal cord injury, and toxicologic syndromes should be kept in mind. However, hypotension always warrants a careful search for occult hemorrhage.

MANAGEMENT

Initial therapy in the setting of acute hemorrhage should involve securing the airway, assuring adequate ventilation and oxygenation, controlling external bleeding (if present), and protecting the spinal cord (if potentially vulnerable). Fluid resuscitation should be determined with the following objectives in mind: (1) restoring intravascular volume sufficiently to reverse systemic hypoperfusion and limit regional hypoperfusion; (2) maintaining adequate oxygen-carrying capacity so that tissue oxygen delivery meets critical tissue oxygen demand; and (3) limiting ongoing loss of circulating RBCs. Unfortunately, there are no readily available precise parameters that allow the clinician to optimally balance these three objectives in the midst of the dynamic physiologic changes seen in acute hemorrhage and resuscitation. Nonetheless, the patient will most likely benefit from the clinician's best efforts to maintain this balance until surgical control of ongoing hemorrhage can be achieved.

Airway Control, Ventilation, and Oxygenation

The first step, as always, in patient care is assuring that the airway is patent, or securing the airway as necessary. Assuring adequate spontaneous ventilation or providing ventilation (partially or completely) logically follows. Providing oxygen is the third crucial step. Supplemental oxygen therapy aimed at achieving a fraction of inspired oxygen (FiO_2) as close to 100 percent as possible is an appropriate objective in the initial management of the patient in hemorrhagic shock. Trauma patients may have associated pulmonary injuries or underlying lung disease that may limit oxygenation of blood as it passes through the lungs. The principal objective in the treatment of hemorrhagic shock is to maintain adequate tissue oxygen delivery, so every effort should be made in the respiratory management of hemorrhagic shock patients to maximize tissue oxygen delivery by optimizing arterial hemoglobin oxygen saturation. Positive pressure ventilation in the setting of hypovolemia may significantly diminish venous return and, thereby, have the adverse effect of decreasing cardiac output. Therefore, adequate ventilation and optimal oxygenation should be sought while avoiding overzealous positive pressure ventilation. Evaluation for potentially immediately treatable injuries that can compromise ventilation and oxygenation, including pneumothorax, tension pneumothorax, hemothorax, and airway foreign body is important.

Vascular Access and Monitoring

Establishing adequate intravenous access should be underway concurrent with airway management. Large-bore peripheral lines may be adequate if two or more can be secured. The rate at which crystalloid can be infused is dependent on the catheter diameter and the driving pressure (Table 31-3). If peripheral lines are not easily achieved or the patient shows evidence of severe hemorrhagic shock, the insertion of a large catheter introducer (8 to 9 Fr) in a femoral vein is appropriate.

TABLE 31-2   Fluid Spaces

Fluid Compartment	% Body Weight* (BW)	% Total Body Water* (TBW)	Volume* (70 kg)
Total body water	60%	100%	42 L
Intracellular	40%	67%	28 L
Extracellular	20%	33%	14 L
Interstitial	15%	25%	10 L
Intravascular	~7–8%	~11–13%	~5–5.5 L
Plasma	~4–4.5%	~7%	~3–3.5 L
Red blood cells†	~3–3.5%	~5%	~2–2.5 L

*Approximate percentage and amount.

†Percentages do not add to 100% because fluid contained within intravascular red blood cells is included within the intracellular fluid compartment.

TABLE 31-3   Isotonic Crystalloid Intravenous Infusion Rates

IV Access	Gravity (80-cm Height)	Pressure (300 mm Hg)
18 g peripheral IV	50–60 mL/min	120–180 mL/min
16 g peripheral IV	90–125 mL/min	200–250 mL/min
14 g peripheral IV	125–160 mL/min	250–300 mL/min
8.5 Fr central venous introducer	200 mL/min	400–500 mL/min

The subclavian and jugular veins can also be used but with the understanding that in the setting of significant hypovolemia they may be partially collapsed. An iatrogenic pneumothorax during attempted cannulation could lead to hemodynamic decompensation. In profound hemorrhagic shock with impending cardiovascular collapse, saphenous vein cutdown at the ankle or the proximal anteromedial thigh is also a reasonable option. Vascular access above the diaphragm is prudent if there is concern of major vascular injury in the area of the abdomen or pelvis. With initial vascular access, a full set of blood tubes should be drawn for appropriate laboratory studies and blood bank procedures (Table 31-4).

The patient should have continuous electrocardiographic heart rate monitoring, continuous pulse oximetry, and, if possible, continuous end-tidal carbon dioxide monitoring. Frequent checks of arterial blood pressure are also warranted. In severe hemorrhage, insertion of an arterial line is reasonable to allow for continuous arterial blood pressure monitoring and ease of arterial blood sampling. Serial arterial blood gas (ABG) and arterial lactate analyses yield important information about respiratory and metabolic status. For example, assessing the severity and trend in base deficit and lactate are helpful in determining the presence of ongoing systemic hypoperfusion that needs further intervention. A urinary catheter should be inserted to initiate urine output monitoring. The urine should be checked for blood and a urine pregnancy test should be performed on female patients of potential childbearing age. Insertion of a central venous line allows for central venous pressure (CVP) monitoring and assessment of central venous oxygen saturation. CVP measurements can be used to assess response to fluid administration; low central venous oxygen saturation is an indication of systemic hypoperfusion. In addition to frequent assessment of vital signs, mental status, and peripheral perfusion signs should be regularly assessed. Various newer monitoring technologies may prove to be very useful in the assessment of patients in hemorrhagic shock. These include pulse contour analysis continuous cardiac output, transcutaneous oximetry, tissue capnometry, and thoracic impedance monitors.

TABLE 31-4   Diagnostic Evaluation in Acute Hemorrhage

Laboratory studies
  Hemoglobin/hematocrit
  Arterial blood gases
  Lactate
  Electrolytes, blood urea nitrogen, creatinine, glucose, calcium
  Coagulation studies
  Platelet count
  Type and cross-match
Studies to evaluate sources of blood loss (as indicated)
  Chest radiograph
  Pelvic radiograph
  Abdominal/pelvic CT
  Abdominal ultrasonography
  Chest CT
  GI endoscopy
  Bronchoscopy
  Vascular radiology

Abbreviations: CT = computed tomography; GI = gastrointestinal.

Fluid Resuscitation

Intravascular volume replacement to treat hemorrhage has been the accepted dogma for decades. The goal of restoring normal intravascular volume and normal arterial blood pressure was generally accepted for most of this time. The major area of controversy was the optimal resuscitation fluid. However, over the past decade the accepted practice of resuscitating patients to a normal blood pressure has been questioned. The early studies that supported aggressive volume replacement were performed in laboratory models of controlled hemorrhage. In such a circumstance, rapidly restoring normovolemia optimized outcome and had no appreciable adverse effects. However, this laboratory model does not accurately reflect the clinical situation. Most hemorrhagic shock patients have not had control of their bleeding achieved prior to initiation of fluid resuscitation. This fact raised concern that fluid resuscitation to a normal blood pressure might actually be deleterious by exacerbating ongoing hemorrhage and ultimately worsening outcome. Formation of clots at areas of vascular injury is facilitated by the lower blood pressure that results during hemorrhage. Increased blood pressure may dislodge these fragile developing clots. Because crystalloid solutions have essentially no oxygen-carrying capacity, any exacerbation of hemorrhage resulting from their infusion will lower the oxygen-carrying capacity of the circulating blood. Laboratory models of acute vascular injury with uncontrolled hemorrhage verified that raising the arterial blood pressure to the normal range increased the rate of ongoing bleeding. This led to the concept of limited volume or "hypotensive" resuscitation.[3]

The goal of this limited approach is to provide sufficient fluid resuscitation to maintain vital organ perfusion and avoid cardiovascular collapse while keeping the arterial blood pressure relatively low (e.g., mean arterial pressure of 60 mm Hg) in the hope of limiting further loss of red blood cells until surgical control of bleeding can be achieved. The potential adverse effect of this approach is that it accepts the presence of regional hypoperfusion, the effects of which are dependent on both the severity and duration of the hypoperfusion. Splanchnic hypoperfusion is especially of concern because this may be a major contributor to the development of subsequent multiple organ dysfunction.[1] Unfortunately, accurate clinical assessment of regional hypoperfusion is not presently possible. Thus, the optimal resuscitation end point is not clear and likely varies with the individual patient. A randomized clinical study that aimed to evaluate hypotensive resuscitation to a systolic blood pressure of 70 mm Hg did not show any mortality benefit for this approach.[4] However, the target pressure of 70 mm Hg was difficult to maintain, with the systolic blood pressure in the hypotensive group reaching an average of 100 mm Hg. This demonstrates the difficulty of achieving and maintaining a specific hypotensive blood pressure target in the dynamic setting of hemorrhagic shock resuscitation. At present, this is still a concept that has not been clearly shown to improve survival. However, it seems reasonable to keep this concept in mind and to avoid excessive fluid resuscitation.

Even more radical than the concept of low volume or hypotensive resuscitation is the suggestion that no fluid should be administered in some cases of acute hemorrhage until surgical repair is ready to begin. A randomized study of hypotensive patients with penetrating torso injuries found that delaying fluid resuscitation until surgical hemostasis improved survival.[5] The full consequences of this bold approach to acute hemorrhage have not been adequately evaluated. It seems that for some patients that are able to adequately compensate for their blood loss, this may be an acceptable approach. However, in the setting of ongoing hemorrhage with impending cardiovascular collapse, it is difficult to justify this approach.

Despite numerous laboratory and clinical investigations, the choice of resuscitation fluid remains controversial (Table 31-5). Crystalloid solutions and various colloids have both been widely used, but studies comparing these two fluid types have yielded varying results. An extensive meta-analysis of available clinical trials found no difference in survival

TABLE 31-5   Resuscitation Fluids

Isotonic crystalloid
    Normal saline (NS)
    Lactated Ringer's (LR) solution
    Ringer's acetate
Colloids
    Albumin: 5% and 25% concentrations
    Fresh-frozen plasma
    Hetastarch: 6% hydroxyethyl starch concentration
    Dextran -40 (molecular weight 40 kDa) 10% solution
    Dextran -70 (molecular weight 70 kDa) 6% solution
    Gelatin
Hypertonic solutions
    Saline: 7.0 to 7.5% NaCl
    Saline and dextran: 7.5% NaCl and 6% Dextran-70
Oxygen carrying resuscitation fluids
    Hemoglobin-based oxygen carriers
    Fluorocarbon-based oxygen carriers
Blood
    Packed red blood cells

comparing crystalloid with colloid resuscitation.[6] The cost of colloid agents tips the recommendation for fluid choice to crystalloid solutions.

Isotonic Crystalloid Solution

Isotonic crystalloid solutions, normal saline (NS) or lactated Ringer's (LR) solution, have been the preferred resuscitation fluid in the United States for many years. Crystalloid solutions are hypo-oncotic because they lack the large protein molecules present in the plasma. This causes a substantial amount of the crystalloid solution administered to shift in to the extravascular space corresponding to the relative size of the intravascular and interstitial fluid compartments (Table 31-6). This is the physiologic basis for the 3:1 ratio for isotonic crystalloid volume replacement: for every amount of blood lost, three times that amount of isotonic crystalloid is required to store intravascular volume because, at best, about 30 percent of the infused fluid stays intravascular. Based on this rule, a loss of 1 L of blood (approximately 15 to 20 percent of total circulating blood volume) would require about 3 L of isotonic crystalloid to restore normovolemia. Bearing this in mind, the recommendations for initial fluid resuscitation have been to administer 2 to 3 L of crystalloid solution in acute hemorrhage and then assess the response. If this amount of crystalloid solution has not stabilized the patient's hemodynamic status, it suggests that blood loss either exceeds 15 to 20 percent of total blood volume, or that there is significant ongoing blood loss, or both.

The choice of NS versus LR solution has been the focus of controversy over time. However, there is no clear evidence that either of these crystalloid solutions is superior to the other. Concerns have been raised about each fluid: (1) infusion of large volumes of either causes increased neutrophil activation; (2) LR solution also increases cytokine release and may increase lactic acidosis when given in large

TABLE 31-6   Theoretical Volemic Effect of 1 L of Fluid Administration on Fluid Compartments

	Intracellular	Interstitial	Plasma
D5W	660 mL	255 mL	85 mL
NS or LR	−100 mL	825 mL	275 mL
7.5% Saline	−2950 mL	2960 mL	990 mL
5% Albumin	0	500 mL	500 mL
Whole blood	0	0	1000 mL

Abbreviations: D5W = 5% dextrose in water; LR = lactated Ringer's solution; NS = normal saline.

volumes; and (3) NS exacerbates intracellular potassium depletion and causes hyperchloremic acidosis.

Blood Transfusion

There are no clearly defined parameters that trigger the switch from crystalloid to blood resuscitation. However, it is generally accepted that a patient in shock that demonstrates minimal or only modest hemodynamic improvement after rapid infusion of 2 to 3 L of crystalloid is in need of blood transfusion. However, it would be acceptable to start blood immediately if it is clear that the patient has suffered profound blood loss and is on the verge of cardiovascular collapse. Some patients may have an adequate hemodynamic response to initial crystalloid therapy that is transient. In such cases, continued crystalloid infusion beyond the first 2 to 3 L might be used for hemodynamic support so long as attention is paid to progressive hemodilution and its effect on tissue oxygen delivery. This hemodilution also lowers the concentration of clotting factors and platelets needed for intrinsic hemostasis at bleeding sites. Serial assessment of blood hemoglobin concentration is useful in such a situation. An American Society of Anesthesiologists task force review found that a blood hemoglobin concentration >10 g/dL (hematocrit >30 percent) very seldom requires blood transfusion, whereas a level <6 g/dL (hematocrit <18 percent) almost always requires blood transfusion.[7] This leaves a rather wide intermediate range of hemoglobin—between 6 and 10 g/dL—where the decision to administer blood is significantly influenced by other factors, such as the presence of underlying disease processes that are sensitive to decreased tissue oxygen delivery and the rate of continued blood loss, if present. Understandably, as the hemoglobin concentration decreases, especially to 8 g/dL or less, the likelihood of needing blood markedly increases.

When possible, typed and cross-matched blood is preferable. However, in the acute setting where time does not permit full cross-matching, type-specific blood is the next best option followed by low-titer O-negative blood. Blood can be administered as whole blood or packed RBC preparations. In U.S. blood banks, whole blood is not stocked, and only packed RBCs are available. In the setting of massive hemorrhage with large volumes of crystalloid and blood resuscitation, fresh-frozen plasma and platelet transfusions may be needed to reverse the associated dilutional coagulopathy.

Red blood cell transfusion obviously restores lost hemoglobin, but stored blood components may also not be fully functional and can have adverse effects, which appear to be exacerbated with longer storage time.[8] Using current preservatives, RBCs can be stored for up to 42 days and it has been reported that the average age of a unit of blood administered in the United States is approximately 21 days old. Stored RBCs can lose deformability, which can limit their ability to pass normally through capillary beds, or can cause capillary plugging. The oxygen dissociation curve is altered by loss of 2,3-diphosphoglycerate in the erythrocyte, which adversely affects the off-loading of oxygen at the tissue level. Clinical studies report worsening of splanchnic ischemia and an increased incidence of multiple-organ dysfunction associated with transfusion of RBCs that have been stored for longer than 2 weeks.[9,10] Therefore, RBC transfusion, although a critical intervention in severe hemorrhagic shock, has limitations and potential adverse effects that should be kept in mind.

Colloid Resuscitation

Several colloid agents have been studied experimentally and used clinically for the treatment of hemorrhagic shock (see Table 31-5). Colloids have larger molecular weight particles with plasma oncotic pressures similar to normal plasma proteins. Therefore, colloids would be expected to remain in the intravascular space, replacing plasma proteins lost as a consequence of hemorrhage, and more effectively restore circulating blood volume than crystalloid solutions. An argument favoring the use of colloids has been the concern that extravascular shift of infused crystalloid solutions has potential adverse effects, including pulmonary interstitial edema with impaired oxygen diffusion and intraabdominal edema with diminished bowel perfusion. However, pathologic conditions, such as hemorrhagic shock and sepsis, lead to increased vascular permeability that can allow for extravascular leakage of these larger colloid molecules.

The colloids that have been used as resuscitation fluids are a heterogeneous group of agents with widely varying characteristics and effects. These agents have been compared to each other as well as to crystalloids. A systematic review of the use of albumin in critically ill patients found an increased relative risk of death, as compared to use of crystalloids or no albumin.[11] The value of other colloid agents such as hetastarch, modified gelatin, and dextran, has not been clearly demonstrated. An extensive review and meta-analysis of clinical studies comparing crystalloids and colloids for fluid resuscitation failed to show any evidence of improved outcome with the use of colloids.[6] Furthermore, a review of different colloids did not demonstrate that any particular colloid product is superior to the others, although confidence intervals were wide, making this conclusion less certain.[12] Given the much greater cost of colloid products, there is no clear basis for the choice of these agents over crystalloid solutions for fluid resuscitation.

Hypertonic Resuscitation Fluids

Hypertonic saline has been proposed as a potential crystalloid solution alternative that would limit the tissue edema effects that are of concern with isotonic crystalloid solutions. Hypertonic saline has been shown to rapidly expand intravascular volume and enhance tissue perfusion with hemodynamic effects beyond the degree of intravascular volume expansion. The intravascular shift of fluid from the extravascular space may be potentially beneficial in head trauma patients by limiting cerebral edema, lowering intracranial pressure, and improving cerebral perfusion. This effect may also limit pulmonary interstitial fluid shift that could potentially adversely affect oxygen diffusion. In early studies, it was noted that the effect of hypertonic saline alone was often transient. The addition of dextran to hypertonic saline was aimed at sustaining the hemodynamic effect of the hypertonic saline. The volume of hypertonic saline solution that can be given during resuscitation is limited due to the potential for hypernatremia.

Laboratory studies show beneficial hemodynamic effects and decreases in intracranial pressure. However, clinical studies comparing hypertonic saline and hypertonic saline/dextran do not show clear evidence of improved outcome, although a trend toward benefit has been suggested for seriously injured trauma patients.[13] The military has a particularly strong interest in hypertonic resuscitation solutions because of the logistics of battlefield care. Recent recommendations have advocated the use of hypertonic saline for battlefield resuscitation.[14]

Oxygen-Carrying Resuscitation Fluid

A major limitation of all crystalloid and colloid resuscitation fluids is that none of these products restores the oxygen-carrying capacity of the lost red blood cells. Tissue oxygen delivery may be improved as a result of improved tissue perfusion but with severe and ongoing hemorrhage loss of hemoglobin becomes critical requiring blood transfusion. The problems of blood availability, transfusion reaction, viral infection, and loss of normal oxygen delivery properties with packed RBCs has led to a search for products that can serve as a substitute for blood transfusion, at least on a temporary basis.

Two classes of agents, hemoglobin-based oxygen carriers and fluorocarbon-based oxygen carriers, have been under development in recent decades to try to meet this demand.[15] Ideally, such an oxygen-carrying resuscitation fluid would have tissue-oxygen-delivery properties comparable to native red blood cell hemoglobin, temperature sta-

bility, long shelf-life, no preparation requirements, and no adverse side effects. None of the oxygen therapeutic agents presently approaching clinical availability meets all these ideal characteristics but some of the hemoglobin-based oxygen carriers have proven sufficiently effective and safe to be close to approval for clinical use. However, the use of large volumes of such products in the setting of severe hemorrhage has not been adequately studied. Furthermore, despite repletion of oxygen-carrying capacity, these products do not restore coagulation components and the lowered viscosity because of loss of cellular elements can further diminish hemostasis at sites of ongoing bleeding. Therefore, the value of oxygen therapeutic agents may be primarily as an "oxygen bridge" until surgical hemostasis can be achieved and normal blood components can be, at least partially, restored.

Hemoglobin-based oxygen carriers have been developed from human hemoglobin (outdated blood units), bovine blood, and recombinant DNA technology. The hemoglobin is free of cellular stroma and must be polymerized or cross-linked to maintain the hemoglobin tetramer intact (two α chains and two β chains) that will adequately carry oxygen and stay within the circulation for a reasonable time. Lack of 2,3-diphosphoglycerate in acellular hemoglobin solution shifts the oxygen dissociation curve toward increased oxygen affinity, which decreases off-loading of oxygen at the tissues. This requires chemical alteration of the oxygen-binding sites to promote effective tissue oxygen delivery. Hemoglobin-based oxygen carriers have been shown to result in significant vasoconstriction. This is a characteristic that must be considered if these products are to be used in the treatment of hemorrhagic shock because blood pressure may be increased disproportionately for the level of intravascular volume replacement. To date, no hemoglobin-based fluid has proven both effective and safe; a multicenter trial of diaspirin cross-linked hemoglobin (DCLHB) for traumatic hemorrhagic shock was prematurely halted when interim analysis found a higher mortality in patients receiving DCLHB. Despite the theoretical attractiveness of such a product, even if a hemoglobin-based solution is proven both effective and safe for human use, the cost of the product may be prohibitively expensive.

Fluorocarbon-based oxygen carriers are emulsions that dissolve respiratory gases in direct proportion to the partial pressure of the respiratory gas (i.e., oxygen). Unlike the S-shaped oxygen dissociation curve of hemoglobin, the relationship for fluorocarbons is linear. Unfortunately, an F_{IO_2} of greater than 70 percent is required before these fluorocarbons carry physiologically useful concentrations of oxygen. Fluorocarbon emulsions have been studied in laboratory models of hemorrhage, but the toxicity to the reticuloendothelial system from these agents at higher doses and the requirement for sustained levels of F_{IO_2} limits their potential for use in the setting of severe hemorrhage. Limited replacement of surgical blood loss may be possible with these products, but large volume resuscitation presently appears doubtful.

Assessing Response to Resuscitation

One of the greatest limitations in the early management of hemorrhagic shock is the lack of adequate, easily measurable parameters that accurately reflect the physiologic status of the patient both prior to and during the course of fluid resuscitation. It is widely recognized that arterial blood pressure does not adequately reflect cardiac output or regional hypoperfusion. Clinical evidence of peripheral hypoperfusion is useful in alerting the clinician to ongoing hypoperfusion but is not quantitative. Monitoring modalities noted previously but not commonly used in the emergency department may be useful in the management of acute hemorrhagic shock patients.

Central venous pressure response to fluid administration is useful in assessing volume status. The principle is that if the CVP does not rise after infusion of a quantity of fluid—typically isotonic crystalloid 250 to 500 mL—then the vascular system is still very compliant (on the flat portion of the pressure-volume compliance curve) and is not "full." If the CVP rises appreciably (>5 to 7 mm Hg) after fluid infusion, then the vascular system has reached the limits of easily distensibility (on the steep portion of the pressure-volume compliance curve) and is therefore "full."

Central venous oxygen saturation (ScvO$_2$) has been shown to correlate with pulmonary artery mixed venous oxygen saturation (SmvO$_2$) and central venous catheterization is much more feasible than pulmonary artery catheterization in the ED.[16] Thus, central venous oximetry is an available and useful parameter for assessing global oxygen supply-demand balance. Low ScvO$_2$ (<50 percent) indicates global hypoperfusion leading to high tissue oxygen extraction in response to inadequate tissue oxygen delivery. However, ScvO$_2$ may not be sensitive enough to identify regional hypoperfusion (e.g., splanchnic hypoperfusion) unless it is severe or fairly widespread, recognizing that regional and global hypoperfusion are on a continuum.

Simultaneous arterial and central venous blood gases allow for the calculation of systemic oxygen extraction ratio (OER, normally about 25 percent). An elevated OER, especially greater than 50 percent, indicates oxygen supply-demand imbalance consistent with global or significant regional hypoperfusion. The relatively recent availability of arterial pulse contour analysis catheters allows for continuous cardiac output measurement via an arterial line. This, in addition to central venous oximetry, could prove very helpful in assessing the dynamic changes and adjusting therapy during resuscitation. End-tidal CO$_2$ is predictive of eventual outcome in severely hypoperfused trauma patients, but it is not yet clear how effective this parameter is in assessing patients with lesser degrees of hypoperfusion.[17] Serial assessment of metabolic parameters, especially lactate and base deficit, can be useful in assessing the correction of systemic metabolic acidosis because of hypoperfusion.[18,19]

All of the monitoring parameters noted above are indicators of global or systemic perfusion status. It would be advantageous to have a means of assessing regional perfusion, especially in the splanchnic circulation, which is particularly vulnerable during hemorrhagic shock caused by compensatory redistribution of blood flow and its potential major role in the subsequent development of multiple organ dysfunction. Gastric intramucosal pH has been suggested as a parameter that reflects splanchnic perfusion. Recently, gastric tissue oxygen saturation, measured using near-infrared spectroscopy, has been reported to rapidly and accurately reflect splanchnic perfusion in a laboratory model of hemorrhagic shock.[20] These are promising parameters that might significantly influence clinical decisions in fluid resuscitation.

REFERENCES

1. Reilly PM, Wilkins KB, Fuh KC, et al: The mesenteric hemodynamic response to circulatory shock: An overview. *Shock* 15:329, 2001.
2. American College of Surgeons Committee on Trauma: *Advanced Trauma Life Support for Doctors Manual.* Chicago: American College of Surgeons, 1997, pp. 97–107.
3. Stern SA: Low-volume fluid resuscitation for presumed hemorrhagic shock: Helpful or harmful? *Curr Opin Crit Care* 7:422, 2001.
4. Dutton RP, Mackenzie CF, Scalea TM: Hypotensive resuscitation during active hemorrhage: Impact on in-hospital mortality. *J Trauma* 52:1141, 2002.
5. Bickell WM, Wall MJ, Pepe PE, et al: Immediate versus delayed fluid resuscitation for hypotensive patients with penetrating torso injuries. *New Engl J Med* 331:1105, 1994.
6. Alderson P, Schierhout G, Roberts I, et al: Colloids versus crystalloids for fluid resuscitation in critically ill patients. *Cochrane Database Syst Rev* (2):CD000567, 2000.
7. American Society of Anesthesiologists Task Force: Practice guidelines for blood component therapy. *Anesthesiology* 84:732, 1996.
8. Zallen G, Offner PJ, Moore EE, et al: Age of transfused blood is an independent risk factor of postinjury multiple organ failure. *Am J Surg* 178:570, 1999.
9. Marik PE, Sibbald WJ: Effect of stored-blood transfusion on oxygen delivery in patients with sepsis. *JAMA* 269:3024, 1993.
10. Moore FA, Moore EE, Sauaia A: Blood transfusion: An independent risk factor for postinjury multiple organ failure. *Arch Surg* 132:620, 1997.
11. Cochrane Injuries Group Albumin Reviewers: Human albumin administration in critically ill patients: Systematic review of randomized controlled trials. *BMJ* 317:235, 1998.
12. Bunn F, Alderson P, Hawkins V: Colloid solutions for fluid resuscitation. *Cochrane Database Syst Rev* (2):CD001319, 2001.
13. Bunn R, Roberts I, Tasker R, et al: Hypertonic versus isotonic crystalloid for fluid resuscitation in critically ill patients. *Cochrane Database Syst Rev* (1):CD002045, 2002.
14. Institute of Medicine, Committee on Fluid Resuscitation for Combat Casualties: *Fluid Resuscitation: State of the Science for Treating Combat Casualties and Civilian Injuries.* Washington, DC: National Academy Press, 1999.
15. Arnoldo BD, Minei JP: Potential of hemoglobin-based oxygen carriers in trauma patients. *Curr Opin Crit Care* 7:431, 2001.
16. Rady MY, Rivers EP, Martin GD, et al: Continuous central venous oximetry and shock index in the emergency department: Use in the evaluation of clinical shock. *Am J Emerg Med* 10:538, 1992.
17. Tyburski JG, Collinge JD, Wilson RF, et al: End-tidal CO$_2$-derived values during emergency trauma surgery correlated with outcome: A prospective study. *J Trauma* 53:738, 2002.
18. Porter JM, Ivatury RR: In search of the optimal end points of resuscitation in trauma patients: A review. *J Trauma* 44:908, 1998.
19. Rutherford EJ, Morris JA, Reed GW, et al: Base deficit stratifies mortality and determines therapy. *J Trauma* 33:417, 1992.
20. Cohn SM, Varela JE, Giannotti G, et al: Splanchnic perfusion evaluation during hemorrhage and resuscitation with gastric near-infrared spectroscopy. *J Trauma* 50:629, 2001.

32 SEPTIC SHOCK
Jonathan Jui

Sepsis is a heterogeneous clinical syndrome that can be caused by any class of microorganism. Although gram-negative and gram-positive bacteria account for most sepsis cases, fungi, mycobacteria, rickettsia, viruses, or protozoans can cause similar presentations. Microbial blood invasion is not essential to the development of sepsis.

EPIDEMIOLOGY

An extrapolation from hospital discharge data from 1995 in seven U.S. states yielded a national estimate of 751,000 cases of severe sepsis per year, or about 3.0 cases per 1000 population and 2.26 cases per 100 hospital discharges.[1] The rate per hospital discharge agrees with a study from eight academic medical centers that reported an incidence of 2 cases of sepsis per 100 hospital admissions.[2] Of these cases, 55 percent occurred in the intensive care unit (ICU), 12 percent in the emergency department, and 33 percent in a non-intensive patient care unit. Up to half of sepsis patients develop shock, with an overall mortality rate of about 45 percent, but with a wide range of 20 to 80 percent depending on host age and comorbidities. Clinical studies in patients with bacteremia indicated that gram-positive and gram-negative bacteria are the etiology of the sepsis in 35 to 40 percent and 55 to 60 percent of the episodes, respectively. The most frequent sites of infection are the lungs, abdomen, and the urinary tract. Factors that predispose to gram-negative bacteremia include diabetes mellitus, lymphoproliferative diseases, cirrhosis of the liver, burns, invasive procedures or devices, and chemotherapy. Major gram-positive bacteremia risk factors include vascular catheters, indwelling mechanical devices, burns, and injection drug use. Fungemia most often occurs in immunocompromised patients.

Although there is no reason to suspect that the occurrence of septic shock would differ according to the patient's gender, studies have found a slightly higher incidence of sepsis in men.[1] This slight difference may reflect a higher rate of preceding surgical procedures in men as opposed to women. Sepsis is more common in older adults; the mean age reported is 55 to 60 years. Older patients are more likely to have conditions that predispose to bacterial infection, such as diabetes, surgical procedures, and cancer.

DEFINITIONS AND RISK CATEGORIZATION

In 1991, the American College of Chest Physicians and the Society of Critical Care proposed a set of definitions that could be applied to patients with sepsis and its sequelae (Table 32-1).[3] The primary goals of this classification were to provide a conceptual and practical framework of the systemic inflammatory response to infection; to improve the ability of clinicians to make early bedside detection of sepsis, thus allowing early therapeutic intervention; and to standardize the definition which would allow better comparison and analysis of research protocols.

The identification of systemic inflammatory response syndrome (SIRS) does not confirm a diagnosis of infection or sepsis, because the features of SIRS can be seen in many other conditions, such as trauma, pancreatitis, burns, or infection (Figure 32-1). Systemic inflammatory response syndrome is not a diagnosis, nor is it a good indicator of outcome. The SIRS criteria may be considered a crude stratification for patients with systemic inflammation. In a prospective study of the epidemiology of SIRS in medical and surgical patients, mortality rates were 3 percent in patients without SIRS, 6 percent in those with two criteria, 10 percent in those with three positive criteria, and 17 percent in those meeting all four criteria.[4] Death rates were similar for patients with culture-negative SIRS and those with culture-positive SIRS. A complementary method of classification of sepsis based primarily on physiologic abnormalities such as the Third Acute Physiology and Chronic Health Evaluation acuity system has been developed. Multivariate analysis using initial Acute Physiology and Chronic Health

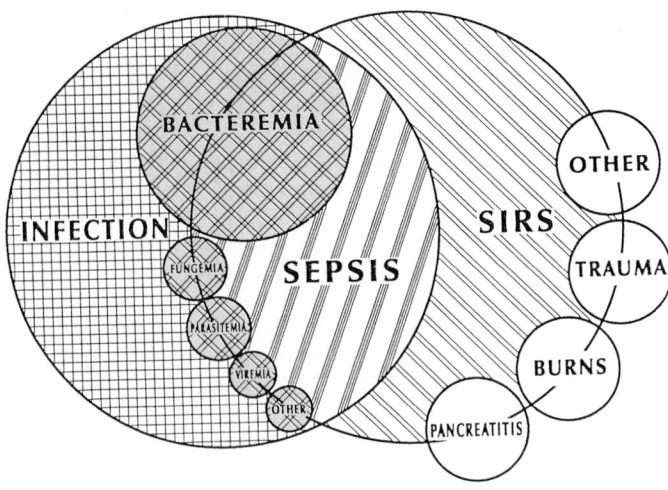

BLOOD BORNE INFECTION

FIG. 32-1. The interrelationship between systemic inflammatory response syndrome (SIRS), sepsis, and infection. (Reproduced with permission from American College of Chest Physicians/Society of Critical Care Medicine: American College of Chest Physicians/Society of Critical Care Medicine consensus conference: Definitions for sepsis and organ failure and guidelines for the use of innovative therapies in sepsis. *Chest* 101:1644, 1992.)

Evaluation score, etiology of sepsis (urosepsis or other), and treatment location before ICU admission enables the risk of hospital death from sepsis to be predicted.

PATHOPHYSIOLOGY

Sepsis starts as a focus of infection (urinary tract infection, pneumonia, cellulitis, abscess, or indwelling prosthetic device) resulting in blood stream invasion or a proliferation of organisms at the infected site (Figure 32-2). These growing organisms release a large amount of exogenous toxins consisting of endotoxins, exotoxins, and other components of the organism's structural components. The host's reaction to these toxins results in the release of endogenous mediators and activation of other humoral defense mechanisms including complement, kinins, and coagulation factors. Among the most prominent of the endogenous mediators are the cytokines [e.g., tumor necrosis factor α (TNF-α) and interleukins (ILs)], platelet-activating factor (PAF), arachidonic acid metabolites, and myocardial depressant substances. Release of myocardial depressant substances results in the depression of myocardial function, dilation of the ventricles, and vasodilation.

Molecular Mediators in the Pathophysiology of Sepsis

Until recently, septic shock and its morbid consequences were attributed to the direct result of endogenous proteins and phospholipid mediators secreted by the infected individual.[5] However, the evidence of overstimulated immune response to microbial infection in sepsis is not as convincing as originally thought. Although some sepsis conditions, such as meningococcemia, have high levels of circulating cytokines that correlate with mortality, generally fewer than 25 percent of patients with sepsis from other organisms have elevated cytokines. Conversely, the presence of elevated cytokines in sepsis correlates with an increased rate of circulatory shock and overall mortality. Cytokine pathophysiology of sepsis can be divided into three phases: induction, cytokine synthesis and secretion, and cascade.

The induction of cytokines involves the interaction of certain microbial molecules that, when recognized by the host, results in the production of mediators that amplify and transmit the microbial signal to

TABLE 32-1 Definitions

Infection = microbial phenomenon characterized by an inflammatory response to the presence of microorganisms or the invasion of normally sterile host tissue by those organisms.

Bacteremia = the presence of viable bacteria in the blood.

Systemic inflammatory response syndrome = the systemic inflammatory response to a variety of severe clinical insults. The response is manifested by two or more of the following conditions: (1) temperature >38°C or <36°C; (2) heart rate >90 beats/min; (3) respiratory rate >20 breaths/min or $Paco_2$ <32 mm Hg; and (4) white blood cell count >12,000/μL, <4000/μL, or >10% immature (band) forms.

Sepsis = the systemic response to infection, manifested by two or more of the following conditions as a result of infection: (1) temperature >38°C or <36°C; (2) heart rate >90 beats/min; (3) respiratory rate >20 breaths/min or $Paco_2$ <32 mm Hg; and (4) white blood cell count >12,000/μL, <4000/μL, or >10% immature (band) forms.

Severe sepsis = sepsis associated with organ dysfunction, hypoperfusion, or hypotension. Hypoperfusion and perfusion abnormalities may include, but are not limited to lactic acidosis, oliguria, or an acute alteration in mental status.

Septic shock = sepsis-induced hypotension despite adequate fluid resuscitation along with the presence of perfusion abnormalities that may include, but are not limited to, lactic acidosis, oliguria, or an acute alteration in mental status. Patients who are receiving inotropic or vasopressor agents may not be hypotensive at the time that perfusion abnormalities are measured.

Sepsis-induced hypotension = a systolic blood pressure <90 mm Hg or a reduction of ≥40 mm Hg from baseline in the absence of other causes for hypotension.

Multiple organ dysfunction syndrome = presence of altered organ function in an acutely ill patient such that homeostasis cannot be maintained without intervention.

Abbreviation: $Paco_2$ = arterial partial pressure of carbon dioxide.

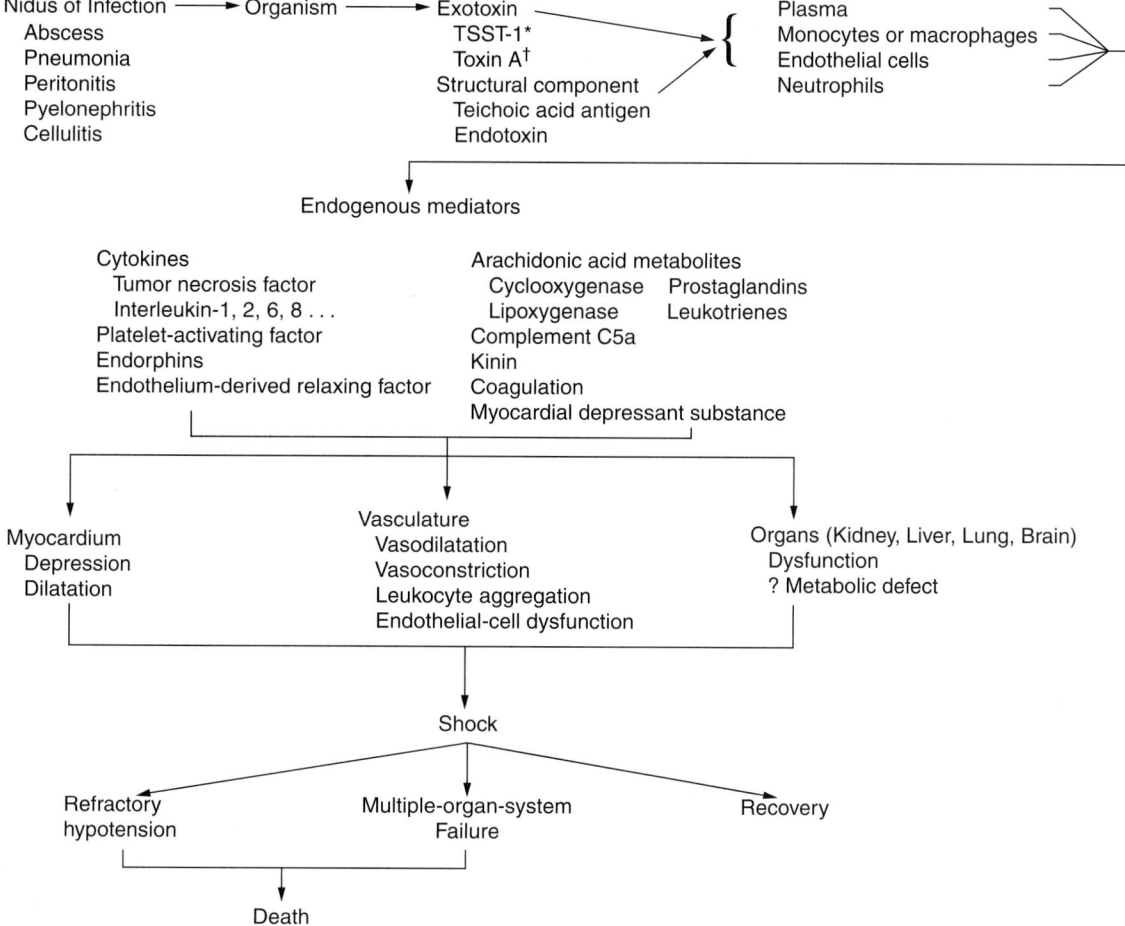

FIG. 32-2. Pathogenic sequence of the events in septic shock. *TSST-1 = toxic shock syndrome toxin 1; †Toxin A = *Pseudomonas aeruginosa* toxin A.

other cells and tissues. For example, in a gram-negative infection, the host is not only exposed to membrane bound lipopolysaccharides (LPSs) at the site of infection but also is systemically exposed to the free endotoxin on fragments of bacterial outer membrane commonly shed during bacterial growth and replication. Lipopolysaccharide binds to LPS-binding protein, forming an LPS–LPS-binding protein complex. This complex is 1000-fold more potent than LPS alone in inducing TNF-α production by macrophages. The receptor for this complex is the CD14 molecule that is found on monocytes, macrophages, and neutrophils. The peptidoglycan and lipoteichoic acids of gram-positive bacteria, certain polysaccharides, extracellular enzymes, and toxins induce cytokine synthesis in manner similar to LPS.

Cytokine synthesis and secretion involves several regulated steps: (1) transcription (synthesis of messenger RNA from the DNA template), (2) translation of mRNA into protein, (3) post-translational processing, and (4) secretion of protein. For example, when the LPS–LPS-binding protein complex interacts with the CD14 receptor in vitro, transcription of the TNF gene increases threefold, with levels of TNF mRNA increasing 100-fold. Biosynthesis and secretion of TNF-α, however, increase over 10,000-fold, primarily due to increased translational efficiency of preformed TNF mRNA and efficient translation of newly transcribed TNF mRNA.

The cytokine cascade in sepsis results from the activation and release of a central mediator (TNF-α, IL-1), which results in the secretion of various secondary mediators (IL-6, IL-8, PAF, prostaglandins, and leukotrienes); the activation of neutrophils, the complement system, and vascular endothelial cells; and synthesis of acute phase reactants. Lipopolysaccharide and TNF-α probably pro-

mote intravascular coagulation initially by inducing blood monocytes to express tissue factor, by initiating the release of plasminogen activator inhibitor type 1, and inhibiting the expression of thrombomodulin and plasminogen activator by vascular endothelial cells. The physiologic outcome of this complex cascade produces the physiologic changes recognized as the SIRS.

Parallel to SIRS is the body's intrinsic anti-inflammatory response. This response, termed the *compensatory anti-inflammatory response syndrome* (CARS), attempts to down-regulate the SIRS response. Agents identified as participating in CARS include interleukins (IL-4, IL-10), transforming growth factor β, colony-stimulating factor, soluble receptors to tumor necrosis factor, and antagonists to TNF-α and IL-1 receptors. These mediators inhibit T- and B-lymphocyte activities and decrease antigen-presenting activity on the monocyte. The body normally maintains a delicate balance between SIRS and CARS. Uncontrolled SIRS leads to profound hypotension, inadequate perfusion, and death. If the CARS reaction is severe, it will manifest clinically as anergy and increase susceptibility to infection.

Vasoactive Mediators in the Pathophysiology of Sepsis

One of the most important of the vasoactive mediators is nitric oxide. Nitric oxide is a low-molecular-weight membrane-permeable gas with harmful and beneficial effects in shock. Under normal conditions, this gas is produced in the endothelium by a calcium- and calmodulin-dependent nitric oxide synthase (NOS), which converts L-arginine and O_2 to L-citrulline and nitric oxide. This pathway is normally well regulated by signal transduction pathways linked to cell-surface receptors for vasodilators such as acetylcholine and histamine. However, inflammatory mediators induce a calcium-independent form of NOS that is not controlled by this mechanism. This form may rise to abnormal amounts of nitric oxide in septic patients and patients given IL-2 for cancer treatment.

Three distinct NOS enzyme complexes have been described. The first, neuronal NOS, is found in central nervous system cells and is thought to support a neurotransmitter function. The second, constitutive NOS, is found in endothelial cells and is thought to play a role in the maintenance of normal vascular tone. The third, a high-output inducible NOS (iNOS), is found in many cell types, including endothelial cells, vascular smooth muscle cells, and macrophages.

Nitric oxide actions include functioning as a neurotransmitter, regulating vascular tone, and inhibiting platelet aggregation and leukocyte adhesion. At higher doses, nitric oxide has antitumor and antimicrobial activities thought to have a beneficial role in sepsis. Nitric oxide is important in maintaining visceral and microvascular blood flow by acting as a counter-regulatory mechanism to the vasoconstriction mediators (thromboxane and endothelin 1) released in inflammation. Nitric oxide is thought to be an important free radical scavenger that prevents microvascular stasis and thrombosis by blocking platelet aggregation and leukocyte adhesion.

However, excess or sustained levels of nitric oxide may have several harmful effects in sepsis. Nitric oxide has been implicated as a major mediator for vasodilation and hypotension in septic shock. Inflammatory mediators, including TNF-α and IL-1, stimulate iNOS. Once induced, iNOS is likely to persist for many hours to days. Peroxynitrite, which is formed from the reaction between superoxide radicals and nitric oxide, may cause direct cellular injury. Nitric oxide also may contribute to the myocardial depression and increased permeability seen in septic shock.

CLINICAL FEATURES

Constitutional

Hyperthermia or hypothermia, tachycardia, wide pulse pressure, tachypnea, and mental status changes are early systemic signs of infection and septic shock. Endotoxin, TNF-α, IL-1, and interferon-α have been shown to elicit febrile responses in humans. Acute hyperventilation with respiratory alkalosis (arterial partial pressure of carbon dioxide $\leq$30 mm Hg) is common in sepsis. The etiological mechanism of this tachypnea is thought to be due to the direct effects of endotoxins or secondary to kallikreins, bradykinin, prostaglandins, or complement activation.

The most frequent mental status change in sepsis is mental obtundation. The neurologic findings are nonfocal and range from mild disorientation to confusion, lethargy, agitation, and coma. The pathophysiology is still unknown; an altered state of amino acid metabolism producing a state similar to portosystemic encephalopathy or decreased cerebral blood flow with secondary disruption of the blood-brain barrier are proposed mechanisms.

Cardiovascular

In the early stages of septic shock, the vasodilatory mediators predominate, and patients present with warm extremities. Cardiac output and stroke volume are usually well maintained. Frequently, cardiac output is increased concomitantly with tachycardia. Hemodynamic measurements during the first 24 h show that the characteristic pattern of septic shock consists of an initial decrease in left and right ventricular ejection fractions, with an increase in end-diastolic and end-systolic volume indices, normal stroke volume, and decreased peripheral vascular resistance. In survivors, the changes are reversible, and the ventricular function and size return to normal by 7 to 10 days

after septic shock onset. Patients with septic shock have been shown to have markedly diminished cardiac response to volume administration, with only minor increments in end-diastolic volume index and left ventricular stroke work index.

Myocardial depression is present in early septic shock. The hypothesis that coronary hypoperfusion with secondary ischemic myocardial dysfunction is the cause of the myocardial depression is not supported by studies showing that the perfusion of the coronary arteries in patients with septic shock are equal to or greater than that in controls. Significant evidence points toward the existence of several active circulating myocardial depressant substances.

Substances that have demonstrated myocardial depressant activity include TNF-α (when IL-1β is present), nitric oxide, PAF, oxygen free radicals, interferon-γ, and arachidonic acid metabolites. The compounds that have received the most scrutiny are the combination of TNF-α, IL-1β, and nitric oxide. Tumor necrosis factor α, in the presence of IL-1β, has been shown to produce significant myocardial depression in vitro. Another major contributor to the prolonged myocardial depression is the stimulation of constitutive NOS and the induction of iNOS in myocytes by TNF-α, IL-1, possibly IL-2, and activated macrophages. Constitutive NOS appears to be involved in the physiologic regulation of myocardial contractility through the interaction between endothelial cells and cardiac myocytes. The inflammatory stimulus of sepsis is sustained at higher capacity through iNOS, which is responsible for a large portion of the prolonged myocardial depression in sepsis.

Pulmonary

Sepsis remains the most common condition associated with adult respiratory distress syndrome (ARDS). Adult respiratory distress syndrome is a physiologic syndrome characterized acutely by lung edema resulting from increased alveolar and capillary permeability resulting from global microcirculatory injury. In trauma and sepsis, this microvascular injury affects capillary beds throughout the body concurrently. The lung is a conspicuous organ, because, when increased microvascular permeability develops in the lung, alveolar flooding occurs, causing dyspnea, hypoxemia, and abnormal opacities on chest radiographs. The appearance of ARDS varies from minutes to hours after the onset of sepsis. Although there are no specific and sensitive markers for ARDS, diagnostic criteria for ARDS include bilateral pulmonary infiltrates, pulmonary artery occlusion pressure (PAOP or "wedge" pressure) below 18 mm Hg, a ratio of arterial to alveolar partial pressure of oxygen less than 0.2, and static airway compliance of less than 40 mL/cm H_2O. Clinically, severe refractory hypoxemia, noncompliant "heavy" lungs, and a chest radiograph showing bilateral pulmonary alveolar infiltrates should suggest the presence of ARDS. The hypoxemia is due to perfusion of the underventilated alveoli; right-to-left shunting has been reported as high as 30 to 50 percent in this syndrome. Pathogenic factors implicated in the global microcirculatory injury are endotoxin, TNF-α, IL-1, IL-6, IL-8, and bacteriocidal/permeability-increasing (BPI) protein.

Renal

Renal manifestations of septic shock include acute renal failure (ARF) with azotemia, oliguria, and active urinary sediment. Factors associated with the development of ARF in septic shock include hypotension, dehydration, aminoglycoside administration, and pigmenturia. Within the kidney, vasoconstrictive and vasodilator mediators are generated, and their balance dictates renal hemodynamics. Renal ischemic injury from hypoperfusion is considered to be a major factor in the pathogenesis of ARF in sepsis. Toxic products resulting from neutrophil-endothelial interactions, endothelial damage by various mediators, reperfusion injury, and microvascular thrombosis in the kidney also contribute to renal dysfunction. In patients without shock, infection may produce renal insufficiency as a consequence of glomerulonephritis or interstitial nephritis. Glomerular disease in the setting of sepsis has been reported in subacute bacterial endocarditis, pyogenic visceral abscesses, and other non-renal distant infections. Urine sediment in glomerular disease contains red blood cells, casts (red, white, or pigmented), and protein. Renal biopsy usually shows proliferative changes. Immune complex deposition with glomerular deposits of immunoglobulin G (IgG), IgM, C3, bacterial antigens, and antibodies to these antigens has been reported. Tubulointerstitial disease has been associated with *Streptococcus pneumoniae, Staphylococcus pyogenes, Legionella pneumophila,* salmonellosis, brucellosis, and diphtheria infections. Acute interstitial nephritis secondary to allergic reaction from antibiotics (most commonly methicillin) usually produces eosinophilia and eosinophiluria.

Hepatic

Liver dysfunction is frequently seen in patients with sepsis; the most frequent abnormality is cholestatic jaundice. Increases in transaminase, alkaline phosphatase (one to three times normal), and bilirubin concentrations (usually not >10 mg/dL) are frequently noted. The proposed mechanism for bilirubin elevation involves hemolysis of red blood cells and hepatocellular dysfunction due to endotoxin, cytokines, or immune complex disease. Prolonged or severe hypotension may induce acute hepatic injury or ischemic bowel necrosis.

Hematologic

Major blood loss secondary to upper gastrointestinal bleeding occurs in only a small percentage of patients with sepsis. However, minor blood loss within 24 h of developing a severe infection is common as patients develop painless 1- to 2-mm erosions in the mucosal layer of the stomach and/or duodenum. Proposed mechanisms for these ulcerations include decrease in the blood flow, hypoxia of the mucosal cells, interruption of the gastric mucosal barrier, and release of mucosal lysozyme.

The most frequent hematologic changes in the septic patient are neutropenia or neutrophilia, thrombocytopenia, and disseminated intravascular coagulation (DIC). Sepsis most frequently produces a neutrophilic leukocytosis with a "left shift." These early changes result from demargination and release of less mature granulocytes from the marrow storage pools. One proposed mechanism for demargination and bone marrow release is the presence of endotoxin or other similar substances and activation by complement (C3a) causing the release of a neutrophil-releasing substance. The sustained neutrophilia that accompanies chronic infection is thought to be secondary to colony-stimulating factors. These glycoproteins increase granulocyte production by activating committed stem cells. Infection increases the colony-stimulating factor elaboration by macrophages, lymphocytes, and other tissues. In certain cases of sepsis, leukemoid reactions with leukocyte counts of 50,000 to 100,000/μL have been reported.

Neutropenia, occurring rarely, is associated with an increase in mortality. The etiology of this neutropenia includes increased peripheral use of neutrophils, damage to neutrophils by bacterial byproducts, or depression of marrow granulocyte production by inflammatory mediators. Morphologic and functional changes to neutrophils have been reported in sepsis. The most commonly reported morphologic changes include the presence of toxic granulations, Dohle bodies, and vacuolization. Functional changes reported in sepsis include increased phagocytic and cytotoxic activities. Eosinophilia occurring in the presence of sepsis has been attributed to the effect of margination or migration of these cells from the vascular space.

Red cell number and morphologic characteristics are not usually affected by sepsis. However, red cell production and survival are decreased during sepsis. Decreased production and survival usually do not cause anemia unless the infection is prolonged. Septic patients generally possess low serum iron concentrations. Sepsis and its intermediaries cause a rapid iron flux into the liver and other parts of the reticuloendothelial cells, with the serum iron concentration decreasing by 50 percent or more within a period of hours, and this effect may last days. An attractive hypothesis is that this represents a host defense mechanism, because the addition of iron to normal human serum enhances the growth of organisms, and iron in the reticuloendothelial system may be beneficial to the host cells in detoxifying bacterial activity.

Thrombocytopenia frequently arises as a consequence of DIC, although isolated thrombocytopenia is present in more than 30 percent of cases of sepsis. Thrombocytopenia may be an early clue to bacteremia and may be useful in observing patient's response to therapy. The proposed mechanisms for the thrombocytopenia include inhibition of thrombopoiesis, increased platelet turnover, increased endothelial adherence, and increased destruction secondary to immunologic mechanisms.

Disseminated intravascular coagulation is a condition in which the clotting and fibrinolytic systems are systemically activated, leading to the consumption of many coagulation factors and platelets. Disseminated intravascular coagulation, with disseminated fibrin deposition in the microcirculation of various organ systems, is a frequent finding in patients with septic shock. The activation of the hemostatic (clotting) system is due primarily to the activation of the extrinsic pathway of clotting. This cascade is triggered by multiple sources, including bacteria (gram-negative and gram-positive), viruses, fungi, endotoxins, and exotoxins (see Figure 32-2). Gram-negative infections precipitate DIC more readily than does gram-positive infections. The fibrinolytic system is also activated in sepsis and plays an important role in limiting fibrin deposition in the microcirculation. Studies of septic patients have demonstrated the release of tissue type plasminogen activator, which activates the fibrinolytic system, at least initially in sepsis. As sepsis progresses, there is an increased release of plasminogen activator inhibitor type 1, which blocks plasmin generation and thus contributes to fibrin deposition in the microcirculation and subsequent multiple-organ failure.

Disseminated intravascular coagulation can be categorized into two forms. The compensated form of DIC is characterized by a "slower" generalized activation of the hemostatic system. Although platelets and coagulation factors are consumed more rapidly than normal, bleeding is prevented by increasing coagulation factor production in the liver, by the release of the platelets from reserve storage sites, and by the synthesis of inhibitors at an accelerated rate. Patients with decompensated DIC will have clinical bleeding and/or thrombosis. Laboratory studies suggesting the presence of DIC include thrombocytopenia, prolonged prothrombin and activated partial thromboplastin values, decreased fibrinogen and antithrombin (AT) III levels, and increased fibrin monomer, fibrin split products, and D-dimer levels.

Endocrine

Hyperglycemia may be seen in septic patients, even without a history of diabetes. Proposed pathogeneses include increased amounts of catecholamines, increased cortisol and glucagon in the circulation, peripheral insulin resistance, impaired glucose use, and decreased insulin secretion. Uncontrolled hyperglycemia is a significant risk for adverse outcome.[6] Hypoglycemia with glucose levels as low as 10 to 20 mg/dL has been reported but is a relatively uncommon manifestation of sepsis. Bacterial infections associated with hypoglycemia include *S. aureus, S. pyogenes, S. pneumoniae, Listeria monocytogenes, Haemophilus influenzae, Neisseria meningitidis,* and *Enterobacteriaceae.* The proposed pathogenesis of hypoglycemia includes the depletion of hepatitic glycogen and inhibition of gluconeogeneses.

Acid-Base

Blood gas analysis performed early in the course of septic shock usually finds respiratory alkalosis. Relative or absolute hypoxemia is often present due to ventilation perfusion mismatches. The development of metabolic acidosis reflects inadequate tissue perfusion, increased glycolysis in peripheral tissues, and impaired hepatic clearance of lactate and pyruvate. As perfusion worsens and continues, tissue hypoxia generates more lactic acid and metabolic acidosis worsens.

Cutaneous

Cutaneous lesions that occur as a result of sepsis can be divided into three categories: direct bacterial involvement of the skin and underlying soft tissues (cellulitis, erysipelas, and fasciitis); lesions that occur as a consequence of sepsis, hypotension, and/or DIC (acrocyanosis and necrosis of peripheral tissues); and lesions secondary to intravascular infections (microemboli and/or immune complex vasculitis).

DIAGNOSIS

Septic shock should be suspected in any individual with a temperature above 38°C or below 36°C and a systolic blood pressure below 90 mm Hg with evidence of inadequate organ perfusion. The hypotension should not reverse with rapid volume replacement of at least 1 L of isotonic crystalloid. Frequently, the diagnosis is straightforward, with the patient presenting with hypotension, inadequate perfusion, and complaints attributable to a serious infection such as pneumonia, acute pyelonephritis, or an acute peritonitis. Other early clinical features of sepsis include mental obtundation; hyperventilation; hot, flushed skin; and a widened pulse pressure. In the elderly, very young, or immunocompromised patient, the clinical presentation may be atypical, with no fever or localized source of infection.

The differential diagnosis of septic shock includes the other nonseptic causes of shock such as cardiogenic, hypovolemic, anaphylactic, neurogenic, obstructive (pulmonary embolism, tamponade), and endocrine (adrenal insufficiency, thyroid storm) causes.

History and physical examination with some basic laboratory or radiologic investigations are usually successful in the initial assessment and identification of a presumptive source of sepsis. Particular attention should be focused on infections in these organ systems: central nervous system, pulmonary, intra-abdominal, urinary tract, skin, and soft tissue.

Acute bacterial meningitis is the central nervous system infection most commonly associated with shock. Community-acquired meningitis with shock is usually due to *S. pneumoniae* or *N. meningitidis*. Most patients present with nuchal rigidity and a depressed level of consciousness. Chest radiographs may show pneumonia with secondary bacteremia due to *S. pneumoniae*. Disseminated meningococcemia may present only with shock without meningismus. Frequently, these patients possess a "new petechial rash," which is the major clue to the etiology of shock. Brain abscesses, subdural or epidural empyemas, and viral central nervous system infections are seldom associated with shock on the initial presentation. Shock is also unusual in neurosurgical patients with *S. aureus* or enteric gram-negative meningitis secondary to neurosurgical procedure or skull fracture.

The major pulmonary entity commonly leading to septic shock is acute bacterial pneumonia. The most frequent organisms are *S. pneumoniae*, *S. aureus*, gram-negative bacilli, and *L. pneumophila*. The physical examination and chest radiograph almost always indicates the presence of pneumonia.

Intra-abdominal processes are the source of infection leading to septic shock in the largest proportion of patients. Acute pancreatitis with or without infection can result in a presentation identical to septic shock. Suppurative cholangitis and empyema of the gallbladder are the primary considerations for the biliary tree. In women of childbearing age, septic abortion and postpartum endometritis or myometritis are the dominating presenting infections leading to septic shock. Acute pyelonephritis secondary to gram-negative enteric bacteria or enterococci occasionally can present with shock. Ureteric obstruction is often present in these syndromes.

The most common skin and soft tissue infection associated with septic shock is cellulitis due to *S. aureus* or *S. pyogenes*. Soft tissue infections secondary to gram-negative organisms are indistinguishable from those due to primary infection by staphylococci or streptococci. Shock associated with soft tissue infections is frequently associated with bacteremia. Shock associated with a generalized erythematous macular rash may represent toxic shock syndrome. Necrotizing soft tissue infections are usually seen in immunocompromised patients, diabetics, or in patients with history of poor vascular circulation.

Individuals without obvious source of septic shock may have a primary bacteremia, or endocarditis. The most prevalent etiologies of primary bacteremias in outpatients are *S. aureus*, *S. pneumoniae*, and *N. meningitidis*. Encapsulated species such as *Salmonella* or *H. influenzae* are important pathogens in individuals who are asplenic. *Pseudomonas aeruginosa* and other gram-negative bacteria are occasional etiologies of bacteremia and endocarditis in injection drug users.

Ancillary Studies

Although there is no specific laboratory test for the diagnosis of septic shock, tests are useful because they (1) assess the general hematologic and metabolic state of the patient, (2) provide results that suggest the potential for occult bacterial infection, and (3) detect a specific microbial etiology for infection. Basic laboratory studies should include a complete blood count including platelet count; DIC panel (prothrombin time, activated partial thromboplastin time, fibrinogen, D-dimer, ATIII concentration); serum electrolytes (including magnesium, calcium, phosphate, and glucose); liver function panel (bilirubin, alkaline phosphate, and alanine aminotransferase); renal function panel (blood urea nitrogen and creatinine); arterial blood gas analysis; and urinalysis. Blood should be typed and crossed if low hematocrit is suspected. A chest radiograph should be part of the basic evaluation. Flat and upright abdominal films are helpful in patients in whom there is a potential abdominal source of infection and should be considered in every patient except individuals with a completely benign abdomen or an obvious alternate source. Any patient with a clinical presentation compatible with meningitis should undergo a lumbar puncture with cerebrospinal fluid collected for analysis without delay in the emergency department. In individuals with papilledema, focal neurologic deficits, or the potential for brain abscess or epidural or subdural empyema, the lumbar puncture should be deferred until an imaging study is performed. However, if meningitis is an important consideration, empiric antimicrobial therapy should be initiated prior to the imaging study.

Bacterial cultures of blood and urine should be obtained from all septic patients. At least two separate sets of blood cultures from different venipuncture sites should be obtained. Gram stain and culture of secretions from any potential site of infection should be performed. Gram stain and other means of rapid identification of microbial etiologies are generally the only immediately available tests useful in selection of antimicrobial therapy.

Laboratory markers of sepsis are subjects of intense interest. Only a few candidates with clinical utility are currently available: C-reactive protein, lactate, pro-calcitonin, and semiquantitative IL-6 levels.[7,8] Comparisons of C-reactive protein and pro-calcitonin in the same patients have shown that pro-calcitonin has greater sensitivity, specificity, overall accuracy, and better predictive power in sepsis and septic shock than does C-reactive protein.[9,10]

STANDARD TREATMENT

Airway and Respiratory Management

Immediate assessment of oxygenation and ventilation status is the first priority in the management. Oxygen by mask and consideration of endotracheal intubation should be done immediately if the patient's airway is not secure or if respirations are inadequate. In addition, patients with hypotension not responding acutely to rapid fluid resuscitation should be intubated to avoid respiratory arrest from fatigue of the respiratory muscles due to inadequate perfusion of these muscles. There is no consensus concerning acceptable levels of oxygen saturation or tensions; however, most experts recommend maintaining oxygen saturations above 90 percent in a septic patient.

Hemodynamic Stabilization

FLUID ADMINISTRATION Correction or stabilization of hypotension and inadequate perfusion is the second goal of resuscitation.[11] Rapid fluid administration at a rate of 0.5 L (10 mL/kg in children) of normal saline or similar isotonic crystalloid should be administered every 5 to 10 min, as needed; it is not unusual for the patient to require 4 to 6 L (60 mL/kg in children) or more of crystalloid in the initial phase of resuscitation. Stabilization of the patient's mentation, blood pressure, respiration, pulse rate, skin perfusion, and central venous pressure, with urine output greater than 30 mL per h (1 mL/kg per h in pediatric patients) are useful clinical parameters in monitoring the response to fluid administration.

INOTROPIC SUPPORT If no response to the fluid infusion is noted after 3 to 4 L of fluid, or if there are signs of fluid overload (elevated central venous pressure or pulmonary edema), an infusion of dopamine can be started.[11] If the patient has a pulmonary artery catheter in place during this resuscitation, dopamine should be added in the setting of a PAOP of 15 to 18 mm Hg or if there are marked increases of the PAOP with additional fluids. Doses of dopamine often required are 5 to 20 μg/kg per min, resulting in β_1-adrenergic inotropic and α-adrenergic vasopressor activities. If the patient does not adequately respond to a rate of 20 μg/kg per min, norepinephrine should be started with the goal of keeping the mean blood pressure at least at 60 mm Hg. Once the blood pressure and perfusion have been stabilized by norepinephrine, the lowest dosage that maintains blood pressure should be used to minimize the complications of vasoconstriction. In addition, data from the canine model have suggested that the use of low-dose dopamine or dobutamine (1 to 4 μg/kg per min) in patients on norepinephrine results in significantly higher renal blood flow and reduced renal vascular resistance. The effect of norepinephrine on survival from septic shock is debatable, but survival rates of up to 40 percent have been reported.

Vasodilators are rarely used in the emergency department, but they have been used in the ICUs in situations of severe myocardial depression, increased system vascular resistance, and adequate blood pressure. Several investigators have published the results of short-term vasopressin infusion (0.04 units/min for 4 to 16 h) in patients with vasodilatory septic shock. Although the numbers of patients were small, all studies to date have suggested a beneficial response of vasopressin with a decreased catecholamine requirement and increase in urine output.[12–14]

HEMODYNAMIC END POINTS There is good evidence for hemodynamic goal-directed therapy in sepsis and septic shock.[15] Rivers and associates used a standardized protocol for fluid resuscitation, vasopressors, inotropes, mechanical ventilation, maintenance of central venous pressure between 8 and 12 mm Hg, hematocrit of 30 percent, and central venous oxygen saturation of at least 70 percent in 130 patients with severe sepsis and septic shock. They found a reduction in hospital mortality from 44% in the control group to 29% in the intervention group [absolute reduction 15%; 95% CI 3.6 to 26.6%].[15] They concluded that early goal-directed therapy initiated in the emergency department provides significant benefit and improves outcome in patients with severe sepsis and septic shock.

Empiric Antimicrobial Therapy

All patients with septic shock should receive empiric antimicrobial therapy as soon as possible. Whenever possible, samples of blood or fluids from potential sites of infection should be obtained before the initiation of antimicrobial therapy. Selection of antibiotics should be based on the adequate coverage of potential pathogens from the potential infection sites and the anticipated antimicrobial susceptibility patterns of the bacterial isolate(s). Survival in septic shock correlates with the initial administration of antibiotics effective against the infecting organism (Table 32-2). In general, empiric therapy should be effective against gram-positive organisms (*Streptococcus* spp. and *Staphylococcus* spp.) and gram-negative bacteria. The route of administration should be intravenous in the maximum doses allowed.

Removal of Source of Infection

If a focal source of sepsis is identified, removal of the nidus of infection is absolutely mandatory for successful treatment. Indwelling intravenous catheters should be removed, and the tips should be sent for quantitative culture. Urinary drainage catheters should be replaced if obstructed. Intra-abdominal or soft tissue sites of pus require urgent drainage.

Initial Baseline Assessment

Hemodynamic and laboratory monitoring is critical to the resuscitation of a patient in septic shock. Some clinicians advocate following the serum lactate as a monitor of response to therapy. Arterial blood gas should be obtained to monitor adequacy of ventilation and perfusion. Septic shock patients should have at least two large-bore intravenous catheters for administration of fluids and vasoactive drugs. Early placement of a central venous catheter (ideally with a 8.5-French catheter introducer) may help in the monitoring of fluid resuscitation. Placement of a flow-directed thermal-dilution pulmonary artery catheter should be considered in patients requiring vasoactive therapy, in whom there is difficulty in assessing volume status, or ongoing hemodynamic instability is present. In general, the placement of this catheter can wait until the patient is in the ICU.

There are several noninvasive methods of patient monitoring for use in severe sepsis and septic shock: sublingual capnography, gastric pH tonometry, muscle oximetry, and bioimpedance determination of cardiac output. Other techniques, such a near-infrared spectroscopy and transcranial Doppler measurement to assess intracerebral oxygenation and evaluation of blood flow velocities in some cerebral arteries, are the current research tools.

NEW INNOVATIVE THERAPIES

Advances in molecular biology and immunology suggest that the host's inflammatory response to infection contributes to the development of severe sepsis and septic shock. Despite aggressive hemodynamic support, broad-spectrum potent antibiotics, and surgical treatment, the mortality rate of septic shock remains high. The development of new interventions is based on the premise that neutralizing bacterial toxins, cytokines, and other mediators could stop or slow this syndrome (Table 32-3).[5]

Currently, only a few randomized controlled trials have shown efficacy of these innovative therapies in the treatment of septic shock in humans. In the cases of interventions directed at endogenous cytokines, none of the studies has produced unequivocal benefit in the treatment of sepsis. Great potential danger exists in altering the natural balance of inflammatory mediators. These mediators perform important functions, such as clearing bacterial toxins and the mobilization of the host defenses that control the infection. Attempting to block the harmful effect of inflammatory mediators may compromise host

TABLE 32-2 Empiric Antibiotic Selection in Severe Sepsis and Septic Shock

Host	Potential Pathogens	Initial Antibiotic Selection
Neonates <1 wk	Group B streptococci *Escherichia coli, Klebsiella, Enterobacter*	Ampicillin plus cefotaxime
Neonates 1–4 wk	Group B streptococci *E. coli, Klebsiella, Enterobacter,* *Haemophilus influenzae, S. epidermidis*	Ampicillin plus cefotaxime Ampicillin plus ceftriaxone
Infants 1–3 mo	*E. coli, Klebsiella, Enterobacter, H. influenzae,* *Streptococcus pneumoniae,* *Neisseria meningitidis*	Cefotaxime Ceftriaxone
Children (non-neutropenic) >3 mo	*S. pneumoniae, N. meningitidis,* *H. influenzae, Staphylococcus aureus*	Cefotaxime Ceftriaxone Cefuroxime
Adults (non-neutropenic) without an obvious source of infection	Gram-negative bacilli, as shown Gram-positive cocci	Antipseudomonal penicillin/β-lactamase inhibitor (e.g., piperacillin/tazobactam) plus Third-generation cephalosporin (e.g., cefotaxime) Some experts advise the addition of an aminoglycoside (tobramycin, gentamicin, or amikacin) Alternatively, imipenem or meropenem alone is acceptable
Neutropenic children and adults	Gram-negative bacilli, especially *Pseudomonas aeruginosa* *S. aureus*	Cefepime, imipenem, or meropenem alone Antipseudomonal aminoglycoside (e.g., gentamicin) plus ceftazidime Antipseudomonal aminoglycoside (e.g., gentamicin) plus antipseudomonal penicillin/β-lactamase inhibitor (e.g., piperacillin/tazobactam)
Patients with history of injection drug use	*S. aureus*	Nafcillin or vancomycin (if MRSA is suspected) should be added to the regimen
Anaerobic source is suspected: intra-abdominal, biliary, female genital tract, necrotizing cellulitis, odontogenic infection, or an anaerobic soft tissue infection	Anaerobic bacteria plus gram-negative bacilli	Metronidazole or clindamycin should be added to the regimen
Patients with indwelling vascular devices	Coagulase-negative staphylococcus	Vancomycin should be added to the regimen
Potential for *Legionella* species infection		Azithromycin or erythromycin should be added to the regimen
Asplenic patients	*S. pneumoniae, N. meningitidis,* *H. influenzae, Capnocytophaga*	Cefotaxime Ceftriaxone

Abbreviation: MRSA = Methicillin-resistant *S. aureus.*
Source: The Sanford Guide to Antimicrobial Therapy, 33rd ed, 2003.

defenses and ultimately worsen the outcome.[5] Successful therapeutic approaches may depend on determining which inflammatory mediators should be inhibited or augmented and when to do so. In almost all the animal models, anti-endotoxin therapy is effective only if given before or simultaneously with endotoxin challenge. Thus, it is very unlikely that anti-endotoxin treatment alone will change outcome in patients in shock and with organ failure. The situations in which these agents may be the most effective are those in which the patients are in early gram-negative sepsis or as a prophylaxis for high-risk patients.

Coagulation Modulation Therapy

The management of DIC has three basic approaches: elimination of the underlying disorder or source of infection, replacement of coagulation constituents lost in the clotting process, and arrest of the intravascular clotting process. If the patient is actively bleeding and decompensated DIC is present, urgent replacement of coagulation factors and platelets is indicated with the rapid infusion of fresh frozen plasma and/or platelets. Reasonable guidelines in the actively bleeding patient with DIC include the transfusion of platelets to maintain a concentration of 50,000/μL and cryoprecipitate and fresh frozen plasma to keep the coagulation parameters (fibrinogen, prothrombin time, and activated thromboplastin time) close to normal.

Interruption of the activated hemostatic system has been attempted by the use of heparin, primarily outside the United States, with mixed results. Currently, no conclusive evidence is available to suggest that heparin therapy reduces morbidity or mortality in septic patients with DIC. Inhibitors of systemic fibrinolysis, such as ε-aminocaproic acid, have been advocated in DIC without clear evidence of benefit.

Several procoagulation mechanisms have been associated with decreased survival in patients with sepsis, including elevated levels of plasminogen activator inhibitor type 1 and decreased levels of antithrombin III and protein C.

Activated protein C inhibits factors Va and VIIa, activates fibrinolysis, inhibits thrombin production, and has additional anti-inflammatory effects. In one study, recombinant human activated protein C [drotrecogin-α (activated)] reduced 28-day mortality from 31% in the control group to 25% in the intervention group (absolute reduction 6.1%; 95% CI 1.9 to 10.4%) in patients with severe sepsis.[16] Treatment was effective regardless of age, severity of illness, the number of dysfunctional organs or systems, the site of infection, and the type of infecting organisms. Notably, 70 percent of the patients were in shock, with 75 percent receiving mechanical ventilation. The investigators noted a 1.5 percent increase in the risk of serious bleeding (3.5% in treated patients and 2% in control patients). Patients were eligible if they met these criteria within a 24-h period: three or more

TABLE 32-3 Selective Innovative Therapies in Sepsis

Coagulation modulation	
Replace deficient hemostatic factors in decompensated DIC	Cryoprecipitate
	Fresh frozen plasma
	Platelets
Deactivate uncontrolled systemic hemostasis	Heparin
	Activated protein C*
	Antithrombin III
Deactivate uncontrolled systemic fibrinolysis	Epsilon aminocaproic acid
Anti-endotoxin therapy	
Anti-endotoxin antibodies	J5
	E5
	MAB-T88
	HA-1A
Endotoxin analogues	E5531
Endotoxin elimination	Hemadsorption
	Hemofiltration
	Hemodialysis
Endotoxin neutralizing protein	Recombinant bactericidal/permeability-increasing protein 21
Anticytokine therapy	
Anti-TNF-α antibodies	TNF-α monoclonal antibody MAK 195F or afelimomab
	BAY 1351
Anti-TNF-α receptor antibodies	TNFR55-IgG₁ or lenercept
Anti–IL-1 receptor antibody	Recombinant human IL-1 receptor antagonist
Anti-neutrophil therapy	
Inhibit neutrophil–endothelial cell adhesion	Monoclonal antibodies against the CD11/CD18 integrin (Hu23F2G or LeukArrest)
	Pentoxifylline
Immunostimulant therapy	
Immunoglobulin	Intravenous immunoglobulin
Granulocyte CSF	Recombinant human granulocyte–macrophage CSF
	Recombinant granulocyte CSF
Nonspecific interventions	
Corticosteroid therapy	High dose
	Low-dose replacement in patients with relative adrenal insufficiency*
Nitric oxide synthetase inhibitors	L-arginine analogue (monomethyl-L-arginine)
	Methylene blue
Cyclooxygenase inhibitors	Ibuprofen
	Ketoconazole
Glucose control	Intensive insulin therapy*

*Consistent benefit to routinely recommend in severe sepsis and septic shock.
Abbreviations: CSF = colony-stimulating factor; DIC = disseminated intravascular coagulation; IL = interleukin; TNF = tumor necrosis factor.

signs of systemic inflammation and sepsis induced dysfunction of at least one organ or system that lasted no longer than 24 h. Excluded subjects included patients with chronic liver disease, those with chronic renal failure on dialysis, those with recent surgery, those with organ transplant, those with thrombocytopenia (platelet count <30,000/μL), and those taking acetylsalicylic acid at a dose larger than 650 mg per d within 3 days before the study. Most experts now recommend that administration of activated protein C should be seriously considered in patients who meet these inclusion criteria.[5]

Administration of a natural anticoagulant, such as ATIII, may arrest clotting without concomitant risk of bleeding. Antithrombin III is a single-chain glycopeptide that is produced by the liver and is an important regulator of hemostasis by inhibiting several serine proteases of the coagulation system, predominately thrombin and factor Xa. Plasma ATIII levels decrease in septic patients with DIC; in healthy in-

dividuals, the half-life of ATIII is approximately 60 h; but in patients with sepsis and septic shock, this half-life may be shortened to 4 to 6 h. The possibility that replacement of ATIII neutralizes excess thrombin and dampens the intravascular coagulation process has prompted several experimental and clinical studies. In several animal models of DIC, infusion of ATIII concentrates shortened the duration of DIC and reduced multiple organ failure and mortality. However, results of human clinical studies have been mixed. A large multicenter trial of high-dose ATIII (30,000 IU in total over 4 days) administered within 6 h in severe sepsis found no difference in overall 28-day mortality: 38.7 percent in the placebo group and 38.9 percent in the ATIII-treated group.[17] High-dose ATIII was associated with increased risk of hemorrhage (from 13.5 to 23.8 percent) when administered with heparin. There was a trend toward improved survival with ATIII in a subgroup of patients not receiving heparin. At this point, some experts have recommended that patients with DIC secondary to a septic process receive replacement of ATIII to a level of 70 to 80 percent of normal. Other investigators have suggested that a much higher level of ATIII (140 to 150 percent) is required for efficacy.

Anti-Endotoxin Therapies

The most studied exogenous mediator is endotoxin. This macromolecule is found in gram-negative bacteria as one of the integral components of the outer bacterial LPS cell wall. The molecule can be functionally divided into three parts: a highly variable O-polysaccharide side chain that provides the heat-stable serologic specificity of gram-negative bacteria and is the basis for the O (somatic) antigen-type scheme; an oligosaccharide or R-core region composed of approximately 10 monosaccharides; and a lipid backbone referred to as *lipid A*. The lipid A portion of endotoxin is responsible for the majority of the molecule's toxicity; this portion is also highly conserved and is essentially invariable and ubiquitous.

Experimental studies of the administration of endotoxin have produced physiologic changes paralleling those of sepsis and septic shock. The cellular basis for the pathophysiologic response to endotoxin is that endotoxin, an LPS-binding protein (LBP), and CD14 (a protein found on the surface of monocytes and macrophages) form a complex that activates the cell and triggers the cascade of events leading to septic shock. Many strategies have been developed to manipulate this complex, including enhanced endotoxin clearance (anti-endotoxin antibodies, direct removal of endotoxin via hemadsorption, hemofiltration, or hemodialysis), direct neutralization of circulating endotoxin (anti-endotoxin antibodies and endotoxin neutralizing proteins), and inhibition of the endotoxin-LBP complex.

Use of dialysis, adsorption, or filtration therapy to remove circulating endotoxin or cytokines has been proposed. In general, the benefits are controversial, and there is no randomized trial data to support the routine use of plasma filtration or hemodialysis in sepsis.[18]

ANTI-ENDOTOXIN ANTIBODIES At least four anti-endotoxin antibodies have been developed and studied in human trials of severe sepsis and septic shock: J5 (a polyclonal antibody), E5 (a murine-murine hybridoma-derived monoclonal antibody), MAB-T88 (a human-derived monoclonal antibody), and HA-1A (a human-murine hybridoma-derived monoclonal antibody). Despite initial promise, trials using J5 found no improved survival in sepsis or septic shock. Trials of E5 found no overall improvement in mortality, but there appeared to be a more rapid resolution of organ failure in patients with gram-negative sepsis without hypotension or shock. Overall, the benefits of E5 are too limited to justify the expense of routine use. After limited phase I trials, MAB-T88 has not been studied further for its outcome effect in sepsis and septic shock in humans. Human trials with HA-1A have not found improved survival and suggested that mortality is worsened in patients without gram-negative bacteremia. The multicenter European Pediatric Meningococcal Septic Shock Trial found no benefit with HA-1A (6 mg/kg of body weight intravenously;

maximum, 100 mg) in children presenting with meningococcal septic shock; the 28-day mortality rates were 27% in the control group and 18.5% in the treatment group (absolute reduction 8.6%; 95% CI −1.4 to 18.5%).[19]

ENDOTOXIN-NEUTRALIZING PROTEIN   A number of endotoxin-neutralizing proteins has been described, of which BPI, a 55-kD neutrophil-derived polypeptide, has been studied most extensively. A recombinant 21-kD modified fragment of human BPI (rBPI21) was studied as an adjunctive treatment for children with severe meningococcal sepsis.[20] Overall survival was not improved (9.9% in the control group and 7.4% in the treated group), but treatment reduced the incidence of amputations and improved functional outcome.

LIPID A ANALOGUES   Inhibition of the endotoxin-LBP interaction is an attractive and potential method of intervention. Analogues can be developed based on the structure of lipid A that will bind to LBP but result in reduced or absent cellular toxicity. These compounds can block endotoxin binding to cells and inhibit LPS-induced TNF-α release. A lipid A analogue, E5531, inhibited physiologic response to experimental endotoxin infusion.[21] No human trials of a lipid A analogue in the treatment of sepsis and septic shock have been reported.

SUMMARY OF ANTI-ENDOTOXIN THERAPY   Anti-endotoxin antibodies have not shown an overall survival benefit for patients with sepsis. The anti-endotoxin antibody HA-1A and the modified human BPI (rBPI21) have shown some benefit as adjunctive treatment for children with severe meningococcal sepsis.

Anti-Cytokine Therapy

Cytokines are peptides that function as cellular signals to regulate the amplitude and duration of the host's inflammatory response and play protective roles in the host's immune response to infection. The host's response to these cytokines consists of recruited and activated neutrophils, macrophages and lymphocytes, increased gene expression, and release of granulocyte colony-stimulating factors. Two cytokines, TNF-α and IL-1, have been studied extensively in patients with sepsis.

TUMOR NECROSIS FACTOR AND TNF-α RECEPTOR   Tumor necrosis factor α is a polypeptide hormone that can stimulate the release of other mediators, including IL-1, IL-6, and PAF. It also promotes the metabolism of arachidonic acid, leading to eicosanoid formation. Tumor necrosis factor α is directly toxic to endothelial cells, increases the adhesion of polymorphonuclear leukocytes to the endothelial cells, and enhances the phagocytic activity of these cells. It also reduces the transmembrane potential of muscle cells, depresses myocardial function, and activates coagulation.

Administration of TNF-α to experimental animals and healthy human subjects duplicates many of the signs and symptoms of sepsis. Injection of TNF-α into animals results in hemodynamic collapse, multiple-organ injury, and a life-threatening vascular leak syndrome. In humans, injection of TNF-α produces hypotension, chills, fever, headache, and malaise synchronously with the time of the peak serum TNF-α level. In addition, rapid and sustained activation of the common pathway of the coagulation system occurs.

Numerous studies have reported a positive correlation between level of serum concentrations of TNF-α and clinical outcome in patients with sepsis. Significantly higher levels of TNF-α were found in non-survivors of meningococcemia, sepsis, children with infectious purpura, and ARDS. Absolute TNF-α levels were a significant predictive factor for morbidity and mortality in patients with septic shock. Perhaps the most compelling evidence that TNF-α is a causal rather than an associative factor are animal studies demonstrating that antibodies to TNF-α enhance survival and reduce physiologic derangements after challenge with endotoxin or live bacteria.

However, human studies with anti-TNF-α therapy have been disappointing.[22] A variety of anti-TNF-α antibodies have been developed, such as TNF-α monoclonal antibody, MAK195F or afelimomab, and BAY 1351. Even though individual trials have found different results, the greatest benefit was a slight 3 to 4 percent non-statistical improvement in survival with anti-TNF-α antibody treatment.[22] Attempts to determine subgroups of septic patients who would be more likely to benefit from anti-TNF-α antibody therapy have not been successful. Investigations using infusion of a TNF-α receptor-IgG1 fusion protein (TNFR55-IgG1) to "trap and eliminate" circulating TNF-α have not improved survival.[23]

INTERLEUKIN 1   Interleukin-1β is also present in the blood of patients with septic shock. Both TNF and IL-1β induce hypotension, and a combination of these cytokines is a more potent inducer of shock than either cytokine alone. Both cytokines induce IL-6, a nonlethal cytokine that serves as an excellent marker of cytokine activity in patients with sepsis. An IL-1 receptor antagonist has been shown to block the hemodynamic consequences of *Escherichia coli* endotoxin and heat-killed *Staphylococcus epidermidis* in experimental animals. However, human studies on the efficacy of recombinant human IL-1 receptor antagonist in patients with sepsis syndrome found no consistent reduction in 28-day mortality.[24]

SUMMARY OF ANTI-CYTOKINE THERAPY   Most investigators believe that TNF-α is a key and perhaps central mediator in sepsis. To date, anti-TNF-α and anti-IL-1 agents have not been shown to consistently improve outcome in the treatment of septic patients.

Neutrophil-Directed Therapy

Evidence suggests that the neutrophil has beneficial and harmful effects in sepsis and septic shock. The neutrophil is a key component of the host defense. Data from neutropenic animals and humans have suggested that augmented neutrophil count and function reduce the risk of infection. Conversely, studies have shown that the neutrophil and its toxic byproducts produce tissue injury and organ dysfunction in sepsis and septic shock.

One area of intense interest is the leukocyte-endothelium interaction that appears to be a crucial step in activated neutrophil migration into an area of inflammation. A neutrophil membrane glycoprotein complex, termed CD11/CD18, and an endothelial cell-expressed intercellular adhesion molecule 1 are involved in transendothelial neutrophil migration. Monoclonal antibodies against the CD11/CD18 complex, in vitro and in vivo, prevent endotoxin, TNF-α, and complement-induced neutrophil adhesion; neutrophil-mediated injury to endothelial cells; and neutrophil extravascular migration. Monoclonal anti-CD11/CD18 antibody therapy in animal models of sepsis have produced conflicting results and suggest that efforts to inhibit neutrophil function by blocking the CD11/CD18 complex may lead to more tissue injury and more adverse outcomes.

Pentoxifylline, a methylxanthine derivative, inhibits cytokine activation of neutrophils and the production of TNF-α by endotoxin-exposed monocytes. This prevents the adherence of neutrophils to endothelium and the release of toxic degranulation products. The mechanism of this action is believed to be via increasing cyclic adenosine monophosphate concentrations. Animal experiments have suggested that treatment with pentoxifylline decreases mortality rate and prevents lung injury by inhibiting migration of neutrophils through the pulmonary capillary endothelium. In small studies, improved survival using pentoxifylline infusion has been seen in adults with severe sepsis and premature neonates with blood culture positive sepsis.[25,26]

Intravenous Immunoglobulin

The role and efficacy of intravenous polyclonal or monoclonal immunoglobulin (IVIG) in the treatment of septic shock remains undefined and is not routinely recommended, but two studies have suggested a role in some circumstances. The Canadian Streptococcal Study Group performed an open-label study on the use of IVIG in patients with streptococcal toxic shock syndrome. The 30-day survival was 34.4% in the control group and 66.7% in the treated group (absolute increase 32.3%; 95% CI 6.3 to 58.3%).[27] Postulated beneficial mechanisms for IVIG therapy are the enhanced ability of the patient's plasma to neutralize bacterial mitogenicity, reduced T-cell production of IL-6 and TNF-α, Fcγ receptor blockade, accelerated clearance of endogenous pathogenic auto-antibodies, inhibition of components of the complement cascade, neutralization of super-antigens and bacterial toxins, and anti-cytokine and anti-idiotype effects. A systemic review of IVIG for sepsis and septic shock found a significant trend toward reduction in mortality (relative risk, 0.91; CI, 0.86 to 0.96).[28] The investigators concluded that "polyclonal IVIG significantly reduced mortality and is a promising adjuvant in the treatment of sepsis and septic shock." They also noted that "the trials were small and the totality of evidence is insufficient to support a robust conclusion of benefit. Adjunctive therapy with monoclonal IVIG remains experimental."

Corticosteroids

Although some animal models have shown that high-dose corticosteroid therapy is effective, large clinical trials have shown (1) no differences in mortality between patients treated with high-dose corticosteroid and control patients, and (2) an increased rate of superinfection in corticosteroid treated patients.[29,30] Conversely, recent studies have associated septic shock with relative adrenal insufficiency and glucocorticoid peripheral resistance. A multicenter trial with low-dose corticosteroid (hydrocortisone 50 mg IV every 6 h, and fludrocortisone 50 μg PO once per day for 7 days) in patients in septic shock significantly reduced the risk of death in patients with septic shock who were relatively adrenal insufficient from 63.5% in the control group to 52.6% in the treated group (absolute reduction 10.9%; 95% CI −1.9 to 23.6%).[31] No significant increase in adverse effects was noted. Thus the primary role of steroids in sepsis and septic shock is in patients with suspected or documented adrenal insufficiency. Adrenal insufficiency should be considered in septic patients with fulminant *N. meningitidis* bacteremia, disseminated tuberculosis, acquired immunodeficiency syndrome, prior glucocorticoid use, or refractory hypotension.

Nitric Oxide Synthase Inhibitors

There is good evidence from a large number of studies that humans with sepsis syndrome also have increased systemic nitric oxide production. The higher the nitric oxide level, the more pronounced the septic hypotension.

Animal studies using NOS inhibitors have shown mixed results. A handful of studies using an NOS antagonist, such as the arginine analogue monomethyl-L-arginine, in septic patients has shown transient improvements in blood pressure but no effect on overall mortality. A small study in 20 patients on the effects of a continuous infusion of methylene blue, an inhibitor of the nitric oxide pathway, on the hemodynamics and organ function in human septic shock found improved cardiac function and a reduced need for inotropic support.[32] Survival rates were 30% in the control group and 50% in the methylene blue-treated group (absolute reduction 20%; 95% CI −22 to 62%). In summary, the role of nitric oxide in septic shock warrants further investigation. To date, only nonselective nitric oxide synthetase inhibitors that block both forms of NOS inhibitors have been studied extensively. Future research most likely will be performed with selective inhibitors.

Cyclooxygenase Inhibitors

There are two principal pathways of arachidonic acid metabolism: the lipoxygenase pathway leads to the production of leukotrienes, which are potent leukocyte chemoattractants, and the cyclooxygenase pathway results in the release of thromboxanes and prostaglandins, which are important regulators of vascular tone.

Ibuprofen is a cyclooxygenase inhibitor. In animal models of endotoxin shock and shock from peritoneal implantation or intravenous infusion of bacteria, ibuprofen administered before or after the septic insult decreased mortality, reversed hemodynamic, metabolic, and blood coagulation abnormalities, improved pulmonary gas exchange, and attenuated the development of increase in microvascular permeability. The Ibuprofen in Sepsis Study Group found that intravenous ibuprofen (10 mg/kg of body weight given every 6 h for a total of eight doses) produced significant declines in temperature, heart rate, oxygen consumption, lactic acidosis, and urinary levels of prostacyclin and thromboxane.[33] However, ibuprofen did not reduce the incidence or duration of shock or ARDS and did not significantly reduce 30-day mortality rate. Subgroup analysis of the 10 percent of study patients who were hypothermic found a significant reduction in 30-day mortality, from 90% in the control group to 54% in the treated group (absolute reduction 36%; 95% CI 12 to 60%).[34] No increase in adverse events (renal dysfunction or gastrointestinal bleeding) was noted in the ibuprofen group. Human and animal studies to date have suggested that ibuprofen decreases the metabolic demand on patients with sepsis.

Miscellaneous

Hyperglycemia is a significant risk factor for developing an infection, and persistent hyperglycemia results in increased morbidity and reduced survival. Tight glucose control (between 80 and 100 mg/dL) with intensive insulin therapy reduced mortality from multiorgan failure in patients with sepsis, regardless of a history of prior diabetes.[6] Studies investigating PAF, bradykinin antagonists, anti-oxidant therapy using *N*-acetylcysteine, interferon-γ, and granulocyte colony-stimulating factor have not shown conclusive evidence of efficacy with reduced mortality or morbidity.

Summary of Potential New Therapies

To date, the only potential new therapies that produce significant benefit as adjuncts to standard treatment have been (1) early goal-directed hemodynamic resuscitation, (2) tight control of blood glucose with insulin, and (3) treatment with activated protein C.[5,6,16]

REFERENCES

1. Angus DC, Linde-Zwirble WT, Lidicker J, et al: Epidemiology of severe sepsis in the United States: Analysis of incidence, outcome, and associated cost of care. *Crit Care Med* 29:1303, 2001.
2. Sands KE, Bates DW, Lanken PN, et al: Epidemiology of sepsis syndrome in 8 academic medical centers. *JAMA* 278:234, 1997.
3. Bone RC, Balk RA, Cerra FB, et al: Definitions for sepsis and organ failure and guidelines for the use of innovative therapies in sepsis. The ACCP/SCCM Consensus Conference Committee. *Chest* 101:1644, 1992.
4. Rangel-Frausto NS, Pittet D, Costigan M, et al: The natural history of the systemic inflammatory response syndrome (SIRS): A prospective study. *JAMA* 273:117, 1995.
5. Hotchkiss RS, Karl IE: The pathophysiology and treatment of sepsis. *New Engl J Med* 348:138, 2003.
6. van den Berghe G, Wouters P, Weekers F, et al: Intensive insulin therapy in the critically ill patients. *New Engl J Med* 345:1359, 2001.
7. Povoa P: C-reactive protein: A valuable marker of sepsis. *Intens Care Med* 28:235, 2002.
8. Reinhart K, Karzai W, Meisner M: Procalcitonin as a marker of the systemic inflammatory response to infection. *Intens Care Med* 26:1193, 2000.
9. Tugrul S, Esen F, Celebi S, et al: Reliability of procalcitonin as a severity marker in critically ill patients with inflammatory response. *Anaesth Intens Care* 30:747, 2002.
10. Guven H, Altintop L, Baydin A, et al: Diagnostic value of procalcitonin levels as an early indicator of sepsis. *Am J Emerg Med* 20:202, 2002.

11. Task Force of the American College of Critical Care Medicine, Society of Critical Care Medicine: Practice parameters for hemodynamic support of sepsis in adult patients in sepsis. *Crit Care Med* 27:639, 1999.

12. Tsuneyoshi I, Yamada H, Kakihana Y, et al: Hemodynamic and metabolic effects of low-dose vasopressin infusions in vasodilatory septic shock. *Crit Care Med* 29:487, 2001.

13. Patel BM, Chittock DR, Russell JA, Walley KR: Beneficial effects of short-term vasopressin infusion during severe septic shock. *Anesthesiology* 96:576, 2002.

14. O'Brien A, Clapp L, Singer M: Terlipressin for norepinephrine-resistant septic shock. *Lancet* 359:1209, 2002.

15. Rivers E, Nguyen B, Havstad S, et al: Early goal-directed therapy in the treatment of severe sepsis and septic shock. *New Engl J Med* 345:1368, 2001.

16. Bernard GR, Vincent JL, Laterre PF, et al: Efficacy and safety of recombinant human activated protein C for severe sepsis. *New Engl J Med* 344:699, 2001.

17. Warren BL, Eid A, Singer P, et al: Caring for the critically ill patient. High-dose antithrombin III in severe sepsis: A randomized controlled trial. *JAMA* 286:1869, 2001.

18. Cole L, Bellomo R, Hart G, et al: A phase II randomized, controlled trial of continuous hemofiltration in sepsis. *Crit Care Med* 30:100, 2002.

19. Derkx B, Wittes J, McCloskey R: Randomized, placebo-controlled trial of HA-1A, a human monoclonal antibody to endotoxin, in children with meningococcal septic shock. European Pediatric Meningococcal Septic Shock Trial Study Group. *Clin Infect Dis* 28:770, 1999.

20. Levin M, Quint PA, Goldstein B, et al: Recombinant bactericidal/permeability-increasing protein (rBPI21) as adjunctive treatment for children with severe meningococcal sepsis: A randomized trial. RBPI21 Meningococcal Sepsis Study Group. *Lancet* 356:961, 2000.

21. Bunnell E, Lynn M, Habet K, et al: A lipid A analog, E5531, blocks the endotoxin response in human volunteers with experimental endotoxemia. *Crit Care Med* 28:2713, 2000.

22. Reinhart K, Karzai W: Anti-tumor necrosis factor therapy in sepsis: An update on clinical trials and lessons learned. *Crit Care Med* 29(suppl):S121, 2001.

23. Abraham E, Laterre PF, Garbino J, et al: Lenercept (p55 tumor necrosis factor receptor fusion protein) in severe sepsis and early septic shock: A randomized, double-blind, placebo-controlled, multicenter phase III trial with 1,342 patients. *Crit Care Med* 29:503, 2001.

24. Opal SM, Fisher CJ, Dhainaut JF, et al: Confirmatory interlukin-1 receptor antagonist trial in severe sepsis: A phase III, randomized, double-blind, placebo-controlled, multicenter trial. The Interlukin-1 Receptor Antagonist Sepsis Investigator Group. *Crit Care Med* 25:1115, 1997.

25. Staubach KH, Schroder J, Stuber F, et al: Effect of pentoxifylline in severe sepsis: Results of a randomized, double-blind, placebo-controlled study. *Arch Surg* 133:94, 1998.

26. Lauterbach R, Pawlik D, Kowalczyk D, et al: Effect of the immunomodulating agent, pentoxifylline, in the treatment of sepsis in prematurely delivered infants: A placebo-controlled, double-blind trial. *Crit Care Med* 27:807, 1999.

27. Kaul R, McGeer A, Norrby-Teglund A, et al: Intravenous immunoglobulin therapy for streptococcal toxic shock syndrome-A comparative observational study. The Canadian Streptococcal Study Group. *Clin Infect Dis* 28:800, 1999.

28. Alejandria MM, Lansang MA, Dans LF, Mantaring JB: Intravenous immunoglobulin for treating sepsis and septic shock. *Cochrane Database Syst Rev* 1:CD001090, 2002.

29. Cronin L, Cook DJ, Carlet J, et al: Corticosteroid treatment for sepsis: A critical appraisal and meta-analysis of the literature. *Crit Care Med* 23:1430, 1995.

30. Lefering R, Neugebauer EAM: Steroid controversy in sepsis and septic shock: A meta-analysis. *Crit Care Med* 23:1294, 1995.

31. Annane D, Sebille V, Charpentier C, et al: Effect of treatment with low doses of hydrocortisone and fludrocortisone on mortality in patients with septic shock. *JAMA* 288:862, 2002.

32. Kirov MY, Evgenov OV, Evgenov NV, et al: Infusion of methylene blue in human septic shock: A pilot, randomized, controlled study. *Crit Care Med* 29:1860, 2001.

33. Bernard GR, Wheeler AP, Russell JA, et al: The effects of ibuprofen on the physiology and survival of patients with sepsis. The Ibuprofen in Sepsis Study Group. *New Engl J Med* 336:912, 1997.

34. Arons MM, Wheeler AP, Bernard GR, et al: Effects of ibuprofen on the physiology and survival of hypothermic sepsis. Ibuprofen in Sepsis Study Group. *Crit Care Med* 27:699, 1999.

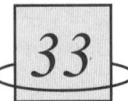

CARDIOGENIC SHOCK

W. Franklin Peacock IV
Jim Edward Weber

Cardiogenic shock is defined as a state of decreased cardiac output (CO) producing inadequate tissue perfusion despite adequate or excessive circulating volume.[1] Clinical signs of cardiogenic shock include evidence of poor CO with tissue hypoperfusion (hypotension, mental status changes, cool mottled skin) and evidence of volume overload (dyspnea, rales). Hemodynamic criteria for cardiogenic shock include (1) sustained hypotension [systolic blood pressure (BP) <90 mm Hg], (2) reduced cardiac index (<2.2 L/min per m^2), and (3) an elevated (>18 mm Hg) pulmonary artery occlusion pressure. Cardiogenic shock is a true emergency that needs aggressive intervention to avert an extremely high mortality rate.[2,3] Although usually caused by contractile failure of the myocardium, other processes may impair CO to produce shock (Table 33-1).

ETIOLOGY

Cardiogenic shock usually results from an acute myocardial infarction (AMI) that affects over 40 percent of the left ventricular myocardium. Cardiogenic shock is the most common cause of AMI-related in-hospital death, with an overall mortality of 50 to 90 percent and accounting for 50,000 to 70,000 deaths each year in the United States. The overall incidence of cardiogenic shock in AMI is 6 to 8 percent, a rate that remained constant from 1975 to 1997.[3,4] Although some patients have cardiogenic shock on initial presentation, the median time from the onset of infarction to the development of shock is 8 h.[5]

Risk factors for post-AMI cardiogenic shock have been identified (Table 33-2). The more risk factors that present, the greater the amount of vulnerable myocardium and the greater the likelihood of cardiogenic shock. Early identification of increased risk may suggest more aggressive reperfusion strategies to prevent cardiogenic shock.

PATHOPHYSIOLOGY

Cardiogenic shock most often is the end result of acute myocardial ischemia and infarction affecting the left ventricle (LV). Acute heart failure may occur with loss of systolic contraction of at least 25 percent of the LV. If over 40 percent of the LV loses contractile function, clinical cardiogenic shock ensues. Most cases of AMI-related cardiogenic shock have ST-segment elevation on the initial electrocardiogram (ST-segment elevation myocardial infarction, or STEMI) that in

TABLE 33-1   Etiologies of Cardiogenic Shock

Acute myocardial infarction
   Pump failure
   Mechanical complications
      Acute mitral regurgitation secondary to papillary muscle rupture
      Ventricular septal defect
      Free-wall rupture
Right ventricular infarction
Severe depression of cardiac contractility
   Sepsis
   Myocarditis
   Myocardial contusion
Mechanical obstruction to forward blood flow
   Aortic stenosis
   Hypertrophic cardiomyopathy
   Mitral stenosis
   Left atrial myxoma
Regurgitation of left ventricular output
   Chordal rupture
   Acute aortic insufficiency

TABLE 33-2 Risk Factors for Cardiogenic Shock

Elderly
Female
Promote current ischemic event
  Impaired ejection fraction
  Extensive infarct (evidence of large myocellular leak)
  Proximal left anterior descending coronary artery occlusion
  Anterior myocardial infarction location
  Associated with multivessel disease
Prior medical history
  Previous myocardial infarction
  Congestive heart failure
  Diabetes

time will evolve Q waves in the same leads. Prior LV dysfunction can affect these percentages; a relatively small AMI may cause cardiogenic shock in a patient with pre-existing heart failure. Cardiogenic shock can develop from mechanical complications of an AMI: myocardial free-wall rupture, acute ventricular septal defect (VSD), or mitral regurgitation from valvular dysfunction or papillary muscle rupture. Less common causes of cardiogenic shock include myocardial depression from conditions such as sepsis or myocarditis, LV outflow obstruction (e.g., aortic stenosis), and severe regurgitation of LV output (acute aortic regurgitation or mitral valve chordae rupture).

Some patients presenting with decompensated congestive heart failure (CHF) may have occult cardiogenic shock and may be clinically indistinguishable from those with mildly decompensated CHF and stable CHF.[6] Central venous oximetry and serum lactate measurements are required to detect those with occult cardiogenic shock.

In post-AMI cardiogenic shock, myocytes in the ischemic border zone demonstrate various stages of cell death, probably from inadequate collateral blood flow. Cellular dysfunction at the edge of the ischemic myocardium is further exacerbated by hypotension. Apoptosis (programmed cell death) may activate inflammatory pathways, increase oxidative stress, and further worsen the dysfunction.[7] With progression, areas of focal necrosis develop throughout the heart, producing further loss of contractile function and hypotension. With arterial hypotension, coronary perfusion pressure declines and worsens already impaired myocardial oxygen delivery. If pulmonary edema develops, hypoxia and acidosis further diminish myocardial contractility. These processes contribute to a rapidly progressive cycle of deterioration leading to irreversible shock.

The severe reduction in CO and subsequent compensatory mechanisms have systemic consequences: oliguria, hepatic failure, gastrointestinal ischemia, anaerobic metabolism, lactic acidosis, and hypoxia. Although LV mass loss is the major predictor for developing cardio-genic shock, disease in non-infarct-related coronary arteries, diastolic dysfunction, or arrhythmia can amplify the negative impact and result in cardiogenic shock with lesser insult.

To compensate for decreased stroke volume, tachycardia develops. The combination of hypotension and tachycardia drastically reduces coronary artery flow by decreasing perfusion pressure and diastolic filling time (when the majority of coronary flow takes place). This results in further ischemia and myocardial dysfunction.

With AMI, neurohormonal mechanisms are triggered to maintain CO and tissue perfusion. Sympathetic nervous system activation leads to increased heart rate, systemic vasoconstriction, and enhanced myocardial contractility. Increased contractility is seen as hyperkinesis in the uninvolved myocardium. Absence of hyperkinesis, from fibrosis or diffuse coronary artery disease, results in end-systolic LV volume increases and is associated with increased cardiogenic shock risk. Another neurohormonal reflex that occurs is activation of the renin-angiotensin aldosterone system as a result of inadequate renal perfusion pressure. Increased angiotensin II leads to peripheral vasoconstriction and aldosterone synthesis. Aldosterone causes retention of sodium and water, which increases blood volume. The net effect of sympathetic nervous system and renin-angiotensin activation may preserve CO and maintain end-organ perfusion, but at the cost of increased systemic vascular resistance (SVR) and higher myocardial oxygen consumption.

Right ventricular (RV) infarction complicates up to 30 percent of inferior wall AMI.[8] Although hypotension is not rare with an RV infarct, shock is much less common and accounts for only 3 to 4 percent of cardiogenic shock cases. The major determinate of cardiogenic shock with RV infarction is the presence of LV dysfunction. With decreased LV contractility, systolic septal function is impaired and RV stroke volume is reduced. With a smaller volume coursing through the RV, LV preload is reduced and LV stroke volume is decreased, producing more arterial hypotension and further reducing coronary perfusion pressure.

Hemodynamic assessment by pulmonary artery catheterization in AMI patients has identified four profiles based on CO and LV preload that are strong predictors of mortality independent of reperfusion therapy (Table 33-3).[9] Patients in cardiogenic shock typically have low cardiac index (<2.2 L/min per m^2) and elevated LV end-diastolic pressure (pulmonary artery occlusion pressure > 18 mm Hg).

CLINICAL FEATURES

History

History can be difficult to obtain due to the severity of the clinical presentation; mental obtundation or confusion may preclude patient cooperation. Emergency medical service personnel, family, or the

TABLE 33-3 Mean Hemodynamic Values in Subsets of Acute Myocardial Infarction[9]

Class	Description	Cardiac Index, L/min per m^2	Pulmonary Artery Occlusion Pressure, mm Hg	Approximate Mortality, %	Comments
I	No congestion or peripheral hypoperfusion	2.7 (normal)	12 (normal)	2	Good prognosis
II	Isolated congestion	2.3 (low to normal)	23 (elevated)	10	Vasodilation and diuresis result in clinical improvement
III	Isolated peripheral hypoperfusion	1.9 (decreased)	12 (normal)	22	There is relative or absolute volume deficiency; cardiac output can be improved by fluid infusions that increase stroke volume according to the Frank-Starling relation
IV	Congestion and peripheral hypoperfusion	1.7 (decreased)	27 (elevated)	55	Clinical shock is typically present

medical record may offer historical information. Patients commonly complain of breathlessness. When AMI is the cause of cardiogenic shock, patients may report chest pain or an ischemic equivalent. The history should attempt to exclude other causes of shock, such as sepsis, gastrointestinal hemorrhage, or massive pulmonary embolism; ask about a history of pre-existing valvular disease or injection drug use.

Physical Examination

Shock is characterized by hypoperfusion and is often, but not always, accompanied by hypotension. Systolic BP is usually below 90 mm Hg, although it can be higher with pre-existing hypertension. A higher BP may reflect compensatory increases in SVR. A pulse pressure less than 20 mm Hg may be evident, due to extreme vasoconstriction. Compensatory sinus tachycardia is common. Unless the patient has advanced to the stage of respiratory fatigue or agonal respirations, tachypnea is common. The lung examination demonstrates rales due to the presence of pulmonary edema. Jugular venous distention and a positive abdominal jugular reflex are usually present. However, with RV infarction, the lung fields may be clear despite hypotension and jugular venous distention. Cool, pale extremities with skin mottling indicates poor perfusion. Peripheral edema suggests pre-existing heart failure. Diaphoresis indicates activation of the sympathetic nervous system.

If the cardiac point of maximal impulse is normally located, shock is likely due to an acute event. If the point of maximal impulse is laterally shifted and diffuse from cardiac remodeling and enlargement, long-standing cardiac disease can be presumed. Loud or new systolic murmurs suggest mechanical dysfunction. Acute mitral regurgitation can occur from chordae tendinea rupture or papillary muscle dysfunction. Chordae tendinea rupture is characterized by a soft holosystolic murmur at the apex radiating to the axilla but is often obscured by rales. With papillary muscle dysfunction, the murmur starts with the first heart sound but terminates before the second. An acute VSD is associated with a new loud holosystolic left parasternal murmur, often with a palpable thrill, that decreases in intensity as the intraventricular pressures equalize.

ANCILLARY STUDIES

Electrocardiogram (ECG)

The ECG is necessary to detect ischemia or infarction, evaluate for arrhythmia, and provide evidence of electrolytic abnormality (e.g., hypokalemia) or drug toxicity (e.g., digoxin). Left ventricular hypertrophy suggests chronic heart failure or hypertension. ST-segment elevation in two or more contiguous ECG leads supports the diagnosis of AMI. Right ventricular infarction complicating inferior MI is detected by ST-segment elevation in the right precordial ECG leads (usually V_4R). Right ventricular infarction complicating inferior MI increases mortality from about 6 percent (without RV involvement) to 31 percent (with RV involvement).[8]

Chest Radiography

A chest radiograph is indicated in all unstable patients. It typically shows pulmonary congestion or edema, Kerley lines, increased pulmonary vascularity, alveolar infiltrates, and pleural effusion. However, these findings may lag the clinical appearance by hours, so their absence does not exclude cardiogenic shock. Another confounder to interpreting the chest radiograph is underlying disease; pulmonary edema is difficult to detect on chest radiography in patients with severe chronic obstructive lung disease. Cardiomegaly is the end result of long-standing myocardial remodeling, and its presence may not explain the acute symptoms. Obtaining prior radiographs may help. The chest radiograph can suggest alternative or confounding diagnoses,

such as pneumonia, pneumothorax, aortic dissection, or pericardial effusion (globular cardiac shape).

Laboratory

The level of serum B-type natriuretic peptide (BNP) correlates with LV end-diastolic pressure and ventricular stretch. BNP has good direct correlation with pulmonary artery occlusion pressures as measured by a pulmonary artery catheter. BNP also is an excellent predictor of the clinical development of heart failure after AMI.[10] Normal serum BNP levels are less than 100 pg/mL.

In cardiogenic shock, cardiac markers of acute injury are needed. Acute MI can be diagnosed, but not excluded, by a single measurement. Arterial blood gas measurements help identify those at risk of CO_2 retention, quantify the presence and severity of acidosis, and determine the contribution of metabolic or respiratory components. An elevated serum lactate may detect unsuspected hypoperfusion. Electrolytes, which change rapidly with acidosis, pulmonary and perfusion changes, and renal dysfunction, should be evaluated. Serum magnesium should be measured with arrhythmia or severe hypokalemia. A complete blood cell count excludes anemia, which can contribute to cardiac ischemia. Obtaining specific drug levels (i.e. digoxin, ethanol, or illicit drugs) is guided by the clinical presentation.

Echocardiography

Transthoracic echocardiography (TTE) is a useful technique for documenting impaired LV contractility and supporting the diagnosis of cardiogenic shock.[4] Echocardiography provides information on ventricular dysfunction (e.g., regional hypokinesis, akinesis, or dyskinesis) and can identify early myocardial dysfunction by visualizing a lack of compensatory hyperkinesis in uninvolved cardiac segments. With the addition of color flow Doppler, TTE can define the mechanical causes of cardiogenic shock, such as acute mitral regurgitation or VSD.

Transthoracic echocardiography is useful for determining other causes of decreased CO. Acute RV dilatation, tricuspid insufficiency, paradoxical systolic septal motion, and high estimated pulmonary artery and RV pressures suggest pulmonary hypertension, as occurs with pulmonary embolus. Loss of RV contractility, RV dilatation, and normal estimated pulmonary pressures occur more commonly with RV infarction. Pericardial effusion, with diastolic collapse of the right atrium or right ventricle, indicates hemodynamically significant cardiac tamponade. Further, TTE may allow for visualization of aortic root dissection, although transesophageal echocardiography is better for sonographic detection of aortic dissection.

Mechanical Catastrophe Diagnosis

With mechanical catastrophe, patients are usually in extremis, and emergent echocardiography may be the best tool for the diagnosis. In the case of myocardial free-wall rupture, death is probable, unless a pseudoaneurysm forms, which may be detected as an acute pericardial effusion on echocardiography. An acute VSD is confirmed by echocardiography or right heart catheterization demonstrating an O_2 saturation step-up from the right atrium to the RV. Acute mitral regurgitation, from papillary muscle rupture or dysfunction, can complicate AMI. Because the murmur may be undetectable by auscultation, echocardiography is a very useful test to detect this treatable cause of cardiogenic shock.

Hemodynamic Monitoring

In patients at risk for cardiogenic shock, there is fair correlation between clinical and hemodynamic assessments of CO and LV preload during AMI. Patients with cardiogenic shock have decreased CO and increased LV pressures (see Table 33-3). However, imprecision in clinical assessment between the different classes limits therapy based solely on clinical criteria. Invasive hemodynamic monitoring with a pulmonary artery catheter can provide confirmatory data and guide treatment, but it is typically unavailable to most emergency physicians.[9]

Noninvasive hemodynamic monitoring shows promise. One technique uses bioimpedance to measure systolic stroke volume and multiplies this value by heart rate to calculate cardiac output. Approved by the U.S. Food and Drug Administration, bioimpedance monitoring is reasonably accurate, is useful for diagnosis, and may be used to exclude other causes of shock, such as volume depletion or septic shock.[11] Bioimpedance collects data by the application of two ECG-type electrodes to the neck and thorax. The signal is then analyzed and coupled with BP and ECG data to provide real-time CO, SVR, and thoracic fluid content values.[11,12]

DIFFERENTIAL DIAGNOSIS

In suspected cardiogenic shock, AMI is always a possibility. Dyspnea in cardiogenic shock is common, so pulmonary embolus, emphysema exacerbation, and pneumonia are considered. Hypertension, peripheral vasoconstriction, and dyspnea suggest acute pulmonary edema. Although diffuse ST-T changes can be seen with acute pericarditis or myocarditis, a nondiagnostic ECG should prompt the consideration of other causes of hypotension. These include aortic dissection, pulmonary embolus, pericardial tamponade, acute valvular insufficiency, hemorrhage, or sepsis. Overdose by a toxin with negative inotropic or chronotropic effects (e.g. β-blocker, calcium channel blocker, or digoxin overdose) should be considered.

TREATMENT

Medical therapy should be considered a temporizing measure while arranging for definitive treatment to re-establish coronary patency.[4] In the prehospital setting, EMS should consider directing the suspected cardiogenic shock patient to a facility that has intraaortic balloon pump (IABP) and 24-h emergency cardiac revascularization capability (i.e., cardiac bypass team). Initial management focuses on airway stability and improving myocardial pump function. Diagnostic and therapeutic interventions should proceed simultaneously in unstable patients.

Airway

Therapy begins with supplemental oxygen to reduce dyspnea and hypoxic anxiety. Because hypoxia is a greater risk than hypercarbia, supplemental oxygen is not withheld due to concerns about CO_2 retention. Impending or acute respiratory failure requires immediate mechanical ventilation. Failure to anticipate airway and ventilatory requirements may result in rapid cardiovascular collapse. Noninvasive ventilation techniques (e.g., continuous positive airway pressure or bilevel positive airway pressure) can serve as temporary airway support for patients with respiratory distress. However, these methods require a hemodynamically stable, cooperative patient, which excludes most with cardiogenic shock.

Endotracheal intubation is often necessary to maintain oxygenation and ventilation. However, the change to positive pressure ventilation may further decrease preload and CO and worsen hypotension. The physician should anticipate this occurrence and be prepared to administer a fluid bolus, in the absence of pulmonary congestion, or initiate the appropriate vasopressor or inotrope.

Stabilization

Cardiac monitoring and intravenous access are necessary. Hypoxia, hypovolemia, rhythm disturbances, electrolyte abnormalities, and acid-base alterations should be corrected as soon as possible. An arte-

rial line, although not mandatory, helps for frequent arterial blood gases and BP monitoring. A urinary drainage catheter may be used to monitor urine output in response to therapy. Pulmonary artery catheter and hemodynamic monitoring should be considered in all unstable patients.

In AMI, aspirin and full-dose heparin should be given unless there is an absolute contraindication.[4] If there is adequate BP, chest pain may be relieved by careful use of intravenous nitroglycerin or morphine. β-blockers and angiotensin-converting enzyme inhibitors should be withheld until the patient's condition is stable. Similarly, other vasodilators cannot be used in most cases when hypotension is present.

Hypotension

Initial therapy must be guided by clinical findings. Because some patients with cardiogenic shock develop hypotension without pulmonary congestion, a small fluid challenge (NS 100 to 250 mL) may be appropriate. If there is pulmonary congestion, this volume infusion should be omitted. If there is no improvement in perfusion with the fluid bolus, or there is hypotension with pulmonary congestion, inotropes are considered.

Inotropes do not change outcome but can temporize while ED personnel arrange interventions to restore coronary artery perfusion and LV function.[13,14] Inotrope selection depends on the suspected etiology of hypotension. If hemodynamics stabilize after inotropes are started, therapy for pulmonary congestion may be started (i.e., diuretics) while arranging admission to the intensive care unit.

Pure vasoconstrictors, such as phenylephrine, are generally contraindicated, because they increase cardiac afterload without augmenting cardiac contractility. Dopamine is used if there is hypotension but may increase cardiac work by increasing heart rate. It may also increase LV end-diastolic pressure by its α-agonist effect. Dobutamine may be effective in increasing cardiac contractility, but it generally should be avoided when systolic BP is below 90 mm Hg, because of its vasodilator potential. Phosphodiesterase inhibitors (e.g., milrinone) augment contractility, but have significant vasodilatory properties, and can decrease BP even greater then dobutamine. Combination therapy with a vasopressor (i.e., dopamine) and an inotrope (i.e., dobutamine) may be more effective than use of either agent alone, although hemodynamic data from a pulmonary artery catheter may best guide these decisions.

In RV infarct with hypotension, fluid infusion should be the first action. In the absence of profound hypotension, dobutamine is a mainstay of initial pharmacologic treatment.[13] With systolic BP below 70 mm Hg, dopamine is preferred as a single agent or in combination with dobutamine. When shock persists despite use of these agents, mechanical inotropic support with an IABP is required.[4,15,16]

In acute mitral regurgitation, hemodynamic support can be initiated with dobutamine and nitroprusside. This treatment supports contractility and provides afterload reduction, respectively, and promotes forward systemic blood flow. The IABP is also beneficial for temporary support.[4] Acute VSD is treated with dobutamine, nitroprusside, and an IABP.[4] Confirmatory evidence for these emergent conditions with two-dimensional echocardiography should be sought, concomitant with emergency consultation from the cardiac surgical team.

REPERFUSION FOR CARDIOGENIC SHOCK

Thrombolytic Therapy

Recent data suggest that patients in cardiogenic shock treated with thrombolytics have better outcomes than those not treated with thrombolytics.[16] The lowest mortality rate was observed with treatment using thrombolytics followed by revascularization.[17] Incomplete lysis in the infarct-related artery and the high frequency of multivessel disease in patients with cardiogenic shock may limit the efficacy of thrombolytic therapy.[18]

Intraaortic Balloon Counterpulsation

The IAPB provides hemodynamic support by decreasing afterload (which lowers myocardial oxygen consumption) and increasing diastolic BP (which augments coronary perfusion) and should be considered in patients presenting with cardiogenic shock.[4,15,16] Recent data suggest that IABP improves survival after thrombolytic therapy by augmenting diastolic perfusion pressure and unloading the LV.[17-19] The IABP does not improve survival without successful revascularization or surgical correction of an acute mechanical catastrophe.[18]

Early Revascularization

In cardiogenic shock, early revascularization with percutaneous coronary intervention or coronary artery bypass graft is the most important life-saving intervention.[4,17,18,20] The greatest short-term benefit is reported in patients younger than 75 years, those with previous MI, and those treated within 6 h of symptom onset. Patients older than 75 years have better survival with medical management.[4,17] Coronary artery bypass graft requires extensive surgical and medical resources and poses significant operative risk for these seriously ill patients, thereby limiting its use. However, outcome studies support that early revascularization should be performed in most patients younger than 75 years with cardiogenic shock.[17,18] Mechanical complications (e.g., acute VSD or mitral regurgitation) producing cardiogenic shock require temporary inotropic support with IABP, followed by early surgical repair.[4]

INOTROPIC MEDICATIONS

Dopamine

Dopamine, a first-line agent for cardiogenic shock, has dose-dependent effects. At infusion rates slower than 2.5 μg/kg per min, dopaminergic stimulation dilates renal, cardiac, and splanchnic vessels. At rates between 2.5 and 5 μg/kg per min, β_1-adrenergic effects predominate, with increased heart rate and cardiac contractility. At rates between 5 and 10 μg/kg per min, α- and β_1-adrenergic effects occur. At rates faster than 10 μg/kg per min, α-adrenergic tone progressively increases with increased BP and systemic vascular resistance. Dosing usually begins at 3 to 5 μg/kg per min and is titrated up to 20 to 50 μg/kg per min to maintain BP (Table 33-4). Complications include arrhythmias, extremity gangrene, and tachycardia at high doses (which increases myocardial oxygen demand and may extend ischemia). Consequently, the lowest possible dose of dopamine should be used.

TABLE 33-4 Inotropic Medications for Cardiogenic Shock*

Drug	Dose	Comments
Dopamine	3–5 μg/kg per min, titrated up to 20–50 μg/kg per min as needed	Use lowest effective dose
Dobutamine	2–5 μg/kg per min, titrated up to 20 μg/kg per min	May need dopamine also
Norepinephrine	2 μg/min, titrate to response	
Milrinone	50 μg/kg IV over 10 min Maintainance infusion of 0.5 μg/kg per min	

*Best with hemodynamic monitoring.

Dobutamine

Dobutamine usually is used for signs of poor perfusion when systolic BP is higher than 90 mm Hg. Primarily a selective β_1-adrenergic agonist, it also has mild α_1- and β_2-adrenergic effects. This sympathomimetic agent improves myocardial contractility and augments diastolic coronary blood flow without inducing excessive tachycardia. The net effect is increased CO, lowered SVR, and reduced LV filling pressure, with little BP change. Dobutamine is started at 2 to 5 μg/kg per min, and it is titrated up to 20 μg/kg per min according to clinical and hemodynamic responses. Complications include arrhythmias, nausea, and headache. If there is an inadequate response to this agent alone, dopamine may be added to support blood pressure.

Norepinephrine

Norepinephrine is used when there is inadequate response to other pressors. Primarily an α_1-agonist, norepinephrine infusion is started at 2 μg per min and titrated according to response. Complications are similar to those with high-dose dopamine.

Milrinone

Milrinone is a phosphodiesterase inhibitor that increases cyclic adenosine monophosphate, increases contractility and CO, and causes peripheral vasodilation. The drop in SVR may require additional therapy with vasopressors to maintain BP, so milrinone use in cardiogenic shock is best guided by hemodynamic measurements from a pulmonary artery catheter. Milrinone is administered with a loading dose of 50 μg/kg IV over 10 min, followed by a maintenance infusion of 0.5 μg/kg per min.

DISPOSITION

Patients in cardiogenic shock are best treated in an institution with invasive revascularization capability. Transfer should be accomplished as quickly as possible. In a large cardiogenic shock registry, mortality rates were 77 percent without thrombolytic therapy or IABP, 63 percent with thrombolytic therapy alone, 57 percent with IABP alone, and 47 percent with thrombolytic therapy and IABP.[18] Although those with IABP were more likely to receive invasive revascularization, there was no outcome difference as long as IABP was begun within 6 h. Although further study is needed, these observations suggest that the best results may be obtained by thrombolytic therapy and IABP, if possible, and early transfer.[4]

All patients with cardiogenic shock requiring hemodynamic monitoring, thrombolytic or inotropic therapy, or an IABP require admission to the intensive care unit. The rare stable patient without multiple comorbidities or a history of heart failure and who does not require hemodynamic monitoring or inotropic support is appropriate for admission to a monitored setting. Not all patients will benefit from aggressive care, particularly elderly patients with multiple comorbid conditions. The decision to perform or withhold therapies should be made in conjunction with the patient's wishes. Factors that may influence the decision to pursue aggressive therapy include advanced age and diminished functional status.

REFERENCES

1. Hollenberg SM, Kavinsky CJ, Parrillo JE: Cardiogenic shock. *Ann Intern Med* 131:47, 1999.
2. Barry WL, Sarembock IJ: Cardiogenic shock: Therapy and prevention. *Clin Cardiol* 21:72, 1998.
3. Goldberg RJ, Samad NA, Yarzebski J, et al: Temporal trends in cardiogenic shock complicating acute myocardial infarction. *New Engl J Med* 340:1162, 1999.
4. Menon V, Hochman JS: Management of cardiogenic shock complicating acute myocardial infarction. *Heart* 88:531, 2002.

5. Califf RM, Bengtson JR: Cardiogenic shock. *New Engl J Med* 330:1724, 1994.
6. Ander DS, Jaggi M, Rivers E, et al: Undetected cardiogenic shock in patients with congestive heart failure presenting to the emergency department. *Am J Cardiol* 82:888, 1998.
7. Bartling B, Holtz J, Darmer D: Contribution of myocyte apoptosis to myocardial infarction? *Basic Res Cardiol* 93:71, 1998.
8. Zehender M, Kasper W, Kauder E, et al: Right ventricular infarction as an independent predictor of prognosis after acute inferior myocardial infarction. *New Engl J Med* 328:981, 1993.
9. Forrester JS, Diamond GA, Swan HJC: Correlative classification of clinical and hemodynamic function after acute myocardial infarction. *Am J Cardiol* 39:137, 1977.
10. Sabatine MS, Morrow DA, de Lemos JA, et al: Multimarker approach to risk stratification in non-ST elevation acute coronary syndromes: Simultaneous assessment of troponin I, C-reactive protein, and B-type natriuretic peptide. *Circulation* 105:1760, 2002.
11. Shoemaker WC, Belzberg H, Wo CC, et al: Multicenter study of noninvasive monitoring systems as alternatives to invasive monitoring of acutely ill emergency patients. *Chest* 114:1643, 1998.
12. Peacock WF, Kies P, Albert NM, et al: Bioimpedance monitoring for detecting pulmonary fluid in heart failure: Equal to chest radiography? *Congest Heart Fail* 6:86, 2000.
13. McGhie AI, Goldstein RA: Pathogenesis and management of acute heart failure and cardiogenic shock: Role of inotropic therapy. *Chest* 102(suppl 2):626S, 1992.
14. Garber PJ, Mathieson AL, Ducas J, et al: Thrombolytic therapy in cardiogenic shock: Effect of increased aortic pressure and rapid tPA administration. *Can J Cardiol* 11:30, 1995.
15. Anderson RD, Ohman EM, Holmes DR, et al: Use of intra-aortic balloon counterpulsation in patients presenting with cardiogenic shock: Observations from the GUSTO-I study. *J Am Coll Card* 30:708, 1997.
16. Webb JG: Interventional management of cardiogenic shock. *Can J Cardiol* 14:233, 1998.
17. Hochman JS, Sleeper LA, White HD, et al: One-year survival following early revascularization for cardiogenic shock. *JAMA* 285:190, 2001.
18. Sanborn TA, Sleeper LA, Bates ER, et al: Impact of thrombolysis, intra-aortic balloon pump counterpulsation, and their combination in cardiogenic shock complicating acute myocardial infarction: A report from the SHOCK trial registry. Should we emergently revascularize occluded coronaries for cardiogenic shock? *J Am Coll Cardiol* 36(suppl A):1123, 2000.
19. Kovack PJ, Rasak MA, Bates ER, et al: Thrombolysis plus aortic counterpulsation: Improved survival in patients who present to community hospitals with cardiogenic shock. *J Am Coll Cardiol* 29:1454, 1997.
20. Hochman JS, Sleeper LA, Webb JG, et al: Early revascularization in acute myocardial infarction complicated by cardiogenic shock. *New Engl J Med* 341:625, 1999.

34 — ANAPHYLAXIS AND ACUTE ALLERGIC REACTIONS
Brian H. Rowe
Stuart Carr

DEFINITIONS

Anaphylaxis is a severe systemic hypersensitivity reaction characterized by multisystem involvement, which may include hypotension or airway compromise. Anaphylaxis is a potentially life-threatening cascade caused by the release of mediators from mast cells and basophils in an IgE-dependent fashion. *Anaphylactoid* describes responses that are clinically indistinguishable from anaphylaxis, which are not IgE mediated, and which do not require a sensitizing exposure.[1] Research shows that the final pathway in "classic" anaphylactic and anaphylactoid reactions is identical, and *anaphylaxis* is now used to refer to both IgE and non-IgE reactions.[2] Hypersensitivity describes an inappropriate immune response to generally harmless antigens, while anaphylaxis represents the most dramatic and severe form of immediate hy-

persensitivity. That being said, it is critical to remember that even apparently mild acute allergic reactions may progress to this severe systemic response, anaphylaxis, and death.

EPIDEMIOLOGY

Neither age, occupation, race, gender, nor geographic factors increase the risk of anaphylaxis. Most studies indicate that atopic individuals are at no greater risk for anaphylaxis from insect stings or drug reactions than are non-atopic individuals.[1] Poorly controlled asthma and previous anaphylaxis is a risk factor for fatal or near-fatal anaphylaxis.[1] The only other factors known to increase the risk of anaphylaxis are a previous exposure to a sensitizing antigen and previous anaphylaxis. Notably, anaphylaxis recurrence risks are not 100 percent for reexposure. The reoccurrence rate is 40 to 60 percent for insect stings, 20 to 40 percent for radiocontrast agents, and 10 to 20 percent for penicillin.

Limited data are available on the epidemiology of allergic reactions in the ED. The prevalence of anaphylaxis ranges from as high as 5 per 1000 to as low as 2 per 10,000 ED visits.[1,3,4] The prevalence of less-severe allergic reactions in the emergency department is much higher, but data are infrequently reported. Currently, the most common causes of serious anaphylaxis are antibiotics, such as penicillin, insects, and food.[1,5] β-Lactam antibiotics are estimated to cause 400 to 800 deaths in the United States annually, with a systemic allergic reaction occurring in 1 per 10,000 exposures.[1] Hymenoptera stings constitute the next most common cause of anaphylaxis, with fewer than 100 deaths in the United States annually.[1] Table 34-1 contains a partial list of the more common causative agents; however, the causes vary with age.[6] Pediatric surveillance studies have shown food allergy to be a very common cause of anaphylaxis in children.[6,7] Latex hypersensitivity is also increasing in prevalence in the general population, with a resultant risk for anaphylaxis.

PATHOPHYSIOLOGY

The basic mechanism underlying allergic reactions is mast cell and basophil degranulation and mediator release.[8] The causes of cell degranulation include IgE cross-linking, complement activation, nonimmunologic or direct activation, modulation of arachidonic acid

TABLE 34-1 Common Causes for Anaphylaxis and Anaphylactoid and Allergic Reactions

DRUGS
β-Lactam antibiotics
Acetylsalicylic acid (ASA)
Trimethoprim-sulfamethoxazole
Vancomycin
Nonsteroidal anti-inflammatory drugs (NSAIDs)
Virtually any drug

FOODS AND ADDITIVES
Shellfish
Soybeans
Nuts
Wheat
Milk
Eggs
Salicylates
Seeds
Sulfites

OTHERS
Hymenoptera stings
Insect parts and molds
Radiographic contrast material
Latex

metabolism, exercise or temperature-dependent effects, and idiopathic causes.[8]

Consensus on classification of hypersensitivity has been elusive, significant overlap may exist in some cases, and some clinical reactions do not fit classification. The four classic mechanisms of hypersensitivity are (1) cross-linking of two adjacent IgE molecules on a mast cell or basophil by a multivalent antigen; (2) reaction of IgG and IgM to cell-surface antigens, resulting in complement activation and cytotoxicity; (3) soluble antigen-antibody complexes that activate the complement system; and (4) activation of T lymphocytes. The first three mechanisms have been mentioned in the literature in relation to anaphylaxis.[1]

The "classic" anaphylaxis (IgE-mediated hypersensitivity) pathway requires two separate exposures to either an antigen or a hapten-protein antigenic complex. An antigen is a molecule, usually a protein, that can stimulate an immune response on its own. Haptens are small molecules, such as penicillin, that are incapable of stimulating an immune response, unless they are bound to endogenous proteins (e.g., albumin), resulting in an antigenic complex large enough to be recognized.

On first exposure, the antigen or hapten-protein complex is processed by macrophages and dendritic cells, and then presented externally on the cell surface bound to the major histocompatibility complex (MHC)-2. T helper cells recognize the antigen-MHC-2 complex and subsequently induce proliferation and differentiation of antibody-producing plasma cells. In the presence of interleukin (IL)-4, secreted from proallergic T-2 cells, these plasma cells produce and release IgE antibody into the bloodstream. The IgE antibody (like all antibodies) has a variable and a constant region. The variable region is specific for the antigen that induced the immune response, and the constant region binds to high-affinity IgE receptors present in vast quantities on mast cells and basophils, resulting in cells covered with antigen-specific IgE molecules. This sensitizing process takes days to weeks, resulting in a latent period during which no clinical response to antigen occurs. After the latent period, on antigen reexposure the variable regions on the IgE bind the antigen, resulting in bridging of adjacent IgE molecules on the mast cell surface. This IgE-antigen-IgE bridging results in activation of cell degranulation with release of chemical mediators.[1] Examples of IgE-mediated reaction triggers include antibiotics, foods, and Hymenoptera stings.

Complement-mediated anaphylactic reactions occur after the administration of blood products secondary to the formation of immune complexes. Immune complex formation results in activation of the complement pathway and formation of the anaphylatoxins C3a and C5a, which directly cause cell degranulation.[8] Immune complexes include IgG aggregates and IgA-IgG from human immunoglobulin therapy, and IgE-IgA complexes formed in selective IgA-deficient patients (1 in 700 people) who have been given blood products repeatedly. Administration of mismatched blood also causes complement activation secondary to the production of IgG and IgM antibodies against transfused red blood cells, resulting in cell lysis, agglutination, anaphylatoxin generation, and subsequent anaphylaxis.

Nonimmunologic anaphylaxis occurs when an exogenous substance results in mast cell degranulation either by direct stimulation of the mast cell or by unknown mechanisms. These reactions are often referred to as anaphylactoid.[1] Substances that cause anaphylactoid reactions include radiocontrast dyes, muscular depolarizing drugs, opiates, and dextrans. The mechanism of radiocontrast reactions is uncertain but is believed to be caused by the activation of the complement and coagulation systems, related in part to the high osmolarity of these dyes. Since the advent of nonionic contrast dyes, the incidence of reactions has dramatically decreased. Opiates and neuromuscular depolarizing drugs cause direct release of mediators from cells.

Aspirin and other nonsteroidal drugs cause anaphylactic symptoms by a non-mast cell process. The mechanism is not precisely known; however, it is thought to involve modulation of the cyclooxygenase-arachidonic acid metabolism pathway, specifically an alteration in prostaglandin and leukotrione synthesis. Five to ten percent of asthmatics have these reactions, which include bronchospasm, bronchorrhea, rhinorrhea, and, rarely, hypotension. Nonasthmatics may experience urticaria, angioedema, and hypotension. New, highly selective COX-2 inhibitors appear to be safe for aspirin-sensitive asthmatics in challenge studies.[9]

Idiopathic anaphylaxis is a diagnosis of exclusion, occurring when no causative agent can be identified for anaphylaxis. Patients suffer recurrent attacks, with no trigger identified after extensive allergy evaluation. They often need prolonged treatment with alternate-day prednisone to maintain remission from attacks.[10]

CLINICAL FEATURES

Anaphylaxis is the most severe life-threatening form of a systemic allergic reaction, often involving respiratory or cardiovascular compromise. The clinical signs of systemic allergic reactions include diffuse urticaria and angioedema. At times, these major symptoms are accompanied by any of the following: abdominal pain or cramping, nausea, vomiting, diarrhea, bronchospasm, rhinorrhea, conjunctivitis, dysrhythmias, and/or hypotension.[1] The clinician should be aware that even mild, localized urticaria can progress to full anaphylaxis, and even to death.

The "classic" presentation of anaphylaxis begins with pruritus, cutaneous flushing, and urticaria. These symptoms are followed by a sense of fullness in the throat, anxiety, a sensation of chest tightness, shortness of breath, and lightheadedness. As the cascade progresses, decreased level of consciousness, respiratory distress, and circulatory collapse may ensue. In its severest form, loss of consciousness and cardiorespiratory arrest may result. A complaint of a "lump in the throat" and hoarseness heralds life-threatening laryngeal edema in a patient with symptoms of anaphylaxis.

In the vast majority of patients, signs and symptoms begin within 60 min of exposure. In general, the faster the onset of symptoms, the more severe the reaction, as evidenced by the fact that one-half of anaphylactic fatalities occur within the first hour. After the initial signs and symptoms have abated, patients are at risk for a recurrence of symptoms. This biphasic phenomenon occurs in 3 to 20 percent of patients.[3] The effect is caused by a second phase of mediator release, peaking 4 to 8 h after the initial exposure and exhibiting itself clinically 3 to 4 h after the initial clinical manifestations have cleared. The late-phase allergic reaction is primarily mediated by the release of newly generated cysteinyl leukotrienes, the former "slow-reacting substance of anaphylaxis."[3]

DIAGNOSIS

The diagnosis of anaphylaxis is made by history and physical examination. Anaphylaxis should be considered clinically when involvement of any two or more body systems is observed, with or without hypotension or airway compromise (e.g., some combination of cutaneous, respiratory, gastrointestinal or cardiovascular systems). The diagnosis is easily made with a clear history of exposure, such as a bee sting, shortly followed by the multisystemic signs and symptoms described above. Unfortunately, diagnosis is not always easy or clear, because symptom onset is delayed more than 1 h in a small percentage of cases. Often, such as in food allergy, the inciting substance may not be known.

The differential diagnosis of anaphylactic reactions is extensive, including vasovagal reactions; myocardial ischemia; arrhythmias; status asthmaticus; seizure; epiglottitis; hereditary angioedema; foreign-body airway obstruction; carcinoid; mastocytosis; vocal cord dysfunction; and non-IgE-mediated drug reactions.[1] The most common anaphylaxis imitator is a vasovagal reaction, which is characterized by hypotension, pallor, bradycardia, diaphoresis, and weakness, and sometimes by syncope.

Because the diagnosis of anaphylaxis is made clinically, laboratory investigations have no role to play. Histamine levels, elevated for 5 to 30 min postreaction, are unhelpful because they decline by presentation to the ED. Tryptase is a neutral protease of unknown function in anaphylaxis that is found only in mast cell granules and is released with degranulation. Serum tryptase levels are elevated for several hours and are useful for later confirmation of a suspected anaphylactic episode.[1]

TREATMENT

Emergency Treatment

Given the possible development of life-threatening complications, all acute allergic reactions should be triaged expeditiously. Anaphylaxis, as defined by airway compromise or hypotension, is obviously a true medical emergency and must be rapidly assessed and treated. With *suspected* anaphylaxis, the single most important step in treatment is the rapid administration of epinephrine. Moreover, with this rapid administration, many of the secondary measures discussed below may not be necessary.

First-Line Therapy

Emergency management starts with the ABC (airway, breathing, circulation) of resuscitation. The first-line therapies for anaphylaxis (e.g., epinephrine, intravenous fluids, and oxygen) have immediate effect during the acute stage of anaphylaxis. Vital signs, intravenous access, oxygen, cardiac monitoring, and pulse oximetry measurements should be obtained immediately.

AIRWAY AND OXYGENATION   Securing the airway is the first priority. The airway should be examined for signs and symptoms of angioedema (e.g., uvula edema, stridor, respiratory distress, hypoxia). If angioedema is producing respiratory distress, intubation should be completed early, because delay may result in complete airway obstruction secondary to progression of angioedema. The patient should be given sufficient oxygen to maintain arterial oxygen saturation greater than 90 percent.

DECONTAMINATION   Exposure to the causative agent, if identified, should be terminated; however, gastric lavage is not recommended for food-borne allergens.

EPINEPHRINE   Epinephrine is the cornerstone of treatment for anaphylactic reactions; however, research suggests that epinephrine in anaphylaxis is underused.[4,7] If the patient has signs of cardiovascular compromise or collapse, epinephrine may be delivered intravenously. Initially, epinephrine 100 μg (0.1 mg) IV should be given as a 1:100,000 dilution. This can be done by placing epinephrine 0.1 mg (0.1 mL of the 1:1000 dilution) in 10 mL of NS solution and infusing it over 5 to 10 min (a rate of 1 to 2 mL/min).[2] If the patient is refractory to the initial bolus, then an epinephrine infusion can be started, by placing epinephrine 1 mg (1.0 mL of the 1:1000 dilution) in 500 mL of D5W or NS and running at a rate of 1 to 4 μg/min (0.5 to 2 mL/min), titrating to effect. Physicians are often hesitant to give intravenous epinephrine because of its side effects (e.g., tachycardia, arrhythmia, tremor). It should be stressed that the initial adult dose is very dilute, is given over 5 to 10 min, and can be stopped immediately if arrhythmias or chest pain occur.

For less-severe symptoms, intramuscular epinephrine can be given.[11] The dose is epinephrine 0.3 to 0.5 mg (0.3 to 0.5 mL of the 1:1000 dilution) repeated every 5 to 10 min according to response or relapse. Most patients do not need more than a single dose. Intramuscular dosing provides higher, more consistent, and more rapid peak blood epinephrine levels than subcutaneous administration, and

should now be the treatment of choice for adults and children.[12,13] Moreover, injections into the thigh are more effective at achieving peak blood levels than are injections into the deltoid area.[12] If the patient is refractory to treatment despite repeated intramuscular epinephrine, then an epinephrine infusion should be instituted. Caution is warranted in patients taking β-blockers, because epinephrine use may result in severe hypertension secondary to unopposed α-adrenergic stimulation.

CRYSTALLOIDS   If hypotension is present, it is generally the result of distributive shock and responds to fluid resuscitation. Patients should receive a NS bolus of 1 to 2 L (10 to 20 mL/kg in children) concurrently with the epinephrine infusion.

Second-Line Therapy

The second-line anaphylaxis treatments include corticosteroids, antihistamines, asthma medications, and glucagon.[1] These drugs are used to treat anaphylaxis refractory to the first-line treatments or associated with complications, and also to prevent recurrences.

CORTICOSTEROIDS   All patients with anaphylaxis should receive corticosteroids. Methylprednisolone 125 mg IV (2 mg/kg in children; up to 125 mg) or hydrocortisone 250 to 500 mg IV (5 to 10 mg/kg in children; up to 500 mg) are appropriate. Methylprednisolone produces less fluid retention than does hydrocortisone and is preferred for elderly patients and for those patients in whom fluid retention would be problematic (e.g., renal and cardiac impairment).

ANTIHISTAMINES   All patients with anaphylaxis should receive histamine-1 (H$_1$) blockers, such as diphenhydramine 25 to 50 mg IV.[2,14] Because the histamine-2 (H$_2$) blockers are effective in shock refractory to epinephrine, fluids, steroids, and H$_1$ blockers, it is recommended that H$_2$ antihistamines be considered as well.[2,14] Use of H$_2$ antihistamines is common in refractory urticaria; however, clear evidence of benefit from controlled trials is lacking. If considered, H$_2$ blockers such as ranitidine and cimetidine may be used in anaphylaxis. Cimetidine should not be used for patients who are elderly (side effects), with multiple comorbidities (interference with metabolism of many drugs) have renal or hepatic impairment, or whose anaphylaxis is complicated by β-blocker use (prolongs metabolism of β-blockers and may prolong anaphylactic state). After the initial intravenous dose of steroids and antihistamines, the patient may be switched to oral medication (Table 34-2).

AGENTS FOR ALLERGIC BRONCHOSPASM   If wheezing is present, a selective bronchodilator, such as intermittent or continuous nebulized albuterol, should be instituted. As might be expected, asthmatics are often more refractory to the treatment of allergic bronchospasm. For severe bronchospasm refractory to the abovementioned treatments, other treatments such as anticholinergics and magnesium sulfate can be added.[15] Anticholinergic agents should be added to the nebulized albuterol (ipratropium bromide 250 to 500 μg/dose) in severe acute bronchospasm. Magnesium sulfate improves pulmonary functions and reduces admissions when administered in severe acute asthma.[15] It is inexpensive and free of major side effects when used in single doses of magnesium sulfate 2 g IV over 20 to 30 min in adults and 25 to 50 mg/kg in children. Bronchodilator and stimulant agents should be used with caution (lower dose and slower rate) in elderly patients. Intravenous aminophylline and β-agonists have no role to play in the early management of acute bronchospasm because their benefit is marginal, as compared to other agents, and their side-effect profile is impressive. There are no data yet on the role of leukotriene receptor antagonists in the treatment of anaphylaxis, although this area warrants further study, given the proven role of the cysteinyl leukotrienes in late-phase allergic responses.

TABLE 34-2   Anaphylaxis and Allergic Reactions Drug Dosing

Drug	Adult Dose	Pediatric Dose
Epinephrine	IV single dose: 100 μg over 5–10 min; 1:100,000 dilution given as 0.1 mg in 10 mL at 1 mL per min IV infusion: 1–4 μg per min IM: 0.3–0.5 mg (0.3–0.5 mL of 1:1000 dilution)	IV infusion: 0.1–0.3 μg/kg per min; maximum 1.5 μg/kg per min IM: 0.01 mg/kg (0.01 mL/kg of 1:1000 dilution)
IV fluids: NS or LR	1–2 L bolus	10–15 mL/kg bolus
Diphenhydramine	25–50 mg q6h IV, IM, or PO	1 mg/kg q6h IV, IM, or PO
Ranitidine	50 mg IV over 5 min	0.5 mg/kg IV over 5 min
Cimetidine	300 mg IV	4–8 mg/kg IV
Hydrocortisone	250–500 mg IV	5–10 mg/kg IV (max: 500 mg)
Methylprednisolone	125 mg IV	1–2 mg/kg IV (max: 125 mg)
Albuterol	Single treatment: 2.5–5.0 mg nebulized (0.5–1.0 mL of 0.5% solution) Continuous nebulization: 5–10 mg per h	Single treatment: 1.25–2.5 mg nebulized (0.25–0.5 mL of 0.5% solution) Continuous nebulization: 3–5 mg per h
Ipratropium bromide	Single treatment: 250–500 μg nebulized	Single treatment: 125–250 μg nebulized
Magnesium sulfate	2 g IV over 20 min	25–50 mg/kg IV over 20 min
Glucagon	1 mg IV q5min until hypotension resolves, followed by 5–15 μg per min infusion	50 μg/kg IV q5min
Prednisone	40–60 mg per d PO divided bid or qd (for outpatients: 3–5 days; tapering not required)	1–2 mg per d PO divided bid or qd (for outpatients: 3–5 days; tapering not required)

GLUCAGON   Concurrent use of β-blocking drugs by the patient is a risk factor for severe prolonged anaphylaxis. In one study, 3 of 5 patients who had severe protracted reactions were being treated with β-blocking drugs.[3] For patients taking β-blockers with hypotension refractory to fluids and epinephrine, glucagon should be used in a dose of 1 mg IV every 5 min until hypotension resolves, followed by an infusion of 5 to 15 μg/min.[1] The side effects of glucagon include nausea, vomiting, hypokalemia, dizziness, and hyperglycemia.

DISPOSITION

Admission

An unstable patient with anaphylaxis refractory to treatment should be admitted to the intensive care unit. All patients who receive epinephrine should be observed; however, the timing of observation is based on experience rather than clear evidence. If the patient remains symptom free after appropriate treatment following 4 h of observation, the patient can be discharged home.[3] Late recurrence is rare, but should be considered in patients with a past history of severe reaction and those using β-blockers. Other factors to consider in discharge planning include distance from medical care, whether the patient lives alone, significant comorbidity (including but not limited to asthma), and age.[3]

Outpatient Care and Prevention

Emergency physicians should provide discharge plans for patients that reduce the chance of recurrence and reduce the frequency and severity of future episodes. For all allergic reactions, the patient should be instructed on how to avoid future exposure to the causative agent, if possible. A prescription and clear instructions on the use of an epinephrine autoinjector should be provided to patients with serious allergic reactions or anaphylaxis when the risk of another reaction is judged to be substantial. All patients with severe or frequent allergic reactions warrant referral to an allergist for in-depth preventive management and attempts at allergen identification.[8] Patients with anaphylactic reactions should be encouraged to wear personal identification of this condition (e.g., Medic-Alert™ bracelets). Any anaphylactic patient on a β-blocker should be switched to another antihypertensive drug.

Treatment in the outpatient setting should include antihistamines and a short course of corticosteroids, although the evidence for this is weak. Prolonged corticosteroid treatment should not be required for most cases; however, an aggressive longer-term approach does reduce the frequency of relapses in patients with idiopathic anaphylaxis.[10] The evidence to treat less-severe allergic reactions with corticosteroids awaits further research. All patients should be provided with a patient information sheet detailing signs and symptoms to watch for and clear instructions for follow-up and immediate return if there is any recurrence of symptoms. Finally, a written action plan on steps to take in the event of future allergen exposure or symptom development may reduce the severity of future attacks.

URTICARIA AND ANGIOEDEMA

Urticaria, or hives, is a cutaneous reaction marked by the development of pruritic, erythremic wheals of varying size that generally are described as "fleeting." Erythema multiforme is a more pronounced variation of urticaria, characterized by typical target skin lesions. Angioedema is believed to be a similar but deeper reaction characterized by edema formation in the dermis, most generally involving the face and neck, and distal extremities. These manifestations may accompany many allergic reactions, but also may be nonallergic in nature. As with all allergic manifestations, a detailed history should be obtained. If an etiologic agent can be identified, future reactions may be avoided, although the majority of acute urticarial reactions are viral in nature. This is especially true in children, or with any hives persisting or recurring for more than 24 h. Treatment of these reactions is generally supportive and symptomatic, with attempts to identify and remove the offending agent. Antihistamines, without or without steroids, are usually sufficient, although epinephrine can be considered in severe or refractory cases. The addition of an H_2 receptor blocker, such as ranitidine, may also be useful in more severe, chronic, or unresponsive cases. Cold compresses may be soothing to affected areas. Referral to an allergy specialist is again indicated in severe, recurrent, or refractory cases.

Angioedema of the tongue, lips, and face is another cause of presentation to the ED with the potential for airway obstruction. Angioedema is caused by a variety of agents; however, use of angiotensin-converting enzyme (ACE) inhibitor is a common trigger with angioedema occurring in 0.1 to 0.7 percent of patients taking ACE inhibitors. Fortunately, most cases are mild and transient. Management is supportive, with special attention to the airway, which can become occluded rapidly and unpredictably.[16] Typical allergic-reaction drugs, such as antihistamines and steroids, are not proven to be beneficial because ACE-inhibitor angioedema is not associated with an increase in IgE. Epinephrine, antihistamines, and steroids are often still used; however, their benefits have not been clearly demonstrated in the literature.

Immediate withdrawal from the ACE inhibitor is indicated, and another antihypertensive should be prescribed with the important exception that angiotensin II receptor-blocking agents should not be used. Patients with mild swelling and no evidence of airway obstruction can be observed in the ED and discharged if swelling diminishes. Rebound or recurrent swelling will not occur unless the patient takes an ACE inhibitor again. Patients with moderate-to-severe swelling, dysphagia, or respiratory distress are best admitted for close observation.

Hereditary angioedema is an autosomal dominant disorder with a characteristic complement pathway defect: low levels of C1 esterase inhibitor or elevated levels of dysfunctional C1 esterase inhibitor with low levels of C4 between acute attacks.[17] Reactions often involve the upper respiratory tract and gastrointestinal tract. Attacks can last from a few hours to 1 to 2 days. Minor trauma often precipitates a reaction. Many of the typical treatments of allergic reactions, such as epinephrine, steroids, and antihistamines, have been ineffective. Prophylaxis of acute attacks may be possible with attenuated androgens, such as stanozolol 2 mg/d or danazol 200 mg/d. Acute attacks can be shortened by C1 esterase inhibitor (C1INH inhibitor) replacement by a concentrate. Treatment of patients is complex and best done in coordination with the appropriate specialist.

OTHER COMMON ALLERGIC PROBLEMS

Food Allergy

Hypersensitivity reactions to ingested foods are generally caused by IgE-mediated reactions to food proteins, and, rarely, by additives; their frequency is rising for unknown reasons.[18] IgE-coated mast cells lining the gastrointestinal tract react to presented allergens in ingested foods and produce clinical findings associated with the release of biologic mediators, as previously described. Non-IgE-mediated food allergy reactions have also been described. Dairy products, eggs, nuts, and shellfish are some of the most commonly implicated foods.

A detailed dietary history within the 24 h of allergic symptoms may provide the best clues to food allergy, with particular attention to other allergic history and prior reactions. Diagnosis is often difficult, however, and it may require multiple episodes before an offending agent is identified. Symptoms of food allergy include swelling and itching of the lips, mouth, and pharynx; nausea; abdominal cramps; vomiting; and diarrhea. Cutaneous manifestations, such as angioedema and urticaria, as well as anaphylaxis, can occur. Treatment for mild reactions is supportive, with the administration of antihistamines to lessen symptoms. More severe reactions or anaphylaxis are managed as previously described.

Insect Sting Allergy

Insect stings can produce significant, and sometimes fatal, reactions, particularly in sensitized patients. True stinging insects belong to the order Hymenoptera, which includes three families: Apidae (honeybees), Formicidae (fire ants), and Vespidae (wasps, yellow jackets, and hornets) (see Chap. 194). The venoms of each family are unique, although all have similar types of components, mostly proteins. This difference accounts for the limited cross-reactivity seen between the insect families, although cross-reactivity among the vespids is common. The normal, toxin-mediated reaction to these stings includes localized pain, pruritus, swelling, and redness. Often this is confused with cellulitis; and antibiotic treatment, alone or in combination with allergy medications, may be inappropriately initiated. Sensitized individuals may have exaggerated local reactions with or without systemic manifestations. Systemic reactions run from mild to angioedema, or anaphylaxis.

Diagnosis depends on clinical history, with particular attention to past reactions, and an examination to locate the site of the sting. Treatment is symptomatic and supportive. Mild local reactions can be managed with application of ice and oral antihistamines. More generalized reactions or local reactions of the head and neck may benefit from a short course of corticosteroids. Severe reactions are managed as previously described. Patients with severe reactions should be advised to carry self-administered epinephrine and antihistamines.

Drug Allergy

Although adverse reactions to drugs are a common clinical problem, true hypersensitivity reactions probably account for less than 10 percent of these problems.[19] Because most drugs are small organic molecules, they are generally unable to stimulate an immune response alone. However, when a drug or metabolite becomes protein-bound, either in serum or on cell surfaces, the drug-protein complex can become an allergen and stimulate immune system responses. Thus, the ability of a drug or its metabolites to sensitize the immune system depends on the ability to bind to tissue proteins. Penicillin is the drug most commonly implicated in eliciting true allergic reactions and accounts for approximately 90 percent of all allergic drug reactions. Of those patients with fatal anaphylactic drug reactions, more than 95 percent reacted to penicillin. Overall, less than 25 percent of patients who die of penicillin anaphylaxis exhibited allergic reactions during previous treatment with the drug. Parenteral penicillin administration is more than twice as likely to produce fatal allergic reactions than is oral administration. The cross reactivity of penicillin allergy with cephalosporins is about 7 percent. Patients with a previous life-threatening or anaphylactic reaction to penicillin should not be given cephalosporins.[20]

The clinical manifestations of drug allergy vary widely. A generalized reaction similar to immune-complex or serum sickness reactions is very common, especially with common agents like trimethoprim-sulfamethoxazole and certain cephalosporins (cefaclor being the most frequent). Although data are conflicting on the crossreactivity of sulfonamide antibiotics with other sulfa-containing compounds, it is best to avoid the latter in patients with allergy to sulfonamide antibiotics (Table 34–3).[21] Beginning usually in the first or second week after the

TABLE 34-3   Some Products Containing Sulfonamides

Trimethoprim-sulfamethoxazole
Furosemide
Glipizide
Thiazides
Diazoxide
Silver sulfadiazine
Mafenide acetate
Bumetanide
Celecoxib

administration of the drug, this reaction may take many weeks to subside after drug withdrawal. Generalized malaise, arthralgias, arthritis, pruritus, urticarial eruptions, and fever are common symptoms; adenopathy and hepatosplenomegaly may be identified on examination. Drug fever may occur without other associated clinical findings and may also occur without an immunologic basis. Circulating immune complexes are probably responsible for the lupus-like reactions caused by some drugs. Cytotoxic reactions, such as penicillin-induced hemolytic anemia, can occur. Skin eruptions may include erythema, pruritus, urticaria, angioedema, erythema multiforme, and photosensitivity, and severe reactions, such as those seen in Stevens-Johnson syndrome and toxic epidermal necrolysis may also occur. Pulmonary complications, including bronchospasm and airway obstruction, can occur.

Delayed hypersensitivity reactions may be manifested as a contact dermatitis from drugs applied topically. Diagnosis is best determined by a careful and thorough history. Treatment is supportive, with oral or parenteral antihistamines, glucocorticoids, and β-adrenergic agents, as discussed above. Immediate drug withdrawal is important; however, reactions can continue or recur after a period of abstinence. Referral to an allergy specialist is indicated in these cases.

REFERENCES

1. Kemp SF, Lockey RF: Anaphylaxis: A review of causes and mechanisms. *J Allergy Clin Immunol* 110:341, 2002.
2. Brown AFT: Therapeutic controversies in the management of acute anaphylaxis. *J Accid Emerg Med* 15:89, 1998.
3. Brady WJ, Luber S, Carter T, et al: Multiphasic anaphylaxis: An uncommon event in the emergency department. *Acad Emerg Med* 4:193, 1997.
4. Stewart AG, Ewan PW: The incidence, aetiology and management of anaphylaxis presenting to an accident and emergency department. *Q J Med* 89:859, 1996.
5. Brown AF, McKinnon D, Chu K: Emergency department anaphylaxis: A review of 1 single year. *J Allergy Clin Immunol* 108:861, 2001.
6. Alves B, Sheikh A: Age specific aetiology of anaphylaxis. *Arch Dis Child* 85:349, 2001.
7. Simons FE, Chad ZH, Gold M: Real-time reporting of anaphylaxis in infants, children and adolescents by physicians involved in the Canadian Pediatric Surveillance Program. *J Allergy Clin Immunol* 109:s181, 2002.
8. Ewan PW: ABC of allergies. *BMJ* 316:1442, 1998.
9. Szczeklik A, Nizankowska E, Bochenek G, et al: Safety of a specific COX-2 inhibitor in aspirin-induced asthma. *Clin Exp Allergy* 31:219, 2001.
10. Ring J, Darsow U: Idiopathic anaphylaxis. *Curr Allergy Asthma Rep* 2:40, 2002.
11. Rowe BH, Bretzlaff JA, Bourdon C, et al: Intravenous magnesium sulfate treatment for acute asthma in the emergency department. *Cochrane Database Syst Rev* 2:CD001490, 2000.
12. Simons FER, Gu X, Simons KJ: Epinephrine absorption in adults: Intramuscular versus subcutaneous injection. *J Allergy Clin Immunol* 108:871, 2001.
13. Simons FE, Roberts JR, Gu X, et al: Epinephrine absorption in children with a history of anaphylaxis. *J Allergy Clin Immunol* 110:33, 1998.
14. Winbery SL, Lieberman PL: Histamine and antihistamines in anaphylaxis. *Clin Allergy Immunol* 17:287, 2002.
15. Plotnick LH, Ducharme FM: Should inhaled anticholinergics be added to β-agonists for treating acute childhood and adolescent asthma? A systematic review. *BMJ* 317:971, 1998.
16. Chiu AG, Newkirk KA, Davidson BJ, et al: Angiotensin-converting enzyme inhibitor-induced angioedema: A multicenter review and an algorithm for airway management. *Ann Otol Rhinol Laryngol* 110:834, 2001.
17. Ebo DG, Stevens WJ: Hereditary angioneurotic edema: A review of the literature. *Acta Clin Belg* 55:22, 2000.
18. O'Leary PF, Shanahan F: Food allergies. *Curr Gastroenterol Rep* 4:373, 2002.
19. Babu KS, Belgi G: Management of cutaneous drug reactions. *Curr Allergy Asthma Rep* 2:26, 2002.
20. Kelkar PS, Li JT-C: Cephalosporin allergy. *New Engl J Med.* 345:808, 2001.
21. Wilholm BE: Identification of sulfonamide-like adverse drug reactions to celecoxib in the World Health Organization database. *Curr Med Res Opin* 17:210, 2001.

NEUROGENIC SHOCK
Brian Euerle
Thomas M. Scalea

Neurogenic shock, characterized by hypotension and bradycardia, occurs after an acute spinal cord injury that disrupts sympathetic outflow, leaving unopposed vagal tone.[1] The term neurogenic shock must be carefully differentiated from another that has a very different meaning—namely, *spinal shock.* Spinal shock refers to the temporary loss of spinal reflex activity that occurs below a total or near total spinal cord injury.[2] These terms are not interchangeable.

The vast majority of patients who sustain a spinal cord injury are initially evaluated in an ED.[3] Although the definitive care of these patients is provided by a variety of specialists, the emergency physician usually performs the initial evaluation, resuscitation, stabilization, and transfer. The patient's prognosis and eventual outcome often depend on initial ED care. Early recognition of the potential injury, along with early spinal immobilization, will help prevent any possible worsening of an injury. For high-dose methylprednisolone therapy to be effective, it should be given within 8 h of injury.[4] The search for associated injuries must be done early, often by the emergency physician.

EPIDEMIOLOGY

Acute spinal cord injury is usually caused by blunt trauma; penetrating trauma causes only 10 to 15 percent of cases.[1,3] The majority of penetrating wounds that produce acute spinal cord injury are caused by gunshot wounds, with a small minority caused by stab wounds.[1] Of the blunt trauma causes, automobile accidents are the most frequent, followed by falls and sports.[5,6] The cervical region is the most commonly injured, followed by the thoracolumbar junction, the thoracic region, and the lumbar segments.[6] Each year, in the United States, approximately 10,000 people sustain spinal cord injury.[5]

PATHOPHYSIOLOGY

The spinal column is composed of 33 bony vertebrae with interspersed cartilaginous intervertebral disks. The typical vertebra consists of an anterior vertebral body and a posterior vertebral arch. These elements form the borders of the vertebral foramen, which contains and protects the spinal cord. The superior and inferior articular processes arising from most vertebrae allow the spine to be a strong yet flexible structure. The pedicles and laminae form the sides of the vertebral arch and are notched to allow for the passage of nerves and blood vessels.

The spinal cord is a cylindrical structure arising at the base of the brain and passing through the skull at the foramen magnum. It is surrounded and protected by three layers of meninges as well as cerebrospinal fluid. Thirty-one pairs of spinal nerves exit the spinal column via the intervertebral foramen. The spinal nerves are formed by the junction of the anterior and posterior nerve roots as they exit from the spinal cord.

The spinal cord consists of both white and gray matter. In general, the white matter is the outer covering of the cord. It contains the nerve fibers running up and down the spinal cord in tracts. The gray matter is made up of nerve cells and is formed in the shape of an H when viewed on cross section (Figure 35-1).

The autonomic nervous system, which maintains the internal balance of the body's many systems, has two main divisions: the sympathetic and parasympathetic. The sympathetic nervous system activates the "fight or flight" response, increasing the heart rate and blood pressure and constricting arterioles of the skin and intestines in order to redistribute blood flow, preferentially to the brain, heart, and skeletal muscle. The parasympathetic nervous system has the opposite effect, slowing the heart rate, decreasing blood pressure, and increasing the peristaltic activity of the gastrointestinal tract.

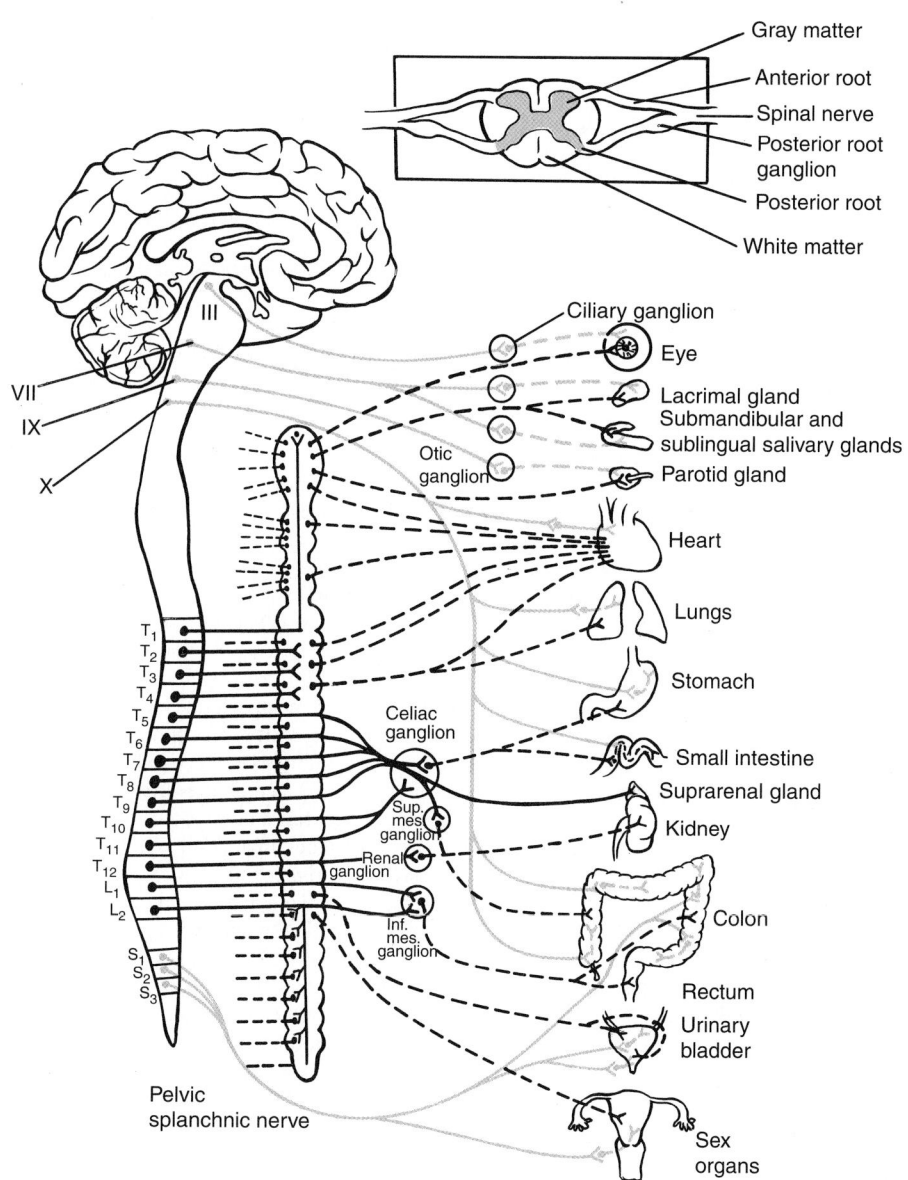

Gray matter
Anterior root
Spinal nerve
Posterior root ganglion
Posterior root
White matter

Ciliary ganglion
Eye
Lacrimal gland
Submandibular and sublingual salivary glands
Otic ganglion
Parotid gland
Heart
Lungs
Stomach
Celiac ganglion
Small intestine
Suprarenal gland
Sup. mes. ganglion
Kidney
Renal ganglion
Inf. mes. ganglion
Colon
Rectum
Urinary bladder
Pelvic splanchnic nerve
Sex organs

FIG. 35-1. Section of the spinal cord, showing the white and gray matter, spinal roots, and spinal nerve (adapted with permission from Snell RS: *Clinical Anatomy for Medical Students.* Philadelphia, Lippincott-Raven, 1973, p. 828), as well as the efferent portion of the autonomic nervous system (used with permission from Snell RS: *Clinical Neuroanatomy for Medical Students.* 4th ed. Philadelphia, Lippincott-Raven, 1997, p. 463).

The anatomy of the autonomic nervous system is quite complex (see Figure 35-1). The outflow portion of the sympathetic system starts with neuron cell bodies located in the lateral gray horns of the first thoracic to the second lumbar segments. In some cases, they may extend to the third lumbar segment. These cells are controlled by the hypothalamus via descending tracts of the reticular formation. The axons from the sympathetic nerve cells in the lateral gray horns leave the spinal cord in the anterior nerve roots and connect to the ganglia of the paraspinal sympathetic trunk. The sympathetic trunk is located along each side of the spinal column and extends along the entire length of the vertebral column. Axons arising from neurons in the sympathetic ganglia then travel throughout the body. The sympathetic fibers that innervate the heart arise primarily from the second to fourth thoracic segments.

The anatomy of the parasympathetic system is very different. The majority of the parasympathetic system is carried along the cranial nerves, although there is a portion that involves the second to fourth sacral segments of the spinal cord. The parasympathetic axons synapse with the cranial nerves in peripheral ganglia close to or within the target organ. The parasympathetic axons from the sacral segments form the pelvic splanchnic nerves. The portion of the parasympathetic system that innervates the heart originates in the dorsal nucleus of the vagus nerve and travels to the heart via the vagus nerves.

In evaluating patients with spinal cord injuries, the concepts of primary and secondary cord injury are important. When the spinal cord is initially injured, the pathologic picture may be relatively benign, showing some scattered hemorrhages and edema.[7] Several weeks later, the appearance is much worse, with large cavities surrounded by gliosis and fibrosis.[7]

These primary or initial changes are caused by the traumatic event, which can cause compression, laceration, or stretching of the cord.[5] Over several days to weeks, the initial injury evolves to what is termed *secondary cord injury.* Spinal cord ischemia has been suggested as the principal etiology of secondary changes, although other mechanisms may exist.[5–7] Ischemia of the spinal cord can be caused by a variety of events. The blood supply to the spinal cord is, in general, not very substantial, and can be easily disrupted by either local trauma to the small anterior and posterior spinal arteries or injury and thrombosis to a large regional vessel, such as the great radicular artery of Adamkiewicz. General systemic hypotension and shock, if severe enough, can cause a low-flow state such that blood flow to the cord is compromised, even with an intact arterial supply.

The clinical relevance of secondary injury is that a patient's presentation can change in the period following the traumatic event. An incomplete lesion can evolve to a complete injury, or the level of injury can become higher because of the cord changes that occur during secondary cord injury.

CLINICAL FEATURES

The initial cardiovascular response after spinal cord injury may include hypertension, widened pulse pressure, and tachycardia.[1] In animal experiments, the hypotension that is characteristic of neurogenic shock generally begins within 5 min of the acute spinal cord injury and lasts 2 to 3 min.[8]

Patients with neurogenic shock are hypotensive and usually have warm, dry skin.[8] Bradycardia is characteristic but not universal. The patient may lose the ability to redirect blood from the periphery to the core because of the loss of sympathetic tone resulting in excessive loss of heat from the skin, with subsequent hypothermia.[8]

These symptoms of neurogenic shock can be expected to last from 1 to 3 weeks.[9] In some cases, significant rehabilitation using elastic stockings, an abdominal binder, and a tilt table may be required to prevent an orthostatic drop in blood pressure when the patient is placed upright.[10]

The anatomic level of the spinal cord injury influences the likelihood and severity of neurogenic shock. Any injury above T1 should be capable of disrupting the spinal tracts that control the entire sympathetic system. Any injury from T1 to L3 has the potential to partially disrupt the sympathetic outflow; intuitively, the higher the injury in this zone, the more likely or more severe the resulting neurogenic shock.[1]

Incomplete spinal cord injury may also cause neurogenic shock. In a large study of 408 patients with cervical cord/column injuries, Soderstrom and Ducker reported a near equal incidence of neurogenic shock in patients with incomplete versus complete lesions; 31.6 percent versus 20.7 percent, respectively.[11] The explanation for this is not entirely clear. Guha and Tator, working with an acute spinal cord injury model in rats, suggest that the decline in cardiac output following acute cord injury is not a result of decreased sympathetic tone alone, but may also be caused by direct myocardial injury, similar to that seen after head injury or subarachnoid hemorrhage.[12]

An interesting difference was found with regard to incidence of neurogenic shock between patients with blunt versus penetrating spinal cord injuries. In a study of patients with blunt cervical spine/cord injury, neurogenic shock alone was believed to be responsible in 69 percent of all patients in shock.[13] In Zipnick's study of patients with penetrating spinal injury at various anatomic levels, neurogenic shock was thought to be responsible in only 22 percent of patients in shock.[1] The reason for the difference is unclear, but is probably related to the fact that the two groups were not equivalent: blunt trauma patients had only cervical injuries, while the penetrating injury patients had injuries at all levels of the spinal cord. Also, part of the difference may stem from the fact that patients with penetrating trauma are more likely to have associated injuries.

TREATMENT

Evaluation and treatment of patients with spinal injury and neurogenic shock starts with the "ABCDEs" of trauma assessment: the "A" is not only for airway but also includes cervical spine protection, and the "D" represents disability, or neurologic evaluation (Table 35-1).[5,9] Cervical spine protection and neurologic evaluation are not discussed further here except to say that they form the cornerstone of all further management of patients with neurogenic shock.

It is impossible to separate the initial evaluation and management of the patient with neurogenic shock from that of the general trauma patient. In essence, the diagnosis of neurogenic shock should be one of exclusion. Certain clues—such as bradycardia and warm, dry skin—may be evident, but hypotension in the trauma patient can never be presumed to be caused by neurogenic shock until all other possible sources of hypotension have been eliminated.[1] Again, a difference has been noted between blunt and penetrating spinal injuries, but a large percentage of these patients will have significant concomitant injuries, causing blood loss, which will explain their hypotension.[1,13] It is only

TABLE 35-1   Treatment of Neurogenic Shock

ABCDE:
   Airway with cervical spine protection
   Breathing
   Circulation
   Disability (neurologic evaluation)
   Exposure
Fluid resuscitation with crystalloid—consider pulmonary artery catheter to avoid over hydration.
Carefully search for and treat any possible causes of hypotension and blood loss.
Maintain mean arterial pressure at 85–90 mm Hg.
Transfer patient, after resuscitation, to regional spine or trauma center.

after these other injuries have been excluded that neurogenic shock can be said to be present.

Once the ABCDEs have been attended to and all other possible sources of hypotension have been investigated and treated, treatment focuses on the hypotension and bradycardia of neurogenic shock.

Hypotension is treated by rapid infusion of crystalloid; this is usually effective in treating neurogenic shock.[6,9] During neurogenic shock, blood pools in the distal circulation because of the loss of sympathetic innervation. Infusion of intravenous crystalloid will correct this relative hypovolemia. Adequate fluid resuscitation should be undertaken with the aim of keeping the mean arterial blood pressure at 85–90 mm Hg for the first 7 days after acute spine injury.[14] This level of blood pressure is a bit arbitrary and has been arrived at by clinical experience. It is thought that this level of pressure provides adequate perfusion and minimizes the effects of secondary cord injury.

The use of fluids in neurogenic shock must, however, be judicious. There is a danger of excessive fluid replacement, with resultant heart failure and pulmonary edema.[15] The placement of a pulmonary artery catheter and its resultant pressure measurements can be of tremendous benefit and help prevent excess fluid administration. If intravenous fluids are not adequate to maintain organ perfusion, the use of positive inotropic pressor agents such as dopamine or dobutamine may be beneficial.[9] These agents will improve cardiac output and raise perfusion pressure. The doses required are variable and should be titrated to the patient's hemodynamic response.

Bradycardia, when present, usually occurs within the first few hours or days of spinal cord injury because of a predominance of vagal tone to the heart.[12] In severe cases, and when the patient's hemodynamics warrant, atropine can be used for treatment. In some patients who may present with heart block or asystole, a pacemaker may be required.[12]

The use of steroids in spinal cord injury is discussed in Chap. 256. Steroids are not indicated for the treatment of neurogenic shock per se.

DISPOSITION

Any patient with neurogenic shock has suffered a severe traumatic injury will obviously be admitted to the hospital. In general, the patient with a spinal cord injury is best cared for at a trauma or spine center. Most areas have a regional spine care center, centralizing the extensive resources needed for the care of these patients and standardizing patient care.

While in the ED, the patient with a spinal cord injury and neurogenic shock can benefit from early consultation and involvement of the appropriate specialty services, namely neurosurgery, trauma surgery, and orthopedics.[16] Early consultation and the consideration of transfer is most important for the patient with continuing or worsening hypotension, an evolving deficit, or a progressing level of injury.

REFERENCES

1. Zipnick RI, Scalea TM, Trooskin SZ, et al: Hemodynamic responses to penetrating spinal cord injuries. *J Trauma* 35:578, 1993.

2. Atkinson PP, Atkinson JLD: Spinal shock. *Mayo Clin Proc* 71:384, 1996.

3. Savitsky E, Votey S: Emergency department approach to acute thoracolumbar spine injury. *J Emerg Med* 15:49, 1997.

4. Bracken MB: Steroids for acute spinal cord injury. *Cochrane Database Syst Rev* 3:CD001046, 2002.

5. McDonald JW, Sadowsky C: Spinal-cord injury. *Lancet* 359:417, 2002.

6. Kirshblum SC, Groah SL, McKinley WO, et al: Spinal cord injury medicine. 1. Etiology, classification, and acute medical management. *Arch Phys Med Rehabil* 83:S50, S90, 2002.

7. Tator CH: Experimental and clinical studies of the pathophysiology and management of acute spinal cord injury. *J Spinal Cord Med* 19:206, 1996.

8. Gilson GJ, Miller AC, Clevenger FW, Curet LB: Acute spinal cord injury and neurogenic shock in pregnancy. *Obstet Gynecol Surv* 50:556, 1995.

9. Ball PA: Critical care of spinal cord injury. *Spine* 26:S27, 2002.

10. McKinley WO, Gittler MS, Kirshblum SC, et al: Spinal cord injury medicine. 2. Medical complications after spinal cord injury: identification and management. *Arch Phys Med Rehabil* 83:S58, S90, 2002.

11. Soderstrom CA, Ducker TB: Increased susceptibility of patients with cervical cord lesions to peptic gastrointestinal complications. *J Trauma* 25:1030, 1985.

12. Guha AB, Tator CH: Acute cardiovascular effects of experimental spinal cord injury. *J Trauma* 28:481, 1988.

13. Soderstrom CA, McArdle DQ, Ducker TB, Militello PR: The diagnosis of intraabdominal injury in patients with cervical cord trauma. *J Trauma* 23:1061, 1983.

14. Anonymous: Blood pressure management after acute spinal cord injury. *Neurosurgery* 50(3 suppl):558, 2002.

15. Wilson RH, Whiteside MCR, Moorehead RJ: Problems in diagnosis and management of hypovolaemia in spinal injury. *Br J Clin Pract* 47:224, 1993.

16. Trivedi JM: Spinal trauma: Therapy – options and outcomes. *Eur J Radiol* 42:127, 2002.

ANALGESIA, ANESTHESIA, AND SEDATION

36 ACUTE PAIN MANAGEMENT IN THE ADULT PATIENT
Gary D. Zimmer

Acute pain accompanies 50 to 60 percent of ED patient visits in the United States and Great Britain. Longstanding tradition and common practice have limited the assessment and treatment of pain in ED patients. Fortunately, resistance to treating acute pain in the ED is diminishing as physicians have become educated and comfortable with the benefits of treating pain in this patient population. "Oligo-analgesia" first appeared in the medical literature in 1973 and in the emergency medicine literature in 1989. Variation in analgesic use among ED patients has been correlated with ethnicity, age, and gender[1–3] (Table 36-1). Although the source of pain varies greatly based on disease process, specific measures should be taken to address the *pain* and *suffering* in addition to its underlying cause.

The route of administration of analgesics is less important than the need for adequate dosing and rapid onset. In selected patients, oral or intramuscular injection of analgesics is adequate, but most patients with severe pain are best served by titrated doses of intravenous analgesics, anxiolytics, and comfort measures.

Guidelines and standards for acute pain management have been published by the Agency for Health Care Policy and Research and the Joint Commission on Accreditation of Healthcare Organizations.[4,5] These documents are a useful guide but should be supplemented with more detailed and current information as appropriate.

PATHOPHYSIOLOGY

Pain is the physiologic response to a noxious stimulus, whereas suffering reflects the perception of pain. Acute pain management is best accomplished with analgesia and anxiolysis. The experience of pain is determined by many factors, including medical condition, physical and emotional maturity, cognitive state, meaning of pain, family attitudes, culture, and environment. Fear and anxiety accentuate physical pain.

Pain involves the release of potent mediators of inflammation and is modulated by neurocognitive factors resulting in an unpleasant sensory and emotional experience. The peripheral nervous system (e.g., nociceptors, C fibers, A-δ fibers, and free nerve endings) is responsible for somatic pain. It registers the original noxious stimulus and conducts it to the central nervous system. The primary afferent peripheral nociceptors have poorly differentiated nerve fiber terminals with slow conduction velocities (ranging from 2.5 ms^{-1} for C fibers to 2.5 to 20.0 ms^{-1} for A-δ fibers) and are normally activated by stimuli of strong to noxious intensity. Stimulation of these peripheral nociceptors releases several neurotransmitters. Glutamate, an excitatory amino acid released from these nociceptors, elicits fast synaptic responses in second-order neurons that are mediated by at least two excitatory amino acid receptor subtypes. Some primary afferent nerve fibers also express and synthesize neuropeptides (substance P, neurokinin A, and calcitonin gene-related peptide) that are coreleased with glutamate within the spinal cord.[6]

The dorsal horn of the spinal cord (e.g., dorsal root ganglion, inhibitory interneurons, and ascending pain tracts) integrates and modulates pain and other sensory stimuli. Supraspinal centers (e.g., hypothalamic centers, thalamic nuclei, the limbic system and reticular activating system) integrate and process pain information, allowing detection and perception of pain. Cognitive interpretation, localization, identification of pain, and triggering of emotional and physiologic reactions also occur at this site. Unlike somatic pain, which is easily localized, visceral pain pathways are more complex and differ in structure from somatic pain pathways, which may explain the poor localization of visceral pain.

Opioid analgesics work by binding to the pain receptors in the spinal cord and brain. There are three main opioid receptors and different agents bind to and stimulate them to different degrees. Stimulation of the μ1 receptor produces supraspinal analgesia, euphoria, miosis, and urinary retention. Stimulation of the μ2 receptor is responsible for respiratory depression, gastrointestinal slowing, and cardiovascular depression and is the likely source of addiction. The κ receptor produces dysphoria and spinal-level analgesia. Unfortunately, there are no pure μ1 agonists. If such an agent were developed, many of the concerns about analgesic abuse and adverse reactions would be mitigated.

EVALUATION

Pain assessment in the ED involves determining its duration, location, quality, severity, exacerbation, and mitigation. Because pain is dynamic and changes with time, its severity requires frequent reassessment, ideally involving the use of validated objective and subjective pain assessment instruments. Documentation of initial pain assessment and progress over time is important for clear communication of successful pain management strategies. There are several assessment scales useful for standard documentation.

Non-Self-Report Measurement

Variation in respiratory and cardiovascular signs and changes in patient expression and movement can occur due to pain. However, factors other than pain can cause or inhibit the same changes, making interpretation difficult. Physiologic parameters may be more useful to confirm a clinical impression than as a primary assessment tool. Non-self-report tools are more commonly used in the pediatric setting (see Chap. 134).

Self-Report Measurement

Self-report tools are the mainstay of pain assessment. Several instruments have been derived and validated in patients with acute pain and usually require only a verbal response (Table 36-2). It is important to understand the limitations of the tool used, so that the response to intervention can be adequately measured. The ideal pain assessment tool would be easy to administer, reliable, valid, and applicable to all patients, irrespective of education, culture, or psychological or developmental level. Naturally, there is no perfect tool. However, several visual scales exist that can be used to monitor pain. The most important element to these tools is that they need to be applied at the onset of intervention and then re-evaluated frequently after an intervention.

The end point for pain management is clinically significant pain relief. The interpretation of pain is variable, and the only relevant goal is to satisfy the needs of the patient. It is not acceptable to look for signs of pain relief without clearly eliciting whether the patient's symptoms have been relieved. All visual scales allow for thresholds for statistically significant decrease in pain, but *clinical significance* is the relevant end point.[7] Therefore, each of these tools should be used in conjunction with an ongoing dialog with the patient regarding satisfaction with the attempted pain relief.

TABLE 36-1   Barriers to Adequate Emergency Department Pain Control

Patient related
   Ethnicity: African-American, Hispanic
   Age: elderly
   Gender: male
   Cognitive level: inability to verbalize pain
   Terminal illness: acceptance of continued pain
Provider related
   Education: inadequate understanding of pain
   Fear of adverse events

ADJECTIVE RATING SCALE   This is a simple, descriptive pain-intensity scale presented graphically or verbally as a linear list of pain descriptors. The labels range from *no pain* to *worst possible pain,* and the instrument allows for marks between discrete labels (Figure 36-1).

VISUAL ANALOG SCALE   The Visual Analog Scale (VAS) is a 10-cm linear scale marked at one end with a term such as *no pain* and at the other end with *worst imaginable pain* (Figure 36-2). The patient places a mark on the line at the point that best represents the pain. The VAS is scored by measuring the distance of the patient's mark from either end. The VAS has been validated in trauma patients and general ED patients with acute pain.[8,9] A change of 13 mm along this scale has been shown to be clinically and statistically significant in groups of patients, although results with individual patients will certainly vary. A disadvantage of the VAS is that it requires visual, manual, and some conceptual skill.

NUMERICAL RATING SCALE   The Numerical Rating Scale (NRS) can be presented as a verbal or graphic scale to describe pain intensity. The patient is asked to self-report pain on a scale from 0 (no pain) to 10 (worst possible pain) and mark it off graphically; self-report verbally; or, when language or speech is difficult, indicate the numerical value with upheld fingers (Figure 36-3). Although not as precise as the VAS, the NRS requires no visual or manual skill and is easy to use.

FIVE-POINT GLOBAL SCALE   This scale is simple to administer and does not require any significant patient interpretation. By limiting the results to five gradations of pain, however, it fails to detect small changes in perceived pain.

VERBAL QUANTITATIVE SCALE   This is one of the most commonly used verbal pain scales. Patients are asked to rate their pain on a scale from 1 to 10 without descriptors, as opposed to the NRS. Patients are familiar with the concept and usually comfortable assigning a number. It is important to remember that the value assigned by a patient is not an absolute value but rather a reference point on which to base pain control. For example, some patients with chest pain during acute myocardial infarction only report the pain as 2 to 3, whereas those with less life-threatening pain may rate it as 10.

GLOBAL SATISFACTION QUESTION   The global satisfaction question is an important part of the management of all forms of pain. It does not adequately follow the improvement in pain over the course of therapy. Rather, it allows the user to know when pain relief is adequate for an individual patient.

UNIQUE PATIENT POPULATIONS

The awake, cooperative, competent patient can describe and locate pain and be assessed easily and reliably. Patients who have difficulty communicating are at risk of inadequate pain management. Patients who are cognitively impaired, psychotic, extremely young or old, or who are unable to communicate with their caregivers are at particular risk. In addition, language barriers or extreme cultural or educational disparity between the patient and the caregiver increases the risk of inadequate pain management. These scenarios require a rigorous approach to pain and the use of translators, family members, and validated, objective measurements of pain.

Extremes of Age

For comprehensive assessment of pain in the pediatric patient, age-appropriate, developmentally specific techniques are essential, and assessment is enhanced by the involvement of the parents or caregiver (see Chap. 134).

The elderly often report pain very differently from younger patients, because of physiologic, psychological, and cultural changes associated with aging. The high prevalence of visual, hearing, motor, and cognitive impairments among the elderly can be barriers to effective pain assessment, thus affecting the reliability of traditional pain assessment instruments.

Gender and Culture

Women are more likely to express pain and to actively seek treatment. However, gender-related differences in reporting of pain intensity are equivocal. Yet, physicians have a tendency to underestimate and un-

TABLE 36-2   Pain Scales

Scale	Method	Comments
Adjective Rating Scale	Patient rates pain by choosing from a linear list of pain descriptors (Figure 36-1)	
Visual Analog Scale	Patient places a mark that best describes pain intensity along a10-cm linear scale marked at one end with a term such as *no pain* and at the other end with *worst imaginable pain* (Figure 36-2)	Pain intensity measured in millimeters from one end. Change of greater than 13 mm significant
Numerical Rating Scale	The patient is asked to self-report pain on a scale of 0 to 10 with descriptors (Figure 36-3)	Can be used in patients with visual, speech, or manual dexterity difficulties
5-Point Global Scale	Patient rates pain as: 0 = none 1 = a little 2 = some 3 = a lot 4 = worst possible	A decrease of one point is a large change; other scales allow monitoring of small changes in pain and may be more sensitive
Verbal Quantitative Scale	The patient is asked to self-report pain on a scale of 0 to 10 without descriptors	Most commonly used scale, easy to administer
Global Satisfaction Question	"Are you satisfied with the pain relief?"	May be clouded by non-pain concerns

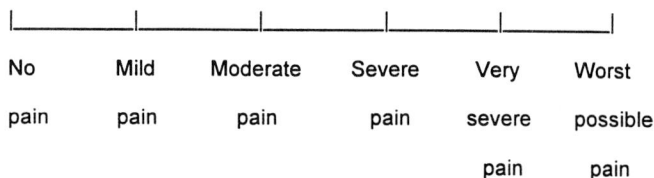

FIG. 36-1. Adjective Rating Scale.

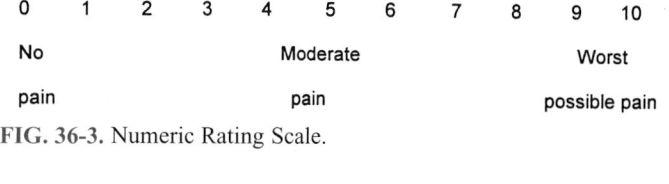

FIG. 36-3. Numeric Rating Scale.

dertreat pain in female patients. Ethnicity has a bearing on different cultural concepts of pain and on the characteristics of culturally appropriate pain-related behaviors. There is also an interplay between the ethnicity of the patient and that of the physician. Most pain instruments are, to some extent, language dependent. In practical consideration of language difficulties and cross-cultural measurement, the VAS is the preferred modality for assessment of pain.

MODALITIES OF PAIN MANAGEMENT

Effective management of acute pain includes pharmacologic agents in addition to nonpharmacologic, cognitive-behavioral, and physical techniques. The key to effective pain management in the ED is prompt onset of analgesic activity, ease of administration, safety, and efficacy (Table 36-3).

Pharmacologic Modalities

The primary agents for the control of pain are the opioids, nonsteroidal anti-inflammatory drugs (NSAIDs), and acetaminophen. Adjuncts, such as anxiolytics and antiemetics, have significant synergy but should not be used without one of the primary analgesics. Adequate control of pain with an analgesic has a mild anxiolytic effect. Using an anxiolytic alone for the control of pain has a less than expected result, because the ongoing pain serves as a nidus for additional anxiety.

A tiered approach should be used. Agents such as NSAIDs should be considered for mild pain, and systemic opioids and/or NSAIDs should be considered for moderate to severe pain. Local or regional neural blockade is a useful technique to minimize the use of narcotic agents (Table 36-4).

Although opioid analgesics are occasionally associated with adverse drug events, the biggest problem is their improper use. Several small case series have found that the incidence of overmedication is comparable to that of undermedication. This finding suggests that undermedication is actually more common, because overmedication is more likely to be recognized and documented.[10]

Opioid Agonists

Opioid analgesics are the cornerstone of pharmacologic management of moderate to severe acute pain (Table 36-5). Proper use of opioids requires careful and deliberate planning:

1. Route of administration
2. Suitable initial dose
3. Frequency of administration titrated against analgesic response
4. Optimal use of nonopioid analgesics and adjunctive agents
5. Incidence and severity of side effects
6. Whether the analgesic will be continued in an inpatient or ambulatory setting

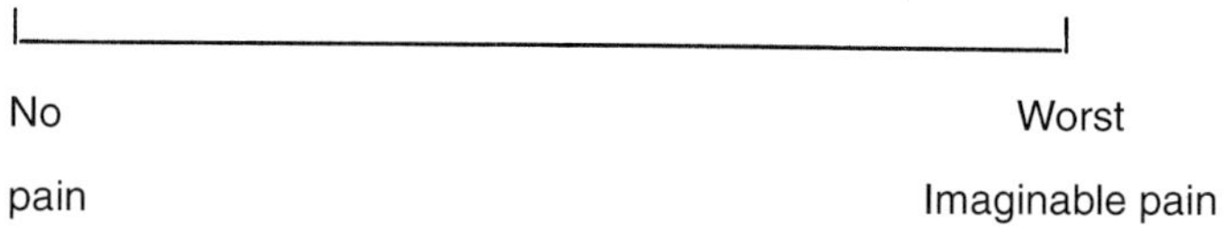

Patients differ greatly in their responses to opioid analgesics; these variations are related to age, body mass, and previous or chronic exposure to opioids. Relative potency estimates provide a rational basis for selecting the appropriate starting dose to initiate analgesic therapy, changing the route of administration (e.g., from parenteral to oral), or switching to another opioid (Table 36-6). The classes of opioids include the phenanthrene derivatives, the phenylpiperidine derivatives, and the diphenylheptane derivatives (Table 36-7). Opiate hypersensitivity is uncommon and true allergic reactions are extremely rare. There is too little data to determine if there is clinical cross-sensitivity within opioid classes. Possible cross-sensitivity has been suggested among the phenylpiperidine class (fentanyl, alfentanil, sufentanil, and meperidine). Until more is known, it would be prudent to switch to a drug from a different opioid class if a patient develops a hypersensitivity reaction to an opiate. When they are used in equianalgesic doses, there is no compelling evidence to recommend one opioid over another. As much as possible, avoid using multiple agents. Become comfortable with a few agents and, whenever possible, titrate a single drug to effect in each individual. Caution is advised with the use of meperidine and codeine; although both agents are capable of producing adequate analgesia at high doses, adverse effects are more common with these two drugs compared with other opioids.

Meperidine was once the mainstay of pain management in EDs. Meperidine should no longer be routinely used for acute pain management, for several reasons: (1) it is the lowest potency opioid and, as a result, often is underdosed; (2) normeperidine, the metabolite of meperidine, has been shown to cause central nervous system toxicity in patients with compromised renal function or those taking monoamine oxidase inhibitors; (3) normeperidine can produce prolonged states of sedation (up to 48 h in rare cases); and (4) meperidine is reported to produce more euphoria and may have an increased risk for addiction when compared with other opioids.

Codeine produces more nausea, vomiting, and dysphoria than other opioids. The standard oral dose of 30 to 60 mg produces little analgesic effect above that of acetaminophen or NSAIDs.

Adverse effects of opioids include nausea, vomiting, constipation, pruritus, urinary retention, confusion, and respiratory depression. Pruritus, urinary retention, confusion, and respiratory depression are more common with intravenous, transmucosal, and epidural administrations as opposed to oral administration. As a practical matter, opioids should be withheld with respiratory depression (fewer than 10 breaths/min in an adult).

Opioids are frequently combined with adjunctive drugs (hydroxyzine or benzodiazepines), which may provide pain relief at a lower opiate dose than using an opiate alone (Table 36-8), yet the data supporting such action are scarce, and polypharmacy may produce unexpected results. Prophylactic dosing of adjuncts before treatment with analgesics is not appropriate as the incidence of adverse side effects is small.[11] However, symptom-targeted therapy with anxiolytics and antiemetics is sometimes necessary.

No pain _____ Worst Imaginable pain

FIG. 36-2. Visual Analog Scale.

TABLE 36-3 Goals of Pain Management

Efficacy
No significant interference with evaluation of the underlying disease process
Rapidity of onset
Ease of administration

TABLE 36-4   Comparison of Pharmacologic Classes

Class	Route	Advantages	Disadvantages
NSAIDs	Oral	Mild/moderate somatic pain plus severe colicky pain	Use caution in the elderly and in those with renal, GI, and hematologic disorders
	Parenteral	Does not require GI absorption	No more effective than oral (well-known placebo effect); costly
Opioids	Oral	Can be effective if adequately dosed	Variable absorption
	Intramuscular	No IV access required	Painful injections; unreliable absorption
	Intravenous	Ideal for titrated dosing	May require monitoring; potential for overdose
Local anesthetics	Infiltration	Technical ease	Limited duration of action
	Peripheral nerve block	Opioid sparing	Technical difficulty
	Regional anesthesia	Opioid and general anesthetic sparing	Risk of autonomic instability, hemodynamic collapse

Abbreviations: GI = gastrointestinal; NSAIDs = nonsteroidal anti-inflammatory drugs.

Concerns have been raised about delayed-release transdermal formulations, because of delayed onset and prolonged duration of action. Transdermal fentanyl preparations are used in the chronic pain and oncology setting. In general, transdermal fentanyl should be avoided for acute pain management.

Opioid Agonist-Antagonists

Opioid agonist-antagonists comprise a group of synthetic analgesics that was developed to minimize some of the adverse effects of pure opioid agonists. The major benefit has been a ceiling on respiratory depression: no further reduction in respiration with increasing doses past a set amount. Concern has been expressed about the possible ceiling effect for analgesia, but the significance of this potential problem is not clear. The variability in efficacy relates to each particular agent's affinity for the various central pain receptors. These agents should be used with extreme caution in patients with opioid addiction because they may precipitate withdrawal symptoms.

Nonopioid Agents

Acetaminophen is an effective analgesic that is adequate for mild to moderate pain. Acetaminophen does not affect platelet aggregation, and it is not an anti-inflammatory (Table 36-9). Dosing is constant throughout life, and no change is required for renal or mild hepatic impairment. The recommended maximal adult daily dose for repetitive use is 4 g per day.

The *NSAIDs,* including aspirin, naproxen, indomethacin, ibuprofen, and ketorolac, are excellent analgesics and anti-inflammatory agents. In therapeutic doses, these agents decrease inflammatory mediators generated at the site of tissue injury. They do not cause sedation, respiratory depression or interfere with bowel or bladder function. Even when insufficient alone, NSAIDs have significant opioid dose-sparing effects. There are oral, rectal, intravenous, and topical preparations. Ketorolac is the only parenteral agent available in the United States. Topical NSAIDs, effective in acute musculoskeletal injuries and chronic pain, are associated with the lowest side effect pro-

TABLE 36-5   Initial Dosing of Common Opioid Analgesics for Acute, Severe Pain

Drug	Adult Dose	Pharmacokinetics	Toxicity

Morphine	0.1 mg/kg IV
	
	10 mg IM
	0.3 mg/kg PO
		Onset: 5 min IV and
		  10–15 min IM/SC
		Peak effect: 15–30 min
		Duration: 1–2 h IV and
		  3–4 h IM/SC
			Histamine release may result in anaphylactoid reaction

Hydromorphone	0.015 mg/kg IV 1–2 mg IM	Same as morphine	
Fentanyl	0.5–3 µg/kg IV	Onset: almost immediately Peak effect: 1–5 min Duration: 30–40 min	High doses can cause chest wall rigidity (>5 µg/kg IV)
Meperidine	1–1.5 mg/kg IV/IM	Duration: 2–3 h	Not recommended; see text
Oxycodone	5–10 mg PO 30 mg PR	Duration: 3–6 h	Lower incidence of nausea Possible inadvertent acetaminophen overdose with combination agents
Hydrocodone	5–10 mg PO	Duration: 3–6 h	Lower incidence of nausea Possible inadvertent acetaminophen overdose with combination agents
Codeine	30–60 mg PO 30–100 mg IM	Duration: 4 h	High incidence of nausea Small portion is metabolized to morphine Low potency results in underdosing Possible inadvertent acetaminophen overdose with combination agents

TABLE 36-6   Equipotent Opioid Doses

Drug	Equipotent IV dose	Equipotent PO Dose
Morphine	1.0	3
Fentanyl	0.01	0.02 (transmucosal)
Hydromorphone	0.2	0.6
Meperidine	5	15
Oxycodone		1.5
Hydrocodone		2.0
Codeine	13	20

file, but are not widely available in the United States.[11] Adverse effects of NSAIDs include platelet dysfunction, impaired coagulation, and gastrointestinal irritation and bleeding. Therefore, they should be used with caution in patients with thrombocytopenia or coagulopathies and in those at risk for bleeding or gastric ulceration. Acute renal failure has been reported and may be precipitated in elderly patients, those who are volume depleted or have lost more than 10 percent of their blood volume, have preexisting renal or cardiac disease, or are taking loop diuretics.

Corticosteroids are potent inhibitors of inflammation and are excellent analgesics for visceral, orthopedic, and neuropathic pain. They are well absorbed from oral and parenteral routes. There are numerous long-term side effects of systemic corticosteroids, thus limiting their efficacy. For short-term pain management, corticosteroids are effective and safe. Dexamethasone is a good agent, because of its minimal mineralocorticoid effects.

Other Agents

Ketamine and nitrous oxide are two agents that have been used widely for brief analgesic therapy; these agents also have sedative properties. Tricyclic antidepressants and anticonvulsants are useful in treating neuropathic pain.

KETAMINE   A phencyclidine derivative, ketamine produces analgesia and dissociative anesthesia with the advantage of causing minimal respiratory depression. The ability of ketamine to produce amnesia makes it a good agent for brief, minor procedures such as wound repair. Adverse effects include increased intracranial pressure, increased intraocular pressure, hypersalivation, and reemergence phenomena (disagreeable dreams or hallucinations upon awakening). It should be avoided in patients with closed head injuries or other conditions associated with increased intracranial pressure. It is a useful agent in the pediatric ED (see Chap. 134).

NITROUS OXIDE   Nitrous oxide is a fast-onset, short-acting analgesic and sedative inhalational agent useful for wound dressing and brief, minor procedures. The primary adverse effects are nausea and vomiting. Barriers to ED use of nitrous oxide include the need for patient cooperation and an effective scavenging system. In addition, it cannot be used in patients with altered mental status, head injury, suspected pneumothorax, or perforated abdominal viscus. Severe pulmonary disease also may alter the respiratory elimination of nitrous oxide.

TABLE 36-7   Classification of Opioid Analgesics

Phenanthrene	Morphine, hydromorphone, nalbuphine, oxycodone, codeine, butorphanol, levorphanol, nalbuphine
Phenylpiperidine	Fentanyl, alfentanil, meperidine, sufentanil
Diphenylheptane	Methadone, propoxyphene

TRICYCLIC ANTIDEPRESSANTS AND ANTICONVULSANTS   Patients with neuropathic pain are difficult to treat with standard analgesics and are often quite resistant to opioids. Amitriptyline and gabapentin have been effective in treating this type of pain.[13,14]

Route of Administration

Systemic pain medications can be given orally, rectally, intravenously, intramuscularly, transmucosally, transdermally, by inhalation, or by epidural administration (Table 36-10). Intravenous opioids are suitable for bolus administration or continuous infusion and are preferred to intermittent intramuscular injections. Repeated intramuscular injections themselves can cause pain and trauma and may deter patients from requesting pain medication. Patient-controlled intravenous analgesic systems do have a role in the ED for the stabilized patient who is to be admitted. Oral administration is convenient and inexpensive and is appropriate once the patient can tolerate oral intake; it is a mainstay of pain management in the ambulatory ED population.

Nonsystemic agents can be delivered transdermally, transmucosally, by infiltrative local and regional injection, or IV for specific regional blocks. Alternative delivery techniques such as iontophoresis and single-dose jet injectors have been available for several years but have not yet emerged as practical, cost-effective products for routine use.

Dosage and Precautions

BASIC DOSING GUIDELINES   The key principle for safe and effective use of opioids is to titrate the dose toward the desired effect while minimizing unwanted effects. In excessive or inappropriate doses, opioids can result in respiratory depression and hypotension. Relative potency estimates provide a rational basis for selecting the appropriate dose. In the setting of comorbidity, such as altered mental status, hemodynamic instability, respiratory dysfunction, or multisystem trauma, initial dosing should be decreased. However, these patients may still require large doses of analgesics, so titration becomes even more important.

EXTREMES OF AGE   Patients at the extremes of age are at risk for inadequate analgesia and pharmacotherapy complications. For the comprehensive management of pediatric pain, age-appropriate assessment techniques and medication dosages and developmentally specific nonpharmacologic adjuncts are essential (see Chap. 134). Elderly patients may have more than one source of pain and comorbidity and are at increased risk for interactions between drugs and between the drug and the disease. The elderly, especially opioid-naive patients, are more sensitive to the analgesic effects of opioid drugs, because they experience a higher peak and longer duration of pain relief. Moreover, they are more sensitive to sedation, respiratory depression, and cognitive and neuropsychiatric dysfunction.

ADDICTION   The appropriate use of opioid analgesics has not been shown to produce dependence after a short duration of therapy for acute pain.[15] Care must be used in the patient with concern for addiction, but reassurance and appropriate dosing guidelines should be used rather than withholding appropriate agents.

Dosing Adjustments

RENAL AND HEPATIC DYSFUNCTION   Because most analgesics are metabolized by the liver or kidney, caution is required when using opioids in patients with altered hepatic or renal function. Renal excretion is a major route of elimination for such pharmacologically active opioid metabolites as norpropoxyphene, normeperidine, morphine-6-glucuronide, and dihydrocodeine. Mild renal failure can impede

TABLE 36-8   Analgesic Adjuncts

Drug	Initial Dosing	Pharmacokinetics	Comments
Anxiolytics			
Lorazepam	0.5–2 mg IV/IM	Duration: 2–6 h	Respiratory depression Synergy with opiates Idiosyncratic agitation
Midazolam	0.5–2 mg IV/IM	Duration: 0.5–2 h	Same
Diazepam	5–10 mg IV/IM	Duration: 4–6 h	Repeated doses can prolong sedation
Oxazepam	15–30 mg PO	Duration: 4–8 h	Not recommended in this setting
Antiemetics			
Prochlorperazine	5–10 mg IV/IM	Duration: 4–6 h	Can cause extrapyramidal reaction
Promethazine	25–50 mg IV/IM	Duration: 4–6 h	Same
Metoclopramide	5–10 mg IV/IM	Duration: 4–6 h	Somewhat less effective Primary action is gastric emptying
Hydroxyzine	25–50 mg IM	Duration: 4–6 h	Reported to potentiate narcotics Limited to IM use Benefit not proven

excretion of the metabolites of many opioids, resulting in clinically significant narcosis and respiratory depression. Mild hepatic dysfunction has little effect on analgesic metabolism. In patients with severe hepatic dysfunction, titration of low doses of analgesics will minimize the risk of overdose.

RESPIRATORY INSUFFICIENCY   Patients with respiratory insufficiency and those with chronic obstructive pulmonary disease, cystic fibrosis, and neuromuscular disorders affecting respiratory effort (e.g., muscular dystrophy and myasthenia gravis) are particularly vulnerable to the respiratory depressant effects of opioids and nitrous oxide. Appropriate monitoring of respiratory function and adequacy of gas exchange is necessary.

DRUG INTERACTIONS   Opioids may have adverse synergistic sedative effects in patients with psychiatric illnesses taking anxiolytics or other psychoactive drugs. The use of monoamine oxidase inhibitors with meperidine has been associated with severe adverse reactions, including death through mechanisms that mimic malignant hyperthermia. The tricyclic antidepressants clomipramine and amitriptyline may increase morphine levels.

Nonpharmacologic Modalities

Traditionally, nonpharmacologic techniques of pain management in the ED are limited to application of heat or cold and immobilization and elevation of injured extremities. Other techniques may prove to have a role in the ED and post-ED setting. Examples include cognitive-behavioral techniques, which are effective in reducing pain and anxiety, may control mild pain when used alone, and enhance patient satisfaction. These techniques include reassurance, explanation, relaxation, music, psychoprophylaxis, biofeedback, guided imagery, hypnosis, and distraction. They are a useful adjunct to pharmacologic management of moderate to severe pain. Successful application of these therapies requires a cognitively intact patient and skilled personnel, but many of the techniques require only a few minutes to teach the patient.

Physical nonpharmacologic agents are becoming increasingly relevant to ED pain management. In addition to the traditional techniques noted above, the less commonly used physical modalities such as transcutaneous electrical nerve stimulation and acupuncture may have some potential role in the ED in the future. Although specific technical skills and equipment are required, there is no need for intravenous access, and there is no systemic effect such as respiratory depression or altered mental status.

Specific Situations

There are a number of situations in which the ideal ED analgesic management approach is complex or controversial. Acute abdominal pain, migraine, and trauma are such situations.

ABDOMINAL PAIN   The 20th edition of *Cope's Early Diagnosis of the Acute Abdomen* marks a historic change in the traditional view of pain management in patients with abdominal pain: "The realization, likely erroneous, that narcotics can obscure the clinical picture has given rise to the unfortunate dictum that these drugs should never be given until a diagnosis has been firmly established. With the numer-

TABLE 36-9   Nonopioid Analgesics

Drug	Adult Dose	Toxicity
Acetaminophen	650–1000 mg PO q4h 1–2 g PR q4h	Toxic dose: 140 mg/kg in 24 h
Aspirin	650–1000 mg PO q4h	Reye syndrome in children, tinnitus
Ibuprofen	400–800 mg PO q4–6h	GI upset, platelet dysfunction, renal dysfunction, bronchospasm
Naproxen	250 mg PO q6–8h 500–1000 mg PR q 6–8h	Same as ibuprofen plus interacts with protein-bound drugs
Indomethacin	25–50 mg PO q12h 100 mg PR q24h	Same as ibuprofen
Ketorolac	30–60 mg IV q6h 60 mg IM	Same as ibuprofen

Abbreviation: GI = gastrointestinal.

TABLE 36-10   Delivery Routes of Systemic Analgesia

Method	Advantages	Disadvantages
Oral	Ease Painless Minimal cost No technical skill required Patient acceptability	Unreliable gastrointestinal absorption Requires gastric motility Slow onset Titration less reliable
Intravenous	Rapid onset Titratable Usually easier to reverse Can use medications with short half-life	Venous access required Potential for overdose
Intramuscular or subcutaneous	Convenient More rapid onset than oral route	Painful Titration difficult and requires repeated injections Absorption variable More expensive than oral route
Rectal (transmucosal)	No first-pass hepatic metabolism No reliance on gastric motility	Requires patient acceptance and cooperation Variable absorption
Buccal/nasal (transmucosal)	Ease Painless	Difficult to control dose Can irritate nasal mucosa
Transdermal	Ease Painless	Variable dose and duration Difficult to titrate Slow onset Prolonged duration after removal
Inhalational	Rapid onset and offset	Requires patient cooperation Scavenger equipment required

ous layers of triage nurses, medical students, residents, and attending physicians in modern emergency units, and with the addition of time-consuming tests often done before an adequate history *and* physical examination, the suffering patient is sometimes forced to wait for many hours before any relief is offered. This cruel practice is to be condemned, but I suspect that it will take many generations to eliminate it because the rule has become so firmly ingrained in the minds of physicians."[16]

Cope's book, originally published nearly a century ago, continued to advise until the 1990s against the administration of analgesics during the evaluation of acute abdominal pain. This dogma has been challenged and is without scientific basis. Early administration of intravenous opioids has been shown to be a safe and effective analgesic in patients with acute abdominal pain in the ED and does not have adverse effects on the accuracy of the evaluation, diagnosis, and management.[17] The one valid concern regarding analgesia and abdominal pain concerns the patient who will not be imaged or held for serial abdominal examinations. In the absence of a diagnostic plan, the indiscriminate use of opioids is potentially dangerous.

MIGRAINE   There is no obvious, best analgesic agent for the management of a patient with migraine headache in the ED. Success rates as high as 95 percent have been reported using promethazine, chlorpromazine, and prochlorperazine.[18] 5-Hydroxytryptamine agonists are very effective in aborting early migraine but have limited effect after the initial prodrome. Migraine recurrence is 20 to 50 percent within 48 h with all of these agents. Headache rate at 24 h was significantly higher for patients who left the ED with persisting headache than in those who left with no pain.[19] More aggressive ED treatment may result in higher successful treatment rates but also may be associated with more adverse effects from the therapy.

Dopamine antagonists, antiemetics, metoclopramide, phenothiazine, haloperidol, sumatriptan, dihydroergotamine, NSAIDs, acetaminophen, and opioids have been studied in acute migraine. The relative benefit of these agents or combinations of therapies remains unclear. Opioid use has lost favor due to poor performance in clinical trials and the potential association with drug-seeking behavior.

TRAUMA   Patients in shock and those with trauma, burns, and hemodynamic or respiratory instability mandate judicious use of narcotics. Titration of short-acting, intravenous opioid analgesics, such as fentanyl, and maximal use of regional analgesia are recommended. The intramuscular route has poor and variable absorption and bioavailability in this setting and should be avoided. If patients require parenteral analgesia, they warrant close observation for occult injuries.

Use of analgesic therapy also must allow for continuous monitoring of neurologic status after a head injury and neurovascular status after limb injury. In the setting of closed head injury or multiple injuries, maximal use of regional and nonpharmacologic modalities is desirable. Although of value in the patient with minor trauma, the use of NSAIDs in the major trauma patient remains controversial. Risks include (1) excessive bleeding from platelet dysfunction and gastric stress ulcers, and (2) the potential for acute renal failure in the volume-depleted patient, minimizing their usefulness for this patient group.

DISPOSITION

Although pain control alone occasionally is an adequate indication for admission, such severe pain often is associated with an underlying condition that is the primary reason for the admission. Most patients may be safely discharged with a plan for the management of their pain. Communication with a primary care provider is important to allow for the continued monitoring of pain control. Patients at risk for serious pathology should not be discharged to an unmonitored setting with opioids. This is the scenario where patients could be harmed by their analgesics, because they self-medicate and may fail to seek appropriate follow-up. Disposition is affected by knowledge of the underlying pathologic diagnosis and an awareness of the home environment and support system.

Awareness of the duration of action of analgesic medications and the time of offset with respect to discharge planning and disposition is essential. In general, shorter-acting agents are preferable, because they allow for more frequent reassessments of ongoing pain. Patients should be counseled to take subsequent doses on a regular basis or when their pain begins to return, rather than when it approaches its peak. In addition, recent recommendations from the Food and Drug Administration have strongly discouraged the use of long-acting agents (such as sustained release oxycodone; OxyContin) for acute pain, because of the serious risk of abuse.

Written discharge instructions detailing specific medication procedures will help patients to take their medications correctly and enhance patients' awareness of side effects. This information should include names of medications, dosages and frequencies, and adverse effects.

REFERENCES

1. Todd KH, Deaton C, D'Adamo AP, Goe L: Ethnicity and analgesic practice. *Ann Emerg Med* 35:11, 2000.
2. Jones JS, Johnson K, McNinch M: Age as a risk factor for inadequate emergency department analgesia. *Am J Emerg Med* 14:157, 1996.
3. Raftery KA, Smith-Coggins R, Chen AH: Gender-associated differences in emergency department pain management. *Ann Emerg Med* 26:414, 1995.
4. Acute Pain Management Guideline Panel: *Acute Pain Management: Operative or Medical Procedures and Trauma. Guideline Report.* Agency for Health Care Policy and Research Publication No. 92-002. Rockville, MD, Agency for Health Care Policy and Research, Public Health Service, US Department of Health and Human Services, 1993.
5. Joint Commission on Accreditation of Healthcare: *Pain Management Standards.* Available at: http://www.jcaho.org.
6. Grubb BD: Peripheral and central mechanisms of pain. *Br J Anaesth* 81:8, 1998.
7. Todd KH: Clinical versus statistical significance in the assessment of pain relief. *Ann Emerg Med* 27:439, 1996.
8. McCormack HM, Home DJ, Sheather S: Clinical applications of visual analog scales: A critical review. *Psychol Med* 19:1007, 1988.
9. Gallagher EJ, Liebman M, Bijur PE: Prospective validation of clinically important changes in pain severity measured on a visual analog scale. *Ann Emerg Med* 38:633, 2001.
10. Bates DW, Cullen DJ, Laird N, et al: Incidence of adverse drug events and potential adverse drug events: Implications for prevention. *JAMA* 274:29, 1995.
11. Paoloni P, Talbot-Stern J: Low incidence of nausea and vomiting with intravenous opiate analgesia in the ED. *Am J Emerg Med* 20:604, 2002.
12. Moore RA, Tramer MR, Carroll D, et al: Quantitative systematic review of topically applied nonsteroidal anti-inflammatory drugs. *Br Med J* 316:333, 1998.
13. McQuay HJ, Tramer M, Nye BA, et al: A systematic review of antidepressants in neuropathic pain. *Pain* 68:217, 1996.
14. Hansen HC: Treatment of chronic pain with antiepileptic drugs: A new era. *South Med J* 92:642,1999
15. Portenoy RK, Dole V, Joseph H, et al: Pain management and chemical dependency: evolving perspectives. *JAMA* 278:592, 1997.
16. Silen W: *Cope's Early Diagnosis of the Acute Abdomen,* 20th ed. New York, Oxford University Press, 2000 p. 5.
17. McHale PM, LoVecchio F: Narcotic analgesia in the acute abdomen—A review of prospective trials. *Eur J Emerg Med* 8:131, 2001.
18. Snow V, Weiss K, Weil EM, Mottor-Pilsor G: Pharmacologic management of acute attacks of migraine and prevention of migraine headache. *Ann Intern Med* 137:840, 2002.
19. Ducharme J, Beveridge RC, Lee J, Beaulieu S: Emergency management of migraine: Is the headache really over? *Acad Emerg Med* 5:899, 1998.

37 LOCAL AND REGIONAL ANESTHESIA
Eric Higginbotham
Robert J. Vissers

Local anesthesia, as it is known today, is the result of the discovery of suitable drugs and delivery methods. Cocaine was first isolated in Europe between 1859 and 1860 and introduced into clinical practice about 25 years later. Simultaneously, the advent of a precise syringe that allowed the delivery of an exact amount of a pharmaceutical agent was being developed concomitantly in Scotland and Lyon, France.[1] Together these discoveries led to the invention of local anesthesia.

Impure cocaine's toxic and addictive effects were rapidly noticed as its use spread throughout Europe, resulting in many deaths among patients and addicted medical staff. Newer, safer agents were developed in the late 19th and 20th centuries, the ester local anesthetics (e.g., tropocaine, eucaine, benzocaine, procaine, and tetracaine) and the amide local anesthetics (e.g., lidocaine, mepivacaine, prilocaine, and bupivacaine). Overall, these drugs are less toxic than cocaine but still possess central nervous system (CNS) and cardiovascular (CV) system toxicity.

Local and regional anesthetics are essential tools in the ED for procedure- and trauma-related pain management. Local anesthetic (LA) techniques provide short-term pain relief by (1) infiltration or application of LA directly into the area to be anesthetized, (2) infiltration of LA into the region of peripheral nerves supplying the area, or (3) infusion of LA into the venous system of an extremity. Specific skills and anatomic knowledge for regional anesthesia techniques are necessary for the effectiveness of LA procedures, and knowledge of the dosages, actions, and toxicity of the LA medications are required for safe use of these agents.

LOCAL ANESTHETICS

Local Anesthetic Agents

Almost all LA agents are synthetic drugs derived from cocaine (except diphenhydramine and benzyl alcohol, which are discussed separately). The chemical structure includes hydrophilic and hydrophobic regions and a linkage (amide or ester) region. Local anesthetics are weak bases supplied as a salt (usually HCl) in an acidic pH solution to increase stability, solubility, and shelf life. The most commonly used pharmacologic agents for local infiltrative and regional anesthesia are the amide agents, with lidocaine and bupivacaine being most often used. Lidocaine has a shorter duration of action than does bupivacaine, but it possesses a lower toxicity profile. Mepivacaine, with an onset of action close to that of lidocaine, with a longer duration of action and devoid of bupivacaine toxicity, is becoming an increasingly recognized alternative.[2] Tetracaine, an ester LA, is frequently used in topical anesthetic preparations. Ester LAs are hydrolyzed by cholinesterase enzymes in plasma. Amide LAs are metabolized by hepatic microsomal enzymes. The metabolism rates of the amide LA (prilocaine > lidocaine > mepivacaine > bupivacaine) are slower overall than those of ester LA, creating the potential for sustained plasma levels and cumulative effects of amide LA. Maximum doses and duration of action of various anesthetics are shown in Table 37-1.

The anesthetic action of LA is produced when the drug molecules occupy enough sodium channels within the axon to interrupt activity and temporarily stop conduction. Local anesthetics bind to receptor sites on the voltage-gated sodium channels (a four-subunit transmembrane protein) in the neuronal membrane and impair or block sodium influx. As LAs increasingly occupy sodium channels, there is a decrease in the rate and degree of depolarization and repolarization, a decrease in conduction velocity, and a prolongation of the refractory period of the neural action potential.[3]

The pharmacologic activity of the LA agents is based on several of their biochemical properties; lipid solubility, pK_a, and protein binding are the key characteristics. Potency is related to lipid solubility; LAs that are more lipid-soluble easily penetrate the nerve cell wall and result in higher intracellular concentrations and thus more blockade. The pK_a, the pH at which 50 percent of the drug exists in the basic or non-ionized state, determines the speed of onset of conduction block. The base form is more lipid-soluble than the ionized form. Therefore, the lower the pK_a for a specific LA, the more uncharged form of the drug is present at tissue pH, and the faster it traverses lipid layers to the

TABLE 37-1 Local Anesthetic Doses for Infiltration

| | | | | Maximum Dose* | | | |
| | | | | Without Epinephrine | | With Epinephrine | |
Drug	Concentration for Infiltration (%)†	Onset (min)	Duration (min)	mg/kg	Total mg	mg/kg	Total mg
Esters							
Procaine	1	2–5	15–45	7	500	9	600
Amides							
Lidocaine‡	1	2–5	30–60	4.5	300	7	500
Bupivacaine#	0.25	3–7	90–360	2	175	3	225
Mepivacaine	1	3–7	90–180	5	400	7	500
Others							
Diphenhydramine	0.5–1	<2	20–30	1.25–1.7	90	§	
Benzyl alcohol	0.9	2–5	Unknown	**	**	**	

*Maximum dose based on a 70-kg patient.
†Percentage of solution defined as the number of grams per deciliter: 0.25% = 2.5 mg/mL, 0.5% = 5 mg/mL, and 1.0% = 10 mg/mL.
‡Lidocaine dose can be repeated in 2 to 4 h.
#Bupivacaine can be repeated every 4 to 6 h (maximum daily dose, 400 mg per d).
§Not given with epinephrine.
**See text.

axoplasm. Protein binding is the affinity an LA has for the sodium channel, and duration of action is related to this affinity; the longer the LA binds to the sodium channel and effects conduction block, the longer the duration of the anesthesia.

Addition of epinephrine (usually in a concentration of 1:100,000, or 10 μg/mL) provides a longer duration of anesthesia, promotes wound hemostasis, and slows systemic absorption, thereby decreasing the potential for toxicity and allowing a greater volume of agent to be used for extensive laceration repair.[4] Epinephrine can increase the pain of infiltration, because it lowers the overall pH of the solution. Epinephrine acts through vasoconstriction to achieve these actions ("chemical tourniquet"). Because of this vasoconstriction, epinephrine has traditionally been avoided in an end-arterial field (e.g., digits, pinna, nose, and penis), although a recent comprehensive review found no cases of digital ischemia since the advent of commercial lidocaine with epinephrine (introduced in 1948).[5] If epinephrine is inadvertently injected into an end-arteriole field, 1 in. of topical nitroglycerin paste applied to the affected area will quickly restore perfusion. Blood pressure should be checked to make sure hypotension does not occur, though it is unlikely. Vasospasm and ischemia from end-arteriole or arterial injection can also be reversed with local or intravascular injection of phentolamine 1.5 to 5 mg. The main side effect of phentolamine, hypotension, is unlikely in this setting.

Toxicity

Toxicity of LA is related to the potency (i.e., lipid solubility) and duration of action (i.e., protein binding) as expressed in the target organ. Toxicity correlates with the amount of nonionized and unbound LA present. It is also related to the total dose of LA and the rate of plasma increase of the LA, with more rapid accumulation being more toxic. The relative absorption of LA is dependent on the vascularity of the site. The absorption therefore, from most rapid to slowest, is: intercostal/intratracheal > epidural/caudal > brachial plexus > mucosal > distal peripheral nerve > subcutaneous. Caution should be exercised with intercostal blocks: the recommended LA dose for intercostal blocks is one-tenth maximum for peripheral blocks. Serious adverse reactions, including systemic toxic reactions, are more frequently encountered with the use of amide rather than with the use of ester LA agents, due in part to the slower amide metabolism. However, patients with atypical plasma cholinesterase may be prone to systemic toxicity

from ester LA. The systemic toxicity of LA is enhanced by hypercarbia, hypoxemia, and acidosis. Systemic toxicity is usually the result of rapid inadvertent intravenous injection or delivery of an excessive total dose of LA. Serious systemic toxicity primarily involves the CNS and CV system (Table 37-2).

CENTRAL NERVOUS SYSTEM TOXICITY Central nervous system toxicity is due to conduction block that occurs within CNS structures. The CNS toxic effects are directly related to lipid solubility; therefore, the agents that are the most effective LAs also carry the greatest CNS toxicity. The more protein bound the agent is, the narrower the gap is between the initial milder symptoms of CNS toxicity and the more catastrophic cardiovascular reactions to LA. Toxicity is due to a combination of central excitatory and depressant activities of the LA, ranging from perioral tingling and numbness to confusion, seizure, and coma. Vigilance for the subtle symptoms of CNS toxicity is important, because the therapeutic-to-toxic ratios are often narrow with these agents. Seizure, although ominous, should be viewed as a warning for impending ventricular arrhythmias and cardiovascular collapse. Because toxicity of the LA agents is potentiated by hypoxia, hypercarbia,

TABLE 37-2 Toxicity of Local Anesthetics

	Toxic Effects
Central nervous system	Mild: visual disturbance, tongue numbness, lightheadedness, apprehension, restlessness Moderate: perioral paresthesia, muscle twitching, slurred speech, excitability, drowsiness Severe: seizures, cardiorespiratory depression, coma
Cardiovascular system	Palpitations, vasodilation, hypertension, ventricular dysrhythmias (particularly bupivacaine), myocardial depression, hypotension, bradycardia, cardiovascular collapse
Respiratory system	Hypoventilation, respiratory arrest
Allergy	Amides (rare) Esters (more common) associated with para-aminobenzoic acid metabolite
Methemoglobinemia	Cyanosis, dyspnea, dizziness, lethargy; children more susceptible

and acidosis, seizures with resultant compromise or loss of the airway can hasten life-threatening CV toxicity.[3]

CARDIOVASCULAR TOXICITY All LAs have a dose-dependent CV toxic effect that is mediated through sodium channel blockade within the heart. This blockade results in two main types of CV toxicity: myocardial depression and dysrhythmias. All LAs have CV toxicity, although the drugs with the highest lipid solubility have the highest incidence of significant CV toxicity (e.g., bupivacaine). In addition, bupivacaine has a "fast-in, slow-out" kinetic pattern that results in accumulation of the drug within the conduction system that increases as heart rate increases. These pharmacologic properties make bupivacaine particularly cardiotoxic and, for this reason, is contraindicated for intravenous regional anesthesia. When the primary cardiac conduction system is blocked, there is increased activity in re-entrant pathways that predisposes the heart to ventricular arrhythmias. Ventricular fibrillation or tachycardia from LA toxicity can be refractory to treatment due to the degree of sodium channel blockade. Pregnancy has been noted to worsen the toxicity of LA, bupivacaine in particular, which is probably mediated through progesterone and the adverse effects of pregnancy on venous return.

METHEMOGLOBINEMIA Prilocaine and benzocaine can cause the oxidation of the ferric form of hemoglobin to the ferrous form, creating methemoglobin. When the methemoglobin concentration exceeds 1.5 g/dL, visible cyanosis results. This cyanosis is usually benign, but when oxygen transport needs to be preserved or signs of hypoxia occur, specific treatment may be necessary (see Chap. 189).

ALLERGIC REACTIONS True allergic reactions to local anesthetics are rare and usually due to the metabolite para-aminobenzoic acid, in the case of ester anesthetics, or the preservative methylparaben, which is structurally similar to para-aminobenzoic acid, in the case of amide anesthetics. Esters are more commonly associated with allergic reactions than are amides. If a true allergy is suspected based on history or documentation, the optimal approach is to use a preservative-free agent from the other class. Diphenhydramine (0.5 to 1.0%) and benzyl alcohol are alternative anesthetic choices in patients allergic to either amide and/or ester-type anesthetics.

MANAGEMENT Management of systemic LA toxicity follows standard advanced life-support protocols (ensure a patent airway, oxygen, and ventilatory and circulatory support), immediate discontinuation of the administration of LA and prompt treatment of the CNS and CV complications. Correcting hypoxia, hypercarbia, and metabolic acidosis is paramount, because these conditions enhance the toxicity of LA. Incremental doses of intravenous benzodiazepines are usually effective to control seizures, and standard protocols should be followed for the management of ventricular arrhythmias. Arrhythmias refractory to standard advanced cardiac life-support protocols have met with anecdotal success with the use of bretylium and cardiopulmonary bypass.

Specific Agents

AMIDE LOCAL ANESTHETICS

Lidocaine Lidocaine is an amide anesthetic available in 0.5, 1.0, and 2% concentrations for injection. It is the most commonly used anesthetic in the ED, because of its excellent efficacy and low toxicity profile. Lidocaine has a rapid onset of action and intermediate duration. It has a pK_a of 7.9, with a pH in commercial preparations of 5.0 to 7.0. Lidocaine with epinephrine has a pH within 3.3 to 5.5 (necessitating bicarbonate buffering to decrease pain during infiltration). The elimination half-life is 45 to 60 min. Metabolism is predominantly hepatic,

with high plasma levels occurring due to hepatic failure and decreased hepatic blood flow (e.g., congestive cardiac failure). Caution should be exercised if these conditions exist.

Bupivacaine Bupivacaine is an amide anesthetic that is highly protein bound. The concentration appropriate for local anesthetic use is 0.25%. It has a pK_a of 8.1 and in commercial preparations has a pH of 3.3 to 5.5. Alkalinization with bicarbonate can cause precipitation at a pH of 6.8 or higher. Some studies suggest that its injection is more painful, possibly owing to the lower pH. It has a slow onset, long duration, and a higher CV toxicity potential. The duration of action is 4 to 6 h. Bupivacaine is preferred for prolonged procedures (such as ingrown toenail removal), when longer postprocedural analgesia is desired, and for peripheral nerve regional blocks. Bupivacaine is contraindicated for intravenous regional blocks due to its cardiac toxicity, from which fatalities have been reported. Bupivacaine also should be used very cautiously in any condition affecting hepatic metabolism.

Mepivacaine Mepivacaine is an amide anesthetic, with a pK_a of 7.6 and a pH of 4.5 to 6.8 in commercial preparations. It has a rapid onset, intermediate duration, and intermediate toxicity. Toxicity, which was once thought to approximate the level of bupivacaine, has been for the most part repudiated.[2] Local infiltration with a 1% concentration has been associated with anesthesia of 1.5 to 3 h in duration. Redosing for longer procedures does not cause tachyphylaxis, and cumulative toxicity is low.[3]

Prilocaine Prilocaine, an amide LA with pK_a of 7.9, has a lower cardiac toxicity profile than does lidocaine or bupivacaine, with similar anesthetic potency. It has rapid onset and intermediate duration. After intravenous injection, its CNS toxicity is less than that of lidocaine due to a lower blood level, because of differences in its distribution and peripheral uptake. It is also broken down by amidases in the liver more rapidly than is lidocaine, resulting in a shorter duration of toxic effects. Prilocaine may lead to methemoglobinemia after a large intravenous bolus (or total dose >600 mg) due to the oxidative properties of one of its metabolites, o-toluidine. Clinical uses include infiltration with up to a 1% solution with an anesthetic duration of 60 to 120 min. Due to its lower toxicity, a 0.25 to 0.5% concentration is commonly used in Australia for intravenous regional arm blocks. Prilocaine and lidocaine are the active agents in a cream consisting of an eutectic mixture of LAs (EMLA) for topical use on intact skin.

ESTER LOCAL ANESTHETICS

Procaine Procaine is a short-acting ester LA, with a pK_a of 8.9. Commercially prepared solutions have a pH of 5.5 to 6.0. Procaine has a slow onset and very short blood half-life (approximately 20 s) owing to the rapid hydrolysis by plasma cholinesterase; hence, little toxicity is associated with this agent. Procaine can be used for patients who are allergic to the amide anesthetics (e.g., lidocaine).

Tetracaine Tetracaine is an ester local anesthetic, with a pK_a of 8.6. In liquid form, the pH can vary from 4.5 to 6.5. It has a slow onset, short plasma half-life (2.5 to 4 min), and long duration of action. Injectable tetracaine 0.2% is used most commonly in spinal anesthesia. In addition, it is used for topical anesthesia of the eye (0.5%) mucous membranes (2%), and skin (4% gel or cream). When applied to the larynx, anesthesia of the airway will persist for a very long duration, with absent airway reflexes. The potential for rapid uptake from mucous membranes does exist with the risk for systemic toxicity. The toxic dose is believed to be approximately 2 mg/kg.

ALTERNATIVE AGENTS Diphenhydramine 0.5 to 1.0% and benzyl alcohol 0.9% are alternative anesthetic choices in patients with true allergies to the amides and/or ester-type anesthetics.[6,7] Although diphenhydramine is an effective local anesthetic, its injection is more painful than lidocaine and can cause tissue irritation and even skin necrosis.[6] Thus, its role for local anesthesia is extremely specific and limited to those patients who have true allergies to ester or amide anesthetics, which are quite rare. Benzyl alcohol 0.9% with epinephrine (1:100,000) is as effective as lidocaine and superior to diphenhydramine as an LA.[6,7] However, the duration of action is short, and about 30 percent of patients need additional anesthetic injection during the procedure.[7]

LOCAL ANESTHETIC INFILTRATION

The most common usage of LA in the ED is local infiltration for wound repair and invasive procedures. Local infiltration has a rapid onset and low risk of systemic toxicity. Infiltration can be into the wound margins or as a field block in a "diamond-shaped wheal" of LA surrounding the wound or procedure site. Lidocaine is the drug of choice for LA infiltration for brief procedures. Bupivacaine or mepivacaine is preferable for longer procedures due to their longer duration of action, but with due caution regarding the increased toxicity. Epinephrine can be added to enhance safety and efficacy, and bicarbonate can be added to minimize pain of infiltration. The maximal dosages commonly cited apply to infiltration of LA, in contrast to the lower maximal dosages for most regional procedures (Tables 37-1 and 37-3).

Additives and Adjuncts to Minimize Pain of Infiltration

Many variables influence the degree of pain experienced with LA infiltration. The depth and rate of injection and the temperature and buffering of the agent are considerations in the attempt to make infiltration painless. Slow infiltration of the anesthetic (30 s/mL) with a 27- or 30-gauge needle will decrease the pain as compared with rapid injection with a larger needle, probably due to less rapid distention of local tissue.

Numerous clinical studies have demonstrated attenuation of pain on infiltration with buffered lidocaine.[8] Buffered lidocaine is prepared

TABLE 37-3 Suggested Volumes for Regional Nerve Blocks in Adults (Weight >40 kg)

Location	Total Volume Lidocaine 1% or Bupivacaine 0.25%
Median nerve	3–5 mL
Ulnar nerve	5–7 mL
Radial nerve	5–10 mL
Digital	3–4 mL
Metacarpal	2–3 mL
Posterior tibial	3–7 mL
Sural nerve	3–5 mL
Saphenous nerve	3–5 mL
Superficial peroneal nerve	3–5 mL
Deep peroneal nerve	3–5 mL
Great toe	4–6 mL
Lesser toes	2–3 mL
Forehead	3–6 mL
Inferior alveolar nerve	1–2 mL
Mental nerve	1–2 mL (intraoral), 2–4 mL (extraoral)
Infraorbital	2–3 mL
Femoral nerve	10–20 mL
Intercostal nerve (per segment)	3–5 mL

by mixing a solution of 9 mL of lidocaine 1% (with or without epinephrine) with 1 mL of sodium bicarbonate 8.4% (1 mEq/mL). The resultant mixture can be prepared ahead of time and stored for future use. Bicarbonate can cause precipitation of bupivacaine and should not be added to this anesthetic unless it can be used immediately. It is prepared by mixing a solution of 29 mL of bupivacaine 0.25% with 1 mL of sodium bicarbonate 8.4% (1 mEq/mL). The exact mechanisms by which buffering of lidocaine reduces pain is not clear. Buffering increases the pH of these acidically packaged anesthetics, bringing the mixture's pH closer to the drug's pK_a, resulting in a higher percentage of the uncharged species. The higher percentage of uncharged molecules allows faster diffusion into the nerve fiber, resulting in more rapid sensory nerve blockade. Buffering to a higher pH also may reduce direct tissue irritation by reducing the acidity of the agent. Because buffered lidocaine undergoes biodegradation at room temperature, its shelf life is limited; studies suggest that efficacy is maintained from 7 to 30 days.

Studies evaluating the efficacy of warm lidocaine (anywhere from 37°C to 42°C) to decrease injection pain have yielded equivocal results.[8] It is postulated that warming the anesthetic causes faster diffusion into tissues and reduces or avoids stimulation of cold receptors, thereby increasing the rate of onset of neuronal block. Lidocaine can be warmed in dry heat (blanket warmers) or in temperature-regulated water baths at 37°C. From a practical standpoint, anesthetics should be administered at least at room temperature. Unlike buffered lidocaine, heated lidocaine undergoes no chemical denaturation, so there are no limitations on shelf life.

Injection through the margins of a wound rather than through intact skin surrounding it greatly reduces the pain associated with infiltration.[9] Use of long needles reduces the number of puncture sites. To prevent breakage, no more than two thirds of the needle should be inserted. The smallest appropriate syringe allows for greater control over the volume and rate of injection.

The nuances of local wound infiltration should be mentioned and in most ways is more important than the agent selected in obtaining a desirable outcome. If the caregiver attempts to establish rapport and allay fears early in the encounter, anxious and uncooperative patients can be calmed and much of their evaluation completed before anesthetic infiltration has occurred. The neurologic examination should be demonstrated on an uninvolved, uninjured area first, to reassure the patient that the examiner will not inflict pain. Distraction techniques are beneficial, including the use of music, skin pressure, or pinching. The needle should be hidden from view of the patient, if possible. The analogy of a bee sting or insect bite should be avoided; most patients are terrified of insect bites, and for most children that has been the most painful experience in their memory. Although unstudied, a topical anesthetic application followed by infiltration may be less painful and better tolerated in selected patients.

To summarize, the least painful method of infiltration is deep, slow injection through the wound margins using a warm, buffered solution with the use of a 27- or 30-gauge needle and a concerted effort to minimize the anxiety surrounding the process.

TOPICAL ANESTHETICS

Topical anesthetics can be used to reduce the discomfort of local procedures and may eliminate or decrease the need for local infiltrative injection.[10] When compared with local infiltration, topical anesthetics can be applied painlessly, do not distort wound edges, and may provide good hemostasis if the formulation includes a vasoconstrictive agent. In general, topical anesthetics work better on the head and neck than on the extremities, have a slower onset, and are less efficacious than injectable LAs. There a number of available formulations in common use: TAC (tetracaine, adrenaline, and cocaine), LET (lidocaine, epinephrine, and tetracaine), and EMLA (lidocaine and prilocaine).

Tetracaine, Adrenaline, and Cocaine

The TAC (original formulation: tetracaine 0.5%, adrenaline 0.05%, and cocaine 11.8%) solution has been largely replaced by other mixtures that are less likely to cause toxicity, cost less, and do not have the regulatory issues associated with a controlled substance. The TAC solution has been associated with seizures, respiratory arrest, and, rarely, death in children due to inadvertent systemic absorption of cocaine. Systemic absorption was most common when used on mucosal surfaces or in large amounts. Other agents such as LET have been found to be equally efficacious and have a more desirable safety profile.[11]

Lidocaine, Epinephrine, and Tetracaine

The LET (lidocaine 4%, epinephrine 0.1%, and tetracaine 0.5%) solution should be prepared in single-use 5-mL vials.[10] It may be applied to the wound directly as drops from a syringe, and then the remainder of the solution is soaked into a cotton ball or gauze, which is then held against the wound. The individual applying the LET should use gloves in order to prevent topical absorption to the caregiver. The LET solution should be applied for at least 20 to 30 min to achieve adequate anesthesia.[11] Contact with mucous membranes, fingers and toes, the ear pinna, the penis, and the tip of the nose should be avoided. It also can be used in a gel form by adding 150 mg of methylcellulose to 3 mL of LET solution. The gel may be applied directly to the wound with a cotton applicator and irrigated off after 20 min. The gel form is more likely to remain in the wound and may be associated with a higher rate of complete anesthesia.

Eutectic Mixture of Local Anesthetics (EMLA)

The EMLA cream contains lidocaine 2.5% and prilocaine 2.5%.[10,12] The EMLA cream has been shown to be effective in relieving the pain associated with venipuncture, port access, arterial puncture, lumbar puncture, and superficial skin procedures. It has been investigated as an anesthetic for open wounds; however, the available preparation is not sterile, and its use is presently recommended only for application on intact skin. Systemic reactions are rare; however, the prilocaine may cause methemoglobinemia, particularly in children younger than 3 months. The EMLA cream should be used sparingly and with caution in infants younger than 3 months (1 g maximum dose for 1 h) and avoided in patients predisposed to methemoglobinemia. EMLA cream in adults is applied by squeezing a dollop of about 2g directly onto the skin and covering the area with an occlusive dressing; the cream layer should be left thick and not massaged or rubbed into the skin. The depth of anesthesia is related to the duration of contact, with satisfactory analgesia achieved at 1 h, peak effect at 2 h, and duration for 1 h after removal.

Lidocaine

Lidocaine is available in solution, ointment, cream, and jelly preparations in concentrations from 1 to 30%. It is commonly used to facilitate the placement of urinary catheters, nasogastric tubes, and the passage of oral and nasal fiberoptic scopes. Two percent viscous lidocaine in an oral solution has been used to provide temporary relief of stomatitis, but the patient must be cautioned to use the solution sparingly (not to exceed 1 teaspoon every 3 h) and expectorate the excess anesthetic. Lidocaine 4% solution applied intranasally with a disposable atomizer has been shown to reduce the discomfort of nasogastric tube placement, even in addition to lidocaine jelly.[13] Plasma levels after topical mucosal applications are similar to those associated with intravenous use, and doses should not exceed 4.5 mg/kg.

The anesthetic ELA-Max is a 4% liposomal lidocaine cream.[12] The lidocaine is encapsulated in liposomes, which enhances the rate and amount of absorption in intact skin and resists rapid metabolism,

thereby prolonging its effects. Compared with EMLA, the onset is approximately twice as fast and does not require occlusion.[12] Similar to EMAL, ELA-Max should be applied in a thick layer (like cake frosting) and should not be rubbed into the skin. It is not recommended for mucosal application.

Other Topical Anesthetic Agents

A number of topical anesthetic combinations have been studied, mainly in comparison with TAC, and have demonstrated different degrees of efficacy. These preparations include prilocaine, tetracaine, or bupivacaine in combination with a vasoconstrictor, such as phenylephrine. It is unclear whether any of these have significant advantages over LET.

Benzocaine is available as a 20% liquid, gel, or spray formulation for mucosal anesthesia. It is used to relieve the pain from oral ulcers, wounds, and inflammation and to facilitate the passage of oral nasogastric tubes and endoscopy. Benzocaine rarely may precipitate methemoglobinemia. A topical combination of antipyrine and benzocaine is used to temporarily relieve the pain of otitis media or externa.

Iontophoresis is a method of delivering a topical anesthetic with a mild electric current. The device is bulky and may cause an uncomfortable electrical sensation. Presently, it has limited use in the emergency setting.

Ethyl Chloride

Ethyl chloride is not an LA but rather a skin refrigerant or vapocoolant delivered by a spray. Upon contact with the skin, it vaporizes, causing a transient drop in temperature to $-20°C$, temporarily freezing it, and causing anesthesia through nerve desensitization. It is useful for venipuncture, injections, and incisions of small abscesses.

Ethyl chloride is applied by inverting the bottle at a distance of 10 to 30 cm from the skin and spraying for 3 to 7 s. The affected area will turn white. Anesthesia is present for only 30 to 60 s. Prolonged spraying could cause chemical frostbite and skin ulceration, and it should not be used on mucosal surfaces. Ethyl chloride should not be inhaled, because it may cause general anesthetic and opioid effects. It is also flammable.

REGIONAL ANESTHETIC PROCEDURES

Regional anesthetic procedures performed in the ED include peripheral nerve blocks, hematoma blocks, and intravenous (Bier's) blocks. In addition to their utility during invasive procedures, these techniques can minimize opiate use and decrease the need for procedural sedation or general anesthesia. The safety and effectiveness of LA for regional anesthetic procedures depends on proper dosage, correct technique, adequate precautions, and preparations to deal with emergencies, if they arise. Regional procedures with LA should be employed only by clinicians who are well-versed in diagnosis and management of LA dose-related toxicity and other acute emergencies that might result from inadvertent systemic absorption of the LA or intra-arterial injection of an epinephrine-containing LA solution. The setting should have resuscitative measures immediately available, if necessary. LA should be administered in the lowest dosage that results in an effective block. Epinephrine can be added to some blocks to enhance the duration, quality, efficacy, reliability, and safety of a block. However, epinephrine is contraindicated in nerve blocks in end-arterial areas except, perhaps, digital nerve blocks.

Peripheral Nerve Blocks

Peripheral nerve blocks are advantageous in the ED environment, particularly for procedures on the digits, hand, or foot. They require less total LA medication, and the site of drug delivery often is less painful than that for local infiltration.[14] It is imperative to document neurovascular status before application of the block, to prevent masking a primary traumatic neurovascular injury. During needle insertion, if the patient reports paresthesia in the nerve distribution, that sensation can be taken as a sign of proper localization for LA injection. The onset of anesthesia with peripheral nerve blocks is more delayed than by direct infiltration and may be up to 15 min. Lidocaine 1% or bupivacaine 0.25% can be used to achieve peripheral nerve blockade (see Table 37-3). The duration depends on the agent used and the amount of drug injected. Complications of nerve blocks include nerve injury and systemic LA toxicity. During injection, severe pain suggests that contact has been made with the nerve. In this circumstance, the needle must be withdrawn and repositioned before anesthetic is injected. Intravascular injection can result in limb and systemic toxicity. Local anesthetic dose exceeding the maximum may result in systemic toxicity, primarily cardiac and CNS. To minimize the likelihood of intravascular injection, the plunger on the needle syringe apparatus should be drawn back in all nerve block procedures before infiltration; if blood is withdrawn, the needle should be repositioned. Total doses of the agent should be calculated in all cases and doubled-checked against the concentration to prevent inadvertent overdosing of a specific LA available in more than one concentration (see Table 37-1).

Wrist Blocks

MEDIAN NERVE   The median nerve provides sensation to the lateral two thirds of the palm of the hand, palmar surfaces of the lateral three and one half digits, and their fingertips. The palmar branches of the median digital nerves extend dorsally over the digit to supply the dorsum of the thumb, the index finger, the middle finger, and lateral half of the ring finger distal to the proximal interphalangeal joint and including the nail and the nail bed (Figure 37-1). The median nerve enters the hand through the carpal tunnel, deep to the flexor retinaculum, between the tendons of the flexor digitorum superficialis and the flexor carpi radialis.

For lacerations of the hand, regional blocks at the wrist are performed at the level of proximal volar skin crease (Figure 37-2). The median nerve is anesthetized by inserting a 27-gauge needle perpendicular to the skin between the tendons of the palmaris longus and flexor carpi radialis muscles at the midpoint of the distal volar crease and injecting 3 to 5 mL of the LA solution with epinephrine (1:100,000).[14]

ULNAR NERVE   The ulnar nerve can be blocked at the elbow or the wrist to provide anesthesia to the medial aspect of the hand and the small finger, including its nail and nail bed (see Figure 37-1). Just

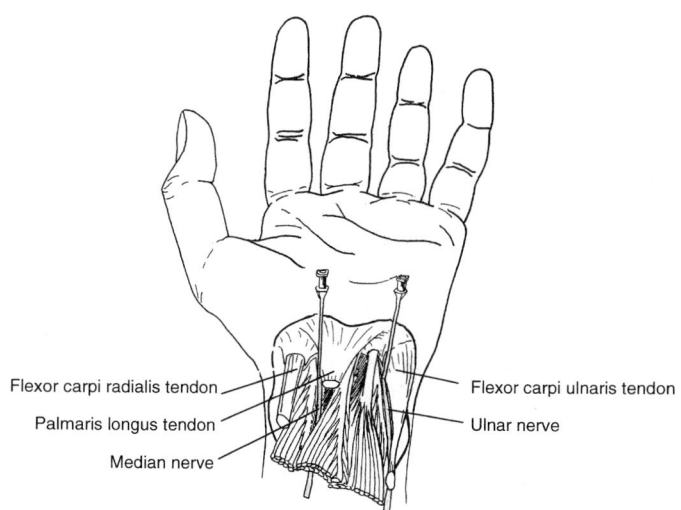

FIG. 37-2. Palmar view of the left hand demonstrating sites for median and ulnar nerve blocks at the wrist.

proximal to the wrist, the ulnar nerve gives off a palmar cutaneous branch, which passes superficially to the flexor retinaculum and palmar aponeurosis to supply the skin of the ulnar side of the palm. It also gives off a dorsal cutaneous branch that supplies the ulnar half of the dorsum of the hand, the small finger, and the ulnar half of the ring finger. The ulnar nerve ends by dividing into a superficial and a deep branch. The superficial branch supplies cutaneous fibers to the anterior surfaces of the small finger and the ulnar half of the ring finger. In the small finger, the dorsal digital nerve extends to the tip of the digit.

A regional block of the ulnar nerve at the wrist is accomplished by passing a 27-gauge needle between the ulnar artery and the flexor carpi ulnaris at the level of the proximal volar skin crease (see Figure 37-2). Alternatively, the needle can be inserted underneath the flexor carpi ulnaris on the ulnar side of the wrist and directed toward the radial side. Once the needle is positioned and especially if the patient reports paresthesia, 5 to 7 mL of LA solution with epinephrine (1:100,000) is injected slowly.[14]

RADIAL NERVE   The radial nerve provides sensation to the lateral two thirds of the dorsum of the hand; the proximal aspect of the dorsum of the thumb, index, and long finger; and the lateral aspect of the dorsum of the ring finger, excluding the nails and nail beds of these digits (see Figure 37-1). The superficial branch of the radial nerve is the direct continuation of the radial nerve along the anterolateral side of the forearm and is entirely sensory.

The superficial rami of the radial nerve can be blocked by raising a subcutaneous wheal with 5 to 10 mL of LA solution with epinephrine (1:100,000), beginning at the level of the tendon of the extensor carpi radialis and extending around the dorsum of the wrist to the styloid process, a distance of about 6 to 8 cm (Figure 37-3).[14]

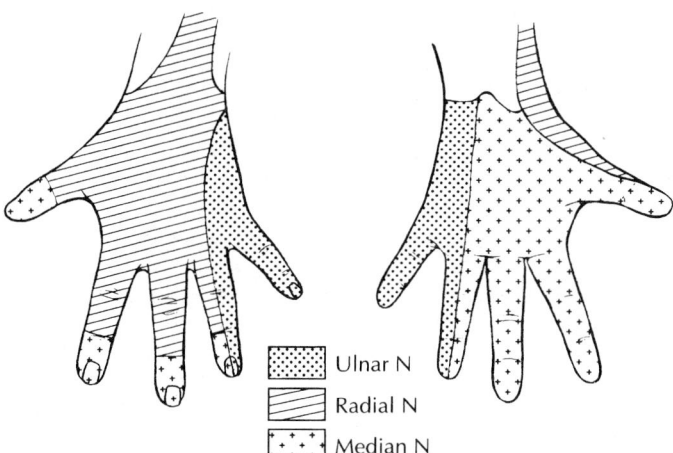

FIG. 37-1. Sensory distribution of the major nerves of the hand.

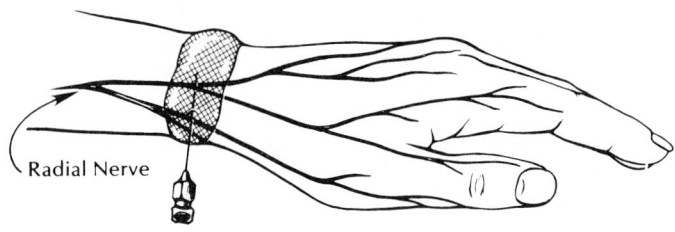

FIG. 37-3. Radial view of the left hand demonstrating location for radial nerve block at the wrist.

Digital Blocks

DIGITAL NERVE BLOCK   The digital nerve block provides excellent anesthesia for fingers and has a more rapid onset than the metacarpal block. It is commonly used for laceration repair, incision and drainage of paronychia, and finger or toenail removal or repair. Preparation with EMLA or ethyl chloride can minimize the pain of injection for these blocks. Epinephrine traditionally has been avoided for digital blocks, although there is no evidence to support this practice.[5] Contraindications to performing this block are any compromise to the digits' blood supply. Complications are few, but large volumes of anesthetic can result in a compartment syndrome. Each digit is supplied by a palmar (volar) and a dorsal digital nerve on each side of the digit, superficial to the digital arteries (Figure 37-4A).

A 27- or 30-gauge needle is inserted through the skin into one side of the extensor tendon of the affected finger just proximal to the web (see Figure 37-4B, 1). After aspirating, approximately 1 mL of LA solution is injected superficially into the subcutaneous tissue lying on the dorsal surface of the extensor tendon to block the dorsal digital nerve. The needle is then advanced toward the palm until its tip is palpable beneath the volar skin at the base of the finger, just distal to the web (see Figure 37-4B, 2). After aspirating, another 1 mL of the anesthetic solution is injected to block the palmar digital nerve. Before removing the needle, it is redirected across the extensor tendon to the opposite side of the finger, and approximately 1 mL of the anesthetic solution is injected into the tissue overlying the other dorsal digital nerve (see Figure 37-4B, 3). Five minutes later, the needle is reintroduced in the anesthetized skin on the opposite side of the finger and advanced to block the palmar digital nerve on that side of the digit (see Figure 37-4B, 4). The total volume of the anesthetic agent should not exceed 4 mL.

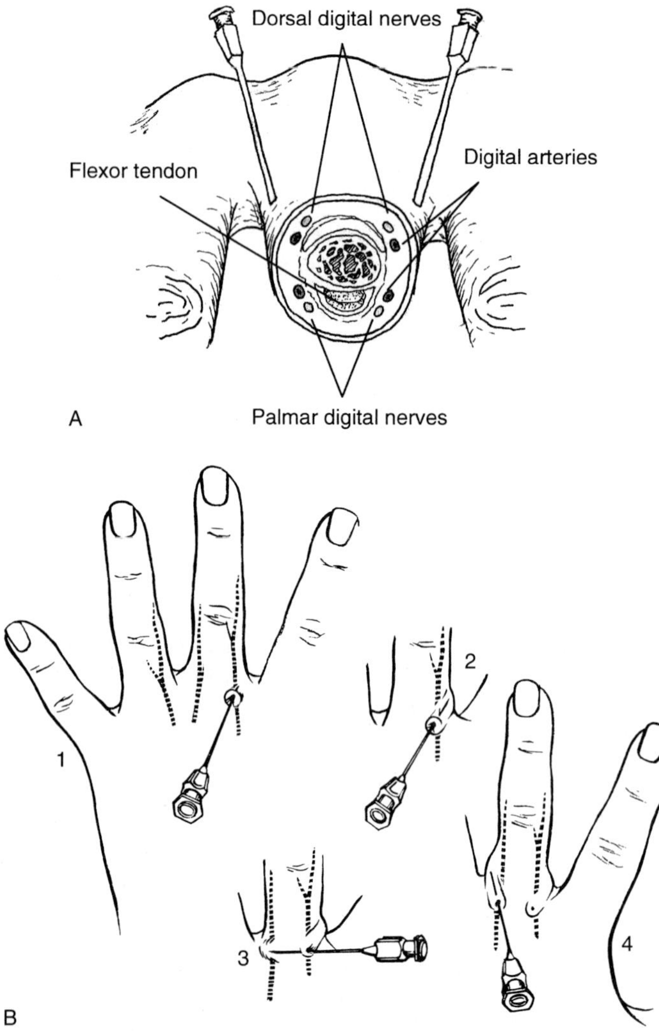

METACARPAL BLOCK   Metacarpal blocks can be used to anesthetize the index, long, ring, or small finger, although digital blocks are preferred. The block is performed on each side of the affected finger by inserting a 27-gauge needle at a 90-degree angle to the dorsum of the hand approximately 1 cm proximal to the metacarpophalangeal joint midway between each metacarpal bone. The needle is then advanced at a 90-degree angle to the skin until its tip is at the level of the lateral volar surface of the metacarpal head or until resistance of the palmar aponeurosis is detected. After aspirating, 3 mL of LA solution is injected slowly.[14]

Toe Blocks

Digital nerve blocks of the toe are used for laceration repair and minor surgical procedures of the toes. Epinephrine is avoided as an adjunct to lidocaine, because of the largely theoretical risk of irreversible ischemic injury. For the lesser toes, a 27- or 30-gauge needle should be introduced through the skin on the dorsal aspect of the base of the midpoint of the involved toe (Figure 37-5B). The needle should be angled around the bone until it induces blanching of the skin on the plantar surface. As the needle is withdrawn, approximately 1.5 mL of LA solution is injected. Before the needle is withdrawn completely from the skin, it should be redirected to the opposite side of the injured toe to inject the LA agent in a similar manner. The total volume of the injected LA agent should not exceed 3 mL.

For the hallux (great toe), a modified collar (ring) block is used (see Figure 37-5A) because of the frequency of occurrence of accessory nerves over the dorsum of the great toe. The 27-gauge needle is inserted through the skin on the dorsolateral aspect of the base of the toe until it blanches the plantar skin. As the needle is withdrawn, 1.5 mL of LA solution is injected into the tissues. Before the needle is removed completely from the skin, the needle is passed under the skin on the dorsal aspect of the toe, and 1.5 mL of LA solution is injected as the needle is withdrawn from the skin. The needle is then introduced through the anesthetized skin on the dorsomedial aspect of the toe and advanced until it produces blanching of the plantar skin, at which time the needle is withdrawn and 1.5 mL of LA solution is injected. To complete the collar block, the needle is inserted at the plantar and medial aspect and advanced to the lateral side until it blanches the skin, and then withdrawn as an additional 1.5 mL of LA solution is injected. Approximately 6 mL of LA solution is needed to anesthetize the hallux.[15]

Foot Blocks

These regional nerve blocks are used for anesthesia of surgical procedures of the foot. There are five nerves that supply sensation to the foot. Most foot blocks involve a block of at least two nerves; it is unusual in the ED setting to need to block the whole foot. The sole of the foot is a commonly injured area, and local infiltration directly into the sole is extremely painful, difficult to perform effectively, and is not recommended. Regional nerve blocks are the preferred LA technique. Buffered lidocaine 1% and bupivacaine 0.25% are the LA agents of choice. Epinephrine is contraindicated, and these blocks should not be used in patients with peripheral vascular disease or traumatic circulatory compromise. All peripheral nerves involved in blocks of the foot

FIG. 37-4. A. Digit cross-section showing location of digital nerves. **B.** Needle positions for digital nerve block. **1.** Initial injection to block dorsal digital nerve. **2.** Needle is advanced to block palmar digital nerve on same side. **3.** Needle is directed across dorsum of digit to block dorsal digital nerve on opposite side. **4.** Needle is inserted to complete block of palmar digital nerve on opposite side of initial injection.

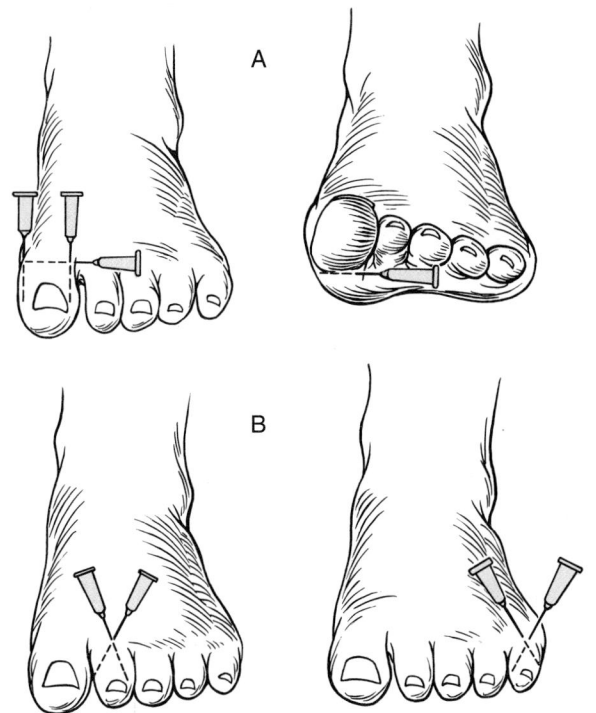

FIG. 37-5. A. Regional block of the great toe using collar infiltration technique. **B.** Digital nerve block of the lesser toes.

are branches of the sciatic nerve, except for the saphenous nerve (a branch of the femoral nerve; Figure 37-6).

The sensory innervations of the plantar surface of the foot are primarily the two main branches of the tibial nerve (posterior tibial and sural nerves) and a small contribution from the saphenous nerve medially. The sensory innervations of the dorsum of the foot are predominantly from the two main branches of the common peroneal nerve (the superficial and deep peroneal nerves), with contribution from the sural nerve laterally and the saphenous nerve medially. The saphenous nerve is the only branch of the femoral nerve below the knee. It becomes subcutaneous at the medial side of the knee joint and then follows the saphenous vein to a site anterior to the medial malleolus. It provides sensory innervation to the skin over the medial malleolus and extends to the skin over the medial side of the foot to the base of the great toe. The superficial peroneal nerve becomes the dorsal digital nerves. It descends toward the ankle in the lateral compartment, entering the ankle just lateral to the extensor digitorum longus, and pro-

vides the cutaneous supply to the dorsum of the foot and all five toes, except for the adjacent sides of the first and second toes (deep peroneal nerve) and lateral side of the fifth toe (sural nerve; see Figure 37-6). It also supplies the peroneus longus and brevis muscles. The sensory supply of the deep peroneal nerve is limited to the 1-cm area of web space between the first and second toes. Thus, blocks of the deep peroneal nerve are not reasonable or practical to perform.[15]

The three nerves that supply the sole of the foot are the posterior tibial nerve (most of the sole and heel), the sural nerve (posterolateral sole), and the saphenous nerve (small area, medially over the arch; see Figure 37-6). The posterior tibial nerve is located along the medial aspect of the ankle, lying between the medial malleolus and the Achilles tendon, just posterior and slightly deeper than the posterior tibial artery (Figure 37-7A) and gives off the three terminal branches, the medial calcaneal branch and the medial and lateral plantar nerves. The sural nerve travels with the short saphenous vein, posterior and inferior to the lateral malleolus; it terminates as the dorsal lateral cutaneous nerve. The saphenous nerve follows the great saphenous vein to the medial malleolus.

POSTERIOR TIBIAL NERVE BLOCK   A posterior tibial nerve block is best performed with the patient in the prone position. The posterior tibial nerve is blocked by injecting the LA solution between the posterior tibial artery and Achilles tendon, at the level of the upper border of the medial malleolus (see Figure 37-7B).[15] Careful aspiration is necessary to ensure no inadvertent intravascular access. Paresthesia upon needle insertion is a sign of correct placement, and adequate block is achieved with 3 to 5 mL of LA solution. If no paresthesia is encountered, then 5 to 7 mL of LA solution should be injected as the needle is withdrawn. Onset of anesthesia should occur within about 5 to 10 min if paresthesia has been elicited and in about 30 min if it has not.

SURAL NERVE BLOCK   The sural nerve is blocked between the lateral malleolus and the Achilles tendon (see Figure 37-7). It is superficial, lying just anterior to the short saphenous vein, and is blocked by superficially injecting 3 to 5 mL of LA solution in a fanlike distribution just lateral to the Achilles tendon 1 cm above the lateral malleolus.[15]

SAPHENOUS NERVE BLOCK   The saphenous nerve lies superficially between the medial malleolus and the anterior tibial tendon (Figure 37-8) and is blocked anteriorly by infiltration of 3 to 5 mL of LA between these landmarks as the needle is withdrawn.[15]

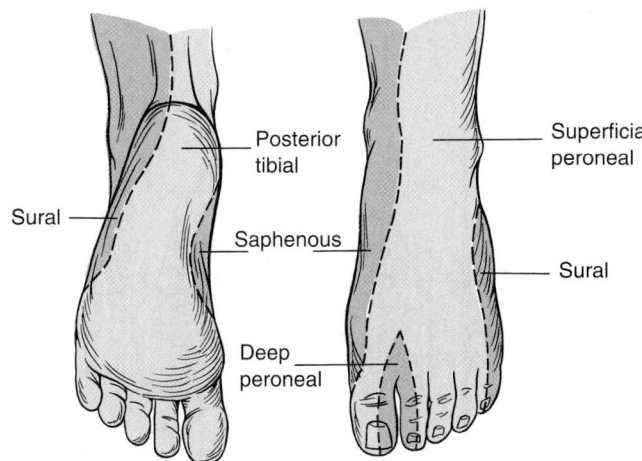

FIG. 37-6. Sensory innervation of the foot and ankle.

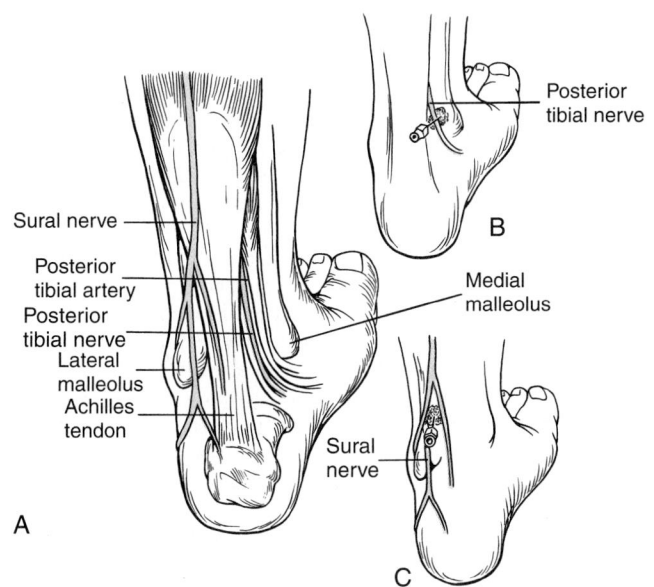

FIG. 37-7. Posterior view of the left foot demonstrating sites for posterior tibial and sural nerve blocks.

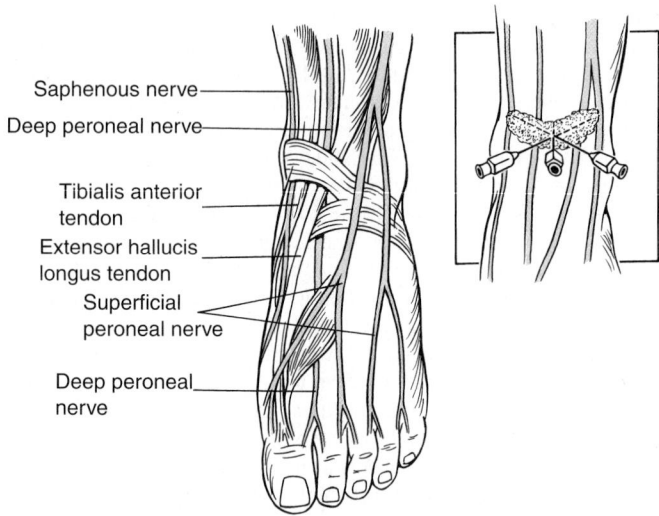

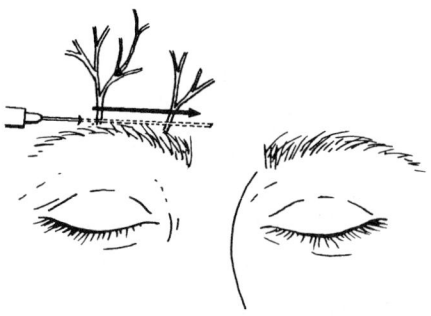

FIG. 37-8. Anterior view of the left foot demonstrating sites for superficial peroneal, saphenous, and deep peroneal nerve blocks.

PERONEAL NERVE BLOCKS   Regional block of the dorsum of the foot has fewer ED applications than do blocks for the sole of the foot, because direct infiltration of the dorsum is more easily performed. The superficial peroneal nerve primarily supplies the sensory innervation of the dorsum of the foot, with contributions from the deep peroneal nerve over the first web space, the sural nerve laterally extending to the lateral malleolus, and the saphenous nerve extending medially over the arch and the medial malleolus (see Figure 37-8).

Peroneal nerve block is best performed with the patient in the supine position. With a 30-gauge needle, a small wheal of LA is raised just above the level of the talocrural joint in the midline anteriorly, between the extensor digitorum longus and the extensor hallucis longus. The superficial peroneal nerve is then blocked by infiltration of 3 to 5 mL of buffered LA solution in a large wheal extending from this point just superior to the talocrural joint at the anterior border of the tibia to the lateral malleolus (see Figure 37-8).[15] The deep peroneal nerve can be blocked by infiltrating 5 mL of buffered LA solution between the tendons of the tibialis anterior and the extensor hallucis longus just above the talocrural joint.[15] However, the area supplied by the deep peroneal nerve is so small that a digital block or local infiltration would achieve the same effect.

Facial and Oral Blocks

Facial blocks are ideal anesthesia techniques for commonly injured areas such as the forehead, chin, lips, nose, tongue, and ear, where local infiltration is often not possible, extremely painful, or results in tissue distortion or potential tissue necrosis. These blocks, similar to foot blocks, often require blockade of more than one nerve to provide for adequate regional anesthesia. For all intraoral routes of infiltration, a small amount of 2% viscous lidocaine should be applied to the mucosa before injection. The needle should not be inserted to its full length during an intraoral procedure nor should the direction of the needle be changed while it is deep in tissue; if inadvertent breakage occurs, retrieval may be difficult. Injection should be slow to minimize pain, and careful aspiration should occur before any injection.[16,17] For percutaneous routes of infiltration, topical EMLA cream, topical ELA-Max cream, or refrigerant sprays should be applied before injection.

FOREHEAD   The sensory innervation of the forehead (anterior aspect from eyebrows extending posteriorly to the lambdoid suture) is supplied by the lateral and medial branches of the frontal (or supraorbital) nerve, the supratrochlear nerve, and fibers from the ophthalmic branch of the trigeminal nerve (Figure 37-9). Regional nerve block of

FIG. 37-9. Regional block of the frontal nerve above the eyebrow.

the forehead can be achieved by infiltration of 3 to 6 mL of LA solution with a 27-gauge needle into the skin immediately above the full length of the eyebrow.[16,17]

LOWER LIP AND CHIN   Direct infiltration to the lip is very painful and causes tissue distortion, which can interfere with the quality of the repair of lacerations. The skin of the chin and lower lip is supplied by the mental nerve (branch of the inferior alveolar nerve). A block of the inferior alveolar nerve as it enters the mandibular foramen, medial and just behind the anterior border of the ramus of the mandible, is performed by the intraoral route (Figure 37-10). Block of the mental nerve can be performed by an intraoral or extraoral percutaneous route (Figure 37-11). The mental foramen is located at the mucosal reflection of the lower lip and gum, inferior to the second premolar (tooth number 20 or 29; see Chap. 242).

The landmark for the inferior alveolar nerve block is the medial surface of the mandibular ramus posterior to and 1 cm above the occlusal surface of the third molar. The physician first identifies the anterior border of the ramus and the oblique alveolar ridge by palpation with the tip of the thumb. The buccal tissues then can be pulled laterally away from the mandible by the pad of the thumb, with the index finger placed externally behind the ramus to stabilize the mandible. The mucosal injection site, 1 cm above the occlusal surface of the third molar, should be anesthetized with a topical agent. A 27-gauge needle is directed from the other side of the mouth, typically between the opposite first and second premolars, and inserted slowly until the needle point touches the bony surface of the medial surface of the ramus (see Figure 37-10). The needle is withdrawn slightly, and 1 to 2 mL of LA solution (with or without epinephrine) is infiltrated.[16]

For the intraoral approach to the mental nerve, the lip is retracted with the thumb and index finger, and topical anesthetic is applied to the mucosa (see Figure 37-11). A 27-gauge needle is inserted at the mucosal junction of the lower lip and gum beneath the second premolar, and 1 to 2 mL of LA solution (with or without epinephrine) is infiltrated while taking care that the needle is not introduced into the mental foramen to avoid neural injury. For the extraoral percutaneous

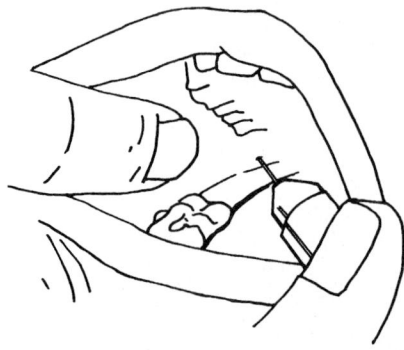

FIG. 37-10. Intraoral approach for inferior alveolar and lingual nerve blocks.

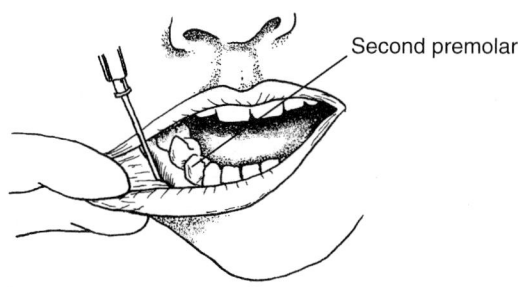

FIG. 37-11. Intraoral approach for mental nerve block.

approach, the mental foramen is located, and percutaneous infiltration of 2 to 4 mL of LA solution close to that location is done.[16,17] The intraoral approach is less painful than the percutaneous approach.

TONGUE   Direct infiltration into the sensate tongue is painful and poorly effective, and a regional block is preferred. The lingual nerve provides sensory innervation to the anterior two thirds of the tongue, the floor of the mouth, and gums. It lies in close proximity to the inferior alveolar nerve at the entrance to the mandibular foramen. The lingual nerve can be blocked by the intraoral route similarly to that for the inferior alveolar nerve (see Figure 37-10).

From an intraoral approach, the vertical ridge of the anterior border of the ramus of the mandible is identified by palpation with the index finger. After the mucosal injection site is anesthetized topically, the procedure for an inferior alveolar nerve block (same as above) is followed. Infiltration of the LA solution as the needle is withdrawn will anesthetize the lingual nerve. Alternatively, the lingual nerve can be anesthetized by injecting 2 to 3 mL of LA solution into the lateral floor of the mouth adjacent to the premolar teeth.[16]

CHEEK, LOWER EYELID, UPPER LIP, AND LATERAL ASPECT OF THE NOSE   The infraorbital nerve supplies sensory innervation to the cheek, lower eyelid, upper lip, and lateral aspect of the side of the nose. A regional block of the infraorbital nerve can be performed by an intraoral approach (Figure 37-12) or extraoral percutaneous approach. The duration of action is more prolonged with the intraoral approach. To identify the infraorbital foramen, the midpoint of the lower margin of the orbit is palpated; approximately 1 cm inferior to this point, the infraorbital nerve exits the infraorbital foramen. For the in-

traoral approach, a palpating finger is positioned over the infraorbital foramen (see Figure 37-12). The cheek is retracted cephalad with the thumb and index finger, and a 27-gauge needle with syringe, held in the other hand, is directed through the mucosa at the reflection of the upper gum opposite and parallel to the long axis of the upper premolar tooth. The needle is then advanced until it is palpated near the infraorbital foramen, approximately a depth of 2.5 cm.[16,17] Caution should be used so as not to introduce the needle directly into the infraorbital foramen, to avoid neural injury. Also, caution should be used so as not to direct the needle too far superiorly or posteriorly, to avoid inadvertently entering the orbit. The syringe should be aspirated to ensure that the facial artery and vein are avoided. Then 2 to 3 mL of LA solution is instilled adjacent to the foramen. The extraoral (percutaneous) approach uses the same landmarks for identification of the infraorbital foramen. Epinephrine is best avoided due to the proximity of the facial artery.[16]

NOSE   The ophthalmic and maxillary branches of the trigeminal nerve also supply the sensory supply of the nose; block of the infraorbital nerve alone will not provide adequate anesthesia of the nose. The mucosal surface of the nose can be anesthetized by topical application of LA spray or gel. The ophthalmic branch of the trigeminal nerve (infratrochlear and external nasal nerves) provides sensation to the majority of the external nose in the midline. These nerves can be blocked by percutaneous infiltration of LA at the sites of their emergence from bony foramina. The remaining aspects of the nose are supplied by the maxillary branch of the trigeminal nerve, the infraorbital nerve for the lateral aspect (see above for intraoral and extraoral block technique), and the posterior nasal and nasopalatine nerves for the septum and inferior midline. The posterior nasal and nasopalatine nerves are best approached intraorally in the midline from the mucosal surface of the reflection of the upper lip.

EAR   The sensory innervation to the external ear is supplied anteriorly by the auriculotemporal nerve (mandibular branch of the trigeminal nerve) and posteriorly by the greater auricular nerve and the mastoid branch of the lesser occipital nerve (branches of the cervical plexus; Figure 37-13A). Direct infiltration of the pinna should be avoided due to the risk of tissue necrosis. Regional block of the ear is

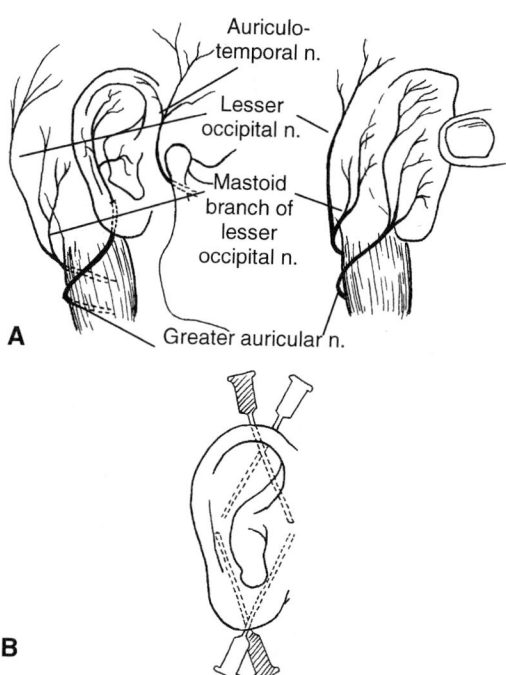

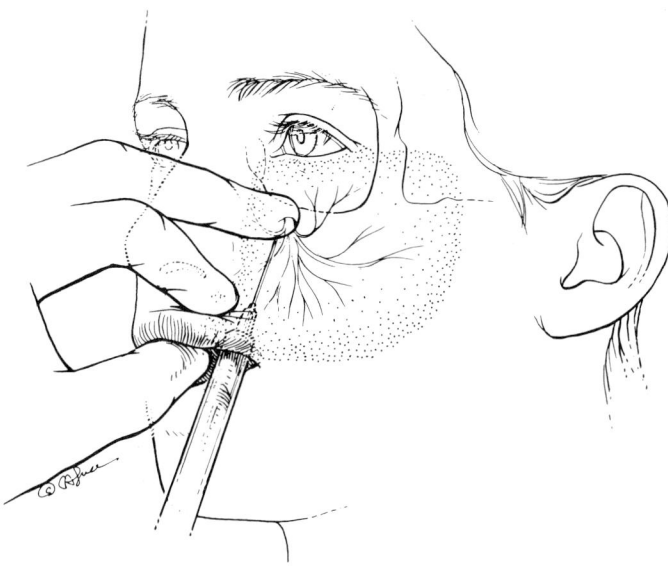

FIG. 37-12. Intraoral approach for infraorbital nerve block.

FIG. 37-13. A. Sensory nerve supply to the auricle. **B.** Technique for regional anesthesia of the auricle.

achieved by infiltration of LA solution via a 27- or 30-gauge needle at the base of the ear from an inferior and superior direction, anteriorly and posteriorly (see Figure 37-13B).

Femoral Nerve Block

Femoral nerve block is an effective technique for relieving pain of a femoral shaft fracture and is useful in the multiple trauma patient when minimizing opiates is important. The femoral nerve is lateral to the femoral artery at the inguinal ligament and innervates the anterior thigh, the periosteum of the femur, and the knee joint (Figure 37-14). Bupivacaine 0.25 to 0.5% is suggested as the preferred LA agent, because of its longer duration of action. A sterile field is prepared over and surrounding the femoral triangle. The femoral artery is located midway between the anterior superior iliac crest and the pubic tubercle. The femoral artery is compressed 1 to 2 cm below the inguinal ligament with the nondominant hand. A wheal of LA is raised in the skin and subcutaneous tissues lateral to the artery; the needle is then introduced at an angle 45 to 60 degrees to the skin lateral and parallel to the femoral artery and directed cephalad. A double loss of resistance, or "pop," is felt as the needle traverses the fascia overlying the femoral nerve. Ten to 20 mL of LA without epinephrine is slowly injected. Onset of anesthesia is 10 to 20 min, and the duration is 3 to 8 h.

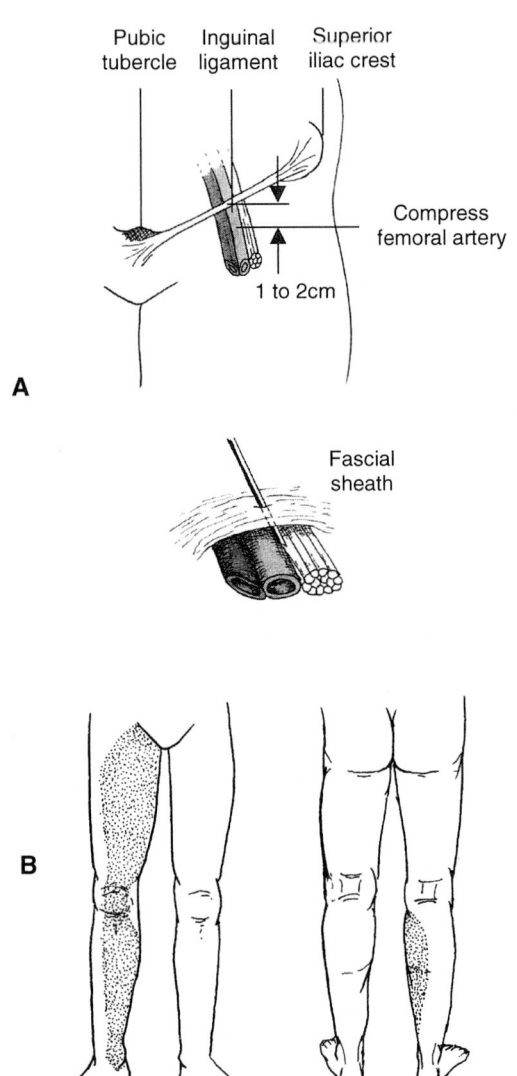

FIG. 37-14. A. Location for femoral nerve block. **B.** Sensory innervation for the femoral nerve (shaded area).

Intercostal Block

Intercostal block is valuable for the management of pain after chest trauma (typically rib fracture) or discomfort from a chest tube. It is a simple block; however, caution should be exercised due to the rapid and high systemic absorption of LA at this site. Contraindications are local soft tissue disease and contralateral pneumothorax. Complications include pneumothorax and systemic toxicity. The intercostal nerves run anteriorly within the neurovascular bundle along the inferior portion of the rib. Addition of epinephrine enhances the safety of this block. The LA dosage range for an adult is 3 to 5 mL per segment (pediatric dosage, 1 to 3 mL). To perform this procedure, the landmarks are the palpable intercostal spaces and the midaxillary line. The intercostal space is identified by palpation. On the upper margin of this space, the inferior border of the upper rib is palpated. At the mid or posterior axillary line, the needle is inserted and advanced at a 90-degree angle until the rib is reached. The needle is withdrawn slightly and redirected caudally to the inferior aspect of this upper rib (Figure 37-15).

HEMATOMA BLOCKS

Hematoma blocks are a simple, quick, and effective mode of regional anesthesia for isolated closed fracture reduction. Although hematoma blocks are safe, the anesthesia that they provide is not as efficacious as the intravenous regional (Bier's) block.[18] The hematoma block is a useful alternative when the intravenous block is contraindicated.

Superficial anesthesia is obtained with local infiltration or other technique such as EMLA applied to the skin over the fracture site. An analgesic dose of opiate also can be given, if deemed appropriate. The fracture site is identified and, using sterile technique, the hematoma is aspirated with a 10-mL syringe and a 20- to 22-gauge needle. Lidocaine 1% without epinephrine is infiltrated to a dose of 3 to 10 mL into the fracture cavity and around the periosteum. The block is effective within 5 to 10 min, with several hours' duration.

INTRAVENOUS REGIONAL BLOCK (BIER'S BLOCK)

The intravenous regional block is an anesthetic procedure involving intravenous infusion of LA distal to an inflated pneumatic tourniquet.[19] It is useful for fracture reductions, large laceration repairs, and foreign body removal. Duration of regional anesthesia is 30 to 60 min. In addition to routine monitoring and resuscitation equipment, the procedure requires a double-cuff tourniquet with a constant pressure gas source. A standard blood pressure cuff is not acceptable and can result in catastrophic systemic leakage of LA. Contraindications include peripheral vascular disease, Raynaud syndrome, sickle cell disease, cardiac conduction abnormalities, hypertension, cellulitis, and children

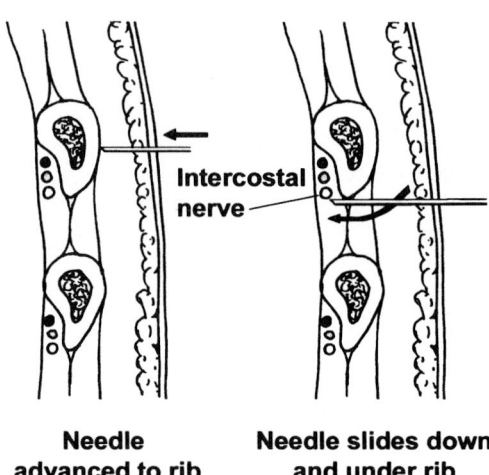

FIG. 37-15. Intercostal nerve block.

younger than 5 years. The need for patients to have nothing by mouth for 4 h before the procedure also may limit the usefulness of the technique. Intravenous regional blocks are used most commonly for upper extremity procedures. Less frequently, this technique has been applied to the lower limb in children.

Lidocaine (3 mg/kg or 0.6 mL/kg of 0.5% solution) without epinephrine is used. In Australia and the United Kingdom, prilocaine (3 mg/kg or 0.6 mL/kg of 0.5% solution) is used. Increased efficacy has been shown with the addition of intravenous ketorolac (60 mg) or fentanyl (1 μg/kg) to the lidocaine.[20] Bupivacaine is absolutely contraindicated due to cardiac toxicity. A "minidose" block with lidocaine (1 to 1.5 mg/kg) has been used effectively in children.

Vital signs and limb neurologic status and perfusion should be monitored and recorded. Intravenous access should be established in both upper limbs, distal to the fracture site on the affected limb. Standard resuscitation equipment and medications should be available. A small dose of intravenous opiate may allay apprehension and the pain of the cuff, which usually occurs after 15 to 30 min. The injured extremity is elevated, and an Esmarch bandage may be applied (distal to proximal) to exsanguinate the limb. Protective padding is then applied to the upper arm to minimize cuff discomfort. Pneumatic double cuffs are then positioned over the padding on the upper arm. The proximal cuff is inflated to 50 to 100 mm Hg above systolic pressure. A venous tourniquet may be positioned just proximal to the fracture site to contain the intravenous local anesthetic to this site. The lidocaine (or prilocaine) 0.5% solution is injected slowly over 2 min into the intravenous cannula in the affected limb. Mottling of the affected limb should occur within 2 to 5 min, followed by anesthesia and paresis of the limb, usually within 10 to 20 min. After 10 min, the distal cuff should be inflated (the area under this cuff should now be anesthetized); once the distal cuff is securely inflated, the proximal cuff can be deflated to minimize cuff pain. The distal cuff should not be deflated until at least 30 min has elapsed from the time of LA injection for tissue binding of the LA agent to occur and thus to minimize the potential for toxicity. Loss of tourniquet pressure before this time will result in a systemic bolus of LA and potential systemic cardiac and CNS toxicity. After completion of the procedure, deflation of the distal cuff should be cycled to prevent the bolus infusion of the LA into the systemic circulation. The cuff is deflated for 5 s, followed by inflation for 1 to 2 min. This cycling action should be repeated three to four times.

REFERENCES

1. Ruetsch YA, Böni T, Borgeat A: From cocaine to ropivacaine: The history of local anesthetic drugs. *Curr Topics Med Chem* 1:175, 2001.
2. Tagariello V, Caporuscio A, De Tommaso O: Mepivacaine: Update on an evergreen local anaesthetic. *Minerva Anesthesiol* 67(suppl 1):5, 2001.
3. Tetzlaff JE: The pharmacology of local anesthetics. *Anesthesiol Clin North Am* 18:217, 2000.
4. Metaxotos NG, Asplund O, Hayes M: The efficacy of bupivacaine with adrenaline in reducing pain and bleeding associated with breast reduction: A prospective trial. *Br J Plast Surg* 52:290, 1999.
5. Denkler K: A comprehensive review of epinephrine in the finger: To do or not to do. *Plast Reconstr Surg* 18:114, 2001.
6. Bartfield JM, Jandreau SW, Raccio-Robak N: A randomized trial of diphenhydramine vs. benzyl alcohol with epinephrine as an alternative to lidocaine local anesthesia. *Ann Emerg Med* 32:650, 1998.
7. Bartfield JM, May-Wheeling HE, Raccio-Robak N, Lai SY: Benzyl alcohol with epinephrine as an alternative to lidocaine with epinephrine. *J Emerg Med* 21:375, 2001.
8. Howell JM, Chisholm CD: Wound care. *Emerg Med Clin North Am* 15:417, 1997.
9. Knapp JF: Updates in wound management for the pediatrician. *Pediatr Clin North Am* 46:1201, 1999.
10. Singer AJ, Stark MJ: EMLA versus LET for pretreating lacerations. A randomized trial. *Acad Emerg Med* 8:223, 2001.
11. Schilling CG, Bank DE, Borchert BA, et al: Tetracaine, epinephrine (adrenalin), and cocaine (TAC) versus lidocaine, epinephrine, and tetracaine (LET) for anesthesia of lacerations in children. *Ann Emerg Med* 25:203, 1995.
12. Eichenfield LF, Funk A, Fallon-Friedlander S, et al: A clinical study to evaluate the efficacy of ELA-Max (4% liposomal lidocaine) as compared with eutectic mixture of local anesthetics cream for pain reduction of venipuncture in children. *Pediatrics* 109:1093, 2002.
13. Wolfe TR, Fosnocht DE, Linscott MS: Atomized lidocaine as a topical anesthesia for nasogastric tube placement: A randomized, double-blind, placebo-controlled trial. *Ann Emerg Med* 35:421, 2000.
14. Gerancher JC: Upper extremity nerve blocks. *Anesthesiol Clin North Am* 18:297, 2000.
15. Dilger JA: Lower extremity nerve blocks. *Anesthesiol Clin North Am* 18:319, 2000.
16. Simpson S: Regional nerve blocks. Part 2—The face and scalp. *Aust Fam Phys* 30:565, 2001.
17. Eaton JS, Grekin RC: Regional anesthesia of the face. *Dermatol Surg* 27:1006, 2001.
18. Furia JP, Alioto RJ, Marquardt JD: The efficacy and safety of the hematoma block for fracture reduction in closed, isolated fractures. *Orthopedics* 20:423, 1997.
19. Simpson S: Regional nerve blocks. Part 5—Bier's block (intravenous regional anesthesia). *Aust Fam Phys* 30:875, 2001.
20. Reuben SS, Steinberg RB, Kreitzer JM, Duprat KM: Intravenous regional anesthesia using lidocaine and ketorolac. *Anesth Analg* 81:110, 1995.

PROCEDURAL SEDATION AND ANALGESIA
David D. Nicolaou

Pain is the chief complaint in approximately 50 percent of patients who seek care in the ED.[1] In addition, physical examination, diagnostic tests, and therapeutic procedures in the ED are often painful. Sedation and analgesia for these painful circumstances is useful to reduce patient pain and anxiety and enhance the success of ED evaluation and treatment.

DEFINITIONS

Pain is a noxious sensation transmitted by specialized nervous structures to the brain, where its perception is modified by cognition and emotion.[2] Analgesic and anesthetic techniques may modulate pain at the level of the peripheral nerves, spinal cord, thalamus, or cortex.

Analgesia is "relief of perception of pain without intentional production of a sedated state. Altered mental status may be a secondary effect of medications administered for this purpose."[3] Agents for pain relief interrupt axonal action potential propagation (e.g., local anesthetics), modulate the inflammatory cascade (e.g., ibuprofen), or modulate central nervous system (CNS) responses to pain (e.g., enkephalins and opioids).

Anxiolysis is the reduction of apprehension without alterations in the level of consciousness.[3] A kind approach to the patient, a realistic and unhurried explanation of what may be expected, distracting conversation, and music have anxiolytic properties.[4]

Neurolepsis is quiescence, indifference to surroundings, and reduced motor activity. Agents used for this purpose include haloperidol and droperidol.

Dissociation is characterized by amnesia, analgesia, sedation, and maintenance of muscle tone. Ketamine is the only commonly used dissociative agent.

Sedation is controlled reduction of environmental awareness.[3] It is not so much a specific level of consciousness as a continuum incorporating anxiolysis or light sedation at one extreme and general anesthesia at the other. The agent or agents chosen, the rate of delivery, the pharmacokinetics of CNS uptake and redistribution, the kinetics of metabolic and elimination pathways, and the degree of patient stimulation may result in different degrees of sedation over time. The level of sedation is dynamic within a given patient and must be continually assessed to detect changes in its depth.

The term *conscious sedation* has been abandoned in favor of *procedural sedation and analgesia* (PSA).[5] The levels of sedation and analgesia defined by the Joint Commission on Accreditation of Health Care Organizations (JCAHO) are:[6]

1. Minimal sedation (anxiolysis): A drug-induced state during which individuals respond normally to verbal commands. Although cognitive function and coordination may be impaired, ventilatory and cardiovascular functions are unaffected.
2. Moderate sedation and analgesia (previously termed "conscious sedation"): A drug-induced depression of consciousness during which individuals respond purposefully to verbal commands alone or accompanied by light tactile stimulation. No interventions are required to maintain a patent airway, and spontaneous ventilation is adequate. Cardiovascular function is usually maintained.
3. Deep sedation and analgesia: A drug-induced depression of consciousness during which individuals cannot be easily aroused but respond purposefully after repeated or painful stimulation. The ability to independently maintain ventilatory function may be impaired. Individuals may require assistance in maintaining a patent airway and spontaneous ventilation may be inadequate. Cardiovascular function is usually maintained.
4. Anesthesia: Consists of general anesthesia and spinal or major regional anesthesia. It does *not* include local anesthesia. General anesthesia is a drug-induced loss of consciousness during which individuals cannot be aroused, even by painful stimulation. The ability to independently maintain ventilatory function is often impaired. Individuals often require assistance in maintaining a patent airway, and positive pressure ventilation may be required because of depressed spontaneous ventilation or drug-induced depression of neuromuscular function. Cardiovascular function may be impaired.

PRINCIPLES OF PSA

The indications for PSA include the treatment of severe pain, attenuation of the pain and anxiety associated with procedures, rapid tranquilization, and the need to perform a diagnostic procedure. No single regimen fits all patients and their clinical problems, so agents and amounts used should be individualized. The physician must integrate the nature of the planned procedure with an assessment of the patient's wishes and physical status, the physician's skills, the patient's intended disposition, the available resources, and a sound knowledge of the pharmacology of the available drugs to formulate a management plan.

The agents used for PSA often have a relatively narrow therapeutic index. *They should therefore be given in small incremental intravenous doses, allowing adequate time for the development and assessment of peak effect.* If the desired effect seems unusually difficult or easy to achieve, no additional medication should be administered and the patient should be carefully monitored until the cause is determined (Table 38-1). Monitoring of patients and medication administration should be performed by another provider who understands the pharmacology of the agents used, possesses sound advanced airway-management skills, and will not be distracted by other tasks during the period when the patient's ability to independently maintain their airway is in doubt.

Ideally, a dedicated area for PSA should be established, with well-labeled supplies and equipment always in a consistent location (Table 38-2). A supply cart or cabinet can easily be stocked with drugs and labels, resuscitation and monitoring equipment, and equipment for common procedures. Drug dosages and documentation tools may be kept in one location, thereby improving risk management and quality-improvement efforts.

The use of pulse oximetry during PSA is important. By 1990, more than 80 deaths had been reported after the use of midazolam, commonly in conjunction with an opioid, for sedation.[7] Co-administration of midazolam (0.05 mg/kg) and fentanyl (2.0 mg/kg) to 12 healthy

TABLE 38-1 Differential Diagnosis of Unexpected Drug Effects by Phase of Drug Disposition

Phase of Disposition	Clinical Effect	
	Less Than Expected	More Than Expected
Delivery	Blood pressure cuff/ tourniquet up IV catheter dislodged IV line clamped/kinked IV bag empty Syringe dose less than intended	Syringe dose more than intended
Uptake and distribution	Hypovolemia Acidosis (opioids) Elevated acute-phase reactants (fentanyl)	Alkalosis (opioids) Hypoproteinemia (protein-bound drugs) Pregnancy (fentanyl)
Redistribution	Obesity (fentanyl)	Reperfusion of muscle (after large doses of fentanyl)
Metabolism	Alcohol use P450 enzyme underexpression (codeine)	P-450 enzyme inhibitors (e.g., cimetidine) P-450 enzyme substrates which compete for metabolism (e.g., erythromycin, lidocaine, midazolam, opioids) Liver disease (morphine)
Elimination		Renal disease Hypovolemia (especially fentanyl) Advanced age (especially fentanyl)
Other	Tolerance	Use of other drugs Delirium Metabolic encephalopathy

volunteers produced hypoxemia (oxygen saturation <90 percent for longer than 10 s) in 11 and apnea in six.[7] A study of pulse oximetry and nasal end-tidal CO_2 values in 27 ED patients who were sedated with benzodiazepines and/or opiates for a painful procedure noted that one patient developed clinically significant apnea and eight developed clinically silent hypoxemia.[8] The American Medical Association's Council on Scientific Affairs subsequently called for the development of standards by specialty societies for the use of pulse oximetry during PSA.[9] Several investigators have noted that, when oxygen supplementation is given, extreme ventilatory insufficiency may develop in the absence of hypoxemia. The clinical significance of hypoxemia during sedation is still uncertain, but abnormal pulse oximetry certainly counsels providers to evaluate the patient carefully.

ASSESSMENT OF PATIENTS

A patient's general physical status can be described conveniently by using the American Society of Anesthesiologists' classification (Table 38-3). Any medications or intoxicants should be solicited and their effects considered when selecting medications. The patient's airway should be systematically evaluated by the provider who will be responsible for its management during PSA (Chap. 19).

It is important to recognize that not every patient can or should undergo PSA in the ED. Depending on clinical circumstances, a patient with an anticipated difficult airway or an American Society of Anesthesiologists classification of III or IV may require consultation with an anesthesiologist. Patients with underlying neurologic diseases such as cerebral palsy, myasthenia gravis, or mental retardation may be much more sensitive to sedatives, and consultation is suggested in such cases.

TABLE 38-2 Suggested Equipment for Procedural Sedation and Analgesia

High-flow oxygen source*
Suction source with large-bore catheters*
Vascular access equipment*
Airway-management equipment*
Monitoring equipment
    Electrocardiography
    Pulse oximeter*
    Blood pressure*
    Capnography
Resuscitation drugs*
Reversal agents (appropriate to drugs being used*)
Adequate staff for monitoring and documentation*

*Suggested minimum equipment. Not all equipment is required for all patients, procedures, and regimens.

Procedural sedation and analgesia requires careful assessment of its risks and benefits based on the clinical scenario and the agents to be used. Patients should be fully informed of the risks of the procedure and the alternatives available. The patient's expectations should be carefully explored and should be corrected when these are not reasonable. Clarify to the patient that PSA is not general anesthesia and that no surety of complete amnesia and analgesia can be offered. Written informed consent for PSA, separately or as part of the procedural consent, is important, as is the physician's documentation of the discussion with the patient.

PHARMACOLOGY

Analgesics

Opioids are the most common analgesics used in PSA. Classes of opioid analgesics include natural (e.g., morphine) and semisynthetic (e.g., codeine, hydromorphone, oxycodone) 5-ring opium derivatives (phenanthrene) and synthetic 3-ring compounds. Of the semisynthetic opioids, phenylpiperidines (e.g., meperidine, fentanyl, sufentanil, and alfentanil) are the only compounds commonly used for PSA (Table 38-4). The analgesic activity of a drug is traditionally referenced to morphine (Table 38-4). After systemic administration, morphine analgesia is mediated through supraspinal μ_1 receptors (possibly by activating descending inhibitory pathways to the dorsal horn cells, and possibly by activating more rostral mechanisms in the brainstem). Spinal cord analgesia is mediated by μ_2 receptors. All opioids have analgesic, sedative, and antitussive effects; they do not reliably produce amnesia when given in doses commonly used for PSA. Opioids also may pro-

TABLE 38-3 American Society of Anesthesiologists Physical Status Classification

Class	Description	Examples
I	Normal, healthy patient	—
II	Mild systemic disease	Asthma, controlled diabetes
III	Moderate systemic disease	Stable angina, diabetes with hyperglycemia, moderate chronic obstructive pulmonary disease
IV	Severe systemic disease	Unstable angina, diabetic ketoacidosis
V	Moribund	—
+E	Modifier added to any classification indicating "emergency" status	All emergency department patients

duce muscle rigidity, pruritus, nausea, vomiting, and constipation and impair ventilation. Respiratory depression is potentiated in the presence of other CNS depressants. The two opioids in common use for ED PSA are morphine and fentanyl.

Morphine is a naturally occurring opioid that is approximately 35 percent protein bound, 77 percent ionized at pH 7.4, and is poorly lipid soluble. It therefore is slow to penetrate the blood-brain barrier and, after small bolus injections, 10 to 30 min is required before its peak effects are seen. Doses of 0.2 mg/kg result in peak effects in less than 1 h that may last for 4 to 6 h. Morphine releases histamine and therefore may produce hypotension, especially in preload-dependent patients. Its analgesic effects and its respiratory depression have been shown to be potentiated by coadministration of hydroxyzine in postoperative patients[10]; the significance of this finding for ED PSA is uncertain, especially because hydroxyzine is not recommended for intravenous use. Morphine undergoes hepatic glucuronidation to morphine-3-glucuronide and morphine-6-glucuronide; the latter is four times as potent as morphine and has a duration of action approximately double that of its parent. The daughter compounds are renally excreted and accumulate in renal insufficiency.

Fentanyl is a synthetic phenylpiperidine derivative that is approximately 80 to 85 percent protein bound and 92 percent ionized at pH 7.4. However, it is highly lipid soluble, resulting in rapid CNS uptake with an effect onset half-time of 6.4 min. Fentanyl is also distributed into adipose tissue, creating a "reservoir" of fentanyl. The size of this reservoir is dose dependent, with higher doses resulting in a progressively increasing duration of effect as the drug is released from tissue stores and then eliminated. Further, distribution from plasma may not result in drug levels below those associated with clinical effects and respiratory depression. Thus, the use of relatively high doses of fentanyl (i.e., in the range of 10 µg/kg) results in greatly prolonged clinical effects and elimination half-times. Fentanyl is metabolized in the liver to inactive compounds.

Fentanyl has been shown to have a low complication rate when used for PSA in the ED. Chudnofsky and colleagues noted six cases of respiratory depression (largely in patients who were intoxicated or had received other drugs) and three cases of hypotension among 841 ED patients receiving fentanyl.[11] Respiratory depression occurs at significantly lower fentanyl doses when another respiratory depressant, such as alcohol or midazolam, is present. Chest wall rigidity may occur in a dose-dependent fashion after fentanyl administration; approximately half of healthy volunteers develop chest wall rigidity in response to 15 µg/kg, a dose not usually used in PSA in the ED. Rigidity and apnea, however, may occur with even small doses of fentanyl, resulting in respiratory insufficiency. The rigidity is not reliably antagonized by naloxone and may require neuromuscular blockade and intubation to enable adequate ventilation. Fentanyl does not release histamine, which mediates most of the peripheral vascular effects of opioids, so it rarely produces hypotension.[12]

Meperidine is a poor choice for ED analgesia in general. It causes more histamine release than morphine or fentanyl.[12] Its primary metabolite, normeperidine, is bioactive and toxic. Normeperidine causes CNS excitation, including tremors, myoclonus, and seizures, effects that are not antagonized by naloxone. Normeperidine is excreted by the kidneys and therefore accumulates in renal insufficiency and with repeated doses. Meperidine also may cause a fatal reaction when coadministered with monoamine oxidase inhibitors. This reaction may be excitatory (agitation, rigidity, hyperpyrexia, seizures, and coma) or depressive (respiratory depression, hypotension, and coma). For these reasons, there are better choices than meperidine for treatment of pain with opioid analgesics.

Anxiolytics

The prototypical anxiolytics in common use for PSA in the ED are the benzodiazepines, which potentiate the inhibitory activity of

TABLE 38-4 Drugs Used for Procedural Sedation and Analgesia

Drug	Dose*	Peak Effect	Duration of Effect	Notes
Morphine	0.05–0.1 mg/kg IV	10–30 min	2–4 h	Releases histamine
Fentanyl	1–2 μg/kg IV	2.5–10 min	30–90 min	Does not release histamine
Midazolam	0.01 mg/kg IV	1–2 min	60 min	Respiratory depression
Propofol	0.2 mg/kg per min infusion	6–7 min	5–10 min	Respiratory depression, deep sedation
Etomidate	0.1 mg/kg IV	20–30 s	2–3 min	Respiratory depression, deep sedation
Ketamine	1–2 mg/kg IV	5 min	30–60 min	Avoid with elevated intracranial pressure
Methohexital	1 mg/kg IV	30–60 s	10 min	Avoid in patients with seizure disorders

*Incremental doses, given in small intravenous amounts, allow adequate time for the development and assessment of peak effect.

γ-aminobutyric acid (GABA) in the CNS by binding to benzodiazepine-specific receptors on the $GABA_A$-benzodiazepine receptor complex. This binding induces a conformational change that potentiates GABA-mediated chloride influx, resulting in sedation, amnesia, anxiolysis, and anticonvulsant effects and respiratory depression. The benzodiazepine most commonly used for PSA in the ED is midazolam, which produces earlier sedation, more frequent amnesia, less pain on injection, and improved 90 min alertness and readiness for discharge when compared with diazepam.[13]

Midazolam has a number of characteristics favorable for use in ED PSA. Its diazepine ring opens at pH values below 4, in which form it is quite water soluble. At physiologic pH, the ring closes, rendering midazolam highly lipid soluble, with associated rapid CNS uptake producing peak effects within a few minutes of intravenous administration. Midazolam's relatively high volume of distribution compared with other benzodiazepines derives from its lipophilicity. This characteristic is greatly amplified in obese patients, resulting in an increase in plasma half-life from 2.7 to 8.4 h. Midazolam is cleared by hepatic hydroxylation to 1-hydroxymidazolam (which is pharmacologically active) and to 4-hydroxymidazolam and 1,4-dihydroxymidazolam, which are conjugated and excreted in the urine.

The combination of midazolam with alcohol or opioids greatly increases sedative and respiratory-depressant effects and increases the risk of cardiovascular depression. Midazolam should be used cautiously in such cases, with careful monitoring of respiratory and hemodynamic status. The dose of midazolam should be individualized. Midazolam should be given in small incremental doses until the desired effect is achieved. Aliquots of 0.25 to 0.5 mg given every 3 to 5 min in healthy adults, or 0.1 to 0.25 mg every 5 to 10 min in the intoxicated or elderly patient, is a reasonable starting point. Chronic alcohol users who do not have cirrhosis may require relatively high doses of midazolam to achieve the clinical effects desired.

Anesthetic Agents

Some agents traditionally used for induction of general anesthesia are also used for PSA: propofol, etomidate, ketamine and methohexital.

Propofol (2,6-diisopropylphenol) is a lipid-soluble anesthetic agent that is supplied in an emulsion of soybean oil and purified egg phosphatide, which most egg-allergic patients should tolerate, because it contains no protein. The emulsion is responsible for frequent burning on injection and contains no preservatives, resulting in the risk of bacterial growth in improperly handled solutions. When given by infusion, the onset of sedation is rapid (6 to 7 min), and it resolves rapidly (5 to 10 min) upon discontinuation of the infusion.[14] Amnesia, however, is not reliably produced in doses used for sedation. The drug possesses antiemetic properties. Propofol produces significant cardiovascular depression, with dose-related declines in systolic blood pressure of up to 25 to 40 percent when given in induction doses. This effect is more pronounced in those with impaired hemodynamic status and in the elderly.

The use of propofol for ED PSA is controversial, and its use outside the operating room by nonanesthesia personnel may be restricted by hospital policy. Limited studies using propofol for ED PSA in children and adults have found a rapid onset of sedation, rapid recovery, and high patient and physician satisfaction scores.[14] Propofol is an attractive agent for ED PSA, because it rapidly produces sedation that quickly abates when the infusion is discontinued. In doses usually used for PSA, however, analgesic and amnestic agents may be required, which may result in hypoventilation and potentiate the already significant hemodynamic effects of propofol. The research agenda and issues surrounding propofol use by the emergency physician have been delineated.[15]

Etomidate is an imidazole derivative that has sedative and hypnotic properties but no analgesic activity; its effects, although not fully understood, may be mediated through the GABA complex. Etomidate reliably produces hypnosis of about 100 s in duration for each 0.1 mg/kg administered by bolus injection. It is rapidly metabolized in the liver to largely inactive compounds, with a short elimination half-life, but redistribution (also rapid) is responsible for the resolution of hypnosis. Etomidate itself is highly (75 percent) protein bound, producing exaggerated effects in hypoproteinemic patients. It produces little alteration in hemodynamics, cerebral blood flow, respiratory function, or coronary oxygenation. Reported adverse effects include nausea and vomiting, myoclonus, and suppression of adrenal steroid synthesis after long-term infusion.[16] The dose used for induction of anesthesia is 0.2 to 0.6 mg/kg as a bolus; doses used for PSA include titrated boluses of 0.1 mg/kg or an infusion of 5 to 8 μg/kg per min, with or without opioid analgesic supplementation. The use of opioids increases the frequency of respiratory depression.

Experience with etomidate for PSA in the ED is limited. Small prospective trials in adults and children and retrospective reviews of the use of etomidate for PSA have suggested that the agent is promising.[16] These studies found a low risk of apnea, intubation, and hemodynamic compromise with good patient acceptance; however, deep sedation frequently occurred.[16]

Ketamine is a phencyclidine derivative that has analgesic and anesthetic properties. Ketamine anesthesia is often called "dissociative," reflecting electroencephalographically demonstrable discontinuity of the corticothalamic and limbic systems. The patient's eyes often remain open, with spontaneous horizontal and vertical nystagmus. Muscle tone may be increased, and corneal reflexes and spontaneous swallowing are preserved; occasional purposeful movements unrelated to the environment occur. Emergence reactions, characterized by disturbing dreams and vivid, sometimes frightening hallucinations, occur in 5 to 30 percent of patients. Patients at greatest risk for emergence reactions are older than 16 years, female, normally dream, have personality disorders, or receive droperidol or atropine. These phenomena may be attenuated with benzodiazepines given before or at the completion of the procedure.

Ketamine is highly lipid soluble and has a pKa of 7.5, accounting for the rapid (within 1 min) onset of hypnosis after intravenous injection. Peak brain and plasma concentrations develop within 1 min; rapid redistribution to peripheral tissues results in a mean hypnosis time of 6 min (1.0 mg/kg) to 10 min (2.0 mg/kg). Ketamine is metabolized by the hepatic P-450 system to several active metabolites, the chief among which is norketamine. Norketamine appears within 2 min of a bolus injection and is one-tenth to one-third less potent than the parent drug, but does not appear to penetrate the CNS in quantities sufficient to produce hypnosis. Subsequent metabolites are conjugated and renally excreted, but, because they are much less active, the dose appears not to require adjustment in patients with renal insufficiency. Drugs that induce the P-450 system increase the metabolism of ketamine, whereas inhibitors prolong the duration of effect.

The hemodynamic response to ketamine is complex. It is a direct myocardial depressant and vasodilator, but these effects are typically overshadowed by stimulation of significant CNS sympathetic outflow, resulting in tachycardia and vasoconstriction. (My experience is that fentanyl 1 to 2 μg/kg given 3 to 5 min before the procedure, attenuates this effect but increases the frequency of hypoxemia, especially when ketamine is given rapidly and/or midazolam is also used.) However, profoundly hypovolemic patients or those with little sympathetic reserve (e.g., cocaine users) may develop hypotension, particularly at rapid rates of injection.

The pulmonary effects of ketamine make it an appealing agent. Although it produces bronchodilation and bronchorrhea, it rarely causes significant respiratory depression unless given by rapid injection (over less than 60 s) or coadministered with other agents. Patients nearly always retain protective airway reflexes, but this is not a certainty.[17] Careful monitoring is therefore necessary when ketamine is used, especially with other agents or for deep sedation.

Before giving ketamine, it is important to consider the drug's likely nontherapeutic effects. If a hyperdynamic state or bronchorrhea may not be well tolerated, then appropriate premedication (opioids or glycopyrrolate) should be given or another agent chosen. A specific discussion of the emergence phenomenon with the patient, family, and friends will reduce the impact of this occasionally dramatic event.

The dose of ketamine commonly used for analgesia is 0.5 to 1.0 mg/kg IV over 60 s. Anesthesia is produced by doses of 1 to 2 mg/kg. When relatively larger doses are administered, midazolam should be given during the emergence phase to attenuate emergence phenomena.

Methohexital is a highly lipophilic short-acting barbiturate with a rapid onset of sedative action, typically 30 to 60 s. Intravenous doses of 1 mg/kg produce sedation for about 10 min. Cumulative doses of 4 to 5 mg/kg are commonly used for procedures with a relative low incidence of complications. In contrast to other barbiturates, methohexital may worsen or precipitate seizures, and it is prudent to avoid methohexital in patients with known seizure disorders

Adjunctive Agents

Antiemetic agents are useful in the treatment of nausea and vomiting accompanying opioid therapy. Their value as "potentiators" of opioids is not clear, and they should not be used routinely for this purpose.

Antidotal Agents

Agents to reverse the effects of opioids and benzodiazepine should be available, but with careful titration of the drugs used for PSA, reversal agents should infrequently be needed.

Naloxone, a competitive antagonist of opioids at μ receptors, is indicated for reversal of unwanted respiratory depression after opioid administration. Naloxone may not reverse chest wall rigidity caused by fentanyl. Patients who are opioid dependent may develop withdrawal or pain after the administration of naloxone, and when circumstances permit they should be given titrated doses (0.1 to 0.2 mg IV every 1 to 2 min) rather than large bolus doses until the desired effect is achieved. Because patients who receive long-acting opioids or who

metabolize opioids slowly may redevelop respiratory depression after clearing all or part of an effective dose of naloxone, continual patient reassessment is required after naloxone administration.

Flumazenil, which is a competitive antagonist of benzodiazepines, is given in intravenous aliquots of 0.1 to 0.2 mg every 1 to 2 min until the desired effect is achieved. It has a half-life of 45 to 104 min, rendering relapse of sedation a possibility if the effects of a long-acting benzodiazepine are reversed with flumazenil. Flumazenil should be used with caution in benzodiazepine-dependent patients. In one study of 133 ED patients,[18] flumazenil was found to reverse midazolam-induced sedation safely and effectively. However, the time from completion of the procedure to discharge from the ED was no shorter in the group treated with flumazenil than in the control group.[18] Flumazenil is indicated for reversal of respiratory depression caused by benzodiazepine during PSA, but its routine use to "awaken" patients cannot be recommended.

DISCHARGE

Patients receiving PSA require a period of observation to allow the sedative and analgesic effects to resolve sufficiently before discharge (Table 38-5). Guidelines for safe discharge may require modification based on the patient's age, clinical circumstances, the agents used, and the patient's social situation. Patients must not be permitted to drive or operate heavy machinery for at least 24 h after PSA. The agents used for PSA often produce anterograde amnesia, which may be present even when consciousness appears otherwise normal. It is therefore vital to evaluate the patient's ability to retain information before discharge.

Discharge planning is an important component of PSA and should be part of the pre-procedure evaluation process. A patient who is likely to require prolonged post-procedure monitoring or treatment should be considered for hospital admission. If a companion is required for discharge, he or she should be identified before beginning PSA.

POLICY ISSUES

Clinical Standards and Documentation

The increasingly widespread use of PSA outside the operating room has garnered the attention of various organizations. The clinician's decisions regarding PSA are increasingly subject to regulations and standards, and these in turn are evolving in parallel with local and national PSA experience. The development of guidelines concerning ED PSA has been hampered by the lack of high-quality clinical evidence, such as clinical trials, supporting particular practices. As a result, few evidence-based standards exist.

The JCAHO standard specifies that a uniform standard of care must be provided throughout an accredited institution. This means that situations in which protective airway reflexes are typically expected to be lost might be held to the standard of care provided in the operating room. The American College of Emergency Physicians[19] and the American Society of Anesthesiologists[20] have begun to promulgate guidelines. Each ED should develop standards for PSA that are carefully reconciled with JCAHO, hospital, evidence-based, and peer

TABLE 38-5 Discharge Criteria for Patients Receiving Procedural Sedation and Analgesia

Vital signs stable for at least 30 min
No evidence of respiratory distress
Minimal or no nausea, vomiting, or dizziness
Alert, oriented, and able to retain information
Able to take fluids and medications by mouth
Ambulation consistent with preprocedure status
Receives, comprehends, and retains discharge instructions
Responsible person present to accompany patient

requirements and practices and then strive to provide and document care consistent with that standard.

REFERENCES

1. Cordell WH, Keene KK, Giles BK, et al: The high prevalence of pain in emergency medical care. *Am J Emerg Med* 20:165, 2002.
2. Lewis LM, Lasater LC, Brooks CB: Are emergency physicians too stingy with analgesics? *South Med J* 87:7, 1994.
3. Sacchetti A, Schafermeyer R, Gerardi M, et al: Pediatric analgesia and sedation. *Ann Emerg Med* 23:237, 1994.
4. Menegazzi JJ, Paris PM, Kersteen CH, et al: A randomized, controlled trial of the use of music during laceration repair. *Ann Emerg Med* 20:348, 1991.
5. Green SM, Krauss B: Procedural sedation terminology: Moving beyond "conscious sedation." *Ann Emerg Med* 39:433, 2002.
6. Joint Commission on Accreditation of Healthcare Organizations. *2001 Sedation and Anesthesia Care Standards.* Available at: http://www.jcaho.org/accredited+organizations/behavioral+health+care/standards/revisions/2001/sedation+and+anesthesia.htm. Accessed June 28, 2002.
7. Bailey PL, Pace NL, Ashburn MA, et al: Frequent hypoxemia and apnea after sedation with midazolam and fentanyl. *Anesthesiology* 73:826, 1990.
8. Wright SW: Conscious sedation in the emergency department: The value of capnography and pulse oximetry. *Ann Emerg Med* 21:551, 1992.
9. Council on Scientific Affairs, American Medical Association: The use of pulse oximetry during conscious sedation. *JAMA* 270:1463, 1993.
10. Hupert CP, Yacoub M, Turgeon LR: Effect of hydroxyzine on morphine analgesia for the treatment of postoperative pain. *Anesth Analg* 59:690, 1980.
11. Chudnofsky CR, Wright SW, Dronen SC, et al: The safety of fentanyl use in the emergency department. *Ann Emerg Med* 18:635, 1989.
12. Flacke JW, Flacke WE, Bloor BC, et al: Histamine release by four narcotics: A double-blind study in humans. *Anesth Analg* 66:723, 1987.
13. Wright SW, Chudnofsky CR, Dronen SC, et al: Comparison of midazolam and diazepam for conscious sedation in the emergency department. *Ann Emerg Med* 22:201, 1993.
14. Havel CJ, Strait RT, Hennes H: A clinical trial of propofol vs midazolam for procedural sedation in a pediatric emergency department. *Acad Emerg Med* 6:989, 1999.
15. Green SM: Propofol for emergency department procedural sedation-not yet ready for prime time [editorial]. *Acad Emerg Med* 6:975, 1999.
16. Vinson DR, Bradbury DR: Etomidate for procedural sedation in emergency medicine. *Ann Emerg Med* 39:592, 2002.
17. Green SM, Denmark TK, Cline J, et al: Ketamine sedation for pediatric critical care procedures. *Pediatr Emerg Care* 17:244, 2001.
18. Chudnofsky CR: Safety and efficacy of flumazenil in reversing conscious sedation in the emergency department. *Acad Emerg Med* 4:944, 1997.
19. American College of Emergency Physicians: Clinical policy for procedural sedation and analgesia in the emergency department. *Ann Emerg Med* 31:663, 1998.
20. American Society of Anesthesiology: Practice guidelines for sedation and analgesia by non-anesthesiologists. A report by the American Society of Anesthesiologists task force on sedation and analgesia by non-anesthesiologists. *Anesthesiology* 84:459, 1996.

39

MANAGEMENT OF PATIENTS WITH CHRONIC PAIN
David M. Cline

Chronic pain is defined as a painful condition that lasts longer than 3 months, a pain that persists beyond the reasonable time for an injury to heal, or a pain that persists 1 month beyond the usual course of an acute disease. There are four basic types of chronic pain: pain persisting beyond the normal healing time for a disease or injury, pain related to a chronic degenerative disease or persistent neurologic condition, cancer-related pain, and pain that emerges or persists without an identifiable cause. Chronic pain differs from acute pain in its function. Acute pain is an essential biologic signal to warn the individual to stop a potentially injurious activity or to prompt one to seek medical care.

Chronic pain serves no obvious biologic function. Chronic pain patients presenting to the ED have not been well studied, despite their apparent numbers.

Complete eradication of pain is not a reasonable end point in most cases. Rather, the goal of therapy is pain reduction and return to functional status. Chronic pain syndromes discussed in this chapter include myofascial headaches, "transformed" migraine headaches, fibromyalgia, myofascial chest pain, back pain, complex regional pain types I and II, postherpetic neuralgia, and phantom limb pain. Drug-seeking patients are also covered.

EPIDEMIOLOGY

Chronic pain affects about one-third of the U.S. population at least once during an individual's lifetime, with an estimated annual cost of 80 to 90 billion dollars in health care payments and lawsuit settlements. Chronic pain may be associated with a chronic pathologic process in the musculoskeletal or vascular system, a chronic pathologic process in one of the organ systems, a prolonged dysfunction in the peripheral or central nervous system, or a psychological or environmental disorder. Discussion of the numerous epidemiologic factors that have been associated with various chronic pain syndromes is beyond the scope of this chapter. In general, patients who attribute their chronic pain to a specific traumatic event experience more emotional distress, more life interference, and more severe pain than those with other causes.[1]

PATHOPHYSIOLOGY

The pathophysiology of chronic pain can be divided into three basic types: nociceptive pain is associated with ongoing tissue damage, neuropathic pain is associated with nervous system dysfunction in the absence of ongoing tissue damage, and psychogenic pain has no identifiable cause.[2] Many chronic pain states begin with an episode of nociceptive pain and then continue with neuropathic or psychogenic pain. For example, an acute injury with fracture involves nociceptive pain, but an associated nerve injury may lead to neuropathic pain, and chronic disability may lead to psychogenic pain. Nociceptive pain results from the stimulation of nociceptors in tissues or organs by noxious mechanical, thermal, or chemical stimuli. Chemical mediators of inflammation, such as bradykinins and prostaglandins, are essential elements in the pathophysiology of nociceptive pain. Examples of chronic nociceptive pain are cancer pain and pain due to chronic pancreatitis. Patients with nociceptive pain usually respond well to centrally acting analgesics. Neuropathic pain is caused by disease of the central or peripheral nervous system. Examples of neuropathic pain include complex regional pain type II (causalgia), postherpetic neuralgia, and phantom limb pain. Neuropathic pain responds poorly to common analgesics, including opioids. Psychogenic pain is a diagnosis of exclusion and can be difficult to establish in the ED. Patients with psychogenic pain believe their pain is physical and tend to strongly reject the concept that it is psychological.

CLINICAL FEATURES

To better define the psychology of chronic pain, psychiatrists have divided patients' characteristics into two groups. The first group has normal psychological function at baseline. However, continued pain and its effects, such as inability to work or altered body image, result in psychological dysfunction. The second group has primary psychopathology that predates the onset of chronic pain. Hypochondriacal, hysterical, pain-prone, and depressive personalities are included in this group. The "seven Ds" (Table 39-1) summarize the clinical features of this second group.

The following set of historical inquiries may prove helpful in the ED. The patients should be asked to describe the nature of the current

TABLE 39-1   Psychological Characteristics of Chronic Pain Patients

Characteristic	Features
Drugs	Misuse of opioids or other medications
Doctors	Tendency to "doctor shop" and play one physician against another
Dysfunction	Bodily impairment related to the physical and emotional factors
Disability	Inability to work or hold a job
Dependance	Loss of self-reliance and helplessness
Dramatization	Exaggeration, acting out by verbalization or by body language
Depression	Despair and negative attitudes

Source: Brena SF, Chapman SL: The "learned pain syndrome": Decoding a patient's pain signals. *Postgrad Med* 69:53, 1981.

pain and the initiating and exacerbating or relieving factors. Other useful information includes determination of the chronic nature of the pain, quantification of similar episodes, and sources and modes of treatment, including medications and dosages for physician-prescribed, over-the-counter, or alternative medications. Outcomes of previous therapeutic efforts and the effect of the condition on the patient's functional status are also important. Addiction to drugs or alcohol or experience with detoxification programs should be noted. A review of systems should be done to rule out other conditions. Substance abuse is a frequent problem in chronic pain patients. Drug detoxification is often the first step of the therapeutic plan for new patients referred to a pain clinic.

Objective findings of acute pain include tachycardia, hypertension, diaphoresis, and muscle spasms on stimulation. Objective evidence of chronic pain includes muscle atrophy in the distribution of pain due to disuse, skin temperature changes due to the effects of the sympathetic nervous system after disuse or secondary to nerve injury, and trigger points, which are focal points of muscle tenderness and tension. How-

ever, these findings do not have to be present for the pain to be factual (Table 39-2).

Myofascial Headaches and Transformed Migraine

Myofascial headache is a variant of tension headache characterized by the presence of trigger points on the scalp; constant, squeezing pain; and occasionally shooting pain. Nausea, vomiting, neck pain, and neck tenderness may be present. It is important to differentiate this disorder from common tension headache, because myofascial headache may benefit from referral for injection of trigger points. *Transformed migraine* is a syndrome in which classic migraine headaches change over time and develop into a chronic pain syndrome. One cause of this change is frequent treatment with opioids. In this regard, patients who initially have "vascular symptoms" eventually have predominantly muscular symptoms: non-throbbing, squeezing, bandlike pain associated with muscle tenderness and tension. Nausea and vomiting or failure of oral antimigraine medications often prompts an ED visit.

Fibromyalgia and Chronic Myofascial Chest Pain

Fibromyalgia is classified by the American College of Rheumatology as the presence of 11 of 18 specific tender points, non-restorative sleep, muscle stiffness, and generalized aching pain, with symptoms persisting for longer than 3 months (www.rheumatology.org). *Chronic myofascial chest pain* classically is a dull, constant pain associated with trigger points on the chest wall. Symptoms may mimic ischemic myocardial-type chest pain but usually is not provoked by exercise (unless the movement involves the use of chest or arm muscles) and is not completely relieved by rest.

Back Pain

Risk factors for chronic back pain after an acute episode include male sex, advanced age, evidence of nonorganic disease, leg pain, prolonged initial episode, and significant disability at onset.[3] Chronic back pain symptoms and causes can be divided into myofascial or muscular, articular, and neurogenic types. Myofascial back pain is

TABLE 39-2   Signs and Symptoms of Chronic Pain Syndromes

Disorder	Pain Symptoms	Signs
Myofascial headache	Constant dull pain, occasional shooting pain	Trigger points on scalp, muscle tenderness, and tension
Transformed migraine	Initially migraine-like, becomes constant, dull; nausea, vomiting	Muscle tenderness and tension, normal neurologic examination
Fibromyalgia	Diffuse muscle pain, stiffness, fatigue, sleep disturbance	Diffuse muscle tenderness, >11 trigger points
Myofascial chest pain	Constant dull pain, occasional shooting pain	Trigger points in area of pain
Myofascial back pain syndrome	Constant dull pain, occasional shooting pain, does not follow nerve distribution	Trigger points in area of pain, usually no muscle atrophy, poor ROM in involved muscle
Articular back pain	Constant or sharp pain exacerbated by movement	Local muscle spasm
Neurogenic back pain	Constant or intermittent, burning or aching, shooting or electric shock-like; may follow dermatome; leg pain > back pain	Possible muscle atrophy in area of pain, possible reflex changes
Complex regional pain type I (RSD)	Burning persistent pain, allodynia, associated with immobilization or disuse	Early: edema, warmth, local sweating Late: above alternates with cold; pale, cyanosis, eventually atrophic changes
Complex regional pain type II (causalgia)	Burning persistent pain, allodynia, associated with peripheral nerve injury	Early: edema, warmth, local sweating Late: above alternates with cold; pale, cyanosis, eventually atrophic changes
Postherpetic neuralgia	Allodynia; shooting, lancinating pain	Sensory changes in the involved dermatome
Phantom limb pain	Variable: aching, cramping, burning, squeezing or tearing sensation	None

Abbreviations: ROM = range of motion; RSD = reflex sympathetic dystrophy.

characterized by constant dull and occasional shooting pain that does not follow a classic nerve distribution. Pain may or may not be exacerbated by movement. Usually trigger points can be found at the site of greatest pain, and muscle atrophy is not found. Range of motion of the involved muscle is reduced, but there is no actual muscle weakness. Previous recommendations for bedrest in the treatment of back pain have proven counterproductive.[4] Exercise programs have been found to be more helpful in chronic low back pain.[5] Articular back pain is characterized by constant or sharp pain that is exacerbated by movement and associated with local muscle spasm. Myofascial and articular back pain may be indistinguishable from each other except by advanced imaging techniques beyond the usual scope of practice in the ED. Neurogenic back pain is classically characterized by constant or intermittent pain that is burning, shooting, or aching. The pain is usually more severe in the leg than in the back and follows a dermatome. Muscle atrophy and reflex changes can be seen over time.

Complex Regional Pain

Patients with complex regional pain type I, also known as reflex sympathetic dystrophy, and complex regional pain type II, also known as causalgia, may be seen in the ED as early as the second week after treatment of an acute injury.[6] These disorders cannot be differentiated from one another on the basis of signs and symptoms. Type I occurs because of prolonged immobilization or disuse, and type II occurs because of a peripheral nerve injury. These disorders should be suspected when a patient presents with classic symptoms: allodynia (pain provoked with a gentle touch of the skin) and a persistent burning or shooting pain. Associated signs early in the course of the disease include edema, warmth, and localized sweating. Therefore, it may be difficult to distinguish this disorder from an underlying wound infection or osteomyelitis. Later signs include periods of edema and warmth that alternate with cold, pale, cyanotic skin and eventually atrophic changes. Complex regional pain is an important diagnosis to make, because early steroid treatment may reduce ongoing symptoms. Further, when complex regional pain is associated with a cast, pin, or external fixation apparatus, the device may need to be removed.[6]

Postherpetic Neuralgia

The classic pain of postherpetic neuralgia may follow the course of an acute episode of herpes zoster in 8 to 70 percent of cases; increased incidence is seen with advancing age. Pain is characterized by allodynia and shooting, lancinating (tearing or sharply cutting) pain. Often patients have hyperesthesia in the involved dermatome. Occasionally there are pigmentation changes in the distribution of the involved dermatome, but this is not unique to postherpetic neuralgia.

Phantom Limb Pain

Phantom limb pain is quite variable in presentation but is more frequent in patients who had pain in the extremity before amputation. Pain may be aching, cramping, burning, tearing, or squeezing. Failure to respond to any treatment, including opioids, is common.

DIAGNOSIS

The most important task of the emergency physician is to distinguish an exacerbation of chronic pain from a presentation that heralds a life- or limb-threatening condition. The history and physical examination should confirm the chronic condition or point to the need for further evaluation when unexpected signs or symptoms are elicited. Because chronic pain patients may be frequent visitors to the ED, the entire staff may prejudge the complaint as chronic or factitious. Physicians should insist that routine procedures be followed, including a full triage assessment and a complete set of vital signs.

Rarely is a provisional diagnosis of a chronic pain condition made for the first time in the ED. The exception is a form of post-nerve injury pain, complex regional pain. The sharp pain from acute injuries, including fractures, rarely continues beyond 2 weeks' duration. Pain in an injured body part beyond this period should alert the clinician to the possibility of nerve injury, and proper treatment (Table 39-3) should be instituted.

Definitive diagnostic testing of chronic pain conditions is difficult and requires expert opinion and often expensive procedures such as

TABLE 39-3   Management of Selected Chronic Pain Syndromes

Disorder	Primary ED Treatment	Secondary Treatment*	Possible Referral Outcome
Cancer pain	NSAIDs, opiates	Long-acting opiates	Optimization of medical therapy
Myofascial, headache	NSAIDs, cyclobenzaprine	Antidepressants, phenothiazines	Trigger point injections, optimization of medical therapy
Transformed migraine	NSAIDs, cyclobenzaprine	Antidepressants	Optimization of medical therapy, opioid withdrawal
Fibromyalgia	NSAIDs	Antidepressants, exercise program	Optimization of medical therapy, dedicated exercise program
Myofascial, chest pain	NSAIDs	Antidepressants	Trigger point injections, optimization of medical therapy
Myofascial, back pain syndrome	NSAIDs, stay active	Antidepressants	Trigger point injections, optimization of medical therapy
Articular back pain	NSAIDs		Surgery, physical therapy
Neurogenic back pain	Acute: tapered prednisolone or prednisone	NSAIDs, muscle relaxants	Epidural steroids, surgery, exercise program
Complex regional pain types I and II (RSD and causalgia)	Prednisone 60 mg/d × 4 d and then taper to include 3 wk of therapy	Calcitonin, antidepressants, anticonvulsants	Spinal cord stimulation, intrathecal baclofen, sympathetic nerve blocks, spinal analgesia
Postherpetic neuralgia	Simple analgesics	Gabapentin, antidepressants	Regional nerve blockade
Phantom limb pain	Simple analgesics	Antidepressants, anticonvulsants	TENS, sympathectomy

*If started in the ED, consultation and/or follow-up with a pain specialist or personal physician is recommended.
Abbreviations: NSAIDs = nonsteroidal anti-inflammatory drugs; RSD = reflex sympathetic dystrophy; TENS = transcutaneous electrical nerve stimulation.

magnetic resonance imaging, computed tomography, and thermography. Therefore, referral back to the primary source of care and eventual specialist referral are warranted to confirm the diagnosis.

TREATMENT

The management of chronic pain conditions uses a multitude of modalities; some are listed in Table 39-3. Emergency physicians must avoid both labeling patients with pain as drug seekers or legitimate patients deserving opioids for pain relief. With these labels, emergency physicians may exacerbate the problem and promote the learned pain response, in which patients believe that they must come to the ED for pain relief. Chronic pain patients often request opioids, although the lure of going to the ED can be just as strong without receiving opioids. Any drug that alters sensorium can exacerbate the learned pain response. The external rewards of visiting the ED for medication or evaluation are many: attention and comforting from family and nursing staff, status as a special patient who must go the ED for pain control, avoiding responsibilities at work and at home, potential money if litigation is involved, and potential income if a disability claim is pending.

Opioids

Before approximately 1990, the use of opioids for chronic pain was discouraged by pain specialists. Since that time, pain specialists have recommended opioids as an important option in a well-integrated treatment program.[7] In a general medical population, 44 percent of those with chronic pain were being managed in part with opioid analgesics.[8] Data from the Drug Abuse Warning Network showed the national trend of increased medical use of opioid analgesics without a concomitant increase in opioid addiction.[9] However, treatment with opiates frequently contributes to the psychopathologic aspects of chronic pain. Further, many types of chronic pain are poorly controlled by opiates, and yet the side effects remain. There are two essential points that affect the use of opioids in the ED: opioids should be used for chronic pain only if they enhance function at home and at work, and one practitioner should be the sole prescriber of opioids or should be aware of their administration by others. A previous opioid addiction is a relative contraindication to the use of opioids in chronic pain; when such patients are treated with opioids, addiction relapse rates approach 50 percent.[10]

Long-acting opioids, such as methadone or transdermal fentanyl, may be more effective than the short-acting agents. Controlled release oxycodone (OxyContin, Purdue Pharma, Stamford, CT) has received considerable attention as a drug frequently abused and diverted for illegal sale. The drug can be easily altered to compromise its controlled release properties. The U.S. Drug Enforcement Administration initiated a comprehensive effort in February 2001 to prevent the diversion of OxyContin. Pain specialists defend its continued use for chronic pain provided potential patients are appropriately screened and monitored.[11]

Nonsteroidal Anti-Inflammatory Drugs

Although nonsteroidal anti-inflammatory drugs (NSAIDs) are most helpful in conditions in which there is ongoing tissue injury, such as chronic inflammatory arthritis or cancer-related nerve or bone damage, they are also helpful in many cases of chronic pain in which no evidence of tissue damage or inflammation is evident. Nonsteroidal anti-inflammatory drugs have been shown to be more helpful in acute than in chronic pain[12]; however, NSAIDs have been found to be the most frequently used analgesic for the treatment of chronic pain in a general population.[8] Standard dosing procedures may be followed except in the elderly patients with a history of GI bleeding, those with renal insufficiency, or salicylate hypersensitivity.

Antidepressants

Antidepressants and, most commonly, the tricyclic antidepressant drugs are the most frequently used drugs for the management of chronic pain. Often effective pain control can be achieved at doses lower than those typically required for relief of depression.[2] An evidence-based review found antidepressants effective in chronic low back pain, fibromyalgia, osteoarthritis, and neuropathic pain.[13] A separate meta-analysis found tricyclic antidepressants more effective in states in which symptoms were unexplained, such as fibromyalgia.[14] A meta-analysis looking at the efficacy of selective serotonin reuptake inhibitors in chronic pain found them effective for mixed chronic pain but less effective for migraine headache, fibromyalgia, tension headaches, and diabetic neuropathy.[15] When antidepressants are prescribed in the ED, a follow-up plan should be in place and discussion with a pain specialist is often beneficial. The most common drug and initial dose is amitriptyline, 10 to 25 mg, 2 h before bedtime.

Anticonvulsants

Anticonvulsants are used for several pain disorders, especially neuropathic pain. Anticonvulsants prevent bursts of action potentials, which may prevent the severe lancinating pain of certain neuropathic syndromes. Carbamazepine (starting at 100 to 200 mg twice daily), valproic acid (starting at 15 mg/kg daily divided into two doses), and clonazepam (starting at 0.5 mg thrice daily) are frequently used. Gabapentin, a structural analog of γ-aminobutyric acid, has been shown to be effective in postherpetic neuralgia[16] and painful diabetic neuropathy[17] and may have some benefit in complex regional pain syndromes. Gabapentin is started with an initial dose of 300 mg per d and is increased up to 1200 mg thrice daily according to the patient's response.

Other Agents

A meta-analysis has found calcitonin to be effective in the treatment of complex regional pain, type I (reflex sympathetic dystrophy).[18] Calcitonin can be given at a dose of 100 IU/d as an intranasal spray. Prednisone at 60 mg per d also has been recommended for complex regional pain, types I and II, when first recognized after an injury. Muscle relaxants, such as cyclobenzaprine 10 mg every 8 h, have been useful for chronic pain patients, but sedating effects may limit their success. Tramadol is an atypical centrally active analgesic. It produces less respiratory depression, less tolerance, and less potential abuse than do opiates. Tramadol has been used with success in patients with fibromyalgia, migraine headaches, low back pain, and neuropathic pain. The dose of tramadol is 50 to 100 mg every 4 to 6 h by mouth.

Chronic Pain in the Elderly

Elderly patients frequently complain of chronic pain. Unfortunately, many of the commonly used medications for pain have higher complication rates in the elderly. In particular, the NSAIDs are associated with higher rates of gastrointestinal bleeding and renal disease in the elderly. Opioids also may cause debilitating sedation and/or constipation in the elderly; however, opioids may produce fewer serious side effects than NSAIDs. Doses of many agents should be reduced when treating the elderly to avoid side effects, and it is essential that a follow-up plan be in place at the time of discharge. There is a perception that the elderly are undermedicated for pain control. This may be true, but the elderly do not seem to be undermedicated more than any other age group.

DISPOSITION

Referral to an appropriate specialist is one of the most productive means of aiding in the care of chronic pain patients who present to the ED. Chronic pain clinics have been successful in changing the lives of patients by eliminating opioid use, decreasing medication use by two-thirds and pain levels by one-third, and increasing work hours twofold. Patients' compliance with pain clinics may improve if the benefits are explained. Admission to the hospital is rarely indicated for chronic pain patients. However, occasionally patients may be admitted for pain control, possibly using self-controlled analgesic administration.

MANAGEMENT OF PATIENTS WITH DRUG-SEEKING BEHAVIOR

There are few controlled studies on "drug-seeking behavior." The spectrum of drug-seeking patients includes those who have chronic pain and have been prescribed limited opioids, the drug addict who is trying to supplement a habit, and the "hustler" who is obtaining prescription drugs to sell on the street. Patients may move from chronic pain patient to addict to hustler as their social and financial supports deteriorate.

Epidemiology

It is impossible to separate prescription drug abuse from other forms of substance abuse. Opioids, stimulants, depressants, and unexpected drugs of abuse, such as antibiotics (used to treat patients with suspected injection drug use infections) and β-blockers (used to limit debilitating subjective anxiety), are examples of abused agents. The Drug Abuse Warning Network tracked drug-related visits in a sampling of U.S. EDs and found that the incidence of visits to the ED involving abuse of opioid analgesics or combinations rose 85 percent between 1994 and 2000.[19] Physicians have been well implicated in this process. The "four Ds" have been used by the American Medical Association to describe physicians who contribute to prescription drug abuse: the disabled (impaired) doctor, the dishonest ("script") doctor who illegally sells drugs, the duped doctor who unwittingly prescribes drugs of abuse to drug-seeking patients and the dated doctor whose obsolete prescribing practices may lend themselves to drug dependency or abuse. Drug-seeking patients are very persistent and suc-

cessful. A study conducted in Portland found that drug-seeking patients presented to the ED 12.6 times per year, visited 4.1 different hospitals, and used 2.2 different aliases.[20] Patients who were refused opioids at one facility were successful in obtaining opioids at another facility 93 percent of the time and were later successful at obtaining opioids from the same facility 71 percent of the time.[20]

Clinical Features

Because of the spectrum of drug-seeking patients, the history given may be factual or fraudulent. Drug seekers may be demanding, intimidating, or flattering. In one ED study, the most common complaints of patients who were drug seeking were (in decreasing order): back pain, headache, extremity pain, and dental pain.[20] Patients may complain of panic disorder or drug withdrawal symptoms and request benzodiazepines (Table 39-4). In some cases, observations of vital signs and physical examination findings will help the physician identify factitious illness, but even experienced clinicians are frequently misled.[20]

Patients should be examined for signs of injection drug use, including needle marks and healed or active superficial cutaneous abscesses, and the heart should be examined for evidence of a new murmur and other signs of endocarditis. Patients attempting to simulate nephrolithiasis can falsify hematuria by biting their buccal mucosa and spitting into the urine sample or by pricking their finger and dipping it into the urine sample. Patients who are suspected of factitious hematuria can have a repeat urine sample collected during observation. Patients with factitious acute injury may massage old deformities to create the appearance of erythema and swelling, but this will dissipate over time if the clinician stops the patient from holding the extremity. Patients may self-mutilate, usually with the dominant hand, and seek opioids. Patients may have evidence of chronic pain or, most commonly, have completely normal physical examination findings. Widespread anecdotal experience of ED personnel has indicated that such patients will relate an "allergy" to alternative pharmacotherapy and insist that only one or two specific opioids are effective.

TABLE 39-4 Common Fraudulent Techniques Used by Drug Seekers and Their Management

Technique	Characteristics	Management
Lost prescription	Calls or returns stating that opioid prescription was lost before being filled	Establish a policy; no opioid prescriptions refilled Notify all patients at discharge as they receive prescriptions
Impending surgery	Wants temporizing opioids, doctor "unavailable," previous surgery, patient from out of town	Call physician Check medical records Offer substitute for opioid
Carries own records and x-rays	Suspicious or forged records, doctor's written permission to receive opioids, patient from out of town	Make phone calls Check records Offer substitute for opioid
Factitious hematuria with complaint of kidney stones	Appears comfortable or overacting, pricked finger dipped in urine, lip/cheek bitten and blood spit into urine	Examine fingers and mouth Obtain witnessed urinalysis Use ketorolac intravenously Obtain confirmatory test before giving opioid
Self-mutilation	Done with dominant hand, requests opioids for pain	Use bupivacaine for local block Do not prescribe opioids without indications Offer substitute for opioids
Dental pain	Dental caries only	Give local nerve block with bupivacaine Refer to dentist
Factitious injury	Old injury, old deformity, self-massaged to produce erythema, patient from out of town	X-ray before treatment Check records Check for erythema that dissipates over time
Partner waiting near telephone at home	"Call my doctor," handwritten number offered, partner answers: "Doctor so-and-so"	Question respondent for medical knowledge Verify number with telephone company
Partner in emergency department	Confirms history, urges opioids	Check records Send to waiting room if verbally abusive

Diagnosis

The diagnosis of drug-seeking behavior may not be possible in the ED. The medical record can provide a wealth of information about the patient, including documentation proving that the patient is supplying false information. Often the diagnosis is suspected in the ED but cannot be confirmed. In such cases, a notation should be made in the chart listing the physician's concerns, but physicians should be careful when using diagnoses such as "drug-seeking behavior" without solid evidence. A listing or card file at the nurses' desk of "drug seekers" violates confidentiality between patient and physician unless it is part of the patient's permanent medical record and subject to the same controls restricting access. Drug-seeking behaviors can be divided into two groups: predictive and less predictive (Table 39-5). The predictive behaviors are illegal in many states and form a solid basis to refuse opioids to the patient. Even so, the patient may have pain and should be evaluated for a medical or surgical illness and possibly treated with a non-opioid drug.

Schedule drug registries and other computerized tracking systems may help emergency physicians identify patients who are abusing or overusing prescription drugs. For example, Kentucky has initiated the Kentucky All Scheduled Prescription Electronic Registry that tracks the dispensing of all scheduled drugs in that state. Turn-around time is not immediate, and information lags 2 to 3 weeks after prescriptions are filled, but the information is valuable to track repeat patients. Pharmacy chains maintain computerized records, and occasionally pharmacists can help physicians make assessments of patients' controlled substance use.

Specific Issues: Legal Implications

The Drug Enforcement Agency (in addition to state agencies) licenses physicians to administer or dispense controlled substances. However, state law determines most prescribing regulations. Physicians should be aware of state laws regulating controlled substances prescribed in their practice setting. Prescribing opioids to a known drug addict could result in restriction of the physician's medical license in some states. However, if a patient refuses to acknowledge an addiction, the physician cannot be held accountable unless medical records at the facility where the patient presents document the addiction. In all states, it is illegal for patients to forge or alter prescriptions. In some states, it is illegal for patients to use aliases or factitious illness to obtain opioids. Further, in some states, concealing previous or recent prescriptions for opioids when requesting opioids from a new practitioner is illegal.

Treatment and Disposition

The treatment of drug-seeking behavior is to refuse the controlled substance, consider the need for alternative medication or treatment, and consider referral for drug counseling. The patient who complains of multiple drug allergies can be difficult. Occasionally the medical record will show previous administration of the drug in question (usually an opioid substitute) with no adverse reaction other than no pain relief. When confronted with a physician's discovery of their fraudulent behavior, many drug-seeking patients become verbally abusive, and hospital security may be required to escort the patient out of the ED. Alternatives to opioids can be offered, and patients should be told that refusal to prescribe opioids is not a refusal of care.

When drug-seeking behavior is confirmed or suspected in the ED, it should be documented in the chart, with careful attention to the facts. When physicians are notified by a pharmacist of forged or altered prescriptions, law enforcement authorities should be called, and physicians should cooperate with the legal investigation. The prosecution of many fraudulent behaviors, such as using aliases to obtain opioids, requires the involvement of the state bureau of investigation or a similar state agency. Physicians may inquire about the legal proceedings with the hospital attorney or the police.

TABLE 39-5   Characteristics of Drug-Seeking Behavior

Behaviors predictive of drug-seeking behavior*
  Sells prescription drugs
  Forges/alters prescriptions
  Factitious illness, requests opioids
  Uses aliases to receive opioids
  Admits to illicit drug addiction
  Conceals multiple physicians prescribing opioids
  Conceals multiple emergency department visits receiving opioids
Less predictive of drug-seeking behavior
  Admits to multiple doctors prescribing opioids
  Admits to multiple prescriptions for opioids
  Abusive when refused
  Multiple drug allergies
  Uses excessive flattery
  From out of town
  Asks for drugs by name

*Behaviors in this category are unlawful in many states.

REFERENCES

1. Turk DC, Okifuji A: Perception of traumatic onset, compensation status, and physical findings: Impact on pain severity, emotional distress, and disability in chronic pain patients. *J Behav Med* 14:435, 1996.
2. Garcia J, Altman RD: Chronic pain states: Pathophysiology and medical therapy. *Semin Arthritis Rheum* 27:1, 1997.
3. Valat JP, Goupille P, Vedere V: Low back pain: Risk factors for chronicity. *Rev Rheum Engl Ed* 64:189, 1997.
4. Waddell G, Feder G, Lewis M: Systemic reviews of bed rest and advice to stay active for acute low back pain. *Br J Gen Pract* 47:647, 1997.
5. Faas A: Exercises: Which ones are worth trying, for which patients, and when. *Spine* 21:2874, 1996.
6. Cooney WP: Somatic versus sympathetic mediated chronic limb pain: Experiences and treatment options. *Hand Clin* 13:355, 1997.
7. Khouzam RH: Chronic pain and its management in primary care. *South Med J* 93:946, 2000.
8. Clark JD: Chronic pain prevalence and analgesic prescribing in a general medical practice. *J Pain Symptom Manage* 23:131, 2002.
9. Joranson DE, Ryan KM, Gilson AM, et al: Trends in medical use and abuse of opioid analgesics. *JAMA* 283:1710, 2000.
10. Dunbar SA, Katz NP: Chronic opioid therapy for nonmalignant pain in patients with a history of substance abuse. *J Pain Symptom Manage* 11:163, 1996.
11. Passik SD: Responding rationally to recent reports of abuse/diversion of OxyContin. *J Pain Symptom Manage* 21:359, 2001.
12. Deyo RA: Drug therapy for back pain: Which drugs help which patients. *Spine* 21:2840, 1996.
13. Fishbain D: Evidence-based data on pain relief with antidepressants. *Ann Med* 32:305, 2000.
14. O'Malley PG, Jackson JL, Santoro J, et al: Antidepressant therapy for unexplained symptoms and symptom syndromes. *J Fam Pract* 48:980, 1999.
15. Jung AC, Staiger T, Sullivan M: The efficacy of selective serotonin reuptake inhibitors for the management of chronic pain. *J Gen Intern Med* 12:384, 1997.
16. Rowbotham M, Harden N, Stacey B, et al: Gabapentin for the treatment of postherpetic neuralgia. *JAMA* 280:1837, 1998.
17. Backonja M, Beydoun A, Edwards KR, et al: Gabapentin for symptomatic treatment of painful diabetic neuropathy in patients with diabetes mellitus. *JAMA* 280:1831, 1998.
18. Perez RSGM, Kwakkel G, Zuurmond WWA, et al: Treatment of reflex sympathetic dystrophy (CRPS Type 1): A research synthesis of 21 randomized controlled trials. *J Pain Symptom Manage* 21:511, 2001.
19. *Emergency Department Trends From the Drug Abuse Warning Network, Preliminary Estimates January–June 2001 With Revised Estimates 1994–2000.* Rockville, MD, National Clearinghouse for Alcohol and Drug Information, 2002.
20. Zechnich AD, Hedges JR: Community-wide emergency department visits by patients suspected of drug seeking behavior. *Acad Emerg Med* 3:312, 1996.

EMERGENCY WOUND MANAGEMENT

40

EVALUATION OF WOUNDS
Judd E. Hollander
Adam J. Singer

EPIDEMIOLOGY

In 2000, over 8 million traumatic wounds were evaluated in emergency departments across the United States, accounting for about 7 percent of all ED visits.[1] The face, scalp, fingers, and hands are the most commonly involved areas of injury.[2] Approximately 40 percent of traumatic lacerations seen in the ED are caused by blunt objects.[2] Wounds on children differ from wounds on adults; lacerations in children are more likely to be located on the head, linear, shorter, less contaminated, and more often caused by blunt trauma.[3,4]

INITIAL EVALUATION

Evaluation of the patient with a traumatic wound should begin with an overall assessment of the patient. Practitioners should exclude less obvious but more serious life-threatening injuries before directing attention to wound management. Initial wound management should be conducted in concert with ascertainment of the patient's past medical history and circumstances surrounding the injury.[5]

External bleeding can usually be controlled by application of pressure over the bleeding site. Tourniquet application is not recommended for routine wound care. When possible, skin flaps should be returned to their original position prior to application of pressure in order to prevent worsening vascular compromise. When amputated fingers or extremities are recovered, they should be covered with a moist, sterile, protective dressing, placed in a waterproof bag, and then placed in a container of ice water for preservation and consideration of future reattachment. Constricting rings or other jewelry that encircle the injured body part should be removed as soon as possible to prevent circumferential objects from acting as constricting bands when swelling progresses. Clothing over the injured area should be removed to reduce the potential for contamination.

Patient comfort should be considered a priority. Pain can initially be minimized by compassionate and professional evaluation of the patient. Before wound exploration, cleansing, and repair, most patients will need some form of anesthesia.[6] Preparing the local anesthetic out of the sight of the patient will help reduce anxiety caused by seeing the needle. Systemic analgesia or procedural sedation may be required (see Chap. 38).

Medical History

Proper wound management begins with a thorough patient history (Table 40-1). The practitioner should ascertain the presence or absence of various factors that can have adverse effects on wound healing. Host factors such as patient age, diabetes mellitus, chronic renal failure, obesity, malnutrition, and the use of immunosuppressive medications may increase the risk of wound infection and impair wound healing.[7] The presence of connective tissue disorders such as Ehlers-Danlos syndrome, Marfan syndrome, osteogenesis imperfecta, and protein and vitamin C deficiencies can also impact wound healing.[8] The tendency of patients to form keloids should be ascertained by both history and examination, since past keloid formation may predict poor scar formation. Both Black and Asian patients are prone to keloid formation.[8] Keloids grow beyond the original wound boundaries compared

to hypertropic scars, which stay within the original wound boundaries and are usually due to tissue tension during healing.

A detailed history of any allergies to anesthetic agents or antibiotics is essential. With the increased incidence of severe reactions to latex products, one must also review any prior allergies to latex.[9] The history of prior tetanus immunization and the need for further tetanus vaccination should be determined (see Chap. 48).

Identification of the mechanism of injury will help identify the presence of any potential wound contaminants and foreign bodies. Bite wounds are at high risk for infection and must be managed differently than other lacerations (see Chap. 47). Patients should be questioned about the presence of a foreign body. Patients with a foreign body sensation are more likely to have a retained foreign body than those without (sensitivity = 43%, specificity = 83%, LR(+) = 2.49, and LR(−) = 0.69).[10] Both foreign body retention and visible contamination increase the risk of infection.[11] Organic and inorganic components of soil can cause infection; wounds contaminated by soil can become infected by very small doses of bacterial inoculum. The major inorganic soil components that cause infection are the clay fractions; sand grains and black dirt from roadways are relatively inert.

The type of forces applied at the time of injury also helps predict the likelihood of infection.[11] The most common mechanism of injury is application of a blunt force such as bumping the head against a stationary object. The skin is crushed against an underlying bone, and it splits. Sharp objects that cut through the skin produce shear forces. Crush injuries are more susceptible to infection than wounds resulting from shearing forces, because they tend to cause greater tissue devitalization.[12]

Low-energy impact injuries may not result in lacerations; instead they may disrupt vessels, leading to ecchymosis or hematoma formation. Some hematomas spontaneously resorb. Those that become encapsulated usually require treatment by aspiration or incision and drainage.

The practitioner should determine the time that the injury occurred. The time interval from injury to closure of a laceration is directly related to the growth of the bacterial inoculum that presumably leads to an increased incidence of wound infection. However, the length of time from injury to closure that results in an clinically relevant increase in the incidence of infection is less clear[8,11] (Table 40-2). A widely quoted study from Jamaica used healing, defined as epithelialization without infection, as the main outcome.[14] This study of 204 lacerations found that head lacerations healed well regardless of the time to closure, even up to 100 h. In contrast, lacerations of the trunk or extremities had lower rates of healing, particularly if they were closed more than 19 h after injury. Other studies have not found a correlation between time from injury to closure and postrepair wound infection.[4,11] Therefore time from injury until presentation is only one element to be considered, in addition to the wound etiology, location, degree of contamination, host risk factors, and the importance of cosmetic appearance, before determining whether or not to perform primary wound closure. Wounds that are not closed primarily because of a high risk of infection should be considered for delayed primary closure after 4 days. After 4 days of open wound management, the risk of infection after closure substantially decreases.

The patient should be asked whether the wound was sustained from an intentional act (e.g., assault or self-inflected) or unintentional event. Most states have regulations that require the reporting of intentional injuries, and patients with self-inflicted injuries should be considered for psychiatric evaluation. Occupational injuries may require alternative follow-up arrangements, so their presence should be ascertained.

TABLE 40-1   Pertinent Medical History

Symptoms
  Pain, swelling, paresthesias, motor function
Type of force causing injury
  Crush or shear
  Bite or puncture
Elements of contamination
  Time elapsed from injury until initial cleansing
  Time elapsed from injury until presentation
  Wound care performed prior to ED arrival
  Object that caused injury (glass, wood, etc.)
  Cleanliness of body and environment at time of injury and afterwards
Factors resulting in injury
  Intentional versus unintentional
  Occupation or non-occupational related
  Assault or self-inflicted
Foreign body potential
  Did the object break or shatter?
  Foreign body sensation
  Removal of portion of object
Function
  Occupation and handedness
Allergies
  Anesthetics, analgesics, antibiotics, and latex
Medications
Chronic medical conditions that increase risk of infection
Chronic medical conditions that increase likelihood of poor wound healing
Previous scar formation (hypertrophic scars or keloids)

Many patients may have already attempted to cleanse or care for their wound. The clinician should inquire about any treatments or home remedies that the patient has used to self-manage the laceration, including solutions or cleansing agents that may have been applied.

The anatomic location of the injury helps predict the clinical outcome, both in terms of infection risk and cosmetic result[4,11,15] (Table 40-3). The risk of infection is determined largely by the interplay between baseline bacterial colonization and vascular blood supply. With respect to bacterial colonization, the density of the bacterial population is low on the upper arms, legs, and torso. Conversely, moist areas of the body, such as the axilla, perineum, toe webs, and intertriginous areas harbor millions of bacteria per square centimeter, including anaerobes. Obviously, any wounds with human or animal fecal contaminants run a high risk of infection, even with therapeutic intervention.

In addition to bacterial flora, anatomical variation in regional blood flow also plays a role in determining the likelihood of infection. Wounds located on highly vascular areas, such as the face or scalp, are less likely to be infected than wounds located in less vascular areas.[4,11,14] The in-

creased vascularity of the area more than offsets the high bacterial inoculum found in the scalp. Lacerations of the scalp and face have a very low infection rate regardless of the intensity of cleansing.[16]

Wound Examination

Wound examination should be conducted when the patient is calm and cooperative and positioned appropriately, with optimal lighting conditions, and with little or no residual bleeding. Cursory examination under poor lighting or when the depths of the wound are obscured by blood will occasionally result in poor detection of foreign bodies and possibly damage to important structures. If bleeding is a problem, epinephrine-containing anesthetic solutions may be helpful, when not contraindicated. Finger tourniquets may be used to obtain a bloodless field, but they should not be used for more than 30 to 60 min. Missed tendon and nerve injuries and retained foreign bodies are common wound-related causes of litigation. The likelihood of these complications can be minimized by performing a compulsory complete physical examination. Lacerations over joints may have penetrated the joint capsule and often the joint should be injected to ensure that there is no communication between the joint space and the laceration. Lacerations over the metacarpophalangeal joints are suspicious for having occurred during a fight (clenched fist injury) and should be treated as though they are human bites.

Adjunctive Testing

Although most lacerations will not require any diagnostic testing, on occasion, wound imaging for detection of foreign bodies may be necessary. Most foreign bodies commonly found in wounds are much denser than the surrounding tissue and are readily apparent on plain radiographs. Metal, bone, teeth, pencil graphite, certain plastics, glass, gravel, sand, some fish bones, some painted wood, and most aluminum are visible on plain radiographs (see Chap. 46). Almost all (>95 percent) glass fragments are visible on radiographs if they are 2 mm or larger in size.[17] If the wound was caused by metal or glass and no foreign body is found on wound exploration or on plain films, it is unlikely that a foreign body exists.[10] Radiopaque skin markers such as paper clips can be placed around the wound entrance so the position of the object can be determined relative to these markers. Some objects will not be identifiable with plain radiography. Computed tomography (CT) and magnetic resonance (MR) imaging are useful for identifying and locating objects that have densities similar to soft tissue. Sonography may also be useful, particularly for wooden foreign bodies, although the sensitivity of sonography is inadequate to reliably exclude small (<2.5 mm) wood fragments.

TABLE 40-2   Risk of Wound Infection as Function of Time from Injury to Closure

	Comments	Distinction Between Early and Late Closure	Infection Rate/Inadequate Healing with Early Closure	Infection Rate/Inadequate Healing with Late Closure	Percent Difference (95% CI)
Morgan 1980[13]	Hand and forearm, all patients received IM penicillin and half received PO clindamycin	4 h	10/148 (7%)	14/69 (21%)	13.5% (3.2 to 23.9%)
Baker 1990[4]	Children, 59% head and neck location	6 h	32/2665 (1.2%)	2/147 (1.3%)	−0.16% (−1.76 to 2.08%)
Berk 1988[14]	All locations	19 h	8/97 (8.2%)	25/107 (23.4%)	15.1% (5.4 to 24.8%)
	Head	19 h	2/44 (5%)	1/36 (3%)	−1.8% (−9.9 to 6.4%)
	Trunk and extremities	19 h	6/53 (11.3%)	24/71 (33.8%)	22.5% (8.6 to 36.4%)

TABLE 40-3   **Risk of Wound Infection as a Function of Anatomic Location**

Location	Risk of Infection
Head and neck	1-2%
Upper extremity	4%
Lower extremity	7%

Patient Education

Patients should be carefully educated regarding the expected cosmetic outcome; they should be informed that there will be some scarring, and if predisposed, possible keloid formation.[15] Some indication of the maximal width of the scar can be predicted based upon wound location, whether the laceration is aligned parallel or perpendicular with lines of minimal tension, and how gaping the wound is while at rest (static tension) or when put through a range of motion (dynamic tension).[15,18] Lacerations over joints (which have more dynamic tension) will have wider scars than similar lacerations subject to less tension. Wounds that deviate from the lines of skin tension will also be prone to greater scar formation after suturing than wounds which are more closely aligned with skin tension.[18] The most important determinant of cosmetic outcome under control of the treating physician is meticulous wound repair with approximation of viable wound edges under little tension. If this is not possible, patients should clearly understand that all lacerations result in some scarring.

REFERENCES

1. Singer AJ, Thode HC: National epidemiology of lacerations. *Ann Emerg Med* 40:541, 2002.
2. Hollander JE, Singer AJ, Valentine S, Henry MC: Wound registry: Development and validation. *Ann Emerg Med* 25:675, 1995.
3. Hollander JE, Singer AJ, Valentine SM: Comparison of wound care practices in pediatric and adult lacerations repaired in the emergency department. *Pediatr Emerg Care* 15:15, 1998.
4. Baker MD, Lanuti M: The management and outcome of lacerations in urban children. *Ann Emerg Med* 19:1001, 1990.
5. Hollander JE: Patient and wound assessment: Basic concepts of the history and physical examination, in Singer AJ, Hollander JE (eds): *Lacerations and Acute Wounds: An Evidence-Based Guide.* Philadelphia, FA Davis Company, 2003, p. 9.
6. Bartfield JM: Wound anesthesia, in Singer AJ, Hollander JE (eds): *Lacerations and Acute Wounds: An Evidence-Based Guide* Philadelphia, FA Davis Company, 2003, p. 23.
7. Cruse PJE, Foord R: A five-year prospective study of 23,649 surgical wounds. *Arch Surg* 107:206, 1973.
8. Singer AJ, Hollander JE, Quinn JV: Evaluation and management of traumatic lacerations. *New Engl J Med* 337:1142, 1997.
9. Charous BL, Blanco C, Tarlo S, et al: Natural rubber latex allergy after 12 years: Recommendations and perspectives. *J Allergy Clin Immunol* 109:31, 2002.
10. Steele MT, Tran LV, Watson WA, Muelleman RL: Retained glass foreign bodies in wounds: Predictive value of wound characteristics, patient perception, and wound exploration. *Am J Emerg Med* 16:627, 1998.
11. Hollander JE, Singer AJ, Valentine SM, Shofer FS: Risk factors for infection in patients with traumatic lacerations. *Acad Emerg Med* 8:716, 2001.
12. Cardany CR, Rodeheaver G, Thacker J, et al: The crush injury: A high risk wound. *JACEP* 5:965, 1976.
13. Morgan WJ, Hutchison D, Johnson HM: The delayed treatment of wounds of the hand and forearm under antibiotic cover. *Br J Surg* 67:140, 1980.
14. Berk WA, Osbourne DD, Taylor DD: Evaluation of the "golden period" for wound repair: 204 cases from a third world emergency department. *Ann Emerg Med* 17:496, 1988.
15. Singer AJ, Quinn JV, Thode HC, Hollander JE: Determinants of poor outcome after laceration and surgical incision repair. *Plast Reconstr Surg* 110:429, 2002.
16. Hollander JE, Richman PB, Werblud M, et al: Irrigation in facial and scalp lacerations: Does it alter outcome? *Ann Emerg Med* 31:73, 1998.
17. Lammers R: Foreign bodies in wounds, in Singer AJ, Hollander JE (eds): *Lacerations and Acute Wounds: An Evidence-Based Guide.* Philadelphia, FA Davis Co, 2003, p. 147.
18. Simon HK, Zempsky WT, Burns TB: Lacerations against Langer's lines: To glue or suture? *J Emerg Med* 16:185, 1998.

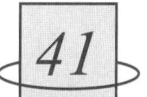

WOUND PREPARATION
Susan Stone
Wallace A. Carter

Wound preparation is the single most important step in treating a traumatic wound. Proper preparation helps set the stage for restoring both the integrity and function of the injured tissue and minimizes the risk of infection and assures the best possible cosmetic result. The majority (80 to 90 percent) of wounds treated in EDs heal with a good outcome. However, careful preparation is particularly important when underlying medical conditions affecting wound healing are present; patients with these conditions have a higher risk of infection (Table 41-1). Many traditional methods of wound preparation have surprisingly little scientific validation.[1,2] This chapter reviews the basic principles of wound preparation, using available experimental models and prospective clinical studies, where available, to justify these techniques.

STERILE TECHNIQUE

While adoption of aseptic technique represented a major advance in medical care, the extent required for ED wound repair remains unclear. Most physicians use sterile gloves alone for ED laceration closure. The use of full sterile technique—with the physician wearing a face mask and hair-covering cap in addition to sterile gloves—does not reduce the incidence of wound infection compared to the use of sterile gloves alone.[3] Conversely, the use of clean, nonsterile examination gloves for suturing does not appreciably increase the incidence of wound infection compared to the use of sterile gloves.[4] Nevertheless, adherence to sterile technique remains the standard of care.

ANESTHESIA

In general, pain control should be provided before extensive wound preparation. Not only is this more humane, the administration of anesthesia and analgesia will enable better preparation and treatment if patients are relaxed and able to cooperate without undue anxiety and pain. Prior to the administration of local or regional anesthetic, the sensory, motor, and vascular examination should be performed.

HEMOSTASIS

Control of bleeding is necessary for proper evaluation of a wound. Diffuse bleeding most often occurs from the subdermal plexus and superficial veins. Direct pressure with saline-soaked sponges or gauze is usually effective in stopping this type of bleeding.

Bleeding from an exposed lacerated vessel is best controlled by direct pressure applied with a gloved fingertip directly on the vessel. Once bleeding is halted, more permanent control can be achieved by clamping the involved vessel, isolating a short length, and ligating it with absorbable synthetic suture (typically 5-0). This approach is most useful for bleeding minor vessels in the extremities, but major arteries of an extremity should not be ligated. Extreme caution must be exercised in the face because of the proximity of important facial structures. Scalp lacerations can bleed extensively from the wound edges due to the highly vascular subcutaneous layer. This bleeding can be

TABLE 41-1   Risk Factors for Poor Wound Repair Outcome

Immunosuppression
   Diabetes
   Chemotherapeutic agents
   Steroids
   Chronic renal failure
   Hematologic malignancies
   Congenital immunodeficiencies
Tissue ischemia
   Peripheral vascular disease
   Anemia
   Vasculitis
Poor wound repair
   Elderly
   Malnourished
   Connective tissue disorders
Wound factors
   Crush injuries
   Tissue loss
   Contamination
   Foreign bodies
   Location

controlled by the use of specially designed clips applied along the wound edges. For bleeding wounds where the involved vessel is not visible, a figure-of-eight or horizontal mattress suture applied adjacent to the wound edge near the site of bleeding will sometimes achieve control. However, this technique may impair blood flow and leave nonviable tissue in the wound.

Chemical means of hemostasis include injected epinephrine, Gelfoam, Oxycel, and Actifoam. Most commonly, epinephrine is mixed with local anesthetics in concentrations of 1:100,000 or 1:200,000 and injected into the wound area. This will induce local vasoconstriction that will allow a longer duration of anesthesia and a larger total local anesthetic dose due to the depot effect of the vasoconstriction. Current practice avoids the use of epinephrine in end organs such as fingers, toes, and tip of nose, ears, and penis, although that practice has been challenged regarding the use of epinephrine mixed with local anesthetics for digital nerve blocks.[5] If epinephrine with lidocaine is inadvertently injected into a digit, nitropaste 1″ can be applied topically to the digit until the effect of epinephrine has dissipated. Blood pressure should be checked to ensure that hypotension does not result. No increase in wound infection has been observed with the addition of epinephrine to local anesthetics used in the ED. Gelfoam, made from denatured gelatin, has no intrinsic hemostatic properties and works by the pressure it exerts as it becomes a fluid-filled sponge. Oxycel, a cellulose derivative, and Actifoam, a collagen sponge, react with blood, forming an artificial clot. These products are not particularly effective for actively bleeding wounds, as the blood can wash them out.

Bipolar electrocautery can achieve hemostasis in blood vessels smaller than 2 mm in diameter, but if improperly or too extensively applied, results in tissue necrosis. Electrocautery units are not routinely available in many EDs. Battery-powered hand-held cautery units are more readily available but do not generate sufficient heat to produce coagulation in vessels larger than capillaries.

Extremity wounds that are refractory to direct pressure, ligation, or cautery may require a tourniquet. Although helpful in stopping exsanguination, tourniquets may compress and damage underlying blood vessels and nerves, reducing tissue viability. The simplest tourniquet to use in an ED is a blood pressure cuff placed proximal to the wound and inflated above the patient's systolic pressure. Elevating the extremity to reduce venous blood volume prior to cuff inflation is useful. If an extremity tourniquet is needed to control bleeding, the patient is best explored and repaired in the operating room.

FOREIGN-BODY REMOVAL

Obvious foreign debris should be carefully removed from the wound, using forceps to avoid injury to the physician from sharp edges or points. Probing wounds with a gloved fingertip to detect foreign bodies by palpation is discouraged. Clinical clues to the presence of a foreign body include foreign body sensation, point tenderness, or increased pain on range of motion. Visual wound inspection, down to the full depth and along the full course of the wound, is the most important method for detecting foreign bodies. Imaging modalities-plain radiology, ultrasound, computed tomography (CT), and magnetic resonance (MR) imaging-have a role in selected patients (see Chap. 46).

SKIN DISINFECTION

A common practice is to disinfect intact skin around the wound with either a povidone-iodine based or chlorhexidine-containing agent. While these agents suppress bacterial growth on intact skin, they impair host defenses and promote bacterial growth in the wound itself. When used, skin disinfectants should be applied from the wound edges outward and care taken to avoid spillage into the wound.

HAIR REMOVAL

Hair can interfere with wound closure, become entangled in sutures or staples, and act as a foreign body, potentially increasing the risk of wound infection. Conversely, in well perfused tissues (e.g., scalp) wounds closed without prior hair removal heal with no apparent increase in infection.[6] If necessary, hair should be removed by clipping 1 to 2 mm above the skin with scissors.[1,2] Shaving the area with a razor damages the hair follicle, allowing bacterial invasion, and is associated with a tenfold increase in infection rates when compared with clipping. An alternative method to clipping is to use ointment or saline to allow hair to be parted away from wound edges. Hair should never be removed from the eyebrows, because of the potential for that hair to not regenerate or to grow back abnormally. Likewise, hair may provide good landmarks for alignment of wound edges during suturing, and removal at the skin-hair interface (eyebrows or scalp) should be avoided when possible.

IRRIGATION

Effective irrigation decreases bacterial count and helps to remove foreign bodies, thereby reducing the risk of wound infection.[1,2] Because of the discomfort involved, local anesthetic is usually necessary prior to irrigation. Irrigation pressures of 5 to 8 psi are recommended, which are easily achieved using a 19-gauge needle with either a 35-mL or 65-mL syringe.[7] Sufficient pressures will not be generated using a bulb syringe or fluid directly from the intravenous fluid bags. Although the exact volume of irrigant required is not known, a common recommendation is to use 60 mL per cm of wound length, although a large observational study found no correlation between the incidence of infection and the volume of irrigation, provided at least 200 mL was used.[8]

Wound soaking is not effective in cleansing contaminated wounds and may actually increase wound bacterial counts.[9] Routine scrubbing of traumatic wounds with a sponge is ineffective, inflicting trauma and impairing resistance to infection.

Sterile normal saline, the most commonly used irrigant, also has the lowest toxicity. There is no added benefit to the addition of an antiseptic (such as povidone-iodine or hydrogen peroxide) to the irrigant.[10] Recent studies have found that tap water irrigation of simple cutaneous lacerations is as safe and efficacious as sterile normal saline.[11] In addition, tap water is easily obtained in large quantities at almost no cost.

Universal Precautions should be observed while participating in wound care. Contaminated fluid can easily be splashed onto health care workers during irrigation, so barrier protection should be used. Irrigation shields attached to the irrigation system may prevent some of the splashing associated with irrigation, but are no substitute for Universal Precautions.

Recently, the need for routine irrigation of traumatic wounds has been questioned, particularly for simple non-bite, non-contaminated wounds in highly vascular areas, such as the scalp and face, and in wounds closed with skin tapes instead of sutures.[12,13]

DEBRIDEMENT

The next step in wound preparation is debridement of nonviable tissue.[1,2] Devitalized tissue may increase the risk of infection and delay healing by acting as a culture medium and inhibiting leukocyte phagocytosis. Debridement not only removes foreign matter, bacteria, and devitalized tissue, but it also creates a clean wound edge that is easier to repair. After debridement is completed, wounds should be re-irrigated.

The most effective type of debridement is excision, because it converts a contaminated wound into a clean surgical wound. A standard surgical blade is recommended. Tissue that has a narrow base or lacks capillary refill will require excision. The goal of debridement is to reestablish a margin of normal tissue at wound edges. The easiest technique for excisional debridement is to mark an elliptical area around the sides of the wound, and then use a surgical blade to cut only through the epidermis. Skin lines should be respected, and extensive excision should be avoided.

Wounds with an extensive amount of nonviable tissue or heavy contamination are more problematic. They may require a large amount of tissue removal and will need more delayed wound closure or grafting. In general, a surgeon should be consulted to manage these wounds.

Debridement has become such a standard in wound care, it is difficult to conceive of a situation in which it should not be applied. However, in cases of wounds that were not sutured (e.g., low-velocity civilian gunshot wounds to the extremities), conservative wound care (irrigation and cleaning) had the same incidence of wound infection as routine wound debridement.[14]

PROPHYLACTIC ANTIBIOTICS

Infections occur in approximately 3 to 5 percent of traumatic wounds repaired in EDs, although this rate varies widely according to mechanism, location, and patient factors.[3] Wound location, extremes of age, crush injuries, puncture or avulsion wounds, retained foreign bodies, and contamination are all risk factors for infection. Less vascular areas, moist areas (axilla and perineum), and exposed areas (feet and hands) also tend to be at higher risk for infection. Crush or puncture wounds are more prone to infection due to the tensile and compressive forces generated that increase the potential for devitalized tissue. The most important step in prevention of a wound infection is adequate irrigation and debridement.

To reduce the incidence of wound infections, antibiotics have been commonly used for years, although there is no clear evidence that antibiotic prophylaxis prevents wound infections in most patients whose wounds are closed in the ED[3,15] (see Chap. 48). Antibiotic prophylaxis has been studied and well accepted in some surgical procedures.[16] The principles learned from these studies are that effectiveness requires the achievement of antimicrobial blood levels prior to or rapidly after wound contamination, and there is no benefit for continuing antibiotics past 24 h in most cases. If used, antibiotic prophylaxis for traumatic wounds in an ED should be (1) initiated before significant tissue manipulation is done; (2) performed with agents that are effective against predicted pathogens; and (3) administered by routes that rapidly achieve desired blood levels. There are no studies that compare the common practice of intravenous administration of the initial dose of prophylactic antibiotics with oral administration. Based on the above principles, the oral route may be as effective if administered before manipulation using an agent with appropriate spectrum and rapid oral absorption.

For wounds contaminated by debris or feces or caused by punctures or bites, wounds with tissue destruction or in avascular areas, and neglected wounds, sufficient bacteria may be present to cause infection, and prophylactic antibiotics are often administered. Since most non-bite wound infections are due to staphylococci or streptococci, amoxicillin-clavolanate or a first-generation cephalosporin provides reasonable coverage. For human bites in all locations and for mammalian bites on the hands, amoxicillin-clavulanate should be used to cover both *Pasteurella* and *Eikenella*. Prophylactic antibiotics do not reduce the incidence of wound infection following dog or cat bites on areas other than the hands.[17,18] Full-thickness oral lacerations should receive penicillin.[19] Wounds contaminated by fresh water and plantar puncture wounds through athletic shoes, should include *Pseudomonas* coverage.

The duration for antibiotic prophylaxis is unknown; most physicians use 3 to 5 days for non-bite wounds and 5 to 7 days for bite wounds. Patients with established wound infections usually require longer treatment. A wound warranting antibiotics should be reevaluated at 24 to 48 h, or patients should be given clear instructions to return at the earliest sign of infection. Contaminated wounds, or those with undetected foreign bodies, may still develop infection despite antibiotic prophylaxis.

REFERENCES

1. Singer A, Hollander JE, Quinn JV: Evaluation and management of traumatic lacerations. *New Engl J Med* 337:1142, 1997.
2. Hollander JE, Singer AJ: Laceration management. *Ann Emerg Med* 34:356, 1999.
3. Hollander JE, Singer AJ, Valentine SM, Shofer FS: Risk factors of infection in patients with traumatic lacerations. *Acad Emerg Med* 8:716, 2001.
4. Whorl GJ: Repairing skin lacerations. *Can Fam Physician* 33:1185, 1987.
5. Wilhelmi BJ, Blackwell SJ, Miller JH, et al: Do not use epinephrine in digital blocks: Myth or truth? *Plast Reconstr Surg* 107:393, 2001.
6. Howell JM, Morgan JA: Scalp laceration repair without prior hair removal. *Am J Emerg Med* 6:7, 1988.
7. Singer AJ, Hollander JE, Subramanian S, et al: Pressure dynamics of various irrigation techniques commonly used in the emergency department. *Ann Emerg Med* 24:36, 1994.
8. Singer AJ, Hollander JE, Cassara G, et al: Level of training, wound care practices, and infection rates. *Am J Emerg Med* 13:265, 1995.
9. Lammers RL, Fourre M, Callaham ML, Boone T: Effect of povidone-iodine and saline soaking on bacterial counts in acute traumatic contaminated wounds. *Ann Emerg Med* 19:709, 1990.
10. Dire DJ, Welch AP: A comparison of wound irrigation solutions used in the emergency department. *Ann Emerg Med* 19:704, 1990.
11. Bansal BC, Wiebe RA, Perkins SD, Abramo TJ: Tap water for irrigation of lacerations. *Am J Emerg Med* 20:469, 2002.
12. Hollander JE, Richman PB, Werblud M, et al: Irrigation in facial and scalp lacerations: Does it alter outcome? *Ann Emerg Med* 31:73, 1998.
13. Maharaj D, Sharma D, Ramdass M, Naraynsingh V: Closure of traumatic wounds without cleaning and suturing. *Postgrad Med J* 78:281, 2002.
14. Brunner RG, Fallon WF: A prospective, randomized clinical trial of wound debridement versus conservative wound care in soft-tissue injury from civilian gunshot wounds. *Am Surg* 56:104, 1990.
15. Cummings P, Del Beccaro MA: Antibiotics to prevent infection of simple wounds: A meta-analysis of randomized studies. *Am J Emerg Med* 13:396, 1995.
16. McDonald M, Grabsch E, Marshall C, Forbes A: Single - versus multiple-dose antimicrobial prophylaxis for major surgery: A systematic review. *Aust NZ J Surg* 68:388, 1998.
17. Medeiros I, Saconato H: Antibiotic prophylaxis for mammalian bites. *Cochrane Database Syst Rev* 2:CD001738, 2001.
18. Dire DJ, Hogan RE, Riggs MW: A prospective evaluation of risk factors for infections from dog-bite wounds. *Acad Emerg Med* 1:258, 1994.
19. Steele MT, Sainsbury CR, Robinson WA, et al: Prophylactic penicillin for intraoral wounds. *Ann Emerg Med* 18:847, 1989.

METHODS FOR WOUND CLOSURE
Adam J. Singer
Judd E. Hollander

The skin is the largest organ in the human body; its primary function is to serve as a barrier between the organism and the external environment. The major goal of wound closure is to restore the skin's integrity in order to reduce the risk of infection, scarring, and impaired function.[1] This may be achieved by one of three methods. With primary closure, the wound is immediately closed by approximating its edges. The main advantage of primary closure is a reduction in healing time in comparison with other closure methods. Rapid wound closure also may reduce bleeding and discomfort often associated with open wounds. Secondary wound closure, in which the wound is left open and allowed to close on its own, is particularly well suited for highly contaminated or infected wounds as well as in patients at high risk of infection. While this method may reduce the risk of infection, it is relatively slow and uncomfortable and leaves a larger scar than primary closure. Delayed primary (or tertiary) closure combines the advantages of both primary and secondary closure. With this method the wound is left open for a period of 4 to 5 days after which it may be closed if no infection supervenes. A recent small study of simple hand and finger lacerations challenges the principle of primary closure.[2] Wounds randomized to secondary closure healed as fast as those closed primarily with no notable differences in appearance and function.[2] However, since this study was limited to short, superficial hand lacerations it cannot be widely recommended for all wounds and lacerations at this time.

OVERVIEW OF WOUND CLOSURE METHODS

Lacerations may be closed by one of four commonly available methods or devices: sutures, staples, adhesive tapes, or tissue adhesives. Each method has advantages and disadvantages (Table 42-1). Choice of the wound closure method and timing should take into account both patient and wound characteristics (Table 42-2). Cosmetic outcome is more

TABLE 42-1   Advantages and Disadvantages of Wound Closure Devices

Technique	Advantages	Disadvantages
Suture	Time-honored Meticulous closure Greatest tensile strength Lowest dehiscence rate	Requires removal Requires anesthesia Greatest tissue reactivity Highest cost Slowest application
Staples	Rapid application Low tissue reactivity Low cost Low risk of needle-stick	Less meticulous closure May interfere with some imaging techniques (CT, MRI)
Tissue adhesives	Rapid application Patient comfort Resistant to bacterial growth No need for removal Low cost No risk of needle-stick	Lower tensile strength than 5-0 or larger sutures Dehiscence over high tension areas (joints) Not useful on hands Cannot bathe or swim (can shower)
Adhesive tapes	Least reactive Lowest infection rates Rapid application Patient comfort Low cost No risk of needle-stick	Frequently fall off Lower tensile strength than sutures Highest rate of dehiscence Require use of toxic adjuncts Cannot be used in areas with hair Cannot get wet

Source: Adapted with permission from Hollander JE, Singer AJ: Laceration management. *Ann Emerg Med* 34:356, 1999.

TABLE 42-2   Patient and Wound Considerations that Affect Wound Healing

Patient Characteristics	Clinical Implications
Age	Increased infection rates at the extremes Impaired healing in elderly or with peripheral vascular disease
Immunocompromising conditions: Diabetes mellitus, renal failure, AIDS, splenectomy, etc.	Increased infection rates
Medications	Increased infection rates with systemic steroids and other immunocompromising agents

Wound Characteristics	Clinical Implications
Time from injury	Increased bacterial counts with time; "golden period" (time during which it is safe to close wounds) is highly variable
Location	Increased infection rates with extremity lacerations Very low infection rates with scalp and facial lacerations
Etiology	Increased infection rates with bites, presence of foreign bodies or debris
Mechanism of injury	Increased infection rates and poorer scarring with crush injuries
Laceration width	Increased infection rates and poorer scarring with wider lacerations

closely related to practitioner technique and the patient's own healing characteristics than to any specific closure method or device.

One of the most important considerations when choosing a wound closure method is the amount of tension on the wound, both static (at rest) and dynamic (with motion). *Linear lacerations subject to little tension* can usually be closed by any one of the four closure methods. In this case, the practitioner should take into consideration patient characteristics and preferences such as compliance, the availability to return for follow-up and device removal, and overall level of anxiety. *With low-tension irregular lacerations,* sutures may be the best alternative, allowing the greatest degree of precision with accurate wound approximation. With *lacerations subject to high tension* (static and/or dynamic) it is vital to relieve the amount of tension on the wound in order to avoid early dehiscence or gradual widening of the scar.[3] Relief of tension is best achieved by careful undermining, placement of deep dermal sutures, and wound immobilization (when appropriate). After placement of deep, tension-relieving sutures, the superficial epidermal layer may be closed by any of the aforementioned closure methods.

With patients at risk of keloid formation, it is best to relieve tension and minimize the amount of foreign material introduced into the wound.

SUTURES

Sutures are the most commonly used method to close lacerations.[4] Sutures are the strongest of all closure devices and allow the most accurate approximation of wound edges, regardless of its shape. However, sutures are the most time consuming and operator dependent of all wound closure methods. In general, sutures may be divided into absorbable and nonabsorbable. By definition, *nonabsorbable sutures* retain their tensile strength for at least 60 days. They are most often used to close the outermost layer of the skin or for repair of tendons. Nonabsorbable sutures are classified based on their origin and configuration (Table 42-3). Monofilament synthetic sutures (such as nylon or

TABLE 42-3   Nonabsorbable Suture Characteristics

Suture	Structure	Raw Material	Tensile Strength Retention In Vivo	Tissue Reactivity	Common ED Uses
Silk	Braided	Organic protein called fibroin	Degradation of fiber results in loss of strength over many months	Significant inflammatory reaction	Intraoral mucosal surfaces for comfort
Nylon (Ethilon, Dermalon)	Monofilament	Polyamide polymer	Hydrolysis results in loss of strength over years	Minimal	Soft tissue and skin reapproximation
Polypropylene (Prolene, Surgipro)	Monofilament	Polypropylene polymer	No degradation or weakening	Least	Soft tissue and skin reapproximation
Polyester (Mersilene, Ticron)	Braided and monofilament	Polyethylene terephthalate	No degradation or weakening	Minimal	Tendon repair using undyed (white) color
Polybutester (Novafil)	Monofilament	Poly (butylene) and poly (tetramethylene ether) glycol terephthalate	No degradation or weakening	Minimal	Soft tissue approximation, easy handling, and knot security

Source: Reproduced with permission from Hollander JE, Singer AJ, in AJ Singer, JE Hollander (eds): *Lacerations and Acute Wounds. An Evidence-Based Guide.* Philadelphia, FA Davis, 2003.

polypropylene) have the lowest rates of infection and are the most commonly used nonabsorbable sutures in the ED. Specific choice of the suture type should be left to individual preferences. *Absorbable sutures* lose most of their tensile strength in less than 60 days. As a result, they are best suited for closure of deep structures such as the dermis and fascia. Due to their strength, handling, and relatively low tissue reactivity, synthetic monofilament sutures are preferred (Table 42-4). Rapidly absorbing sutures (e.g., Vicryl Rapide) can also be used to close the superficial skin layers, especially when avoidance of suture removal is desirable.[5] Lacerations in the hand and fingers should be closed with 5-0 sutures while facial lacerations should be closed with 5-0 or 6-0 sutures. For lacerations in most other locations a 4-0 suture is most appropriate.

Improper tissue handling further traumatizes the tissues and results in an increased risk of infection and poor scarring.[6] Gentle tissue handling using either skin hooks or the open limb of fine forceps is encouraged (Figure 42-1). Hemostasis is best achieved by direct pressure with or without a topical vasoconstrictor (such as epinephrine 1:1000). With injury to vessels larger than 2 mm in diameter, careful and selective placement of a ligature tie is often necessary. Bipolar electrocautery should only rarely be used since this increases the risk of infection and scarring.[6]

The best cosmetic outcome is achieved by carefully matching each layer of the wound with its corresponding counterpart on the opposite side, ensuring eversion of the wound edges, and minimizing the amount of tension on the wound. As the wound heals and the swelling subsides, the wound will eventually flatten, becoming flush with the surrounding skin surface. Inadvertent inversion of the wound edges may result in an unsightly depressed scar. Suggested indications for the most commonly used suturing methods are presented in Table 42-5.

Simple Interrupted Percutaneous Sutures   These are the most basic and most commonly used sutures in the ED. With this method individual sutures are placed, sequentially bisecting the original wound into smaller segments until adequate coaptation of the edges is achieved. The needle is introduced through the outer layer of the skin and exits at the level of the dermis on one side of the wound. The needle is then inserted through the opposite wound edge starting at the level of the dermis and exiting superficially (Figure 42-2). In order to ensure proper wound edge eversion, the needle should enter and exit the skin at equal distances and at an angle of 90 degrees. Taking a larger bite at the depth of the wound than through the more superficial layers helps achieve wound eversion. Generally, the number of ties

should correspond to the suture size (i.e., 4 ties for a 4-0 suture, 5 ties for a 5-0 suture, etc.).

Continuous (Running) Percutaneous Sutures   The major advantage of this method is its rapidity, since the entire wound is closed before dividing the suture material. It is most appropriate for long linear wounds. Because it does not allow perfect wound edge apposition it should be avoided in irregular lacerations. With this method the first suture is placed similarly to an interrupted percutaneous suture. However, the suture is not cut and the needle is reintroduced into the skin on the opposite side so the suture crosses the wound superficially at a 65 degree angle (Figure 42-3). The needle then crosses the depth of the wound in a circular motion perpendicular to the wound, exiting on the opposite side approximately 3 to 5 mm from the wound edge. This process is repeated as needed until the entire wound is approximated.

Deep Dermal Sutures   The major role of these sutures is to reduce tension. They are also used to close dead spaces. However, their presence increases the risk of infection in contaminated wounds.[7] Sutures through adipose tissue do not hold tension, increase infection rates, and should be avoided.[8] With deep dermal sutures, the needle is first inserted at the level of the mid dermis on one side of the wound and then exits more superficially below the dermal-epidermal junction (Figure 42-4). The needle is then introduced below the dermal epidermal junction on the opposite wound side and exits at the level of the mid dermis. Thus the knot becomes buried in the depth of the tissue when tying of the suture is completed. The first suture is placed at the center of the laceration, while additional sutures then sequentially bisect the wound. The number of deep sutures should be minimized.

Continuous Subcuticular Sutures   Rarely used in the ED setting, this is one of the most complex methods of wound closure. The major advantage of this method is that it results in fairly good wound approximation without requiring any more superficial wound closure devices. One may use either absorbable or nonabsorbable sutures with this method. However, nonabsorbable sutures require removal. With this method, after anchoring the suture in the deep dermis, sequential horizontally oriented "bites" are taken immediately below the dermal-epidermal junction until the wound is adequately approximated (Figure 42-5).

Horizontal Half-Buried Mattress Sutures   These sutures are particularly well suited for closing the tip of skin flaps since they minimize

TABLE 42-4 Absorbable Sutures

Suture	Types	Material	Tensile Strength Retention In Vivo	Absorption Rate	Tissue Reactivity	Common ED Uses
Surgical gut	Plain	Collagen derived from bovine intestine	Retains 50% tensile strength for 5–7 days	Absorbed by proteolytic processes in weeks	Moderate reactivity	Rarely, for intraoral wounds
Chromic gut	Chromium coating	Collagen derived from bovine intestine	Retains 50% tensile strength for 10–14 days	Absorbed by proteolytic processes in weeks	Moderate reactivity	Rarely, for subcutaneous closures and intraoral wounds
Polyglycolic acid (Dexon)	Braided	Polymer of glycolic acid	Retains 65% tensile strength at 2 weeks, 35% at 3 weeks	Completely absorbed by slow hydrolysis by 60–90 days	Minimal	Approximation of deep soft tissue structures (i.e., dermis), for ligation
Polyglactin 910 (Vicryl)	Braided	Copolymer of lactide and glycolide coated with polyglactin 370 and calcium stearate	Retains 65% tensile strength at 2 weeks, 40% at 3 weeks	Completely absorbed by slow hydrolysis by 56–70 days	Minimal	Approximation of deep soft tissue structures, (i.e., dermis). for ligation
Polyglactin 910 (Vicryl Rapide)	Braided	Copolymer of glycolide and lactide coated with polyglactin 370 and calcum stearate	Retains 50% tensile strength for 5 days; all lost by 2 weeks	Absorbed by hydrolysis; usually complete by 42 days	Minimal to moderate	Skin approximation when absorbable sutures used
Polyglactin 910 (Lactomer)	Braided	Copolymer of glycolide and lactide coated with caprolactone and glycolide	Retains 40% tensile strength for 3 weeks	Absorbed by hydrolysis; usually complete by 56–70 days	Minimal	Subcutaneous soft tissue approximation
Polydioxanone (PDS II)	Monofilament	Polyester polymer	Retain 50% tensile strength for 4 weeks; 25% for 6 weeks	Minimal until 90 days, complete by 6 months	Slight	Subcutaneous soft tissue approximation where more prolonged strength is needed
Poliglecaprone 25 (Monocryl)	Monofilament	Copolymer of glycolide and epsilon-caprolactine	Retains 60% tensile strength for 1 week; 30% at 2 weeks	Absorbed by hydrolysis within 3–4 months	Minimal	Subcutaneous soft tissue approximation where more prolonged strength is needed
Glycomer 631	Monofilament	Terpolymer of glycolide, trimethylene carbonate and dioxanone	Retains 70% tensile strength 28 days; 13% at 56 days	Complete by 90–110 days	Slight	Subcutaneous soft tissue approximation where more prolonged strength is needed
Lactide glycolide (Panacryl)	Braided	Copolymer of lactide and glycolide	Retains 80% tensile strength at 3 months, 60% at 6 months, 20% at 1 year	Complete within 1.5–2.5 years	Minimal	Subcutaneous soft tissue approximation (e.g., fascia) where more prolonged strength is needed, excellent handling
Polyglyconate (Maxon)	Monofilament	Polyglyconate polymer	Retains 70% tensile strength 28 days; 13% at 56 days	Complete by 90–110 days	Slight	Subcutaneous soft tissue approximation where more prolonged strength is needed

Source: Reproduced with permission from Hollander JE, Singer AJ, in AJ Singer, JE Hollander (eds): *Lacreations and Acute Wounds. An Evidence-Based Guide.* Philadelphia, FA Davis, 2003.

FIG. 42-1. Handling of the skin with skin hook *(left)* and open limb of fine forceps *(right)*. [Reproduced with permission from Singer AJ, Hollander JE (eds): *Lacerations and Acute Wounds. An Evidence-Based Guide.* Philadelphia, PA: FA Davis, 2003, p. 109.]

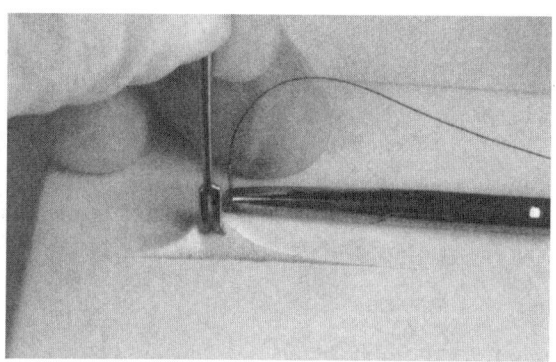 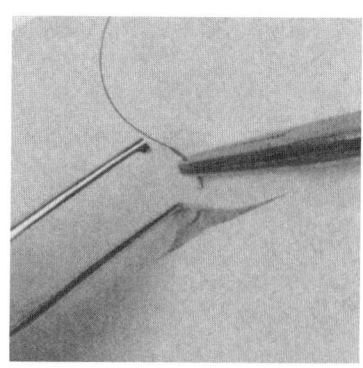

strangulation of the tip. The needle is introduced percutaneously through one side of the wound, then horizontally through the flap tip at the level of the dermis. The suture is completed by exiting through the remaining wound side from dermis to epidermis (Figure 42-6).

Vertical Mattress Sutures These sutures combine some of the advantages of deep and percutaneous sutures. They also result in excellent wound edge eversion. Vertical mattress sutures are particularly useful in very thin or lax skin, and in areas where the deep subcutaneous tissues are too fragile to be used for anchoring tension-reducing sutures (e.g., over the shin). After taking a large deep bite from both sides of the wound, the direction of the needle is reversed and a smaller superficial bite is taken from both sides of the laceration (Figure 42-7). Care should be taken since vertical mattress sutures may result in too much tension on the more superficial skin edges, which reduces blood supply to the skin.

STAPLES

The major advantages of staples are their speed and relative ease of use.[9–11] They are also cost effective, especially when devices containing fewer staples are used in the ED, where most lacerations are relatively short. However, of all closure devices, staples allow the least precision in wound approximation. As a result their use should be limited to linear, nonfacial lacerations. They are particularly useful for scalp lacerations.[10] However, deep sutures may be required to close lacerations of the galea aponeurotica, while percutaneous sutures are always desirable when hemostasis is problematic. In experimental animal models, staples result in less tissue reactivity than sutures;[12] however, infection rates and cosmetic outcome are similar to sutures in the clinical setting.[9–11] Staple removal is more painful than removal of sutures.[11] While a variety of stapling devices are commercially available, there are few practical differences between them from the standpoint of the emergency practitioner.

TABLE 42-5   Selecting Closure Method Based on Wound Type

Suture Type	Advantages	Disadvantages	Frequent Uses
Interrupted percutaneous	Excellent approximation	Time-consuming May strangulate tissues	Low-tension wounds May be used with deep sutures for high-tension wounds
Continuous percutaneous	Rapid closure Accommodates edema	Less meticulous closure than interrupted sutures If a single knot unravels the wound may dehisce (if no deep sutures are placed)	Percutaneous closure in conjunction with deep sutures
Interrupted dermal	Reduces tension on wound surface Allows early removal of percutaneous sutures, avoiding hatch marking May reduce scar width	May increase infection in contaminated wounds	High-tension wounds Closure of dead space
Continuous dermal	Rapid Reduces tension on wound surface Allows early removal of percutaneous sutures, avoiding hatch marking May reduce scar width	Technically difficult Less accurate approximation than interrupted sutures If a single knot unravels, the wound may dehisce	High-tension wounds require interrupted dermal sutures Closure of dead space
Vertical mattress	Excellent wound edge eversion Combines advantages of deep and superficial sutures	May cause tissue strangulation	Thin or lax skin with little dermal or fascial tissue High-tension areas (e.g., extremities)
Horizontal mattress	More rapid than simple interrupted sutures Excellent wound edge eversion	May cause tissue strangulation	Bleeding scalp wounds Initial approximation of high-tension wounds
Half-buried, horizontal mattress	Less compromising to flap perfusion	Time-consuming Technically difficult	Corner stitches and flaps

Source: Reproduced with permission from Singer AJ, Rosenberg L, in AJ Singer, JE Hollander (eds): *Lacerations and Acute Wounds. An Evidence-Based Guide.* Philadelphia, FA Davis, 2003.

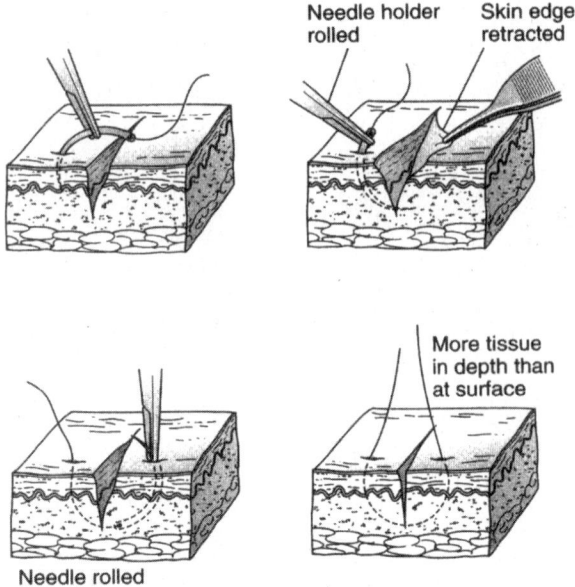

FIG. 42-2. Placement of simple interrupted percutaneous sutures. The distance of the suture from the wound edge is greater at the depth of the wound than at the surface, promoting wound edge eversion when tightened. [Reproduced with permission from Singer AJ, Hollander JE (eds): *Lacerations and Acute Wounds. An Evidence-Based Guide.* Philadelphia, PA: FA Davis, 2003, p. 115.]

ADHESIVE TAPES

Adhesive tapes are the least reactive of all wound closure devices.[12] Their application is simple, painless, and rapid. They are also inexpensive and do not require formal removal. However, they tend to slough off when exposed to any tension or moisture. As a result their

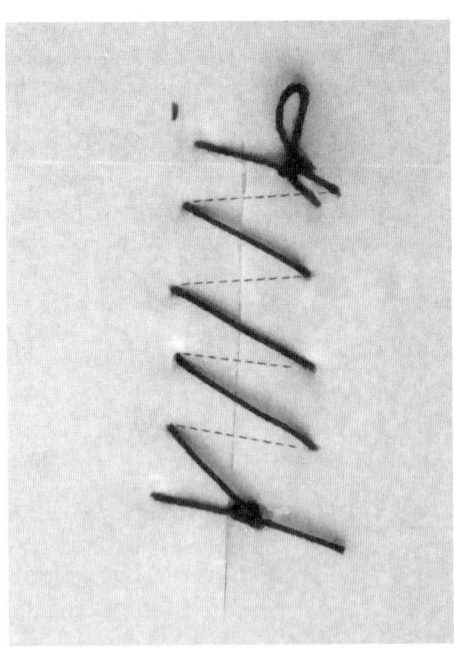

FIG. 42-3. Placement of continuous percutaneous sutures. The suture crosses the wound superficially at a 65° angle and traverses the depth of the wound at a 90° angle, perpendicular to the wound. [Reproduced with permission from Singer AJ, Hollander JE (eds): *Lacerations and Acute Wounds. An Evidence-Based Guide.* Philadelphia, PA: FA Davis, 2003, p. 122.]

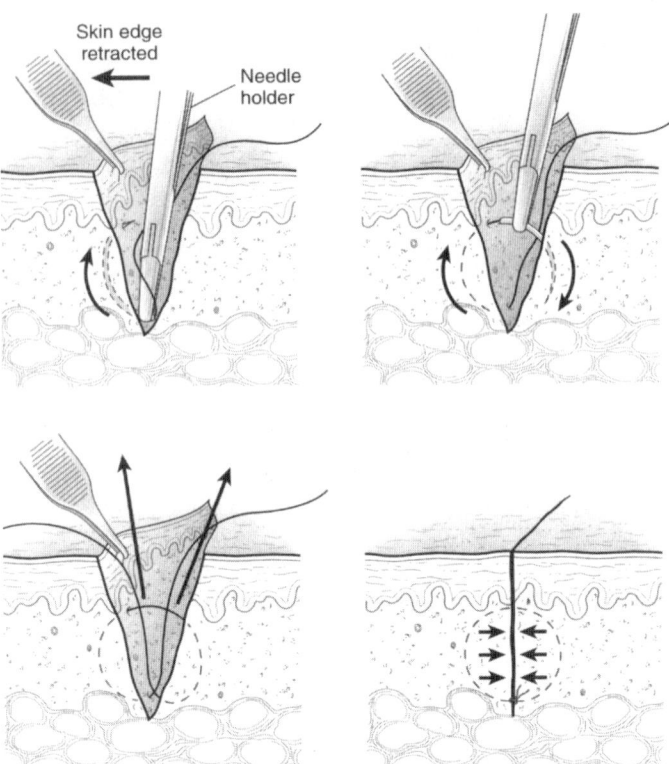

FIG. 42-4. Placement of deep dermal sutures. The needle is inserted at the depth of the dermis and directed upward, exiting beneath the dermal-epidermal junction. Then the needle is inserted across the wound and directed downward, exiting at the wound base. The suture knot is then placed deep in the wound. [Reproduced with permission from Singer AJ, Hollander JE (eds): *Lacerations and Acute Wounds. An Evidence-Based Guide.* Philadelphia, PA: FA Davis, 2003, p. 121.]

use is limited to very low-tension simple wounds or for closure of fragile skin subject to low tension. They are also of little use in noncompliant patients since they are so easy to remove. In order to increase their adhesiveness skin tapes should be used in conjunction with an adhesive adjunct such as mastisol or tincture of benzoin that is gently painted on either side of the wound edges. Since these adhesive adjuncts are toxic to wounds, care must be taken to avoid their introduction into the wound itself. The tapes should be placed perpendicular to the wound edges approximately 2 to 3 mm apart. With long lac-

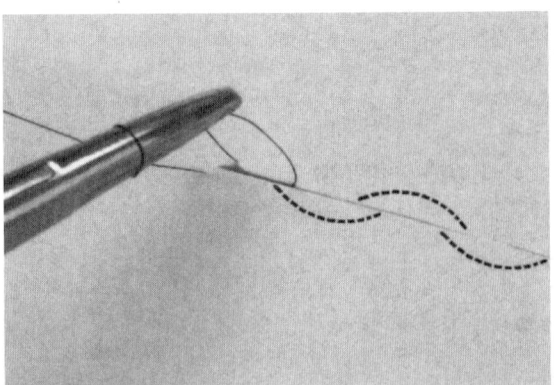

FIG. 42-5. Placement of continuous subcuticular sutures. Small horizontal bites are taken beneath the dermal-epidermal junction. Slight backtracking of the needle path should be performed to ensure wound coaptation. [Reproduced with permission from Singer AJ, Hollander JE (eds): *Lacerations and Acute Wounds. An Evidence-Based Guide.* Philadelphia, PA: FA Davis, 2003, p. 125.]

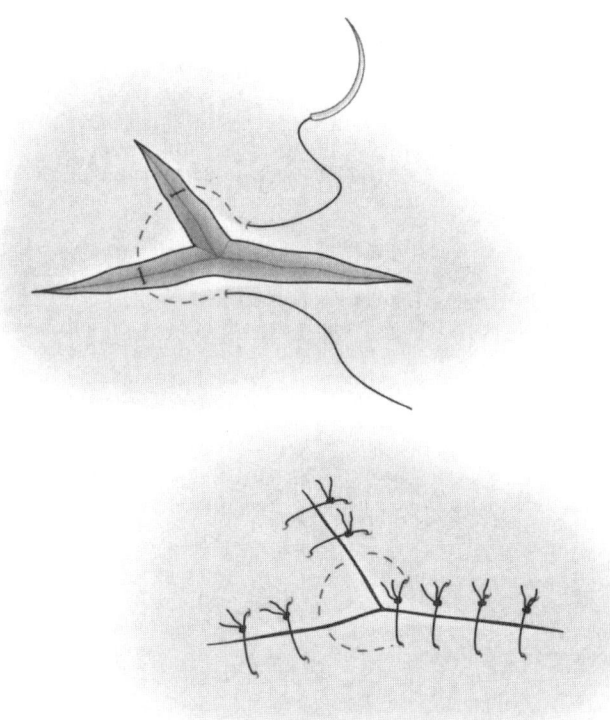

FIG. 42-6. Placement of horizontal half-buried mattress sutures. The needle enters the skin on one side of the laceration, passes across the gap, traverses the tip of the flap underneath the epidermis, crosses the gap at the other side, and then exits the skin from the other side. [Reproduced with permission from Singer AJ, Hollander JE (eds): *Lacerations and Acute Wounds. An Evidence-Based Guide.* Philadelphia, PA: FA Davis, 2003, p. 130.]

erations, the first strip of tape should be placed across the center of the wound followed by additional strips on either side of the wound center. To reduce the possibility of skin blistering or premature dislodgement, additional strips should be placed over the ends of the other strips, parallel to the laceration. With the introduction of more durable skin tissue adhesives, tapes are mostly used to reinforce lacerations after suture or staple removal. The cosmetic results and dehiscence rates after closure of small and superficial facial lacerations with tapes is similar to cyanoacrylate tissue adhesives.[13]

CYANOACRYLATE TISSUE ADHESIVES

The cyanoacrylate tissue adhesives have been used to close lacerations and surgical incisions for several decades, but have only recently become available in the United States. The cyanoacrylate tissue adhesives are liquid monomers that polymerize into a stable bond when they come into contact with moisture. They are applied topically to the apposed wound edges and should not be introduced into the wound. The tissue adhesives offer many advantages over standard wound closure devices. They may be applied rapidly and painlessly to any easily approximated laceration. Because they slough off spontaneously within 5 to 10 days, they do not require removal. They are equivalent in strength to 5-0 sutures, and thus should not be used alone for high-tension wounds. They can be used in conjunction with deep sutures and/or immobilization aimed at reducing wound tension. The cyanoacrylates form an occlusive dressing that serves as a barrier to microbial penetration and have been shown to reduce infection rates in experimental animal models.[14,15]

Currently, the only FDA-approved tissue adhesives are Dermabond (Ethicon Inc., Somerville, NJ), an octyl-cyanoacrylate (OCA)-based adhesive, and Indermil (Dimensional Analysis Systems, Inc., Leonia, NJ), a butyl-cyanoacrylate-based adhesive. The tensile strength of octyl-cyanoacrylate is three times greater than that of butyl-cyanoacrylates. Furthermore, it is more flexible than the butyls, allowing its use on irregular surfaces and for long lacerations.

The first randomized clinical trial comparing octyl-cyanoacrylate to sutures for closing 136 facial (as well as selected extremity and torso) lacerations in adults was reported by Quinn et al in 1997.[16] At 3 months there were no differences between the groups in the visual analogue cosmesis scores or the percentage of wounds receiving optimal wound evaluation scores. Wound closure with the adhesive was found to be faster and less painful than with sutures. The cosmetic results were also comparable after 1 year of follow-up.

The largest prospective randomized clinical trial to date evaluating octyl-cyanoacrylate for wound closure has recently been published.[17] This study included data from ten clinical sites that included urgent care centers, ED, and a variety of operating room settings (general, orthopedic, dermatologic, and gynecologic surgery). Enrolled patients had a variety of traumatic lacerations, surgical incisions as well as surgical excisional wounds. Wounds ranged in size from 0.1 to 14 cm with over 100 wounds greater than 4 cm in length. These wounds were located on a wide range of body areas including the head and neck, trunk, and extremities. This study concluded that wound closure with OCA was faster than with standard wound closure devices, and had comparable rates of infection, dehiscence, and optimal cosmetic appearance.[17]

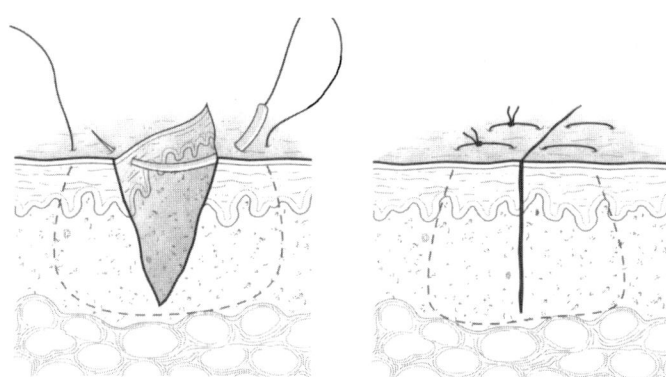

FIG. 42-7. Placement of vertical mattress sutures. The first bite is taken far from the wound, the needle is reversed, and the second bite is taken close to the wound edge. The wound edges evert as the knot is tied. [Reproduced with permission from Singer AJ, Hollander JE (eds): *Lacerations and Acute Wounds. An Evidence-Based Guide.* Philadelphia, PA: FA Davis, 2003, p. 127.]

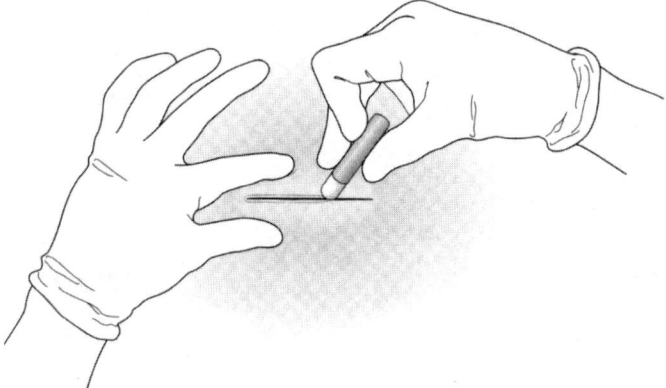

FIG. 42-8. Application of tissue adhesive. The wound edges are held in apposition with the fingers of the nondominant hand as the tissue adhesive is applied. [Reproduced with permission from Singer AJ, Hollander JE (eds): *Lacerations and Acute Wounds. An Evidence-Based Guide.* Philadelphia, PA: FA Davis, 2003, p. 90.]

TABLE 42-6 Avoiding Potential Pitfalls of Tissue Adhesives

Problem	Ways To Avoid the Problem
Runoff	Position patient with wound parallel to floor Circumscribe wound with ointment
Spillage into eyes	Cover eyes with gauze barrier Position patient so wound is not above eye Apply petrolatum jelly barrier before applying adhesive
Wound dehiscence	Avoid adhesive use for high-tension wounds Avoid frequent exposure to friction or moisture Use deep sutures or immobilization for high-tension wounds
Wound infection	Use adhesives only for properly selected wounds Use proper wound preparation, including irrigation, exploration, and when necessary, debridement Use proper application technique
Getting stuck to the wound	Practice expressing small amounts of adhesive and controlling runoff Alternate the hand used to appose wound edges prior to complete polymerization of the adhesive

Source: Reproduced with permission from Singer AJ, Quinn JV, in AJ Singer, JE Hollander (eds): *Lacerations and Acute Wounds. An Evidence-Based Guide.* Philadelphia: FA Davis, 2003.

The Cochrane Library published a systematic review on the use of tissue adhesives in 2002. The authors concluded that (1) there is no significant difference in cosmetic result between tissue adhesives and standard wound closure, (2) patient-reported pain scores and physician-reported procedure time were significantly lower with tissue adhesives, and (3) there is a small increase (absolute difference = 4 percent, 95% CI 1 to 7 percent) in wound dehiscence using tissue adhesives.[18]

While there are many studies evaluating different cyanoacrylates individually and in comparison with sutures, few studies have directly compared the various cyanoacrylate tissue adhesives against each other. A recent comparison of OCA and a butyl-cyanoacrylate (Histoacryl Blue) demonstrated comparable cosmetic results after closure of selected, short, simple facial lacerations in children.[19] In contrast, a study comparing OCA and the same butyl-cyanoacrylate for closure of pediatric operative wounds found that OCA was superior in terms of dehiscence rates.[20]

In order to ensure optimal results, tissue adhesives should only be used when laceration edges are easily approximated with the practitioner's hands or forceps. Occasionally an assistant can be valuable in helping to ensure constant and meticulous wound edge apposition while the adhesive is applied. The adhesive is carefully expressed through the tip of the applicator and gently brushed over the wound surface in a continuous steady motion (Figure 42-8). The adhesive should cover the entire wound as well as an area extending 5 to 10 mm on either side of the wound edges. After allowing the first layer of the adhesive to polymerize for 30 to 45 s, 2 to 3 additional layers of the adhesive are similarly brushed onto the surface of the wound, waiting 5 to 10 s between successive layers. Care in application will reduce some of the commonly reported pitfalls associated with tissue adhesives (Table 42-6). A new high viscosity octyl-cyanoacrylate that is six times thicker than the current octyl-cyanoacrylate formulation is now available that reduces runoff and spillage.

REFERENCES

1. Singer AJ, Clark RAF: Advances in cutaneous wound healing. *New Engl J Med* 341:738, 1999.
2. Quinn J, Cummings S, Callaham M, Sellers K: Suturing versus conservative management of lacerations of the hand: Randomised controlled trial. *BMJ* 325:299, 2002.
3. Wray RC: Force required for wound closure and scar appearance. *Plast Reconstr Surg* 72:380, 1983.
4. Hollander JE, Singer AJ, Valentine S, Henry MC: Wound registry: Development and validation. *Ann Emerg Med* 25:675, 1995.
5. Canarelli JP, Ricard J, Collet LM, Marasse E: Use of fast absorbing material for skin closure in young children. *Int Surg* 73:151, 1988.
6. Singer AJ, Quinn JV, Thode HC, Hollander JE: Determinants of poor outcome after laceration and incision repair. *Plast Reconstr Surg* 110:429, 2002.
7. Mehta PH, Dunn KA, Bradfield JF, Austin PE: Contaminated wounds: Infection rates with subcutaneous sutures. *Ann Emerg Med* 27:43, 1996.
8. Milewski PJ, Thomson H: Is a fat stitch necessary? *Br J Surg* 67:393, 1980.
9. Ritchie AJ, Rocke LG: Staples versus sutures in the closure of scalp wounds: A prospective, double-blind, randomized trial. *Injury* 20:217, 1989.
10. Hollander JE, Giarrusso E, Cassara G, Valentine S, Singer AJ: Comparison of staples and sutures for closure of scalp lacerations (abstract). *Acad Emerg Med* 4:460, 1997.
11. George TK, Simpson DC: Skin wound closure with staples in the accident and emergency department. *J Roy Coll Surg Edinburgh* 30:54, 1985.
12. Edlich RF, Rodeheaver G, Kuphal J, et al: Technique of closure: Contaminated wounds. *JACEP* 3:375, 1974.
13. Zempsky WT, Grem C, Nichols J, Parrotti D: Prospective comparison of cosmetic outcomes of facial lacerations closed with steri-strips or dermabond (abstract). *Acad Emerg Med* 8:438, 2001.
14. Singer AJ, Nable M, Cameau P, Singer DD, McClain SA: Evaluation of a liquid occlusive dressing for excisional wounds. *Wound Rep Regen* 11:181, 2003.
15. Quinn J, Maw J, Ramotar K, Wenckebach G, Wells G: Octyl cyanoacrylate tissue adhesive versus suture wound repair in a contaminated wound model. *Surgery* 122:69, 1997.
16. Quinn J, Wells G, Sutcliffe T, et al: A randomized trial comparing octyl-cyanoacrylate tissue adhesive and sutures in the management of lacerations. *JAMA* 277:1527, 1997.
17. Singer AJ, Quinn JV, Hollander JE, Clark RE: Closure of lacerations and incisions with octyl cyanoacrylate: A multi-center randomized clinical trial. *Surgery* 131:270, 2002.
18. Farion K, Osmond MH, Hartling L, et al: Tissue adhesives for traumatic lacerations in children and adults. *Cochrane Database Syst Rev* CD003326, 2002.
19. Osmond MH, Quinn JV, Sutcliffe T, Jarmuske M, Klassen TP: A randomized, clinical trial comparing butylcyanoacrylate with octylcyanoacrylate in the management of selected pediatric facial lacerations. *Acad Emerg Med* 6:171, 1999.
20. Steiner Z, Mogilner J: Histoacryl vs. Dermabond cyanoacrylate glue for closing small operative wounds. *Harefuah* 139:409, 2000.

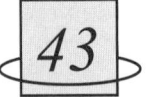

43 LACERATIONS TO THE FACE AND SCALP
Wendy C. Coates

EPIDEMIOLOGY

Lacerations to the face and scalp account for approximately 50 percent of the wounds treated in EDs in the United States.[1] The most cosmetically apparent wounds are those that appear on the face; therefore careful evaluation and meticulous repair technique are important for excellent results. The emergency physician can repair the majority of facial lacerations; however, because of the cosmetic impact of these wounds, consultation with specialists is encouraged when the technical aspects of closure exceed the physician's ability.[2] Wounds to the face that involve areas of tissue avulsion may best be repaired primarily in the operating room so flaps or grafts can be applied. When the emergency physician initially evaluates the wound, it should be cleaned and properly irrigated even if a delayed repair by a specialist is anticipated.

In today's society, a growing number of victims of domestic violence are identified in the ED. Anyone with facial trauma should be questioned about the possibility of domestic violence and appropriate authorities should be notified (Table 43-1).[3,4]

TABLE 43-1   Maxillofacial Injuries and Domestic Violence in the ED

Most victims of domestic violence have maxillofacial injuries
Women more commonly affected than men
Fist is most common weapon
Left side of face is most common site of injury
Nasal bone commonly fractured

PATHOPHYSIOLOGY

Facial and scalp wounds are most often caused by a combination of sharp and blunt mechanisms. For example, a victim of a motor vehicle accident may bluntly strike the windshield and be cut by the glass as it shatters. People involved in interpersonal trauma or falls may have a similar pattern of injury. Lacerations caused by sharp objects are likely to have more discrete edges, but may be deeper and involve underlying structures such as the muscles of facial expression, nerves, and arteries. Wounds caused by blunt forces burst the skin open, damage cells, and produce tissue edema, which slows the wound-healing process. As a result, it takes an average of ten times fewer bacteria to cause an infection in a blunt wound compared to a sharp wound. Blunt forces are more likely to cause diffuse underlying damage, such as fractures of the facial bones or skull. The presence of foreign bodies such as soil, glass, or wood fragments further complicates the potential for good healing.[5]

SCALP AND FOREHEAD

Anatomy

The scalp and forehead have a similar structure (Figure 43-1). The skin is thick, and on the scalp it has abundant hair follicles and sebaceous glands. There is a rich network of blood vessels: the arterial supply to each side of the scalp includes three branches off the external carotid artery (occipital, superficial temporal, and posterior auricular arteries) and two branches from the internal carotid artery (supraorbital and supratrochlear arteries).[6] Since the dermal tissue is so fibrous, vessel retraction is limited following injury, and significant hemorrhage can result. The potential space between the periosteum and the galea aponeurosis allows for easy movement of the scalp over the cranium. However, hematoma and infection can collect and spread within this space to involve the entire forehead and scalp. This high degree of mobility sometimes leads to a scalping injury, in which a large segment of the scalp is torn off in one piece.

Evaluation

For many patients with scalp and forehead lacerations, the wound may be only a minor part of the overall injury; prior to definitive wound care, airway, breathing, circulation, hemorrhage control, and spinal and neurologic injury should be addressed. In some cases it may be necessary to control scalp hemorrhage urgently by applying direct pressure or clamping the involved vessel(s) at the wound edges (e.g., using Raney clips).

Routine lacerations should be inspected and gently palpated to determine their depth, noting whether the galea is lacerated or if there is an underlying depressed skull fracture. Palpable depressions in the outer table of the skull should be evaluated further with computed tomography. Orientation of forehead lacerations has important cosmetic implications; in general, wounds that fall along the lines of skin tension have better cosmetic results. Skin tension lines are perpendicular to the underlying muscles. As an obvious example, the horizontal lines seen on the forehead when the brow is raised are perpendicular to the frontalis muscle underneath (Figure 43-2). Forehead lacerations that extend to other structures, such as the eyebrow, nose, or ear must be evaluated and managed with the cosmetic result of these structures in mind.

Wound Preparation

For wound preparation and closure in pediatric patients, sedation may be required during the procedure (see Chap. 134). Anesthesia can be provided by topical, local, or regional infiltration. A supraorbital block can be used to anesthetize one side of the forehead and anterior third of the scalp. The advantage of a regional block in the face is that the volume of locally instilled anesthetic does not distort the wound (see Chap. 37). Local anesthetics containing epinephrine are often used in highly vascular wounds to help control hemorrhage from small vessels.[7] Topical agents such as LET (lidocaine-epinephrine-tetracaine) or EMLA (eutectic mixture of local anesthetics) may provide adequate anesthesia alone in about 50 percent of patients and reduce the pain of local anesthetic injection in those who require it.[8,9] TAC (tetracaine-adrenaline-cocaine) is not recommended because of the potential for systemic absorption and cocaine toxicity.

All traumatic wounds are irrigated to reduce contamination and lessen the risk of wound infection. However, in nonbite, noncontaminated facial and scalp wounds presenting within 6 h, routine irrigation does not alter the rate of infection or subsequent cosmetic appearance after suture repair.[10]

Repair of Scalp Lacerations

It is not necessary to shave or cut scalp hair prior to wound closure; shaving increases the likelihood of a wound infection.[11] In most cases,

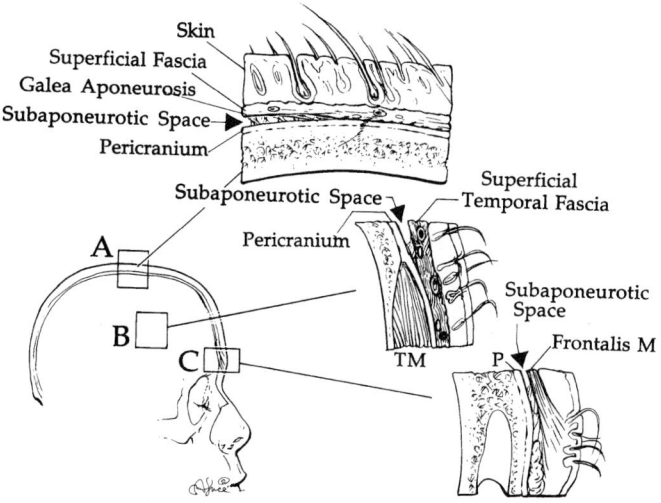

FIG. 43-1. The layers of the **A.** scalp, **B.** temporal region, and **C.** eyebrow. TM = temporalis muscle.

Skin
Superficial Fascia
Galea Aponeurosis
Subaponeurotic Space
Pericranium

Subaponeurotic Space
Superficial Temporal Fascia
Pericranium
Subaponeurotic Space
Frontalis M
TM   P

A
B
C

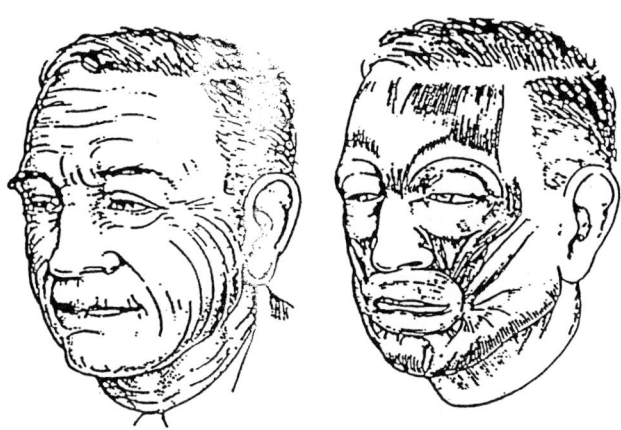

FIG. 43-2. Skin tension lines are perpendicular to underlying muscles.

the hair can be brushed aside or an ointment such as bacitracin zinc or petrolatum can be applied to mat down the hair adjacent to the laceration.

Large galeal defects should be sutured if possible to prevent a wide, depressed appearance of the final scar and to minimize the development of a subgaleal hematoma. Buried 4-0 nonabsorbable monofilament nylon or polypropylene interrupted or horizontal mattress sutures may be used (Table 43-2). In large wounds, the muscle layer may be approximated with 4-0 absorbable monofilament or multifilament in a simple interrupted fashion. This reduces the apparent width and depth of the final scar. Conversely, the skin and muscle layers can be closed with a single suture layer through both structures. The skin can be closed with surgical staples or by simple interrupted nylon or rapidly absorbable braided sutures. It is helpful to leave the tails long and use sutures of a color different than the hair to facilitate removal. Superficial scalp lacerations without galeal injury can be closed with staples alone.[12,13]

Hair braiding has been described as an alternate closure technique for scalp lacerations.[14] While tissue adhesive alone is not recommended for the scalp, recently a technique combining hair apposition and tissue adhesive has been described for closure of scalp lacerations.[15] In this technique, 4 to 5 strands of hair from opposite sides of the wound are brought together, twisted once, and secured with tissue adhesive.

A pressure dressing should be considered for the first 24 h on a deep scalp laceration to prevent the formation of a hematoma. Patients who have sustained a significant scalping injury should be sent to the operating room for definitive repair.

Repair of Forehead Lacerations

The deep layers of the forehead may be approximated in a similar fashion to the scalp. In this area, unrepaired muscle layers are more likely to produce noticeable scars, especially when the facial muscles of expression are involved. The skin may be closed with 6-0 nonabsorbable interrupted suture or tissue adhesive. For deep wounds under tension, a buried 5-0 intradermal, absorbable monofilament or multifilament suture can be used. The epidermal layer can be closed with 6-0 nonabsorbable sutures in a simple, interrupted fashion; with skin closure strips over adhesive adjuncts; or with tissue adhesive[16] (Table 43-3). Alternate methods of closure are especially attractive if the patient is at risk to develop keloids or hypertrophic scars. Care should be taken in the forehead to approximate the skin tension lines and hairline precisely (Figure 43-3).

Repair of Eyebrow Lacerations

The eyebrow marks the lowest portion of the forehead. The eyebrows should never be clipped or shaved because their delicate contour and form are valuable landmarks for the meticulous reapproximation of the wound edges. If shaved it is also unlikely that they will grow back in exactly the same fashion as they had been prior to the injury. If debridement in any hairy area must take place, the scalpel should cut at an angle parallel to the hair follicles to minimize the area of subsequent alopecia. When repairing a laceration that involves the eyebrow, the hair margins must be lined up exactly. It is helpful to use sutures that are a different color from the hair and to leave long tails to facilitate removal.

Disposition

Patients whose overall medical condition does not warrant surgery or admission to the hospital can be discharged with routine wound-care instructions and, if the injury resulted from a major blunt impact, closed head injury precautions. Removal of scalp sutures or staples should take place in 7 to 10 days, while nonabsorbable sutures in the face should be removed in 3 to 5 days.

EYELIDS

Anatomy

The eyelid is a thin tissue that covers the globe and is composed of five layers: skin, subcutaneous tissue, orbicularis oculi muscle, tarsal plate, and conjunctiva. The muscular layer controls lid closure and forms both the medial and lateral canthus; fibers of the orbicularis oculi wrap

TABLE 43-2   Suturing Guidelines for the Face and Scalp

Area	Suture	Size	Anesthetic	Removal
Scalp and face				
Galea	Nylon	4-0	Local or supraorbital	Not removed
Muscle	Monofilament or braided absorbable	4-0	Local or supraorbital	Not removed
Skin	Staples	Standard	Local or supraorbital	7–10 days
	Nylon	4-0		
	Rapidly absorbing	4-0		
Forehead	Coated or plain nylon	6-0	Local or supraorbital	5 days
	Tissue adhesive	May need deep layer		
Face	Coated or plain nylon	6-0	Local, infraorbital, or mandibular	5 days
	Tissue adhesive	May need deep layer		
Eyelids	Coated or plain nylon	6-0 or 7-0	Supra- or infraorbital	3 days
Nose				
Cartilage	Braided absorbable	5-0	Intranasal pack (no epinephrine)	Not removed
Skin	Coated or plain nylon	6-0	Intranasal pack (no epinephrine)	3–5 days
Ears				
Cartilage	Coated nylon	6-0	Auricular block (no epinephrine)	Not removed
Skin	Coated nylon	6-0	Auricular block (no epinephrine)	5 days
Lips				
Mucosa	Rapidly absorbing	5-0	Local, infraorbital, or mandibular	Not removed
Muscle	Monofilament or braided absorbable	4-0 or 5-0	Local, infraorbital, or mandibular	Not removed
Skin	Plain or coated nylon	6-0	Local, infraorbital, or mandibular	3–5 days

TABLE 43-3   Indications for Tissue Adhesives on the Face

Minimal tension
Avoid hairy areas
Epidermal closure only (no mucosa)
Do not use on human or animal bites

around the lacrimal system. Nerve supply to the eyelid arises from the temporal and zygomatic branches of the facial nerve. The tarsal plate forms the main body of the lower half of the lid and consists of elastic tissue in a dense matrix of connective tissue. Embedded in the tarsal plate are the Meibomian glands, which open into the white line just in front of the conjunctival edge of the lid margin. In the lid margin, the eyelashes are arranged in three irregular rows with their follicles extending obliquely into the tarsal plate.

The lacrimal system begins at the upper and lower puncta as they form the canaliculi. The nasolacrimal duct extends 3 to 5 mm above the level of the medial canthus. It is responsible for tear drainage.[6]

Evaluation

The structures surrounding the eye and eyelids are very delicate and are cosmetically and functionally important. A high degree of suspicion for injury to these structures from periorbital trauma is required and the emergency physician should have a low threshold for referring these lacerations to an ophthalmologist or oculoplastic specialist for definitive treatment.

The eyelids are very thin and do not offer any protection from penetrating injuries to the globe. A complete examination of the eye's structure and function and a search for foreign bodies must be completed before wound care is carried out. Once the integrity of the globe and muscular structures is verified, the lid should be examined for involvement of the canthi, the lacrimal system, or penetration through the tarsal plate or lid margin. The following injuries should be referred to an ophthalmologist or oculoplastic specialist: (1) involving the inner surface of the lid, (2) involving the lid margins, (3) involving the lacrimal duct, (4) associated with ptosis, or (5) extending into the tarsal plate. Poor approximation of the lid margins leads to a notched appearance. Failure to recognize and properly repair the lacrimal system can result in chronic tearing (epiphora). In general, wounds that

are superficial and especially those parallel to the lid margins may be carefully repaired by the emergency physician (Figure 43-4).

Treatment and Disposition

Gentle irrigation with normal saline should be performed after anesthesia. Closure with 6-0 or 7-0 nonabsorbable simple interrupted nylon suture or polypropylene is preferred. Extreme care should be taken to avoid deep penetration of the needle through the lid and into the underlying globe; small bites only through the skin layer should be taken. Tissue adhesive is contraindicated near the eye. In the event of inadvertent tissue adhesive contact with the eye, copious irrigation and/or application of a petrolatum ointment is indicated. Routine evaluation and treatment of the subsequent corneal abrasion should follow. Sutures should be removed in 3 to 5 days. A thin layer of antibiotic ointment may be applied in place of a dressing.

NOSE

Anatomy

As a protuberant structure, the nose is especially vulnerable to blunt trauma. It is the most common fracture in victims of domestic violence and assault.[4] The nose is composed of cartilaginous and osseous structures that support the overlying skin and musculature and the underlying mucosa. It is separated into halves by the septum. Two C-shaped alar cartilages that are covered directly by skin form the tip of the nose. The interior of the nose is covered by specialized skin with mucus-producing cells and thick, long hairs near the end, while the proximal portion of the nasal lining is made up of ciliated pseudostratified columnar epithelial cells.[6]

Evaluation

The most important assessment of nasal lacerations is to determine their depth and the involvement of the deeper tissue layers.[17] Exposed

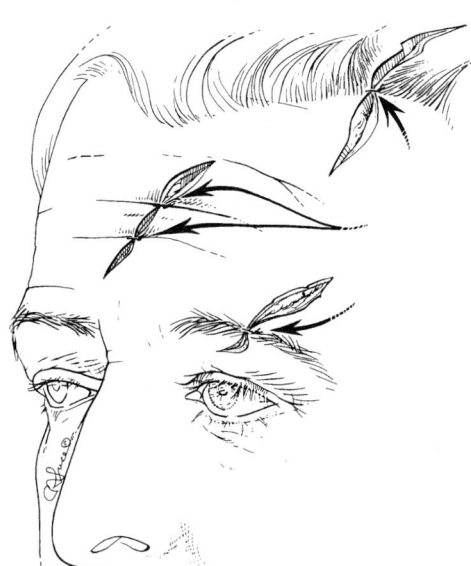

FIG. 43-3. Key stitches in the forehead.

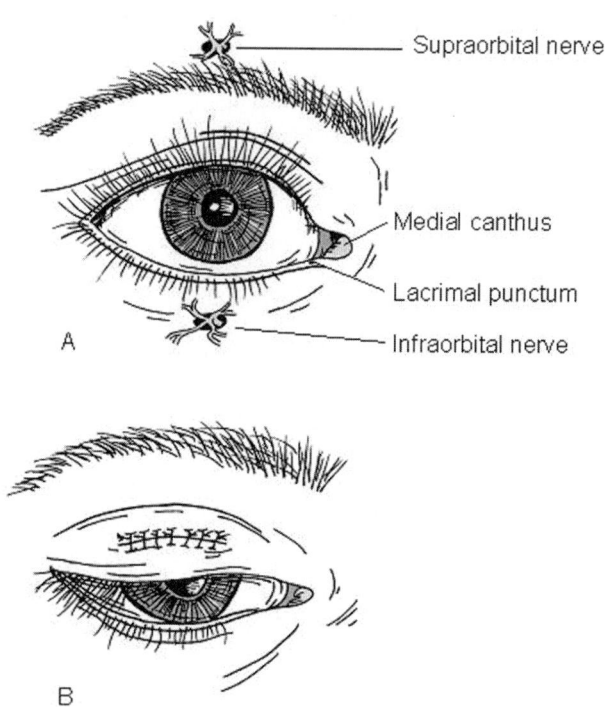

FIG. 43-4. Eyelid anatomy. **A.** External landmarks. **B.** Simple closure of a superficial laceration of the upper lid.

cartilage or penetration through all tissue layers increases the risk of infection. When there is septal trauma, the presence of a hematoma underneath the cartilage and its protective mucoperichondrial layer may eventually lead to permanent thickening of the septum, causing partial airway obstruction of the nasal passage. Alternatively, the pressure exerted by a large, untreated septal hematoma may cause necrosis and subsequent erosion of the septum, enabling communication between the nasal passageways. Besides the annoyance to the patient, it may lead to a cosmetic saddle-nose deformity. If the mechanism of injury includes blunt force delivered to the nose, the possibility of a cribriform plate fracture with cerebrospinal fluid rhinorrhea should be considered.

Treatment and Disposition

Local anesthesia of the nose may be attempted but is difficult because of the tightly adhering skin. Injection of epinephrine-containing anesthetics should be avoided on the tip of the nose. Regional anesthetic injection is difficult, but topical application of lidocaine into the nasal cavity may provide sufficient anesthesia. Insertion of multiple cotton-tipped swabs or plain nasal packing gauze soaked in the 4% lidocaine solution is usually sufficient (Figure 43-5). After several minutes and prior to repair, the swabs or gauze should be removed.

Superficial lacerations to the skin layer may be closed with 6-0 nonabsorbable monofilament simple interrupted sutures, which may be removed in 3 to 5 days. Lacerations over exposed cartilage should be closed promptly. Small pieces of cartilage that may be present should be preserved under the skin to provide the optimal cosmetic result. Future revision by a plastic surgeon will be easier if there is abundant tissue available for reconstruction.

If the laceration extends through all tissue layers, closure should begin with a 5-0 monofilament synthetic suture that aligns the skin surrounding the entrance to the nasal canals at the alar rim (Figure 43-5). Initially, the ends can be left untied and long to facilitate the closure of the deeper structures. *Gentle* traction on this suture provides alignment of the mucosa and cartilage layers. The mucosal layer is closed with 5-0 rapidly absorbable interrupted sutures and the area is reirrigated gently from the outside. The cartilage may rarely need to be approximated with a minimal number of 5-0 absorbable sutures. In sharply demarcated linear lacerations, closure of the overlying skin is usually sufficient. Finally, the initial stitch at the alar margin should be reevaluated for precise alignment and tied; then the remainder of the skin should be sutured with 6-0 monofilament nonabsorbable material. Removal of the external sutures may take place in 3 to 5 days.

Septal hematomas should be drained. For a small, unilateral hematoma, the clot can often be aspirated through an 18-gauge needle. Larger hematomas require a horizontal incision at the base (Figure 43-5). Following the procedure, nasal packing prevents the reaccumulation of blood. A brief course of prophylactic antibiotics is recommended to prevent infection of the cartilage. The packing may be removed in 2 to 3 days. Bilateral hematomas are often drained in the operating room.

LIPS

Anatomy

The external surfaces of the lips have three distinct regions: the skin, the vermilion, and the oral mucosa. The cosmetically important junction of the skin and the red portion of the lip is called the *vermilion border*. The orbicularis oris muscle surrounds the mouth. Its integrity is responsible for retaining the saliva inside the mouth, producing the bilabial sounds of speech, and providing important facial expressions.

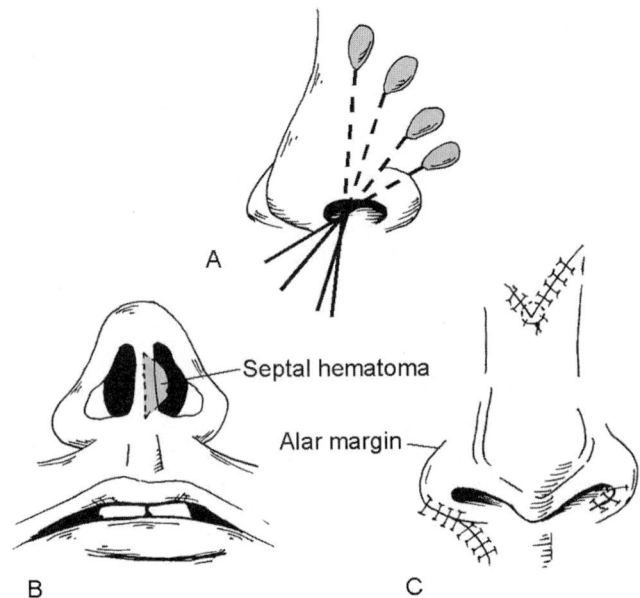

FIG. 43-5. The nose. **A.** Nasal anesthetic technique using cotton-tipped applicators. **B.** Septal hematoma and lateral anatomy. **C.** Frontal view showing closure of skin edges.

The infraorbital nerve supplies the upper lip and the mental nerve supplies the lower lip. Both are branches of the trigeminal nerve and can easily be blocked by regional anesthetic techniques. The lips are richly supplied by the labial arteries.[6]

Evaluation

External as well as intraoral examination is required to appreciate the complete injury. Lacerations should be fully explored. Missing, impacted, or fractured teeth; involvement of the parotid (Stensen) duct; or exposed bone of the maxilla or mandible should be noted. Lacerations that cross the vermilion border are of the utmost cosmetic importance.

Treatment and Disposition

Isolated intraoral mucosal lacerations may not need to be sutured, or if closed, a rapidly absorbable suture is recommended. Through-and-through lacerations that do not include the vermilion border can be closed in layers. The mucosal layer is closed with a 5-0 rapidly absorbable suture followed by gentle reirrigation from the outside. Next, the orbicularis oris muscle is approximated with 5-0 absorbable suture material with a simple interrupted or horizontal mattress technique. Finally, the skin is sutured with 6-0 nonabsorbable monofilament sutures in a simple interrupted fashion. The sutures should be removed in 5 days. Alternatively, the skin can be approximated with tissue adhesive.

Wounds that cross the vermilion border should be repaired by placing the first stitch to precisely approximate the edges of the vermilion border (Figure 43-6). Even 1 mm of step-off will be cosmetically unappealing. Following this first stitch, the repair can proceed as previously described. In some cases, it is helpful to place this crucial suture and leave it untied until the remainder of the skin is sutured. Gentle traction on the ends can help approximate underlying tissue to provide optimal cosmesis. Care should be taken to avoid pulling the suture through the skin in this delicate area. Patients with sutured intraoral lacerations should receive prophylactic antibiotics, usually penicillin.

FIG. 43-6. Irregular-edged vertical laceration of the upper lip. **A.** Traction is applied to the lips and closure of the wound is begun first at the vermilion-skin junction. **B.** The orbicularis oris muscle is then repaired with interrupted, absorbable 4-0 synthetic sutures. **C.** The irregular edges of the skin are then approximated.

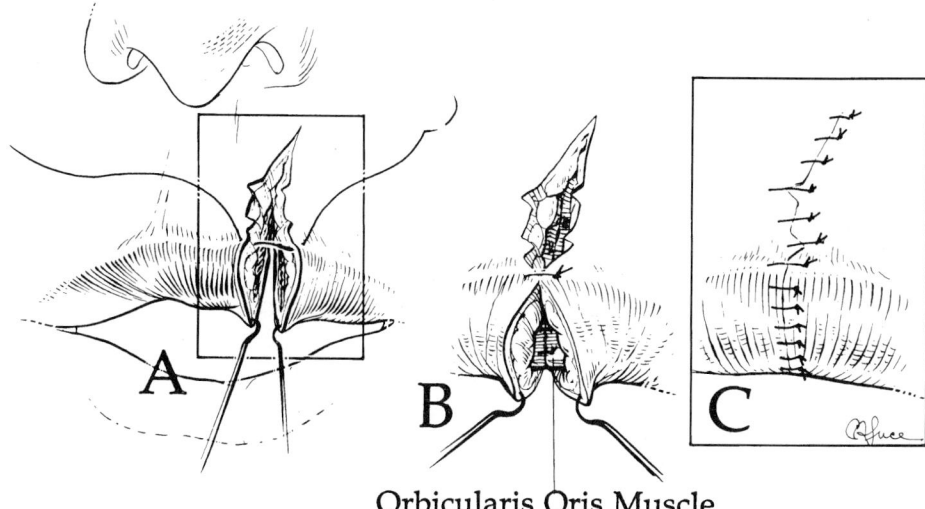

Orbicularis Oris Muscle

EARS

Anatomy

The external ear begins with the external auditory canal and extends to the fibrocartilaginous framework of the auricle and the soft fatty tissue of the earlobe. The blood supply to the ear arises from the superficial temporal and posterior auricular arteries. The majority of the sensory innervation is from the anterior and posterior branches of the greater auricular nerve. The auricular branches of the vagus nerve supply the posterior wall of the external auditory canal, so lacerations that involve this area cannot be anesthetized with auricular nerve blocks.[6]

Evaluation

Lacerations caused by blunt forces to the ear can rupture the tympanic membrane or produce a subchondral hematoma. Hematomas can form even in the absence of a laceration. Lacerations caused by blunt or shear forces may involve the cartilage.[17] The presence of cerebrospinal fluid otorrhea signals a basilar skull fracture.

Treatment and Disposition

During routine wound preparation, a cotton plug can be inserted into the ear canal during irrigation. If a wound extends deep into the canal, the integrity of the tympanic membrane should be verified. Regional anesthesia by auricular nerve block is ideal. Epinephrine should be avoided in lacerations involving the auricle. Impeccable hemostasis prior to repair of an auricular laceration is required to prevent the formation of a hematoma.

Superficial lacerations to the skin can be closed with 6-0 monofilament interrupted sutures (Figure 43-7). Any exposed cartilage should be covered to prevent subsequent infection. If an injury produces several crushed pieces of cartilage under the skin, they should not be removed; remaining cartilage will be beneficial if reconstructive surgery is necessary. Debridement of skin is not advisable, since there is very little excess skin available to cover the existing cartilage. In most through-and-through lacerations of the auricle, the skin can be approximated and the underlying cartilage will be supported adequately. In a large, gaping wound, one or two 6-0 nonabsorbable coated nylon stitches can be used to approximate the edges of cartilage. The knots should be tied so they will not cause an obvious deformity through the skin. If the overlying skin is avulsed, referral to a plastic surgeon for repair using a flap is recommended.[18]

Following repair of the simple ear laceration, a small piece of nonadherent gauze may be applied over the laceration only and a pressure dressing applied. Gauze squares are placed behind the ear to apply pressure and the head is wrapped circumferentially with gauze. The dressing may be tied into place by cutting the last portion of the gauze longitudinally (Figure 43-8). Sutures should be removed in 5 days. Complete avulsion of the ear must be urgently referred to a plastic surgeon.

If an auricular hematoma is suspected, consultation with a plastic surgeon or otolaryngologist is recommended. Proper treatment requires the complete and permanent evacuation of the hematoma and definitive control of the bleeding that caused it. Neglecting to treat an auricular hematoma may produce a cauliflower-ear type cosmetic defect of the cartilage.

THE CHEEKS AND FACE

Lacerations that involve the surface of the face may be repaired carefully using standard wound-care techniques. In general, facial lacerations are closed with 6-0 monofilament simple interrupted sutures that are removed in 5 days. Tissue adhesive may be used in superficial wounds after proper irrigation. If there is significant ten-

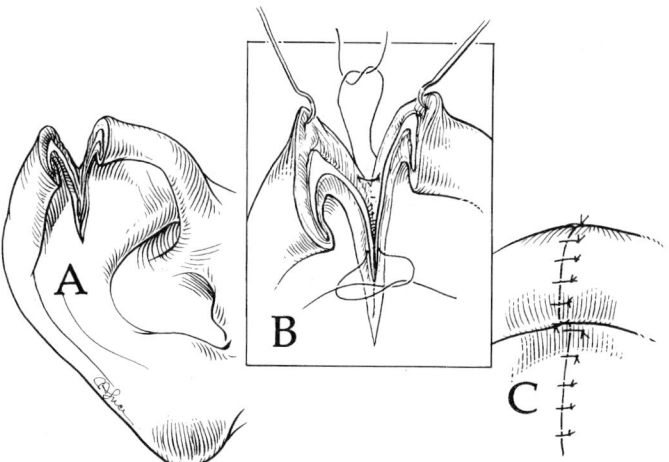

FIG. 43-7. A. Laceration through auricle. **B.** One or two interrupted, 6-0 coated nylon sutures will approximate divided edges of cartilage. **C.** Interrupted nonabsorbable 6-0 synthetic sutures approximate the skin edges.

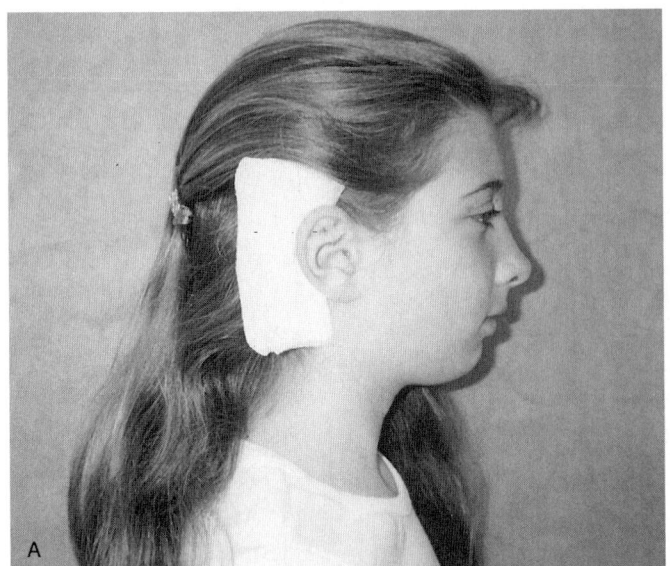

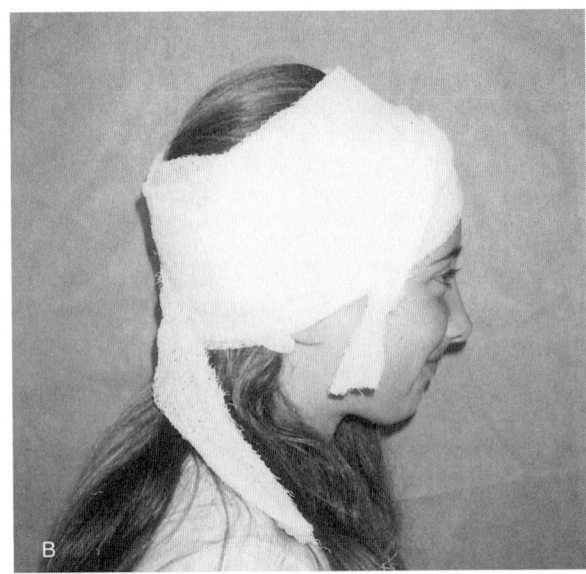

FIG. 43-8. Pressure dressing for ear lacerations. **A.** Gauze placed behind auricle. **B.** Bandage wrapped around head with two ends cut for tying. **C.** Ends tied.

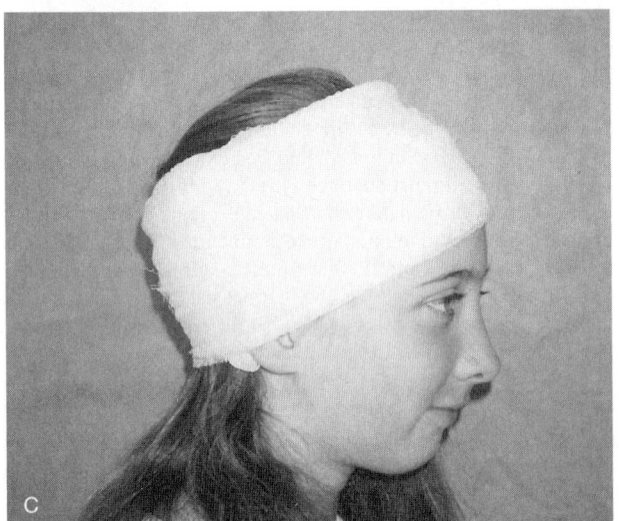

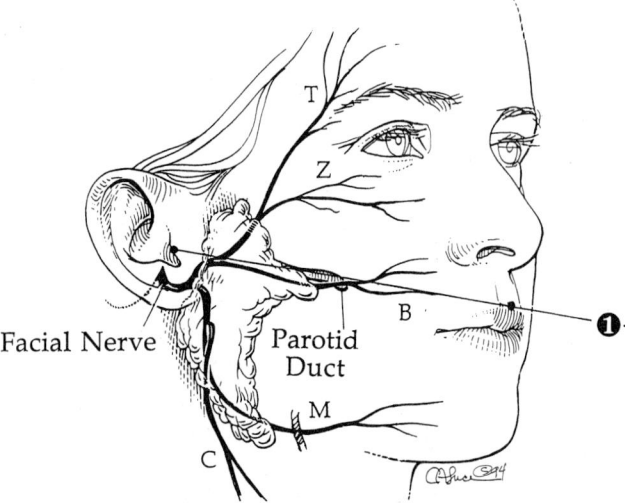

FIG. 43-9. Anatomic structures of the cheek. (1): The course of the parotid duct is deep to a line drawn from the tragus of the ear to the midportion of the upper lip. Branches of the facial nerve: temporal **(T)**, zygomatic **(Z)**, buccal **(B)**, mental **(M)**, and cervical **(C)**.

sion, an underlying layer of 4-0 absorbable suture closure is indicated. Attention to underlying anatomic structures including the facial nerve and parotid gland is important (Figure 43-9).[6] If these structures are involved, operative repair is indicated.

REFERENCES

1. Hollander JE, Singer AJ, Valentine S, Henry MC: Wound registry: Development and validation. *Ann Emerg Med* 25:675, 1995.
2. Hollander JE, Singer AJ: Laceration management. *Ann Emerg Med* 34:356, 1999.
3. Salber PR, Talieferro E: *The Physician's Guide to Domestic Violence: How to Ask the Right Questions and Recognize Abuse-Another Way to Save a Life.* Volcano, CA: Volcano Press, 1995.
4. Le BT, Dierks EJ, Ueek BA, et al: Maxillofacial injuries associated with domestic violence. *J Oral Maxillofac Surg* 59:1277, 2001.
5. Hollander JE, Singer AJ, Valentine S, Shofer FS: Risk factors for infections in patients with traumatic lacerations. *Acad Emerg Med* 8:716, 2001.
6. Moore KL: *Clinically Oriented Anatomy,* 4th ed. Philadelphia: Lippincott, Williams & Wilkins, 1999.
7. Metaxotos NG, Asplund O, Hayes M: The efficacy of bupivacaine with adrenaline in reducing pain and bleeding associated with breast reduction: A prospective trial. *Br J Plastic Surg* 52:290, 1999.

8. Adler AJ, Dubinisky I, Eisen J: Does the use of topical lidocaine, epinephrine, and tetracaine solution provide sufficient anesthesia for laceration repair? *Acad Emerg Med* 5:108, 1988.
9. Singer AJ, Stark MJ: LET versus EMLA for pretreating lacerations: A randomized trial. *Acad Emerg Med* 8:223, 2001.
10. Hollander JE, Richman PB, Werblud M, et al: Irrigation in facial and scalp lacerations: Does it alter outcome? *Ann Emerg Med* 31:73, 1998.
11. Howell JM, Morgan JA: Scalp laceration repair without prior hair removal. *Am J Emerg Med* 6:7, 1988.
12. Hogg K, Carley: Staples or sutures for repair of scalp laceration in adults. *Emerg Med J* 19:327, 2002.
13. Hogg K, Carley S: Staples or sutures in children with scalp lacerations. *Emerg Med J* 19:328, 2002.
14. Aoki N, Oikawa A, Sakai T: Hair braiding closure for superficial wounds. *Surg Neurol* 46:150, 1996.
15. Hock M, Ooi SBS, Saw SM, Lim SH: A randomized controlled trial comparing the hair apposition technique with tissue glue to standard suturing in scalp lacerations (HAT study). *Ann Emerg Med* 40:19, 2002.
16. Singer AJ, Quinn JV, Clark RE, et al: Closure of lacerations and incisions with octyl cyanoacrylate: A multicenter randomized controlled trial. *Surgery* 131:270, 2002.
17. Hochberg J, Ardenghy M, Toledo S, et al: Soft tissue injuries to face and neck: Early assessment and repair. *World J Surg* 25:1023, 2001.
18. Gur E, Barnea Y, Leshem D, et al: Walk through injuries: Glass door facial injuries. *Ann Plast Surg* 46:613, 2001.

44

INJURIES TO THE ARM, HAND, FINGERTIP, AND NAIL

Fiona E. Gallahue
Wallace A. Carter

Soft tissue upper extremity injuries account for about 35 percent of the wounds and lacerations evaluated in the ED.[1] Specific issues relative to wounds and lacerations of the arm and hand include: (1) the potential of injury to the arteries, nerves, and tendons that lie close to the skin, and (2) the importance of hand function in daily and occupational life. Injuries may be classified as closed crush, simple lacerations, open crush with partial amputation, and complete amputation.[2,3] The approach to treatment depends on multiple factors: the mechanism of injury; location of the injury; injury to adjacent arteries, nerves, and tendons; patient's age, sex, handedness, occupation and concurrent medical problems; presence of exposed bone; and anticipated future use of the hand.

GENERAL MANAGEMENT PRINCIPLES

History and Examination

The majority of hand and arm injuries are isolated injuries and can be managed in the ED. Complex or extensive injuries calling for skin grafting or technically advanced skills require consultation with a specialist. Specific considerations in the history include age (potential for underlying bony injury and likelihood for healing and functional recovery), occupation (necessity for arm and hand function), and hand dominance.

Examination of arm and hand injuries includes inspection, evaluation of motor nerve and tendon function, evaluation of sensory nerve function, and evaluation of perfusion.

During inspection, note the position and stance of the arm, hand, and digits. Note if the wound is adjacent to major arteries, nerves, and tendons. Is there exposed tendon or bone? Does the wound contain foreign bodies, debris, or visible contamination? Has there been avulsion of soft tissue or loss of length?

Examining active motion and resistance to passive movement assesses motor function. Patients with a painful injury may be unwilling to move the hand; providing appropriate anesthesia after checking sensory nerve function may provide enough comfort to obtain an adequate motor exam. Despite some overlap, there are pure motor functions of each nerve that should be tested against resistance (Table 44-1). Each tendon in or adjacent to the injured area should be individually assessed. For injuries to the hand and fingers, the extensor digitorum (ED), flexor digitorum profundus (FDP), and the flexor digitorum superficialis (FDS) to each digit is examined individually. The FDS, which splits and inserts at the proximal interphalangeal (PIP) joint, can be examined by holding all other digits in extension and flexing the PIP joint against resistance. The FDP, which runs below the FDS past the split to attach at the distal interphalangeal (DIP) joint, can be examined by holding the PIP joint in extension and flexing the DIP joint against resistance. Limited or painful movement suggests partial involvement of a tendon.[3] Abnormality in motor nerve or tendon function testing warrants a more in-depth examination including visual inspection and appropriate consultation.

Sensation should be assessed in the median, ulnar, and radial nerve distribution (Table 44-2 and Figure 44-1). For injuries distal to the mid-palm, the digital nerves should be assessed by static two-point discrimination longitudinally along the ulnar and radial aspect of the volar pad of the potentially involved digits. Static two-point discrimination is evaluated by using ECG calipers or a paper clip bent into a "V" shape with the two ends separated by approximately 5 to 6 mm. During testing, the two points should not cross the midline and each stimulus should be 3 to 4 s apart. Normal two-point discrimination is defined as <6 mm; good is 6 to 10 mm; fair is 11 to 15 mm; and poor is >15 mm. Two-point spatial acuity of touch diminishes with age; young (18 to 33 years) patients have a mean two-point acuity of 2 mm while elderly (>66 years) patients have a mean acuity of 5 mm.[4] The two most important areas to maintain sensation are the ulnar side of the thumb and the radial side of the index volar pads in order to preserve pinch sensation.

Intact radial and ulnar pulses and capillary refill are usually adequate to exclude significant vascular injury. However, an arterial injury proximal to the wrist may not be obvious due to good collateral circulation. For forearm wounds proximal to the wrist, an Allen test should be performed. A Doppler probe is useful to detect a diminished pulse, detect flow in digital arteries, and to calculate an arterial pressure index (API = the ratio of the systolic blood pressure between the injured and the uninjured side). In the absence of a diminished pulse or a ratio less than 1.0, the likelihood of a clinically significant occult arterial injury is exceedingly small. Lack of obvious arterial bleeding does not rule out arterial injury since cleanly transected arteries may contract and prevent obvious bleeding.[2]

Imaging Studies

Radiographic evaluation with anteroposterior (AP) and lateral films is indicated if bony injuries, retained radiopaque foreign bodies, or joint penetration are suspected. Oblique views of the hands and digits are useful to visualize small areas with overlapping bones. For finger injuries, isolated radiographs of the involved digit(s) are better because the detail on hand films alone is often not adequate for complete evaluation.

Where there is suspicion for a radiolucent retained foreign body, especially wood, another imaging study (ultrasound, computed

TABLE 44-1 Motor Testing of the Peripheral Nerves of the Upper Extremity

Nerve	Motor Exam
Radial	Dorsiflexion of wrist
Median	Thumb abduction away from the palm Thumb interphalangeal joint flexion
Ulnar	Adduction/abduction of digits

TABLE 44-2 Sensory Testing of Peripheral Nerves in the Upper Extremity

Sensory Nerve	Area of Test
Radial	First dorsal web space
Median	Volar tip of index finger
Ulnar	Volar tip of little finger

tomography [CT], or magnetic resonance [MR]) may be necessary (see Chap. 46). Ultrasound may detect radiolucent objects such as vegetative matter as small as 1 × 2 mm, but requires operator skill and experience. CT can also identify radiolucent objects and localizes a foreign body in relationship to the surrounding anatomy. MR has similar capabilities as CT but cannot be used for metal objects.

Adequate Visualization

Since wounds and the adjacent structures are often small, patient positioning, adequate lighting, and a bloodless field are necessary for wound evaluation.

For some injuries, a bloodless field may require a proximal tourniquet to temporarily halt arterial inflow. The two most commonly used tourniquets are the rubber (Penrose) drain for finger injuries and the pneumatic tourniquet placed around the upper arm for forearm and hand injuries.

For a rubber tourniquet for digital injuries, a 1-inch Penrose drain is placed around the base of the finger, stretched away from the hand, and secured with a clamp or hemostat. If time allows, the digit can be exsanguinated prior to tourniquet placement by wrapping the digit with the Penrose drain from distal to proximal, then carefully removing the drain from distal to proximal before securing it around the base of the digit. Excessively high pressures and duration, which can cause neurovascular damage, may be avoided by limiting the stretch of the drain to no more than 50 percent of the original length for 15- to 20-min periods.[3,5]

For more proximal injuries, especially those with brisk arterial bleeding, a pneumatic tourniquet using the manual blood pressure cuff is useful. Esmarch's technique is to elevate the injured extremity and apply an elastic bandage starting distally and proceeding proximally to the area where the cuff is to be applied. This will help to exsanguinate the limb and prevent backflow bleeding. The cuff is applied around the upper arm and inflated to pressures above the systolic blood pressure of the patient, but not to exceed 250 mm Hg.[3] The cuff tubing is clamped with a hemostat instead of closing the air release valve in order to prevent slow air leakage. The maximum cuff inflation time is

1 h, although a limit of 30 min is recommended to ensure patient safety.

Once adequate visualization is obtained, the injury can be examined for foreign bodies and tendon and joint capsule injuries. It is important to examine the arm and hand in the position of injury in order to avoid missing injuries that may have moved out of the field of view when examined in a neutral position.

Lacerations in proximity to joints should be carefully examined for potential violation of the joint capsule. If the depth of the injury raises the question of extension into the joint capsule, joint injection is warranted. After antiseptic preparation of the area, the joint is injected with normal saline from an area away from the laceration site. Fluid dripping from the joint indicates an open joint capsule and requires specialty consultation.[6] For small joints or questionable exams, a few drops of fluorescein may be added to the injected saline and the joint examined with a Wood's lamp for evidence of fluorescent effluent. Methylene blue, once used to aid in this diagnosis, is discouraged due to the staining of the intra-articular surfaces.

Wound Dressing and Postrepair Care

Once the injury is repaired, antibiotic ointment should be applied to the repaired incision and sutures and the wound covered with a nonadherent dressing (see Chap. 48). The area should always be wrapped loosely in a soft dressing to allow for adequate circulation. Where possible, the fingernail or volar pad should remain visible so capillary refill can be followed. Depending on the size or nature of the injury, especially injuries in close proximity to a joint or with tendon involvement, splinting may be advisable for protection and avoidance of painful stimulation (see Chap. 267). Isolated digital lacerations may be better served with a padded aluminum splint. The extremity should be kept elevated above the level of the heart to reduce edema and adequate analgesia should be provided. A follow-up wound check is recommended within 48 to 72 h. Sutures are usually removed 8 to 10 days after the injury.

Prophylactic antibiotics are not routinely indicated, but may be considered in wounds that are contaminated, due to mammalian bites, for injuries that are more than 12 h old, in the presence of exposed bone, or in patients with concurrent medical problems that may affect wound healing (i.e., those with diabetes or renal or peripheral vascular disease) (see Chap. 48). Antibiotics should be chosen to cover suspected contaminants and pathogens and given early by a route that quickly achieves high blood and tissue levels.

Indications for admission to the hospital include injuries that require repair in the operating room, those that require a course of intravenous antibiotics, or the presence of social issues such as homelessness or the patient's inability to follow basic aftercare instructions.

SPECIAL CONSIDERATIONS

High Pressure Injection Injuries

Injuries to the hand from high-pressure injectors have potentially devastating consequences. Substances such as grease and oil-based compounds do not produce an inflammatory response until much later due to their high viscosity. These injuries often go unsuspected since they usually present with an initially benign appearance, most commonly an isolated puncture wound to the index finger of the nondominant hand.[7] The patient and physician may not be aware that they have an injected substance subcutaneously until radiographs are obtained. The severity of these injuries is based on several factors: properties of the injected material, amount of injected material, velocity of the injectant, anatomy of the injection site, spread of the injectant, and time to diagnosis and treatment. Injection injuries should be referred immediately to a hand specialist or plastic surgeon for operative debridement. The amputation rate for these injuries ranges from 16 to 55 percent.[7]

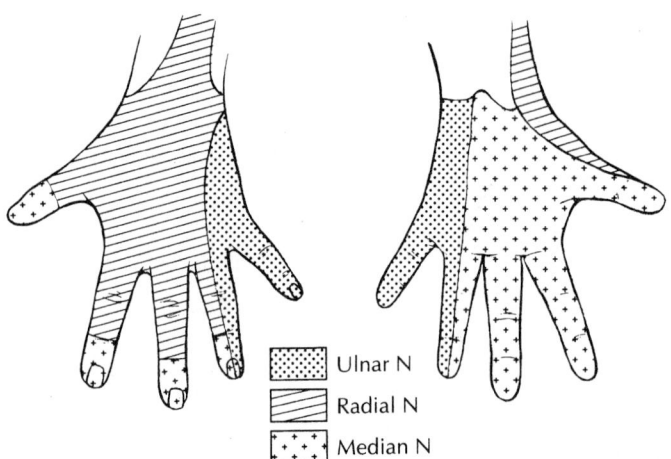

Ulnar N

Radial N

Median N

FIG. 44-1. Sensory innervation to the hand.

Injuries in Children

In a child, identifying a fracture with plain radiographs may be difficult owing to an open epiphysis. It is often necessary to obtain radiographs of the opposite side for comparison. If a surgical procedure is indicated and the child is unable to tolerate the procedure after local anesthesia alone, procedural sedation may be required.

Keeping dressings intact on children poses a problem because of their continuous activity, rendering a routine hand dressing and protective finger splint ineffective. If the dressing is essential to wound healing, the child should be placed in a long arm cast.[8]

SPECIFIC TREATMENT STRATEGIES

Forearm and Wrist Lacerations

Patients with wrist lacerations should be questioned about suicidal gestures or attempts. Patients with suicidal intent require psychiatric evaluation after wound repair.

Tendons and nerves distal to the wound should be individually examined. The forearm has six extensor compartments located dorsally, innervated by the radial nerve (Table 44-3). Located on the volar surface of the forearm and crossing the wrist are the 12 flexor tendons innervated by the median and ulnar nerves (Table 44-4).

Injuries about the elbow may affect the radial and ulnar nerves, which are in close proximity to the lateral and medial epicondyles, respectively. The radial nerve emanates from the spiral groove in the humerus approximately 10 cm proximal to the lateral epicondyle. The ulnar nerve travels behind the medial epicondyle as it runs between the two heads of the flexor carpi ulnaris into the forearm. The median nerve is more protected in the elbow region as it runs in close proximity with the brachial artery, crossing anteriorly to the ulnar artery at the origin of the anterior interosseous nerve in the forearm. Though injuries to these nerves are more common in fractures and dislocations, these nerves can be compromised by simple soft tissue injuries at the elbow due to their location and lack of overlying protective soft tissue in this area.[9]

For most simple lacerations to the forearm and wrist, 4-0 or 5-0 nonabsorbable monofilament sutures such as nylon or polypropylene should be used. For gaping injuries or injuries under high stress, deep sutures using 4-0 absorbable material may be required. Injuries that involve more than one parallel laceration, classic for suicide attempts,

TABLE 44-3   Extensor Compartments in the Forearm

Extensors in the Forearm	Function
First compartment	
Abductor pollicis longus	Abducts and extends thumb
Extensor pollicis brevis	Extends thumb at MCP joint
Second compartment	
Extensor carpi radialis longus	Extends and radially deviates
Extensor carpi radialis brevis	wrist (both)
Third compartment	
Extensor pollicis longus	Extends thumb at IP joint
Fourth compartment	
Extensor digitorum communis	Splits into four tendons at level of the wrist.
	Extends index, long, ring, and little digits
Extensor indicis proprius	Extends index finger
Fifth compartment	
Extensor digiti minimi	Extends little finger at MCP joint
Sixth compartment	
Extensor carpi ulnaris	Extends and radially deviates wrist

Abbreviations: IP = interphalangeal; MCP = metacarpophalangeal.

TABLE 44-4   Flexor Tendons in the Forearm

Flexor Tendon	Function
Flexor carpi radialis	Flexes and radially deviates wrist
Flexor carpi ulnaris	Flexes and ulnarly deviates wrist
Palmaris longus	Flexes wrist
Flexor pollicis longus	Flexes thumb at MCP and IP joint
At index, middle, ring and little fingers:	
Flexor digitorum superficialis	Flexes digits at MCP and PIP joints
Flexor digitorum profundus	Flexes digits at MCP, PIP, and DIP joints

Abbreviations: DIP = distal interphalangeal; PIP = proximal interphalangeal; IP = interphalangeal; MCP = metacarpophalangeal.

may require horizontal mattress sutures to cross all lacerations for closure to prevent compromising the vascular supply of the island of skin located between incisions (Figure 44-2). Adhesive tapes or tissue adhesives in conjunction with sutures or alone for closure may also be useful.[10]

Palm Lacerations

The palmar skin surface is adapted for contact with objects in the environment; it is thicker with an underlying connective tissue layer of fascia, making it much more adherent to bone than dorsal skin. The thenar, palmar, and digital creases are connections between the skin and underlying fascia without intervening adipose tissue.[3] These creases should be carefully approximated during closures. The thickness of palmar skin makes eversion of the edges especially difficult. For this reason, interrupted horizontal mattress sutures with 5-0 nonabsorbable monofilament suture are recommended to ensure that these sutures do not pull through.[10]

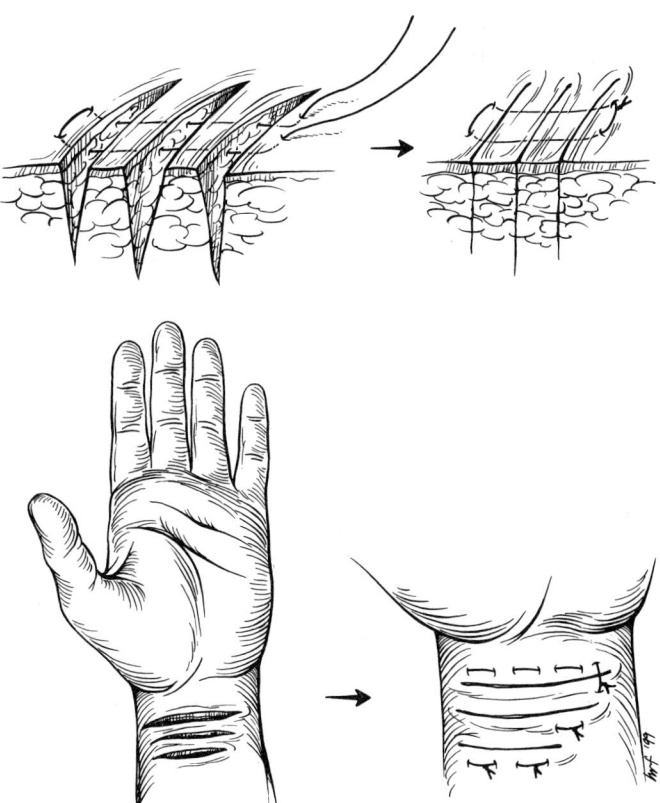

FIG. 44-2. Horizontal mattress sutures for multiple parallel lacerations.

Dorsal Hand Lacerations

CLENCHED FIST INJURIES   Patients with injuries to the dorsum of the hand should be questioned about the possibility of a clenched fist injury (CFI) with a human bite. These wounds generally produce a small laceration (3 to 5 mm) over the dorsal MCP joint.[11] After contact is made, the patient is likely to extend the hand, which deeply inoculates oral bacteria into the wound. Human saliva contains as many as 50 species of bacteria with a microbe concentration of 1×10^8 organisms per mL. *Staphylococcus aureus* is the most common bacterial species isolated from human bite wounds followed by *Streptococcus* spp., *Corynebacterium* spp., and *Eikenella corrodens*. Human bites have been documented to transmit herpes, actinomycosis, syphilis, tetanus, and hepatitis B and C.[11] HBIG and Hepatitis B vaccine should be given if indicated. In CFI infections, polymicrobial involvement is the rule.

Radiography should be performed in these injuries to evaluate for embedded teeth, air in the joint or soft tissues, or fractures. For patients who delay evaluation and develop obvious infection, exploration, open irrigation, and debridement in the operating room are required followed by admission for intravenous antibiotics and elevation. If the patient presents soon after the injury and without evident infection, evaluation, exploration, irrigation, and debridement can be done in the ED with appropriate equipment and physician expertise. It is important to visualize the full extent of the wound, evaluate the hand through full range of motion, and exclude injury to the extensor tendon or joint capsule. If no injury to these structures is seen, the wound should be copiously irrigated and dressed with a nonadherent dressing. The hand should be splinted in a position of function. A 3- to 5-day course of prophylactic antibiotics should be prescribed, usually amoxicillin-clavulanate, (see Chap. 48). The patient should be instructed to elevate the extremity and re-evaluation within 24 to 48 h is recommended. If there are any issues of patient compliance, comorbid illness causing immunocompromise, current evidence of infection, or joint or tendon involvement, a hand surgeon should be consulted and the patient admitted for observation and IV antibiotics, usually ampicillin-sulbactam or cefoxitin.

SKIN LACERATIONS   The dorsal skin of the hand is thin and freely mobile, allowing for extensive range of motion for all joints. Because of the mobility of the skin and superficial nature of the extensor tendons, a careful examination through a full range of motion at the site of injury as well as in the position of injury is necessary to avoid missing a tendon injury. The thinness and lack of underlying tissue allows skin avulsion to occur easily, making skin approximation difficult.[3,10] Simple 5-0 nonabsorbable sutures should be adequate for closure. To provide better cosmesis for injuries to the dorsum of the hand, subcuticular stitches with 5-0 absorbable, a pull-through subcuticular closure with nonabsorbable suture for linear lacerations, or a corner stitch for a V-shaped laceration may be considered[10] (Figure 44-3).

Extensor Tendon Lacerations

The proximity of the extensor tendons to the surface makes them vulnerable to any open injury. An emergency physician who is experienced and comfortable with the procedure can repair extensor tendon injuries between the distal wrist and metacarpophalangeal joints. However, it is good practice to discuss these cases with the consulting hand surgeon for treatment preferences and continuity of care. Extensor tendon injuries of the thumb or those with severe contamination should be referred to a hand surgeon. Small partial extensor tendon injuries (<50 percent transected) should be repaired with absorbable synthetic material.[3,12] Larger partial tendon injuries (>50 percent transected) and complete extensor tendon lacerations should be sutured with 4-0 (5-0 for smaller tendons) colorless nonabsorbable material such as polypropylene or nylon, and the skin closed with 5-0

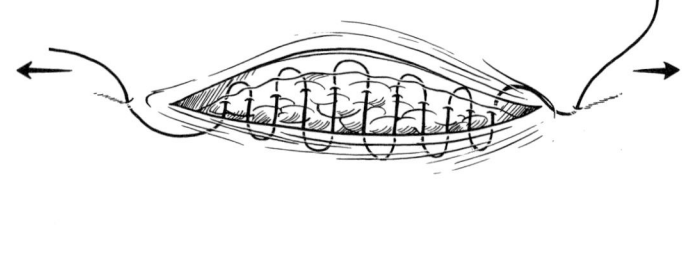
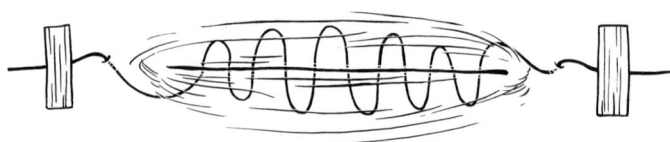

FIG. 44-3. Pull-through subcuticular suture.

nonabsorbable suture material.[3,12] A figure-of-eight stitch with the knot placed at the edge of the tendon is recommended to repair lacerated extensors[3,12] (Figure 44-4). After repair of the tendon and overlying skin, the hand or digit should be splinted in position of function with instructions to maintain elevation of the extremity. Follow-up with a hand surgeon is recommended within 7 days.

Certain complications can be seen with disrupted extensor mechanisms. A swan neck deformity or mallet finger deformity is caused by the complete disruption of the terminal extensor mechanism and subsequent proximal and dorsal displacement of the lateral bands (Figure 44-5A). A boutonniere deformity is usually a delayed complication after injury to the PIP joint. The central slip becomes disrupted and there is unopposed action of the FDS tendon, forcing the lateral bands to move volarly and operate as flexors (Figure 44-5B). If open, these injuries require operative repair. If they are closed injuries, they require splinting in extension for up to 6 weeks or operative repair, and referral to a hand surgeon.[3]

Flexor Tendon Lacerations

Flexor tendon injuries are usually repaired in the operating room by a hand surgeon because of the complexity required. Early consultation is important because many surgeons will repair complete flexor tendon lacerations no later than 12 to 24 h after injury.[3] If operative repair of the flexor tendon is going to be delayed, as a temporizing measure the wound should be appropriately cleaned, the skin closed, and the hand splinted in flexion to prevent contraction of the surrounding muscles. The hand surgeon can follow-up the patient in 2 to 3 days and schedule the flexor tendon repair within 7 days. Postinjury scarring and tendon retraction make flexor tendon repairs more difficult after 10 to 14 days.

Finger Lacerations

In general, isolated finger lacerations are straightforward injuries to examine and repair. Vascular status is checked by capillary refill and sensory nerve status is checked by static two-point discrimination. Motor function of the extensor and two flexor mechanisms should be examined. Simple interrupted sutures with 5-0 nonabsorbable suture provide adequate closure for most digital lacerations.[10]

Deep finger lacerations may include partial or complete amputations of the digit. These injuries should involve the consultation of a hand surgeon to discuss the possibility of replantation. Guidelines for digit replantation are only that-general principles and not absolute criteria. Relative indications for replantation are injuries in children, injuries to the thumb, multiple digit amputation, and single digit am-

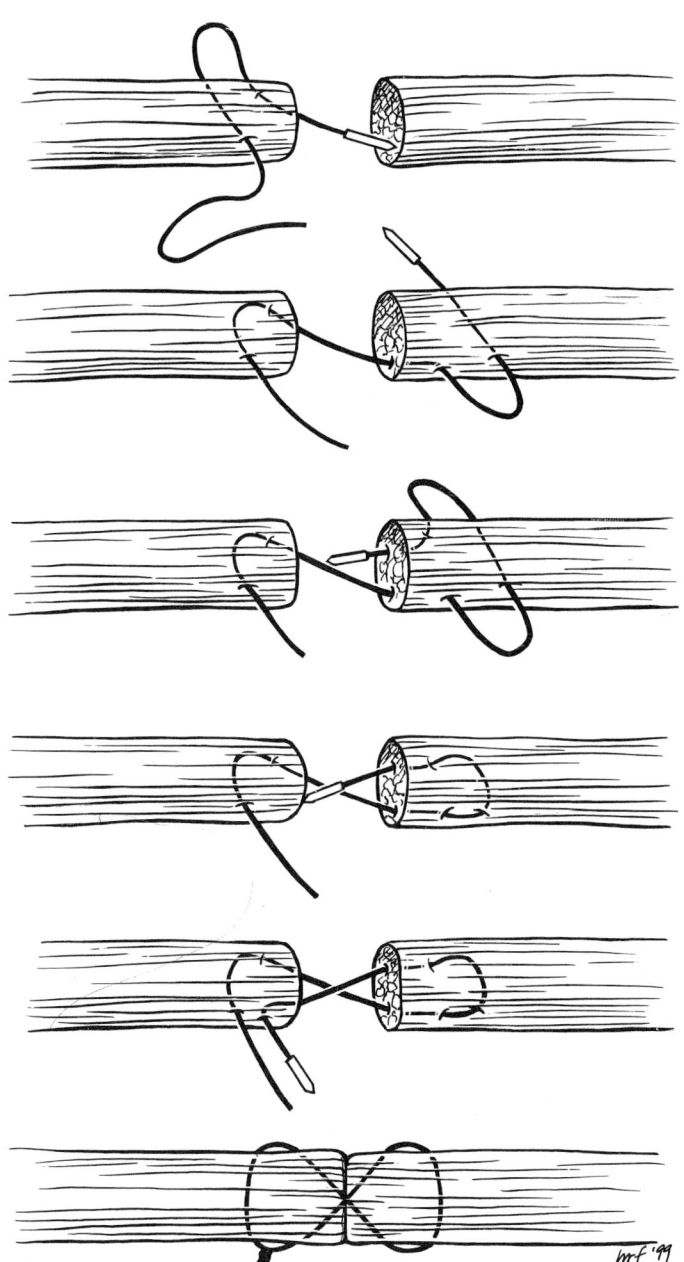

FIG. 44-4. Extensor tendon laceration repair with a figure-of-eight stitch.

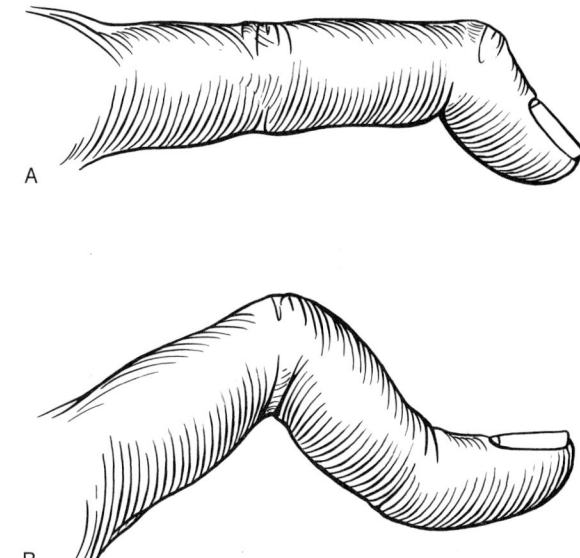

FIG. 44-5. A. Mallet finger. **B.** Boutonniere deformity.

Digital Nerve Injuries

Injuries to the digital nerve can be classified as contusion (neuropraxia), crush (axonotmesis), or transection (neurotmesis). Digital nerve injuries are suspected when static two-point discrimination is distinctly greater on one side of the volar pad than the other, or when it is >10 mm. Digital nerve injuries can be repaired using microsurgical techniques either acutely or days to weeks after the injury. Concomitant injuries and wound contamination are typical indications for delayed repair. Prognosis depends on the specific injury and age of the patient. Neuropraxias heal in 12 days to 6 months. Transection injuries do slightly better than crush injuries, but even with microsurgical repair, recovery is often incomplete.

Fingertip Injuries

Fingertip injuries are those that occur distal to the insertion of the flexor and extensor tendons about at the level of the lunula. These injuries are among the most frequently injured parts of the hand and such injuries may involve the skin, pulp tissue, distal phalanx, and the perionychium, which is made up of the nail, nail bed, and surrounding structures.[14,15] (Figure 44-6). The goals of healing are to maintain length and cosmetic appearance, have the fingertip approach normal sensation and function, and have as short and uncomplicated a healing period as possible.

putation proximal to the insertion of the FDS.[3,13] The strongest contraindications to replantation are crush injuries and avulsion injuries since the neurovascular damage to the amputated digit is significant and offers a poor prognosis. Other relative contraindications include multiple levels of injury to the amputated part, long ischemia time (>24 h) of the amputated part, patients in poor health, or significant comorbid factors such as diabetes or severe pulmonary or cardiac disease which may lead to significant perioperative mortality.[3,13] Another relative contraindication is a smoking history since replants in smokers are prone to profound vasospasm leading to loss of the replanted digit. The final relative contraindication for replantation is injuries between the MCP joint and the mid-level of the middle phalanx. Fingers replanted at this level are often stiff due to recurrent tendon adhesions between the FDS and FDP tendons, limiting the function of the adjacent uninjured fingers.[8]

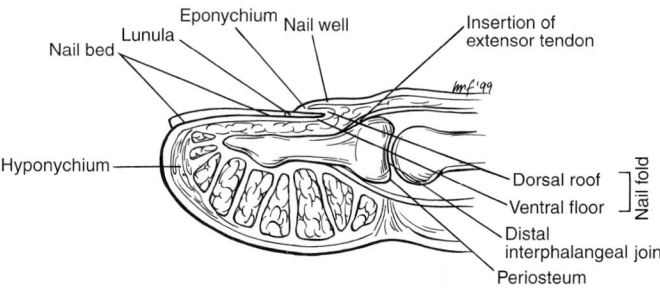

FIG. 44-6. Anatomy of the perionychium. [Reproduced with permission from Zook EG: The perionychium, in DP Green, (ed): *Operative Hand Surgery,* 2d ed. New York, NY: Churchill Livingstone, 1988, p. 1332.]

DIGITAL TIP INJURIES WITH SKIN AND PULP TISSUE LOSS ONLY

Distal fingertip amputations that are 1 cm^2 or less in size without exposed bone can usually be treated conservatively with serial dressing changes alone (Figure 44-7A).[14,15] This is a desirable option, because healing occurs by secondary intention and results in very little scarring. Follow-up is arranged in 2 days for wound check and the patient is made aware that wound care is vital to the success of this technique. The patient is instructed to soak the injured fingertip in warm water to which an antibacterial soap has been added once a day for 10 min, followed by tap-water irrigation and application of a sterile nonadherent dressing. This procedure is performed daily for the first 10 to 15 days and every other day thereafter. On average, complete healing may take 4 to 8 weeks, and both the cosmetic appearance and sensibility of the fingertip are quite satisfactory with this technique. Conservative management is advocated in children less than 12 years of age, since they have greater regenerative potential than do adults.[11]

In cases in which the severed skin tip is available, an alternative means of treatment is to use the amputated portion as a full-thickness skin graft. The amputated tissue is cleaned and debrided of nonviable tissue, the undersurface of the skin is then defatted with sharp scissors, and the graft is sutured to the defect using nylon sutures. Sutures are left long and tied over a 2 × 2 cm gauze stent dressing to compress the graft firmly against the fingertip. Appropriate follow-up is made and unless obvious purulence ensues, the stented dressing is left undisturbed for 7 to 12 days.

A split- or full-thickness skin graft harvested from a distant site is another means of wound closure. This procedure may be indicated in situations in which the severed skin tip is either not available or nonviable, significant pulp tissue loss is greater than 1 cm^2, or the patient's desire to have full use of the hand precludes waiting the 4 to 8 weeks necessary for healing by secondary intention. In these cases, consultation with a specialist is appropriate.

Many authors agree that conservative management of fingertip injuries without bone exposure, as opposed to the above techniques, is superior in terms of cosmetic appearance, improved function, and sensibility of the involved digit.[8,14,15]

DIGITAL TIP INJURIES WITH EXPOSED BONE

If a significant loss of tissue to the fingertip causes exposure of the tuft of the distal phalanx, skin grafting will be unsuccessful since bone does not provide adequate vascularity to support the donor tissue.[14,15] Several treatment options exist, always keeping in mind the important goals of preserving digit

length, especially with regard to the thumb and index finger, as well as sensitivity and functionality of the fingertip. The size and geometry of the injury, the angle of tip amputation, and the availability of the amputated tip will determine the options available for wound closure.

If the bony protuberance is less than 0.5 cm in length and the soft tissue defect is less than 1 cm^2, the bone may be trimmed back using a rongeur and the wound left to heal by secondary intention as previously described. A dorsal obliquely angulated wound may be treated in the ED with bone shortening followed by primary closure of the wound using the adjacent volar tissue (see Figure 44-7D). An injury of this type has a favorable prognosis because the sensate volar skin is intact. Fat from the local tissue may need to be trimmed to allow wound closure without tension. The nail should be removed and attention paid to associated injuries to the nail bed and surrounding structures. Although results are comparable to those following conservative management, shortcomings include loss of length as well as tenderness of the fingertip and some degree of functional disability.

Amputations that are angled either in a transverse or volar direction have less favorable outcomes because they do not always have adequate soft tissue and skin coverage to allow for primary closure and preservation of length (see Figures 44-7B and C). Consultation with a plastic or hand surgeon is necessary, as these injuries often require techniques beyond the scope of practice of most emergency physicians.

Incomplete digital tip amputations, defined by the retention of the neurovascular bundle as well as portions of the underlying bone, are among the most difficult injuries to reconstruct and require consultation with a specialist. If adequate circulation is retained in the tip, the injury is treated with fracture reduction, internal pin fixation, and repair of the soft tissue injury. This procedure is optimally performed in the operating room.

In all patients with a complete amputation that occurs proximal to the lunula, consultation with a hand or plastic surgeon is recommended for possible replantation in the operating room.[13] Conversely, in the adult patient, replantation of a complete amputation distal to the lunula is not usually advocated. This is because the procedure is technically demanding owing to the arborization of the neurovascular bundle at this location, and carries a poor prognosis. However, consultation with the surgical specialist is clearly indicated in all patients with specific occupational concerns and when the injured digit is the thumb or index finger.

Although fingertip injuries are quite common in children, most require only conservative management because of the rapid healing process.[8] Repairs should be done using absorbable sutures. Surgical procedures such as grafts and advancement flaps should be avoided where possible. A completely amputated composite tip may be reattached to serve solely as a biologic dressing, and parents should be informed that the tip might necrose, dry up, and turn black as the underlying wound continues to heal. In children less than 6 years of age, replantation and revascularization of the composite tip may be a viable treatment option when performed by the surgical specialist.

INJURIES INVOLVING THE PERIONYCHIUM

The nail, nail bed, and surrounding soft tissue make up the perionychium (see Figure 44-6). The nail bed is made up of the germinal and sterile matrix. The germinal matrix begins 3 to 5 mm proximal and deep to the eponychium and extends distally to the lunula. From there, the sterile matrix extends distally to the hyponychium. Nail injuries can be described as simple nail bed laceration, stellate laceration, severe crush, and complete avulsion. Injury to the perionychium is most commonly due to closure of the fingertip in a door, and is usually in the distal portion of the nail bed. The mechanism of injury is a force directed to the dorsum of the nail, causing it to bend or break and crushing the nail bed against the unyielding tuft of the distal phalanx. There is an associated distal tuft fracture in approximately 50 percent of nail bed injuries; thus all patients require the standard three radiographic views of the involved digit(s). Nail plate deformity permanently affecting nail growth is the most common complication resulting from lack of treatment.

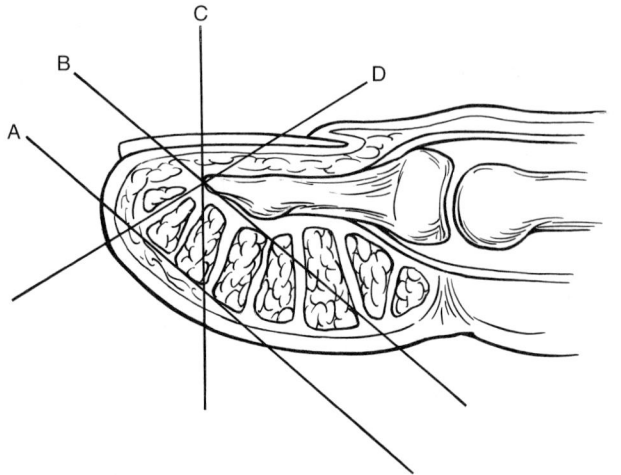

FIG. 44-7. Fingertip amputations. **A.** Volar angulation without bone exposure. **B.** Volar angulation with bone exposure. **C.** Transverse or perpendicular angulation with bone exposure. **D.** Dorsal angulation with bone exposure. [Reproduced with permission from Russell RC: Fingertip injuries, in J McCarthy (ed): *Plastic Surgery.* Philadelphia, PA: Saunders, 1990, p. 4479.]

Subungual Hematoma   These are injuries due to disruption of the blood vessels of the nail bed. The area of the hematoma is directly proportional to the degree of vascular damage. If the subungual hematoma covers greater than 50 percent, treatment can be accomplished with trephination of the nail plate to allow for adequate decompression and drainage of the hematoma. Various tools have been used effectively for this purpose, including a heated paper clip, electric nail drill, electrocautery, 18-gauge needle, and scalpel. The disadvantages of the heated paper clip include coagulation of the hematoma and introduction of carbon particles called "lampblack" into the nail bed, which may delay healing and cause tattooing. Use of a needle, scalpel, or nail drill can be painful and may necessitate local anesthesia. A hand-held electrocautery device permits rapid and painless trephination and is sterile and disposable. However, not every ED will be equipped with such a tool, and emergency physicians will likely perform nail trephination using tools they are familiar with. Patients are discharged with local wound care instructions to soak the affected finger in warm water containing antibacterial soap two to three times a day for 7 days.

Previously, it was commonly recommended that for a subungual hematoma occupying more than 50 percent of the nail bed area, the nail be removed in order to evaluate the nail bed and repair any underlying laceration. This practice has fallen out of favor with recent prospective studies showing that simple trephination produces a good to excellent outcome in most patients with subungual hematoma regardless of size, injury mechanism, or the presence of fracture.[16,17] Nail removal is recommended only if there is associated nail avulsion or surrounding nail fold disruption.

Nail removal can be accomplished with adequate anesthesia, digit tourniquet, nail elevation off the nail bed using iris scissors, elevation of the eponychium off the nail, and then removal by gentle longitudinal traction with a hemostat. Lacerations of the nail bed are carefully repaired using 6-0 absorbable sutures. Crush injuries often result in stellate lacerations, which may require extensive meticulous repair using a magnifying loupe for visualization. The nail is gently cleaned with saline, taking care not to damage the germinal matrix; it is then trephinated and secured in its anatomic position. This is accomplished by placing a 5-0 nonabsorbable suture through the proximal end of the nail plate and then passing it underneath and through the center of the eponychial fold. Once the nail plate is returned to its anatomic position, the suture is tied down over the nail. The replaced nail acts as a natural splint to the terminal phalanx, prevents formation of synechiae, and protects the sensitive nail bed. If the nail is not available, nonbiologic stents or a sterile piece of the aluminum foil used to wrap suture materials may be fashioned to resemble the avulsed nail and inserted under the eponychium. The fingertip is then dressed in nonadherent gauze and placed in a volar splint to limit movement at the DIP joint. Patients are given postoperative wound care instructions (e.g., as to hand elevation as well as neurovascular checks) and are given adequate pain relief. Unless obvious purulence is noted, the dressing is left undisturbed for 5 to 7 days, after which the site is examined for new hematoma formation. The suture attached to the nail is removed after 3 weeks and the existing nail will be dislodged by the new ingrowing nail after 1 to 3 months.

If an associated distal phalanx fracture coexists with a nail bed laceration, it usually manifests as an avulsion of the nail out of the proximal eponychial fold. If this happens, the nail is removed, the fracture is stabilized by manual reduction, and the nail bed is repaired as previously described. The nail replaced in its anatomic position serves as a biologic splint to maintain fracture reduction, owing to its proximity to the underlying bone. Unstable reductions require consultation with a plastic or hand surgeon for internal fixation using Kirschner wires to prevent deformity of the nail bed.

Nail Bed Avulsion Injuries   An avulsion or crush injury may tear the nail completely away from the digit, with fragments of matrix tissue left on the underside of the avulsed nail. These matrix fragments should be preserved for use as free grafts, and when possible attached to the nail bed using 6-0 or 7-0 absorbable sutures. When the nail or avulsed nail bed fragments are not available, or in the case of a large defect, a full-thickness nail bed graft can be harvested from the patient's toe and sutured into the nail bed of the affected finger. As these injuries are complex and their repair is technically challenging, consultation with a hand or plastic surgeon is appropriate. In addition, avulsion injuries to the nail bed have the poorest prognosis of any fingertip injury.

Avulsion injuries may also incompletely tear the proximal portion of the nail out from under the eponychium. Management entails replacement of the nail root into its anatomic position using a series of three horizontal mattress sutures (Figure 44-8). One suture is placed through the center and one in each corner of the eponychial fold. The sutures are then passed through the proximal portion of the corresponding segment of avulsed germinal matrix and then back out through the nail fold, pulling the matrix back to its anatomic position.

Ring Tourniquet Syndrome

A tight ring encircling the proximal phalanx may become entrapped because of distal swelling. Such swelling may be the result of trauma, infections, skin disorders, allergic reactions, or the tight ring alone. As the digit expands, venous outflow is restricted by the tight ring, producing more swelling. This vicious cycle may lead to nerve damage, ischemia, and digital gangrene. The presence of impaired sensation (diminished static two-point discrimination) or diminished perfusion (delayed capillary refill) indicates significant constriction; rapid ring removal is then warranted. Rapid removal usually requires cutting the ring. If sensation and perfusion are intact, removal can be attempted with slower techniques that preserve the ring. The exception to ring preservation methods arises when there is an underlying phalangeal fracture; it is then prudent to cut the ring off. After removal, sensation and perfusion should be reassessed.

In all methods, the hand should be elevated to encourage venous and lymphatic drainage, thus reducing swelling. Alternatively, the finger can be circumferentially wrapped with a $\frac{1}{2}$- to 1-inch elastic band (e.g., Penrose drain), starting from the distal tip and winding the band tightly around the finger, progressing toward the proximal phalanx to reduce swelling. The wrap is left in place for several minutes before it is unwrapped and the ring is removed by one of the methods described

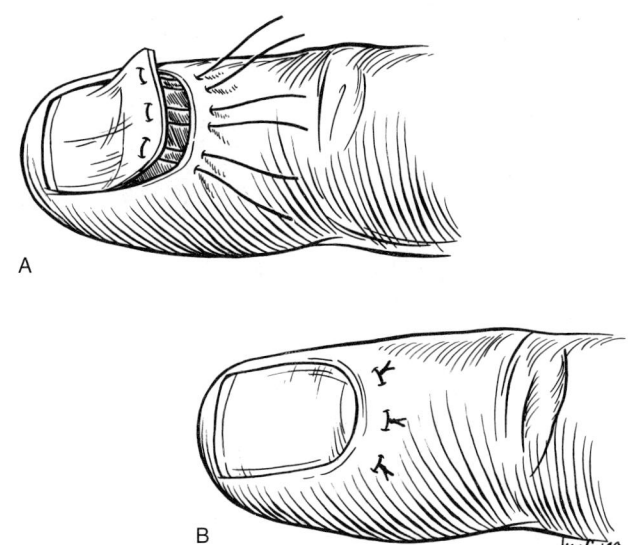

FIG. 44-8. Technique for repair of an avulsion of the germinal matrix using three horizontal mattress sutures. (Reproduced with permission from Chudnofsky CR, Sebastian S: Special wounds—Nail bed, plantar puncture, and cartilage. *Emerg Med Clin North Am* 10:808, 1992.)

below. Regional anesthesia is often required, particularly in patients who cannot tolerate the pain of circumferential compression. The metacarpal block is ideal because it produces less swelling of the finger than a digital block (see Chap. 37).

The simplest technique is lubrication. A variety of water-soluble lubricants can be applied to the digit and the ring removed with circular motion and traction.

The string technique uses a length of string wound circumferentially around the finger. When the string is unwrapped, the ring is advanced toward and off the distal tip of the finger. Either string, umbilical tape, or 0-gauge silk sutures can be used. Synthetic monofilament sutures should not be used because they tend to cut the skin. The required length depends on the diameter of the string and the size of the finger; up to 100 in. of string may be required. The method starts by passing one end of the string under the ring and then wrapping the finger, starting next to the ring and winding clockwise, with each loop snug against the previous one, from proximal to distal. With each loop, the tissue underneath is compressed. When it is completely wrapped, the finger should be entirely covered by the string with no tissue showing between the loops (Figure 44-9A). Wrapping and compression is a painful process and usually requires regional anesthesia. To remove the ring, the proximal end of the string is slowly unwrapped in a counterclockwise manner, advancing the ring toward the distal end as the string unwinds (see Figure 44-9B). The PIP region is the widest portion of the finger and is the most difficult site over which to maneuver the ring. Abrasions are commonly produced with the string method.

A variety of modifications to the string technique have been described. One involves wrapping from distal to proximal so as to reduce distal edema. Elastic band compression to reduce digital edema can be combined with a blood pressure cuff inflated above systolic pressure to prevent reaccumulation of edema once the elastic band is removed.[18] Another method uses a self-adherent compression bandage.[19]

The rubber band technique uses a 3- to 4-mm rubber band that is passed between the ring and skin; the two ends of the rubber band are then picked up by a clamp and used to place distal traction on the ring. The finger and ring are then lubricated. Traction is applied to the rubber band as it is moved circumferentially around the ring, slowly pulling it distal.[20]

Ring cutters are available in both manual and power models. The cutter has a small guard that fits underneath the ring and contains a channel allowing the circular blade to cut down through the ring without coming in contact with the skin. Sometimes, the swelling is so severe that the guard cannot slip under the ring. In these cases, reducing edema by using an elastic band as noted above may be successful. Alternatively, the circular ring may be deformed into an oval, creating a gap on the long axis of the ring. Rings should be cut in the thinnest and most accessible site. Thick rings cannot easily be bent; such rings may need to be cut in two locations, opposite each other, separating the ring into two halves.

REFERENCES

1. Hollander JE, Singer AJ, Valentine S, Henry MC: Wound registry: Development and validation. *Ann Emerg Med* 25:675, 1995.
2. Modrall JG, Weaver FA, Yellin AE: Contemporary issues in trauma: Diagnosis and management of penetrating vascular trauma and the injured extremity. *Emerg Med Clin North Am* 16:129, 1998.
3. Harrison BP, Hilliard MW: Emergency department evaluation and treatment of hand injuries. *Emerg Med Clin North Am* 17:793, 1999.
4. Stevens JC: Aging and spatial acuity of touch. *J Gerontol* 47:P35, 1992.
5. Shaw JA, DeMuth WW, Gillespy AW: Guidelines for the use of digital tourniquets based on physiologic pressure measurements. *J Bone Joint Surg Am* 67:1086, 1985.
6. Voit G, Irvine G, Beals RK: Saline load test for penetration of periarticular laceration. *J Bone Joint Surg Br* 78:732, 1996.
7. Vasilevski D, Noorbergen M, Depierreux M, et al: High-pressure injection injuries to the hand. *Am J Emerg Med* 18:820, 2000.
8. Herndon JH: Hand injuries-special considerations in children. *Emerg Med Clin North Am* 3:405, 1985.
9. Nelson AJ, Izzi JA, Green A, et al: Elbow trauma and reconstruction: Traumatic nerve injuries about the elbow. *Orthop Clin North Am* 30:91, 1999.
10. Coates WC: Lacerations and wound care, in Hart RG, Uehara DT, Wagner MJ (eds): *Emergency and Primary Care of The Hand.* Dallas: American College of Emergency Physicians, 2001, p. 51.
11. Perron AD, Miller MD, Brady MJ: Orthopedic pitfalls in the ED: Fight bite. *Am J Emerg Med* 20:114, 2002.
12. Wolford RW, White JM: Extensor tendon injuries, in Hart RG, Uehara DT, Wagner MJ (eds): *Emergency and Primary Care of The Hand.* Dallas: American College of Emergency Physicians, 2001, p. 175.
13. Alkdred BN: Amputations, in Hart RG, Uehara DT, Wagner MJ (eds): *Emergency and Primary Care of The Hand.* Dallas: American College of Emergency Physicians, 2001, p. 211.
14. Hart RG, Kleinert HE: Fingertip and nail bed injuries. *Emerg Med Clin North Am* 11:755, 1993.
15. Brown RE: Acute nail bed injuries. *Hand Clin* 18:561, 2002.
16. Seaberg DC, Angelos WJ, Paris PM: Treatment of subungual hematomas with nail trephination: A prospective study. *Am J Emerg Med* 9:209, 1991.
17. Roser SE, Gellman H: Comparison of nail bed repair versus nail trephination for subungual hematomas in children. *J Hand Surg [Am]* 24:1166, 1999.
18. Cresap CR: Removal of hardened steel ring from an extremely swollen finger. *Am J Emerg Med* 13:318, 1995.
19. Mullett ST: Ring removal from the oedematous finger: An alternative method. *J Hand Surg [Br]* 20:496, 1995.
20. McElfresch EC, Peterson-Elijah RC: Removal of a tight ring by the rubber band. *J Hand Surg [Br]* 16:225, 1991.

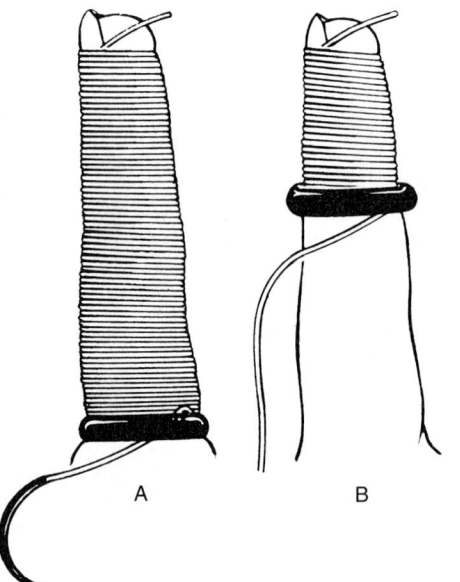

FIG. 44-9. String technique for ring removal. **A.** Completely wrapped. **B.** Unwrapping with ring advancing off with the string.

45

LACERATIONS OF THE LEG AND FOOT
Earl J. Reisdorff

EPIDEMIOLOGY

Injuries to the leg and foot account for about 13 percent of traumatic wounds evaluated in the ED, distributed roughly into a third each for the foot, calf, and knee and thigh regions.[1] Any injury to the lower extremity (especially the foot) jeopardizes the ability to walk. Traumatic wounds to the foot can be sustained in a variety of ways, from simple plantar puncture wounds to catastrophic lawn mower injuries. The leg or foot is commonly injured in sports and recreational activities.[2] Urban children can sustain foot lacerations while playing in water from fire hydrants, mostly due to stepping on broken glass.[3] Bicycle spoke injuries result in complex lacerations with marked surrounding abrasions and even tissue loss, usually occurring over the Achilles tendon area.[4] Lawn mower injuries are usually sustained from the blades of push mowers, often when being pulled backwards.[5] Lawn mower-induced lacerations are heavily contaminated with multiple organisms. Lawn mower-induced foot lacerations can also be sustained from debris flying out from the undercarriage. Unfortunately, footwear does not provide protection from such injury. Metal lawn and garden edging is associated with plantar and knee lacerations.[6] Hockey skates are associated with boot-top injuries; typically these consist of a small cutaneous laceration with injury to the underlying tibialis anterior tendon, extensor hallucis tendon, and dorsalis pedis artery and nerve.[7] High-pressure water spray cleaning systems cause complex laceration-injection injuries. Blunt-force wounds often have irregular edges and are more likely to be associated with an underlying fracture. These characteristics increase the likelihood of wound infection compared to wounds caused by sharp objects.[8] Given the proximity of the foot and ankle to the ground, soil contamination of lacerations is common, increasing the risk of infection, worsening scarring, and slowing healing. Due to the biomechanical importance of the foot and the enhanced risk of infection with wounds to the foot, lacerations must be treated properly to avoid complications.

PATHOPHYSIOLOGY

During standing and walking, the soles of the feet are in contact with the ground. This relatively small area of contact surface tells the body about its position, as well as detailed information about the terrain being traversed. The tough plantar epidermis and dermis are thick, except in the arch area. This thick skin is able to withstand the numerous forces that a moving body produces, but is also quite sensitive to two-point discrimination and pressure. The primary "shock absorber" in the sole of the foot is a modified layer of fat. The heel has an 18-mm-thick modified pad of fat separated into chambers by fibrous septa. There is an additional broad internal fibrous arch, called the inner cup ligament, that helps maintain the shape of the heel. The skin of the sole readily hypertrophies and can become quite thickened, especially in people who walk barefoot. The blood and lymphatic vessels of the foot are under high hydrostatic pressure. As a consequence, edema easily results from injury and can retard healing.

The dorsal aspect of the foot and the entire ankle provides little protection for underlying tendons, nerves, and blood vessels. The dorsum of the foot and the ankle is particularly vulnerable to work-related injuries such as when heavy objects are dropped on the foot. The shin is especially vulnerable when struck.

The pattern of pedal tendons roughly approximates that of the hand. One important location is just posterior to the lateral malleolus, where the peroneus longus tendon runs and can easily be lacerated at this location. Lacerations of the shin rarely involve vital nerves or tendons. However, in the infrapatellar area, lacerations can transect the patellar tendon, resulting in inability to extend the leg.

The dense fibrous fatty tissue of the ball of the foot and heel makes wound exploration and visualization difficult in the ED. However, lacerations to the arch, although more uncommon, are more readily explored. Most lacerations about the ankle are easily explored, except for posterior ankle lacerations, an unfortunate limitation when a partial laceration of the Achilles tendon is considered. Lacerations involving the shin, calf, and thigh present few problems regarding wound exploration and visualization.

CLINICAL FEATURES

History

The time interval from injury to evaluation is important to note because of the increased incidence of infection, especially with delayed presentations. The mechanism of the injury determines the likelihood of injury to underlying tissue, the risk of a retained foreign body, and degree of potential contamination. For example, the following circumstances are associated with specific pathogens: (1) farming accidents (*Clostridium perfringens*), (2) wading in a freshwater stream (*Aeromonas hydrophila*), (3) high-pressure water systems used for cleaning surfaces (*Acinetobacter calcoaceticus*), and (4) animal bites (*Pasteurella multocida* and *Capnocytophaga canimorsus*). The complaint of any new paresthesia, anesthesia, weakness, or loss of function suggests a nerve, vascular, or tendon injury, prompting a careful examination of the affected site.

The past medical history should include questions about tetanus immunization status and conditions that increase the risk for infection or delayed wound healing (diabetes mellitus, immunosuppression), and risk of bacteremia (valvular heart disease, asplenia).

Physical Examination

Physical examination should determine the location, length, depth, and shape of the wound. A wound on the weight-bearing surface is important to note because the wound care plan should consider avoiding weight bearing. As with all lacerations, the distal sensory nerve function, motor function, and vascular integrity (as assessed by pallor and capillary refill) should be evaluated prior to the administration of local or regional anesthesia, if possible. Nerves and tendons are easily involved in lacerations of the foot and ankle (Figure 45-1). If a nerve laceration is suspected, both light touch and static two-point discrimination should tested in the foot and toes, and compared to the uninjured side (Figure 45-2) Motor function may be easier to assess after anesthesia or reduction of an associated fracture or dislocation. The superficial peroneal nerve is responsible for foot eversion, the deep peroneal nerve causes foot inversion and ankle dorsiflexion, and the posterior tibial nerve produces ankle plantarflexion. The wound should be inspected for foreign bodies during the general examination as well as during sterile inspection with a bloodless field just prior to wound closure. The loose thin skin over the dorsum of the foot allows for adequate visual, digital, and instrument exploration for tendon lacerations, as well as for foreign body discovery. Direct visualization of the tendon should be attempted because a partially lacerated tendon can mimic normal function, especially with the Achilles and patellar tendons. The dense tissue of the plantar surface of the foot severely limits wound visualization and the risk of creating new or further injury limits exploration at weight-bearing sites. The exception to this general policy of limited exploration on weight-bearing plantar surfaces is in an infected wound with suspected foreign body.

Ancillary Studies

While the most important parameter to monitor in a wound infection is the clinical appearance, a white blood cell count may assist in determining the degree of inflammation and the effectiveness of antibiotic therapy. Some clinicians also measure an erythrocyte sedimentation rate and C-reactive protein if underlying osteomyelitis is considered. Blood cultures should be obtained if bacteremia is anticipated.

Radiographic imaging is useful when a fracture, radiopaque foreign body, or joint penetration is suspected. Soft tissue radiography is not required for the initial evaluation of every laceration at risk for containing a foreign body. If the clinician feels that adequate wound exploration has reasonably excluded the presence of a foreign body, the wound can be irrigated and closed, forgoing radiographic evaluation.

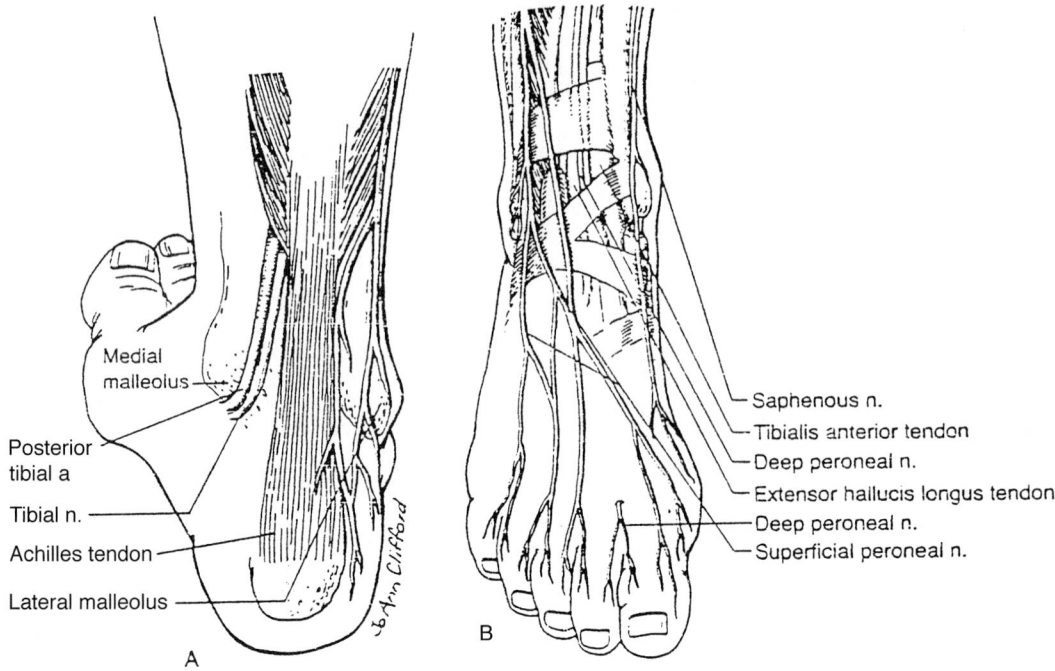

FIG. 45-1. Anatomy of the ankle and foot.

With radiopaque material, standard plain-film radiographs suffice; glass fragments larger than 2 mm and gravel larger than 1 mm are typically seen (>95 percent sensitivity) (see Chap. 46). For radiolucent material, the wound site can be marked with a radiodense marker and the retained material may be seen from distortion of soft tissue shadows around the foreign body. For some types of highly reactive organic material with a high risk of infection and complications, computed tomography or magnetic resonance imaging is required. Retained foreign bodies can be visualized on ultrasound, although experience using this modality on the foot is limited.

Lacerations over the ankle and knee should be examined for joint capsule integrity. The clinical detection of joint penetration by physical examination alone is often incorrect.[9] Air within the joint space on plain radiographs is a sign of joint penetration. The other method to evaluate joint capsule integrity is to inject sterile saline into the joint space, in an amount sufficient to cause synovial distension using a

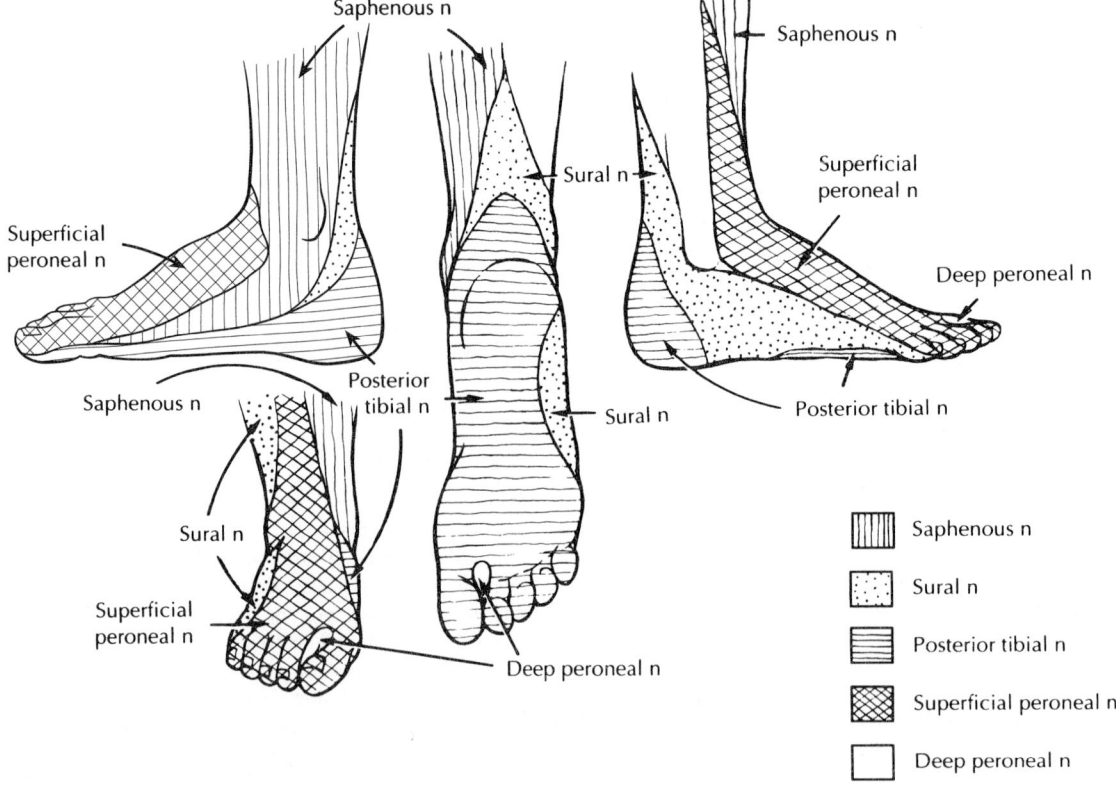

FIG. 45-2. Sensory innervation to the foot.

standard arthrocentesis approach at a site separate from the laceration. Fluid leaking from the wound indicates joint penetration.[9]

TREATMENT

Age Considerations

Elderly patients tend to have thin skin and decreased subcutaneous fat, especially over the anterior shin, making wound edges more difficult to appose, resulting in closure under tension. Elderly patients are more likely to have medical conditions that can delay wound healing and are less likely to be adequately immunized against tetanus.

The preverbal child may have difficulty limiting movement of the injured extremity, and is more likely to contaminate the wound. Generous dressings aid in protecting any lower extremity laceration; the general rule to follow is "the smaller the child, the larger the dressing."

Wound Anesthesia

The sensory examination should precede the administration of anesthesia. Lacerations to the dorsum of the foot can be sufficiently anesthetized by infiltration of local anesthetic, usually with epinephrine. Certain areas of the foot, especially the plantar surface, are particularly sensitive to the infiltration of a local anesthetic, so nerve blocks are very useful (see Chap. 37). The toes can be anesthetized using standard digital blocks. Epinephrine-containing local anesthetics are traditionally avoided in toes because of the potential risk of digital ischemia. For extensive plantar lacerations, regional nerve blocks are useful, with supplemental local infiltration as required. The two most commonly used foot nerve blocks are the sural nerve block and the posterior tibial nerve block. The lateral aspect of the sole is anesthetized using a sural nerve block, by depositing a generous band-like deposit of lidocaine 1 cm posterior to the distal aspect of the lateral malleolus. The posterior tibial nerve block numbs most of the sole, and is accomplished by infiltrating the area next to the posterior tibial artery, just posterior to the distal aspect of the medial malleolus. Procedural sedation should be considered for plantar surface lacerations in children (see Chap. 134).

Topical anesthetic preparations, such as lidocaine-epinephrine-tetracaine (LET) or eutectic mixture of local anesthetics (EMLA) are poorly effective on the dense epidermis of the sole, especially at the contact areas. Conversely, adequate anesthesia with topical preparations can usually be achieved on the dorsum of the foot and elsewhere on the leg.[10] If topical preparations are used, the blood coagulum is first removed and the solution-soaked cotton or gauze pledget is placed firmly into the wound.

Wound Preparation and Repair

The repair of lower extremity lacerations, and especially plantar surface foot lacerations, has been poorly studied and only recently have observational outcome studies been published. Too few randomized studies evaluating various methods of wound preparation or closure for foot and leg lacerations have been done to scientifically direct clinical practice. Most recommendations are based on reasonable extrapolations from the existing studies and common sense clinical judgment.

Due to the inherent risk of infection with foot lacerations, wound irrigation with copious amounts of saline at pressures of 5 to 8 psi is important. The ideal time to perform a thorough dry-field exploration evaluating tendon integrity and detecting foreign bodies is when the wound is completely anesthetized and after irrigation.

Lacerations of the lower extremity tend to be under increased wound tension compared to other anatomic sites. Lacerations under significant tension should be repaired with a multiple-layered closure using buried deep 3-0 or 4-0 absorbable sutures followed by simple in-

terrupted 3-0 or 4-0 nonabsorbable monofilament sutures. Simple interrupted sutures of 4-0 nonabsorbable suture material may be used for skin closure in lacerations under minimal tension. Horizontal mattress sutures are ideal for wounds under moderate tension in the lower extremity. Wounds proximal to the knee and in areas that are usually covered (i.e., where cosmesis is not an issue) can be closed with skin staples. In wounds that are prone to infection, deep absorbable material is avoided and skin staples or horizontal mattress sutures are used. For large thigh lacerations (e.g., a chain saw injury), running sutures are avoided so if there is an infection, selected sutures can be removed.

Debridement to remove devitalized tissue is considered an important aspect of wound care to reduce the risk of wound complications. Nonetheless, debridement should be limited on the plantar surface because the thick, dense, fibrous tissue is not pliable, and any defect resulting from debridement is thus closed under tension across the laceration. Likewise, anterior shin lacerations should undergo minimal debridement.

Lacerations associated with nail injuries require close attention. On the dorsum of the phalanx, the skin is attached directly to the periosteum with no intervening layer of subcutaneous tissue. Therefore, a laceration to the nail bed places the underlying bone at risk for bacterial contamination.

The timing of closure should also be considered. The foot is a body area with a high concentration of bacteria. Therefore the risk of foot infection increases significantly with delay in closure. The "golden period" during which a wound may be closed with minimal risk of infection is unknown. The common recommendation of limiting primary closure to lower extremity wounds less than 6 h old is without much support in the limited number of studies that address this issue (see Chap. 40). Each wound should be evaluated on its individual merits and the decision to undertake primary closure made encompassing all the factors. A delayed primary closure should be considered in cases of delayed presentation or contamination. For delayed primary closure, the wound is packed with saline-soaked gauze and the patient is placed on an antistaphylococcal antibiotic. At 4 days after injury, the wound is reevaluated, and if not clinically infected, closed using interrupted nonabsorbable monofilament sutures.

Plantar Lacerations

Repairing a laceration on the plantar surface is best done with the patient placed in a prone position, with the foot overhanging the cart or elevated by placing a pillow beneath the ankle. Heavy, large suture needles and thick thread are required to penetrate the hypertrophied epidermis and dermis of the sole of the foot, typically 3-0 and sometimes 4-0 suture with a large curved cutting needle. Simple interrupted sutures usually suffice. The advantage of interrupted sutures is that if the foot becomes infected, individual sutures can be selectively removed. If there is tissue loss or the site is under tension, a vertical mattress suture may be required. In the arch area, achieving tissue eversion can be difficult. Adhesive tapes, tissue adhesives, and staples are avoided on the plantar surface.

Dorsal Lacerations

Dorsal surface lacerations are repaired almost exclusively with nonabsorbable monofilament suture material, most commonly 4-0 or 5-0 for small lacerations. Running sutures are acceptable on the dorsal surface. Under select circumstances adhesive tapes or tissue adhesives with splints to restrict movement during the first 5 to 7 days can be used.[11]

Interdigital Lacerations

Lacerations between the toes are difficult to repair; the interdigital space is confined within a deep web space. Having an assistant gently separate the toes enhances the exploration and repair of interdigital lacerations. The use of simple interrupted sutures often leads to skin inversion and risk of failure of the initial wound repair. The more effective closure technique, albeit somewhat more difficult to perform, is to place horizontal or vertical mattress sutures. This is best accomplished with 5-0 monofilament nonabsorbable suture on a small cutting needle. In young children, monofilament absorbable suture can be used, thus avoiding suture removal. When a web space laceration involves the neurovascular bundle, the skin is usually closed without any subsequent consideration to repairing the neurovascular injury.

Shin Lacerations

Wounds over the anterior tibial surface are under considerable tension. Whenever possible, they should be approximated with a multiple-layered closure, first using buried deep 3-0 or 4-0 absorbable sutures followed by simple interrupted or horizontal mattress 4-0 nonabsorbable sutures. In elderly patients, the skin may be extremely thin, creating difficulty for closure. Deep closure with absorbable material should first be attempted. The skin is closed with wide horizontal mattress sutures using 4-0 nonabsorbable material. Occasionally, the 4-0 suture is too fine and cuts through the skin, requiring 3-0 monofilament suture. Broad adhesive strips (one-half inch) can be placed with adhesive adjunct (e.g., tincture of benzoin) over the suture site to minimize dynamic tension across the wound. An elastic bandage is placed over a generous dressing. Weight-bearing should be limited for the first 5 days of wound healing if there is significant wound tension.

Alternatively, a new technique using deep reinforced sutures placed through adhesive strips laid down parallel to the wound edges has been recently described.[12] This technique is useful for both linear and flap lacerations and limits tearing by the suture material of the often fragile skin over the shin.

Knee Lacerations

For lacerations about the knee, potential joint capsule penetration and laceration of the patellar and quadriceps tendons should be assessed. The common peroneal nerve is prone to injury as it runs over the head of the fibula laterally, and distal function should be assessed (inversion, eversion, and dorsiflexion). Deep popliteal wounds can injure the popliteal artery and tibial nerve. Popliteal artery injuries are serious because the leg has minimal collateral circulation distal to the knee.

Simple lacerations about the knee can be closed with 4-0 nonabsorbable material, using simple interrupted or horizontal mattress sutures because of the marked active skin tension in this area. Skin staples are an alternative in patients subject to poor wound healing. The knee should be splinted or placed in a knee immobilizer to decrease active tension and promote better wound healing. Limited experience suggests that lacerations about the knee in children can be closed with tissue adhesives and splints to restrict movement.[11]

Tendon Lacerations

The decision to repair tendon lacerations in the foot depends on the functional impairment caused by the injury compared to the benefits of repair.[13–15] Many extensor tendon lacerations involving the midfoot and forefoot can go unrepaired without sacrificing any necessary foot function; the skin is closed and the foot splinted.[15] However, any laceration of the extensor hallucis longus or tibialis anterior requires discussion with an orthopedist since dorsiflexion of the great toe and foot can be important in walking or running.[15] Flexor tendon lacerations across the toes (excluding the great toe) can be left unrepaired without significant functional sequelae. Occasionally, a hammer toe or claw toe deformity results from the failure to repair a tendon (usually flexor tendon) laceration.[14] Although lacerations of the flexor hallucis longus are frequently repaired, no long-term evaluation has determined that

this is essential.[15] In fact, there are limited data indicating that unrepaired flexor hallucis longus tendon lacerations do not result in a functional deficit, even among athletes.[15]

Since the Achilles tendon is not the only tendon responsible for plantarflexion of the foot, its individual function may be difficult to assess. The Achilles tendon is first palpated for defects. A complete laceration produces a conspicuous absence of the tendon at the posterior ankle. The patient then lies prone on the examination cart with the foot hanging over the edge of the bed and the mid calf is squeezed by the examiner (Thompson test). If the Achilles tendon is intact, the foot plantarflexes. Comparison to the unaffected calf can be helpful. If the Achilles tendon injury results from a laceration, the Achilles tendon may easily be seen with simple exploration through the open wound.

Significant tendon lacerations of the lower extremity are usually repaired a few days to weeks after the initial injury. Treatment in the ED consists of skin closure; splinting of the foot, ankle, and leg; initiation of prophylactic antibiotics; instruction for non-weight-bearing crutch use; and arrangement for the patient to follow-up with an orthopedist.

Tissue Loss and Amputation

Certain injuries can lead to major tissue loss as well as toe or foot amputation (e.g., motorcycle, lawn mower, and antipersonnel land mine injuries). Tissue grafts and flap reconstruction by an orthopedist or plastic surgeon may be required. Reimplantation of a severed toe is not typically performed. Reattachment of an amputated great toe, forefoot, or entire foot is occasionally done, although it is extremely complex. Immediate consultation with a reimplantation surgeon is essential in such circumstances. Any severed part should be gently washed (not scrubbed) with sterile saline to remove gross debris, wrapped in saline-soaked gauze, and placed in a plastic bag that is then closed and placed in an ice water bath.

Retained Foreign Bodies

Retained (nonreactive) foreign bodies such as glass can pose a problem. Chronic pain, especially during walking, can occur if the material is not removed. In the absence of chronic discomfort, inert foreign bodies can remain in the foot. The material typically becomes encapsulated, as is sometimes seen with insulin needles retained in the feet of patients with diabetic neuropathy. Conversely, reactive organic material must be aggressively sought and removed. Deep foreign bodies in the foot can be extremely difficult to remove in the ED. Fluoroscopy can be useful to help locate and remove radiopaque foreign bodies.

Hair Tourniquet Syndrome

Hair tourniquet syndrome is an unusual type of toe injury that is seen during infancy.[16,17] A long strand of hair becomes wrapped around a toe, often producing strangulation and digital ischemia. This can be an occult source of irritability for infants. Removal must be complete to restore perfusion. Moreover, complete removal eliminates any further circumferential laceration of the skin around the toe. The standard approach to salvage the compromised digit is to make a midline longitudinal incision along the extensor surface of the toe.[17] The incision should be deep enough to split the fibers of the extensor ligament without transecting the fibers. The multiple strands of hair are then removed using fine forceps without teeth. Unfortunately, the toe often retains the initial appearance, making one uncertain whether all of the strands have been removed or cut. A novel approach to removal involves the use of hair-dissolving compounds, although this approach has not been studied sufficiently to routinely recommend it.

Despite the unusual nature of this injury, the consensus in the medical literature is that hair tourniquet syndrome is not the result of intentional injury and does not warrant reporting as suspected child abuse.

DISPOSITION

A bulky dressing is applied to the plantar surface to cushion any plantar laceration. For large lacerations on the plantar surface, weight-bearing is avoided for at least 5 days. However, infants will naturally step on the injured site. Since crutches are too difficult to use in children younger than age 7 years, young children may need to be carried. Elevation of the extremity decreases swelling and infection risk. Sutures are typically removed in 10 to 14 days.

Prophylactic Antibiotic Use

While infection occurs in 3 to 8 percent of lower extremity lacerations[8,18] and up to 34 percent of plantar lacerations,[3] there is no evidence that prophylactic antibiotics reduce the frequency of postrepair wound infections[19] (see Chap. 48). Therefore, the decision to use prophylactic antibiotics is made using clinical judgment according to the degree of contamination, the presence of foreign debris, the presence of associated injuries, and host factors that predispose to infection. At one extreme, clean, small lacerations to the dorsum of the foot do not require antibiotic prophylaxis. At the other extreme, patients with grossly contaminated lawn mower-induced wounds should have it.

Animal bites to the leg and foot require coverage against *Staphylococcus, Streptococcus,* and *Pasteurella.* Asplenic or immunocompromised patients who sustain a dog bite should receive coverage against *C. canimorsus.* Amoxicillin-clavulanate will cover all four organisms. Lacerations sustained when wading in freshwater streams should receive antibiotic prophylaxis for *Aeromonas hydrophila* (a gram-negative bacillus) with a fluoroquinolone. *Aeromonas* infections occur 8 to 48 h after inoculation and are rapidly progressive. Fascia, tendon, muscle, bone, or joint involvement occurs in 39 percent of cases.[20] Compartment syndrome, myonecrosis, and foot amputation can result. Effective antibiotic coverage against *Aeromonas* includes aminoglycosides, trimethoprim-sulfamethoxazole, and fluoroquinolones. Open fractures are most commonly infected by *S. aureus,* so patients should receive antibiotic prophylaxis with a first-generation cephalosporin and an aminoglycoside in the ED.

REFERENCES

1. Hollander JE, Singer AJ, Valentine S, Henry MC: Wound registry: Development and validation. *Ann Emerg Med* 25:675, 1995.
2. Nonfatal sports- and recreation-related injuries treated in emergency departments-United States, July 2000-June 2001. *MMWR* 51:736, 2002.
3. Joffe M, Torrey SB, Baker D: Fire hydrant play: Injuries and their prevention. *Pediatrics* 87:900, 1991.
4. Mine R, Fukui M, Nishimura G: Bicycle spoke injuries in the lower extremity. *Plast Reconstr Surg* 106:1501, 2000.
5. Anger DM, Ledbetter BR, Stasikelis PJ, Calhoun JH: Injuries of the foot related to the use of lawn mowers. *J Bone Joint Surg Am* 77:719, 1995.
6. Rittichier KK, Bassett KE: Metal lawn and garden edging: The hidden knife? *Pediatr Emerg Care* 17:28, 2001.
7. Simonet WT, Sim L: Boot-top tendon lacerations in ice hockey. *J Trauma* 38:30, 1995.
8. Singer AJ, Quinn JV, Thode HC, Hollander JE: Determinants of poor outcome after laceration and surgical incision repair. *Plast Reconstr Surg* 110:429, 2002.
9. Voit G, Irvine G, Beals RK: Saline load test for penetration of periarticular laceration. *J Bone Joint Surg Br* 78:732, 1996.
10. Zempsky WT, Karasic RB: EMLA versus TAC for topical anesthesia of extremity wounds in children. *Ann Emerg Med* 30:163, 1997.
11. Saxena AK, Willital GH: Octyl cyanoacrylate tissue adhesive in the repair of pediatric extremity lacerations. *Am Surg* 65:470, 1999.
12. Silk J: A new approach to the management of pretibial lacerations. *Injury* 32:373, 2001.
13. Yancey HA Jr: Lacerations of the plantar aspect of the foot. *Clin Orthop* 122:46, 1977.
14. Floyd DW, Heckman JD, Rockwood CA: Tendon lacerations in the foot. *Foot Ankle* 4:8, 1983.
15. Scaduto AA, Cracchiolo A: Lacerations and ruptures of the flexor or extensor hallucis longus tendon. *Foot Ankle Clin* 5:725, 2000.
16. Liow RY, Budny P, Regan PJ: Hair thread tourniquet syndrome. *J Accid Emerg Med* 13:138, 1996.
17. Harris EJ: Acute digital ischemia in infants: The hair-thread tourniquet syndrome-a report of two cases. *J Foot Ankle Surg* 41:112, 2002.
18. Baker MD, Lanuti M: The management and outcome of lacerations in urban children. *Ann Emerg Med* 19:1001, 1991.
19. Stamou SC, Malterzou HC, Psaltipoulou T, et al: Wound infections after minor limb lacerations: Risk factors and the role of antimicrobial agents. *J Trauma* 46:1078, 1999.
20. Semel JD, Trenholme G: *Aeromonas hydrophila* water-associated traumatic wound infections: A review. *J Trauma* 30:324, 1990.

SOFT TISSUE FOREIGN BODIES
Richard L. Lammers

Soft tissue foreign bodies may be encountered when managing new wounds or evaluating complications of old wounds. When evaluating fresh injuries, the physician is responsible for detecting foreign bodies and for deciding if removal is urgent, can be delayed, or is even necessary. Many foreign bodies should be removed in the ED; for example, all foreign material within the cavities of fresh lacerations should be irrigated away, debrided, or extracted with instruments. The decision to remove foreign bodies embedded below the dermal layer of skin depends on the size, location, composition, accessibility, and anticipated mechanical and inflammatory effects of the object. Occasionally, patients with subcutaneous foreign bodies should be referred to appropriate physicians for delayed removal.

Many foreign bodies are detectable during clinical examination, but some will not be apparent to the sight or touch of the examining physician. Various imaging studies can be used to evaluate wounds when nothing is found during exploration but the probability of a concealed object remains high. Some foreign bodies, however, may be invisible to radiographic or sonographic study. Consequently, liability for missed foreign bodies will continue to plague emergency physicians.

PATHOPHYSIOLOGY

Transient inflammation is an integral part of normal wound healing. A small amount of foreign debris in a wound provokes an inflammatory response in an effort to eliminate or contain the invader. When large quantities of devitalized tissue, foreign debris, bacteria, or other irritants are present within a wound, this protective response intensifies. Excessive or prolonged inflammation may delay wound healing or destroy surrounding soft tissue and bone, producing periosteal reactions, osteolytic lesions, synovitis, and arthritis. If the body fails to dissolve or extrude foreign material, it will become encapsulated within a fibrous capsule. Many granulomas result from chronic inflammation caused by foreign bodies that inflammation could not eliminate. Once a retained foreign body is encapsulated, inflammation subsides.

The type and intensity of an inflammatory reaction is determined primarily by the chemical composition and physical form of the foreign object. Material that is inert—such as glass, metal, or plastic—may not elicit any abnormal tissue response. Objects with smooth, nonporous surfaces produce less inflammation and fibrosis than those with rough surfaces. Most metals are inert, but those that oxidize will cause mild to moderate inflammation. Earrings with studs dipped in gold paint cause earlobe swelling and inflammation when the paint flakes off. Vegetative foreign bodies, such as wood, thorns, and spines, trigger the most severe inflammatory reactions. Sea urchin spines, other marine foreign bodies, and hair may cause chronic inflammation with granuloma formation.

In some cases, inflammation is caused by a local toxic reaction. For example, blackthorns contain an alkaloid that produces intense inflammation. The oils and resins in redwood and cedar splinters also cause considerable inflammation. Sea urchin spines and catfish spines contain venom that causes severe burning pain at the puncture site and a variety of systemic symptoms (see Chap. 196). A sudden, local inflammatory reaction from a rose thorn or cactus spine may be an allergic response to fungi on the plant. Some cacti cause a delayed hypersensitivity reaction. Systemic toxic and allergic reactions are unusual but serious complications of foreign bodies. Foreign bodies containing lead have the potential to produce systemic lead poisoning, particularly if they are in contact with pleural, peritoneal, cerebrospinal, or joint fluid.[1]

Infections are the most common complication of retained foreign bodies, even when the foreign material itself is not contaminated. Foreign bodies may incite a variety of soft tissue infections, including local wound infection, cellulitis, abscess formation, lymphangitis, tenosynovitis, bursitis, and osteomyelitis. These infections are characteristically resistant to therapy; antibiotics, antiinflammatory drugs, and steroids may produce a partial regression of symptoms but seldom eradicate the infection. Some infections will resolve spontaneously once the foreign bodies are removed. Vegetative foreign bodies may cause fungal infections, particularly in immunosuppressed patients.

Foreign objects can also cause mechanical damage by compressing or lacerating anatomic structures or occluding vessels. Repeated movement of tissue containing a foreign object increases the fibrous reaction.

CLINICAL FEATURES

History

Every wound has the potential for concealing a foreign body, but only a small percentage of lacerations and puncture wounds actually contain them.[2,3] Certain historical factors are associated with a higher risk for a retained foreign body: the mechanism of injury, composition and shape of the wounding object, and the shape and location of the resulting wound.[2,3] Objects that shatter, splinter, or break in the process of causing a wound often leave remnants behind. For example, a wound caused by glass that broke on the skin is more likely to contain shards than a wound caused by previously-broken glass. Dental fractures following a blow to the mouth serve as a warning that fragments of teeth may be embedded in the lip or tongue of the patient or in the hand of the assailant. Thorns, spines, and sharp wooden branches are usually brittle and tend to penetrate deeply into puncture wounds before breaking. Wood splinters are notorious for fragmenting when they are pulled out of a puncture wound. Patients impaled by long, thin metallic objects such as hypodermic or sewing needles may remove them without realizing that a portion of the object broke off beneath the skin surface. Both remnants of a needle and impurities in street drugs can cause persistent pain or abscess formation at the site of intravenous drug use. Nails that penetrate socks and shoes may drive leather, rubber, or cloth into the plantar surface of a patient's foot. Blunt objects with a diameter greater than 4.5 mm may push a plug of skin deep into a wound, resulting in an epidermal inclusion cyst. If any object pulled from a wound does not appear intact, the wound should be explored for further contaminants.

The patient's perception of a foreign body sensation in a fresh wound with an actual foreign body is modestly useful [sensitivity = 43%, specificity = 83%, LR(+) = 2.49, and LR(−) = 0.69].[3]

Patients with retained foreign bodies may present to the ED after a wound heals, complaining of sharp pain with movement or with pressure over the site. Failure to heal a wound also may be evidence of a retained irritant. Chronic, delayed, and recurrent infections also can be associated with retained foreign bodies. New puncture wounds that become infected and infections that are resistant to antibiotic therapy suggest that a foreign body has been missed. Arthritis in a joint near an old puncture wound may be a thorn-induced synovitis. Delayed nerve, vessel, or tendon injuries also require further investigation.

Physical Examination

Physicians are occasionally surprised by foreign bodies that can be embedded in small or seemingly superficial wounds.[2] Several physical findings indicate the presence of a foreign body. A discoloration or visible mass under the epidermis makes the diagnosis obvious. Sometimes a mass cannot be seen but can be palpated. Sharp, well-localized pain with palpation over a puncture wound is a useful sign. If passive range of motion of a joint near a wound is limited, a foreign body may be responsible.

Old wounds with retained foreign bodies may have a persistent purulent drainage, a chronic draining sinus, or a chronic granulomatous reaction. A sterile abscess that complicates wound healing may be the result of a foreign body.

Some foreign bodies are discovered in wounds unexpectedly, but most are found during a deliberate and careful exploration of wounds considered to be at risk.[2,3] Adequate lighting, good hemostasis, complete local anesthesia, and patient cooperation are essential. Every effort should be made to visually inspect all recesses of a wound. Wounds deeper than 5 mm and wounds whose depth cannot be visualized have a higher association with foreign bodies.[2] If punctures and other narrow wounds make direct visualization difficult and the physician is concerned about the possibility of a foreign body below the surface, the wound margins should be extended with a scalpel (Figure 46-1). However, wounds that penetrate deeply into adipose tissue are difficult to explore and easily hide foreign material. Blind probing with a hemostat is a less effective but sometimes acceptable alternative to wound exploration when the wound is narrow and deep and extending the wound is not desirable. This method is used frequently to evaluate plantar puncture wounds caused by nails and to search for clear glass, which is difficult to see in a wound. A closed hemostat should be introduced into the wound and either used as a probe or spread open and then withdrawn. If an instrument strikes a metallic or glass foreign body, it will produce a grating sensation. The instrument should not be used to grasp blindly in hopes of clamping an unseen object. This technique is especially dangerous in hands, feet, or faces, where direct visualization is the preferred method of exploration.

DIAGNOSIS

Imaging studies should be ordered in most cases in which a retained foreign body is suspected but not found during wound exploration or when exploration is technically impossible. They are also useful after initial removal of multiple foreign bodies to determine if all the pieces were found.

A number of imaging modalities are available. The ability of any of these modalities to find a foreign body depends on the characteristics of the study as well as the object's size, shape, density, and orientation relative to the imaging beam. Materials that are the same density as surrounding soft tissue are difficult to see with any type of radiographic or sonographic technique.

Plain Radiography

It is fortunate that many foreign bodies are radiopaque; most foreign bodies that can be missed during the initial clinical evaluation can be seen on plain films.[4] Plain films are readily available but must be obtained with appropriate technique and inspected carefully to detect small and faint foreign bodies. Metal, mammalian bone, some types of fish bones (cod, haddock, grey mullet, red snapper, and sole), teeth, pencil graphite, certain plastics, glass, gravel, sand, and aluminum are visible on plain radiographs[4–10] (Table 46-1). Almost all glass is visible on radiographs if it is 2 mm or larger, and contrary to myth, glass does not have to contain lead to be visible on plain films.[4,5,7,8] A radiopaque fragment is more easily seen if it is positioned parallel to the central ray of the x-ray beam, which increases its apparent density.

Radiographs should be obtained with an underpenetrated soft tissue technique, producing a lighter film that increases the contrast between the foreign body and surrounding tissue. The contrast and brightness of digital radiographs can be adjusted to achieve the same

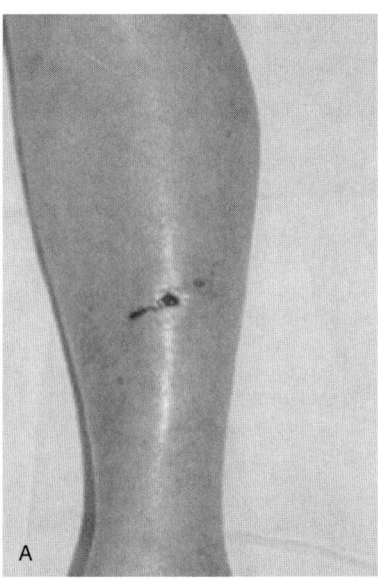 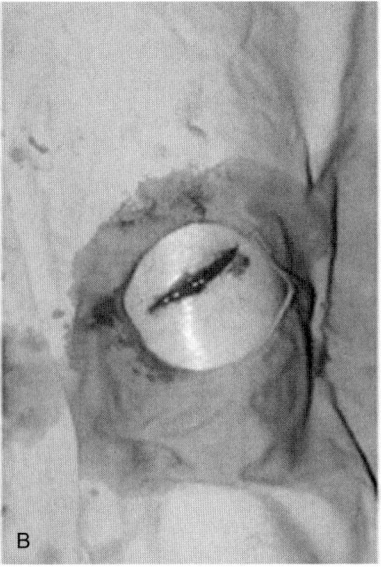 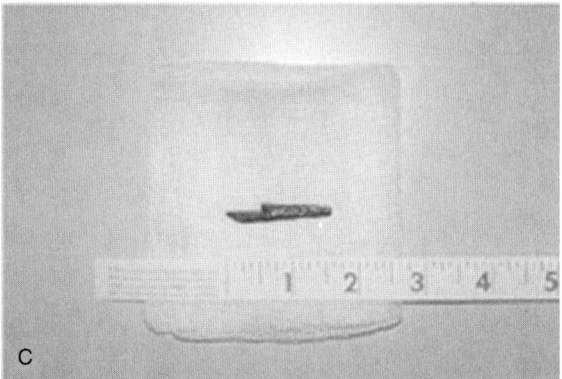

FIG. 46-1. A. This patient's leg was punctured by a wooden stake 2 days prior to presentation. Surrounding cellulitis and point tenderness lateral to the wound indicated the probability of a retained foreign body. **B.** The entrance to the wound was extended. **C.** A 1.5-cm piece of wood was removed from a 3.5-cm-deep wound.

effect as an underpenetrated film.[7] Plain films should be taken in multiple projections to separate the shadow of the foreign body from underlying bone and to help gauge the depth of the object in the tissue. Chronic inflammatory changes may create secondary bony changes such as osteolytic and osteoblastic lesions, pseudotumor formation, and periosteal reaction, revealing the object's location.

Many common or highly reactive materials such as wood, thorns, cactus spines, some fish bones, other organic matter, and most plastics are not visible on plain films.[4,7,8,10] Sometimes there is indirect evidence of their presence; a radiolucent filling defect may occur when the object is less dense than surrounding tissue. However, even radiopaque foreign bodies may be invisible on plain films if they are obscured by or impacted in bone.

Computed Tomography (CT)

CT is capable of detecting more types of foreign materials than plain-film radiography because it is 100 times more sensitive in differentiating densities.[4,8] Subtle density differences can be distinguished with a narrow radiographic density window adjustment, particularly if a computer workstation is used to vary the gain and contrast settings.[8] Thorns, spines, wood toothpicks, fish bones, and plastic foreign bodies have been identified with this method.[4,8,11] CT may detect objects embedded in bone, and isodense objects may be outlined by surrounding

air within the wound. Digital edge enhancement can further improve the visibility of these objects.[9] CT images can be created in multiple planes and can demonstrate the relationship of a foreign object to important anatomic structures. The principal disadvantages of CT are its cost, higher radiation dose, and the fact that with time, wood and other organic material absorb water from the surrounding tissue, becoming isodense and difficult to distinguish from surrounding tissue.

Ultrasonography

Sonography has been described in clinical series and studied in experimental models to identify soft tissue foreign bodies such as wood, fish bones, sea urchin spines, other organic material, fiber, and plastic.[12–19] Most authors have reported greater than 90 percent sensitivity with ultrasound for detection of foreign bodies larger than 4 to 5 mm (Table 46-2). In clinical practice, variation in detection rates may be due to the size and sonographic nature of the foreign body, the presence of confounding factors (e.g., bone, blood, air, purulence, scars, old sutures) associated with the foreign body, and operator skill and experience. A hyperechoic rim around or acoustic shadowing behind the foreign body may help to localize it.[14] Areas with many echogenic structures such as calcifications, sesamoid bones, and tendons may hide foreign bodies within their acoustic shadows, so these areas must be scanned slowly to detect foreign bodies that are small or oriented

TABLE 46-1   Experimental Studies Using Plain Radiography to Detect Radiopaque Objects

Material, Author, Reference	Object Size (Approximate)	N (Number of Observations)	Sensitivity (95% CI)
Aluminum			
Ellis[6]	0.5–4 mm	6	100% (54–100%)
Glass			
Courter[5]	0.5 mm	150	61% (53–69%)
Courter[5]	1 mm	150	83% (76–88%)
Courter[5]	2 mm	150	99% (95–100%)
Manthey[17]	2 mm	20	95% (75–100%)
Gravel			
Chisholm[9]	0.5 mm	120	72% (63–80%)
Chisholm[9]	1 mm	120	99% (95–100%)
Chisholm[9]	2 mm	120	94% (88–97%)
Manthey[17]	5 mm	20	100% (96–100%)

TABLE 46-2   Experimental Studies Using Ultrasound to Detect Radiolucent Objects

Material, Author, Reference	Object Size (Approximate)	N (Number of Observations)	Sensitivity (95% CI)
Plastic			
Schlager[16]	1 × 2 mm	10	100% (92–100%)
Manthey[17]	10 mm length	20	40% (19–64%)
Wood			
Jacobson[15]	1.0 × 2.5 mm	30	87% (69–96%)
Jacobson[15]	1.0 × 5.0 mm	30	93% (78–99%)
Manthey[17]	10 mm length	20	50% (27–73%)
Schlager[16]	15 mm length	10	100% (92–100%)
Bray[19]	1 × 4 mm	28	96% (82–100%)
Bray[19]	2 × 5 mm	28	100% (88–100%)
Mixed			
Harcke[18]	3 to 30 mm	60	97% (88–100%)
Cactus spine			
Manthey[17]	10 mm	10	30% (12–54%)
Schlager[16]	Agave spine	10	100% (92–100%)

perpendicular to the skin surface. Some areas of the body that are prone to foreign body penetration, such as the web spaces of the hands or toes, may not accommodate an ultrasound probe.

Once a foreign body is confirmed by plain films or CT studies, sonography can be used in place of fluoroscopy to guide an instrument to the object during retrieval.[20–21] The scanning beam should be oriented parallel to the long axis of a hemostat, which can be directed toward the long axis of the foreign body. Transverse and longitudinal scans provide views in multiple planes. A 7.5-MHz linear-array transducer can be used to find objects that are small and superficial (up to 3 cm deep), and a 5.0-MHz transducer can be used for larger and deeper objects. The linear scan is preferred for localization, and the sector scan for retrieval.[20] The primary advantage of ultrasonography is the avoidance of radiation exposure.

Xeroradiography

Xeroradiographs enhance soft tissue images, improving images already visible on plain films. However, this modality fails to detect radiolucent foreign bodies and has been supplanted by other imaging techniques.[5]

Magnetic Resonance Imaging (MRI)

MRI can detect nonmetallic radiolucent foreign bodies and in limited comparison studies is more accurate than any other modality in identifying wood, plastic, spines, and thorns.[5] MRI should not be used with gravel or metal-containing foreign bodies because ferromagnetic streaks obscure visualization. MRI may prove more effective than CT in visualizing organic foreign bodies, but comparison studies are needed.

Fluoroscopy

Bedside fluoroscopy accurately detects radiopaque (metal, gravel, glass, and pencil graphite) foreign bodies as small as 3 mm.[22,23] Theoretical advantages of fluoroscopy compared to conventional plain film radiography are convenience, reduced cost, shortened ED time, and less radiation exposure. Fluoroscopy can be used to assist foreign body removal by helping guide the instrument.

Selecting an Imaging Study

If a foreign body is suspected but not found during exploration of a wound, a plain film should be ordered first, since plain radiography will detect as many as 80 to 90 percent of all foreign bodies. It is pru-

dent to order films if a patient believes there is a retained object. If the wound was caused by metal, glass, or gravel and no foreign body was found on plain films or wound exploration, the physician can end the search. For objects not routinely visible on plain radiography, CT scans are the modality of choice. Ultrasound is not as reliable as CT in confirming the presence or absence of nonradiopaque foreign bodies.

TREATMENT

General Principles

Once a soft tissue foreign body is discovered, the physician must weigh the risk of leaving the foreign body in place against the potential harm of attempting to remove it. Not all foreign bodies must be removed, and not all that require removal must be extracted in the ED. However, every effort should be made to identify their presence during the initial visit. General indications for foreign body removal include potential for later infection, toxicity, injury, and functional problems (Table 46-3). Usually, objects that are small, inert, deeply embedded, and causing no symptoms can be left in place. A common question concerns bullets that come to rest deep within a muscle belly; they are usually not removed because the procedure can cause more

TABLE 46-3   Indications for Foreign Body Removal

Potential for inflammation or infection
    Vegetative or chemically reactive material
    Heavy bacterial contamination (e.g., teeth, soil)
    Proximity to fractured bone
    Established infection
    Allergic reaction
Toxicity
    Spines with venom
    Heavy metals
Functional and cosmetic problems
    Impingement on nerves, vessels, or tendons
    Restriction of joint mobility
    Proximity to tendons
    Impairment of gait
    Persistent pain
    Cosmetic deformity (e.g., tattooing)
    Psychological distress
Potential for later injury
    Intraarticular location
    Intravascular location
    Migration toward important structures

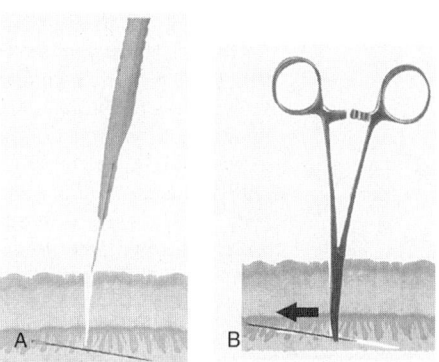

FIG. 46-2. A. An incision is made perpendicular to the needle at its midpoint. **B.** The needle is grasped through the incision with a hemostat and backed out of the puncture wound.

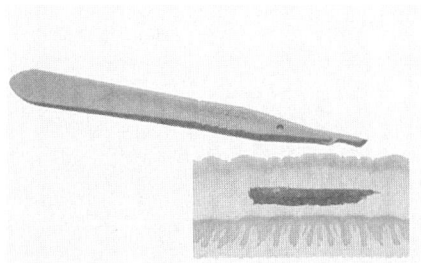

FIG. 46-4. To remove a friable foreign body such as a wood splinter that is parallel to the skin surface, an incision is made along its long axis. The object can be lifted out and the entire length of the wound inspected for remnants.

damage than leaving the foreign object in place. Projectiles may drag bits of clothing or skin into the wound, so the entrance wound deserves cleaning and debridement. Bullet migration and embolization are rare but possible complications. Bullets near vessels can enter the systemic circulation. Bullets that cause distal ischemia, thrombus formation, or wall erosion or that lie within the lumen of a blood vessel require immediate removal in the operating room.

Thorns, spines, wood splinters, and other vegetative materials require immediate removal because they cause intense and excessive inflammation. Foreign objects that are heavily contaminated, such as fractured teeth and soil-covered objects, should be removed as soon as possible; antibiotic treatment will not take the place of foreign body removal. Glass, metal, and plastic are relatively inert, and removal can be postponed if necessary. Glass foreign bodies in hands or feet can cause persistent pain with gripping or walking, and they can sever nerves or tendons years after the initial injury. Patients with deep, sharp foreign bodies in these locations should be referred to appropriate specialists for eventual removal.

Sometimes harmless foreign bodies are psychologically distressing to patients, particularly when they are visible under the skin surface or produce a lump. Patient concern may be a justification for elective removal.

Successful removal of foreign bodies requires adequate local or regional anesthesia and good lighting. Depending on location and depth, tourniquet control of bleeding and assistance may be needed. Depth and accessibility of the object and physician time are the limiting factors for removal of foreign bodies by the emergency physician. Foreign bodies buried deeply in adipose tissue or muscle are difficult to locate. Most foreign bodies in hands should be removed because the hand is mobile and sensitive. Deep exploration of hands by the emergency physician is not recommended because magnification and experience are needed to avoid injury to numerous closely spaced vital structures.

The emergency physician may not be able to devote more than about 15 to 30 min to the removal procedure, particularly when other seriously ill or injured patients demand attention. This amount of time is sufficient for locating most foreign bodies. The patient should be informed before

the procedure that the duration of the exploration will be limited. If more time is required, the patient should be referred to a surgeon.

Methods of Localization

Accurate localization of a foreign body prior to removal is important because blind searching is time consuming and can cause further injury. However, it is usually easier to detect the presence of a foreign body than to locate its exact position. If a foreign body is radiopaque, one can estimate its location and depth by taping radiopaque skin markers such as lead circles or paper clips on the skin at the wound entrance or directly over the object. With multiple projections the object can be seen in relation to the markers. Hypodermic needles can be used as skin markers. Two or three needles are inserted into the skin near the object at approximately 90 degrees to each other to provide a frame of reference around the object. Plain films taken in multiple projections allow the physician to gauge the distance of the object from the closest needle or its distance between two needles.

The limitations of this technique are that it does not provide a true three-dimensional image and that images on radiographs are distorted by divergence and parallax. Tendons and other structures may block the most accessible path to the foreign body. Alternatively, the site of injury can be rotated under fluoroscopy to visualize the object between the markers.[22,23] Radiation exposure should be minimized by brief, intermittent imaging and appropriate shielding. An incision is made between needles or markers, or dissection is carried along the path of the closest needle.

Ultrasound can be useful in directing exploration and foreign body removal.[21,22]

Specific Foreign Bodies and Removal Procedures

METALLIC NEEDLES   Long, thin foreign bodies such as sewing and hypodermic needles may be difficult to locate in soft tissue. Two techniques are available for removing needles that are parallel to the surface of the skin. If the needle is superficial enough to be palpable, an

FIG. 46-3. A. The entrance site is enlarged with a skin incision. **B.** If the incision passes to the side of the object, the skin is undermined. **C.** Pressure on the skin edges displaces the foreign body into the center of the wound.

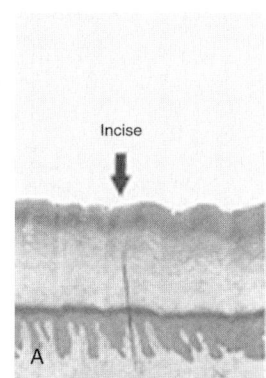

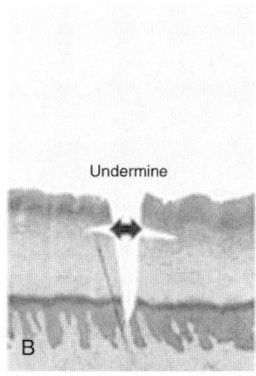

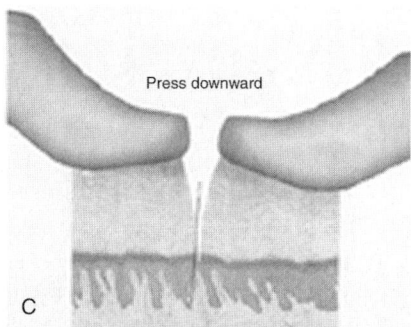

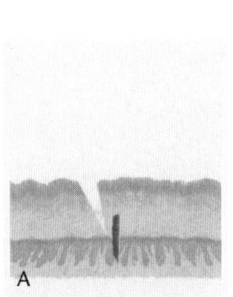 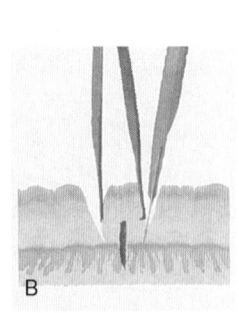 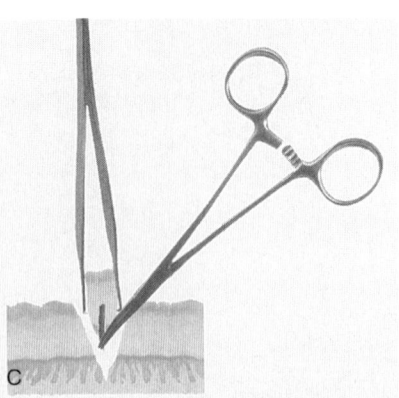

FIG. 46-5. Block excision is effective for foreign bodies that are friable, difficult to find, buried in fatty tissue, or stain surrounding tissue. **A.** A small, elliptical incision is made around the original wound. **B.** The incision is undercut until contact is made with the foreign body. **C.** The block of tissue is grasped with a forceps, the foreign body is clamped with a hemostat, and both are removed.

incision is made at one end to expose and grasp it with a hemostat. If the needle is deep, an incision is made perpendicular to the needle at its midpoint, where it can be clamped with a hemostat and pushed out of the entrance of the original wound (Figure 46-2).

Long, thin foreign bodies that are oriented perpendicular to the skin surface can be elusive. If a needle can be reached with an alligator forceps or hemostat, it can be pulled straight out. If a needle lies beyond the reach of a hemostat, the entrance wound must be enlarged with a skin incision (Figure 46-3). However, the incision can easily pass to the side of the object, so the skin edges should be undermined, and pressure applied on the skin edges may displace the foreign body into the center of the wound, where it can be seen and grasped. Once removed, the needle and the wound should be inspected to ensure that the object was removed in its entirety.

WOOD SPLINTERS AND ORGANIC SPINES
Solid foreign bodies can be pulled out of puncture wounds with forceps, but wood splinters and organic spines (e.g., cactus, sea urchin, and fish) may disintegrate with this technique. Only superficial splinters that are a few millimeters long can be grasped and removed with a fine-point splinter forceps. A splinter parallel to the skin surface should be lifted out of the wound after incising the skin along the long axis of the object (Figure 46-4). If the splinter is lodged in the subcutaneous tissue, the entrance wound must be enlarged with a skin incision so the foreign body can be grasped under direct visualization. Wood fragments may be impossible to locate precisely. One solution is to create an elliptical incision around the puncture wound and extract the fragment in a block of tissue (Figure 46-5). The physician should avoid incorporating nerves, vessels, or tendons within the excised block. Either technique creates a larger wound but allows a better inspection and more thorough cleaning after removal.

Subungual splinters must be removed because subsequent infection is almost inevitable, and the distal phalanx is at risk for osteomyelitis. If the splinter is underneath the distal end of the nail, it can be grasped by a splinter forceps or hooked by a hypodermic needle bent at its tip. More proximal splinters can be reached by anesthetizing the finger and removing a wedge of the nail overlying part of the foreign body (Figure 46-6). If pieces of the splinter remain, the entire nail can be removed.

Numerous, tiny cactus spines in the dermis can be plucked out individually with forceps or extracted together with depilatory wax, professional-quality facial gel, rubber cement, or household glue. Larger spines and thorns should be removed with incision or excision techniques.

FISHHOOKS
Fishhooks have a variety of sizes and shapes based on a common pattern (Figure 46-7). The barb, which is a projection extending backward from the point of the hook, keeps the point embedded in the fish's mouth and makes removal from skin a challenging task. Most injuries with fishhooks involve the hand, head, or face.

Several methods for removing fishhooks in skin have been reported. The best strategy depends primarily on the depth of the hook. If the hook has multiple barbs, precautions should be taken to avoid impaling the treating physician, bystanders, or the patient (a second time) during removal by taping or cutting off the exposed barbs. With any technique, the skin should be prepared and anesthetized at the entry site. If the hook is superficial, gentle downward pressure is placed on the shank while the hook is simply pulled in a retrograde direction along the path of entry (Figure 46-8).

The *string-pull method* is a variation on the retrograde technique. String is wrapped around the bend of the hook where it enters the skin.

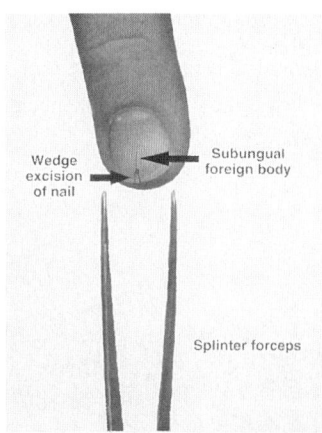

FIG. 46-6. Subungual foreign bodies that are beyond the reach of a splinter forceps can be exposed by excising a wedge of the overlying nail.

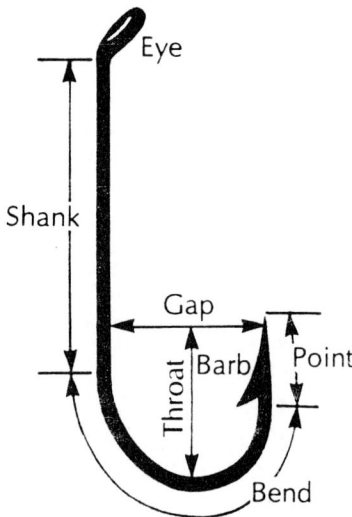

FIG. 46-7. Anatomy of a fishhook.

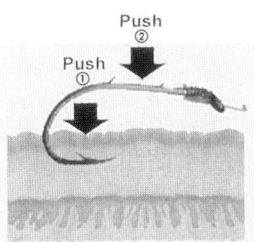

FIG. 46-8. Simple retrograde technique. While pressing the skin over the tip of the hook to disengage the barb and applying gentle downward pressure on the shank, the physician backs the hook out of the skin. If the barb catches on skin fibers, other techniques must be used.

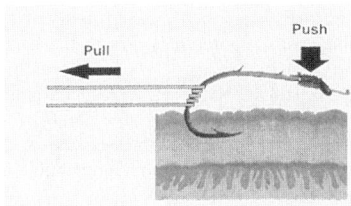

FIG. 46-9. String-pull technique. String or suture material is tied to the curve of the hook. The hook is positioned as described in the simple retrograde technique, and a quick pull on the string will dislodge the hook.

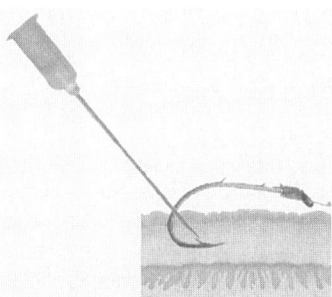

FIG. 46-10. Needle-cover technique. The area is anesthetized, and an 18-gauge needle is inserted into the entrance wound along the hook. The lumen of the needle is placed over the barb to cover it, and both the hook and needle are backed out of the wound.

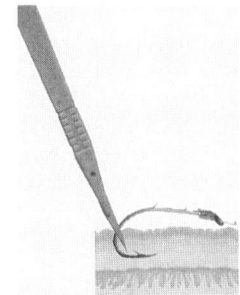

FIG. 46-12. Incision technique. The area is anesthetized, and a small incision is made along the shaft of the hook to the barb. The hook is withdrawn through the incision.

The end of the shank is depressed with one hand to disengage the barb from deeper tissue. The other hand then gives a quick pull on the string, extracting the hook (Figure 46-9). The disadvantages of this technique are that failure can cause further pain to the patient and success can result in ripped tissue or a sharp, blood-contaminated object flying uncontrollably across the room.

The *needle-cover technique* requires physician dexterity. An 18-gauge needle is inserted into the entrance wound alongside the shank of the hook. The needle follows the bend of the hook until the lumen of the needle can be placed over the barb to sheathe it. The hook and needle are then withdrawn from the wound as a unit (Figure 46-10).

The *advance-and-cut technique* is useful for deeply penetrated and larger fishhooks (Figure 46-11). The tip of the hook is advanced through the skin surface. Once exposed, the point and barb are cut with wire cutters, and the remaining part of the hook is rotated back out of the original wound. If barbs along the shank are embedded beneath the dermis, the shank can be clipped near the hook's eye. The remaining part of the hook is then passed antegrade through the skin. Since the advance-and-cut method further traumatizes and contaminates tissue, it probably should be reserved for wilderness situations. However, this may be an effective method in the ED if the barb has nearly or already penetrated the surface of the skin or is embedded within a joint, cartilage, or tendon.

A fifth technique is a modification of the needle cover technique for fishhooks embedded in the dermis. The entrance wound is enlarged to 2 to 3 mm with a no. 11 scalpel blade. The incision is carried along the bend of the hook to the barb until the barb is disengaged from the soft tissue. The hook can then be withdrawn easily through the larger entrance (Figure 46-12). If necessary, the barb can be grasped with a hemostat to prevent it from snagging tissue on the way out. There are two major benefits to enlarging puncture wounds containing foreign bodies. First, the wound is more easily inspected for additional foreign bodies. In the case of fishhook impalement, the wound may be harboring the bait that was on the hook. Second, the wound tract is more easily irrigated through a larger opening. However, the physician must avoid injuring tendons, nerves, or vessels with the scalpel.

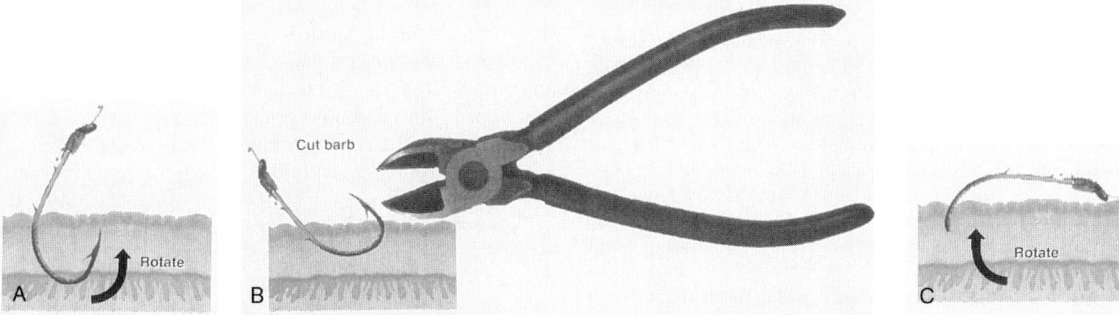

FIG. 46-11. Advance-and-cut technique. The area is anesthetized, and the tip of the hook is advanced through the skin surface (**A**), the barb is cut (**B**), and the hook is rotated back out of the original wound (**C**).

TRAUMATIC DERMAL TATTOOING Foreign particulates may be embedded in the epidermal and dermal layers of skin by an abrasion, which permanently stains or "tattoos" the surrounding tissue. If vigorous scrubbing does not remove the particulates, the patient can be referred to specialists for dermabrasion or block excision. The graphite from pencil lead can produce a pigmentation that will never dissolve, and graphite tattoos should be excised in cosmetic areas.

DISPOSITION

Postremoval Treatment

After removal of a foreign body, the wound should be irrigated thoroughly. A puncture wound is difficult to clean adequately because either the small wound diameter prevents the irrigation fluid from reaching the wounded tissue or the fluid enters the wound but does not completely drain. If the puncture is contaminated, the entrance wound can be enlarged to allow more effective cleaning. If foreign debris is impregnated in tissue, the contaminated area can be debrided or excised. If multiple radiopaque objects were removed, a postprocedure plain film should be obtained. The decision to close lacerations, incisions, and block excisions depends on the potential for infection; wounds in which all foreign contaminants can be removed and those in locations with good blood supply can be closed primarily. Otherwise, delayed primary closure is preferred to immediate closure. Necessary tetanus immunization should be provided. If a foreign body is deliberately left in place, the patient should be informed. If foreign material was removed, the patient should be warned that there is always a possibility that not all pieces were found.

Delayed Removal

Many patients must be referred to surgical specialists for delayed removal of foreign bodies. It is important to inform the patient that the object is present but unlikely to cause harm before it is removed. The benefit of prophylactic antibiotics for uninfected wounds containing foreign bodies has not been studied. Antibiotics are justified for infected wounds, particularly when removal must be postponed, even though removal allows infections to clear rapidly. If a foreign body is near a joint or highly mobile region, the affected area should be splinted prior to removal to prevent further injury or migration of the object.

REFERENCES

1. Farrell SE, Vandevander P, Lee D, et al.: Elevated serum lead levels in ED patients with retained lead foreign bodies [abstr]. *Acad Emerg Med* 3:418, 1996.
2. Avner JR, Baker MD: Lacerations involving glass: The role of routine roentgenograms. *Am J Dis Child* 146:600, 1992.
3. Steele MT, Tran LV, Watson WA, Muelleman RL: Retained glass foreign bodies in wounds: Predictive value of wound characteristics, patient perception, and wound exploration. *Am J Emerg Med* 16:627, 1998.
4. Russell RC, Williamson DA, Sullivan JW, et al: Detection of foreign bodies in the hand. *J Hand Surg Am* 16A:2, 1991.
5. Courter BJ: Radiographic screening for glass foreign bodies: What does a "negative" foreign body series really mean? *Ann Emerg Med* 19:997, 1990.
6. Ellis G: Are aluminum foreign bodies detectable radiographically? *Am J Emerg Med* 11:12, 1993.
7. Roobottom CA, Weston MJ: The detection of foreign bodies in soft tissue: Comparison of conventional and digital radiography. *Clin Radiol* 49:330, 1994.
8. Reiner B, Siegel E, McLaurin T, et al: Evaluation of soft-tissue foreign bodies: Comparing conventional plain film radiography, computed radiography printed on film, and computed tomography displayed on a computer workstation. *Am J Roentgenol* 167:141, 1996.
9. Chisholm CD, Wood CO, Chua G, et al: Radiographic detection of gravel in soft tissue. *Ann Emerg Med* 29:725, 1997.
10. Ell SR, Sprigg A, Parker AJ: A multi-observer study examining the radiographic visibility of fishbone foreign bodies. *J R Soc Med* 89:31, 1996.
11. Lue AJ, Fang WD, Manolidis S: Use of plain radiography and computed tomography to identify fish bone foreign bodies. *Otolaryngol Head Neck Surg* 123:435, 2000.
12. Graham DD: Ultrasound in the emergency department: Detection of wooden foreign bodies in the soft tissues. *J Emerg Med* 22:75, 2002.
13. Blankstein A, Cohen I, Heiman Z, et al: Ultrasonography as a diagnostic modality and therapeutic adjuvant in the management of soft tissue foreign bodies in the lower extremities. *Isr Med Assoc J* 3:411, 2001.
14. Boyse TD, Fessell DP, Jacobson JA, et al: US of soft-tissue foreign bodies and associated complications with surgical correlation. *Radiographics* 21:1251, 2001.
15. Jacobson JA, Powell A, Craig JG, et al: Wooden foreign bodies in soft tissue: Detection at ultrasound. *Radiology* 206:45, 1998.
16. Schlager D, Sanders AB, Wiggins D, et al: Ultrasound for the detection of foreign bodies. *Ann Emerg Med* 20:189, 1991.
17. Manthey DE, Storrow AB, Milbourn JM, et al: Ultrasound versus radiography in the detection of soft-tissue foreign bodies. *Ann Emerg Med* 28:7, 1996.
18. Harcke HT, Levy AD, Lonergan GJ: The sonographic appearance and detectability of nonopaque and semiopaque materials of military origin. *Mil Med* 167:459, 2002.
19. Bray PW, Mahoney JL, Campbell JP: Sensitivity and specificity of ultrasound in the diagnosis of foreign bodies in the hand. *J Hand Surg Am* 20A:661, 1995.
20. Turner J, Wilde CH, Hughes KC, et al: Ultrasound-guided retrieval of small foreign objects in subcutaneous tissue. *Ann Emerg Med* 29:731, 1997.
21. Blankstein A, Cohen I, Heiman Z, et al: Localization, detection, and guided removal of soft tissue in the hand using sonography. *Arch Orthop Trauma Surg* 120:514, 2000.
22. Wyn T, Jones J, McNinch D, Neacox R: Bedside fluoroscopy for the detection of foreign bodies. *Acad Emerg Med* 2:979, 1995.
23. Cohen DM, Garcia CT, Dietrich AM, Hickey RW: Miniature C-arm imaging: An in vitro study of detecting foreign bodies in the emergency department. *Pediatr Emerg Care* 13:247, 1997.

47 PUNCTURE WOUNDS AND MAMMALIAN BITES
Robert A. Schwab
Robert D. Powers

PUNCTURE WOUNDS

Puncture wounds can be loosely defined as wounds whose depth exceeds the diameter of the visible surface injury. They usually involve the plantar surface of the foot; punctures to the leg and upper extremity occur less often.[1] The relatively innocuous-appearing skin wound belies the potential for injury to underlying structures and infection. Punctures caused by high-pressure injection equipment, mammalian bites, and those involving exposure to body fluids each have the potential for unique complications that affects evaluation and management.

Pathophysiology

In puncture wounds, shear forces between the missile and tissue result in tissue disruption, producing hemorrhage and devitalization of skin and underlying tissues. Inoculation of organisms from the missile (with or without a foreign body) or from the skin surface into the deeper tissues is followed by relatively rapid closure of the small skin wound, creating an environment favorable for the development of infection, which is reported to occur in 6 to 11 percent of puncture wounds.[2]

Most soft-tissue infections from puncture wounds are caused by gram-positive organisms; *Staphylococcus aureus* predominates, followed by other staphylococcal and streptococcal species.[2] Puncture wounds over joints can penetrate the joint capsule and produce septic arthritis, while penetration of cartilage, periosteum, and bone can lead to osteomyelitis. *Pseudomonas aeruginosa* is the most frequent pathogen isolated from plantar puncture wound-related osteomyelitis, particularly when the injury occurs through the rubber sole of an athletic shoe.[3]

The incidence of puncture wound infection is increased in the presence of host factors that inhibit wound healing; diabetes mellitus, peripheral vascular disease, or immunosuppression by disease or chronic immunosuppressive therapy (see Table 42–2).[4]

Clinical characteristics associated with higher complication rates include patients seen more than 6 h after injury, wounds obviously contaminated with debris, wounds occurring outdoors, puncture wounds through footwear, wounds from longer objects with deeper penetration, and host factors inhibiting wound healing.

Most literature related to plantar puncture wounds identifies forefoot injuries as inherently high-risk. Theoretically, since most of the body weight is transmitted to the metatarsal heads during walking, a puncture in this area might penetrate deeply. A published case series of patients hospitalized with infected plantar puncture wounds seemed to confirm this theory.[5] However, although a majority of these patients had sustained forefoot injuries, neither this study nor any other has prospectively followed enough forefoot injuries to definitively determine the incidence of complications from this injury and the assertion that forefoot injuries are higher risk for infection has not been proven.

Clinical Features

Important historical features related to puncture wounds include the time of injury as well as circumstances leading up to the injury. A history of jumping or falling onto an object suggests deeper penetration than other mechanisms. The footwear (for plantar wounds) or clothing through which the missile passed will help assess the potential for foreign body and infection. The patient's estimate of depth as well as foreign body sensation should be elicited, as should the postinjury care rendered prior to presentation. The medical history will disclose host factors predisposing to infection.

The characteristics of the missile are important in predicting risk of foreign body and infection. Materials such as wood, glass, and plastic are prone to break or splinter, leaving retained fragments in the wound. Thin objects such as needles or pins can break off beneath the skin surface.

Physical examination of puncture wounds should assess wound characteristics as well as function of underlying structures. In punctures of the hand, distal function of tendons and nerves and integrity of distal perfusion should be assessed. Puncture wounds should be carefully inspected for their proximity to underlying structures, the condition of the surrounding skin, and the presence of foreign matter or devitalized tissue. Wound infection is suggested by severe pain, swelling, erythema, warmth, fluctuance, drainage, or pain with motion of tendons or joints.

Because the entire depth of a puncture wound cannot be reliably explored, assessment for the presence of a foreign body is problematic. Patient perception of a foreign body is modestly useful in predicting the presence of one [sensitivity = 43%, specificity = 83%, LR(+) = 2.49 and LR(−) = 0.69].[6] Probing of the wound with a blunt instrument has been recommended as a means of blindly assessing for depth and for the presence of a foreign body, but the benefit of this practice is unproven.

Diagnostic Studies

Plain-film radiographs utilizing soft-tissue visualization techniques are indicated in all infected puncture wounds, in wounds caused by materials prone to fragment, and whenever the patient reports a foreign body sensation. Plain radiographs will detect more than 90 percent of radiopaque foreign bodies larger than 1.0 mm in diameter (see Chap. 46). Most organic substances such as wood, thorns, and other plant matter have radiodensities close to that of soft tissue and cannot be identified with plain radiographs.

Ultrasonography can identify soft-tissue foreign bodies, but the ability to detect small objects that would be anticipated to be introduced through a puncture wound is limited (see Chap. 46). Computed tomography (CT) can accurately detect radiolucent foreign bodies, and is the method of choice for patients with suspected occult foreign body following a puncture wound. Magnetic resonance imaging (MRI) provides excellent visualization of foreign bodies, but cannot be used to image metallic objects or objects containing certain minerals due to the production of ferromagnetic artifact. CT or MRI should done on patients with deep-space infection, persistent pain after a puncture wound, or with superficial infections that fail to respond to therapy.

Treatment

Treatment recommendations for puncture wounds are largely based on anecdotal evidence and reviews of uncontrolled case series.[2] The small entrance wound, often closed at the time of presentation, makes traditional wound cleansing techniques ineffective. Therefore aggressive debridement and irrigation are sometimes recommended. However, these recommendations for aggressive wound debridement ignore the benign course of the overwhelming majority of these injuries in an attempt to avoid rare but potentially catastrophic complications.[1]

Uncomplicated clean punctures presenting less than 6 h after injury require superficial wound cleansing and tetanus prophylaxis as indicated. Soaking of the wound has no proven benefit. Low-pressure (e.g., 0.5 psi) irrigation of wounds will assist in surface cleansing and allow visualization of the entrance site, whereas high-pressure (e.g., 7 psi) injection of irrigation fluid into the wound has no proven benefit and theoretically could force foreign matter and bacteria deeper into the surrounding tissue.

Debridement or coring of the wound tract in clean wounds has been recommended, but has not been proven to reduce infection or to facilitate accurate diagnosis of deeper structural injury. Without clear evidence of benefit, it is difficult to endorse a procedure that is painful and time consuming, particularly when it leaves the patient with a wound larger than the initial puncture.

Perhaps the greatest controversy in the management of puncture wounds concerns the role of prophylactic antibiotics. There is no proven benefit of prophylactic antibiotics in any type of puncture, although many authorities recommend their use in high-risk patients with plantar puncture wounds. "High-risk" includes patients with impaired host defenses, and may also include forefoot injuries and patients sustaining punctures through athletic shoes. The only published study on prophylactic antibiotics for plantar puncture wounds that compared treated with untreated patients during the same study period was an observational nonrandomized trial using a variety of oral antibiotics.[7] This study found that none of the 18 patients treated with prophylactic antibiotics within 24 h of injury developed an infection compared to 18 patients who developed infections out of 62 individuals who did not receive prophylactic antibiotics within 24 h (absolute reduction in infection 29%; 95% CI 18 to 40%). A recent review of available evidence concluded that because there were no randomized clinical studies, no evidence-based recommendations can be made regarding the use of prophylactic antibiotics for plantar puncture wounds, and physicians are counseled to "follow local advice" in deciding when or if to treat.[8]

If prophylactic antibiotics are used, an oral fluoroquinolone (ciprofloxacin or levofloxacin) seems sensible although expensive. These broad-spectrum antibiotics achieve high blood levels rapidly after ingestion and possess antipseudomonal activity. Alternative agents, such as dicloxacillin, cephalexin, or erythromycin may be effective despite the theoretical disadvantage of no antipseudomonal coverage.[7] If antipseudomonal coverage is desired and oral fluoroquinolones are contraindicated, a combination of oral antistaphylococcal and parenteral antipseudomonal antibiotics (e.g., ticarcillin, ceftazidime, or gentamicin) would be an acceptable albeit inconvenient choice.

Complications

Skin tattooing from foreign material can lead to undesirable cosmetic outcomes, but meticulous wound cleansing can prevent this problem. Two more serious complications are retained foreign body and infection. The hallmark of both of these complications is pain. Any patient with significant pain more than 48 h after the initial injury should undergo a thorough evaluation for missed foreign body or infection; if no definitive infection is found, the use of prophylactic antibiotics in this subgroup of patients is a reasonable if unproven strategy.[2] Infections that develop after puncture wounds include cellulitis, local abscess, deeper spreading soft tissue infection, and infections of bone or cartilage.

CELLULITIS   This localized infection of the dermis surrounding the puncture wound usually becomes clinically detectable within the first 4 days after the injury. The patient typically presents due to persistent pain causing inability to bear weight. The patient may also note swelling. Physical examination usually reveals erythema, warmth, and tenderness surrounding the area of injury. Swelling may be present, but swelling or erythema in areas not contiguous with the injury is absent. Radiographs, if not done at the time of injury, are indicated to exclude a radiopaque foreign body. These infections are generally caused by streptococcal and staphylococcal skin flora, and usually respond to a 7- to 10-day course of a first-generation cephalosporin.

LOCALIZED ABSCESS   This complication is usually associated with a retained foreign body. The patient presents due to pain, and may also complain of a foreign body sensation or drainage from the wound site. On examination, a tender, warm, fluctuant mass is palpable at the site of injury, but again no abnormalities are noted in areas not initially affected by the injury. Radiographs are indicated if not done at the time of injury. Incision and drainage will often disclose a foreign body, and is curative. A short course of antibiotics is indicated if there is significant cellulitis in conjunction with the abscess.

Outpatient management of cellulitis and localized abscesses is the rule. Patients should be instructed to apply warm compresses or use warm soaks, avoid weight-bearing on plantar puncture wounds, and to elevate the affected extremity. Appropriate analgesia should be prescribed as well as antibiotics. Routine follow-up within 48 h is recommended.

DEEP SOFT TISSUE INFECTION   Patients present with pain that is generally more severe than with cellulitis or localized abscess. Redness, swelling, and drainage at the wound site may be seen. The key physical examination finding is pain, redness, or swelling at a site remote from the puncture site. With plantar puncture wounds, signs of infection on the dorsum of the foot should alert the clinician to the presence of a more serious complication. Radiographs should be performed to identify foreign bodies and to look for gas in the soft tissue planes. These infections may involve gram-negative and anaerobic bacteria, and always require parenteral antibiotics and immediate referral to a specialist for surgical management.

OSTEOMYELITIS   Bone and joint infections are the most disastrous sequelae of puncture wounds. The overall incidence following plantar puncture wounds is between 0.1 and 2%, and may be somewhat higher in patients sustaining forefoot punctures through athletic shoes.[2] These patients present somewhat later than those with other complications, often after a period of symptomatic improvement. Pain, swelling, redness, and drainage may all occur, but pain is the presenting complaint in nearly every case. Examination may reveal erythema, swelling, and drainage, or may be deceptively normal. Radiographs may also be normal in the early stages of osteomyelitis. An elevated white blood cell count or an elevated erythrocyte sedimentation rate supports the diagnosis of osteomyelitis, but neither test is sensitive enough to absolutely exclude bony infection.[9] The definitive diagnostic study is a bone scan, which will demonstrate osteomyelitis within 72 h of the onset of symptoms. Once the diagnosis is made, immediate surgical referral should be made; antibiotic administration should be withheld pending discussion with the consultant, since pathogen identification is best done from cultures obtained during operative debridement. If antibiotics are administered before surgery, coverage against staphylococcal and pseudomonal species is recommended.

NEEDLE-STICK INJURIES

Needle-stick injuries are common among health care professionals; a recent survey of emergency medicine residents found that over 50% reported at least one occupational exposure to blood during their training.[10] Most of these exposures involved a puncture with a hollow needle or other sharp object.

Like other punctures, these injuries carry the risk of infection with hepatitis and human immunodeficiency virus (HIV). The risk of clinical infection after an inadvertent needle stick from an infectious source has been estimated to be negligible for hepatitis A, 6 percent for hepatitis B, 2 percent for hepatitis C, and 0.3 percent for HIV.[11]

Preexposure prophylaxis is available for hepatitis B. Postexposure prophylaxis is available for hepatitis B and HIV. Postexposure prophylaxis of hepatitis C is no longer recommended.[11] The specific recommendations for postexposure prophylaxis of HIV are updated regularly by the Centers for Disease Control and Prevention: (http://www.cdc.gov/health/needlesticks.htm); PEPline: 1.888.HIV.4911). The latest update, in June 2001 (*Morb Mortal Wkly Rep* 50:RR-11, 2001), emphasized the use of rapid HIV testing on source patients, and 48- to 72-h follow-up when rapid testing is not available, so overuse of antiretroviral therapy can be avoided. Recommendations for management are complex and change frequently; each hospital should have a predetermined needle-stick protocol endorsed by local infectious disease specialists. See Chap. 154 for detailed discussion.

HIGH-PRESSURE INJECTION INJURIES

High-pressure injection injuries are caused by industrial equipment designed to force paint, grease, or other liquids through a small-diameter nozzle at pressures several times higher than that required to penetrate intact skin. Although a significant amount of energy is dissipated in overcoming skin resistance, the material still spreads widely along fascial planes. The type, amount, and viscosity of material injected will determine the degree of tissue inflammatory response, and in less distensible tissue compartments sudden pressure elevations produce vascular injuries, ischemic necrosis, and gangrene.[12]

Most injuries occur in the nondominant hand of an operator using a high-pressure gun. The injury may initially cause little pain, leading to delays in presentation or misdiagnosis of the extent of injury. Within hours, pain typically becomes severe and evidence of ischemia or widespread inflammation is manifest. Unfortunately, delays in initial management increase the risk of amputation or disability.[12]

The apparent lack of significant external injury can be misleading when the patient is first evaluated; the small entrance wound with some surrounding edema suggests only a minor injury. However, the history alone should prompt aggressive treatment and immediate surgical consultation.

ED evaluation should include assessment of neurovascular integrity and tendon function, aggressive pain management utilizing intravenous opioids, prophylactic antibiotic coverage against skin flora, and tetanus prophylaxis as indicated. Radiographs will often demonstrate wide dissemination of radiopaque material as well as injected air along fascial planes. Digital nerve blocks should be avoided, as they may further increase pressure in finger compartments.

Early surgical debridement is necessary to avoid amputation and minimize disability.[12] A hand specialist should be consulted without delay.

MAMMALIAN BITES

Most patients presenting for ED care of bite injuries have been bitten by domestic dogs or cats. The United States has more than 50 million dogs and 100 million cats; in a typical year they inflict more than 12,000 bites each day. Of the nearly 4 million Americans who are bitten each year, just under 500,000 seek medical attention in EDs and 10 to 20 will die of their injuries.[13,14] The economic cost in homeowners insurance payouts and medical care expenditures exceeds $100 million. Children seek care for bites more often than adults. Dogs that are specifically trained for guard duty (pit bulls, rottweilers, German shepherds) cause a disproportionate number of serious injuries and deaths.[13,14]

General Principles of Bite Wound Management

Considerations in caring for patients with bite wounds include the injury inflicted by the bite, prevention or treatment of local bacterial infection, and prevention, recognition, and management of subsequent systemic illness.

In the initial assessment of the injured patient, attention should be paid to the potential for a life-threatening injury. A large animal, or multiple animals attacking a child or small adult can inflict severe injuries, including vascular damage and blunt or penetrating trauma. Standard assessment and resuscitation protocols for trauma victims should be employed in the rare circumstance in which the patient is seriously injured. In the more typical case of an isolated soft tissue injury, wound management and prevention of infectious complications become paramount.

Meticulous examination and wound cleansing measures including aggressive irrigation and debridement of devitalized tissue are important. Care should be taken to determine the extent of underlying tissue damage, with special attention to the potential for penetration into joint spaces and tendon sheaths. Management of wounds involving the face, hands, or perineum will be problematic due to the close proximity of delicate structures. If there is suspicion of foreign material in the wound, imaging may be indicated.

Some bite lacerations can be safely and cosmetically sutured primarily. If closure is desirable for cosmetic or functional reasons, a skilled practitioner should perform this procedure under optimum conditions.[15,16] Delayed primary closure is a technique that has been used successfully in contaminated wounds, and should be considered in the management of bite injuries. Wounds that are already infected should be managed without closure, as should wounds occurring in immunocompromised hosts. Puncture-type bite wounds, wounds greater than 6 h old, and most wounds on the hand and foot should be left open.

Microbiology and Therapy of Infections from Cat and Dog Bites

Mammalian saliva contains large concentrations of microorganisms, and all bite wounds should be considered to be contaminated with pathogenic bacteria. Their proliferation in tissue can lead to serious cellulitis, tenosynovitis, and pyarthrosis. Despite the presumably large inoculum of bacteria, only about 5 to 6 percent of untreated dog bites will become infected; this infection rate approximates that found with lacerations from nonbite mechanisms.[17,18] Cats have narrower, sharper teeth than dogs, and the ability to deliver infectious agents deep into a small-bore puncture wound. It is not surprising that as many as 60 to 80 percent of cat bites will become infected.[17,18]

Infection following a cat bite is likely due to *Pasteurella multocida,* particularly if the infection has a rapid onset. Infected dog bites are also likely to contain *Pasteurella,* as well as anaerobes, streptococcal, and staphylococcal species.

The use of antibiotics in postexposure prophylaxis of bite wounds is controversial. A structured review of eight randomized clinical trials has found evidence lacking for efficacy in dog and cat wounds overall, but the power of the analysis was limited by the small number of patients and the suboptimal spectrum of agents utilized.[18] The only significant benefit was for dog or cat bites of the hands, where the infection rate was reduced by prophylactic antibiotics from 28 percent in the control group to 2 percent in the treated group (absolute reduction 26%, 95% CI 2 to 50%). Only one small, randomized clinical trial of 11 patients total analyzed the effect of prophylactic antibiotics after cat bite; 67 percent (4/6) of control patients developed an infection compared to 0 percent (0/5) of treated patients. However, because of the small number of patients studied, the difference is not statistically significant.

A prudent approach is to treat all infected wounds and to prescribe prophylactic antibiotics for high-risk uninfected wounds. These would include all cat bites, all bites in immunocompromised hosts, deep dog bite puncture wounds, hand wounds, and any laceration that is being sutured. An initial 5- to 7-day course of an appropriate antimicrobial should be sufficient. The patient should receive a follow-up wound check in all but the most trivial cases. In lower-risk situations, counsel and advice regarding relative risk of treatment in addition to wound precautions are warranted.

Amoxicillin-clavulanate is the medication most commonly recommended for therapy and prophylaxis.[15,17] However, penicillin or ampicillin should be adequate for *Pasteurella multocida* infections, and represent logical lower-cost alternatives for prophylaxis of cat bites. Penicillin-allergic patients require therapy with doxycycline or cefuroxime for cat bites, and clindamycin plus a fluoroquinolone for dog bites. Cephalexin, dicloxacillin, erythromycin, or clindamycin should not be used alone, as their spectrum does not include *Pasteurella* species.

Systemic Bacterial Infections Following Dog and Cat Bites

There are a few serious systemic sequelae of dog and cat bite infections. These febrile illnesses can develop days after the bite, and are not necessarily accompanied by local bite wound infection. *Capnocytophaga canimorsus* causes a rare but fulminant bacteremic illness following a dog bite. Fatal multiorgan failure can occur, particularly in splenectomized patients, or those with alcoholism or other immunosuppressive disorders. Diagnosis is confirmed with positive blood cultures; broad-spectrum therapy with penicillin and other agents is indicated in concert with aggressive support.[19] The virulence of this infection provides some justification for the prophylactic use of penicillins in all immunocompromised patients bitten by dogs.

Cat-scratch disease is a clinical syndrome of regional lymphadenopathy developing 7 to 12 days after a cat bite or scratch. This chronic indolent infection caused by *Bartonella henselae* can result in painful, matted masses of lymph nodes lasting up to 4 months. Diagnosis is made by serology or biopsy; therapy consisting of pain relief, reassurance, and aspiration of symptomatic buboes is usually successful. Azithromycin may speed resolution of adenopathy.[20]

Human Bites

Human bites deserve special consideration, as they tend to be more serious than those from domestic animals. The low incidence of these injuries has hampered prospective study, but experience suggests that they have a high rate of complication. All should be treated as contaminated puncture wounds; many will present late due to the circumstances leading to the injury. Of particular concern is the closed-fist injury (CFI), incurred when a flexed knuckle strikes a human tooth in the course of an altercation. The subsequent tenosynovitis and pyarthrosis generally require operative management and intravenous antibiotics.

Human bite wound infections are polymicrobial; staphylococcal and streptococcal species are common; other pathogens include the species-specific gram-negative rod *Eikenella corrodens.* Amoxicillin-clavulanate is recommended for treatment and prophylaxis following all but the most trivial human bites.[18] Parenteral agents of choice include ampicillin-sulbactam, cefoxitin, or piperacillin-tazobactam. Herpes simplex virus can cause local infection following a human bite or contact with infected saliva. The resultant herpetic whitlow is a painful coalescence of pustules, typically on the distal phalanx. Incision and drainage are contraindicated; therapy with acyclovir or other appropriate antiviral is recommended.

Rodents, Livestock, Exotic and Wild Animals

Patients often seek care or consultation after being bitten by a rodent. The injury is usually trivial, the risk of infection is low, and rodents are not known to carry or transmit rabies, so standard wound care and reassurance should suffice. Rat-bite fever consists of two similar febrile illnesses following a small percentage of bites from rats or other rodents. Diagnosis is confirmed by blood cultures positive for *Streptobacillus moniliformis* or *Spirillum minus;* penicillin or streptomycin is appropriate therapy.

Livestock and large game animals can inflict serious tissue injury with their powerful jaws and grinding teeth. In addition, the risk of wound infection and systemic illnesses such as brucellosis, leptospirosis, and tularemia is significant. Aggressive wound care and prophylactic broad-spectrum antibiotics are recommended in these situations; a febrile illness following such a bite usually requires inpatient antibiotic therapy guided by blood culture results.

Systemic Infections: Spirochetes; Rabies and Other Viruses

Disseminated spirochetal and viral illnesses that can result from mammalian bites include syphilis, rabies, hepatitis, and infection with herpes B or human immunodeficiency virus. Spirochetes are present in infectious quantities in the saliva of patients with early syphilis; transmission of the disease can occur via biting or kissing.

Rabies is a rare disease in developed countries; most of the 35,000 cases per year worldwide are concentrated in lesser-developed countries (see Chap. 147). In the United States, there were approximately two cases each year in the latter half of the twentieth century. Many of these were acquired from contact with domestic bats, or from dog bites sustained while traveling abroad. Postexposure prophylaxis with immunoglobulin and vaccine is necessary for patients at risk. Significant North American reservoirs of animal rabies exist in bats, skunks, raccoons, and foxes. All carnivores and omnivores can transmit rabies, whereas rodents, hares, and rabbits are extremely unlikely to harbor the disease. Local public health agencies are a good source of information regarding the rabies risk from contact with specific indigenous animals. In certain parts of the world, notably South Asia, monkeys are presumed to be at high risk for carriage and transmission of rabies.

Herpes B virus, also called *Herpesvirus simiae,* can be transmitted by bites from monkeys and other nonhuman primates. Myelitis and hemorrhagic encephalitis can occur in humans and death occurs in 68 percent of infected individuals. Wound care of the bite location should include scrubbing with povidone-iodine for 15 min followed by copious irrigation. Early therapy with acyclovir 800 mg PO five times per day beginning immediately after injury can prevent or ameliorate these manifestations.

Viral hepatitis and HIV can both be transmitted by a human bite, although HIV concentration in nonbloody saliva is thought to be relatively low. Use of a protocol similar to that for an occupational needle-stick injury should be used when a patient sustains a bite from a high-risk source.

REFERENCES

1. Baldwin G, Colbourne M: Puncture wounds. *Pediatr Rev* 20:21-23, 1999.
2. Schwab RA, Powers RD: Conservative therapy of plantar puncture wounds. *J Emerg Med* 13:291, 1995.
3. Inaba AS, Zukin DD, Perro M: An update on the evaluation and management of plantar puncture wounds and *Pseudomonas* osteomyelitis. *Pediatr Emerg Care* 8:38, 1992.
4. Armstrong DG, Lavery LA, Quebedeaux TL, et al: Surgical morbidity and the risk of amputation due to infected puncture wounds in diabetics and nondiabetic adults. *J Am Podiatr Med Assoc* 87:321, 1997.
5. Patzakis MJ, Wilkins J, Brien WW, et al: Wound site as a predictor of complications following deep nail punctures to the foot. *West J Med* 150:545, 1989.
6. Steele MT, Tran LV, Watson WA, Muelleman RT: Retained glass foreign bodies in wounds: Predictive value of wound characteristics, patient perception, and wound exploration. *Am J Emerg Med* 16:627, 1998.
7. Pennycook A, Makower R, O'Donnell A-M: Puncture wounds of the foot: Can infective complications be avoided? *J Roy Soc Med* 87:581, 1994.
8. Harrison M, Thomas M: Antibiotics after puncture wounds to the foot. *Emerg Med J* 19:49, 2002.
9. Lavery LA, Armstrong DG, Quebedeaux TL, et al: Puncture wounds: Normal laboratory values in the face of severe infection in diabetics and nondiabetics. *Am J Med* 101:521, 1996.
10. Lee CH, Carter WA, Chiang WK, et al: Occupational exposures to blood among emergency medicine residents. *Acad Emerg Med* 6:1036, 1999.
11. Mikulich VJ, Schriger DL: Abridged version of the updated US Public Health Service guidelines for the management of occupational exposures to hepatitis B virus, hepatitis C virus, and human immunodeficiency virus and recommendations for postexposure prophylaxis. *Ann Emerg Med* 39:321, 2002.
12. Vasilevski D, Noorbergen M, Depierreux M, et al: High-pressure injection injuries to the hand. *Am J Emerg Med* 18:820, 2000.
13. McCaig LF, Ly N: National Hospital Ambulatory Care Survey: 2000 Emergency Department Summary. Atlanta, GA: Centers for Disease Control and Prevention, 2002.
14. Centers for Disease Control and Prevention: Dog bite related fatalities-United States 1995-96. *MMWR* 46:463, 1997.
15. Fleisher G: The management of bite wounds. *New Engl J Med* 340:138, 1999.
16. Chen E, Hornig S, Shepherd SM, Hollander JE: Primary closure of mammalian bites. *Acad Emerg Med* 7:157, 2000.
17. Talan DA, Citron DM, Abrahamian FM, et al: Bacteriologic analysis of infected dog and cat bites. *New Engl J Med* 340:85, 1999.
18. Medeiros I, Saconato H: Antibiotic prophylaxis for mammalian bites. *Cochrane Database Syst Rev* 2:CD001738, 2001.
19. Lion C, Escande F, Burdin JC: *Capnocytophaga canimorsus* infections in humans: Review of the literature and case report. *Eur J Epidemiol* 12:521, 1996.
20. Bass JW, Freitas BD, Sisier CL, et al: Prospective randomized double-blind placebo-controlled evaluation of azithromycin for treatment of cat scratch disease. *Pediatr Infect Dis J* 17:447, 1998.

POSTREPAIR WOUND CARE
Adam J. Singer
Judd E. Hollander

Postoperative care begins immediately following laceration repair in the ED. Continued care and instructions should be provided so that the outcome of wound repair is optimized and complications are minimized. Immediately following repair, the injured area should be gently cleansed with normal saline to remove any residual blood products or contamination. Postoperative considerations that should be individually considered for each patient in the ED include the use of dressings, topical antibiotics, systemic antibiotics, need for splinting, and evaluation of tetanus status. Prior to ED release, the patient should be counseled regarding wound cleansing, pain control, signs of infection, and short-term and long-term cosmetic expectations.

USE OF DRESSINGS

Postoperative wound care should optimize healing. It must be tailored to both the type of wound and method of wound closure. Many sutured or stapled lacerations should be covered with a protective, nonadherent dressing for 24 to 48 h. Maintaining a warm, moist environment increases the rate of reepithelialization and occluded wounds heal faster than those exposed to air.[1] Although leaving lacerations exposed to air may result in slightly lower healing rate, it does not result in an increased rate of infection.[2] Therefore, although dressings are one strategy that can be used to maintain a moist wound environment, they have never been shown to decrease the infection rate.

Semipermeable films are manufactured from transparent polyurethane or similar synthetic films, coated on one surface with a water-resistant hypoallergenic adhesive. They are highly elastic, conform easily to body parts, and are generally resistant to shear and tear. They are permeable to moisture vapor and oxygen but impermeable to water and bacteria. Common types of dressings are OpSite, Bioclusive, and Tegaderm. The disadvantages of these materials are that they cannot absorb large amounts of fluid and exudate and they do not adhere well in very moist states.

An alternative to the use of commercial dressings to maintain a moist environment is the use of topical antibiotics for this purpose. Topical antibiotics can be used to maintain a moist environment in sutured or stapled lacerations, but not lacerations repaired with tissue adhesives. As an added benefit, topical antibiotics may help reduce infection rates and may also prevent scab formation.[3] However, patients whose lacerations are closed with tissue adhesives should not use topical ointments because they will loosen the adhesive and may result in dehiscence. Tissue adhesives serve as their own antimicrobial barrier and do not require supplementary dressings.

PATIENT POSITIONING AFTER WOUND REPAIR

When possible, the site of injury should be elevated above the patient's heart to limit the accumulation of fluid in the wound interstitial spaces. Wounds with little edema heal more rapidly than those with marked edema. Splints can be used for extremity injuries since they will decrease movement of the injured part, are associated with reductions in edema, and increase the attention paid to the injured body part. Although few wounds actually require splinting, splints are quite useful for extremity injuries, especially over joints. They can also be used to decrease the pain associated with soft-tissue injury.

Pressure dressings can be used to minimize the accumulation of intercellular fluid in the dead space. Pressure dressings are most useful for ear and scalp lacerations. For scalp lacerations that have a tendency to bleed, short-term use of a pressure dressing will help resolve the bleeding. For ear lacerations that might be prone to auricular hematoma formation, pressure dressings help reduce the likelihood of developing a cauliflower deformity. However, excessive pressure should be avoided, especially in the extremities where it may compromise circulation.

PROPHYLACTIC ANTIBIOTICS

Topical antibiotic ointments are commonly used by emergency physicians: one survey found that 71 percent of emergency physicians use topical antibiotics on recently repaired wounds.[4] Despite the frequent use of topical antibiotics, there are surprisingly few studies that assess the efficacy of topical antibiotics on the suture line after closure. As noted, one randomized study found a reduced infection rate with antibiotic ointment compared to petrolatum control.[3] Topical antibiotics provide a warm, moist environment that is beneficial for wound healing; therefore it is reasonable to use them for many lacerations.

On the other hand, the use of prophylactic oral antibiotics is not indicated except for select clinical circumstances. Several studies and a meta-analysis have all found no benefit to prophylactic antibiotics for routine laceration repair.[5] The use of antibiotics should be individualized based on the degree of bacterial contamination, the presence of infection-potentiating factors (e.g., soil), the mechanism of injury, and the presence or absence of host predisposition to infection.[6,7] In general, compulsive wound cleansing is far more important than anti-

otics. Inappropriate use of prophylactic antibiotics will not reduce the overall risk of infection. Rather, it will skew the microbiology toward more unusual or resistant pathogens.

Prophylactic antibiotics should be used for human bites, dog or cat bites on the extremities, intraoral lacerations, open fractures, and wounds with exposed joints or tendons.[6,7] Additionally, patients with grossly contaminated lacerations who are prone to the development of infective endocarditis, have prosthetic joints or other permanent "hardware," and patients with lymphedema should receive prophylactic antimicrobial therapy. It is recommended that patients at high risk for systemic complications such as endocarditis be given intravenous antibiotics before care of contaminated wounds.

The specific antibiotics used for prophylaxis are similar to those used for treatment of established infections (Table 48-1). For most patients, a first-generation cephalosporin or antistaphylococcal penicillin (e.g., dicloxacillin) is reasonable. Penicillin, which is active against most oral pathogens, should be used for intraoral wounds. Amoxicillin-clavulanate is the preferred prophylactic treatment for high-risk mammalian bite wounds. For open fractures or joints, a parenteral antistaphylococcal agent and an aminoglycoside should be used. There is no clear evidence that patients who receive oral antibiotic prophylaxis benefit from an intravenous dose in the ED, despite this common practice. For antibiotic prophylaxis, a 3 to 5 day course of oral antibiotics for nonbite injuries and 5 to 7 day course for bite wounds is adequate.

TETANUS PROPHYLAXIS

Two-thirds of the recent tetanus cases in the United States have followed lacerations, puncture wounds, and crush injuries. For every wounded patient, information about the mechanism of injury, the characteristics of the wound and its age, previous active immunization status, history of a neurologic or severe hypersensitivity reaction after a previous immunization treatment, and plans for follow-up if primary series should be obtained. Recommendations on tetanus prophylaxis are based on the condition of the wound and the patient's immunization history (Table 48-2). Passive immunization with tetanus immune globulin (TIG) should be considered for each patient, especially those without a history of a primary series of three tetanus immunizations.

The only contraindication to tetanus toxoid is a history of neurologic or severe systemic reaction after a previous dose. Local self-limited reactions such as erythema, induration, and pain at the injection site are common and self-limited after tetanus vaccination. These local side effects do not preclude future tetanus immunization. Exaggerated local reactions occur occasionally following tetanus toxoid and involve extensive pain and swelling of the entire extremity. Exaggerated local reactions occur most often in adults with high serum tetanus antitoxin levels who have received frequent doses of tetanus toxoid. These patients should not receive tetanus toxoid more frequently than every 10 years. Severe systemic reactions to tetanus immunization include generalized urticaria, anaphylaxis, or neurologic complications including peripheral neuropathy and Guillain-Barré syndrome. A severe allergic reaction including acute respiratory distress or cardiovascular collapse following a dose of tetanus toxoid is a contraindication to further immunization. A moderate or severe acute illness is also a reason to defer routine immunization, although a minor illness is not. If the use of a tetanus toxoid is contraindicated, passive immunization with TIG against tetanus should be considered in a tetanus-prone wound.

WOUND CLEANSING

Sutured or stapled wounds should be gently washed and cleansed as early as 8 h after closure.[8] The use of soap and tap water to cleanse lacerations is not associated with an increased infection rate. Gentle blotting should be used to dry the area; aggressive wiping could result in wound dehiscence. Patients with dressings should remove their dressing

TABLE 48-1 Empiric Antibiotics for Wound Infections

Clinical Situation	First-Line Agent	Alternative Therapy	Comment
Uncomplicated cellulitis	First-generation cephalosporin or antistaphylococcal penicillin	Macrolide	
Patient with underlying immunodeficiency	Amoxicillin-clavulanate or second-generation cephalosporin	Clindamycin plus a fluoroquinolone	
Patient with prosthetic heart valve or orthopedic implant	Consider adding vancomycin to standard regimen		Give prophylaxis before manipulating abscesses
Barnyard injuries, fecal contamination	Amoxicillin-clavulanate or second-generation cephalosporin	Fluoroquinolone plus either clindamycin or metronidazole	
Saltwater exposure	Third-generation cephalosporin ± doxycycline	Fluoroquinolone	*Vibrio* may cause hemorrhagic, bullous lesions
Freshwater exposure	Antipseudomonal aminoglycoside or antipseudomonal penicillin	Fluoroquinolone	*Aeromonas* or *Pseudomonas* may be involved
Abscesses, infections due to intravenous drug use	Amoxicillin-clavulanate or second-generation cephalosporin	Clindamycin	Antibiotics usually not necessary, incision and drainage essential
Necrotizing fasciitis	Imipenem or meropenem	Oxacillin plus gentamicin plus clindamycin	
Bite wounds	Amoxicillin-clavulanate or cefoxitin/cefotetan	Clindamycin plus either a fluoroquinolone or trimethoprim-sulfamethoxazole	
Open fracture	First-generation cephalosporin or antistaphylococcal penicillin	Vancomycin	
Plantar puncture wound osteomyelitis	Ceftazidime	Ciprofloxacin	

Source: Reproduced with permission from Singer AJ, Hollander JE (eds): *Lacerations and Acute Wounds. An Evidence-Based Guide,* Philadelphia, FA Davis.

after 24 to 48 h, cleanse the wound, and examine it for signs of infection.

Daily cleansing ensures that the patient examines the laceration for early signs of infection. Patients should be instructed to observe the wound for redness, warmth, swelling, and drainage, as these findings may indicate infection. Patients who notice signs of infection should initiate contact with the health care system. Standardized wound care instructions improves patient compliance and understanding.[7]

TABLE 48-2 Recommendations for Tetanus Prophylaxis

| History of Tetanus Immunization | CLEAN MINOR WOUNDS | | ALL OTHER WOUNDS* | |
	Administer Tetanus Toxoid[†]	Administer TIG[‡]	Administer Tetanus Toxoid	Administer TIG
<3 or uncertain doses	Yes	No	Yes	Yes
≥3 doses				
Last dose within 5 years	No	No	No	No
Last dose within 5–10 years	No	No	Yes	No
Last dose >10 years	Yes	No	Yes	No

*Especially if older than 6 h, deep (>1 cm), grossly contaminated, exposed to saliva or feces, stellate, ischemic or infected, avulsions, punctures, or crush injuries.

†Tetanus toxoid: Td if older than 7 years and DT if younger than 7 years, preferably administered into the deltoid.

‡Tetanus immune globulin: adult dose 250–500 IU administered into deltoid opposite the Td immunization site.

Abbreviations: DT = diphtheria-tetanus toxoid; Td = tetanus-diphtheria toxoid.

Reapplication of topical antibiotics for 3 to 5 days will decrease scab formation, thereby preventing wound-edge separation. Patients with tissue adhesives may shower, but they should avoid bathing and swimming because prolonged moisture will loosen the adhesive bond.

WOUND DRAINS

Drains are placed in wounds and surgical incisions under three circumstances: (1) to drain interstitial fluid or blood and prevent their accumulation into a seroma or hematoma, respectively; (2) maintain a tract so pus can drain from an infected area; or (3) allow for drainage from a contaminated location and prevent an abscess from forming. Drains allow for near complete wound closure in many circumstances in which closure would otherwise be impeded by fluid, pus, or blood accumulation. Drains can be categorized as (1) gauze packing to maintain open drainage and collect the exudate, (2) open systems using soft rubber (e.g., Penrose drain) or silicone tubing to direct drainage onto external gauze dressings, or (3) closed systems using silicone tubing and attached fluid collection reservoirs. Drains can be placed either through the suture line of the initial wound or incision, or through an adjacent incision made specifically for drain access.

The most common type of wound drain placed in the ED is $\frac{1}{4}$- to 1-inch ribbon gauze used to pack an abscess cavity after incision and drainage. Dressings over draining abscesses may initially require frequent changes. The internal packing should be replaced daily as long as the wound continues to produce exudate. Once the purulence stops, internal packing is no longer required, and daily cleaning with external dressing changes should continue until enough granulation tissue forms and the wound becomes dry. Maintaining a moist, clean environment promotes wound healing.

Open drainage using soft rubber tubing (e.g., Penrose drains) has been used for years to drain infected or contaminated wounds that have been partially or completely closed. A safety pin placed through the tubing can prevent the drain from inappropriately advancing into the wound. As the exudate diminishes and the wound heals, the Penrose drain can be pulled out a portion each day to allow the wound to heal from the "bottom up." The disadvantage of open drains such as the Penrose is the access they provide for bacteria into the wound.

For most purposes, especially postsurgery, closed drainage systems are preferred to open wound drains because closed systems prevent access of bacteria into the wound. The collection reservoir for closed drainage systems often has self-inflating ability so it can be squeezed before attachment to the tubing in order to place vacuum suction in the wound to enhance drainage (e.g., Jackson-Pratt, Hemovac, VacuDrain, and Constavac). Assessment of the tubing and emptying of the reservoir should be done with sterile technique (similar to dressing changes for indwelling lines). If a drainage tube is accidentally pulled out, it should not be reinserted. The reservoir may require emptying several times per day, depending on the drainage volume. It is common practice to remove closed drains when the amount of fluid drained each day reaches low levels (typically 30 to 40 mL per d).

PAIN CONTROL

Abrasions and some lacerations can be quite painful. Patients should be educated regarding the expected degree of pain and measures that may help reduce pain. Splints can be used to reduce swelling and pain for extremity lacerations. Appropriate analgesic medications and anti-inflammatory agents will help control pain. The pain from lacerations generally decreases after the initial 48 h and opiate analgesics are rarely necessary after that time. On the other hand, some patients with lacerations have concurrent contusions (such as victims of motor vehicle crashes), and they will often report worsening pain 24 to 48 h after the initial injury.

HEALTH CARE PROVIDER FOLLOW-UP

Patients should be instructed when and with whom to follow-up for suture removal or wound examination.[9] Sutures or staples in most locations should be removed after approximately 7 to 10 days (Table 48-3). Facial sutures should be removed within 3 to 5 days to avoid formation of unsightly sinus tracts and hatch marks.[10] Sutures over the joints or in the hands should be left in place for 10 to 14 days, since they may be subject to high tension during movement. When removing sutures, care should be taken to avoid applying tension in a direction that would tend to cause dehiscence. Any scab or crusting over the

TABLE 48-3 Time from Wound Closure Until Removal of Sutures or Staples

Location	Number of Days
Face	3–5
Scalp	7
Chest	8–10
Back	10–14
Forearm	10–14
Fingers	8–10
Hand	8–10
Lower extremity	8–12
Foot	10–12

Source: Singer AJ, Hollander JE (eds): *Lacerations and Acute Wounds. An Evidence-Based Guide.* Philadelphia, FA Davis, 2002, p. 188.

sutures may be debrided prior to suture removal by gently applying hydrogen peroxide with gauze.

Tissue adhesives will slough off, typically within 5 to 10 days of application. They do not usually require removal by a health care practitioner. When 2-octylcyanoacrylate is used, the patient should be careful to avoid picking at or scrubbing the area or exposing it to water for more than brief periods. When tissue adhesives remain on the skin for prolonged periods, antibiotic ointment, petroleum jelly, or bathing can accelerate removal.

Most patients do not require mandatory "wound checks." This practice might be useful in high-risk patients, high-risk wounds, or patients unable to identify signs of infection. Since many healing wounds may develop erythema and patients are not able to correctly identify wound infections, prescription of antibiotics without a reevaluation is inappropriate and often unnecessary.[11] Patients with wound infections should be treated with antibiotics as outlined earlier (see Table 48-1). Patients who require further tetanus immunization to complete their primary series should have the second dose 1 to 2 months later and the third dose 6 to 12 months after the second dose.

PATIENT EDUCATION ABOUT LONG-TERM COSMETIC OUTCOME

Although patients should be educated about the expected outcome before wound closure, the time of suture or staple removal or wound follow-up is another excellent time for patient education. Patients should understand that all traumatic lacerations result in some scarring. They should also understand that the short-term cosmetic appearance is not highly predictive of the ultimate cosmetic outcome.[12] Healing lacerations and abrasions should not be exposed to the sun, since sun exposure can result in permanent hyperpigmentation.[13] Injured skin should be protected with a sun-blocking agent for at least 6 to 12 months after injury.

REFERENCES

1. Hinman CD, Maibach H: Effect of air exposure and occlusion on experimental human skin wounds. *Nature* 200:377, 1963.
2. Howells CHL, Young HB: A study of completely undressed surgical wounds. *Br J Surg* 53:436, 1966.
3. Dire DJ, Coppola M, Dwyer DA, et al: A prospective evaluation of topical antibiotics for preventing infections in uncomplicated soft-tissue wounds repaired in the ED. *Acad Emerg Med* 2:4, 1995.
4. Howell JM, Chisholm CD: Outpatient wound preparation and care: A national survey. *Ann Emerg Med* 21:976, 1992.
5. Cummings P, Del Beccaro MA: Antibiotics to prevent infection of simple wounds: A meta-analysis of randomized studies. *Am J Emerg Med* 13:396, 1995.
6. Singer AJ, Hollander JE, Quinn JV: Evaluation and management of traumatic lacerations. *New Engl J Med* 337:1142, 1997.
7. Hollander JE, Singer AJ: Laceration management. *Ann Emerg Med* 34:356, 1999.
8. Goldberg HM, Rosenthal SAE, Nemetz JC: Effect of washing closed head and neck wounds on wound healing and infection. *Am J Surg* 141:358, 1981.
9. Austin PE, Matlack R II, Dun KA, et al: Discharge instructions: Do illustrations help our patients understand them? *Ann Emerg Med* 25:317, 1995.
10. Crikelair GF: Skin suture marks. *Am J Surg* 96:631, 1958.
11. Seaman M, Lammers R: Inability of patients to self diagnose wound infections. *J Emerg Med* 9:215, 1991.
12. Hollander JE, Blasko B, Singer AJ, et al: Poor correlation of short and long term appearance of repaired lacerations. *Acad Emerg Med* 2:983, 1995.
13. Ship AG, Weiss PR: Pigmentation after dermabrasion: An avoidable complication. *Plast Reconstr Surg* 75:528, 1985.

APPROACH TO CHEST PAIN
Gary B. Green
Peter M. Hill

OVERVIEW

Approximately 5 percent of all U.S. ED visits, or about 5 million visits a year, are for chest pain, but accurate diagnosis remains a challenge.[1,2] This chapter covers the approach to acute chest pain, with attention to identifying patients with potentially serious disorders.

Pathophysiology of Chest Pain

Stimulation of visceral or somatic afferent pain fibers results in two distinct pain syndromes. The dermis and parietal pleura are innervated by somatic pain fibers, which enter the spinal cord at specific levels and are arranged in dermatomal patterns. Visceral pain fibers are found in internal organs, such as the heart and blood vessels, the esophagus, and the visceral pleura. These visceral pain fibers enter the spinal cord at multiple levels and map to areas on the parietal cortex corresponding to the cord levels shared with the somatic fibers. Pain from somatic fibers is usually easily described, precisely located, and experienced as a sharp sensation, whereas pain from visceral fibers is more difficult to describe and is imprecisely localized. Accordingly, those experiencing visceral pain are more likely to use terms such as *discomfort, heaviness,* or *aching.* Patients frequently misinterpret the origin of visceral pain, because it is often referred to a different area of the body corresponding to an adjacent somatic nerve. For example, diaphragmatic irritation can present as shoulder pain, and arm pain may actually represent myocardial ischemia.

Gender, age, comorbidities, medications, drugs, and alcohol may interact with psychological and cultural influences to affect the patient's perception and communication of pain.

Definitions

The phrase *acute chest pain,* commonly used in emergency medicine, deserves definition. The term *acute* means of sudden or recent onset. While there is no precise time period defined, in common practice acute means that the patient stops his or her usual activity to seek medical attention, typically within minutes to hours. Some studies of acute chest pain patients in the ED limit entry to those with chest pain of less than 24-h duration. The term *chest* in this context means a location described by the patient on the anterior thorax, from xiphoid to suprasternal notch and between the right and left midaxillary lines. This is because the major serious thoracic disorders typically manifest symptoms localized to the anterior thorax. While it is true that pain localized to the back, between the base of the neck and the lumbar region, is on the thorax cage, in isolation, pain localized to this region is approached differently (see Chap. 282). That said, there are occasional patients with serious and life-threatening intrathoracic disorders who will manifest a location of their most intense pain outside the boundaries noted above. In addition, some patients may have migratory pain that has moved out of the anterior chest by the time the patient reaches medical attention. Therefore, clinicians are encouraged to include within their differential diagnosis important and significant intrathoracic disorders when patients describe pain in adjacent regions; e.g., epigastric, neck and jaw, and arm. The term *pain* describes a noxious uncomfortable sensation. However, pain perception and description

vary widely, and patients may use terms such as *ache* or *discomfort.* Alternative descriptions are common in the elderly. Similar to alternative locations, clinicians should be attuned to variation in the patient's description of the noxious sensation. In summary, acute chest pain refers to (1) recent onset, typically less than 24 h, that causes the patient to seek prompt medical attention, (2) location described on the anterior thorax, and (3) a noxious uncomfortable sensation distressing to the patient.

INITIAL APPROACH

The initial approach to acute chest pain recognizes that some causes are serious and life-threatening, and prompt medical attention may prevent death and limit morbidity. Therefore, patients should be triaged promptly. Patients with visceral-type chest pain (defined below), significantly abnormal pulse or blood pressure measurements, or with dyspnea should be placed directly into a treatment bed, a cardiac monitor initiated, an intravenous line established, oxygen administered, and an ECG ordered. Other less well-defined patients also deserve expeditious evaluation, and experienced triage officers and nurses often have a "gut" feeling about certain patients; that insight should be respected.

The initial evaluation should focus on immediate life threats: ensuring adequate airway, breathing, and circulation. The vital signs should be assessed and repeated at regular intervals as determined by the patient's condition. The initial history should focus on specific questions concerning the character of the chest pain, the presence of associated symptoms, and a history of cardiopulmonary conditions. The patient is asked to grade pain intensity in order to follow response to therapy. A 0 to 10 scale is commonly used, with 10 being the worst pain the patient can imagine and 0 being no pain at all. Focused cardiac, pulmonary, and vascular examinations should follow.

If immediate life threats are not detected or have already been addressed, a more extensive evaluation can be preformed. This "secondary survey" consists of a history that defines symptoms more precisely. Chest pain should be assessed like other pain syndromes, with specific questions concerning quality, location, radiation or migration, severity, time and character of onset, progression, provoking factors, relieving factors, and associated symptoms. If the pain has been episodic, the frequency of pain episodes should be assessed over the past weeks to better determine progression. Risk factors for cardiopulmonary disease should be assessed. The physical examination during this phase should complete those body systems not evaluated initially as well as rechecking abnormalities noted before. Many organizations have developed structured history and physician examination forms for acute chest pain to direct the information-gathering process and organize the diagnostic approach. Such structured records are particularly helpful to less experienced physicians. Further diagnostic testing is directed by the history and physical examination.

Categorization

A useful initial approach is to classify patients into three categories: (1) chest wall pain, (2) pleuritic or respiratory chest pain, and (3) visceral chest pain. Chest wall pain is a somatic pain, usually described as sharp in quality, that can be precisely localized (often with one fingertip) and is reproducible by direct palpation and/or chest wall movement during stretching or twisting. Pleuritic chest pain is also a somatic pain, usually described as sharp in quality that is distinctly worsened by breathing or coughing. The term *pleuritic* is potentially confusing; more than the pleura moves during respiration, and disorders other than "pleurisy" may be worse with respiration. Visceral chest pain is poorly localized and usually described as aching or heaviness. Important causes of chest pain within each category are noted in Table 49-1.

A very useful principle in the clinical assessment of acute chest pain is that, with rare exception, chest pain diagnosis is a composite picture, no one fact or observation make the diagnosis. The challenge to the clinician is to take the often-confusing history and nondiagnostic physician examination and select the useful features that guide further assessment, management, and disposition.

Assessment of risk factors for cardiovascular disease can play a role in patient assessment. Specifically, the presence of risk factors for coronary artery disease (cigarette smoking, diabetes, hypertension, hypercholesterolemia, family history), aortic dissection (middle aged, male gender, hypertension, Marfan syndrome), and pulmonary embolism (hypercoagulable diathesis, malignancy, recent immobilization or surgery) are useful in judging the probability of these diagnoses. Likewise, age can be used to assess the probability of atherosclerotic disease; clinically significant coronary artery disease is rare in patients under the age of 30. Acute cocaine use has been associated with acute myocardial infarction, and chronic cocaine use is associated with accelerated atherosclerosis and severe coronary artery disease (see Chap. 168). However, youth or absence of risk factors does not completely eliminate any potentially serious cause of acute chest pain.

The patient's medical record should be reviewed. The current ECG should be compared with previous tracings. Results of prior cardiac studies (echocardiograms, stress testing, or catheterizations), esophageal studies (endoscopy, oral contrast swallowing studies), gastrointestinal studies (ultrasound, computed tomography), or pulmonary studies (spirometry) should be reviewed and present symptoms interpreted in comparison with these results. In general, cardiac stress studies within the previous 6 months and coronary angiography within the prior 2 years are considered to likely reflect the current state of the coronary circulation.

A practice to be decried is the use of therapeutic trials in acute chest pain; usually in the form of (1) a "gastrointestinal (GI) cocktail" containing an antacid, antispasmodic, and local anesthetic for gastroesophageal reflux, (2) nitroglycerin for myocardial ischemia, and (3) nonsteroidal anti-inflammatories for chest wall pain. The placebo effect makes it difficult to interpret a positive response; patients with definite myocardial ischemia have been reported as experiencing complete pain relief with a GI cocktail. In addition, nitroglycerin is a smooth muscle dilator and may produce relief in esophageal spasm and biliary colic as well as myocardial ischemia. The analgesic properties of nonsteroidal anti-inflammatories are not specific for any location.

TABLE 49-1 Important Causes of Acute Chest Pain

Chest Wall Pain	Pleuritic Pain	Visceral Pain
Costosternal syndrome	Pulmonary embolism	Typical exertional angina
Costochrondritis (Tietze syndrome)	Pneumonia	
	Spontaneous pneumothorax	Atypical (nonexertional) angina
Precordial catch syndrome		
Slipping rib syndrome	Pericarditis	
Xiphodynia	Pleurisy	Unstable angina
Radicular syndromes		Acute myocardial infarction
Intercostal nerve syndromes		Aortic dissection
Fibromyalgia		Pericarditis
		Esophageal reflux or spasm
		Esophageal rupture
		Mitral valve prolapse

Ischemic Equivalents

A confounding observation is that many patients with acute coronary syndrome (ACS, defined below), perhaps as high as 40 percent, do not describe chest pain as their predominant symptom.[3] The absence of chest pain leads to delayed or inadequate anti-ischemic therapy and increased inhospital mortality.[4]

Truly silent myocardial ischemia does occur, but these patients are not likely to come to the ED. For those that do, ischemic equivalents or atypical presentations are important to note: dyspnea at rest or with less exertion compared to the patient's previous baseline; shoulder, arm, or jaw discomfort; nausea; lightheadedness; generalized weakness; acute change in mental status; or diaphoresis. Epigastric or upper abdominal discomfort can be the presenting symptom of myocardial ischemia. Patients with sensory impairment due to diabetes, advanced age, psychiatric disease, or altered mental status are more likely to present with atypical symptoms with ACS. Atypical presentations of ACS also occur more frequently in women and non-white populations compared to white males.[5]

Differential Diagnosis

When patients present with acute chest pain due to myocardial ischemia, the term *acute coronary syndrome,* or ACS, is used because, on initial assessment, it is not possible to determine if the patient has an acute myocardial infarction (AMI) or unstable angina (UA). ACS is a common cause of acute chest pain; in a typical ED population of adults over the age of 30 presenting with visceral-type chest pain, about 15 percent will have AMI and 25 to 30 percent will have UA.[1]

The pain of myocardial ischemia is almost always retrosternal and diffuse, usually described as a heaviness or pressure, and commonly radiates, usually to the neck or left arm (see Chap. 50). In exertional angina, the pain is episodic, lasting minutes (usually <10 min and not seconds or hours), provoked by exertion, and relieved by rest or sublingual nitroglycerin. Exertional angina is most often due to atherosclerotic disease of the epicardial coronary arteries that restricts blood flow. In atypical angina, the pain is the same as that with exertional angina, but pain occurs at rest. Atypical angina appears to be caused by coronary artery spasm. In about two-thirds of patients with atypical angina, coronary artery lesions are seen, and patients may have exertional as well as rest pain. In both exertional angina and atypical angina, the pattern is stable in terms of frequency of episodes, severity, ease of provocation, and response to rest or nitroglycerin. In UA, the episodic anginal pain has changed its pattern; it is either (1) of new onset (less than 1 to 2 months), (2) more frequent, easily provoked, more severe, or difficult to relieve, or (3) occurring at rest for prolonged spells (>20 min). UA is a potentially serious condition and patients are at high risk for early AMI or death. In AMI, the pain is usually persistent (>20 min), severe, and associated with symptoms of dyspnea, diaphoresis, or nausea.

In ACS, the most useful test is an ECG for both detecting myocardial ischemia and risk stratification. Using the initial ECG, the incidence of AMI is approximately 80 percent for patients with new ST-segment elevation greater than 1 mm in two contiguous leads, about 20 percent in patients with new ST-segment depression or T-wave inversion, but less than 4 percent in patients without either of these two patterns.

Pulmonary embolism is common and life-threatening and is a diagnosis that can be missed in the ED due to the frequently atypical nature of its presentation. Pulmonary embolism can manifest with any combination of chest pain, dyspnea, syncope, shock, and/or hypoxia (see Chap. 56). The pain associated with a PE occurs when inflammation of the parietal pleura overlying the infarction causes chest pain that is generally sharp and related to respiration. Dyspnea, fever, cough, and/or hemoptysis also may be present, and the chest wall may be tender to palpation. Patients with massive PEs often present with unstable vital signs and the classic presentation of sharp, pleuritic chest pain and dyspnea associated with tachypnea, tachycardia, and hypoxemia. A clinical scoring system maybe useful in categorizing patients into low (about 10 percent), intermediate (about 40 percent), and high (about 80 percent) prevalence for PE.[6]

Risk factors for *aortic dissection* include atherosclerosis, uncontrolled hypertension, coarctation of the aorta, bicuspid aortic valves, aortic stenosis, Marfan syndrome, Ehlers-Danlos syndrome, and pregnancy (see Chap. 58). The pain of aortic dissection, i.e., midline substernal chest pain, is classically described as tearing, ripping, or searing and radiating to the interscapular area of the back. Typically, the pain is at its worst at symptom onset and is often felt above and below the diaphragm. Symptoms of "secondary" pathologies resulting from arterial branch occlusions, such as stroke, AMI, or limb ischemia, may overshadow the clinical presentation of the dissection and make an accurate diagnosis difficult. No combination of clinical factors or chest radiography findings are adequate to exclude the diagnosis of aortic dissection, and specific imaging studies are usually required.[7]

Spontaneous pneumothorax may occur due to sudden changes in barometric pressure, in smokers or patients with chronic obstructive pulmonary disease or idiopathic pleural bleb disease, or in those with another pulmonary pathology (see Chap. 66). Patients usually complain of a sudden, sharp, lancinating, pleuritic chest pain and dyspnea. Auscultation of the lungs may reveal absence of breath sounds on the ipsilateral side and hyperresonance to percussion, but clinical impression alone is unreliable. Diagnosis of a simple pneumothorax is made by chest radiography.

Esophageal rupture (Boerhaave syndrome) is a rare but potentially life-threatening cause of chest pain. Patients classically present with a history of substernal, sharp chest pain of sudden onset that occurs immediately after an episode of forceful vomiting (see Chap. 75). The patient is usually ill-appearing, dyspneic, and diaphoretic. The physical examination is often normal but may reveal evidence of pneumothorax or subcutaneous air. Chest radiography may be normal or may demonstrate pleural effusion (left more common than right), pneumothorax, pneumomediastinum, pneumoperitoneum, and/or subcutaneous air. The diagnosis can be confirmed by a study with water-soluble contrast.

The pain of *acute pericarditis* is typically acute, sharp, severe, and constant (see Chap. 55). It is usually described as substernal, with radiation to the back, neck, or shoulders, and is exacerbated by lying down and by inspiration. It is classically described as being relieved by leaning forward. A pericardial friction rub is the most important diagnostic finding. The ECG may show diffuse ST-segment elevation and T-wave inversion. In addition, depression of the PR segment is a highly specific ECG finding for pericarditis.

Pneumonia can produce chest pain or discomfort that is usually sharp and pleuritic (see Chap. 63). It is usually associated with fever, cough, and possibly hypoxia. Physical examination may reveal rales over the affected lobes, decreased breath sounds, and signs of consolidation (i.e., bronchial breath sounds). A chest radiograph confirms the diagnosis.

Mitral valve prolapse (MVP) is the most frequently diagnosed cardiac valvular abnormality and is more commonly diagnosed in women than in men. The discomfort of MVP often occurs at rest, is atypical for myocardial ischemia, and can be associated with dizziness, hyperventilation, anxiety, depression, palpitations, and fatigue (see Chap. 54). The discomfort may be related to papillary muscle tension, and many patients benefit from the administration of β-adrenergic blocking agents. Two-dimensional echocardiography is the diagnostic tool of choice and, with physical examination findings, helps to stratify patients into high- and low-risk categories for developing serious complications. Palpitations and every type of supraventricular or ventricular dysrhythmia have been associated with MVP.

Musculoskeletal or chest wall pain syndromes are characterized by highly localized, sharp, positional chest pain. Pain that is completely reproducible by light to moderate palpation of a discrete area of the chest wall often represents pain of musculoskeletal origin, although chest wall tenderness occurs in some patients with PE and myocardial ischemia. Costochondritis is an inflammation of the costal cartilages and/or their sternal articulations and causes chest pain that is variably sharp, dull, and/or increased with respirations. *Tietze syndrome* is a particular cause of costochondral pain related to fusiform swelling in one or more upper costal cartilages and has a pain pattern similar to that of other costochondral syndromes. Xiphodynia is another inflammatory process that causes sharp, pleuritic chest pain reproduced by light palpation over the xiphoid process. Texidor twinge or precordial catch syndrome is described as a short, lancinating chest discomfort that occurs in episodic bunches lasting 1 to 2 min near the cardiac apex associated with inspiration and poor posture and inactivity.

Gastrointestinal disorders cannot be reliably discriminated from myocardial ischemia by history and examination alone. Dyspepsia syndromes, including gastroesophageal reflux, often produce pain described as burning or gnawing, usually in the lower half of the chest, and often accompanied by a brackish or acidic taste in the back of the mouth (see Chap. 75). The recumbent position usually exacerbates the symptoms, and although the pain is typically relieved with antacids, this therapeutic response also can be observed in myocardial ischemia. *Esophageal spasm* is often associated with reflux disease and is characterized by a sudden onset of dull, tight, or gripping substernal chest pain, frequently precipitated by the consumption of hot or cold liquids or a large food bolus and often lasting for hours (see Chap. 75). The pain also responds to sublingual nitroglycerin (although supposedly with a slight delay).

Peptic ulcer disease is classically characterized as a postprandial, dull, boring pain in the midepigastric region (see Chap. 77). Patients often describe being awakened from sleep by discomfort. Duodenal ulcer pain is usually relieved after eating food, in contrast to gastric ulcer symptoms, which are often exacerbated by eating. Symptomatic relief is usually achieved by antacid medications. Acute pancreatitis and biliary tract disease present with right upper quadrant or epigastric pain and tenderness but also can present with chest pain.

Panic disorder (PD) is defined as a syndrome characterized by recurrent unexpected panic attacks (discrete periods of intense fear or discomfort) with at least four of the following symptoms: palpitations, diaphoresis, tremor, dyspnea, choking, chest pain or discomfort, nausea, dizziness, derealization or depersonalization, fear of losing control or dying, paresthesias, chills or hot flushes (see Chap. 292). The diagnosis can be made only in the absence of direct physiologic effects of a substance disorder, a general medical condition, or symptoms better accounted for by another mental disorder. Several studies have used standardized screening tools to evaluate ED chest pain patients for PD and have reported an incidence of 17 to 32 percent. In a small trial, investigators found that ED physicians can successfully diagnose PD by using a brief screening procedure, and they suggested that PD patients could benefit from the initiation of specific pharmacologic therapy (serotonin reuptake inhibitors) in the ED.[8] Many patients with PD and other anxiety disorders have elevated baseline sympathetic tone, that may be an independent risk factor for coronary artery disease (CAD). In fact, when all ED chest pain patients were screened for PD, 25 percent of those screening positive had a discharge diagnosis of ACS (9.3 percent) or stable angina pectoris (15.7 percent).[9] Thus, PD always must be considered a diagnosis of exclusion.

ANCILLARY TESTING

Ancillary testing in acute chest pain generally utilizes electrocardiography, measurement of serum markers of myocardial injury, and/or imaging studies to detect intrathoracic pathology. The specific studies are chosen according to the clinical circumstances. That said, because ACS is the most common potentially serious cause of acute chest pain, clinical studies and common practice focus on the use of the ECG and serum marker measurement to detect or exclude acute myocardial injury. The remainder of this chapter will focus on this topic. The use of ancillary tests in other conditions are discussed in their respective chapters.

Electrocardiography

Due to the importance of early diagnosis of AMI (and, hence, reduced delay of thrombolytic treatment), the American College of Cardiology/American Heart Association (ACC/AHA) guidelines for management of patients with AMI recommend standing orders that all patients with "ischemic-type pain" have a 12-lead ECG performed within 10 min of arrival and that the ECG be handed directly to the treating physician for immediate interpretation.[10] Considering the difficulty of defining "ischemic-type" pain and the frequency of atypical presentations, it may be prudent to extend this protocol to *all* adult patients with chest pain or other symptoms of possible ischemia.

The normal myocardium depolarizes from endocardium to epicardium and repolarizes in the opposite direction. Ischemic myocardium remains electrically less positive than nonischemic myocardium at the end of depolarization. This creates an electrical potential between normal and ischemic myocardium during depolarization and results in ST-segment elevation in an overlying electrode. Conversely, if the electrode is located over normal myocardium opposite an ischemic region, ST-segment depression will be seen. If ischemia is limited to the subendocardial area, an overlying electrode will be separated from the ischemic tissue by a layer of normal myocardium, resulting in an electrical potential pointed inward from the normal to ischemic tissue, resulting in ST-segment depression.

Myocardial ischemia can also delay the repolarization process. In extensive or transmural ischemia, the direction of repolarization is reversed so that recovery occurs from endocardium to epicardium, resulting in T-wave inversions in an overlying electrode. In subendocardial ischemia, the delay does not alter the normal recovery process (epicardium to endocardium), so T waves are not inverted. However, because normal epicardium repolarization is unopposed due to delayed subendocardial repolarization, the T wave in an overlying electrode may be larger than normal (called *hyperacute T waves*)

After infarction, the area of necrosis is electrically silent, not able to depolarize. During ventricular depolarization, initial electrical activity will be generated in normal myocardium, away from the infarcted area. This results in an electrical potential directed from the infarcted area toward normal myocardium, causing an abnormal initial negative deflection (pathologic Q waves) in the QRS complex of overlying electrodes. Occasionally, small Q waves (called septal Q waves) are seen in the limb or lateral precordial ECG leads. Pathologic Q-waves are distinguished by their duration (greater than 40 ms) and depth (greater than 25 percent of the corresponding R wave).

The ECG is an important tool in the detection of acute infarction and conduction blocks.[11] Also, the ECG can help identify the infarct-related artery and help predict reperfusion. The sensitivity of the initial ECG for the diagnosis of AMI has been extensively studied. Approximately half of patients with AMI have diagnostic changes on their initial ECG with new ST-segment elevation greater than 1 mm in two contiguous leads. Another 20 to 30 percent will have new ST-segment or T-wave inversion suggestive of myocardial ischemia. About 10 to 20 percent will have ST-segment depressions and T-wave inversions similar to that seen on previous tracings. About 10 percent have nonspecific ST-segment and T-wave abnormalities. Only about 1 to 5 percent of AMI patients will have a truly normal initial ECG.

The sensitivity of the initial ECG in unstable angina is less well defined, probably because the diagnosis is clinical as there is no "gold standard" against which to evaluate a diagnostic test. In addition, the initial ECG would not be expected to be abnormal if a patient with UA presents during a pain-free period.

The positive predictive value of the different ECG patterns has also been studied. For new ST-segment elevation, the positive predictive value for AMI is about 80 percent. For new ST-segment depression and T-wave inversions, the positive predictive value is about 20 percent for AMI and between 14 and 43 percent for UA. With acute chest pain and an initial ECG showing preexisting ST-segment depressions and T-wave inversions, the positive predictive value is about 4 percent for AMI and 21 to 48 percent for UA. Thus, the standard 12-lead ECG is useful in conjunction with the clinical history for detection of ACS.

Variations on the standard 12-lead ECG have been proposed. One approach uses a continuous 12-lead ECG monitor that records (but does not print) a new 12-lead ECG every 20 s. When the ST-segment baseline is altered from the previous tracing, an alarm is raised and a copy of the new ECG is shared or printed. This technology is potentially useful for monitoring patients with ongoing pain and a nondiagnostic initial ECG.[12] Because of the costs, concerns regarding labile ST-segment and T-wave changes from patient movement and respiration, and a lack of ED-based prospective studies, continuous 12-lead ECG monitoring cannot be recommended for routine use.

Electrocardiograms with added leads—for a total of 15, 18, and 22 leads—have been studied. In general, adding more leads increases the sensitivity for AMI detection, but reduces specificity. The only generally agreed upon extension to the standard 12-lead ECG is the use of right-sided precordial leads in the setting of acute inferior myocardial infarction in order to detect right ventricular involvement.[13]

Risk stratification based on the initial ED ECG also has been suggested as a way of improving ED decision making. Although the initial ECG cannot exclude AMI, stable ED patients whose initial ECG is without ischemic changes are at low risk of subsequent life-threatening complications and usually can be managed in a nonintensive-care setting. Conversely, patients whose initial ECG demonstrates ischemic changes (ST-segment depression or T-wave inversion), even in the absence of confirmed AMI, are at significantly greater risk of short- and long-term morbidity and mortality and should be managed accordingly.

Serum Markers of Myocardial Injury

CREATINE KINASE, CREATINE KINASE ISOENZYMES, AND ISO-FORMS Creatine kinase (CK; adenosine triphosphate creatine *N*-phosphotransferase) is an intracellular enzyme involved in the transfer of high-energy phosphate groups from ATP to creatine. Although found in small quantities in many tissues, CK is present in large concentrations in cardiac and skeletal muscle and the brain. The enzyme is a dimer composed of two subunits, each of which may be the M (muscle) type or the B (brain) type, thus creating three distinct dimers, or isoenzymes: CK-BB, CK-MM, and CK-MB. Type CK-BB predominates in brain tissue, whereas skeletal muscle consists mostly of CK-MM, in addition to CK-MB in small amounts. The "cardiac isoenzyme," CK-MB, accounts for 14 to 42 percent of total cardiac muscle enzyme activity, thus the predominant enzyme in the heart is actually CK-MM.

The quantitative and temporal patterns of appearance and disappearance of CK and its isoenzymes in the blood occur in a reproducible manner but can vary considerably depending on the amount of CK released from cells, the amount of perfusion of damaged tissues, and the rate of clearance by the reticuloendothelial system. The CK levels usually become abnormally high within 4 to 8 h after coronary artery occlusion (onset of symptoms), peak between 12 and 24 h, and return to normal between 3 and 4 days (Figure 49-1). Reports of the sensitivity of total CK vary from 93 to 100 percent, whereas the specificity is lower (57 to 86 percent), owing to the presence of CK in other tissues. Thus, this marker's usefulness is limited. The CK-MB isoenzyme curve parallels the total CK curve, with levels detectable 4 to 8 h after onset of symptoms (see Figure 49-1). Type CK-MB may peak

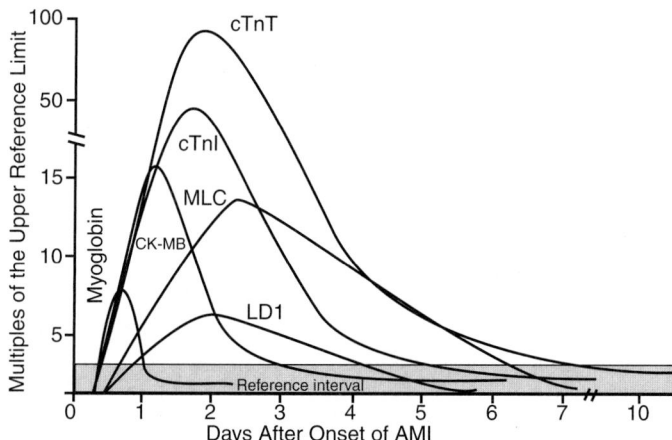

FIG. 49-1. Typical pattern of serum marker elevation after AMI. *Abbreviations:* CK-MB = creatine kinase-MB isoenzyme; cTnI = cardiac troponin I; cTnT = cardiac troponin T; LD1 = lactate dehydrogenase isoenzyme 1; MLC = myosin light chain.

slightly earlier than total CK, and it is cleared more rapidly, usually within 48 h (vs. 72 to 96 h). Using CK-MB and the ratio of CK-MB to total CK, most studies have reported sensitivity and specificity to be greater than 95 percent. Cutoff values vary between techniques, laboratories, and populations, but CK-MB values in healthy controls may be up to 5 μg/L and up to 5 percent of total CK. Historically, CK-MB had been universally adopted as the gold standard for diagnosis of AMI. Although specificity is generally improved over total CK, 37 conditions other than AMI have been associated with elevated CK-MB levels (Table 49-2). Fortunately, most of these conditions can be easily differentiated from AMI on clinical grounds. The relatively rapid return of elevated CK-MB levels to normal is another potential disadvantage, because of the possibility of missing the diagnosis in patients presenting later in the course of AMI. However, this rapid clearance may be used to a different advantage, because it enables the identification of infarct extension and reinfarction.

The 4- to 8-h delay in CK-MB detection after onset of symptoms has been overcome in part with the development of rapid assays for CK-MB isoforms (subforms). The isoenzymes CK-MM, CK-MB, and CK-BB are dimeric molecules consisting of three different combinations of two monomers, M and B. On its release from damaged cells, the M monomer found in tissue CK (M_t) is acted on by an enzyme present in serum, carboxypeptidase N, which cleaves off the C-terminal lysine. This action results in its conversion into the M monomer found in serum CK (M_s). Newly released unmodified CK-M_tB (or CK-MB$_2$) is enzymatically changed into CK-M_sB (or CK-MB$_1$). Because the rate of this conversion is limited, CK-MB$_2$ activity reflects new recent release into the serum. By measuring MB$_2$ activity (>1 U/L) and the MB$_2$:MB$_1$ ratio (>1.5), infarction can be detected before the total level of CK-MB exceeds the normal range. Although this method has reported early (<6 h of symptom onset) sensitivity and specificity for AMI of 95.7 percent and 93.9 percent, respectively, technical difficulties with the assay system have thus far limited clinical acceptance.[14]

MYOGLOBIN   Myoglobin is a small (17,500 Da), heme-containing protein found in striated (skeletal) and cardiac muscle cells. When disrupted, these cells rapidly release myoglobin into the serum. After AMI, serum myoglobin levels begin to rise within 3 h of onset of symptoms and are abnormally elevated in 80 to 100 percent of patients at 6 to 8 h, peak at 4 to 9 h (see Figure 49-1), and with normal kidney function return to baseline within 24 h from symptom onset. A false-negative result may occur if the test is performed after myoglobin has already been cleared from the serum. False positives also abound, because the myoglobin found in myocardium is indistinguishable from that found in skeletal muscle. Fortunately, conditions that also result in myoglobin release usually can be clinically diagnosed. By excluding those patients with known trauma, renal failure, or cocaine use, one study found myoglobin's "clinical specificity" to be equivalent to that of CK-MB and troponin.[15]

TROPONINS I AND T   The troponin complex is the main regulatory protein of the thin filament of the myofibrils that regulate the Ca²⁺-dependent ATP hydrolysis of actomyosin. The troponin complex consists of three subunits: an inhibitory subunit (troponin I), a tropomyosin-binding subunit (troponin T), and a calcium-binding subunit (troponin C). Immunoassays based on the significant heterogeneity in amino acid sequences can detect the specific isoforms. The cardiac isoform of troponin I is not found in skeletal muscle during any stage of development and therefore is associated only with myocardial necrosis.

After AMI, cardiac troponin I (cTnI) and troponin T (cTnT) become elevated after approximately 6 h, peak at 12 h, and remain elevated for 7 to 10 days. Both have a higher specificity for myocardial necrosis than CK-MB in selected subsets of patients, such as those presenting late in the course of AMI or those with recent surgery, a cocaine habit, or skeletal muscle disease. Both troponins have been

TABLE 49-2   Conditions Associated with Elevated CK-MB Levels

Common	Uncommon	Rare	Unclear
Unstable angina, acute coronary ischemia	Congestive heart failure	Isolated case in normal person	Acromegaly
Inflammatory heart diseases	Coronary artery disease after stress test		Hypothermia
Cardiomyopathies	Angina pectoris		Rocky Mountain spotted fever
Circulatory failure and shock	Valvular defects		Typhoid fever
Cardiac surgery	Tachycardia		Chronic bronchitis
Cardiac trauma	Cardiac catheterization		Lumbago
Skeletal muscle trauma (severe)	Electrical countershock		Febrile disorder
Dermatomyositis, polymyositis	Noncardiac surgery		
Myopathic disorders	Brain and head trauma		
Muscular dystrophy, especially Duchenne	Peripartum period		
Extreme exercise	Miscellaneous drug overdoses		
Malignant hyperthermia	CO poisoning		
Reye syndrome	Prostatic cancer		
Rhabdomyolysis of any cause			
Delirium tremens			
Ethanol poisoning (chronic)			

Abbreviation: CK-MB = creatine kinase, subunits muscle and brain.

shown to have high sensitivity and specificity for AMI in ED patients with chest pain and among those with possible ischemic equivalents. Elevation of either cardiac troponin also predicts subsequent cardiovascular complications independent of CK-MB and the ECG.[16]

Interpretation of troponin results in the presence of renal failure is an area of controversy. Although only troponin T has been found in skeletal muscle biopsies of patients with renal failure, troponins I and T are sometimes elevated in renal patients without other evidence of cardiac disease. Further, there have been conflicting reports as to the prognostic significance of elevated levels of either troponin in patients with renal failure.

OTHER MARKERS   Other markers of myocardial ischemia or infarction are currently being evaluated for utility: myoglobin/carbonic anhydrase III combinations, glycogen phosphorylase BB, and myosin light chains, to name three. In addition, markers of inflammation (e.g., C-reactive protein), platelet activation and adhesion (e.g., P-selectin and other integrins), and cardiac function (B-type natriuretic peptide, or BNP) are theoretically attractive as indicators of ACS. C-reactive protein and BNP have some prognostic value in patients with possible ACS, but their overall role in diagnosis remains to be determined.

Clinical Applications of Myocardial Marker Measurements

The current literature supports the inclusion of myocardial marker measurements in protocols governing the ED evaluation of patients with chest pain for four distinct purposes. The first three applications are discussed below, while the fourth use of an accelerated marker curve is discussed later in Chap. 50.

EARLY DIAGNOSIS OF AMI   In those patients whose initial ECG is diagnostic for AMI, no further marker testing is required before initiation of appropriate interventions. In patients with a nondiagnostic ECG, AMI cannot be definitively excluded within the first few hours from symptom onset. However, some AMI patients with nondiagnostic initial ECGs will have positive marker tests upon ED arrival, and many more will develop positive tests during the first few hours after presentation.

In AMI, the initial CK-MB measurement obtained upon ED arrival is elevated in about 30 to 50 percent of patients.[17] By serial measures at 2- to 3-h intervals, diagnostic increases in CK-MB can be obtained in 80 to 96 percent of AMI patients during the initial six hours. The same principle can be applied with serial measurements of cTnI and cTnT. Owing to its earlier release into serum after coronary artery occlusion, myoglobin has a potential advantage over CK-MB and troponin for early diagnosis of AMI. Using a panel of markers (myoglobin, CK-MB, and cTnI) performed upon arrival and after 3 h, it is possible to detect over 90 percent of AMI patients.[17,18]

IDENTIFYING "MISSED MI" PATIENTS   Single-sample myocardial marker measurements cannot be used to exclude the diagnosis of AMI in the ED. However, routine incorporation of marker testing into patient-care algorithms for those patients deemed sufficiently low risk so that they are slated for discharge without definitive AMI rule-out has been shown to identify some patients (admitted and discharged from the ED) with unsuspected MI.[19] Further, a strategy using two CK-MB measurements drawn 3 h apart for patients selected for discharge will identify ACS patients. Although these strategies have not been validated, these and several other studies suggest that ED patients slated for discharge after evaluation for chest pain and ischemic equivalents may benefit from at least one myocardial marker measurement.

EARLY RISK STRATIFICATION   Increased use of newer anti-ischemic therapies (angiographic interventions and antiplatelet and antithrombotic drugs), although improving outcomes, carries risks and high costs. Thus, a selective approach to their use is required. Several investigations have suggested that markers of myocardial injury can be used successfully in the ED to rapidly identify those patients most likely to benefit from a more aggressive approach. Numerous investigations have demonstrated that early ED testing of CK-MB, myoglobin, troponin T, or troponin I yields clinically useful prognostic data for adverse events, and that simultaneous testing of troponin and CK-MB may identify additional high-risk patients as opposed to testing for one marker.

After reviewing this evidence, the Joint European Society of Cardiology/American College of Cardiology Committee for the Redefinition of MI reported in 2000 that there is "no discernible threshold below which an elevated value for cardiac troponin would be deemed harmless. All elevated values are associated with a worsened prognosis."[20] Unfortunately, the threshold values historically suggested by the manufacturers of laboratory assays for CK-MB, troponin, and other myocardial markers have been determined based on the traditional definition of MI and are therefore inadequate for risk stratification. Recognizing this, the joint committee went on to recommend that new threshold values for each marker be established at the 99th percentile of the values for an appropriate reference control (normal) group. Because this recommendation has not been uniformly accepted and implemented by hospital laboratories, to optimally use the prognostic information offered by ED myocardial marker testing, emergency physicians should be aware of the appropriate threshold values for risk stratification and for MI diagnosis in their individual institutions.

POINT OF CARE TESTING   With current monoclonal antibody technology, qualitative and quantitative cardiac marker panels for CK-MB, troponin I and T, and myoglobin are available for use at the bedside. A quantitative assay for BNP has also been developed for bedside use. Most point of care cardiac marker testing panels provide results within 15 to 20 min, generally faster than most hospital laboratories. Rapid bedside results would be theoretically useful when the results would affect early therapy (e.g., initiation of glycoprotein IIb/IIIa inhibitors) or alter disposition (e.g., primary percutaneous coronary intervention instead of medical therapy). Rapid bedside cardiac marker assessment may also be useful when the initial ECG is rendered difficult to evaluate due to preexisting ventricular conduction blocks or chronic ventricular pacing. The overall value of rapid bedside cardiac marker detection remains to be determined.

COMPUTERIZED DECISION AIDS

To facilitate more accurate disposition decisions and thereby reduce mounting health care costs, several investigators tried to develop computerized decision aids or computer-based triage protocols for ED patients with chest pain. Unfortunately, no simple algorithm has proven both safe and effective for ED-based triage of acute chest pain patients.

Other methods, such as multivariate analysis and artificial neural networks, have been used to develop predictive instruments. Actual clinical use of the most studied of these decision aids, the Acute Cardiac Ischemia Time-Insensitive Predictive Instrument (ACI-TIPI), resulted in a decrease of 26 percent in cardiac care unit admissions and an increase of 47 percent in ED discharges to home without increasing the number of missed AMIs. The ACI-TIPI uses a logistic regression formula that evaluates the probability of acute ischemia by analyzing specific history and ECG characteristics. The instrument has been incorporated into computerized ECG machines in the ED, and the result is printed directly onto the ECG tracing.[21]

An artificial neural network is a nonlinear statistical program that can recognize complex patterns and maintain accuracy even when some of the required data are missing. This theoretically enables users to apply the tool in real time even when they do not have all of the required data elements called for in the stratification model. The accuracy of one such tool was hypothetically tested in 2204 patients. The network demonstrated a significant improvement over physician decision making, with a sensitivity of 94.5 percent and a specificity of 95.5 percent for the diagnosis of AMI.[22] A more recent instrument has been developed to include diagnoses in the overall spectrum of myocardial ischemia.[23]

Despite the demonstration of diagnostic superiority and improved cost-effectiveness compared with physician decision making alone, these instruments have not been embraced by clinicians. Among the barriers cited to acceptance of decision aids into clinical practice are medicolegal concerns, slow adoption of new technology, and physicians' fear of losing autonomy. Thus, additional work in this area must now focus on physician behavior and the interface between human and machine.

APPROACH TO LOW PROBABILITY OF ISCHEMIA

Patients identified as having ST-segment elevation MI or recognized as having a high potential for an ACS are addressed as discussed in Chap. 50. Other patients may be classified as having a very low, low, or moderate probability of acute ischemia based on clinical information available within the initial hours of their ED visit. Many investigators now recommend the use of a five-subgroup classification scheme for this initial risk stratification (Table 49-3). However, there is still no consensus regarding optimal risk subgroupings, criteria for such stratification, or agreement as to the most effective evaluation and treatment protocols after initial categorization. There is consensus on two issues regarding lower-risk patients: **history alone is inadequate to exclude the presence of acute ischemia,** and the goal should always be "zero tolerance" for missed AMI. It is also accepted that some form of systematic approach based on objective data is required to accurately and efficiently pursue further diagnostic evaluation to an appropriate end point in each patient (Figure 49-2).[10]

**TABLE 49-3   Prognosis-Based Classification System
for ED Chest Pain Patients***

   I. Acute myocardial infarction: immediate revascularization candidate
  II. Probable acute ischemia: high risk for adverse events
        Any of the following
          Evidence of clinical instability (i.e., pulmonary edema, hypotension, arrhythmia)
          Ongoing pain thought to be ischemic
          Pain at rest associated with ischemic ECG changes
          One or more positive myocardial marker measurements
          Positive perfusion imaging study
 III. Possible acute ischemia: intermediate risk for adverse events
        History suggestive of ischemia with any of the following
          Rest pain, now resolved
          New onset of pain
          Crescendo pattern of pain
          Ischemic pattern on ECG not associated with pain
 IV. A. Probably not ischemia: low risk for adverse events
        Requires all of the following
          History not strongly suggestive of ischemia
          ECG normal, unchanged from previous, or nonspecific changes
          Negative myocardial marker measurement
      B. Stable angina pectoris: low risk for adverse events
        Requires all of the following
          More than 2 wk of unchanged symptom pattern or longstanding
            symptoms with only mild change in exertional pain threshold
          ECG normal, unchanged from previous, or nonspecific changes
          Negative initial myocardial marker measurement
  V. Definitely not ischemia: very low risk for adverse events
        Requires all of the following
          Clear objective evidence of non-ischemic symptom etiology
          ECG normal, unchanged from previous, or nonspecific changes
          Negative initial myocardial marker mesurement

*Authors' analyses from multiple sources.
Abbreviation: ECG = electrocardiogram.

Interpretation of the many diagnostic tests now available to assist in diagnosis and risk stratification of ED patients with possible ACS increasingly has become the responsibility of the emergency physician.

Common Diagnostic Tests Used in Emergency Cardiac Care

ECG-BASED (STANDARD) EXERCISE STRESS TESTING   In the ED setting, exercise testing has been recommended for patients applied as the final component of a chest pain observation protocol after the exclusion of AMI or, in selected low-risk patients, soon after presentation as an alternative to an extended observation period.[24]

Many variations exist in the equipment, procedures, and interpretive algorithms used. Treadmills are used more commonly in the United States, because many patients cannot reach the desired point of maximum oxygen uptake by using cycles or other devices. In appropriate patients, stress testing is safe: dysrhythmia, AMI, and death occur at rates of 4.8, 3.6, and 0.5 per 10,000 tests, respectively.

No consensus exists on the preferred protocol, although the Bruce protocol is the most common and best studied. Depending on the protocol followed, exercise is terminated when the subject reaches a predetermined percentage of predicted maximum heart rate (i.e., 85 percent) or when another defined end point is reached. The most commonly used definition of a positive exercise test result from an ECG standpoint is greater than or equal to 1 mm of horizontal or downsloping ST-segment depression or elevation for at least 60 to 80 ms after the end of the QRS complex.

Exercise stress testing may be contraindicated for various reasons (Table 49-4). If the patient has physical limitations preventing exercise but no other contraindications, a pharmacologic stress test using a chronotropic drug (i.e., dobutamine) may be appropriate. Exercise testing may not be safe for patients at high risk for acute ischemia or those with other uncontrolled cardiovascular or pulmonary pathologies. Further, patients with an abnormal baseline ECG, such as those with left ventricular hypertrophy, bundle-branch block, or digoxin effect, are less likely to benefit from standard exercise testing owing to difficulties in interpretation of exercise-induced ECG changes.

The clinical utility of ED stress testing depends on the test result's ability to modify the pretest probability of the diagnosis and to change treatment and disposition. Emergency department stress testing is particularly difficult to quantify, because test sensitivity and specificity are greatly influenced by the population being tested. As the pretest probability of significant CAD increases, the likelihood of a false-negative test also increases. Conversely, when a population with a very low pretest probability of disease is tested, the likelihood of a false-positive result increases. Therefore, based on current data, **diagnostic stress testing is recommended for patients with a low pretest probability of CAD but is unlikely to be helpful in those at very low risk** (<5 percent) or moderate to high risk (>30 percent). The pretest probability of disease can be determined semiquantitatively based on demographic, historical, and ECG data with any of the validated decision aids previously described.

Emergency department stress testing may be of further value when applied to a broader range of patients, if the goal of testing is to predict prognosis rather than diagnosis. Many studies have confirmed that ED stress testing of selected patients can reliably predict short-term (<1 y) prognosis.

Myocardial Imaging

ECHOCARDIOGRAPHY   Advantages of *echocardiography* include its noninvasive, dynamic nature, its lack of radioactive materials, and that even sophisticated machines can be used at the bedside in the ED.[24] Further, it can assess the potential for other etiologies of chest pain, including aortic dissection, pericardial pathology, valvular disease, and possibly PE (see Chap. 61).

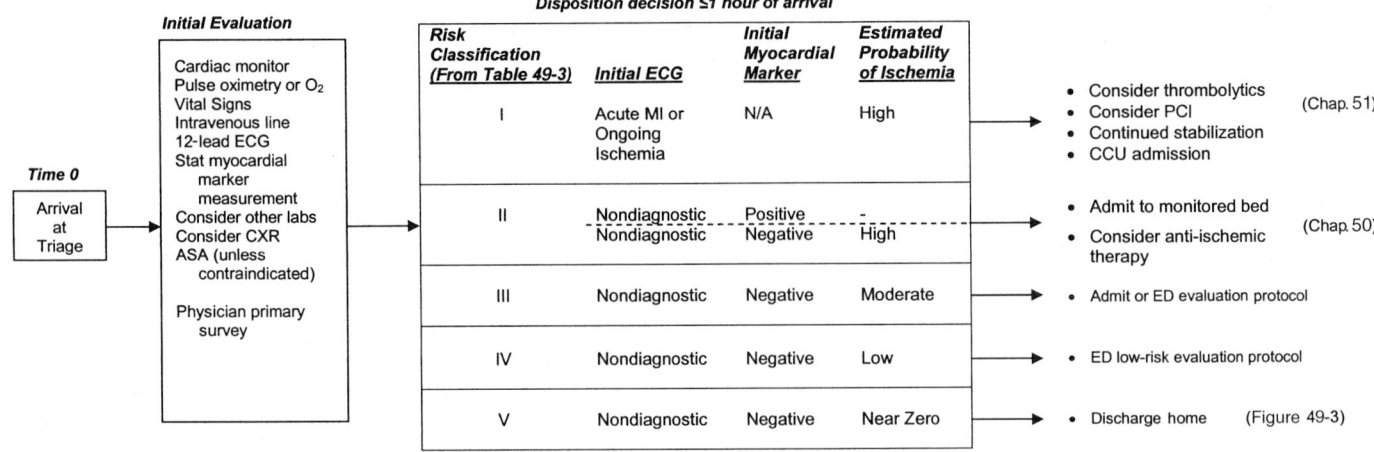

FIG. 49-2. Algorithm for risk-based decision-making. *Abbreviation:* PCI = percutaneous coronary intervention.

The value of echocardiography in evaluating ischemic heart disease is based largely on the experimental finding in animal and human studies that acute myocardial ischemia reliably and rapidly results in observable wall motion abnormalities. Thus, theoretically, a normal echocardiogram during chest pain should exclude the presence of ischemia. Unfortunately, this finding is limited by several factors. Because the effects of adjacent wall segments commonly lead to false-positive and false-negative interpretations of wall motion abnormalities, systolic wall thickening is used as a more specific indicator of ischemia. However, detection of wall-thickening abnormalities is highly dependent on imaging technique and interpretative skills, with up to 10 percent of tests being technically inadequate. Further, the echocardiogram cannot distinguish between myocardial ischemia and acute infarction, cannot reliably detect subendocardial ischemia, and may be falsely interpreted as positive in the presence of several conditions (conduction disturbances, volume overload, heart surgery, or trauma). Timing of the test relative to the onset of symptoms is critical, because transient wall motion abnormalities may resolve within minutes of an ischemic episode. Indeed, one prospective study of ED patients found that resting echo within 12 h of ED arrival does not provide additional predictive value for MI over myocardial markers alone. Thus, a normal resting echocardiogram in the ED should not be used to exclude ACS.[25]

Stress echocardiography combines a standard ECG stress test with cardiac imaging at rest and after exercise (or during pharmacologically induced tachycardia). Thus, it is superior to standard stress testing. When evaluated among low-risk ED patients, three studies have reported negative predictive values for subsequent cardiac events to be 97 to 100 percent, comparable to that of stress testing using nuclear imaging techniques.[25]

Contrast echocardiography using physiologically safe microbubbles is a newer technique that holds future promise but is not routinely used in clinical practice. Studies have suggested that this technique significantly improves the detection of regional wall motion abnormalities and wall thickening as compared with conventional sonography. In one study, 28 percent of standard stress echoes performed were inconclusive due to difficulties in interpretation but were decisively normal or abnormal with the use of contrast. In the future, contrast echocardiography may be able to directly assess coronary vessel patency, even at the microvascular level, with sensitivity similar to or greater than that of nuclear perfusion imaging.[25]

PERFUSION IMAGING *Myocardial perfusion imaging* uses an intravenously injected radioactive tracer that is distributed throughout the coronary circulation (see Chap. 61). Local myocardial uptake and, subsequently, myocardial imaging therefore are dependent on adequate regional coronary flow and myocardial cell integrity. Tracer uptake occurs in direct proportion to regional myocardial blood flow.[24]

Thallium 201 is the oldest and most studied tracer in common use today. Thallium is rapidly redistributed after initial uptake. The image represents blood flow at the moment of imaging. Areas of positive uptake reflect adequate coronary flow and viable myocardium, whereas areas without uptake represent infarcted or ischemic myocardium. On repeat imaging several hours later, continued lack of perfusion ("irreversible defect") indicates an area of infarction, whereas areas with tracer uptake only on delayed images ("reversible defect") represent previously ischemic myocardium. Combined with conventional ECG-based stress testing, thallium imaging offers improved sensitivity and specificity for detection of significant CAD over ECG-based testing alone. Further, thallium testing (or other perfusion imaging) is likely to be of value in patients who would not otherwise benefit from stress testing due to a confounding or potentially masking abnormal baseline ECG.

There are several limitations of thallium testing. Imaging must be performed soon after injection, making it impractical for use in pa-

TABLE 49-4   Contraindications to Exercise Testing

Absolute
  Acute myocardial infarction (within 2 d)
  Unstable angina not previously stabilized by medical therapy
  Uncontrolled cardiac dysrhythmias causing symptoms or hemodynamic
    compromise
  Symptomatic severe aortic stenosis
  Uncontrolled symptomatic heart failure
  Acute pulmonary embolus or pulmonary infarction
  Acute myocarditis or pericarditis
  Acute aortic dissection
Relative*
  Left main coronary stenosis
  Moderate stenotic valvular heart disease
  Electrolyte abnormalities
  Severe arterial hypertension†
  Tachydysrhythmias or bradydysrhythmias
  Hypertrophic cardiomyopathy and other forms of outflow tract obstruction
  Mental or physical impairment leading to inability to exercise adequately
  High-degree atrioventricular block

*Relative contraindications can be superseded if the benefits of exercise outweigh the risks.

†In the absence of definitive evidence, the AHA committee suggests systolic blood pressure of >200 mm Hg and/or diastolic blood pressure of >110 mm Hg.

Source: Fletcher GF, Balady G, Froelicher VF, et al: Exercise standards: A statement for healthcare professionals from the American Heart Association Writing Group. Special Report. *Circulation* 91:580, 1995.

tients with ongoing chest pain. Moreover, because of a long half-life, the injected dose of thallium must be kept low to avoid excessive radiation exposure. This and other properties of the tracer result in a relatively poor image quality and the frequent occurrence of artifactual perfusion defects (false positives) due to overlying tissue attenuation. This is particularly common in women and obese patients. Due to these limitations and the lack of ED-based efficacy studies, thallium-201 imaging alone is not an ideal agent for use in the ED.

Myocardial perfusion imaging using *technetium 99m* (^{99m}Tc)-labeled agents such as sestamibi offers advantages over thallium for ED use. Because the half-life of ^{99m}Tc is much shorter than that of thallium (6 vs. 73 h), a larger dosage can be injected without harm to the patient. This results in the superior image quality, decreased tissue attenuation-related artifacts, and higher specificity for sestamibi imaging. Newer ^{99m}Tc agents being introduced continue to improve image quality. In addition, in contrast to thallium, the initial distribution of ^{99m}Tc agents is stable for several hours. Therefore, accurate imaging can occur up to 3 h after injection. The image represents the blood flow at the moment of injection. By using "gated" image acquisition technology, sestamibi scanning can yield an accurate estimation of ejection fraction. As with thallium, resting and stress (exercise or pharmacologic) images can be compared to yield additional data.

Dual isotope stress testing using thallium and sestamibi is an increasingly common component of ED ACS evaluation protocols. In this technique, a resting thallium scan is first performed. Those patients without resting defects can then immediately undergo stress testing with sestamibi imaging, thereby avoiding the delay usually required for isotope "washout" in single isotope techniques. In a recent prospective study, a strategy using this method reliably identified or excluded ACS among 1775 low-risk ED patients.[26]

The use of *electron-beam computed tomography* for the detection of coronary artery calcification has shown promise as a noninvasive alternative for the diagnosis of CAD. A "calcium score" is generated and is directly related to the likelihood of having CAD (within a given demographic group). Electron-beam computed tomography has a number of limitations. It cannot identify the minority of plaques that do not contain calcium, and it does not demonstrate microvascular or vasospastic disease. Although this technique shows promise as an alternative to the previously discussed imaging techniques, its role in ED evaluation remains undefined.[27]

Low-Risk Patient Protocols

INPATIENT ADMISSION In settings where extended observation and definitive diagnostic testing are not available in the ED, all patients whose presentations suggest a reasonable plausibility of an acute ischemic event should be admitted to an inpatient bed. Once the need for inpatient admission has been determined, further stratification based on assessment of the patient's short-term risk of morbidity or mortality can be made based on the patient's history and physical examination, initial ECG, and early myocardial marker measurement. Patients with a prior history of CAD, evidence of congestive heart failure on physical examination, recurrent chest pain in the ED, or new or presumed new ischemic ECG changes are at higher short-term risk and may be more appropriately managed in an intermediate-care (step-down) unit. Conversely, patients whose initial ED ECG is normal or unchanged from a previous ECG have a very low risk of adverse events and can safely be evaluated on a monitored floor or telemetry bed. Those with nonspecific changes on the initial ECG represent an intermediate-risk group. A single myocardial marker measurement soon after ED presentation also can identify those patients at greater risk from among those with atypical presentations.

ED OBSERVATION/MONITORING In 1991, the Multicenter Chest Pain Study Group reported that the diagnosis of infarction could have been safely excluded within a 12-h observation period among a

subgroup of patients admitted for chest pain but identified at presentation as having a low probability of AMI.[28] The investigators also suggested routine predischarge stress testing of these patients to reduce the risk of discharging patients with unstable coronary syndromes prematurely. Gibler and colleagues later refined this approach.[29] Patients with symptoms consistent but weakly suggestive of acute ischemia were observed for 9 h with continuous 12-lead ST-segment ECG monitoring and serial CK-MB testing at 0, 3, 6, and 9 h after presentation. Those who completed a negative 9-h evaluation subsequently underwent echocardiography followed by graded exercise stress testing in the ED before discharge. With this approach, 82.1 percent of patients were released home from the cardiac evaluation unit.[29]

Although there is no consensus on the best approach, many studies have documented clinical safety and efficacy and cost savings associated with use of an ED-based Cardiac Evaluation Unit protocol compared with traditional inpatient admission, and their use has continued to expand.

Normal serial ECGs and myocardial marker measurements do not preclude the presence of other ACSs (i.e., unstable angina), which may still put the patient at high risk for a subsequent adverse event. Therefore, further evaluation is generally recommended before discharge (Figure 49-3). The various forms of stress testing (with or without myocardial imaging) currently offer the best noninvasive method to predict the presence of CAD and assess prognosis. Over the past decade, numerous published reports have confirmed the safety, clinical utility, and cost-effectiveness of various versions of this accelerated MI rule-out/early risk stratification concept, and this strategy has been incorporated into the ACC/AHA 2002 guideline update for the management of patients with unstable angina and non-ST-segment elevation MI.[10]

DISPOSITION

The assessment of acute chest pain patients is difficult, and the processes and approaches discussed in this chapter are not perfect. This is best illustrated in AMI, where the "miss" rate for AMI in patients evaluated in the emergency department using history, physical examination, ECG, and serum markers is currently about 2 percent; these patients were discharged and upon follow-up were determined to have sustained an AMI. The good news is that the use of serial marker measurements, evaluation or observation units, myocardial imaging studies, and stress testing has the potential to reduce this "missed-MI" rate to close to zero. Unfortunately, UA sometimes remains an elusive and difficult diagnosis. There is little information on the ED "miss rate" for the important diagnoses of aortic dissection and pulmonary embolism. Despite advances in serum marker technology and imaging studies, the physician must still exercise clinical judgment when evaluating acute chest pain patients. To make the best possible decisions, clinicians should collect adequate information first before exercising their judgment. The ability to make good decisions when faced with incomplete or uncertain information is an important skill.

The disposition of patients who have a defined diagnosis as the cause of their chest pain is relatively straightforward. Those patients without a specific diagnosis—so-called atypical chest pain—pose more of a problem. A useful principle in these patients with atypical chest pain is the use of a composite picture to assign patients to a category where the potential for ACS or other serious causes of chest pain is vanishingly small, and such patients can be safely discharged. These patients often have pain described as sharp; well localized; reproducible by position, breathing, or palpation; and have no prior diagnosis of angina or AMI. The pretest probability of ACS or other serious conditions is so low that ancillary testing is usually not indicated and patients can be discharged after the history and physical examination. Conversely, patients with unexplained visceral chest pain should not be discharged unless potentially serious conditions have been excluded using appropriate ancillary testing.

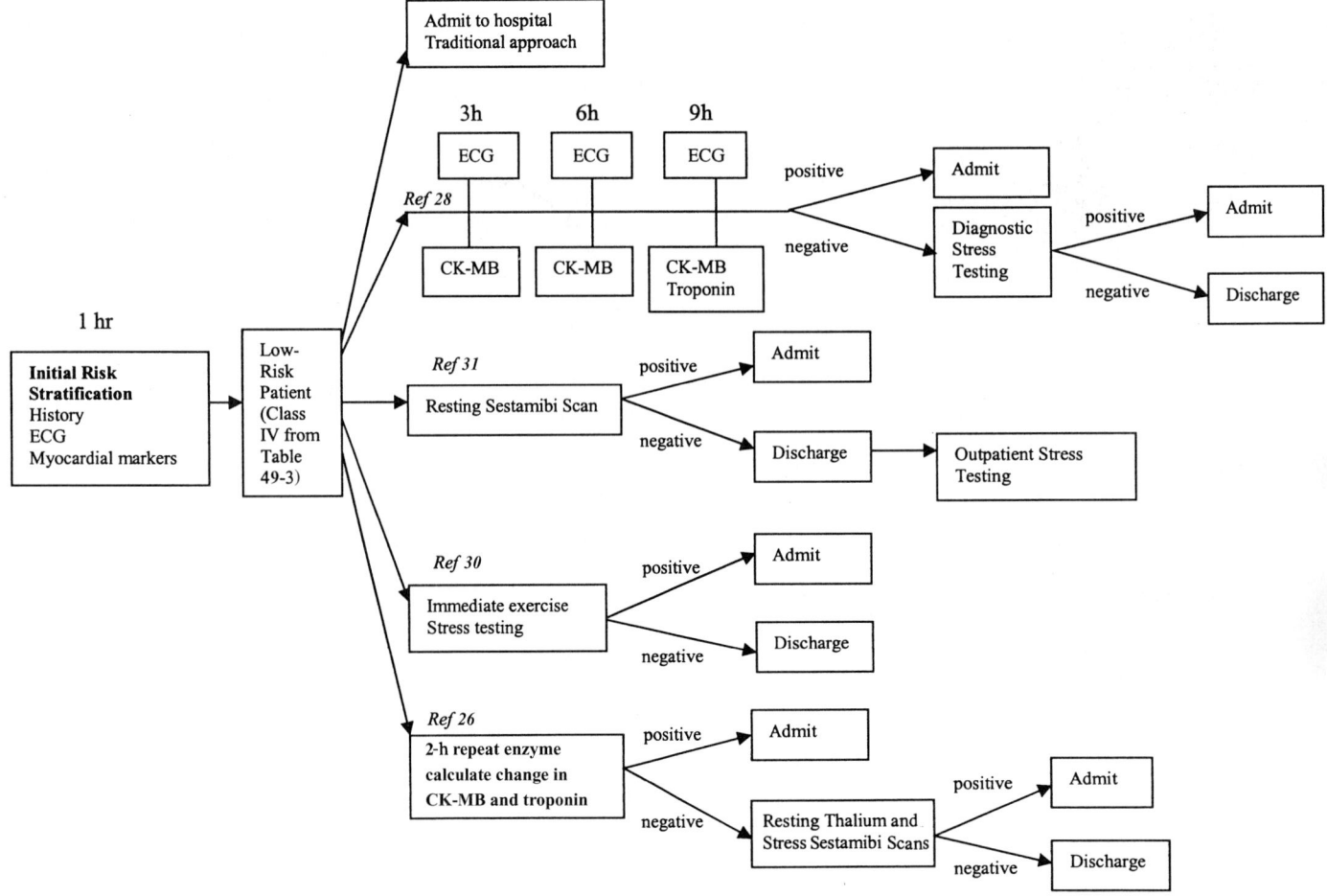

FIG. 49-3. Alternative risk stratification protocols for low-risk patients.

Discharged patients should receive appropriate instructions regarding medications and follow-up directions. They should also be instructed to seek prompt attention or return for recurrent or worsening chest pain or other serious symptoms. Some institutions have instituted chest pain clinics to ensure that patients receive appropriate follow-up after their discharge from the ED.

REFERENCES

1. Lee TH, Goldman L: Evaluation of the patient with acute chest pain. *New Engl J Med* 342:1187, 2000.
2. Panju AA, Hemmelgarn BR, Guyatt GH, Simel DL: Is this patient having a myocardial infarction? *JAMA* 280:1256, 1998.
3. Gupta M, Tabas JA, Kohn MA: Presenting complaint among patients with myocardial infarction who present to an urban, public hospital emergency department. *Ann Emerg Med* 40:180, 2002.
4. Canto JG, Shlipak MG, Rogers WJ, et al: Prevalence, clinical characteristics, and mortality among patients with myocardial infarction presenting without chest pain. *JAMA* 283;3227, 2002.
5. Douglas PS, Ginsburg GS: The evaluation of chest pain in women. *New Engl J Med* 334:1311, 1996.
6. Wicki J, Perneger TV, Junod AF, et al: Assessing clinical probability of pulmonary embolism in the emergency ward. *Arch Intern Med* 161:92, 2001.
7. Klompas M: Does this patient have an acute thoracic aortic dissection? *JAMA* 287:2262, 2002.
8. Wulsin L, Liu T, Storrow A, et al: A randomized, controlled trial of panic disorder treatment initiation in an emergency department chest pain center. *Ann Emerg Med* 39:139, 2002.
9. Fleet RP, Dupuis G, Marchand A, et al: Panic disorder in ED chest pain patients: Prevalence, comorbidity, suicidal ideation and physician recognition. *Am J Med* 101:371, 1996.
10. Braumwald E, Antman EM, Beasley JW, et al: ACC/AHA 2002 guideline update for the management of patients with unstable angina and non-ST-segment elevation myocardial infarction: A report of the ACC/AHA Task Force on Practice Guidelines (Committee on the Management of Patients with Unstable Angina), 2002. Available at www.acc.org/clinical/guidelines/unstable/unstable.pdf.
11. Zimetbaum PJ, Josephson ME: Use of the electrocardiogram in acute myocardial infarction. *New Engl J Med* 348:933, 2003.
12. Silber SH, Leo PJ, Katapadi M: Serial electrocardiograms for chest pain patients with initial nondiagnostic electrocardiograms: Implications for thrombolytic therapy. *Acad Emerg Med* 3:147, 1996.
13. Selker HP, Zalenski RJ, Antman EM, et al: An evaluation of technologies for identification of acute cardiac ischemia in the emergency department: A report from the National Heart Attack Alert Program Working Group. *Ann Emerg Med* 29:13, 1997.
14. Puleo PR, Meyer D, Wathen C, et al: Use of a rapid assay of subforms of creatine kinase-MB to diagnose or rule out acute myocardial infarction. *New Engl J Med* 331:561, 1994.
15. Green GB, Skarbek-Borosky GW, Chan DW, et al: Myoglobin for early risk stratification of ED patients with possible myocardial ischemia. *Acad Emerg Med* 7:625, 2000.
16. Green GB, Li DJ, Bessman ES, et al: The prognostic significance of troponin I and troponin T. *Acad Emerg Med* 5:758, 1998.
17. Malasky BR, Alpert JS: Diagnosis of myocardial injury by biochemical markers: Problems and promises. *Cardiol Rev* 10:306, 2002.
18. Fesmire FM: Improved identification of acute coronary syndromes with delta cardiac serum marker measurements during emergency department evaluation of chest pain patients. *Cardiovasc Toxicol* 1:117, 2001.
19. Green GB, Hansen KW, Chan DW, et al: Potential utility of a rapid CK-MB assay in evaluating emergency department patients with possible myocardial infarction. *Ann Emerg Med* 20:954, 1991.
20. Alpert JS, Thygesen K, Antman E, et al: Myocardial infarction redefined – A consensus document of the Joint European Society of Cardiology/Amer-

ican College of Cardiology Committee for the Redefinition of MI. *J Am Coll Cardiol* 36:959, 2000.

21. Selker HP, Beschansky JR, Griffith JL, et al: Use of the Acute Cardiac Ischemia Time-Insensitive Predictive Instrument (ACI-TIPI) to assist with triage of patients with chest pain or other symptoms suggestive of acute cardiac ischemia. *Ann Intern Med* 129:845, 1998.

22. Baxt WG, Shofer FS, Sites FD, Hollander JE: A neural computational aid to the diagnosis of acute myocardial infarction. *Ann Emerg Med* 39:366, 2002.

23. Baxt WG, Shofer FS, Sites FD, Hollander JE: A neural network aid for the early diagnosis of cardiac ischemia in patients presenting to the ED with chest pain. *Ann Emerg Med* 40:575, 2002.

24. Mather PJ, Shah R: Echocardiography, nuclear scintigraphy, and stress testing in the emergency department evaluation of acute coronary syndrome. *Emerg Med Clin North Am* 19:339, 2001.

25. Selker HP, Zalenski RJ, Antman EM, et al: Echocardiogram: In an evaluation of technologies for identification of acute cardiac ischemia in the emergency department: A report from a National Heart Attack Alert Program Working Group. *Ann Emerg Med* 29:69, 1997.

26. Fesmire FM, Hughes AD, Stout PK, et al: Selective dual nuclear scanning in low-risk patients with chest pain to reliably identify and exclude acute coronary syndromes. *Ann Emerg Med* 38:207, 2001.

27. Georgiu D, Budoff MJ, Kaufer E, et al: Screening patients with chest pain in the ED using electron bean tomography: A follow-up study. *J Am Coll Cardiol* 38:105, 2001.

28. Lee TH, Juarez G, Cook F, et al: Ruling out acute myocardial infarction: A prospective multicenter validation of a 12-hour strategy for patients at low risk. *New Engl J Med* 324:1239, 1991.

29. Gibler WB, Runyon JP, Levy RC, et al: A rapid diagnostic and treatment center for patients with chest pain in the emergency department. *Ann Emerg Med* 25:1, 1995.

30. Amsterdam EA, Kirk JD, Diercks DB, et al: Immediate exercise testing to evaluate low-risk patients presenting to the emergency department with chest pain. *J Am Coll Cardiol* 40:251, 2002.

31. Tatum JL, Jesse RL, Kantos MC, et al: Comprehensive strategy for the evaluation and triage of the chest pain patient. *Ann Emerg Med* 29:166, 1997.

ACUTE CORONARY SYNDROMES: ACUTE MYOCARDIAL INFARCTION AND UNSTABLE ANGINA
Judd E. Hollander

Ischemic heart disease is the leading cause of death among adults in the United States, accounting for more than 500,000 deaths annually. Atherosclerotic disease of the epicardial coronary arteries—termed *coronary artery disease,* or CAD—accounts for the vast majority of patients with ischemic heart disease. The predominant symptom of CAD is chest pain, and concern over potential CAD and myocardial ischemia contributes to the over 5 million visits each year to U.S. EDs for acute chest pain. In a typical adult ED population with acute chest pain, about 15 percent of patients will have acute myocardial infarction and about 25 to 30 percent will have unstable angina.

Ischemic heart disease represents a spectrum from chronic stable angina to acute myocardial infarction (AMI). Three categorization schemes are commonly used in ischemic heart disease patients. The first is the Canadian Cardiovascular Society categorization of angina into four classes (Table 50-1). The second is the categorization of unstable angina (UA) into three principal presentations by the Agency for Health Care Policy and Research (Table 50-2).[1] Both of these classifications assume a diagnosis of ischemic heart disease and their utility is problematic in the ED when patients present with acute chest pain that may or may not be due to ischemic heart disease. The third categorization scheme assesses the short-term risk for patients with unstable angina (UA) (Table 50-3).

Acute Coronary Syndrome (ACS) is a term used to describe patients who present with acute chest pain and other symptoms of my-

TABLE 50-1   Canadian Cardiovascular Society Classification of Angina

Class I	Angina occurs only with strenuous, rapid, or prolonged exertion. Ordinary physical activity does not cause angina.
Class II	Slight limitation of ordinary activity. Angina occurs with climbing stairs rapidly, walking uphill, walking after meals, in cold, in wind, or under emotional stress.
Class III	Marked limitations of ordinary physical activity. Angina occurs on walking 1–2 level blocks or climbing one flight of stairs at usual pace.
Class IV	Inability to carry on physical activity without discomfort. Anginal symptoms may be present at rest.

Source: Braunwald E, Mark DB, Jones RH, et al: *Unstable Angina: Diagnosis and Management.* Clincal Practice Guideline No. 10 (amended). AHCPR Publication No. 94-0602. Rockville, MD, Agency for Health Care Policy and Research and the National Health, Lung and Blood Institute, Public Health Service, U.S. Department of Health and Human Services, 1994.

ocardial ischemia, often with diagnostic or suggestive electrocardiographic changes of myocardial ischemia. During the initial assessment, it is often not possible to determine whether the patient has or will sustain permanent damage to the myocardium (necrosis or AMI) or has reversible ischemia (injury or UA). Only in retrospect, after either serial ECG changes and/or serial serum markers of myocardial injury, can this distinction between AMI and UA be made. ACS is a useful concept because the triage, assessment, and initial management of UA and AMI are similar.

ANATOMY

Knowledge of the anatomy of the coronary arteries is essential to understand the effects of myocardial ischemia and why some complications are more common with anterior or inferior wall myocardial infarction (Figure 50-1). The left coronary artery arises from the ascending aorta in the left sinus of the aortic valve. It courses through the atrioventricular sulcus on the left side and divides into the left circumflex and the left anterior descending branch. The left anterior descending branch courses down the anterior aspect of the heart around the inferior margin and anastomoses with the posterior diagonal branch of the right coronary artery. It is the main blood supply to the anterior and septal regions of the heart. The circumflex branch continues around the atrioventricular sulcus, where it anastomoses with the right coronary artery. It supplies blood to some of the anterior wall and a large portion of the lateral wall of the heart. The right coronary artery arises from the right sinus of the aortic valve and runs in the atrioventricular sulcus between the right atrium and right ventricle. It gives off a marginal branch near the lower aspect of the heart and terminates as the right posterior descending artery. The right coronary artery supplies the right side of the heart with blood, and it provides some

TABLE 50-2   Principal Presentations of Unstable Angina

Rest angina	Angina occurring at rest and usually prolonged >20 min occurring within a week of presentation
New-onset angina	Angina of at least CCSC III severity with onset within 2 mo of presentation
Increasing angina	Previously diagnosed angina that is distinctly more frequent, longer in duration, or lower in threshold (increased by at least one CCSC class to at least CCSC III severity).

Abbreviation: CCSC = Canadian Cardiovascular Society Classification.
Source: Braunwald E, Mark DB, Jones RH, et al: *Unstable Angina: Diagnosis and Management.* Clincal Practice Guideline No. 10 (amended). AHCPR Publication No. 94-0602. Rockville, MD, Agency for Health Care Policy and Research and the National Health, Lung and Blood Institute, Public Health Service, U.S. Department of Health and Human Services, 1994.

TABLE 50-3   Short-Term Risk of Death or Nonfatal Myocardial Infarction by Risk Stratification in Patients with Unstable Angina

High Risk	Intermediate Risk	Low Risk
At least one of the following features must be present	*No high-risk feature but must have one of the following*	*No high- or intermediate-risk features but may have any of the following features*
Prolonged ongoing (>20 min) rest pain	Prolonged (>20 min) rest angina, now resolved, with moderate or high likelihood of CAD	Increased angina frequency, severity, or duration
Pulmonary edema, most likely related to ischemia	Rest angina (>20 min) not promptly relieved with rest or sublingual nitroglycerin	Angina provoked at a lower threshold
Angina at rest with dynamic ST changes ≥1 mm	Nocturnal angina	New-onset angina with onset 2 wk to 2 mo before presentation
Angina with new or worsening MR murmur	Angina with dynamic T-wave changes	Normal or unchanged ECG
Angina with S_3 or new or worsening rales	New-onset CCSC III or IV angina in the past 2 wk with moderate or high likelihood of CAD	
Angina with hypotension	Pathologic Q waves or resting ST depression ≤1mm in multiple-lead groups (anterior, inferior, and lateral)	
	Age >65 y	

Abbreviations: CAD = coronary artery disease; CCSC = Canadian Cardiology Society Classification; ECG = electrocardiogram; MR = mitral regurgitation.
Source: Braunwald E, Mark DB, Jones RH, et al: *Unstable Angina: Diagnosis and Management.* Clincal Practice Guideline No. 10 (amended). AHCPR Publication No. 94-0602. Rockville, MD, Agency for Health Care Policy and Research and the National Health, Lung and Blood Institute, Public Health Service, U.S. Department of Health and Human Services, 1994.

perfusion to the inferior aspect of the left ventricle through the posterior descending artery.

The atrioventricular (AV) conduction system receives blood supply from the AV branch of the right coronary artery and the septal perforating branch of the left anterior descending coronary artery. Similarly, the right bundle branch and the left posterior division obtain a dual blood flow from the left anterior descending and right coronary arteries. The posteromedial papillary muscle receives blood supply from one coronary artery, usually the right coronary artery.

PATHOPHYSIOLOGY

Hypoxia is a deficiency in oxygen supply or availability to tissues. Ischemia is oxygen deprivation accompanied by inadequate removal of metabolites due to reduced perfusion. Ischemia and hypoxia are relative terms, because conditions that result in ischemia in one patient may not result in ischemia in another. Ischemia occurs when there is an imbalance between oxygen demand and oxygen supply. Oxygen supply is influenced by the oxygen-carrying capacity of the blood and the coronary artery blood flow. The oxygen-carrying capacity of the blood is determined by the amount of hemoglobin present and oxygen saturation. Coronary artery blood flow is determined by the duration of diastolic relaxation of the heart and peripheral vascular resistance. Humoral, neural, metabolic, and extravascular compressive forces and local autoregulation mechanisms determine the coronary vascular resistance.

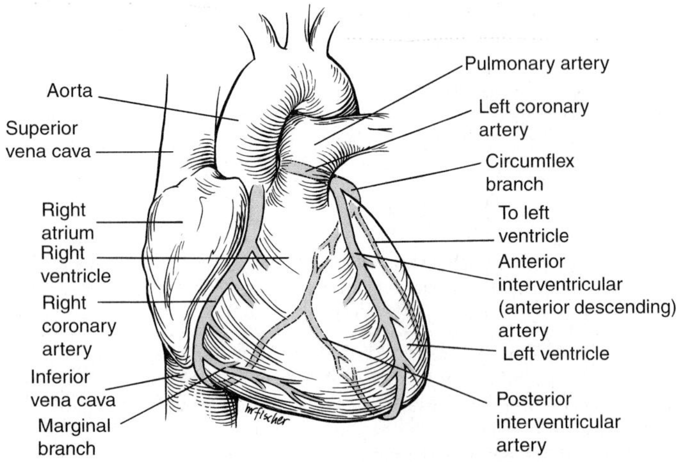

Myocardial ischemia and its sequelae usually occur as a result of fixed atherosclerotic lesions. ACS is caused by secondary reduction in myocardial blood flow due to coronary arterial spasm, disruption of atherosclerotic plaques, and platelet aggregation or thrombus formation at the site of an atherosclerotic lesion. Nonatherosclerotic etiologies of ACS are considerably less common.

Atherosclerotic plaque formation occurs through repetitive injury to the vessel wall. Macrophages and smooth muscle cells are the main cellular elements in plaque development, whereas lipids are predominant in the extracellular milieu. Plaque fissuring and rupture are affected by features inherent to the plaque, such as its composition and shape, and local factors, such as shear forces, coronary arterial tone, coronary arterial perfusion pressure, and movements of the artery in response to myocardial contractions. When plaque rupture occurs, potent thrombogenic substances are exposed to circulating platelets.

The platelet response involves adhesion, activation, and aggregation. Platelet adhesion occurs through the weak platelet interactions with subendothelial adhesion molecules, such as collagen, fibronectin, and laminin, and the binding of the glycoprotein Ib receptor to the subendothelial form of von Willebrand factor. Adherent platelets are strongly thrombogenic because subendothelial collagen is a potent inducer of platelet activation. Lipid-laden macrophages in the plaque core and adventitia of the vessel wall release tissue factor, which stimulates the conversion of prothrombin to thrombin. Thrombin and the local shear forces are also potent platelet activators. Platelet secretion of adenosine diphosphate, thromboxane A_2, and serotonin are autostimulatory agonists of platelet activation. Activated platelet glycoprotein IIb/IIIa receptors become cross-linked by fibrinogen or von Willebrand factor in the final common pathway of platelet aggregation.

The extent of oxygen deprivation and thus clinical presentation of ACS depend on the limitation of O_2 delivery imposed by thrombus adhering to fixed, fissured, or eroded atherosclerotic plaque. Myocardial ischemia can be manifest by chest or epigastric discomfort, dyspnea, characteristic or nonspecific electrocardiographic changes, depressed myocardial function, reduced central and peripheral perfusion, or any combination of the above. In stable angina, ischemia occurs only when

FIG. 50-1. Schematic diagram of the coronary arteries.

activity induces O_2 demands beyond the supply restrictions imposed by a partially occluded coronary vessel. This occurs at a relatively fixed and predictable point and changes slowly over time. Atherosclerotic plaque has not ruptured, and there is little, if any, superimposed thrombus. In ACS, atherosclerotic plaque rupture and platelet-rich thrombus develop. Coronary blood flow is reduced and myocardial ischemia occurs. The degree and duration of the oxygen supply-demand mismatch determines whether the patient develops reversible myocardial ischemia without necrosis (unstable angina) or myocardial ischemia with necrosis (myocardial infarction). More severe and prolonged obstruction increases the likelihood of infarction.

Acute myocardial ischemia may inhibit myocardial contractility, thereby affecting central and peripheral perfusion. In AMI, the fundamental alteration is loss of functioning myocardium. When an area of the myocardium does not receive adequate O_2, the functional deterioration is progressive through four sequentially abnormal contraction patterns. *Dyssynchrony,* the dissociation in time course of contraction of adjacent segments of myocardium, occurs first. *Hypokinesis,* the reduction in the extent of shortening with contraction, occurs next. *Akinesis,* the cessation of shortening with systolic contraction, follows. *Dyskinesis,* the paradoxical expansion of infarcted tissue, occurs during systole. With increasing size of the infarcted myocardium, left ventricular pump function decreases. Left ventricular end-diastolic pressure and left ventricular end-systolic volume increase. Cardiac output, stroke volume, and blood pressure may decrease. When left atrial and pulmonary capillary pressures increase, congestive heart failure or pulmonary edema may develop. Poor perfusion to the brain and kidneys can result in altered mental status and impaired renal function, respectively.

CLINICAL FEATURES

Clinical History

The main symptom of ischemic heart disease is chest pain, and the history should characterize its severity, location, radiation, duration, and quality. In addition, the presence of associated symptoms, such as nausea, vomiting, diaphoresis, dyspnea, lightheadedness, syncope, and palpitations, may be helpful. A history regarding the onset and duration of symptoms, activities that precipitate symptoms, and prior evaluations for similar symptoms should be ascertained.

Symptoms of acute myocardial ischemia often will be described as discomfort rather than as pain. Anginal symptoms include chest pressure, heaviness, tightness, fullness, or squeezing. Less commonly but not infrequently, patients will describe their symptoms as knifelike, sharp, or stabbing. The classic location is substernal or in the left chest. Radiation to the arm, neck, or jaw may occur. Reproducible chest wall tenderness is not uncommon, possibly because the pericardium may become inflamed and it sits beneath the chest wall.

Exercise, stress, or a cold environment classically precipitates angina pectoris. Angina usually has a duration of symptoms of typically <10 min, occasionally lasting up to 10 to 20 min, and usually improves within 2 to 5 min after rest or nitroglycerin. However, early classic descriptions of angina describe episodes as short as 2 min. In contrast, AMI is usually accompanied by more prolonged and severe chest discomfort, more prominent associated symptoms (nausea, diaphoresis, shortness of breath, etc.), and little, if any, response to initial sublingual nitroglycerin. Easy fatigability may be a prominent symptom of ACS.

It is important to know the frequency of anginal episodes and any change in frequency of episodes over the past months. The patient should be questioned to determine any increase in severity or duration of symptoms or whether less effort is required to precipitate them.

Atypical presentations or silent myocardial ischemia are common. Up to 30 percent of patients with AMI identified in large longitudinal studies are clinically unrecognized. Some of these patients have had atypical symptoms for which they did not pursue medical advice. Others cannot recall any symptoms. The prognosis for patients who have atypical symptoms at the time of their infarction is worse than that of patients who had more typical symptoms. Women and the elderly are more likely to have atypical presentations.

Cardiac risk factors are modestly predictive of CAD in asymptomatic patients. **In the ED, cardiac risk factors are poor predictors of cardiac risk for myocardial infarction or other ACS.**[2] Traditional cardiac risk factors for CAD, such as hypertension, diabetes mellitus, tobacco use, family history of CAD at an early age, and hypercholesterolemia, are not predictive of ACS in female ED chest pain patients. In male patients, only diabetes and family history are weakly predictive.[3] The distinction between the utility of cardiac risk factors in the asymptomatic patient and the ED chest pain patient is easy to understand. The cardiac risk factors were derived from population-based longitudinal cohort studies of asymptomatic patients to determine risk of CAD. In contrast, cardiac risk factors for CAD have significantly less predictive value for an acute event than the mere presence of symptoms.

Physical Examination

The physical examination is not helpful in distinguishing patients with ACS from those with noncardiac etiologies when an alternate diagnosis is not clear. Patients with ACSs may appear deceptively well without any clinical signs of distress or may be uncomfortable, pale, cyanotic, and in respiratory distress. The pulse rate may be normal or display bradycardia, tachycardia, or irregular pulses. Bradycardic rhythms are more common with inferior wall myocardial ischemia. In the setting of an anterior wall infarction, bradycardic rhythms or heart block is an extremely poor prognostic sign. Blood pressure can be normal, elevated (due to baseline hypertension, sympathetic stimulation, and anxiety), or decreased (due to pump failure or inadequate preload). Extremes of blood pressure are associated with a worse prognosis.

The first and second heart sounds are often diminished due to poor myocardial contractility. An S_3 is present in 15 to 20 percent of patients with AMI. An S_4 is common in patients with long-standing hypertension or myocardial dysfunction. The presence or absence of the noted heart sounds is not usually helpful in the ED, although an S_3, if truly detected, may imply a failing myocardium. However, the presence of a new systolic murmur is an ominous sign, because it may signify papillary muscle dysfunction, a flail leaflet of the mitral valve with resultant mitral regurgitation, or a ventricular septal defect.

The presence of rales, with or without an S_3 gallop, is associated with left ventricular dysfunction and left-sided congestive heart failure. Jugular venous distention, hepatojugular reflex, and peripheral edema suggest right-sided congestive heart failure. It is important to determine the patient's baseline condition from medical records or from the patient's physician to establish the presence of new findings that may help guide management.

Electrocardiography

The standard 12-lead ECG is the single best test to identify patients with AMI upon ED presentation.[4] **Published consensus guidelines establish a goal that the initial 12-lead ECG be obtained and integrated within 10 min of presentation for patients with acute chest pain or other symptoms suggestive of myocardial ischemia.** Although the ECG is the best immediately available test in the ED, it has relatively low sensitivity for detection of AMI. The ST segment is elevated on the initial ECG in approximately 50 percent of patients; i.e., half of the patients who present to the ED with AMI will not have diagnostic ST-segment changes on the initial ECG. Most other AMI patients without diagnostic ST-segment elevation will have ST-segment depression and/or T-wave inversions, and only 1 to 5 percent of patients with AMI have an entirely normal initial ECG.[5]

Standard diagnostic ECG criteria for AMI are shown in Table 50-4. ST-segment elevations in the distributions shown suggest acute transmural injury. ST-segment depressions in these distributions suggest subendocardial ischemia. **All inferior wall acute myocardial infarctions should have a right-sided lead V_4 (V_{4R}) obtained,** because ST-segment elevation in V_{4R} is highly suggestive of right ventricular infarction.

Reciprocal ST-segment changes (such as ST-segment depressions in the anterior precordial leads in the setting of an inferior wall AMI) predict a larger infarct distribution, an increased severity of underlying CAD, more severe pump failure, a higher likelihood of cardiovascular complications, and increased mortality. In general, the more elevated the ST segments and the more ST segments that are elevated, the more extensive the injury.

The ECG can also be used to predict the infarct-related vessel. Inferior wall myocardial infarctions can result from occlusion of the left circumflex artery or the right coronary artery. In the setting of an inferior wall AMI, ST-segment elevation in at least one lateral lead (V_5, V_6, or aV_L) with an isoelectric or elevated ST segment in lead I is strongly suggestive of a left circumflex lesion. The presence of ST-segment elevation in lead III greater than that in lead II predicts a right coronary artery occlusion. When accompanied by ST-segment elevation in V_1 or a V_{4R}, it predicts a proximal right coronary artery lesion with accompanying right ventricular infarction. Reciprocal anterior ST-segment depressions in V_1 through V_4 are equally prevalent in right coronary and left circumflex inferior wall AMIs.

The main utility of the ECG is to detect AMI. The standard 12-lead ECG is less helpful in the detection of unstable angina. One classification system divides the ECG into six categories:

1. Normal
2. Nonspecific ST-segment or T-wave changes: less than 1 mm ST-segment depression directed toward the baseline, T waves flattened or diphasic
3. Abnormal, but not diagnostic of ischemia or infarction: less than 1 mm ST-segment depression horizontal to the baseline, T waves inverted
4. Ischemia, strain, or infarction known to be old: Q waves, more than 1 mm ST-segment depression horizontal to or directed away from the baseline, and T-wave inversions noted on prior ECGs.
5. Ischemia, strain, or infarction not known to be old: Q waves, more than 1 mm ST-segment depression horizontal to or directed away from the baseline, and T-wave inversions either not noted on prior ECGs or no prior ECG available.
6. Probable AMI: ST-segment elevation greater than 1 mm in two contiguous ECG leads

This classification and others like it have been used to show that patients with more significant ECG abnormalities are more likely to have

AMI, unstable angina, and serious cardiovascular complications. Nonetheless, even patients with normal or nonspecific ECGs have a 1 to 5 percent incidence of AMI and a 4 to 23 percent incidence of unstable angina. Patients with nondiagnostic ECGs or evidence of ischemia that is age-indeterminate have a 4 to 7 percent incidence of AMI and a 21 to 48 percent incidence of unstable angina. Demonstration of new ischemia in ECG increases the risk of AMI from 25 to 73 percent and the unstable angina risk from 14 to 43 percent.[4] Thus, the standard 12-lead ECG is useful for cardiovascular risk stratification of patients with ACSs.[6] It can be used in conjunction with clinical history and cardiac markers to determine admission location for such patients.

The addition of other leads to the standard 12-lead ECG modestly increases sensitivity for detection of AMI, but reduces specificity.[7] The only recommended addition to the standard 12-lead ECG is the use of right-sided precordial leads in the setting of acute inferior myocardial infarction in order to detect right ventricular involvement.[4]

There are several clinical conditions in which ECG interpretation is difficult (Table 50-5). It is occasionally possible that in the setting of paced rhythms and left bundle-branch blocks, acute myocardial ischemia can be identified. In the setting of a left bundle-branch block, the following three ST-segment patterns are indicative of AMI: (1) ST-segment elevation 1 mm or greater and concordant (in the same direction as the main deflection) with the QRS complex (odds ratio 25.2, 95% CI 11.6 – 54.7), (2) ST-segment depression 1 mm or more in leads V_1, V_2, or V_3 (odds ratio 6.0, 95% CI 1.9 – 19.3), and (3) ST-segment elevation 5 mm or greater and discordant (in the opposite direction) with the QRS complex (odds ratio 4.3, 95% CI 1.8 – 10.6).[8]

Right ventricular pacing causes secondary repolarization changes of opposing polarity to that of the predominant QRS complex. Most leads have predominant negative QRS complexes followed by ST-

TABLE 50-4 Electrocardiographic Criteria for Acute Myocardial Infarction

Location	Electrocardiographic findings
Anteroseptal	QS deflections in V_1, V_2, V_3, and possibly V_4
Anterior	rS deflection in V_1 with Q waves in V_2–V_4 or decrease in amplitude of initial R waves in V_1–V_4
Anterolateral	Q waves in V_4–V_6, I, and aV_L
Lateral	Q waves in I and aV_L
Inferior	Q waves in II, III, and aV_F
Inferolateral	Q waves in II, III, aV_F, and V_5 and V_6
True posterior	Initial R waves in V_1 and V_2 >0.04 s and R/S ratio ≥1
Right ventricular	Q waves in II, III, and aV_F and ST elevation in right-side V_4

TABLE 50-5 Some Clinical Conditions in Which the Electrocardiogram Interpretation Can Be Difficult

May have ST-segment elevation in the absence of acute myocardial infarction
  Early repolarization
  Left ventricular hypertrophy
  Pericarditis
  Myocarditis
  Left ventricular aneurysm
  Hypertropic cardiomyopathy
  Hypothermia
  Ventricular paced rhythms
  Left bundle-branch block
May have ST-segment depressions in the absence of ischemia
  Hypokalemia
  Digoxin effect
  Cor pulmonale and right heart strain
  Early repolarization
  Left ventricular hypertrophy
  Ventricular paced rhythms
  Left bundle-branch block
May have T-wave inversions in the absence of ischemia
  Persistent juvenile pattern
  Stokes-Adams syncope or seizures
  Post–tachycardia T-wave inversion
  Post–pacemaker T-wave inversion
  Intracranial pathology (central nervous system hemorrhage)
  Mitral valve prolapse
  Pericarditis
  Primary or secondary myocardial diseases
  Pulmonary embolism or cor pulmonale from other causes
  Spontaneous pneumothorax
  Myocardial contusion
  Left ventricular hypertrophy
  Ventricular paced rhythms
  Left bundle-branch block
  Right bundle-branch block

segment elevation and positive T waves. ST-segment elevation of at least 5 mm is the finding most indicative of AMI in leads with predominantly negative QRS complexes.[9] Any ST-segment elevation concordant to the QRS complex in a predominantly positive QRS complex is highly specific for AMI. The QRS complex is predominantly negative in leads V_1 to V_3 with RV pacing. ST-segment depression in these leads has 80 percent specificity for AMI.[9]

Serum Markers of Myocardial Injury

The utility of serum markers depends on their ability to detect and risk-stratify patients with ACS (Table 50-6). For example, patients with diagnostic ST-segment elevation on their initial ECG do not require serum marker measurement to make appropriate treatment and disposition decisions. Conversely, serum markers are useful in patients with nondiagnostic ECGs for both diagnosis and risk stratification.[10–14] Markers vary in terms of their molecular weight, cellular location, solubility, plasma concentration, clearance, and ability to be detected accurately in serum with rapid immunochemical techniques. In general, serial measurements are more sensitive and accurate than initial single measurements, and serial sampling every 2 to 3 h is a validated practice for the rapid exclusion of AMI in acute chest pain patients.

Serum markers have less utility in the diagnosis of UA, only about half or less of these patients will demonstrate low levels of troponin elevation. Conversely, these low-level troponin elevations are independent risk factors for acute (<30 d) cardiac complications and short-term (<1 y) prognosis in UA.[12–14]

The creatine kinase MB isoenzyme (CK-MB) is the most commonly used serum marker in ACS. A serial rise in CK-MB to above five times baseline followed by a fall back to baseline is considered diagnostic for AMI. Sensitive mass assays are widely available, and quantitative point-of-care testing technology is available to use at the bedside. The typical time course for CK-MB rise following an AMI is a peak value at 12 to 24 h, with a fall back to baseline in 2 to 3 d. CK-MB is useful for detecting recurrent infarction after the initial 1 to 2 d by noting a repeat elevation in its level.

The troponin complex is the main regulatory protein for the actin-myosin myofibrils. This complex consists of three subunits: an inhibitory subunit (troponin I), tropomyosin-binding subunit (troponin T), and a calcium-binding subunit (troponin C). Isoforms of both troponins I and T specific to cardiac muscle have been identified. In fact, the cardiac isoform of troponin I (cTnI) has not been identified in skeletal muscle during any stage of development, whereas low levels of the cardiac isoform of troponin T (cTnT) has been found in various skeletal muscle disorders. Assays for both troponins have undergone several generations of development, and currently available tests are highly specific. The typical time course for troponin rise following an AMI is a peak level in 12 h with a prolonged elevation for 7 to 10 d before returning to baseline. This sustained presence makes either troponin useful for diagnosis of AMI when the patient presents days after symptom onset. However, because of the prolonged elevation, troponins are not useful for detecting recurrent infarction during initial hospitalization.

A rise in serum troponin I or T is now accepted as diagnostic for AMI.[15] Low-level elevations in either troponin correlate with risk for cardiovascular complications in UA, CAD, and renal failure.[12–14]

Cardiac Imaging

Echocardiography and nuclear scintigraphy have a complimentary role in the diagnosis and assessment of ACS patients. Echocardiography, using the criterion of regional wall motion abnormalities, has been reported to have a high sensitivity (above 90 percent) for AMI.[16] However, this imaging study is operator-dependent, many patients have technically inadequate studies, and specificity for AMI is only 50 to 60 percent. Echocardiography is more useful in assessing the extent of myocardial impairment for risk-stratification and detecting complications of acute infarction.[17]

Nuclear scintigraphy using technetium-99m sestamibi is a radionuclide that is taken up by the myocardium in proportion to myocardial blood flow at the time of injection. This allows administration of the isotope during symptomatic episodes but enables imaging after patient stabilization. Technetium sestamibi scanning is highly sensitive and specific for CAD and has short-term (<1 y) predictive value in patients with acute chest pain.[16] Sestamibi scanning is useful in the ACS patient who does not have serial ECG or serum marker changes of AMI and is not a candidate for standard stress testing.

COMPLICATIONS OF MYOCARDIAL INFARCTION AND ISCHEMIA

Myocardial perfusion and cardiac function affect blood flow to the entire body. As a result, any end organ can be damaged when cardiac pump function is decreased. In this section, discussion of the complications of ACS is limited to the direct effects on the heart. The systemic effects of cardiac function are discussed in organ-appropriate

TABLE 50-6 Summary of Predictive Properties of Cardiac Markers of Diagnosis of Acute Myocardial Infarction

Marker	Studies, n	Subjects, n	Sensitivity (95% CI)	Specificity (95% CI)	Diagnostic Odds Ratio (95% CI)
At time of presentation					
CK	12	3195	37 (31–44)	87 (80–91)	3.9 (2.7–5.7)
CK-MB	19	6425	42 (36–48)	97 (95–98)	25 (18–36)
Myoglobin	18	4172	49 (53–55)	91 (87–94)	11 (8–15)
Troponin I	4	1149	39 (10–78)	93 (88–97)	11 (3.4–34)
Troponin T	6	1348	39 (26–53)	93 (90–96)	9.5 (5.7–16)
CK-MB and myoglobin	3	2283	83 (51–96)	82 (68–90)	17 (7.6–40)
Serial markers					
CK	2	786	69–99	68–84	12–220
CK-MB	14	11,625	79 (71–86)	96 (95–97)	140 (65–310)
Myoglobin	10	1277	89 (80–94)	87 (80–92)	84 (44–160)
Troponin I	2	1393	90–100	83–96	230–460
Troponin T	3	904	93 (85–97)	85 (76–91)	83 (33–210)
CK-MB and myoglobin	2	291	100	75–91	4.3–14

Abbreviations: CI = confidence interval; CK = creatine kinase; CK-MB = creatine kinase and muscle and brain subdomains.
Source: Lau J, Ioannidis JPA, Balk EM, et al: Diagnosing acute cardiac ischemia in the emergency department: A systematic review of the accuracy and clincial effect of current technologies. *Ann Emerg Med* 37:453, 2001.

chapters of this book. The treatment of these complications is discussed in Chap. 51.

Dysrhythmias and Conduction Disturbances

The genesis, diagnosis, and treatment of dysrhythmias are presented in Chap. 28. The effect dysrhythmias have in complicating the course of patients with ACSs is the subject of this section.

Dysrhythmias occur in 72 to 100 percent of AMI patients treated in the coronary care unit.[18] Table 50-7 shows the approximate frequency of the various dysrhythmias observed in patients with AMI. Many of these dysrhythmias occur in the prehospital and ED settings. The main consequence of these dysrhythmias is that they may impair hemodynamic performance, compromise myocardial viability by increasing myocardial oxygen requirements, and predispose to even more serious rhythm disturbances by diminishing the ventricular fibrillation threshold.

Early in the course of AMI, patients frequently exhibit evidence of increased autonomic nervous system activity. Sinus bradycardia, atrioventricular block, and hypotension may occur from increased vagal tone. Activation of atrial and ventricular receptors in the myocardium may result in enhanced efferent sympathetic activity, increased circulating catecholamines, and increased local catecholamine release. These increased catecholamines in the setting of a sensitive myocardium form the substrate for the generation of tachyarrhythmias. Electrical instability during AMI results in ventricular premature beats, ventricular tachycardia, ventricular fibrillation, accelerated idioventricular rhythms, and some AV junctional tachycardias.

The hemodynamic consequences of dysrhythmias are dependent on ventricular function. Patients with left ventricular dysfunction have a relatively fixed stroke volume. They depend on changes in heart rate to alter cardiac output. The range of heart rate that is optimal becomes narrowed with increasing dysfunction. Slower or faster heart rates may further depress cardiac output.

In addition, maintenance of the atrial kick is important for patients with AMI. Patients with normal hearts have a loss of 10 to 20 percent of left ventricular output when the atrial kick is eliminated. Patients with reduced left ventricular compliance, as occurs from AMI, have up to 35 percent reduction in stroke volume when the atrial systole is eliminated.

TABLE 50-7 Frequency of Occurrence of Arrhythmias During Acute Myocardial Infarction

Arrhythmia	Frequency of Occurrence, %
Bradydysrhythmias	
Sinus bradycardia	15–40
First-degree AV block	4–14
Second-degree AV block, type I	4–10
Second-degree AV block, type II	<1
Third-degree AV block	5–8
Asystole	1–14
Tachydysrhythmias	
Sinus tachycardia	33
Atrial premature contractions	50
Supraventricular tachycardia	2–11
Atrial fibrillation	10–15
Atrial flutter	1–3
Ventricular premature beats	>90
Accelerated idioventricular rhythm	8–20
Ventricular tachycardia	10–40
Ventricular fibrillation	4–18

Abbreviation: AV = atrioventricular.
Source: Pasternack RC, Braunwald E, Sobel BE: Acute myocardial infarction, in Braunwald E (ed): *Heart Disease. A Textbook of Cardiovascular Medicine,* 4th ed. Philadelphia, WB Saunders, 1992, pp. 1239–1245.

"Pump" failure with resultant increased sympathetic stimulation results in sinus tachycardia, atrial fibrillation or flutter, and supraventricular tachycardias. Conduction disturbances result in bradydysrhythmias, such as sinus bradycardia, junctional escape rhythms, and atrioventricular and idioventricular blocks.

The significance of cardiac dysrhythmias during AMI is the subject of some debate. On the one hand, sinus bradycardia during the early phases of AMI may predispose to hypotension and repetitive ventricular dysrhythmias. On the other hand, it appears to be protective, because it reduces the myocardial oxygen requirement. The net effect is that the presence of sinus bradycardia does not appear to increase mortality during AMI.

Almost all patients with first-degree AV block have infranodal disturbances above the His bundle and will not progress to higher degrees of AV block. Mobitz I (Wenckebach) accounts for 90 percent of second-degree AV block. It generally occurs within the AV node, is associated with narrow QRS complexes, and results from ischemic injury. It is more common with inferior than with anterior AMI, is intermittent usually during the first 72 h after infarction, and rarely progresses to complete heart block or other pathologic rhythm. Conversely, Mobitz II second-degree heart block originates from conduction lesions below the His bundle, is associated with a wide QRS complex, is usually associated with anterior AMI, and does progress to complete heart block.

Complete heart block can occur in patients with anterior and inferior AMI, because the atrioventricular conduction system receives blood supply from the AV branch of the right coronary artery and the septal perforating branch of the left anterior descending coronary artery. Complete heart block occurs in the setting of inferior myocardial infarction; it usually progresses from lesser forms of AV block.[19] This form of third-degree block is usually stable and should resolve. In the absence of right ventricular involvement, the mortality is approximately 15 percent. It rises to greater than 30 percent when right ventricular involvement is present. In contrast, complete heart block in the setting of an anterior MI is seldom benign and portends a grave prognosis. Junctional rhythms are usually transient and occur within 48 h of infarction. Whether they affect long-term prognosis is not clear.

Sinus tachycardia is quite prominent in patients with anterior wall AMI. Because of increased myocardial oxygen use, persistent sinus tachycardia is associated with a poor prognosis. The etiology of the sinus tachycardia should be determined. It may include anxiety, pain, left ventricular failure, fever, pericarditis, hypovolemia, atrial infarction, pulmonary emboli, or use of medications that accelerate heart rate. Similarly, paroxysmal supraventricular tachycardia, atrial fibrillation, and atrial flutter are associated with an increased mortality. Atrial premature contractions are common. They occur in up to 50 percent of AMI patients and are not associated with an increased mortality related to the acute event.

Ventricular premature contractions are common in patients with AMI. They do not appear to have much prognostic ability. Accelerated idioventricular rhythms in patients with AMI have not been shown to have an effect on prognosis. Ventricular tachycardia shortly after AMI is often transient and does not portend a poor prognosis. When ventricular tachycardia occurs late in the course of AMI, it is usually associated with transmural infarction and left ventricular dysfunction, induces hemodynamic deterioration, and is associated with a mortality rate approaching 50 percent. Primary ventricular fibrillation occurring shortly after symptom onset does not appear to have a large effect on mortality and prognosis. Delayed or secondary ventricular fibrillation during hospitalization is associated with severe ventricular dysfunction and a 75 percent in-hospital mortality.

Intraventricular conduction disturbances occur in 10 to 20 percent of patients with AMI. Approximately half of these disturbances are already present at the time of ED presentation and may not represent a new finding. Blood supply to the anterior division of the left bundle branch comes from septal perforators of the left anterior descending coronary artery. The right bundle branch and the posterior division of the left bundle branch obtain a dual blood flow from the left anterior descending and right coronary arteries. For this reason, left anterior hemiblock is more common.

New right bundle-branch block occurs in approximately 2 percent of AMI patients, most commonly anteroseptal AMI, and is associated with an increased mortality, because it often leads to complete AV block. New left bundle-branch block occurs in 5 percent of patients with AMI and is associated with a high mortality. The left posterior fascicle is larger than the left anterior fascicle. Thus, left posterior hemiblock is associated with a higher mortality than is isolated left anterior hemiblock, because it represents a larger area of infarction. Bifascicular block (right bundle-branch block and a left hemiblock) is associated with an increased likelihood of progression to complete heart block; it represents a large infarction and is associated with an increased likelihood of pump failure and mortality.[19] Other combinations of heart block and their treatment are discussed in Chap. 28.

Cardiac Failure

Some 15 to 20 percent of patients with AMI present in some degree of congestive heart failure. One third of these patients have circulatory shock. In the setting of AMI, congestive heart failure can occur through diastolic dysfunction alone or a combination of systolic and diastolic dysfunction. Left ventricular diastolic dysfunction leads to pulmonary congestion. Systolic dysfunction is responsible for decreased forward flow, reduced cardiac output, and reduced ejection fraction. In general, the more severe the degree of left ventricular dysfunction, the higher the mortality. The degree of left ventricular dysfunction in any single patient is dependent on the net effect of prior myocardial dysfunction (prior MI or cardiomyopathy), baseline myocardial hypertrophy, acute myocardial necrosis, and acute reversible myocardial dysfunction ("stunned myocardium").

Patients with AMI can be classified into four subsets based on hemodynamic status (Forrester-Diamond-Swan classification) and clinical status (Killip classification), shown in Tables 50-8 and 50-9. These classifications are useful to guide therapy and predict response to treatment. Patients with decreasing cardiac output or increasing pulmonary congestion have an increasingly higher mortality in the setting of AMI. Class I patients have a mortality of 2 to 5 percent. Class IV patients (i.e., those with cardiogenic shock) are at very high risk of mortality (50 to 80 percent). B-type natriuretic peptide, a powerful predictor of outcome in patients with congestive heart failure, is also useful for risk stratification of patients with non-ST-segment elevation

TABLE 50-8 Forrester-Diamond-Swan Hemodynamic Classification

Class	Cardic Index L/min per m^2	Pulmonary Artery Wedge Pressure, mm Hg	Approximate Mortality, %
I: No pulmonary congestion or hypoperfusion	>2.2	<18	2–3
II: Isolated pulmonary congestion	>2.2	>18	10
III: Isolated peripheral hypoperfusion	<2.2	<18	2–25
IV: Pulmonary congestion and peripheral hypoperfusion	<2.2	>18	50–55

TABLE 50-9 Killip Clinical Classification

Class	Approximate Mortality, %
I: No congestive heart failure	5
II: Mild congestive heart failure (bibasilar rales and an S$_3$)	15–20
III: Frank pulmonary edema	40
IV: Cardiogenic shock	80

myocardial infarction and unstable angina. Elevated levels of BNP early in the hospital course portend a worse 30-day outcome.[20]

The presence of shock in AMI results in a complex spiral relationship. Coronary obstruction leads to myocardial ischemia, which in turn impairs myocardial contractility and ventricular outflow. The resulting reduction in arterial blood pressure leads to further decreases in coronary arterial perfusion, resulting in worsening myocardial ischemia and more severe myocardial necrosis. Interruption of this downward spiral requires careful attention to fluid management and the use of inotropic agents.[21] Resolution of ischemia and preventing or minimizing the area of stunned myocardium that progresses to infarction is imperative.

Mechanical Complications of AMI

Sudden decompensation of previously stable patients should always raise concern of the "mechanical" complications of AMI. As a group, these complications usually involve the tearing or rupture of infarcted tissue. Therefore, they are unlikely to occur in patients with non-AMI ACSs. The clinical presentation of these entities depends on the site of rupture (papillary muscles, interventricular septum, or ventricular free wall).

Free wall rupture occurs in 10 percent of AMI fatalities, usually 1 to 5 days after infarction. Rupture of the left ventricular free wall usually leads to pericardial tamponade and death (in more than 90 percent of cases). Patients may complain of tearing pain or sudden onset of severe pain. They will be hypotensive and tachycardic and may have onset of confusion and agitation. Increased neck veins, decreased heart sounds, and pulsus paradoxus may be present. Echocardiography is the diagnostic test of choice, although near equalization of right atrial, right ventricular mid-diastolic, and right ventricular systolic pressures on pulmonary artery catheterization may also be useful. Treatment is surgical.

Rupture has been attributed to intense necrosis at the distal end of blood supply, poor collateral blood flow, and a thin apical left ventricular wall in conjunction with the shearing effects of muscle contraction. Anti-inflammatory medications, steroids, and late administration of thrombolytic agents have been linked to an increased likelihood of cardiac rupture. However, studies remain contradictory. The elderly appear to be more prone to cardiac rupture. Left ventricular hypertrophy appears to be protective.

Rupture of the interventricular septum is more often detected clinically than rupture of the ventricular free wall, despite the fact that rupture of the ventricular free wall is more commonly detected in autopsy studies. The size of the defect determines the degree of left-to-right shunt and the ultimate prognosis. Clinically, interventricular septal rupture presents with chest pain, dyspnea, and sudden appearance of a new holosystolic murmur. The murmur is usually accompanied by a palpable thrill and is heard best at the lower left sternal border. Doppler echocardiography is the diagnostic procedure of choice. Demonstration of left-to-right shunt by pulmonary catheter blood sampling may be useful. An oxygen step-up of more than 10 percent from right atrial to right ventricular samples is diagnostic. Rupture of the interventricular septum is more common in patients with anterior wall myocardial infarction and patients with extensive (three-vessel) CAD.

Papillary muscle rupture occurs in approximately 1 percent of patients with AMI, is more common with inferior myocardial infarction, and usually occurs 3 to 5 days after AMI. In contrast to rupture of the interventricular septum, papillary muscle rupture often occurs with a small to modest-sized AMI. Patients may have relatively limited CAD. Patients present with acute onset of dyspnea, increasing degree of congestive heart failure, and a new holosystolic murmur consistent with mitral regurgitation. The posteromedial papillary muscle is most commonly ruptured, because it receives blood supply from one coronary artery, usually the right coronary artery. Echocardiography often can distinguish rupture of a portion of the papillary muscle from other etiologies of mitral regurgitation. Treatment is surgical.

Pericarditis

Post-AMI pericarditis occurs in 10 to 20 percent of patients. It is more common in patients with transmural AMI. It results from inflammation adjacent to the pericardium on the epicardial surface of a transmural infarction. It generally occurs 2 to 4 days after AMI. Pericardial friction rubs are detected more often with inferior wall and right ventricular infarction, because the right ventricle lies immediately beneath the chest wall. The pain of pericarditis can be confused with that of infarct extension or post-AMI angina. Classically, the discomfort of pericarditis becomes worse with a deep inspiration and may be somewhat relieved by sitting forward. Echocardiography may demonstrate a pericardial effusion, but pericardial effusions are much more common than pericarditis and often are present in the absence of pericarditis. Similarly, pericarditis can be present in the absence of a pericardial effusion. The resorption rate of post-AMI pericardial effusions is slow, often taking several months. Dressler syndrome (post-AMI syndrome) occurs 2 to 10 weeks after AMI and presents as chest pain, fever, and pleuropericarditis.

Right Ventricular Infarction

Isolated right ventricular infarction is extremely rare, and it is usually seen as a complication of an inferior infarction. The right ventricle most commonly receives its blood supply from the right coronary artery. In patients with left dominant systems, the blood supply may come from the left circumflex. The anterior portion of the right ventricle is supplied by branches of the left anterior diagonal artery. Approximately 30 percent of inferior wall myocardial infarctions involve the right ventricle. The presence of right ventricular infarction is associated with a significant increase in mortality and cardiovascular complications. Right ventricular infarction can be diagnosed by the presence of ST-segment elevation in the precordial V_{4R} lead in the setting of an inferior wall myocardial infarction. The presence of elevated neck veins or hypotension in response to nitroglycerin is also suggestive. Echocardiography or nuclear imaging can be diagnostic, but they are less readily available in the ED.

The most serious complication of right ventricular infarction is shock. The severity of the hemodynamic derangement in the setting of right ventricular infarction is related to the extent of right ventricular dysfunction, the interaction between the ventricles (the right and left ventricles share the interventricular septum), and the interaction between the pericardium and the right ventricle. Right ventricular infarction results in a reduction in right ventricular end-systolic pressure, left ventricular end-diastolic size, cardiac output, and aortic pressure as the right ventricle becomes more of a passive conduit to blood flow. Left ventricular contraction causes bulging of the interventricular septum into the right ventricle, with resultant ejection of blood into the pulmonary circulation. As a result, right ventricular infarction with concurrent left ventricular infarction has a particularly devastating effect on hemodynamic function. Fluid balance and maintenance of adequate preload are critical in the treatment of right ventricular infarction. Treatment of right ventricular infarction is discussed in Chap. 51.

Other Complications

Other complications of AMI that occur but are not usually seen in the ED include left ventricular thrombus formation, arterial embolization, venous thrombosis, pulmonary embolism, postinfarction angina, and infarct extension. With the more rapid discharge of uncomplicated AMI patients, the emergency physician should keep these possibilities in mind for patients who return to the ED shortly after hospital discharge.

SPECIFIC ISSUES

Age, Gender, and Diabetes Mellitus

The patient's age and gender and the presence or absence of diabetes mellitus play a role in the presentation of patients with ACS. Advanced age, female gender, and a history of diabetes mellitus are associated with more atypical presentations. However, there is no evidence that AMI patients should be evaluated differently in the ED as a result of age or gender.

Postprocedure Chest Pain

Patients who present with symptoms of an ACS shortly after percutaneous coronary interventions such as angioplasty or stent placement should be assumed to have had abrupt vessel closure until proven otherwise. Subacute thrombotic occlusion after stent placement occurs in approximately 4 percent of patients 2 to 14 days postprocedure. Although less common than closure after percutaneous transluminal coronary angioplasty, it is associated with a high likelihood of major ischemic complications. Patients should be treated aggressively for an ACS, and cardiology or interventional cardiology consultation should be obtained. Patients with chest pain syndromes after coronary artery bypass grafting also may have abrupt vessel closure; however, symptoms of recurrent ischemia can be confused with post-AMI pericarditis, as discussed above.

Cocaine Chest Pain

Chest pain associated with cocaine use is discussed in Chap. 168.

DISPOSITION

All patients with acute chest pain need to be evaluated for the possibility of ACS.[22] Based on the initial history, physical examination, and ECG, patients can be subclassified into those with and without known CAD. Patients with known CAD should be subclassified further into those who meet criteria for AMI (and may or may not meet criteria for reperfusion therapy), those with a stable anginal pattern who do not require acute intervention, and those with unstable angina. Patients with unstable angina should be treated according to their risk for AMI and death (see Table 50-3).

Patients without known CAD who do not have an obvious myocardial infarction should be evaluated for their likelihood of CAD (Table 50-10) and the possibility of an alternative diagnosis (not ischemic heart disease). Those with a clear alternative diagnosis should be treated accordingly. Those with risks for CAD should be referred for appropriate outpatient evaluation.

Patients at high risk of AMI or death should be admitted to an intensive care unit (ICU). Moderate-risk patients should be admitted to a non-ICU monitored setting. Patients at low risk can be treated in a non-ICU monitored setting or can be observed in an ED observation unit. Emergency department observation units and non-ICU monitored settings are

TABLE 50-10   Likelihood of Significant Coronary Artery Disease in Patients with Symptoms Suggesting Unstable Angina

High Likelihood (85–99%)	Intermediate Likelihood (15–84%)	Low Likelihood (1–14%)
Any of the following features	*Absence of high-likelihood features and any of the following*	*Absence of high- or intermediate-likelihood features but may have*
History of prior AMI, sudden death, or other known history of CAD	Definite angina; males <60 or females <70 years of age	Chest pain classified as probably not angina
Definite angina: males ≥60 or females ≥70 y of age	Probable angina: males ≥60 or females ≥70 y of age	One risk factor other than diabetes
Transient hemodynamic or ECG changes during pain	Chest pain probably not angina in patients with diabetes	T-wave flattening or inversion <1 mm in leads with dominant R waves
Variant angina (pain with reversible ST-segment elevation)	Chest pain probably not angina and 2 or 3 risk factors other than diabetes	Normal ECG
ST-segment elevation or depression ≥1 mm	Extracardiac vascular disease	
Marked symmetric T-wave inversion in multiple precordial leads	ST depression 0.05–1 mm	
	T-wave inversion ≥1 mm in leads with dominant R waves	

Abbreviations: AMI = acute myocardial infarction; CAD = coronary artery disease; ECG = electrocardiogram.
Source: Braunwald E, Mark DB, Jones RH, et al: *Unstable Angina: Diagnosis and Management.* Clincal Practice Guideline No. 10 (amended). AHCPR Publication No. 94-0602. Rockville, MD, Agency for Health Care Policy and Research and the National Health, Lung and Blood Institute, Public Health Service, U.S. Department of Health and Human Services, 1994.

safe and cost-effective for patients with a normal ECG and other low-risk clinical features. Prior invasive and noninvasive assessments of cardiac function should be taken into account in making disposition decisions. Patients known to have severe CAD or depressed left ventricular function might be triaged to a more intensive setting than patients with a similar presentation without such dysfunction.

Results of prior cardiac catheterization are very useful for risk stratification. Patients who have previously been documented to have minimal (<25 percent) stenosis or normal coronary arteriograms have an excellent long-term prognosis. More than 98 percent of patients with this profile are free from myocardial infarction 10 years later.[23] Repeat cardiac catheterizations an average of 9 years later found that approximately 90 percent of patients did not develop even single-vessel CAD. Thus, a recent (within the past 2 years) cardiac catheterization with normal or minimally diseased vessels almost eliminates the possibility of an ACS due to atherosclerosis. It would not eliminate the possibility of vasospasm or small vessel disease (syndrome X). Without other complicating circumstances, even observation protocols are unnecessary.

Stress tests are less useful because the precise results of such tests may not be available. When patients complete all stages of the stress protocol, have no ECG changes, and have normal imaging studies, exercise testing can rule out acute ischemic syndromes with sensitivities in the range of 80 to 90 percent. When patients do not meet their target heart rates, exercise testing has poor sensitivity (<80 percent), leading to false-negative results. Unless the patient reached the maximal heart rate (220 beats/min minus the patient's age), had no ECG changes, and had normal imaging (when done), one cannot rely heavily on the results of prior exercise testing in making disposition decisions. The emergency practitioner should read the actual stress report before accepting that it was a "negative" test. However, a negative exercise stress test that meets these criteria predicts a favorable 1-year survival free of cardiac events.

REFERENCES

1. Braunwald E, Mark DB, Jones RH, et al: *Unstable Angina: Diagnosis and Management.* Clinical Practice Guideline No. 10 (amended). AHCPR Publication No. 94-0602. Rockville, MD, Agency for Health Care Policy and Research and the National Health, Lung and Blood Institute, Public Health Service, U.S. Department of Health and Human Services, 1994.
2. Jayes RL, Beshansky JR, D'Agostino RB, Selker HP: Do patients' coronary risk factor reports predict acute cardiac ischemia in the emergency department? A multicenter study. *J Clin Epidemiol* 45:621, 1992.
3. Lee T, Cook F, Weisberg M, et al: Acute chest pain in the emergency room: Identification and examination of low-risk patients. *Arch Intern Med* 145:65, 1985.
4. Selker HP, Zalenski RJ, Antman EM, et al: An evaluation of technologies for identification of acute cardiac ischemia in the emergency department: A report from a National Heart Attack Alert Program Working Group. *Ann Emerg Med* 29:13, 1997.
5. Slater DK, Hlatky MA, Mark DB, et al: Outcome in suspected acute myocardial infarction with normal or minimally abnormal admission electrocardiographic findings. *Am J Cardiol* 60:766, 1987.
6. Brush JE, Brand DA, Acampora D, et al: Use of the initial electrocardiogram to predict in-hospital complications of acute myocardial infarction. *New Engl J Med* 312:1137, 1985.
7. Zalenski RJ, Cooke D, Rydman R, et al: Assessing the diagnostic value of an ECG containing leads V_{4R}, V_8 and V_9: The 15-lead ECG. *Ann Emerg Med* 22:786, 1993.
8. Sgarbossa EB, Pinski SL, Barbagelata A, et al: Electrocardiographic diagnosis of evolving acute myocardial infarction in the presence of left bundle branch block. *New Engl J Med* 334:481, 1996.
9. Sgarbossa EB, Pinski SL, Gates KB, Wagner GS, for GUSTO-1 Investigators: Early electrocardiographic diagnosis of acute myocardial infarction in the presence of ventricular paced rhythm. *Am J Cardiol* 77:423, 1996.
10. Hedges JR, Young GP, Henkel GF, et al: Early CK-MB elevations predict ischemic events in stable chest pain patients. *Acad Emerg Med* 1:9, 1994.
11. Hoekstra JW, Hedges JR, Gibler WB, et al: Emergency department CK-MB: A predictor of ischemic complications. *Acad Emerg Med* 1:17, 1994.
12. Green GB, Li DJ, Bessman ES, et al: The prognostic significance of troponin I and troponin T. *Acad Emerg Med* 5:758, 1998.
13. Antman EM, Tanasijevic MJ, Thompson B, et al: Cardiac specific troponin I levels predict the risk of mortality in patients with acute coronary syndromes. *New Engl J Med* 335:1342, 1996.
14. Ohman EM, Armstrong PW, Christenson RH, et al: Cardiac troponin-T levels for risk stratification in acute myocardial ischemia. *New Engl J Med* 335:1333, 1996.
15. Alpert JS, Thygesen K, Antman E, et al: Myocardial infarction redefined—A censensus document of the Joint European Society of Cardiology/American College of Cardiology Committee for the redefinition of MI. *J Am Coll Cardiol* 36:959, 2000.

16. Mather PJ, Shah R: Echocardiography, nuclear scientigraphy, and stress testers in the emergency department evaluation of acute coronary artery syndrome. *Emerg Med Clin North Am* 19:339, 2001.

17. Fleischmann KE, Lee TH, Come PC, et al: Echocardiographic prediction of complications in patients with chest pain. *Am J Cardiol* 79:292, 1997.

18. Aufderheide TP: Arrhythmias associated with acute myocardial infarction and thrombolysis. *Emerg Med Clin North Am* 16:583, 1998.

19. Escosteguy CC, Caryalho Mde A, Medronha Rde A, et al: Bundle branch and atrioventricular block as complications of acute myocardial infarction in the thrombolyte era. *Arg Bras Cardiol* 76:291, 2001.

20. DeLemos JA, Morrow DA, Bentley JH, et al: The prognostic value of B-type natriuretic peptide in patients with acute coronary syndromes. *New Engl J Med* 345;1014, 2001.

21. Menon V, Hochman JS: Management of cardiogenic shock complicating acute myocardial infarction. *Heart* 88:531, 2002.

22. Tatum JL, Jesse RL, Kontos MC, et al: Comprehensive strategy for the evaluation and triage of the chest pain patient. *Ann Emerg Med* 29:116, 1997.

23. Pitts WR, Lange RA, Cigarroa JE, Hillis LD: Repeat coronary angiography in patients with chest pain and previously normal coronary angiogram. *Am J Cardiol* 80:1086, 1997.

51 INTERVENTION STRATEGIES FOR ACUTE CORONARY SYNDROMES

Judd E. Hollander

Deborah B. Diercks

The treatment of acute coronary syndromes (ACSs) is individualized based on duration and persistence of symptoms, cardiac history, and findings on physical examination and the initial electrocardiogram. Generally speaking, patients with persistent symptoms and ST-segment elevation myocardial infarction (STEMI) should receive fibrinolytic therapy or mechanical reperfusion (angioplasty). Treatment with antiplatelet agents, anticoagulants, β-antagonists, nitrates, and angiotensin-converting enzyme (ACE) inhibitors should be considered, based on symptoms, vital signs, and the presence or absence of heart failure. Patients with unstable angina or non-STEMI (NSTEMI) should be treated with antiplatelet agents and anticoagulants and possibly β-antagonists and nitrates. Patients refractory to these therapies or patients scheduled to undergo percutaneous coronary intervention (PCI) also benefit from the use of glycoprotein (GP) IIb/IIIa antagonists. Diagnosis of ACS is discussed in Chap. 50.

GENERAL MEASURES

Intravenous access and continued electrocardiographic monitoring should be established in all patients with ACSs. Supplemental oxygen may reduce ST-segment elevation in patients with acute myocardial infarction (AMI). It is therefore reasonable to provide 2 to 4 L of oxygen routinely by nasal cannula, even to patients with normal oxygen saturation. In patients with unstable angina or NSTEMI, O_2 should be provided in patients with signs of hypoxia. Treatment strategies aim to achieve immediate reperfusion and limit infarct size (Table 51-1 and Figure 51-1).

REPERFUSION

Reperfusion therapies can be mechanical or pharmacologic. Angioplasty, coronary stent placement, and atherectomy are the major methods of mechanical reperfusion. Pharmacologic interventions include fibrinolytic and antiplatelet therapy.

Fibrinolytics

Fibrinolytic agents act on the acute thrombosis directly or indirectly as plasminogen activators. Plasminogen, an inactive proteolytic enzyme,

TABLE 51-1   Recommended Doses of Drugs Used in the Emergency Treatment of Acute Coronary Syndromes

Antiplatelet agents	
Aspirin	160–325 mg PO
Clopidogrel	Loading dose of 300 mg PO followed by 75 mg/d
Antithrombins	
Heparin	Bolus of 60–70 units/kg (maximum, 5000 units) followed by infusion of 12–15 units/kg per h (maximum, 1000 units/h) titrated to a PTT 1.5–2.5 times control
Enoxaparin (LMWH)	1 mg/kg SC q12h
Fibrinolytic agents	
Streptokinase	1.5 million units over 60 min
Alteplase (tPA)	Body weight >67 kg: 15 mg initial IV bolus; 50 mg infused over next 30 min; 35 mg infused over next 60 min
	Body weight <67 kg: 15 mg initial IV bolus; 0.75 mg/kg infused over next 30 min; 0.5 mg/kg infused over next 60 min
Reteplase (rPA)	10 mg IV bolus followed by 10 mg IV bolus 30 min later

Tenecteplase (TNKase)	Weight	Dose*
	<60 kg	30 mg
	≥60 but <70 kg	35 mg
	≥70 but <80 kg	40 mg
	≥80 but <90	45 mg
	≥90	50 mg
	*Total dose not to exceed 50 mg	

Glycoprotein IIb/IIIa inhibitors	
Abciximab	0.25 mg/kg bolus followed by infusion of 0.125 μg/kg per min (maximum, 10 μg/min) for 12–24 h
Eptifibatide	180 μg/kg bolus followed by infusion of 2.0 μg/kg per min for 72–96 h
Tirofiban	0.4 μg/kg per min for 30 min followed by infusion of 0.1 μg/kg per min for 48–96 h
Other anti-ischemic therapies	
Nitroglycerin	SL: 0.4 mg q5 min × 3 prn pain
	IV: start at 10 μg/min, titrate to 10% reduction in MAP if normotensive, 30% reduction in MAP if hypertensive
Morphine	2–5 mg IV q5–15 min prn pain
Metoprolol	5 mg IV over 2 min q5 min up to 15 mg, followed by 50 mg PO q6h 15 min after last IV dose
Atenolol	5 mg IV over 5 min, repeat once 10 min later, followed with 50 mg PO

Abbreviation: MAP = mean arterial pressure; PTT = partial thromboplastin time; SL = sublingual.

binds directly to fibrin during thrombus formation to form a plasminogen-fibrin complex. This plasminogen-fibrin complex is more susceptible than plasma plasminogen to activation, and this promotes fibrin proteolysis.

The original randomized controlled clinical trials (RCTs) comparing streptokinase with placebo for treatment of STEMI demonstrated that fibrinolytic therapy improves left ventricular function and short-term and long-term mortalities. A meta-analysis of all nine RCTs found that the net benefit of fibrinolytic treatment in the first 3 h was more than 30 lives saved per thousand patients. The loss of benefit-per-hour delay in fibrinolytic administration was 1.6 lives per 1000 patients per hour.

Fibrinolytic therapy is indicated for patients with symptoms compatible with AMI, if time to treatment is less than 6 to 12 h from symptom onset and the electrocardiogram has at least 1-mm ST-segment elevation in two or more contiguous leads.[1] Therapy is more beneficial if given early and for larger infarctions and anterior infarctions than for smaller or inferior infarctions. In the elderly, the overall risk of

FIG. 51–1. Treatment considerations for patients with acute coronary syndrome. *Preferred antithrombin. AMI = acute myocardial infarction; ECG = electrocardiogram; LBBB = left bundle-branch block; PCI = percutaneous intervention; UFH = unfractionated heparin.

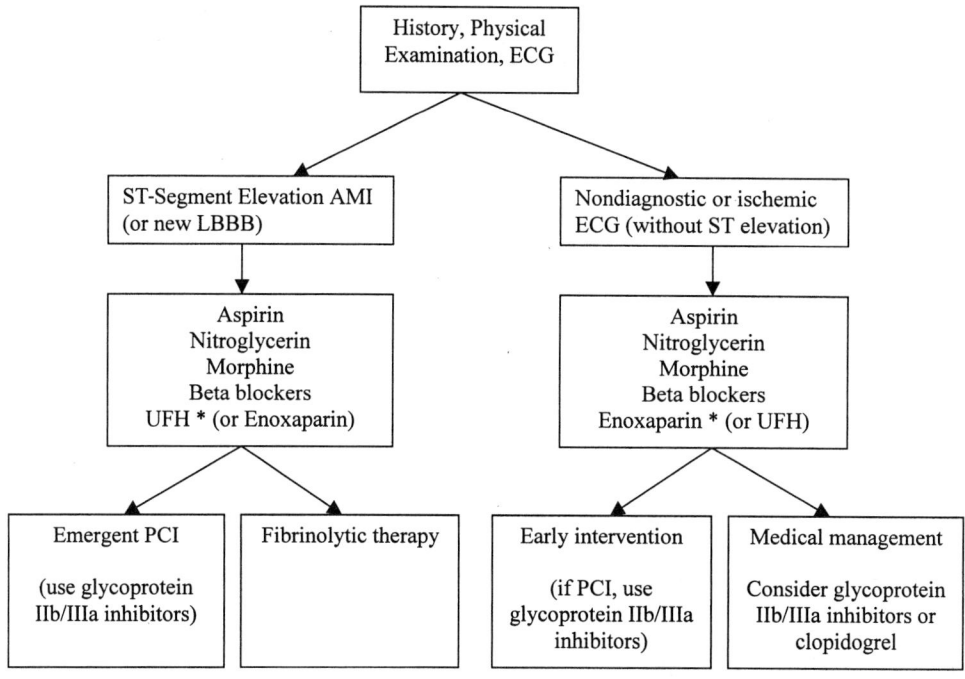

Note: See text for discussion of individual treatment options, indications, and contraindications

mortality from AMI is high. The proportionate reduction in mortality rate appears to be less in patients older than 75 years, but the absolute number of patients who may be saved is still considerable.

Contraindications to fibrinolytic therapy are those that increase the risk of hemorrhage (Table 51-2). The most catastrophic complication is intracranial bleeding. Clinical variables that can be assessed in the ED and predict an increased risk of intracranial hemorrhage are age (>65 years, odds ratio of 2.2), low body weight (<70 kg, odds ratio of 2.1), and hypertension on presentation (odds ratio of 2.0).[2] Intracranial hemorrhage is also more common with tissue plasminogen activator (tPA) than with streptokinase (odds ratio of 1.6). Patients with relative contraindications may still receive fibrinolytic therapy when the benefits of therapy outweigh the risks of the complications, but institutions with direct PCI availability should consider direct angioplasty over fibrinolytic therapy in the presence of relative contraindications. Although fibrinolytic therapy is the standard of care for patients with STEMI, it does have limitations. First, even the most potent fibrinolytic agents do not achieve early and complete restoration of coronary blood flow in 40 to 50 percent of patients. Fibrinolytics are plasminogen activators. When fibrin is lysed, thrombin is exposed. The exposed thrombin is one of the most potent biologic platelet activators known. As a result, the more fibrin that is lysed, the more thrombin is exposed and the more prothrombotic substrate is engendered. The second limitation of fibrinolytic therapy is that approximately 0.5 to 1 percent of patients have intracranial hemorrhage, which usually results in death or disabling stroke.

STREPTOKINASE Streptokinase is a polypeptide derived from β-hemolytic *Streptococcus* cultures. It binds 1:1 to plasminogen, causing a conformational change that activates the plasminogen-streptokinase complex. This complex cleaves peptide bonds on other plasminogen molecules to activate them. This activated complex does not have fibrin specificity. Streptokinase compared with placebo reduces mortality rate and improves left ventricular function in patients with STEMI.

Antibodies may develop after treatment, so retreatment is generally avoided. Streptokinase allergy can be seen in approximately 5 percent of patients treated for the first time, especially those with a recent *Streptococcus* infection. Self-limited allergic reactions usually respond to antihistamines. Fewer than 0.2 percent of patients experience a serious anaphylactic reaction. During intravenous administration, approximately 15 percent of patients will experience hypotension, which usually responds to decreasing the rate of infusion and volume

TABLE 51-2 Contraindications to Fibrinolytic Therapy in Acute Myocardial Infarction

Absolute contraindications
  Previous hemorrhagic stroke at any time
  Bland CVA in past year
  Known intracranial neoplasm
  Active internal bleeding (excluding menses)
  Suspected aortic dissection or pericarditis
Relative contraindications
  Severe uncontrolled blood pressure (>180/100 mm Hg)
  History of chronic severe hypertension
  History of prior CVA of known intracranial pathology not covered in
    contraindications
  Current use of anticoagulants with known INR >2–3
  Known bleeding diathesis
  Recent trauma (past 2 wk)
  Prolonged CPR (>10 min)
  Major surgery (<3 wk)
  Noncompressible vascular punctures (including subclavian and internal
    jugular central lines)
  Recent internal bleeding (2–4 wk)
  Prior streptokinase should not receive streptokinase
  Pregnancy
  Active peptic ulcer disease
  Other medical conditions likely to increase risk of bleeding

Abbreviations: CVA = cerebrovascular accident (stroke); INR = international normalized ratio.

expansion. Streptokinase produces a fibrinolytic state for up to 24 h. Streptokinase is less costly than other fibrinolytic agents.

TISSUE PLASMINOGEN ACTIVATOR Tissue plasminogen activator (tPA) is a naturally occurring enzyme produced by the vascular endothelium and other tissues. It has a binding site for fibrin that allows it to attach to a formed thrombus and trigger fibrinolysis (fibrin specificity). Tissue plasminogen activator achieves higher infarct-related artery patency rates than does streptokinase. Three large RCTs have compared streptokinase with tPA. GISSI-2 (>20,000 patients) found that tPA increases the rate of stroke or death at 5 per 1000 patients in comparison with streptokinase at 30 to 35 days.[2] ISIS-3 (27,000 patients) found a 1 per 1000 patient benefit in favor of tPA.[3] The GUSTO trial found a 5.4 per 1000 patient benefit in favor of tPA, which increased to 9 per 1000 patients when the accelerated tPA regimen was given.[4] As a result, when tPA is used as the fibrinolytic agent, the accelerated regimen is recommended (see Table 51-1).

Meta-analysis of these three mega-trials found no statistical difference between streptokinase and tPA with respect to the composite end point of stroke and death. Based on this analysis, the choice of which fibrinolytic agent to use is probably less relevant than the speed of fibrinolytic administration (which saves an additional 1.6 per 1000 lives per hour earlier when treatment is provided). In addition, it is reasonable to choose streptokinase over tPA when the risk for intracranial hemorrhage is highest (e.g., in the elderly), because tPA has an increased likelihood of resulting in hemorrhagic stroke.[1] Also, streptokinase is less expensive than other fibrinolysis agents.

The mechanism of improved benefit of tPA is early patency of the infarct-related vessel.[5] For tPA, streptokinase and subcutaneous heparin, streptokinase and intravenous heparin, and streptokinase and tPA, the patency rates at 90 min were 81, 56, 61, and 73 percent, respectively.[5] These patency rates were predictive of survival outcomes.

RETEPLASE Reteplase plasminogen activator (rPA) is a genetically engineered modification of tPA, with a prolonged half-life (18 vs 3 min) and reduced fibrin binding. Several smaller studies initially suggested that reteplase has a faster time to reperfusion. However, GUSTO III showed no clinically relevant difference in outcomes (mortality and stroke) between tPA and rPA. Reteplase can be given as a double bolus, 10 mg each, 30 min apart. The easy double-bolus administration is an advantage in the ED.

TENECTEPLASE Tenecteplase (TNK) is another tPA mutant with prolonged half-life, is resistant to endogenous plasminogen activator inhibitor 1 inactivation, and has high fibrin specificity and binding. In animal models, it produces more active and complete fibrinolysis with less risk of intracranial bleeding. In a large RCT study with AMI, there was no difference in 30-day mortality or intracranial hemorrhage rates between TNK and tPA.[6] Single-bolus administration makes this the easiest fibrinolytic agent to administer, but the requirement of weight-based dosing may not always be practical.

The choice of fibrinolytic agent is generally based on institution. Because tPA, rPA, and TNK have similar efficacy and safety profiles, the decision is usually based on other factors, such as ease of administration, cost, and the personal preference of the cardiologist and emergency physician.

Mechanical Reperfusion

Coronary angioplasty with or without stent placement is the most common PCI. Alternatives include atherectomy and laser angioplasty. Balloon angioplasty increases the size of the arterial lumen through endothelial denudation; cracking, splitting, and disruption of atherosclerotic plaque; dehiscence of intima and plaque from underlying media; and stretching or tearing of underlying media and adventitia. With successful dilatation, small amounts of arterial wall dissection and aneurysmal expansion may be seen. The greater the increase in luminal size, the lower is the risk of restenosis. However, more aggressive balloon inflation can be associated with excessive dissection, platelet deposition, thrombus formation, and plaque hemorrhage.

Alternative PCI procedures have been developed in an attempt to limit complications. Directional and rotational coronary atherectomy extract atherosclerotic tissue from the coronary artery. Excimer laser atherectomy vaporizes atheromatous tissue. It results in larger luminal diameters but has not reduced rates of restenosis or other complications associated with percutaneous angioplasty procedures.

Coronary stents are fenestrated stainless-steel tubes that are expanded by a balloon to provide scaffolding within the coronary arteries. The addition of antiplatelet therapies (in particular, GP IIb/IIIa inhibitors and clopidogrel) results in lower adverse events at 6 months compared with patients undergoing percutaneous transluminal coronary angioplasty (PTCA) or stent placement without GP IIb/IIIa inhibitors,[7] and these improved outcomes are apparent up to 3 years after the procedure.

Direct coronary angioplasty has compared favorably with fibrinolytic therapy for the treatment of patients with AMI. In centers with significant expertise in direct angioplasty, primary angioplasty as opposed to fibrinolytic therapy reduces the cardiovascular complication rate in patients with AMI and is considered the optimal treatment by some. In GUSTO IIB, the incidence of death, nonfatal reinfarction, and nonfatal disabling stroke was 33 percent lower in patients who presented within 12 h of AMI onset who received primary angioplasty versus those who received accelerated tPA.[8] There does not appear to be a large benefit of direct angioplasty over fibrinolysis in the community hospital setting.[9]

Primary angioplasty may offer benefits over fibrinolysis in highly specialized centers, with ready availability of cardiac catheterization and skilled operators, that are not apparent with longer delays or less skilled operators. The decision to use primary interventional procedures rather than fibrinolysis should be individualized based on institutional expertise and availability and risk of complications from fibrinolysis.

There have been multiple trials evaluating the benefit of early angioplasty versus conservative medical treatment for patients with unstable angina (UA) or NSTEMI. In the TACTICS-TIMI 18 trial, 2220 patients with UA or NSTEMI were treated with aspirin, low-molecular-weight heparin, and the GP IIb/IIIa inhibitor tirofiban and were randomized to an early invasive strategy with coronary angiography within 48 h or conservative medical therapy.[10] A reduction in death, myocardial infarction (MI), or rehospitalization was found at 6 months in the invasive group (15.9 vs. 19.4 percent). However, in the absence of high-risk features, [cardiac troponin T (cTnT) >0.1 ng/mL, the presence of ST-deviation, or a TIMI score >3],[11] there was no difference in 6-month outcome between the two treatments.

The American Heart Association and American College of Cardiology (AHA/ACC) guidelines for the management of UA/NSTEMI patients recommend early invasive therapy in patients with recurrent angina/ischemia with or without symptoms of congestive heart failure (CHF), elevated cardiac troponins, high-risk findings on noninvasive stress testing, depressed left ventricular function, hemodynamic instability, sustained ventricular tachycardia, PCIs within the previous 6 months, or prior coronary artery bypass grafting (CABG) in addition to the previously mentioned high-risk features.[12] However, there is no consensus on the definition of "early."

ANTIPLATELET AGENTS

Platelets are at the core of coronary artery thrombosis. Platelet activation and adhesion to subendothelial matrix elements occur as a result of plaque rupture. Platelet aggregation may be initiated by shearing forces, fibrinolytics, thrombin, thromboxane A_2, adenosine diphosphate, epinephrine, serotonin, or plasmin. These trigger the arachidonic acid pathway, the protein kinase C pathway, or other pathways that result in platelet aggregation. The final common pathway of platelet activation is exposure of GP IIb/IIIa receptors on the surface of the platelet. Bivalent fibrinogen molecules cross-link activated platelets together by using these receptors.

The GP IIb/IIIa antagonists are considerably stronger antiplatelet agents than aspirin, because they interrupt platelet activation regardless of agonist. In contrast, aspirin only inhibits platelet aggregation stimulated through thromboxane A_2 and mediated through the arachidonic acid pathway.

Glycoprotein IIb/IIIa Inhibitors

Several different GP IIb/IIIa antagonists are available. *Abciximab* is a chimeric antibody that binds irreversibly to the GP IIb/IIIa antagonists. The duration of action is longer than that of the smaller peptide molecules. As a result, benefits may be realized with a shorter duration of infusion. *Eptifibatide* is a synthetic heptapeptide that binds reversibly to the GP IIb/IIIa receptor. *Tirofiban* is a synthetic molecule with reversible binding to the GP IIb/IIIa receptor. All require an intravenous infusion to demonstrate sustained benefits. Reversal of platelet inhibition after cessation of infusion is more rapid with the polypeptide or small molecules, offering an advantage when bleeding complications occur.

The GP IIb/IIIa inhibitors have been evaluated for use in three clinical areas: with PCI; for medical stabilization of patients with ACS; and in combination with low-dose fibrinolysis.

With PCI, GP IIb/IIIa inhibitors are recommended for use in high-risk patients undergoing PCI in the cardiac catheterization laboratory. Six large trials together enrolled more than 10,000 PCI patients and found that patients treated with GP IIb/IIIa inhibitors (in addition to aspirin and heparin) have an approximately 40 percent reduced risk of death or AMI in 30 days. Some of this benefit was sustained for up to 3 years (13 percent reduction).

Medical Stabilization of ACS

Glycoprotein IIb/IIIa antagonists also have been shown to be efficacious for medical stabilization and treatment of patients with ACSs, although the results are less impressive than with PCI patients. Four large trials evaluated GP IIb/IIIa antagonists for the medical stabilization of patients with UA or non-Q-wave AMI.[13-16] The trials evaluated tirofiban and eptifibatide and demonstrated improved outcomes with the use of these agents when a triple composite end point of death, AMI, and recurrent ischemia was used as the main outcome.[13-15] However, abciximab was not found to be of benefit in patients who did not undergo coronary angiography within 48 h.[16] In a meta-analysis of six randomized placebo-controlled trials, a small reduction in the composite end point of death or AMI was noted in patients receiving GP IIb/IIIa inhibitors (11.8 vs. 10.8 percent).[17] There was no difference between placebo and GP IIb/IIIa when the end points of death and AMI were considered individually. Glycoprotein IIa/IIIb inhibitors showed the greatest reduction in patients undergoing PCI. There were not sufficient data in the meta-analysis to determine whether the GP IIb/IIIa inhibitors are effective in patients who do not undergo PCI. **At this time, the greatest benefit from GP IIb/IIIa inhibitors is for patients undergoing PCI.** The AHA/ACC guidelines for the management of UA/NSTEMI patients makes administration of GP IIb/IIIa inhibitors to patients in whom a PCI is planned a class I recommendation.[12] The GP IIb/IIIa inhibitors, eptifibatide and tirofiban, are considered class IIa for ACS patients in whom PCI is not planned. Abciximab is not recommended for patients who will be receiving medical management without PCI.

Combination Therapy: Fibrinolytic Therapy with GP IIb/IIIa Inhibitors

Although much of coronary thrombosis is red clot (fibrin and erythrocytes), central platelet thrombus (white clot) is fully resistant to fibrinolytic therapy. These platelets secrete plasminogen activator inhibitor 1, which is a potent inhibitor of fibrinolysis. In theory, combination therapy with antiplatelet agents and fibrinolytics will attack both components of coronary thrombosis. This is one explanation why even a weak antiplatelet agent reduces mortality rate as much as treatment with streptokinase alone.

Preclinical studies and dose-ranging trials of GP IIb/IIIa antagonists combined with a 50 percent reduced fibrinolytic dose found that fibrinolysis occurred more rapidly and was more stable.[18] Two large RCTs of combination therapy found divergent results. GUSTO-V found no advantage (as measured by death at 30 days) over strategies using rPA.[19] ASSENT-3 found improvement in survival, AMI, and recurrent ischemia with abciximab added to TNK and unfractionated heparin (UFH) without an increase in intracranial hemorrhage and a nonsignificant increase in major bleeding with enoxaparin.[20] **At this time, the use of combination therapy with GP IIb/IIIa inhibitors is unproven as a superior treatment to standard fibrinolytics alone or in combination with low-molecular-weight heparin (LMWH).**

Aspirin

Aspirin should be given as soon as possible to all patients with ACSs. In platelets, aspirin prevents formation of thromboxane A_2, an agonist of platelet aggregation. This inhibition persists for the 9- to 10-day life of the platelet, because platelets are unable to generate new cyclooxygenase. Aspirin alone has been shown to be as efficacious as streptokinase alone. Aspirin alone reduces mortality rate by 23 percent. In conjunction with streptokinase, mortality rate is reduced by 43 percent. Aspirin used in conjunction with fibrinolytic therapy further reduces ischemic events and coronary artery reocclusion. Doses larger than 160 mg cause immediate, nearly complete inhibition of thromboxane A_2. Smaller doses may be effective for long-term prophylaxis but may not be effective for acute use. Aspirin reduces vascular events in patients with AMI and patients with UA.[1] In patients with prior MI or stroke, it reduces vascular events by about 4 percent.[21]

The side effects of aspirin are mainly gastrointestinal and dose related. They can be reduced by using diluted or buffered aspirin solutions, lowest possible doses, or concurrent antacid or H_2 antagonist administration. In the setting of acute ischemia, the delay in absorption of enteric-coated aspirin is best avoided. Due to the substantial benefits of aspirin therapy during ACS, it should not be withheld from patients with minor contraindications (vague allergy, history of remote peptic ulcer, or gastrointestinal bleeding).[1] Other antiplatelet agents, such as clopidogrel, can be substituted if true aspirin allergy or active peptic ulcer disease exists.[12] The aspirin dose should be at least 160 mg.

Adenosine Diphosphate Receptor Antagonists

Ticlopidine and *clopidogrel* are antiplatelet agents that inhibit platelet aggregation induced by a wide range of agonists. Clopidogrel is preferred to ticlopidine in the ACS setting, because it has more rapid inhibition of platelets and limited side effects. The CURE trial randomized 12,562 patients with UA/NSTEMI to clopidogrel (300-mg loading dose and 75-mg daily dose) or placebo.[22] All patients received aspirin. The clopidogrel group had a 20 percent reduction in death, AMI, or stroke between 3 and 12 months. There was an excess of bleeding in the clopidogrel group compared with controls.

Current AHA/ACC guidelines recommend clopidogrel in patients who have aspirin allergy, and early administration in patients in whom noninvasive management or PCI is planned.[18] Because of an increased bleeding risk, it is recommended that this agent be withheld 5 days before CABG, if possible.

The inhibitory effect of ticlopidine is delayed 24 to 48 h after its administration.[1] It is effective in reducing 6-month vascular death and AMI rate in patients with UA. Side effects include neutropenia, which is more common in patients treated for longer than 2 weeks. The dose is 250 mg twice per day. Because clopidogrel has fewer serious side effects and acts more rapidly than ticlopidine, there is little reason to use ticlopidine in the ED.

ANTITHROMBINS

Heparin

Heparin is a specific antithrombin agent. Thrombin generation plays an intricate role in the pathogenesis of coronary artery thrombosis. Thrombin converts soluble fibrinogen to insoluble fibrin; activates coagulation factors V and VIII, which exert positive feedback on coagulation through the prothrombinase complex; and activates factor XIII, which stabilizes thrombus formation by promoting fibrin cross-linking. In addition, thrombin serves as a platelet agonist.

Unfractionated heparin consists of a mixture of molecules with molecular weights varying between 2000 and 20,000. The different-size molecules have different effects on the coagulation system. Heparin complexes with antithrombin III, and this complex inactivates thrombin and activated factor X. The heparin-antithrombin III complex is not effective against clot-bound thrombin.

Heparin reduces the risk of AMI and death during the acute phase of UA. The combination therapy of aspirin and heparin reduces the short-term risk of death or AMI by 56 percent compared with aspirin alone. When heparin is used in combination with aspirin, recurrence of ischemia is diminished after cessation of the heparin infusion.[23] Thus, **combination therapy with aspirin and heparin is indicated for patients with ACSs.**

Unfractionated heparin has some limitations. It has an unpredictable anticoagulant response, because the bioavailability of heparin is variable. It requires careful laboratory monitoring and dose adjustment. The weight-adjusted regimen is recommended, with an initial bolus of 60 to 70 units/kg (maximum, 5000 units) and an infusion of 12 to 15 units/kg per hour (maximum, 1000 units/h).[12]

Low-Molecular-Weight Heparins

The LMWHs have greater bioavailability, lower protein binding, a longer half-life, and achieve a more reliable anticoagulant effect. As a result, they can be administered in a fixed dose subcutaneously once or twice a day and achieve a stable therapeutic response without the need for monitoring anticoagulation.

Several clinical trials have compared LMWH with standard heparin regimens for treatment of ACS. The largest RCT showed that, at 14 and 30 days, the risk of death, AMI, or recurrent angina was at least 15 percent lower in patients with angina/NSTEMI who received (aspirin and) enoxaparin compared with those who received (aspirin and) UFH, without an increase in major bleeding complications among patients with UA or non-Q-wave infarction.[24] The benefit of enoxaparin was related to the TIMI risk score, with a significant decrease in the composite end point of death, AMI, and recurrent ischemia requiring PCI at 14 days in patients with a TIMI risk score above 3.[11] Because the level of anticoagulant activity is not rapidly measured, there is some concern about the use of these agents in patients requiring emergent PCI. However, recent trials have suggested that it is safe in this setting. In patients in whom CABG is planned, it is recommended that LMWH be held and UFH be used in the 12 to 24 h before surgery. The ACC/AHA guidelines consider enoxaparin preferable to UFH for patients with UA/NSTEMI, unless CABG is planned in the next 24 h.[12] Other LMWHs have not had the same efficacy as enoxaparin in clinical trials of UA/NSTEMI patients.

Direct Thrombin Inhibitors

These agents bind to the catalytic site of thrombin, bind to thrombin in clot, and are resistant to agents that degrade heparin. Hirudin, a 65–amino acid peptide, is derived from the medicinal leech and is one of the most potent, naturally occurring anticoagulants. One large clinical trial was terminated because hirudin increased the incidence of intracranial bleeding compared with heparin. *Bivalirudin* (Hirulog) may reduce the short-term risk of postischemic complications relative to high-dose UFH in patients PCI for unstable or postinfarction angina, but benefits do appear to persist long term. Similarly, inogatran does not appear to offer benefits over UFH for the treatment of patients with ACS.[25] Thus, at this time, there is no clearly defined role for direct thrombin inhibitors in the medical management of ACS patients in the ED.

LIMITING INFARCT SIZE

Nitrates

Nitrates relax vascular smooth muscle in arteries, arterioles, and veins through the metabolic conversion of organic nitrates to nitric oxide. The pulmonary capillary wedge pressure, systemic arterial pressure, and left ventricular end-systolic and end-diastolic volumes decrease. Reduction in right and left ventricular filling pressures that result from peripheral dilatation combined with afterload reduction that results from arterial dilatation decrease cardiac work and myocardial oxygen requirements. Nitroglycerin has direct vasodilator effects on the coronary vascular bed and increases global and regional myocardial blood flows. When obstructing atherosclerotic lesions contain intact vascular smooth muscle, nitrates may dilate these vessels, thereby improving blood flow. Platelet aggregation is also inhibited by nitroglycerin.

When nitroglycerin is used in AMI patients not treated with thrombolytics, several clinical trials have demonstrated a reduction in infarct size, improved regional function, and decreased rate of cardiovascular complications. The mortality rate appears to be reduced by 35 percent with the use of nitrates. It is important to note that, in most studies, intravenous nitroglycerin was titrated to 10 percent reduction in mean arterial pressure for normotensive patients and to 30 percent reduction in mean arterial pressure for hypertensive patients. It was not titrated to symptom resolution. Thus, when used for patients with AMI, **intravenous nitroglycerin should be titrated to blood pressure reduction rather than to symptom (chest pain) resolution.** Studies in patients who have received fibrinolytic agents have not found a benefit to the addition of nitroglycerin. Unfortunately, large numbers of the control (non-nitroglycerin) patients were prescribed nitroglycerin by their physicians, thus precluding optimal data interpretation.

The ACC/AHA guidelines recommend the use of intravenous nitroglycerin for the first 24 to 48 h for patients with AMI and recurrent ischemia, congestive heart failure, or hypertension.[1] Benefits are likely to be greatest in patients not receiving concurrent fibrinolytic therapy. The UA/NSTEMI guidelines recommend that intravenous nitroglycerin be used in patients with UA who are not responsive to sublingual nitroglycerin tablets.[12]

The most serious side effect of nitroglycerin is hypotension, which may result in reflex tachycardia and worsening ischemia. Nitrates should not be used for patients with right ventricular infarction.[26] **Nitroglycerin should be used very cautiously for patients with inferior wall ischemia,** because one third of such patients might have right ventricular involvement. Patients with right ventricular infarction are volume dependent. Administration of nitrates reduces preload and commonly results in hypotension in these patients. The development of hypotension is associated with an increased infarct size. When nitroglycerin results in hypotension and bradycardia, the drug should be discontinued, legs should be elevated, and fluid should be administered. Atropine may be necessary in some cases.

β-Blockers

β-Adrenergic antagonists have antiarrhythmic, anti-ischemic, and antihypertensive properties. During AMI, they diminish myocardial oxygen demand by decreasing heart rate, systemic arterial pressure, and myocardial contractility. Prolongation of diastole may augment perfusion to ischemic myocardium. Studies in the mid-1980s set immediate β-antagonist administration in AMI as a standard by reduced chest pain, wall stress, infarct size, incidence of cardiovascular complications, and mortality rate for patients not treated with fibrinolytics. For patients treated with fibrinolytics, β-antagonists decrease the risk of nonfatal reinfarction and recurrent ischemia if given within several hours of symptom onset.

The ACC/AHA guidelines recommend that all patients with STEMI who do not have a contraindication to β-antagonists be treated with these agents within 12 h of onset of infarction, regardless of whether they have received fibrinolytic therapy.[1] Patients with recurrent ischemia and tachyarrhythmias should receive β-antagonist therapy. The AHA/ACC guidelines recommend that patients with UA or NSTEMI receive early treatment with β-antagonists, when not contraindicated.[12]

Relative contraindications to β-adrenergic antagonists are heart rate slower than 60 beats/min, systolic blood pressure below 100 mm Hg, moderate to severe left ventricular failure, signs of peripheral hypoperfusion, PR interval longer than 0.24 s, second-degree or third-degree atrioventricular block, severe chronic obstructive pulmonary disease, history of asthma, severe peripheral vascular disease, and insulin-dependent diabetes mellitus.[1] Use of β-antagonists should be individualized for patients with these conditions.

Angiotensin-Converting Enzyme Inhibitors

Angiotensin-converting enzyme inhibitors reduce left ventricular dysfunction and left ventricular dilatation and slow the development of congestive heart failure during AMI. Studies have consistently shown a reduction in mortality rate for patients treated with oral ACE inhibitors during and soon after AMI. A meta-analysis of 15 trials including more than 100,000 patients supported a 6.5 percent reduction in short-term mortality rate, with an absolute benefit of 4.6 fewer deaths per 1000 patients treated with early ACE inhibitor therapy.[27] Oral administration is recommended; intravenous enalaprilat is associated with increased hypotension.

The ACC/AHA guidelines recommend that patients with STEMI or heart failure receive treatment with ACE inhibitors within the first 24 h (not necessarily in the ED).[1] The UA/NSTEMI guidelines recommend ACE inhibitors when hypertension persists after treatment with nitroglycerin and β-blockers in patients with depressed left ventricular function or CHF.

Contraindications to ACE inhibitors include hypotension, bilateral renal artery stenosis, renal failure, or history of cough or angioedema due to prior ACE inhibitor use. The efficacy of ACE inhibitors in UA has not been well evaluated.

Magnesium

Magnesium produces systemic and coronary vasodilatation, possesses antiplatelet activity, suppresses automaticity, and protects myocytes from calcium influx during reperfusion. Studies, however, are conflicting: some have found mortality rate reduced by about 75 percent, whereas others have showed no benefit at all. The disparity in findings may be related to the interval between symptom onset and magnesium administration and various concurrent therapies (including fibrinolysis). In light of these conflicting data, the ACC/AHA guidelines support correction of documented hypomagnesemia during AMI and treatment of torsades-type ventricular tachycardia with a prolonged QT interval.[1] Magnesium bolus and infusion in high-risk patients, such as the elderly and those in whom reperfusion therapy is not suitable, is considered possibly beneficial.[1]

Calcium Channel Antagonists

Calcium channel blockers have antianginal, vasodilatory, and antihypertensive properties. Calcium antagonists have not been shown to re-

duce mortality rate after AMI. In fact, they may be harmful to some patients with cardiovascular disease.[1] Nifedipine is the most studied of the calcium channel blockers for the treatment of AMI. This short-acting dihydropyridine has been associated with a nonsignificant increase in mortality rate when given during or shortly after AMI in several clinical trials.[28] Immediate-release nifedipine may be harmful as a result of a coronary "steal" syndrome, in which coronary perfusion pressure is reduced through disproportionate dilatation of the coronary arteries adjacent to the ischemic zone and/or reflex activation of the sympathetic nervous system, with a resultant increase in myocardial oxygen demand.

Diltiazem also has been associated with increased mortality rate, particularly for patients with CHF.[29] Similarly, studies evaluating verapamil have not found mortality-rate benefits. Verapamil is detrimental for patients with CHF or bradydysrhythmia. There are no data supporting the use of second-generation dihydropyridines (amlodipine and felodipine) for treatment of AMI.

The ACC/AHA guidelines state that "these agents are still used too frequently in patients with AMI and that beta-adrenoreceptor blocking agents are a more appropriate choice."[1] Verapamil and diltiazem are considered potentially beneficial for use in patients with ongoing ischemia or atrial fibrillation with rapid ventricular response who do not have CHF, left ventricular dysfunction, or atrioventricular block, and when β-adrenergic antagonists are contraindicated.[3,30]

SPECIAL ISSUES IN TREATMENT OF AMI COMPLICATIONS

Recurrent or Refractory Ischemia

Patients unresponsive to medical management with continued ischemia require an individualized approach to treatment. Depending on the infarct distribution and coronary anatomy, decisions could be made regarding continued medical management, rescue angioplasty, or CABG. Emergency cardiology referral should be considered. Refractory ischemia should be investigated with coronary catheterization. Patients with ACS after stent placement should be treated aggressively with anticoagulation and may require urgent coronary catheterization.

Intraaortic balloon counterpulsation delivers phased pulsations synchronized to the electrocardiograph, so that balloon inflation will occur at the time of aortic valve closure and deflation occurs just before onset of systole. The augmented coronary perfusion pressure during diastole enhances coronary blood flow. Balloon deflation during systole allows the left ventricle to eject blood against a lower resistance. The net effect of intraaortic balloon counterpulsation is an increase in cardiac output, reduction in systolic arterial pressure, increase in diastolic arterial pressure, little change in mean arterial pressure, and reduction in heart rate. The reduction in left ventricular afterload leads to reduced myocardial oxygen consumption, thereby decreasing the amount of myocardial ischemia. Intraaortic balloon counterpulsation is recommended for patients with ACS who are refractory to aggressive medical management or are hemodynamically unstable, as a means to bridge a patient's stability en route to definitive treatment.

Cardiogenic Shock

This is discussed in Chap. 33.

Right Ventricular Infarction

One third of patients with inferior wall myocardial infarction have right ventricular involvement. The most serious complication of right ventricular infarction is shock. Right ventricular infarction results in a reduction in right ventricular end-systolic pressure, left ventricular end-diastolic size, cardiac output, and aortic pressure as the right ventricle becomes more of a passive conduit to blood flow. Left ventricular contraction causes bulging of the interventricular septum into the right ventricle, with resultant ejection of blood into the pulmonary circulation. As a result, right ventricular infarction in the setting of a large left ventricular infarction has a particularly devastating effect on hemodynamic function. Factors that reduce preload (volume depletion, diuretics, and nitrates) or decrease right atrial contraction (atrial infarction and loss of atrioventricular synchrony) and factors that increase right ventricular afterload (left ventricular failure) can lead to significant hemodynamic derangements.

Treatment of right ventricular infarction includes maintenance of preload, reduction of right ventricular afterload, and inotropic support of the ischemic right ventricle, in addition to early reperfusion. Patients with right ventricular infarction should not be treated with drugs, such as nitrates, that reduce preload. In the setting of right ventricular infarction, nitrates often will reduce cardiac output and produce hypotension. Instead, patients with marginal preload or hypotension should be treated with volume loading (normal saline). The increased preload will improve right ventricular cardiac output. If cardiac output is not improved after 1 to 2 L of normal saline, inotropic support with dobutamine should be initiated.

High-degree heart block is very common in patients with right ventricular infarction. The loss of right atrial contraction can greatly compromise right ventricular cardiac output. Restitution of atrioventricular synchrony is important. For patients who require pacing in the setting of right ventricular infarction, it may be necessary to establish atrioventricular sequential pacing leads. Patients who do not attain hemodynamic improvement after placement of a ventricular pacer may still improve with atrioventricular sequential pacing.

When right ventricular infarction is accompanied by left ventricular dysfunction, the use of nitroprusside to reduce afterload or intra-aortic balloon counterpulsation may be of benefit. Reduction in left ventricular afterload may help passive movement of blood through the right ventricle.

Selected Dysrhythmias in AMI

ATRIAL FIBRILLATION   Atrial fibrillation associated with AMI most typically occurs in the first 24 h and is usually transient. It more often occurs in patients with excess catecholamine release, hypokalemia, hypomagnesemia, hypoxia, chronic lung disease, and sinus node or left circumflex ischemia. Patients with supraventricular tachycardia, atrial fibrillation, and atrial flutter who have hemodynamic compromise should receive cardioversion with 100 J, 200 to 300 J, and then 360 J, if lower energies fail. Patients without hemodynamic compromise, clinical left ventricular dysfunction, reactive airway disease, or heart block can be treated with β-adrenergic antagonists, such as atenolol (2.5 to 5 mg over 2 min to a total of 10 mg) or metoprolol (2.5 to 5 mg every 2 to 5 min to a total of 15 mg). Patients with contraindications to β-adrenergic antagonists can be treated with digoxin (0.3- to 0.5-mg initial bolus with a repeat in 4 h) or a calcium antagonist such as verapamil or diltiazem. Digoxin will take longer to work but is still preferred by the ACC/AHA guidelines, because of the potential negative inotropic effects of calcium antagonists, their lack of efficacy in reducing mortality during AMI, and potentially harmful effects in some subsets of AMI patients.[30] The AHA/ACC recommend sotalol as the initial antiarrhythmic agent in the setting of ACS based on its β-blocking activity. This medication is contraindicated in patients with CHF. The alternative anti-arrhythmic agent is amiodarone.[30] The etiology of the tachydysrhythmia should also be addressed. Heparin should be given, because atrial fibrillation during AMI is associated with a threefold risk in systemic embolization.

BRADYDYSRHYTHMIAS   The increased mortality in patients with heart block during AMI is related to more extensive myocardial dam-

TABLE 51-3   Indications for Temporary Pacemaker Placement

Temporary transcutaneous pacemaker indications
Unresponsive symptomatic bradycardia
Mobitz II or higher AV blocks
New LBBB and bifascicular blocks
RBBB or LBBB with first-degree block
Some cases with stable bradycardia and new or indeterminate age RBBB

Temporary transvenous pacemaker indications
Asystole
Unresponsive symptomatic bradycardia
Mobitz II or higher AV blocks
New or indeterminate age LBBB
Alternating BBB
RBBB or LBBB with first-degree block
Consider in RBBB with left anterior or posterior hemiblocks
Overdrive pacing in unresponsive VT
Unresponsive recurrent sinus pauses (>3 s)

Abbreviations: AV = atrioventricular; BBB = bundle-branch block; LBBB = left bundle-branch block; RBBB = right bundle-branch block; VT = tidal volume.

age and not to the heart block itself. As a result, pacing has not been shown to reduce mortality in patients with atrioventricular (AV) block or intraventricular conduction delay. Nonetheless, pacing is recommended to protect against sudden hypotension, acute ischemia, and precipitation of ventricular dysrhythmias in certain patients.

The risk of developing third-degree heart block during AMI is increased in the setting of first-degree AV block, both types of second-degree AV block (more likely with Mobitz II), left anterior hemiblock, left posterior hemiblock, right bundle-branch block, and left bundle-branch block. The prognosis is related to the site of infarction, the site of the block (intranodal vs. infranodal), the type of escape rhythm, and the hemodynamic response to the rhythm.

Atropine is recommended for sinus bradycardia when it results in hypotension, ischemia, or ventricular escape rhythms and for treatment of symptomatic AV block occurring at the AV nodal level (second-degree type 1 or third-degree AV block). Atropine will reverse decreases in heart rate, systemic vascular resistance, and blood pressure that are mediated by parasympathetic activity. It should be used cautiously in the setting of AMI, because the parasympathetic tone is protective against infarct extension and ventricular fibrillation and may result in increased myocardial oxygen demand.

Temporary *transcutaneous* pacers are recommended for patients at moderate to high risk of progression to AV block (Table 51-3). *Transvenous* pacing should be considered in patients who require permanent pacing and in patients with a very high likelihood (>30 percent) of requiring permanent pacing (see Table 51-3). Patients with right ventricular infarction who are very dependent on atrial systole may require AV sequential pacing to maintain cardiac output.

REFERENCES

1. Ryan TJ, Antman EM, Brooks NH, et al: 1999 Update: ACC/AHA guidelines for the management of patients with acute myocardial infarction. A report of the American College of Cardiology/American Heart Association Task Force on Practice Guidelines (Committee on Management of Acute Myocardial Infarction). *J Am Coll Cardiol* 34:890, 1999.
2. International Study Group: In-hospital mortality and clinical course of 20,891 patients with suspected acute myocardial infarction randomized between alteplase and streptokinase with or without heparin. *Lancet* 336:71, 1990.
3. ISIS-3 Collaborative Group: A randomized comparison of streptokinase vs tissue plasminogen activator vs anistreplase and of aspirin plus heparin vs aspirin alone among 41,299 cases of suspected acute myocardial infarction: ISIS-3. *Lancet* 339:753, 1992.
4. GUSTO Investigators: An international randomized trial comparing four thrombolytic strategies for acute myocardial infarction. *New Engl J Med* 329:673, 1993.

5. GUSTO Angiographic Investigators: The effects of tissue plasminogen activator, streptokinase, or both on coronary-artery patency, ventricular function, and survival after acute myocardial infarction. *New Engl J Med* 329: 1615, 1993.

6. Assessment of the Safety and Efficacy of a New Thrombolytic Investigators: Single-bolus tenecteplase compared with front-loaded alteplase in acute myocardial infarction: the ASSENT-2 double-blind randomised trial. *Lancet* 354:716, 1999.

7. SoRelle R: Stents are the CADILLAC of care. Controlled abciximab and device investigation to lower late angioplasty complications. *Circulation* 105:e9094, 2002.

8. GUSTO IIB Angioplasty Substudy Investigators: A clinical trial comparing primary coronary angioplasty with tissue plasminogen activator for acute myocardial infarction. *New Engl J Med* 336:1621, 1997.

9. Every NR, Parsons LS, Hlatky M, et al, for MITI Investigators: A comparison of thrombolytic therapy with primary coronary angioplasty for acute myocardial infarction. *New Engl J Med* 335:1253, 1996.

10. Cannon CP, Weintraub WS, Demopoulos LA, et al: Comparison of early invasive and conservative strategies in patients with unstable coronary syndromes treated with the glycoprotein IIb/IIIa inhibitor tirofiban. *New Engl J Med* 344:1879, 2001.

11. Antman EM, Cohen M, Bernink PJ, et al: The TIMI risk score for unstable angina/non-ST elevation MI: A method for prognostication and therapeutic decision making. *JAMA* 284:835, 2000.

12. Braunwald E, Antman EM, Beasley JW, et al: American College of Cardiology/American Heart Association Task Force on Practice Guidelines (Committee on the Management of Patients With Unstable Angina). ACC/AHA guideline update for the management of patients with unstable angina and non-ST-segment elevation myocardial infarction—2002: Summary article: A report of the American College of Cardiology/American Heart Association Task Force on Practice Guidelines (Committee on the Management of Patients With Unstable Angina). *Circulation* 106:1893, 2002.

13. Platelet Receptor Inhibition in Ischemic Syndrome Management (PRISM) Study Investigators: A comparison of aspirin plus tirofiban with aspirin plus heparin for unstable angina. *New Engl J Med* 338:1498, 1998.

14. Platelet Receptor Inhibition in Ischemic Syndrome Management in Patients Limited by Unstable Signs and Symptoms (PRISM-PLUS) Study Investigators: Inhibition of the platelet glycoprotein IIb/IIIa receptor with tirofiban in unstable angina and non-Q-wave myocardial infarction. *New Engl J Med* 338:1488, 1998.

15. PURSUIT Investigators: Inhibition of platelet glycoprotein IIb/IIIa with eptifibatide in patients with acute coronary syndromes. *New Engl J Med* 339:436, 1998.

16. Simoons ML: Effect of glycoprotein IIb/IIIa receptor blocker abciximab on outcome in patients with acute coronary syndromes without early coronary revascularization: The GUSTO IV-ACS randomized trial. *Lancet* 357:1915, 2001.

17. Boersma E, Harrington RA, Moliterno DJ, et al: Platelet glycoprotein IIb/IIIa inhibitors in acute coronary syndromes: A meta-analysis of all major randomised clinical trials. *Lancet* 359:189, 2002.

18. Herrmann HC, Moliterno DJ, Ohman E, et al: Facilitation of early percutaneous coronary intervention after reteplase with or without abciximab in acute myocardial infarction: Results from the SPEED (GUSTO-4 Pilot) trial. *J Am Coll Cardiol* 36:1489, 2000.

19. GUSTO V Investigators: Reperfusion therapy for acute myocardial infarction with fibrinolytic therapy or combination reduced fibrinolytic therapy and platelet glycoprotein IIb/IIa inhibition: The GUSTO V randomized trial. *Lancet* 357:1905, 2001.

20. ASSENT-3 Investigators: Efficacy and safety of tenecteplase in combination with enoxaparin, abciximab or unfractionated heparin: The ASSENT-3 randomized trial in acute myocardial infarction. *Lancet* 358:605, 2001.

21. Collins R, Peto R, Baigent C, Sleight P: Aspirin, heparin, and fibrinolytic therapy in suspected acute myocardial infarction. *New Engl J Med* 336:847, 1997.

22. Yusuf S, Zhao F, Mehta SR, et al: Effects of clopidogrel in addition to aspirin in patients with acute coronary syndromes without ST-segment elevation. *New Engl J Med* 345:494, 2001.

23. Theroux P, Waters D, Qiu S, et al: Aspirin versus heparin to prevent myocardial infarction during the acute phase of unstable angina. *Circulation* 88:2045, 1993.

24. Cohen M, Demers C, Gurfinkel EP, et al: A comparison of low molecular weight heparin with unfractionated heparin for unstable coronary artery disease. *New Engl J Med* 337:447, 1997.

25. Anderson K, Dellborg M, for the TRIM Study Group: Heparin is more effective than inogatran, a low molecular weight thrombin inhibitor, in suppressing ischemia and recurrent angina in unstable coronary disease. *Am J Cardiol* 81:939, 1998.

26. Fergusen JJ, Diver DJ, Boldt M, Pasternak RC: Significance of nitroglycerin-induced hypotension with inferior wall acute myocardial infarction. *Am J Cardiol* 64:311, 1989.

27. Latini R, Maggioni AP, Flather M, et al: ACE inhibitor use in patients with acute myocardial infarction: Summary of evidence from clinical trials. *Circulation* 92:3132, 1995.

28. Furberg CD, Patsy BM, Meyer JV: Nifedipine: Dose-related increase in mortality in patients with coronary heart disease. *Circulation* 92:1326, 1995.

29. Multicenter Diltiazem Postinfarction Trial Research Group: The effect of diltiazem on mortality and reinfarction after myocardial infarction. *New Engl J Med* 319:385, 1988.

30. Fuster V, Ryden LE, Asinger RW, et al: ACC/AHA/ESC Guidelines for the Management of Patients With Atrial Fibrillation: Executive Summary. A Report of the American College of Cardiology/American Heart Association Task Force on Practice Guidelines and the European Society of Cardiology Committee for Practice Guidelines and Policy Conferences (Committee to Develop Guidelines for the Management of Patients With Atrial Fibrillation) developed in Collaboration With the North American Society of Pacing and Electrophysiology. *Circulation* 104:2118, 2001.

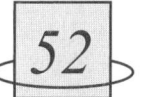

SYNCOPE
Barbara K. Blok
Tina M. Newman

Syncope is a sudden, transient loss of consciousness associated with inability to maintain postural tone. Syncope accounts for approximately 3 percent of ED visits each year. The elderly population has the highest incidence and is at increased risk for morbidity from syncopal episodes.[1] Near-syncope, a premonition of syncope without loss of consciousness, shares the same basic pathophysiologic processes as syncope. Vertigo and dizziness, which lack a premonition of syncope, are not considered near-syncope (see Chap. 231).

PATHOPHYSIOLOGY

The final common pathway of syncope is a lack of vital nutrient delivery to the brainstem reticular activating system, leading to loss of consciousness and postural tone. Most commonly, an inciting event causes a drop in cardiac output, which, unless corrected rapidly, decreases oxygen and substrate delivery to the brain. Less commonly, vasospasm or other alterations in flow singularly reduce central nervous system blood flow. The reclined posture of syncope and the response of autonomic autoregulatory centers reestablish cerebral perfusion, leading to a spontaneous return of consciousness.

ETIOLOGY

The differential diagnosis of syncope is vast and includes everything from common benign disorders to life-threatening processes (Table 52-1). The most common causes of syncope are cardiac dysrhythmia, vasovagal reflex-mediated, and orthostatic hypotension.[2,3] In the Framingham Heart Study, 7814 patients were followed for 17 years, and 822 reported syncope. The causes were: vasovagal (21%), cardiac (10%), orthostatic (9%), unknown (37%).[4]

Reflex-Mediated Syncope

Under normal circumstances a physical or emotional stress leads to increased sympathetic outflow and a subsequent increase in heart rate, blood pressure, and cardiac output. In patients with reflex-mediated

TABLE 52-1   Causes of Syncope

Reflex-mediated	Cardiac*
Vasovagal	Structural cardiopulmonary disease
Situational	Valvular heart disease
Cough	Aortic stenosis
Micturition	Tricuspid stenosis
Defecation	Mitral stenosis
Swallow	Cardiomyopathy
Neuralgia	Pulmonary hypertension
Carotid sinus syndrome	Congenital heart disease
Orthostatic hypotension*	Myxoma
(See text)	Pericardial disease
	Aortic dissection
Psychiatric	Pulmonary embolism
	Myocardial ischemia
Neurologic	Myocardial infarction
Transient ischemic	Dysrhythmias
attacks*	Bradydysrhythmias
Subclavian steal*	Stokes-Adams attack
Migraine	Sinus node disease
	2nd- or 3rd-degree heart block
Medications (Table 52-2)*	Pacemaker malfunction
Breath Holding	Tachydysrhythmias
(pediatric)	Ventricular tachycardia
	Torsade de pointes
	Supraventricular tachycardia
	Atrial fibrillation or flutter

*Etiology that must be considered in the ED. If these etiologies cannot be excluded or the underlying cause readily addressed, the patient should be admitted.

syncope (also termed neurocardiogenic or neurally mediated syncope), the stimulus produces an abnormal autonomic nervous system reflex. Most commonly, an initial increase in sympathetic outflow is inappropriately withdrawn and replaced by increased vagal tone. Hypotension with or without bradycardia follows, leading to decreased cerebral perfusion and syncope. Less commonly, the stimulus leads directly to vagal hyperactivity and symptoms. Prodromal symptoms are varied, but include blurring of vision, dizziness, pallor, nausea, and diaphoresis.

The classic example of reflex-mediated syncope is the vasovagal faint incited by a noxious stimulus (pain, fear) or a characteristic setting. Vasovagal syncope is typically preceded by warning symptoms, which may last several minutes. This diagnosis should not be made without the typical prodromal symptoms. The individual is usually in the vertical position at the time of the event. Attacks are aborted or resolved after reclining, which increases central circulation and cerebral perfusion. Upright tilt table testing can be used to diagnose vasovagal syncope.[5]

Carotid sinus hypersensitivity is another type of reflex-mediated syncope. The carotid body, located at the carotid bifurcation, is a pressure-sensitive organ. The stimulation of an abnormally sensitive carotid body by external pressure may lead to two autonomic responses. Most commonly, there is an abnormal vagal response leading to bradycardia and asystole of greater than 3 s. Less commonly, there is a vasodepressor response leading to a decrease in blood pressure of more than 50 mmHg without a significant change in heart rate. Both responses may occur simultaneously. Carotid sinus hypersensitivity is more common in men, the elderly, and among those with ischemic heart disease, hypertension, and certain head and neck malignancies. Although a number of patients may have a hypersensitive carotid sinus response on testing, unless this response culminates in syncope or recurrence of prodromal symptoms and can be associated with an inciting event, such as shaving or turning of the head, it cannot be definitely diagnosed as the cause of syncope. Approximately 25 percent of patients with carotid sinus hypersensitivity have true carotid sinus syndrome with spontaneous symptoms.[2] Carotid sinus hypersensitivity should be considered in all older patients with recurrent syncope and negative cardiac evaluations.

In situational syncope, there is an abnormal or hypersensitive autonomic reflex response to a specific physical stimulus (see Table 52-1).

Additionally, there may be a component of raised intracranial pressure or increased intrathoracic pressure leading to decreased cerebral perfusion. The physical stimulus may be associated with another underlying disease process: esophageal stricture in swallow syncope, prostatic hypertrophy or bladder neck obstruction with micturition syncope, and constipation with defecation syncope.

Orthostatic Syncope

When a person assumes an upright posture, blood is shifted to the lower part of the body and cardiac output drops. When a drop in cardiac output or blood pressure occurs in a healthy individual, the autonomic nervous system responds with an increase in sympathetic output and a decrease in parasympathetic output. This autonomic nervous system reflex produces an increase in heart rate and peripheral vascular resistance, leading to an increase in both cardiac output and blood pressure, thereby allowing the individual to maintain an upright posture. If the autonomic response is insufficient to counter the drop in cardiac output, decreased cerebral perfusion and syncope may follow if the person remains upright. Symptom onset is usually within the first 3 min after assuming the upright posture, but may be more delayed in some patients. Symptoms are characteristic of decreased cerebral perfusion, with blurred vision, dizziness, and tunnel vision. Orthostatic hypotension is defined as a fall in systolic blood pressure of greater than 20 mm Hg upon assuming the upright posture. Caution should be taken in diagnosing a patient with orthostatic syncope based on orthostatic blood pressure measurements alone, because 5 to 55 percent of patients with other causes of syncope have orthostatic hypotension on physical examination.[6] To establish orthostasis as the cause of syncope, the patient should have recurrence of syncopal symptoms on orthostatic testing.

Autonomic dysfunction may cause severe symptoms, with failure of vasoconstriction during orthostatic stress. Autonomic dysfunction may be a primary disease process or secondary to peripheral neuropathy, certain medications such as ganglionic blockers, spinal cord injury, and a variety of other neurologic diseases. Commonly, orthostatic symptoms are due to other conditions that lead to volume depletion, including gastrointestinal losses, bleeding, and diuresis. Medications commonly contribute to orthostatic syncope by blunting the chronotropic response of the heart to orthostatic stress or by leading to relative or absolute volume depletion. The elderly are more susceptible to orthostatic hypotension for many reasons, including use of diuretics and β-blocking agents, varying degrees of autonomic dysfunction, and other changes related to aging.

Cardiac Syncope

The causes of cardiac syncope are divided into two categories: dysrhythmias and structural cardiopulmonary lesions. In both settings, the heart is unable to provide adequate cardiac output to maintain cerebral perfusion.

Although both brady- and tachydysrythmias may lead to transient cerebral hypoperfusion, there is no absolute high or low heart rate that will produce syncope. Symptoms depend on both the autonomic nervous system's ability to compensate for a decrease in cardiac output and the degree of cerebrovascular atherosclerotic disease. A variety of dysrhythmias may lead to syncope (see Table 52-1). A bradydysrhythmia is more likely to be an incidental finding on electrocardiogram (ECG) rather than the actual cause of syncope.[7] Dysrhythmias are most likely to occur in the setting of underlying structural heart disease, be it congenital disease or an acquired defect such as ischemic heart disease or Lyme disease. They may also occur because of a primary electrolyte imbalance as in hypomagnesemia (torsade de pointes). Dysrhythmias rarely occur in structurally normal hearts, but are seen in the familial disorders of Brugada's syndrome, long QT syndrome and catecholamine polymorphic ventricular tachycardia. Syncope from dysrhythmias is typically sudden, with prodromal symptoms, if any, lasting less than 3 s. Many patients report lack of any warning or premonition when questioned.

A wide variety of cardiopulmonary disorders may lead to syncope. Syncope caused by underlying structural cardiopulmonary disease often occurs in the setting of physical exertion, but also may be seen in response to vasodilation from medication or heat stress. A decrease in systemic vascular resistance is normally compensated by an increase in cardiac output to maintain arterial perfusion. In the presence of obstruction to flow, the upper limit of cardiac output is relatively fixed, limiting the compensation for decreased systemic vascular resistance and leading to a decrease in arterial perfusion. Aortic stenosis should be excluded as a cause of syncope in the elderly. The classic presentation is chest pain, dyspnea on exertion and syncope. Hypertrophic cardiomyopathy is characterized by asymmetric left ventricular hypertrophy and occurs most commonly in the young, although this entity is frequently present in persons older than the age of 60 years. Pulmonary outflow obstruction may also lead to syncope. Up to 13 percent of patients with acute pulmonary embolism develop syncope secondary to the acute obstruction to blood flow by a large embolus.[8]

Medications

Medications may contribute to syncope by a variety of means (Table 52-2).[9] Antihypertensive medications such as β-blockers or calcium channel blockers commonly lead to a blunted heart rate response after orthostatic stress. Diuretics may produce volume depletion and subsequent orthostatic hypotension. Some medications have proarrhythmic properties, increasing the concern for dysrhythmia as the cause of syncope.

Psychiatric Illness

Psychiatric disorders are found in a modest percentage of patients with syncope. In one study, the most frequent psychiatric diagnoses were generalized anxiety disorder and major depressive disorder.[10] Hyperventilation has been used as a provocative maneuver in diagnosing panic disorder and generalized anxiety disorders, and can lead do hypocarbia, cerebral vasoconstriction, and subsequent syncope.[11,12] Hyperventilation may not be obvious to the observer but can be documented by end-tidal CO_2 monitoring.[11] In general, a patient with syncope and a psychiatric disorder is likely to be young, with repeated episodes of syncope, multiple prodromal symptoms, and a generally positive review of symptoms. A psychiatric cause for syncope should be one of exclusion, assigned only after organic causes have been excluded.

Neurovascular Syncope

Cerebrovascular disorders are rarely the primary cause of syncope, but must be considered in any patient with syncope and signs or symptoms indicating central nervous system pathology.

Brainstem ischemia may cause a decrease in blood flow to the reticular activating system, leading to sudden brief episodes of loss of consciousness. These episodes of loss of consciousness are typically associated with other signs and symptoms of posterior circulation ischemia,

TABLE 52-2   Drugs Commonly Implicated in Syncope

Antihypertensives
β-blockers
Cardiac glycosides
Diuretics
Antidysrhythmics
Antipsychotics
Antiparkinsonism drugs
Antidepressants
Phenothiazines
Nitrates
Alcohol
Cocaine

including diplopia, vertigo, and nausea, and possibly vertebrobasilar bruits. Subclavian steal is a rare cause of brainstem ischemia. It is characterized by an abnormal narrowing of the subclavian artery proximal to the origin of the vertebral artery such that with exercise of the ipsilateral arm, blood is shunted, or "stolen," from the vertebrobasilar system to the subclavian artery supplying the arm muscles. Because of anatomy, it is more common on the left. Physical examination may reveal decreased pulse volume and diminished blood pressure in the affected arm. Other causes of brainstem ischemia include vertebrobasilar atherosclerotic disease and basilar artery migraines.

Subarachnoid hemorrhage is a devastating disease process that may present with syncope. Accurate data regarding frequency of syncopal presentation of subarachnoid hemorrhage is not readily available, but it does not seem to be particularly common. As intracranial pressure increases there is a decrease in cerebral perfusion pressure, which may cause syncope. The patient typically complains of sudden severe headache and may have focal neurologic findings.

Syncope in Special Populations

THE ELDERLY   Because of both normal physiologic changes with aging and age-related disease processes, the elderly are at increased risk for syncope. They also are susceptible to increased morbidity from either the trauma of the syncopal episode or from iatrogenic events during subsequent hospital admission.

As a person ages, the blood vessels become calcified and less compliant, leading to diminished flow rates. The left ventricle also becomes less compliant, resulting in increased diastolic filling pressures and an increased dependence on the "atrial kick." There is a general decrease in adrenergic receptor responsiveness of both the heart and the peripheral blood vessels. Decreased adrenergic responsiveness contributes to the diminished chronotropic response seen after orthostatic stresses in the elderly. Incidence of vasovagal syncope actually decreases with age, in part as a consequence of this decreased responsiveness of the autonomic nervous. The elderly also have a less-sensitive thirst mechanism and a decreased endocrine response to volume depletion. Pathophysiologic processes that may contribute to diminished cerebral perfusion include disorders such as hypertension, atherosclerosis, and valvular disease. Chronic hypertension shifts the cerebral autoregulation mechanism to higher pressures. Orthostatic hypotension and postprandial hypotension are more common among the hypertensive elderly. Atherosclerotic disease leads to ischemia and myocardial infarction and subsequent congestive heart failure and dysrhythmias. Aortic stenosis is the most common obstructive cardiac lesion in the elderly, producing a fixed cardiac output. Risk for syncope increases when increased demand for cardiac output cannot be met.[13] Diabetes may lead to autonomic dysfunction and peripheral neuropathy. Finally, medication usage is much more common in the elderly population, again increasing the risk of orthostasis and decreasing autonomic responsiveness to orthostatic stress. It is important to note that syncope in the elderly population is most often multifactorial and the etiology may, therefore, be difficult to establish, particularly in the ED.

PREGNANCY   Pregnancy is associated with numerous physiologic changes including increased heart rate, decreased peripheral resistance, and increased stroke volume. In late pregnancy, the enlarged uterus may compress the inferior vena cava, decreasing venous return. The incidence of cardiac dysrhythmias, especially premature ventricular contractions, increases during normal pregnancy in young healthy women. However, a positive correlation has not been shown between symptoms of presyncope or syncope and cardiac dysrhythmia.[14] Vasovagal syncope is a diagnosis of exclusion.

PEDIATRICS   Syncope in the pediatric population is discussed elsewhere in this text (Chap. 131).

EMERGENCY DEPARTMENT EVALUATION

The goal of the emergency department evaluation of the patient with syncope is to identify those at increased risk for both immediate decompensation as a result of an underlying disease process and for future risk of serious morbidity or sudden death. The core components of the ED evaluation of syncope are a careful history, a thorough physical examination, and the electrocardiogram. The history and physical examination alone will identify the cause of syncope in most patients in whom a diagnosis can be established.[2]

History

Clinical history should be obtained from the patient and any witness of the event. Emphasis should be placed on the events leading up to the loss of consciousness, the characteristics of the loss of consciousness, and symptoms occurring after regaining consciousness. The history should begin with a detailed description of the events preceding the loss of consciousness, including position, environmental stimuli, and the involvement of strenuous activity or arm exercise. All premonitory symptoms should be recorded, looking for neurologic symptoms, such as vertigo or focal weakness, and cardiac symptoms, such as palpitations. Duration of loss of consciousness and symptoms occurring after regaining consciousness should also be documented. Symptoms associated with syncope that should raise concern of an immediately life-threatening diagnosis include chest pain (acute myocardial infarction, aortic dissection, pulmonary embolism, aortic stenosis), headache (subarachnoid hemorrhage), and abdominal or back pain (leaking abdominal aortic aneurysm, ruptured ectopic pregnancy). A sudden event without warning and events associated with exertion should increase suspicion of a cardiac dysrhythmia or structural cardiopulmonary lesion.[16] Antecedent illness or substance use should be documented. The past medical history should include questions regarding underlying structural heart disease including congenital heart disease, valvular heart disease, coronary artery disease, and cardiomyopathy. The past medical history should also include details about prior cardiopulmonary events, including prior myocardial infarction, pulmonary embolism, ventricular dysrhythmias, and congestive heart failure. Any prior history of syncope should also be documented, as patients who have recurrent syncope with more than five episodes in 1 year are more likely to have vasovagal syncope or a psychiatric diagnosis than dysrhythmia as the cause.[2] All medications should be recorded, including over-the-counter medications such as laxatives. Patients aggressively dieting to lose weight may have electrolyte disturbances or be taking amphetamine-like medications. The family history is important in regards to history of prolonged QT syndrome, dysrhythmias, sudden cardiac death, or other cardiac risks.

Special attention should be paid to patients presenting with single-car motor vehicle crashes (especially driving off the road), particularly if the patients are elderly. Clinicians may become preoccupied by the trauma evaluation and miss the possibility of syncopal event.

Seizure is the most common event mistaken as syncope. The two conditions do not share the same pathophysiologic mechanisms. Occasionally, the underlying mechanism that causes syncope may result in an associated seizure (e.g., cerebral hypoperfusion). History is very important in differentiating syncope from seizure.[15] Pre- and postmonitory symptoms may assist in differentiation. A classic aura or postictal confusion and muscle pain indicate seizure while characteristic prodromal symptoms of nausea and diaphoresis suggest reflex-mediated syncope. Witness information of the event may also be useful. Witnessed head turning or unusual posture during the event is consistent with seizure. Extremity movement is less reliable, as the brief asynchronous movements that may follow the loss of consciousness with syncope are often confused with the tonic-clonic movements of seizures. Urinary incontinence is not useful in the distinction. A wide transitory, anion gap acidosis follows a generalized seizure but is not present in simple syncope.

Physical Examination

Evidence of trauma without defensive injuries to the hands or knees should raise suspicion of a sudden event without warning, such as a dysrhythmia. The physical examination should focus on both the cardiovascular and neurologic systems. Blood pressure measurements should be taken in both arms. Unequal blood pressures should increase suspicion of aortic dissection or subclavian steal. The presence of orthostatic hypotension and symptoms should be sought. To appropriately evaluate orthostasis, the patient should be supine for a period of 5 min and then should arise to the standing position. After standing, blood pressure measurements should be taken two to three times over the next few minutes. A decrease in systolic blood pressure greater than 20 mm Hg is considered positive. Cardiac examination may reveal the murmur of hypertrophic cardiomyopathy or aortic stenosis. The neurologic examination may uncover findings of focal neurologic disease or evidence of autonomic instability such as the presence of peripheral neuropathy. Rectal examination should be performed to evaluate for gastrointestinal bleeding.

Electrocardiogram

A 12-lead ECG should be obtained, even though the electrocardiogram and rhythm strip lead to a diagnosis in only a small number of patients.[3] The ECG should be evaluated for evidence of prior cardiopulmonary disease, acute ischemia, dysrhythmia, and heart block, prolonged QT interval. Patients should be monitored for abnormal cardiac activity until a cardiac origin has been reasonably excluded.

Laboratory Testing

Laboratory testing is directed by results of the history and physical examination. For example, a patient with orthostatic symptoms and heme-positive stool test warrants at least a complete blood count (CBC). A reproductive-age female should have a urine pregnancy test. Although electrolyte abnormalities may be implicated as a cause of seizures, they are rarely the cause of syncope.[3] Evidence of an irritable myocardium, profound weakness, dehydration, or diuretic use merits serum electrolyte determination, particularly potassium.

Carotid Massage

Carotid massage is used to diagnose carotid sinus hypersensitivity in the patient with a history suggestive of carotid sinus syndrome. Although not general emergency practice at this time, it can be done at the bedside in the ED with continuous electrocardiographic and blood pressure monitoring after informed consent has been obtained. Each carotid body is separately massaged for 5 to 10 s. The test is considered positive if symptoms are reproduced in the presence of asystole greater than 3 s or fall in systolic blood pressure of >50 mm Hg. Carotid massage should not be done if the patient has known carotid stenosis, if bruits are present, if there is history of recent (<3 months) stroke or myocardial infarction, or if there is a history of ventricular tachycardia or fibrillation. Neurologic deficits resulting from cardiac massage are rare, with deficits lasting more than 24 h in approximately 0.1 percent of patients.[17,18] Only a small number of patients with carotid hypersensitivity will have the true carotid sinus syndrome.

Hyperventilation Maneuver

A hyperventilation maneuver (open-mouthed, slow, deep breaths at a rate of 20 to 30 breaths per minute for 2 to 3 min) can be very useful in the young patient with undiagnosed syncope and suspected psychiatric illness. This can easily be performed in the ED. A recurrence of prodromal symptoms or syncope significantly correlates with psychiatric (anxiety-provoking) causes of syncope.[11]

Neurologic Testing

Studies fail to show any benefit of routine computed tomography (CT) scanning, electroencephalogram (EEG), or lumbar puncture for patients who lack a history or physical examination that supports a neurologic cause of syncope.[3]

DISPOSITION

Figure 52-1 provides a general management strategy.

Diagnosis Established

If a cause of syncope can be determined by the initial history, physical examination and ECG, identification of high-risk patients is simple. Those patients with acute neurologic deficits or life-threatening disorders are at immediate risk of morbidity. Additionally, patients with cardiac causes of syncope represent a high-risk group for major morbidity or death and need further inpatient monitoring and evaluation. In the Framingham Study, the hazard ratios for cardiac syncope were 2, 2.66, and 2 for death from any cause, myocardial infarction or death from coronary heart disease, and fatal or nonfatal stroke, respectively. Patients with reflex-mediated syncope (including vasovagal, orthostatic, and medication-related syncope) had no increased risk of cardiovascular morbidity or mortality.[4] Unfortunately, on evaluation in the ED, a cause of syncope is not identifiable in up to half of patients.[3]

Unexplained Syncope

Patients with an unknown etiology of syncope after the initial ED evaluation need a further inpatient or outpatient medical evaluation that focuses on the identification of risk factors for morbidity and mortality (see Figure 52-1).

The evaluation of the patient with unexplained syncope should focus on identifying those at high risk for a cardiac etiology. Heart disease should be suspected in patients presenting with exertional syncope or an abnormal cardiac history, examination or electrocardiogram. Patients with underlying heart disease, irrespective of cause, are at greatest risk of cardiac arrhythmia and death.[18] This is further supported by a prospective study that focused on risk stratification of patients with syncope based on clinical and electrocardiographic characteristics.[19] **The study found four significant predictors of sudden cardiac death or signifi-**

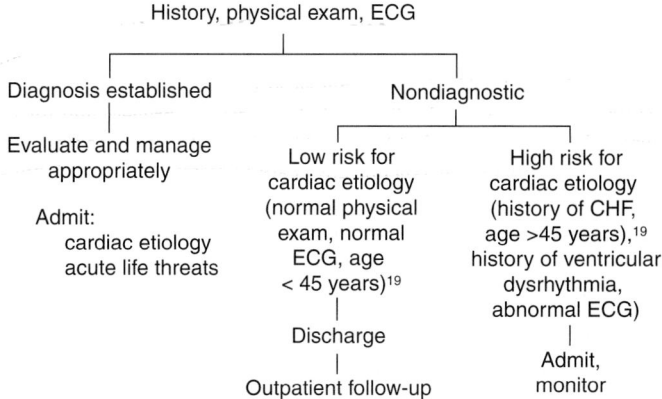

FIG. 52-1. ED management of syncope.

cant dysrhythmia within one year of a syncopal event: abnormal electrocardiogram (anything other than nonspecific ST-T changes), age older than 45 years, history of ventricular dysrhythmia, and history of congestive heart failure. Numbers of predictors are correlated with degree of risk. This is also consistent with prior studies that show that the prognosis of syncope in patients without heart disease is very good.[20,21] The young patient with syncope, a normal physical examination, and a normal electrocardiogram has a very low risk of morbidity.

Indications for hospital admission, therefore, include patients with acute neurologic or life-threatening disorders and patients at risk for a cardiac etiology of syncope (see Figure 52-1). Patients without a clear diagnosis of vasovagal episode who are discharged from the ED should be accompanied by a responsible adult and be advised not to drive, work at heights, or operate machinery until further outpatient evaluation.

POST-ED EVALUATION

Inpatient Evaluation

With the exception of those patients with acute life-threatening diagnoses (stroke, aortic dissection, etc.), the core of the inpatient evaluation is focused on identification of underlying heart disease and detection of dysrhythmias (Table 52-3). All admitted patients require

TABLE 52-3   **Post-ED Testing for Syncope**

Test	Indication	Utility
Cardiac syncope		
Electrocardiographic monitoring	Admission	Cardiac syncope confirmed if recurrent symptoms occur during monitored dysrhythmia; excluded if recurrent symptoms reported during sinus rhythm
	Outpatient event monitor if no significant cardiac disease suspected	
Echocardiography	History, examination or ECG suggestive of structural heart disease	Confirm and quantify suspected structural heart disease
Electrophysiology testing	Documented dysrhythmia or serious underlying heart disease	Identifies inducible tachydysrhythmias and some bradydysrhythmias
Stress testing	Exercise-related syncope	Identifies exercise-induced dysrhythmias and postexercise syncope
Neurologic syncope		
CT/MRA/Carotid Doppler	Neurologic signs or symptoms	Identify cerebrovascular abnormality or subclavian stenosis
Electroencephalography	Suspected seizure	Document underlying seizure disorder
Reflex-mediated syncope		
Tilt table testing	Recurrent syncope, cardiac etiology excluded	Positive test establishes diagnosis of neurocardiogenic syncope
Psychogenic		
Psychiatric testing	Young patient, no underlying heart disease	Identifies underlying psychiatric disorder predisposing to syncope

continuous electrocardiographic monitoring. Dysrhythmia as the cause of syncope is confirmed in the patient with recurrent symptoms during a monitored dysrhythmia and excluded in the patient with recurrent symptoms and sinus rhythm. An echocardiogram should be performed on patients with known or suspected heart disease to evaluate for abnormalities, such as valvular disorders, congenital anomalies and cardiomyopathies, and to determine overall cardiac function. Abnormalities are usually clinically apparent and will seldom be found in patients with a normal cardiac examination and ECG. Stress testing is used to identify exercise-induced dysrhythmias or ischemia, or to reproduce postexertional syncope. It should be performed in patients with exercise-related syncope, once hypertrophic cardiomyopathy has been excluded by echocardiography. Electrophysiology (EP) testing is typically reserved for patients with documented dysrhythmia, preexcitation or underlying heart disease. EP testing involves invasive electrical stimulation and monitoring of the heart to uncover possible conduction abnormalities that predispose patients to tachydysrhythmias (both ventricular and supraventricular). EP studies may also detect bradydysrhythmias, but the yield is lower.

Outpatient Evaluation

Patients undergoing outpatient syncope evaluation are deemed to be at low risk for serious cardiac dysrhythmias. Long-term monitoring, which includes external or implanted loop-event monitors, is useful to further evaluate potential dysrhythmias (see Table 52-3). Tilt table testing is also suggested for patients with recurrent, unexplained syncope. This test is designed to identify reflex-mediated syncope by rapidly moving the patient from a supine position on the tilt table to an upright position of 60 degrees for 45 min. A positive end point is reached if syncope, hypotension, or the patient's typical symptoms are reproduced. Repeat testing with isoproterenol or sublingual nitroglycerin is performed if the initial evaluation is negative. Recurrent reflex-mediated syncope resistant to conservative therapies has been successfully treated with a cardiac pacemaker. Psychiatric referral is recommended for young patients without underlying heart disease who have frequent syncopal events. Generalized anxiety and depressive disorders are the most commonly assigned diagnoses.

REFERENCES

1. Kapoor WN: Syncope in older persons. *J Am Geriatr Soc* 42:426, 1994.
2. Sarasin, FP, Louis-Simonet M, Carballo D, et al: Prospective evaluation of patients with syncope: A population-based study. *Am J Med* 111:177, 2001.
3. Linzer M, Yang EH, Estes NA III, et al: Diagnosing syncope. Part 1: Value of history, physical examination and electrocardiography. The clinical efficacy assessment project of the American College of Physicians. *Ann Intern Med* 126:989, 1997.
4. Soteriades ES, Evans JC, Larson MG, et al: Incidence and prognosis of syncope. *New Engl J Med* 347:878, 2002.
5. Strasberg B, Rechavia E, Sagie A, et al: The head up tilt-table test in patients with syncope of unknown origin. *Am Heart J* 118(5 part 1):923, 1989.
6. Atkins D, Hanusa B, Sefcik T, et al: Syncope and orthostatic hypotension. *Am J Med* 91:179, 1991.
7. McAnulty JH, Rahimtoola SH, Murphy E, et al: Natural history of "high-risk" bundle-branch block: Final report of a prospective study. *New Engl J Med* 307:137, 1982.
8. Thames MD, Alpert JS, Dalen JE: Syncope in patients with pulmonary embolism. *JAMA* 238:2509, 1977.
9. Hanlon JT, Linzer M, MacMillan JP, et al: Syncope and presyncope associated with probable adverse drug reaction. *Arch Intern Med* 150:2309, 1990.
10. Kapoor WN, Fortunato M, Hanusa BH, et al: Psychiatric illness in patients with syncope, *Am J Med* 99:505, 1995.
11. Koenig D, Pontinen G, Divine GW: Syncope in young adults: Evidence for a combined medical and psychiatric approach. *J Intern Med* 232:169, 1992.
12. Naschitz JE, Gaitini L, Mazov I, et al: The capnography-tilt test for the diagnosis of hyperventilation syncope. *QJM* 90:139, 1997.
13. Lindroos M, Kupari M, Heikkila J, et al: Prevalence of aortic valve abnormalities in the elderly: An echocardiographic study of a random population. *J Am Coll Cardiol* 21:1220, 1993.
14. Shotan A, Ostrzega E, Mehra A, et al: Incidence of arrhythmias in normal pregnancy and relation to palpitations, dizziness, and syncope. *Am J Cardiol* 79:1061, 1997.
15. Sheldon R, Rose S, Ritchie D, et al: Historical criteria that distinguish syncope from seizures. *J Am Coll Cardiol* 40:142, 2002.
16. Alboni P, Brignole M, Menozzi C, et al: Diagnostic value of history in patients with syncope with or without heart disease. *J Am Coll Cardiol* 37:1921, 2001.
17. Richardson DA, Bexton R, Shaw F, et al: Complications of carotid sinus massage-a prospective series of older patients. *Age Aging* 29:413, 2000.
18. Kapoor WN, Hanusa BH: Is syncope a risk factor for poor outcomes? Comparison of patients with and without syncope. *Am J Med* 100:646, 1996.
19. Martin TP, Hanusa BH, Kapoor WN: Risk stratification of patients with syncope. *Ann Emerg Med* 29:4, 1997.
20. Eagle KA, Black HR, Cook EF, et al: Evaluation of prognostic classifications for patients with syncope. *Am J Med* 79:455, 1985.
21. Martin GJ, Adams SL, Martin HG, et al: Prospective evaluation of syncope. *Ann Emerg Med* 13:499, 1984.

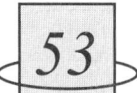

53 CONGESTIVE HEART FAILURE AND ACUTE PULMONARY EDEMA
W. Franklin Peacock IV

With 4.7 million cases and approximately 550,000 new patients each year,[1] the United States is currently experiencing a heart failure (HF) epidemic. Heart failure disproportionally affects the aged. Fewer than 1 percent of Americans younger than 50 years are stricken, but prevalence doubles each decade until, by age 80 years, nearly 10 percent carry the diagnosis. It is the leading cause of hospitalization among those older than 65 years,[1] accounts for nearly 1,000,000 hospitalizations annually, and up to 60 percent of discharged HF patients are rehospitalized within 6 months due to recurrent decompensation.[2] With predictions that the cohort older than 65 years will double in the next 30 years, the impact of HF is expected to increase. The costs of HF are roughly double that of any cancer diagnoses in the United States. In 2002 the estimated direct costs will exceed 15 billion dollars.[2]

PROGNOSIS

Heart failure has a poor prognosis. Once symptomatic, 2-year mortality is about 35 percent and over the next 6 years increases to 80 percent for men and 65 percent for women.[1] Symptom severity predicts outcome. Annual mortality rates are 5 to 10 percent in mild-moderate HF and 30 to 40 percent in severe HF. After the development of pulmonary edema, only 50 percent survive 1 year. After cardiogenic shock, up to 85 percent die within 1 week.

The New York Heart Association (NYHA) HF classification is used as a prognostic scale in most existing studies (Table 53-1). This scale is limited by excluding asymptomatic HF, has poor sensitivity and high interobserver variability, but does predict mortality. One-year mortality exceeds 50 percent in class IV. The American Heart Association scale uses risk factors to determine interventions. This system recognizes that earlier intervention has the greatest potential for morbidity and mortality reductions (see Table 53-1).[3]

PATHOPHYSIOLOGY

Heart failure may present acutely as a result of acute pump dysfunction from acute myocardial infarction. Mechanistically, loss of a critical mass of myocardium results in immediate symptoms. If there is symptomatic hypotension with inadequate perfusion, cardiogenic shock is present (see Chap. 33).

TABLE 53-1 Heart Failure Classifications and Stages

NYHA Class	ACC/AHA Class	Stage	Patient Description	Median BNP (pg/mL)
	A	High risk for developing LVD	Hypertension, coronary artery disease, diabetes mellitus, family history of cardiomyopathy	<100
I	B	Asymptomatic LVD	Previous MI or LV systolic dysfunction, asymptomatic valvular disease, no limitations of physical activity	100
II and III	C	Symptomatic LVD	Known structural heart disease, reduced exercise tolerance, shortness of breath and fatigue with ADL	220 to 450
IV	D	Refractory end-stage heart failure	Marked symptoms at rest despite maximal medical therapy	1000

Abbreviations: ACC/AHA = American College of Cardiology/American Heart Association; ADL = activity of daily living; BNP = B-type natriuretic peptide; LV = left ventricular; LVD = left ventricle dysfunction; MI = myocardial infarction; NYHA = New York Heart Assocation.

Heart failure can present precipitously as acute pulmonary edema (APE). Acute pulmonary edema is the clinical manifestation of a downward spiral of rapidly decreasing cardiac output (CO) and rising systolic vascular resistance (SVR) on the face of underlying cardiac dysfunction. Even relatively small elevations of blood pressure (BP) can result in decreased CO. Decreasing CO triggers increased SVR, which further worsens CO. Acute pulmonary edema can present acutely with severe symptoms, and, if the extremely elevated SVR is not promptly reversed, it will be the terminal event. Heart failure can also present insidiously as the final consequence of a cascade of pathologic neurohormonal and hemodynamic reflexes initiated by myocardial injury or stress. Threats to CO trigger a neurohormonally mediated cascade that includes activation of the renin-angiotensin-aldosterone system and the sympathetic nervous systems. Levels of norepinephrine, vasopressin, endothelin (a potent vasoconstrictor), and tissue necrosis factor-α are increased. Although not available clinically, levels of these hormones directly correlate with mortality in HF patients.

The combined clinical effects of neurohormonal activation are sodium and water retention and increased SVR. These compensatory mechanisms may maintain BP and perfusion, but at the cost of increased myocardial workload, wall tension, and, hence, myocardial oxygen demand. Although some patients are initially asymptomatic, the mechanism of cardiac remodeling, a secondary pathologic process, begins to occur. The type of remodeling determines future hemodynamics and therapies.

Natriuretic peptides (NPs) are the endogenous counterregulatory arm to the pathologic neurohormonal activation of HF. Three types are recognized: atrial NP, primarily secreted from the atria; B-type NP (BNP), secreted mainly from the cardiac ventricle; and CNP, localized in the endothelium. Natriuretic peptides result in vasodilation, natriuresis, decreased levels of endothelin, and inhibition of the renin-angiotensin-aldosterone system and the sympathetic nervous systems. BNP is the only NP for which an assay is currently available. BNP is synthesized as N-terminal pre-pro-BNP, which itself is cleared to two substances, inactive N-terminal pro-BNP, with a half-life of approximately 2 h, and physiologically active BNP, with a half-life of about 20 min.[4]

Because elevated levels of neurohormones portend a worse prognosis in HF, their attenuation provides the theoretical basis for most therapies proven to delay HF morbidity and mortality. These include treatment with angiotensin-converting enzyme inhibitors (ACEIs), angiotensin receptor blockers (ARBs), spironolactone, β-blockers, and nesiritide.

SYSTOLIC VERSUS DIASTOLIC HF

The law of LaPlace describes wall tension as a product of pressure (afterload) and ventricular radius. Increased wall tension is the stimulus

for cardiac remodeling. Initially, myocytes hypertrophy or die (apoptosis) to form scar tissue. The dominant response determines HF type. Many different pathologies can lead to the clinical presentation of HF (Table 53-2).

Heart failure is classified as systolic or diastolic by ejection fraction (EF) measurement, which is normally 60 percent. *Systolic dysfunction,* defined as an EF under 40 percent, is most commonly from ischemic heart disease, but other causes may be considered. Mechanistically, the ventricle has difficulty ejecting blood. Impaired contractility leads to increased intracardiac volumes and pressure and *afterload sensitivity.* With circulatory stress (e.g., walking), failure to

TABLE 53-2 Common Causes of Heart Failure and Pulmonary Edema

Myocardial ischemia: Acute and chronic*
Valvular dysfunction
  Aortic valve disease
    Aortic stenosis
    Aortic insufficiency
      Aortic dissection
      Infectious endocarditis
  Mitral valve disease
    Mitral stenosis
    Mitral regurgitation
      Papillary muscle dysfunction or rupture
      Ruptured chordae tendineae
      Infectious endocarditis
  Prosthetic valve malfunction
Other causes of left ventricular outflow obstruction
  Supravalvular aortic stenosis
  Membranous subvalvular aortic stenosis
Cardiomyopathy*
  Hypertrophic cardiomyopathy
  Dilated†
  Restrictive
Acquired cardiomyopathy
  Toxic: Alcohol, cocaine, doxorubicin
  Metabolic: Thyrotoxicosis, myxedema
Myocarditis: Radiation, infection
Constrictive pericarditis
Cardiac tamponade
Systemic hypertension*
Miscellaneous
  Anemia
  Cardiac dysrhythmias*

*Seen in the ED with higher frequency.
†Includes idiopathic (see Chap. 55).

improve contractility, despite increasing venous return, results in increased cardiac pressures, pulmonary congestion, and edema.

In *diastolic HF,* contractile function is preserved, and the EF is normal or higher. The main pathology is impaired ventricular relaxation, causing an abnormal relation between diastolic pressure and volume. This results in a left ventricle (LV) that has difficulty receiving blood. Decreased LV compliance necessitates higher atrial pressures to ensure adequate diastolic LV filling and results in *preload sensitivity.* The frequency of diastolic dysfunction increases with age. Chronic hypertension and LV hypertrophy are often responsible for this condition (see Table 53-2). Coronary artery disease also contributes, as diastolic dysfunction is an early event in the ischemic cascade.

As many as 30 to 50 percent of elderly HF patients have circulatory congestion on the basis of diastolic dysfunction.[5] Treatment for volume overload, the most common ED presentation, is the same irrespective of EF. Because patients with diastolic dysfunction are preload dependent, excessive diuresis or venodilation may exacerbate the underlying deficit in ventricular filling and cause hypotension. After hemodynamics are stabilized and congestion resolved, treatment of diastolic dysfunction requires consideration of the underlying etiology. Determining HF type is difficult from the history and physical examination. Consequently, an echocardiogram is usually necessary. Determining the etiology for diastolic dysfunction is rarely an ED task, but the workup may be initiated from an observation or acute care unit.

Some differentiate left- from right-side HF. Isolated left-side HF is associated with dyspnea, fatigue, weakness, cough, paroxysmal nocturnal dyspnea, and orthopnea in the absence of peripheral edema, jugular venous distention (JVD), or hepatojugular reflux. Right-side HF has peripheral edema, JVD, right upper quadrant pain, and hepatojugular reflex, without pulmonary symptoms. Abnormal pressure and chamber volumes are eventually reflected to the contralateral side. Untreated or poorly controlled left-side HF eventually may be reflected on the right. With isolated right-side HF (e.g., right ventricular infarct), left-side HF is less likely but can eventually occur. This traditional distinction (right vs. left HF), although often mentioned, does not have great bearing on the ED approach. For example, volume overload is approached in a uniform manner for the most part. This distinction has greatest applicability when there is suspicion of valvular heart disease or right ventricular infarction (see Chaps. 50 and 54).

High output HF can occur when the normally intact myocardium is unable to meet excess functional demands. These instances are relatively few but include anemia, thyrotoxicosis, large atrioventricular shunts, beriberi, and Paget disease of the bone. The appropriate treatment for these conditions is symptomatic and addresses the causative pathology.

DIAGNOSIS

History and Physical Examination

Acute pulmonary edema is characterized by severe respiratory distress, relative hypertension, and cool diaphoretic skin. Rales may be heard over most of the lung fields, JVD is marked, but peripheral edema may or may not be present. In comparison with pulmonary edema, decompensated HF is a difficult diagnosis. It occurs in a population of patients at risk for many comorbidities, and errors in diagnosis are further compounded by a lack of accurate testing available in real time. The ED diagnostic error rate is reported as 12 percent, equally divided between over- and underdiagnosis.[6] Errors occur because neither history nor physical examination are accurate for HF. Dyspnea has a sensitivity and specificity of about 50 percent; orthopnea has a specificity of 88 percent, but with no better sensitivity; and rales have a predictive accuracy of only 70 percent. Edema is even worse as a HF indicator. The best physical finding suggestive of an elevated pulmonary capillary wedge pressure (PCWP) is the S3, with a specificity of 99 percent. However, it is difficult to detect in the ED, and its sensitivity is 20 percent.[6] Similarly, JVD, with a specificity of 94 percent, has a sensitivity of 39 percent. In other studies, reported confounders impeding a correct HF diagnosis include obesity, deconditioning, and female sex.

Chest Radiography

Until recently, ancillary tests available in the ED offered little accuracy improvement over history and physical examination. Even though the HF diagnostic gold standard is echocardiography, because of limitations on technology or performance expertise, it is not used for this purpose in most EDs. Therefore, other measures are used. Chest radiographs (CXR) are easily obtained but are a blunt tool for evaluating cardiopulmonary status. Although a normal CXR cannot exclude abnormal LV function, it helps eliminate other diagnoses (e.g., pneumonia). The radiographic findings of left-side HF are, in descending order of frequency, dilated upper lobe vessels, cardiomegaly, interstitial edema, enlarged pulmonary artery, pleural effusion, alveolar edema, prominent superior vena cava, and Kerley lines.[8] **Because acute abnormalities lag the clinical appearance by up to 6 h, therapy is not withheld pending an CXR.**

In chronic HF, congestive signs have unreliable sensitivity, specificity, and predictive value for identifying patients with high PCWP. Radiographic pulmonary congestion is absent in 53 percent of patients with mild to moderately elevated PCWP (16 to 29 mm Hg) and in 39 percent of those with markedly elevated PCWP (>30 mm Hg).[9]

Cardiomegaly can be helpful for diagnosing HF. However, although a cardiothoracic ratio larger than 60 percent correlates with increased 5-year mortality, CXR sensitivity for cardiomegaly can be poor. This observation is explained by intrathoracic cardiac rotation. In one study of echocardiographically proven cardiomegaly, 22 percent had a normal cardiothoracic ratio.[10]

Pleural effusion can be missed by the CXR, especially if the patient is intubated and supine. In patients with pleural effusions, the sensitivity, specificity, and accuracy of the supine CXR for HF were reported to be 67, 70, and 67 percent, respectively.[11]

The sensitivity for HF with a portable CXR is poor. In mild HF, only the finding of dilated upper lobe vessels was reported in more than 60 percent of patients. Nevertheless, in the ED setting, the CXR is helpful. The frequency that CXR HF parameters are present increases with HF severity. With severe HF, some CXR findings occurred in at least two thirds of patients, except for Kerley lines (11 percent) and prominent vena cava (44 percent).[8] Absence of any associated findings in CXR without significant vital sign or pulse oximetric abnormalities is reassuring.

Natriuretic Peptide Assay

Natriuretic peptide measurement offers improved diagnostic accuracy for HF. These proteins are released by ventricular pressure or volume stimulus and, consequently, correlate with elevated PCWP. As a point-of-care assay, BNP, predicts the presence of HF. In non-HF, BNP levels averaged 38 pg/mL, compared with HF patients whose mean level was 1076 pg/mL.[6] When HF is graded by NYHA class, BNP levels vary directly with severity. BNP is helpful in patients most difficult to diagnose, i.e., those with combined COPD and HF. In dyspnea due to COPD, BNP levels were less than 100 pg/mL, compared with HF patients whose levels exceeded 1000 pg/ml. An analysis of edematous patients found similar results.[6] When signs and symptoms raise suspicion of HF, a BNP level may contribute to an accurate diagnosis.

In ED patients, BNP levels also correlate with subsequent clinical events. Emergency department BNP levels greater than 480 pg/mL were associated with a 40 percent rate of death or HF re-hospitalization within 6 months, compared with 3 percent when levels were lower than 230 pg/mL.[12] Mortality is also predicted by BNP. With BNP levels above 73 pg/mL, mortality is markedly increased in the next 12 months versus those with BNP levels below 73 pg/mL.[13]

The diagnosis of HF is suggested by the proper clinical scenario and a BNP greater than 100 pg/mL. This test has a coefficient of variation of about 10 percent; but in the ranges that BNP occurs clinically, this number is not statistically significant. At the 100 pg/mL level, BNP demonstrates a sensitivity of 90 to 94 percent and a specificity of 76 to 94 percent. The positive and negative predictive values are 79 to 92 percent and 89 to 96 percent, respectively, and the overall accuracy is 83 to 94 percent.[14,15] There are confounders to BNP as an HF test. BNP is increased in the elderly, women, those with cirrhosis or renal failure, possibly those on hormone replacement therapy, and probably those with pulmonary embolus and primary pulmonary hypertension. Consequently, the clinical application of the BNP assay is that a level below 100 pg/mL effectively excludes HF with good reliability, and a markedly elevated BNP is strong evidence of HF. However, lesser elevations (100 to 250 pg/mL) should prompt consideration of other confounding diagnoses and confirmatory testing.

Differential Diagnosis

The differential diagnosis should be considered from two perspectives: (1) conditions that mimic or may be confused with HF, and (2) conditions that precipitate or worsen HF (Table 53-3). Many of the conditions that mimic HF can actually precipitate it. Until excluded, acute myocardial infarction must always be considered as the etiology of the HF exacerbation. Further, breathlessness is a common symptom, so other dyspneic conditions should be considered. A common confounder is coexisting obstructive pulmonary disease. Severe hypertension and peripheral vasoconstriction suggest acute HF, even with audible wheezing. Pneumonia or pulmonary embolus can mimic or exacerbate HF. Differentiating HF from other causes can be challenging. History and physical examination may help, but the CXR is misleading when chronic HF findings are unrelated to the presentation. Comparison views may be helpful here. Edema is seen in HF but is nonspecific, because it is found in hypoproteinemic states, hepatic or renal failure, and vascular diseases.

TABLE 53-3 Differential Diagnoses for Heart Failure

Dyspneic States
  Asthma exacerbation
  Chronic obstructive pulmonary disease exacerbation
  Pleural effusion
  Pneumonia or other pulmonary infection
  Pneumothorax
  Pulmonary embolus
  Physical deconditioning or obesity
Fluid retentive states
  Dependent edema or deep vein thrombosis
  Hypoproteinemia
  Liver failure or cirrhosis
  Portal vein thrombosis
  Renal failure or nephrotic syndrome
Impaired cardiac output states
  Acute myocardial infarction
  Acute valvular insufficiency
  Drug overdose/effect
  Dysrhythmias
  Pericardial tamponade
  Tension hydro- or pneumothorax
  High output state
    Sepsis
    Anemia
    Thyroid dysfunction

TREATMENT

General Measures

The initial approach is driven by the acuity of presentation, volume status, and systemic perfusion. In critical patients, airway management supersedes all else. This is in contrast to the mildly symptomatic patient whose evaluation may precede emergent stabilization procedures.

Initial stabilization is aimed at maintaining airway control and adequate ventilation. Supplemental oxygen use may be guided by pulse oximetry. Because hypoxia is a greater risk than hypercarbia, O_2 is not withheld due to CO_2 retention concerns. Arterial blood gas measurements may be helpful in the critically ill or if CO_2 retention is likely. Endotracheal intubation with mechanical ventilation or support is indicated if stability is unclear.

Noninvasive positive pressure ventilation (NIPPV) is controversial in the HF patient (see Chap. 18). Some investigators report that it temporizes the properly selected patient while awaiting hemodynamic interventions to become effective. Biphasic positive airway pressure (BiPAP) involves delivery of separately controlled inspiratory and expiratory pressures by face mask. Continuous positive airway pressure (CPAP) delivers constant pressure throughout the respiratory cycle. For a trial of NIPPV, close monitoring, hemodynamic stability, and patient cooperation are required. NIPPV may offer a mortality benefit over invasive mechanical ventilation in COPD, but data are controversial in acute pulmonary edema. The use of NIPPV may decrease need for endotracheal intubations; however, mortality appears to be unchanged, and some report that patients on CPAP have higher rates of myocardial infarction than do patients treated with BiPAP,[16] although even this finding is unclear.

Standard initial ED measures include cardiac monitoring, pulse oximetry, 12-lead electrocardiogram, intravenous access, and frequent vital sign assessments. Coronary artery disease is one of the most common underlying conditions associated with HF. As many as 14% of ED patients presenting with acute decompensated HF will have positive serum cardiac markers.[17a] If acute myocardial infarction is suspected, emergent reperfusion therapy is considered. Chest radiography, complete blood cell count, electrolytes, BNP level, and cardiac markers are generally measured.

Other considerations include liver enzymes in the face of hepatomegaly, which may exclude etiologies other than passive congestion. In the presence of widened anion gap acidosis, an elevated lactate level may confirm cardiogenic shock. Testing for drug levels, e.g., digoxin, is guided by the presentation. Ethanol and drug screening may be needed, and assay for Mg^{2+} is considered with arrhythmia or severe hypokalemia. A urinary drainage catheter is placed as needed to monitor fluid status in the severely ill, or if urine output is sufficient to interfere with the patient's ability to rest.

Precipitants of decompensation should be measured (Table 53-4).

Acute Pulmonary Edema

The failing heart is very sensitive to increases in afterload. In some, systolic BP as low as 150 mm Hg can precipitate pulmonary edema. Prompt recognition and afterload reduction can avoid the need for intubation. An initial approach is repeated sublingual administration of nitroglycerin (NTG), 0.4 mg, at rate of up to one per minute, until intravenous NTG (0.2 to 0.4 μg/kg per min) is initiated, or BP declines and symptoms improve. Intravenous NTG is titrated rapidly upward (200 μg/min or higher) until BP is controlled. If pressures remain elevated, and clinical improvement is not achieved, conversion to intravenous nitroprusside may be required. Nesiritide may be an appropriate alternative to NTG in selected patients who do not require immediate endotracheal intubation The critical end point is rapidly lowering the filling pressure to prevent the need for endotracheal intubation.

TABLE 53-4   Precipitants of Decompensated Heart Failure

Noncompliance
  Excess salt*
  Medication noncompliance*
Cardiac causes
  New arrhythmia
  Rapid atrial fibrillation
  Acute coronary syndrome
  Uncontrolled hypertension
Iatrogenic
  Use of calcium channel blocker, β-blocker, or nonsteroidal
    anti-inflammatory drugs
  Inappropriate therapy reduction
  Antiarrhythmic agents within 48 h
Non-cardiac causes
  Exacerbation of comorbidity (e.g., chronic obstructive pulmonary disease)
  Pulmonary embolus
Volume overload
  Renal failure (especially missed dialysis)*

*Very common.

These agents should be administered as soon as vascular access is established. Volume reduction with diuretics is also critical to lower BP and cardiac filling pressures. Intravenous furosemide or bumetanide are the preferred diuretics in the setting of acute pulmonary edema (Table 53-5). Ethacrynic acid is used if there is a serious sulfa allergy. These diuretics share the parameters of rapid onset; diuresis can begin 10 to 15 min after intravenous furosemide. If urine output is inadequate in 20 to 30 min, the diuretic dose is increased and repeated. Diuretics also have an early effect as weak venodilators.

Morphine (2 to 5 mg IV) is also used as a venodilator. Successful management of BP and cardiac filling pressure is reflected by a marked improvement in respiratory status long before any significant diuresis.

Contraindications to Vasodilation

Several pathologic conditions increase the risk of hypotension as a consequence of overly aggressive vasodilation. Physiologically, these are the preload-dependent states and include right ventricular infarction, aortic stenosis, or volume depletion. Hypertrophic cardiomyopathy (HCM) is also a contraindication to vasodilation. Combined with acute pulmonary edema, the latter is a very difficult management problem. Increases in cardiac contractility or heart rate can increase the dynamic outflow obstruction of HCM, and conditions of decreased preload or afterload also worsen the obstructive gradient. Therapy is aimed at decreasing the outflow gradient by slowing heart rate and cardiac contractility. Although this can be accomplished with intravenous β-blockers, it is best done in the intensive care unit (ICU) with hemodynamic guidance. If there is coexistent shock, phenylephrine (40 to 100 μg/min IV) is the preferred pressor, because it results in peripheral vasoconstriction without increasing cardiac contractility.

Decompensated HF

These patients may have stable vital signs, adequate oxygenation, and ventilation. However, patients will have some signs and symptoms (e.g., shortness of breath, orthopnea, JVD, rales, and possibly an S_3). Most require only diuresis, oxygen, and BP control. Selecting optimal treatment requires determining perfusion status and estimating the degree of pulmonary congestion. The worse the decompensation, the closer the management models reflect that required for pulmonary edema, described above. Vasoconstricted patients will benefit from vasodilators; those with congestion require diuretics. The most common presentation of ED HF is the vasoconstricted congested patient; for these patients, treatment with vasodilators and diuretics will generate the best outcomes. In addition, this strategy, by decreasing PCWP, is likely to produce the best clinical results in chronic HF, because mortality rates are linked directly to the PCWP.

Stable HF

Very large trials provide evidence-based data for managing stable outpatient, systolic HF. The principal drugs are β-blockers, ACEIs, ARBs, hydralazine or nitrates, diuretics, digoxin, and spironolactone. In

TABLE 53-5   Treatment Options for Congestive Heart Failure

Diuretics for Heart Failure			
Diuretic	Dose (IV)	Effect	Complications

Furosemide	No prior use: 40 mg IVP
	If prior use: Double last 24-h usage
	  (range, 80–180 mg)
	If no effect by 20–30 mins:
	  re-double dose
		Diuresis starts within 15–20 min
		Duration of action is 4–6 h
			↓ K$^+$, ↓ Mg^{2+}, hyperuricemia, hypovolemia
			Ototoxicity, pre–renal azotemia, sulfa allergy

Bumetanide	1–3 mg	Diuresis starts within 10 min Peak action at 60 min	Same as above
Ethacrynic acid	50 mg	Similar to furosemide	Same as above, ↑ ototoxicity
Vasodilators for Acute Heart Failure			
Vasodilator	Dose	Titration End Point	Complications
SL NTG IV NTG	0.4 mg, q1–5 min 0.2–0.4 μg/kg per min (starting dose)	Blood pressure Symptoms	Hypotension Headache
Nitroprussside	0.3 μg/kg per min (starting dose), 10 μg/kg per min (maximum)	Blood pressure Symptoms	Hypotension, cyanide toxicity, ?coronary steal Thiocyanate toxicity
Nesiritide	2 μg/kg bolus, then infusion of 0.01 μg/kg per min	Titration usually unnecessary	Hypotension
Morphine	2–5 mg IV, q3–5 min	Blood pressure Respiratory rate Symptoms	Respiratory depression Hypotension Altered mental status

Abbreviations: IVP = intravenous push; NTG = nitroglycerin; SL = sublingual.

general, the strategy focuses on maintaining the lowest possible BP for mentation, ambulation, and urination. All HF patients without contraindications should be chronically treated with ACEI and β-blockers (Table 53-6), even in the setting of stable disease and minimal symptoms. The neurohormonal antagonism requirements of HF therapy differ from those of most diseases for which therapy is driven by continuing symptoms. The emphasis on neurohormonal antagonism for HF represents a major management shift. Historically, diuretic relief of congestion was the main thrust of ED therapy. Although diuretics are important for acute symptomatic congestion relief, they do not improve mortality. Neurohormonal antagonism is required for the greatest mortality improvement. If there are no contraindications, ACEI therapy can be initiated for outpatient use from the ED or observation unit. Alternatively, patients already taking medications can have the dosage increased. Consultation with the patient's physician is advisable.

Details of Pharmacotherapy

DIURETICS   Diuretics are indicated for pulmonary edema and decompensated HF. Loop diuretics provide rapid symptomatic relief of congestive symptoms and improve the effects of ACEIs by decreasing intravascular volume. Most ED patients require intravenous dosing because bowel wall edema can prevent proper gastrointestinal absorption. Dosing is guided by symptoms and prior usage. Suggested dosing is listed in Table 53-5. Once congestion is resolved, a fixed maintenance dose is continued to prevent recurrence, but, because there is no mortality benefit, they are not used as monotherapy in HF.[17]

Loop diuretics promote water and sodium excretion and are effective except in severe renal dysfunction. Furosemide is inexpensive and efficacious. If bumetanide is used, 1 mg equals 40 mg of furosemide. Some patients require adding a thiazide diuretic, such as metolazone, for efficacy. Metolazone (5 to 20 mg PO, daily) can be given 20 to 30 min before furosemide in decompensated HF. The effectiveness of combination therapy results from acting on different sites of the nephron. Ethacrynic acid is the only loop diuretic that can be used in patients with a significant sulfa allergy.

Potassium-sparing diuretics, such as spironolactone, are generally reserved for class III and IV HF but not for mild decompensated HF. Aggressive diuresis can result in severe hypokalemia and must be monitored carefully. An increasing QT interval may suggest hypocalcemia, hypokalemia, or hypomagnesemia. Ototoxicity is rare but may occur if used in conjunction with aminoglycoside antibiotics.

Urinary diuretic response requires monitoring. With more symptoms or less response to initial intravenous diuretics, dosing may be doubled and repeated in 20 to 60 min or as needed based on urine output. If output remains inadequate and the patient is in an observation unit, hospitalization should be considered. Adequate output should exceed 500 mL by 2 h, unless the creatinine exceeds 2.5 mg/dL when output goals are halved.[18] Diuretic response correlates with prognosis. Poor diuresis in the setting of acute pulmonary edema has a fourfold increase in acute mortality.[19]

As an outpatient, diuretic use is guided by daily measured body weight. Patients taking diuretics should limit their salt intake to less than 3 g daily. In addition, agents that antagonize diuretic action are discouraged. These agents include nonsteroidal anti-inflammatory drugs and cyclooxygenase-2 inhibitors, especially rofecoxib.

VASODILATORS   Vasodilators are also indicated for pulmonary edema and decompensated HF. The commonly used vasodilators are NTG, nitroprusside, and nesiritide (see Table 53-5). Because all may exert significant hypotensive effects, they are not recommended if there are signs of cardiogenic shock (hypoperfusion or symptomatic hypotension). Before their use, the physician should auscultate for murmurs and inquire about HCM or aortic stenosis, because if these disorders are treated with vasodilators, hypotension may result. In any patient who becomes acutely hypotensive after the administration of vasodilators, the physician should consider the differential diagnoses listed in Table 53-7.

Nitroglycerin   Nitroglycerin can be beneficial in HF provided there is adequate BP, in particular if there is hypertension. A short-acting, rapid-onset, systemic arterial and venous dilator, it decreases mean arterial pressure by reducing afterload and preload. Its coronary vasodilatory effects also may decrease myocardial ischemia and thereby improve cardiac function.

Nitroglycerin is administered intravenously, sublingually, or transdermally. Sublingual NTG can be given as often as needed to reach a desired clinical end point, provided there is adequate BP. Intravenous NTG is initiated at 0.2 to 0.4 μg/kg per min (10 to 30 μg/min), rapidly increased by 5 to 10 μg/min increments, and titrated to BP and symptomatic improvement. High doses may be required in the acute setting.

The most important complication, hypotension, may be seen transiently. If persistent, hypotension is more likely due to volume depletion or right ventricular infarct. It usually resolves after cessation of NTG. If this fails to improve BP, a small fluid bolus (e.g., NS 250 mL) may be required. Headache is frequent, but acetaminophen usually is adequate therapy. Methemoglobinemia has been reported with use of high doses of NTG.

NITROPRUSSIDE   If further afterload reduction is required (i.e., continued high systemic vascular resistance usually manifested by persisting elevated BP despite NTG doses >200 μg), intravenous nitroprusside may be used. A more potent arterial vasodilator than NTG, its hemodynamic effects include decreased BP and LV filling pressure and increased CO. The initial dose is usually 0.3 μg/kg per min and titrated up every 5 to 10 min based on BP and clinical response. The

TABLE 53-6   ACEI and β-Blocker Contraindications

ACEI contraindications
  Angioedema
  Progressive azotemia (creatinine >3 mg/dL, or increasing)
  Bilateral renal artery stenosis
  Systemic hypotension (SBP <80 mm Hg, especially in ambulatory
    patients)
  Hyperkalemia
  Pregnancy
  Hemodynamic instability
  Intolerance secondary to severe cough
β-blocker contraindications
  Unstable hemodynamics, or congested and requiring IV diuresis
    (most ED patients)
  Severe bronchospastic airway disease
  Symptomatic bradycardia
  Advanced heart block
  Acute vascular insufficiency or worsening claudication/rest pain
  Class IV stable HF (therapy should be provided by HF specialist)
  Inotropic therapy or cardiogenic shock
  Severe conduction system disease (unless protected by a pacemaker)

Abbreviations: ACEI = angiotensin-converting enzyme inhibitor; HF = heart failure; SBP = systolic blood pressure.

TABLE 53-7   Causes of Hypotension after Vasodilator Use

Excessive vasodilation
Hypertrophic obstructive cardiomyopathy
Intravascular volume depletion
Right ventricular infarction
Cardiogenic shock
Aortic stenosis
Anaphylaxis

major complication is hypotension. Long-term use (many days at high dose) is associated with thiocyanate toxicity, especially in renal failure.

Nesiritide Identical to endogenous BNP, nesiritide has acutely beneficial hemodynamic effects. It has diuretic and natriuretic properties that result in increased urinary sodium and volume, but without increased urinary potassium or creatinine clearance. Physiologically, it is the counterbalance to pathologic neurohormonal elevations of HF; nesiritide antagonizes the renin-angiotensin-aldosterone system and sympathetic nervous systems and decreases pathologic elevations of neurohormones in HF.

The hemodynamic effects include vasodilation of veins, arteries, and coronaries, which causes a rapid decrease in right atrial pressure, pulmonary artery pressure, PCWP, SVR, mean arterial pressure, and increases stroke volume and CO.[20] Although more expensive, nesiritide results in better PCWP decrease, superior clinical improvement, and less dyspnea by 24 h than does NTG. Complications are similar to those with NTG, but with less headache. In the first 3 h of use, the rate of symptomatic hypotension with nesiritide is about 0.5 percent.[21]

Because the hemodynamic profile of nesiritide, i.e., decreasing myocardial oxygen consumption (MVO_2) and causing coronary vasodilation, suggests safety in suspected acute coronary syndromes, it is not necessary to delay treatment while awaiting cardiac marker results. Small pilot studies suggest superior outcome with nesiritide as compared with NTG for HF patients with a concurrent acute coronary syndrome.

Nesiritide is used in acute decompensated HF without cardiogenic shock. It should be used concurrently with ACEI, β-blockers, and diuretics. Recommended dosing is an initial bolus of 2 μg/kg, followed by a fixed intravenous dose of 0.01 μg/kg per min. The most common complication is dose-dependent hypotension, with an overall rate of 4 percent.

OTHER HF DRUGS

Angiotensin-Converting Enzyme Inhibitors Because they decrease mortality and hospitalizations,[17] in the absence of contraindications (see Table 53-6), all HF patients should be on an ACEI before hospital discharge. Enalapril decreases 1-year mortality in class IV HF by 31 percent and in class II and III HF by 16 percent.[22] For mortality reduction, ACEIs are better than ARBs or the combination of hydralazine and isosorbide.

The ACEI-induced angioedema results from increased bradykinin. Emergent anaphylaxis treatment is outlined in Chap. 34 but should obviously include permanent ACEI cessation. Cough can complicate ACEI therapy but should prompt a search for other causes (e.g., worse HF or infection) before it is considered a side effect. If ACEI related, the cough disappears within 1 to 2 weeks of stopping the drug. If cough is not severe, education of the benefits and encouragement to continue the ACEI are appropriate. Hydralazine/isosorbide is considered if the patient is unable to take ACEIs or ARBs.

Angiotensin-converting enzyme inhibitors can induce hypotension, so therapy may be delayed during aggressive diuresis. Hyponatremia suggests renin-angiotensin-aldosterone system activation and may predict ACEI-induced hypotension. If symptomatic on the first dose of ACEI, diuretics can be decreased and the ACEI continued. Mild azotemia during ACEI use is tolerated as long as the patient does not have bilateral renal artery stenosis, oliguria, or creatinine levels above 3 mg/dL. Potassium and renal function require close follow-up when ACEIs are started.

In general, low doses are started and titrated upward, but even lower than target doses of ACEIs reduce mortality. In addition, because they inhibit neurohormonal pathways, ACEIs may take weeks to months to exert symptomatic benefit. Even in the absence of symptomatic improvement, ACEI therapy should be continued for the long-term effects on LV remodeling and mortality.

ACEI Alternative: Angiotensin Receptor Blockers Angiotensin II promotes aldosterone release, LV remodeling (including apoptosis), arterial vasoconstriction, and renal damage. The angiotensin receptor blockers (ARBs) block angiotensin II receptors by preventing its adverse effects and may cause fewer side effects than ACEIs. Cough and angioedema are reported less frequently with ARBs, but it is unclear whether ARBs should replace ACEIs as first-line HF treatment.

ACEI Alternative: Hydralazine/Isosorbide Dinitrate The combination of hydralazine and isosorbide dinitrate decreases preload and afterload and achieves protective effects against ventricular remodeling. It reduces mortality when compared with placebo, but enalapril-treated patients have better long-term outcomes. Hydralazine/isosorbide dinitrate should be considered second-line therapy and only in patients who have proven ACEI intolerant. Complications include drug-induced lupus, hypotension, gastrointestinal complaints, and headache.

β-Blockers Norepinephrine levels are elevated in HF, contribute to myocardial hypertrophy, increase afterload and coronary vasoconstriction, and are associated with mortality. Beta blockers reduce sympathetic nervous system activity and are used in HF for mortality reduction and symptom relief, with effects comparable to some ACEIs. Metoprolol decreases 1-year mortality as much 34 percent in class II and III chronic HF[23] and decreases sudden death by 41 percent. Other studies have shown benefit in NYHA class II, III, and IV HF.

β-blockers are unlikely to be initiated in the acute setting, except perhaps to control rate-related HF. They are generally reserved for stable patients. All HF patients are considered for β-blockers, except as listed in Table 53-6.

Patients on maintenance β-blockers presenting in an acutely decompensated state represent a difficult management problem. Terminating the β-blockers may cause deterioration from β-blocker withdrawal. However, higher doses may compromise tenuous hemodynamics. The optimal compromise may be a short course of an intravenous inotrope (e.g., milrinone) to support hemodynamics while stabilizing with intravenous diuretics and vasodilators. If there is hypoperfusion or pulmonary edema, the β-blockers may be stopped.

Digoxin This alkaloid inhibits myocardial cellular membrane $Na^+K^+ATPase$. It is used to control ventricular response in atrial fibrillation. However, in HF with atrial fibrillation, β-blockers may be more effective. Digoxin can improve clinical symptoms when ACEIs and β-blockers are initiated and during the time it takes for their clinical effects to manifest, and digoxin is considered if therapy with ACEIs, β-blockers, and diuretics fail to control HF symptoms.

Digoxin is not used unless the patient is receiving other HF therapies. Levels need close monitoring in the elderly, patients with renal insufficiency, and those with electrolyte abnormalities (hypokalemia increases toxicity risk). Digoxin is started at 0.125 mg per d. Using the highest tolerable dose is no longer recommended.

Spironolactone The aldosterone antagonist spironolactone decreases mortality by about 30 percent in class III and IV HF,[24] but is not recommended in patients with NYHA class I or II HF. Adverse effects include hyperkalemia and gynecomastia. Recommended usage of spironolactone is for symptomatic patients, despite ACEI, β-blockers, digoxin, and diuretics. Contraindications are creatinine levels above 2.5 mg/dL or a potassium levels above 5 mEq/L. In general, spironolactone is not initiated from the ED.

Morphine Sulfate Morphine can be used in acute pulmonary edema, provided there is adequate BP. It reduces anxiety, is a venodilator, and treats the chest pain of acute myocardial infarction. Initial dosing is 2 to 5 mg IV and titrated to clinical effect. Despite its long historic use in this setting, there are no studies demonstrating efficacy. Because it is a respiratory and central nervous system depressant, it should be avoided in patients with diminished respiratory effort or altered sensorium. Naloxone should be available, if needed. Complications include hypotension, hypoventilation, sedation, nausea, and vomiting.

Anticoagulation

CHRONIC THERAPY   The risk of thromboembolism in the clinically stable HF outpatient is low, estimated at 1 to 3 percent per year, and is greatest with the lowest EF. Warfarin is used in HF, but there are insufficient data to guide a precise approach. Most investigators recommend warfarin for significant LV dysfunction and atrial fibrillation, LV thrombus, or prior embolic event. Warfarin therapy is unlikely to be initiated solely by the emergency practitioner.

INPATIENT THERAPY   Hospitalized HF patients are at greater risk for sustaining a deep venous thrombosis (DVT) and its complications. In a study of admitted HF patients, subcutaneous enoxaparin decreased venographically documented DVT, from 14.9 to 5.5 percent with 40 mg of enoxaparin daily.[25] This therapy can be initiated in the ED. Empiric DVT prevention in hospitalized, bedridden HF patients must be balanced against the relatively low risk of complications associated with anticoagulant prophylaxis.

Drugs to be Avoided in HF

CALCIUM CHANNEL BLOCKERS   Calcium channel blockers are not routinely recommended in HF. Short-term use may result in pulmonary edema and cardiogenic shock, and long-term use may increase the risk of worsening HF and death.[26] These adverse effects have been attributed to the negative inotropic effects of calcium channel blockers. If necessary, amlodipine, with no clear adverse mortality effect, may be used for compelling clinical reasons (e.g., as an antianginal agent despite maximal therapy with nitrates and β-blockers).

NONSTEROIDAL ANTI-INFLAMMATORY DRUGS   Nonsteroidal anti-inflammatory drugs should be avoided in HF. They inhibit the effects of diuretics and ACEIs and can worsen cardiac and renal function.[17] The routine use of aspirin for coronary artery disease prophylaxis, with concurrent ACEI treatment, is controversial.

ANTIARRHYTHMICS   HF patients are sensitive to the pro-arrhythmic and cardiodepressant effects of antiarrhythmics. Because their use does not prevent sudden cardiac death, suppression of asymptomatic ventricular arrhythmias usually is unnecessary.

Except for immediate treatment of life-threatening ventricular arrhythmias, class I antiarrhythmics (e.g., quinidine, procainamide, and flecainide) should not be used in HF. Some class III agents (e.g., amiodarone) do not increase the risk of sudden death, so these agents are preferred for atrial arrhythmias.[17] However, due to toxicity, amiodarone is not recommended for chronic use to prevent sudden death in patients already treated with mortality reducing drugs (ACEIs or β-blockers).[17]

COMPLICATIONS OF HEART FAILURE

Sudden Death or Ventricular Arrhythmias

HF is an important sudden death risk factor. Ventricular arrhythmias are common, and premature ventricular contractions occur in 95 percent of dilated cardiomyopathy patients. Nonsustained ventricular tachycardia is seen in 30 to 40 percent. Sudden death risk increases in proportion to the decrease in EF and HF severity, occurring in 10 to 40 percent of HF patients. Progressive pump failure is the fatal event in about 50 percent.

Because arrhythmias are common in HF and neither Holter monitoring nor electrophysiologic studies predict sudden death risk, symptoms guide therapy. Syncope, resuscitation after cardiac arrest, and sustained and symptomatic nonsustained ventricular tachycardia suggest aggressive management. In these patients, electrophysiologic testing and consideration for an implantable cardioverter-defibrillator are warranted.[17] **Prophylactic administration of antiarrhythmics is not effective, and may increase mortality.**

DISPOSITION

Acute Pulmonary Edema

Most patients with acute pulmonary edema are likely to require ICU admission. A subset of initially severely hypertensive patients will improve greatly while still in the ED. For these patients, if the hypertension is controlled and dyspnea resolved, admission to a non-ICU monitored bed may be feasible. In more stable patients, the choice of medication may determine disposition. Patients receiving nitroglycerin requiring frequent titration adjustment due to tachyphylaxis should be admitted to an ICU environment. Patients receiving nesiritide can be managed in a telemetry unit. This decision also depends on the underlying etiology. Because even transient hypertension can result in a recurrence of hemodynamic decompensation, close monitoring is needed.

Decompensated HF

These patients usually require hospital admission, intravenous diuresis, vasodilator therapy, oral medication dose titration to target levels, and correction of any of the reversible causes of HF decompensation. If the clinical scenario suggests acute coronary syndrome, ICU admission is warranted.

All patients with new-onset HF, poor social support, hypoxemia, hypercarbia, concurrent infection, respiratory distress, syncope, or symptomatic hypotension should be admitted to the hospital. Stable fluid-overloaded patients with a prior HF diagnosis and without a malignant cause for their exacerbation may be admitted to a nonmonitored setting or an ED observation unit.

Those with mild symptoms secondary to a clearly correctable precipitant (e.g., medication noncompliance), whose symptoms resolve with therapy; have normal laboratory, chest radiograph, and electrocardiographic evaluations; have a strong social situation; and are likely to comply with outpatient follow-up are candidates for ED discharge. More significant symptoms or inadequate response to therapy likely warrant hospital admission.

Admission requirements may correlate with BNP levels. In one study, HF patients requiring hospitalization had BNP levels above 700 pg/mL, whereas those able to be treated as outpatients had BNP levels below 254 pg/mL.[6] In another study, patients with BNP levels above 480 pg/mL had 6-month rates of death and re-hospitalization greater than those with BNP levels below 230 pg/mL.[12] These findings need to be confirmed in larger studies.

Observation, Acute Care, and Short-Stay Unit

Intensive HF management with vasodilators and diuretics has beneficial effects in preventing inpatient hospitalizations and decreasing repeat admissions.[18,27] Protocol-driven therapy improves outcomes, as compared with nonprotocol management, and ensures that the many

TABLE 53-8 Observation/Acute Care/Short-Stay Unit Heart Failure Protocol Entry Guidelines*

History
  Orthopnea
  Dyspnea on exertion
  Paroxysmal nocturnal dyspnea
  Shortness of breath
  Swelling of legs or abdomen
  Weight gain
Physical examination
  JVD or elevation in pulsation
  Positive hepatojugular reflux
  S_3/S_4
  Inspiratory rales
  Peripheral edema
Chest radiograph
  Cardiomegaly
  Pulmonary vascular congestion
  Kerley B lines
  Pulmonary edema
  Pleural effusion
Laboratory
  B-type natriuretic peptide >100 pg/mL

*Must have at least one from each category.

multidisciplinary interactions required for successful HF management occur in a timely fashion.[18] It is important that patients entered into an intensive regimen of diuretics are properly selected. Heart failure management entry and exclusion guidelines are listed in Tables 53-8 and 53-9, respectively.[27] Suggested guidelines for disposition from the observation/acute care unit are listed in Table 53-10. Posttherapy BNP levels may assist in predicting posthospitalization course. Patients whose BNP levels decline with therapy have lower subsequent rehospitalization and death rates than do those whose BNP levels are unchanged or increase despite therapy.

Discharge Home

Discharged patients require outpatient follow-up by a physician knowledgeable in the management of HF. Further, social service evaluation may be helpful to ensure medication compliance, dietary education, and re-enforcing smoking cessation instructions. Smoking cessation has the same mortality effect as the best medication therapies.[28]

TABLE 53-9 Heart Failure Vasodilation and Diuresis Protocol Exclusion Criteria*

Hemodynamic instability
  Unstable vital signs (BP >220/120 mm Hg, RR >25, HR >130 beats/min
  Unstable airway or needing >4 L/min nasal cannula O_2 for Sao_2 ≥90%
  Requiring continuous vasoactive medication (e.g., nitroglycerin, nitroprusside, dobutamine, or milrinone) except nesiritide
  Evidence of cardiogenic shock (systolic BP <90 mm Hg, altered mental status, peripheral vasoconstriction)
  Clinically significant arrhythmia (e.g., nonsustained VT not due to electrolyte imbalance)
Signs of acute coronary syndrome (ECG change or cardiac marker elevation)
Chronic renal failure requiring dialysis
Complex decompensation (underlying precipitant is not clearly cardiac or volume related)
Multiple comorbidities
Acute mental status abnormality

*Any one positive result excludes the patient from the heart failure protocol and suggests inpatient management.
Abbreviations: ECG = electrocardiogram; HR = heart rate; RR = respiratory rate; Sao_2 = arterial oxygen saturation; VT = tidal volume.

TABLE 53-10 Discharge Guidelines from Observation/Acute Care/Short-Stay Units

Patients not meeting all of the following criteria should be considered for inpatient treatment*
  Patient reports subjective improvement
  Ambulatory, without long-suffering orthostasis
  Resting HR <100 beats/min
  Systolic BP >80 mm Hg
  Net urine output >1000 mL and no new decrease in urine output <30 mL/h (or <0.5 mL/kg per h)
  Room air Sao_2 >90% (unless on home O_2)
  All CK-MB <8.8 ng/mL, and troponin T <0.1 μg/L
  No ischemic-type chest pain
  No new clinically significant arrhythmia
  Stable electrolyte profile

*Except as appropriate in the end-stage palliative-care cohort.
Abbreviation: CK-MB = muscle and brain types of creatine kinase; HR = heart rate; Sao_2 = arterial oxygen saturation.

REFERENCES

1. Massie BM, Shah NB: Evolving trends in epidemiologic factors of heart failure: Rationale for preventative strategies and comprehensive disease management. *Am Heart J* 133:703, 1997.
2. American Heart Association: *2002 Heart and Stroke Statistical Update.* Dallas, TX, American Heart Association, 2001.
3. Hunt SA, Baker D, Chin MH, et al: American College of Cardiology/American Heart Association. ACC/AHA guidelines for the evaluation and management of chronic heart failure in the adult: Executive summary. A report of the American College of Cardiology/American Heart Association Task Force on Practice Guidelines (Committee to revise the 1995 Guidelines for the Evaluation and Management of Heart Failure). *J Am Coll Cardiol* 38:2101, 2001.
4. Clemens LE, Almirez RG, Baudouin KA, et al: Pharmacokinetics and biological actions of subcutaneously administered human brain natriuretic peptide. *J Pharmacol Exp Ther* 287:67, 1998.
5. Rich MW: Epidemiology, pathophysiology, and etiology of congestive heart failure in older adults. *J Am Geriatr Soc* 45:968, 1997.
6. Dao Q, Krishnaswamy P, Kazanegra R, et al: Utility of B-type natriuretic peptide in the diagnosis of congestive heart failure in an urgent-care setting. *J Am Coll Cardiol* 37:379, 2001.
7. Remes J, Miettinen H, Reunanen A, et al: Validity of clinical diagnosis of heart failure in primary health care. *Eur Heart J* 12:15, 1991.
8. Chait A, Cohen HE, Meltzer LE, et al: The bedside chest radiograph in the evaluation of incipient heart failure. *Radiology* 105:563, 1972.
9. Chakko S, Woska D, Marinez H, et al: Clinical, radiographic, and hemodynamic correlations in chronic congestive heart failure: Conflicting results may lead to inappropriate care. *Am J Med* 90:353, 1991.
10. Kono T, Suwa M, Hanada H, et al: Clinical significance of normal cardiac silhouette in dilated cardiomyopathy—Evaluation based upon echocardiography and magnetic resonance imaging. *Jpn Circ J* 56:359, 1992.
11. Ruskin JA, Gurney JW, Thorsen MK, et al: Detection of pleural effusions on supine chest radiographs. *AJR* 148:681, 1987.
12. Harrison A, Morrison LK, Krishnaswamy P, et al: B-type natriuretic peptide predicts future cardiac events in patients presenting to the emergency department with dyspnea. *Ann Emerg Med* 39:131, 2002.
13. Tsutamoto T, Wada A, Maeda K, et al: Attenuation of compensation of endogenous cardiac natriuretic peptide system in chronic heart failure: Prognostic role of plasma brain natriuretic peptide concentration in patients with chronic symptomatic left ventricular dysfunction. *Circulation* 96:509, 1997.
14. Peacock WF: The B-type natriuretic peptide assay: A rapid test for heart failure. *Cleve Clin J Med* 69:243, 2002.
15. Maisel AS, Krishnaswamy P, Nowak RM, et al: Rapid measurement of B-type natriuretic peptide in the emergency diagnosis of heart failure. *New Engl J Med* 347:161, 2002.
16. Arroliga AC: Noninvasive positive pressure ventilation in acute respiratory failure: Does it improve outcomes? *Cleve Clin J Med* 68:677, 2001.
17. Packer M, Cohn JN: Consensus recommendations for the management of chronic heart failure. *Am J Cardiol* 83:1A, 1999.

17a. Peacock WF, Emerman CL, Doleh M, et al: The incidence of elevated cardiac enzymes in decompensated heart failure. *Congest Heart Fail* 2003, (in press).

18. Peacock WF IV, Remer EE, Aponte J, et al: Effective observation unit treatment of decompensated heart failure. *Congest Heart Fail* 8:68, 2002.

19. Le Conte P, Coutant V, N'Guyen JM, et al: Prognostic factors in acute cardiogenic pulmonary edema. *Am J Emerg Med* 17:329, 1999.

20. Abraham WT, Lowes BD, Ferguson DA, et al: Systemic hemodynamic, neurohormonal, and renal effects of a steady-state infusion of human brain natriuretic peptide in patients with hemodynamically decompensated heart failure. *J Cardiac Fail* 4:37, 1998.

21. VMAC Investigators: Intravenous nesiritide vs. nitroglycerin for treatment of decompensated congestive heart failure: A randomized controlled trial. *JAMA* 287:1531, 2002.

22. SOLVD Investigators: Effect of enalapril on survival in patients with reduced ventricular ejection fraction and congestive heart failure. *New Engl J Med* 325:293, 1991.

23. MERIT-HF Study Group: Effect of metoprolol CR/XL in chronic heart failure: Metoprolol CR/XL randomized intervention trial in congestive heart failure. *Lancet* 353:2001, 1999.

24. RALES Study Investigators: The effect of spironolactone on morbidity and mortality in patients with severe heart failure. *New Engl J Med* 341:709, 1999.

25. Turpie AG: Thrombosis prophylaxis in the acutely ill medical patient: Insights from the prophylaxis in MEDical patients with ENOXaparin (MEDENOX) trial. *Am J Cardiol* 86:48M, 2000.

26. Advisory Council to Improve Outcomes Nationwide in Heart Failure. Packer M, Cohn JN, (eds): Consensus recommendations for the management of chronic heart failure. *Am J Cardiol* 83:54A, 1999.

27. Peacock WF IV, Albert NM: Observation unit management of heart failure. *Emerg Med Clin North Am* 19:209, 2001.

28. Suskin N, Sheath T, Negassa A, et al. Relationship of current and past smoking to mortality and morbidity in patients with left ventricular dysfunction. *J Am Coll Cardiol* 37:1677, 2001.

54

VALVULAR EMERGENCIES
David M. Cline

Ninety percent of valvular disease is chronic, with decades between the onset of the structural abnormality and symptoms. Through chronic adaptation by dilatation or hypertrophy, cardiac function can be preserved for years, which may delay the diagnosis for one to two decades. In contrast to the more common chronic presentations, acute rupture of a cardiac valve presents with dramatic symptoms. The emergency physician most commonly encounters patients with valvular disease after the diagnosis has been made but is occasionally the first to suspect valvular dysfunction based on the patient's symptoms and examination. Compared with the general population, patients with hemodynamically significant valvular heart disease have a 2.5-fold increased rate of death and a 3.2-fold increased rate of stroke.[1]

The four heart valves prevent retrograde flow of blood during the cardiac cycle, allowing efficient ejection of blood with each contraction of the ventricles. The mitral valve has two cusps, whereas the other three heart valves normally have three cusps. The right and left papillary muscles promote effective closure of the tricuspid and mitral valves, respectively. The papillary muscles are attached to the cusps of the atrioventricular (AV) valves by tendinous cords, the chordae tendineae. Abnormalities of the valvular cusps, the papillary muscles, the chordae tendineae, or the cardiac chambers themselves can cause valvular dysfunction.

DIAGNOSING A NEWLY DISCOVERED MURMUR

The first step in diagnosing a newly discovered murmur is to consider it in the context of the patient's medical condition. Patients with normal cardiac anatomy may have murmurs associated with anemia, thyrotoxicosis, sepsis, fever, renal failure with volume overload, pregnancy, and other conditions associated with increased cardiac output. A diastolic murmur or a new murmur associated with symptoms at rest always should be considered abnormal and warrants referral for cardiology evaluation and echocardiographic study. Figure 54-1 presents an algorithm for the clinical assessment of a newly discovered systolic murmur.[2] The studies referred to by Etchells and colleagues used cardiologists as examiners, and these issues have not been tested in the emergency department setting. However, the algorithm can be expected to prompt the clinician to perform the appropriate examinations and maneuvers to help uncover an abnormal murmur. Whenever the clinician is uncertain of the diagnosis of a newly discovered murmur, referral should be made to a cardiologist or back to the primary care physician. In general, the urgency for an accurate diagnosis and appropriate referral or admission depends on the severity of symptoms, not the presence of the murmur. The exception is a patient with suspected aortic stenosis and syncope who may appear well at rest yet is at risk for another cardiovascular event. See Chap. 145 for admission recommendations in the setting of endocarditis. See Chap. 55 for admission indications in the setting of hypertrophic cardiomyopathy.

New cardiac murmurs, especially those of valvular insufficiency, can also be a sign of endocarditis. Endocarditis is discussed in detail in Chap. 145 and **Table 145-6 lists regimens for antibiotic prophylaxis before procedures, in patients with valvular disease or prosthetic valves.**

A truly innocent (physiologic) murmur is associated with no abnormal symptoms or signs. The soft systolic ejection murmur begins after S_1 and ends before S_2, and the heart sounds are completely normal. The review of systems elicits no symptoms compatible with cardiovascular disease, and other findings on complete physical examination are normal.

Listen for a murmur in the second right intercostal space that radiates to the right carotid artery and determine:

Slow Rate of Rise of Carotid Artery, or Late or Mid Peaking Murmur, or Decreased S2, or Brachioradial Delay, or Effort Induced Syncope	YES → Refer for possible Aortic Stenosis and Possible Admission

If not, listen for a murmur in the fifth intercostal space, mid left thorax, that radiates to the left axilla and determine:

Murmur in Mitral Area, or Late or Holosystolic Murmur, or Any New Murmur with Acute MI	YES → Refer for possible Mitral Regurgitation

If not, also listen for a click in this area:

Systolic Click and Murmur, or Systolic Click, or Nonejection Click	YES → Refer for possible Mitral Valve Prolapse

If not, listen for a murmur in the fifth intercostal space, mid left thorax that radiates to the lower left sternal border and determine:

Decrease Murmur Intensity with Passive Leg Elevation, or Increased Murmur Intensity When Going from Squating to Standing Position	YES → Refer for possible Hypertrophic Cardiomyopathy

If not, listen for a murmur in the lower left sternal border that radiates to the lower right sternal border and determine:

Increased Murmur Intensity During Inspiration, or Increased Murmur Intensity During Sustained Abdominal Pressure	YES → Refer for possible Tricuspid Regurgitation

If not, then:

Refer to a Family Physician to Follow Murmur

FIG. 54-1. Algorithm for evaluation of newly discovered systolic murmur.

MITRAL STENOSIS

Pathophysiology

Despite its declining frequency, rheumatic heart disease is still the most common cause of mitral valve stenosis. Scarring from rheumatic endocarditis causes fusion of the commissures and matting of the chordae tendineae, which interferes with valve closure. Calcification over time makes the valve less mobile. Progressive stenosis may lead to pulmonary hypertension, which may signal the need for surgery. Most patients eventually develop atrial fibrillation because of progressive dilatation of the atria. Pulmonary hypertension may lead to pulmonary and tricuspid valve incompetence. Although the valvular obstruction is slowly progressive, acute symptoms are produced when the obstruction prevents an increase in cardiac output to meet an increased need, such as during exercise.

Clinical Features

Conditions that prompt symptoms in mitral stenosis include exertion, tachycardia, anemia, pregnancy, infection, emotional upset, and atrial fibrillation. As with all valvular diseases, exertional dyspnea is the most common presenting symptom. Paroxysmal nocturnal dyspnea and acute pulmonary edema may occur with more severe disease. In the past, hemoptysis was the second most common presenting symptom but is less common now with earlier recognition and treatment. Hemoptysis may be massive if a bronchial vein ruptures. Other common symptoms and signs include orthopnea and premature atrial contractions. Systemic emboli may occur and result in myocardial, kidney, central nervous system, or peripheral infarction. Embolic stroke is more frequent in the presence of atrial fibrillation. As the disease progresses, symptoms of right-sided heart failure may develop.

Signs of mitral stenosis include a mid-diastolic rumbling murmur, with crescendo toward the S_2. With the onset of atrial fibrillation, the presystolic accentuation of the murmur disappears. Typically the S_1 is loud and is followed by a loud opening snap that is high-pitched and heard best at the right of the apex. The apical impulse is small and tapping, representing an underfilled left ventricle. Systemic blood pressure is typically normal or low. If pulmonary hypertension is present, signs may include a thin body habitus, peripheral cyanosis, and cool extremities because of low cardiac output. With pulmonary hypertension, the auscultatory findings are less evident.

Diagnosis

The electrocardiogram (ECG) may demonstrate notched or biphasic P waves and right-axis deviation. On the chest radiograph, straightening of the left heart border (i.e., loss of the pulmonary window), indicating left atrial enlargement, is a typical early radiographic finding. Eventually, findings of pulmonary congestion are noted: redistribution of flow to the upper lung fields, Kerley B lines, and an increase in vascular markings. The chest radiograph is useful in assessing the degree of pulmonary congestion. The diagnosis of mitral stenosis should be confirmed with echocardiography and/or consultation with a cardiologist. Transesophageal echocardiography yields a more complete analysis of valvular dysfunction, especially of the mitral valve. However, transthoracic echocardiography generally is performed first.[3]

Treatment

The sequelae or complications of mitral stenosis may require emergency department intervention. The medical management of mitral stenosis includes intermittent diuretics to alleviate pulmonary congestion, the treatment of atrial fibrillation (see Chap. 28), and anticoagulation for patients at risk for arterial embolic events. Patients with mitral stenosis and paroxysmal or chronic atrial fibrillation or a history of an embolic event should be on long-term warfarin therapy with an international normalized ratio (INR) goal of 2 to 3.[4] Patients with severe mitral stenosis should be counseled to avoid strenuous physical activity. Hemoptysis may occur in the setting of mitral stenosis and pulmonary hypertension. Bleeding may be severe enough to require blood transfusion, consultation with a thoracic surgeon, and emergency surgery.

MITRAL INCOMPETENCE

Pathophysiology

Infective endocarditis or myocardial infarction can cause acute rupture of the chordae tendineae or papillary muscles or cause perforation of the valve leaflets. Common causes of chronic mitral incompetence include myocardial infarction, mitral valve prolapse syndrome, rheumatic heart disease, coronary artery disease, and collagen-vascular disease. Inferior myocardial infarction due to right coronary occlusion is the most common cause of ischemic mitral valve incompetence. Rarely, trauma may cause acute mitral incompetence. Patients with acute mitral valve rupture deteriorate rapidly. Intermittent mitral incompetence can be due to ischemia, which causes papillary muscle dysfunction. Although an association between appetite-suppressant drugs (fenfluramine and phentermine, or dexfenfluramine alone) and aortic regurgitation generally has been accepted,[5,6] the suspected association of mitral incompetence with the appetite-suppressant drugs remains unclear.[7]

Acute regurgitation into a noncompliant left atrium quickly elevates pressures and causes pulmonary edema. In contrast, in the chronic state, the left atrium dilates so that left atrial pressure rises little, even with a large regurgitant flow. As an adaptation, the total stroke volume of the left ventricle increases so that effective forward flow into the aorta is maintained despite the large regurgitant volume across the mitral valve.

Clinical Features

Acute mitral incompetence presents with dyspnea, tachycardia, and pulmonary edema. Usually an S_3 and S_4 will be heard. Acutely, the harsh apical systolic murmur starts with S_1 and may end before S_2. These patients may deteriorate quickly to cardiogenic shock or cardiac arrest. Intermittent mitral incompetence usually presents with acute episodes of respiratory distress due to pulmonary edema and can be asymptomatic between attacks. The pronounced dyspnea may mask angina that accompanies the ischemia. Patients may have an active apical impulse, systolic thrust, and thrill at the apex.

Chronic mitral incompetence may be tolerated for years or even decades. The first symptom is usually exertional dyspnea, sometimes prompted by atrial fibrillation. If patients are not anticoagulated, systemic emboli occur in 20 percent and are often asymptomatic. Endocarditis is still a feared complication. Signs of chronic mitral incompetence include a late systolic left parasternal lift. There is a high-pitched holosystolic murmur that is best heard in the fifth intercostal space, mid-left thorax, and radiates to the axilla. The first heart sound is soft and often obscured by the murmur. An S_3 is usually heard and is followed by a short diastolic rumble, indicating increased flow into the left ventricle.

Diagnosis

In acute disease, the ECG may show evidence of acute inferior wall infarction (more common than anterior wall infarction in this setting). On the chest radiograph, acute mitral incompetence from papillary muscle rupture may result in a minimally enlarged left atrium and pulmonary edema. Auscultation of acute mitral regurgitation may be difficult in a tachycardic and dyspneic patient. The diagnosis of acute mitral incompetence should be suspected in patients with new-onset pulmonary edema, especially when the heart is smaller than expected on the chest radiograph or when the patient does not respond to conventional therapy. Echocardiography is essential to make the diagnosis with certainty, and emergency bedside echocardiography should be considered for the acutely ill patient. However, transthoracic echocardiography may underestimate lesion severity, and the transesophageal technique should be undertaken as soon as the patient is adequately stable.

In chronic disease, the ECG may demonstrate findings of left atrial enlargement and left ventricular hypertrophy (LVH). On the chest radiograph, chronic mitral incompetence produces left ventricular and atrial enlargement that is proportional to the severity of the regurgitant volume. For patients with chronic but undiagnosed disease, the diagnosis should be confirmed with transthoracic or transesophageal echocardiography as the clinical picture demands, usually on an outpatient basis.

Treatment

In acute severe mitral incompetence, the goal of medical therapy is to diminish the amount of regurgitation, thereby increasing forward flow and reducing pulmonary congestion. Pulmonary edema should be treated initially with oxygen, intubation for failing respiratory effort, diuretics, and nitrates as the patient tolerates (see Chap. 53 for general principles). Nitroprusside increases forward output by increasing aortic flow and partially restoring mitral valve competence as left ventricular size diminishes. Start nitroprusside at 0.3 μg/kg per min IV unless the patient is hypotensive. There may be a subset of patients whose mitral regurgitation is worsened by nitroprusside (those patients who respond with a dilatation of the regurgitant orifice).[8] Thus careful monitoring is essential. Hypotensive patients should receive inotropic agents such as dobutamine titrated from 2.5 to 20 μg/kg per min in addition to nitroprusside.

Aortic balloon counter pulsation increases forward flow and mean arterial pressure while diminishing regurgitant volume and left ventricular filling pressure and can be used to stabilize a patient while awaiting surgery. Emergency surgery should be considered in cases of acute mitral valve rupture. The urgency of the situation may leave little time for intubation, intravenous afterload reducers, echocardiography, and assembling the surgical team for emergency valve replacement. When acute cases of ischemic mitral valve incompetence are suspected, the patient may be treated with nitrates, provided that the patient is not hypotensive. If endocarditis is a potential underlying etiology, the patient will need specific evaluation and treatment. (See Chap. 145 for management of endocarditis).

There is no accepted therapy for asymptomatic mitral regurgitation. Atrial fibrillation should be treated with anticoagulation using heparin and ventricular rate control with β-blockers or calcium channel blockers. Although the risk of embolization is less than in patients with mitral stenosis, patients with mitral incompetence and atrial fibrillation generally are maintained on warfarin therapy with an INR goal of 2 to 3.[9] Patients with acute mitral incompetence or sustained atrial fibrillation in the setting of chronic mitral incompetence generally are hospitalized.

MITRAL VALVE PROLAPSE

Pathophysiology

The etiology of mitral valve prolapse (MVP), or the click-murmur syndrome, is not known but may be congenital. MVP is the most common valvular heart disease in industrialized countries, affecting approximately 2.4 percent of the population.[10] One or both of the mitral valve leaflets prolapse into the atrium during systole, and this may or may not be accompanied by regurgitant flow. Population studies have found no increased risk of atrial fibrillation, syncope, stroke, or sudden death.[10,11] Male sex, age over 45, and the presence of regurgitation, recognized clinically by a short systolic murmur, place the patient in a higher-risk group for complications.[12] Click-murmur syndrome has unique symptoms that differentiate it from other forms of mitral regurgitation.

Clinical Features

Most patients are asymptomatic. Symptoms include atypical chest pain, palpitations, fatigue, and dyspnea unrelated to exertion. Symptoms are more common in those who know they have the syndrome. In patients with MVP without mitral regurgitation at rest, exercise provokes mitral regurgitation in 32 percent of patients and predicts a higher risk for morbid events.[13] The classic cardiac finding is a midsystolic click. The second heart sound may be diminished by the late systolic murmur, with crescendos into S_2 (not present in all patients). Some patients may have pectus excavatum, a straight thoracic spine, or scoliosis.

Diagnosis

The diagnosis is unlikely to be made in the emergency department, nor is it important to do so. The ECG is usually normal, as is the chest radiograph, unless the thoracic cage abnormalities described earlier are seen. Referral to a cardiologist and outpatient echocardiography is recommended to confirm the clinical diagnosis of MVP and to identify any associated mitral regurgitation.[3]

Treatment

Initiating treatment for MVP is rarely required for patients seen in the emergency department. The treatment of asymptomatic MVP is reassurance. Patients with palpitations, chest pain, or anxiety frequently respond to β-blockers. Avoiding alcohol, tobacco, and caffeine also may relieve symptoms. Aspirin 80 to 325 mg orally daily is recommended for MVP patients with focal neurologic events who do not have indications for warfarin therapy. Patients with MVP associated with atrial fibrillation and additional risk factors for embolization such as age greater than 65, mitral regurgitation, hypertension, or heart failure should be on warfarin (INR goal of 2–3).[9] Patients with MVP and atrial fibrillation without the listed additional risk factors can be managed with aspirin 160 mg PO daily.

AORTIC STENOSIS

Pathophysiology

Degenerative heart disease or calcific aortic stenosis is the most common cause of aortic stenosis in adults residing in the United States. Congenital heart disease is the most common cause of aortic stenosis in young adults, with the presence of a bicuspid valve accounting for 50 percent of cases. Rheumatic heart disease is the third most common cause in the United States but remains the most common cause worldwide. The prevalence of critical aortic stenosis is about 3 percent in patients over age 74. Calcification is a common feature of aortic stenosis in older adults regardless of the cause.[14] Blood flow into the aorta is obstructed, producing progressive LVH and low cardiac output. This produces a marked reduction in coronary blood flow.

Clinical Features

The classic triad of aortic stenosis is dyspnea, chest pain, and syncope. Exercise may induce acute symptoms. Symptoms appear late in the course of the disease. In active persons, the symptoms appear more rapidly. Dyspnea is usually the first symptom, followed by paroxysmal nocturnal dyspnea, exertional syncope, angina, and myocardial infarction. Atrial fibrillation is less common than in mitral disease, but 10 percent of patients have atrial fibrillation at the time of surgery. With isolated aortic stenosis, endocarditis occurs in only 2 percent of patients.

The most common signs include a pulse of small amplitude. The carotid pulse can be assessed most accurately and is found to have a slow rate of increase.[2] Blood pressure is normal or low, with a narrow pulse pressure. LVH is common. There is paradoxical splitting of S_2. S_3 and S_4 are commonly present. Classically, there is a harsh systolic ejection murmur that is best heard in the second right intercostal space and that radiates to the right carotid artery. Brachioradial delay is an important finding in aortic stenosis.[15] The examiner palpates simultaneously the right brachial artery of the patient with the thumb and the right radial artery of the patient with the middle or index finger. Any palpable delay between the brachial and radial arteries is considered abnormal.[15] Sudden death, usually from dysrhythmia, occurs in 25 percent of patients. Without surgery, 75 percent of patients with aortic stenosis will be dead within 3 years of the time of diagnosis.[16]

Diagnosis

Syncope in the setting of a new systolic murmur always should raise the possibility of aortic stenosis as the etiology (see Figure 54-1). Other ancillary findings available in the emergency department are nonspecific. The ECG usually demonstrates criteria for LVH and, in 10 percent of patients, left or right bundle branch block. The chest radiograph is normal early, but eventually LVH and findings of congestive heart failure are evident if the patient does not have valve replacement. The patient should be admitted and echocardiography undertaken.

Treatment

Patients presenting with pulmonary edema can be treated with oxygen and diuretics, but nitrates should be used with caution because reducing preload may cause significant hypotension. Nitroprusside is not well tolerated in patients with aortic stenosis. Atrial fibrillation may severely compromise cardiac output. New-onset atrial fibrillation may require anticoagulation with heparin, as well as cardioversion. Negative inotropic drugs may be poorly tolerated. Patients with profound symptoms secondary to aortic stenosis, such as syncope, usually are admitted to the hospital. Patients with aortic stenosis should limit vigorous physical activity.

AORTIC INCOMPETENCE

Pathophysiology

In 20 percent of patients, the cause of aortic incompetence is acute in nature. Infective endocarditis accounts of the majority of acute cases; aortic dissection at the aortic root is the second most common cause. Trauma to the aortic valve may cause acute regurgitation. In acute cases, a sudden increase in backflow of blood into the ventricle raises left ventricular end-diastolic pressure, which may cause acute heart failure. Increased ventricular pressure elevates pressure in the left atrium, and pulmonary congestion results. Calcific degeneration, congenital disease (most notably bicuspid valves), systemic hypertension, myxomatous proliferation, and rheumatic heart disease cause most chronic cases. Marfan syndrome, syphilis, ankylosing spondylitis, Ehlers-Danlos syndrome, and Reiter syndrome are less frequent causes. An association between the appetite-suppressant drugs (fenfluramine and phentermine or dexfenfluramine alone) has been found

for aortic incompetence.[5–7] Chronic disease is more common in males than in females, with a ratio of 3:2. In chronic disease, the ventricle progressively dilates to accommodate the regurgitant blood volume. Wide pulse pressures result from the fall in diastolic pressure, and marked peripheral vasodilation is seen. During exercise and tachycardia, the diastolic filling period shortens, thus decreasing the length of time per minute that regurgitation can occur. Cardiac function is therefore close to normal with exercise early in the course of the disease. In contrast, isometric exercise or stress may precipitate symptoms earlier in the disease process.

Clinical Features

In acute disease, dyspnea is the most common presenting symptom, seen in 50 percent of patients. Many patients have acute pulmonary edema with pink frothy sputum. Patients may complain of fever and chills if endocarditis is the cause. Patients may present with systemic emboli or a persistent sinus tachycardia. Dissection of the ascending aorta typically produces a "tearing" chest pain that may radiate between the shoulder blades. Sudden death is common in patients with both acute and chronic aortic incompetence.

Elevated temperature is common with acute endocarditis. Patients commonly have tachycardia, tachypnea, and rales. Classically, there is a high-pitched blowing diastolic murmur heard immediately after S_2, best heard in the right second or third intercostal parasternal area. In the face of failure, there may be an S_3 with a long diastolic murmur, and there may be associated systolic flow murmur.

In the chronic state, about one-third of patients have palpitations associated with a large stroke volume and/or premature ventricular contractions. Frequently these sensations are noticed in bed. Patients may complain of stabbing chest pain, fatigue, or dyspnea. Two-thirds of patients have no symptoms for up to 20 years despite a hemodynamically significant lesion, defined as a diastolic blood pressure of less than 70 mm Hg. Symptoms of left ventricular failure may occur late in the course of the disease and include dyspnea, pulmonary edema, ischemic chest pain, and sweating.

In the chronic state, signs include a wide pulse pressure with a prominent ventricular impulse, which may be manifested as head bobbing. A "water hammer pulse" may be noted; this is a peripheral pulse that has a quick rise in upstroke followed by a peripheral collapse. Other classic findings include accentuated precordial apical thrust, pulsus biferiens, Duroziez sign (a to-and-fro femoral murmur), and Quincke pulse (capillary pulsations visible/palpable at the proximal nailbed while pressure is applied at the tip).

Diagnosis

In patients with acute regurgitation, the chest radiograph demonstrates acute pulmonary edema with less cardiac enlargement than expected. In chronic aortic incompetence, the ECG demonstrates LVH, and the chest radiograph shows cardiomegaly, aortic dilatation, and possibly evidence of congestive heart failure. Echocardiography is essential for confirming the presence of and evaluating the severity of valvular regurgitation. Bedside transthoracic echocardiography should be undertaken in the unstable patient, who is potentially in need of emergency surgery. Transesophageal echocardiography is needed when aortic dissection is suspected. ECG changes may be seen with aortic dissection, including ischemia or findings of acute inferior myocardial, suggesting involvement of the right coronary artery.

Treatment

In cases of acute aortic regurgitation, death from pulmonary edema, ventricular dysrhythmias, or circulatory collapse is common even with intensive medical management. Pulmonary edema should be treated initially with oxygen and intubation for failing respiratory effort. Diuretics and nitrates can be used but cannot be expected to be effective. Nitroprusside (start at 0.3 µg/kg per min) along with inotropic agents such as dobutamine (start at 2.5 µg/kg per min) or dopamine (start at 2.5 µg/kg per min) can be used to augment forward flow and reduce left ventricular end-diastolic pressure in an attempt to stabilize a patient prior to emergency surgery. Intra-aortic balloon counterpulsation is contraindicated. Although β-blockers are used often in treating aortic dissection, these drugs should be used with great caution, if at all, in the setting of acute aortic valve rupture because they will block the compensatory tachycardia. Emergency surgery may be lifesaving.

Chronic aortic regurgitation typically is treated with vasodilators such as angiotensin-converting enzyme (ACE) inhibitors or nifedipine (initiated by a patient's private physician). In a randomized trial of severe by asymptomatic aortic regurgitation, nifedipine was shown to reduce or delay the need for aortic valve replacement compared with digoxin.[17]

RIGHT-SIDED VALVULAR HEART DISEASE

Pathophysiology

Symptomatic right-sided valvular heart disease is much less common than symptomatic left-sided valvular disease. However, the prevalence of tricuspid regurgitation is 14.8 percent in men and 18.4 percent in woman, the majority of whom are asymptomatic.[18] Drug users with endocarditis due to aggressive organisms, such as *Staphylococcus aureus,* are the largest group of patients with isolated symptomatic tricuspid disease. Chronic obstructive pulmonary disease (COPD) associated with pulmonary hypertension may cause tricuspid regurgitation. Right ventricular failure with dilatation may lead to tricuspid valve incompetence. Rheumatic heart disease may affect more than one valve, and tricuspid valve disease is seen frequently in conjunction with left-sided valvular disease. Rarely, blunt trauma can lead to tricuspid valve incompetence.

Pulmonary valvular incompetence is most commonly due to pulmonary hypertension, and symptoms of pulmonary hypertension dominate the clinical picture. The most common cause of pulmonary stenosis is congenital tetralogy of Fallot, which is usually corrected surgically in infancy.

Clinical Features

The most common presenting symptoms of right-sided valvular disease are dyspnea and orthopnea. As the disease progresses, signs of right-sided heart failure are evident: jugular venous distention with a prominent *a* wave, peripheral edema, hepatomegaly, splenomegaly, and ascites.

In tricuspid valve incompetence, the murmur is soft, blowing, and holosystolic and best heard along the lower left sternal border. In tricuspid valve stenosis, the rumbling crescendo-decrescendo diastolic murmur occurs just prior to S_1. This murmur is best heard along the lower left sternal border. Because of the organisms involved, patients presenting with tricuspid valve incompetence in association with endocarditis are acutely ill with sepsis.

Diagnosis

The diagnosis of right-sided valvular heart disease requires echocardiography. Transesophageal is more accurate than transthoracic.

Treatment

The treatment of right-sided valvular heart disease should first address the underlying cause, such as the treatment for COPD associated with pulmonary hypertension. Diuretics, often in very high doses, are used to manage the effects of elevated venous pressure, such as leg edema and hepatic congestion. Patients may present to the emergency department with complications of diuretic therapy, such as volume depletion or electrolyte abnormalities.

PROSTHETIC VALVE DISEASE

Prosthetic valves are implanted in 40,000 patients per year in the United States. There are approximately 80 types of artificial valves, each with advantages and disadvantages. Patients who receive prosthetic valves are instructed to carry a descriptive card in their wallet. The prosthetic valves can be divided into two basic groups: mechanical, nontissue models and bioprostheses using porcine, bovine, or human valves. Complications of prosthetic valves are more common in patients who have advanced heart disease, including cardiac dilatation, LVH, congestive heart failure, or dysrhythmias, at the time of their original operation. Survival is higher and primary valve failure is lower in patients with mechanical valve replacement, but bleeding is more common than with bioprosthetic valves.[19]

Pathophysiology

Prosthetic valves tend to be slightly stenotic, and a very small amount of regurgitation is common because of incomplete closure. Patients with mechanical valves require continuous anticoagulation. Some bioprostheses do not require long-term anticoagulation, unless atrial fibrillation coexists. Several complications can lead to dysfunction of artificial valves. Thrombi can form on a prosthetic valve and become large enough to obstruct flow or prevent closure. The dysfunction due to thrombi can be acute or slowly progressive. Bioprostheses may degenerate gradually, undergoing gradual thinning, stiffening, and possible tearing, which result in valvular incompetence. The sutures that secure the prosthetic valve may become disrupted, leading to paravalvular regurgitation as a fistula forms at the periphery of the valve. Mechanical models suddenly may fracture or fail. These failures usually bring sudden symptoms and often are fatal before corrective surgery can be accomplished.

Bleeding and systemic embolism originating from a thrombus on the prosthetic valve are the most important complications of mechanical heart valves, occurring at a rate of 1.4 and 1 percent per year, respectively, for patients on warfarin.[20] Lifelong anticoagulation is required to reduce the risk of thromboembolism and valve thrombosis. The optimal anticoagulation regimen is controversial, with disagreement concerning the intensity of warfarin therapy as well as the need for an antiplatelet agent. Embolism is more common after mitral valve replacement. Embolism occurs less frequently with bioprostheses, and bleeding complications depend on the therapy given.

Patients with artificial valves develop endocarditis at a rate of 0.5 percent per year. Infections occur more frequently during the first 2 months after operation. The most common organisms during this period are *Staphylococcus epidermidis* and *S. aureus.* Gram-negative organisms and fungi are also frequent causes of endocarditis during this early period. Late cases of endocarditis are similar to those affecting native valves. The most frequent organism is *Streptococcus viridans,* but *Serratia* and *Pseudomonas* also occur. Patients with prosthetic valves and endocarditis may develop a ring abscess around the valve, which requires valve replacement. Patients with mechanical prostheses have an increased rate of intravascular destruction of red blood cells. Usually the red blood cell loss is easily corrected by the bone marrow. Finally, patients with prosthetic valves may be particularly susceptible to hemodynamic compromise from a new arrhythmia, such as atrial fibrillation.

Clinical Features

Many patients have persistent dyspnea and reduced effort tolerance after successful valve replacement. This is more common in the presence of preexisting heart dysfunction or atrial fibrillation. Many symptoms of valvular dysfunction described in the preceding sections on specific valvular disease may occur in the setting of prosthetic valves. However, in addition to those symptoms, patients with prosthetic valves experience symptoms specific to the presence of the artificial valve.

Large paravalvular leaks usually present with congestive heart failure. Patients with new neurologic symptoms may have thromboembolism associated with the valve thrombi or endocarditis. Minor embolic episodes, such as transient neurologic symptoms, amaurosis fugax, or self-limited ischemic episodes in the extremities or organs in the absence of endocarditis, are common. Patients may present with major embolic events, including stroke, mesenteric infarction, or sudden death. Major bleeding due to anticoagulant therapy also can occur, with hemorrhagic stroke the most common lethal bleeding complication.

Patients with prosthetic valves usually have abnormal cardiac sounds. Mechanical valves have loud, metallic closing sounds. Systolic murmurs are present commonly with mechanical models. Loud diastolic murmurs generally are not present with mechanical valves. Patients with bioprostheses usually have normal S_1 and S_2, with no abnormal opening sounds. The aortic bioprosthesis usually is associated with short midsystolic murmur. Only the mitral bioprosthesis normally is associated with diastolic rumble.

Diagnosis of Prosthetic Valve Dysfunction or Complications

New or progressive symptoms referable to the heart suggest a prosthetic valve disorder. Therefore, new or progressive dyspnea of any form, new onset or worsening of congestive heart failure, decreased exercise tolerance, or a change in chest pain compatible with ischemia all suggest valvular dysfunction. Persistent fever in patients with prosthetic valves should be evaluated for possible endocarditis. Changes in valve position may be noted on chest radiographs if comparison views are available. Blood studies that may be helpful include a complete blood count with red blood cell indices and coagulation studies if the patient is on warfarin. Emergency echocardiographic studies should be requested if there is any question about valve dysfunction. Ultimately, echocardiography and/or cardiac catheterization may be required for diagnosis.

Emergency Department Management and Admission Indications

Patients suspected of having acute prosthetic valvular dysfunction need immediate referral to a cardiac surgeon for possible emergency surgery. Medical management of patients with acute mitral or aortic valvular incompetence should be guided by the preceding section. The need for the intensity of anticoagulation therapy varies with each type of mechanical valve but ranges from an INR goal of 2 to 3.5.[4] Patients with bioprosthetic valves without additional risk factors for embolism should receive aspirin therapy (160 mg/d).[9] Acute prosthetic valvular dysfunction due to thrombotic obstruction has been treated successfully with thrombolytic therapy,[9] but requires consultation with a cardiologist. Lesser degrees of obstruction should be treated with optimization of anticoagulation. Disposition of patients with worsening of symptoms can be problematic, and consultation with the cardiologist may be needed prior to consideration for discharge.

REFERENCES

1. Petty GW, Khandheria BK, Whisnant JP, et al: Predictors of cerebrovascular events and death among patients with valvular heart disease: A population based study. *Stroke* 31:2628, 2000.
2. Etchells E, Bell C, Robb K: Does this patient have an abnormal systolic murmur? *JAMA* 277:564, 1997.
3. Cheitlin MD, Alpert JS, Armstrong WF, et al: ACC/AHA guidelines for the clinical application of echocardiography: A report of the American College of Cardiology/American Heart Association Task Force on Practice Guidelines (Committee on Clinical Application of Echocardiography). *Circulation* 95:1686, 1997.
4. Salem DN, Levine HJ, Pauker SG, et al: Antithrombotic therapy in valvular heart disease. *Chest* 114:590S, 1998.
5. Jollis JG, Landolfo CK, Kisslo J, et al: Fenfluramine and phentermine and cardiovascular findings: Effect of treatment duration and prevalence of valve abnormalities. *Circulation* 101:2071, 2000.
6. Gardin JM, Schumacher D, Constantine G, et al: Valvular abnormalities and cardiovascular status following exposure to dexfenfluramine or phentermine/fenfluramine. *JAMA* 283:1703, 2000.
7. Jick H: Heart valve disorders and appetite suppressant drugs. *JAMA* 283:1738, 2000.
8. Kizilbash AM, Willett DL, Brickner ME, et al: Effects of afterload reduction on vena contracta width in mitral regurgitation. *J Am Coll Cardiol* 32:427, 1998.
9. Bonow RO, Carabello B, de Leon AC Jr, et al: ACC/AHA guidelines for the management of patients with valvular heart disease: A report of the American College of Cardiology/American Heart Association Task Force on Practice Guidelines (Committee on Management of Patients with Valvular Heart Disease). *J Am Coll Cardiol* 32:1486, 1998.
10. Freed LA, Levy D, Levine RA, et al: Prevalence and clinical outcome of mitral-valve prolapse. *New Engl J Med* 341:1, 1999.
11. Gilon D, Buonanno FS, Joffe MM, et al: Lack of evidence of an association between mitral-valve prolapse and stroke in young patients. *New Engl J Med* 341:8, 1999.
12. Zuppiroli A, Rinaldi M, Kramer-Fox R. et al: Natural history of mitral valve prolapse. *J Am Cardiol* 75:1028, 1995.
13. Stoddard MF, Prince CR, Dillon S, et al: Exercise-induced mitral regurgitation is a predictor of morbid events in subjects with mitral valve prolapse. *J Am Coll Cardiol* 25:693, 1995.
14. Stephan PJ, Henry AC, Hebeler RF, et al: Comparison of age, gender, number of or aortic cusps, concomitant coronary artery bypass grafting, and magnitude of left ventricular-systemic arterial peak systolic gradient in adults having aortic valve replacement for isolated aortic valve stenosis. *Am J Cardiol* 79:166, 1997.
15. Leach RM, McBrian DJ: Brachioradial delay: A new clinical indicator of the severity of aortic stenosis. *Lancet* 335:1199, 1990.
16. Lester SJ, Heibron B, Gin K, et al: The natural history and rate of progression of aortic stenosis. *Chest* 113:1109, 1998.
17. Scognamiglio R, Rahimtoola SH, Fasoli G, et al: Nifedipine in asymptomatic patients with severe aortic regurgitation and normal left ventricular function. *New Engl J Med* 331:689, 1994.
18. Singh JP, Evans SC, Levy D, et al: Prevalence and clinical determinant of mitral, tricuspid, and aortic regurgitation. (The Framingham Heart Study). *Am J Cardiol* 83:897, 1999.
19. Hammermeister K, Sethi GK, Henderson WG, et al: Outcomes 15 years after valve replacement with mechanical vs. a bioprosthetic valve: Final report of the Veterans Affairs Trial. *J Am Coll Cardiol* 36:1152, 2000.
20. Cannegieter SC, Rosendaal FR, Briet E: Thromboembolic and bleeding complications in patients with mechanical heart valves. *Circulation* 89:635, 1994.

55 THE CARDIOMYOPATHIES, MYOCARDITIS, AND PERICARDIAL DISEASE
James T. Niemann

THE CARDIOMYOPATHIES

The term *cardiomyopathy* is used to describe a group of diseases that directly alter cardiac structure and impair myocardial function. Four types of cardiomyopathy are currently recognized: (1) dilated cardiomyopathy (DCM), (2) hypertrophic cardiomyopathy (HCM), (3) restrictive cardiomyopathy, and (4) arrhythmogenic right ventricular cardiomyopathy.[1] It is acknowledged that there are some primary heart muscle disorders that do not fit readily into one of these four groups, and these conditions have been termed unclassified cardiomyopathies. Finally, the term *specific cardiomyopathies* is now used to describe heart muscle diseases that are associated with specific cardiac or systemic disorders. They often present with hemodynamic findings similar to those of the idiopathic dilated or restrictive form of cardiomyopathy. Some specific cardiomyopathies are listed in Table 55-1. As a group, the cardiomyopathies are the third most common form of cardiac disease encountered in the United States, following coronary (ischemic) heart disease and hypertensive heart disease. HCM is the second most common cause of sudden cardiac death in the adolescent population and the leading cause of sudden death in competitive athletes.[2]

Dilated Cardiomyopathy

Hemodynamically, DCM is characterized by depressed myocardial systolic function and systolic pump failure. Left ventricular (LV), and often right ventricular (RV), contractile force is diminished, resulting in a low cardiac output and increased end-systolic and end-diastolic ventricular volumes and intracavitary pressures. LV, and often RV, dilatation accompanied by compensatory hypertrophy are the hallmarks of DCM. Histologic findings are nonspecific.

Approximately 80 percent of cases of DCM are of unknown etiology; that is, they are not associated with specific cardiac or systemic disorders (see Table 55-1) and are considered idiopathic.[3] The idiopathic form of DCM is the cause in approximately 25 percent of all cases of congestive heart failure (CHF) and the primary indication for cardiac transplantation in the United States. The prevalence of idiopathic DCM is estimated to be approximately 36 cases per 100,000 population. Blacks and males have a 2.5-fold increase in risk compared to whites and females. Most patients are diagnosed between the ages of 20 and 50 years, and the majority have advanced symptoms of CHF at the time of initial presentation.[3]

CLINICAL FEATURES AND DIAGNOSIS As a result of systolic pump failure, the patient presents with symptoms of CHF: dyspnea on exertion, orthopnea, and paroxysmal nocturnal dyspnea. Depressed ventricular contractile function and dilatation may result in the formation of mural thrombi, and the patient may present with manifestations

TABLE 55-1   Common Causes of Specific Cardiomyopathies

Toxins
  Ethanol
  Chemotherapeutic agents (doxorubicin)
  Antiretroviral drugs (zidovudine, didanosine)
  Phenothiazines
  Cocaine
Infections
  Viruses (coxsackie virus, echovirus, cytomegalovirus, HIV)
  Rickettsia
  Bacteria (diphtheria, rheumatic fever)
  Mycobacteria
  Fungal
  Parasitic (toxoplasmosis, Chagas disease)
Systemic rheumatic disorders
  Scleroderma
  Systemic lupus erythematosus
  Dermatomyositis
Hypersensitivity myocarditis
Peripartum cardiomyopathy
Metabolic
  Nutritional deficiency (thiamine)
  Endocrine (hypothyroidism, Cushing disease, hyperthyroidism)
  Electrolyte disturbances (hypophosphatemia, hypocalcemia)
Neuromuscular disorders (muscular dystrophy, Friedreich ataxia)
Familial cardiomyopathy

of peripheral embolization (e.g., an acute neurologic deficit, flank pain, and hematuria or a pulseless, cyanotic extremity). Chest pain with features of typical angina pectoris occurs in approximately one-third of patients. Chest pain in these patients is felt to be due to limited coronary vascular reserve rather than atherosclerotic coronary artery disease.

Murmurs are frequently heard during cardiac auscultation and are not necessarily indicative of primary valvular disease. Ventricular dilatation and the resultant annular dilatation and displacement of the papillary muscles of the atrioventricular valves inhibit leaflet coaptation and complete valve closure. Holosystolic regurgitant murmurs of mitral and tricuspid valve origin are frequently heard at the apex or lower left sternal border in the patient with biventricular failure. On occasion an apical diastolic rumble may be heard and is due either to accentuated, early-diastolic atrial-to-ventricular flow (the result of mitral regurgitation and left atrial overload) or to a loud summation gallop. An enlarged, pulsatile liver may be found if tricuspid insufficiency is significant. Bibasilar rales and dependent edema are common additional findings.

The chest radiograph invariably shows an enlarged cardiac silhouette and increased cardiothoracic ratio; biventricular enlargement is common. Evidence of pulmonary venous hypertension ("cephalization" of flow and enlarged hila) is also frequent and may serve to differentiate cardiac enlargement due to myocardial failure from that due to a large pericardial effusion.

The electrocardiogram (ECG) is almost always abnormal. Left ventricular hypertrophy and left atrial enlargement are the most common findings. Q or QS waves and poor R-wave progression across the anterior precordium may produce a pseudoinfarction pattern. Atrial fibrillation and ventricular ectopy are common rhythm disturbances.

Echocardiographic studies in a symptomatic patient demonstrate a decreased ejection fraction, increased systolic and diastolic volumes, and ventricular and atrial enlargement.

TREATMENT AND DISPOSITION A timely assessment is indicated in patients who present with newly diagnosed symptomatic CHF, and evaluation typically requires hospitalization. Echocardiography is indicated to exclude known causes of heart failure that may be correctable (e.g., pericardial effusion or valvular disease), to estimate ejection fraction, and to rule out other potential complications (e.g., mural thrombi) that may be amenable to therapy. Symptom-directed therapy is best initiated in the inpatient setting in order to minimize adverse drug effects, although protocols for short stay/observation units are being investigated. Almost all patients will benefit symptomatically from digitalis glycoside therapy and diuretics, but these drugs have not been shown to improve survival rates and may require different doses in men and women. Detailed reviews suggest the use of angiotensin-converting enzyme inhibitors and β-blockers, specifically carvedilol and metoprolol, have been shown to improve survival in patients with DCM and CHF.[4,5] Patients with complex ventricular ectopy who are determined to be at risk for sudden cardiac death may benefit from amiodarone therapy or an implanted cardioverter-defibrillator (ICD).[6]

Patients with a known DCM and chronic CHF may present to the ED with a mild-to-moderate worsening of symptoms. In most instances, the cause is noncompliance with medical therapy or dietary indiscretion.[7] Such patients can often be managed in the ED with intravenous diuretics, reinstitution of prescribed medications, counseling of the patient, and timely referral to the primary care physician. However, other causes of an acute exacerbation of symptoms in a disease characterized by a slow and progressive history must be considered (see Chap. 53) and, if present or suspected, require hospitalization for definitive management.

Hypertrophic Cardiomyopathy

Hypertrophic cardiomyopathy is characterized by LV and/or RV hypertrophy that is usually asymmetrical and involves primarily the interventricular septum. The diagnostic hallmarks of the disease remain echocardiographic asymmetrical septal hypertrophy and histologic hypertrophy associated with myocardial fiber disarray surrounding areas of increased loose connective tissue.[8,9] In approximately 50 percent of cases, it is a familial disease with autosomal dominant inheritance. In the rest, it is sporadic. There is no apparent sex or ethnic predilection. Molecular genetics has demonstrated that HCM is a heterogeneous disease of the sarcomere with many mutations. The most common mutation involves the β-myosin heavy chain. There is evidence that particular genotypes have more rapidly progressive courses. The prevalence in the general population is approximately 1 in 500. The annual mortality rate in the overall HCM population is about 1 percent per annum, but up to 4 to 6 percent in childhood and adolescence.

Hemodynamically, HCM is characterized by abnormal LV diastolic function due to reduced compliance of the hypertrophied left ventricle. This decreased compliance is reflected by an increase in LV filling pressure. Cardiac output, ejection fraction, and end-systolic and end-diastolic volumes are usually normal. During cardiac catheterization and hemodynamic monitoring, a systolic pressure gradient between the body of the left ventricle and the subvalvular outflow tract can be recorded in some patients at rest or after provocation (e.g., exercise or isoproterenol infusion). The majority of clinical symptoms in this heart muscle disease are the result of impaired diastolic relaxation and restricted LV filling.

CLINICAL FEATURES AND DIAGNOSIS   Severity of symptoms in most instances is related to the patient's age; the older the patient, the more severe the symptoms. Dyspnea on exertion is the most frequent initial complaint and is due to exercise-induced sinus tachycardia, which results in an abrupt elevated LV diastolic pressure and pulmonary venous hypertension. Additional symptoms include chest pain, palpitations, and syncope. A family history of death due to cardiac disease, frequently described as "massive heart attack" or "heart failure," is not uncommon. Complaints of paroxysmal nocturnal dyspnea and pedal edema are infrequent.

Chest pain in HCM patients is due to an imbalance between the oxygen demand of the hypertrophied left ventricle and the available myocardial blood flow. In older patients, associated atherosclerotic coronary artery disease may further limit myocardial perfusion. Precordial or retrosternal chest discomfort in HCM may mimic angina pectoris or may be "atypical." Response to nitroglycerin administration is poor and highly variable.

The HCM patient may be aware of forceful ventricular contraction and complain of an abnormal heartbeat or "palpitations." Atrial and ventricular dysrhythmias are not uncommon in these patients; rapid atrial dysrhythmias, especially atrial fibrillation, are particularly poorly tolerated because of the increased importance of the atrial contribution to LV filling in the poorly compliant heart and require aggressive management in hemodynamically unstable patients.

Jugular venous pressure is usually not elevated; however, a prominent *a* wave may be noted on close inspection of the neck veins. The upstroke of the carotid arterial pulse is rapid and frequently biphasic or bifid (pulsus bisferiens). The apical impulse is sustained and hyperdynamic, and a presystolic lift is common.

The first and second heart sounds are usually normal, and a fourth sound (S_4) will be heard in most patients. The characteristic systolic ejection-type murmur of HCM is heard best at the lower left sternal border or at the apex and rarely radiates to the carotid arteries. Easily performed bedside maneuvers can be used to increase the intensity and duration of the murmur (Table 55-2). Interventions that decrease LV filling and the distending pressure in the LV outflow tract or that increase the force of myocardial contraction accentuate the murmur of HCM. Such interventions include standing and during the strain phase of the Valsalva maneuver. The murmur is also louder with the first sinus beat following a premature ventricular contraction. Maneuvers that increase LV filling (squatting, passive leg elevation, and hand grip) have an opposite effect on murmur characteristics. The murmurs of HCM and mitral valve prolapse are similar and are compared in Table 55-2.

ECG findings of LV hypertrophy and left atrial enlargement are found in 30 percent and 25 to 50 percent, respectively, of HCM patients. Evidence of chamber enlargement is most common in patients with large gradients across the LV outflow tract. Q waves of considerable amplitude (more than 0.3 mV), termed septal Q waves, are seen in about 25 percent of patients and may be encountered in the anterior, lateral, or inferior leads. These Q waves may mimic those seen following myocardial infarction (pseudoinfarction pattern). The polarity of the T wave may serve as a diagnostic clue in the differentiation between HCM septal Q waves from Q waves due to myocardial infarction. Upright T waves in those leads with QS or QR complexes are usually found in HCM; T-wave inversion in such leads is highly suggestive of ischemic heart disease.

The chest radiograph is frequently normal, and identifiable abnormalities are largely nonspecific. Many patients do not show radiographic evidence of LV or left atrial enlargement. Evidence of pulmonary venous congestion is unusual.

Echocardiography has played a substantial role in the diagnosis of HCM, in the correlation of the auscultatory and hemodynamic events with LV anatomic changes, and in defining inheritance patterns. The characteristic echocardiographic finding is disproportionate septal hypertrophy. Additional described echocardiographic abnormalities include normal or reduced LV end-diastolic dimensions, systolic anterior motion of the mitral valve, and midsystolic closure of the aortic valve.

TREATMENT AND DISPOSITION   A systematic review reveals that the majority of patients with HCM who seek medical care typically do so because of declining exercise tolerance, chest pain, or syncope.[9] Symptoms may mimic those of ischemic heart disease, or in the young patient, symptoms may be ascribed to a noncardiac cause. The patient who presents complaining of exercise intolerance or chest pain in whom the typical murmur of HCM is heard should be referred for echocardiographic evaluation. Syncope in patients with HCM typically occurs during or immediately after exercise. If HCM is suspected in a patient with syncope, hospitalization is indicated. The work-up in such cases is extensive and includes echocardiographic studies as well as extended ambulatory (Holter) monitoring, exercise stress testing to assess blood pressure response, and tilt testing. Syncope in patients with HCM may be due to one or more factors and may presage sudden cardiac death.[9] Vigorous exercise is discouraged for such patients, and preparticipation screening guidelines have been developed for competitive athletes to minimize the risk of sudden death due to HCM.[10] β-Blockers are the mainstay of therapy for patients with chest pain.

TABLE 55-2   Effect of Bedside Interventions on the Murmur of Hypertrophic Cardiomyopathy Compared to Mitral Valve Prolapse

	Hypertrophic Cardiomyopathy	Mitral Valve Prolapse
Valsalva maneuver (strain phase)	Murmur increased	Click closer to S_1, murmur increased
Standing after squatting	Murmur increased	Click closer to S_1, murmur increased
Passive leg elevation in supine patient	Murmur decreased	Click closer to S_2, murmur decreased
Hand grip	Murmur decreased	Click closer to S_1, murmur increased
Squatting	Murmur decreased	Click closer to S_2, murmur decreased

Restrictive Cardiomyopathy

The restrictive forms are among the least common of the described cardiomyopathies. *Restrictive cardiomyopathy* is defined as heart muscle disease that results in "restricted" ventricular filling, with normal or decreased diastolic volume of either or both ventricles. Systolic function is usually normal, and ventricular wall thickness may be normal or increased, depending on the underlying cause. The hemodynamic hallmarks include (1) elevated LV and RV end-diastolic pressure, (2) normal LV systolic function (ejection fraction greater than 50 percent), and (3) a marked decrease followed by a rapid rise and plateau in early-diastolic ventricular pressure. The rapid rise and abrupt plateau in the early-diastolic ventricular pressure trace produce a characteristic "square-root sign" or "dip-and-plateau" filling pattern due to increased myocardial stiffness. This pattern is not diagnostic, however, and may be seen in constrictive pericarditis, with which restrictive cardiomyopathy is commonly confused. Differentiation between the two is critical because constrictive pericarditis can be cured surgically. The diagnosis of restrictive cardiomyopathy should be considered in a patient presenting with CHF but no evidence of cardiomegaly or systolic dysfunction.[11]

Restrictive cardiomyopathy may result from systemic disorders (amyloidosis, sarcoidosis, hemochromatosis, progressive systemic sclerosis [scleroderma], carcinoid heart disease, endomyocardial fibrosis, hypereosinophilic syndrome), but most cases are idiopathic. The idiopathic form is sometimes familial, with autosomal dominant transmission. There has been no clearly demonstrated predilection for gender or ethnicity.

CLINICAL FEATURES AND DIAGNOSIS   Symptoms are typical of CHF and include dyspnea, orthopnea, and pedal edema. Right-sided manifestations may predominate and result in hepatomegaly, right upper quadrant pain, and ascites. Chest pain is uncommon, except in amyloidosis.

Findings on physical examination depend on the stage or severity of myocardial involvement. An S_3 is almost always present, and an S_4 is often heard if the patient is in sinus rhythm. Pulmonary rales, jugular venous distention, Kussmaul sign (jugular venous pulse rises during inspiration rather than falling), hepatomegaly, pedal edema, and ascites are also typical findings.

The chest radiograph may reveal signs of CHF in the absence of cardiomegaly. Chamber enlargement due to wall thickening, but not dilatation, and nonspecific ST-T-wave changes are usually noted on the ECG. Cardiac conduction disturbances are common in amyloidosis and sarcoidosis. Atrial fibrillation may occur in the setting of atrial enlargement. Low-voltage QRS complexes (QRS amplitude less than 0.7 mV) have been frequently described in patients with restrictive cardiomyopathy secondary to amyloidosis and hemochromatosis.

TREATMENT AND DISPOSITION   Symptoms and signs of CHF, particularly right-sided failure, with a normal-size cardiac silhouette on chest radiograph should prompt a suspicion of underlying restrictive cardiomyopathy. The differential diagnosis includes constrictive pericarditis, or diastolic LV dysfunction (most commonly due to ischemic heart disease, hypertension, or age-related changes in ventricular diastolic compliance). Doppler echocardiographic studies and cardiac catheterization with hemodynamic assessment are often required to differentiate between the above-mentioned entities. Computed tomography and magnetic resonance imaging of the heart are felt to be of value in differentiating constrictive pericarditis and restrictive cardiomyopathy.[11] Timely diagnosis is important because constrictive pericarditis can be surgically corrected and diastolic LV dysfunction not due to restrictive cardiomyopathy usually responds well to drug therapy (β-blockers or calcium-channel blockers). The medical management of restrictive cardiomyopathy is less effective and symptom directed (diuretics and angiotensin-converting enzyme inhibitors) unless due to sarcoidosis (corticosteroid therapy) or he-

mochromatosis (chelation therapy). The need for admission is usually determined by the severity of symptoms and the availability of a timely and usually invasive work-up.

Arrhythmogenic Right Ventricular Cardiomyopathy

Arrhythmogenic cardiomyopathy, or dysplasia, is the rarest of the cardiomyopathies. Familial disease is common with an autosomal dominant inheritance pattern with incomplete penetrance. This cardiomyopathy is characterized by progressive replacement of the RV myocardium with fibrofatty tissue in an eventual global distribution. The left ventricle and septum are usually spared.[12]

CLINICAL FEATURES AND DIAGNOSIS   The typical presentation is that of sudden death or ventricular dysrhythmia in a young or middle-aged patient. The findings upon physical examination are normal. The chest radiograph shows no specific findings, and the heart size is not enlarged. The ECG may show a right bundle branch pattern and precordial T-wave inversion. Echocardiographic studies, radionuclide angiography, and cardiac catheterization are routinely required to confirm the diagnosis. The echocardiogram has the highest sensitivity and positive predictive value for the diagnosis of RV abnormalities and typically shows RV contraction abnormalities and RV enlargement.[12] Magnetic resonance imaging has been shown to detect fatty infiltration of the myocardium and may become the preferred diagnostic test.

TREATMENT AND DISPOSITION   The majority of patients present after aborted sudden cardiac death, with syncope, or with complex ventricular ectopy. Following such presentations, hospitalization is invariable. Ventricular tachycardia can be suppressed with antiarrhythmic drugs, but ablative procedures or implantation of an antiarrhythmic device may be necessary.

MYOCARDITIS

Definition

Myocarditis is broadly but nonspecifically defined as inflammation of the heart muscle and is most frequently characterized pathologically by focal infiltration of the myocardium by lymphocytes, plasma cells, and histiocytes. Varying amounts of myocytolysis and destruction of the interstitial reticulin network are also seen.[13] Because many episodes are mild, they do not always come to medical attention; thus their incidence is unknown. The pathologic changes have been ascribed to a number of infectious agents (Table 55-3), some of which involve the myocardium secondarily as part of a systemic disease process. Myocarditis is frequently accompanied by pericarditis.

Clinical Features and Diagnosis

Fever is common, as is sinus tachycardia, which is usually out of proportion with respect to the extent of temperature elevation. Signs and symptoms depend on the extent of myocardial involvement and resultant depression of myocardial systolic function. In severe cases, progressive heart failure, with its associated symptoms, may be seen. With less extensive myocardial involvement, pericarditis and the clinical manifestations of systemic illness (fever, myalgias, headache, and rigors) may overshadow clinical signs of myocardial dysfunction, and myocarditis may not be suspected. Retrosternal or precordial chest pain is a frequent presenting complaint and is most commonly secondary to associated pericardial inflammation (myopericarditis). This chest pain may mimic angina in its character. A pericardial friction rub is commonly heard in patients with myopericarditis.

The chest roentgenogram is usually normal, and reported abnormalities (cardiomegaly and pulmonary venous hypertension and/or

TABLE 55-3   Common Infectious Causes of Myocarditis

Viral Agents	Bacteria
Coxsackie B virus	*Corynebacterium diphtheriae*
Echovirus	*Neisseria meningitidis*
Influenza virus	*Mycoplasma pneumoniae*
Parainfluenza virus	β-Hemolytic streptococci (rheumatic fever)
Epstein-Barr virus	Lyme disease
Hepatitis B virus	
HIV	

pulmonary edema) vary with disease severity and are nondiagnostic. Reported ECG changes include nonspecific ST-T-wave changes, ST-segment elevation (due to associated pericarditis), atrioventricular block, and prolonged QRS duration. Levels of cardiac enzymes (creatine kinase and CK-MB) and troponin may be elevated.[13] Echocardiographic studies may reveal depressed systolic function in severe cases. Children are not expected to have a different presentation.

TREATMENT AND DISPOSITION   Current therapy in cases of idiopathic or viral myocarditis is largely supportive and symptom-directed. Myocarditis in rheumatic fever and complicating diphtheria or meningococcemia necessitates directed antibiotic therapy. Immunosuppressive therapy may be of value in selected patients.[14] Admission is usually indicated if the patient presents with symptoms of rapidly progressive CHF.

UNEXPLAINED HEART FAILURE AND CARDIOMEGALY: DIFFERENTIAL DIAGNOSIS AND EVALUATION

Symptoms of CHF and associated cardiomegaly or evidence of cardiomegaly in an asymptomatic patient necessitates a directed evaluation. In the vast majority of instances, one of the following five disease entities will eventually be diagnosed. Where appropriate, recognized diagnostic clues are noted.

1. *Hypertensive heart disease.* Systemic arterial hypertension affects 10 to 20 percent of the adult population. This is a disease with a high prevalence that may be diagnosed at a number of stages. Patients with a dilated cardiomyopathy and untreated cardiac failure frequently present with an elevated blood pressure due to autonomically mediated compensatory reflexes. Isolated involvement of the myocardium as the major manifestation of systemic arterial hypertension is rare. A careful search for evidence of other end-organ damage due to arterial hypertension should be undertaken (examination of fundi, assessment of renal function, evaluation for focal neurologic changes, or history of such entities).

2. *Ischemic heart disease (ischemic cardiomyopathy).* Most patients with clinical signs of biventricular heart failure and cardiomegaly due to obstructive coronary arterial disease relate a history of typical anginal pain or documented myocardial infarction. A few do not, and clinical presentation and physical findings in these cases mimics those of an idiopathic dilated cardiomyopathy.

3. *Valvular heart disease.* Although the incidence of rheumatic heart disease in the United States is low, it remains prevalent in underdeveloped countries and is frequently first diagnosed in recent immigrants. The growing geriatric population is prone to calcific aortic stenosis and mitral annular calcification. In addition, bicuspid or unicuspid aortic valve abnormalities remain the most common congenital heart disease. All valvular diseases may present with CHF or incidental cardiac enlargement, and systolic and diastolic murmurs may be noted. Echocardiographic studies are the diagnostic tests of choice in patients with suspected valvular heart disease. Hemodynamic and angiographic studies may be confirmatory.

4. *Myocarditis.* Patients with severe myocarditis may present with signs and symptoms of progressive cardiac insufficiency. Such patients are usually young, have no significant past cardiac history, have few risk factors for atherosclerotic coronary arterial disease, and present with a recent, abrupt onset of symptoms during or immediately following a systemic or viral illness.

5. *Idiopathic cardiomyopathy.* This diagnosis should be considered only if the first four entities have been excluded. A careful search for potential causes should then be undertaken.

PERICARDIAL DISEASE

The pericardium consists of a serous or loose fibrous membrane (visceral pericardium) overlying the epicardium and a dense collagenous sac (parietal pericardium) surrounding the heart. The space between the visceral and parietal pericardium may contain up to 50 mL of fluid under normal conditions, and intrapericardial pressure is normally subatmospheric. Because its layers are serosal surfaces and because of its proximity and attachments to other structures, the pericardium may be involved in a number of systemic or localized disease processes (Table 55-4). A recent review affirmed the clinical presentation of pericardial heart disease is variable and dependent on the pericardium's response to injury and how this response affects cardiac function.[13] In this section the clinical manifestations and evaluation of acute and constrictive pericarditis and nontraumatic cardiac tamponade are discussed.

Acute Pericarditis

CLINICAL FEATURES   The most common symptom is precordial or retrosternal chest pain, which is most frequently described as sharp or stabbing. It may be of sudden or gradual onset and radiate to the back, neck, left shoulder, or arm; referral to the left trapezial ridge (due to inflammation of the joining diaphragmatic pleura) is a particular distinguishing feature. Chest pain due to acute pericarditis may be aggravated by inspiration or movement. *Typically, chest pain is most severe when the patient is supine and is often relieved when the patient sits up and leans forward.* In most instances, these characteristics allow the pain of acute pericarditis to be distinguished from the ischemic pain of angina or acute myocardial infarction.

Associated symptoms include (1) low-grade, intermittent fever, particularly if pericarditis is infectious in origin or of the idiopathic type; (2) dyspnea, due to accentuated pain with inspiration; and (3) dysphagia, ascribed to irritation of the esophagus by the posterior pericardium.

TABLE 55-4   Common Causes of Acute Pericarditis

Idiopathic
Infectious
   Viral (coxsackie virus, echovirus, HIV)
   Bacterial [especially *Staphylococcus, Streptococcus pneumoniae,*
     β-hemolytic streptococci (acute rheumatic fever), *Mycobacterium*
     tuberculosis]
   Fungal (especially *Histoplasma capsulatum*)
Malignancy (leukemia, lymphoma, metastatic breast and lung carcinoma,
   melanoma)
Drug-induced (procainamide, hydralazine)
Systemic rheumatic diseases (systemic lupus erythematosus, rheumatoid
   arthritis, scleroderma, polyarteritis nodosa, dermatomyositis)
Radiation-induced
Postmyocardial infarction (Dressler syndrome)
Uremia
Myxedema

A pericardial friction rub is the most common and important physical finding in pericarditis, but may be difficult to appreciate in a noisy ED. It is best heard with the diaphragm of the stethoscope at the lower left sternal border or apex when the patient is sitting and leaning forward or in the hands-and-knees position. It may be audible only during a certain phase of respiration and characteristically is transient (e.g., heard one hour and not the next). No inference as to the amount of pericardial fluid should be drawn from the presence or absence of a pericardial friction rub.

A pericardial rub is most often triphasic in character, consisting of a systolic component due to ventricular contraction, an early diastolic component occurring during the early phase of ventricular filling, and a presystolic component synchronous with atrial systole. It is less commonly biphasic, with a systolic component with either an early diastolic or presystolic component. A monophasic rub is unusual (18 percent of cases) but is most often systolic.

DIAGNOSIS

Electrocardiogram   Serial ECGs recorded over a number of days may be diagnostic in acute pericarditis. The evolutionary ECG changes during acute pericarditis and convalescence have been divided into four stages. During stage 1, or the acute phase, ST-segment elevation (reflecting associated subepicardial inflammation and/or injury) is prominent in the precordial leads, especially V_5 and V_6, and in standard lead I. PR-segment depression may be noted in leads II, aVF, and V_4 to V_6 (Figure 55-1). In stage 2, the ST segment begins returning to the isoelectric line, and T-wave amplitude decreases. T-wave inversion is rarely seen until stage 3. Stage 3 is characterized by an isoelectric ST segment and T-wave inversion in those leads previously showing ST-segment elevation. Resolution of repolarization abnormalities is the hallmark of stage 4.

If a large pericardial effusion develops during the course of acute pericarditis, additional ECG abnormalities may be noted, including low-voltage QRS complexes and electrical alternans. These phenomena are due to the insulating effect of pericardial fluid, which attenuates electrical signals of myocardial origin, and the pendular motion of the heart within the fluid-filled pericardial space.

Although serial ECG tracings are of diagnostic value in acute pericarditis, sequential ECG assessment is not a diagnostic luxury afforded the emergency physician. Differentiating pericarditis from the normal variant with "early repolarization" is a common problem and can be difficult when only a single 12-lead ECG is available. The ST-T-wave changes present in the early repolarization or normal variant ECG mimic those of pericarditis and have been reported in 2 percent of healthy young adults. Investigations attempting to distinguish these two conditions have yielded conflicting results. However, a simple criterion offers considerable diagnostic utility, namely, the ST-segment/T-wave amplitude ratio in leads V_5, V_6, or I.[15] Using the end of the PR segment as baseline, or 0 mV, the amplitude or height of the ST segment at its onset is measured in one of the aforementioned leads and recorded in millivolts. The height of the T-wave in the same lead is measured from the baseline to the T-wave peak. *If the ratio of ST amplitude* (in millivolts) *to T-wave amplitude* (in millivolts) *is above 0.25, acute pericarditis is likely* and if the ratio is less than 0.25, acute pericarditis is unlikely. Sensitivity at an ST/T ratio >0.25 for acute pericarditis is greater than 0.85 and the specificity more than 0.8 [LR (+) about 4 and LR(−) about 0.2]. This criterion may allow differentiation of acute pericarditis (stage 1) from early repolarization during ED evaluation (see Figure 55-1). Pericarditis alone does not cause significant cardiac rhythm disturbances.

Radiographic Assessment   Conventional posteroanterior and lateral chest radiographs are of limited value. The cardiac silhouette may be of normal size and contour in acute pericarditis and in some instances, the setting of cardiac tamponade. If previous chest radiographs are available for comparison, a recent increase in the size of the cardiac silhouette or an increase in the cardiothoracic ratio without radiographic evidence of pulmonary venous hypertension aids in distinguishing an expanding pericardial effusion from left heart failure. The epicardial "fat-pad sign" is rarely seen on the lateral chest radiograph and has been reported in only 15 percent of cases of acute pericarditis during fluoroscopy with image intensification. If acute pericarditis is suspected on the basis of history, physical examination, or ECG, posteroanterior and lateral chest radiographs, which may demonstrate a pleuropulmonary or mediastinal abnormality, may assist in establishing the underlying cause (e.g., neoplastic or infectious).

Echocardiographic Studies   Echocardiography has become the procedure of choice for the detection, confirmation, and serial follow-up of patients with acute pericarditis and a pericardial effusion.

Normally, the pericardial sac is only a "potential" space, and the myocardium is echocardiographically in direct contact with surrounding thoracic structures. The anterior RV wall is in contact with the chest wall, and the posterior LV wall is in contact with the posterior pericardium and adjacent pleura. When a pericardial effusion is present, the pericardial space fills with echo-free fluid. Echocardiographically, a separation is seen between the right ventricle and the chest wall and between the left ventricle and the posterior pericardium. Quantitation of the size of the effusion is arbitrary and is determined by where the echo-free space is seen (anterior or posterior) and when in the cardiac cycle it occurs. For example, when an echo-free space is seen only posteriorly and only during systole, a small effusion is said to be present.

Ancillary Laboratory Evaluation   The laboratory studies listed in Table 55-5 may be of value in establishing an etiologic diagnosis.[16] Serum CK-MB and troponins may be elevated in acute pericarditis due to associated myocarditis.[17]

TREATMENT AND DISPOSITION   Most patients with idiopathic or presumed viral pericarditis will respond to nonsteroidal anti-inflammatory agents administered for 7 days to 3 weeks. If a specific cause is identified, therapy should be directed toward the underlying disease. Patients with an enlarged cardiac silhouette on chest radiograph should be admitted for early Doppler echocardiography to assess the extent of the effusion and degree of hemodynamic compromise.

Nontraumatic Cardiac Tamponade

PATHOPHYSIOLOGY   An increase in the amount of fluid within the pericardial sac results in an increase in intrapericardial pressure. The normal fibrocollagenous parietal pericardium has elastic properties and stretches to accommodate increases in intrapericardial fluid. The initial portion of the pericardial volume-pressure curve is flat: relatively large increases in volume result in comparatively small changes in intrapericardial pressure. The curve becomes steeper as the parietal pericardium reaches the limits of its distensibility. If fluid continues to accumulate, intrapericardial pressure rises to a level greater than that of the normal filling pressures of the right heart chambers. When this occurs, ventricular filling is restricted and results in cardiac tamponade. The point at which this occurs is determined by the slope of the pericardial volume-pressure curve, which is dependent on the rate of fluid accumulation, pericardial compliance (a thickened parietal pericardium is less distensible), and intravascular volume (hypovolemia lowers ventricular filling pressure). Common causes of cardiac tamponade in nontrauma patients are listed in Table 55-6.

CLINICAL FEATURES AND DIAGNOSIS   Symptoms are nonspecific, and patients most commonly complain of dyspnea and profound exertional intolerance. Additional complaints may be present due to the underlying disease (e.g., uremia) or if the pericardial effusion has

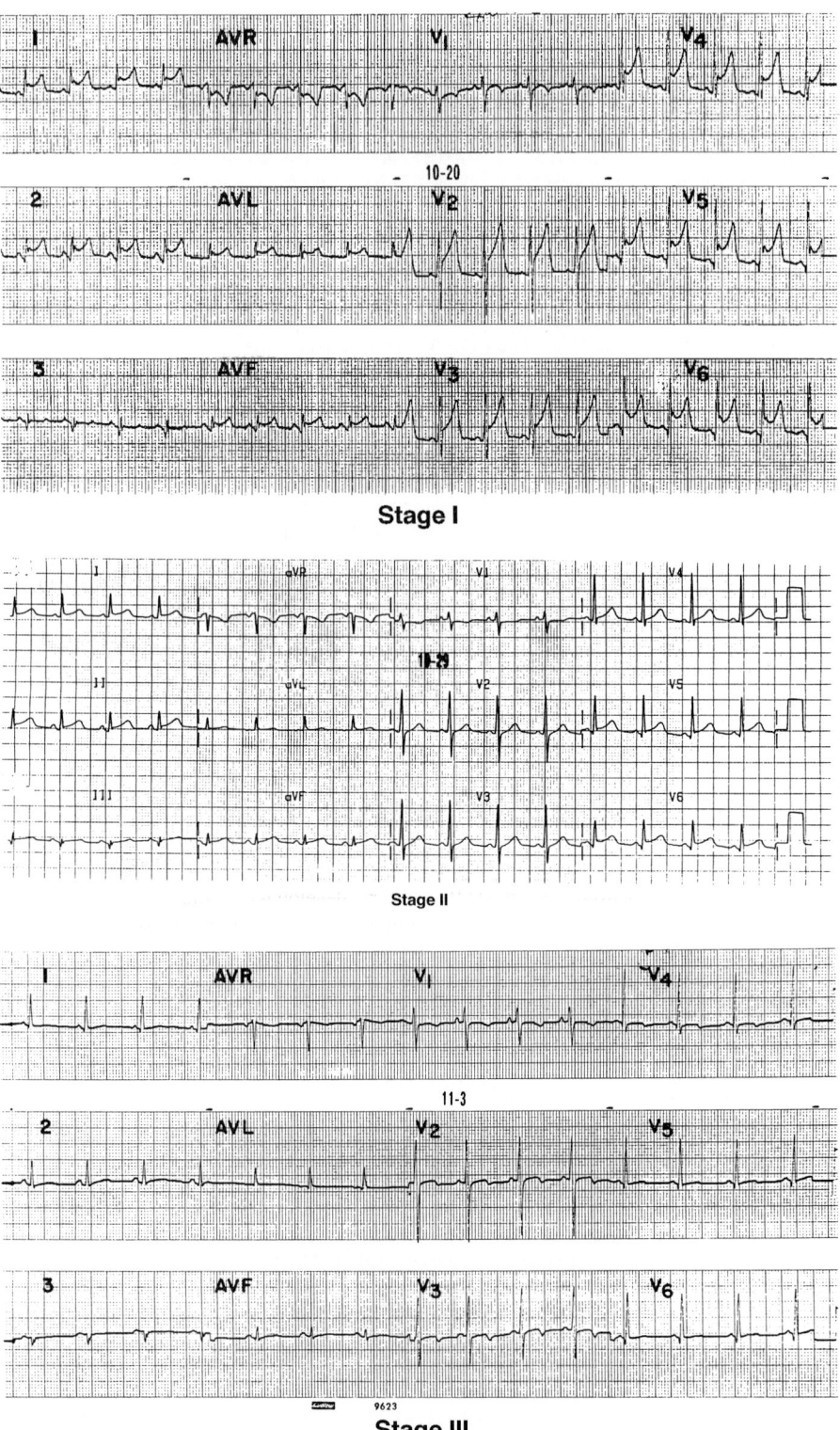

FIG. 55-1. This series of ECGs was recorded in a 28-year-old male who presented complaining of pleuritic retrosternal pain, cough, and fever. The initial ECG (dated 10-20) demonstrates diffuse ST-segment elevation (stage I). The ST-segment to T-wave amplitude ratio measured in V_6 is 5 mm/10 mm, or 0.50, thus meeting criteria for pericarditis rather than early repolarization (see the text). The ECG dated 10-29 demonstrates a return of the ST segment to the isoelectric point in most leads in which they had been elevated (stage II). The third tracing (dated 11-3) demonstrates resolution of ST changes and the appearance of T-wave inversion in the anterior precordial leads (stage III). These evolutionary changes are typical of and diagnostic for pericarditis and usually occur over several weeks.

developed gradually (e.g., tuberculous pericarditis). Such symptoms may include weight loss, pedal edema, ascites, and so on.

Physical examination most commonly reveals tachycardia and low systolic arterial blood pressure with a narrow pulse pressure. Pulsus paradoxus may also be present. A paradoxical arterial pulse is said to be present when the cardiac rhythm is regular and there are apparent dropped beats in the peripheral pulse during inspiration. There is usually a greater than 10 mm Hg decrease in systolic blood pressure during inspiration in the supine position. A value greater than 25 mm Hg usually separates true tamponade from lesser degrees of restricted car-

diac filling.[18] Pulsus paradoxus is not diagnostic of cardiac tamponade and may be noted in other cardiopulmonary processes. In cardiac tamponade, the neck veins are usually distended with an absent *y* descent. The apical impulse is indistinct or tapping in quality. Cardiac auscultation may reveal "distant" or soft heart sounds. Pulmonary rales are usually absent, and there may be right upper quadrant tenderness due to hepatic venous congestion.

The chest radiograph may or may not reveal an enlarged cardiac silhouette, and this finding is dependent on the amount of intrapericardial fluid accumulation. The pulmonary vasculature typically ap-

TABLE 55-5   Ancillary Diagnostic Studies in Acute Pericarditis

Complete blood count and differential white blood cell count	May suggest infection or leukemia
Blood urea nitrogen/creatinine	May suggest a diagnosis of uremic pericarditis
Streptococcal serologic testing (antistreptolysin O, anti-DNAse, antihyaluronidase)	Particularly in patients with a history of rheumatic heart disease or pharyngitis
Blood cultures	If bacterial infection suspected
Serologic studies	Antinuclear antibodies, anti-DNA titers, or rheumatoid factor in patients with systemic symptoms
Erythrocyte sedimentation rate	Will not facilitate an etiologic diagnosis but can be followed serially to assess response to therapy
Acute and convalescent viral antibody titers	
Thyroid function studies	

pears normal. An epicardial fat-pad line, or sign, may occasionally be seen within the cardiac silhouette.

The ECG usually shows low-voltage QRS complexes (less than 0.7 mV) and ST-segment elevation (due to the inflammation of the epicardium) with PR-segment depression, as in pericarditis. Electrical alternans (beat-to-beat variation in the amplitude of the P and R waves unrelated to the respiratory cycles) is a classic but uncommon finding (about 20 percent of cases). Electrical alternans is demonstrated in Figure 55-2.

The diagnosis should be suspected based on the clinical examination and chest radiograph findings. Echocardiographic assessment is the diagnostic test of choice. In addition to a large pericardial fluid volume, typical echocardiographic findings described in cardiac tamponade are right atrial compression, right ventricular diastolic collapse, abnormal respiratory variation in tricuspid and mitral flow velocities (Doppler), and dilated inferior vena cava with lack of inspiratory collapse.

TREATMENT AND DISPOSITION   Volume expansion with a bolus of NS solution (500 to 1000 mL) will increase intravascular volume, facilitate right heart filling, and increase cardiac output and arterial pressure. However, it is a temporary measure, and patients will require pericardiocentesis as initial definitive therapy and for diagnostic evaluation.

Pericardiocentesis is optimally performed in the cardiac catheterization laboratory using echocardiographic guidance. The major potential complications, namely cardiac perforation and coronary artery laceration, can be minimized. In addition, a pigtail catheter can be inserted to allow continuous fluid drainage and prevention of fluid accumulation.

TABLE 55-6   Cardiac Tamponade in Medical (Nontrauma) Patients

Cause	Approximate Frequency, %
Metastatic malignancy	40
Acute idiopathic pericarditis	15
Uremia	10
Bacterial or tubercular pericarditis	10
Chronic idiopathic pericarditis	10
Hemorrhage (anticoagulant)	5
Other (systemic lupus erythematosus, postradiation, myxedema, etc.)	10

Emergency pericardiocentesis might be necessary within the emergency department if dictated by hemodynamic instability. The technique is described in Chap. 259.

If the equipment is available, echocardiographically guided emergency pericardiocentesis can be performed in the emergency department. Definitive management (insertion of an intrapericardial pigtail catheter through a pericardial window) is best undertaken following admission. After pericardiocentesis, patients require admission in a monitored setting.

Constrictive Pericarditis

PATHOPHYSIOLOGY   Constrictive pericarditis is pathologically distinct from acute pericarditis.[19] Following pericardial injury and the resultant inflammatory and reparative process, fibrous thickening of the layers of the pericardium may occur. This fibrous reparative process is most commonly encountered after cardiac trauma with intrapericardial hemorrhage, after pericardiotomy (open-heart surgery, including coronary revascularization), in fungal or tuberculous pericarditis, and in chronic renal failure (uremic pericarditis). When the fibrous and/or collagenous response prevents passive diastolic filling of the normally distensible cardiac chambers, constriction is said to be present. Intrapericardial fluid is not required to produce such a hemodynamic effect. By its nature, constrictive pericarditis is most commonly a slowly progressive process without initial symptoms. However, clinical manifestations may occur early if fluid also accumulates within the thickened, noncompliant pericardial sac (so-called effusive constrictive pericarditis). In the vast majority of cases of constrictive pericarditis that are proved by hemodynamic assessment (see below), a specific cause is never determined.

CLINICAL FEATURES   The symptoms of constrictive pericarditis usually develop gradually and may mimic those of CHF and restrictive cardiomyopathy.[19] If symptoms develop within months of a pericardial injury, a combination of pericardial effusion and constriction should be suspected. Exertional dyspnea and decreased exercise tolerance are common complaints; however, orthopnea, paroxysmal nocturnal dyspnea, and chest pain are unusual. Lower-extremity swelling (pedal edema) and increasing abdominal girth (ascites) are also common complaints and are the result of decreased RV diastolic compliance and the resultant increase in systemic venous pressure.

In most instances, physical findings and their correct interpretation will lead the clinician to suspect constrictive pericarditis. Examination of the neck veins with the torso of the patient at a 45° angle from horizontal will reveal jugular venous distention and a rapid y descent of the cervical venous pulse. Elevated venous pressure is also seen in CHF, but a rapid y descent is infrequently encountered. The Kussmaul sign (inspiratory neck vein distention) is frequently but not invariably noted in constrictive pericarditis but rarely noted in uncompensated CHF. A paradoxical pulse is found in a minority of patients, and thus its absence does not exclude a diagnosis of constrictive pericarditis. On cardiac auscultation, an early diastolic sound, a pericardial "knock," may be heard at the apex 60 to 120 milliseconds after the second heart sound. The pericardial knock sounds like a ventricular gallop but occurs earlier than the S_3 of CHF, which it may mimic. The knock is due to accelerated RV inflow in early diastole and early myocardial distention, followed by an abrupt slowing of further ventricular expansion. There is usually no pericardial friction rub. Hepatomegaly, ascites, and dependent edema of varying severity are usually found.

DIAGNOSIS

Electrocardiogram   Diagnostic ECG changes have not been described in constrictive pericarditis. However, low-voltage QRS complexes and inverted T waves are common.

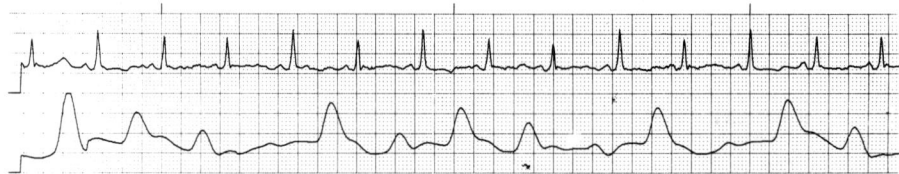

FIG. 55-2. This rhythm strip **(lead II, top tracing)** and plethysmograph **(bottom tracing)** were recorded in a patient who presented with dyspnea, hypotension, and clinical and echocardiographic evidence of cardiac tamponade. A paradoxical pulse was noted on palpation of the radial artery. The amplitude of the R waves varies from beat to beat (electrical alternans). Similar changes are seen in P-wave amplitude. These ECG changes are not related to the respiratory cycle.

Radiographic Assessment Conventional posteroanterior and lateral chest radiographs most commonly demonstrate a normal or slightly enlarged cardiac silhouette, clear lung fields, and little or no evidence of pulmonary venous congestion. Pericardial calcification, which may be evident in up to 50 percent of patients with constrictive pericarditis, is seen best on the lateral chest radiograph but is not diagnostic of constrictive pericarditis. Thoracic computed tomography (CT) and magnetic resonance imaging (MRI) may also demonstrate a thickened pericardium.[20]

Echocardiographic Studies On occasion, two-dimensional echocardiography may demonstrate pericardial thickening and abnormal ventricular septal motion in a patient with suspected constrictive pericarditis. However, its diagnostic utility is much less than in a patient with acute pericarditis. Doppler echocardiography is preferred, and cardiac CT and MRI may also be useful.

TREATMENT AND DISPOSITION In cases of significant constriction and impaired ventricular filling, pericardiectomy is the treatment of choice.

REFERENCES

1. Richardson P, McKenna W, Bristow M, et al: Report of the 1995 World Health Organization/International Society and Federation of Cardiology Task Force on the definition and classification of cardiomyopathies. *Circulation* 93:841, 1996.
2. Liberthson RR: Sudden death from cardiac causes in children and young adults. *New Engl J Med* 334:1039, 1996.
3. Felker GM, Hu W, Hare JM, et al: The spectrum of dilated cardiomyopathy. The Johns Hopkins experience with 1,278 patients. *Medicine* 78:270, 1999.
4. Hunt SA, Baker DW, Chin MH, et al: ACC/AHA guidelines for the evaluation and management of chronic heart failure in the adult: a report of the American College of Cardiology/American Heart Association Task Force on Practice Guidelines (Committee to Revise the 1995 Guidelines for the Evaluation and Management of Heart Failure). *J Am Coll Cardiol* 38:2101, 2001. Also available at: http://www.acc.org/clinical/guidelines/failure/hf_index.htm.
5. Foody JM, Farrell MH, Krumholz HM: β-Blocker therapy in heart failure. A scientific review. *JAMA* 287:883, 2002.
6. Heidenrich PA, Keeffe B, McDonald KM, et al: Overview of randomized trials of antiarrhythmic drugs and devices for the prevention of sudden cardiac death. *Am Heart J* 144:422, 2002.
7. Tsuyuski RT, McKelvie RS, Arnold MO, et al: Acute precipitants of congestive heart failure exacerbations. *Arch Intern Med* 161:2337, 2001.
8. Roberts R, Sigwart U: New concepts in hypertrophic cardiomyopathies, Part I. *Circulation* 104:2113, 2001. Part II. *Circulation* 104:2249, 2001.
9. Maron BJ: Hypertrophic cardiomyopathy. A systematic review. *JAMA* 287:1308, 2002.
10. Maron BJ, Thompson PD, Puffer JC, et al: Cardiovascular preparticipation screening of competitive athletes: A statement for health professionals from the Sudden Death Committee (Clinical Cardiology) and Congenital Cardiac Defects Committee (Cardiovascular Disease in the Young), American Heart Association. *Circulation* 94:850, 1996.
11. Kushwaha SS, Fallon JT, Fuster V: Restrictive cardiomyopathy. *New Engl J Med* 336:267, 1997.
12. Fontaine G, Fountaliran F, Frank R: Arrhythmogenic right ventricular cardiomyopathies: Clinical forms and main differential diagnoses. *Circulation* 97:1532, 1998.
13. Oakley CM: Myocarditis, pericarditis, and other pericardial diseases. *Heart* 84:449, 2000.
14. Parrillo JE: Inflammatory cardiomyopathy (myocarditis). Which patients should be treated with anti-inflammatory therapy? *Circulation* 104:4, 2001.
15. Ginzton LE, Laks MM: The differential diagnosis of acute pericarditis from the normal variant: New electrocardiographic criteria. *Circulation* 65:1004, 1982.
16. Zayas R, Anguita M, Torres F, et al: Incidence of specific etiology and role of methods for specific etiologic diagnosis of primary acute pericarditis. *Am J Cardiol* 75:378, 1995.
17. Brandt RR, Filzmaier K, Hanrath P: Circulating cardiac troponin I in acute pericarditis. *Am J Cardiol* 87:1326, 2001.
18. Curtiss EI, Reddy S, Uretsky BF, et al: Pulsus paradoxus: definition and relation to the severity of cardiac tamponade. *Am Heart J* 115:391, 1988.
19. Myers RB, Spodick DH: Constrictive pericarditis: clinical and pathologic characteristics. *Am Heart J* 138:219, 1999.
20. Breen JF: Imaging of the pericardium. *J Thorac Imaging* 16:47, 2001.

PULMONARY EMBOLISM
Jeffrey A. Kline

Despite recent widening educational efforts toward increasing vigilance for pulmonary embolism (PE) among emergency physicians, the diagnosis is difficult. This chapter discusses pulmonary embolism. Thrombophlebitis is discussed in Chap. 59.

INITIAL APPROACH TO THE PATIENT

Even in the current era of unprecedented recognition of the need for prophylaxis and diagnosis of thrombosis, fatal PE often is not diagnosed, even when the patient has recently seen a physician.[1] Patients with PE usually present with symptoms and findings that mimic many other diseases. Moreover, PE may present with almost no symptoms and may even occur in the complete absence of apparent symptoms. Thus, many clinicians are unsure when to consider this diagnosis within their workup. Although details are discussed below, an appropriate approach is shown in Figure 56-1.

Pathophysiology of Pulmonary Embolism

Appropriate consideration of PE within the differential diagnosis begins with recognition of risk factors that predispose to thrombosis, the precursor to PE. Risk factors are embodied by the triad of factors associated with thrombosis described by Rudolph Virchow: hypercoagulability, stasis, and venous injury (Table 56-1). Hypercoagulability, also referred to as *thrombophilia,* can be broadly classified as malignancy (the most common cause) and nonmalignancy. Malignancies of primary adenocarcinoma or brain origin are the most likely to cause

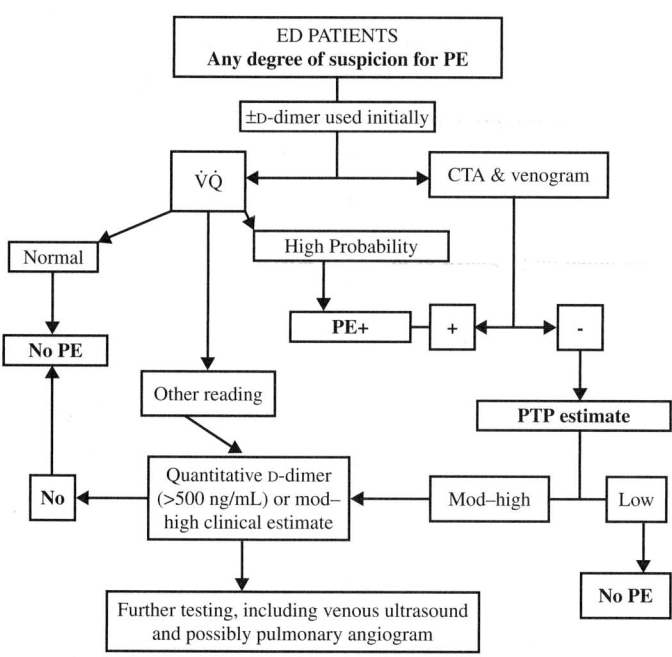

FIG. 56-1. Algorithm for evaluation of suspected PE. *Abbreviation:* CTA = computed tomographic angiogram.

thrombosis. The causes of nonmalignant thrombophilia, listed in descending order of frequency in the ED, include estrogen use, pregnancy, antiphospholipid antibody syndromes, and genomic mutations. The genomic mutations that cause inherited thrombophilia (including the factor V Leiden mutation, the prothrombin mutation, methylenetetrahydrofolate reductase gene mutation, factor VIII mutations, functional or antigenic protein C deficiency, or functional or antigenic protein S deficiency) have been the subject of recent reviews.[2,3] Emergency department patients can be subjected to immobility resulting in stasis for many reasons, including paralysis, debilitating diseases, or recent trauma. Emergency physicians should recognize that ED patients who are recently discharged after surgery maintain a high risk of PE; the thrombotic mechanisms of stasis and venous injury do not vanish when the postoperative patient leaves the hospital.

Although a remote prior history of PE may seem like a potent predictor of present PE, the importance of this factor is not as strong as

TABLE 56-1   Classic Risk Factors for Thrombosis

Hypercoagulability
  Malignancy
  Nonmalignant thrombophilia
    Pregancy
    Postpartum status (<4 wk)
    Estrogen
    Antiphospholipid antibodies
    Genetic mutations
      Factor V Leiden mutation
      Prothrombin mutation
      Methylenetetrahydrofolate reductase gene mutation
      Factor VIII mutations
      Functional or antigenic protein C deficiency
      Functional or antigenic protein S deficiency
Venous stasis
  Bedrest >48 h
  Cast or external fixator
  Recent hospitalization
  Long-distance automobile or air travel
Venous injury
  Recent surgery requiring endotracheal intubation
  Recent trauma requiring hospitalization (especially lower extremity, pelvis)

might be expected. If the patient had a clearly reversible factor (e.g., postoperative or postpartum status) at the time of diagnosis and has no thrombophilia, then he or she is at no greater statistical risk for PE than an age-matched patient who never had a PE.

Clinical Features

The clinical manifestations of PE result from cardiopulmonary stress caused by the clot in the lung. This stress produces the symptoms perceived by the patient and the signs observed by the physician. Shortness of breath is the most common symptom of PE, occurring in approximately 90 percent of patients with established diagnoses. The presence of unexplained dyspnea is sufficient to initiate a diagnostic evaluation. No one is certain of the exact mechanism of dyspnea from PE, but ventilation-perfusion mismatch is an important pathophysiologic cause. At the bedside, ventilation-perfusion mismatch is manifested as hypoxemia and tachypnea. The definitions of hypoxemia and tachypnea vary with age and comorbidity, but, as a rule of thumb, a pulse oximetry reading measuring less than 95 percent or an arterial partial pressure of oxygen less than 80 mm Hg should be considered preliminary evidence of relative hypoxemia (the arbitrary definition of hypoxemia is generally accepted as <60 mm Hg; see Chap. 62). A respiratory rate faster than 20 breaths/min should be considered tachypnea. Unfortunately, the degree of ventilation-perfusion mismatch with PE can be capricious, sometimes being severe with small PE and sometimes being mild with large PE. Also, because of changes in the location of the embolic material within the heart and pulmonary vasculature and reflexive adaptations of the pulmonary vasculature and bronchi, the degree of dyspnea and associated findings can change with time. In other words, **patients with PE can have intermittent shortness of breath.** Also, patients with PE often describe their shortness of breath as exertional, distracting the focus of some clinicians toward a search for cardiogenic dyspnea.

Chest pain represents the second most common symptom of cardiopulmonary stress in patients with PE. However, it must be cautioned that up to one third of patients have PE diagnosed on the basis of isolated dyspnea without any history of chest pain. Upon detailed questioning, others will relate only a vague sensation of chest discomfort. Still other patients with smaller clots, lodged in segmental or smaller pulmonary arteries, will point specifically to one extremely painful, localized area of the chest, usually at the periphery and pleuritic in nature. These patients often go on to develop radiographic evidence of lung parenchymal consolidation in the embolized segment of lung, suggesting the presence of hemorrhagic transformation of the ischemic tissue. With time, some patients with peripheral PE develop hemoptysis and, as such, are declared to have pulmonary infarction. Among all patients with PE, patients with infarction are the most likely with PE to develop fever. Patients with massive PE may complain of substernal or epigastric pain that appears to be associated with subendocardial ischemia in the right ventricle (RV). These patients often present in severe distress, with a systolic blood pressure less than 100 mm Hg or a heart rate that exceeds the systolic blood pressure measurement (i.e., a shock index measurement: heart rate/systolic blood pressure >1.0).

Cardiac arrest might be considered the most extreme form of cardiopulmonary stress and occurs in approximately 2 percent of patients with PE. Some clinicians assume that PE always causes pulseless electrical activity upon arrest secondary to complete pulmonary vascular obstruction. This hypothesis has been examined in some detail by using autopsy registries.[4] These studies suggested that approximately 60 percent of patients who die from PE have pulseless electrical activity (rate >20 beats/min) as the initial arrest rhythm, but about one third have immediate asystole as the proximate cause of arrest. The mechanism of asystole with PE has been postulated as an end effect of inhibited cardiac automaticity from vagal impulses, coupled with infranodal conduction blockade that can occur with very high RV pressures.

Fewer than 10 percent of patients with fatal PE experience ventricular tachycardia or ventricular fibrillation.

Some experts have referred to a spectrum of cardiopulmonary stress from PE, ranging from the peripheral clot causing focal pleuritic chest pain, to the relatively painless syndrome of the dyspneic embolism, to the more rare but devastating massive PE with acute cor pulmonale, to the fatal syndrome of pulseless electrical activity arrest.

Tachycardia represents a cardinal sign of cardiopulmonary stress from PE. As with many other aspects of PE, the etiology of the tachycardia remains obscure and probably results from a combination of factors, including baroreceptor unloading, release of chronotropic agents from the thrombus, and the secondary effects of ventilation-perfusion mismatch, including hypoxemia and perception of dyspnea that leads to anxiety. In most published studies, a heart rate faster than 100 beats/min is used to represent tachycardia. The absence of tachycardia alone does not exclude the presence of PE. About one half of all patients with diagnosed PE have a heart rate slower than 100 beats/min.[5]

Timing of symptom onset carries little prognostic significance in determining who requires an ED evaluation for PE. Similarly, the acuity of onset or lack thereof has no statistical predictive value for the diagnosis. When ED patients are systematically questioned as to their perception of the onset of the first symptom of PE, up to one fourth relate the onset of symptoms over 2 weeks before the date of diagnosis. It is corroborated by the finding that over one half of ED patients with PE have radiographic evidence of more than four clots in their lungs at the time of diagnosis.[6] Autopsy results show that about one half of patients with fatal PE have multiple clots that exhibit pathologic features suggesting a wide range of ages.

More useful than timing and acuity of onset of symptoms to predict PE is the history of dyspnea, pleuritic chest pain, or findings of tachycardia, tachypnea, or hypoxemia with insufficient explanation.[7] As one very specific example, the diagnosis of bronchitis does not adequately explain the combination of cough, chest pain, a respiratory rate of 22 breaths/min, a pulse rate of 102 beats/min, and pulse oximetry of 94 percent in a young patient with a clear chest radiograph. If an ED population appropriate for PE evaluation by competent emergency physicians is statistically analyzed, the factors that predict a final diagnosis of PE can be somewhat surprising (Table 56-2). For example, the presence of existing lung disease (smoking, asthma, or chronic obstructive pulmonary disease) clearly does not protect a patient from PE, but the presence of these diseases effectively lowers the probability of PE in ED patients selected for evaluation, apparently because patients who smoke or have asthma or chronic obstructive pulmonary disease are more likely to have some other pathologic process that shares the clinical features of PE.

Chest pain, tachypnea, and tachycardia are each frequently associated with PE. However, the presence of all three is not all that frequent but, when noted, is highly suggestive of PE, especially in the face of risks. The absence of all three, particularly without other supporting features, such as altered mental status, syncope, or seizure, are strong indicators that the diagnosis rests with another condition.

Pretest Probability Assessment for PE

Multiple factors must be considered simultaneously to arrive at a pretest probability for PE, i.e., the likely prevalence of PE that could be expected in a group of patients who are very similar to the patient at hand. The importance of the pretest probability for PE cannot be underestimated, inasmuch as its influence has a greater impact on the final decision of whether or not a PE is present than the choice of the laboratory or imaging test used to exclude it (Figure 56-2). The pretest probability guides the choice of diagnostic testing and helps determine when to terminate ancillary investigation. In practice, many clinical factors are used to arrive at a rough (empiric) assessment of pretest probability. The problems with empiric assessment include the fact that it requires *gestalt*. Clinicians often disagree about the empiric pretest probability of PE, and accuracy requires clinical experience.[8] Unfortunately, empiric assessment of low-risk patients may not produce a low probability of PE. In a multicenter study in Europe, Sanson and colleagues found that clinicians using empiric pretest methods categorize only 14 percent of patients as low risk for PE, but the posttest occurrence of PE in this low-risk group was 19 percent.[9] To help deal with the shortcomings of empiric assessment, researchers have resorted to the use of decision rules or score systems that incorporate symptoms, signs, and risk factors for PE into scores or algorithms to

TABLE 56-2 Factors That Help Distinguish the Presence or Absence of an Outcome Diagnosis of PE in Outpatients Selected for Evaluation for PE*

	Factors Associated with PE	Factors Associated with Absence of PE	Factors Contributing to the Decision to Evaluate for PE but Do Not Distinguish Presence or Absence of PE
Symptoms	Unexplained dyspnea, hemoptysis	Substernal chest pain, nonspecific dizziness	Pleuritic chest pain, syncope, nonproductive cough, anxiety
Signs	Unilateral leg swelling, heart rate >100 beats/min, hypoxemia (room air pulse oximetry <95% with no history of lung disease)	Wheezing, temperature >102°F, bilateral leg edema, pulse oximetry measured on room air consistently at 100%	Rales, temperature <102°F, respiratory distress, room air pulse oximetry reading of 95–99%
Risk factors	Age >50 y, recent surgery (requiring general anesthesia within past 4 wk), thrombophilia, adenocarcinoma (ovarian, pancreatic, prostate, and gastrointestinal) or brain cancer (especially glioblastoma multiforma), new-onset limb or body immobility >48 h	Age <30 y, COPD, asthma, smoking	Prior PE or DVT with a therapeutic INR and no thrombophilia, pregnancy, estrogen usage, lung or breast cancer, postpartum status, congestive heart failure, or recent travel

*No individual criterion should be used as evidence to not test for PE.
Abbreviations: COPD = chronic obstructive pulmonary disease; DVT = deep vein thrombosis; INR = international normalized ratio; PE = pulmonary embolism.
Source: Kline JA, Nelson RD, Jackson RE, Courtney DM; Criteria for the safe use of D-dimer testing in emergency department patients with suspected pulmonary embolism: A multicenter United States study. *Ann Emerg Med* 39:144, 2002; Wells PS, Anderson DR, Rodger M, et al: Derivation of a simple clinical model to categorize patients' probability of pulmonary embolism: Increasing the model's utility with the SimpliRED D-dimer. *Thromb Haemost,* 83:416, 2000; and Wicki J, Perneger TV, Junod AE, et al: Assessing clinical probability of pulmonary embolism in the emergency ward: A simple score. *Arch Intern Med* 161:92, 2001.

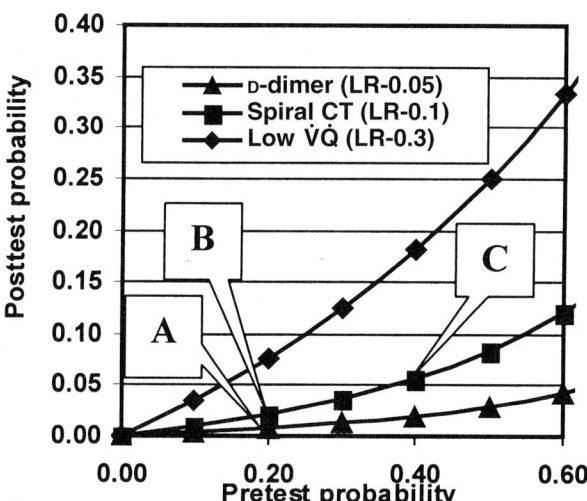

FIG. 56-2. Plot of posttest probability as a function of pretest probability for three diagnostic tests for pulmonary embolism (PE), magnifying the area of the pretest and posttest probability ranges most relevant to screening for PE in the emergency department. The figure shows that the pretest probability can affect the posttest probability to an even greater extent than the diagnostic performance of the test used to exclude the disease. Points A, B, and C show that doubling the pretest probability has greater impact on posttest probability than does halving the likelihood ratio (LR) of a test that is negative for disease. The negative LR [(1 − sensitivity)/specificity] represents a composite measure of diagnostic test performance, and the numbers shown for D-dimer, computed tomography, and a low probability ventilation-perfusion lung scan are approximate. Point A shows that a patient with a pretest probability of 20 percent has a posttest probability of about 1 percent after a negative quantitative D-dimer assay. If a test with a negative LR that is twice as high is used on the same patient (point B), the posttest probability increases to only about 2 percent. However, if the pretest probability is doubled from B to C and the same diagnostic test is used, the posttest probability increases to 6 percent.

categorize individual patients into broad groups. Most systems group patients into these cohorts: low-risk (e.g., <10 percent probability), moderate-risk (11 to 60 percent probability), or high-risk (>60 percent probability).[7,10] Others classify patients into high-risk and non-high-risk categories.[5] The benefits and drawbacks to these rules have been reviewed elsewhere, and it is not the objective of this chapter to state which rule or system to use; rather, it is to inform the reader of their existence.

No evidence has been published to define the threshold at which the pretest probability reaches a level when a workup for PE should be initiated. Certainly, most experts would agree that all patients who have an empiric or decision rule-derived probability of PE of greater than 10 percent or more than low risk should undergo objective testing. However, it must be recognized that over one half of patients evaluated for PE in the ED are deemed low risk.[7,10] The optimal choice of diagnostic testing remains in a state of flux. Several of the more common options are discussed, and each is considered in the context of the pretest probability.

ANCILLARY TESTING

Figure 56-2 illustrates the effect of pretest probability on the final outcome as to whether or not PE is present (posttest probability). The figure compares the effect of three tests with three levels of diagnostic performance and shows how pretest probability can cause a greater impact on posttest probability than even the performance of the diagnostic test, as assessed by its negative likelihood ratio.

The Criterion Standard

Studies of new tests for PE are usually compared against a "gold" reference or criterion standard that represents the best available method to diagnose or exclude the disease. For the past four decades, the gold standard has been selective pulmonary angiography with cineangio-fluoroscopy to evaluate for the presence of a filling defect or arterial cutoff in the pulmonary vascular tree. When performed by an experienced specialist, pulmonary angiography is a safe procedure that can produce brilliant images with resolution of vessels as small as 3 to 4 mm in diameter. Pulmonary angiography also provides pulmonary arterial pressure data and can serve as the prelude to the use of catheter fragmentation to reduce the clot burden. However, pulmonary angiography itself is not perfect. Approximately 1 percent of patients at high risk are diagnosed with PE within a few months after a normal pulmonary arteriogram, although it is unclear whether the PE developed subsequent to the initial visit. Pulmonary angiography may not accurately diagnose very small (subsegmental) PEs owing to a high degree of variability across radiologists interpreting the examinations.[11]

Autopsy is another excellent criterion standard, although it should be noted that most pathologists and medical examiners do not perform meticulous microdissection of the lung vasculature to look for small, diffuse PE that may be the cause of death. In recent years, the criterion standard used in published studies of PE has shifted away from requiring absolute proof of the presence or absence of PE and toward the use of outcomes. Researchers have argued that, if the patient feels well several months after having PE excluded, it makes no difference whether the patient had PE, because the patient did not need treatment. This concept evokes debate and remains unresolved.

Electrocardiography

The electrocardiogram is not a particularly discriminating tool in the clinical evaluation of patients with suspected PE. Sinus tachycardia is frequent but presents in many of the considerations in the differential diagnosis. A "normal" electrocardiogram does not have sufficient sensitivity to effectively exclude PE. Its greatest value may be in consideration of the presence of acute coronary syndromes and in determining whether pulmonary hypertension is present.

Arterial Blood Gases and Pulse Oximetry

Most patients with PE have an arterial partial pressure of oxygen (Pa_{O_2}) less than 80 mm Hg when breathing room air, but up to 25 percent of patients with PE have a Pa_{O_2} >80 mm Hg; a few will have Pa_{O_2} greater than 95 mm Hg. Unless there is a concomitant respiratory acidosis (i.e., CO_2 retention), the A-a gradient will usually be widened. The overall sensitivity of an abnormal Pa_{O_2} or A-a gradient is approximately 90 percent.[12] However, many diseases in the differential diagnosis on PE are also associated with hypoxemia, and so the specificity of the widened A-a gradient is approximately 15 percent, thus limiting its diagnostic utility. Arterial blood gases, however, may help in risk stratification of patients with PE, because Pa_{O_2} appears to correlate with degree of pulmonary vascular occlusion from PE, and severe hypoxemia has been shown to predict poor outcome.[13] Pulse oximetry of 100 percent tends to favor the absence of PE, although it does not exclude it.

D-Dimer Testing

It is important to understand the type of D-dimer assay that is used in the hospital laboratory (see Chap. 59). For example, the diagnostic sensitivity of qualitative D-dimers is approximately 80 to 85 percent (including the erythrocyte agglutination assays and latex agglutination assays), whereas the sensitivity of quantitative D-dimers (including enzyme-linked immunosorbent assays and turbidimetric assays) is approximately 95 percent. Some facilities may not use the more rapidly available tests, thus reducing their value. Most published research has restricted the use of the D-dimer to patients with low pretest probability, although one recent study demonstrated excellent sensitivity (96 percent) and specificity, regardless of pretest probability.[14]

At least three factors contribute to the presence of PE in a low-risk patient with a normal D-dimer concentration. One is the formation of thrombus in the lung more than 72 h before the blood is assayed for the D-dimer and no new clot forming in that interval. The circulating half-life of the D-dimer is less than 8 h, and patients with symptoms from PE of at least 3 days are more likely to have normal D-dimer concentration.[15] Another reason for the diagnosis of PE in a low-risk patient with a normal D-dimer is the presence of subsegmental PE.[16] Moreover, some diagnoses of PE in the presence of normal D-dimer concentrations result from false-positive confirmatory testing. Extensive work by Wells and colleagues has documented the safety of using the combination of a low pretest probability plus a normal qualitative D-dimer (simpliRED) to exclude PE.[7] Other investigators have suggested that the combination of a qualitative D-dimer plus a normal index of gas exchange, including a normal alveolar dead-space measurement or a normal calculated difference between arterial and alveolar partial pressures of oxygen, can exclude PE.[17] It is my opinion that, in the presence of a low pretest probability (using published systems or empiric assessment from an experienced clinician), a patient with a quantitative D-dimer concentration below 500 μg/L does not need to be anticoagulated.

Regardless of the test format or combination of factors used, the clinician must concede that any patient with a positive D-dimer must undergo further testing for PE. The D-dimer will be abnormally high in 75 percent of patients with normal pregnancy and more than 50 percent of patients with active malignancy, postpartum status within 1 week, surgery within the past week, or age older than 80 years. In general, any disease or process that causes increased fibrin deposition or decreased D-dimer clearance can elevate circulatory D-dimer concentration. These conditions include sepsis, hemorrhage, myocardial infarction, stroke, collagen vascular diseases, and liver impairment. Some clinicians argue that D-dimer determination is a waste of time in these patients.

Chest Radiographs

The literature is quite conflicting with regard to the value and findings of plain chest radiographs in ED patients with proven PE and suspected PE, because of patient selection bias. Many of the studies are restricted to inpatients with proven PE. **A normal chest x-ray may be present in fewer than 25 percent.** In the largest sample, cardiomegaly was the most frequent abnormality (27 percent) among those with PE, but most of the patients were inpatients. In the outpatient setting, basilar atelectasis carries the most discriminative value. Because of conflicting findings, the greatest value in plain film chest radiographs is in consideration of the differential diagnosis.

Ventilation-Perfusion Lung Scanning

At present, the ventilation-perfusion ($\dot{V}/\dot{Q}$) scan is a common modality used to image the lungs for PE. The reason it is still used stems primarily from the data afforded by the multicenter study sponsored by the National Institutes of Health, known as PIOPED.[18] The PIOPED study performed $\dot{V}/\dot{Q}$ scanning and pulmonary angiography in 755 patients, 30 percent of whom were enrolled from the ED or a clinic. The PIOPED study plus a massive body of published literature and widespread clinical use over the past three decades have established the normal $\dot{V}/\dot{Q}$ scan as a strong technique to exclude the presence of PE. A *normal $\dot{V}/\dot{Q}$ scan reading* refers to the homogeneous appearance of scintillation activity in the lungs after injection of a radiolabeled material into a peripheral vein, and is also referred to as a *normal perfusion lung scan* (although the scan does not measure lung blood flow or tissue perfusion). A $\dot{V}/\dot{Q}$ scan can be read as normal in the absence of

a ventilation phase. A patient with a normal $\dot{V}/\dot{Q}$ scan has such a low risk of PE that the disease can be effectively excluded, even in the presence of a high pretest probability. As a caveat, up to 4 percent of patients with normal $\dot{V}/\dot{Q}$ scans and suspected PE have confirmed deep vein thrombosis (DVT).[19] Conversely, a high probability reading (Figure 56-2), for all practical purposes, confirms the diagnosis of PE, although, in the presence of a low pretest probability, about one half of patients with a high probability $\dot{V}/\dot{Q}$ scan have a pulmonary angiogram that is negative for PE.

In the ED, about one third of patients who undergo $\dot{V}/\dot{Q}$ scanning have a normal reading and another 10 percent have a high-probability reading, leaving the majority of scans in a gray area, sometimes referred to as the *nondiagnostic category*. At many centers in the Unites States, this category is further broken down into low, moderate, and indeterminate categories (Table 56-3). There is no consensus regarding the lower limit of probability after which further pursuit of the diagnosis is no longer indicated. Each of these $\dot{V}/\dot{Q}$ scan readings must be considered in the context of the patient's pretest probability.

Patients with a low (<10 percent) pretest probability and a low probability $\dot{V}/\dot{Q}$ scan have an approximately 2 percent probability of PE, so many clinicians do not perform further testing with this combination. Patients with a greater than 10 percent pretest probability and a low probability $\dot{V}/\dot{Q}$ scan or any patient with a moderate probability or indeterminate probability $\dot{V}/\dot{Q}$ scan should undergo further testing. One published method is to order a quantitative D-dimer (if the test has not already been done) and use a level below 500 μg/L as evidence to exclude PE.[20] Another option is to exclude the presence of a DVT in the legs by ordering a lower extremity ultrasound. However, if the leg ultrasound is negative for DVT, this finding only confers a marginal reduction in the probability of PE.[21] Most authorities recommend that patients in this category receive a follow-up ultrasound in 3 to 7 days. If the follow-up ultrasound is negative, the added value of performing a third ultrasound is minimal. In the presence of a high pretest probability of PE (>60 percent) and any nondiagnostic $\dot{V}/\dot{Q}$ scan, the patient should undergo another lung imaging test. At some centers, the next step is a formal pulmonary angiography. Other centers use contrast-enhanced helical computed tomography (CT) of the chest as the follow-up to a nondiagnostic $\dot{V}/\dot{Q}$ scan. Ventilation-perfusion scanning is not possible in patients without peripheral venous access and among those who are unable to breathe in aerosolized labeled particles or hold still for imaging.

Computed Tomography

In the past decade, contrast-enhanced helical CT angiogram of the chest has become accepted in some centers as the diagnostic modality of choice for PE. As with many aspects of PE, the diagnostic value of CT angiogram remains controversial and varies from hospital to hospital. The emergency physician should be aware of several technical aspects of the CT angiogram. The CT angiogram requires an intra-

TABLE 56-3   Definition of $\dot{V}/\dot{Q}$ Scan Probabilities

$\dot{V}/\dot{Q}$ Scan Category	Definition
High probability (>80%)	Two or more large mismatched segments or the equivalent
Intermediate probability (20–79%)	One moderate to two large mismatched segments
Low probability (<20%)	Nonsegmental perfusion defects, matched defects
Normal	No perfusion defects

Source: Adapted with permission from Sostman HD, Coleman RE, DeLong DM, et al: Evaluation of revised criteria for ventilation-perfusion scintigraphy in patients with suspected pulmonary embolism. *Radiology* 193:103, 1994.

venous catheter, preferably 20 gauge or larger, into which approximately 150 mL of radio-opaque contrast is injected. Some radiologists are reluctant to administer contrast via a central line. This may be a concern for a 16-gauge Peripherally Inserted Central Catheter (PICC) line but not for a triple-lumen or 7.5-French or larger central line catheter. A timing run with a test dose of 10 mL of contrast would allow determination for the time frame of image acquisition and central line usage. Patients with massive obesity or congestive heart failure can be difficult to image, because the contrast may not opacify the pulmonary arterial tree well. The CT angiogram requires the patient to lie supine with the arms over the head and to breath-hold for about 5 to 10 s. The images are obtained in approximately 3-mm slices from the diaphragm to the apex of the lung. Some centers employ the so-called indirect venography phase by then obtaining 3-cm cuts from the popliteal fossae through the pelvis to image the leg and pelvic veins for DVT. The equipment used to collect and reconstruct the images remains a key issue in the diagnostic accuracy of the CT angiogram.

Although published studies indicate that radiologists' experience has little bearing on their ability to interpret CT angiography, my experience suggests otherwise. Many radiologists believe that the images should be interpreted on the computer screen rather than on the cut films. With the latest generation 16-head multichannel helical (or spiral) ultrafast CT machines (e.g., GE Light Speed QX/I), images can be reconstructed to produce resolution of approximately 2 mm, which is smaller than the purported level of resolution of the pulmonary angiogram. Publications report that radiologists interpret the CT angiogram as positive or negative for PE, although in practice at least 10 percent of scans are read as indeterminate owing to motion artifact or poor vascular opacification. In earlier studies, when the CT angiogram was compared with pulmonary angiography, the aggregated sensitivity of the CT angiogram was approximately 80 percent and the specificity was 85 percent.[12] The major source of false-negative interpretation was the presence of small PEs in subsegmental pulmonary arteries, which could not be imaged with earlier generation CT scans. To my knowledge, the results of CT angiogram have not been compared with autopsy findings. However, several studies demonstrate a 2 percent or lower rate of PE discovered on follow-up after negative CT angiography, although it is unclear if these occurred subsequent to the index study. However, Perrier and associates demonstrated that the rate of PE discovered on follow-up after a negative CT angiogram in ED patients with a positive D-dimer is less than 5 percent.[22]

The sensitivity of the CT angiogram may be significantly improved with the addition of the indirect venography phase. In two U.S. EDs, Richman and colleagues demonstrated that the addition of the indirect venography phase to the imaging protocol detects DVT in the absence of a visible PE in 2 percent of all ED patients imaged.[23] Thus, if the presence of DVT in a patient with symptoms or signs of PE is considered tantamount to the diagnosis of PE (at least in terms of initiating treatment), the indirect venography phase confers an additional 17 percent sensitivity to CT angiography. At present, the authors of the original PIOPED study are completing the PIOPED II study to examine the diagnostic sensitivity and specificity of CT angiography (with indirect venography) for PE.

One of the great advantages of the CT angiogram for ED evaluation is its ability to provide information about the presence of other life-threatening thoracic processes. In one series of more than 1000 ED patients, 7 percent of scans had a non-PE finding that warranted immediate attention and another 10 percent required specific action of follow-up. In many cases, the alternative finding can explain the patient's symptoms.[24]

Several issues influence the diagnostic accuracy of the CT angiogram (Table 56-4). I recommend using the CT angiogram as the procedure of choice if the systems issues and patient issues are favorable. The CT angiogram may also be the test of choice in patients with a chest radiograph that shows a parenchymal infiltrate, for the patient with known emphysema, or a prior nondiagnostic $\dot{V}/\dot{Q}$ scan.

TABLE 56-4 Factors That Affect the Diagnostic Accuracy of Computed Tomography for PE

Systems issues that improve test accuracy
The radiologist has adequate training and comfort in interpreting the images
The hospital has a multichannel helical CT scanner
The radiology technicians have a protocol in place to perform the contrast injection
The indirect venography phase is employed

Individual patient issues that improve test accuracy
The patient has adequate IV access and can tolerate 150 mL of contrast
The patient can hold his or her breath and lie supine with the arms over the head
The patient does not have massive obesity, congestive heart failure, or shock

Factors responsible for false-negative interpretations
Inadequate contrast opacification of the pulmonary vasculature
Inadequate CT scanning equipment to image small vessels
Failure to use reconstructed images
Failure to use the indirect venography phase

Factors responsible for false-positive interpretations
Motion artifact
Interpretation of a filling defect observed in one image as positive for PE
Interpreting a vein or bronchus as an artery with a filling defect
Extrinsic vascular compression from neoplasm or adenopathy

Abbreviations: CT = computed tomography; PE = pulmonary embolism.

TREATMENT

The objectives in treating PE are to eliminate the clot burden and prevent recurrent thrombosis. In most cases, this can be safely accomplished with the combination of heparin (which by itself has little effect on clot burden already present) anticoagulation plus warfarin anticoagulation. Heparin offers several salutary effects. The most important immediate effect of heparin is the initiation of immediate thrombin inhibition, thus preventing thrombus extension. Although heparin has no intrinsic fibrinolytic capacity, by allowing unopposed action of plasmin, it does accelerate clot removal over 48 to 72 h. Heparin also affords a prominent antiplatelet effect, which helps prevent thrombus reoccurrence and reduces the elaboration of vasoconstrictive chemicals from platelets. Heparin also may inhibit inflammatory processes that contribute to vascular remodeling after PE. Heparin also helps to counteract the transient hypercoagulable state caused by a relative deficiency in protein C in the first days of warfarin therapy. Unfractionated or fractionated heparin will yield good results with a low incidence of serious hemorrhage. Table 56-5 shows the doses of heparin regimens approved by the U.S. Food and Drug Administration.

TABLE 56-5 Regimens Approved by the Food and Drug Administration for the Acute Treatment of Pulmonary Embolism

Drug	Dosage
Unfractionated heparin	80 units/kg bolus IV, then 18 units/kg per h to maintain partial thromboplastin time, INR = 2.5–3.0
Fractionated heparin	
Enoxaparin	1 mg/kg SC BID
Fibrinolytic therapy	
Streptokinase	250,000 units IV over 30 min followed by 100,000 units/h for 24 h
Urokinase	4400 units/kg IV over 10 min followed by 4000 units/kg per h for 12 h
Alteplase	15-mg IV bolus followed by 2-h infusion of 85 mg; discontinue heparin during infusion

Abbreviation: INR = international normalized ratio.

There are very few "absolute contraindications" to anticoagulation in a patient with diagnosed PE. Examples include a recent intraparenchymal brain hemorrhage and active gastrointestinal hemorrhage. Recent abdominal, orthopedic, or gynecologic surgery or even neurosurgery should not be considered absolute contraindications to heparin anticoagulation. Metastatic disease per se, including brain metastases, is also not a contraindication unless the lesions are hemorrhagic.

Emergency physicians have the ability to assess the risks of a patient with PE to decide when to treat with therapy more aggressive than heparin anticoagulation. Low arterial blood pressure offers a specific but nonsensitive indicator of the presence of severe PE. Even the authorities who are skeptical of the importance of fibrinolytic therapy believe that a patient with confirmed PE, a sustained systolic blood pressure less than 100 mm Hg, and no contraindications should be administered fibrinolytic therapy.[25] The contraindications to fibrinolysis are the same as those for acute myocardial infarction (see Chap. 51). The Food and Drug Administration has approved three fibrinolytic agents for treatment of PE: streptokinase, urokinase, and alteplase. The approved infusion protocol for alteplase is the same as for the treatment of myocardial infarction, and **heparin should be discontinued only while the fibrinolytic drug is being infused.** In the setting of PE with severe hypotension (systolic blood pressure <80 mm Hg), a bolus injection of alteplase may afford more rapid fibrinolysis with no increased risk of hemorrhage. Systemic infusion is adequate, as intrapulmonary infusion of fibrinolytic therapy does not appear to afford more rapid reduction in clot burden or improve outcome.

In patients with PE, sustained hypotension, and a contraindication to fibrinolytic therapy, the use of catheter fragmentation remains the best option to reduce clot burden at hospitals that have this capacity. In the hands of an experienced thoracic surgeon, surgical thrombectomy can be a lifesaving procedure for patients with large PE and hypotension (with or without a contraindication to thrombolytic therapy). One advantage of surgical thrombectomy is that the patient is placed on right atrial and left atrial or veno-arterial bypass, which effectively bypasses the obstructed pulmonary vasculature to ensure adequate perfusion of vital organs while the clot is removed from the pulmonary vasculature.

The decision-making process becomes more subtle in patients with PE and normal or nearly normal blood pressure. The major question remains as how to accurately and quickly recognize the patient with submassive, "nonhypotensive" PE that is going to cause trouble in the short term. Data are available from a convenience sample of 207 normotensive ED patients diagnosed with PE and treated with heparin at seven urban academic EDs in the United States from 1995 to 1999. An unexpected 4 percent of these initially "stable" patients with PE died within 24 h after diagnosis.

Of all risk-stratification modalities, the largest body of evidence has been published for the use of transthoracic echocardiography to visualize the presence of a dilated, hypokinetic RV as a marker of occult hemodynamic instability. Prospective studies[26] and large registries[27] have demonstrated that fewer than 10 percent of patients with PE and normal RV size and function die or develop respiratory failure or circulatory shock during hospitalization. However, the specificity of RV dilation or hypokinesis is about 40 percent, because many patients with RV dilation with PE have no in-hospital complications with heparin treatment. Clearly, the presence of RV dilation or hypokinesis indicates risk of a bad outcome, but whether this risk rises to a level that warrants the increased risk of serious bleeding that is associated with fibrinolytic therapy remains a source of research. I believe that RV dilation or hypokinesis should not be used in isolation as the sole reason to administer fibrinolytics. Moreover, a normal echocardiogram, an inadequate acoustic window, or unavailability of echocardiography should not be used to challenge the decision to administer fibrinolytic therapy to a patient with an otherwise overwhelming clinical picture of severe PE. Table 56-6 outlines other clinical factors that can be used to

TABLE 56-6   Factors That Can Help Prognose the Short-Term Outcome of Normotensive Patients with Pulmonary Embolism

Good Outcome Likely	Adverse Outcome More Likely
No syncope or seizure at presentation	Syncope or seizure with respiratory distress at presentation
Age <50 y	Age >70 y
Absence of COPD, CHF, or prior PE	Presence of COPD, CHF, or prior PE
<50% pulmonary vascular occlusion	>50% pulmonary vascular occlusion; floating thrombus in the RV or right atrium observed on echocardiography or CT angiography
Normal ECG	ECG with T-wave inversion in V_1–V_4 and a new incomplete right bundle branch block
Heart rate/systolic blood pressure <0.8	Heart rate/systolic blood pressure >1.0
Pulse oximetry reading >94% breathing room air	Pulse oximetry reading <94% breathing room air
Troponin I concentration <0.4 μg/L	Troponin I concentration >1.0 μg/L
Normal RV function and size	RV dilation or hypokinesis, or an estimated RV systolic pressure >40 mm Hg

Abbreviations: CHF = congestive heart failure; COPD = chronic obstructive pulmonary disease; CT = computed tomography; ECG = electrocardiogram; PE = pulmonary embolism; RV = right ventricle.
Sources: Thames MD, Alpert JS, Dalen JE: Syncope in patients with pulmonary embolism. *JAMA* 238:2509, 1997; Daniel KR, Courtney DM, Kline JA: Assessment of cardiac stress from massive pulmonary embolism with 12-lead electrocardiography. *Chest* 120:474, 2001; Courtney DM, Kline JA: Identification of clinical factors associated with outpatient massive pulmonary embolism. *Acad Emerg Med* 8:1136, 2001; Konstantinides S, Geibel A, Olschewski M, et al: Importance of cardiac troponins I and T in risk stratification of patients with acute pulmonary embolism. *Circulation* 106:1263, 2002; and Goldhaber SZ, Visani L, De Rosa M; Acute pulmonary embolism: Clinical outcomes in the international cooperative pulmonary embolism registry (ICOPER). *Lancet* 353:1386, 1999.

prognose the severity of PE. Many of these factors are readily ascertained at the bedside. These factors can be used in conjunction with or instead of echocardiography (when the procedure is not available) to help decide when heparin treatment is not enough.

Recent work indicated that normotensive patients who were randomized to receive alteplase plus heparin were less likely to have a worsening clinical course than were patients who received heparin only.[28] The major drawback to this non-blinded study was that most patients treated with heparin only who were then crossed over to receive alteplase experienced clinical deterioration defined as worsening dyspnea or respiratory distress that did not require intubation. Whether this represents a clinically important or patient-oriented outcome remains uncertain. **To date, no study has shown a survival benefit with thrombolytic therapy for the treatment of PE.**

SPECIAL CIRCUMSTANCES

Recurrent Visits

Many patients who are diagnosed with PE return to the ED with complaints that are perceived as similar to those of the first episode. The first objective is to determine whether the patient exhibits signs of cardiopulmonary stress. If the electrocardiogram, heart rate, and pulse oximetry readings are of no concern and a plain film chest radiograph is normal, the patient does not need to be treated empirically with heparin. The second objective is to determine whether the patient has a therapeutic prothrombin time.

Not every patient with an established diagnosis of PE who is therapeutic on warfarin necessarily needs to be imaged again. However, if the patient does not have a therapeutic prothrombin time (or admitted noncompliance) or has new symptoms or findings (tachycardia, new-onset hypoxemia, unilateral leg swelling, severe unexplained dyspnea, or hemoptysis), then pulmonary vascular imaging should be undertaken, even if the prothrombin time is therapeutic. An effort should be made to determine what imaging modality was used to diagnose the PE the first time and to order that same modality again. For patients with remote history of PE who are not currently being treated, the decision to embark on a diagnostic evaluation hinges on several points. History of PE without an underlying risk or a resolved risk is not associated with recurrence. The clinician is advised to look for other features, shown in Table 56-2, that suggest the presence of PE before testing. This can be an important point, because many patients with prior PE demonstrate abnormal $\dot{V}/\dot{Q}$ scans and difficult-to-interpret CT angiograms.

Massive Obesity

Patients who weigh more than 190 kg (400 lb) may be too large to fit into some CT scanners or to image with $\dot{V}/\dot{Q}$ scanning. Pulmonary angiography or magnetic resonance angiography are also usually not feasible. In most cases, venous ultrasonography can at best demonstrate poor images of the leg veins. One option is to look for alternative causes of disease and, when none is found and if the patient has no contraindications, to initiate empiric anticoagulation. A quantitative D-dimer assay may help in the decision to administer empiric anticoagulation. A D-dimer concentration less than 500 µg/L can be used as evidence to withhold anticoagulation, whereas a D-dimer concentration greater than 2000 µg/L can be used as evidence of thrombosis when PE is suspected and imaging is impossible. No evidence has been published to support this recommendation, and no study has determined the correct dose of enoxaparin to administer to massively obese patients, but some authorities recommend a ceiling dose of 250 mg per d.

Pregnancy

The ED physician who orders an imaging test on a pregnant patient should be certain to involve the patient, the obstetrician, and the radiologist in the decision-making process. Many centers employ half-dose injection of radioactive material to perform a perfusion lung scan. Filling the bladder with fluid using a urinary drainage catheter and intravenous hydration may help reduce fetal exposure to ionizing radiation. If the perfusion scan is homogeneous, no further testing is necessary. Alternatively, a CT angiogram without indirect venography can be performed and the uterus shielded during image acquisition, which may induce less fetal radiation than $\dot{V}/\dot{Q}$ scanning. A D-dimer concentration can be ordered to help select which pregnant patient needs imaging, but the D-dimer is almost always elevated with normal pregnancy. Published studies have indicated that the upper limit of a normal D-dimer increases with each trimester of pregnancy but should not exceed 1000 µg/L at any time.[29]

Another approach is to order Doppler ultrasound of the lower extremities, because this is noninvasive and carries no ionizing radiation risk. If DVT is present, then treatment decisions are the same as those for PE. The risk of this approach is the potential to terminate the further pursuit of the diagnosis simply because the ultrasound was negative.

When to Start Heparin Before Imaging

This question frequently arises. Studies that have measured perfusion defect and pulmonary vascular resistance have indicated that heparin confers little reduction in clot burden during the first 6 h. Whether any observed reduction would occur with time alone remains unknown. However, imaging can take 3 to 4 h to complete, and in vitro studies have shown that clot volume can grow up to 50 percent in this interval. Thus, in the absence of a contraindication and **with a pretest probability that exceeds 50 percent, empiric heparin should be administered.** I believe that all hypotensive patients and all normotensive patients with hypoxemia (pulse oximetry reading <95 percent breathing room air) or tachycardia out of proportion to the systolic blood pressure (i.e., a shock index of heart rate/systolic blood pressure >1.0) should receive heparin before imaging.

When to Draw Blood for Hypercoagulability Workup

Measurement of protein C, antithrombin III, or protein S before heparin therapy can be helpful for the diagnosis of a hypercoagulable state. Extra tubes can be drawn for these analyses. The most important factors to measure are the common genomic mutations factor V Leiden and the prothrombin mutation G20210A (assayed by polymerase chain reaction, which is unaffected by heparin or the presence of thrombosis); the antiphospholipid antibodies, including anticardiolipin antibodies (immunoglobulins M, G, and A); and lupus anticoagulant levels. The latter two protein classes can be spuriously elevated in the presence of thrombosis. Similarly, the antigenic and functional levels of proteins C and S and antithrombin can be spuriously decreased with thrombosis. Accordingly, any declaration of excess or deficiency of these proteins should be based on measurements made during follow-up, when radiographic evidence has confirmed the dissolution of clot in the lungs and legs.

Septic Emboli

The approach to septic emboli is somewhat different (see Chap. 145). The mainstay of treatment is early administration of antibiotics. If based on ultrasound, valvular vegetation is huge, or there is significant valvular damage, immediate anticoagulation seems warranted.

Witnessed Cardiac Arrest

Occasionally, the patient with known PE or who is in transit to or from an imaging procedure for PE sustains cardiac arrest that is managed by the ED. The primary treatment for cardiac arrest for PE is cardiopulmonary resuscitation and standard advanced cardiac life support (ACLS) procedures. If no pulse returns within a few minutes, the next step is to bolus inject 100 mg of alteplase or an equivalent dose of fibrinolytic therapy while cardiopulmonary resuscitation is continued for at least 20 min. If the pulse returns in a young patient who has had an imaging procedure to identify the location of the thrombus in the pulmonary vasculature, the next step is to contact a thoracic surgeon to arrange for surgical thrombectomy. Prior administration of fibrinolytic therapy should not be considered a contraindication to surgery after cardiac arrest.

REFERENCES

1. Pineda LA, Hathwar VS, Grant BJB: Clinical suspicion of fatal pulmonary embolism. *Chest* 120:791, 2001.
2. Lane DA, Mannucci PM, Bauer KA, et al: Inherited thrombophilia: Part 1 [review]. *Thromb Haemost* 76:651, 1996.
3. Murin S, Marelich GP, Arroliga AC, Matthay RA: Hereditary thrombophilia and venous thromboembolism [review]. *Am J Resp Crit Care Med* 158:1369, 1998.
4. Courtney DM, Sasser H, Pincus B, Kline JA: Pulseless electrical activity with witnessed arrest as a predictor of sudden death from massive pulmonary embolism in outpatients. *Resuscitation* 49:265, 2001.
5. Kline JA, Nelson RD, Jackson RE, Courtney DM: Criteria for the safe use of D-dimer testing in emergency department patients with suspected pulmonary embolism: A multicenter United States study. *Ann Emerg Med* 39:144, 2002.

6. Susec O, Boudrow D, Kline J: The clinical features of acute pulmonary embolism in ambulatory patients. *Acad Emerg Med* 4:891, 1997.

7. Wells PS, Anderson DR, Rodger M, et al: Excluding pulmonary embolism at the bedside without diagnostic imaging: Management of patients with suspected pulmonary embolism presenting to the emergency department by using a simple clinical model and D-dimer. *Ann Intern Med* 135:98, 2001.

8. Rosen M, Sands D, Morris J, et al: Does a physician's ability to accurately assess the likelihood of pulmonary embolism increase with training? *Acad Med* 75:1199, 2000.

9. Sanson BJ, Lijmer JG, MacGillavry MR, et al: Comparison of a clinical probability estimate and two clinical models in patients with suspected pulmonary embolism. *Thromb Haemost* 83:199, 2000.

10. Chagnon I, Bounameaux H, Aujesky D, et al: Comparison of two clinical prediction rules and implicit assessment among patients with suspected pulmonary embolism [see comments]. *Am J Med* 113:269, 2002.

11. Stein PD, Henry JW, Gottschalk A: Reassessment of pulmonary angiography for the diagnosis of pulmonary embolism: Relation of interpreter agreement to the order of the involved pulmonary arterial branch. *Radiology* 210:689, 1999.

12. Kline JA, Johns KL, Coluciello SA, Israel EG: New diagnostic tests for pulmonary embolism. *Ann Emerg Med* 35:168, 2000.

13. Kline JA, Hernandez-Nino J, Newgard CD, et al: Use of pulse oximetry to predict in-hospital complications in normotensive patients with pulmonary embolism. *Am J Med.* In press 2003.

14. Dunn KL, Wolf JP, Dorfman DM, Fitzpatrick P: Normal D-dimer levels in emergency department patients suspected of acute pulmonary embolism. *J Am Coll Cardiol* 40:1475, 2002.

15. Brown MD, Rowe BH, Reeves MJ, et al: The accuracy of the enzyme-linked immunoabsorbent assay D-dimer test in the diagnosis of pulmonary embolism: A meta-analysis. *Ann Emerg Med* 40:133, 2002.

16. De Monye W, Sanson BJ, Mac GM, et al: Embolus location affects the sensitivity of a rapid quantitative D-dimer assay in the diagnosis of pulmonary embolism. *Am J Resp Crit Care Med* 165:345, 2002.

17. Kline JA, Israel EG, O'Neil BJ, et al: Diagnostic accuracy of a bedside D-dimer assay and alveolar dead-space measurement for rapid exclusion of pulmonary embolism: A multicenter study. *JAMA* 285:761, 2001.

18. PIOPED Investigators: Value of the ventilation/perfusion scan in acute pulmonary embolism. *JAMA* 263:2753, 1990.

19. van Rossum AB, van Houwelingen HC, Kieft GJ, Pattynama PM: Prevalence of deep vein thrombosis in suspected and proven pulmonary embolism: A meta-analysis. *Br J Radiol* 71:1260, 1998.

20. Perrier A, Desmarais S, Miron M-J, et al: Non-invasive diagnosis of venous thromboembolism in outpatients. *Lancet* 353:190, 1999.

21. Daniel KR, Jackson RE, Kline JA: Utility of the lower extremity venous ultrasound in the diagnosis and exclusion of pulmonary embolism in outpatients. *Ann Emerg Med* 35:547, 2000.

22. Perrier A, Howarth N, Didler D, et al: Performance of helical computed tomography in unselected outpatients with suspected pulmonary embolism. *Ann Intern Med* 135:88, 2001.

23. Richman PB, Wood J, Kasper DM, et al: Contribution of indirect computed tomography venography to computed tomography angiography of the chest for the diagnosis of thromboembolic disease in two United States emergency departments. *J Thromb Haemost* 1:652, 2003.

24. Richman PB, Courtney DM, Wood J, et al: Chest CT angiography (CTA) to rule out pulmonary embolism (PE) frequently reveals clinically significant ancillary findings—A multi-center study of 1025 emergency department patients. *Acad Emerg Med* 10:564, 2003.

25. Dalen JE, Alpert JS, Hirsch J: Thrombolytic therapy for pulmonary embolism: Is it effective? Is it safe? When is it indicated? [review; see comments]. *Arch Intern Med* 157:2550, 1997.

26. Grifoni S, Olivotto I, Cecchini P, et al: Short-term clinical outcome of patients with acute pulmonary embolism, normal blood pressure, and echocardiographic right ventricular dysfunction. *Circulation* 101:2817, 2000.

27. Kasper W, Konstantinides S, Geibel A, et al: Management strategies and determinants of outcome in acute major pulmonary embolism: Results of a multicenter registry. *J Am Coll Cardiol* 30:1165, 1997.

28. Konstantinides S, Geibel A, Heusel G, et al: Heparin plus alteplase compared with heparin alone in patients with submassive pulmonary embolism. *New Engl J Med* 347:1143, 2002.

29. Giavarina D, Mezzena G, Dorizzi RM, Soffiati G: Reference interval of D-dimer in pregnant women. *Clin Biochem* 34:331, 2001.

HYPERTENSION

Melissa M. Wu

Arjun Chanmugam

Hypertension is considered one of the most important modifiable risk factors for cardiovascular disease and is the fourth most prevalent chronic medical condition in the United States.[1] Up to 24 percent of the United States general adult population and 32 percent of African Americans may be affected.[2]

Overall morbidity and mortality rates, and in particular the risk of developing serious cardiovascular, renal, or cerebrovascular disease, increase with poorly controlled blood pressure. Although the public has become more knowledgeable, only two-thirds of Americans with high blood pressure are aware of their diagnosis. Of greater concern is that nearly 75 percent of adult Americans with hypertension are not controlling their blood pressure to below 140/90 mm Hg, and only half are taking their prescription medications as directed.[1,2] In addition, there are a significant number of patients who are under the care of a physician, but either have undiagnosed hypertension or hypertension that is uncontrolled.

Poorly controlled hypertension may become an increasingly common problem in the United States as the demographic makeup of the country changes. The pattern of elevation in systolic blood pressure (SBP) with diastolic blood pressure (DBP) <90 mm Hg predominates not only in the elderly, but also in the middle aged. The lack of control is not confined to the poor, uninsured, or minorities.

The primary responsibilities of emergency physicians in the approach to hypertensive patients are to recognize and treat true emergencies, to manage the complications of chronic disease, and to arrange the most appropriate follow-up for nonemergent cases.

CLASSIFICATION

The Joint National Committee on Prevention, Detection, Evaluation, and Treatment of High Blood Pressure developed a consensus definition of hypertension, which includes a graded classification dependent on risk factors and clinical condition (Table 57-1).[1] In general, either a SBP greater than 140 mm Hg or a DBP greater than 90 mm Hg constitutes hypertension. However, management of hypertension depends more on the individual's clinical condition rather than the absolute systolic or diastolic values. The ED approach is based on four general categories.

Hypertensive Emergency

Hypertensive emergencies, the most serious of these, occur in about 1 percent of all hypertensive patients. *Malignant hypertension* or *hypertensive crisis* have also been used to refer to this category. Target-

TABLE 57-1 Classification of Blood Pressure for Adults Aged 18 Years and Older

Category	Systolic Blood Pressure (mm Hg)	Diastolic Blood Pressure (mm Hg)
Optimal	<120	<80
Normal	<130	<85
High-normal	130–139	85–89
Hypertension		
Stage 1	140–159	90–99
Stage 2	160–179	100–109
Stage 3	≥180	≥110

Note: When systolic and diastolic pressures fall into different categories, the higher category should be used to classify the individual's blood pressure status.
Source: From JNC,[1] with permission.

organ damage is evident when conditions such as hypertensive encephalopathy (see below), intracranial hemorrhage, acute left ventricular failure with pulmonary edema, unstable angina pectoris, acute myocardial infarction, dissecting aortic aneurysm, (worsening) renal failure, and eclampsia exist.[1] A hypertensive emergency is not defined by any absolute pressure measurements. Instead, it is contingent on the presence of relative blood pressure increases combined with evidence of injury to any of the so-called target organs. In fact, a patient with a low baseline pressure can present with "normal" or mildly elevated pressure and be considered to have a true hypertensive emergency, if there is evidence of concurrent related central nervous system (CNS), cardiovascular, or renal dysfunction.

Hypertensive Urgency

Hypertensive urgency is less clearly defined. Most sources concur that hypertensive urgency represents a risk for imminent target-organ damage, although acute organ injury has not yet occurred. In many cases of hypertensive urgency, the presence of preexisting conditions (e.g., renal insufficiency, congestive heart failure, coronary artery disease, CNS disorders, or retinal changes) increases the likelihood of target-organ damage. Again, relative increases in blood pressure are more important than absolute values.

The main challenge for the clinician is differentiating asymptomatic hypertension from a hypertensive urgency. If target-organ dysfunction is not evident, the clinician must judge whether significant risk of such damage is impending without timely intervention. Unfortunately, no evidence-based data exist to guide the practitioner in this regard. If target-organ dysfunction is shown, it must be determined whether this represents chronic disease or an acute deterioration or process. If the latter is the case, then a hypertensive emergency exists. This may be difficult without knowledge of the patient's past medical history, including prior laboratory values and clinical findings. In many cases, the clinician may be obligated to initiate antihypertensive treatment without being certain of the diagnostic classification.

Acute Hypertensive Episode

Acute hypertensive (nonemergency/nonurgency) episode occurs when a patient is found to have stage 3 hypertension (see Table 57-1; systolic pressure of 180 mm Hg or more, and diastolic pressure of 110 mm Hg or more) with no signs or symptoms of evolving or impending target-organ damage.[1] Although many of these patients receive treatment in an effort to prevent target-organ damage, there is some controversy regarding the need for immediate treatment (see below).

Transient Hypertension

Transient hypertension occurs in association with other conditions such as anxiety, alcohol-withdrawal syndromes, sudden cessation of medications, and some toxicologic substances. Treatment is aimed at the underlying cause. One specific type of transient hypertension is "*white-coat hypertension*,"[4] a phenomenon that occurs when a patient has an elevated blood pressure in a clinical setting but has a normal pressure at other times. Such patients are normotensive when followed over a 24-h period with ambulatory blood pressure monitoring. A number of studies have shown that at least 20 percent of newly diagnosed hypertensive individuals are actually normotensive in their regular environment.[4] The cardiovascular morbidity and mortality rates of individuals with white-coat hypertension correlate with their ambulatory blood pressure. Therefore, a single encounter in the ED setting should not be the basis for diagnosis of new-onset hypertension, nor does it constitute an indication to initiate antihypertensive therapy. However, patients do require prompt and close follow-up care for repeat blood pressure testing.

PATHOPHYSIOLOGY

Systemic blood pressure is related to vascular smooth muscle tone. At the cellular level, postsynaptic α_1 and α_2 receptors are stimulated by norepinephrine released from the presynaptic sympathetic nerve ending, ultimately leading to the release of intracellular calcium stores. Calcium release results in smooth muscle contraction via activation of actin and myosin. The increase in smooth muscle tone results in increased peripheral vascular resistance, thereby causing increased blood pressure. When stimulated by norepinephrine, the presynaptic α_2 receptors help to limit this response by preventing further release of norepinephrine through a negative-feedback loop.

There are two major theories to explain how hypertension develops: (1) as a result of alterations in the contractile properties of smooth muscle in arterial walls, and (2) as a response to failure of normal autoregulatory mechanisms. Most individuals with hypertension have elevated peripheral vascular resistance with normal cardiac output. However, some patients may also have elevated cardiac output as a result of increased α-adrenergic and β-adrenergic tone.

The concept of autoregulation is important in the vascular beds of the vital organs, including the heart, kidneys, and brain, but has been most extensively studied in the latter.[5] In the brain, as blood pressure falls, cerebral vasodilation occurs. When blood pressure rises, the autoregulatory response is vasoconstriction, ensuring a stable cerebral blood flow rate across a range of blood pressures. However, autoregulation is effective only within a specific range of blood pressures. Most authorities specify a range of 50 to 150 mm Hg for MAP, within which there is effective autoregulation in the uninjured brain. At pressures beyond this narrow range, the limits of autoregulation are breached, and hypoperfusion or hyperperfusion results. In patients with chronically elevated blood pressure, the narrow range at which autoregulation functions is shifted higher. Thus chronically hypertensive patients can develop symptoms of brain hypoperfusion if their blood pressure is lowered to "normal" levels, because normal levels may be below the limits of the individual's adjusted autoregulation. The lower limit of cerebral autoregulation is generally about 25 percent below a patient's baseline MAP.[5]

When poorly controlled blood pressure is allowed to persist over time, it can cause damage to specific organs and vascular beds. The pathologic change responsible for target-organ damage is fibrinoid necrosis of small arterioles. This process begins when vessels in capillary beds dilate in response to an elevated blood pressure that overwhelms the autoregulatory mechanism. The persistently elevated pressures cause injury to the endothelium, leading to increased vascular permeability and vascular wall injury. Eventually, endothelial damage leads to deposition of fibrin within the vessel walls and causes activation of mediators of coagulation and cell proliferation. A recurrent cycle of vascular reactivity develops, with an increased release of vasoconstrictors, endothelial damage, platelet aggregation, myointimal proliferation, and progressive narrowing of arterioles.

A directly observable example of the vascular changes is *hypertensive retinopathy*. Hypertensive retinopathy is traditionally graded into four categories. In grade I, there is minimal diffuse or focal narrowing of arterioles. In grade II, "copper" and "silver" wiring (increased light reflex) is seen. These are considered relatively mild target-organ effects. In grade III and IV retinopathy, cotton-wool spots (focal ischemia), hard exudates and hemorrhages (vessel leakage), and extensive microvascular changes are seen. Grade IV retinopathy is distinguished by disk edema and in the past has been used to define malignant hypertension or hypertensive crisis. (The term *papilledema* is frequently used, but the disk edema is due to infarction and hypoxia of the optic disk. Thus the term papilledema is best reserved for disk edema associated with elevated cerebrospinal fluid pressure.) Grade I and grade II retinopathy are evidence of chronic hypertension. Grades III and IV are evidence of accelerated retinopathy, particularly in the young. Also grade III and IV changes might not be seen in the elderly. The mechanism of underlying pathology—arteriolar spasm—ultimately leads to degeneration of the muscle of the blood vessel, with subsequent degeneration of the endothelial cells of the vessel lumen. The elderly, who are likely to have arteriosclerotic vessels, are paradoxically protected by the presence of this other underlying pathology.

In the brain, an abrupt, sustained rise in blood pressure exceeding the limits of cerebral autoregulation may be associated with stroke, intracerebral hemorrhage, or hypertensive encephalopathy.[5] Vascular injury caused by an abrupt or persistent elevation in blood pressure may result in ischemia or infarction in vulnerable regions of the brain. Intracerebral bleeding from dilated vessels may result in cerebral or subarachnoid hemorrhage. Hypertensive encephalopathy is characterized by marked vasospasm with ischemia, punctate hemorrhages, and increased vascular permeability, all leading to cerebral edema (a mechanism similar to retinopathy). This mechanism is different from localized cerebral edema in the area of ischemic stroke caused by emboli or thrombi. An increase in blood pressure may be a physiologic response to maintain adequate cerebral perfusion to areas distal to the occlusion and may not justify classification as a hypertensive emergency. Some researchers are even examining the benefit of induced hypertension as a potential treatment of acute stroke.

In the heart, increased afterload occurring after an acute rise in blood pressure results in increased left ventricular wall tension, that in turn increases myocardial oxygen demand. Angina or myocardial infarction occurs when hypertension causes a decrease in coronary blood flow relative to an increased demand. Pulmonary edema occurs when the sudden increase in MAP precipitates acute left ventricular failure, resulting in elevated end-diastolic pressure and filling volume.

In the kidneys, impaired autoregulation due to elevated blood pressure results in decreased renal perfusion. Decreased renal perfusion stimulates the renin-angiotensin (I and II) cascade, ultimately leading to increased vasoconstriction. If this cycle continues, arteriolar necrosis occurs, ultimately leading to renal impairment. Angiotensin II can exacerbate hypertension not only by causing vasoconstriction, but also by promoting sodium retention via direct stimulation of the proximal tubule and by secretion of aldosterone. Sodium retention induces hypertension in susceptible individuals by a variety of mechanisms, including (1) increased sympathetic nervous system activity; (2) decreased response to dopamine; (3) change in calcium and potassium metabolism; (4) resistance to insulin; and (5) inappropriate response of renal vasculature and adrenals to angiotensin II.[6]

Hypertension is associated with major cardiovascular risk factors such as smoking, hyperlipidemia, diabetes mellitus, age older than 60 years, gender (men and postmenopausal women), obesity, and a family history of cardiovascular disease.[1] In addition, dietary sodium excess in salt-sensitive individuals (50 percent of hypertensive patients) can induce hypertension. Although no single cause of hypertension has been identified, a combination of factors such as these are believed to contribute to elevated blood pressure.

Although most cases of hypertension are considered to be essential (i.e., hypertension with no known cause), several specific causes do exist. Of the known causes, renal disease is the most prevalent and includes renal arteriostenosis, fibromuscular disease of the renal arteries, chronic pyelonephritis, and nonspecific glomerulonephritis. Coarctation of the aorta, although uncommon, is also an important cause of secondary hypertension and should be suspected in any patient with the triad of upper extremity hypertension, a systolic murmur best heard over the back, and delayed femoral pulses. Another cause of hypertension is excessive glucocorticoids, seen in Cushing syndrome, but usually due to exogenous steroid therapy. Endogenous overproduction is less common but results from excessive adrenocorticotropic hormone (ACTH) production by a pituitary tumor, ectopic ACTH production by a nonpituitary tumor, or glucocorticoid production by tumors of the adrenal cortex.

Pheochromocytomas are tumors that produce catecholamines, and they arise from cells of the sympathetic nervous system (most commonly from the adrenal medulla) and account for fewer than 1 percent of cases of hypertension. The characteristic features of pheochromocytomas are paroxysms of hypertension associated with palpitations, tachycardia, malaise, apprehension, and sweating. Finally, ingestion of foods containing large amounts of tyramine can raise blood pressure by causing release of norepinephrine stored in nerve endings. This normally transient response may become prolonged in patients taking monoamine oxidase (MAO) inhibitors, since these agents block the enzyme that destroys tyramine.

CLINICAL EVALUATION

Overview

The clinical evaluation of hypertensive patients is aimed at determining the underlying reason for the hypertensive episode and ascertaining the effects on end organs. Management is directed by this assessment. Although patients with hypertension present to the ED relatively frequently, the number of individuals who actually require emergent intervention is small.[7] ED management should begin with an accurate blood pressure measurement, confirmed by **repeat assessment in both arms if the initial value is elevated.** The challenge is to determine whether the presenting blood pressure reading is only a transient circumstantial elevation or is representative of the patient's baseline. The approach to hypertensive patients in the ED is summarized in the algorithm shown in Figure 57-1. Traditional teaching has been that pressure differences between arms >10 mm Hg is abnormal. Recent data indicates that almost 20 percent of hypertensive ED patients may have differences >10 mm Hg between the two arms, without evident pathology.[8]

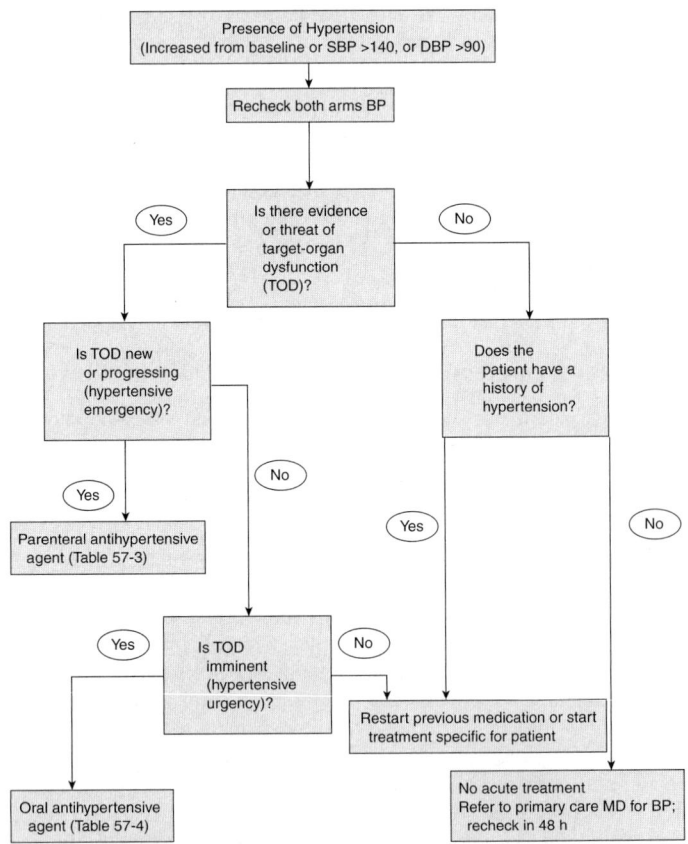

FIG. 57-1. Algorithm for approach to hypertensive patients.

Medical History

Any prior diagnosis of hypertension, including treatment regimens, compliance patterns, and baseline recordings of past blood pressures, are important to ascertain. Elevated blood pressure in the context of several months of noncompliance with antihypertensive medications likely represents a patient's baseline, whereas hypertension after several days of noncompliance could be a more serious abrupt cessation syndrome. A history of all medication use, including over-the-counter and illicit drugs, should be obtained, since many commonly used agents-including cocaine, amphetamines, decongestants, stimulants, oral contraceptives, and nonsteroidal anti-inflammatory drugs (NSAIDs)—may elevate blood pressure. MAO inhibitors in combination with tyramine-containing foods (e.g., beer and aged cheese) or certain drugs (e.g., amphetamines and tricyclic antidepressants) can also precipitate acute blood pressure elevation. Any past medical history of cardiovascular, cerebrovascular, or renal disease; diabetes; hyperlipidemia; chronic obstructive pulmonary disease (COPD); asthma; or gout; or a family history of hypertension or premature heart disease should also be elicited.[1] Patients with elevated pressures should be asked specifically about CNS symptoms (e.g., headache, diplopia, blurred vision, confusion, hemiparesis, and seizures), cardiac symptoms (e.g., chest pain, dyspnea, and palpitations), and renal symptoms (e.g., hematuria and anuria) that may be indicative of progressive end-organ damage.[1]

Physical Examination

The blood pressure should be measured with a cuff of the appropriate size for the patient. The width of the inflatable portion of the cuff should be about 40 percent of the circumference of the limb and the length of the inflatable portion should equal 80 percent of the limb's circumference. Using a cuff that is too short, too narrow, or too loose may cause falsely high readings. The blood pressure should be measured at least twice if the first value is elevated (SBP of more than 140 mm Hg or DBP of more than 90 mm Hg). For severe elevation, measure pressure in both arms and legs, and palpate pulses in all extremities. In adults, a differential in brachial systolic pressures of more than 20 mm Hg may suggest the presence of aortic coarctation, aneurysm, or dissection.

Focus the physical examination on the detection of target-organ damage and determine the acuity. Neurologic examinations that reveal focal findings or mental status changes may indicate hypertensive encephalopathy, subarachnoid hemorrhage, or stroke. A careful funduscopic examination may reveal acute changes such as hemorrhages, cotton-wool exudates, or disk or retinal edema (grade III or IV retinopathy). Alternatively, grade II retinopathy suggests chronic uncontrolled hypertension. Hyperreflexia with peripheral edema in a pregnant woman is suggestive of preeclampsia. This physical finding may also be found in elderly patients with multiple small ischemic strokes (cerebral lacunae).

On cardiovascular examination, auscultate for carotid bruits, right or left sided murmurs, third and fourth heart sounds (S_3 and S_4), and a pericardial rub. An S_3 occurs in association with ventricular failure, whereas an S_4 occurs when there is left ventricular hypertrophy and a noncompliant left ventricle. Left-sided congestive heart failure is associated with unexplained tachycardia as an early finding and pulmonary rales as a late finding. Diminished extremity pulses may be found in patients with coarctation of the aorta or aortic dissection. Signs of aortic insufficiency should be sought (see Chap. 58). The abdomen should be examined for a bruit and a palpable pulsatile mass that may indicate the presence of an abdominal aortic aneurysm.[1]

Diagnostic Studies

Blood urea nitrogen (BUN), creatinine, electrolyte, and glucose levels should be determined, and complete blood count (CBC), an electrocardiogram (ECG), urinalysis, and chest radiograph should be obtained in cases of suspected hypertensive emergencies to look for evidence of target-organ damage.[1] Renal impairment may present as hematuria, proteinuria, or elevations in BUN, creatinine, and potassium levels. Red cell casts suggest glomerulonephritis. The blood glucose level is important because hypoglycemia may simulate hypertensive encephalopathy or stroke. The CBC may reveal microangiopathic hemolytic anemia that may occur as a result of vascular damage after an acute, severe rise in blood pressure. The ECG should be compared with previous tracings. ST-T wave changes may be evidence of ischemia, electrolyte abnormalities, or left ventricular hypertrophy. The chest radiograph may be helpful in showing evidence of left-sided congestive heart failure or aortic dissection. In patients with neurologic symptoms, computed tomography (CT) of the head should be performed to look for evidence of stroke or hemorrhage.

TYPES OF HYPERTENSIVE EMERGENCIES

Hypertensive Encephalopathy

Although no specific blood pressure is pathognomonic, the elevated pressure exceeds the limits of cerebral autoregulation of the low-resistance arteries, resulting in cerebral hyperperfusion with loss of integrity of the blood-brain barrier. In most cases, autoregulation usually cannot accommodate a constant cerebral blood flow above a MAP of 150 to 160 mm Hg.

Hypertensive encephalopathy is usually acute in onset and reversible. It is characterized by severe headaches and nausea and vomiting, and may also include altered mental status. Neurologic symptoms can range from confusion and drowsiness to seizures, decreased visual acuity, focal deficits, or even coma. Since the pathologic mechanisms are the same, accelerated hypertensive retinopathy is often seen. The differential diagnosis is diverse and includes intracranial hemorrhage, stroke, meningoencephalitis, brain tumors, toxidromes, and metabolic coma. If hypertensive encephalopathy is suspected, antihypertensive therapy should be initiated while awaiting the results of certain key studies such as serum chemistry tests and CT scan.

Hypertensive encephalopathy is a true medical emergency, and if left untreated, can progress over hours and lead to coma and death. Treatment involves close cardiac monitoring, supplemental oxygen, intravenous access, and arterial monitoring. Immediate reduction of blood pressure by 20 to 25 percent will help reverse the vasospasm that occurs at these pressures; however, excessive reduction in blood pressure must be avoided in order to prevent hypoperfusion and further cerebral ischemia.[8] The medication of choice is sodium nitroprusside infused at an initial dose of 0.3 µg/kg per min and titrated up to a maximum of 10 µg/kg per min. Intravenous nitroglycerin and labetalol have been successfully used, but they have not replaced nitroprusside as first-line therapy for hypertensive encephalopathy.

Stroke Syndromes (see Chap. 228)

Elevated blood pressure is commonly associated with stroke syndromes and is often the result of a physiologic response to the stroke itself (to maintain adequate cerebral perfusion to the viable but edematous tissue surrounding the ischemic area) and not its immediate cause. In the area of the stroke, cerebral autoregulation is lost, causing tissue blood flow to become directly pressure-dependent. Most patients suffering from embolic or thrombotic strokes without associated hemorrhage do not have substantial elevations in blood pressure and do not need aggressive antihypertensive treatment. Furthermore, if the patient has a longstanding history of hypertension, any rapid reduction in blood pressure may further reduce cerebral blood flow to watershed areas and cause increased ischemia.[9] In the rare case of a stroke patient with extreme blood pressure elevation or sustained diastolic pressure greater than 140 mm Hg, the blood pressure may be reduced in a controlled manner by no more than 20 percent with intravenous labetalol in small doses beginning with 5-mg increments.

In contrast to the relatively minor blood pressure elevations seen with most strokes, intracranial hemorrhage commonly results in profound reactive rise in blood pressure. Causes of intracranial hemorrhage include hypertensive vascular disease, arteriovenous anomalies, arterial aneurysms, bleeding associated with tumors, and trauma. Hypertension associated with hemorrhagic stroke is usually transitory and the result of increased intracranial pressure and irritation of the autonomic nervous system. The acute management of blood pressure associated with intracranial hemorrhage is controversial. In the case of subarachnoid hemorrhage, oral nimodipine (60 mg every 4 h) has been used to reverse the vasospasm associated with subarachnoid blood. Intravenous nicardipine (2-mg boluses followed by a 4- to 15-mg per h infusion) is also now used by some for the management of hypertension during this type of hemorrhage.

Acute Pulmonary Edema

The hypertension associated with acute pulmonary edema is usually a result of increased peripheral vascular resistance caused by elevated catecholamines. In some cases, pulmonary edema occurs because an abrupt rise in blood pressure precipitates acute left ventricular failure. The blood pressure must be lowered to reverse this process, and nitroprusside and intravenous nitroglycerin are the agents of choice, although the latter does not reduce blood pressure as much as nitroprusside. Additional standard therapy for pulmonary edema includes nitrates (to reduce preload and afterload), oxygen, diuretics, and morphine sulfate (see Chap. 53).

Acute Coronary Syndromes

Increased left ventricular end-diastolic pressure increases the workload of the heart. Wall tension is one of the greatest determinants of myocardial oxygen demand. Increases in oxygen requirements secondary to hypertension may result in angina. Myocardial infarction may also develop, particularly among those with fixed lesions in coronary arteries, preventing appropriate delivery of required oxygen. The use of agents that increase myocardial oxygen demand, such as diazoxide, hydralazine, and minoxidil, should be avoided.

In cases of hypertension and angina, immediate blood pressure reduction is indicated to prevent myocardial damage, and therapy should be initiated with nitroglycerin, either sublingually or parenterally. For a greater degree of pressure reduction, sodium nitroprusside may be started.

Aortic Dissection (see Chap. 58)

Because aortic dissection is associated with hypertension in about 90 percent of cases, medical therapy aimed at reducing blood pressure can limit the extent of the dissection. Pathophysiology of aortic dissection is discussed in Chap. 58.

The initial medical therapy for a suspected dissection is aimed at reduction of the ventricular ejection force (rate of change in pressure with time, dp/dt) of the heart. The treatment of choice includes either a combination of a β-adrenergic antagonist (such as esmolol) and sodium nitroprusside, or labetalol alone. Emergency surgical consultation should be obtained for all suspected aortic dissections, although dissections involving the descending aorta are often medically managed. Surgical intervention is indicated in dissections involving the ascending aorta or aortic arch and in cases in which pain and blood pressure cannot be adequately controlled.

Renal Failure

Blood pressure and renal function are intrinsically related. Hypertension may cause acute renal failure or exacerbate chronic renal failure, whereas renal disease may result in hypertension. In patients with renal disease, the control of hypertension can delay the progression of further injury. Worsening renal function in the setting of elevated pressure, with elevation of BUN and creatinine levels, proteinuria, or the presence of red cells and red cell casts in the urine, is considered a hypertensive emergency that requires immediate reduction of blood pressure. Nitroprusside is the preferred agent in these cases. Patients who have known renal failure, are dialysis-dependent, and have volume overload may require emergent dialysis if they present with uncontrolled hypertension with other evidence of end-organ dysfunction.

Preeclampsia and Eclampsia

These are discussed in Chap. 106.

Epistaxis

The association between hypertension and epistaxis remains controversial.[10] A definite conclusion of epistaxis is a manifestation of end-organ dysfunction due to arterial hypertension has not been made. However, studies have confirmed that those patients with active epistaxis presenting to an ED have a greater chance of having increased blood pressure.[11] Some authors have suggested that the presence of active epistaxis should prompt the emergency physician to investigate hypertension as an additional possible diagnosis.[11]

Although the implications for management decisions regarding epistaxis and hypertension remain unclear at this time, hypertension as a possible diagnosis should be considered in the patient that presents to the ED with high blood pressure and an active nosebleed.

Childhood Hypertensive Emergencies

Hypertension is an uncommon problem in children, occurring in less than 5 percent,[12] and is defined as SBP or DBP equal to or greater than the 95th percentile for age and sex. Blood pressure should be measured with a cuff of the appropriate size as noted earlier. In the majority of confirmed cases of hypertension, renal/renovascular disease and pheochromocytoma are the most common etiologies.

Children often will have nonspecific complaints such as throbbing frontal headache or blurred vision. Physical findings associated with hypertension are similar to those found in adults.

The decision to treat is based on the combination of blood pressure and symptoms, but a guideline for urgent treatment is blood pressure that exceeds previous measurements by 30 percent. The goal of treatment, as in adults, is to reduce pressure within 1 h by 25 percent. Nitroprusside (0.3 μg/kg per min) and labetalol (1 to 2 mg/kg per h) are the agents of choice to treat hypertensive emergencies of childhood. Pediatric hypertension that may require intervention in the ED probably mandates consultation and likely admission.

TREATMENT OF HYPERTENSIVE EMERGENCIES

Treatment Goals

The treatment goal in hypertensive emergency is the immediate reduction of mean arterial pressure (MAP = [1/3(SBP − DBP) + DBP]) in a controlled, graded manner, using improvement in the patient's condition as a guide. **Blood pressure reduction should not exceed a 20 to 25 percent reduction within the first 30 to 60 min.**

Agents used in hypertensive emergencies are shown in Table 57-2.

TABLE 57-2   Parenteral Agents for Hypertensive Emergencies

Drug	Mechanism of Action	Initial Dose	Onset of Action	Duration	Contra-Indications	Adverse Effects
Nitroprusside	Vascular smooth muscle dilator	0.3 µg/kg per min IV	Seconds	3–5 min	Hepatic dysfunction	Cyanide toxicity (prolonged use)
Labetalol	α_1,β-Adrenergic blocker	20 mg IV over 10 min	5 min	4–8 h	Asthma, COPD, bradycardia	Bronchoconstriction, bradycardia
Esmolol	β_1-Adrenergic blocker	500 µg/kg IV over 1 min, then 50 µg/kg per min IV	5–30 min	30 min	Asthma, COPD	Bronchoconstriction
Nitroglycerin	Vascular smooth muscle dilator	5–10 µg/min IV	2–5 min	5–10 min		Headache
Hydralazine	Arteriolar dilator	10–20 mg IV *or* 10–50 mg IM	10 min 20 min	4–6 h	Aortic dissection, CAD	Tachycardia, increases catecholamines
Trimethaphan	Ganglionic blocker	0.3 mg per min IV	1–5 min	10 min		Autonomic effects. tachycardia
Enalaprilat	ACE inhibitor	0.625–1.25 mg IV	15 min	6 h	Renal artery stenosis	Acute renal failure, angioedema
Fenoldopam	Dopaminergic receptor agonist	0.05–0.1 mg/kg per min IV	4 min	8–10 min		Headache, flushing
Nicardipine	Calcium-channel blocker	2 mg IV, then 4 mg/h IV	15–30 min	40 min	Aortic stenosis	Headache, tachycardia
Urapidil	α_1-Receptor blocker, 5-HT$_{1A}$-receptor agonist	12.5–25 mg IV	10–20 min	4–6 h		Headache, vertigo

Abbreviations: ACE = angiotensin-converting enzyme; CAD = coronary artery disease; COPD = chronic obstructive pulmonary disease.

Specific Agents

SODIUM NITROPRUSSIDE (NIPRIDE)

Actions and Pharmacology   This rapidly acting arteriolar dilator and venodilator is the drug of choice for hypertensive emergencies and is the standard against which all other agents are compared. It acts by reacting with cysteine to form nitrosocysteine, a potent activator of guanylate cyclase, which in turn stimulates the formation of cyclic guanosine monophosphate (GMP) to relax smooth muscle in both arteries and veins. This decreases preload and afterload, resulting in decreased myocardial oxygen demand. The heart rate may increase slightly secondary to a baroreceptor-mediated reflex, but there is no change in cardiac output or myocardial blood flow unless there is pre-existing coronary artery disease, that can result in a significant reduction in regional blood flow ("coronary steal"; see below). Cerebral blood flow may be affected, decreasing in a dose-dependent manner. Renal blood flow remains unchanged, but plasma renin activity is increased. Pulmonary shunting may occur with nitroprusside use.

The rate of onset is extremely rapid, with a duration of action of 1 to 2 min and a plasma half-life of 3 to 4 min. Nitroprusside is metabolized to thiocyanate in the liver and is excreted slowly by the kidneys. Cyanide is an intermediate metabolite, but cyanide toxicity is rare.

Indications   Sodium nitroprusside is an excellent agent for all hypertensive emergencies except eclampsia prior to delivery (because it crosses the placenta). It is only indicated for postpartum eclampsia or in eclampsia resistant to other interventions.

Use   The MAP should not be reduced by more than 20 to 25 percent within 30 to 60 min. The solution is made by mixing 50 mg of sodium nitroprusside in 500 mL of D5W (0.1 mg/mL). The infusion is usually started at 0.3 µg/kg per min, titrating up to a maximum of 10 µg/kg per min until the desired blood pressure has been achieved. An arterial line will allow blood pressure to be closely monitored. Because of rapid degradation and sensitivity to light, sodium nitroprusside solution should be used within 24 h of mixing and be protected from light by wrapping the solution and tubing in aluminum foil.

Adverse Effects and Contraindications   The most common complication is hypotension. Prolonged infusions may lead to the rare complications of cyanide toxicity, which may occur in patients with hepatic dysfunction, and thiocyanate toxicity, which is associated with renal failure. This rarely occurs in the ED. Because nitroprusside inhibits hypoxia-induced vasoconstriction in the pulmonary vasculature, there may be increased perfusion to nonventilated areas of the lung. Myocardial ischemia may be worsened by a coronary steal syndrome because of dilation of coronary arteries or by the combination of nitroprusside and clonidine. Another consequence of the vasodilatory effect of nitroprusside is increased intracranial pressure.

LABETALOL

Actions and Pharmacology   This antihypertensive agent is a competitive, selective α_1-blocker and a competitive, nonselective β-blocker, with the β-blocking action being 4 to 8 times the α-blocking action. It can be given either PO or IV. It lowers blood pressure by blocking α_1 adrenoreceptors in vascular smooth muscle but, because of the simultaneous β-blockade, causes no reflex tachycardia.

When given intravenously, the distribution to peripheral tissues is rapid, with a large volume of distribution (15.7 L/kg). Onset of action is 5 to 10 min, and the duration of action is 8 h. The elimination half-life is 5.5 h. When taken PO, it is rapidly absorbed, with an absorption half-life of about 12 min and peak plasma concentrations at about 50 min. Labetalol is safe for use in patients with renal insufficiency, because it is predominantly (95 percent) hepatically metabolized. Oral dosing may need to be reduced in patients with hepatic disease. Oral bioavailability is only 25 percent, but increases in the elderly or when taken with food or cimetidine. The elimination half-life after an oral dose is 8 h.

Labetalol reduces systolic arterial pressure and total peripheral vascular resistance. Cardiac output may be slightly decreased or unchanged, pulmonary artery and wedge pressures decrease, and angiotensin II activity decreases, while cerebral blood flow, renal blood flow, and glomerular filtration rates are unchanged. With prolonged use, fluid retention may occur. Labetalol should be used with caution in patients with asthma and COPD, because of its nonselective β-blocking activity, which decreases the forced expiratory volume in 1 s (FEV$_1$) by causing bronchospasm. The use of labetalol should also be avoided in patients with bradycardia and second- or third-degree heart block.

Indications Labetalol can be used intravenously for hypertensive emergencies and be easily converted to the oral formulation as the first-line agent for hypertensive urgencies. It offers the advantages of providing a steady, consistent drop in blood pressure without decreasing cerebral blood flow or producing reflex tachycardia. It can be safely used in patients with cerebral vascular disease and coronary artery disease. Labetalol is ideal for use in syndromes associated with excessive catecholamine stimulation, such as from pheochromocytoma, MAO inhibitor-induced emergencies, and abrupt clonidine withdrawal. It has also been used in pregnancy-induced hypertension. It is a class C drug in pregnancy.

Use Labetalol can be given for hypertensive emergencies with repeated, incremental boluses starting with 20 mg IV, until the target blood pressure is achieved or a total dose of 300 mg is reached. After an intravenous bolus, the blood pressure falls in 5 min, with a maximum response in 10 min, and antihypertensive effect lasting for up to 6 h. After a 20-mg loading dose, labetalol may also be given as a continuous infusion by mixing 200 mg in 200 mL of D5W and running this at 2 mg per min (2 mL per min). The infusion should be stopped when the target pressure has been achieved.

The initial oral dose in hypertensive urgencies is 200 mg. Patients experience the onset of effects within 1 to 3 h.

Adverse Effects and Contraindications Labetalol has a prolonged action because of its large volume of distribution and long elimination half-life. In 5 percent of patients, orthostatic hypotension is a complication of therapy. The nonselective β-blocking action can exacerbate heart failure and induce bronchospasm. A paradoxical hypertensive effect may occur when the drug is used in low doses in catecholamine-induced crisis, because of the predominant β-blockade, leaving relatively unblocked α-receptors for the circulating catecholamines. In addition, patients with ischemic heart disease may experience exacerbation of angina, and in some cases, myocardial infarction after abrupt discontinuation of oral therapy.

ESMOLOL

Actions and Pharmacology This is an ultra-short-acting β$_1$-selective adrenergic blocker, which has rapid distribution and elimination half-lives of 2 and 9 min, respectively. When given as an intravenous bolus, followed by an infusion, 90 percent of β-blockade is achieved within 5 min; however, when given as an infusion without a bolus, steady-state blood levels are reached within 30 min. Within 2 min of discontinuing an infusion, there is a significant decrease in the β-antagonist activity, and generally all blockade will resolve within 30 min. Because of its rapid onset of action, short duration of action, and easy reversibility—properties not found in other β-blockers—esmolol is very useful in acute settings. When compared with sodium nitroprusside, esmolol provides similar rapid control of hypertension without producing the excessive reduction in DBP and reflex tachycardia that are seen with sodium nitroprusside.

Indications Esmolol has been used in the treatment of supraventricular tachycardias; to lower pulse and blood pressure in perioperative patients and in patients with myocardial infarction, unstable angina, and thyrotoxicosis; and to blunt rises in blood pressure associated with intubation. It has also been used for severe hypertension but is not particularly efficacious as monotherapy.

Use A loading dose of 500 μg/kg per min given over 1 min prior to the initiation of an infusion of 50 to 300 μg/kg per min. Esmolol may also be given without a loading dose, but then takes longer to reach a steady state. It is usually used in combination with other agents such as nitroprusside or phentolamine for hypertensive emergencies.

Adverse Effects and Contraindications Because of its β-antagonist activity, the use of esmolol should be avoided in patients with asthma or COPD. It also should not be used to treat patients with cocaine-induced cardiovascular complications, because of the predominant β-blockade, leaving relatively unblocked α-receptors.

INTRAVENOUS NITROGLYCERIN

Actions and Pharmacology This agent acts by causing both arteriolar dilation and venodilation, with a greater effect on the venous system (preload) than on the arterial vasculature (afterload). Onset of action is almost immediate when nitroglycerin is given intravenously, and the half-life is 4 min. The mechanism of action is thought to involve the reduction of sulfhydryl groups at a smooth muscle nitrate receptor, resulting in an increase in cyclic GMP. Nitroglycerin is hepatically metabolized. Cardiac output usually remains unchanged but may decrease slightly.

Indications The main indication for nitroglycerin is in the setting of myocardial ischemia, because it is a better vasodilator of the coronary vessels than is nitroprusside; therefore, it is the agent of choice for moderate hypertension complicating unstable angina, myocardial infarction, or pulmonary edema. It also has a less harmful effect on pulmonary gas exchange than does nitroprusside.

Use The initial infusion rate should be 5 to 10 μg/min with increases every 5 min in 5 μg/min increments until symptoms are improved or adverse effects necessitate stopping the infusion.

Adverse Effects and Contraindications The most common side effects include headache, tachycardia, nausea, vomiting, hypoxia, and hypotension.

HYDRALAZINE

Actions and Pharmacology This agent acts as a direct arteriolar dilator, with onset of action within 10 min when given intravenously and a duration of action of 4 to 6 h. The onset of action increases to 20 min when hydralazine is given intramuscularly and to 30 min after an oral dose. The plasma half-life is 2 to 4 h, but the antihypertensive effect may outlast this time interval. Its mechanisms of action are not well understood, but it is known to directly relax vascular smooth muscle, resulting in vasodilation. Hydralazine is metabolized by acetylation in the liver and gut walls by ring hydroxylation and conjugation. In patients who are "slow acetylators" (50 percent of the United States population), there is a higher incidence of hypotension and toxic complications. Within 24 h, 80 percent of hydralazine and its metabolites are excreted in the urine. Doses need to be decreased in patients with renal insufficiency.

Indications The main indication for use of intravenous hydralazine is pregnancy-induced hypertension.[14] The drug can be used orally and in combination with other drugs.

Use In cases of eclampsia, hydralazine can be given as either a 10- to 20-mg intravenous dose or a 10- to 50-mg IM dose. This dose can be repeated in 30 min.

Adverse Effects and Contraindications Hydralazine should not be used in patients with aortic dissection or a history of coronary artery disease, because it causes reflex tachycardia and increases plasma renin and catecholamines. It also causes sodium and water retention and can cause headaches, nausea, tachycardia, lethargy, and postural hypotension. A lupus-like syndrome can result from chronic oral use.

TRIMETHAPHAN

Actions and Pharmacology This is a ganglionic blocking agent that inhibits both sympathetic and parasympathetic discharge by occupying receptor sites. This acetylcholine blockade results in vasodilation, improved blood flow to some vascular beds, and a decrease in blood pressure. The heart rate may rise in response to the decrease in peripheral vascular resistance. Cardiac output, stroke volume, and left ventricular work decrease. It has a rapid onset of action, and its effects are of short duration.

Indications Historically, trimethaphan had been the drug of choice for acute aortic dissection, especially of the descending type. However, because it causes a number of serious side effects, it has been replaced by the combination of nitroprusside and β-blockade as the therapy of choice. It continues as a second-line agent in this setting.

Use Trimethaphan is given by intravenous infusion at a rate of 0.3 to 3.0 mg per min. It is sometimes used in combination with propranolol (1 to 3 mg IV or 10 to 40 mg PO qid) to reduce the velocity and force of left ventricular ejection.

Adverse Effects and Contraindications A number of serious side effects can occur, including bladder atony with urinary retention, ileus, gastric atony, cycloplegia, severe postural hypotension from blockade of circulatory reflex pathways, and even respiratory arrest. Tolerance develops with continued use; therefore, it is mainly useful for short-term administration such as in patients awaiting surgery or in inoperable patients until oral therapy with another agent can be started.

ENALAPRILAT

Actions and Pharmacology This agent, which is the first intravenous ACE inhibitor approved for clinical use, is the biologically active form of the oral ACE inhibitor enalapril that forms after deesterification in the liver. It is effective in patients with chronic heart failure with left ventricular ejection fractions of 20 to 44 percent, because it causes coronary vasodilation and significant reduction in mean arterial blood pressure and pulmonary capillary wedge pressure. It also improves cardiac index and stroke volume without affecting the heart rate or stroke work index.

The onset of antihypertensive effect is within minutes of an intravenous bolus injection, with the maximal decrease in DBP in 30 min and duration of action up to 6 h. The degree of blood pressure reduction seems to be associated with the degree of pretreatment plasma renin activity, thus suggesting that the mechanism of antihypertensive effect may be renin-angiotensin inhibition. Enalaprilat is excreted primarily by the kidney; therefore its dosage should be decreased in patients with severe renal insufficiency.

Indications Enalaprilat is an effective intravenous antihypertensive agent in hypertensive emergencies that can be easily continued as an oral preparation for long-term maintenance therapy.

Use An initial dose of 0.625 to 1.25 mg by intravenous bolus has been found to be effective in reducing blood pressure and heart rate. Doses of 2.5, 5, and 10 mg, up to a maximum of 40 mg, have been tried in different studies but have not been found to show any appreciable difference in the magnitude of blood pressure reduction with increasing dose.[15] A bolus can be given every 6 h. The onset of hypotensive effects is variable.

Adverse Effects and Contraindications This agent produces complications and effects that are similar to those of other ACE inhibitors, most notably angioneurotic edema and deterioration of renal function.

FENOLDOPAM

Actions and Pharmacology This antihypertensive agent is a selective postsynaptic dopaminergic receptor (DA1) agonist that has potent vasodilatory and natriuretic properties. Recent clinical trials have shown this intravenous agent to be as effective as nitroprusside in the treatment of severe hypertension without causing a change in heart rate.[16] The onset of action is 4 min, with duration of antihypertensive effect of 8 to 10 min.

Indications Fenoldopam has recently been FDA approved for use in treating hypertensive emergencies.

Use The initial dose is 0.05 to 0.1 mg/kg per min and can be increased at increments of 0.1 mg/kg per min to a maximum infusion rate of 1.6 mg/kg per min or to a diastolic pressure of less than 110 mm Hg.

Adverse Effects and Contraindications Mild side effects of headache and flushing occur in about 25 percent of patients. In addition, fenoldopam can cause an increase in intraocular pressure.

NICARDIPINE

Actions and Pharmacology This is a dihydropyridine calcium channel blocker that decreases afterload by reducing total peripheral resistance without reducing cardiac output and without apparent negative inotropic effect on the heart. It improves left ventricular pumping activity in patients with mild to moderate heart failure. Nicardipine also displays a greater vasodilatory effect on coronary than on systemic vessels, and produces a clinically significant decrease in cerebral vasospasm after subarachnoid hemorrhage.[17] The onset of action is 15 to 30 min, with a duration of action of 40 min.

Indications It has been used for the treatment of postoperative hypertension, stable angina, and congestive heart failure, and shows promise for use in patients with subarachnoid hemorrhage.

Use Nicardipine can be given initially as a 2-mg intravenous bolus, followed by a 4- to 15-mg per h infusion.

Adverse Effects and Contraindications Nicardipine does not produce the negative inotropic effects seen with other calcium channel blockers such as nifedipine. Headache occurs as a side effect in 20 to 50 percent of patients. Other less common effects include hypotension, tachycardia, nausea, and vomiting. The use of nicardipine is contraindicated in patients with severe aortic stenosis.

URAPIDIL

Actions and Pharmacology Urapidil is a promising antihypertensive agent that been studied extensively in Europe, but is not yet in use in the United States. It is a peripheral α_1-receptor blocker and central 5-HT$_{1A}$-receptor agonist that has been found to be equally effective in the treatment of hypertensive emergencies as nitroprusside when given intravenously.[19] Its mechanism of action is via peripheral arterial vasodilation. In addition, it induces very little reflex tachycardia because of a nonadrenergic, centrally mediated reduction of peripheral sympathetic tone. In addition, urapidil has no effect on cardiac output or intracranial pressure; therefore it is suitable for patients with preexisting cerebrovascular or cardiovascular disease because of the low risk of hypoperfusion.

The onset of action when given intravenously is 10 to 20 min, with a duration of antihypertensive effect of 4 to 6 h. There is also an oral form that can be used for long-term treatment.

Indications   Urapidil shows promise for use in treating hypertensive emergencies. It appears to be particularly effective in the treatment of pulmonary edema.

Use   The initial dose is 12.5 to 25 mg by intravenous bolus to achieve blood pressure reduction without high risk of severe hypotension. Higher doses can be given, with a maximum of 75 mg.

Adverse Effects and Contraindications   Minor side effects of headache, vertigo, and orthostatic dysregulation occur in a small percentage of patients.

TREATMENT OF HYPERTENSIVE URGENCIES

Treatment Goals

The treatment goal in hypertensive urgencies is the gradual reduction of blood pressure within 24 h by using oral antihypertensive agents (Table 57-3). The recommended duration to achieve blood pressure reduction varies from a few hours to 48 h in the literature. Since a common cause of hypertensive urgency is noncompliance with medications, restarting a patient on a previously established regimen is an acceptable strategy. Follow-up in 24 h should be arranged. Admission decisions depend on the patient's comorbid conditions, and the clinician's impression of the patient's anticipated response to therapy.

Specific Agents

SUBLINGUAL NITROGLYCERIN

Indications   It is the agent of choice for unstable angina, for immediate treatment of pain in acute myocardial infarction, and for the treatment of left ventricular insufficiency and pulmonary edema.

Use   Nitroglycerin is absorbed very quickly through the oral mucosa. It is given as a 0.3- to 0.6-mg tablet or spray under the tongue. The onset of hypotensive effect is in 5 min and can last several hours.

Adverse Effects and Contraindications   The most common side effects include headache, tachycardia, nausea, vomiting, hypoxia, and hypotension. It should be used with caution in patients with aortic stenosis.

CLONIDINE

Actions and Pharmacology   This agent is a centrally acting α_2-adrenergic agonist that decreases central sympathetic activity, lowering plasma catecholamine levels. Clonidine causes little postural hypotension because vasomotor reflexes are unchanged. It also does not increase heart rate or cardiac output and does not change renal blood flow or glomerular filtration rates. Overall, the effect of clonidine is to lower blood pressure, slow the heart rate, and cause sedation.

The onset of action is 30 to 60 min after an oral dose, with peak effect in 2 to 4 h. The duration of action is 6 to 8 h. Clonidine crosses the blood-brain barrier. Because approximately 50 percent is excreted unchanged in the urine in the first 24 h, it can accumulate in patients with renal insufficiency and is not dialyzable; however, in cases of renal failure, it is excreted in the feces.

Indications   This is considered to be a second-line agent for the treatment of hypertensive urgencies. It can be used safely in the elderly and in renal failure. It is a good choice for hypertensive urgency associated with cocaine withdrawal. However, because it sometimes requires up to 6 h for an adequate response, it is not ideal for ED use.

Use   The initial dose is 0.1 to 0.2 mg, with additional doses of 0.1 mg every hour until the diastolic pressure is below 115 mm Hg or a maximum dose of 0.7 mg has been given. A patient who is given clonidine in the ED setting does not need to be discharged on this specific agent long term.

Adverse Effects and Contraindications   The most common side effects include dry mouth, drowsiness, and constipation. Rarely, bradycardia can occur in patients with sick sinus syndrome. Clonidine may interact with other drugs, causing adverse effects such as orthostatic hypotension in patients taking diuretics, decreased anti-

TABLE 57-3   Oral Agents for Hypertensive Urgencies

Drug	Mechanism of Action	Dose	Onset of Action	Duration	Contra-indications	Adverse Effects
Nitroglycerin	Vascular smooth muscle dilator	0.3–0.6 mg SL	5 min	5–10 min	Aortic stenosis	Headache
Labetalol	α_1,β-Adrenergic blocker	200–400 mg PO, repeat every 2–3 h	30–120 min	6–12 h	Asthma, COPD, bradycardia	Bronchoconstriction, bradycardia
Clonidine	Central α_2 agonist	0.1–0.2 mg PO, repeat 0.1 mg every hour	30–60 min	6–8 h	CHF, 2nd- or 3rd-degree heart block	Drowsiness, sedation, tachycardia, dry mouth
Captopril	ACE inhibitor	25 mg PO	15–30 min	4–6 h	Renal artery stenosis	Acute renal failure, angioedema
Nifedipine (extended release)	Calcium channel blocker	10 mg PO, may repeat q30–60 min	5–15 min	3–6 h	Angina, acute hypertension	MI, CVA, syncope, heart block, CHF
Losartan	Angiotensin II receptor antagonist	50 mg PO	60 min	12–24 h	2nd and 3rd trimesters of pregnancy	Allergic (rare)

Abbreviations: ACE = angiotensin-converting enzyme; CHF = congestive heart failure; COPD = chronic obstructive pulmonary disease; CVA = cerebrovascular accident; MI = myocardial infarction; SL = sublingual.

hypertensive effects with cyclic antidepressants, increased sedation with alcohol, and bradyarrhythmias or other dysrhythmias with negative inotropic agents. When high doses of clonidine are abruptly stopped, the well-documented phenomenon of clonidine withdrawal with severe rebound hypertension, tachycardia, flushing, and abdominal symptoms may be seen. If this syndrome occurs, the pa-tient should be given clonidine therapy promptly. The use of β-blockers should be avoided because they may worsen the withdrawal symptoms.

CAPTOPRIL

Actions and Pharmacology   This is an ACE inhibitor that is rapidly absorbed PO, with an onset of action within 15 to 30 min, peak effects of blood pressure reduction between 50 and 90 min, and duration of antihypertensive effect of 4 to 6 h. It causes no change in cardiac output, heart rate, or cerebral blood flow. Since captopril is metabolized by the kidneys, its dosing must be decreased in patients with renal insufficiency. Postural hypotension is a rare problem, because it has no effect on baroreceptor reflexes.

Indications   Captopril is effective in cases of refractory acute congestive heart failure and is also useful in treating hypertensive urgencies with known renovascular hypertension.

Use   The usual oral dose is 25 mg. The dose-response curve for captopril is flat; therefore increasing doses generally do not cause greater reductions in blood pressure.

Adverse Effects and Contraindications   Several common side effects include skin rash, cough, and loss of taste. Laboratory abnormalities that can occur include leukopenia, proteinuria, and hyperkalemia. Captopril should not be used in combination with potassium-sparing diuretics. It also should not be given to patients with bilateral renal artery stenosis or unilateral stenosis with one kidney, because of the risk of acute renal failure. In patients with chronic renal failure or collagen vascular disease, there is an increased risk of side effects. A potentially life-threatening complication of this therapeutic agent is angioneurotic edema, which can result in airway compromise.

NIFEDIPINE   This dihydropyridine calcium-channel antagonist has been one of the most extensively studied agents for rapid control of blood pressure. Until the last few years, when awareness of serious side effects became more widespread, it had been the most frequently used agent for acute blood pressure lowering in hospitalized patients.

The US Food and Drug Administration (FDA) has never specifically approved the use of short-acting nifedipine for the treatment of hypertension of any kind. Because of the risks of serious adverse reactions, such as acute coronary events or an ischemic stroke, the US National Heart, Lung, and Blood Institute issued a warning in 1995 stating that **this agent should not be used in the treatment of hypertension, angina, and myocardial infarction.**[18]

LOSARTAN

Actions and Pharmacology   Losartan is a promising new agent that is a highly selective angiotensin II-receptor antagonist. It blocks the vasoconstrictor and aldosterone-secreting effects of angiotensin II. It selectively blocks the binding of angiotensin II to specific receptors found in vascular smooth muscle and the adrenal gland. It undergoes substantial first-pass metabolism by cytochrome P-450 enzymes and is converted to an active metabolite. The half-life of losartan is about 2 h

and of the metabolite about 6 to 9 h. Peak concentrations of losartan and its active metabolite are reached in 1 h and in 3 to 4 h, respectively.

Indications   Losartan has been used in clinical trials in the treatment of hypertensive urgency.

Use   It is available as 10-, 25-, or 50-mg tablets. The 50-mg dose has been found in studies to produce better results than the lower doses, but higher doses do not produce a more significant blood pressure reduction.

Adverse Effects and Contraindications   Because of potential fetal injury, the use of **losartan should be avoided in the second and third trimesters of pregnancy.** Dosing should be decreased in patients with hepatic insufficiency.

TREATMENT OF ACUTE HYPERTENSIVE EPISODE

As noted, there is a paucity of evidence that acute intervention in blood pressure in the ED is warranted. Rather, there is evidence that in some cases acute interventions may actually be harmful.[3] In chronically hypertensive individuals, complications of acute blood pressure reduction can include altered sensorium, seizures, transient ischemic attacks, and amaurosis as well as other visual changes. In addition, there is no evidence of a beneficial effect of acute blood pressure reduction on long-term control or on the chronic effects of hypertension. In general, these patients require no acute ED intervention but should be referred to a primary care physician for follow-up and initiation of therapy. If these patients have previously been diagnosed as hypertensive but have been noncompliant with medications, a reasonable strategy would be to restart the patients on their previous treatment regimen and then refer for appropriate follow-up care within 24 to 48 h.

SELECTION OF CLASS OF ANTIHYPERTENSIVE AGENT

Table 57-4 summarizes guidelines for the selection of an antihypertensive agent for patients in an ambulatory setting with various coexisting conditions.[13] Diuretics should be the agents of first choice in patients with renal disease and congestive heart failure who are judged to be volume overloaded. Because of their greater prevalence of stage 3 hypertension (SBP of 180 mm Hg or more, and DBP of 110 mm Hg or more), African-American patients may require multidrug therapy. For treatment of patients with angina pectoris or postmyocardial infarction, β-blockers are indicated. They are also indicated for those patients with a history of migraines, atrial fibrillation with rapid ventricular response, paroxysmal supraventricular tachycardia, and senile tremor. The use of β-blockers is safe in the latter part of pregnancy, but their use should be avoided in early pregnancy because of an association with fetal growth restriction. Angiotensin-converting enzyme (ACE) inhibitors should be used in patients with congestive heart failure (see Chap. 53) and can also be used in patients with a history of diabetes mellitus, especially those with diabetic nephropathy. The use of ACE inhibitors should be avoided in pregnant women.

In the elderly, diuretics are the first choice for antihypertensive therapy because the pathophysiology of their hypertension is usually related to total peripheral resistance rather than cardiac output. Beta-blockers are also recommended as alternative therapy. Use of agents that cause significant orthostatic changes (e.g., calcium channel blockers, peripheral α1-adrenergic blockers), as well as drugs that cause cognitive dysfunction (e.g., central α2 agonists) should be avoided in the elderly.

TABLE 57-4 Antihypertensive Treatment Regimens for Specific Populations

Coexisting Condition	Diuretic	β-Blocker	Angiotensin-Converting Enzyme Inhibitor	α₁-Blocker	Calcium Channel Blocker
Older age	++	+/−	+	+	+
Black race	++	+/−	+/−	+	++
Angina pectoris	+	++	+	+	++
Postmyocardial infarction	+	++	+	+	−
Congestive heart failure with systolic dysfunction	++	−	++	+	−
Cerebrovascular disease	+	+	+	+/−	+
Renal disease (Cr >2.3 mg/dL)	++	+/−	−	+	+
Diabetes mellitus with nephropathy	+	+/−	+	+	+
Migraine	+	++	+	+	+
Atrial fibrillation (with rapid ventricular response)	+	++	+	+	+
Paroxysmal supraventricular tachycardia	+	++	+	+	+
Senile tremor	+	++	+	+	+

Symbols: ++, preferred; +, suitable; +/−, usually not preferred; −, usually contraindicated.
Abbreviation: Cr = serum creatinine.
Source: From Kaplan and Gifford,[13] with permission.

REFERENCES

1. Joint National Committee (JNC) on Prevention, Detection, Evaluation, and Treatment of High Blood Pressure: The sixth report of the Joint National Committee on Prevention, Detection, Evaluation, and Treatment of High Blood Pressure (JNC-6). *Arch Intern Med* 157:2413, 1997.
2. Burt VL, Whelton P, Roccella EJ, et al: Prevalence of hypertension in the U.S. adult population: Results from the Third Health and Nutrition Examination Survey, 1988-1991. *Hypertension* 25:305, 1995.
3. Hyman DJ, Pavlik VN: Characteristics of patients with uncontrolled hypertension in the United States. *New Engl J Med* 345:479, 2001.
4. Pierdomenico SD, Mezzetti A: White coat hypertension in patients with newly diagnosed hypertension: Evaluation of prevalence by ambulatory monitoring and impact on cost of health care. *Eur Heart J* 16:692, 1995.
5. Strandgaard S: Autoregulation of cerebral blood flow in hypertensive patients: The modifying influence of prolonged anti-hypertensive treatment on the tolerance of acute, drug-induced hypotension. *Circulation* 53:720, 1976.
6. Grossman E, Messerli FH: High blood pressure: A side effect of drugs, poisons, and food. *Arch Intern Med* 155:450, 1995.
7. Zampaglione B, Pascale C: Hypertensive urgencies and emergencies: Prevalence and clinical presentation. *Hypertension* 27:144, 1996.
8. Pesola GR, Pesola HR, Lin M, et al: The normal difference in bilateral indirect blood pressure recording in hypertensive individuals. *Acad Emerg Med* 9:342, 2002.
9. Graham DI: Ischaemic brain following emergency blood pressure lowering in hypertensive patients, *Acta Med Scand* 678(Suppl):61, 1983.
10. Temmel AF, Quint C, Toth J: Debate about blood pressure and epistaxis will continue. *BMJ* 12:322, 2001.
11. Herkner H, Havel C, Mullner M, et al: Active epistaxis at ED presentation is associated with arterial hypertension *Am J Emerg Med* 20:92-95, 2002.
12. Sinaiko AR: Hypertension in children. *N Engl J Med* 335:1968, 1996.
13. Kaplan NM, Gifford RW: Choice of initial therapy for hypertension. *JAMA* 275:1577, 1996.
14. Lowe SA, Rubin PC: The pharmacologic management of hypertension in pregnancy. *J Hypertens* 10:201, 1992.
15. Hirschl MM, Binder M, Bur A, et al: Clinical evaluation of different doses of intravenous enalaprilat in patients with hypertensive crisis. *Arch Intern Med* 155:2217, 1995.
16. Vaughn CJ, Delanty N: Hypertensive emergencies. *Lancet* 356:411, 2000.
17. Haley EC Jr, Kassell NF, Torner JC: A randomized controlled trial of high-dose intravenous nicardipine in aneurysmal subarachnoid hemorrhage. *J Neurosurg* 78:537, 1993.
18. McCarthy M: US NIH issues warning on nifedipine. *Lancet* 346:689, 1995.
19. Hirschl MM, Binder M, Bur A, et al: Safety and efficacy of urapidil and sodium nitroprusside in the treatment of hypertensive emergencies. *Intensive Care Med* 23:885, 1997.

AORTIC DISSECTION AND ANEURYSMS

Louise A. Prince
Gary A. Johnson

Thoracic and abdominal aneurysmal disease comprises a significant subset of emergencies. A ruptured aneurysm or dissecting aneurysm is a prominent cause of sudden death as well as severe abdominal, chest, or back pain. These diseases disproportionately affect the elderly. As our patient population becomes older, the incidence of presentations for aneurysms will continue to increase.[1]

Abdominal aortic aneurysms (AAA) have a clear familial trend. Eighteen percent of patients with AAA have a family history of aneurysm (a first-degree relative) compared with less than 3 percent of controls. Patients with Marfan syndrome have been found to have mutations in the *FBN1* gene on chromosome 15.[1] Other genetic abnormalities have been investigated as well.[1]

The incidence of AAA increases with age, and the disease rarely presents before age 50. Most patients are older than age 60, and males have an increased risk of disease. Patients with other aneurysms and peripheral arterial disease are at increased risk as well.

PATHOGENESIS

Risk factors for aneurysms include connective tissue disorders, familial history of aneurysm, and atherosclerotic risk factors (i.e., age, smoking, hypertension, hyperlipidemia, and diabetes). These risk factors combine to increase the expansile force on the aortic wall or to impair the patient's ability to withstand these forces. The Laplace law [wall tension = (pressure × radius)] dictates that as the aorta dilates, the force on the aortic wall increases, therefore causing further aortic dilatation.

Destruction of the media of the aorta is a prominent feature in aneurysm pathogenesis. Elastin and collagen are markedly reduced in the aneurysmal aorta, and fibrolamellar units are dramatically decreased. In addition, the normal abdominal aorta has a decreasing number of elastic lamellae as the aorta becomes more distal. This may help account for the prominent infrarenal location of aneurysm in many patients.

Histologic examination of an aneurysmal wall will show an intima that is infiltrated by atherosclerosis and a thinned media. There may be intraluminal thrombus, and the adventitia often has been infiltrated by inflammatory cells. Patients with saccular outpouchings (blisters) may have an increased risk of rupture. Such blisters have been shown to increase the incidence of rupture of small (<5 cm) aneurysms.[2]

Rate of aneurysmal dilatation is variable. As a consequence of the LaPlace law, larger aneurysms will expand more quickly than smaller ones. An average rate may be 0.25 to 0.5 cm per year.[2] Patients with known aneurysms must be followed closely for unpredictably fast expansion.

Dissecting Aneurysms

Aortic dissections occur from a violation of the intima that allows blood to enter the media and dissect between the intimal and the adventitial layers. Common sites for tear include the ascending aorta and the region of the ligamentum arteriosum. The dissecting column of blood ruptures the intima and thus maintains a true and false lumen. The dissection may extend proximally, distally, or both. The patient's symptoms may cease abruptly when the dissection reenters the intima; this may suggest a spontaneous cure clinically. Alternatively, blood may dissect through the adventitia and nearly always will be fatal.

Aortic dissection presents in a bimodal fashion. One group consists of younger patients with specific predisposing conditions. The predominant group consists of patients above age 50 (mean age 63) with hypertension. Two-thirds of patients are male, and 72 percent have hypertension.[3] Atherosclerosis is only a minor contributor to the pathogenesis of dissection.

Predisposing conditions for dissection include multiple forms of congenital heart disease, connective tissue disease, and pregnancy. Approximately 25 to 30 percent of patients with Marfan syndrome develop a dissection. Dissection also may be induced iatrogenically from aortic catheterization or cardiac surgery.

Aortic dissections have been classified by two separate systems. The Stanford classification considers any involvement of the ascending aorta a type A dissection and dissections restricted to the descending aorta type B. DeBakey classified type I dissections as those which simultaneously involve the ascending aorta, the arch, and the descending aorta. Type II involves only the ascending aorta and type III only the descending aorta.

Pseudoaneurysms

Pseudoaneurysms (or false aneurysms) may occur when there is a violation of the intima that creates an ulcer into the aortic media. This type of lesion may dilate slowly or cause a deepening of the ulcer and form a pseudoaneurysm; it occurs most commonly in the descending thoracic aorta. Pseudoaneurysms do not evolve commonly into dissections and rupture rarely.[4]

Other Aneurysms

Patients may have aneurysms at anastomoses from prior vascular reconstruction. The aneurysm occurs at the site where the graft is sewn to the artery. Anastomotic aneurysms may occur in the aortic, iliac, or femoral arteries. These aneurysms commonly rupture and cause catastrophic bleeding; however, they also may present with smaller sentinel hemorrhages. Anastomotic aneurysms may erode into the adjacent intestine and form an aortoenteric fistula.

CLINICAL FEATURES

Abdominal Aortic Aneurysms

Symptomatic abdominal aortic aneurysms may present as syncope, back or abdominal pain, shock, or sudden death. Sudden death most commonly occurs from intraperitoneal rupture of the aneurysm. These ruptures lead to massive, rapid blood loss, and it will not be possible to resuscitate the patient. History that is often cited as classic for acute rupture of the abdominal aneurysm is syncope with no warning symptoms followed by severe abdominal or back pain. Syncope is caused by rapid blood loss and a lack of cerebral perfusion. Patients often regain consciousness after their own compensatory mechanisms have been invoked, but they most often will slip again into shock without prompt medical intervention.

In general, pain is the most common presenting symptom. The pain is described more often as severe and abrupt in onset, and it may be located in the back or abdomen.

Approximately 50 percent of patients describe a ripping or tearing pain.[3] Syncope may be present in 10 to 12 percent of patients. Many patients present with atypical sites of pain: flank, groin, isolated quadrants of the abdomen, and hip. Other symptoms such as bladder pain, tenesmus, nausea, and vomiting many complicate the presentation. Constitutional symptoms such as nausea and vomiting are present commonly.

Physical examination of a patient with acute rupture of an aortic aneurysm may detect the aneurysm. Tenderness to palpation of an aneurysm is commonly interpreted as a sign of rupture. However, a lack of tenderness cannot imply an intact aorta. Patients with an obese abdomen are difficult to examine for the presence of an aortic aneurysm. Very thin patients may have an aorta that is easily palpable, and the diameter of the aorta should be measurable.

Evidence of retroperitoneal hematoma may be seen as periumbilical ecchymosis (Cullen sign) or flank ecchymosis (Grey-Turner sign). Retroperitoneal blood also may dissect into the perineum or groin. Scrotal hematomas or inguinal masses may be seen on examination. Retroperitoneal blood also may irritate the psoas muscle and produce an iliopsoas sign. Blood may compress the femoral nerve and present as a neuropathy. The presence or rupture of an AAA typically does not alter femoral arterial pulsations.[5]

Aortoenteric fistulas should be considered in all patients with unexplained gastrointestinal bleeding. A history of aortic graft placement should increase the clinical suspicion of fistula.[6] The duodenum is involved most frequently, and therefore, bleeding may manifest as hematemesis, melenemesis, melena, or (if there is rapid transport) hematochezia. These fistulas commonly present as massive, life-threatening bleeding. However, mild "sentinel" bleeding may precede a full-blown rupture. Aortic aneurysms also may erode into the venous vasculature and form aortovenous fistulas, which may present as high-output cardiac failure, decreased arterial blood flow distal to the fistula, and increased central venous volume.

AAAs uncommonly may present as chronic contained ruptures. A retroperitoneal rupture may cause enough fibrosis to limit blood loss. The inflammatory response commonly causes pain, which may continue for a significant length of time. Despite the seriousness of this pathology, the patient may appear remarkably well.

An asymptomatic aneurysm may be found on physical examination or radiologic evaluation. Any aneurysm that is found should be referred for follow-up. **Aneurysms greater than 5 cm in diameter are at an increased risk of rupture (size is measured outer wall to outer wall). Aneurysms of less than 5 cm are less likely to rupture.** However, patients with such asymptomatic aneurysms must be followed closely by their primary care physicians or surgeons. The management of patients with small, asymptomatic aneurysms (including the timing of surgery) is a controversial topic.[1,7] Symptomatic aneurysms of any size should be considered emergent.

Thoracic Aortic Aneurysm

Thoracic aortic aneurysms may become symptomatic by compressing or eroding into adjacent structures. Presenting symptoms can include esophageal, tracheal, bronchial, or even neurologic disorders. A thoracic aneurysm that erodes to an adjacent structure is generally immediately fatal. Rare patients may survive with the assistance of hemodynamic resuscitation.

Dissecting Aortic Aneurysms

Aortic dissections commonly present (>85 percent) with abrupt and severe pain in the chest or between the scapulae. Recent literature suggests that back pain is a less common presentation than previously thought.[3] One half of all patients often describe the pain as tearing or ripping. Pain in the anterior chest often is associated with involvement of the ascending aorta (70 percent). Back pain may indicate involvement of the descending aorta (63 percent). Dissection often presents with dynamic pathology; therefore, pain patterns often change as the anatomic injury migrates.[3]

The aortic dissection will cause a spectrum of symptoms based on the anatomic course of the lesion. Dissection into a carotid artery may lead to a classic stroke presentation. Forty percent of patients with dissection will have some neurologic sequelae.[3] Paraplegia may occur if the arterial blood supply to the spinal cord is interrupted. Abdominal or flank pain may be caused by dissection into the abdominal aorta, renal arteries, or iliac arteries. Dissection of the aortic root may lead to pericardial tamponade.

Systemic constitutional symptoms may occur with the dissection. Nausea, vomiting, and diaphoresis are common. Patients frequently are apprehensive and express feelings of impending doom.

Physical examination may help to eliminate some differential diagnoses but most likely will reveal a normal heart and lung examination. The diastolic murmur of aortic insufficiency may be heard. Decreased pulsation in the radial, femoral, and/or carotid arteries should significantly raise the suspicion of an aortic lesion but is present in less than 20 percent of patients.[3] Specific threshold values of blood pressure changes between extremities have not been defined. Hypertension and tachycardia are commonly present, but the dissection also may cause hypotension. Hypotension may accompany pericardial tamponade or coronary artery interruption. Tamponade may result in muffled heart tones, elevated jugular venous pressure, and pulsus paradoxus. Compression of the recurrent laryngeal nerve or the superior cervical sympathetic ganglion may cause either hoarseness of the voice or Horner syndrome, respectively.

DIAGNOSIS

Abdominal Aortic Aneurysms

The differential diagnoses for AAAs include the causes of syncope, abdominal pain, chest pain, back pain, and shock. The presentation of syncope with back pain or shock should strongly suggest aortic disease. However, the diagnosis will be difficult to make in shock or syncope without a significant complaint of pain. Other cardiac, abdominal, and retroperitoneal diseases need to be considered, including renal disorders, hepatobiliary disorders, and pancreatic disease. Unfortunately, some patients may appear well enough to receive benign diagnoses such as musculoskeletal back pain or enteritis and be discharged from the ED.

The diagnosis may be further confused by coexisting pathology. Coronary artery disease and chronic lung disease are often present, and these features may distract the physician from the diagnosis of aneurysmal disease. This is especially true in patients without significant pain.

Aneurysms of large arteries other than the aorta may expand or rupture. Iliac artery aneurysms are notoriously difficult to diagnose because they may be confused with urologic, bowel, or groin disorders. Splenic artery aneurysms may present as undifferentiated shock or intra-abdominal catastrophe. A rupture of the splenic artery has a poor prognosis owing to its intraperitoneal location.

Radiologic studies may be very helpful in confirming a ruptured AAA, but since radiographs often unnecessarily delay operative repair, the decision to obtain confirmatory studies must be made carefully.

Radiologic evaluation may include plain radiography (Figure 58-1A, B), ultrasound (Figure 58-2), computed tomographic (CT) scanning (Figure 58-3), or magnetic resonance imaging. Plain abdominal films may show a calcified and bulging aortic contour, implying the presence of an aneurysm. Approximately 65 percent of patients with symptomatic aortic aneurysmal disease will have a calcified aorta. Some propose that a cross-table lateral film of the abdominal aorta will have a higher yield for calcifications. The lateral view will allow the aorta to be visualized without overlying the vertebral column. An anteroposterior projection may show an arch of calcification, most commonly on the patient's left. Rarely, a chronic aneurysm may erode into a vertebral body. Plain film cannot exclude the presence of AAA.

Rapid bedside ultrasonography (see Figure 58-2) is ideal for unstable patients who cannot undergo CT scanning. A technically adequate ultrasound study has virtually 100 percent sensitivity for demonstrating the presence of an aneurysm and measuring its diameter. Obesity or bowel gas may make the study difficult to perform. Rupture cannot be seen reliably on ultrasound.

CT scanning with intravenous contrast material (see Figure 58-3) is useful to demonstrate the anatomic details of the aneurysm and associated retroperitoneal hemorrhage. CT scanning should be obtained on stable patients. Should unusual circumstances occur (such as the presence of other prominent acute abdominal conditions) and a CT scan becomes necessary, the patient should be accompanied by the surgeon, who could expedite an emergent operation if necessary.

Dissecting Aneurysms

The ischemic end-organ manifestations associated with many dissections may confuse the differential diagnosis, which includes myocardial infarction, pericardial disease, pulmonary disorders, stroke, musculoskeletal disease of the extremities, spinal cord injuries, and intra-abdominal disorders. Ischemic manifestations may change with time (as the dissection progresses), distracting the physician from making the correct diagnosis. Rupture of the dissection into the true lumen may cause a cessation of symptoms, and the correct diagnosis may then be dismissed inappropriately.

Thoracic dissecting aneurysms most commonly (90 percent) will have an abnormality on chest radiography.[3] Widening of the mediastinum, an abnormal aortic contour, pleural effusions, or deviation of the trachea, mainstem bronchi, or esophagus may be seen (Figure 58-4). Intimal calcium may be visible and distant from the edge of the aortic contour (calcium sign).

CT scanning may reliably make the diagnosis of aortic dissection[8] (Figure 58-5). Sensitivity for dissection ranges from 83 to 100 percent, and specificity ranges from 87 to 100 percent.[8] Spiral CT scanning with rapid intravenous boluses of radiopaque contrast material may be more sensitive. However, CT scanning cannot reliably give anatomic details of other arterial branches emanating from the aorta and cannot address aortic valve competence.

Angiography is still considered the "gold standard" for diagnosis by many and will provide more anatomic detail than a CT scan.[8] Aortography also will reliably show complications of dissection, including involvement of branch vessels, aortic valve incompetence, and coronary artery involvement. However, the angiogram is not a perfect study. Erbel[9] found aortography to have a specificity of 94 percent and a sensitivity of 88 percent. Risks of the procedure include the use of intravenous contrast agents and the delay in assembling an angiography team.

Magnetic resonance angiography (MRA) is comparable to angiography and CT angiography, but is not readily available or practical for most ED patients. CT remains the modality of choice in unstable patients.

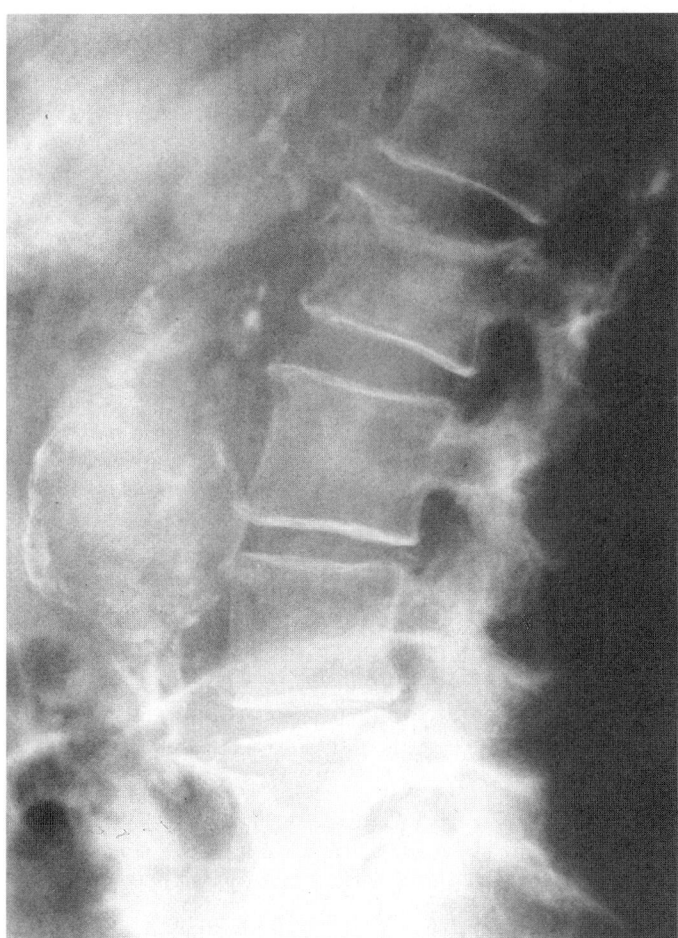

A

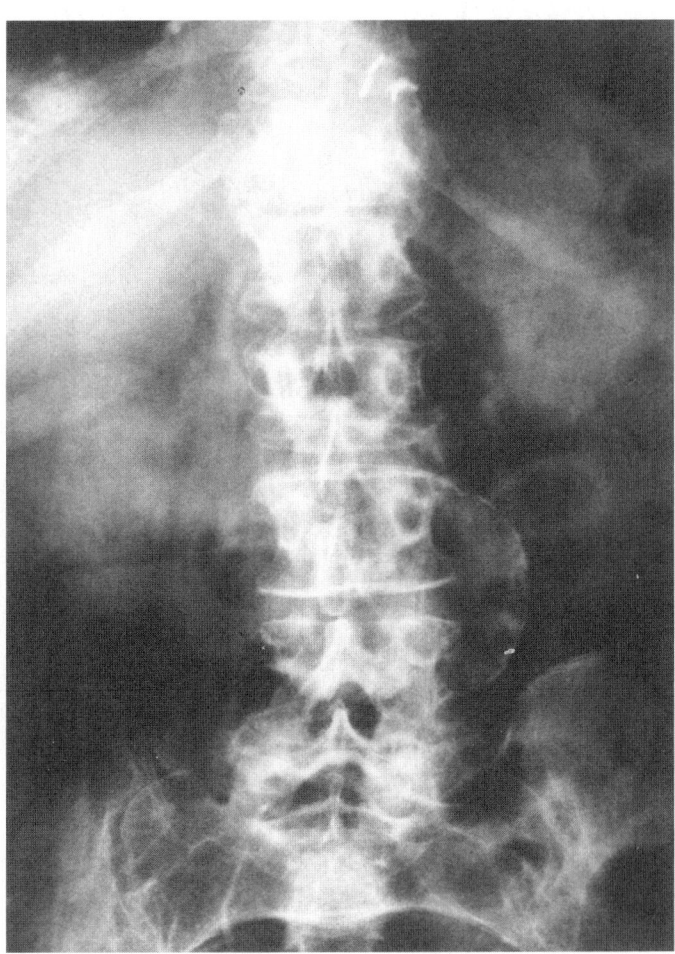

B

FIG. 58-1. A. Lateral view of a calcified infrarenal aortic aneurysm. **B.** Posteroanterior view of a calcified infrarenal aortic aneurysm.

In experienced hands, a transesophageal echocardiogram (TEE) may be as sensitive and specific as angiography.[10–12] Sensitivity for dissection ranges from 97 to 100 percent, and specificity ranges from 97 to 99 percent. Some 3 percent of patients cannot tolerate the procedure, which should be performed under sedation or general anesthesia. Known esophageal disease is a relative contraindication. Disrup-

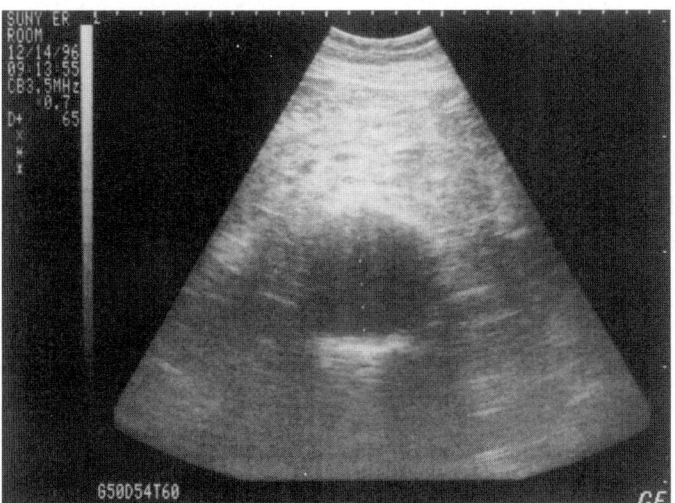

FIG. 58-2. Bedside ultrasound image of an AAA. This aneurysm measures 6.5 cm.

tion of sound transmission by air in the trachea or left bronchi may cause difficulty in evaluating the ascending aorta. Among the imaging techniques mentioned earlier, TEE has the highest diagnostic variability between operators or observers. Therefore, the imaging procedure of choice may vary between institutions. In contrast with AAAs, suspected dissections must be confirmed radiologically prior to operative repair.

Thoracic aortic saccular aneurysms generally are identified on chest radiography. Rarely, the presence of thoracic, pleural, or parenchymal densities may make the diagnosis more difficult. CT scanning will delineate these aneurysms reliably.

EMERGENCY DEPARTMENT TREATMENT

Ruptured Abdominal Aortic Aneurysm

All symptomatic aneurysms require urgent surgical consultation. The emergency physician's role in the care of a patient with an acute rupture of an AAA lies largely in making the diagnosis and assisting with rapid transfer to the operating room.

Any suspected ruptured aneurysm requires immediate operative repair. One-half of patients with a ruptured aneurysm who reach the operating room die.[7] **Imaging modalities should be restricted to patients who are considered unlikely to have a ruptured AAA.** Standard resuscitative maneuvers (two large-bore intravenous catheters, a cardiac monitor, and supplemental oxygen) are required. The patient suspected of having an AAA may require resuscitation for blood loss.

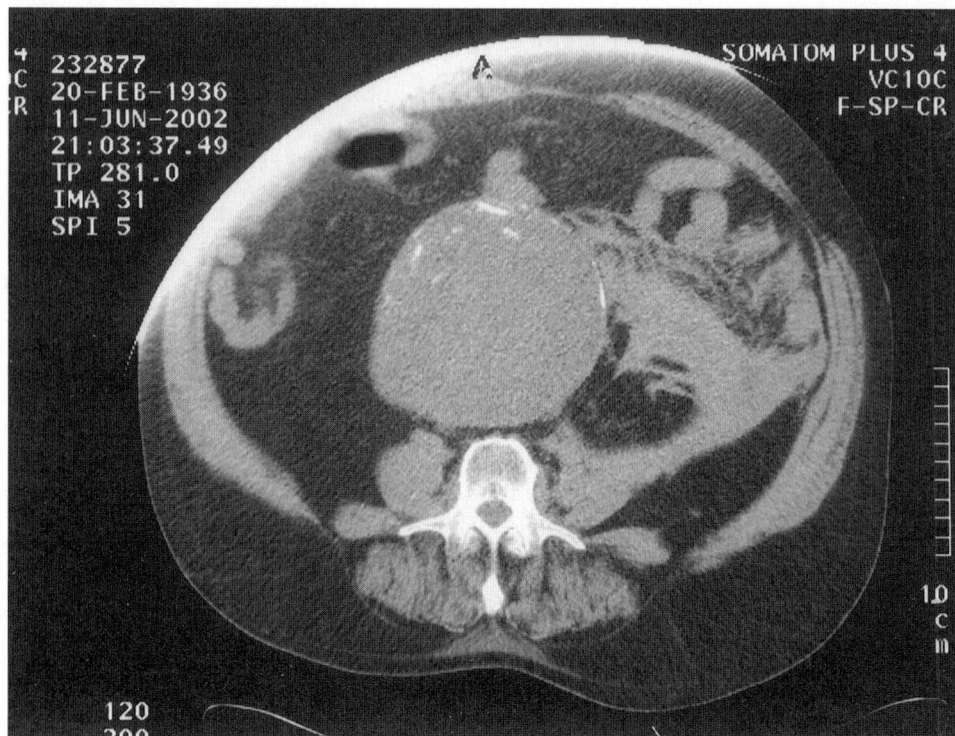

FIG. 58-3. CT scan of a patient with a 12-cm abdominal aortic aneurysm. Calcification of the wall is seen. Evidence of hemorrhage and surrounding inflammation is seen in the left side of the abdomen.

However, overly vigorous fluid resuscitation may be harmful, and the appropriate amount of intravenous fluids to be given is controversial.

Aortic Dissection

Patients with suspected aortic dissection commonly will require antihypertensive treatment, which must be provided without increasing the shear force on the intimal flap of the aorta. Therefore, medications with negative inotropic effects must be given initially. β-blockers (e.g., esmolol, metoprolol, or propranolol) are used commonly for this purpose. The optimal blood pressure is undefined and must be tailored to each patient. However, a systolic pressure of 120 to 130 mm Hg may be a convenient starting point.

Esmolol may be given as an initial bolus of 500 μg/kg over 1 min, followed by an infusion of 50 to 150 μg/kg per min. Metoprolol may be given IV in three 5-mg doses every 2 min, followed by 2 to 5 mg/h

IV infusion. Labetalol is given as an initial dose of 20 mg IV, with repeat doses of 40 to 80 mg every 10 min to desired effect or a total dose of 300 mg. Calcium channel blockers may be used if a contraindication to β-blockers is present.

Vasodilators (such as nitroprusside) may be added for further antihypertensive treatment after successful administration of a negative inotrope. Nitroprusside may be infused at an initial dose of 0.3 μg/kg per min IV. Patients should have clear evidence of adequate β-receptor or calcium channel blockade prior to starting a vasodilator. Close monitoring of the pulse rate is required because this is a convenient indicator of blockade in most patients. Aortic dissections may cause hypotension, which requires fluid or blood product resuscitation.

Rapid referral to a surgeon is mandatory. Dissections with involvement of the ascending aorta require prompt surgical repair. Patients with dissecting aneurysms of only the descending aorta are worse surgical risks, and indications for repair are controversial.

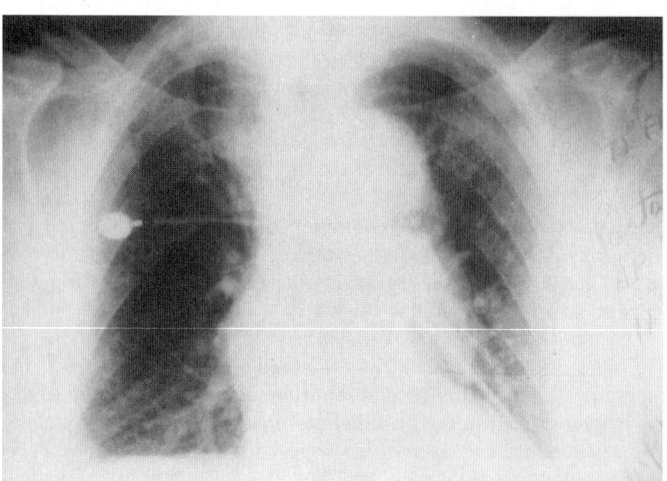

FIG. 58-4. Chest x-ray of a dissecting thoracic aneurysm.

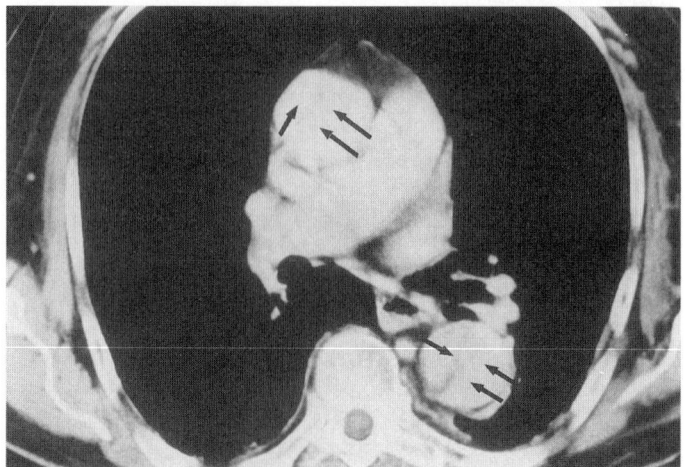

FIG. 58-5. CT scan of patient in Figure 58-3 revealing false *(double arrows)* and true aortic lumens in both ascending and descending aorta.

Asymptomatic abdominal and thoracic aortic aneurysms require prompt outpatient referral. Other interventions generally are not needed.

REFERENCES

1. Henney AM, Adiseshiah M, Poulter N, et al: Abdominal aortic aneurysm: Report of a meeting of physicians and scientists, University College London Medical School. *Lancet* 341:215, 1993.
2. Faggioli GL, Stella A, Gargiulo M, et al: Morphology of small aneurysms: Definition and impact on risk of rupture. *Am J Surg* 168:131, 1994.
3. Hagan P, Nienaber C, Isselbacher EM, et al: The International Registry of Acute Aortic Dissection (IRAD): New insights into an old disease. *JAMA* 283:897, 2000.
4. Harris JA, Kostaki G, Glover J, et al: Penetrating atherosclerotic ulcers of the aorta. *J Vasc Surg* 19:90, 1994.
5. Satta J, Laara E, Immonen K, et al: The rupture type determines the outcome for ruptured abdominal aortic aneurysm patients. *Ann Chir Gynaecol* 86:24, 1997.
6. Batounis E, Georgopoulos S, Maltezos C, et al: The validity of current vascular imaging methods in the evaluation of aortic anastomotic aneurysms developing after abdominal aortic aneurysm repair. *Ann Vasc Surg* 10:537, 1996.
7. Nevitt MP, Ballard DJ, Hallett JW Jr: Prognosis of abdominal aortic aneurysms: A population-based study. *New Engl J Med* 321:1009, 1989.
7a. Kuhn M, Bonnin RLL, Davey MJ, et al: Emergency ultrasound scanning for abdominal aortic aneurysm: Accessible accurate, and advantageous. *Ann Emerg Med* 36:219, 2000.
8. Cigarroa JE, Isselbacher EM, DeSanctis RW, et al: Medical progress: Diagnostic imaging in the evaluation of suspected aortic dissection. Old standards and new directions. *New Engl J Med* 328:35, 1993.
9. Erbel R, Engberding R, Daniel W, et al: Echocardiography in diagnosis of aortic dissection. *Lancet* 1:457, 1989.
10. Erbel R, Oelert H, Meyer J, et al: Effect of medical and surgical therapy on aortic dissection evaluated by transesophageal echocardiography: Implications for prognosis and therapy. *Circulation* 87:1604, 1993.
11. Blanchard DG, Kimura BJ, Dittrich HC, et al: Transesophageal echocardiography of the aorta. *JAMA* 272:546, 1994.
12. Hartnell G, Costello P, Goldstein S, et al: The diagnosis of thoracic aortic dissection by noninvasive imaging procedures. *New Engl J Med* 328:1637, 1993.

59

THROMBOPHLEBITIS AND OCCLUSIVE ARTERIAL DISEASE
Anil Chopra

THROMBOPHLEBITIS

Deep venous thrombosis (DVT) is a common condition, with potentially life-threatening sequelae. The true incidence, however, is not known because much of DVT is occult. The admission rate for DVT has declined greatly owing to the widespread use of newer outpatient treatments. The most common life-threatening consequence of DVT is pulmonary embolism (PE), with more than 200,000 cases diagnosed every year in the United States, and PE is associated with a 7-day mortality of 25 percent.[1] The recognition and early treatment of a presumed or known DVT is paramount to reducing the morbidity and mortality from its local and thromboembolic sequelae. Pulmonary embolism is discussed in Chap. 56.

Pathophysiology

The formation of venous clots is related to the presence of at least one of Virchow's triad of factors: venous stasis, injury to the vessel wall, and hypercoagulable state. Table 59-1 outlines the clinical risk factors predisposing to DVT, which can be remembered by the mnemonic *thrombosis;* Table 59-2 provides a detailed list of associated condi-

TABLE 59-1   Clinical Risk Factors for Deep Venous Thrombosis

T	Trauma, travel
H	Hypercoagulable, hormone replacement
R	Recreational drugs (intravenous drugs)
O	Old (age >60 y)
M	Malignancy
B	Birth control pill, blood group A
O	Obesity, obstetrics
S	Surgery, smoking
I	Immobilization
S	Sickness

tions. The highest risk of venous thrombosis occurs with major surgery or trauma, prolonged immobilization, malignancy or other hypercoagulable state, and prior thromboembolic disease. Trauma may be caused by major head injury, spinal injury, pelvic fractures, lower extremity fractures, and burns. Recent literature has suggested a fourfold increase in the incidence of DVT with travel longer than 4 h by air and land.[2] This travel risk may be related not only to immobility but also to posture, decreased fluid intake and urine output with hemoconcentration, and decreased fibrinolysis with lower ambient oxygen with air travel. Compression leg stockings, salicylic acid, and low-molecular-weight heparin (LMWH) before travel in high-risk individuals substantially reduces this risk.

The most common cause of hereditary thrombophilia is factor V Leiden due to a gene mutation on factor V. Other hypercoagulable states are listed in Table 59-2. Obstetric risk occurs not only during pregnancy but also in the postpartum period. Medications that predispose to thrombosis include second- and third-generation oral contraceptives and replacement hormones. Surgery risk is diminished with prophylactic subcutaneous unfractionated heparin (UFH), LMWH, or fondaparinux postoperatively. Illnesses with an increased risk includes myocardial infarction, congestive heart failure, cerebrovascular accident, nephrotic syndrome, inflammatory bowel disease, and vasculitis (lupus, Behçet syndrome). Presence of liver disease may decrease the risk of DVT by 90 percent.[1]

Thrombi most commonly form at the venous cusps of deep veins in the lower extremities, where altered or static blood flow initiates clot formation. Alternatively, an intimal defect anywhere along a vein resulting from injury or central catheters can be the nidus of a clot. Blood clots are composed primarily of red cells, fibrin, and platelets. An immature thrombus may propagate, dissolve, or embolize, depending on various local and systemic factors related to thrombogenesis (in particular venous stasis and activation of the coagulation pathway) and the body's defenses responsible for clot lysis (antithrombin III, protein C, plasmin, and other factors). The signs and symptoms of DVT are typically due to a partly or totally occluded vein, leading to venous outflow obstruction and/or the variable inflammatory response to a clot adhering to endothelium. Pulmonary embolism sometimes may be the first and only clinical indication of an existing DVT.

A postphlebitic syndrome (PPS) may develop after the resolution of a DVT and is related to valvular incompetence, persistent venous outflow obstruction, and abnormal microcirculation. The true incidence of PPS is unknown and depends on the criteria used for diagnosis, but studies have reported incidences of 23 percent 2 years and 28 percent 5 years after a first episode of proximal DVT.[3] There is no relation between the extent of the initial thrombosis and subsequent development of PPS.

Superficial Thrombophlebitis

Thrombosis can occur in any superficial vein. There is predilection for varicosities at the saphenous vein or its tributaries. It is a common, benign, self-limiting process but can cause significant incapacitation. Local pain, redness, and tenderness of a cord along the course of the

TABLE 59-2 **Conditions Associated with Deep Venous Thrombosis**

Hereditary
  Factor V Leiden*
  Prothrombin mutation (factor II)
  Deficiencies
    Antithrombin III
    Protein C or S
  Elevations
    Factors VIII, IX, and XI
    Fibrinogen
  Dysfibrinogenemia
  Homozygous homocysteinemia
  Polycythemia vera
  Primary thrombocytosis
General
  Age >60 y
  Blood group A
  Obesity
  Pregnancy and postpartum period
  Previous thromboembolism*
  Smoking
Acquired
  Antiphospholipid antibodies*
  Heparin-induced thrombocytopenia
  Hyperhomocysteinemia
  Hormones
    Oral contraceptives
    Replacement therapy
  Immobilization*
    Cast
    Illness
    Long travel
  Malignancy*
  Medical illness
    Congestive heart failure
    Inflammatory disease (bowel, vasculitis)
    Myocardial infarction
    Nephrotic syndrome
    Sepsis
    Stroke
  Resistance to protein C
  Surgery*
    Brain or spinal
    Extensive abdominal or pelvic
    Hip or lower extremity
    Thoracic
  Trauma*
    Brain or spinal
    Burns
    Multisystem
    Pelvic or lower extremity
  Vascular injury
    Central line
    Intravenous drugs
    Transvenous pacemaker

*Particularly high risk.

involved vein are typical findings. Bruising or bleeding may also be noted at the involved site. Doppler ultrasound may be used to confirm the diagnosis if there is any ambiguity or if an alternative diagnosis such as a DVT, cellulitis, or lymphangitis is possible. Demonstration of flow within the involved vein reliably excludes superficial venous thrombosis.

Mild cases can be treated with warm compresses, analgesia, and elastic supports for the involved extremity, with the patient continuing daily activities as tolerated. Severe thrombophlebitis, where the patient is functionally debilitated by symptoms, should be managed with periods of bedrest, elevation of the extremity, support stockings, and analgesia. Anti-inflammatory medications are commonly used to treat superficial thrombophlebitis. Antibiotics and anticoagulants are of no proven benefit unless septic thrombophlebitis is suspected, such as may occur among intravenous drug users. The incidence of DVT from extension of a superficial thrombus is about 3 percent, but the incidence of embolization is extremely low.[4] Most thromboses in the proximal greater saphenous vein that extend into the deep system will do so in 1 week. Thus, a follow-up ultrasound examination to exclude extension should occur at that time. Improvement with aggressive therapy can be painfully slow, and symptoms may persist for weeks. Definitive treatment for refractory or recurrent disease is ligation and excision of the involved vein. Patients with recurrent or migratory thrombophlebitis should be investigated to exclude a malignancy or other hypercoagulable state.

Deep Venous Thrombosis

CLINICAL FEATURES   The clinical examination is unreliable for the detection or exclusion of DVT. Suspicion of DVT by symptoms alone is sufficient to initiate objective investigations, even with a negative physical examination. The constellation of pain, redness, swelling, warmth, and tenderness is present in less than half of patients with confirmed DVT. Sensitivities are relatively poor for the presence of calf pain (66 to 91 percent), leg swelling (35 to 97 percent), and calf tenderness (56 to 82 percent).[5] The specificities of any of these findings are even poorer. Although some patients with DVT may have a low-grade fever, one should be careful to exclude an infectious process, such as cellulitis. Pain in the calf with forced dorsiflexion of the ankle and the leg straight (Homans sign) is not reliable for DVT. The physical findings with DVT depend on its location and the degree of venous obstruction, inflammation, and collateral blood flow. For example, significant iliofemoral vein occlusion can present with minimal to absent clinical findings but can result in a catastrophic PE.

Despite the problem with individual clinical findings or lack thereof, several investigators have developed instruments to risk-stratify patients suspected of having a venous thrombosis. One such clinical model developed and validated by Wells and colleagues has been shown to be reliable in predicting the probability of DVT, which was ultimately confirmed by venogram in that study group.[6] This model incorporates nine predictors (Table 59-3) to categorize patients as having a low, moderate, or high probability of DVT. With this instrument, the likelihoods of DVT are 5, 33, and 85 percent in the low (0 point), moderate (1 or 2 points), and high (≥3 points) pretest probability groups, respectively.

Symptomatic DVT will be in the popliteal or more proximal veins in more than 80 percent of cases. An isolated calf DVT will extend proxi-

TABLE 59-3 **Predictors of Deep Vein Thrombosis**

Clinical Feature	Score
Active cancer (treatment ongoing, palliative)	1
Paralysis, paresis, or recent plaster immobilization of lower extremities	1
Recently bedridden >3 d or major surgery within 4 wk	1
Localized tenderness along the distribution of the deep venous system	1
Entire leg swollen	1
Calf swelling >3 cm on the asymptomatic side (10 cm below tibial tuberosity)	1
Pitting edema confined to the symptomatic leg	1
Collateral superficial veins (non-varicose)	1
Alternative diagnosis as likely or greater than that of deep vein thrombosis	−2

Source: Wells PS, Anderson DR, Ginsberg J: Assessment of deep vein thrombosis or pulmonary embolism by the combined use of clinical model and noninvasive diagnostic tests. *Semin Thromb Hemost* 26:643, 2000.

mally only 20 percent of the time, usually within 1 week of presentation.[7] Unlike proximal DVT, nonextending calf DVT will rarely cause a PE.

Uncommon presentations of DVT include *phlegmasia cerulea dolens* (painful blue inflammation) and *phlegmasia alba dolens* ("milk leg"). In the former, the patient presents with an extensively swollen, cyanotic leg from venous engorgement due to massive iliofemoral thrombosis. This high-grade obstruction can compromise perfusion to the foot from high compartment pressures and lead to venous gangrene.[8] Petechiae and bullae may be present on the skin. *Phlegmasia alba dolens,* usually seen in association with pregnancy, is also due to massive iliofemoral thrombosis, but the patient's leg is pale or white secondary to associated arterial spasm. Dorsalis pedis and posterior tibial pulses may be diminished or absent, which can lead to a false diagnosis of arterial occlusion. The arterial spasm with milk leg is transient and often followed by venous engorgement, suggesting the correct diagnosis. Patients with large iliofemoral thromboses are at significant risk of shock, gangrene, and major PE.

The PPS is manifest by signs and symptoms that can be difficult to differentiate from recurrent DVT. Pain, swelling, and occasionally ulceration of the skin can occur months to years after the resolution of DVT. Patients with postphlebitic venous insufficiency can have an acute exacerbation of pain and swelling likely secondary to venous dilatation and hypertension. Long-term follow-up of patients reveals that the PPS can occur in up to a third of patients who have had a previous proximal or calf DVT.[3]

Diagnosis

Owing to the poor accuracy of clinical methods in identifying DVT, **all patients with any signs or symptoms suggesting DVT should undergo an objective diagnostic evaluation.** Less than one third of patients with clinically suspected DVT are found to have the disease after objective investigation.[7] Several investigative techniques are available to search for a deep thrombus, including plasma D-dimer level, impedance plethysmography (IPG), Doppler ultrasound (duplex), contrast venography, computed tomographic venography, radionuclide scintigraphy, and magnetic resonance imaging (MRI; Table 59-4).

Venography has represented the historical "gold standard" for the detection of DVT but is rarely required owing to the accuracy of noninvasive testing. It can be useful for patients with a high clinical probability of DVT when noninvasive tests are inconclusive, negative, or impossible to perform. Because it is the reference standard, venography, by definition, has a 100 percent sensitivity and specificity for detection of limb DVT. However, it is an invasive, often painful, and expensive test that is difficult to perform and may cause contrast-related reactions or iatrogenic phlebitis and DVT in about 1 to 3 percent of patients. When contrast is seen throughout the deep venous system (not possible in 5 to 10 percent of tests), a venogram reliably excludes DVT. Inadequate visualization of the deep venous system can occur due to difficulties with venous access (e.g., obesity, severe edema, and cellulitis), dilution of contrast in the proximal lower limb, or a previous thrombus. Computed tomographic venography is a more expensive but less sensitive test for DVT than plain venography or ultrasound and is not recommended.[9]

The choice test used to identify a DVT in North America is ultrasonography. Compression ultrasound (real-time B-mode imaging) produces two-dimensional images of a vein and its surrounding structures and can directly visualize a clot, whereas Doppler flow capacity, when combined with color images, provides a visual and audible evaluation of blood flow for venous obstruction. B-mode ultrasonography combined with Doppler flow is termed a *duplex*. A duplex scan with or without color flow has high sensitivity and specificity for a symptomatic, proximal DVT (clot proximal to the popliteal veins) of 97 percent and 94 percent, respectively, when compared with venography.[7] Ultrasound is less accurate for detecting pelvic DVT (see below), and its sensitivity for a calf DVT is only 73 percent. It is also often difficult to distinguish an acute from chronic DVT by ultrasound.

Compared with IPG, ultrasound has higher sensitivity and positive predictive value for DVT. Both of these tests are portable, noninvasive, operator-dependent, safe, quick, readily accessible, and provide immediate information. Ultrasound requires more expertise (due to subjective interpretation) and is more expensive, but it remains the test of choice for DVT owing to its higher accuracy. Both tests are insensitive for calf DVTs, and serial testing is required to exclude the extension of clot to proximal veins (see below). Some centers will not routinely scan the leg for a calf DVT, choosing instead to do a more time-limited study looking only for the more significant proximal clots. An additional advantage of ultrasound is its ability to detect alternative pathologies, such as a Baker cyst, hematoma, lymphadenopathy, arterial aneurysm, abscess, and superficial thrombophlebitis.

TABLE 59-4   Diagnostic Tests for DVT

	Indication	Sensitivity (Proximal DVT)	Advantage	Disadvantage
Duplex	Extremity DVT	97%	Noninvasive, portable, detects alternative etiology	Poor sensitivity for calf DVT, serial testing needed
IPG	Duplex not available	>80%	Portable, inexpensive	Poor sensitivity, false-positives, serial testing needed
Venography	Duplex inconclusive or unavailable	100%	Readily available, highly accurate, visualizes calf DVT	Invasive, painful, contrast needed, may cause phlebitis
Radionuclide studies	Inpatients with inconclusive tests and contraindication to contrast	Variable	None	Delayed results, expensive
MRI	Duplex inconclusive, suspected pelvic DVT, PE also suspected	>95%	Noninvasive, highly accurate, safe during pregnancy, detects alternative etiology, distinguishes acute from chronic DVT	Expensive, not readily available, contraindicated with ferromagnetic prosthesis
D-Dimers	Ancillary test	Variable	Readily available	Poor specificity
ELISA		97%	Highly sensitive	Expensive, time-consuming
Latex agglutination		<80%	Inexpensive	Poor sensitivity
SimpliRED		84–94%	Bedside test	Interobserver variability

Abbreviations: duplex = Doppler ultrasound; DVT = deep vein thrombosis; ELISA = enzyme-linked immunosorbent assay; IPG = impedance plethysmography; MRI = magnetic resonance imaging; PE = pulmonary embolism.

Impedance plethysmography has been rapidly supplanted by ultrasound for evaluation of patients suspected of having DVT. IPG measures changes in electrical resistance in response to changes in calf volume secondary to venous obstruction. Meta-analysis of studies has shown that IPG has a sensitivity of 73 to 96 percent, specificity of 83 to 95 percent for proximal DVT, but a high negative predictive value of about 97 percent.[5,7] False-positives can occur with PPS, abdominal or pelvic neoplasms, congestive heart failure, and pregnancy.

Radioisotopes have been used to detect DVT but are not particularly useful in the ED. Several radioisotopes are available, including [111]In- or ^{99m}Tc-labeled antifibrin monoclonal antibodies, ^{125}I-labeled fibrinogen, and ^{99m}Tc-labeled red blood cells or macroaggregated albumin. These radioisotopes are incorporated into actively forming thrombi and can be detected by scanning the extremity hours or days after injection. The sensitivity of this technique is poor for proximal DVT, in particular pelvic veins, but about 90 percent for calf DVT, although with a high false-positive rate. Radioisotope evaluation for DVT is reserved primarily for inpatient assessment of diagnostically difficult patients with indeterminate results from other noninvasive tests and positive D-dimers. Radionuclide venography is expensive; time-consuming, results are not available for 24 to 72 h; and is not as accurate as IPG or a duplex for proximal DVT.

Magnetic resonance imaging is being recommended with increasing frequency as the alternative gold standard to venography for imaging the venous system. It is at least as accurate as any other investigational modality and can detect a filling defect in the entire extremity (including calf veins) and pelvic veins, which are not well visualized by ultrasonography or even venography. It is noninvasive, relatively fast, uses no ionizing radiation or contrast material, can distinguish acute from chronic DVT, and can be used to detect thromboembolic disease in pregnancy. An MRI visualizes both extremities simultaneously and can identify alternative causes of extremity swelling, such as cysts, aneurysms, hematomas, tumors, superficial phlebitis, joint effusions, and other masses. Some of the limitations of MRI include its cost, lack of ready availability, lack of portability, and inability to be used in patients harboring ferromagnetic objects (e.g., prostheses and pacemakers).

Recent literature has reported the usefulness of magnetic resonance direct thrombus imaging. This modality allows for direct visualization of the clot rather than of a filling defect. Magnetic resonance direct thrombus imaging detects methemoglobin in the thrombus and distinguishes it from blood and fat without the use of intravenous contrast. With an overall sensitivity of 95 percent for DVT compared with venography (91 percent for calf DVT), it can detect iliofemoral DVT with nearly 100 percent accuracy (compared with venography).[10] As MRI scanning becomes more available and accessible, and scanning speed increases, its associated costs are likely to decline, making it a more attractive tool for DVT detection.

D-Dimer fragments, which are degradation products of fibrin, can be measured as an indicator of the presence or absence of DVT or PE. The reference standard against which all other assays are compared is the quantitative enzyme-linked immunosorbent assay (ELISA). Based on numerous studies, this test has a *mean* sensitivity of 97 percent and specificity of 35 percent for proximal DVT.[11] In low-risk patients, the sensitivity is 99 percent. At a discriminate level of less than 500 ng/mL (μg/L) by ELISA, the likelihood of DVT is less than 1 percent, so it is helpful to exclude a venous thrombosis, but the test is expensive and takes several hours to perform. This limits the usefulness of the standard ELISA as a practical ED tool. To overcome this shortcoming, newer rapid quantitative and qualitative ELISA are now available that have similar sensitivities as the standard ELISA, but with a turnaround time of less than 1 h. A second type of D-dimer assay, latex agglutination, is rapid and inexpensive, but not clinically useful due to a sensitivity of less than 80 percent for detecting DVT.[6] All D-dimer assays are fairly nonspecific tests, as many other conditions, such as sepsis, surgery, trauma, hemorrhage, pregnancy, cardiovascular disease (myo-

cardial infarction, stroke), collagen vascular disease, liver disease, and cancer, are associated with an elevated level. Therefore, it follows that **a D-dimer level is useful only when it is low.**

The most common D-dimer assays recently studied are the third type based on whole blood agglutination. A particularly popular bedside assay, SimpliRED, uses monoclonal antibodies directed against D-dimer and red blood cell surface. This test requires only a drop of blood and provides a result in less than 5 min. The sensitivity of this assay in clinical trials has varied between 84 and 94 percent.[6] A notable concern with qualitative bedside tests such as the SimpliRED is the potential for interobserver variability due to ambiguity in interpretation of a visual marking. The Joint Commission on the Accreditation of Healthcare Organizations also requires strict quality control for bedside testing.

Clinical Approach to Establishing the Diagnosis

Assessing the pretest clinical probability with a validated instrument such as the Wells model (see Table 59-3) allows for accurate risk stratification of patients and helps guide an appropriate diagnostic strategy. Serial testing and the combination of tests have become the norm in many institutions and are supported by numerous proposed algorithms in the literature. However, the approach at any given institution is dependent on availability of resources, physicians' preferences, and local expertise.

Figure 59-1 outlines a practical, cost-effective approach to diagnosing DVT. Some basic assumptions and facts were used in the formulation of this algorithm. Because the diagnosis of DVT is difficult to establish based solely on history or physical examination, some type of objective testing is necessary. Unless a rapid ELISA D-dimer assay is readily available, a duplex scan will be required as the initial imaging of choice. In low- to moderate-risk patients, a negative ELISA accurately excludes DVT, with a negative predictive value above 99 percent.[11] Use of the SimpliRED test alone to exclude DVT in low-risk patients is controversial and not universally accepted due to variable sensitivities reported in the literature. A recent study did indicate a 100 percent negative predictive value of the SimpliRED assay in low-risk emergency patients, but the prevalence of DVT was only 13 percent in the study population.[12] Patients with a negative duplex scan can be managed in a variety of ways: (1) no further testing in low-risk patients, (2) D-dimer assay (whole blood agglutination or ELISA), or (3) repeat duplex in 1 week. An initial negative duplex scan in low-risk patients or two negative duplex scans 1 week apart carry a less than 1 percent risk of symptomatic proximal DVT or PE at 3 months

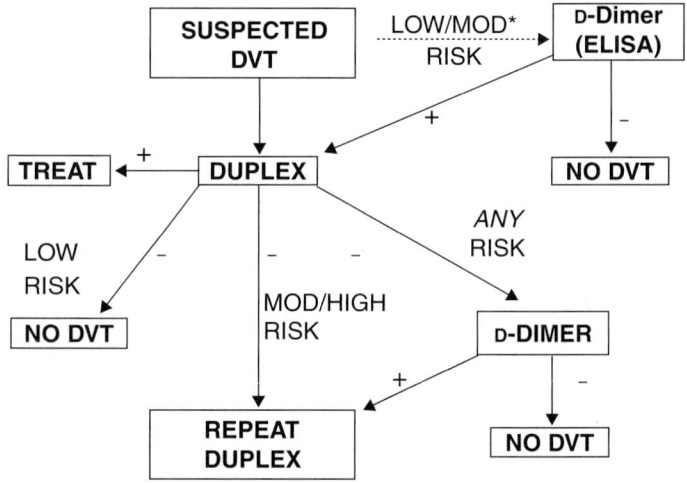

FIG. 59-1. Diagnosis of deep vein thrombosis (DVT). *If available and rapid. Duplex = Doppler ultrasound; ELISA = enzyme-linked immunosorbent assay.

follow-up.[6,12] Serial duplex scanning, however, is costly and inconvenient for patients with a positive yield of only 1 percent for proximal DVT if all patients with an initial negative ultrasound are rescanned. The negative predictive value of a low D-dimer assay and negative initial duplex scan or IPG is 99 percent or greater for proximal DVT and only slightly lower for calf DVT.[6,7,13]

In patients with risk factors and in whom duplex or IPG is positive, anticoagulation therapy may be initiated, if there are no contraindications. If the diagnosis is equivocal or there is potential for false-positive or false-negative results, contrast venography or MRI can be performed.

Treatment

Traditional therapeutic measures, including bed rest, continuous leg elevation, and elastic stockings, are of unproven benefit when used in addition to anticoagulation in the management of a DVT. Aggressive anticoagulation will prevent extension of clot and allow for its lysis by the intrinsic fibrinolytic pathways. Early ambulation with appropriate analgesia, as needed, after adequate anticoagulation with heparin is a practical and safe approach. The PPS can be treated with periodic leg elevation, compression stockings, and pain medications, as required.

Prevention of PE is the primary objective in treating DVT. Several studies have documented the accuracy of serial duplex examinations and the safety of withholding anticoagulation in patients clinically suspected of having DVT but with a normal initial ultrasound.[6,7,13] A repeat duplex should be done in these patients 7 days after initial examination. If the second duplex scan is negative, the patient need not be imaged again unless symptoms or signs progress. The risk of a PE within 7 days of a normal duplex scan in patients with symptoms of DVT of the lower extremity is nearly zero. The probability of detecting a proximal DVT on a second ultrasound when there is a normal duplex scan from the week before is approximately 1 percent.[11] Subsequent thromboembolism (typically nonfatal) within 3 months of two normal serial duplex studies occurs in about 0.6 percent of patients, which is comparable to the outcome in patients with normal venograms.[13] Thus, withholding anticoagulation in patients with negative serial ultrasounds is safe, accurate, and cost-effective. However, anticoagulation is recommended for nonextending calf DVT in high-risk groups such as patients with a history of a previous proximal DVT or PE, significant cardiovascular comorbidity (higher risk of fatal PE), a persistent hypercoagulable state, or continued immobilization.

Proven proximal DVT requires immediate anticoagulation to reduce local morbidity and prevent thromboembolism. The preferred treatment is LMWH, such as ardeparin, dalteparin, enoxaparin, nadroparin, reviparin, or tinzaparin. These are *weight adjusted* and given once or twice daily subcutaneously until oral anticoagulation reaches the therapeutic range. The three most commonly used LMWHs for treatment of DVT in North America are dalteparin (200 units/kg every 24 h; maximum, 18,000 units), enoxaparin (1.5 mg/kg every 24 h; maximum, 180 mg), and tinzaparin (175 units/kg every 24 h; maximum, 18,000 units), with dosage based on actual rather than on ideal body weight. The available LMWH agents are *not* simply interchangeable due to differing pharmacokinetic and pharmacodynamic profiles. Despite the recommended maximum daily doses by the manufacturers of these drugs, it is not uncommon for physicians to use higher doses for overweight patients. These drugs have several advantages over UFH, including a more predictable anticoagulant effect, ease of administration, longer half-life, lack of a need to monitor the anticoagulation effect, and a lower incidence of major bleeding and heparin-induced thrombocytopenia (HIT).[14] Low-molecular-weight heparin has a preferential inhibitory effect on factor Xa rather than on factor IIa (thrombin), and the partial thromboplastin time (PTT) cannot be used to monitor its effect. Measurement of anti-Xa levels is expensive, not readily available,

and unnecessary given the very predictable effect of these heparins. However, because all LMWHs are cleared by the kidneys, there is a prolonged effect, with a higher risk of bleeding in renal failure patients unless anti-Xa levels are closely monitored. For this reason, LMWH generally should be avoided in outpatients with a creatinine level higher than 180 μmol/L (2.03 mg/dL). These patients will require UFH or dose adjustments of LMWH based on anti-Xa levels. Reviparin need not be adjusted in renal patients if given in standard prophylactic doses. **One need not wait for the creatinine result before initiating LMWH therapy,** but subsequent doses should be adjusted with evidence of renal insufficiency.

The once-daily use of LMWH in outpatient treatment has revolutionized the management of DVT and is at least as effective and safe as UFH in the treatment of DVT or PE.[14] Several meta-analyses comparing intravenous UFH with subcutaneous LMWH for treatment of DVT have noted a lower mortality, less major bleeding, reduction in clot extension, and fewer recurrent thromboembolic events in favor of LMWH.[15] The ability to discharge most patients home from the ED after an initial dose of LMWH with next-day follow-up is clearly a safe, practical, and cost-effective strategy that is acceptable to the vast majority of physicians and patients. The treatment plan must be discussed with the continuing care physician, including follow-up in 24 h and institution of warfarin at the same time as LMWH. The patient or the caregiver also will require education regarding administration of LMWH. This can be done during the follow-up visit.

Indications for admission include instability to ambulate, poor social support, unreliable follow-up, difficulty with education for drug administration, need for lytic or invasive therapy, and an alternative serious diagnosis under investigation or that requires treatment (e.g., arterial ischemia, cellulitis, or pelvic mass).

If LMWH is not available or contraindicated, a continuous infusion of UFH can be started until LMWH is initiated or oral anticoagulation reaches therapeutic levels. Weight-adjusted dosing of 80 units/kg bolus followed by an infusion of 18 units/kg per h will rapidly achieve a therapeutic activated PTT (aPTT). (Traditional dosing of a 5000-units bolus followed by an infusion of 1000 units per h will result in subtherapeutic aPTT at 6 h in two thirds of treated patients.) The infusion is adjusted to keep the aPTT between 55 and 80 s (1.5 to 2.5 times normal).

Close monitoring of patients is required to detect bleeding, HIT, and thrombosis. Serious bleeding due to LMWH is very unusual, but, if it occurs, the anti-Xa effect cannot be completely reversed. Protamine can counteract the minor antithrombin effect of LMWH and has been useful to reverse bleeding complications, although its use has been associated with hypotension and anaphylactoid reactions. In the uncommon scenario when heparin is contraindicated in the acute management of DVT, as in patients with HIT, a thrombin inhibitor, such as lepirudin, is an effective alternative. Lepirudin is administered as a 0.4-mg/kg slow bolus over 15 to 20 s (maximum, 44 mg), reduced in half for renal patients. Subsequent infusion is 0.1 to 0.15 mg/kg per h (maximum, 11 mg per h) to keep PPT at 1.5 to 2.5 times normal. In pregnant patients, danaparoid is the preferred agent when heparin cannot be used (1500 to 2250 units SC every 12 h). **Monitoring is not required except in the presence of renal disease.**

It is a common and accepted practice to start heparin (including LMWH[16]) and warfarin simultaneously, because early warfarin administration has been shown to be safe and effective. The procoagulant effect before reduction of prothrombin concentrations, particularly in patients with protein C or S deficiency, is controlled by the simultaneous administration of heparin. A loading dose of warfarin is unnecessary. An initial daily dose of 5 mg of warfarin is adjusted to maintain the INR between 2 and 3. A lower initial dose of warfarin may be used in the elderly (4 mg) and in patients with liver disease or at higher risk of bleeding. Heparin is typically continued until the INR is in the therapeutic range for 2 consecutive days (usually 5 to 7 days).

Warfarin is associated with some serious potential adverse effects and should not be used in certain circumstances. The most common adverse effect is bleeding, usually related to the degree of anticoagulation, and typically responds to dose reduction. Skin necrosis secondary to warfarin occurs primarily in patients with a deficiency of protein C or S. The necrosis is due to thrombotic occlusion of small vessels, usually 3 to 8 days after initiation of this drug. Warfarin is contraindicated in patients who are pregnant, have a serious or active bleeding diathesis, or have had very recent major surgery (thoracoabdominal, nervous system, spine, or eye). It causes fetal bleeding and is teratogenic. (Neither UFH nor LMWH crosses the placenta, and both are safe for the fetus.) Low-molecular-weight heparin is the preferred drug for the treatment of a DVT in pregnancy and is continued until delivery. Warfarin can be safely started in the postpartum period, even in breast-feeding women, and is usually continued for 4 to 8 weeks.[17]

The duration of warfarin treatment has to be individualized and depends on a history of previous DVT or PE, reversibility of previous thromboembolic risk factors, the effectiveness of warfarin to resolve thrombosis, and the risk of bleeding. Oral anticoagulation should be continued for 3 months for patients with proximal DVT when reversible risk factors are identified. There is no evidence that a longer course of warfarin is needed for patients with PE. For patients with idiopathic DVT or recurrent thromboembolic disease, prolonged anticoagulation for at least 6 months is recommended.[18] Life-long anticoagulation may be necessary in patients with ongoing risk factors, such as hypercoagulable states and malignancy. The recurrence of thromboembolic disease is related to patient-specific risk factors but is estimated to be 6 percent at 1 year and 13 percent at 5 years, despite adequate anticoagulation therapy for the initial DVT. Patients who present with a new or progressive clot despite adequate anticoagulation with warfarin should have LMWH initiated and be investigated for a hypercoagulable state on an urgent outpatient basis. Warfarin resistance is commonly seen in patients with metastatic disease.

The issue of initiating anticoagulation and interference with evaluation for possible hypercoagulability occasionally arises. Because **LMWH does not alter the ability to investigate hypercoagulable states,** there is no need to procure additional blood samples beyond routine coagulation studies in patients with a straightforward DVT. Further, acute-phase reactants can alter blood results with an acute DVT or PE. Initiation of UFH therapy is likely to interfere with the evaluation of hypercoagulability. However, such investigations for the underlying etiology of a DVT typically do not alter management. Thus, patients may be investigated at a later date, when anticoagulation is completed. When a patient is seen in follow-up, hematologic testing includes factor V Leiden, prothrombin molecular tests, screening for antiphospholipid anticoagulants, and a fasting homocysteine level. Upon completion of anticoagulation, further evaluation includes antithrombin III, protein C, protein S, and factor VIII levels, plus other patient-specific tests, as required. When a patient presents with a refractory or progressive clot despite warfarin treatment, LMWH should be initiated, and an urgent referral to a hematologist is necessary. If, for some reason, UFH is used to treat a patient with warfarin-refractory DVT, then at least two extra blood tubes should be obtained before initiation of treatment, and those samples should be held for further testing by the hematologist.

Thrombolytic and Mechanical Therapy

Currently, no controlled clinical trials have shown a survival benefit of thrombolytics over heparin and warfarin. Despite the fact that thrombolysis results in better early vein patency and venous valve integrity, a reduction in the risk of PPS is unproven.[19] In practice, thrombolytic drugs are rarely used to treat DVT. Thrombolytics have a significantly greater bleeding risk, including fatal intracerebral hemorrhage, than does heparin or warfarin. There is a greater risk of bleeding with thrombolytic use in DVT than in myocardial infarction, likely related to the longer duration of therapy for DVT. The appropriate role of catheter-directed therapy in DVT is unknown, because adequate studies have not been done, but appears reasonable for patients with *phlegmasia cerulea dolens.*

Thrombolysis for DVT, in general, can be considered for extensive iliofemoral thrombosis and upper extremity DVT in patients with a low risk of bleeding. A standard systemic regimen of streptokinase is a loading dose of 250,000 units over 30 min, followed by an infusion of 100,000 units per h for 72 h. For alteplase (tPA), infusions of 0.05 to 0.5 mg/kg per h have been used for variable lengths of time, from hours to days.[19] Catheter-directed thrombolysis with a catheter placed in the popliteal or femoral vein can be done with a tPA bolus of 2 to 10 mg followed by an infusion of 1 to 4 mg per h for 4 to 12 h. Unfractionated heparin should not be given with streptokinase but is optional concurrently with tPA infusions.

An inferior vena cava filter can be placed to prevent a PE when oral anticoagulation is contraindicated, a major complication of anticoagulation occurs (e.g. bleeding, HIT), a DVT persists or propagates despite adequate medical treatment, or embolization occurs after 1 to 2 weeks of therapeutic anticoagulation. Given the ease of insertion, low complication rate, and greater than 95 percent patency rate of a Greenfield filter at 1 year after placement, its indications may be expanded. A free-floating, nonadherent iliofemoral thrombus larger than 5 cm has an up to 60 percent chance of forming a PE; in such cases, filter placement should be considered. These devices reduce the rate of PE but have not been shown to improve early or late survival. After filter placement, there is risk of recurrent DVT unless anticoagulation is initiated.

Surgical thrombectomy was enthusiastically received in previous decades, but owing to high rates of rethrombosis and failure to prevent postphlebitic sequelae, it is rarely considered today. When conventional therapy for DVT is contraindicated or ineffective, thrombectomy followed by heparin and warfarin can achieve long-term patency. Surgical treatment of a DVT is typically reserved for patients when limb viability is jeopardized by a massive venous clot, such as a persistently ischemic leg secondary to *phlegmasia cerulea dolens.*

The ED management of patients who are adequately anticoagulated but present with propagation or a new clot is fairly straightforward. These patients should be started on LMWH with urgent follow-up (or, if otherwise indicated, admission). If they fail LMWH or have large free-floating thrombi, a Greenfield filter should be emergently placed by an interventional radiologist or vascular surgeon. The investigation of these patients for a hypercoagulable state or malignancy need not be initiated in the ED. There is no evidence in the literature that increasing anticoagulation beyond an INR of 3 is effective in treating refractory DVT.

Pelvic Vein Thrombosis

Thrombosis of the pelvic veins typically occurs as an extension from the femoral vein. An isolated pelvic vein clot is extremely uncommon but can occur as a complication in the postpartum period, with pelvic inflammatory disease, and after pelvic surgery or trauma. Clinical presentation of an isolated pelvic vein thrombosis can be difficult to recognize, because the patient may present with nonspecific abdominal symptoms of pain and vomiting without any significant leg findings. Septic pelvic vein thrombophlebitis is a rare but life-threatening condition that may occur with postpartum endometritis and can lead to septic pulmonary emboli. Diagnosis can be difficult because ultrasound and even contrast venography are less accurate than MR venography and computed tomography (CT) with contrast. Treatment of pelvic vein thrombosis is similar to therapy for lower extremity DVT, and surgical clot evacuation is usually unnecessary except in cases of associated pelvic infection.

Axillary and Subclavian Vein Thromboses

Although up to 90 percent of all DVTs occur in the lower extremities, 2 to 4 percent develop in the axillary or subclavian vein. The risk factors for developing a venous thrombus in the upper extremity are outlined in Table 59-2, with a higher incidence being associated with current or recent central venous catheters or transvenous pacemakers, intravenous drug use, excessive or unusual exercise (effort thrombosis), malignancy, and other hypercoagulable states. A predisposing venous stricture or chronic compression (cervical rib, hypertrophied scalene muscle, congenital web, etc.) is commonly detected as a causal factor. Presentation can be an abrupt or gradual onset of swelling in the arm, associated with dilated veins in the hand and forearm. The arm may feel heavy, with pain on physical activity that is relieved with rest. Sudden onset of severe pain and swelling with a change in the color of the arm is a rare presentation. The initial imaging study for investigating a suspected venous thrombosis of an upper limb is by duplex scanning, which has a sensitivity of 56 to 100 percent.[20] Venography or MRI may be required when there is high clinical suspicion of DVT, despite a negative duplex.

It is estimated that a PE occurs in 5 to 10 percent of cases involving axillary or subclavian DVTs, although a rate as high as 36 percent has been reported with catheter-associated upper extremity DVT.[5] Current treatment options include anticoagulation alone or preceded by catheter-directed thrombolysis. The choice of therapy should be discussed with the consulting vascular surgeon and invasive radiologist but should be individualized. The underlying cause, duration of symptoms, comorbidity, and contraindications to thrombolytic agents or anticoagulants can help guide the choice of the most appropriate therapy. Resolution of symptoms and signs depends not only on therapy but also on the development of collateral flow. After initial therapy, an underlying compressive abnormality or venous stenosis, if present, must be corrected (e.g., rib resection and balloon angioplasty).

OCCLUSIVE ARTERIAL DISEASE

Acute limb ischemia secondary to thrombosis or embolism is a true emergency requiring immediate therapy to salvage the limb. Despite improvements in management, mortality is in excess of 25 percent, and amputation is required in 20 percent of survivors. The emergency physician must urgently initiate treatment and investigation of a threatened limb in collaboration with the radiologist and vascular surgeon. An understanding of the pathophysiology, etiology, and clinical pre-sentation of peripheral vascular disease will help guide management in the effort to restore blood flow to the affected limb.

Epidemiology

Intermittent claudication has a prevalence of between 2 and 6 percent for men older than 55 years. With objective noninvasive testing, however, peripheral arterial disease is noted in 11 to 27 percent of elderly men and women equally.[21] Symptoms of this disease increase with age and are two to four times more common in men than in women. Most of these patients have a long history of smoking, although diabetes, hyperlipidemia, hypertension, and hyperhomocysteinemia are significant risk factors. There has been an increase in the incidence of chronic limb ischemia and arterial embolic disease in the past two decades. At least half of these patients have coronary or cerebrovascular disease. The severity of peripheral vascular disease is closely linked to the risk of myocardial infarction, ischemic stroke, and death from vascular disease.[21] The most frequently diseased arteries leading to limb ischemia include, in order of occurrence, femoropopliteal and tibial, aortoiliac, and brachiocephalic vessels. Embolic occlusion of an artery also occurs primarily in elderly men and postmenopausal women, given the higher prevalence in this group of heart disease, which is the major source of thromboemboli.

Pathophysiology

Acute limb ischemia results from a blood supply that is inadequate to meet tissue oxygen and nutrient requirements. Ultimately, it will lead to cell death and irreversible tissue damage. Even after perfusion is partly or completely restored, reperfusion injury can occur as oxygen radicals form and cause further cell injury. Reperfusion may not be fully attainable with prolonged arterial obstruction due to distal edema and thrombi forming in the microcirculation. The extent of injury depends on the duration and location of the arterial blockage, the amount of collateral flow, and the previous health of the involved limb. Also, some tissues are more susceptible than others to anoxia, presumably on the basis of differences in cellular respiration and oxygen requirements. Peripheral nerves and skeletal muscle are very sensitive to ischemia, and irreversible changes occur in these tissues within 6 h of anoxia at room temperature.

Nonembolic limb ischemia is secondary to atherosclerosis in the vast majority of patients. Plaque formation within the intima of an artery results from lipid accumulation, proliferation of smooth muscle cells, and fibrogenesis. Further narrowing of the vascular lumen occurs with progression of the atheromatous plaque. Complete or high-grade obstruction can occur at this site of stenosis secondary to plaque rupture or endothelial erosion, which triggers a thrombus formation. Progression of ischemic injury can occur through several mechanisms: (1) propagation of clot to occlude collateral vessels, (2) ischemia-related distal edema leading to high compartment pressures (compartment syndrome), (3) fragmentation of clot into the microcirculation, and (4) edema of the microvasculature cells. Obstruction of the microvasculature can result in distal perfusion impairment despite successful large vessel reperfusion. Uncommonly, arterial thrombosis is noted in an apparently normal vessel with absence of a preexisting atherosclerotic plaque prompting a hypercoagulable workup, but subclinical injury or early atherosclerosis may still underline these events.

An atherosclerotic vessel can give rise to an aneurysm because of its weakened walls. A true aneurysm, involving dilatation of its entire wall, can present clinically with thrombosis, rupture, and hemorrhaging or by its mass effect on adjacent structures.

Etiology

Contrary to previous thought, the recent literature indicates that thrombotic occlusion is a significantly more common cause of acute limb ischemia than is embolism. In the lower limbs, embolic occlusion accounts for fewer than 20 percent of all cases.[22] In the upper limbs, most cases of acute limb ischemia are thrombotic and about one third are due to embolism and nearly one fourth secondary to arteritis.[23] Nevertheless, the distinction between a thrombotic and embolic etiology in any given patient is fraught with inaccuracy. Bypass graft thrombosis is occuring with increasing frequency as the rate of revascularization procedures increase for chronic lower limb ischemia.

Emboli originate from the heart in 80 to 90 percent of cases. Atrial fibrillation is associated with at least two thirds of all peripheral emboli, and clot is found most commonly in the left atrial appendage. Mural thrombus in the ventricle after recent myocardial infarction is the second most frequent source, accounting for about 20 percent of all limb emboli. With adequate anticoagulation, the incidence of an embolus originating from a mechanical valve has greatly diminished. Rare cardiac sources of emboli include tumor emboli from atrial myxomas, vegetations from valve leaflets, and parts of prosthetic devices, such as mechanical valves.

Noncardiac sources of arterial emboli include thrombi from aneurysms and atheromatous plaques. Mural thrombus in aneurysms of aortoiliac, femoral, popliteal, and subclavian arteries are the most notable sources. Atheroemboli result from plaque fragmentation and cause obstruction of the microcirculation, thereby producing symptoms in the feet ("blue toe syndrome"), hands, or cerebral circulation (transient ischemic attack). Iatrogenic embolization during angiographic procedures of the aorta and larger vessels is another likely source of atheroemboli and can be showered to multiple parts of the body. In addition, paradoxical embolization can occur when a venous clot passes from the right to the left side of the heart through an intracardiac shunt, most commonly a patent foramen ovale.

The natural history of an embolus is to fragment and embolize distally or to propagate locally into a larger clot, although associated venous thrombosis can occur, possibly secondary to local ischemia, decreased venous flow, and inflammation. Two thirds of all noncerebral emboli enter vessels of the lower limbs and locate where vessels branch or taper. The most common location for an embolus in the leg is the bifurcation of the common femoral artery followed by the popliteal artery. In the upper limb, the brachial artery is the most common location for an embolism to lodge.

Thrombosis unrelated to atherosclerotic disease can occur at an area of vessel injury, as with invasive catheters, balloons, sites of bypass grafting, or intraarterial drug injection, and with hypercoagulable states. All are potential sources of embolization. Femoral artery catheterization for coronary angiography or angioplasty and vascular access can result in ischemia of an extremity secondary to thrombosis or expanding hematoma; symptoms may be altered by preexisting aortoiliac or femoropopliteal plaques. Radial artery injury during blood gas analysis or the placement of arterial lines rarely leads to tissue ischemia, given the excellent collateral supply from the ulnar artery. Intentional or accidental intraarterial drug injections by medical personnel or for illicit drugs can result in local vasospasm, infectious arteritis, thrombosis, pseudoaneurysms, and mycotic aneurysms. Inert particles or drug crystals can embolize to obstruct end arteries, leading to gangrene of digits, especially as drug users tend to delay seeking medical attention.

Peripheral arterial supply also can be obstructed by vasospastic or inflammatory conditions. *Raynaud disease* involves vasospasm in small arteries and arterioles in response to a stressor, such as cold temperature or emotional stress. Symptoms of local pain, pallor followed by cyanosis, numbness, and paresthesias usually involve the fingers and hands and generally resolve within 30 to 60 min, especially with rewarming. Inflammation of arteries in the limb can occur with collagen vascular diseases, such as rheumatoid arthritis, lupus, and polyarteritis nodosa. When clinically active, these vasculitides are often associated with systemic symptoms and multiorgan involvement. Necrosis of blood vessels and loss of limb tissue is always a possibility. *Thromboangiitis obliterans* (Buerger disease) is an idiopathic occlusive disease resulting from segmental inflammation of arteries in all extremities. It occurs almost exclusively in young smokers (age 20 to 40 years), predominantly males, and is characterized by painful, tender nodules in the limbs with decreased distal flow.

Limb ischemia may occur with nonembolic central causes. A thoracic aortic dissection can propagate into the carotid, subclavian, and iliofemoral systems and present with neurologic and extremity findings. The false lumen created by the dissection occludes flow in the involved artery. *Takayasu arteritis,* which primarily occurs in Asian females, involves the aortic arch and its branches and has a "pulseless phase" when peripheral ischemia and necrosis can develop.

More commonly, low cardiac output states with cardiogenic or hypovolemic shock may present with extremity ischemia in the presence of previous existing arterial disease. Severe left ventricular dysfunction, which can occur with ischemic cardiomyopathy, valvular heart disease, and cardiac tamponade, acutely threatens limb blood flow, particularly in elderly patients with preexisting atherosclerosis. Acute hemorrhage similarly reduces perfusion to the limbs but, with acute intervention, may be reversible.

Clinical Features

Patients with acute limb ischemia will exhibit one or more of the "six Ps": pain, pallor, polar (for cold), pulselessness, paresthesias, and paralysis. However, a lack of one or more of these findings does not exclude ischemia. Further, total occlusion of a severely diseased artery in patients with peripheral vascular disease with well-developed collateral blood supply may not be a dramatic event and is occasionally silent. Pain alone may be the earliest symptom of ischemia, localized in the limb distal to the site of obstruction. High clinical suspicion is paramount to early intervention to save a limb. Complete arterial obstruction results in visible skin changes, with initial pallor that may be followed by blotchy, mottled areas of cyanosis and associated petechiae and blisters. Livedo reticulosis may be evident. Severe, steady pain in the involved extremity associated with decreased skin temperature is expected. Hypoesthesia or hyperesthesia due to ischemic neuropathy is typically an early finding, as is muscle weakness. An absent palpable pulse distal to the arterial obstruction is not very helpful. It may be an abrupt new sign of an occlusive clot or a longstanding finding of chronic vascular disease. However, an abrupt loss of a previously strong pulse strongly suggests an embolus. As ischemic injury progresses, anesthesia and paralysis become evident and foreshadow impending gangrene. Preservation of light touch on skin testing is a good guide to tissue viability. Necrosis of skin and fat is a late finding.

Despite the generally held belief that limb salvage is possible with reperfusion within 4 to 6 h, tissue loss can occur with significantly shorter occlusion times. As important, mild to severe limb dysfunction is possible even with an injury involving only brief anoxia, with potential for lasting disability. The poor predictability of functional outcome after ischemic injury underscores the need to attain rapid reperfusion and not rely on a probable safe interval until resolution of occlusion. Disability and tissue loss are inevitable after 6 h of occlusive anoxic injury.

Microemboli present clinically with pain and cyanosis in the involved digit, petechiae, and local muscle pain and tenderness at the site of infarction. Several different small areas can be affected with a shower of microemboli originating from a large or unstable source. Although mottling and decreased function may occur, pulses are preserved.

Chronic peripheral arterial insufficiency is characterized by intermittent claudication, which may progress to intermittent ischemic pain at rest. Femoral and popliteal disease often causes reproducible calf pain with activity that is relieved with rest. Pain at rest typically localizes to the foot and is aggravated by leg elevation, improves with standing, and is poorly controlled with analgesics. Shiny, hyperpigmented skin with hair loss and ulceration, thickened nails, muscle atrophy, vascular bruits, and poor pulses are the hallmark of chronic vascular disease. Complete arterial occlusion from thrombosis of a limb in these patients may present subacutely owing to a well-developed collateral circulation.

Diagnosis

Clinical evaluation is the most useful diagnostic tool for the assessment of occlusive arterial disease. A history of an abruptly ischemic limb in a patient with atrial fibrillation or recent myocardial infarction is strongly suggestive of an embolus. Acute ischemia in the limb of a patient known to have advanced peripheral vascular disease is more likely due to thrombosis or a low cardiac output state. In a patient with embolic obstruction, it is unusual to have a history of claudication, and an examination of the uninvolved limb often reveals no evidence of occlusive disease.

At the bedside, blanching the involved extremity with finger pressure and noting a delay in the return of blood as compared with the uninvolved extremity indicates decreased perfusion. However, several factors can influence capillary refill; thus, one cannot rely on the presence or absence of this finding alone.

A hand-held Doppler can document the amplitude of flow or its absence when held over the dorsalis pedis, posterior tibial, popliteal, or femoral arteries in the lower limb and over the radial, ulnar, brachial, or axillary arteries in the arm. If Doppler flow is detected in the affected limb, an ankle-brachial index (ABI) and segmental leg pressures should be checked. The ABI is the ratio of the systolic blood pressure with the cuff just above the malleoli (with the Doppler probe over the posterior tibial or dorsalis pedis artery) to the brachial pressure in the arm. Patients with chronic peripheral vascular disease have an ABI less than 1.0. With acute arterial obstruction, there is a significant difference in the ABI of the involved (usually <0.5) and uninvolved lower extremities. Segmental blood pressures with Doppler on the posterior tibial or dorsalis pedis and the cuff placed below the knee, above the knee, and high thigh are also useful. **A difference of 30 mm Hg or more between any adjacent levels accurately localizes the site of obstruction.** With successful reperfusion, the ABI and segmental pressures begin to return to baseline or normalize if no residual obstruction remains after clot dissolution.

If time permits or the diagnosis of arterial occlusion is in question, duplex ultrasonography can be undertaken to detect an obstruction to flow. It is very accurate for detecting obstruction in the common femoral, superficial femoral, and popliteal vessels and at previous bypass grafts. Sensitivity declines for localization of thromboembolic occlusion at calf level and below. In patients with severe peripheral vascular disease (PVD), duplex ultrasonography can detect even incomplete obstruction with a sensitivity greater than 85 percent. Similarly, duplex ultrasonography has high sensitivity for detecting obstruction in the axillary, subclavian, and brachial arteries. Nevertheless, the diagnostic modality of choice is usually arteriography. Cardiac monitoring and an electrocardiogram will detect a dysrhythmia, and an echocardiogram can be done to look for an intracardiac thrombus, if such is clinically suspected.

In consultation with a vascular surgeon and during the period of preoperative and/or medical management, an arteriogram can be done to confirm the diagnosis, define the vascular anatomy and perfusion, and guide aggressive management. A particular advantage of arteriography is the ability to perform this test on the operating room table before and during surgery. Use of magnetic resonance arteriography for a limb, although accurate and noninvasive, usually is not practical, given the time constraints, in the face of an acutely ischemic limb. However, when an aortic dissection or sources of microemboli, such as aortoiliac or femoral aneurysms, are suspected, an aortogram, CT, or MRI can be useful. Computed tomography, which is the most readily available among these in most EDs, has a sensitivity similar to that of aortography. Magnetic resonance imaging has higher sensitivity and specificity but is not readily available. Transesophageal echocardiography is also an accurate modality for detecting cardiac or aortic root pathology.

Treatment

The goals of therapy for acute arterial obstruction include restoration of blood flow, preservation of limb and life, and prevention of recurrent thrombosis or embolism. Although no studies to date have established an unequivocal beneficial role of any generally administered antithrombotic agent for acute arterial occlusion, when the diagnosis of acute limb ischemia is known or suspected, current practice is the immediate administration of intravenous UFH, if no contraindications exist. Several authorities suggest that a larger initial bolus be given. Dosing is the same as for DVT. This may help prevent clot extension, recurrent emboli, venous thrombosis, the appearance of microthrombi distal to the obstruction, and reocclusion after reperfusion.[24] It is still unclear whether heparin improves outcome in the clinical circumstances of thrombosis in a plaque-laden artery.

Fluid resuscitation and treatment of heart failure and dysrhythmias are sometimes necessary to improve limb perfusion.

Definitive treatment of an obstructing clot should be done in conjunction with a vascular surgeon. Choices for treatment include throm-

bolysis, percutaneous mechanical thrombectomy, and standard surgery. Prompt surgical embolectomy is the optimal therapy for an acute arterial embolism causing limb-threatening ischemia. Catheter embolectomy has been the preferred technique for removal of clot ever since the development of the Fogarty balloon catheter in 1963. It has reduced mortality from arterial emboli by 50 percent and need for amputation by 35 percent.[24] Overall mortality from an arterial embolus is about 15 percent and is usually due to the underlying cardiovascular disease. The limb salvage rate ranges from 62 to 96 percent. Similarly, balloon catheters are usually effective in thrombotic occlusions. For bypass graft occlusions, replacement of the graft is preferred to thrombectomy by most vascular surgeons.

Use of thrombolytics as the sole or part of combination therapy for acute limb ischemia is still quite controversial. Catheter-directed, intraarterial thrombolysis is associated with better reperfusion rates than is systemic thrombolysis for arterial clots.[24] Ample literature documents the use of streptokinase and tPA infused for hours to days as an alternative to surgery, with a rate of successful reperfusion of 50 to 85 percent.[24] Drawbacks to the use of thrombolytics include delay of reperfusion, which may be hours after initiation of drug, and the significant risk of local and systemic bleeding, including fatal intracerebral hemorrhage.

Randomized, multicenter trials have compared thrombolysis with surgery in the management of acute arterial obstruction, and the results do not show decreased mortality, better limb salvage, improved safety, or lowered costs of treatment. Thus, thrombolysis cannot be considered a standard for routine use. However, it is an attractive option for selected patients who may be poor surgical candidates or for distal thromboembolic occlusion in small arteries (such as in the hands, legs, and feet) that are surgically inaccessible and for acute thrombosis in a limb with chronic arterial insufficiency and adequate collateral flow.[24]

Thrombotic occlusion in arteries with advanced atherosclerosis and a well-developed collateral blood supply often will present subacutely. Management of this condition therefore is more conservative, with heparin alone. An angiogram is helpful to direct therapy and exclude embolic occlusion (radiologically seen as an abrupt cutoff of blood flow in a disease-free or minimally diseased vessel) when limb viability is acutely threatened.

Upper Extremity Ischemia

Acute arterial occlusion in the upper extremities is significantly less common than in the lower limbs. With a well-developed collateral circulation around the shoulder and elbow, arterial occlusion is much better tolerated. Ischemic rest pain and gangrene are rare in the upper limb in the absence of distal embolization. Etiology of upper limb ischemia includes vasospasm, arteritis, trauma, atherosclerotic plaque rupture, embolism, iatrogenic injury (e.g., brachial artery access for cardiac catheterization), thoracic outlet syndromes, aneurysms, and hypercoagulable states. After clinical examination, further investigation of suspected ischemia is done with segmental blood pressure measurements above and below the elbow, Doppler evaluation, duplex ultrasonography, and arteriography. Treatment of acute limb-threatening ischemia of the hand and forearm includes heparinization and emergent surgical thromboembolectomy.

Aneurysms of the Extremity

The incidence of aneurysms in the leg appears to be increasing, likely related to the aging population and better detection methods. Femoral and popliteal aneurysms account for the vast majority of peripheral arterial aneurysms and are due predominantly to atherosclerosis. More than 95 percent of patients with these aneurysms are elderly males. Aneurysms can give rise to local pain, limb edema, and ischemic complications. Acute symptoms can develop with thrombosis or distal embolization, and rupture is rare. False aneurysms of the femoral artery, consisting of encapsulated hematomas adjoining the vessel lumen, arise from iatrogenic injury and occur more frequently than do true femoral aneurysms. Duplex ultrasonography, CT, or MRI can confirm the clinical diagnosis and detect mural thrombus. Arteriography is of limited value in the diagnosis of an occluded aneurysm due to poor contrast filling.

The risk of ischemic complications from an asymptomatic popliteal aneurysm ranges from 8 to 100 percent (mean, 36 percent).[25] Thus, elective surgery after arteriography is recommended for all cases.[25] Because 37 percent of patients with a single popliteal aneurysm have an aortic aneurysm and half have a contralateral popliteal aneurysm, a thorough search is indicated after detection of a single aneurysm. Nonoperative management is acceptable for asymptomatic femoral aneurysms given their low incidence of complications.

Subclavian artery aneurysms occur from atherosclerosis, trauma, or thoracic outlet obstruction and much less commonly from syphilis or cystic medial necrosis. Thromboembolism gives rise to signs and symptoms typical of distal ischemia, but it also may produce central neurologic deficits from retrograde propagation of clot into the vertebral and carotid circulation. Because of their severe potential morbidity, these aneurysms should be surgically removed promptly after diagnosis.

REFERENCES

1. Heit JA, Silverstein MD, Mohr DN, et al: The epidemiology of venous thromboembolism in the community. *Thromb Haemost* 86:452, 2001.
2. Ferrari E, Chevallier T, Chapelier A, et al: Travel as a risk factor for venous thromboembolic disease: A case-control study. *Chest* 115:440, 1999.
3. Prandoni P, Lensing AWA, Cogo A, et al: The long-term clinical course of acute deep venous thrombosis. *Ann Intern Med* 125:1, 1996.
4. Chengelis DL, Bendick PJ, Glover JL, et al: Progression of superficial venous thrombosis to deep vein thrombosis. *J Vasc Surg* 24:745, 1996.
5. American Thoracic Society: The diagnostic approach to acute venous thromboembolism. *Am J Respir Crit Care Med* 160:1043, 1999.
6. Wells PS, Anderson DR, Ginsberg J: Assessment of deep vein thrombosis or pulmonary embolism by the combined use of clinical model and noninvasive diagnostic tests. *Semin Thromb Hemost* 26:643, 2000.
7. Kearon C, Julian JA, Newman TE, et al: Noninvasive diagnosis of deep venous thrombosis. *Ann Intern Med* 128:663, 1998.
8. Garg SK: Developing venous gangrene in deep vein thrombosis: Intraarterial low-dose burst therapy with urokinase: Case reports. *Angiology* 50(2): 157, 1999.
9. Peterson DA, Kazerooni EA, Wakefield TW, et al: Computed tomographic venography is specific but not sensitive for diagnosis of acute lower-extremity deep venous thrombosis in patients with suspected pulmonary embolus. *J Vasc Surg* 34:798, 2001.
10. Fraser DGW, Moody AR, Morgan PS, et al: Diagnosis of lower-limb deep venous thrombosis: A prospective blinded study of magnetic resonance direct thrombus imaging. *Ann Intern Med* 136:89, 2002.
11. Perrier A, Bounameaux H: Cost-effective diagnosis of deep vein thrombosis and pulmonary embolism. *Thromb Haemost* 86:475, 2001.
12. Anderson DR, Wells PS, Stiell I, et al: Management of patients with suspected deep vein thrombosis in the emergency department: Combining use of a clinical diagnosis model with D-dimer testing. *J Emerg Med* 19:225, 2000.
13. Birdwell BG, Raskob GE, Whitsett TL, et al: The clinical validity of normal compression ultrasonography in outpatients suspected of having deep venous thrombosis. *Ann Intern Med* 128:1, 1998.
14. Hirsh J, Warkentin TE, Shaughnessy SG, et al: Heparin and low-molecular-weight heparin. *Chest* 119:64S, 2001.
15. Gould MK, Dembitzer AD, Doyle RL, et al: Low-molecular-weight heparins compared with unfractionated heparin for the treatment of acute deep venous thrombosis: A meta-analysis of randomized controlled trials. *Ann Intern Med* 130:800, 1999.
16. Hyers TM, Agnelli G, Hull RD, et al: Antithrombotic therapy for venous thromboembolic disease. *Chest* 119:176S, 2001.
17. American College of Obstetrics and Gynecology: Clinical management guidelines for obstetrician-gynecologist. ACOG Practice Bulletin no. 19. *Obstet Gynecol* 19:1, 2000.
18. Hirsh, J, Dalen JE, Anderson DR, et al: Oral anticoagulants: Mechanism of action, clinical effectiveness, and optimal therapeutic range. *Chest* 119:8S, 2001.
19. Wells, PS, Forster AJ: Thrombolysis in deep vein thrombosis: Is there still an indication? *Thromb Haemost* 86:499, 2001.
20. Mustafa BO, Rathbun SW, Whitsett TL, et al: Sensitivity and specificity of ultrasonography in the diagnosis of upper extremity deep vein thrombosis. *Arch Intern Med* 162:401, 2002.
21. Hiatt WR: Medical treatment of peripheral arterial disease and claudication. *New Engl J Med* 344:1608, 2001.
22. Ouriel K, Veith FJ, Sasahara AA: A comparison of recombinant urokinase with vascular surgery as initial treatment for acute arterial occlusion of the legs. *New Engl J Med* 338:1105, 1998.
23. Sultan E, Evoy D, Eldin AS, et al: Atraumatic acute upper limb ischemia: A series of 64 patients in Middle East tertiary vascular center and literature review. *J Vasc Surg* 35:181, 2001.
24. Jackson MR, Clagett GP: Antithrombotic therapy in peripheral arterial occlusive disease. *Chest* 119:283S, 2001.
25. Dawson I, Sie RB, vanBockel JH: Atherosclerotic popliteal aneurysm. *Br J Surg* 84:293, 1997.

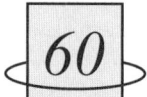

60 | CARDIAC TRANSPLANTATION
Michael R. Mill
Michelle S. Mill

The first clinically successful cardiac transplant was performed in December 1967. Since then, advances in the immunosuppression and postoperative care of these patients have resulted in dramatically improved patient survival. This has been accompanied by a tremendous growth in the number of procedures performed. Data from the registry of the International Society of Heart and Lung Transplantation (ISHLT) and the United Network for Organ Sharing (UNOS) reveal that 61,533 heart transplants were performed at 328 centers throughout the world between January 1, 1983, and December 31, 2001.[1,2] This total includes more than 2000 heart transplants per year in the United States since 1990. The actuarial survival after transplantation reported by UNOS is 85 percent at 1 year, with 3- and 5-year actuarial survivals of 77 and 69 percent, respectively.[3] Given the increased number of patients undergoing transplantation and their excellent long-term survival, these patients will come to the attention of physicians in the ED with increasing frequency.

TRANSPLANT RECIPIENTS

Cardiac transplantation has been applied successfully to patients of all ages, from newborns through persons in their late sixties. Heart transplantation is indicated for patients with end-stage heart failure not remediable by standard medical or surgical therapy. The etiology of heart failure in transplant recipients as reported by the ISHLT/UNOS registry is listed in Tables 60-1 and 60-2.[1,2] The majority of adult patients have either idiopathic dilated cardiomyopathies or end-stage coronary artery disease (see Table 60-1). Many in the latter group will

TABLE 60-1   Etiology of Heart Failure in Adult Transplant Recipients

Adult	Occurrence
Coronary artery disease	45%
Dilated cardiomyopathies	45%
Valvular	4%
Retransplantation	2%
Congenital	2%
Miscellaneous	2%

TABLE 60-2 Etiology of Heart Failure in Pediatric Treatment Recipients

Diagnosis	AGE		
	<1 yr	1–10 yrs	11–17 yrs
Congenital artery disease	75%	37%	24%
Dilated cardiomyopathies	20%	50%	62%
Retransplantation	1%	5%	4%
Other	4%	8%	10%

Source: From Boucek MM, et al.[2]

have undergone previous coronary artery bypass surgery. The predominant diagnoses in children undergoing transplantation are dilated cardiomyopathies and congenital heart disease (see Table 60-2). Many of the children with congenital heart disease will have undergone previous palliative or corrective operations. Patients are evaluated carefully for other irreversible end-organ dysfunction and other systemic illnesses that would separately limit survival.

CARDIAC PHYSIOLOGY AFTER TRANSPLANTATION

The physiologic basis on which cardiac transplantation is grounded is the ability of the denervated heart to support normal circulation. The lack of sympathetic and parasympathetic innervation does, however, induce an altered physiologic state. The denervated heart has a normal sinus rhythm with a heart rate between 90 and 100 beats/min. Denervation results in the absence of the initial centrally mediated tachycardia in response to stress or exercise. The heart remains responsive to circulating catecholamines of either endogenous or exogenous origin. The cardiac response to stress or exertion therefore is blunted. With the onset of exercise, the heart rate initially remains unchanged and then increases gradually to a level of approximately 80 percent of predicted over 10 to 15 min. After termination of exercise, this exercise-induced tachycardia will persist for approximately 20 to 30 min before

slowly returning to the patient's baseline rate. Patients may complain of fatigue or shortness of breath with the onset of exercise that resolves with continued exertion as an appropriate tachycardia develops.

Cardiac hemodynamics after transplantation as measured by cardiac catheterization reveal a normal to mildly depressed cardiac output at rest. With exercise, cardiac output increases in response to increased venous return (preload) and circulating catecholamines. Maximal cardiac outputs of 80 to 100 percent of normal have been measured. Patients are able to resume normal activity levels, including vigorous exercise, following transplantation. A number of posttransplant patients have completed marathons and participated in other rigorous physical activities, and at least one such individual has competed as a professional athlete.

Cardiac denervation results in an altered response to some medications used in emergency resuscitation.[4] In patients with supraventricular tachycardias, the lack of sympathetic innervation obviates the utility of carotid sinus massage. Atropine, which acts by abolishing reflex vagal slowing, will have no effect on heart rate in patients with symptomatic bradyarrhythmias. Conversely, denervated hearts are quite sensitive to the chronotropic effects of β-adrenergic agents such as isoproterenol, dopamine, and dobutamine. Because these are normal hearts, they are resistant to the proarrhythmic effects of these drugs. Isoproterenol (1-4 μg/min administered by continuous intravenous infusion) is used preferentially to increase donor heart rates because it has the greatest chronotropic effects and can be titrated easily to achieve the desired heart rate.

CARDIAC EVALUATION OF THE POSTTRANSPLANT PATIENT

Electrocardiograms (ECGs) obtained on transplant recipients should demonstrate normal sinus rhythm. The donor heart is implanted with its own sinus node intact to preserve normal atrioventricular conduction. The technique of cardiac transplantation also results in preservation of the recipient's sinus node at the superior cavoatrial junction. The atrial suture line renders the two sinus nodes electrically isolated from each other. Thus **ECGs frequently will have two distinct P waves** (Figure 60-1). The sinus node of the donor heart is easily identified by its constant 1:1 relationship to the QRS complex,

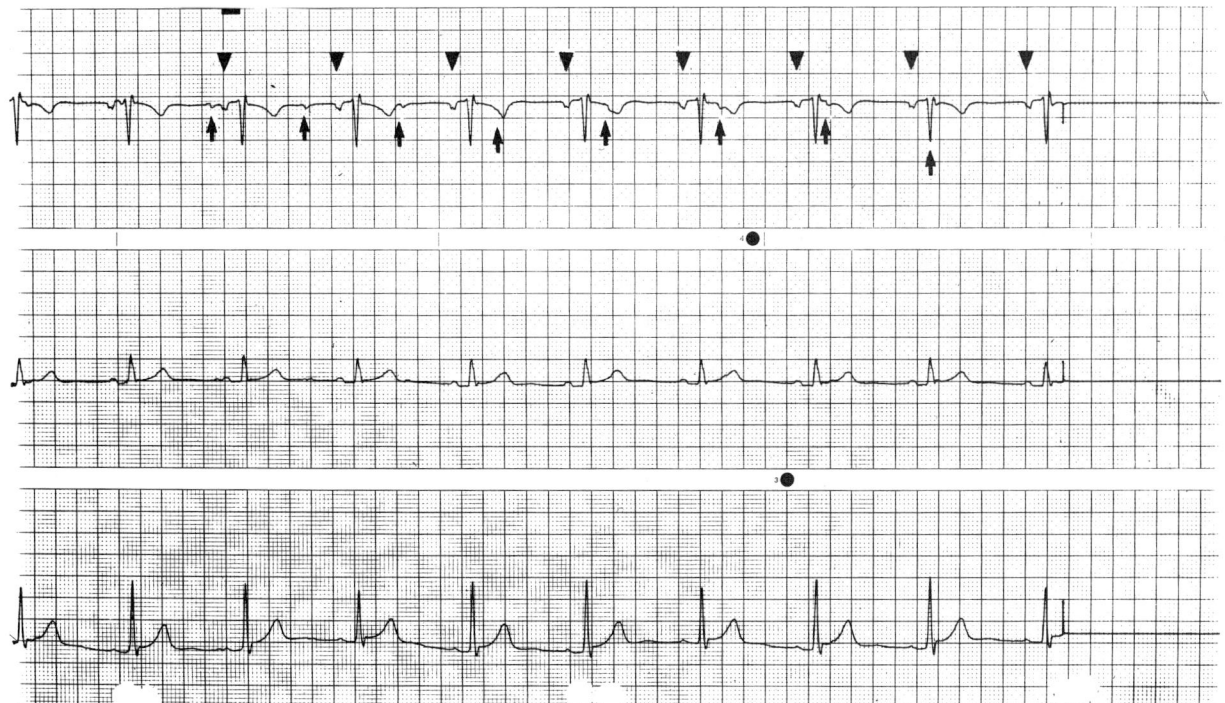

FIG. 60-1. Electrocardiogram demonstrating donor and recipient P waves (▼ = donor P wave; ↑ = recipient P wave).

whereas the native P wave marches through the donor heart rhythm independently. The presence of the two separate P waves may lead to confusion about the patient's rhythm. The ECGs may be interpreted erroneously as showing atrial fibrillation, atrial flutter, or frequent premature atrial complexes. The use of calipers aids in definition of the two distinct P waves. Sinus node dysfunction in the posttransplant heart occurs in approximately 4 to 5 percent of patients and is manifest by either sinus brachycardia with heart rates of equal to or less than 50 beats/min or sinus standstill with a junctional escape rhythm with heart rates of 60 to 70 beats/min. This dysfunction occurs in the early postoperative period and resolves spontaneously in most patients. For patients in whom sinus node dysfunction persists, treatment consists of either theophylline, which accelerates the sinus bradycardia in some patients, or implantation of a permanent transvenous pacemaker. The type of pacemaker implanted varies depending on institutional preference but generally is either an atrial pacemaker programmed in the AAIR mode or a ventricular pacemaker programmed in the VVIR mode. Use of an atrial rate-responsive pacemaker preserves atrioventricular conduction in addition to providing physiologic rate responsiveness.

Posttransplant chest radiographs show evidence of a prior sternotomy but otherwise generally are normal. Some patients may have evidence of "cardiomegaly" related to the transplantation of a heart from a donor who was larger than the recipient (Figure 60-2).

Echocardiography is a useful tool for evaluating cardiac function after transplantation. Interpretation of the echocardiogram is routine, with the exception of evaluation of atrial size. Because the atrial anastomoses incorporate the posterior walls of the recipient's native atria, echocardiography will show atrial enlargement, but this has no significant effect on cardiac function. Early rejection results in diastolic dysfunction, although the echocardiographic indices may be subtle and difficult to detect. Severe rejection will be accompanied by signs of biventricular enlargement with global hypocontractility and significant atrioventricular valve regurgitation.

IMMUNOSUPPRESSION FOR CARDIAC TRANSPLANTATION

As with all types of solid-organ transplantation, lifelong immunosuppression is required to prevent acute graft rejection. One of the most significant challenges of clinical transplantation is to maintain an adequate level of immunosuppression to prevent rejection while preserving adequate immunocompetence to avoid serious infectious complications. Since the mid-1980s, standard immunosuppression has employed a triple-drug regimen consisting of cyclosporine (Sandimmune, Neoral), prednisone, and azathioprine (Imuran). Recently, generic formulations of cyclosporine have become available. Care should be taken to maintain patients on the same preparation to prevent alterations in drug levels. The combination of these agents has resulted in superior graft and patient survival rates, has decreased the mortality from infectious complications, and has minimized the side effects of the individual agents. Recently, the newer immunosuppressive agents tacrolimus (Prograf) and mycophenolate mofetil (Cellcept) have been used in place of cyclosporine and azathioprine, respectively. In addition, some programs use induction therapy in the early postoperative period, employing cytotoxic antibody preparations targeted against the T lymphocytes. The most commonly used agents include OKT3, a murine monoclonal antibody, and polyclonal preparations such as antilymphocyte serum (ALS) and antilymphocyte globulin (ALG). Newer induction agents include daclizumab (Zenapax) and basilixamab (Simulect). These therapies are monospecific humanized mouse antibodies targeted against the interleukin 2 (IL-2) receptor of the T cell. With fewer side effects than other induction therapies, they are being used by many transplant programs, especially in patients with perioperative renal insufficiency.[5]

Cyclosporine remains one of the mainstays of immunosuppressive regimens. This fungal metabolite is a potent inhibitor of T-lymphocyte activity and interferes with the generation of IL-2. It is a lipophilic substance that is metabolized in the liver by the cytochrome P450 system. Cyclosporine is usually taken twice daily, and doses are adjusted based on serial blood levels. Target trough levels vary depending on the specific laboratory assay used. Levels are maintained in the range of 300 to 400 ng/dL early after transplantation and then lowered to approximately 150 ng/dL long term. The list of drugs that interact with cyclosporine (Table 60-3) continues to grow yearly, and careful consideration is required before adding or withdrawing medications for an individual patient. Such changes always should be made with the knowledge and input of the patient's transplant physician. Acute increases in cyclosporine levels may be associated with severe renal dys-

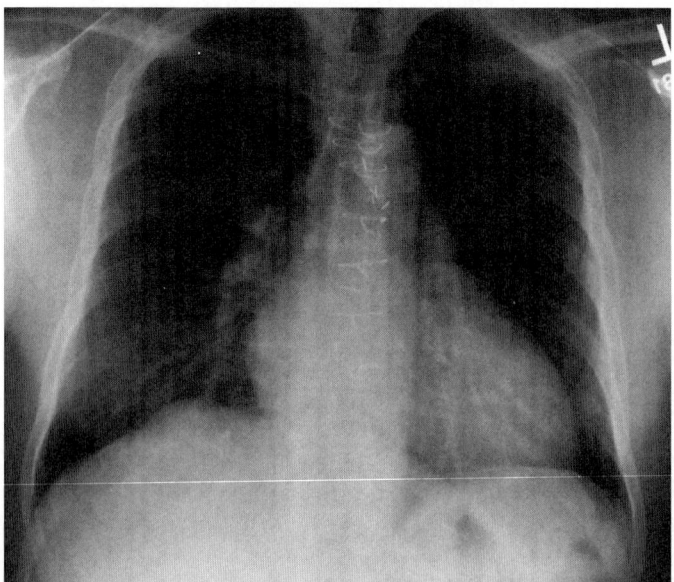

FIG. 60-2. Chest radiograph of healthy posttransplant patient with typical postoperative changes.

TABLE 60-3   Cyclosporine and Tacrolimus Drug Interactions

Drugs increasing blood levels
    Clarithromycin
    Diltiazem
    Erythromycin
    Fluconazole
    Itraconazole
    Josamycin
    Ketoconazole
    Methylprednisolone
    Metoclopramide
    Nicardipine
    Verapamil
Drugs decreasing blood levels
    Carbamazepine
    Phenobarbital
    Phenytoin
    Rifampin
    Ticlopidine
Drugs causing enhanced/additive nephrotoxicity
    Acyclovir
    Amphotericin B
    Ganciclovir
    Gentamicin
    Nonsteroidal anti-inflammatory drugs
    Trimethoprim/sulfamethoxazole
    Tobramycin

function, and acute decreases may result in the development of acute rejection.

Commonly encountered side effects of cyclosporine are listed in Table 60-4. Hypertension occurs in the majority of patients and frequently requires combination therapy to achieve adequate control. Renal insufficiency is also quite common and is mediated at least in part by the vasoconstrictive effects of cyclosporine on the proximal renal tubule. Management of cyclosporine-induced renal insufficiency requires careful monitoring because worsening renal insufficiency results in elevated cyclosporine levels, thus creating a vicious cycle. Although early renal insufficiency is frequently reversible, some patients have developed end-stage renal disease requiring dialysis or renal transplantation.

Formally known as FK-506, tacrolimus is a macrolide antibiotic with an immunosuppressive mechanism similar to that of cyclosporine. Tacrolimus prevents rejection of the transplanted organ by inhibiting the expression of IL-2 in T cells and inhibiting T-cell growth and proliferation. Studies show that replacing cyclosporine with tacrolimus as a primary or rescue immunosuppressant may result in fewer episodes of rejection, less clinically relevant hypertension, and lower doses of maintenance corticosteroids.[6] Initial studies with tacrolimus after cardiac transplantation suggest that tacrolimus is a safe and effective immunosuppressant alternative to cyclosporine. Oral doses of tacrolimus are typically 0.1 to 0.15 mg/kg divided every 12 h. Doses are adjusted to achieve a goal trough blood level of 10 to 15 ng/dL for the first several months after transplantation and then 5 to 10 ng/dL long term. The most common side effects of tacrolimus are similar to those of cyclosporine, as shown in Table 60-4, with the exception of hirsutism and gingival hyperplasia, which have not been reported. Based on the mechanism by which tacrolimus is metabolized, drugs known to interact with cyclosporine and erythromycin should be considered potential interactants for tacrolimus until proven otherwise.

Azathioprine is a 6-mercaptopurine derivative that acts as a false metabolite in the proliferation of bone marrow stem cells. The typical dose is 1 to 2 mg/kg per d, adjusted to maintain a white blood cell count greater than $5000/\mu L$. The most common side effect is bone marrow suppression, manifested as neutropenia. In some patients, anemia and thrombocytopenia may be present. The most common drug interaction is with allopurinol, which may be prescribed to treat acute gouty arthritis, itself a side effect of cyclosporine therapy. If allopurinol is to be prescribed, the dose of azathioprine should be decreased to half, and frequent follow-up white blood cell counts should be obtained to avoid profound bone marrow suppression.

Mycophenolate mofetil (MMF), another new immunosuppressant, is a potent inhibitor of de novo purine synthesis inhibiting T- and B-lymphocyte proliferation.[5] MMF has been approved by the Food and Drug Administration (FDA) for the prophylaxis of organ rejection in renal transplantation when used concomitantly with cyclosporine

and prednisone. MMF is being promoted as an improvement over azathioprine, replacing it in the standard triple-drug immunosuppressive regimen. Clinical studies of MMF after cardiac transplantation suggest that it is a safe and effective alternative to azathioprine in maintenance immunotherapy and possibly more effective in the treatment of refractory and persistent rejection.[7] Dosing of MMF is typically 1.0 to 1.5 g twice daily. The most common side effects include nausea, vomiting, diarrhea, leukopenia, and an increase in opportunistic infections, especially involving cytomegalovirus (CMV), both tissue-invasive disease and viremia.[8] Should neutropenia develop, the MMF dosage should be adjusted or the therapy discontinued. Drugs that interact with MMF include antacids and cholestyramine, which decrease absorption of MMF and therefore should not be taken at the same time.

Steroids remain an integral part of posttransplant immunosuppression. Prednisone is begun initially at high doses (1.0-1.5 mg/kg per d) after transplantation and weaned over 4 to 6 weeks to a maintenance dose of 0.2 mg/kg per d (about 15 mg/d in the average adult recipient). Many programs now attempt to wean steroids in an effort to avoid the well-known deleterious effects of chronic therapy. Steroid withdrawal is successful in approximately 50 percent of cases.

REJECTION

Rejection after cardiac transplantation is a lifelong risk, although the incidence of rejection decreases with time. Rejection can be divided into three types, based on mechanism of rejection and time after transplantation. *Hyperacute rejection* is mediated by preformed anti-HLA antibodies directed against the donor tissue. Hyperacute rejection results in immediate and irreversible donor heart failure and is a fatal complication unless the patient can be maintained with a mechanical assist device until a new donor heart is located. With the use of ABO blood group-compatible donors and screening of transplant candidates for elevated levels of preformed anti-HLA antibodies, hyperacute rejection is very rare in cardiac transplantation.

Acute rejection, the most common type of rejection encountered, occurs in approximately 75 percent of all patients at some time after transplantation. The incidence of acute rejection is greatest within the first 6 weeks after transplantation as immunosuppressive medications are weaned to chronic maintenance levels. Acute rejection can occur at any time after transplantation. Late episodes usually can be correlated with some change in the patient's immunosuppressive status, such as an acute illness or noncompliance with medications. Acute rejection is a cellular phenomenon resulting in the infiltration of lymphocytes into the myocardium, with subsequent destruction of individual myocytes. Because most episodes of rejection do not cause clinically detectable graft dysfunction, surveillance endomyocardial biopsies are performed on a routine basis after transplantation. Biopsy specimens are examined histologically and graded according to a grading system (Table 60-5) developed by a working group of the ISHLT.[9] Mild to

TABLE 60-4 Common Cyclosporine and Tacrolimus Side Effects

Hypertension
Renal insufficiency
Hirsutism*
Tremor
Gingival hyperplasia*
Hyperkalemia
Hypomagnesemia
Hyperruricemia
Glucose intolerance
Seizures
Headache
Nausea and diarrhea (esp. tacrolimus)

*Cyclosporine only.

TABLE 60-5 Standardized Cardiac Biopsy Grading System

Grade	Histologic Description
0	No rejection
1	A = focal (perivascular or interstitial) infiltrate without necrosis B = diffuse but sparse infiltrate without necrosis
2	One focus only with aggressive infiltration and/or focal myocyte damage
3	A = multifocal aggressive infiltrates and/or myocyte damage B = diffuse inflammatory process with necrosis
4	Diffuse aggressive polymorphous infiltrate ± edema, ± hemorrhage, ± vasculitis, with necrosis

moderate episodes of rejection (grades 0-2) generally are not accompanied by clinical symptoms or hemodynamic changes. Severe rejection (grade 4) can result in profound myocardial dysfunction and death. Patients with grade 2 or higher rejection are treated with augmented steroids or cytotoxic therapy, as outlined below.

Although most episodes of acute rejection are asymptomatic, symptoms can occur. The most common presenting symptoms are dysrhythmias and generalized fatigue. **The development of either atrial or ventricular dysrhythmias in a cardiac transplant recipient must be assumed to be due to acute rejection until proven otherwise.** Arrangements should be made for prompt performance of an endomyocardial biopsy. If patients are hemodynamically compromised by their dysrhythmias, empirical therapy for rejection with methylprednisolone, 1 g IV, may be given. If the diagnosis of rejection is confirmed, standard antirejection therapy should be completed. Atrial dysrhythmias may respond to treatment with digoxin or calcium channel blockers. Ventricular dysrhythmias may respond to lidocaine or other class Ic agents. Frequently, the dysrhythmias will be controlled only with antirejection therapy.

Untreated acute cardiac rejection results in progressive myocardial dysfunction. Diastolic dysfunction occurs first, followed by systolic dysfunction as the degree of myocardial damage increases. Diastolic dysfunction causes symptoms of congestive heart failure with shortness of breath, fatigue, and malaise. Progressive myocardial dysfunction results in low-output syndrome, with symptoms including nausea, vomiting, and/or diarrhea. Severe rejection leads to hypotension and circulatory collapse. Symptoms of rejection may be mistakenly attributed to a viral syndrome or gastroenteritis. Physical examination reveals signs of heart failure, including distended neck veins, an S_3 gallop on cardiac auscultation, rales on pulmonary auscultation, and occasionally, the presence of ascites or peripheral edema. Chest radiographs show enlargement of the cardiac silhouette and pulmonary vascular congestion. ECGs may demonstrate—in addition to dysrhythmias—a decrease in amplitude and widening of the QRS complex.

Patients with signs or symptoms suggestive of acute rejection should be admitted to the hospital with continuous ECG monitoring. Arrangements should be made for performance of an endomyocardial biopsy at the earliest possible time. If facilities for obtaining and interpreting biopsy specimens are not available, transfer to the nearest transplant center should be arranged. Low-output syndrome and/or hypotension should be treated with inotropic agents such as dopamine or dobutamine while specific treatment for rejection is instituted. *Treatment for rejection without biopsy confirmation is contraindicated except when the patient is hemodynamically unstable.* This is especially true in patients whose symptoms are due to an occult infection because of the potential adverse consequences of high-dose steroid therapy. Empirical treatment for rejection should be employed only after consultation with the patient's transplant center.

Standard therapy for acute rejection includes intravenous methylprednisolone 1 g/d for 3 days. In patients with refractory rejection, treatment with specific T-cell cytotoxic agents such as OKT3, ALS, or ALG is required. Occasionally, patients have been supported successfully with mechanical assist devices for profound circulatory collapse while undergoing therapy for rejection, with resulting complete recovery of normal ventricular function.

Chronic rejection is believed to be manifested in the heart by the development of graft atherosclerosis. This antibody-mediated phenomenon is thought to result in injury to the endothelial lining of the coronary arteries, with the subsequent development of intimal hypertrophy. The lesions may be focal but more often are diffuse and concentric, involving the entire length of the epicardial and intramyocardial vessels. Because the heart is denervated, *myocardial ischemia does not present with angina.* Instead, recipients present with heart failure secondary to silent myocardial infarctions or with sudden death. Transplant recipients who present with new-onset shortness of breath, chest fullness, or symptoms of congestive heart failure should

be evaluated for the presence of myocardial ischemia or infarction. This is done in routine fashion with ECG and serial cardiac enzyme determinations. Echocardiography can be used to look for segmental wall motion abnormalities. If evidence for myocardial ischemia or infarction is found, cardiac catheterization with ventriculography and coronary angiography is indicated. The rate of development of graft coronary disease is quite variable, occurring months to years after transplantation; consequently, cardiac transplant programs employ annual follow-up coronary angiograms to detect its presence. The diffuse nature of graft coronary artery disease generally precludes standard methods of myocardial revascularization such as percutaneous transluminal coronary angioplasty, stent implantation, or coronary artery bypass surgery. Retransplantation is the most effective treatment.

INFECTIOUS COMPLICATIONS AFTER CARDIAC TRANSPLANTATION

Infectious complications are fairly common after transplantation, particularly in the early posttransplant period, when the highest doses of immunosuppressive medications are employed. The infectious complications after cardiac transplantation are similar to those following all types of solid-organ transplantation and those in other immunocompromised hosts.[10] The infections encountered most commonly are listed in Table 60-6. Prophylactic regimens are employed by most transplant centers. Pretransplantation, patients are vaccinated with pneumococcal, *Haemophilus influenzae,* and hepatitis B vaccines. Perioperatively, routine antistaphylococcal antibiotics are used. Postoperatively, antifungal mouthwash is used to prevent oral and esophageal candidiasis while the patients are on high-dose steroids and is reinstituted when augmented steroid therapy is required to treat rejection. *Toxoplasma gondii* can infect the transplanted heart; it may result from reactivation of a latent recipient infection or be transmitted with the donor organ. *Toxoplasma* titers are measured in all recipients and donors, and pyrimethamine is administered prophylactically for 6 weeks after transplantation if titers are elevated. Beginning approximately 2 months after transplantation, trimethoprim-sulfamethoxazole is used as prophylaxis against *Pneumocystis carinii* pneumonia (PCP). Antibiotic prophylaxis for any invasive procedure (e.g., dental work, endoscopy, or surgical procedures) is recommended for the lifetime of the patient. Annual flu shots are recommended. *Measles, mumps, rubella, and other live attenuated virus vaccines are contraindicated in transplant recipients.*

Any patient with a history of solid-organ transplantation who presents with symptoms of an infection must be evaluated in an aggressive and thorough manner. Appropriate stains and cultures should be obtained to allow identification of bacterial, fungal, and viral

TABLE 60-6   Common Infections after Cardiac Transplantation

Early posttransplant infections (first month)
   Pneumonia: gram-negative bacilli
   Mediastinitis: *Staphylococcus epidermidis, Staphylococcus aureus,* gram-negative bacilli
   Intravenous lines: *Staphylococcus epidermidis, S. aureus,* gram-negative bacilli, *Candida albicans*
   Urinary tract infections: Gram-negative bacilli, enterococcus, *C. albicans*
   Skin: herpes simplex virus
Late posttransplant infections (after first month) and for duration of immunosuppression
   Viral: cytomegalovirus (CMV), herpes simplex, varicella-zoster, non-A, non-B hepatitis
   Bacteria: *Listeria, Nocardia, Legionella, Mycobacterium*
   Fungi: *Aspergillus, Cryptococcus, Candida, Mucor (Phycomyces)*
   Protozoa: *Pneumocystis carinii, Toxoplasma gondii*

Source: Horn JE, Barlett JG: Infectious complications following heart transplantation, in Baumgartner WA, Reitz BA, Achuff SC, (eds): *Heart and Heart-Lung Transplantation.* Philadelphia, WB Saunders, 1990, p 223.

pathogens. There should be a low threshold for instituting antimicrobial therapy while awaiting culture results and for admitting patients to the hospital for further evaluation and intravenous antibiotics. Patients with evidence of pulmonary infiltrates but without productive sputum require bronchoscopy with bronchoalveolar lavage and transbronchial biopsy for definitive diagnosis. Pulmonary infections that are encountered frequently include *P. carinii, Nocardia, Legionella pneumophilia,* and *Aspergillus;* these require special stains and studies for accurate diagnosis. Patients with gastroenteritis and nausea, vomiting, and/or diarrhea require special attention. Inability to ingest or adequately absorb immunosuppressive medications may result in the development of an episode of acute rejection. If there is any question about a recipient's ability to maintain adequate oral intake, the patient should be hospitalized and immunosuppressive medications administered intravenously.

Antibiotic therapy for documented infections should be guided by appropriate culture and sensitivities and must take into account underlying renal insufficiency and potential interactions with cyclosporine or tacrolimus.

Of special note is the risk of CMV infection after cardiac transplantation. CMV is a common virus to which the majority of adults have been exposed, as demonstrated by the presence of anti-CMV IgG antibodies in the serum. After transplantation, CMV infections can occur due either to the reactivation of latent virus in a previously infected recipient or the development of a new infection with a different viral strain transmitted with the donor organ. The latter situation is much more serious and potentially life-threatening, particularly in recipients who were CMV-negative prior to transplantation. Routine posttransplant surveillance for CMV infection is performed using serial IgG and IgM antibody testing, and now CMV antigenemia testing is available for early detection of CMV infection. Ganciclovir, available in both intravenous and oral preparations, is used for CMV prophylaxis in high-risk recipients (CMV-negative prior to transplant) as well as moderate-risk recipients (CMV-positive prior to transplant).[5]

CMV disease can occur in either a mild or severe form. Mild disease is manifested by a flulike illness with low-grade fever, fatigue, malaise, and nausea. Severe disease may include profound leukopenia; pneumonitis; gastroenteritis including epigastric pain, vomiting, and diarrhea; and hepatitis with elevated transaminases. CMV pneumonitis carries a mortality of greater than 50 percent. CMV infection typically occurs 4 to 12 weeks after transplantation. The diagnosis is made by the demonstration of cytoplasmic inclusion bodies in biopsy specimens of affected organs. Treatment includes the use of intravenous ganciclovir and, in severe cases, intravenous immunoglobulin infusions. Of particular concern is the documented increased incidence of acute rejection complicating acute CMV infections. Therefore, patients with active CMV disease must be monitored carefully for signs and symptoms of rejection. An endomyocardial biopsy should be performed if there is any suspicion of rejection.

NONINFECTIOUS COMPLICATIONS OF CARDIAC TRANSPLANTATION

In addition to common forms of cancer, those malignancies associated with chronic immunosuppression also occur in cardiac transplant recipients. These include posttransplant lymphoproliferative disorders (PTLDs), which are usually B-cell lymphomas and have been related to the Epstein-Barr virus. PTLDs may occur as early as 1 month after transplantation and may present with a variety of nonspecific symptoms. If diagnosed in their early stages, they may respond to decreased levels of immunosuppression, chemotherapy, and/or radiation therapy, with long-term survival reported.

Aseptic necrosis of the femoral heads and thoracic and lumbar spine compression fractures are not uncommon manifestations of long-term steroid therapy. The development of hip pain referred to the medial thigh or knee is often indicative of early aseptic necrosis. Magnetic resonance imaging (MRI) is the most sensitive means of detection, and patients should be referred for orthopedic evaluation if this diagnosis is suspected.

PEDIATRIC CARDIAC TRANSPLANTATION

The care and evaluation of pediatric heart transplant recipients is similar to that of adults, with a few special considerations. Rejection surveillance in infants and small children is done primarily with serial echocardiograms. Difficulties with vascular access and the need for anesthesia make serial endomyocardial biopsy procedures impractical. Acute rejection is heralded more frequently by symptoms in children than in adults. Children will present with a low-grade fever, fussiness, and poor feeding. Echocardiography will demonstrate decreased ventricular contractility, thickening of the posterior wall of the left ventricle, cardiac enlargement, and mitral and tricuspid valve insufficiency. Because the signs of rejection may be subtle and difficult to quantify, serial echocardiographic studies are required throughout the postoperative period to establish each patient's baseline echocardiographic characteristics.

Immunosuppression for children is based on standard triple therapy. Because of the more rapid metabolism of cyclosporine and tacrolimus, higher doses and more frequent (thrice daily) dosing often are needed in children. Steroids are withdrawn whenever possible to avoid their deleterious effects on somatic growth.

Childhood infections are encountered frequently and should be treated according to routine practice. Vaccinations with live attenuated virus are avoided. Exposure to chickenpox (varicella) is avoided if possible. If exposure does occur in a recipient without a history of previous infection, treatment with varicella-zoster immune globulin (VZIG) is indicated. Recipients who develop chickenpox are treated with intravenous acyclovir.

EMERGENCY DEPARTMENT EVALUATION AND TREATMENT OF THE POSTTRANSPLANT PATIENT

Cardiac transplant recipients are susceptible to all the acute illnesses that affect the general population. These patients should be treated in the same way as any other acutely ill or traumatized patient. In the assessment of such patients, however, the possibility that symptoms may be due to rejection, infection, or side effects of their immunosuppressive medications always must be considered. Patients taking steroids long term will have adrenal suppression and may need stress coverage if they are severely ill or in need of surgical intervention. Uninterrupted administration of immunosuppressive medications must be ensured to avoid the development of acute rejection. **Nonsteroidal antiinflammatory drugs (NSAIDs) should be used with extreme caution** because of the potential exacerbation of underlying renal insufficiency secondary to cyclosporine or tacrolimus use.

The evaluation of patients presenting with signs and symptoms of congestive heart failure should include the consideration of rejection, myocardial ischemia, and fluid overload due to renal insufficiency. Echocardiography provides important information regarding cardiac performance and may demonstrate findings suggestive of rejection (global dysfunction) or ischemic dysfunction (segmental wall motion abnormality). Results of routine annual cardiac evaluations are useful in assessing whether echocardiographic abnormalities represent acute changes or chronic conditions. Similarly, the availability of old laboratory test results will aid in assessing the importance and acuity of renal impairment.

Any transplant patient presenting with an acute febrile illness warrants aggressive and complete evaluation. If a specific diagnosis cannot be established by history, physical examination, and readily available laboratory and radiographic tests in the ED, consultation with the infectious disease or transplant service is indicated. The patient should be admitted to the hospital for further invasive tests and broad-spectrum intravenous antibiotics until culture results are available and a specific diagnosis is made.

In the event that a transplant recipient presents to the ED in extremis, standard cardiopulmonary resuscitation should be performed. Etiologies for hemodynamic collapse related to the posttransplant state include severe acute rejection and myocardial ischemia due to advanced graft coronary disease. Sudden death due to a dysrhythmia also may result from rejection or ischemia. Because of sympathetic denervation, vagally induced bradycardias do not occur; therefore, **atropine has no role in the resuscitation of these patients.** The empirical administration of high-dose steroids (methylprednisolone 1 g IV) may be beneficial if rejection is present. Finally, hyperkalemia due to chronic renal insufficiency may result in acute dysrhythmias and should be corrected with standard pharmacologic intervention.

REFERENCES

1. Hertz MI, Taylor DO, Trulock EP, et al: The Registry of the International Society for Heart and Lung Transplantation: Nineteenth Official Report—2002. *J Heart Lung Transplant* 21:950, 2002.
2. Boucek MM, Edwards LB, Keck BM, et al: The Registry of the International Society for Heart and Lung Transplantation: Fifth Official Pediatric Report—2001–2002. *J Heart Lung Transplant* 21:827, 2002.
3. UNOS: United Network for Organ Sharing, Richmond, VA. Web site: http://www.optn.org/latestdata/step2.asp.
4. Farrell TG, Camm AJ: Action of drugs in the denervated heart. *Semin Thorac Cardiovasc Surg* 2:279, 1990.
5. Stuart FP, Abecassis MM, Kaufman DB: *Organ Transplantation.* Georgetown, TX, Landes Bioscience, 2000.
6. Kelly PA, Burckart GJ, Venkatarmanan R: Tacrolimus: A new immunosuppressive agent. *Am J Health Syst Pharm* 52:1521, 1995.
7. Kirklin JK, Bourge RC, Naftel DC, et al: Treatment of recurrent heart rejection with mycophenolate mofetil (RS-61443): Initial clinical experience. *J Heart Lung Transplant* 13:444, 1994.
8. Hood KA, Zarembski DG: Mycophenolate mofetil: A unique immunosuppressive agent. *Am J Health Syst Pharm* 54:285, 1997.
9. Billingham ME, Cary NRB, Hammond ME, et al: A working formulation for the standardization of nomenclature in the diagnosis of heart and lung rejection: Heart Rejection Study Group. *J Heart Transplant* 9:587, 1990.
10. Baumgartner WA, Reitz BA, Achuff SC (eds): *Heart and Heart-Lung Transplantation.* Philadelphia, WB Saunders, 1990.

61 NONINVASIVE MYOCARDIAL IMAGING

David A. Bluemke

Bennett Chin

Joao A. C. Lima

Malek Tebache

Imaging for myocardial disease has advanced substantially in sophistication. Recent developments include new scintigraphic diagnostic contrast agents in nuclear medicine, Doppler methods in echocardiography, and rapid magnetic resonance imaging (MRI) of the heart. Because the cost of these diagnostic tests is relatively high, it is essential that the "correct" test be selected to arrive at the most accurate diagnosis in a short period, with few false positives or negatives.

CHEST X-RAY

Chest x-ray is often the first imaging test obtained for patients with suspected cardiovascular disease. Ideally, lateral and posteroanterior (PA) views of the chest are obtained, with film exposure at a distance of 6 ft

(1.8 m). Patients should be upright and have a moderately deep inspiration. For patients who are too ill to stand, semi-erect x-rays are obtained with an anteroposterior (AP) film exposure. The AP film has two disadvantages: the heart demonstrates magnification, and the pulmonary vessels, which show information regarding the extent of congestive failure, are somewhat blurred because of longer exposure times.

Cardiac size can be measured from the chest x-ray with an error of ±10 percent. Factors such as depth of inspiration, conformation of the chest wall, and pulmonary diseases may affect the appearance of heart size on chest x-ray. The cardiothoracic ratio is the ratio between the transverse diameter of the heart on a PA chest x-ray and the greatest internal diameter of the thorax. Although there are other formulas for measuring cardiac size, this method is the quickest and easiest. The normal adult heart measures 50 percent or less of the transverse diameter of the chest. In adults, a cardiothoracic ratio greater than 50 percent is considered diagnostic for cardiomegaly. In children, the normal cardiothoracic ratio is 65 percent in the first year and decreases to 50 percent by age 5 years.

The heart and major vessels are visualized in the middle mediastinum and are readily recognized on chest x-ray. The heart and the great vessels appear to have the same density relative to the radiolucent lungs. On the left side, there is usually air around the cardiac border; on the right side, the heart blends in with the density of the liver. In normal individuals, two thirds of the heart lies to the left of the midline.

Chest X-Ray Interpretation

On the PA view of the chest, there are three visible cardiac segments (Figure 61-1A). The lowermost segment, adjacent to the diaphragm, consists of the lateral and apical walls of the left ventricle. A small rounded density may be lateral to the cardiac apex; this represents the epicardial fat pad. Superior to the left ventricle is a rounded short segment that varies considerably in size. This is the pulmonary artery and its left main branch. Prominence of the pulmonary artery is normal in young women. Just below this level, the left atrial appendage forms a short portion of the lateral portion of the left heart border. Conditions that result in left atrial enlargement will cause a convex bulge in this portion of the cardiac silhouette. The third and most superior portion of the left edge of the cardiac silhouette is formed by the transverse aortic arch. On a properly exposed chest film, the descending aorta can be seen descending behind the heart shadow. On the right side of the cardiovascular silhouette, the lower rounded portion is due to the lateral border of the right atrium. The upper segment is formed by the superior vena cava. In older adults in whom the ascending aorta becomes more rounded and dilated, the upper segment of the right heart border may become convex, representing the lateral border of the ascending aorta.

On the lateral view of the chest, the anterior and superior-most shadow of the cardiac silhouette is formed first by the ascending aorta, then the pulmonary artery and the pulmonary artery outflow tract, and then the anterior border of the right ventricle (Figure 61-1B). Posteriorly, the superior shadow is due to the left atrium, with the left ventricle forming the cardiac silhouette inferiorly.

Early left ventricular failure is reflected on the chest x-ray by a "redistribution" pattern of blood flow. Normally, the most prominent pulmonary veins are at the lung bases. With the redistribution phase, the vascularity in the upper lung fields is increased relative to that in the lower lung fields.

As pulmonary capillary wedge pressure elevates to 20 to 25 mm Hg (Figure 61-2), fluid moves from the vascular bed into the interstitial spaces of the lung. The chest x-ray appears hazy at this stage, with short lines appearing perpendicular to the pleura (Kerley B lines). As pulmonary capillary wedge pressure increases to 30 to 35 mm Hg, frank alveolar edema ensues due to massive fluid movement from the vasculature to the alveolar spaces.

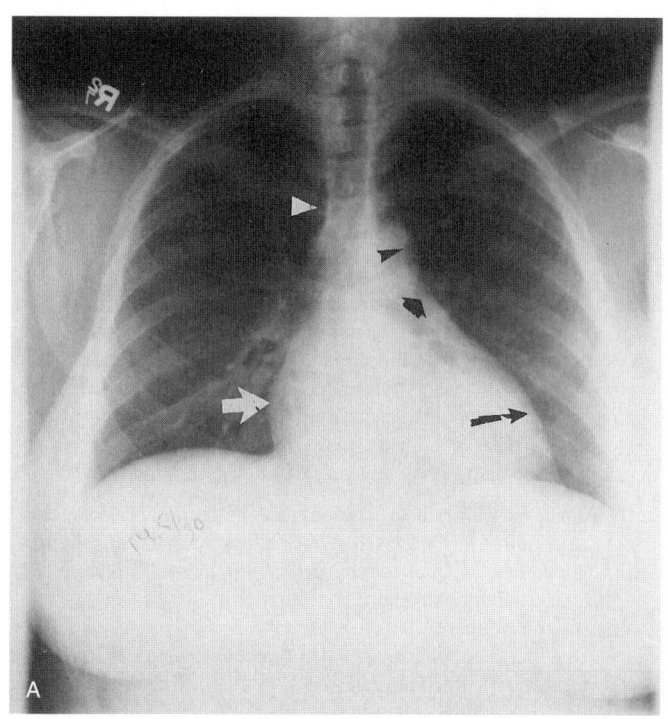

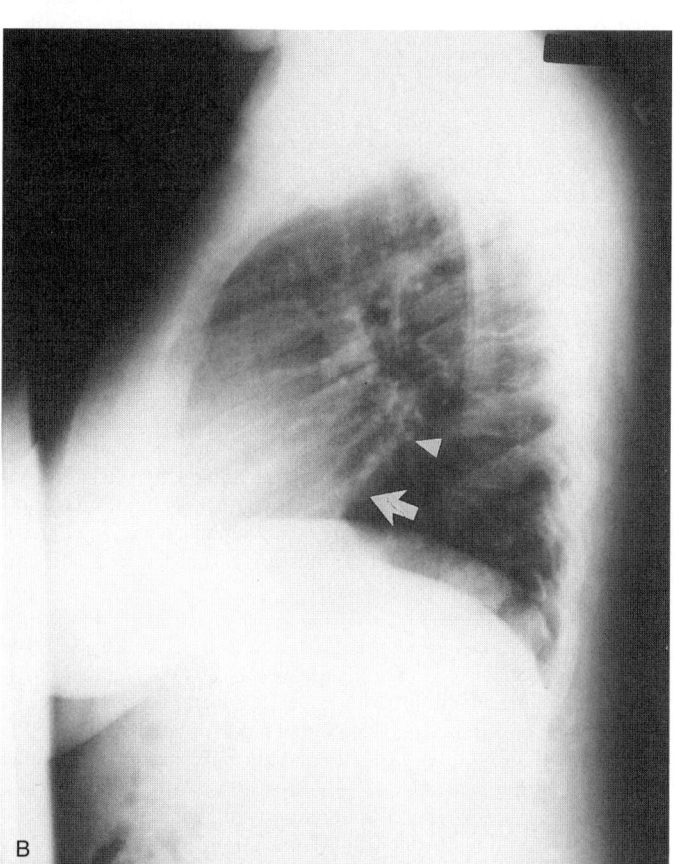

FIG. 61-1. Normal cardiac size and lung fields. **A.** Frontal view. The lateral wall of the left ventricle *(long black arrow)*, the pulmonary artery *(short black arrow)*, and the aortic arch *(black arrowhead)* form three visible cardiac segments on the left side. On the right side, the right atrium *(white arrow)* and superior vena cava *(white arrowhead)* form lower and upper borders, respectively. **B.** Lateral view. The left ventricle *(arrow)* forms the lower posterior cardiac border, and the left atrium is superior to it *(arrowhead)*.

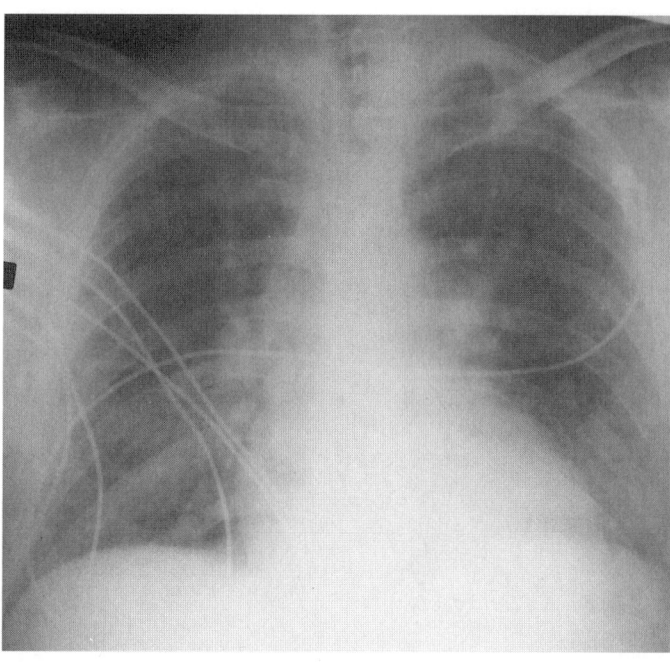

FIG. 61-2. Pulmonary vascular congestion. Bilateral increased lung markings are present, particularly in the lower lung fields, with prominent interstitial lung markings. The pulmonary hila are also enlarged.

Cardiac Chamber Enlargement

LEFT VENTRICLE Increased workload by the left ventricle initially results in dilatation of the ventricle, but, if it is sustained, hypertrophy of the left ventricular wall occurs. Hypertrophy is a normal response to increased workload. Chest x-ray findings at this time are usually normal. As the ventricle begins to fail, dilatation results, and the cardiothoracic ratio increases. The apex of the heart also becomes more rounded in appearance. The most marked increases in size of the left ventricle result from hypertension, aortic insufficiency, and cardiomyopathy. Pericardial effusion results in generalized cardiac enlargement (Figure 61-3).

RIGHT VENTRICLE The right ventricle enlarges from processes that increase the work of this chamber, such as pulmonary diseases or pulmonary artery hypertension. Mitral valve disease will also eventually result in right ventricle enlargement. The outflow tract of the right ventricle enlarges first; chest x-ray findings are subtle but include straightening or convexity of the pulmonary artery segment below the aortic knob in the frontal view. Multichamber enlargement is frequent, so that the relative involvement of each cardiac chamber is not easily distinguished on chest x-ray.

LEFT ATRIUM Common cases of left atrial enlargement include mitral valve disease from rheumatic fever and congenital defects resulting in left-to-right shunts. The normal left atrium is posterior and does not form any portion of the cardiac silhouette in a normal patient. Moderate enlargement causes the left atrial appendage to become larger and causes a bulge or straightening of the left cardiac border below the pulmonary artery segment. Further enlargement may cause the right-side border of the left atrium to extend beyond the normal upper aspect of the right atrium and superior vena cava. A double cardiac border is seen on the frontal view on the right side. If the left atrial enlargement is less extreme, a double border may still be seen, because of the increased radiodensity of the left atrium. On the lateral view, the upper posterior border of the cardiac silhouette projects more posteriorly than normal.

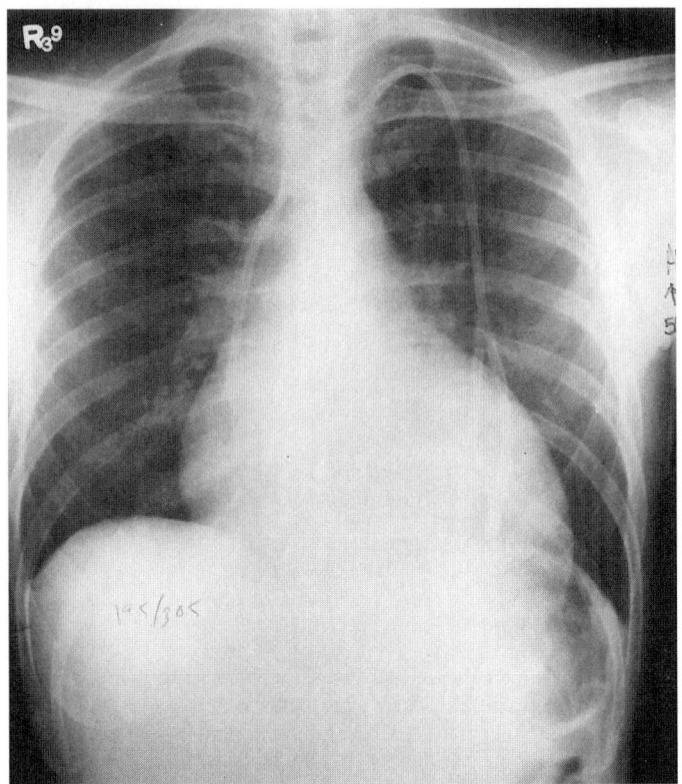

FIG. 61-3. Pericardial effusion. Generalized dilatation of the heart is present, with the cardiothoracic ratio measuring greater than 50 percent. Although a similar cardiac silhouette would be present in patients with dilated cardiomyopathy, this patient had documented pericardial effusion.

RIGHT ATRIUM   Enlargement of the right atrium causes enlargement of the lower right cardiac contour with increased convexity. Diseases resulting in right atrial enlargement include atrial septal defect, tricuspid stenosis and insufficiency, and right ventricular failure. In multichamber disease, right atrial enlargement is not identified separately.

COMPUTED TOMOGRAPHY

In evaluation of the heart, the primary role of conventional computed tomography (CT) has been to exclude other abnormalities, such as aortic dissection, that may secondarily affect cardiac function. Because of excellent anatomic resolution, CT is also useful in depicting paracardiac disease processes that involve the myocardium.

Advantages of CT examination of myocardial structures include good resolution at 0.1 to 0.5 mm^2 and rapid imaging times of 5 min or shorter for the chest. The low-density epicardial fat usually provides excellent contrast to the higher density of the cardiac structures. Calcifications, present at the site of ventricular aneurysms, of the coronary arteries, or of atherosclerotic change, are easily depicted. With the advent of helical CT scanners, a full three-dimensional (3D) set of images is obtained, allowing multiplanar reconstruction and 3D viewing. Although conventional CT scanners provide one image slice every 2 to 5 s, helical CT is increasingly available to EDs. *Helical CT* and *spiral CT* are synonymous.

Helical Computed Tomography

In conventional (nonhelical) CT scanning, the image acquisition is as follows: scan a slice, move the patient, scan a slice, etc. Thus, there are two distinct parts to the process: turn on the x-ray beam, usually for about 1 to 2 s, and then move the patient to the next table position.

Patient motion to the next position may take an additional 2 to 4 s. Therefore, each slice can take approximately 5 s (1 s of scanning and 4 s of motion), only 20 percent (1 s/5 s) of which is actually imaging time.

In its most basic form, helical CT consists of scanning a patient *continuously* while tracing a helix along the patient's body while the patient is being moved continuously through the CT gantry. In this mode, the x-ray beam is on for perhaps 20 s or longer, and the patient is moved for this same duration. The efficiency of scanning is 100 percent. Most recent technical developments have made available multi-detector-row CT (MDCT). Multidetector-row CT has a four-slice detector array and a rotation time of 500 ms. This innovative technology allows the entire heart to be scanned with thin slices (1.25 mm), in a breath-hold of 35 s, and with a temporal resolution of 250 ms. Retrospective or prospective electrocardiogram (ECG) gating is available.

Helical CT data sets are truly 3D. Instead of scanning a series of slices, a volume data set is acquired, with the following results.

Vastly improved multiplanar and 3D reconstructions. Because data sets are acquired in one breath-hold, respiratory misregistration is eliminated. Data appear "smoother," with fewer "stair-step" artifacts in sagittal and coronal reconstructions.

Reconstruction of slices at arbitrary intervals. Because of the 3D nature of helical scanning, images can be reconstructed at small intervals, e.g., 2 to 3 mm. This reduces stair-step artifacts in 3D reconstructions.

Rapid acquisition. Complete helical data sets of a patient's examination are typically acquired within 20 to 30 s, and the patient is then done with the examination.

Electron-Beam Computed Tomography

Electron-beam CT technology (Imatron, South San Francisco, CA) operates by a technology different from helical and conventional CT. With those methods, a large detector array and x-ray unit rotate around the patient. The sheer mass of the x-ray apparatus limits the rate of rotation to about once every 0.5 to 1.0 s. With electron-beam CT, electrons are generated and deflected electromagnetically onto tungsten target rings located in the gantry below the patient. X-rays are generated by the electron bombardment of the target rings. The x-rays are then tightly collimated and directed to pass through the patient onto a double ring of detectors in the gantry above the patient. Because mechanical motion is not involved, imaging times are very rapid: images can be acquired every 58 ms (17 images/s). Similar to helical CT, image resolution is excellent: 0.1 to 0.5 mm^2. At this rate of image formation, very little blurring of cardiac structures takes place. Calcifications involving the coronary arteries are easily detected, and cine images of the myocardium are available.

Electron-beam CT and helical CT require injection of an iodinated contrast medium to enhance blood in the vessels and myocardial cavities relative to the myocardium itself. With helical CT, approximately 120 mL of iodinated contrast is delivered intravenously at a rate of 3 mL/s. With electron-beam CT, 40 to 80 mL of contrast is given at 2 to 10 mL/s. In both cases, a power injector is used, necessitating large-bore intravenous access.

Radiation exposure is a consideration with all CT scanning methods. With conventional or helical CT, radiation levels are 2 to 4 cGy (2 to 4 rad) per CT slice. If multiple slices are taken at the same level of the heart, then the radiation increases directly in proportion to the number of slices. Electron-beam CT requires less exposure to radiation for the patient: each slice has an exposure of 0.54 cGy (540 mrad). However, more imaging slices are acquired with electron-beam CT in obtaining a cine sequence of the heart, so that 10 cine frames would result in an exposure of 5.4 rad. For comparison purposes, one x-ray of the lumbar spine is approximately equivalent to 1 cGy (1 rad), whereas radiation exposure from a chest x-ray is 0.06 cGy (60 mrad).

Applications

Electron-beam CT is available in only a very few centers across the United States. A major nonemergent application is the detection of coronary artery calcification. The degree of coronary artery calcification bears a strong relation to the presence of significant coronary artery stenosis. Cardiac anatomy, the relation between the chambers of the heart and great vessels, is readily determined with this modality. Because electron-beam CT can obtain cine images of the heart, cardiac function and focal wall motion abnormalities can be determined. Due to the limited availability of this modality, however, the remaining discussion focuses on non-electron-beam methods.

Although helical CT offers very rapid scanning, it is not well suited to assess cardiac function, given its need for contrast medium and radiation, when compared with echo imaging and MRI. Cardiac anatomy, however, is well assessed. Focal abnormalities of the myocardial wall are indicative of cardiac tumor or thrombus (Figure 61-4). Differentiation of these possibilities usually requires cine imaging, so that patients with such masses are referred for echocardiography or MRI.

Computed tomography offers a good depiction of pericardial disease (Figure 61-5). Simple pericardial effusions appear as low density relative to the myocardium, and the extent of effusion can be readily quantified, if necessary. The presence of calcifications of the pericardium is an important factor in the diagnosis of constrictive pericarditis and, with the correct symptoms, improves the specificity of this diagnosis. High-density pericardial fluid collections are likely to represent localized hematomas from trauma or surgery.

Helical CT after intravenous administration of contrast is an excellent modality for assessing diseases of the pulmonary arteries. Pulmonary artery emboli appear as low-attenuation defects in the opacified pulmonary arteries. Helical CT can demonstrate emboli not only in the main pulmonary arteries but also in the third- and fourth-order branches, because of high spatial resolution and cross-sectional imaging of these vessels.

Plain MDCT scans detect and quantify coronary calcifications. This capacity may have a role in ruling out coronary artery disease in patients with atypical chest pain or asymptomatic patients with high cardiovascular risk factors. Enhanced MDCT scans produce high-resolution studies of the cardiac chambers and the valve planes. It may be competitive with transesophageal echocardiography in searching for cardiac thrombi or quantifying valve stenosis. Multidetector-row

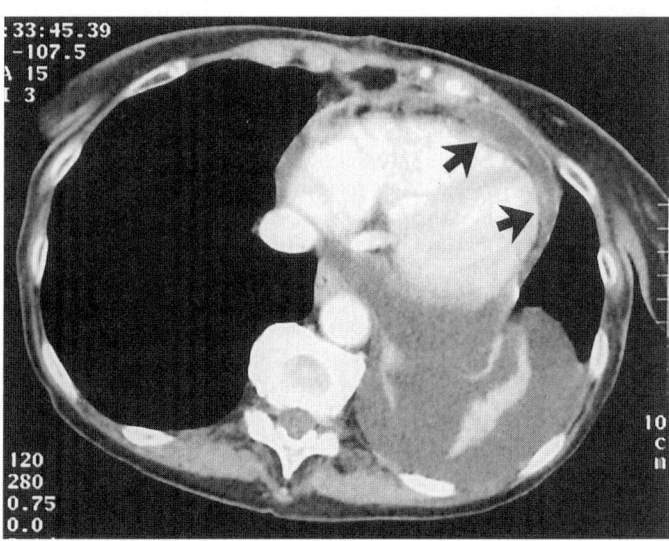

FIG. 61-5. Computed tomography after intravenous contrast administration shows pericardial effusion and enhancement *(arrows)* due to pericarditis, with left pleural effusion and left lower lobe atelectasis. [Reprinted with permission from Bluemke DA, Boxerman JL: MRI of acquired cardiac disease, in Stark DD, Bradley WGJ (eds): *Magnetic Resonance Imaging,* 3rd ed. Philadelphia, CV Mosby, 1998, pp. 409–438.]

CT angioscan may demonstrate the coronary anatomy (origin and proximal course), thus allowing one to look for anomalous coronary anatomy and to assess and follow the patency of venous bypass grafts, coronary stents, or percutaneous coronary angioplasty.[1]

NUCLEAR MEDICINE

Nuclear medicine examinations of the heart represent the study of cardiac function and physiology rather than of anatomy. Because of higher spatial resolution, MRI and CT are better suited to anatomic evaluation of the heart. Nevertheless, nuclear medicine examinations of the heart remain a primary means for assessing cardiovascular function; in particular, gated radionuclide angiography of the heart is a mainstay of cardiovascular imaging.

Radiopharmaceuticals and Imaging Techniques

ASSESSMENT OF CARDIAC PERFUSION

Thallium-201   Thallium is a potassium analogue that is transported by the $Na^+K^+ATPase$ system in cells in direct proportion to regional blood flow. Approximately 85 percent of each "pass" of the contrast agent is extracted from the blood across the capillary bed. Thallium is initially extracted by myocardial cells but is then redistributed to maintain equilibrium with the blood at a rate that is proportional to that of regional blood flow. Thus, the early images from a thallium scan reflect blood flow, and the later images (redistribution phase) reflect the intracellular K^+ blood pool. The intracellular K^+ blood pool in turn reflects cellular viability. The redistribution phase is usually imaged 4 to 24 h after the initial injection of thallium.

In combination with exercise or pharmacologically induced coronary hyperemia (from dipyridamole or adenosine), thallium imaging is able to distinguish normal blood flow, ischemia, infarction, and hibernating myocardium. Myocardial tissues distal to a physiologic coronary artery stenosis are unable to increase their blood supply during stress conditions or hyperemia and thus have low radiotracer activity. On 4-h delayed images, however, the thallium redistributes to these areas, and the

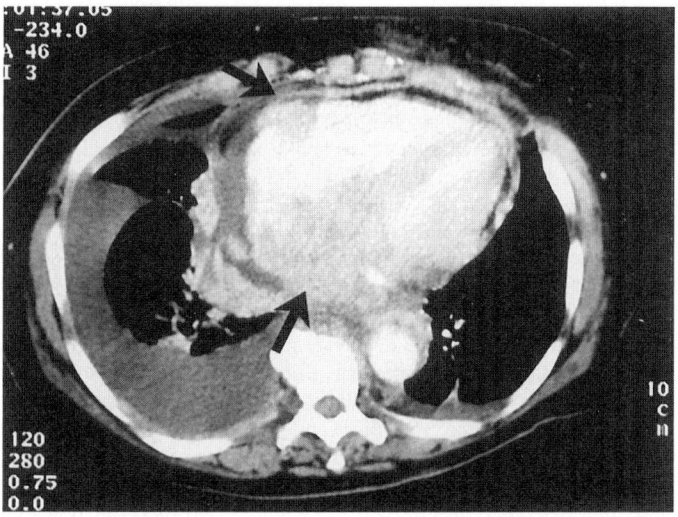

FIG. 61-4. High-grade malignant neoplasm. Helical computed tomography demonstrates right pleural effusion, pericardial effusion, and thickening of the septum and left atrium *(arrows)*. [Reprinted with permission from Bluemke DA, Boxerman JL: MRI of acquired cardiac disease, in Stark DD, Bradley WGJ (eds): *Magnetic Resonance Imaging,* 3rd ed. Philadelphia, CV Mosby, 1998, pp. 409–438.]

radiotracer activity of the myocardium becomes more uniform. With infarction, delayed images show no evidence of radiotracer redistribution, reflecting the lack of intracellular K^+ blood in the area of infarction. With hibernating myocardium, redistribution occurs by 24 h.

Technetium   Technetium radionuclides offer greater ease of use and availability for nuclear medicine departments. Whereas thallium requires a cyclotron to produce, technetium agents are widely available and produced by a generator in each nuclear medicine laboratory. The most commonly used technetium agent is technetium-99m sestamibi (^{99m}Tc-sestamibi). This agent is taken up by the myocardium in direct proportion to myocardial blood flow. At this point, the sestamibi molecule becomes trapped within the myocardium and does not redistribute (contrary to the behavior of thallium). Thus, the initial uptake by the myocardium reflects blood flow at the time of injection. Typically, ^{99m}Tc-sestamibi is initially injected at peak exercise or during the period of maximum coronary vasodilatation (induced by dipyridamole or adenosine).

^{99m}Tc-sestamibi does not redistribute on delayed images. Myocardial infarction and decreased flow from physiologically significant coronary stenosis appear as myocardial defects on images. To differentiate these two possibilities, a second dose of ^{99m}Tc-sestamibi is given while the patient is at rest. If the rest images show uniform radiotracer distribution, then the defect seen on stress images is due to ischemia. Persistent areas of absent radiotracer on rest images indicate areas of myocardial infarction.

Gated Radionuclide Angiography

Gated radionuclide angiography (RNA) has remained a clinical gold standard for overall assessment of left ventricular function. This test has the advantage of being applicable to nearly all patients, regardless of body habitus or underlying illness. In addition, unlike echocardiography, RNA is relatively operator independent. Radiation exposure is present but insufficient to prevent serial examination of cardiac function in the same patient.

In RNA, a blood sample is labeled with a technetium-based radionuclide, and a series of images of the heart is acquired. These images are gated to the R wave of the ECG. Function and measurement of ejection fraction involve measuring radioactivity counts at multiple time points throughout the cardiac cycle. The number of radioactive counts is directly proportional to the blood volume in the cardiac chamber. Thus, the method is insensitive to the precise geometry of the left ventricle, because only the overall count rates, and thus volumes, are measured. Other than segmentation of the left ventricle from other cardiac cavities, no geometric assumptions regarding left ventricular anatomy are necessary with the technique. By using gated techniques, with display of images as a cine loop, it is possible to assess segmental function of the heart. However, the resolution of the images is limited, and the strength of the examination relies primarily on accurate quantitation of the global left ventricular function.

Ventricular function is assessed by qualitative evaluation of cardiac wall motion, and quantitative assessment of radionuclide counts as a function of time. Computer-generated curves are verified by an experienced observer's interpretation of regional wall motion determined by gated RNA studies. Radionuclide angiography allows particularly good views of the lateral wall of the left ventricle, where there is no overlap from other cardiac segments. Although systolic function is easily assessed, diastolic function of the left ventricle is more commonly performed by echocardiography.

First-Pass Cardiac Studies

If the radionuclide is rapidly injected, and the acquisition speed of the nuclear images is rapid, the "first pass" of the radionuclide can be tracked as it passes through the heart. This method relies on tracking of the radionuclide bolus as it passes through the ventricular cavities

immediately after contrast injection. In this technique, the acquisition time is very rapid (30 s), although very few heartbeats are evaluated, thus limiting spatial resolution.

Left ventricular ejection fraction measurement is determined by following the passage of the radiotracer between the left and right ventricles. The injection of the radiotracer must be rapid, or poor separation of radiotracer between the two sides of the heart occurs. Patients with dysrhythmias, atrial septal defect, or significant regurgitation across the mitral or tricuspid valves will have poor ejection fraction estimates when using this method. First-pass studies using ^{99m}Tc-sestamibi enable cardiac function and perfusion to be assessed in the same study.

Gated Perfusion Imaging

After injection of ^{99m}Tc-sestamibi, images can be collected such that multiple time points, or cine frames, during the cardiac cycle can be independently collected by gating data acquisition to the cardiac cycle. In this manner, a cine loop, or movie of the cardiac cycle, can be generated. The function of the heart can be qualitatively reviewed to assess for wall thickening or segmental dysfunction. Thus, the perfusion of the heart can be assessed in the same setting as cardiac function. Functional imaging aids in discriminating between true mild perfusion defects and imaging artifacts, such as those due to attenuation from overlying breast tissue or the diaphragm. When severe perfusion defects are present, due to infarct or significant coronary artery narrowing, accurate estimation of ejection fraction is difficult to measure.

Applications

Myocardial perfusion scintigraphy is a noninvasive modality with high sensitivity for the diagnosis and evaluation of coronary artery disease. Physiologically significant coronary stenoses may be evaluated in populations with known or suspected coronary disease, after therapeutic interventions, preoperatively for risk assessment, and for prognostication after acute ischemia or infarction.

A more recent application of this technique has been made to the patients presenting to the ED with chest pain. In a subset of patients with an intermediate or low probability of coronary artery disease and chest pain (unstable angina), the missed diagnosis of acute coronary syndrome (ACS) has been reported to be as high as 5 to 8 percent. Several centers around the country have used myocardial perfusion scintigraphy to further classify this subset into high-risk and low-risk categories to reduce the incidence of missed ACS and the number of unnecessary hospital admissions for noncardiac chest pain. In a large study at the Medical College of Virginia involving 1187 patients, ^{99m}Tc-sestamibi perfusion imaging was used in defining the critical pathways in this population.[2] Used with established clinical criteria, the cardiac event rate at 1-year follow-up for patients with abnormal scan findings was 42 percent versus 3 percent (revascularization) for those with normal scan findings. In those with abnormal scan findings, 11 percent experienced myocardial infarction and 8 percent suffered cardiac death; in those with normal scan findings, none had myocardial infarction or death. Other centers around the country have reported similarly favorable results.[3,4]

The nuclear perfusion imaging protocol performed in the ED is very similar to conventional myocardial perfusion stress protocols, with the exception that the injections are performed at rest during chest pain. Preliminary reports indicate that timing of injection during chest pain may improve diagnostic sensitivity; however, other centers have reported good results with injections performed up to within 12 h of the chest pain.[5] ^{99m}Tc-sestamibi and tetrofosmin are used because of their favorable imaging properties of minimal redistribution and lower radiation dosimetry compared with ^{201}Tl chloride. After intravenous injection, these ^{99m}Tc tracers are highly extracted and retained for several hours within the myocardium in a distribution proportional to coronary blood flow. This permits imaging several hours later after additional ED evaluation or intervention. Because of the more favorable dosimetry of ^{99m}Tc tracers, a higher dosage approaching 7 to 10 times the injected dose of ^{201}Tl is typically used. This permits high-quality tomographic imaging (single-photon emission CT) and ECG gating, which provides additional information, including assessment of wall motion, wall thickening, and left ventricular ejection fraction. In patients with normal findings on resting perfusion study, further evaluation with a stress myocardial perfusion study may be performed on an outpatient basis. Preliminary studies have shown the cost effectiveness of this risk stratification, and further studies are currently in progress. Figures 61-6, 61-7, and 61-8 illustrate the utility of myocardial perfusion scintigraphy in a patient with acute chest pain.

ECHOCARDIOGRAPHY

Echocardiography is the use of ultrasound to image the heart and great vessels. This general term includes the techniques of M-mode, two-dimensional (2D) imaging, pulsed wave, and color Doppler studies. Frequently, an examination of the heart will apply a combination of these ultrasound methods to the clinical problem at hand.

Echocardiography, after the chest x-ray, represents one of the most commonly applied methods for cardiac diagnosis. In the ED it is particularly useful in trauma to identify hemopericardium as part of the FAST examination (see Chap. 251) and to evaluate pulseless electrical activity. Other standard applications include assessment of cardiac chamber size and function, patterns of flow within the ventricles, pericardial assessment, and identification of cardiac masses, including tumors, valve vegetations or calcification, and thrombi (Figure 61-9). Advantages for this technique include its relatively low cost, portability of the ultrasound equipment, good patient comfort, and safety.

Although the use of echocardiography is extremely widespread, there are limitations to the technique. The method is highly operator dependent. Patient positioning relative to the ultrasound probe is crucial, and specific machine adjustments must be made to optimize the examination to a particular patient. These adjustments may substantially alter the diagnostic ability of the examination. Certain patients have poor "acoustic windows," through which the ultrasound beam "looks" to see the cardiac structures. This limits examination quality in patients with chronic obstructive lung disease, obesity, and some musculoskeletal deformities. The use of transesophageal echocardiography, in part, alleviates the limitations of the technique for these patient populations.

Acoustic Impedance

The physics of sonography are discussed in detail in Chap. 303. At tissue interfaces, sound waves are reflected back to the transducer (specular interface) or scattered into many different directions. The endocardial border represents a specular interface; sound waves are maximally reflected back from this interface when they are incident upon the interface at a 90-degree angle. As the sound waves become more parallel to the endocardium, the reflected waves weaken.

Incident ultrasound waves that are scattered as they reflect from red blood cells may be used to assess the Doppler phenomenon and thus measure the velocity of the red blood cells. The *Doppler phenomenon* refers to increased frequency of the ultrasound wave, when the motion of the red blood cells is toward the transducer, and decreased frequency, when the motion is away from the transducer (the Doppler shift). In Doppler display mode, blood flowing toward the transducer is coded red; blood flow away from the transducer is shown as blue. The intensity of the red or blue is displayed as proportional to the

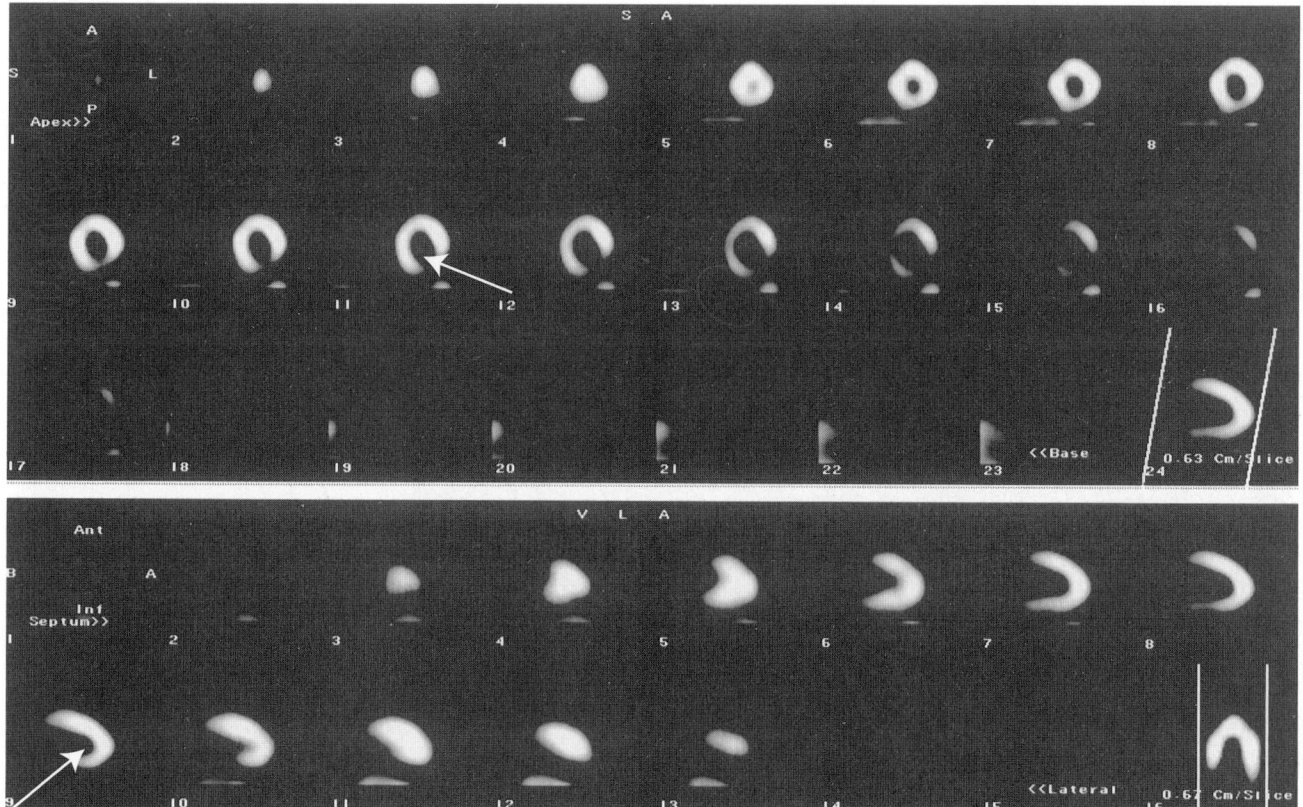

FIG. 61-6. A 59-year-old white hypertensive man who arrived at the emergency department with 6 h of intermittent chest pain. Findings on physical examination and electrocardiography were unremarkable. Initial cardiac enzyme levels (CK-MB, myoglobin, and troponin T) were normal. ^{99m}Tc-sestamibi single-photon emission computed tomographic perfusion images show a moderate area *(arrow)* of hypoperfusion in the middle and proximal inferolateral wall. The patient went directly to catheterization, which showed a 95 percent circumflex marginal stenosis that was successfully treated by angioplasty. (Courtesy of Ethan Spiegler, MD.)

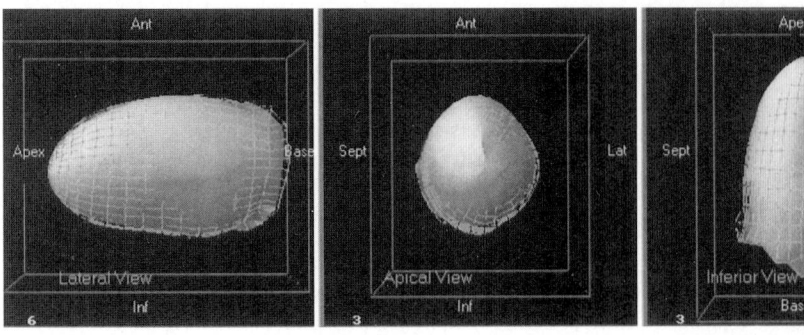

FIG. 61-7. Three-dimensional representation of gated single-photon emission computed tomography data at end diastole.

velocity. Velocities are most accurate when the angle between the ultrasound beam and blood flow is close to zero. Pulsed wave ultrasound techniques may be used to assess blood velocity: a series of rapid pulses is sent into the tissue, followed by a short segment of time for receiving the reflected waves.

M-Mode Display

M-mode display is unique in medical imaging to echocardiography. The primary advantage of this display mode is that high time resolution, to approximately one thousandth of a second, can be displayed on the time axis. Compared with this, traditional 2D displays are updated only approximately 30 times per second. Thus, M-mode display has excellent time resolution and can be used to display the periodic motion of, for example, cardiac valves or vegetations. In this display mode, a 2D display is typically first selected. A single line, or slice, of the 2D display is then selected, often across a valve plane. M-mode

displays then show the reflected ultrasound signal along this single line, with continual updating every millisecond.

Applications

MYOCARDIAL INFARCTION   Use of echocardiography for evaluation of ACS is limited in the ED. However, applications previously outside of the realm of the ED are now more common with the proliferation of ED-based "chest pain" or "cardiac evaluation" units. Echocardiography is more sensitive and specific than history and ECG findings in diagnosing myocardial infarction in patients presenting with chest pain. In several clinical series, left ventricular wall motion abnormalities were observed in 89 to 100 percent of patients with transmural infarction.[6] The sensitivity of echocardiography in detecting a nontransmural infarction is somewhat less and depends on the transmural thickness of the infarcted myocardial segment. In addition, patients who had no echocardiographically detected wall motion abnormalities had smaller infarctions and fewer complications.[6]

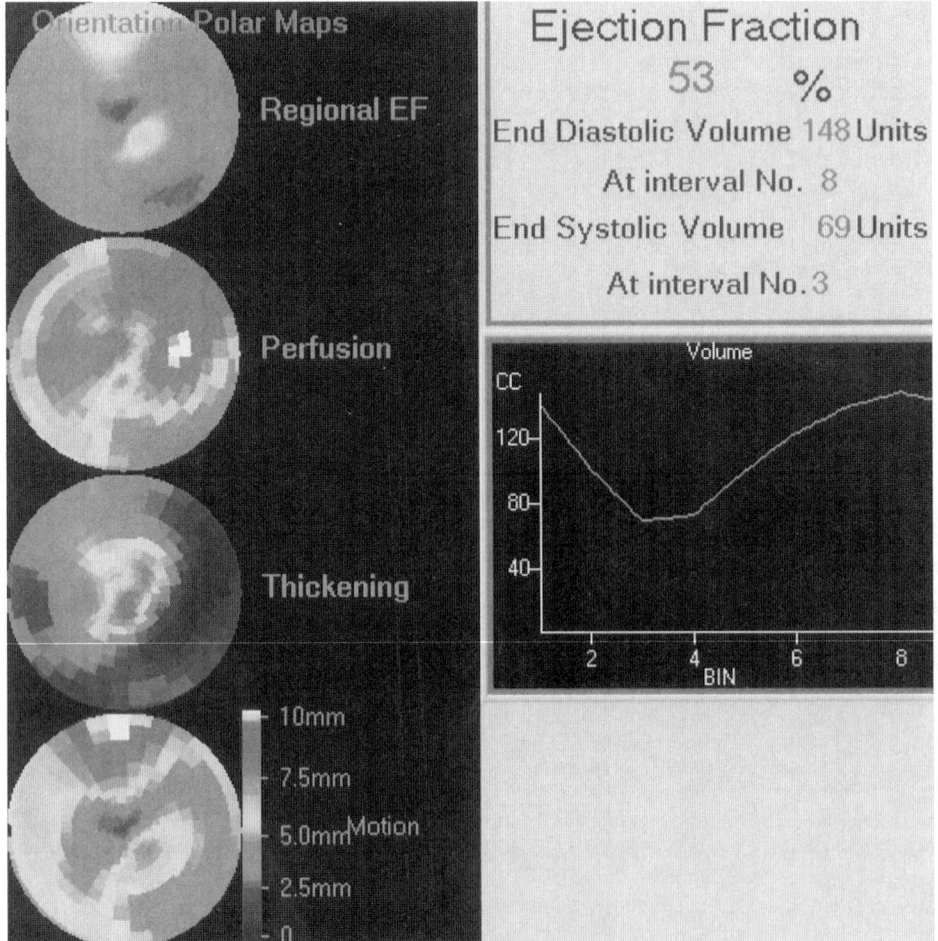

FIG. 61-8. Bull's-eye representation of gated single-photon emission computed tomographic data. Hypoperfusion of the proximal inferolateral wall, mild hypokinesis, and diminished wall thickening are visible. There is preserved global left ventricular function.

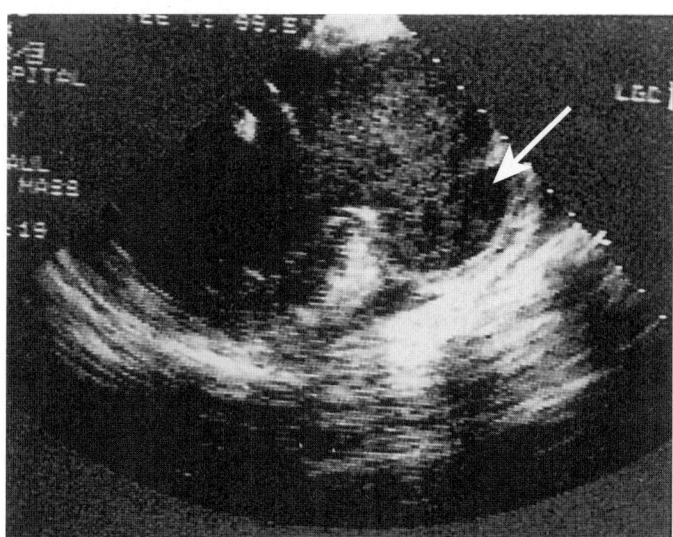

FIG. 61-9. Echocardiography of inferior wall pseudoaneurysm due to prior rupture of the left ventricular wall. [Reprinted with permission from Burton AA, Lima JAC: Echocardiography in patients with acute myocardial infarction, in Lima JAC (ed): *Diagnostic Imaging in Clinical Cardiology.* London, Martin Dunitz, 1998, p. 53.]

Echocardiography is also useful in the diagnosis and management of chest pain due to causes other than myocardial infarction. Patients with chest pain due to myocardial ischemia usually have echocardiographically detectable wall motion abnormalities with pain, even in the absence of infarction. Other causes of chest pain, including aortic dissection, hypertrophic cardiomyopathy, valvular heart disease, pericarditis, and pulmonary embolism, can frequently be identified or suspected based on transthoracic echocardiography.

In addition to facilitating diagnosis, echocardiography early in the course of acute myocardial infarction provides information important in guiding early management and determining short-term prognosis. The location and size of wall motion abnormalities correlate well with the coronary artery involved in an infarction. Obstruction of the left anterior descending coronary artery usually causes abnormal function in the anterior, septal, and apical segments of the left ventricle. Akinesis of the basal anterior segment predicts occlusion of the left anterior descending coronary artery, proximal to the first septal perforator, a finding of prognostic significance. There is overlap in the areas of abnormal wall motion in myocardial infarcts involving the left circumflex and right coronary arteries. Occlusion of either vessel can cause abnormal motion in the middle and basilar segments of the posterior and inferior walls. Wall motion abnormalities confined to the posterior and lateral walls are usually caused by obstruction of the circumflex, whereas abnormalities confined to the inferior basal segment are characteristic of obstruction of the right coronary artery.

A number of factors, including the presence of ischemia, stunning, or overload, confound the relation between the size of regional wall motion abnormalities and the amount of infarcted myocardium. When compared with pathologic examination, echocardiography tends to overestimate the amount of necrosed myocardium early in the course of myocardial infarction. Despite this limitation, echocardiographic estimation of the extent of myocardial infarction correlates well with infarct size as determined by peak creatine kinase, radionuclide imaging, and contrast ventriculography. Echocardiographic evaluation of left ventricular function early in the course of myocardial infarction has been found to be a better predictor of in-hospital mortality than the prognostically strongest clinical parameters. An echocardiographically determined ejection fraction of greater than 40 percent has correlated with a low short-term mortality and might be used to select low-risk patients for early discharge.[7] In contrast, a tall peaked E wave on

Doppler evaluation of left ventricular filling has been correlated with elevated left ventricular end-diastolic pressure and worse prognosis.

Echocardiography has been used to assess the efficacy of thrombolytic therapy. The time required for improvement of left ventricular function after reperfusion is related to the duration of ischemia and size of the ischemic zone. In patients with successful reperfusion induced by thrombolytic agents or direct angioplasty, echocardiographically detectable improvement in contractility can occur in the first 24 h. The delay in recovery of function, even after successful reperfusion, limits the utility of echocardiography in acutely assessing the success of thrombolytic therapy.

The widespread use of echocardiography early in the course of myocardial infarction reflects the clinical utility, availability, and safety of this technique. Echocardiography does have a number of potential shortcomings in the early diagnosis and management of acute myocardial infarction. The quality of echocardiographic images depends on the skill of the operator and the habitus of the patient. Images adequate for evaluation of wall motion cannot be obtained in 5 to 15 percent of patients in clinical studies of myocardial infarction.[6] Abnormal wall motion can be present in patients with Wolff-Parkinson-White syndrome, bundle branch block, right ventricular overload, and after cardiac surgery. However, in contrast to patients with myocardial infarction, in these patients, wall thickening is usually preserved. Conversely, myocarditis may cause regional loss of wall thickening and be indistinguishable from infarction by echocardiography. In addition, it is sometimes difficult to differentiate new wall motion abnormalities from preexisting ones by echocardiography. The value of screening cardiac ultrasonography as part of ED evaluation has been too slow to be superior to clinical evaluation and prognostic for hospital stay.[8]

ACUTE MITRAL REGURGITATION   This disorder often requires emergent surgery and has a higher mortality rate than that of chronic mitral valve disease. Etiologies include endocarditis, acute ischemia or myocardial infarction, prosthetic valve failure, and chordal rupture due to myxomatous mitral disease or trauma.

Echocardiographic signs in acute mitral regurgitation include the "snake" sign, corresponding to high-frequency fluttering of a ruptured chord in the left atrium. Rupture of the papillary muscle may cause disconnection of the involved tip from the body of the muscle. The direction of the mitral regurgitant distinguishes anterior from posterior flail leaflet: anterior leaflet failure is associated with posteriorly directed jet, and posterior leaflet failure shows anteriorly directed jet. Transesophageal echocardiography appears to be superior to transthoracic imaging for determining the size and etiology of the valvular disorder.

ACUTE AORTIC REGURGITATION   Acute aortic regurgitation results from trauma, endocarditis, or aortic dissection. This condition is rapidly fatal and requires immediate surgical repair. Transesophageal echocardiography may be necessary to delineate disruption of valvular or annular architecture in this condition.

For chronic aortic regurgitation, color Doppler demonstrates a regurgitant jet in the left ventricle. In the acute case, however, rapid equilibration of pressures in the aorta and the normal-size left ventricle causes a small, or no, Doppler jet. The spectral pattern of the continuous wave Doppler will have a low peak velocity and an extremely rapid deceleration slope. These findings correspond to the inaudibility of the murmur of acute regurgitation. In the most severe case, there is little diastolic flow into the ventricle, because the aorta and left ventricle become a continuous chamber. Early closure of the mitral valve or diastolic mitral regurgitation on M-mode or 2D echocardiography is an ominous prognostic sign. Early mitral valve closure indicates severe and acute decompensated aortic insufficiency.

MAGNETIC RESONANCE IMAGING

Magnetic resonance imaging is rapidly becoming the gold standard for noninvasive assessment of cardiac structure and function. The high contrast between moving blood and the myocardium by MRI, the high spatial resolution (Figure 61-10), and lack of ionizing radiation result in a superb technique for myocardial assessment. Dedicated cardiovascular MR scanners are now widely available at major medical centers, and experience with critically ill patients is becoming widespread. Lack of immediate access to an MR scanner may be limiting in an emergency situation but likely will become increasingly available in cardiac evaluation centers. More commonly patients will be triaged to receive MR studies based on indeterminate echocardiography or CT examinations. Nevertheless, the ED physician should un-derstand the increasingly important role of MRI for patients that have unresolved questions based on initial imaging results. Magnetic resonance imaging is the most definitive study for problems involving the right side of the heart, the paracardiac structures, and morphologic abnormalities of the myocardium itself. An emerging area of use of MRI is the detection of myocardial infarction in the setting of chest pain with indeterminate ECG or serum enzymes.

This section reviews principles and specific applications of MRI to provide a basis for emergency medicine professionals in requesting and evaluating MR studies.

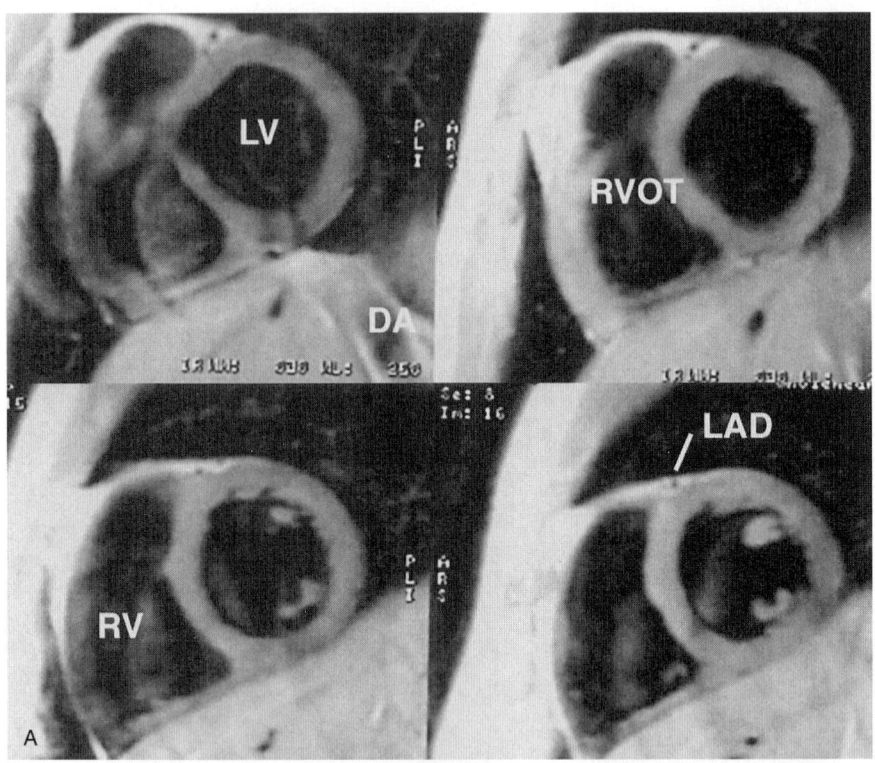

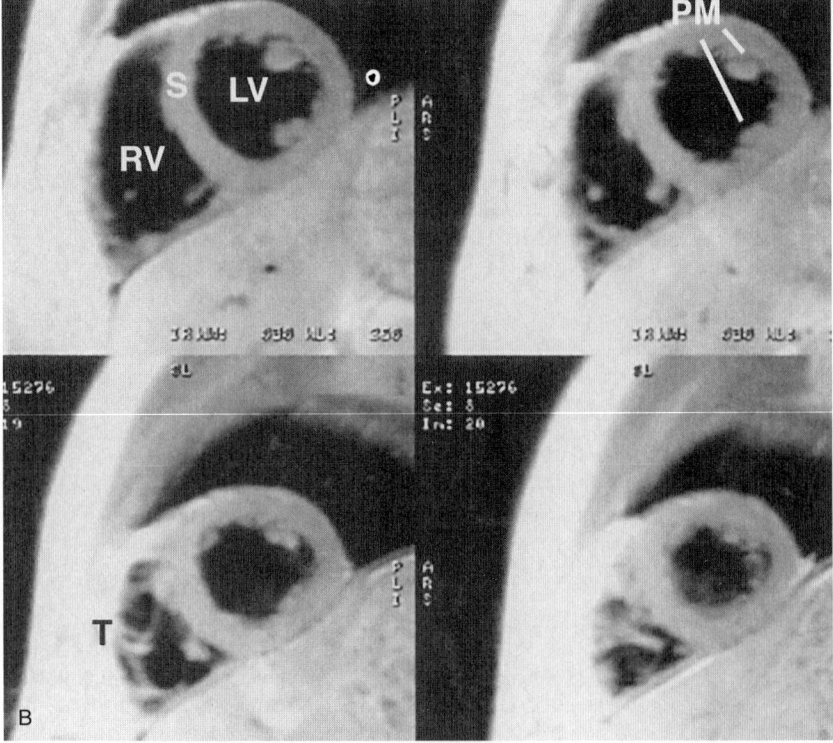

FIG. 61-10. Magnetic resonance imaging of normal short-axis cardiac anatomy from the base of the heart **(A)** through the cardiac apex **(B)**. Successive images are displayed left to right, top to bottom. LAD = left anterior descending coronary artery; LV = left ventricle; PM = papillary muscles; RV = right ventricle; RVOT = right ventricular outflow tract; S = septum; T = trabeculations in the right ventricle. [Reprinted with permission from Bluemke DA, Boxerman JL: MRI of acquired cardiac disease, in Stark DD, Bradley WGJ (eds): *Magnetic Resonance Imaging,* 3rd ed. Philadelphia, CV Mosby, 1998, pp. 409–438.]

Principles of Magnetic Resonance Imaging

T1-weighted images (see Chap. 305) are generally those that help define the *anatomy* that is being viewed (Figure 61-11). *T2 images* are those that better define the *pathology* of the tissue. *Proton-density images* may also be generated, in which the image intensity is proportional to the number of protons present. Images can be generated that are sensitive to flowing blood (*bright blood images* or MR angiograms). It is the unique property and strength of MRI that four different physical factors (T1, T2, proton density, and blood flow) can be used to derive a variety of imaging results. In contrast, for CT scanning or echocardiography, only one factor (x-ray attenuation or acoustic attenuation, respectively) is used to generate contrast in images. Magnetic resonance enhances the power of the technique for detecting subtle changes in pathologic tissues relative to normal tissues.

Two parameters are particularly helpful in determining MRI contrast: time to repetition (TR) describes the time between radiofrequency pulses, and time to echo (TE) describes the time after each radiofrequency pulse when the MR scanner "listens" for a signal from the patient. By changing the TR and TE values, different types of image contrast are obtained (see Table 305-1). For more detailed information regarding MR physics, the reader is referred to standard textbooks on the subject, such as that by Berning and Steensgaard- Hansen.[9]

Magnetic Resonance Pulse Sequences

CONVENTIONAL SPIN ECHO IMAGING   The most common pulse sequence traditionally used for cardiac imaging is a conventional spin echo sequence gated to the cardiac cycle. In this technique, the TR is equal to the duration of the RR interval. Because the T1 time of the myocardium is on the order of 800 ms, only moderate T1 weighting is achieved (Figure 61-12). Image quality is only moderate and is highly dependent on consistent ECG gating and lack of patient motion during the relatively long acquisition times. However, the contrast difference between the heart, the epicardial fat, and the ventricular cavities is relatively good.

T2 weighting for spin echo images is achieved by gating at several multiples of the RR interval. Imaging times are quite long if conventional spin echo techniques are used. The image quality of T2-weighted images is lower than that of T1 images, because of lower signal-to-noise ratios typically associated with T2 images. Also, artifacts due to respiratory and cardiac motion may be pronounced because of long imaging times. T2-weighted images usually are not necessary for *anatomic* evaluation of the heart but are more helpful for characterization of cardiac or paracardiac masses (see Figure 61-11B). In these cases, the mass frequently has somewhat restricted motion relative to the myocardium, so that image quality is often adequate. *Fast spin echo* or *turbo spin echo* T2-weighted pulse sequences are available on most new MR sequences. These methods reduce imaging time for T2-weighted images. Because of the high signal intensity of fat on fast spin echo images, an additional radiofrequency pulse is often added to cause fat to be very dark. This in turn helps to highlight nonfatty structures.

CINE IMAGING   Cine imaging for cardiac MRI consists of a motion picture loop of various phases of the cardiac cycle (Figure 61-13). To generate cine images, images must be gated to the cardiac cycle. In cine acquisitions, the imaging pulse is triggered, or gated, to begin based on

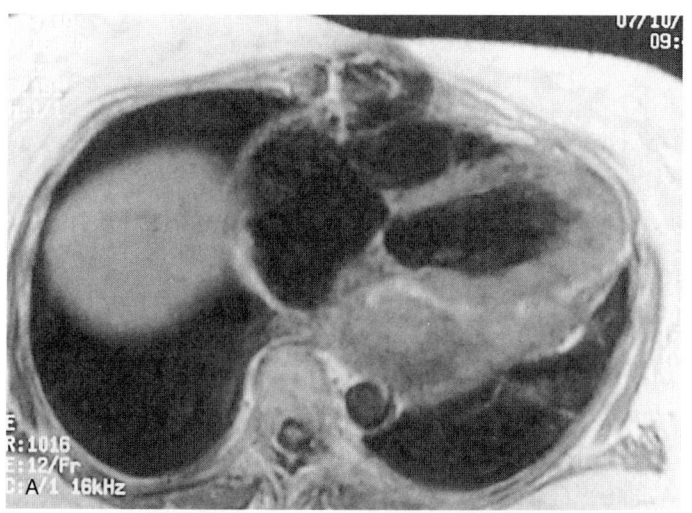

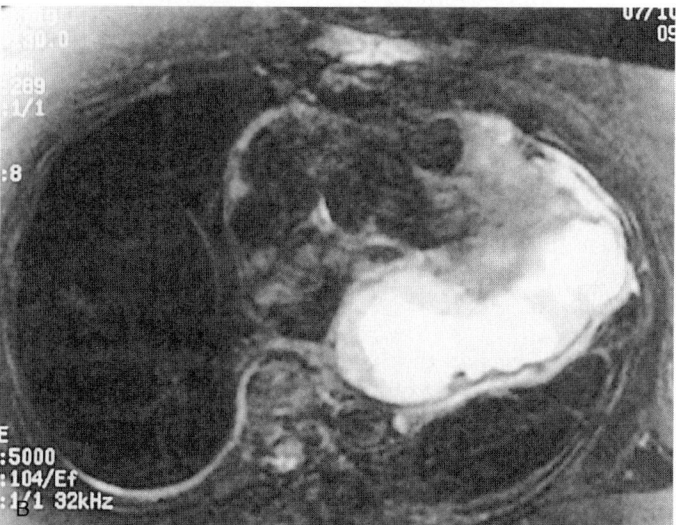

FIG. 61-11. Paracardiac mass demonstrated by magnetic resonance imaging. Axial images of the chest demonstrating a mass posterior to the left ventricle. **A.** T1-weighted image, showing thickening of the posterior wall of the left ventricle. **B.** T2-weighted image, showing bright increased signal in the mass. Biopsy revealed hemangiopericytoma. [Reprinted with permission from Bluemke DA, Boxerman JL: MRI of acquired cardiac disease, in Stark DD, Bradley WGJ (eds): *Magnetic Resonance Imaging,* 3rd ed. Philadelphia, CV Mosby, 1998, pp. 409–438.]

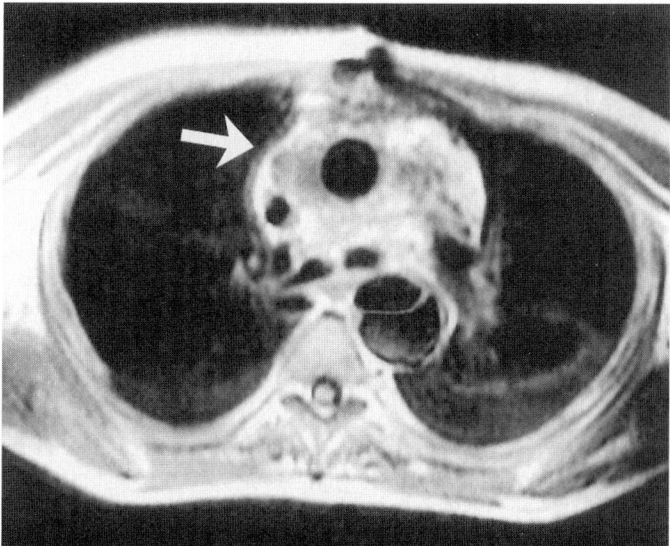

FIG. 61-12. Magnetic resonance imaging of aortic dissection. Axial T1-weighted image shows the site of prior repair of the ascending aorta after dissection. There is residual soft tissue thickening around the ascending aorta *(arrow)*. A residual dissection remains in the descending aorta. The patient had a history of Marfan disease.

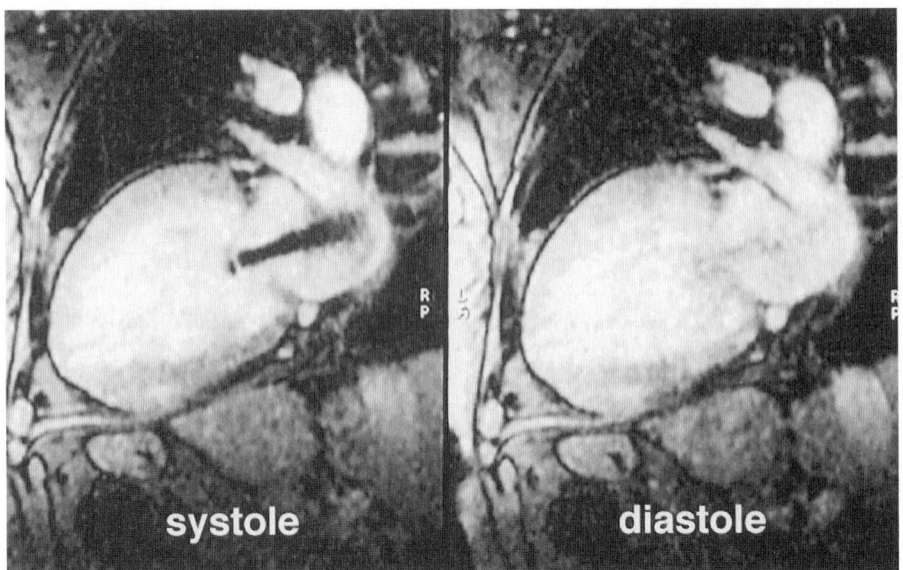

FIG. 61-13. Magnetic resonance imaging of mitral valve dysfunction. Images during systole and diastole show a dark regurgitant jet extending from the valve plane to the left atrium during systole, compatible with mitral valve regurgitation. [Reprinted with permission from Bluemke DA, Boxerman JL: MRI of acquired cardiac disease, in Stark DD, Bradley WGJ (eds): *Magnetic Resonance Imaging*, 3rd ed. Philadelphia, CV Mosby, 1998, pp. 409–438.]

the R wave of the ECG. A complete cine sequence of the heart is acquired within a breath-hold of 12 to 18 heartbeats. The physics of this technique result in saturation of background stationary tissues, whereas flowing blood has a higher and brighter signal. Breath-hold cine imaging of the heart can be performed in any anatomic plane, e.g., parallel to the long axis and short axis of the heart.

Specific Applications of Magnetic Resonance Imaging

CARDIAC AND PARACARDIAC MASSES Patients with cardiac and paracardiac masses may be assessed in the ED or referred for outpatient MRI under variable circumstances. The suspicion may arise from incidental findings from chest plain film or echocardiography. Magnetic resonance imaging, with its high spatial and temporal resolutions, is well suited to image the cardiac anatomy. It benefits from a large field of view and defines the relations of the lesion to the cardiac chambers walls, the valves, the pericardium, the outflow tracts, and the vessels. White-blood (gradient echo) and black-blood (spin echo) ECG-gated sequences can be obtained in any desired plane. Even if a specific diagnosis is difficult to obtain, MRI may characterize certain components of the mass (fat, blood, and fluid), identify their location and extent, and show the degree of vascularization.

LEFT VENTRICULAR ANEURYSM Left ventricular aneurysm is a potential complication of acute transmural myocardial infarction. Usually it is located in the anteroseptal or apical region. Patients may suffer from arrhythmias, thromboembolic episodes, and congestive heart failure.

Left ventricular pseudoaneurysm consists of a cardiac rupture contained by adherent pericardium or scar tissue. This condition may be induced by myocardial infarction, cardiac surgery, trauma, and infection. Unlike true aneurysm, it arises from inferior myocardial infarction and thus takes place on the lateral, apical, or inferior surface. Electrocardiogram and chest plain films are nonspecific tests for the diagnosis of these conditions.

Transesophageal echocardiography and MRI are the reasonable next steps when a high index of suspicion is present. Transesophageal echocardiography is more uncomfortable for the patient and does not provide a large field of view as compared with MRI. Also, MRI provides preoperative morphology and functional information to the cardiac surgeon.

ANOMALOUS CORONARY ARTERY The diagnosis of anomalous coronary artery origin should be considered in unexplained syncope (and myocardial infarct and sudden death) among young adults. The pathophysiologic mechanism seems to be the impingement of the anomalous vessel in its path between the aorta and the pulmonary trunk. Conventional angiography generates 2D projections of the coronary anatomy, whereas MRI identifies the relations of coronary arteries, origins, and proximal courses with the great vessels, thereby allowing a more accurate diagnosis and identifying the risk of cardiac morbidity or mortality in function by the type of anomalous coronary course.

CARDIOMYOPATHY Patients with cardiomyopathy and presenting to the ED may suffer from syncope, atrial or ventricular arrhythmias, and episodes of cardiac failure or sudden death. Cardiomyopathy may result from ischemia, infection, arterial hypertension, valvular disease, genetic affection, or may be idiopathic. Magnetic resonance imaging can evaluate morphology and function in these conditions. It accurately defines the location and the extent of the thickened myocardium, quantifies ventricular mass, and demonstrates the effect of the hypertrophic muscle on chamber volume and ventricular function.

Magnetic resonance imaging is well suited to assess treatment effects, such as radiofrequency ablation of a subaortic septal hypertrophic cardiomyopathy. Restrictive cardiomyopathy and constrictive pericarditis are frequently well evaluated by MRI. Both conditions share the same clinical features. The underlying pathologic process is diastolic dysfunction due to myocardial stiffness for restrictive disease and pericardial thickening for the constriction. The differential diagnosis is crucial, because constrictive pericarditis is treated surgically, whereas restrictive disease is treated medically or with transplantation.

CORONARY HEART DISEASE

Myocardial Ischemia and Noninvasive Coronary Artery Disease Identification Stress-perfusion MRI combines administration of a pharmacologic vasodilator with intravenous injection of a gadolinium MRI contrast agent. First-pass MRI myocardial perfusion evaluates coronary flow reserve. Coronary flow reserve is defined as the ratio of blood flow at maximal vasodilatation, divided by flow at rest. The ratio typically ranges from 3 to 5 in normal individuals. In the presence of fixed coronary stenoses, coronary flow reserve is markedly reduced,[10] and this induces perfusion heterogeneity. In fact, the myocardium perfused by a stenotic coronary vessel will receive less blood flow than the neighboring normal myocardium in maximal vasodilatation.

This indicates that patients with microvascular dysfunction from epicardial vascular disease or diseases altering the microvasculature, such as hypertension or diabetes, may be assessed with these methods.[11]

An alternative to perfusion MRI, in screening for coronary artery disease, is to evaluate the *function* of the myocardium during inotropic stimulation.[12] Dobutamine stress MRI is highly analogous to dobutamine stress echocardiography. In this method, MR cine images of the myocardium are imaged during constant infusion of increasing doses of dobutamine. Dobutamine is an inotropic and chronotropic agent inducing an increase in oxygen demand. High-dose dobutamine stress tests may cause wall motion abnormalities in territories perfused by a coronary vessel with a hemodynamically significant stenosis. These wall motion abnormalities are identified in the MR images.

Myocardial Infarction and Viability The ischemic myocardium may appear dysfunctional. This state may be due to myocardial infarction, stunning, or hibernation. Infarct is a nonviable area, whereas stunned or hibernating myocardium is a viable region with depressed function. It is crucial to differentiate between these conditions, for assessing the prognosis after myocardial infarction and for identifying patients who would benefit from surgical revascularization. Indeed, performing coronary bypass to treat a nonviable myocardial segment is pointless and brings unnecessary risks to the patient.

Nuclear imaging and echocardiography are routinely used to look for viability of any dysfunctional myocardial region during stress tests, mainly with low- or medium-dose dobutamine infusion. Recovery of normal function during stress demonstrates the viability. The same approach is done with MRI,[13] which is well suited to assess the pattern of myocardial contraction.

The temporal resolution of an up-to-date MR unit (40 ms) is sufficient to obtain perfusion images encompassing the entire left ventricle every one to two heartbeats. Rapid injection of a small volume of contrast is performed by a power injector to achieve first-pass images showing myocardial blood flow. Magnetic resonance images show contrast passage through the right ventricle, the pulmonary arteries, the left ventricle chamber, and then through the left and right ventricular myocardia. The washin and washout of the contrast agent distinguishes pathologic tissue, such as infarct, from normal myocardium.

In acute myocardial infarction, MR images show a subendocardial perfusion abnormality (Figure 61-14). This "core" of the infarct is af-fected by microvascular obstruction, despite patency of the major epicardial coronary artery. The presence of microvascular obstruction is associated with long-term cardiovascular complications,[14] such as recurrent myocardial infarction, congestive heart failure, and stroke. In addition to perfusion imaging, late enhancement is analyzed. About 20 min after the intravenous injection of gadolinium-DTPA, myocardial infarction is depicted by a delayed area of tissue enhancement relative to normal, unaffected myocardium.[15] This method readily defines the size of the infarct and its transmural extent (Figure 61-15).

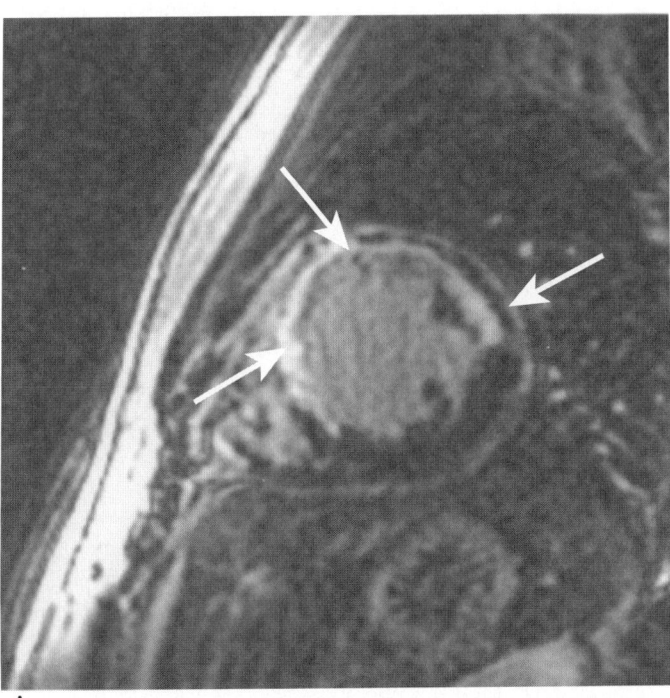

A

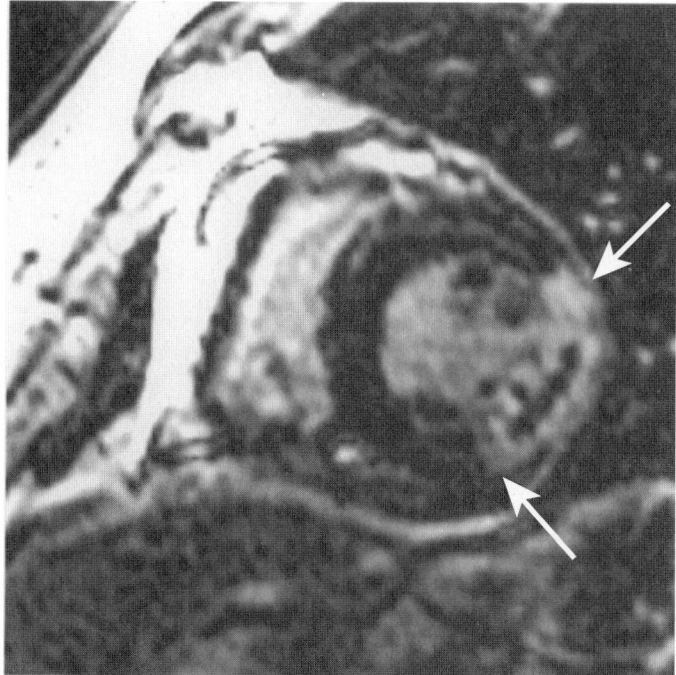

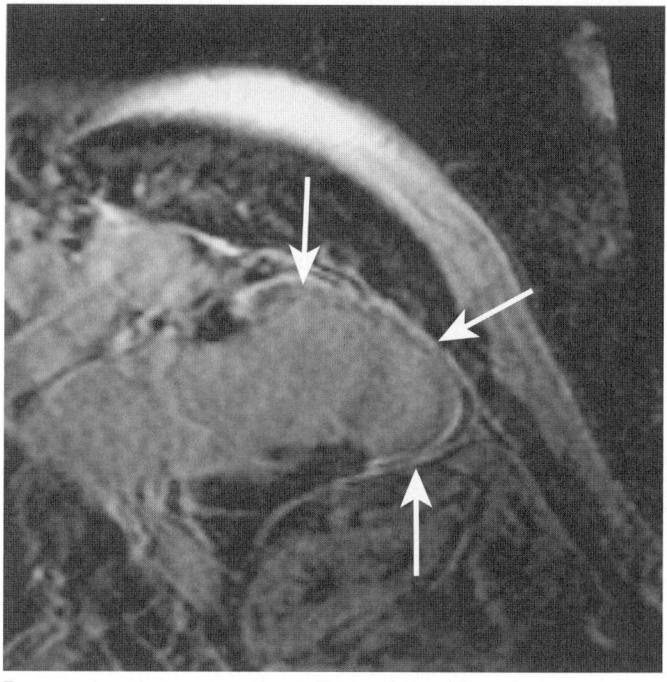

B

FIG. 61-14. Midventricular (left ventricle) short axis view obtained with the delayed enhanced technique. The enhanced *(arrows)* area indicates a transmural circumflex artery territory infarct. The ischemic insult appears as a subendocardial hypointense region consisting of microvascular obstruction (no-reflow zone).

FIG. 61-15. Midventricular short-axis **(A)** and long-axis **(B)** views of left ventricle in a patient with huge septal, anterior, apical, and inferior infarct. Images were obtained with the delayed enhanced technique. The hyperenhanced circular area defines the infarct extent *(arrows),* which is transmural in its septal and inferior components.

In doing so, this method of imaging clarifies the prognosis of the myocardial ischemic insult and may help the clinician and patient with atypical chest pain.

Observation of patients at low risk for ACS has become routine in the case of indeterminate ECG or serum enzyme results. Magnetic resonance methods for myocardial infarction detection have been used recently for evaluating ED patients with indeterminate ECG or serum enzyme results. These methods currently remain confined to major medical centers. Nevertheless, the potential of MR infarct imaging to reduce hospital costs related to patient triage is actively being evaluated.

REFERENCES

1. Becker CR, Ohnesorge BM, Schoepf UJ, et al: Current development of cardiac imaging with multidetector-row CT. *Eur J Radiol* 36:97, 2000.
2. Tatum JL, Jesse RL, Kontos MC, et al: Comprehensive strategy for the evaluation and triage of the chest pain patient. *Ann Emerg Med* 29:116, 1997.
3. Spiegler EJ, Civelek AC, Bahr R, et al: The use of technetium-99m sestamibi in the emergency room: Can it assist in the triage of patients with chest pain? *Clin Nucl Med* 18:807, 1993.
4. Hilton TC, Thompson RC, Williams HJ, et al: Technetium-99m sestamibi myocardial perfusion imaging in the emergency room evaluation of chest pain. *J Am Coll Cardiol* 23:1016, 1994.
5. Varetto T, Cantalupi D, Altieri A, et al: Emergency room technetium sestamibi imaging to rule out acute myocardial ischemic events in patients with nondiagnostic electrocardiograms. *J Am Coll Cardiol* 22:1804, 1993.
6. Peels CH, Visser CA, Kupper AJ, et al: Usefulness of two-dimensional echocardiography for immediate detection of myocardial ischemia in the emergency room. *Am J Cardiol* 65:687, 1990.
7. Berning J, Steensgaard-Hansen F: Early estimation of risk by echocardiographic determination of wall motion index in an unselected population with acute myocardial infarction. *Am J Cardiol* 65:567, 1990.
8. Kimura BJ, Bocchicchio M, Willis CL, et al: Screening cardiac ultrasonographic examination in patients with suspected cardiac disease in the emergency department. *Am Heart J* 142:324, 2001.
9. Stark DD, Bradley WG Jr (eds): *Magnetic Resonance Imaging.* Philadelphia, CV Mosby, 1998.
10. Wilke N, Simm C, Zhang J, et al: Contrast-enhanced first pass myocardial perfusion imaging: Correlation between myocardial blood flow in dogs at rest and during hyperemia. *Magn Reson Med* 29:485, 1993.
11. Wilke N, Jerosch-Herold M, Wang Y, et al: Myocardial perfusion reserve: Assessment with multisection, quantitative, first-pass MR imaging. *Radiology* 204:373, 1997.
12. Nagel E, Lehmkuhl HB, Bocksch W, et al: Noninvasive diagnosis of ischemia induced wall motion abnormalities with the use of high dose dobutamine stress echocardiography. *Circulation* 99:763, 1999.
13. Gerber BL, Bluemke DA, Lima JA, et al: Relation between Gd-DTPA contrast enhancement and regional inotropic response in the periphery and center of myocardial infarction. *Circulation* 104:998, 2001.
14. Wu KC, Zerhouni EA, Judd RM, et al: Prognostic significance of microvascular obstruction by magnetic resonance imaging in patients with acute myocardial infarction. *Circulation* 97:765, 1998.
15. Kim RJ, Simonetti O, Judd RM, et al: The use of contrast-enhanced magnetic resonance imaging to identify reversible myocardial dysfunction. *New Engl J Med* 343:1445, 2000.

RESPIRATORY DISTRESS
J. Stephan Stapczynski

Common respiratory symptoms that bring patients to the ED include dyspnea (with the associated findings of hypoxia and hypercapnia), wheezing, and cough. Hiccups are an infrequent presenting symptom, but when persistent, they are very distressing to the patient. Cyanosis can be associated with pulmonary and vascular, as well as hematologic conditions. Pleural effusion can be caused by a variety of pulmonary and cardiac diseases. This chapter discusses these symptoms, signs, and disorders as they relate to evaluation of emergency patients. It is worth noting that, despite the increasing availability of and reliance on ancillary tests, the assessment of patients still begins with an accurate history and a careful physical examination in order to make the wisest use of ancillary tests.[1]

DYSPNEA

Dyspnea is a subjective feeling of difficult, labored, or uncomfortable breathing. This common emergency department complaint is often described as "shortness of breath," "breathlessness," "not getting enough air," and a variety of other phrases. Dyspnea does not result from a single pathophysiologic mechanism and may result from many disorders. Approximately two-thirds of patients presenting to the ED with dyspnea have either a cardiac or a pulmonary disorder. An emergency physician can usually distinguish these on the basis of history, physical examination, and, occasionally, ancillary tests.

Dyspnea is distinguished from other respiratory symptoms. Tachypnea is rapid breathing; it may or may not be associated with dyspnea, and dyspnea is not always accompanied by tachypnea. Orthopnea is dyspnea in the recumbent position. It is most often the result of left ventricular failure and may be associated with diaphragmatic paralysis or chronic obstructive pulmonary disease (COPD). Paroxysmal nocturnal dyspnea is orthopnea that awakens the patient from sleep. Trepopnea is dyspnea associated with only one of several recumbent positions. Trepopnea can occur with unilateral diaphragmatic paralysis, with ball-valve airway obstruction, or after surgical pneumonectomy. Platypnea is the opposite of orthopnea: dyspnea in the upright position. Platypnea results from the loss of abdominal wall muscular tone and, in rare cases, from right-to-left intracardiac shunting, as occurs from a patent foramen ovale. Hyperpnea is essentially hyperventilation and is defined as minute ventilation in excess of metabolic demand. Hyperpnea may not be associated with dyspnea, and dyspnea is not always associated with increased minute ventilation.

Pathophysiology

Dyspnea is a complex sensation that involves both objective and subjective elements. Unlike other noxious sensations, dyspnea does not have a defined neural pathway, and the perceived difficulty probably arises from the interaction of several pathophysiologic mechanisms.[2] The following processes are involved in the sensation of dyspnea:

1. A conscious sense of the voluntary peripheral skeletal and respiratory muscular effort that occurs with increased work of breathing.
2. Stimulation of upper airway mechanical and thermal receptors.
3. Decreased stimulation of chest wall afferents.
4. Stimulation of central hypercapnic chemoreceptors in the central medulla.
5. Stimulation of peripheral hypoxic chemoreceptors, primarily in the carotid body in concert with those in the aortic arch.
6. Stimulation of a variety of lung receptors, including intraparenchymal pulmonary stretch receptors, airway irritant receptors, and unmyelinated receptors that respond to interstitial edema or a change in compliance.
7. Stimulation of peripheral vascular receptors, including the right atrial and left atrial mechanoreceptor and the pulmonary artery baroreceptor.

Input from any or all of these receptors is integrated in a complex manner in the central nervous system (CNS) at both the subcortical and cortical level. Many authors believe that dyspnea results from afferent mismatch, when feedback from these peripheral receptors indicates that the work of breathing is greater than would be expected by the patient's level of activity.[3]

Clinical Features

Dyspnea has many causes but can be divided into general categories (Table 62-1). Because of its mainly subjective component, the presence or degree of dyspnea is difficult to measure, although categorical scales (e.g., the Borg or Fletcher scales) and visual analogue scales can be used in individual patients to gauge changes in the degree of distress in response to therapy.[4] The initial assessment of any patient with dyspnea should be directed toward identifying imminent respiratory failure. The physician should specifically evaluate for tachypnea, tachycardia, stridor, and use of the accessory respiratory muscles, including the sternocleidomastoid, sternoclavicular, and intercostals. Other signs and symptoms of imminent respiratory failure are inability to speak as a consequence of the breathlessness, agitation or lethargy as a consequence of hypoxia, and paradoxical abdominal wall movement (abdominal wall retracts inward) with inspiration, indicating diaphragmatic fatigue. In patients with any of these signs or symptoms, oxygen should be administered and the need for airway control and mechanical ventilation anticipated. Lesser degrees of dyspnea allow for a more detailed medical history, physical examination, and indicated ancillary tests.

Diagnosis

A detailed medical history often identifies the primary process resulting in dyspnea. Patients often have underlying chronic disorders and can frequently specifically and accurately self-diagnose their exacerbations. The medical history should include recent infectious and environmental exposures that may impair respiratory function. Patients who require daily medications for symptom control should be questioned carefully about compliance and possible drug interactions.

A number of ancillary tests aid in determining the severity and specific cause of dyspnea. Pulse oximetry is a rapid but insensitive screening test for disorders of gas exchange, and results may be normal in acute dyspnea. Arterial blood gas (ABG) analysis is more sensitive for detecting impaired gas exchange, but results may also be normal in acute dyspnea, and ABG analysis cannot evaluate the work of breathing. Rarely, patients who appear dyspneic or tachypneic but who exhibit no evidence of hypoxia or pulmonary disease are shown to be hyperventilating from metabolic acidosis on ABG testing. A chest radiograph may indicate the general category of primary disease; infiltrate, effusion, and pneumothorax. Bedside spirometric analysis (peak expiratory flow, or PEF) before and after bronchodilator therapy

TABLE 62-1   Causes of Dyspnea

Most Common Causes	Most Immediately Life-Threatening
Obstructive airway disease: asthma, COPD	Upper airway obstruction: foreign body, angioedema, hemorrhage
Congestive heart failure/ cardiogenic pulmonary edema	Tension pneumothorax
Ischemic heart disease: unstable angina and myocardial infarction	Pulmonary embolism
Pneumonia	Neuromuscular weakness: myasthenia gravis, Guillain-Barré syndrome, botulism
Psychogenic	

can be used to diagnose and treat dyspnea resulting from asthma or COPD, although it requires voluntary effort that might be difficult for dyspneic patients. B-type natriuretic peptide (BNP) serum levels >100 pg/mL can be used to diagnose congestive heart failure in patients with acute dyspnea in the ED.[5] Other potentially useful tests include an electrocardiogram and determination of hemoglobin level. Uncommonly, the cause of dyspnea cannot be identified by the history, the physical examination, and these ancillary tests, and specialized testing, including cardiac stress testing, echocardiography, formal pulmonary function testing, computed tomography scanning of the chest, or combined cardiopulmonary exercise testing, is indicated.

Treatment

Just as there is no single cause of dyspnea, there is no single treatment. In severe dyspnea, the primary treatment goal is maintenance of the airway and oxygenation with a Pa_{O_2} (partial pressure of arterial oxygen) >60 mm Hg and/or arterial oxygen saturation (Sa_{O_2}) ≥90 percent. After this is ensured, or for patients with lesser degrees of dyspnea, disorder-specific treatment can be provided. Patients with unrelieved dyspnea at rest, particularly those with terminal malignancies, may benefit from opioids or benzodiazepines.[6]

HYPOXEMIA

Hypoxia is insufficient delivery of oxygen to the tissues. The amount of oxygen available to the tissues is a function of the arterial oxygen content (Ca_{O_2}) and blood flow.

$$Ca_{O_2} = 0.0031 \times Pa_{O_2} + 1.38 \times Hb \times Sa_{O_2}$$

Tissue hypoxia occurs in states of low cardiac output, low hemoglobin (Hb) concentration, or low Sa_{O_2}. The percent oxygen saturation of arterial hemoglobin is, in turn, dependent on the Pa_{O_2}, as described by the oxygen-hemoglobin dissociation curve. Hypoxemia is an abnormally low arterial oxygen tension. Under most situations, cardiac output is within a normal range, and hypoxemia is the most common cause of hypoxia. Although the terms *hypoxia* and *hypoxemia* are generally used interchangeably, one can occur without the other. For example, in states of low Pa_{O_2} (hypoxemia) with concomitant polycythemia, the patient may have no tissue hypoxia. Alternatively, very anemic patients may suffer tissue hypoxia despite a normal Pa_{O_2}. Hypoxemia is arbitrarily defined as a Pa_{O_2} <60 mm Hg. As noted above, patients with hypoxemia may not necessarily have dyspnea, and patients with dyspnea may not have hypoxemia.

Relative hypoxemia is the term used when the arterial oxygen tension is lower than expected for a given level of inhaled oxygen. The degree of relative hypoxemia can be assessed by calculating the alveolar-arterial (A-a) oxygen partial pressure gradient. This A-a O_2 gradient measures how well alveolar oxygen is transferred from the lungs to the

circulation. Alveolar oxygen partial pressure is determined by the inhaled oxygen concentration (21 percent for room air), atmospheric pressure (760 mm Hg at sea level), and displacement by water vapor (47 mm Hg for full saturation) and carbon dioxide. Gas in the alveolus is fully saturated with water vapor, and the amount of alveolar oxygen is further reduced by carbon dioxide that freely diffuses from the pulmonary capillaries in an amount determined by the ratio between oxygen consumption and carbon dioxide production, termed the respiratory quotient (R). On a typical diet, the respiratory quotient is 0.8. Thus, alveolar oxygen from breathing room air at sea level has a $Pa_{O_2} = 0.21 \times (760 - 47) - Pa_{CO_2}/0.8$. The A-a gradient at sea level for room air is $P(A-a)_{O_2} = 149 - Pa_{CO_2}/0.8 - Pa_{O_2}$. **A simplified formula is often used is $P(A-a)_{O_2} = 145 - Pa_{CO_2} - Pa_{O_2}$. A normal $P(A-a)_{O_2}$ is under 10 mm Hg in young, healthy patients, and increases with age, predicted by the formula $P(A-a)_{O_2} = 2.5 + 0.21$ (age in years) (± 11).** This value for the normal A-a gradient is for healthy, asymptomatic individuals measured in an upright or sitting position. The supine position alone, as well as many chronic cardiac or pulmonary diseases, may raise the A-a gradient. Thus, many patients seen in the emergency department already have an elevated A-a gradient due to position or underlying chronic diseases, making it difficult to evaluate increases in the gradient that may be due to an acute pathologic condition.

Pathophysiology

Hypoxemia results from any combination of five distinct mechanisms.

1. *Hypoventilation.* Hypoventilation from a variety of disorders may result in hypoxemia. Regardless of its specific etiology, hypoxemia resulting from hypoventilation alone is always associated with an increased Pa_{CO_2}, and a normal A-a O_2 gradient. In the case of pure hypoventilation, the additional CO_2 displaces the inhaled oxygen and lowers the amount in the alveolus. This lowered oxygen content, however, diffuses and mixes normally into the arterial blood.

2. *Right-to-left shunt.* Right-to-left shunting occurs when blood enters the systemic arteries without traversing ventilated lung. There is always a small degree of right-to-left shunting because of the direct left ventricular return of deoxygenated blood from both the coronary veins and the bronchial arteries. Increased right-to-left shunting occurs in a variety of conditions, including pulmonary consolidation, pulmonary atelectasis, and vascular malformations. Regardless of the specific cause of the right-to-left shunt, there is always an increase in the A-a O_2 gradient. Right-to-left shunting does not increase Pa_{CO_2}, and patients with a right-to-left shunt may have an abnormally low Pa_{CO_2} because of hyperventilation. A hallmark of significant right-to-left shunting is the failure of arterial oxygen levels to increase in response to supplemental oxygen. Although a small improvement is observed with supplemental oxygen, hypoxemia is never fully eliminated because of the continuing mixture of deoxygenated blood into the systemic circulation.

3. *Ventilation-perfusion mismatch.* Ideal pulmonary gas exchange depends on a balance of ventilation and perfusion. Any abnormality resulting in a regional alteration of either ventilation or perfusion can adversely affect pulmonary gas exchange, resulting in hypoxemia. A wide variety of etiologies may result in these regional impairments, including pulmonary emboli, pneumonia, asthma, COPD, and even extrinsic vascular compression. Regardless of its specific etiology, hypoxemia from ventilation-perfusion mismatch is associated with an increased A-a O_2 gradient and hypoxemia improves with supplemental oxygen.

4. *Diffusion impairment.* Pulmonary gas exchange also depends on diffusion across the alveolar-blood barrier. Any condition that influences this diffusion may result in hypoxemia. Regardless of the specific cause of the diffusion impairment, the A-a O_2 gradient is increased and hypoxemia improves with supplemental oxygen. From

a practical standpoint, diffusion impairment alone does not produce clinically significant hypoxemia in humans.

5. *Low inspired oxygen.* Decreased ambient oxygen pressure results in hypoxemia. This is most commonly seen at high altitude or in nonobstructive asphyxia. The A-a O_2 gradient is normal and hypoxemia improves with supplemental oxygen. For example, Denver, at 5400 ft above sea level, has an atmospheric pressure of 620 mm Hg and an inhaled oxygen partial pressure of only $0.21 \times 620 = 130$ mm Hg, as opposed to 160 mm Hg at sea level.

There are three distinct acute compensatory mechanisms for hypoxemia. Initially, minute ventilation increases. Next, pulmonary arterial vasoconstriction decreases perfusion to hypoxic alveoli. While vasoconstriction balances ventilation and perfusion in order to restore arterial oxygenation, it may also cause acute right heart failure and is ineffective with diffuse lung disease. Finally, sympathetic tone increases and improves oxygen delivery by increasing cardiac output, usually with an increased heart rate. Chronic compensatory mechanisms include an increased red blood cell mass and decreased tissue oxygen demands. These compensatory mechanisms appear to be activated at different levels of hypoxemia for different individuals. However, the acute compensatory mechanisms are always activated when Pao_2 reaches 60 mm Hg, and compensatory mechanisms fail when Pao_2 falls below 20 mm Hg.

Clinical Features

The signs and symptoms of hypoxemia are nonspecific. CNS manifestations include agitation, headache, somnolence, coma, and seizures. While tachypnea and hyperventilation are often present, at a Pao_2 <20 mm Hg, there is a central depression of respiratory drive. Cyanosis is not a sensitive or specific indicator of hypoxemia. Patients with chronic compensatory mechanisms may display polycythemia or alterations in body habitus (e.g., pulmonary cachexia). Using a combination of clinical signs, it is possible to predict hypoxemia in children with acute respiratory tract infections with a reasonable accuracy.[7]

Diagnosis

The diagnosis of arterial hypoxemia requires objective measurement. Because hypoxemia is defined as a Pao_2 <60 mm Hg, formal diagnosis requires ABG analysis. Although pulse oximetry is useful for screening purposes and decreased Sao_2 readings accurately predict significant hypoxemia, normal oxygen saturation readings do not exclude hypoxemia.

Treatment

Regardless of the specific cause of hypoxemia, the initial approach remains the same: ensuring a patent airway and providing supplemental oxygenation with a goal of maintaining a Pao_2 >60 mm Hg. Except in patients with right-to-left shunts, arterial oxygenation responds to supplemental oxygen.

HYPERCAPNIA

Hypercapnia is exclusively caused by alveolar hypoventilation and is arbitrarily defined as a $Paco_2$ >45 mm Hg. Alveolar hypoventilation can be a result of a variety of disorders, including rapid shallow breathing, small tidal volumes, underventilation of the lung, or reduced respiratory drive; it is never a result of increased CO_2 production (Table 62-2).

Pathophysiology

A portion of each tidal volume remains in the non-gas-exchange portion of the respiratory system—termed the "dead space"—and is usu-

TABLE 62-2   Causes of Hypercapnia

Depressed central respiratory drive
Structural CNS disease: brainstem lesions
Drug depression of respiratory center: opioids, sedatives, anesthetics
Endogenous toxins: tetanus
Thoracic cage disorders
Kyphoscoliosis
Morbid obesity
Neuromuscular impairment
Neuromuscular disease: myasthenia gravis, Guillain-Barré syndrome
Neuromuscular toxin: organophosphate poisoning, botulism
Intrinsic lung disease associated with increased dead space
COPD
Upper airway obstruction

ally determined by the anatomic size of the conducting airways (trachea and bronchi). The portion of the tidal volume that reaches the alveoli is that which remains after the dead space volume is subtracted: Ta (alveolar volume) = TV (tidal volume) −Td (dead space). Alveolar ventilation per minute is the volume multiplied by the rate: A = Ta × R (respiratory rate) = (TV −Td) × R. Alveolar hypoventilation can result from a decrease in respiratory rate, a decrease in tidal volume, or an increase in dead space. Under some conditions, dead space volume can increase above that caused by the anatomic size of the conducting airways. This increase is a result of ventilation of lung portions with deficient or absent perfusion; these ventilated portions do not participate fully in gas exchange because of inadequate blood flow.

Because the medullary chemoreceptors stimulate both respiratory rate and tidal volume in response to increased CO_2, alveolar ventilation is finely controlled to maintain $Paco_2$ within a narrow range under most circumstances. In essence, alveolar ventilation is balanced relative to the production of CO_2 to maintain the $Paco_2$ within a narrow range. Decreased respiratory drive is associated with CNS lesions and toxic depression (see Table 62-2). Thoracic cage and neuromuscular disorders produce hypoventilation by slowing respiratory rate and/or decreasing tidal volume relative to the production of CO_2. Intrinsic lung diseases, such as COPD, produce alveolar hypoventilation because of an increase in dead space.

Clinical Features

The signs and symptoms of hypercapnia depend on the absolute value of $Paco_2$ and its rate of change. Acute elevations result in increased intracranial pressure, and patients may complain of headache, confusion, or lethargy. With severe hypercapnia, seizures and coma can result. Extreme hypercapnia can result in cardiovascular collapse, but this is usually seen only with acute elevations of $Paco_2$ >100 mm Hg. As opposed to acute hypercapnia, chronic hypercapnia, even >80 mm Hg, may be well tolerated.

Diagnosis

Diagnosis of hypercapnia requires ABG analysis. Depending on other factors, pulse oximetry analysis can be normal. With acute hypercapnia, the serum bicarbonate level increases slightly as a result of mass action through the CO_2-bicarbonate equilibrium: bicarbonate increases about 1 mEq/L for each increase of 10 mm Hg in the $Paco_2$. Patients with chronic hypercapnia have an elevated serum bicarbonate concentration due to the renal response to increased $Paco_2$: the serum bicarbonate concentration increases about 3.5 mEq/L for each increase of 10 mm Hg in the $Paco_2$.

Treatment

Treatment of hypercapnia requires maneuvers to increase minute ventilation, both the rate and the tidal volume as appropriate. This involves ensuring a patent airway and may require mechanical ventilation or a respiratory stimulant such as doxapram.[8] The disposition of hypercapnic patients depends primarily on the underlying cause and severity. In general, patients with hypercapnia that causes CNS symptoms should be hospitalized. Also, patients with neuromuscular disease—either congenital or acquired—who present with acute hypercapnia should be hospitalized. Some COPD patients have chronic hypercapnia and do not require admission provided they are stable. Conversely, patients with COPD who display worsening hypercapnia despite maximal therapy require hospital admission.

WHEEZING

Wheezes are adventitious lung sounds that can be best described as "musical," produced by airflow through the central and distal airways.[9] Wheezes have sinusoidal acoustics, over a wide frequency range, typically 100 to 1000 Hz. The duration is prolonged, typically longer than 80 ms. Wheezes differ from the other two main adventitial lung sounds: rhonchi and crackles (rales). Rhonchi are a series of damped sinusoidal sounds of lower frequency (<300 Hz) and prolonged duration (>100 ms). Crackles are a series of intermittent individual sounds, typically of less than 20 ms duration.

Pathophysiology

The current theory is that wheezes are produced by airway flutter and vortex shedding from the central and distal airways, although movement of airway secretions may play a small role. While flutter and vortex shedding are possible in normal airways, these processes are more pronounced in obstructed airways. Airway obstruction is associated with the processes of bronchial smooth muscle contraction (bronchospasm), smooth muscle hypertrophy, increased mucus secretion, and peribronchial inflammation.

Clinical Features

Wheezing is not synonymous with airflow obstruction as evidenced by the observation that wheezing can occur during quiet inspiration in some normal children and adults, and with forced expiration in many more. Conversely, patients with airflow obstruction may not have wheezing; the sensitivity of wheezing in detecting bronchial hyperreactivity with airflow limitation of greater than 20 percent is at best 75 percent, and patients with profound obstruction (<20 percent of normal) may have not enough gas movement to generate a sound. These facts notwithstanding, wheezing is usually associated with asthma and other obstructive pulmonary diseases characterized by bronchial obstruction caused by muscular spasm and inflammation (Table 62-3).

The duration of wheezing, or, more precisely, that portion of the expiratory phase occupied by wheezing, has been used to quantify the severity of airflow obstruction in moderate-to-severe acute asthma. As noted above, patients with the most profound obstruction may not wheeze, but their condition can be detected by noting markedly decreased lung sounds.

Most patients with bronchospastic disease (either asthma or COPD) relate a history of previous attacks and response to bronchodilators. The finding of wheezing in a symptomatic patient without such a history is a clue that another process may be present.

Diagnosis

Airflow obstruction can be assessed by bedside spirometric analysis using portable machines; either PEF or forced expiratory volume in 1 s (FEV_1) is measured. Accurate measurement requires a cooperative patient and several (usually three) maximal-effort expirations. Severely dyspneic patients are often not able to perform the maneuver. Likewise, children may not understand the directions well enough to give a maximal effort. Because this test is effort dependent, only the maximal value should be reported. The obtained value should be compared to predicted normal values, dependent primarily on age, gender, and height, with only a small and clinically inconsequential adjustment for weight and ethnic background. For practical purposes, PEF or FEV_1 values >80 percent of the predicted value are within the normal range. Values between 50 and 80 percent of the predicted value constitute mild airflow obstruction, values between 25 and 50 percent constitute moderate airflow obstruction, and values <25 percent constitute severe airflow obstruction. However, the severity of clinical symptoms is dependent as much on the rapidity of the development of obstruction as on its absolute value. Conversely, relief of symptoms is correlated more closely with the relative degree of airflow improvement than with the absolute value.

Spirometric analysis can also be used to monitor response to treatment. Because of variations in effort and measurement, a change in spirometric value of up to 6 percent can be within the error range of the test. Thus, a significant change in PEF or FEV_1 is more than 8 to 10 percent from one measurement to another.

A chest radiograph may be useful in assessing wheezing, particularly for patients without a history of asthma. As noted elsewhere, patients with uncomplicated acute asthma do not require routine chest radiographs during their ED assessment and treatment. Conversely, patients with COPD and congestive heart failure who present with dyspnea and wheezing should have chest radiographs to evaluate for severity and complications.

ABG analysis is useful if clinical examination suggests hypoxemia, hypercapnia, or metabolic acidosis. The ABG analysis may also provide baseline values for further testing and treatment. However, most patients with mild-to-moderate asthma and wheezing can be assessed by spirometric analysis and do not require routine ABG analysis.

Treatment

Treatment of wheezing is directed by the underlying disorder and often involves aerosols of β_2-agonists (e.g., albuterol) and/or anticholinergics (e.g., ipratropium bromide). Patients with peribronchial inflammation are often treated with systemic (oral or intravenous) or inhaled steroids.

COUGH

Cough is a common and nonspecific symptom that may bring patients to the ED, particularly if the cough interferes with activity or sleep.

Pathophysiology

Cough is a protective reflex that acts to clear secretions and foreign debris from the tracheobronchial tree.[10] Coughing is initiated by stimu-

---

TABLE 62-3   Causes of Wheezing

Upper airway (more likely to be stridor, may have element of wheezing)
    Angioedema: allergic, ACE inhibitor, idiopathic
    Foreign body
    Infection: croup, epiglottis, tracheitis
Lower airway
    Asthma
    Transient airway hyperreactivity (usually caused by infection or irritation)
    Bronchiolitis
    COPD
    Foreign body
Cardiovascular
    Cardiogenic pulmonary edema ("cardiac asthma")
    Noncardiogenic pulmonary edema (ARDS)
    Pulmonary embolus (rare)
Psychogenic

Abbreviations: ACE = angiotensin-converting enzyme; ARDS = acute respiratory distress syndrome.

lation of irritant receptors located largely in the larynx, trachea, and major bronchi. These receptors are stimulated by inhaled irritants (e.g., dust), allergens (e.g., ragweed pollen), toxic substances (e.g., gastric acid), hypo- or hyperosmotic liquids, inflammation (e.g., asthma), cold air, instrumentation, and excess pulmonary secretions. Minor cough receptors located in the upper respiratory tract (sinuses and pharynx) and chest (pleura, pericardium, and diaphragm) may stimulate coughing. Signals from these receptors travel via the vagus, phrenic, and other nerves to the cough center in the medulla.

Once stimulated, the cough center initiates the stereotypical cough pattern: a deep inspiration followed by attempted expiration against a closed glottis that suddenly opens, providing for a forceful exhalation of gas, secretions, and foreign debris from the tracheobronchial tree. Extremely high peak airway velocities have been measured with coughing. The coughing sound is generated at the larynx and resonates in the nasal cavity and the lungs.[10]

Coughing patterns vary widely according to the underlying pathologic condition of the lung, the presence or absence of secretions, and whether the cough is voluntary or involuntary. Thus, it is not surprising that the frequency, duration, and quality of coughing vary among patients.

Clinical Features

For the purposes of differential diagnosis, cough has been subdivided into acute and chronic, primarily used to separate the self-limited syndromes of acute bronchitis and upper respiratory infection (URI) from other causes (Table 62-4). Chronic cough is defined as a cough that is present for more than 3 weeks without any periods of resolution. Cough has also been divided into nonproductive and productive with excess sputum production. That distinction may be artificial because, at least for cases of chronic cough, the same disorders produce both nonproductive and productive coughing; the distinction is without diagnostic utility.

Excluding environmental exposures, acute cough is most often caused by URI, lower respiratory tract infection, and allergic reactions. Common URIs are associated with a combination of rhinorrhea, sinusitis, pharyngitis, and laryngitis, with the cough a result of drainage from the nasopharynx onto cough receptors in the pharynx and larynx. A productive cough is the hallmark of acute bronchitis. While pneumonia generally produces a cough, pulmonary secretions may be scant and the cough nonproductive. Mycobacterial and fungal pulmonary infections may produce cough, but the presentation is usually more

subacute or chronic. Acute asthma is often associated with cough, but symptoms of wheezing and dyspnea usually dominate. Occasionally, a patient with asthma may present with coughing, as opposed to wheezing, as the principle manifestation of airflow obstruction.

Chronic cough is caused by a wide variety of disorders, but studies have found that most patients have chronic cough because of (1) smoking, often with chronic bronchitis, (2) postnasal discharge, (3) asthma, (4) gastroesophageal (GE) reflux, and (5) angiotensin-converting enzyme (ACE) inhibitor or angiotensin II receptor blocker therapy (see Table 62-4).[11–13] The association of smoking, chronic bronchitis, and persistent cough is so obvious as to merit little discussion, other than to firmly point it out to patients. Smoking-induced coughing is usually worse in the morning and, with chronic bronchitis, usually productive. Rhinitis with postnasal discharge is associated with mucus drainage from the nose, a history of "allergies or sinus problems," and frequent clearing of the throat or swallowing of mucus. Chronic cough associated with asthma is usually worse at night, exacerbated by irritants, and associated with episodic wheezing and dyspnea. Asthma can be exacerbated by β-blocker therapy and presents with nocturnal coughing. Cough associated with GE reflux often has a history of heartburn, is worse when lying down, and improves with antiacid therapy (antacids, H_2 blockers, or proton-pump blockers). The incidence of ACE inhibitor cough is approximately 10 to 12 percent, although higher values have been published.[14] All ACE inhibitors and angiotensin II receptor blockers have been reported to induce cough and it is not clear whether certain agents have a higher likelihood of inducing cough than others. ACE inhibitor cough is thought to result when the blockade of ACE leads to accumulation of bradykinin and substance P, which stimulate the pulmonary cough receptors and enhance the formation of irritating prostaglandin metabolites. Extreme variability characterizes ACE inhibitor cough: early (1 week) or later (1 year) onset after starting treatment, only slightly bothersome to debilitating symptoms, and variation during the day. The association of pertussis in adults with persistent cough (>2 weeks) was documented from a convenience sample from one emergency department and in isolated outbreaks.[15]

Diagnosis

Most causes of acute cough do not warrant routine ancillary tests. A chest radiograph may be used in patients with purulent sputum and/or fever, and spirometric analysis may be used to document the presence of airflow obstruction in patients with asthma.

Patients with chronic cough are usually treated based on clinical assessment first, and ancillary tests are performed only if symptoms persist. Nasolaryngoscopy can be used to document the presence of mucosal inflammation and excessive mucus drainage. Sinus radiographs or computed tomography scanning can document the presence of sinusitis. A chest radiograph can detect focal or diffuse lung disease. Spirometric analysis can identify airflow obstruction, although, in cases of asthma-associated cough, the spirometric values are normal between attacks. GE reflux can be documented by a number of methods; esophageal pH monitoring is probably the most useful.

Treatment

In addition to disease-specific therapy, patients with acute cough may occasionally benefit from antitussives, which block the cough reflex at various locations.[16] The effectiveness of medicinal and herbal antitussives is controversial, and the majority of benefit may be a placebo effect or demulcent effect. The most effective cough suppressants are the opioids, such as dextromethorphan, codeine, and oxycodone. While cough suppressants are usually restricted to patients with a dry cough and avoided in patients with significant sputum production, there is only tradition to support this practice. Demulcents, part of most proprietary cough preparations, soothe the pharynx and somewhat suppress the cough reflex. Of the herbal agents, menthol and the pungent

TABLE 62-4   Causes of Cough

Acute	Chronic: Common	Chronic: Less Common
Upper respiratory infection: rhinitis, sinusitis	Smoking and/or chronic bronchitis	Congestive heart failure
Lower respiratory tract infection: bronchitis, pneumonia	Postnasal discharge	Bronchiectasis
Allergic reaction	Asthma: reactive airways disease	Lung cancer or other intrathoracic mass
Asthma	Gastroesophageal reflux	Emphysema
Environmental irritants	Angiotensin-converting enzyme inhibitor	Occupational and environmental irritants
Transient airway hyperresponsiveness	Angiotensin II receptor blocker	Recurrent aspiration or chronic foreign body
Foreign body		Miscellaneous: cystic fibrosis, interstitial lung disease

spices (e.g., pepper, mustard, garlic, radish, and onions) have an antitussive effect.[16]

Because chronic cough is most often the result of a few common disorders, an algorithmic approach to treatment using sequential steps appears to be effective:[13,17]

 1. Reduce exposure to lung irritants (e.g., smoking) and discontinue ACE inhibitors, angiotensin II receptor blockers, and β-blockers.
2. Treat for postnasal discharge with an oral antihistamine-decongestant and/or an inhaled nasal steroid. If the cough improves, continue treatment and evaluate for sinus disease with imaging studies.
3. Evaluate and treat for asthma.
4. Obtain chest and sinus radiographs if not already done.
5. Evaluate and treat for GE reflux.
6. Refer the patient for bronchoscopy.

By using a sequential approach, tailoring treatment to the clinical symptoms and the patient's responses, more than 95 percent of patients achieve resolution of their cough.[17]

HICCUPS

Hiccup, or singultus, is an involuntary respiratory reflex with spastic contraction of the inspiratory muscles against a closed glottis, producing the characteristic sound. As opposed to coughing, where the reflex serves the useful purpose of expelling secretions and debris from the pulmonary tree, a specific protective purpose has not be elucidated for hiccups.[18]

Pathophysiology

The afferent arm of the hiccup reflex consists of the phrenic and vagus nerves as well as the thoracic sympathetic chain. There is no well-defined central hiccup center; instead, there is an intensive interconnection among the hypothalamus, medullary reticular formation, respiratory center, and cranial nerve nuclei. The efferent limb of the reflux uses the phrenic nerve, the recurrent laryngeal branch of the vagus nerve, and the motor nerves to the anterior scalene and intercostal muscles.

As noted above, hiccups are produced by spasmodic contraction of the inspiratory muscles (diaphragm and intercostals) against a closed glottis, a breakdown in the normal relationship between inspiration and glottic closure. Inspiration normally inhibits glottic closure and maintains an open airway. During swallowing, the stimulation of glottic closure inhibits inspiration, preventing aspiration. In some manner, the hiccup reflex disrupts the connection between these two processes so that 30 to 40 ms after the onset of inspiration, glottic closure is stimulated. In most cases where a specific cause can be assigned, hiccups appear to result from stimulation, inflammation, or injury to one of the nerves of the reflex arc.

Clinical Features

For diagnostic classification, hiccups are divided into benign self-limited and persistent, or intractable (Table 62-5).[18]

Benign hiccups are generally initiated by gastric distention from food, drinking (especially carbonated beverages), or air. Alcohol ingestion appears to precipitate hiccups by relaxing the relationship between inspiration and glottic closure, making it easier for other stimuli to trigger the reflex. Excessive smoking, a sudden change in environmental temperature, and psychogenic events (excitement or stress) are sometimes associated with hiccups.

Persistent hiccups are usually a result of damage or irritation to a branch of the vagus or phrenic nerve. A wide variety of events have been implicated in producing persistent hiccups. One rare but readily treatable stimulus is a foreign body (often a hair) in the external auditory canal that is pressing against the tympanic membrane and stimu-

TABLE 62-5 Causes of Hiccups

Acute: Benign, Self-limited	Chronic: Persistent, Intractable
Gastric distention	Central nervous system structural lesions
Alcohol intoxication	Vagal or phrenic nerve irritation
Excessive smoking	Metabolic: uremia, hyperglycemia
Abrupt change in environmental temperature	General anesthesia
Psychogenic	Surgical procedures: thoracic, abdominal, prostate and urinary tract, craniotomy

lating the auricular branch of the vagus nerve. Several drugs—usually steroids and benzodiazepines—are implicated in inducing hiccups, but the evidence is weak.[19]

Diagnosis

Most patients with benign hiccups resolve spontaneously or with simple maneuvers, do not seek medical attention, and do not require specific diagnosis. Patients with persistent hiccups often seek medical attention, occasionally in the ED.

The evaluation of persistent hiccups should start with a history to determine whether a specific event was associated with the onset. Are the hiccups persistent during sleep? Persistence during sleep suggests an organic cause, and resolution during sleep suggests a psychogenic cause, although this distinction is not absolute. Inquiries should be made concerning general anesthesia, surgical procedures, and several metabolic diseases that are associated with persistent hiccups. As noted above, the external auditory canal should be carefully examined. A chest radiograph should be done to evaluate for possible intrathoracic pathology. Fluoroscopy can be useful to evaluate for unilateral versus bilateral diaphragmatic movement during hiccups.

Treatment

A wide variety of physical maneuvers have been used to terminate an acute episode of hiccups. Many of these measures are based on the concept that stimulating the pharynx will block the vagal portion of the reflex arc and abolish the hiccups.[20] No one method appears to be more effective than another. Swallowing a teaspoon of granulated sugar dry is about as effective as others and does not involve the infliction of noxious or painful stimulation.

Drug treatment also works by inhibiting the reflex arc.[20] A large number of agents have been described as effective, but mostly only as case reports. Of the recommended drugs, only chlorpromazine has been tried enough to have achieved U.S. Food and Drug Administration approval for treatment of intractable hiccups. The recommended dose is 25 to 50 mg IV, with a repeated dose in 2 to 4 h if needed. If improvement is noted, oral therapy with 25 to 50 mg tid or qid should be given. Metoclopramide 10 mg IV or IM and, if effective, followed by 10 to 20 mg qid for 10 days, appears to be effective. Unlike with other agents, the effectiveness of both these drugs is usually evident within 30 min. The major disadvantages are extrapyramidal symptoms with both drugs and hypotension with chlorpromazine.

For more gradual control and with perhaps less risk of adverse reactions, oral treatment can be initiated with nifedipine 10 to 20 mg tid or qid, valproic acid 15 mg/kg per d taken tid, or baclofen 10 mg tid. Initiation and maintenance of these agents is best done in concert with a primary care physician who will follow up with the patient.

CYANOSIS

Cyanosis is a bluish color of the skin and mucous membranes that results from an increased amount of reduced hemoglobin (deoxyhemoglobin) or hemoglobin derivatives. The detection of cyanosis can be highly subjective and is not considered a sensitive indicator of the state of arterial oxygenation. In fact, cyanosis is determined by the absolute amount of deoxygenated hemoglobin in the blood; the amount of oxygenated hemoglobin is of little influence.

Pathophysiology

Traditional teaching has been that cyanosis is usually present when deoxygenated hemoglobin exceeds 5 g/dL. However, this figure is questionable because central cyanosis can be detected with deoxyhemoglobin concentration as low as 1.5 g/dL. In some instances, cyanosis can be detected when Sao_2 has fallen to 85 percent; in others, it may not be detected until Sao_2 is 75 percent.

Various physiologic, anatomic, and physical factors other than the amount of reduced hemoglobin may influence the appearance of cyanosis, making an accurate clinical detection of the degree or even the presence of cyanosis difficult. Physiologic factors include the oxygen content of the blood, level of tissue oxygenation, degree of oxygen extraction, and oxyhemoglobin dissociation curve. Anatomic factors include the status of the cutaneous microcirculation, pigmentation, and thickness of the skin. Physical factors include the lighting under which the patient is examined and the skill of the physician. The tongue is considered one of the most sensitive sites for observing central cyanosis, and the earlobes, conjunctivae, and nail beds are considered to be much-less reliable.

Clinical Features

Clinically, the presence of cyanosis suggests the possibility of tissue hypoxia, and possible causes for hypoxia should be considered. Unexplained cyanosis, particularly in association with normal arterial oxygen tension (Pao_2), suggests the possibility of abnormal hemoglobin, such as methemoglobin.

Cyanosis is traditionally divided into two categories: central and peripheral. The central type is seen under conditions with unsaturated arterial blood or abnormal hemoglobin. The mucous membranes and skin are both affected. In contrast, peripheral cyanosis is caused by the slowing of blood flow to an area and an abnormally great extraction of oxygen from normally saturated arterial blood. Congestive heart failure, peripheral vascular disease, shock states, and cold exposure all create states of vasoconstriction and decreased peripheral blood flow. The differentiation between central and peripheral cyanosis may not be possible in conditions where both mechanisms are present (Table 62-6).

Diagnosis

The presence of cyanosis suggests the possibility of hypoxemia, and pulse oximetry analysis is readily available to assist the physician in the early diagnosis of hypoxemia and provide continuous oxygen saturation measurements. However, an exception occurs when the hemoglobin is in a state in which it is unable to bind to oxygen (i.e., methemoglobin or carboxyhemoglobin). In such situations, pulse oximetry analysis not only overestimates the oxygen saturation but also reflects a diminished response to any supplemental oxygen. ABG analysis with co-oximetry is still the gold standard in the assessment of any patient with suspected cyanosis. In central cyanosis, the oxygen saturation measured from the ABG is decreased because of the underlying hypoxemia. In peripheral cyanosis, assuming normal cardiopulmonary and hemoglobin status, the oxygen saturation should be normal. If methemoglobinemia or carboxyhemoglobinemia is suspected, the

TABLE 62-6   Causes of Cyanosis

Central Cyanosis	Peripheral Cyanosis
Hypoxemia	Reduced cardiac output
Decreased Fio_2: high altitude	Cold extremities
Hypoventilation	Maldistribution of blood flow:
Ventilation–perfusion mismatch	distributive forms of shock
Right-to-left shunt: congenital	Arterial or venous obstruction
heart disease, pulmonary	
arteriovenous fistulas, multiple	
intrapulmonary shunts	
Hemoglobin abnormalities	
Methemoglobinemia: hereditary,	
acquired	
Sulfhemoglobinemia: acquired	
Carboxyhemoglobinemia	
(not true cyanosis)	

Abbreviation: Fio_2 = fraction of inspired oxygen.

ABG analysis will show a normal Pao_2 (reflecting a normal amount of dissolved oxygen in the plasma), a normal calculated oxygen saturation (from the normal Pao_2), and a decrease in measured oxygen saturation (because of a decreased number of oxygen binding sites).

Few tests are as vulnerable to errors introduced by improper sampling, handling, and storage as are ABG analyses. The technical difficulties with obtaining an arterial sample via percutaneous puncture accounts for much of the high preanalytic error rate for isolated ABG samples obtained in the emergency department, compared to a low error rate for samples obtained from an indwelling arterial catheter.

Special attention should be given to the following sources of preanalytic error with ABG samples. Heparin is the anticoagulant of choice, and one should make sure that the syringe is flushed with heparin and then emptied thoroughly. This will allow adequate anticoagulation of a 2- to 4-mL blood sample with assurance that the results will not be altered by the anticoagulant. Excessive heparin affects the pH, Pco_2, and Po_2 as well as the hemoglobin determination. Air bubbles that mix with the blood sample will result in gas equilibration, significantly lowering the Pco_2 values with an increase in pH and Po_2. Any sample obtained with more than minor air bubbles should be discarded. Reducing the temperature of the blood by placing the sample immediately in ice slush will significantly deter changes in the Pco_2 and pH for a period of several hours. As a general rule, arterial blood samples should be analyzed within 10 min or cooled immediately. Failure to properly cool the sample is a common source of preanalytic error.

Hypoxemia, anemia, and polycythemia can be diagnosed by means of hemoglobin and ABG determination. The red cyanosis of polycythemia vera occurs because the increase in the number of red blood cells and the hemoglobin concentration results in sludging of blood flow in cutaneous capillaries and venules. Similarly, cyanosis is enhanced in chronic hypoxemia accompanied by polycythemia.

If the measured Pao_2 and the hemoglobin concentration are normal, the cyanosis may be a result of abnormal skin pigmentation or abnormal hemoglobin. The term pseudocyanosis is used to describe a blue, gray, or purple cutaneous discoloration that may mimic cyanosis. Pseudocyanosis can be caused by heavy metals [e.g., iron (hemochromatosis), gold, silver, lead, and arsenic] or drugs (e.g., phenothiazine, minocycline, amiodarone, and chloroquine). Chrysiasis is a specific type of pseudocyanosis that is characterized by a gray, blue, or purple pigmentation of areas exposed to light. It is a rare dose-dependent complication of gold treatment that tends to cause permanent discoloration of the skin. Another example of pseudocyanosis is argyria, which is a slate blue-to-gray coloration of the skin resulting from either chronic ingestion or chronic local application of silver salts or colloidal silver. In pseudocyanosis the skin does not blanch with pressure, in contrast to true cyanotic skin, which does blanch. Carboxyhemoglobinemia does not cause cyanosis. Occasionally, however, carboxyhemoglobinemia does produce a cherry-red flush of the skin, retina, or mucous membranes.

Cyanosis can be caused by methemoglobinemia and sulfhemoglobinemia. Most cases are caused by chemicals or medications. Although a wide range of drugs can produce methemoglobinemia, benzocaine, nitrates, and nitrites are the most common agents implicated in drug-induced methemoglobinemia. Sulfhemoglobinemia most commonly results from either phenacetin or acetanilid. Industrial aniline compounds may produce either sulfhemoglobinemia or methemoglobinemia.

The incidence of acquired methemoglobinemia secondary to industrial exposure to aniline dyes and aromatic amino and nitro compounds has decreased with improvement in occupational health standards. Hereditary methemoglobinemia is a rare genetic disorder affecting the enzyme NADH [nicotinamide adenine dinucleotide (reduced form)]-methemoglobin reductase, resulting in structural alterations of the hemoglobin molecule. This enzyme is the major pathway responsible for converting methemoglobin to its reduced state. This pathway plays a clinically significant role in the treatment of methemoglobinemia because it is the pathway by which the antidote, methylene blue, is able to enhance the reduction of methemoglobin. Patients with NADH-methemoglobin reductase deficiency appear cyanotic but are usually compensated and asymptomatic.

Methemoglobinemia produces visible cyanosis with as little as 1.5 g/dL. Because methemoglobin is incapable of binding with oxygen, the symptoms of methemoglobinemia are secondary to hypoxia, and the severity is related to the quantity of methemoglobin present, the rapidity of onset, and the patient's cardiopulmonary system. Cyanotic patients without cardiovascular or pulmonary disease should be suspected of having methemoglobinemia, especially if cyanosis is not relieved by oxygen administration. An additional clue is that venous blood will appear chocolate brown. Spectrophotometric analysis is required for identification of the pigment and its quantity.

Sulfhemoglobin is inert as an oxygen carrier and can produce deep cyanosis at a level of less than 0.5 g/dL. Unlike methemoglobinemia, sulfhemoglobinemia is irreversible. Treatment is directed toward symptomatic and supportive care as well as the identification and removal of suspected causes.

Treatment

Patients with central cyanosis should be started on supplemental oxygen. Failure to improve suggests impaired circulation (shock), abnormal hemoglobin, or pseudocyanosis. In acquired methemoglobinemia, no treatment is necessary unless signs of hypoxia (i.e., angina, arrhythmias, hypotension, stupor, or coma) are present. Methylene blue 1 to 2 mg/kg of body weight given intravenously over 5 min is the antidote for acquired methemoglobinemia (see Chap. 189). Caution should be taken whenever methylene blue is used; by itself, at high doses, it can cause hemolysis or even precipitate methemoglobinemia and possibly worsen the patient's condition.

PLEURAL EFFUSION

Pleural effusions result from fluid accumulating in the potential space between the visceral and parietal pleurae. While pleural effusions can result from many causes, in developed countries, the most common causes are congestive heart failure, pneumonia, and cancer (Table 62-7).

Pathophysiology

Normally, a small amount of fluid is secreted from the parietal pleural into the pleural space where it is absorbed by the visceral pleural microcirculation. This small amount of pleural fluid reduces friction between the pleural layers and allows for smooth lung expansion and contraction with respiration. Any process that increases fluid production or

TABLE 62-7   Causes of Pleural Effusion

Common	Less Common
TRANSUDATES	
Congestive heart failure	Cirrhosis with ascites
	Peritoneal dialysis
	Nephrotic syndrome
EXUDATES	
Cancer: primary or metastatic	Viral, fungal, mycobacterial, or parasitic infection
Bacterial pneumonia with parapneumonic effusion	Systemic rheumatologic disorders: systemic lupus erythematosus, rheumatoid arthritis
Pulmonary embolism	Uremia, pancreatitis
	Postcardiac surgery or radiotherapy
	Drug-related: amiodarone
EITHER TRANSUDATES OR EXUDATES	
Transudates after diuretic therapy	Pulmonary embolism

interferes with fluid absorption will result in accumulation in the pleural space. Pleural effusions are traditionally divided into exudates or transudates based on mechanism.[21] Exudative effusions result from pleural disease, usually inflammation or neoplasia, that results in active fluid secretion or leakage with high protein content. Transudative effusions result from an imbalance in hydrostatic (e.g., congestive heart failure) or oncotic (e.g., nephrotic syndrome) pressure and produce an ultrafiltrate across the pleural membrane with low protein content.

Clinical Features

A pleural effusion may be clinically silent, or come to detection from either symptoms of an underlying disease, an increase in volume of the effusion with the production of dyspnea, or the development of inflammation and associated pain with respiration. Physical findings of a pleural effusion include percussion dullness and decreased breath sounds. Because pleural fluid typically pools in the dependent portions of the hemithorax, small or moderate size effusions have percussion dullness and decreased breath sounds at the lung base with relatively normal lung findings above the level of fluid. With large or massive effusions, it may be impossible to distinguish a fluid level on clinical examination.

Diagnosis

In an adult, 150 to 200 mL of pleural fluid in the hemithorax is required to produce signs on upright chest radiography. When taken in the supine position, chest radiographs may demonstrate only a hazy appearance of pleural fluid in the posterior pleural space. Small free-flowing pleural effusions can be visualized on decubitus radiographic views. Ultrasonography can be used to image pleural effusions, although accuracy depends on operator technique and the quality of interpretation. A significant pleural effusion is large enough to produce a pleural fluid strip more than 10 mm wide on lateral decubitus radiographic views or by ultrasonography.[21]

Diagnostic thoracentesis is done to obtain pleural fluid for analysis in cases without a clearly evident cause, to confirm a suspected diagnosis, or to detect pleural space infection. For example, because the largest single cause of pleural effusion is congestive heart failure, if a patient presents with a typical appearance (cardiomegaly, roughly equal in size bilateral effusions), then a period of treatment with monitoring for pleural fluid resolution is indicated, and routine thoracentesis is reserved for those patients who do not resolve in 3 to 4 days. Otherwise, diagnostic thoracentesis and pleural fluid analysis is indicated.

Light and colleagues developed the most widely used criteria to differentiate transudate from exudates using serum and pleural fluid

TABLE 62-8   Pleural Fluid Diagnostic Tests

DETECTION OF EXUDATIVE PLEURAL EFFUSION

Light[21] and colleagues criteria for pleural exudate: one or more of the following present (modified)

Pleural fluid/serum protein ratio >0.5,
or
Pleural fluid/serum LDH ratio >0.6,
or
Pleural fluid LDH greater than two-thirds of the upper limit for serum LDH

ADDITIONAL TESTS ON EXUDATIVE EFFUSIONS

Gram stain and culture to detect bacterial infection
Cell count
   Neutrophil predominance: parapneumonic, pulmonary embolism, pancreatitis
   Lymphocytic predominance: cancer, tuberculosis, postcardiac surgery
Glucose: low glucose seen in parapneumonic, malignant, tuberculosis, and rheumatoid arthritis causes of pleural effusions
Cytology for malignancy: highest yield is with adenocarcinoma, much lower with squamous cell, lymphoma, or mesothelioma
Pleural fluid pH: normal pleural fluid pH around 7.64. In parapneumonic effusions, a pleural fluid pH <7.10 predicts development of empyema or persistence and indicates need for thoracostomy tube drainage
Pleural fluid amylase: elevated in pleural effusions due to pancreatitis or esophageal rupture
Mycobacterial and fungal stains and cultures: as suggested clinically
Tuberculosis pleural fluid markers: polymerase chain reaction for mycobacterial DNA, pleural fluid adenosine deaminase, or pleural fluid interferon-γ

Abbreviation: LDH = lactate dehydrogenase.

---

protein and lactate dehydrogenase (LDH) levels (Table 62-8).[21] Several modifications to the original criteria have been proposed.[22] Regardless, the sensitivity of these criteria for the detection of an exudative pleural effusion in 98 to 99 percent with specificity from 65 to 86 percent. If the clinical circumstances suggest that the effusion is likely to be transudative, the only tests indicated are pleural fluid and serum protein content and LDH levels. If the pleural effusion is exudative, additional tests are indicated (see Table 62-8).

The distinction between exudates and transudates may be obscured by the effect of diuretic therapy in patients with transudative pleural effusions; during diuresis, the resorption of water is faster than that of protein, so that protein concentration rises into the range consistent with an exudative etiology. A serum to pleural albumin difference of greater than 1.2 g/dL has been proposed to help in this scenario, but this approach will reduce the sensitivity of exudative pleural effusion detection by more than 10 percent.[21,22]

Treatment

If the patient has dyspnea at rest, therapeutic thoracentesis with drainage of 1 to 1.5 L of fluid is indicated. Patients with pleural empyema (gross pus or organisms on Gram stain) require drainage with large bore thoracostomy tubes. Treatment of parapneumonic effusions is controversial (see Chap. 63). Consensus guidelines recommend thoracostomy tube drainage of parapneumonic effusions with positive cultures, positive Gram stain, or pleural fluid pH below 7.10. Diuretic therapy typically resolves more than 75 percent of effusions due to of congestive heart failure within 2 to 3 days.

REFERENCES

1. Sharma OP: Symptoms and signs in pulmonary medicine: Old observations and new interpretations. *Dis Mon* 41:577, 1995.
2. Scano G, Ambrosion N: Pathophysiology of dyspnea. *Lung* 180:131, 2002.
3. American Thoracic Society: Dyspnea. Mechanism, assessment, and management: A consensus statement. *Am J Respir Care Med* 159:321, 1999.
4. Cullen DL, Rodak B: Clinical utility of measures of breathlessness. *Respir Care* 47:986, 2002.
5. McCullough PA, Nowak RM, McCord J, et al: B-type natriuretic peptide and clinical judgment in emergency diagnosis of heart failure: Analysis from Breathing Not Properly (BNP) Multinational Study. *Circulation* 106:416, 2002.
6. Thomas JR, von Gunten CF: Clinical management of dyspnoea. *Lancet Oncol* 3:223, 2002.
7. Usen S, Webert M: Clinical signs of hypoxaemia in children with acute lower respiratory infection: Indicators of oxygen therapy. *Int J Tuberc Lung Dis* 5:505, 2001.
8. Greenstone M: Doxapram for ventilatory failure due to exacerbations of chronic obstructive pulmonary disease. *Cochrane Database Syst Rev* (2): CD000223, 2000.
9. Pasterknap H, Kraman SS, Wodicka GR: Respiratory sounds: Advances beyond the stethoscope. *Am J Respir Crit Care Med* 156:974, 1997.
10. Piirila P, Sovijarvi ARA: Objective assessment of cough. *Eur Respir J* 8:1949, 1995.
11. Smyrnios NA, Irwin RS, Curley FJ, French CL: From a prospective study of chronic cough: Diagnostic and therapeutic aspects in older adults. *Arch Intern Med* 158:1222, 1998.
12. Morice AH: Epidemiology of cough. *Pulm Pharmacol Ther* 15:253, 2002.
13. D'Urzo A, Jugovic P: Chronic cough. Three most common causes. *Can Fam Physician* 48:1311, 2002.
14. Pylypchuk GB: ACE inhibitor versus angiotensin II blocker-induced cough and angioedema. *Ann Pharmacother* 32:1060, 1998.
15. Skaggs P, Jennings C, Hunt K, et al: Pertussis outbreak among adults at an oil refinery—Illinois, August–October 2002. *MMWR* 52:1, 2003.
16. Ziment I: Herbal antitussives. *Pulm Pharmacol Ther* 15:327, 2002.
17. Pratter MR, Bartter T, Akers S, DuBois J: An algorithmic approach to chronic cough. *Ann Intern Med* 119:977, 1993.
18. Launois S, Bizec JL, Whitelaw WA, et al: Hiccup in adults: An overview. *Eur Respir J* 6:563, 1993.
19. Thompson DF, Landry JP: Drug-induced hiccups. *Ann Pharmacother* 31:367, 1997.
20. Friedman NL: Hiccups: A treatment review. *Pharmacotherapy* 16:986, 1996.
21. Light RW: Pleural effusion. *New Engl J Med* 346:1971, 2002.
22. Tarn AC, Lapworth R: Biochemical analysis of pleural fluid: What should we measure? *Ann Clin Biochem* 38:311, 2001.

63

BRONCHITIS, PNEUMONIA, AND PLEURAL EMPYEMA
Donald A. Moffa, Jr.
Charles L. Emerman

ACUTE BRONCHITIS

Epidemiology

Uncomplicated acute bronchitis (UAB) refers to an acute respiratory tract infection in which cough, occasionally with phlegm, is the predominant feature, and which is not caused by pneumonia or chronic bronchitis.[1] UAB usually lasts 1 to 3 weeks typically, but may last longer. Approximately 5 percent of adults in the United States report an episode of UAB each year, typically between October and March.

Pathophysiology

Microbiologic studies of UAB have successfully identified pathogens in 16 to 55 percent of cases; more than one pathogen may be identified in up to 10 percent.[2] Respiratory viruses cause the vast majority of cases of UAB: influenza B, influenza A, parainfluenza, and respiratory syncytial virus are most often implicated, but viruses that commonly produce upper respiratory tract infection (coronavirus, adenovirus, rhinoviruses, and coxsackievirus) have also been identified.

Bordetella pertussis, Mycoplasma pneumoniae, Chlamydia pneumoniae, and *Legionella* species are reported in 5 to 25 percent of cases of UAB.[1,3] Acute bronchitis in adults from *Bordetella pertussis* and parapertussis does not produce the characteristic whooping cough as these infections do in children.[3] *Bordetella pertussis, Mycoplasma pneumoniae,* and *Chlamydia pneumoniae* are recovered in 10 to 20 percent of adults with chronic or persistent cough lasting more than 2 to 3 weeks.[1] *Streptococcus pneumoniae, Haemophilus influenzae,* and *Moraxella catarrhalis* have been found in sputum of 7 to 44 percent of patients with UAB, but because they are part of the normal oropharyngeal flora, their significance in causing UAB is unknown.[3]

Clinical Features

The cough of UAB is commonly productive, and in as many as 20 percent of patients may last as long as 2 months.[1] The presence of purulent sputum is unimportant in diagnosing or treating UAB unless other symptoms and clinical findings suggest pneumonia. Fever >38°C (100.4°F), heart rate >100 beats/min, respiratory rate >24 breaths/min, focal chest pain or lung findings, and the absence of rhinorrhea or sore throat suggest pneumonia. Less than 10 percent of patients with UAB are febrile. UAB overlaps with symptoms of other common upper respiratory tract infections. The strongest positive independent predictors for UAB are cough and wheezing, and nausea is the strongest negative independent predictor that the diagnosis is not UAB.[4] Transient bronchial hyperresponsiveness appears to be the predominant mechanism for the cough of UAB, and differentiating it from asthma may be a challenge since abnormal spirometry will be present in both.[1] In fact, approximately one-third of patients presenting with symptoms of UAB may have asthma.[5]

Diagnosis

Clinical diagnosis of UAB is appropriately made with the following: (1) acute cough (less than 1 to 2 weeks), (2) no prior lung disease, and (3) no auscultatory abnormalities that suggest pneumonia. Pulse oximetry is indicated if the patient describes dyspnea or appears to be short of breath. Bedside spirometry (peak expiratory flow or forced expiratory volume in 1 s) is indicated if the patient describes wheezing or wheezing is heard on examination.

Since most cases of UAB are viral in etiology and because sputum Gram stain and culture do not reliably detect the most common nonviral pathogens (*Mycoplasma pneumoniae, Chlamydia pneumoniae,* and *Bordetella pertussis*), sputum Gram stain and culture are not recommended in evaluation of patients with UAB.[1] In previously healthy, nonelderly adults, chest radiography is not indicated unless the cough has been present 3 weeks or longer or if evidence of pneumonia as found.

Treatment

Many patients receive antibiotics for UAB, although studies have failed to show significant improvement unless treating pertussis is a consideration.[1] Some studies have found pertussis in up to 20 percent of patients with a cough lasting longer than 2 to 3 weeks, but no clinical features allow clinicians to distinguish adults with a cough due to pertussis from other pathogens.[1] At best, antibiotic therapy may decrease duration of cough, decrease purulent sputum production, and return patients to work by less than 1 day each.[1,3] Even when atypical pathogens are identified in causing the UAB, treatment with the antibiotics amoxicillin, erythromycin, or a fluoroquinolone does not affect outcome, and treatment with antibiotics is significantly more likely to cause side effects including nausea, vomiting, headache, skin rash, or vaginitis.[2]

Patients with airflow obstruction suggested by wheezing during UAB are more likely to benefit from inhaled bronchodilators than patients who simply have a cough without wheezing.[6] There is no evidence to support using β_2-agonists in children with acute cough and without evidence of airflow obstruction.[6] Inhaled bronchodilator treatment is not without side effects; up to two-thirds of adults receiving them report tremor, shaking, or nervousness.[6]

Acute Exacerbation of Chronic Bronchitis (AECB)

Approximately two-thirds of AECB cases are bacterial in origin, with nontypeable *H. influenzae, Streptococcus pneumoniae,* and *Moraxella catarrhalis* the most common organisms identified.[7] High-risk patients are the elderly and those with poor lung function or structural lung disease, poor performance status, other comorbid illnesses, and those having frequent exacerbations requiring corticosteroids. AECB is characterized by increased dyspnea, increased cough and sputum production, and increasing sputum purulence in a patient with underlying chronic obstructive pulmonary disease (COPD). During AECB, an increased number of bacteria, neutrophils, and inflammatory mediators may be seen in the patient's sputum, and an acute antibody response in serum may be present.

In AECB patients with at least two of the following (1) increased dyspnea, (2) increased sputum volume, or (3) increased sputum purulence, treatment with a broad-spectrum antibiotic such as doxycycline, extended-spectrum oral cephalosporin, an advanced-generation macrolide, amoxicillin-clavulanate, or a fluoroquinolone leads to a modest improvement in clinical outcome, fewer therapeutic failures, and a more rapid recovery of lung function compared to treatment with placebo.[7] The greatest benefit is seen in patients with more severe disease, including those who are older, who have poorer lung function, more comorbid diseases, and more frequent exacerbations.

PNEUMONIA

Epidemiology

Community-acquired pneumonia (CAP) is a common medical problem, accounting for about 4 million cases and 1 million hospitalizations per year in the United States.[8] It is the sixth leading cause of death, particularly among older adults, in whom the disease is more common. Whereas older studies of pneumonia pointed to pneumococci as the most common cause of pneumonia, there is an increasing frequency of atypical or opportunistic infections. The classic presentation of pneumococcal pneumonia is generally apparent, but atypical infections, infections in compromised hosts, and infections in patients at the extremes of age may present with more subtle findings. Older patients may present with a change in mental status or a decline in function without the typical respiratory symptoms.

Pathophysiology

Pneumonia may occur through a variety of routes of infection. Pathogenic organisms may be inhaled or aspirated directly into the lungs. Alternatively, some bacteria, such as *Staphylococcus aureus* or *Pneumococcus,* may produce pneumonia as a result of hematogenous seeding. With this in mind, patients most at risk for pneumonia are those with a predisposition to aspiration, impaired mucociliary clearance, or risk of bacteremia (Table 63-1).

Pneumonia is an infection of the alveolar or gas-exchanging portions of the lung. Some forms of pneumonia produce an intense inflammatory response within the alveoli that leads to filling of the air space with organisms, exudate, and white blood cells. Pneumonia can spread throughout the lung via the bronchial tree or through the pores of Kohn. Bacterial pneumonia, with an intense inflammatory response, tends to cause a productive cough, whereas other atypical organisms do not lead to such an intense inflammatory response and may only be associated with mild nonproductive cough.

TABLE 63-1 Risk Factors for Pneumonia

Aspiration risk
    Swallowing and esophageal motility disorders
    Stroke
    Nasogastric tube
    Intubation
    Seizure and syncope
Bacteremia risk
    Indwelling vascular devices
    Intrathoracic devices (e.g., chest tube)
Debilitation
    Alcoholism
    Extremes of age
    Neoplasia
    Immunosuppression
Chronic diseases
    Diabetes
    Renal failure
    Liver failure
    Valvular heart disease
    Congestive heart failure
Pulmonary disorders
    Chronic obstructive pulmonary disease
    Chest wall disorders
    Skeletal muscle disorders
    Bronchial obstruction
    Bronchoscopy
    Viral lung infections

Prospective studies of both inpatients and outpatients with CAP fail to identify a specific pathogen in 40 to 60 percent of patients. When an etiology is found, pneumococcus is still the most common single agent, followed by viruses and the atypical agents such as *Mycoplasma, Chlamydia,* and *Legionella.* In up to 5 percent, multiple agents are identified. Special populations, including nursing-home residents, chronic alcoholics, and HIV-infected patients, have a somewhat different etiologic spectrum.

Clinical Features

Patients with pneumonia usually present with cough, dyspnea, sputum production, fever and pleuritic chest pain.[8] However, there is variability in the individual symptoms and physical findings that may make clinical diagnosis difficult.[9] The typical presentation of pneumococcal pneumonia is a sudden onset of illness with fever, rigors, dyspnea, bloody sputum production, chest pain, tachycardia, tachypnea, and abnormal findings on lung examination. Most other types of pneumonia do not have such a sudden and characteristic presentation. Pneumonia may be preceded by symptoms of a viral upper respiratory infection with coryza, low-grade fever, rhinorrhea, or nonproductive cough. Weight loss, malaise, dizziness, and weakness may be associated with pneumonia. Some of the atypical agents are associated with dramatic presentations of headache or gastrointestinal (GI) illness. Occasionally, pneumonia is associated with extrapulmonary symptoms, including joint pain, hematuria, or skin rashes.

The physical examination may show evidence of alveolar fluid (inspiratory rales), consolidation (bronchial breath sounds), pleural effusion (dullness and decreased breath sounds), or bronchial congestion (rhonchi and wheezing).[9] Tachypnea, tachycardia, fever, and hypotension are associated with severe illness.

PNEUMOCOCCAL PNEUMONIA *Streptococcus pneumoniae* is particularly prevalent at the extremes of age and in the chronically ill; persons at highest risk for infection are the elderly, children under 2 years old, minorities, children who attend group day-care centers, and persons with underlying medical conditions including HIV infection and sickle-cell disease. Classically, patients with pneumococcal pneu-

monia present with sudden onset of disease with rigors, bloody sputum, high fever, and chest pain. In this setting, patients will frequently have lobar pneumonia, with parapneumonic pleural effusions occurring in about 25 percent of patients. Patients with functional or anatomic asplenia or patients being treated with immunosuppressive drugs, such as transplant patients, may have a very rapid progression of disease, with acute prostration and septic shock progressing to multisystem organ failure. Patients with chronic lung disease, nursing-home patients, or otherwise healthy elderly patients tend to have a slower progression of the disease. They may present with malaise associated with minimal cough or sputum production. Along with the frequent finding of leukocytosis, elevation of the serum bilirubin or other liver enzymes may be seen. In addition, hyponatremia may be a finding in many causes of pneumonia, including pneumococcal pneumonia.

Pneumococcal pneumonia will respond to a variety of antibiotics, although there is an increased incidence of penicillin-resistant pneumococci. The risk factors for penicillin resistance include patients at the extremes of age, day-care attendance, immunosuppression from alcoholism or cancer, and recent use of broad-spectrum antibiotics or travel to areas where penicillin resistance is common, especially the Mediterranean region. In addition to penicillin resistance, there is increasing resistance to other common antibiotics, including tetracycline and trimethoprim-sulfamethoxazole (TMP-SMX). Patients with intermediate penicillin-resistant pneumococci may still be effectively treated with routine antibiotics so long as an adequate dose is administered.[10] Patients with highly penicillin-resistant pneumococci may require treatment with either vancomycin, imipenem, or a newer fluoroquinolone.

OTHER BACTERIAL PNEUMONIA *Staphylococcus aureus* is a consideration in patients with chronic lung disease, patients with laryngeal cancer, immunosuppressed patients, nursing-home patients, or others at risk for aspiration pneumonia. *S. aureus* pneumonia may occur in otherwise healthy patients following viral illness, such as during an influenza epidemic, although pneumococcus is still more common. Patients with staphylococcal pneumonia typically have an insidious onset of disease with low-grade fever, sputum production, and dyspnea. The chest radiograph usually demonstrates extensive disease with empyema, pleural effusions, and multiple areas of infiltrate.

Klebsiella pneumonia usually occurs in compromised patients: patients at risk of aspiration, alcoholics, the elderly, and other patients with chronic lung disease. In contrast to *S. aureus,* patients with *Klebsiella* have acute onset of severe disease with fever, rigors, and chest pain. Herpes labialis is occasionally associated with *Klebsiella* pneumonia. Patients with *Klebsiella* may develop abscesses, although more commonly they have a lobar infiltrate.

Pseudomonas causes a severe pneumonia with cyanosis, confusion, and other signs of systemic illness. The chest radiograph usually shows bilateral lower lobe infiltrates, occasionally associated with empyema. *Pseudomonas* is not a typical cause of CAP, but may be seen in patients who have had a prolonged hospitalization, have been on broad-spectrum antibiotics, have been on high-dose steroid therapy, have structural lung disease, or are nursing-home residents.

Haemophilus influenzae pneumonia may be seen in the elderly and should be considered in patients with chronic lung disease, sickle cell disease, or immunocompromised disorders and in alcoholics and diabetics. Routine vaccination of children has markedly reduced the incidence of *H. influenzae* pneumonia in the pediatric population. Patients may either have a gradual progression of disease with low-grade fever and sputum production or occasionally have the sudden onset of chest pain, dyspnea, and sputum production. Bacteremia may be seen in older adults. Pleural effusions and multilobar infiltrates are common findings in *H. influenzae* pneumonia.

Moraxella catarrhalis pneumonia has clinical features similar in spectrum to those of *H. influenzae.* Typically, patients with *M. catarrhalis* present with an indolent course of cough and sputum production. Fever and pleuritic chest pain are common clinical symptoms. The chest radiograph usually shows diffuse infiltrates.

ATYPICAL PNEUMONIA   Atypical agents are being recognized more frequently as a cause of pneumonia in older children, in young adults, and in the elderly. Because these agents lack a cell wall, they do not respond to beta-lactam antibiotics, and current recommendations for empiric antibiotic treatment of CAP take this into account, using either a macrolide or a newer-generation fluoroquinolone.

Legionella can cause a range of illness from benign self-limited disease to multisystem organ failure with acute respiratory distress syndrome. Patients at particular risk include cigarette smokers, patients with chronic lung disease, transplant patients, and immunosuppressed patients. There is no seasonality to *Legionella* pneumonia, making it a more common cause of pneumonia in the summer. *Legionella* pneumonia is commonly complicated by GI symptoms, including abdominal pain, vomiting, and diarrhea. In addition, *Legionella* can affect other organ systems, causing sinusitis, pancreatitis, myocarditis, and pyelonephritis. The chest radiograph frequently shows a patchy infiltrate, with the occasional appearance of hilar adenopathy and pleural effusions.

Chlamydia pneumonia is a common cause of respiratory infection, with about half of the population demonstrating antibodies by the age of 15. Infection with *Chlamydia* usually causes a mild subacute illness with sore throat, mild fever, and nonproductive cough, although occasionally patients have a more severe course. Patients with *Chlamydia* pneumonia frequently have abnormal physical examination findings, with rales or rhonchi. The chest radiograph usually shows a patchy subsegmental infiltrate. Chlamydial infection has been associated with the development of adult-onset asthma.

Mycoplasma pneumonia also occurs year round, although it tends to cluster in epidemics every 4 to 8 years. As is the case with *Chlamydia,* it may cause a subacute respiratory illness with cough, sore throat, and headache. *Mycoplasma* pneumonia is frequently associated with retrosternal chest pain. Unlike *Legionella,* *Mycoplasma* usually is not associated with GI symptoms. The chest radiograph shows patchy infiltrates, with the common occurrence of hilar adenopathy and pleural effusions. *Mycoplasma* occasionally causes extrapulmonary symptoms, including bullous myringitis, rash, neurologic symptoms, arthritis and arthralgia, hematologic abnormalities, and rarely, renal failure.

Diagnosis

Pneumonia is suspected based on a constellation of symptoms and signs, but individual symptoms and clinical findings lack accuracy for precise diagnosis.[9] Attempts have been made to combine some of the symptoms and signs into a scoring system that predicts the probability of pneumonia for the purposes of determining the need for chest radiography in adult outpatients (Table 63-2). The results of these attempts have produced scoring criteria with modest likelihood ratios. These

TABLE 63-2   Prediction Rules for Pneumonia in Adult Patients with Cough

Author and Rule	Threshold Score	Sensitivity %	Specificity %	Positive Likelihood Ratio LR(+)	Negative Likelihood Ratio LR(−)
Diehr et al	0	67	67	2.0	0.50
Points:					
−2 for rhinorrhea					
−1 for sore throat					
1 for night sweats					
1 for myalgia					
1 for sputum all day					
2 for respiratory rate >25					
2 for temperature >38°C (100°F)					
Total score, −3 to 7					
Singal et al	All three, cough and fever, or cough and rales	76	55	1.7	0.44
Probability = (1 + e^{-y}), Where y = 3.095 + 1.214 (cough) + 1.007 (fever) + 0.823 (rales) Each variable = 1 if present and 0 if absent					
Gennis et al	Any abnormality	62	76	2.6	0.50
Positive, if any:					
T >37.8°C (100.04°F)					
Heart rate >100					
Respiratory rate >20					
Heckerling et al	+2	71	67	2.2	0.43
Points (one each for):					
Absence of asthma					
Temperature >37.8°C (100.4°F)					
Heart rate >100					
Decreased breath sounds					
Rales					
Total score, 0 to 5					

Sources: Diehr P, Wood RW, Bushyhead J, et al: Prediction of pneumonia in outpatients with acute cough—A statistical approach. *J Chronic Dis* 37:215, 1984; Singal BM, Hedges JR, Radack KL: Decision rules and clinical prediction of pneumonia: Evaluation of low-yield criteria. *Ann Emerg Med* 18:13, 1989; Gennis P, Gallagher J, Falvo C, et al: Clinical criteria for the detection of pneumonia in adults: Guidelines for ordering chest roentgenograms in the emergency department. *J Emerg Med* 7:263, 1989; and Heckerling PS, Tape TG, Wigton RS, et al: Clinical prediction rule for pulmonary infiltrates. *Ann Intern Med* 113:664, 1990.

clinical criteria are most useful for excluding pneumonia when the prevalence is very low, <5 to 7 percent; that is, if a patient has none of the positive predictors, the probability of pneumonia is very low, from 1 to 4 percent. However, clinical criteria are inadequate for including pneumonia; even if a patient has all of the positive clinical predictors, these scoring systems predict pneumonia with a maximal accuracy of 40 to 50 percent.[9] Thus for accurate diagnosis, a chest radiograph is required, although in practice high-risk patients are sometimes treated empirically.

Patients with complaints of dyspnea or physical signs of respiratory distress should have oxygen saturation measured by pulse oximetry. In otherwise healthy, mildly ill, ambulatory patients, no further ancillary testing may be necessary. If a patient requires admission, additional tests may be necessary, including complete blood count and determination of serum electrolytes, blood urea nitrogen, creatinine, and glucose levels. Evaluation of arterial blood gas is indicated if patients are markedly desaturated or have severe respiratory distress. No single set of recommendations for diagnostic testing can encompass all patients, and additional ancillary studies should be obtained according to appropriate indications.

In patients with fever, cough, and radiographic abnormalities, the etiology of the infection can be confirmed, at times, by identification of a pathogenic organism from the blood, sputum, or pleural fluid. Atypical agents may be demonstrated by a variety of sophisticated laboratory techniques, including evaluation of titers from acute and convalescence sera or by direct fluorescent antibody testing. Most patients do not require identification of a specific organism.

In hospitalized patients with CAP, the incidence of positive blood cultures increases with increasing disease severity.[11] The incidence of positive blood cultures in nonhospitalized patients with CAP is lower, pathogen identification does not alter treatment, and the overwhelming majority of patients respond to empiric antibiotic treatment. Thus blood cultures are recommended only for patients who require hospitalization.

The value of sputum examination in CAP has been debated. Many patients are unable to produce adequate sputum, the Gram stain is frequently negative, and the results rarely change therapy.[12]

The differential diagnosis of patients with cough and radiographic abnormality includes disorders such as lung cancer, tuberculosis, pulmonary embolism, chemical or hypersensitivity pneumonitis, connective tissue disorders, granulomatous disease, and fungal infections. While the radiographic appearance may suggest the underlying microbial etiology, the overlapping variations in radiographic signs between different organisms may lead to misclassification. Pneumococcal pneumonia typically presents with lobar segmental pneumonia. Occasionally, patients may present with the so-called round infiltrate of pneumococcal pneumonia. In general, patients with bacterial pneumonia are more likely to have unilobar or focal infiltrates than patients with viral or atypical pneumonia. Hilar adenopathy is more common in patients with atypical pneumonia. Pleural effusions occur more commonly in patients with bacterial pneumonia, although occasionally patients with viral pneumonia or atypical agents may have small effusions. Cavitary lesions occur in patients with bacterial or tuberculous lesions. Lung abscesses are rare complications of pneumonia in the antibiotic era, but they sometimes occur due to *S. aureus* or *Klebsiella*. Pneumonia may mimic the appearance of lung masses, particularly when the cause is pneumococcal or staphylococcal. Other atypical pneumonia such as Q fever and tularemia may present as discrete masses.

Pneumonia in Special Populations

PNEUMONIA IN ALCOHOLICS   Alcoholics have a significantly higher incidence of many lung diseases including pneumonia, tuberculosis, pleurisy, bronchitis, empyema, and COPD, compared to non-alcoholics. Alcoholics are more likely than the general population to have poor nutrition, to develop aspiration pneumonitis, to be heavy smokers, and to have sequelae of alcoholic cirrhosis and portal hypertension. Compared to the nonalcoholic, the alcoholic has greater oropharyngeal colonization with gram-negative bacteria and is more likely to have pulmonary function abnormalities, including reduced long volumes, increased airway resistance, and decreased diffusion capacity. In addition, alcoholism depresses granulocyte and lymphocyte counts and impairs delivery of neutrophils to sites of infection.

Streptococcus pneumoniae is still the most common pathogen causing pneumonia in alcoholics, but *Klebsiella* species and *Haemophilus* species are also important agents of infection. In general, rates of pneumonia and death from pneumonia are higher in alcoholics compared to nonalcoholic patients.

PNEUMONIA IN DIABETICS   Diabetes mellitus is an independent risk factor for pneumonia. Diabetic patients between the ages of 25 and 64 are four times more likely to have pneumonia and influenza, and diabetics are two to three times more likely than nondiabetics to die with pneumonia and influenza as an underlying cause of death. Pathogens that occur with increased frequency in diabetic patients include *Staphylococcus aureus,* gram-negative bacteria, *Mucor,* and *Mycobacterium tuberculosis*. Infections due to *Streptococcus pneumoniae, Legionella pneumophila,* and influenza are associated with increased morbidity and mortality in diabetic patients.

PNEUMONIA IN PREGNANCY   Community-acquired pneumonia in pregnancy is one of the most serious nonobstetric infections complicating pregnancy. Maternal anemia and asthma are risk factors for pneumonia, and pregnant women with pneumonia are more likely to experience preterm labor, have a preterm delivery, and deliver a low birthweight infant compared to the expectant mother without pneumonia.[13] Maternal mortality from antepartum pneumonia is approximately 3 percent. Pregnancy does not seem to alter the course of bacterial pneumonia, but viral pneumonia during pregnancy carries a worse prognosis than in the nonpregnant patient.

Varicella pneumonia may be a particular problem in pregnancy. Pregnant women who develop varicella pneumonia are five times more likely to be smokers, and approximately 16 times more likely to have skin lesions suggestive of the disease. Chest radiography is recommended for patients with symptoms of respiratory tract infection and varicella exposure. An arterial blood gas may be helpful in identifying patients with early respiratory compromise. Intravenous acyclovir may be started in the ED, although there is little evidence that the timing of administration affects outcome.

Pneumocystis carinii pneumonia (PCP) is the most common cause of AIDS-related death in pregnant women in the United States, with a mortality rate around 50 percent. Respiratory failure requiring mechanical ventilation may be experienced by over half of these patients. Combination treatment with pentamidine, steroids, and eflornithine improves survival compared to those patients treated with TMP-SMX alone.

PNEUMONIA IN THE ELDERLY   Pneumonia is the most common infection and represents the fifth leading cause of death among the elderly.[14] The incidence of lower respiratory tract infection in the elderly ranges from 25 to 44 cases per 1000 in the general population, with a mortality rate approaching 40 percent. COPD, congestive heart failure (CHF), cardiovascular and cerebrovascular disease, lung cancer, dementia, diminished gag reflex, and other disorders that predispose the elderly to aspiration make them more susceptible to infection.

The elderly are three times more likely to have pneumococcal bacteremia than younger patients. The mortality from pneumococcal pneumonia is three to five times greater in the elderly (up to 40 percent) than in those younger than age 65. Although becoming recognized more frequently in the elderly, atypical pathogens such as *Mycoplasma* are still more common in younger populations. *Legionella* is the most common atypical agent in the elderly and is responsible for up to 10 percent of cases of CAP. Influenza is the most common serious viral infection in the elderly. Postinfluenza bacterial pneumonia is most commonly caused by *S. pneumoniae, S. aureus,* and *H. influenzae.*

Elderly patients with pneumonia may complain about falling, weakness, tremulousness, functional decline, or GI symptoms, and may exhibit delirium or confusion. Elderly patients are more likely to be afebrile on presentation, but are more likely than younger adults to have a serious bacterial infection when the temperature is higher than 38.3°C (100.9°F).

Up to one-third of elderly patients with CAP will not manifest leukocytosis. Poor prognostic indicators for pneumonia in the elderly include hypothermia or a temperature greater than 38.3°C (100.9°F), a low white blood cell count, immunosuppression, gram-negative or staphylococcal infection, cardiac disease, bilateral infiltrates, and extrapulmonary disease. Elderly patients with pneumonia frequently require hospitalization and about 10 percent may require intensive care.

PNEUMONIA IN NURSING-HOME PATIENTS Pneumonia is a major cause of morbidity, mortality, and hospitalization among nursing home residents.[14,15] Nursing home-acquired pneumonia (NHAP) affects patients who are significantly older, have more cerebrovascular disease, and have higher mortality risk scores at hospital presentation.

These patients are less likely to have a productive cough or pleuritic chest pain, but more likely to be confused and have poorer functional status and more severe disease.[15] Eight variables are significant independent predictors of pneumonia in nursing home patients: increased pulse rate, respiratory rate greater than or equal to 30/min, temperature greater than or equal to 38°C (100.4°F), somnolence or decreased alertness, presence of acute confusion, lung crackles on auscultation, the absence of wheezes, and an increased leukocyte count. A patient with one of these variables has a 33 percent chance of having pneumonia, while three or more variables suggest a 50 percent likelihood of pneumonia.[16] Fewer than 10 percent of nursing home patients with pneumonia will have no respiratory symptoms.[16] Fever, although nonspecific, is present in approximately 40 percent of cases of NHAP.[16]

The most frequently reported pathogens among patients with NHAP are *Streptococcus pneumoniae*, gram-negative bacilli, and *Haemophilus influenzae*. Because nursing home patients live in close proximity, residents are subject to outbreaks of influenza. Unfortunately, vaccination against influenza is only approximately 33 to 55 percent effective in preventing postinfluenzal pneumonia in nursing home patients. *Mycoplasma pneumoniae* and *Legionella* are uncommon causes of pneumonia in nursing home patients.

NHAP is often treated in the hospital, although some studies have suggested that patients can be treated in nursing homes with either intramuscular or oral antibiotics.[17]

PNEUMONIA IN HIV PATIENTS Among HIV seropositive individuals, the incidence of bacterial pneumonia is 5.5 per 100 person-years, an incidence higher than that of *Pneumocystis carinii* pneumonia in this population.[18] Among hospitalized patients with HIV, the incidence of bacterial pneumonia is as high as 12.5 per 100 person-years.[18] CAP accounts for roughly three-quarters of bacterial pneumonia diagnosed in patients hospitalized with HIV infection. Compared to HIV seropositive patients hospitalized *without* pneumonia, those admitted *with* pneumonia generally have a lower CD4+ T-cell count, a higher APACHE II score, a longer length of hospital stay, a greater chance of ICU admission, and higher case-fatality rate.[18]

Streptococcus pneumoniae is the most common cause of bacterial pneumonia in patients with HIV and may be recovered on blood culture in 60 percent of patients with HIV compared to 15 to 30 percent of patients without HIV infection who have pneumococcal pneumonia.[18] *Pseudomonas aeruginosa* infection has traditionally been asso-

ciated with neutropenia, hospitalization, central venous catheters, burn wounds, bronchiectasis, and cystic fibrosis, but *Pseudomonas aeruginosa* is a common cause of bacterial pneumonia in HIV-positive patients.[18] HIV-positive patients with *Pseudomonas aeruginosa* pneumonia are more likely to have a lower leukocyte and CD4+ T-cell count, longer hospital stay, but similar case fatality rate.[18]

Opportunistic infections are more likely to occur with lower CD4+ count. Bacterial infections are more likely to cause pneumonia when the CD4+ count is above 800 cells/μL. Between 250 and 500 cells/μL, infection from *Mycobacterium tuberculosis, Cryptococcus neoformans,* or *Histoplasma capsulatum* poses a greater risk. The risk of *Pneumocystis carinii* pneumonia is more likely when the CD4+ count is below 200 cells/μL.

Bacterial pneumonia produces a pleural effusion in up to about 60 percent of patients with AIDS, most commonly due to *Streptococcus pneumoniae* and *Staphylococcus aureus.* Non-Hodgkin lymphoma, Kaposi sarcoma, and adenocarcinoma of lung are the three leading noninfectious causes of pleural effusion in HIV patients. Patients with Kaposi sarcoma, cytomegalovirus (CMV) pneumonia, and hydrostatic pulmonary edema may present with alveolar hemorrhage as seen by bloody fluid on bronchoalveolar lavage or frank hemoptysis. Pulmonary nodules in the HIV patient are most commonly caused by opportunistic infection, bacterial pneumonia, and tuberculosis. Fever, cough, and a nodule size of less than 1 cm are independent predictors of an opportunistic infection. Miliary pneumonia on CT scan or chest radiograph may represent varicella pneumonia.

PNEUMONIA IN TRANSPLANT PATIENTS Bacterial pneumonia is less common after renal transplantation, but more common in patients receiving liver, heart, or lung transplants during the first 3 months after surgery, compared to other surgical patients. Gram-negative bacilli (especially *Pseudomonas aeruginosa* associated with mechanical ventilation), *Staphylococcus aureus,* and *Legionella* predominate in the first 3 months posttransplantation. *Klebsiella pneumoniae, Escherichia coli,* and fungi may also cause pneumonia in this time period. These early onset nosocomial bacterial pneumonias carry a substantial mortality rate, approximately 33 percent. CMV, *Pneumocystis carinii,* and fungal infections, especially *Aspergillus* species, are opportunistic infections, which may be seen in the first 6 months postsurgery. After 6 months posttransplant, bacteria more typical of CAP (*Streptococcus pneumoniae, Haemophilus influenzae*) are the most likely pathogens and portend considerably less mortality.

Treatment of Community-Acquired Pneumonia

Emergency physicians will most often initiate empiric treatment for outpatients who have CAP. Many different specialty societies and task forces have developed guidelines for the treatment of adults with CAP, including the American Thoracic Society (ATS), The British Thoracic Society, the CDC Working Group, the Canadian Infectious Disease Society, and the Infectious Disease Society of America.[8,19] Some differences exist between the guidelines, particularly regarding etiologic diagnosis and antimicrobial therapy. All guidelines recognize that although pneumococcal pneumonia is still the single most common cause of CAP, atypical agents are increasingly recognized in adults and adolescents such that empiric therapy should include antibiotics that are active against organisms that lack a cell wall (Table 63-3).

Recommended agents for outpatient therapy include doxycycline, a newer macrolide, or one of the newer fluoroquinolones orally for a varying duration depending on the agent. Other agents or regimens may be effective in individual cases, but these recommendations are thought to provide the broadest coverage for empiric therapy of outpatients. Doxycycline is useful because of its tolerance, bioavailability, and low cost. Erythromycin is a very cost-effective agent for CAP, but is associated with GI side effects in about 25 percent of adult patients.

TABLE 63-3 Antibiotics Commonly Used in Adults with Community-Acquired Pneumonia

Drug	Class	Oral	Intravenous
Doxycycline	Tetracycline	100 mg bid	100 mg q12h
Clarithromycin XL	Macrolide	500 mg qd	
Azithromycin	Macrolide	500 mg on day 1 and 250 mg on days 2–5	500 mg qd
Ampicillin-clavulanate	Penicillin + β-lactamase inhibitor	875/125 mg bid	
Ampicillin-sulbactam	Penicillin + β-lactamase inhibitor		1.5–3.0 g q6h
Piperacillin/tazobactam	Penicillin + β-lactamase inhibitor		3.375 g q6h
Moxifloxacin	Fluoroquinolone	400 mg qd	400 mg qd
Levofloxacin	Fluoroquinolone	500 mg qd	500 mg qd
Gatifloxacin	Fluoroquinolone	400 mg qd	400 mg qd
Cefuroxime	Second-generation cephalosporin		750 mg q8h
Cefpodoxime	Third-generation cephalosporin	200 mg bid	
Cefoperazone	Third-generation cephalosporin		1–2 g q12h
Cefotaxime	Third-generation cephalosporin		1–2 g q8h
Ceftazidime	Third-generation cephalosporin		500–1000 mg q8h
Ceftriaxone	Third-generation cephalosporin		1–2 g qd
Cefepime	Fourth-generation cephalosporin		1–2 g q12h
Imipenem/cilastatin	Carbapenem		500 mg q6h
Meropenem	Carbapenem		1.0 g q8h
Vancomycin	Miscellaneous		1.0 g q12h
Clindamycin	Miscellaneous		600–900 mg q8h

Clarithromycin has fewer GI side effects, although some patients may complain about the taste. Azithromycin has the advantage of once-a-day dosing. The newer fluoroquinolone agents, including moxifloxacin, levofloxacin, and gatifloxacin, have extended coverage that includes both common bacterial agents and atypical agents, along with the advantage of once-a-day dosing. The Centers for Disease Control's Working Group has expressed concern about the development of fluoroquinolone resistance and has recommended that these agents be reserved for patients who cannot tolerate other agents, have documented pneumococcal resistance, or have failed other therapies. Outpatients with CAP are typically treated until afebrile for 3 to 5 days; usually a total treatment of 7 to 14 days.

Emergency physicians play a prominent role in the initiation of treatment for patients being hospitalized with CAP. Recent evidence indicates that early administration of antibiotics, within the first 8 h of presentation, leads to a lower mortality rate and a shorter hospital stay. Although the yield is low, admitting physicians may benefit from the results of the sputum Gram stain, sputum culture, or blood culture obtained in the ED. For patients hospitalized with CAP, therapy should be initiated with a second- or third-generation cephalosporin or penicillin plus a beta-lactamase inhibitor, with a macrolide to provide coverage against *Legionella* or other atypical agents. Ceftriaxone and cefotaxime provide adequate coverage against most strains of *S. pneumoniae*. Coverage can also be provided by a fluoroquinolone such as levofloxacin, moxifloxacin, or gatifloxacin. The efficacy of monotherapy with fluoroquinolones alone has not been clearly established in patients with severe pneumonia who require ICU admission, and those patients should receive dual therapy. Patients at risk for *Pseudomonas* include those with structural lung disease and those recently treated with high-dose steroids or broad-spectrum antibiotics. In addition to the therapy discussed above, these patients should receive antipseudomonal coverage with antipseudomonal cephalosporins such as cefepime, a carbapenem such as meropenem, a fluoroquinolone with adequate coverage such as ciprofloxacin, an aminoglycoside such as gentamycin, or other antibiotics with antipseudomonal activity.

Disposition

An estimated 75 percent of patients with CAP do not require hospitalization.[8,19] Many factors influence the prognosis and outcome of CAP. In general, physicians tend to overestimate the risk of pneumonia mortality. Fine and coworkers have developed a decision rule that can be used to estimate the risk of death and ICU placement from pneumonia (Tables 63-4, 63-5, and 63-6). Others have used this rule to guide the need for hospitalization. With this decision rule, patients are assigned to one of five risk categories, with the lowest category having a mortality rate of around 0.1 percent. Although not a prominent part of this decision rule, patients who are immunocompromised as a result of AIDS or chronic alcohol use may require hospitalization. Other factors such as social situation or unusual medical conditions may also play a role in the admission decision. In addition, a chest radiograph that demonstrates bilateral effusions, bilateral infiltrates, moderately large pleural effusions, or extensive pulmonary involvement is associated with a higher risk of mortality. Patients should be considered for admission to an intensive care unit if they are markedly tachypneic or have high oxygen requirements, evidence of shock, or very extensive pulmonary involvement (more than 50 percent of the lung). For patients in risk category III, the admission decision may be made based on the presence of relative hypoxemia, social factors, and the inability to complete a course of oral antibiotics. A brief hospitalization or observation may be considered in these patients.

Emergency physicians play a role in educating patients about their disease. Most patients will achieve some measure of resolution within 3 to 5 days after the initiation of antibiotics. Many hospitalized patients can be switched to oral antibiotics at around 3 days and then subsequently discharged to complete a course of therapy. Large population studies have demonstrated, however, that many patients are still symptomatic at 30 days, with a significant minority of patients experiencing chest pain, malaise, or mild dyspnea even 2 to 3 months after treatment. Patients should be educated about the importance of smoking cessation and moderation of alcohol use. Patients may benefit from instructions about rest, nutrition, hydration, and follow-up. Patients at risk should be educated about the importance of vaccination against pneumococcus and influenza.

PLEURAL EMPYEMA

Epidemiology

Pleural empyema has been defined as pus in the pleural space.[20] Many authors expand that definition to include pleural space infections as evidenced by positive Gram stain or culture results or effusions associated with pneumonia (parapneumonic) without pleural fluid sampling.

TABLE 63-4   Assignment to Risk Class I

Age ≤50 years
No comorbid conditions
   Neoplastic disease
   Congestive heart failure
   Renal disease
   Liver disease
No physical examination abnormalities
   Altered mental status
   Pulse >125
   Systolic blood pressure <90 mm Hg
   Temperature <35°C (95°F) or 40°C (104°F)

Source: Adapted with permission from Fine MJ, Auble TE, Yealy DM, et al: A prediction rule to identify low-risk patients with community-acquired pneumonia. *New Engl J Med* 336:243, 1997.

Pleural effusions are present on the chest x-ray of 20 to 60 percent of patients with bacterial pneumonia and often resolve with antibiotic therapy.[21] Other causes of pleural empyema include complications of penetrating chest trauma, blunt abdominal and chest trauma, perforated esophagus, complication of lung abscess, direct extension from a sub-diaphragmatic infection, vertebral osteomyelitis, other near-pleural infections, and infected hemothorax, hydrothorax, or chylothorax.[20]

Risk factors for pleural empyema include aspiration pneumonia and its attendant risk factors, immunocompromised patients with gram-negative bacillary infections, fungal infections, tuberculosis, or malignancy. Chronic alcoholics, because of their predisposition to aspiration and *Klebsiella* infections, are at risk to develop pleural empyema. *S. aureus* or mixed anaerobic bacteria are also commonly cultured from pleural empyema.[20]

Pathophysiology

Pleural empyema has three stages of development.[20] The *exudative stage* is characterized by free-flowing pleural fluid. This stage is very amenable to treatment with closed tube drainage since the infected

TABLE 63-5   Assignment to Risk Classes II to V

Criteria	Points
Demographics	
Female gender	−10
Nursing home resident	10
Coexistent illness	
Neoplastic disease	30
Congestive heart failure	20
Cerebrovascular accident	10
Renal disease	10
Liver disease	10
Physical examination	
Abnormal mental status	20
Pulse ≥125	20
RR ≥30	20
Blood pressure (≤90 mm Hg)	15
Temperature <35°C (95°F) or >40°C (104°F)	10
Ancillary studies	
pH <7.35	30
Blood urea nitrogen ≥30 mg/dL	20
Na ≤130 mEq/L	20
Glucose ≥250 mg/dL	10
Hematocrit <30%	10
Pao$_2$ <60 mm Hg	10
Pleural effusion	10

Source: Adapted with permission from Fine MJ, Auble TE, Yealy DM, et al: A prediction rule to identify low-risk patients with community-acquired pneumonia. *New Engl J Med* 336:243, 1997.

TABLE 63-6   Prediction of Mortality from Pneumonia

Class	Points	Mortality, %	Treatment Recommendation
I	No predictors	0.1	Outpatient
II	<70	0.6	Outpatient
III	71–90	2.8	Inpatient (briefly)
IV	91–130	8.2	Inpatient
V	>130	29.2	Inpatient

Source: Adapted with permission from Fine MJ, Auble TE, Yealy DM, et al: A prediction rule to identify low-risk patients with community-acquired pneumonia. *New Engl J Med* 336:243, 1997.

fluid is free flowing. The exudative stage may be short lived, often with less than a 48-h duration. The *fibrinopurulent stage* is characterized by the formation of fibrin strands through the pleural fluid. This results in loculations throughout the pleural space, making adequate drainage with a single chest tube unlikely. This deposition of fibrin along the parietal pleura will inhibit the resorption of pleural fluid, and restrict access to lymphatics, which also hampers fluid resorption and can ultimately interfere with chest wall mechanics. In the *organizational stage*, which takes several weeks to develop, fibrosis is much more extensive, forming a pleural peel that restricts lung expansion even if the fluid can be evacuated.

Empyema can be a slow indolent process and many patients may have symptoms for several weeks before seeking medical attention. By that time, they have already reached the fibrinopurulent or organizational stage and will require more extensive treatment. Patients who are treated earlier in the course of this illness will tend to require less invasive, less painful, and less expensive therapeutic interventions.

Clinical Features

Patients with empyema will usually have a preceding pulmonary infection. Many will have symptoms of pneumonia that have not resolved; fever, shortness of breath, pleuritic chest pain, cough, and general malaise are common symptoms. Weight loss may occur and anemia from chronic infection may develop. Often these patients appear chronically ill with risk factors as previously discussed: alcoholism, cancer, and other immunocompromising states.

Physical examination will reveal decreased breath sounds and dullness to percussion on the involved side. Patients may be splinting with respirations secondary to pain because of the inflammatory nature of the empyema. Rales and rhonchi are often heard because of an underlying pulmonary infection, but these incidental findings are not diagnostic of pleural empyema.

Diagnosis

A standard chest radiograph will indicate the presence of pleural fluid, but will not make the diagnosis of pleural empyema. Decubitus films will be helpful in determining if the fluid is free flowing or loculated. Aspiration and evaluation of pleural fluid will confirm the diagnosis. The more difficult loculated effusions may require thoracentesis performed with CT or ultrasound guidance. A major advantage of ultrasound over plain radiography is its ability to rapidly differentiate solid (tumor, fibrous peel) from liquid components in the pleural process. Laboratory and microbiologic evaluation of the fluid will allow confirmation of the diagnosis of pleural empyema. Pleural fluid that is gross pus or fluid with positive cultures or Gram stain is considered pleural empyema. Other pleural findings indicative of infection include pleural fluid pH <7.1, glucose <40 mg/dL, and lactate dehydrogenase >1000 IU/L.[21]

Treatment

The basic principles of pleural empyema treatment are drainage of pus, reexpansion of the lung, and eradication of the infection.[22] However, parapneumonic effusions do not always require drainage, particularly if no bacteria are found in the pleural fluid.[22] The decision concerning pleural drainage is made through consideration of the patient's general condition, presence of comorbidities, virulence of the infecting pathogen, extent of the pneumonia, and pleural fluid characteristics.[22]

Pleural empyema in the exudative stage can be treated with chest tube thoracostomy and antibiotics.[20] Treatment in the fibrinopurulent stage may require intrapleural fibrinolytic agents and should be done in consultation with a thoracic surgeon or pulmonary specialist. Urokinase is slightly more efficacious and has fewer side effects than streptokinase in the treatment of pleural empyema.[23] To adequately treat loculated effusions, surgical therapy is often required. Video assisted thoracoscopic surgery (VATS) appears to be superior to chest tube drainage and streptokinase to drain the pleural cavity and break up loculations.[24] Treatment of the organizational stage requires surgical intervention with removal of the fibrous peel. Other surgical options include decortication and rib resection to facilitate chronic drainage to prevent recurrent sepsis.

Initial antibiotic treatment should provide coverage for expected pathogens. A typical regimen for an acute, usually parapneumonic, empyema would include a third-generation cephalosporin (cefotaxime or ceftriaxone) *and* vancomycin. Antibiotic therapy can be adjusted according to culture results. Initial antibiotic treatment for subacute or chronic empyema should include anaerobic coverage, and a typical regimen would be clindamycin *and* a third-generation cephalosporin (cefotaxime or ceftriaxone).

Disposition

Patients with a diagnosis of pleural empyema should be admitted to the hospital for drainage of the empyema, intravenous antibiotics, and further evaluation of the extent of their disease. Modification of risk factors (i.e., alcoholism, drug abuse, immunocompromising states) and evaluation for cancer can be addressed during the admission.

REFERENCES

1. Gonzales R, Bartlett JG, Besser RE, et al: Principles of appropriate antibiotic use for treatment of uncomplicated acute bronchitis: Background. *Ann Intern Med* 134:521, 2001.
2. Macfarlane J, Holmes W, Gard P, et al: Prospect study of the incidence, etiology and outcome of adult lower respiratory tract illness in the community. *Thorax* 56:109, 2001.
3. Bent S, Saint S, Vittinghoff E, Grady D: Antibiotics in acute bronchitis: A meta-analysis. *Am J Med* 107:62, 1999.
4. Hueston W, Mainous A, Dacus E, et al: Does acute bronchitis really exist? A reconceptualization of acute viral respiratory infections. *J Fam Pract* 49:401, 2000.
5. Thaidens H, Postma D, deBock G, et al: Asthma in adult patients presenting with symptoms of acute bronchitis in general practice. *Scand J Primary Health Care* 18:188, 2000.
6. Smucny J, Flynn C, Becker L, Glazier R: Are beta 2-agonists effective treatment for acute bronchitis or acute cough in patients without underlying pulmonary disease? A systematic review. *J Fam Pract* 15:945, 2001.
7. Dever LL, Shashikumar K, Johanson WG: Antibiotics in the treatment of acute exacerbations of chronic bronchitis. *Expert Opin Investig Drugs* 11:911, 2002.
8. Halm EA, Teirstein AS: Management of community acquired pneumonia. *New Engl J Med* 347:2039, 2002.
9. Metlay J, Kapoor W, Fine M: Does this patient have community-acquired pneumonia? Diagnosing pneumonia by history and physical examination. *JAMA* 278:1440, 1997.
10. Metlay JP: Update on community-acquired pneumonia: Impact of antibiotic resistance on clinical outcomes. *Curr Opin Infect Dis* 15:163, 2002.
11. Waterer GW, Wunderink RG: The influence of the severity of community-acquired pneumonia on the usefulness of blood cultures. *Respir Med* 95:78, 2001.
12. Theerthakarai R, El-Halees W, Ismail M, et al: Nonvalue of the initial microbiological studies in the management of nonsevere community-acquired pneumonia. *Chest* 119:181, 2001.
13. Ramsey PS, Ramin KD: Pneumonia in pregnancy. *Obstet Gynecol Clin North Am* 28:553, 2001.
14. Meehan TP, Chua-Reyes JM, Tate J, et al: Process of care performance, patient characteristics, and outcomes in elderly patients hospitalized with community-acquired or nursing home-acquired pneumonia. *Chest* 117:1378, 2000.
15. Lim WS, Macfarlane JT: A prospective comparison of nursing home acquired pneumonia with community-acquired pneumonia. *Eur Respir J* 18:362, 2001.
16. Mehr DR, Binder EF, Kruse RL, et al: Clinical findings associated with radiographic pneumonia in nursing home residents. *J Fam Pract* 50:931, 2001.
17. Naughton B, Mylotte J: Treatment guideline for nursing home-acquired pneumonia based on community practice. *J Am Geriatrics Soc* 48:82, 2000.
18. Afessa B, Green B: Bacterial pneumonia in hospitalized patients with HIV infection: The Pulmonary Complications, ICU Support, and Prognostic Factors of Hospitalized Patients with HIV (PIP) Study. *Chest* 117:1017, 2000.
19. Niederman MS, Mandell LA, Anzueto A, et al: Guidelines for the management of adults with community-acquired pneumonia. Diagnosis, assessment of severity, antimicrobial therapy, and prevention. *Am J Respir Crit Care Med* 163:1730, 2001.
20. de Hoyos A, Sundaresan S: Thoracic empyema. *Surg Clin North Am* 82:643, 2002.
21. Hamm H, Light RW: Parapneumonic effusion and empyema. *Eur Respir J* 10:1150, 1997.
22. Heffner JE: Indications for draining a parapneumonic effusion: An evidence-based approach. *Semin Respir Infect* 14:48, 1999.
23. Cameron R: Intra-pleural fibrinolytic therapy vs. conservative management in the treatment of parapneumonic effusions and empyema. *Cochrane Database Syst Rev* 3:CD002312, 2000.
24. Coote N: Surgical versus non-surgical management of pleural empyema. *Cochrane Database Syst Rev* 2:CD001956, 2002.

64
ASPIRATION PNEUMONIA AND LUNG ABSCESS
Eric Anderson

ASPIRATION PNEUMONITIS AND PNEUMONIA

Epidemiology

Aspiration pneumonia is an alveolar space infection resulting from the inhalation of pathogenic material from the oropharynx. Conversely, aspiration pneumonitis is an inflammatory chemical injury of the tracheobronchial tree and pulmonary parenchyma produced from the inhalation of regurgitated sterile gastric contents.[1] Aspiration pneumonitis can lead to aspiration pneumonia due to the breakdown of the pulmonary defense mechanisms caused by the chemical irritation. The exact incidence of aspiration pneumonia has been difficult to quantitate. It is estimated that 5 to 15 percent of community-acquired pneumonia (CAP), up to 20 percent of CAP in the elderly, and the majority of nursing home-acquired pneumonia is due to aspiration.[1–3] The true incidence of aspiration pneumonia may even be higher, because of the observation that approximately 50 percent of normal adults and 70 percent of the elderly with CAP aspirate during sleep.[2,4]

Another population at high risk for aspiration and aspiration pneumonia is the critically ill patient in an intensive care unit.[1] Gastroesophageal reflux and pulmonary aspiration is very common in this population due to a prolonged supine position, gastroparesis from the underlying illness, endotracheal intubation for ventilatory support, and nasogastric or orogastric tubes for gastric decompression and nutrition.

Aspiration pneumonitis is usually associated with depressed level of consciousness that allows for the regurgitation of gastric contents and inhibits the protective upper airway reflexes from preventing aspiration. The classic patient is young, has a depressed mental status due to recreational or therapeutic drugs, and regurgitates a significant volume of gastric contents.

Risk factors for aspiration pneumonia include conditions that promote oropharyngeal colonization with pathogenic bacteria or conditions that impair the swallowing or gag mechanisms (Table 64-1). The incidence of aspiration is highest in patients with dementia or stroke, and the risk of infection is compounded by poor oral care, leading to oropharyngeal colonization, the placement of nasogastric or gastric feeding tubes, and the use of sedative and neuroleptic drugs.[5–9] Although many of these patients have evidence of aspiration with dysphagia or emesis or coughing while eating, up to one third of those who aspirate have silent aspiration without evidence of cough or gag. Aspiration has a significant impact on morbidity and mortality in patients in long-term care facilities.

PATHOPHYSIOLOGY

The development of aspiration pneumonitis depends on the volume and pH of the aspirate. General consensus is that aspiration of gastric contents with pH less than 2.5 and an aspirated volume of 0.3 to 0.4 mL/kg (20 to 30 mL in adults) are required to develop aspiration pneumonitis.[1] The injury produced by acid aspiration is initially a direct, caustic effect followed by an inflammatory response that peaks in 4 to 6 h. Many of the symptoms of aspiration are elicited by the inflammatory response to the infectious or irritative material. Proinflammatory cytokines increase capillary permeability and cause fluid and inflammatory cells to enter the area of irritation. These reactions may manifest clinically as cough, pleuritic chest pain, fever, and radiographic findings. Aspiration of solid or very viscous material blocking the airway may result in precipitous asphyxiation.

The potential to aspirate pathogenic bacteria is increased in patients with periodontal disease, with chronic colonization of the upper airways, and when conditions such as small bowel obstruction, tube

TABLE 64-1 Risk Factors for Aspiration Pneumonia and Lung Abscess

Intoxicants	Alcohol and illicit drugs
	Therapeutic drug overdose
	Sedative drug use
	Procedural sedation
	General anesthesia
Neurologic	Stroke, especially brain-stem involvement with dysphagia
	Seizure
	Head trauma
	Chronic debilitating neurologic condition, especially dementia
Oropharyngeal	Impaired glottic functions
	Emergent intubation
	Periodontal disease and poor oral hygiene
Gastrointestinal	High gastric pressures: prior meal, bag-mask ventilation
	Gastroesophageal reflux
	Esophageal dysmotility or obstruction
	Nasogastric, orogastric, and percutaneous gastric tube
	Tracheobronchial fistula
Other	Supine position
	Rapid sequence intubation
	Advanced age
	Chronic debility
	Extension neck contractures

feeding, H_2-receptor blockers, or proton pump inhibitors make gastric colonization with pathogenic bacteria possible.[1] The tracheobronchial tree is normally able to handle small amounts of aspirated oropharyngeal contents, because the mucociliary escalator transports the aspirated material back up to the oropharynx, where it is expectorated or swallowed. Alveolar macrophages, polymorphonuclear leukocytes, or lymphocytes destroy infectious particles that are small enough to reach the alveoli. Aspiration of food, various liquids or chemicals, dirt, sand, or other objects result in mechanical or chemical injury to these defense mechanisms and predispose the lungs to infection.

Typical bacterial species involved in aspiration pneumonia include *Streptococcus pneumoniae, Staphylococcus aureus, Haemophilus influenzae,* and *Enterobacteriaceae* in community-acquired aspiration pneumonia and *Pseudomonas aeruginosa* and gram-negative organisms in hospital-acquired aspiration pneumonia.[1] Anaerobic bacteria were thought to play a significant role in aspiration pneumonia, but studies conducted in the 1990s using special collection techniques demonstrated that anaerobes are not found in the cultures of the lower respiratory tract in patients with aspiration pneumonia.[10,11]

Characteristic radiographic locations have been described for aspiration pneumonitis and pneumonia.[12] In recumbent patients, the common lung segments involved are those most dependent when supine: the posterior segments of the upper lobes and the superior segments of the lower lobes. In upright patients, the most dependent portions of the lungs are the basal segments of the lower lobes. The inflammatory injury may include, bilateral, patchy, interstitial, or alveolar inflates, particularly in aspiration of large volumes, as in near drowning.[12]

CLINICAL PRESENTATION

Witnessed or suspected aspiration is a key feature in the diagnosis of aspiration pneumonitis or pneumonia. A witnessed aspiration of solid or liquid material while eating, during a therapeutic procedure, or after being submerged while swimming or working in water is an obvious clue.[13,14] Patients with known swallowing or esophageal motility disorders, esophageal obstruction, or enteral tube feedings should be considered risks for aspiration.[6] Silent aspirators are more difficult to detect. Historical features that suggest silent aspiration include general debility, recurrent cough, hoarseness, or dysphagia. History may be difficult to obtain in chronically debilitated or otherwise noncommunicative patients.

The patient with aspiration pneumonitis may have only minor symptoms, such as nonproductive cough and tachypnea. Aspiration of larger or more acidic gastric contents may produce tracheobronchitis with bronchospasm, bloody or frothy sputum, and respiratory distress. Aspiration of large volumes or very caustic material may result in respiratory failure.

The clinical symptoms of aspiration pneumonia include fever, dyspnea, and productive cough. Other symptoms of systemic infection in the elderly and debilitated patients may be present, including a change in mental status or function, lethargy, or nausea and vomiting.[2,3] The physical examination may reveal signs classic for pneumonia: tachycardia, tachypnea, fever, rales, or decreased breath sounds in an ill-appearing patient. Patients with underlying pulmonary disease may decompensate rapidly and have more symptoms and signs of respiratory distress.

Chest radiographs in aspiration pneumonia usually show unilateral focal or patchy consolidations in the dependent lung segments, as noted above.[12] Occasionally, bilateral or interstitial patterns can be seen. The right lower lobe is the most common area of consolidation when the aspiration occurs when the patient is upright (Figure 64-1).

Laboratory values will be of little diagnostic value. Early in the course, the white blood cell count may or may not be elevated. Arterial blood gases may reflect hypoxia or hypoventilation, but this may be secondary to the patient's underlying lung disease, and comparison with previous blood gas results would be helpful. Expectorated spu-

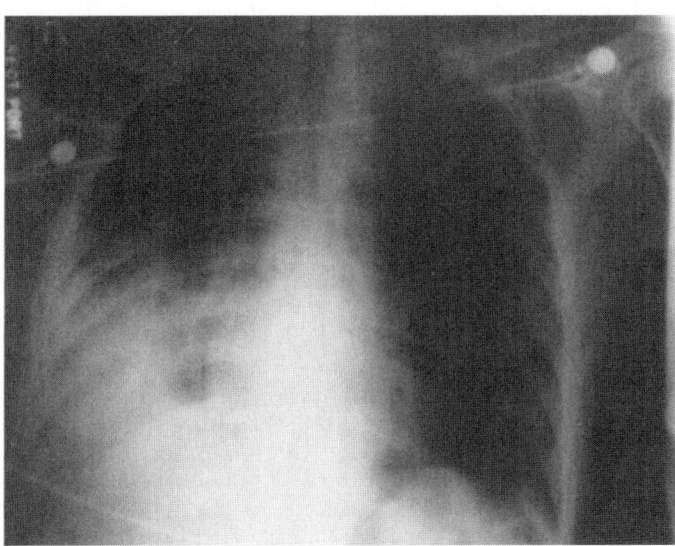

FIG. 64-1. Aspiration pneumonia of the right lower lobe.

tum cultures are of low yield, because of the increased rate of contamination from oropharyngeal colonization in most patients with aspiration pneumonia.

Treatment

Patients who have a witnessed aspiration from regurgitation of a large volume of gastric contents should have prompt suctioning of the upper airway. Endotracheal tube placement should be considered, as should placement of an orogastric or nasogastric tube for gastric decompression. Patients who aspirate large volumes of solid material or tenacious material may require suctioning of the tracheobronchial tree or bronchoalveolar lavage to clear the airway. Bronchodilators may be required for aspiration-induced bronchospasm. Prophylactic antibiotics are not recommended, and there is no evidence that corticosteroids prevent lung injury.[1]

Healthy persons who aspirate small volumes of nontoxic material may be observed for short time, approximately 1 h, and, if stable and reliable, discharged with instructions to return for worsening symptoms. Antibiotic treatment is not necessary. However, previously healthy patients whose symptoms of aspiration pneumonitis fail to resolve in 24 to 48 h should be treated with broad-spectrum antibiotics[1] (Table 64-2).

Chronically ill or nursing home patients who have a witnessed episode of aspiration followed by respiratory symptoms (cough, dyspnea, tachypnea, or wheezing) are more problematic. These patients are often sent to the ED for evaluation, by which time their symptoms have improved or resolved. These patients are at greater risk for aspiration pneumonia due to their oropharyngeal colonization from pathogenic bacteria. It is not possible to differentiate which patients will be able to spontaneously resolve their symptoms, from those who will progress to aspiration pneumonitis, or aspiration pneumonia. A reasonable, although not validated, approach would be to observe a stable patient (no respiratory distress, no fever, normal or baseline oxygen saturation, no new radiographic infiltrate). A stable patient can be discharged back to the monitored chronic care or nursing home facility. Patients who remain symptomatic or have a new radiographic infiltrate should be considered for admission or continued observation. There is no firm evidence regarding the benefits of antibiotic treatment in this population, and some discourage it because of the potential of selecting resistant organisms in a patient with an otherwise uncomplicated chemical pneumonitis.[1] Nursing home patients with worsening symptoms, fever, cough or sputum production, hypoxemia, or radiographic infiltrate should be considered as developing aspiration pneumonia and receive antibiotic treatment in the hospital or nursing home.[15]

Empiric broad-spectrum antibiotic therapy is indicated in patients with aspiration pneumonia. The specific agents are chosen according to the potential pathogens as determined by the patient's general health and location[1] (see Table 64-2). Agents that treat predominately anaerobes (penicillin or clindamycin) are not sufficient to cover the spectrum of bacteria involved in most aspiration pneumonias and should not be used alone.[1,10,11]

Disposition

Reliable patients who have a witnessed episode of aspiration and who are otherwise healthy and exhibit no signs of infection or respiratory compromise may be discharged home with instructions to follow up

TABLE 64-2   Empiric Antibiotics Recommended for Common Aspiration Syndromes

Syndrome and Clinical Situation	Antibiotic (Usual Dose)*
Aspiration pneumonitis	
Signs or symptoms lasting >48 h	Levofloxacin 500 mg per d[†] *or* Ceftriaxone 1–2 g per d
Small bowel obstruction or use of antacids or antisecretory agents	Levofloxacin 500 mg per d[†] *or* Ceftriaxone 1–2 g per d, *or* Ciprofloxacin 400 mg every 12 h *or* Piperacillin–tazobactam 3.375 g every 6 h *or* Ceftazidime 2 g every 8 h
Aspiration pneumonia	
Community-acquired	Levofloxacin 500 mg per d† *or* Ceftriaxone 1–2 g per d
Residence in a long-term care facility	Levofloxacin 500 mg per d† *or* Piperacillin–tazobactam 3.375 g every 6 h *or* Ceftazidime 2 g every 8 h
Severe periodontal disease, putrid sputum, or alcoholism	Piperacillin–tazobactam 3.375 g every 6 h *or* Imipenem 0.5–1.0 g every 6–8 h *or* Levofloxacin 500 mg per d† plus clindamycin 600 mg every 8 h *or* metronidazole 500 mg every 8 h *or* Ciprofloxacin 400 mg every 12 h plus clindamycin 600 mg every 8 h or metronidazole 500 mg every 8 h *or* Ceftriaxone 1–2 g per d plus clindamycin 600 mg every 8 h *or* metronidazole 500 mg every 8 h

*The doses listed are those for patients with normal renal function.
†Levofloxacin is given by slow infusion over 60 min. Levofloxacin 500 mg per d, may be replaced by gatifloxacin 400 mg per d.
Source: Marik PE: Aspiration pneumonitis and aspiration pneumonia. *New Engl J Med* 344:669, 2001.

with their primary care physician in the next few days. They should be instructed to watch for shortness of breath, fever, chest pain, unusual fatigue, or the development of a persistent cough and to return promptly to the ED or their primary care physician if any of these symptoms develop.

Patients who appear stable but have risk factors for worsening or very aggressive disease (e.g., diabetes, advanced age, renal dialysis, recent stroke, chronic pulmonary disease, active cancer, and human immunodeficiency virus) should be admitted to a hospital or an observation unit. Oxygen and possibly antibiotics should be started, and the patient should be observed carefully for 12 to 24 h. If stable after 12 to 24 h of treatment and observation, such patients can be sent home and instructed to follow up, as described above, and to return if any signs of deterioration develop. Patients with definite evidence of infection should have antibiotic treatment initiated and then admitted, or selected patients can be treated in the nursing home provided that the nursing home has the ability to monitor and treat these patients.[1,15] Patients who exhibit hemodynamic or respiratory instability require admission to an intensive care unit.

LUNG ABSCESS

Epidemiology

Lung abscess is defined as a localized suppurative necrotizing process occurring within the pulmonary parenchyma.[16] Lung abscess typically is caused by a suppurative pulmonary bacterial infection secondary to aspiration pneumonia. Lung abscess also can be caused by bacterial infection in an area of lung infarct or as a result of an infected pulmonary pneumocyst. Other causes of cavitary lung lesions include fungal infections, parasitic infections, inflammatory conditions, and primary and metastatic neoplasias (Table 64-3). The incidence of lung abscess has declined tenfold over the past four decades, presumably secondary to improved treatment regimes for pneumonia. The mortality from lung abscesses also has decreased but remains between 2 and

TABLE 64-3 Cavitary Lung Lesions

Infectious	
Bacterial	Anaerobic abscess (immunocompetent)
	Aerobic abscess (immunocompromised)
	Infected bullae
	Infected pulmonary infarct
	Tuberculosis
	Actinomycosis
	Pleural empyema
Fungal	Coccidioidomycosis
	Histoplasmosis
	Blastomycosis
	Aspergillosis
	Cryptococcosis
Parasitic	Echinococcosis
	Amebiasis
Neoplastic	Bronchogenic carcinoma (squamous cell or adenocarcinoma)
	Metastatic cancer (colorectal or renal)
	Lymphoma or Hodgkin's disease
Inflammatory	Wegner granulomatosus
	Sarcoidosis

Source: Cassiere HA, Niederman MS: Aspiration pneumonia, lipoid pneumonia, and lung abscess, in Baum GL, Celli BR, Crapo JD, Karlinsky JB (eds): *Textbook of Pulmonary Diseases,* 6th ed. Philadelphia, Lippincott-Raven, 1998, p. 651.

10 percent for community-acquired lung abscess but up to 60 percent for hospital-acquired lung abscess.

Pathophysiology

Lung abscess typically is caused by a breakdown of the usual pulmonary defense mechanisms that allows a parenchymal infection to evolve into an abscess. A lung abscess that evolves from aspiration pneumonia takes approximately 8 to 14 days to form after the aspiratory event. Anaerobic bacteria are the most common isolates from lung abscesses in immunocompetent patients.[17] Aerobic bacteria are found more commonly from lung abscesses in immunocompromised patients and include *S. aureus, Escherichia coli, Klebsiella pneumoniae, P. aeruginosa, Streptococcus pyogenes, P. pseudomallei, H. influenzae, Legionella pneumophillia, Nocardia asteroides, Actinomyces* species, and, rarely, pneumococci.[16,17]

Medical conditions that predispose for the development of pulmonary abscess include those conditions that predispose to aspiration pneumonia, including poor dentition, gingival disease, chronic alcoholism, chronic debility with extension neck contractures, and chronically depressed mental status (see Table 64-1).

Infectious lung abscesses typically occur in the basal segments of the lower lobes or the posterior segments of the upper lobes. When abscesses occur in the anterior portion of the lungs, a neoplastic etiology should be considered more likely. Cancer causes 8 to 18 percent of lung abscesses at all ages, but the percentage is closer to 30 percent in those older than 45 years.

Clinical Features

Patients with lung abscess classically present with an indolent course of cough, fever, pleuritic chest pain, weight loss, and night sweats. The typical patient will present after having the symptoms for approximately 14 days. There may be cough productive of putrid sputum that layers out when allowed to stand. Hemoptysis can be seen in up to 25 percent of cases. Because the infection is more indolent, vital sign abnormalities typical of an acute infection (tachycardia or tachypnea) are often absent. Laboratory findings usually are nonspecific but commonly include an elevated white blood cell count and erythrocyte sedimentation rate.

Diagnosis

The diagnosis is usually made by a chest radiograph showing an area of dense consolidation with an air-fluid level inside of a cavitary lesion (Figure 64-2), indicating that the abscess cavity communicates with a bronchiole, as occurs in about three fourths of patients with lung abscesses. In the other fourth, the abscess will appear as an area of very dense consolidation on chest radiograph and require a chest computed tomography to disclose the presence of a cavitary lesion. Multiple abscesses are unusual.

The differential diagnosis of cavitary lesions with air-fluid levels seen on chest radiographs includes (1) an infected bullae in a patient with bullous emphysema (infected bullae will have thin walls), (2) a pleural fluid collection with a bronchopleural fistula resulting in a pleural air-fluid level (the pleural air-fluid level will extend to the chest wall and taper at the apex), and (3) a loop of bowel extending through a diaphragmatic hernia (there may nausea or vomiting due to incarceration or audible bowel sounds on the chest wall at the site of the hernia).

Treatment

Medical management will successfully treat 85 to 90 percent of lung abscesses.[16,18,19] Historically, penicillin was the treatment of choice, but studies have demonstrated that clindamycin is superior in efficacy,

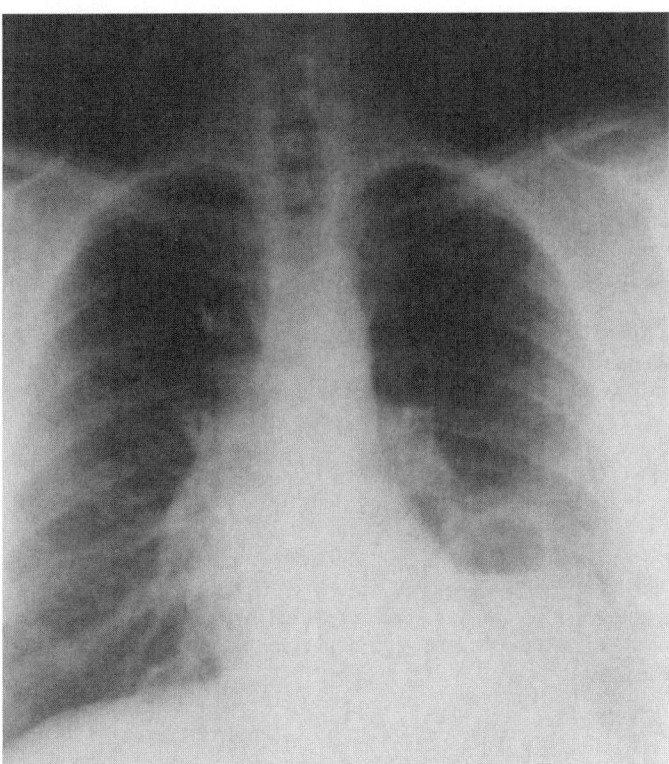

FIG. 64-2. Lung abscess of the left lower lobe demonstrating an air-fluid level.

time to symptom resolution, and side effect profile. Appropriate treatment consists of (1) clindamycin in a dosage of 600 mg IV every 6 to 8 h for adults or (2) an aminopenicillin/β-lactamase inhibitor such as ampicillin/sulbactam 1.5 to 3.0 g IV every 6 h for those who cannot take clindamycin.[16,18] Concern that clindamycin has only gram-positive coverage has led to the consideration that combination treatment with the addition of a second-generation cephalosporin.[18] Typically, parenteral treatment is initiated until the patient is afebrile and clinically improved, usually in 4 to 8 days. Therapy may be continued with oral clindamycin or amoxicillin/clavulanate.

Drainage usually occurs spontaneously from communication of the abscess cavity with the tracheobronchial tree. This is signaled by the development of an air-fluid level on chest radiographs. Attempts at postural drainage or bronchoscopic drainage of the abscess cavity should be discouraged, because these actions may result in seeding other parts of the lungs with infectious material. Some patients fail medical treatment (Table 64-4). Another reason for failure of medical

TABLE 64-4 Factors Associated with Failure of Medical Therapy in Lung Abscess

Recurrent aspiration
Large cavity (>6 cm)
Prolonged symptom complex before presentation
Abscess associated with an obstructing lesion
Presence of thick-walled cavities
Underlying serious comorbidity
Development of empyema

Source: Cassiere HA, Niederman MS: Aspiration pneumonia, lipoid pneumonia, and lung abscess, in Baum GL, Celli BR, Crapo JD, Karlinksy JB (eds): *Textbook of Pulmonary Diseases,* 6th ed. Philadelphia, Lippincott-Raven, 1998, p. 653.

treatment is a nonbacterial cause of the abscess, i.e., neoplastic, fungal, inflammatory, or parasitic. Surgical treatments for nondraining lung abscess include image-guided percutaneous drainage or thoracotomy and pulmonary resection.[20,21]

Disposition

Patients with lung abscess typically will respond to parenteral antibiotics and management of the other medical conditions that predisposed to the development of the abscess. After resolution of symptoms, these patients can be discharged on oral antibiotics for 4 to 8 weeks. Chest radiographic findings will lag behind clinical progress and on average take more than 2 months to resolve.[16]

Complications of lung abscess include empyema, massive hemoptysis, contamination of uninvolved lung, and failure of the abscess cavity to resolve. Approximately 10 percent of lung abscesses will require surgical intervention.[19–21]

REFERENCES

1. Marik PE: Aspiration pneumonitis and aspiration pneumonia. *New Engl J Med* 344:665, 2001.
2. Marrie TJ: Community-acquired pneumonia in the elderly. *Clin Infect Dis* 31:1066, 2000.
3. Mylotte JM: Nursing home-acquired pneumonia. *Clin Infect Dis* 35:1205, 2002.
4. Gleeson K, Eggli DF, Maxwell SL: Quantitative aspiration during sleep in normal subjects. *Chest* 111:1266, 1997.
5. Daniels SK, Brailey K Preistly DH et al: Aspiration in patients with acute stroke. *Arch Phys Med Rehabil* 79:14, 1998.
6. Langmore SE, Skarupski KA, Park PS, Fries BE: Predictors of aspiration pneumonia in nursing home residents. *Dysphagia* 17:298, 2002.
7. Wada H, Nakojoh K, Satoh-Nakagawa T, et al: Risk factors of aspiration pneumonia in Alzheimer's disease. *Gerontology* 47:271, 2001.
8. Taylor HM: Pneumonia frequencies with different enteral tube feeding access sites. *Am J Ment Retard* 107:175, 2002.
9. Vergis EN, Brennen C, Wagener M, Muder RR: Pneumonia in long-term care: A prospective case-control study of risk factors and impact on survival. *Arch Intern Med* 161:2378, 2001.
10. Mier L, Dreyfuss D, Darchy B, et al: Is penicillin G an adequate initial treatment for aspiration pneumonia? A prospective evaluation using a protected specimen brush and quantitative cultures. *Intensive Care Med* 19:279, 1993.
11. Marik PE, Careau P: The role of anaerobes in patients with ventilator associated pneumonia and aspiration pneumonia: A prospective study. *Chest* 115:178, 1999.
12. Franquet T, Gimenez A, Roson N, et al: Aspiration diseases: Findings, pitfalls, and differential diagnosis. *Radiographics* 20:673, 2000.
13. Thibodeau LG, Verdile VP, Bartfield JM: Incidence of aspiration after urgent intubation. *Am J Emerg Med* 15:562, 1997.
14. Green SM, Krauss B: Pulmonary aspiration risk during emergency department procedural sedation-An examination of the role of fasting and sedation depth. *Acad Emerg Med* 9:35, 2002.
15. Hutt E, Kramer AM: Evidence-based guidelines for management of nursing home-acquired pneumonia. *J Fam Pract* 51:709, 2002.
16. Wiedemann HP, Rice TW: Lung abscess and empyema. *Semin Thorac Cardiovasc Surg* 7:119, 1995.
17. Mansharamani N, Balachandran D, Delaney D, et al: Lung abscess in adults: Clinical comparison of immunocompromised to non-immunocompromised patients. *Respir Med* 96:178, 2002.
18. Ewig S, Schafer H: Treatment of community-acquired lung abscess associated with aspiration. *Pneumologie* 55:431, 2001.
19. Mwandumba HC, Beeching NJ: Pyogenic lung infections: Factors for predicting clinical outcome of lung abscess and thoracic empyema. *Curr Opin Pulm Med* 6:234, 2000.
20. Wali SO, Shugaeri A, Samman YS, Abdelaziz M: Percutaneous drainage of pyogenic lung abscess. *Scand J Infect Dis* 34:673, 2002.
21. Tseng YL, Wu MH, Lin MY, et al: Surgery for lung abscess in immunocompetent and immunocompromised children. *J Pediatr Surg* 36:470, 2001.

65 TUBERCULOSIS
Janet M. Poponick

EPIDEMIOLOGY

Tuberculosis remains an important infectious disease in the world today; more than one third of the world's population has tuberculosis. It causes 8 million new cases per year, with 2 million deaths per year.[1] In the United States, new cases of tuberculosis steadily declined from the late 1800s until 1984, followed by increases at alarming rates until 1992. Factors believed to be responsible for this resurgence of tuberculosis include an increase in the number of homeless persons, the human immunodeficiency virus (HIV) epidemic, drug abuse, increased immigration, the inability of local and state governments to maintain tuberculosis control programs, and the increase of multidrug-resistant tuberculosis.[2]

From 1993 to 2000, tuberculosis was once again on the decline in the U.S., primarily due to stronger tuberculosis control programs, which targeted high-risk individuals. In 2000 there were 16,377 cases of tuberculosis reported (5.8 cases per 100,000 population), which represents a 45 percent decrease from 1992, when tuberculosis cases peaked (10.5 cases per 100,000 population).[3] Tuberculosis remains more common in urban areas. The case rate for foreign-born persons has increased, whereas the case rate for U.S.-born persons has decreased; in 2000, 46 percent of the cases were in foreign-born persons.[3,4]

Continued improvement in tuberculosis control and prevention requires recognition and treatment of high-risk populations (Table 65-1), continued funding of programs for surveillance and treatment of noncompliant patients, aggressive screening of foreign-born persons, continued basic research into the pathogenesis and immunologic response, and continued development of new pharmacologic agents.[3]

PATHOPHYSIOLOGY

Mycobacterium tuberculosis is a slow-growing aerobic rod that has a unique, multilayered cell wall that contains a variety of lipids that account for its acid-fast property. Transmission occurs through inhalation of droplet nuclei into the lungs. Persons with active tuberculosis who excrete stainable mycobacteria in saliva or sputum are the most infectious.[5]

Once the organisms reach the lungs, host defenses are activated.[1,5] In immunocompetent persons, such defenses may kill off the inhaled mycobacteria and prevent infection. Some organisms may survive, however, and be transported to the regional lymph nodes, where the host's cell-mediated immunity is further activated to contain the infection. Granulomas, known as *tubercles,* may form as a result of this process, which involves activated macrophages. Tubercles are a sign of primary infection and may progress to caseation necrosis and calcification leading to the Ghon complex.[5] In most cases, the bacteria are contained in the tubercles, but some organisms enter the thoracic duct and spread throughout the body, where they may remain dormant for many years. This is referred to as *latent infection* and is manifested by a positive tuberculin skin test.[1] In most cases of dissemination in immunocompetent hosts, the organisms do not find a suitable area to proliferate. Survival is favored in areas of high oxygen content or blood flow, such as the apical and posterior segments of the upper lobe and the superior segment of the lower lobe of the lung, the renal cortex, the

TABLE 65-1 Patients with a High Prevalence of Tuberculosis

Elderly and nursing home patients
Immigrants from high-prevalence countries
Patients with the human immunodeficiency virus
Alcoholics and illicit drug users
Residents and staff of prisons or shelters for the homeless

meninges, the epiphyses of long bones, and the vertebrae.[5] In immunocompromised hosts, hematogenous spread occurs early, because normal host defenses are unable to contain the organisms, and disseminated disease occurs.[5]

The latent infection may reactivate when a host's immune system is no longer capable of containing the foci of previous hematogenous spread.[1] The young, the elderly, or patients with other chronic debilitating diseases are at higher risk for such reactivation disease. In 5 percent of persons, latent infection may progress to active disease within 2 years after initial exposure, with another 5 percent developing disease over a lifetime.[1] The population at risk for HIV infection is also at risk for tuberculosis. As the host defense system weakens, latent infection may progress to active tuberculosis. The incidence of progression to active disease in HIV patients is reported at 7 to 10 percent per year.[1] Other groups at risk for developing active tuberculosis include those immunocompromised from carcinoma of solid organs, leukemias, transplantation and those with diabetes, chronic renal failure requiring hemodialysis, and silicosis.[6]

Current research emphasizes the basic science involved in the host response to mycobacteria. The key cells are the alveolar macrophages and T lymphocytes, especially the T-helper cells, and the various cytokines and interleukins that are released. With successful treatment, local tumor necrosis factor-α secretion decreases whereas interferon-γ secretion increases.[7]

CLINICAL FEATURES

Primary Tuberculosis

The initial infection is usually asymptomatic and only identified by a positive reaction to purified protein derivative (PPD).[1] Infrequently, a pneumonitis may result that is similar to a viral or bacterial infection. Hilar adenopathy is present but rarely massive. In some cases, especially in immunocompromised patients, the primary infection may be rapidly progressive and fatal.

Reactivation Tuberculosis

When latent infection progresses to active tuberculosis, symptoms can be divided into systemic and pulmonary. The most common symptom is fever, followed by night sweats, malaise, fatigue, and weight loss. Productive cough, hemoptysis, and pleuritic chest pain develop as the infection spreads within the lungs. When the infection is extensive, shortness of breath may develop. The results of a physical examination are generally unremarkable, but rales may be noted over areas of pulmonary infection. Although most cases of tuberculosis are pulmonary, up to 15 percent of cases will have extrapulmonary manifestations.[1] Common sites include the adrenal glands, bones and joints, gastrointestinal tract, genitourinary tract, lymph nodes, meninges, pericardium, peritoneum, and pleura.

Miliary tuberculosis is the result of wide hematogenous spread during the primary infection or secondary seeding of the other organs in an immunocompromised host. Fever, cough, weight loss, hepatomegaly, splenomegaly, lymphadenopathy, and signs of multisystem illness should cause one to suspect miliary disease. Laboratory abnormalities include hyponatremia, anemia, thrombocytopenia, and leukopenia. The chest radiograph shows numerous small nodular lesions.

The most common extrapulmonary site of tuberculosis is the lymphatic system and may involve any of the lymph nodes. Fever is usually absent, and the lymphadenopathy is painless. The nodes may develop draining sinuses.

A tuberculous pleural effusion usually occurs after primary infection, when a subpleural node ruptures into the pleura.[5] Some cases occur during hematogenous spread. Symptoms are usually fever, shortness of breath, and pleuritic chest pain. The fluid is exudative in nature, and the organisms may not be visible on acid-fast staining. A pleural biopsy is often necessary to confirm diagnosis.

Pericarditis and peritonitis as a result of tuberculosis are difficult to diagnose and often require biopsy. Complications of tuberculous pericarditis include tamponade and constrictive pericarditis.[5]

The central nervous system may become seeded during primary infection, leading to tuberculous (Rich) foci in the meninges, spinal cord, or the brain parenchyma. Rupture of a Rich focus into the subarachnoid space may result in meningitis. In children, the disease is acute, whereas a more indolent course is noted in adults. Fever, signs of meningeal irritation, and cranial nerve deficits are seen. Typical cerebrospinal fluid analysis reveals mononuclear cells and a low glucose level, but early samples may show a predominance of neutrophils.[5]

Pediatric Tuberculosis

Tuberculosis in the pediatric population occurs in the same risk groups as in the adult population (see Table 65-1). Primary tuberculosis is usually an asymptomatic disease and generally found during school screening or household screening programs.[5] The classic symptoms of fever, night sweats, and weight loss may be seen in older children, but, in those younger than age 5, presentation may be that of miliary tuberculosis, meningitis, or a pneumonia that does not respond to therapy.[5,8] The most common radiographic findings include hilar adenopathy, mediastinal lymphadenopathy, or consolidated pneumonia. The most common extrapulmonary presentation is cervical lymphadenitis, but meningitis, bone, and joint involvement also may occur.[8]

Tuberculosis and HIV

Tuberculosis (pulmonary and extrapulmonary) often can be the initial clinical manifestation of immunodeficiency and is considered an illness that defines acquired immunodeficiency syndrome (AIDS). Infection with HIV increases the risk of latent disease and the likelihood that initial infection will result in active disease.[1,9] The incidence of tuberculosis in HIV-positive patients varies according to community prevalence but is much higher than in the general population. Physicians considering a diagnosis of tuberculosis should offer patients HIV testing, which may provide early diagnosis and therapy.

Pulmonary involvement may be difficult to distinguish from other HIV-associated lung disorders. Tuberculosis must be in the differential of any HIV-associated respiratory disorder and can present atypically on chest radiographs. The incidence of extrapulmonary tuberculosis is higher in patients diagnosed with HIV infection with the potential to involve any organ system. The most commonly reported extrapulmonary sites are the lymph nodes, pleura, and bones or joints.

Treatment of tuberculosis in HIV-positive individuals is generally effective, but some reports have indicated higher mortality rates in coinfected patients, especially in those severely immunocompromised.[9] The incidence of adverse drug reactions to antituberculosis chemotherapy is higher in HIV-positive than in HIV-negative patients. Due to the number of medications taken by patients with HIV, potential drug interactions also must be of concern.

Multidrug-Resistant Tuberculosis

The incidence of multidrug-resistant tuberculosis (MDR-TB) peaked during the resurgence of tuberculosis. During that period, most cases involved those coinfected with HIV and were associated with a high mortality rate. With the increased surveillance of high-risk groups, the overall incidence of drug resistance has decreased.[3] However, MDR-TB remains a problem in foreign-born persons, accounting for 72 percent of the MDR-TB cases reported in 2000.[3] *Mycobacterium tuberculosis* becomes resistant by spontaneous genetic mutation, often as a

result of inadequate drug therapy or noncompliance with initial treatment.[2,10] The most powerful predictors of drug resistance remain a history of previous tuberculosis, cavitary lung disease, and positive sputum smears.[10–12]

In the HIV-positive population, the most common pattern is resistance to both isoniazid and rifampin.[5] Available data suggest no difference in isoniazid monoresistance among those patients with or without HIV. Rifampin monoresistant tuberculosis has become a problem, especially in those with AIDS.[13] Cases with rifampin monoresistance were more commonly seen in patients who previously had tuberculosis, a history of diarrhea, rifabutin use, or antifungal therapy.[13]

For those HIV-negative patients treated for MDR-TB strains, a long-term response rate ranging from 56 to 96 percent has been reported. When MDR-TB is diagnosed early and appropriately treated, the cure rate is higher. Recent reports stress the importance of aggressive contact investigation and treatment in specialized centers to appropriately control the spread of MDR-TB.[11,12] One study from Turkey reported an overall success rate of 77 percent when using aggressive surveillance and treatment protocols.[14] In that study, a mean number of 5.5 drugs were used, some of which are considered second-line treatment.

Treatment of MDR-TB remains challenging and depends on the sensitivity patterns from culture. Most regimens include four to six drugs, with treatment as long as 18 to 24 months after sputum conversion. The fluoroquinolones have been used successfully in treatment of MDR-TB.[10,14] Side effects of multiple-drug regimens are a common problem. When drug therapy fails, resectional surgery may be necessary to eradicate the disease.

DIAGNOSIS

The diagnosis of tuberculosis can present a challenge to emergency physicians. In the past, physicians mainly considered the diagnosis when presented with a patient with reactivation infection. With the increased incidence of tuberculosis and the appearance of multidrug-resistant strains, one must consider the diagnosis in a wider range of patients. The variable clinical presentation and the time required to culture the organism make emergent diagnosis difficult. A heightened awareness of the disease and the potential of new rapid diagnostic tests can ensure that these patients are not returned to the community without proper therapy.

All prehospital and ED personnel should be trained to suspect tuberculosis, institute appropriate precautions, and notify health care providers of their suspicions. Triage workers should ask appropriate questions to detect potential cases. Patients with suspected tuberculosis should be placed in separate waiting areas, wear surgical masks, and be instructed to cover the mouth and nose when coughing. Any immunocompromised patient with respiratory symptoms should be isolated until tuberculosis can be excluded. Prompt evaluation will ensure a minimal amount of time spent in the ambulatory care setting and a minimal risk of exposure to health care providers and other patients.[15]

Skin Test

The most common method to detect exposure to *M. tuberculosis* is a skin test. The Mantoux test, which involves the intracutaneous injection of 0.1 mL of PPD into the forearm, relies on a delayed-type hypersensitivity reaction that is triggered if past infection with tuberculosis has occurred. The test is read between 48 and 72 h after administration by measuring the extent of skin induration at the test site; erythema or other skin changes are not assessed (Table 65-2).[6] All persons with a positive PPD reaction or recent conversion should be referred for possible treatment of latent tuberculosis.

In a few situations, however, the PPD test may be nondiagnostic. Individuals who have received Bacille Calmette-Guérin immunization

TABLE 65-2 Interpretation of Purified Protein Derivative Skin Test*

1. ≥5 mm induration is positive in
   a. Patients with the human immunodeficiency virus
   b. Patients with close contact with a tuberculosis-infected individual
   c. Patients with abnormal chest radiograph suggestive of healed tuberculosis
   d. Patients with organ transplants and other immunosuppressed patients receiving the equivalent of prednisone >15 mg per d for greater than 1 month
2. ≥10 mm induration is positive in patients not meeting the above criteria but who have other risks
   a. Injection drug users
   b. High-prevalence groups (immigrants, long-term–care facility residents, persons in local high-risk areas)
   c. Patients with conditions that increase the risk of progression to active disease (silicosis, diabetes, carcinoma of the head, neck, or lung)
   d. Children <4 y of age
3. ≥15 mm induration is positive in all others
4. Detection of newly infected persons in a screening program
   a. ≥10 mm induration increase within any 2 y period is positive if younger than 35 y
   b. ≥15 mm induration increase within any 2 y period is positive if 35 y or older
5. If the patient is anergic, other epidemiologic factors must be considered

*A positive reaction does not necessarily indicate disease.

for tuberculosis prevention would be expected to have a positive response. Exposure to nontuberculosis mycobacteria also can result in a false-positive PPD reaction.[6]

A competent immune system is required to yield a positive response to the PPD if there has been infection with *M. tuberculosis*. Therefore, individuals with abnormal immune systems, such as in AIDS, may lose their ability to mount a delayed-type hypersensitivity reaction required to produce a positive PPD reaction. Although the Centers for Disease Control and Prevention (CDC) no longer recommend routine anergy testing among HIV-positive individuals, some clinicians use control agents, such as mumps or *Candida*, to assess at-risk patients for anergy. However, reacting to controls does not exclude the diagnosis of tuberculosis, and a negative skin test in a patient suspected of disease requires further evaluation.[16] False negatives have been demonstrated with improper PPD administration. Nonreactivity to a PPD has been occasionally reported in patients with active culture-positive tuberculosis; therefore, a PPD test occasionally may be unreliable in acute stages of the disease.

Chest Radiograph

The chest radiograph is used to screen for disease in individuals with positive PPD skin test and for those with signs and symptoms of active infection. In the past, the classic findings of tuberculosis were those associated with reactivation infection: cavitary or noncavitary lesions in the upper lobe or superior segment of the lower lobe of the lungs.[17] Cavitation can be associated with increased infectivity.[5] Calcification of the lesions may be a later finding.

With the resurgence of tuberculosis, radiographic findings of primary disease are becoming more common. In primary infection, parenchymal infiltrates in any area of the lung may be found. Isolated ipsilateral hilar or mediastinal adenopathy is sometimes the only finding. Miliary tuberculosis as primary or reactivation disease frequently shows small (1 to 3 mm) nodules throughout the lung fields. Pleural effusions, which are usually unilateral, can occur alone or in association with parenchymal disease. Atelectasis, fibrotic scarring, tracheal deviation, and signs of prior thoracic surgery are other findings. Because tuberculosis has a wide variety of appearances on chest radi-

ographs, comparison with previous films is extremely helpful in determining the significance of an abnormal or unusual finding.

Immunocompromised patients, such as those with advanced HIV, are more likely to have radiographs typical of primary infection or with atypical findings as opposed to classic cavitary lesions. Normal radiographs in the presence of active disease are seen more frequently in HIV-positive patients.[9,17]

Microbiology

Culture for tuberculosis is the "gold standard" for diagnosis.[5] Sputum is commonly collected to detect the presence of *M. tuberculosis* by culture and smear. In the absence of a satisfactory sputum sample, gastric aspirates, pleural and other body fluids, and tissue samples may be used for culture and other diagnostic tests. Staining of the specimen for acid fastness (i.e., Ziehl-Neelsen stain) or a fluorochrome procedure is the quickest and least expensive method to provide a presumptive diagnosis of tuberculosis. Approximately 60 percent of culture-positive cases of tuberculosis will have smears in which acid-fast bacilli are detected, although this may be lower in individuals with HIV.[9]

Newer methods are under development to aid in the speed and sensitivity of diagnosing tuberculosis. Although not widely available, techniques that use radiometric technology, DNA probes, polymerase chain reaction, reverse transcription, or other technologies may someday provide definitive results in a matter of hours.[5] At this time, the technology is used for a DNA fingerprint to understand transmission of disease for epidemiologic purposes.[18]

TREATMENT

Because of the possibility of resistance, the treatment of active tuberculosis involves the use of a combination of antimycobacterial medications.[1,19] Initial therapy usually consists of three or four-drugs [isoniazid (INH), rifampin (RIF), pyrazinamide (PZA), ethambutol (EMB)] for 8 weeks, followed by two-drug continuation treatment for 18 to 31 weeks. The recommended CDC regimens are:[19]

1. Daily four-drug (INH, RIF, PZA, EMB) therapy for 8 weeks, followed by either INH/RIF or INH/rifapentine for 18 weeks.
2. Daily four-drug therapy for 2 weeks, followed by two times per week for 6 weeks, with subsequent INH/RIF or INH/RPT for 18 weeks.
3. Three times weekly four-drug therapy for 8 weeks, followed by INH/RIF three times weekly for 18 weeks.
4. Daily three-drug (INH, RIF, EMB) for 8 weeks followed by INH/RIF for 31 weeks.

More prolonged therapy is recommended for immunocompromised patients, such as those with HIV or extrapulmonary disease. Initial therapy may be modified once drug susceptibilities are available. The importance of directly observed therapy (DOT), where patients are observed taking their antituberculosis medications to ensure compliance, cannot be overstated. The CDC recommends that all regimens of two or three times per week should be given by DOT.[1,6,11,12,19]

Although the standard medications used to treat tuberculosis are generally efficacious and safe, occasionally side effects or drug interactions may be significant (Table 65-3). Isoniazid, the most frequently used antituberculosis agent, has hepatitis as its major toxicity. Advancing age is thought to be a significant risk factor for the development of hepatitis.[5] Pre-existing liver disease, pregnancy, ethanol use, HIV, and hepatitis C infection have been associated with an increased risk for hepatotoxicity from INH.[6] In addition, those with pre-existing medical conditions requiring multiple medications may be at higher risk for drug interactions with antimycobacterial agents.[19]

TABLE 65-3   Dosages and Common Side Effects of Some Drugs Used in Tuberculosis (Adults)

Drug	Daily (Maximum)	3 Times Weekly DOT (Maximum)	2 Times Weekly DOT (Maximum)	Potential Side Effects and Comments
Isoniazid (INH)	5 mg/kg PO (300 mg)	15 mg/kg PO (900 mg)	15 mg/kg PO (900 mg)	Hepatitis, peripheral neuropathy, drug interactions
Rifampin (RIF)	10 mg/kg PO (600 mg)	10 mg/kg PO (600 mg)	10 mg/kg PO (600 mg)	Hepatitis, thrombocytopenia, GI disturbances, drug interactions
Rifabutin	5 mg/kg PO (300 mg)	5 mg/kg PO (300 mg)	5 mg/kg PO (300 mg)	Similar to RIF, used for patients who cannot tolerate RIF
Rifapentine (RPT)	ND	ND	10 mg/kg PO (600 mg) once per week	Similar to RIF, used with INH for once weekly continuation phase treatment
Ethambutol (EMB)	15–20 mg/kg PO (1.6 g)	25–30 mg/kg PO (2.4 g)	50 mg/kg PO (4 g)	Retrobulbar neuritis, peripheral neuropathy
Pyrazinamide (PZA)	15–30 mg/kg PO (2 g)	50–70 mg/kg PO (3 g)	50–70 mg/kg PO (4 g)	Hepatitis, arthralgia, hyperuricemia
Cycloserine	10–15 mg/kg per d PO divided bid	ND	ND	CNS disturbances, seizures, peripheral neuropathy
Ethionamide	10–15 mg/kg per d PO divided bid	ND	ND	Nausea, vomiting diarrhea, abdominal cramps, anorexia
Streptomycin	15 mg/kg IM (1 g)	15 mg/kg IM (1 g)	15 mg/kg IM (1 g)	Ototoxicity, nephrotoxicity
Capreomycin	15 mg/kg IM (1 g)	15 mg/kg IM (1 g)	15 mg/kg IM (1 g)	Nephrotoxicity, ototoxicity
Para-aminosalicylic acid	8–12 g per d, divided into two or three doses	ND	ND	GI disturbances, hypothyroidism, hepatitis
Levofloxacin	500–1000 mg per d PO	ND	ND	GI disturbances, dizziness, rash

Abbreviations: CNS = central nervous system; DOT = directly observed therapy; GI = gastrointestinal; ND = no data to support this dosing regimen.
Source: MMWR 52 (RR-11):4, July 20, 2003.

With the emergence of multidrug resistance, other treatment modalities have been used to treat infection that does not respond to antimycobacterial chemotherapy. Among them, surgical resection for MDR-TB is a treatment modality that has been shown to have good results, with cure rates of up to 90 percent.[10,14]

Treatment of latent infection with INH should be considered for patients with recent conversion to PPD-positive status, for persons who have been in close contact with an individual with active tuberculosis, and for anergic individuals with known tuberculosis contact.[6] The decision to institute therapy should be based on the likelihood that the positive PPD reaction represents true exposure to *M. tuberculosis,* the risk of progression to active disease, and the likelihood of INH-induced hepatitis. Therapy should continue for a minimum of 9 months for adults, children, and HIV-infected persons.[6] Those at risk for INH hepatotoxicity should be monitored closely for its development, if treatment is elected. For those exposed to INH-resistant strains or those who are intolerant to its use, rifampin and pyrazinamide for 2 months have been used with success.[6] However, careful monitoring for signs of liver failure are mandatory. Rifampin for 4 months is an alternative treatment.[6]

DISPOSITION

Admission

All hospitalized patients with suspected tuberculosis must be placed in respiratory isolation until the diagnosis is certain. Admission is important in cases in which the social situation makes it difficult to obtain a proper diagnosis and for therapy to be instituted. When a patient is proven to have active MDR-TB, hospital admission is also indicated to institute therapy and observe for drug toxicity. Other indications for admission include uncertain diagnosis or patient noncompliance. Physicians should be aware of local laws regarding involuntary hospitalization and treatment. However, less restrictive means, such as court-mandated DOT, are very effective and should be attempted before confinement.[20]

Outpatient Treatment

The vast majority of patients with tuberculosis can be treated initially as outpatients.[19] Emergency physicians should contact physicians or public health services providing long-term care before discharge. Discharge instructions include home isolation procedures and sites of medication (if DOT is used) and ongoing care. Antituberculosis medications should be instituted by health care professionals who will coordinate the treatment and monitor adverse effects of the medication. Such medications should not be routinely instituted in the emergency department without these measures.

PREVENTION

Prevention of tuberculosis transmission in health care facilities is extremely important. Guidelines for prevention of transmission have been published and are available through the CDC (www.cdc.gov). These recommendations include early detection and treatment of active cases, education and screening of health care workers, and engineering controls (Table 65-4).[15] Ambulatory care facilities that frequently see tuberculosis patients will need isolation rooms available. Personnel who work in emergency or ambulatory settings where patients with tuberculosis are treated should have routine PPD testing to detect occupational exposure and be offered appropriate treatment.[6,15]

TABLE 65-4   Engineering Controls to Reduce the Transmission of Tuberculosis

High airflow (at least six room air changes per hour) with external exhaust
High-efficiency particulate filters on ventilation system
Ultraviolet germicidal irradiation
Negative-pressure isolation rooms
Personal respiratory protection: high-efficiency particulate filter masks or respirators

REFERENCES

1. Small PM, Fujiwara PI: Management of tuberculosis in the United States. *New Engl J Med* 345:189, 2001.
2. Brudney K, Dobkin J: Resurgent tuberculosis in New York City. *Am Rev Respir Dis* 144:745, 1991.
3. Centers for Disease Control: Tuberculosis morbidity among U.S.-born and foreign-born populations-United States, 2000. *MMWR* 51:101, 2002.
4. Geng E, Kreiswirth B, Driver C, et al: Changes in the transmission of tuberculosis in New York City from 1990 to 1999. *New Engl J Med* 346:1453, 2002.
5. Rossman MD, MacGregor RR: *Tuberculosis.* New York, McGraw-Hill, 1995.
6. American Thoracic Society: Targeted tuberculin testing and treatment of latent tuberculosis infection. *Am J Respir Crit Care Med* 161:S221, 2000.
7. Condos R, Rom WN, Liu YK, Schluger NW: Local immune responses correlate with presentation and outcome in tuberculosis. *Am J Respir Crit Care Med* 157:729, 1998.
8. Maltezou HC, Spyridis P, Kafetzis DA: Extra-pulmonary tuberculosis in children. *Arch Dis Child* 83:342, 2000.
9. Havlir DV, Barnes, PF: Tuberculosis in patients with human immunodeficiency virus infection. *New Engl J Med* 340:367, 1999.
10. Iseman MD: Treatment of multidrug-resistant tuberculosis. *New Engl J Med* 329:784, 1993.
11. Narita M, Alonso P, Lauzardo M, et al: Treatment experience of multidrug-resistant tuberculosis in Florida, 1994-1997. *Chest* 120:343, 2001.
12. Nitta AT, Knowles KS, Kim J, et al: Limited transmission of multidrug-resistant tuberculosis despite a high proportion of infectious cases in Los Angeles County, California. *Am J Respir Crit Care Med* 165:812, 2002.
13. Ridzon R, Whitney CG, McKenna MT, et al: Risk factors for rifampin monoresistant tuberculosis. *Am J Respir Crit Care Med* 157:1881, 1998.
14. Tahaoglu K, Torun T, Sevim T, et al: The treatment of multidrug-resistant tuberculosis in Turkey. *New Engl J Med* 345:170, 2001.
15. Behrman AJ, Shofer FS: Tuberculosis exposure and control in an urban emergency department. *Ann Emerg Med* 31:370, 1998.
16. Slovis BS, Plitman JD, Haas DW: The case against anergy testing as a routine adjunct to tuberculin skin testing. *JAMA* 283:2003, 2000.
17. Gharib AM, Stern EJ: Radiology of pneumonia. *Med Clin North Am* 85:1461, 2001.
18. Van Soolingen D: Molecular epidemiology of tuberculosis and other mycobacterial infections: main methodologies and achievements. *J Intern Med* 249:1, 2001.
19. American Thoracic Society, CDC, and Infectious Diseases Society of America: Treatment of tuberculosis. *MMWR* 52 (RR-11):1, July 20, 2003.
20. Gasner MR, Maw KL, Feldman GE, et al: The use of legal action in New York City to ensure treatment of tuberculosis. *New Engl J Med* 340:359, 1999.

SPONTANEOUS AND IATROGENIC PNEUMOTHORAX
William Franklin Young, Jr.
Roger L. Humphries

Pneumothorax occurs when air enters the potential space between the visceral and parietal pleura as a consequence of blunt trauma, penetrating trauma, or spontaneous occurrence. Iatrogenic pneumothorax occurs secondary to a diagnostic or therapeutic procedure and is really a subset of penetrating traumatic pneumothorax. Primary spontaneous pneumothorax occurs in individuals without known lung disease and accounts for two-thirds of spontaneous pneumothoraces. Secondary spontaneous pneumothorax occurs in patients with underlying lung disease, especially chronic obstructive pulmonary disease. Emergency department evaluation and management of pneumothorax centers on immediate management of complications such as tension pneumothorax or ventilatory failure, and then on eliminating the intrapleural air and optimizing pleural healing.

SPONTANEOUS PNEUMOTHORAX

Epidemiology

An estimated 20,000 new spontaneous pneumothoraces occur each year in the United States, and there is evidence that the rate is increasing.[1,2] However, the true incidence of spontaneous pneumothorax is unknown, with estimates that up to 20 percent of such patients do not seek medical help.[3] Spontaneous pneumothorax is primarily a disease of male smokers who have greater height-to-weight ratios. Male sex carries a 6:1 relative risk as compared with the risk for females, although more recent studies show a trend to increased cases among women, perhaps because of smoking trends.[2] Smoking is an important risk factor, with an overall greater than 20:1 relative risk as compared with nonsmokers.[4] Spontaneous pneumothorax has three age-related occurrence peaks: among neonates (because of hyaline membrane disease or aspiration), among 20- to 40-year-olds (such cases tend to be primary), and among those older than age 40 years (typically secondary cases).[4] A genetic component is evidenced in the 11 percent of patients who have family members with spontaneous pneumothorax. Contrary to common belief, only 10 to 20 percent of cases occur with exertion. Spontaneous pneumothorax may rarely be associated with menses (catamenial).

Pathophysiology

The pleurae are serous membranes that surround each lung: the parietal pleura lines the thoracic wall and abuts the visceral pleura closely applied to the lung surface. At the hilum of each lung, the parietal and visceral pleurae meet in a continuous reflection around the hilar vessels and bronchus. The intrapleural space has subatmospheric pressure caused by the inherent tendency of the chest wall to expand and the lung to collapse from elastic recoil.

Primary spontaneous pneumothorax seems to result from rupture of a subpleural bleb, usually in an upper lobe.[5] These blebs are usually multiple and have increased wall tension, allowing distention and eventual rupture. The mechanism of bleb formation remains unknown, but higher upper lobe transpulmonary pressure, local ischemia from decreased upper lobe blood flow, and subclinical emphysema-like changes have been postulated.[3,5]

Chronic obstructive pulmonary disease (COPD) accounts for most cases of secondary spontaneous pneumothorax. Other causes include cystic fibrosis, pulmonary infections, interstitial lung disease, AIDS, neoplasms, and drug use. Pneumothorax occurs in 5 percent of AIDS patients, is associated with subpleural necrosis from *Pneumocystis* infection, and carries a high mortality.[6] Because of necrosis of lung tissue and continued air leak, simple aspiration and nondrainage techniques fail in this group of patients.

Regardless of the inciting event, once there is a break in the pleura, air travels down a pressure gradient into the intrapleural space until pressure equilibrium occurs with partial or total lung collapse. Altered ventilation perfusion relationships and decreased vital capacity then contribute to dyspnea and hypoxemia.

Clinical Features

Symptoms are related to the size of the pneumothorax, rate of development, and underlying clinical status of the patient. Patients with mild symptoms may not come for evaluation, whereas those with underlying lung disease may arrive in extremis. Patients with secondary spontaneous pneumothoraces present more dramatically than those with primary pneumothoraces. Tension pneumothorax is rare in either primary or secondary spontaneous pneumothorax. Pneumothorax is an important differential diagnosis in patients with chest pain, because it can mimic ischemia causing ST changes and T-wave inversion on the electrocardiogram (ECG).[3]

Acute pleuritic chest pain occurs in 95 percent of patients and localizes to the side of the pneumothorax in >90 percent of cases. Dyspnea occurs in 80 percent of patients, and predicts a larger pneumothorax. Patients with COPD who develop a spontaneous pneumothorax may acutely decompensate, with 1 to 17 percent mortality. Decreased breath sounds occur over the affected lung 85 percent of the time, but only 5 percent have tachypnea of more than 24 breaths/min or tachycardia of more than 120 beats/min. Hyperresonance occurs in fewer than one-third. Tracheal deviation and hemodynamic compromise are the hallmarks of tension pneumothorax that demand immediate treatment.

Diagnosis

Tension pneumothorax diagnosed on clinical grounds requires immediate treatment by needle decompression and expeditious chest tube thoracostomy before radiographic evaluation. The traditional "gold standard" for diagnosis of pneumothorax continues to be the 6-foot upright posteroanterior chest radiograph, although the sensitivity of this examination is 83 percent.[7] The radiographic hallmark of a pneumothorax is visualization of the visceral pleural line with an overlying radiolucent area without vascular or lung markings between the visceral pleural line and chest wall. Pseudo-pneumothorax caused by a skin fold, scapular border, or tubing, is differentiated from true pneumothorax by looking for vascular markings inside the confines of the radiolucent area and the blending of these lines into the chest wall, rather than following the borders of a collapsed lung. Large bullae have been mistaken for pneumothoraces, but bullae and cysts have concave inner margins and rounded edges. Pneumothorax is much more difficult to detect on a supine anteroposterior radiograph. On the anteroposterior view, a deep sulcus sign, representing a deep lateral costophrenic angle, sometimes is a clue to a pneumothorax.[7]

Expiratory radiographs by themselves are no more sensitive than inspiratory films and provide inferior evaluation of lung parenchyma.[7] In approximately 5 percent of patients, a pneumothorax is better visualized on the expiratory view than on the inspiratory view.[7] Comparison of paired inspiratory and expiratory films may be more sensitive than either view alone.[8]

Chest computed tomography (CT) may be more sensitive than plain radiographs in detection of pneumothorax and may be helpful in equivocal cases, but most studies comparing supine chest x-ray (CXR) film with chest CT have been in the setting of trauma.

Ultrasonography, although portable and easy to perform, has traditionally been considered an imaging modality incapable of adequately visualizing the lung parenchyma and therefore of little use in the detection of pneumothorax. Ultrasound waves do not transmit well through air and this is a common cause of sonographic artifact and poor quality ultrasonographic imaging in any application. However, European experience with ultrasonography has found this technique capable of detecting pneumothorax after ultrasound-guided pleural or lung biopsy and pneumothorax associated with ventilatory-induced barotrauma with a sensitivity approaching 100 percent.[9] Ultrasonography has been used to detect traumatic pneumothorax, also with a sensitivity approaching 100 percent.[10] Sonographic signs of a pneumothorax include (1) absence of lung sliding as assessed on the time-motion view (the normal granulous pattern is replaced by multiple horizontal artifact lines termed "A-lines"); (2) the demonstration of a "lung point" on the time-motion view, in which, during inspiration, at one transducer position, the normal granulous pattern of the lung in contact with the chest wall, is replaced by the multiple horizontal artifact lines as the lung collapses away from the chest wall; and (3) absence of vertical comet-tail artifacts arising from the pleural line on a B-mode two-dimensional view.[9] As with any ultrasonographic application, the technical ability of the operator and the quality of the interpretation determines the clinical utility of this imaging modality.

Spontaneous pneumothorax should be included in the differential diagnosis of acute chest pain or acute deterioration in a patient with COPD. ST-segment and T-wave changes may be mistaken for ischemia. Occasionally, severe bullous COPD may mimic pneumothorax, and careful review of the CXR is needed with confirmatory CT, if the patient is stable. A thoracostomy with the chest tube inserted into a bulla mistaken for a pneumothorax results in a large pneumothorax, associated bronchopulmonary fistula, and its complications.[3]

The size of the pneumothorax may be calculated, and some physicians use size as a guide to therapy. Radiologist "best guess" estimates show substantial interobserver disagreement and lack of reproducibility. Most published formulae show only a modest correlation to actual pneumothorax size (R = 0.7).[11,12] Chest CT volume measurements represent the current "gold standard," but the patient's clinical status more than the pneumothorax size, should determine treatment options. A more pragmatic approach is to classify pneumothorax size as small (<3 cm apex to cupola) or large (≥3 cm apex to cupola).[13]

Treatment

Treatment goals are the elimination of intrapleural air, optimization of pleural healing, and prevention of recurrences. There is marked practice variation, but attempts at consensus have been made with varying degrees of application.[13–15] Observation, oxygen, catheter aspiration (either single or sequential), tube thoracostomy (either minicatheter or standard chest tube), pleurodesis, video-assisted thorascopy (VAT), and thoracotomy are all options, but only the latter three procedures reduce the risk of future pneumothorax recurrence.

Because 1.25 percent of intrapleural air is reabsorbed each day, stable patients with a small primary spontaneous pneumothorax may be observed for 3 to 6 h. Concomitant oxygen administration at 3 to 4 L/min increases pleural air resorption three- to fourfold and should be used.[1] If a repeat chest radiograph shows no increase in pneumothorax size, the patient can be discharged with instructions to return if symptoms develop or worsen. A repeat chest radiograph in 12 to 48 h is recommended. Extended outpatient observation is sometimes needed because a 25 percent pneumothorax would take approximately 20 days to resolve. Critics of this treatment plan point to the 23 to 40 percent of patients treated by observation who eventually require tube thoracostomy.[1] Observation may also be a reasonable approach for those patients with a contraindication to invasive therapy, such as coagulopathy.

Catheter aspiration is underused for treatment of spontaneous pneumothorax and may be as effective as chest tube thoracostomy in primary spontaneous pneumothorax.[16] Multiple techniques, equipment, and protocols are described, making a consensus statement difficult. Success rates from 37 to 75 percent are described with the greater success seen in primary spontaneous pneumothoraces.[1] Techniques include simple one-time aspiration with small plastic 16- to 18-gauge intravenous catheters, repeated aspirations through the same catheter, and small-caliber chest tube with aspiration. Minicatheter tube placement uses a specially designed catheter with multiple side ports, eliminating the problem of single-lumen obstruction seen with intravenous catheters. The technique involves placing a small catheter either into the second anterior intercostal space in the midclavicular line or laterally at the fourth or fifth intercostal space in the anterior axillary line after local anesthesia and sterile preparation. A three-way stopcock is applied, and a 60-mL syringe is used to aspirate the pleural space until resistance is met and the patient coughs. The stopcock is closed, the tube is secured, and a chest radiograph is obtained to assure reexpansion. Aspiration of more than 4 L suggests continued air leak and failure of simple aspiration. Failure to fully expand warrants another aspiration attempt, addition of a Heimlich valve, or formal tube thoracostomy. If the procedure is successful, patients should be observed for 6 h and, if no recurrence is seen, the catheter is removed and the patient discharged with close follow-up within 24 h.

Standard chest tube thoracostomy with underwater seal drainage is the most commonly used therapy and remains the standard in many hospitals. Proponents point to a low complication rate and a high success rate of 95 percent.[17] If there is a low risk of air leak, a small <14 Fr tube suffices, otherwise use a 24 to 28 Fr tube with water seal (no suction).[18] Patients with secondary spontaneous pneumothorax, those with recurrent pneumothorax, and those with abnormal vital signs should have chest tube thoracostomy.

Short-term complications of spontaneous pneumothorax include tension pneumothorax, failure to reexpand, persistent air leak, and complications related to the removal of intrapleural air, such as infection, technical errors, and reexpansion pulmonary edema. Reexpansion pulmonary edema is multifactorial, poorly studied, and more often seen in younger patients aged 20 to 39 years, with larger pneumothoraces present for >72 h, rapidly expanded with suction.[18] Pulmonary edema generally occurs on the side of the reexpanded lung. Treatment is supportive and mirrors that for noncardiogenic pulmonary edema.

Disposition

After successful treatment of a spontaneous pneumothorax, referral and consultation regarding potential definitive management with pleurodesis with or without VAT or thoracotomy should be done. Some authors recommend thorascopic surgery for the first spontaneous pneumothorax because of the relatively high rate of pneumothorax recurrence, lower overall cost, success rate of the procedure, and better long-term quality of life.[19] However, the procedure is not risk free, is invasive, and recurrence after VAT requires open thoracotomy with pleurectomy or pleural scarification. Most guidelines recommend definitive treatment only after second recurrence.

Recurrence of pneumothorax is the major long-term complication and the reason that all patients with spontaneous pneumothorax require referral for potential definitive therapy. Primary spontaneous pneumothorax recurs in approximately 20 to 30 percent of patients and is independent of the method chosen to remove the intrapleural air.[20] Almost all recurrences occur within 2 years.[20] Smoking cessation reduces this risk by half.[2] Secondary spontaneous pneumothorax recurs in 40 to 50 percent of patients.

IATROGENIC PNEUMOTHORAX

Iatrogenic pneumothorax occurs more often than spontaneous pneumothorax and is a subset of traumatic penetrating pneumothorax. Transthoracic needle procedures (transthoracic needle biopsy and thoracentesis) account for approximately half and subclavian vein catheterization accounts for a fourth of iatrogenic pneumothoraces. Given that one central venous line is placed every minute in the United States, and that pneumothorax occurs after 2 to 6 percent of subclavian line attempts, iatrogenic pneumothorax must be common.[21] Some of the factors increasing the frequency of iatrogenic pneumothorax include the patient population, underlying disease, body habitus, and experience of the operator. Ultrasound guidance for thoracentesis significantly reduces the pneumothorax complication rate and appears promising for reducing the incidence of pneumothorax with central venous line placement.

Chest radiograph is standard after central line placement or transthoracic needle procedures, but may miss an iatrogenic pneumothorax because of the use of a supine technique or inadequate time for the pneumothorax to develop. Delayed pneumothoraces are common after subclavian line placement; up to a third are not seen on the initial postprocedural chest radiograph.[21]

Treatment for iatrogenic pneumothorax parallels that for spontaneous pneumothorax, with some important caveats. Patients with res-

piratory distress or on mechanical ventilation require large-bore tube thoracostomy. Conversely, patients sustaining a small pneumothorax after a needle puncture and not receiving positive pressure ventilation can be initially treated with simple catheter aspiration with or without a Heimlich valve, which will be adequate in 60 to 80 percent of patients.[21] Stable patients with a small pneumothorax can be observed and selected patients can be followed as outpatients.[21] Because prolonged air leak may occur in some patients, usually after pleural or lung biopsy-induced pneumothorax or difficult subclavian vein catheterization attempt, hospitalization is recommended in these patients. Long-term recurrence is not an issue with iatrogenic pneumothorax.

REFERENCES

1. Baumann MH, Strange C: Treatment of spontaneous pneumothorax: A more aggressive approach? *Chest* 112:789, 1997.
2. Sadikot RT, Greene T, Meadows K, Arnold AG: Recurrence of spontaneous pneumothorax. *Thorax* 52:805, 1997.
3. Kirby TJ, Ginsberg RJ: Management of the pneumothorax and barotrauma. *Clin Chest Med* 13:97, 1992.
4. Schramel FM, Postmus PE, Vanerschueren RG: Current aspects of spontaneous pneumothorax. *Eur Respir J* 10:1372, 1997.
5. Baumann MH, Strange C: The clinician's perspective on pneumothorax management. *Chest* 112:822, 1997.
6. Light RW, Hamm H: Pleural disease and acquired immune deficiency syndrome. *Eur Respir J* 10:2638, 1997.
7. Seow A, Kazerooni EA, Pernicano PG, Neary M: Comparison of upright inspiratory and expiratory chest radiographs for detecting pneumothoraces. *AJR Am J Roentgenol* 166:313, 1996.
8. Aitchison F, Bleetman A, Munro P, et al: Detection of pneumothorax by accident and emergency officers and radiologists on single chest film. *Arch Emerg Med* 10:343, 1993.
9. Lichtenstein DA: Lung ultrasound in the intensive care unit. *Recent Res Devel Resp Crit Care Med* 1:83, 2001.
10. Rowan KR, Kirkpatrick AW, Liu D, et al: Traumatic pneumothorax detection with thoracic US: Correlation with chest radiography and CT—Initial experience. *Radiology* 225:210, 2002.
11. Collins CD, Lopez A, Mathie A, et al: Quantification of pneumothorax size on chest radiographs using interpleural distances: Regression analysis based on volume measurements from helical CT. *AJR* 165:1127, 1995.
12. Choi BG, Park SH, Yun EH, et al: Pneumothorax size: Correlation of supine anteroposterior with erect posteroanterior chest radiographs. *Radiology* 209:567, 1998.
13. Baumann MH, Strange C, Heffner JE, et al: Management of spontaneous pneumothorax: An American College of Chest Physicians Delphi consensus statement. *Chest* 119:590, 2001.
14. Miller AC, Harvey JE: Guidelines for the management of spontaneous pneumothorax. Standards of Care Committee, British Thoracic Society. *BMJ* 307:114, 1993.
15. Mendis D, El-Shanawany A, Mathur, et al: Management of spontaneous pneumothorax: Are British Thoracic Society guidelines being followed? *Postgrad Med J* 78:80, 2002.
16. Noppen M, Alexander P, Driesen P: Manual aspiration versus chest tube drainage in first episodes of primary spontaneous pneumothorax. *Am J Respir Crit Care Med* 165:1240, 2002.
17. Light RW: Management of spontaneous pneumothorax. *Am Rev Respir Dis* 148:245, 1993.
18. Karnik AM. Management of pneumothorax and barotrauma: Current concepts. *Compr Ther* 27:311, 2001.
19. Morimoto T, Fukui T, Kayama H, et al: Optimal strategy for the first episode of primary spontaneous pneumothorax in young men. *J Gen Intern Med* 17:193, 2002.
20. Vernejoux J-M, Raherison C, Combe P, et al: Spontaneous pneumothorax: Pragmatic management and long-term outcome. *Respir Med* 95:857, 2001.
21. Laronga C, Meric F, Truong MT, et al: A treatment algorithm for pneumothoraces complicating central venous catheter insertion. *Am J Surg* 180:523, 2000.

HEMOPTYSIS
William Franklin Young, Jr.
Michael Stava

Hemoptysis is expectoration of blood from the respiratory tract below the level of the larynx. The causes of hemoptysis vary from simple bronchitis to life-threatening pulmonary embolism.[1] Most causes are not life-threatening, but the symptoms are quite frightening to patients and cause them to seek emergent evaluation. Even with careful evaluation, a cause is not identified in up to 25 percent. Priorities in the evaluation of hemoptysis are: (1) ensuring adequate oxygenation and ventilation, (2) confirming a pulmonary source of bleeding, (3) attempting to identify the cause of hemoptysis through appropriate diagnostic evaluation, and (4) appropriate disposition.

EPIDEMIOLOGY

The true incidence of hemoptysis is unknown because many cases are unreported. Before the 1960s, most cases of hemoptysis were caused by tuberculosis, followed by bronchiectasis and lung neoplasia. With the introduction of antibiotics and the increases in cigarette smoking, bronchitis and lung neoplasia have become more common. A retrospective meta-analysis of six prior studies of hemoptysis found an infectious nontubercular cause in approximately 25 percent of hemoptysis cases, tuberculosis caused approximately 5 percent, neoplasia accounted for 28 percent, and miscellaneous and multiple causes accounted for 13 percent.[2] Of note, 28 percent of hemoptysis cases had an undetermined cause, often referred to as *cryptogenic hemoptysis.* These percentages vary according to patient demographics and location.[3–6] Cardiovascular causes account for 3 percent of total hemoptysis cases, of which three of four are congestive heart failure. Trauma accounts for fewer than 3 percent of hemoptysis cases. In summary, for industrialized countries, of every four cases of hemoptysis, expect about one neoplasm, one nontubercular infectious case, one miscellaneous case, and one idiopathic case.

Hemoptysis has a 60:40 male predominance, and occurs in all age groups. Lifestyle activities such as smoking predispose patients to lung disease and an increased risk of hemoptysis. Male gender, age older than 40 years, and history of smoking are risk factors for a neoplastic cause of hemoptysis.[2] Hemoptysis in children is rare and most often due to cystic fibrosis, congenital heart disease, infection (pneumonia, tracheobronchitis), and tracheostomy complications.[7]

PATHOPHYSIOLOGY

The causes of hemoptysis are numerous (Table 67-1). The lung has a dual blood supply consisting of the bronchial and the pulmonary vessels, and bleeding may occur from either or both. The bronchial vessels are under systemic circulatory pressure and supply the supporting structures of the lung, and the pulmonary vessels are under low pressure and supply the alveoli. Bleeding from either source may occur by three mechanisms: pulmonary hypertension, erosion into a pulmonary or bronchial blood vessel, and as a complication of a bleeding diathesis. Hemoptysis arising from increases in pulmonary vascular pressure most often results from primary cardiac abnormalities, such left-sided congestive heart failure (comprising 75 percent of cardiac cases) or mitral stenosis.

Infectious causes include bronchitis, pneumonia, lung abscesses, and fungal infections. Inflammatory causes include bronchiectasis and cystic fibrosis. Malignant lesions producing hemoptysis can be primary lung neoplasms or metastatic tumors. Although classically associated with pulmonary embolism, hemoptysis is seen in only 3 to 20 percent of cases. Hemoptysis from vasculitis is usually alveolar in location and part of a larger systemic vasculopathy, such as systemic lupus erythematosus, Wegener granulomatosus, polyarteritis, or Goodpasture syndrome.

TABLE 67-1 Common Causes of Hemoptysis

Infectious: bronchitis, pneumonia, lung abscess, tuberculosis
Neoplastic: lung cancer, bronchial adenoma
Cardiovascular: pulmonary embolism, mitral stenosis, congestive heart failure, pulmonary hypertension, pulmonary angiodysplasia
Alveolar hemorrhage syndromes: Beçhet syndrome, Goodpasture syndrome, Wegener granulomatosus
Hematologic: uremia, platelet dysfunction, anticoagulant therapy
Traumatic: foreign body aspiration, ruptured bronchus, arteriotracheobronchial fistula (aortic aneurysm)
Iatrogenic: bronchoscopy, lung biopsy
Inflammatory: bronchiectasis, cystic fibrosis

Hemophilia, thrombocytopenia, inherited coagulopathy, and iatrogenic use of anticoagulants and thrombolytics may cause hemoptysis. Thrombolytic-induced hemoptysis occurs in fewer than 1 percent of patients receiving thrombolysis and is usually self-limited.[8]

The erosion of bronchial vessels under systemic circulatory pressures from tuberculosis or bronchiectasis can produce severe hemoptysis[8] (Table 67-2). Severe hemorrhage from the pulmonary circulation can occur from mycetomas, lung abscess, and cavitary lung cancer.

CLINICAL FEATURES

Hemoptysis may be defined as mild, moderate, or severe. Mild hemoptysis is usually defined as less than 20 mL of blood in 24 h, moderate hemoptysis is defined as 20 to 600 mL in 24 h, and severe or massive hemoptysis is defined as more than 600 mL in 24 h.[1] Often patients are unable to accurately estimate the degree of bleeding. The exact amount of hemoptysis required for each categorization is arbitrary, not evidence based, does not predict mortality (except in the severe category), and involves longer time frames than seen in the emergency department. A reasonable categorization for the ED might include scant or blood-streaked sputum, frank hemoptysis, and massive hemoptysis interfering with respiration.

A careful history and physical examination have only moderate roles in identifying a specific etiology.[9] An abrupt onset of cough with bloody purulent sputum, with or without fever, may indicate acute pneumonia or bronchitis. Hemoptysis is an insensitive marker for pulmonary embolism, and pulmonary infarction secondary to pulmonary embolism causing hemoptysis is often overshadowed by anxiety, dyspnea, and chest pain. A chronic productive cough may reflect chronic bronchitis or bronchiectasis. Fevers, night sweats, and weight loss suggest tubercular infection. Chronic weight loss and change in cough may reflect bronchogenic carcinoma. About 80 percent of neoplasm-caused hemoptysis lasts longer than 1 week. Alveolar hemorrhage syndromes from vasculitis present with dyspnea and mild hemoptysis associated with renal disease and hematuria.

Physical examination is useful in determining the severity of hemoptysis but is unreliable in localizing the site of bleeding.[9] Fever usually indicates infection. Tachypnea may reflect respiratory compromise with hypoxemia from intrapulmonary blood interfering with gas exchange or from underlying lung disease with altered ventilation and perfusion. Blood pressure usually is not changed, except in massive hemoptysis. The nasal cavity and oropharynx should be carefully examined for extrapulmonary causes of expectorated blood (pseudohemoptysis) and signs

TABLE 67-2 Common Causes of Massive Hemoptysis

Bronchiectasis
Tuberculosis
Lung cancer (typically cavitary)
Lung abscess
Arteriotracheobronchial fistula (e.g., aortic aneurysm)
Pulmonary angiodysplasia

of extrapulmonary vasculitis.[10] The cardiac examination may show valvular heart disease (e.g., the diastolic murmur of mitral stenosis). The pulmonary examination may show fine inspiratory crackles associated with alveolar blood or inspiratory and expiratory crackles associated with airway secretions and blood. There may be wheezing from bronchial narrowing. Digital clubbing should be assessed as a sign of chronic lung disease. Muscle wasting or adenopathy may indicate neoplasia.

DIAGNOSTIC EVALUATION

Diagnostic evaluation should first center on the patient's respiratory stability with the assurance of adequate oxygenation and ventilation. Massive hemoptysis requires immediate intervention with supplemental oxygen, intravenous access, typed and cross-matched blood, and urgent consultation with a pulmonologist or thoracic surgeon.[8] Airway control might necessitate intubation. Patients who are stable should have their sputum evaluated for the degree of hemoptysis and to differentiate true hemoptysis from pseudohemoptysis due to a nasopharyngeal or gastrointestinal source. True hemoptysis often displays a bright red color, frothy appearance, alkaline pH, and the presence of macrophages. Gastrointestinal blood typically is acidic and dark red, although swallowed epistaxis may have similar characteristics. Approximately 10 percent of patients with apparent hemoptysis are identified as having bleeding due to lesions of the upper aerodigestive tract.[10]

It is generally agreed that all patients with true hemoptysis require radiographic imaging, starting with a chest radiograph.[1,2,9] Approximately 80 to 90 percent of individuals with neoplasm as a cause of hemoptysis have an abnormal chest radiograph. Overall, 15 to 30 percent of patients presenting with hemoptysis have a normal chest radiograph, most of whom have hemoptysis from nonspecific bronchitis.[11] After chest radiography, further diagnostic options include computed tomography (CT) and bronchoscopy.

Bronchoscopy allows for direct visualization of the more central airways, is better at identifying luminal lesions such as tumors or areas of inflammation, allows for any required biopsy specimens to be obtained, and facilitates placement of selective lung ventilation devices.[1,12] Patients unstable due to airway obstruction from massive hemoptysis have traditionally undergone rigid bronchoscopy to evacuate clots and determine the source of bleeding. In stable patients with less bleeding, fiberoptic bronchoscopy is generally done.[13] Although early fiberoptic bronchoscopy has not been shown to appreciably affect the clinical outcome, many researchers recommend this study for individuals with hemoptysis and a normal or nonlocalizing chest x-ray. Because bronchoscopy is an invasive procedure, it carries a higher rate of complications as compared with CT.

Chest CT is noninvasive, more readily available on an urgent basis, more effectively delineates abnormalities in the peripheral airways, and has greater sensitivity in detecting bronchiectasis and nodular lesions such as carcinomas.[2,14] Limited data suggest that CT is more efficient than bronchoscopy at identifying the cause of bleeding in patients with large or massive hemoptysis.[15] Often, CT and bronchoscopy are performed in the evaluation of hemoptysis, especially in the high-risk patient presenting with hemoptysis, i.e., one who is male, older than 40 years, and has a history of tobacco use.[2] Close consultation with the follow-up physician is important to determine individual physician preference and to coordinate the timing of these evaluations. In general, patients with hemoptysis and an abnormal chest radiograph require an emergency department chest CT (Figure 67-1).

The laboratory evaluation should be guided by clinical suspicion and might include complete blood cell count, coagulation studies, blood gas analysis, sputum stains and cultures, and evaluation of renal function.

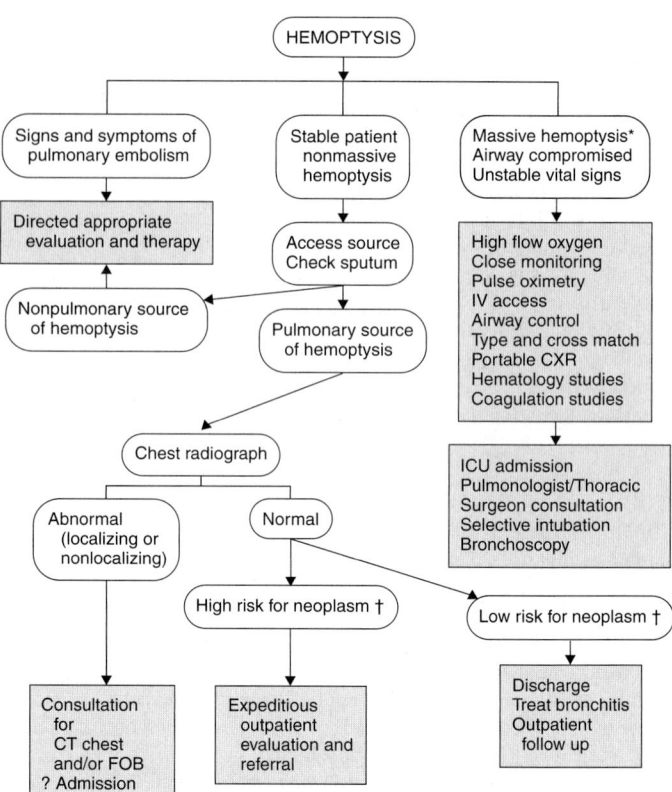

FIG. 67-1. Evaluation of hemoptysis.
†High risk for neoplasm: male, age >40 y, smoking history.

TREATMENT

Treatment in the ED depends on the severity of the hemoptysis. All patients with moderate or severe hemoptysis will require admission and should have intravenous access established, supplemental oxygen provided, laboratory testing initiated and type and cross for potential blood transfusion done.[1,8]

Patients with ongoing massive hemoptysis are commonly positioned with the bleeding lung down, to minimize soiling of the contralateral normal lung. This belief is theoretical, not based on clinical studies, and a prone head-down position has been advocated as promoting better ventilation and perfusion matching in such patients.[8,16] Tracheal intubation with a large-diameter endotracheal tube (8 mm or larger to allow for bronchoscopy) is indicated if there is respiratory failure or if the patient is unable to clear blood from the airways. If bleeding persists despite initial measures, an endotracheal tube may be advanced to the mainstem bronchus of the nonbleeding lung to minimize further aspiration of blood and provide ventilation.[8] The right mainstem bronchus is easily entered by advancing a standard orotracheal tube. Inserting the tube will occlude the right upper lobe tertiary bronchus and ventilate the right middle and right lower lobes only. The left mainstem bronchus is more sharply angled from the trachea, and selective intubation usually requires special equipment and technique. Double-lumen endotracheal tubes usually require fiberoptic bronchoscopy for placement, and their small lumen diameters limit suctioning and airway clearance. Recently, a technique for blind insertion of a 37-French double-lumen endotracheal tube has been described in patients undergoing elective thoracic surgery, with the implication that this technique may be useful in emergency situations.[17] However, there is no published experience with the use of this technique in patients with massive hemoptysis. After intubation, mechanical ventilation should be instituted, as necessary, to support ventilation.

Fresh-frozen plasma and/or platelet concentrates should be administered to correct identified coagulopathies. Tranexamic acid has been recommended based on anecdotal reports, but a recent randomized double-blinded, placebo-controlled trial found no benefit in reducing days of bleeding.[18] Cough suppression with codeine or opioids might be helpful to prevent dislodging of hemostatic clots.

Emergency consultation is needed with a pulmonologist and thoracic surgeon for patients with massive hemoptysis to facilitate bronchoscopy or bronchial artery angiography to localize the specific bleeding site.[8,13] Approximately 90 percent of massive hemoptysis cases originate from the bronchial circulation, and catheter-directed bronchial artery embolization has proven very effective in controlling the hemorrhage.[19] For patients with massive hemoptysis from localized lesions who continue to bleed despite medical treatment, surgical resection should be considered.[20] Massive hemoptysis is less common in children, but similar evaluation and management are appropriate.

PATIENT DISPOSITION

Patients with continuing moderate or severe hemoptysis require admission, often to an intensive care unit.[13] Patients with massive hemoptysis that has subsided are at high risk for recurrence and require similar intensive management and hospital admission, usually to an intensive care unit. Overall, the in-hospital mortality for patients with massive hemoptysis is about 20 to 25 percent.[20] Patients with certain disease processes also will require admission (congestive heart failure, pulmonary embolus), even if hemoptysis is mild. If appropriate specialists are not available, medical stabilization is essential before considering transfer to a hospital that provides such services.

Patients with minor hemoptysis due to bronchitis should be treated for the underlying disease, as appropriate. In those patients with mild hemoptysis, an abnormal chest radiograph, and a benign CT scan, disposition should be decided in close consultation with a pulmonary care specialist. Further evaluation of patients with a normal chest radiograph is important, because of the 5 to 20 percent risk for occult neoplasms of the lungs, trachea, or pharynx, and these patients should be directed to close follow-up with their primary care physician or a pulmonary specialist.[11,21]

REFERENCES

1. Lenner RA, Schilero GJ, Lesser M: Hemoptysis: Diagnosis and management. *Compr Ther* 28:7, 2002.
2. Marshall TJ, Flower CDR, Jackson JE: Review—The role of radiology in the investigation and management of patients with haemoptysis. *Clin Radiol* 51:391, 1996.
3. Haro Estarriol M, Vizcaya Sanches M, Jimenez Lopez J, Tornero Molina A: Etiology of hemoptysis: Prospective analysis of 752 cases. *Rev Clin Esp* 201:696, 2001.
4. Abal AT, Nair PC, Cherian J: Haemoptysis: Aetiology, evaluation and outcome—A prospective study in a third-world country. *Respir Med* 95:548, 2001.
5. Boulay F, Berthier F, Sisteron O, et al: Season variation in cryptogenic and noncryptogenic hemoptysis hospitalizations in France. *Chest* 118:440, 2000.
6. Fidan A, Ozdogan S, Oruc O, et al: Hemoptysis: A retrospective analysis of 108 cases. *Respir Med* 96:677, 2002.
7. Coss-Bu JA, Sachdeva RC, Bricker JT, et al: Hemoptysis: A 10-year retrospective study. *Pediatrics* 100:E7, 1997.
8. Jean-Baptiste E: Clinical assessment and management of massive hemoptysis. *Crit Care Med* 28:1642, 2000.
9. Haro Estarriol M, Vizcaya Sanchez M, Rubio Goday M, et al: Utility of the clinical history, physical examination and radiography in the localization of bleeding in patients with hemoptysis. *An Med Interna* 19:289, 2002.
10. DiLeo MD, Amedee RG, Butcher RB: Hemoptysis and pseudohemoptysis: The patient expectorating blood. *Ear Nose Throat J* 74:822, 1995.
11. Kaminski J: Frequency and causes of hemoptysis and role of bronchoscopy in patients with normal chest roentgenogram hospitalized in the Department of Physiopneumonology Silesian Medical University in the years 1961–1996. *Pneumonol Alergol Pol* 69:663, 2001.
12. Karmy-Jones R, Cuschieri J, Vallieres E: Role of bronchoscopy in massive hemoptysis. *Chest Surg Clin North Am* 11:873, 2001.
13. Haponik EF, Fein A, Chin R: Managing life-threatening hemoptysis: Has anything really changed? *Chest* 118:1431, 2000.
14. Tak S, Ahluealia G, Sharma SK, et al: Haemoptysis in patients with a normal chest radiograph: Bronchoscopy–CT correlation. *Australas Radiol* 43: 451, 1999.
15. Revel MP, Fournier LS, Hennebicque AS, et al: Can CT replace bronchoscopy in the detection of the site and cause of bleeding in patients with large or massive hemoptysis? *AJR* 179:1217, 2002.
16. Savage R: Prone, head down for pulmonary hemorrhage. *Br J Anaesth* 89:185, 2002.
17. Bahk JH, Lim YJ, Kim CS: Positioning of a double-lumen endobronchial tube without the aid of any instruments: An implication for emergency management. *J Trauma* 49:899, 2000.
18. Tscheikuna J, Chvaychoo B, Naruman C, Maranetra N: Tranexamic acid in patients with hemoptysis. *J Med Assoc Thai* 85:399, 2002.
19. Yoon W, Kim JK, Kim YH, et al: Bronchial and nonbronchial systemic artery embolization for life-threatening hemoptysis: A comprehensive review. *Radiographics* 22:1395, 2002.
20. Jougon J, Ballester M, Delcambre F, et al: Massive hemoptysis: What place for medical and surgical treatment. *Eur J Cardiothorac Surg* 22:345, 2002.
21. Herth F, Ernst A, Becker HD: Long-term outcome and lung cancer incidence in patients with hemoptysis of unknown origin. *Chest* 120:1592, 2001.

ACUTE ASTHMA IN ADULTS
Rita K. Cydulka

Asthma is a chronic inflammatory disorder characterized by increased responsiveness of the airways to multiple stimuli. Many cells and cellular elements, such as mast cells, eosinophils, T lymphocytes, macrophages, neutrophils, and epithelial cells, play a role in the development of the inflammatory response. In susceptible individuals, the inflammation causes recurrent episodes of wheezing, breathlessness, chest tightness, and coughing, particularly at night or in the early morning. These episodes usually are associated with widespread, but variable, airflow obstruction that is often reversible spontaneously or with treatment.

Most acute attacks are reversible and improve spontaneously or within minutes to hours with treatment. Although patients appear to recover completely clinically, evidence suggests that asthmatic patients develop chronic airflow limitation. The recognition that asthma is a chronic inflammatory disorder of the airways has significant implications for the diagnosis, management, and potential prevention of its acute exacerbation.

EPIDEMIOLOGY

Asthma affects approximately 4 to 5 percent of the population in the United States.[1] It is the most common chronic disease of childhood, with a prevalence of 5 to 10 percent. On the other end of the spectrum, asthma affects 7 to 10 percent of the elderly, accounting for 68,000 admissions to hospitals in 1991.[2] About one-half of cases of asthma develop before the age of 10 years and another one-third before the age of 40 years. The 2:1 male-to-female preponderance of asthma in childhood equalizes by age 30 years. Self-reported prevalence rates for asthma in the United States increased by 74 percent from 1980 to 1996.[1] Similar prevalence rates are reported in developed nations throughout the world. From 1980 to 1999, the estimated annual number of office visits for asthma in the United States increased by 83 percent, from 5.9 million to 10.4 million. Whereas the number of ED visits increased by 36 percent (from 1.5 million to 2 million) between 1992 and 1999, the number of hospitalizations and deaths seems to have declined since 1995.[1] In the United States alone, the estimated direct and indirect costs of asthma in all age groups was 6.2 billion dollars in 1990.[3]

PATHOPHYSIOLOGY

Asthma is characterized by inflammation of the airways, with an abnormal accumulation of eosinophils, lymphocytes, mast cells, macrophages, dendritic cells, and myofibroblasts. The pathophysiologic hallmark of asthma is a reduction in airway diameter caused by smooth muscle contraction, vascular congestion, bronchial wall edema, and thick secretions. These changes are reflected in pulmonary function changes, increased work of breathing, and abnormal distribution of pulmonary blood flow (Table 68-1). Large and small airways often contain plugs composed of mucus, serum proteins, inflammatory cells, and cellular debris. On a microscopic level, airways are infiltrated with eosinophils and mononuclear cells. Evidence of microvascular leakage, epithelial disruption, and vasodilation is frequently noted. The airway smooth muscle is hypertrophied and characterized by new vessel formation, an increased number of epithelial goblet cells, and deposition of interstitial collagen beneath the epithelium. Subepithelial fibrosis, an increase in the thickness of the reticular layer of the basement membrane, is characteristically increased in the large and small airways. Data collected from transbronchial biopsy, alveolar lavage, and specialized airway imaging techniques suggest that inflammation affects all bronchial pulmonary structures.

Current hypothesis states that airway inflammation may be acute, subacute, or chronic. The acute response is determined by early recruitment of cells to the airway. Antigens come in contact with mast cells in the submucosa and cause elaboration of mediators, such as histamine, leukotrienes (including leukotriene B4), chemokines, tryptase, interleukin 5, interleukin 8, proinflammatory cytokines, and interleukin 4, that produce an intense inflammatory reaction, with bronchoconstriction, vascular congestion, edema formation, increased mucus production, and impaired mucociliary transport. Eosinophils, platelets, and polymorphonuclear leukocytes are recruited to the site, activated, and contribute further to the inflammatory cycle that has already been initiated. The IgE response is controlled by T and B lymphocytes and activated by the interaction of antigen with the mast cell-bound IgE molecules. In the subacute or late phase, recruited and resident cells are activated, causing a more persistent pattern of inflammation.

Chronic inflammation is characterized by persistent cell damage and an ongoing repair process, contributing to some of the microscopic changes seen in the airway. Mediators target ciliated airway epithelium to cause injury or disruption. As a consequence, epithelial cells and myofibroblasts, present beneath the epithelial layer, proliferate and begin to deposit interstitial collagen in the lamina reticularis of the basement membrane. Fibroblasts contribute to the process by releasing cytokines and chemokines, which may be important in initiating and maintaining the level of airway inflammation and may explain the apparent basement membrane thickening and irreversible airway changes seen in some asthmatics. Clearly, the inflammatory process is multicellular, redundant, and self-amplifying.

Allergic asthma is frequently associated with a personal or family history of allergic diseases, such as rhinitis, urticaria, and eczema. Idiosyncratic, or nonallergic, asthma is associated with no family or personal history of allergy and normal serum levels of IgE. Many stimuli have been noted to provoke an increase in airway responsiveness. Viral respiratory infections are among the most common of the stimuli that invoke acute asthma exacerbation.[4] Increased airway responsiveness secondary to infection may last anywhere from 2 to 8 weeks.[4] Exercise is another common precipitant of acute asthma. Unlike other precipitants of acute exacerbation, long-term sequelae is not noted as a result of exercise. Environmental conditions, such as atmospheric pollutants and antigens noted in heavy industrial or densely populated urban areas, are associated with higher incidence and severity of asthma. In addition, indoor antigens, such as mold, house dust mites, cockroaches, and animal dander, are associated with acute asthma. Occupational exposures, such as metal salt, wood and vegetable dust, pharmaceutical, industrial chemical and plastic, biological enzyme, vapors, gases, and aerosols, also may stimulate an asthma attack. Multiple pharmaceutical agents, such as aspirin, β-blockers (including topical β-blockers), nonsteroidal anti-inflammatory agents, sulfating agents, tartrazine dyes, and food additives and preservatives, have been implicated in acute asthma. As in exercise-induced asthma, exposure to cold air alone can induce acute bronchospasm. Recent evidence indicates that endocrine factors, such as changing levels of estradiols and progesterone during the normal menstrual cycle and pregnancy, may contribute to the level of airway reactivity.[5] Emotional stress also can produce an asthma attack.

CLINICAL FEATURES

The symptoms of asthma consist of a triad of dyspnea, wheezing, and cough. Many patients will relay the history of asthma upon presentation, but some will not. Early in the attack, patients will complain of a sensation of chest constriction and cough. As the exacerbation progresses, wheezing becomes apparent, expiration becomes prolonged, and accessory muscle use may become evident. Key historical points should be obtained on asthmatics presenting with exacerbation to EDs (Table 68-2). Acute asthma exacerbation can be categorized based on clinical features (Table 68-3).

Physical examination findings are variable. Patients presenting with a severe asthma attack may be in obvious respiratory distress, with rapid breathing and loud wheezing, whereas patients with mild exacerbation may present with only cough and end-expiratory wheezing. At times, wheezing may be audible without a stethoscope. Other conditions may present with wheezing and mimic asthma (Table 68-4). The use of accessory muscles of inspiration indicates diaphragmatic fatigue, whereas the appearance of paradoxical respirations reflects impending ventilatory failure. Alteration in the mental status (e.g., lethargy, exhaustion, agitation, or confusion) also heralds respiratory arrest.

Directed physical examination reveals hyperresonance to percussion, decreased intensity of breath sounds, and prolongation of the expiratory phase, usually with wheezing. Although wheezing results from the movement of air through narrowed airways, the intensity of the wheeze may not correlate with the severity of airflow obstruction. The "silent chest" reflects very severe airflow obstruction, with air movement insufficient to promote a wheeze. A pulsus paradoxus above 20 mm Hg is also indicative of severe asthma. Although tachycardia and tachypnea are usually seen with acute asthma, vital signs normalize very quickly as airflow obstruction improves. Therefore, a normal heart rate, respiratory rate, and the absence of a pulsus paradoxus do not indicate complete relief of airway obstruction.

TABLE 68-1 Physiologic Consequences of Airflow Obstruction

Increased airway resistance
Decreased maximum expiratory flow rates
Air trapping
Increased airway pressure
  Barotrauma
  Adverse hemodynamic effects
Ventilation–perfusion imbalance
  Hypoxemia
  Hypercarbia
Increased work of breathing
  Pulsus paradoxus
  Respiratory muscle fatigue with ventilatory failure

TABLE 68-2   Key Historical Elements When Obtaining a History from Patients with Acute Asthma Exacerbation

Symptoms
  Cough
  Wheezing
  Shortness of breath
  Chest tightness
  Sputum production
  Fever
Pattern of symptoms
  Perennial and/or seasonal
  Continual or episodic
  Onset
  Duration
  Frequency
Aggravating factors
History of disease
  Age of onset and method of diagnosis
  Course of disease
  Present management and medications
  History of oral corticosteroid use
  Intensive care unit admissions
  History of intubation for asthma exacerbation
  Other medical diseases
Family history
Social history
  Condition of home
  Exposure to allergens
  Smoking
  Identification of participating causes
Exacerbation profile
  Usual pattern of exacerbation and outcome
Best spirometry measures
Risk factors for death from asthma
  Past history of sudden severe exacerbations
  Prior intubation for asthma
  Prior admission for asthma to an intensive care unit
  Two or more hospitalizations for asthma in the past year
  Three or more emergency care visits for asthma in the past year
  Hospitalization or emergency care visit for asthma within the past month
  Use of more than two canisters per month of inhaled short-acting β_2-agonist
  Current use of systemic corticosteroids or recent withdrawal from systemic corticosteroids
  Difficulty perceiving airflow obstruction or its severity
  Comorbidity, as from cardiovascular diseases or chronic obstructive pulmonary disease
  Serious psychiatric illness or psychosocial problems
  Low socioeconomic status in urban residents
  Illicit drug use

Source: Adapted from the National Asthma Education and Prevention Program, Expert Panel Report II: *Guidelines for the Diagnosis and Management of Asthma.* Publication 97-4051. Bethesda, MD, National Institutes of Health, 1997.

DIAGNOSIS

Bedside spirometry provides a rapid, objective assessment of patients and serves as a guide to the effectiveness of therapy. The forced expiratory volume in 1 s (FEV_1) and the peak expiratory flow rate (PEFR) directly measure the degree of large airway obstruction. Patient cooperation is essential for these tests to be reliable. Sequential measurements help emergency physicians assess severity and determine response to therapy. Signs on physical examination and a patient's report of symptoms of asthma do not necessarily correlate well with the severity of airflow obstruction. When possible, management decisions should be based on a patient's personal best PEFR or FEV_1 or, if unknown, the percentage of predicted spirometric values in addition to other physiologic and historical factors.

Pulse oximetry is a useful and convenient method for assessing oxygenation and monitoring oxygen saturation during treatment. Determination of arterial blood gas is not indicated in most patients with mild to moderate asthma exacerbation. The main reason to determine arterial blood gas during an asthma attack is to assess for hypoventilation with carbon dioxide retention and respiratory acidosis. Such patients almost always have clinical evidence of severe attacks or spirometry demonstrating a PEFR or FEV_1 of less than 25 percent predicted.[6] With acute attacks, ventilation is stimulated, resulting in a decrease in partial pressure of carbon dioxide ($PaCO_2$). Therefore, a normal or slightly elevated $PaCO_2$ (e.g., ≥ 42 mm Hg) indicates extreme airway obstruction and fatigue and may herald the onset of acute ventilatory failure.

Routine radiography is unnecessary but is indicated in patients with asthma exacerbation if there is clinical indication of a complication such as pneumothorax, pneumomediastinum, pneumonia, or other medical concern. For patients with asthma exacerbations requiring admission, up to one-third of patients will demonstrate an abnormality on chest radiograph.

A routine complete blood cell count is not indicated and likely will show modest leukocytosis secondary to administration of β-agonist therapy or corticosteroid treatment. In patients taking theophylline before ED presentation, a serum theophylline level should be determined. Routine electrocardiogram is also unnecessary but may reveal right ventricular strain, abnormal P waves, or nonspecific ST- and T-wave abnormalities, which resolve with treatment. Older patients, especially those with coexisting heart disease, should have cardiac monitoring during treatment. Asthma index scores have failed to predict outcome better than clinical judgment.

TREATMENT

The goal of treatment of acute asthma in the ED is to reverse airflow obstruction rapidly by repetitive or continuous administration of inhaled β_2-agonists, ensure adequate oxygenation, and relieve inflammation. The National Asthma Education and Prevention Program (NAEPP) Expert Panel has developed guidelines for emergency treatment of asthma (Figure 68-1),[7] as have other organizations around the world. The following categories of medications are used in the treatment of acute asthma: β-adrenergic agonists, anticholinergics, and glucocorticoids. Magnesium, heliox (mixture of helium and oxygen), and ketamine may be considered when the aforementioned medications fail to relieve bronchospasm. Mast cell-stabilizing agents, methylxanthines, and leukotriene modifiers are currently reserved for maintenance therapy only.

Adrenergic Agents

β-Adrenergic agonists are the preferred initial rescue medication for acute bronchospasm. β-Adrenergic receptors are divided into two types, β_1 and β_2. Stimulation of β_1-receptors increases rate and force of cardiac contraction and decreases small intestine motility and tone, whereas β_2-adrenergic stimulation promotes bronchodilation, vasodilation, uterine relaxation, and skeletal muscle tremor.

The mechanism of bronchodilator action of β-adrenergic drugs involves stimulation of the enzyme adenyl cyclase, which converts intracellular adenosine triphosphate into cyclic adenosine monophosphate. This action enhances the binding of intracellular calcium to cell membranes, reducing the myoplasmic calcium concentration, and results in relaxation of bronchial smooth muscle. In addition to bronchodilation, β-adrenergic drugs inhibit mediator release and promote mucociliary clearance.

The most common side effect of β-adrenergic drugs is skeletal muscle tremor. Patients also may experience nervousness, anxiety, insomnia, headache, hyperglycemia, palpitations, tachycardia, and hypertension. Despite earlier concerns over potential cardiotoxicity, especially when these drugs were used in combination with theophylline, clinical experience has not shown significant problems.

TABLE 68-3 Classifying Severity of Asthma Exacerbations*

	Mild	Moderate	Severe	Respiratory Arrest Imminent
Symptoms				
Breathlessness	While walking	While talking	While at rest	
Position	Can lie down	Prefers sitting	Sits upright	
Talks in	Sentences	Phrases	Words	
Alertness	May be agitated	Usually agitated	Usually agitated	Drowsy or confused
Signs				
Respiratory rate	Increased	Increased	Often >30/min	
Use of accessory muscles; suprasternal retractions	Usually not	Commonly	Usually	Paradoxical thoracoabdominal movement
Wheeze	Moderate, often only end expiratory	Loud; throughout exhalation	Usually loud; throughout inhalation and exhalation	Absent
Pulse per min	<100	100–120	>120	Bradycardia
Pulsus paradoxus	Absent <10 mm Hg	May be present 10–25 mm Hg	Often present >25 mm Hg (adult) 20–40 mm Hg (child)	Absence suggests respiratory muscle fatigue
Functional assessment				
Peak expiratory flow % predicted or % personal best	80%	~50–80%	<50% or response lasts <2 h	
Pa_{O_2} (on air)	Normal (test not usually necessary)	>60 mm Hg (test not usually necessary)	<60 mm Hg: possible cyanosis	
Pa_{CO_2}	<42 mm Hg (test not usually necessary)	<42 mm Hg (test not usually necessary)	≥42 mm Hg: possible respiratory failure (see text)	
Sa_{O_2}% (on air) at sea level	>95%	91–95%	<91%	

*The presence of several parameters, but not necessarily all, indicates the general classification of the exacerbation. Many of these parameters have not been systemically studied, so they serve only as general guides. Hypercapnia (hypoventilation) develops more readily in young children than in adults and adolescents.
Abbreviations: Pa_{CO_2} = partial pressure of carbon dioxide, arterial; Pa_{O_2} = partial pressure of oxygen, arterial; Sa_{O_2} = arterial oxygen saturation.
Source: Adapted from the National Asthma Education and Prevention Program, Expert Panel Report II: *Guidelines for the Diagnosis and Management of Asthma.* Publication No. 97-4051. Bethesda, MD, National Institutes of Health, 1997.

Arrhythmias and evidence of myocardial ischemia are rare, especially in patients without prior histories of coronary artery disease.

The β-adrenergic agonists used today are analogues of naturally occurring sympathomimetics (Table 68-5). The ideal bronchodilator in this class of drugs would possess pure β_2-receptor activity bronchodilation without cardiac effects. The older catecholamine bronchodilators, isoproterenol and epinephrine, are not β_2 specific and have a short duration of action. Isoetharine is more β_2 selective but still has a short duration of action. Newer agents produced by chemical modification of the parent compound have nearly replaced these drugs. The resorcinol bronchodilators (metaproterenol, terbutaline, and fenoterol) and saligenin bronchodilators (albuterol and carbuterol) share greater β_2 specificity and longer duration of action and effectiveness through the oral route due to resistance to intestinal sulfatases.

Aerosol therapy with β_2-adrenergic drugs produces excellent bronchodilation and is favored over the oral and parenteral routes. The aerosol route achieves topical administration of a relatively small dose of drug, thereby producing local effects with minimum systemic absorption and fewer side effects. Aerosol delivery may be achieved with a metered dose inhaler (MDI) with a spacing device or a compressor-driven nebulizer. A spacing device attached to the inhaler can improve drug deposition when patient technique is inadequate. Even with opti-

mum technique, however, a maximum of 15 percent of the drug dose is retained in the lungs, regardless of the aerosol method used. Dry-powder delivery devices and MDIs using hydrofluoroalkane as the propellant have recently replaced devices run by chlorinated fluorocarbon.

Aerosol treatments may be administered every 15 to 20 min or on a continuous basis. Epinephrine or terbutaline may be administered SC to patients unable to coordinate aerosolized or MDI treatments. Intravenous β-agonist infusions offer no advantage over aerosolized or MDI-delivered agents and carry potential risk.[8]

Salmeterol xinafoate is a β_2-adrenoreceptor agonist that binds with greater affinity to the β_2-receptor site than does albuterol. *It is indicated for twice-daily maintenance therapy, should never be used more frequently, and is to be avoided for treatment of acute exacerbation.* Its bronchodilator effect lasts at least 12 h, and tachyphylaxis has not been reported with long-term use. It is an effective treatment for long-term control of asthma, especially nocturnal asthma. Short-acting β_2-adrenoreceptor agonists are generally added for symptoms that occur despite the use of salmeterol.

Corticosteroids

Corticosteroids are highly effective drugs in asthma exacerbation and form one of the cornerstones of treatment. Although the mechanism of action is unknown, many believe that steroids produce beneficial effects by restoring β-adrenergic responsiveness and reducing inflammation. The onset of anti-inflammatory effect is delayed at least 4 to 8 h after intravenous or oral administration.

Evidence suggests that corticosteroids administered within 1 h of arrival in the ED reduces the need for hospitalization.[9] Although there is considerable disagreement over what constitutes the optimal dose in acute asthma, an initial dose of oral prednisone 40 to 60 mg, or an intravenous bolus of methylprednisolone 60 to 125 mg IV in patients unable to tolerate oral medications, is sufficient. High-dose corticosteroid

TABLE 68-4 Asthma Mimickers

Congestive heart failure ("cardiac asthma")
Upper airway obstruction
Aspiration of foreign body or gastric acid
Bronchogenic carcinoma with endobronchial obstruction
Metastatic carcinoma with lymphangitic metastasis
Sarcoidosis with endobronchial obstruction
Vocal cord dysfunction
Multiple pulmonary emboli (rare)

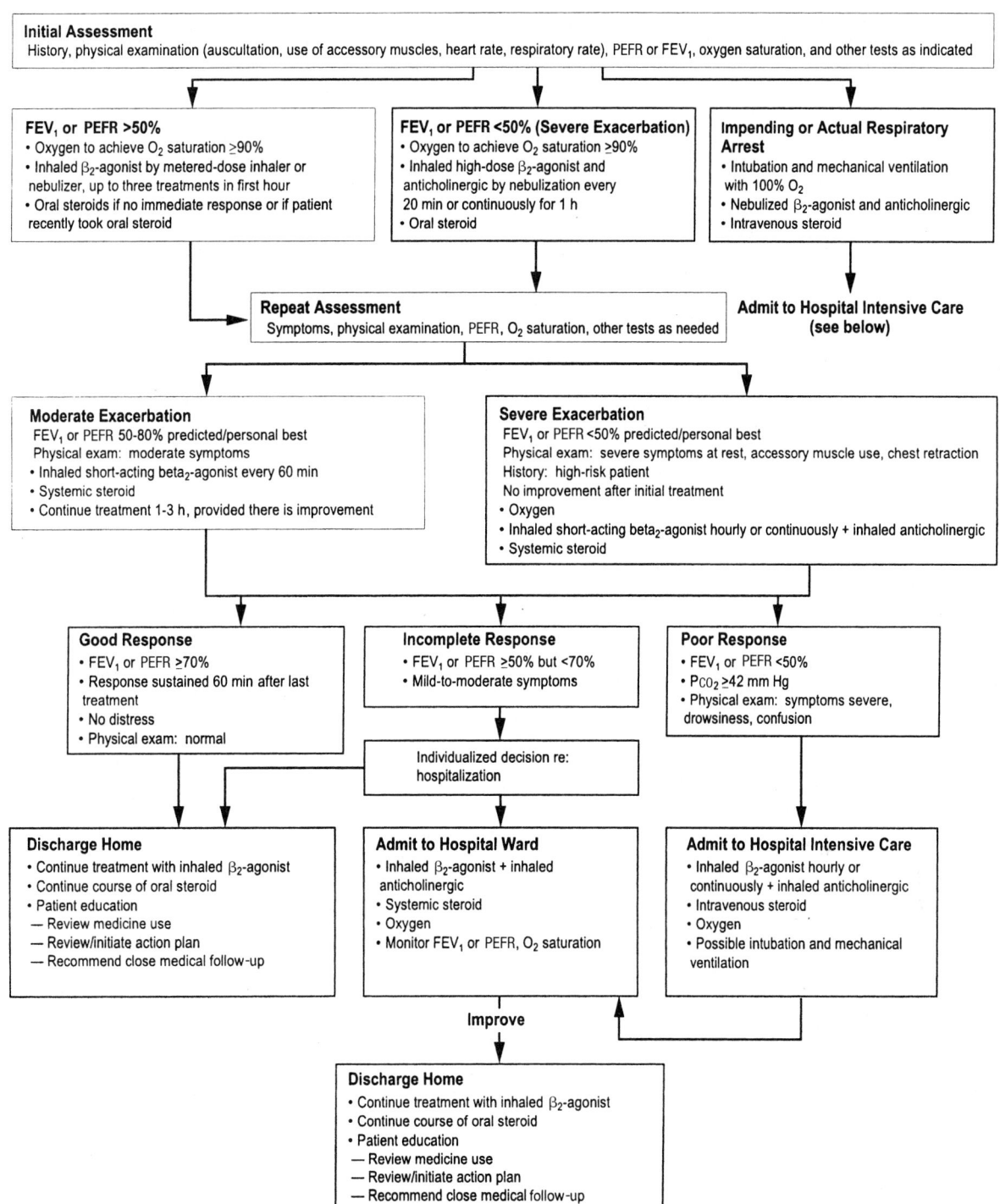

FIG. 68-1. Management of asthma exacerbations: emergency department and hospital-based care. (Adapted with permission from the National Asthma Education and Prevention Program, Expert Panel Report II: *Practical Guide for the Diagnosis and Management of Asthma.* Publication 97-4053. Bethesda, MD, National Institutes of Health, 1997.)

therapy offers no advantage.[10] Additional doses should be given every 4 to 6 h until significant subjective and objective improvements are achieved. Patients who are being discharged home with an FEV_1 or PEFR of less than 70 percent predicted after aggressive ED treatment should be prescribed a 3- to 10-day non-tapering burst of oral steroids, prednisone 40 to 60 mg per d, or its equivalent.[11]

Current recommendations favor maintaining all patients with mild persistent asthma or more severe asthma with inhaled corticosteroids.[12] Therefore, consideration should be given to discharging all

patients with mild persistent or more severe asthma on maintenance inhaled corticosteroids in addition to a burst of oral corticosteroids.[11]

Anticholinergics

Plants containing anticholinergic alkaloids have been smoked for hundreds, if not thousands, of years to treat respiratory disorders. In recent years, anticholinergics have been rediscovered as potent bronchodilators in patients with asthma and other forms of obstructive lung

TABLE 68-5 Dosages of Drugs for Asthma Exacerbations in Emergency Medical Care or Hospital

Medications	Adult Dosages	Comments
Inhaled short-acting β_2 agonists		
Albuterol		
Nebulizer solution (5 mg/mL)	2.5–5.0 mg every 20 min for 3 doses, then 2.5–10 mg every 1–4 h as needed *or* 10–15 mg per h continuously	Only selective β_2 agonists are recommended; for optimal delivery, dilute aerosols to minimum of 4 mL at gas flow of 6–8 L per min
MDI (90 μg/puff)	4–8 puffs every 20 min up to 4 h, then every 1–4 h as needed	As effective as nebulized therapy if patient is able to coordinate inhalation maneuver; use spacer/holding chamber
Bitolterol		
Nebulizer solution (2 mg/mL)	See albuterol dose	Has not been studied in severe asthma exacerbations; do not mix with other drugs
MDI (370 μg/puff)	See albuterol dose	Has not been studied in severe asthma exacerbations
Pirbuterol		
MDI (200 μg/puff)	See albuterol dose	Has not been studied in severe asthma exacerbations
Systemic (injected), β_2 agonists		
Epinephrine (1:1000 or 1 mg/mL)	0.3–0.5 mg SC every 20 min for 3 doses	No proven advantage of systemic therapy over aerosol
Terbutaline (1 mg/mL)	0.25 mg SC every 20 min for 3 doses	No proven advantage of systemic therapy over aerosol
Anticholinergics		
Ipratropium bromide		
Nebulizer solution (0.2 mg/mL)	0.5 mg every 30 min for 3 doses, then every 2–4 h as needed	Should not be used as first-line therapy; should be added to β_2 agonist therapy; may mix in same nebulizer with albuterol
MDI (18 μg/puff)	4–8 puffs every 6–8 h	Dose delivered from MDI is low and has not been studied in asthma exacerbations
Corticosteroids		
Prednisone Methylprednisolone Prednisolone	120–180 mg per d in 3 or 4 divided doses for 48 h, then 60–80 mg per d until FEV$_1$, or PEFR reaches 70% of predicted or personal best*	For outpatient "burst," use 40–60 mg per d, for 3–10 d in adults

*Dosage for admitted patients.
Abbreviations: FEV$_1$ = forced expiratory volume in 1 sec; MDI = metered dose inhaler; PEFR = peak expiratory flow rate; SC = subcutaneous.
Source: Adapted from the National Asthma Education and Prevention Program, Expert Panel Report II: *Guidelines for the Diagnosis and Management of Asthma.* Publication 97-4051. Bethesda, MD, National Institutes of Health, 1997.

disease. Although comparisons of bronchodilator response between anticholinergics and β-adrenergic agonists have produced conflicting results, the effects of the drugs used in combination is additive. This effect is plausible, because anticholinergics affect large, central airways, whereas β-adrenergic drugs dilate smaller airways.

Anticholinergic drugs competitively antagonize acetylcholine at the postganglionic junction between the parasympathetic nerve terminal and effector cell. This process blocks the bronchoconstriction induced by vagal cholinergic-mediated innervation to the larger central airways. In addition, concentrations of cyclic guanosine monophosphate in airway smooth muscle are reduced, further promoting bronchodilation.

Because of significant systemic side effects, atropine sulfate, once the major nebulized anticholinergic used in the United States, has been virtually replaced by the synthetic quaternary derivative: ipratropium bromide. This drug causes far fewer systemic side effects and is very well tolerated. Ipratropium is currently available as a nebulized solution and an MDI (see Table 68-5).

Aerosolized ipratropium bromide 0.5 mg, should be administered to patients with severe exacerbation.[7] Potential side effects with nebulized anticholinergics include dry mouth, thirst, and difficulty swallowing. Less commonly, tachycardia, restlessness, irritability, confusion, difficulty in micturition, ileus, blurring of vision, or an increase in intraocular pressure is noted.

Theophylline

Theophylline is no longer considered a first-line treatment for acute asthma.[7] Studies have shown that theophylline, in combination with inhaled β$_2$-adrenergic drugs, appears to increase the toxicity, but not the efficacy, of treatment.[13] Theoretically, theophylline may be a useful adjunct by providing a more sustained bronchodilator effect, contributing to small airway bronchodilation, improving respiratory muscle endurance, and improving resistance to fatigue. Recent data suggest an anti-inflammatory mechanism of action.

The mechanism of action of theophylline remains unknown; 90 percent of theophylline metabolism is hepatic, and the remainder is excreted unchanged through the kidneys. A serum theophylline level should be determined for patients who regularly use theophylline. The most common side effects of theophylline are nervousness, nausea, vomiting, anorexia, and headache. At plasma levels greater than 30 μg/mL, there is a risk of seizures and cardiac arrhythmias.

Magnesium

Intravenous magnesium sulfate is indicated in the management of acute, very severe asthma (i.e., FEV$_1$ <25 percent predicted), but its usefulness in mild and moderate exacerbation has not been established.[14] Although the bronchodilating properties of magnesium sulfate can be helpful, it should not be substituted for standard therapy regimens. The dose is 1 to 2 g IV over 30 min.

Heliox, Ketamine, and Halothane

Although several studies have demonstrated that a mixture of 80 percent helium and 20 percent oxygen (heliox) can lower airway resistance and act as an adjunct in the treatment of very severe asthma exacerbation, other studies have failed to demonstrate these effects.[15,16] Therefore, heliox currently is not indicated for use in mild or moderate bronchospasm.

Several investigators have reported success with ketamine and halothane in cases in which all other treatment modalities have failed. Controlled trials substantiating these claims are lacking.

Mast Cell Modifiers

Cromolyn and nedocromil exert their anti-inflammatory action by blockage of chlorine channels, thus modulating mast cell mediator release and eosinophil recruitment. These agents also inhibit early and late responses to allergen challenge and exercise. Neither is indicated for treatment of acute bronchospasm.

Leukotriene Modifiers

Leukotrienes are potent proinflammatory mediators that contract airway smooth muscle, increase microvascular permeability, stimulate mucus secretion, decrease mucociliary clearance, and recruit eosinophils into the airway. Several leukotriene modifiers, namely montelukast, zafirlukast, and zileuton, are currently available as oral tablets for the treatment of asthma. Leukotriene modifiers improve lung function, diminish symptoms, and diminish the need for short-acting β_2-agonists. They may be used as an alternative to low-dose inhaled corticosteroid therapy in mild persistent asthmatics and as steroid-sparing agents with inhaled corticosteroids in moderate persistent asthmatics.[12] Although one trial found that intravenous montelukast can cause rapid bronchodilation when used as adjuvant therapy for acute asthma,[17] it would be premature to recommend its use in the treatment of acute bronchospasm. Currently, there is no indication for the use of any of the leukotriene modifiers in the ED.

Mechanical Ventilation

When, despite the emergency physician's best effort to treat an acute asthma exacerbation, the patient begins to exhibit signs of acute ventilatory failure, noninvasive positive-pressure ventilation may be attempted. However, if the patient manifests progressive hypercarbia and acidosis or becomes exhausted or confused, intubation and mechanical ventilation are necessary to prevent respiratory arrest. Mechanical ventilation does not relieve the airflow obstruction; it merely eliminates the work of breathing and enables the patient to rest while the airflow obstruction is resolved. Fortunately, fewer than 1 percent of asthmatics ever require mechanical ventilation. Direct oral intubation is preferred over the nasotracheal route.

The potential complications of mechanical ventilation in asthmatic patients are numerous. Increased airway resistance may lead to extremely high peak airway pressures, barotrauma, and hemodynamic impairment. Mucous plugging is frequent, often leading to increased airway resistance, atelectasis, and pulmonary infection. Due to the severity of airflow obstruction during the early phases of treatment, the tidal volume may be larger than the returned volume, leading to air trapping and increased residual volume (intrinsic positive end-expiratory pressure). These effects may be avoided in part by using rapid inspiratory flow rates at a reduced respiratory frequency (12 to 14 breaths/min) and allowing adequate time for the expiratory phase. One can achieve the goal of ventilatory support, that is, maintenance of adequate arterial oxygen saturation (≥ 90 percent), without concern for "normalizing" the hypercarbic acidosis. This approach is called *controlled mechanical hypoventilation* or *permissive hypoventilation*. All patients requiring mechanical ventilation must be admitted to an intensive care unit.

SPECIFIC ISSUES THAT AFFECT DIAGNOSIS, EVALUATION, AND TREATMENT

Age

Although newly diagnosed asthma in older populations is not uncommon, differentiation of the etiology of wheezing in older asthmatics may present a challenge. Historical data may help differentiate between congestive heart failure, pulmonary malignancy, and obstructive airway disease, but distinguishing between chronic obstructive pulmonary disease and acute asthma is often difficult.[2] Treatment of older asthmatics should proceed in the same manner as treatment of younger asthmatics. Age-related changes in pulmonary function must be considered when determining response to treatment in older asthmatics, and care should be taken to avoid medication interactions.

Gender

Men and women interpret changes in pulmonary function differently. Women express a sensation of dyspnea at higher percentage-predicted PEFR than do men.[18] In addition, cyclic hormonal changes may influence pulmonary function in women.[5]

Pregnancy

Asthma complicates approximately 4 percent of pregnancies. Studies indicate that as many as 42 percent of pregnant asthmatics require hospitalization and that an additional 11 to 18 percent have one or more visits to the ED for exacerbation.[5]

In 1993, the NAEPP Expert Panel developed guidelines for the treatment of asthma exacerbation during pregnancy. The principles of managing acute asthma exacerbation are similar to those of managing exacerbation in a nonpregnant state. They consist of repetitive lung function measurements, maintenance of oxygen saturation at greater than 95 percent, administration of repetitive inhaled β_2-agonist, and early administration of systemic corticosteroids, in addition to fetal monitoring. Early intervention during acute exacerbation is key to the prevention of impaired maternal and fetal oxygenation. Uncontrolled asthma is associated with a variety of maternal and fetal complications, including hyperemesis, hypertension, toxemia, vaginal hemorrhage, complicated labor, intrauterine growth restriction, preterm birth, increased perinatal mortality, and neonatal hypoxemia. Although no asthma medication labeled to date qualifies for Food and Drug Administration use-in-pregnancy category A rating (for which adequate well-controlled studies in pregnant women have failed to demonstrate risk to the fetus), problems as a result of routine treatment of asthma in the ED have not been reported.

Hyperventilation of pregnancy leads to a higher Pa_{O_2} and a diminished Pa_{CO_2}. Thus, a Pa_{O_2} of less than 70 mm Hg in pregnant women with acute asthma represents fairly severe hypoxemia, and a Pa_{CO_2} of greater than 35 mm Hg represents respiratory failure. During asthma exacerbation, the normal alkalosis of pregnancy is aggravated, leading to a decrease in placental blood flow. Hypoxemia is usually more severe in the fetus than in the mother.

β_2-Agonists and inhaled corticosteroids are considered safe during pregnancy and are recommended as a routine part of asthma management. As in nonpregnant patients, a short burst of oral steroid (prednisone 40 to 60 mg per d) or its equivalent, and inhaled corticosteroids in patients with mild persistent or more severe asthma should be considered for pregnant asthmatics discharged from the ED after treatment for an exacerbation.

DISPOSITION

Disposition decisions should take into account a combination of subjective parameters, such as resolution of wheezing and improvement in air exchange, as assessed by auscultation and patient opinion, objective measures, such as normalization of FEV_1 or PEFR, and historical factors, such as compliance, history of ED use, and hospitalization. The ideal combination of elements needed for successful discharge without risk of early relapse has not yet been determined.[19] Some degree of residual airflow obstruction, airway lability, and inflammation persists after treatment and discharge from the ED.

No single treatment program can be recommended for all patients discharged home from the ED after treatment of exacerbation.

TABLE 68-6 Hospital Discharge Checklist for Patients with Asthma Exacerbations

Intervention	Dose/Timing	Education/Advise	MD/RN Initials
Inhaled medications (metered dose inhaler + spacer/holding chamber) β_2-agonist Corticosteroids	Select agent, dose, and frequency (e.g., albuterol) 2–6 puffs q4h 2 puffs qid	Teach purpose Teach technique Emphasize need for spacer/holding chamber Check patient technique	
Oral medications	Select agent, dose, and frequency (e.g., prednisone 20 mg bid for 3–10 d)	Teach purpose Teach side effects	
Peak flow meter	Measure A.M. and P.M. PEFR and record best of three tries each time	Teach purpose Teach technique Distribute peak flow diary	
Follow-up visit	Make appointment for follow-up with primary clinician or asthma specialist	Advise patient (or caregiver) of date, time, and location of appointment within 7 d of hospital discharge	
Action plan	Before or at discharge	Instruct patient (or caregiver) on simple plan for actions to be taken when symptoms, signs, and peak expiratory flow values suggest recurrent airflow obstruction	

Abbreviation: PEFR = peak expiratory flow rate.
Source: Adapted from the National Asthma Education and Prevention Program, Expert Panel Report II: *Guidelines for the Diagnosis and Management of Asthma.* Publication 97-4051. Bethesda, MD, National Institutes of Health, 1997.

Although several studies have demonstrated that a short course of oral steroids and β_2-agonist bronchodilators reduce relapse rates among discharged patients, other studies have reported high relapse rates regardless of ED management and use of steroids.[19] Patients with histories of previous ED visits and hospitalization are at highest risk of relapse, regardless of management.[19]

Current guidelines help to determine hospitalization and discharge criteria based on response to aggressive treatment. A good response to treatment is demonstrated by complete resolution of symptoms and a PEFR or FEV_1 of greater than 70 percent predicted. Such individuals can be safely discharged home. Patients with a poor response to treatment are defined as those with persistent symptoms and FEV_1 or PEFR of less than 50 percent predicted. Such patients are likely to have persistent wheezing and dyspnea at rest despite intensive treatment in the ED and should be admitted. An incomplete response to treatment, the middle ground, is defined as some persistence of symptoms and a PEFR or FEV_1 between 50 and 70 percent predicted. Most asthmatics treated in the ED fall into this category. They may be discharged home safely, provided they have no risk factors for death from asthma (see Table 68-2).[7] Patients who fail to improve adequately over a period of several hours, because they are in the late phase of their exacerbation, and those with significant risk factors for death from asthma should be admitted to an observation unit or the hospital.[7]

The role of observation units in the care of acute asthma exacerbation is currently being determined. Although early studies indicated no reduction in hospitalization rates after treatment in ED observation units, more recent studies indicated that 59 percent of asthmatics admitted to observation units, where strict care protocols are followed, are successfully treated and discharged.[20]

Follow-up care must be arranged after an acute exacerbation to ensure resolution and to review the long-term medication plan for the chronic management of asthma. High relapse rates, despite the routine use of steroids, strongly suggest the need for follow-up within days of the ED visit. Patients with asthma should have an appropriate written plan of action that addresses routine care and care of worsening symptoms.

Education of patients should become an integral part of ED care. The ED personnel should provide basic education on asthma and help link patients with primary care providers or asthma specialists while providing discharge instructions. Review of the patient's discharge medication, use of inhaler technique, and the use of peak flow monitoring are just some of the issues ED physicians can teach and emphasize (Table 68-6).

REFERENCES

1. Mannino DM, Homa DM, Akinbami LJ, et al: Surveillance for asthma-United States, 1980-1999. *MMWR Surveill Summ* 51:1, 2002.
2. Cydulka RK, McFadden ER Jr, Emerman CL, et al: Patterns of hospitalization in elderly patients with asthma and chronic obstructive pulmonary disease. *Am J Respir Crit Care Med* 156:1807, 1997.
3. Weiss KB, Gergen PJ, Hodgson TA: An economic evaluation of asthma in the United States. *New Engl J Med* 326:862, 1992.
4. Busse WW, Gern JE: Viruses in asthma. *J Allergy Clin Immunol* 100:147, 1997.
5. Schatz M: Interrelationships between asthma and pregnancy: A literature review. *J Allergy Clin Immunol* 103:S330, 1999.
6. Martin TG, Elenbaas RM, Pingleton SH: Use of peak expiratory flow rates to eliminate unnecessary arterial blood gases in acute asthma. *Ann Emerg Med* 11:70, 1982.
7. National Asthma Education and Prevention Program, Expert Panel Report II: *Guidelines for the Diagnosis and Management of Asthma.* Publication 97-4051. Bethesda, MD, National Institutes of Health, 1997.
8. Salmeron S, Brochard L, Mal H, et al: Nebulized versus intravenous albuterol in hypercapnic acute asthma. A multicenter, double-blind, randomized study. *Am J Respir Crit Care Med* 149:1466, 1994.
9. Rowe BH, Spooner C, Ducharme FM, et al: Early emergency department treatment of acute asthma with systemic corticosteroids. *Cochrane Database Syst Rev* 1:CD002178, 2001.
10. Emerman CL, Cydulka RK: A randomized comparison of 100-mg vs 500-mg dose of methylprednisolone in the treatment of acute asthma. *Chest* 107:1559, 1995.
11. Rowe BH, Spooner CH, Ducharme FM, et al: Corticosteroids for preventing relapse following acute exacerbations of asthma. *Cochrane Database Syst Rev* 1:CD000195, 2001.
12. National Asthma Education and Prevention Program, Expert Panel Report: Guidelines for the diagnosis and management of asthma-Update on selected topics 2002. *J Allergy Clin Immunology* 110(5 pt 2):7A, 2002.
13. Parameswaran K, Belda J, Rowe BH: Addition of intravenous aminophylline to beta2-agonists in adults with acute asthma. *Cochrane Database Syst Rev* 4:CD002742, 2000.
14. Rowe BH, Bretzlaff JA, Bourdon C, et al: Magnesium sulfate for treating exacerbations of acute asthma in the emergency department. *Cochrane Database Syst Rev* 2:CD001490, 2000.

15. Carter ER: Heliox for acute severe asthma. *Chest* 117:1212, 2000.

16. Dorfman TA, Shipley ER, Burton JH, et al: Inhaled heliox does not benefit ED patients with moderate to severe asthma. *Am J Emerg Med* 18:495, 2000.

17. Camargo CA, Smithline HA, Malice MP, et al: Rapid bronchodilator response to intravenous montelukast in acute asthma. *Am J Respir Crit Care Med* 167:528, 2003.

18. Cydulka RK, Emerman CL, Rowe BH, et al: Differences between men and women in reporting of symptoms during an asthma exacerbation. *Ann Emerg Med* 38:123, 2001.

19. Emerman CL, Woodruff PG, Cydulka RK, et al: Prospective multicenter study of relapse following treatment for acute asthma among adults presenting to the emergency department. *Chest* 115:919, 1999.

20. Rydman RJ, Isola ML, Roberts RR, et al: Emergency department observation unit versus hospital inpatient care for a chronic asthmatic population: A randomized trial of health status outcome and cost. *Med Care* 36:599, 1998.

69 CHRONIC OBSTRUCTIVE PULMONARY DISEASE

Rita K. Cydulka

Mohak Dave

Management of patients with chronic obstructive pulmonary disease (COPD) can be challenging and frustrating. Although many advances in the treatment of other disease entities have emerged over the past several decades, research and progress in the treatment of COPD remain limited. Recent efforts to improve public awareness and research in COPD worldwide have resulted in the recent release of at least five sets of guidelines directed at the evaluation and treatment of COPD.[1-6]

According the U.S. National Heart, Lung, and Blood Institute and the World Health Organization's Global Initiative for Chronic Obstructive Lung Disease (GOLD), COPD is characterized by airflow limitation that is not fully reversible. The airflow obstruction is generally progressive and associated with an abnormal inflammatory response to noxious particles or gases.[5] A diagnosis of COPD should be considered in any patient who complains of chronic cough, sputum production or dyspnea, and/or exposure to risk factors for the disease. The diagnosis may be confirmed with spirometric evaluation: a postbronchodilator forced expiratory volume in 1 s (FEV_1) of less than 80 percent predicted in combination with a ratio of FEV_1 to forced vital capacity of less than 70 percent.[5] About 85 percent of patients with COPD suffer from chronic bronchitis, and 15 percent suffer primarily from emphysema.[6] Chronic bronchitis is defined as the presence of chronic productive cough for 3 months in each of 2 successive years in a patient in whom other causes of chronic cough have been excluded. Emphysema is defined as abnormal, permanent enlargement of the airspaces distal to the terminal bronchioles, accompanied by destruction of their walls and without obvious fibrosis. Chronic bronchitis is defined in clinical terms, and emphysema is defined in terms of anatomic pathology. In contrast, the GOLD definition does not distinguish between chronic bronchitis and emphysema.[5]

EPIDEMIOLOGY

Chronic obstructive pulmonary disease is a major worldwide respiratory health problem. It is the sixth leading cause of death in the world, the fourth most common cause of death in the United States, the third most common cause of hospitalization, and the only leading cause of death that is increasing in prevalence.

In North America, COPD is rare in persons younger than 40 years but very common among older individuals, with a prevalence of approximately 10 percent in those 55 to 85 years of age. The disease is more common in men than in women, but the prevalence of COPD in women has doubled in the past few decades, a reflection of increased smoking behavior of women and increased recognition of COPD in women as a diagnostic possibility by physicians. The prevalence of COPD is highest in those countries that have the greatest cigarette use.

The mortality of patients while hospitalized for a COPD exacerbation is approximately 5 to 14 percent.[7] Mortality of COPD patients patients admitted to an intensive care unit for exacerbation is 24 percent. For patients 65 years or older and discharged from the intensive care unit after treatment of a COPD exacerbation, the 1-year mortality is 59 percent, nearly double the expected 30 percent.

Chronic obstructive pulmonary disease is an expensive public health problem in terms of direct economic costs (such as hospital admissions and outpatient treatments), indirect economic costs (such as lost years of life, disability, and loss of working capacity), and reduction in quality of life. Estimations on the annual cost of COPD in the United States reached more than 30 billion dollars in 1995. The use of health care resources by elderly patients with COPD is immense during hospitalization and after discharge.[8]

PATHOPHYSIOLOGY

Cigarette smoking accounts for an estimated 80 to 90 percent of the risk of developing COPD. Age of starting, total pack-years, and current smoking status are predictive of COPD mortality.[2] Of note, only 15 percent of smokers develop clinically significant COPD. A variety of other environmental risk factors, such as respiratory infections, occupational exposures, ambient air pollution, passive smoke exposure, and diet, have been suggested as other risk factors. The only proven genetic risk factor is α_1-antitrypsin deficiency, although this accounts for fewer than 1 percent of COPD patients.

The earliest objective changes in the evolution of COPD are clinically imperceptible and are measured as small increases in peripheral airway resistance or lung compliance. The slow, insidious appearance of dyspnea and hypersecretion often requires several decades of disease. The recently released GOLD guideline stages COPD by severity. The use of this staging system may prove helpful in diagnosing and treating COPD earlier (Table 69-1).

The sedentary habits of many cigarette smokers result in failure to unmask exertional dyspnea, and denial results in suppression of symptoms or attribution of such symptoms to aging, poor conditioning, obesity, or allergies. Further, the respiratory consequences of cigarette smoking are a continuum of slowly evolving and latent effects, unique to each individual, in a complex dose-response relationship. Early in disease evolution, abstinence from smoking may eliminate symptoms and result in physiologic improvement. Once well established, however, abnormalities persist and may progress despite abstinence.

Pathologic specimens from patients with early disease demonstrate minor metaplasia of bronchial epithelium and an increase in bronchial gland number and size. As disease evolves, such findings are exaggerated, acute and chronic inflammatory changes in the epithelium are more notable, and acinar expansion, destruction, and coalescence are seen. Elements of emphysematous disease are invariably present in concert with those of bronchitic disease, although one often predominates.

Despite recognition of causative factors, what determines the clinical onset and rate of progression of chronic airflow obstruction and the direction toward emphysematous or bronchitic patterns are uncertain. Clearly, there is a great deal of variability in disease pattern and severity among individuals with a seemingly similar predisposition to disease.

The central element in the pathophysiology of chronic airflow obstruction is impedance to airflow, especially expiratory airflow, due to increased resistance or decreased caliber throughout the small bronchi and bronchioles. The majority of airway inflammation and obstruction occurs in bronchioles and lung parenchyma. Airflow obstruction results from a combination of airway secretions, mucosal edema, bronchospasm, and bronchoconstriction from impaired elasticity. Impedance to airflow alone accounts substantially for the abnormal physiology of the disease.

TABLE 69-1 Classification of Chronic Obstructive Pulmonary Disease by Severity

Stage	Characteristics
0. At risk	Normal spirometry Chronic symptoms (cough, sputum production)
I. Mild COPD	$FEV_1/FVC <70\%$ $FEV_1 \geq 80\%$ predicted With or without chronic symptoms (cough, sputum production)
II. Moderate COPD IIA IIB	$FEV_1/FVC <70\%$ $30\% \geq FEV_1 <80\%$ predicted $50\% \leq FEV_1 <80\%$ predicted $30\% \leq FEV_1 <50\%$ predicted With or without chronic symptoms (cough, sputum production)
III. Severe COPD	$FEV_1/FVC <70\%$ $FEV_1 <30\%$ predicted or $<50\%$ predicted plus respiratory failure or clinical signs of right heart failure

Abbreviations: COPD = chronic obstructive pulmonary disease; FEV_1 = forced expiratory volume in 1 s; FVC = forced vital capacity; respiratory failure = arterial partial pressure of onxgen <60 mm Hg (8.0 kPa) with or without arterial partial pressure of carbon dioxide >50 mm Hg (6.7 kPa) while breathing air at sea level.
Source: Adapted from Pauwels RA, Buist AS, Calverley PM, et al: Global strategy for the diagnosis, management, and prevention of chronic obstructive pulmonary disease. NHLBI/WHO Global Initiative for Chronic Obstructive Lung Disease (GOLD) Workshop summary. *Am J Respir Crit Care Med* 163:1256, 2001.

Exaggerated airway resistance reduces total minute ventilation or increases respiratory work. To the degree that alveolar hypoventilation occurs, hypoxemia and hypercarbia result. Even without hypoventilation, hypoxemia occurs due to ventilation-perfusion mismatching.

In addition to obstruction of peripheral airways, all forms of advanced chronic airflow obstruction involve other pathophysiologic elements to complete the overall picture. For example, in dominantly emphysematous disease, destruction and coalescence of alveolar architecture reduce the total "matched" alveolar and capillary surface areas for diffusion of gas, and vascular destruction results in "unmatched" regions where ventilation is wasted. In addition, neurochemical and proprioceptive ventilatory responses in chronic airflow obstruction may be aberrant. For example, ventilatory response to hypercarbia may be blunted during sleep, and ventilatory drive and dyspnea may be exaggerated despite normal pulmonary inflation. The composition of muscle fiber types, breathing patterns, and resistance to fatigue of respiratory muscles are also altered in advanced disease. Moreover, pulmonary arterial hypertension supervenes as chronic airflow obstruction progresses. The right ventricle transiently hypertrophies and then dilates with the evolution of overt cor pulmonale. A low-output state in the pulmonary circulation translates into low left ventricular output. Arterial hypoxemia increases as the effects of right-to-left shunt on poorly oxygenated mixed venous blood are exaggerated. Right ventricular pressure overload is associated with atrial and ventricular arrhythmias.

Although COPD is increasingly becoming recognized as a chronic inflammatory disease, there is no mention in the current guidelines of lower airway inflammation in the definition of COPD.[1-6]

CLINICAL FEATURES

Chronic, Compensated COPD

Despite the pathophysiologic segregation of chronic airflow obstruction into categories of pulmonary emphysema, chronic bronchitis, and bronchiectasis, none of these exist as a pure entity in clinical medicine.

Most patients demonstrate a mixture of symptoms and signs. The hallmark symptoms are exertional dyspnea and cough. Chronic, productive cough is common, and minor hemoptysis is frequent, especially in chronic bronchitis and bronchiectasis.

Physical findings include tachypnea, accessory respiratory muscle use, and pursed-lip exhalation. Airflow obstruction causes wheezing during exhalation, especially during maximum forced exhalation, and prolongation of the expiratory time. In dominantly bronchitic disease, coarse crackles are heard as uncleared secretions move about the central airways. In dominantly emphysematous disease, there is expansion of the thorax, impeded diaphragmatic motion, and global diminution of breath sounds. Weight loss is frequent due to poor dietary intake and excessive caloric expenditure for the work of breathing. Plethora due to secondary polycythemia and cyanosis and tremor, somnolence, and confusion due to hypercarbia may be seen in advanced disease. Findings of secondary pulmonary hypertension with or without cor pulmonale may be present. The physical signs of ventricular dysfunction are often disguised or underestimated by the seemingly more overwhelming signs of respiratory disease, or because pulmonary hyperinflation prohibits adequate auscultation.

Acute Exacerbations of COPD

Decompensation is usually due to worsening of airflow obstruction resulting from superimposed respiratory infection, increased bronchospasm, or other respiratory pathology, such as pulmonary embolism, interference with respiratory drive, cardiovascular deterioration, smoking, noncompliance with medications, noxious environmental exposures, use of medications that prevent bronchorrhea, and adverse responses to medication. Disordered ventilatory drive may arise from misuse of oxygen therapy, hypnotics, or tranquilizers. Metabolic disturbances and inadequate oxygen delivery independent of respiratory function may cause decompensated COPD.

Exacerbations of COPD frequently result in progressive hypoxemia. Signs of hypoxemia include tachypnea, tachycardia, systemic hypertension, cyanosis, and a change in mental status. The most life-threatening feature of decompensation is hypoxemia, where arterial saturation falls below 90 percent. With increased work of breathing, muscle production of carbon dioxide increases, and alveolar ventilation is often unable to increase to prevent carbon dioxide retention and respiratory acidosis. Signs of hypercapnia include mental status changes and hypopnea.

Upon presentation to the ED, patients usually complain of dyspnea and orthopnea. The intensified effort to ventilate is further dramatized by the sitting-up-and-forward position, pursed-lip exhalation, accessory muscle use, and diaphoresis. Pulsus paradoxus may be noted during blood pressure recording. Complications such as pneumonia, pneumothorax, pulmonary embolism, or an acute abdomen may be neglected or minimized by the patient's generalized respiratory distress, tachypnea, or global diminution of breath sounds. The physician should maintain a broad differential diagnosis for other disease entities that may be present with similar symptoms of dyspnea, such as asthma, congestive heart failure, pneumonia, pulmonary embolism, tuberculosis, and metabolic disturbances.

DIAGNOSIS

Chronic, Compensated COPD

The most valuable tool in characterizing disease severity is pulmonary function testing. In addition, examination of lung mechanics, analysis of arterial blood gases, description of ventilatory response patterns, tests of respiratory muscle performance, metabolic assessment, and noninvasive survey of hemodynamic reserve can be performed. The ratio of FEV_1 to forced vital capacity should be used to diagnose mild COPD. However, once the disease progresses, the percentage of predicted FEV_1 is a better measure of disease severity.[1-6] Various guidelines characterize COPD severity as mild, moderate, or severe, although agreement on precise FEV_1 standards remains arbitrary.[1-6]

In the early stages of COPD, arterial blood gas measurements reveal mild-to-moderate hypoxemia without evidence of hypercapnia. As the disease progresses in severity (especially when the FEV_1 falls below 1 L), hypoxemia becomes more more severe and the development of hypercapnia becomes more evident. Arterial blood gas measurements worsen during acute exacerbations and may worsen during exercise and sleep.

Radiographic examination is often misleading; mild chronic airflow obstruction is not likely to be radiographically apparent. Dominantly bronchitic disease may be associated with subtle or absent x-ray findings. In contrast, dominantly emphysematous disease may be associated with remarkable signs of hyperaeration, such as increased anteroposterior diameter, flattened diaphragms, increased parenchymal lucency, and attenuation of pulmonary arterial vascular shadows, despite only mild-to-moderate physiologic alterations. Right or left ventricular enlargement may not produce relative enlargement of the cardiac silhouette. Certainly, radiography is of unquestionable value in diagnosing complications such as pneumothorax, pneumonia, pleural effusion, and pulmonary neoplasia.

Diagnosing heart failure and assessing ventricular function in patients with COPD is difficult, although the use of B-natriuretic peptide may aid in this differentiation.[9] Echocardiography or gated nuclear scans to estimate ejection fractions may also be helpful. Electrocardiograms are useful to identify arrhythmias or ischemic injury but do not accurately assess the severity of pulmonary hypertension or right ventricular dysfunction.

Acute Exacerbations of COPD

Assessment of the patient with COPD exacerbation includes a thorough medical history and a thorough history of the patient's recent COPD history, assessment of oxygenation, physical examination, bedside pulmonary function tests (if possible), assessment of sputum, and chest radiography.

Assessing oxygenation is essential. Although pulse oximetry may identify hypoxemia, it cannot identify hypercapnia or acid-base disturbances. Further, unlike asthma, a correlation between FEV_1 and oxygenation does not exist. Therefore, the spirometric criteria that have been used to eliminate the need for arterial blood gases in asthmatic patients cannot be safely applied to patients with COPD.[10] A partial pressure of oxygen, arterial (PaO_2) of less than 60 mm Hg or an arterial oxygen saturation (SaO_2) of less than 90 percent in room air indicates respiratory failure. In addition, a patient who is hypercapnic or who has a pH of less than 7.30 likely is experiencing a life-threatening episode of ventilatory failure and needs intensive management in the emergency department and in the intensive care unit.

Bedside pulmonary function tests can provide a rapid, objective assessment of patients and serve as a guide to the effectiveness of therapy; however, patient cooperation is essential for these tests to be reliable. Frequently, patients with COPD exacerbation are too dyspneic to cooperate with these tests. As a result, some guidelines do not recommend using these measurements during acute exacerbation.[3-6] If the patient is able to cooperate, a peak expiratory flow rate (PEFR) of less than 100 L per min or an FEV_1 of less than 1.00 L in a patient without chronic severe obstruction indicates a severe exacerbation. Sequential measurements can be very helpful in determining response to therapy. Signs on physical examination and physician estimates of pulmonary function are highly inaccurate.[11] Measurement of FEV_1 is preferred to PEFR, because FEV_1 allows comparison with baseline studies and published guidelines.

Assessment of sputum includes questions about changes in volume and color, especially an increase in purulence. An increase in sputum volume and color changes suggest a bacterial etiology for the exacerbation and indicate a need for antibiotic therapy.[12] Recommendations for obtaining sputum cultures vary among various guidelines.[1-6]

Radiographic abnormalities are common in COPD exacerbation and may elucidate the underlying etiology of the exacerbation, such as pneumonia, or may identify an alternative diagnosis, such as congestive heart failure. Therefore, radiographs should be strongly considered when evaluating a patient with COPD exacerbation.[13]

Electrocardiograms may reveal concurrent disease processes, such as ischemia or acute myocardial infarction, signs of cor pulmonale, and arrhythmias, such as multifocal atrial tachycardia. Theophylline levels should be measured in patients who take theophylline. Other tests, such as complete blood cell counts, electrolytes, B-natriuretic peptide, spiral computed tomography, and D-dimers should be obtained based on the clinical picture.

TREATMENT

Chronic, Compensated COPD

The appropriate and optimal management of decompensated chronic airflow obstruction in an emergency department setting requires an appreciation of chronic day-to-day therapy. Specific management limits further insults to the respiratory system, treats reversible bronchospasm, and prevents or treats complications.

HEALTHY LIFESTYLE   Elements include regular exercise, weight control, and smoking cessation. Smoking cessation is the only therapeutic intervention that can reduce the accelerated decline in lung function.[14] Smoking cessation (and long-term oxygen therapy) has been shown to reduce COPD mortality.[1-6] Pulmonary rehabilitation can improve exercise capacity and quality of life and is recommended in those patients with moderate to severe COPD. Although there is some controversy regarding the pneumococcal vaccine in COPD patients, it is currently recommended by the American Thoracic Society.[2]

OXYGEN   The primary goal of long-term oxygen therapy (LTOT) is to increase baseline PaO_2 to at least 60 mm Hg or an SaO_2 of at least 90 percent at rest. The use of long-term oxygen therapy in patients with chronic respiratory failure has been demonstrated to reduce COPD mortality. Long-term oxygen therapy should be started in patients in whom arterial blood gases demonstrate a PaO_2 of 55 mm Hg or less, an SaO_2 below 88 percent, or a PaO_2 between 56 and 59 mm Hg when signs of pulmonary hypertension, cor pulmonale, or polycythemia are present.[5] Home oxygen therapy accounts for approximately 30 percent of all COPD-related costs in the United States.

PHARMACOTHERAPY   Although there is no evidence that pharmacotherapy alters the progression of COPD, it is used to provide symptomatic relief, control exacerbations, improve quality of life, and improve exercise performance. Inhaled bronchodilators are used on an as-needed basis for mild to moderately obstructed patients with intermittent symptoms or on a regular basis to prevent or decrease symptoms, although they probably only chronically improve FEV_1 by 10 percent in COPD.

β_2-Agonists relax smooth muscle by stimulating β_2-adrenergic receptors. The use of long-acting inhaled β_2-agonists, such as salmeterol and formoterol, may improve overall symptoms and health status.[15] The use of short-acting β_2-agonists also improve exercise capacity but may be less convenient to use.

Anticholinergic agents facilitate bronchodilation by blocking the effect of acetylcholine on muscarinic-3 receptors. In those patients with persistent symptoms, who are refractory to β_2-adrenergic agents, or who are bothered by side effects, ipratropium bromide is the drug of choice. The regular use of inhaled ipratropium also has been shown to improve health status.

Consideration should be given to combining β_2-agonists with ipratropium, because the combination may improve bronchodilation more than either drug alone.[14] With increasing symptoms, even after optimization of the above two classes of bronchodilators, theophylline may be helpful.

Evidence is currently lacking to recommend the use of long-term systemic corticosteroid therapy for all patients with COPD.[14] Only about 20 to 30 percent of patients with COPD improve when given chronic oral steroids. Initiating corticosteroid therapy requires careful analysis so as not to subject a nonresponder to the side effects unnecessarily.

Data from large trials studying the effects of inhaled corticosteroids in COPD showed that regular treatment with inhaled corticosteroids is indicated only for patients with a documented spirometric response to inhaled corticosteroids, those with an FEV_1 of less than 50 percent, or those with predicted and recurrent exacerbations requiring antibiotic treatment or systemic corticosteroids.[5]

Although some studies support the use of theophylline in stable COPD patients, most current COPD guidelines consider it an adjunct therapy.[1-6]

MOBILIZATION OF SECRETIONS   Assurance of generous oral fluid intake and atmospheric humidification, avoidance of antihistamine and decongestant agents, and limitation of antitussive use help mobilize respiratory secretions. The efficacy of specific expectorant products is dubious.

Acute Exacerbations of COPD

The goals of emergency therapy in exacerbation of COPD are to correct tissue oxygenation, alleviate reversible bronchospasm, and treat the underlying etiology of the exacerbation (Table 69-2). Factors that influence therapy in the ED include (1) the patient's mental status; (2) degree of reversible bronchospasm; (3) recent medication usage and evidence of potential toxicity; (4) prior history of exacerbation courses, hospitalization, and intubation; (5) the presence of contraindications to any drug or class of drugs; and (6) specific causes or complications related to the exacerbation.

OXYGEN   The first goal in the treatment of COPD is to correct or prevent life-threatening hypoxemia, aiming for a PaO_2 greater than 60 mm Hg or an SaO_2 greater than 90 percent. This can be accomplished in the ED with any of the following devices: standard dual-prong nasal cannula, simple face mask, Venturi mask, and non-rebreathing mask with reservoir and one-way valve. The need to increase PaO_2 must be balanced against the possibility of producing hypercapnia, so monitoring of oxygenation and CO_2 levels with arterial blood gases is imperative. Improvement after administration of supplemental oxygen may take 20 to 30 min to achieve a steady state. If adequate oxygenation is not achieved or respiratory acidosis ensues, assisted ventilation may be required.

β_2-ADRENERGIC AGONISTS β_2-Agonists and anticholinergic agents are first-line therapies in the management of acute, severe COPD recommended by most guidelines.[1-6] Aerosolized forms, via nebulizer or metered dose inhalers, are preferred because they minimize systemic toxicity, although limited data exist regarding the optimal dose and frequency of administration. According to American Thoracic Society guidelines, β_2-agonist agents may be administered every 30 to 60 min, if tolerated.[2] Nebulized aerosols administered every 20 min may result in more rapid improvement of FEV_1, but the incidence of side effects is greater.[16] Side effects of β_2-agonists include tremor, anxiety, and palpitations. β_2-Agonists should be accompanied by heart monitoring in patients known to have or are suspected of having coexisting heart disease.

ANTICHOLINERGICS   Anticholinergic agents, such as ipratropium and glycopyrrolate, produce similar short-term improvements in airflow obstruction measured by FEV_1 and PEFR, as do β_2-agonists.[3-6] Whereas some guidelines favor β_2-agonists as a first-line therapy, oth-

TABLE 69-2   Summary for Emergency Department Management of Exacerbations in Chronic Obstructive Pulmonary Disease

Assess severity of symptom
   Administer controlled oxygen therapy
   Perform arterial blood gas measurement after 20–30 min if SaO_2 remains
      <90% or if concerned about symptomatic hypercapnia
Administer bronchodilators
   β_2-agonists and/or anticholinergic agents by nebulization or MDI with
      spacer
Consider adding intravenous methylxanthine, if needed
Add corticosteroids
   Oral or intravenous
Consider antibiotics
   If increased sputum volume, change in sputum color, fever, or suspicion of
      infectious etiology of exacerbation
Consider noninvasive mechanical ventilation
Laboratory evaluation
   Chest x-ray
   CBC with differential
   Electrolytes
   Arterial blood gases
   ECG as needed
At all times
   Monitor fluid balance
   Consider subcutaneous heparin (venous thrombosis prophylaxis)
   Identify and treat associated conditions (e.g., heart failure, arrhythmias)
   Closely monitor condition of the patient

Abbreviations: CBC = complete blood cell count; ECG = electrocardiogram; MDI = metered dose inhaler; SaO_2 = arterial oxygen saturation.
Source: Adapted from Pauwels RA, Buist AS, Calverley PM, et al: Global strategy for the diagnosis, management, and prevention of chronic obstructive pulmonary disease. NHLBI/WHO Global Initiative for Chronic Obstructive Lung Disease (GOLD) Workshop summary. *Am J Respir Crit Care Med* 163:1256, 2001.

ers favor anticholinergic agents. Ipratropium bromide given by metered dose inhaler with a spacer or as an inhalant solution by nebulization (0.5 mg or 2.5 mL of the 0.02% inhalant solution) is the usual agent of choice, although aerosolized glycopyrrolate 2 mg in 10 mL of saline, has been shown to be effective. The timing of repeat doses of anticholinergic agents has not been well studied. Side effects are minimal and appear to be limited to dry mouth and an occasional metallic taste.

Evidence regarding the efficacy of the combination of a β_2-adrenergic agent and an anticholinergic agent compared with a single agent alone is conflicting, although many physicians favor using this combination initially and some favor using it if the response to maximal doses of a single bronchodilator is poor.

CORTICOSTEROIDS   The use of a short course (7 to 14 days) of systemic steroids appears more effective than placebo in improving FEV_1 in acute severe exacerbations of COPD, although their role in mild-to-moderate exacerbations needs to be delineated further.[17,18] If used, the optimal effective dose ranges from one to three times the maximal physiologic adrenal secretion rate (i.e., the equivalent of prednisone, 60 to 180 mg per d). Hyperglycemia is the most common adverse effect.

ANTIBIOTICS   All current guidelines recommend antibiotics for the treatment of COPD exacerbation if there is evidence of infection, such as change in volume of sputum and increased purulence of sputum. Saint's meta-analysis demonstrated a small, but statistically significant, benefit for antibiotics in terms of resolution of obstruction and symptoms.[12] The benefits are more apparent in more severe exacerbations.[6] Antibiotic choices should be directed at the most common pathogens known to be associated with COPD exacerbation, namely

Streptococcus pneumoniae, Haemophilus influenzae, and *Moraxella catarrhalis.* There is little evidence regarding the duration of treatment; 3 to 14 days is typical in these studies.

METHYLXANTHINES The role of methylxanthines, such as theophylline and aminophylline, in the treatment of COPD exacerbation remains controversial. Current evidence does not support the routine use of methylxanthines for COPD exacerbations, although most guidelines suggest their use in certain situations, such as severe exacerbation when other therapy has failed or in patients already using methylxanthines who have subtherapeutic drug levels.[3–5] The bronchodilation effect of aminophylline is limited, and its therapeutic range is narrow.

The intravenous loading dose usually required to obtain an initial serum concentration of 8 to 12 μg/mL is 5 to 6 mg/kg ideal body weight in patients not currently receiving the drug. In patients who regularly use theophylline, a mini-loading dose should be administered: (target concentration−currently assayed concentration) × volume of distribution (i.e., 0.5 times ideal body weight in liters). With the mini-load method, the target concentration should be between 10 and 15 μg/mL. The intravenous maintenance infusion rate is 0.2 to 0.8 mg/kg ideal body weight per h. It is important to lower maintenance rates when treating patients with lower clearance rates due to congestive heart failure or hepatic insufficiency and raise maintenance rates in patients with higher clearance rates, such as smokers.

Maintenance theophylline infusion in patients on chronic oral therapy is complicated, because it is difficult to account for enteric drug yet to be absorbed. Loading and maintenance doses may need to be reduced to minimize the risk of "summation toxicity" due to continued enteric absorption. Standard-release preparations may continue to be absorbed for up to 6 h, and sustained-release preparations may require up to 12 h. Therefore, maintenance infusion rates should be reduced for 6 h after ingestion of a standard-release formulation and 12 h after ingestion of a sustained-release preparation (including 24-h release forms). Theophylline and aminophylline should not be given orally in an emergency setting unless decompensation is not severe, alimentary motility is assured, and forthcoming ambulatory care is imminent.

ASSISTED VENTILATION Mechanical ventilation is indicated in patients with COPD exacerbation if there is evidence of respiratory muscle fatigue, worsening respiratory acidosis, deteriorating mental status, and in those with clinically significant hypoxemia refractory to supplemental oxygen by usual techniques (Table 69-3). The main goals of assisted ventilation are to rest ventilatory muscles and to restore gas exchange to a stable baseline.

Noninvasive positive pressure ventilation (NIPPV) can be delivered via a nasal mask, full face mask, or mouthpiece. No particular mode of ventilation or ventilatory device has been shown to be clearly superior. Studies have demonstrated better outcomes in terms of intubation rates, short-term mortality rates, symptomatic improvement, and length of hospitalization in patients with respiratory failure who receive NIPPV.[19] Disadvantages of NIPPV include slower correction of gas-exchange abnormalities, risk of aspiration, inability to control airway secretions directly, and possible complications of gastric distention and skin necrosis. Contraindications to the use of NIPPV include an uncooperative or obtunded patient, inability of the patient to clear airway secretions, hemodynamic instability, respiratory arrest, recent facial or gastroesophageal surgery, burns, poor mask fit, or extreme obesity.

Invasive ventilation should be considered in patients with ventilatory or respiratory failure who do not qualify for NIPPV. The methods most commonly used are assisted control ventilation, pressure support ventilation, or pressure support ventilation in combination with intermittent mandatory ventilation. Adverse events associated with invasive ventilation include pneumonia, barotrauma, and failure to wean.

OTHER OPTIONS There is currently little evidence to support the use of a mixture of helium and oxygen or magnesium in the treatment of acute COPD exacerbation. Factors underlying the exacerbation, comorbidities, and other etiologies of dyspnea should be identified and treated.

Future Considerations and New Therapies

Bronchodilators play an important role in the long-term management of patients with COPD, but they do not alter the progression of COPD. Major advances include the development of long-acting anticholinergic agents, such as tiotropium bromide. Tiotropium bromide has the benefit of once-daily dosing. Inflammation is being investigated more closely in the pathogenesis of COPD, especially the role of neutrophils. Corticosteroids, chemokine (interleukin 8) inhibitors, leukotriene B$_4$ inhibitors, adhesion molecule inhibitors, and phosphodiesterase inhibitors are being studied with the goal of inhibiting neutrophil activity. Surfactant replacement and lung reduction therapies are also under investigation. Evidence suggests that the imbalance between proteases in COPD patients may be restored by inhibiting proteolytic enzymes, such as neutrophil elastase inhibitors, cathepsin inhibitors, matrix metalloproteinase inhibitors, and secretory leukoprotease inhibitors, or by increasing antiproteases, such as α_1-antitrypsin. Evidence also exists that oxidative stress is increased in patients with COPD, and that reactive oxygen species are involved in the pathogenesis of COPD. Therefore, antioxidants such as *N*-acetyl

---

TABLE 69-3 Indications for Invasive Mechanical Ventilation

Severe dyspnea with use of accessory muscles and paradoxical abdominal motion

Respiratory frequency >35 breaths per min

Life-threatening hypoxemia: Pao$_2$ <50 mm Hg (<5.3 kPa) or Pao$_2$/Fio$_2$ <200 mm Hg

Severe acidosis (pH <7.25) and hypercapnia (Paco$_2$ >60 mm Hg or >8.0 kPa)

Respiratory arrest

Somnolence, impaired mental status

Cardiovascular complications (hypotension, shock, heart failure)

NIPPV failure

Abbreviations: Fio$_2$ = fraction of inspired oxygen; NIPPV = noninvasive positive pressure ventilation; Paco$_2$ = partial pressure of carbon dioxide, arterial; Pao$_2$ = partial pressure of oxygen, arterial.

Source: Adapted from Pauwels RA, Buist AS, Calverley PM, et al: Global strategy for the diagnosis, management, and prevention of chronic obstructive pulmonary disease. NHLBI/WHO Global Initiative for Chronic Obstructive Lung Disease (GOLD) Workshop summary. *Am J Respir Crit Care Med* 163:1256, 2001.

TABLE 69-4 Indications for Hospital Admission for Acute Exacerbations of Chronic Obstructive Pulmonary Disease

Marked increase in intensity of symptoms, such as sudden development of resting dyspnea

Severe background of chronic obstructive pulmonary disease

Onset of new physical signs (e.g., cyanosis, peripheral edema)

Failure of exacerbation to respond to initial medical management

Significant comorbidities

Newly occurring arrhythmias

Diagnostic uncertainty

Older age

Insufficient home support

Source: Adapted from Pauwels RA, Buist AS, Calverley PM, et al: Global strategy for the diagnosis, management, and prevention of chronic obstructive pulmonary disease. NHLBI/WHO Global Initiative for Chronic Obstructive Lung Disease (GOLD) Workshop summary. *Am J Respir Crit Care Med* 163:1256, 2001.

TABLE 69-5   Indications for Intensive Care Admission of Patients with Acute Exacerbations of Chronic Obstructive Pulmonary Disease

Severe dyspnea that responds inadequately to initial emergency therapy
Confusion, lethargy, coma
Persistent or worsening hypoxemia: PaO_2 <50 mm Hg (<6.7 kPa)
Severe or worsening hypercapnia: $PaCO_2$ >70 mm Hg (>9.3 kPa)
Severe or worsening respiratory acidosis (pH <7.30) despite supplemental oxygen and NIPPV

Abbreviations: NIPPV = noninvasive positive pressure ventilation; $PaCO_2$ = partial pressure of carbon dioxide, arterial; PaO_2 = partial pressure of oxygen, arterial.
Source: Adapted from Pauwels RA, Buist AS, Calverley PM, et al: Global strategy for the diagnosis, management, and prevention of chronic obstructive pulmonary disease. NHLBI/WHO Global Initiative for Chronic Obstructive Lung Disease (GOLD) Workshop summary. *Am J Respir Crit Care Med* 163:1256, 2001.

cysteine and spin-trap antioxidants such as α-phenyl-*N*-tertbutyl nitrone may be useful. Pulmonary vasodilators, such as prostacyclin analogues, nitric oxide donors, endothelial antagonists, and angiotensin antagonists, are being studied in the hope of preventing the progression of pulmonary hypertension and cor pulmonale. Mucus regulators, such as tachykinin antagonists, sensory neuropeptide-release inhibitors, mediator and enzyme inhibitors, MUC gene suppressors, and mucolytic agents, may inhibit the hypersecretion of mucus, without affecting normal mucus secretion and normal mucociliary clearance.

DISPOSITION

Admission Criteria

Patients who fail to improve adequately or deteriorate despite medical therapy, have significant comorbid illnesses, or are without an intact social support system at home should be hospitalized. Unfortunately, objective criteria regarding hospital admission, observation unit stay, and ED discharge are lacking. The GOLD guidelines offer criteria that may help guide the emergency physician's disposition decision-making process (Tables 69-4 and 69-5). Although Emerman and colleagues found that patients with an $FEV_1 \geq 40$ percent predicted and no clinical evidence of respiratory distress after treatment have a low rate of relapse and may be safely discharged home,[20] current data indicate that 43 percent of patients with COPD exacerbation discharged home from the ED have ongoing symptoms at 2 weeks and 43 percent have a relapse of symptoms.[21] The primary goals of hospitalization are to manage the acute exacerbation, prevent further deterioration, and educate patients about disease management.

Discharge

If the patient is deemed stable enough for discharge to home, the following should be arranged: (1) adequate supply of home oxygen, if needed; (2) adequate and appropriate bronchodilator treatment; (3) consideration of a short course of oral corticosteroids;[18] and (4) a follow-up appointment with their physician.

REFERENCES

1. COPD Guidelines Group of the Standards of Care Committee of the BTS: BTS guidelines for the management of chronic obstructive pulmonary disease. *Thorax* 52(suppl 5):S1, 1997.
2. American Thoracic Society: Standards for the diagnosis and care of patients with chronic obstructive pulmonary disease. *Am J Respir Crit Care Med* 152:S77, 1995.
3. Snow V, Lascher S, Mottur-Pilson C: Evidence base for management of acute exacerbations of chronic obstructive pulmonary disease. *Ann Intern Med* 134:595, 2001.
4. Siafakas NM, Vermeire P, Pride NB, et al: Optimal assessment and management of chronic obstructive pulmonary disease (COPD). The European Respiratory Society Task Force. *Eur Respir J* 8:1398, 1995.
5. Pauwels RA, Buist AS, Calverley PM, et al: Global strategy for the diagnosis, management, and prevention of chronic obstructive pulmonary disease. NHLBI/WHO Global Initiative for Chronic Obstructive Lung Disease (GOLD) Workshop summary. *Am J Respir Crit Care Med* 163:1256, 2001.
6. Bach PB, Brown C, Gelfand SE, McCrory DC: Management of acute exacerbations of chronic obstructive pulmonary disease: A summary and appraisal of published evidence. *Ann Intern Med* 134:600, 2001.
7. Connors AF Jr, Dawson NV, Thomas C, et al: Outcomes following acute exacerbation of severe chronic obstructive lung disease. The SUPPORT investigators (Study to Understand Prognoses and Preferences for Outcomes and Risks of Treatments). *Am J Respir Crit Care Med.* 154:959, 1996. Published erratum: *Am J Respir Crit Care Med* 155:386, 1997.
8. Cydulka RK, McFadden ER Jr, Emerman CL, et al: Patterns of hospitalization in elderly patients with asthma and chronic obstructive pulmonary disease. *Am J Respir Crit Care Med* 156:1807, 1997.
9. Morrison LK, Harrison A, Krishnaswamy P, et al: Utility of a rapid B-natriuretic peptide assay in differentiating congestive heart failure from lung disease in patients presenting with dyspnea. *J Am Coll Cardiol* 39:202, 2002.
10. Emerman CL, Connors AF, Lukens TW, et al: Relationship between arterial blood gases and spirometry in acute exacerbations of chronic obstructive pulmonary disease. *Ann Emerg Med* 18:523, 1989.
11. Emerman CL, Lukens TW, Effron D: Physician estimation of FEV_1 in acute exacerbation of COPD. *Chest* 105:1709, 1994.
12. Saint S, Bent S, Vittinghoff E, Grady D: Antibiotics in chronic obstructive pulmonary disease exacerbations. A meta-analysis. *JAMA* 273:957, 1995.
13. Emerman CL, Cydulka RK: Evaluation of high-yield criteria for chest radiography in acute exacerbation of chronic obstructive pulmonary disease. *Ann Emerg Med* 22:680, 1993.
14. COMBIVENT Inhalation Solution Study Group: Routine nebulized ipratropium and albuterol together are better than either alone in COPD. *Chest* 112:1514, 1997.
15. Boyd G, Morice AH, Pounsford JC, et al: An evaluation of salmeterol in the treatment of chronic obstructive pulmonary disease (COPD). *Eur Respir J* 10:815, 1997.
16. Emerman CL, Cydulka RK: Effect of different albuterol dosing regimens in the treatment of acute exacerbation of chronic obstructive pulmonary disease. *Ann Emerg Med* 29:474, 1997.
17. Singh JM, Palda VA, Stanbrook MB, Chapman KR: Corticosteroid therapy for patients with acute exacerbations of chronic obstructive pulmonary disease. A systematic review. *Arch Intern Med* 162:2527, 2002.
18. Aaron SD, Vandemheen KL, Hebert P, et al: Outpatient oral prednisone after emergency treatment of chronic obstructive pulmonary disease. *New Engl J Med* 348:2618, 2003.
19. Mehta S, Hill NS: Noninvasive ventilation. *Am J Respir Crit Care Med* 163:540, 2001.
20. Emerman CL, Effron D, Lukens TW: Spirometric criteria for hospital admission of patients with acute exacerbation of COPD. *Chest* 99:595, 1991.
21. Kim S, Emerman CE, Cydulka RK, et al: Prospective multicenter study of relapse following treatment for asthma/COPD among adults presenting to the emergency department. *Acad Emerg Med* 8:533, 2001.

70 THE LUNG TRANSPLANT PATIENT
Thomas P. Noeller

Since the first successful single-lung transplant in 1983 and the first successful double-lung transplant in 1986, lung transplantation has become a viable therapeutic modality for end-stage pulmonary disease. Currently, about 75 centers in the United States perform lung transplants, and in 2002 a total of 1042 patients underwent lung transplant nationally.[1] On April 29, 2003, the United Network for Organ Sharing listed 3843 patients on a waiting list for lung transplantation and noted that 481 patients had been removed from a waiting list owing to death during 2002.[1] In 2001, 21 percent of lung transplant recipients were transplanted within 6 months of listing on the waiting list and 38 percent were on the waiting list longer than 2 y before transplant.[2] Overall survival rates are 77 and 42 percent at 1 and 5 years, respectively.[2] The long-term survival rates were slightly higher at centers performing more than 30 lung transplants per year. Single- and double-lung transplants and heart-and-lung transplants are most commonly performed for cystic fibrosis, idiopathic pulmonary fibrosis, and emphysema, including α_1-antitrypsin deficiency.[3] Primary pulmonary hypertension, congenital heart disease, and Eisenmenger's complex also may be indications for heart-and-lung transplantation. Living donor lobar transplantation, performed for 290 patients from 1991 through 2001, primarily for cystic fibrosis, is now an option for some patients.

MANAGEMENT OF PRETRANSPLANT PATIENTS

Pretransplant patients are likely to present with exacerbations of their underlying disease; assessment and management should be targeted to these processes. The transplant coordinator should always be contacted early in the course of evaluation and treatment to aid in timely disposition (Table 70-1).

Important features to note are the respiratory rate, pulse oximetry measurement, and physical findings of cyanosis, diaphoresis, use of accessory muscles, signs of congestive heart failure, and adequacy of peripheral perfusion. Supplemental oxygen should be applied, intravenous access obtained, and the patient placed on a cardiac monitor. A chest radiograph should be obtained to identify infiltrates or pneumothorax, and an arterial blood gas analysis should be performed when adequacy of ventilation is in question. β_2-Agonists, anticholinergics, and antibiotics should be given as indicated.

Although the perioperative use of corticosteroids was formerly considered a contraindication to transplantation, this notion has changed somewhat. A maintenance dose of prednisone, 0.2 to 0.3 mg/kg per d, is acceptable to most centers. If the patient requires a corticosteroid burst or an increase in the maintenance dose to treat an acute exacerbation, the transplant coordinator should be contacted. A dose of prednisone larger than 20 mg per d may result in the patient being suspended from the transplant list until such time that the dose can safely be tapered down to 20 mg per d or less. In primary pulmonary hypertension and Eisenmenger complex, consideration should be given to therapies that may help to decrease pulmonary vascular resistance, such as morphine sulfate, nitrates, and furosemide. For patients with respiratory failure, noninvasive ventilation or endotracheal intubation with mechanical ventilation may be required, thereby increasing the risk of barotrauma. Ventilator dependence has generally been regarded as a relative contraindication to lung transplantation. Successes have been reported, but ventilator-dependent patients have a much higher mortality after transplantation.[4]

Idiopathic pulmonary fibrosis is a common indication for lung transplantation and has a worse 1- and 5-y posttransplant survival compared to other lung diseases. Treatment with high-dose steroids is rarely successful at achieving a remission, and supportive therapy is the mainstay of acute management. The transplant team may recommend cytotoxic drugs, such as cyclophosphamide and azathioprine, for their steroid-sparing effect.

Chronic infection, especially common in patients with cystic fibrosis, is a major issue with regard to eligibility for transplantation. Patients with cystic fibrosis tend to be infected with multiple organisms by the time transplantation is considered. The most common organisms include *Pseudomonas* spp., *Burkholderia cepacia, Aspergillus,* and nontuberculous mycobacteria. *Aspergillus* and mycobacterial infections have not been associated with worse outcomes in posttransplant patients. However, infection with *B. cepacia* and pan-resistant *Pseudomonas* spp. has been associated with poor outcomes and is considered a contraindication to transplantation in some centers. Therefore, emergency physicians need to pay particular attention to infection-control measures and antibiotic selection in pretransplant patients with cystic fibrosis. In general, those patients requiring antibiotics for acute infections require admission for broad spectrum, multiple-drug regimens to prevent the development of pan-resistant strains.

In patients with primary pulmonary hypertension, survival correlates with the New York Heart Association (NYHA) classification. Prostacyclin has been approved for treatment of NYHA class III or IV patients, in whom it has been shown to improve hemodynamics and exercise tolerance and survival. Calcium channel blockers are the main treatment for NYHA class I and II patients. In acute decompensation, morphine, nitrates, and furosemide may reduce pulmonary vascular resistance and improve dyspnea.

MANAGEMENT OF POTENTIAL DONORS

Identification and early management of potential donors have become part of the practice of emergency medicine. The establishment of brain death is generally not done in the ED; however several steps need to be taken to maximize organ retrieval in appropriate patients. Most organ procurement organizations work closely with their local EDs by providing education in the various facets of organ procurement. Early communication with the organ procurement organization is encouraged, because it can help to identify factors that may qualify or disqualify a potential donor, provide assistance in speaking with families about organ donation, and guide the clinicians through the complicated process.

Initial management is focused on maintaining the integrity of potential donor lungs by optimizing hemodynamics and preventing aspiration. Accepting centers generally require a clear chest radiograph, partial pressure of arterial oxygen greater than 450 mm Hg on 100 percent fraction of inspired oxygen, and no obvious infection on bronchoscopic evaluation. Mechanical ventilation should maintain arterial Pa_{O_2} at greater than 80 mm Hg, Pa_{CO_2} between 35 and 45 mm Hg, and a pH between 7.30 and 7.45. Hemodynamics should be monitored, with a desirable central venous pressure greater than 10 mm Hg. If systemic blood pressure cannot be maintained with fluid resuscitation alone without causing pulmonary edema, then dopamine may be used. Transfusions may be used to maintain a hematocrit above 30 percent to optimize tissue oxygenation. However, it is crucial to specify the use of blood that is cytomegalovirus (CMV) negative so as not to infect a CMV-negative recipient. Although these criteria are used to determine acceptability for donation, it has been observed that aggressive management of lung donors generally considered unacceptable produces identical 30-day and 1-year mortality rates among recipients when compared with recipients who received transplants from traditionally acceptable donors.[5]

MANAGEMENT OF POSTTRANSPLANT PATIENTS

Transplant patients are managed by a multidisciplinary team composed of transplant surgeons, pulmonologists, nurse coordinators, pharmacists,

TABLE 70-1 Indications for Hospital Admission

Pretransplant patients
  Respiratory failure
  Infiltrate
  Systemic infection
  Decompensated congestive heart failure or pulmonary edema
  Pneumothorax
Posttransplant patients
  Respiratory failure
  Acute rejection
  Rapidly progressive airflow limitation (FEV_1 fall >10% over 48 h)
  Infiltrate
  Systemic infection
  Febrile neutropenia
  Pneumothorax

Abbreviation: FEV_1 = forced expiratory volume in 1 s.

physical therapists, dietitians, psychologists, and social workers. At each transplant center, a nurse coordinator is on call to address concerns regarding the care of posttransplant patients in the ED. Patients tend to be well educated and well informed about their disease, but the nurse coordinator may be able to provide additional information regarding recent infection history, medication doses, rejection history, and potential complications in a specific patient. Coordinators should always be called early in the course of patient assessment and management.

Posttransplant patients are at risk for several complications related to their underlying disease, medication side effects, and immunocompromised state. Most centers use cyclosporine or tacrolimus, azathioprine or mycophenolate mofetil, and prednisone for maintenance immunosuppression. In addition, prophylaxis against *Pneumocystis carinii* pneumonia is undertaken with trimethoprim-sulfamethoxazole (TMP-SMX).[6] Prophylaxis against herpes simplex virus (HSV) and CMV is indicated based on the specific immunologic status of the donor and the recipient. Inhaled cyclosporine and corticosteroids are used to help prevent the development of bronchiolitis obliterans.

Patients learn to measure their pulmonary function (FEV$_1$, forced expiratory volume in 1 s; and forced vital capacity), systemic blood pressure, and temperature daily. They carry a diary with vital signs, present medications and doses, names of hospital contacts, and guidelines for contacting the nurse coordinator. Because most patients return to their home communities 2 to 3 months after surgery, they may be initially treated and stabilized in their hometown ED before transfer back to the transplant center. Common warning signs of a fever, cough, sputum, or FEV$_1$ decline by more than 10 percent for over 48 h should prompt a call or visit to the transplant center.

The most frequent complications prompting ED presentation are infection and rejection, which can be difficult to differentiate clinically. When these diagnoses are suspected, the patient should be placed in respiratory isolation. Initial assessment is similar to that in the pretransplant patient with regard to stabilization and supportive care. In addition to the standard evaluation of airway, respiratory, and circulatory status, initial assessment should include a chest radiograph, arterial blood gases, FEV$_1$ measurement, complete blood cell count with differential, serum electrolytes, magnesium, creatinine, and appropriate drug levels. Bronchoscopy is necessary to diagnose subclinical rejection and infection. Each transplant center has a protocol concerning bronchoscopy indications.

Early Complications

REJECTION   Acute rejection is common and may occur three to six times in the first postoperative year. After the first year, the frequency of acute rejection decreases, but it can occur for several years after transplant. Signs of rejection include cough, chest tightness, fever ($\geq 0.5°C$ above baseline), hypoxemia, decline in FEV$_1$ (≥ 10 percent), and the development of infiltrates on the chest radiograph. Radiographic abnormalities are less common more than 6 weeks posttransplant, and an acute rejection episode actually may be "radiographically silent" after this period. Clinically, acute rejection may be difficult to distinguish from infection. Therefore, bronchoscopy with transbronchial biopsy is frequently necessary to make the definitive diagnosis. During episodes of acute rejection in patients with single-lung transplants, there is a proportional decrease in blood flow to the transplanted lung, which can be monitored with radionuclide perfusion scans.

Acute rejection is treated with large doses of intravenous methylprednisolone 500 to 1000 mg on day 1, followed by 500 mg IV every day on days 2 an 3. Clinical response is gauged by improvements in oxygenation, spirometry, and radiographic appearance and typically occurs within 24 to 48 h after treatment is initiated. Failure to do so should suggest infection as an alternative diagnosis. After clinical improvement, the maintenance dose of prednisone is increased, with a slow taper back to baseline.

INFECTION   Infectious complications are the most common cause of morbidity and mortality in lung transplant patients.[7–9] Infections may be due to bacteria, fungi, or viruses and most commonly affect the allograft. Bacterial pneumonia is the most common complication in the first 3 months after transplant due to decreased mucociliary clearance, diminished cough reflex, disrupted lymphatics, reperfusion injury, and immunosuppression. Late or recurrent infections are associated with an increased risk of bronchiolitis obliterans. Infectious agents may be present in the donor lung, generating infection in the posttransplant immunosuppressed host. The vast majority of washings from a donor before retrieval will grow at least one organism. Perioperative antibiotics based on culture and sensitivity results have decreased the rate of invasive infection significantly. Infection with panresistant *Pseudomonas* spp. or *B. cepacia* is associated with increased morbidity and mortality and is generally associated with a higher risk of bronchiolitis obliterans. *Pneumocystis carinii* pneumonia is now rare due to common prophylaxis with TMP-SMX.[6] Other commonly encountered infectious agents include gram-negative and gram-positive bacteria, *Mycobacterium* spp., *Aspergillus,* CMV, HSV, and Epstein-Barr virus (EBV).

Cytomegalovirus is the most commonly encountered viral agent implicated in posttransplant pulmonary infection. Its clinical spectrum is broad, ranging from asymptomatic shedding to CMV pneumonitis. The risk of infection is directly related to the donor's and recipient's pretransplant immune status. Donor-positive, recipient-negative status is universally associated with the development of CMV infection in the recipient unless aggressive prophylaxis is undertaken with ganciclovir, acyclovir, and intravenous immunoglobulin. If the recipient is CMV positive, a regimen of ganciclovir followed by acyclovir is used. If the donor and recipient are CMV negative and either the donor or recipient is HSV positive, only acyclovir is used. Cytomegalovirus matching has not altered long-term outcome in lung transplant patients, so most centers will transplant regardless of CMV status.

Cytomegalovirus infections occur most commonly between 14 and 100 days posttransplant and can manifest as either a flulike syndrome or severe multisystem disease, including pneumonitis, hepatitis, bone marrow suppression, gastritis, and colitis. Key laboratory features include neutropenia with or without thrombocytopenia, conversion of anti-CMV IgM to positive, and positive CMV cultures from urine, buffy coat, or bronchoalveolar lavage. Definitive diagnosis of CMV pneumonitis requires histopathologic confirmation of tissue obtained by transbronchial biopsy. After confirmation of diagnosis, treatment with ganciclovir or foscarnet is indicated. Cytomegalovirus pneumonitis may be complicated by acute rejection or by bacterial or fungal pneumonia.

Other viral agents, in particular HSV and EBV, have been implicated in posttransplant infections. Herpes simplex virus has a presentation similar to that of CMV, with diagnosis based on viral culture and differential staining of biopsy specimens. Treatment is with acyclovir. Epstein-Barr virus may present as a mononucleosis-type syndrome but is also associated with the development of posttransplant lymphomas.

Fungal infections are less common but carry a relatively high risk of associated morbidity and mortality. *Candida albicans* is a common airway colonizer but a much less common pathogen. Systemic candidiasis is usually associated with prolonged courses of broad-spectrum antibiotics. The treatment for *C. albicans* is fluconazole, but other *Candida* species may require treatment with amphotericin B. *Aspergillus* spp. also may colonize the airways; this does not require treatment unless associated with invasive disease, as demonstrated by ulcerations, or histologic evidence of invasion. Itraconazole with amphotericin B is frequently successful in treating early infections, but disseminated disease is usually fatal.

Lung transplant patients are subject to bacterial endocarditis because, during the transplant operation, the donor pulmonary veins are attached to the atrium by the establishment of a cuff. Therefore, antimicrobial prophylaxis is necessary before dental and other invasive procedures associated with risk for bacteremia.

OTHER PULMONARY COMPLICATIONS Airway dehiscence and stenosis are now uncommon postoperative complications.[10] Airway dehiscence typically occurs within 3 weeks of transplantation, while the patient is still in the hospital. Bronchial stenosis limits clearance of secretions and leads to pneumonia. Treatment is with stenting or laser therapy. Spontaneous pneumothorax necessitates the placement of a thoracostomy tube and evaluation of the airways by bronchoscopy.

MEDICATION EFFECTS Various induction agents are used in the perioperative and immediate postoperative periods. These agents include high-dose corticosteroids and T-cell lytic therapy with equine-derived antithymocyte globulin, a polyclonal thymocyte preparation, or OKT-3, a murine monoclonal antibody. The most common posttransplant immunosuppressive agents include cyclosporine, azathioprine, and prednisone. Recently, two new drugs have come into common use: tacrolimus and mycophenolate mofetil (MMF). These medications have significant toxicity (see Table 99–2).

Tacrolimus and cyclosporine work in a similar fashion, by inhibiting transcription of genes leading to T-cell activation. Each drug has a narrow therapeutic window, making it necessary to monitor drug levels frequently. Recent studies have suggested that tacrolimus may be more effective than cyclosporine at preventing acute rejection, leading to wider use of this agent in immunosuppressive regimens.[11]

Mycophenolate mofetil inhibits lymphocyte proliferation by interfering with purine synthesis. It has been compared with azathioprine, the immunosuppressive mechanism of which is not entirely known. Recent trials have suggested superiority of MMF over azathioprine in preventing acute rejection episodes and possibly decreasing the incidence and severity of bronchiolitis obliterans.[11]

Glucocorticoids and cyclosporine can exacerbate glucose intolerance, worsen osteoporosis, and cause myopathy and systemic hypertension. Cyclosporine and tacrolimus have similar side-effect profiles. Commonly, chronic cyclosporine or tacrolimus use at the levels employed in lung transplant immunosuppression results in renal insufficiency by decreasing renal blood flow and by a direct effect on the renal tubules, thereby causing hyperkalemia and hypomagnesemia. Nonsteroidal anti-inflammatory drugs should be avoided, because these will act synergistically with cyclosporine to further reduce glomerular filtration. Neutropenia often may result from azathioprine or CMV infection. The primary side effects of MMF are gastrointestinal.

Drugs that are metabolized by the P-450 system will interact with cyclosporine and tacrolimus metabolism (see Table 99–3). Drugs that induce these enzymes (e.g., phenytoin, rifampin, and phenobarbital) may lower cyclosporine and tacrolimus levels acutely, possibly precipitating rejection. Drugs that inhibit cyclosporine and tacrolimus metabolism (e.g., erythromycin, ketoconazole, cimetidine, and the calcium channel blockers) may elevate levels into the toxic range and should be avoided unless appropriate changes in dosing are made to compensate. Azathioprine-induced bone marrow suppression can be enhanced with concomitant use of allopurinol. Mycophenolate mofetil absorption may be affected by antacids and cholestyramine, and renal excretion may be affected by competing drugs, such as acyclovir and ganciclovir, in the setting of renal insufficiency.

Late Complications

BRONCHIOLITIS OBLITERANS The most frequent cause of death after the second posttransplant year is bronchiolitis obliterans, which is characterized by chronic allograft dysfunction and airflow limitation.[12] Current evidence suggests that chronic rejection plays the most important role in the development of bronchiolitis obliterans, but other factors, such as CMV infection, toxic fume inhalation, and chronic foreign body exposure caused by abnormal mucociliary clearance, may contribute. Diagnostically, the yield from bronchoscopy and biopsy is low. Therefore, diagnosis rests on clinical criteria (i.e., ≤ 20 percent fall in FEV_1 without any other identifiable cause). Be-

cause the large airways become bronchiectatic as the small airways are obliterated, episodes of bacterial bronchitis are common. Typically the chest radiograph is clear of infiltrates. Current treatment for bronchiolitis obliterans is augmentation of immunosuppression, including high-dose steroids. The prevalence of bronchiolitis obliterans in long-term survivors is 20 to 50 percent. The course of the disease is highly variable, with some patients stabilizing at a lower level of pulmonary function and others progressing to respiratory failure and death.

POSTTRANSPLANT LYMPHOPROLIFERATIVE DISEASE Posttransplant lymphoproliferative disease (PTLD) can be a consequence of T-cell suppression with long-term cyclosporine use. The overall incidence in lung transplant patients is approximately 8 percent. The disease tends to occur with primary EBV infection after lung transplant. Because younger patients are more likely to be EBV negative at the time of transplantation, they tend to develop EBV infection and PTLD at a higher rate, especially among Caucasian males.[13] Presenting features include isolated lymphadenopathy, painful otitis media (secondary to tonsillar involvement), or a viral-like syndrome. The occurrence of PTLD within 1 year of transplantation is usually localized and can be successfully treated with reduced immunosuppression and high-dose acyclovir, with a relatively good prognosis. In contrast, PTLD after 1 year tends to be disseminated, unresponsive to treatment, and usually fatal.

REFERENCES

1. United Network for Organ Sharing: Home page. Accessed on April 30, 2003. Available at: www.unos.org.
2. Organ Procurement and Transplantation Network: Data: 2002 Annual Report. Available at: www.optn.org/data/annualReport.asp. Accessed on April 30, 2003.
3. DeMeo DL, Ginns LC: Clinical status of lung transplantation. *Transplantation* 72:1713, 2001.
4. Meyers BF, Lynch JP, Battafarano RJ, et al: Lung transplantation is warranted for stable, ventilator-dependent recipients. *Ann Thorac Surg* 70:1675, 2000.
5. Straznicka M, Follette DM, Eisner MD, et al: Aggressive management of lung donors classified as unacceptable: Excellent recipient survival one year after transplantation. J *Thorac Cardiovasc Surg* 124:250, 2002.
6. Fishman JA: Prevention of infection caused by *Pneumocystis carinii* in transplant recipients. *Clin Infect Dis* 33:1397, 2001.
7. Alexander BD, Tapson VF: Infectious complications of lung transplantation. *Transpl Infect Dis* 3:128, 2001.
8. Speich R, Van der Bij W: Epidemiology and management of infections after lung transplantation. *Clin Infect Dis* 33(suppl 1):S58, 2001.
9. Catalla R, Leaf HL: Aspects of pulmonary infections after solid organ transplantation. *Curr Infect Dis Rep* 2:201, 2000.
10. Alvarez A, Algar J, Santos F, et al: Airway complications after lung transplantation: A review of 151 anastomoses. *Eur J Cardiothorac Surg* 19:381, 2001.
11. Speich R, Boehler A, Zalunardo MP, et al: Improved results after lung transplantation—Analysis of factors. *Swiss Med Wkly* 131:238, 2001.
12. Estenne M, Hertz MI: Bronchiolitis obliterans after human lung transplantation. *Am J Respir Crit Care Med* 166:440, 2002.
13. Dharnidharka VR, Tejani AH, Ho PL, Harmon WE: Post-transplant lymphoproliferative disorders in the United States: Young Caucasian males are at highest risk. *Am J Transpl* 2:993, 2002.

71

PULMONARY IMAGING
Janet M. Poponick

Imaging of the chest is common practice in the evaluation of patients with dyspnea, chest pain, or trauma. This chapter reviews the use of plain chest radiography, ventilation-perfusion scans, computed tomography, and thoracic ultrasonography in the ED. The value of an imaging study depends on the technical quality of the procedure and the ability of the physician to interpret the image. Although many studies and findings may have excellent interobserver reliability, others do not. Thus, clinical decisions should be based on knowledge of the value and limitations of image interpretation.

PLAIN RADIOGRAPHY

Chest radiography, which is the most commonly ordered radiologic examination, evaluates the lung parenchyma, cardiac and mediastinal size, and the bony structures of the chest wall. The examination is preferably done in the radiology department with the patient in the standing position with the x-ray beam passing posterior to anterior [posterior-anterior (PA) view]. The patient must be able to take a deep breath and hold while the picture is taken. A "good inspiration" is defined as visualizing the ninth rib above the diaphragm. Adding the lateral film visualizes the posterior lung bases and the retrosternal area, and also helps to localize infiltrates and masses anatomically.

For unstable patients, portable chest radiography is performed at the bedside, with patients sitting upright. Portable chest radiography is limited by the low power of the equipment and variations in radiographic technique. The bedside study is obtained as an anterior-posterior (AP) view, with the x-ray beam passing anterior to posterior, which magnifies the mediastinal structures. For a trauma victim on a backboard, the portable film may be more difficult to interpret. Skinfolds and clothing under a patient may mimic a pneumothorax. In the supine position, air rises anteriorly, making the diagnosis of a small pneumothorax very difficult.[1] Fluid collections layer posteriorly in supine patients, causing a diffuse haziness in the lung fields, which can be confused with infiltrate or contusion. The magnification of the mediastinal structures produced by AP imaging may mimic a mediastinal hematoma suggesting aortic injury. Therefore, chest radiographs are limited by a patient's overall condition, the patient's ability to cooperate with directions, and the technique chosen. The PA and lateral chest radiographs remain the best views.

Occasionally, other techniques and views may be useful. While inspiratory and expiratory chest radiographs are equally sensitive for pneumothorax detection, an expiratory film may accentuate a free air-lung interface, enabling the diagnosis of a small pneumothorax not seen on the inspiratory view.[2] In suspected foreign-body aspiration, the expiratory film may show hyperinflation on the affected side as air is trapped behind the foreign body. Lateral decubitus views can be used to demonstrate a freely flowing pleural effusion with the affected side down and can visualize a small pneumothorax with the affected side up. Apical lordotic views can be used to better visualize the lung apices in cases with possible infiltrate or tumor in that region.

The chest radiograph should be systematically analyzed so as not to miss key information. Specific abnormalities to note on the chest radiograph are pulmonary edema, infiltrates, lung nodules and masses, hilar size and contour, cardiac size and configuration, pleural effusions, and pneumothorax. Identify the study by patient name to ensure that the radiograph is of the correct patient. Assess the technique and the quality of the study. In a good-quality study, the trachea is visible in the midline, the medial borders of the clavicle are centrally located over the superior mediastinum, and the thoracic spine is visible through the mediastinal structures. Identify and note the positioning of all lines, the endotracheal tube, and the nasogastric tube. The trachea should be followed to the left and right main-stem bronchi and to the mediastinal structures. Look at the mediastinum for evidence of free air, for density behind the heart, and for cardiac size (which should be less than 55 percent of the thoracic size on the erect view and less than 58 percent on the supine view). Assess position of the diaphragms, looking at position, contour, and subdiaphragmatic free air: the right hemidiaphragm should be slightly elevated when compared with the left (0.5 to 2.5 cm is normal). Assess the lung fields and pleura, looking for masses, infiltrates, free air, or effusions. Finally, assess the soft tissue and bones, looking for subcutaneous air or fractures.

Aortic injuries are often suspected in the trauma patient with a deceleration mechanism of injury. Radiographic findings of a mediasti-

nal hematoma have traditionally been used as a screening study for aortic injury: mediastinal widening, deviation of the nasogastric tube or endotracheal tube to the right, loss of aortic knob contour, and apical capping. While mediastinal widening is often subjectively estimated, a mediastinal width of greater than 8 cm at the carina, or a mediastinal width at the carina of greater than 25% of the thoracic diameter have been commonly used to identify a wide mediastinum. Because of patient position and technique, supine portable AP chest radiographs often have a wide mediastinum that is normal when the chest radiograph is obtained by upright PA technique. A reverse Trendelenburg radiograph is helpful in this situation because tilting the bed to 45 degrees approximates the anatomy of an upright radiograph.[3] This technique can be used in the trauma resuscitation room while the patient is fully immobilized by elevating the head of the stretcher 45 degrees. This technique reduces the need for further aortic studies by about 25 percent.

Pneumothorax may be difficult to visualize in the supine position due to air layering anteriorly. A pneumothorax is usually visualized and its size reasonably well estimated on the upright PA chest radiograph.[4] If visible on the supine view, the size of a pneumothorax can also be estimated on a supine film by using the average intrapleural distance and a nomogram.[5]

VENTILATION-PERFUSION SCANS

The ventilation-perfusion (V/Q) scan is often the initial screening test for patients with suspected pulmonary embolism (PE).[6-8] The study has a low incidence of adverse reactions, is noninvasive, and requires little advance patient preparation.[6]

The V/Q scan is a two-step process. First, the perfusion study is performed in which technetium-99m (^{99m}Tc)-macroaggregated albumin is injected intravenously and becomes trapped within the pulmonary circulation. Images are obtained with the patient in multiple positions. If the perfusion study is normal, the ventilation portion of the test may be avoided.[6,9] The ventilation portion of the examination is performed with the patient breathing an aerosolized solution of ^{99m}Tc diethylenetriaminepentaacetic acid (DTPA). The aerosol is deposited deep into the lungs in proportion to alveolar ventilation. Images are obtained from different projections. Procedural problems arise when a patient is unable to lie still. The ventilation study may be limited if a patient cannot take a deep breath, follow instructions, or is on a ventilator. A problem with central deposition of the aerosol may occur in patients with chronic obstructive pulmonary disease. Newer agents, such as Tc99m Technegas, which distribute more diffusely to all areas of lung ventilation, have been developed.[6]

Diagnosis of PE on V/Q scan is based on documenting perfusion defects in an area of normal ventilation, a mismatched defect. Perfusion defects in areas of associated ventilation abnormalities, or matched defects, may be seen with parenchymal lung disease, making interpretation difficult. The V/Q scan is correlated with the chest radiograph and assigned one of three readings: normal or near-normal, high probability, and nondiagnostic.[6] The high probability scan is one with large segmental mismatches (intact ventilation but absent perfusion). The nondiagnostic category has both perfusion and ventilation abnormalities, which are neither normal nor high probability. This new system of V/Q reporting is less cumbersome than previous systems, which used high, intermediate, and low probability categories developed from the Prospective Investigation of Pulmonary Embolus Diagnosis (PIOPED) study.[10]

The test characteristics (sensitivity and specificity) of the V/Q scan vary according to the interpretation and the utility of this test depends on the pretest clinical suspicion of PE.[8,9] A V/Q scan result other than normal or near-normal has a sensitivity of 98 percent [95% CI, 95 to 99%] for PE. Thus a normal or near-normal V/Q scan excludes PE and is sufficient to withhold further diagnostic study or treatment. The PIOPED study found that a normal V/Q scan had a 4 percent overall prevalence of PE found on angiography.[10] But perhaps more importantly, patients in this category were followed and had no demonstrable morbidity or mortality. Conversely, a high-probability V/Q scan has a specificity of 98 percent (95% CI; 96 to 99%); this result is sufficient to diagnose and treat PE. The PIOPED study found that a high-probability V/Q scan had an 87 percent overall prevalence of PE found on angiography.[10] Unfortunately, 50 to 70 percent of V/Q scans fall into the nondiagnostic category. For this group, the next diagnostic test would be pulmonary angiography, which would identify PE in approximately 25 percent of cases.[10]

PULMONARY ANGIOGRAPHY

Pulmonary angiography remains the gold standard for accurately diagnosing PE.[6,8] A pulmonary angiogram is performed by a flexible catheter advanced from a peripheral large vein, typically the femoral vein, through the right atrium and ventricle, and into the pulmonary artery. Selective injections of contrast media are made into the lobar pulmonary arteries by using the results of the V/Q scan to guide which lobar arteries should be inspected first. A PE is definitely identified by an intraluminal filling defect in two views or an abrupt cutoff of dye. Narrowing or luminal irregularities can be caused by other processes and are not considered diagnostic for PE.

In the PIOPED study, pulmonary angiography had good interobserver reliability: review of study angiograms by another radiologist reached the same diagnosis in 92 percent of cases. Interobserver agreement was best for lobar (98 percent) and segmental (90 percent) PE. However, at the subsegmental level, interobserver agreement was only 66 percent.[11] Despite this variation, pulmonary angiography remains the gold standard to which newer technologies in CT and magnetic resonance imaging (MRI) are compared.

Complications of pulmonary angiography include (1) fatalities in 0.5 percent; (2) major nonfatal complications such as renal failure, significant hematoma, or respiratory distress in 17 percent; and (3) minor complications such as angina, urticaria, or bronchospasm in 5 percent. Those with a known left bundle-branch block require a temporary pacemaker during the procedure to avoid complete heart block. Those with known renal insufficiency should be adequately hydrated before and after the procedure. Disadvantages of the procedure include patient discomfort, high cost, and the need for an experienced invasive radiologist. Newer noninvasive techniques are replacing pulmonary angiography in many centers.

COMPUTED TOMOGRAPHY

CT provides sharp cross-sectional anatomic displays, which enable identification of fluid collections and distinction between soft tissue structures. The chest CT eliminates overlap of tissues and delineates mediastinal structures very well. Chest CT is usually obtained with intravenous radiocontrast agents. Improved computer technology has enhanced the ability to obtain good quality scans in a short period of time. The current programs have made it possible to evaluate pulmonary nodules and interstitial lung disease more accurately.[12,13] Computer programs using helical CT scans allow accurate airway visualization, similar to a bronchoscopy.[7] In the ED, helical CT scans are useful in assessing the mediastinum of a patient with blunt trauma for aortic injury, in assessing the patient with a possible aortic dissection, or evaluating the patient with pulmonary embolism. The disadvantages of chest CT include cost, radiation exposure, and adverse reactions to intravascular radiocontrast media. Transporting the unstable patient should be done with cardiac monitoring and appropriate personnel.

Blunt trauma to the chest and abdomen often requires further evaluation by CT.[14] In many cases, pneumothorax is diagnosed by looking at the upper cuts of the abdominal CT scan, often identifying a small pneumothorax not seen on supine chest radiograph.[1,15] The risk of progression is small and most small (minuscule) and moderate (anterior) radiographically occult pneumothoraces can be managed without initial placement of a thoracostomy tube if the patient is not to undergo positive pressure ventilation.[16]

Helical CT scanning with intravenous radiocontrast can be useful to evaluate trauma patients for possible aortic injury. Some investigators recommend helical CT for all patients with high-speed deceleration injury even if the initial chest radiograph is normal because approximately 50 percent of such patients with a normal chest radiograph have been found to have multiple injuries on CT scan.[17]

Helical CT scan of the chest is helpful in patients with signs and symptoms of aortic dissection: an accurate diagnosis of dissection will be obtained in more than 96 percent of such patients.[14] Helical CT scan can accurately identify dissection by visualizing an intimal flap with opacification of the true and false lumens. In patients with type B (descending aorta) dissection, no other study is necessary. A disadvantage of helical CT scan in type A (ascending aorta) dissection is that aortography is still required to assess the aortic valve and major arterial vessels prior to surgery.

In many centers, the helical CT scan has become the initial noninvasive test for the evaluation of possible PE.[7,8,18] The helical CT scan can be performed in minutes, provides imaging of other pulmonary disorders that may produce dyspnea, has overall good test characteristics (86 percent sensitivity and 93 percent specificity), and has a very low frequency of nondiagnostic or uninterpretable studies (less than 8 percent).[8,18] The disadvantages of helical CT include the use of radiocontrast media, radiation exposure, and the special expertise needed to interpret the test. In patients with abnormal chest radiographs and underlying pulmonary disease, the V/Q scan is usually nondiagnostic and the helical CT scan is a cost-effective means of evaluating such patients.

After intravenous injection of approximately 120 mL of radiocontrast dye, the scan is performed from the aortic arch to the diaphragms. Patients must be able to hold their breath, typically for 20 to 24 s, although faster CT scanners may require only 10 s of breath-holding to image. Breath holding may be difficult for dyspneic patients and motion artifact leads to a nondiagnostic study in 2 to 4 percent. While intravenous radiocontrast dye may be a disadvantage, it can also be used to scan for deep venous thrombosis (DVT) by obtaining CT cuts from the knees to the mid-abdomen. The combined helical CT scan of the chest and contrast venography of the lower extremities is convenient and easy to do while the patient is in the radiology suite.[18]

An acute embolus is diagnosed when thrombus is seen central within the vessel with distention of the involved vessel. Chronic emboli are eccentric and contiguous with the vessel wall.[18] Interpretations of scans are extremely accurate for central embolus (sensitivity approaching 100 percent), but significantly less at the subsegmental level (sensitivity 53 to 91 percent).[8] The prevalence and clinical consequence of these small subsegmental PE among outpatients is unknown.

There is still debate over the use of helical CT scan or V/Q scan as the initial noninvasive test for evaluation of PE. Both a normal or near-normal V/Q lung scan or normal helical CT scan have excellent sensitivities and clinically exclude PE. Because of the large number of nondiagnostic V/Q lung scans seen in patients with underlying lung disease or radiographic infiltrates, the CT scan may be the appropriate first test in such patients.

THORACIC ULTRASONOGRAPHY

Thoracic ultrasonography can be used to image pleural diseases (effusion, pneumothorax), parenchymal lung diseases (pneumonia, tumors), and chest wall problems (tumor, rib fracture), and to assess diaphragmatic movement.[19] Ultrasonography is less expensive and more conveniently brought to the patient than CT. Ultrasonography provides real-time immediate images as opposed to other imaging modalities.

Ultrasonography can be used to guide placement of drains, aspirations, and biopsies. As with other ultrasonographic applications, operator technique and the quality of the interpretation is key to overall accuracy.

In the ED, one application of bedside thoracic ultrasonography is to detect traumatic pneumothorax and hemothorax in the supine patient. The ultrasonographic viewing areas for a pneumothorax are the anterior second to fourth intercostal spaces and the sixth to eighth intercostal spaces in the midaxillary line on both the right and left sides for a total of four imaging areas. Pneumothorax is identified by disappearance of lung sliding with respiration and loss of the comet-tail artifact at the pleural interface. The ultrasonographic viewing areas for a hemothorax (pleural fluid) are the right and left intercostal oblique views. Fluid in the pleural space was identified as an anechoic space distal to the hyperechoic line representing the diaphragm. Bedside ultrasonography has a sensitivity approaching 100 percent in detecting traumatic pneumothorax and a sensitivity of approximately 96 percent in detecting traumatic hemothorax.[20,21]

MAGNETIC RESONANCE ANGIOGRAPHY

Recent improvements in technology make magnetic resonance angiography (MRA) a possibility in the evaluation of patients with PE.[7] The focus has been on the development of a fast, three-dimensional gadolinium-enhanced scan, which has been reliable in small studies to the segmental vessels (negative predictive value 100 percent). DVT may also be assessed at the same time, similar to the protocol described using CT angiography. For those with CT contrast allergy or renal insufficiency, MRA is a promising alternative for evaluation of PE.

REFERENCES

1. Holmes JF, Brant WE, Bogren HG, et al: Prevalence and importance of pneumothoraces visualized on abdominal computed tomographic scan in children with blunt trauma. *J Trauma* 50:516, 2001.
2. Seow A, Kazerooni EA, Pernicano PG, Neary M: Comparison of upright inspiratory and expiratory chest radiographs for detecting pneumothoraces. *AJR* 166:313, 1996.
3. Barker DE, Crabtree JD, White JE, et al: Mediastinal evaluation utilizing the reverse Trendelenburg radiograph. *Am Surg* 65:484, 1999.
4. Collins CD, Lopez A, Mathie A, et al: Quantification of pneumothorax size on chest radiographs using interpleural distances: Regression analysis based on volume measurements from helical CT. *AJR* 165:1127, 1995.
5. Choi, BG, Park SH, Yun EH, et al: Pneumothorax size: Correlation of supine anteroposterior with erect posteroanterior chest radiographs. *Radiology* 209:567, 1998.
6. Worsley DF, Alavi A: Radionuclide imaging of acute pulmonary embolism. *Radiol Clin North Am* 39:1035, 2001.
7. Maki DD, Gefter WB, Alavi A: Recent advances in pulmonary imaging. *Chest* 116:1388, 1999.
8. Kline JA, Johns KL, Colucciello SA, Israel EG: New diagnostic tests for pulmonary embolism. *Ann Emerg Med* 35:168, 2000.
9. Miniati M, Pistolesi M, Marini C, et al: Value of perfusion lung scan in the diagnosis of pulmonary embolism: Results of the Prospective Investigative Study of Acute Pulmonary Embolism Diagnosis (PISA-PED). *Am J Respir Crit Care Med* 154:1387, 1996.
10. PIOPED Investigators: Value of ventilation/perfusion scan in acute pulmonary embolism: Results of the Prospective Investigation of Pulmonary Embolism Diagnosis (PIOPED). *JAMA* 263:2753, 1990.
11. Stein PD, Henry JW, Gottschalk A: Reassessment of pulmonary angiography for the diagnosis of pulmonary embolism: Relation of interpreter agreement to the order of the involved pulmonary arterial branch. *Radiology* 210:689, 1999.
12. Griffin CB, Primack SL: High-resolution CT: Normal anatomy, techniques, and pitfalls. *Radiol Clin North Am* 39: 1073, 2001.
13. Collins J: CT signs and patterns of lung disease. *Radiol Clin North Am* 39: 1115, 2001.
14. Novelline RA, Rhea JT, Rao PM, Stuk JL: Helical CT in emergency radiology. *Radiology* 213:321, 1999.
15. Exadaktylos AK, Sclabas G, Schmid SW, et al: Do we really need routine computed tomographic scanning in the primary evaluation of blunt chest trauma in patients with "normal" chest radiograph? *J Trauma* 51: 1173, 2001.
16. Wolfman NT, Myers WS, Glauser SJ, et al: Validity of CT classification on management of occult pneumothorax: A prospective study. *AJR* 171:1317, 1998.
17. Demetriades D, Gomez H, Velmahos GC, et al: Routine helical computed tomographic evaluation of the mediastinum in high-risk blunt trauma patients. *Arch Surg* 133:1084, 1998.
18. Garg K: CT of pulmonary thromboembolic disease. *Radiol Clin North Am* 40:111, 2002.
19. Koh DM, Burke S, Davies N, Padley SP: Transthoracic US of the chest: Clinical uses and applications. *Radiographics* 22:e1, 2002.
20. Rowan KR, Kirkpatrick AW, Liu D, et al: Traumatic pneumothorax detection with thoracic US: Correlation with chest radiography and CT-Initial experience. *Radiology* 225:210, 2002.
21. Ma OJ, Mateer JR: Trauma ultrasound examination versus chest radiography in the detection of hemothorax. *Ann Emerg Med* 29:312, 1997.

ACUTE ABDOMINAL PAIN
E. John Gallagher

SCOPE AND DEFINITIONS

Acute abdominal pain is commonly defined as pain of less than 1 week's duration.[1] This chapter discusses nontraumatic acute abdominal pain in postpubescent males and females. Abdominal pain in women in the third trimester of pregnancy or the first month postpartum is discussed in Chaps. 102, 105.

EPIDEMIOLOGY

Data from the U.S. National Center for Health Statistics indicate that stomach and abdominal pain was the principal reason offered by patients for visiting EDs in 2000 (annual incidence approximately 63/1000 ED visits).[2] Admission rates for abdominal pain vary markedly, ranging from 18 to 42 percent, with rates as high as 63 percent reported in patients over 65 years of age.

PATHOPHYSIOLOGY

Abdominal pain is traditionally divided into three categories: visceral, parietal, and referred. In general, visceral (autonomic) and parietal (somatic) are considered the two basic causes of abdominal pain. Referred pain can be considered separately as a cortical misperception of either visceral or parietal afferent stimuli. Although each type of pain is thought to have a different neuropathophysiology, the categories are not entirely discrete. For example, visceral pain often blends with parietal pain as a pathologic process evolves. Still, these distinctions are clinically useful ways of thinking about abdominal pain.

Visceral Pain

Visceral abdominal pain is usually caused by stretching of fibers innervating the walls or capsules of hollow or solid organs, respectively. Less commonly, it is caused by early ischemia or inflammation. Severity ranges from a steady ache or vague discomfort to excruciating or colicky pain. Because the visceral afferents follow a segmental distribution, visceral pain can be localized by the sensory cortex to an approximate spinal cord level determined by the embryologic origin of the organ involved. For example, foregut organs (stomach, duodenum, biliary tract) produce pain in the epigastric region; midgut organs (most small bowel, appendix, cecum) cause periumbilical pain; and hindgut organs (most of colon, including sigmoid) as well as the intraperitoneal portions of the genitourinary tract cause pain initially in the suprapubic or hypogastric area.

Because intraperitoneal organs are bilaterally innervated, stimuli are sent to both sides of the spinal cord, causing intraperitoneal visceral pain to be felt in the midline, independent of its right- or left-sided anatomic origin. For example, stimuli from visceral fibers in the wall of the appendix enter the spinal cord at about T10. When obstruction causes appendiceal distention in early appendicitis, pain is initially perceived as midline periumbilical area, corresponding roughly to the location of the T10 cutaneous dermatome.

Parietal Pain

Parietal or somatic abdominal pain is caused by irritation of fibers that innervate the parietal peritoneum, usually the portion covering the anterior abdominal wall. Because parietal afferent signals are sent from a specific area of peritoneum, parietal pain—in contrast to visceral pain—can be localized to the dermatome superficial to the site of the painful stimulus. As the underlying disease process evolves, the symptoms of visceral pain give way to the signs of parietal pain, causing tenderness and guarding. As localized peritonitis develops further, rigidity and rebound appear.

Referred Pain

Referred pain is felt at a location distant from the diseased organ. Similar to visceral pain, and in contrast to parietal pain, referred pain produces symptoms, not signs. Unlike visceral pain, referred pain is usually ipsilateral to the involved organ and is felt in the midline only if the pathologic process is also located in the midline. This is because referred pain, in contrast to visceral pain, is not mediated by fibers providing bilateral innervation to the cord. Similar to visceral pain, referred pain patterns are based upon developmental embryology. For example, the ureter and the testes were once anatomically contiguous, and therefore share the same segmental innervation, supplying afferent fibers to the lower thoracic and upper lumbar segments of the spinal cord. Thus acute ureteral obstruction is often associated with ipsilateral testicular pain. Other sites of referred pain reflect similar dermatomal sharing, providing explanations for otherwise puzzling associations, e.g., supra- or subdiaphragmatic irritation and ipsilateral supraclavicular or shoulder pain; gynecologic pathology and back or proximal lower extremity pain; biliary tract disease and right infrascapular pain; and myocardial ischemia and midepigastric, neck, jaw, or upper extremity pain.

CLINICAL FEATURES

Conceptual Framework

CLASSIFICATION   The classification scheme divides abdominal pain into two main categories: Intraabdominal (i.e., arising from within the abdominal cavity or retroperitoneum) and extraabdominal. Intraabdominal causes are divided by organ system into the "3-G's": GI (gastrointestinal), GU (genitourinary), and GYN (gynecologic), plus a fourth, less common but often catastrophic group of VASCULAR emergencies. Each of these four is further subdivided into specific diagnoses within that organ system. Pain of extraabdominal origin, which is substantially less common, is similarly divided into four broad etiologic categories of cardiopulmonary, abdominal wall, toxic-metabolic, and neurogenic. A systematic evaluation is necessary in the assessment of acute abdominal pain.

Finally, nonspecific abdominal pain (NSAP), which is the most common cause of abdominal pain among ED patients, is listed as a third category. Nonspecific abdominal pain stands alone since it is not known to what extent it may represent an underlying intra- vs. extraabdominal problem.

ABDOMINAL TOPOGRAPHY   By combining the four-quadrant approach traditionally used by U.S. physicians with selected aspects of a strategy widely employed throughout Europe and Asia, a simple model of abdominal topography can be developed. In addition to the four standard quadrants (RUQ, RLQ, LUQ, LLQ), this model includes four areas of the abdomen that are not discrete, but rather constitute combinations of all or part of two or more quadrants: (1) upper half of

colicky

abdomen (UHA), which includes an area of pain as small as the mid-epigastrium, or as large as the RUQ + LUQ combined; (2) lower half of abdomen (LHA), which similarly includes an area of pain as small as the midhypogastrium or as large as the RLQ + LLQ combined; (3) central (CTL), which includes an area of pain composed of the centermost "quarters" of all four discrete quadrants, such that carving out these areas from each quadrant defines a periumbilical or central quadrant; and (4) generalized (GEN), which includes poorly localized pain encompassing much, perhaps most, of the abdomen, including at least some portion of all four discrete quadrants.

This topographic configuration incorporates both the early (visceral, poorly localized) and late (parietal, better localized) pain of an evolving intraabdominal pathological process, as well as the more generalized pain associated with toxic-metabolic derangements.

However, the association between the location of overlying pain or tenderness and underlying disease is so variable that about one case of abdominal pain in every three that comes to operation presents in a fashion that clinicians retrospectively regard as atypical. Failure to appreciate this may represent the largest single reason that error in the clinical diagnosis of abdominal pain is so common.

Historical Features

Historical data can be conveniently divided into attributes of pain, associated symptoms, and past history.

PAIN ATTRIBUTES   The principal characteristics of abdominal pain include location, quality, severity, onset, duration, aggravating and alleviating factors, and change in any of these features over time.

ASSOCIATED SYMPTOMS   These can be subdivided into one of the four main organ systems associated with intraabdominal pain.

Gastrointestinal Symptoms   Anorexia, nausea, and vomiting (unless bloody) are among the least helpful symptoms in altering the conditional probability that a patient does or does not have a GI cause of abdominal pain. For example, vomiting has been reported in over 40 percent of patients with salpingitis, and in over 60 percent of patients with renal colic. Lower GI symptoms such as nonbloody diarrhea or constipation are similarly too insensitive and nonspecific to significantly alter the probability of a GI cause of abdominal pain.

Genitourinary Symptoms   The hallmark of abdominal pain of GU origin is the concomitant development of some, often subtle, alteration in micturition, e.g., dysuria, frequency, urgency, hematuria, incomplete emptying, or incontinence (usually overflow). Non-GU pathology may develop in organs contiguous to the GU system, giving the appearance of an intrinsic GU problem. For example, an inflamed appendix lying across the bladder may cause urinary frequency.

Gynecologic Symptoms   Distinguishing GI from GYN causes of acute abdominal pain is one of the most challenging clinical dilemmas in emergency practice. A thorough gynecologic history is indicated, including menses, mode of contraception, fertility, sexual activity, sexually transmitted diseases, vaginal discharge, recent dyspareunia, and a past gynecologic history, to include pregnancies, deliveries, abortions, ectopics, cysts, fibroids, pelvic inflammatory disease, and laparoscopy.

Vascular Symptoms   History of MI, other ischemic heart disease or cardiomyopathy, atrial fibrillation, anticoagulation, congestive failure, peripheral vascular disease, or a family history of aortic aneurysm are all pertinent historical features in older patients.

PAST MEDICAL HISTORY   This includes a history of recent and current medications (including nonsteroidal antiinflammatory drugs and antibiotics), past hospitalizations, in- or outpatient surgeries, diabetes, other chronic diseases (including HIV status and risk factors), and any history of recent trauma. A social history that includes habits (tobacco, alcohol, and other drug use), occupation, possible toxic exposures, and living circumstances (homeless, dwelling heated, running water, living alone, other family members ill with similar symptoms) provides important background and context in which to place the presenting complaint of acute abdominal pain.

Physical Examination

GENERAL   The patient's general appearance, including facial expression, diaphoresis, pallor, and degree of agitation provides information about the severity of pain. Although this is critically important in determining the need for analgesia, intensity of abdominal pain may bear no relationship to the severity of illness. For example, the pain of early mesenteric ischemia may be a vague discomfort, in contrast to the excruciating pain of ureteral colic. Nevertheless, uncomplicated kidney stones have no short-term mortality, while the majority of patients with ischemic small bowel go on to die.

Patients with colicky pain, which is characteristically visceral due to distention of a hollow organ, are often unable to lie still, while those with peritonitis prefer to remain immobile.

VITAL SIGNS   A reliable means of obtaining a core temperature is important, although absence of fever, especially in the elderly, has no predictive value. Careful counting of rate and observation of depth of respirations for 15 s is often overlooked. However, it can provide crucial information about tachypnea or hyperpnea, which may be subtle. Pulse and blood pressure should include orthostatic changes if, after obtaining the history, there is any reason to suspect intravascular volume contraction. A pulse increase of thirty points lying to standing at 1 minute (or the development of symptoms of presyncope) has been shown to be highly specific for the loss of a liter of blood or its equivalent (roughly 3 L of NS). Changes in blood pressure have not been shown to be discriminatory, probably because they are late findings representing failure of a reflex tachycardia to maintain cardiac output. The tilt-test threshold of thirty points of pulse change may not be applicable to patients on medications such as beta-blockers, diabetics (who may have an autonomic neuropathy), and among the elderly, due to the effects of aging on the cardiac conducting system.

ABDOMEN

Inspection   The abdomen should be inspected for distention (with air or fluid), scars, and masses.

Auscultation   Contrary to conventional teaching, absent or diminished bowel sounds provide little clinically useful information. Patients with operative confirmation of peritonitis due to perforation of peptic ulcer have been noted to have normal or increased bowel sounds preoperatively. Hyperactive or obstructive bowel sounds, although of limited value, are somewhat more helpful for the diagnosis of small bowel obstruction (SBO). However, many with SBO can also have absent or diminished bowel sounds. It appears, therefore, that only hyperactive or obstructive bowel sounds have clinical utility, increasing the likelihood of SBO by about fivefold; however, normal or absent bowel sounds appear very nearly valueless, as evidenced by their occurrence with roughly the same frequency in both SBO and perforated peptic ulcer.

Palpation   The vast majority of clinical information obtained from examination of the abdomen is acquired through gentle palpation, using the middle three fingers, and beginning at a distance from the area of maximum pain. Voluntary guarding (contraction of the abdominal musculature in anticipation of or in response to palpation) can be diminished by asking patients to flex their knees. Those who remain guarded following this maneuver will often relax if the clinician's hand is placed over the patient's, and the patient is then asked to use their own hand to palpate their abdomen. In contrast to the symptom of pain, tenderness is a *sign* in which pain is produced by palpation. Optimally, the patient's tenderness will be confined to one of the four discrete quadrants. However, this is often not the case, and one finds more diffuse tenderness encompassing one or more of the four combined areas noted above. Peritoneal irritation is suggested by rigidity (involuntary guarding or reflex spasm of abdominal muscles), as is pain referred to the point of maximum tenderness when palpating an adjacent quadrant.

Rebound tenderness, often regarded as the clinical criterion standard for peritonitis, has several important limitations. In patients with peritonitis, the combination of rigidity, referred tenderness, and especially pain with coughing usually provides sufficient diagnostic confirmation that little additional information is gained by eliciting the unnecessary pain of rebound. False positives occur in about one patient in four without peritonitis, perhaps due to a nonspecific startle response. Based on this, one might reasonably question whether rebound has sufficient predictive value to justify the discomfort it causes patients.

Enlargement of the liver or spleen, and other masses, including a distended bladder, should be sought. One should also examine for hernias in both men and women, particularly those that are tender, suggesting incarceration or strangulation.

In women, the pelvic examination—like the pregnancy test—may provide the clinician with relevant information that would not have been expected on the basis of the history. For this reason, it is wise to perform a pelvic examination in the evaluation of abdominal pain, particularly in women of reproductive age.

Although the rectal examination is widely regarded as an essential component in the assessment of abdominal pain, particularly in suspected appendicitis, there is little evidence that rectal tenderness in patients with RLQ pain provides useful incremental information beyond what has already been obtained by other components of the physical examination. Grossly melanotic, maroon, or bloody stool indicates GI bleeding. The test for occult blood, although routinely done, loses sensitivity if not performed serially over several days. Conversely, repeated rectal examinations performed over several hours by multiple examiners tends to reduce the specificity of the test for occult blood, presumably due to local trauma. Among patients with a final diagnosis on follow-up of NSAP, 10 percent had a positive stool test for occult blood.

Basic Laboratory and Radiographic Tests

The complete blood count and plain abdominal film are among the most overutilized tests in emergency practice. Neither test offers sufficiently powerful likelihood ratios (see below) to revise disease probability. One approach to the use of both these tests is to take note only of high threshold abnormalities, e.g., a very elevated WBC ($>20,000/mm^3$), but to resist the temptation to draw *any* reassurance from a "normal" WBC or a "nonspecific bowel gas pattern."

COMPLETE BLOOD COUNT   The limited clinical utility of the CBC can be demonstrated most readily by examining its performance characteristics in the three most common causes of abdominal pain: Appendicitis, biliary tract disease (principally cholecystitis), and NSAP. Based upon a metaanalysis of three studies containing a total of over 1800 patients, a WBC exceeding the threshold value of $10,000/\mu L$ only doubled the odds of appendicitis, while a WBC below this cutoff point reduced the odds by only about half. As noted below in the discussion of likelihood ratios (LRs), an LR (+) = 2 and an LR (−) = 0.4 are of marginal clinical value.

For acute cholecystitis, the LRs of the WBC count are virtually identical to those seen in appendicitis, and of equally limited clinical utility.

In one large, well-conducted series of patients with NSAP, 28 percent (95% CI; 22 to 34%) of patients were reported to have WBC counts $>10,500/\mu L$. In the development of a decision rule for identification of NSAP, investigators did not find the CBC to be of value in distinguishing patients with NSAP from other, more serious diagnoses. Because of the design of studies on NSAP, it is not possible to calculate a specificity or likelihood ratios for the performance of the WBC count in this setting. However, using 28 percent as the approximate sensitivity of the test, it is possible to estimate that, in order for leukocytosis to be of any value in NSAP (defined as producing LRs that deviate significantly from 1), the WBC count would have to demonstrate substantially better specificity than was seen in either appendicitis or cholecystitis.

All of the above refers only to individual WBC counts. There is some evidence that serial counts may assist in the identification of appendicitis. However, in this setting, it would seem wiser to obtain a CT rather than risk a perforation or other complication while obtaining serial WBCs and waiting for development of leukocytosis.

PLAIN ABDOMINAL RADIOGRAPH   The plain abdominal radiograph (PAR) is often ordered as an "abdominal series," the meaning of which is variously defined. In some institutions, this includes an upright abdomen, in others an upright chest; in still others, only a single supine film is obtained. The utility of the erect abdominal film, when added to the combination of the supine abdominal and erect chest film, is generally low and does not impact management. Abdominal films in suspected appendicitis, NSAP, or urinary tract infection are also unlikely to be helpful, and can be misleading.

An additional limitation of the plain abdominal radiograph is poor interrater reliability for commonly used radiographic signs.

Restriction of PARs to patients with suspected obstruction or perforation would reduce utilization by over 80 percent with no adverse impact on management. Ultrasound may be a more sensitive test for detection of free air than the combination of upright chest and left lateral decubitus plain films (93 vs. 79 percent), which is one of the principal uses for plain radiography in abdominal pain.[3] Ultrasound can be extremely helpful, particularly as a rapid bedside screening test, but it is highly operator-dependent and limited by overlying gas and obesity. Computed tomography (CT) is markedly superior for identifying virtually any abnormality that could be seen on plain films, particularly SBO and renal colic (Tables 72-1 and 72-2). Bedside sonography, combined with computed tomography would seem to be the key to obviating the need for continued use of the PAR in the future.

DIAGNOSIS AND TESTING

Diagnosis is now more closely linked to appropriate disposition and treatment than was the case when the only interventions in abdominal pain were laparotomy or observation with medical management.

Accurate diagnosis is extremely difficult using only clinical information and basic laboratory tests. When initial and final diagnoses are compared, diagnostic accuracy falls somewhere between 50 and 65 percent overall. Diagnostic error in adults with abdominal pain increases in proportion to age, ranging from a low of 20 percent if only young adults are considered, to a high of 70 percent in the very elderly.

Although some improvement in clinical diagnostic accuracy occurs with experience, most is due to diagnostic imaging.

Performance Characteristics of Diagnostic Tests

Tables 72-1, 72-2, 72-4–72-11 provide a summary of the performance of diagnostic tests used in the ED work-up of acute abdominal pain. These test properties are displayed as sensitivity, specificity, and likelihood ratios. When derived from a metaanalysis of several studies,

TABLE 72-1   Diagnostic Tests for Small Bowel Obstruction

Target Diagnosis	Test	Sensitivity (Range)	Specificity (Range)	LR (+)	LR (−)
Small bowel obstruction (SBO)	Plain abdominal films	63% (44–71%)	54% (38–65%)	1	0.7
SBO high-grade	CT with IV +/− PO contrast	90% (81–97%)	96% (85–98%)	22	0.1
SBO low- & high-grade	CT with IV +/− PO contrast	64% (55–85%)	79% (68–88%)	3	0.5
SBO with ischemia	CT with IV +/− PO contrast	83% (32–100%)	88% (61–100%)	7	0.2

sensitivity and specificity, bounded by 95 percent confidence intervals (CIs), are calculated using the Summary Receiver Operating Characteristics (SROC) methodology, which adjusts for interstudy variation in diagnostic threshold.[4] Under conditions where merged studies are too clinically or statistically heterogenous for valid metaanalysis, aggregate sensitivity and specificity are calculated as weighted means, bounded by ranges.

DEFINITION OF LIKELIHOOD RATIOS (LR'S)[5]   In the far right-hand columns of Tables 72-1, 72-2, 72-4–72-11, test performance is expressed using positive and negative likelihood ratios (LRs).

LRs are often divided into positive and negative LRs, expressed as follows: LR of a positive test = (TPR/FPR) = [(true positive rate)/(false positive rate)] = [sensitivity/(1 − specificity)]. LR of a negative test = (FNR/TNR) = [(false negative rate)/(true negative rate)] = [(1 − sensitivity)/specificity]. LR calculations derived from sensitivities or specificities of 100 percent are calculated conservatively by using the midpoint of the 95% CI surrounding the estimate of sensitivity or specificity in order to avoid obtaining a clinically meaningless LR (+) of ∞ or an LR (−) of 0.

The formal definition of an LR (+) is simply a special case of the general definition of LRs: An LR (+) is the likelihood that a *positive* test result would be found in a patient *with* the target disorder, compared to the likelihood of a *positive* test result occurring in a patient *without* the target disorder. The definition of an LR (−) is the likelihood that a *negative* test result would be found in a patient *with* the target disorder, compared to the likelihood of a *negative* test result occurring in a patient *without* the target disorder.

INTERPRETATION OF LR'S   In general, an LR (+) of 1 to 2, or an LR (−) of 0.5 to 1, alters disease probability by a small and clinically insignificant degree. In contrast, LR (+)s >10, or LR (−)s <0.1 may have a very substantial impact on clinical decision-making through meaningful revision of disease probability. LR (+)s of 2 to 10, or LR (−)s of 0.5 to 0.1 may still make some small contribution to management, depending on their magnitude and the clinical context in which they are applied. Because LRs are odds, a diagnostic test with an LR (−) = 0.1 is as powerful as a diagnostic test with an LR (+) = 10.

CLINICAL APPLICATION OF LR'S   Likelihood ratios (LRs) combine the stability of sensitivity and specificity with the utility of predictive values, resulting in an index of test performance that can be applied directly to a particular patient at the bedside. This is done by multiplying an LR (+) or LR (−) times the pretest odds of disease, resulting, respectively, in an increase or decrease in post-test odds of disease. The larger the LR (+) or the smaller the LR (−), the more powerful the test is to revise the posttest probability of a given target disorder.

Although odds (O) and probabilities (p) are mathematically different, they are conceptually similar and easily interconverted according to the following formulas: O = p/(1 − p), and p = O/(O + 1). Thus, if O = 1:1, p = 1/(1 + 1) = 1/2 = .5 or 50 percent probability; conversely, if p = 0.5 or 50 percent , O = .5/(1 − .5) = .5/.5 = 1:1.

Once determined, an LR can be incorporated directly into the calculation of posttest probability by employing Bayes' theorem: (LR) × (clinically estimated pretest odds of disease) = (posttest odds of disease). This simple equation illustrates a convergence between the central strategy underlying diagnostic testing, i.e., the revision of disease probability, and the fundamental nature of likelihood ratios.

The performance characteristics of the various tests shown in Tables 72-1, 72-2, 72-4–72-11 are incorporated into the discussion of specific diagnoses below.

SPECIFIC DIAGNOSES

The data in Table 72-3 were drawn from a combined series of over 8500 cases of acute abdominal pain (<1 week duration) presenting to over 200 EDs in 17 countries during a 10-year period. The data were collected on a highly standardized instrument.

TABLE 72-2   Diagnostic Tests for Renal Colic

Test	Sensitivity [95% CI] (Range)	Specificity [95% CI] (Range)	LR (+)	LR (−)
Microscopic Urinalysis	84% [81–87%]*	48% [43–53%]	2	0.3
Plain abdominal film	58% (39–68%)	74% [47–88%]	2	0.6
Unenhanced helical CT (criterion standard)	—	—	—	—
Intravenous pyelogram (IVP)	78% [67–88%]	95% [91–99%]	16	0.2
Ultrasonography (without Doppler)	74% (19–100%)	95% (90–100%)	15	0.3
Doppler ultrasound (resistive index)	90% [79–97%]	100% [94–100%]	30	0.1

* Brackets indicate 95% CI; parentheses indicate range.

TABLE 72-3   Causes of Acute Abdominal Pain Stratified by Age

Final Diagnosis	≥50 Years (N = 2406)	<50 Years (N = 6317)
Biliary tract disease	21%	6%
Nonspecific abdominal pain (NSAP)	16%	40%
Appendicitis	15%	32%
Bowel obstruction	12%	2%
Pancreatitis	7%	2%
Diverticular disease	6%	<.1%
Cancer	4%	<.1%
Hernia	3%	<.1%
Vascular	2%	<.1%
Gynecologic	<.1%	4%
Other	13%	13%

In virtually all large series of acute abdominal pain in adults, the substantial majority of final diagnoses include nonspecific abdominal pain (NSAP), appendicitis, and biliary tract disease (usually cholecystitis), in that order, accounting for nearly 75 percent of all acute abdominal pain. However, as shown in Table 72-3, as patients age, the triad remains, but the order changes to: biliary tract disease (again, usually cholecystitis), followed by NSAP and appendicitis.

Intraabdominal Diagnoses by Organ System

GASTROINTESTINAL

Appendicitis In spite of a large number of algorithms and decision rules incorporating many different clinical and laboratory features, an accurate preoperative diagnosis of appendicitis has remained elusive for more than a century. In at least 20 percent of patients with appendicitis, the diagnosis is missed; conversely, normal appendices are found in 15 to 40 percent of all operations performed for suspected appendicitis. Thus the diagnosis of appendicitis turns out to be either a false positive or false negative just about as often as it turns out to be correct.[6]

Among patients presenting to an ED with acute abdominal pain, the pretest probability, or prevalence, of appendicitis is roughly 10 to 25 percent. Converting this to odds to facilitate multiplication by LRs, the pretest odds of appendicitis in patients with undifferentiated acute abdominal pain is roughly between 0.1 and 0.3. Five clinical features appear to have sufficiently powerful LR (+)s that the presence of *any one* should drive up the clinical odds to the point that an imaging procedure is indicated. Those clinical features with some predictive value include: Pain located in the RLQ [LR (+) = 8]; pain migration from the periumbilical area to the RLQ [LR (+) = 3]; rigidity [LR (+) = 4]; pain before vomiting [LR (+) = 2 to 3]; and a positive psoas sign [LR (+) = 2]. Anorexia is not a useful symptom. In fact, about one patient in three with surgically documented appendicitis is *not* anorectic preoperatively.

In excluding the diagnosis of appendicitis, the absence of RLQ pain [LR (−) = 0.2], presence of similar previous pain [LR (−) = 0.3], and absence of typical pain migration to the RLQ [LR (−) = 0.5] are only somewhat helpful. This is because no single historical or physical finding is sufficiently powerful to exclude the diagnosis. Therefore, to clinically rule out appendicitis, one relies upon the absence of several key features, or the presence of a strong competing alternative diagnosis. Lacking either of these conditions, an imaging procedure, usually a CT, should be obtained.

Although sonography is an option in suspected appendicitis, the **CT is generally preferred in adults and nonpregnant women** with a working diagnosis of appendicitis because ultrasound of the appendix is technically challenging, highly operator-dependent, and often unavailable after hours. Additionally, although ultrasound has a sufficiently powerful LR (+) that a positive finding usually results in surgery, its poor LR (−) precludes its use as a screening (rule-out) test. Color-flow Doppler added to the standard graded compression grayscale sonography improves test performance by detecting appendiceal and periappendiceal inflammation. However, the increment in LRs is insufficient to change the clinical implications of the test results, i.e., a positive finding still favors surgical intervention, and a negative result fails to exclude the diagnosis.

As shown in Table 72-4, CT of suspected appendicitis can be targeted at the RLQ or include the entire abdomen and pelvis. It can be performed as an unenhanced (noncontrast) study, or may be done with various combinations of PO, IV, or colonic contrast. Although the focused appendiceal CT obtained with colonic contrast appears to have excellent test properties and has been shown to alter management in the majority (59 percent) of cases,[7] these targeted examinations are not commonly performed because they are so narrowly focused on the RLQ that a negative result often requires a repeat abdominopelvic CT. Evidence of appendicitis on any type of abdominal CT has such a high

LR (+) that it almost invariably drives surgical intervention. Although the LR (−) is sufficiently strong to reduce the odds of appendicitis by about tenfold, it is not as strong as the LR (+). Absence of evidence of appendicitis on CT, or even visualization of an apparently normal appendix therefore does not exclude the diagnosis with the same degree of certainty that a positive CT confirms it.

For example, if the clinician is working with a 50 percent pretest probability of appendicitis (not an unreasonable estimate, given the prevalence of the disease in the population), a negative CT reduces that posttest probability to just under 10 percent. While this finding, depending upon the clinical picture, might be sufficient to stay the surgeon's hand, logical application of Bayes' theorem does not support use of a negative CT as grounds for discharging the patient from the ED. In order to make such a disposition, the prior probability of appendicitis would have to be substantially lower than 50 percent. This example also assumes the optimal conditions under which the studies used to generate the contents of Table 72-4 were conducted, i.e., complete filling of the entire appendiceal lumen in order to exclude distal appendicitis, a helical machine with narrowly collimated beams (optimally 5-mm cuts), and an experienced radiologist trained in body CT available to read the images. The relative rarity of such conditions may help to explain the observation that, in spite of several well-conducted clinical trials demonstrating the salutary impact of advances in abdominal imaging on diagnostic accuracy in appendicitis, the population-based incidence of misdiagnosis and perforation have not changed over the past decade.[8]

Biliary Tract Disease This is the most common diagnosis in ED patients ≥50 years old. Among those found to have pathologically-confirmed acute cholecystitis, the majority lack fever and about 40 percent lack a leukocytosis. Recognition that the diagnoses of cholecystitis, "biliary colic," and symptomatic common duct obstruction may represent pathologically distinct entities that cannot be reliably distinguished from one another on clinical grounds, has led some authors to redefine the *clinical* target disorder as simply "biliary tract disease." Although there is an association between symptomatic biliary tract disease and steady postprandial upper abdominal pain that radiates to the upper back, the likelihood ratios of individual signs, symptoms, and combinations of signs and symptoms are relatively weak discriminators. Just over one-third of patients have pain isolated to the RUQ, although about two-thirds have tenderness in that location. Most of the remainder complain of diffuse pain in the upper half of the abdomen, and among those with pain in the lower abdomen, it is almost invariably in the RLQ. Among the one-third who do not have RUQ tenderness, the distribution is about equally divided among the upper half, the right side, and generalized tenderness throughout the belly.

As shown in Table 72-5, sonography is the initial test of choice for patients with suspected biliary tract disease. In many institutions, this can be performed rapidly at the bedside by the ED physician as an extension of the clinical assessment. Ultrasound is better in the identification of cholecystitis than in the detection of common duct obstruction. Cholescintigraphy (radionuclide scanning) of the biliary tree is a more sensitive test than sonography for the diagnosis of both these conditions.[9] At present, CT does not have a major role in the initial work-up of biliary tract disease, although it will often identify unexpected abnormalities of the gallbladder on an abdominopelvic double contrast CT obtained for other reasons, particularly if thinly collimated cuts are obtained. MR cholangiography has shown extremely good sensitivity and specificity in identifying stones and other obstructions of the common duct.[10]

Small Bowel Obstruction The central issues in small bowel obstruction (SBO) are diagnosis of the primary disorder and early detection of secondary strangulation or ischemia, when present. Only two historical features (previous abdominal surgery and intermittent/colicky pain) and two physical findings (abdominal distention and abnormal bowel sounds) appear to have predictive value. Although about

TABLE 72-4   Diagnostic Tests for Appendicitis

Test	Sensitivity [95% CI] (Range)	Specificity [95% CI] (Range)	LR (+)	LR (−)
Plain abdominal radiograph	48% [41–54%]	58% [54–62%]	1	0.9
Abdominopelvic ultrasound (real-time, graded compression, gray-scale)	55% [48–62%]	95% [93–97%]	11	0.5
Abdominopelvic ultrasound (color Doppler added to gray-scale)	84% [77–91%]	96% [88–100%]	21	0.2
Abdominopelvic unenhanced helical CT (no PO, IV, or colonic contrast)	88% [82–94%]	97% [94–99%]	29	0.1
Abdominopelvic helical CT (double [PO + IV] contrast; no colonic contrast)	91% [81–98%]	95% [90–98%]	18	0.1
Focused appendiceal (RLQ) unenhanced helical CT (no PO, IV, or colonic contrast)	87% [78–93%]	97% [92–99%]	29	0.1
Focused appendiceal (RLQ) helical CT (PO contrast only; no IV or colonic contrast)	76% [62–87%]	95% [90–98%]	15	0.3
Focused appendiceal (RLQ) helical CT (PO + colonic contrast; no IV contrast)	100% [94–100%]	95% [84–99%]	21	0.03
Focused appendiceal (RLQ) helical CT (colonic contrast only; no PO or IV contrast)	98% [90–100%]	98% [89–100%]	49	0.02
MRI (gadolinium-enhanced)	97% [85–100%]	92% [75–99%]	12	0.03

two-thirds of SBO presents with generalized or central abdominal pain, and about half have generalized tenderness, the LRs of these findings alone or in combination are such that SBO is another diagnosis that requires imaging confirmation. The general limitations of bowel sounds have been noted previously. As shown in Table 72-1, and also discussed above, the plain abdominal film is hampered by a large number of indeterminate readings, leaving it with LRs that are of marginal utility. The CT is far superior to the plain film in detection of high-grade SBO, but is limited in its ability to identify low-grade obstruction, which may require small-bowel follow-through.[11]

Those patients with ischemic bowel secondary to strangulation are extremely difficult to detect clinically or with plain radiography. Here the CT is useful in altering the likelihood of ischemia, and has been shown to have a substantial impact on treatment.

Acute Pancreatitis   About 80 percent of acute pancreatitis in the United States is caused by alcohol or gallstones, with one etiology predominating over the other depending on the population studied. The pain and tenderness of acute pancreatitis are limited to the anatomic area of the pancreas in the upper half of the abdomen in only a minority of instances. Most patients' pain and tenderness include this area, but in about half the pain extends well beyond the upper abdomen to cause generalized tenderness. This may be related to the absence of a capsule that might otherwise contain the inflammation, and to the difficulty of localizing pathology that—much like that of an abdominal aortic aneurysm—resides deep in the belly and extends into the retroperitoneum. Other features of the history and physical exam, such as quality of pain—which is steady and severe in the majority of patients—or vomiting, have not been shown to have sufficient discriminatory power

TABLE 72-5   Diagnostic Tests for Biliary Tract Disease

Target Diagnosis	Test	Sensitivity [95% CI] (Range)	Specificity [95% CI] (Range)	LR (+)	LR (−)
Cholelithiasis	Plain abdominal radiograph	64% [59–68%]	68% [52–83%]	2	0.5
Cholelithiasis	Ultrasound (US)	91% [84–97%]	97% [95–99%]	30	0.1
Cholelithiasis	CT	85% (77–96%)	97% (86–99%)	28	0.2
Acute cholecystitis	US	86% (65–97%)	97% (87–100%)	29	0.1
Acute cholecystitis	Color velocity imaging & power Doppler US	93% (77–100%)	97% (88–100%)	31	0.1
Acute cholecystitis	Radionuclide scanning	95% [91–98%]	90% [86–94%]	10	.05
Common duct obstruction	US	90% (38–95%)	92% (48–97%)	11	0.1
Common duct obstruction	CT	83% (51–90%)	87% (44–94%)	6	0.2
Common duct obstruction	Radionuclide scanning	93% (81–99%)	92% (84–100%)	12	0.1
Common duct obstruction	MR cholangiography	95% (85–96%)	97% (85–99%)	32	0.05
Common duct stone	US	85% (19–76%)	89% (52–98%)	8	0.2
Common duct stone	CT	71% (29–82%)	86% (55–92%)	5	0.3
Common duct stone	MR cholangiography	95% (86–100%)	96% (87–100%)	24	0.05

to make them clinically useful. Thus most patients with upper, central, or generalized abdominal pain and tenderness, who lack an alternative explanation for their presentation will require further testing.

As lipase assays have improved in accuracy and speed over the last several years, serum lipase has begun to replace amylase as the preferred ED screening test for suspected acute pancreatitis. By setting the threshold for a positive test at twice the upper limit of normal serum lipase, the likelihood ratios for lipase are better than twice as powerful as those of serum amylase in confirming or excluding the diagnosis of acute pancreatitis (Table 72-6).[12] Preliminary reports that ratios of urine to serum amylase or of lipase to amylase improve diagnostic accuracy have not been validated. Like amylase, the accuracy of serum lipase in the diagnosis of acute pancreatitis is inversely related to the time elapsed between symptom onset and presentation.

Depending upon institutional custom, a diagnosis of acute pancreatitis may be sufficient to determine the appropriate admitting service. However, in settings where not all pancreatitis is admitted to a single service, or where it is expected that the ED will make a monitored vs. unmonitored bed admitting decision, it may be necessary for the ED to assess the patient for biliary pancreatitis and for the likelihood of peripancreatic complications, such as necrosis, hemorrhage, or drainable fluid collections. Although the height of pancreatic enzyme elevations do not have prognostic value, a double contrast helical CT stages severity and predicts mortality earlier than the Ranson criteria.

Because timely identification of biliary pancreatitis is important, early assessment for common bile duct obstruction is necessary, particularly among patients over 50 years old. All patients with an ALT >150 U/L (about 3× normal), including alcoholics, are at increased risk of biliary pancreatitis (see Table 72-6). Because elevations in transaminase due to alcoholic hepatitis may mask an increased ALT secondary to obstruction, this subset of alcoholic patients warrants evaluation for common duct obstruction. Unfortunately, there are no blood tests or imaging modalities short of MR cholangiography that possess a sufficiently powerful LR (−) to exclude common duct obstruction in all patients (see Table 72-6). Depending on availability, a double contrast helical CT is usually performed first to examine the pancreas and identify peripancreatic complications. Contingent upon the CT protocol used—principally the thinness of the collimated beam—the common bile duct may be adequately visualized. Usually, however, it is necessary to follow the CT with a sonogram of the biliary tree because the LR (−) of ultrasound is superior to CT in this setting (see Table 72-6).[13] If sonography is unavailable, a radionuclide scan is a reasonable alternative test for the detection of *complete* obstruction. In the future, the problem of distinguishing primary inflammatory (usually alcoholic) pancreatitis from secondary obstructive (usually biliary) pancreatitis may be resolved through wider availability of MR cholangiopancreatography (MRCP). This test simultaneously and noninvasively images the pancreas and common bile duct, and may ultimately obviate the need for purely diagnostic ERCP.

Diverticulitis Clinical diagnostic accuracy in one large study of colonic diverticulitis was only 34 percent [95% CI; 26 to 42%]. When the "possible/equivocal" clinical diagnoses were removed from analysis, and only those patients with a pretest diagnosis of either "highly suspected" or "very unlikely" were included as clinical positives and negatives respectively, the LR (+) was 2 to 3, and the LR (−) was 0.4, neither of which offers much help in the revision of disease probability. Of those patients with diverticular abscesses, diagnostic performance was somewhat better, with 70 percent categorized as "highly suspected" and the remainder as "possible/equivocal." No documented abscesses were categorized clinically as "very unlikely."

Pain in diverticulitis was confined to the LLQ in less than one-fourth of documented cases, and to the lower half of the abdomen in only an additional one-third of patients. With respect to tenderness, it was as likely to be generalized as it was to be limited to the lower half of the abdomen or to the LLQ. About 10 percent of patients with operatively confirmed diverticulitis lacked abdominal pain and 20 percent had no abdominal tenderness whatsoever, most of whom were elderly. Older patients are also at risk for a severe and often fatal complication of diverticulitis only rarely seen in younger age groups: free perforation of the colon.

As shown in Table 72-7, CT with colonic contrast is the test of choice for diverticulitis, demonstrating excellent performance characteristics that are superior to ultrasound. Sonography relies on identification of an inflamed diverticulum to make the diagnosis, which is often obscured in patients with complicated diverticulitis.[14] In contrast, CT accurately identifies abscesses and other complications, informing surgical management strategies.[15]

GENITOURINARY

Renal Colic As in appendicitis, a number of clinical decision rules have been developed to identify patients with the preimaging diagnosis of ureterolithiasis. Most algorithms include features of the pain, e.g., location (unilateral flank), onset (abrupt), quality (colicky), and radiation (groin/testicle/labia). Although hematuria and plain abdomi-

TABLE 72-6 Diagnostic Tests for Acute Pancreatitis

Target Diagnosis	Test	Sensitivity (Range)	Specificity (Range)	LR (+)	LR (−)
Inflammation	Serum amylase	82% (72–93%)	85% (78–94%)	5	0.2
Inflammation	Serum lipase >2× normal	90% (79–99%)	92% (85–98%)	11	0.1
Pancreatic necrosis	CT with PO & bolus IV contrast	92% (75–100%)	95% (92–100%)	18	0.1
Drainable collections	Transabdominal ultrasound (US)	54% (23–83%)	88% (47–100%)	4	0.5
Drainable collections	CT with PO & bolus IV contrast	90% (72–100%)	48% (32–85%)	2	0.2
Drainable collections	MRI (unenhanced)	92% (66–100%)	88% (79–100%)	8	0.1
Acute hemorrhagic pancreatitis	Unenhanced CT (criterion standard)	—	—	—	—
Biliary pancreatitis	Serum alanine aminotransferase (ALT) >3× normal	54% (38–73%)	92% (77–96%)	7	0.5
Common bile duct obstruction	US	90% (38–95%)	92% (48–97%)	11	0.1
Common bile duct obstruction	CT	83% (51–90%)	87% (44–94%)	6	0.2
Common bile duct obstruction	Radionuclide scanning	93% (81–99%)	92% (84–100%)	12	0.1
Common bile duct obstruction	MR cholangiography	95% (85–96%)	97% (85–99%)	32	0.05

TABLE 72-7 Diagnostic Tests for Acute Diverticulitis

Target Diagnosis	Test	Sensitivity (Range)	Specificity (Range)	LR (+)	LR (−)
Inflammation or abscess	Ultrasonography (high resolution, graded compression)	83% (77–91%)	95% (86–99%)	17	0.2
Inflammation or abscess	Helical CT with colonic contrast only (no IV or PO contrast)	98% (88–99%)	99% (96–100%)	98	0.02

nal films still appear in many clinical algorithms, the weak LRs of both tests, as shown in Table 72-2, do not provide strong support for their continued inclusion in the diagnostic evaluation of suspected renal colic.[16]

Although the IVP has a specificity comparable to unenhanced helical CT, because of the IVP's poor sensitivity, demonstrated in head-to-head comparison, noncontrast helical CT has become the criterion standard for the diagnosis of renal colic. Traditional sonography has performance characteristics that are similar to those of the IVP (see Table 72-2). However, with the addition of Doppler ultrasound, elevation of the "renal resistive index" in one kidney relative to the other may identify the presence of a stone in the ipsilateral ureter. Based on preliminary data, this test appears to have a strong LR (+), but its LR (−), though good, is not as powerful as that of unenhanced helical CT (see Table 72-2). Because this test requires specialized equipment and a skilled operator, its availability to the ED is not comparable to CT.

In older patients, any presentation that resembles renal colic, with or without hematuria, mandates the exclusion of an abdominal aortic aneurysm (AAA). This is yet another reason to obtain a noncontrast helical CT, since it performs extremely well in the detection of both ureteral stones and AAAs.

Because the GU tract is mostly retroperitoneal, it only uncommonly causes significant anterior abdominal tenderness. A notable exception to this is an impacted stone at the ureterovesical (U-V) junction where the ureter enters the bladder, producing ipsilateral lower quadrant pain and tenderness. Because stones at the U-V junction (like those at the uretero-pelvic [U-P] junction) are less likely to produce colicky pain than are stones located between the top and bottom of the ureter, impaction of a stone at the U-V junction on the right may easily mimic appendicitis, and will require a noncontrast CT to identify stone disease. If this shows neither a stone nor evidence of other intraabdominal pathology, a double contrast abdominopelvic CT should be obtained, searching for evidence of appendicitis.

Acute Urinary Retention Another common GU cause of abdominal pain is acute urethral obstruction, producing a distended bladder. When the obstruction is truly acute, the tense bladder often feels like a solid mass rather than a fluid-filled hollow viscus. However, if one always considers this common entity when confronted with a midline mass of variable tenderness arising from the lower half of the abdomen, insertion of a urethral catheter easily makes the diagnosis and treats the immediate problem.

GYNECOLOGIC PAIN

Acute Pelvic Inflammatory Disease Absence of a criterion standard has further confounded the already clinically difficult diagnosis of acute pelvic inflammatory disease (PID). Laparoscopic and histopathologic findings, both of which have been proposed as diagnostic standards, are discordant. Because gross laparoscopic findings have historically been used as the standard in most well-designed studies, the LRs of clinical features, laboratory results, and sonographic findings that follow have been measured against direct macroscopic inspection of the adnexa, unless otherwise noted.

Symptoms such as lower abdominal pain, which would be expected to have a high LR (−) for PID, have not been studied because they typically represent inclusion criteria for study enrollment. To date, there have been no historical features associated with laparoscopic PID that demonstrate clinically useful LRs in more than one study population. Similar to lower abdominal pain, signs such as adnexal and cervical motion tenderness have not been well-studied because they have also been used as inclusion criteria in most investigations. The only physical finding associated with laparoscopic PID across more than one study population is an abnormal vaginal discharge. In spite of this statistical association, the LRs of vaginal discharge range from 0.5 to 2.5, representing very limited power to alter disease probability. Elevated temperature and a palpable mass have been inconsistently associated with PID. The white blood cell count has not been found to be helpful in any of the studies that examined it. For the performance characteristics of other laboratory tests that have been associated with PID (e.g., the erythrocyte sedimentation rate [ESR] and C-reactive protein [CRP]), see Table 72-8. An examination of this table suggests that the best noninvasive test presently available for suspected PID is transvaginal sonography, in which a positive test result, such as a thickened tubal wall, increases the likelihood of PID about 18 times. If this is supplemented by transvaginal power Doppler, a negative test result, such as absence of the hyperemia associated with tubal inflammation, will decrease the likelihood of PID by about tenfold.[17]

As in the evaluation of ectopic pregnancy (see below), the role of culdocentesis in the diagnosis of PID is *not* well-supported by evidence.

Ectopic Pregnancy In ruptured ectopic pregnancy, abdominal pain is almost universally present. However, as emphasis in ectopic pregnancy has shifted to identification of patients prior to rupture—with the goal of preserving fertility—pain may be absent at this earlier stage, with a sentinel complaint of only vaginal bleeding. Therefore, any woman of childbearing age who presents to the ED with abdominal pain *or* abnormal vaginal bleeding should receive a qualitative pregnancy test (either urine or serum) as a screening measure.

The poor predictive performance of historical features, such as "risk factors," and of the physical examination (sensitivity 19 percent, LR [−] = 0.8 for ectopic pregnancy among women with high hCG levels), argue persuasively that this diagnosis cannot be excluded on clinical grounds.

For this reason, the results of a urine or serum pregnancy test, independent of other data, will determine if further testing is indicated to exclude an ectopic. All commercial pregnancy tests are highly accurate, with excellent LRs (Table 72-9). If the qualitative hCG is positive, the preferred test is bedside transvaginal sonography (TVS), targeted solely at answering the question: Is this pregnancy in the uterus? In patients not undergoing treatment for infertility, clear visualization of an intrauterine pregnancy (IUP) in two perpendicular views essentially excludes an ectopic pregnancy. If an IUP is not seen, this must be interpreted in the context of the discriminatory zone (DZ) of the quantitative hCG. The DZ is the threshold level of serum HCG, above which a *normal* IUP should be seen on sonography. The accuracy of TVS permits reduction of the DZ to an operator-dependent level of 1500 mIU/mL. The performance of the TVS in the identification or exclusion of intrauterine and ectopic pregnancy is shown as a func-

TABLE 72-8 Diagnostic Tests for Acute Pelvic Inflammatory Disease

Target Diagnosis	Test	Sensitivity [95% CI] (Range)	Specificity [95% CI] (Range)	LR (+)	LR (−)
Salpingitis (macroscopic laparoscopy)	Erythrocyte sedimentation rate >15 mm per h	78% (45–81%)	44% (25–57%)	1	0.5
Salpingitis (macroscopic laparoscopy)	C-reactive protein	70% (54–93%)	59% (48–90%)	2	0.5
Salpingitis (macroscopic laparoscopy)	Endometrial biopsy	80% (70–89%)	76% (67–89%)	3	0.3
Salpingitis (macroscopic laparoscopy)	*Gonococcus* or *Chlamydia* cultured from upper genital tract	65% [41–85%]	100% [75–100%]	5	0.4
Salpingitis (macroscopic laparoscopy)	Transvaginal power Doppler	100% [83–100%]	80% (56–94%)	5	0.1
Endometritis (endometrial biopsy)	Conventional transvaginal sonography	85% [54–98%]	100% [91–100%]	18	0.2
Salpingitis (fimbrial minibiopsy)	Laparoscopy (macroscopic)	50% [29–71%]	80% [66–90%]	2	0.6
Endometritis (endometrial biopsy)	Laparoscopy (macroscopic)	93% [68–100%]	67% [41–87%]	3	0.1
Salpingitis/endometritis (fimbrial minibiopsy or endometrial biopsy)	Laparoscopy (macroscopic)	48% [30–67%]	79% [66–88%]	2	0.7
Chlamydia cultured from upper genital tract	Laparoscopy (macroscopic)	53% [28–77%]	67% [22–96%]	2	0.7

tion of hCG levels in Table 72-9.[18] Although there is a broad range of normal variation in hCG kinetics, failure of levels to increase by about 66 percent within 48 h in first-trimester pregnancy suggests an abnormal gestation. This will not distinguish a threatened miscarriage or blighted pregnancy from an ectopic. However, it does signal a potential problem that requires tracking of serial hCGs over time and subsequent investigation with TVS. If a diagnosis cannot be firmly established, laparoscopy is indicated.

Progesterone levels may be helpful if >22 ng/mL, since this markedly reduces the likelihood of an ectopic. A serum progesterone below this threshold, however, is not helpful (LR [+] = 1), since most pregnant women with levels <22 ng/mL will not be harboring an ectopic.[19]

As shown in Table 72-9, culdocentesis compares poorly to TVS performed by an experienced sonographer above the DZ, both in the identification of ectopic pregnancy and in distinguishing ruptured from unruptured ectopics. Indeed, LRs associated with culdocentesis, analyzed under conditions that optimize test performance by excluding nondiagnostic (dry) taps, range between 0.4 and 3, indicating poor discrimination. These data suggest that, with the widespread availability of quantitative hCG measurement and experienced TVS, there is little justification for performing this invasive and painful procedure.

VASCULAR

Abdominal Aortic Aneurysm Although abdominal aortic aneurysms (AAAs) have little in common with aortic dissections, these two major forms of catastrophic disease of the aorta are often lumped together. Dissections are uncommon causes of abdominal pain and, because they almost invariably originate in the thoracic aorta,

TABLE 72-9 Diagnostic Tests for Ectopic Pregnancy

Target Diagnosis	Test	Sensitivity [95% CI] (Range)	Specificity [95% CI] (Range)	LR (+)	LR (−)
Pregnancy	Serum hCG [≥10 mIU/mL = (+)]	99% [92–100%]	98% [94–100%]	50	.01
Pregnancy	Serum hCG [≥25 mIU/mL = (+)]	98% [91–100%]	99% [94–100%]	98	.02
Pregnancy	Urine hCG [>20 mIU/mL = (+)]	98% [96–100%]	98% [96–99%]	49	.02
Pregnancy	Urine hCG [>50 mIU/mL = (+)]	95% [90–98%]	99% [97–99%]	95	.05
IUP	TVS on all patients w/ (+) hCG	94% [90–97%]	93% [88–97%]	13	.06
IUP	TVS on patients w/ hCG <1500 mIU/mL	33% [10–65%]	98% [90–100%]	16	0.7
IUP	TVS on patients w/ hCG ≥1500 mIU/mL	98% [95–99%]	90% [81–96%]	10	0.2
Ectopic	TVS on all patients w/ (+) hCG	56% [35–76%]	99% [97–100%]	56	0.4
Ectopic	TVS on patients w/ hCG <1500 mIU/mL	25% [5–57%]	96% [87–99%]	6	0.8
Ectopic	TVS on patients w/ hCG >1500 mIU/mL	80% [52–96%]	99% [97–100%]	80	0.2
Ectopic	Progesterone <22 ng/mL	98% [96–100%]	29% [27–31%]	1	.07
Ectopic	Culdocentesis	56% (38–81%)	70% (20–86%)	2	0.6
Ruptured ectopic	Culdocentesis	68% (52–84%)	76% (39–93%)	3	0.4

usually produce chest or upper back pain before migrating into the abdomen as the dissection moves distally.

AAAs on the other hand tend to enlarge, become aneurysmal over years, and rather than dissect, leak and rupture. Fewer than half of AAAs present with the triad of hypotension, abdominal or back pain, and a pulsatile abdominal mass; over three-quarters are normotensive. Spontaneous containment of bleeding is the principal determinant of prehospital survival and degree of hypotension, if any, on arrival. Absence of abdominal pain or tenderness is entirely compatible with a contained leak extending into the retroperitoneum. Neither the presence or absence of femoral pulses or an abdominal bruit have LRs that deviate very far from 1, and therefore are not helpful clinically. In fact, palpation is the only feature of the physical exam that has been shown to have some clinical utility. As might be expected, the LR (−) for palpation is poor, ranging from 0.5 to 0.7 in a recent pooled analysis. The LR (+), however, ranges from 12 to 16 as the size of the aneurysm increases from >3 cm to >4 cm.[20] Thus, inability to palpate an enlarged aorta in a patient with suspected AAA should not deter one from obtaining an imaging procedure in a stable patient or moving directly to the OR if the patient is unstable. Conversely, palpation of an enlarged aorta in the same patient should only serve to increase the urgency with which imaging or surgical intervention occurs as the next step, again contingent upon hemodynamic instability.

In emergency practice, this means that any stable patient, particularly one over 50 years old, presenting with recent onset of abdominal/flank/low back pain is likely to require either a normal aortic sonogram (performed by an experienced operator) or a noncontrast helical CT (criterion standard) before an AAA can be excluded from the differential diagnosis. Although sonography has the advantage of ready availability at the bedside in many EDs, in contrast to the CT it can only identify an AAA, and cannot provide additional information about leakage or rupture (Table 72-10). In unstable patients, if a bedside sonogram can be obtained during resuscitation, visualization of an enlarged aorta in the setting of a suggestive clinical picture is taken as de facto evidence of leakage or rupture, requiring immediate surgery.

Because MRI is limited in its ability to identify fresh bleeding, MR technology, including MR angiography, is not an appropriate emergency procedure.

As noted earlier, the appearance of "renal colic" in older patients should be regarded as representing an AAA until the CT proves otherwise. Fortunately, the important distinction between a kidney stone and an AAA can be readily made by obtaining a helical unenhanced abdominopelvic CT.

Mesenteric Ischemia Mesenteric ischemia can be divided into arterial and venous disease (mesenteric venous thrombosis [MVT]). Arterial disease can be subdivided into occlusive and nonocclusive (NOMI or low-flow state). Finally, occlusive arterial disease (generally understood to mean superior mesenteric artery occlusion) may be further categorized into thrombotic or embolic. Several features combine to produce a very high mortality associated with mesenteric ischemia: (1) Unless young patients have an arrhythmia (usually atrial fibrillation causing embolization) or a hypercoagulable state (causing MVT), individuals with mesenteric ischemia tend to be older with substantial age-related comorbidity; (2) the small bowel, which is supplied by the superior mesenteric artery, has a warm ischemia time of only 2 to 3 h; (3) the clinical picture is characterized initially by poorly localized visceral-type abdominal pain, without tenderness; (4) patients may become transiently better after a few hours of ischemia at the time of onset of mucosal infarction, only to develop peritoneal findings as full-thickness necrosis of the bowel wall becomes clinically apparent over several more hours; and (5) timely diagnosis requires that conventional angiography, an invasive procedure, be obtained early in older, often fragile patients who may not appear initially to be as ill as they are.

There are some distinctions that can be made among the four major forms of mesenteric ischemia: (1) embolic disease is the most abrupt in onset, and MVT the most indolent, with the temporal profile of arterial thrombosis somewhere in between; (2) NOMI is usually accompanied by clinical evidence of a low-flow state, typically due to cardiac disease, which responds to improvement in cardiac output; (3) MVT may be more amenable to noninvasive diagnosis with CT, occurs in younger patients, has a lower mortality, and can be treated with immediate anticoagulation; (4) following diagnosis, arteriography with papaverine infusion may be an important component of treatment in patients with splanchnic vasoconstriction.

Elevation of serum phosphate was initially thought to be a sensitive marker for mesenteric ischemia, but this has not been supported by subsequent work. As shown in Table 72-11, serial serum lactates that remain *persistently* normal reduce the likelihood of mesenteric ischemia by more than tenfold. Unfortunately the test has a weak LR (+) because lactate is elevated in many other conditions, and therefore lacks adequate power to increase the probability of mesenteric ischemia in any clinically important way. Conventional invasive angiography is the diagnostic and initial therapeutic procedure of choice at the present time (see Table 72-11).[21]

Ischemic Colitis As is characteristic of all vascular diseases, ischemic colitis is predominantly a disease of older patients. About 80 percent of individuals have diffuse or lower abdominal visceral pain, accompanied by diarrhea in about 60 percent, often mixed with blood. In contrast to mesenteric ischemia, ischemic colitis is not generally due to large-vessel occlusive disease, angiography is not usually indicated, and if performed is often normal. The diagnosis is typically made by colonoscopy, which is preferred to sigmoidoscopy. Color Doppler sonography can also be used for diagnosis. Rectal sparing, in contrast to ulcerative colitis, is a typical finding in ischemic colitis. Not surprisingly, the severity of the presentation is related to the extent

TABLE 72-10   Diagnostic Tests for Abdominal Aortic Aneurysm

Target Diagnosis	Test	Sensitivity (Range)	Specificity (Range)	LR (+)	LR (−)
Uncomplicated abdominal aortic aneurysm (AAA)	Sonography	92% (81–100%)	89% (85–100%)	9	0.1
Leaking/ ruptured AAA (intra- or retro-peritoneal)	Sonography	12% (4–52%)	84% (34–100%)	1	1
Uncomplicated or leaking/ruptured AAA (intra- or retro-peritoneal)	CT	97% (82–100%)	95% (86–100%)	19	.03
Detailed preoperative anatomy	Conventional angiography	No longer a preferred emergency procedure			
Detailed preoperative anatomy	MRI/MRA	Not a preferred emergency procedure at this time			

TABLE 72-11   Diagnostic Tests for Ischemia of the Small and Large Bowel

Target Diagnosis	Test	Sensitivity [95% CI] (Range)	Specificity [95% CI] (Range)	LR (+)	LR (−)
Small bowel ischemia	Conventional angiography	88% (62–98%)	95% (93–100%)	18	0.1
Small bowel ischemia	CT & CT angiography (including multi-detector row image acquisition with 3D reformatting)	77% (57–92%)	85% (71–100%)	5	0.3
Small bowel ischemia	Gadolinium-enhanced MRA (including 3D reformatting)	83% (78–100%)	89% (71–99%)	8	0.2
Small bowel ischemia/infarction	Serum lactate (persistent elevation without alternative explanation)	90% (66–100%)	62% (42–77%)	2	0.2
Ischemic colitis	Colonoscopy	93% (82–100%)	90% (85–100%)	9	0.1
Large bowel infarction	Color Doppler sonography	82% [48–98%]	92% [64–100%]	10	0.2

of occlusion and ischemia. In the majority of cases, only segmental portions of the mucosa and submucosa slough. These then go on to heal uneventfully with conservative management. At the opposite end of the spectrum is full-thickness infarction of the colon, occurring in about 20 percent of cases. Bowel necrosis, whether segmental or pancolitic, causes peritonitis, requiring partial or complete colectomy.

In between mucosal/submucosal ischemia and full-thickness infarction of the large bowel is an intermediate form of ischemic colitis involving portions of the muscular layer of the large bowel. These areas of deep but incomplete ischemia may later heal with stricture formation, placing the patient at risk for subsequent large bowel obstruction or chronic segmental colitis. In many instances, the attack of ischemic colitis that led to stricture formation may have been so mild that medical care was not sought at the time, and the episode forgotten entirely by the patient.

Extraabdominal Diagnoses

CARDIOPULMONARY   If the patient is complaining of pain in the upper half of the abdomen (with or without tenderness), the chest should be examined for basilar involvement of lung parenchyma or pleura. Because the stethoscope exam is neither sensitive nor specific for the diagnosis of pneumonia, pulmonary infarction, small pleural effusions, or small pneumothoraces, a chest film should be obtained. Whether a decubitus or expiratory film is requested depends on clinical suspicion of effusion or pneumothorax, respectively. A negative film, especially if the pain is pleuritic in quality, introduces pulmonary embolism into the differential diagnosis.

If the pain is epigastric, and the patient is in an age/gender group in whom coronary artery disease is prevalent, a further cardiac history and ECG should be obtained. Ischemic cardiac pain referred to the epigastrium is not associated with significant tenderness, although cutaneous dysesthesia may be present, similar to that found in the upper extremity in other ischemic cardiac pain patterns.

ABDOMINAL WALL   Pain originating from the abdominal wall may be confused with visceral pain because superficial innervation from the lower thoracic roots enter the spinal cord via the same dorsal horn as the deeper visceral afferents. A useful and underutilized test is the sit-up test, also known as Carnett's sign. Following identification of the site of maximum abdominal tenderness, patients are asked to fold their arms across their chest and sit up halfway. The examiner maintains a finger on the tender area, and if palpation in the semi-sit-up position produces the same or increased tenderness, the test is said to be positive for an abdominal wall syndrome. The logic of this is that tensing of the abdominal muscles would be likely to protect the underlying peritoneum and intraabdominal organs, thus reducing tenderness if the cause of pain were deep. In patients unable to perform a sit-up,

simply asking them to raise their head and shoulders off the bed is usually sufficient to tense the abdominal muscles.

Abdominal wall syndromes overlap with hernias, neuropathic causes of abdominal pain, and NSAP.

HERNIAS   Hernias represent a special type of abdominal wall syndrome, characterized by a defect through which intraabdominal contents protrude, often intermittently, during transient increases in intraabdominal pressure. Uncomplicated hernias are ordinarily asymptomatic or at worst, aching and uncomfortable, but do not generally cause significant pain unless they have become incarcerated or strangulated. Although the vast majority of hernias are inguinal, there are many other types that must be considered, including incisional, periumbilical, and particularly in women, femoral hernias. Sonography of the abdominal wall is helpful in identifying hernias and other causes of abdominal wall pain.

OTHER ABDOMINAL WALL SYNDROMES   Other causes of abdominal wall pain include rectus sheath hematomas and trauma to other portions of the abdominal wall. In older patients or in those on anticoagulants, the trauma may be minor and forgotten. In circumstances in which the injury is due to stretching, causing tearing of muscle fibers, the overlying skin will not show any evidence of bruising that might otherwise provide a clue to the presence of bleeding into the abdominal wall.

TOXIC-METABOLIC

Toxic   A large number of infectious agents irritate the GI tract, producing pain that is usually crampy. Concomitant vomiting or diarrhea suggests a gastroenteritis or enterocolitis. Although many agents cause both upper and lower GI tract symptoms, in adults usually one symptom complex predominates over the other. Because most of these infections are confined to the mucosa of the GI tract, there is an absence of significant tenderness. This is because the parietal peritoneum is not irritated by mucosal disease. If infarction, penetration, or perforation of the bowel wall occurs, as may happen with some of the invasive dysenteries (e.g., *Salmonella*), peritoneal tenderness follows. This is the reason that abdominal tenderness of any significance should never be attributed to uncomplicated "gastroenteritis." Furthermore, because the overall incidence of symptomatic mucosal GI infections declines markedly with age (with the exception of antibiotic-associated diarrhea), the probability of "gastroenteritis" as the basis for abdominal complaints, particularly pain, in the elderly is very low indeed.

Other infections are associated with abdominal pain, although their pathophysiology is less clear. These include group A beta-hemolytic streptococcal pharyngitis, with or without associated scarlet fever, Rocky Mountain spotted fever, and early toxic shock syndrome.

The other major category of toxic causes of abdominal pain are those secondary to poisoning and overdose. These are numerous and tend to be nonspecific/nondiagnostic in most instances. An exception to this is envenomation by the female black widow spider, which is said to mimic peritonitis. This might represent a diagnostic dilemma if no history was taken and only the abdomen was examined. However, because the rigid abdomen following envenomation is due to muscular spasm, which begins at the site of the bite and gradually spreads to involve other large muscle groups of the back and proximal extremities, the prominence of extraabdominal signs and symptoms, as well as their historical evolution, should point the clinician away from a primary intraabdominal process. Isopropanol-induced hemorrhagic gastritis may be associated with cramping pain. Cocaine-induced intestinal ischemia progressing to infarction and perforation has been reported. Iron poisoning produces abdominal pain, and may cause hematemesis due to its direct corrosive effects on the GI tract. Large amounts of iron left in the stomach may also cause perforation. Mercury salts cause severe corrosion of the GI tract, associated with shock. *Acute* inorganic lead toxicity is typically associated with severe, crampy, abdominal pain. This is in contrast to *chronic* lead toxicity in which abdominal pain, if present, is usually less severe and often associated with constipation. The development of abdominal pain following electrical injury suggests a potentially serious complication and the need for admission. Opioid withdrawal produces abdominal pain, usually crampy in character, associated with diaphoresis and piloerection. In some individuals, the abdominal skin is dysesthetic, but significant tenderness should not be present. Mushroom toxicity, though rarely fatal, is commonly accompanied by a chemical gastroenteritis and severe abdominal pain out of proportion to tenderness.

Metabolic Anion-gap metabolic acidoses, particularly those seen in diabetic (DKA) and alcoholic (AKA) ketoacidosis, are common causes of abdominal pain. Although the discomfort associated with DKA and AKA has been attributed to gastric distention and paralytic ileus, this has not been clearly substantiated. In DKA or AKA, it is critical to consider the possibility that an underlying abdominal problem may have triggered the ketoacidosis, rather than the reverse. This is a particularly challenging clinical problem when amylase or lipase levels are elevated, since both AKA and DKA can be a consequence or a cause of acute pancreatitis. If the acidosis is resistant to standard treatment, or the pain persists after normalization of the pH, intraabdominal disease should be suspected.

Of the endocrinopathies associated with abdominal pain, adrenal crisis is the most striking. Patients are often shocky and diffusely peritoneal. The syndrome appears to be related to hypocortisolism rather than hypoaldosteronism. Without a history of similar prior episodes following reduced intake or absorption of adrenal steroids, these patients may be indistinguishable from those with an intraabdominal catastrophe. Other endocrinopathies and electrolyte abnormalities associated with abdominal pain include thyroid storm and hypo- and hypercalcemia. This pain is generally crampy, and tenderness is absent unless the hyperthyroid state has caused acute hepatomegaly and distention of the liver capsule. Hypoglycemia has been reportedly associated with abdominal pain, but the evidence supporting this is unconvincing.

A painful sickle cell crisis is a common cause of abdominal pain, second only to musculoskeletal pain as the most common manifestation of a vasoocclusive crisis in homozygous (SS) disease. Occasionally, patients with SC disease and other symptomatic heterozygous forms may present with abdominal pain due to splenomegaly or splenic infarct. Those with heterozygous sickle trait (SA) are almost invariably asymptomatic. The most reliable means of determining whether the abdominal pain is part of a crisis or secondary to an underlying intraabdominal problem is to ask the patient whether or not this is the pain of a typical crisis or whether it represents a pattern break. If the latter, the problem is usually localized to the RUQ, either

secondary to biliary tract disease (about 75 percent of those with SS have bilirubin stones due to chronic hemolysis) or hepatomegaly due to sinusoidal sludging of sickled cells. Additional considerations for SS patients include pancreatitis, *Salmonella* infection, and mesenteric venous thrombosis.

Less common "metabolic" entities associated with abdominal pain include virtually all forms of vasculitis, especially systemic lupus and Henoch-Schînlein purpura, porphyria, and familial Mediterranean fever. Each of these may produce peritonitis.

NEUROGENIC The hallmark of neurogenic abdominal pain is a dysesthetic sensation, particularly in response to light touch in the area of discomfort. This has been characterized by one author as the "hover" sign, in which the patient shows signs of discomfort when the examining hand is hovering just above or is passed very lightly over the area of dysesthesia. A positive hover sign may be mistakenly interpreted as indicating a generally hyperreactive patient, rather than a normal physiologic response to a dysesthetic or anticipated dysesthetic stimulus.

Because deep and superficial nerve fibers from the same area of the abdomen may enter the cord together, dysesthesias have also been reported with other, more serious, intraabdominal disease, such as appendicitis. In the latter, however, the problem is usually more acute, and either upon presentation or subsequently, is accompanied by tenderness (in contrast to dysesthesia alone). This category includes neural entrapment syndromes such as rectus nerve entrapment and iliohypogastric entrapment following a Pfannelstiel incision. A number of other incisional entrapment syndromes have been described. Many of these patients will have a positive Carnett's test, but the hover sign is probably more indicative of neurogenic abdominal pain.

Radicular problems causing abdominal pain include diabetic or zosteriform radiculopathy, the latter characterized by dysesthesias outlining a dermatome, usually with some "spillover" into contiguous dermatomes on either side of the involved root. The dysesthesias may present as lancinating, ticlike bouts of shooting pain or continuous burning. Accompanying vesicles confirm the diagnosis, although the pain may precede the cutaneous eruption by several days. Diabetic neuropathic involvement of a root, plexus, or nerve can be confirmed by electromyography.

There is evidence that greater attention to the examination of the abdominal wall reduces the frequency with which the diagnosis of NSAP is made. In one report, about 25 percent of patients with the diagnosis of NSAP were found to have abdominal wall syndromes.

Nonspecific Abdominal Pain (NSAP)

Despite a thorough work-up, the largest single group of patients seen in the ED will have no definite diagnosis, and will receive the designation of nonspecific abdominal pain (NSAP). It is essential that diagnostic terms with specific meanings, such as gastroenteritis or gastritis, not be used as catch-all phrases to describe patients with NSAP.

Although NSAP is a diagnosis of exclusion, there are some clinical features characteristically associated with it. Nausea, present in nearly half the patients, is the most common symptom after abdominal pain. Pain location is usually mid-epigastric or in the lower half of the abdomen. Tenderness is not usually severe, is absent in about one-third of the patients, and localized to the RLQ or mid-epigastrium in another one-third. Laboratory tests are usually normal, although a mild leukocytosis is entirely compatible with NSAP. Abdominal radiographs are virtually always normal or nonspecific. The key to confirming NSAP is reexamination over time (see below).

Special Considerations

Diagnostic accuracy of acute abdominal pain in those ≥50 years old is less than 50 percent, reaching a low of about 30 percent in octogenarians. For a detailed discussion of diagnosing abdominal pain in the elderly, see Chap. 73.

The causes of abdominal pain in elderly patients differ substantially from those seen in younger patients. For example, as shown in Table 72-12, the most common cause of abdominal pain in virtually all consecutive series of adults presenting to the ED is NSAP. However, when ED patients are dichotomized by age at 50 years old, NSAP remains at the top of the list of diagnoses in the younger cohort, but among older patients is markedly diminished in prevalence to <20 percent (see Table 72-3).

There are a number of serious vascular causes of abdominal pain seen almost exclusively among patients ≥50 years old, such as mesenteric ischemia, ischemic colitis, and AAA.

Among common causes of abdominal pain in both young and old, the nature of the presentation and evolution of the same illness is often very different. Using appendicitis as the most common example, those ≥50 years old are much more likely to have generalized pain and tenderness (about 14 percent) than are younger patients (about 2 percent). The absence of localization to an area of maximum pain or tenderness may help to account for the nearly tenfold difference in perforation rate (4 percent vs. 37 percent) in those >60 years old when compared to their younger counterparts. Later presentation in the course of their illness may also contribute to the increased perforation rate (75 percent of the elderly with appendicitis have >24 h of symptoms before seeking care), as may the higher frequency of distention in older patients, making the physical examination more difficult.

An additional contributor to the high incidence of perforation in appendicitis in the elderly is an understandable but unfortunate reluctance to operate on frail elderly patients without clear-cut signs of peritoneal irritation. This is reflected in the well-established inverse association between negative laparotomies and perforated appendices. At about the age of 45 years, the negative laparotomy rate begins to decrease in parallel with the increase in perforations until each plateaus at about 80 years of age. Thus, the negative laparotomy rate for appendicitis is lowest in the oldest, who are the group most likely to perforate, and therefore most in need of early, expedient surgery.

Therefore, one must assume that the elderly patient with abdominal pain has surgical disease. In support of this is the observation that about 40 percent of all patients >65 years old presenting to the ED with abdominal pain ultimately require surgery.

HIV/AIDS   There are several features of HIV/AIDS patients presenting to the ED with abdominal pain that merit special attention. Abdominal pain is rarely the index event that identifies a patient with HIV. Rather, most patients presenting with HIV-associated acute abdominal pain will have previously met criteria for AIDS and be aware of their diagnosis.

Distinguishing acuity of pain from an extensive background of severe, chronic illness represents the principal challenge in the evaluation of abdominal pain in HIV-positive patients. Identifying a precise infectious etiology for the pain at the time of presentation is well beyond the purview of emergency medicine.

Enterocolitis is the most common cause of abdominal pain in AIDS patients. It is typically accompanied by profuse diarrhea and dehydration. If associated with fecal leukocytes, it is more often accompanied by bacteremia than in immunocompetent patients. Perforation, when it occurs, tends to be large bowel perforation, often caused by cytomegalovirus (CMV). Obstruction presents in a typical fashion, but may be due to an unusual cause such as Kaposi sarcoma, lymphoma, or atypical mycobacteria.

Biliary tract disease is very common in AIDS patients, presenting in one of two unique forms: (1) AIDS-related cholangiopathy, caused principally by CMV or *Cryptosporidium* spp. (this can be treated with sphincterotomy), and (2) AIDS-associated cholecystitis, which is usually acalculous and has a propensity for early perforation.

TREATMENT

General Strategies

HYPOTENSION   Clinically important decreases in cardiac output are commonly underdiagnosed in the elderly. This is because many older patients have chronic systolic hypertension, making the traditional threshold value of 100 mm Hg systolic an insensitive marker for shock in the elderly. Conversely, healthy young women with abdominal pain, particularly if pregnant, may run systolic BPs that rarely reach 100 mm Hg. Thus in abdominal pain, as in all other clinical circumstances, hypotension is relative; the BP must be interpreted in context if it is to provide meaningful information.

In abdominal pain with relative hypotension, management depends on the presumed etiology. In the absence of heavy GI bleeding, which is not usually accompanied by abdominal pain, younger patients are most likely to be volume-contracted from vomiting, diarrhea, decreased oral intake, or third-spacing into the GI tract or peritoneum. Treatment is isotonic crystalloid.

In a smaller number of young patients, hypotension may be the result of abdominal sepsis. In this setting, in addition to appropriate antibiotics (see below) and isotonic crystalloid, pressors may be necessary to sustain BP until more definitive intervention can be undertaken. Vasoconstrictors are indicated in septic (vasodilatory) shock, with norepinephrine bitartrate (Levophed) or high-dose dopamine as the usual choice of agents.

In older patients, in addition to volume contraction and a higher incidence of abdominal sepsis, associated cardiovascular disease represents a third possible cause of decreased cardiac output. Indeed, in nonocclusive mesenteric ischemia, diminished cardiac output is the cause, rather than the consequence, of the presenting abdominal pain. In this circumstance, if the problem is acute myocardial ischemia, an aortic balloon pump may be necessary to buy time until the underlying problem can be corrected with angioplasty or bypass. If the decreased cardiac output is secondary to congestive failure, appropriate treatment for CHF is indicated with the caveat that digoxin is thought to be contraindicated in mesenteric ischemia because of a theoretical concern about worsening vasoconstriction. If pump failure appears to be the problem, dolbutamine may be used while slowly administering isotonic crystalloid. Arterial or venous pH and lactate levels are a more accurate means of monitoring end-organ perfusion and shock than is the BP.

TABLE 72-12   Most Common Causes of Acute Abdominal Pain

Final Diagnosis	Proportion of >10,000 Patients	
Nonspecific abdominal pain (NSAP)	34%	
Appendicitis	28%	
Biliary tract disease	10%	
Small bowel obstruction	4%	
Acute gynecologic disease	4%	
	Salpingitis	68%
	Ovarian cyst	21%
	Ectopic	6%
	Incomplete abortion	5%
Pancreatitis	3%	
Renal colic	3%	
Perforated peptic ulcer	3%	
Cancer	2%	
Diverticular disease	2%	
Other (<1% each)	6%	

ANALGESICS In the U.S., analgesia is usually withheld from patients with acute abdominal pain until a firm treatment plan is formulated. There is no evidence to support this longstanding practice, which has been attributed to Sir Zachary Cope. More than 75 years ago, Dr. Cope wrote that provision of analgesia to patients with abdominal pain might obscure the diagnosis, with dire consequences. There are many reasons why this may have been sage advice in 1921, not the least of them being the likely outcome of perforation and sepsis in the preantibiotic era. However, much has changed since that time in both the diagnosis and treatment of abdominal pain: (1) There have been major advances in diagnostic technology, the accuracy of which—in contrast to the serial clinical examination—is largely independent of the patient's degree of evolving pain and tenderness; (2) There have been parallel advances in therapeutic technology, including the universal availability of antibiotics and sophisticated intra- and perioperative monitoring.

There are at least five published randomized clinical trials, too heterogeneous for metaanalysis, but each consistent with the hypothesis that administration of opioids to patients with abdominal pain is at least safe. Although none of these trials answers the question definitively, at least one of them suggests that diagnosis and management of abdominal pain may, if anything, be facilitated by opioids. The plausibility of this is supported by an improved ability to obtain a history from a patient relieved of severe pain, and the enhanced localization of tenderness through reduction of guarding. In spite of these data, about 75 percent of emergency physicians recently surveyed indicated that they did not administer opioids until after a surgeon had seen the patient.[22]

The information on the safety of opioids cannot be extrapolated to nonsteroidal antiinflammatories (NSAIDs) such as parenteral ketorolac, because NSAIDs are not pure analgesics and have the potential to mask evidence of early peritoneal inflammation. At the present time all available evidence, and the recent recommendation of the Agency for Healthcare Research and Quality (AHRQ),[23] favors judicious use of opioid analgesia in the ED management of acute abdominal pain.

ANTIEMETICS Metoclopramide (Reglan) appears to be a more effective antiemetic than prochlorperazine (Compazine). Most patients will respond within 10 min to 10 to 20 mg of intravenous metoclopramide given slowly to minimize extrapyramidal side effects. In many institutions, 25 to 50 mg of intravenous diphenhydramine (Benadryl) is administered as prophylaxis against dystonias. Liberal use of antiemetics may obviate the need for insertion of a nasogastric tube, whose therapeutic value in abdominal pain has never been convincingly demonstrated.

ANTIBIOTICS Antibiotics are indicated in suspected abdominal sepsis and in most patients with localized, and all patients with diffuse, peritonitis. Endogenous gut flora cause abdominal infections in the GI or GU tract. Primary gynecologic infections, of which PID is the prototype, behave differently and will be discussed separately under the treatment of suspected PID, below. In all intraabdominal nongynecologic infections, minimal coverage should be targeted at anaerobes and facultative aerobic gram-negatives. An exception to this generalization is the need to provide additional coverage for gram-positive aerobes (e.g., *Pneumococcus*) in spontaneous bacterial peritonitis (SBP). SBP, also known as primary peritonitis, occurs in patients with cirrhosis and ascites, probably due to spontaneous bacteremic seeding of ascitic fluid. The modifier "primary" is used to distinguish SBP from the more common peritonitis secondary to intraabdominal organ inflammation, ischemia, leakage, or perforation.

Historically, a two-drug regimen, attacking gram-negative aerobes with an aminoglycoside (gentamicin or tobramycin, 1.5 mg/kg IV q8h, or amikacin 5 mg/kg IV q8h) and anaerobes with metronidazole (1 g intravenous loading dose, followed by 500 mg IV q6h, given slowly) or clindamycin (900 mg IV q8h) has been used to obtain the requisite coverage for intraabdominal infections. While dual therapy may still be necessary for sicker, older, immunocompromised, or hypotensive patients, monotherapy with a second-generation cephalosporin, such as cefoxitin (2 g IV q6h) or cefotetan (2 g IV q6h) is often adequate for those who are less ill. Alternative "combined" monotherapy includes ampicillin-sulbactam (3 g IV q6h) or ticarcillin-clavulanate (3.1 g IV q6h). For patients requiring a more potent regimen, but in whom one is reluctant to use an aminoglycoside, the combination of piperacillin-tazobactam (3.3 g IV q6h) appears to be at least as effective as imipenem-cilastatin (1 g IV q6h, maximum dose), particularly in treatment of suspected biliary sepsis, and is less likely to cause seizures.

For patients with a history of severe allergy to penicillins or cephalosporins, aztreonam (2 g IV q6h, maximum dose) and clindamycin or metronidazole is a safe alternative. In SBP, monotherapy with a third-generation cephalosporin such as ceftriaxone (2 g IV q12h, maximum dose) or cefotaxime (2 g IV q4h, maximum dose) broadens the spectrum sufficiently to cover for *Pneumococcus* in addition to the gram-negative enteric bacteria, such as *E. coli*.

Gynecologic infections differ from those of the GI and GU tract in several important respects: (1) They do not generally cause a septic syndrome; (2) elderly patients, who are most likely to suffer mortality from delay in the treatment of abdominal infections or sepsis, do not generally present with primary gynecologic infections as the cause of their abdominal pain; and (3) treatment of PID requires different antibiotic combinations than do GI and GU infections.

For outpatient treatment of PID, the combination of a single dose of ceftriaxone 250 mg IM plus azithromycin 1 g PO given under direct observation, has become standard in many EDs. However, the CDC still recommends ceftriaxone 250 mg IM plus doxycycline 100 mg PO bid for 14 days rather than azithromycin for outpatient PID. For inpatient treatment, the recommendation remains cefoxitin 2 g IV q6h plus doxycycline 100 mg q12h IV until improvement, then 100 mg PO bid to complete 14 days. However, many inpatient physicians are also using azithromycin in preference to doxycycline. If there is evidence of a tubo-ovarian abscess, the cure rate may be increased with use of triple antibiotic coverage: clindamycin 900 mg IV q8h plus gentamicin 1.5 mg/kg IV q8h plus ampicillin 1 g IV q6h. Doses of all aminoglycosides recommended assume normal renal function, and must be adjusted for decreased glomerular filtration rate.

DISPOSITION

General Indications for Admission

In addition to those with a specific diagnosis requiring admission, the following patients should be seriously considered as candidates for hospitalization: those who appear ill; any elderly or immunocompromised (including HIV-positive) patient (with or without comorbidity) in whom the diagnosis is unclear; young, apparently healthy patients in whom the diagnosis is unclear and all potentially serious causes of abdominal pain have not been reasonably excluded; intractable pain or vomiting; acute or chronically altered mental status; inability to follow discharge or follow-up instructions; undomiciled, living in a shelter, or otherwise lacking social supports; and alcohol or other drug use.

Nonspecific Abdominal Pain

A substantial number of patients who are discharged with the diagnosis of NSAP are initially admitted as suspected appendicitis. This may be the reason that there appears to be an unexplained predominance of RLQ pain among patients discharged with the diagnosis of NSAP.

Although this entity is poorly understood pathophysiologically, follow-up among patients discharged from the ED with this diagnosis has found that nearly 90 percent are better or asymptomatic at 2 to 3 weeks. Similarly, follow-up of patients discharged from inpatient services with the diagnosis of NSAP has shown that about 80 percent have no further problems and are asymptomatic at 5 years. Of the remainder, about one-third are rehospitalized, of whom one-third of these have appendicitis. Some of these individuals probably had early appendicitis on their prior admission, with spontaneous resolution due to disimpaction of the appendiceal lumen. Of this group, it is plausible that some later developed recurrent appendicitis and required appendectomy. The remaining two-thirds of patients who were neither rehospitalized nor asymptomatic, turned out to have benign gynecologic and colonic problems, most commonly irritable bowel.

The key to confirming NSAP as a working diagnosis is reexamination in 24 h, repeated as necessary over time if patients remain symptomatic. Whether this occurs on the inpatient service, in an ED observation unit, or follow-up in the ED depends on the culture of the institution, the clinician's degree of uncertainty about the diagnosis, and the presence of facilities for reliable outpatient follow-up.

REFERENCES

1. American College of Emergency Physicians: Clinical policy: Critical issues for the initial evaluation and management of patients presenting with a chief complaint of nontraumatic acute abdominal pain. *Ann Emerg Med* 36:406, 2000.

2. McCaig LF, Nghi L: National Hospital Ambulatory Medical Care Survey: 2000 Emergency Department Summary. Advance data from vital and health statistics, no. 326. Hyattsville, MD: National Center for Health Statistics, 2002, p. 14.

3. Chen SC, Wang HP, Chen WJ, et al: Selective use of ultrasonography for the detection of pneumoperitoneum. *Acad Emerg Med* 9:643, 2002.

4. Irwig LI, Tosteson ANA, Gatsonis C, et al: Guidelines for meta-analyses evaluating diagnostic tests. *Ann Intern Med* 120:667, 1994.

5. Gallagher EJ: Clinical utility of likelihood ratios. *Ann Emerg Med* 31:391, 1998.

6. McColl I: More precision in diagnosing appendicitis. *New Engl J Med* 338:190, 1998.

7. Rao PM, Rhea JT, Novelline RA, et al: Effect of computed tomography of the appendix on treatment of patients and use of hospital resources. *New Engl J Med* 338:141, 1998.

8. Flum DR, Morris A, Koepsell T, et al: Has misdiagnosis of appendicitis decreased over time? A population-based analysis. *JAMA* 286:1748, 2001.

9. Kalimi R, Gecelter GR, Caplin D, et al: Diagnosis of acute cholecystitis: Sensitivity of sonography, cholescintigraphy, and combined sonography-cholescintigraphy. *J Am Coll Surg* 193:609, 2001.

10. Magnuson TH, Bender JS, Duncan MD, et al: Utility of magnetic resonance cholangiography in the evaluation of biliary obstruction. *J Am Coll Surg* 189:63, 1999.

11. Burkill GJ, Bell JR, Healy JC: The utility of computed tomography in acute small bowel obstruction. *Clin Radiol* 56:350, 2001.

12. Vissers RJ, Abu-Laban RB, McHugh DF: Amylase and lipase in the emergency department evaluation of acute pancreatitis. *J Emerg Med* 17:1027, 1999.

13. Harvey RT, Miller WT: Acute biliary disease: Initial CT and follow-up US versus initial US and follow-up CT. *Radiology* 213:831, 1999.

14. Hollerweger A, Macheiner P, Rettenbacher T, et al: Colonic diverticulitis: diagnostic value and appearance of inflamed diverticula-sonographic evaluation. *Eur Radiol* 11:1956, 2001.

15. Kircher MF, Rhea JT, Kihiczak D, et al: Frequency, sensitivity, and specificity of individual signs of diverticulitis on thin-section helical CT with colonic contrast material: Experience with 312 cases. *AJR* 178:1313, 2002.

16. Luchs JS, Katz DS, Lane MJ, et al: Utility of hematuria testing in patients with suspected renal colic: Correlation with unenhanced helical CT results. *Urology* 59:839, 2002.

17. Molander P, Sjoberg J, Paavonen J, et al: Transvaginal power Doppler findings in laparoscopically proven acute pelvic inflammatory disease. *Ultrasound Obstet Gynecol* 17:233, 2001.

18. Barnhart KT, Simhan H, Kamelle SA: Diagnostic accuracy of ultrasound above and below the beta-hCG discriminatory zone. *Obstet Gynecol* 94:583, 1999.

19. Buckley RG, King KJ, Disney JD, et al: Serum progesterone testing to predict ectopic pregnancy in symptomatic first-trimester patients. *Ann Emerg Med* 36:95, 2000.

20. Lederle FA, Simel DL: The rational clinical examination. Does this patient have abdominal aortic aneurysm? *JAMA* 281:77, 1999.

21. Horton KM, Fishman EK: Volume-rendered 3D CT of the mesenteric vasculature: Normal anatomy, anatomic variants, and pathologic conditions. *Radiographics* 22:161, 2002.

22. Wolfe JM, Lein DY, Lenkoski K, et al: Analgesic administration to patients with an acute abdomen: A survey of emergency physicians. *Am J Emerg Med* 18:250, 2000.

23. Brownfield E: Pain management: Use of analgesics in the acute abdomen. Agency for Healthcare Research and Quality (AHRQ). http://www.AHRQ. GOV/CLINIC/PTSAFETY/CHAP37A.HTM37.1; Accessed June 11, 2002.

73 ABDOMINAL PAIN IN THE ELDERLY
Robert McNamara

EPIDEMIOLOGY

A recent study of 10 northern New Jersey EDs reported that 4.2 percent of the visits for those age 65 and greater were for abdominal pain.[1] In the United States, the elderly (age 65 and up) accounted for 15.1 percent of the 108 million ED encounters in 2000.[2] Regardless of the current frequency of ED visits for abdominal pain in the elderly, one can count on a steadily rising volume of such cases. Current projections predict that the number of those aged 65 and older will rise from 13 percent of the population in the year 2000 to approximately 20 percent by the year 2030.[3] Practicing emergency physicians rate abdominal pain as the most challenging clinical situation in this population.[3] Over half of the patients aged 65 or greater who present to the ED with abdominal pain require admission, and one-quarter to one-third will require surgical intervention at some point during their hospital stay.[4,5] The mortality rate across all causes of abdominal pain in the elderly is 11 to 14 percent, justifying its anxiety-provoking reputation.[5,6] The mortality rate can double if the diagnosis rendered in the ED is incorrect.[6,7]

PATHOPHYSIOLOGY

The approach to acute abdominal pain in all age groups requires an understanding of the visceral and somatic pathways of pain perception. Neural pathways are not rerouted as we age; however, it is an accepted axiom that the perception of abdominal pain or at least the reporting of it is altered in the elderly.[7] There is limited proof of this axiom for abdominal pain; however, it is fairly clear that ischemic heart disease is associated with altered pain perception or reporting in the elderly. Other factors such as fear, stoicism, and communication problems may affect the reporting of abdominal pain in older persons.[7,8]

Aging is associated with several factors that influence the prevalence and spectrum of abdominal conditions encountered in this population (Table 73-1). For example, older patients have a statistically increased frequency of abdominal aortic aneurysms. The presence of

TABLE 73-1 Influence of Aging on Abdominal Pain

Increased Risk in the Elderly	Resultant Disease
ASCVD	AAA, mesenteric ischemic, ischemic colitis
Cholelithiasis	Cholecystitis, pancreatitis
Carcinoma	Large bowel obstruction, intussusception
Immobility	Colonic volvulus, Ogilvie's syndrome
Medications	Peptic ulcer disease, pancreatitis
Prior surgery	Small bowel obstruction

Abbreviations: AAA = abdominal aortic aneurysm; ASCUD = atherosclerotic cardiovascular disease.

comorbid diseases and their associated therapy contributes to the complexity of care. Other important pathophysiologic features include decreased cardiopulmonary reserve, lowered tolerance for hypovolemic shock, and the treatment issues of altered pharmacodynamics and pharmacokinetics.

CLINICAL FEATURES

The History

History taking in older patients with abdominal pain should follow the same general sequence and rules as in younger patients. Unfortunately, an accurate history may be difficult to obtain in this age group. Serious abdominal disease may cause an acute mental status change or distract the patient's attention. Memory deficits or underlying dementia can obscure important aspects, such as the time and nature of the onset of pain.[8] The noise and pace of the ED are often inconsistent with the needs of the older patient who is attempting to relay historical information about his or her abdominal pain. The following historical aspects should be covered:

1. *Time of onset:* Pain awakening the patient from sleep should always be considered significant.
2. *Mode of onset:* Sudden, severe pain suggests serious disease, including a ruptured abdominal aortic aneurysm, aortic dissection, superior mesenteric artery embolus, perforation of a peptic ulcer, or volvulus. However, these disorders may present without a sudden onset. For example, in one prospective series of patients over the age of 70 with perforated ulcers, only 47 percent reported a sudden onset of pain.[6]
3. *Progression since onset:* Steady improvement is reassuring; worsening is not.
4. *Location of the pain:* In general, this seems to be reliable in the elderly. For example, appendicitis in this age group, although diagnostically difficult, generally presents with right-lower-quadrant pain.[9]
5. *Character of the pain:* Severe pain should be taken as an indicator of serious disease. Think of mesenteric ischemia, perforation of a gastric ulcer, vascular accidents, and volvulus.
6. *Referral or radiation of the pain:* As with location, this aspect of abdominal pain should not change with aging. For example, the referral pattern is helpful in diagnosing older patients with biliary tract disease.[8]
7. *Precipitating and relieving factors:* Pain with movement suggests irritation of the parietal peritoneum. The results of any self-treatment should be determined.
8. *Prior episodes:* This generally suggests a medical cause with the notable exceptions of mesenteric ischemia (intestinal angina) and cholecystitis.
9. *Associated symptoms:* Anorexia, vomiting, bowel habits, and urinary symptoms are key areas to cover. In general, pain almost always precedes vomiting in surgical causes of abdominal pain, while the converse is true in 75 percent of patients with gastroenteritis or a nonspecific cause of abdominal pain.[4]
10. *Further history:* A detailed review of systems is desirable to seek other causes of abdominal pain, especially those of a cardiopulmonary nature. Do not neglect a careful review of medications, including over-the-counter nonsteroidal antiinflammatory agents. Underlying alcohol abuse must also be a consideration in this age group.

The Physical Examination

As with the history, the abdominal examination in the older patient proceeds in the same manner as for younger patients. Complicating factors may include the patient's stoicism or inability to report pain

and the less pronounced muscular response to inflammation.[7,8] The following should be addressed:

1. *General appearance:* An ill-appearing older patient with abdominal pain should cause immediate concern, given the high mortality rate in general case series of elderly patients with abdominal pain.[4–6] On the other hand, the clinician can be misled by a deceptively "well" appearance in the face of serious underlying disease.[8]
2. *Vital signs:* Reflexively think of a ruptured abdominal aortic aneurysm in the hypotensive older patient with abdominal pain.[10] Determination of a core temperature is advisable; however, lack of fever commonly occurs with serious infectious causes of abdominal pain. Tachypnea and tachycardia are nonspecific findings but should raise the possibility of a cardiopulmonary disorder or sepsis.
3. *Inspection and auscultation:* Distention is common in large bowel obstruction, including sigmoid and cecal volvulus.[11] High-pitched "rushes" suggest small bowel obstruction.
4. *Abdominal palpation:* In general, the location of tenderness is generally reliable in the older patient. Appendicitis usually manifests right-lower-quadrant tenderness,[6,9,12] while cholecystitis and pancreatitis generally cause tenderness in the expected location.[8] Unfortunately, abdominal guarding or muscular rigidity may be lacking despite the presence of chemical or infectious peritoneal irritation. This is partially attributed to the relatively thin abdominal musculature of older patients.[7,8] Disturbingly, of patients over the age of 70 with a perforated ulcer, only 21 percent had epigastric rigidity.[6]
5. *Rectal examination:* This should be performed routinely, and the detection of occult blood should receive follow-up evaluation. In one series of patients over the age of 50, about 10 percent of those discharged from the ED with a diagnosis of nonspecific abdominal pain were diagnosed with cancer, principally of the large bowel, within a year.[13]
6. *Further examination:* There should be careful inspection for hernias, particularly of the femoral canal in the older female patient. Aortic dissection may manifest with unequal femoral pulses. The back should be inspected for herpes zoster. Genital and pelvic examinations may reveal the cause of pain. Assessment of the heart and lungs may yield clues to a nonabdominal cause of the pain.

SPECIFIC DIAGNOSES AND ISSUES

This section reviews the major diagnostic causes of abdominal pain in the older patient and points out specific diagnostic issues to consider in this population. The frequency of each particular disease varies in the reported case series of elderly patients presenting to the ED with abdominal pain. Cholecystitis (12 to 41 percent) is generally the most frequently encountered disease of a surgical nature, followed by bowel obstruction (7 to 14 percent). Nonspecific abdominal pain is also a frequent diagnosis (10 to 23 percent). Perforated viscus, appendicitis, diverticulitis, and pancreatitis each generally represent around 4 to 7 percent, depending on the case series. Aortic aneurysms and mesenteric ischemia are less common.[4,6,8] General coverage of the following conditions can also be found in other chapters.

Appendicitis

Diagnostic problems surrounding appendicitis in the elderly are well known in emergency medicine. In one series, only 51 percent of patients over the age of 60 with proven appendicitis had that diagnosis made during the ED phase of their care.[13] Delayed presentation is common and contributes to the higher perforation and complication rate. One must be careful not to exclude appendicitis because of prolonged symptoms, as a small but significant percentage of the elderly will wait more than a week to seek care for this condition (see Chap. 78).

The abdominal pain is generally reported to be in the right lower quadrant; however, the description may be vague or the pain poorly localized.[9,13] Migration has been reported from a low of 5 percent to as high as 64 percent of elderly patients with appendicitis.[9] Anorexia, an expected finding in younger patients, may be lacking (reported in 19 to 44 percent), while nausea and vomiting are reported in roughly half of elderly patients with appendicitis.[8,9,13] Diarrhea and urinary tract symptoms do not exclude the disease.

Fever may be absent in one-third or more. Tenderness in the right lower quadrant is a frequent finding occurring in 80 to 90 percent. The presence of rigidity and rebound tenderness ranges from 20 percent to more than 80 percent.[8,9] Laboratory assessment is potentially misleading, as most studies indicate that 20 percent or more will have a white blood cell count below 10,000.[9,13] Up to 17 percent of the elderly with appendicitis have hyperbilirubinemia.[12] Abdominal radiographs rarely add to the diagnostic process and can lead one astray by suggesting small bowel obstruction.[8]

It is prudent to include appendicitis in the differential diagnosis of any elderly patient with abdominal pain who has not undergone an appendectomy. The clinician must not expect a neat diagnostic package. In one series, only 20 percent of older patients with appendicitis had all of fever, nausea or vomiting, tenderness in the right lower quadrant, and an elevated white blood cell count.[13]

Acute Cholecystitis

Acute cholecystitis (see Chap. 85) is the most common surgical emergency in older patients with abdominal pain. Fortunately, physicians have a record of high diagnostic accuracy for this condition in the elderly.[6] The presenting features of acute cholecystitis in the older population are similar to those in younger patients. Right-upper-quadrant or epigastric pain is present in most, while radiation to the back or shoulder area occurs in about one-third. Roughly half will report nausea or vomiting, and jaundice will occur in 10 to 30 percent. Fever may be absent in over half of these patients. Laboratory testing may be misleading, as 30 to 40 percent can have a normal white blood cell count. Plain radiographs are of little value; the diagnostic study of choice is ultrasonography. Computed tomography is generally of limited usefulness.[8,14]

Conservative management is generally unsuccessful and operative delay increases the complication rate. The older patient can appear deceptively well with acute cholecystitis; however, the overall mortality rate is approximately 10 percent.[15] Additionally, a clinical picture of fever, jaundice, and altered mental status without significant abdominal findings has been described in a subset of elderly patients with acute cholecystitis.

Small Bowel Obstruction

The diagnosis of small bowel obstruction is usually straightforward in the older patient (see Chap. 79). Colicky pain, distention, and vomiting that progresses from gastric contents to bile-stained to feculent are the cardinal features. Prior surgery is still the principal risk factor in this age group, and the physician should conduct a careful search for hernias. The mortality rate for small bowel obstruction in the elderly ranges from 14 to 45 percent. Errors in management most frequently relate to misinterpretation of radiographic studies and excessive delays in operative management.[7]

Perforated Peptic Ulcer

Although peptic ulcer disease most frequently presents as gastrointestinal bleeding, perforation is an important cause of abdominal pain in the older patient (see Chap. 77). The expected description of a sudden, acute onset of epigastric pain is reported in only one-half of patients over age 70 with a perforated ulcer.[6] The pain has usually been present only for a matter of hours and is generally severe, constant, and present to some degree in the epigastrium. Free intraperitoneal perforation can cause generalized pain or lower-quadrant symptoms.[8] Vomiting is infrequent. The physical examination is expected to reveal epigastric tenderness, although muscular guarding is variable. In one study, only 21 percent of the elderly with a perforated ulcer had epigastric rigidity.[6] Fever is generally not present early on.

The key diagnostic mistake is excluding this diagnosis because of a lack of free air on plain radiographs. Roughly 40 percent of patients with perforated ulcers will not have this finding on their initial chest radiograph. The left lateral decubitus view or the lateral view of the upright chest radiograph may help to detect the presence of free air. Repeat radiographs after instillation of 500 mL of air via a nasogastric tube can increase the diagnostic yield of plain radiographs, although its use is somewhat controversial. Computed tomography is capable of detecting small amounts of air in the peritoneal cavity. In one series, missed perforated ulcer was the leading cause of death in elderly patients with abdominal pain, and in each case the plain radiographs did not reveal free air.[7]

Large Bowel Obstruction

A carcinoma is the leading cause of large bowel obstruction, while volvulus and diverticulitis account for most of the remaining cases. All of these precipitating conditions are more common in the elderly. The overall mortality rate approximates 40 percent. Distention is common, and vomiting and constipation are reported in about half of the patients. Importantly, a significant percentage (up to 20 percent) will report diarrhea. A history of rectal bleeding, altered bowel habits, or weight loss may be present with underlying carcinoma.[11] The pain is usually gradual in onset; however, cecal volvulus can present with the acute onset of severe, colicky pain.[16] Sigmoid volvulus is two to three times more frequent than cecal volvulus and more commonly presents with a gradual onset of pain. Fever or the presence of peritoneal irritation suggests a perforation or gangrenous bowel.

The principal diagnostic study is plain abdominal radiography; however, cecal volvulus may appear as small bowel obstruction and require a barium enema to make the diagnosis.[16] In one large series, a cecal diameter of 10 cm was not useful in predicting perforation. In fact, cecal diameters of up to 20 cm responded to routine decompression methods.[11] Colonic pseudo-obstruction, also known as Ogilvie syndrome, can present in a manner similar to that of large bowel obstruction. This is massive gaseous distention of the colon, generally occurring in chronically ill, immobilized older patients. It is thought to be a result of an imbalance in the regulation of the colonic motor function by the autonomic nervous system.[17] The abdomen is distended and tympanitic but usually nontender. A cavernous rectal vault is an important clue on physical examination. Old medical records frequently reveal several such presentations. It is important to avoid surgery in these patients as there is no underlying mechanical blockage. Neostigmine (2.0 mg IV) has a high success rate in the treatment of this condition.[17]

Diverticulitis

The presence of diverticula increases with age, and acute inflammation, diverticulitis, is a common cause of abdominal pain in the older patient (see Chap. 81). Computed tomography is the diagnostic study of choice, as a barium enema or colonoscopy can precipitate perforation. Also, diverticulitis can be mistaken for a pelvic mass of gynecologic origin in the older female.

Acute Mesenteric Infarction

The management of mesenteric ischemia is complicated by diagnostic delays that are often associated with a fatal outcome. Early diagnosis markedly improves the chances of survival,[18] and in a recent series it was the leading diagnosis in only 25 percent of those admitted with mesenteric infarction.[19] The key to making the correct diagnosis is to consider this possibility in the elderly patient with abdominal pain and risk factors for the disease. Classically, superior mesenteric artery occlusion by an embolus or thrombus accounted for the majority of cases, but infarction resulting from low flow states is becoming more common.[19] Inferior mesenteric artery occlusion, venous thrombosis, arteritis, and dissection are other causes of this condition.

The specific risk factors are listed in Table 73-2. The principal manifestation of mesenteric infarction is severe abdominal pain, often refractory to narcotic analgesics. Severe pain, with gradually increasing intensity, combined with a relatively normal abdominal examination, is considered the sine qua non of early mesenteric infarction. If an embolus is the cause, sudden, severe pain may be reported.[18] There may be a history of prior episodes of spontaneously resolving pain, particularly with mesenteric arterial thrombosis. Associated gastrointestinal symptoms are very common. Nausea, anorexia, and vomiting are common, and up to half will report diarrhea. Objective findings on physical examination represent intestinal necrosis and possible perforation. Theoretically, the stool should be guaiac-negative early on. Patients will inevitably develop guaiac-positive stools. Laboratory abnormalities such as metabolic acidosis and extreme leukocytosis are likewise indicators of advanced, perhaps irreversible disease.

The critical aspect of care is to pursue mesenteric angiography based on the history and physical examination without waiting for hard evidence from the exam or diagnostic studies. One series reported a 90 percent survival rate when angiography was performed prior to the onset of peritonitis.[18] The usual survival rate is 30 percent or less.

Abdominal Aortic Aneurysm

Rupture of an abdominal aortic aneurysm is a lethal condition that will be more frequently encountered as the population ages (see Chap. 58). The incidence of abdominal aortic aneurysm in men increases rapidly after age 55 and peaks at the age of 80 at 5.9 percent. In women, the incidence rises quickly after age 70, peaking at 4.5 percent at age 90.[20] With rupture, the mortality rate among those who reach the hospital is generally on the order of 50 percent or higher. A favorable outcome depends on a rapid diagnosis and early operative intervention. Unfortunately, initial misdiagnosis is common, occurring in 30 percent of patients in one series.[10]

The most common symptom is abdominal pain, occurring in 70 to 80 percent, and not back pain, which is noted by just over half. The typical pain is sudden and significant. Atypical locations include the hips, inguinal area, and external genitalia. Syncope may be part of the presenting picture with or without significant blood loss from the aneurysm. Because of the lethal nature of this condition, the diagnosis should be considered in any older patient, especially male, with back, flank, or abdominal pain. Hypotension occurs at some point in the majority of these patients. Palpation of a tender, enlarged (>5 cm) aorta is the key physical finding. Unfortunately, the size of the aorta is often difficult to determine on examination.

TABLE 73-2   Risk Factors for Mesenteric Ischemia

Mesenteric Condition	Risk Factors
SMA embolus	Atrial fibrillation, recent MI
SMA thrombosis	Atherosclerosis, low CO states
Nonocclusive infarction	Low CO states (esp. CHF), digoxin therapy
Venous thrombosis	Hypercoagulability, prior DVT, liver disease

Abbreviations: CHF = congestive heart failure; CO = cardiac output; DVT = deep venous thrombosis; MI = myocardial infarction; SMA = superior mesenteric artery.

Management of the unstable patient with a clinically suspected ruptured abdominal aortic aneurysm involves immediate operative intervention without confirmatory testing. A supine plain radiograph of the abdomen will often reveal a clue to the diagnosis, such as a calcified aortic outline or loss of the renal or psoas outline. In the stable patient, ultrasonography can delineate the size of the aorta, while computed tomography gives more information regarding actual rupture.[20] Any such testing must include careful monitoring of the patient's condition, with appropriate alerting of the operating theater and surgical team.

The most common diagnostic mistake is to diagnose renal colic in these patients. This is understandable given the severe pain and the location of the pain. Furthermore, abdominal aortic aneurysm may present with hematuria. It should be axiomatic that aortic aneurysm be strongly considered in any patient over the age of 50 suspected of having renal colic. An episode of hypotension is often wrongly ascribed to developing sepsis or a "vagal" reaction in the patient initially misdiagnosed as having renal colic.[10]

Other Conditions and Causes

The list presented above is certainly not comprehensive for abdominal pain in the elderly. Aortic dissection is common in this age group and may cause abdominal pain directly or by causing ischemia of intraabdominal organs, including the bowel. The diagnosis of pancreatitis in this age group is generally straightforward. Tumors can serve as lead points for intussusception in elderly patients. Acute gastric volvulus should be considered in the older patient with sudden epigastric pain, repetitive nonproductive retching, and inability to pass a nasogastric tube. Older patients with underlying vascular disease may develop ischemic colitis, which can be difficult to distinguish from other forms of colitis.

The list of other conditions that can cause abdominal pain in the older patient is extensive, highlighting the need for the comprehensive evaluation of such patients. The most important disease to suspect is acute myocardial ischemia. Virtually all other "chest" diseases can cause abdominal pain, including pneumonia, pulmonary embolism, empyema, tuberculosis, congestive heart failure, esophageal rupture, and endocarditis. Genitourinary disease including renal colic, pyelonephritis, epididymitis, and testicular torsion is a possible cause of abdominal pain in the elderly. Diabetic ketoacidosis, herpes zoster, hypercalcemia, addisonian crisis, hemochromatosis, and retroperitoneal or rectus sheath hematomas secondary to anticoagulant therapy are examples of "medical" causes of abdominal pain in the elderly.

DISPOSITION

A period of observation with serial examinations should be considered in the elderly patient with undifferentiated abdominal pain. Depending on the circumstances, this could occur in the ED, an observation unit, or in an inpatient unit. Patients with severe pain or worsening pain while in the ED should generally not be sent home. Resolved pain is generally reassuring, and such patients who are discharged should receive routine follow-up with their primary care providers. Biliary tract disease and underlying cancer are possibilities in this circumstance.[13]

If an older patient is to be discharged with abdominal pain, the patient should be instructed to return if the symptoms worsen or do not resolve in a brief period of time (6 to 8 h). Vomiting after discharge should prompt reevaluation.

REFERENCES

1. Ciccone A, Allegra JR, Cochrane DG, et al: Age related differences in diagnoses within the elderly population. *Am J Emerg Med* 16:43, 1998.
2. McCaig LF, Ly N: National Hospital Ambulatory Medical Care Survey: 2000 Emergency Department Summary. Advance data from vital and health statistics, no. 326. Hyattsville, MD: National Center for Health Statistics, 2002.

PUD → 1° cause of GI bleeding

3. McNamara RM, Rousseau E, Sanders AB: Geriatric emergency medicine: A survey of practicing emergency physicians. *Ann Emerg Med* 21:796, 1992.
4. Brewer RJ, Golden GT, Hitch DC, et al: Abdominal pain: An analysis of 1,000 consecutive cases in a university hospital emergency room. *Am J Surg* 131:219, 1976.
5. Kizer KW, Vassar MJ: Emergency department diagnosis of abdominal disorders in the elderly. *Am J Emerg Med* 16:357, 1998.
6. Fenyo G: Acute abdominal disease in the elderly: Experience from two series in Stockholm. *Am J Surg* 143:751, 1982.
7. Bender JS: Approach to the acute abdomen. *Med Clin North Am* 73:1413, 1989.
8. Fenyo G: Diagnostic problems of acute abdominal pain in the aged. *Acta Chir Scand* 140:396, 1974.
9. Kraemer M, Franke C, Ohmann C, et al: Acute appendicitis in late adulthood: Incidence, presentation, and outcome. Results of a prospective multicenter acute abdominal pain study and a review of the literature. *Langenbeck's Arch Surg* 385:470, 2000.
10. Marston WA, Ahlquist R, Johnson G, et al: Misdiagnosis of ruptured abdominal aortic aneurysms. *J Vasc Surg* 16:17, 1992.
11. Greenlee HB, Pienkos EJ, Vanderbilt PC, et al: Acute large bowel obstruction. *Arch Surg* 108:470, 1974.
12. Horattas MC, Guyton DP, Wu D: A reappraisal of appendicitis in the elderly. *Am J Surg* 160:291, 1990.
13. DeDombal FT, Matharu SS, Staniland JR, et al: Presentation of cancer to hospital as "acute abdominal pain." *Br J Surg* 67:413, 1980.
14. Parker LJ, Vukov LF, Wollan PC: Emergency department evaluation of geriatric patients with acute cholecystitis. *Acad Emerg Med* 4:51, 1997.
15. Glenn F: Surgical management of acute cholecystitis in patients 65 years of age and older. *Ann Surg* 193:56, 1981.
16. Andersson A, Bergdahl L, Van Der Linden W: Volvulus of the cecum. *Ann Surg* 181:876, 1976.
17. Ponec RJ, Saunders MD, Kimmey MB: Neostigmine for the treatment of acute colonic pseudo-obstruction. *New Engl J Med* 341:137, 1999.
18. Boley SJ, Sprayregan S, Siegelman SS, et al: Initial results from an aggressive roentgenological and surgical approach to acute mesenteric ischemia. *Surgery* 82:848, 1977.
19. Newman TS, Magnuson TH, Ahrendt SA, et al: The changing face of mesenteric infarction. *Am Surgeon* 64:611, 1998.
20. Ernst CB: Abdominal aortic aneurysm. *New Engl J Med* 328:1167, 1993.

74

GASTROINTESTINAL BLEEDING
David T. Overton

Gastrointestinal (GI) bleeding is a common problem in emergency medical practice and should be considered potentially life threatening until proven otherwise.

Acute upper GI bleeding in adults has an overall annual incidence of approximately 100 per 100,000. It is more common among males and markedly more common among the elderly. Its associated mortality rises with age.[1,2] Lower GI bleeding is somewhat less common, with an annual incidence of approximately 20 per 100,000. It, too, is more common among males and among the elderly.[3]

As with all true emergencies, the traditional triad of medical history, physical examination, and diagnosis often must be accomplished simultaneously with resuscitation and stabilization. **Factors associated with a high morbidity rate are hemodynamic instability, repeated hematemesis or hematochezia, failure to clear with gastric lavage, age older than 60 years, and coexistent organ system disease.**

PATHOPHYSIOLOGY

Causes of Upper Gastrointestinal Bleeding

Upper GI bleeding is defined as that originating proximal to the ligament of Treitz, whereas lower GI bleeding originates more distally.

PEPTIC ULCER DISEASE Peptic ulcer disease, including gastric, duodenal, and stomal ulcers, remains the most common etiology for upper GI hemorrhage, encompassing approximately 60 percent of all cases.[2] Duodenal ulcers, which comprise approximately 29 percent of all ulcers, will rebleed in approximately 10 percent of cases, usually within 24 to 48 h. Gastric ulcers, which comprise approximately 16 percent of all cases, are more likely to rebleed. Stomal ulcers are uncommon (fewer than 5 percent of all upper GI bleeds) and are present in only one-third of bleeding patients with a history of peptic ulcer surgery.

EROSIVE GASTRITIS AND ESOPHAGITIS Erosive gastritis, esophagitis, and duodenitis together are responsible for approximately 15 percent of all cases of upper GI hemorrhage. Irritative factors, such as alcohol, salicylates, and nonsteroidal anti-inflammatory agents, are predisposing factors.

ESOPHAGEAL AND GASTRIC VARICES Esophageal and gastric varices result from portal hypertension and, in the United States, are most often a result of alcoholic liver disease. Although varices account for only about 6 percent of all cases of upper GI hemorrhage, they are highly likely to rebleed and carry a high mortality rate. Nevertheless, many patients with end-stage cirrhosis never develop varices, many patients with documented varices never bleed, and many patients with a documented history of varices presenting with upper GI bleeding will bleed from nonvariceal sites.

MALLORY-WEISS SYNDROME Mallory-Weiss syndrome is upper GI bleeding secondary to a longitudinal mucosal tear in the cardioesophageal region. The classic history is repeated retching followed by bright red hematemesis, but coughing and seizures also have been reported as etiologic factors.

OTHER ETIOLOGIES Stress ulcer, arteriovenous malformation, and malignancy are other etiologies of upper GI hemorrhage. Ear, nose, and throat sources of bleeding can also masquerade as GI hemorrhage. An aortoenteric fistula secondary to an aortic graft is an unusual but important cause of bleeding to keep in mind. Classically, this will present as a self-limited "herald" bleed preceding a subsequent massive hemorrhage.

Causes of Lower Gastrointestinal Bleeding

The most common cause of what initially appears to be lower GI bleeding is actually upper GI bleeding. Thus, proximal etiologies should be sought.

Among patients with an established lower GI source of their bleeding, the most common etiology is hemorrhoids. Among those with nonhemorrhoidal bleeding, angiodysplasia and diverticular disease are most common, followed by adenomatous polyps and malignancies.[4]

DIVERTICULOSIS Diverticular bleeding is usually painless and is thought to result from erosion into the penetrating artery of the diverticulum. Diverticular bleeding may be massive. Patients are often elderly with underlying medical illnesses that contribute to morbidity and mortality rates.

ANGIODYSPLASIA Arteriovenous malformations (angiodysplasia), usually of the right colon, are a common etiology of obscure lower GI bleeding, particularly in the elderly population. They are thought to be more common in patients with hypertension and aortic stenosis.

OTHER ETIOLOGIES Numerous other lesions may result in lower GI hemorrhage. Whereas carcinoma and hemorrhoids are relatively common causes of bleeding, massive hemorrhage is unusual. Similarly, inflammatory bowel disease, polyps, and infectious gastroenteritis rarely cause severe bleeding. In addition, Meckel diverticulum is an unusual but important etiology to keep in mind.

DIAGNOSIS

Medical History

Although the medical history may suggest the source of bleeding, it is often misleading. Thus, clinicians should strive to maintain a broad differential and clinical approach. Although most patients will volunteer complaints of hematemesis, hematochezia, or melena, GI bleeding may have more subtle presentations. Patients who present with hypotension, tachycardia, angina, syncope, weakness, confusion, or even cardiac arrest may harbor occult, underlying GI hemorrhage.

Historical features such as hematemesis, coffee-ground emesis, melena, or hematochezia should be sought. Classically, hematemesis or coffee-ground emesis suggests a source proximal to the right colon, and hematochezia indicates a more distal colorectal lesion. However, exceptions to these rules occur. Weight loss and changes in bowel habits are classic symptoms of malignancy. Vomiting and retching, followed by hematemesis, is suggestive of a Mallory-Weiss tear. A history of an aortic graft should suggest the possibility of an aortoenteric fistula. A history of medication use should be determined, in particular salicylates, glucocorticoids, nonsteroidal anti-inflammatory agents, and anticoagulants. Alcohol abuse is strongly associated with a number of causes of GI bleeding, including peptic ulcer disease, erosive gastritis, and esophageal varices. Ingestion of iron or bismuth can simulate melena, and certain foods, such as beets, can simulate hematochezia. In such instances, stool guaiac testing will be negative. A history of GI bleeding should be sought, although recurrent bleeding episodes often originate from different sources.

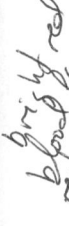

Physical Examination

The vital signs may reveal obvious hypotension and tachycardia or more subtle manifestations such as a decreased pulse pressure or tachypnea. Clinicians should remember that some patients can tolerate substantial volume losses with minimal or no changes in vital signs. Similarly, paradoxical bradycardia can occur in the face of profound hypovolemia.

Skin findings should be noted. Cool, clammy skin is an obvious sign of shock. Spider angiomata, palmar erythema, jaundice, and gynecomastia suggest underlying liver disease. Petechiae and purpura suggest an underlying coagulopathy. Skin findings may be suggestive of Peutz-Jeghers, Rendu-Osler-Weber, or Gardner syndrome. A careful ear, nose, and throat examination occasionally may reveal an occult bleeding source that has resulted in swallowed blood and subsequent coffee-ground emesis or melena. The abdominal examination may disclose tenderness, masses, ascites, or organomegaly. A rectal examination is indicated to detect the presence of blood, its appearance (bright red, maroon, or melanotic), and the presence of masses.

Laboratory Data

In patients with significant GI bleeding, the most important laboratory test is to type and cross-match blood. Another important laboratory test is the complete blood count. In addition, blood urea nitrogen (BUN), creatinine, electrolyte, glucose, coagulation studies and liver function studies should be considered. The initial hematocrit level often will not reflect the actual amount of blood loss. Upper tract hemorrhage may elevate BUN levels through digestion and absorption of hemoglobin. Coagulation studies, including prothrombin time, partial thromboplastin time, and platelet count, are of obvious benefit in patients taking anticoagulants or those with underlying hepatic disease. An electrocardiogram should be considered in patients statistically likely to have coronary artery disease. Silent ischemia can occur secondary to the decreased oxygen delivery accompanying significant GI bleeding; thus, supplemental oxygen is advised for such patients.

Diagnostic Studies

Routine abdominal radiographs are often obtained in patients with GI bleeding. In the absence of specific indications, they are of limited value. Similarly, routine admission chest x-rays for patients with acute GI hemorrhage, even those admitted to the intensive care unit, have been shown to be of limited utility in the absence of known pulmonary disease or abnormal findings on lung examination.[5] Barium contrast studies similarly are of limited diagnostic value in an emergency setting. Further, barium limits the use of subsequent endoscopy or angiography.

Angiography sometimes can detect the site of bleeding, particularly in cases of obscure lower tract hemorrhage. Moreover, angiography permits therapeutic options such as transcatheter arterial embolization or the infusion of vasoconstrictive agents. However, to be diagnostic, **angiography requires a relatively brisk bleeding rate (0.5 to 2.0 mL per min).**

Technetium-labeled red cell scans also have been used to localize the site of bleeding in obscure hemorrhage. Such localization can be used to map the therapeutic approach, whether via angiography or operatively. **Scintigraphy appears more sensitive than angiography and can localize the site of bleeding at a rate of 0.1 mL per min.**

Another approach is colonoscopy, which may be not only diagnostic but, through the use of endoscopic hemostasis, also therapeutic. In most circumstances, endoscopy is more accurate than arteriography or scintigraphy.

Controversy in the literature remains as to whether scintigraphy, angiography, or colonoscopy, and in which order, should be the initial diagnostic procedure of choice in the evaluation of lower GI bleeding.[6–9] Thus, these decisions are often based on local availability and consultant preference.

TREATMENT

Primary

Immediate resuscitative measures take priority. Patients with profuse upper GI hemorrhage may require definitive airway management to prevent aspiration of blood. Oxygen should be administered, and cardiac monitoring is indicated. Volume replacement should be initiated with crystalloids via large-bore intravenous lines. The decision to administer blood should be based on the clinical findings of volume depletion or continued bleeding rather than on initial hematocrit values. General guidelines for initiation of blood transfusion are continued active bleeding and failure to improve perfusion and vital signs after the infusion of 2 L of crystalloid. The threshold for blood transfusion should be lower in the elderly. Coagulation factors should be replaced as needed. A urinary catheter is indicated in patients with hypotension.

A nasogastric (NG) tube should be placed in all patients with significant GI bleeding, regardless of the presumed source. **Concerns that NG tube passage may provoke bleeding in patients with varices are unwarranted.** Bright red or maroon blood per rectum unexpectedly originates from upper GI sources approximately 14 percent of the time.[10] A negative gastric aspirate does not conclusively exclude an upper GI etiology and may result from intermittent bleeding, pyloric spasm, or edema preventing reflux of duodenal blood. If bright red blood or clots are found on NG aspiration, gentle gastric lavage should be performed. To be effective, a large-bore tube, usually oral, must be used. Room temperature water is the preferred irrigant, because iced solutions have no proven benefit and have theoretical disadvantages. The addition of levarterenol to the lavage solution is similarly of unproven benefit. Overvigorous suction should be avoided, because it may produce gastric erosions that can confuse findings on subsequent endoscopy.

Secondary

ENDOSCOPY Upper GI endoscopy is the most accurate technique for the identification of upper tract bleeding sites. It predicts morbidity and, with the advent of therapeutic endoscopy, is associated with improved outcomes. Early therapeutic endoscopy, where available, should be considered the treatment of choice for significant upper GI bleeding. Thus, early consultation for potential endoscopy should be considered in patients with significant hemorrhage.

Esophageal varices can be endoscopically treated by band ligation or injection sclerotherapy. Sclerotherapy, which controls acute hemorrhage in up to 90 percent of patients, may decrease the duration of hospitalization and the amount of blood transfused when compared with portal-caval shunting. However, complications of sclerotherapy include perforation, sepsis, stricture formation, and portal and mesenteric venous thrombosis. Endoscopic band ligation appears to be as effective as sclerotherapy, but with a decreased incidence of complications, in particular rebleeding and esophageal stricture formation.[11] In addition, band ligation appears superior to sclerotherapy in the long-term management of varices.[12]

Endoscopic hemostasis (with injection sclerotherapy, electrocoagulation, heater probes, and lasers) also has been used successfully in a variety of nonvariceal etiologies of upper GI bleeding.

In lower GI bleeding, proctoscopy is often diagnostic in patients with anorectal sources of bleeding, such as hemorrhoids. If an anorectal source is suspected, the patient should be evaluated carefully for significant volume loss or more dangerous proximal sources of bleeding mimicking anorectal bleeding. Colonoscopy can be diagnostic in other forms of lower tract hemorrhage, such as diverticulosis or angiodysplasia, and may allow ablation of bleeding sites by using the aforementioned technologies.

DRUG THERAPY Infusions of somatostatin and its synthetic, longer-acting derivative, octreotide, have been shown to be effective in reducing bleeding from varices and peptic ulcer disease. Octreotide has been shown to be as effective as sclerotherapy in acute variceal bleeding.[13] Both agents, when used in addition to sclerotherapy, are more effective than sclerotherapy alone.[14,15] These agents possess the advantages of vasopressin, with considerably fewer side effects. They should be considered useful adjuncts before endoscopy or when endoscopy is unsuccessful, contraindicated, or unavailable.[16] The dose of octreotide is 50 μg IV bolus, followed by 50 μg 8–24h; the dose of somatostatin is 250–500 μg IV bolus followed by 250–500 μg per h. See Chap. 86 for detailed discussion of somatostatin and octreotide.

Vasopressin has been used to control GI bleeding, most commonly from varices. However, adverse reactions are common, including hypertension, dysrhythmias, myocardial and splanchnic ischemia, decreased cardiac output, and gangrene from local infiltration. Although the concomitant use of nitroglycerin has been shown to reduce the incidence of these side effects, the use of vasopressin has been largely supplanted by the use of somatostatin, octreotide, and therapeutic endoscopy.

Studies have also suggested that the proton-pump inhibitor omeprazole may be useful to reduce rebleeding, transfusion requirements, and the need for surgery in the treatment of bleeding peptic ulcers.[17,18]

Other drugs may be of benefit in patients with GI hemorrhage, but are of less concern in the initial emergency department management. For instance, beta-blocker therapy has been shown to be beneficial in patients with varices in preventing initial variceal bleeds and rebleeding.[19,20] In addition, the treatment of *Helicobacter pylori* infection with antibiotics reduces the recurrence of peptic ulcer and rebleeding.[21] However, the use of H2 antagonists in acute upper GI hemorrhage remains of unproven benefit, with no conclusive evidence for reduction in the rates of rebleeding, surgery, or death.

BALLOON TAMPONADE Balloon tamponade with the Sengstaken-Blakemore tube or its variants can provide therapeutic benefit and presumptive diagnostic information. It can control documented variceal hemorrhage in 40 to 80 percent of patients. The device consists of gastric and esophageal balloons and, depending on the variation, may include gastric and/or esophageal aspiration ports. The gastric balloon should be inflated first. If bleeding does not cease, the esophageal balloon should then be inflated by using a manometer to ensure that the pressure does not exceed 40 to 50 mm Hg. Radiologic confirmation of proper balloon placement is suggested. The device should be kept in place 24 h after bleeding has ceased. Some authors recommend deflating the esophageal balloon for 30 to 60 min every 8 h to prevent mucosal ulceration.

Like vasopressin therapy, balloon tamponade is frequently associated with adverse reactions, often severe. Mucosal ulceration, esophageal or gastric rupture, asphyxiation from dislodged balloons, tracheal compression secondary to balloon inflation, and aspiration pneumonia have been reported. Many authors recommend routine prophylactic endotracheal intubation to prevent pulmonary complications. Because of the incidence of adverse reactions, the use of balloon tamponade has decreased considerably and should be considered an adjunctive or temporizing measure supplementing the more definitive modalities of band ligation or sclerotherapy.

SURGERY With patients who do not respond to medical therapy and in whom endoscopic hemostasis, if available, fails, emergency surgical intervention is indicated. Surgical consultation on any patient admitted to the hospital for GI bleeding is prudent in case uncontrollable rebleeding occurs.

DISPOSITION

Patients with significant GI hemorrhage will require hospital admission, and early referral to an endoscopist is advisable. Corley and colleagues found five variables to be independent predictors of adverse outcomes in upper GI bleeding: initial hematocrit less than 30 percent, initial systolic blood pressure lower than 100 mm Hg, red blood in the NG lavage, history of cirrhosis or ascites on examination, and a history of vomiting red blood.[22] Such patients are more likely to require a greater intensity of inpatient care.

In contrast, certain subsets of patients with upper GI bleeding are low risk and potentially eligible for early discharge. Patients are risk stratified by clinical and endoscopic criteria, so endoscopy must still be performed before discharge. Rockall and coworkers developed a risk score for variceal upper GI bleeding based on age, presence of shock, comorbidity, diagnosis, and endoscopic findings.[23] Longstreth and associates developed similar guidelines.[24] A randomized controlled trial found no difference in outcome between admitted and discharged low-risk patients. Adoption of such guidelines requires close coordination between the emergency physician and gastroenterologist.

REFERENCES

1. Rockall TA, Logan RF, Devlin HB, et al: Incidence of and mortality from acute upper gastrointestinal hemorrhage in the United Kingdom: Steering Committee and members of the National Audit of Acute Upper Gastrointestinal Haemorrhage. *BMJ* 311:222, 1995.
2. Longstreth GF: Epidemiology and outcome of patients hospitalized with acute lower gastrointestinal hemorrhage: A population-based study. *Am J Gastroenterol* 92:419, 1997.
3. Longstreth GF: Epidemiology of hospitalization for acute upper gastrointestinal hemorrhage: A population-based study. *Am J Gastroenterol* 90:206, 1995.
4. Machicado GA, Jensen DM: Acute and chronic management of lower gastrointestinal bleeding: Cost-effective approaches. *Gastroenterologist* 5:189, 1997.
5. Tobin K, Klein J, Barbieri C, et al: Utility of routine admission chest radiographs in patients with acute gastrointestinal hemorrhage admitted to an intensive care unit. *Am J Med* 101:349, 1996.
6. Suzman MS, Talmor M, Jennis R, et al: Accurate localization and surgical management of active lower gastrointestinal hemorrhage with technetium-labeled erythrocyte scintigraphy. *Ann Surg* 224:29, 1996.

7. Vernava AM, Moore BA, Longo WE, et al: Lower gastrointestinal bleeding. *Dis Colon Rectum* 40:846, 1997.

8. Richter JM, Christensen MR, Kaplan LM, et al: Effective of current technology in the diagnosis and management of lower gastrointestinal hemorrhage. *Gastrointest Endosc* 41:93, 1995.

9. Ng DA, Opekla FG, Beck DE, et al: Predictive value of technetium Tc 99m-labelled red blood cell scintigraphy for positive angiogram in massive lower gastrointestinal hemorrhage. *Dis Colon Rectum* 40:471, 1997.

10. Wilcox CM, Alexander LN, Cotsonis G: A prospective characterization of upper gastrointestinal hemorrhage presenting with hematochezia. *Am J Gastroenterol* 92:231, 1997.

11. Cello JP: Endoscopy management of esophageal variceal hemorrhage: Injection, banding, glue, octreotide or a combination? *Semin Gastrointest Dis* 8:179, 1997.

12. Avgerinos A, Armonis A, Manokakopoulos S, et al: Endoscopic sclerotherapy versus variceal ligation in the long-term management of patients with cirrhosis after variceal bleeding: A prospective randomized study. *J Hepatol* 26:1034, 1997.

13. Jenkins SA, Shields R, Davies M, et al: A multicenter randomized trial comparing octreotide and injection sclerotherapy in the management and outcome of acute variceal hemorrhage. *Gut* 41:526, 1997.

14. Avgerinos A, Nevens F, Raptis S, et al: Early administration of somatostatin and efficacy of sclerotherapy in acute oesophageal variceal bleeds: The European Acute Bleeding Oesophageal Variceal Episodes (ABOVE) randomized trial. *Lancet* 350:1495, 1997.

15. Beeson I, Ingrand P, Person B, et al: Sclerotherapy with or without octreotide for acute variceal bleeding. *New Engl J Med* 333:555, 1995.

16. Imperiale TF, Birgisson S: Somatostatin or octreotide compared with H2 antagonists and placebo in the management of acute nonvariceal upper gastrointestinal hemorrhage: A meta-analysis. *Ann Intern Med* 127:1062, 1997.

17. Khuroo MS, Yattoo GN, Javid G, et al: A comparison of omeprazole and placebo for bleeding peptic ulcer. *New Engl J Med* 336:1054, 1997.

18. Schaffalitzky de Muckadell OB, Havelund T, Harding H, et al: Effect of omeprazole on the outcome of endoscopically treated bleeding peptic ulcers: Randomized double-blind placebo-controlled multicentre study. *Scand J Gastroenterol* 32:320, 1997.

19. Grace ND: Diagnosis and treatment of gastrointestinal bleeding secondary to portal hypertension: American College of Gastroenterology Practice Parameters Committee. *Am J Gastroenterol* 92:1081, 1997.

20. Avgerinos A, Rekoumis G, Klonis C, et al: Propranolol in the prevention of recurrent upper gastrointestinal bleeding in patients with cirrhosis undergoing endoscopic sclerotherapy: A randomized controlled trial. *J Hepatol* 19:301, 1993.

21. Santander C, Gravalos RG, Gomez-Cedenilla A, et al: Antimicrobial therapy for *Helicobacter pylori* infection versus long-term maintenance antisecretion treatment in the prevention of recurrent hemorrhage from peptic ulcer: Prospective nonrandomized trial on 125 patients. *Am J Gastroenterol* 91:1549, 1996.

22. Corley DA, Stefan AM, Wolf M, et al: Early indicators of prognosis in upper gastrointestinal hemorrhage. *Am J Gastroenterol* 93:336, 1998.

23. Rockall TA, Logan RF, Devlin HB, et al: Selection of patients for early discharge or outpatient care after acute upper gastrointestinal haemorrhage: National Audit of Acute Upper Gastrointestinal Haemorrhage. *Lancet* 347:1138, 1996.

24. Longstreth GF, Feitelberg SP: Outpatient care of selected patients with acute non-variceal upper gastrointestinal haemorrhage. *Lancet* 345:108, 1995.

ESOPHAGEAL EMERGENCIES
75
Moss H. Mendelson

Patients develop a wide variety of problems related to the esophagus. The complaints of dysphagia, odynophagia, or ingested foreign body immediately implicate the esophagus. The esophagus also is often the site of pathology in patients presenting with chest pain, upper gastrointestinal bleeding, malignancy, and mediastinitis. Many diseases of the esophagus can be evaluated over time in an outpatient setting, but several, such as variceal bleeding and esophageal perforation, can be

fulminant and rapidly fatal, requiring a unique knowledge base for effective, emergent intervention.

ANATOMY AND PHYSIOLOGY

The esophagus is a muscular tube approximately 20 to 25 cm long. The majority of the esophagus is located in the mediastinum, posterior and slightly lateral to the trachea, with smaller cervical and abdominal components as well, as shown in Figure 75-1. There is an outer longitudinal muscle layer and an inner circular muscle layer. The upper third of the esophagus is made up of striated muscle. From the lower half down, the esophagus is all smooth muscle [including the lower esophageal sphincter (LES)]. The esophagus is lined with stratified squamous epithelial cells that have no secretory function.

Two sphincters regulate the passage of material into and out of the esophagus. The upper esophageal sphincter (UES) prevents air from entering the esophagus and food from refluxing out of the esophagus into the pharynx. The LES regulates the passage of food into the stomach and prevents stomach contents from refluxing into the esophagus. The UES is composed primarily of the cricopharyngeus muscle. Additional tone is variably provided by the inferior pharyngeal constrictor and the cervical esophagus.[1] The UES has a resting pressure of around 100 mm Hg. The LES is not discretely identifiable on an anatomic basis. The smooth muscle of the lower 1 to 2 cm of the esophagus, in combination with the skeletal muscle of the diaphragmatic hiatus, functions as the sphincter, with a resting pressure of

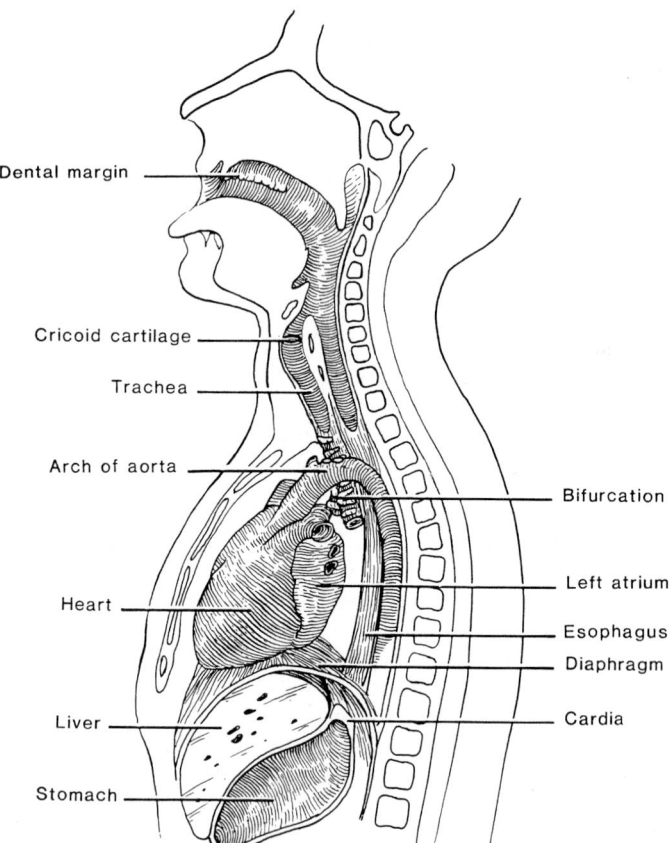

FIG. 75-1. Anatomic relations of the esophagus (seen from the left side). The esophagus is about 25 cm (10 in.) long. The distance from the upper incisor teeth to the beginning of the esophagus (cricoid cartilage) is about 15 cm (6 in.); from the upper incisors to the level of the bronchi, 22 to 23 cm (9 in.); to the cardia, 40 cm (16 in.). Structures contiguous to the esophagus that affect esophageal function are demonstrated.

25 mm Hg. The pressure within the resting body of the esophagus closely approximates intrathoracic pressure. Dysfunction of the LES is a major source of esophageal symptoms and is discussed below.

Three major anatomic constrictions exist within the esophagus and are important when faced with an esophageal foreign body or food bolus impaction, discussed below. The constrictions occur at the cricopharyngeus muscle, the level of the aortic arch/left main stem bronchus, and the gastroesophageal junction. An empty, collapsed esophagus has no apparent constrictions; the narrow areas are only apparent with esophageal filling.

The innervation of the heart mirrors that of the esophagus, and a convergence of visceral and somatic stimuli occurs within the sympathetic system. This is the anatomic basis that makes esophageal and cardiac chest pain notoriously similar, as discussed below.[2]

The esophageal blood supply is derived from several arterial sources. The inferior thyroid artery, small branches of the thoracic aorta, and ascending branches from the left gastric and inferior phrenic arteries supply the esophagus throughout its length. The esophageal venous circulation includes a submucosal plexus of veins that drains into another plexus of veins surrounding the outside of the esophagus. Blood flows from this outer plexus into the inferior thyroid, azygos, coronary, and gastric venous systems, the latter an important link between portal and systemic circulation. Variceal dilatation of the submucosal system can lead to massive upper gastrointestinal (GI) bleeding, reviewed below.[3]

DYSPHAGIA

Dysphagia is defined as difficulty with swallowing. The vast majority of patients with dysphagia will have an identifiable, organic process causing their symptoms.

Patients with dysphagia can be classified into two broad pathophysiologic groups; those with transfer dysphagia and those with transport dysphagia.[4] Transfer dysphagia occurs very early in the swallowing process (as the food bolus moves from the oropharynx through the UES) and is often reported as difficulty in initiating a swallow. In transport dysphagia, there is impaired movement of the bolus down the esophagus and through the LES. Transport dysphagia is perceived later in the swallowing process, usually 2 to 4 s or more after swallowing is initiated, and most commonly results in the feeling of food "getting stuck." This initial differentiation between transfer and transport dysphagia provides valuable information regarding the likely underlying esophageal pathology, as noted in Table 75-1. Another useful classification scheme divides dysphagia into obstructive

disease versus motor dysfunction. Functional or motility disorders usually cause dysphagia that is intermittent and variable. Mechanical or obstructive disease is usually progressive (solids, then liquids).

Clinical Features

Historical information is key to the diagnosis of dysphagia. Though often occurring as an independent symptom, dysphagia can be associated with odynophagia, which is painful swallowing (suggesting an inflammatory process), or with chest pain that is esophageal in nature and suggests gastroesophageal reflux disease (GERD) or a motility disorder. Additional pertinent historical features to elicit in a patient complaining of dysphagia include the following: Has this been an acute, subacute, or chronic course? Is the dysphagia present for solids, liquids, or both? Is it intermittent or progressive? Is there a sensation of the food being stuck in the esophagus, and where? Is there any past history of esophageal disease? Transport dysphagia that is present for solids only generally suggests a mechanical or obstructive process. Motility disorders typically cause transport dysphagia for solids and liquids.

A poorly chewed meat bolus that impacts in the esophagus is a well-recognized complication of esophageal disease. A preceding history of dysphagia may or may not be present. An impacted food bolus can be the presenting complaint for a variety of underlying esophageal pathologies. The bolus may be well localized by the patient; in general, patients able to identify a level of dysphagia below the neck are usually anatomically accurate, whereas those complaining of dysphagia in the neck may be reporting sensations referred from elsewhere in the esophagus.[5] Esophageal filling proximal to the impacted bolus can cause inability to swallow secretions and can present an airway/aspiration risk.

Physical examination of patients with dysphagia should focus on the head and neck and the neurologic exam. Signs of previous cerebrovascular accident, muscle disease, or Parkinson's disease can be present. Cachexia and cervical or supraclavicular nodes can be observed in patients with cancer of the esophagus. Watching the patient take a small sip of water can also provide very valuable information. Unfortunately, the physical examination is often normal in patients with dysphagia, despite the high-yield nature of this complaint.

Diagnosis

The diagnosis of the underlying pathology of dysphagia is most often made outside of the ED. The work-up is dependent on whether transfer or transport dysphagia is thought to be present, as noted above.

TABLE 75-1 Dysphagia

Transfer Dysphagia (Oropharyngeal)	Transport Dysphagia (Esophageal)
Discoordination in transferring bolus from pharynx to esophagus	Improper transfer of the bolus from the upper esophagus into the stomach
Swallowing symptoms—gagging, coughing, nasal regurgitation, inability to initiate swallow, need for repeated swallows	Swallowing symptoms—food "sticking," restrosternal fullness with solids (and eventually liquids), possibly odynophagia
Risk of aspiration present	Risk of aspiration present, generally less pronounced than in transfer dysphagia
Long term—weight loss, malnutrition, chronic bronchitis, asthma, multiple episodes of pneumonia	Long term—malnutrition, dehydration, weight loss, systemic effects of cancer
Neuromuscular disease (80%)—cerebrovascular accident; polymyositis and dermatomyositis, scleroderma, myasthenia gravis, tetanus; Parkinson's disease, botulism, lead poisoning, thyroid disease	Obstructive disease (85%)—foreign body; carcinoma, webs, strictures, thyroid enlargement, diverticulum, congenital or acquired large vessel abnormalities
Localized disease—pharyngitis; aphthous ulcers; candidal infection; peritonsillar and retropharyngeal abscesses; carcinoma of tongue, pharynx, larynx; Zenker diverticulum; cricopharyngeal bar; cervical osteophytes	Motor disorder—achalasia, peristaltic dysfunction (nutcracker esophagus), diffuse esophageal spasm, scleroderma
Inadequate lubrication—scleroderma	Inflammatory disease

Initial evaluation of dysphagia in the ED can include anteroposterior (AP) and lateral neck radiographs, which can be helpful in transfer dysphagia and cases in which the transport dysfunction seems proximal. Chest radiography should be obtained in patients thought to have transport dysphagia. Direct laryngoscopy can be used to identify structural lesions.

Ultimately, oropharyngeal dysphagia is best worked up with video-esophagography, a specialized form of a barium swallow study in which videotaped images are reviewed at low-speed playback to allow detailed analysis. Traditional barium swallow is usually the first test for patients with transport dysphagia. Manometry and esophagoscopy are also employed, depending on the clinical picture. If a foreign body is suspected, the diagnostic evaluation takes yet another path (see Chap. 76).

Selected Structural or Obstructive Causes

Neoplasms are a common cause of transfer and transport dysphagia. The esophagus or surrounding structures can be the primary site. Esophageal cancer is diagnosed in about 10,000 people a year in the United States. Ninety-five percent of esophageal neoplasms are squamous cell; the remaining 5 percent are adenocarcinomas. Men are affected three times as often as women. Risk factors for squamous cell disease include alcohol, smoking, achalasia, and previous caustic ingestion with lye. Barrett's esophagus predisposes to adenocarcinoma, which has shown an increase in incidence in recent years.[6] There is usually a fairly rapid progression of dysphagia from solids to liquids (6 months). In addition to dysphagia, patients with neoplasm may present with bleeding. Early diagnosis impacts outcome, and for this reason the emergency physician should assume a neoplastic cause in patients over age 40 who present with new-onset dysphagia. These patients need an expedient work-up to rule out malignancy. Definitive diagnosis is made by endoscopy with biopsy. Survival is dismal; the median is less than 1 year.

Esophageal stricture occurs as a result of scarring from GERD or other chronic inflammation. Generally strictures occur in the distal esophagus, proximal to the gastroesophageal (GE) junction and may interfere with LES function. Symptoms may build over years and are often noted solely with solids. Stricture can serve as a barrier to reflux, so heartburn may decrease as dysphagia increases. Evaluation involves ruling out malignancy and treatment is dilatation.[7]

Schatzki ring is the most common cause of intermittent dysphagia with solids. This fibrous, diaphragm-like stricture near the GE junction is present in up to 15 percent of the population, the majority of whom are asymptomatic. The etiology is debated; a ring may form over time in response to GERD.[8] Steakhouse syndrome (food impaction in the esophagus due to poorly chewed meat) is a frequent presentation for patients with this obstructive phenomenon. Treatment of Schatzki ring is dilatation.

Esophageal webs are thin structures of mucosa and submucosa found most often in the mid or proximal esophagus. They can be congenital or acquired. Esophageal webs also occur as a component of Plummer-Vinson syndrome (along with iron-deficiency anemia), and can be seen in patients with pemphigoid and epidermolysis bullosa. Treatment, again, is dilatation.

Diverticula may be found throughout the esophagus. Pharyngoesophageal, or Zenker diverticulum is a progressive outpouching of pharyngeal mucosa, just above the UES, caused by increased pressures during the hypopharyngeal phase of swallowing.[5] Presentation is usually after age 50, as this is an acquired disease. Patients complain of typical transfer dysfunction; additionally, they may have halitosis and the feeling of a neck mass. Diverticula can also be seen in the body of the esophagus, usually in association with a motility disorder.

Selected Motor Lesions Causing Dysphagia

Neuromuscular disorders typically result in misdirection of the food bolus, with repeated swallowing attempts. Liquids, especially at the extremes of temperature, are generally more difficult to handle than solids. Symptoms are often intermittent in nature. Cerebrovascular accident (CVA) is the most common cause in this category. Oropharyngeal muscle weakness is often the mechanism, though there can be poor function of the UES as well. Polymyositis and dermatomyositis are the second most common causes of transfer dysphagia in this category.

Achalasia is a dysmotility disorder of unknown cause and the most common motility disorder producing dysphagia. Impaired swallowing-induced relaxation of the LES is noted, along with the absence of esophageal peristalsis. Most patients present between 20 and 40 years of age. Achalasia may be associated with esophageal spasm and chest pain and with odynophagia. Associated symptoms can include regurgitation and weight loss. Dilatation of the esophagus can be massive enough to impinge on the trachea and cause airway symptoms.[9] Therapy involves decreasing the LES pressure by oral medications, the endoscopic injection of botulinum toxin into the muscle of the sphincter, dilatations, or surgical myotomy.

Diffuse esophageal spasm refers to normal peristalsis that is periodically interrupted by simultaneous (nonperistaltic) contraction. Dysphagia is intermittent and does not progress over time. These patients also commonly complain of chest pain, discussed below. Therapy involves controlling any reflux that might be present and consideration of smooth muscle relaxants and/or antidepressants, though no data convincingly show that medications are efficacious.[10]

CHEST PAIN OF ESOPHAGEAL ORIGIN

Most esophageal causes of chest pain are not immediate threats to life; however, differentiating esophageal pain from ischemic chest pain can be impossible in the ED. Patients with esophageal pain can report spontaneous onset of pain or pain at night, regurgitation, odynophagia, dysphagia, or meal-induced heartburn; however, these symptoms are also found in patients with coronary artery disease (CAD), and there is no historical feature that is sensitive or specific enough to routinely make a differentiation between the two.

To minimize missing patients with acute coronary syndrome (ACS), the emergency physician's default assumption is that the pain is cardiac in nature and not esophageal. The high rate of admission for chest pain of noncardiac etiology is well publicized and appropriate. Ultimately, esophageal disease is often found to be the underlying pathology; the incidence of esophageal disease in patients with chest pain and normal coronary arteries has been reported as ranging from 20 to 60 percent.[5] The use of ED observation units can help sort these patients out by providing time for a protocol-driven, rapid rule-out of acute myocardial infarction, followed by risk stratification for underlying ACS with stress or radionuclide testing, all done on an outpatient basis (see Chap. 49 for further discussion). At a minimum, an electrocardiogram (ECG) and chest radiographs should be obtained in all patients with ambiguous presentations.

If chest pain is determined to be noncardiac in nature, treatment aimed at esophageal disease is often initiated empirically. There are no reliable data on which to base a therapeutic plan for these patients.[11] Outpatient options beyond 6 to 8 weeks of empiric treatment for GERD include an acid infusion test, esophagoscopy, and/or manometry to help clarify pain of esophageal origin.

Gastroesophageal Reflux Disease (GERD)

Reflux of gastric contents into the esophagus causes a wide array of symptoms and long-term effects. It affects up to 25 percent of the adult population, possibly with even higher rates in elderly populations.[12] Classically, a weak LES has been the mechanism held responsible for reflux, and this is seen in some patients. However, transient relaxation of the LES complex (with normal tone in between periods of relaxation) is the primary mechanism causing reflux. Patients with moderate to severe reflux also often have concomitant hiatal hernia.[13] Prolonged gastric emptying, agents that decrease LES pressure, and impaired esophageal motility predispose to reflux. Table 75-2 highlights some common contributors.

As noted, differentiating esophageal symptoms from acute ischemic coronary symptoms is often not possible in the ED. Heartburn is the classic symptom of GERD, and chest discomfort may be the sole manifestation of the disease. The burning nature of the discomfort is probably due to localized lower esophageal mucosal inflammation. Many GERD patients will report other associated gastrointestinal symptoms, such as odynophagia, dysphagia, acid regurgitation, and hypersalivation. The association of pain with meals can be helpful in identifying pain that is due to GERD. Postural changes in pain can also be useful: increasing intraabdominal pressure or negating the advantage of gravity can exacerbate reflux symptoms dramatically. Antacid-induced relief of symptoms is often noted in reflux disease, though the pain can return after the transient antacid effect wears off, and a certain number of patients with ischemic disease also report improvement with the same therapy. Unfortunately, like cardiac pain, GERD pain may be squeezing, pressure-like, and include a history of onset with exertion and offset with rest. Both types of pain may be accompanied by diaphoresis, pallor, and nausea and vomiting. Radiation of esophageal pain can occur in one or both arms, the neck, the shoulders, or the back. Given the serious outcome of unrecognized ischemic disease compared with the relatively benign nature of esophageal pain, a cautious approach to these patients is warranted.

Over time, GERD can cause complications: strictures can develop, with associated dysphagia as discussed above, and inflammatory esophagitis can develop, also discussed below. A severe consequence of GERD, Barrett esophagus, is present in up to 10 percent of patients with GERD.[14] This condition is identified by biopsy; simple columnar epithelium replaces the normal stratified squamous epithelium in the distal esophagus. Metaplasia and ulceration can be present. Barrett esophagus is considered a premalignant condition, with a well-reported association between the development of metaplasia and the onset of adenocarcinoma.[15]

Less obvious presentations of GERD also occur. Pulmonary symptoms, especially asthma exacerbations, and multiple ear/nose/throat symptoms are well described. GERD is present in many asthmatics, and can contribute to their disease by aspiration of minute amounts of gastric contents, with subsequent inflammation and bronchospasm, and by esophageal activation of reflex vagal tone with consequent bronchospasm. Unfortunately, identifying asthmatic patients with GERD who will benefit with antireflux therapy remains difficult.[15,16] GERD has been implicated in the etiology of dental erosion, vocal cord ulcers and granulomas, laryngitis with hoarseness, chronic sinusitis, and chronic cough.[17,18]

Comprehensive treatment of reflux disease involves decreasing acid production in the stomach, enhancing upper tract motility, and eliminating risk factors for the disease. As noted above, mild disease is often treated empirically. H2 blockers or proton-pump inhibitors are mainstays of therapy. Dosage is titrated for each patient. A prokinetic drug may also greatly decrease symptoms. Simple ED discharge instructions should be given to all patients thought to be experiencing reflux-related symptoms: Avoid agents that exacerbate GERD (ethanol, caffeine, nicotine, chocolate, fatty foods), sleep with the head of the bed elevated (30°), and avoid eating within 3 h of going to bed at night. Management of Barrett's esophagus includes intensive treatment of the underlying GERD with proton-pump inhibition. Often, laser or photodynamic ablation therapy and surgical treatment are employed as well. Close monitoring for dysplastic change is essential.

Esophagitis

Esophagitis can cause prolonged periods of chest pain and almost always causes odynophagia as well. Diagnosis of advanced esophagitis is by endoscopy. Low-grade disease can be seen by histopathologic examination.

INFLAMMATORY ESOPHAGITIS   GERD may induce an inflammatory response in the lower esophageal mucosa. Over time, this can progress to esophageal ulcerations, scarring, and stricture formation. The presence of reflux-induced esophagitis warrants aggressive pharmacologic therapy with acid-suppressive medications. If this treatment regimen is not sufficient, surgical options are considered.[15] Ingested medications can also be a source for inflammatory esophagitis, usually from prolonged contact of the medication with the esophageal mucosa. Ulceration can be associated with this process. Multiple medications have been implicated. Common offenders include nonsteroidal and other antiinflammatory drugs, potassium chloride, and especially antibiotics (e.g., doxycycline, tetracycline, and clindamycin).[19] Risk factors for pill-induced esophageal injury include swallowing position, fluid intake, capsule size, and age. Withdrawal of the offending agent is generally curative.

INFECTIOUS ESOPHAGITIS   Patients with immunosuppression [acquired immunodeficiency syndrome (AIDS), iatrogenic causes, cancer] can develop an infectious esophagitis. AIDS has made esophageal infection more routine in the ED. The diagnosis of infectious esophagitis in an otherwise seemingly healthy host should prompt a search for underlying immunocompromise. Candidal species are the most common pathogens, often associated with dysphagia as a primary symptom. Herpes simplex, cytomegalovirus, and aphthous ulceration are also seen and may be more frequently associated with odynophagia. Other agents are rare and include other fungal infections, mycobacteria, and other viral pathogens such as varicella zoster and Epstein-Barr virus. Endoscopy with biopsy and culture is used to establish this diagnosis.[20]

Esophageal Motility Disorders

Esophageal dysmotility is the excessive, uncoordinated contraction of esophageal smooth muscle. Debate continues over the correlation between symptoms (pain) and observed motor events during manometry, a primary diagnostic modality for these disorders.[10] Achalasia and diffuse esophageal spasm were discussed above. The other motility disorders commonly recognized include ineffective esophageal motility, hypertensive LES, and nutcracker esophagus.

Clinically, chest pain is the presenting symptom in the majority of patients with these disorders. The onset is usually in the fifth decade. The pain often occurs at rest and is dull or colicky in nature. Stress or ingestion of liquids at the extremes of temperature may serve as a trigger. An acute episode of pain may be followed by hours of dull, achy, residual discomfort. Many patients will also experience dysphagia, which is usually intermittent. Pain from spasm may respond to

TABLE 75-2   Causes of Gastroesophageal Reflux Disease

Decreased Pressure of Lower Esophageal Sphincter	Decreased Esophageal Motility	Prolonged Gastric Emptying
High-fat food	Achalsia	Medicines (anticholinergics)
Nicotine	Scleroderma	Outlet obstruction
Ethanol	Presbyesophagus	Diabetic gastroparesis
Caffeine	Diabetes mellitus	High-fat food
Medicines (nitrates, calcium channel blockers, anticholinergics, progesterone, estrogen)		
Pregnancy		

nitroglycerin. Calcium channel blockers and anticholinergic agents can also be employed.

"*Nutcracker esophagus*" is a motility disorder in which there are high-amplitude, long-duration peristaltic contractions in the distal body of the esophagus or the LES. Manometric criteria require readings of >180 mm Hg. The cause of nutcracker esophagus is unknown. The disease is the most common motility disorder found in patients with noncardiac chest pain.[10] Patients with this disorder frequently have associated psychiatric disorders and about one-third have GERD.

ESOPHAGEAL PERFORATION

Perforation of the esophagus can occur secondary to a number of disparate processes[21] as noted in Table 75-3. Iatrogenic injury is the most frequent cause of esophageal injury, accounting for up to 75 percent of all perforations. Endoscopy, a prime offender, has a lower rate of perforation when performed on an esophagus free of disease than on a diseased esophagus. Dilation of strictures increases the risk of perforation greatly. Other intraluminal procedures, such as variceal therapy and palliative laser treatment for cancer, are also associated with perforation. A well-recognized clinical scenario of postemetic perforation, Boerhaave syndrome, is responsible for roughly 10 to 15 percent of esophageal perforations and is discussed below.

Perforation causes a dramatic presentation if esophageal contents leak into the mediastinum. A fulminant, necrotizing mediastinitis with polymicrobial infection that rapidly leads to shock and death can ensue. Perforation into the pleural or peritoneal spaces can occur as well, and contamination of these large potential spaces also tends to result in rapidly progressive infection and shock. If the perforation is small and leakage is contained by contiguous structures, the course may be significantly more indolent. Most spontaneous perforations occur through the left posterolateral wall of the distal esophagus.[22] Proximal perforation, seen mostly with instrumentation, tends to be less severe than distal perforation and can be contained locally as a periesophageal abscess with minimal systemic toxicity.

Pain is classically described as acute, severe, unrelenting and diffuse, and is reported in the chest, neck, and abdomen. Pain can radiate to the back and shoulders, or back pain may be the predominant symptom. Pain is often exacerbated by swallowing. Dysphagia, dyspnea, hematemesis, and cyanosis can be present as well. Less acute and atypical presentations are also described. Esophageal perforation is of-

TABLE 75-3   Causes of Esophageal Perforation

Causes of Perforation	Comments
Iatrogenic	Intraluminal procedures 　Endoscopy 　Dilatation 　Variceal therapy 　Gastric intubation Intraoperative injury
Boerhaave syndrome	"Spontaneous" usually associated with transient increase in intraesophageal pressure
Trauma	Penetrating Blunt (rare) Caustic ingestion
Foreign body	Includes pill-related injury
Infection	Rare
Tumor	May be intrinsic or extrinsic cancer
Aortic pathology	Aneurysm Aberrant right subclavian artery
Miscellaneous	Barrett esophagus Zollinger-Ellison syndrome

ten ascribed to acute myocardial infarction (MI), pulmonary embolus, peptic ulcer disease, aortic catastrophe, or acute abdomen, resulting in critical delays in diagnosis, the most important factor in determining morbidity and mortality outcome.

Physical examination varies with the severity of the rupture and the elapsed time between the rupture and presentation. Abdominal rigidity with hypotension and fever often occur early. Tachycardia and tachypnea are common. Cervical subcutaneous emphysema is common in cervical esophageal perforations. Mediastinal emphysema takes time to develop. It is less commonly detected by examination or radiography in lower esophageal perforation, and its absence does not rule out perforation.[23] Hammon crunch, caused by air in the mediastinum being moved by the beating heart, can sometimes be auscultated. Pleural effusion develops in half of patients with intrathoracic perforations and is uncommon in those with cervical perforations. Pleural fluid can be due to either direct contamination of the pleural space or a sympathetic serous effusion from mediastinitis.

Making the correct diagnosis in a timely manner in an ill patient with esophageal perforation requires suspicion on the clinician's part. Chest x-ray can suggest the diagnosis. If a pleural effusion is aspirated, elevated amylase in the pleural fluid suggests esophageal perforation. Computed tomography (CT) of the chest or emergency endoscopy are most often used to confirm the diagnosis. Selection of the procedure depends upon the clinical setting and the local resources available.

Perforation of the esophagus is associated with a high mortality rate regardless of the underlying cause. The elapsed time between perforation and the initiation of therapy, the location of the perforation, and the etiology all affect outcome. Rapid, aggressive management is key to minimizing the morbidity and mortality associated with esophageal perforation. In the ED, resuscitation of shock, broadspectrum parenteral antibiotics, and emergent surgical consultation should be obtained as soon as the diagnosis is seriously entertained. Patients with systemic symptoms and signs after perforation need operative management. Criteria are developing for the nonoperative management of perforation in select patients.[21]

Instrumentation, especially endoscopic dilatation, has a relatively high rate of perforation; therefore it is patients with strictures who sustain these injuries, usually perforating distally around the level of the obstruction. A patient with a relatively healthy esophagus undergoing instrumentation will more commonly perforate proximally. Perforation from other instrumentation, including nasogastric tube placement, has been reported.[24]

Boerhaave syndrome refers to full-thickness perforation of the esophagus following a sudden rise in intraesophageal pressure. The mechanism is sudden, forceful emesis in about three-fourths of the cases; coughing, straining, seizures, and childbirth have been reported as causing perforations as well. Alcohol is frequently an antecedent to this syndrome, which is seen more commonly in males. The perforation is usually in the distal esophagus on the left side.

Trauma to the esophagus accounts for roughly 10 percent of all esophageal perforations. Rupture from blunt injury is rare. Penetrating wounds to the esophagus from neck trauma occur but are often masked by more rapidly fatal injuries to the surrounding critical structures, such as the airway and major vessels. A combination of esophagography and esophagoscopy is used to assess patients for potential esophageal injury.

Foreign-body ingestion may result in perforation of the esophagus as well. The perforation is almost always at one of the sites of anatomic narrowing, where foreign bodies become wedged. The injury can be due to pressure necrosis from the object (coin), penetration from the object (pin, bones), or chemical irritation from the object (battery, pill).

ESOPHAGEAL BLEEDING

The general approach to upper gastrointestinal bleeding (UGIB) from an esophageal source does not differ from the approach for bleeding from other sources and is addressed in more depth in Chaps. 74 and

86. Resuscitation proceeds concurrently with the diagnostic effort of history, physical examination, and laboratory evaluation. Gastric lavage through a nasogastric tube or larger-bore gastric tube is generally accepted, and early airway management should be considered. Prompt mobilization of resources-including blood products, gastroenterology consult for endoscopy, and an appropriate inpatient level of care—is important.

About 60 percent of variceal bleeding will resolve with supportive care alone. The rate of spontaneous cessation is higher for nonvariceal sources of UGIB (up to 80 percent). Patients who continue to bleed need specific intervention. Early endoscopy is generally accepted in patients with UGIB for its diagnostic and therapeutic applications. Multiple pharmacotherapeutic agents (somatostatin analogues) have a role in controlling variceal bleeding, but efficacy in nonvariceal bleeding is less certain. Balloon tamponade is generally considered a last-resort therapy when pharmacologic management has failed and endoscopy is either not feasible secondary to massive bleeding or is ineffective. Surgical treatment can also be considered for patients who fail endoscopic and medical intervention.

Varices develop in patients with chronic liver disease in response to portal hypertension. Around 60 percent of patients with chronic liver disease will develop varices. Of patients who develop varices, 25 to 30 percent experience hemorrhage.[25] Patients who develop varices from alcohol abuse have a higher risk of bleeding, especially if there is ongoing alcohol consumption. About two-thirds of patients who have an index bleed experience recurrent hemorrhage, 50 percent occurring within 6 weeks of the initial episode.

With variceal bleeding, endoscopic therapy is often first-line in attempts to control the hemorrhage. Sclerotherapy and ligation are the main alternatives, though the use of injected Histoacryl (a tissue adhesive) to obstruct the variceal lumen has gained popularity. Some authors consider the combination of a vasoactive drug (e.g., octreotide or terlipressin) with endoscopic therapy to be superior to endoscopy alone. More recent review seems to support a trial of medical therapy alone for variceal bleeding in cirrhotics, with results comparable to primary sclerotherapy.[26,27] Shunting procedures performed transvenously or by surgical approach can also be considered.[28] Despite progress in treating variceal bleeding, mortality remains high. Concurrent hepatic failure is a risk factor for poor outcome.

Mallory-Weiss syndrome is arterial bleeding from longitudinal mucosal lacerations of the distal esophagus/proximal stomach. The majority of these lacerations are located at the GE junction, with only 10 percent found in the lower esophagus proper. Mallory-Weiss tears are responsible for between 5 and 15 percent of upper GI hemorrhages. They can occur at any age but are most common in the fourth through sixth decades. The pathophysiology of Mallory-Weiss syndrome is thought to be a transient, large pressure gradient between thorax and stomach, experienced maximally at the GE junction.

Acute onset of upper GI bleeding is the usual presentation, though some patients can present with melena or hematochezia. Rarely the presentation will be one of isolated abdominal pain or syncope. Less than half of patients with Mallory-Weiss tears will report a history of vomiting prior to hematemesis. The spectrum of severity of bleeding is broad, but overall a low relative incidence of surgical intervention or adverse outcome is seen. Initial treatment is supportive as the vast majority of Mallory-Weiss tears stop bleeding spontaneously. Ongoing hemorrhage can require treatment with electrocoagulation, sclerotherapy, and laser photocoagulation. Angiographic embolization or surgical intervention remain options as well.

Esophageal cancer often results in heme-positive stools but is an uncommon cause of significant upper or lower GI bleeding.

REFERENCES

1. Lang IM, Shaker R: Anatomy and physiology of the upper esophageal sphincter. *Am J Med* 103:50S, 1997.

2. Moore KL, Dalley AF: *Clinically Oriented Anatomy,* 4th ed. Baltimore, MD: Lippincott Williams & Wilkins, 1999.

3. Pope CEN: The esophagus for the nonesophagologist. *Am J Med* 103:19S, 1997.

4. Trate DM, Parkman HP, Fisher RS: Dysphagia: Evaluation, diagnosis, and treatment. *Primary Care* 23:417, 1996.

5. Falk GW, Richter JE: Approach to the patient with acute dysphagia, odynophagia and noncardiac chest pain, in Taylor MB (ed): *Gastrointestinal Emergencies.* Baltimore, MD: Williams & Wilkins, 1997.

6. Pera M, Cameron AJ, Trastek VF, et al: Increasing incidence of adenocarcinoma of the esophagus and esophagogastric junction. *Gastroenterology* 104:510, 1993.

7. Swann LA, Munter DW: Esophageal emergencies. *Emerg Med Clin North Am* 14:557, 1996.

8. Marshall JB, Kretschmar JM, Diaz-Arias AA: Gastroesophageal reflux as a pathogenic factor in the development of symptomatic lower esophageal rings. *Arch Intern Med* 150:1669, 1990.

9. Turkot S, Golzman B, Kogan J, et al: Acute upper-airway obstruction in a patient with achalasia. *Ann Emerg Med* 29:687, 1997.

10. Richter JE: Oesophageal motility disorders. *Lancet* 358:823, 2001.

11. Ho K: Noncardiac chest pain and abdominal pain. *Ann Emerg Med* 27:457, 1996.

12. Richter JE: Typical and atypical presentations of gastroesophageal reflux disease: The role of esophageal testing in diagnosis and management. *Gastroenterol Clin North Am* 25:75, 1996.

13. Dent J: Patterns of lower esophageal sphincter function associated with gastroesophageal reflux. *Am J Med* 103(5A):29S, 1997.

14. Barbezat GO: Recent advances: Gastroenterology. *BMJ* 316:125, 1998.

15. Gibson PG, Henry RL, Coughlan JL: Gastro-oesophageal reflux treatment for asthma in adults and children (Cochrane Review), in *The Cochrane Library,* Issue 2. Oxford: Update Software, 2002.

16. Sontag SJ: Gastroesophageal reflux and asthma. *Am J Med* 103:84S, 1997.

17. Hogan WJ: Spectrum of supraesophageal complications of gastroesophageal reflux disease. *Am J Med* 103:77S, 1997.

18. de Caestecker J: Medical therapy for supraesophageal complications of gastroesophageal reflux. *Am J Med* 103(5A):138S, 1997.

19. Arora AS, Murray JA: Iatrogenic esophagitis. *Curr Gastroenterol Rep* 2:224, 2000.

20. Varghese GK, Crane LR: Evaluation and treatment of HIV-related illnesses in the emergency department. *Ann Emerg Med* 24:503, 1994.

21. Williamson WA, Ellis FHJ: Esophageal perforation, in Taylor MB (ed): *Gastrointestinal Emergencies.* Baltimore, MD: Williams & Wilkins, 1997.

22. Levy F, Mysko WK, Kelen GD: Spontaneous esophageal perforation presenting with right-sided pleural effusion. *J Emerg Med* 13:321, 1995.

23. Janjua KJ: Boerhaave's syndrome. *Postgrad Med J* 73:265, 1997.

24. Ahmed A, Aggarwal M, Watson E: Esophageal perforation: A complication of nasogastric tube placement. *Am J Emerg Med* 16:64, 1998.

25. Polio J, Groszmann RJ, Taylor MB: Acute management of portal hypertensive hemorrhage from the upper gastrointestinal tract, in Taylor MB (ed): *Gastrointestinal Emergencies.* Baltimore, MD: Williams & Wilkins, 1997.

26. Banares R, Albillos A, Rincon D, et al: Endoscopic treatment versus endoscopic plus pharmacologic treatment for acute variceal bleeding: A meta-analysis. *Hepatology* 3:609, 2002.

27. D'Amico G, Pietrosi G, Tarantino I, Pagliaro L: Emergency sclerotherapy versus medical interventions for bleeding oesophageal varices in cirrhotic patients (Cochrane Review), in *The Cochrane Library,* Issue 2. Oxford: Update Software, 2002.

28. Rossle M, Siegersetter V, Huber M, Ochs A: The first decade of the transjugular intrahepatic portosystemic shunt (TIPS): State of the art. *Liver* 18:73, 1998.

SWALLOWED FOREIGN BODIES
Wade R. Gaasch
Robert A. Barish

Swallowed foreign bodies, a common presentation in emergency departments, can be innocuous or life threatening. In the United States, approximately 1500 people die yearly as a result of ingesting foreign bodies.[1] Often thought to be confined to the pediatric population, foreign body ingestion occurs in all age groups. The pediatric age group accounts for approximately 80 percent of all cases, followed by edentulous adults, prisoners, and psychiatric patients. The presence of dentures eliminates the tactile sensitivity of the palatal surface vital to the identification of small items. A correlation exists between age groups and specific types of ingested material. Children most often ingest coins, toys, crayons, and ballpoint pen caps; adults tend to have problems with meat and bones.[2] In addition, psychiatric patients and prison inmates may ingest such unlikely objects as spoons and razor blades.

PATHOPHYSIOLOGY

Most objects pass spontaneously, but 10 to 20 percent require some intervention, and only 1 percent demand surgical treatment.[3] Ingested foreign bodies may be found anywhere throughout the digestive tract, but the majority of articles tend to lodge in several physiologic "narrow spaces." The pediatric esophagus has five areas of constriction where coins and other objects may become trapped: cricopharyngeal narrowing (C6), the most common site; the thoracic inlet (T1); the aortic arch (T4); the tracheal bifurcation (T6); and the hiatal narrowing (T10-11). Most pediatric obstructions occur in the proximal esophagus; the vast majority of adult impactions arise from esophageal disease in the distal esophagus. Because 97 percent of adults presenting with meat impaction harbor pathologic esophageal conditions, barium swallow must be performed to confirm foreign body clearance and evaluate possible underlying disease.

Once an object has traversed the pylorus, it usually continues to the rectum and is passed in the stool. If, however, the object has irregular or sharp edges, it may become lodged anywhere in the gastrointestinal tract. Objects that lodge in the esophagus (not necessarily limited to those with sharp or irregular contour) can result in airway obstruction, stricture, or perforation with resulting mediastinitis, cardiac tamponade, paraesophageal abscess, or aortotracheoesophageal fistula. Perforation may be the result of direct mechanical erosion, as with bones, or chemical corrosion, as with button batteries.

CLINICAL PRESENTATION

Objects lodged in the esophagus generally produce anxiety and discomfort. Adult patients often complain of retrosternal pain. Patients are likely to retch or vomit and experience dysphagia, resulting in choking, coughing, or aspiration if they attempt to wash down the object. Eventually, patients may be unable to swallow their own secretions. In the adult, the history often provides all the pertinent information necessary for diagnosis and treatment. However, this is often not true for children. In those 16 years and younger, symptoms include refusal to eat, vomiting (with or without hematemesis), gagging, choking, stridor ("pseudoasthma"), neck or throat pain, inability to swallow, increased salivation, and foreign body sensation in the chest.

The differential diagnosis for patients suspected of having swallowed a foreign body (Table 76-1) includes dysphagia, esophageal carcinoma, and gastroesophageal reflux disease.[4]

Physical examination must include careful evaluation of the nasopharynx, oropharynx, neck, and subcutaneous tissues for air resulting from perforation of a hollow viscus. Laryngoscopy, direct or indi-rect, should be done, especially when the patient complains of a sticking sensation or has ingested a bone. Although physical signs are not always present, findings consistent with foreign body ingestion in 16 years and younger consist of red throat, dysphagia, palatal abrasion, temperature elevation, anxiety and distress, and peritoneal signs.

EMERGENCY DEPARTMENT MANAGEMENT

General Care

Because the great majority of ingested foreign bodies traverse the entire gastrointestinal tract without any problems, treatment can be expectant once the object has passed through the pylorus.[5] If, however, a foreign body obstructs the esophagus, prevention of aspiration is paramount. This can be accomplished by inserting a tube above the obstructing body to remove unswallowed fluids above the impaction. Conditions warranting consultation with an endoscopist and possible hospital admission are listed in Table 76-2. In almost all cases, endoscopy allows removal of a foreign body without complications.[6]

The offending object can be located in several ways. A radiopaque object will be demonstrated on standard x-ray films of the neck or abdomen. The procedure of choice for finding and then extracting a foreign body in the esophagus is endoscopy.[7] This procedure has a high success rate and thus avoids progression to surgery.[8] It is also time efficient.[9] Although many other diagnostic methods are available, they are not as reliable and thorough as endoscopy, so the time spent in arranging for and conducting such tests may not be time well spent for a frightened, uncomfortable patient.

If endoscopic equipment and expertise are not available, an esophagogram can be performed. Consultation with an endoscopist is strongly recommended before initiation of any contrast study, because direct visualization of the foreign body after contrast administration may not be possible because of interference from swallowed contrast medium.

The type of contrast agent must be chosen based on the anticipated clinical findings and course.[10] If perforation is suspected, a water-soluble contrast agent (Gastrografin) should be used. However, because water-soluble agents are pulmonary irritants, barium should be used if aspiration is possible. The least amount of barium possible should be instilled, because barium will block the endoscopic field. If perforation and aspiration are possible, a nonionic contrast agent is indicated.

Progress of the object through the gastrointestinal tract must be monitored with repeat abdominal x-ray films, usually 2 to 4 h apart. The use of metal detectors, if available, has been advocated as a means of localizing and tracking the progression of metal objects, thereby avoiding repeated radiation exposure. Abdominal examinations should be done frequently to detect early signs of developing peritonitis should perforation occur. Virtually all symptomatic patients will require observation and esophagoscopy. If a nonfood object becomes lodged in the esophagus or is unable to pass through the pylorus, it must be removed as soon as possible with the use of esophagogastroscopy. Fatal lead encephalopathy has been reported in a child who ingested a lead curtain weight, which supposedly had been in the stomach for an extended period.[11]

TABLE 76-1   Differential Diagnosis of Swallowed Foreign Body

Dysphagia
Odynophagia
Esophageal carcinoma
Esophageal stricture
Gastroesophageal reflux disease
Bowel obstruction
Intestinal perforation
Peritonitis secondary to other pathologies
Pneumomediastinum
Tracheal foreign body

TABLE 76-2   Esophageal Foreign Bodies Warranting Endoscopy Consultation

Sharp or elongated objects
Multiple foreign bodies
Button batteries
Evidence of perforation
Child with a nickel or quarter at the level of the cricopharyngeus muscle
Airway compromise
Presence of foreign body for more than 24 h

Source: Adapted from Munter DW: Disorders of the esophagus, in Howell JM, et al (eds): *Emergency Medicine.* Philadelphia: Saunders, 1998, p. 318.

Food Impaction

Meat impaction may be treated expectantly, provided the patient can manage the secretions. Time and sedation often will allow the meat to pass into the stomach, but the bolus should not be allowed to remain impacted longer than 12 h. Endoscopy is the preferred method for removal. Alternatives have been suggested if endoscopy is not available.

The use of proteolytic enzymes, such as an aqueous solution of papain (e.g., Adolph's Meat Tenderizer), to dissolve a meat bolus is *not* recommended, because of the number of reported complications and because of increasing availability of and expertise in endoscopy. Several reports in the literature have described esophageal perforation secondary to the enzymatic action of the solution. Mucosal ischemia resulting from distention of the esophageal wall renders the esophagus more susceptible to enzymatic degradation. Hemorrhagic pulmonary edema also has been reported after aspiration of Adolph's Meat Tenderizer.

Intravenous administration of glucagon to relax esophageal smooth muscle also has been suggested as a method of treating food impaction. A test dose should be given to ensure that hypersensitivity does not exist; then the recommended dose is 1 mg. If the food bolus is not passed in 20 min, an additional 2 mg is given IV. An esophagogram must be performed after treatment to ensure passage. This strategy was questioned by Tibbling and associates who found no statistical difference in disimpaction rates between patients given spasmolytic drugs and those given placebo.[12] For patients with esophageal obstruction caused by food, more efficient approaches to treatment are endoscopy and esophagoscopy.

Bell and Eibling reported the successful use of nifedipine, which reduces lower esophageal sphincter pressure and the amplitude of the sphincter contractions without changing the amplitude of contractions in the body of the esophagus.[12] By this mechanism, a bolus of food lodged in the vicinity of the gastroesophageal junction may pass. The recommended dose is 10 mg administered sublingually. Sublingual nitroglycerin also has been used successfully, but it can cause hypotension.

Coin Ingestion

Because as many as 35 percent of children with a coin lodged in their esophagus will be asymptomatic, some authors recommend that radiographs be performed in *all* children suspected of swallowing coins to determine the presence and location of the object. However, Caravati and colleagues noted no difference in 5-day morbidity rates between children who underwent radiographic evaluation and those who did not after coin ingestion.[14] Coins in the esophagus lie in the frontal plane with the flat side visible on an anteroposterior radiograph; coins in the trachea lie in the sagittal plane (Figure 76-1).

The use of a Foley catheter, initially reported in the late 1960s, has been promoted as a safe and effective technique for removal when the coin has been impacted for fewer than 24 h. Before attempting extraction, the airway must be secured with endotracheal intubation. The catheter is passed down the esophagus beyond the object and the balloon is inflated. As the catheter is slowly withdrawn, the object is withdrawn along with it. Retrieval of a coin by this technique is less effective after 24 h. Most clinicians prefer using the Foley catheter under fluoroscopic guidance. Foley catheter retrieval of foreign bodies may be complicated by aspiration, and personnel and equipment for airway control must be immediately available. If endoscopic expertise is readily available, Foley catheterization retrieval should be a secondary option.

Button Battery Ingestion

A button battery lodged in the esophagus is a true emergency, because of the extremely rapid action of the alkaline substance on the mucosa. Burns to the esophagus have been reported to occur in as few as 4 h, with perforation as soon as 6 h after ingestion. Button batteries in the esophagus require emergency removal if significant morbidity is to be averted. Outcome does not appear to be affected by battery discharge state but is affected by chemical composition.[15] Lithium cells are associated disproportionately with adverse outcome. Mercuric oxide cells tend to fragment more frequently than other cells; however, the threat of heavy metal poisoning has not been supported by the literature or clinical experience. This fact notwithstanding, blood and urine mercury levels should be measured whenever a mercury-containing cell is observed to have split while in the gastrointestinal tract.

Button ingestion can be managed along two main pathways (Figure 76-2). If the button battery is lodged in the esophagus, its location should be documented by radiograph; then emergent endoscopic removal is mandatory. Given the widespread expertise with endoscopy, we cannot recommend alternative techniques, many of which are associated with significant complications. Ipecac has no place in the management of button battery ingestion.[15] Button batteries that have passed the esophagus need not be retrieved in the asymptomatic patient unless the cell is not passing through the pylorus after 48 h of observation. This is rarely the case unless the battery is of large diameter and the patient is younger than 6 years. In this case, endoscopic

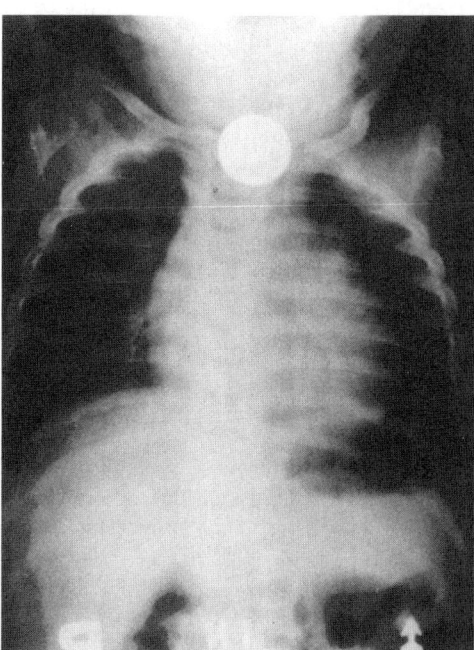
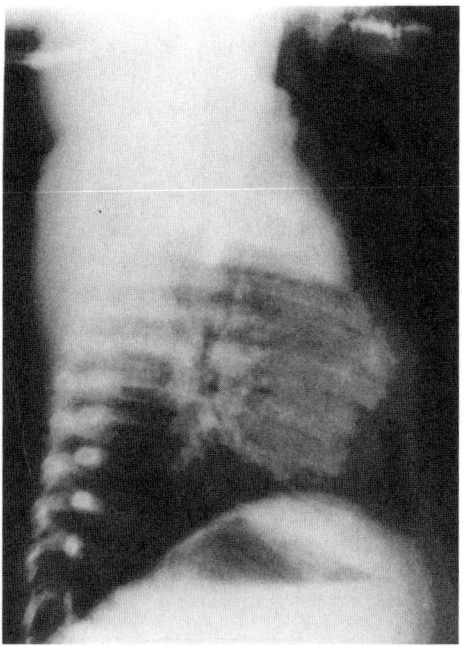

FIG. 76-1. A coin lodged in a child's esophagus is visible on an anteroposterior radiograph. [Reproduced with permission from Effron D (ed): *Pediatric Photo and X-Ray Stimuli for Emergency Medicine,* volume II. Columbus, Ohio Chapter of the American College of Emergency Physicians, 1997, case 27.]

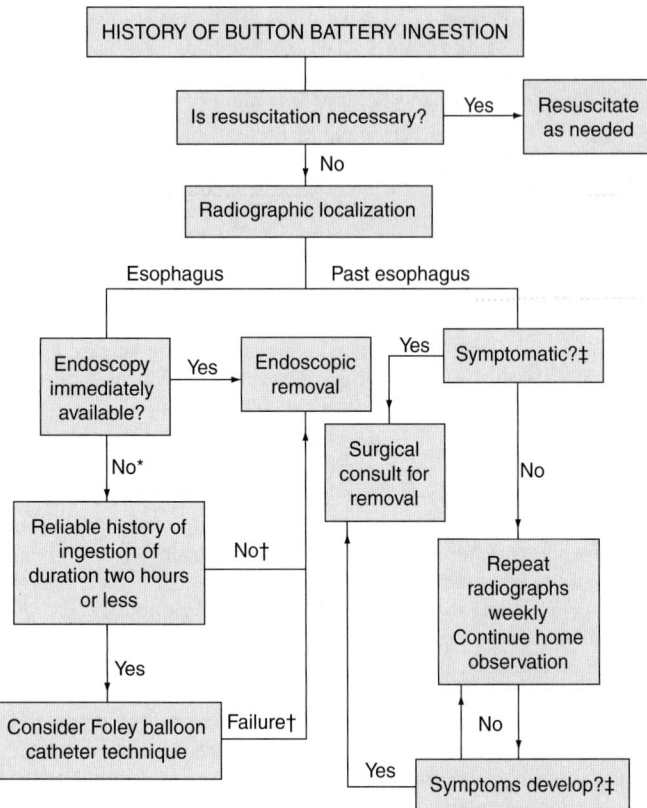

FIG. 76-2. Algorithm for management of button battery ingestion. *Button batteries in the esophagus must be removed. Endoscopy should be used, if available. The balloon catheter technique can be used if the ingestion occurred no more than 2 h previously, but it should not be used after this period, because it may increase the amount of damage to the weakened esophagus. †When the Foley technique fails or is contraindicated because more than 2 h have elapsed, the button battery should be removed endoscopically. This may require transfer of the patient. ‡Acute abdomen, tarry or bloody stools, fever, persistent vomiting. (Adapted from Kuhns DW, Dire DJ: Button battery ingestions. *Ann Emerg Med* 18:293, 1989.)

retrieval is the preferred option. Most batteries pass completely through the body within 48 to 72 h, although passage has been reported to take as long as 14 days. All patients with signs and symptoms of gastrointestinal tract injury require immediate surgical consultation. Assistance with cell identification may be obtained by calling the National Button Battery Ingestion Hotline (National Capital Poison Center, Washington, DC) at 1-202-625-3333.

Ingestion of Sharp Objects

Management of ingested sharp and pointed foreign bodies is controversial. Objects longer than 5 cm and wider than 2 cm rarely will pass the stomach. Objects of that size and those with extremely pointed edges, such as open safety pins or razor blades, must be removed before they pass from the stomach because 15 to 35 percent will cause intestinal perforation, usually in the ileocecal valve.

Paul and Jaffe recommended the following management for children who have swallowed sharp objects.[16] All patients should have an initial radiograph and physical examination. If the patient is symptomatic or has ingested a sewing needle, surgical consultation for possible endoscopy and laparotomy is indicated. Children who have swallowed a sharp object (other than sewing needles) but are asymptomatic can be managed on an expectant basis. Progression of the sharp object should be documented with serial radiographs. If progression past the stomach

is not seen, a water-soluble contrast film may document gastrointestinal perforation. At the first sign of perforation, the object should be removed even if the patient remains asymptomatic. If the object does not progress through the gastrointestinal tract, surgical retrieval is indicated.

Cocaine Ingestion

Cocaine ingestion is an increasingly widespread problem. Carriers will ingest multiple small packets of cocaine in attempts to conceal the drug. A favored packet is the condom, which may hold up to 5 g of cocaine. Rupture of even one such packet may be fatal. Webb recommended surgery as the safest method of recovery to avoid the likelihood of packet rupture during endoscopic retrieval.[2] If the packet appears to be passing intact through the intestinal tract, the clinician may choose to observe the patient and wait for the packet to be delivered spontaneously through the rectum.

REFERENCES

1. Schwartz GF, Polsky HS: Ingested foreign bodies of the gastrointestinal tract. *Am Surg* 42:236, 1976.
2. Webb WA: Management of foreign bodies of the upper gastrointestinal tract: Update. *Gastrointest Endosc* 41:39, 1995.
3. American Society for Gastrointestinal Endoscopy: Guideline for the management of ingested foreign bodies. *Gastrointest Endosc* 41:622, 1995.
4. Klaus A, Swain JM, Hinder RA: Laparoscopic antireflux surgery for supraesophageal complications of gastroesophageal reflux disease. *Am J Med* 111(suppl 8A):202S, 2001.
5. Binder L, Anderson WA: Pediatric gastrointestinal foreign body ingestions. *Ann Emerg Med* 13:112, 1984.
6. Mosca S, Manes G, Martino R, et al: Endoscopic management of foreign bodies in the upper gastrointestinal tract: Report on a series of 414 adult patients. *Endoscopy* 33:692, 2001.
7. Ginsberg GG: Management of ingested foreign objects and food bolus impactions. *Gastrointest Endosc* 41:33, 1995.
8. Blair SR, Graeber GM, Cruzzavala JL, et al: Current management of esophageal impactions. *Chest* 104:1205, 1993.
9. Stack LB, Munter DW: Foreign bodies in the gastrointestinal tract. *Emerg Med Clin North Am* 14:493, 1996.
10. Barsan WG, Lowell JM, Wolf LR: Disorders of the upper gastrointestinal tract, in Rosen P, Barkin R, Danzl DF, et al (eds): *Emergency Medicine: Concepts and Clinical Practice.* St. Louis, Mosby-Year Book, 1998, pp. 1958.
11. Hugelmeyer CD, Moorhead JC, Horenblas L, Bayer MJ: Fatal lead encephalopathy following foreign body ingestion: Case report. *J Emerg Med* 6:397, 1988.
12. Tibbling L, Bjorkhoel A, Jansson E, Stenkvist M: Effect of spasmolytic drugs on esophageal foreign bodies. *Dysphagia* 10:126, 1995.
13. Bell AF, Eibling DE: Nifedipine in the treatment of distal esophageal food impaction. *Arch Otolaryngol Head Neck Surg* 114:682, 1988.
14. Caravati EM, Bennett DL, McElwee NE: Pediatric coin ingestion: A prospective study on the utility of routine roentgenograms. *Am J Dis Child* 143:549, 1989.
15. Litovitz T, Schmitz BF: Ingestion of cylindrical and button batteries: An analysis of 2382 cases. *Pediatrics* 89:747, 1992.
16. Paul RI, Jaffe DM: Sharp object ingestions in children: Illustrative case and literature review. *Pediatr Emerg Care* 4:245, 1988.

PEPTIC ULCER DISEASE AND GASTRITIS
Matthew C. Gratton

Peptic ulcer disease is a chronic illness manifested by recurrent ulcerations in the stomach and proximal duodenum. Acid and pepsin are thought to be crucial to ulcer development, but it is now recognized that the great majority of peptic ulcers are directly related to infection with *Helicobacter pylori* or nonsteroidal anti-inflammatory drug

(NSAID) use.[1,2] Gastritis is acute or chronic inflammation of the gastric mucosa and has various etiologies. Dyspepsia is continuous or recurrent upper abdominal pain or discomfort with or without associated symptoms (nausea, bloating, regurgitation, etc.).[3] Dyspepsia may be caused by a number of diseases or may be functional.

EPIDEMIOLOGY

Approximately 10 percent of the U.S. population older than 17 years have peptic ulcer disease at some time. One third of them report an active ulcer within the past year.[4] Peptic ulcer disease has a high rate of morbidity, with 8 million physicians' visits and 275,000 hospitalizations per year and a high cost to society of $5.65 billion per year in lost wages and medical care.[4] The prevalence of *H. pylori* infection in white Americans younger than 35 years is about 10 percent, rising to almost 80 percent by age 75. Forty-five percent of black Americans younger than 25 years are infected.[5] Presumably because of improvements in the standard of living, the prevalence of *H. pylori* is decreasing in most developed countries.[6] The prevalence of dyspepsia is 25 to 30 percent in the United States.[3,7]

PATHOPHYSIOLOGY

Hydrochloric acid and pepsin destroy gastric and duodenal mucosa. Mucous and bicarbonate ion secretions protect mucosa. Prostaglandins protect mucosa by enhancing mucous and bicarbonate production and by enhancing mucosal blood flow, thereby supporting metabolism. The balance between these protective and destructive forces determines whether peptic ulcer disease will occur. *Helicobacter pylori* infection or NSAIDs are thought to be the causal agents of peptic ulcer disease in almost all cases.[1,2] *Helicobacter pylori* infection is present in 95 percent of duodenal ulcers and 80 percent of gastric ulcers.[8] Although traditional treatment of peptic ulcers by various modalities heals most ulcers, eradication of *H. pylori* reduces recurrence rates from 80 to 15 percent for duodenal ulcers and from 50 to 10 percent for gastric ulcers.[8] *Helicobacter pylori* is a spiral, urease-producing, flagellated bacterium that is found living between the mucous gel and the mucosa primarily in the gastric antrum.[5] The production of urease, cytotoxins, proteases, and other compounds is thought to disturb the mucous gel and cause tissue injury.[2,5] In the presence of acid and pepsin, ulceration may occur. Chronic active (usually asymptomatic) gastritis is an almost universal finding with *H. pylori* infection, but only 10 to 20 percent of infected people develop peptic ulcer disease.[5,9] It is unclear why most infected persons do not develop symptomatic peptic ulcer disease, but it most likely reflects an interaction of factors, including host and pathogen (different virulence of strains of bacteria).[9]

Helicobacter pylori has been linked to mucosa-associated lymphoid tissue lymphoma, and regression has been documented with eradication of infection. In addition, *H. pylori* infection is considered a definite risk factor for adenocarcinoma of the stomach. However, because the prevalence of gastric cancer in the United States is very low and the *H. pylori* infection rate is very high, other factors undoubtedly are involved.[5]

Nonsteroidal anti-inflammatory drugs inhibit prostaglandin synthesis, thereby decreasing mucous and bicarbonate production and mucosal blood flow, allowing ulcer formation.[2] Gastrin-secreting tumors produce ulceration due to high levels of acid and pepsin production, but acid alone rarely causes ulceration. However, inhibition of acid secretion may allow ulcers to heal and is the basis for traditional ulcer treatments.

Hereditary factors cause a predisposition to peptic ulcer disease. There is an association between chronic renal failure, renal transplantation, cirrhosis, chronic obstructive pulmonary disease, and peptic ulceration, but the precise mechanism is unclear. Cigarette smoking is a predisposing factor for peptic ulcer disease, perhaps due to an inhibi-

tion of bicarbonate ion production or to increased gastric emptying (but not to increased acid production). Emotional stress may predispose to peptic ulcer disease, but diet and alcohol use do not.

Acute gastritis may be related to ischemia from severe illness (shock, trauma, severe burns, organ failure, etc.) or the direct toxic effects of agents (NSAIDs, alcohol, bile acids, etc.). *Helicobacter pylori* infection causes acute and chronic gastritis (both usually asymptomatic). Chronic gastritis may also be caused by autoimmune factors that destroy gastric parietal cells, resulting in the loss of acid production and the loss of intrinsic factor production, which in turn cause malabsorption of vitamin B_{12} and, hence, pernicious anemia.

CLINICAL FEATURES

Burning epigastric pain is the most classic symptom of peptic ulcer disease. The pain also may be described as sharp, dull, an ache, or an "empty" or "hungry" feeling. Pain may be relieved by milk, food, or antacids, presumably due to buffering and/or dilution of acid. Pain recurs as the gastric contents empty, and the recurrent pain may classically awaken the patient at night. Pain tends to occur daily for weeks, resolve, and then reoccur in weeks to months. Although no symptoms allow complete discrimination, Talley and colleagues found that peptic ulceration is more likely than nonulcer dyspepsia or cholelithiasis in the presence of night pain; pain relieved by food, milk, or antacids; and a shorter duration of pain.[7] Postprandial pain, food intolerance, nausea, retrosternal pain, and belching are not related to peptic ulcer disease.[10] Atypical presentations are common in those older than 65 years, including no pain, epigastric pain not relieved by eating, nausea, vomiting, anorexia, weight loss, and bleeding.[11]

A change in the character of the patient's typical pain may herald a complication. Abrupt onset of severe or generalized pain may indicate perforation with spillage of gastric or duodenal contents and resulting peritonitis. Rapid onset of mid-back pain may be due to posterior penetration into the pancreas, with the development of pancreatitis. Nausea and vomiting may indicate gastric outlet obstruction from scarring or edema. Vomiting bright red blood or coffee-ground emesis or passing tarry or melanotic stool or hematochezia indicates ulcer bleeding.

On physical examination, the only positive finding in patients with uncomplicated peptic ulcer disease may be epigastric tenderness. This finding is neither sensitive nor specific for the diagnosis.[7] Other physical findings may be indicative of complications: a rigid abdomen consistent with peritonitis in perforation; abdominal distention or a succussion splash due to obstruction; occult or gross blood per rectum or nasogastric tube with ulcer bleeding.

Epigastric pain, nausea, and vomiting may be present with acute gastritis, but the most common presentation is gastrointestinal bleeding, ranging from occult blood loss in the stool to massive upper gastrointestinal hemorrhage. Physical findings may be normal, may reflect only the gastrointestinal bleeding, or may reflect a severe underlying associated illness (as listed above).

DIAGNOSIS

A definitive diagnosis of peptic ulcer disease cannot be made on clinical grounds alone.[10] Uncomplicated peptic ulcer disease can be strongly suspected in the presence of a "classic" history, including epigastric burning pain; relief of pain with milk, food, or antacids; and night pain accompanied by "benign" physical examination findings, including normal vital signs with or without mild epigastric tenderness. The differential diagnosis of epigastric pain is extensive and, in addition to peptic ulcer disease, includes gastritis, gastroesophageal reflux disease, cholelithiasis, pancreatitis, hepatitis, abdominal aortic aneurysm (AAA), gastroparesis, and "functional" dyspepsia. A careful history may elicit features that point away from peptic ulcer disease: burning pain radiating into the chest, water brash, and belching may suggest gastroesophageal reflux disease; more severe pain radiating to the right upper quadrant and around the right or left side suggests cholelithiasis; radiation through to the back indicates pancreatitis or AAA; chronic pain, anorexia, or weight loss may indicate gastric cancer. Myocardial ischemic pain may also present as epigastric pain and should be strongly considered in the appropriate clinical setting.

Physical examination findings may suggest other diagnoses: right upper quadrant tenderness points to cholelithiasis or hepatitis, an epigastric mass to pancreatitis (pseudocyst), a pulsatile mass to AAA, jaundice to hepatitis, and peritoneal findings to an acute abdomen.

In a patient presenting with epigastric pain, a number of ancillary tests may be helpful to exclude peptic ulcer disease complications and to narrow the differential diagnosis. A normal complete blood count will rule out anemia from chronic gastrointestinal bleeding due to peptic ulcer disease, gastritis, or cancer (but does not rule out acute blood loss). Elevated liver function test results may indicate hepatitis, and elevated lipase levels may indicate pancreatitis. An acute abdominal series may show free air associated with perforation. A "limited" emergency department ultrasound examination may show gallstones or an AAA. An electrocardiogram and cardiac enzyme determination are indicated if there is a suspicion of myocardial ischemic pain.

The definitive diagnosis of peptic ulcer disease is made by visualization of the ulcer via upper gastrointestinal barium contrast radiography or via upper gastrointestinal endoscopy. Endoscopy has a higher yield rate for ulcer and other mucosal pathologic conditions, which may affect clinical care[1] (Table 77-1). However, endoscopy also has a higher cost and complication rate.[1]

Because most peptic ulcers are caused by *H. pylori* infection and eradication of *H. pylori* dramatically decreases ulcer recurrence rate, it is important to note how to diagnose infection. *Helicobacter pylori* can be diagnosed by endoscopic tests, including the rapid urease test, histologic study, or culture, and noninvasive tests, including serologic tests, urea breath tests, and stool antigen tests.[1,6,9,12,13] The rapid urease test (also know as the *Campylobacter*-like organism test) detects the presence of urease in a biopsy specimen (presumptive evidence of *H. pylori* infection) with 90 to 95 percent sensitivity and 90 to 100 percent specificity and a cost of $6 to $20. Histologic study using special stains has a sensitivity and specificity above 90 percent and costs $60 to $250. Culture is difficult and has a sensitivity no better than that of histologic studies (although it has 100 percent specificity if results are positive). *The aforementioned costs do not include the cost of endoscopy.* Serologic studies detect immunoglobulin G antibodies to *H. pylori* via latex agglutination or enzyme-linked immunosorbent assay tests with high sensitivity and specificity at a cost of $10 to $100 (higher sensitivity, specificity, and cost with enzyme-linked immunosorbent assay). Serologic studies are not useful as a test of cure, because antibodies remain for several years after eradication of infection. The urea breath test also relies on the presence of urease produced by *H. pylori*. Urea, labeled with ^{13}C or ^{14}C instead of ^{12}C, is ingested and, in the presence of bacterial urease, is broken down into labeled carbon dioxide and ammonia. The labeled carbon dioxide is detected in the breath 30 min later. Sensitivity and specificity are greater than 90 percent, and the cost is $250 to $350 for ^{13}C and $20 to $65 for ^{14}C (^{14}C is radioactive and, hence, is contraindicated in children and women of childbearing potential). This test is ideal for con-

firming cure of infection. *Helicobacter pylori* antigens can be detected in the stool with 80 to 100 percent sensitivity. Testing performed 4 weeks or more after completion of *H. pylori* eradication therapy may prove useful as a test of cure.

TREATMENT

After peptic ulcer disease is diagnosed, the goal of treatment is to heal the ulcer while relieving pain and preventing complications and recurrence. Traditional ulcer therapy heals, relieves pain, and prevents complications, but does not prevent recurrence. Treatment of *H. pylori* infection, when present, dramatically decreases the recurrence rate.[8] If NSAID-associated ulcers are present, the offending agent must be stopped to reduce the recurrence rate.

Traditional therapy includes proton pump inhibitors (PPIs), histamine (H$_2$) receptor antagonists (H$_2$RAs), sucralfate, and antacids[1,14] (Table 77-2). Proton pump inhibitors decrease acid production by irreversibly (covalent bond) binding with a sulfhydryl group of a H$^+$K$^+$ATPase molecule (proton pump) located on the gastric parietal cell, thus blocking hydrogen ion secretion. Proton pump inhibitors generally heal ulcers faster than do H$_2$RAs and also have some in vitro inhibitory effect against *H. pylori*.[1,14] They are metabolized in the liver by the cytochrome P450 system and therefore may decrease the metabolism of many other drugs. In addition, PPIs may inhibit the absorption of drugs that rely on gastric acidity. Serious side effects are rare. Histamine receptor antagonists competitively inhibit the actions

TABLE 77-2   Traditional Drugs for Peptic Ulcers

Drug	Dosage (PO)	Comments
H$_2$ receptor antagonists		Serious adverse reactions rare with all in class; dosages should be decreased in renal failure
Cimetidine	400 mg bid	More likely to have drug interactions due to more inhibition of cytochrome system
Famotidine	20 mg bid	
Nizatidine	150 mg bid	
Ranitidine	150 mg bid	
Proton pump inhibitors		Serious adverse reactions rare with all in class
Lansoprazole	15 mg qd	
Omeprazole	20 mg qd	
Rabeprazole	20 mg qd	
Other drugs		
Sucralfate	1 g qid	Facilitates aluminum absorption (should not be used with aluminum-containing antacids in patients with renal failure)
Misoprostol*	200 μg qid	Contraindicated in pregnancy (abortifacient)
Antacids		Avoid aluminum-containing antacids in renal failure
Magnesium hydroxide		
Aluminum hydroxide		
Simethecone		
Maalox Extra Strength	15–30 mL	
Antacid (Ciba)	qid	
Mylanta Double Strength (J & J Merck)	2 tablets qid	

*Approved by the Food and Drug Administration only for prevention of ulcers associated with nonsteroidal anti-inflammatory drugs.
Source: Drugs for treatment of peptic ulcers. *Med Lett* 39:1, 1997.

TABLE 77-1   "Alarm" Features Suggesting Need for Endoscopy Referral

Age older than 45–50 y
Weight loss
Long history of symptoms
Anemia
Persistent anorexia
Early satiety
Persistent vomiting
Gastrointestinal bleeding

of histamine on the H_2 receptors of the gastric parietal cells. All four drugs heal ulcers approximately equally and are available in over-the-counter preparations.[1,14] Because of renal excretion, dosage adjustments must be made in patients with renal failure. Side effects are uncommon, but cimetidine has more significant drug interactions than do the other three due to inhibition of cytochrome P450 activity.[14] Sucralfate appears to protect the ulcer from acid exposure (by forming a sticky gel that adheres to the ulcer crater) and allows healing to occur about as well as H_2RAs.[1] Sucralfate has few side effects but does inhibit absorption of a number of medications.[14] Antacids heal ulcers by buffering gastric acid and are as effective as H_2RAs.[1] Magnesium- and aluminum-containing antacids can inhibit absorption of drugs. In renal failure, aluminum can accumulate and cause osteoporosis and encephalopathy, so aluminum-containing antacids should be avoided. Due to the simplicity of H_2RA, PPI, and sucralfate dosing requirements, antacids currently are used mainly on an as-needed basis for ulcer pain until healing occurs.

Although NSAIDs should be stopped in patients with peptic ulcer disease whenever possible, misoprostol may prevent ulcer formation in those on concurrent NSAID therapy. Misoprostol is a prostaglandin analogue that may act by increasing mucous and bicarbonate production and by increasing mucosal blood flow.

If *H. pylori* infection is diagnosed in the presence of peptic ulcer disease, eradication is clearly indicated.[14] Multiple regimens have been proposed and studied, mainly by using combinations of a PPI (or ranitidine bismuth citrate) and two antibiotics, most commonly clarithromycin and amoxicillin or metronidazole.[12,15,16] Cure rates of 80 to 90 percent are typical.[12] Although some European studies demonstrate that 7-day regimens are sufficient for cure, authorities in the United States recommend 10- to 14-day regimens for the best cure rates.[12,15] A typical 14-day regimen of lansoprazole, clarithromycin, and amoxicillin would cost approximately $228.[16]

Patients generally do not present to the emergency department with a definitive diagnosis of peptic ulcer disease but rather with a symptom, such as epigastric pain. If appropriate history, physical examination, and laboratory evaluation result in a physician's impression of "possible peptic ulcer disease" or "dyspepsia," the physician is left with three main options: empiric treatment with conventional antiulcer medication, immediate referral for definite diagnosis (endoscopic or radiologic study), or noninvasive testing for *H. pylori* followed by antibiotic therapy for patients with positive test results.[1,9]

Traditional emergency department treatment would entail initiating a trial of antacids and/or H_2RAs and early referral to a primary care provider to direct evaluation and subsequent treatment. This remains a reasonable option. Immediate referral for definite diagnosis is mandated if certain "alarm" features are present: age older than 45 to 50 years, weight loss, long history of symptoms, anemia, persistent anorexia, early satiety, persistent vomiting, or gastrointestinal bleeding.[1,9,12,15] Cost-effectiveness analysis and consensus statements support treatment of *H. pylori*-positive dyspeptic patients with antimicrobial and antisecretory therapy followed by endoscopic study only in those with persistent symptoms.[1,12,15,17] It also would be reasonable for the emergency department physician to begin symptomatic therapy, order serologic testing for *H. pylori,* and refer for early follow-up with a primary care provider for initiation of antibacterial therapy if the test results are positive.

COMPLICATIONS

Hemorrhage

In the United States, about 150,000 patients per year are admitted to the hospital with gastrointestinal bleeding due to peptic ulcer disease.[18] Factors predicting death include large initial bleed, continued or recurrent bleeding, older age, and comorbid illness.[18] The mortality rate is 2 to 3 percent for the 80 to 85 percent of patients who do not rebleed, compared with 20 percent or greater for those who do bleed while hospitalized.[18] Shock, low initial hematocrit, red blood in the emesis or stool, and failure of blood to clear with lavage predict further bleeding.[18]

Treatment for ulcer bleeding should focus on restoring hemodynamic stability by intravenous administration of isotonic saline solution and packed red blood cells. Appropriate blood work should be performed, including a complete blood count and type and cross-matching for several units of packed red cells. Two large-bore intravenous lines should be started, and the patient should be placed on oxygen and a cardiac monitor. A nasogastric tube should be inserted and lavaged with water until clear. This does not slow bleeding but does allow monitoring of ongoing bleeding and clears the stomach for endoscopy. An H_2RA or PPI can be started, but there is no proof that either reduces rebleeding rates.

Most patients should undergo upper gastrointestinal endoscopy for diagnostic, prognostic, and treatment purposes. An actively bleeding vessel seen on endoscopy heralds a 35 percent chance of emergency surgery and an 11 percent mortality rate. Morbidity and mortality decrease with findings of a nonbleeding visible vessel, an adherent clot and a flat, pigmented spot. A low of 0.5 percent emergency surgery and a 2 percent mortality rate is realized if a clear base is found.[18] Treatment through endoscopy includes injection therapy with epinephrine, alcohol, or combinations; heat probe or bipolar electrical coagulation; or laser therapy. All of these treatments stop bleeding, prevent recurrences, and decrease transfusion rates and length of hospital stay. The technique chosen depends on the equipment available and the experience of the endoscopist.[18]

The rebleeding rate after endoscopic therapy is about 20 percent and can be treated by repeat endoscopy or emergency surgery. Surgery is also indicated if bleeding cannot be controlled by initial endoscopy. Angiography with arterial vasopressin or embolization can be considered if endoscopy has failed and surgery is thought to be very high risk.[18]

Hospitalization in an intensive care setting is indicated for all patients with significant upper gastrointestinal bleeding due to peptic ulcers. If clinical and endoscopic features suggest a low risk of rebleeding, a ward bed may be acceptable.

Perforation

Perforation is heralded by the abrupt onset of severe epigastric pain as gastric or duodenal contents spill into the peritoneal cavity, followed by the development of chemical and then bacterial peritonitis. Patients may not have a prior history of peptic ulcer disease and may in fact have no antecedent history of ulcer-like symptoms. Elderly patients may not have dramatic pain or impressive peritoneal findings.

When the diagnosis is suspected, appropriate laboratory tests, including a complete blood count, type, and cross-match, and a lipase level determination, should be performed; two large-bore intravenous lines started; oxygen and a monitor placed; a nasogastric tube inserted and placed on suction; and an acute abdominal series obtained. Free air is not always present. Some authorities suggest instillation of air into the stomach through the nasogastric tube to detect perforation. This procedure may open a sealed perforation, causing more spillage, and nonvisualization of free air does not rule out a perforation; thus, it is not recommended. Broad-spectrum antibiotics should be given and a surgical consult promptly obtained. In some cases, nonsurgical therapy has been successful, but operative intervention is the standard in the United States.

Obstruction

Obstruction occurs because of scarring of the gastric outlet due to chronic peptic ulcer disease, edema due to an active ulcer, or some combination of both. Resulting symptoms include abdominal fullness, nausea, and vomiting, and signs may include abdominal distention and a succussion splash. Dehydration and electrolyte imbalances may occur. Treatment includes rehydration with intravenous fluids, correction of electrolyte abnormalities, and relief of distention with nasogastric suction. Hospitalization is almost always indicated. The outlet may open as edema subsides, but surgical correction is often necessary.

DISPOSITION

Patients with complications always require consultation, and most require admission to an appropriate inpatient unit based on the diagnosis and hemodynamic stability. Most patients with epigastric pain or dyspepsia do not leave the emergency department with a definitive diagnosis, but, if critical diagnoses (e.g., AAA or myocardial ischemia) are still in the differential, consultation for admission and appropriate workup is indicated. When uncomplicated peptic ulcer disease, gastritis, or dyspepsia is strongly suspected, the great majority of patients can be discharged with antacids and an H$_2$RA, with or without a serologic test for *H. pylori,* and close follow-up with their primary care provider. If "alarm" features (indicating possible cancer or bleeding) are present, consultation for early endoscopy is indicated.

Discharge instructions should include an explanation of the diagnosis and home treatment, specific follow-up instructions, and warning symptoms that should prompt immediate reevaluation. The explanation of the diagnosis should specify that peptic ulcer disease is a presumptive diagnosis and that more definitive diagnostic testing may be necessary. Home treatment should include a reminder to take medications as directed; a warning against use of alcohol, tobacco products, and aspirin or other NSAIDs; and a recommendation to avoid foods that appear to upset the individual's "stomach." Specific follow-up should include a name and phone number of the appropriate provider whenever possible and a time frame for reevaluation, generally 24 to 48 h, if not improving, or 1 to 2 weeks, if improving. Warning symptoms that merit immediate reevaluation include those that may be attributed to ulcer complications or confounding illness: worsening pain, increased vomiting, hematemesis or melena, weakness or syncope, fever, chest pain, radiation of pain to the neck or back, and shortness of breath.

REFERENCES

1. Soll AH: Medical treatment of peptic ulcer disease: Practice guidelines. *JAMA* 275:622, 1996.
2. Sontag SJ: Guilty as charged: Bugs and drugs in gastric ulcer. *Am J Gastroenterol* 92:1255, 1997.
3. Talley NJ, Weaver AL, Tesmer DL, Zinsmeister AR: Lack of discriminant value of dyspepsia subgroups in patients referred for upper endoscopy. *Gastroenterology* 105:1378, 1993.
4. Sonnenberg A, Everhart JE: Health impact of peptic ulcer in the United States. *Am J Gastroenterol* 92:614, 1997.
5. Damianos AJ, McGarrity TJ: Treatment strategies for *Helicobacter pylori* infection. *Am Fam Phys* 55:2765, 1997.
6. Logan RPH, Walker MM: Epidemiology and diagnosis of *Helicobacter pylori* infection. *BMJ* 323:920, 2001.
7. Talley NJ, McNeil D, Piper DW: Discriminant value of dyspeptic symptoms: A study of the clinical presentation of 221 patients with dyspepsia of unknown cause, peptic ulceration, and cholelithiasis. *Gut* 28:40, 1987.
8. Forbes GM: Review: *Helicobacter pylori:* Current issues and new directions. *J Gastroenterol Hepatol* 12:419, 1997.
9. Falk GW: *H. pylori* 1997: Testing and treatment options. *Cleve Clin J Med* 64:187, 1997.
10. Werdmuller BFM, Van der Putten ABMM, Loffeld RJLF: Review: The clinical presentation of peptic ulcer disease. *Neth J Med* 50:115,1997.
11. Kemppainen H, Raiha I, Sourander L: Clinical presentation of peptic ulcer in the elderly. *Gerontology* 43:283, 1997.
12. Peterson WL, Fendrick AM, Cave DR, et al: *Helicobacter pylori*-related disease: guidelines for testing and treatment. *Arch Intern Med* 160: 1285, 2000.
13. Howden CW, Hunt RH: Guidelines for the management of *Helicobacter pylori* infection. *Am J Gastrol* 93: 2330, 1998
14. Drugs for treatment of peptic ulcers. *Med Lett* 39:1, 1997.
15. Malfertheiner P, Megraud F, O'Morain C, et al: Current concepts in the management of *Helicobacter pylori* infection—The Maastricht 2-2000 consensus report. *Aliment Pharmacol Ther* 16:167, 2002.
16. Godshall CJ: Treatment of *Helicobacter pylori* infection in patients with peptic ulcer disease. *Am J Surg* 183: 2, 2002.
17. Ofman JJ, Etchason J, Fullerton S, et al: Management strategies for *Helicobacter pylori* seropositive patients with dyspepsia: Clinical and economic consequences. *Ann Intern Med* 126:280, 1997.
18. Jiranek GC, Kozarek RA: A cost-effective approach to the patient with peptic ulcer bleeding. *Surg Clin North Am* 76:83, 1996.

ACUTE APPENDICITIS
Denis J. FitzGerald
Arthur M. Pancioli

EPIDEMIOLOGY

While reports on the stability of the incidence of acute appendicitis vary, the incidence of appendectomy appears to be declining due to more accurate preoperative diagnosis.[1-3] Still, despite the introduction of newer imaging techniques, acute appendicitis can be extremely difficult to diagnose.

PATHOPHYSIOLOGY

Acute appendicitis is thought to begin with an obstruction of the lumen. The obstruction can result from food matter, adhesions, or lymphoid hyperplasia. Despite the obstruction, mucosal secretion continues, leading to an increase in intraluminal pressure. This pressure eventually will exceed capillary perfusion pressure and will obstruct venous and lymphatic drainage. With such vascular compromise, the epithelial mucosa begins to break down, allowing bacterial invasion by bowel flora. The subsequent inflammatory response and edema further exacerbate the increased intraluminal pressure. Eventually, this increased pressure leads to arterial stasis and tissue infarction. The end result is perforation and spillage of the infected appendiceal contents into the peritoneum.

In order to understand the clinical presentation and the clinical progression of acute appendicitis, it is important to consider the innervation and anatomic variability of the appendix. Presumably, the initial luminal distention triggers the visceral afferent pain fibers from the appendix, which enter the spinal cord at the tenth thoracic vertebra. As is characteristic of visceral afferent innervation, this pain is generally vague and poorly localized. Based on the anatomic level of these afferent fibers at the tenth thoracic level, the pain generally is perceived by the patient at the periumbilical or epigastric region. Eventually, as the inflammatory process continues, the appendiceal serosa and adjacent structures become inflamed. This inflammation triggers the somatic pain fibers, which innervate the peritoneal structures, typically localizing the pain in the right lower quadrant. This explains the migration of pain from the periumbilical area to the right lower quadrant, classically associated with acute appendicitis.

However, there are many exceptions to the classic presentation. These exceptions are often due to the variability of the anatomic location of the appendix. In a study of 71,000 human appendix specimens removed over a 40-year period, 26 percent were retrocecal, and 4 percent were located in the right upper quadrant.[4] **With the retrocecal appendix, the pain of acute appendicitis may localize to the flank rather than the right lower quadrant.** Similarly, in pregnant patients, the gravid uterus may displace the appendix, leading to a presentation of right upper quadrant or flank pain. In male patients, a retroileal appendicitis may irritate the ureter, causing pain in the testicle. A pelvic appendix may irritate the bladder or rectum and cause suprapubic pain, pain with urination, or the feeling of a need to defecate. These anatomically based variations in presentation help to explain the difficulty in making the diagnosis of acute appendicitis.

CLINICAL FEATURES

History

The primary symptom in acute appendicitis is abdominal pain. In approximately one-half to two-thirds of patients with appendicitis, the pain evolves in a classic pattern. Beginning in the epigastrium or periumbilical region early in the illness, the pain is vague initially and difficult to localize. Patients may describe their discomfort as indigestion or as a feeling of the need to defecate or pass flatus. In the classic presentation, periumbilical pain is followed by anorexia, nausea, and vomiting. As the illness progresses, the pain becomes more localized, typically in the right lower quadrant. In one meta-analysis, right lower quadrant pain was 81 percent sensitive and 53 percent specific for the diagnosis of acute appendicitis. Similarly, migration of the pain from initial periumbilical pain to the right lower quadrant was 64 percent sensitive and 82 percent specific for the diagnosis of acute appendicitis.[5]

In addition to abdominal pain, the classic symptoms in appendicitis include anorexia, nausea, and vomiting. In acute appendicitis, these symptoms typically appear after the onset of vague abdominal pain. Anorexia is the most common of these symptoms, with 68 percent sensitivity and 36 percent specificity.[5] Vomiting is more variable in acute appendicitis, occurring in about half of patients with acute appendicitis.[5] The significance of the temporal relationship between abdominal pain and onset of vomiting as a predictor of acute appendicitis has not yet been established. Table 78-1 provides a summary of the sensitivity and specificity of many symptoms associated with appendicitis.

Physical Examination

Like the history, the findings on physical examination of a patient with acute appendicitis depend on the duration of the illness prior to the examination. Early in the course of acute appendicitis, the patient may not have localized tenderness. As the illness progresses, the patient typically develops tenderness, especially to deep palpation, over

McBurney's point. This is a point just below the middle of a line connecting the umbilicus and the anterosuperior iliac spine. Pain in the right lower quadrant with palpation of the left lower quadrant (Rovsing sign) also may be elicited. As with the subjective pain, the localization of tenderness varies with the anatomic position of the appendix. If the patient has a pelvic appendix, the patient's tenderness may be most pronounced on rectal examination. With a retrocecal appendix, tenderness to palpation may be attenuated by the overlying cecum or may be most pronounced in the right flank.

Additional components of the physical examination that may help in the diagnosis include rebound tenderness, voluntary guarding, local muscular rigidity over the inflamed area (involuntary guarding), and tenderness on rectal examination. The sensitivity and specificity of these findings are seen in Table 78-1.

Special maneuvers that can aid in the diagnosis of acute appendicitis include the psoas sign and the obturator sign. The examiner checks for a *psoas sign* by placing the patient in the left lateral decubitus position and extending the right leg at the hip. If an inflamed appendix is overlying the psoas muscle, this maneuver will cause an increase in the patient's pain, thereby eliciting a positive psoas sign. The *obturator sign* is evaluated by passively flexing the right hip and knee and internally rotating the hip. This action will stretch the obturator muscle. An inflamed appendix may irritate the obturator muscle, and this maneuver will increase pain, indicating a positive obturator sign.

Fever is another relatively late physical finding in acute appendicitis. At the onset of pain, the patient's temperature probably will be normal. If the temperature is taken frequently during the progression of the illness, it will usually rise 1 to 2°C. Temperatures above 39°C (102.2°F) are uncommon in the first 24 h of the illness but not uncommon after rupture of an appendix.

DIAGNOSIS

The diagnosis of acute appendicitis should be suspected in any individual with epigastric, periumbilical, right flank, or right-sided abdominal pain who has not had an appendectomy. Women of childbearing age should have a pelvic examination and pregnancy test to exclude gynecologic causes of pain. The evaluation of abdominal pain in women is difficult and is discussed in detail in Chap. 102. Additional studies including a complete blood count (CBC), urinalysis

TABLE 78-1   Summary of Clinical Examination Operating Characteristics for Appendicitis*

Procedure	Sensitivity	Specificity	LR(+) [95% CI]	LR(−) [95% CI]
Right lower quadrant pain	0.81	0.53	7.31–8.46†	0–0.28†
Rigidity	0.27	0.83	3.76 (2.96–4.78)	0.82 (0.79–0.85)
Migration	0.64	0.82	3.18 (2.41–4.21)	0.50 (0.42–0.59)
Pain before vomiting‡	1.00	0.64	2.76 (1.94–3.94)	NA
Psoas sign	0.16	0.95	2.38 (1.21–4.67)	0.90 (0.83–0.98)
Fever	0.67	0.79	1.94 (1.63–2.32)	0.58 (0.51–0.67)
Rebound tenderness test	0.63	0.69	1.10–6.30†	0–0.86†
Guarding	0.74	0.57	1.65–1.78†	0–0.54†
No similar pain previously	0.81	0.41	1.50 (1.36–1.66)	0.323 (0.246–0.424)
Rectal tenderness	0.41	0.77	0.83–5.34†	0.36–1.15†
Anorexia	0.68	0.36	1.27 (1.16–1.38)	0.64 (0.54–0.75)
Nausea	0.58	0.37	0.69–1.20†	0.70–0.84†
Vomiting	0.51	0.45	0.92 (0.82–1.04)	1.12 (0.95–1.33)

*LR(+) indicates the positive likelihood ratio with its 95% CI; LR(−), the negative likelihood ratio with its 95% CI.
†In heterogeneous studies, the LRs are reported as ranges.
‡Only one study on this is included in the meta-analysis.
Source: From Wagner J, McKinney WP, Carpenter JL: Does this patient have appendicitis? *JAMA* 276:1589, 1996, with permission.

(UA), and imaging studies are often needed to help make the diagnosis. Clinical observation is another common diagnostic modality.

Complete Blood Count

The WBC is of limited value.[6,7] The sensitivity of an elevated WBC above 10,000/μL in acute appendicitis is 70 to 90 percent, but the specificity is very low.[7] More important, the positive and negative predictive values of an elevated WBC in acute appendicitis are 92 and 50 percent, respectively.[8] The diagnostic value of C-reactive protein and erythrocyte sedimentation rate have been studied in acute appendicitis with mixed results.[9]

Urinalysis

Abnormal urinalysis results, excluding proteinuria, are found in 19 to 40 percent of patients with acute appendicitis.[10,11] Abnormalities include pyuria, hematuria, and bacteriuria, possibly related to the extension of appendiceal inflammation to the ureter. The presence of greater than 20 white blood cells per high-powered field (without epithelial cells) in the urine should elevate consideration of urinary tract pathology in the differential diagnosis.[10]

Imaging Studies

Imaging studies performed in the evaluation of possible acute appendicitis include plain radiographs, ultrasound studies, and computed tomographic (CT) scans. Plain radiographs of the abdomen are abnormal in 24 to 95 percent of patients with acute appendicitis.[7] Radiographic indicators of possible acute appendicitis include appendiceal fecalith, appendiceal gas, localized paralytic ileus, blurred right psoas muscle, and free air. Since many of these signs are seen in multiple other processes, abdominal radiographs have limited diagnostic value in acute appendicitis.

Graded compression ultrasonography is reported to have a sensitivity of 94.7 percent with a specificity of 88.9 percent.[12] The principle of this technique is the fact that normal bowel loops and a normal appendix can be compressed with the application of moderate pressure, whereas an inflamed appendix cannot be compressed. The diagnostic criteria for acute appendicitis include the visualization of a noncompressible appendix that has a diameter of 6 mm or greater, demonstration of an appendicolith, or demonstration of a periappendiceal abscess. This technique has limitations with a retrocecal appendix, in that the overlying bowel may limit visualization and compression testing. In addition, an early perforation may be missed because the diameter of the appendix may be normal after perforation.[13] Finally, color Doppler ultrasound studies may be helpful when the appendix is well visualized but equivocal in size. With this technique, hyperemia in the wall of the appendix has been found to be a sensitive indicator of inflammation.[14]

Given its wide availability and usefulness in establishing alternative diagnoses, a CT scan is probably the best choice as initial imaging study, although its radiation exposure limits its application in pregnant women and children. In one study that directly compared CT scan with ultrasound in 100 patients, the CT scan had greater sensitivity (96 vs. 76 percent), greater accuracy (94 vs. 83 percent), and a greater negative predictive value (95 vs. 76 percent). In this study, there was no significant difference when CT scan was compared with ultrasound with regard to specificity or positive predictive value.[15] CT scan findings suggesting acute appendicitis include pericecal inflammation, abscess, periappendiceal phlegmon, and fluid collections. Even if the appendix is not directly visible, localized fat stranding in the right lower quadrant can still reliably point to the diagnosis. A recent trend in CT technology involves the use of a focused appendiceal approach to evaluate patients for appendicitis.[16] The purported advantages of this approach include less scanning time, less radiation, and often no intravenous contrast material. However, there remains debate over whether focused appendiceal CT scan or traditional nonfocused abdominal CT scan is the better choice.[16,17] **CT scanning does appear to change management decisions and decreases unnecessary appendectomies in women. It is not as useful for changing management decisions in men.**[18]

Clinical Observation

For patients presenting atypically with suspicion for appendicitis, clinical observation in the emergency department with serial abdominal examinations is another method for identifying evolving cases of appendicitis.[19]

SPECIFIC ISSUES THAT AFFECT DIAGNOSIS, EVALUATION, AND TREATMENT

Special Populations

Certain groups of patients (e.g., very young, very old, pregnant, AIDS patients) present atypically and more often have delayed diagnoses as a result, with a concomitant increase in complications, such as appendiceal perforation. Very young patients present insidiously. The rate of misdiagnosis is high, with a consequent increase in the perforation rate, particularly in children under 5 years of age.[20] Diagnosis in children can be confounded by difficulty with communication and atypical symptoms, including concurrent respiratory symptoms or suspected gastroenteritis.[20] Peritonitis in children can present with varied signs such as lethargy, inactivity, and hypothermia. A high index of suspicion and early surgical consultation are recommended for children. Ultrasound and CT scan also can be used to assist in diagnosis.[21,22]

Misdiagnosis rates in the elderly can exceed 50 percent, with a high incidence of perforation ranging from 40 to 70 percent.[23] Mortality rates for patients over age 70 with acute appendicitis approach 30 percent.[24] In addition to late presentation with an advanced course, anatomic changes in the appendix involving the vascular bed and reduced mural thickness are thought to contribute to the fulminant course of appendicitis seen in the elderly. One study found that the most significant predictors of acute appendicitis in the aged were tenderness, rigidity, pain at diagnosis, fever, and previous abdominal surgery.[25] Since extensive laboratory studies may obscure the diagnosis in patients with other concurrent medical problems, a high index of clinical suspicion is needed in management of the elderly.

Appendicitis remains the most common extrauterine surgical emergency in pregnancy, and fetal mortality rates can be four times higher if the appendicitis is complicated by perforation and peritonitis.[26] Consequently, the diagnosis of appendicitis must be entertained in any gravid patient presenting with abdominal pain and gastrointestinal symptoms. Ultrasound can be used to aid in diagnosis, particularly in differentiating obstetric causes of pain from appendicitis.

Patients with AIDS are particularly susceptible to complications from appendicitis. Although symptoms are no different for appendicitis in this population,[27] diagnosis can be delayed because of the baseline frequency of gastrointestinal symptoms unrelated to appendicitis and the occurrence of nonsurgical opportunistic pathologic conditions with similar presentations. One study noted a higher incidence of perforation in this population, possibly related to the delay in presentation or to the immunocompromised state.[27] One clear difference in management relates to the WBC, which is generally not elevated even in acute appendicitis.

TREATMENT

Appendectomy is the standard of care for acute appendicitis. Patients who are being prepared for appendectomy should be given nothing by mouth, have intravenous (IV) fluid resuscitation, and be given preoperative antibiotics. Antibiotics are most effective when given prior to surgery. In patients with uncomplicated appendicitis, antibiotics decrease the incidence of postoperative wound infections.[28] In patients with perforation, early antibiotics have been shown to decrease post-operative abscess formation.[28] There are multiple acceptable approaches to antimicrobial therapy as long as the regimen covers anaerobic flora, enterococci, and gram-negative intestinal flora.[28] One such sample regimen is monotherapy with either tazobactam-piperacillin 3.375 g IV or ampicillin-sulbactam 3.00 g IV.

Analgesia should be given to treat acute abdominal pain.[29] A short-acting parenteral narcotic such as fentanyl administered IV is a good choice for pain management.

DISPOSITION

In general, patients with abdominal pain can be stratified into four groups with respect to their potential for appendicitis. The first group is composed of patients who demonstrate the classic presentation for acute appendicitis. The management of these patients is straightforward, involving prompt surgical consultation and subsequent appendectomy. The emergency department course is focused on preoperative preparation, as outlined previously.

The second group includes patients with signs and symptoms that are suspicious but not diagnostic for appendicitis. This group of patients most likely would benefit from imaging studies, either CT scan or ultrasound, to elucidate the diagnosis. Observation for a 4- to 6-h period with serial examinations may clarify the diagnosis. Surgical consultation is clearly indicated in patients in whom the examination becomes progressively more characteristic of appendicitis or if a surgical finding is identified on an imaging study.

The third group involves patients with abdominal pain in whom appendicitis is considered to be a remote diagnostic possibility. These patients should be observed in the ED for a period with serial examinations. If the course remains benign and no other contraindications to discharge exist, the discharge diagnosis should be *nonspecific abdominal pain*. Patients should be told that no clear cause for their symptoms was found but that over time their symptoms will either abate or coalesce into a recognizable pattern. Follow-up instructions should include a description of worrisome symptoms that suggest progressive disease and warrant return to the emergency department. Patients should be reevaluated in 12 to 24 h by their primary physician or by the emergency department to ensure resolution of symptoms. Patients should be cautioned to avoid strong analgesics that might mask evolving pathologic processes; instead, they should be instructed to return if their pain increases. In this fashion, the emergency physician establishes a clear continuity of care for the patient with guidelines that minimize the likelihood of an adverse outcome.

The fourth group is composed of all high-risk special populations presenting with abdominal pain. This group includes elderly, pediatric, pregnant, and immunocompromised patients. As emphasized earlier, these patients require a high index of clinical suspicion and a low threshold for imaging studies and surgical consultation to avoid morbidity and mortality from undetected appendicitis.

REFERENCES

1. Williams NM, Jackson D, Everson NW, et al: Is the incidence of acute appendicitis really falling? *Ann R Coll Surg* 80(2);122, 1998.
2. Korner H, Soreide, JA, Pederson EJ, et al: Stability in incidence of acute appendicits: A population-based longitudinal study. *Dig Surg* 18(1):61, 2001.
3. Rao PM, Rhea JT, Rattner DW, et al: Introduction of appendiceal CT: Impact on negative appendectomy and appendiceal perforation rates. *Ann Surg* 229(3):344, 1999.
4. Collins DC: 71,000 human appendix specimens: A final report, summarizing forty years' study. *Am J Proctol* 14:365, 1963.
5. Wagner J, McKinney WP, Carpenter JL: Does this patient have appendicitis? *JAMA* 276:1589, 1996.
6. Vermeulen B, Morabia A, Unger PF: Influence of white cell count on surgical decision making in patients with abdominal pain in the right lower quadrant. *Eur J Surg* 161:483, 1995.
7. Hoffmann J, Rausmussen O: Aids in the diagnosis of acute appendicitis. *Br J Surg* 76:774, 1989.
8. Marchand A, Van Lente F, Galen RS: The assessment of laboratory tests in the diagnosis of acute appendicitis. *Am J Clin Pathol* 80:369, 1983.
9. Jaye DL, Waites KB: Clinical applications of C-reactive protein in pediatrics. *Pediatr Infect Dis J* 16:735, 1997.
10. Kretchmar LH, McDonald DF: The urine sediment in acute appendicitis. *Arch Surg* 87:209, 1963.
11. Puskar D, Bedalov G, Fridrih S, et al: Urinalysis, ultrasound analysis, and renal dynamic scintigraphy in acute appendicitis. *Urology* 45:108, 1995.
12. Douglas CD, Macpherson NE, Davidson PM, et al: Randomised controlled trial of ultrasonography in diagnosis of acute appendicitis, incorporating the Alvarado score. *Br Med J* 321:1–7, 2000.
13. Jeffrey RB, Jain KA, Ngheim HV: Sonographic diagnosis of acute appendicitis: Interpretive pitfalls. *AJR* 162:55, 1994.
14. Lim HK, Lee WJ, Kim TH: Appendicitis: Usefulness of color Doppler US. *Radiology* 201:221, 1996.
15. Balthazar EJ, Birnbaum BA, Yee J: Acute appendicitis: CT and US correlation in 100 patients. *Radiology* 190:31, 1994.
16. Wijetunga R, Tan BS, Rouse JC, et al: Diagnostic accuracy of focused appendiceal CT in clinically equivocal cases of acute appendicitis. *Radiology* 221:747, 2001.
17. Jacobs JE, Birnbaum BA, Macari M, et al: Acute appendicitis: Comparison of helical CT diagnosis-focused technique with oral contrast material versus nonfocused technique with oral and intravenous contrast material. *Radiology* 220:683, 2001.
18. Paulson EK, Kalady MF, Pappas TN; Suspected appendicitis. *NEJM* 348: 236, 2003.
19. Graff L, Radford MJ, Werne C: Probability of appendicitis before and after observation. *Ann Emerg Med* 20:503, 1991.
20. Cappendijik VC, Hazebroek FWJ: The impact of diagnostic delay on the course of acute appendicitis. *Arch Dis Child* 83:64, 2000.
21. Kaiser S, Frenckner B, Jorulf HK: Suspected appendicitis in children: US and CT. A prospective randomized study. *Radiology* 223:633, 2002.
22. Applegate KE, Sivit CJ, Salvator AE, et al: Effect of cross-sectional imaging on negative appendectomy and perforation rates in children. *Radiology* 220:103, 2001.
23. Klein SR, Layden L, Wright JF, et al: Appendicitis in the elderly. *Postgrad Med* 83:247, 1988.
24. Franz M, Norman J, Fabri PJ: Increased mortality of appendicitis with advancing age. *Am Surg* 61:40, 1995.
25. Eskelinen M, Ikonen J, Lipponen P: The value of history-taking, physical examination, and computer assistance in the diagnosis of acute appendicitis in patients more than 50 years old. *Scand J Gastroenterol* 30:349, 1995.
26. Mahmoodian S: Appendicitis complicating pregnancy. *South Med J* 85:19, 1992.
27. Flum DR, Steinberg SD, Sarkis AY, et al: Appendicitis in patients with acquired immunodeficiency syndrome. *J Am Coll Surg* 184:481, 1997.
28. Andersen BR, Kallehave FL, Andersen HK: Antibiotics versus placebo for prevention of postoperative infection after appendicectomy (Cochrane Review). *The Cochrane Library* Issue 1, 2003, Oxford: Update Software.
29. Mackway-Jones K: Analgesia and assessment of abdominal pain. *J Accid Emerg Med* 17:128, 2000.

79

INTESTINAL OBSTRUCTION
Salvator J. Vicario
Timothy G. Price

Intestinal obstruction is the inability of the intestinal tract to allow for regular passage of food and bowel contents secondary to mechanical obstruction or adynamic ileus. Adynamic ileus (paralytic ileus) is the more common entity but is usually self-limiting and does not require surgical intervention. Mechanical obstruction can be caused by either intrinsic or extrinsic factors and generally requires definitive intervention in a relatively short period of time to determine the cause and minimize subsequent morbidity and mortality.

Both large and small intestines may be obstructed by various pathologic processes (Table 79-1). Extrinsic, intrinsic, or intraluminal processes precipitate mechanical obstruction. Differentiating small bowel obstruction (SBO) from large bowel obstruction (LBO) is

TABLE 79-1   Common Causes of Intestinal Obstruction

Duodenum	Small Bowel	Colon
Stenosis	Adhesions	Carcinoma
Foreign body (Bezoars)	Hernia	Fecal impaction
Stricture	Intussusception	Ulcerative colitis
Superior mesenteric artery syndrome	Lymphoma	Volvulus
	Stricture	Diverticulitis (stricture, abscess)
		Intussusception
		Pseudo-obstruction

important because the incidence, clinical presentation, and modes of therapy vary depending on the anatomic site of the obstruction. The small intestine is characterized by transverse linear densities that extend completely across the bowel lumen (plicae circulares). The colon is situated peripherally in the abdomen, is larger in diameter, and contains short, blunt, and thick projections (haustra) that arise from the bowel wall and extend only partially into the lumen. Haustra are less numerous and situated farther apart than plicae circulares.

SMALL BOWEL OBSTRUCTION

The most common cause of SBO is adhesions following abdominal surgery.[1] Although in most cases several months to years have passed from the time of the previous surgery, SBO may occur within the first few weeks following surgery.[2] The second most common cause of SBO is incarceration of a groin hernia[1] (see Chap. 80). This can occur in infants as well as adults and should be suspected anytime there is a complaint of a "knot" or growth in the inguinal region that fails to reduce with manipulation. Other sites that occasionally are responsible for SBO secondary to hernia include the umbilicus, femoral canal, and rarely, the obturator foramen. Umbilical hernias are more readily apparent and occur in any age group. Obturator or femoral hernias are much less common. Elderly females are particularly susceptible to these hernias, which may present with femoral or medial thigh pain. Finally, a defect in the mesentery itself may cause intestinal obstruction.

Other causes of SBO are much less common and generally are the result of intraluminal or intramural processes. Primary small bowel lesions include polyps, lymphoma, or adenocarcinoma. An unusual cause of intraluminal obstruction is gallstone ileus. In this situation, a gallstone has eroded from the gallbladder through the bowel wall and can cause obstruction at the ileocecal valve. Besides the findings of bowel obstruction, one may note air in the biliary tree on abdominal radiographs. Lymphomas may be the leading point of intussusception and present as SBO. Bezoars are most commonly composed of vegetable matter or pulp from persimmons. Patients who have undergone gastrointestinal pyloroplasty or pyloric resection are most susceptible to intraluminal obstruction by bezoars.

Inflammatory bowel disease also may affect the small bowel at various sites. Likewise, infectious processes including abscesses may obstruct the bowel. Radiation enteritis is also a possible cause of SBO in patients who have undergone radiation therapy.

LARGE BOWEL OBSTRUCTION

Colonic obstruction is almost never caused by hernia or surgical adhesions. Neoplasms are by far the most common cause of LBO.[3,4] Therefore, anyone who has symptoms of colonic obstruction should be evaluated for a neoplasm. Diverticulitis may create significant secondary obstruction and mesenteric edema. Stricture formation may occur with chronic inflammation and scarring. Fecal impaction is a common problem in elderly, debilitated patients and may present with symptoms of colonic obstruction.

The next most frequent cause of LBO after cancer and diverticulitis is sigmoid volvulus. Elderly, bedridden, or psychiatric patients who are taking anticholinergic medication are most often subject to this mechanical problem. A history of constipation may precede the volvulus and presenting symptoms. Radiographic appearance is usually classic (Figure 79-1). Finally, although much less common, cecal volvulus also may cause LBO. There is a higher incidence of cecal volvulus in gravid patients.[5]

PATHOPHYSIOLOGY

Normal bowel contains gas as well as gastric secretions and food. Intraluminal accumulation of gastric, biliary, and pancreatic secretions continues even if there is no oral intake. As obstruction develops, the bowel becomes congested, and there is failure of intestinal contents to be absorbed. Vomiting and decreased oral intake follow. The combination of decreased absorption, vomiting, and reduced intake leads to volume depletion with hemoconcentration and electrolyte imbalance and ultimately can cause renal failure or shock.[4]

Bowel distention often accompanies mechanical obstruction. Distention is due to the accumulation of fluids in the bowel lumen, an increase in intraluminal pressure with enhanced peristaltic contractions, and air swallowing. When intraluminal pressure exceeds capillary and venous pressure in the bowel wall, absorption and lymphatic drainage decrease. At this stage, bacteria may enter the bloodstream, the bowel becomes ischemic, and septicemia and bowel necrosis can develop. Shock ensues rapidly. Mortality approaches 70 percent if bowel obstruction has been allowed to progress this far. With a *closed-loop ob-*

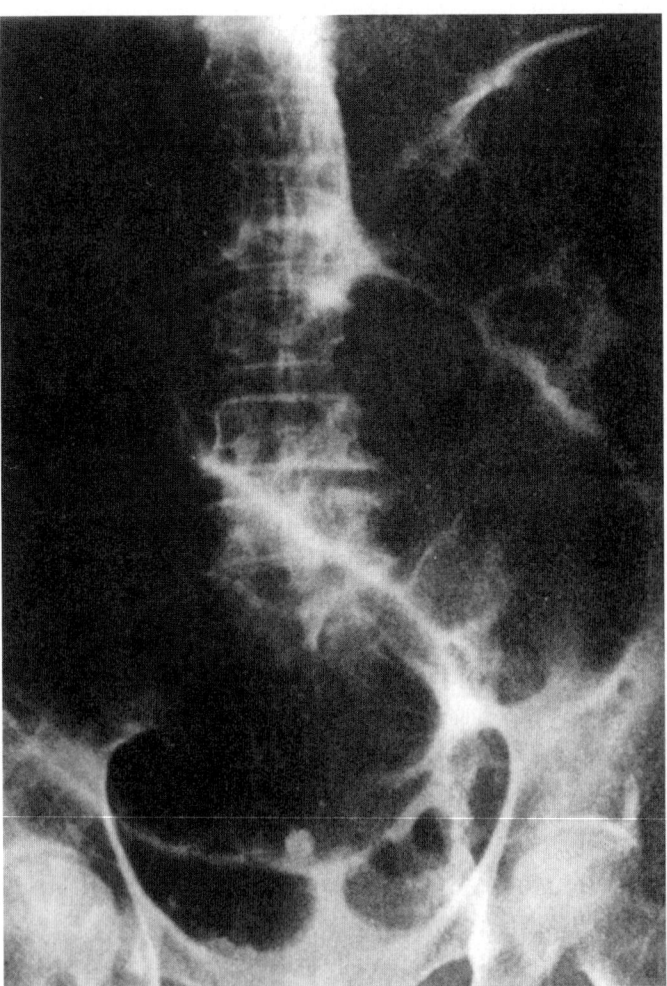

FIG. 79-1. Sigmoid volvulus. Note distention of large bowel and central stripe, giving a "coffee bean" appearance.

SBO → episodic, few min ; perium/diffuse ; vomiting
∅ Bd
∅ flatus | LBO → hypogastric, feculent vomitus

79 • INTESTINAL OBSTRUCTION   525

struction, this sequence of events may occur more rapidly. In this instance, there is no proximal escape for bowel contents. Examples of closed-loop obstruction include an incarcerated hernia and complete colon obstruction in the presence of a closed ileocecal valve.

CLINICAL FEATURES

The site and nature of the obstruction and the preexisting condition of the patient will determine the clinical presentation. Almost all patients will have abdominal pain.[3] The pain generally is described as crampy and intermittent. Pain of mechanical SBO is often episodic, usually lasting for a few minutes at a time, and it may be periumbilical or more diffuse. In adynamic ileus, the pain tends to be less intense and more constant. If the obstruction is proximal, vomiting is usually present. The vomitus in proximal obstruction is usually bilious but is feculent in distal ileal obstruction. The pain of LBO is usually hypogastric. LBOs may be associated with feculent vomitus.

Other features that are consistently present with obstruction of small bowel or colon include the inability to have a bowel movement or pass flatus. Care should be taken to avoid the diagnosis of constipation because this symptom is secondary to partial or complete obstruction. Partial bowel obstruction, however, is often associated with regular passage of stool and flatus.

Physical findings vary depending on the site, duration, and etiology of the pathologic process. Early symptoms usually are associated with some abdominal distention, often impressive with colonic obstruction yet not readily apparent in cases of incarcerated hernia. Abdominal tenderness may be minimal and diffuse or localized and severe.[2,3] Patients who have developed peritonitis will have severe tenderness. The abdomen may be tympanitic to percussion. Mechanical obstruction will produce active, high-pitched bowel sounds with occasional "rushes." If obstruction has been present for several hours, peristaltic waves and bowel sounds may be diminished. Patients with an adynamic ileus may have some abdominal distention associated with diminished or absent bowel sounds. Careful search for localized or rebound tenderness is essential to rule out the possibility of gangrenous or perforated bowel, which requires immediate surgical intervention.

Elderly patients have signs and symptoms that are similar to younger patients with intestinal obstruction. Adhesions and hernias are common causes for SBO in this age group, whereas carcinomas are the most likely etiology of LBO because of the increased likelihood of cancer as people age.[6] Elderly patients who are debilitated or confused or who are on multiple medications may be unable to give a detailed history. Patients over 60 years old are more likely to succumb secondary to complications of bowel obstruction.[2] Careful examination for characteristic bowel sounds and masses or blood in stool and radiographic investigation often will distinguish bowel obstruction from ileus. Emptiness of the left iliac fossa has been reported to be a reliable sign of sigmoid volvulus.[7]

All patients with abdominal pain or distention should be examined for signs of organomegaly or masses that may suggest a cause of the obstruction. A rectal examination may identify fecal impaction, rectal carcinoma, occult blood, or stricture. The absence of stool or air in the vault may aid in the diagnosis of bowel obstruction, but its presence does not eliminate a more proximal obstruction because patients may not be able to evacuate preexisting rectal contents. A pelvic examination should be performed to identify any gynecologic pathology causing obstruction. A vaginal pessary can cause colonic obstruction due to extrinsic compression of the colon.[8]

LABORATORY AND RADIOGRAPHIC FINDINGS

All patients with suspected obstruction should have flat and upright abdominal radiographs and upright chest x-ray or a lateral decubitus view if the patient cannot be upright. An abdominal radiograph can confirm the diagnosis, identify free air or masses, and localize the site to large or small bowel (Figure 79-2A,B). Laboratory studies usually

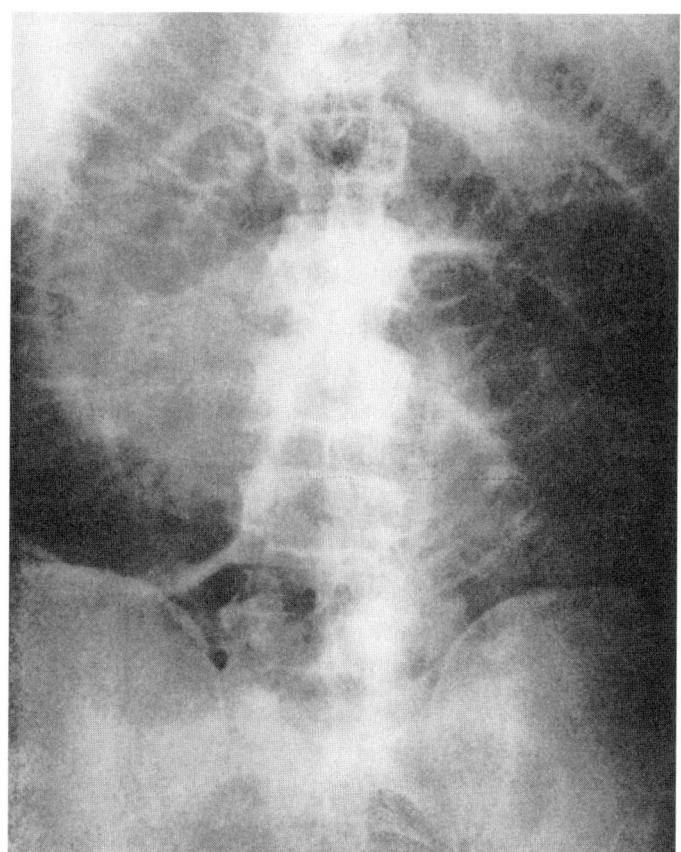

A

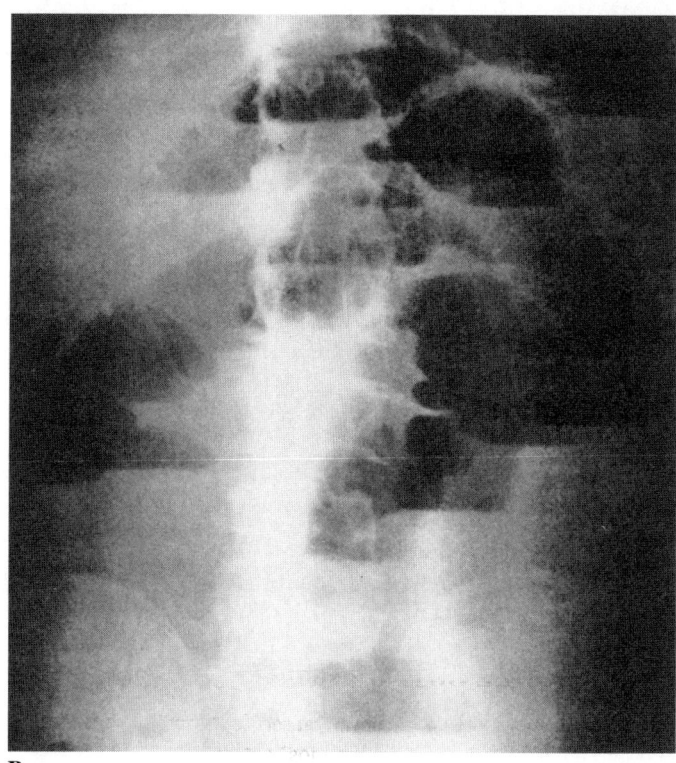

B

FIG. 79-2. A. Flat-plate abdominal film illustrates distended loops of small bowel. **B.** Upright film demonstrates multiple air-fluid levels and "stepladder" appearance. (From Harris JH, Harris WH: *The Radiology of Emergency Medicine,* 3d ed. Baltimore, Williams and Wilkins, 1993, p. 843, with permission.)

include a complete blood count and electrolyte levels. Depending on the duration of symptoms and site of obstruction or whether there is bowel necrosis, one may find a wide range in white blood cell (WBC) counts and hemoglobin, hematocrit, and electrolyte values. A white count greater than 20,000/L or left shift should make one suspect bowel gangrene, intra-abdominal abscess, or peritonitis.[4] Extreme WBC elevation (>40,000/L) suggests mesenteric vascular occlusion. The serum amylase and lipase levels may be mildly elevated. Levels of serum electrolytes usually are normal or mildly reduced,[3] depending on whether the obstruction is of short or long duration or whether there is associated emesis. Increases in hematocrit, blood urea nitrogen (BUN), and creatinine are consistent with volume depletion and dehydration. Other indications of the severity of obstruction or secondary complications include increased urine specific gravity, ketonuria, elevated lactate levels, and metabolic acidosis.

Further investigations to determine the site or etiology of obstruction include sigmoidoscopy or barium enema. Upper gastrointestinal studies are rarely indicated. Barium enema can determine the cause and site of LBO (Figure 79-3). Sigmoidoscopy can identify friable mucosa, intraluminal lesions, or the dark-blue gangrenous mucosa associated with dead bowel. If the diagnosis is unclear, repeated examination, preferably by the same examiner, will be necessary. The use of contrast-enhanced computed tomography (CT) has been advocated to delineate partial from complete bowel obstruction.[9,10]

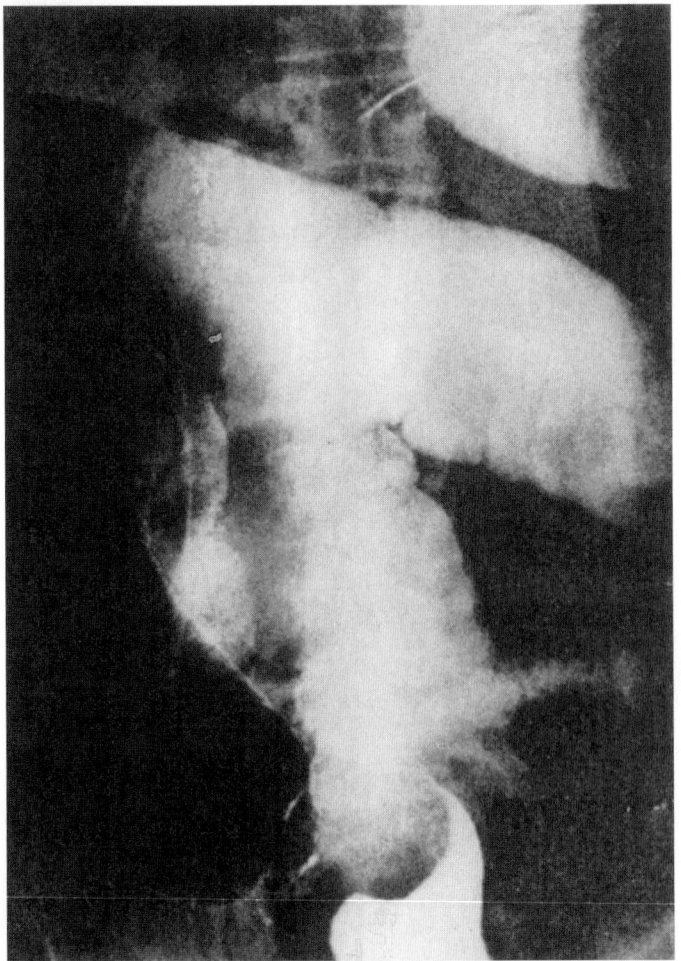

FIG. 79-3. Barium enema examination demonstrating incomplete filling of the sigmoid secondary to volvulus. Note the "parrot beak" appearance of the point of the volvulus. (From Schwartz GR: *Principles and Practice of Emergency Medicine,* 3d ed. Malvern, PA, Lea & Febiger, 1992, p. 1720, with permission.)

TREATMENT

If a true mechanical obstruction is diagnosed, then surgical intervention is often required. Prior to surgical intervention, a nasogastric tube should be inserted to remove excess bowel contents and air. Intravenous fluid replacement is needed because of loss of absorptive capacity, decreased oral intake, and vomiting. Patients can be monitored prior to surgical intervention by the response of blood pressure and heart rate and measurement of urine output. Surgery should not be delayed unnecessarily by attempting to use long intestinal tubes (Baker, Cantor, or Miller-Abbott) or excessive testing. A volvulus of the sigmoid colon usually will decompress via sigmoidoscopy and insertion of a rectal tube. Should a closed-loop obstruction, bowel necrosis, or cecal volvulus be suspected, then surgical intervention should be performed without delay.[3] All patients with mechanical obstruction require broad-spectrum antibiotic coverage preoperatively because the risk of infection and septicemia is significant in most conditions.[9] There are many possible regimens. Monotherapy could be tazobactam-piperacillin 3.375 g IV q6h or ampicillin-sulbactam 3.00 g IV q6h.

If adynamic ileus is the primary problem or the diagnosis is uncertain, conservative measures, including intravenous fluids, nasogastric decompression, and observation, generally are effective in allowing the bowel to resume normal activity and function. Any medication that inhibits bowel mobility should be discontinued. Abdominal CT contrast radiography is used commonly to distinguish partial SBO from ileus or for the differentiation of strangulated from simple SBO.[6,13]

PSEUDO-OBSTRUCTION

Intestinal pseudo-obstruction (Ogilvie syndrome) also may mimic bowel obstruction. Although any segment of bowel may be affected, low colonic obstruction is the most common clinical presentation. Large amounts of gas will be present in the large intestine. Radiographs reveal a dilated colon with well-defined septa and haustral markings and very little fluid, making air-fluid levels uncommon.[14] Patients may be using anticholinergic or tricyclic antidepressants, which depress motility. One must avoid the use of barium studies because the patient may be unable to evacuate the barium. Preference should be given to colonoscopy after digital rectal examination as an early intervention to rule out true obstruction or significant lesions. Colonoscopy also will treat the pseudo-obstruction by decompression. Surgery usually is not helpful and may be harmful.[14] Neostigmine infusion is reported to be effective at relieving pseudo-obstruction in patients who had not responded to conservative means.[15]

REFERENCES

1. Leffall LD, Syphax B: Clinical aids in strangulation intestinal obstruction. *Arch Surg* 117:334, 1982.
2. Becker WF: Intestinal obstruction: An analysis of 1007 cases. *South Med J* 48:41, 1955.
3. Shatila AH, Chamberlain BE, Webb WR: Current status of diagnosis and management of strangulation obstruction of the small bowel. *Am J Surg* 132:299, 1976.
4. Cheadle WC, Garr FE, Richardson JD: The importance of early diagnosis of small bowel obstruction. *Am Surg* 54:565, 1988.
5. Tarraza HM, Moore RD: Gynecologic causes of the acute abdomen and the acute abdomen in pregnancy. *Surg Clin North Am* 77(6):1371, 1997.
6. Frager D, Baer JW, et al: Detection of intestinal ischemia in patients with acute small bowel obstruction due to adhesions or hernia: Efficacy of CT. *AJR* 166:67, 1991.
7. Raveenthiran V: Emptiness of the left iliac fossa: A new clinical sign of sigmoid volvulus. *Postgrad Med J* 76:638, 2000.
8. Roberge RJ, Keller C, Garfinkel M: Vaginal pessary-induced mechanical bowel obstruction. *J Emerg Med* 30(4):367, 2001.
9. Maglinte DT, Peterson LA, et al: Enterolysis in partial small bowel obstruction. *Am J Surg* 147:325, 1984.
10. Ha HK, Him JS: Differentiation of simple and strangulated small bowel obstructions: Usefulness of known CT criteria. *Radiology* 204:507, 1997.

11. Daneshmand S, Hedley CG, Stain SC: The utility and reliability of computed tomography scan in the diagnosis of small bowel obstruction. *Am Surg* 65:922, 1999.
12. Moore CJ, Corl FM, Fishman EK: CT of cecal volvulus: Unraveling the image. *AJR* 177:95, 2001.
13. Maglinte DD, Reyes BC, et al: Reliability and role of plain film radiography and CT in the diagnosis of small bowel obstruction. *AJR* 167:1451, 1996.
14. Vanek VW, Al-Salti M: Acute pseudo-obstruction of the colon (Ogilvie's syndrome): An analysis of 400 cases. *Dis Colon Rectum* 29:203, 1986.
15. Ponec RJ, Saunders MD, Kimmey MB: Neostigmine for the treatment of acute colonic psuedo-obstruction. *New Engl J Med* 341(3):137, 1999.

80

HERNIA IN ADULTS AND CHILDREN

Frank W. Lavoie

Mary Harkins Becker

A *hernia* is defined as the protrusion of any body part from its natural cavity. The protrusion may be internal or external and in a wide range of locations. However, the usual use of the term *hernia* refers to external herniation through the abdominal wall. Hernias also may be interparietal, within the layers of the abdominal wall. Abdominal wall hernias occur in adults and children and may be subdivided further into groin (inguinal or femoral), umbilical, anterior abdominal, pelvic, or lumbar locations.

PATHOPHYSIOLOGY

General Characteristics

Essential to the understanding of hernias are the anatomic characteristics of the abdominal cavity and, in particular, its fascial and aponeurotic layers. Embryologic development produces localized areas of inherent weakness in the abdominal wall. These include areas where extraperitoneal structures penetrate (as in the inguinal, femoral, and obturator canals, the sciatic foramen, and the umbilical region) and areas devoid of strong multilayer structural support (as in the anterior abdominal wall's linea alba and semilunar line). In addition, surgical incision and trauma may produce areas of abdominal wall weakness.

A hernia may contain preperitoneal fat, intraperitoneal structures such as omentum and bowel, and occasionally retroperitoneal organs. A hernia sac is composed of peritoneum and any intraperitoneal structures that accompany it.

If the contents of a hernia can be returned to their natural cavity by external manipulation, the hernia is termed *reducible;* if they cannot, it is termed *irreducible* or *incarcerated.* Incarcerated hernias are subject to inflammatory and edematous changes and are at risk for strangulation. *Strangulation* of a hernia refers to vascular compromise of the incarcerated contents. When strangulation is not rapidly relieved, necrosis and gangrene develop.

The presence of a hernia in and of itself is not an emergency condition. It is when the hernial sac becomes incarcerated or stuck that a surgical emergency is present.

Risk Factors

Lack of developmental maturity of anatomic structures is known to predispose to the formation of hernias, as in indirect inguinal and umbilical hernias in premature infants. Family history, undescended testis, and genitourinary abnormalities are additional risks for inguinal hernia. Conditions that increase intra-abdominal pressure such as ascites, peritoneal dialysis, ventriculoperitoneal shunt, cystic fibrosis, chronic obstructive pulmonary disease, and pregnancy are thought to be associated with abdominal wall hernia.

Specific Hernia Types

INDIRECT INGUINAL HERNIA The inguinal canal is a tract through muscle and fascial layers in the abdominal wall that forms during fetal development to allow for the passage of the gubernaculum, the testis, and the spermatic cord in males and the round ligament in females. The canal is defined by an internal ring defect in the transversalis fascia and transverses the abdominus aponeurosis lateral to the inferior epigastric vessels and a more medial ring defect in the external oblique aponeurosis (Figures 80-1 and 80-2).

The reproductive organs develop in the peritoneal cavity and then pass through the inguinal canal via an evagination of the peritoneum. This outpouching of peritoneum is called the *processus vaginalis.* After passage of these organs, the processus vaginalis is normally reabsorbed, thus preventing future travel of intraperitoneal contents through the inguinal canal. A congenitally persistent processus vaginalis is the etiology for all indirect inguinal hernias. Latent passage of contents through a persistent patent processus vaginalis along the inguinal canal is called an *indirect inguinal hernia.* Acquired myoaponeurotic defects also may contribute to indirect inguinal hernia in adults.

Passage of the testis is thought to enlarge the canal and increase the likelihood of inguinal hernia in males. It is more common on the right side due to later passage of the right testis. Indirect inguinal hernias frequently incarcerate and strangulate, particularly in the first year of life and in females.[1]

DIRECT INGUINAL HERNIA These hernias are protrusions directly through the transversalis fascia and the external inguinal ring, medial to the inferior epigastric vessels (see Figures 80-1 and 80-3). Direct inguinal hernias are acquired defects that do not involve passage through the inguinal canal. They occur predominantly in adults and rarely incarcerate and strangulate. Recurrence after repair is more frequent than for an indirect inguinal hernia.

FEMORAL HERNIA A femoral hernia is a protrusion below the inguinal ligament and adjacent to the femoral vessels in the femoral canal (see Figure 80-1). Femoral hernias are more common in women due to the different anatomic structure of the pelvis. Femoral hernias are far less common than inguinal hernias, but they more frequently incarcerate and strangulate.[2]

UMBILICAL HERNIA Congenital umbilical hernias occur commonly, especially in children of African descent (Figure 80-4). In utero contraction of the umbilical cord insertion forms a fibromuscular umbilical

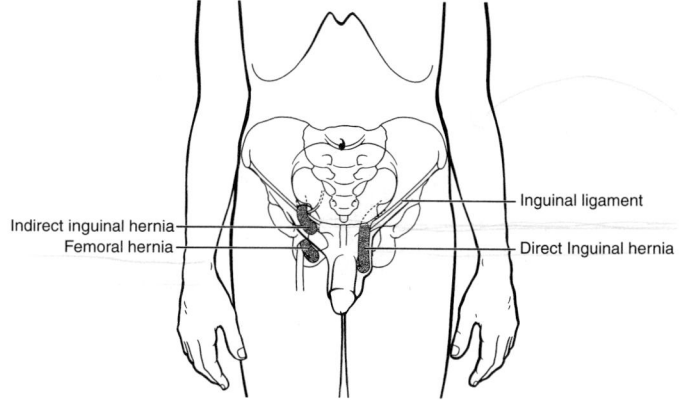

FIG. 80-1. Groin hernias.

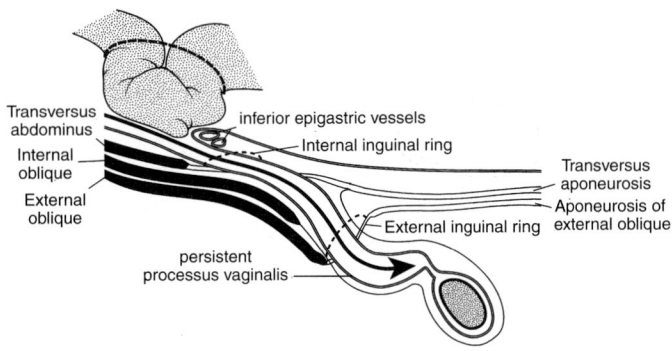

FIG. 80-2. Indirect inguinal hernia.

ring. Incomplete development or weakness of this ring allows herniation of abdominal contents. These hernias rarely incarcerate and usually spontaneously seal over time.[1,3]

Umbilical hernias also may develop in adults. This acquired defect is more common in women and is associated with obesity, pregnancy, and ascites. Unlike congenital umbilical hernias, acquired umbilical hernias frequently incarcerate.

EPIGASTRIC HERNIA An epigastric hernia involves herniation through the linea alba of the rectus sheath, above the umbilicus (see Figure 80-4).

SPIGELIAN HERNIA Herniation at the site of the semilunar or arcuate line, just lateral to the rectus muscle, through the combined aponeurosis of the transversus abdominis and internal oblique muscles is known as a *spigelian* or *lateral ventral hernia*. This hernia is frequently interparietal, making diagnosis difficult (see Figure 80-4).

PELVIC HERNIA Pelvic hernias are rare. They occur internally and cannot be palpated on examination. There are *sciatic hernias,* passing through sciatic foramen; *perineal hernias,* passing between perineal muscles; and *obturator hernias,* passing through the obturator canal with the obturator vessels. Obturator hernias frequently incarcerate.[4]

LUMBAR HERNIA Herniation rarely may occur through the inferior or superior lumbar triangles.

INCISIONAL HERNIA Herniation through a surgical incision is a frequent complication of abdominal surgery occurring in 10 to 20 percent of patients who have undergone laparotomy. Obesity and postoperative wound infections are known risk factors. Incarceration of the bowel can occur. Elective repair is recommended, but recurrence rates after repair are high.[5]

EPIDEMIOLOGY

The incidence of abdominal hernia is estimated to be from 10 to 20 per 1000 births and is greater among premature infants.[6] In the screening

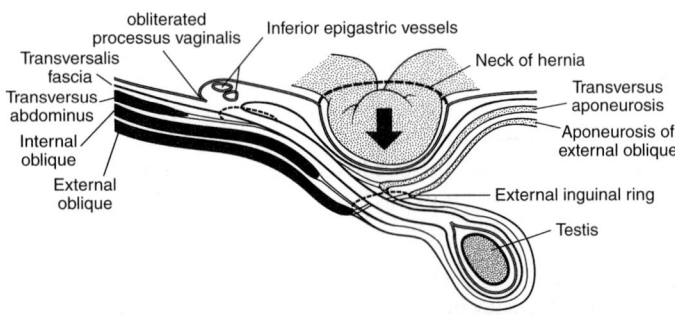

FIG. 80-3. Direct inguinal hernia.

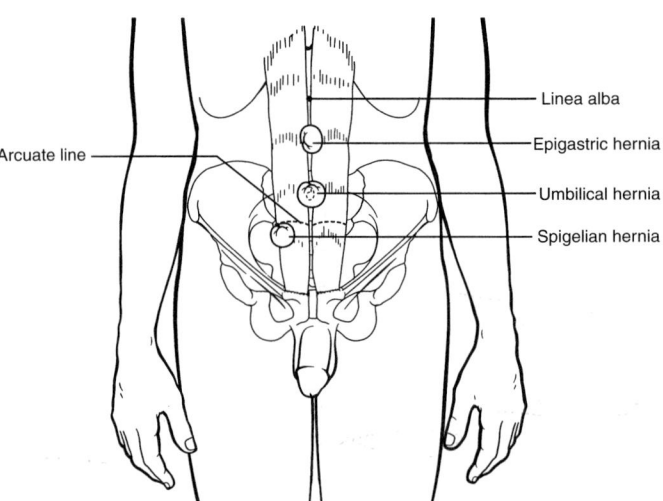

FIG. 80-4. Anterior abdominal wall hernias.

of otherwise healthy young adult military recruits, approximately 3 percent are determined to have groin hernias.[7] Approximately 750,000 herniorrhaphies are performed annually in the United States on inguinal hernias alone, most on an outpatient basis.[8]

All inguinal hernias occur more commonly in males than in females. Femoral hernias are more common in females and hernias of the anterior abdominal wall are of similar incidence. Indirect inguinal hernia is the most common hernia in both sexes. The distribution of hernia types by sex is shown in Figures 80-5 and 80-6.

Indirect inguinal hernias have a bimodal distribution, with peaks in the first year of life and after the age of 40 years.[9] Direct inguinal hernias are characteristically seen in adults, with a large male preponderance after 40 years of age. The incidence and distribution of other uncommon hernias are less clear.

CLINICAL FEATURES

Most hernias are detected on routine physical examination or as an asymptomatic lump by the patient. Some patients note soreness in the area, but significant pain is not common unless incarceration has occurred.

Patients with incarceration frequently present a history of hernia that on presentation will no longer reduce. If incarceration occurs, pain may develop suddenly. With infants, irritability may be the only presenting complaint. Incarceration may be accompanied by nausea and vomiting if bowel obstruction has occurred. Incarcerated hernias are a leading cause of bowel obstruction, second only to postoperative adhesions.

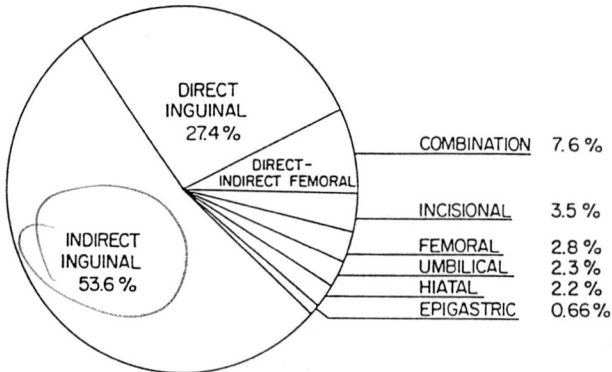

FIG. 80-5. The relative distribution of common hernias seen in 1655 men in 1965 and 1967. The high proportion of indirect and direct inguinal hernias is striking. (Reproduced with permission from Ponka JL: *Hernias of the Abdominal Wall.* Philadelphia, Saunders, 1980, p. 85.)

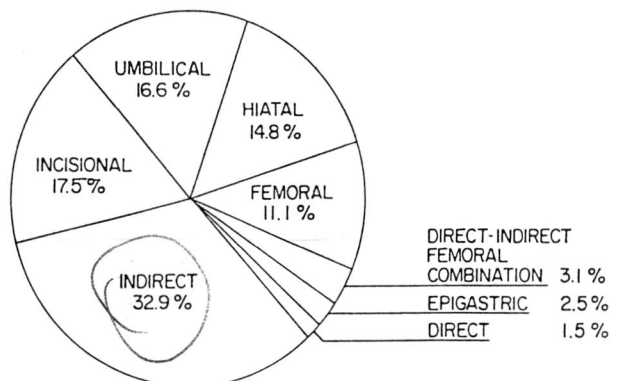

FIG. 80-6. The distribution of common hernias in 325 women in 1965 and 1967. Note the relatively greater frequency of incisional, umbilical, hiatal, and femoral hernias in the female. (Reproduced with permission from Ponka JL: *Hernias of the Abdominal Wall.* Philadelphia, Saunders, 1980, p. 85.)

If strangulation occurs, the patient may be toxic. Unrelieved strangulation may result in perforation, abscess formation, peritonitis, or septic shock.[10]

Physical examination of the patient with a hernia may reveal an abnormal soft tissue mass. In inguinal hernias in males, swelling may extend into the scrotum. The consistency of the mass varies depending on the content of the hernial sac. If incarceration is present, the mass is usually tender due to inflammation of the bowel wall or omentum and surrounding tissues. Tachycardia and mild temperature elevation also may be present.

Pain and hypesthesia along the medial aspect of the thigh to the knee are associated with obturator hernias. These patients also may have intermittent bouts of small bowel obstruction of several years' duration.

DIAGNOSIS OF INGUINAL HERNIAS

Patients frequently present to the emergency department with a complaint of groin pain. In males, palpation of the inguinal canal is easily performed by inversion of scrotal skin and passage of a finger through the external ring. The patient is then asked to cough or perform Valsalva. If an inguinal hernia is present, the examiner should feel a tapping sensation at the tip of the finger.

In females, the external ring is generally narrower and the skin of the labium majora is not easily inverted, making passage of a finger difficult. Therefore, failure to palpate a hernial sac in women is not foolproof.

Groin hernias have a large number of differential diagnostic possibilities (Table 80-1). They most commonly are confused with tender lymph nodes and hydroceles. Lymph nodes are generally movable, firm, and multiple. Hydroceles may transilluminate and are not tender. Incarcerated hernias will not transilluminate and are tender. If bowel is contained in the hernia sac, bowel sounds may be heard and peristalsis may be seen. Testicular torsion or tumor may be confused with in-

carcerated inguinal hernias. In children, retractile or undescended testes may be mistaken for hernias.

Laboratory studies may be helpful if incarceration has occurred. The white blood cell count may be elevated, with a shift to the left. Electrolyte abnormalities and elevation of the serum urea nitrogen level may occur as a reflection of the patient's state of hydration and toxicity. In the elderly and immunocompromised, laboratory studies may not be reliable indicators of the patient's condition. Occasionally, as part of a diagnostic evaluation for abdominal pain, a hernia is detected on barium enema.

Abdominal x-rays are recommended if bowel obstruction or perforation is suspected. Free air may be seen under the diaphragm on an upright chest film. Flat and upright films of the abdomen, including the groin, should be obtained to assess for air-fluid levels and other signs of obstruction. Loops of bowel may be seen entering a hernial sac.

Suspicion of spigelian or pelvic hernias often necessitates use of sonography or computed tomography for diagnosis,[11–13] because detection of herniation is frequently difficult and confusion with other masses is possible.

TREATMENT

Incarcerated hernias require immediate attention. If there is a reliable history that the incarceration is of recent onset, an attempt may be made to reduce the hernia. **If there is any question of the duration of the incarceration, no attempt at reduction should be made so that dead bowel is not introduced into the abdominal cavity.**

Before an attempt is made to reduce the hernia, the patient should be placed in the Trendelenburg position. Pain medication or anxiolytics should be considered and administered as needed to allow the patient's abdominal musculature to relax. A warm compress over the area also may be useful. Only gentle compression of the hernia should be used, and nothing should be forced.

The treatment for an incarcerated hernia that cannot be manually reduced is surgical fixation. If strangulation is suspected or shock is present, broad-spectrum antibiotics and fluid resuscitation are also necessary. Mortality is high in the elderly when emergency surgery is necessary.

Most asymptomatic or reducible hernias are repaired electively. Elective treatment has changed significantly over the past 20 years. Historically, hernias were repaired by using an open technique and primary closure with sutures. Currently, there are many accepted techniques, including mesh closures and laparoscopic approaches. Outpatient surgery is the norm, and local anesthesia is an adequate option for many patients. Complication and recurrence rates vary greatly and are operator dependent. The need for repair of all groin hernias has recently come into question.[14]

DISPOSITION

Any acutely incarcerated hernia that cannot be reduced, regardless of type or the patient's age, requires immediate surgical evaluation and repair.

Adult patients with reducible hernias may be discharged and referred for discussion of elective surgical repair. They should be advised to avoid conditions that increase intra-abdominal pressure, such as heavy lifting. Return to the emergency department is necessary if the patient has recurrence and is unable to reduce the hernia promptly. After surgical evaluation, patients who are not candidates for operative repair may be fitted with trusses.

In children, inguinal hernias have a high risk of incarceration, particularly in the first year of life. These hernias should be electively repaired shortly after diagnosis and therefore require emergency surgical consultation. Infants with inguinal hernias reduced in the emergency department should generally have repair within a few days.[15]

Umbilical hernias in children very rarely incarcerate. Spontaneous closure of the umbilical ring occurs in 80 percent of these children by

TABLE 80-1 Differential Considerations in Groin Hernia

Direct inguinal hernia	Testicular torsion
Indirect inguinal hernia	Retractile or undescended testis
Femoral hernia	Epididymitis
Lymph nodes	Groin cellulitis
Hydrocele	Femoral thrombophlebitis
Spermatic cord tumor	Femoral artery aneurysm
Testicular tumor	

age 3 or 4 years. Discharge and primary care observation are the standard of care for young children with hernias smaller than 2.0 cm in diameter. Children older than 4 years or with larger hernias should be referred for surgical evaluation.

REFERENCES

1. Skinner MA, Grosfeld JL: Inguinal and umbilical hernia repair in infants and children. *Surg Clin North Am* 73:439, 1993.
2. Gallegos NC, Dawson J, Jarvis M, et al: Risk of strangulation in groin hernias. *Br J Surg* 78:1171, 1991.
3. Scherer LR, Grosfeld JL: Inguinal hernia and umbilical anomalies. *Pediatr Clin North Am* 40:1121, 1993.
4. Bergstein JM, Condon RE: Obturator hernia: Current diagnosis and treatment. *Surgery* 119:133, 1996.
5. Luijendijk RW, Hop WCJ, et al: A comparison of suture repair with mesh repair for incisional hernia. *New Engl J Med* 343:392, 2000.
6. Mensching JJ, Musielewicz AJ: Abdominal wall hernias. *Emerg Med Clin North Am* 14:739, 1996.
7. Akin ML, Karakaya M, Batkin A, et al: Prevalence of inguinal hernia in otherwise healthy males of 20 to 22 years of age. *J R Army Med Corps* 143:101, 1997.
8. Rutkow IM: Epidemiologic, economic, and sociologic aspects of hernia surgery in the United States in the 19990s. *Surg Clin North Am* 78:941, 1998.
9. Millikan KW, Deziel DJ: The management of hernia: Considerations in cost effectiveness. *Surg Clin North Am* 76:105, 1996.
10. Primatesta P, Goldacre MJ: Inguinal hernia repair: Incidence of elective and emergency surgery, readmission and mortality. *Int J Epidemiol* 25:835, 1996.
11. Torzilli G, Carmana G, Lumachi V, et al: The usefulness of ultrasonography in the diagnosis of the spigelian hernia. *Int Surg* 80:280, 1995.
12. Mufid MM, Abu-Yousef MM, Kakish ME, et al: Spigelian hernia: Diagnosis by high-resolution real-time sonography. *J Ultrasound Med* 16:183, 1997.
13. Hojer AM, Rygaard H, Jess P: CT in the diagnosis of abdominal wall hernias: A preliminary study. *Eur Radiol* 7:1416, 1997.
14. Crawford DL, Phillips EH: Laparoscopic repair and groin hernia surgery. *Surg Clin North Am* 78:1047, 1998.
15. Gahukamble DE, Khamage AS: Early versus delayed repair of reduced incarcerated inguinal hernias in the pediatric population. *J Pediatr Surg* 31:1218, 1996.

81   ILEITIS, COLITIS, AND DIVERTICULITIS
Howard A. Werman
Hagop S. Mekhjian
Douglas A. Rund

CROHN DISEASE

Crohn disease is a chronic granulomatous inflammatory disease of the gastrointestinal (GI) tract; the exact cause is still unknown. **Crohn disease can involve any part of the GI tract from the mouth to the anus.** The ileum is involved in the majority of cases. In 20 percent, the disease is confined to the colon, making differentiation from ulcerative colitis difficult. The terms *regional enteritis, terminal ileitis, granulomatous ileocolitis,* and *Crohn disease* are all used to describe the same disease process.

Etiology and Pathogenesis

Environmental, genetic, infectious, and host factors have all been implicated as a cause of both Crohn disease and ulcerative colitis. Immunologic factors undoubtedly play a major role. Several mechanisms have been proposed, including autoimmune destruction of the gut mu-

cosal cells as the result of cross-reactivity with antigens from enteric bacteria; and nonspecific immunologic injury to the gut mucosa as the result of a chronic inflammatory process for both ulcerative colitis and Crohn disease. Cytokines, including interleukins and tumor necrosis factor, have been invoked in the perpetuation of the inflammatory response. The efficacy of anti-tumor necrosis factor such as infliximab (Remicade) in active Crohn disease and fistulizing Crohn disease supports the role of immunologic factors. Whether immune factors play a primary or secondary role in the pathogenesis of these diseases is not known. Extraintestinal manifestations suggest a role for immune complexes or an autoantibody response at various involved sites.

Epidemiology

The peak incidence of Crohn disease occurs between 16 and 22 years of age, with a secondary peak from 55 to 60 years. There is a 20 to 30 percent increased risk of Crohn disease among women as compared with men. The disease has a worldwide distribution but is more common in people of European extraction. It is four times more common among Jews than non-Jews and is more common in whites than blacks, Asians, or Native Americans. A family history of inflammatory bowel disease is present in 10 to 15 percent of patients, particularly with early onset of disease. Ulcerative colitis as well as Crohn disease may be present in other family members, and siblings of patients with Crohn disease have a higher incidence of the disease.

Pathology

The most important pathologic feature of Crohn disease is the involvement of all the layers of the bowel and extension into mesenteric lymph nodes. In addition, the disease is discontinuous, with normal areas of bowel ("skip areas") located between one or more involved areas. The appearance of the mucosa varies with the extent and severity of the disease. Longitudinal, deep ulcerations are characteristic. These often penetrate the bowel wall, resulting in fissures, fistulas, and abscesses. Late in the disease, a cobblestone appearance of the mucosa results from the criss-crossing of these ulcers with intervening normal mucosa.

Clinical Features

The clinical course of Crohn disease varies and in the individual patient is unpredictable. Abdominal pain, anorexia, diarrhea, and weight loss are present in most cases. Chronic abdominal pain, fever, and diarrhea may be present for several years before the definitive diagnosis is established. Approximately one-third of patients develop perianal fissures or fistulas, abscesses, or rectal prolapse, particularly when there is colonic involvement. Finally, patients may also present with complications of the disease, such as obstruction with vomiting, crampy abdominal pain, and obstipation, or an intraabdominal abscess with fever, abdominal pain, and a palpable mass. In 10 to 20 percent of patients, the extraintestinal manifestations of arthritis, uveitis, or liver disease may be presenting symptoms. Crohn disease should also be considered in the differential diagnosis of patients with fever of unknown etiology.

The clinical course and manifestations of the disease appear to be related, partly because of its anatomic distribution; in 30 percent the disease involves only the small bowel; in 20 percent only the colon is involved; and in 50 percent both the small bowel and colon are involved. A small percentage of patients present with disease involving the mouth, esophagus, and stomach. Patients with Crohn's disease of the stomach may demonstrate symptoms similar to those associated with peptic ulcer disease (see Chap. 77).

The recurrence rate for patients with Crohn disease is 25 to 50 percent within 1 year for patients whose disease has responded to medical management; the recurrence rate is higher for patients who require surgery. Patients with ileocolitis have the highest recurrence rate following surgery. The incidence of hematochezia and perianal disease is higher when the colon is involved, as in ileocolitis or Crohn colitis. A slight increase in the incidence of arthritis may be associated with Crohn colitis. Except for the additional concern of growth retardation, childhood-onset Crohn disease seems to have a course similar to that of adult-onset disease.

Extraintestinal manifestations are seen in 25 to 30 percent of patients with Crohn disease (Table 81-1), and the incidence of these complications does not differ between patients with Crohn disease and those with ulcerative colitis. Extraintestinal manifestations are divided among arthritic (19 percent), dermatologic (4 percent), hepatobiliary (4 percent), and vascular (1.3 percent) complications. Peripheral arthropathies are commonly seen in both ulcerative colitis and Crohn disease and tend to manifest during exacerbations of the underlying disease process. Ankylosing spondylitis can be detected in up to 20 percent of patients with inflammatory bowel disease. Symptoms may occur before, during, and after bouts of Crohn disease or ulcerative colitis.

Dermatologic complications include erythema nodosum and pyoderma gangrenosum. Ocular manifestations include episcleritis and uveitis.

Hepatobiliary disease is common in patients with inflammatory bowel disease and includes pericholangitis, chronic active hepatitis, primary sclerosing cholangitis, and cholangiocarcinoma. Gallstones are detected in up to 33 percent of patients with Crohn disease. The incidence of acute and chronic pancreatitis is increased in patients with Crohn disease and ulcerative colitis.

Vascular manifestations include thromboembolic disease, vasculitis, and arteritis. Patients with thromboembolic complications have a mortality rate of approximately 25 percent. Thromboembolic disease is the result of a hypercoagulable state induced in patients with both Crohn disease and ulcerative colitis and ranks as the third leading cause of death in patients afflicted with these conditions, behind peritonitis and malignancy. Malnutrition and chronic anemia are seen in many patients with longstanding Crohn disease. Growth retardation can be seen in children.

Hyperoxaluria is a common and potentially treatable occurrence in patients with ileal disease and steatorrhea. This results from increased colonic absorption of dietary oxalate and accounts for the occurrence of nephrolithiasis in 20 to 25 percent of patients with ileal disease. Finally, myelodysplastic disease, osteomyelitis, and osteonecrosis have been reported as rare complications of ulcerative colitis, and in particular, Crohn disease.

Complications

More than three out of four patients with Crohn disease will require surgery within the first 20 years of the onset of initial symptoms. Abscess and fissure formation is seen in approximately 30 percent of patients. Abscesses can be characterized as intraperitoneal, retroperitoneal, interloop, or intramesenteric. These patients present with abdominal pain and tenderness typical of their underlying disease, but may also have fever spikes and a palpable mass. Patients with retroperitoneal abscesses may present with hip or back pain and difficulty ambulating. Liver abscesses have also been reported in patients with Crohn disease.

Fistulas are the result of extension of the intestinal fissures seen in Crohn disease into adjacent structures. The most common sites are between the ileum and the sigmoid colon, the cecum, another ileal segment, or the skin. Internal fistulas should be suspected when there are

TABLE 81-1   Extraintestinal Manifestations of Inflammatory Bowel Disease

Manifestation	Description
ARTHRITIC	
Peripheral arthritis	Migratory monarticular or polyarticular pain in peripheral joints (hip, knee, ankle, wrist) with effusion
Ankylosing spondylitis	Pain and stiffness of spine, hips, neck, and rib cage with limitation in truncal motion, loss of lumbar lordosis; decreased chest expansion and forward cervical flexion in advanced disease
Sacroiliitis	Low back pain with morning stiffness, relieved by exercise; progressive joint sclerosis
OCULAR	
Episcleritis	Eye burning or itching without visual changes or pain; scleral and conjunctival hyperemia
Uveitis	Acute blurring of vision, photophobia and pain; perilimbic scleral injection
DERMATOLOGIC	
Erythema nodosum	Painful, red, raised nodules on extensor surfaces of arms or legs
Pyoderma gangrenosum	Ulcerative lesions with a necrotic center and violaceous skin typically found in pretibial region or trunk
HEPATOBILIARY	
Cholelithiasis	Varies from asymptomatic stones to right upper quadrant pain, fever, vomiting
Fatty liver	Mild right upper quadrant pain; hepatomegaly
Pericholangitis	Mild elevation in serum alkaline phosphatase, asymptomatic
Chronic active hepatitis	Autoimmune elevation of liver aminotransferase enzymes, may progress to cirrhosis
Primary sclerosing cholangitis	Pruritus progressing to jaundice, fatigue, and lethargy; laboratory findings vary from mild elevations of alkaline phosphatase to cirrhosis, portal hypertension, and liver failure; male predominance
Cholangiocarcinoma	Extrahepatic biliary mass, evidence of biliary obstruction, jaundice, right upper quadrant pain, fever, malaise
Pancreatitis	Varies from painless elevation of serum amylase to clinically apparent central abdominal pain radiating to back; may be associated with drugs such as azathioprine, 6-mercaptopurine, sulfasalazine, mesalamine, olsalazine, metronidazole
VASCULAR	
Thromboembolic disease	Symptoms of deep venous thrombosis and pulmonary emboli; portal vein, mesenteric vein, and hepatic venous thrombosis reported
OTHER	
Malnutrition	Fatigue, malaise, muscular wasting, cachexia
Chronic anemia	Fatigue, malaise, pallor, dyspnea; may be microcytic (blood loss), macrocytic (B_{12} deficiency) or autoimmune hemolytic
Nephrolithiasis	Flank pain, nausea, vomiting, hematuria; stones result from increased dietary oxylate absorption (calcium oxylate stones) and dehydration (urate stones)

changes in the patient's symptom complex, including bowel movement frequency, amount of pain, or weight loss. Enterovesical fistulas are rare complications of Crohn disease.

Obstruction is the result of both stricture formation due to the inflammatory process and of edema of the bowel wall. The distal small bowel is the most common site of obstruction. Symptoms include crampy abdominal pain, distention, nausea, and bloating.

Perianal complications are seen in one-third of patients with Crohn disease and include perianal or ischiorectal abscesses, fissures, fistulas, rectovaginal fistulas, and rectal prolapse. These are more commonly seen in patients with colonic involvement.

While gastrointestinal bleeding is common in patients with Crohn disease, only about 1 percent of patients develop life-threatening hemorrhage.[1] In patients with Crohn disease, bleeding is the result of erosion into a vessel in the bowel wall. Toxic megacolon occurs in 6 percent of all cases of Crohn disease and is associated with massive gastrointestinal bleeding in over half the cases. Fifty percent of all cases of toxic megacolon occur in patients with Crohn disease. Free perforation, however, rarely occurs.

When bowel symptoms are present, malnutrition, malabsorption, hypocalcemia, and vitamin deficiency can be severe. In addition to the complications of the disease itself are complications associated with the treatment of the disease with sulfasalazine, steroids, immunosuppressive agents, and antibiotics. These include leukopenia, thrombocytopenia, fever, infection, profuse diarrhea, pancreatitis, renal insufficiency and liver failure.

The incidence of malignant neoplasm of the GI tract is three times higher in patients with Crohn disease than for the general population.

Diagnosis

In the majority of patients, the definitive diagnosis of Crohn disease is established months or years after the onset of symptoms. Occasionally, the initial presenting complaint is not related to the GI tract but is an extraintestinal manifestation such as arthritis or uveitis. A provisional diagnosis of appendicitis or pelvic inflammatory disease may change to Crohn disease at the time of surgery. A careful and detailed history for previous bowel symptoms that preceded the onset of acute right lower quadrant pain and the absence of true guarding or rebound in patients with Crohn disease may provide clues to the correct diagnosis before surgery.

A definitive diagnosis of Crohn disease is confirmed by an upper GI series, an air-contrast barium enema, and colonoscopy. Oral barium studies with fluoroscopy are fairly sensitive and specific for detecting ileal involvement. The characteristic radiographic findings in the small intestine include segmental narrowing, destruction of the normal mucosal pattern, and fistulas. Segmental involvement of the colon (right-sided colitis) with rectal sparing is the usual feature.

Colonoscopy is the most sensitive technique for examining patients with Crohn colitis. This technique is useful in detecting early mucosal lesions, in defining the extent of colonic involvement, and in surveillance for the occurrence of colon cancer. As mentioned earlier, rectal sparing with involvement of the proximal colon helps to differentiate Crohn colitis from ulcerative colitis. Abdominal CT scanning is the most useful diagnostic test in patients with acute symptoms who have known or suspected Crohn disease. Findings such as bowel wall thickening, mesenteric edema, and local abscess formation suggest the diagnosis of Crohn disease. Extraintestinal complications such as gallstones, renal calculi, hydronephrosis, sacroiliitis, and osteomyelitis can also be seen on CT scan. Intraabdominal abscesses, mesenteric inflammation, and fistulas are also diagnosed using computed tomography.

Differential Diagnosis

Diseases that should be considered in the differential diagnosis of Crohn disease (Table 81-2) include lymphoma, ileocecal amebiasis, sarcoidosis, deep chronic mycotic infections involving the GI tract, gastrointestinal tuberculosis, Kaposi's sarcoma, *Campylobacter* enteritis, and *Yersinia* ileocolitis. Fortunately, most of these are uncommon conditions and can be differentiated by appropriate laboratory tests. *Yersinia* ileocolitis and *Campylobacter* enteritis may cause chronic abdominal pain and diarrhea similar to Crohn disease, but can be diagnosed by appropriate stool cultures. Acute ileitis should not be confused with Crohn disease. Young patients with acute ileitis usually recover without sequelae and should not undergo surgery. When Crohn disease is confined to the colon, ischemic bowel disease (particularly in the elderly) and pseudomembranous enterocolitis as well as ulcerative colitis must be included in the differential diagnosis.

Treatment

The aim of therapy includes relief of symptoms, induction of remission, maintenance of remission, prevention of complications, optimizing timing of surgery, and maintenance of nutrition. In a disease that is virtually incurable, the emphasis should be on relief of symptoms and prevention of complications. The pharmacologic agents available for the management of Crohn disease include symptomatic agents, antiinflammatory agents, antibiotics, and immunomodulators. Treatment guidelines have been developed for adult patients with Crohn disease.[2,3] Initial evaluation in the ED should focus on determining the severity of the attack; identifying significant complications such as obstruction, intraabdominal abscess, life-threatening hemorrhage, or toxic megacolon; and eliminating other possible causes of the patient's complaints. Laboratory evaluation should include a CBC, serum electrolytes, BUN, creatinine, and a type and cross-match where appropriate. Plain radiographs of the abdomen may reveal evidence of obstruction, perforation, or toxic megacolon. Initial treatment

TABLE 81-2 Differential Diagnosis of Ileitis, Colitis, and Diverticulitis

Acute appendicitis
Peptic ulcer disease
Pelvic inflammatory disease
Endometriosis
Ischemic colitis
Leaking aortic aneurysm
Renal calculus
Irritable bowel syndrome
Lactate intolerance
Carcinoma of the colon
Intestinal lymphoma
Kaposi's sarcoma
Gay bowel syndrome
Sarcoidosis
Infectious causes
    Campylobacter enteritis
    Shigella enteritis
    Salmonella enteritis
    Yersinia ileocolitis
    Hemorrhagic *Escherichia coli* enteritis
    Intestinal tuberculosis
    Amebiasis
    Lymphogranuloma venereum
    Gonorrheal proctitis
    Syphilis
    Actinomycosis
    Entamoeba histolytica
    Cytomegalovirus
    Herpes simplex virus
Irradiation colitis
Postirradiation proctosigmoiditis
Fecal impaction
Foreign-body granuloma
Collagen vascular disease

(Table 81-3) consists of adequate fluid resuscitation and restoration of electrolyte balance. Nasogastric decompression should be initiated in any patient with evidence of obstruction, peritonitis, or toxic mega-colon. Broad-spectrum antibiotics (ampicillin or a cephalosporin, an aminoglycoside, and metronidazole) should be used in patients with fulminant colitis or peritonitis. Patients with severe disease should receive intravenous steroids such as hydrocortisone 300 mg per d or an equivalent dose of methylprednisolone (48 mg per d) or prednisolone (60 mg per d).

Sulfasalazine (Azulfidine), 3 to 4 g per d, has been shown to be effective in treating patients with mild to moderate active Crohn disease. The mechanism of action is not known but is presumed to be through the topical action of 5-aminosalicylic acid, which is released by the action of colonic bacteria on sulfasalazine. Sulfapyridine is also a by-product of this breakdown. Many of the toxic side effects of sulfasalazine are attributable to sulfapyrizine. These include nausea, vomiting, anorexia, epigastric distress, arthralgias, headache, diarrhea, male infertility, and hypersensitivity reactions (pericarditis, pleuritis, pancreatitis, arthritis, and rash). Because of the toxicity profile associated with sulfasalazine 5-aminosalicylic acid derivative agents are now available for either oral or topical use. A slow, timed-release mesalamine (Pentasa) 4 g per d or a pH-dependent release mesalamine (Asacol, Claversal, Salofalk) 2 to 4 g per d have the primary advantage of delivery into the colon. Olsalazine (Dipentum) 1 g per d is a derivative of the sodium salt of 5-aminosalicylic acid, which is converted to two 5-aminosalicylic molecules in the colon and has identical antiinflammatory properties. Balsalazide (Colazide) 1.5 to 6 g per d has the 5-aminosalicylic acid moiety bound to an inert molecule. The mesalamine formulations are most effective in colonic disease. The topical preparations have limited usefulness and are effective only in the management of Crohn disease limited to the rectum or the distal 40 cm of rectosigmoid.

Oral glucocorticoids such as prednisone (40 to 60 mg per d) are reserved for more severely affected patients and are effective primarily in small intestinal disease as well as in ileocolitis. Alternatively, an ileal-released form of budesonide (9 mg per d) may be beneficial in these patients. Immunosuppressive drugs such as 6-mercaptopurine (6-MP) (1 to 1.5 mg/kg per d) or azathioprine (2 to 2.5 mg/kg per d) are useful as steroid-sparing agents, in healing fistulas, and in patients in whom there are serious contraindications to surgery. Recent evidence suggests that they are also effective as maintenance agents. Both agents have been associated with leukopenia, fever, hepatitis, and pancreatitis, necessitating the need for close follow-up, particularly during the initial phase of therapy. Thioguanine (6-TG), the active metabolite of azathioprine and 6-MP may offer a safer alternative.[4] The response to immunosuppressives should not be expected before 3 to 6 months following the initiation of therapy. Cyclosporine (4 mg/kg per d for 7 to 10 d) and methotrexate (15 to 25 mg per week) have been used in refractory cases.

Metronidazole (10 to 20 mg/kg per d) has been shown to be effective in controlled clinical trials and is particularly useful in treatment of patients with perianal complications and fistulous disease. Ciprofloxacin (1.0 to 1.5 mg/kg per d) has also been used in this setting as well as in active Crohn's ileitis and ileocolitis.

Patients with medically-resistant moderate to severe Crohn's disease may benefit from the anti-tumor necrosis factor antibody infliximab (Remicade) 5 mg/kg intravenously.[5] Active tuberculosis can develop after initiation of treatment with infliximab. Before initiation of treatment, patients should be screened for tuberculosis.[6] In addition, patients with perianal disease have been shown to respond to repeated infusions of 5 mg/kg at 0, 2, and 6 weeks.[7] Newer agents such as CDP571 (Cellcept), etanercept, thalidomide, and interleukin therapy may also be beneficial in these settings.

Maintenance therapy and the effectiveness of various therapeutic agents in Crohn disease is variable. Glucocorticoids should not be used for maintaining a remission because of the lack of sufficient evidence of their efficacy and the potential for long-term complications. When a patient is responsive to immunosuppressive therapy, it would seem advisable to continue this in a reduced dose for the maintenance of remission. Similarly, a reduced dose of 5-aminosalicyclic acid derivatives is appropriate for the maintenance of remission of colonic disease. The addition of sulfasalazine, azathioprine, and 6-mercaptopurine to prednisone does not improve the response rate and increases the risk of side effects.

Diarrhea can be controlled by the use of loperamide (Imodium) 4 to 16 mg per d, diphenoxylate (Lomotil) 5 to 20 mg per d, and in some cases, cholestyramine (Questran) 4 g 1 to 6 times a day. The latter is particularly useful as an exchange resin in patients who have limited ileal disease or resection, no bowel obstruction, and mild steatorrhea. The mechanism of action is binding bile acids and eliminating their known cathartic action. The primary aim of dietary therapy is the maintenance of nutrition and the alleviation of diarrhea. Elimination of lactose from the diet is of benefit in patients with lactose intolerance. Reduction in dietary oxalate should be considered in every patient. In addition, supplementation of trace metals, fat-soluble vitamins, and medium-chain triglycerides should be considered in selected patients.

Disposition

Patients who demonstrate signs of fulminant colitis, peritonitis, or complications such as obstruction, significant gastrointestinal hemorrhage, severe dehydration, or fluid/electrolyte imbalance should be hospitalized under the care of a gastroenterologist or surgeon. Hospital admission should be considered in less severe cases that fail outpatient management. Surgical intervention is indicated in those patients with complications of the disease, including intestinal obstruction or hemorrhage, perforation, abscess or fistula formation, toxic megacolon, and perianal disease. In addition, surgery may be indicated in those patients who fail medical therapy. The recurrence rate after surgery approaches 100 percent.

When patients with Crohn disease are discharged from the ED, alterations in their therapeutic regimen should be discussed with a consulting gastroenterologist. Close follow-up of these patients must be assured prior to discharge.

TABLE 81-3 Treatment of Fulminant Colitis

Restore fluid and electrolyte balance
Nothing by mouth
Nasogastric suction for
  Obstruction
  Adynamic ileus
  Suspected toxic megacolon
Parenteral corticosteroids
  ACTH 120 U per d (if not receiving prior steroids)
  Hydrocortisone 300 mg per d or methylprednisolone 48 mg per d or
    prednisolone 60 mg per d
Broad-spectrum antibiotics
  Ampicillin or cephalosporin
  Aminoglycoside (gentamicin or tobramycin)
  Metronidazole or clindamycin
Observe for complications
  Obstruction
  Perforation
  Toxic megacolon
  Life-threatening hemorrhage
  Intraabdominal abscess
Out Patient Management (non toxic patients)
  Liquids only for first 48 h
Oral Antibiotics
  Ampicillin, TMP/SMX, Ciprofloxacin, or Cefalexin
  and
  Metranidazole or Clindamycin

ULCERATIVE COLITIS

Ulcerative colitis is a chronic inflammatory disease of the colon. The inflammation tends to be progressively more severe from proximal to the distal colon. The rectum is involved nearly 100 percent of the time. Clinically, the characteristic symptom is bloody diarrhea. The etiology, like that of Crohn disease, remains unknown.

Epidemiology

Epidemiologic considerations are similar to those of Crohn disease; the disease is more prevalent in the United States and northern Europe, and peak incidence occurs in the second and the third decades of life. There is a slight predominance of men among patients with the disease. First-degree relatives of patients with ulcerative colitis have a 15-fold risk of developing ulcerative colitis and a 3.5-fold risk of developing Crohn disease.

Pathology

Ulcerative colitis involves primarily the mucosa and submucosa. Microscopically, the disease is characterized by mucosal inflammation with the formation of crypt abscesses, epithelial necrosis, and mucosal ulceration. The submucosa, muscular layer, and serosa are usually spared. In the usual case, the disease increases in severity more distally, the rectosigmoid being involved in 95 percent of cases. In the early stages of the disease, the mucous membranes appear finely granular and friable. In more severe cases, the mucosa appears as a red, spongy surface dotted with small ulcerations oozing blood and purulent exudate. In very advanced disease, one sees large, oozing ulcerations and pseudopolyps (areas of hyperplastic overgrowth surrounded by inflamed mucosa).

Clinical Features

The clinical features and course of ulcerative colitis vary but are somewhat dependent on the anatomical distribution of the disease in the colon. The disease is classified as mild, moderate, or severe depending on the clinical manifestations. Patients with mild disease have fewer than four bowel movements per day, no systemic symptoms, and few extraintestinal manifestations. Of all patients with ulcerative colitis, 60 percent have mild disease; in 80 percent of cases, the disease is limited to the rectum. Occasionally, constipation and rectal bleeding are the presenting complaints. Progression to pancolitis occurs in 10 to 15 percent of patients with mild disease.

Patients with severe disease constitute 15 percent of those with ulcerative colitis. Severe disease is associated with frequent bowel movements, anemia, fever, weight loss, tachycardia, low serum albumin, and more frequent extraintestinal manifestations. Patients with severe disease account for 90 percent of the mortality from ulcerative colitis. Virtually all severely affected patients have pancolitis.

Moderate disease is seen in 25 percent of patients. The clinical manifestations are less severe and patients demonstrate a good response to therapy. These patients usually have colitis extending to the splenic flexure (left-sided colitis), but may develop pancolitis.

Most commonly, ulcerative colitis is characterized by intermittent attacks of acute disease with complete remission between attacks. Such a pattern occurs in the majority of patients. In other patients, the first attack is followed by a prolonged period of inactivity. Infrequently, patients run a chronically active course. The factors associated with an unfavorable prognosis and increased mortality include higher severity and extent of disease, a short interval between attacks, and onset of the disease after 60 years of age.

Extraintestinal complications of ulcerative colitis include peripheral arthritis, ankylosing spondylitis, episcleritis, uveitis, pyoderma gangrenosum, and erythema nodosum (see Table 81-1). Clinically apparent liver disease may occur in 5 to 10 percent of patients. The manifestations of liver disease may include any of the following: pericholangitis, chronic active hepatitis, fatty liver or cirrhosis, cholelithiasis, sclerosing cholangitis, and bile duct carcinoma.

Complications

Although blood loss from sustained hemorrhage may be the most common complication of the illness, toxic megacolon is an associated clinical entity that must not be missed.

Toxic megacolon develops in advanced cases of colitis when the disease process begins to extend through all layers of the colon. The result is a loss of muscular tone within the colon, with dilatation and localized peritonitis. If the colon continues to dilate without treatment, signs of toxicity will develop. Plain radiography of the abdomen demonstrates a long, continuous segment of air-filled colon greater than 6 cm in diameter. Loss of colonic haustra and "thumbprinting," representing bowel wall edema, may also be seen. The distended portion of the atonic colon can perforate, causing peritonitis and septicemia. Mortality from this complication is approximately 50 percent if perforation occurs, but less than 10 percent if surgery is undertaken prior to perforation.

A patient with toxic megacolon appears severely ill; the abdomen is distended, tender, and tympanitic. Severe diarrhea (more than 10 bowel movements per day) is often seen but may have ceased prior to onset. Fever, tachycardia, and signs of hypovolemia are typically part of the clinical picture. Leukocytosis, anemia, electrolyte disturbances, and hypoalbuminemia are the supporting laboratory results.

Some of the more prominent features of toxic megacolon, such as leukocytosis and peritonitis, can be masked in the patient taking corticosteroids. When such therapy is being administered, greater suspicion is required to make the diagnosis. Antidiarrheal agents, hypokalemia, narcotics, cathartics, pregnancy, enemas, and recent colonoscopy have been implicated as precipitating factors in toxic megacolon. Medical therapy with nasogastric suction, intravenous prednisolone 60 mg per d, or hydrocortisone 300 mg per d, parenteral broad-spectrum antibiotics active against coliforms and anaerobes, and intravenous fluids should be attempted as initial therapy and in preparing the patient for possible surgery. However, prolonged medical treatment of these patients increases mortality; therefore early surgical consultation must be sought with the aim of performing a colectomy if clinical improvement is not noted in 24 to 48 h with medical treatment.

Perirectal fistulas and abscesses may occur in up to 20 percent of patients with ulcerative colitis. Massive gastrointestinal hemorrhage, obstruction secondary to stricture formation, and acute perforation are other complications of the disease.

There is a 10- to 30-fold increase in the development of carcinoma of the colon in patients with ulcerative colitis. The major risk factors for the development of carcinoma of the colon are extensive involvement and prolonged duration of the disease. The cumulative risk of cancer after 20 and 30 years is 5 to 10 percent and 12 to 20 percent, respectively. Additional factors that constitute increased risk of cancer in patients with ulcerative colitis include early onset of the disease and a family history of colon cancer. The availability of fiberoptic colonoscopy allows surveillance of ulcerative colitis patients with periodic colonoscopies and biopsies to detect the high-grade dysplasia thought to predict the development or association of colon cancer. In patients with pancolitis, such surveillance should start 8 to 10 years after the onset of the disease.[8]

Diagnosis

Laboratory findings in patients with ulcerative colitis are nonspecific; they may include leukocytosis, anemia, thrombocytosis, decreased serum albumin, and abnormal liver function studies. Therefore, the diagnosis of ulcerative colitis rests on the following: a history of abdominal cramps and diarrhea, mucoid stools, stool examination negative for ova and parasites, stool cultures negative for enteric pathogens, and confirmation by sigmoidoscopic or colonoscopic examination. The results of the latter examination are abnormal in 95 percent of the patients with ulcerative colitis. The observed pathologic changes vary depending on the severity and duration of the disease. Granularity, friability, ulceration of the mucosa, and, in more advanced cases, pseudopolyposis are quite characteristic.

Sigmoidoscopy may be done in the office or the ED to confirm the clinical suspicion, but the appearance is not specific. Biopsy may help differentiate acute from chronic colitis (crypt distortion) and diseases caused by specific etiology, such as amebiasis (see "Pathology," above). Barium enema examination may be useful in differentiating ulcerative colitis from Crohn disease and defining the extent of involvement of the colon. Colonoscopy, however, is the most sensitive method for making the diagnosis and defining the extent and severity of the disease. In addition, colonoscopy is extremely useful in the evaluation of the patient for the development of dysplasia or colon cancer. Barium enema examination should be done with caution or postponed in moderately ill patients. Rigid or fiberoptic proctosigmoidoscopy can be used, however, even in the severely ill patient, provided that it is done gently and without the administration of any enemas or laxatives.

Differential Diagnosis

The major diseases that should be considered in the differential diagnosis of ulcerative colitis include infectious colitis, Crohn colitis, ischemic colitis, radiation colitis, toxic colitis from antineoplastic agents, and pseudomembranous colitis (see Table 81-2). When the disease is limited to the rectum, particular attention should be paid to sexually acquired diseases, which are frequently seen in the male homosexual population (gay bowel disease). Some of the more common diseases in this category include rectal syphilis, gonococcal proctitis, lymphogranuloma venereum, and inflammations caused by herpes simplex virus, *Entamoeba histolytica, Shigella,* and *Campylobacter.*

Treatment

Patients with severe ulcerative colitis should be treated with intravenous steroids, replacement of fluids, correction of electrolyte abnormalities, and broad-spectrum antibiotics active against coliforms and anaerobes (ampicillin and clindamycin or metronidazole); hyperalimentation may be considered for the individual patient (see Table 81-3). Steroid options include hydrocortisone 300 mg per d IV or an equivalent dose of methylprednisolone (48 mg per d IV or PO) or prednisolone (60 mg per d PO). Recently, cyclosporine (4 mg/kg per d) has been advocated for cases of fulminant colitis that have failed treatment with intravenous corticosteroids.[9] The use of complete bowel rest and routine administration of parenteral nutrition remains controversial in patients with fulminant disease.[10] When toxic megacolon is suspected, nasogastric suction should be initiated, a surgical consultation obtained, and the patient observed by frequent examinations and flat films of the abdomen. When the diagnosis of toxic megacolon is established and the patient fails to show dramatic clinical improvement within 24 to 48 h, emergency surgery should be considered.

The majority of those with mild and moderate disease can be treated as outpatients. Glucocorticoids are effective in inducing a remission in the majority of cases and constitute the mainstay of therapy in an acute attack. Daily doses of 40 to 60 mg of prednisone are usually sufficient and can be adjusted depending on the severity of the disease. In the treatment of patients with active proctitis, proctosigmoiditis, and left-sided colitis (less than 60 cm of active disease), 5-aminosalicylic acid enemas have been used with great success. Topical steroid preparations (beclomethasone, hydrocortisone, tixocortol, and budesonide) have also been successful and offer the benefit of fewer systemic side effects. This therapy has also been used to maintain remission in these patients. Once clinical remission is achieved, steroids should be slowly tapered and dis-

continued. There is no evidence that maintenance dosages of steroids reduce the incidence of relapses.

Sulfasalazine has been used in the treatment of acute attacks but is probably inferior to steroids, especially in the more severe cases. Its primary usefulness is in the form of adjunctive therapy and in the maintenance of a remission. Maintenance doses of 1.5 to 2 g per d significantly reduce the recurrence rate of the disease.

In addition to sulfasalazine, the newer 5-aminosalicylic derivatives are quite effective in inducing remission of ulcerative colitis as well as maintaining it. The main advantage of the newer agents is reduced side effects from the sulfapyridine moiety of sulfasalazine. The choice of agents available for the treatment of ulcerative colitis is very similar to that in Crohn disease [mesalamine (Pentasa, Asacol), olsalazine (Dipentum), and balasalazide]. Topical glucocorticoid enemas or 5-aminosalicylic enemas (Rowasa, 2 to 4 g/60 mL per d for 3 weeks) or suppositories (500 mg bid) are quite effective in distal protosigmoiditis and have lower systemic side-effect profiles. In refractory cases, a combination of glucocorticoids and immunomodulators such as 6-mercaptopurine (1 to 1.5 mg/kg per d) or azathioprine (2 mg/kg per d) should be considered. The beneficial effects of this combination therapy will not be seen before 3 to 6 months, somewhat limiting its usefulness in very sick patients. For these reasons, surgical intervention with elective proctocolectomy may be necessary. Newer agents under investigation for the treatment of ulcerative colitis include nicotine, heparin, biological therapies, and immunomodulating drugs including infliximab (Remicade).

Supportive measures in the treatment of mild to moderately sick patients include the replenishment of iron stores, a nutritious diet with the elimination of lactose, and adequate physical and psychological rest. Hydrophilic bulk agents such as psyllium (Metamucil) can be used in some patients to improve stool consistency. Antidiarrheal agents should be used with caution in ill patients because they may precipitate toxic megacolon and because they are generally ineffective.

Disposition

Patients with fulminant attacks of ulcerative colitis should be hospitalized for aggressive fluid and electrolyte resuscitation and careful observation for the development of complications. Patients with complications such as gastrointestinal hemorrhage, toxic megacolon, and bowel perforation should also be admitted with consultation to both a gastroenterologist and a surgeon. In addition to toxic megacolon, the indications for surgery include colonic perforation, massive lower gastrointestinal bleeding, suspicion of colon cancer, and disease that is refractory to medical therapy (large doses of steroids required to control the disease). Age and patient acceptance often influence the choice of surgical procedure, with the increased performance of continent procedures.

Patients with mild to moderate disease can be discharged from the ED. Close follow-up should be arranged with the patient's physician or gastroenterologist, and any adjustment in medical therapy discussed. In addition, the patient should be instructed to eat a low-residue diet. Patients should be instructed to return if symptoms do not improve or worsen. Particular attention should focus on the quantity of diarrhea, toleration of oral intake, and associated symptoms such as fever, rectal bleeding, or abdominal pain.

PSEUDOMEMBRANOUS ENTEROCOLITIS

Pseudomembranous enterocolitis is an inflammatory bowel disorder in which membrane-like yellowish plaques of exudate overlie and replace necrotic intestinal mucosa.

Epidemiology

Clostridium difficile is a spore-forming obligate anaerobic bacillus that causes pseudomembranous colitis. Three different syndromes have been described: neonatal pseudomembranous enterocolitis, post-operative pseudomembranous enterocolitis, and antibiotic-associated pseudomembranous colitis. Recent antibiotic use, gastrointestinal surgery or manipulation, severe underlying medical illness, and advancing age have all been identified as risk factors for developing pseudomembranous colitis. Transmission of the organism has been implicated from direct human contact as well as contact with inanimate objects (commodes, telephones, rectal thermometers).

Pathophysiology

Hospitalized patients are colonized with *C. difficile* in 10 to 25 percent of cases, so the development of diarrhea in recently discharged patients should suggest consideration of *C. difficile*. There is a linear relationship between the length of hospital stay, colonization with *C. difficile* and the development of *C. difficile* diarrhea.[11] Broad-spectrum antibiotics—most notably clindamycin, cephalosporins, and ampicillin/amoxicillin—alter the gut flora in such a way that toxin-producing *C. difficile* can flourish within the colon, producing clinical manifestations of pseudomembranous colitis. However, almost any antibiotic (including metronidazole and vancomycin) can lead to pseudomembranous colitis, and chemotherapeutic agents and antiviral agents have also been implicated. Bowel ischemia, recent bowel surgery, uremia, malnutrition, shock, and Hirschsprung disease also contribute to the development of pseudomembranous colitis. Most disease-producing strains of *C. difficile* produce two toxins: toxin A, an enterotoxin, and toxin B, a cytotoxin, that interact in a complex and not completely understood manner to produce pseudomembranous colitis and its associated symptoms.

Clinical Features

Pseudomembranous colitis results in a spectrum of clinical manifestations that vary from frequent, mucoid, watery stools to a toxic picture that includes profuse diarrhea (20 to 30 stools per day), crampy abdominal pain, fever, leukocytosis, dehydration, and hypovolemia. Examination of the stool may reveal the presence of fecal leukocytes. These are not generally found in more benign forms of antibiotic-induced diarrhea.[12] Complications of the disease include severe electrolyte imbalance, hypotension, and anasarca from decreased serum albumin. In 1 to 3 percent of patients, toxic megacolon or colonic perforation may occur in patients with pseudomembranous colitis.[13] The disease typically begins 7 to 10 days after the institution of antibiotic therapy, although symptoms may develop within a few days or up to several weeks after the antibiotic is discontinued. Extraintestinal complications are rare and include arthritis, visceral abscesses, cellulitis, necrotizing fasciitis, osteomyelitis, and prosthetic device infection.[14]

Diagnosis

The diagnosis is suggested by a history of diarrhea that develops during administration of antibiotics or within 2 weeks of their discontinuation. The diagnosis may be confirmed by stool examination for the *C. difficile* toxin and colonoscopy.

The diagnosis is confirmed by the demonstration of *C. difficile* in the stool and by the detection of the toxin in stool filtrates. The organism is best identified by stool culture using a selective growth medium. This technique has a sensitivity approaching 100 percent, but lacks specificity because the presence of *C. difficile* does not necessarily mean it causes disease. In addition, culture results take between 28 and 72 h, thus limiting their utilization in establishing the diagnosis in patients with suspected pseudomembranous colitis.

Instead, *C. difficile* toxins are detected directly using a number of techniques including tissue-culture assay, enzyme-linked immunosorbent assays (ELISA), latex agglutination, dot-immunobinding assays, and polymerase chain reaction (PCR). Tests vary in their sensitivity, specificity, and time to completion. While tissue-culture assays are considered the gold standard, most laboratories utilize the ELISA technique to detect the clostridial toxins; it has a sensitivity of 63 to 94 percent and a specificity of 75 to 100 percent.[15] Five to twenty percent of patients require more than one stool specimen to detect toxin.

Colonoscopy reveals characteristic yellowish plaques within the intestinal lumen. Lesions may be seen throughout the entire alimentary tract, although they are typically limited to the right colon. Colonoscopy is not routinely needed to establish a diagnosis of pseudomembranous colitis. It may be used in patients who require a rapid diagnosis and those who cannot produce a stool specimen due to ileus.

Treatment

The treatment of pseudomembranous colitis includes discontinuing antibiotic therapy and instituting supportive measures such as the administration of fluids and the correction of electrolyte abnormalities. Twenty-five percent of patients will respond to these measures alone. For those patients with mild to moderate disease who do not respond to supportive measures, metronidazole 250 mg qid is the therapy of choice.[12] Vancomycin 125 to 250 mg qid is an alternative regimen, although it is considerably more expensive than metronidazole, and metronidazole is just as effective. Vancomycin should be reserved for cases in which the patient has not responded to or is intolerant of metronidazole, the organism is resistant to metronidazole, or in children or pregnant patients.

Severely ill persons must be hospitalized. Oral vancomycin, 125 to 250 mg qid for 10 days, is effective in the majority of severely ill patients. The symptoms usually resolve within a few days. Rarely, emergency colectomy may be required for patients with toxic dilatation of the colon or colonic perforation.

Relapses occur in 10 to 20 percent of patients. The use of antidiarrheal agents may prolong or worsen symptoms in patients with pseudomembranous colitis and should be avoided. Steroids and surgical intervention are rarely needed.

Disposition

Patients with severe diarrhea, symptoms that persist despite appropriate outpatient management, or those with a systemic response (fever, leukocytosis, severe abdominal pain) should be hospitalized. Patients with pseudomembranous colitis who are suspected of having a toxic megacolon, intestinal perforation, or those who fail to respond to appropriate medical therapy should have an immediate surgical consultation. For those patients who are discharged, discontinuation of any antibiotics and good oral intake must be encouraged. Metronidazole or vancomycin are equally effective in the treatment of antibiotic-induced colitis.

DIVERTICULITIS

Diverticulitis is an acute inflammation of the wall of a diverticulum and surrounding tissue caused by either a micro- or macroperforation.

Epidemiology

Acquired diverticular disease of the colon has become an increasingly common disorder of industrialized nations. Radiologic studies have suggested that one-third of the population will have acquired the disease by age 50 and two-thirds by age 85. Diverticula are rare in individuals under age 20.

Diverticulitis is estimated to occur in 10 to 25 percent of patients with known diverticulosis. The incidence of diverticulitis increases with age. Only 2 to 4 percent of patients with diverticulitis are under the age of 40. Diverticulitis in the younger age group tends to be a more virulent form of the disease, with frequent complications requiring earlier surgical intervention. Although the frequency of the disease is higher in men, there is an increasing incidence of diverticulitis in women.

Pathophysiology

Colonic diverticula are false diverticula because they do not include all layers of the bowel wall. They consist of mucosa and submucosa with a peritoneal covering that has herniated through a defect in the circular muscle layer of the wall. The sites of herniation are located between the mesenteric and antimesenteric taenia, where intramural blood vessels penetrate the muscularis. Cecal diverticuli, on the other hand, are true diverticula.

The cause of diverticular disease is not known. It is still unresolved whether diverticular disease is a disorder of colonic motility, a colonic muscle abnormality, a connective tissue disorder, or a normal concomitant of aging. Low-residue diets have been implicated as a major factor in the pathogenesis of diverticular disease. The most common hypothesis is that acquired diverticula arise because of high intraluminal pressures in areas of relative weakness of the colonic wall. This is based on observations that the majority of patients have diverticula located within the sigmoid colon. Laplace's law states that the tension on the wall of a hollow cylinder is inversely proportional to the radius of the cylinder multiplied by the pressure within the cylinder. This suggests that the intraluminal pressure in the colon is greatest where the lumen is narrowest. The diameter of the colon is smallest in the sigmoid region, and thus this region of the colon is the most likely location for the development of diverticula.

The acute complications of diverticular disease can be divided into two broad categories: (1) inflammation and its associated complications, and (2) bleeding (see Chap. 74).

Inflammation, or diverticulitis, is the most common complication of diverticular disease. It was thought to occur when fecal material became inspissated in the neck of an acquired diverticulum, resulting in obstruction of the neck of the diverticulum and subsequent proliferation of colonic bacteria, mucous secretion, and distention of the diverticulum. The latter mechanism probably contributes to a small percentage of cases of diverticulitis. More commonly, clinical diverticulitis results from high pressure in the colon, erosion of the wall of the diverticulum, and microperforation and inflammation of pericolonic tissue. Fortunately, fecal contamination of the peritoneum is usually limited because perforation of a diverticulum occurs into the leaves of the mesentery or because the contamination is walled off by the mobile loops of the sigmoid colon or small bowel and adjacent pelvic structures. Free perforation may occur with generalized peritonitis, but it is uncommon. Other complications include intestinal obstruction and fistula formation between the diverticula and the bladder in a male or vagina in a female.

Clinical Features

The most common symptom of diverticulitis is pain. This is commonly described as a steady, deep discomfort in the left lower quadrant. Patients will frequently complain of a change in bowel habits, either in the form of diarrhea or increasing constipation. Tenesmus is another common symptom. The involved diverticulum may irritate the bladder or ureter, causing the patient to have urinary frequency, dysuria, or pyuria. If a fistula develops between the colon and the bladder, the patient may present with recurrent urinary tract infections or pneumaturia. Paralytic ileus with abdominal distention, nausea, and vomiting may develop secondary to intraabdominal irritation and peritonitis. Small bowel obstruction may also occur as an adjacent loop of small bowel becomes kinked or narrowed in the inflammatory mass.

The clinical presentation may be indistinguishable from acute appendicitis. This may occur when the patient has a redundant sigmoid colon lying on the right side of the abdomen or a cecal diverticulum that becomes inflamed. The possibility of diverticulitis or appendicitis should always be considered in the patient 50 years of age or older with right lower abdominal pain. Cases of diverticulitis in the cecum or ascending colon have also been reported.

Perforation is characterized by sudden lower abdominal pain progressing to generalized abdominal involvement. Prior steroid use predisposes the patient to perforation and may mask some of the typical signs and symptoms.

Physical examination frequently demonstrates a low-grade fever, around 38°C (100.4°F). However, the temperature may be more elevated in patients with generalized peritonitis or in those who have formed an abscess. The abdominal examination reveals localized tenderness, often with voluntary guarding and rebound tenderness. With careful palpation, one may be able to appreciate a fullness or mass over the involved segment of the colon. Rectal examination will often reveal tenderness on the left side. Occult blood may be present in the stool. When free perforation does occur, diffuse abdominal tenderness, rigidity, guarding, and rebound tenderness may be noted. In the female patient, a pelvic examination should always be carried out to eliminate a gynecologic source of symptoms.

Diagnosis

The diagnosis is usually suspected by the clinical history and the findings on physical examination. The presence of peritoneal signs or generalized peritonitis should suggest free perforation or rupture of a peridiverticular abscess. The presence of an abdominal mass associated with occult blood in the stool could indicate colon cancer. Colonic or small bowel obstruction, though uncommon, may necessitate surgical intervention.

The acute abdominal series may be normal or may demonstrate associated ileus, partial small bowel obstruction, free air indicating bowel perforation, or extraluminal collections of air that might indicate a walled-off abscess. Abdominal ultrasonography is an inexpensive noninvasive method but is operator-dependent and lacks specificity. Abdominal CT is the diagnostic procedure of choice.[16] It can demonstrate inflammation of pericolic fat, presence of diverticula, thickening of the bowel wall, or peridiverticular abscess. Colon cancer is best ruled out by sigmoidoscopy or colonoscopy.

Barium contrast studies can easily demonstrate diverticula but are insensitive in detecting the presence of diverticulitis. In addition, barium introduced under high pressure carries the risk of precipitating a colonic perforation. Water soluble contrast enemas have also been used in some centers to establish the diagnosis.

Laboratory studies should include routine screening blood tests, urinalysis, and an acute abdominal series. However, these all lack sensitivity and specificity for the diagnosis. Leukocytosis was seen in only 36 percent of patients with acute diverticulitis.[17] Sigmoidoscopy or colonoscopy are generally performed only after the acute inflammatory process has subsided.

Differential Diagnosis

In patients over the age of 40 presenting with complaints of abdominal pain, a change in bowel habits, and urinary symptoms, a diagnosis of colonic diverticulitis should be entertained. These symptoms, however, are nonspecific, and a number of pathologic entities may present with similar signs and symptoms (see Table 81-2). Some of the most important are discussed below.

Symptoms of irritable bowel syndrome include diffuse crampy or colicky abdominal pain, brought on by meals or emotional upset. The patients may also describe a bloated or distended sensation in the abdomen. The symptoms are usually intermittent and chronic. The passage of flatus or a bowel movement may bring relief. The disease is characterized by alternating bouts of constipation and diarrhea. On physical examination, the patient is afebrile and a cordlike mass may be appreciated in the left lower quadrant corresponding to the sigmoid colon. Signs of localized or generalized peritonitis are not seen. Laboratory studies are normal.

Patients who have colon carcinoma may present with a change in bowel habits, either diarrhea or constipation, and/or abdominal pain that can mimic symptoms of diverticular disease. There may be blood mixed with the patient's stools and weight loss. Physical examination may reveal a palpable mass, usually nontender. Fever and chills are less common, and laboratory studies may demonstrate anemia without evidence of leukocytosis. An acute abdominal series may demonstrate findings of colonic obstruction. This can be produced by an inflamed diverticulum or a carcinoma in an area of the bowel with underlying diverticulosis. Fiberoptic colonoscopy can be useful in differentiating diverticular disease from carcinoma. A perforated colonic carcinoma may mimic acute diverticulitis.

Pelvic inflammatory disease may present with abdominal pain, fever, and leukocytosis. The disease is usually found in young women. A careful pelvic examination should be carried out in all female patients with lower abdominal pain. A history of irregular menses and the finding of vaginal discharge should aid in the diagnosis.

Ischemic colitis can present with a broad range of clinical manifestations. Mild transient ischemia may result in mucosal sloughing and painless rectal bleeding. If the disease progresses to gangrene, the patient develops severe abdominal pain and peritonitis. Pain may be out of proportion to physical findings. A plain film of the abdomen may reveal thumbprinting in the region of the involved colonic segment. In more advanced cases, there may be gas within the bowel wall, or, if perforation has occurred, free air in the abdomen. Cautious endoscopic evaluation and contrast x-ray studies are helpful in distinguishing ischemic colitis from diverticulitis.

Treatment

Initial resuscitation of patients with acute diverticulitis should focus on determining the severity of the illness, eliminating other causes of symptoms, and appropriate fluid and electrolyte resuscitation (Table 81-4). In patients who demonstrate signs of toxicity such as fever, tachycardia, leukocytosis, and severe abdominal pain, intravenous antibiotics are administered. These should include an aminoglycoside (gentamicin or tobramycin 1.5 mg/kg IV) and either clindamycin 300 to 600 mg IV or metronidazole 500 mg IV, or ticarcillin-clavulanic acid or imipenem. The patient is placed on bowel rest, but in this case, nothing by mouth is given and intravenous fluids are administered.

TABLE 81-4   Treatment of Acute Diverticulitis

Restore fluid and electrolyte balance
Nothing by mouth
Nasogastric suction for
    Obstruction
    Adynamic ileus
Broad-spectrum antibiotics
    Aminoglycoside (gentamicin or tobramycin)
    Metronidazole or clindamycin
    Ticarcillin-clavulanic acid or imipenem (alternative therapy)
Observe for complications
    Obstruction
    Perforation
    Intraabdominal abscess
Outpatient Management (nontoxic patients)
    Liquids only for first 48 h
Oral Antibiotics:
    Ampicillin, TMP/SMX, Ciprofloxacin, or Cefalexin
    and
    Metronidazole or Clindamycin

Nasogastric suction is necessary only if the patient manifests signs of bowel obstruction or an adynamic ileus.

Outpatient treatment consists of bowel rest and broad-spectrum oral antibiotic therapy. Patients are instructed to limit activity and to maintain a liquid diet for 48 h. If symptoms improve, low-residue foods are added to the diet. Broad-spectrum antibiotics covering both aerobic and anaerobic bacteria are given. Predominant colonic aerobes include *Escherichia coli, Klebsiella,* and *Enterobacter,* while *Bacteroides fragilis, Peptostreptococcus,* and *Clostridium* are the predominant colonic anaerobes. Common oral antibiotic agents effective against aerobic organisms include ampicillin (500 mg q6h), trimethoprim-sulfamethoxazole (2 tablets q12h), ciprofloxacin (500 mg q12h), or a cephalosporin such as cefalexin (500 mg q6h). One of these agents is taken in combination with metronidazole (Flagyl 500 mg q8h), or clindamycin (Cleocin 300 mg q6h), which are utilized to treat the anaerobic organisms. Practice guidelines have been developed for the care of patients with sigmoid diverticulitis.[18]

Disposition

Patients who have localized pain without signs and symptoms of local peritonitis and without evidence of systemic infection may be treated on an outpatient basis. Careful follow-up should be arranged with the patient's primary physician. Patients should be instructed to return if fever develops, if they are unable to tolerate oral intake, or if there is worsening abdominal pain.

If a patient has systemic signs and symptoms of infection, has failed outpatient management, or demonstrates signs of localized peritonitis, hospitalization is necessary. Surgical consultation should be obtained at the time of hospitalization. Urgent surgical consultation is indicated if free perforation, intestinal obstruction, abscess, or fistulas are found. In addition, early surgical involvement is indicated in immunocompromised patients and patients under the age of 45 years with diverticulitis.

REFERENCES

1. Robert JR, Sachar DB, Greenstein AJ: Severe gastrointestinal hemorrhage in Crohn's disease. *Ann Surg* 213:207, 1991.
2. Hanauer SB, Sandborn W, The Practice Parameters Committee of the American College of Gastroenterology: Management of Crohn's disease in adults. *Am J Gastroenterol* 96:635, 2001.
3. Podolsky DK: Inflammatory bowel disease. *New Engl J Med* 347:417, 2002.
4. Dubinsky MC, Hassard PV, Abreu MT, et al: Thioguanine (6-TG): A therapeutic alternative in a subgroup of IBD patients failing 6-mercaptopurine. *Gastroenterology* 118:A891, 2000.
5. Targan SR, Hanauer SB, Ven Deventer SJH, et al: A short-term study of chimeric monoclonal antibody CA2 to tumor necrosis factor α for Crohn's disease. *New Engl J Med* 337:1029, 1997.
6. Keane J, Gershon S, Wise RP, et al: Tuberculosis associated with infliximab, a tumor necrosis factor α-neutralizing agent. *New Engl J Med* 345:1098, 2001.
7. Present DH, Rutgeerts P, Targan S, et al: Infliximab for the treatment of fistulas in patients with Crohn's disease. *New Engl J Med* 340:1398, 1999.
8. Kornbluth A, Sachar DB: Ulcerative colitis practice guidelines in adults. *Am J Gastroenterol* 92:204, 1997.
9. Lichtiger S, Present DH, Kornbluth A, et al: Cyclosporine in severe ulcerative colitis refractory to steroid therapy. *New Engl J Med* 330:1841, 1994.
10. Gonzales-Huix F, Fernandez-Banares F, Esteve-Comas M, et al: Enteral versus parenteral nutrition as adjunct therapy in acute ulcerative colitis. *Am J Gastroenterol* 88:227, 1993.
11. Johnson S, Gerding DN: *Clostridium difficile*-associated diarrhea. *Clin Infect Dis* 26:1027, 1998.
12. Bartlett JG: Antibiotic-associated diarrhea. *New Engl J Med* 346:334, 2002.
13. Kelly CP, LaMont JT: *Clostridium difficile* infection. *Ann Rev* 49:375–390, 1998.
14. Jacobs A, Barnard K, Fishel R, Gradon JD: Extracolonic manifestations of *Clostridium difficile* infections: Presentation of 2 cases and review of the literature. *Medicine* 80:88, 2001.

15. Gerding DN, Johnson S, Peterson LR, et al: *Clostridium difficile*-associated diarrhea and colitis. *Infect Control Hosp Epidemiol* 16:459, 1995.

16. Johnson CD, Baker ME, Rice RP: Diagnosis of acute colonic diverticulitis: Comparison of barium enema and CT. *Am J Radiol* 148:541, 1987.

17. Ferzoco LB, Raptopoulos V, Sileu W: Acute diverticulitis. *New Engl J Med* 338:1521, 1998.

18. Standards Task Force of the American Society of Colon and Rectal Surgeons: Practice parameters for the treatment of sigmoid diverticulitis. *Dis Colon Rectum* 43:289, 2000.

ANORECTAL DISORDERS
82
Brian E. Burgess
James K. Bouzoukis

Anorectal disorders range from simple to complex, may be varied and multiple, and at times can manifest signs and symptoms of underlying serious local or systemic disorders that may be life-threatening.

ANATOMY

The rectum is an anatomic structure that begins at the S3 vertebral body and descends for about 13 to 15 cm. This entodermal intestine unites with and opens into an orifice of ectodermal origin, the anal canal, which is about 4 cm long. The junction of these two embryonic structures is the dentate line, which marks the anatomic beginning of the anal canal and is in continuity more distally with the perianal skin at the anal verge. The mucosa of the anal canal consists of stratified squamous epithelium but contains no hair follicles or sweat glands. At the anal verge, the anoderm thickens and includes in its structure hair follicles and other cutaneous appendages. Proximal to the dentate line, the rectal ampulla narrows to conform to the opening of the anal canal; in doing so its mucosa takes on a pleated appearance, forming 8 to 14 convoluted longitudinal folds: the columns of Morgagni. Each adjacent column is connected at the dentate line by a flap of mucosa that forms a small anal crypt, normally 1 to 3 mm in longitudinal depth. Connected to the crypts are a number of glands that lubricate the stool for passage. Inflammation, obstruction, and infection of these crypts and glands become the source of anal sepsis, as characterized by the development of cryptitis, perianal abscesses, and fistulas. The anal wall, from its mucosal lining to the intersphincteric space, which separates the internal from the external sphincters, is a continuation of the usual layers of the wall of the colon and rectum. The innermost lining, the mucosa, continues to the anal verge, undergoing a transition just proximal to the dentate line from rectal columnar to cuboidal to squamous epithelium. The submucosa, which normally contains the bulk of the bowel's blood vessels (and autonomic nerves), thickens considerably proximal to the dentate line. The hemorrhoidal arteries supply the anorectum, while the venous network in this area is referred to as the internal hemorrhoidal plexus. The superior (internal) hemorrhoidal veins drain into the portal system, whereas the inferior (external) hemorrhoidal veins drain into the inferior vena cava. The inner circular muscle layer of the rectum thickens considerably as it terminates distally in the anorectum to form the internal sphincter muscles. The more attenuated longitudinal muscles of the rectum extend caudally, blending with fibers of voluntary skeletal muscles from the levator ani and external sphincter groups, to form the intersphincteric space (Figure 82-1).

Additional sphincteric support is provided by an outer layer of voluntary skeletal muscles which make up the external sphincters, and are divided into three parts: deep, superficial, and subcutaneous. The external sphincters are actually a caudal extension of the puborectalis muscle, which interacts with the levator ani muscle, forming the pelvic floor. The puborectalis, the proximal external sphincters, and the internal sphincters form the ring of muscles that one palpates when performing a digital examination of the anorectum.

Lateral to the external sphincters is the ischiorectal space, and superior to the levator ani is the supralevator (pelvirectal) space, where deep, life-threatening infections can occur.

Inferior mesenteric nodes drain the proximal two-thirds of the rectum, whereas the lower one-third of the rectum and proximal anal canal are drained by both the inferior mesenteric nodes and the internal iliac nodes. The inguinal nodes usually drain lymphatics distal to the dentate line.

Parasympathetic nervous stimulation (S2-S4) supports elimination via rectal wall contraction with concomitant internal anal sphincter relaxation, while sympathetic stimulation (L1-L3) maintains continence through rectal wall inhibition and contraction of the internal anal sphincter.

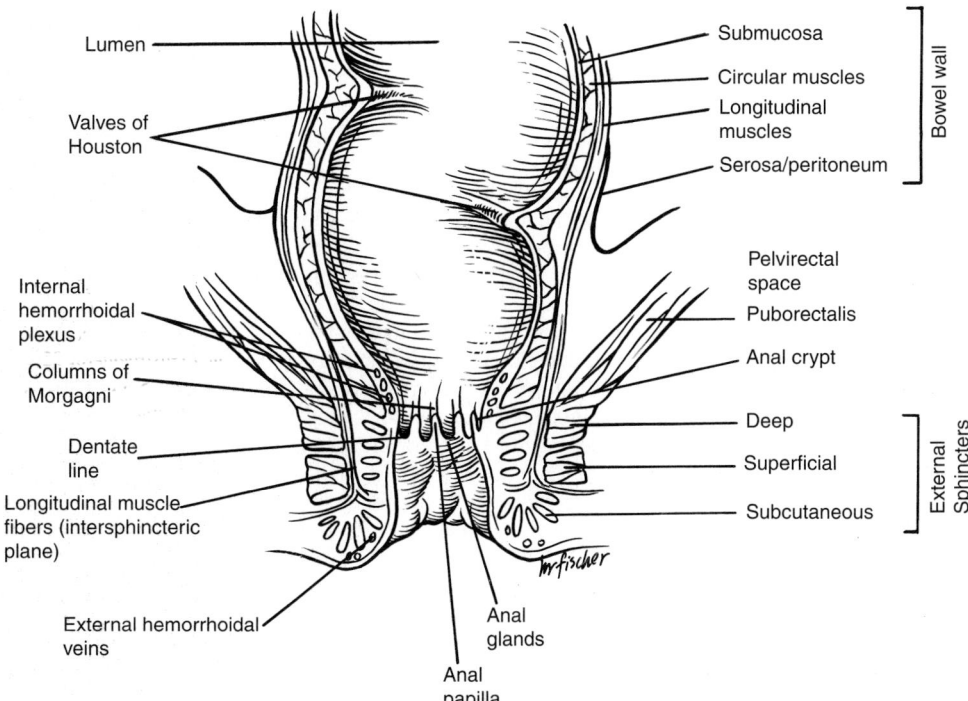

FIG. 82-1. Coronal section of the anorectum.

Lumen

Valves of Houston

Internal hemorrhoidal plexus

Columns of Morgagni

Dentate line

Longitudinal muscle fibers (intersphincteric plane)

External hemorrhoidal veins

Anal papilla

Anal glands

Submucosa

Circular muscles

Longitudinal muscles

Serosa/peritoneum

Bowel wall

Pelvirectal space

Puborectalis

Anal crypt

Deep

Superficial

Subcutaneous

External Sphincters

EXAMINATION OF THE PATIENT

No matter how much historical information is obtained, no definitive diagnosis can be made without a careful examination of the anus and rectum, including anoscopy and, if necessary, proctoscopy. Patient education before and during the examination will be helpful in obtaining maximal cooperation.

The lateral or Sims position, performed with the appropriately draped patient lying on his or her left side, with the left leg extended and the right knee and hip flexed, is probably the most commonly used approach for performing a routine digital rectal examination and is the preferred position for elderly or pregnant patients. From the Sims position, one should elevate the upper buttock to provide better exposure of the perianal area; if needed, endoscopic examination of the anus and distal rectum can be performed with the patient in this position. In debilitated patients, one may have to perform the examination with the patient in a supine, lithotomy position.

Examining a patient placed in the knee-chest position requires a cooperative patient who is not too ill or in too much distress. This provides for a thorough inspection of the perianal area and is convenient for anoscopy and proctoscopy. Thighs should be at right angles to the table with the feet extended over the end of the table.

A digital examination should always be performed before doing any endoscopic procedure. After performing a digital examination and determining that the patient will tolerate passage of an anoscope, introduce a well-lubricated, lighted anoscope, remove the obturator, and gently rotate as needed to view the anorectum circumferentially. No bowel preparation is needed to perform an anoscopic examination. It is usually difficult to perform a proper sigmoidoscopic examination in an ED setting. Ordinarily, the lower bowel must be prepped; a natural bowel movement, spontaneous or induced 1 to 2 h before examination, is usually sufficient preparation. In some acute situations, such as trying to determine the source of lower GI bleeding or obtaining cultures in a case of suppurative proctitis, emergency proctoscopy may be performed. A rigid sigmoidoscope should be utilized with the patient placed in a Sims position. An inexperienced endoscopist should not attempt to pass the sigmoidoscope beyond the rectosigmoid junction, where the lumen is greatly angulated, because of the risk of perforation.

HEMORRHOIDS

The anorectal area is drained by the internal and external hemorrhoidal venous systems. The internal hemorrhoidal veins, which in essence are submucosal vascular cushions that may contribute to anal continence, are located proximal to the dentate line and drain into the portal system through the superior rectal veins and the inferior mesenteric vein. They also communicate freely with the external hemorrhoidal veins, which are subcutaneous to the anoderm and drain primarily through the pudendal and iliac venous systems. When these hemorrhoidal plexuses become excessively engorged, prolapsed, or thrombosed, they are referred to as hemorrhoids—one of the most common problems afflicting human beings. Internal hemorrhoids course along the terminal branches of the superior rectal artery and are constant in their location, coursing longitudinally at the right posterolateral, right anterolateral, and left lateral positions (at the 2-, 5-, and 9-o'clock positions when the patient is viewed prone) (Figure 82-2). Internal hemorrhoids are not readily palpable and can best be visualized through an anoscope. Their appearance is consistent with the columnar epithelial surface of the surrounding anal canal. External hemorrhoids, which are located distal to the dentate line, form as a result of dilatation of veins at the anal verge and can be seen at external inspection. Their appearance is consistent with the stratified squamous epithelium of the surrounding anoderm with exquisite sensory innervation.

Although the cause of enlarged hemorrhoids is not always known, there is an association with constipation and straining at stool. Hem-

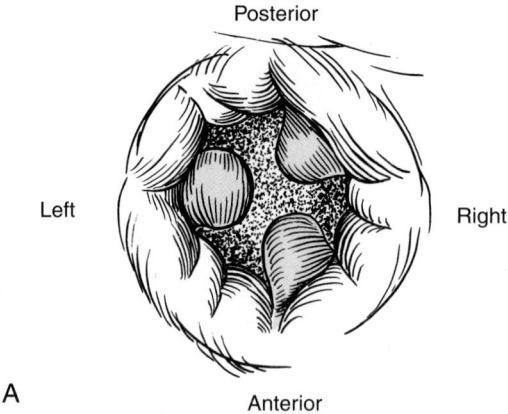

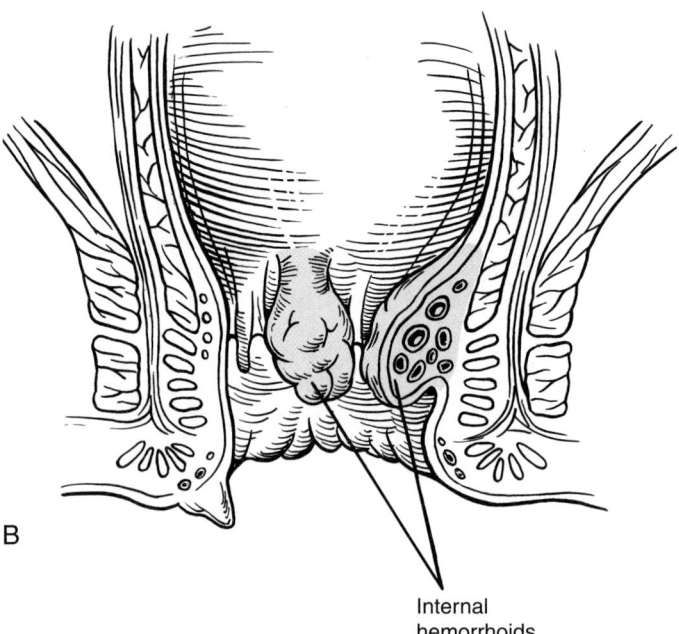

FIG. 82-2. Common sites of hemorrhoids. **A.** Internal hemorrhoids at 2, 5, and 9 o'clock. **B.** Protrusion of anal cushions.

orrhoidal veins are devoid of valves and with age they lose supportive connective tissue surrounding the vasculature which may contribute to the formation of hemorrhoids. They are prevalent during pregnancy and may be the result of sustained increased pressure on the venous drainage of the rectum. One of the physiologic shunts of the portal system involves the hemorrhoidal veins. Consequently, increased portal pressure, occurring as a result of chronic liver disease, may produce marked dilatation and varix formation of the hemorrhoids. The bleeding that can result is extremely difficult to control.

Tumors of the rectum and sigmoid colon, often associated with constipation, tenesmus, and incomplete evacuation, may cause hemorrhoids and must be ruled out in all cases of rectal bleeding in patients over the age of 40. Ascites, ovarian tumors, distended bladders, and excessive fibrosis from radiation therapy may contribute to the formation of external hemorrhoids.

Clinical Features

Hemorrhoids may become more prominent as one strains, whereby a few localized curvilinear swellings may appear. Uncomplicated internal hemorrhoids are painless due to lack of sensory innervation, and the chief complaint is painless, bright-red rectal bleeding with defecation. Bleeding is usually limited, with the blood being found on the surface of the stool, on the toilet tissue, or dripping into the toilet bowl. Internal hemorrhoids may be palpable on digital examination when thrombosed or prolapsed.[1] Nonreducible, prolapsed internal hemorrhoids may become thrombosed and gangrenous, exhibiting exquisite pain. Painless bleeding may also occur with external hemorrhoidal bleeding; however, pain is usually present when the external hemorrhoids become thrombosed. External thrombosed hemorrhoids usually exhibit a bluish-purple discoloration. Pain, when present, may be noted with palpation, can be quite severe at the time of defecation, and usually subsides with time. Although the most common cause of rectal bleeding is hemorrhoids, other, more serious causes should be sought in all patients who present with bleeding as the chief complaint. Clinical signs cannot reliably differentiate colonic lesions from hemorrhoids.[2] Chronic, slow blood loss may go unnoticed, but can result in significant anemia. As they increase in size, hemorrhoids may prolapse, requiring periodic reduction by the patient. Internal hemorrhoids may be classified as first degree, which do not prolapse; second degree, which prolapse and spontaneously reduce; third degree, which prolapse and require manual reduction; and fourth degree, which prolapse and are not reducible. When prolapse occurs, the patient may develop a mucous discharge and pruritus ani.

If the prolapse cannot be reduced, strangulation can result. Other complications include severe bleeding, thrombosis, infarction, gangrene, sepsis, and hepatic abscess formation. Both strangulation and thrombosis are extremely painful and are accompanied by significant edema that must be treated before surgical intervention. Ulceration of the overlying mucosa may also occur. External skin tags from old thrombosed external hemorrhoids may occasionally be noted on examination.[1]

Treatment

Most treatment is local and nonsurgical unless a complication such as acute thrombosis and gangrene is present. This conservative therapy is suggested for mild to moderate symptomatic patients with first- to third-degree hemorrhoids. Manual reduction of an uncomplicated, prolapsed internal hemorrhoid in a patient with minimal symptoms, along with warm sitz baths (decreasing sphincter pressures) for at least 15 min three times a day and after each bowel movement are the most effective way to relieve pain. Following the bath, the anus must be dried gently but thoroughly to avoid maceration of the perianal skin. Topical analgesics and steroid-containing ointments may provide relief. The patient should not sit on the commode for a prolonged period. Bulk laxatives, such as psyllium seed compounds, or other stool softeners should be used after the acute phase is treated. Laxatives causing liquid stool must be avoided; this can result in cryptitis and anal sepsis. The addition of bran or other forms of roughage to the patient's diet should help to prevent future problems.

As a rule, internal hemorrhoids will bleed and treatment most often involves conservative observation with the addition of stool softeners and a high-fiber diet. Surgical consultation in the emergency department should be obtained for fourth-degree incarcerated internal hemorrhoids.

External hemorrhoidal hematoma formation is usually self-limiting with resolution in 1 week. External hemorrhoids may thrombose and selection of therapy for thrombosed external hemorrhoids depends on the severity of symptoms. If the thrombosis has been present more than 48 h, the swelling is not tense, and the pain is tolerable, the patient may be treated with sitz baths and bulk laxatives. Suppositories, which are placed proximal to the anorectal ring, are of no help. If, on the other hand, thrombosis is acute, has lasted less than 48 h, and is extremely painful, significant relief can be provided by excising the clots. With the patient in side-lying or prone position, the area of the overlying skin to be incised is infiltrated with a local anesthetic such

as bupivacaine (Marcaine) 0.5 percent with epinephrine (1:200,000) and bicarbonate using a 30-gauge needle.[1] While applying gentle traction to the skin adjacent to the thrombosed hemorrhoid, an elliptical incision distal to the anal verge is made in the overlying skin, exposing the thrombosis, which is then locally excised through the opening (Figure 82-3). Because of the multiloculated clots that are invariably present, the technique of unroofing a thrombosed hemorrhoid with an elliptical incision and removing the overlying skin gives far better results than the simple incision and evacuation of a clot. Bleeding is controlled by tucking the corner of a small piece of gauze into the wound and leaving it in place for a few hours. A small pressure dressing may be applied external to the gauze and removed when the patient takes the first sitz bath 6 to 12 h after the drainage procedure. Narcotics may be prescribed, but only judiciously, since they cause constipation and may produce more problems. Complications such as continued bleeding, recurrence, infection, fistula, and abscess formation may occur and close follow-up care is therefore suggested. Referral for definitive hemorrhoidectomy is also prudent. Emergent surgical consultation and intervention for hemorrhoids is indicated for: continued and severe bleeding, incarceration and/or strangulation (fourth-degree hemorrhoids), and intractable pain. Incarcerated hemorrhoids are quite painful, may become infected, develop necrosis, and may be associated with urinary retention.[1] In general, for less urgent hemorrhoids surgical treatment, usually as a referral, can consist of sclerosing injections, the use of rubber-band ligation,[3] photocoagulation, cryotherapy, electrocautery, or excision. Up to 5 percent of patients undergoing rubber-band ligation may develop acute thrombosis of external hemorrhoids, and immunocompromised patients so treated may develop pelvic sepsis. Excision should not be performed in the ED on immunocompromised patients, pediatric patients, pregnant patients, patients with portal hypertension, and those who are anticoagulated.

CRYPTITIS

Anal crypts are the superficial mucosal pockets that lie between the columns of Morgagni (Figure 82-4). They are formed by the puckering action of the sphincter muscles and normally flatten out during the passage of a stool. Sphincter spasm and superficial trauma caused by repeated bouts of diarrhea, or trauma produced by evacuation of large, hard stools associated with constipation cause breakdown in the mucosal lining of the crypts. This permits infecting organisms to enter pockets and inflammation to extend into the lymphoid tissue of both the crypts and anal glands. Cryptitis could well be the common denominator for the development of fissure in ano, fistula in ano, and perirectal abscesses.

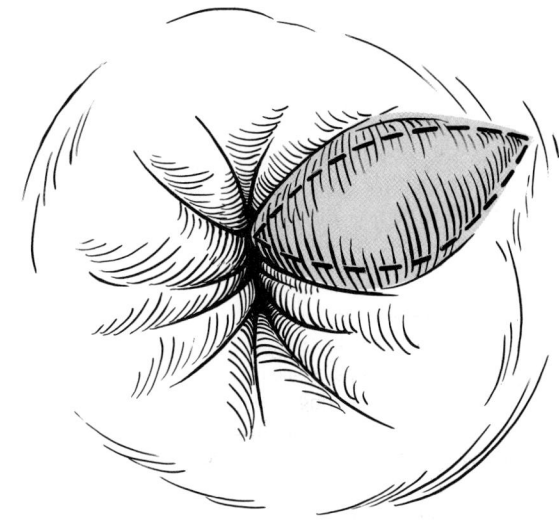

FIG. 82-3. Elliptical excision of thrombosed external hemorrhoid.

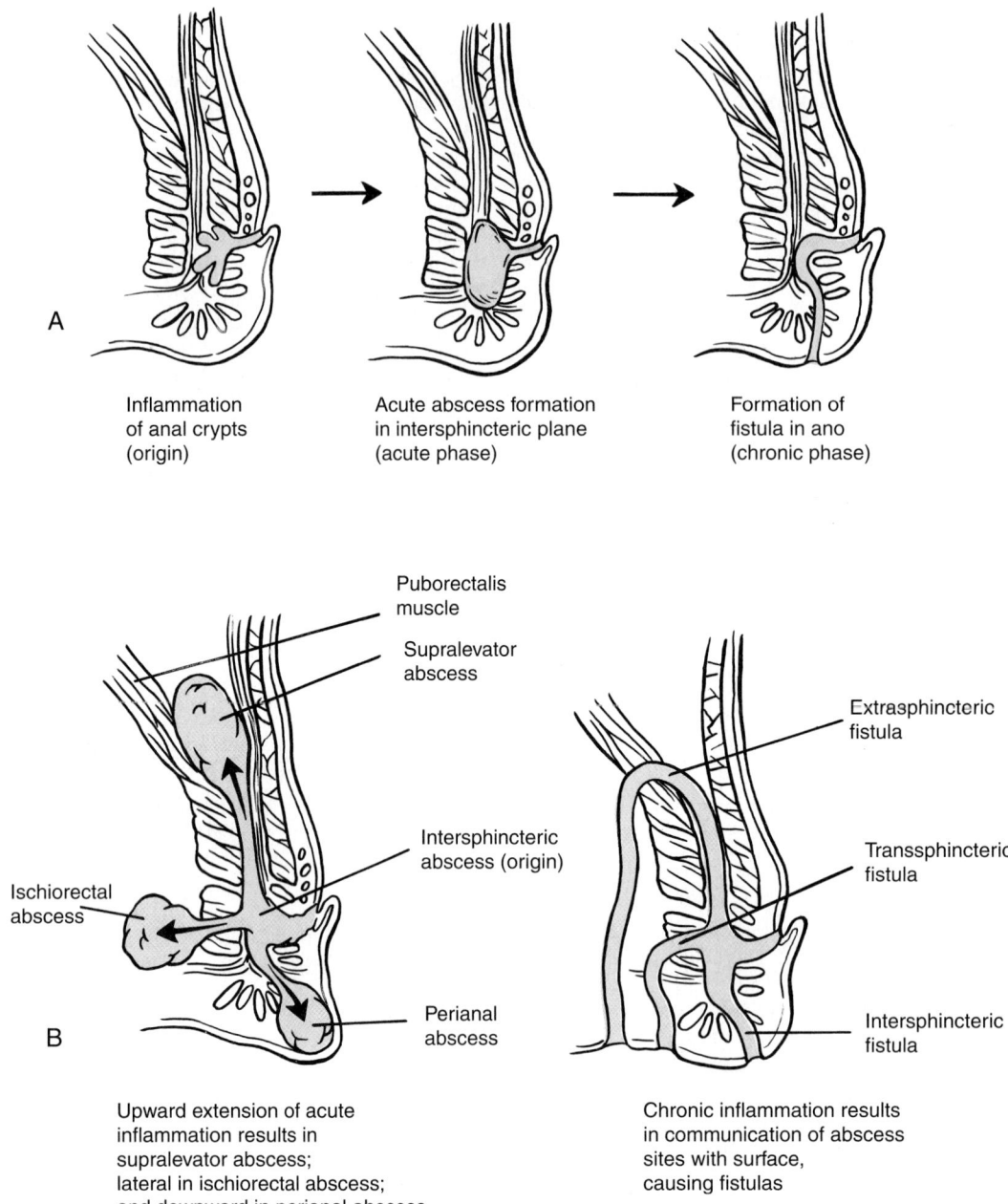

FIG. 82-4. Illustration of mechanism for anorectal abscess and fistula formation.

Associated with cryptitis is the development of hypertrophied anal papillae, which lie between adjacent crypts. When hypertrophy occurs, the papillae may be palpated as small, hard nodules along the wall of the anal canal. Rarely, papillae may hypertrophy and present as a prolapsing polypoid tumor. The crypts most commonly involved are in the posterior half of the anal ring, and in most cases, in the posterior midline, the same location where anal fissures occur.

Clinical Features

Initially, the locally inflamed crypts produce no symptoms, but as the trauma from recurrent diarrhea or passage of large, hard stools continues, the inflammation of the crypts extends to the adjacent papillae, producing an edematous swelling of the sensitive anoderm that lines this part of the canal. At this stage the patient will experience pain with bowel movements, and if there is an associated papillitis or fissure in ano, there will also be a small amount of bleeding. Anal pain, spasm, and itching with or without bleeding are the cardinal signs and symptoms of cryptitis.

Treatment

Treatment of anal cryptitis, which should be conservative, is based on establishing a definitive diagnosis and ruling out the possibility of more serious anorectal problems. The diagnosis can be suspected clinically from the history and the palpation of the tender, swollen crypt and its associated hypertrophied papillae. Definitive diagnosis of cryptitis is made by anoscopic examination.

The goal of treatment is to control the trauma of abnormal bowel movements and thus enable the inflammation to subside. Bulk laxatives and additional roughage added to the diet to produce formed, soft stools and hot sitz baths both enhance healing by keeping the anus clean and the crypts empty.

Surgical referral is indicated when the infection has progressed and there is a deep, redundant crypt that will not drain adequately on its own. Gentle insertion of a hooked probe into the crypts brought into view through the anoscope will reveal the involved crypt(s) to be deeper than normal and definitely more tender. In these cases, the roof

FIG
anal

(mucosal surface), as outlined by the passage of a hooked probe, should be infiltrated with local anesthetic and excised. Thus what had been a deep pocket is converted into an open wound that should heal with proper control of bowel movements and frequent sitz baths.

FISSURE IN ANO (ANAL FISSURE)

This disorder is the result of a superficial linear tear of the anal canal beginning at or just below the dentate line and extending distally along the anal canal, to the anal verge (see Figure 82-4). The epithelium in this area consists of anoderm, which has a rich supply of somatic sensory nerve fibers. Consequently, anal fissures are the most common cause of painful rectal bleeding. Anal fissures are common among children and young adults and are the most frequent cause of rectal bleeding in infants.[4]

in
(se
wh
tha
cia
sei
bo
fo
po
in
(F
an
ca

C

A
n
ri
al
n
o
u
q
U
c
a
c

Anal fissures, as they become more chronic, are often associated with swelling of the surrounding tissues and raised edges, producing hypertrophic papillae proximally and the characteristic sentinel pile distally. The latter is frequently misdiagnosed as an external hemorrhoid when in actuality it is the result of edema and fibrosis secondary to the ulcerating fissure. In more than 90 percent of cases, anal fissures occur in the midline posteriorly. In 10 percent to 40 percent of women but in only 1 percent of men it may be in the midline anteriorly. This almost constant location of anal fissures may be because of the posterior angulation of the rectum on the anus where the posterior midline of the anorectal canal becomes the "lesser curvature" for the passage of stool. Women may develop anterior fissures postpartum. A fissure not located in the midline should arouse suspicion that another, potentially life-threatening cause may be involved. Such diagnostic possibilities include Crohn disease, chronic ulcerative colitis, squamous cell carcinoma of the anus, adenocarcinoma of the rectum invading the anal canal, localized anal cancers such as Bowen disease and extramammary Paget disease, leukemia, lymphoma, syphilitic fissures, chlamydia, gonorrhea, and a tuberculous ulcer. Such patients must be referred for a diagnostic biopsy of the ulcer edge, culture of the anal canal, and a systemic evaluation. Interestingly, fissures due to Crohn disease and tuberculosis are often painless whereas fissures associated with AIDS are painful and may be associated with incontinence. Painless fissures associated with Crohn disease are often associated with external skin tags.[4]

Most often, the traditional midline anal fissure is caused by the trauma produced by the passage of a particularly hard and large fecal mass, but it is also seen after frequent acute episodes of diarrhea. Children with constipation will commonly complain of painful defecation only to find an anal fissure upon closer inspection. Fissures persist because of the severe, chronic internal sphincter spasm that occurs along with the secondary infection of its base.

Clinical Features

Pain of the sharp, cutting variety is the most common symptom. Typically, the pain is most severe during and immediately after a bowel movement. The pain may persist as a dull ache for a few hours after each bowel movement, but invariably it subsides between movements, which is a feature that distinguishes fissures from other forms of painful anorectal disease. The bleeding is bright red and small in quantity, usually being noticed only on the toilet paper. In infants, the presence of small amounts of bright blood on the stool or toilet paper is usually the presenting complaint for an anal fissure. Sphincter spasm and pain may be severe enough to make the patient retain stool and avoid defecation.

The diagnosis of anal fissure is usually suggested by the history; however, the anal area must be examined in all cases. With proper exposure, the sentinel pile, if present, and frequently the distal end of the fissure itself, may be seen. The mere retraction of the buttocks and the anal skin may cause considerable discomfort; sphincter spasm may be so severe that the patient will not permit digital examination. Application of a topical anesthetic may provide some relief. If the fissure can be visualized and is present in the posterior midline, rectal examination can be deferred until the patient is having less spasm and pain.

Treatment

Treatment is aimed at providing symptomatic relief, relieving the anal sphincter spasm, and preventing stricture formation. Hot sitz baths for at least 15 min three to four times a day and after each bowel movement will relax the sphincter and provide symptomatic relief. The addition of bran to the diet will serve to prevent stricture formation by providing a bulky stool. Local analgesic ointments provide symptomatic relief. The use of hydrocortisone-containing ointments does provide relief and helps with healing. In a study that compared the effectiveness of these three modalities, most rapid healing of fissures occurred with sitz baths and a diet rich in bran, though healing was aided by both, an analgesic ointment or a hydrocortisone-containing ointment. Meticulous anal hygiene is imperative; following defecation, the anus must be cleaned thoroughly. Healing is by the development of granulation tissue and the reepithelialization of the ulcerated area. Relapse rate after medical treatment for chronic anal fissures has been noted as high as 50 percent. If healing does not occur in a reasonable amount of time or relapses are frequent, anal dilatation or operative treatment consisting of partial sphincterotomy and excision of the fissure may be required.

ANORECTAL ABSCESSES

Abscesses are frequently encountered in the perianal and perirectal region. Almost all begin with involvement of an anal crypt and its gland. The mechanism involves obstruction of an anal gland that opens in the base of an anal crypt which normally drains into the anal canal. When obstruction occurs, the gland orifice is blocked, resulting in infection and abscess formation. The abscesses are typically polymicrobial with both aerobic and anaerobic bacteria. As they persist fistula formation may develop as a common chronic sequela. From there, the infection can progress to involve any of the potential spaces that are normally filled with fatty areolar tissue and have little inherent resistance to the progression of infection. These spaces, which can become infected alone or in combination with each other, are as follows: the perianal space, the intersphincteric space, the ischiorectal space, the deep postanal space (connecting the ischiorectal space on each side posteriorly), and the supralevator or pelvirectal space (Figures 82-4 and 82-5). An element of cryptitis can frequently be identified by anoscopic examination.

The perianal abscess is most common and the supralevator abscess occurs least often. It presents close to the anal verge, posterior midline, as a superficial tender mass, which may or may not be fluctuant. In contradistinction, ischiorectal abscesses, which are second most common, tend to be larger, indurated, well circumscribed, and are present more laterally, on the medial aspect of the buttocks. Usually the patient will exhibit swelling, fever, and anorexia. Deeper perirectal abscesses may not manifest cutaneous signs, but rectal pain and tenderness are invariably present. The isolated perianal abscess not associated with deeper, perirectal abscesses is the only type of anorectal abscess that can be adequately treated in an ED setting. Although clinical evaluation of abscesses is usually sufficient, if pain is out of proportion to physical findings or if the extent of the abscess is uncertain, ultrasonography can be helpful.[5]

Ischiorectal and other deep abscesses pose a different problem. The ischiorectal fossa forms a large potential space on either side of the rectum, communicating behind it through the deep postanal space, and in males has extensions anteriorly above the perineal membrane to the prostate. Intersphincteric, submucous, and supralevator abscesses may not present with swelling, though they usually exhibit constitutional

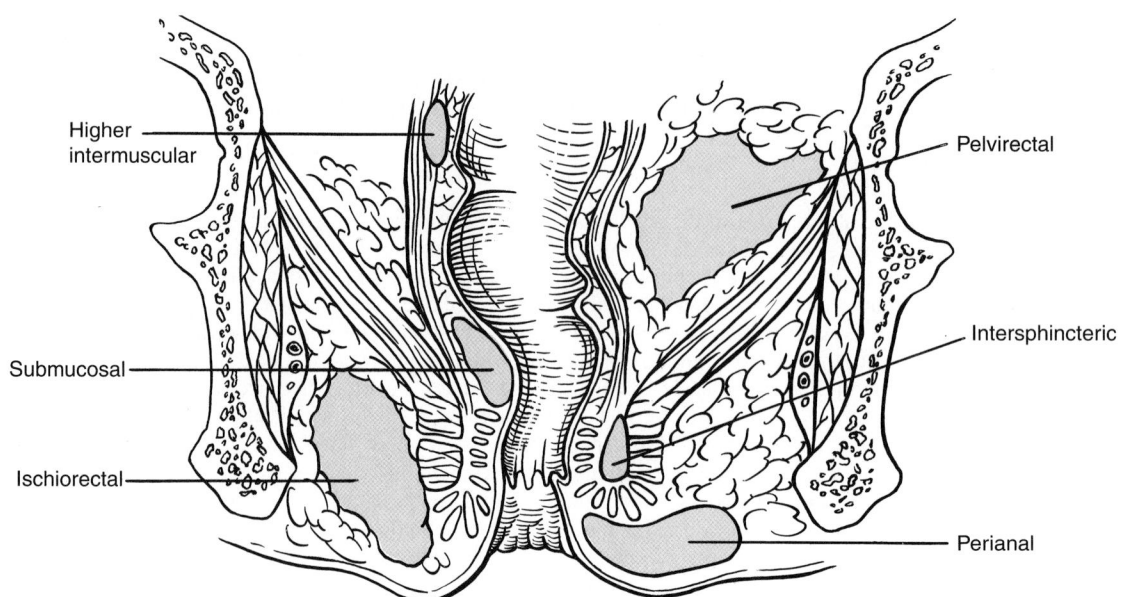

FIG. 82-5. Anatomical classification of common anorectal abscesses.

symptoms. Infections in this area are insidious and extensive and can spread to an area some distance from the anal verge. These abscesses can be large, and yet only a diffuse, nonfluctuant, tender "mass" may be palpable either through the rectal wall or the overlying skin. If only induration is present, endorectal ultrasonography,[5] needle localization, exam under anesthesia, CT scanning, or magnetic resonance imaging (MRI) may be needed to confirm the diagnosis. Ultrasound may be more useful to diagnose intersphincteric and submucosal abscesses, whereas CT or MRI are capable of detecting those as well as deeper abscess formations such as supralevator and ischiorectal rectal abscesses.

A variety of diseases and other conditions are associated with the development of fistulous abscesses, including Crohn's disease; carcinoma of adjacent organs; radiation fibrosis; trauma; Hodgkin's disease; tuberculosis; gonococcal proctitis; lymphogranuloma venereum; immunocompromised states; and infections by *Chlamydia, Actinomyces,* Herpes, *Staphylococcus aureus, Streptococcus* spp., *E. coli, Proteus,* and *Bacteroides..*

Clinical Features

Anorectal abscesses are more common in young middle-aged males. Initially, the patient notices a dull, aching, or throbbing pain that becomes worse immediately before defecation, is lessened after defecation, but persists between bowel movements. The pain, significantly increased by the increased pressure in the rectum, occurs just before defecation. Acute prostatis is in the differential diagnosis. Perianal abscesses, easily palpable, are usually not accompanied by fever, leukocytosis, and sepsis in the immunocompetent patient.

As the abscess spreads, increases in size, and comes nearer to the surface, the associated pain becomes more intense. Pain will be aggravated by straining, coughing, or sneezing. As the abscess progresses, pain and tenderness interfere with walking or sitting. Ischiorectal abscesses are painful and may express fewer outward signs upon examination; however, as they become larger, they may become indurated and erythematous more lateral to the anal verge compared to the perianal abscess. The patient appears markedly uncomfortable and may be febrile. A tender mass may be present upon rectal examination or there may be a tender, erythematous area with or without fluctuance. Leukocytosis may be present. Intersphincteric abscesses exhibit pain with defecation, may be associated with rectal discharge and fever, and a tender mass may be palpable on digital examination. Supralevator abscesses in contrast often present with few outward

signs as the patient complains of buttock or perirectal pain. Fever, leukocytosis, and at times urinary retention are not uncommon.[1]

Treatment

Treatment is surgical and should be performed as soon as the diagnosis is made, before the abscesses become fluctuant. Drainage should be both early and extensive. All perirectal abscesses (supralevator, intersphincteric, and complicated ischiorectal) should be drained in the operating room. Despite apparently adequate incision and drainage under local anesthesia, there is a relatively high incidence of recurrent abscess formation requiring a second procedure.

Isolated, simple, fluctuant perianal abscesses that are not associated with the presence of any deeper abscesses may be drained using local anesthetics and often, procedural sedation, in an ED setting. The local anesthetic should be administered with the finest-gauge needle available (30-gauge) and should be accompanied by the administration of systemic analgesia or conscious sedation. Needle aspiration over the painful region may be done to localize the pus if needed. If a simple, linear drainage incision is made, the abscess is more likely to recur because of premature closure of skin edges. Whenever this technique is used the abscess cavity must be packed initially with strips of gauze for at least 24 h. These patients will require closer follow-up care and definitive surgical repair should be considered. To ensure adequate drainage, a cruciate incision can be made over the fluctuant part of the abscess (Figures 82-6A and B). No packing is required, but if it is used it should be removed in 24 h. The wound should be covered with a bulk dressing; sitz baths should be started the next day.

As a rule, antibiotics are not necessary after an abscess has been adequately drained. On the other hand, patients with fever, leukocytosis, valvular heart disease, or those with cellulitis should be given broad-spectrum antibiotics. Patients whose immune system may be compromised by diabetes mellitus, inflammatory bowel disease, AIDS, malignancies, and chemotherapy should be given broad-spectrum antibiotics. Surgical consultation and strong consideration for admission would be prudent. Current tetanus immunization should be noted. Delay in appropriate treatment may lead to sphincter dysfunction.

FISTULA IN ANO

An anal fistula is an abnormal tract that connects the anal canal with the skin and is lined with epithelium and granulation tissue. A fistula

FIG. 82-6. Technique of drainage of perianal abscess.

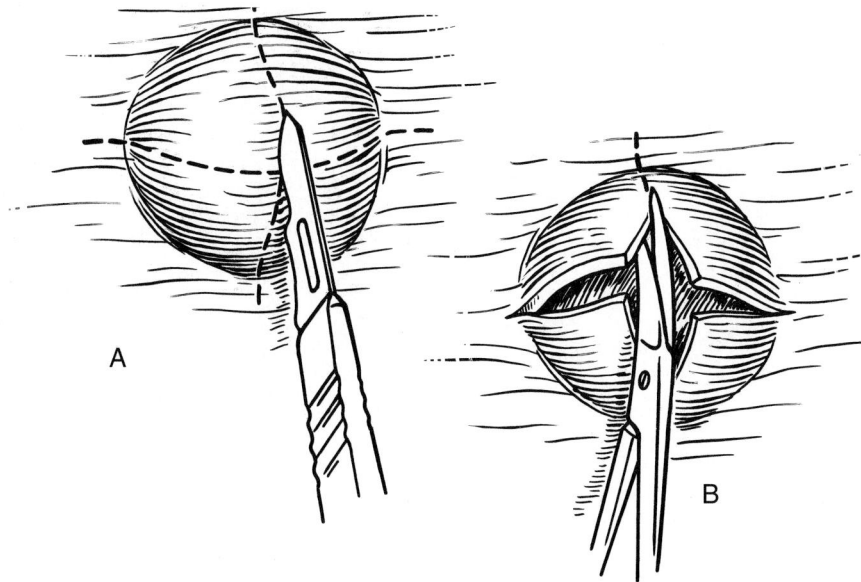

in ano most commonly results from a perianal or ischiorectal abscess (see Figure 82-4). These abscesses usually originate in the glands, which are located in the intersphincteric space and have drainage ducts that empty at the level of the dentate line. These fistulae may be associated with ulcerative colitis, Crohn disease, colonic malignancies, sexually transmitted disease, actinomycosis, anal fissures, foreign bodies, or tuberculosis. Although anterior-opening fistulas tend to follow a simple, direct course to the anal canal (Goodsall's rule), posterior-opening fistulas may follow a devious, curving path, including some that are horseshoe-shaped, opening in the posterior midline (Figure 82-7). Crohn disease should be considered in patients with anorectal disorders when rectal strictures, painless fissures, skin tags, cavitating ulcers, and complex fistulae are present.

Clinical Features

As long as the tract remains open, there is a persistent, blood-stained, malodorous discharge. More commonly, the tract becomes blocked periodically, producing bouts of inflammation and even local, recurrent abscess formation that is relieved by spontaneous rupture. An abscess may be the only sign of fistula in ano. This underscores the importance of an accurate diagnosis for successful treatment. Ultrasound has been used to identify intersphincteric fistula development, though inadequate focal length precludes sufficient examination of deeper fistulae. Ultrasound utilizing a 7-MHz endoprobe and enhanced with a 3 percent hydrogen peroxide solution has been used to identify fistula in ano, and appears to be superior, increasing accuracy from 62 to 95 percent compared to traditional perianal ultrasound.[6] (Figures 82-8A and

B). High-resolution MRI and possibly endoluminal MRI are often the tests of choice for detecting simple fistulae as well as more complex interconnecting and deeper fistulae.

Treatment

The only definitive treatment is surgical excision. Improperly excised fistulas may result in permanent fecal incontinence.

VENEREAL PROCTITIS

Sexually transmitted diseases (STDs) of the anorectum are not uncommon among patients who practice anal sex. The infecting organisms that cause AIDS, gonorrhea, and syphilis are essentially the same ones that are transmitted via vaginal coitus; infection is transmitted and perpetuated almost entirely by men who fail to use condoms (Table 82-1). Exceptions to this are seen in women whose lymphogranuloma venereum (LGV) due to chlamydial infection extends directly to the rectum from the vagina, and on occasions when there is contamination of the anus by gonococcal-laden discharge emanating from the urethra or cervix.

As a rule, if the patient has an anorectal infection caused by one of the STD organisms, the assumption must be made that another STD may be present; appropriate blood tests must be obtained, and patients should be anoscoped or proctoscoped in order to obtain specimens for Gram stain as well as for viral and bacterial cultures.

Clinical Features

Most venereal diseases involving the anorectal area manifest themselves initially with itching, seepage, and mild pain or irritation. Some infections may persist with mild to minimal symptoms, rendering the patient a carrier of the disease. Most venereal infections, however, will produce significant symptoms of pain, bleeding, and discharge in addition to bothersome pruritus.

CONDYLOMATA ACUMINATA Condylomata acuminata, commonly known as anal warts, are caused by a papillomavirus and are probably sexually transmitted in more than 90 percent of cases. They begin as discrete, soft, fleshy growths on the skin of the perianal area as well as on the squamous epithelium of the anal canal. Occasionally, the mucosa of the lower rectum becomes involved. Patients usually first notice the presence of a growth in the perianal area as well as

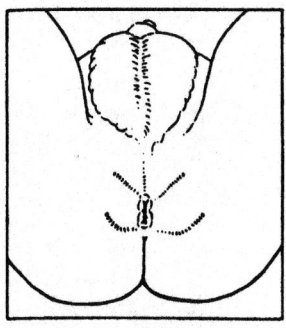
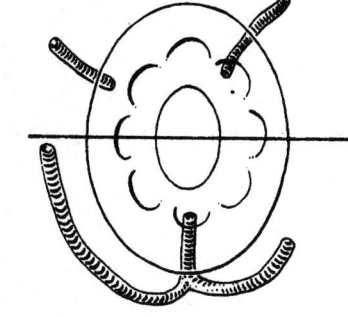

FIG. 82-7. Goodsall's rule.

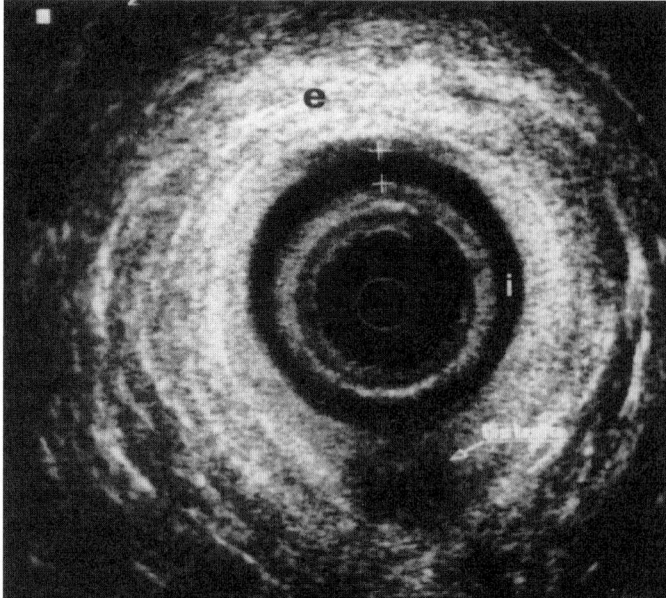

A

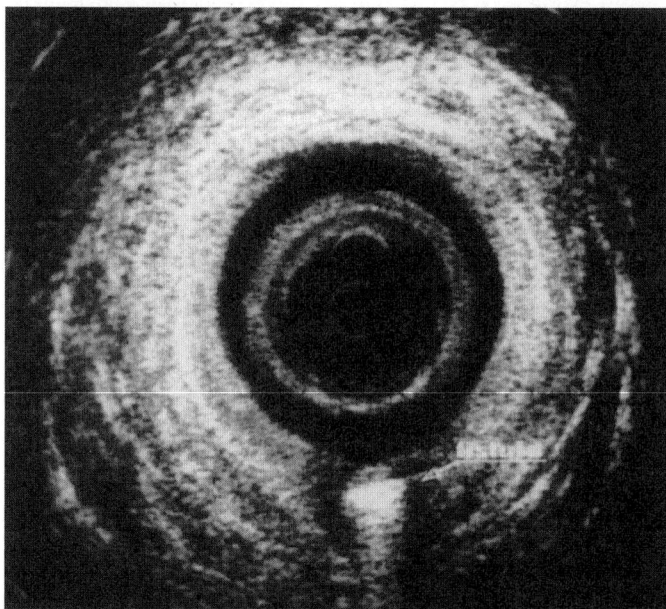

B

FIG. 82-8. A. Transanal ultrasound of a simple transsphincteric fistula. The dark hypoechoic area *(arrow)* is visible dorsally in the external anal sphincter. **B.** Transanal ultrasound after infusion of hydrogen peroxide revealing a hyperechoic fistula. E = external sphincter; I = internal sphincter.

associated pruritus and varying degrees of anal pain. With time, bleeding and anal discharge become part of the symptom complex. Evaluation of a patient with condyloma acuminata should include screening for HIV, *Chlamydia,* syphilis, gonorrhea, herpes, hepatitis, cytomegalovirus, and *Giardia.* Topical podophyllum and chemotherapy have been used in the past but the recurrence rate is significant. These patients should be referred to an appropriate specialist for definitive treatment involving laser ablation, cryotherapy, electrocautery, immunotherapy, and surgical excision. Overall recurrence remains at about 40 percent. Because cases of squamous cell carcinoma arising in association with condyloma acuminata have been reported, multiple biopsies must be taken.

TABLE 82-1 Anorectal Sexually Transmitted Diseases

Bacteria
   Neisseria gonorrhoeae
   Chlamydia trachomatis
   Treponema pallidum
Viruses
   Herpes simplex type 2
   Human immunodeficiency virus
   Papillomavirus

GONORRHEA Symptoms of gonococcal proctitis vary, ranging from none to the more common symptoms of severe rectal pain with profuse yellow, bloody discharge. The symptoms usually start about 1 week after exposure. Patients in the acute phase generally have mild burning and/or pruritus with some purulent seepage. Anoscopic examination during this phase of the disease reveals marked hyperemia and edema of the rectal mucosa and diffuse inflammation with purulent discharge from the anal crypts. Unlike nonvenereal cryptitis, infection is not confined to the posterior crypt. Diagnosis is made by Gram stain and cultures. Dissemination involving the heart, liver, CNS, and joints should be considered.

CHLAMYDIAL INFECTIONS *Chlamydia trachomatis* is an obligate human intracellular parasite that causes, among other conditions, both urogenital and anorectal infections. The lymphogranulomatous (LGV) variety occurs mainly in tropical and subtropical climates. Infection can involve the rectum by perirectal lymphatic invasion from vaginal seeding or from direct anorectal mucosal infections. The non-LGV chlamydial organisms may infect the rectal mucosa, although they do not cause the extensive rectal scarring and stricturing that its lymph gland–invading cousin from the tropics does. A patient with chlamydial proctitis may be asymptomatic or may present with nonspecific symptoms, including anal pruritus, pain, and purulent discharge. Tenesmus and bleeding may also be present.

The more severe form of proctitis occurring with this infection is usually due to the LGV type of chlamydia. Acutely painful anal ulcerations associated with prominent unilateral lymph node enlargement can be noted. Fever and constitutional flulike symptoms may be seen. In addition to rectal scarring which is a late sequela, infection of the perirectal tissue results in perirectal abscesses and chronic fistulas.

Red, friable mucosa may be seen on anoscopy. *Chlamydia* may be identified by culture. The LGV forms may be distinguished from the non-LGV variety by the Frei intradermal test or the LGV complement fixation test. Immunofluorescent antibody testing is the diagnostic test of choice. Treatments for the non-LGV chlamydial proctitis include the standard treatments for *Chlamydia.* Treatment for LGV chlamydial infections should be maintained for at least 21 days.

SYPHILIS The causative agent is the spirochete *Treponema pallidum.* Chancres that form a few weeks after infection are the characteristic lesion of primary syphilis and usually manifest themselves at the anal verge or in the anal canal. Rarely will a chancre involve the rectal mucosa, although proctitis due to syphilis can occur in the absence of a chancre. Syphilitic chancres are typically painless, although anal chancres are often very painful. If they are not identified and treated, they will resolve and the patient will proceed to develop secondary and tertiary syphilis. Condylomata lata, which are flatter and firmer than condylomata acuminata, appear in the perianal region as a manifestation of the secondary stage of syphilis. The fluorescent treponemal antibody (FTA) test becomes positive in about 1 month, and the rapid plasma regain (RPR) and the Venereal Disease Research Laboratory (VDRL) tests are also commonly used to diagnose syphilis. AIDS patients may remain nonreactive and CNS infections are not uncommon.

HERPES Anorectal herpes is almost always caused by the type 2 herpes simplex virus (HSV-2). Symptoms occur within a few weeks after exposure and consist of itching and soreness in the perianal area, progressing to severe anorectal pain. Initially, the virus manifests itself as small, discrete groups of vesicles superimposed on an erythematous base. These vesicles enlarge, coalesce, and rupture, forming exquisitely tender aphthous ulcers that appear on the perianal skin, the anoderm, and even the rectal mucosa. The pain and tenesmus from these lesions may be so intense that the patient is reluctant to have a bowel movement, resulting in constipation and possibly fecal impaction. The patient may develop a flulike illness with inguinal adenopathy noted on examination during the initial course of the illness. Symptoms persist for 1 to 2 weeks and are frequently recurrent, though less pronounced, during the ensuing year. Topical analgesia may be needed for adequate examination. Viral cultures and immunofluorescent testing are helpful for diagnosis. Treatment consisting of adequate pain medication, stool softeners, and acyclovir is in order.

AIDS-RELATED INFECTIONS   Ironically, infection of the rectum by the human immunodeficiency virus (HIV) per se does not cause any local reaction or symptoms, but its effect on the patient inoculated with this virus can be devastating. Patients who have been rendered immunodeficient by HIV are subject to a variety of opportunistic infections that affect the intestinal, anorectal, and other body systems. Infections with herpes simplex type 1 as well as type 2 are commonly seen in AIDS patients. Protozoal infections involving *Entamoeba histolytica* and *Giardia lamblia* may affect the homosexual population following oral-anal sex. Crampy, abdominal pain with diarrhea, occasionally bloody and malodorous, is frequently present with both. Testing stool for ova and parasites confirms the diagnosis. Table 82-2 lists other common enteric organisms that infect AIDS patients. Severe rectal pain, diarrhea, and hematochezia are common presenting symptoms.

Treatment

Success in the management of patients with acute venereal proctitis depends on suspecting the diagnosis, obtaining specimens to confirm the diagnosis, and initiating therapy as expeditiously as possible. Patients presenting with symptoms of anorectal pain, rectal discharge, and/or tenesmus should be considered to have proctitis until proven otherwise. Anoscopy or proctoscopy and a Gram stain should be performed to document the presence of acute proctitis. In addition to the appropriate culture specimens, blood should be drawn to check for syphilis.

Antibiotic therapy should not be delayed pending the results of cultures. Empirical therapy aimed at eradicating gonorrhea, non-LGV chlamydia, and incubating syphilis should be initiated for any patient presenting with symptoms and physical signs suggestive of acute proctitis. This therapy should be administered to all patients with acute proctitis even if there are concomitant lesions suggestive of herpetic or papillomavirus infections. As is the case for STDs in general, these patients must be referred for appropriate follow-up to ensure completion of therapy and eradication of disease.

RECTAL PROLAPSE

Rectal prolapse, known as procidentia, is the circumferential protrusion of part or all layers of the rectum through the anal canal. There

TABLE 82-2   Anorectal AIDS-Related Infections

Herpes simplex type 1
Mycobacterium avium-intracellulare
Cytomegalovirus
Salmonella enterocolitis
Shigella
Campylobacter
Entamoeba
Giardia

are three classes of rectal prolapse: (1) prolapse involving the rectal mucosa only, (2) prolapse involving all layers of the rectum, and (3) intussusception of the upper rectum into and through the lower rectum so that the apex of the intussusception protrudes through the anus.

In the first group, seen primarily in children under the age of 2, the prolapse occurs because of the loose attachment of the mucosa to the submucosal layers, and there is an associated weakness of the anal sphincter. In the second and third groups, prolapse occurs because of the laxity of the pelvic fascia and muscles in addition to a generalized weakening of the anal sphincters. In all cases, the rectum does not conform with, but lies anterior to the sacral concavity, thus obliterating the angulation that normally occurs between rectum and anus. The prolapsing mucosa of a partial prolapse rarely protrudes more than 4 cm beyond the anal verge; the mucosal folds emanate in a radial fashion from the central lumen of the prolapsed mucosa. Mucosal prolapse is frequently associated with third- and fourth-degree hemorrhoids. Complete rectal prolapse (procidentia) occurs at the extremes of life, most commonly in elderly women.

Clinical Features

Most patients are able to detect the presence of a mass, especially following defecation or strenuous activity. In more advanced cases, this may be present when they stand or walk. Irritation to the rectal mucosa caused by recurrent prolapse results in a mucous discharge with some associated bleeding. Some patients may present because of blood-stained mucus on their undergarments; others because of fecal incontinence caused by associated anal sphincter weakness. Patients may complain of a dull, aching pain with the inability to completely evacuate during defecation. In pediatric patients, parents often mistakenly believe that the prolapsed mucosa is hemorrhoids.

Treatment

In young children, after appropriate analgesia and sedation, prolapse can be reduced manually by replacing the protruding mucosa proximal to the anorectal ring of sphincter muscles. Every effort should be made to prevent the child from becoming constipated, and the child should be referred for further evaluation.

Surgical intervention is generally indicated in all other age groups unless the prolapse is minimal. A variety of effective surgical procedures are available and may be used depending on the degree of prolapse and the general health of the patient. All patients should be referred to have a least a proctosigmoidoscopic examination or a colonoscopy to rule out tumor, polyps, or diagnose inflammatory bowel disease. In addition, one should check for the possibility of an anterior rectal wall ulcer that may occur in patients with recurrent prolapse.

If vascular compromise appears to have occurred, reduction may be necessary on an emergency basis. Because of the risk of having reduced ischemic bowel that could perforate, these patients must be hospitalized.

ANORECTAL TUMORS

Carcinoma of the anal area represents less than 5 percent of all large bowel malignancies. At the level of the dentate line and extending approximately 1 cm proximal is a transitional zone of epithelium connecting the squamous cell epithelium of the anoderm with the columnar epithelium of the rectum. This transition zone includes columnar, cuboidal, transitional, and squamous epithelial cells that represent the source for a variety of malignancies that arise in the anal canal. For the purpose of grading malignancies, the United Nations World Health Organization has divided the anal canal into two regions: (1) malignancies of the portion proximal to the dentate line and including the transitional zone are referred to as anal canal neoplasms, and (2) tumors arising in the anoderm distal to the dentate line are referred to as anal margin neoplasms.

Anal margin neoplasms, including Bowen disease, squamous cell carcinoma, basal cell carcinoma, and Paget disease, have a low-grade malignant potential and are slow to metastasize. Anal canal neoplasms, including adenocarcinoma of glands and ducts, transitional carcinoma, melanoma, Kaposi sarcoma, and villous adenoma on the other hand are far more virulent, metastasize early, and have a poor prognosis. Squamous cell carcinoma of the anal canal has a much poorer prognosis than its anal margin counterpart. Anal canal malignancies metastasize not only to mesenteric lymph nodes and the portal circulation, but also to the regional inguinal nodes and via the systemic circulation.

Included among the anal canal neoplasms is Kaposi sarcoma, the most common AIDS-related malignancy. The anal canal is the third most common site for malignant melanoma (after the skin and the eye) which when it occurs there, may not be pigmented and is frequently overlooked.

Clinical Features

Early anal canal malignancies usually cause nonspecific symptoms such as pruritus, pain, and bleeding admixed with stool. The sensation and presence of a lump in the anal canal may be erroneously diagnosed as a hemorrhoid. As the neoplasm progresses, the patient experiences anorexia, weight loss, diarrhea, constipation, narrowing of the caliber of the stool, and eventually tenesmus with or without bowel movement. They may be ulcerative and involve part of the canal; however, complete obstruction may also occur.

Anal canal tumors may produce partial rectal prolapse; hemorrhoidal dilatation and prolapse may also occur. More advanced malignancies may present as perirectal abscesses or fistulas.

Villous adenomas, which arise from the rectal columnar epithelium, frequently produce diarrhea and a profuse rectal discharge, with secondary excoriation of skin and pruritus. Patients may suffer a significant loss of electrolytes, resulting in a clinically significant hypokalemia and/or hyponatremia.

Treatment

The anal margin neoplasms tend to be circumferential and may present as persistent ulcers or as chronic dermatologic conditions such as eczema or mycotic infections. Any ulcer that fails to heal within 30 days or any discrete skin lesion that fails to improve with appropriate therapy must be biopsied to rule out the presence of malignancy.

Virtually all anorectal tumors can be detected by careful visual examination of the perianal area, digital palpation of the distal rectum and anal canal, and procto- or sigmoidoscopic examination. The emergency physician should suspect these lesions when the clinical history is suspicious, and complete a thorough physical examination, including digital and anoscopic examination. Appropriate surgical consultation and referral is imperative. Failure to look, feel, and think would be the only reason not to suspect the presence of these curable but life-threatening lesions.

RECTAL FOREIGN BODIES

The medical literature is replete with the variety of foreign bodies that have been reported to have been inserted into the rectum. Most foreign bodies are in the rectal ampulla and are therefore palpable through digital examination and detectable on proctoscopic examination. More proximal foreign bodies are usually not palpable. Any patient presenting with an intrarectal foreign body must have x-rays of the abdomen taken to demonstrate not only the position, shapes, and number of foreign bodies, but also the possible presence of free air. Perforation of the rectum or colon is the most frequent and most serious complication. Perforation of the rectum below the peritoneal reflection often causes retroperitoneal injuries and may yield extraperitoneal air along

the psoas muscles on a flat plate radiograph. Perforation above the peritoneal reflection usually reveals intraperitoneal free air under the diaphragm noted on an upright CXR. Fever, leukocytosis, abdominal pain, peritoneal signs, and rectal bleeding are clinical manifestations suggestive of perforation. Both can result in life-threatening sepsis, although perforation below the peritoneal reflection may be managed with more conservative therapy.

Treatment

Although some foreign bodies can be removed in the ED, many require surgical intervention, particularly if they are made of glass or have sharp edges. If the foreign body is removed in the emergency department and is of a size or shape that could cause perforation, a follow-up proctoscopic examination and x-ray studies must be performed. In questionable cases, observations for at least 12 h should be done to ensure that perforation has not occurred. Rectal and anal lacerations may be present and require repair.

Sphincter relaxation is mandatory for removal of large foreign bodies. If the patient's sphincters are taut or otherwise not sufficiently relaxed, local infiltrative anesthesia must be administered to achieve proper relaxation. Intravenous sedation should be considered. After the patient has been sedated and placed in the lithotomy position, local anesthetic is injected through a fine, 30-gauge needle to raise an intradermal wheal at the 6 and 12 o'clock positions. The index finger of the physician's nondominant hand is then inserted into the anal canal to act as a guide for a $1\frac{1}{2}$-in. larger-gauge needle through which anesthetic is injected circumferentially along the internal sphincter muscles as they course along the anal canal. Five milliliters of anesthetic should suffice for each quadrant of infiltration. Large bulbar objects create a vacuum-like effect in the rectal ampulla, making it difficult to retrieve the object by simple traction. The vacuum can be overcome by passing a catheter beyond the object and injecting air. A modification of this technique is to insert Foley catheters around the foreign body and, after the vacuum is relieved by injecting air, to inflate the balloon of the Foley catheter and use the catheters as traction devices to deliver the foreign body or manipulate it into a more accessible position.

If there is a risk of perforation or if excess manipulation (potential for bacteremia) will be needed to remove the foreign body, the patient should be prepared for emergency surgery, which includes obtaining appropriate laboratory studies, initiating intravenous therapy with crystalloid solution, and administering a loading dose of a broad-spectrum antibiotic (such as a third-generation cephalosporin) with adequate coverage for anaerobic as well as aerobic bacteria.

PRURITUS ANI

Pruritus ani is a symptom complex that occurs secondary to a variety of anal and systemic problems. It is not in itself a specific disease process. It affects men far more often than women, and it occurs most commonly during the fifth and sixth decades of life.

There is an entity of primary or idiopathic pruritus ani, the etiology of which is unknown. To make such a diagnosis, one has to rule out the many specific, known causes of secondary pruritus ani such as local infections, local irritants, systemic illnesses, and psychogenic causes. Even so, idiopathic pruritus ani may occur in association with or be precipitated by secondary pruritus ani. Table 82-3 lists the major categories of the various likely causes of secondary pruritus ani.

The etiology of pruritus ani includes many of the various categories that have been discussed in this chapter. The pruritus that accompanies such conditions as fissures, fistulas, hemorrhoids, and prolapses occurs as a result of the perianal skin being exposed to and macerated by constant mucous and purulent discharge. It is probably the increased perianal moisture caused by these conditions that results in itching. The itching triggers a vicious cycle of scratching, excoriation, and more itching.

TABLE 82-3 Pruritus Ani

Anorectal disease
Dietary factors
Local infection
Local irritants
Dermatologic conditions
Systemic illness
Psychogenic factors

Numerous dietary factors have been implicated and are associated with secondary pruritus ani, although proof of cause is lacking for most of them. Those dietary factors most commonly listed include excessive consumption of caffeine-containing liquids (such as coffee, tea, or colas) and beer, although there have been conflicting reports demonstrating a correlation between pruritus ani and alcohol consumption. Milk, chocolate, tomatoes, and citrus fruits are other food products that allegedly contribute to pruritus ani. Likewise, certain drugs, such as colchicine and mineral oil, have been associated with pruritus ani. Ingestion of these products can result in increased liquidity and seepage of fecal material, which in itself is a probable cause of pruritus ani.

Infectious agents that have to be considered as causes of pruritus ani include bacteria, viruses, fungi, spirochetes, and parasites. More common bacterial infections, such as staphylococci and streptococci, in addition to all sexually transmitted organisms, will cause pruritus, if not actual pain. Pinworms (*Enterobius vermicularis*) are the most common cause of anal pruritus in children (see Chap. 49). *Candida albicans* is commonly found on the perianal skin but is not usually associated with pruritus; the *Trichophyton* species, on the other hand, are always associated with pruritus.

Local irritants, if not the initial cause, commonly contribute to the incidence of pruritus. Fecal contamination resulting from poor anal hygiene is by far the most common irritant to the perianal skin. Lysozyme from intestinal mucous secretions, acting together with bacterial exotoxins to raise the stool and skin pH, will cause pruritus. Ironically, patients who compulsively clean their anus, particularly if they use perfumed toilet tissue, soaps, detergents, or hygiene sprays can cause pruritic reactions. Also, wearing of synthetic, tight-fitting underwear retains moisture that normally exudes from the perianal area, another leading cause of pruritus.

Dermatologic conditions contributing to this symptom complex include atopic dermatitis, lichen planus, psoriasis, and seborrheic der-

matitis. Any of the anal margin neoplasms, particularly Bowen's disease and extramammary Paget's disease, may initially manifest itself as pruritus.

Finally, systemic conditions, such as diabetes mellitus, lymphoma, and certain vitamin deficiencies (vitamins A and D and niacin), because of their secondary effect on the perianal skin, will cause pruritus.

Clinical Features

Appearance of the perianal skin will depend on the severity and chronicity of the underlying conditions that are causing the pruritus. The skin will appear normal with early, mild cases. With acute, more severe exacerbations, the perianal skin will appear reddened, edematous, and moist; frequently, there are excoriations caused by scratching. In chronic cases, the perianal skin takes on a thickened, almost leathery, depigmented appearance. The normal radiating folds of skin thicken into rugae and may include factitiously induced superficial fissures.

Treatment

Pruritus, like any other symptom, suggests the presence of an underlying cause that should be diagnosed and treated appropriately. Thus excision of malignancies or surgical correction of fistulas, prolapses, or hemorrhoids would be the definitive treatment for patients with those conditions.

In most cases, specific anorectal lesions are not apparent, and the patient must be referred to a proctologist or dermatologist for probable long-term management.

In the meantime, the patient should be advised to make certain dietary changes, if appropriate, and should be instructed about proper anal hygiene. Scratching of the area must be avoided; if necessary, the patient should be advised to wear gloves at bedtime, when most of the scratching is likely to occur. Patients with maceration of perianal skin should use moist cotton rather than toilet paper. Soaps should be avoided, and the patient should take sitz baths for at least 15 min two to three times a day. The skin should then be thoroughly dried by gently blotting with a soft cloth. Zinc oxide ointment can provide a protective covering for the perianal skin and may enhance healing. Fungicidal creams should be prescribed for patients with secondary fungal infections. One percent hydrocortisone cream is effective for the allergic component of the inflammation. Finally, as an adjunct to providing

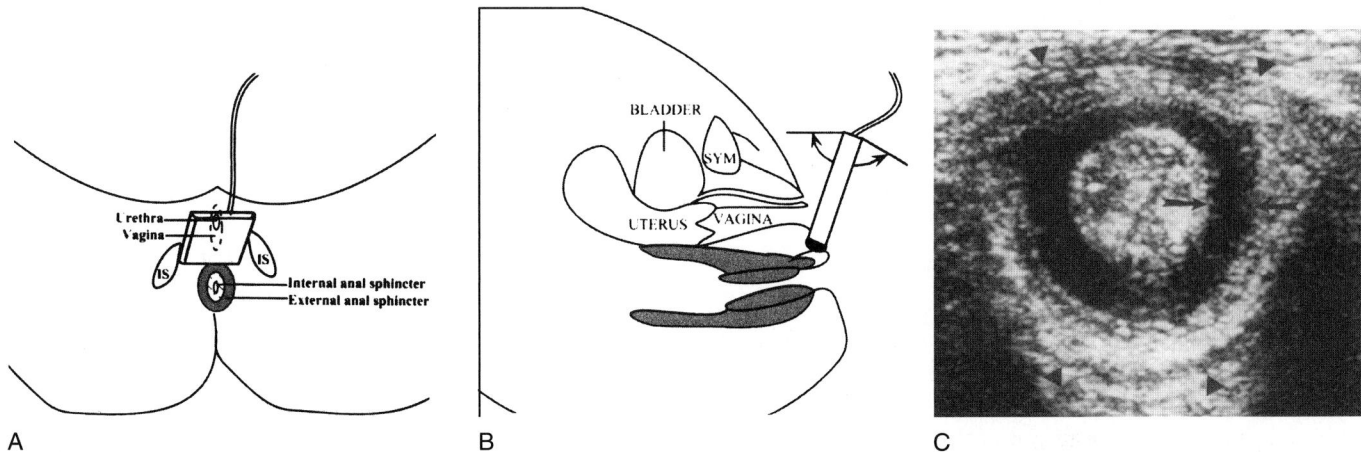

FIG. 82-9. Sonographic technique for axial imaging. Transducer may be a 5- to 10-MHz linear array, curved linear array, or sector scanner, operating at highest penetrating frequency. Patient in dorsal lithotomy position. **A.** Drawing shows female positioning; male positioning identical, with scrotum elevated. Transducer is placed directly on the perineal body between vagina (anterior) and rectum (posterior). Transducer is pressed posteriorly and angled cranially to caudally. IS = ischium. **B.** Sagittal diagram shows transducer position with respect to anterior sphincter apparatus. SYM = symphysis pubis. **C.** Axial sonogram with patient supine shows well-defined 3-mm hypoechoic internal sphincter *(arrows)* and 3.5-mm echogenic striated external sphincter *(arrowheads)*.

symptomatic relief, consider prescribing hydroxyzine hydrochloride (Atarax) as an effective bedtime sedative.

PILONIDAL SINUS

Pilonidal sinus has nothing to do with the anorectum, anatomically or embryologically. Pilonidal sinuses or cysts occur in the midline in the upper part of the natal cleft overlying the lower sacrum and coccyx. Because of their proximity to the anus, infected pilonidal cysts (abscesses) are sometimes mistakenly diagnosed as perirectal abscesses. An abscessed pilonidal sinus is always located in the posterior midline over the sacrum and coccyx (although there may be secondary fistulous openings on either side of the midline) and does not communicate with the anorectum. On the other hand, long, horseshoe-type fistulas emanating from a perirectal abscess may drain close to the location of a pilonidal sinus but not in the midline.

Although once thought to be congenital in nature, pilonidal sinus is now considered an acquired problem. The sinus is formed by the penetration of the skin by ingrowing hair, which causes a foreign body granuloma reaction. The sinus is perpetuated by the presence of the hair and repeated bouts of infection. Although pilonidal sinuses or infected pilonidal cysts occur most commonly in white men before the fourth decade of life, a small portion of patients may develop this problem in their fourth decade. Pilonidal sinus and abscess formation should be considered a chronic and recurring disease.

Carcinoma is a rare complication of chronic, recurring pilonidal sinus disease. It is more frequent in men and is usually a well-differentiated dermal-type squamous cell carcinoma.

Treatment of pilonidal sinus is described in detail in Chap. 152, under Cutaneous Abscesses.

PROCTALGIA FUGAX

This painful condition, which lasts intermittently for a few months, is thought to occur as a result of transient perianal muscle spasm causing exquisite pain in the lower rectum and anus. The pain is often acute, can be quite severe, usually lasts for a few seconds, and may be associated with irritable bowel syndrome. A thorough examination is required to exclude structural causes, although there is usually no significant cause for this condition.[4]

HIDRADENITIS SUPPURATIVA

The perianal surface containing the apocrine sweat glands, in association with the perineal, groin, and axillary regions often become the sites of significant edema, superficial fistulae, and small superficial abscesses. Chronic inflammation, edema, tissue induration, and watery discharge may occur. Postpubescent patients are commonly affected as the apocrine ducts become blocked. Good hygiene, warm soaks, intermittent antibiotics, incision and drainage, and at times extensive surgery with skin grafts are needed for effective treatment.

PERIANAL ULTRASOUND AND MRI

Diagnostic imaging has expanded greatly over the last 10 to 20 years. Older tests utilizing barium contrast and fistulograms have given way to ultrasound, CT scanning, and MRI. Traditionally, distal rectum and anal ultrasonic evaluations were performed utilizing endorectal sonography. Endorectal ultrasound has been used for the diagnosis and management of certain perirectal abscesses, rectal tumor evaluation and staging, and anal sphincter evaluation for incontinence. More recently transperineal sonography is being utilized, providing equivalent information with better patient tolerance.[7] Views in both the axial and longitudinal planes provide significant information about perirectal anatomic structures (Figures 82-9 and 82-10). Limitations such as decreased ultrasonic penetration above the distal 5 cm of rectum and pos-

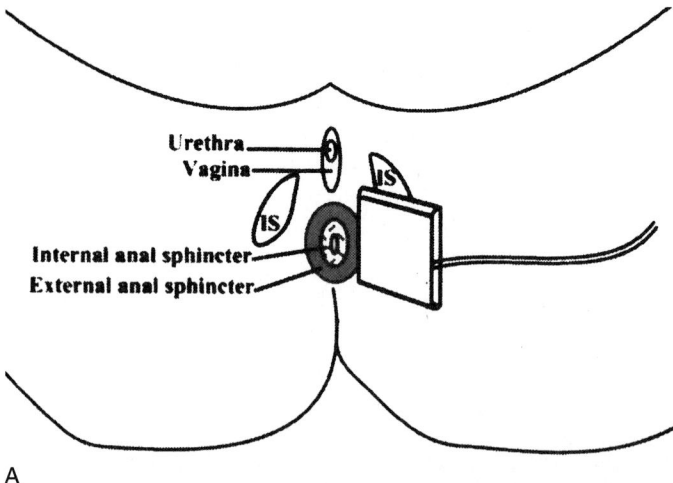

A

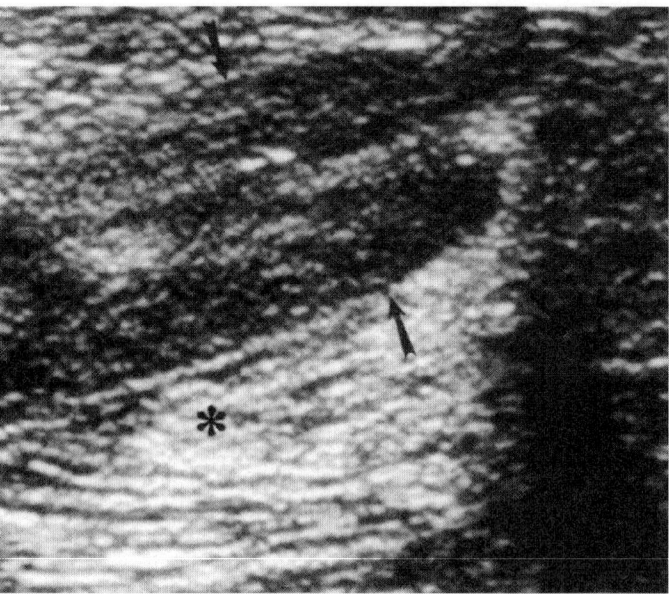

B

FIG. 82-10. Longitudinal sonography. **A.** Drawing shows transducer in parasaggital plane, adjacent to rectum and parallel to vaginal opening. Transducer can be angled laterally or medially. With medial and caudal angulation, the oblique coronal plane can be achieved. IS = ischium. **B.** Oblique sagittal sonogram shows hypoechoic internal sphincter *(arrows)* and mixed-echogenicity external sphincter *(asterisk)* as imaged from left of rectum. Transducer, 9 MHz.

sible difficulty with skin contact due to structural anatomic variances may hinder adequate views. The technique involves utilization of a 5 to 10 MHz curved linear array transducer in both the axial and longitudinal planes with the patient in the supine position. The probe can be moved in a fanlike fashion to provide a more panoramic view of the perirectal region. Normally, the hypoechoic internal sphincter is about 3 mm thick and surrounds the rectal mucosa, which is more echogenic. More peripherally, the external sphincter is about 5 mm thick, and has mixed echogenicity. This technique may be used to identify some perirectal abscesses, fistula tracts, and local tumors.[7] The transperineal technique is often better tolerated by the patient compared to the transrectal or endoanal approach. Perianal evaluations using a cone-shaped 10-MHz probe may be utilized. Other techniques may be utilized for evaluation such as a pelvic ultrasound (limited to females) and are slightly more invasive. Endorectal ultrasound with a condom-covered transducer is an uncomfortable, somewhat invasive technique which may require sedation. Drawbacks to this technique include patient discomfort, ultrasound scatter from air bubbles within the condom and incomplete preparation with stool present. CT scan and MRI may be used and are thought to be complementary, though cost and availability are possible concerns.[7] Endoluminal MRI has been used to detect anal sphincter invasion with an accuracy of 92 percent compared to endosonography at 50 percent.[8] Endoanal ultrasound has been used to detect sphincter damage and anal malignancy staging; however, the primary use in the emergency department is to detect abscess and fistula formation in the appropriate presentation. As such, the abscess and fistulous tract will present as a hypoechoic shadow. In fact, endoanal ultrasound has been found to be superior to CT and digital examination for the detection of fistulous tracts and abscesses.[9] Caution must be taken as ultrasound may miss extension of the fistulas into the ischiorectal and supralevator regions. Difficulty in distinguishing abscess cavities, granulation tracts, and scar tissue has been described. MRI, used to detect granulation, is quite useful for detecting fistulae. New MRI endoprobes are being developed and may further enhance the ability to detect these fistulae.[9]

BIBLIOGRAPHY

Condon ER (ed): Colon, in Zuideme GD (ed): *Shackelford's Surgery of the Alimentary Tract,* 4th ed. Philadelphia, PA: Saunders, 1996, p. 275.

Schecter WP, Albo RJ: Removal of rectal foreign bodies, in Baker RJ, Fischer JE (eds): *Mastery of Surgery,* 4th ed. Philadelphia, PA: Lippincott Williams & Wilkins, 2001, p. 1633.

Keighley MRB: Anorectal disorders, in Baker RJ, Fischer JE (eds): *Mastery of Surgery,* 4th ed. Philadelphia, PA: Lippincott Williams & Wilkins, 2001, p. 1638.

REFERENCES

1. Janicke DM, Pundt MR: Anorectal disorders. *Emerg Med Clin North Am* 14:757, 1996.
2. Segal WN, Greenberg PD, Rochay DC, et al: The outpatient evaluation of hematochezia. *Am J Gastroenterol* 93:179, 1998.
3. Bayer I, Nysloraty B, Picovsky BM: Rubber band ligation of hemorrhoids. *J Clin Gastroenterol* 23:50, 1996.
4. Maltz C, Black A: Anorectal disorders. *Emerg Med* 33:11, 2001.
5. Cataldo PA, Scenagore AJ, Luchtfeld MA: Intrarectal ultrasound in the evaluation of perirectal abscesses. *Dis Colon Rectum* 36:554, 1993.
6. Poen AC, Felt-Bersma RJF, Eijsbouts QAJ, et al: Hydrogen peroxide-enhanced transanal ultrasound in the assessment of fistula-in-ano. *Dis Colon Rectum* 41:1147, 1998.
7. Rubens DJ, Strang JG, Bogineni-Misra S, et al: Tranperineal sonography of the rectum: Anatomy and pathology revealed by sonography compared with CT and MR imaging. *AJR* 170:637, 1998.
8. Stoker J, Rociu E, Wiersma TG, et al: Imaging of anorectal disease. *Br J Surg* 87:10, 2000.
9. Kumar A, Scholefield JH: Endosonography of the anal canal and rectum. *World J Surg* 24:208, 2000.

VOMITING, DIARRHEA, AND CONSTIPATION
Annie T. Sadosty
Jennifer J. Hess

Vomiting, diarrhea, and constipation are among the most common complaints of patients presenting to emergency departments. Gastrointestinal dysfunction is the final common pathway for a variety of diseases. Therefore, many patients complaining of vomiting, diarrhea, or constipation have a cause for their symptoms remote from the gastrointestinal system. Emergency physicians must consider not only the gastrointestinal emergencies manifested as vomiting, diarrhea, or con-

stipation but also the nongastrointestinal emergencies manifested as gastrointestinal dysfunction.

An important and often difficult step in the evaluation of patients with vomiting, diarrhea, or constipation is having the patient define the illness. The lay person's definitions of *vomiting, diarrhea,* and *constipation* often differ tremendously from the medical definitions. For example, patients often say "vomiting" when they really mean "coughing up sputum." Some patients complain of "constipation" and mean that they are straining to defecate. Defining the complaint allows the physician to treat patients correctly and in turn increases patients' satisfaction. A complete history of the current illness is the first step toward the correct diagnosis.

After defining the illness, the emergency physician's next step is to determine whether the illness represents an emergency. At the end of the emergency department evaluation, the cause of the patient's symptoms may not be clear. Nevertheless, the physician must decide, based on limited information, whether a patient may be discharged safely and what the initial treatment plan will be.

VOMITING

Pathophysiology

Vomiting is a complex, highly coordinated activity involving the gastrointestinal tract, the central nervous system, and the vestibular system. In 1952, Wang and Borison identified a medullary vomiting center.[1] The proximity of the medullary vomiting center to other central nervous system nuclei allows for the coordinated activity of vomiting.[1] Three stages of vomiting have been described: nausea, retching, and emesis.[2] Nausea is the subjective feeling that immediately precedes vomiting and is accompanied by hypersalivation and tachycardia. Retching occurs when the pylorus contracts and the fundus relaxes, thereby moving food to the gastric cardia. Emesis occurs when the powerful abdominal muscles contract simultaneously and thus eject food or gastric secretions from the stomach.

Clinical Features

HISTORY   There are various causes of vomiting (Table 83-1). Fortunately, the patient's history often leads the physician to the correct diagnosis. Asking the right questions will help to uncover the etiology.

First, define the vomitus. Is it bloody, bilious or nonbilious, feculent or posttussive? Hematemesis is seen with gastritis, peptic ulcer disease, gastric and esophageal tumors, and Mallory-Weiss tears. Nonbilious emesis occurs with gastric outlet obstruction, as in patients with pyloric strictures secondary to ulcer disease or infants with pyloric stenosis.

Second, determine what symptoms accompany the vomiting. Is the patient febrile? Fever could point toward an infectious or inflammatory source, or it could represent a toxicologic cause, such as salicylate intoxication. Is there associated abdominal pain, back pain, headache, or chest pain that may point to a specific cause? Pancreatitis, cholecystitis, peptic ulcer disease, appendicitis, and pelvic inflammatory disease typically cause abdominal pain. Back pain usually accompanies aortic dissections, rupturing aortic aneurysm, pyelonephritis, and biliary or renal colic. Vomiting is one of the signs of increased intracranial or intraocular pressure and may be a foreboding sign in patients complaining of headache. The complaint of vomiting associated with chest or epigastric pain might suggest a diagnosis of myocardial ischemia. In female patients, obstetric and gynecologic causes of vomiting should always be considered. In a pregnant woman, epigastric pain and vomiting accompanying hypertension may indicate preeclampsia.

Learning more about the patient is as important as defining the illness. What complicating medical conditions does the patient have? Is

TABLE 83-1 Vomiting and Diarrhea: The GASTROENTERITIS Mnemonic

	Vomiting	Diarrhea
Gastrointestinal	Obstruction: tumor, stricture, hernia, volvulus, intussusception, foreign body, bezoar, extrinsic compression (SMA syndrome), fecal impaction Dysmotility: achalasia, scleroderma, gastroparesis, GERD, Ogilvie syndrome, postvagotomy, diabetes, etc. Inflammation: esophagitis, gastritis, PUD, biliary colic, cholecystitis, pancreatitis, hepatitis, inflammatory bowel disease, diverticulitis	Obstruction: fecal impaction with overflow Dysmotility: irritable bowel syndrome, postvagotomy, short bowel syndrome Inflammation: inflammatory bowel disease, diverticulitis, sprue, radiation enteritis Malabsorption (pancreatic exocrine dysfunction) Lactose intolerance GI bleeding
Appendicitis or aorta	Appendicitis/aortic aneurysm or dissection	Appendicitis
Specific diseases	Glaucoma Torsion of testis or ovary	
Trauma	Obstruction (duodenal hematoma) Dysmotility (ileus secondary to lumbar compression fractures) Inflammation (pancreatitis)	
Rx (prescription)	Medication side effect (naloxone, opioid analgesics, erythromycin, chemotherapy, ipecac)	Medication side effect (antibiotics, chemotherapy, laxatives, antacids, sorbitol, colchicine)
Obstetrics and gynecology	Pregnancy (ectopic, uterine, molar) Preeclampsia Hyperemesis gravidarum	
Endocrine or metabolic	Adrenal insufficiency Thyrotoxicosis Diabetic ketoacidosis Alcoholic ketoacidosis Reye syndrome Uremia	Adrenal insufficiency Thyrotoxicosis Uremia
Neurologic	Autonomic neuropathy (gastroparesis in diabetes) Vestibular disorders (cranial nerve VIII) Migraine headache Hypertensive encephalopathy Hydrocephalus Increased ICP (intracranial neoplasms, subdural or epidural hematoma, subarachnoid hemorrhage, cerebral edema)	Autonomic neuropathy (diabetes)

(continued)

the patient diabetic? If so, could the vomiting be a manifestation of diabetic ketoacidosis? In a patient with a history of peripheral vascular disease, vomiting may be a sign of mesenteric ischemia. Patients with a history of multiple abdominal surgeries are at risk for intestinal obstruction due to adhesions. Knowledge of the medications to which the patient has access is also critical, because intentional and unintentional poisonings often present first with emesis. Physicians should be suspicious of drug-induced toxicity in patients taking medicines known to have gastrointestinal toxicity (e.g., lithium, digoxin, or theophylline). The social history provides clues, too. Vomiting in a person who enjoys mushroom hunting may well represent *Amanita* poisoning.

PHYSICAL EXAMINATION Clinical clues also may assist in making the diagnosis. In addition to evaluating the ABCs, much of the physician's initial attention should be directed toward the assessment of hydration status. Severely volume-depleted patients require immediate intervention, lest circulatory collapse be imminent. The abdominal, genitourinary, and pelvic examinations are often revealing. Physicians should search carefully for tenderness, peritoneal signs, hernias, masses, and evidence of obstruction or torsion. The findings of a careful physical examination may point toward unsuspected causes of vomiting, such as bulimia (scars on the dorsum of hands), pneumonia (consolidative findings on lung examination), or Addison disease (hyperpigmentation). The rectal examination is important. An anal fistula may be the only clue to Crohn disease in an otherwise healthy teenager with vomiting or a hard stool mass in the rectal vault may indicate fecal impaction.

Acquire data selectively and smartly. Order diagnostic tests according to the differential diagnosis. In the vomiting, premenopausal woman, consider pregnancy high on the differential diagnosis, and rule it in or out with a pregnancy test. Other laboratory tests that may be of assistance are determination of blood urea nitrogen, creatinine, and amylase levels; liver function tests; determination of blood alcohol and drug levels; and urinalysis. Addisonian crisis can present with vomiting, and the laboratory results may show hyperkalemia and hyponatremia. An electrocardiogram can help if the physician is considering the diagnosis of myocardial ischemia. Chest and abdominal radiography can assist in the determination of the presence or absence of pneumoperitoneum, pneumonia, or intestinal obstruction.

Treatment

Initial management of the acutely ill, vomiting patient is the same, regardless of cause. The ABCs always take precedence. For patients with circulatory collapse secondary to severe dehydration, aggressive volume repletion must begin immediately upon arrival. Two large-bore intravenous catheters should be placed, and crystalloid should be administered aggressively to restore circulation quickly.

For patients with less acute conditions, treatment hinges on making the correct diagnosis. A vomiting patient with diabetic ketoacidosis will not respond to symptomatic therapy with antiemetics: vomiting continues until the underlying illness is treated. It is important, therefore, to recognize the illnesses that are not self-limited and to treat them appropriately. However, not all patients with the chief complaint of vomiting

TABLE 83-1   Vomiting and Diarrhea: The GASTROENTERITIS Mnemonic (*Continued*)

	Vomiting	Diarrhea
Toxicology	Acetaminophen Heavy metals (arsenic, mercury, iron, lithium) Alcohol Mushrooms Nicotine Chlorinated hydrocarbon insecticides Organophosphate or carbamates Digoxin Salicylate Isoniazid Theophylline or caffeine	Heavy metals (arsenic, mercury, iron, lithium) Ergot alkaloids Theophylline or caffeine Mushrooms Nicotine Chlorinated hydrocarbon insecticides Thyroid replacement hormone overdose Organophosphate or carbamates
Environmental	Food poisoning Envenomation (e.g., black widow, *Hymenoptera,* scorpion) High-altitude illness Acute radiation syndrome	Food poisoning Envenomation (black widow, snake, *Hymenoptera*) Acute radiation syndrome
Renal	Obstructive uropathy Renal colic	
Infection	Infectious gastroenteritis (viral, bacterial, parasitic) Pyelonephritis Pneumonia (i.e., pertussis) Pelvic inflammatory disease Meningitis Hepatitis	Infectious gastroenteritis (viral, bacterial, parasitic) Pseudomembranous colitis Pneumonia (e.g., *Legionella*) HIV
Tumors	Gastrinoma	Medullary carcinoma of the thyroid Villous adenoma APUD tumors (glucagonoma, gastrinoma, carcinoid, VIPoma)
Ischemia	Myocardial infarction Mesenteric ischemia	Mesenteric ischemia Ischemic colitis
Supratentorial	Bulimia	Psychosocial stress

Abbreviations: APUD = amine precursor uptake and decarboxylation; GERD = gastroesophageal reflux disease; HIV = human immunodeficiency virus; ICP = intracranial pressure; PUD = peptic ulcer disease; SMA = superior mesenteric artery; VIPoma = vasoactive intestinal peptide tumor.

are discharged from the emergency department with a clear diagnosis. These patients should be treated symptomatically, and follow-up should be ensured. For patients with mild to moderate dehydration who are actively vomiting, we recommend intravenous rehydration and antiemetic therapy directed toward the mechanism involved in eliciting the emesis (Table 83-2). For instance, vertigo and motion sickness will respond best to pharmacologic treatment with anticholinergics and antihistamines. The treatment of nausea from visceral distention involves blocking vagal afferents with serotonin (5-HT$_3$) receptor agonists. It is also important to note the form of drug delivery to ensure successful administration of the medication in the ED or upon dismissal.

Disposition

Patients with life-threatening causes of vomiting should be admitted to the hospital, as should severely dehydrated patients with presumably self-limited causes of emesis. The patient in whom the diagnosis is unclear, but who the physician feels confident does not have a life-threatening cause of emesis, may be discharged safely, provided the patient tolerates fluids in the ED and that follow-up the next day, if vomiting continues, is ensured. A dehydrated patient who cannot tolerate oral intake should not be discharged.

DIARRHEA

Epidemiology

At the turn of the twentieth century, diarrhea was one of the leading causes of death in the United States. In the 1990s, however, diarrhea accounted for fewer than 0.5 percent of all deaths in the United States.[3] Most diarrheal deaths occur in the elderly and the young.[3,4] Worldwide, however, diarrhea remains one of the leading causes of death. In fact, in 1990, diarrhea was listed as the fourth leading cause of death globally and was responsible for a total of 2.9 million deaths.[5] Despite the low U.S. mortality rate, diarrhea causes significant morbidity. It is the second most common reason for work absenteeism and is estimated to cost $608 million in lost productivity per year.[6,7]

Pathophysiology

There are four basic mechanisms of diarrhea: increased intestinal secretion, decreased intestinal absorption, increased osmotic load, and abnormal intestinal motility. Knowledge of normal intestinal function assists in understanding these various mechanisms. Normally, the jejunum receives between 6 and 8 L per d of fluid in the form of oral intake and gastric, pancreatic, and biliary secretions. Dietary intake actually constitutes a small portion of the jejunal load (1.5 L). A healthy small intestine absorbs nearly 75 percent of the fluid to which it is exposed. The 2 L of fluid not absorbed by the small intestine then enters the colon, where fluid is absorbed at an even higher rate. The absorptive power of the colon approaches 90 percent efficiency and far exceeds that of the small intestine. In fact, the colon can make up for a decrease in small intestinal absorption. Under normal conditions, very little fluid (<100 mL) is lost in the stool each day.[8]

In diarrheal states, normal intestinal physiology is disrupted. At a cellular level, intestinal absorption occurs through the villi, and secretion occurs through the crypts. Fluids are absorbed via two mechanisms: passively with the transport of sodium and actively with the

TABLE 83-2   Pharmacologic Therapy for Nausea and Vomiting

Mechanism	Generic Name	Trade Name	Dosing and Route	Clinical Stimuli Targeted	Side Effects
(M$_{1-5}$) Muscarinic antagonist	Scopolamine	Transderm Scōp	0.5 mg TD patch q24h	Motion sickness; prophylaxis	Dry mouth, drowsiness, vision disturbance, confusion, restlessness, narrow-angle glaucoma
H$_1$ histaminergic antagonists	Meclizine Diphenhydramine Dimenhydrinate	Antivert Benadryl Dramamine	12.5–50 mg PO qd 25–50 mg PO/IV/IM q6h prn 50–100 mg PO/IV/IM q4–6h	Motion sickness, labyrinthe tumors or infections, Meniere's disease	Drowsiness, HA, fatigue, constipation, dry mouth, paradoxical CNS stimulation
H$_1$ histaminergic, M$_1$ muscarinic, and D$_1$ dopaminergic antagonists	Promethazine Prochlorperazine	Phenergan Compazine	12.5–25 mg q4h PO/IM/IV q12h PR 5–10 mg PO/IM tid/qid, 2.5–10 mg IV q3–4h, 25 mg PR q12h	Motion sickness, space sickness (in flight), sea sickness, labyrinthine tumors or infections, Meniere's disease, migraines, GI disorders, chemotherapy, radiation therapy, medications (opiates, digoxin, and others), metabolic disturbances (uremia, hypercalcemia, DKA)	Common: sedation, dry mouth, dizziness, blurred vision, extrapyramidal effects, hypotension Serious: tardive dyskinesia, respiratory depression, bradycardia, neuroleptic malignant syndrome
Peripheral D$_2$ dopaminergic antagonist and weak 5-HT$_3$ blockade	Metoclopramide	Reglan	5–10 mg PO/IV/IM q6–8h	Chemotherapy, gastroparesis (stimulates gastric smooth muscle cells and hastens gastric emptying), GERD (increases LES tone)	Common: drowsiness, restlessness, dizziness, akathisia, extrapyramidal effects, disorientation, hypotension Serious: seizures, bronchospasm, acute dystonia, tardive dyskinesia, neuroleptic malignant syndrome, arrhythmias
5-HT$_3$ receptor antagonist	Ondansetron	Zofran Zofran ODT	4–8 mg IV with up to 24 mg for use with chemotherapy 4 and 8 mg PO disintegrating tablet	Gastric irritants (*Staphylococcus* enterotoxin, salicylates), nongastric stimuli (colonic, biliary, or intestinal distension, peritonitis, mesenteric occlusion), chemotherapy, abdominal irradiation, pharyngeal stimulation	Mild headache, asthenia, constipation, dizziness; hypotension or heart block (rare) with >32 mg

Abbreviations: CNS = central nervous system, DKA = diabetic ketoacidosis; GERD = gastroesophageal reflux disease; 5-HT$_3$ = serotonin 3; HA = headache; LES = lower esophageal sphincter; TD = transdermal.

absorption of glucose. Selected enterotoxins block the passive sodium resorption and specifically stimulate sodium excretion, resulting in a net loss of fluid. The glucose-dependent mechanism of water absorption, however, is unaffected by these toxins and can be exploited by including glucose in the rehydration treatments. The composition of oral rehydration therapies recommended by the World Health Organization is based largely on this physiology. In addition, diarrheal states, enterotoxins, inflammation, or ischemia disrupt the structure of the intestinal villi preferentially to the crypts. As a result, diarrhea occurs because of diminished intestinal villi absorption *and* unopposed crypt secretion (the crypts are more resilient after injury).[9] Diarrhea also accompanies the delivery of an osmotic load to the intestine. For example, administration of a laxative results in the collection of an osmotically active, nondigestible agent within the intestinal lumen. Osmosis occurs, drawing fluid into the intestinal lumen, and results in diarrhea. Increased intestinal motility causes diarrhea, as in patients with irritable bowel syndrome, neuropathies, or a shortened intestine secondary to surgery.

Clinical Features

HISTORY   The definition of diarrhea varies within the medical literature, so it is not surprising that patients' definitions vary, too. Many patients come to the emergency department complaining of "diarrhea" when what they really have is soft stools or two stools per day compared with their usual one. Strictly speaking, diarrhea is present when the daily stool weight exceeds 200 g.[10] Practically speaking, however, diarrhea is present when the patient is making more stools of lesser consistency more frequently.

Once a true diarrheal illness is confirmed, the physician's focus should change toward attempting to ascertain the cause of the diarrhea. There are many causes of diarrhea. Fortunately, the history usually leads the physician to the etiology. The first step is to determine whether the diarrhea is acute (<3 weeks) or chronic (>3 weeks). The acute diarrheas are of greatest concern to the emergency physician, for they are more apt to be a manifestation of an immediately life-threatening illness (infection, ischemia, intoxication, or inflammation).[10]

The next step is to define the diarrhea. Is it bloody or melanotic? Is it associated with possible food poisoning (see Chap. 150), or the ingestion of certain foods, such as milk or sorbitol? Does it resolve or persist with fasting? This can indicate an osmotic or secretory diarrhea, respectively. Are the stools of smaller volume localizing to the large intestine or of larger volume indicating small intestine pathology? What symptoms accompany the diarrhea? Is there fever or abdominal pain, which may suggest diverticulitis or infectious gastroenteritis? Seizures accompanying diarrhea often point toward shigellosis but could also indicate theophylline toxicity. Does the patient have heat intolerance and anxiety, suggesting thyrotoxicosis, or paresthesias and reverse temperature sensation, suggesting ciguatera?

Define the host. A patient's medical and surgical history often assists in narrowing the differential diagnosis. For example, diarrhea resulting from malabsorption secondary to pancreatic exocrine insufficiency need not be considered in an otherwise healthy host. Conversely, the differential diagnosis for diarrhea is broadened for a patient with acquired immunodeficiency syndrome. Medications commonly have diarrhea as a side effect or sequela. Is the patient taking medication that may have contributed to the diarrhea (e.g., antibiotics, lithium, chemotherapy, colchicine, and laxatives)? Has the patient traveled outside the United States or to the countryside recently? Rural hiking places the patient at risk for *Giardia,* particularly if water-purification procedures were not strictly followed, and travel to Third World countries increases the chances of parasitic infection and traveler's diarrhea. Sexual and occupational histories are also important. A patient's sexual preference or occupation may be the physician's only clue to a diagnosis of "gay" bowel disease or organophosphate poisoning.

PHYSICAL EXAMINATION   As with a vomiting patient, the examination begins with the ABCs. Thus, assessment of hydration status occurs shortly after the physician arrives at the bedside. Like the history, a careful physical examination can help narrow the differential diagnosis. Only by doing a thyroid examination can the physician discover a thyroid mass that may be contributing to diarrhea. Several other findings may be helpful in uncovering the underlying cause of the diarrhea, especially if it is more chronic in nature. These examination findings include oral ulcers, erythema nodosum, episcleritis, or an anal fissure, which would point toward inflammatory bowel disease. Reiter's syndrome, the triad of arthritis, conjunctivitis, and urethritis or cervicitis, should raise thoughts of *Salmonella, Shigella, Campylobacter,* or *Yersinia.* **Abdominal and rectal examinations are critical. Especially in the elderly, fecal impaction may result in diarrhea as liquid stool passes around the impaction.** Special attention should be given to the presence or absence of surgical scars, tenderness, masses, or peritoneal signs. Checking the stool for the presence or absence of blood is also important, because bloody diarrhea can be caused by inflammation, infection, or ischemia. An elderly patient with bloody diarrhea and abdominal pain out of proportion to the physical examination may have mesenteric ischemia—a true emergency.

DIAGNOSTIC STOOL EVALUATION   Tests specific to the emergency department evaluation of a patient with diarrhea include Wright stain for fecal leukocytes; stool culture for bacteria, ova, and parasites; and stool analysis for *Clostridium difficile* toxin. Diagnostic testing, although rarely helpful to the emergency physician, occasionally is helpful to the primary care physician. Who should be tested? Stool cultures for bacteria should be obtained in children, toxic patients, patients with a protracted diarrheal illness lasting longer than 3 days, and immunocompromised patients in whom infectious diarrhea is suspected. A request for an ova and parasite evaluation can be made for patients at risk for parasitic disease. In addition, patients at risk for *C. difficile* colitis should have a stool sample sent for *C. difficile* toxin assay.

Wright Stain   When applied to a stool sample, Wright stain allows detection of fecal leukocytes. A positive Wright stain has a sensitivity of 82 percent and a specificity of 83 percent for the presence of bacterial pathogen.[11] Historically, Wright stain for fecal leukocytes has been used to differentiate invasive from noninvasive infectious diarrheas. In the past, this was an important distinction: physicians were reluctant to prescribe antibiotics for patients with infectious diarrhea, because of the fear of prolonging the *Salmonella* carrier state. They therefore reserved antimicrobial treatment for the toxic patients who they felt *truly* had invasive diarrhea. Recently, this dictum has been questioned, and many physicians now treat patients with diarrheal illness with antibiotics regardless of whether or not the diarrhea is invasive or bacterial in origin.[12] Therefore, ascertaining the presence or absence of fecal leukocytes is superfluous.

Bacterial Stool Culture   Bacterial stool culture is an expensive and labor-intensive diagnostic test that plays a minor role in the emergency department evaluation of a patient with diarrhea. Most laboratories culture for only three common bacterial pathogens: *Salmonella, Shigella,* and *Campylobacter.* Because of a low sensitivity for detecting pathogens, each positive routine stool culture costs the laboratory approximately $950 to $1200, depending on the number of samples tested and the number of tests run on each sample.[9] To limit cost and increase yield, diagnostic testing should be limited to patients with high pretest probabilities of bacterial disease: severely dehydrated or toxic patients, children, immunocompromised patients, and patients with diarrhea lasting longer than 3 days.[9] In addition, if other enteric pathogens are suspected, the laboratory should be notified so that appropriate testing may be performed.

Ova and Parasitic Evaluation   Patients in whom a parasitic cause of diarrhea is suspected should have stool sent for evaluation for ova and parasites. These tests lack sensitivity, because many parasites are fastidious and shedding of the organisms is intermittent. Multiple samples may need to be collected to be sufficient to yield a positive result. Recently, direct immunofluorescence staining has been shown to improve the sensitivity for detecting *Giardia* and *Cryptosporidium.*[13]

***Clostridium difficile* Toxin Assay**   Diarrhea in a patient with an antecedent history of antibiotic use or hospitalization may be caused by pseudomembranous colitis from *C. difficile* infection. This is diagnosed with the *C. difficile* toxin assay. Unfortunately, this assay has a 10 percent false-negative rate and is rarely available to the emergency physician, because the turnaround time on the test approaches 24 h.[14]

Other Diagnostic Tests   If diarrhea is not felt to be infectious in origin, data acquisition should be dictated by the differential diagnosis. Rarely are serum chemistry results or complete blood count results diagnostic or necessary. Electrolyte measurements are warranted in severely dehydrated patients, regardless of the cause of dehydration. These measurements also can be helpful in patients experiencing an Addisonian crisis. Serum drug levels can assist the physician in making the diagnosis of theophylline, lithium, or heavy metal intoxication. In patients with a history of abdominal surgery, abdominal films may help rule out partial obstruction as a cause of diarrhea. A chest radiograph may help diagnose an occult pneumonia (i.e., *Legionella*) in a patient with diarrhea and a cough. For patients in whom mesenteric ischemia is suspected, mesenteric angiography is the test of choice.

Treatment

Initial treatment of any patient begins with the ABCs. Rehydration of severely dehydrated patients should begin immediately after large-bore intravenous access is achieved. Thereafter, treatment is dictated by the differential diagnosis. The emergency medicine approach to a patient with diarrhea, therefore, hinges on treating or excluding the life-threatening causes of diarrhea. Because infectious diarrhea is the most common cause of acute diarrhea, after the differential diagnosis is considered, physicians most commonly are left considering that diagnosis.

NONINFECTIOUS DIARRHEA   Almost all true diarrheal emergencies (e.g., gastrointestinal bleed, adrenal insufficiency, thyroid storm, toxicologic exposures, acute radiation syndrome, and mesenteric ischemia, all discussed elsewhere in this textbook) are of noninfectious origin. The emergency physician must be ever mindful of them, because patients with those conditions require intensive treatment and hospitalization. The less emergent, noninfectious causes of diarrhea are listed in Table 83-1.

ANTIBIOTIC OR DRUG-ASSOCIATED DIARRHEA   Drugs have many direct and indirect effects on gastrointestinal function. For example, erythromycin accelerates the rate of gastric emptying, clavulanate stimulates small bowel motility, and antibiotics may reduce fecal anaerobes. Fecal anaerobes are important for carbohydrate metabolism and bile acid breakdown. Gut carbohydrates can cause osmotic diarrhea, and bile acids are colonic secretory agents. Nonantibiotics that can cause diarrhea include laxatives, antacids, oral contrast agents, lactose, sorbitol, nonsteroidal anti-inflammatory agents, and cholinergics.

Antibiotic-associated diarrhea is usually moderate in severity, without cramps, fever, or fecal leukocytes. Stool assays for pathogens are negative. Symptoms resolve upon withdrawal of the antibiotic or drug. Metronidazole or vancomycin are not indicated.

INFECTIOUS DIARRHEA   Viruses cause the vast majority of infectious diarrheas, followed by bacterial and parasitic organisms. Treatment of infectious diarrhea involves antibiotic therapy, antimotility agents, restoration of fluid balance, and avoidance of agents that worsen diarrhea (Table 83-3). See Chap. 81 for a discussion of *C. difficile* colitis.

For the past 30 years, two pervasive myths involving the use of antibiotics and antimotility agents in the treatment of infectious diarrhea have dictated the management of large numbers of patients with diarrhea. These myths are discussed in detail below, and a discussion of the modern medical approach to infectious diarrhea follows.

Antibiotics

MYTH   For years, physicians avoided antibiotic use in the treatment of infectious diarrhea because of a fear of prolonging the *Salmonella* carrier state. This fear arose from an article published in 1969 in which the duration of *Salmonella* excretion after a salmonellosis epidemic was studied.[15] The study compared the length of excretion in patients who received antibiotics (ampicillin or chloramphenicol) with that of patients who were not treated and found that *Salmonella* excretion was longer in the cohort that received antibiotics. The authors concluded that, because of a prolonged carrier state, antibiotics should not be given to patients suspected of having a diarrheal illness due to *Salmonella*.

MODERN MEDICINE   For adults with domestically acquired diarrhea in whom the origin is felt to be infectious, antibiotics (500 mg of ciprofloxacin by mouth as a single dose for onset of travelers' diarrhea or twice daily for 3 days)[12,16] shorten the duration of illness by approximately 24 h. Regardless of the causative agent, all patients—even those who had a negative Wright's stain, negative stool culture, and a low diarrheal illness score, suggesting less clinically significant disease and/or a viral cause—improved on ciprofloxacin.[17] Even though most infectious diarrheas are self-limited, because of the inconveniencing and occasionally life-threatening nature of the disease, **we recommend ciprofloxacin treatment for all patients believed to have an infectious diarrhea who do not have a contraindication to antimicrobial treatment** (e.g., pediatric age group, allergy, pregnancy, or drug interaction). Trimethoprim/sulfamethoxazole (Bactrim DS; one tablet by mouth as a single dose or twice daily for 3 days) also shortens the duration of infectious diarrhea in adults but was proven to be inferior to a course of ciprofloxacin secondary to resistant organisms.[17]

Antimotility Agents

MYTH   Since the early 1960s, the use of antimotility agents in the treatment of diarrhea has been denounced by most of the medical community. This dictum emerged out of a 1963 study published by Formal and colleagues.[18] In this study, guinea pigs were starved and poisoned to make them susceptible to *Shigella* infection (an organism to which

TABLE 83-3   Empiric Treatment of Traveler's Diarrhea in the Adult

Rehydration
   Fluids: chicken broth with fruit juices, Gatorade, noncaffeinated sodas, packages of salts and glucose to be reconstituted with boiled or treated water, Ceralyte 90, Pedialyte
   Foods: complex carbohydrates (bananas, bread, rice, apple juice, and tortillas), potatoes, crackers, *Lactobacillus*-containing yogurt

	Trade Name	Dosage	Comments
Antimotility Agents			
Bismuth subsalicylate	Pepto Bismol	30 mL or 2 tablets every 30 min for 8 doses; repeat on day 2	Salicylate toxicity may occur with excessive dosing; may cause bismuth encephalopathy in HIV patients
Loperamide	Imodium	4 mg initially, then 2 mg after each unformed stool for no more than 2 d; maximum, 16 mg per d	Preferred first-line agent for antimotility, with minimal central opiate effects
Diphenoxylate and atropine	Lomotil	4 mg qid for ≤2 d	Recommended as a second-line agent with more central opiate effects (narcotic related to meperidine); may potentiate the action of barbiturates, tranquilizers, and alcohol
Antibiotics			
Ciprofloxacin	Cipro	500 mg single dose or 500 mg bid for 3 d	Indicated for moderately severe illness; complete 3-d course if single dose fails; significant drug–drug interactions may occur
Trimethoprim/sulfamethoxazole	Bactrim	160 mg/800 mg for single dose, 160 mg/800 mg bid for 3 d	Indicated for moderately severe illness; resistance limits reliable effectiveness
Bismuth subsalicylate	Pepto Bismol	30 mL or 2 tablets every 30 min for 8 doses; repeat on day 2 Prophylaxis: 2 tablets chewed with each meal and at bedtime	Indicated for mild illness and prophylaxis; see comments above

Abbreviation: HIV = human immunodeficiency virus.

guinea pigs are not usually susceptible). They were then inoculated with *Shigella,* and a subset of the study was then given opium. The authors discovered an association between opium administration and fatal *Shigella* infection. From these data, the authors concluded that a major defense mechanism of the guinea pig is its peristaltic activity and that antimotility agents (opium) might increase susceptibility to enteric infection.

A study in 1973 on human volunteers perpetuated the myth. In this study, DuPont and Hornick examined, among other things, the effect of diphenoxylate and atropine (Lomotil) on shigellosis.[19] The authors found that Lomotil seemed to diminish the number of unformed stools but in so doing may have increased patients' susceptibility to invasive infection, because fever was prolonged only in the patients receiving Lomotil. However, the sample size in this study was 25, and there were four treatment arms, making the number of patients in each treatment arm approximately six. The authors admitted that the study was inconclusive due to its small sample size and suggested that further investigation occur before conclusions could be made regarding the use of Lomotil in infectious diarrhea. Nevertheless, the two studies led to a nearly universal avoidance of the use of antimotility agents in patients with infectious diarrhea.

MODERN MEDICINE In 1990, Ericsson and colleagues[20] published a paper that addressed the use of loperamide (Imodium) in the treatment of traveler's diarrhea. In a study of 227 adults with acute diarrhea, combination treatment with Bactrim and loperamide was proven to be safe and effective in treating traveler's diarrhea. In 1993, a randomized, placebo-controlled, double-blind study was performed in Thailand comparing the use of ciprofloxacin and loperamide with ciprofloxacin and placebo in the treatment of adults with bacillary dysentery.[21] The study showed that loperamide combined with ciprofloxacin decreased the number of diarrheal stools and shortened the duration of illness in adult patients with dysentery due to *Shigella* or enteroinvasive *Escherichia coli.* No complications were seen in the group treated with loperamide. Although the study size was small ($n = 88$), it was much larger than in the 1973 study by DuPont and Hornick,[19] and it was the first of its kind to suggest the safety of antimotility agents in the treatment of adult invasive diarrheas. We therefore recommend the prescription of loperamide (see Table 83-3 for dosing), because it has clearly been proven to shorten duration of symptoms when combined with an antibiotic regimen. Diphenoxylate and atropine (Lomotil) is a more potent antidiarrheal whose modern-day safety is less well studied. For patients with severely inconveniencing diarrhea refractory to loperamide, diphenoxylate and atropine may be helpful. It should be used with caution, however, in patients with a history of constipation or cardiac disease.

Rehydration For patients presenting to the emergency department with significant dehydration, intravenous fluid therapy is indicated. For a mildly dehydrated patient who is not vomiting, oral rehydration therapy is recommended. Glucose-containing, caffeine-free beverages are the fluids of choice. Recall that it is the glucose transport mechanism that is unaffected by the enterotoxins, allowing for water absorption in the small intestine. For patients who can afford to buy it, Gatorade is a good rehydration choice with mild dehydration. The World Health Organization recommends a solution with a higher sodium concentration well suited to more extensive dehydration. Mildly dehydrated patients should aim to drink 30 to 50 mL/kg over the next 4 h. For moderate dehydration, patients should drink 100 mL/kg over the next 4 h.[10]

Dietary Restrictions Patients should be counseled to avoid caffeine, which stimulates gastric motility, and sorbitol-containing chewing gum or raw fruits, which can exacerbate an osmotic diarrhea. Lactose should be avoided initially until the colonic villi are able to recover and produce the necessary digestive enzymes. Patients should be encouraged to attempt early solid food intake with these restrictions, because this has been shown to expedite the recovery from diarrheal illnesses.[22]

Disposition

Patients with the noninfectious emergencies outlined above warrant hospitalization. Most other patients can be discharged home safely. When deciding whether to admit a patient with diarrhea, conservatism should be the rule with the young and the elderly. They do have higher morbidity and mortality rates and should be evaluated with a careful eye. Regardless of age, any toxic patient should be admitted, as should any patient who cannot convincingly comply with oral rehydration guidelines. Upon discharge, patients with infectious diarrhea should be counseled on limiting the spread of disease through the use of judicious hand washing. Work excuses should be given liberally to patients employed in the food, day-care, and health care industries. Prevention strategies for infectious diarrhea can be reiterated for those who acquired the diarrhea with foreign travel. A quick, but helpful phrase that can be shared for prevention is, "Peel it, boil it, cook it, or forget it!" For tourists tempted with luscious foods of the native land, this remains a difficult task!

CONSTIPATION

Epidemiology

Constipation is the most common digestive complaint in the United States and accounts for more than 2.5 million physician visits per year.[23,24] There is an age-related increase in the incidence of constipation, with 30 to 40 percent of adults older than 65 years citing constipation as a problem.[24,25]

Pathophysiology

The cause of constipation is usually multifactorial. Dietary intake affects bowel motility. Diminishing intake of fiber associated with decreased fluid intake can result in constipation. In addition, exercise, medical conditions, and medications affect gut motility. Sedentary patients often become constipated. Medical conditions such as hypothyroidism, hyperparathyroidism, lead poisoning, and chronic neurologic disorders are well-known causes. Some anal pathologic conditions cause painful defecation and in turn can result in constipation due to consequent fear, particularly in children. Patients confined to a hospital bed after an orthopedic injury, for example, may become constipated due to their inability to use a bedpan successfully. Certain medications, such as calcium-channel blockers, iron, narcotic analgesics, and antipsychotics, are also common causes of constipation. Indeed, constipation is a complicated condition with multiple causes (Table 83-4).

TABLE 83-4   Differential Diagnosis of Constipation

ACUTE OR SUBACUTE

Gastrointestinal: obstructing cancer, volvulus, stricture, hernia, adhesion, pelvic or abdominal masses, inflammation
Medicinal: addition of new medicine (e.g., antipsychotic, anticholinergic, narcotic analgesic, antacids)
Environmental: change in defecation regimen (e.g., forced to use bedpan)
Exercise and diet: decrease in level of exercise, fiber intake, fluid intake

CHRONIC

Gastrointestinal: slowly growing tumor, colonic dysmotility, anal pathology
Medicinal: chronic laxative abuse, antipsychotics, anticholinergics, narcotic analgesics
Neurologic: neuropathy, Parkinson disease, paraplegia, cerebral palsy
Endocrine: diabetes, hypothyroidism, hyperparathyroidism
Rheumatologic: scleroderma
Toxicologic: lead poisoning

Clinical Features

HISTORY The easiest, most practical definition of *constipation* is the following: the presence of hard stools that are difficult to pass. Some patients become bowel fixated and feel they are constipated if they do not have a daily bowel movement. They are not.

The differential diagnosis of constipation is broad. Determining the onset of the constipation helps narrow the differential diagnosis. Acute constipation represents intestinal obstruction until proven otherwise. Tumors, strictures, and volvuloses can present as acute constipation. Physicians often mistake subacute for chronic constipation. The important distinction here is to determine exactly when bowel habits changed. In general, acute and subacute conditions have the same differential diagnosis. Chronic constipation, that is, a lifelong or persistent habit, is usually less ominous and, if uncomplicated, can often be managed on an outpatient basis. The presence or absence of associated symptoms may help guide decision-making. Vomiting rarely accompanies benign constipation. Inability to pass flatus also raises concern about obstruction. A history of gradually diminishing stool caliber may suggest colon cancer, especially if accompanied by weight loss. The physician should ask the patient about recent changes in dietary fiber or fluid intake. What other medical problems does the patient have? Is there a history of hypothyroidism or diabetes? An antecedent history of diverticulitis may point toward inflammatory stricture. A history of nephrolithiasis could suggest hyperparathyroidism as a cause for constipation. A quick review of the patient's medication list also may point to the culprit.

PHYSICAL EXAMINATION The physical examination should concentrate on ruling out organic causes of constipation. First and foremost, intestinal obstruction must be ruled out. The patient should be examined carefully for the presence or absence of hernias and abdominal or pelvic masses. Rectal and pelvic examinations are necessary. In addition to detecting the presence or absence of an obstructing rectal mass, rectal examination enables the physician to ascertain whether there is fecal impaction. Anal fissures are also detected during the rectal examination. In addition, rectal examination allows the physician to determine whether the stools are bloody. Guaiac-positive stools can be seen in functional constipation and constipation resulting from colon cancer. With constipation resulting in fecal impaction, one can develop pressure necrosis of the rectal mucosa that forms stercoral ulcers on the rectal walls. These ulcers may yield guaiac-positive stools or be revealed by fecaliths on an abdominal plain film. With constipation caused by tumor, stools are also often guaiac positive. Constipation and new ascites in postmenopausal women should prompt evaluation for ovarian or uterine carcinoma. Signs of hypothyroidism may also be evident during the physical examination.

The evaluation of a constipated patient depends on the clinician's level of concern for organic causes of constipation. Patients with a long-standing history of constipation often require little, if any, data acquisition, provided the history and physical examination do not point toward an organic process. An upright chest film and abdominal flat and erect films should be obtained in patients who are at risk for intestinal obstruction: patients with prior abdominal surgery, associated vomiting, significant abdominal distention, abdominal pain, and an acute or subacute history of constipation. In addition to assessing the presence or absence of intestinal obstruction, abdominal films allow the physician to assess stool burden. In patients in whom an organic cause for constipation is suspected, a complete blood count should be obtained to screen for anemia. In addition, thyroid function tests may be helpful with patients in whom the physician suspects hypothyroidism. Electrolyte abnormalities, specifically hypokalemia and hypercalcemia, can be associated with constipation and are worth checking in patients suspected of having an organic cause.

TABLE 83-5 Medical Adjuncts Used in the Treatment of Constipation (Listed from Least to Most Potent)

Type	Generic Name	Trade Name	Prn Doses	Side Effects	Mechanism
Fiber	Bran	NA	1 cup qd	Bloating, flatulence	Increase stool bulk or transit time, increase gut motility
	Psyllium	Metamucil	1 tsp tid	Bloating, flatulence	
Emollient	Docusate sodium	Colace	100 mg qd bid	Cramping	Facilitates mixture of stool fat and water
Stimulants	Bisacodyl	Dulcolax	10 mg PR tid	Incontinence, rectal burning	Stimulates the myenteric plexus, thereby increasing intestinal motility
	Anthraquinones	Peri-Colace	1–2 tablets PO qd/bid	Melanosis coli, degeneration of myenteric plexus	
	Senna	Senokot, Ex-lax	2 tablets PO qd/bid or 15–30 mL qd/bid	Laxative abuse, nausea, melanosis coli, cramping	
Saline laxative	Magnesium	Milk of magnesia	15–30 mL qd/bid	Magnesium toxicity	Colonic transit time is shortened
		Magnesium citrate	100–240 mL qd/bid	Cramping, flatulence, hypermagnesemia	
Suppository	Glycerin suppository	NA	1 PR qd	Rectal irritation	Local rectal stimulation prompts defecation
Hyperosmolar agents	Lactulose	NA	15–30 mL qd/bid	Cramps, flatulence, belching, nausea	Osmotically active nonabsorbable sugars pull fluid into the gut
	Sorbitol	NA	15–30 mL qd/bid	Cramps, flatulence	
	Polyethylene glycol	Golytely	1 gal/4 h	Nausea, cramping, anal irritation	
Enemas	Tap water	NA	500 mL PR	Local trauma	Colonic distention encourages evacuation
	Soap suds	NA	1500 mL PR	Local trauma	
	Monophosphate	Fleets	1 U PR	Local trauma, hyperphosphatemia (especially in patients with renal failure)	

Abbreviation: NA = not applicable.

Treatment

FUNCTIONAL CONSTIPATION The treatment of functional (chronic) constipation involves a multidisciplinary approach. Many patients come to the emergency department looking for medication. Medications often employed in the treatment of constipation are listed in Table 83-5. However, the most important part of treatment is dietary and behavior modification. The most important prescription a patient with constipation receives is for a strict dietary and exercise regimen, because, without adequate fluid (1.5 L per d), fiber (10 g per d), and exercise, medicinal methods usually fail.[24] In addition, patients should be urged to take advantage of the gastrocolic reflex by attempting to defecate daily after a certain meal.

In its extreme form, functional constipation can result in a variety of potentially life-threatening complications. Fecal impaction and intestinal pseudo-obstruction are two sequelae of which the emergency physician should be acutely aware.

Fecal Impaction Patients with fecal impaction must be disimpacted manually before leaving the emergency department. Manual disimpaction is not a glamorous procedure, and, as a result, many physicians avoid doing it. This is unfortunate, because enemas, the alternative therapy, rarely work for fecal impaction. It must be remembered that manual disimpaction can be a painful procedure for which patients at times require sedation. After disimpaction, a host of medicines may be used to assist the patient in achieving normal fecal flow. The agents in Table 83-5 are listed in the order most easily tolerated by patients.

Intestinal Pseudo-Obstruction Intestinal pseudo-obstruction is a condition seen in patients with a long-standing history of colonic dysmotility. Patients present in a manner that mimics intestinal obstruction: abdominal distention, crampy abdominal pain, and obstipation. Abdominal x-ray films may reveal a severely dilated colon. Treatment is varied and is best determined in consultation with a surgeon. Sometimes the symptoms resolve with conservative management. Other times, however, patients require operative or colonoscopic decompression of the very dilated intestine.

ORGANIC CONSTIPATION The treatment of organic constipation is dictated by the cause of the constipation. In the emergency department, the precise cause of the constipation is not always known. Emergency physicians often suspect organic causes, such as hypothyroidism and hyperparathyroidism, but seldom actually confirm these diagnoses in the emergency department. Patients in whom an organic cause of constipation is suspected and who are without evidence of obstruction may start a bowel-cleansing regimen. Fecal impaction also occurs with organic constipation (i.e., hypothyroidism or hyperparathyroidism) and must be managed aggressively, as outlined above.

Constipation caused by intestinal obstruction is an emergency. Definitive treatment is dictated by the cause of the obstruction. For example, sigmoid volvulus often can be reduced by means of rigid sigmoidoscopy. Large-bowel obstruction resulting from colon cancer requires operative management. Regardless of the cause, intestinal obstruction warrants surgical consultation to assist with management decisions.

Disposition

Many constipated patients can be safely discharged from the emergency department with the caveat that certain key aspects have been adequately addressed (Table 83-6).[25] Patients with functional constipation with or without fecal impaction can be managed safely as outpatients provided patients with fecal impaction are disimpacted manually before discharge. Patients with organic constipation of a nonobstructive cause also can be managed safely as outpatients. The primary care provider should be contacted to ensure follow-up and to communicate concern for an organic process. If thyroid function tests

TABLE 83-6 Key Aspects to Address Before Discharging a Constipated Patient

1. Possible obstructing lesion
2. Systemic illness
3. Electrolyte imbalance
4. Potential for intestinal perforation with self-administered enemas

Source: Adapted from Holson et al.[26]

were performed, the primary care doctor should be informed so that they may be followed up.

Referral to a gastroenterologist is warranted for patients with nonorganic constipation of recent onset; chronic constipation associated with weight loss, anemia, or change in stool caliber; refractory constipation; and constipation requiring chronic laxative use.[21] Patients with organic constipation of obstructive origin require hospitalization and surgical evaluation.

REFERENCES

1. Wang SC, Borison HL: A new concept of organization of the central emetic mechanism: Recent studies on the sites of action of apomorphine, copper sulfate and cardiac glycosides. *Gastroenterology* 22:1, 1952.
2. Lumsden K, Holden WS: The act of vomiting in man. *Gut* 10:173, 1969.
3. Lew JF, Glass RI, Gangarosa RE, et al: Diarrheal deaths in the United States, 1979 through 1987. *JAMA* 265:3280, 1991.
4. Bennett RG, Greenough WB: Approach to acute diarrhea in the elderly. *Gastroenterol Clin North Am* 22:517, 1993.
5. Murray CJL, Lopez AD: Mortality by cause for eight regions of the world: Global Burden of Disease Study. *Lancet* 349:1269, 1997.
6. Siegel D, Cohen PT, Neighbor M, et al: Predictive value of stool examination in acute diarrhea. *Arch Pathol Lab Med* 111:715, 1987.
7. Brownlee HJ: Introduction: Management of acute nonspecific diarrhea. *Am J Med* 88(suppl 6A):1S, 1990.
8. Binder HJ: Pathophysiology of acute diarrhea. *Am J Med* 88(suppl 6A):2S, 1990.
9. Park SI, Giannella RA: Approach to the adult patient with acute diarrhea. *Gastroenterol Clin North Am* 22:483, 1993.
10. Kroser JA, Metz DC: Evaluation of the adult patient with diarrhea. *Primary Care* 23: 629, 1996.
11. DuBois D, Binder L, Nelson B: Usefulness of the stool Wright's stain in the emergency department. *J Emerg Med* 6:483, 1988.
12. Salam I, Katelaris P, Leigh-Smith S, et al: Randomized trial of single-dose ciprofloxacin for travellers' diarrhoea. *Lancet* 344:1537, 1994.
13. Hines J, Nachamkin I: Effective use of the clinical microbiology laboratory for diagnosing diarrheal diseases. *Clin Infect Dis* 23:1292, 1996.
14. Bartlett JG: Antibiotic-associated diarrhea. *New Engl J Med* 346:334, 2002.
15. Aserkoff B, Bennett JV: Effect of antibiotic therapy in acute salmonellosis on the fecal excretion of *Salmonellae. New Engl J Med* 281:636, 1969.
16. Akalin HE: Role of quinolones in the treatment of diarrhoeal diseases. *Drugs* 49(suppl 2):128, 1995.
17. Goodman LJ, Trenholme GM, Kaplan RL, et al: Empiric antimicrobial therapy of domestically acquired acute diarrhea in urban adults. *Arch Intern Med* 150:541, 1990.
18. Formal SB, Abrams GD, Schneider H, et al: Experimental *Shigella* infections: Role of the small intestine in an experimental infection in guinea pigs. *J Bacteriol* 85:119, 1963.
19. DuPont HL, Hornick RB: Adverse effect of Lomotil therapy in shigellosis. *JAMA* 226:1525, 1973.
20. Ericsson CD, DuPont HL, Mathewson JJ, et al: Treatment of traveler's diarrhea with sulfamethoxazole and trimethoprim and loperamide. *JAMA* 263:257, 1990.
21. Murphy GS, Bodhidatta L, Echeverria P, et al: Ciprofloxacin and loperamide in the treatment of bacillary dysentery. *Ann Intern Med* 118:582, 1993.
22. Sullivan P: Nutritional management of acute diarrhea. *Nutrition* 14:758, 1998.
23. Sonnenberg A, Koch TR: Physician visits in the United States for constipation: 1958 to 1986. *Dig Dis Sci* 34:606, 1989.
24. Romero Y, Evans JM, Fleming KC, et al: Constipation and fecal incontinence in the elderly population. *Mayo Clin Proc* 71:81, 1996.
25. Abyad A, Mourad F: Constipation: Common sense care of the older patient. *Geriatrics* 51:28, 1996.
26. Holson D, Oster N: Constipation. *eMed J* 2:111, 2001.

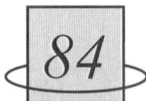

JAUNDICE
Richard O. Shields, Jr.

Jaundice is a physical finding that emergency physicians see as a presenting complaint and as an abnormal finding during the evaluation of other complaints and symptoms. Except in neonates, jaundice itself causes no adverse effects; it serves as a clinical marker of a defect in the metabolism and excretion of bilirubin. The task is to initiate laboratory evaluation or imaging studies, identify the underlying cause of jaundice, and determine whether admission or outpatient care is needed.

PATHOPHYSIOLOGY

Jaundice or icterus is the yellowish discoloration of the sclera, skin, and mucous membranes caused by the deposition of bile pigments associated with elevated levels of bilirubin in the blood (hyperbilirubinemia). Jaundice usually can be detected clinically when serum bilirubin levels reach 2.0 to 2.5 mg/dL or above, about twice the upper level of normal. It is usually first noticed in the sclera, because scleral tissue contains a large amount of elastin, which has a high affinity for bilirubin. Jaundice is easier to detect in people with light complexions and in the presence of significant anemia. The brownish discoloration of the sclerae in many people with darker complexions may be confused with scleral icterus and makes it more difficult to detect. A greenish tint to the skin indicates longstanding jaundice during which some of the bilirubin deposited in the skin has been metabolized to biliverdin. A yellow-orange discoloration of the skin can be caused by the presence of high levels of carotene in the blood (resulting from the dietary intake of large amounts of β-carotene) or by longstanding hemochromatosis. Neither will discolor the sclera.

Bilirubin, a breakdown product of hemoglobin from injured or senescent red blood cells and other heme-containing proteins, is produced in the reticuloendothelial system and then released into the plasma, where it is bound to albumin. Hepatocytes take up the bilirubin, conjugate it (mostly as mono- and diglucuronides), and excrete it through the bile channels into the small intestine. In the gut, bacterial enzymes release some of the bilirubin and reduce it to urobilinogen and the other pigments that give fecal material its typical color. Some urobilinogen is reabsorbed into the portal circulation, where most is taken up by the liver and re-excreted into the bile. A small amount reaches the kidneys and is excreted unchanged into the urine. Hyperbilirubinemia and jaundice, therefore, can be produced by an overproduction of bilirubin in the reticuloendothelial system, a failure of hepatocyte uptake of bilirubin, a failure of the hepatocyte to conjugate or excrete bilirubin, or an obstruction of biliary excretion into the intestine.

Depending on whether the defect occurs before or after the conjugation phase in the hepatocyte, two types of hyperbilirubinemia can be produced: unconjugated and conjugated. If increased production of bilirubin exceeds the ability of the liver to process it or if there is a defect in bilirubin uptake or conjugation, then levels of the unconjugated form will rise, producing unconjugated hyperbilirubinemia. Causes include hemolysis from hemoglobinopathies, hemolytic anemias or transfusion reactions, and in-born errors of bilirubin metabolism.

If the liver can produce but not normally excrete conjugated bilirubin because of a metabolic defect or intra- or extrahepatic obstruction, conjugated hyperbilirubinemia and cholestasis result. Intrahepatic cholestasis is caused by decreased excretion of conjugated bilirubin, hepatocellular damage, or damage to the biliary endothelium. Obstruction of biliary outflow by a congenital defect, inflammation, a mass lesion, or gallstones produces extrahepatic cholestasis.

It is helpful clinically to categorize conditions that produce jaundice as disorders of bilirubin metabolism (e.g., hemolysis and in-born errors), hepatocellular disorders (e.g., viral hepatitis and drug toxic-

ity), or bile duct obstruction (e.g., gallstones and tumor).[1] More than one type can be present in a given patient (Table 84-1).

CLINICAL FEATURES

A careful history and physical examination and select laboratory studies should enable the diagnosis. Often, however, more extensive diagnostic procedures, such as ultrasonography, computed tomography, or biopsy, are needed.

A family history of jaundice or a history of recurrent mild jaundice that resolves spontaneously is most consistent with a familial disorder of bilirubin metabolism, such as Gilbert, Rotor, Crigler-Najjar, or Dubin-Johnson syndrome. Most patients with sickle cell disease develop chronic jaundice from ongoing hemolysis, but in the presence of abdominal pain, vomiting, and fever, acute cholecystitis or biliary obstruction must be strongly suspected. The patient should also be asked about other hemoglobinopathies or prior episodes of hemolysis.

Hepatic causes of jaundice can be acute or chronic. The sudden appearance of jaundice in a previously healthy young person, especially if preceded by a brief prodrome of fever, malaise, and myalgias, is likely to be caused by a viral hepatitis. Inquire about body fluid exposure over the previous few months, including transfusion of blood products, intimate contact with someone with hepatitis or jaundice,

TABLE 84-1 Causes of Jaundice

Disorders of bilirubin metabolism
  Neonatal jaundice
  Hemolysis
  Hemoglobinopathy
  Transfusion reaction
  In-born errors of metabolism
Hepatocellular causes
  Infections
    Viral hepatitis
    Leptospirosis
    Infectious mononucleosis
  Drugs and toxins
    Ethanol
    Acetaminophen
    Amanita toxin
    Carbon tetrachloride
    Anabolic steroids
    Chlorpromazine
    Isoniazid
  Metabolic
    Wilson disease
    Reye syndrome
    Hemochromatosis
  Granulomatous
    Wegener granulomatosis
    Sarcoidosis
    Lymphoma
    Mycobacterial
  Miscellaneous
    Fatty liver of pregnancy
    Ischemia
    Primary biliary cirrhosis
    Benign recurrent intrahepatic cholestasis
    Postoperative cholestasis
    Amyloidosis
Bile duct obstruction
  Gallstones
  Cholangiopathy due to acquired immunodeficiency syndrome
  Primary sclerosing cholangitis
  Bile duct stricture
  Pancreatic tumors or cysts
  Pancreatitis
  Cholangiocarcinoma

promiscuous sexual activity, intravenous drug use, accidental needle-stick injuries or mucosal contact with body fluids, travel to countries where hepatitis is prevalent, raw shellfish ingestion, and recent tattoos or body piercing. Many times, however, no history of exposure can be elicited. Right upper quadrant pain and tenderness and hepatomegaly may be present, but pruritus is usually absent. Examine for needle tracks, because patients may not volunteer a history of drug use. Jaundice caused by drugs and hepatotoxins also may appear suddenly. Toxic hepatitis should be suspected if a history of ingestion or exposure to such substances is obtained. Signs of hepatocellular damage may be present with toxicity from agents such as acetaminophen, halothane, methyldopa, isoniazid, or phenytoin. Cholestatic changes predominate in toxicity from anabolic steroids, oral contraceptives, and chlorpromazine. *Amanita* mushroom poisoning, carbon tetrachloride, and phosphorus can produce massive hepatic necrosis.[2]

Jaundice that develops gradually may fall into the hepatic or bile duct obstruction categories. Alcoholic liver disease and cirrhosis are likely if jaundice is accompanied by weakness, peripheral muscle wasting, ascites, spider angiomata, pruritus, and symptoms of portal hypertension. A reliable history of sustained, significant alcohol intake should be sought from the patient or from family and friends. A history of any previous episodes of jaundice, pancreatitis, or hematemesis should be obtained. Fever, vomiting, and right upper quadrant tenderness accompany episodes of alcoholic hepatitis. The presence of asterixis, fetor hepaticus, or encephalopathy indicates advanced disease.

Jaundice that develops acutely with abdominal pain, vomiting, fever, and right upper quadrant tenderness is strongly suggestive of acute cholangitis, most commonly from choledocholithiasis. A history of fatty food intolerance and typical biliary colic is supportive. Cholecystitis alone does not produce jaundice. Painless jaundice in an older patient, especially if accompanied by an epigastric mass and weight loss, strongly suggests biliary obstruction from a malignancy. A history of known gastrointestinal malignancy accompanied by a hard, nodular liver indicates metastatic disease as the cause of jaundice. A history of prior biliary tract surgery, pancreatitis, cholangitis, acquired immunodeficiency syndrome, or inflammatory bowel disease should be elicited, because these conditions may be associated with the development of biliary obstruction.

Hepatomegaly with pedal edema, jugular venous distention, and a gallop rhythm makes congestive cardiac failure the likely cause of jaundice.

LABORATORY EVALUATION

The initial laboratory evaluation of the jaundiced patient should include determinations of the serum bilirubin level (total and the direct-reacting fraction), the serum liver aminotransferase levels, and the serum alkaline phosphatase level; urinalysis for bilirubin and urobilinogen; a complete blood count; prothrombin time; and any other pertinent tests suggested by the physical examination and history (e.g., determinations of serum amylase or lipase levels). The serum bilirubin level is measured by the van den Bergh reaction with the use of two techniques to measure total bilirubin and conjugated bilirubin (the direct fraction). The indirect fraction can then be calculated by subtracting the direct fraction from the total.

If the patient has unconjugated hyperbilirubinemia, the bilirubin is usually only mildly elevated and consists predominately (>85 percent) of the indirect fraction. Because unconjugated bilirubin is tightly bound to albumin, it does not appear in the urine. Liver aminotransferase levels will be normal, and the blood count and smear may show evidence of anemia or hemolysis. A Coombs test and hemoglobin electrophoresis may be helpful if no history of hemolytic anemia or hemoglobinopathy is known. Gilbert's syndrome is the most common cause of mild unconjugated hyperbilirubinemia. This is an inherited deficiency in bilirubin conjugation that produces no symptoms other than variable elevations of bilirubin and no adverse effects. Factors

that can cause bilirubin to rise include fever, heavy physical exertion, fasting, surgery, and heavy alcohol consumption.

A direct-reacting fraction of at least 30 percent (and usually much higher) is present with conjugated hyperbilirubinemia. Conjugated bilirubin is water soluble and appears in the urine at very low serum concentrations. Urobilinogen will be absent from the urine if significant cholestasis is present. If liver enzyme levels are normal, the jaundice is caused by sepsis or recent systemic infection, in-born errors of bilirubin metabolism (such as Rotor syndrome or Dubin-Johnson syndrome), or pregnancy, rather than by primary hepatic disease. If liver enzyme levels are abnormal, which is much more common, the pattern of abnormality suggests the cause. Predominance of aminotransferase elevation is more suggestive of hepatocellular disease, such as viral or toxic hepatitis or cirrhosis, whereas marked elevations of alkaline phosphatase (two to three times normal) and γ-glutamyl transpeptidase suggest intra- or extrahepatic obstruction, such as malignancy or gallstones.

Further laboratory testing and imaging studies should be undertaken next, directed by which type of jaundice is present. If the initial laboratory studies suggest hepatocellular disease and the clinical examination suggests viral hepatitis, then serologic studies for viral hepatitis should be done. If the clinical picture points to alcoholic liver disease or other toxins, then platelet count and serum albumin levels should be determined to help estimate the degree of liver injury. If results of the serologic studies are negative, there is no improvement with withdrawal of the suspected toxic agent, or there is no other obvious etiology, liver biopsy should be considered.

If the clinical examination and initial laboratory findings suggest intrahepatic cholestasis or extrahepatic biliary obstruction, ultrasound studies should be performed to look for gallstones, dilated extrahepatic biliary ducts, or masses in the liver, pancreas, or portal area. Computed tomography also can be used but is usually more costly, involves radiation exposure, and is less sensitive than is ultrasound at detecting stones in the gallbladder.

DISPOSITION

Jaundice alone is not an indication for admission. A hemodynamically stable patient with new-onset jaundice without evidence of liver failure or acute biliary obstruction can be discharged from the emergency department, if the appropriate laboratory studies have been ordered and follow-up has been arranged. Surgical consultation should be obtained if extrahepatic biliary obstruction is suspected. For other admission indicators, refer to the appropriate chapters in this text.

REFERENCES

1. Feldman M, Friedman L, Sleisenger M, Scharschmidt B (eds): *Sleisenger & Fordtran's Gastrointestinal and Liver Disease,* 7th ed. Philadelphia, W.B. Saunders, 2002.
2. Lewis JH, Zimmerman HJ: Drug- and chemical-induced cholestasis. *Clin Liver Dis* 3:433, 1999.

85

CHOLECYSTITIS AND BILIARY COLIC

William J. Brady

Thomas P. Aufderheide

Judith E. Tintinalli

Biliary tract emergencies result primarily from obstruction by biliary calculi in the gallbladder and bile ducts. The four major biliary tract emergencies related to gallstones include biliary colic (symptomatic cholelithiasis), cholecystitis, gallstone pancreatitis, and ascending cholangitis. While gallstones are common, most are asymptomatic. The incidence of new-onset biliary pain among patients with previously asymptomatic gallstones is about 2 percent per year for the first 5 years and 15 percent at 10 years.[1] Although the classic patient with symptomatic biliary tract disease is an obese female aged 20 to 40 years, the disease occurs in all age groups and must be especially considered in diabetics and the elderly.[2] Upper abdominal pain is the chief complaint most predictive of biliary colic or cholecystitis.[3]

Certain patient subpopulations exhibit gallstone-related illness at differing rates and in differing fashion. Cholelithiasis can occur in children, albeit infrequently. Gallstones in this age group may be idiopathic or may develop due to hemolytic disorders, cystic fibrosis, obesity, ileal resection, or long-term use of total parenteral nutrition. Among pregnant patients, recent reports support a strong association between pregnancy and gallstone formation. Valdivieso and colleagues[4] studied the natural history of gallstones during pregnancy. Using ultrasound, they reported that 12 percent of the recently pregnant women had gallstones versus 1.3 percent of the nonpregnant control group. Maringhini et al[5] demonstrated not only an increase in the incidence of biliary sludge and gallstones as pregnancy progressed, but the resolution of these same stones postpartum. While pregnancy seems to predispose to cholelithiasis, cholecystitis remains uncommon.[6] The elderly have a reasonably high incidence of symptomatic gallstones and related complications; the overall frequency of gallstone disease in the elderly has been estimated to be between 14 and 27 percent based on large population studies.[7] Elderly patients with acute cholecystitis are more likely than younger patients to have biliary sepsis and gangrenous changes in the gallbladder, resulting in increased perioperative morbidity. The increased severity of cholecystitis in the elderly is thought to be secondary to impaired immune defense mechanisms, delays in diagnosis, and comorbidities common to this age group. Mortality rates of 19 percent have been reported.[8]

A number of risk factors (Table 85-1), including familial tendency, are associated with cholecystitis and calculi. Clinical characteristics associated with an increased risk of the development of pigment stones are Asian descent, chronic biliary tract infection, parasitic infection (e.g., *Ascaris lumbricoides*), chronic liver disease (particularly related to alcohol), and chronic intravascular hemolysis (sickle cell anemia and hereditary spherocytosis). Hepatitis A, B, C, and E viruses; HIV; and the herpesviruses are associated with viral cholangitis and hepatitis.[9]

TABLE 85-1 Risk Factors for the Development of Gallstones

Increased age
Female sex
Parity
Obesity
Profound weight loss
Prolonged fasting
Cystic fibrosis
Hypertriglyceridemia
Total parenteral nutrition
Pregnancy
High spinal cord injury
Medications
    Oral contraceptives
    Octreotide
    Estrogens/progesterones
    Ceftriaxone
    Clofibrate
Ethnicity
    Pima Indian tribe
    Scandinavia
Chronic intravascular hemolysis
Liver disease
Chronic parasitic infections

PATHOPHYSIOLOGY

Bile is manufactured in and secreted from hepatocytes and transported to the gallbladder for storage via the canaliculi, ductiles, and bile ducts. The bile ducts become progressively larger and eventually coalesce to form the right and left hepatic ducts, which unite to form the common hepatic duct. The common hepatic duct joins with the cystic duct from the gallbladder to form the common bile duct, which empties into the duodenum through the ampulla of Vater. The pancreatic duct often merges with the common bile duct immediately prior to entering the duodenum. The wall of the gallbladder is innervated with sympathetic and parasympathetic nerves from the celiac plexus.[10]

Bile is composed primarily of water (80 percent), bile acids (10 percent), lecithin and other phospholipids (4 to 5 percent), cholesterol (1 percent), conjugated bilirubin, electrolytes, mucus, and various proteins. The major stimulus for release of bile is the gastrointestinal hormone cholecystokinin, which is secreted from the small intestinal mucosal cells when fats and amino acids enter the duodenum. Cholecystokinin causes forceful contraction of the gallbladder, relaxation of the sphincter of Oddi, increased hepatic bile production, and ultimately release of bile into the duodenum for digestion of a meal. Approximately 95 percent of bile is conserved via enterohepatic circulation.

Gallstones, crystalline structures formed from both normal and abnormal bile components, are divided into three major types: cholesterol (70 percent), pigment (20 percent), and mixed (10 percent). Cholesterol stones, the most commonly encountered gallstones, contain more than 70 percent cholesterol monohydrate. The formation of such stones is complex, involving cholesterol supersaturation of the bile; the formation of monohydrate crystals, with aggregation into successively larger structures; and delayed gallbladder emptying with bile stasis. Pigment stones are subdivided into black and brown varieties. Black stones are noted in patients with advanced liver disease and hemolytic disorders, while brown stones are found commonly in patients of Asian descent, usually resulting from bacterial or parasitic infection. Both subtypes of pigment stones result from abnormal solubilization of unconjugated bilirubin coupled with the precipitation of calcium salts. The calcium content of cholesterol stones is much lower than that of pigment stones, making cholesterol stones most frequently radiolucent and pigment stones radiopaque. Anatomically, cholesterol gallstones are found in the gallbladder, cystic duct, intrahepatic ducts, and common bile duct. Brown pigment stones have a distribution similar to that of cholesterol gallstones, while black stones occur exclusively in the gallbladder.

The pathogenesis of symptomatic cholelithiasis involves stone migration from the gallbladder into the biliary tract and eventual obstruction. The stone, once lodged in either the cystic or common bile duct, produces increased intraluminal pressure and distention of the hollow viscus, resulting in pain, nausea, and vomiting. Forceful, repetitive contractions of the entire biliary system may relieve the obstruction. If obstruction persists, particularly in either the cystic duct or the infundibulum of the gallbladder, acute cholecystitis may develop. The inflammatory response in acute cholecystitis results from a combination of three factors: mechanical, chemical, and infectious. The mechanical factor produces the rise in intraluminal pressure and distention of the viscus, which culminates in visceral ischemia. Chemical inflammation occurs with the release of various mediators (lysolecithin, phospholipase A, and prostaglandins), resulting in direct mucosal injury. The contribution to the inflammatory response by bacterial agents is variable, occurring in 50 to 80 percent of patients with acute cholecystitis. Bacterial pathogens include Enterobacteriaceae (70 percent, particularly *Escherichia coli* and *Klebsiella* species), enterococci (15 percent), *Bacteroides* (10 percent), *Clostridium* species (10 percent), group D *Streptococcus,* and *Staphylococcus* species. The inflammatory process may progress to gangrene of the gallbladder wall with or without perforation.

Gallstone pancreatitis is similarly multifactorial, since it is experimentally produced by injecting bile, bacteria, and trypsin under pressure.[11]

CLINICAL FEATURES

Gallbladder diseases is a continuum, ranging from asymptomatic cholelithiasis, to biliary colic, to acute cholecystitis. Location, radiation, and duration of pain are all poor discriminators of gallbladder disease. There is overlap of signs and symptoms with peptic ulcer disease, gastritis, esophageal reflux, and nonspecific dyspepsia. In addition, it has been difficult to determine which symptoms are attributable to biliary tract disease.[12,13] RUQ pain is a common symptom in patients with and without gallstones.[3,14] Up to 25 percent of post-cholecystectomy patients may experience RUQ pain of unknown cause. Upper abdominal or epigastric pain is the predominant symptom of biliary tract disease[3,14] thus accounting for the difficulty in using clinical signs and symptoms to make or exclude the diagnosis. Radiation of pain to the left upper back appears to be more commonly associated with biliary tract disease than with other upper gastrointestinal disorders, with a likelihood ratio of 4.0 for gallbladder pathology.[14] In fact, no single clinical finding has a negative LR sufficient to rule out the diagnosis.[15]

The duration and character of the pain are also nonspecific, but the pain of biliary colic is reported to persist for 2 to 6 h. Pain quality is generally persistent, not colicky, and pain episodes are infrequent, occurring at intervals of more than a week.[9] Gallstone pain is not related to meals in at least one-third of patients,[14,16] and clinical studies have not been able to identify an association with fatty food intolerance that is different from its association with a number of other upper gastrointestinal disorders.[3,14,16] Investigators have noted a circadian rhythm to biliary colic,[16] with a peak of symptoms occurring around midnight to 1 a.m., and a time distribution from 9 P.M. to 4 A.M. Attacks tend to recur at the same time. This circadian rhythm has obvious diagnostic implications for patients who present with upper abdominal pain during the midnight shift.

Acute cholecystitis usually begins with pain similar to that of biliary colic but that persists beyond the typical 6 h. Associated nausea, vomiting, and anorexia are noted; a history of fever and/or chills is not uncommon. Patients may have either a history of similar attacks or documented gallstones. As the inflammatory process progresses, the patient's pain changes in character and location from visceral (dull and poorly localized mid-upper abdominal) to parietal (sharp and localized RUQ). The examination reveals a patient in moderate-to-severe distress with signs of systemic toxicity, including tachycardia and fever. The abdomen is tender in the RUQ, at times with evidence of localized peritoneal irritation, distention, and hypoactive bowel sounds. Generalized peritonitis with rigidity is rare and, if found, suggests perforation. The Murphy sign—worsened pain or inspiratory arrest resulting from deep, subcostal palpation on inspiration—has been estimated to be 97 percent sensitive for acute cholecystitis.[3] However, a recent metaanalysis[3] of 17 studies calculated a sensitivity of 65 percent and specificity of 87 percent, an LR (+) of 2.8 (95% CI 0.8–8.6) and an LR (−) of 0.5 (95% CI 0.2–1.0) for Murphy sign. Volume depletion is frequently found. Jaundice, usually not present, may be found in patients with prolonged biliary obstruction with late onset of inflammation or in cases of chronic intravascular hemolysis.

Acalculous cholecystitis, which occurs in 5 to 10 percent of patients with acute cholecystitis, tends to have a more rapid, malignant course. Patients frequently are elderly and have a history of diabetes mellitus. Other risk factors include multiple trauma, extensive burn injury, prolonged labor, major surgery, gallbladder torsion, systemic vasculitic states, and bacterial or parasitic infections of the biliary tract. Patients with acalculous cholecystitis are indistinguishable from those with calculous cholecystitis with two major exceptions: acalculous cholecystitis frequently occurs as a complication of another process

TABLE 85-2   Clinical Manifestations of Gallbladder Disease

Cholelithiasis
   Right upper quadrant or epigastric pain, often colicky and postprandial
   Pain may radiate to shoulder or around waist
   Nausea and vomiting may be present
Cholecystitis
   Same manifestations as those for cholelithiasis, plus
   Murphy sign present
   Fever and chills may be present
Cholangitis
   Same manifestations as those for cholecystitis, plus
   Jaundice
   Altered mental status
   Shock

(e.g., multiple trauma or extensive burns), and patients frequently are gravely ill on initial presentation.

Refer to Table 85-2 for a comparison of the clinical manifestations of the continuum of gallbladder disease.

DIFFERENTIAL DIAGNOSIS

The differential diagnosis of biliary colic includes other conditions associated with upper abdominal pain, including gastritis, gastroesophageal reflux, pancreatitis, hepatitis, and peptic ulcer disease. Atypical myocardial infarction should be considered in older patients. Acute renal colic can be associated with upper abdominal and upper back pain. Both conditions can also be associated with flank tenderness, nausea, and vomiting. Renal colic does not have a circadian rhythm, and the pain is colicky, not continuous as in biliary colic. Nonetheless, it can be difficult to distinguish biliary from renal colic, and definitive imaging studies may be needed to make the correct diagnosis. Acute pyelonephritis, like cholecystitis, can be associated with flank and upper quadrant pain, but pyuria confirms the former diagnosis. Appendicitis can sometimes be associated with RUQ pain, especially in pregnancy or in patients with a retrocecal or redundant appendix. In women of childbearing age, the differential diagnosis is expanded to include a wide variety of gynecologic disorders, including pelvic inflammatory disease, perihepatitis (Fitzhugh-Curtis syndrome), and ectopic pregnancy. Pregnancy testing, gynecologic history, and pelvic examination should focus on the correct diagnosis. Finally, pneumonia or pleural effusion can be associated with RUQ pain. Diagnosis is confirmed by chest x-ray. However, pancreatitis can also be associated with pleural effusions, usually on the right.

DIAGNOSTIC STUDIES

Because of the poor predictive value of history, physical examination, and laboratory findings for cholecystitis, the most important features for diagnosis are a high clinical suspicion and ultrasound imaging.[3] Results of laboratory studies in patients with biliary colic are frequently normal.[3] The hemogram may reveal chronic anemia with or without evidence of hemolysis in patients with pigment stones. The white blood cell count, serum bilirubin level, alkaline phosphatase level, and aminotransferase levels are often normal. The serum lipase level should be obtained to rule out pancreatitis. The urine must be examined to exclude other causes of abdominal pain. In females, serum or urine pregnancy testing should be performed to rule out obstetric causes of abdominal pain. A negative pregnancy test result also enables one to proceed safely with radiologic studies, if indicated.

The presence of leukocytosis or abnormal liver function study results or lipase levels are often used as indicators for the diagnosis of acute cholecystitis. However, no single test or combination of laboratory tests has a sufficiently high sensitivity to detect acute cholecystitis.[3,17] A retrospective review of ED patients with acute cholecystitis found that 32 percent lacked a white blood cell count greater than 11,000 cells/mL.[18] Typical signs, symptoms, and laboratory findings may not be present in patients over age 60. The sensitivity of Murphy sign was only 48 percent in the elderly.[19] In a cohort of geriatric emergency department patients with abdominal pain who were determined at surgery to have acute cholecystitis, 56 percent were afebrile, 41 percent had no leukocytosis, and 13 percent were both afebrile and had normal values on routine laboratory tests.[20]

Additional studies in patients with biliary colic may be performed to support the diagnosis and rule out other causes of upper abdominal pain with nausea. Plain film radiographs of the abdomen demonstrate gallstones in only 10 to 20 percent of cases. The majority of stones are cholesterol and therefore radiolucent. Pigment and mixed stones containing at least 4 percent calcium by weight are radiopaque. Abdominal films are more useful in excluding other causes of pain. A chest radiograph should be obtained to identify right lower lobe pneumonia or pleural effusions. A 12-lead electrocardiogram should be considered in older patients to exclude an acute coronary syndrome.

Ultrasonography is now the initial diagnostic modality of choice. It may show the presence of stones as small as 2 mm, gallbladder distention, wall thickening, and pericholecystic fluid, and during the procedure a sonographic Murphy sign may be elicited. Ultrasonography has an unadjusted sensitivity of 94 percent and a specificity of 78 percent for the diagnosis of acute cholecystitis,[21] and when adjusted for spectrum bias, sensitivity is 88 and 80 percent. These figures can be replicated by emergency-physician-performed ultrasound examinations.[22,23] The sonographic Murphy's sign was found to be present in emergency physician examinations (sensitivity, 75 percent) more often than in radiological examinations (sensitivity, 45 percent). The decreased accuracy of emergency physicians in determining pericholecystic fluid, wall thickness, air in the gallbladder, and ductal dilatation did not result in any adverse outcomes. The reduction in length of ED stay from 223 min to 180 min was the major advantage of emergency physician ultrasound.[22] A recent prospective study[24] investigated the use of ultrasound by the emergency physician (EP) in the evaluation of the right upper quadrant pain. In this study, EPs performed ultrasound examinations on 116 such patients. Using formal abdominal ultrasound performed by radiology as the gold standard, EP exhibited reasonably high rates of agreement for detecting cholelithiasis and lesser rates of agreement for the diagnosis of cholecystitis. The authors concluded that ultrasound performed by the EP may be used to exclude cholelithiasis. They cautioned, however, that EPs with limited experience must interpret scans revealing possible cholecystitis with caution and advise that a confirmatory test is warranted before cholecystectomy.[24]

Computed tomography (CT) scanning can be most useful in the diagnosis of acute cholecystitis when other intraabdominal disorders are considerations in the differential diagnosis. Wall thickening, pericholecystic fluid, and subserosal edema can be identified. However, the sensitivity of CT scanning is insufficient (as low as 50 percent) for it to replace ultrasonography as the diagnostic procedure of choice.[25]

Radioisotope cholescintigraphy using technetium-iminoacetic acid analogues (HIDA) has a sensitivity and specificity of 97 and 90 percent, respectively.[21] The study is performed by injecting radioisotopes intravenously. The material is absorbed by the hepatocytes and secreted into the biliary tract. A normal patient will have a clearly outlined gallbladder and cystic duct within 1 h. Failure to demonstrate the gallbladder within this time frame is consistent with cystic duct obstruction. The HIDA scan can only be used in patients with a serum bilirubin level of less than 5 mg/dL. With serum bilirubin above this level, an alternative radioisotope study, the DISIDA scan, is preferred.

COMPLICATIONS

Fluid and electrolyte deficits due to protracted vomiting and anorexia, and upper gastrointestinal hemorrhage from emesis-related Mallory-Weiss tears can coexist with biliary tract emergencies. Complications associated with cholelithiasis include gallstone pancreatitis, ascending cholangitis, and cholecystitis. Patients with cholecystitis may further develop a number of serious complications, including gallbladder empyema and emphysematous (gangrenous) cholecystitis.

Approximately 70 percent of cases of acute pancreatitis are due to either gallstones or alcohol. Depending on the population studied, gallstones are involved in 30 to 70 percent of patients with acute pancreatitis. Of all patients with gallstones, 15 to 20 percent will develop pancreatitis as a result of biliary calculi. Patients with pancreatitis due to gallstones will present similarly to patients with pancreatic inflammation caused by ethanol, with epigastric or diffuse abdominal pain radiating to the back, associated with nausea and vomiting. Patients may manifest symptoms of both acute cholecystitis and acute pancreatitis. Management includes intravenous fluids, nasogastric decompression, analgesics, and parenteral antibiotics (Table 85-3) with subsequent surgery. In patients who present in extremis or in those who demonstrate clinical deterioration, urgent biliary decompression (surgical or endoscopic) is mandatory.

Ascending cholangitis is a life-threatening emergency with a mortality rate approaching 100 percent in untreated or improperly treated patients. The process results from complete biliary obstruction in the presence of bacteria (gram-negative organisms as well as enterococcal and various anaerobic species). As the obstruction persists, intraluminal pressure increases, resulting in reflux of bacteria into the lymphatic vessels and hepatic veins, with eventual entrance into the systemic circulation. The obstruction most often is due to choledocholithiasis (gallstone obstruction of the common bile duct) and less often to biliary tract strictures, surgical anastomotic strictures, various postprocedural complications, and extrinsic compression from malignancy. Patients present with jaundice, fever, RUQ pain, mental confusion, and shock. The classic Charcot triad of fever, jaundice, and RUQ pain is noted in only 25 percent of patients. Management includes initial volume resuscitation with vasopressor support in cases unresponsive to crystalloid infusion alone, broad-spectrum parenteral antibiotics, and rapid decompression (surgical or endoscopic) of the biliary tree.

Gallbladder empyema, a life-threatening complication of cholecystitis, results from complete obstruction of the cystic duct with bacterial infection of the stagnant bile and abscess formation within the gallbladder wall. Risk factors include age, diabetes mellitus, trauma, burns, vasculitis, and bacterial or parasitic infections of the biliary tract. The presentation is similar to cholangitis, with fever, RUQ pain, altered mentation, and hypotension. Patients frequently develop gram-negative sepsis and require immediate broad-spectrum antibiotic coverage, fluid resuscitation, and urgent surgical consultation for cholecystectomy. The outcome is poor without prompt definitive care.

Gangrene of the gallbladder wall may be focal or diffuse. Focal gangrene results from segmental ischemia of the gallbladder wall caused by severe distention, acute inflammation, empyema, torsion with arterial compromise, or coexisting vasculitis. Patients with diabetes mellitus are at risk for this complication. Perforation of the wall may occur in a contained fashion (into the omentum) or free (into the peritoneal cavity).

TABLE 85-3 Antibiotic Choices for Acute Cholecystitis with Sepsis and Ascending Cholangitis

Ampicillin, gentamicin, and metronidazole
Ciprofloxacin and/or metronidazole
Piperacillin-tazobactam
Ampicillin-sulbactam
Ticarcillin-clavulanate
Imipenem
Third-generation cephalosporin and metronidazole or clindamycin
Aztreonam and clindamycin

Gangrene of the entire gallbladder, also known as emphysematous cholecystitis, is an uncommon complication, occurring in approximately 1 percent of patients with cholecystitis. Emphysematous cholecystitis is acalculous in 30 percent of patients. The gallbladder wall becomes ischemic, with eventual bacterial infection and gangrene. Patients present in extremis with fever, RUQ pain, and septic shock. Plain-film radiographs may demonstrate air in the gallbladder itself, the gallbladder wall, or the biliary tree because of the frequent presence of gas-forming organisms. An abdominal CT scan is the suggested imaging study. The bacteriology of either focal or diffuse gallbladder gangrene includes gram-negative, gram-positive, and anaerobic organisms. Polymicrobial infection is common. Management is similar to that of gallbladder empyema. Mortality rates for gangrenous cholecystitis are very high because of associated sepsis and attendant comorbidity in the typical elderly diabetic patient.

TREATMENT

Patients with accurately diagnosed uncomplicated symptomatic cholelithiasis do not necessarily require immediate surgical intervention. Patients presenting with biliary colic and emesis are best treated with antispasmodic agents (glycopyrrolate), opiate analgesics (meperidine), and antiemetics (promethazine). Meperidine is the analgesic of choice because it produces significantly less spasm of the sphincter of Oddi than do other narcotic agents, such as morphine. Ketorolac tromethamine has been shown effective in relieving the pain of gallbladder distention. This distention causes the release of prostaglandins, which are associated with the production of pain. Ketorolac inhibits the production of prostaglandins, which may explain why it is effective in this situation. It is not as effective in relieving pain in the presence of infection. Gastric decompression with nasogastric suction may be warranted for protracted vomiting. Volume deficits and electrolyte imbalance can be corrected with isotonic intravenous fluids. With an accurate diagnosis, resolution of symptoms, correction of intravascular volume deficits, and a demonstrated ability to maintain hydration orally, the patient may be discharged from the ED. Prior to discharge, the case should be discussed with a surgical consultant or the patient's primary care physician to arrange for timely outpatient follow-up. Patients may be given oral narcotic-acetaminophen pain medication for the common residual abdominal aching. If the symptoms do not resolve within a 4- to 6-h period in the ED, the diagnosis of biliary colic must be questioned. Such prolonged pain may represent early, acute cholecystitis.

Patients with uncomplicated symptomatic cholelithiasis have several options for definitive treatment, including open or laparoscopic cholecystectomy, medical dissolution therapy, and gallstone lithotripsy. Open cholecystectomy with intraoperative cholangiogram provides definitive cure for patients with biliary colic. The laparoscopic technique is rapidly replacing the traditional open cholecystectomy as the procedure of choice. Patients with frequent or severe attacks of biliary colic, a history of associated complications of gallstones, large biliary calculi (>2 cm in diameter), a congenitally abnormal hepatobiliary system, diabetes mellitus, or a desire for rapid cure are best managed with open or laparoscopic cholecystectomy or endoscopic retrograde cholangiopancreatography with possible endoscopic sphincterotomy (ES). Approximately 5 percent of patients have complications from cholecystectomy. The majority of these adverse outcomes are wound infections. Abscess, hemorrhage, bile leakage, and fistula formation are infrequent. Approximately 8 percent of patients develop complications from ES. Pancreatitis and hemorrhage are the most common complications within 30 days of the procedure. Complications occurring months to years later, such as recurrent stones and cholangitis, are seen in about 10 percent of patients. Medical dissolution therapy with oral bile acid treatment is an option for those with small radiolucent stones (about 10 percent of patients).

Treatment of calculous and acalculous acute cholecystitis is surgical. Basic supportive medical therapy occurs in the emergency department prior to hospital admission and/or surgery. As with biliary colic, patients with acute cholecystitis require volume resuscitation with intravenous isotonic fluid, pain control with opiate analgesics, and bowel rest with nasogastric suction and antiemetic agents. Antibiotic treatment is recommended despite the questionable role of acute infection in all cases of early acute cholecystitis. In patients presenting without sepsis, single-agent therapy with a third-generation cephalosporin is adequate. In patients with sepsis, a widened spectrum of antibiotic therapy is recommended (see Table 85-3).

Patients with obvious infection should receive broadened coverage with ampicillin, gentamicin, and clindamycin, or the equivalent (see Table 85-3). A minority of patients (usually those with either acalculous or emphysematous cholecystitis or a complication of cholecystitis) present in septic shock and require aggressive resuscitation. All patients with acute cholecystitis must be admitted to the hospital for continued intravenous fluid therapy and antibiotics. Approximately 75 percent of patients treated medically have a complete remission of symptoms within 2 to 7 d of hospitalization; the remainder of patients experience either a progression of the inflammatory process or a complication of acute cholecystitis within this time frame. Most often, surgery is performed 24 to 72 h after admission, once symptoms have resolved. Surgical options include open or laparoscopic cholecystectomy. Patients with a toxic presentation or clinical deterioration require immediate surgery.

REFERENCES

1. Gracie WA, Ransohoff DF: The natural history of silent gallstones: The innocent gallstone is not a myth. *New Engl J Med* 307:798, 1982.
2. Ikard RW: Gallstones, cholecystitis, and diabetes. *Surg Gynecol Obstet* 171:528, 1990.
3. Berger MY, van der Velden JJ, Lijmer G, et al: Abdominal symptoms: Do they predict gallstones? A systematic review. *Scand J Gastroenterol* 35:70, 2000.
4. Valdivieso V, Covarrobias C, Seigel F, et al: Pregnancy and cholelithiasis: Pathogenesis and natural course of gallstones diagnosed in early puerperium. *Hepatology* 17:1, 1993.
5. Maringhini A, Ciambra M, Baccelliere P, et al: Biliary sludge and gallstones in pregnancy: Incidence, risk factors, and natural history. *Ann Intern Med* 119:116, 1993.
6. Landers D, Carmona R, Cromblehome W: Acute cholecystitis in pregnancy. *Obstet Gynecol* 69:131, 1987.
7. Ross SO, Forsmark CE: Pancreatic and biliary disorders in the elderly. *Gastroenterology Clin* 30:531, 2001.
8. Rosenthal RA, Anderson DK: Surgery in the elderly: Observations on the pathophysiology and treatment of choledocholithiasis. *Exp Gerontol* 28:459, 1993.
9. Burgart LJ: Cholangitis in viral disease. *Mayo Clin Proc* 73:479, 1998.
10. Snell RS, Smith MS: Clinical anatomy for emergency medicine. St. Louis: Mosby, 1994, p. 431.
11. Mergener K, Baillie J: Fortnightly review: Acute pancreatitis. *BMJ* 316:44, 1998.
12. Sondenaa K, Nesvik I, Solhaug O, et al: Randomization to surgery or observation in patients with symptomatic gallbladder stone disease: The problem of evidence-based medicine in clinical practice. *Scand J Gastroenterol* 32:611, 1997.
13. Fenstr LF, Lonborg R, Thirlby R, et al: What symptoms does cholecystectomy cure? *Am J Surg* 169:533, 1995.
14. Diehl AK, Sugarek NJ, Todd K: Clinical evaluation for gallstone disease: Usefulness of symptoms and signs in diagnosis. *Am J Med* 89:29, 1990.
15. Trowbridge RL, Rutkowski NK, Shojania KG: "Does this patient have acute cholecystitis." *JAMA* 289(1):80, 2003.
16. Rigas B, Torosis J, McDougall C, et al: The circadian rhythm of biliary colic. *J Clin Gastroenterol* 12:409, 1990.
17. Singer AJ, McCracken G, Henry MC: Correlation among clinical, laboratory, and hepatobiliary scanning findings in patients with suspected acute cholecystitis. *Ann Emerg Med* 28:267, 1996.
18. Gruber PJ, Silverman RA, Gottesfield S, et al: Presence of fever and leukocytosis in acute cholecystitis. *Ann Emerg Med* 28:273, 1996.

19. Adedji OA, McAdam A: Murphy's sign, acute cholecystitis, and elderly people. *J R Coll Surg Edinburgh* 41:88, 1996.
20. Parker LJ, Vukov LF, Woolan PC: Emergency department evaluation of geriatric patients with acute cholecystitis. *Acad Emerg Med* 4:51, 1997.
21. Shea JA, Berlin JA, Escarce JJ, et al: Revised estimates of diagnostic test sensitivity and specificity in suspected biliary tract disease. *Arch Intern Med* 154(22):2573, 1994.
22. Kendall JL, Shimp RJ: Performance and interpretation of focused right upper quadrant ultrasound by emergency physicians. *J Emerg Med* 21:7, 2001.
23. Lanoix R, Leak LV, Gaeta T, Gernsheimer JR: A preliminary evaluation of emergency ultrasound in the setting of an emergency medicine training program. *Am J Emerg Med* 18:41, 2000.
24. Rosen CL, Brown DFM, Chang Y, et al: Ultrasonography by emergency physicians in patients with suspected cholecystitis. *Am J Emerg Med* 19:32, 2001.
25. Fidler J, Paulson EK, Layfield L: CT evaluation of acute cholecystitis: Findings and usefulness in diagnosis. *AJR* 166:1085, 1996.

86 HEPATIC DISORDERS AND HEPATIC FAILURE

Joshua S. Broder
Rawden Evans

This chapter will review the epidemiology, pathophysiology, and clinical presentations of acute and chronic liver failure. It will summarize laboratory testing and evidence-based emergency diagnosis and management of complications of hepatic failure, including gastrointestinal hemorrhage, spontaneous bacterial peritonitis, hepatorenal syndrome, and hepatic encephalopathy. The differential diagnosis of jaundice is discussed in Chap. 84, and cholecystitis and biliary colic are discussed in Chap. 85.

ACUTE AND CHRONIC LIVER DISEASE

Epidemiology

In the year 2000, chronic liver disease was the twelfth leading cause of death in the United States and the tenth leading cause of death among U.S. men, accounting for 17,214 deaths (1.5 percent).[1–3] Despite the high toll of *chronic* liver disease, new infections with hepatitis viruses A, B, and C actually declined in the last decade in the United States (Table 86-1).

About one-third of the U.S. population has acquired immunity to hepatitis A virus (HAV). There are approximately 125,000 to 200,000 cases of HAV infection reported yearly, with an estimated 100 related deaths. Fulminant liver failure is a rare complication of HAV infection, and chronic infection does not occur.[4,5]

Vaccination against hepatitis B virus (HBV) has reduced the incidence of fulminant hepatic failure by as much as three-quarters in some studies.[6] Chronic infection occurs in only 6 to 10 percent of cases of hepatitis B. In contrast, chronic hepatitis C occurs in 85 percent of those infected, with 70 percent developing resulting chronic liver disease.[7,8]

The hepatitis D virus (HDV) is uncommon and is described as a defective agent because infection depends on concomitant or preexisting chronic infection by HBV. In individuals with chronic HBV infection, superinfection with HDV often results in a rapidly progressive or fulminant form of liver disease carrying a high short-term mortality rate. This variety of infection is most commonly associated with intravenous drug use.[9]

Acute illness with liver function test abnormalities also occurs with infection by other hepatotropic viruses such as cytomegalovirus (CMV), herpes simplex virus (HSV), Coxsackie virus, and Epstein-Barr virus (EBV), although these agents are unlikely to cause clinically evident hepatitis and jaundice in otherwise healthy individuals.

TABLE 86-1 Hepatitis Disease Burden in the United States, 2000–2001

	Hepatitis A		Hepatitis B		Hepatitis C	
	2001	2000	2001	2000	2001	2000
Reported acute cases	10,616	13,397	7,844	8,036	—	—
Estimated acute cases	45,000	57,000	22,000	22,000	4,000	5,700
Estimated new infections	93,000	143,000	78,000	81,000	25,000	35,000
Chronic infections		—	1.25 million		2.7 million	
Estimated yearly chronic liver disease deaths		—	5000		8,000–10,000	
Percent current U.S. population ever infected	31.3		4.9		1.8	

Source: National Center for Infectious Diseases. Viral Hepatitis Surveillance. Disease Burden from Hepatitis A, B, and C in the United States. http://www.cdc.gov/ncidod/diseases/hepatitis/resource/dz_burden02.htm.

Alcoholic liver disease and viral hepatitis comprise the vast majority of cases of acute and chronic liver disease. Other causes include a variety of toxins, idiosyncratic drug reactions, and autoimmune and metabolic hepatobiliary diseases.[4,10–12]

Pathophysiology

Hepatobiliary diseases are classified according to the main pathologic processes involved and include hepatocellular, cholestatic, immunologic, and infiltrative disorders. Considerable overlap occurs among these different processes, with a common result being progressive hepatic dysfunction.

Hepatic cirrhosis results from fibrous scarring mixed with hepatocyte regeneration in response to sustained inflammatory, toxic, or metabolic insults. Over time, the functional anatomy of the liver is replaced by scar tissue, isolating nodules of regenerating hepatocytes. These isolated foci are less efficient at performing the metabolic functions of the normal, highly structured liver. In addition to causing progressive loss of synthetic and metabolic function, scarring increases resistance to blood flow from the splanchnic circulation, leading to portal hypertension and portal-systemic shunting. Reduced blood flow through the liver deprives the remaining hepatocytes of substrate for synthesis of essential proteins and degradation of toxins, worsening the metabolic deficiencies of chronic liver disease. Portal hypertension results in splenomegaly and the development of gastroesophageal varices. Varices are thin-walled submucosal vessels prone to ulceration and hemorrhage. Splenomegaly contributes to anemia and thrombocytopenia.

Ascites develops secondary to portal hypertension. Abnormalities in renal sodium and water excretion [caused by diminished glomerular filtration rate (GFR) and elevations in both aldosterone and antidiuretic hormone] also contribute to ascites. Ascites worsens chronic fatigue and compromises respiratory function. It sets the stage for recurrent episodes of spontaneous bacterial peritonitis. Encephalopathy results from the accumulation of a variety of neurotoxic substances. Each of these complications will be further addressed below.[10]

Clinical Features

Clinical presentation of acute liver disease is variable. Symptoms of hepatocellular necrosis accompanying viral hepatitis include anorexia, nausea, vomiting, and low-grade fever. Cholestatic disease is accompanied by jaundice, pruritus, clay-colored stools, and dark urine. Cholestasis resulting from intrahepatic processes and infiltrative disease presents more insidiously with the slow development of jaundice and few other constitutional complaints.

Chronic liver disease often presents with complications of advancing cirrhosis and portal hypertension that include abdominal pain, ascites, gastrointestinal bleeding, fever, and altered mental status. However, progressive generalized fatigue may be the only symptom of chronic liver disease in the absence of supervening complications.

Features of history are sometimes useful: sexual behaviors, travel, volume and duration of alcohol use, illicit drug use, consumption of nutritional supplements (vitamin A), history of blood transfusions, needle-stick blood exposures, herbal remedies, mushroom ingestion, or raw oyster consumption.

Family history can identify some hereditary conditions that cause only mild symptoms or laboratory abnormalities (e.g., Gilbert syndrome, Dubin-Johnson, or Rotor syndrome). Other familial disorders can lead to severe, premature, chronic liver failure. Examples include Wilson disease, hemochromatosis, or α_1-antitrypsin deficiency.

Physical findings of acute hepatitis often are limited to moderate liver enlargement and tenderness, with or without jaundice. Chronic liver disease is accompanied by a host of physical findings, including sallow complexion, extremity muscle atrophy, palmar erythema, cutaneous spider nevi, parotid gland enlargement, and testicular atrophy and gynecomastia. The liver may be uniformly enlarged and firm or, in advanced cirrhosis, shrunken and grossly nodular. Splenomegaly and ascites accompany portal hypertension.

Liver Function Tests

Laboratory tests for hepatobiliary disease can be divided into three general categories: (1) markers of acute hepatocyte injury and death, (2) measures of hepatocyte synthetic function, and (3) indicators of hepatocyte catabolic activity. Traditional liver function tests are actually a mix of markers of hepatocyte injury, including aspartate aminotransferase (AST or SGPT), alanine aminotransferase (ALT or SGOT), and alkaline phosphatase, and indicators of hepatocyte catabolic activity (direct and indirect bilirubin). Tests that reflect hepatocyte synthetic function include prothrombin time and albumin. Ammonia reflects catabolic function of the liver, although levels do not correlate accurately to clinical status.

BILIRUBIN Bilirubin is a metabolite of heme proteins, including hemoglobin, myoglobin, and cytochromes. Laboratory tests for bilirubin are conducted by an assay that differentiates the conjugated form (direct bilirubin) from the unconjugated form (indirect bilirubin). Unconjugated bilirubin has poor water solubility and is carried in serum tightly bound to albumin. This complex is taken up by hepatocytes, which conjugate the bilirubin, increasing its water solubility, before secretion it into the bile. Bilirubin is then excreted in the stool, with a small percentage undergoing enterohepatic recirculation. Normally, the total serum bilirubin level is less than 1.1 mg/dL, with 70 percent being unconjugated.

An increase in the supply of unconjugated bilirubin reaching the liver (e.g., due to erythrocyte hemolysis) may temporarily exceed the capacity of hepatocytes to conjugate bilirubin, increasing both the indirect and total values. As hepatocytes conjugate the excess substrate, the direct bilirubin also will increase.

Similarly, decreased hepatocyte metabolic capacity (e.g., due to chronic or acute hepatocyte injury) can increase indirect and total bilirubin. Bilirubin is also elevated in states of biliary stasis or obstruction (e.g., due to an obstructing gallstone).

TRANSAMINASES Transaminases are intracellular enzymes found in hepatocytes and some other cell types. Hepatocyte injury or necrosis results in release of these enzymes into the circulation, just as cre-

atine phosphokinase and troponin are released in conditions of myocyte injury and death. Elevated levels may result from any hepatocyte injury, whether induced by infection, ischemia, or toxins such as alcohol, acetaminophen, carbon tetrachloride, or hepatotoxic mushrooms. Elevations in the hundreds of units per liter suggest mild injury, whereas levels in the thousands suggest extensive acute hepatic necrosis. This test may be near normal in end-stage liver failure, where no acute hepatocyte injury occurs.

Commonly measured transaminases include AST and ALT. AST is a nonspecific marker because it is found not only in liver but also in heart, smooth muscle, kidney, and brain. Elevated AST also may be due to medications, including acetaminophen, nonsteroidal anti-inflammatory drugs, angiotensin-converting enzyme (ACE) inhibitors, nicotinic acid, isoniazid, sulfonamides, erythromycin, griseofulvin, and fluconazole. ALT is a more specific marker of hepatocyte injury.

Calculation of the AST-ALT ratio may suggest the etiology of hepatic injury. A ratio of greater than 2 is common in alcoholic hepatitis because alcohol stimulates AST production. A ratio of less than 1 is typical of acute or chronic viral hepatitis. In the absence of active alcohol use, mild elevations of AST and ALT and a ratio greater than 1 suggest underlying cirrhosis.

ALKALINE PHOSPHATASE Elevated alkaline phosphatase (AP) is associated with biliary obstruction and cholestasis. Mild to moderate elevations accompany virtually all hepatobiliary disease; however, elevations greater than four times normal strongly suggest cholestasis. AP is a nonspecific marker, also derived from bone, placenta, intestine, kidneys, and leukocytes. The specificity of AP for cholestasis can be improved by comeasurement of the enzyme γ-glutamyl transpeptidase (GGTP), which when elevated supports the diagnosis of cholestasis. However, like AST, GGTP production is stimulated by alcohol consumption and is also elevated by drugs inducing hepatic microsomal enzyme activity such as phenobarbital and warfarin. GGTP may rise in acute and chronic pancreatitis, acute myocardial infarction, uremia, chronic obstructive pulmonary disease, rheumatoid arthritis, and diabetes mellitus.

Isolated significant elevation of AP without marked hyperbilirubinemia (AP-bilirubin ratio of 1000:1) is characteristic of infiltrative and granulomatous liver disease such as lymphoma, fungal infections, sarcoidosis, and tuberculosis. The uncommon conditions primary biliary cirrhosis and primary sclerosing cholangitis elevate AP disproportionately to bilirubin levels.

AP levels in healthy children are often two- to threefold higher than the upper limit of normal for adults. Doubling of AP levels is common and normal in pregnancy. Incidental findings of three- to fivefold elevations in transaminase levels and doubling of AP in otherwise healthy diabetics and the obese suggest the presence of nonalcoholic steatohepatitis (NASH). Other conditions associated with NASH include jejunoileal bypass, total parenteral nutrition, hyper- and hypothyroidism, and the antiarrhythmic drug amiodarone.[14]

LACTATE DEHYDROGENASE Lactate dehydrogenase (LDH) is often included in liver test panels, although its lack of specificity is limiting. Moderate elevations are seen in all hepatocellular disorders and cirrhosis but less so in purely cholestatic conditions. LDH may become significantly elevated as a result of hemolysis and accompany a related increase in unconjugated bilirubin. The isoenzyme LDH-5 is specific to the liver, and tests for it are sometimes useful, although not widely available.

AMMONIA Metabolism of nitrogen-containing compounds results in the generation of ammonia, which is further metabolized to urea via the Krebs cycle in the liver. An elevated serum ammonia level may occur in acute and chronic liver disease as a manifestation of hepatic metabolic failure. Very high ammonia levels are seen in fulminant liver failure, contributing to overall toxicity and signifying poor prognosis.

In cirrhosis with worsening portal hypertension and isolation of remaining functional hepatic tissue, ammonia formed by colonic bacteria is carried into the general circulation. This process is worsened by large intestinal protein loads such as occur with gastrointestinal bleeding. However, elevated serum ammonia levels do not reliably correlate with acute worsening of hepatic function in the cirrhotic and serve more as a marker of generalized decline than as a useful diagnostic tool or therapeutic end point.

PROTHROMBIN TIME   Prolongation of the prothrombin time (PT) in liver disease reflects the decreased synthesis of the vitamin K-dependent coagulation factors II, VII, IX, and X and as such serves as a real measure of liver function. Prolonged PT is a common complication of advancing cirrhosis, although it also may be seen in acute hepatitis and exacerbations of chronic compensated liver disease. When present in acute viral hepatitis, prolonged PT often indicates severe disease with widespread hepatocellular necrosis. There is some correlation between the extent of PT prolongation and clinical outcome in fulminant liver disease.

Although PT is often used as a marker of hepatic function, abnormal values may occur in the presence of a normal liver. Abnormalities in PT also result from fat malabsorption by the gut because vitamin K is fat-soluble. Cholestatic syndromes interfere with fat absorption and thereby promote vitamin K deficiency. Vitamin K deficiency can be distinguished from liver synthetic dysfunction by administration of parenteral vitamin K (phytonadione 10 mg IM). A 30 percent reduction in PT within 24 h should occur in vitamin-deficiency states.

ALBUMIN   Like PT, the albumin level reflects liver synthetic function. It may decrease in advancing cirrhosis or severe acute hepatitis, marking a poor short-term prognosis. Albumin is less useful in evaluating fulminant liver disease because its serum half-life is approximately 3 weeks, whereas PT becomes prolonged in a matter of days. Serum albumin also reflects overall nutritional status, and a low value may be nonspecific in a chronically ill individual.

VIRAL HEPATITIS SEROLOGY   Serum testing for viral hepatitis is often offered as screening panels by hospital laboratories. In hepatitis A, IgM anti-HAV is detectable at the onset of clinical illness. Hepatitis B serology is somewhat more complicated. Hepatitis B surface antigen (HBsAg) is measurable *before* clinical illness and elevations in transaminases are seen and remain elevated for 1 to 2 months. Antibodies to the hepatitis B core antigen (anti-HBc) appear 2 weeks after HBsAg, and their presence is useful in defining the so-called "window period" before antibody to the surface antigen (anti-HBsAg) appears. Anti-HBc may be the only reliably positive test in the window period and also provides a rough estimate of the time of exposure for epidemiologic purposes. Antibody testing for hepatitis C has become standardized in recent years and is now part of all viral hepatitis screening panels. The alphabetized nomenclature is expanding as more infectious agents responsible for acute and chronic liver disease are recognized. However, hepatitis A, B, and C remain the principal varieties of concern to practitioners in North America.[5,9]

Nonhepatic Causes of Abnormal Liver Tests

Multiple nonhepatic causes may lead to abnormal liver function tests. Abnormal liver test results occur in up to one-third of those screened. Only 1 percent of these indicate clinically significant liver disease.[15,16] Hypoalbuminemia accompanies protein wasting enteropathies, malnutrition, and nephrotic syndrome. AP elevations occur with a variety of bone diseases, pregnancy, and malignancies. AST elevations accompany acute myocardial infarction and rhabdomyolysis. Bilirubin elevations occur in severe hemolysis, sepsis, and syndromes involving abnormal erythropoiesis. PT elevations occur in vitamin K deficiency, chronic antibiotic use, warfarin therapy, and long-standing steatorrhea.

SPECIFIC CLINICAL SYNDROMES

Cirrhosis and Complications of End-Stage Liver Disease

The evaluation and treatment of patients with acute or chronic liver failure are primarily supportive. The goals are (1) to identify and eliminate any reversible cause of liver injury and (2) to identify and treat complications of hepatic dysfunction (Table 86-2). Treatment and admission criteria for liver failure patients are usually similar to those for patients without liver disease presenting with the complication in question. A few specific therapies are now emerging.

End-stage liver disease has three major consequences: loss of hepatic synthetic function, loss of hepatic degradative capacity, and portal hypertension. Complications of end-stage liver disease result from one or more of these. For example, gastrointestinal hemorrhage results from altered portal blood flow but is complicated by loss of hepatic synthetic function, with resulting coagulopathy. Life-threatening complications of end-stage liver disease include variceal hemorrhage, spontaneous bacterial peritonitis, hepatorenal syndrome, and hepatic encephalopathy, each of which will be discussed below.

Gastroesophageal Varices and Hemorrhage

Gastroesophageal varices form as intrahepatic fibrosis increases resistance to blood flow from the portal vein to the inferior vena cava. Blood flow increases through collateral vessels, including thin-walled gastric and esophageal vessels, which are prone to bleeding due to their superficial location and lack of supporting connective tissue.

TABLE 86-2   Fulminant Liver Failure

Presentation	Causes/Associations	Complications

Acute hepatocellular necrosis with rapid development of encephalopathy and liver failure developing in <8 weeks	Hepatitis B, C, D
	Hepatitis A (rare)
	Hepatotoxins
	    Acetominophen
	    Isoniazid
	    Halothane
	    Valproic acid
	    Mushrooms
	    Carbon tetrachloride
	(Reye syndrome and acute fatty liver of pregnancy resemble fulminant liver failure, but microvesicular fatty infiltation occurs without hepatocellular necrosis)
		Encephalopathy
		Hypoglycemia
		Hyponatremia
		Hypokalemia
		GI hemorrhage
		Renal failure
		Cerebral edema
		Sepsis
		Spontaneous bacterial peritonitis

The prevalence of asymptomatic esophageal varices in patients with cirrhosis correlates with the Child-Turcotte-Pugh class, reaching 35 percent in mild (class A) cases and 60 percent in moderate to severe cases (classes B and C). The prevalence of *large* varices, which may be most likely to bleed, is roughly equal among these classes (29, 24, and 24 percent, respectively).[17]

Mortality associated with variceal hemorrhage has decreased with the wider availability of endoscopic and pharmacologic therapy but remains high. A Veterans Administration study found that 30-day mortality in patients with variceal hemorrhage decreased from 29.6 to 20.8 percent over an 11-year period from 1981 to 1991, whereas 6-year mortality declined from 74.5 to 69.7 percent. Sclerotherapy decreased mortality in the late group to 17 and 68 percent at 30 days and 6 years, respectively.[18]

CLINICAL FEATURES Bleeding symptoms may include hematemesis, "coffee-grounds" emesis, melena, or (with massive hemorrhage) even bright red blood per rectum. Symptoms may be more occult, such as light-headedness, generalized weakness, or fatigue. Vital-sign abnormalities may be masked by coexisting medical conditions and medications. Patients with end-stage liver disease may have baseline hypotension due to decreased intravascular oncotic pressure, and beta blockers may prevent reflex tachycardia.

Variceal bleeding should be suspected in any patient with melena or hematemesis and a history of liver disease. Gastric lavage should be performed to identify ongoing hemorrhage and determine the need for immediate endoscopy. Patients with hemodynamic instability or continued bleeding despite lavage deserve emergent endoscopy. Known or suspected gastroesophageal varices are not a contraindication to naso- or orogastric tube placement. Review of the medical literature **shows no evidence of increased risk of iatrogenic hemorrhage from placement of naso- or orogastric catheters.**

TREATMENT Hemodynamic and airway stabilization take priority over precise diagnosis. Large-bore intravenous access should be obtained immediately, and packed red blood cells and fresh frozen plasma should be ordered in anticipation of coexisting coagulopathy. In the patient with hematemesis, hemodynamic instability, or altered mental status, early intubation should be considered.

Endoscopy Endoscopy provides definitive diagnosis of the source of bleeding and can provide direct hemostasis by banding or sclerother-apy. Endoscopy has been shown to reduce mortality in some studies.[18] However, a recent Cochrane review found *no advantage* to early endoscopy compared with pharmacologic therapy for treatment of acute variceal bleeding. Patients treated with endoscopy or one of several vasoactive drugs had similar rates of failure to achieve initial hemostasis, rebleeding, blood transfusion, and mortality. Endoscopy was associated with a greater complication rate than was pharmacotherapy.[19]

Balloon tamponade with inflated gastroesophageal obturators such as the Sengstaken-Blakemore tube is used infrequently because of the high rate of complications and the increasing effectiveness and availability of pharmacotherapy and endoscopic sclerotherapy. Principal complications of these devices include bronchopulmonary aspiration and esophageal rupture. β-Blockers and portosystemic shunt surgery or transjugular intrahepatic portosystemic shunts (TIPS) are effective prophylactic mea-sures in some patients with gastroesophageal varices but have no proven role in the management of acute gastro-esophageal hemorrhage.

Pharmacotherapy A number of pharmacologic therapies are temporizing measures while awaiting assistance from a gastroenterologist or transfer of the patient to a tertiary care facility.

VASOACTIVE DRUGS As indicated earlier, sclerotherapy and vasoactive medications have similar efficacy in establishing initial hemostasis.[19] However, in patients with variceal bleeding, addition of vasoactive agents to endoscopy improves initial hemostasis.[20] The two classes of vasoactive drugs are somatostatin and octreotide and vasopressin and terlipressin. Somatostatin and octreotide are preferred because they do not have serious side effects (Table 86-3).

Somatostatin and its synthetic analogue octreotide cause specific *relaxation* of mesenteric vascular smooth muscle, reducing portal venous pressure without arterial vasospasm. Octreotide should be considered for initial therapy due to its proven efficacy and minimal side effects. Several recent randomized, controlled studies have demonstrated similar efficacy of octreotide and sclerotherapy in the initial management of variceal bleeding.[21–24] Somatostatin and octreotide reduce transfusion requirements by approximately 1 unit per patient treated and slightly improve initial hemostasis.[25] Side effects from octreotide appear less common than with vasopressin or terlipressin therapy.[26] However, somatostatin and octreotide do not appear to reduce rebleeding, need for balloon tamponade, or overall mortality.[25]

TABLE 86-3 Pharmacologic Therapy for Acute Variceal Hemorrhage

Agent	Dosing	Mechanism	Advantages	Disadvantages
Octreotide	50 μg IV bolus, then 50 μg per h continuous IV infusion	Synthetic analogue of somatostatin	Reduces transfusion requirement As effective as endoscopy Additive benefit with sclerotherapy	Minimal

Antibiotics
  piperacillin/tazobactam
  or
  quinolone
 	
  Plus clindamycin/flagyl
  or
  cephalosporin
 	
  Plus clindamycin/flagyl
  or
  ampicillin
  Plus clindamycin
	3.375/g IV
	
	(levofloxacin 500 mg IV *or*
	  ciprofloxacin 400 mg IV *or*
	  gatifloxacin 400 mg IV)
	
	(ceftriaxone 2 g IV q24
	   or cefotaxime 2 g IV q8)
	
	2 g IV plus gentamycin
	900 mg IV			

Somatostatin
  (endogenous
  hormone)
	250–500 μg IV bolus, then 250–500 μg per h continuous IV infusion	Decreases portal pressure by specific relaxation of mesenteric vascular smooth muscle	—	Minimal

Vasopressin and its synthetic analogue terlipressin act by nonspecific *arterial vasoconstriction,* reducing inflow through the mesenteric circulation and thereby reducing portal pressure. Side effects of end-organ ischemia are potentially severe, including stroke, myocardial infarction or arrhythmia, mesenteric infarction, or limb ischemia. Because of its adverse-effect profile, vasopressin generally is not given in the ED; terlipressin generally is not available in the United States.[27]

ANTIBIOTICS   A recent Cochrane review found that antibiotic therapy reduced all-cause mortality from variceal bleeding by 27 percent and infections by 60 percent with minimal side effects. Empirical therapy should cover enteric organisms.[28]

Ascites and Spontaneous Bacterial Peritonitis

Ascites and anasarca commonly develop in cirrhotic patients due to the combination of portal hypertension, hypoalbuminemia, and poor renal excretion of sodium and water. These factors increase the transportal hydrostatic pressure gradient and decrease the intravascular oncotic pressure, leading to transit of water into the extracellular space and peritoneum. Patients may complain of abdominal pain and dyspnea due to abdominal distention that may limit diaphragmatic movement. Moreover, hydrothorax may occur in the presence of diaphragmatic hernias, and abdominal contents may herniate into the thorax.

Spontaneous bacterial peritonitis occurs as normal bowel flora translocate across the bowel wall, a process facilitated by bowel wall edema and poor production of immunologically active proteins by the liver. Once in the peritoneum, bacteria benefit from a poorly defended site with an ample growth medium, ascites. Antibiotic therapy must target normal bowel flora, including anaerobes and gram-negative rods.

CLINICAL FEATURES   The most common life-threatening complication of ascites is spontaneous bacterial peritonitis (SBP), classically presenting with fever and diffuse abdominal pain and tenderness. However, fever may be absent. In patients with known ascites, the 1-year incidence of spontaneous bacterial peritonitis is 29 percent. Recurrence of SBP is as high as 44 percent, and survival in patients with a first episode of SBP is low (68.1 percent at 1 month and 30.8 percent at 6 months), probably a result both of acute infection and coexisting illness.[29] Abdominal paracentesis is necessary to obtain ascitic fluid analysis in cases of suspected spontaneous bacterial peritonitis. However, physical examination has poor and variable sensitivity for the detection of ascites (50–90 percent).[30] Blind paracentesis of the left lower quadrant has a reported average success rate of 58 percent.[31]

PARACENTESIS: PROCEDURE   A scrupulously sterile technique must be used to avoid introducing skin flora into the peritoneum, causing iatrogenic infection. Classically, the patient is positioned supine. Most patients undergoing this procedure in the ED will have moderate to tense ascites on examination (hence the suspicion for SBP). An appropriate position for needle placement can be located by percussion dullness in either lower lateral abdominal quadrant. Regions with prior abdominal surgery should be avoided because postoperative adhesions may result in adherence of bowel to the parietal peritoneum, leading to iatrogenic bowel perforation during paracentesis. The patient's bladder should be emptied either by catheterization or by spontaneous voiding just before the procedure.

Sterile skin preparation with Betadine solution is performed, and sterile drapes are applied. Anesthesia is obtained by local infiltration with 1% lidocaine. Although special paracentesis trays are available commercially, an 18- or 20-gauge angiocatheter and 20-mL syringe are adequate for the procedure. To avoid postprocedure leakage of ascites from the puncture site, aspiration should follow a Z track: First, the initial skin puncture is performed. Second, traction is applied to the skin and needle, displacing the skin puncture to a location over the distal parietal peritoneum. Third, the needle is advanced through the peritoneum with continuous aspiration performed. The needle should be advanced only as far as is necessary to initiate flow of ascites. Finally, when the needle is removed and traction is no longer applied, the skin puncture should no longer overlie the peritoneal puncture site, limiting ascites leakage.

ULTRASOUND-GUIDED PARACENTESIS   No studies to date have directly compared the safety of ED paracentesis with ultrasound guidance versus blind paracentesis. In patients with malignant ascites, ultrasound-guided paracentesis has a high reported success rate with low complications (hypotension 2.6 percent, mortality 1.6 percent).[32]

One study demonstrated free fluid volumes in descending order in the following locations: perihepatic space, pericystic space, right paracolic gutter, and left lower quadrant. This same study demonstrated air-filled bowel loops in the projected path of a left lower quadrant paracentesis needle. Based on these findings, investigators have suggested that ultrasound could improve the safety and efficacy of paracentesis.[33]

LARGE-VOLUME PARACENTESIS   Secondary indications for abdominal paracentesis in patients presenting with tense ascites include symptomatic relief of abdominal pain, anorexia, and dyspnea. Patients who have tense ascites despite high-dose diuretic therapy may require frequent paracentesis for temporary relief. Discussion with the patient's primary care physician or gastroenterologist may help to guide therapy.

Large-volume paracentesis can be safe and effective, and volumes as great as 6 to 9 L have been removed without complication. Some studies suggest that volume expanders such as exogenous albumin or dextran or reinfused concentrated albumin (prepared by dialysis of the patient's ascitic fluid) may reduce the incidence of renal dysfunction. Other studies show that large-volume paracentesis does not worsen existing hyponatremia or renal failure.[34–36]

LABORATORY TESTING OF ASCITIC FLUID   Once ascitic fluid is obtained, it should be sent for a white blood cell count with differential, glucose and protein determinations, Gram stain, and bacterial culture and sensitivity. A total white blood cell count greater than $1000/\mu L$ or a neutrophil count greater than $250/\mu L$ is diagnostic of spontaneous bacterial peritonitis. Low glucose or high protein values are suggestive of infection. Gram stains and culture results may be negative (30–40 percent), and empirical therapy should be initiated in the ED based on clinical suspicion. Culture sensitivity may be increased by the addition of 10 mL of ascites to blood culture bottles. Additional studies that may be of value to the inpatient evaluation include cytology, albumin, LDH, and tumor markers.

ANTIBIOTIC AND ADJUNCTIVE THERAPY OF SBP   Empirical therapy should cover typical enteric flora. Studies demonstrate the usual organisms in SBP to be Enterobacteriaceae (63 percent), *Streptococcus pneumoniae* (15 percent), enteroccoci (6–10 percent), and anaerobes (<1 percent). Suggested regimens are shown in Table 86-4. There is no compelling evidence for the superiority of cefotaxime over ampicillin-tobramycin for SBP, and oral quinolones have not been shown effective for clinically mild SBP.[28]

Patients may have had prior infections with resistant organisms, so microbiologic sensitivities from prior admissions should be reviewed, if available. For resistant *Escherichia coli* or *Klebsiella,* imipenem or meropenem or a fluoroquinolone should be added. Addition of intravenous albumin (1.5 g/kg at diagnosis, 1 g/kg on day 3) to antibiotic therapy may reduce renal failure and hospital mortality in patients with SBP.[37]

Hepatorenal Syndrome

Hepatorenal syndrome is the development of acute renal failure in a patient with histologically normal kidneys in the presence of preexist-

TABLE 86-4 Diagnosis and Treatment of Spontaneous Bacterial Peritonitis

Clinical Setting	Cirrhosis with Ascites
Presentation	Any of the following: fever, abdominal pain and tenderness, worsening encephalopathy
Diagnosis	Ascitic fluid WBC >1000/mL PMN >250/mL
Treatment	Any of: Cefotaxime 2.0 g IV q8h, q4h if life-threatening Ticarcillin-clavulanic acid 3.1 g IV q6h Pipariacillin-tazobactam 3.375 g IV q6h Ampicillin-sulbactam 3.0 g IV q6h Ceftriaxone 2.0 g IV q24h PLUS Albumin 1.5 g/kg IV at diagnosis and 1 g/kg IV on day 3
Disposition	Hospitalize, unless clinically well, compliant, with access to timely follow-up

ing chronic or acute hepatic failure. Renal function may recover after liver transplantation, and kidneys from hepatorenal syndrome patients can perform normally when transplanted into patients with renal failure from other causes.[38]

The precise cause of renal dysfunction in cirrhotic patients is unknown, although new studies have found links to cytokines, endothelin, and the renin-angiotensin-aldosterone system. Disruption of normal renal blood flow has been demonstrated using Doppler ultrasound techniques.

The presence of new renal failure in a cirrhotic patient should be viewed as a marker of extreme morbidity. Median survival for hepatorenal syndrome is approximately 21 days with intensive medical therapy. One should undertake an urgent search for reversible causes of renal failure, such as intravascular volume depletion (prerenal azotemia), intrinsic renal disease (such as drug-induced interstitial nephritis), postrenal obstruction, or infection.

Recent studies of terlipressin with albumin infusion found improved renal function and survival; future studies are necessary to substantiate these findings.[39,40]

Hepatic Encephalopathy

Hepatic encephalopathy is a poorly understood syndrome thought to be due to accumulation of nitrogenous waste products normally metabolized by the liver. These products may be chemically similar to normal neuropeptides, resulting in an altered level of consciousness and characteristic motor findings. Hepatic encephalopathy spans a spectrum of illness from chronic fatigue to acute lethargy. Characteristic motor findings include asterixis, a repetitive tonic-clonic wrist flexion elicited after forced wrist hyperextension.

The development of hepatic encephalopathy in a patient with chronic liver disease suggests a shift in the existing balance between the liver's ability to metabolize waste products and the supply of those products to the liver and brain. Sources of nitrogenous wastes include protein metabolism from dietary sources and protein load from occult gastrointestinal bleeding. In addition, the production of nitrogenous wastes depends in part on gastrointestinal flora. Changes in gut flora due to addition or removal of antibiotic therapy may precipitate hepatic encephalopathy.

Changes in the liver's metabolic capacity may result from worsening of the patient's underlying liver condition, hypoperfusion states such as sepsis, or iatrogenic interventions. For example, hepatic en-

cephalopathy is a common complication following TIPS, a procedure in which portal blood is shunted to the inferior vena cava, bypassing the liver. Although this procedure may succeed in reducing portal hypertension and esophageal varix bleeding, it also reduces hepatic metabolism of nitrogenous wastes by reducing hepatic blood flow.

To appreciate the presence or worsening of encephalopathy, determine if there are changes in personality, worsening dementia, alterations in levels of consciousness, or declining neuromuscular function. Table 86-5 lists clinical stages of encephalopathy. Asterixis characterizes stage II and is elicited by having the patient hold the arms straight up and extending the wrists. The hands begin to flap repetitively. Another manifestation of asterixis is back-and-forth tongue movement when the tongue is extended. A patient with known encephalopathy in stage I or II who is otherwise well and has no other acute comorbidities can be managed as an outpatient generally after consultation with the primary care physician or gastroenterologist.

Hepatic encephalopathy is a diagnosis of exclusion. In the cirrhotic patient presenting with altered mental status or lethargy, multiple other causes must first be ruled out, even in the presence of an elevated serum ammonia level. Patients with end-stage liver disease are often coagulopathic and may have spontaneous or traumatic subdural hematoma. Decreased hepatic gluconeogenesis and glycogen stores and poor nutritional status increase the risk of hypoglycemia and nutritional encephalopathies such as Wernecke-Korsakoff syndrome. Cirrhotic patients often are treated with diuretics, increasing the risk of symptomatic hyper- or hyponatremia. Patients also may have decreased hepatic clearance of drugs such as benzodiazepines, prolonging their effect and leading to accidental overdose. Renal failure and sepsis from any source (spontaneous bacterial peritonitis, pneumonia, urinary tract infection, bacteremia, meningitis) are other considerations. Gastrointestinal bleeding always should be excluded as a precipitant of hepatic encephalopathy.

TREATMENT After the preceding comorbidities have been excluded, treatment is aimed at reducing the production of nitrogenous wastes by reducing protein intake and the metabolic activity of intestinal bacteria (Table 86-6).

Lactulose is the current mainstay of therapy. Lactulose is a synthetic disaccharide containing one molecule of galactose and one of fructose. It is minimally absorbed into the bloodstream. In the colon it is degraded primarily into lactic acid. By acidifying the gastrointestinal environment, ammonia is trapped and is excreted in the stool. Blood ammonia levels can be reduced up to 50 percent. Lactulose also inhibits glutamine-dependent ammonia production in the gut wall.

Lactulose can be given orally or rectally. The oral dose is 20 g in a glass of water, fruit juice, or carbonated citrus beverage. For rectal administration, 300 mL of lactulose syrup is diluted with 700 mL of water or normal saline. The enema should be retained for 30 min.

Other agents such as antibiotics and benzodiazepine receptor antagonists generally are not administered in the ED. Antibiotics such as neomycin and rifaximin directly inhibit bacterial growth and protein metabolism, so they are not given intravenously for hepatic encephalopathy. Neomycin can cause nephro- and ototoxicity, whereas Rifaximin apparently does not. Flumazenil may have short-term benefit in some patients with hepatic encephalopathy but has no effect on survival or long-term recovery.[41]

TABLE 86-5 Staging of Hepatic Encephalopathy

Stages	Features
I	General apathy
II	Lethargy, drowsiness, variable orientation, asterixis
III	Stupor with hyperreflexia, extensor plantar reflexes
IV	Coma

TABLE 86-6 Pharmacologic Therapy of Hepatic Encephalopathy

Medication	Dose	Mechanism
Lactulose	20 g (30 mL) PO *or* 300-mL retention enema q4–6h	Alters GI pH, trapping NH₃ and stimulating nitrogen-fixing bacteria

Vascular Disease of the Liver

Vascular diseases of the liver are relatively uncommon when compared with the preceding conditions, but they warrant brief inclusion because their consideration is key to timely diagnosis, treatment, and ultimately improved outcome. These conditions include portal vein thrombosis, hepatic vein thrombosis (Budd-Chiari syndrome), and nonthrombotic venoocclusive disease.

Portal vein thrombosis can result as a late complication of abdominal trauma, sepsis, pancreatitis, and hypercoagulable states and in neonates with umbilical vein infection. Portal hypertension and related complications develop in a subacute manner. Splenomegaly may occur in the absence of hepatomegaly, and liver histology is normal. The diagnosis is made by angiography, and therapy is surgical.[42]

Hepatic vein thrombosis, or Budd-Chiari syndrome, has both acute and chronic presentations that include abdominal pain, hepatomegaly, ascites, and usually mild alterations in liver function studies. Causes and associations include a history of abdominal trauma, oral contraceptive use, polycythemia vera, paroxysmal nocturnal hemoglobinuria, hypercoagulable states, and congenital webs of the vena cava. Diagnosis can be made by Doppler ultrasound of the hepatic veins, and therapy includes anticoagulation.[43]

Nonthrombotic occlusion of hepatic venules creating a small-vessel variant of Budd-Chiari syndrome is associated with the ingestion of certain medicinal teas containing pyrrolozidine alkaloids. These alkaloids are found in *Senecio* and *Crotalia* genera of plants.[44] Veno-occlusive hepatic disease also occurs rarely as a complication of chemotherapy and bone marrow transplantation.

REFERENCES

1. Minino AM, Arias E, Kochanek KD, et al: Deaths: Final data for 2000. *Natl Vital Stat Rep* 50, 2002.
2. 1999 National Hospital Discharge Survey: Annual Summary with Detailed Diagnosis and Procedure Data. *Vital Health and Statistics Report.* Series 13, no. 151. Washington, U.S. Department of Health and Human Services, Centers for Disease Control and Prevention.
3. Anderson RN: Deaths: Leading causes for 2000. *Natl Vital Stat Rep* 50, 2002.
4. Koff R: Hepatitis A. *Lancet* 351:1643, 1998.
5. Centers for Disease Control and Prevention: Hepatitis home page: *www.cdc.gov/ncidod/diseases/hepatitis/index.htm.*
6. Kao JH, Chen DS: Global control of hepatitis B virus infection. *Lancet Infect Dis* 2:395, 2002.
7. Lee WM: Medical progress: Hepatitis B virus infection. *New Engl J Med* 337:1733, 1997.
8. Lee M, Walker BD: Medical progress: Hepatitis C infection. *New Engl J Med* 345:41, 2001.
9. Bondesson JD, Saperston AR: Hepatitis. *Emerg Med Clin North Am* 14: 695, 1996.
10. Williams EJ, Iredale JP: Liver cirrhosis. *Postgrad Med J* 74:193, 1998.
11. Lee WM: Medical progress: Drug-induced hepatotoxicity. *New Engl J Med* 333:1118, 1995
12. Krawitt EL: Medical progress: Autoimmune hepatitis. *New Engl J Med* 334:897, 1996.
13. Kaplan MM: Medical progress: Primary biliary cirrhosis. *New Engl J Med* 335:1570, 1996.
14. Angulo P. Nonalcoholic fatty liver disease. *New Engl J Med* 346:1221, 2002
15. Kamath PS: Clinical approach to the patient with abnormal liver test results. *Mayo Clin Proc* 71:1089, 1996.
16. Aranda-Michel J, Sherman KE: Tests of the liver: Use and misuse. *Gastroenterologist* 6:34, 1998.
17. Madhotra R, Mulcahy HE, Willner I, Reuben A: Prediction of esophageal varices in patients with cirrhosis. *J Clin Gastroenterol* 34:4, 2002.
18. El-Serag HB, Everhart JE: Improved survival after variceal hemorrhage over an 11-year period in the Department of Veterans Affairs. *Am J Gastroenterol* 95:3566, 2000.
19. D'Amico G, Pietrosi G, Tarantino I, Pagliaro L: Emergency sclerotherapy versus medical interventions for bleeding oesophageal varices in cirrhotic patients (Cochrane Review), in *The Cochrane Library,* Issue 4. Oxford: Update Software, 2002.
20. Banares R, Albillos A, Rincon D, et al: Endoscopic treatment versus endoscopic plus pharmacologic treatment for acute variceal bleeding: A meta-analysis. *Hepatology* 35:609, 2002.
21. Freitas DS, Sofia C, Pontes JM, et al: Octreotide in acute bleeding esophageal varices: A prospective randomized study. *Hepatogastroenterology* 47:1310, 2000.
22. Bildozola M, Kravetz D, Argonz J, et al: Efficacy of octreotide and sclerotherapy in the treatment of acute variceal bleeding in cirrhotic patients: A prospective, multicentric, and randomized clinical trial. *Scand J Gastroenterol* 35:419, 2000.
23. Zuberi BF, Baloch Q: Comparison of endoscopic variceal sclerotherapy alone and in combination with octreotide in controlling acute variceal hemorrhage and early rebleeding in patients with low-risk cirrhosis. *Am J Gastroenterol* 95:768, 2000.
24. Sivri B, Oksuzoglu G, Bayraktar Y, Kayhan B: A prospective randomized trial from Turkey comparing octreotide versus injection sclerotherapy in acute variceal bleeding. *Hepatogastroenterology* 47:168, 2000.
25. Gøtzsche PC: Somatostatin analogues for acute bleeding oesophageal varices (Cochrane Review), in *The Cochrane Library,* Issue 4. Oxford: Update Software, 2002.
26. Corley DA, Cello JP, Adkisson W, et al: Octreotide for acute esophageal variceal bleeding: A meta-analysis. *Gastroenterology* 120:946, 2001.
27. Ioannou G, Doust J, Rockey DC: Terlipressin for acute esophageal variceal hemorrhage (Cochrane Review), in *The Cochrane Library,* Issue 4. Oxford: Update Software, 2002.
28. Soares-Weiser K, Brezis M, Tur-Kaspa R, Leibovici L: Antibiotic prophylaxis for cirrhotic patients with gastrointestinal bleeding (Cochrane Review), in *The Cochrane Library,* Issue 4. Oxford: Update Software, 2002.
29. Franca AV, De Souza JB, Silva CM, Soares EC: Long-term prognosis of cirrhosis after spontaneous bacterial peritonitis treated with ceftriaxone. *J Clin Gastroenterol* 33:295, 2001.
30. Cattau EL Jr, Benjamin SB, Knuff TE, Castell DO: The accuracy of the physical examination in the diagnosis of suspected ascites. *JAMA* 26;247:1164, 1982.
31. Cappell MS, Shetty V: A multicenter, case-controlled study of the clinical presentation and etiology of ascites and of the safety and clinical efficacy of diagnostic abdominal paracentesis in HIV seropositive patients. *Am J Gastroenterol* 89:2172, 1994.
32. Ross GJ, Kessler HB, Clair MR, et al: Sonographically guided paracentesis for palliation of symptomatic malignant ascites. *AJR* 153:1309, 1989.
33. Bard C, Lafortune M, Breton G: Ascites: Ultrasound guidance or blind paracentesis? *Can Med Assoc J* 135:209, 1986.
34. Vila MC, Coll S, Sola R, et al: Total paracentesis in cirrhotic patients with tense ascites and dilutional hyponatremia. *Am J Gastroenterol* 94:2219, 1999.
35. Graziotto A, Rossaro L, Inturri P, Salvagnini M: Reinfusion of concentrated ascitic fluid versus total paracentesis: A randomized prospective trial. *Dig Dis Sci* 42:1708, 1997.
36. Forouzandeh B, Konicek F, Sheagren JN: Large-volume paracentesis in the treatment of cirrhotic patients with refractory ascites: The role of postparacentesis plasma volume expansion. *J Clin Gastroenterol* 22:207, 1996.
37. Sort P, Navasa M, Arroyo V, et al: Effect of intravenous albumin on renal impairment and mortality in patients with cirrhosis and spontaneous bacterial peritonitis. *New Engl J Med* 341:403, 1999.
38. Jeyarajah DR, Gonwa TA, McBride M, et al: Hepatorenal syndrome: Combined liver kidney transplants versus isolated liver transplant. *Transplantation* 27;64:1760, 1997.
39. Wong F: Hepatorenal syndrome: Is it truly the end of the road? *Hepatology* 36:1292, 2002.
40. Ortega R, Gines P, Uriz J, Cardenas A, et al: Terlipressin therapy with and without albumin for patients with hepatorenal syndrome: Results of a prospective, nonrandomized study. *Hepatology* 36(4 pt 1):941, 2002.

41. Goulenok C, Bernard B, Cadranel JF, et al: Flumazenil versus placebo in hepatic encephalopathy in patients with cirrhosis: A meta-analysis. *Aliment Pharmacol Ther* 16:361, 2002.
42. Cohen J, Edelman RR, Chopra S: Portal vein thrombosis: A review. *Am J Med* 92:173, 1992.
43. Shill M, Henderson JM, Tavil AS: The Budd-Chiari syndrome revisited. *Gastroenterologist* 2:27, 1994.
44. Ernst E: Harmless herbs? A review of the recent literature. *Am J Med* 104:170, 1998.

87

ACUTE AND CHRONIC PANCREATITIS

Robert J. Vissers
Riyad B. Abu-Laban

ACUTE PANCREATITIS

Pancreatitis is a common cause of abdominal pain, and the lack of a pathognomonic clinical presentation and the absence of a diagnostic "gold standard" make this disease a diagnostic challenge. Its clinical presentation can vary from mild abdominal pain to refractory shock, and many of its signs and symptoms are shared by other intra-abdominal conditions.

Epidemiology

Acute pancreatitis is secondary to cholelithiasis or alcohol abuse in up to 90 percent of cases in the United States, but the etiology varies in different countries.[1] The overall prevalence is estimated to be 0.5 percent, but this also depends on the setting and patient population. Patients with biliary pancreatitis are more commonly female and over 50 years of age and represent the most common form of pancreatitis in a community hospital setting. Alcoholic pancreatitis presents more frequently to urban emergency departments and is seen most commonly in men between the ages of 35 and 45.[2]

The list of other factors associated with the development of acute pancreatitis is extensive, including drugs, infection, inflammation, trauma, and metabolic disturbances. Drugs account for up to half the remaining cases after alcohol and biliary diseases have been excluded (Table 87-1).

Pathophysiology

Although there are many distinct etiologies for acute pancreatitis, the specific mechanism that leads to the disease state remains unclear. The central pathophysiologic cause is believed to be the activation of digestive zymogens in the pancreatic acinar cells instead of the small intestine and subsequent autodigestion of the pancreas.[1,3,4] A number of factors (e.g., endotoxins, toxins, ischemia, infections, and anoxia) are believed to trigger the activation of proenzymes. Activated proteolytic enzymes, such as trypsin, then digest cellular membranes within the pancreas and cause edema, interstitial hemorrhage, vascular damage, coagulation, and cellular necrosis.[1] This noninfectious destruction of the pancreatic parenchyma rapidly causes a local inflammatory reaction that further contributes to the vascular dilatation, permeability, and edema.

Adult pancreatitis is distinguished from most other intra-abdominal diseases by its propensity to cause remote systemic effects. It is believed that this represents an extension of the localized process into a generalized systemic inflammatory response.[4] This may lead to shock, acute respiratory distress syndrome (ARDS), and eventually, multisystem organ failure. Recently, pancreatitis research has focused on the identification of systemic inflammatory mediators. A number of compounds have been implicated, including bradykinin, compliment,

TABLE 87-1 Drugs Associated with Acute Pancreatitis*

Antiarrhythmics: Amiodarone, amlodipine
Antiasthmatic: Montelukast
Antibiotics: Erythromycin, azithromycin, clarithromycin, sulfamethoxazole, quinolones, pentamidine, paromomycin, rifampin, dalfopristin-quinupristin
Antiepileptics: Carbamazepine, valproic acid, topiramate
Antifungals: Metronidazole
Antihypertensives: Diazoxide, indapamide, methyldopa
Antilipemic agents: All types
Antineoplastic agents: L-Asparaginase, pegaspargase, cytarabine, tamoxifen, mycophenolate, vinorelbine, anagrelide, interleukin[2] (IL-2) analogues, interferons
Antipsychotics: Risperidone
Antiretrovirals: All types
Diphenoxylate (opiate agonist)
Diuretics: Thiazides, furosemide, ethacrynic acid, metolazone
Ergotamines
Estrogens: All types
Etanercept (anti-TNF)
Ethanol
Gastrointestinal agents: Cholestyramine, cimetidine, octreotide, ranitidine, proton pump inhibitors
Glucocorticoids: All types
Hydroxyurea
Nonsteroidal anti-inflammatory agents: All types
Retinoic acid derivatives
Salicylates
Somatropin (growth hormone)

*Clinical Pharmacology, http://cpip.gsm.com.

platelet-activating factor, nitrous oxide, and most recently, inflammatory cytokines.[4] Inflammatory mediators presently hold the most promise for the identification of better prognostic markers and potential therapies for acute pancreatitis; however, their clinical usefulness remains to be seen.[5]

Clinical Features

The major symptom of acute pancreatitis is midepigastric or left upper quadrant pain. It is described most commonly as a constant, boring pain that often radiates to the back as well as the flanks, chest, or lower abdomen. Although usually described as severe, the intensity can be extremely variable and does not correlate with the severity of the disease.[1] The pain is exacerbated in the supine position and can be relieved when sitting with the trunk and knees flexed. Colicky discomfort is atypical and suggests another etiology. Nausea and vomiting are common, and abdominal bloating from gastric and intestinal hypomotility is a frequent complaint.

Physical examination usually reveals a patient in moderate distress. Low-grade fevers and tachycardia are frequently present, and hypotension is not unusual.[1] About 10 percent of patients have respiratory symptoms secondary to atelectasis, pleural effusion (usually left sided), and rarely, ARDS. Abdominal examination is notable for epigastric tenderness. Peritonitis is a late finding, presumably due to the retroperitoneal location of the organ. Bowel sounds may be diminished from an associated ileus. Cullen sign, a bluish discoloration around the umbilicus, and Grey Turner sign, a bluish discoloration of the flanks, are characteristic but rare signs of hemorrhagic pancreatitis.

Patients with pancreatitis may present in hypovolemic shock and multisystem organ failure. Hypotension can result from fluid third-spacing, hemorrhage, increased vascular permeability, vasodilatation, cardiac depression, and vomiting.[2]

Diagnosis

The absence of a pathognomonic clinical syndrome often precludes a diagnosis based solely on presentation. Unfortunately, the only diagnostic "gold standard" is pathologic examination of the pancreas. Laboratory and radiographic investigations can be helpful in the diagnosis of acute pancreatitis, but both suffer from limited diagnostic accuracy.

LABORATORY TESTS   Serum amylase and lipase are the most widely used laboratory tests in the evaluation of acute pancreatitis (Table 87-2). Both enzyme markers, released during pancreatic inflammation, lack the sensitivity and specificity to be the sole indicators of disease and must be interpreted in the context of the clinical setting.[6–8]

Amylase   This digestive enzyme, used to cleave starch into smaller carbohydrates, is found primarily in the pancreas and salivary glands. Low levels of amylase also can be found in numerous other tissues, including the fallopian tubes, ovaries, testes, adipose tissue, small bowel, lung, thyroid, skeletal muscle, and certain neoplasms. As a result, serum amylase can be elevated in many conditions, making this test relatively nonspecific.

Amylase levels are expressed in either Somogyi units (SU) or international units (IU), with the normal ranges generally reported as 60 to 160 SU/100 mL or 110 to 300 IU/L, respectively.[8] Amylase has a half-life of about 2 h, and although its elimination is incompletely understood, it is at least partially cleared by the kidneys, leading to elevated levels in renal failure.

Not only are there many extrapancreatic causes of an elevated amylase, but serum amylase levels may be normal in proven cases of acute pancreatitis.[9] The lack of a diagnostic "gold standard" has made estimates of the sensitivity of this test difficult, but most studies suggest a sensitivity of 80 to 90 percent if blood is sampled within 36 h of symptom onset.[8] **Amylase rises quickly but, because of its short half-life, returns to normal in 3 to 4 days (even in the presence of ongoing inflammation),** making it less sensitive after the first 36 h.

The main difficulty in using serum amylase for the diagnosis of acute pancreatitis is its poor specificity. Depending on the cutoff used, the specificity of amylase ranges from 40 percent when the normal range is used to greater than 90 percent at a cutoff of five times the upper limit of normal. The best accuracy appears to occur at a cutoff of three times the upper limit of normal, which improves the specificity to 75 percent without greatly compromising the sensitivity.[7,8]

Lipase   This enzyme, which catalyzes the breakdown of triglycerides into free fatty acids, is found predominantly in the pancreas, but lipase activity is present in the gastric and intestinal mucosa and in the liver. An elevated serum lipase level has been noted in a number of nonpancreatic diseases, most of which are intestinal or hepatobiliary disorders.[7,10] Heparin may cause a release of endothelial membrane-bound lipase into the serum, resulting in a measurable increase in lipase activity within minutes of heparin administration. Lipase is cleared by the kidneys and can be elevated to three times the upper limit of normal in renal failure. The half-life is approximately 7 h, and serum lipase will remain elevated for several days after amylase has returned

to baseline. Lipase activity is expressed in units per liter, and the normal range varies greatly depending on the assay used.

The addition of colipase to these assays has improved the specificity to greater than 90 percent (specificity ranges from 80 to 99 percent depending on the cutoff used). In addition, the sensitivity of lipase is at least as good as amylase (>90 percent). The most appropriate cutoff in the emergency department appears to be two times the upper limit of normal.[7,8] Lipase is a more accurate test than amylase in the diagnosis of acute pancreatitis. Although lipase suffers from imperfect sensitivity, a recent study of over 5000 patients in whom both amylase and lipase tests were ordered found that the addition of amylase was not warranted.[11] **It is not cost-effective to order amylase or lipase determinations indiscriminately in all cases of undifferentiated abdominal pain.**[6]

Other enzymatic markers have been investigated, including isoenzymes of amylase, but variables such as time, cost, and test accuracy have prevented their use in clinical practice.[8] Lipase-amylase ratios and amylase-creatinine clearance ratios add little to the diagnosis of acute pancreatitis beyond lipase determination alone.[2,3]

RADIOLOGY   Plain radiographs of the chest and abdomen are most useful in excluding other diseases that may be confused with pancreatitis. Calcification of the gland is suggestive of chronic pancreatitis. A sentinel loop secondary to small bowel ileus or a colon-cutoff sign suggesting local colonic ileus may be present, but neither is diagnostic. Chest radiographs may reveal an elevated hemidiaphragm or a pleural or pericardial effusion.

Ultrasonography is most helpful in the identification of gallstones or dilatation of the biliary tree, which has both diagnostic and therapeutic implications in pancreatic disease. Although pancreatic edema and associated pseudocysts may be visualized on ultrasound, it is generally an insensitive test for the diagnosis of acute pancreatitis, particularly in nonbiliary etiologies. Overlying bowel gas or adipose tissue and the retroperitoneal location of the pancreas frequently impair adequate imaging.[2]

Because of better anatomic definition, computed tomographic (CT) scanning may facilitate grading the severity of the disease and enable better prognostication and is the primary imaging modality used in acute pancreatitis.[12] CT scan cannot be used to rule out pancreatitis because it is insensitive in early or mild disease.

Endoscopic retrograde cholangiopancreatography (ERCP) is employed rarely in emergency department evaluation but can be very useful for patients in whom the etiology of the pancreatitis remains unclear after initial assessment. Magnetic resonance imaging (MRI), particularly magnetic resonance pancreatography (MRP), is being used for the evaluation of pancreatic carcinoma and chronic pancreatitis. MRP may be used as an alternative to ERCP, but its utility in acute pancreatitis is unclear.[13]

Prognostic Markers

For most patients, acute pancreatitis is a self-limited disease, but 5 to 10 percent suffer from significant associated morbidity and mortality.[2,14] It can be difficult to identify patients at risk, although signs of a systemic response suggest a more complicated course. Ranson has identified multiple diagnostic criteria to predict patient outcome.[15] The criteria on admission are age >55 years; BS >200 mg/dL; white blood cell count (WBC) >16,000/L; serum glutamic-oxaloacetic transaminase (SGOT) >250 units/L; and lactate dehydrogenase (LDH) >700 IU/L. The number of factors present is then used to predict mortality. Although they serve as a reminder of features that portend a worse prognosis, **the Ranson criteria have poor predictive value in the acute setting** that does not improve on clinical judgment.[15] Other scoring systems have been used to predict severity in pancreatitis, such as the acute physiology and chronic health evaluation (APACHE II) score, but complexity and poor sensitivity on initial

TABLE 87-2   Laboratory Utilization in Suspected Acute Pancreatitis

Test Characteristic	Amylase	Lipase
Sensitivity	80–90%	90%
Specificity	75%	90%
Suggested best cutoff	3× upper limit of normal	2× upper limit of normal
Prognostic value	Poor	Poor
Rate of rise	Rapid	Rapid
Return to baseline	3–4 days	7–14 days
Other	No additional benefit to ordering both amylase and lipase.	

presentation limit their role in the emergency department.[1] In general, the presence of extra-abdominal complications or comorbid conditions indicates an increased mortality risk. Hypotension, tachycardia of more than 130 beats/min, a Po_2 of less than 60 mm Hg, oliguria, increasing blood urea nitrogen (BUN) or creatinine, and hypocalcemia are key indicators of a potentially complicated course.[1,3,14] **The absolute level of serum amylase or lipase does not correlate with severity.**[3,7,8]

A CT scan, particularly if contrast-enhanced, may provide valuable estimates of the severity and prognosis in cases of moderate to severe acute pancreatitis.[12] Complications include phlegmons, abscesses, or pseudocysts,[16] usually in the first 2 to 3 weeks after the onset of pancreatitis. Systemic complications include pulmonary, cardiovascular, renal, hematologic, central nervous system, and metabolic abnormalities[14] (Table 87-3).

Treatment

Of patients with acute pancreatitis, 90 percent recover without complications and require supportive measures only.[1] The general principle is to "rest the pancreas." Although the use of a nasogastric tube has been widely advocated, no studies have demonstrated that nasogastric suction alters the course of the illness, and it should not be used in routine management. It is traditionally recommended to withhold all oral intake, but clear liquids do not appear to be harmful in mild to moderate disease.

The mainstay of treatment for acute pancreatitis is fluid resuscitation. A balanced electrolyte solution, such as normal saline, should be administered for rehydration. Amounts should be given to ensure renal perfusion and good urine output of about 100 mL per h. In unstable patients, hemodynamic monitoring may be required, and pressors are indicated for persistent hypotension despite adequate fluid resuscitation.

Other aspects of supportive care include parenteral narcotics and antiemetics.

In biliary pancreatitis, urgent decompression is indicated if there is persistent biliary obstruction, ideally by endoscopic sphincterotomy of the ampulla of Vater.[1,2] If the obstruction is transient, most patients can be managed with supportive care, and elective cholecystectomy may be performed once inflammation subsides.

Empiric antibiotics are not indicated in mild to moderate pancreatitis but should be considered in severe disease. Approximately 20 percent of acute pancreatitis cases develop a severe course characterized by pancreatic necrosis and local and systemic complications. Almost half of these cases are complicated by infected pancreatic necrosis within the first 2 weeks of illness. Since needle aspiration is the only method of distinguishing between infected and sterile necrosis, evidence of a complicated, severe course is an indication for treatment. Infections are thought to occur from direct transmural spread from the colon. Infections are often polymicrobial and predominantly gram-negative bacteria such as *E. coli, Pseudomonas* spp., *Klebsiella* spp., and gram-positive staphylococci and enterococci accounting for the remainder. Antibiotic choice should be guided by suspected etiologic bacteria and the ability to penetrate pancreatic tissue. The traditionally utilized penicillins, first-generation and second-generation cephalosporins, and aminoglycosides have poor penetration and should not be used in prophylaxis or treatment. Intravenous imipenem or a quinolone (ofloxacin or ciprofloxacin) in combination with metronidazole are recommended and have demonstrated high tissue levels as well as bactericidal activity. Controversy exists over whether antibiotic therapy alone may preclude surgical intervention in infected necrotizing pancreatitis. Although many other drugs have been used as potential therapeutic agents in acute pancreatitis, such as H_2 blockers, steroids, nonsteroidal anti-inflammatory drugs, and glucagon, none has demonstrated benefit in controlled, prospective trials.[2]

Peritoneal lavage may provide short-term clinical improvement but does not appear to alter clinical outcome. Acute fluid collections are rarely symptomatic and frequently resolve spontaneously. Laparotomy is indicated for hemorrhage control and abscess drainage. Abscesses and pseudocysts also may be drained radiologically or endoscopically, if indicated.

Disposition

Patients with mild pancreatitis, no evidence of systemic complications, and a low likelihood of biliary tract disease may be managed as outpatients if they are able to tolerate oral fluids and their pain is well controlled. A clear-liquid diet is recommended, oral analgesics should be prescribed, and follow-up in 24 to 48 h is needed. All other patients with acute pancreatitis should be admitted to the hospital. Patients with significant systemic complications, shock, or extensive pancreatic necrosis will need an intensive care setting. Evidence of a pancreatic abscess requires surgical consultation.

CHRONIC PANCREATITIS

Chronic pancreatitis is a chronic inflammatory condition that causes irreversible damage to pancreatic structure and function.

Epidemiology

Table 87-4 lists the causes of chronic pancreatitis. Of these, alcohol abuse is the most important, accounting for 70 to 80 percent of cases.[16] Most of the remaining cases are idiopathic. The mean ages of onset and death in chronic pancreatitis are 42 and 52 years, respectively. Because the disease can be undiagnosed, the true prevalence is unknown, with estimates ranging from 0.04 to 5 percent.[17] As with alcohol abuse, chronic pancreatitis is most common in men. Gallstones are not a cause of chronic pancreatitis despite their role in the acute form of the disease.[18,19] It is believed that acute pancreatitis does not

---

TABLE 87-3   Complications of Acute Pancreatitis

Pulmonary
  Pleural effusions, usually left sided
  Atelectasis
  Hypoxemia
  Acute respiratory distress syndrome (>50% mortality)
Cardiovascular
  Myocardial depression
  Hemorrhage, hypovolemia, and myocardial depressant factor
Metabolic
  Hypocalcemia
  Hyperglycemia
  Hyperlipidemia
  Coagulopathy, disseminated intravascular coagulopathy
Other
  Hemorrhage
  Colonic perforation
  Renal failure
  Erythema-nodosum dermatitis
  Arthritis
  Pseudocyst
  Abscess

TABLE 87-4   Causes of Chronic Pancreatitis

Alcohol abuse
Malnutrition ("tropical pancreatitis")
Hyperparathyroidism
Pancreas divisum
Ampullary stenosis
Cystic fibrosis
Hereditary
Trauma
Idiopathic

progress to chronic disease unless complications such as pseudocysts or ductal strictures are present.[17]

Pathophysiology

The pathophysiology of chronic pancreatitis remains poorly understood.[17] In contrast to acute pancreatitis, the pancreas is pathologically abnormal in chronic pancreatitis, both before and after exacerbation. In alcohol-induced disease, it is thought that alcohol either is directly toxic to acinar cells or induces pathologic changes in secretory function.[18] The risk of alcohol-induced chronic pancreatitis is clearly related to the amount and duration of alcohol consumption.[16] Once established, the disease may progress despite abstinence, although the mortality rate is reduced.[18] Chronic pancreatitis, regardless of the etiology, results in interstitial inflammation with duct obstruction and dilatation leading to parenchymal loss and fibrosis. This causes pain and eventual impairment of both exocrine and endocrine pancreatic functions, with endocrine impairment occurring later in the disease process.[17] Clinically significant malabsorption does not occur until more than 90 percent of glandular function is lost.[16] The etiology of pain is likely multifactorial and may include parenchymal inflammation, pressure on acinar tissue or small ducts, perineural inflammation, and duodenal or common bile duct stenosis.[18] It is controversial whether pain "burns out" as chronic pancreatitis progresses.[17]

Clinical Features

The hallmark of chronic pancreatitis is abdominal pain, but in about 10 percent of cases the disease may be painless.[19] As in acute pancreatitis, pain is usually midepigastric and may radiate to the back, although abdominal tenderness is often less prominent.[2] Nausea and vomiting may be present. In the early stages of chronic pancreatitis, discrete attacks of pain (formerly called *relapsing pancreatitis*) occur, lasting days to weeks.[16] Pain is frequently worse after alcohol ingestion or a fatty meal. As the disease progresses, pain-free periods become less frequent and often disappear completely.[2] In distinction to acute pancreatitis, patients with chronic pancreatitis appear chronically ill and may have signs and symptoms of pancreatic insufficiency, including weight loss, steatorrhea, clubbing, and polyuria. Stigmata of chronic liver disease may be present if the etiology is alcohol abuse.

Diagnosis

Differentiating acute and chronic pancreatitis may be difficult during an exacerbation because the primary distinction is based on disease reversibility.[2] Laboratory investigations are nonspecific in chronic pancreatitis. Amylase and lipase levels may be elevated but have no prognostic significance and are usually normal, particularly when fibrosis is advanced. Glucose tolerance is often impaired, occasionally with an elevated fasting blood sugar level. In 5 to 10 percent of patients with chronic pancreatitis, compression of the intrahepatic portion of the bile duct leads to elevations of bilirubin and alkaline phosphatase levels.[17] Pancreatic calcification on abdominal radiographs is considered pathognomonic for chronic pancreatitis and is present in some 30 percent of patients, particularly those with alcohol-induced disease.[16,20] Lists of diagnostic criteria for chronic pancreatitis have been developed because no single "gold standard" exists.[21] Either CT scan or ultrasound may be indicated to identify local complications of chronic pancreatitis, such as abscess or pseudocyst. The differentiation between chronic pancreatitis and pancreatic cancer can be challenging and is an essential component of imaging interpretation. Both MRP and endoscopic ultrasonography are being used in the diagnosis and differentiation of chronic pancreatitis. Their role is still being defined, but they appear to be less sensitive than ERCP in mild disease and have limited indications in the emergency setting.[13,21]

Treatment

The management of chronic pancreatitis in the ED involves ruling out other diagnoses or complications and includes supportive care. Intravenous narcotic analgesics and antiemetics usually are required. Fluid and electrolyte abnormalities should be corrected. The long-term goals of treatment are pain control, relief of mechanical obstruction or complications, correction of malabsorption, and alteration of the disease course. Pancreatic extracts frequently are administered to improve absorption and reduce pain. Cessation of alcohol ingestion is essential because the 5-year mortality rate of chronic pancreatitis in patients who continue to abuse alcohol is 50 percent.[16] If pain is increasing or intractable, imaging should be performed to assess for complications such as pseudocyst or mechanical obstruction. Surgery, either open or endoscopic, can be helpful in such cases. Other complications include mechanical obstruction of the duodenum or common bile duct, fistulas, ascites or pleural effusions, splenic vein thrombosis, and pseudoaneurysm. Celiac plexus nerve block is performed frequently for long-term pain control.

Disposition

Many patients with chronic pancreatitis can be discharged safely from the ED once complications have been ruled out or addressed. Appropriate follow-up is particularly important if pain management is poor or significant weight loss or symptom changes have occurred. Hospital admission may be required during severe pain exacerbation.

REFERENCES

1. Mergener K, Baillic J: Fortnightly review: Acute pancreatitis. *Br Med J* 316:44, 1998.
2. Moscati RM: Pancreatitis. *Emerg Med Clin North Am* 14:719, 1996.
3. Steinberg W, Tenner S: Acute pancreatitis. *New Engl J Med* 330:1198, 1994.
4. Karne S, Gorelick FS: Etiopathogenesis of acute pancreatitis. *Surg Clin North Am* 79:699, 1999.
5. Lipsett PA: Serum, cytokines, proteins and receptors in acute pancreatitis: Mediators, markers, or more of the same? *Crit Care Med* 29:1642, 2001.
6. Hoffman JR, Jaber AJ, Schriger DL: Serum amylase determination in the emergency department evaluation of abdominal pain. *J Clin Gastroenterol* 13:401, 1991.
7. Tietz NW: Support of the diagnosis of pancreatitis by enzymatic tests: Old problems, new techniques. *Clin Chem* 257:85, 1997.
8. Vissers RJ, Abu-Laban RB, McHugh DF: Amylase and lipase in the emergency department evaluation of acute pancreatitis. *J Emerg Med* 17:1027, 1999.
9. Orebaugh S: Normal amylase levels in the presence of acute pancreatitis. *Am J Emerg Med* 12:21, 1994.
10. Rosenblum J: Serum lipase is increased in disease states other than acute pancreatitis: Amylase revisited. *Clin Chem* 37:315, 1991.
11. Vissers RJ, Dagnone J, Abu-Laban R, Walls RM: Serum amylase offers no additional benefit to serum lipase in the ED diagnosis of acute pancreatitis. *Acad Emerg Med* 4:396, 1998.
12. Balthazar E: Acute pancreatitis: Assessment of severity with clinical and CT evaluation. *Radiology* 223:603, 2002.
13. Megibow AJ, Lavelle MT, Rofsky NM: MR imaging of the pancreas. *Surg Clin North Am* 81:307, 2001.
14. Pitchumoni S, Agarwal N, Jain NK: Systemic complications of acute pancreatitis. *Am J Gastroenterol* 83:597, 1988.
15. De Bernardinis M, Violi V, Roncoroni L, et al: Discriminant power and information content of Ranson's prognostic signs in acute pancreatitis: A meta-analytic study. *Crit Care Med* 27:2272, 1999.
16. Mergener K, Baillie J: Chronic pancreatitis. *Lancet* 350:1379, 1997.
17. Steer ML, Waxman I, Freedman S: Medical progress: Chronic pancreatitis. *N Engl J Med* 332:1482, 1995.
18. Holt S: Chronic pancreatitis. *South Med J* 86:201, 1993.
19. Naruse S, Kitagawa M, Ishiguro H, et al: Chronic pancreatitis: Overview of medical aspects. *Pancreas* 16:323, 1998.

20. Amman RW: The natural history of chronic pancreatitis. *Intern Med* 40:368, 2001.
21. Etemad B: Chronic pancreatitis: Diagnosis, classification, and new genetic developments. *Gastroenterology* 120:682, 2001.

COMPLICATIONS OF GENERAL SURGICAL PROCEDURES
Edmond A. Hooker

Outpatient surgical procedures are commonplace, and, with increasing pressure for cost containment, admitted patients are being discharged earlier in their postoperative course. As a result, more patients are presenting to the ED with postoperative fever, respiratory complications, genitourinary complaints, wound infections, vascular problems, and complications of drug therapy (Table 88-1). This chapter reviews the complications common to all surgical procedures and those specific to one procedure.

The operating surgeon should be called when one of his or her patients appears in the ED with a surgical complication. This is not just courtesy but provides continuity of care important for the patient's well-being.

FEVER

Fever is a common presenting complaint (Table 88-2). A mnemonic for the common causes of postoperative fever is the "five Ws": wind (atelectasis or pneumonia), water (urinary tract infection), wound, walking (deep vein thrombosis), and wonder drugs (drug fever or pseudomembranous colitis).[1] Fever during the initial 24 h is usually caused by atelectasis; however, necrotizing streptococcal and clostridial infections also occur in surgical wounds early in the postoperative course. Respiratory complications, such as pneumonia and atelectasis, and intravenous catheter-related problems, such as thrombophlebitis, are the predominant causes of fever in the 24- to 72-h period.

Urinary tract infections become evident 3 to 5 days postoperatively. Seven to 10 days postoperatively, clinical manifestations of wound infections develop. Deep venous thrombosis can result in fever any time but usually not until the fifth postoperative day. Antibiotic-induced pseudomembranous colitis occurs up to 6 weeks postoperatively. An approach for evaluating and managing fever in postoperative patients is presented in Table 88-3. It is important to remember that leukocytosis can be absent in up to one-third of patients with clinically significant infections.[2]

RESPIRATORY COMPLICATIONS

Respiratory complications occur in many surgical patients and range from atelectasis and pneumonia to pneumothorax or pulmonary embolism.

Atelectasis

Atelectasis, the collapse of pulmonary alveoli, is very common. Contributing factors include inadequate clearance of secretions after general anesthesia, decreased intra-alveolar pressure, and postoperative pain, which results in hypoventilation. Although atelectasis can occur after any procedure, it frequently occurs after upper abdominal and thoracic surgery. The presentation varies from an isolated fever to tachypnea, dyspnea, and tachycardia.

Evaluation includes a chest radiograph, pulse oximetry, and a complete blood count (CBC). Chest radiographs may be normal or show platelike linear densities, triangular densities, or lobar consolidation. Mild hypoxemia from ventilation and perfusion mismatch is common, but hypercarbia is uncommon. Patients with mild atelectasis and no evidence of hypoxemia may be managed as outpatients with pain control

and increased deep breathing. Admission is indicated for aggressive pulmonary toilet and supplemental oxygenation in debilitated patients, patients with underlying lung disease, patients with hypoxemia, or those in whom the diagnosis is in question.

Pneumonia

Pneumonia usually presents between 24 and 96 h postoperatively. Predisposing factors include prolonged ventilatory support and atelectasis.

TABLE 88-1   Complications of General Surgical Procedures

Complication	Important Points
Fever	Wind, water, wound, walking, wonder drugs
Pulmonary complications	
Atelectasis	<24 h, treat with pulmonary toilet, discharge unless ill or hypoxemic
Pneumonia	24–96 h, polymicrobial, most require admission
Pneumothorax	Multiple causes, consider expiratory views, consider needle aspiration
Pulmonary embolism	Dyspnea is main symptom, high index of suspicion
Gastrointestinal complications	
Intestinal obstruction	Obtain radiographs, search for causes
Intraabdominal abscess	CT diagnosis, early broad-spectrum antibiotics
Pancreatitis	Always consider in postoperative patients with abdominal pain
Cholecystitis	Usually in older patients, can be acalculous
Fistulas	Can be high output, admit if concerns over output
Genitourinary complications	
Urinary tract infection	3–5 d, oral antibiotics, most discharged
Urinary retention	Rapid catheter drainage, most discharged
Acute renal failure	Prerenal, renal, and postrenal causes, most admitted
Wound complications	
Hematoma	Caused by poor hemostasis, can drain most, but be careful with neck hematomas and hematomas after vascular surgery
Seroma	Painless swelling, clear fluid, drain and discharge
Infection	Open, drain, and culture; be careful with wounds associated with respiratory, gastrointestinal tract, genitourinary tract, or secondary to trauma
Necrotizing fasciitis	Pain out of proportion to physical findings
Dehiscence	Careful with abdominal incisions (evisceration)
Vascular complications	
Superficial thrombophlebitis	Usually aseptic, local therapy and discharge
Deep venous thrombosis	Upper and lower extremity, Doppler studies
Complications of drug therapy	
Diarrhea	Consider pseudomembranous colitis
Drug fever	Many drugs implicated, requires admission
Tetanus	Can occur after gastrointestinal surgery
Procedure-specific complications	See text

Abbreviation: CT = computed tomography.

TABLE 88-2 Common Causes of Postoperative Fevers in General Surgical Patients

Atelectasis	Pseudomembranous colitis
Pneumonia	Hepatitis
Urinary tract infections	Peritonitis
Skin and soft tissue injury	Pulmonary embolism
Thrombophlebitis (septic and sterile)	Transfusion reaction
Deep vein thrombosis	
Intraabdominal abscesses	
Unrelated bacterial infection	

Presenting symptoms can include dyspnea, chest pain, productive cough, fever, and tachypnea. Postoperative pneumonia is likely to be polymicrobial. After cultures of sputum and blood are obtained, parenteral antimicrobial therapy with an aminoglycoside and an antipseudomonal penicillin should be administered. Admission to the hospital is generally indicated.

Pneumothorax

Pneumothorax can occur as a complication of thoracic wall surgery, breast biopsy, laparoscopic abdominal surgery, abdominal paracentesis, nasogastric and feeding tube insertion, thoracic surgery, central venous catheter insertion, endoscopic procedures, shoulder arthros-copy, and tracheostomy. The pathophysiology varies with these different procedures, but clinical features are similar. Patients complain of chest pain, shoulder pain, or dyspnea. Physical findings can include tachypnea, hyperresonance to percussion, and decreased breath sounds on the affected side. Diagnosis is confirmed by chest x-ray with expiratory views.

TABLE 88-3 Evaluation and Management of Postoperative Fever

HISTORY

Presenting signs and symptoms
Onset of symptoms, time since procedure
Procedures performed and complications
Medications
History of blood transfusion

PHYSICAL EXAMINATION

Particular attention to
  Operative sites and contiguous areas
  Sites of catheters and invasive monitors
  Signs of deep venous thrombosis and pulmonary embolism
  Decubiti
  Lungs

ANCILLARY STUDIES

Complete blood count with differential
Chest radiograph
Gram stain and culture of wound exudate
Urinalysis (culture if infected)
Sputum gram stain and culture
Blood cultures
If diarrhea present, consider immunoassay of specimen for *Clostridium difficile* toxin
Further tests as indicated (e.g., computed tomography, radionuclide studies, venography, arteriograms)

TREATMENT

If source identified, start antibiotics; admission based on condition of patient
If no source identified, consider admission, change and culture all catheters, stop all medication that might cause fever

Pulmonary Embolus

Pulmonary embolism may present any time during the postoperative period. A lower extremity or pelvic thrombus dislodges and migrates to the pulmonary vasculature. The presenting signs and symptoms depend on the size of embolus and the underlying cardiopulmonary status of the patient. Patients have different degrees of dyspnea, chest pain, cough, and anxiety. Hemoptysis is usually seen only late in a patient's course and with massive pulmonary embolism. The patient may have essentially normal vital signs or be tachypneic and tachycardic.

Diagnosis of pulmonary embolism is difficult because of the poor sensitivity of noninvasive tests. Although hypoxemia and a widened alveolar-arterial oxygen gradient are frequently found with larger emboli, patients may have normal oxygen content and a normal alveolar-arterial gradient. Diagnosis requires venous Doppler ultrasonography, ventilation-perfusion scan, pulmonary computed tomography (CT), or pulmonary angiography. Patients with low clinical suspicion, normal vital signs, good oxygenation, and a low probability scan can be discharged, provided other causes of their symptoms have been addressed.

GENITOURINARY COMPLICATIONS

The most common postoperative genitourinary complication is urinary tract infection. However, patients may present with acute urinary retention and acute renal failure (ARF).

Urinary Tract Infection

Urinary tract infections can occur after any surgical procedure. However, there is an increased incidence in patients who have had instrumentation of the genitourinary tract or bladder catheterization. The cause is direct contamination of the urinary bladder, most commonly with *Escherichia coli*. Other organisms isolated include *Staphylococcus aureus, Staphylococcus epidermidis, Proteus mirabilis, Klebsiella, Pseudomonas,* and enterococci. Oral antibiotics are appropriate for most infections; however, elderly or debilitated patients and patients with evidence of sepsis require admission for parenteral antibiotics.

Urinary Retention

Acute urinary retention occurs in about 4 percent of all surgical patients.[3] It is postulated that urinary retention occurs as the result of catecholamine stimulation of α-adrenergic receptors in the bladder neck and urethral smooth muscle. Increased incidence of urinary retention is likely to occur in elderly males, with excessive fluid administration during surgery, and with the use of spinal or epidural anesthesia.

Patients with urinary retention present with lower abdominal discomfort, urinary urgency, and inability to void. The diagnosis is confirmed by placement of a Foley catheter. The bladder can be safely drained quickly without clamping, because there appears to be no foundation for the fears of hematuria, postobstructive diuresis, and hypotension.[4] For patients with normal renal function and no anatomic obstruction, continued catheter drainage is not necessary. For patients with retention after genitourinary procedures, the urologist must be consulted before disposition. Prophylactic antibiotics can be given if the genitourinary tract has been instrumented, if retention is prolonged, or if the patient is at risk for infection.

Acute Renal Failure

Acute renal failure is classified according to the primary cause: prerenal, intrinsic, or postrenal. Volume depletion is the most common prerenal cause. Intrinsic causes include acute tubular necrosis and drug nephrotoxicity. Obstructive uropathy is the cause of postrenal ARF. Patients with ARF have oliguria or anuria and, depending on the degree of ARF, may have signs of uremia and electrolyte abnormalities.

Patients should be examined for signs of hypovolemia and have a urinary catheter placed. Indwelling urinary catheters must be irrigated or replaced. If the patient is hypotensive, a fluid bolus is given to determine whether the cause is prerenal. In patients with urinary outlet obstruction, the urinary catheter is diagnostic and therapeutic. If there is doubt about the cause of the renal failure, central venous pressure and pulmonary capillary wedge pressure measurements can be helpful. The presence of postobstructive uropathy above the urinary bladder can be confirmed with abdominal ultrasound. When no prerenal or postrenal cause can be identified, there is likely to be an intrinsic cause of ARF.

WOUND COMPLICATIONS

Wound complications are frequent and include hematomas, seromas, infections, necrotizing fasciitis, and dehiscence. The patient's surgeon should be notified of all wound complications.

Hematomas

Wound hematomas result from unrecognized inadequate hemostasis. Patients have pain, pressure, and swelling within the wound. Patients with wound hematomas may be febrile and have sanguineous or serous wound drainage. Differentiating between hematoma and wound infection can be difficult. A few sutures are removed to allow the hematoma to drain, and cultures are obtained. If there is no evidence of infection and hemostasis can be maintained, the patient can be discharged. In patients with a hematoma of the neck or who have undergone vascular surgery, extreme caution and consultation are appropriate.

Seromas

A seroma, a collection of serous fluid, is usually the result of inadequate control of lymphatics during dissection but can occur under split-thickness skin grafts and areas with large dead spaces (e.g., axilla, groin, neck, or pelvis). Patients have painless swelling below the wound or graft, and needle aspiration yields a serous fluid. Aspiration confirms the diagnosis and alleviates the problem, although aspiration may have to be repeated later.

Infection

Systemic factors (e.g., extremes of age, poor nutrition, or diabetes) contribute to wound infections; however, local factors (e.g., necrotic tissue, poor perfusion, foreign bodies, and hematomas) are of greatest significance. In nontraumatic, uninfected operative wounds in which the respiratory, alimentary, and genitourinary tracts were not entered, infection rates are low. In these cases, the infecting organism is usually from the skin but can originate from remote infected sources (e.g., urinary tract infection). If there is a remote infected source, the organism is probably the same in both infections. Wounds associated with entering the respiratory, alimentary, or genitourinary tract or secondary to trauma have a higher risk of infection.

Presenting signs and symptoms of wound infections include increasing pain, erythema, swelling, drainage, and tenderness at the incision site. Wounds not involving the perineum and not associated with entry into the gastrointestinal or biliary tract are most often infected with *S. aureus* or streptococci. Such wounds can be safely managed with drainage, culture of the wound, irrigation, loose packing with gauze, and outpatient antibiotics. Wounds involving the perineum or associated with the gastrointestinal or biliary tract are often infected with multiple organisms, including gram-negative bacteria and anaerobes. Parenteral broad-spectrum antibiotics are administered, and admission is necessary.

Necrotizing Fasciitis

Necrotizing fasciitis is a feared complication. The usual cause is direct contamination of the wound with group A streptococcus or *S. aureus;* however, mixed aerobic and anaerobic infections have been reported. Risk factors include diabetes mellitus, alcoholism, immunosuppression, and peripheral vascular disease, but necrotizing fasciitis also occurs in young, otherwise healthy individuals. Early clinical differentiation from cellulitis can be difficult. CT may show asymmetric fascial thickening, gas tracking along fascial planes, or focal fluid collections; however, the actual sensitivity and specificity of CT in the diagnosis of necrotizing fasciitis has not been defined.[5] Magnetic resonance imaging has been shown to be highly sensitive but not totally specific for necrotizing fasciitis and can be a useful adjunct.[6] The presence of marked systemic toxicity and pain out of proportion to local findings indicate fasciitis. In more advanced cases, there may be deep pain with patchy areas of surface hypesthesia, crepitance, or bullae. Treatment should include antibiotics and immediate surgical debridement. Antibiotic choice is controversial but probably should include penicillin or cephalosporin, an aminoglycoside, and clindamycin.[7]

Wound Dehiscence

Wound dehiscence can be superficial or can extend into the deeper fascial planes. Dehiscence is caused by inadequate closure or intrinsic host factors, such as malnutrition, glucocorticoid use, or diabetes. The patient may have serosanguineous fluid leaking from the wound. Dehiscence of abdominal incisions has the potential for evisceration. If evisceration is not present, conservative management using abdominal binders is appropriate. However, if there is any uncertainty, operative exploration is indicated.

VASCULAR COMPLICATIONS

Postoperative vascular complications include thrombophlebitis and deep venous thrombosis. Superficial thrombophlebitis usually occurs in the upper extremities, secondary to prolonged cannulation of the vein or infusion of irritating fluids. Deep venous thrombosis is secondary to stasis, endothelial damage, or hypercoagulopathy.

Superficial Thrombophlebitis

Superficial thrombophlebitis of the lower extremities is most frequently secondary to stasis in varicose veins. It is usually aseptic. The patient complains of redness and warmth of the affected vein. If there is no evidence of surrounding cellulitis or lymphangitis, the patient is treated with local heat and elevation. Suppurative superficial thrombophlebitis is characterized by erythema, palpable tender cord, lymphangitis, and pain. Suppurative thrombophlebitis requires excision of the affected vein.

Deep Venous Thrombosis

When lower extremity superficial thrombophlebitis is seen, the possibility of concurrent deep venous thrombosis must be considered. Swelling of the extremity is the most specific physical sign, and its presence requires diagnostic evaluation. Doppler ultrasonography is generally the preferred diagnostic test. Patients with normal color-flow study results should be treated with elevation and bedrest. Repeat color-flow Doppler ultrasound studies should be performed in 3 days if symptoms persist but sooner if symptoms worsen.

COMPLICATIONS OF DRUG THERAPY

Many medicines have been reported to cause drug fever (Table 88-4).[8] The mechanisms proposed are hypersensitivity reactions, pyogenic effect, and disturbed thermoregulation. In patients in whom no source for the fever can be found, it is appropriate to consider stopping medications known to cause drug fever.

TABLE 88-4 Some Medications Associated with Drug Fever

Allopurinol	Lysergic acid
Aminoglycosides	Mebendazole
Amphetamine	Methyldopa
Amphotericin B	Metoclopramide
Antihistamines	Nifedipine
Asparaginase	Nitrofurantoin sodium
Azathioprine	Nomifensine
Barbiturates	Oxprenolol
Benztropine	Para-aminosalicylic acid
Bleomycin sulfate	Penicillins
Carbamazepine	Phenytoin sodium
Cephalosporins	Procainamide
Chlorpromazine	Propafenone
Cimetidine	Propylthiouracil
Clofibrate	Prostaglandin E_2
Cocaine derivatives	Quinidine sulfate
Dobutamine	Rifampin
Folate	Ritodrine
Heparin	Salicylates
Haloperidol	Streptokinase
Hydralazine	Streptomycin sulfate
Hydroxyurea	Sulfonamides
Ibuprofen	Tetracycline
Interferon	Thioridazine
Iodides	Tolmetin
Isoniazid	Triamterene
Levamisole	Trifluoperazine
Lincomycin	Vancomycin

Many antibiotics can cause diarrhea; however, the greatest concern in postoperative patients is pseudomembranous colitis. Pseudomembranous colitis is due to the toxin produced by the bacterium *Clostridium difficile*. Pseudomembranous colitis is related to antibiotic use, which destroys the normal enteric bacterial flora, allowing an overgrowth of the *C. difficile*. Even short courses of antibiotics have been associated with pseudomembranous colitis. Patients have watery and sometimes bloody diarrhea, elevated temperature, and crampy abdominal pain. Although tissue culture for *C. difficile* is the diagnostic gold standard, the diagnosis is usually made by detecting *C. difficile* cytotoxin in the stool.[1] This immunoassay is slightly less sensitive than is the tissue culture, but it is technically easier to do and provides an answer within 2 to 3 h. If results on the first specimen are negative and the diagnosis is still suspected, a second sample should be sent for immunoassay. When severe illness is present, consider empiric therapy with metronidazole while awaiting diagnostic studies.

COMPLICATIONS OF BREAST SURGERY

Breast biopsy is a common procedure. Although complications are infrequent, patients can develop minor wound infections and hematomas. Rarely, pneumothorax has been reported. Wound hematomas frequently require operative control for proper evacuation and hemostasis.

Early complications seen with mastectomies include wound infection, necrosis of skin flaps, and the accumulation of seromas. The most common late complication is lymphedema of the arm. The incidence of postmastectomy lymphedema ranges from a low of 5.5 percent to a high of 80 percent. Most patients can be managed by using a combination of fitted compression garments, nighttime elevation, and minor activity restrictions.[9]

COMPLICATIONS OF GASTROINTESTINAL SURGERY

Patients who have undergone any gastrointestinal surgery may have intestinal obstruction, intra-abdominal abscess, pancreatitis, cholecystitis, fistulas, and tetanus. Certain procedures, such as anastomoses, gastric surgery, placement of gastrostomy tubes, biliary tract surgery, other laparoscopic surgery, stomas, colonoscopy, and rectal surgery have specific complications.

General Considerations

INTESTINAL OBSTRUCTION Ileus, a functional obstruction of the bowel, is postulated to be the result of stimulation of the splanchnic nerves, leading to neuronal inhibition of coordinated intrinsic bowel wall motor activity. It is expected after any operation in which the peritoneal cavity is violated. After gastrointestinal surgery, small bowel tone usually returns to normal within 24 h, and colonic function returns within 3 to 5 days.[10] Ileus can also occur after nongastrointestinal procedures, is usually secondary to anesthetic agents, and function returns to normal after 24 h. Prolonged ileus can be caused by peritonitis, intra-abdominal abscess, hemoperitoneum, pneumonia, electrolyte imbalance, sepsis, and medications.

Presenting symptoms of ileus include nausea, vomiting, obstipation, constipation, abdominal distention, and abdominal pain. When these symptoms are present in the first few days after surgery, they are most often due to adynamic ileus. The symptoms of adynamic ileus are most often mild and respond to nasogastric suction, bowel rest, and intravenous hydration. However, in cases of prolonged ileus, the physician must always look for an underlying cause. Evaluation of patients with suspected ileus includes abdominal radiographs to identify air-fluid levels, chest x-ray, CBC, electrolytes, and urinalysis for secondary causes of ileus.

Mechanical ileus of the bowel is most often secondary to adhesions. Small bowel obstruction above the ligament of Treitz is associated with frequent bouts of bilious emesis. In cases of more distal obstruction, pain and distention become more severe, the frequency and volume of vomiting decrease, and emesis becomes more feculent. Abdominal radiographs demonstrate multiple air-fluid levels and a paucity of gas in the colon; however, with high obstruction, above the ligament of Treitz, there may be no air-fluid levels. In the ED, differentiating between functional ileus and mechanical bowel obstruction can be difficult. Both disorders result in different degrees of abdominal pain, distention, nausea, vomiting, and constipation. Once the diagnosis of mechanical obstruction is confirmed or suspected, surgical consultation is indicated.

INTRA-ABDOMINAL ABSCESS Intra-abdominal abscess is caused most frequently by preoperative contamination, spillage of bowel contents during surgery, contamination of a hematoma, or postoperative anastomotic leaks. Patients may have abdominal pain, nausea, vomiting, ileus, abdominal distention, fever, chills, anorexia, and abdominal tenderness. If the diagnosis is suspected, CT or ultrasound studies of the abdomen are required. The patient should receive broad-spectrum antibiotics. Although some abscesses are amenable to percutaneous drainage, many patients require surgical exploration.

PANCREATITIS Pancreatitis after abdominal surgery is secondary to direct manipulation or retraction of the pancreatic duct. It most commonly occurs after gastric resection, biliary tract surgery, and endoscopic retrograde cholangiopancreatography (ERCP). Clinical presentation varies from mild nausea, vomiting, and abdominal discomfort to intractable vomiting, leukocytosis, and left pleural effusion. Severe hemorrhagic presentation can cause lumbar pain accompanied by blue-gray discoloration of the skin in the flank area (Turner sign) or similar changes around the umbilicus (Cullen sign). Although the serum amylase level rises in acute pancreatitis, it is also elevated in patients with severe cholecystitis, renal insufficiency, intestinal obstruction, perforated ulcer, or ischemic bowel. A serum lipase measurement may help to identify those with true pancreatitis, although it may be elevated in a patient with a perforated viscus. Abdominal radiographs may show localized ileus in the region of the pancreas (sentinel loop). CT is useful in defining pancreatic fluid collections or abscesses. In general, the treatment of postoperative pancreatitis is similar to the treatment of nonoperative pancreatitis: bowel rest, antiemetics, and nasogastric suction.

CHOLECYSTITIS Patients may present during the postoperative period with biliary colic, acute calculous cholecystitis, or acute acalculous cholecystitis. The etiology of these disorders in the postoperative period is not clear. Ultrasound studies of the gallbladder and pancreas should be performed to aid in the diagnosis.

Acalculous cholecystitis is of particular concern in the postoperative period. Although it may occur in any age group, it seems to be more common in elderly males. Signs and symptoms are similar to those for calculous cholecystitis, but ultrasound studies fail to reveal gallstones. Liver function studies and the neutrophil count may be normal. Important findings on ultrasonography include gallbladder enlargement, wall thickening, and pericholecystic fluid collection. Hepatobiliary scintigraphy may be helpful. Early diagnosis is critical, because early operative intervention can reduce morbidity and mortality rates.

FISTULAS Enterocutaneous fistulas can occur almost anywhere in the gastrointestinal tract and are usually the result of technical complications or direct bowel injury. High-output fistulas can result in electrolyte abnormalities and volume depletion. Fistulas involving the proximal gastrointestinal tract are frequently high output and are of the greatest concern. Sepsis is the other major complication. Most patients require admission, although many fistulas ultimately close spontaneously.

TETANUS Although most cases of tetanus in the United States occur after minor trauma, there have been numerous reports of tetanus after general surgical procedures. *Clostridium tetani* is found in the gastrointestinal tract of 1 percent of the population.[11] During gastrointestinal surgery, there is spillage of *C. tetani*. Proliferation of the organism is facilitated by the presence of devitalized tissue, blood clots, and surgical suture. Incubation can take from 0 to 73 days, at which time the toxin leads to clinical tetanus.[12] The classic symptoms of tetanus, trismus, and opisthotonos may not be manifest at initial presentation. Patients may present with nonspecific symptoms of abdominal discomfort, fever, and abdominal wall rigidity. Diagnosis is based on physical examination and a history of inadequate immunization.

Specific Considerations

ANASTOMOSIS Anastomotic leaks occur most frequently after esophageal and colonic surgeries and least frequently after gastric and small intestinal anastomoses. The cause of anastomotic leakage is related mainly to surgical technique.

Intrathoracic esophageal anastomotic leaks usually manifest within 10 days of surgery. The presentation is dramatic, with fever, chest pain, tachypnea, tachycardia, and possibly shock. Chest x-ray may reveal a pneumothorax with pleural effusion. Disruption can be confirmed by contrast esophagography using a water-soluble contrast agent. Even with immediate reoperation, morbidity and mortality rates are high.

The signs and symptoms of gastric anastomotic leaks include abdominal pain, fever, leukocytosis, gastric outlet obstruction, hyperamylasemia, hyperbilirubinemia, peritonitis, and shock. Plain radiographs may reveal pneumoperitoneum or air-fluid levels. The patient should have immediate volume resuscitation, parenteral broad-spectrum antibiotics, and nasogastric tube drainage. Immediate surgery is required.

Small intestinal anastomoses infrequently leak because of the excellent blood supply and rapid healing of the area. However, if a leak occurs, the patient usually presents with local abscess formation or peritonitis. Treatment is immediate reoperation.

Colorectal anastomoses are prone to disruption because of the large number of pathogenic bacteria, propensity for colonic distention, and a single thin layer of circular muscle to support sutures. The patients usually present 7 to 14 days postoperatively with evidence of intra-abdominal or pelvic abscess. CT can be helpful in diagnosis. Patients should receive broad-spectrum parenteral antibiotics, nasogastric tube drainage, and adequate fluid resuscitation in preparation for surgery.

GASTRIC SURGERY Patients who have undergone partial or complete gastrectomy can present with a few distinct syndromes: dumping syndrome, alkaline reflux gastritis, afferent loop syndrome, and postvagotomy diarrhea. Although these complications are rare, the symptoms can be disabling.

Dumping syndrome can occur early or late after a meal. Although the precise etiology of dumping symptoms is unclear, it occurs when the pylorus is bypassed or removed. The hyperosmolar chyme contents of the stomach are dumped into the jejunum, resulting in rapid influx of extracellular fluid and an autonomic response.

Patients experience nausea, epigastric discomfort, palpitations, abdominal colic, diaphoresis, and, in some cases, dizziness and syncope. Patients with early dumping symptoms experience diarrhea, whereas those with late dumping symptoms, 2 to 4 h postprandially, usually do not. The late dumping syndrome is believed to be due to a reactive hypoglycemia. The mainstay of treatment is dietary modification; eating small, dry meals; and separating solids from liquids. In refractory cases, pyloroplasty can be tried. Most of these patients do not require admission.

Patients with reflux gastritis present with continual burning epigastric pain that is aggravated by meals and unrelieved by vomiting. The syndrome is caused by reflux of bile into the stomach. Diagnosis is made by endoscopic examination.

Patients with afferent loop syndrome also present with severe epigastric pain 1 to 2 h after eating, which is relieved by vomiting. The vomitus will be bilious, without food. The syndrome occurs in patients who have undergone gastroenterostomy (Billroth II) reconstruction after partial gastrectomy. Diagnosis is made by contrast radiography or endoscopy. Operative reconstruction is required.

Whereas most patients undergoing truncal vagotomy have increased bowel movements, some will have diarrhea. The precise etiology is not clear. Patients present with diarrhea that is variable in its occurrence and not associated with food intake. It is often unpredictable and explosive, which can lead to weight loss, malnutrition, and severe social complications. The incidence of the diarrhea decreases with time, and treatment is mostly symptomatic.

GASTROSTOMY TUBES Most gastrostomy tubes are now placed by an endoscopist via percutaneous endoscopy or by a radiologist via percutaneous fluoroscopy. If the patient has undergone a laparotomy, the general surgeon may place a gastrostomy tube at the time of surgery. If the tube was placed by the surgeon and has not been replaced, it will have a bumper holding the tube in place. The tube has to be cut and the bumper allowed to pass, or the bumper has to be removed by endoscopic technique. For further discussion, see Chap. 89, "Complications of Gastrointestinal Devices."

BILIARY TRACT SURGERY More than 50 percent of all cholecystectomies are now performed laparoscopically. There are complications seen after open and laparoscopic cholecystectomies (Table 88-5) and complications related to the laparoscopic technique (Table 88-6).[13,14] Patients are likely to present to the ED with nonspecific abdominal symptoms.

The evaluation of abdominal pain after cholecystectomy depends on the clinical condition of the patient. If there are signs of peritoneal irritation or fever, an injury to the biliary system is likely. The patient should have an abdominal CT in addition to a CBC, electrolyte measurements,

TABLE 88-5   Complications of Cholecystectomy

Bile leak
Bile duct stricture
Bleeding
Bowel injury
Intraabdominal abscess
Myocardial infarction
Pancreatitis
Pulmonary complications
Retained common duct stones or stones spilled into peritoneum
Umbilical hernia
Wound infection

liver function tests, and a serum lipase test. Endoscopic retrograde cholangiopancreatography will be required to identify the site of the injury; however, a collection of bile can be seen on CT. Depending on the ERCP results, reoperation may be necessary. Small collections of bile may require only observation or percutaneous drainage.

Patients presenting soon after cholecystectomy with pain, pancreatitis, and/or jaundice may have retained common duct stones. If CT does not reveal an intra-abdominal collection of fluid, an ERCP should be performed. Endoscopic sphincterotomy is usually an effective means of dealing with retained stones. Patients presenting late after cholecystectomy with fever, pain, and jaundice may have bile duct stricture. Diagnosis requires ERCP. Stents are usually tried first, but surgical repair may be necessary. A more recent concern has been the spillage of gallstones into the peritoneal cavity at the time of surgery. Initially, such stones were thought to be innocuous. However, they have been linked to abdominal pain, pelvic pain, dysmenorrhea, intraabdominal abscess, colocutaneous fistula, and implantation into the ovary with subsequent infertility.[15]

OTHER LAPAROSCOPIC SURGERIES   Laparoscopic techniques are now being used for an increasing number of procedures. In addition to cholecystectomy, they have been used for appendectomy, colon resection, antireflux surgery, herniorrhaphy, fundoplication, and most gynecologic surgical procedures, including hysterectomy. The complications associated with these procedures have not been completely identified; however, they are likely to be similar to those seen with cholecystectomy.

TABLE 88-6   Complications of Laparoscopy

RELATED TO PNEUMOPERITONEUM
Cardiac arrhythmias during the procedure
Subcutaneous emphysema
Pneumothorax
Pneumomediastinum
CO_2 embolization

RELATED TO INSERTION OF NEEDLE AND TROCAR
Bleeding from trocar site
Gastrointestinal tract injuries
Laceration
Intestinal burns
Genitourinary tract injuries
Major vessel injuries
Hernia from trocar site
Wound infection

MISCELLANEOUS
Retained intraabdominal gallstones
Biliary cutaneous fistula
Chronic pain
Infertility
Cholelithiasis
Metastases to the trocar site

STOMAS   The two most common stomas placed are the ileostomy and the colostomy. Problems with these stomas can be quite debilitating. Most complications are related to technical errors as to where the stomas are placed; however, there can be problems of new disease within the stoma (e.g., Crohn disease or cancer). Possible complications include ischemia and stomal necrosis, peristomal skin irritation, peristomal hernia, and stomal prolapse.

Ischemia and stomal necrosis are manifested very early in the postoperative course. The cause is inadequate blood supply to the stoma. Normally, the stoma is pink, without evidence of cyanosis. Any evidence of compromised blood flow requires surgical evaluation.

Peristomal maceration and skin destruction are most likely secondary to a poor seal of the stomal appliance. Consultation with an enterostomal therapist for a properly fitting appliance is indicated.

Prolapse can occur with ileostomies and colostomies. The cause is usually inadequate fixation of the intra-abdominal portion or too large an abdominal wall opening. Patients present with the stoma protrusion, with or without pain. The stoma must be examined to determine viability. The stoma should be pink and painless. Reduction should be attempted if the tissue is viable, followed by consultation with a surgeon. Definitive therapy requires surgical revision.

Parastomal hernias are secondary to too large an abdominal wall opening. As with any hernia, the physician should determine whether the hernia is incarcerated, attempt reduction, and consult a surgeon. Definitive therapy requires local reconstruction of the orifice.

COLONOSCOPY   Potential complications of colonoscopy include hemorrhage, perforation, retroperitoneal abscess, pneumoscrotum, pneumothorax, volvulus, postcolonoscopy distention, bacteremia, and infection.

Hemorrhage is the most common complication and can be secondary to the polypectomy procedures, biopsies, laceration of the mucosa by the instrument, or tearing of the mesentery or spleen.[16] If the bleeding is intraluminal, the patient will present with rectal bleeding. Patients with mesenteric or splenic injury will present with signs of intraabdominal bleeding. Treatment of intraluminal bleeding depends on the magnitude of hemorrhage. Signs of intra-abdominal bleeding require emergency laparotomy.

Perforation of the colon with pneumoperitoneum usually is evident immediately but can take several hours to manifest.[17] Perforation is usually secondary to intrinsic disease of the colon (e.g., diverticulitis) or to vigorous manipulation during the procedure. Most patients will require immediate laparotomy; however, in some patients presenting late (1 to 2 days later) without signs of peritonitis, expectant management may be appropriate.

RECTAL SURGERY   Patients who have undergone hemorrhoidectomy frequently have problems with postoperative urinary retention, the management of which has been discussed previously. Three other problems that can occur are constipation, rectal hemorrhage, and rectal prolapse.

The management of constipation in a patient who has undergone rectal surgery is no different from that of any other patient with constipation. Gentle rectal examination is indicated, and enemas can still be used. Posthemorrhoidectomy rectal hemorrhage can occur immediately postoperatively but may be delayed (4 ± 2 days).[18] Proposed causes of delayed bleeding include sepsis of the pedicle, disruption of a clot, and sloughing of tissue.[19] The patient may present with minimal bleeding or massive hemorrhage. Although ligation of the affected vessel is needed, a temporary tamponade with a Foley catheter may be helpful.

Patients may present with mucosal prolapse or complete rectal prolapse. Mucosal prolapse occurs when the surgeon has not removed all redundant mucosa during hemorrhoidectomy and is much more common than rectal prolapse. Local treatment by a surgeon is usually corrective. Rectal prolapse can occur after any anorectal surgical procedure and likely is related to injury of the puborectalis muscle. The patient will present with the sensation of protrusion and may complain of pain. The treatment is reduction and surgical consultation.

Infection after anorectal surgery is surprisingly uncommon. The patient usually complains of increasing pain and fever. Examination of the area is necessary to detect an abscess or cellulitis. Fournier's gangrene may follow anorectal surgery. If this is suspected, broad-spectrum parenteral antibiotics are given immediately. The patient requires immediate surgical debridement.

REFERENCES

1. O'Grady NP, Barie PS, Bartlett J, et al: Practice parameters for evaluating new fever in critically ill adult patients. Task Force of the American College of Critical Care Medicine of the Society of Critical Care Medicine in collaboration with the Infectious Disease Society of America. *Crit Care Med* 26:392, 1998.
2. Crabtree TD, Pelletier SJ, Antevil JL, et al: Cohort study of fever and leukocytosis as diagnostic and prognostic indicators in infected surgical patients. *World J Surg* 25:739, 2001.
3. Tammela T, Kontturi M, Lukkarinen O: Postoperative urinary retention. I. Incidence and predisposing factors. *Scand J Urol Nephrol* 20:197, 1986.
4. Nyman MA, Schwenk NM, Silverstein MD: Management of urinary retention: Rapid versus gradual decompression and risk of complications. *Mayo Clin Proc* 72:951, 1997.
5. Wysoki MG, Santora TA, Shah RM, et al: Necrotizing fasciitis: CT characteristics. *Radiology* 203:859, 1997.
6. Schmid MR, Kossmann T, Duewell S: Differentiation of necrotizing fasciitis and cellulitis using MR imaging. *AJR* 170:615, 1998.
7. Childers BJ, Potyondy LD, Nachreiner R, et al: Necrotizing fasciitis: A fourteen-year retrospective study of 163 consecutive patients. *Am Surg* 68:109, 2002.
8. Cunha BA: Antibiotic side effects. *Med Clin North Am* 85:149, 2001.
9. Brennan MJ, Miller LT: Overview of treatment options and review of the current role and use of compression garments, intermittent pumps, and exercise in the management of lymphedema. *Cancer* 83:2821, 1998.
10. Nachlas MM, Younis MT, Roda CP, et al: Gastrointestinal motility studies as a guide to postoperative management. *Ann Surg* 175:510, 1972.
11. Meyer KA, Spector BK: The incidence of tetanus bacilli in the stools and on the regional skin of one hundred urban herniotomy cases. *Surg Gynecol Obstet* 54:785, 1932.
12. Bardenheier B, Prevots DR, Khetsuriani N, et al: Tetanus surveillance-United States, 1995-1997. *Morb Mortal Wkly Rep CDC Surveill Summ* 47:1, 1998.
13. Callery MP, Strasberg SM, Soper NJ: Complications of laparoscopic general surgery. *Gastrointest Endosc Clin North Am* 6:423, 1996.
14. Lujan JA, Parrilla P, Robles R, et al: Laparoscopic cholecystectomy vs open cholecystectomy in the treatment of acute cholecystitis: a prospective study. *Arch Surg* 133:173, 1998.
15. Patterson EJ, Nagy AG: Don't cry over spilled stones? Complications of gallstones spilled during laparoscopic cholecystectomy: Case report and literature review. *Can J Surg* 40:300, 1997.
16. Dafnis G, Ekbom A, Pahlman L, et al: Complications of diagnostic and therapeutic colonoscopy within a defined population in Sweden. *Gastrointest Endosc* 54:302, 2001.
17. Araghizadeh FY, Timmcke AE, Opelka FG, et al: Colonoscopic perforations. *Dis Colon Rectum* 44:713, 2001.
18. Basso L, Pescatori M: Outcome of delayed hemorrhage following surgical hemorrhoidectomy. *Dis Colon Rectum* 37:288, 1994.
19. Rosen L, Sipe P, Stasik JJ, et al: Outcome of delayed hemorrhage following surgical hemorrhoidectomy. *Dis Colon Rectum* 36:743, 1993.

COMPLICATIONS OF GASTROINTESTINAL DEVICES
Edmond A. Hooker

The gastrointestinal (GI) device that is most commonly used by emergency physicians is the nasogastric (NG) tube. Other GI devices encountered in the emergency department include large-bore orogastric tubes, small-bore nasointestinal ("feeding") tubes, and transabdominal feeding tubes (gastrostomy, jejunostomy, and gastrojejunostomy tubes). Although complications from the use of these are rare, they must be anticipated and prevented, if possible.

NASOGASTRIC TUBES

The NG tube is probably the most common device placed in the GI tract. Tubes range in size from 6 to 18 F (1 F = 0.3 mm). These devices are relatively easy to place blindly in an alert, cooperative patient. Obtunded patients or those without an active gag reflex may require endotracheal intubation before NG insertion. It is important to note that the presence of an endotracheal tube with an inflated balloon does not prevent passage of these tubes into the respiratory tract.

Major complications have been reported with the use of NG tubes (Table 89-1). Improper placement is the principal cause of these complications, and different techniques have been proposed to help identify improper placement of NG tubes (Table 89-2).[1] However, according to published research, none of the techniques have proven effective. The technique that is probably most commonly used, insufflation of air into the NG tube while listening over the stomach, has many reported failures. A recently proposed technique used capnography with excellent results.[2]

Placement of the NG tube into the respiratory tract can result in pneumonia or pneumothorax. If charcoal is instilled, the outcome can be fatal. Although not the standard of care, chest radiographs may aid in the confirmation of NG placement before instilling charcoal or other medications. If the tube is identified in the chest cavity, it must be determined whether it entered through the lungs or through the esophagus. All possible charcoal should be removed by suctioning before removing the NG tube or, in the case of charcoal thorax, by chest tube drainage.

There are numerous reports of intracranial placement of NG tubes. Most cases have been reported in trauma patients; however, there is at least one report of intracranial placement in a nontrauma patient. As with any catheter insertion, force should never be used, and NG tubes should be inserted through the mouth in trauma patients who may have facial or basilar skull fractures. Any time a NG tube is placed and cannot be easily removed, an x-ray should be obtained to determine the location of the tube.

OROGASTRIC LAVAGE TUBES

Large-bore tubes (28 to 40 F) are used for gastric decontamination and charcoal instillation. The use of these tubes has come into relative disfavor in recent years.[3] This was not because of complications but rather because of a lack of proven efficacy. Complications have only been rarely reported with the use of the tubes but have included esophageal tears and inability to remove the tube secondary to esophageal spasm. If an orogastric lavage tube cannot easily be removed, the patient should undergo fluoroscopic examination with contrast to determine its exact location and any kinking. If the tube is simply stuck because of esophageal spasm, glucagon can be given to assist in its removal.[4]

TABLE 89-1 Complications of Placement of Nasogastric and Nasoenteric Tubes

Epistaxis
Intracranial placement
Bronchial placement
Pharyngeal placement
Esophageal obstruction or rupture
Bronchial or alveolar perforation
Pneumothorax
Charcoal instillation into the lungs and pleural cavity
Gastric or duodenal rupture
Vocal cord paralysis
Pneumomediastinum
Laryngeal injuries
Knotting-preventing removal

TABLE 89-2 Techniques for Identifying Nasogastric and Nasointestinal Feeding Tube Placement

Indicates gastric placement
  Epigastric auscultation of air insufflated through the tube
  Aspiration of visually recognizable gastrointestinal secretions
  pH testing of aspirates (pH ≤6 indicates gastric placement)
  Failure to detect end-tidal carbon dioxide pattern using capnograph
Indicates tracheobronchial placement
  Coughing or choking
  Inability to speak
  Air bubbles when proximal end of tube is placed in water

NASOINTESTINAL TUBES

The small-bore nasointestinal tubes (more commonly called feeding tubes) are usually placed to support nutrition. Complications of these tubes include all of those described with NG tubes (see Table 89-1), but the former are also more easily dislodged and clogged. With numerous reports of placement of these tubes into the respiratory tract and subsequent intrapulmonary instillation of tube feedings, most institutions require radiographic confirmation of tube placement.[5,6] A novel technique using a magnetic detector has been introduced recently and may help obviate a radiograph.[7] Because patients can easily dislodge these tubes after initial confirmation of placement, some recommend pH testing before each use.[8]

Replacement of a dislodged tube should be performed according to the manufacturer's instructions and radiographic confirmation should be obtained (Table 89-3). When one of these tubes is clogged from buildup of sediment, the physician can attempt to unclog the tube by instilling saline or cola drink into the tube and leaving it for 30 min; however, replacement frequently will be necessary.[9]

TRANSABDOMINAL FEEDING TUBES

Although the techniques for the initial placement of transabdominal feeding tubes (gastrostomy, jejunostomy, and gastrojejunostomy) are beyond the scope of emergency physicians, complications related to these tubes need to be recognized (Table 89-4). These tubes can be placed by a surgeon via open technique, by a gastroenterologist via endoscopic technique (percutaneous endoscopic gastrostomy), or by a radiologist via percutaneous techniques. The radiographic technique has been associated with fewer complications than has open or endoscopically assisted placement.[10,11]

Frequent minor complications are associated with the use of these tubes, including purulent drainage and leakage around the stomal site, clogging, dislodgement, and vomiting and diarrhea.

Drainage from the stomal site is a common finding and represents a foreign-body reaction due to the catheter. As long as there is no evidence of cellulitis or necrotizing fasciitis, local skin care with hydro-

TABLE 89-3 Method for Inserting a Nasointestinal Feeding Tube*

Step 1: Prepare nares with topical anesthetic and lubricant. Restrain uncooperative patients. Lubricate and insert the stylet into the feeding tube (ensure that the stylet does not protrude beyond tip of tube).
Step 2: Place tube through nares into hypopharynx. If patient starts coughing or choking, tube may be in respiratory tract or coiled up in hypopharynx. The cooperative patient may swallow liquids to assist passage.
Step 3: After successful passage, remove stylet from tube and obtain a chest x-ray that includes the epigastric area. If tube is in proper position, start feedings.

Warnings: Never reinsert a stylet into a feeding tube while the tube is still in the patient and never use a feeding tube before radiographic confirmation of placement.

TABLE 89-4 Complications Seen with Transabdominal Feeding Tubes

Complication	Initial Considerations
Purulent drainage from stoma	Local care with hydrogen peroxide unless cellulitis is present
Leakage from stoma	Carefully replace with larger tube
Tube occlusion	Attempt irrigation, most often just replace
Dislodged tubes	Gently replace, confirm placement with x-rays
Pneumothorax	High index of suspicion, consider needle aspiration
Bacteremia	Consider as potential source in septic patient
Bleeding from tract	If recently inserted, consider local injection, consult
Bleeding from granuloma buildup	Local therapy with silver nitrate
Infection of surrounding skin	Consultation, pull tube, IV antibiotics
Necrotizing fasciitis	Consider MRI to help confirm, surgical debridement
Peritonitis	Determine if fistula exists, consultation, IV antibiotics
Pulmonary aspiration of feedings	Reduce flow rate, half-strength feeds, consider J tube
Vomiting or diarrhea	Reduce flow rate, half-strength feeds, stop feeds
Gastroesophageal reflux	Reduce flow rate, half-strength feeds, consider J tube
Intestinal obstruction	Step feedings, NPO, admit and observe
Gastric outlet obstruction	Reposition tube
Gastric volvulus	Surgical consult
Gastric perforation	Surgical consult
Esophageal perforation	Surgical consult
Colonic perforation	Surgical consult
Colocutaneous fistula	Surgical consult
Electrolyte abnormalities	Change feedings or increase free water
Gastrointestinal bleeding	Endoscopy and therapy directed at cause

Abbreviation: NPO = non per os.

gen peroxide and warm water usually will clear up the problem. If there is granuloma formation with localized bleeding from friable skin, local treatment with silver nitrate usually will help.

Leakage of gastric contents can become a problem. This is managed by careful insertion of a larger tube. Care should be used not to force too large a tube into the stoma, because this can cause separation of the stomach wall from the abdominal wall.

Prevention is the best treatment for clogging of gastrostomy (G) and jejunostomy (J) tubes. Frequent flushing with water and careful crushing of pills usually can prevent this problem. Vomiting and diarrhea can be relieved by decreasing the amount of the feedings and/or diluting the feedings.

If the tube cannot be unclogged or if it has fallen out, replacement will be necessary. If the tube was placed by a surgeon or gastroenterologist and has not been replaced, it probably will have a bolster (also called a mushroom) holding the tube in place (Figure 89-1). This will prevent the tube from being removed. The bolster must be removed endoscopically or the tube may be cut off and the bolster allowed to pass through the GI tract.[12] The latter technique is generally safe in adults; however, its use in children has been associated with

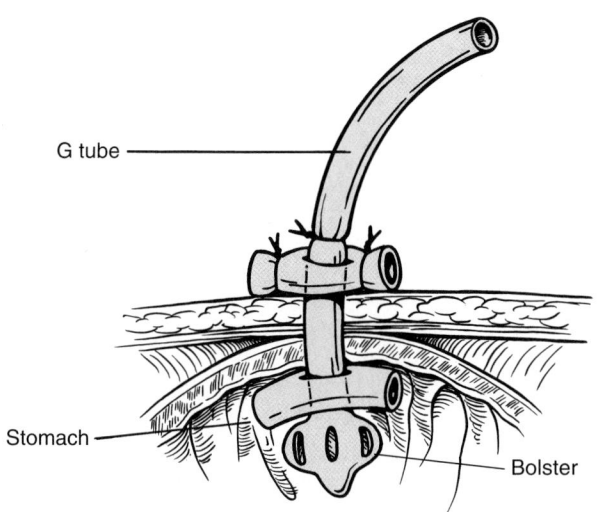

FIG. 89-1. Percutaneous endoscopic gastrostomy tube with a mushroom bolster in place. (Adapted with permission from Gauderer MWL, Ponsky JL: A simplified technique for constructing a tube feeding gastrostomy. *Surg Gynecol Obstet* 152:83, 1981.)

more frequent complications.[13] Endoscopic removal is advisable when there is suspected or potential obstructive disease of the GI tract, such as pyloric stenosis, intestinal pseudoobstruction, and intestinal stricture (e.g., due to radiation, ischemia, or inflammatory bowel disease). If the tube is cut, an abdominal radiograph should be obtained 1 week later to confirm passage of the internal component. Most reported complications from a retained internal bolster have occurred when the bolster did not pass within 1 to 2 weeks.[14]

When the feeding tube has already been replaced or was originally placed via radiographic technique, it should have a balloon holding it in place. The balloon usually can be deflated and the tube easily removed. If there is a problem with removal, the tube can be cut off halfway down; this usually will allow the balloon to deflate. If the catheter still cannot be removed easily, it can be cut off at the skin and the internal component allowed to pass. **It should be replaced as quickly as possible to prevent closure of the tract.** Although there is no published research stating how long it takes for a tract to mature, tracts that are 7 to 10 days old probably will remain open long enough to allow replacement. The physician first must determine, if possible, which type of tube is being used. If the tube is available, replacement with the same size is usually possible. If the tube is not available, it can be difficult to determine whether the tract is for a J or G tube. Location on the abdominal wall is not helpful. A tract for a G tube is usually larger. Old records may be useful and should be obtained, if possible. After determining the type of tract and size of tube used previously, insertion should be performed by the physician with a water-soluble lubricant. If the size of the tube being replaced cannot be ascertained, it is reasonable to start with a 16-F replacement G tube or Foley catheter. The lubricated tube should pass easily into the stoma without additional equipment. If resistance is met, the attempt should be abandoned. A smaller tube can be tried to keep the tract open. After replacing the tube, a 20- to 30-mL bolus of a water-soluble contrast material (e.g., Gastrografin) should be instilled through the tube, and a supine abdominal x-ray should be obtained within 1 to 2 min.[15] The x-ray should demonstrate rugae of the stomach for a G tube and flow into a small bowel for a J tube. If there is any question of improper placement, immediate consultation should be obtained.

A special caution regarding J tubes should be noted. Jejunostomy tracts are smaller, and smaller tubes are used (8 to 14 F). These tubes usually are not sutured in place and frequently become dislodged. They can be replaced with catheters made specifically for jejunostomies or with Foley catheters. **If a Foley catheter is used to replace a lost J catheter, the balloon should never be inflated** because it can cause a bowel obstruction or damage the jejunum. The tube is lubricated, inserted into the stoma, and advanced 20 cm. These tubes are easily replaced if the tract is mature: however, if resistance is met, referral to a radiologist for fluoroscopic placement using guidewires is recommended.[16]

REFERENCES

1. Metheny NA, Titler MG: Assessing placement of feeding tubes. *Am J Nurs* 101:36, 2001.
2. White NA: Confirmation of placement of fine-bore nasogastric tubes. *Anaesthesia* 56:1123, 2001.
3. Vale JA: Position statement: Gastric lavage. American Academy of Clinical Toxicology; European Association of Poisons Centres and Clinical Toxicologists. *J Toxicol Clin Toxicol* 35:711, 1997.
4. Thoma ME, Glauser JM: Use of glucagon for removal of an orogastric lavage tube. *Am J Emerg Med* 13:219, 1995.
5. Bankier AA, Wiesmayr MN, Henk C, et al: Radiographic detection of intrabronchial malpositions of nasogastric tubes and subsequent complications in intensive care unit patients. *Intens Care Med* 23:406, 1997.
6. Lipman TO, Kessler T, Arabian A: Nasopulmonary intubation with feeding tubes: Case reports and review of the literature. *J Parenter Enteral Nutr* 9:618, 1985.
7. Tobin RW, Gonzales AJ, Golden RN, et al: Magnetic detection to position human nasogastric tubes. *Biomed Instrum Technol* 34:432, 2000.
8. Metheny NA, Smith L, Stewart BJ: Development of a reliable and valid bedside test for bilirubin and its utility for improving prediction of feeding tube location. *Nurs Res* 49:302, 2000.
9. Nicholson LJ: Declogging small-bore feeding tubes. *J Parenter Enter Nutr* 11:594, 1987.
10. Wollman B, D'Agostino HB: Percutaneous radiologic and endoscopic gastrostomy: A 3-year institutional analysis of procedure performance. *Am J Roentgenol* 169:1551, 1997.
11. Wollman B, D'Agostino HB, Walus-Wigle JR, et al: Radiologic, endoscopic, and surgical gastrostomy: An institutional evaluation and meta-analysis of the literature. *Radiology* 197:699, 1995.
12. Korula J, Harma C: A simple and inexpensive method of removal or replacement of gastrostomy tubes. *JAMA* 265:1426, 1991.
13. Chait PG, Weinberg J, Connolly BL, et al: Retrograde percutaneous gastrostomy and gastrojejunostomy in 505 children: A 4 $\frac{1}{2}$-year experience. *Radiology* 201:691, 1996.
14. Yaseen M, Steele MI, Grunow JE: Nonendoscopic removal of percutaneous endoscopic gastrostomy tubes: Morbidity and mortality in children. *Gastrointest Endosc* 44:235, 1996.
15. Wolf EL, Frager D, Beneventano TC: Radiologic demonstration of important gastrostomy tube complications. *Gastrointest Radiol* 11:20, 1986.
16. Boland MP, Patrick J, Stoski DS, et al: Permanent enteral feeding in cystic fibrosis: Advantages of a replaceable jejunostomy tube. *J Pediatr Surg* 22:843, 1987.

THE LIVER TRANSPLANT PATIENT
Steven Kronick

DEMOGRAPHICS AND SURVIVAL

More than 70,000 liver transplantations have been performed worldwide. In the United States, 5181 liver transplantations were performed at 123 centers in 2001. At present, the number of transplantations performed is limited only by the availability of organ donors. The use of living donors has expanded the potential for liver transplantation.[1] In October of 2002, more than 17,000 patients in the United States were on the liver transplant waiting list. Improvements in surgical techniques, immunosuppression protocols, and patient selection have increased mean patient survival to 87 percent at 1 year and 80.9 percent at 3 years.[2]

Transplantation is the treatment of choice for end-stage liver disease (ESLD) refractory to all other interventions and is considered an effective means to improve quality of life as well as survival.[3] Indications for liver transplantation are listed in Table 90-1. The incidence of transplant-related problems is high (Table 90-2), and evaluation is made difficult by the fact that many of the complications present with similar signs, symptoms, and laboratory abnormalities. Most transplant-related problems will require, at a minimum, direct communication with the transplant center for consultation and follow-up.[4]

TRANSPLANT PROCEDURE

The harvested liver can tolerate ischemia up to 24 h, but it functions best if ischemia time is less than 8 h. The risk of preservation injury increases after this time. Most patients undergo bilateral subcostal incision with upper midline extension to the xiphoid process. After recipient hepatectomy, the donor liver is placed in the recipient, typically in the same (orthotopic) location as the liver it is replacing. Venovenous bypass, used by some centers, may predispose the patient to thrombosis and pulmonary embolism. Normal color and consistency return to the organ in approximately 15 min. Early bile production after vascular reanastomosis is most indicative of graft function. The preferred method for biliary tract reconstruction is an end-to-end choledochocholedochostomy. The use of a percutaneous biliary drain varies by center, and when it is used, it may stay in place for several weeks to months. In children with biliary atresia and in adults whose anatomy will not allow choledochocholedochostomy, Roux-en-Y choledochojejunostomy is performed.[5] Newer techniques being used increasingly in pediatric patients include reduced-size liver transplant, split-liver transplant, and living-related transplantation.[6]

POSTOPERATIVE COMPLICATIONS

Immediate postoperative complications are not seen in the emergency department because patients typically remain hospitalized for approximately 1 to 2 weeks. Postoperative problems seen in the emergency department relate most commonly to bleeding, biliary, vascular, and wound complications.[7]

Bleeding Complications

The vast majority of postoperative bleeding complications in patients will occur in the first week and will not be seen in the ED. Gastrointestinal bleeding can develop after discharge. It should be managed in the usual fashion but may signal graft dysfunction and be accompanied by profound hypoglycemia and progressive coagulopathy.[4] Portal hypertension is reversed by liver transplantation, and gastrointestinal (GI) bleeding from varices postoperatively may be indicative of portal

TABLE 90-1   Indications for Liver Transplantation

Primary biliary cirrhosis
Primary sclerosing cholangitis
Fulminant and subfulminant hepatitis
Cirrhosis due to hepatitis B or C virus
Alcoholic cirrhosis
Children: biliary atresia (accounts for >50%)
           selected inborn errors of metabolism
Controversial indications
Hepatocellular carcinoma
Contraindications
Extrahepatic malignancy
Liver metastases
Extrahepatic organ failure
Noncompliance
Active substance abuse
AIDS

TABLE 90-2   Common Complications Following Liver Transplantation

Complication	Percent with Complication
Infection	>60
Rejection	>50
Neurologic	≤47
Vascular clot, stenosis	≤30
Renal insufficiency	≤25
Hemorrhage	≤20
Biliary stenosis, leak	≤20
GI	≤15
PTLD	4

Abbreviation: PTL = posttransplant lymphoproliferative disorder.

vein thrombosis. Another contributing factor that may predispose patients to GI bleeding is high-dose steroids. Cytomegalovirus (CMV), herpes simplex virus (HSV), and candidal infection also can lead to significant bleeding.

Biliary Complications

Biliary problems account for a significant proportion of complications, and incidence may be as high as 28 percent.[8] Leaks, strictures (ductal narrowing), and obstruction (ductal blockage) account for 80 percent of these complications. In general, leaks occur early, with 38 percent in the first 30 days and most (80 percent) within the first 6 months.[9] Early leaks tend to be more severe owing to duct disruption and higher immunosuppression, notoriously difficult to treat, and generally due to hepatic artery thrombosis or other technical causes. Leaks after the first month are invariably associated with either elective or inadvertent removal of an indwelling biliary catheter.[10] In children, stricture and obstruction are responsible for 90 percent of complications.[9] For patients with Roux-en-Y procedures, the leak tends to occur at the anastomosis, whereas for the majority of patients who have choledochocholedochostomy, the leak is at the anastomosis early or the T-tube site later.[5] The cause of biliary injury is either immunologic or preservation injury, infection, or ischemia. Biliary leaks present most commonly with peritonitis, fever, abdominal pain, constipation, and abdominal distention, but signs and symptoms may be subtle or masked due to the use of immunosuppressive agents. Laboratory abnormalities are often nonspecific and include leukocytosis, hyperbilirubinemia, and increased alkaline phosphatase. If abdominal drains are still in place, one may see bile in the drain, or if a T-tube is present, bile may appear at the tube site.[7] Evaluation should include right upper quadrant ultrasound, although sensitivity for biliary abnormality may be only 50 percent. Since there is an association of biliary abnormality with hepatic artery thrombosis (HAT), Doppler ultrasonography should be performed to evaluate vascular flow to the graft. Treatment of the leak includes drainage of abscess, if present, and intravenous antibiotics. Broad-spectrum antibiotic coverage should be directed against gram-positive, gram-negative, and anaerobic organisms.[8] Bacterial infections tend to be polymicrobial and include *Enterobacter, Enterococcus, Bacteroides, Clostridium,* and *Pseudomonas* species.[4]

After 12 months, stricture and/or obstruction accounts for the vast majority of biliary complications. Development of a biliary complication is heralded by three typical presentations. Most common is intermittent episodes of fever and fluctuating liver function tests. The second presentation is gradual asymptomatic worsening of liver function tests. Finally, biliary complication may present as acute bacterial cholangitis with fever, chills, abdominal pain, jaundice, and bacteremia. Stricture or narrowing of the bile duct frequently develops insidiously.[10] The presentation of biliary complications can be difficult to distinguish clinically from rejection, HAT, CMV infection, or a recurrence of a preexisting disease (especially hepatitis).

Liver transplant recipients with suspected biliary complications should be referred to the transplant center. All patients should have a complete blood count (CBC) with platelet count and differential; serum chemistries, including electrolytes, blood urea nitrogen (BUN), creatinine, basic coagulation studies, liver function tests, amylase, and lipase levels; cultures of blood, urine, bile, and ascites, if present; chest x-ray; and abdominal ultrasonography with Doppler flow studies. Ultrasound rules out the presence of fluid collections, screens for the presence of thrombosis of the hepatic artery or portal vein, and identifies any dilatation of the biliary tree, although the absence of biliary dilatation does not rule out obstruction or other posttransplantation pathology. The intrahepatic ductal system rarely appears dilated appreciably by ultrasound, even in the presence of complete obstruction. Patients often require cholangiography for complete evaluation. Patients with choledochocholedochostomy may be best evaluated by endoscopic retrograde cholangiopancreatography (ERCP) because it permits both a radiographic diagnosis and the potential for nonoperative intervention. Patients who have Roux-en-Y hepaticojejunostomy or those who cannot have ERCP must undergo percutaneous cholangiography. Early broad-spectrum prophylactic antibiotics should be administered prior to any biliary tract manipulation.

Vascular Complications

Vascular complications are less common than biliary complications but are associated with high morbidity, mortality, and graft failure. Hepatic artery thrombosis (HAT) is the most common vascular complication and tends to occur within the first 3 weeks after transplantation.[11] The incidence reported is between 5 and 40 percent and tends to be higher in children.[12] For this reason, children are frequently treated prophylactically with antiplatelet agents.

The presentation of HAT in the early postoperative period may be signaled by elevated prothrombin (PT) and transaminase levels, little or no bile production, liver abscess, or unexplained sepsis or as a biliary tract problem (leak, obstruction, abscess, or breakdown of the anastomosis). HAT may present with massive hepatic necrosis, sepsis, fever, and bacteremia after early thrombosis, bile leak because the hepatic artery is the sole blood supply, or relapsing fever with bacteremia secondary to focal abscesses or biloma, or it can be asymptomatic if collaterals have formed.[7] HAT is ominous and frequently requires retransplantation. Occasionally, if diagnosed early, immediate thrombectomy and revision of the anastomosis may preclude the need for retransplantation. Pediatric patients are more susceptible to HAT and have a much more varied presentation, with an incidence as high as 26 percent in children and 31 percent in neonates. Duplex ultrasonography has a sensitivity of 92 percent for the diagnosis of HAT.[13] If ultrasound is not diagnostic and suspicion remains, one should proceed to angiography. Hepatic artery rupture is uncommon and generally associated with intra-abdominal sepsis and poor prognosis.[7] Portal vein thrombosis is less common and affects 2 to 3 percent of patients. The diagnosis is suggested by variceal hemorrhage, massive ascites, or other signs of portal hypertension. Initially, effort is directed toward reducing the portosystemic pressure gradient, but retransplantation may be necessary.

Wound Complications

Wound problems are probably underreported and include infection, hematomas, and seromas as the most common complications. Presentation may be subtle. Fever, chills, incisional pain, swelling, erythema, or drainage may not always be present due to immunosuppressive diminution of signs of inflammation. Infection can lead to necrotizing

fasciitis. An increased degree of suspicion is necessary. Adequate drainage and early broad-spectrum antibiotic coverage should be considered.

REJECTION

Acute allograft rejection is seen most commonly at 7 to 14 days. The incidence of acute rejection varies from 40 to 80 percent during the first posttransplant year. After several months, the incidence of acute rejection decreases steadily, but it may be triggered at any time by tapering of immunosuppressive agents. Although frequently subtle in presentation, symptoms of rejection include fever, liver tenderness, lymphocytosis, eosinophilia, liver enzyme elevation, and a change in bile color or production. In the perioperative period, the differential diagnosis must include infection, acute biliary obstruction, and vascular insufficiency. The diagnosis can be made with certainty only by excluding other causes of graft dysfunction and biopsy, which usually requires referral back to the transplant center for management and follow-up. Acute rejection typically is treated by a high-dose glucocorticosteroid bolus followed by a rapid taper over 5 to 7 days. This treatment is effective in 65 to 80 percent of transplant recipients.[4] Secondary therapy includes the infusion of antilymphocyte globulin (e.g., OKT3), which is accompanied by a variety of potential side effects. Both these therapies are best managed at an experienced transplant center.

Chronic allograft rejection occurs in approximately 5 to 10 percent of recipients and is a major cause of late graft failure. The primary manifestation of chronic rejection is a persistently cholestatic liver injury pattern with elevated serum alkaline phosphatase and bilirubin, which can be associated with pruritus. Significant loss of hepatic synthetic function is often not evident until late in the course of chronic rejection. The diagnosis is made by biopsy.

INFECTION

General Considerations

The vast majority of liver transplant recipients have at least one episode of infection at some time after their transplantation, and many have more than one episode. Infections or their complications are believed to account for a large number of deaths. Vigilance for infection must remain high because immunosuppression-induced blunting of the inflammatory response may mask the classic signs and symptoms of infection.

Timing of infection after transplantation can be organized into three segments: less than 1 month, 1 to 6 months, and greater than 6 months (see Table 99-3).[14]

INFECTION IN THE FIRST 30 DAYS   Infection in the first 30 postoperative days is primarily from bacteria and fungi. The patient is typically at the greatest level of immunosuppression, and the anastomoses are at their most vulnerable. The vast majority of infectious agents seen in less than 1 month are the same nosocomial agents seen in similar surgical patients. Opportunistic organisms are notably absent in the first month. CMV is discussed below.

During the first postoperative month, intra-abdominal infections—including cholangitis, peritonitis, and liver and other intra-abdominal abscesses—predominate. Presentation is marked by fever, abdominal pain and distension, ascites, and occasionally, jaundice. Workup should include a CBC with differential, liver function tests, urinalysis, chest x-ray, abdominal ultrasound, and blood and fluid cultures. Evaluation may include ultrasound, computed tomographic (CT) scan, T-tube cholangiography, ERCP, liver biopsy, and cultures of blood, urine, or aspirated fluid. The organisms responsible tend to be enterococci, gram-negative aerobes, anaerobes, *Staphylococcus,* and *Candida* species. Patients also may present with pneumonia or urinary tract infections related to intubation or indwelling bladder catheterization while hospitalized.

INFECTIONS AFTER 30 DAYS From 1 to 6 months, most infection is from viruses [reactivation, donor transmission, Epstein-Barr virus (EBV)] or opportunistic organisms. Special cultures must be obtained if less common organisms such as fungi, viruses, CMV, *Nocardia* species, and *Mycobacterium tuberculosis* are suspected.

After 6 months, the incidence of serious infection declines, with cholangitis predominating. Risk of infection after 6 months approaches that of the general population, although morbidity and mortality may be higher. A high index of suspicion should be maintained whenever immunosuppression is high. Close monitoring is essential because rapid deterioration can take place while the patient is still in the ED.

Bacterial Infection

Bacterial infection is most common in the first month. Although gram-negative organisms predominate (especially *Pseudomonas aeruginosa*), gram-positive and anaerobic organisms are not uncommon. Broad-spectrum antibiotics should be considered early in the patient's course. Bacterial infection is frequently associated with the vascular or biliary anastomosis, especially HAT but also portal vein thrombosis. Ischemia may lead to bile leak and abscess or deep soft tissue infection. After the first month, the incidence of bacterial infections decreases and the incidence of opportunistic infection increases, but vigilance for bacterial illnesses should remain high. Community-acquired pneumonia is most likely due to *Streptococcus pneumoniae* and *Haemophilus influenzae*. Meningitis shows a high preponderance of *Listeria monocytogenes* as well as *S. pneumoniae, Staphylococcus aureus,* and gram-negative rods. Empirical antibiotic coverage should be aimed at these flora.

Fungal Infection

Although uncommon, fungal disease is seen most within the first 2 months; it can be disseminated and is accompanied by high mortality. Fungal disease can present with multiple organ involvement, peritonitis, fungemia, pneumonitis, or asymptomatic colonization. The incidence of fungal disease is continuing to decrease, but mortality remains high. Mortality is up to 78 percent if disease is systemic. *Candida* species are responsible for up to 75 percent of fungal illnesses. The diagnosis is by culture or biopsy, and the fungus may be difficult to isolate. Disseminated infection is present when infection is found in two or more sites and is associated with even higher mortality. Fungal infection becomes more likely with retransplantation, the Roux-en-Y procedure, preoperative steroid use, accompanying vascular complications, the use of three or more intravenous antibiotics, and when the transplant is performed emergently. Endemic mycoses (coccidioidomycoses, histoplasmosis, blastomycosis) are always possible in the immunocompromised host but are seen rarely in liver transplant patients.[4]

Viral Infection

Viral illnesses tend to present within the first few months. Viral and bacterial illnesses are often seen concurrently.

CYTOMEGALOVIRUS INFECTION The most common viral agent and the most common cause of infection after transplantation is cytomegalovirus (CMV), a herpesvirus. It is reported to occur in between 23 and 85 percent of all liver transplant patients. Despite its high incidence and morbidity, it is rarely fatal unless disseminated and rarely has a significant effect on graft survival. It generally occurs

within the first 3 months, with the peak incidence in the third and fourth weeks. Later occurrence generally is related to the need to increase immunosuppression for the treatment of a prolonged episode of rejection. CMV can cause primary infection, or the infection can be a reactivation. Infection has three basic effects. First, it can produce a mononucleosis-like syndrome with spiking fever, arthralgias, malaise, neutropenia, atypical lymphocytes, and thrombocytopenia, with mild or moderate elevation in transaminase levels. Jaundice is rare. Second, CMV is frequently associated with opportunistic infection, which may be due to an additional immunosuppressive effect of its own. Finally, there is an increased propensity for allograft rejection.

CMV pneumonitis is characterized by bilateral interstitial infiltrates that may lead to acute respiratory distress syndrome. Diagnosis may require bronchoalveolar lavage, but the appearance of the chest x-ray and the clinical picture may be suggestive enough for diagnosis. CMV pneumonitis may be seen in conjunction with *Pneumocystis carinii* pneumonia (PCP).

CMV hepatitis may present similarly to rejection, with fever, malaise, anorexia, abdominal pain, hepatomegaly, and liver dysfunction. Liver biopsy is frequently needed for diagnosis but still may not be able to distinguish CMV disease from rejection. Disseminated disease is frequently associated with an increase in immunosuppression, especially with treatment with OKT3.

CMV chorioretinitis may present with decreased visual acuity, photophobia, scotomata, floaters, eye redness, or pain. Its presence signals a poor prognosis and the presence of profound immunosuppression.

There are three patterns of CMV infection. The patient at greatest risk is the seronegative recipient of a seropositive donor. Disease also may be caused by reactivation of latent virus that replicates after the initiation of immunosuppression—typically in the seropositive recipient of a liver from a seronegative donor. Finally, a seropositive recipient may receive a liver from a seropositive donor, which may produce either reactivation or superinfection, although it is clinically impossible and irrelevant to distinguish between them.

Effective treatment depends on rapid diagnosis. Treatment is with intravenous ganciclovir for 2 to 4 weeks. Diagnosis traditionally has been based on histology and culture. Standard fibroblast tube cell culture, however, can require 10 to 14 days for incubation. Serologic markers are too insensitive in the immunosuppressed patient, and electron microscopy is cumbersome. The shell-vial technique can detect the presence of CMV after 16 h of incubation. It is an indirect immunofluorescence testing method that uses a monoclonal antibody directed at an early antigen of the virus. Early detection and high antigenemia correlate positively with the severity of the infection.

OTHER VIRUSES Other viruses may cause illnesses in the posttransplant patient. Up to 34 percent of all transplant patients develop HSV, and half of these present within the first 3 weeks. Mucocutaneous or genital disease is generally due to reactivation of latent infection. It is usually not severe, and diagnosis can be made with Tzanck smear or culture. EBV can cause primary infection in children or the more common reactivated infection in adults. The disease can be self-limited and cause a mononucleosis-like syndrome, with fever, tonsillitis, and lymphadenopathy, or it may progress to a polymorphous, multiorgan B cell infiltrative process with high mortality. Finally, it may produce a localized solid tumor. EBV plays a role in the development of a posttransplantation lymphoproliferative disorder and has a high incidence (20 to 30 percent) in patients maintained on immunosuppression and higher (80 percent) in patients who have received antithymocyte antibody. Adenovirus and enteroviruses may cause systemic illness but are uncommon.

Parasitic Infection

Parasites are not common. PCP may present concomitantly with CMV or by itself. Diagnosis may require bronchoalveolar or transbronchial biopsy. Prophylaxis with trimethoprim-sulfamethoxazole (Bactrim) for the first 3 months has greatly reduced the incidence of PCP. *Toxoplasma gondii* is also uncommon but may cause a meningoencephalitis or single or multiple mass lesions. *Toxoplasma* infection may cause fever, mental status changes, focal neurologic signs, seizures, or visual changes.

COMPLICATIONS OF IMMUNOSUPPRESSIVE AGENTS

Therapeutic immunosuppression is accompanied by a number of side effects and complications. Common and most life-threatening are the infections that occur with the suppression of cell-mediated immunity. The agents of immunosuppression also have a number of nonspecific toxicities that complicate their use (see Table 70-2). Combined toxicities can produce or worsen preexisting renal insufficiency, hypertension, and hyperglycemia. Hypertension is perhaps the best example of combined toxicity.

Azathioprine interferes with both B and T cell responses to antigenic stimulation. Generalized myelosuppression is a common side effect resulting in leukopenia and, to varying degrees, thrombocytopenia and anemia (megaloblastic) and generally is seen within the first few weeks. Other observed toxicities include hepatitis, cholestasis, HAT, pancreatitis, dermatitis, and alopecia. Prolonged use also predisposes to malignancies such as squamous cell carcinoma of the skin and lip, cervical carcinoma, and lymphoproliferative disorder. Mycophenolate mofetil is a new antiproliferative agent often used to replace azathioprine. Again, leukopenia is a common toxicity, although GI distress is seen as well.

Glucocorticoids act primarily by inhibiting T cell and macrophage function. In addition to immune suppression, long-term use of glucocorticoids suppresses endogenous adrenal function, which may produce Cushing syndrome and cause hypertension, glucose intolerance, osteoporosis, avascular necrosis of the hip, cataracts, pancreatitis, peptic ulcer disease, delayed wound healing, behavioral disorders, and malignancies.

Cyclosporine and FK506 inhibit T cell proliferation. Nephrotoxicity is a common and usually reversible side effect manifest by elevated serum creatinine levels, hypertension, hyperkalemia, hyperuricemia, and gout. Patients are sensitive to dehydration. Other side effects include headache, hirsutism, gingival hyperplasia, hyperglycemia, hypomagnesemia, hypercholesterolemia, hypertriglyceridemia, hepatotoxicity, and hemolytic uremic syndrome. Unlike those of other immunosuppressive agents, blood levels of cyclosporine and FK506 can be monitored along with serum creatinine to avoid serious toxicity; however, random levels are rarely helpful, and the dose is adjusted based on trough levels.[4]

Nonsteroidal anti-inflammatory agents should be avoided because they may increase nephrotoxicity.

There are numerous drug interactions to consider with a patient taking immunosuppressive agents, and it is suggested that before starting any new drug, interactions with the patient's immunosuppressants should be determined. Some of these interactions and adverse effects are summarized in Tables 99-2 and 99-3.

INCIDENTAL PROBLEMS

Immunization

All live virus vaccines are contraindicated in immunosuppressed patients. Vaccines consisting of denatured protein, carbohydrate, or killed virus are safe, so diphtheria-pertussis-tetanus (DPT), inactivated polio, *H. influenzae* Pittman type, and Heptavax are all safe. Live viral or bacterial vaccines are absolutely contraindicated (oral polio, measles, mumps, rubella, yellow fever, bacille Calmette-Guérin, TY21a typhoid, and varicella). All of these may produce clinical disease.

Surgery

If surgery for problems other than those related to the graft is necessary, complications secondary to chronic steroids and immunosuppression should be anticipated. Also, caution must be taken in the presence of a coagulopathy. It is recommended that immunosuppression not be stopped unless there is sepsis, in which case the doses of immunosuppressive agents might need to be reduced. Two series looking at cardiac and general surgery showed no documented decline in graft function and no need for stress dosing of steroids.[15,16]

Bone Disease

Skeletal complications are responsible for significant morbidity and, because of increased survival times in transplant recipients, are becoming more prevalent. Osteopenia and osteonecrosis can occur due to immobility, poor nutritional status, decreased muscle mass, steroid use, and immunosuppressive drugs. The first 3 to 6 months after transplantation are accompanied by accelerated bone loss (mostly trabecular). Fractures are common in the first year postoperatively, particularly at sites of trabecular bone (vertebrae and ribs), although long bone and pelvic fractures are also seen. The incidence of vertebral compression fracture may be as high as 38 percent. Patients may develop avascular necrosis of the femoral head from steroid use. Fractures should be treated in the standard fashion.

Neurologic Complications

It is reported that between 9 and 42 percent of all adult liver transplant patients have a neurologic complication at some time during their posttransplant course.[17] Neurologic complications in children, however, are much less common. Common presenting problems include headache, seizures, and mental status changes. The etiology is more likely to be noninfectious than infectious. Common noninfectious etiologies are immunosuppressive toxicity, metabolic derangement, and hemorrhage.

Central nervous system (CNS) infection is most common in the first few months, with viral and fungal etiologies predominating. CNS CMV infection is rare, and CNS herpesvirus infection is seen with the same frequency as in the general population. Bacterial etiologies include *Listeria, Klebsiella, S. aureus, Nocardia,* and *Escherichia coli. Aspergillus, Candida,* and *Cryptococcus* species are the more common fungal agents involved. Cryptococcal disease is most common between 2 and 7 months. Patients presenting with headache, seizures, or mental status changes need to evaluated for the presence of metabolic derangement as well as hemorrhage or infection. They often will require CT scan of the head and lumbar puncture to rule out these etiologies. Neuropathic pain may be seen and is poorly responsive to opioids. It may respond to tricyclic antidepressants.

Cardiovascular Disease

Cardiovascular complications are the leading late cause of death in liver transplant patients. Liver transplant patients are at risk for the development of diabetes, hyperlipidemia, and hypertension, so their risk of cardiovascular disease also increases. Their relative risk, however, still surpasses that of age- and sex-matched patients.[15,18]

Malignancy

The second leading cause of late death in liver transplant patients is de novo malignancy. There is an increased risk of new malignancy including squamous cell carcinoma, lymphomas, AND posttransplant lymphoproliferative disorder (PTLD). There is no increased risk of lung, colon, breast, or prostate cancer.[19] The most common posttransplant malignancy is squamous cell cancer of the skin, but sarcoma,

Kaposi sarcoma, and hepatobiliary cancer occur. PTLD accounts for 20 to 50 percent of de novo tumors after liver transplant and is more frequent in pediatric liver transplant recipients. Immunosuppression and EBV infection have been implicated.

REFERENCES

1. Trotter J, Wachs M, Everson G, et al: Adult-to-adult transplantation of the right hepatic lobe from a living donor. *New Engl J Med* 346(14):1076, 2002.
2. The United Network for Organ Sharing (UNOS) Web site (http://www.unos.org), 2002.
3. Geevarghese S, Bradley A, Wright K, et al: Outcomes analysis in 100 liver transplant patients. *Am J Surg* 175:348, 1998.
4. Savitsky E, Uner A, Votey S: Evaluation of orthotopic liver transplant recipients presenting to the emergency department. *Ann Emerg Med* 31:507, 1998.
5. Patenaude Y, Dubois J, Sinsky A, et al: Liver transplantation: Review of the literature. 1. Anatomic features and current concepts. *Can Assoc Radiol J* 48:171, 1997.
6. Wood R, Ozaki C, Katz S, Monsour H, et al: Liver transplantation: The last ten years. *Surg Clin North Am* 74:1133, 1994.
7. Ozaki C, Katz S, Monsour H, Dyer C, Wood R: Surgical complications of liver transplantation. *Surg Clin North Am* 74:1155, 1994.
8. Nemec P, Ondrasek J, Studenik P, et al: Biliary complications in liver transplantation. *Ann Transplant* 6(2):24, 2001.
9. Greif F, Bronsther O, Van Thiel D, et al: The incidence, timing and management of biliary tract complications after orthotopic liver transplantation. *Ann Surg* 219:40, 1994.
10. Porayko M, Kondo M, Steers J: Liver transplantation: Late complications of the biliary tract and their management. *Semin Liver Dis* 15:139, 1995.
11. Pastacaldi S, Teixeira R, Montalto P, et al: Hepatic artery thrombosis after orthotopic liver transplantation: A review of nonsurgical causes. *Liver Transplant* 7(2):75, 2001.
12. Stafford-Johnson D, Hamilton B, Dong Q, et al: Vascular complications of liver transplantation: Evaluation with gadolinium-enhanced MR angiography. *Radiology* 207:153, 1998.
13. Nolten A, Sproat I: Hepatic artery thrombosis after liver transplantation: Temporal accuracy of diagnosis with duplex US and the syndrome of impending thrombosis. *Radiology* 198:553, 1996.
14. Fishman J, Rubin R: Infection in organ-transplant recipients. *New Engl J Med* 338:1741, 1998.
15. Prabhakar G, Testa G, Abbasoglu O, et al: The safety of cardiac operations in the liver transplant recipient. *Ann Thorac Surg* 65:1060, 1998.
16. Testa G, Goldstein R, Toughanipour A, et al: Guidelines for surgical procedures after liver transplantation. *Ann Surg* 227:590, 1998.
17. Bronster D, Boccagni E, Sheiner P, et al: Central nervous system complications in liver transplant recipients: Incidence, timing and long-term follow-up. *Clin Transplant* 14:1, 2000.
18. Rabkin J, Corless C, Rose H, et al: Immmunosuppression impact on long-term cardiovascular complications after liver transplantation. *Am J Surg* 183:595, 2002.
19. Fung J, Jain A, Kwak E, et al: De novo malignancies after liver transplantation: A major cause of late death. *Liver Transplant* 7(11 suppl 1):S109, 2001.

91 | GASTROINTESTINAL IMAGING
Michael J. Bono

BASIC IMAGING TECHNIQUES

Plain Film Radiography

Plain films remain the workhorse imaging study for the emergency department evaluating a patient with abdominal pain. Plain films can be obtained quickly, cause no discomfort to the patient, and are relatively inexpensive compared with other gastrointestinal (GI) imaging modalities. The emergency physician can interpret plain films. Unlike the chest, where the organs have great differences in water and air content

and, hence, in radiodensity, the abdomen contains structures of similar radiodensities. Only the presence of air and fat in the bowel or other structures allows identification of organ boundaries, and the air is transient. A plain film of the abdomen represents a "snapshot" of a dynamic system and should be examined systematically. A time-honored technique is to first examine the bones (spine, ribs, pelvis, and hips); the upper quadrants, flanks, and mid-abdomen for organ masses and calcifications; and then the lower abdomen. The physician should attempt to look at the area of special interest last.

At most centers, an "acute abdominal series" includes a supine film centered at the iliac crest, an upright film centered at the crest, and an upright posteroanterior chest film. The supine film detects fluid or blood in the peritoneum and gas in the bowel, and the upright film displays any air-fluid levels. If the patient is too ill to stand, a left lateral decubitus (left side down) view is acceptable, but a right lateral decubitus is not. On a left lateral decubitus view, free air can be detected between the liver and the peritoneum; this is not possible in a right lateral decubitus view (right side down) because air in the bowel loops will contact the peritoneum. The standard upright posteroanterior chest view is best for demonstrating free air in the peritoneal cavity and other pathologic conditions of the chest that cause abdominal pain, such as pneumonia, pneumothorax, or atelectasis.

Contrast Radiography

Barium sulfate remains the standard substance for contrast GI imaging. Barium is an insoluble material that is suspended in different carriers by different manufacturers. It has high viscosity and is not absorbed by the GI tract. Gastrograffin is a water-soluble substance, has low viscosity, and, like barium, is not absorbed by the GI tract in most normal adult patients. It is absorbed slightly by the gut in children. Gastrograffin draws substantial amounts of fluid into the bowel lumen, and its low viscosity causes rapid transit through the small bowel into the colon. It therefore has a considerable laxative effect. Gastrograffin is not a recommended oral contrast agent in children, in particular neonates and infants, because the fluid shifts and laxative effect may cause significant fluid and electrolyte disturbances.

Computed Tomography

Computed tomography (CT) provides imaging of solid organs and, very importantly, a view into the retroperitoneum. Unlike plain radiographs, CT is not dependent on the amount of air and gas in the bowel. Oral contrast material is given to identify bowel, and intravenous contrast material enhances the density of blood vessels. The introduction of the helical CT scan (spiral CT) has made a significant impact on abdominal imaging due to the speed of the procedure. Routine CT scanning of the abdomen usually requires the patient to lie motionless for 15 to 30 min, whereas the helical CT scan may be finished in a single breath hold. The radiation dose to the patient is unchanged. Another advantage of helical CT is improved vascular opacification, which allows excellent imaging of the thoracoabdominal aorta and renal arteries. Data obtained from helical CT can be reformatted in several ways, revealing three-dimensional surface anatomy and obviating arteriography.

Radionuclide Scanning

Radionuclide scanning has been virtually replaced by ultrasonography for emergency department patients with right upper quadrant pain. Technetium-99m-labeled iminodiacetic acid (IDA) is injected intravenously, is taken up by hepatocytes, is secreted into the bile canaliculi, and then flows into the small bowel. Normally there is a small amount of reflux into the cystic duct and gallbladder, but in cholecystitis the cystic duct is frequently occluded. The gallbladder, hepatic duct, and common duct should be visualized within 1 h of iminodiacetic acid administration, but total test time may be several hours.

Ultrasonography

Ultrasound is a valuable tool for the diagnosis of select conditions in the ED. It is noninvasive and inexpensive and should be readily available to the ED physician. Improvements in transducer technology have greatly improved ultrasound imaging. Ultrasound is somewhat operator dependent, and the images are difficult to interpret in obese patients or patients with large amounts of intestinal air or gas. Air is a poor conductor of ultrasound, because it scatters, refracts, and reflects the sound waves. Fluid-filled structures transmit sound exceedingly well, and because most soft tissues are composed of different amounts of water, ultrasound is feasible throughout the GI tract and pelvis. A full bladder is an acoustic window into the pelvis, and the liver helps transmit ultrasound in the right upper quadrant.

SPECIFIC GASTROINTESTINAL CONDITIONS

Plain Film Radiography

In the past, tradition dictated the routine use of plain films to screen patients with acute abdominal pain.[1] Routine plain-film screening of patients with acute abdominal pain is not advisable, because the yield of positive findings that would change clinical management is low, in the range of 10 to 40 percent.[2] However, in the proper clinical setting, plain abdominal radiographs are entirely appropriate and are still considered the first test of choice. In patients with a suspected perforated ulcer or free air in the abdomen, plain films demonstrate free air, if present, in a large percentage of patients.[3] Plain films may demonstrate as little as 1 to 2 mL of air.[4] In patients with suspected small bowel obstruction, plain films are the initial method of imaging. Plain films have a sensitivity of 69 to 82 percent for revealing high-grade small bowel obstruction, but, when combined with barium contrast studies, the sensitivity rate may approach 100 percent.[5,6] Low-grade small bowel obstruction is difficult to demonstrate on plain films and has much lower diagnostic rates.[7] Other appropriate conditions for the use of plain film radiographs include moderate or severe abdominal tenderness, suspicion of bowel ischemia, ingestion of radiopaque foreign bodies, and penetrating foreign bodies, such as gunshot wounds.

Abdominal Computed Tomography

Computed tomography is the diagnostic tool of choice for many acute abdominal conditions. It is the first imaging study of choice for patients with suspected diverticulitis, pancreatitis, pancreatic pseudocyst, aortic aneurysm, blunt trauma, and appendicitis. The diagnosis of appendicitis can be made on clinical evaluation, but CT has been proven remarkably sensitive and specific in confirming the diagnosis.[8] Patients with signs and symptoms consistent with acute appendicitis who are otherwise healthy may undergo CT without oral or intravenous contrast, although the sensitivity and specificity are inferior to those of contrast CT.[9–11] CT is a useful adjunct to plain films in suspected cases of intestinal ischemia, where specific findings may include pneumatosis intestinalis, portal venous gas, mesenteric vessel occlusion, and enlargement of a thrombosed vein.[12] Although patients with suspected small bowel obstruction should be imaged initially with plain radiographs, CT has similar sensitivity in revealing high- and low-grade obstructions. When CT correctly showed a small bowel obstruction, the cause of the obstruction was demonstrated in 95 percent of cases. CT offers another advantage to the emergency physician evaluating the patient with multiple potential causes for acute abdominal pain. Although never advocated as a "screening tool," CT scanning can pinpoint a diagnosis in 95 percent of cases where clinical judgment and other imaging studies fail to narrow a wide range of potential diagnoses.[13]

Ultrasonography

Ultrasound is the initial imaging study of choice for evaluation of patients with right upper quadrant pain. By using the liver as an acoustic window, ultrasound can detect cholelithiasis, cholecystitis, choledocholithiasis, biliary duct dilation, and pancreatic masses, both solid and cystic. Ultrasound is also the modality of choice for evaluating patients with pelvic pain. Transvaginal scanning has supplemented the transabdominal approach because of better visualization with higher-frequency endovaginal probe transducers (see Chap. 113, "Pelvic Ultrasonography"). Ultrasonography of the genitourinary system is discussed in Chap. 100, "Renal Imaging."

Graded-compression ultrasound imaging for acute appendicitis has been studied extensively. Sensitivities for appendicitis range from 68 to 93 percent and specificities between 73 and 100 percent, with accuracy in the 95 percent range.[14] Graded-compression ultrasonography can reduce negative laparotomy rates.[15] The ultrasonographer is searching for a tubular structure off the cecum that is compressible without pain and is no larger than 6 mm in diameter. An infected, inflamed appendix is tender, larger than 6 mm in diameter, fluid filled, and noncompressible. The appendix is difficult to visualize, and the examination is best left to experienced ultrasonographers, which is the reason CT has replaced ultrasound for evaluation of the appendix in many institutions. Negative ultrasound results in the face of a strong clinical suspicion should never delay surgical intervention. The false-negative rate for graded-compression ultrasonography is from 6 to 14 percent. Other disease processes that can confuse the clinical picture are cecal diverticulitis, inflammatory bowel disease involving the terminal ileum, and periappendiceal phlegmon. Graded-compression ultrasonography is most helpful in the evaluation of patients with atypical right lower quadrant pain and a suspicion of appendicitis.

Air Contrast or Barium Enema

For children with signs and symptoms suggestive of intussusception, air contrast enema is preferred over barium enema to avoid the potential risk of barium spillage into the peritoneal cavity. Plain films may demonstrate signs of intestinal obstruction, such as distended loops, air-fluid levels, and a paucity of bowel gas in the right lower quadrant, the so-called Dance sign. A barium enema may be useful for the diagnosis of bowel obstruction, volvulus, appendicitis, and diverticulitis, usually in consultation with surgical colleagues, although its emergency use has been supplanted by CT scanning.

Angiography

Computed tomography has replaced angiography for imaging patients with suspected abdominal aortic aneurysm. Angiography may be helpful in evaluating patients with lower GI bleeding, particularly when combined with colonoscopy to pinpoint the bleeding lesion.[16]

Radionuclide Scanning

Radionuclide scanning can be a useful adjunct to ultrasonography for patients with right upper quadrant abdominal pain. When the ultrasound results are negative or inconclusive in a patient with suspected cholecystitis or cystic duct obstruction, radionuclide scanning may be diagnostic in the absence of stones. It may take several hours for the radioisotope to localize to the affected area.

Magnetic Resonance Imaging

Magnetic resonance imaging currently has no role in imaging the GI tract in the emergency department patient. Magnetic resonance imaging is outstanding for imaging the central nervous system and musculoskeletal system, but cost, time in the scanner, and poor image quality due to movement of the bowel limit applicability. Magnetic resonance imaging is being evaluated as a tool for imaging relatively stationary GI structures, such as the appendix and biliary tree, and has shown some promise.[17,18]

REFERENCES

1. Martin RF: The acute abdomen: An overview and algorithms. *Surg Clin North Am* 77:1235, 1997.
2. Campbell JP: Abdominal radiographs and acute pain. *Br J Surg* 75:554, 1998.
3. Grassi R, Pinto A, Cioffi A, et al: Sixty-one consecutive patients with gastrointestinal perforation: Comparison of conventional radiology, ultrasonography, and computerized tomography, in terms of timing of the study. *Radiol Med (Torino)* 91:247, 1996.
4. Miller RE: The roentgenologic demonstration of tiny amounts of free intraperitoneal gas: Experimental and clinical studies. *AJR* 112:574, 1971.
5. Maglinte DD, Harmon BH, Kelvin FM, et al: Reliability and role of plain film radiography and CT in the diagnosis of small bowel obstruction. *AJR* 167:1451, 1996.
6. Anderson CA: Contrast radiography in small bowel obstruction: A prospective, randomized trial. *Mil Med* 162:749, 1997.
7. Maglinte DD, Balthazar EJ, Kelvin FM, Megibow AJ: The role of radiography in the diagnosis of small bowel obstruction. *AJR* 168:1171, 1997.
8. Balthazar EJ, Birnbaum BA, Yee J, et al: Acute appendicitis: CT and US correlation in 100 patients. *Radiology* 190:31, 1994.
9. Lane MJ, Huynh MD, Jeffrey RB Jr, et al: Suspected acute appendicitis: Nonenhanced CT in 300 consecutive patients. *Radiology* 213:341, 1999.
10. Peck J, Peck C, Peck J: The clinical role of noncontrast helical computed tomography in the diagnosis of acute appendicitis. *Am J Surg* 180:133, 2000.
11. Pickuth D: Unenhanced spiral CT for evaluating acute appendicitis in daily routine. A prospective study. *Hepatogastroenterology* 48:140, 2001.
12. Castellone JA: Ischemic bowel syndromes: A comprehensive, state of the art approach to emergency diagnosis and management. *Emerg Med Rep* 18:189, 1997.
13. Taourel P, Baron MP, Pradel J, et al: Acute abdomen of unknown origin: Impact of CT on diagnosis and management. *Gastrointest Radiol* 17:287, 1992.
14. Orr RK, Hartmann D: Ultrasonography to evaluate adults for appendicitis: Decision-making based on meta-analysis and problematic reasoning. *Acad Emerg Med* 2:644, 1995.
15. Schwerk WB, Wichtrup B, Rothmund M, Rüschaft J: Ultrasonography in the diagnosis of acute appendicitis: A prospective study. *Gastroenterology* 97:630, 1989.
16. Bono MJ: Lower gastrointestinal tract bleeding. *Emerg Clin North Am* 14:547, 1996.
17. Incesu L, Coskun A, Selcuk MB, et al: Acute appendicitis: MR imaging and sonographic correlation. *AJR* 168:669, 1997.
18. Reinhold C: Current status of MR cholangiopancreatography. *AJR* 166:1285, 1996.

ACUTE RENAL FAILURE
Richard Sinert
Peter R. Peacock, Jr.

Acute renal failure (ARF) is the deterioration of renal function over hours or days resulting in the accumulation of toxic wastes and the loss of internal homeostasis. Clinicians have only indirect measures of glomerular filtration rate (GFR) to define ARF, such as a 50 percent decline in creatinine clearance or a 50 percent increase in serum creatinine from baseline. The diagnosis of ARF is complicated by the fact that acute declines in GFR, especially early in their course, are asymptomatic.

With the advent of advanced critical care, treatment of streptococcal infection, and other advances, ARF is increasingly a disease of the critically ill rather than of ambulatory patients. The most clinically significant aspect of ARF is usually the underlying primary multi-organ disease process that has triggered it, rather than any primary renal disease. The emergency physician is in the unique position to identify patients at risk for ARF and ameliorate ongoing renal damage or prevent iatrogenic injury.

EPIDEMIOLOGY

The distinction between community- and hospital-acquired ARF is important for the differential diagnosis, treatment, and eventual outcome of patients with ARF (Table 92-1). The annual incidence of community-acquired ARF is approximately 100 per 1 million population[1] and will be diagnosed in only 1 percent of hospital admissions at presentation,[2] whereas hospital-acquired ARF will occur in as many as 4 percent of hospital admissions and 20 percent of critical care admissions.[3] This increased incidence of hospital-acquired ARF is multifactorial, related to an aging population with increased risk of ARF,[4] the high prevalence of nephrotoxic exposures possible in a hospital setting, and increasing severity of illness.

Because the majority of community-acquired ARF is secondary to volume depletion, it has been estimated that as many as 90 percent of cases presenting to the ED have a potentially reversible cause.[2] Hospital-acquired ARF often occurs in an intensive care unit and is commonly the end result of multi-organ failure. This dichotomy in the etiology of ARF explains the higher mortality, dialysis requirements, and rates of progression to end-stage renal failure seen in hospital- as opposed to community-acquired ARF.

Mortality rates for ARF are approximately 50 percent and have changed little since the advent of dialysis. This curious statistic simply reflects the changing demographics of ARF from community- to hospital-acquired settings. Currently, the mortality rate for hospital-acquired ARF is reported to be as high as 70 percent and is directly correlated to the severity of the patient's other disease processes. Mortality among patients presenting to the ED with prerenal ARF may be as low as 7 percent.[3] With the advent of dialysis, the most common causes of death associated with ARF are sepsis and cardiac and pulmonary failure. Interestingly, patients older than 80 years with ARF have mortality rates similar to those of younger adult patients.[4] Pediatric patients with ARF represent a different set of etiologies and have mortality rates averaging 25 percent.[5]

PATHOPHYSIOLOGY

The driving force for glomerular filtration is the pressure gradient across the glomerulus to Bowman's space of the proximal tubule. Glomerular capillary pressure depends on renal blood flow (RBF), which is maintained by cardiac output and autoregulated by the combined resistances of the renal afferent and efferent arterioles.

Regardless of the cause, global or regional decrease in RBF is the final common pathway in ARF. The relation between reductions in RBF and GFR is most straightforward in prerenal failure, in which tubular and glomerular function are normal, and GFR is depressed by compromised renal perfusion. Intrinsic renal failure occurs with diseases of the glomerulus, interstitium, or tubule and is associated with the release of renal vasoconstrictors. Postobstructive renal failure initially results in an increase in tubular pressure decreasing the filtration driving force. This pressure gradient soon equalizes, and the maintenance of depressed GFR depends on vasoconstrictors.

Under normal circumstances, the kidneys receive 25 percent of cardiac output, and even then the partial pressure of oxygen in the outer medulla is typically 5 to 15 mm Hg. After an ischemic insult of any sort, total RBF normalizes, but the outer medulla is affected by a marked regional decrease in perfusion.[6] Microvascular congestion, resulting from edema, red blood cell trapping, and activation of the coagulation cascade and leukocyte adherence, amplifies the ischemic injury.[7] Part of the physiologic response to this insult is persistent preglomerular capillary vasoconstriction, resulting in depressed GFR. This response is likely to be adaptive, thereby allowing the body to preserve volume that would be lost due to the decreased reabsorptive capacity of the injured tubules, and has been appropriately referred to as *acute renal success*.[8]

Injured renal tubular cells lose their brush border, polarity, and cell-to-cell and cell-to-matrix connections, including tight junctions. Some tubular cells slough off into the tubule, forming casts. These events further depress GFR in the affected nephrons via back-leak of ultrafiltrate and tubular obstruction.

During the period of depressed RBF, the kidneys are especially vulnerable to further insults. Exposure to known nephrotoxins such as radiocontrast agents, aminoglycosides, and nonsteroidal anti-inflammatory drugs at this time explains the high rate of iatrogenic ARF.

Recovery from ARF is first dependent on restoration of RBF. In prerenal failure, restoration of circulating blood volume is usually sufficient. Rapid relief of urinary obstruction in postrenal failure results in a prompt decrease of vasoconstriction. Clearance of tubular toxins and initiation of therapy for glomerular diseases decrease vasoconstriction and restore RBF in patients with intrinsic renal failure.

Once RBF is restored, the remaining functional nephrons will increase their filtration and eventually hypertrophy. Depending on the size of this remnant nephron pool, GFR will proportionally recover. If the number of remaining nephrons is below some critical number, continued hyperfiltration results in progressive glomerular sclerosis, eventually leading to nephron loss. A vicious cycle then ensues until complete renal failure occurs. This sequence explains the commonly observed scenario in which progressive renal failure occurs after the initial recovery from ARF.[6]

DIFFERENTIAL DIAGNOSIS

The differential diagnosis of ARF is classified according to pathophysiologic terms: prerenal, intrinsic renal, and postrenal etiologies. Prerenal is the most common etiology of ARF presenting to the ED, followed by intrinsic renal and postrenal. These percentages change dramatically when examining in-hospital ARF (see Table 92-1). Acute renal failure has a different spectrum in the pediatric population: a

TABLE 92-1   Etiology of Community-Acquired and Hospital-Acquired ARF

Community-Acquired		Hospital-Acquired	
Prerenal	70%	Prerenal	20%
Intrinsic	20%	Acute Tubular Necrosis	70%
Postrenal	10%	Postrenal	10%

higher incidence of intrinsic renal causes for ARF (45 percent) secondary to diseases such as glomerulonephritis and hemolytic-uremic syndrome. Elderly male patients are more likely to suffer ARF from obstruction and infection.

Prerenal Failure

The differential diagnosis for prerenal azotemia can be broken down into volume loss, fluid sequestration, decreased cardiac output, and diseases of the large and small renal arteries (Table 92-2). Besides being an independent cause of ARF, prerenal failure is a common precursor to ischemic and nephrotoxic causes of intrinsic renal failure.

Postrenal Failure

Postrenal or obstructive ARF accounts for 5 to 17 percent of all community-acquired ARF, and in the elderly population, the rate is as high as 22 percent (Table 92-3). Risk factors include both extremes of age, male sex, malignancy, nephrolithiasis, and retroperitoneal disease. Timely relief of obstruction is essential for the return of normal renal function; significant permanent loss of renal function happens over the course of 10 to 14 days in the setting of complete urinary obstruction. The risk of permanent renal failure is significantly greater if obstruction is complicated by urinary tract infection.

Intrinsic Renal Failure

Intrinsic ARF is less common in community-acquired ARF, but it is the most common cause in hospitalized patients. Intrinsic renal failure

TABLE 92-2   Differential Diagnosis of Prerenal Failure

Volume loss
  Hemorrhagic shock
  Vomiting
  Diarrhea
  Diuretics
  Primary hypoaldosteronism
  Salt-losing nephropathy
  Postobstructive diuresis
Decreased cardiac output
  Myocardial ischemia/infarction
  Valvular heart disease
  Cardiomyopathy
  Pericardial tamponade
  β-blockers
  High-output failure (thyrotoxicosis, thiamine deficiency, Paget disease, arteriovenous fistula)
Renal artery and small vessel disease
  Cyclosporine and tacrolimus
  Embolic disease (septic, cholesterol)
  Malignant hypertension
  Transplant rejection
  Sickle cell disease
  Preeclampsia
  Hypercalcemia
  Hemolytic-uremic syndrome
  Vasculitis

TABLE 92-3   Differential Diagnosis of Postobstructive Renal Failure

Infants and children
  Urethra and bladder outlet
    Urethral atresia
    Phimosis
    Ureterocele
    Meatal stenosis
    Anterior and posterior urethral valves (males)
    Calculus (Southeast Asia)
    Neurogenic bladder
    Blood clot
  Ureter
    Vesicoureteral reflux (female preponderance)
    Ureterovesical junction obstruction
    Ureterocele
    Megaureter (prune belly) syndrome
    Retrocaval ureter
    Retroperitoneal tumor
    Blood clot
Adults
  Urethra and bladder outlet
    Phimosis or urethral stricture (male preponderance)
    Benign prostate hypertrophy
    Cancer of prostate, bladder, cervix, or colon
    Neurogenic bladder: diabetes mellitus, spinal cord disease, multiple sclerosis, Parkinson's disease, anticholinergic drugs and α-adrenergic antagonists
    Miscellaneous: trauma, blood clot, calculi
  Ureter
    Vesicoureteral reflux (female preponderance)
    Calculi, uric acid crystals
    Papillary necrosis: sickle cell disease, diabetes mellitus, pyelonephritis
    Tumor: carcinoma of ureter, uterus, prostate, bladder, colon, rectum, retroperitoneal lymphoma, uterine leiomyomata
    Retroperitoneal fibrosis: idiopathic, tuberculosis, sarcoidosis, methylsergide, propranolol
    Stricture: tuberculosis, radiation, schistosomiasis, nonsteroidal anti-inflammatory drugs
    Miscellaneous: aortic aneurysm, pregnant uterus, inflammatory bowel disease, blood clot, trauma, accidental surgical ligation
  Intrarenal
    Crystals: uric acid, sulfonamide, acyclovir, indinavir
    Protein casts: multiple myeloma, amyloidosis

can result from injury to the glomerulus, tubule, interstitium, and vasculature (Table 92-4). In community-acquired intrinsic ARF, drugs and infection are common precipitants, whereas in the hospital, toxic and ischemic insults cause the majority of cases (Table 92-5).[1,2]

Radiocontrast-induced nephropathy is a common cause of in-hospital ARF, with a typical course of increasing creatinine over 3 to 5 days, followed by complete resolution. The occurrence of radiocontrast-induced nephropathy has been linked to increased in-hospital mortality. Risk factors include chronic renal insufficiency (CRI), diabetes (in particular the insulin-dependent type), age, hypovolemia, hypoalbuminemia, myeloma, and type and dose of contrast.

Crystal-induced nephropathy involves precipitation of crystals within the renal tubules, resulting in mechanical and inflammatory injuries of the tubular epithelium. Chronic renal insufficiency and hypovolemia predispose patients to this form of renal injury, and urinary pH affects the formation of many of these crystals. Uric acid in the setting of tumor lysis syndrome and medications, in particular acyclovir, sulfonamides, indinavir, and triamterene, are the most common causes of this form of ARF.

Angiotensin-converting enzyme inhibitors (ACEIs) may precipitate ARF in rare patients. By dilating postglomerular capillaries, they increase RBF and decrease GFR. These changes naturally result in a modest (10 to 20 percent) increase in serum creatinine, but in rare

TABLE 92-4 Differential Diagnosis of Intrinsic Renal Failure

Tubular diseases
  Ischemic acute tubular necrosis (ATN)
  Nephrotoxins: aminoglycosides, radiocontrast, cisplatin, myeloma light
    chains
  Heme pigments: rhabdomyolysis, massive hemolysis
Interstitial diseases
  Acute interstitial nephritis (drug reactions)
  Infiltrative disease: sarcoidosis, lymphoma
  Autoimmune diseases: SLE
  Infectious agents: Legionnaire disease, hanta virus
Glomerular diseases
  Rapidly progressive glomerulonephritis: Goodpasture syndrome,
    Wegener granulomatosis, Henoch-Schönlein purpura, SLE,
    membranoproliferative glomerulonephritis
  Postinfectious glomerulonephritis
Vascular diseases
  Malignant hypertension
  Scleroderma
  Thrombotic thrombocytopenic purpura
  Hemolytic uremic syndrome
  Renal vein thrombosis
  Polyarteritis nodosa

Abbreviation: SLE = systemic lupus erythematosus.

cases the increase can be more dramatic; in both circumstances the changes are observed shortly after initiation of ACEI therapy.[9] Acute renal failure occurring in the setting of ACEI initiation should prompt consideration of bilateral renal vascular stenosis, in which case maintenance of GFR is dependent on postglomerular arteriole vasoconstriction. Volume depletion and concomitant vasoconstricting medications are other common precipitants for ACEI-induced ARF. Angiotensin receptor blockers also have the potential to precipitate ARF.[10] Hyperkalemia, usually mild, is a relatively common complication of ACEI administration.

Cyclooxygenase inhibitors (most nonsteroidal anti-inflammatory drugs) comprise another family of medications frequently implicated in ARF. Renal effects of selective cyclooxygenase II inhibitors seem to be very similar to those of nonselective inhibitors.[11] Risk factors for adverse reactions to these medications are age, CRI, congestive heart failure, diabetes, volume depletion, and use of diuretics or ACEIs. Edema and ARF are typically observed early in the course of treatment

TABLE 92-5 Drugs Associated with Acute Renal Failure

Reduction in renal perfusion through alteration in intrarenal hemodynamics
  NSAIDs, angiotensin-converting enzyme inhibitors, cyclosporine,
    tacrolimus, radiocontrast agents, amphotericin B, interleukin 2
Direct tubular toxicity
  Aminoglycoside antibiotics, radiocontrast agents, cisplatin, cyclosporine,
    tacrolimus, amphotericin B, methotrexate, foscarnet, pentamidine,
    organic solvents, heavy metals, intravenous immunoglobulin
Heme-pigment–induced tubular toxicity (rhabdomyolysis)
  Cocaine, ethanol, lovastatin
Intratubular obstruction by precipitation of the agent, its metabolites, or
  byproducts
  Acyclovir, sulfonamides, ethylene glycol, chemotherapeutic agents,
    methotrexate
Allergic interstitial nephritis
  Penicillins, cephalosporins, sulfonamides, rifampin, ciprofloxacin,
    NSAIDs, thiazide diuretics, furosemide, cimetidine, phenytoin,
    allopurinol
Hemolytic-uremic syndrome
  Cyclosporine, tacrolimus, mitomycin, cocaine, quinine, conjugated
    estrogens

Abbreviation: NSAIDs = nonsteroidal anti-inflammatory drugs.
Source: Reproduced with permission from Thadhani R, Pascual M, Bonventre JV: Acute renal failure. *New Engl J Med* 334:1451, 1996.

and are dose dependent. In reported cases, ARF has resolved with discontinuation of the medication.

Aminoglycosides are another important cause of iatrogenic renal injury. The trough concentration seems to be more relevant than the peak concentration in predicting renal injury, and once-daily dosing has been shown to reduce the incidence of nephrotoxicity.[12]

Hemoglobin and myoglobin in the settings of hemolysis or rhabdomyolysis are deposited and concentrated in the renal tubules. Renal injury in these settings occurs through obstruction and direct tubular toxicity, the latter being dependent in part on low urine pH. Myeloma light-chain nephropathy may be similar. In patients with myoglobinuric ARF induced by crush injury, the incidence of hyperkalemia among patients surviving to the hospital was 42 percent, and mortality was 15 percent in the same population.

CLINICAL FEATURES

History

Acute renal failure itself has few symptoms until severe uremia has developed. At that time, nausea, vomiting, drowsiness, fatigue, confusion, and coma are common findings. Patients are more likely to present with symptoms related to the cause of their ARF.

Patients with prerenal ARF commonly present with thirst, orthostatic lightheadedness, and decreasing urine output. Excessive vomiting, diarrhea, urination, hemorrhage, fever, or sweating can reduce circulating volume enough to precipitate ARF. Causes of endothelial leak and third spacing, such as sepsis, pancreatitis, burns, and hepatic failure, can result in prerenal ARF. Progression of heart failure from whatever cause or overdiuresis of the compensated congestive heart failure patient can result in ARF. Decreased fluid intake from physical or cognitive disability can result in hypovolemia sufficient to cause ARF, and ARF is a common finding among elderly patients presenting with vague mental status change.

Intrinsic renal diseases can be anticipated because of symptoms of their precipitant cause. Ischemic acute tubular necrosis (ATN) is uncommon in community-acquired ARF but might be expected in the setting of cardiac arrest or other cause of prolonged hypotension. Crystal-induced nephropathy can present with flank pain and hematuria, as can nephrolithiasis and papillary necrosis. Pigment-induced ARF should be suspected in patients with possible rhabdomyolysis (e.g., muscle tenderness, recent coma, seizures, drug abuse, alcohol, excessive exercise, or limb ischemia) and with hemolysis (e.g., recent blood transfusion). Darkening urine and edema with or without constitutional symptoms, such as fever, malaise, and rash, should raise suspicion of acute glomerulonephritis, which may have been preceded by pharyngitis or cutaneous infection. Fever, arthralgia, and rash are common with acute interstitial nephritis. Cough, dyspnea, and hemoptysis raise the possibility of the pulmonary-renal syndromes (Goodpasture disease or Wegener granulomatosis).

Postrenal failure should be suspected in patients with appropriate risk factors. Symptoms of urethral obstruction often are not communicated to the physician because of their gradual onset. Anuria strongly suggests obstruction, although vascular obstruction and fulminant renal disease are also possible. Alternating oliguria and polyuria are virtually pathognomonic of obstruction.

Physical Examination

The patient's volume status should be assessed. Hypotension and tachycardia are obvious clues to decreased renal perfusion, but blood pressure and pulse are insensitive indicators of hypovolemia. It is important to recognize that a normal blood pressure may be relatively hypotensive for a chronically hypertensive patient. Evaluation of mucosal membrane moisture, tissue turgor, and an orthostatic pulse increase may suggest hypovolemia. Base deficit, lactate, central venous pressure, and central venous oxygen saturation may be more sensitive and reliable indicators of hypovolemia. There is growing evidence that use of early invasive hemodynamic monitoring may improve resuscitation outcomes.[13]

Fever suggests infectious or autoimmune causes. Examination of the skin (e.g., livedo reticularis, digital ischemia, butterfly rash, palpable purpura, and petechiae) may suggest a systemic vasculitis, atheroembolic disease, or endocarditis. Maculopapular rashes raise the possibility of allergic interstitial nephritis, and stigmata of intravenous drug abuse should suggest endocarditis.

Examination of the eyes may find evidence of autoimmune vasculitis (keratitis, iritis, uveitis, and dry conjunctiva), liver disease (jaundice), multiple myeloma (band keratopathy from hypercalcemia), diabetes mellitus, hypertension, or atheroemboli (retinopathy).

The cardiac examination may find signs suggesting peripheral arterial emboli (atrial fibrillation), endocarditis (murmurs), and heart failure (jugular venous distention, hepatojugular reflux, or S₃ gallop). The pulmonary examination may suggest heart failure, Goodpasture syndrome, or Wegener granulomatosis (rales). The abdominal examination may find evidence of aortic aneurysm, nephrolithiasis, crystal nephropathy or papillary necrosis (flank tenderness), or urinary obstruction (pelvic, rectal masses, prostatic hypertrophy, and bladder distention). Examination of the extremities may suggest rhabdomyolysis (limb cyanosis, pulselessness, and edema), vasculitis (palpable purpura), or atherosclerotic disease (diminished pulses).

DIAGNOSTIC SEQUENCE/CLINICAL APPROACH

In the critically ill patient with ARF, resuscitation is the first priority, and multiple diagnostic and therapeutic processes can proceed simultaneously. Electrocardiography is often the fastest screening test for significant hyperkalemia, although it may not always show abnormalities, even in the setting of critically high potassium levels. Chest radiography helps evaluate for increased volume, effusions, and pneumonia, all of which can result from or precipitate ARF. After obvious intravascular volume deficits are corrected, the remainder of the initial diagnostic sequence focuses on the exclusion of urinary obstruction and interpretation of basic blood and urine tests.

After having the patient void, a urinary catheter should be placed. A properly positioned bladder catheter is diagnostic of and therapeutic for obstruction below the level of the bladder. If no urine is obtained, catheter placement should be tested by irrigation or ultrasound. If irrigation fluid returns freely, the catheter tip is most probably in the bladder, and obstruction above the bladder should be investigated. Large postvoid residuals (more than 125 mL) on catheterization suggest obstruction below the bladder, and catheter drainage will need to be maintained until the obstruction is relieved. Urine will need to be sent for urinalysis with microscopy, electrolytes, osmolality, and culture.

It has traditionally been recommended that the catheter be clamped intermittently to prevent hypotension and hematuria during drainage of a distended bladder, but experimental and clinical evidence provides no support for this practice. Hematuria upon catheter drainage of a distended bladder is related to the degree of bladder wall damage before relief of obstruction and is not correlated with the rate of emptying. Urine should be completely and rapidly drained from an obstructed bladder, because prolonged urine stasis predisposes the patient to urinary tract infection, urosepsis, and renal failure. Urine output has limitations in the estimation of blood volume; in the setting of ARF, its use is particularly problematic.

Concerns about postobstructive diuresis, however, are appropriate. Many investigators recommend admission of patients with persistent diuresis greater than 250 mL per h for more than 2 h in otherwise uncomplicated urethral obstruction. The syndrome of postobstructive diuresis is important to recognize, because it can result in sig-

nificant volume loss and even death. This complication of obstruction typically occurs when the obstruction has been prolonged and has resulted in ARF or significant volume overload.

ANCILLARY TESTS

Imaging

Once obstruction below the bladder level has been investigated, obstruction in the upper urinary tract should be investigated. Imaging studies can reliably identify hydronephrosis, but it is important to realize that, in intermittent or partial obstruction, hydronephrosis may not be present and may be absent in complete obstruction with retroperitoneal fibrosis. Further, functional dilatation can occur in the setting of chronic reflux. Renal ultrasound is considered the test of choice, with approximately 90 percent sensitivity and specificity for detecting hydronephrosis due to mechanical obstruction. The addition of Doppler and other advanced ultrasound techniques will allow evaluation of RBF and may suggest specific etiologies. If the renal ultrasound detects hydronephrosis, a secondary imaging study to define the location of obstruction is required. Intravenous pyelogram had been the gold standard for evaluation of the urinary tract for obstruction, but its dependence on radiocontrast and the availability of other modalities limit its value in the setting of ARF. Noncontrast computed tomography and magnetic resonance imaging have significant utility for this indication. Noncontrast computed tomography is widely available, has sensitivity for hydronephrosis that is equivalent to that with ultrasound, and has the added advantage of describing the site and often the cause of obstruction. Magnetic resonance pyelography has performed well in published studies, with 100 percent sensitivity and 98 percent specificity when compared with the combination of ultrasound and contrast pyelography. If functional obstruction is a consideration in the presence of a dilated genitourinary tract, radionuclide scans and magnetic resonance urography before and after diuretics can be obtained.

Chemistry and Urine Analysis

In combination, microscopic urinalysis and serum and urine chemistries have a great utility in determining the etiology of ARF. **However, the diagnosis must first be suspected, and without knowledge of a patient's baseline blood urea nitrogen (BUN) and creatinine (Cr), it is possible to overlook evidence of significant renal injury.** A patient with a very low baseline Cr can lose more than half of functioning nephrons before developing an elevated Cr. Serum urea nitrogen is depressed in patients with malnutrition and hepatic synthetic dysfunction and can be increased in the setting of protein loading, gastrointestinal hemorrhage, or trauma.

Creatinine provides the most accurate and consistent estimation of GFR (Table 92-6). Creatinine is a breakdown product of the skeletal muscle protein creatine, and its level is thus linked to muscle mass. Therefore, patients with lower muscle mass (e.g., older patients and women) have lower GFRs for any given Cr level. Several conditions can interfere with the correlation of serum Cr and GFR. Glomerulonephritis causes increased tubular secretion, whereas trimethoprim, cimetidine, and salicylates cause decreased secretion, thus altering the Cr level independently of the GFR. The rate of increase in serum Cr can be used to estimate GFR. In patients with no renal function (GFR = 0), serum Cr will increase 1 to 3 mg/dL a day. Lesser increases in Cr indicate residual GFR, whereas faster increases suggest muscle breakdown (e.g., rhabdomyolysis).

The ratio of BUN to Cr can suggest hypovolemia, because of differences in the way each is handled in the nephron. Both substances are passively filtered at the glomerulus; however, whereas Cr remains within the tubule, urea is highly permeable to renal tubules and is pas-

TABLE 92-6   Estimation of Glomerular Filtration Rate by Serum Creatinine

Serum Cr (mg/dL)	GFR (mL/min)
1.0	Normal baseline
2.0	50% reduction
4.0	70–85% reduction
8.0	90–99% reduction

Abbreviations: Cr = creatinine; GFR = glomerular filtration rate.

sively reabsorbed with sodium. Therefore, in the setting of avid sodium retention, urea clearance is as low as 30 percent of GFR, whereas in the setting of adequate volume and sodium, urea clearance can increase to 70 to 100 percent of GFR. Thus, if the patient has normal concentrating ability, in the setting of prerenal failure, the serum ratio of BUN to Cr is typically greater than 20.

The fractional excretion of sodium ($Fe_{Na} = U_{Na}/P_{Na} \div U_{Cr}/P_{Cr}$) is another test that is commonly used to identify hypovolemia as the cause of ARF, but it has a few limitations. For example, in the setting of intrinsic renal failure in which tubular concentrating capacity is retained, as in the case of glomerulonephritis, the Fe_{Na} may be depressed, just as it will be in the setting of normal kidneys under a prerenal stress. In the setting of tubular injury, such as ischemic or toxic ATN, the loss of concentrating ability results in a dilute urine, with an Fe_{Na} above 1 percent (Table 92-7).

Microscopic examination of urine is very useful in establishing the differential diagnosis of ARF (Table 92-7). In the setting of acute glomerulonephritis, red blood cells enter the filtrate at the glomerulus and, on the urinalysis, appear as casts and dysmorphic cells due to the increased tonicity of the renal medulla. In the setting of ATN, the tubular epithelium breaks down and there is significant protein leak into the filtrate and tubular epithelial cells in the sediment.

Cast formation is a common feature in many causes of ARF, and the composition of the casts offers clues to the cause. Hyaline casts are common in prerenal failure, whereas pigmented granular casts are common with ischemic or toxic tubular injury. Brown granular casts are a common finding in the setting of pigment nephropathy (e.g., hemoglobin or myoglobinuria). Crystals may be seen on conventional urinalysis but are best seen with polarized light microscopy. An "active sediment," with red cell casts and proteinuria, should prompt investigation of a primary glomerulonephritis or some underlying autoimmune disease.

Renal Biopsy

Renal biopsy should be considered in all causes of intrinsic ARF, especially in the estimated 10 to 25 percent of patients with ARF in whom the cause cannot be clinically diagnosed. Retrospective studies have shown that the results of the renal biopsy significantly changed the diagnosis and management of ARF in 40 percent of cases. The most common complication of renal biopsy is hematuria, which occurs in almost all patients. Serious complications, defined as the need for blood transfusion, nephrectomy, puncture of other organs, or perinephric hematomas, occur at a rate of 2 percent. Overall mortality for renal biopsy is 0.1 percent.

TREATMENT

Fluid Administration

Patients with ARF present challenging fluid-management problems. Hypovolemia potentiates and exacerbates all forms of ARF. The reversal of hypovolemia by rapid fluid infusion is often sufficient to treat and/or ameliorate many forms of ARF, but rapid fluid infusion can result in life-threatening fluid overload in patients with ARF. Accurate determination of these patients' volume status is essential and often requires invasive hemodynamic monitoring, particularly in the setting of cardiac dysfunction. Crystalloids are the resuscitation fluid of choice, and, among colloids, albumin should specifically be avoided, because of the possibility of additive renal injury.[14]

Medications

Because patients with nonoliguric as opposed to oliguric ARF have improved mortality and renal function recovery rates, many investigators recommend diuretics in an effort to "convert" oliguric to nonoliguric ARF. However, randomized double-blind controlled trials have failed to show a benefit in administering diuretics to patients with ARF.[15] These studies concluded that diuretics are useful only in the management of volume-overloaded patients, a setting in which venodilators and dialysis may be more effective. The prevalence of prerenal physiology in the ED and the association of high-dose furosemide with long-term hearing deficits also should be considered before using diuretics.

Renal vascular vasodilators in ARF have theoretical and experimental support. Low ("renal")-dose dopamine (1 to 5 μg/kg per min) was widely used for many years to treat ARF. In this setting, dopamine does increase urine output, but there is no evidence that dopamine

TABLE 92-7   Typical Urine Findings in Conditions That Cause Acute Renal Failure

Condition	Dipstick Test	Sediment Analysis	Urine Osmolality (mOsm/kg)	Fractional Excretion of Sodium (%)
Prerenal azotemia	Trace to no proteinuria	A few hyaline casts possible	>500	<1
Renal azotemia Tubular injury				
Ischemia	Mild to moderate proteinuria	Pigmented granular casts	<350	>1
Nephrotoxins	Mild to moderate proteinuria	Pigmented granular casts	<350	>1
Acute interstitial nephritis	Mild to moderate proteinuria; hemoglobin, leukocytes	White cells and white cell casts; eosinophils and eosinophil casts; red cells	<350	>1
Acute glomerulonephritis	Moderate to severe proteinuria; hemoglobin	Red cells and red cell casts; red cells can be dysmorphic	>500	<1
Postrenal azotemia	Trace to no proteinuria; can have hemoglobin and leukocytes	Crystals, red cells, and white cells possible	<350	>1

Source: Reproduced with permission from Thadhani R, Pascual M, Bonventre JV: Acute renal failure. *New Engl J Med* 334:1451, 1996.

produces a significant improvement in either renal recovery or mortality.[16] Dopamine is pro-arrhythmic, and its diuretic effect may come at the cost of increased medullary oxygen consumption without increased oxygen delivery.

In animal models, calcium channel blockers are protective against ARF if given before the renal insult. In humans, their major benefit has been in preventing ARF in renal transplant patients taking cyclosporine, but they have not found wider use.

There are no controlled studies of mannitol showing benefit in patients with established ARF. In fact, mannitol, given in high doses, has been identified as a cause of ARF. There are also significant risks of fluid overload and hyperkalemia associated with administering large doses of mannitol to ARF patients.

In the setting of pigment nephropathy (myoglobinuric ARF), early large-volume crystalloid infusion is the cornerstone of treatment. Mannitol is also routinely recommended in this setting, in which it may have rheologic and dilutional effects. Sodium bicarbonate dosed to accomplish urine alkalinization is also recommended. Tubular acidosis has been shown to be a potent cofactor in the tubular toxicity of myoglobin.

Urinary pH plays an important role in most drug-associated crystal nephropathies, and alkalinization is used for some of them. Even though some crystal nephropathies theoretically could benefit from urine acidification, the risks associated with acid infusion outweigh its benefit, even in this setting. Volume resuscitation and discontinuation of any offending medication are most important.

Several interventions have been shown to be useful in the prevention of radiocontrast nephropathy. Acetylcysteine reduced the rate of ARF in a high-risk population, from 21 to 2 percent.[17] Fenoldopam reduced the incidence of ARF by almost half in patients with CRI undergoing angiography.[18] Crystalloid infusion also may reduce the risk of this common complication of radiocontrast administration.

Although there has been no demonstration that interventions directed toward prevention or arrest of the pathophysiology of ischemic ATN improve outcomes, growing understanding of these mechanisms continues to increase the hope that such interventions will soon be available. Strategies directed toward interrupting the ischemic or inflammatory cascade at multiple steps may prove more effective than more focused interventions. Specific strategies may include arginine-glycine-aspartic acid peptides, antioxidants, phosphodiesterase inhibitors, growth factors, adenosine receptor antagonists, and targeting of cell-to-cell adhesion molecules.

Renal Replacement Therapy

The advent of renal replacement therapy (RRT) has had a significant impact on the treatment of life-threatening fluid and electrolyte complications of ARF. It is not clear, however, whether it plays a role in renal recovery, whether the timing of initiation affects outcome, or which of several methods is best in ARF. In recognition of the fact that there is little evidence on which to base guidelines regarding RRT in ARF, several notable contributors to this literature started the Acute Dialysis Quality Initiative in 2000 to guide future research and develop evidence-based practice guidelines.

The principal methods of RRT are intermittent hemodialysis (IHD), continuous venovenous hemofiltration (CVVH), and peritoneal dialysis. Each has advantages and limitations. Intermittent hemodialysis is widely available, has only moderate technical difficulty, and is the most efficient way of removing volume or solute from the vascular compartment quickly. Unfortunately, dialysis-associated hypotension may adversely affect remaining renal function, particularly in the critically ill. Continuous venovenous hemofiltration is more expensive and not universally available but, in addition to avoiding hypotension, is believed to achieve better control of uremia and clearance of solute from the extravascular compartment. Because it continues around the clock, CVVH is able to remove larger fluid volumes, which is a significant advantage with critical care patients on parenteral nutrition and multiple infusions. Continuous venovenous hemofiltration also may better preserve cerebral perfusion pressure. A theoretical but contested advantage of CVVH is the clearance of mediators of the inflammatory cascade. Several studies have sought to directly compare CVVH with IHD; none has found a convincing advantage for one therapy over the other. Nevertheless, many authorities assert that the choice of IHD over CVVH in the setting of shock would be inappropriate and unethical. Peritoneal dialysis is inexpensive, widely available, and does not result in hypotension. However, it cannot remove large volumes of fluid or solute. Its use may be most common in children.

Indications for and timing of initiation of RRT are also important, if somewhat controversial, subjects. Widely accepted indications for initiation of RRT include volume overload, hyperkalemia (K^+ >6.5 or rising), acid-base imbalance, "symptomatic uremia" (pericarditis, encephalopathy, bleeding dyscrasia, nausea, vomiting, or pruritus), uremia (BUN >100), and dialyzable intoxications. Severe dysnatremia (<115 or >165) and dysthermia also may be appropriate indications for RRT. Significant intoxications with a dialyzable agent (e.g., methanol, ethylene glycol, theophylline, aspirin, and lithium) may be the strongest indication for emergent dialysis, because there are other effective temporizing therapeutic interventions for most other complications of ARF. Volume overload can be treated with nitrates and phlebotomy; hyperkalemia can be treated with calcium, insulin, glucose, bicarbonate, binding resins, and β-adrenergic agonists.

The timing of initiation of RRT in the absence of these indications is more controversial, although there may be growing consensus that RRT itself contributes to the resolution of ARF. Intensity of RRT is another area of active controversy and research; two recent studies have suggested that more is better. In a study of CVVH intensity in which patients with ARF were randomized to standard or supernormal levels of ultrafiltration, the patients with more intense RRT had significantly lower mortality.[19] Another randomized trial compared daily with traditional every-other-day IHD in ARF patients and found that mortality (28 vs. 46 percent) and speed of renal recovery (9 vs. 16 days) were significantly improved.[20]

DISPOSITION

Patients with ARF require admission to the hospital, often to an intensive care setting, where their fluid and medical management can be monitored on an hour-to-hour basis. An appropriate specialist (nephrologist, intensive care specialist, or internist) should be consulted early.

REFERENCES

1. Liano F, Pascual J, Madrid Acute Renal Failure Study Group: Epidemiology of acute renal failure: A prospective, multicenter, community-based study. *Kidney Int* 50:811, 1996.
2. Kaufman J, Dhakai M, Balubhai P, Hamburger R: Community-acquired acute renal failure. *Am J Kidney Dis* 17:191, 1991.
3. Thadhani R, Pascual M, Bonventre JV: Acute renal failure. *New Engl J Med* 334:1448, 1996.
4. Akposso K, Hertig A, Couprie R, et al: Acute renal failure in patients over 80 years old: 25 years' experience. *Intens Care Med* 26:400, 2000.
5. Moghal NE, Brocklebank JT, Meadow SR: A review of acute renal failure in children: Incidence, etiology and outcome. *Clin Nephrol* 49:91, 1998.
6. Molitoris BA, Sandoval R, Sutton TA: Endothelial injury and dysfunction in ischemic acute renal failure. *Crit Care Med* 30:S235, 2002.
7. Molitoris BA, Marrs J: The role of cell adhesion molecules in ischemic acute renal failure. *Am J Med* 106:583, 1999.
8. Thurau K, Boylan JW: Acute renal success. The unexpected logic of oliguria in acute renal failure. *Am J Med* 61:308, 1976.
9. Schoolwerth AC, Sica DA, Ballermann BJ, Wilcox CS: Renal considerations in angiotensin converting enzyme inhibitor therapy. *Circulation* 104:1985, 2001.

10. Toto R: Angiotensin II subtype 1-receptor blockers and renal function. *Arch Intern Med* 161:1492, 2001.
11. Harris RC: Cyclooxygenase-2 inhibition and renal physiology. *Am J Cardiol* 89:10D, 2002.
12. Barza M, Ioannidis JP, Cappelleri JC, Lau J: Single or multiple daily doses of aminoglycosides: A meta-analysis. *BMJ* 312:338, 1996.
13. Rivers E, Nguyen B, Havstad S, et al: Early goal-directed therapy in the treatment of severe sepsis and septic shock. *New Engl J Med* 345:1368, 2001.
14. Ragaller MJ, Theilen H, Koch R: Volume replacement in critically ill patients with acute renal failure. *J Am Soc Nephrol* 12(suppl 17):S33, 2001.
15. Shilliday IR, Quinn KJ, Allison ME: Loop diuretics in the management of acute renal failure: A prospective, double-blind, placebo-controlled, randomized study. *Nephrol Dial Transplant* 12:2592, 1997.
16. Kellum JA, Decker J: Use of dopamine in acute renal failure: A meta-analysis. *Crit Care Med* 29:1526, 2001.
17. Tepel M, Van Der Geit M, Schwarzfeld C, et al: Prevention of radiographic-contrast-agent-induced reductions in renal function by acetylcysteine. *New Engl J Med* 343:180, 2000.
18. Tumlin JA, Wang A, Murray PT, Mathur VS: Fenoldopam mesylate blocks reductions in renal plasma flow after radiocontrast dye infusion: A pilot trial in the prevention of contrast nephropathy. *Am Heart J* 143:894, 2002.
19. Ronco C, Bellomo R, Homel P, et al: Effects of different doses in continuous veno-venous haemofiltration on outcomes of acute renal failure: A prospective randomized trial. *Lancet* 356:26, 2000.
20. Schiffl H, Lang SM, Fischer R: Daily hemodialysis and the outcome of acute renal failure. *New Engl J Med* 346:305, 2002.

93 EMERGENCIES IN RENAL FAILURE AND DIALYSIS PATIENTS
Richard Sinert
Mark Spektor

End-stage renal disease (ESRD) is the irreversible loss of renal function, resulting in the accumulation of toxins and the loss of internal homeostasis. Uremia, the clinical syndrome resulting from ESRD, is universally fatal without some form of renal replacement therapy (RRT). At present, RRT consists of two basic modalities: renal transplant and dialysis therapy. This chapter discusses the pathophysiology and clinical features of uremia and the specific techniques and complications related to hemodialysis (HD) and peritoneal dialysis (PD).

EPIDEMIOLOGY

The 2001 annual report of the United States Renal Data System (USRDS) noted that, for 1999, there were 89,252 new cases of ESRD, with 424,179 patients being treated for ESRD.[1] End-stage renal disease is a disease of the elderly, with patients older than age 65 years comprising 47.9 percent of new cases of ESRD and accounting for 37.2 percent of all living patients with ESRD. Diabetes mellitus is the most common disease (42.8 percent) responsible for ESRD, followed by hypertension (25.9 percent), glomerulonephritis (9.0 percent), cystic kidney disease (2.3 percent), and other causes (20.0 percent). The USRDS projects a 6 to 7 percent growth per year in the incidence of ESRD. An expanding incidence and life span will result in an expected increasing prevalence of ESRD of 8 to 9 percent per year.

The use of RRT for ESRD is divided into 70.1 percent on dialysis therapy and 29.9 percent with renal transplants. Of the patients on dialysis, 89 percent are on HD and 11 percent are on PD. Pediatric patients (ages 0 to 19 years) have higher rates of renal transplantation (77.7 percent) and PD (12.1 percent) than do other age groups.

One-, two-, and five-year survival rates (adjusted for age, race, sex, and primary disease) for ESRD are 79.6, 64.9, and 34.4 percent, respectively. Cardiac causes account for approximately 50 percent of all cases of ESRD death. Infectious causes of death occur in 10 to 25 percent of patients. Cerebrovascular events make up 6 percent of ESRD

deaths, with malignancy accounting for another 1 to 4 percent. Approximately 20 percent of dialysis patients withdraw from therapy before death. Patients older than 65 years have the highest withdrawal rate (25 percent). The increasing incidence of withdrawal with age is linked to progressive severity of comorbid conditions affecting patients' quality of life on RRT.

PATHOPHYSIOLOGY OF UREMIA

In 1840, Piorry was the first to use the term *uremia,* contamination of the blood with urine, to describe the clinical syndrome from ESRD. The concept that uremia is from an excretory failure resulting in toxin accumulation is reinforced by the continued use of the term *azotemia,* the buildup of blood nitrogen.

Excretory Failure

Excretory failure leads to elevated levels of more than 70 chemicals in uremic plasma, leading to the hypothesis that these toxins, individually or in combination, cause uremic organ dysfunction and produce the symptoms of uremia. For more than 100 years, limiting protein intake markedly has been noted to improve the symptoms of uremia. Urea, the major break-down product of proteins, reproduces a few of the neurobehavioral uremic symptoms, but only at very high concentrations. Other potential uremic toxins include cyanate, guanidine, polyamines, and β_2-microglobulin.

Although toxins from ESRD excretory failure are definitely a factor in uremia, they cannot explain all its clinical features. In addition, if uremia were simply a toxidrome, then dialysis would reverse all its untoward effects. Because many uremic organ dysfunctions persist after dialysis, other processes are clearly important.

Biosynthetic Failure

Biosynthetic failure refers to the aspects of uremia from loss of the renal hormones $1,25(OH)_3$ vitamin D_3 and erythropoietin. The kidneys are primarily responsible for the secretion of erythropoietin and 1-α-hydroxylase, which is necessary to produce the active form of vitamin D_3. Because 85 percent of erythropoietin is produced in the kidneys, ESRD patients have depressed levels, thereby contributing to anemia. Vitamin D_3 deficiency results in decreased gastrointestinal (GI) calcium absorption, thereby inducing secondary hyperparathyroidism, which is responsible for the development of renal bone disease.

Regulatory Failure

Regulatory failure results in an over-secretion of hormones, leading to uremia by disruption of normal feedback mechanisms after renal failure. In response to the accumulation of ions and other waste products with ESRD, the maintenance of internal homeostasis depends on a variety of extrarenal processes. These homeostatic responses, although adaptive to one toxin, may have untoward effects outside the system they are attempting to regulate. The "tradeoff" hypothesis, first proposed by Bricker,[2] was initially postulated to explain how hyperparathyroidism in ESRD was a tradeoff for the beneficial effects of high parathyroid hormone (PTH) levels on controlling phosphate levels. The tradeoff for the maintenance of normal calcium and phosphate levels is hyperparathyroidism, which causes increased bone turnover and leads to renal bone disease. Bricker extended this tradeoff hypothesis to sodium regulation in ESRD. As the glomerular filtration rate (GFR) decreases in ESRD patients, increasing fractional sodium excretion prevents salt retention. Bricker postulated that the tradeoff for this natriuretic factor is a generalized inhibition of sodium transport, which explains many aspects of uremic organ dysfunction.

Although Bricker's tradeoff hypothesis is still controversial, sodium transport abnormalities have been well documented in uremia.

Na^+K^+ATPase activity is reduced in the red blood cells, leukocytes, intestinal epithelium, cardiac muscle, and skeletal muscle in uremic patients. Inhibition of Na^+K^+ATPase activity results in partial cellular depolarization and increased calcium entry, which are linked to the high prevalence of hypertension and heart failure in ESRD. Recently, an endogenous dialyzable digitalis-like inhibitor of Na^+K^+ATPase activity has been isolated in uremic plasma. This defect in Na^+K^+ATPase activity is reversed by dialysis.

The uremic state produces excess free oxygen radicals, which react with carbohydrates, lipids, and amino acids, to create advanced glycation end products (AGEs), which have been linked to atherosclerosis and amyloidosis in ESRD patients.[3] Unfortunately, AGEs are largely protein bound and not cleared by dialysis, which may explain the progressive nature of atherosclerosis and amyloidosis seen in ESRD patients.[4]

CLINICAL FEATURES OF UREMIA

Uremia should be viewed only as a clinical syndrome; no single symptom, sign, or laboratory test is reliable in diagnosing all aspects of uremia. Although a correlation exists between the symptoms of uremia and low GFR (8 to 10 mL per min), available laboratory tests (e.g., determinations of serum urea nitrogen and serum creatinine) are inaccurate markers of the clinical syndrome of uremia. The decision to start chronic dialysis should be a clinical one based on the symptoms of uremia (Table 93-1).

Neurologic Complications

Subdural hematoma occurs in approximately 3.5 percent of HD patients, presumably related to head trauma, bleeding dyscrasias, anticoagulants, excessive ultrafiltration, and hypertension. Bilateral subdural hematomas commonly present without focal neurologic deficits and should be considered in the differential in any ESRD patient with a change in mental status.

TABLE 93-1   Clinical Features of Uremia

Neurologic
  Uremic encephalopathy: cognitive defects, memory loss, decreased
    attentiveness, slurred speech, reversal of sleep–wake cycle, asterixis,
    seizure, coma, symptomatic improvement with dialysis
  Dialysis dementia: progressive neurologic decline, fatal, fails to improve
    with dialysis
  Subdural hematoma: headache, focal neurologic deficits, seizure, and coma
  Peripheral neuropathy: singultus (hiccups), restless leg syndrome,
    sensorimotor neuropathy, autonomic neuropathy
Cardiovascular
  Coronary artery disease
  Hypertension: essential hypertension, glomerulonephritis, renal artery
    stenosis, fluid overload
  Heart failure: high-output AV fistula, uremic cardiomyopathy, fluid
    overload
  Pericarditis: uremic, dialysis-related, pericardial tamponade
Hematologic
  Anemia, decreased red blood cell survival, decreased erythropoietin levels
  Bleeding diathesis
  Immunodeficiency (humoral and cellular)
Gastrointestinal
  Anorexia, metallic taste, nausea, vomiting
  GI bleeding
  Diverticulosis, diverticulitis
  Ascites
Renal Bone Disease
  Metastatic calcification (calciphylaxis)
  Hyperparathyroidism (osteitis fibrosa cystica)
  Vitamin D_3 deficiency and aluminum intoxication (osteomalacia)

Abbreviations: AV = arteriovenous; GI = gastrointestinal.

Uremic encephalopathy is a constellation of nonspecific central neurologic symptoms associated with renal failure that respond, in large part, to RRT. Uremic encephalopathy should remain a diagnosis of exclusion after structural, vascular, infectious, toxic, and metabolic causes of neurologic dysfunction have been investigated. Objective findings of uremic encephalopathy include a significant increase in slow delta waves on the electroencephalogram and consistently low scores on psychometric testing. Magnetic resonance imaging may reveal increased signal intensity bilaterally in the cortical and subcortical areas of the occipital and parietal lobes.[5]

The objective findings of neurologic dysfunction have been linked to inhibition of Na^+K^+ATPase activity and increases in brain calcium from elevated PTH levels or abnormal calcium transport in uremic brains. Symptomatic and objective neurologic findings of uremic encephalopathy improve with dialysis and can be followed to judge the adequacy of RRT.

Dialysis dementia is similar to uremic encephalopathy, consisting of a nonspecific set of neuropsychiatric dysfunctions that, unlike uremic encephalopathy, are progressive and eventually fatal. This disorder usually becomes evident after at least 2 years on dialysis and fails to respond to increases in dialysis frequency or renal transplantation. Electroencephalographic findings can differentiate uremic encephalopathy from dialysis dementia. High brain aluminum levels from oral ingestion of aluminum or high levels of aluminum in dialysate water have been correlated with the development of dialysis dementia. Some improvement with desferrioxamine binding of aluminum has been demonstrated.

Peripheral neuropathy is one of the most frequent neurologic manifestations of ESRD, occurring in more than 50 percent of HD patients. The symptoms of peripheral neuropathy generally respond poorly to dialysis but can be reversed by renal transplantation. Failure of vibration sense usually is the earliest clinical manifestation. Patients can have asymmetric (mononeuropathies) and symmetric (polyneuropathies) peripheral deficits. Another common deficit is "glove-and-stocking" sensory involvement, presenting with pain or anesthesia affecting the most distal nerves. Electrophysiologic testing of patients with uremia shows depression of motor and sensory nerve conduction. No single pathologic correlate has been identified for peripheral uremic neuropathy, although inactivation of axons by long-term exposure to toxins and subsequent "dying back" phenomenon has been postulated.[6]

Autonomic dysfunction as demonstrated by impotence, postural dizziness, gastric fullness, bowel dysfunction, and reduced sweating are common complaints in many ESRD patients. Objective testing for autonomic dysfunction in ESRD has found reduced heart rate variability and baroreceptor control impairment. Autonomic dysfunction does not seem to explain intradialytic hypotension,[7] but it is common in a subset of chronically hypotensive ESRD patients whose blood pressures do not respond to volume challenges.[8] Hemodialysis does not seem to improve autonomic dysfunction.[9]

Cardiovascular Complications

The prevalence of cardiovascular disease (CVD) is significantly greater in ESRD patients than in the general population. Coronary artery disease, left ventricular (LV) hypertrophy, and congestive heart failure (CHF) are estimated to occur in 12, 20, and 5 percent, respectively, in the general population. In dialysis patients, these prevalences increase to 40, 75, and 40 percent.[10]

The etiology of CVD in ESRD patients is multifactorial, related to pre-existing conditions (e.g., hypertension, diabetes, etc.), uremia (e.g., uremic toxins, hyperlipidemias, homocysteine, hyperparathyroidism, etc.), and dialysis-related conditions (e.g., hypotension, dialysis membrane reactions, hypoalbuminemia, etc.). In addition, increased levels of AGEs represent a unique risk for advanced atherosclerosis in ESRD patients.[11]

The diagnosis of ischemic CVD in ESRD patients often has been clouded by the misconception that the traditional serum protein markers of myocardial damage (creatine protein kinase and troponin) are unreliable in dialysis patients. Creatine protein kinase and MB, troponin I, and troponin T are not significantly elevated in ESRD patients undergoing regular dialysis and have been shown to be specific markers of myocardial ischemia in these patients.[12,13]

Hypertension is present in 80 to 90 percent of patients starting dialysis. Hemodynamic profiles of hypertensive ESRD patients show that maintenance of hypertension depends on increases in total peripheral resistance. The etiology of the increase in total peripheral resistance appears to be multifactorial. Increases in blood volume, the vasopressor effects of native kidneys, the renin-angiotensin system, and the sympathetic nervous system have been shown to play roles in ESRD hypertension.

Management of hypertension in ESRD patients should begin with the control of blood volume. If that is unsuccessful, most patients' hypertension can be controlled with adrenergic-blocking agents, angiotensin-converting enzyme inhibitors, or vasodilating agents, such as hydralazine or minoxidil. Bilateral nephrectomy is rarely necessary for blood pressure control.

Congestive heart failure occurs for many of the same reasons in ESRD patients as in other patients; hypertension is the most common cause of CHF in ESRD patients, followed by coronary artery disease and valvular defects. Causes of CHF unique to ESRD include uremic cardiomyopathy, fluid overload, and arteriovenous (AV) fistula-related high-output failure (see Complications of Vascular Access).

Uremic cardiomyopathy should be a diagnosis of exclusion when all other causes of CHF have been ruled out. In most uremic patients, LV dysfunction is related to ischemic heart disease, hypertension, and hypoalbuminemia rather than to a uremic toxin. Dialysis rarely improves LV function in uremic patients with CHF. However, PTH has been linked to decreased LV function in uremia by studies showing marked improvement of LV function after parathyroidectomy.

Pulmonary edema in ESRD patients is commonly ascribed to fluid overload, but other differentials should always be investigated. Acute myocardial ischemia can cause depressed LV function, causing pulmonary edema even in patients at or below their postdialysis ("dry") weight.

Management of pulmonary edema in ESRD patients is generally similar to treatment in non-ESRD patients. Cornerstones of therapy in both types of patients include oxygen, nitrates, angiotensin-converting enzyme inhibitors,[14] and morphine. **Diuretics, such as furosemide, are still effective in treating CHF in ESRD patients, even with minimal urine output.**[15] In pulmonary edema, intravenous furosemide in doses of 60 to 100 mg provides pulmonary vasodilatation, thus improving oxygenation. Preload reduction in ESRD patients also can be accomplished by inducing diarrhea with sorbitol and by phlebotomy. Although not a first-line therapy, phlebotomy of as little as 150 mL of blood is safe and effective in treating pulmonary edema.[16] For example, phlebotomy of 150 mL in a patient with a hematocrit of 20 percent results in the loss of 120 mL of plasma and 30 mL of packed red blood cells (10 g of hemoglobin). The improved oxygenation by phlebotomy will more than offset the decrease in oxygen-carrying capacity due to the decrease in hemoglobin. Phlebotomized blood should be collected in transfusion bags, enabling plasma to be extracted by the blood bank and transfusion of red blood cells later during dialysis. Hemodialysis is the ultimate treatment for fluid overload in ESRD patients. Peritoneal dialysis does not remove volume fast enough to have a significant impact on pulmonary edema.

Cardiac tamponade is the main concern in all patients with pericarditis and should be considered in the differential diagnosis of any critically ill ESRD patient. **Patients with ESRD and tamponade rarely present with the classic signs of Beck's triad.** Instead, ESRD patients may present with changes in mental status, hypotension, or shortness of breath. Increased interdialytic weight gain, increased edema, and intradialytic hypotension suggest the early diagnosis of tamponade. Two other findings include moderate hypotension and an increasing heart size on chest radiograph. Echocardiography can detect the pericardial effusion and may detect evidence of tamponade. Hemodynamically significant pericardial effusions require pericardiocentesis under fluoroscopic or ultrasonographic guidance. Pericardiocentesis, because of its high complication rate, should be used only in hemodynamically unstable patients.

Pericarditis in ESRD patients is usually due to uremia, but patients should be evaluated carefully for other causes. Approximately 20 percent of uremic patients requiring chronic dialysis develop uremic pericarditis or dialysis-related pericarditis.

Uremic pericarditis is more common of the two and represents approximately 75 percent of cases. Uremic pericarditis is most common when the other symptoms of uremia are most severe. The etiology of uremic pericarditis has been linked to fluid overload, abnormal platelet function, and increased fibrinolytic and inflammatory cell activities. Pericardial contents are sterile unless infected and are abundant with fibrin and inflammatory cells.

Uremic pericarditis causes pericardial friction rubs, which are louder than in most other forms of pericarditis, often palpable, and frequently persist for some time after metabolic abnormalities have been corrected. Serum urea nitrogen is nearly always over 60 mg/dL. One of the unique features of uninfected uremic pericarditis is that the inflammatory cells do not penetrate into the myocardium, so typical electrocardiographic changes of acute pericarditis are absent. Most often, the ECG may demonstrate associated abnormalities, such as LV hypertrophy, ischemia, and metabolic abnormalities (e.g., hyperkalemia and hypocalcemia). When the ECG is typical of acute pericarditis, infection should be suspected.

Dialysis-related pericarditis also seems related to the general uremic milieu. This form of pericarditis is most common during periods of increased catabolism (trauma and sepsis) or inadequate dialysis due to missed sessions or vascular access problems. The pathophysiology of dialysis-related pericarditis has been linked to the buildup of middle molecules and hyperparathyroidism.

Dialysis-related pericarditis is more common during HD than during PD and fortunately is becoming less frequent because of improved dialytic techniques. Constitutional symptoms, such as fever, are more common and severe than in uremic pericarditis. Effusion, with and without hemorrhage, is the most important complication and tends to be recurrent. Due to the recurrent nature of dialysis pericarditis, adhesions and fluid loculations are more common, which complicate echocardiography and other imaging modalities.

Mortality rates for ESRD patients with pericarditis are as high as 8 percent, and average survival without dialysis is approximately 1 month. Management of uremic and dialysis-related pericarditis in hemodynamically stable patients is by intensive dialysis therapy. Hemodialysis is preferred over PD because of its higher clearance rates, but the risks of heparin and rapid fluid shifts precipitating tamponade must be taken into account. This therapy is effective in more than 55 percent of cases of dialysis-related pericarditis, usually after 10 to 14 days. Indomethacin and steroids are of questionable value for ESRD pericarditis. If pericardial effusion persists for more than 10 to 14 days with intensive dialysis, the treatment is considered a failure. Most centers now recommend anterior pericardectomy as the treatment of choice in this condition. Total pericardectomy is reserved for constrictive pericarditis.

Hematologic Complications

Anemia in ESRD patients is of multifactorial origin, secondary to decreased erythropoietin, blood loss from dialysis, and decreased red blood cell survival times. In addition, wide fluctuations in plasma blood volume seen in dialysis patients often cause factitious anemia. Without treatment, the hematocrit in ESRD patients usually will stabilize at 15 to 20 percent, with normocytic and normochromic red blood cells. Bone marrow will show erythroid hypoplasia, with little effect on leukopoiesis or megakaryocytopoiesis. Management of anemia is by the infusion of human recombinant erythropoietin on a regular basis. Erythropoietin replacement therapy has markedly improved the quality of life for ESRD patients by increasing exercise capacity and tolerance.

The *bleeding diathesis* seen in ESRD patients produces increased risks of GI tract bleeding, subdural hematomas, subcapsular liver hematomas, and intraocular bleeding. Abnormal hemostasis in ESRD is multifactorial in origin. Several mechanisms, including decreased platelet function, abnormal platelet-vessel wall interactions, altered von Willebrand factor, anemia, and abnormal guanidinosuccinic acid-dependent production of nitric oxide, are contributors to uremic bleeding.

The skin-bleeding test is the best predictor of clinically important defects in hemostasis. Improvements in bleeding times can be obtained by infusion of desmopressin, conjugated estrogens, and erythropoietin (see Chap. 219 for further discussion). A 6-day course of oral tranexamic acid also has been shown to result in significant shortening or normalization of bleeding time in 67 percent of uremic patients.

Immunologic deficiency in ESRD patients produces a high mortality rate from infectious diseases. Leukocyte chemotaxis and phagocytosis are depressed in uremic patients secondary to anemia, malnutrition, and zinc, selenium, and vitamin deficiency. Increased intracellular calcium concentration and low- and high-molecular-weight uremic toxins also have been proposed as a cause for impaired function.[17] Abnormal T-cell activation also has been noted in ESRD patients secondary to reduction in interleukin-2 production.

Dialysis therapy does not appear to improve the immune function of leukocytes or T cells. In fact, HD may even exacerbate immunodeficiency by complement activation after exposure to the HD filter membrane. However, addition of Vitamin E to the membrane reduces complement activation.[18] Parathyroid hormone has been proposed as the culprit in increasing the intracellular calcium concentration in uremia. Calcium channel blockers interfere with the effect of PTH on polymorphonuclear leukocytes and have been associated with improvement in metabolism and phagocytosis in neutrophils.[19]

Gastrointestinal Complications

Anorexia, nausea, and vomiting are common symptoms of uremia and often are used as an indication to initiate dialysis and to follow the adequacy of RRT. There is an increased incidence of gastritis and upper GI bleeding in ESRD patients, but the incidence of gastric and duodenal ulcers is similar in ESRD patients and the general population. The increased incidence of GI bleeding and re-bleeding and the higher mortality rates from GI hemorrhage in ESRD patients are functions more of the bleeding dyscrasias than of a primary GI disease. In addition, ESRD patients are at increased risk from bleeding from angiodysplasias. Successful prevention of recurrent bleeding from GI angiodysplasias has been obtained by use of tranexamic acid and conjugated estrogens, which decrease bleeding time.

Chronic constipation is common among ESRD patients secondary to decreased fluid intake and the use of phosphate-bonding gels. End-stage renal disease patients have an increased incidence of diverticular disease and colonic perforation, especially patients with polycystic kidney disease.

Dialysis-related ascites is an idiopathic form of ascites secondary to fluid overload, portal hypertension from polycystic liver disease, and osmotic disequilibrium. Treatment of refractory ascites is possible with peritoneovenous shunts.

Renal Bone Disease

SYSTEMIC CALCIFICATION   As the GFR falls, phosphate excretion decreases, resulting in increased serum phosphate levels. When the calcium-phosphate product [Ca (mg/dL) $\times$ PO$_4$ (mg/dL)] is greater than 70 to 80, metastatic calcification can ensue. Patients typically present with complaints of pseudogout secondary to metastatic calcification of synovial-lined joints. Metastatic calcification in small vessels results in skin and finger necrosis. Life-threatening calcifications can occur in the cardiac and pulmonary systems. An increased mortality rate has been observed in ESRD patients with a calcium-phosphate product greater than 72. Treatment consists of the use of low-calcium dialysate and phosphate-binding gels.

HYPERPARATHYROIDISM (OSTEITIS FIBROSA CYSTICA)   As ESRD progresses, the combination of calciphylaxis and vitamin D$_3$ deficiency results in depressed ionized calcium levels and stimulation of the parathyroid gland. The increased production of PTH results in high bone turnover. Patients present with weakened bones highly susceptible to fracture. In addition, patients with osteitis fibrosa cystica often complain of bone pain and muscle weakness. High alkaline phosphatase and PTH levels make the diagnosis. Treatment consists of control of serum phosphate with binding gels, vitamin D$_3$ replacement, and, if necessary, subtotal parathyroidectomy.

VITAMIN D$_3$ DEFICIENCY AND ALUMINUM INTOXICATION (OSTEOMALACIA)   A subset of ESRD patients develops osteomalacia, a defect in bone calcification. Once vitamin D$_3$ replacement became universally available, aluminum intoxication became the major cause of osteomalacia in ESRD patients. Sources of aluminum are dialysate diluent and phosphate-binding gels. The signs and symptoms are weakened bones, bone pain, and muscle weakness, similar to those for hyperparathyroidism. Osteomalacia has low-to-normal alkaline phosphatase levels and low PTH levels. Elevated serum aluminum and bone aluminum levels are useful for confirming the diagnosis. Treatment with desferrioxamine has been shown to be effective in aluminum bone disease.

β$_2$-MICROGLOBULIN AMYLOIDOSIS   Dialysis-related amyloidosis, or β$_2$-microglobulin amyloidosis, is seen commonly in dialysis patients older than 50 years and on dialysis for more than 10 years. Advanced glycation end products appear central to the chronic inflammatory condition leading to amyloidosis in ESRD patients. Amyloid deposits are found in the GI tract, bones, and joints. Complications include GI perforations, bone cysts with pathologic fractures, and arthropathies, including carpal tunnel syndrome and rotator cuff tears. Patients with amyloidosis have significantly higher mortality rates than do those without this disorder.

HEMODIALYSIS

HD in humans was made possible by the invention of the rotating-drum artificial kidney by Kolff and colleagues in 1943. Access to the patient's bloodstream was not practical until the development of the external AV shunt by Scribner in 1960. Brescia and Cimino in 1966 developed the subcutaneous AV fistula, which made HD safer and more acceptable. Renal replacement therapy became widely available after 1973, when the U.S. Congress authorized Medicare funding for the treatment of ESRD.

Technical Aspects of Hemodialysis

The nephron removes toxins and maintains internal homeostasis through an elegant combination of glomerular filtration followed by selective reabsorption and secretion of water and solutes. Hemodialysis uses the brute force techniques of ultrafiltration and clearance to replace the functions of the nephron. Hemodialysis substitutes a hemodialyzer filter for the glomerulus to produce an ultrafiltrate of plasma. Adjustment of the pressure gradient across the hemodialyzer filter during HD controls the amount of fluid removal (ultrafiltration).

Solute removal (clearance) during HD depends on the filter pore size, the amount of ultrafiltration (solute drag), and the concentration gradient across the filter (diffusion). Solute diffusion of chemical gradients from the blood to the dialysis fluid (dialysate) determines their final blood concentration. Because hemodialyzer pore size prevents the filtration of proteins, dialysate consists only of electrolytes (Na^+, K^+, Cl^-, HCO_3^-, Ca^{2+}, and Mg^{2+}) and glucose, whose concentrations are varied to control their clearance.

During HD, blood is removed from the vascular access site by large-bore needles (typically 15 gauge), circulated through the dialysis machine at rates of 300 to 500 mL per min, and returned to the patient. The dialysate usually flows at a rate of 500 to 800 mL per min through the dialysis filter in the direction opposite to blood flow. Small amounts of intravenous heparin, 1000 to 2000 units, are typically used to prevent thrombosis at the vascular access site. HD sessions typically take 3 to 4 h.

Complications of Vascular Access

Long-term successful HD depends on reliable access to the patient's circulation. In cases in which a native artery or vein are not suitable for fistula creation, an interposing vascular graft made of an autologous vein, polytetrafluoroethylene, or bovine carotid artery must be used for vascular access. These grafts generally have a higher complication rate and shorter functional life expectancies than do natural AV fistulas. The third form of vascular access for HD is tunnel-cuffed catheters (e.g., Hickman, Neostar, Quinton) placed using a surgically created tunnel. The most common site for tunnel-cuffed catheter placement is the right internal jugular vein. Because of the cuff, these catheters cannot and should not be removed by pulling. Vascular access is the Achilles heel of HD, and complications of the vascular access account for more inpatient hospital days than do any other complication of HD.

Thrombosis and stenosis of the vascular access are the most common complications. Grafts generally have a higher rate of stenosis, secondary to endothelial hyperplasia, than do fistulas. Stenosis or thrombosis presents with loss of bruit and thrill over the access. Stenosis and even thrombosis are not emergencies and can be treated within 24 h by angiographic clot removal or angioplasty. Thrombosis of vascular access can also be treated with direct injection of alteplase 2.2 mg into the access.

Vascular access infections occur in 2 to 5 percent of AV fistulas and about 10 percent of vascular grafts over their functional lifetime. Patients with an infected access often present with signs of systemic sepsis, such as fever, hypotension, or an elevated white blood cell count. Classic signs of pain, erythema, swelling, and discharge from an infected vascular access are often missing. The most common organism is *Staphylococcus aureus,* followed by gram-negative bacteria. Patients with access infections usually require hospital admission. Vancomycin is the drug of choice (1 g IV), because of its effectiveness in methicillin-resistant organisms and long half-life (5 to 7 days) in dialysis patients. An aminoglycoside (gentamicin 100 mg IV initially and after each dialysis) is usually added empirically to cover gram-negative organisms.

Hemorrhage from a vascular access can produce life-threatening blood loss. Hemorrhage can result from aneurysms, anastomosis rupture, or over-anticoagulation. Bleeding that requires the patient to come to the emergency department should immediately be controlled with digital pressure at the puncture sites for 5 to 10 min, and the patient should be observed for 1 to 2 h thereafter. Continued or life-threatening hemorrhage may require the placement of a tourniquet proximal to the access. A vascular surgeon should be consulted if bleeding cannot quickly be brought under control. If over-anticoagulation is a concern, the effects of heparin can be reversed by protamine given at a dose of 0.01 mg/units heparin dispensed during dialysis. If the dose of heparin is unknown, protamine, 10 to 20 mg, will be suf-

ficient to reverse heparin, 1000 to 2000 units. If bleeding stops, the patient should be observed for 1 to 2 h for rebleeding or thrombosis. Occasionally, a newly inserted vascular access will continue to ooze at the insertion despite pressure. Small pieces of gelfoam soaked in reconstituted thrombin can be placed onto oozing sites. Desmopressin acetate (0.3 μg/kg IV, maximum dose 20 mg) can be administered as an adjunct. If the emergency physician is unfamiliar with the use of desmopressin acetate in this situation, the nephrologist should be consulted.

Vascular access aneurysms result from repeated puncturing, leading to bulging of the wall. True aneurysms are very rare, occurring in fewer than 4 percent of fistulas or grafts. Most aneurysms are asymptomatic, with patients occasionally complaining of pain or an associated peripheral impingement neuropathy. Aneurysms rarely rupture.

Vascular access pseudoaneurysms result from subcutaneous extravasation of blood from puncture sites. Patients commonly present with bleeding and infections at access sites. Bleeding from the puncture site is usually controlled by digital pressure or a subcutaneous suture carefully placed at the puncture site. Vascular surgery may be required for continued bleeding or infection.

Vascular insufficiency of the extremity distal to the vascular access occurs in approximately 1 percent of all patients. The so-called "steal syndrome" is the result of preferential shunting of arterial blood away from nutrient arteries to the low-pressure venous side of the access. Patients present with exercise pain, nonhealing ulcers, and cool, pulseless digits. Steal syndrome is diagnosed by Doppler ultrasound or angiography and is repaired surgically.

High-output heart failure can occur when greater than 20 percent of the cardiac output is diverted through the access. Branham sign, a drop in heart rate after temporary access occlusion, is useful for detecting this complication.[20] Doppler ultrasound can accurately measure access flow rate and establish the diagnosis. Surgical banding of the access is the treatment of choice to decrease flow and treat heart failure.

Complications During Hemodialysis

Hypotension is the most frequent complication of HD, occurring during 10 to 20 percent of treatments (Table 93-2). Fluid removal during HD averages 1 to 3 L over a 4-h session, but removal of up to 2 L per h is possible. Maintenance of a normal blood pressure during ultrafiltration depends on cardiovascular compensatory mechanisms and refilling of the vascular space by fluid shifts from the interstitial and intracellular compartments. Excessive ultrafiltration from underestimation of the patient's ideal blood volume (dry weight) is the most common cause of intradialytic hypotension. In fact, dry weight is often clinically defined when hypotension prevents further fluid removal.

Cardiac compensation for fluid loss often is inhibited by diastolic dysfunction common in ESRD patients. Myocardial dysfunction from ischemia, hypoxia, arrhythmias, and early pericardial tamponade also should be included in the differential of intradialytic hypotension. Abnormalities of vascular tone during HD may occur in patients with

TABLE 93-2 Differential Diagnosis of Peridialytic Hypotension

Excessive ultrafiltration
Clearance simultaneous with ultrafiltration
Predialytic volume loss (GI losses, decreased oral intake)
Intradialytic volume loss (tube and hemodialyzer blood losses)
Postdialytic volume loss (vascular access blood loss)
Medication effects (antihypertensives, opiates)
Decreased vascular tone (sepsis, food, dialysate temperature >37°C or 98.6°F)
Cardiac dysfunction (LVH, ischemia, hypoxia, arrhythmia)
Pericardial disease (effusion, tamponade)

Abbreviations: GI = gastrointestinal; LVH = left ventricular hypertrophy.

sepsis, overproduction of nitric oxide, and antihypertensive medications. Refilling of the vascular tree can be inhibited by hypoalbuminemia and concurrent removal of solutes with ultrafiltration. Vascular refilling can be enhanced by improved nutrition, performing ultrafiltration before dialysis, and increasing the sodium concentration of the dialysate solution.

The timing of intradialytic hypotension is often helpful in the differential diagnosis. Hypotension early in the dialysis session is usually due to pre-existing hypovolemia. Predialysis losses should be suspected when the patient starts HD below their dry weight and is usually due to GI bleeding, sepsis, vomiting, diarrhea, or decreased intake of salt and water. Intradialytic blood loss can occur from blood tubing or hemodialyzer filter leaks. Hypotension near the end of dialysis is usually the result of excessive ultrafiltration, but pericardial or cardiac disease is still a possibility.

Intradialytic hypotension produces nausea, vomiting, and anxiety. Orthostatic hypotension, tachycardia, dizziness, and even syncope may occur. Treatment of intradialytic hypotension includes halting HD and placing the patient in the Trendelenburg position. If hypotension persists, the patient is given salt by mouth (broth) or NS, 100 to 200 mL IV. If these conservative measures fail, excessive ultrafiltration is very unlikely, and a more extensive evaluation is justified. These patients are commonly transferred to the ED for further evaluation.

The emergency physician should focus on immediate and potential life threats. The patient should be evaluated for adequacy of volume status, impairment of cardiac function, pericardial disease, infection, and GI bleeding. All of these entities may be producing or contributing to hypotension. Remember that estimation of the patient's blood volume by clinical criteria has already failed in the dialysis unit. The decision to undertake further volume expansion or administer vasopressors to support blood pressure may require invasive hemodynamic monitoring in an intensive care setting.

Dialysis disequilibrium is a clinical syndrome occurring at the end of dialysis and is characterized by nausea, vomiting, and hypertension, which can progress to seizure, coma, and death. This syndrome should be distinguished from other neurologic disorders, such as subdural hematoma, stroke, hypertensive crisis, hypoxia, and seizures. Dialysis disequilibrium is produced when large solute clearances occur during HD, as during the patient's first dialysis session or in hypercatabolic patients. The cause of dialysis disequilibrium is believed to be cerebral edema from an osmolar imbalance between the brain and the blood. During high solute removal, the blood has a transiently lower osmolality than the brain, favoring water movement into the brain and causing cerebral edema. This condition can be prevented by limiting solute clearance when initiating HD. Treatment consists of stopping dialysis and administering mannitol IV to increase serum osmolality.

Air embolism is always a risk when blood is pumped through an extracorporeal circuit. The clinical presentation depends on the patient's body habitus at the time of the air embolism. If the patient was sitting, air will pass retrogradely through the internal jugular vein to the cerebral circulation, causing neurologic symptoms due to increase intracranial pressure. In a recumbent position, air will go into the right ventricle and pulmonary circulation, causing pulmonary hypertension and systemic hypotension. The passage of air through a right-to-left (e.g., patent foramen ovale) creates an arterial air embolism, which can lodge in the coronary or cerebral circulation, causing myocardial infarction or stoke.

Patients with an air embolism typically present with symptoms of acute dyspnea, chest tightness, and unconsciousness, sometimes progressing to full cardiac arrest. Physical examination may show cyanosis and a churning sound in the heart from air bubbles in the blood.

Treatment consists of clamping the venous bloodline and placing the patient supine. Traditional recommendations have often included the Trendelenburg position with the left side down, presumably to favor air trapping in the right ventricle. However, experimental and anecdotal clinical evidence does not indicate any special benefit of this position. Oxygen, administered by 100 percent non-rebreather mask, should be applied to aid reabsorption of the air. Other suggested therapies for vascular air embolism include percutaneous aspiration of air from the right ventricle, intravenous steroids, full heparinization, and hyperbaric oxygen treatment.

Electrolyte abnormalities can occur from errors in mixing the dialysate concentrate with water, resulting in rapid osmolar shifts and hemolysis. In some communities, water contains high concentrations of calcium and magnesium and produces a final dialysate high in these minerals. This dialysate can result in the "hard water syndrome," characterized by clinically significant hypercalcemia and hypermagnesemia in HD patients. These patients present with nausea, vomiting, headaches, burning skin, muscle weakness, lethargy, and hypertension. Treatment consists of properly filtering the dialysis water to lower calcium and magnesium concentrations.

Hypoglycemia has been reported in diabetic and nondiabetic ESRD patients. In addition to drug-induced hypoglycemia, malnutrition and sepsis are important causes of hypoglycemia that carry significant mortality.[21]

Evaluation of Hemodialysis Patients

Patients on HD may present to the ED for complications related to their ESRD or HD, or these conditions may be incidental to the reason for the visit. The medical history is very important in HD patients, because many of the same diseases that caused ESRD (e.g., hypertension, diabetes, etc.) persist after the patient's kidneys have failed. Questions should be asked about the patient's ESRD and HD (Table 93-3). Repeated episodes of intradialytic hypotension may provide important early clues to pericardial tamponade or myocardial ischemia. Repeated access infections may represent a worsening immunologic status.

Patients should be asked about their HD schedule. Most HD patients in the United States are on an every-other-day schedule (Monday, Wednesday, and Friday or Tuesday, Thursday, and Saturday), with each session lasting approximately 4 h. Certain centers have begun using high-flux HD machines with higher blood flows, allowing shorter HD sessions. The physician should document all recent missed sessions and the patient's explanations for missing them. Such history taking may provide important clues concerning worsening medical or social issues that need to be addressed outside the patient's chief complaint.

Dialysis patients are often quite knowledgeable about their dry weights and baseline laboratory test results. If the patient is not forthcoming with these data, the emergency physician can contact the HD center and ask about the dry weight, average interdialytic weight gains, and any recent HD complications. In addition, the dialysis nurses and technicians are very devoted to their patients and can provide a great deal of "soft data" concerning the patient. Query the patient in detail with regard to uremic symptoms as markers of inadequate HD. Patients should be asked whether they retain their native kidneys, which can be continued sources of hypertension, infection, and nephrolithiasis.

The physical examination of HD patients should always include a careful examination of the vascular access (Table 93-4). The vascular

TABLE 93-3   Key Historical Elements for Hemodialysis Patients

Etiology of ESRD
Dialysis schedule: any missed dialysis sessions?
Recent complications of HD
Dry weight, baseline laboratory values, and vital signs
Average intradialytic weight gain
Does patient usually make dry weight by end of HD?
Does patient experience intradialysis hypotension? (Timing of hypotension?)
Which vascular access is currently functioning?
Symptoms of uremia
Retention of native kidneys?
Still producing urine?

Abbreviations: ESRD = end-stage renal disease; HD = hemodialysis.

TABLE 93-4 Key Elements of Physical Examination of Hemodialysis Patients

Vital signs
Vascular access: bruit, thrill, erythema, warmth, swelling, tenderness, discharge, bleeding, Branham's sign
Cardiac: signs of heart failure, murmurs, muffled (distant) heart sounds
Neurologic: mental status, peripheral neuropathy, and asterixis

access is the patient's lifeline and Achilles heel, complications of which are responsible for the majority of ESRD inpatient days. Flow through the access can be established by the presence of a bruit and thrill over the access site. The classic signs of infection, erythema, swelling, tenderness, and purulent discharge, are commonly limited until the infection is far advanced. The bedside Branham sign may detect patients with CHF due to high-output fistula-related heart failure. The cardiac examination of HD patients deserves some special attention. Signs of CHF, such as peripheral edema, HJR, and JVD, may misleadingly suggest the diagnosis of fluid overload when pericardial tamponade is present. A loud cardiac murmur in HD patients may just represent increased flow secondary to anemia or the AV access. Neurologic dysfunction in HD patients is generally diffuse and nonfocal. Any findings suggestive of a focal neurologic deficit should be investigated for structural, vascular, and infectious causes. Rectal examination to detect GI bleeding is always recommended.

PERITONEAL DIALYSIS

Ganter accomplished the first PD in 1923. Practical long-term RRT with PD did not become available until 1976, when Popovich and Moncrief worked out the basic concepts of continuous ambulatory peritoneal dialysis (CAPD). Their work was significantly aided by the development of a practical silicon rubber catheter by Tenckhoff in 1968, which is still in use today. Because of its simplicity, PD is the most common form of RRT used outside the United States and Canada.

Technical Aspects of Peritoneal Dialysis

Similarly to HD, PD relies on the separate processes of clearance (solute removal) and ultrafiltration (fluid removal) to replace the functions of the nephron. In PD, the peritoneal membrane serves as the blood-dialysate interface. Most solute removal occurs via diffusion down chemical gradients established by altering dialysate electrolyte concentrations. The amount of ultrafiltration is determined by osmotic pressure differences between the blood and dialysate, which are manipulated by changing the dialysate glucose concentration. Dialysate is supplied in a 1.5 or 4.25 percent glucose formulation, which can be alternated to increase or decrease ultrafiltration.

Typical CAPD regimens use four exchanges daily, with 2 L of dialysate infused and left in place for several hours before draining. During the day, approximately 8 L is infused and about 10 L is drained, for a removal of approximately 2 L per d of fluid. Peritoneal dialysis can be accomplished in an acute setting, chronically via exchanges of solution throughout the day (CAPD), or through multiple exchanges at night while the patient sleeps (continuous cyclic peritoneal dialysis).

Complications of CAPD

Peritonitis is the most common complication of PD. The incidence of peritonitis is about one episode every 15 to 18 patient-months. Mortality rates with peritonitis have been reported as between 2.5 and 12.5 percent, depending on the center studied. Symptoms and signs of peritonitis in PD patients are no different from those for other patients with peritonitis: fever, abdominal pain, and rebound tenderness. Cloudy effluent suggests the diagnosis of peritonitis. Patients often will bring in a sample of the cloudy dialysate fluid, which should be

sent for cell count, Gram's stain, and culture. The cell count in PD-related peritonitis is usually more than 100 leukocytes, with more than 50 percent neutrophils. Results of the Gram stain are positive in only 10 to 40 percent of cases of culture-proven PD-related peritonitis. Organisms isolated in PD-related peritonitis are *Staphylococcus epidermidis* (about 40 percent), *S. aureus* (10 percent), *Streptococcus* species (15 to 20 percent), gram-negative bacteria (15 to 20 percent), anaerobic bacteria (5 percent), and fungi (5 percent).

Empiric therapy should begin with a few rapid exchanges of fluid lavaged quickly in and out to decrease the number of inflammatory cells in the peritoneum. The addition of heparin (500 to 1000 U/L dialysate) will decrease fibrin clot formation. Empiric antibiotics are selected to treat the expected gram-positive and gram-negative organisms. Peritonitis related to PD can be treated with antibiotics added to the dialysate; parenteral administration is not required. A first-generation cephalosporin (e.g., cephalothin) can be mixed with the dialysate, 500 mg/L with the first exchange and 200 mg/L with subsequent exchanges. In penicillin-allergic patients, vancomycin can be substituted, with an initial dose of 500 mg/L and maintenance doses of 50 mg/L per exchange. Gentamicin can be added, with a loading dose of 100 mg/L and maintenance doses of 4 to 8 mg/L per exchange. Most protocols recommend treating for 7 days after the first negative culture results, usually for a total of 10 days. The decision to admit these patients or treat them as outpatients is a clinical decision based on how ill the patient appears.

Infections around a PD catheter are much less well defined than peritonitis. Patients present with pain, erythema, swelling, and discharge around the catheter exit site. The most common bacteria are *S. aureus* and *Pseudomonas aeruginosa*. Empiric therapy consists of a first-generation cephalosporin or ciprofloxacin for outpatient therapy. Patients should be referred back to their CAPD centers for follow-up the next day.

Abdominal wall hernias occur in 10 to 15 percent of PD patients. The literature recommends immediate surgical repair of pericatheter hernias, which have the highest risk of developing an incarceration.

Evaluation of Peritoneal Dialysis Patient

When a PD patient arrives in the emergency department, certain historical elements are important (Table 93-5). As with HD patients, the disease that caused the renal failure frequently persists. The type of PD and the person who performs the daily care may provide information about the risks of infection. The date of the patient's last episode of peritonitis should be ascertained; frequent relapses may signify a fungal etiology or tunnel infection. The patient should be asked about baseline weight and laboratory values; PD patients are selected for their knowledge about their condition and their ability to perform the procedure and monitor their care away from professional supervision. Weight gain may signal heart failure from ischemia or pericardial effusion. Weight gain also may be from ultrafiltration failure, a late sign of peritonitis.

The physical examination of PD patients should focus on the abdomen. The physician should focus on signs of infection of the peritoneum, tunnel, and exit site (Table 93-6).

TABLE 93-5 Key Historical Elements for Peritoneal Dialysis Patients

Etiology of ESRD
Type of peritoneal dialysis (CAPD vs. CCPD)
PD schedule: concentration, number of exchanges per day
Recent complications of PD
Baseline weight, laboratory values, and vital signs
Symptoms of uremia
Retention of native kidneys?
Still producing urine?

Abbreviations: CAPD = continuous ambulatory peritoneal dialysis; CCPD = continuous cyclic peritoneal dialysis; ESRD = end-stage renal disease; PD = peritoneal dialysis.

TABLE 93-6   Key Elements of Physical Examination of Peritoneal Dialysis Patients

Abdominal examination: inspection for hernia, auscultation of bowel sounds, test for rebound tenderness

Peritoneal catheter: examination of surrounding skin, palpation of tunnel

REFERENCES

1. U.S. Renal Data System: *USRDS 2001 Annual Data Report: Atlas of End-Stage Renal Disease in the United States.* Bethesda, MD, National Institutes of Health, National Institute of Diabetes and Digestive and Kidney Diseases, 2001. (*The data reported here have been supplied by the USRDS. The interpretation and reporting of these data are the responsibility of the author(s) and in no way should be seen as an official policy or interpretation of the U.S. government.*)
2. Bricker NS: On the pathogenesis of the uremic state: An exposition of the "trade-off" hypothesis. *New Engl J Med* 286:1093, 1972.
3. Miyata T, van Ypersele de Strihou C, et al: Alterations in nonenzymatic biochemistry in uremia: Origin and significance of "carbonyl stress" in long-term uremic complications. *Kidney Int* 55:389, 1999.
4. Miyata T, Ueda Y, Yoshida A, et al: Clearance of pentosidine, an advanced glycation end product, by different modalities of renal replacement therapy. *Kidney Int* 51:880, 1997.
5. Schmidt M, Sitter T, Lederer SR, et al: Reversible MRI changes in a patient with uremic encephalopathy. *J Nephrol* 14:424, 2001.
6. Mansouri B, Adybeig B, Rayegani M, et al: Uremic neuropathy and the analysis of electrophysiological changes. *Electromyogr Clin Neurophysiol* 41:107, 2001.
7. Straver B, De Vries PM, ten Voorde BJ, et al: Intradialytic hypotension in relation to pre-existent autonomic dysfunction in hemodialysis patients. *Int J Artif Organs* 21:794, 1998.
8. Stojceva-Taneva O, Majin G, Polenakovic M, et al: Autonomic nervous system dysfunction and volume nonresponsive hypotension in hemodialysis patients. *Am J Nephrol* 11:123, 1991.
9. Vita G, Savica V, Puglisi RM, et al: The course of autonomic neural function in chronic uraemic patients during haemodialysis treatment. *Nephrol Dial Transplant* 7:1022, 1992.
10. Levey AS, Eknoyan G: Cardiovascular disease in chronic renal disease. *Nephrol Dial Transplant* 14:828, 1999.
11. Kitiyakara C, Gonin J, Massy Z, Wilcox CS: Non-traditional cardiovascular disease risk factors in end-stage renal disease: Oxidate stress and hyperhomocystinemia. *Curr Opin Nephrol Hypertens* 9:477, 2000.
12. Tun A, Khan IA, Win MT, et al: Specificity of cardiac troponin I and creatine kinase-MB isoenzyme in asymptomatic long-term hemodialysis patients and effect of hemodialysis on these cardiac markers. *Cardiology* 90:280, 1998.
13. Aviles RJ, Askari AT, Lindahl B, et al: Troponin T levels in patients with acute coronary syndromes, with or without renal dysfunction. *New Engl J Med* 346:2047, 2002.
14. Hruby, ZW,Kuzniar J, Szewczyk Z: Captopril in temporary, non-dialytic management of pulmonary edema in end-stage renal disease. *Mater Med Pol* 21:134, 1989.
15. Russo D, Memoli B, Andreucci VE: The place of loop diuretics in the treatment of acute and chronic renal failure. *Clin Nephrol* 38(suppl 1):S69, 1992.
16. Eiser AR, Lieber JJ, Neff MS: Phlebotomy for pulmonary edema in dialysis patients. *Clin Nephrol* 47:47, 1997.
17. Horl WH: Neutrophil function and infections in uremia. *Am J Kidney Dis* 33:xlv, 1999.
18. Tsuruoka S, Kawaguchi A, Nishiki K, et al: Vitamin E-bonded hemodialyzer improves neutrophil function and oxidative stress in patients with end-stage renal failure. *Am J Kidney Dis* 39:127, 2002.
19. Massry S, Smogorzewski M: Dysfunction of polymorphonuclear leukocytes in uremia: Role of parathyroid hormone. *Kidney Int* 78(suppl):S195, 2001.
20. Longo T, Brusoni B, Merlo L, Marchetti GV: Haemodynamics at rest and under effort in chronic arteriovenous fistulae (AVFs). *J Cardiovasc Surg (Torino)* 18:509, 1977.
21. Haviv YS, Sharkia M, Safadi R: Hypoglycemia in patients with renal failure. *Ren Fail* 22:219, 2000.

URINARY TRACT INFECTIONS
David S. Howes
Mark P. Bogner

Urinary tract infection (UTI) is defined as significant bacteriuria in the presence of symptoms, such as painful urination (dysuria), hematuria, increased urinary frequency, urgency, hesitancy, suprapubic discomfort, and costovertebral angle (CVA) tenderness. Uncomplicated acute UTI in otherwise healthy, nonpregnant, nonobstructed young females is generally regarded as a benign illness if treated appropriately. Conversely, there can be very significant long-term sequelae of UTI, in particular recurrent or obstructive UTI, in pregnant patients, children, older patients, and patients with significant comorbidities (e.g., human immunodeficiency virus and acquired immunodeficiency syndrome [HIV/AIDS], diabetes mellitus, or other chronic illnesses). In the elderly population, UTI is a major cause of nosocomial gram-negative sepsis, with a significant associated mortality rate.

Many classification schemes exist and are used to describe UTI. As the above discussion suggests, one practical scheme is to divide UTI into two major categories, complicated and uncomplicated. The distinction is clinically useful, because extensive testing and anatomic evaluation are rarely necessary in cases of uncomplicated UTI. However, increasing resistance to traditional first-line antibiotics require attention to local resistance patterns when selecting antibiotics to treat uncomplicated UTI. Conversely, complicated UTI often poses significant challenges in diagnosis and treatment to account for other host factors and comorbidities contributing to the expected potential severity and sequelae of the infection.

EPIDEMIOLOGY

Urinary tract infection affects an estimated 20 percent of women at some point in their lives, and in the United States accounts for at least 1 million emergency department visits, 7 million office visits, and 100,000 hospitalizations every year. It is the second most common form of infection, representing up to 25 percent of all infections and more than 20 percent of all hospital acquired infections. The estimated U.S. annual cost of community-acquired UTI is approximately 1.6 billion dollars.[1]

The epidemiology of UTI differs with age and sex. There are four groups at increased risk for infection: neonates, girls, young women, and older men. In neonates, a UTI occurs more often in males (1.5:1 male:female ratio) and is often part of the syndrome of gram-negative sepsis. The incidence of UTI in preschool children is approximately 2 percent, and the incidence in girls is at least 10 times greater than the incidence in boys. In school-age children, UTI incidence rises to 5 percent, almost exclusively occurring in girls. The incidence of infection in postmenopausal women also increases with age. The prevalence of bacteriuria among elderly women in nursing homes exceeds 40 percent.

Bacteriuria is rare in males younger than 50 years, and symptoms of dysuria or urinary frequency are usually due to a sexually transmitted disease-related infection of the urethra or prostate. However, in men older than 50 years, the incidence of UTI rises dramatically, because of prostatic obstruction or subsequent instrumentation. By their eighth decade over one-third of men will have had an episode of bacteriuria and one-fourth will have been diagnosed with prostatitis.[2]

Dysuria in females is a common symptom and usually due to infection. Urinary tract infection is a frequent problem in otherwise healthy young women, and the incidence of UTI in this population has been shown to increase as a result of the following risk factors: sexual activity, specifically increased intercourse frequency in the past month; spermicide and/or diaphragm use; a new sex partner within the past 12 months; age younger than 15 years at first UTI; and history of UTI in the patient's mother.[3] Conversely, oral contraceptive use independent of sexual activity, personal hygiene habits, and postcoital voiding have not been clearly demonstrated as significant risk factors for UTI.[3] The relation between intercourse and UTI is sufficiently strong that recurrent UTI has been proposed as a possible marker for teenage sex.

The infecting organisms in UTI are generally those found colonizing the perineum. In women with a traditional "positive" culture of 10^5 colony-forming units (CFU) per milliliter of urine, *Escherichia coli* is responsible for approximately 80 to 90 percent of infections. However, up to one-half of cases of dysuria in young women is characterized by low bacterial concentration (10^2 to 10^4 CFU/mL), which has been termed the *acute urethral syndrome*. It is now believed that these patients have low-grade or early urinary tract infection due to *E. coli*, *Staphylococcus saprophyticus,* or *Chlamydia trachomatis*. The more than 10^5 CFU/mL definition for UTI was based on studies of upper urinary tract infection that established this degree of bacterial concentration as indicative of "significant bacteriuria." Subsequent research suggested that, with regard to lower urinary tract infections in the presence of symptoms, a colony count of at least 100 CFU/mL may represent significant bacteriuria and merit treatment.

Asymptomatic bacteriuria (ABU) is defined by the presence of more than 10^5 CFU/mL of one bacterial species on two successive urine cultures in a patient without symptoms. This requirement for two positive cultures is to eliminate those individuals with transient colonization of the urinary tract. Asymptomatic bacteriuria occurs in up to 30 percent of pregnant women and in up to 40 percent of female nursing-home residents. Asymptomatic bacteriuria is also common in patients with indwelling urinary catheters and disorders that prevent complete emptying of the bladder. In otherwise healthy, nonpregnant, sexually active women ages 18 through 40 years, the prevalence of ABU is approximately 5 percent.[4] Persistence of ABU is uncommon; however, the presence of ABU is a strong predictor of subsequent UTI, which occurs within 1 week approximately eight times more frequently in patients with ABU than in those without ABU.[4]

Urinary tract infections in women recur because of relapse or reinfection. Relapse is caused by the same organism, and symptoms recurring within 1 month represent treatment failure. When symptoms recur in 1 to 6 months, it is generally due to reinfection. Reinfection is usually from a different enteric organism or a different serotype of the same organism, and may represent a defect in the defense mechanisms of the host. If a patient has a cluster of infections with more than three recurrences in 1 year, a more complete workup may be warranted to look for the presence of structural abnormalities, tumor, renal calculi, or associated systemic illness, such as diabetes mellitus.

Urinary tract infection during pregnancy poses special problems. If untreated, ABU may progress to symptomatic UTI or pyelonephritis, especially in the third trimester, and may lead to preeclampsia, sepsis, or miscarriage. This is the single setting in which treatment of ABU is definitely indicated.[5]

PATHOPHYSIOLOGY

Uncomplicated UTI is generally thought of as UTI occurring in otherwise healthy, young, female, sexually active but nonpregnant patients without an underlying defect in urinary anatomy or renal function.[6] Most other cases will fall under the classification of complicated UTI: occurring in patients with underlying renal or neurologic disease, ureteral stone or other obstructive pathology; recurrent UTI history, pregnancy, advanced or very young age, impaired immune function (e.g., HIV/AIDS, chemotherapy patients), and other significant co-morbidities. The most common urinary pathogen remains *E. coli* (Table 94-1). Uropathogenic organisms often have adhesins, fibrillae, or pili that allow for bacterial adherence to the uroepithelium. Anaerobic organisms do not grow well in urine and are rarely pathogenic. Whereas complicated UTIs can be caused by *E. coli,* they are more likely to be caused by unusual pathogens, such as *Pseudomonas* spp. or enterococcus.

TABLE 94-1 Etiologic Agents in Uncomplicated Urinary Tract Infection

Organism	Incidence
Escherichia coli	>80%
Klebsiella spp.	5–20%
Proteus spp.	5–20%
Enterobacter spp.	5–20%
Pseudomonas spp.	5–20%
Group D streptococci	<5%
*Chlamydia trachomatis**	<5%
*Staphylococcus saprophyticus**	<5%

*Much more common in the "dysuria pyuria" syndrome in which sterile or low colony count culture results are obtained. *Staphylococcus saprophyticus* may account for up to 15% of acute lower tract infection in young, sexually active females but rarely progresses to involve the upper tract.

Depending on its pH and chemical constituents, urine is generally a good culture medium. Factors unfavorable to bacterial growth are a low pH (≤ 5.5); a high concentration of urea; and the presence of organic acids derived from a diet including fruit juice and methionine, a breakdown product of ingested protein that enhances acidification of the urine. A thin film of urine remains in the bladder after voiding. An intact bladder mucosa removes organisms from the film, probably by the production of organic acids by the mucosal cells and not by antibody formation or phagocytosis. Incomplete bladder emptying renders this mechanism ineffective and is responsible for the increased frequency of infection in patients with a neurogenic bladder and in postmenopausal women with bladder or uterine prolapse. The latter group also has marked changes in vaginal microflora due to lack of estrogen, with loss of lactobacilli and increased colonization by *E. coli*.

Frequent and complete voiding has been associated with the reduction in recurrence of UTI.[7] Studies have found that the concentration of bacteria in the bladder may increase tenfold after sexual intercourse due to a "milking action" of the female urethra during intercourse. The use of a diaphragm and spermicide is also associated with recurrent UTI, probably because the spermicide enhances vaginal colonization with *E. coli*.[3,4,6] It has long been recommended, although unproved, that prompt voiding after intercourse may lessen the frequency of UTI.[7]

Susceptibility to UTIs may have a genetic basis. Women who do not secrete blood group antigens (nonsecretors) have been shown to have a higher incidence of recurrent infection. This higher incidence appears to be due to the presence of specific uroepithelial cell *E. coli*-binding glycolipids that promote fecal coliform colonization of the vagina.[6]

Most UTIs occur as one of three clinical syndromes: acute cystitis, subclinical pyelonephritis, or acute pyelonephritis. The simplest and most common UTI is acute cystitis, in which infection is isolated to the bladder. Competent ureteral valves prevent ascent of the bacteria into the kidneys in most cases.

Subclinical pyelonephritis is characterized by bacterial infection in the upper urinary tract and detected by bladder washout techniques, selective ureteral catheterization, or the presence of antibody-coated bacteria in the urine. However, subclinical pyelonephritis is clinically indistinguishable from acute cystitis, and it has been estimated that approximately 25 to 30 percent of patients with the acute cystitis syndrome actually have subclinical pyelonephritis. Several epidemiologic factors correlate with increased risk for subclinical pyelonephritis: lower socioeconomic status; pregnancy; structural urinary tract abnormality; urinary stone; history of relapse after treatment for a UTI; prior history of acute pyelonephritis; frequent UTIs; symptoms lasting longer than 7 days; or diabetes or other immunosuppressing conditions.[6,10]

Acute pyelonephritis is characterized by the presence of bacteria in the kidney with localized pain and CVA tenderness, with systemic symptoms of infection (fever, chills, nausea, vomiting, and prostration). The infective process of acute pyelonephritis can progress into three patterns of renal infection not commonly considered part of the UTI spectrum: acute bacterial nephritis, renal abscess, and emphysematous pyelonephritis.[8] These tend to be diagnoses made on imaging studies performed on patients who have an inadequate or atypical response to treatment for presumed acute pyelonephritis. On ultrasound or computed tomography, acute pyelonephritis is seen as a diffusely enlarged kidney without focal abnormalities. Acute bacterial nephritis produces ill-defined focal areas, sometimes striated or wedge-shaped, of decreased density.[8] Renal abscesses appear as well-defined areas of decreased density. Emphysematous pyelonephritis is a rare gas-forming infection within the kidney, nearly always occurring in diabetics (70 to 90 percent of patients).[9] These patients usually have symptoms and signs of a severe infection, often with dehydration and pyelonephritis.[9] Nephrectomy is required to adequately treat emphysematous pyelonephritis.

CLINICAL FEATURES

The presence of four specific symptoms and one sign has been shown to significantly increase the clinical probability of UTI: dysuria, frequency, visible (gross) hematuria, and CVA tenderness. Conversely, the probability of UTI is significantly decreased in the absence of dysuria and/or back pain, particularly if the patient complains of vaginal discharge or irritation or has vaginal discharge on physical examination.[10] Self-diagnosis also has been shown to significantly increase the probability of UTI.[11]

Unfortunately, the correlation between symptoms and the presence of infection is inexact, because only 50 to 60 percent of women with dysuria have significant bacteriuria. Internal dysuria, a burning suprapubic pain during urination associated with bladder tenderness, is more associated with UTIs than is external dysuria, the burning sensation as urine passes over inflamed perineal tissue. In females, external dysuria or a history of vaginal discharge or irritation more often is associated with vaginitis, cervicitis, or pelvic inflammatory disease than with a UTI. The presence of specific symptom combinations (e.g., dysuria and frequency) and the absence of vaginal discharge or irritation increase the probability of uncomplicated UTI in otherwise healthy, nonpregnant, sexually active young women to approximately 90 percent. It is important to note that, when a patient presents with one or more of these symptoms, further history, physical examination, and urinalysis cannot provide sufficient strength of evidence to lower the posttest probability of UTI to a point where it can be safely "ruled out." As such, these data support the case for empiric treatment of uncomplicated UTI in selected cases (discussed later).[10]

Flank pain, costovertebral angle tenderness, or specific renal tenderness to deep palpation may be associated with cystitis because of referred pain. However, when these findings occur in association with fever, chills, nausea, vomiting, and prostration, the clinical diagnosis is acute pyelonephritis.

In the male, dysuria with a urethral discharge indicates urethritis.[1,6] Gram stain of the discharge may reveal gram-negative intracellular diplococci, which is virtually diagnostic of gonococcal urethritis. If Gram stain is inconclusive, the diagnosis is most likely nonspecific urethritis, which is mainly chlamydial or another sexually transmitted infection. In both cases, laboratory tests for gonorrhea and chlamydia should be obtained and possibly a serologic test for syphilis. It should be emphasized to the emergency department triage personnel that UTI in young adult males is extremely rare; therefore, a urine specimen should not be obtained until after examination by a physician. On the one hand, withholding urination may enhance the likelihood of a positive urethral swab in the male patient with minimal discharge. On the other hand, several investigators have demonstrated that the presence of urinary leukocytes is more sensitive than urethral Gram stain in detecting patients who were later found to have chlamydial infection as confirmed by culture. If bacteriuria is present and not clinically associated with urethritis or prostatitis, then treatment, followed by urologic referral, is indicated.

DIAGNOSIS

Independent predictors of a UTI in a patient with dysuria include advanced age, history of a prior UTI, back pain, pyuria, hematuria, and bacteriuria.[10] Among sexually active women, the incidence of symptomatic UTIs is high, and the risk is independently associated with sexual intercourse, use of spermicides and/or a diaphragm, and previous history of a UTI.[3,4,7]

The first step in diagnosis is the careful collection of urine for a urinalysis and potentially for culture. The midstream voiding specimen is as accurate as urine obtained by catheterization if the patient is given and follows careful instructions. Instruct the woman to remove her underwear, sit facing the back of the toilet, spread the labia with one hand, cleanse from front to back with antiseptic towelettes or swabs, pass a small amount of urine into the toilet, and then urinate into a sterile cup. Instruct the man to carefully clean the urethral meatus, retract the foreskin if present, and obtain a midstream specimen, as described above.

If the sample is properly collected, it should contain no or few epithelial cells. The many sources of contamination include material in the collection bottle, menses, vaginal discharge, urethral or periurethral tissue, and organisms multiplying in the urine after collection. Bacteria in urine double each hour at room temperature; therefore, urine should be refrigerated if not sent directly to the laboratory. In addition to special care in cleaning, the use of a tampon helps women to obtain a clean-catch specimen if menstruation or profuse discharge is present.

Catheterization is indicated if the patient cannot void spontaneously, is too ill or immobilized, or is extremely obese. It also may be performed as part of a urologic evaluation and to relieve obstruction. Many researchers have promoted the ease and accuracy of "minicath" kits to obtain urine in women, especially with a vaginal discharge or bleeding. However, unnecessary catheterization should be avoided because 1 to 2 percent of patients develop UTI after one catheter insertion, especially if it is done just before delivery in pregnant patients.

Visual inspection or the smell of the urine is generally not helpful in determining infection. Cloudiness is usually not due to white blood cells (WBCs) or bacteria, but to large amounts of protein or amorphous phosphate crystals. Malodorous urine may be caused by diet or medications and is not a reliable sign of infection.

Current emphasis is on the detection of pyuria and bacteriuria in the initial examination of the urine to confirm the diagnosis of a UTI. However, the assessment of pyuria is imperfect. Variables include the specific gravity of the urine, method of centrifuging the specimen, the amount of supernatant in which the sediment is resuspended, and the final volume of urine under the coverslip that is examined. Laboratories that use a WBC counting chamber diminish some of this variability and increase accuracy in assessing centrifuged and non-centrifuged urine. When using a WBC counting chamber, abnormal pyuria can be defined as the presence of at least eight leukocytes per milliliter of non-centrifuged urine. This figure roughly corresponds to two to five leukocytes per high-power field (HPF; or 400×) from a centrifuged specimen.

Whereas some investigators feel that low-level pyuria (<10 WBCs/HPF) is clinically important, others have suggested that pyuria in women is significant only if there are more than 10 WBCs/HPF, and only if bacteria are also present on the microscopic examination. Although the combination of pyuria and bacteriuria is likely to be true with typical coliform infection, lower degrees of pyuria with or without bacteriuria may be significant, especially with regard to infection with *Chlamydia*.

It is clear that women with symptoms and low-level pyuria (<10 WBCs/HPF) do have significant infection that will symptomatically and bacteriologically respond to antimicrobial therapy. In the past, these women were not treated initially, and their cultures often did not contain more than 10^5 CFU/mL. Sensitivity to causes of lower UTI other than typical coliforms has brought the designation of the *dysuria-pyuria syndrome* (also referred to as the *acute urethral syndrome*), which almost always benefits from treatment.[1,6] It is in this subgroup of women that the urinalysis may well be more useful than the urine culture. In addition, if the patient has dysuria-pyuria syndrome caused by *Chlamydia* infection, then the urine culture will be negative in any case.

In men, more than 1 to 2 WBCs/HPF can be significant in the presence of bacteria.[2,6] It must be remembered that urethritis and prostatitis are far more likely causes of pyuria in young males who are sexually active and complain of dysuria, regardless of the presence or absence of urethral discharge.

Bacteriuria is also felt to be a sensitive tool for detection of UTI in the symptomatic patient. **The presence of any bacteria on a Gram stain of non-centrifuged urine (more than one bacterium per oil-power field, or 1000×) is significant** and strongly correlates with culture results of more than 10^5 CFU/mL. For Gram-stained centrifuged specimens, more than 15 bacteria/oil-power field (1000×) are significant. Both methods fail to detect low colony-count UTI or infection caused by *Chlamydia*. False-positive results can occur when vaginal or fecal contamination is present.

Several studies have evaluated urinary dipstick nitrite and leukocyte esterase tests in the diagnosis of UTIs and correlated the results with urinalysis.[12,13] The urine nitrite reaction has a very high specificity (>90 percent), and a positive result is very useful in confirming the diagnosis of a UTI and is highly predictive of the absence of pure enterococcal bacteriuria.[13] Unfortunately urine nitrite sensitivity is low (about 50 percent), rendering it much less useful as a screening examination, and a negative result does not exclude the diagnosis of a UTI. Initial reports of high sensitivity (nearly 88 percent) for leukocyte esterase as a screening tool for pyuria were obtained in symptomatic women with high levels of pyuria. Studies from the emergency department found a low sensitivity (48 percent) for leukocyte esterase with more common levels of pyuria (6 to 20 WBCs/HPF). Fortunately, specificity for leukocyte esterase is good (80 to 90 percent). In summary, a positive urinary dipstick nitrite or leukocyte esterase test supports the diagnosis of UTI, but a negative test does not exclude it.

Sometimes, women will have dysuria, without pyuria or demonstrable pathogen on culture, and will not respond to antimicrobial treatment. The absence of pyuria in these patients is useful, because it indicates that antimicrobial treatment is probably unnecessary. Presuming that vulvovaginitis or cervicitis (gonorrhea, chlamydia, and herpes) has been excluded, causes of dysuria may include inflammation of the urethra from physical trauma or due to the use of chemical agents, such as spermicides, cleansing douches, or other feminine hygiene products.

In a symptomatic patient who has fewer than 2 to 5 WBCs/HPF, other causes of false-negative pyuria should be considered, such as ingestion of large amounts of fluids, which washes out the bladder and produces a dilute urine; systemic leukopenia; or self-medication with consequent partly treated UTI-caused by patients often using old or leftover medications from previous UTIs or medications prescribed to another person. It should be remembered that pyuria may be intermittent or absent if the patient has an obstructed and infected kidney.

For the patient with typical symptoms of an uncomplicated UTI and a "positive" urinalysis evident as pyuria on microscopic examination, positive leukocyte esterase test, bacteriuria on Gram stain, and/or positive urine nitrite test, urine culture is not required. The vast majority of these patients respond to empiric therapy. In fact, a current trend in the diagnosis and treatment of uncomplicated UTI is to treat on the basis of history alone and without obtaining any urine tests, in many cases by telephone management and self-diagnosis or "patient-initiated treatment" protocols, which have been shown to be at least as effective as traditional approaches, less expensive, more convenient for patients, and without deterioration in quality of care.[14,15] Given the frequency of visits to clinics and emergency departments for UTI and the enormous cost of diagnosing and treating UTI, it seems worthwhile to consider these new approaches in managing acute, uncomplicated UTI with empiric treatment on the basis of history and perhaps limited physical examination when patients present to the ED.

Most investigators agree that a urine culture should be obtained in the following settings: acute pyelonephritis; patients with epidemiologic risk factors for subclinical pyelonephritis; any patient who needs to be hospitalized; those patients who have a chronic indwelling catheter; and all pregnant women, children, and adult males.[1,2,5,10] If the patient is symptomatic, one positive culture is significant. For ABU, two or three positive cultures are necessary before treatment is undertaken, with the exception that treatment for ABU is always indicated in pregnancy.

In addition to urine cultures, blood cultures are commonly recommended in cases of acute pyelonephritis; and although they are positive in about 30 percent of patients, the results rarely change management.[16] Renal imaging studies are not indicated in otherwise healthy patients with acute pyelonephritis that can be managed on an outpatient basis. Elderly, diabetic, or severely ill patients with acute pyelonephritis should be considered for imaging, particularly if there is a poor initial response to antibiotic therapy. The kidneys can be imaged with portable ultrasound at the bedside for the evaluation of obstruction and focal parenchymal abnormalities.[8] Plain film radiology and ultrasound have poor sensitivity for detection of intrarenal gas formation in emphysematous pyelonephritis; in suspected cases (e.g., diabetic patients with fever and flank pain), computed tomography is the best imaging modality.[8,9]

TREATMENT

Acute Cystitis

The selection of antibiotics depends on the suspected bacteriology of the infection, the patient's compliance, potential drug toxicity, and cost.[17] In uncomplicated UTIs, *E. coli* is the offending microorganism in the vast majority of cases, and this and other typical coliform pathogens remain largely susceptible to a variety of agents, e.g., trimethoprim (TMP), TMP and sulfamethoxazole (TMP/SMX), nitrofurantoin macrocrystals, and the fluoroquinolones (Table 94-2). Most uncomplicated UTIs can be treated with a short (3 day) course of antibiotics.

Trimethoprim or TMP/SMX are still recommended as first-line agents in most cases, because these are inexpensive and effective.[6,18,19] However, resistance to TMP/SMX has increased dramatically in recent years. There is wide regional variation in TMP/SMX resistance, and this must be considered when choosing TMP or TMP/SMX as an empiric treatment choice. Resistance to TMP/SMX has been reported at over 30 percent in the western United States, up to 14 percent in the mid-west, and around 7 percent in the east.[20] Currently, recommendations are to avoid TMP/SMX (unless treating on the basis of urine culture with sensitivities) as the first-line empiric agent of choice when local resistance exceeds 20 percent. It may even be prudent to do so when resistance gets above 10 percent. The cost of treatment failures when using TMP/SMX where resistance is known to exceed 10 to 20 percent probably obviates any savings from choosing to use TMP/SMX as a less expensive medication. The need for repeat visits, retesting, retreatment and, in most cases, longer treatment courses with more expensive agents, and potential development of complicated UTI and/or pyelonephritis possibly necessitating hospital admission are good

TABLE 94-2 Guidelines for Outpatient Management of Uncomplicated Urinary Tract Infection

Patient	UTI Type	Clinical Characteristics	Antimicrobial Regimens	Comments
Adult female	Lower	Uncomplicated UTI = not pregnant, few prior UTI episodes, brief duration of symptoms (<7 d), and no risk factors for subclinical pyelonephritis	TMP/SMX DS (160/800 mg) 1 tab bid × 3 d *or* Trimethoprim 200 mg bid × 3 d If community resistance to these agents is high (>10–20%) or patient allergic, then Ciprofloxacin 250 mg bid × 3 d *or* Ofloxacin 200 mg bid × 3 d *or* Levofloxacin 250 mg qd × 3 d *or* Nitrofurantoin 100 mg qid × 5 d* *or* Amoxicillin/clavulanate 875/125 mg bid × 5 d	No initial culture is required. If using a short course regimen, good follow-up is important. TMP/SMX or TMP remains first line unless community resistance is high (>10–20%). β-Lactams and nitrofurantoin are less effective than others when used for only 3 d.
Adult female	Lower/upper	Risk of subclinical pyelonephritis: prolonged symptoms, relapse or recurrent UTI, diabetes mellitus, urinary tract abnormalities, recent pyelonephritis, indigent patients	Ciprofloxacin 250–500 mg bid *or* Ofloxacin 200–400 mg bid *or* Levofloxacin 250–500 mg qd If susceptibilities are known, consider: TMP/SMX DS (160/800 mg) 1 tab bid Nitrofurantoin 100 mg qid Amoxicillin/clavulanate 875/125 mg bid	Urine culture is advised. Coliforms are common. Treat for at least 10 (mild symptoms) or 14 (more severe symptoms) d. Admit if patient very ill or pregnant.
Adult male	Lower/upper	Suspect underlying anatomic abnormality; consider urethritis and prostatitis	Ciprofloxacin 250–500 mg bid *or* Ofloxacin 200–400 mg bid *or* Levofloxacin 250–500 mg qd If susceptibilities are known, consider TMP/SMX DS (160/800 mg) 1 tab bid Nitrofurantoin 100 mg qid* Amoxicillin/clavulanate 875/125 mg bid	Urine culture is advised. Coliforms are common. Treat for at least 10 (mild symptoms) or 14 (more severe symptoms) d. Admit if patient very ill.
Adult female	Lower	Stuttering symptoms, new sexual partner or partner with urethritis, signs and symptoms of cervicitis, pyuria without bacteriuria	Ofloxacin 400 mg bid × 14 d *or* Levofloxacin 500 mg qd × 14 d (covers common pathogens, gonorrhea, and *Chlamydia* at this dose) Doxycycline 100 mg bid × 14 d (covers *Chlamydia* but not gonorrhea; thus, potential cost savings uncertain without culture and treatment failure rate is high) Erythromycin 500 mg qid × 14 d (if pregnant, will only eradicate *Chlamydia,* not gonorrhea)	Culture for gonococcus and chlamydia. Consider consultation with patient's obstetrician, if pregnant. Gonorrhea resistance to quinolones is rising.

*Compliance falls with qid medications. Nitrofurantoin sustained release (Macrobid) is a bid alternative (no generic yet).
Abbreviations: DS = double strength; tab = tablet; TMP/SMX = trimethoprim/sulfamethoxazole; UTI = urinary tract infection.

arguments for considering other agents (e.g., fluoroquinolones such as ciprofloxacin) as first-line agents when resistance to TMP/SMX is known to be high. Many experts feel that TMP/SMX soon will be ineffective as a first-line agent for UTI in any part of the United States.[8,18–20]

Nitrofurantoin is also a generally effective agent for treating UTI, although compliance with frequent dosing (qid) is a problem, and nitrofurantoin is not effective against *S. saprophyticus.* There is a twice-daily formulation of nitrofurantoin (Macrobid), but it is expensive and not currently available in generic form. It is a favorite antibiotic among obstetricians for ABU and otherwise uncomplicated UTI in pregnant patients.[5,12] Nitrofurantoin has not been well studied in the many trials demonstrating the effectiveness of short courses of antibiotics for UTI (e.g., 3-day regimens), and what data there are suggest that nitrofurantoin may be less effective at eradicating bacteriuria and infection than TMP/SMX or fluoroquinolones when used in short courses.[18]

Nitrofurantoin does has a favorable resistance profile in many regions as compared with TMP/SMX, it is a generally safe alternative, and the brand name twice-daily form (Macrobid) is slightly less expensive than most fluoroquinolones. Because nitrofurantoin is not currently a proven agent for short course regimens, it should probably be used only when a longer treatment course is already indicated, when the patient is pregnant, or when urine cultures showing sensitivity to nitrofurantoin are readily available.[18]

Because of greatly increased bacterial resistance, extended-spectrum penicillins (e.g., amoxicillin and other β-lactams) and cephalosporins have become less acceptable alternatives. If cultures and sensitivities are available, these agents are reasonable choices, but this is rarely the case in the emergency department. Further, there is evidence that short course regimens using β-lactams and cephalosporins have a higher failure rate as compared with TMP/SMX and fluoroquinolones.[6]

In cases of treatment failure, or in the host with a structural or immunologic defect, use of amoxicillin with clavulanic acid or one of the fluoroquinolones should be considered. Urine cultures with sensitivities should be obtained and used to guide treatment. Short course regimens are not an option in these cases. Concern about the emergence of resistant organisms and expense has and should continue to preclude indiscriminate use of fluoroquinolones. Nonetheless, where TMP/SMX resistance is known to be greater than 10 to 20 percent and empiric short course (3 day) therapy is indicated, fluoroquinolones are the only remaining reasonable first choice.[21] Unfortunately, fluoroquinolone-resistant UTI is already becoming a problem and is expected to increase dramatically in the coming years.

In uncomplicated UTIs, the urine should be free of bacteria in 24 to 48 h, with substantial relief of symptoms within the same period. The offer of 1 to 2 days of an oral bladder analgesic, such as phenazopyridine, is considerate when urination is painful for the patient. Within the past decade, multiple studies of shorter treatment regimens for uncomplicated infections in nonpregnant adult women have been published, and 3-day regimens have become the recommended standard of care.[6,17,18] Short duration treatment regimens offer a number of advantages: cost and side effects are substantially reduced, compliance improves, and the development of resistant strains of bacteria is less likely. However, 20 to 30 percent of patients given short duration therapy fail treatment and/or quickly relapse. In addition, 3-day regimens are not adequate for all patients, and a 7-day course is recommended for pregnant women, those with symptoms lasting longer than 1 week, patients with diabetes, individuals who had a previous, recent UTI, those who are older than 65 years, and women who use spermicides or a diaphragm.[6,17,18]

The recommendations and increased use of 3-day treatment regimens have generated concerns that that an increased incidence of treatment failures would result because of unsuspected subclinical pyelonephritis. Several studies of patients with apparently simple cystitis exhibiting kidney involvement as demonstrated by the presence of antibody-coated bacteria did not respond to short-term therapy when compared with patients with antibody-coated bacteria who received 10 to 14 days of treatment. The current paradigm is to use short course treatment for apparently uncomplicated acute cystitis, with the expectation of cure in the majority. Those patients with recurrence of symptoms, pyuria, and bacteriuria will be promptly identified as having subclinical renal infection necessitating 14 days of subsequent therapy.[6,18]

In ED settings serving indigent populations, in which there is delay in seeking care, the incidence of subclinical pyelonephritis may approach 70 percent of patients. In this circumstance, short course therapy is difficult to justify. Before the ED physician decides to use a 3-day course of treatment, the patient's ability to follow-up within 1 week or return if symptoms persist must be assessed. If follow-up compliance is not expected, or the epidemiologic risk of subclinical pyelonephritis is great, then the patient should be placed on a 10- to 14-day regimen of appropriate antibiotics.

One should be suspicious that *Chlamydia* is responsible for symptoms in the following settings: a woman with a new sexual partner; a partner with urethritis; examination findings of cervicitis; or when there is low-grade pyuria with no bacteria seen on urinalysis. Concurrent infection with gonorrhea is common with chlamydia infections. If the patient has UTI symptoms and suspicion of a chlamydia and gonorrhea infection (cervicitis and/or salpingitis), antibiotic treatment is more complex. If the patient is not sufficiently ill to require admission and is not pregnant, one initial treatment approach is to use ofloxacin, 400 mg bid for 14 days; ofloxacin effectively covers all common UTI pathogens, chlamydia and gonorrhea. If salpingitis is clinically evident, metronidazole 500 mg bid for 14 days, should complete treatment. This approach is expensive, but the cost of the medication should be balanced against the long-term costs of treatment failures and morbidity associated with untreated cervicitis and salpingitis.

When treating a young teenage patient with recurrent UTI, the emergency physician should take a sexual history and, if the patient is sexually active, consider counseling of the patient regarding contraception and prevention of sexually transmitted disease.[10] Assistance from a social worker may be useful.

Recurrent infection is often due to a new serotype of *E. coli,* or it may be due to newly resistant organisms that develop as a result of antibiotics excreted into the gastrointestinal tract. If empiric therapy is considered for recurrent infections, it probably should use fluoroquinolones unless community resistance to TMP/SMX is known to be low. However, successful management in cases of recurrent UTI depends on urine culture and sensitivity testing.[6,10,18] In addition to evaluation of the urinary tract, chronic suppressive therapy is usually instituted. Up to 80 percent of women who have had one UTI develop another one later on. Because many factors are involved in reinfection and some of these are correctable, appropriate referral is important in patients with recurrent UTIs.

In patients discharged from the ED with treatment plans for UTI, adjunctive therapy should include plenty of fluids to enhance diuresis, fruit juices containing vitamin C to acidify the urine, a proper diet, and frequent voiding (at least every 2 h) to diminish tissue contact with bacteria. The effectiveness of cranberry juice in preventing UTI is curiously controversial, and careful review of the literature provides rather weak support for promoting cranberry juice as a UTI prophylaxis. Nevertheless, many studies have suggested at least some benefit from cranberry juice in preventing UTI, and there is certainly no harm in drinking it.[22] Women should be reminded that postcoital voiding also may be helpful in reducing recurrent infection. Although no panacea, these adjunctive measures have long been recommended by physicians and are loudly proclaimed as significant in popular women's magazines and Internet-based public health information sites. Because they are unlikely to cause harm, may help, and stating otherwise to patients is likely to create confusion and potential aggravation for the emergency physician, continuing to recommend these measures is reasonable.

Aggressive therapy is warranted for pregnant women with pyuria or bacteriuria, whether or not associated symptoms are present. Urine culture with sensitivities is always indicated in these patients. Most clinicians prefer nitrofurantoin or a cephalosporin for initial outpatient treatment. Trimethoprim and SMX may be considered except in the first trimester, when TMP is contraindicated, within 2 weeks of the estimated delivery date, and in those with glucose-6-phosphate dehydrogenase deficiency. Fluoroquinolones are contraindicated in pregnancy. Amoxicillin is generally safe, but resistance and, hence, treatment failure rates are high. All regimens should be continued for at least 7 days, and the patient should be referred to her obstetrician for follow-up within 48 h. If the patient is greater than 20 weeks' estimated gestation, the emergency physician should contact the patient's obstetrician to discuss treatment options, if possible. Inpatient management is stressed for suspected pyelonephritis, because the incidence is higher in pregnancy, with subsequent maternal and fetal morbidity.

Acute Pyelonephritis

Classically, acute pyelonephritis is characterized by shaking chills, fever, flank pain, and CVA tenderness after several days of dysuria and frequency.[18] The urine often demonstrates WBC casts and clumps and bacteria. Sometimes the presentation may not be dramatic, and it might be difficult to distinguish lower from upper UTI.

Factors associated with an increased risk for pyelonephritis include advanced age, pregnancy, prolonged symptoms before seeking care, three or more UTIs in the past year, immunocompromised state, poor general health and comorbidities, morbid obesity, institutionalization, chronic indwelling urinary catheter or the need for self-catheterization, and diabetes mellitus. Less often, the patient may have a congenital or acquired anatomic urinary tract abnormality, neurogenic problems that result in incomplete bladder emptying, recent urinary tract instrumentation, renal calculi and nephrocalcinosis, prostatic hypertrophy, or prostatitis as precipitating factors for acute pyelonephritis.[18]

Young, otherwise healthy females with uncomplicated acute pyelonephritis may be candidates for outpatient management.[18,23] Conversely, oral outpatient treatment cannot be recommended for patients who are immunocompromised, pregnant, diabetic, or chronically ill. Although unproved, a popular regimen at many institutions is to treat the patient with antipyretics, intravenous fluids, analgesics, and the first dose of antibiotic (oral or parenteral) while undergoing a brief period of observation in the ED to ensure that further oral therapy will be tolerated, which is assessed by having the patient drink water. As compared with traditional inpatient treatment for pyelonephritis, outpatient therapy for selected patients (young, otherwise healthy, nonpregnant, able to keep down fluids and antibiotics) is equally safe and effective and considerably less expensive.[6,10,18] Fluoroquinolones are now the recommended first-line agents for the outpatient management of acute pyelonephritis.[18,23] If urine culture and sensitivity results are available and demonstrate sensitivity to other medications (e.g., TMP/SMX, β-lactams, cephalosporins, and nitrofurantoin), these also can be used safely. Treatment should be continued for 10 to 14 days. Patients should be instructed to return with increasing pain, fever, or vomiting. Prescriptions for analgesics (e.g., hydrocodone plus acetaminophen) should be provided. Overall, 80 to 90 percent of selected patients with acute pyelonephritis will respond well to outpatient oral therapy.[23]

The decision to admit a patient with acute pyelonephritis is based on age, host factors, and response to initial emergency department interventions. Fluid replacement and parenteral antibiotics are necessary if the patient is vomiting or dehydrated and has unremitting fever and/or loss of vasomotor tone. In an otherwise healthy host with no prior or recent history of UTI, the typical infecting bacteria would be *E. coli* or another coliform bacteria. Acceptable first-line intravenous antibiotic regimens include a fluoroquinolone (ciprofloxacin, levofloxacin, or ofloxacin), ampicillin plus gentamicin, a third-generation cephalosporin (cefotaxime, ceftazidime, or ceftriaxone), or extended spectrum penicillin plus β-lactamase inhibitor (ticarcillin plus clavulanate or ampicillin plus sulbactam).[17] Urine culture with sensitivities is mandatory in these cases. When selecting the antibiotic for administration, the physician also should consider cost differences and local sensitivity patterns. In most cases, single drug therapy with a fluoroquinolone is the best initial option.

Overall, about 1 to 3 percent of patients with acute pyelonephritis will die from the infection, with younger patients experiencing the fewest complications. Factors associated with an unfavorable prognosis are advanced age and general debility, renal calculi or obstruction, a recent history of hospitalization or instrumentation, diabetes mellitus, evidence of chronic nephropathy, sickle cell anemia, underlying carcinoma, and immunocompromised states (e.g., chemotherapy, HIV/AIDS). In patients with these factors, broad-spectrum antibiotic coverage to include *Pseudomonas* spp. should be provided. A fluoroquinolone is a good initial choice.

Dangerous complications of acute pyelonephritis include acute papillary necrosis with possible ureter obstruction, septic shock, perinephric abscesses, and emphysematous pyelonephritis. Imaging studies (usually computed tomography) are necessary to detect these complications. Adequate fluid resuscitation, pain and fever control, antiemetics, and early initiation of appropriate antibiotics are critical.

HIV/AIDS Patients

In patients with HIV/AIDS, TMP/SMX resistance is increased largely due to its use in *Pneumocystis carinii* prophylaxis. Fluoroquinolones should be the initial antibiotic used in UTI with these patients, unless urine culture and sensitivity results are available to guide therapy. Most UTIs in HIV/AIDS patients are caused by typical pathogens or common sexually transmitted organisms. *Mycobacterium tuberculosis* is an infrequent cause of UTI in the HIV/AIDS population. Close outpatient follow-up and possible infectious disease consultation are warranted when treating UTI in this population.[24]

REFERENCES

1. Foxman B: Epidemiology of urinary tract infections: Incidence, morbidity, and economic costs. *Am J Med* 113(suppl 1A):55, 2002.
2. Lipsky BA: Prostatitis and urinary tract infection in men: What's new; what's true? *Am J Med* 106:327, 1999.
3. Scholes D, Hooton TM, Roberts PL, et al: Risk factors for recurrent urinary tract infection in young women. *J Infect Dis* 182:1177, 2000.
4. Hooton TM, Scholes D, Stapleton AE, et al: A prospective study of asymptomatic bacteriuria in sexually active young women. *New Engl J Med* 343:992, 2000.
5. Connolly A, Thorp JM Jr: Urinary tract infections in pregnancy. *Urol Clin North Am* 26:779, 1999.
6. Krieger JN: Urinary tract infections: What's new? *J Urol* 168:2531, 2002.
7. Hooton TM, Scholes D, Hughes JP, et al: A prospective study of risk factors for symptomatic urinary tract infection in young women. *New Engl J Med* 335:468, 1996.
8. Huang JJ, Sung JM, Chen KW, et al: Acute bacterial nephritis: A clinicoradiologic correlation based on computed tomography. *Am J Med* 93:289, 1992.
9. Stapleton A: Urinary tract infections in patients with diabetes. *Am J Med* 113(suppl 1A):80s, 2002.
10. Bent S, Nallamothu BK, Simel DL, et al: Does this woman have an acute uncomplicated urinary tract infection? *JAMA* 287:2701, 2002.
11. Gupta K, Hooton TM, Roberts PL, Stamm WE: Patient-initiated treatment of uncomplicated recurrent urinary tract infections in young women. *Ann Intern Med* 135:9, 2001.
12. Van Nostrand JD, Junkins AD, Bartholdi RK: Poor predictive ability of urinalysis and microscopic evaluation to detect urinary tract infection. *Am J Clin Pathol* 113:709, 2000.
13. Holloway J, Joshi N, O'Bryan T: Positive urine nitrite test: An accurate predictor of absence of pure enterococcal bacteriuria. *South Med J* 93:681, 2000.
14. Saint S, Scholes D, Fihn SD, et al: The effectiveness of a clinical practice guideline for the management of presumed uncomplicated urinary tract infection in women. *Am J Med* 106:636, 1999.
15. Bent S, Saint S: The optimal use of diagnostic testing in women with acute uncomplicated cystitis. *Am J Med* 113(suppl 1A):20s, 2002.
16. Thanassi M: Utility of urine and blood cultures in pyelonephritis. *Acad Emerg Med* 4:797, 1997.
17. Nicolle LE: Urinary tract infection: Traditional pharmacologic therapies. *Dis Mon* 49:111, 2003.
18. Warren JW, Abrutyn E, Hebel JR, et al: Guidelines for antimicrobial treatment of uncomplicated acute bacterial cystitis and acute pyelonephritis in women. *Clin Infect Dis* 29:745, 1999.
19. Gupta K, Hooton TM, Stamm WE: Increasing antimicrobial resistance and the management of uncomplicated community-acquired urinary tract infections. *Ann Intern Med* 135:41, 2001.
20. Talan DA, Stamm WE, Hooton TM, et al: Comparison of ciprofloxacin (7 days) and trimethoprim-sulfamethoxazole (14 days) for acute uncomplicated pyelonephritis in women: A randomized trial. *JAMA* 283:153, 2000.
21. Schaeffer AJ: The expanding role of fluoroquinolones. *Am J Med* 113(suppl 1A):45s, 2002.
22. Kontiokari T, Sundqvist K, Nuutinen M, et al: Randomized trial of cranberry-lingonberry juice and *Lactobacillus* GG drink for the prevention of urinary tract infections in women. *BMJ* 322:1571, 2001.
23. Pinson AG, Philbrick JT, Lindbeck GH, Schorling JB: Oral antibiotic therapy for acute pyelonephritis: A methodologic review of the literature. *J Gen Intern Med* 7:544, 1992.
24. Lee LK, Dinneen MD, Ahmad S: The urologist and the patient with human immunodeficiency virus or with acquired immunodeficiency syndrome. *BJU Int* 88:500, 2001.

MALE GENITAL PROBLEMS
Robert E. Schneider

95

One of the most anxiety-provoking problems presenting to an emergency department is the male with an acute genital disorders. Further, the extensive sensory innervation of this area can produce severe symptoms. The close relations of the abdominal and genital sensory afferent pathways in the male account for the common association of abdominal pain with some acute genitourinary disorders.

ANATOMY

Penis

The penis is composed of three cylindrical bodies: the two corpora cavernosa, which form the main bulk of the penis, and the corpus spongiosum, which surrounds the urethra (Figure 95-1). The corpora cavernosa are the major erectile bodies, extending distally from the pubic rami and capped by the glans penis. These two cylindrical structures are encased in a thick tunic of dense connective tissue, the tunica albuginea. All three cylinders are collectively covered by a thinner Buck's fascia, which fuses with Colles' fascia at the level of the urogenital diaphragm.

The blood supply is primarily from the internal pudendal artery, which branches to form the deep and superficial penile arteries. Lymphatic drainage is into the deep and superficial inguinal nodes.

Scrotum

The prepubertal scrotal skin is thin and thickens with subsequent hormonal stimulation. Immediately beneath the skin are the smooth muscle and elastic tissue layers of Dartos' fascia, similar to the superficial fatty layer (Camper's fascia) of the abdominal wall. The deep membranous layer (Scarpa's fascia) of the abdominal wall extends into the perineum, where it is referred to as Colles' fascia, and forms part of the scrotal wall (Figure 95-2). The blood supply is derived primarily from branches of the femoral and internal pudendal arteries. Lymphatics from the scrotum drain into the inguinal and femoral nodes.

Testes

The testes usually lie in an upright position, with the superior portion tipped slightly forward and outward. The average size is between 4 and

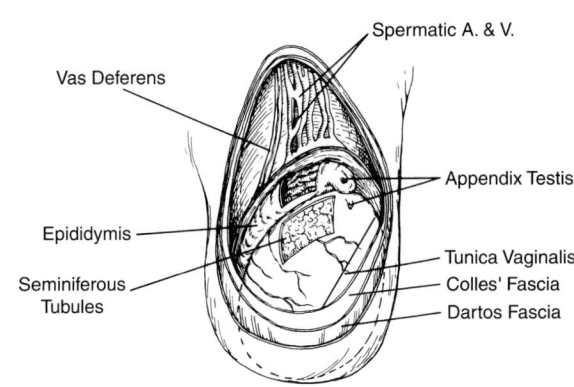

FIG. 95-2. Anatomy of the scrotum and the testis.

5 cm in length and approximately 3 cm in width and depth. The overall volume is about 25 mL. Each testis is encased in a thick fibrous tunica albuginea except posterolaterally, where it is in tight apposition with the epididymis. The enveloping tunica vaginalis covers the anterior and lateral aspects of the testes and attaches to the posterior scrotal wall. Superiorly, the testes are suspended from the spermatic cord; inferiorly, the testis is anchored to the scrotum by the scrotal ligament (gubernaculum). Maldevelopment with lack of firm posterior fixation of the tunica vaginalis leaves the testes and epididymis at risk for torsion. The posterior (visceral) leaf of the tunica vaginalis is adherent with the tunica albuginea of the anterior testicular surface. A potential space exists between this visceral leaf and the anterior (parietal) tunica vaginalis. Any traumatic or inflammatory event will impede the normal parietal tunica vaginalis from absorbing viscerally secreted fluid, resulting in a hydrocele (Figure 95-3).

The blood supply is by the internal spermatic and external spermatic arteries, which travel together in the spermatic cord. Venous return is primarily by the internal spermatic, epigastric, internal circumflex, and scrotal veins. The lymphatics drain toward the external, common iliac, and periaortic nodes.

The epididymis is a single, fine, tubular structure approximately 4 to 5 m long compressed into an area of about 5 cm. The function of the epididymis is to promote sperm maturation and motility. Vestigial embryonic structures, the appendix epididymis and the appendix testis, which have no known physiologic function, are often associated with the testes and epididymis. The appendix epididymis, a remnant of the epigenitales, is found attached to the head of the epididymis, or globus major. The appendix testis, a pear-shaped structure of Müllerian duct

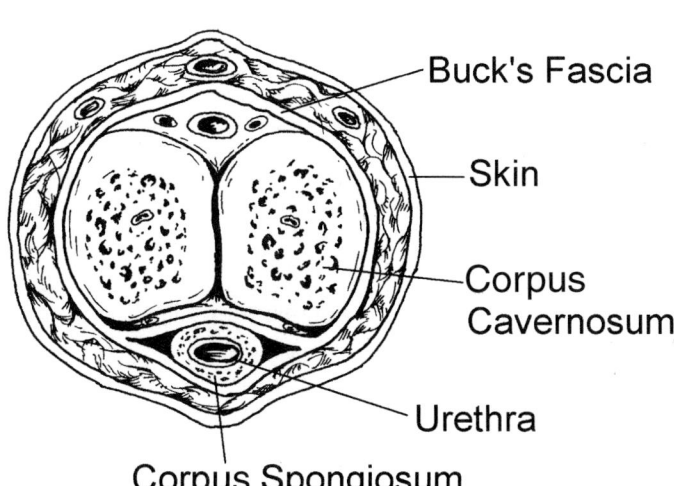

FIG. 95-1. Cross section of the penis.

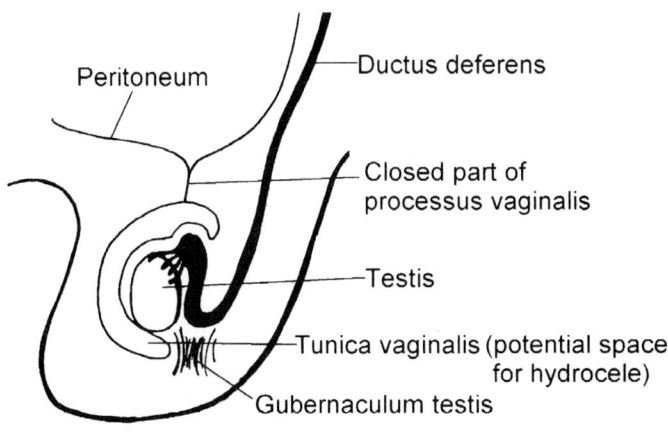

FIG. 95-3. Embryonic retroperitoneal testis descends into the scrotum and invaginates into the tunica vaginalis, which anchors it to the posterior scrotal wall. Note the potential space in the tunica vaginalis for development of a hydrocele.

origin, is usually situated on the uppermost portion of the testis at the junction of the testis and the globus major of the epididymis.

The vas deferens, a prominent part of the adnexa of the scrotal contents, is a distinct muscular tube that is easily palpable within the scrotal sac. It extends cephalad in the spermatic cord from the tail of the epididymis (globus minor), traverses the inguinal canal, and crosses medially behind the bladder over the ureters to form the ampullae of the vas, where it joins with the seminal vesicles to form the paired ejaculatory ducts in the prostatic urethra.

Prostate

The prostate originates from the urogenital sinus at approximately the third month of embryonic life. It is continually enlarging and in the young male is approximately 10 to 15 g, often not definable on rectal examination. As a man matures, the prostate may enlarge dramatically, resulting in significant bladder outlet obstruction. The prostate is divided into five lobes: anterior, median, posterior, and two lateral lobes.

PHYSICAL EXAMINATION

Physical examination should be performed with the patient in the supine and upright positions in a well-illuminated, warm room. If the scrotum is contracted despite proper room temperature, a warm towel placed over the genitalia permits the scrotum to relax and the testes to descend and be comfortably examined.

Examination should always begin with visual inspection. In uncircumcised males, the foreskin should be fully retracted to inspect the glans, coronal sulcus, and preputial areas for ulceration or malignant lesions. The location of the urethral meatus and presence of discharge should be noted. The penile shaft should be carefully palpated for plaques, cysts, or early abscesses.

The supine or modified lithotomy (frogleg) position is more comfortable for the patient and the examiner and allows a more thorough examination of each testis, epididymis, the prostate, seminal vesicles, and rectal ampulla. During the critical evaluation of a scrotal mass, the patient's relaxation and cooperation in the supine position are paramount. Testicular nodularity or firmness should be considered carcinoma until proven otherwise. The epididymis usually lies on the posterolateral aspect of the testis and, if not inflamed or involved with other pathologic entities, has a soft, fleshy feel similar to that of the earlobe. Many males experience pain and tenderness with palpation of a normal globus major (head), body, and globus minor (tail) of the epididymis. All males experience some discomfort during palpation of a normal prostate. The supine position helps prevent an infrequent vasovagal response to the scrotal or prostate examination. The prostate has a heart-shaped contour, with its apex located more distally, abutting the urogenital diaphragm (anatomic soft spot). The consistency of the normal prostate has the same resiliency as the cartilaginous tip of the nose, whereas suspicious carcinogenic areas feel more like the bony prominence of the chin. The posterior lobe is small and thin, allowing palpation of the median raphe that distinguishes the two lateral lobes. A rectal prostate examination cannot assess the anterior or median lobes. The seminal vesicles, lying just superior to the prostate, cannot normally be distinguished unless there is inflammation, induration, or enlargement.

Examination of the inguinal canals for hernias and the scrotal spermatic cords for varicoceles is best done in the upright position, with the patient straining at the designated time. When the patient is upright, it should be determined whether the testes are aligned along a vertical or horizontal axis; horizontally aligned testes are at greater risk for torsion.

Some genital disorders may require urine collection and analysis. The uncircumcised male should retract his foreskin and wash the glans penis with cleansing towels before collecting a midstream specimen. Failure to do so will result in preputial contamination. The often described three-cup specimen used to localize male lower urinary tract

infections is time consuming and requires the patient's compliance, factors that tend to limit its usefulness in the emergency department.

COMMON GENITOURINARY DISORDERS

Scrotum

Because the scrotal skin is loose and elastic, dramatic enlargement of the scrotum may occur secondary to scrotal or testicular pathology.

SCROTAL EDEMA   Simple, isolated scrotal edema is uncommon. It usually occurs secondary to insect or human bites, contact dermatitis, or, in young boys, idiopathic scrotal edema. Contiguous scrotal and penile edema occurs in older men in conjunction with lower extremity edema in fluid overload states (congestive heart failure), hypoalbuminemia, and generalized anasarca. Idiopathic scrotal edema presents as unilateral pain with unilateral scrotal, perineal, and inguinal swelling and erythema in boys between 3 and 9 years.[1] Ultrasound findings include thickened scrotal wall, increased peri-testicular blood flow, and reactive hydrocele. Episodes resolve in 1 to 4 days, although recurrences occur in 10 to 20 percent of patients.

SCROTAL ABSCESS   The important distinction with a scrotal abscess is whether the phlegmon is localized to the scrotal wall, i.e., simple hair follicle abscess, or involves, and even perhaps originates from, infection in one of the primary intrascrotal organs, i.e., testis, epididymis, or bulbous urethra. This distinction can be very difficult late in the course of the infective process, when a scrotal mass may be the only discernible finding.

A simple hair follicle scrotal wall abscess can be managed by incision and drainage. Oftentimes wound care can be simplified by circumferential excision of the entire roof of the abscess. This allows access for wound care and sitz baths and assures healing from the base outward. Antibiotics are rarely needed in an immunocompetent male.

Contiguous involvement of the scrotal skin by an inflammatory mass in the testis or epididymis is best evaluated by ultrasound. A retrograde urethrogram will delineate the integrity of the urethra. Definitive care of any complex abscesses should be referred to a urologist.

FOURNIER GANGRENE   Fournier gangrene is a polymicrobial, synergistic, necrotizing infection of the perineal subcutaneous fascia and male genitalia that originates from the skin, urethra, or rectum. This infectious process typically begins as a benign infection or simple abscess that quickly becomes virulent, especially in an immunocompromised host, and leads to end-artery thrombosis in the subcutaneous tissue that promotes widespread necrosis of previously healthy tissue (Figure 95-4).

The diabetic male seems to be most at risk. Prompt recognition of Fournier gangrene in its early stages should prevent extensive tissue loss that accompanies delayed diagnosis. Aggressive fluid resuscitation; gram-positive, gram-negative, and anaerobic antibiotic coverage; and wide surgical debridement sometimes in conjunction with pre- and postoperative hyperbaric oxygen therapy are the mainstays of treatment.[2] Overall mortality is about 20 percent. Urologic consultation is often required when periurethral abscess is the inciting event, or when other etiologies have secondarily invaded the urinary tract and supravesical urinary drainage is needed. Emergency physicians should maintain a high index of suspicion for this entity in immunocompromised patients who present complaining of scrotal, rectal, or any genitalia pain out of proportion to their physical examination findings of infection (warmth, erythema, and swelling).

Penis

BALANOPOSTHITIS   *Balanitis* is inflammation of the glans penis, *posthitis* is inflammation of the foreskin, and *balanoposthitis* is in-

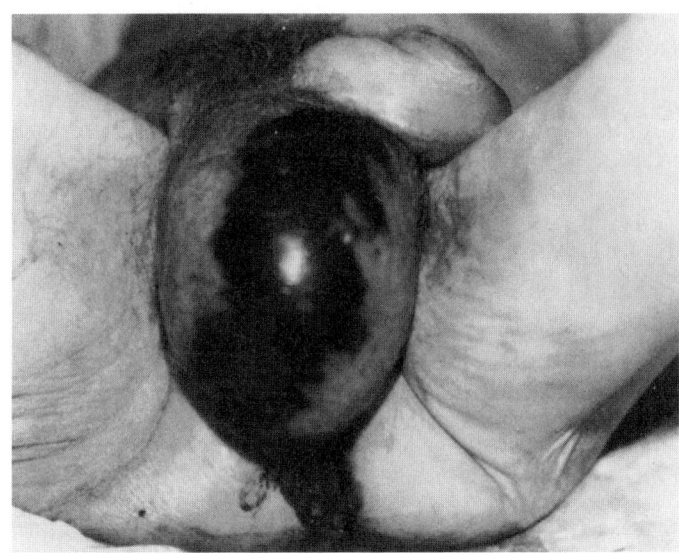

FIG. 95-4. A patient with Fournier's gangrene of the scrotum. Note the sharp demarcation of gangrenous changes and the marked edema of the scrotum and the penis.

Phimosis

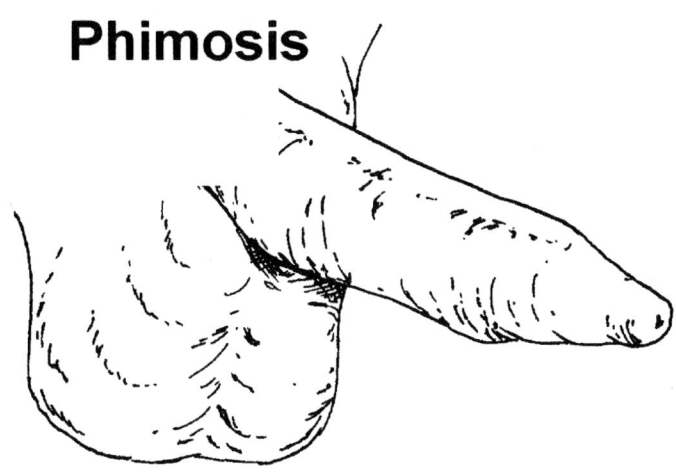

Paraphimosis

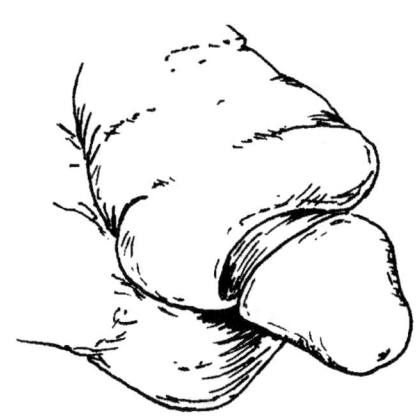

FIG. 95-5. Phimosis and paraphimosis.

flammation of the glans and foreskin.[3] When foreskin retraction is attempted, the glans and apposing prepuce appear purulent, excoriated, malodorous, and tender. **Recurrent balanoposthitis can be the sole presenting sign of diabetes.** Many cases are caused by infection, most commonly *Candida* followed by *Gardnerella* and anaerobes. Treatment consists of cleansing the area with mild soap, ensuring adequate dryness, application of antifungal creams (nystatin or clotrimazole), treatment with an oral azole (fluconazole), and possibly circumcision.[4] Bacterial infection is suggested by warmth, erythema, and edema of the glans, foreskin, and penile shaft. If these signs are present, a broad-spectrum antibiotic, usually a first- or second-generation oral cephalosporin, should be prescribed. Cases that persist warrant culture for potential infective causes or biopsy.[3]

PHIMOSIS   *Phimosis* is the inability to retract the foreskin proximally and posterior to the glans penis (Figure 95-5). Causes include infection, poor hygiene, or previous preputial injury with scarring. Scarring at the tip of the foreskin can occlude the preputial meatus, infrequently causing urinary retention. Hemostatic dilation of the preputial ostium can be done to temporarily relieve the urinary retention. Definitive treatment has traditionally been circumcision. Recently, topical steroid treatment (triamcinolone 0.025% bid, or betamethasone 0.05% qd) applied from the tip of the foreskin to the glandis corona for 4 to 6 weeks has been shown to be 70 to 90 percent effective in treating phimosis to allow for some degree of foreskin retraction and avert circumcision.[5]

PARAPHIMOSIS   *Paraphimosis* is the inability to reduce the proximal edematous foreskin distally over the glans penis into its naturally occurring position (see Figure 95-5). The resulting glans edema and venous engorgement can progress to arterial compromise and gangrene.

Paraphimosis is a true urologic emergency.[6] Paraphimosis often can be reduced by compression of the glans for several minutes to reduce edema and allow for successful reduction of the foreskin back over the now smaller glans. Tightly wrapping the glans with a 2-in. elastic bandage for 5 min is one method to reduce edema. Infrequently, several puncture wounds with a small needle (22 to 25 gauge) can help edema fluid be expressed out of the glans. A local anesthetic block of the penis is also helpful if the patient cannot tolerate the pain of compression. If these methods are unsuccessful, local infiltration of the constricting band with lidocaine 1 percent without epinephrine fol-

lowed by superficial dorsal incision of the band will decompress the glans and allow foreskin reduction. In cases with impaired perfusion to the glans, an emergency physician should do this procedure unless a urologist is immediately available.

ENTRAPMENT INJURIES   Various objects can be placed around the penis, initially occluding the venous, and subsequently the arterial, blood supply. String, metal rings, and wire have been wrapped around the penis for sexual, experimental, or accidental reasons. Removal of the offending object often requires ingenuity and care. One of the most insidious objects that can become entrapped behind the coronal ridge is human hair, usually found in young circumcised boys age 2 to 5 years, termed the *penile hair-tourniquet syndrome* (Figure 95-6). The child presents with swelling of the glans. The offending hair may be invisible within the edematous coronal sulcus. If the hair has been present for some time, the urethra and dorsal nerve supply of the penis may be partly or completely involved. In this case, urethral integrity (retrograde urethrogram) and distal penile arterial blood supply (Doppler) should be ensured before emergency department discharge. Despite the appearance, the consensus from the medical literature is that penile hair-tourniquet syndrome is not a sign of child abuse.

FRACTURE OF THE PENIS   An acute tear or rupture of the corpus cavernosa tunica albuginea is an uncommon condition.[7] The penis is acutely swollen but flaccid, discolored, and tender. The history is of trauma during intercourse or other sexual activity, when a sudden "snapping sound" occurs. Most patients are between 30 and 40 years.

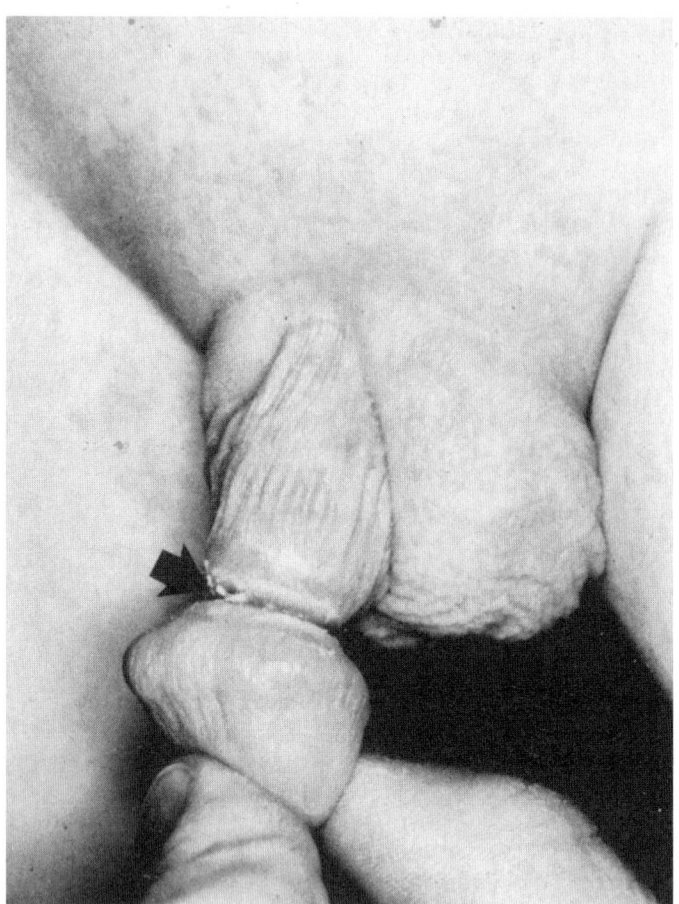

FIG. 95-6. Hair is entrapped behind the coronal sulcus *(arrow)*, constricting and progressively amputating the glans.

Even though the urethra is infrequently injured, a retrograde urethrogram may be necessary to assure urethral integrity. Surgical treatment consists of hematoma evacuation and suture apposition of the disrupted tunica albuginea.

PEYRONIE DISEASE   Peyronie disease produces progressive penile deformity, typically curvature with erections, that is painful and may result in erectile dysfunction or preclude successful vaginal penetration during intercourse.[8] Examination of the penile shaft will disclose a thickened plaque, typically on the dorsum, involving the tunica albuginea of the corpora bodies. Reassurance and urologic referral are warranted. Peyronie disease of the penis has been noted in association with Dupuytren's contractures of the hand.

PRIAPISM   Priapism is a urologic emergency that presents as a persistent, usually painful, pathologic erection in which both corpora cavernosa are engorged with stagnant blood.[9] Even though the glans penis and the corpus spongiosum are characteristically soft and uninvolved, urinary retention may develop. Impotence has been reported to occur in 35 percent of cases with sustained erections for prolonged periods; thus, expedient treatment and early urologic consultation are required.

Many cases of priapism in adults are pharmacologically related to intracavernosal injection of vasoactive substances for impotence (papaverine, prostaglandin E_1) or use of oral agents for hypertension (hydralazine, prazosin, or calcium channel blockers) or mental disorders (chlorpromazine, trazodone, thioridazine).[9] Most cases of priapism in children are due to hematologic disorders, usually sickle cell disease. Case reports have attempted to relate a variety of other drugs, metabolic conditions, and trauma to priapism, although the pathophysiologic mechanisms are speculative in most cases.

Priapism is classified into high-flow (nonischemic) priapism and low-flow (ischemic) priapism. High-flow (nonischemic) priapism is rare, most often nonpainful, and usually results from traumatic fistulae between the cavernosal artery and the corpus cavernosum. It is readily diagnosed by color Doppler ultrasound and successfully treated by embolization. Low-flow (ischemic) priapism is more common, is usually quite painful, and is diagnosed by the aspiration of dark acidic intracavernosal blood from the corpus cavernosum.

Adequate analgesia should be given. Regardless of specific etiology, initial therapy with terbutaline, 0.25 to 0.5 mg SC in the deltoid area, repeated in 20 to 30 min as needed, is the most effective therapy. Traditional therapies of sedation or ice water enemas are ineffective. Pseudoephedrine, 60 to 120 mg PO, has been reported as effective in some cases that present early (within 4 h). Priapism due to sickle cell disease is most consistently reversed by simple or exchange transfusion. Corporal aspiration followed by irrigation (with plain saline or α-adrenergic agonists, i.e., phenylephrine) is the primary treatment method for persistent priapism. The urologic consultant usually performs this procedure, but if one is not readily available, the emergency physician may need to intervene under the direction of a urologist. If medical treatment or phenylephrine infusion fails to produce detumescence, surgery may be required.

CARCINOMA   Carcinoma of the penis is a rare disease occurring in about 1 of every 100,000 malignancies reported, usually appearing in the fifth or sixth decade in an uncircumcised male. Carcinoma may appear as a nontender ulcer or warty growth beneath the foreskin in the area of the coronal sulcus or glans penis and is often hidden by an inflamed phimotic foreskin.

Testes and Epididymis

TESTICULAR TORSION   The differential diagnosis of acute scrotal pain includes testicular torsion, torsion of the testicular appendages, and epididymitis.[10] Because of the potential for infarction and infertility, testicular torsion must be the primary consideration.[11] Although the peak incidence of intravaginal torsion occurs at puberty in conjunction with maximal hormonal stimulation, it may occur at any age.

Torsion of the testis or spermatic cord results from maldevelopment (usually bilateral) of fixation between the enveloping tunica vaginalis and the posterior scrotal wall. Characteristically, the at-risk testis is aligned along a horizontal rather than a vertical axis. The axis of alignment can be determined only with the patient in an upright position, and even then the determination may be difficult.

Frequently there is a history of an athletic event, strenuous physical activity, or trauma just before the onset of scrotal pain. However, a fair number occur during sleep, when unilateral cremaster muscle contraction results in testicular torsion. The pain usually occurs suddenly, is severe, and is usually felt in the lower abdominal quadrant, the inguinal canal, or the testis. Although the pain may be constant or intermittent, it is not positional in nature, because testicular torsion is primarily an ischemic event that becomes inflammatory only after the testis has infarcted.

On examination, the involved testis is firm, tender, and often higher in the scrotum when examined with the patient standing. The epididymis may be displaced and not found in its normal posterolateral position. The cremasteric reflex is typically absent. Exacerbation or relief of pain with elevation of the affected testicle (Prehn sign) cannot reliably distinguish torsion from epididymitis.

In obvious cases of testicular torsion, emergent urologic consultation and surgical exploration are recommended. The often quoted 4-h warm-ischemia time for greater than 90 percent testicular salvage comes from controlled animal studies and cannot be extrapolated to clinical medicine. There are no readily available clinical or laboratory parameters to judge the degree or duration of testicular ischemia.

Therefore, no matter how long the patient has been symptomatic and no matter what the presenting physical examination suggests, if testicular torsion cannot be excluded by history, physical examination, and imaging studies, emergency scrotal exploration is the definitive procedure of choice.

Color-flow duplex Doppler ultrasound and radionuclide scintigraphy are two imaging modalities used to evaluate patients with indeterminate clinical presentations.[10,12,13] Both may be useful, but their routine clinical use is limited by timely availability and operator experience in interpreting the images. These studies are considered "positive" for testicular torsion when they demonstrate absent or clearly reduced intratesticular blood flow to the painful side when compared with the opposite testicle, and "negative" when flow is normal or increased. Both studies have nearly identical reported sensitivity (80 to 90 percent) and specificity (75 to 95 percent) for testicular torsion. Ultrasound has the advantage of demonstrating scrotal anatomy (which may indicate an alternative diagnosis) but has the disadvantage of the greater number of indeterminate results when compared with scintigraphy. Within these limitations, both modalities may be useful when promptly available for patients with unclear clinical presentations but should never delay attempted manual detorsion and scrotal exploration.

For emergent or preoperative treatment, the emergency physician should consider manual detorsion of the affected testis.[14,15] Most testes twist in a lateral to medial fashion; therefore, detorsion initially should be done in a medial to lateral motion. It must be explained to the patient that detorsion is a painful procedure and, although local anesthesia of the affected spermatic cord can initially make the patient more comfortable, it also removes an important end point of the detorsion maneuver, i.e., relief of pain. Detorsion is done in a manner similar to opening a book (Figure 95-7A). If one were to stand at the pa-

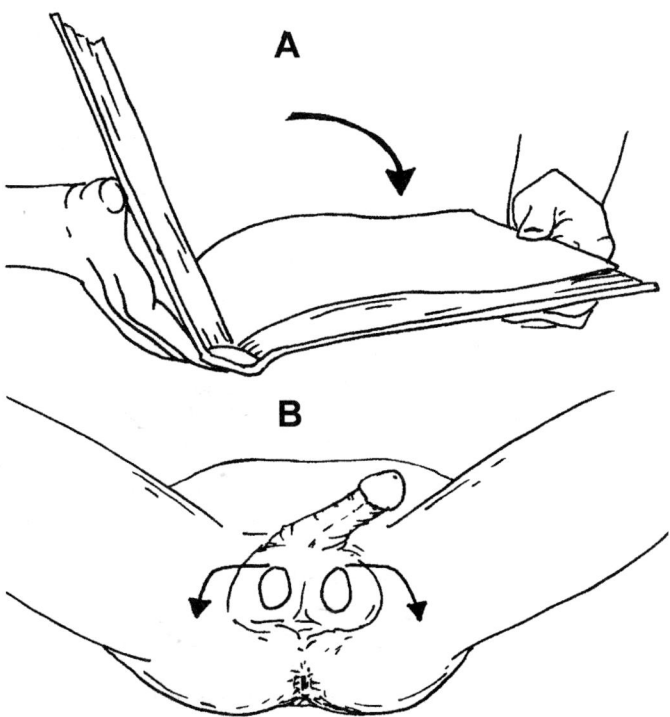

View from below

FIG. 95-7. Testicular detorsion. This procedure is best done standing at the foot of or on the right side of the patient's bed. **A.** The torsed testis is detorsed in a fashion similar to opening a book. **B.** The patient's right testis is rotated counterclockwise, and the left testis is rotated clockwise.

tient's feet, the patient's right testis would be rotated in a counterclockwise fashion and the patient's left testis in a clockwise fashion (Figure 95-7B). The initial attempt should include one and one half rotations (540°). Any relief of pain is a positive end point, and the success of the maneuver can be assessed with Doppler ultrasound demonstrating restoration of blood flow.[15] An occasional patient will require manipulation beyond the initial one and one half rotations. A worsening of the patient's pain would dictate that detorsion be done in the opposite direction. Successful detorsion converts an emergent procedure to an elective one.[14] The timing of the elective surgical correction should depend on the patient's compliance and responsibility.

Young boys may present to the ED with nonspecific abdominal pain suggestive of gastroenteritis only to return 1 to 2 days later with testicular torsion. Whether these patients had undisclosed testicular torsion at their initial evaluation is not known, but emergency physicians should think about testicular torsion in the differential diagnosis of any male presenting with a complaint of abdominal pain.

TORSION OF THE APPENDAGES   The four testicular appendages, appendix testis, appendix epididymis, paradidymis (organ of Giraldes), and vas aberrans, have no known physiologic function. These pedunculated structures are, however, capable of torsion and, in prepubertal boys, probably twist more often than the testes. The appendix testes and appendix epididymis account for about 90 and 8 percent of appendage torsion, respectively. If the patient is seen early, the pain is more intense near the head of the epididymis or testis, and an isolated tender nodule can often be palpated.[16] When the involved infarcted appendage is brought close to the thin, prepubertal, nonhormonally stimulated scrotal skin, a small dark or blue spot may be seen when light shines on or transilluminates the scrotum. This "blue dot sign" is pathognomonic of torsion of the appendix testis or epididymis. If the diagnosis can be assured and confirmed by color Doppler ultrasound showing normal intratesticular blood flow to the involved testis, surgical exploration is not necessary, and most appendages will calcify or degenerate over 10 to 14 days without causing harm. If late in the process and testicular swelling is present, or if the color Doppler ultrasound is equivocal, then urologic consultation and surgical exploration may be necessary to exclude testicular torsion.[10]

EPIDIDYMITIS   The onset of pain in epididymitis or epididymo-orchitis is usually more gradual than that of testicular torsion because of its inflammatory etiology. Bacterial infection is the most common cause and tends to depend on age.[17] In young boys, epididymitis or epididymo-orchitis is due to coliform bacteria, often with congenital anomalies of the lower urinary tract that promote urinary reflux into the globus minor (tail of the epididymis). In patients younger than 35 years, epididymitis is due primarily to sexually transmitted diseases (STD) or their complications, i.e., urethral stricture. In homosexual men with epididymitis or epididymo-orchitis, fungal infection of the lower urinary tract in addition to the more common STD organisms must be considered. In patients older than 40 years, epididymitis is caused by common urinary pathogens such as *Escherichia coli* and *Klebsiella*. These patients most often will have pyuria on urinalysis, but the absence of white cells or bacteria does not exclude the diagnosis. Older men with epididymitis due to infected urine must be evaluated for the cause of their lower urinary tract infection, i.e., benign prostatic hypertrophy or urethral stricture. Oftentimes the answer may be found by passing a 14- or 16-French Foley or Coudé catheter into the bladder; easy passage precludes a stricture. Large residual urine should alert the physician to outlet obstruction as the cause of the patient's infection. Chemical epididymitis can occur due to reflux of sterile urine and should be considered when the patient has prolonged symptoms despite appropriate antibiotic treatment.

Epididymitis causes lower abdominal, inguinal canal, scrotal, or testicular pain alone or in combination. The retrograde progression of infection from the prostatic urethra to the epididymis explains the location and progression of pain. Patients with epididymitis are more prone to lower urinary tract irritative voiding symptoms and may note transient relief of their pain in the recumbent position with scrotal elevation (positive Prehn sign). Initially, isolated firmness and nodularity of the affected globus minor are noted on examination. As the disease progresses, the sulcus between the epididymis and testis becomes obliterated, and the inflammatory epididymal mass may become contiguous with the testis, producing a large, tender scrotal mass (epididymo-orchitis) that may be difficult to differentiate from testicular torsion or abscess.

Urinalysis may show pyuria in about half of patients. Culture or DNA probe for gonorrhea and *Chlamydia* should be done if urethral discharge is present or in patients younger than 35 to 40 years. Urine culture should be done in children and older patients. Adjunctive diagnostic modalities such as color-flow duplex Doppler sonography or radionuclide scintigraphy will demonstrate increased or preserved blood flow to the testes. A reactive hydrocele may be seen on ultrasound.

Most cases of epididymitis can be managed as outpatient cases with oral antibiotics for 10 to 14 days[18] (Table 95-1). Admission criteria for epididymitis include fever with elevated white blood cell count and subjective toxicity, which can be indicative of epididymal or testicular abscess formation. Inpatient management includes: (1) bedrest for the first 24 to 48 h, with scrotal elevation and ice application (10 to 15 min every 4 to 6 h) to the involved testis or epididymis; (2) nonsteroidal anti-inflammatory drugs; (3) intravenous antibiotics based on presumed etiology; and (4) opiates for pain control. The ambulatory patient should wear a scrotal supporter, being careful not to lift heavy objects or strain when having a bowel movement, both of which will increase intra-abdominal pressure and exacerbate the inflammatory cycle. A urologist will need to re-evaluate the patient in 5 to 7 days and then ultimately decide when the patient may return to work based on his job description, i.e., a sedentary worker would be able to return sooner than a laborer.

ORCHITIS   Isolated orchitis, or inflammation of the testicle, is quite rare and usually occurs in conjunction with other systemic infections, such as mumps or other viral illnesses (coxsackie, Epstein-Barr virus, varicella, or echovirus). Mumps orchitis presents with unilateral involvement in 70 percent of cases, followed by contralateral involvement in 1 to 9 days. Bacterial orchitis is almost always associated with epididymitis. Immunocompromised patients have been reported to have orchitis due to mycobacteriosis, cryptococcosis, toxoplasmosis, or candidiasis. Patients with orchitis usually present with testicular tenderness and swelling over a few days' duration. History and physical examination are usually adequate for diagnosis, but ultrasound may be useful to exclude testicular torsion or abscess. Treatment is symptomatic and disease specific.

TESTICULAR MALIGNANCY   Any asymptomatic testicular mass, firmness, or induration is the hallmark of testicular carcinoma. Ten percent of tumors will present with pain secondary to acute hemor-

rhage within the tumor. Metastatic testicular tumors can be insidious and must be suspected in any male with unexplained supraclavicular lymphadenopathy, abdominal mass, or chronic nonproductive cough from a lung metastasis; testicular examination may disclose a primary tumor. Although not a urologic emergency, any unexplained testicular mass must be approached as a possible tumor with urgent urologic referral.

Acute Prostatitis

Acute prostatitis is bacterial inflammation of the prostate gland. It is characterized by low back pain; perineal, suprapubic, or genital discomfort; obstructive lower urinary tract voiding symptoms; perineal pain with ejaculation; frequency or dysuria; and fever or chills. Risk factors include anatomic or neurophysiologic lower urinary tract obstruction; acute epididymitis or urethritis; unprotected rectal intercourse; phimosis; intraprostatic ductal reflux; and indwelling urethral catheter or condom drainage. The causative organism is *E. coli* in most cases, with *Pseudomonas, Klebsiella, Enterobacter, Serratia,* or *Staphylococcus* in the remainder.

Clinical findings include perineal tenderness, rectal sphincter spasm, and prostatic tenderness or bogginess. The diagnosis is clinical as urinalysis and urine culture may or may not be positive. Prostatic massage is not necessary to make the diagnosis. Urethral cultures should be obtained to test for the presence of gonorrhea and chlamydia.

Favored initial treatment is ciprofloxacin 500 mg PO bid for 30 days. If drug cost is an issue, trimethoprim-sulfamethoxazole (TMP/SMX) DS one tablet PO bid for 30 days is an alternative, although cure rates are lower for TMP/SMX than for ciprofloxacin.

Most patients can be treated as outpatients, although if there is evidence of sepsis or other risk factors for sepsis such as diabetes or immunosuppression, admission will be necessary. Urologic follow-up should be provided for discharged patients, to ensure eradication of infection and to provide continuity of care in case of relapse.

Urethra

URETHRITIS   Urethritis is characterized by purulent or mucopurulent urethral discharge. Diagnosis is clinical, although it can be confirmed by evidence of pyuria or bacteriuria in a first void urine specimen. Most cases are due to *N. gonorrhoeae* or *C. trachomatis*. HSV, *U. urealyticum,* or *Trichomonas vaginalis* are less frequent causes.

Physical examination should exclude other disorders such as epididymitis, disseminated gonococcemia, or Reiter syndrome. Treatment is ceftriaxone 125 mg IM and azithromycin 1 g PO or doxycycline 100 mg PO bid × 7 d. Failure to respond suggests re-infection or re-exposure or infection with *T. vaginalis* or doxycycline-resistant *U. urealyticum*. For the former, metronidazole should be given, for the latter, azithromycin. See Chap. 141 for further discussion of STDs.

URETHRAL STRICTURE   Urethral strictures are becoming more prevalent secondary to the rising incidence of STDs. Increasingly, in teenagers and young adults, gonococcal and chlamydial infections result in bulbous urethral strictures (Figure 95-8). Urethral strictures from trauma and instrumentation are less common and tend to be localized to areas where a traumatic event has occurred. In the older population, postendoscopy meatal stenosis or localized urethral strictures are more common.[19]

If a patient requires measurement of his residual urine, has difficulty voiding, or is in urinary retention, and a 14- or 16-French Foley or Coudé catheter cannot be easily placed into the bladder, the differential diagnostic possibilities include urethral stricture, voluntary external sphincter spasm, bladder neck contracture, or benign prostatic hypertrophy. If time permits, retrograde urethrography can be done, which will define the location and extent of a urethral stricture. Only

---

TABLE 95-1 Empiric Outpatient Treatment of Epididymitis and Epididymo-Orchitis

Age <35–40 y: Treat for gonorrhea and *Chlamydia*
Ceftriaxone 250 mg IM, plus doxycycline 100 mg PO bid × 10 d
Ofloxacin 300 mg PO bid × 10 d
Age >35–40 y: Treat for gram-negative bacilli
Ciprofloxacin 500 mg PO bid × 10–14 d
Levofloxacin 250 mg PO per d × 10–14 d
Trimethoprim/sulfamethoxazole 160/800 mg (DS) PO bid × 10–14 d
Antibiotic treatment should be adjusted depending on culture results

Abbreviation: DS = double strength.

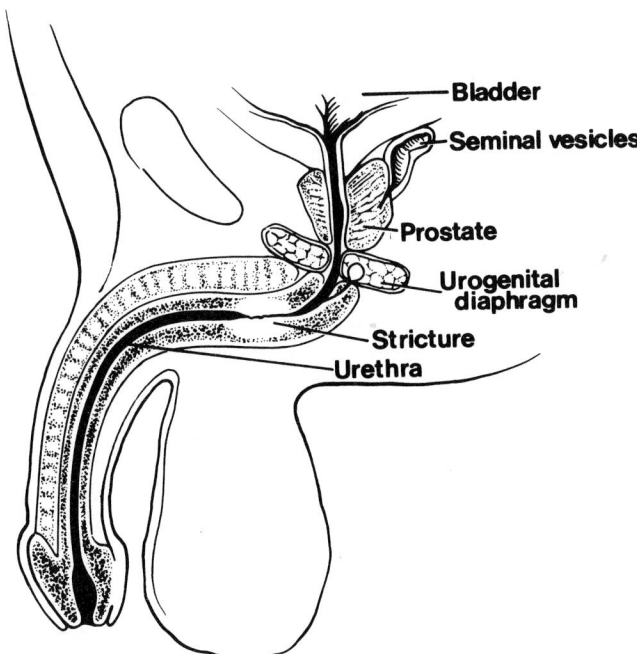

FIG. 95-8. Stricture of the bulbous urethra.

endoscopy can confirm a bladder neck contracture or the extent of an obstructing prostate gland. Suspected voluntary external sphincter spasm can be overcome by holding the penis upright and encouraging the patient to relax his perineum and breathe slowly during urinary catheter insertion.

When a urethral stricture is encountered, copious anesthetic lubrication is placed intraurethrally after the foreskin has been controlled with a folded 4 × 4. This latter maneuver is especially important in uncircumcised patients. A 12- or 14-French Coudé catheter may negotiate the strictured area, because this catheter has an angled bend near its tip. If there are previous false passages from attempts at dilation or unsuccessful instrumentation, passage of the Coudé catheter may be difficult. Further urethral manipulation may create new false passages, leading to unnecessary hemorrhage and possible gram-negative bacteremia. If two or three gentle attempts to pass the catheter fail, urologic consultation is indicated. A catheter guide or urethral sound should be used only by a urologist.

For emergency bladder decompression, a suprapubic cystostomy using Seldinger technique can be performed in the ED. The infraumbilical and suprapubic area is prepped with antiseptic (i.e., povidone iodine) solution. A 25- to 27-gauge spinal needle is used to locate the bladder. This step is especially important in cases of previous lower abdominal surgery in which normal anatomic relationships may be distorted. Alternatively, bedside ultrasound can be used to locate the bladder. Commercially available introducer cystostomy kits are readily available for temporary drainage. After the bladder has been accessed with a syringe and needle, the syringe is removed and a guidewire is passed through the needle into the bladder. The needle is then removed, and the fascial dilator with an overlying 14- to 18-French peel away sheath is passed over the wire into the bladder. The wire and dilator are then removed, leaving the hollow peel-away sheath. An appropriate-size Foley balloon catheter is passed through the peel-away sheath into the bladder, urine is aspirated from the catheter to ensure proper placement, and the balloon is inflated with water. The sheath is then removed from the bladder and peeled away, leaving the indwelling catheter, which should be withdrawn until it snugly approximates the cystostomy site. Appropriate urologic follow-up is necessary in 2 to 3 days.

URETHRAL FOREIGN BODIES Patients of all ages, but especially young children, may be victims of innocent urethral exploration or attempts to heighten sexual experiences by using a variety of foreign bodies such as bobby pins; long, thin paint brushes; or ball point pens.[20] Bloody urine combined with infection and slow, painful urination should suggest a possible foreign body in the lower urinary tract. An x-ray of the bladder and urethral areas may disclose the presence of a radiopaque foreign body.

Foreign bodies often require endoscopic removal or even open cystotomy. Occasionally a gentle milking action of the proximal end of the urethral foreign body by an experienced examiner will allow its retrieval from the distal urethral meatus. Even then, retrograde urethrography or endoscopic confirmation of an intact urethra is indicated.

Urinary Retention

Bladder outlet obstruction causes a variety of signs and symptoms; overt urinary retention represents one end of the spectrum, and symptoms of insidious overflow incontinence often will fool an unsuspecting examiner.[21] Urinary retention may be suggested if chronic systemic medical illnesses or carcinomas that have as sequelae sensory or motor neurogenic side effects or complications are present. A detailed medication history, including over-the-counter cold and dietary medications, may reveal the ingestion of a sympathomimetic agonist that has secondarily caused outlet obstruction due to its muscle-constricting effect on the abundant α-agonistic fibers in the bladder neck. Inconvenient, and therefore infrequent, voiding during a prolonged car trip by a vacationing patient with borderline obstructive symptoms may be just enough to result in urinary retention. Mechanical causes of bladder outlet obstruction include meatal stenosis, urethral stricture, bladder neck stricture, and benign prostatic hypertrophy.

A voiding history begins with questions regarding problems holding or initiating the urinary stream, voiding completely with one continuous stream rather than starting and stopping of the stream, a feeling of complete bladder emptying as opposed to incomplete emptying and postvoid residual, and the relative frequency of nocturia. Most men do not void as well or completely empty their bladders when sitting down to urinate, which happens most often during the night. Infrequent ejaculation may lead to secondary prostatic congestion and subsequent spurious symptoms of irritation and outlet obstruction.

The most difficult evaluation involves the patient with silent prostatism. Historically, voiding symptoms have gradually worsened over the years, but at such a pace that the patient often makes adjustments and then perceives each worsening state as "normal" for him. The ultimate result is urinary retention, with a large palpable bladder and often 1600 to 2000 mL of residual urine upon urinary catheterization. An intact sensory examination, anal sphincter, and bulbocavernosus reflex differentiate chronic outlet obstruction from the sensory or motor neurogenic bladder.

Appropriate physical examination requires inspection of the meatus for stenosis; palpation of the entire urethral length for masses or fistulas consistent with urethral stricture disease or abscess formation; lower abdominal examination for palpation of a suprapubic mass; and rectal examination to evaluate anal sphincter tone and the size and consistency of the prostate. Outlet obstruction due to a large intravesical prostate can result in a palpably normal prostate on rectal examination. Similarly, rectal examination in a patient in urinary retention initially may reveal a spuriously enlarged, nodular prostate that will shrink considerably once bladder decompression is achieved. Bedside ultrasonography is a noninvasive, accurate way to determine bladder distention and significant postvoid residual.

Most patients with acute urinary retention are in distress, and passage of a urethral catheter using lubricant with Lidocaine (Lidocaine Jelly) alleviates their pain and urinary retention. If attempts at passage of a straight 16-French Foley catheter fail, a 16-French Coudé catheter should be passed. The catheter should be passed to its fullest extent to obtain a free flow of urine, and only then can the catheter balloon be inflated. This will prevent balloon inflation in the prostatic urethra. If the catheter drainage holes become obstructed with lubricating jelly, gentle irrigation with sterile saline or water will quickly establish urinary drainage. Spontaneous, complete drainage of a distended bladder can be accomplished rapidly without the need for repeated clamping of the catheter. Occasionally, when a bladder has been chronically distended, bladder mucosal edema develops. Rapid decompression after catheter placement may result in transient gross hematuria. The transient hematuria is usually self-limited, of little consequence, and responds to orally induced diuresis. Post-micturitional or bladder decompression syncope is rare and should be treated symptomatically.

The catheter should be left indwelling and connected to a portable leg drainage bag. The patient or his family must be instructed in the care and drainage of this simple device. Antibiotics should be initiated if there is evidence of urinary infection. The patient or a family member should be instructed on Foley balloon deflation in case emergent removal of the catheter is necessary.

If urinary retention has been chronic or insidious, postobstructive diuresis may occur secondary to osmotic diuresis or interstitial tubular dysfunction. Postobstructive diuresis may occur in the presence of normal serum urea nitrogen and creatinine levels and may become an emergency if the patient suddenly becomes hypovolemic or hypotensive without warning. Thus, close monitoring of urine output is essential, with appropriate fluid replacement. For these reasons, all patients with chronic or insidious obstructive voiding symptoms and urinary retention should be observed for 4 to 6 h or be admitted, with particular attention paid to hourly intake, urinary output, vital signs, and urine and serum electrolytes. Osmotic diuresis will dissipate or the dysfunctional tubules will recover within 24 to 48 h. In all cases of urinary retention, consultation and follow-up with a urologist for a genitourinary evaluation are necessary.

REFERENCES

1. Klin B, Lotan G, Efrati Y, et al: Acute idiopathic scrotal edema in children- Revisited. *J Pediatr Surg* 37:1200, 2002.
2. Dahm P, Roland FH, Vaslef SN, et al: Outcome analysis in patients with primary necrotizing fasciitis of the male genitalia. *Urology* 56:31, 2000.
3. Edwards S: Balanitis and balanoposthitis: A review. *Genitourin Med* 72: 155, 1996.
4. Edwards SK: European guideline for the management of balanoposthitis. *Int J STD AIDS* 12(suppl 3):68, 2001.
5. Webster TM, Leonard MP: Topical steroid therapy for phimosis. *Can J Urol* 9:1492, 2002.
6. Choe JM: Paraphimosis: Current treatment options. *Am Fam Phys* 62:2623, 2000.
7. Eke N: Fracture of the penis. *Br J Surg* 89:555, 2002.
8. Lischer GH, Nehra A: New advances in Peyronie's disease. *Curr Opin Urol* 11:631, 2001.
9. Keoghane SR, Sullivan ME, Miller MA: The aetiology, pathogenesis and management of priapism. *BJU Int* 90:149, 2002.
10. Marcozzi D, Suner S: The nontraumatic, acute scrotum. *Emerg Med Clin North Am* 19:547, 2001.
11. Cuckow PM, Frank JD: Torsion of the testis. *BJU Int* 86:349, 2000.
12. Baker LA, Sigman D, Mathews RI, et al: An analysis of clinical outcomes using color Doppler testicular ultrasound for testicular torsion. *Pediatrics* 105(pt 1):604, 2000.
13. Blaivas M, Sierzenski P, Lambert M: Emergency evaluation of patients presenting with acute scrotum using bedside ultrasonography. *Acad Emerg Med* 8:90, 2001.
14. Cornel EB, Karthaus HF: Manual derotation of the twisted spermatic cord. *BJU Int* 83:672, 1999.
15. Garel L, Dubois J, Azzie G, et al: Preoperative detorsion of the spermatic cord with Doppler ultrasound monitoring in patients with intravaginal acute testicular torsion. *Pediatr Radiol* 30:41, 2000.
16. Kadisk HA, Bolte RG: A retrospective review of pediatric patients with epididymitis, testicular torsion, and torsion of the testicular appendages. *Pediatrics* 102(pt 1):73, 1998.
17. Chan PT, Schlegel PN: Inflammatory conditions of the male excurrent ductal system. Part I. *J Androl* 23:453, 2002.
18. Naber KG, Bergman B, Bishop MC, et al: EAU guidelines for the management of urinary and male genital infections. *Eur Urol* 40:576, 2001.
19. Andrich DE, Mundy AR: Urethral strictures and their surgical management. *BJU Int* 86:571, 2000.
20. van Ophoven A, deKernion JB: Clinical management of foreign bodies of the genitourinary tract. *J Urol* 164:274, 2000.
21. Curtis LA, Dolan TS, Cespedes RD: Acute urinary retention and urinary incontinence. *Emerg Med Clin North Am* 91:591, 2001.

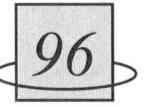

96   UROLOGIC STONE DISEASE
Rakesh Engineer
W. Franklin Peacock IV

RENAL AND URETERAL STONES

Epidemiology

Urologic stone disease is a common condition, with an incidence estimated as high as 12 percent.[1] Stones occur three times more often in males, usually in the third to fifth decades of life. Some hereditary diseases (e.g., renal tubular acidosis, hyperparathyroidism, and cystinuria) predispose patients to kidney stones.

Lifestyle factors can augment stone growth. Patients in mountainous, desert, or tropical regions and those in sedentary jobs have a higher frequency of stone disease.[2] There is also an increased incidence during the warmest 3 months of the year for any geographic location. Increased water intake is associated with a decreased incidence of calculi.[1]

Some medications predispose to stone disease. The protease inhibitor, indinavir sulfate, used to treat the human immunodeficiency virus, is associated with a 4 percent incidence of symptomatic urolithiasis. Carbonic anhydrase inhibitors, triamterene, and laxative abuse also increase the prevalence of renal stones.[2,3]

Children younger than 16 years constitute approximately 7 percent of all renal stone cases. Unique to children is a 1:1 sex distribution.[4] The most common causes in pediatrics involve metabolic abnormalities (50 percent), urologic anomalies (20 percent), infection (15 percent), and immobilization syndrome (5 percent). The remainder are considered idiopathic.

In patients with a history of a renal stone, up to a third suffer recurrence within 1 year. The 5-year recurrence rate nears 50 percent, probably due to the persistence of the underlying abnormality creating the first stone.

Pathophysiology

Stone formation is a multistep process that begins with supersaturation of urine with urinary solutes.[1,2] Crystals eventually precipitate out as more solute is added. Once crystals form, their growth into a stone is prevented by inhibitory substances (e.g., citrate and pyrophosphate) and, more importantly, the free flow of urine. Thus, stone formation requires three key elements: supersaturation, a relative lack of inhibitors, and stasis.[1,2] Urinary stasis from physical anomaly, neurogenic bladder or catheter placement, and the presence of foreign bodies (e.g., surgical suture) may provide the environment for stone growth.

Approximately 75 percent of calculi are composed of calcium, occurring in conjunction with oxalate, phosphate, or a combination of both. These stones may develop as a result of increased urinary excretion of a given solute. Calcium excretion is elevated in conditions that include hyperparathyroidism, absorptive and renal hypercalciuria, and immobilization syndrome. Oxalate excretion is enhanced in patients with inflammatory bowel disease and as a result of small bowel resection or jejunoileal bypass. Ten percent of stones are struvite (magnesium-ammonium-phosphate). These stones often are associated with infection by urea-splitting bacteria and are the most common cause of staghorn calculi, large stones that form a cast of the renal pelvis. Antibiotic penetration into staghorn calculi is poor, and the potential for urosepsis exists as long as the stones remain. Consequently, surgical treatment is recommended for staghorn calculi. Uric acid causes 10 percent of uroliths. Cystine and other uncommon minerals comprise the remainder. Certain groups of patients are identified as high risk for preventable stone formation secondary to their underlying medical illness (Table 96-1). With appropriate evaluation, 90 percent of patients will have a cause identified, and 85 percent of calcium oxalate stone recurrences can be prevented.[3]

Passage of stones through the urinary tract may be slowed or halted by areas of anatomic narrowing or bending. Progressing proximally to distally, common areas of impaction include the renal calyx, the renal ureteropelvic junction (UPJ), where the ureter passes over the pelvic brim and iliac vessels, and the ureterovesical junction (UVJ). The UVJ has the smallest diameter of the urinary tract and is a common location for impacted stones. Another location in women is the posterior pelvis, where the ureter is crossed anteriorly by the pelvic blood vessels and broad ligament.

With acute ureteral obstruction, after an initial rise of renal blood flow and intraureteral pressure, both parameters decline and glomerular filtration falls. Concurrently, there is a proportional increase in blood flow to the contralateral kidney. These effects are reversible if the obstruction is relieved. However, after prolonged obstruction (several weeks), irreversible renal damage occurs. Because the contralateral kidney usually can maintain excretory requirements, serum urea nitrogen and creatinine levels do not rise, even though there may be only one functional kidney.

The probability of spontaneous passage of stones is determined by multiple factors, including size, shape, location, and degree of ureteral obstruction (Table 96-2). Bizarre or irregularly shaped stones with spicules or sharp edges have a lower passage rate. With complete obstruction, there is a lower rate of spontaneous passage than if the blockage is partial.

Clinical Features

Uroliths may be asymptomatic until there is at least partial obstruction of the urinary tract. The typical episode occurs while the patient is sedentary or at rest. Ureteral distention and peristalsis cause the acute onset of remarkably severe, episodic visceral pain and little, if any, tenderness on examination. Although subacute presentations occur, the usual rapidity of symptom onset is in contradistinction to many other diagnoses that may mimic renal colic.

Typically pain originates in either flank, radiates anteroinferiorly around the abdomen, and progresses toward the ipsilateral testicle or labium majorum. The discomfort can be intense and may be associated with nausea, vomiting, or diaphoresis. Patients may be unable to find a comfortable position to relieve their symptoms. Consequently, they may be anxious, pacing, and reluctant to lie still on the examining table. The "writhing of renal colic" is a useful point in the construction of a differential diagnosis.

TABLE 96-1   Some Conditions at Risk for Preventable Renal Stone Formation

Hypercalciuria: absorptive, resorptive (primary hyperparathyroidism), renal leak
Hyperoxaluria: primary genetic disorder, malabsorption associated with chronic diarrhea or short bowel syndrome
Hyperuricosuria: gout
Cystinuria: primary genetic disorder
Struvite stones: infection

TABLE 96-2   Probability of Spontaneous Renal Stone Passage

Characteristic	Probability
Size	
<4 mm	90%
4–6 mm	50%
>6 mm	10%
Location in ureter at first diagnosis	
Proximal	20%
Middle	50%
Distal	70%

The characteristic radiating pattern of renal colic results from autonomic nerve fibers serving the kidney and ipsilateral gonad. Atypical presentations of pain referral to the hip, thigh, or knee are rarely reported. As a stone progresses to the mid-ureter, anterior abdominal pain may radiate back toward the flank. With passage near the bladder, the patient may develop urinary frequency and urgency. Symptoms can be remarkably episodic due to intermittent obstruction of the urinary tract. If the stone passes or the obstruction is temporarily relieved, the patient has immediate symptom relief. Patients are frequently cool and diaphoretic, and a history of fever is unusual. Fever should prompt an investigation for urinary tract infection or other causes of febrile illness.

In children, symptoms vary with age. Older children are more likely to present with typical adult symptoms. Younger children may have a more nonspecific presentation, such as abdominal or pelvic pain. Although renal colic is rare in infants, symptoms may be mistakenly attributed to intestinal colic.[4] Overall, 20 to 30 percent of children may have only painless hematuria with urologic stone disease.

Patients with known stone disease may present after treatment with extracorporeal shock wave lithotripsy. Extracorporeal shock wave lithotripsy fractures stones into small particles with the use of focused sound waves. The resulting "sludge" is passed in the urine. When there are large fragments, an acute episode of renal colic occurs. The clinical presentation is identical to that of "de novo" renal colic.

Diagnosis

PHYSICAL EXAMINATION   Special attention is given to the abdominal and cardiovascular examinations so that potential catastrophes mimicking acute renal colic can be excluded. Elevations of blood pressure and pulse secondary to severe discomfort are common. The presence of fever or hypotension suggests the possibility of concurrent infection or an alternative diagnosis.

The abdominal examination is extremely important. Auscultation of a bruit or palpation of a pulsatile mass suggests a rupturing or dissecting aortic aneurysm. Distal pulses in the extremities should be carefully examined; diminished, absent, or asymmetric pulses suggest a potential vascular emergency. However, lack of abnormal physical findings does not exclude aortic disease, and elderly, hypertensive patients without a prior history of renal colic should be considered at risk for an abdominal aortic aneurysm (AAA).

Mild tenderness may be noted over the site of an impacted stone. However, peritoneal findings (e.g., guarding or rebound) or abdominal distention is not a usual component of acute renal colic, but if present, other pathologies should be considered.

The genitourinary examination is also important. Costovertebral angle tenderness is not unusual but, if present with fever or other symptoms of urinary tract infection, suggests pyelonephritis. Pyelonephritis can occur simultaneously with stone disease. In addition, because the radiating pattern of discomfort in renal colic includes the testicle or labium majorum, these areas should be evaluated for a potential incarcerated hernia. In a male patient, the testicles should be examined to exclude torsion or infection. A pelvic examination is not indicated in females with a consistent evaluation (typical flank pain, microscopic hematuria, and a "positive" imaging study), but should be considered when the diagnosis is unclear.

The general physical examination should address the cardiac, respiratory, musculoskeletal, and dermatologic systems. An abnormal chest examination may suggest an alternative diagnosis, such as lobar pneumonia or pulmonary embolus. Musculoskeletal complaints may result in flank pain similar to that with renal stones. The presence of a vesicular rash over a flank dermatome may represent herpes zoster.

LABORATORY TESTS   A urinalysis should be performed in patients with suspected renal colic to identify hematuria or infection. The finding of hematuria supports the diagnosis of renal colic, but there is no correlation between the amount of hematuria and the degree of urinary tract obstruction. A few patients may demonstrate gross hematuria, and in up to 15 percent, microscopic hematuria is absent.[5] A urine test strip detects hemoglobin, myoglobin, or porphyrins as blood. A microscopic urinalysis can confirm hematuria by demonstrating the presence of red blood cells. A urine culture and sensitivity should be obtained if the test strip is positive for leukocyte esterase or nitrates or if the microscopic urinalysis shows bacteria or pyuria. The presence of oxalate or urate stones on microscopic urinalysis can be an aid to identifying stone composition. However, because crystals may be seen without renal stones, their presence is not diagnostic and should be interpreted cautiously. An elevated urine pH (>7.6) is associated with infection and may indicate the presence of a urea-splitting organism. Alkaline urine is also seen in renal tubular acidosis or after ingestion of large amounts of alkali. Collected urine should be strained to detect any passed stones, and all collected stones should be retained for pathologic analysis.

A pregnancy test should be performed in women of reproductive age. A positive result suggests a possible ectopic pregnancy and affects the choice of imaging study to confirm a renal colic diagnosis. A complete blood cell count is not indicated in routine renal colic but should be considered if the presentation suggests the possibility of anemia, infection, or AAA.

Other laboratory testing can be individualized. Renal evaluation (e.g., blood urea nitrogen and creatinine) may be required in patients at risk for nephrotoxicity (the elderly and those with renal insufficiency, diabetes, or hypovolemia) if a radiocontrast media (RCM) study is planned. There is a higher incidence of RCM nephropathy in diabetics with serum creatinine levels above 1.5 mg/dL and in patients with chronic renal insufficiency and serum creatinine levels above 2.5 mg/dL. Diabetics also may require a serum glucose measurement, because the stress of renal colic may cause significant hyperglycemia or nausea, and vomiting may produce hypoglycemia.

DIAGNOSTIC IMAGING   **Helical computed tomography (CT) is generally the preferred imaging modality to diagnose renal colic.**[1,6] Ultrasound is preferred in pregnant women to minimize radiation exposure.[1,2] Other modalities that may assist in the diagnosis include intravenous urography, radionuclide renal scan, and plain abdominal radiographs (Table 96-3).

Imaging confirms the presence of a ureteral stone, rules out other diagnoses, identifies complications, defines stone location, and assists with management if the stone fails to pass spontaneously.[1] It is unclear if all patients require ED imaging for suspected renal colic. For young, healthy patients in whom the diagnosis is clinically clear, imaging can be conducted later on an outpatient basis if symptoms dictate.[7] In women, imaging can be helpful to exclude gastrointestinal or gynecologic disorders. In older patients, disorders such as renal cell carcinoma, acute appendicitis, or AAA can be excluded by proper imaging studies.

COMPUTED TOMOGRAPHY   The noncontrast helical CT scan is sensitive and specific, with "diagnostic" positive and negative likelihood ratios for detection of renal stones[6] (see Table 96-3). Images are obtained from the top of the kidney to the bladder base. Secondary signs of ureteral obstruction, such as ureteral dilatation, stranding of perinephric fat, dilatation of the collecting system, and renal enlargement, can be helpful in making the diagnosis. In combination, unilateral ureteral dilatation and perinephric stranding have a positive predictive value of 96 percent for stone disease.[8] If both are absent, the negative predictive value is 93 to 97 percent.[8]

Noncontrast helical CT has advantages over other imaging modalities, including superior speed, the avoidance of RCM, and greater ability to identify other pathologies. However, because RCM are not used, the specificity and sensitivity for other diagnoses (e.g., AAA, appendicitis, or perinephric abscess) are not as great as with imaging protocols using contrast. The helical CT scan has a few disadvantages. Helical CT does not evaluate renal function or provide information on the degree of obstruction.

INTRAVENOUS UROGRAPHY   Intravenous urography (or intravenous pyelogram) yields information on renal function and anatomy. It detects calculi with modest sensitivity but excellent specificity[6,9] (see Table 96-3). When performing the study, maintaining adequate urine output by giving intravenous fluids before RCM infusion may decrease the risk of contrast-induced renal injury. An initial scout film is obtained, followed by RCM administration, with repeat films at 5, 10, and 20 min. The first and most reliable indication of ureteral obstruction is a delayed nephrogram. Because the ureter is peristaltic, it is usually not completely seen on one film. Visualization of the entire ureter is suggestive of obstruction.

TABLE 96-3   Ancillary Tests in Urologic Stone Disease

Test	Sensitivity	Specificity	LR(+)	LR(−)	Comments
Noncontrast computed tomography	94–97%	96–99%	24–∞	0.02–0.04	Advantages: speed, no RCM, detects other diagnoses Disadvantages: radiation, no evaluation of renal function
Intravenous urogram	64–90%	94–100%	15–∞	0.11–0.15	Advantage: evaluates renal function Disadvantage: RCM (allergy, nephrotoxicity, metformin)
Ultrasound	63–85%	79–100%	10–∞	0.10–0.34	Advantages: pregnancy, no RCM, no radiation, no known side effects Disadvantages: insensitive in middle third of the ureter, may miss smaller stones (<5 mm)
Plain abdominal radiograph	29–58%	69–74%	1.9–2.0	0.58–0.64	Advantage: may be used to follow stones Disadvantage: poor sensitivity and specificity
Urine test strip	80%	35%	1.2	0.57	Rapid screening test but can miss complete obstruction if hematuria is absent, provides additional information on the possibility of infection
Microscopic urinalysis >0 RBC/HPF	89%	29%	1.3	0.38	

Abbreviations: HPF = high-power field; LR(+) = positive likelihood ratio; LR(−) = negative likelihood ratio; RBC = red blood cell; RCM = radiocontrast media.

The location of a radiolucent obstructing stone often can be determined by a ureteral contrast column cutoff. Adjuncts to the diagnosis of renal colic include the presence of a prolonged nephrogram, renal enlargement, dilatation of the collecting system, and contrast extravasation.[10] Extravasation suggests obstruction that decompressed into the perinephric tissue. Extra-urinary tract urine (urinoma) has the potential for infection and abscess formation.

A postvoid film can identify stones at the UVJ or distal ureter that are otherwise obscured by a full bladder. In patients with high-grade or complete obstruction, delayed films taken at 1- to 2-h intervals may be required to precisely determine the level of obstruction.

The advantage of intravenous urography over other imaging modalities is that it provides information on renal function. It can be an adjunct to CT if functional information and knowledge of the degree of obstruction are required. The main disadvantage of intravenous urography is the RCM administration, which has possible side effects of allergic reaction and nephrotoxicity. The patient should be closely questioned for possible allergy to contrast media, and appropriate material for managing acute anaphylaxis should be immediately available.

Radiocontrast media nephrotoxicity is seen in approximately 9 percent of patients with pre-existing renal insufficiency or diabetes mellitus[10] (Table 96-4). With risk for nephrotoxicity, RCM administration should be deferred until normal blood urea nitrogen and creatinine are documented. Nonionic contrast agents may result in a lower rate of kidney damage. Radiocontrast media should be used with caution in patients on metformin, because this drug has been associated with severe lactic acidosis and RCM nephrotoxicity.[11]

Other disadvantages of intravenous urography include time required to complete delayed films and the lack of bowel preparation, which may affect the final interpretation. A false-negative study can occur if the stone is small, radiolucent, partially obstructing, or if it passes into the bladder before the contrast is excreted by the kidneys. If this happens, the patient experiences nearly complete relief of pain. The intravenous pyelogram may show evidence of ureteral spasm after stone passage.

ULTRASOUND If patients are not candidates for CT or intravenous urography due to concerns of radiation (e.g., during pregnancy or in children), ultrasound can assist in the diagnosis.[9,12] It is useful in the detection of larger stones; however, it may miss smaller (<5 mm in diameter) ureteral stones.[12] Ultrasound is helpful in diagnosing stones in the proximal and distal ureters but is insensitive for mid-ureteral stones. Overall, ultrasound has only modest sensitivity and specificity for detecting renal stones (see Table 96-3) but is 98 percent sensitive for detecting hydronephrosis. However, up to 22 percent of hydronephroses diagnosed by ultrasound do not represent obstruction.[10] Causes of false-positive hydronephrosis include normal anatomic variation, full bladder, and renal cysts. Ultrasound studies provide information on renal size and, with Doppler scanning, renal blood and urine flow. Limited information may be obtained about other pathologic conditions mimicking urologic stone disease.

Ultrasound has many advantages: it is noninvasive, uses no dye or radiation, and has no known side effects. It may also be superior to intravenous urography for detecting UVJ stones. However, it is limited to anatomic findings; and whereas the Doppler study provides information about renal blood flow, ultrasound yields no information on renal excretory function. In addition, accuracy is operator and equipment dependent. Obesity may interfere with obtaining good-quality scans, and ultrasound can miss early obstructive signs. Rapid bolus infusion of crystalloid can result in a false-positive finding of hydroureter.

PLAIN ABDOMINAL RADIOGRAPHS About 90 percent of urinary calculi are radiopaque because calcium phosphate and calcium oxalate stones have a density similar to that of bone. Magnesium-ammonium-phosphate (struvite) is slightly less radiodense, followed by cystine, which is only partly radiodense. Uric acid and matrix stones are essentially radiolucent, as are most stones associated with medications.[13] Unfortunately, because of small size and overlapping soft tissue and bone shadows, urinary stones are visible much less frequently on plain films. Plain abdominal radiographs have poor sensitivity and specificity for detecting renal stones[9,14] (see Table 96-3). The weak likelihood ratios indicate that plain radiographs are of little value in the diagnosis of renal colic. Although a plain abdominal radiograph can localize some large radiopaque stones, its greatest utility is exclusion of other conditions, and it may be used to follow known radiopaque stones.

Differential Diagnosis

Many diagnoses can be confused with renal colic (Table 96-5). History and physical examination can be difficult because the patient's discomfort may interfere with adequate information collection. The most critical diagnosis to consider is aortic dissection or ruptured AAA. Renal colic and AAA may have similar presentations. Focal abdominal tenderness, abdominal distention, pulse disparity, and hemodynamic instability are not found in renal colic and suggest a leaking or ruptured AAA.

Pyelonephritis may cause flank pain; however, the prodrome is less acute and the discomfort not as severe as with renal colic. Fever is not a finding with kidney stones. In renal colic without concomitant infection, urinalysis does not demonstrate bacteriuria or pyuria. If renal obstruction is suspected with pyelonephritis, obstruction should be excluded by intravenous urography, CT, or ultrasound. Antibiotics have poor penetration into an obstructed kidney, and if infection and obstruction are confirmed, emergency urologic consultation for obstruction relief is indicated.

TABLE 96-4 Radiocontrast Media Nephrotoxicity Risk Factors

Pre-existing renal insufficiency
Diabetes mellitus
Hypovolemia
Hypotension
Age older than 70 years
Multiple myeloma
Hyperuricemia
Hypertension (uncontrolled)
Radiocontrast media within past 72 h

TABLE 96-5 Differential Diagnosis of Renal Colic

Vascular	Aortic abdominal aneurysm
	Aortic dissection
Renal	Pyelonephritis
	Papillary necrosis
	Renal infarction
	Renal vein thrombosis
	Renal cell carcinoma
Gastrointestinal	Mesenteric ischemia
	Biliary colic
	Pancreatitis
	Perforated peptic ulcer
	Appendicitis
	Ventral/inguinal hernia
	Diverticulitis
Gynecologic	Ectopic pregnancy
	Salpingitis
	Tubo-ovarian abscess
	Ovarian cyst
Genitourinary	Testicular torsion
	Epididymitis
Miscellaneous	Drug seeking

Papillary necrosis presents similarly to renal stones. It is most frequent in sickle cell disease, diabetes, nonsteroidal analgesic abuse, or infection. The urinalysis may demonstrate hematuria and pyuria. Intravenous urography or CT can demonstrate the sloughed renal papillae as lucency within the renal pelvis. Urologic consultation and hospitalization are usually required.

Renal infarction, from vascular dissection or arterial embolus, may present with acute flank pain and hematuria. The noncontrast CT scan likely will show no abnormality. Diagnosis requires evidence of impaired excretion (intravenous urography) or diminished blood flow (Doppler ultrasound or renal angiography). In renal vein thrombosis, there is increased kidney size and decreased function with proteinuria and microscopic hematuria.

Other pathologic conditions may cause ureteral compression or obstruction, producing symptoms similar to renal colic. Any intraabdominal mass can cause ureteral obstruction. If within the urinary system, it may cause obstruction and pain from expanding size or in association with hemorrhage or necrosis.

Patients with pain out of proportion to the findings on the physical examination raise suspicion of mesenteric ischemia. Other gastrointestinal conditions may mimic renal colic but usually have significant abdominal tenderness. Gynecologic disorders may mimic renal colic. Ruptured ectopic pregnancy can present with acute pelvic and flank pain. Salpingitis usually has a more insidious onset, with cervical motion tenderness and purulent discharge on the pelvic examination. Although renal colic can cause pain radiating to the testicle, the testicle itself is normal; the presence of testicular tenderness, redness, or swelling on examination should indicate another cause.

Drug seekers may present with factitious renal colic, they are remarkably inventive in the complexity of their ruse, and there is no specific method for detection. A history of multiple medical allergies to non-opiate analgesics and RCM is frequently given. They may report a known radiolucent stone and can simulate hematuria by placing blood in their urine. The vital signs may suggest this behavior if changes in blood pressure and heart rate do not match the extreme discomfort demonstrated. When the clinician is unsure, it is better to give analgesia than to deprive a patient suffering from renal colic.

Treatment

The mainstay of ED treatment is pain control. Because, in most cases, the diagnosis is clinical, a rapid urine test strip positive for blood may provide sufficient information, coupled with clinical findings, to start analgesics. **Pain medication should not be delayed pending test results.** Relief frequently requires multiple doses of intravenous opiates, titrated to the level of discomfort. Opiates may be accompanied by nonsteroidal anti-inflammatory drugs (NSAIDs). Because time of onset for NSAIDs is slower than that for intravenous opiates, they are not effective monotherapy. However, their use in combination with opiates may result in earlier ED discharge.[15] NSAIDs should be used with caution in patients with suspected renal insufficiency (e.g., diabetics) so as not to precipitate or accelerate a decline in renal function. An antiemetic is helpful if there is emesis, or when nausea complicates opiate use. Intravenous fluids, usually NS, can be given for hypovolemia, vomiting, or if a RCM study is planned.

If there is evidence of associated infection, urine culture should be obtained and parenteral antibiotics given promptly, while the patient is still in the ED.

Disposition

Patients with infection and concurrent obstruction have the potential for severe systemic toxicity and represent a urologic emergency; urologic consultation and admission are required (Table 96-6). In addition, disposition should be discussed with a urologist if there is (1) renal insufficiency, (2) severe underlying disease, (3) an intravenous urogram showing extravasation or complete obstruction, (4) multiple ED visits, (5) a large stone, or (6) sloughed renal papillae. Because of lower rates of spontaneous passage, patients with large (>5 mm), irregular, or proximal stones should be considered for admission. In severe concurrent underlying disease (e.g., angina or chronic obstructive pulmonary disease) or in the fragile elderly, who may be unable to tolerate the stress of renal colic, a lower admission threshold is indicated. Patients who return with continued pain require a careful history and physical examination to ensure the diagnosis is correct, but repeat imaging is probably unnecessary.

In most situations, excluding pain, unilateral renal obstruction has minimal acute or permanent effects. Discharge is appropriate in those with smaller, rounded stones; in the absence of infection; and when pain is controlled by oral analgesics.[16] Patients should be given a urinary strainer with instructions to save any stones they pass for pathologic evaluation. Average time for stone passage varies according to size and location, but may range up to 7 to 20 days for stones 5 to 6 mm in diameter.[17] Patients should be counseled to return promptly for fever, vomiting, or uncontrolled pain, and a prescription for an oral opiate and NSAIDs should be provided. There is limited evidence that the addition of sustained-release calcium channel blockers (nifedipine) and steroids (prednisone or deflazacort) added to standard outpatient treatment with opioids and NSAIDs enhances stone passage rate and reduces lost work days, repeat ED visits, and surgical interventions.[17,18] Follow-up with a urologist within 7 days should be recommended.[16]

If the stone passes in the ED, no further treatment is required. Elective urologic consultation is recommended so that the etiology of the stone is evaluated and a prophylactic strategy can be arranged. Patients with hematuria, negative imaging studies, and no other attributable source require outpatient urologic follow-up to determine the cause of their hematuria.

Protease-inhibitor-induced urolithiasis management is similar to that with other causes of stone disease; however, adequate hydration is particularly important.[13] In addition, discontinuation of the offending agent for a short period may be necessary. Such a decision should be made in consultation with a urologist and infectious disease specialist.

BLADDER (VESICAL) STONES

Vesical calculi account for about 5 percent of urinary calculi, and in developed countries usually are associated with bladder foreign bodies, bladder outlet obstruction, or infection.[19] Bladder stones are endemic in some developing countries, and historically the vast majority occur in males and develop in early childhood. In developed countries, 90 percent occur in males, with 80 percent in those older than 50 years. Calculi are associated with outflow obstruction or neuropathic bladder disease in 70 percent of cases. Urinary tract infection, vesical diverticuli, and foreign body (e.g., sutures, catheters, or implants) predispose to bladder calculi. Consequently, bladder calculi are reported in children and adults as a urologic surgery complication.[19] Calcium oxalate is the most common constituent of bladder stones, but urate and struvite stones also occur. Usually solitary, multiple bladder stones are found in 25 percent of cases.

Bladder calculi may be asymptomatic, especially in patients with underlying prostatic obstruction. Typical symptoms are intermittent dysuria and terminal hematuria. The greatest discomfort usually oc-

TABLE 96-6 Indications for Admission

Infection with concurrent obstruction
Solitary or transplanted kidney with obstruction
Uncontrolled pain
Intractable emesis

Source: Rivers K, Shetty S, Menon M: When and how to evaluate a patient with nephrolithiasis. *Urol Clin North Am* 27:203, 2000.

curs at the end of micturition, as the stone impinges upon the bladder neck. In bladder outlet obstruction, there is interruption of the urinary stream, with frequency and urgency commonly reported. There may be associated dull, aching, low abdominal pain unrelated to urination that is exacerbated by exercise and abrupt movement. Pain usually is referred to the penile tip or scrotum by the second and third sacral nerves. Occasionally pain is referred to the low back or heel.

Physical examination is of little diagnostic help. Rarely, exceptionally large stones are palpated during rectal, vaginal, or abdominal examination. Urinalysis may demonstrate hematuria, pyuria, or bacteriuria. Plain radiographs detect vesical stones in approximately 50 percent of cases. Although ultrasound may demonstrate bladder stones, cystoscopic examination is the most accurate detection method.

Other bladder pathology can mimic vesical stones, including foreign body, carcinoma, neurogenic bladder, bladder diverticula, or fistula. Complications include chronic bladder irritation, fistulas, and urethral obstruction. Pericystitis may develop, if chronic, and can result in adherence of the bladder to the adjacent pelvic fat. Bladder perforation is a rare complication.

Bladder calculi require emergency therapy when they result in urinary obstruction or with associated infection. Acute urethral obstruction requires stone removal or catheter placement. Very distal stones may be gently milked from the penis or removed by forceps. More proximal stones require emergency urologic consultation. If there is coexistent infection, antibiotics should be administered in the ED. Patients with symptomatic nonobstructing bladder stones may be discharged with urology referral, because most vesical calculi require cystoscopic removal.

REFERENCES

1. Manthey DE, Teichman J: Nephrolithiasis. *Emerg Med Clin North Am* 19:633, 2001.
2. Shokeir AA: Renal colic: New concepts related to pathophysiology, diagnosis and treatment. *Curr Opin Urol* 12:263, 2002.
3. Rivers K, Shetty S, Menon M: When and how to evaluate a patient with nephrolithiasis. *Urol Clin North Am* 27:203, 2000.
4. Minevich E: Pediatric urolithiasis. *Pediatr Clin North Am* 48:1571, 2001.
5. Bove P, Kaplan D, Dalrymple N, et al: Reexamining the value of hematuria testing in patients with acute flank pain. *J Urol* 162(pt 1):685, 1999.
6. Worster A, Preyra I, Weaver B, Haines T: The accuracy of noncontrast helical computed tomography versus intravenous pyelography in the diagnosis of suspected acute urolithiasis: A meta-analysis. *Ann Emerg Med* 40: 280, 2002.
7. Tasso SR, Shields CP, Rosenberg CR, et al: Effectiveness of selective use of intravenous pyelography in patients presenting to the emergency department with ureteral colic. *Acad Emerg Med* 4:780, 1997.
8. Smith RC, Verga M, Dalrymple NC, et al: Acute ureteral obstruction: Value of secondary signs on helical unenhanced CT. *AJR* 167:1109, 1996.
9. Svedstrom E, Alanen A, Nurmi M: Radiologic evaluation of renal colic: The role of plain films, excretory urography, and sonography. *Eur J Radiol* 11:180, 1990.
10. Koelliker SL, Cronan JJ: Acute urinary tract obstruction: Imaging update. *Urol Clin North Am* 24:571, 1997.
11. Calabrese AT, Coley KC, DaPos SV, et al: Evaluation of prescribing practices: Risk of lactic acidosis with metformin therapy. *Arch Intern Med* 162:434, 2002.
12. Fowler KA, Locken JA, Duchesne JH, Williamson MR: US for detecting renal calculi with nonenhanced CT as a reference standard. *Radiology* 222:109, 2002.
13. Gentle DL, Stoller ML, Jarrett TW, et al: Protease inhibitor-induced urolithiasis. *Urology* 50:508, 1997.
14. Boyd R, Gray AJ: Role of the plain radiograph and urinalysis in acute ureteral colic. *J Accid Emerg Med* 13:390, 1996.
15. Larkin GL, Peacock WF, Pearl SM, et al: Efficacy of detorolac tromethamine versus meperidine in the ED treatment of acute renal colic. *Am J Emerg Med* 17:6, 1999.
16. Singal RK, Denstedt JD: Contemporary management of ureteral stones. *Urol Clin North Am* 24:59, 1997.
17. Porpiglia F, Destefanis P, Fiori C, Fontana D: Effectiveness of nifedipine and deflazacort in the management of distal ureter stone. *Urology* 56:579, 2000.
18. Cooper JT, Stack GM, Cooper TP: Intensive medical management of ureteral calculi. *Urology* 56:575, 2000.
19. Schwartz BF, Stoller ML: The vesical calculus. *Urol Clin North Am* 27:333, 2000.

HEMATURIA AND HEMATOSPERMIA

David S. Howes
Mark P. Bogner

HEMATURIA

Normal urine contains a small number of red blood cells (RBCs), usually too small to be detected by routine chemical test strip testing or microscopic urinalysis. Hematuria that should concern the clinician may be visible to the eye (gross or frank hematuria) or invisible (microscopic hematuria). Gross hematuria often motivates the patient to come to the ED while microscopic hematuria is usually detected in the course of evaluating other symptoms. Hematuria may be associated with pain during urination and often accompanies urinary tract infections. Painless hematuria is more often a result of neoplastic, hyperplastic, and vascular causes. Whether gross or microscopic, hematuria warrants an attempt at definitive diagnosis, because underlying disease can be found in a substantial percentage of cases. The emergency physician's task is to exclude a life-threatening cause, make a diagnosis if possible, initiate treatment, educate the patient, and ensure appropriate treatment, disposition, follow-up, and referral.

Epidemiology

Gross hematuria is easy to define: the urine appears red. However, other pigments, particularly myoglobin, may discolor the urine, or bleeding from a nonurinary source may contaminate the urine. It takes approximately 1 mL of whole blood per liter of urine to result in visible hematuria. Gross hematuria may also result in false proteinuria, because 1 mL of whole blood contains approximately 50 mg of albumin. This must be taken into account when protein-losing diseases (e.g., nephritic or nephrotic syndromes) are considered in the differential diagnosis. Approximately 3 percent of the general population reports at least one prior episode of gross hematuria.[1] The incidence is higher in women (because of urinary tract infections), older adults (because of neoplasia), and older men (because of prostatic hyperplasia).

Microscopic hematuria is less-well defined. Approximately 1 million RBCs typically pass into the urine each day. This small amount will be reflected as 1 to 3 RBCs/high-power field (hpf) (400×) on microscopic examination of centrifuged urine sediment. The American Urological Association Best Practice Policy Panel on Asymptomatic Microscopic Hematuria (AMH) defines AMH as ≥3 RBCs/hpf from two of three properly collected urinalysis specimens.[2] This definition allows for some degree of AMH in normal patients. **A practical definition of microscopic hematuria for use in the ED is >5 RBCs/hpf on a single sample;** avoiding impractical attempts at obtaining multiple urine samples on a single visit. Population-based studies of healthy young individuals have found at least one episode of transient microscopic hematuria in up to 40 percent of men and 13 percent of women.[2–5] The incidence of microscopic hematuria in children and adolescents is up to 6 percent for one specimen and 1 percent to 2 percent for two positive specimens.[6,7]

Pathophysiology

Any process that results in infection, inflammation, or injury to the kidneys, ureters, bladder, prostate, male genitalia, or urethra may result in hematuria (Tables 97-1 and 97-2).[8,9] In false hematuria, the urine appears bloody, but dipstick test results are negative for blood, and there are no RBCs on microscopic evaluation (Table 97-3). Free hemoglobin, myoglobin, or porphyrins in the urine result in a positive urine test strip reaction for blood without RBCs on microscopic evaluation.

Clinical Features

It is useful to identify when the blood appears during micturition. Initial hematuria is the appearance of blood at the beginning of micturition, with subsequent clearing, and suggests urethral disease. Hematuria occurring between voiding and noticed only as staining of underclothes with blood, while voided urine is clear, indicates lesions at the distal urethra or the meatus. Total hematuria is visible throughout micturition and corresponds to disease of the kidneys, ureters, or bladder. Terminal hematuria, occurring at the end of micturition after initially voiding clear urine, occurs with disease at the bladder neck or prostatic urethra.

Gross hematuria more often indicates a lower-tract cause, while microscopic hematuria tends to occur with kidney disease. Brown or smoky-colored urine along with RBC casts and proteinuria suggest a glomerular source. Red, clotted blood in the urine indicates a source below the kidneys. Hematuria that varies with menstruation and is associated with severe dysmenorrhea may indicate endometriosis involving the urinary tract.

In younger patients, microscopic hematuria is most often caused by nephrolithiasis or urinary tract infection.[1] It is also important to consider such disorders as glomerulonephritis, immune complex disease, Goodpasture syndrome, Henoch-Schönlein purpura and Wilms tumor in children, and sickle cell anemia or trait. Poststreptococcal glomerulonephritis is more common in children and typically follows a throat or skin infection. Symptoms appear 7 to 14 days after the primary infection, and the subsequent findings can vary from isolated hematuria to severe nephritis. Treatment of the primary streptococcal infection with antibiotics does not reduce the incidence of poststreptococcal glomerulonephritis. IgA nephropathy develops several days after a viral respiratory infection and is often accompanied by proteinuria secondary to glomerular damage from immune-complex deposition.

In older patients, infections and nephrolithiasis remain common causes of hematuria. Nonetheless, hematuria in patients older than 40 years—even with a clear diagnosis of urinary tract infection or stone—warrants close follow-up and retesting of urine because renal, bladder, and prostate cancer increase in frequency and may coexist with urinary tract infection or kidney stone.[10] Risk factors for uroepithelial cancer in addition to age greater than 40 years include excessive analgesic use, tobacco use, occupational exposures (e.g., to dyes, benzenes, or aromatic amines), pelvic irradiation, and cyclophosphamide use.[10] Similarly, hematuria in a patient on oral anticoagulants should not be attributed to the anticoagulant alone, because the inci-

TABLE 97-1 Common Causes of Hematuria

Etiology	Associated Age
Infections	Any
Nephrolithiasis	Usually >20 years
Neoplasms	Typically >40 years (except Wilms')
Benign prostatic hypertrophy	Males >40 years
Glomerulonephritis	Mostly young patients and children
Schistosomiasis	Any; most common cause worldwide

TABLE 97-2 Differential Diagnosis of Hematuria

Urologic (lower tract)
  Any location
    Iatrogenic/postprocedure
    Trauma
    Infection
    Stones/calculi
    Erosion or mechanical obstruction by tumor
  Ureter(s)
    Dilatation of stricture
  Bladder
    Transitional cell carcinoma
    Vascular lesions or malformations
    Chemical or radiation cystitis
  Prostate
    Benign prostatic hypertrophy
    Prostatitis
  Urethra
    Stricture
    Diverticulosis
    Foreign body
    Endometriosis (cyclic hematuria with menstrual pain)
Renal (upper tract)
  Glomerular
    Glomerulonephritis
    IgA nephropathy (Berger disease)
    Lupus nephritis
    Hereditary nephritis (Alport syndrome)
    Toxemia of pregnancy
    Serum sickness
    Erythema multiforme
  Nonglomerular
    Interstitial nephritis
    Pyelonephritis
    Papillary necrosis: sickle cell disease, diabetes, NSAIDs
    Vascular: AV malformations, emboli, aortocaval fistula
    Malignancy
    Polycystic kidney disease
    Medullary sponge disease
    Tuberculosis
    Renal trauma
Hematologic
  Primary coagulopathy (e.g., hemophilia)
  Pharmacologic anticoagulation
  Sickle cell disease
Miscellaneous
  Eroding abdominal aortic aneurysm
  Malignant hypertension
  Loin pain-hematuria syndrome
  Renal vein thrombosis
  Exercise-induced hematuria
  Cantharidin (Spanish fly) poisoning
  Bites or stings by insects and reptiles having venom with anticoagulant properties

Abbreviations: AV = atrioventricular; IgA = immunoglobulin A; NSAID = nonsteroidal anti-inflammatory drug.

dence of underlying disease may be as high as 80 percent.[11] Expanding abdominal aortic aneurysms (AAA) may erode into the urogenital tract and produce hematuria.

Malignant hypertension, embolic renal infarction, and renal vein thrombosis (RVT) are other serious diagnoses that can cause hematuria. Pregnancy, dehydration, nephrotic syndrome, lymphoma, and renal cell or other types of carcinoma are all predisposing disorders for RVT. RVT is commonly asymptomatic, with minimal or no pain. Children with RVT are typically volume depleted and have some other cause of a hypercoagulable state. In adults with RVT, there is usually underlying nephropathy and obvious nephrotic syndrome. In pregnancy, hematuria can be associated with urinary tract infection, nephrolithiasis, or preeclampsia.

TABLE 97-3   False Hematuria (Discolored Urine)

Medications
　Rifampin, phenazopyridine, phenophthalein
Foods/dyes
　Beets, berries, rhubarb
Disinfectants
　Iodide, bromide

Abbreviation: NSAID = nonsteroidal anti-inflammatory drug.

The reported incidence of hematuria in HIV-infected patients is 18 to 50 percent.[12] Causes include subclinical viral renal infection, early glomerulonephritis, urinary tract infection, chlamydial and gonococcal urethritis, chronic hepatitis B infection, neurogenic bladder, thrombocytopenia, subclinical uroepithelial Kaposi sarcoma, and urethral trauma. However, up to 80 percent of HIV-positive patients with an episode of asymptomatic hematuria have no specific etiology found after complete urologic evaluation.[12]

Diagnosis

Potential causes for hematuria are sometimes suggested by considering the patient's age, gender, demographic characteristics, habits, potential risk factors for urologic cancer, recent genitourinary instrumentation, and comorbidity.[3,8]

The symptom should be clarified: is the hematuria traumatic or atraumatic; gross or microscopic; initial, terminal, or total? When did it start? Are there associated symptoms, such as menstruation; flank, back, or abdominal pain; dysuria; nausea; or fever? Is the patient pregnant? Are there risk factors for cancer or RVT? Has the patient had a recent respiratory or other infection that might predispose to IgA nephropathy or poststreptococcal glomerulonephritis? Has the patient recently traveled outside the United States, particularly to the Middle East or Africa, raising the risk of schistosomiasis? Was there recent instrumentation of the urinary tract or urinary or renal disease? Are there comorbid conditions, such as diabetes, hypertension, sickle cell disease, HIV, tuberculosis, cancers, lupus, or other diseases associated with vasculitis? A complete medication history is important to identify the use of anticoagulants or nephrotoxic agents. Strenuous exercise is a common cause of benign hematuria in healthy young individuals.[13]

The physical examination should note the vital signs and the patient's appearance. A younger and otherwise healthy patient without fever, writhing in pain on the cart, unable to find a comfortable position, and complaining of severe flank pain radiating to the perineum most likely has nephrolithiasis. Hypertension and edema imply nephrotic syndrome. A new heart murmur (endocarditis) or atrial fibrillation increases the likelihood of embolic disease and renal infarction. Dysuria and suprapubic pain and tenderness with or without fever suggest hemorrhagic cystitis. Perineal pain, dysuria, and a tender, boggy prostate in older men indicate prostatitis. A nodular prostate suggests the possibility of cancer. Flank or back pain with fever and costovertebral angle tenderness suggests pyelonephritis. Flank or back pain without fever suggests nephrolithiasis, AAA, renal infarction, or obstruction secondary to tumor. In an older patient, the examiner should palpate for a pulsatile abdominal mass and listen carefully for bruits. Hematuria with rash, arthritis, and abdominal pain may be the result of Henoch-Schönlein purpura in children. Polycystic kidney disease or renal malignancy may result in a large, palpable kidney. External genitalia in males should be examined for obvious tumor or trauma. A pelvic examination should be performed to exclude a vulvar or vaginal source of hematuria.

A clean-catch midstream urine collection is appropriate for most patients. Catheter-collected specimens are recommended for women with a vaginal discharge, menstrual or vaginal bleeding, or perineal disease. While urethral catheterization may induce hematuria in approximately 15 percent of patients, the amount rarely exceeds 3 RBCs/hpf.[14]

Convenient, commercially available bedside urine dipstick and pregnancy tests provide useful initial screening examinations.[8] A urine test strip test for blood can detect as little as 150 μg/L of free hemoglobin, corresponding to 5 to 20 intact RBCs/μL on microscopic analysis. False-negative results may be obtained with urine dipstick tests for blood if the urine has a high concentration of ascorbic acid (more than 5 mg/dL) or a high specific gravity. False-positive results occur when oxidizing agents are present (e.g., household bleach used in cleaning containers) and in the presence of free hemoglobin, myoglobin, or porphyrins. Povidone-iodine may also result in a false-positive urine dipstick test result for blood. The urine dipstick test also provides useful information regarding infection (positive leukocyte esterase or nitrite test results), proteinuria, glycosuria, and ketonuria.

When results of the initial urine test strip screening examination are positive or unavailable, or the clinical picture is highly suspicious for a urinary tract cause, a microscopic urinalysis is indicated. Abnormal RBC morphologic characteristics, RBC casts, and proteinuria suggest a glomerular source and the need for further nephrologic or hematologic workup.[8,10] Such patients typically do not require emergent renal imaging. The finding of normal RBCs on microscopic examination of the urine together with bacteriuria and leukocytes in a young healthy patient supports urinary tract infection as the probable cause of hematuria. If leukocytes are plentiful [more than 20 white blood cells (WBCs)/hpf] and clumped, and the patient also has back pain and fever, then pyelonephritis is likely. The presence of normal RBCs without evidence of infection should prompt further urologic evaluation to determine the site of bleeding.

Strenuous exercise is a frequent cause of hematuria, and follow-up is recommended even in cases of prompt resolution.[1,13] Patients taking anticoagulants should have appropriate coagulation studies performed in the ED with imaging studies indicated in follow-up for most older patients in order to exclude malignancy.[10,11]

A minority of patients (5 to 15 percent) with acute symptomatic urinary lithiasis have no hematuria, as measured by a urine test strip or formal urinalysis.[15] Thus, patients with a clinical picture indicative of nephrolithiasis but without hematuria still require further evaluation. Further laboratory examination depends on the results of the history, physical examination, and presumptive differential diagnosis.

Renal imaging is done with one of three complementary studies: intravenous pyelography (IVP), helical computed tomography (CT) scanning, or renal ultrasound.[16,17] The advantage of an IVP is that this study clearly delineates most renal tumors, obstruction, or stones and their precise location.[16] The disadvantage is the use of radiocontrast media with attendant risk. Serum creatinine should be measured in older patients, diabetics, and those with preexisting renal disease before administering radiocontrast. In addition, the IVP does not directly assess the aorta, retroperitoneum, and pelvis.

Helical (ultrafast) CT scanning without contrast material is highly sensitive and specific in identifying nephrolithiasis.[17] In cases in which no stone is identified, intravenous contrast infusion may also be performed and other intra-abdominal or retroperitoneal structures evaluated at the same time; i.e., AAA and appendicitis can often be excluded simultaneously. Helical CT scanning with or without intravenous contrast is faster and simpler when compared to IVP. The amount of intravenous contrast used is less than with IVP, making helical CT more useful when renal function is suboptimal. These facts together with increased availability of helical CT scanners in hospitals and reduced costs have made it the initial study of choice in most cases, largely replacing IVP.

Renal ultrasound is useful when screening for obstruction, hydronephrosis, or AAA. It is the study of choice in pregnant patients with suspected nephrolithiasis.[18] The presence of two kidneys can be confirmed, and they can be measured and screened for tumors or cysts. The pelvis, abdomen, and retroperitoneum can be scanned for free fluid, mass, or aneurysm. However, renal ultrasound rarely identifies or locates stones in the ureters that are not large enough to give findings of obstruction. Renal ultrasound also does not provide any assessment of renal function—normal enhancing and excretion of contrast by both kidneys—whereas both helical CT with contrast and IVP do provide such important information.

Gross hematuria in patients with blunt or penetrating trauma to the abdomen, flank, or back warrants an aggressive approach to identify the source of bleeding and to guide management (see Chap. 261).[19] Some trauma centers use the degree of hematuria, quantified as the number of red blood cells per high-power field, to decide which patients with posttraumatic microscopic hematuria to image. While such an approach is not universally accepted, the studies indicate that patients with relatively minor blunt trauma to the back or flank (e.g., punched, kicked, fall of less than 10 ft) with low levels of microscopic hematuria (less than 20 RBCs/hpf) rarely have significant urinary injury. If they are stable, such patients can be discharged with careful return instructions and referred for repeat urinalysis.

Treatment and Disposition

Treatment of hematuria is directed at the cause. Urinary tract infections should be treated with appropriate antibiotics. Nephrolithiasis should be treated with hydration and analgesics. Systemic diseases should be appropriately treated. Outpatient management and referral for follow-up are appropriate in hemodynamically stable patients without an apparent life-threatening cause of the hematuria. Patients who are discharged should have no or minimal symptoms; be able to tolerate oral fluids, antibiotics, and analgesics as indicated; and have no significant comorbid conditions. Discharged patients should not have significant anemia or acute renal insufficiency.

Patients younger than 40 years of age should be referred to a primary care physician for repeat urinalysis 1 to 2 weeks after treatment. Transient asymptomatic microscopic hematuria (AMH) is so common, particularly with increasing age, that it might be considered a normal variant unless it persists or is associated with other risk factors.[8] Persistent hematuria warrants urologic evaluation. Stable patients older than age 40 years with risk factors for urologic cancer should be referred to a urologist for more expeditious outpatient workup.

In the general population, AMH alone is not associated with an increased risk of urologic malignancy, but it is associated with a twofold increased risk of later developing renal failure.[8] A thorough investigation of AMH in high-risk populations, particularly older men, occasionally discovers malignancies, most commonly transitional cell carcinoma of the bladder.[8] Proteinuria is a sign of prognostically significant glomerular disease. Consequently, any degree of proteinuria accompanying microscopic hematuria, regardless of age or other risk factors, requires further investigation within a reasonable time frame.[8] Children with hematuria should have pediatric referral. HIV-positive patients with asymptomatic microscopic hematuria who have a benign urologic history and normal renal function can be safely referred for outpatient follow-up and repeat urinalysis.

Gross hematuria may lead to intravesical clot formation and bladder outlet obstruction. This is treated by placing a triple-lumen urinary drainage catheter and starting intermittent or continuous bladder irrigation with normal saline. Manual irrigation using a syringe may be initially necessary if the catheter does not drain after initial placement. Once drainage is present, irrigation using gravity is started to wash clots out of the bladder. The rate of irrigant flow is determined by the appearance of the output; the goal is clear to only slightly pink tinged drainage. If placement of the triple-lumen catheter is unsuccessful, cystoscopy may be required for clot removal.

Patients with intractable pain, intolerance of oral fluids and medications, significant comorbid illness, bladder outlet obstruction, evidence of hemodynamic instability, or possibly life-threatening causes of hematuria should be admitted. Patients with suspected or newly diagnosed glomerulonephritis are at high risk of developing complications, such as pulmonary edema, volume overload, azotemia, or hypertensive emergency, and should be admitted. In pregnant women, hematuria can accompany preeclampsia, pyelonephritis, or obstructing nephrolithiasis; consultation and admission are indicated.

HEMATOSPERMIA

Hemospermia, or hematospermia, is a disturbing symptom that produces extreme anxiety in sexually active males. Most seek medical attention after one or two occurrences. Any process that results in trauma or other injury (e.g., tumor with erosion), inflammation, or infection of the male ejaculatory system may result in bloody semen.[20] Two of the most common causes of hematospermia are iatrogenic trauma from instrumentation of the urinary tract or radiation therapy. In patients older than age 40 years, tumors of the prostate or elsewhere in the ejaculatory system and benign prostatic hypertrophy are considerations. In patients younger than age 40 years, common causes are infections and inflammatory conditions, including prostatitis, seminal vesiculitis, urethritis, sexually transmitted diseases, epididymoorchitis, calculi with inflammation, and tuberculosis. Testicular tumors occur in the younger population. Vascular abnormalities and cysts causing ductal obstruction are less common causes. As with hematuria, systemic factors may cause hematospermia, including hemophilia, other coagulopathies, oral anticoagulation, severe hypertension, leukemia or other hematologic disease, lymphoma, and scurvy.

A careful history, including sexual history, recent urologic procedures, medications, and HIV and tuberculosis risk factors, should be obtained. The patient's general health and condition, vital signs, abdomen, external genitalia, and prostate should be examined. Because hematospermia may be the initial and only presenting complaint in underlying urologic disease, a urinalysis is generally warranted, and treatment and disposition are directed by the urinalysis findings.

Hematospermia has long been considered a benign condition and is usually diagnosed as idiopathic after a complete urologic evaluation. It is not uncommon after vigorous sexual activity. Infection, including sexually transmitted disease, should be treated appropriately. In the absence of other reasons for an expedited workup or admission, patients should be referred to a urologist for follow-up and further outpatient evaluation. Patients younger than age 40 years can be reassured that the vast majority of cases of hematospermia in their age group are benign, self-limited, and idiopathic. While all patients with hematospermia should be referred to a urologist, those older than age 40 years are at higher risk for cancer and should be strongly advised to seek further evaluation by a urologist, even when there is spontaneous resolution of hematospermia.

REFERENCES

1. Sutton JM: Evaluation of hematuria in adults. *JAMA* 263:2475, 1990.
2. Grossfeld GD, Litwin MS, Wolf JS, et al: Evaluation of asymptomatic microscopic hematuria in adults: The American Urological Association best practice policy—Part I: definition, detection, prevalence, and etiology; Part II: patient evaluation, cytology, voided markers, imaging, cystoscopy, nephrology evaluation and follow-up. *Urology* 57:599, 604, 2001.
3. Ahmed Z, Lee J: Asymptomatic urinary abnormalities: Hematuria and proteinuria. *Med Clin North Am* 81:641, 1997.
4. Clarkson AR: Microscopic hematuria: Whom to investigate. *Aust N Z J Med* 26:7, 1996.
5. Fogazzi G, Ponticelli C: Microscopic hematuria: Diagnosis and management. *Nephron* 72:125, 1996.
6. Feld LG, Waz WR, Perez LM, Joseph DB: Hematuria: An integrated medical and surgical approach. *Pediatr Clin North Am* 44:1191, 1997.
7. Mahan JD, Turman MA, Mentser M: Evaluation of hematuria, proteinuria, and hypertension in adolescents. *Pediatr Clin North Am* 44:1573, 1997.
8. Tomson C, Porter T: Asymptomatic microscopic or dipstick haematuria in adults: Which investigations for which patients? A review of the evidence. *BJU Int* 90:185, 2002.
9. Sokolosky MC: Hematuria. *Emerg Med Clin North Am* 19:621, 2001.

10. Summerton N, Mann S, Rigby AS, et al: Patients with new onset haematuria: Assessing the discriminant value of clinical information in relation to urologic malignancies. *Br J Gen Pract* 52:284, 2002.

11. Van Savage JG, Fried FA: Anticoagulant associated hematuria: A prospective study. *J Urol* 153:1594, 1995.

12. Cespedes RD, Peretsman SJ, Blatt SP: The significance of hematuria in patients infected with the human immunodeficiency virus. *J Urol* 154:1455, 1995.

13. Jones GR, Newhouse I: Sport-related hematuria: A review. *Clin J Sport Med* 7:119, 1997.

14. Hockberger RS, Schwartz B, Connor J: Hematuria induced by urethral catheterization. *Ann Emerg Med* 16:550, 1987.

15. Press SM, Smith AD: Incidence of negative hematuria in patients with acute urinary lithiasis presenting to the emergency room with flank pain. *Urology* 45:753, 1995.

16. Chen MY, Zagoria RJ, Dyer RB: Radiologic findings in acute urinary tract obstruction. *J Emerg Med* 15:339, 1997.

17. Colistro R, Torreggiani WC, Lynburn ID, et al: Unenhanced helical CT in the investigation of acute flank pain. *Clin Radiol* 57:435, 2002.

18. Swanson SK, Heilman RL, Eversman WG: Urinary tract stones in pregnancy. *Surg Clin North Am* 75:123, 1995.

19. Miller KS, McAninch JW: Radiographic assessment of renal trauma: Our 15-year experience. *J Urol* 154:352, 1995.

20. Munkelwitz R, Krasnokutsky S, Lie J, et al: Current perspectives on hematospermia: A review. *J Androl* 18:6, 1997.

98
COMPLICATIONS OF UROLOGIC PROCEDURES AND DEVICES

Elaine B. Josephson
Jatinder Singh

Urologic surgical procedures are increasingly performed with outpatients or inpatients who are discharged from the hospital earlier in their postoperative course. Thus, patients often come to the ED with specific problems due to common urologic surgeries involving the renal or ureteral system, vasectomies, and the prostate. Similarly, because urologic devices, ranging from urinary (Foley) catheters, artificial urinary sphincters, nephrostomy tubes and stents, to objects used for erectile dysfunction and genital piercing, are in more widespread usage, complications arising from their presence also may bring patients to the ED. In general, a urology consult should be obtained for complications arising from urologic procedures and devices, and whenever possible, the urologist who performed the original operation should be contacted.

LITHOTRIPSY

Extracorporeal shock wave lithotripsy (ESWL) involves the use of high-intensity sound waves to break up calculi within the genitourinary system. The main advantage of this technique is to noninvasively treat a large obstructing calculus. Overall morbidity with ESWL is quite low. Typically patients with post-ESWL complications may come to the ED with the following signs and symptoms: abdominal and flank pain, nausea, vomiting (especially 48 h postprocedure), skin ecchymosis, or ureteral colic and fever. Hematuria is a common occurrence after lithotripsy but is generally self-limited (<24 h). Although symptomatic treatment is often required, it is important to note that these presenting complaints also may be the indication of more serious problems.[1,2]

Potentially more serious post-ESWL entities, although rare, are the perinephric and renal hematomas (usually secondary to subcapsular renal hemorrhage). The diagnosis is suspected when there is significant and severe flank pain and evidence of hemorrhage (flank hematoma or fall in hematocrit). Patients also may present with hypotension or syncope secondary to the bleeding. The diagnosis is made

with computed tomography or ultrasound. Acute management may include fluid resuscitation, blood transfusions, analgesics, and antibiotics. Most patients are managed conservatively, with close monitoring of hemodynamic status and laboratory studies to assess for decreasing hematocrit and renal function. A urology consult should be obtained early on, because treatments, such as embolization and nephrectomy, may be required.[1,2]

Steinstrasse ("street of stone") refers to the post-ESWL dispersal of stone fragments, usually within the ureters. When an accumulation of these calculi, or one large fragment, becomes lodged, flank or groin pain, urinary obstruction, and superimposed infection can ensue. Patients can be asymptomatic or may present with flank pain, nausea, vomiting, fever, hematuria, or dysuria. Steinstrasse can be visualized on plain abdominal radiographs. Treatment options may include conservative management, repeat ESWL, or percutaneous nephrostomy.[2]

There are some case reports of rare events in which ESWL caused injury to other abdominal viscera secondary to the high energy used and close proximity of the other organs to the kidney. Complications reported included bowel perforation, gastrointestinal mucosal erosions and hemorrhages, ureteric perforations, and splenic trauma in the form of rupture, hemorrhage, and abscess. Patients may present with abdominal pain, signs of peritonitis, and fall in hematocrit. Diagnosis usually requires imaging: computed tomography or ultrasound. Surgery and urology consultation should be obtained for definitive treatment.[3,4]

In managing all postprocedural complications of ESWL patients, supportive therapy is important: intravenous fluid hydration, antiemetics (if needed), analgesics, and antibiotic treatment, if indicated. In addition, prompt urologic consultation should be obtained, when there is concern regarding complicated steinstrasse, a renal hematoma, or in conjunction with the surgeon if there is suspicion that other abdominal organs may be involved.

VASECTOMIES

Vasectomies are often done in an outpatient setting. In general, this surgical procedure is a safe method of contraception, with a low failure rate and risk of side effects. However, acute postoperative complications that may present to the ED can include bleeding and scrotal hematoma, local wound infections (cellulitis and abscess), epididymitis, and painful sperm granulomas. Some patients may present months to years later with chronic complications, such as persistent testicular pain, or congestive epididymitis (pain and testicular tenderness on the affected side).[5]

In the ED, patients should receive appropriate pain management and antibiotics, when indicated, especially in cases of immunosuppression. When there is no evidence of bleeding or wound infection, treatment options for postvasectomy epididymitis include ice packs, scrotal support, and analgesia with nonsteroidal anti-inflammatory agents or opiates. For patients with suspicion of testicular abscess (diffuse pain and swelling, often with fever), a scrotal ultrasound should be used. An urologist should be consulted for testicular abscess or scrotal hematoma.

PROSTATE SURGICAL PROCEDURES

Prostate surgery is usually performed for benign prostatic hyperplasia or prostate cancer. Common surgical techniques include transurethral resection of the prostate, transurethral incision of the prostate, transurethral electrovaporization of the prostate, transurethral microwave thermotherapy of the prostate, transurethral needle ablation of the prostate, and visually assisted laser prostatectomy.[6,7]

Surgical procedures of the prostate typically involve direct manipulation of the urinary outflow tract. Therefore, common complications include hematuria, urinary blood clots with subsequent retention and failure to void, urethral strictures, and urinary tract infections. Some patients experience obstructive or irritative voiding symptoms that may include incontinence, hesitancy, dribbling, urgency, and frequency.[6,7]

The overall rate of serious hemorrhage is low.[6,7] If bleeding is significant, patients should be evaluated for hemodynamic instability, intravenous fluids administered, and appropriate laboratory studies ordered (complete blood cell count, renal function from serum urea nitrogen and creatinine levels, and urinalysis). Outflow obstruction should be relieved by placing a urethral catheter (triple-lumen) and irrigating with saline to remove clots. If infection is present, antibiotics should be administered.

COMPLICATIONS OF URINARY CATHETERS

Urinary catheters are used for a multitude of indications. Short-term catheterization is initially done for patients with acute urinary retention, for hospitalized patients who have urologic surgery or spinal cord injuries, and for monitoring the urinary output in critical patients. Long-term catheterization (>30 days) is used for patients with bladder outlet obstruction not treatable otherwise, for severely incontinent patients who are terminally ill or cannot care for themselves, and for some patients with neurogenic incontinence. Such a prolonged form of catheterization is often used for chronically ill patients in nursing homes. Problems relating to the use of urinary catheters include infection, obstruction, and leakage, and traumatic complications that can occur during catheter placement.

Infection

Catheter-associated urinary tract infections (CAUTIs) are one of the most common causes of nosocomial infections. The risk of infection is related to a number of factors; chief among them are duration of catheterization and patient comorbid factors. Duration of catheterization is one of the more important predictors of risk of infection. The risk of infection is about 1 to 2 percent with a catheter in place for less than 24 h, with the prevalence of bacteriuria reaching almost 100 percent for long-term catheterization (longer than 28 to 30 days). There is about a 3 to 10 percent incidence of bacteriuria for each day the catheter is in place. Comorbid patient problems, which increase the risk of CAUTI, include female sex, men with obstruction secondary to an enlarged prostate, renal disease, diabetes, and those who are elderly and debilitated. Another important contributing risk factor for CAUTI is the use of unsterile techniques during initial insertion of the catheter and subsequent handling during its drainage.[8]

Microbial factors associated with an incidence of CAUTI include the source of the organisms, the specific bacteria, the route of invasion, and the duration of catheterization. The organisms may be part of the patient's endogenous intestinal flora or may be acquired from outside sources such as other patients, hospital personnel, or unsterile equipment. Bacteria may be able to gain access to the urinary tract through the catheter lumen (intraluminal) or along the catheter surface (extraluminal). An infection from the extraluminal route begins with the formation of a film on the catheter surface consisting of urinary electrolytes, host proteins, and other urinary substances. Bacteria adhere to this film and transform it into a biofilm formed of products of bacterial metabolism and urinary components. Bacteria become embedded within the biofilm and gain protection from antibiotics.[8]

The microbiology of CAUTI varies according to the duration of catheter placement. During short-term catheterization, infections are usually due to single organisms, most commonly *Escherichia coli,* followed by *Klebsiella, Pseudomonas, Enterobacter,* and gram-positive cocci such as staphylococci. With long-term catheterization, CAUTIs are usually polymicrobial from *E. coli, Proteus mirabilis, Pseudomonas,* and *Morganella morgagni,* and *Candida* spp. These infections are usually difficult to treat due to antibiotic resistance by the infecting bacteria.[8]

Bacteriuria may be present without symptoms. Asymptomatic bacteriuria usually occurs with short-term catheterization, and removal of the catheter clears the bacteriuria. Antibiotic treatment of asymptomatic bacteriuria in a patient with a short-term indwelling urinary catheter is controversial: some argue that treatment only promotes resistance and some advocate a short course of antibiotics. However, bacteriuria with a fever and other signs of systemic illness in association with urinary catheters (especially long term) requires aggressive workup for the cause for the fever and early institution of antibiotic therapy. The most common location for CAUTI with fever is pyelonephritis; other sites include prostatitis, epididymitis, and scrotal abscess. Urine cultures should be obtained to guide antibiotic therapy, and blood cultures should be obtained if the patient is septic or immunocompromised. Antibiotics should be instituted promptly, because a delay in treatment can lead to the development of serious complications.[8,9]

The duration of antibiotic therapy for CAUTI varies from 5 to 14 days. Most can be treated with a single agent. However, those with the possibility of polymicrobial infection or who are seriously ill should be started on a broad-spectrum agent, e.g., ampicillin plus an aminoglycoside, anti-pseudomonal penicillin, carbapenem, or a fluoroquinolone.[9]

Obstruction and Leakage

Urethral catheters can become obstructed for many reasons, most commonly from the formation of intraluminal encrustations during long-term placement. These concretions are composed of compounds, such as ammonium magnesium sulfate (struvite) and calcium phosphate (apatite), often with urease splitting organisms, such as *Protease* and *Morganella.* Such encrustations can increase the risk of formation of infectious stones and cause bladder trauma leading to blood clots. A catheter obstruction may lead to urinary leakage around the catheter and acute urinary retention. Management options include repeated bladder irrigations, methenamine treatment, and removal of the catheter if the other methods fail. Infections should be treated with antibiotics.[9] Mechanical obstruction also can occur due to a nondeflation of the retention balloon on the catheter. Removal usually requires urologic intervention and potential cystoscopy.

Periurethral (or pericatheter) leakage can occur secondary to bladder spasms or catheter obstruction. The two can be differentiated by attempting to flush the catheter; if it does not flush, the catheter is probably obstructed. Treatment options include the use of antispasmodics, such as oxybutynin, flavoxate, and dicyclomine for bladder spasms and catheter irrigation and/or removal in case of obstruction.[9]

Traumatic Complications

Adequate lubrication and proper catheter size selection help to minimize the risk of trauma to the urethra during urinary catheter insertion. The urethra can be injured from inflation of the retention balloon within the urethra. Forceful attempts at catheter removal with an inflated balloon can cause edema and tears to the urethra. During insertion, a false lumen can be created, especially in patients with underlying urethral strictures or prostate enlargement, when excessive force is applied. Subsequently, the patient may develop bleeding, pain, and a lack of urine output from intraurethral clot formation or urethral disruption. Surgical intervention by the urologist may be required. To avoid possible traumatic complications, a Coudé tipped or large-size catheter should be tried with less force when there is a problem with insertion in these patients. Although uncommon, bladder perforation should be suspected in patients with peritoneal signs, pyuria, hematuria, and diminished urine output. This warrants a diagnostic cystogram and urgent urologic consultation for definitive care, if the bladder is perforated.

Alternatives to Indwelling Catheters

Alternatives to long-term urethral catheters have a lower rate of complications and should be considered, if feasible. One option is the use of intermittent catheterization, which involves insertion and removal of a urinary catheter several times a day at periodic intervals. It is especially useful for patients with bladder emptying dysfunction and children with neurogenic bladders. For male patients, condom catheters are a noninvasive approach to incontinence with a lower risk of infection when compared with urethral catheters. Complications from condom catheters include penile skin erosion and penile strangulation.[8]

Suprapubic catheterization places a catheter directly into the bladder through the anterior abdominal wall. Compared with urethral catheterization, suprapubic catheterization is associated with a lesser incidence of bacteriuria, because the abdominal wall has a lower concentration of bacteria than the periurethral area. However, the suprapubic route carries risks of cellulitis, hematoma formation, and persistent leakage.[9]

COMPLICATIONS OF PERCUTANEOUS NEPHROSTOMY TUBES

Percutaneous nephrostomy is a urinary drainage procedure used for supravesical or ureteral obstruction secondary to malignancy, pyonephrosis, genitourinary stones, and ureteral strictures. It is also used as an adjunctive therapy with ESWL and ureteral stents. Nephrostomy tubes are also used for urinary diversion associated with vesical fistula, ureteral transaction, and trauma. Patients may present to the ED from postoperative complications related to the procedure or days and months after the procedure. In general, the risk of complications is low and includes bleeding, infection, mechanical complications related to the catheter (dislodgement or obstruction), and accidental punctures of adjacent organs.

During insertion, injury can occur to the lungs (pneumothorax), liver, spleen, and the bowel (perforation). The risk may be higher in patients with an enlarged liver or spleen. The complication usually is clinically apparent during or immediately after the procedure, but recognition may be delayed a few days.[10]

Bleeding and hemorrhage can occur, especially if the patient has a coagulopathy. The hemoglobin, hematocrit, and renal function should be checked. Coagulation studies (prothrombin time, partial thromboplastin time, and platelet count) and type and crossmatch should be obtained if bleeding is excessive or the patient has a suspected coagulopathy. Most bleeding episodes are mild and can be managed with irrigation to clear nephrostomy tube blood clots. More severe bleeding can be handled by catheter tamponade, a procedure undertaken by the urologist and radiologist. Sometimes, bleeding can be severe enough to cause hemodynamic compromise. Severe hemorrhage occurs from vascular injury, such as laceration of an artery, formation of an arteriovenous fistula, or bleeding from a pseudoaneurysm, and may occur in the retroperitoneal space or perirenal areas. In such cases, fluid resuscitation and blood transfusion, in addition to more definitive interventions, are required. Angiographic studies with possible embolization may be needed to ascertain the site of bleeding and effect treatment.[10]

Infectious complications from nephrostomy tubes include simple bacteriuria, pyelonephritis, renal abscess, bacteremia, and urosepsis. The patient may present with fever, chills, rigors, pain, and purulent drainage at the site or from the tube. Urine and wound drainage (if present) cultures should be obtained, and antibiotics should be started in consultation with the urologist.[10]

Mechanical complications, such as catheter dislodgement and tube blockage, can occur with these devices. The risk of catheter dislodgement increases with increasing duration of the nephrostomy. Dislodgement occurring in the early postoperative period usually requires creation of a new tract at a different site. Dislodgement occurring after some period may be treated by recannulation under fluoroscopic guidance. Tube blockage can occur secondary to encrustations and kinking. The urologist has several techniques available to re-establish access to an obstructed nephrostomy tube.[10]

COMPLICATIONS OF ARTIFICIAL URINARY SPHINCTERS

The artificial urinary sphincter (AUS) is a device used for urinary incontinence secondary to sphincter disturbance, postsurgical incontinence, neurogenic bladder and incontinence, trauma to the urethra, and congenital conditions associated with bladder dysfunction, such as meningomyelocele, exstrophy, and epispadias. Many different models (the AMS 800, a current example) have been introduced over the years, with successive revisions. The basic principle of the AUS is to increase the resistance around the urethra and thus provide urinary continence. Mechanical parts of the AUS include a pump, an inflatable cuff that encircles the urethra, and a pressure regulating reservoir balloon. These are connected by a set of two tubes. Continence occurs when fluid is moved from the balloon to the cuff. To allow urination, the cuff is emptied of the fluid, which moves to the reservoir. Both activities are controlled by the pump, which is implanted in the scrotum of males or the pelvis of females.[11]

Postoperative complications of the AUS device include bleeding, infection, and malfunctions. A common problem associated with AUS implantation is the formation of a hematoma. These hematomas usually occur in the scrotum or the labia and most resolve spontaneously. Larger hematomas may need to be drained to aid with the healing process.[11,12]

Infections are the most serious complication of the AUS. Periprosthetic infection can present early or late after AUS implantation. Infections occurring early after implantation are usually due to skin flora. Later infections are usually due to gram-negative organisms of the urinary tract. Symptoms and signs of infection can range from pain, swelling, and induration of the site to localized erythema of the pump or cuff site. More serious infections can present with fever, local abscess formation, drainage from incision sites, and erosion of the pump or the cuff. Infections can cause the components (e.g., cuff) to externalize out onto the skin or erode the urethra.[12]

Treatment of periprosthetic infection requires antibiotics and removal of the sphincter. Patients with an AUS in place should get antibiotic prophylaxis when undergoing procedures that may cause hematogenous seeding of the device, such as dental procedures.[11,12]

Retained air bubbles, fluid leaks, and tube kinking are some of the mechanical complications that can occur with the AUS. Design modifications over time have decreased some of the mechanical complications. Air bubbles can cause blockage of the pump, leading to filling defects and thus incontinence. Ineffective device functioning secondary to fluid leakage also can lead to sudden onset of incontinence. Tube kinking, a rare complication, can result in fluid blockage, thereby leading to urinary retention. A careful history may provide clues to malfunction. A pump that is difficult to squeeze implies blockage due to any cause, whereas a pump that remains compressed after squeezing signifies pressure loss or fluid leakage. Plain radiographs of the pelvis and other imaging studies are used to assess continuity of the mechanical components.[11]

Urethral erosion secondary to infection or excessive cuff pressure around the urethra is another serious complication, and one that is seen most commonly 3 to 4 months after the implantation. Patients may present with pain, swelling along the urethra and in the perineum, urinary incontinence, bloody urethral discharge, and infection. Cystourethroscopy and cuff removal are necessary for management of erosions.[11]

Recurrent incontinence after AUS placement can have many etiologies; infection, cuff erosion, fistulas due to surgical injuries, and mechanical failure are the most common causes. Evaluation requires urodynamic studies to accurately define the cause. Acute urinary retention in a patient with an AUS implant may occur as a result of bladder neck contractures, urethral strictures, or cuff erosion. Evaluation usually requires imaging studies, such as cystourethrography and endoscopic viewing of the urinary system.[12]

Evaluation in the ED of complications related to the AUS requires a thorough history noting the model type and make and symptom assessment and a detailed physical examination, urinalysis, and appropriate imaging studies. **No attempt should be made to introduce a urethral urinary drainage catheter through an AUS.** A urologist should be consulted for further evaluation and management.

COMPLICATIONS OF URETERAL STENTS

Ureteral stents are used primarily in patients to relieve ureteral obstruction and maintain ureteral lumen patency. Obstruction to the ureter may result from causes such as stones, strictures, trauma, malignancies, or retroperitoneal fibrosis. Stents are also used during surgery involving the genitourinary tract to maintain urinary patency and drainage and as adjuncts to lithotripsy in the management of nephrolithiasis. The use of stents has increased during the past three decades, and more complications secondary to their use are being reported now. Side effects seen early (first week) after stent insertion include fever, infection, irritative bladder symptoms, and hematuria.[13,14]

Many factors contribute to stent-related urinary tract infections. Stents induce a foreign body reaction, which increases the risk for infections. Encrustation of stents in the presence of infection with urea-splitting organisms also promotes infection. More serious infections, such as pyelonephritis and sepsis, can occur but are less common.

Most minor infections can be managed with outpatient antibiotics and do not require removal of the stent. If pyelonephritis or a systemic infection is suspected, intravenous antibiotics, imaging studies to determine the position of the stent, and urologic consultation are required. Stents usually can be visualized by plain abdominal x-rays due to the presence of radiodense marking imbedded within the catheters.[14]

Symptoms, such as mild flank pain, and signs suggestive of an irritative bladder, such as dysuria, urgency, frequency, and pain during voiding, occur commonly in patients with ureteral stents. Treatment options for these symptoms can include analgesics, anticholinergic medications, or, in severe cases, belladonna alkaloid and opioid suppositories. New complaints and symptoms, such as severe flank pain, require evaluation for stent migration, infection, or obstruction. Asymptomatic microscopic hematuria is usually of no clinical significance, whereas gross hematuria may indicate a more serious pathology, such as stent migration or erosion of the urinary tract, requiring imaging studies to locate the stent position.[14]

Serious problems, such as stent migration and stent fragmentation, are usually late complications seen with long-term stent placements. Stent migration can occur upward above the ureteropelvic junction or downward below this junction. Such migration can lead to obstruction and infections. These patients initially may present to the emergency department with new-onset abdominal pain, fever, and irritative bladder symptoms.[13,14] Most serious complications require urgent consultation with a urologist.

COMPLICATIONS OF DEVICES USED FOR ERECTILE DYSFUNCTION

About 20 million American males suffer from erectile dysfunction. The most common causes are diabetes, medications, post-prostate surgery, spinal cord dysfunction, and psychogenic. Although oral medication therapy currently exists for erectile dysfunction, some patients with erectile dysfunction are treated with devices or procedures, such as vacuum therapy, penile injections, external penile splints, and implantable penile prostheses.

Vacuum devices work by use of negative pressure and the use of a constriction ring to cause venous and arterial congestion, thus causing penile tumescence. The most common complaint reported is pain during application of the device and during ejaculation secondary to inappropriate pressure rise. Both symptoms can be resolved with proper use of device. Local skin cyanosis secondary to a drop in penile blood flow from the negative pressure may also be seen. Serious complications from the use of a vacuum device include penile skin necrosis, urethral bleeding, ischemia, and subcutaneous hemorrhage with ecchymosis. Peyronie disease and Fournier gangrene have also been reported.[15]

The external penile splint consists of two steel support rods in a silicone cover that have a support loop at the distal end, to loop around the subcoronal sulcus, and support rings at the proximal end, to position around the base of the penis. Aside from occasional dislodgement during sexual intercourse, these splints are relatively free of side effects.[15]

Two forms of injection therapy for erectile dysfunction are available: intracavernosal and intraurethral. The intracavernosal injections are given along the lateral aspect of the penis, directly into the corpora cavernosa. The basic mechanism involves vasodilation of arteries and veins leading to corporal smooth muscle relaxation and penile erection. Drugs used are papaverine, phentolamine, and alprostadil, a prostaglandin E_1 analogue, singly or in combination. Side effects include penile pain, prolonged erections (4 to 6 h), priapism (painful erection for longer than 6 h), and localized hematoma. Of these, priapism is the most urgent complication. Treatment includes the use of terbutaline, α-adrenergic agonists such as phenylephedrine, and corporal aspiration of blood with emergent urology consultation.[16]

Intraurethral injections use alprostadil to produce penile tumescence. One marketed product, the MUSE (medicated transurethral system for erection), uses a medicated pellet via an applicator that allows insertion of the drug into the urethra. The basic mechanism of intraurethral administration is similar to intracavernosal injections; the drug is absorbed from the urethra and through the local communicating vessels and exerts its actions on the corpora. Side effects are few and can include penile pain, urethral bleeding, laceration of the cavernosal artery, and dizziness. Very rarely priapism can occur. Intraurethral administration is usually free of any major systemic side effects, but syncope secondary to a vasovagal reaction due to the anxiety of the injection and the vasodilatory effects of the drug can occur.[16]

Several different types of implantable penile prostheses are used: the rigid rod prosthesis, the malleable or semirigid device, and the inflatable device. The inflatable device is composed of a pair of inflatable cylinders inserted in the cavernosa, a scrotal pump, and an abdominal fluid reservoir. Infection is the most devastating of all penile prosthesis complications and usually occurs soon after the primary surgery for implantation. Late infections can occur years after the procedure secondary to seeding via the bloodstream. Infection usually occurs in the periprosthetic space, the area between the prosthesis and the secondary capsule formed around it, due to a foreign body type reaction of the body to the foreign material. The surface of the device is a site for bacterial adherence and the formation of a biofilm. This film allows bacteria to grow on the prosthetic surface and limit antibiotic penetration. Organisms causing penile prosthesis infection are *Staphylococcus epidermidis, Staphylococcus aureus,* and gram-negative bacilli. Infections present as pain along the device (e.g., in the scrotum or along the penis), erosion, and purulent urethral discharge. Treatment requires removal of the entire device by the urologist and antibiotics.[17]

Migration and erosion of the prosthesis occur most commonly due to infection. Migration may occur proximally or distally, presenting as extrusion through the urethral meatus. Migration most often requires removal. Penile ischemia and necrosis are rare but serious complications occurring mainly in patients with predisposing factors, such as diabetes and vascular disease. Mechanical failures, such as tubing fracture, cylinder rupture, and reservoir leakage, have decreased over time due to device improvement. Evaluation of mechanical problems requires an assessment of the device by a urologist.[17]

COMPLICATIONS OF GENITAL PIERCINGS AND PENILE FOREIGN BODIES

Body piercing is the use of needles, rings, and other ornaments to pierce the skin for fashion and cultural practices. Although the earlobe traditionally is the most common site used, the piercing of other body parts, such as the navel and genitalia, are now becoming more prevalent in Western society. With this trend come risks of medical complications. In evaluating cases of genital piercings, information regarding where the procedure was performed and by whom, the composition of the jewelry used, the presence of comorbid conditions, and postprocedure care should be ascertained.[18]

Body piercing is not a benign procedure. Piercing can result in damage to deeper structures. Frequently, an unlicensed person who may use an unsterile technique or instruments, thus increasing the risk of infections, trauma, and other complications, performs the piercing.[19] Sometimes, embarrassment about the use of piercing leads to delay in seeking medical attention for problems.

Complications from body and genital piercings have been described mostly in case reports; there are no prospective studies of the incidence or frequency of these events. Some complications are unique to the body part involved, e.g., paraphimosis or urethral injury from encircling penile foreign bodies. Local and systemic reactions can be related to the material in the jewelry used, e.g., contact dermatitis or asthma from metal allergies (most commonly nickel). Silver has been reported to produce localized argyria or systemic silver poisoning. Embedded jewelry and migration of jewelry are other problems that can occur after piercing procedures.[18]

Infections usually present with redness, swelling, and/or purulent drainage at the affected site. Infectious complications such as local cellulitis, sepsis, toxic shock syndrome, and endocarditis have been reported. An increased risk for infection occurs in immunosuppressed patients, such as those with diabetes or the human immunodeficiency virus. Similarly, patients with a history of valvular heart disease may be at increased risk of endocarditis. Most infections are bacterial and usually due to *Staphylococcus aureus*. Hepatitis B, C, and D have been reported after piercing. Treatment requires local wound care, antibiotic therapy, and, in some cases, removal of the piercing object.[18]

Because genital piercing is essentially an invasive procedure, trauma due initially to the procedure itself and later secondary to traction on the object can produce local edema, hematoma, tissue tearing, and bleeding. Urethral rupture, tears, and paraphimosis have been reported from penile piercing.[18] Granulomatous reactions resembling sarcoid, hypertrophic scars, and keloids, and inguinal lymphadenopathy are delayed complications reported from piercing.[19]

Penile strangulation due to an encircling object, such as a ring or similar device, can lead to edema and vascular compromise, eventually causing ulceration, necrosis, and gangrene of the penis. Penile strangulation grades have been described: grade 1: distal penis edema, no skin ulceration or urethral injury; grade 2, distal penile edema with decreased sensation, skin injury and constriction of corpus spongiosum, no urethral injury; grade 3: loss of distal penile sensation, injury to skin and urethra, but no urethral fistula; grade 4: loss of distal penile sensation with complete division of the corpus spongiosum leading to urethral fistula and constriction of the corpus cavernosum; and grade 5: gangrene, necrosis, or complete amputation of distal penis. The relief of strangulation requires prompt removal of the device from the penis. Evaluation involves assessment of penile temperature, color, and sensation; ability to void; presence of pulses (Doppler ultrasound); and urethral integrity. Urologic consultation is indicated for evidence of penile ischemia, potential urethral injury, and when it is not possible to remove the object from the penis in the ED.

REFERENCES

1. Auge BK, Preminger GM: Update on shock wave lithotripsy technology. *Curr Opin Urol* 12:287, 2002.
2. Sayed MAB, El-Taher AM, Aboul-Ella HA, et al: Steinstrasse after extracorporeal shockwave lithotripsy: Aeitiology, prevention and treatment. *BJU Int* 88:675, 2001.
3. Klug R, Kurz F, Dunzinger M, et al: Small bowel perforation after extracorporeal shockwave lithotripsy of an ureter stone. *Dig Surg* 18:241, 2001.
4. Fugita OE, Trigo-Rocha F, Mitre AI, et al: Splenic rupture and abscess after extracorporeal shock wave lithotripsy. *Urology* 52:322, 1998.
5. Schwingl PJ, Guess HA: Safety and effectiveness of vasectomy. *Fertil Steril* 73:923, 2000.
6. Jepsen JV, Bruskewitz RC: Recent developments in the surgical management of benign prostatic hyperplasia. *Urology* 51(suppl 4A):23, 1998.
7. Borboroglu PG, Kane CJ, Ward JF, et al: Immediate and postoperative complications of transurethral prostatectomy in the 1990s. *J Urol* 162: 1307, 1999.
8. Sedor J, Mulholland SG: Hospital-acquired urinary tract infections associated with the indwelling catheter. *Urol Clin North Am* 26:821, 1999.
9. Cravens DD, Zweig S: Urinary catheter management. *Am Fam Phys* 61:369, 2000.
10. Millward SF: Percutaneous nephrostomy: A practical approach. *J Intervasc Radiat* 11:955, 2000.
11. Diana M, Schettini M, Gallucci M: Evaluation and management of malfunctionings following implantation of the artificial urinary sphincter. *Int Surg* 84:241, 1999.
12. Hajivassiliou CA: A review of the complications and results of implantation of the AMS artificial urinary sphincter. *Eur Urol* 35:36, 1999.
13. Richter S, Ringel A, Shalev M, Nissenkorn I: The indwelling ureteric stent: A 'friendly' procedure with unfriendly high morbidity. *BJU Int* 85:408, 2000.
14. Adams J: Renal stents. *Emerg Med Clin North Am* 12:750, 1994.
15. Levine LA, Dimitriou RJ: Vacuum constriction and external erection devices in erectile dysfunction. *Urol Clin North Am* 28:335, 2001.
16. Leungwattanakij S, Flynn V Jr., Hellstrom WJG: Intracavernosal injection and intraurethral therapy for erectile dysfunction. *Urol Clin North Am* 28:343, 2001.
17. Evans C: The use of penile prosthesis in the treatment of impotence. *Br J Urol* 81:591, 1998.
18. Koenig LM, Carnes M: Body piercing: Medical concerns with cutting-edge fashion. *J Gen Intern Med* 14:379, 1999.
19. Folz BJ, Lippert BM, Kuelkens C, et al: Hazards of piercing and facial body art: A report of three cases and literature review. *Ann Plast Surg* 45:374, 2000.

THE RENAL TRANSPLANT PATIENT
Richard Sinert
Mert Erogul

Since the first transplantation of a kidney from one human to another in 1954, the procedure has evolved from the realm of experimental medicine to the routine. Renal transplantation has become the preferred treatment for end-stage renal disease. With more than 200,000 living kidney recipients, emergency physicians can expect to encounter these patients, and should become familiar with the issues regarding organ rejection and complications of immunosuppressive therapy. Special emphasis should be given to the evaluation of the renal transplant patient with infections and acute renal failure (ARF).

EPIDEMIOLOGY

Renal transplants account for the majority of solid-organ transplants in the United States; in 2001, there were 23,848 solid organs transplanted, of which 14,024 were kidneys.[1] At the same time, approximately 51,000 patients were waiting for a kidney transplant, and approximately 2900 patients died while on the waiting list.[1]

Approximately 60 percent of kidneys are obtained from cadaveric donors, many of whom may be initially identified in an ED setting.[1] Traditionally, cadaveric donors have been victims of head injury or intracranial hemorrhage with unsurvivable neurologic injury, but do have preserved cardiovascular function. The "wet ischemia" time—that is, the time from cessation of circulation to removal of the organ and its placement in cold storage—should be no longer than 30 min. This reality, as well as other practical and logistical factors, stands in the way of using ED "code victims" as solid-organ donors. Absolute contraindications for organ donation include HIV, sepsis, and malignancy [with the exception of primary central nervous system (CNS) tumors]. Advanced age is a relative contraindication; most organ procurement organizations (OPOs) do not harvest solid organs from individuals older than 75 years of age. However, any questions concerning suitability for donation should be referred to the OPO representative.

While potential donors may be identified in the emergency department, the determination of neurologic death is usually not completed there. While there is still no global consensus on the definition of brain death, most accepted definitions require (1) the elimination of multiple masquerading conditions such as drug intoxication, hypothermia, and endocrinopathies, and (2) demonstration of complete and irreversible loss of brain and brainstem function, including cerebral unresponsiveness, brainstem areflexia, and apnea. Many definitions of brain death require a repeat assessment of the patient's neurologic status after a span of a number of hours.

Following brain death, a number of physiologic changes occur that necessitate intervention to preserve donor organ perfusion. Increasing cerebral edema after trauma or a cerebrovascular accident initially results in elevated catecholamine release and hypertension. With brainstem necrosis, catecholamine levels drop rapidly to 10 percent of normal values, causing hypotension that must be corrected with fluids and vasopressors as needed. Pituitary necrosis occurs in approximately 75 percent of organ donors, resulting in diabetes insipidus, which can cause significant hypovolemia if untreated. Antidiuretic hormone and free-water deficits should be rapidly replaced in these patients. Approximately 85 percent of donors become hypothermic from ischemia to their hypothalamus. Hypothermia has many detrimental effects on potential donor organs, including coagulopathy, shifting of the oxygen-hemoglobin dissociation curve, and hepatic and cardiac dysfunction. Potential brain-dead donors should be quickly admitted to an intensive care unit so that their cardiorespiratory status is maintained against the onslaught of physiologic insults that ensue once neurologic function has ceased.

Once an appropriate patient has been identified, consent must be obtained from the family. This is best done by an agent of the regional organ procurement organization, a list of which may be obtained from the American Association for Organ Procurement (www.aopo.org). Emergency physicians should be familiar with their departmental policies on brain death and organ procurement. Telephone and beeper numbers for the regional organ procurement organization should be readily available. OPOs should be notified early of potential organ donors, even before the formal declaration of brain death.

The Uniform Anatomical Gift Act of 1987 gives competent adults the legal authority to consent to organ donation after their death, often by simply signing a statement on the back of their driver's license. In practice, the OPO representative will often forego donation if a family opposes donation, even if the donor has provided consent prior to his or her death. The need to obtain consent from family members invariably comes at a time of great sadness and stress, and family members refuse approximately 50 percent of potential donations.[2] Experience shows that discussion of organ donation with the family is best done separately from discussion and acceptance of brain death. Once brain death has been declared, the OPO coordinator, who is highly trained for this delicate discussion, should broach the subject of organ donation. For multiple reasons, families may perceive a mixed message if the physicians caring for their seriously ill relative also initiates discussion of organ donation before the patients are "officially dead." The emergency physician should focus on identifying possible donor candidates and giving the family a realistic prognosis for the patient.[3] Consent rates for donation are highest when the family initiates the discussion of organ donation and are higher if the discussion about organ donation is decoupled from the explanation of brain death.

MORBIDITY AND MORTALITY

Renal Graft Prognosis

Graft prognosis is directly related to the source of the donor kidney: recipients of cadaveric kidneys generally have more episodes of rejection and lower graft survival rates. The graft survival rate for kidneys from living donors is approximately 95 percent at 1 year and 76 percent at 5 years, whereas the graft survival rate for kidneys from cadaveric donors is 89 percent at 1 year and 61 percent at 5 years.[4] The major causes of morbidity after renal transplant are hypertension (75 to 85 percent of all renal transplants), hyperlipidemia (60 percent), cardiovascular disease (15.8 to 23 percent), diabetes mellitus (16.9 to 19.9 percent), osteoporosis (60 percent), and malignant neoplasm (14 percent).[5]

Recipient Prognosis

Predictably, recipients from living, related donors have lower mortality rates than recipients from cadaveric donors. This is likely related to fewer rejection episodes and thus lower immunosuppression requirements. Patients' survival rate after transplantation from a living donor is 98 percent at 1 year and 91 percent at 5 years, as compared to survival after cadaveric donation of 95 percent at 1 year and 81 percent at 5 years.[4] Common causes of death include coronary artery disease (30.4 percent), sepsis (27.1 percent), neoplasm (13 percent), and stroke (8 percent).[6] During the first year, most deaths are from infectious causes. Long-term mortality rates are more closely related to the development of coronary artery disease.

GRAFT FAILURE

Acute renal failure (ARF) in transplant patients is defined as a 20 percent rise from baseline serum creatinine levels, as opposed to a 50 percent rise in other patients with ARF. Causes of ARF range from graft rejection to nephrotoxicity from immunosuppressive agents such as cyclosporine and tacrolimus, urinary tract infection or obstruction, renal vascular stenosis or thrombosis, and recurrent renal disease from hypertension, diabetes, or other causes (Table 99-1).

Renal Vascular Stenosis and Thrombosis

Renal artery stenosis (RAS) is a treatable cause of graft failure that occurs in up to 12 percent of posttransplant cases from the second postoperative month onward, although usually after a year. It may arise because of stricture at the site of anastomosis or arteriosclerosis elsewhere along the course of the artery. RAS should be suspected in the patient who develops uncontrolled hypertension or whose renal function deteriorates, particularly after initiation of angiotensin-converting enzyme (ACE) inhibitors. *Renal artery thrombosis* is a very early complication thought to be associated with technical surgical considerations, while *renal vein thrombosis* generally occurs during the first month after transplant and may present to an ED setting.

TABLE 99-1 Differential Diagnosis of ARF Unique to Renal Transplant Patients

Complications of surgery
    Renal artery stenosis or thrombosis
    Urinary tract obstruction
    Renal vein thrombosis
Rejection syndromes
    Hyperacute rejection
    Acute rejection
    Chronic rejection
Cyclosporine and tacrolimus nephrotoxicity
Recurrent renal disease

Thrombosis of the artery or vein may be diagnosed by ultrasonography, although both are associated with poor outcome and often lead to transplant nephrectomy.

Transplant Rejection

Graft rejection occurs when the host immune system recognizes a donated organ as foreign and attacks it through both cellular and humoral immune pathways. From 30 to 50 percent of transplant recipients will experience an episode of rejection, and 15 to 20 percent will experience recurrent rejection episodes.[7] Rejection episodes may be separated into hyperacute, acute, and chronic mechanisms.

Hyperacute rejection is a rare event that occurs within minutes to hours of transplantation and generally results in immediate transplant nephrectomy. It is caused by ABO incompatibility or by some other critical human leukocyte antigen (HLA) mismatch that went unrecognized during the pretransplant tissue typing.

Acute rejection occurs from days to decades after transplantation, but most commonly in the first 3 months. Rejection is related to activation of T cells, which, in turn, stimulate specific antibody production against the graft. The clinical presentation of acute rejection is notoriously unreliable, but may include hypertension and decreasing urine output. With severe rejection episodes, fever, leukocytosis, and pain over the graft site may also be seen. Measurement of serum creatinine is the best way to detect an acute change in renal function related to rejection. Instances of acute rejection have been shown to disproportionately affect the long-term graft survival; they are the greatest predictor for the development of chronic rejection, so the focus has shifted from treating acute rejection to preventing it by front loading immunosuppression during the initial vulnerable period. Consequently, patients are most prone to opportunistic infection during this early period.

The differential diagnosis of acute rejection includes cyclosporine or tacrolimus toxicity, acute tubular necrosis, renal artery stenosis, urinary tract obstruction, and urinary tract infection. Patients should undergo renal ultrasonography to rule out obstruction. Cyclosporine and other immunosuppressive drug levels should be drawn to gauge the potential for drug toxicity, and urine should be sent for analysis and culture. The treatment of acute graft rejection initially involves hospitalization for high doses of intravenous steroids. Patients who do not respond to this steroid pulse should be considered for renal biopsy.

Chronic rejection occurs after the initial peak of immunosuppression has been tapered to a maintenance regimen. It is more correctly termed *chronic allograft dysfunction* because the pathophysiologic mechanisms underlying chronic rejection include immunologic causes as well as nonimmunologic factors such as hypertension, hyperlipidemia, and cyclosporine toxicity. This condition manifests clinically by a gradual increase in creatinine over 4 to 6 months accompanied by low-grade proteinuria and progressive hypertension. Immunosuppressive therapy is not considered helpful unless the patient recently discontinued or precipitously tapered their medicine. Currently, only nonimmunologic interventions such as blood pressure control and hyperlipidemia treatment may be offered to patients with chronic allograft dysfunction.

IMMUNOSUPPRESSIVE AGENTS

Patients generally begin their posttransplant course with an induction regimen of immunosuppression that is then modified to a maintenance regimen after an initial 3- to 6-month period in which the rejection risk is greatest. These regimens are typically combinations of some of the drugs listed below at dosages designed to balance immunosuppression with unwanted side effects. Episodes of acute rejection may be treated with any one of a number of sequential rescue protocols that usually commence with pulse doses of steroids.

Corticosteroids have been a cornerstone of immunosuppressive therapy since the earliest solid-organ transplants. They function by

TABLE 99-2 Important Adverse Effects of Antirejection Medications

MORE COMMON	LESS COMMON
Cyclosporine	
Nephrotoxicity—renal insufficiency	Hyperkalemia
Hypertension	Convulsions—often with
Tremor	hypomagnesemia
Headache	Hypomagnesemia
Gingival hyperplasia	Dizziness
GI disturbance—anorexia, nausea,	Paresthesias
dyspepsia	Glucose intolerance—hyperglycemia
Hirsutism	Hyperlipidemia
	Bone marrow suppression—
	thrombocytopenia
	Thrombotic thrombocytopenic purpura
Tacrolimus	
Nephrotoxicity—renal insufficiency	Paresthesias
Hypertension	Hypokalemia
Tremor	Hypomagnesemia
Headache	Hyperlipidemia
GI disturbance—nausea, vomiting,	Bone marrow suppression—anemia,
diarrhea, abdominal pain,	leukopenia
constipation	
Glucose intolerance—	
hyperglycemia	
Hyperkalemia	
Azathioprine	
Bone marrow suppression—	Anemia
leukopenia, thrombocytopenia	Cholestatic jaundice
Increased susceptibility to	Pancreatitis
infection	Alopecia
Mycophenolate mofetil	
GI disturbance—diarrhea, vomiting	Peripheral edema
Bone marrow suppression—	GI hemorrhage—mucosal ulcerations
anemia, leukopenia,	Opportunistic infections—tissue
thrombocytopenia	invasive CMV infection
Headache	Pulmonary edema
Prednisone	
Cushing syndrome	Myopathy
Glucose intolerance—	Cataracts
hyperglycemia	
Osteoporosis	
Adrenal suppression	
Hypertension	
Hyperlipidemia	

inhibiting antigen stimulated T-lymphocyte proliferation and lymphokine production. A major drawback of the use of steroids is the nonselectivity of their immunosuppression—they affect both cellular and humoral immunity, resulting in a significantly increased risk of infection. Other deleterious effects of steroids are common (Table 99-2). For these reasons, initial steroid doses are tapered and sometimes discontinued entirely as the risk of acute rejection abates. Patients on maintenance steroid therapy who present to the emergency department with suspicion of infection or other significant physiologic stress should receive intravenous stress doses of steroids.

Cyclosporine is a macrolide antibiotic that blocks the phosphatase action of calcineurin thereby inhibiting the release of interleukin (IL)-2 and the subsequent proliferation of helper and cytotoxic T cells. Since its introduction in 1971, cyclosporine has become a mainstay of immunosuppressive regimens and has contributed to a steady improvement in graft survival percentages. Cyclosporine has significant side effects (see Table 99-2). As a consequence, cyclosporine levels must be strictly maintained in a range that balances graft rejection with adverse effects; trough levels between 150 and 300 ng/mL are associated with improved graft survival. Because cyclosporine is metabolized by the hepatic P450 system, its clearance is affected by many other drugs (Table 99-3).

Tacrolimus is a newer agent that works similarly to cyclosporine, has a comparable side-effect profile, and appears to be more effective in preventing episodes of acute rejection (see Table 99–2).[8] Additionally, tacrolimus appears to have a steroid-sparing effect that allows up to 60 percent of patients to taper off steroids completely. Tacrolimus has numerous drug interactions (see Table 99-3).

Sirolimus is the newest macrolide antibiotic with immunosuppressive properties. It compares favorably to tacrolimus from the standpoint of graft rejection, but does not induce hypertension, diabetes or neurologic adverse effects. The major side effects are bone marrow suppression and hyperlipidemia.[9]

Azathioprine is a purine analogue that was once a mainstay of transplant immunosuppression, but has been largely supplanted by newer agents. The immunosuppressant action of azathioprine occurs through blocking gene activation of stimulated T lymphocytes. The major adverse effect of azathioprine is bone marrow suppression (see Table 99-2).

Mycophenolate mofetil inhibits de novo purine biosynthesis during cell division and thereby affects both T- and B-lymphocyte cell lines. Side effects include dose-related pancytopenia and diarrhea (see Table 99-2).

Monoclonal antibodies against the IL-2 receptor have emerged as recent promising supplements to traditional immunosuppressive regimens. Although costly, the relative lack of side effects make them especially attractive agents.

INFECTIOUS COMPLICATIONS

Infection is the most common cause of mortality and morbidity for transplant patients in the first year.[10] Between 40 and 80 percent of transplant patients experience at least one infection during the first posttransplant year, although these numbers are decreasing as more transplant recipients undergo preoperative immunizations and take posttransplantation antibiotic prophylaxis.[11] Infections most commonly are mucocutaneous (41 percent), urinary tract (17.2 percent), and respiratory tract (13.9 percent).[11] The most common infective agents are bacterial (45.9 percent), viral (40.6 percent), fungal (12.5 percent), and protozoan (1 percent). Among the viral illnesses, cytomegalovirus (CMV) (31.5 percent), herpes simplex (23.4 percent), and herpes zoster (23.4 percent) are the most frequent organisms. Death is most commonly caused by infection (32 percent) with pneumonias accounting for about half of the deaths from infection.

The number and type of infection depends largely on time since surgery and the transplant recipient's current state of immunosuppression (Table 99-4).[12] During the first month posttransplant, patients are likely to encounter typical infections associated with any surgical procedure, such as urinary tract infections, pneumonias, intravenous line sepsis, and wound infection. Unexplained fever during this initial postoperative period should draw suspicion to the possibility of perinephric abscess or other local surgical complication. One exception to this is the development of significant herpesvirus disease in the first month, as detailed below.

The second through sixth months after surgery are regarded as the critical period when opportunistic pathogens associated with compromised cellular immunity manifest themselves; CMV, pneumocystis, toxoplasmosis, and various fungal infections. Reactivation of latent mycobacterial disease may also occur. Patients who present during this period—or during bouts of acute rejection for which they are receiving supplemental immunosuppression—should undergo an aggressive diagnostic workup for relatively subtle presentations.

After immunosuppression is curtailed at 6 months posttransplantation, patients with well-functioning grafts on minimal immunosuppression typically have infection profiles comparable to those of the

TABLE 99-3 Cyclosporine and Tacrolimus Drug Interactions

INCREASES LEVELS	DECREASES LEVELS	ENHANCES NEPHROTOXICITY
Cyclosporine		
Calcium channel blockers—diltiazem, verapamil, nifedipine, nicardipine	Antibiotics—nafcillin, rifampin	Antibiotics—gentamicin, tobramycin, vancomycin, trimethoprim-sulfamethoxazole
Antibiotics—erythromycin, clarithromycin, doxycycline	Anticonvulsants—phenytoin, phenobarbital, carbamazepine	Nonsteroidal anti-inflammatories—all formulations colchicine
Antifungals—ketoconazole	Miscellaneous—St. John's wort, ticlopidine	Antivirals—acyclovir
GI agents—metoclopramide		Antifungals—ketoconazole, amphotericin
Miscellaneous—amiodarone, allopurinol, grapefruit and grapefruit juice		GI agents—cimetidine, ranitidine
		Tacrolimus
Tacrolimus		
Calcium channel blockers—diltiazem, verapamil, nifedipine, nicardipine	Antibiotics—rifampin	Antibiotics—aminoglycosides
Antibiotics—erythromycin, clarithromycin	Anticonvulsants—phenytoin, phenobarbital, carbamazepine	Antifungals—amphotericin B
Antifungals—ketoconazole, fluconazole	Miscellaneous—St. John's wort	Antineoplastics—cisplatin
GI agents—metoclopramide, cimetidine, omeprazole		Cyclosporine
HIV protease inhibitors		
Miscellaneous—methylprednisolone, grapefruit and grapefruit juice		

TABLE 99-4 Etiology of Infection According to Time from Transplant

First posttransplant month: infections related to surgery
  Urinary tract infections *(Escherichia coli)*
  Intravenous lines and wound infections *(Staphylococus aureus, Streptococcus viridans)*
  Pneumonia *(Streptococcus pneumoniae)*
1–6 Posttransplant months: highest incidence of opportunistic infections
  Viremia (cytomegalovirus, Epstein–Barr virus)
  Pneumonia *(Pneumocystis carinii)*
  Meningitis *(Listeria monocytogenes)*
  Sepsis *(Aspergillus fumigatus)*
After 6 posttransplant months: patients divide into three subgroups
  Patients with good graft function on minimal immunosuppressants have the same risk of infection as the general population.
  Patients chronically infected with latent viruses (e.g., cytomegalovirus, Epstein–Barr virus, hepatitis B & C) often have significant and ongoing end-organ damage (e.g., cirrhosis) secondary to these infections.
  Patients with poorly functioning grafts who have sustained multiple episodes of rejection, now requiring large dosages of immunosuppressants commonly have acute and chronic opportunistic infections (e.g., *P. carinii, Candida*)

general community, with the exceptions of a higher than normal incidence of CMV retinitis, herpes zoster and cryptococcal disease. Patients who have chronic persistent viral infections with CMV, Epstein-Barr virus (EBV), or hepatitis B or C may demonstrate end-organ damage referable to this chronic infection.

Viral Infections

Viral infections produce significant morbidity and mortality in the renal transplant recipient and present diagnostic challenges because viral cultures are not very sensitive.[13]

The most common viral infections are caused by the herpes group of viruses: CMV, EBV, herpes simplex virus (HSV), and varicella-zoster virus (VZV). Transplant patients are also more susceptible to, and have a worse outcome from, infections with other viruses such as adenovirus, influenza virus, and hepatitis virus.

CMV is the most important viral agent to cause infection in renal transplant recipients, accounting for more than two-thirds of febrile episodes in the first 6 months posttransplant. Transmission of CMV occurs with an organ transplant from a seropositive donor. With primary CMV infection, patients often present with fever spikes and malaise, and sometimes arthralgias, myalgias, and lymphadenopathy. Tissue-invasive disease such as hepatitis, pneumonitis, primary chorioretinitis, or gastrointestinal (GI) tract ulceration may also occur. In addition to causing an infectious syndrome, CMV can cause a leukopenia and depressed cellular-mediated immunity, which increases the incidence of opportunistic infections such as *Pneumocystis carinii, Listeria,* and *Aspergillus.* CMV is linked to distinct allograft nephropathy, both acute and chronic, and is associated with decreased long-term patient survival. Diagnosis of CMV infection is best established by DNA capture hybrid assays or quantitative polymerase chain reaction (PCR). Untreated CMV is associated with 10 to 15 percent mortality rates, and patients diagnosed with CMV should generally be treated with ganciclovir or foscarnet despite the potential for adverse side effects. CMV seronegative transplant recipients requiring blood transfusion should receive CMV-seronegative, filtered, or leukocyte-poor blood products.

EBV infection in the renal transplant patient can present as two distinct clinical syndromes, either as the typical uncomplicated mononucleosis syndrome (characterized by fever, mild hepatitis, and leukopenia with atypical lymphocytosis) or as posttransplant lymphoproliferative disease (PTLD). The latter is an EBV-induced activation of B cells with expansion of lymphoid tissue, most frequently occurring in the CNS, renal allograft, or GI tract. PTLD occurs in approximately 1 percent of renal transplant recipients and can range from a mild benign polyclonal disease to a rapidly progressive monoclonal form, which carries a poor prognosis. Other symptoms and signs of EBV are fever of unknown origin, weight loss, hepatotoxicity, pulmonary infiltrates, and gastrointestinal bleeding and perforation. Diagnosis of EBV is generally serologic, although suspicion of PTLD warrants biopsy and histologic examination of affected tissue. Primary EBV infection is treated by reducing immunosuppression and administering intravenous acyclovir. Treatment of PTLD involves excision, radiation, antiviral therapy, and, occasionally, chemotherapy, although there continues to be a substantial mortality rate.

VZV also presents with two distinct clinical syndromes in the renal transplant patient. Most patients will have been exposed to VZV before transplantation, either through primary chickenpox or through pretransplant immunization. These patients are most likely to present with the typical reactivation-type infection limited to skin eruptions. Patients with no prior VZV exposure are at risk of developing primary VZV infection, usually contracted when tissue from a seropositive donor is transplanted to a seronegative host. This primary VZV infection can produce a simple chickenpox syndrome or can progress to virulent disease ranging from hemorrhagic pneumonia to encephalitis, hepatitis, and pancreatitis, with a high mortality rate. Direct immunofluorescence or viral culture is required to make the diagnosis of VZV. Acyclovir, valacyclovir, and famciclovir are indicated for both primary and reactivated VZV, although dosages must be increased as compared to those for HSV infection. Immunization with the attenuated virus is contraindicated after transplant, and seronegative patients who are exposed to VZV should receive varicella immunoglobulin within 96 h as postexposure prophylaxis.

HSV infection is relatively common during the first transplant month, and is largely a reactivation disease presenting with typical mucocutaneous ulcerations. Primary HSV, frequently contracted from the donor organ, may also present during the initial month as a life-threatening hepatitis, pneumonitis, or meningoencephalitis. Classic herpes lesions are the exception rather than the rule in these instances, and diagnosis depends on high index of suspicion, and attention to the timing of symptoms after transplant. Orolabial or anogenital lesions may be more ulcerative than vesicular, and if the diagnosis is unclear, immunofluorescence techniques or PCR may be helpful. Oral acyclovir, valacyclovir, or famciclovir are effective in mucocutaneous disease, whereas treatment with intravenous acyclovir may be indicated in disease that is more widespread.

Hepatitis viruses B and C may be contracted from an infected donor, or may reactivate with immunosuppression following renal transplantation. Immunosuppressive therapy directly stimulates viral replication, and seropositive patients frequently progress to active hepatitis, cirrhosis or hepatocellular carcinoma. In addition, infection with these viruses can suppress the host's immune defenses. Diagnosis is based on serologic and histologic studies. Therapy with interferon and lamivudine has shown limited success.

Respiratory viruses such as influenza and parainfluenza virus do not cause serious disease in transplant patients, although patients should receive routine immunization against influenza and treatment with neuraminidase inhibitors is warranted in symptomatic patients who test positive for influenza during epidemics. Adenovirus has become recognized as an important cause of pneumonia and hemorrhagic cystitis. Respiratory syncytial virus (RSV) has been implicated in pneumonia, and parvovirus in bone marrow suppression.

Bacterial Infections

Urinary tract infections (UTIs) are very common after renal transplantation, occurring in 30 to 40 percent of patients, and are responsible for 60 percent of the gram-negative bacteremias in these patients.[14] Prophylactic treatment during the first 6 months with trimethoprim-sulfamethoxazole (TMP/SMX) or fluoroquinolone is standard in many transplant centers, and is effective in reducing the incidence of UTIs to between 5 and 10 percent, as well as opportunistic organisms such as *Pneumocystis, Listeria,* and *Nocardia.*[15] The organisms responsible for UTIs in transplant patients are similar to those in nontransplant patients: *Escherichia coli,* enterococci, and *Pseudomonas aeruginosa,* although gram-positive organisms may be encountered in the immediate postoperative period because of urinary tract catheterization and instrumentation. UTIs in the first 6 months posttransplant frequently progress to pyelonephritis and urosepsis, and warrant longer courses of treatment (10 to 14 days) with a fluoroquinolone, as well as investigation for the possibility of complicating obstruction and stone formation. Infections in men should be treated for 4 to 6 weeks followed by long-term prophylaxis because of the possibility for prostatic seeding. Infections occurring after the initial 6-month postoperative period can be treated for shorter periods with less-intensive courses.

The gastrointestinal tract is the next most common source of bacterial infection in the renal transplant patient. Acute bacterial gastroenteritis secondary to *Salmonella, Campylobacter,* and *Listeria* is common in these patients, and significant diarrhea warrants evaluation with stool cultures. Diverticulitis, often complicated by perforation, is another common gastrointestinal infection encountered in transplant patients. Patients commonly present with findings of vague abdominal pain as the only symptom of this potentially life-threatening disease. A high index of suspicion should be maintained when evaluating transplant recipients with abdominal pain.

Among the common opportunistic bacterial pathogens, *Listeria* and *Nocardia* deserve special mention, although the incidence of these infections has decreased with the advent of prophylactic antibiotics. *Listeria monocytogenes* is a common opportunistic bacterial infection usually acquired by ingesting contaminated foods. Presentation is with diarrhea and abdominal cramps, which can quickly progress to pneumonia, endophthalmitis, and meningitis. Treatment consists of ampicillin and gentamicin, or TMP/SMX. *Nocardia asteroides* in renal transplant patients typically presents with fever, cough, and pulmonary infiltrates, eventually spreading to skin and central nervous system. *Nocardia* may also be effectively treated with TMP/SMX.

Tuberculosis occurs in renal transplant patients both as a primary and as a reactivation disease, and while it occurs in only approximately 5 percent of transplant patients, half of those cases present as disseminated disease.[16] There is no typical presentation for a transplant patient with tuberculosis; instead, a highly variable presentation has been described, including cavitary pulmonary disease, miliary disease, and multiorgan involvement. Diagnosis is rarely aided by tuberculin skin testing. Definitive diagnosis is by organism identification and culture from sputum, pleural effusions, and bronchoalveolar lavage, lung, or bone marrow biopsy. Therapeutic options are complicated because of cyclosporine drug interactions with many antituberculosis medications.

Fungal Infections

Fungal infections affect 2 to 14 percent of renal transplant patients and can occur at every stage of the posttransplant course.[17] Specific tests (fungal cultures) are necessary to make their diagnosis.

Candida albicans infection is the result of immunosuppression (especially from steroid use) causing overgrowth of an endogenous gut flora. Mucocutaneous disease affecting the oropharynx, esophagus, or vagina is the most common presentation. Candidal urinary tract infections, usually associated with indwelling catheters, can run a benign course with just cystitis or spread to pyelonephritis. Disseminated candidiasis often results in endocarditis, aortitis, osteomyelitis, meningitis, and brain abscess. Finding the organism in tissues, blood, or urine makes the diagnosis, but specific fungal cultures must be requested. Treatment of mucocutaneous candidiasis is with nystatin, clotrimazole, or oral fluconazole. Amphotericin is an effective agent for dis-

seminated disease, but intravenous fluconazole may be preferable because of decreased nephrotoxicity.

Cryptococcosis occurs in approximately 3 percent of renal transplant patients. *Cryptococcus neoformans* enters through the lung and can spread to the skin and central nervous system, resulting in meningitis. Diagnosis is made by testing for cryptococcal antigen in serum and/or cerebrospinal fluid. Treatment consists of a combination of amphotericin and fluconazole.

Patients living in endemic areas are at risk for infection with *Coccidioides immitis, Histoplasma capsulatum,* and *Blastomyces dermatitidis.* The most common symptoms are nonproductive cough and fever.

Aspergillus fumigatus and *Aspergillus flavus* may cause infections of the lungs, skin, and central nervous system in renal transplant patients, but generally presents with pulmonary symptoms.[12] Risk factors for infection include steroid use, CMV infection, and neutropenia. Diagnosis is by organism identification from sputum culture, bronchoalveolar lavage or lung biopsy. Treatment is with amphotericin and surgical débridement of isolated lung focus if found.

Mucormycosis is caused by infections from fungi of *Rhizopus, Absidia,* and *Mucor* species. Risk factors include diabetes mellitus, steroid use, and deferoxamine therapy. The most feared complication is invasive rhinocerebral disease, which is associated with a high mortality despite aggressive treatment with amphotericin and wide surgical resection.

Parasitic Infections

Pneumocystis carinii pneumonia (PCP) occurred in up to 10 percent of renal transplant patients before the advent of prophylactic therapy, but is less common now. Risk factors for infection include recent increases in immunosuppression and concurrent CMV infections. PCP most often presents during the first 6 months posttransplant with fever, dry cough, dyspnea on exertion, and interstitial pulmonary infiltrates. Diagnosis is based on recovery of the organism on induced sputum or bronchoalveolar lavage, although treatment should begin based on presenting symptoms and clinical suspicion.

OTHER COMPLICATIONS/ SPECIAL CONSIDERATIONS

Cardiovascular Disease

Overall, the risk of coronary artery disease posttransplant is three- to fivefold that for age- and sex-matched control subjects.[18] Risk factors for coronary artery disease include (1) pretransplant coronary artery disease; (2) hyperlipidemia secondary to antirejection medications; (3) hypertension; (4) corticosteroid therapy; (5) insulin-dependent diabetes mellitus; (6) erythrocytosis with increased blood viscosity; (7) smoking; and (8) frequent rejection episodes. Hypertension is found in approximately 50 percent of all transplant patients. Possible causes of hypertension include (1) graft rejection; (2) cyclosporine toxicity; (3) glomerulonephritis (recurrent and de novo); (4) graft renal artery stenosis; (5) essential hypertension from native kidneys; (6) hypercalcemia; and (7) steroids. Calcium channel blockers (CCBs) are particularly efficacious in treating hypertension in renal transplant patients on cyclosporine, although CCBs interfere with cyclosporine metabolism (see Table 99-3).

Chronic Liver Disease

Chronic liver disease is an important cause of morbidity and mortality for renal transplant patients. Causes of hepatic dysfunction include (1) viral hepatitis (CMV is leading cause, followed by hepatitis C and B) and (2) antirejection drugs (both azathioprine and cyclosporine cause cholestatic jaundice).

Malignancy

Transplant patients are at significantly higher risk for cancers than the general population because of (1) chronic immunosuppression; (2) chronic antigenic stimulation; (3) increased susceptibility to oncogenic viral infections; and (4) direct neoplastic action of immunosuppressants. Transplant patients suffer a significant overall two- to five-fold excess risk in both sexes for cancers of the colon, larynx, lung, and bladder, and in men for cancers of the prostate and testis. A ten- to thirtyfold excess risk exists for cancers of the lip, skin (non-melanoma), kidney, endocrine glands, and non-Hodgkin lymphoma, and in women, cancers of the cervix and vulva-vagina.[19]

Blood Transfusion

Immunosuppressed patients requiring blood transfusion should receive CMV seronegative blood. If this product is not available, they should be transfused through a leukocyte filter.

PATIENT EVALUATION

History

Because many of the clinical rejection syndromes are correlated with the age of the graft, the date of the transplant surgery should always be obtained (Table 99-5). The donor source is also an important consideration because cadaveric kidneys have higher incidences of ARF and rejection. The patient's immunization status against infectious agents and any information regarding transmissible agents carried by the donor can help target diagnostic and therapeutic interventions. A history of recent and repeated infections gives important clues to the patient's level of immunosuppression. In patients with infections, it is common practice to decrease immunosuppression, which increases the risk of rejection. A complete drug history is very important because many medications affect the levels and toxicity of cyclosporine (see Table 99-3).

The most common reason for a transplant recipient to present to the emergency department is fever, and while fever is the most common symptom of infection, it may be masked by immunosuppressive agents which limit the inflammatory response, and by steroids, uremia, and hyperglycemia, which suppress baseline body temperature. While the absence of fever should not be used to rule out possible infection in a transplant patient, the presence of fever may be caused by factors other than infection, such as hypersensitivity reaction, rejection, or malignancy. That said, fever in a transplant patient should occasion an aggressive workup, even for relatively subtle presentations. This is especially true during the critical period between the first and sixth postoperative months when immunosuppression is at its highest, or during bouts of acute rejection when immunosuppression has been augmented. A history of recent or repeated rejections may also suggest the presence of increased intensity of immunosuppression because these drugs are commonly increased during periods of rejection. The degree of immunosuppression should direct clinical suspicion toward various opportunistic organisms (see Table 99-4).

Physical Examination

The physical findings of renal failure may be subtle or absent (Table 99-6). Peripheral edema in these patients is often a misleading sign of fluid overload that can occur in hypovolemic patients because of hypoalbuminemia or venous stasis. The vital signs, patient weight, skin turgor, orthostatic pulse, and blood pressure changes may be helpful in identifying hypovolemia. Examination of the renal graft may disclose swelling and tenderness associated with acute rejection, renal vein thrombosis, and obstruction.

A high index of suspicion is required to find infections in unusual sites in an immunocompromised patient. In addition to the common sites of infection (skin, pulmonary tract, and genitourinary tract), the head, neck, rectum, and abdomen should be closely scrutinized for infection. Infections during the first 4 weeks posttransplant are most commonly related to the surgical procedure of engraftment. Special attention should be given to the renal graft looking for signs of wound infection, pyelonephritis, and urine leakage with infection.

TABLE 99-5 Key Historical Elements in Renal Transplant Patients

History of recent temperature elevations?
Date of transplantation surgery?
Graft source: donor living related vs. cadaveric?
Rejection history: Number of rejection episodes? Date of last rejection episode? Note any recent changes in dosages of antirejection medications.
History of immunizations, chronic infections (CMV, EBV, hepatitis B & C viruses, etc.) and recent exposure to patients with infections (chickenpox, CMV, TB, etc.)
A complete list of and compliance with immunosuppressive medications.
Complete list of all medications, including those that are unrelated to renal transplant and all over-the-counter medications.
Baseline: blood pressure, body weight, serum creatinine, and cyclosporine or tacrolimus level.

Abbreviations: CMV = cytomegalovirus; EBV = Epstein–Barr virus; TB = tuberculosis.

TABLE 99-6 Key Physical Examination Elements in Renal Transplant Patients

Mental Status / Neurologic Examination: cyclosporine/tacrolimus neurotoxicity, steroid psychosis, HSV encephalitis, *Listeria* meningitis/encephalitis, cryptococcal meningitis.
Volume Status: Often invasive hemodynamic monitoring (pulmonary artery catheterization) is the only reliable means of determining volume status in renal transplant patients.
HEENT: Periorbital edema (glomerulonephritis), retina (CMV or toxoplasmic chorioretinitis, *Listeria* endophthalmitis), sinuses (*Staphylococcus aureus,* mucormycosis, and invasive fungal disease), mouth (*Candida,* HSV), neck (meningismus, retropharyngeal abscess), lymphadenopathy (CMV, EBV, hepatitis)
Skin: Rashes are commonly seen in viral syndromes (hepatitis B and EBV), cellulitis from indwelling catheter sites, nocardial cutaneous lesions.
Lung: Pneumonia is a common source of infections in transplant patients. *Streptococcus pneumoniae* and other community-acquired agents are still common sources, but opportunistic infections such as PCP, *Aspergillus,* TB, coccidioidomycosis, and viral pneumonias should be suspected.
Heart: Pericardial friction rubs as a complication of uremia and a wide range of viral infections.
Abdomen: Peritonitis without a defined source is one of the most common sites for infection in transplant patients. RUQ tenderness associated with hepatitis B & C, CMV, and EBV. VZV causes pancreatitis. If left in place, peritoneal dialysis catheters can be sources of infection.
Renal Graft: Usually placed in abdominal flap; inspection (look for signs of wound infection), palpation (graft tenderness and swelling are often seen in acute rejection, outflow obstruction, and pyelonephritis), and auscultation (bruits suggest renal artery stenosis and AV malformations).
Rectal: Perirectal abscess is a common, yet often-overlooked, source of infection in transplant patients.
Extremities: Access sites for hemodialysis can be sources of infection. Peripheral edema in renal transplant patient can represent a number of different etiologies: recurrent vs. de novo glomerulonephritis, graft failure, cirrhosis, nephrotic syndrome (from native kidneys), renal vein thrombosis, malnutrition, and heart failure.

Abbreviations: AV = atrioventricular; CMV = cytomegalovirus; EBV = Epstein–Barr virus; HEENT = head, ears, eyes, nose, and throat; HSV = herpes simplex virus; PCP = *Pneumocystis carinii* pneumonia; RUQ = right upper quadrant; TB = tuberculosis; VZV = varicella-zoster virus.

Ancillary Tests

The serum creatinine level is the most valuable prognostic marker of graft function at all times after transplantation, and should be obtained whenever renal failure or infection is suspected (Table 99-7).[20] The urinalysis provides important clues to acute changes in graft viability. Red blood cell casts and proteinuria are commonly seen in recurrent or de novo glomerulonephritis. The presence of white blood cells, bacteria, and nitrites is helpful in diagnosing UTIs. Significant proteinuria may signal rejection, drug toxicity, glomerular disease, or other graft nephropathy, although proteinuria from the native kidney should also be considered. Cyclosporine or tacrolimus blood levels should be determined for all patients.

The evaluation of a renal transplant patient with suspected infection should include routine testing as well as additional tests based on the patient's presenting complaint, history, and physical examination (see Table 99-7). Leukocytosis or left shift of the white blood cell count may be blunted by immunosuppressive agents and, conversely, leukopenia with an increase in atypical lymphocytes is commonly seen with viral infections, especially CMV. Liver function tests may show mild transaminase elevations with CMV and EBV infections, and much higher elevations with hepatotropic viruses such as hepatitis B and C viruses. Urine *Legionella* antigen should be ordered prior to treatment of patients with pneumonia or GI complaints. Bacterial cultures and fungal cultures of blood and urine should be obtained on all patients. Because viral cultures are not very sensitive, clinicians should rely on their acumen to order organism-specific antigen assays and antibody titers when contemplating viral or parasitic infections.

Renal ultrasonography is the best test to detect urinary obstruction and color duplex imaging of the renal artery and vein are helpful in assessing renal vascular stenosis or thrombosis. Renal graft ultrasonography should be obtained in patients suspected of having urinary obstruction, pyelonephritis, perinephric abscess, urine leak, wound infection, or an episode of rejection. Renal biopsy is the gold standard for diagnosing rejection.

DISPOSITION

Transplant patients are chronically immunosuppressed, attempting to balance between under-immunosuppression, with the risk of graft rejection, and overimmunosuppression, with the risk of infection. When these patients present to the emergency department with fever, increasing edema, decreased urine output, graft pain or swelling, or increasing fatigue, they should be evaluated for infection and renal graft function. These patients are complex, and it is often difficult to determine on initial assessment the presence of a serious infection or complication. It is recommended that the patient's physician or transplant coordinator be consulted to help the emergency physician in making the disposition decision.

TABLE 99-7   Possible Ancillary Tests for the Evaluation of a Renal Transplant Patient

Serum creatinine
Urinalysis
Chest radiograph (posterior–anterior and lateral)
Complete blood count
Electrolytes
Liver function tests
Cyclosporine or tacrolimus level
Cultures: mouth, sputum, urine, blood, stool, access and wound sites
Serology: cytomegalovirus, Epstein–Barr virus, hepatitis, toxoplasmosis, cryptococcosis
Ultrasonography of the renal graft
Renal biopsy

REFERENCES

1. URREA; UNOS. 2002 Annual Report of the U.S. Organ Procurement and Transplantation Network and the Scientific Registry of Transplant Recipients: Transplant Data 1992–2001 [Internet]. Rockville, MD: HHS/HRSA/OSP/DOT; 2003. Available from: http://www.optn.org/data/annualReport.asp.
2. Klaussen AC, Klassen DK: Who are the donors in organ donation? The family's perspective in mandated choice. *Ann Intern Med* 125:70, 1996.
3. Olsen JC, Buenefe ML, Falco WD: Death in the emergency department. *Ann Emerg Med* 31:758, 1998.
4. Gjertson DW: A multi-factor analysis of kidney graft outcomes at one and five years posttransplantation, in Cecka JM, Terasaki PI (eds): *Clinical Transplants 1996*. Los Angeles: UCLA Tissue Typing Laboratory, 1997.
5. Cohen D, Galbraith C: General health management and long-term care of the renal transplant recipient. *Am J Kidney Dis* 38(Suppl 6):S10, 2001.
6. Howard RJ, Reed AI, Hemming AW, et al: Graft loss and death: Changing causes after kidney transplantation. *Transplant Proc* 33:3416, 2001.
7. Chan L, Gaston R, Hariharan S: Evolution of immunosuppression and continued importance of acute rejection in renal transplantation. *Am J Kidney Dis* 38:(Suppl 6):S2, 2001.
8. Knoll GA, Bell RC: Tacrolimus versus cyclosporin for immunosuppression in renal transplantation: Meta-analysis of randomized trials. *BMJ* 318:1104, 1999.
9. Nashan B: Early clinical experience with a novel rapamycin derivative. *Ther Drug Monit* 24:53, 2002.
10. Tanphaichit NT, Brennan DC: Infectious complications in renal transplant recipients. *Adv Ren Replace Ther* 7:131, 2000.
11. Kim HC, Park SB: Infection in the renal transplant recipient. *Transplant Proc* 32:1974, 2000.
12. Patel R: Infections in recipients of kidney transplants. *Infect Dis Clin North Am* 15:901, 2001.
13. Smith SR: Viral infection after renal transplantation. *Am J Kidney Dis* 37:659, 2001.
14. Glazier DB, Jacobs MG, Lyman NW, et al: Urinary tract infection associated with ureteral stents in renal transplantation. *Can J Urol* 5:462, 1998.
15. Conrad S, Schneider AW, Gonnermann D, et al: [Urologic complications after kidney transplantation. Experiences in a center with 539 recipients]. *Urologe A* 33:392, 1994.
16. Aguado JM, Herrero JA, Gavalda J, et al: Clinical presentation and outcome of tuberculosis in kidney, liver, and heart transplant recipients in Spain. Spanish Transplantation Infection Study Group, GESITRA [published erratum appears in *Transplantation* 64:942, 1997]. *Transplantation* 63:1278, 1997.
17. Paya CV: Fungal infections in solid-organ transplantation. *Clin Infect Dis* 16:677, 1993.
18. Kasiske BL: Epidemiology of cardiovascular disease after renal transplantation. *Transplantation* 72(6 Suppl):S5, 2001.
19. Birkeland SA, Storm HH, Lamm LU, et al: Cancer risk after renal transplantation in the Nordic countries, 1964–1986. *Int J Cancer* 60:183, 1995.
20. Kasiske BL, Vazquez MA, Harmon WE, et al: Recommendations for the outpatient surveillance of renal transplant recipients. American Society of Transplantation. *J Am Soc Nephrol* 11(Suppl 15):S1, 2000.

RENAL IMAGING
Daniel E. Wiener
Emily H. Sheffer

The recent years have seen an explosion in the modalities available to the emergency physician to image the urinary system. This chapter reviews the different methods and discusses their role in the management of patients in the ED.

IMAGING MODALITIES

Plain-Film Radiography

The KUB (kidneys, ureters, and bladder) is a plain full-length film of the abdomen. The kidneys can be visualized because the perinephric fat gives them a lucent outline. Renal calculi can usually be visualized, but small ureteral calculi may be hidden by bowel shadows. Calculi in the lower ureters may be confused with phleboliths. The KUB by itself rarely adds to patient care in the ED and is most useful in conjunction with ultrasonography or intravenous pyelography (IVP).

Ultrasonography

Ultrasonography is a rapid, painless method to visualize the urinary tract.[1] The patient requires no preparation and is not exposed to the potentially harmful effects of radiation or contrast material. The limitations of this modality include poor visualization of the ureter and difficulty in imaging obese patients. The quality of the study is both operator- and equipment-dependent. Ultrasonography is an anatomic study and provides no data regarding kidney function. Renal ultrasonography can document the presence, location, and size of the kidneys and detect focal parenchymal lesions such as cysts and tumors. Hydronephrosis, and on occasion dilated ureters and calculi, can be demonstrated (Figure 100-1). Fluid collections surrounding the kidney can also be seen. With Doppler flow capability, reduced renal blood flow can be identified.

Ultrasonography is performed using a 3.5-MHz transducer. With the patient in a supine position, the transducer is placed subcostally from the lateral approach. The operator sweeps the ultrasound plane to locate the kidney. Rotation of the probe permits documentation of the longitudinal and transverse renal axes. The liver is usually used as an acoustic window to visualize the right kidney and the spleen to visualize the left. Images on the right are technically superior to those on the left because the liver provides a better acoustic window than does the spleen. An air-filled stomach and dilated loops of bowel can hinder visualization. The kidneys move with respiration, and having patients hold their breath after a maximal inhalation often enhances visualization.

Gerota fascia, the renal cortex, the collecting system, and the renal sinus, as well as proximal and distal calculi, can be visualized. Gerota fascia is associated with perinephric fat and is visualized as a bright area surrounding the kidney. The renal cortex is homogeneous in appearance and more reflective (brighter) than the renal medulla. The renal pelvis is centrally located and appears echogenic. Dilation of the collecting system by fluid (echo-free) is thus readily apparent. The normal ureter is not visualized, but the dilated ureter can sometimes be seen. In the longitudinal plane, the normal kidney is oblong-shaped and measures 9 to 12 cm. In the transverse plane, the normal kidney is C-shaped and measures 4 to 5 cm. The kidneys normally measure within 2 cm of each other in the longitudinal axis.

Intravenous Pyelography

Intravenous pyelography (IVP) provides both anatomic and functional information about the kidney. It is most commonly used in the setting of flank pain and hematuria, and has long been considered the "gold standard" for visualizing renal calculi. The disadvantages of the study include the necessity of transporting the patient to the radiology department, the time demand of the study, and the administration of contrast material. Concern regarding potentially poor images in ED patients because of the lack of bowel preparation is unwarranted.[2]

Before initiation of the IVP, the patient is asked to void and the abdomen is compressed by an inflatable belt to enhance visualization of the calyx and renal pelvis. The standard series of films taken during an IVP include the following:

1. The scout film, a plain radiograph from the level of the kidneys to the bladder prior to the administration of contrast. This allows visualization of stones that may be obscured by contrast material.
2. The nephrogram, a coned view of the kidneys obtained 1 min after injection of contrast material. This film is examined for the absence or delay in visualization, homogeneity, and duration of the nephrogram.
3. The pyelogram, two films taken 5 and 10 min after injection of contrast material. Calyceal dilation or effacement, ureteral dilation, intraluminal filling defects, and the extravasation of contrast material can be seen. The compression device is typically deflated after these images.
4. The bladder film, taken 20 min after injection of contrast material.
5. The postvoid film, used to evaluate postvoid residual bladder volume and to visualize any retained contrast or distal ureteral stone that may have been hidden by the full bladder. Multiple views and tomograms are often used to enhance the quality of the study. When a ureteral obstruction is suspected, two views are required to distinguish a peristaltic contraction from a tumor or a stricture.
6. Delayed views over 1 to 4 h may be necessary in instances of obstruction or nonvisualization.

Computed Tomography

Computed tomography (CT) scanning provides both anatomic and functional information about the kidney. The renal parenchyma, collecting system, extrarenal space, ureters, and bladder can all be visualized. Renal perfusion can be assessed with the administration of contrast material. CT can identify extrarenal pathology or injury not clinically suspected. The disadvantage of CT is the necessity of transporting the patient to the device, the time required to perform the study, and the need to administer contrast if optimal results are to be obtained.

With CT, images of the kidney and urinary system are reconstructed from information collected by focused x-ray beams arranged on a plane that cuts through the patient's body in a transverse or horizontal direction as the patient passes through the CT gantry on a movable table. As these beams pass through the patient, they are absorbed by a ring of detectors on the opposite side of the gantry. The intensity of the x-ray beam that reaches the detector is dependent on the absorption characteristics of the intervening tissue. The radiodensity of a small area of tissue can then be calculated from the absorption pattern of multiple beams crossing the area from different directions.

During helical CT, the x-ray tube is in continuous rotation while the patient is moved smoothly, at a constant speed, through the scanning field. This technique improves the detection of small lesions, as scanning is performed during a single breath-hold, thus reducing the movement of intra-abdominal organs and motion artifact, which occurs when imaging is performed during respiration. Data from multiple scanning planes can be used to produce three-dimensional reconstruction of lesions. In addition, shaded surface displays allow volume surface analysis of parenchymal organs and maximal-intensity projections provide analysis of the vasculature. The selected slice thickness of a scan depends on the clinical presentation. Trauma scans are usually 8- to 10-mm thick and are obtained from the diaphragm down to

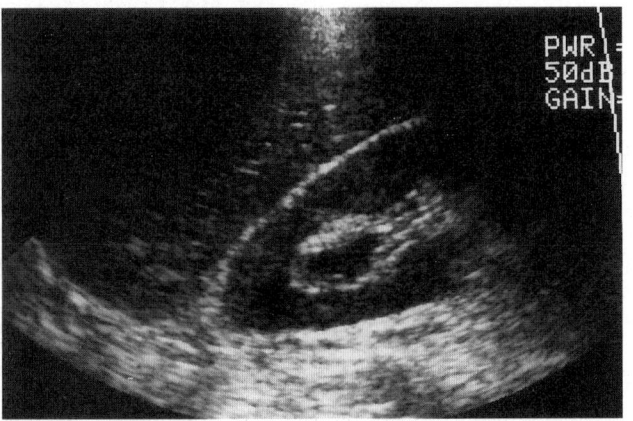

FIG. 100-1. Sonogram showing hydronephrosis from a right uretero-vesicular junction stone. (Photograph courtesy of David Frager, MD.)

the bottom of the pelvis. CT scans for renal colic use 5-mm slices from the top of the kidneys down to the bladder. If there is an area of subtle or equivocal findings, the radiologist may elect to make smaller cuts for clarification.

A CT cystogram is performed by instilling at least 350 mL of diluted contrast material into the bladder via a urinary catheter, the catheter is then clamped and contiguous axial images are obtained from the dome of the diaphragm to the perineum. The clamp is then released and additional images may be obtained after the bladder is emptied.

Intravenous Contrast Enhancement

IVP and CT use intravenous radiocontrast material containing iodinated compounds that absorb x-rays. These agents allow vessels and organs to be more easily differentiated from adjacent nonenhancing structures. A typical imaging protocol involves the administration of 150 mL of intravenous radiocontrast by a power injector into an intravenous catheter of adequate size, typically an 18-gauge catheter in the antecubital vein.

Intravenous radiocontrast media are classified according to two characteristics: ionic versus nonionic and high osmolar versus low osmolar. Nonionic media are approximately 10 times more expensive then ionic media but have only a fourth the incidence of adverse reactions compared to ionic media. High-osmolar contrast media (HOCM) are all ionic, as opposed to low-osmolar contrast media (LOCM), which can be ionic or nonionic. Intravenous contrast media are nephrotoxic; the least nephrotoxic is nonionic LOCM. In patients with normal renal function, there is no measurable impairment of renal function with the use of either HOCM or LOCM.[3] However, in patients with preexisting renal insufficiency and diabetes, nonionic LOCM causes less impairment to renal function than does HOCM. Therefore, LOCM should be considered as the first choice of contrast media in patients with the following risk factors: age greater than 50 years, debilitation, known severe cardiovascular disease, asthma, previous reaction to contrast, preexisting renal insufficiency, and/or diabetes.

The following agents have demonstrated some efficacy in reducing the severity of radiocontrast nephrotoxicity: (1) prostaglandin E1 20 ng/kg per min infusion started 1 h before contrast administration and continued for 6 h afterwards; (2) acetylcysteine 600 mg PO twice daily started the day before contrast administration and continued for 2 days afterwards; (3) theophylline 200 mg IV 30 min before contrast administration; and (4) fenoldopam mesylate 0.1 μg/kg per min infusion for at least 1 h before contrast administration.[4–7] To date, studies have been small in size and the effects have been modest. There is no consensus regarding the routine use of these agents in patients at risk for radiocontrast nephrotoxicity.

Oral-Contrast Enhancement

Oral contrast is used with the abdominal CT scan for a patient suspected of having intra-abdominal pathology. This barium- or iodine-based solution markedly increases the density of the gastrointestinal tract, differentiating bowel from other pathology. When there is a suspicion of renal injury, both oral and intravenous contrast is used. **Oral contrast poses no threat to the kidneys** and can be used in patients with depressed renal function.

Dynamic CT Scanning

In dynamic CT scanning, a series of rapid images using helical CT is obtained during peak vessel contrast enhancement. As with IVP, the kidney is visualized in the (1) vascular phase, when major vessels are visualized; (2) nephrogram phase, when contrast reaches the tubules and medullary opacification occurs; and (3) pyelogram phase, when calyceal and pelvic filling is observed. Dynamic CT is useful in demonstrating impaired of parenchymal perfusion and can also differentiate abscesses and hematomas.

Retrograde Urethrogram

The retrograde urethrogram is used to assess urethral injury (usually from trauma) or strictures, and occasionally used to evaluate urethral foreign bodies. It is an invasive procedure requiring the use of contrast material.

Using sterile procedure, the foreskin is retracted and the penis is stretched perpendicularly across the patient's thigh to prevent urethral folding. Radiocontrast solution is injected into the penis using the catheter tip of a 60-mL syringe or through a nonlubricated 16- or 18-Fr balloon-tipped urinary catheter inserted just inside the urethral meatus. If a catheter is used, the balloon of the catheter is inserted 2 to 3 cm past the meatus and 1 to 2 mL of saline is injected into the balloon to secure the catheter in the fossa navicularis. In the direct syringe technique, slow constant pressure is used to inject 50 to 60 mL of contrast material. With the catheter technique, gravity is used to infuse the contrast medium from the filled syringe with the plunger removed and attached to the catheter, held above the patient's bed. If the medium will not flow, slow, constant pressure can be used, as with the direct syringe approach. The examination is best performed under fluoroscopic visualization, although fixed or portable radiographic equipment can be used with the image taken during the injection of approximately the last 10 mL of contrast.

In instances when a urinary catheter has already been inserted into the bladder and there is a suspected urethral injury, it may be necessary to confirm that the urethra is intact and the catheter is in the bladder. The catheter should not be removed; instead, the urethrogram should be performed around it. Using a lubricated pediatric feeding tube placed alongside the existing catheter, contrast material can slowly be injected to demonstrate the presence or absence of extravasation.

Cystogram

Cystography using radiocontrast solution is the standard examination for bladder pathology. An anteroposterior (AP) pelvic or KUB film should be obtained as a scout film before contrast material is introduced.

Using sterile technique, a 16- or 18-Fr urinary catheter is carefully placed into the bladder. A 60-mL pistonless catheter-tip syringe is attached to the catheter and contrast material is poured into the syringe. Contrast is then allowed to enter the bladder via gravity as the syringe is placed above the level of the patient's bladder. The bladder is allowed to fill until extravasation occurs if done using fluoroscopy or the bladder is filled (400 mL). If bladder contraction occurs during filling, an additional 50 mL is injected by hand. In children younger than age 11 years, estimated bladder capacity is calculated based on the formula (age in years +2) × 30. Incomplete filling of the bladder can limit the quality of the study. To accurately exclude bladder rupture and extravasation, the bladder must be filled with at least 250 mL of contrast material.

Cystograms should be done using fluoroscopy or plain films in the AP, oblique, and lateral projections. If there is an associated pelvic fracture, the patient should be kept in the supine position to avoid possible disruption of any retropubic hematomas. To detect retrovesical extravasation, an AP film should always be obtained after bladder drainage.

Angiography

Angiography is a test to define vascular injuries of the kidney. It is highly invasive, requiring cannulation of the femoral artery and the use of intravascular radiocontrast material. Indications include the absence of a functioning kidney on IVP or CT, findings of a large retroperitoneal hematoma, major renal fractures, or segmental areas of renal non-enhancement. In some instances injuries to the parenchyma and arteries can be treated using interventional angiography to stop hemorrhage.

The femoral artery is accessed by the Seldinger technique (flexible catheter advanced over a guidewire). The tip of the catheter is placed in the aorta and a midstream aortogram obtained to evaluate the number and status of the renal arteries. The catheter tip is then placed at the upper level of the proximal artery and films are obtained to capture the arterial, capillary, and venous phases.

Renal Cortical Scintigraphy

Renal cortical scintigraphy (RCS), using dimercaptosuccinic acid (DMSA), is a radionuclear study that evaluates kidney function. RCS is most commonly used in the evaluation of children with suspected pyelonephritis and, occasionally, assessment of a renal transplant.

Two hours after administration of ^{99m}Tc-DMSA, scanning is performed using a gamma camera. DMSA binds to the renal tubules and accumulates in the functioning renal cortex. Intrarenal blood flow and proximal tubular cell membrane transport determine cortical uptake. Focal or diffuse areas of decreased DMSA cortical uptake without any loss of volume indicate the presence of pyelonephritis. Areas of decreased uptake with volume loss indicate old scars. Images are evaluated for the size of the kidneys, their shape and location, and differential renal function as well as the distribution of cortical uptake.

CONDITIONS

Renal Colic

The ideal imaging study in renal colic would (1) determine the size and location of the stone, (2) define the presence and degree of ureteral obstruction, and (3) identify other causes of flank pain and hematuria when renal calculi have been excluded.

Some 90 percent of renal calculi are radiopaque and theoretically visible on plain radiographs. Studies in the 1930s and more recent textbooks report visualization of stones in 85 to 90 percent of cases. These studies did not specify whether the visualized "stone" was related to the patient's symptoms or confirmed by other radiographic studies. Recent comparisons between plain-film radiography and IVP or CT (the "gold standard") found that plain radiography had a sensitivity of about 45 to 60 percent.[8] Plain radiography alone has low utility and should not be used alone in the evaluation of patients with suspected renal colic; it does, however, play a role as an adjunct to IVP and ultrasonography.

IVP has long been considered the "gold standard" for the evaluation of renal colic. The location of a calculus can be seen by a radiocontrast cutoff in the ureter, the size of the calculus can usually be determined, and ureteral obstruction is suggested by visualization of the entire ureter secondary to a lack of peristaltic contractions. Identifying stones at the ureterovesical (UV) junction or the distal ureter can be difficult but is enhanced by assessment of the postvoid film. Secondary findings of stone disease include delay in the appearance of the nephrogram, distention of the renal pelvis, calyceal distortion, or radiocontrast extravasation.

Recent studies have compared the efficacy of ultrasonography to IVP or CT in the diagnosis of renal stones in ED patients presenting with renal colic (Table 100-1).[9–11] These sonographic studies used detection of the stone and/or evidence of hydronephrosis as a positive test result for the diagnosis of renal calculi. Both ultrasonography and IVP are slightly better at identifying obstruction than at localizing a stone. Using either stone identification or detection of obstruction, both modalities have essentially the same range of sensitivity and specificity, although ultrasound has a wider range of sensitivity, reflecting the greater dependence on operator skill and limitations of the modality. Use of Doppler ultrasonography to compare resistive indices of urinary jets entering the bladder has been reported to increase sensitivity. Plain-film radiographs can be used as road maps to focus the ultrasonograph study. Theoretically, ultrasonography has an advantage in imaging radiolucent stones (approximately 10 to 20 percent of urinary calculi), but if there is no dilation of the ureter, it becomes more difficult to place the visualized density correctly. Furthermore, ultrasonography has particular difficulty in visualizing dilations of the upper and mid-ureter. The distal ureter is more accessible, because the bladder acts as an acoustic window. Ultrasonography may also be limited by the delayed appearance of hydronephrosis; in a patients with renal calculi causing ureteral obstruction, the initial sonogram may be negative in up to a fourth but show hydronephrosis when repeated 8 to 12 h later.[10]

Published studies indicate that emergency physicians can perform bedside ultrasound examinations in patients with renal colic and detect hydronephrosis with more than 90 percent sensitivity, as compared with an IVP. The availability of ultrasound equipment for use in the ED, and the training of more emergency physicians in the use of this equipment, has the potential to expand the use of this modality and reduce the use of IVP studies for patients with acute renal colic.

Selecting ultrasonography instead of IVP or CT for an individual patient requires some clinical judgment. Certainly, patients with contraindications to radiation should have an ultrasonogram. The clinician will have to further weigh the importance of ascertaining functional information about the kidney, as well as the increased likelihood of identifying the location of the stone using radiocontrast media versus the added time and radiation exposure necessary to complete an IVP or CT. One approach is to obtain an ultrasonogram in all patients presenting with signs and symptoms of renal colic and only proceed to IVP or CT if the patient is deemed to require surgical intervention or if the diagnosis remains unclear.

Helical CT without intravenous contrast material has become the imaging modality of choice in many institutions for patients with acute renal colic.[11] The helical CT takes only 5 min to perform and can identify the presence and location of calculi of all compositions except pure indinavir stones, not only providing prompt and accurate diagnosis in most patients with calculi but also identifying extrarenal disorders in patients without calculi. The average dose of radiation at the skin from a helical CT is 3 to 5 cGy, comparable to 1.5 to 3 cGy (0.25 to 0.3 cGy per radiograph) from an IVP. One limitation of the helical CT is that it does not provide functional information about the degree of ureteral obstruction.

TABLE 100-1 Imaging Modalities in Renal Colic: Approximate Sensitivities and Specificities

	Identification of Stone or Hydronephrosis		Identification of Stone		Identification of Hydronephrosis	
	Sensitivity	Specificity	Sensitivity	Specificity	Sensitivity	Specificity
IVP	80–85%	95%	60–80%	95%	90%	95%
Ultrasonography	65–93%	90–95%	65–93%	95%	85%	95%
Helical CT	95–98%	95%	90%	95%	85–90%	90–95%

Abbreviations: CT = computed tomography; IVP = intravenous pyelography.

Studies demonstrate that helical CT has excellent sensitivity and specificity in the diagnosis of renal colic (see Table 100-1).[11] It can detect stones as small as 1 mm in diameter. One limitation is distinguishing phleboliths from renal calculi, but secondary signs can be used to help make this distinction. For renal colic, these signs include ureteral dilation (sensitivity 90 percent and specificity 93 percent), perinephric stranding (sensitivity 82 percent and specificity 93 percent), collecting system dilation (sensitivity 83 percent and specificity 94 percent), and renal enlargement (sensitivity 71 percent and specificity 89 percent). The presence of ureteral dilation and perinephric stranding had a positive predictive value of 99 percent, and the absence of both had a negative predictive value of 95 percent. Edema of the ureteral wall surrounding the calculus (rim sign) is up to 100 percent sensitive and 94 percent specific in distinguishing renal stones from phleboliths. Helical CT should be considered positive for calculi when any of the following are seen: (1) a stone, (2) both ureteral dilation and perinephric stranding, or (3) a tissue rim sign. These are of particular importance when indinavir stones are considered. Urologists were able to use helical CT without further imaging in almost 90 percent of patients who underwent lithotripsy or endoscopic stone removal.[12]

Renal Transplant

Renal transplant failure can be secondary to graft rejection or renovascular complications. Modalities available to evaluate the transplanted kidney include angiography, ultrasonography with color-flow Doppler and duplex Doppler, and renal cortical scintigraphy. The choice of modality will depend on the clinician's index of suspicion for graft rejection or vascular compromise.

The most common vascular complication of transplant is renal artery stenosis (RAS), with an incidence of 3 to 15 percent in the first 3 years after transplant. Renal artery and vein thromboses are rare, usually occur in the perioperative period, and are generally catastrophic, resulting in loss of the renal graft. In contrast, identification and treatment of RAS can result in graft salvage. Patients with RAS often present with hypertension and worsening renal function. While posttransplant patients are reported to have a 50 to 60 percent incidence of hypertension unrelated to RAS, a renal transplant patient with hypertension that is progressive or difficult to control with medical therapy should be considered at risk for RAS. The gold standard for diagnosing RAS is angiography. However, angiography is limited by its invasive nature, the use of nephrotoxic contrast agents, the risk of an adverse reaction to contrast media, and complication rates of 0.5 to 2.3 percent (hemorrhage, intimal flaps, and arteriovenous fistulas). Gadolinium-enhanced magnetic resonance angiography (MRA) has several advantages over angiography, including short acquisition time (30 s), no risk of nephrotoxicity secondary to contrast agents, and avoiding hospitalization. MRA has a reported 100 percent sensitivity and 93 to 100 percent specificity for RAS.[13] However, contrast-enhanced MRA is an anatomic test that provides little information about the functional significance of a stenosis.

The conventional sonogram has limited utility but may detect some anatomic abnormalities suggesting a vascular or nonvascular diagnosis.[1] Duplex and color-flow Doppler have been used to evaluate the renal artery, but are technically difficult and the subject of controversy in the literature about their diagnostic accuracy. Color-flow Doppler has the advantage of sampling long segments of vessels but cannot accurately quantitate flow disturbances. Flow disturbances can be quantified by duplex Doppler. Using peak flow rates, studies have attempted to define a rate of flow that can accurately predict RAS. The threshold flow-rate value that provides the best combination of sensitivity and specificity is controversial. Peak systolic velocity of 190 to 250 cm/s has a sensitivity of 90 to 100 percent for RAS greater than 50 percent luminal narrowing. However, specificity varies from as low as 55 percent to as high as 95 percent. The overall accuracy can be improved by using peak systolic velocity in conjunction with analysis of the waveform (rounded, smaller-amplitude waveform with stenosis) in detecting significant proximal RAS.

Renal scintigraphy is a test of vascular perfusion, parenchymal extraction, and excretion. Abnormal findings from this study include (1) impaired uptake and visualization, which is consistent with vascular obstruction or hyperacute rejection and is a poor prognostic sign; (2) normal uptake and visualization but with parenchymal retention, which is associated with poor urine flow and the retention of the secreted isotope in the tubules; and (3) decreased uptake with normal parenchymal transit time and absent or minimal cortical retention, which is consistent with chronic rejection or renovascular hypertension. Unfortunately, the effects of renal artery stenosis, graft rejection, and cyclosporine toxicity cannot be distinguished by using renal scintigraphy.

Captopril-augmented RCS has been used to distinguish physiologic from nonphysiologic RAS. Patients with normal captopril-augmented RCS are not likely to respond to angioplasty, while patients with abnormal studies will likely have a significant improvement following angioplasty. Captopril-augmented RCS can replace renal vein renin sampling in identifying patients with lesions amenable to intervention.

Urinary Tract Infection

There is consderable controversy regarding the appropriate imaging of children with urinary tract infection (UTI) to identify predisposing functional and anatomic abnormalities.[14] Sometimes, an emergency evaluation is required because of diagnostic confusion based on atypical presentations, a negative urinalysis, or treatment failure based on persistent fever and toxicity 72 h following the initiation of therapy.

RCS using ^{99m}Tc-DMSA is the most sensitive imaging modality for establishing the diagnosis of pyelonephritis with a sensitivity of 90 percent and specificity of 100 percent.[14,15] Controversy exists concerning the necessity of documenting renal scarring and pyelonephritis in a child with an apparently simple UTI. Because patients with vesicoureteral reflux do not always demonstrate scarring on RCS, the American Academy of Pediatrics currently recommends both ultrasonography and voiding cystourethrogram (VCUG) evaluation for all children ages 2 to 24 months with their first documented UTI.[16] Conversely, a significant proportion of children without reflux demonstrate renal scarring, validating the importance of RCS evaluation despite a negative VCUG.[17] An advantage of RCS is that it can be used in children and neonates with poor renal function. Up to 17 percent of pediatric end-stage renal disease be attributed to chronic VUR and renal scarring.[16,18] Conversely, there are currently no long-term studies that determine the risk of developing ESRD in infants with VUR and no scarring.

The voiding cystogram is used to demonstrate VUR, the most common abnormality found in the urinary tract of children, which is seen in approximately 35 percent of children with UTI. Children at risk for VUR include those with a family history of reflux and whites. Voiding cystography can be done by radiographic or radionuclide technique. The radionuclide voiding cystogram using technetium pertechnetate no longer has the advantage of less radiation exposure when compared to VCUG using low frequency, pulsed, and grid-based fluoroscopy. Radionuclide technique also has the disadvantage of poor visualization of urethral and bladder abnormalities, including posterior urethral valves, which are commonly seen in boys. Thus, boys should undergo radiographic VCUG. Contrary to previous beliefs, VCUG performed at the time of infection does not result in falsely elevated rates of reflux. Furthermore, performing VCUG early prevents the failure to diagnose VUR secondary to poor compliance and loss to follow up.[19]

Ultrasonography is an insensitive method for diagnosing pyelonephritis or VUR but can provide anatomic information unavailable in other modalities. It can visualize renal abscesses, hydronephrosis, strictures, and obstruction at either the ureterovesical or ureteropelvic junction. Of patients with UTI, 40 to 50 percent of infants, and 30 percent of older children will have an anatomic abnormality. The sensitivity and specificity of ultrasonography for children with posterior urethral valves is 87 and 98 percent, respectively.[20] Recently, the practice of prenatal renal ultrasonography has led to earlier diagnosis of urinary tract abnormalities.[15] This may ultimately decrease the associated morbidity of hypertension and ESRD.

MRI may be comparable to RCS for detecting pyelonephritis. Using RCS as the gold standard, MRI has a reported sensitivity of 100 percent and a specificity of 78 percent.[21] CT signs of pyelonephritis include renal enlargement, poor corticomedullary definition, and patchy areas of decreased definition. Renal and perinephric abscesses are well visualized on CT. CT is not recommended in children because of the proximity of the gonads and their radiosensitivity before puberty. Adults with pyelonephritis only require imaging studies if there is suspicion of complications, including obstruction and perinephric abscess.

REFERENCES

1. Mostbeck GH, Zomtsich T, Turetschek K: Ultrasound of the kidney: Obstruction and medical diseases. *Eur Radiol* 11:1878–1889, 2001.
2. Schuster GA, Nazos D, Lewis GA: Preparation of outpatients for excretory urography: Is bowel preparation with laxatives and dietary restrictions necessary? *AJR* 164:1425, 1995.
3. Barrett BJ, Carlisle EJ: Meta-analysis of the relative nephrotoxicity of high- and low-osmolality iodinated contrast media. *Radiology* 188:171, 1993.
4. Sketch MH, Whelton A, Schollmayer E, et al: Prevention of contrast media-induced renal dysfunction with prostaglandin E1: A randomized, double-blind, placebo-controlled study. *Am J Ther* 8:155, 2001.
5. Tepel M, van der Giet M, Schwarzfeld C, et al: Prevention of radiographic contrast-agent-induced reductions in renal function by acetylcysteine. *New Eng J Med* 343:180, 2000.
6. Huber W, Ilgmann K, Page M, et al: Effect of theophylline on contrast material-nephropathy in patients with chronic renal insufficiency: Controlled, randomized, double-blinded study. *Radiology* 223:772, 2002.
7. Tumlin JA, Wand A, Murrary PT, Mathur VS: Fenoldopam mesylate blocks reductions in renal plasma flow after radiocontrast dye infusion: A pilot trial in the prevention of contrast nephropathy. *Am Heart J* 143:894, 2002.
8. Levine JA, Neitlich J, Verga M: Ureteral calculi in patients with flank pain: Correlation of plain radiography with unenhanced helical CT. *Radiology* 204:27, 1997.
9. Patlas M, Farkas A, Fisher D, et al: Ultrasound vs CT for the detection of ureteric stones in patients with renal colic. *Br J Radiol* 74:901, 2001.
10. Andresen R, Wegner HEH: Intravenous urography revisited in the age of ultrasound and computerized tomography: Diagnostic yield in cases of renal colic, suspected pelvic and abdominal malignancies, suspected renal mass, and acute pyelonephritis. *Urol Int* 58:221, 1997.
11. Colistro R, Torreggiani WC, Lynburn ID, et al: Unenhanced helical CT in the investigation of acute flank pain. *Clin Radiol* 57:435, 2002.
12. Preminger GM, Vieweg J, Leder RA, et al: Urolithiasis: Detection and management with unenhanced spiral CT—A urologic perspective. *Radiology* 207:308, 1998.
13. Huber A, Heuck A, Scheidler J, et al: Contrast-enhanced MR angiography in patients after kidney transplant. *Eur Radiol* 11:2488, 2001.
14. Santen SA, Altieri, MF: Pediatric urinary tract infection. *Emerg Med Clin North Am* 19:675, 2001.
15. Kraus SJ: Genitourinary imaging in children. *Pediatr Clin North Am* 48:1381, 2001.
16. Downs SM: Technical report: Urinary tract infections in febrile infants and young children. The Urinary Tract Subcommittee of the American Academy of Pediatrics Committee on Quality Improvement. *Pediatrics* 103:e54, 1999.
17. Belman AB: Vesicoureteral reflux. *Pediatr Clin North Am* 44:1171, 1997.
18. Craig JC Irwig LM, Knight JF, Roy LP: Does treatment of vesicoureteral reflux in childhood prevent end-stage renal disease attributable to reflux nephropathy? *Pediatrics* 105:1236, 2000.
19. Mahant S, To T, Friedman J: Timing of voiding cystourethrogram in the investigation of urinary tract infection. *J Pediatr* 139:568, 2001.
20. Williams CR, Perez, LM, Joseph, DB: Accuracy of renal-bladder ultrasonography as a screening method to suggest posterior urethral valves. *J Urol* 165(Pt 2):2245, 2001.
21. Chan YL, Chan KW, Yeung CK, et al: Potential utility of MRI in the evaluation of children at risk of renal scarring. *Pediatr Radiol* 29:856, 1999.

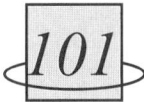

VAGINAL BLEEDING IN THE NONPREGNANT PATIENT
Laurie J. Morrison
Julie M. Spence

EPIDEMIOLOGY

ED visits for vaginal bleeding by women of reproductive-age are common. An estimated 5 percent of women aged 30 to 49 years will consult a physician for treatment of menorrhagia.

PHYSIOLOGY

Normal Menstrual Cycle

Ten years of age tends to be the lower limit for menarche, and the mean age in North America is 12.5 years. Most children develop secondary breast changes 2 years prior to the onset of menarche. At the time of ovarian stimulation, a white or yellow vaginal discharge, which is both nonodorous and nonirritating, may appear. Early cycles are anovulatory and irregular, but unlike adult anovulatory cycles, bleeding is generally not excessive. The hypothalamic pituitary axis takes 1 to 5 years to reach full maturity, and the average time to establish ovulatory cycles is 2 years after menarche.

The normal menstrual cycle is 28 days and is divided into four phases: follicular, ovulation, luteal or secretory, and menses. The first 14 days are the follicular phase, during which the ovary matures an oocyte for ovulation, and the granulosa cells, lining the follicle, produce estrogen. This stimulates the endometrium to proliferate and thicken (Figure 101-1). In response to the rising estrogen levels, the pituitary gland secretes follicle-stimulating hormone (FSH) and luteinizing hormone (LH), which stimulate the release of the mature oocyte. The residual follicular capsule forms the corpus luteum. During the luteal phase, the corpus luteum secretes estrogen and progesterone, which maintain the endometrium and make it more receptive to implantation. If fertilization and implantation occur, the developing embryo secretes human chorionic gonadotropin (hCG) into the bloodstream, signaling the corpus luteum to continue the production of progesterone and estrogen necessary to support early pregnancy. In the absence of hCG, the corpus luteum involutes, and estrogen and progesterone levels fall. Hormonal withdrawal causes vasoconstriction in the spiral arterioles of the endometrium. This leads to the final phase, or menses, when the ischemic endometrial lining becomes necrotic and sloughs. The vaginal effluvium contains blood, endometrial tissue, and fluid. The estimated amount of menstrual blood loss ranges from 25 to 60 mL. Judging the amount of bleeding in a menstrual cycle may be difficult. The average tampon or pad absorbs 20 to 30 mL of vaginal effluent, although the number of pads or tampons used is unreliable, as personal habits vary greatly among women. In a normal cycle, fibrinolysis occurs in the uterine cavity and the cervix. In women with heavy bleeding, there may be insufficient time for fibrinolysis, and blood clots may occur. Definitions of terminology commonly used in gynecology have been included in Table 101-1.

Menopause

Menopause on average occurs at age 51 years. During the transition phase, or perimenopausal period, there is lengthening or marked variation in the intermenstrual intervals. By age 45 years, only a few primordial cells remain, and the production of estrogen decreases. As a result, the pituitary continuously produces large quantities of FSH and LH. There is no midcycle rise in estrogen to trigger a further surge of pituitary hormones for ovulation. Estrogens continue to be produced in lower, subcritical levels for a short time after menopause, until the remaining follicles become atretic, and production falls to almost zero.

DIFFERENTIAL DIAGNOSIS OF ABNORMAL VAGINAL BLEEDING

The gynecologic causes of abnormal vaginal bleeding in nonpregnant, reproductive-age females can be broadly grouped into three categories: ovulatory abnormal bleeding, anovulatory abnormal bleeding, and nonuterine bleeding. Abnormal ovulatory bleeding usually results in menorrhagia and intermenstrual bleeding. Nonovulatory cycles may be irregular and heavy (menometrorrhagia) or frequent and light (polymenorrhea) bleeding. Nongynecologic causes of bleeding should also be considered.

Table 101-2 lists causes of bleeding by approximate frequency and age group.

Ovulatory Bleeding

Ovulatory bleeding is associated with regular menstrual periods that are preceded by breast tenderness, abdominal bloating, and dysmenorrhea. Abnormal bleeding may occur during ovulation as a result of low estrogen levels. Intermenstrual bleeding may also be caused by structural and inflammatory lesions, including cervical polyps, vaginal lacerations, cervicitis, invasive cervical cancer, endometrial cancer, and fibroids. Premenstrual spotting or delayed menses frequently results from an inadequate luteal phase or persistent corpus luteum. Abnormal or heavy menstrual bleeding may be due to pelvic diseases, such as endometriosis, pelvic inflammatory disease (PID), and ovarian neoplasms. Uterine causes include leiomyomas, endometrial polyps, endometrial hyperplasia or malignancy, and adenomyosis. Finally, iatrogenic factors, pregnancy and postpartum complications, and bleeding dyscrasias may result in abnormal bleeding in the woman with ovulatory cycles. Idiopathic heavy menstrual bleeding in the absence of pathology responds to medical therapy at best in 50 percent of cases.

Anovulatory Bleeding

Menorrhagia secondary to anovulation is seen in 10 to 15 percent of all gynecologic patients. It is common in perimenarchal and perimenopausal women, as well as in patients with endocrine disorders, polycystic ovary syndrome, exogenous hormone use, and liver or renal disease.

Anovulatory uterine bleeding in adolescence is secondary to the immature hypothalamic–pituitary–ovarian axis. The amount of bleeding is usually minimal and painless. The findings on pelvic and rectovaginal examination are likely to be normal. Investigations are warranted when bleeding persists after 9 days, recurs at intervals of less than 21 days, or produces anemia. In some cases the blood loss can be considerable, with monthly losses of 100 to 200 mL, resulting in iron deficiency, marrow depletion, and anemia. If bleeding at the onset of menarche is considerable or necessitates blood transfusions, a coagulopathy should be excluded. Acute menorrhagia can generally be controlled with estrogen therapy or the oral contraceptive pill (OCP) (Table 101-3). Dilatation and curettage (D&C) is rarely required.

Anovulatory bleeding in the reproductive-age female may be regular but more often is irregular because of fluctuating estrogen levels

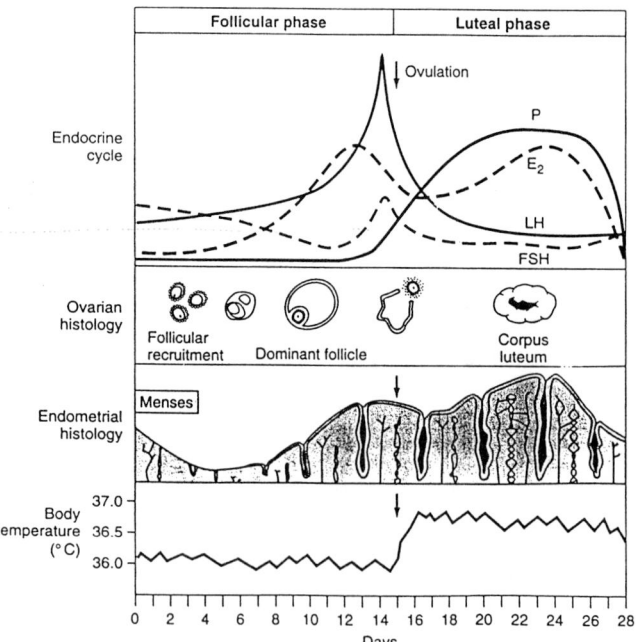

FIG. 101-1. The hormonal, ovarian, endometrial, and basal body temperature changes and relationships throughout the normal menstrual cycle. (Reproduced with permission from Carr BR, Wilson JD: Disorders of the ovary and female reproductive tract, in Isselbacher KJ, Braunwald E, Wilson JD, et al (eds): *Harrison's Principles of Internal Medicine,* 13th ed. New York, McGraw-Hill, 1998, p 2101.)

below the critical level required to maintain endometrial growth. The level of estrogen depends on the age, number, and activity of ovarian follicles. As some follicles degenerate, others resume the production of estrogen and the endometrium continues to proliferate for weeks to months, which may cause glandular hyperplasia ("Swiss cheese" hyperplasia). This estrogen steady state is insufficient to meet the growing needs of the endometrium and produces a relative estrogen insufficiency, and vaginal bleeding ensues. Alternatively, when follicle degeneration and stimulation are not balanced, absolute estrogen levels fall and withdrawal bleeding occurs. Characteristically, anovulatory cycles present as prolonged amenorrhea with periodic menorrhagia. Because of the lack of progesterone-mediated myometrial contractions and arteriolar vasospasm, anovulatory cycles are rarely associated with cramping. This pattern of bleeding increases the risk of endometrial hyperplasia and adenocarcinoma.

OCP use remains the most common cause of midcycle bleeding. Eating disorders, excessive weight loss, stress, and exercise can cause abnormal uterine bleeding. Additionally, medications (e.g., antiseizure medications) that increase the P450 system of the liver may increase

the metabolism of endogenous hormonal glucocorticoids and may cause withdrawal bleeding.

In perimenopausal and menopausal patients, it is important to distinguish true pathology from dysfunctional bleeding. Malignancy should always be considered, since it is the most important, although not the most common, diagnosis.[1] The amount of bleeding does not correlate with the severity of disease. Postmenopausal bleeding warrants prompt referral for evaluation. Older patients may not be able to accurately describe the location of pain or bleeding in the proximity of the bladder, uterus, or rectosigmoid. The vagina and cervix must be adequately visualized on pelvic examination. Bleeding from a vaginal source is uncommon but may be associated with the use of pessaries and douche solutions, which can irritate the mucosa. Cervical polyps may be a source of bleeding. However, an endometrial biopsy is ultimately required to rule out other serious causes of bleeding (Table 101-4).

Although bleeding is frequently caused by an unstable or atrophic endometrium, other causes must be considered. Important conditions in the differential diagnosis include submucosal leiomyomas, endometrial polyps, endometrial hyperplasia, adenomyosis, and tumors. Emergency therapy should be directed at investigating and treating obvious causes of bleeding. Outpatient ultrasound and endometrial biopsy can then be arranged for stable patients.

Nonuterine Bleeding

Nonuterine causes of vaginal bleeding must be included in the differential diagnosis, systematically addressed during the history taking and physical examination, and pursued with relevant investigations and consultations, if indicated. Primary coagulation disorders account for almost 20 percent of acute menorrhagia in adolescents. von Willebrand disease (vWD) is the most common; however, myeloproliferative disorders and immune thrombocytopenia are also possibilities.

Potential sources of nonuterine bleeding include the cervix, vagina, lower urinary tract, and lower gastrointestinal (GI) tract. Cervical causes include carcinoma, polyps, condylomata, eversion of squamocolumnar junction associated with OCP use or pregnancy, trauma, and some infections. Vaginal sources of bleeding include carcinoma, sarcoma, adenosis, lacerations, infections, and retained foreign bodies.

Lower urinary tract lesions, such as urethral caruncles and infected urethral diverticula, may mimic vaginal bleeding. Some patients may not be able to determine the source of bleeding, and lower GI causes may need to be investigated.

CLINICAL FEATURES

History

Adolescent and adult patients presenting to the ED with vaginal bleeding share many common elements of the history and physical examination. Key points that should be routinely addressed when taking the clinical history are age of menarche, menstrual history, date of the last menstrual period (LMP), pattern of abnormal bleeding or discharge, and the presence of dysmenorrhea. Complications related to pregnancy are always possible, and routine inquiries are both appropriate and necessary. Sexually active patients should be asked about contraception, current sexual activity, use of barrier protection, HIV and hepatitis status, and history of PID, sexually transmitted diseases (STDs), or ectopic pregnancy. Signs and symptoms of a coagulopathy, including nosebleeds, petechiae, and ecchymoses, and a family and surgical history should be recorded.

Patients who present with pain should be asked about its quality, timing, location, radiation, and aggravating or alleviating factors. Associated symptoms of the urinary, GI, and musculoskeletal systems, as well as the presence of fever or syncope, should be documented. A his-

TABLE 101-1 Definitions Related to Vaginal Bleeding

Vaginal bleeding	Defined temporally as midcycle (ovulatory), premenstrual, menstrual, and postmenstrual
Abnormal vaginal bleeding	Vaginal bleeding occurring outside the regular cycle
Menorrhagia	Menses >7 days, or menstruation >60 mL, or <21-day recurrence, from any cause
Metrorrhagia	Irregular vaginal bleeding outside the normal cycle
Menometrorrhagia	Excessive irregular vaginal bleeding
Dysfunctional uterine bleeding	Abnormal vaginal bleeding due to anovulation
Postcoital bleeding	Vaginal bleeding after intercourse, suggesting cervical pathology
Postmenopausal bleeding	Any bleeding that occurs more than 6 months after cessation of menstruation

TABLE 101-2 Causes of Bleeding by Approximate Frequency and Age Group*

		BLEEDING	
Adolescent	Reproductive	Perimenopausal	Postmenopausal
Anovulation	Pregnancy	Anovulation	Endometrial lesions, including cancer (30%)
Pregnancy	Anovulation	Uterine leiomyomas	Exogenous hormone use (30%)
Exogenous hormone use	Exogenous hormone use	Cervical and endometrial polyps	Atrophic vaginitis (30%)
Coagulopathy	Uterine leiomyomas	Thyroid dysfunction	Other tumor—vulvar, vaginal, cervical (10%)
	Cervical and endometrial polyps		
	Thyroid dysfunction		

*Prepubertal bleeding is discussed in Chap. 139.

Sources: Modified from Hillard PA: Benign diseases of the female reproductive tract: Symptoms and signs, in Berek JS, Adashi EY, Hillard PA (eds): *Novak's Gynecology,* 12th ed. Baltimore, MD, Williams & Wilkins, 1996, p. 333; and Hacker NF, Moore JG: *Essentials of Obstetrics and Gynecology.* Philadelphia, WB Saunders, 1998, p. 467.

tory of recent illness, psychological stress, weight change, or endocrine problems, including thyroid disease and pituitary tumors, should be obtained.

Taking the history of adolescent girls is challenging. Honest responses to questioning will require assurances of confidentiality by the physician. If the patient requests a female physician, the request should be honored, if at all possible. Always interview the patient without the parent present. Questions regarding STDs and sexual activity can be very disturbing for adolescents. It is important historical information and should be obtained in a nonjudgmental, gentle way that in itself will be educational. It may not be possible to obtain an accurate history about the occurrence of periods early in menarche, as the cycle is usually irregular for the first 1 to 2 years and perhaps as long as 5 years.

Physical Examination

Vital signs should be assessed in all patients. In cases of heavy bleeding, any postural changes in vital signs should be recorded. A complete ex-

TABLE 101-3 Short-Term Medical Management of Hemodynamically Stable Uterine Bleeding

Estrogen therapy
  Oral conjugated estrogen (e.g., Premarin) 10 mg/d (2.5 mg qid) or 25 mg IV every 2 to 4 h for 24 h. Note: the efficacy of oral and intravenous estrogens are similar.
  When bleeding subsides, add medroxyprogesterone acetate (Provera) 10 mg/d.
  Continue both the conjugated estrogen and the medroxyprogesterone for 7 to 10 days.
  Stop for synchronized withdrawal bleed.
Oral contraceptive pill
  Ethinyl estradiol 35 μg and norethindrone 1 mg—4 tabs for 7 days
    or
  Slow taper (ethinyl estradiol 35 μg and norethindrone 1 mg)
    4 tabs for 2 days
    3 tabs for 2 days
    2 tabs for 2 days
    1 tab for 3 days
Progesterone
  Medroxyprogesterone acetate (e.g., Provera) 10 mg/d is used for 10 days.
Antifibrinolytic therapy
  Tranexamic acid:
    0.3–1.0 g PO every 8 h for 3 days.

Sources: Coulter A, Kelland J, Peto V, Rees MCP: Treating menorrhagia in primary care: An overview of drug trials and a survey of prescribing practice. *Int J Technol Assess Health Care* 11:456–471, 1995 (0.5 g); and Lethaby A, Farquhar C, Cooke I: Antifibrinolytics for heavy menstrual bleeding. Cochrane Menstrual Disorders and Subfertility Group. *Cochrane Database Syst Rev* Nov. 27, 2001.

amination should include a careful abdominal examination to rule out nongynecologic causes of vaginal bleeding. Femoral and inguinal nodes should be examined for size and tenderness. Signs of other illnesses, including hypothyroidism, galactorrhea, and obesity associated with hirsutism, should be documented.

Male physicians should have a chaperone during gynecologic examinations. Female physicians are equally well advised to have a chaperone. Prior to beginning the examination, a simple explanation should be given and verbal consent obtained. Adolescents should be examined without their parents or guardians. The patient should be allowed to empty her bladder and remove any tampons prior to the examination. Positioning and draping should allow the patient to see the physician during the examination. Occasional eye contact is reassuring.

The examination of nonvirginal patients includes a speculum examination, a vaginoabdominal examination (bimanual), and a rectovaginal examination. The vulva and urethral opening should be inspected prior to inserting the warmed and lubricated speculum into the vagina. The site of abnormal bleeding should be determined through careful examination of the perineum, urethra, vulva, and perianal region. The vagina should be inspected for signs of lacerations, fissures, lesions, infection, and foreign bodies. The cervix should be well visualized to rule out polyps, inflammation, infection, ulcers, and evidence of cancer. Cultures are generally taken as part of the examination if a mucopurulent discharge is found. The cervical os should be inspected for blood, tissue, an intrauterine device (IUD), pedunculated leiomyomata or polyps, and signs of infection.

On bimanual vaginoabdominal examination, the softness and patency of the cervical os, and pain on movement should be documented. The ovaries and uterus are palpated for size, consistency, pain, and the presence of associated masses. The adnexa and periuterine area should also be carefully examined. The rectovaginal examination is essential and should be done in every patient, especially if the patient cannot tolerate a bimanual examination. The rectovaginal examination enables evaluation of the posterior cul-de-sac for ovarian masses, the posterior wall of the uterus for size and consistency, and the uterosacral ligaments for metastatic nodules or ectopic endometriosis. Stool should be evaluated for the presence of blood.

Virginal patients with menstrual cramps, mittelschmerz, or vaginal discharge do not require a full pelvic examination, because a rectovaginal examination is generally sufficient. In the case of trauma and abnormal vaginal bleeding, a vaginal examination is necessary. Adolescents with intact hymen can generally tolerate a speculum examination if a narrow Pederson-type adolescent or Huffman pediatric speculum is used. Conscious sedation or full anesthesia may be required, depending on psychological response of the patient, the circumstances and the extent of the injury or disease.

Older patients with a history of bleeding should undergo a full gynecologic examination. Degenerative changes to the lumbar spine and hips may make the traditional lithotomy position difficult. Alternatively,

TABLE 101-4   Factors Frequently Used to Determine the Cause of Abnormal Bleeding in Perimenopausal Women

Test	CAUSE OF BLEEDING					
	Perimenopause	Neoplasia	Fibroid	Adenomyosis	Polyp	Pregnancy Related
History						
Associated hot flashes	Yes	No	No	No	No	No
Increased cramping	No	Sometimes	Sometimes	Yes	No	Sometimes
Bleeding pattern						
Skips and misses	Yes	Possible	No	No	No	—
Amenorrhea	Yes	No	No	No	No	Yes
Regular but shorter interval	Yes	No	No	No	No	No
Regular but heavy	No	No	Yes	Yes	Yes	No
Irregular	Yes	Possible	No	No	Yes	Yes
Physical examination						
Enlarged uterus	No	Sometimes	Yes	Yes	No	Yes
Enlarged and tender uterus	No	No	No	Yes	No	Possible
Ultrasonography						
Enlarged uterus	No	No	Yes	Yes	No	No
Enlarged uterus with intrauterine mass	No	Yes	Sometimes	No	Yes	Yes
Laboratory tests						
FSH	Elevated	Normal	Normal	Normal	Normal	Normal
CBC	Usually normal	Normal/low	Normal/low	Normal/low	Normal/low	Normal/low
hCG	Negative	Negative	Negative	Negative	Negative	Positive

Abbreviations: CBC = complete blood count; FSH = follicle-stimulating hormone; hCG = human chorionic gonadotropin.
Source: Reproduced with permission from Pearlman MD: Menopause, in Pearlman MD, Tintinalli JE (eds): *Emergency Care of the Woman.* New York, McGraw-Hill, 1998, p. 625.

the patient may be examined supine with knees flexed and legs dropped to the side, or lying on her side with the lower arm behind her back and thighs flexed (the Sims position). A small speculum (e.g., a 1- to 1.5-cm Pederson) should be used if the vulva and vagina appear atrophic. Physicians must remember that the vaginal walls may become adherent in individuals who are not sexually active, and a gentle digital examination may be required to ensure that a speculum examination is possible. Vaginal examination is generally well tolerated in women who are on estrogen replacement. Documentation of the size, shape, and mobility of the uterus is especially important when making a diagnosis in this population. The normal ovary should not be palpable 5 years after menopause, and any enlargement should be considered abnormal.

LABORATORY STUDIES AND IMAGING

Pregnancy tests should be ordered routinely in women of childbearing age to rule out pregnancy as a cause of bleeding. A complete blood count is essential in most cases of vaginal bleeding. Coagulation studies are ordered only when indicated by the history and physical examination. In individuals with suspected endocrine disorders, determination of thyroid-stimulating hormone and prolactin levels may be helpful, but the levels are rarely available for ED evaluation.

Ultrasonography is an important imaging modality for gynecologic conditions such as vaginal bleeding, adnexal or uterine masses, or pain. In nonpregnant patients, a formal ultrasonographic evaluation is used to determine uterine size and the characteristics of the endometrium, as well as the presence of leiomyoma, ovarian cysts, hydrosalpinx, pelvic adhesions, tuboovarian abscesses (TOAs), endometriosis, and tumors. Transvaginal (i.e., endovaginal) ultrasonography may be particularly helpful in further delineating ovarian cysts and fluid in the cul-de-sac. Depending on the degree of pain and findings on physical examination, ultrasonography may be done on an emergency basis, or deferred for outpatient evaluation.

Computed tomography is used primarily in the ED for the evaluation of acute abdominal or pelvic pain (see Chap. 102) Magnetic resonance imaging is used primarily for cancer staging.

Referral for follow-up will usually lead to endometrial biopsy in women who are at risk for endometrial cancer and are not pregnant. This procedure is generally indicated for women older than age 35 years with abnormal uterine bleeding or women younger than age 35 years with risk factors for endometrial cancer such as obesity and chronic anovulation. Hysteroscopy is a valuable test that affords a more complete examination of the surface of the endometrium than D&C, which may miss 10 to 25 percent of lesions.[2]

Hormone replacement therapy (HRT) is commonly used to relieve symptoms associated with menopause and to reduce the risk of cardiovascular disease. Recent trials have called this practice into question, citing no benefit for primary and secondary prevention of cardiovascular disease and excessive risk of endometrial, breast and colorectal cancer and thromboembolism.[3,4] Perimenopausal women with abnormal uterine bleeding should have an endometrial biopsy prior to the initiation of HRT. Bleeding after 6 months of continuous combined HRT, or unexpected bleeding with cyclic HRT, prompt referral for evaluation. In patients receiving continuous therapy, 40 percent will have abnormal bleeding in the initial 4 to 6 months. There are no acceptable criteria for "abnormal bleeding" on these therapies, and investigations are warranted if bleeding continues beyond 6 months or recurs after amenorrhea is established. Most frequently implicated in patients on HRT are poor compliance, poor GI absorption, drug interactions, failure to synchronize therapy with endogenous ovarian activity, and coagulation disorders.

TREATMENT

General Approach

The main approach to nonpregnant patients with established vaginal bleeding is to determine whether the condition requires general (e.g., resuscitation) or specific ED-based evaluation or intervention. In patients who present primarily with vaginal bleeding, the main issue is to determine whether there has been significant blood loss, and whether a condition exists (such as traumatic injury or bleeding dyscrasia) that places the patient at risk for uncontrolled or significant bleeding. If the bleeding has not led to hemodynamic compromise (and is unlikely to), then, after pregnancy has been ruled out, the only diagnoses that need to be absolutely established in the ED are trauma (including sexual abuse and assault), bleeding dyscrasia, infection and foreign bodies. Otherwise, patients can be referred for outpatient investigation, with the timing based on the urgency of the presentation.

Short-Term Management

HEMODYNAMICALLY UNSTABLE Patients who are hemodynamically unstable because of bleeding must be resuscitated according to standard protocols. Attempts should be made to localize the source of bleeding. In women with severe, persistent uterine bleeding, immediate D&C is usually indicated. Uterine packing should be avoided, because it increases the risk of infection and may hide ongoing blood loss. Conjugated estrogens may be useful in the ED treatment of life-threatening hemorrhage not caused by pregnancy or tumor or amenable to surgical intervention.

HEMODYNAMICALLY STABLE Medical management should be considered in hemodynamically stable patients provided the diagnosis is clear. Short-term hormonal manipulation allows the endometrium to stabilize, which, in turn, will slow or stop acute bleeding. Estrogen may be used to stimulate growth when ultrasonographic examination has revealed a thin endometrium. With the regimen outlined in Table 101-3, subsequent bleeding may be heavy but should not be prolonged. Oral contraceptives may be used in women who are not pregnant and have no anatomic abnormalities. The progesterone in the OCP decreases the number of available estrogen receptors and, as a result, bleeding may not stop as quickly as when estrogen is used alone. Side effects include nausea and vomiting. Two treatment regimens have been developed using a fixed-dosage pill, with 35 μg ethinyl estradiol and 1 mg norethindrone (see Table 101-3). In individuals with persistent light bleeding associated with anovulation, progesterone alone can be used to stabilize an immature endometrium. Bleeding occurs 3 to 10 days after discontinuation and may be heavy as a consequence of the large amount of tissue being sloughed. If the diagnosis is unclear, the patient should be referred for further investigation involving formal ultrasonographic evaluation and outpatient management.

Long-Term Management

Many therapies are available for the long-term management of vaginal bleeding. Expectant management is appropriate if episodes of heavy or irregular bleeding are infrequent. The OCP is an excellent choice if contraception is required. Ovulatory menorrhagia is decreased by 50 percent, with a similar reduction in the degree of dysmenorrhea. This therapy may be effective in the treatment of patients with fibroids.

Nonsteroidal anti-inflammatory drugs (NSAIDs) are helpful in the treatment of both ovulatory and anovulatory bleeding and dysmenorrhea. All of these medications have the same basic mechanism of action and inhibit cyclooxygenase in the arachidonic acid cascade. The prostaglandin inhibitors alter the ratio of prostaglandin $F_{2\alpha}$, which causes vasoconstriction, and prostaglandin E_2, which causes vasodilation. NSAIDs also increase levels of thromboxane A_2, which causes vasoconstriction and increases platelet aggregation. These medications may reduce blood loss by 20 to 50 percent and reduce dysmenorrhea. They have a mild side-effect profile and are inexpensive. Not all women will respond, although 75 percent of patients report a 30 percent decrease in blood loss.[5] NSAIDs are less useful in patients with uterine leiomyomas.[5] Mefenamic acid (500 mg tid) and naproxen (500 mg bid) are the most well studied, and ibuprofen (400 mg q6h) has been shown to reduce menstrual bleeding in IUD users. NSAIDs should be started on the first day of the period and continued until bleeding stops and pain resolves.

Although virtually never initiated in the ED, clomiphene citrate may be used to decrease bleeding as well as to induce ovulation if pregnancy is desired. If there is no contraindication to estrogen usage, oral medroxyprogesterone acetate 10 mg daily for 10 days can be used to produce scheduled bleeding. Intrauterine progesterone release is also available. Danazol may be used to decrease bleeding significantly, although it is expensive. Patient acceptance is similar to that of patients on NSAIDs, and reduction of bleeding may be greater. Side effects include musculoskeletal pain, flushing vertigo, backache, breast atrophy, and hirsutism.[5] Patients may still ovulate when using this medication. Gonadotropin-releasing hormone agonists may play a role in the induction of amenorrhea, and women on this therapy become menopausal. Other drawbacks include medication expense and bone loss when used for longer than 6 months. Tranexamic acid, a fibrinolytic, reduces objective signs of vaginal bleeding without any increase in side effects and better quality of life when compared to hormone therapy and NSAIDS. Data on thromboembolic events are not available.[6] Overall there is insufficient evidence to define optimal medical management.[7,8]

Hysteroscopy is both diagnostic and therapeutic. It can be used to sample the endometrium, as well as to resect polyps and myoma. Endometrial ablation may be performed in patients who do not desire fertility, have no pathologic diagnosis, and for whom medical therapy has failed. This may be performed using laser, electrocautery, or rollerball ablation. Amenorrhea is seen in approximately 50 percent of women treated, and decreased flow is seen in another 35 percent.[9] Improvement of symptoms of dysmenorrhea is reported in up to 80 percent of patients. Myomectomy may be useful in patients with symptomatic fibroids. Hysterectomy is reserved for selected patient populations. Evidence based on large case series suggests that uterine embolization may be an effective nonsurgical option for the management of bleeding caused by fibroids.

CLINICAL CONDITIONS

Genital Trauma

Vaginal injuries following intercourse are not uncommon. The majority of coital injuries result from vigorous voluntary sexual activity, although violent involuntary sexual activity should be considered. The most common site of injury is the posterior vaginal fornix. Misdiagnosis of coital injuries occurs frequently because either the physician fails to take an adequate history or the patient does not admit to antecedent sexual activity. Most coital injuries are minor, but severe injuries may lead to hemorrhagic shock.

Adenomyosis

In patients with adenomyosis, dysmenorrhea occurs just prior to or at the time of menstruation. In this condition, endometrial glands grow deeply into the underlying myometrium. Menorrhagia is common and is felt to be a result of aberrant tissue impairing the normal uterine contractility. Symptoms gradually increase in the fourth and fifth decades of life. On pelvic examination, there may be a large fibroid-like mass, or adenomyoma, but more commonly it is a diffuse, infiltrative process. Therapy is symptomatic, and simple analgesics are prescribed. Some cases require surgical management.

Leiomyomas

Leiomyomas (fibroids) are benign tumors of muscle cell origin and are the most frequently occurring pelvic tumor. They are found in 25 percent of white women and in 50 percent of African American women, and are usually multiple. The etiology is unclear, and theories include the proliferation from a single muscle cell from a small embryonic rest or a defined region of tissue with a higher level of estrogen receptors. Leiomyomas decrease in size during menopause, and enlarge early in pregnancy and, in some cases, OCP use. Up to 30 percent of patients with leiomyomas experience pelvic pain and abnormal bleeding. Acute pain is rare, but severe pain may be experienced with torsion or degeneration. Degeneration is a result of rapid growth and loss of blood supply, almost exclusively seen in early pregnancy.

Leiomyomas are diagnosed on examination and by imaging. A mass or multiple masses are palpable. In patients with acute degeneration, tenderness, rebound guarding, a fever, and elevated white blood cell count (WBC) may be seen. Pedunculated subserosal leiomyomas may undergo torsion or cause uterine cramping. Rapid growth at any age or growth after menopause is highly suspicious for malignant transformation. Treatment depends on size and symptoms. Medical management includes administration of NSAIDs, medroxyprogesterone acetate or depomedroxyprogesterone acetate, and gonadotropin-releasing hormone agonists. Pedunculated intracavitary leiomyomas may be removed by hysteroscopy. Surgical removal is associated with a 25 to 30 percent rate of recurrence and significant bleeding complications. A percutaneous interventional technique involving uterine artery embolization shows promise in observational trials. Embolization appears to alleviate symptoms and cause fibroid shrinkage.[10]

Blood Dyscrasias

Bleeding disorders may become apparent with an initial presentation of abnormal menstrual bleeding. Uterine hemostasis is not well understood, and any disorder of blood vessels, platelet abnormalities, and coagulation disorders, including vWD, may result in excessive menstrual bleeding. Of historical interest, the first described case of vWD was in a 13-year-old who died as a result of uncontrollable uterine bleeding.[11] The prevalence of objectively confirmed abnormal uterine bleeding is increased in patients with vWD, carriers of hemophilia, and factor XI deficiency, at 73, 57, and 59 percent, respectively, when compared with a 9 to 11 percent rate in a population-based sample. Treatment options include use of antifibrinolytics and the OCP. The latter raises factor VIII and vWF levels and is an effective and popular form of therapy. Antifibrinolytics such as tranexamic acid reduce both plasminogen activator activity and plasmin activity to reduce the amount of bleeding. Desmopressin acetate (DDAVP) stimulates endogenous release of factor VIII and vWF and may be used prophylactically for minor procedures or treatment of bleeding episodes and menorrhagia. DDAVP is given intranasally, parenterally, or by subcutaneous injection. It is important that the blood of vWD patients is typed and screened for antibodies prior to instituting DDAVP, because DDAVP may induce thrombocytopenia in certain subgroups. NSAIDs are ineffective and may increase blood loss.

Polycystic Ovary Syndrome

Polycystic ovary syndrome, one of the most common endocrine disorders, is the association of hyperandrogenism and anovulation without underlying disease of the adrenal or pituitary glands. A triad of obesity, hirsutism, and oligomenorrhea is classically described, although obesity is not universally seen. When menses occurs, it is heavy and prolonged.[12] The syndrome is further characterized by acne, androgen-dependent alopecia, elevated serum concentrations of androgens, and hypersecretion of LH with a normal or low FSH level. Typical ovarian morphology, which may be seen by ultrasonography, is not necessary for the diagnosis and may in fact represent a response of the ovary to chronic anovulation. The differential diagnosis includes hyperprolactinemia, acromegaly, congenital adrenal hyperplasia, and androgen-secreting tumors of the ovary or adrenal gland. Management of menorrhagia in women who do not desire fertility includes low-dose oral contraceptives or cyclic progestin administration.

Other Conditions

Periods of physical or psychological stress, illness, malnutrition, rapid weight gain or loss, and intense physical regimens affect the hypothalamus and disrupt the normal pattern of gonadotropin release. This usually causes amenorrhea but may result in irregular, heavy bleeding. In obese women, menorrhagia may be a result of increased circulating levels of estrogen from peripheral conversion of androstenedione to estrone in fatty tissue. Patients with liver and renal disease may also develop irregular bleeding.

SPECIAL CONSIDERATIONS

The Legalities of Treating Adolescents Without Parental Consent

Consent is not required to evaluate and initiate treatment in an emergency. State consent statutes and case law vary; so emergency physicians should know and follow their state law and hospital policy with respect to consent. There should be a mechanism in place to obtain consent from the courts when necessary. Figure 101-2 summarizes the American College of Emergency Physicians policy on consent. All states allow minors to consent to diagnosis and treatment of STDs and drug abuse without parental consent. Many states have similar statutes allowing minors independent direct access to prenatal care, termination of pregnancy, and medical care for crime-related injuries. Special considerations are included in some state legislation for emancipated and mature minors. Common sense and appropriate documentation should prevail above all with respect to issues of consent. An a priori awareness of the statutes and policies and established liaisons with local child protection services and the courts should assist emergency physicians in the ongoing provision of timely emergency care.

HIV-Infected Women

In general, there is no need to change the approach to vaginal bleeding in HIV-positive women. Physicians must look for associated infections and complications of chronic illness. The rate of vaginal and pelvic infections and cervical dysplasia is high in this cohort of patients. In a cross-sectional survey of 386 women younger than age 50

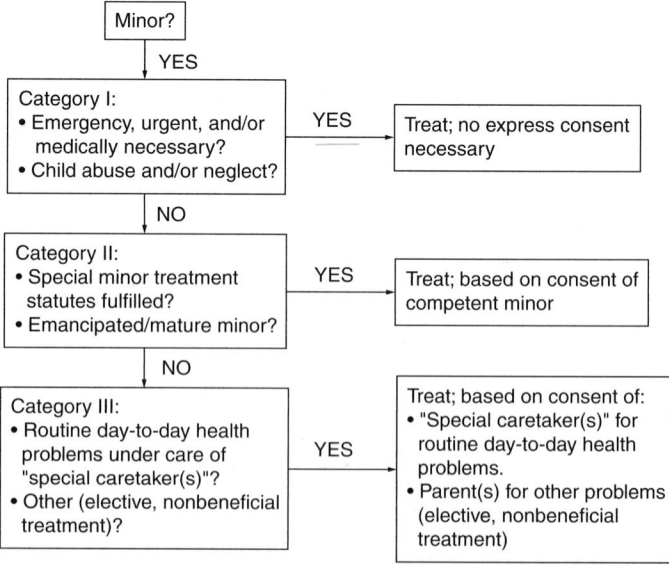

FIG. 101-2. Initial approach to consent for treatment. (Reproduced with permission from Tsai AK, Schafermeyer RW, Kalifon D, et al: Evaluation and treatment of minors: Reference on consent. *Ann Emerg Med* 22:1212, 1993.)

years, with and without HIV, neither infection nor immunosuppression affected menstruation or the rate of abnormal vaginal bleeding.[13] This was also seen in a study of 85 seropositive women, although the power of the study was low.[14]

REFERENCES

1. Brenner PF: Differential diagnosis of abnormal uterine bleeding. *Am J Obstet Gynecol* 175:166, 1996.
2. Gimpelson R, Rappold H: A comparative study between panoramic hysteroscopy with directed biopsies and dilation and curettage. *Am J Obstet Gynecol* 158:489, 1988.
3. Grady D, Herrington D, Bittner V, et al: Cardiovascular disease outcomes during 6.8 years of hormone therapy: Heart and Estrogen/Progestin Replacement Study follow-up (HERS II). *JAMA* 288(1):99, 2002.
4. Women's Health Initiative Investigators: Risks and benefits of estrogen plus progestin in healthy postmenopausal women: Principal results from the Women's Health Initiative randomized controlled trial. *JAMA* 288(3):321, 2002.
5. Duncan KM, Hart LL: Nonsteroidal antiinflammatory drugs in menorrhagia. *Ann Pharmacother* 27:1353, 1993.
6. Lethaby A, Farquhar C, Cooke I: Antifibrinolytics for heavy menstrual bleeding. Cochrane Menstrual Disorders and Subfertility Group. *Cochrane Database Syst Rev* 1, 2003.
7. Iyer V, Farquhar C, Jepson R: Oral contraceptive pills for heavy menstrual bleeding. Cochrane Menstrual Disorders and Subfertility Group. *Cochrane Database Syst Rev* 1, 2003.
8. Lethaby A, Augood C, Duckitt K: Nonsteroidal anti-inflammatory drugs for heavy menstrual bleeding. Cochrane Menstrual Disorders and Subfertility Group. *Cochrane Database Syst Rev* 1, 2003.
9. Carlson KJ, Schiff I: Alternatives to hysterectomy for menorrhagia. *New Engl J Med* 335:198, 1996.
10. Worthington-Kirsch RL, Popky GL, Hutchins FL: Uterine arterial embolization for the management of leiomyomas: Quality of life assessment and clinical response. *Radiology* 208:625, 1998.
11. Anonymous: A meeting held in London, 12–13 January 1998, to discuss bleeding disorders in women. *Hemophilia* 4:145, 1998.
12. Franks S: Medical progress: Polycystic ovary syndrome. *New Engl J Med* 333:853, 1995.
13. Ellerbrock TV, Wright T, Bush T, et al: Characteristics of menstruation in women infected with human immunodeficiency virus. *Obstet Gynecol* 87:1030, 1996.
14. Shah PN, Smith JR, Wells C, et al: Menstrual symptoms in women infected by the human immunodeficiency virus. *Obstet Gynecol* 83:397, 1994.

102 ABDOMINAL AND PELVIC PAIN IN THE NONPREGNANT PATIENT
Reb Close

This chapter provides an overview of the approach to a nonpregnant female who presents to the ED with abdominal and/or pelvic pain. Pregnancy-associated abdominal and pelvic complaints are discussed in Chap. 106. The reader is directed to Chap. 72 as well as standard references for more specific discussion on gastrointestinal disorders causing abdominal pain in both men and women. The clinical presentation, ED evaluation, and workup are integral in determining which patients need admission, which require surgery, and which can be safely discharged home.[1]

PHYSIOLOGY

Understanding the types and etiology of pain helps the examiner use information obtained through the history and physical examination to narrow the differential diagnosis.

Visceral pain results when obstruction of a hollow organ causes stretch of the smooth muscle wall. Stretch and associated inflammation or ischemia stimulate autonomic nerve fibers resulting in diffuse,

cramping, poorly localized pain. Pain is typically midline and difficult for the patient to describe. Visceral pain is common in early appendicitis, bowel obstruction, renal colic, and early pelvic inflammatory disease (PID).

Somatic pain fibers are found in the skin, abdominal wall and musculature, and in the parietal peritoneum. Inflammation or irritation in these areas can be from direct injury or bacterial or chemical contact. The resulting pain is typically well localized, sharp, and constant. Tenderness is elicited at the area of peritoneal inflammation. Somatic pain is seen as appendicitis and PID progress. Contamination of the peritoneal cavity by blood, urine, pus, and cystic or gastric fluid also results in somatic pain, which can be diffuse in nature.

Referred pain describes pain that originates in one organ but is described by the patient as located in a distant area. Visceral nerve fibers that innervate the diseased organ enter the spinal cord at the same level as somatic nerve fibers that innervate the areas of referred pain. As somatic pain is better localized than visceral pain, the patient may emphasize the area of referred pain. Typical examples are inner thigh pain seen with appendicitis or PID, or groin and labial pain with renal colic. Table 102-1 lists the nerves that innervate the lower abdominal and pelvic organs.

Females of any age can present with pelvic pain and associated symptoms. The differential diagnosis changes dramatically with the onset of both puberty and sexual activity.

CLINICAL FEATURES

History

A standard history regarding the pain characteristics (location, migration, radiation, quality, onset, severity, and exacerbating and relieving factors) and associated symptoms should be followed by a complete gynecologic, obstetric, and sexual history. The examiner must keep in mind that a negative history for pregnancy is unreliable.[1] In one study, about 7 percent of patients who stated that their last menstrual period was entirely normal and who denied any chance of pregnancy were

TABLE 102-1   Nerves Carrying Pain Impulses from the Pelvic Organs

Organ	Spinal Segments	Nerves
Perineum, vulva, lower vagina	S2–S4	Pudendal, inguinal, genitofemoral, posterofemoral, cutaneous
Upper vagina, cervix, lower uterine segment, posterior urethra, bladder trigone, uterosacral and cardinal ligaments, rectosigmoid, lower ureters	S2–S4	Sacral afferents traveling through the pelvic plexus
Uterine fundus, proximal fallopian tubes, broad ligaments, upper bladder, cecum, appendix, terminal large bowel	T11–T12, L1	Thoracolumbar splanchnic nerves through uterine and hypogastric plexus
Outer two-thirds of fallopian tubes, upper ureter	T9–T10	Thoracolumbar splanchnic nerves through mesenteric plexus
Ovaries	T9–T10	Thoracolumbar splanchnic nerves traveling with ovarian vessels via renal and aortic plexus and celiac and mesenteric ganglia

indeed pregnant.[2] Past medical history [sexually transmitted diseases (STDs), gallstones, kidney stones], surgical history, history of trauma, and history of similar episodes are important and often narrow the differential diagnosis. Specific risk factors for PID (late adolescence, multiple sex partners, frequent douching, recent IUD insertion, prior history, and cigarette smoking) should be ascertained.[3] Recent and current medications and allergies should be documented. Family history of breast or ovarian neoplasms should be identified, as patients with such a family history may have unspoken anxieties about these disorders that can bias or confound the evaluation of acute abdominal pain. Screening for domestic violence or sexual assault should also be part of the history taking.

Pain Characteristics

The location of pain coupled with a description of its migration and radiation patterns helps to make a diagnosis. Pain moving from the epigastrium or umbilicus to the right lower quadrant suggests appendicitis. Pain originating in the flank that radiates to the lower abdomen or groin suggests renal colic or pyelonephritis.

Questions about the quality of the pain can be helpful. True colicky pain is of a visceral origin and is associated with stretch of hollow organs. Bowel obstruction, biliary colic, renal colic, and fallopian tube obstruction due to ectopic pregnancy or ovarian torsion are examples. Renal colic represents an atypical presentation of colicky pain in that one wave of pain has typically not resolved before the next wave begins. This pattern of atypical colicky pain may also be seen with obstruction of other hollow organs. Sharp, well-localized pain indicates peritoneal inflammation and can be a late finding seen with appendicitis and PID.

The severity and onset of pain can guide the differential diagnosis. Pain that awakens a patient from sleep is generally associated with acute obstruction, ischemia, inflammation, or perforation of an organ. This can be seen with ovarian torsion or fallopian tube rupture. Severe, sudden-onset pain may be associated with life-threatening pathology, for example with organ rupture, but there are instances in which severe pain may have a typically benign etiology, as seen with nephrolithiasis.

Factors that exacerbate and relieve pain can provide information about the etiology. Pain with movement or pain elicited by tapping the heel suggests peritonitis. Pain that changes with eating, vomiting, or belching suggests gastrointestinal etiology.

Associated gastrointestinal symptoms such as nausea, vomiting, anorexia, diarrhea, or constipation are often nonspecific, as they can coexist with genitourinary and gynecologic disorders as well. Absence of anorexia is unusual in gastrointestinal disorders. Genitourinary symptoms such as dysuria, frequency, urgency, and hematuria suggest urinary tract infection or renal stone. However, dysuria and lower abdominal pain radiating to the groin can also be present with gynecologic disorders and gastrointestinal pathology such as appendicitis. Vaginal discharge, irregular bleeding, and dyspareunia are more common with gynecologic disorders, but can also be seen with other pathology.

Adolescents should always be interviewed without the parent present. This can be accomplished by asking the parent to leave the room for the physical examination. As accuracy of the history is paramount to diagnosis and treatment, it is very important to approach history regarding sexual activity, STDs, and pregnancy in a nonjudgmental manner while reassuring the patient regarding confidentiality.

Physical Examination

Obtaining vital signs and assessment of volume status, including orthostatic signs to detect hypovolemia, is the first step in examination.

A patient may have normal vital signs early in the course of very serious disease, and the presence or absence of fever has never been shown to aid in the delineation of medical versus surgical pathology.[1]

The patient's general appearance and position of comfort should be noted. A patient with peritoneal irritation tends to lie perfectly still as movement exacerbates the pain. The knees may be drawn toward the abdomen in an attempt to reduce intraabdominal pressure.

Examination of the abdomen and pelvis should concentrate on quality and frequency of bowel sounds, presence of peritoneal findings (involuntary guarding, rebound tenderness), point of maximal pain, and masses. Absence of rebound tenderness should not be used as evidence that the patient is free of a medical or surgical emergency. Early torsion and PID are both diagnoses in which rebound tenderness is unlikely, but in which early surgical or medical treatment is critical to preserve fertility.[1]

Rectal Examination

Perirectal abscesses and fistulae are often seen with inflammatory bowel disease. Stool that is grossly bloody, melanotic, or positive for occult blood strongly suggests gastrointestinal pathology. Tenderness in the right lower quadrant elicited by rectal examination can be seen in appendicitis, PID, and ectopic pregnancy, but the overall sensitivity of the rectal examination for diagnosing pathology is low.[1,4]

Pelvic Examination

All physicians should always have a chaperone present for the gynecologic examination. An assistant also facilitates obtaining specimens. A speculum examination should be performed in nonvirginal patients complaining of pelvic pain, bleeding, or vaginal discharge. The external genitalia, vagina, and cervix should be inspected for discharge, inflammation, lacerations, ulcers, and tumors. A wet mount and cultures for gonorrhea and *Chlamydia* are generally obtained during the speculum examination, especially if there is mucopurulent discharge or other evidence of inflammation.

RELIABILITY AND VALIDITY OF PELVIC EXAMINATION   Despite the common performance of the pelvic examination and the historical use of the results for making clinical decisions, few studies have addressed its reliability and validity. Bimanual pelvic examinations performed by experienced emergency physicians in the ED have been found to have poor interobserver agreement for the evaluation of uterine size, uterine tenderness, adnexal tenderness or masses, and cervical motion tenderness.[5] Padilla and associates found bimanual examinations performed under general anesthesia by medical students, gynecology residents, and attending gynecologists to be inaccurate for detecting adnexal masses that were confirmed surgically. They also found no statistically significant difference in accuracy between the medical students, residents, and attending physicians.[6] Several studies that have compared bimanual pelvic examination to pelvic ultrasonography and laparotomy have shown accuracy of pelvic examination to be poor, especially when the results are thought to be "normal."[7,8] Many texts and articles cite pelvic examination findings that confirm disease states (for example, cervical motion tenderness confirming a diagnosis of PID). Since the reliability of this examination is poor, then its positive or negative findings should not be the sole criterion for diagnosis.[5] Findings on pelvic examination appear related to examiner experience, patient cooperation, patient body habitus, prior abdominal surgery, and the limitations of the examination itself. Furthermore, criteria have not been standardized for the production of, or scoring of, cervical motion or adnexal tenderness. In addition, infection or inflammation of the peritoneum, urologic, pelvic, or gastrointestinal organs can cause pelvic tenderness.

Therefore, given the current uncertainty about the validity and reliability of the pelvic examination, further diagnostic testing is generally necessary for more precision in diagnosis. There are no validated clinical decision pathways for acute abdominal pain in women, and clinical decisions depend upon results from history and physical examination, as well as age and risk factors for specific disease processes. Burstin and colleagues published consensus guidelines for the evaluation of abdominal pain, but these are one-step guidelines based on clinical context and have not been validated.[9]

DIAGNOSIS

Abdominal and pelvic pain in women can be of gastrointestinal, genitourinary, or gynecologic etiologies. Gastrointestinal, genitourinary, pregnancy-associated pain, and pain associated with vaginal bleeding are covered in Chaps. 72, 96, 106, and 101, respectively. Table 102-2 lists some common causes of abdominal and pelvic pain. Specific

etiologies are discussed later in this chapter. The differential can be narrowed by aspects of the history and physical examination, and by using some ancillary tests and diagnostic imaging.

Laboratory Evaluation

URINE AND SERUM PREGNANCY TESTS   A quantitative urine enzyme-linked immunosorbent assay (ELISA) pregnancy test will detect beta-human chorionic gonadotropin (β-hCG) at levels greater than 20 mIU/mL[1,10] and will detect urine β-hCG at about day 21 of the menstrual cycle.[10] If point-of-care testing is done in the ED,

TABLE 102-2   Differential Diagnoses of Nontraumatic Pelvic Pain in Nonpregnant Adolescents and Adults

	History	Physical Examination	Ancillary Studies	Special Procedures
Ovarian cysts (rupture, hemorrhage, torsion, infection)*	Sudden-onset unilateral pelvic pain; can be preceded by activity or trauma	Tenderness to palpation; peritoneal signs if rupture	Pregnancy test; hematocrit if suspected rupture with blood loss; urinalysis; pelvic ultrasound	Laparoscopy
Adnexal torsion*	Possible history of adnexal cyst or tumor; sudden-onset unilateral pelvic pain; can be preceded by activity or trauma	Tenderness to palpation; peritoneal signs if rupture	Pregnancy test; hematocrit if suspected rupture with blood loss; urinalysis; ultrasound with Doppler flow	Laparoscopy
Pelvic inflammatory disease*	Lower abdominal or pelvic pain, dull, often bilateral; vaginal bleeding or discharge; urinary symptoms; fever	Fever; tenderness on abdominal and pelvic examinations; cervical motion tenderness; mucopurulent cervical discharge	Pregnancy test; WBC of limited value; cervical cultures for gonorrhea, *Chlamydia*, wet mount; ultrasound to rule out TOA	
Endometriosis	Dysmenorrhea; chronic pelvic pain; onset typically in third or fourth decades	Normal or may reveal pelvic tenderness or ovarian tenderness or enlargement	Pregnancy test; hematocrit with menometrorrhagia and suspected significant blood loss; urinalysis; ultrasound	Laparoscopy
Adenomyosis	Dysmenorrhea; menorrhagia; onset typically in third or fourth decades	Symmetrically enlarged uterus or fibroid-like mass	Pregnancy test; hematocrit with menometrorrhagia and suspected significant blood loss; ultrasound	Laparoscopy
Leiomyomas	Pelvic pain or pelvic mass	Pelvic or abdominal tenderness; pelvic or abdominal mass	Pregnancy test; ultrasound	
Tuboovarian abscess*	Fever; unilateral lower abdominal or pelvic pain; vaginal bleeding or discharge	Fever; lower abdominal or adnexal tenderness or fullness; possible CMT	Pregnancy test; WBC of limited value; cervical cultures for gonorrhea, *Chlamydia*, and wet mount; ultrasound	Laparoscopy
Appendicitis*	Periumbilical abdominal pain that migrates to right lower quadrant; fever, anorexia, nausea, vomiting	Right lower quadrant tenderness with possible rebound and guarding; fever; Rovsing sign†; psoas and obturator signs	Pregnancy test; CT scan; ultrasound in select patients	Laparoscopy
Diverticulitis*	Left lower quadrant abdominal pain; history of constipation; nausea, vomiting, fever	Tenderness in the left lower quadrant with possible rebound and guarding; peritonitis and sepsis if perforated	CT of the abdomen and pelvis with IV and PO contrast; abdominal series if suspected perforation	
Incarcerated hernia*	Abdominal, pelvic, or inguinal pain; mass; abdominal distention and vomiting; symptoms of bowel obstruction	Distention; palpable mass that is unable to be reduced	X-rays to evaluate obstruction; ultrasound may be used to evaluate the mass; CT of abdomen and pelvis	

*Diagnoses that must be considered as part of ED evaluation.
†Pressure applied to left lower quadrant elicits right lower quadrant pain.
Abbreviations: CMT = cervical motion tenderness; TOA = tubo-ovarian abscess; WBC = white blood cell count.

timing must be exact, or false-negative results can occur. A screening urine pregnancy test should be performed on all women of childbearing age with abdominal and pelvic pain, because a positive result will change the differential diagnosis and management options (e.g., medications and radiologic procedures).

COMPLETE BLOOD COUNT   An elevated white blood cell (WBC) count is neither sensitive nor specific for the diagnosis of an acute surgical condition. Sellors and colleagues found no difference in WBC count in patients with or without inflammatory disease diagnosed by endometrial biopsy and/or laparoscopy.[11] In the patient with vaginal bleeding, the hematocrit may not accurately reflect acute blood loss, although serial determinations of the hematocrit can be of value.

URINALYSIS   Positive findings have variable sensitivity and are not specific for urinary pathology. Urinalysis may be falsely positive with hematuria or evidence of infection in patients with appendicitis, likely due to periappendiceal inflammation. Positive urinalysis can similarly be seen with gynecologic infections. The sensitivity of urinalysis for hematuria varies, depending on the pathology and on the definition of positive results [≥1 RBC per high-power field (RBC/hpf) vs. ≥5 RBC/hpf considered positive]. Sensitivity of hematuria is only about 84 percent in patients suspected of renal colic with CT-proven nephrolithiasis.[12] Also, hematuria (defined as 1 RBC/hpf on microscopic urinalysis) may be present in over 50 percent of patients presenting with flank pain, but without nephrolithiasis as documented on CT.[13]

Depending on the cutoff for diagnosis of urinary tract infection (UTI) (nitrite-positive, leukocyte esterase–positive, and/or positive microscopic evaluation for bacteria and WBC), the sensitivity of urine reagent strip results varies.[14] In a study by Lammers and associates, if urine reagent strip results are defined as positive when leukocyte esterase or nitrite is positive or blood is more than trace, the overtreatment rate was 47 percent and the undertreatment rate was 13 percent, when compared to the results of urine culture. When the results were considered positive, WBCs >3 per high-power field or RBCs >5 per high-power field, the overtreatment rate was 44 percent and the undertreatment rate was 11 percent.[14] Also, since infection is a risk factor for nephrolithiasis, both conditions may coexist.[1] Urine culture and sensitivities should therefore be obtained to confirm the diagnosis when there is a moderate to high pretest probability of UTI (see Chap. 94).

TESTING FOR GONORRHEA AND CHLAMYDIA   Positive STD test results have public health implications and increase patient risk for future infertility and ectopic pregnancy. Many studies have shown a very high rate of asymptomatic infection in ED patients, especially teenagers and young adults.[15] Newer modalities of testing include first-catch urine (not practical in the ED, as many patients void the first daily urine before entering the ED), random urine, and patient-obtained vaginal swabs. Each of these has been shown to have high accuracy when compared to the gold standard of culture and are better tolerated by the asymptomatic patient, including the young.[16–20] Individual laboratory capabilities vary by institution.

Radiologic Evaluation

Pelvic ultrasonography with Doppler flow analysis can be utilized in the evaluation of a patient with lower abdominal pain in whom PID, torsion, tuboovarian abscess (TOA), leiomyoma, and ovarian cysts are all possible diagnoses.[1,21] Whether the study is done in the ED or as an outpatient depends on the patient's clinical status and availability of outpatient procedures. Ultrasonography has been shown to have high sensitivity and specificity for evaluation of surgically confirmed pelvic masses and is routinely the test of choice for evaluating suspected pelvic and gynecologic pathology.[1,7,22,23] Comparison with CT for accuracy in the evaluation of pelvic organs has not yet been performed. MRI and CT are available for evaluation of abdominal and pelvic complaints, and CT has recently been evaluated for differ-

entiating appendicitis and acute gynecologic conditions, with sensitivities of 100 percent and 87 percent, and specificities of 97 percent and 100 percent for appendicitis and acute gynecologic conditions, respectively.[24]

Diagnostic Laparoscopy

Laparoscopy is the gold standard for diagnosing PID and has been shown to aid in the diagnosis and surgical treatment if necessary for ovarian torsion, TOA, and adnexal masses.[3,25]

TREATMENT

The approach to the nonpregnant patient with pelvic pain is to determine if true emergent conditions exist that require immediate management. Once pregnancy and its associated complications have been excluded, the remaining emergent conditions include infection, torsion, and nongynecologic surgical etiologies. Rarely, a ruptured functional cyst may result in hemodynamic compromise and severe pain. Clinical suspicion, laboratory analysis, ultrasonography, and CT can all be used to determine if a condition requiring emergent management exists.

Pain management is one of the most important cornerstones in patient care. Treating pain is humane, safe, and aids in patient evaluation. Patients with surgical conditions are easier to evaluate when their pain is at least partially controlled, and short-acting parenteral narcotic analgesics can be used to decrease pain and anxiety and to facilitate abdominal examination.[1,26] Consensus should be reached between emergency services and gynecologic and surgical consultants regarding the necessity of acute pain management.

For patients who are unlikely to have surgical conditions, many other analgesics may be used in the treatment of pain. Nonsteroidal anti-inflammatory drugs (NSAIDs) are typically very helpful with visceral pain and pain associated with inflammation, but should be avoided in the elderly, the diabetic, those with renal dysfunction, and those taking angiotensin-converting enzyme (ACE) inhibitors.

Repeat Evaluation

Very often the etiology of abdominal and pelvic pain will not be clear on initial evaluation. Progression or resolution of pathology can dramatically change the examination findings. Serial examinations over 6 to 12 h can be instrumental in the ultimate diagnosis of abdominal pain.

Disposition

Patients with a diagnosis that requires surgical or medical intervention obviously need admission. Patients with severe pain unable to be controlled with oral medications must be admitted for pain control and further diagnostic evaluation. Patients with persistent volume depletion or vomiting unresponsive to the administration of antiemetics and fluids must also be admitted. With thorough history, physical examination, and laboratory and radiologic evaluation, along with a period of observation, a diagnosis can usually be established for most women with acute pelvic pain. In some, the cause of pain will not be established, and in others the initial diagnosis may be incorrect. For this reason, patients not being admitted to the hospital must have follow-up arranged in 12 to 24 h, and the discharge instructions should include clear signs or symptoms that require immediate return to the emergency department.

SPECIFIC DIAGNOSES IN NONPREGNANT ADOLESCENTS AND ADULTS

Functional Ovarian Cysts

Rupture, hemorrhage, torsion, or infection of an ovarian cyst results in the typical presentation of sudden unilateral pelvic pain. Pain may be preceded by exercise, intercourse, or trauma. Tenderness may be elicited on the side of the cyst, and peritoneal signs may be present if the cyst has ruptured or is causing peritoneal inflammation. Hemorrhage may be significant. A patient may or may not give a history of past ovarian cysts. Ultrasonography aids in the diagnosis and helps quantitate blood loss in the acutely ill patient. As patients with cyst pain may present very similarly to patients with an ectopic pregnancy, rapid determination of pregnancy status is critical. Ovarian cysts that are less than 8 cm, unilocular, and unilateral are generally observed. The natural history of functional cysts is generally spontaneous resolution within two cycles, with or without hormone administration. Multiloculated, solid, or large cysts (>5 cm) should be considered ovarian endometriomas, dermoid cysts, or potentially neoplastic until proven otherwise.[22,27] Because of the lack of sensitivity and specificity of the pelvic examination, women with acute abdominal pain and a negative pregnancy test should have ultrasonography to confirm the diagnosis of a functional ovarian cyst. Whether this is accomplished in the ED or during outpatient gynecology follow-up depends upon a number of factors, including the degree of patient discomfort, the physician's comfort with the diagnostic pretest probability of a functional cyst, and the emergency availability of high-quality pelvic ultrasonography.

Adnexal Torsion

Adnexal torsion is a surgical emergency, both for relief of pain and to preserve ovarian function. Ischemia results from twisting of the vascular pedicle. Patients can either present with sudden onset of severe, unilateral pelvic pain or present with dull, aching pain with acute and sharp exacerbations if the torsion is intermittent. Patients with ovarian masses (cysts or tumors) are at increased risk for torsion, as are patients with pelvic adhesions. The onset of pain may occur after trauma, intercourse, or exercise. Tenderness may be elicited on the side of the twisted adnexa with rebound and guarding. Ultrasound with Doppler flow evaluation is used for diagnosis. Early gynecologic consultation and preparation for surgery are important for adnexal salvage. In a 15-year retrospective chart review of ovarian torsion, only 25 percent of patients had a history of an ovarian cyst, pain characteristics were variable, and objective findings on pelvic examination were uncommon.[28] These features confirm the difficulty in making the diagnosis.

Pelvic Inflammatory Disease

PID is discussed in detail in Chap. 109.

Endometriosis

The true incidence of endometriosis is unknown, but it is estimated that 15 percent of females have some degree of the disease. It is second only to dysmenorrhea as the etiology for cyclic pain in females of reproductive age. Patients typically present in the third decade with pelvic pain related to menses. Endometrial glands and stroma are typically located on the ovaries and pelvic peritoneum, but may be located in sites distant to the pelvis. As the disease progresses and forms pelvic adhesions, a chronic, constant pain syndrome may develop. There are many theories for the development of endometriosis. The most accepted at this point is retrograde menstruation with seeding of endometrial glands to distant sites. Other theories include lymphatic and hematogenous spread.

Primary diagnosis is rarely if ever established during an ED visit. Physical examination may be completely normal or demonstrate pelvic tenderness, ovarian tenderness, or enlargement, but typically does not narrow the differential diagnosis. Ultrasound may reveal endometriomas (endometriosis within the ovarian capsule, also known as chocolate cysts), but is not diagnostic. Diagnosis is confirmed by direct visualization during laparoscopy. Various hormonal therapies may be initiated, with relief of pain for certain patients. Pregnancy can lead to remission and sometimes cure.

Adenomyosis

Adenomyosis occurs when the endometrial glands and stroma extend into the uterine musculature. An adenomyoma occurs when the adenomyosis is confined to one portion of the myometrium. Patients typically present in the third and fourth decades, with secondary dysmenorrhea and menorrhagia. Physical examination may reveal a symmetrically enlarged uterus or a fibroid-like mass. Diagnosis often requires endometrial biopsy to rule out endometrial cancer as an etiology for menorrhagia. No specific ED intervention is required if this diagnosis is established. Initial treatment includes simple analgesics and hormonal therapies, and hysterectomy may be ultimately necessary in refractory cases.

Leiomyomas

Uterine leiomyomas (fibroids) are the most common pelvic tumor and the most common indication for major surgery in women. Fibroids become more common by the age of 40, and there is both an increased incidence and increased rate of growth in black women. The etiology is unclear, but current theories include proliferation of smooth muscle or connective tissue cells. The cells are estrogen-dependent and generally enlarge during pregnancy, potentially causing serious pregnancy-related complications. They are rarely seen before menarche, and typically do not develop or enlarge after menopause unless stimulated by exogenous estrogen. There is an increased frequency of endometrial cancer in patients with leiomyomas.

Leiomyomas may be subserosal, intramural, or submucosal. Both subserosal and submucosal leiomyomas may be pedunculated. Although they appear discrete in outline, there is no cellular capsule. Very few blood vessels are able to traverse the fibrous "pseudocapsule," making degeneration a common etiology of pain associated with leiomyomas, specifically with the rapid growth that occurs during pregnancy. Severe, acute pain may be experienced with degeneration or with torsion of a pedunculated fibroid.

Patients with leiomyomas are typically asymptomatic, but may present with acute pain, insidious onset of pelvic pain, or with an abdominal mass. Physical examination often reveals pelvic or abdominal masses. With acute degeneration, the patient may have severe localized tenderness, rebound tenderness, guarding, and fever. Ultrasound is used to delineate the leiomyomas and helps exclude other etiologies for pain. No specific ED intervention is required if this diagnosis is established. Treatment involves analgesia and occasionally hormonal therapies. Myomectomy and hysterectomy are indicated in those whose symptoms are refractory to conservative management.

REFERENCES

1. American College of Emergency Physicians: Clinical policy: Critical issues for the initial evaluation and management of patients presenting with a chief complaint of nontraumatic acute abdominal pain. *Ann Emerg Med* 36:406, 2000.
2. Ramosa EA, Sacchetti AD, Nepp M: Reliability of patient history in determining the possibility of pregnancy. *Ann Emerg Med* 18:48, 1989.
3. McCormack WM: Pelvic inflammatory disease. *New Engl J Med* 330:115, 1994.
4. Dixon JM, Elton RA, Rainey JB, et al: Rectal examination in patients with pain in the right lower quadrant of the abdomen. *BMJ* 302:386, 1991.
5. Close R, Sachs C, Dyne P: Reliability of bimanual pelvic examinations performed in emergency departments. *West J Med* 175:240, 2001.
6. Padilla L, Radosevich DM, Milad MP: Accuracy of the pelvic examination in detecting adnexal masses. *Obstet Gynecol* 96:593, 2000.
7. Carter J, Fowler J, Carson L: How accurate is the pelvic examination as compared to transvaginal sonography? *J Reprod Med* 39:32, 1994.
8. Andolf E, Jorgensen C: Prospective comparison of clinical ultrasound and operative examination of the female pelvis. *J Ultrasound Med* 7:617, 1988.
9. Burstin HR, Conn A, Setnik G, et al: Benchmarking and quality improvement: The Harvard Emergency Department Quality Study. *Am J Med* 107:437, 1999.

10. Lipscomb GH, Spellman JR, Ling FW: The effect of same-day pregnancy testing on the incidence of luteal phase pregnancy. *Obstet Gynecol* 82:411, 1993.

11. Sellors J, Mahony J, Goldsmith C, et al: Accuracy of clinical findings and laparoscopy in pelvic inflammatory disease. *Am J Obstet Gynecol* 164:113, 1991.

12. Luch JS: Utility of hematuria testing on patients with suspected renal colic: Correlation with unenhanced helical CT results. *Urology* 59:839, 2002.

13. Bove P, Kaplan D, Dalrymple N, et al: Reexamining the value of hematuria testing in patients with acute flank pain. *J Urol* 162:165, 1999.

14. Lammers RL, Gibson S, Kovacs D, et al: Comparison of test characteristics of urine dipstick and urinalysis at various test cutoff points. *Ann Emerg Med* 38:505, 2001.

15. Mehta SD, Rothman RE, Kelen GD, et al: Unsuspected gonorrhea and chlamydia in patients of an urban adult emergency department: A critical population for STD control intervention. *Sex Transm Dis* 28:33, 2001.

16. Oh MK, Smith KR, O'Cain M, et al: Urine-based screening of adolescents in detention to guide treatment for gonococcal and chlamydial infections. Translating research into intervention. *Arch Pediatr Adolesc Med* 152:53, 1998.

17. Hook EW 3rd, Smith K, Mullen C, et al: Diagnosis of genitourinary *Chlamydia trachomatis* infections by using the ligase chain reaction on patient-obtained vaginal swabs. *J Clin Microbiol* 35:2133, 1997.

18. Hook EW 3rd, Ching SF, Stephens J, et al: Diagnosis of *Neisseria gonorrhoeae* infections by using the ligase chain reaction on patient-obtained vaginal swabs. *J Clin Microbiol* 35:2129, 1997.

19. Embling ML, Monroe KW, Oh MK, et al: Opportunistic urine ligase chain reaction screening for sexually transmitted diseases in adolescents seeking care in an urban emergency department. *Ann Emerg Med* 36:28, 2000.

20. Oh MK, Richey CM, Pate MS, et al: High prevalence of *Chlamydia trachomatis* infections in adolescent females not having pelvic examinations: Utility of PCR-based urine screening in urban adolescent clinic setting. *J Adolesc Health* 21:80, 1997.

21. Cacciatore B, Leminen A, Ingman-Friberg S: Transvaginal sonographic findings in ambulatory patients with suspected pelvic inflammatory disease. *Obstet Gynecol* 80:912, 1992.

22. Jermy K, Luise C, Bourne T: The characterization of common ovarian cysts in premenopausal women. *Ultrasound Obstet Gynecol* 17:140, 2001.

23. Mikkelsen AL, Felding C: Laparoscopy and ultrasound examination in women with acute pelvic pain. *Gynecol Obstet Invest* 30:162, 1990.

24. Rao PM, Feltmate CM, Rhea JT, et al: Helical computed tomography in differentiating appendicitis and acute gynecologic conditions. *Obstet Gynecol* 93:417, 1999.

25. Porpora MG, Gomel V: The role of laparoscopy in the management of pelvic pain in women of reproductive age. *Fertil Steril* 70:592, 1998.

26. Brewster GS, Herbert ME, Hoffman JR: Medical myth: Analgesia should not be given to patients with an acute abdomen because it obscures the diagnosis. *West J Med* 172:209, 2000.

27. MacKenna A, Fabres C, Alam V, et al: Clinical management of functional ovarian cysts: A prospective and randomized study. *Hum Reprod* 15:2567, 2000.

28. Houry D, Abbott JT: Ovarian torsion: A fifteen-year review. *Ann Emerg Med* 38:156, 2001.

ECTOPIC PREGNANCY
Richard S. Krause
David M. Janicke

Ectopic pregnancy (EP) occurs when a conceptus is implanted outside of the uterine cavity. EP is the leading cause of first-trimester pregnancy-related maternal death in the United States. Today, earlier diagnosis and hence decreased morbidity and mortality have been made possible by transvaginal sonography and improved sensitivity of serum pregnancy markers. As a result more patients may be eligible for conservative medical and surgical therapies.

EPIDEMIOLOGY

The incidence of EP increased from 4.5 per 1000 reported pregnancies (0.45 percent) in 1970 to 19.7 per 1000 reported pregnancies (nearly

2 percent) in 1992, the last year for official reporting in the United States.[1] Reported pregnancies include live births, legally induced abortions, and ectopic pregnancies. An overestimation of the incidence of EP is possible, since the denominator, reported pregnancies, could be biased by lack of reporting of illegally terminated pregnancies or undetected spontaneous abortions. Some possible reasons postulated for the increased incidence of EP include the increased incidence of sexually transmitted tubal infections, unsuccessful tubal sterilizations, assisted reproductive techniques, previous pelvic surgery, and more sensitive and earlier diagnostic techniques.

The case-fatality rate per 10,000 ectopic pregnancies decreased from 35.5 in 1970 to 8.8 in 1980 to 3.8 in 1989. This trend was observed in both white and nonwhite women. However, nonwhite women overall had a 3.4 times greater risk of death than white women. Teenagers were the age group with the highest mortality rate. The observed decreased mortality is attributed largely to improved diagnostics and also a heightened awareness among medical personnel. However, EP remains the leading cause of maternal death in the first trimester of pregnancy and is the second leading cause of maternal mortality overall.[1]

PATHOPHYSIOLOGY

Fertilization of the oocyte usually occurs in the ampullary segment of the fallopian tube. In normal pregnancy, after fertilization, the zygote passes along the fallopian tube and implants into the endometrium of the uterus. An EP occurs when the zygote implants in any location other than the uterus. The vast majority of ectopic pregnancies occur in the fallopian tube. Extratubal sites include the abdominal cavity, cervix, and ovary. Abdominal ectopic pregnancies most commonly derive from early rupture or abortion of a tubal pregnancy, with subsequent reimplantation in the peritoneal cavity.

A normal placenta is uncommon in ectopic pregnancies, possibly accounting for the much higher incidence of a blighted ovum in EP. Tubal abortion occurs when the vascular supply to the placenta is disrupted, with bleeding into the fallopian tube and hematoma formation. Intermittent distention of the fallopian tube with blood can occur with leakage of blood from the fimbriated end of the fallopian tube into the peritoneal cavity. The aborting EP and associated hematoma can be completely or partially extruded out of the end of the fallopian tube or through a rupture site in the tubal wall. Tubal rupture is usually spontaneous; however, in anecdotal accounts, precipitating factors include trauma associated with coitus or a bimanual examination.

Meta-analysis of risk factors for ectopic pregnancy indicates that conditions causing damage to the fallopian tube pose the highest risk for subsequent EP.[2] Major risk factors are shown in Table 103-1. When pregnancy occurs in a patient with prior tubal surgery for sterilization it should be assumed to be an EP until proven otherwise.

CLINICAL FEATURES

History

The classic triad of symptoms in EP is abdominal pain with vaginal bleeding or spotting in a woman with amenorrhea. The positive predictive value of this triad is low, as it is more commonly seen in threatened

TABLE 103-1   Major Risk Factors for Ectopic Pregnancy

Pelvic inflammatory disease
History of tubal surgery
Use of intrauterine device
In-utero exposure to diethylstilbestrol
Assisted reproduction techniques
Previous ectopic pregnancy

or spontaneous abortion than in EP, and may occur due to other causes in nonpregnant women. Many other presentations occur, and range from sudden abdominal pain with life-threatening hypovolemic shock to an asymptomatic EP discovered incidentally on ultrasound exam. To achieve the goal of early diagnosis in as many cases as possible, **EP should be considered in all women of childbearing age who present with abdominal or pelvic complaints or with unexplained signs or symptoms of hypovolemia.**

Identified risk factors for EP are often absent (see Table 103-1), and are useful only for raising clinical suspicion.

Abdominal pain or discomfort is the most common symptom of EP, and is reported in 90 percent of EP patients.[3] Pain is due to tubal distention or rupture. The classic pain of rupture is lateralized, sudden, sharp, and severe. However, shoulder pain secondary to diaphragmatic irritation from a ruptured EP can also occur. Any lateral or bilateral abdominal discomfort or tenderness in a woman of childbearing age requires consideration of EP.

The menstrual history is often, but not always, abnormal. The classic sign if amenorrhea from 4 to 12 weeks after the last normal period, reported in 70 percent of EP cases.[3] No missed menses are reported in 15 percent of EP cases.[3] Vaginal bleeding is reported in 50 to 80 percent of EP.[3] While bleeding is often scant, heavy bleeding does not exclude an EP. The differential diagnosis of vaginal bleeding in early pregnancy includes EP; threatened, inevitable, missed, or incomplete abortion; implantation bleeding; cervicitis; cervical conditions such as polyp or ectropion; bleeding from the urinary or gastrointestinal tracts; or cervical carcinoma.

Typical early pregnancy symptoms may occur and may not differ from symptoms of previous normal intrauterine pregnancies.[3]

Physical Examination

The physical examination in EP is highly variable and EP is difficult to diagnose or exclude based upon physical examination. In cases of ruptured EP, patients may present in shock, with peritoneal signs and an adnexal mass and tenderness. Relative bradycardia may occur as a consequence of vagal stimulation. There is poor correlation between the volume of hemoperitoneum and vital signs in ruptured EP.[4] In cases of rupture without hemodynamically significant bleeding, less prominent peritonitis without significant alteration of vital signs is expected. Fever is rare.

In the more common situation of an unruptured EP, the vital signs are likely to be normal. If an adnexal mass or fullness with tenderness is detected, it may be due to EP or to a corpus luteum cyst. Cervical motion tenderness may be seen and blood is often present in the vaginal vault. The cervix may have a blue coloration, as in a normal pregnancy. Uterine size for estimated gestational age, is most often normal. Pelvic examination may be completely normal in cases of ectopic pregnancy. Patients with unruptured EP compared to those with normal intrauterine pregnancies are expected to have similar clinical characteristics. A study which attempted to develop a clinical prediction model for EP reported that only the rare findings of Doppler fetal heart tones or tissue extruding from the cervical os were reliable signs for excluding EP.[5]

DIAGNOSIS

The differential diagnosis for women of childbearing potential who present with abdominal or pelvic symptoms or abnormal vaginal bleeding is broad (Table 103-2). However, once pregnancy is established, the differential narrows and no combination of signs or symptoms has sufficient negative predictive value to rule out ectopic pregnancy. Pregnancy testing is therefore mandatory. If pregnancy is detected, EP remains in the differential diagnosis until it can be either confirmed or excluded with conviction.

TABLE 103-2 Differential Diagnosis of Ectopic Pregnancy

All Patients (Pregnancy Not Established)	Pregnant Patients
Appendicitis	Normal (intrauterine pregnancy)
Inflammatory bowel disease	Threatened abortion
Ovarian pathology Cyst Torsion	Inevitable abortion
Pelvic inflammatory disease	Molar pregnancy
Endometriosis	Heterotopic pregnancy*
Sexual assault/trauma	Implantation bleeding
Urinary tract infection	Corpus luteum cyst
Ureteral colic	

*Heterotopic pregnancy = combined IUP and EP.

Pregnancy Testing

The diagnosis of pregnancy is central to the diagnosis of possible EP. Pregnancy tests currently in use rely on the detection of the β subunit of human chorionic gonadotropin (βhCG) in the urine or serum. Human chorionic gonadotropin (hCG) is a hormone produced by the trophoblast. Intact hCG consists of the α and β subunits. Tests based on detection of the intact molecule or the α subunit can cross-react on immunologic assays with hormones found in the nonpregnant individual and are thus less specific then tests for the βhCG subunit.

Human chorionic gonadotropin preparations are currently standardized in relation to the International Reference Preparation (IRP). Other standard preparations are not equivalent. A preparation often referred to in earlier literature is the Second International Standard (Second IS). The IRP is roughly equal to 1.7 times the Second IS. To avoid confusion when interpreting the literature, attention must be paid to the standard used. In this chapter, hCG and βhCG concentrations are in reference to the IRP unless otherwise noted.

Very early in either an intrauterine pregnancy (IUP) or an EP, detectable amounts of βhCG are released into the serum and filtered into the urine. The concentration of βhCG is fairly closely correlated in the urine and serum, with urinary concentration also depending upon urine specific gravity. Qualitative urine and serum tests for pregnancy usually use the enzyme-linked immunosorbent assay (ELISA) methodology. In the laboratory setting, ELISA tests can detect βhCG at concentrations below 1 mIU/mL.

Qualitative tests in clinical use are typically reported as "positive" when the βhCG concentration is ≥20 mIU/mL in urine and ≥10 mIU/mL in serum. A positive qualitative test therefore implies that βhCG is present in at least this concentration. At this level of detection, the false-negative rate for detection of pregnancy will not be more than 1 percent for urine and 0.5 percent or less for serum. In clinical use, the performance of urine qualitative testing has been found to be from 95 to 100 percent sensitive and specific as compared with serum tests.

Urine tests can be performed rapidly at the bedside, and kits from some manufacturers may be used for either urine or serum. A bedside test for urine is therefore the best first test for pregnancy when EP is suspected. **Dilute urine may cause a false-negative urine pregnancy test,** particularly early in pregnancy when βhCG levels are low (<50 mIU/mL).

When a bedside urine test is negative and EP is still being considered, a quantitative serum test should be performed. The sensitivity of quantitative serum testing for the diagnosis of pregnancy is virtually 100 percent when an assay capable of detecting ≥5 mIU/mL of βhCG is used.[6]

Laboratory Tests and Ectopic Pregnancy

The definitive diagnosis of EP is made either by ultrasound (US), direct visualization via the laparoscope, or at surgery. No single diagnostic test or combination of laboratory tests are currently considered to have sufficient negative predictive or positive predictive value to completely exclude EP or to definitively establish the diagnosis.

Differences in the dynamics of βhCG production in normal and pathologic pregnancy are useful in the diagnosis of EP. Early in normal pregnancy, βhCG levels rise rapidly. βhCG levels decline in non-viable pregnancies and in successfully treated EP. Absolute levels of βhCG tend to be lower in pathologic pregnancies than in IUP, but there is much overlap. Owing to the variability in absolute levels and the overlap between normal and pathologic pregnancies, **no single bhCG level can reliably distinguish between a normal and a pathologic pregnancy.** *Doubling time* refers to the time needed for βhCG concentration in the serum to double. In normal pregnancy, serum levels of βhCG increase by at least 66 percent every 48 h in 85 percent of patients. Absolute levels of βhCG are lower and doubling times longer in EP and other abnormal pregnancies. This and many other observations has lead to the widely used rule of thumb stating that the serum concentration of βhCG approximately doubles every 2 days early in a normal pregnancy, and that longer doubling times indicate pathologic pregnancy. Varying degrees of sensitivity (36 to 75 percent) and specificity (63 to 93 percent) are obtained using different criteria for evaluating the rate of increase of βhCG levels. A serum βhCG that fails to double in 48 h is thus suggestive but not diagnostic of an EP or an abnormal IUP.

Even in EP, approximately 13 percent of patients will have an increase in serum βhCG of at least 66 percent in 2 days. In stable patients serial measurements of βhCG are therefore used to either heighten or lower the suspicion for EP, but are not diagnostic.[7] The American College of Emergency Physicians does recommend that a repeat serum βhCG measurement made at least 2 days after the initial presentation is useful in characterizing the risk of ectopic pregnancy and the probability of a viable IUP (Table 103-3).[8]

Progesterone (P) is a steroid hormone secreted by the ovaries, adrenal glands, and placenta during pregnancy. During the first 8 to 10 weeks of pregnancy, ovarian production of P predominates and serum levels remain relatively constant. After the tenth week of pregnancy, placental production increases and serum levels rise. Absolute levels of P are lower in pathologic pregnancies and fall when a pregnancy fails. This observation has led multiple authors to propose various P levels as a diagnostic aid in differentiating an early normal from a pathologic pregnancy. Most pathologic pregnancies have P levels ≤10 ng/mL. For P ≤5 ng/mL, nearly 100 percent of pregnancies will be pathologic; there are no normal pregnancies reported with P ≤2.5 ng/mL. Progesterone levels >25 ng/mL have 97 percent sensitivity for viable IUP. In a recent study of patients with P ≤5.0 ng/mL, an empty uterus or nonspecific fluid collection on ultrasound was found to be highly predictive of abnormal IUP or EP. None of 82 patients with an empty uterus and 1 of 29 with nonspecific fluid had a normal IUP.[9]

There is considerable overlap between P levels in normal and pathologic pregnancy. Very low values for serum P thus should increase the clinical suspicion for EP or abnormal IUP, but as with βhCG levels, no value is diagnostic or can completely exclude or definitively diagnose EP. Certain authors strongly advocate protocols using serum P levels instead of or as an adjunct to quantitative βhCG levels.

However, P levels may not be routinely available on an urgent basis and, as noted, many patients have intermediate values, thus limiting the usefulness of the test. Consequently, the role of serum progesterone assays is currently unclear and it is undergoing further evolution and evaluation.

Numerous other serum markers for the diagnosis of EP have been investigated. These include secretory endometrial protein, estradiol, the pregnancy-associated proteins A to D, and others, as well as routine laboratory tests such as amylase, creatine kinase, erythrocyte sedimentation rate, and others. None have been accepted as equal or superior to βhCG measurements at this time.

TABLE 103-3 Summary of ACEP Clinical Policy Regarding Evaluation and Management of Patients in Early Pregnancy

Clinical Issue	Recommendation	Level of Recommendation*
Use of TVU to detect IUP when serum βhCG <1000 mIU/mL	Consider	Level C
Use of TVU to detect EP when serum βhCG <1000 mIU/mL	Consider	Level C
Role of serial quantitative βhCG to diagnose or exclude EP	Obtain after initial presentation; considered useful in characterizing risk of EP and probability of viable IUP	Level B
Serum βhCG level by which absence of IUP by TVU implies EP	Follow-up patients with serum βhCG >2000 mIU/mL with nondiagnostic TVU; increased likelihood of EP	Level B
Methotrexate in EP	Single dose treatment failure can occur in up to 36%; GI symptoms should not be attributed to drug side effect before treatment failure is excluded	Level C
Anti-Rh₀ (D) immune globulin for EP	50 μg Rhogam for all Rh(−) women in loss of established first-trimester pregnancy	Level B

*Level A: reflects high degree of clinical certainty. Level B: reflects moderate clinical certainty. Level C: reflects preliminary or conflicting evidence or based on consensus.
Abbreviations: EP = Ectopic pregnancy; IUP = intrauterine pregnancy; TVU = transvaginal ultrasound.
Source: American College of Emergency Physicians.[8]

Sonography and Ectopic Pregnancy

Sonography plays an essential role in the diagnosis of EP. The primary goal of sonography in suspected EP is to determine if an IUP is present. Sonographic findings may also be useful in planning therapy when an EP is discovered. Noninvasive therapies are often reserved for EPs in which no cardiac activity is seen or those in which the mass is less than a specified size, though this area is undergoing rapid change. In addition, sonography provides information regarding fetal age and viability when an IUP is present.

It has previously been assumed that if an IUP exists, the diagnosis of EP has been excluded. This assumption is based on the historical incidence of heterotopic pregnancy (combined IUP and EP), reported to occur once per 30,000 pregnancies. This is no longer a completely safe assumption, with heterotopic pregnancy now occurring in up to 1 in 3000 pregnancies in the general population. In vitro fertilization and other efforts to enhance fertility with the use of ovulation-inducing drugs have resulted in a higher incidence of heterotopic pregnancy. A recent study of 725 in vitro fertilization pregnancies found 4 percent EP with 2 of 29 heterotopic gestations.[10] Heterotopic pregnancy should be considered even when sonography demonstrates an IUP in the assisted reproduction population. For other patients, demonstrating an IUP still provides a high degree of confidence in ruling out EP. This confidence should be somewhat tempered when a patient has risk factors for EP.

Advances in sonographic imaging include improved portability, decreased cost, and improved image quality of newer machines. Use of transvaginal (TV) scanning allows earlier detection of an IUP or an EP. These advances have contributed to increasing use of real-time, bedside sonography in the ED performed by emergency physicians. ED sonography has the further advantage of allowing a potentially unstable patient to remain under continuous observation in the ED. Bedside ED sonography in the first trimester of pregnancy has been shown to be accurate and to contribute to earlier diagnosis and treatment of EP. However, sonography remains an operator-dependent procedure and there is limited validation in the community setting of the positive results obtained in academic teaching hospitals. Therefore the limitations of the procedure, equipment, and operator experience must be kept in mind.[11,12]

The sequencing of transabdominal (TA) versus TV sonography is situation and operator dependent. Usually, TA scanning is performed first. Among other differences, TA scanning is less invasive and offers a wider field of view and easier orientation to the pelvic organs. A full bladder is required for an appropriate acoustic window. When TA sonography is not diagnostic, TV scanning should be performed. A full bladder is not required. The shallower depth of field and higher frequencies made possible by the lack of interposed abdominal fat allows better visualization of small structures such as early pregnancies. Orientation to the pelvic organs is more difficult with TV scanning than with TA. There are reports of negative TV but positive TA sonography in cases of EP, so both studies should be performed if the study performed first is not diagnostic.

When sonography reveals an unequivocal IUP and no other abnormalities, EP is effectively excluded unless the patient is at high risk for heterotopic pregnancy. An embryo with cardiac activity seen within the uterine cavity is referred to as a viable IUP. When an embryo without cardiac activity is visualized within the uterus, the diagnosis of fetal demise can be entertained, provided that the crown-rump length is at least 5 mm. Sonographic findings related to age of gestation are discussed in Chap. 113. Briefly, TV scanning can usually visualize the early sonographic signs of pregnancy, the gestational sac, yolk sac, and fetal pole at 4.5, 5.5, and 6 weeks respectively (see Figures 113–13 through 113–16). Visualization by TA can be done approximately 1 week later.

No further diagnostic testing is needed when sonographic findings confirm or are highly suggestive of EP. An empty uterus with embryonic cardiac activity visualized outside the uterus is diagnostic of EP. This is seen in less than 10 percent of EPs using TA scanning, but in up to 25 percent of cases when the TV approach is used. When a pelvic mass or free pelvic fluid is seen in conjunction with an empty uterus, EP is considered highly likely. The combination of an echogenic adnexal mass with free fluid in the setting of an empty uterus confers a risk of EP near 100 percent, while a large amount of free fluid alone has a 86 percent risk and a mass alone a 70 percent risk (Table 103-4). In addition to a living extrauterine pregnancy, an extrauterine gestational sac is highly predictive of EP. Any adnexal mass (other than a simple cyst) seen with US also has high positive predictive value for the diagnosis of EP.[13,14] It has also been suggested that increased

thickness of the endometrial stripe is predictive of EP when no other diagnostic findings are noted on sonography. However, the wide overlap between endometrial stripe thickness in normal and EP limits the usefulness of this observation.[15]

If sonography fails to reveal a definite IUP or fails to show findings strongly suggestive or diagnostic of an EP, the test should be considered indeterminate and interpreted in light of quantitative serum βhCG levels. The concept of the "discriminatory zone" was developed by Kadar and colleagues to relate βhCG levels and sonography findings in a clinically useful way.[16] The discriminatory zone is the level of βhCG at which findings of an IUP are expected on sonography. If the βhCG level is higher than the discriminatory zone and the uterus is empty, this is interpreted as suggestive of an EP. An empty uterus with a βhCG level below the discriminatory zone or interpreted as indeterminate, neither confirms nor negates the diagnosis of EP. The actual level of βhCG representing the discriminatory zone is operator and technique dependent. With TV scanning, the discriminatory zone is often considered to be 1500 mIU/mL, or even lower. For TA scanning, an IUP should be detectable when the βhCG level reaches about 6000 mIU/mL. Clinicians should understand this concept and collaborate closely with imaging specialists in equivocal cases to avoid confusion. **When EP is suspected, sonography should be performed even in patients with low βhCG levels,** as EP can occur even at very low (<500 mIU/mL) βhCG levels. Cacciatore and colleagues identified IUP with 100 percent accuracy in patients with βhCG >1000 mIU/mL using TV sonography. Patients with IUP and even lower βhCG levels are often identified.[17]

Diagnostic algorithms using the concept of the discriminatory zone have been proposed and validated. A study of 1263 consecutive ED patients with clinically suspected EP by Braffman and associates found 205 cases of EP, of whom 81.5 percent were hemodynamically stable. In stable patients, they correctly diagnosed 49.1 percent of EP and 96 percent of IUP on the initial visit with a combination of βhCG levels and TV sonography. A level of 1500 mIU/mL was used as the discriminatory zone. If the βhCG level was >1500 mIU/mL and the uterus was empty, dilation and curettage (D&C) or laparoscopy was used to diagnose EP. (A D&C was performed on patients not wishing to continue the pregnancy.) If chorionic villi were present, IUP was considered confirmed. When the βhCG level was <1500 mIU/mL and the uterus was empty, serial βhCG measurements were repeated every 2 days. If βhCG failed to increase by at least 66 percent in a 2-day period, an operative procedure was used to diagnose possible EP. TV sonography was repeated if the βhCG level was >1500 mIU/mL. With use of this protocol, 100 percent of EPs were identified without any complications (sensitivity = 100 percent).[18] Other reports using similar protocols confirm these results.

Magnetic resonance imaging (MRI) has also been investigated for the early diagnosis of EP. Small studies have shown high sensitivity and specificity. But cost, availability, and the time to perform the study make this of only theoretical interest at the present time.

Invasive Diagnostic Techniques

Culdocentesis has been largely supplanted by tests for βhCG in combination with sonography, but it may have use when sonography is unavailable. Laparoscopy may be both diagnostic and therapeutic. D&C may provide a definitive diagnosis of IUP, thus excluding EP except in cases of heterotopic pregnancy.

CULDOCENTESIS   Because of the changes in technology, emergency practitioners have either not been trained in culdocentesis or experience has waned during the better part of the last two decades. This procedure is now rarely performed for the diagnosis of EP, even by experienced gynecologist/obstetrician specialists.

Although culdocentesis is less useful than noninvasive tests for the diagnosis of EP, one indication remains. Culdocentesis may be considered

TABLE 103-4   Ancillary Ultrasound Findings Suggestive of Ectopic Pregnancy in High-Risk Patients

Ancillary Findings	Risk of Ectopic Pregnancy
Small amount of free pelvic fluid	52%
Echogenic adnexal mass	70%
Moderate/large amount of free pelvic fluid	86%
Any mass plus echogenic fluid	97%

for both stable and unstable patients when sonography is unavailable. In this setting, a positive test would facilitate an appropriate, rapid surgical intervention.

Possible results include a dry aspiration, which has no diagnostic value. If clear, nonbloody peritoneal fluid is aspirated, the tap is considered negative. Aspiration of nonclotting blood constitutes a positive tap, considered indicative of an EP. However, there is no consensus regarding the criteria for a positive test. Various authors have proposed volumes between 0.3 mL and 10 mL with hematocrit from 3 to 15 percent. The pathophysiologic basis for culdocentesis is that a ruptured EP will bleed into the pelvic peritoneal cavity. Some 85 to 90 percent of patients with a ruptured EP will have a positive culdocentesis. Surprisingly, up to 70 percent of patients with an unruptured EP will also have a positive result. A basic limitation of the technique is that it is less sensitive in the diagnosis of nonruptured than ruptured EP. Another cause of false-negative results is that in cases of rapid bleeding, intraperitoneal blood may clot due to the lack of sufficient dwell time to produce defibrination. False-positive results occur because of technical errors (entering a vein or other vascular structure with the needle) or a ruptured corpus luteum cyst. Aspiration of purulent material may indicate another diagnosis, such as pelvic inflammatory disease.

LAPAROSCOPY Laparoscopy is primarily useful in patients with suspected EP and a nondiagnostic sonogram. It may provide an earlier diagnosis and a possible route for definitive treatment when compared with serial βhCG measurements and sonography. Laparoscopy is an accurate technique for the diagnosis of EP with low false-negative rates. False-positive rates are somewhat greater, but still considered to be rare. As with other invasive techniques, results will vary with the skill of the operator and the quality of the available equipment. If a laparoscopist is available who is skilled in the diagnosis and laparoscopic treatment of EP, laparoscopy is a viable alternative that may be accomplished rapidly and with low morbidity.

DILATATION AND CURETTAGE Uterine curettage (D&C) provides a method for the definitive diagnosis of an IUP when chorionic villi are obtained from the uterine cavity. EP is thus excluded unless a heterotopic pregnancy is present. The procedure can be performed in an outpatient setting with intravenous sedation. D&C terminates an IUP if present and is thus applicable only when termination of pregnancy is desired or when a nonviable pregnancy has been documented. A progesterone level of ≤5 ng/mL or stable or falling βhCG levels provide good, though not certain, evidence of nonviability. The specimen obtained at D&C is examined for the presence of chorionic villi. This may be done at the bedside by suspending the specimen in saline. Villi float, and absence of material that floats is presumptive evidence of absent villi and thus suggestive of an EP. However, there are false-negative as well as false-positive observations with this technique, thus formal histologic exam is required.

TREATMENT

The traditional treatment of EP has been laparotomy and salpingectomy. Over the last two decades, more conservative surgical and medical approaches have been developed that allow fallopian tube preservation, outpatient treatment, or shorter hospital admissions, and decreased medical expenditures. The treatment of EP can be divided into surgical, medical, and expectant approaches. Most authors would agree that if laparoscopy is needed for diagnosis, a surgical approach is most appropriate. For unruptured EP, the most frequently used surgical approach is laparoscopic salpingostomy; the most frequently used medical approach is systemic methotrexate treatment. For ruptured EP, laparotomy is the treatment of choice in hemodynamically unstable patients, although laparoscopic approaches have been utilized even in patients with large-volume hemoperitoneum.

Surgical Approach

Laparoscopy, as opposed to laparotomy, has emerged as the preferred surgical approach in the treatment of EP in a hemodynamically stable patient. Laparoscopic salpingostomy is preferred over laparoscopic salpingectomy for the treatment of unruptured tubal EP in patients in whom future fertility is desired. Although salpingostomy may be associated with an increased incidence of persistent and recurrent EP, it permits a higher rate of subsequent IUP by allowing preservation of the fallopian tube. Specific indications for laparoscopic salpingostomy include hemodynamic stability, ectopic size ≤5 cm, unruptured or minimally ruptured fallopian tube, appropriate tubal location of the conceptus, and patient desire to preserve reproductive potential.

Laparoscopic salpingostomy is performed by a linear incision over the antimesenteric side of the fallopian tube adjacent to the EP. The products of conception are removed and the tube usually left open to heal by secondary intention.

Currently, laparotomy is reserved for cases that are too difficult for laparoscopic surgery, for hemodynamically unstable patients, and when the operator is inexperienced with operative laparoscopy. A laparotomy for EP may be followed by either salpingectomy or salpingostomy, depending on the clinical circumstances.

To assess for a persistent EP following laparoscopic salpingostomy, a weekly βhCG level is obtained. By the second postoperative week, the βhCG level should be undetectable or less than 20 mIU/mL. Persistent trophoblastic tissue (suspected based on elevated βhCG levels) is most commonly found in the proximal portion of the fallopian tube and may be treated by surgical reoperation, methotrexate treatment, or expectant management.

Medical Treatment

Pharmaceutical agents including methotrexate (MTX), prostaglandins, hyperosmolar glucose, potassium chloride, and mifepristone have been used as systemic agents or for local injection treatment of EP. Expectant management with serial βhCG levels and ultrasound is also a medical option.

MTX is the only drug currently recommended as a medical alternative to surgical treatment of EP. MTX inhibits cell division in rapidly growing tissues such as those in the trophoblast. Different methotrexate regimens have been used, including both systemic intramuscular injections and direct injection into the ectopic gestational sac. Systemic intramuscular administration of MTX is the most commonly used approach, eliminating the need for laparoscopy or ultrasound guidance for local injection therapy. The largest study of systemic MTX to date revealed a success rate of 91.5 percent.[19]

The most common side effects associated with MTX include abdominal pain after treatment (up to 75 percent of patients) followed by flatulence and then stomatitis. Lower abdominal pain lasting up to 12 h is common 3 to 7 days after MTX treatment and is thought to be secondary to MTX-induced tubal abortion or tubal distention due to hematoma formation. The pain is usually self limited and may respond to NSAIDs.

Abdominal pain after MTX treatment can represent a clinical dilemma. It is difficult to differentiate expected pain from therapeutic tubal abortion and pain from rupturing persistent EP. Suggested evaluation of patients presenting with abdominal pain in this time frame following methotrexate administration includes a complete blood count and abdominopelvic US to rule out EP rupture[7] and significant hemoperitoneum, and consideration of other causes of abdominal pain. Such patients may need admission to the hospital for observation. Hemodynamic instability and/or falling hematocrit require consideration for surgical intervention. Prognostic factors associated with a higher failure rate for MTX treatment include larger tubal diameter, higher initial βhCG levels, severe abdominal pain, and fetal cardiac activity.[19]

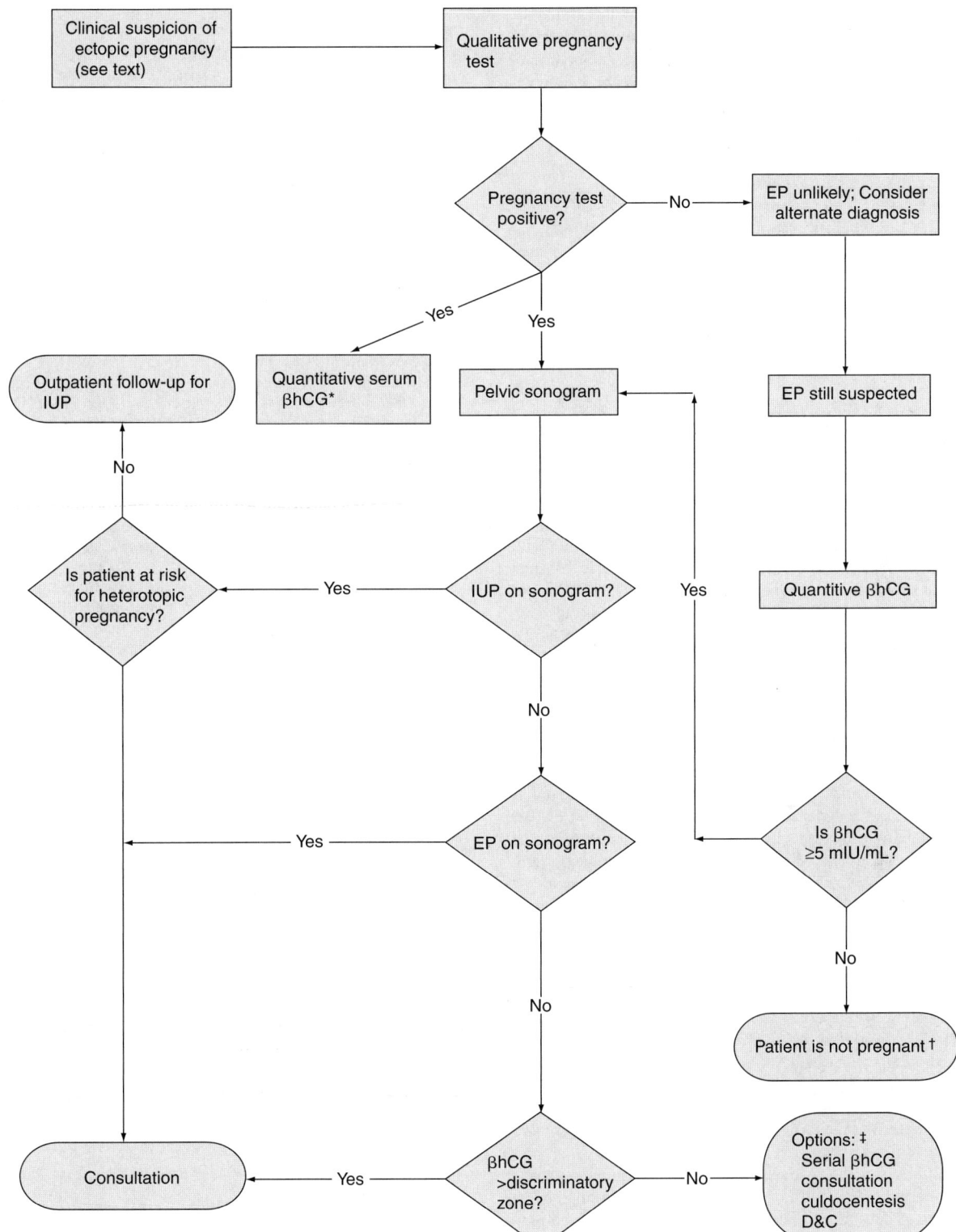

FIG. 103-1. Diagnostic algorithm for suspected ectopic pregnancy *(Courtesy of Richard S. Krause, MD).*

*Quantitative βhCG measurement *prior* to sonography may facilitate rapid patient disposition by saving time.

†There have been extremely rare reports of pregnancy with βhCG <5 mIU/mL.

‡Serial outpatient βhCG measurements are recommended only for stable patients judged to be at low risk for ruptured EP (see text).

MTX administration in properly selected patients with EP may be initiated in the ED, clinic, or OB/GYN office. Treatment initiated in the ED should be in close conjunction with an obstetrician/gynecologist or other physician capable of providing follow-up care. Pelvic examinations after MTX treatment should be kept to a minimum to decrease the risk of tubal rupture. Patient instruction on discharge should include the following points.

1. Treatment failure occurs in up to 36 percent of cases.[20]
2. Elective or emergency surgical treatment may be necessary if medical therapy fails or tubal rupture occurs (~5 percent of cases).
3. Vaginal bleeding, abdominal pain, weakness, dizziness, or syncope following treatment should be evaluated immediately as possible signs of tubal rupture (see Table 103-3).
4. Patients should refrain from sexual intercourse for 14 to 21 days following treatment (until βhCG levels are undetectable) as it may increase the risk of tubal rupture.

Rh Seroconversion and Indications for Anti-D Immunoglobulin

Rh_0 (D) antigen can be detected as early as 5.5 weeks and certainly by 6 weeks of gestation. Alloimmunization can occur with as little as 0.1 mL of fetal blood admixing with the mother's. There is strong evidence in the literature that alloimmunization can occur as a result of ectopic pregnancy. Circulating blood volume of the fetus is less than 5 mL in the first trimester. Accordingly, both the American College of Emergency Physicians (ACEP) and the American College of Obstetricians and Gynecologists recommend treatment of 50 μg of anti-Rh_0 (D) immunoglobulin for Rh-negative women with ectopic pregnancy.

DISPOSITION

When a patient with signs or symptoms suggestive of EP is found to be pregnant, further testing to determine if the pregnancy is intrauterine should be undertaken (Figure 103-1). The nature and timing of additional diagnostic measures depends on the clinical condition of the patient. Unstable patients with suspected EP should receive resuscitation, urgent consultation, and operative intervention. Surgery may be both diagnostic and therapeutic if an EP is found, or may reveal another cause for the patient's condition. When bedside ED sonography is available, it may be valuable even in unstable patients, as it should not interfere with resuscitation, consultation, and rapid transfer to the operating room.

Ideally, all pregnant patients with suspected EP should receive immediate sonography. However, issues of availability during off hours may make this impractical. Stable patients who are judged to be at low risk for EP can be considered for discharge and outpatient follow-up. Such patients should have a quantitative βhCG level obtained to facilitate subsequent management. Culdocentesis remains an option where sonography is unavailable, but currently is used rarely due to limitations of the technique and the unfamiliarity of many emergency physicians with the technique.

Stable patients with βhCG levels above the discriminatory zone and an empty uterus on US, with or without other US findings of an EP, are presumed to have an EP. These patients should receive consultation in the ED.

Management options for stable patients with a βhCG level below the discriminatory zone and indeterminate sonography include consultation in the ED or discharge for follow-up in 2 days for reexamination and repeat βhCG levels. Culdocentesis, D&C, and laparoscopy are also options in this circumstance. Figure 103-1 illustrates a suggested diagnostic approach.

REFERENCES

1. Leads From the Morbidity and Mortality Weekly Report: Ectopic Pregnancy—United States, 1990–1992. *JAMA* 273:533, 1995.
2. Ankum WM, Mol BWJ, Van der Veen F, et al: Risk factors for ectopic pregnancy: A meta-analysis. *Fertil Steril* 65:1093, 1996.
3. Stovall TG, Kellerman AL, Ling FW, et al: Emergency department diagnosis of ectopic pregnancy. *Ann Emerg Med* 19:1098, 1990.
4. Hick JL, Rodgerson JD, Heegard WG, et al: Vital signs fail to correlate with hemoperitoneum from ruptured ectopic pregnancy. *Am J Emerg Med* 19:488, 2001.
5. Buckley RG, King KJ, Disney JD, et al: History and physical exam to estimate the risk of ectopic pregnancy: Validation of a clinical prediction model. *Ann Emerg Med* 34:589, 1999.
6. Kaplan BC, Dart RG, Moskos M, et al: Ectopic pregnancy: Prospective study with improved diagnostic accuracy. *Ann Emerg Med* 28:10, 1996.
7. Dart RG, Mitterando J, Dart LM: Rate of change of serial βhCG values as a predictor of ectopic pregnancy in patients with indeterminate transvaginal ultrasound findings. *Ann Emerg Med* 34:703, 1999.
8. American College of Emergency Physicians: Clinical policy: Critical issues in the initial evaluation and management of patients presenting to the emergency department in early pregnancy. *Ann Emerg Med* 41:123, 2003.
9. Dart R, Ramanujum P, Dart L: Progesterone as a predictor of ectopic pregnancy when the ultrasound is indeterminate. *Am J Emerg Med* 20:575, 2002.
10. Strandell A, Thorburn J, Hamburger L: Risk factors for ectopic pregnancy in assisted reproduction. *Fertil Steril* 71:282, 1999.
11. Burgher SW, Tandy TK, Dawdy MR: Transvaginal ultrasonography by emergency physicians decreases patient time in the emergency department. *Acad Emerg Med* 5:802, 1998.
12. Mateer JR, Aiman EJ, Brown MH, et al: Ultrasonographic examination by emergency physicians of patients at risk for ectopic pregnancy. *Acad Emerg Med* 2:867, 1995.
13. Brown DL, Doubilet PM: Transvaginal sonography for the diagnosis of ectopic pregnancy: Positivity and performance characteristics. *J Ultrasound Med* 13:259, 1994.
14. Aleem FA, DeFazio M, Gintautas J: Endovaginal sonography for the early diagnosis of intrauterine and ectopic pregnancies. *Hum Reprod* 5:755, 1990.
15. Levgur M, Tsai T, Kang K, et al: Endometrial stripe thickness in tubal and intrauterine pregnancies. *Fertil Steril* 74:889, 2000.
16. Kadar N, DeVore G, Romero R: Discriminatory hCG zone: Its use in the sonographic evaluation for ectopic pregnancy. *Obstet Gynecol* 58:156, 1981.
17. Cacciatore B, Stenman U, Ylosato P: Diagnosis of ectopic pregnancy by vaginal ultrasonography in combination with a discriminatory serum hCG level of 1000 IU/L (IRP). *Br J Obstet Gynecol* 97:904, 1990.
18. Braffman BH, Coleman BG, Ramchandani P, et al: Emergency department screening for ectopic pregnancy: A prospective US study. *Radiology* 190:797, 1994.
19. Lipscomb G, Bran D, McCord M, et al: Analysis of 315 ectopic pregnancies treated with single dose methotrexate. *Am J Obstet Gynecol* 178:1354, 1998.
20. Jiminez-Caballo A, Rodriguea-Donoso G: A 6-year clinical trail of methotrexate therapy in the treatment on ectopic pregnancy. *Eur J Obstet Gynecol Reprod Biol* 79:167, 1998.

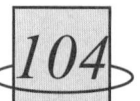

104 NORMAL PREGNANCY
Christina E. Hantsch
Donna L. Seger

Regardless of the chief complaint, the possibility of pregnancy must be considered in every woman of reproductive age who presents to the ED. In one study pregnancy was documented in over 7 percent of women who stated there was no chance they were pregnant and reported an on-time normal last menstrual period.[1] The use of barrier methods (condoms, diaphragms, etc.), contraceptives, or tubal sterilization does not guarantee pregnancy prevention. The failure rates of barrier methods are variable. Although the failure rate with compliant use of oral contraceptives is less than 1 per 100, nearly 30 percent of women who rely solely on oral contraceptives to prevent pregnancy are not consistently compliant.[2] During the first 5 years of therapy with levonorgestrel implants, the annual pregnancy rate is 0.8 per 100. The failure rate of implants increases with time.[3] Tubal sterilization is a more reliable means of pregnancy prevention, with the failure rate depending on the surgical technique. Partial salpingectomy achieves pregnancy prevention with a failure rate of only 0.75 percent.[4]

TERMINOLOGY

Gravidity denotes the total number of pregnancies regardless of duration and outcome. *Parity* denotes the number of pregnancies completed to delivery during the viable period. Parity is not increased for a pregnancy resulting in multiple births or decreased for a stillborn fetus. Notation of obstetric history typically lists the gravidity (G) followed by the appropriate number and then the parity (P) followed by the appropriate number. After the gravidity and parity, there may be a listing of the number of term deliveries, preterm deliveries, abortions, and living children. The latter four numbers are separated by hyphens and listed in parentheses. For example, the obstetric history of a woman during her seventh pregnancy who has had four term deliveries, one preterm delivery, and one abortion and has five living children is abbreviated G7 P5 (4-1-1-5).

The duration of pregnancy is approximately 40 weeks. By convention, gestational age (or menstrual age) is calculated from the first day of the last normal menstrual period. Ovulation normally occurs around day 14 of the menstrual cycle. After ovulation, the ovocyte remains capable of being successfully fertilized for up to 12 h. Fertilization usually takes place in the ampulla of the oviduct. The fertilized ovocyte (zygote) transforms into the morula as it travels toward the uterus. By 6 days after fertilization, it enters the uterine cavity and implants in the endometrium. Weeks 2 through 8 (after fertilization) are the embryonic period. Week 9 is the start of the fetal period.

Pregnancy is typically divided into three trimesters of approximately equal length. The first trimester is from conception to 14 weeks, the second trimester is from 14 to 28 weeks, and the third trimester is from 28 to 42 weeks. A term pregnancy requires completion of at least 37 weeks of gestation.

PHYSIOLOGY

Cardiovascular System

Maternal cardiovascular changes during pregnancy include a 40 to 45 percent increase in circulating blood volume, a 43 percent increase in cardiac output, and a 17 percent increase in resting heart rate.[5] Systemic vascular resistance is 20 percent lower. Blood pressure decreases to a nadir during the second trimester. The diastolic decrement (10–15 mm Hg) is greater than the systolic decrement (5–10 mm Hg). Hemodynamic measurements should be taken with the patient in the left lateral decubitus position because body position has a significant influence on hemodynamic values. The left lateral position increases venous return by relieving the pressure of the uterus on the inferior vena cava. The increase in cardiac output is detectable from the first trimester until after delivery when readings are taken with the patient in this position.[6]

Elevation of the diaphragm displaces the heart superiorly and to the left. This displacement produces a larger cardiac silhouette on chest radiograph and a slight left-axis deviation on the electrocardiogram. A small, benign pericardial effusion also may contribute to the enlarged cardiac silhouette.

Respiratory System

Many women experience dyspnea during pregnancy. Although the respiratory rate is unchanged, this symptom may be the result of a hormone-induced 40 percent increase in tidal volume and the attendant P_{CO_2} decrease (normal value in pregnancy, 30 mm Hg). Functional residual capacity is decreased because of a rise in the level of the diaphragm.[7]

Gastrointestinal System

Pregnancy-induced changes in the gastrointestinal system are due to both progressive displacement of the abdominal viscera and hormone-mediated functional alterations. Gastric reflux commonly occurs as a result of delayed gastric emptying, decreased intestinal motility, and decreased lower esophageal sphincter tone. The size and morphologic characteristics of the liver are not altered by pregnancy, but the presence of placental alkaline phosphatase may increase maternal serum alkaline phosphatase concentration. Bilirubin concentration and aspartate aminotransferase and alanine aminotransferase activities are unaltered. Hepatic enzyme systems are induced during pregnancy. Gallbladder emptying is delayed and less efficient, and pregnancy therefore increases the risk of cholesterol gallstones.

Urinary System

Pregnancy-related renal changes include increases in kidney size, renal blood flow, and glomerular filtration rate (GFR). By the second trimester, the GFR may increase by 50 percent. Consequently, blood urea nitrogen and creatinine levels decrease. Dilatation of ureteral and renal calyces or pelves due to ureteral compression are also seen frequently on imaging studies. These changes are often less pronounced on the left side because the sigmoid colon cushions the left ureter from the pressure of the enlarging uterus.

Hematopoietic System

During pregnancy, circulating blood volume expands by an average of 40 to 45 percent due to an increase in both plasma volume and the number of erythrocytes.[6] Hemoglobin concentration decreases due to dilutional intravascular volume expansion but should not fall below 11 g/dL. Maternal erythropoiesis combined with fetal erythropoiesis produce the high iron requirements of pregnancy. Reticulocyte count is also slightly increased during the second half of pregnancy, the period of marked erythropoiesis. Leukocyte counts during pregnancy range from 5000 to 12,000 cells/μL. Dilutional effects on blood volume also may contribute to the variation in leukocyte counts. Beginning in the second trimester, leukocyte function is usually depressed, and increased susceptibility to infection may occur.[8] Patients with chronic autoimmune conditions may improve clinically. Circulating coagulation factor concentrations and erythrocyte sedimentation rate increase during pregnancy. Platelet count may decrease slightly due to increased consumption. However, thrombocytopenia should prompt further evaluation for a pathologic cause.

Endocrine System

Pregnancy-related hormonal changes and feedback mechanism adjustments are incompletely understood. Characteristic changes in carbohydrate metabolism lead to hyperinsulinemia and fasting hypoglycemia. The altered response to glucose ingestion produces postprandial hyperglycemia and ensures a sustained glucose supply to the fetus. Mineral (especially iron), protein, and fat metabolism are also changed. Thyroid alterations include increased vascularity and mild hyperplasia, but clinically detectable goiter is not a normal finding in pregnancy. To assess thyroid function during pregnancy, free thyroxine and thyroid-stimulating hormone concentrations should be measured because they are not affected by physiologic changes of normal pregnancy.

Uterus

Uterine weight and intrauterine volume increase during pregnancy from 70 to 1100 g and from 10 to 5000 mL, respectively. These changes occur through marked stretching and hypertrophy of existing muscle cells rather than formation of new cells. By 12 weeks of gestational age, the uterus exceeds the capacity of the pelvis and expands into the abdominal cavity. There is a progressive increase in uterine blood flow to approximately 450 to 650 mL/min by term.

Breasts

Many women note breast tenderness and tingling from early in the first trimester. The breasts enlarge and become more nodular. Nipple size and pigmentation increase. Striations similar to those often seen on the abdominal wall may develop on the breasts.

HISTORY AND PHYSICAL EXAMINATION

Obstetric and gynecologic history, including menstrual status and contraceptive use, should be obtained on every woman of reproductive age. Cessation of menses, nausea, vomiting, fatigue, and urinary frequency may be suggestive of pregnancy. The date of the last normal menstrual period aids in determination of gestational age (although it may be misleading if, for example, contraceptive use was discontinued recently). Quickening, the first maternal perception of fetal movement, helps establish gestational age. Primigravida women note fetal movement between 18 and 20 weeks' gestation. With subsequent pregnancies, quickening typically occurs about 2 weeks earlier (i.e., between 16 and 18 weeks' gestation). The patient's history of prenatal care and the course of current and past pregnancies, as well as the essential components of any medical history, should be obtained. Physical examination should include routine assessment of maternal well-being as well as an evaluation of fetal status. Fetal heart tones can be heard with a fetal stethoscope by 16 to 19 weeks' gestation. The normal fetal heart rate ranges from 120 to 160 beats/min. Since the fetus easily changes position, the site on the maternal abdomen where the fetal heart tones are best detected varies. Pulsation of the maternal aorta should be distinguished from the fetal heart tones.

A pelvic examination should be performed whenever pregnancy is part of the differential diagnosis. Appearance of the cervix and the presence of discharge or blood in the vaginal vault should be noted. Wet preparation and culture for *Neisseria gonorrhoeae* and *Chlamydia trachomatis* may be indicated. Bimanual examination determines size and tenderness of the uterus and adnexa.

By the end of the first trimester, the size of the uterus also can be assessed by abdominal examination. At 12 weeks' gestation, the fundus should be palpable at the level of the symphysis pubis. At 16 weeks, the fundus should be midway between the symphysis and the umbilicus; at 20 weeks, it should be at the umbilicus. From 20 to 32 weeks, the height (in centimeters) of the fundus above the symphysis approximates the gestational age for a singleton pregnancy. For an accurate measurement, the pregnant patient should have an empty bladder when fundal height is determined. Later in pregnancy, the presenting part of the fetus also should be determined by palpating the maternal abdomen.

DIAGNOSIS

Standard analytical techniques screen blood or urine for human chorionic gonadotropin (HCG), a glycoprotein produced by the trophoblast after implantation. Since implantation occurs about 1 week after conception, these screening tests are particularly helpful in establishing or excluding early pregnancy. At 4 to 5 weeks' gestation and beyond, definitive diagnosis can be made by sonographic visualization of the embryo or fetus (see Chap. 113). Alternatively, in later stages, detection (by fetal stethoscope or sonogram) of fetal heart activity distinct from maternal heart activity or detection of palpable fetal movement may confirm pregnancy.

Analytical Techniques

HCG is composed of α and β subunits. The HCG α subunit is indistinct from the α subunit of several other glycoproteins, including luteinizing hormone. The β subunit is unique to HCG. Qualitative enzyme-linked immunosorbent assays (ELISAs) that detect β-HCG in urine can be completed in minutes at the patient's bedside. Available commercial tests can detect β-HCG concentrations as low as 10 to 20 mIU/mL. These tests have a false-negative rate of only 1 percent in detecting pregnancy as early as 1 week after conception. However, to achieve this level of sensitivity, the analysis must be performed on a urine specimen that is not dilute. When urine is dilute, a false-negative result may be obtained for women with early pregnancy (serum HCG <50 IU/mL).[9] Serum analysis should be performed in clinical situations where pregnancy is a concern but the urine result is questionable. Quantitative serum values are obtained by ELISA technique and can be completed in 1 to 2 h. There are several international standards for serum β-HCG, and the specific reference range should be appropriate for the standard employed.

A positive result on a pregnancy test, whether qualitative or quantitative, does not confirm a normal intrauterine pregnancy. Ectopic pregnancy, recent spontaneous or induced abortion, and HCG-secreting tumors (e.g., molar pregnancy) also may produce a positive result. A single quantitative β-HCG determination in combination with pelvic ultrasonography may differentiate intrauterine pregnancy from these conditions (see Chap. 113). Serial quantitative serum β-HCG determinations may be useful in some outpatient situations because serum β-HCG levels approximately double (66%) every 1.4 to 2.0 days following implantation in early normal pregnancy. Failure of the HCG concentration to double in this time period suggests an ectopic or a nonviable pregnancy.

Pelvic Ultrasonography

More detailed discussions of ultrasonography and its application can be found in Chap. 113. The earliest definitive sonographic finding in pregnancy is a gestational sac. Using transabdominal technique, the gestational sac can be detected at 5.5 to 6 weeks' gestation. With transvaginal technique, the gestational sac can be detected at 4 to 5 weeks' gestation. Other ultrasound markers of pregnancy and the gestational age at which they may be detected by transvaginal ultrasound include the yolk sac at 5 to 5.5 weeks' gestation, the fetal pole at 5.5 to 6 weeks, and cardiac activity at 6 weeks. Correlation of these markers with specific, quantitative serum β-HCG values varies with the capabilities of the ultrasound equipment and the skill of the ultrasonographer.

SPECIFIC ISSUES IN PREGNANCY

Abdominal Discomfort

Many pregnant women experience abdominal discomfort. The differential diagnosis of abdominal pain varies with the stage of gestation and must include all the possibilities in a nonpregnant patient (see Chap. 102) as well as those unique to pregnancy. Ectopic pregnancy and threatened abortion should be considered when abdominal pain occurs during the first trimester. Premature labor, abruption, and uterine rupture should be considered when abdominal pain occurs during late second and third trimesters.

Vascular congestion of pelvic tissue and round ligament tension may cause lower abdominal discomfort early in pregnancy. Round ligament tension produces sharp pain (bilateral or unilateral) that is often precipitated by movement.

Braxton-Hicks contractions are irregular, palpable contractions that may occur particularly during late pregnancy.

Appendicitis, cholecystitis, and other acute abdominal surgical diseases can complicate pregnancy. The incidence of appendicitis is unchanged during pregnancy, but the diagnosis may be more difficult. Symptoms of appendicitis such as nausea, vomiting, and anorexia may be attributed to the pregnancy; location of abdominal pain caused by the inflamed appendix may be altered due to upward and rightward displacement of the appendix, especially in the third trimester. Physiologic gastrointestinal changes result in an increased risk of cholelithiasis throughout pregnancy. Cholelithiasis may be asymptomatic or cause cholecystitis or pancreatitis.

Syncope

Many women experience palpitations, dizziness, near-syncope, or syncope during pregnancy. The differential diagnosis includes anemia, electrolyte imbalance, dehydration, pulmonary embolism, and arrhythmia, but the etiology of these symptoms is often unclear. The incidence of arrhythmias, especially premature atrial and ventricular beats, is increased in pregnancy. In one study, however, only 10 percent of symptomatic episodes of palpitations, dizziness, near-syncope, or syncope were associated with arrhythmias. These may occur in pregnant patients with or without identifiable heart disease.[10]

Medication Use

Multiple factors, including gestational age and stage of development, dose and duration of exposure, and individual susceptibility, influence the potential effects of drug exposure during pregnancy. Teratogenesis is defined as the structural or functional dysgenesis of fetal organs. Typical manifestations include restricted growth, fetal death, carcinogenesis, and malformations. The fetus is most vulnerable to teratogenic effects at 4 to 12 weeks' gestation, the period of organogenesis. Administration of drugs early during the period of organogenesis, will affect the organs developing then, such as the heart or neural tube. Closer to the end of the classic teratogenic period, the ear and palate are forming and may thus be affected. Before 4 weeks, exposure to a teratogen produces an all-or-none effect, i.e. either the conceptus survives without anomalies, or does not survive at all. If the organism remains viable, organ-specific anomalies do not develop because repair or replacement permits normal development. A similar insult at a later stage may produce organ-specific defects. Thus, drug exposure early in pregnancy may lead to spontaneous abortion. Drug exposure later in pregnancy may cause teratogenesis by altering placental blood flow and/or directly affecting the fetus. Medication use during pregnancy also may cause neonatal central nervous system (CNS) depression, seizures, respiratory depression, kernicterus, or premature closure of the ductus arteriosus. Manifestations depend on the specific medication. Neonatal withdrawal may occur after maternal use of opiates or benzodiazepines during pregnancy. Finally, the adverse effects of fetal exposure to some medications (e.g., tetracyclines, which produce discoloration of teeth and bone, and diethylstilbestrol, which produces female genital tract abnormalities) may not be evident until later in the life of the child.

Pharmaceutical companies do not test drugs in pregnant women to determine potential fetal effects. Much of the available information on teratogenesis is based on animal studies, inadvertent human exposure during unrecognized pregnancies, and case reports or epidemiologic studies of pregnancy outcome after therapeutic drug administration. Manufacturer labeling and drug reference books often contain ambiguous statements concerning use of drugs in pregnancy. The U.S. Food and Drug Administration (FDA) classifies drugs into five risk categories based on available information (Table 104-1). Because of ambiguity and potential inaccuracy within this system, alternative ways of outlining estimated fetal risk for both physicians and the general population are being investigated. Table 104-2 lists common medications generally considered safe on pregnancy.

TABLE 104-1 Food and Drug Administration Categorization of Drug Risk in Pregnancy*

Drug Category	Risk During Pregnancy
A	Controlled studies have failed to demonstrate a fetal risk in the first trimester (and there is no evidence of risk in later trimesters), and the possibility of fetal harm is remote.
B	*Either* animal studies have not demonstrated a fetal risk but there are no controlled human studies, *or* animal studies have demonstrated an adverse effect that was not confirmed in controlled human studies in women in the first trimester (and there is no evidence of risk in later trimesters).
C	*Either* animal studies have revealed adverse effects on the fetus (teratogenic or embryocidal) and there are no controlled studies in humans, *or* no human or animal studies are available. Drugs should only be used if the potential benefit justifies the potential fetal risk.
D	Evidence of human fetal risk exists, but the benefits of use in pregnant women may be acceptable despite the risk.
X	Studies in animals or humans have demonstrated fetal risk, or there is evidence of fetal risk based on human experience. The risk of use in pregnancy clearly outweighs any possible benefit. Drugs are contraindicated for use in women who are or may become pregnant.

*Source: http://www.fda.gov/ohrms/dockets/ac102/slides/3902$1-09-miller/ts/d009.htm (accessed May 2003).

ANTIMICROBIAL AGENTS Antimicrobial medications are used frequently during pregnancy. All these agents enter the fetal circulation to some extent. The potential teratogenic effects are unknown for some antimicrobials. Information on the safety of newer extended-spectrum or late-generation agents is limited.[11] Table 105-1 includes known pregnancy-related contraindications to some frequently used antibiotics.

Penicillin and cephalosporins generally are regarded as safe for use in any trimester. Neither group has been associated with teratogenesis in either animals or humans. Erythromycin does not cause known adverse fetal effects, but the estolate formulation is contraindicated in pregnancy because it may cause maternal cholestatic hepatitis. Sulfonamides (including the sulfamethoxazole component of trimethoprim-sulfamethoxazole) are not known human teratogens. Maternal use close to term, however, may cause complications in the neonate. Sulfonamides compete with bilirubin for albumin binding. The fetus clears free bilirubin via the placenta, but in the neonate, free bilirubin accumulates and may cause kernicterus. Trimethoprim, the other component of this combination antibiotic, should be avoided in the first trimester because it is a folate antagonist, and decreased folate may cause neural tube abnormalities. If trimethoprim-sulfamethoxazole offers a clear advantage over other antibiotics, it is reasonable to use; however, the period of gestation should be considered in making such a decision. Tetracyclines are contraindicated in pregnancy because they chelate calcium, cause abnormalities in fetal bone development, discolor teeth, and cause maternal hepatic and renal toxicity. Fluoroquinolones have caused fetal cartilage abnormalities in animals and as of this writing remain contraindicated throughout pregnancy.[11]

ANALGESIC AGENTS **Acetaminophen is the agent of choice** for analgesia or antipyresis in pregnancy. Aspirin should be avoided during pregnancy. Although evidence is conflicting, aspirin use in the first trimester has been associated with congenital defects. Use later in pregnancy may cause coagulation abnormalities with hemorrhagic complications in both the neonate and the mother. Premature ductus

TABLE 104-2   Medications Generally Considered Safe During Pregnancy

Agent
Antimicrobial agents
Cephalosporins
Erythromycin and azithromycin*
Nitrofurantoin
Penicillins
Analgesic agents
Acetaminophen
Gastrointestinal agents
Promethazine
Prochlorperazine
Metoclopramide
Ondansetron
Tums, Rolaids
Cimetidine
Ranitidine
Antihistamines
Diphenhydramine
Cold preparations
Pseudoephedrine
Dextromethorphan
Guaifenesin
Anaesthetics
Lidocaine

*Not erythromycin estolate (hepatotoxicity risk), or clarithromycin.

arteriosus closure and cardiovascular complications in the neonate also may be a result of maternal aspirin use late in pregnancy. Aspirin and other nonsteroidal anti-inflammatory drugs (NSAIDs) may prolong gestation and labor through inhibition of cyclooxygenase. Unfortunately, nonaspirin NSAIDs cannot be employed as tocolytic agents because they, like aspirin, cause premature ductus closure and subsequent pulmonary hypertension. Use of NSAIDs (especially indomethacin) also has been associated with oligohydramnios, intestinal perforation, hydrops fetalis, and renal failure.

GASTROINTESTINAL AGENTS   Many pregnant women, particularly those in the first trimester, suffer nausea and vomiting. Conservative measures, such as reduced meal size and avoidance of specific foods, frequently ease symptoms. Intravenous fluids and electrolyte replacement may alleviate symptoms, but in some cases medications may be necessary.

The safety of antiemetics has not been studied in prospective human trials, but the benefit of improved metabolic conditions and maternal well-being should be considered in the management decision.[12] Phenothiazines, such as promethazine and prochlorperazine, may be considered. Several other antiemetics, including metoclopramide (5–10 mg PO, IV, IM every 8 h) and ondansetron (8 mg PO every 8 h), are presumed safe based on animal study data.

Physiologic changes in pregnancy often lead to dyspepsia during the third trimester. Most over-the-counter antacid preparations are acceptable. The histamine antagonists cimetidine and ranitidine have no known teratogenic effect in animals. Although they have not been evaluated in humans, their use in general is considered safe.

COLD PREPARATIONS   Over-the-counter cold preparations are frequently combination medications containing sympathomimetic agents. All sympathomimetic drugs have vasoconstrictive properties and may lead to vascular-mediated congenital defects. Data on spe-

cific agents and their teratogenic potential are inconclusive. Conservative measures for control of symptoms during upper respiratory infections are preferred. When medication is necessary, each component of a combination preparation should be considered before a choice is made. First-trimester exposure to dextromethorphan or guaifenesin has not been associated with adverse fetal effects.

ANESTHETICS   Proper use of most agents for local or regional anesthesia, including subcutaneous infiltration of **lidocaine, has not been associated with detrimental fetal effects.** Combination preparations such as tetracaine, adrenaline-epinephrine, and cocaine (TAC) and lidocaine, adrenaline, and tetracaine (LAT) should not be used due to the potential risks of absorbed cocaine and adrenaline-epinephrine.

CONTRACEPTIVES   Pregnancy may occur in women taking oral contraceptive agents due either to a failure of therapy or to noncompliance. While there is no demonstrated risk of fetal malformation due to contraceptive use in early pregnancy, they should be discontinued as soon as pregnancy is recognized.[3]

Radiation Exposure

Complicating effects of radiation are discussed in Chap. 105.

Immunizations

Live-virus vaccines, including measles, mumps, rubella, poliomyelitis, and varicella, should be avoided in all trimesters of pregnancy as well as for 3 months before conception.[13] Inactivated (killed-virus) vaccines, including the influenza vaccine, can be administered during pregnancy. In fact, the Advisory Committee on Immunization Practices of the Centers for Disease Control and Prevention recommends vaccination against influenza for women who will be in the second or third trimester during the influenza season[13] because women at those stages of pregnancy are at increased risk of influenza-related complications. **Tetanus toxoid alone or in combination with diphtheria toxoid can be given during pregnancy.** Immunoglobulins, including tetanus, hepatitis, rabies, and varicella immunoglobulin, can be administered when indicated regardless of the stage of gestation.[13]

PREVENTIVE MEDICINE AND COUNSELING

Nutrition and Nutritional Supplementation

Nutrition is important to pregnancy outcome. Total weight gain as well as the pattern of weight gain affects newborn birth weight. Maternal weight gain begins in the first trimester and is most significant during the first half of pregnancy. Average total gain is 12.5 kg (28 lb). Routine supplementation with a multivitamin is not necessary with a balanced diet. Since folic acid supplementation before and during early pregnancy may prevent neural tube defects, supplementation of 1 mg/d should be started as soon as pregnancy is established.[14] For women with a previous pregnancy affected by neural tube defect, the supplementation should be further increased to 4 mg/d.[14] Appropriate use of vitamin preparations is not harmful, but excess intake of some vitamins (e.g., A, D, C, and B_6) may lead to congenital defects.

Since most women of childbearing age have poor iron stores and normal dietary intake cannot meet the increased demand during pregnancy, iron supplementation is recommended, but other mineral supplementation is not. Zinc deficiency may be associated with neural tube defects. Daily intake of zinc during pregnancy should be 15 mg.[14]

Caffeine

Results of human studies on the effects of caffeine use during pregnancy are conflicting. Some evidence suggests an increased risk of spontaneous abortion in nonsmokers who experience nausea during pregnancy and consume 500 mg (equivalent to 5 cups of coffee) per day or more of caffeine.[15]

Aspartame

Aspartame (Nutrasweet) is metabolized to phenylalanine. Phenylalanine crosses into fetal circulation and at very high concentrations can lead to mental retardation. Except in cases of excessive maternal dietary intake or maternal heterozygous carriers of phenylketonuria, fetal toxicity is unlikely.

Substance Abuse

Illicit substance abuse, as well as alcohol and tobacco use, may affect the fetus and/or the mother and is one of the greatest threats to normal pregnancy. Frequently, multiple substances are involved.

ILLICIT SUBSTANCES   Use of cocaine, opiates, or amphetamines is associated with multiple complications of pregnancy and congenital abnormalities. Data on other substances, such as hallucinogens and "designer drugs," is inconclusive. Effects of abused substances as well as the general health and well-being of the mother are of concern when treating a pregnant substance abuser. A multidisciplinary approach is important.

NICOTINE   Cigarette smoking, a habit to which 25 to 30 percent of reproductive-age women admit, increases the risk of many pregnancy complications. Only 20 percent of smokers quit by the time of the first prenatal evaluation.[16] Although the mechanism by which nicotine produces some of these adverse outcomes is incompletely understood, exposure to nicotine is associated with higher rates of spontaneous abortion, abruption, preterm labor, and low birth weight. Smoking cessation by 16 weeks' gestation may ameliorate adverse effects. Attempts at cessation should first be made without pharmacologic intervention. Recommendations for the use of nicotine gum (pregnancy category C) and nicotine patches (pregnancy category D) should be individualized. Prior cessation attempts and total number of cigarettes per day should be considered in assessing the potential risks and benefits of such interventions.[16]

ALCOHOL   Ethanol readily crosses the placenta and enters the CNS of the developing fetus. Fetal exposure to ethanol produces a characteristic clinical condition known as *fetal alcohol syndrome,* which includes CNS dysfunction, growth retardation, and facial abnormalities. CNS abnormalities including microcephaly, mental retardation, and behavioral disorders are typically the most severe. This syndrome may result from ethanol use during any period of gestation; however, the greatest risk is with first-trimester exposure. Furthermore, although evidence supports a dose-related response to ethanol exposure, there is no established safe quantity of alcohol that may be consumed.

Travel

In general, a normal pregnancy does not prevent women from traveling to reasonable destinations. Immunization requirements and the possibility of travel-related diseases or development of complications while in remote areas are issues that should be addressed before travel is begun. High-altitude stays of a few days' duration have not been associated with risk to the fetus, but exposure for longer duration increases the chance of fetal growth retardation, maternal high blood pressure, and premature delivery. Travel in pressurized aircraft has not been associated with adverse outcome in an otherwise uncomplicated pregnancy. Some commercial airlines, however, enforce restrictions limiting travel during the third trimester. Frequent ambulation is important during travel of long duration regardless of the period of ges-

TABLE 104-3   Symptoms and Signs in Pregnancy that Need Prompt Evaluation

Change in fetal movement pattern
Fever, chills
Refractory emesis
Visual disturbance
Abdominal pain
Significant headache
Anasarca
Dysuria
Vaginal bleeding and fluid loss
Abnormal vaginal discharge

tation. Protective restraint devices should be used at all times in automobiles and airplanes. Lap belts should have a snug, comfortable fit under the abdomen and across the hipbones.[17,18]

Exercise

The effects of physical exertion on pregnancy outcome are not known. In general, uncomplicated pregnancy should not limit the ability to engage in moderate physical exercise. The American College of Obstetricians and Gynecologists recommends some modifications in exercise routines in view of the physiologic and morphologic changes of gestation.[6] Non-weight-bearing activity and activities that minimize the chance of even mild abdominal trauma are preferable. Scuba diving should be avoided due to the increased fetal risk for decompression sickness.[19] Exercise in the supine position should be avoided completely after the first trimester due to potential for decreased cardiac output. Although there does not appear to be a need to alter goal intensity as judged by heart rate, exercise should be stopped at the onset of fatigue rather than continuing to exhaustion. Regular activity is preferable to sporadic exertion. Exercise may be beneficial in the prevention of gestational diabetes. Subjective benefits of exercise both before conception and during early pregnancy have been reported.[20] Specific recommendations for exercise during pregnancy need to be individualized and made with the knowledge that there is no conclusive evidence on which to base recommendations.

DISPOSITION

Timely access to prenatal care should be arranged. Recommendations for prenatal care for a normal pregnancy include an initial obstetric evaluation no later than 6 to 8 weeks' gestation. Discharge instructions should include recommendations about symptoms and signs for which the patient should be urgently reevaluated (Table 104-3). Recommendations on activities, lifestyle, and appropriate use of prescription and over-the-counter medications should be given.

Obstetric consultation should be obtained whenever there is uncertainty regarding issues, such as specific travel, immunization, medication, or management options. Gestational age, fetal heart tones (expected if gestational age is greater than 16 to 19 weeks), analytical values, parity, and general maternal information should be provided to the consultant.

REFERENCES

1. Ramoska EA, Sacchetti AD, Nepp M: Reliability of patient history in determining the possibility of pregnancy. *Ann Emerg Med* 18:48, 1989.
2. US Department of Health and Human Services: Fertility, Family Planning, and Women's Health: New Data from the 1995 National Survey of Family Growth. DHHS publication PHS 97, 1995.
3. American College of Obstetricians and Gynecologists: Hormonal contraception. Technical bulletin 198. *Int J Gynaecol Obstet* 48:115, 1995.
4. Peterson HB, Xia Z, Hughes JM, et al: The risk of pregnancy after tubal sterilization: Findings from the US Collaborative Review of Sterilization. *Am J Obstet Gynecol* 174:1161, 1996.

5. Clark SL, Cotton DB, Lee W, et al: Central hemodynamic assessment of normal term pregnancy. *Am J Obstet Gynecol* 161:1439, 1989.

6. Whittaker PG, Macphail S, Lind T: Serial hematologic changes and pregnancy outcome. *Obstet Gynecol* 88:33, 1996.

7. American College of Obstetricians and Gynecologists: Exercise during pregnancy and the postpartum period. Washington, Technical bulletin 189, 1994.

8. Krause PJ, Ingirdia CJ, Pontius LT: Host defense during pregnancy: Neutrophil chemotaxis and adherence. *Am J Obstet Gynecol* 157:274, 1987.

9. Gibbon BN, Hemphill RR, Santen SA: Do we still have to worry when the urine is dilute? *Ann Emerg Med* 32:287, 1998.

10. Shotan A. Ostrzega E, Mehra A, et al: Incidence of arrhythmias in normal pregnancy and relation to palpitations, dizziness, and syncope. *Am J Cardiol* 79:1061, 1997.

11. American College of Obstetricians and Gynecologists: Antimicrobial therapy for obstetric patients. Washington, Educational bulletin 245, 1998.

12. Nelson-Piercy C: Treatment of nausea and vomiting in pregnancy. *Drug Safety* 19:155, 1998.

13. Faix RG: Immunization during pregnancy. *Clin Obstet Gynecol* 45:42, 2002.

14. American College of Obstetricians and Gynecologists: Nutrition and women. Washington, Educational bulletin 229, 1996.

15. Cnattingius S, Signorello LB, Anneren G, et al: Caffeine intake and the risk of first-trimester spontaneous abortion. *New Engl J Med* 343:1839, 2000.

16. American College of Obstetricians and Gynecologists: Smoking and women's health. Educational bulletin 240. *Int J Gynaecol Obstet* 60:71, 1997.

17. American College of Obstetricians and Gynecologists: Air travel during pregnancy. Washington, Committee opinion 264, 2001.

18. Rose SR: Pregnancy and travel. *Emerg Med Clin North Am* 15:93, 1997.

19. American College of Obstetricians and Gynecologists: Exercise during pregnancy and the postpartum period. Washington, Committee opinion 267, 2002.

20. Wang TW, Apgar BS: Exercise during pregnancy. *Am Fam Phys* 57:1846, 1998.

105 COMORBID DISEASES IN PREGNANCY

Jessica L. Bienstock

Harold E. Fox

DIABETES

Diabetes mellitus complicates approximately 2 to 3 percent of all pregnancies. Diabetes in pregnancy falls into two categories: Approximately 90 percent of pregnant diabetic patients have gestational diabetes, and 10 percent have diabetes that predates the pregnancy. Those with gestational diabetes are subdivided into classes A_1 and A_2, the former being controlled by diet alone and the latter requiring insulin therapy. Patients with preexisting diabetes, even if they were managed previously with oral hypoglycemic agents, are all treated with insulin therapy during pregnancy. **Oral hypoglycemic agents are not used during pregnancy** because they do not provide an adequate level of glucose control. In addition, some of these agents have been associated with an increased risk of congenital anomalies, hyperbilirubinemia, and irreversible β-cell hyperplasia in exposed infants. Pregnant diabetic patients are at increased risk for fetal death in utero, particularly patients with preexisting vascular disease and preeclampsia, as well as those with poor glycemic control.

The goals of glucose control for all patients with gestational diabetes is a fasting plasma glucose level of less than 90 mg/dL and 1-h postprandial blood glucose levels of less than 140 mg/dL. Patients with gestational diabetes who are managed by diet alone rarely develop acute glycemic complications because their glucose values rarely reach levels consistent with diabetic ketoacidosis.

Among patients with insulin-dependent diabetes, the need for insulin tends to increase throughout the course of pregnancy. In general,

during the first trimester, the initial insulin requirement is 0.7 units/kg per d. By late pregnancy, patients generally require 1 unit/kg per d. Generally, two-thirds of the total insulin dose is given in the morning and one-third in the evening. Usually, two-thirds of the morning dose consists of NPH and one-third of regular insulin. The evening dose consists of half NPH and half regular insulin. Occasionally, this regimen may result in nocturnal hypoglycemia between 1 and 3 A.M. Administering the predinner NPH at bedtime has been suggested as a way of remedying the problem.

Pregnant diabetics are at increased risk for several pregnancy complications, including hypertensive diseases, preterm labor, spontaneous abortion, and pyelonephritis, in addition to hypoglycemia and diabetic ketoacidos (DKA).

About 10 percent of insulin-dependent diabetics will develop ketoacidosis at some point during pregnancy.[1] Ketoacidosis has been reported to occur more rapidly and at lower glucose levels in pregnant patients as compared with nonpregnant patients. While classically the diagnosis of ketoacidosis requires a plasma glucose level of greater than 300 mg/dL, DKA may develop in pregnancy at lower glucose values. β-sympathomimetic agents used for tocolysis, such as ritodrene and terbutaline, have been associated with an increased risk of diabetic ketoacidosis. Pregnant women in DKA are treated with a constant low-dose insulin infusion. General management guidelines are the same as for nonpregnant patients (see Chap. 211).

With contemporary medical management, fetal loss is less frequent, although the literature reports a high fetal mortality rate in patients treated for DKA. It is not uncommon to find pathologic patterns of fetal heart rate during DKA; these tend, however, to improve as maternal status improves. Steps should be taken to improve uterine blood flow, such as administration of oxygen and left lateral uterine displacement.

Up to 45 percent of insulin-dependent diabetics will require evaluation for severe hypoglycemia at some time during the course of their pregnancy.[2] Hypoglycemia generally presents as sweating, tremors, blurred or double vision, weakness, hunger, confusion, paraesthesias, anxiety, palpitations, nausea, headache, or stupor. Hypoglycemic episodes generally are well tolerated by the fetus. Mild hypoglycemia—that is, a glucose level of less than 70 mg/dL—in a patient who is able to follow commands can be treated by administration of 1 cup of low-fat milk together with bread or crackers every 15 min. This regimen is preferred over more highly concentrated glucose solutions because it avoids "overshoot" and subsequent hyperglycemia. In patients who are unable to cooperate with oral therapy owing to severe hypoglycemia, parenteral therapy may be begun using one ampule (50 mL) of a D50W solution given via intravenous push. Alternatively, the patient may be treated using glucagon 1 to 2 mg IM or SQ. In addition, intravenous therapy should be instituted with D5W at a rate of 50 to 100 mL/h. Consideration should be given to the avoidance of subsequent hyperglycemia from glycogen mobilization with acute glucose administration. The goal is normoglycemic control without wide swings.

HYPERTHYROIDISM

Hyperthyroidism in pregnancy is associated with an increased risk of preeclampsia and neonatal morbidity, including low birth weight and possibly congenital malformations. Symptoms of hyperthyroidism closely mimic symptoms of normal pregnancy and may consist of nervousness, palpitations, heat intolerance, and inability to gain weight despite a good appetite. Thyrotoxicosis in pregnancy also may present as hyperemesis gravidarum.

Hyperthyroidism in pregnancy is treated with propylthiouracil (PTU). The time to onset of action of PTU is generally 4 to 6 weeks to achieve maximum effect. PTU is started at a dose of 100 to 150 mg three times a day and increased as needed to a maximum dose of up to 200 mg three times a day. The goal of therapy is to maintain a free triiodothyroxine (T_4) level at the upper range of normal. Approximately

2 percent of patients taking PTU will experience a mild purpuric skin rash within the first 4 weeks of therapy. If this occurs, the PTU should be stopped and replaced with methimazole. Agranulocytosis occurs in about 0.3 percent of patients treated with PTU. If agranulocytosis develops, the PTU should be stopped, and methimazole should not be started.

THYROID STORM

Patients with thyroid storm present with fever, volume depletion, cardiac decompensation. Thyroid storm has been associated with a mortality rate of up to 25 percent. Patients are treated with IV fluids, oxygen, antipyretic agents, and PTU 400 mg PO every 8 h and sodium iodide 1 g in 500 mL of IV fluid each day. Long-term use (>10 days) of sodium iodide results in a high incidence of fetal goiter and hypothyroidism. Propranolol 40 mg PO every 6 h is administered unless evidence of cardiac failure is present. Acetaminophen is used for treatment of hyperthermia; a cooling blanket also may be used. Steps should be taken to improve uterine blood flow, such as administration of oxygen as well as maintenance of adequate maternal hydration and left lateral uterine displacement. **Radioactive iodine therapy is not used** because the fetus will concentrate iodine-131 after the tenth to twelfth week of gestation, and congenital hypothyroidism results.

HYPERTENSION

Hypertension in pregnancy can be divided into chronic hypertension and preeclampsia. In addition, patients with chronic hypertension not uncommonly develop superimposed preeclampsia. Preeclampsia is discussed elsewhere (see Chap. 106).

Chronic hypertension complicates 4 to 5 percent of all pregnancies. It is diagnosed by sustained elevation of arterial blood pressure to greater than 140/90 mm Hg before the twentieth week of gestation. Pharmacotherapy for pregnant hypertensive patients generally is started when the systolic blood pressure exceeds 160 mm Hg or the diastolic blood pressure exceeds 100 mm Hg. Commonly used agents for the treatment of chronic hypertension in pregnancy include α-methyldopa (Aldomet), labetalol, and nifedipine. Antihypertensive agents that generally are not used in pregnancy include diuretics, because of their association with a reduction of uteral placental blood flow, and angiotensin-converting enzyme (ACE) inhibitors, owing to their teratogenic effects as well as fetal/neonatal hypotension and anuria. Maternal mortality associated with chronic hypertension is usually the result of severe hypertension and associated congestive heart failure or cerebrovascular accident. Fetal perinatal outcome is associated most closely with the development of superimposed preeclampsia or placental abruption. However, antihypertensive therapy has not been shown to alter the incidence of fetal complications.

Management of an acute hypertensive crisis in pregnancy is accomplished most commonly with IV labetalol (10 mg every 5 to 10 min up to a total dose of 300 mg). Hydralazine (5–10 mg every 15 min) given as IV bolus injections is an alternative still used by many obstetricians. The aim of antihypertensive therapy in pregnancy is to maintain the blood pressure between 140 and 150 mm Hg systolic and 90 and 100 mm Hg diastolic. Persistent blood pressure levels below this range may jeopardize placental perfusion. Acute intervention for blood pressure control should include fetal monitoring as well as careful assessment of fetal well-being. In all chronic hypertensives, the possibility of superimposed preeclampsia always must be considered (see Chap. 106).

DYSRHYTHMIAS

Significant cardiac dysrhythmias are rare in pregnancy. However, medications such as lidocaine, digoxin, and procainamide may be used for the usual indications and in the usual therapeutic doses and have not been shown to be harmful to the fetus. Use of β-blockers for acute tachydysrhythmias has not been associated with adverse neonatal outcomes,[3] but maintenance β-blockers are class C drugs that should be prescribed only in consultation with a cardiologist and obstetrician. Verapamil has been shown to be effective in the conversion of supraventricular tachycardia to sinus rhythm without adverse fetal effects. Anticoagulation using unfractionated or low-molecular-weight heparin for the treatment of atrial fibrillation in pregnancy appears safe and may be used if the patient meets the criteria for anticoagulation described for nonpregnant patients. Cardioversion also appears safe for the fetus.[4] The presence of an artificial pacemaker has not been shown to affect the course of pregnancy.[5]

THROMBOEMBOLISM

The incidence of deep venous thrombosis (DVT) in pregnancy ranges between 0.5 and 0.7 percent.[6] Factors associated with an increased risk of venous thromboembolism in pregnancy include advanced maternal age, increasing parity, multiple gestation, operative delivery, bed rest, obesity, history of previous thromboembolism, antithrombin III deficiency, protein S or protein C deficiency, and the lupus anticoagulant syndrome. Both DVT and PE occur during the antenatal period more than twice as often as during the post partum period[6,7] and up to 30 percent may not have any identifiable risk.[6] Those over 35 years also appear to be at greater risk.[6,7]

The clinical diagnosis of DVT is similar in pregnant patients to that in nonpregnant patients. Pregnant patients commonly complain of swelling and leg discomfort; duplex Doppler studies should be done to confirm the diagnosis. Impedance plethysmography also may be used safely in pregnancy. **Iodine-125 fibrinogen scanning should not be used** because unbound iodine crosses the placental barrier and enters the fetal circulation, where it may concentrate in the fetal thyroid. Radionuclide venography using particles of technetium-99m is of no risk to the fetus and can be used to obtain studies of the lower extremity as well as to perform perfusion lung scans.

Diagnosis of pulmonary embolism in pregnancy is similar to that in the nonpregnant patient. Ventilation perfusion scans may be performed safely in pregnancy. No adverse fetal effects of xenon-133 or technetium-99m lung scanning have been reported. Pulmonary arteriography also may be performed in pregnant women if scanning is indeterminant. The diagnostic efficiency of spiral computed tomographic (CT) scanning has not been studied in pregnancy. Treatment for both DVT and pulmonary embolism in pregnancy is with intravenous heparin, with the goal of maintaining the partial thromboplastin time (PTT) of 11/2 to 2 times control. Low-molecular-weight heparin also may be used for both the prophylaxis and treatment of thromboembolic disease at a dose of 1 mg/kg enoxaparin SQ twice a day. Warfarin is not used in pregnancy because it crosses the placenta and is associated with embryopathy in the first trimester; in the second and third trimesters it may lead to a variety of central nervous system (CNS) and ophthamalogic abnormalities. Protamine sulfate may be used safely in pregnancy for patients who require rapid reversal of their heparin anticoagulation. Although there is minimal experience with the use thrombolytic therapy in pregnancy, its use may be entertained in life-threatening situations.

ASTHMA

Asthma complicates between 0.4 and 1.3 percent of all pregnancies. In general, however, there are no differences in the outcome of pregnancies in well-controlled asthmatics versus the general population. Severe asthmatics with poorly controlled disease, however, do have a slight increase in the risk of preterm birth, stillbirth, and low-birth-weight babies. In approximately one-third of patients, asthma worsen in pregnancy; approximately one-third remain stable, and one-third improve.[8]

The presentation of asthma in pregnancy is similar to that of the nonpregnant state, with the usual triad of cough, wheezing, and dyspnea. Unfortunately, pulmonary embolism (PE) also can present with a similar symptom complex, and—as noted, because of the hypercoagulable state of pregnancy—pregnant women are at increased risk for PE. Therapeutic agents that are used safely in pregnancy include inhaled glucocorticoids, such as beclomethasone, and cromolyn sodium by inhaler. These agents are used as preventive therapy. For acute therapy of asthma exacerbations β_2-agonists such as salbutamol, metaproterenol, albuterol, and isoproterenol may be given via nebulizer. Intravenous methylprednisolone and oral prednisone can be used in pregnancy because they do not cross the placenta. Any time glucocorticoids are used, maternal hyperglycemia should be expected and considered in acute management (see "Diabetes" above). Epinephrine 0.3 mL (1:1000 dilution) can be given subcutaneously. Oxygen should be administered and titrated to maintain an arterial P_{O_2} of 65 mm Hg or greater. Fetal monitoring should be done after 20 weeks of gestation.

Clinical management of a pregnant asthmatic patient is best guided by the use of the peak expiratory flow rate to assess the severity of the obstruction and monitor the response to therapy. Peak expiratory flow rate is not altered, with mean peak expiratory flow rates in normal pregnant women ranging between 380 and 550 L per min. Peak expiratory flow rates do not change significantly as pregnancy progresses.[9] Peak expiratory flow rates of less than 100 L per min or that demonstrate less than 10 percent improvement with treatment are a sign of a potentially poor prognosis. Aggressive management is warranted.

Normal values of arterial blood gases are changed during pregnancy. The normal maternal P_{O_2} ranges between 101 and 108 mm Hg early in pregnancy and falls to 90 to 100 mm Hg near term. The normal Pa_{CO_2} in pregnancy ranges from 27 to 32 mm Hg, and the normal pH ranges from 7.40 to 7.45. The patient should be placed in a near-sitting position with a leftward tilt because up to 25 percent of normal pregnant women in the third trimester with develop moderate hypoxia in the supine position. There should be a low threshold for obtaining arterial blood gas assessment as part of the evaluation of pregnant women with asthma, particularly patients who present with obvious hypoventilation and cyanosis whose asthma does not improve after initial therapy or who have a peak flow of less than 200 L/min.[9] Goals of therapy include maintenance of a P_{O_2} at greater than 65 mm Hg or an oxygen saturation of greater than 95 percent on an $F_{I_{O_2}}$ of 35 to 60 percent.

Indications for intubation of the pregnant asthmatic with status asthmaticus include (1) inability to maintain the Pa_{O_2} at greater than 65 mm Hg (90 percent hemoglobin saturation) despite supplemental oxygen, (2) inability to maintain a Pa_{CO_2} at less than 40 mm Hg, (3) evidence of maternal exhaustion, (4) significant respiratory acidosis (pH <7.20–7.25) refractory to initial management with bronchodilator therapy, and (5) altered mental status.[10] Standard agents for rapid-sequence intubation can be used.

Medications for asthma that may have adverse fetal effects include iodides, which may be associated with neonatal hypothyroidism and goiter, as well as sodium bicarbonate, which, without adequate ventilation, can diminish the transfer of carbon dioxide from the fetus to the mother. Glucocorticoids also may cause alterations in carbohydrate metabolism, although this is a secondary concern in the acute setting. Essentially, acute management should be guided by consideration for the mother. The best outcome for the developing fetus is based on optimal treatment of the mother.

CHRONIC RENAL DISEASE

Maternal risks associated with renal disease are linked to the degree of renal compromise. As renal function diminishes, fertility decreases. Pregnancy rarely occurs in women who have a preconception serum creatine level of greater than 3 mg/dL. Preterm delivery and superim-posed preeclampsia frequently complicate pregnancies of patients with underlying renal disease. Patients with chronic pyelonephritis may have an increased number of recurrences due to bacteriuria, increased glucosuria, and mechanical compression of the ureter in the third trimester. Those with a history of reflux nephropathy are at increased risk of sudden escalating hypertension and worsening renal function. Urolithiasis is associated with more frequent urinary tract infections. Patients with lupus nephropathy are at greatly increased risk for exacerbations of the disease and superimposed preeclampsia, particularly if their disease was not in remission for at least 6 months prior to conception.

CYSTITIS AND PYELONEPHRITIS

The increased urinary stasis associated with pregnancy makes the urinary tract the most common point of infection during pregnancy. After midpregnancy, mild right-sided hydronephrosis can be found in 75 percent of patients, and mild left-sided hydronephrosis is seen in 33 percent of patients. Asymptomatic bacteriuria is present in between 2 and 10 percent of pregnant women.[11,12] Acute cystitis occurs in about 1 to 2 percent of pregnant women,[13] acute pyelonephritis occurs in approximately the same percent of all pregnancies.[14] The presentation of both cystitis and pyelonephritis is similar in pregnant and nonpregnant women. Causative organisms are similar to those in the general population, with *Escherichia coli* being the etiology in approximately 75 percent and *Klebsiella pneumoniae* or *Proteus* being responsible for 10 to 15 percent. It is not uncommon for acute pyelonephritis to precipitate preterm labor. Therefore, prompt therapy is needed. In addition, pregnant women are at increased risk for the development of bacteremia and septic shock as compared with the nonpregnant population.[14]

Patients with simple cystitis may be treated with a 3-day course of oral nitrofurantoin, ampicillin, or a cephalosporin. Because of the low prevalence of resistance of urinary pathogens to nitrofurantoin, this agent is generally the preferred method of therapy. Trimethoprin, a folate antagonist, is used by many obstetricians after the first trimester. **Single-dose antibiotic therapy is not used for the treatment of cystitis in pregnant patients** owing to the high rate of treatment failure.

Treatment of pregnant patients with pyelonephritis is much more intense than that of nonpregnant patients. Approximately 10 to 15 percent of pregnant patients with pyelonephritis become bacteremic,[15] and 2 to 8 percent will develop respiratory insufficiency from acute lung injury.[16] Due to the high rate of complications, patients are generally hospitalized, aggressively hydrated, and treated with intravenous antibiotics. The intravenous antibiotics of choice are generally a second or third generation cephalosporin. Intravenous antibiotics are continued until the patient is afebrile for at least 48 h, and costovertebral angle tenderness has resolved. Patients are then discharged home on oral antibiotics to complete a 10-day course of therapy. Many providers choose to continue women with a history of pyelonephritis during the course of their pregnancy on antibiotic suppression for the remainder of their pregnancy. This generally is accomplished using nitrofurantoin at a dose of 50 to 100 mg per d.

INFLAMMATORY BOWEL DISEASE

Pregnant patients with inflammatory bowel disease are at increased risk for nutritional and metabolic abnormalities that may put the fetus at increased risk for intrauterine growth restriction. Pregnancy itself, however, seems to have little effect on inflammatory bowel disease. When an exacerbation does occur during pregnancy, it happens most frequently in either the first trimester or the postpartum period. It is hypothesized that this is due to a correlation with levels of circulating corticosteroids during pregnancy.

In general, treatment of the pregnant patient with inflammatory bowel disease is the same as that of the nonpregnant patient. Antidiarrheal drugs including codeine, opium, paregoric, and Lomotil also may be used safely in pregnancy. While sulfasalazine and corticosteroids may be used safely in pregnancy, the possibility of the development of gestational diabetes must be considered in all patients on steroid therapy. Sulfa drugs are theoretically contraindicated in the third trimester due to concerns about neonatal hyperbilirubinemia, but they are used fairly commonly by obstetricians without adverse effect. It is important to supplement women who are taking sulfasalazine with folic acid because sulfasalazine is known to inhibit the absorption and metabolism of folate. The use of suppressive therapy with azathioprine or 6-mercaptopurine has been reported to be safe during pregnancy, but experience with these agents is very limited. Total parental nutrition is a potentially useful adjunct to therapy in some patients who have severe nutritional deficiencies, and it may be used safely in pregnancy. Metronidazole for the treatment of perianal fistulas in patients with Crohn disease is generally not recommended until after completion of the first trimester.

SICKLE CELL DISEASE

Women with sickle cell disease are at increased risk for miscarriage, preterm labor, and other complications due to impaired oxygen supply and sickling infarcts in the placental circulation. Pregnant women are at increased risk for vascular occlusive events, particularly during the third trimester and the postpartum period. Painful crises present similarly in the pregnant and the nonpregnant state. Treatment of painful crises in pregnancy is similar to that for nonpregnant patients. Cornerstones of management include aggressive hydration and analgesic therapy. Both oral and intravenous narcotics can be used. Caution should be exercised when using nonsteroidal anti-inflammatory agents, particularly after 32 weeks of gestation, because of oligohydramnios and a significant risk of premature closure of the fetal ductus arteriosus. Hydroxyurea should not be used in pregnancy because of its teratogenic effects. Sickle cell crisis that does not respond to conservative management is commonly managed using partial exchange transfusion via automated erythrocytapheresis. Simple transfusion alone can be helpful when the hemoglobin level is less than 6 g/dL.[17] The incidence of fetal death in utero can be minimized during sickle cell crisis by using information from continuous electronic fetal monitoring in a woman with a potentially viable fetus. While fetal heart rate patterns frequently are nonreassuring during the acute episode of vasoocclusive crisis, fetal heart rate patterns tend to normalize as the crisis improves. In utero resuscitation (oxygen, intravenous hydration, left lateral uterine displacement) should be initiated prior to consideration of emergency delivery.

While the majority of sickle cell crises in pregnancy are vasoocclusive crises, aplastic crises present a unique problem because they usually are caused by parvovirus B19 infection, which has been associated with hydrops fetalis. This disease thus presents a risk to both the pregnant woman and her fetus. Careful sonographic fetal assessment should be performed to evaluate the fetus for evidence of parvovirus infection. Once patients with sickle cell disease has been exposed to parvovirus B19, they are unlikely to acquire the infection a second time due to acquired immunity.[18] Thus, the pregnant patient with a past history of aplastic crisis is unlikely to experience it again.

MIGRAINE

Pregnancy usually improves classic migraines. However, when migraines do occur, they are difficult to treat because ergot alkaloids should not be used and there has been little experience with the use of sumatriptan in pregnancy. Treatment therefore rests on the use of analgesics and antiemetic agents. Acetaminophen, codeine, and meperidine all have been shown to be safe for use in pregnancy.

Prophylactic therapy using β-blockers such as propanol (40–160 mg per d) or atenolol (50–100 mg per d) also effective.

SEIZURE DISORDERS

Seizure disorders occur in 0.15 to 1.0 percent of all women of childbearing age. Seizure frequency tends to increase slightly in pregnancy because of the increased volume of distribution, an increase in plasma clearance, and poor medication compliance. Management of a pregnant patient with a known seizure does not differ from that of a nonpregnant woman. Consideration of potential adverse effects of antiseizure medication mandates the use of single-drug therapy when possible. About half of patients will experience an increase in seizure frequency during pregnancy. Medication doses may need to be increased in pregnancy; however, the serum therapeutic levels do not change. The use of valproic acid generally is avoided in early pregnancy because of its association with 1 to 3 percent risk of neural tube defects.

A single maternal grand mal seizure may be followed by fetal bradycardia lasting for up to 20 min. While transient maternal hypoxia and acidosis are potential threats to the fetus, there is usually no apparent harm caused by isolated seizures. Steps should be taken to optimize the intrauterine environment, including administration of oxygen and left lateral uterine displacement. In contrast, status epilepticus poses a real threat to both mother and the fetus, with 50 percent of fetuses and 33 percent of mothers not surviving the event. Aggressive management with intubation and ventilation should be considered early in the management of pregnant women with status epilepticus.

HUMAN IMMUNODEFICIENCY VIRUS (HIV) INFECTION

All pregnant HIV-infected patients beyond 14 weeks' gestation should be on zidovudine therapy in an effort to decrease the risk of vertical transmission. Randomized clinical trials of zidovudine have documented a reduction in the vertical transmission rate from 25 to 8 percent.[19] Pregnancy does not appear to alter the natural course of HIV disease,[19] nor do uninfected babies born to HIV-positive women appear to be at increased risk for neonatal complications when compared with appropriate control patients. Patients with CD4$^+$ T-cell counts of less than 200/μL should be maintained on prophylaxis for *Pneumocystis carinii* pneumonia using trimethoprim-sulfamethoxazole (TMP-SMX; Bactrim DS). The risks and benefits of TMP-SMX therapy should be weighed if needed during the first trimester. Folate supplementation may be appropriate if benefit appears to outweigh risk. Alternatively, aerosolized pentamidine also may be used in pregnant patients. Treatment of overt opportunistic infections in HIV-infected pregnant women should be addressed just as in those who are not pregnant. Patients may present with respiratory insufficiency. The prompt initiation of artificial ventilation in such patients may improve the intrauterine environment and therefore the outcome for the fetus.

SUBSTANCE ABUSE

All pregnant women identified in the ED as substance abusers should be referred to a high-risk obstetrics clinic and be offered substance-abuse counseling.[20,21] The incidence of a positive urine toxicology test for cocaine ranges from 4 to 76 percent in urban and suburban hospitals. However, when hair analysis is employed, cocaine exposure can be identified by up to four times more.[22,23] Cocaine use has been associated with an increased risk of placental abruption and fetal death in utero as well as an increased risk of intrauterine growth restriction, preterm labor, premature rupture of membranes, spontaneous abortion, and cerebral infarcts in the fetus. Maternal complications of cocaine use include myocardial infarction, hypertension (which can result in aortic dissection), pulmonary edema, and cardiac dysrhythmias. Subarachnoid hemorrhage, ruptured aneurysms, and strokes all have been reported in cocaine users and are most likely related to transient hypertension. Treatment of acute cocaine intoxication is handled in the usual manner.

Pregnant women in opiate withdrawal are currently treated with methadone or clonidine. There is currently insufficient evidence regarding the use of buprenorphine in pregnancy. Pregnant women should not have methadone discontinued during pregnancy because it may increase the risk of fetal death in utero and tends to decrease compliance with prenatal care. Patients in withdrawal may be treated with clonidine 0.1 to 0.2 mg sublingually every hour up to 0.8 mg until signs of withdrawal resolve. The maintenance dose is then 0.8 to 1.2 mg per d in divided doses for the first 7 days and tapering for the following 3 days.

The incidence of alcohol abuse during pregnancy is difficult to determine because most studies have been limited to single hospitals or urban settings, but it probably ranges between 1 and 2 percent. In the largest study, almost 7 percent of women had detectable alcohol in urine samples taken at the time of delivery.[24] It is felt that two or more drinks a day may contribute to increased rates of spontaneous abortion, low-birth-weight infants, preterm deliveries, and perinatal mortality. Alcohol use in pregnancy can result in fetal alcohol syndrome. The incidence of fetal alcohol syndrome is difficult to characterize due to significant differences in patient populations studied and methods used. However, it is likely in the range of 0.1 to 0.3 percent of live births. Patients who present in coma due to acute alcohol intoxication or in alcohol withdrawal are managed similarly to nonpregnant patients. Short-acting barbiturates such as pentobarbital can be used for withdrawal, although benzodiazepines should be avoided in early pregnancy if at all possible because of possible teratogenicity. Disulfiram (Antabuse) is a potential teratogen and should be avoided in pregnancy.

DOMESTIC VIOLENCE

Between 14 and 17 percent of pregnant women experience domestic violence during the course of their pregnancy.[25,26] It is a particularly vulnerable time during which "intimate violence" may escalate. Late entry into prenatal care, unintended pregnancy, drug and alcohol use, depression, and housing problems have all been associate with an increased risk of domestic violence. Pregnant women who are the victims of domestic violence are at an increased risk for placental abruption, fetal fractures, uterine rupture, and preterm labor. It is imperative to keep a high index of suspicion and be prepared to initiate appropriate referrals to social service and law enforcement agencies. In addition, for Rh-negative women who have experienced blunt abdominal trauma, consideration should be given to the administration of Rhogam to prevent isoimmunization (see Chap. 106 for a detailed discussion).

MEDICATIONS FOR CONCURRENT ILLNESS DURING PREGNANCY AND LACTATION

The classic teratogenic period is from day 31 after the first day of the last menstrual period (LMP) in a 28-day cycle to 71 days from the LMP. During this critical time, organs are forming, and teratogens may cause overt malformation. Administration of drugs early in the period of organogenesis will affect the organs developing then, such as the heart or neural tube. Closer to the end of the classic teratogenic period, the ear and palate are forming and may be affected by a teratogen.

Before day 31, exposure to a teratogen produces an all-or-none effect. With exposure around conception, the conceptus usually either does not survive or survives without anomalies. If the organism remains viable, organ-specific anomalies do not develop because repair or replacement permits normal development. A similar insult at a later stage may produce organ-specific defects; after the first trimester, chronic exposure may produce growth restriction.

The Food and Drug Administration (FDA) lists five categories of labeling for drug use in pregnancy (see Table 104-1 in Chap. 104).

Table 105-1 lists medications for acute or chronic illness to be avoided in pregnancy. Table 104-2 briefly summarizes medications that are generally considered safe during pregnancy. Table 105-2 lists medications to be avoided during lactation, as well as those generally considered safe during breastfeeding.

COMPLICATING EFFECTS OF RADIATION

The major factor determining the degree of risk to the fetus in an imaging technique is the amount of ionizing radiation involved in the test. Exposure to ionizing radiation occurs with plain x-ray films, angiography, fluoroscopy, nuclear medicine, and computed tomography (CT). Nonionizing studies include magnetic resonance imaging (MRI) and ultrasound.

The risks of radiation exposure vary with gestational age. The predominant deterministic effect due to exposure during the first 2 weeks of pregnancy is resorption of the embryo. The second to eighth week postconception is the period of organogenesis. Significant x-ray exposure during this period may result in teratogenesis (birth defects). Examples include gross malformation and growth restriction, the latter of which can occur both at term and later at adulthood. Neuropathology and small head size also may occur as a result of significant exposures during weeks 2 to 8.

The embryo has developed into a fetus at about the seventh to eighth week, and neurologic development occurs during the next 7 weeks. Significant x-ray exposure at this time (between weeks 8 and

TABLE 105-1 Therapeutic Agents Commonly Used in Emergency Settings with Known Adverse Effects in Human Pregnancy

Drug	Effect
ACE inhibitors	Renal failure, oligohydramnios
Aminoglycosides	Ototoxicity
Androgenic steroids	Masculinize female fetus
Antibiotics	
Erythromycin estolate	Maternal hepatotoxicity
Fluoroquinolones	Fetal catilage abnormality
Kanamycin	Fetal cranial nerve VIII damage
Metronidazole	Fetal midline facial defects (1st trimester)
Streptomycin	Fetal cranial nerve VIII damage
Sulfonamides	Fetal hemolysis, neonatal kernicterus (near term)
Tetracyclines	Fetal teeth and bone abnormalities
Trimethoprim	Folate antagonist (1st trimester)
Anticonvulsants	Dysmorphic syndrome, anomalies
Antithyroid agents	Fetal goiter
Aspirin	Bleeding, antepartum and postpartum
Cytotoxic agents, i.e., methotrexate	Multiple anomalies
Isotretinoin	Hydrocephalus, deafness, anomalies
Lithium	Congenital heart disease (Ebstein anomaly)
Methotrexate	Anomalies
Nonsteroidal anti-inflammatory drugs (prolonged use after 32 weeks)	Oligohydramnios, constriction of fetal ductus arteriosus
Thalidomide	Phocomelia
Warfarin	Embryopathy—nasal hypoplasia, optic atrophy

TABLE 105-2 Medication Use During Breast-Feeding

CONTRAINDICATED DRUGS

Amphetamines
Aspirin (high doses)
Bromocriptine (Parlodel)
Cytotoxic agents
Ergotamine
Lithium
Radiopharmaceuticals

EFFECTS ON NURSING INFANTS UNKNOWN BUT OF POTENTIAL CONCERN

Metronidazole (Flagyl)
Psychotropic drugs
Antianxiety drugs
Antidepressant drugs
Antipsychotic drugs

DRUG AFFECTING THE MILK SUPPLY

Decongestants
Diuretics
Combination oral contraceptives

DRUGS USUALLY CONSIDERED COMPATIBLE WITH BREAST-FEEDING

Analgesics	Antihypertensives
Antiasthmatics	Antithyroid agents
Antibiotics (most)	Corticosteroids
Anticoagulants	Digoxin
Anticonvulsants	Narcotics
Antiemetics	Oral contraceptives
Antihistamines	Sedatives

Source: Adapted in part from: American Academy of Pediatrics Policy Statement. The transfer of drugs and other chemicals into human milk. *Pediatrics* 108:776, 2001.

TABLE 105-3 Radiation Exposure to the Uterus/Fetus

Dosage, rad	Procedure
0.00005	Chest radiography (two views) with shielding of the maternal abdomen.
0.686–1.398	Intravenous pyelogram full series; in the case of a suspected stone a one-shot pyelogram should be used when a renal ultrasound is inconclusive or unavailable
.1	Kidney, ureter, bladder—single abdominal film
0.51–0.126	Lumbar spine series (three films)
0.168–0.359	Lumbosacral spine series (three films)
0.007–0.02	Mammography—diagnostic for suspected breast cancers
0.01	Cerebral angiography
0.056	Upper gastrointestinal series
1.9–3.9	Barium enema
<0.1	Head computed tomography (CT)
<1	Chest CT
3.5	Abdominal CT
3.5	Lumbar spine CT
0.25	Pelvimetry CT
3.6	IVP

Sources: Brent RL, Gorson RO: Radiation exposure in pregnancy. In: Current Problems in Radiology. Technic of pneumoencephalography. Chicago: Year Book Medical, 1972; National Council on Radiation Protection and Measurements: *Medical radiation exposure of pregnant and potentially pregnant women.* NCRP Report no 54. Bethesda, MD, The Council, 1977; Cunningham FG, MacDonald PC, Gant NF, et al (eds). *William Obstetrics,* 20th ed. Stamford, CN; Appleton & Lange, 1997; American College of Obstetricians and Gynecologists, Committee on Obstetric Practice: *Guidelines for diagnostic imaging during pregnancy.* ACOG Committee opinion no 158. Washington, DC, ACOG, 1995; and Gray JE: Safety (risk) of diagnostic radiology exposures. In: American College of Radiology. Radiation risk: A primer. Reston, VA, American College of Radiology, 1996.

15) may result in mental restriction, small head size, and decreased IQ. Other possible but less likely effects due to significant exposure during this period include growth restriction as an adult and sterility. Even less likely but still possible are cataracts, neuropathology, and growth restriction at term.

Most of the deterministic effects just mentioned are either not observed or observed much less frequently when the fetus receives a significant radiation dose beyond 15 weeks after conception. Mental retardation has been observed as a result of significant exposure during the eighth to twenty-fifth weeks but not beyond. Other effects that have been observed because of exposure after week 15 include sterility and growth restriction as an adult. Less likely effects that have been demonstrated are cataracts, neuropathology, and growth retardation at term.

The most recent evidence suggests that 10 rad is a threshold for human teratogenesis, and the fetus appears to be most vulnerable at 8 to 15 weeks' gestation.[27] However, cumulative doses from multiple procedures may enter the harmful range. The radiation doses involved in commonly used diagnostic tests are given in Table 105-3.

A common nuclear medicine imaging study used by the ED physician is the ventilation-perfusion scan. Total fetal exposure to xenon-133 and technetium-99m is about 0.5 rad, and they can be used safely in pregnancy. Fetal exposure from other studies using technetium-99 range from 0.03 to 0.06 rad/mCi and is safe in pregnancy. Because the excretion of these radionuclide particles is often via the maternal bladder, which is close to the fetus, hydration and frequent voiding need to be encouraged.

The two nonionizing imaging studies used frequently are ultrasound and MRI. Ultrasound has been extensively studied over the past 25 years and has no known teratogenic effect. There is much less experience with MRI, but thus far there are no known harmful effects.

REFERENCES

1. Cousins L: Pregnancy complications among diabetic women 1965–1985. *Obstet Gynecol Surv* 42:140, 1987.
2. Coustan DR, Reece RA, Sherwin R, et al: A randomized clinical trial of insulin pump vs intensive conventional therapy in diabetic pregnancies. *JAMA* 255:631, 1986.
3. Frishman WH, Chesner M: Beta-adrenergic blockers in pregnancy. *Am Heart J* 115:147, 1988.
4. Schroeder JS, Harrison DC: Repeated cardioversion during pregnancy. *Am J Cardiol* 27:445, 1971.
5. Jaffe R, Gruber A, Fejgin M, et al: Pregnancy with an artificial pacemaker. *Obstet Gynecol Surv* 42:137, 1987.
6. McColl MD, Ramsay JE, Tait RC, et al: Risk factors for pregnancy-associated venous thromboembolism. *Thromb Haemost* 78(4):1183, 1997.
7. Macklon NS, Greer IA: Venous thromboembolic disease in obstetrics and gynaecology. The Scottish experience. *Scot Med J* 41:83, 1996.
8. Clark SL and the National Asthma Education Program Working Group on Asthma in Pregnancy, National Institutes of Health, NHBLI: Asthma in pregnancy. *Obstet Gynecol* 82:1036, 1993.
9. Brancazio LR, Laifer SA, Schwartz T: Peak expiratory flow rate in normal pregnancy. *Obstet Gynecol* 89:383, 1997.
10. National Asthma Education Working Group: *Management of Asthma during Pregnancy: Report of the Working Group on Asthma and Pregnancy.* NIH publication no 93-3279. Bethesda, MD, National Heart Lung and Blood Institute, NIH, US Department of Health and Human Services, 1993.
11. Lucas MJ, Cunningham FG: Urinary tract infection during pregnancy. *Clin Obstet Gynecol* 36:855, 1993.
12. Whalley P: Bacteriuria of pregnancy. *Am J Obstet Gynecol* 97:732, 1967.

13. Harris RE, Gilstrap LC III: Cystitis during pregnancy. A distinct clinical entity. *Obstet Gynecol* 57:578, 1981.

14. Gilstrap LC, Cunningham FG, Whalley PJ: Acute pyelonephritis in pregnancy. An anterospective study. *Obstet Gynecol* 57:409, 1981.

15. Fein AM, Duvivier R: Sepsis in pregnancy. *Clin Chest Medicine* 13:709, 1992.

16. Towers CV, Kaminskas CM, Garite TJ, et al: Pulmonary injury, associated with antepartum pyelonephritis. Can patients at risk be identified? *Am J Obstet Gynecol* 164:974, 1991.

17. Koshy M, Burd L, Wallace D, et al: Prophylactic red cell transfusion in pregnant patients with sickle cell disease. *New Engl J Med* 319:1447, 1988.

18. Serjeant GR, Serjeant BE, Thomas PW, et al: Human parvovirus in homozygous sickle cell disease. *Lancet* 341:1237, 1993.

19. Recommendations of the USPHS task force on the use of zidovudine to reduce the perinatal transmission of HIV. *MMWR* 43:1, 1994.

20. Shiono PH, Klebanoff MA, Nugent RP, et al: The impact of cocaine and marijuana use on low birth weight and preterm birth: A multicenter study. *Am J Obstet Gynecol* 172:19, 1995.

21. Bauer CR, Shankaran S, Bada HS, et al: The Maternal Lifestyle Study: Drug exposure during pregnancy and short-term maternal outcomes. *Am J Obstet Gynecol* 186:487, 2002.

22. Markovic N, Ness RB, Cefilli D, et al: Substance use measures among women in early pregnancy. *Am J Obstet Gynecol* 183:627, 2000.

23. Kline J, Ng SK, Schittini M, et al: Cocaine use during pregnancy: Sensitive detection by hair assay. *Am J Public Health* 87(3):352.

24. Vega WA, Kolady B, Hung J, et al: Prevalence and magnitude of perinatal substance exposure in California. *New Engl J Med* 329:852, 1993.

25. Mayer L, Liebschutz: Domestic violence in the pregnant patient: Obstetric and behavioral interventions. *Obstet Gynecol Surv* 53:627, 1998.

26. Rhodes KV, Lauderdale DS, He T, et al: Between me and the computer: Increased detection of intimate partner violence using a computer questionnaire. *Am Emerg Med* 40:476, 2002.

27. American College of Obstetricians and Gynecologists, Committee on Obstetric Practice. Guidelines for diagnostic imaging during pregnancy. ACOG Committee opinion no. 158. Washington, DC: ACOG, 1995.

106 EMERGENCIES DURING PREGNANCY AND THE POSTPARTUM PERIOD
Gloria J. Kuhn

While the majority of pregnancies in the United States result in the delivery of a healthy infant from a healthy mother, there are conditions that can complicate the natural course of pregnancy. The birth rate in 2000 was 14.8 births per 1000 population, an increase of 2 percent from 1999.[1] This translates to a large population of patients who may require emergency care. This chapter discusses diseases that have the potential of complicating pregnancy and increasing morbidity and mortality rates for either the mother or the fetus.

MORTALITY AND MORBIDITY RATES

One of the national health objectives for the year 2000 was to reduce the overall *maternal mortality ratio* (MMR), defined as the number of maternal deaths per 100,000 live-born infants, to no more than 3.3. However, during 1982–1996, the MMR remained at approximately 7.5.[2] An increase was seen among women of all races. A higher risk of pregnancy-related death is associated with increasing maternal age, increasing live-birth order, absent prenatal care, unmarried status,[3] and minority race.[2]

Direct maternal death includes the death of the mother due to obstetric complications of pregnancy, labor, or the puerperium. Indirect maternal death includes death not directly due to obstetric causes but resulting from previously existing disease or a disease that developed during the gravid period or was exacerbated by the pregnancy.

The black-white mortality rate differential is greatest for diseases seen in the first trimester: ectopic pregnancy, spontaneous abortion,

induced abortion, and gestational trophoblastic disease (GTD). Maternal mortality rates remain stable despite evidence that many maternal deaths are preventable.[4] The leading causes of pregnancy-related deaths are hemorrhage, pulmonary embolism (mostly thromboembolic), and hypertensive disorders of pregnancy (leading to cerebrovascular accident).[3]

EMERGENCIES DURING THE FIRST HALF OF PREGNANCY

While pregnancy is usually considered in terms of trimesters, when discussing patterns of emergencies, dividing pregnancy into halves is advantageous. Emergencies during the first half include ectopic pregnancy, vaginal bleeding, GTD, urinary tract infection (UTI), and hyperemesis gravadarum.

Vaginal Bleeding

The differential diagnosis of vaginal bleeding during the first trimester is shown in Table 106-1. Any woman of childbearing age who presents with a chief complaint of abdominal pain or vaginal bleeding and has not had a hysterectomy should be tested for pregnancy. If a serum or urine pregnancy test result is positive, further evaluation, particularly for ectopic pregnancy or spontaneous abortion, is indicated. Ectopic pregnancy is discussed in Chap. 103. Women of childbearing age with syncope, hypotension, or mental status changes should have pregnancy testing and ectopic pregnancy considered within the differential diagnosis.

Abortion

The World Health Organization (WHO) defines spontaneous abortion as loss of pregnancy before 20 weeks or loss of a fetus weighing less than 500 g. Estimates of pregnancies that abort spontaneously range from 20 to 40 percent. About 75 percent of spontaneous abortions occur before 8 weeks of gestation. *Threatened abortion* is defined as pregnancy-related bloody vaginal discharge or frank bleeding during the first half of pregnancy without cervical dilatation. *Inevitable abortion* will occur in the face of vaginal bleeding and dilatation of the cervix. *Incomplete abortion* is defined as passage of only parts of the products of conception and is more likely to occur between 6 and 14 weeks of pregnancy. *Complete abortion* is passage of all fetal tissue, including trophoblast and all products of conception, before 20 weeks of conception. *Missed abortion* is a fetal death at less than 20 weeks without passage of any fetal tissue for 4 weeks after fetal death. *Septic abortion* is evidence of infection during any stage of abortion.

The most common cause of fetal wastage is chromosomal abnormalities, accounting for 50 to 60 percent of all losses. Related and other risk factors include advanced maternal age, prior poor obstetric history, concurrent medical disorders, previous abortion, certain infections (including syphilis and HIV), and some anatomic abnormalities of the upper genital tract. Exposure to some agents, such as certain anesthetic agents, certain heavy metals, and tobacco, is also thought to contribute to the incidence of abortion.

A pelvic examination is mandatory as part of the history and physical examination in order to define the type of abortion, determine the

TABLE 106-1   Common Causes of Bleeding During the First Trimester of Pregnancy

Abortion*
Ectopic pregnancy
Gestational trophoblastic disease
Implantation bleeding (physiologic)
Cervical ectropion cervicitis infection

*Very common.

amount and site of bleeding, whether the cervix has dilated, and whether any tissue has been passed. The amount of bleeding as pads used per hour, last menstrual period, and past medical and obstetric history should be part of the history obtained.

A complete blood count (CBC), blood type, Rh factor and antibody screen, urinalysis (UTI has been associated with increased fetal wastage), and quantitative serum beta human chorionic gonadotropin (β-hCG) level should be obtained. Vaginal ultrasound studies should be performed to rule out ectopic pregnancy, as a prognostic tool for fetal viability, and to diagnose retained products of conception.

If the patient is bleeding heavily, a Yankauer suction tip is useful to suction blood from the vaginal vault. All material in the vaginal vault should be examined to determine whether it is blood clot or products of conception. Products of conception should be sent for pathologic examination. If tissue is protruding from the cervical os, its careful removal with ring forceps may allow the os to close and decrease bleeding. However, care must be taken to ensure that the tissue is not the rare cervical ectopic pregnancy. If profuse bleeding continues in the face of inevitable abortion, 20 units of oxytocin can be added to 1 L of NS solution and infused at 150 to 200 mL per h to obtain hemostasis until dilatation and curettage (D&C) can be arranged. If hemodynamic instability is present, fluid resuscitation should be started immediately.

The quantitative β-hCG analysis may be very helpful. The beta-subunit of hCG is first detectable as early as 9 to 11 days following ovulation (usually 24 days after the last menstrual period) and reaches 200 IU/mL at the expected time of menses.[5] An abnormally high β-hCG level suggests advanced pregnancy, multiple gestation, GTD, or rarely, an ovarian tumor.

Ultrasound studies combined with determinations of β-hCG levels can be both diagnostic and prognostic. If the β-hCG level is greater than 1,500 IU/mL, an intrauterine gestation should be visible using transvaginal technique. (Note: The 1500 IU/mL is somewhat arbitrary and the value is set at each institution. In some institutions, the value is set at 1000 IU/mL or even lower.) A yolk sac is seen at 36 days, and a heartbeat is noted 41 to 47 days after the last menstrual period. Gestational sacs with a mean diameter greater than 25 mm without an embryo or greater than 20 mm without a yolk sac are definitely abnormal, and loss of pregnancy will result.[5]

Patients with a diagnosis of threatened abortion can be discharged safely if close follow-up is ensured. While low level of activity and even bed rest are sometimes advised, there is no proven effectiveness of this practice. Generally speaking, a miscarriage cannot be avoided. Intercourse and tampons are to be avoided to minimize likelihood of infection. The patient with an incomplete abortion should have the uterus evacuated. The patient with a complete abortion, as shown by ultrasound and/or complete passage of products of conception, can be discharged safely after follow-up is ensured to ascertain that the bleeding has stopped. If there is any doubt, obstetrics consultation for possible D&C should be initiated. The patient with a nonviable fetus can be either admitted or discharged to be followed up within a week by her physician, depending on the comfort level of the patient and physician with this decision. Warnings should be given to return immediately if there is heavy bleeding (more than one pad per hour for 6 h), pain, or fever.

If unsensitized, all pregnant patients with vaginal bleeding who are Rh-negative should be treated with Rh_0 (D) immune globulin (Rhogam). Because the total fetal blood volume at 12 weeks is less than 4.2 mL, the volume of fetal blood for admixture during the first trimester is small. Some authorities suggest using only 150 µg Rhogam, and others recommend a dose as small as 50 µg. There is no uniform agreement, and many continue to recommend the full dose. This is discussed in detail in Chap. 254. Ideally, Rhogam should be administered prior to discharge, but it also can be administered within 72 h by the primary care physician or obstetrician when the woman presents several days or weeks after vaginal bleeding has begun.

Gestational Trophoblastic Disease

GTD consists of a broad spectrum of conditions ranging from an uncomplicated partial hydatidiform molar pregnancy to stage IV choriocarcinoma with cerebral metastases. It is a neoplasm that arises in the trophoblastic cells of the placenta. It complicates 1 in 1700 pregnancies in North America and is more common in Asian women. The noninvasive form of the disease is the hydatidiform mole, which is either complete or partial. Complete moles are more common, and in this form there is no actual fetus, whereas in the partial mole a deformed, nonviable fetus is present. Both moles and invasive forms of GTD are composed of trophoblasts that produce β-hCG. Patients with a history of hydatidiform molar pregnancy are at increased risk of future molar pregnancies, with a risk of 1 percent in subsequent gestations after one molar pregnancy and a risk as high as 23 percent after two molar gestations.

Symptoms include vaginal bleeding in the first or second trimester (75 to 95 percent of cases) and hyperemesis (26 percent). GTDs, or molar pregnancies, that persist into the second trimester are associated with preeclampsia. When pregnancy-induced hypertension is seen prior to 24 weeks of gestation, the possibility of a molar pregnancy should be considered. The uterus is excessive in size for gestational age and shows a placenta with many lucent areas interspersed with brighter areas on ultrasound study. Since not all molar pregnancies are found on ultrasonography, all tissue extracted from the uterus on suction curettage or during pelvic examination should be sent for histologic examination.[6] If GTD is suspected because of abnormally high β-hCG levels, a uterine size either larger or smaller than expected, and ultrasound findings suggestive of the diagnosis, obstetric consultation should be obtained. Treatment is by suction curettage in the hospital setting because of risk of hemorrhage. β-hCG levels that fail to decrease after evaluation are evidence of persistent or invasive disease necessitating chemotherapy. Metastasis to lung, liver, and brain may occur, but the prognosis for most patients is very good. Trophoblastic embolization, although extremely rare, may occur, with resulting rapid onset of respiratory distress resembling amniotic fluid embolus.

Nausea, Vomiting, and Hyperemesis Gravidarum

Nausea and vomiting of pregnancy (NVP) generally are seen in the first 12 weeks and affect 60 and 80 percent, respectively. Most cases are usually mild. The etiology is unknown, but NVP is thought to be associated with a protective function because some studies have shown a lower rate of miscarriages in women with NVP.[7] Severe NVP is known as *hyperemesis gravidarum* and is defined as intractable vomiting with weight loss, volume depletion, and laboratory values showing hypokalemia or ketonemia. It occurs in up to 2 percent of all pregnancies. Patients with GTD also may present with intractable vomiting. The cause is not known. Women who lose more than 5 percent of prepregnancy body weight have an increased risk of intrauterine growth restriction and low-birth-weight infants.

The presence of abdominal pain in NVP or hyperemesis gravidarum is highly unusual and should suggest another diagnosis. Ruptured ectopic pregnancies occasionally present with nausea and vomiting as well as diarrhea and abdominal pain. After the first trimester, the volume of the gallbladder increases during fasting and after contraction after a meal. Also, biliary sludge seems to increase in pregnancy in 30 percent, predisposing to stone formation. Cholelithiasis and cholecystitis are more common in pregnant women than in women of comparable age and health status who are not pregnant. Differential diagnosis of vomiting or vomiting with abdominal pain should include cholecystitis, cholelithiasis, gastroenteritis, pancreatitis, hepatitis, peptic ulcer, pyelonephritis, ectopic pregnancy, and fatty liver of pregnancy, and HELLP syndrome (see below).

Findings on physical examination in NVP are usually normal except for signs of volume depletion. Laboratory tests to consider include

CBC, determination of serum electrolytes, BUN, creatinine, and urinalysis. The finding of ketonuria is important because it is an early sign of starvation. However, there is no evidence in the literature that ketosis per se is harmful to the fetus. Serial measurements of urinary ketones can be used to determine success of therapy.

Treatment consists of intravenous fluids containing 5% glucose in either LR or NS to replete volume and reverse ketonuria. A number of antiemetic drugs can be used (Table 106-2) for patients who remain nauseated or continue to vomit. Initially, the patient should be given nothing by mouth. Oral fluids should be started after the nausea and vomiting are controlled but prior to discharge.

The patient may be discharged after reversal of ketonuria, correction of electrolyte imbalance, and a successful trial of oral fluids. Discharge with antiemetic medication is usually necessary. There is no clear drug of choice.

Phenothiazines have the disadvantage of causing drowsiness or dystonic reactions in some patients. Ondansetron (Zofran) (8 mg IV or 4 mg PO three times daily) can cause headache, constipation, diarrhea, or light-headedness. It does not cause dystonia. Its chief disadvantage is cost. It is apparently no more effective than promethazine.[8] Bendectin (doxylamine and pyridoxine), a mainstay of therapy in the past, was discontinued due to fears of teratogenicity, but recent information suggests it does not represent an increase in fetal risk.[9]

Admission guidelines include uncertain diagnosis, intractable vomiting, persistent ketone or electrolyte abnormalities after volume repletion, and weight loss of over 10 percent of prepregnancy weight.

EMERGENCIES DURING THE SECOND HALF OF PREGNANCY

Hypertension, Preeclampsia, Eclampsia, and HELLP Syndrome

Hypertensive disorders of pregnancy remain the second most common cause of maternal death in the United States (after thromboembolic disease), accounting for 15 percent of maternal deaths. Hypertension is also implicated in abruptio placentae and in the birth of preterm and low-birth-weight infants. Hypertension during pregnancy is defined as a blood pressure of 140/90 mm Hg or greater or a 20-mm Hg rise in the systolic or 10-mm Hg rise in the diastolic blood pressure. Thus **a normal-appearing blood pressure may in fact be in the preeclampsia range for a given patient.** Hypertension during pregnancy may be classified as (1) chronic hypertension, (2) preeclampsia superimposed on chronic hypertension, (3) transient hypertension, and (4) preeclampsia or eclampsia. Transient hypertension develops after the midtrimester, is mild, does not compromise the pregnancy, and regresses postpartum but may return in subsequent gestations.

Preeclampsia is the combination of hypertension and proteinuria with or without pathologic edema that occurs in the second half of pregnancy. The cause of preeclampsia is not known, but recent research suggests that there are fewer placental cytotrophoblasts in women who will develop preeclampsia. These do not invade as deeply, remaining in an early stage and failing to take on the characteristics of blood vessel cells.[10] Whatever the placental abnormality, the end result is widespread vasospasm and endothelial injury. There is no test to detect women at risk for the disease, nor is there effective therapy to prevent preeclampsia. The disease complicates 5 to 10 percent of pregnancies. There are multiple risk factors (Table 106-3). It is a clinical diagnosis that includes persistent elevation of blood pressure to 140/90 mm Hg or higher after 20 weeks' gestation, proteinuria (urine protein concentration of 0.1 g/L or more in at least two random urine specimens collected 6 h or more apart or 0.3 g per d in a 24-h collection), and usually edema (Table 106-4). From the ED perspective, even a single blood pressure reading of 140/90 mm Hg or higher is sufficient to indicate further ED evaluation of preeclampsia (see below). Presenting complaints may include headache, visual disturbances, edema, or abdominal pain. It always occurs after 20 weeks of gestation unless GTD is present. **The treatment for preeclampsia is delivery of the fetus.** In mild preeclampsia (asymptomatic, trace protein only) the decision regarding delivery is more complicated. When the woman is less than 37 weeks' gestation, the question of whether the fetus is mature enough for delivery without significant morbidity arises. The decision is further complicated by the fact that uteroplacental blood flow is already reduced by about 50 percent by the time the patient develops clinical signs of preeclampsia. There are currently few data that have shown the value of antihypertensive medication to improve either maternal or fetal outcome in mild preeclampsia.

TABLE 106-2 Antiemetics

Antiemetic	Brand Name	FDA Category	Oral	Rectal	Intravenous
ACUTE INTERVENTION FOR BOTH N/V AND HG					
Promethazine	Phenergan	C	25 mg q4h	25 mg q4h	25–50 mg IV push 50 mg in 500 mL NS over 2 h
Prochlorperazine	Compazine		10 mg q6–8h	25 mg q12h	10 mg over 2 min Maximum of 40 mg q24h
Chlorpromazine	Thorazine	C	10–25 mg q4–6h	100 mg q6–8h	25 mg in 500 mL NS at 250 mL/h
MAINTENANCE THERAPY FOR N/V					
Doxylamine with pyridoxine	Unisom Vitamin B$_6$		25 mg every evening 25 mg q8h		
Diphenhydramine	Benadryl	B	26–50 mg q6h		
Cisapride	Propulsid	C	10 mg q6h		
MAINTENANCE THERAPY FOR HG					
Metoclopramide	Reglan	B			10 mg over 1–2 min q4–6h or 1 mg/kg in 50 mL D5 1/2 NS, over 30 min
Trimethobenzamide	Tigan	C	250 mg q6–8h	200 mg q6–8h	Should not be given IV May be given 200 mg IM q6–8h
Ondansetron	Zofran	B	4–8 mg bid	—	8 mg IV over 5 min

Abbreviations: FDA = US Food and Drug Adminstration; HG = hyperemesis gravidarum; N/V = nausea and vomiting of pregnancy.
Source: From Pearlman M, Tintinalli JE (eds): *Emergency Care of the Woman.* New York, McGraw-Hill, 1998, with permission.

TABLE 106-3   Risk Factors for Development of Hypertension during Pregnancy

Nulliparity
Age >40 years
Prepregnancy hypertension
Chronic renal disease
African-American heritage
Diabetes mellitus
Multiple gestation
Gestational trophoblastic disease
Obesity
Previous history of preeclampsia

Severe preeclampsia is a systolic blood pressure of 160 mm Hg or greater systolic or 110 mm Hg or greater diastolic, proteinuria of at least 5 g/24 h, microangiopathic hemolysis, thrombocyopenia, elevated serum transaminase levels, uterine growth restriction, or symptoms of end-organ involvement such as headache, visual disturbances, or abdominal pain.

Eclampsia is the superimposition of seizures on preeclampsia or aggravated hypertension. Seizures are defined as eclamptic if they occur from the twentieth week of gestation to 7 days after delivery but have been reported as late as 1 month after delivery. All chronic hypertensive disorders, regardless of their cause, predispose to the development of preeclampsia or eclampsia. Blood pressure alone is not always a dependable indicator of severity of disease and must be evaluated in the context of other signs and symptoms.[11] It should be remembered that during normal pregnancy, blood pressure decreases gradually to a nadir between 14 and 24 weeks and then increases to prepregnancy values in the third trimester.

The *HELLP syndrome* (an acronym for *h*emolysis, *e*levated *l*iver enzymes, and *l*ow *p*latelets) is an important clinical variant of preeclampsia that has a predilection for the multigravid patient (in contrast with the primigravida, in whom preeclampsia is more common). In the HELLP syndrome, the blood pressure is variable and may not be elevated initially. This fact, combined with the usual complaint of epigastric or right upper quadrant pain, makes it easy to mistake the HELLP syndrome for other causes of abdominal pain, such as gastroenteritis, hepatitis, pancreatitis, or pyelonephritis. The HELLP syndrome should be considered in any pregnant or postpartum patient who presents to the ED with a chief complaint of abdominal pain. The diagnosis can be made based on clinical findings coupled with laboratory results (Table 106-5).

All patients with a sustained blood pressure of 140/90 mm Hg or greater and any symptoms that may be secondary to hypertension need emergency obstetric consultation and consideration for hospitalization. A patient with severe hypertension whose blood pressure is greater than 140/90 mm Hg and who has epigastric or liver tenderness, visual disturbance, or severe headache is managed in the same way as a patient with eclampsia, i.e., with administration of magnesium sulfate, antihypertensive drugs as needed, and delivery of the fetus. The dose of IV magnesium sulfate is 4 to 6 g over 15 min, followed by IV infusion of 1 to 2 g per h. Reflexes and serum magnesium

TABLE 106-4   Criteria for Hypertension, Preeclampsia, and Eclampsia

Hypertension	BP >140/90 measured twice at least 6 h apart
Transient hypertension	BP >140/90 without other signs of preeclampsia or eclampsia
Preeclampsia	BP >140/90, or >20 mm Hg rise in systolic, or >10 mm Hg rise in diastolic BP
	Proteinuria (300 mg/24 h or 1 g/mL)
	Generalized or pedal edema or weight gain of at least 5 lb over 1 week
Eclampsia	Above findings plus generalized seizure

TABLE 106-5   Laboratory Evaluation for Suspected Preeclampsia or HELLP Syndrome

Test	Findings in HELLP Syndrome
CBC and peripheral smear	Schistocytes
Platelet count	<100,000 but suspicious if <150,000
Liver function tests (AST, ALT)	Elevated but below levels usually seen in viral hepatitis (<500 IU/L)
Renal function tests	Normal or elevated BUN and creatinine levels
Coagulation profile	Abnormal

Abbreviations: ALT = alanine aminotransferase; AST = aspartate aminotransferase; BUN = blood urea nitrogen.

levels should be followed to avoid neuromuscular depression. Angiotensin-converting enzyme (ACE) inhibitors never should be used because of fetal side effects.

Complications of severe preeclampsia, HELLP syndrome, and eclampsia include spontaneous hepatic and splenic hemorrhage, end-organ failure, abruptio placentae, intracranial bleeding, and death of the fetus. Emergency obstetric consultation should be obtained, or transfer to a tertiary care hospital should be arranged as soon as the patient is stabilized.

Methyldopa is the drug used most often to treat pregnant patients with chronic hypertension because use of this drug does not adversely affect the fetus.[11] Dosage can be started at 250 mg every 6 h and titrated for control of blood pressure. Sedation may occur during initiation of therapy or when dosage is increased but usually is transient. Obstetric consultation should be obtained before beginning therapy because there is controversy over the efficacy of treatment of hypertension in the prevention of complications to mother and fetus.

Vaginal Bleeding During the Second Half of Pregnancy

The differential diagnosis of vaginal bleeding during the second half of pregnancy includes abruptio placentae, placenta previa, preterm labor, and bleeding from various lesions of the cervix and lower genital tract. One-third of fetuses die when vaginal bleeding occurs after 20 weeks of gestation.[12]

ABRUPTIO PLACENTAE   *Abruptio placentae,* premature separation of the normally implanted placenta from the uterine wall, occurs in 1 percent of all pregnancies. It is one of the most dangerous complications for mother and fetus. It should be suspected when a gravid patient presents with the triad of sudden onset of antepartum vaginal bleeding, a tender uterus with increased resting tone, and hypertonic or hyperactive uterine contractions. However, patients may complain of nausea and vomiting or dizziness. Some patients have only mild abdominal cramping. This complication can occur either spontaneously or as the result of trauma to the abdomen. The spontaneous form is far more common, with hypertension the most common risk factor. Other risk factors include maternal trauma, increased maternal age, multiparity, smoking, cocaine use, and previous abruptions. Abruption can be complete, partial, or concealed. If the abruption is concealed (blood does not reach the cervical os), there may be only mild or no vaginal bleeding. Clinical signs and symptoms depend on the size of the abruption, the amount of blood loss, and whether bleeding is evident.

Fetal distress, hypotension, and disseminated intravascular coagulation can develop. Abruptio placentae frequently is misdiagnosed as preterm labor. Complications include fetal death, maternal death from hemorrhage or disseminated intravascular coagulation (DIC), fetomaternal transfusion, and amniotic fluid embolism. Separation of 50 percent or more of the total effective placental area usually results in fetal demise. Ultrasonography will allow the exclusion of placenta previa as an etiology of vaginal bleeding but may not be diagnostic of abruption. Therefore, a high index of suspicion must be maintained in women with shock, an abnormally tender uterus, or hypertonic contractions. Laboratory tests that should be ordered include a CBC, type and crossmatch, coagulation profile, and renal function studies. Approximately 50 percent of patients will have laboratory evidence of a coagulopathy, as shown by thrombocyopenia, prolonged prothrombin time, hypofibrinogenemia, and elevated fibrin split products. A fibrinogen level of less than 200 mg/dL is abnormal, and bleeding may appear when the level is less than 100 mg/dL. DIC should be expected when the fibrinogen level is 150 mg/dL. Crystalloids should be given to maintain maternal volume status and fresh frozen plasma should be given for coagulopathy. Emergency obstetric consultation is necessary whenever abruption is suspected. Cardiotocodynamometry and ultrasound studies are used to monitor fetal well-being, and emergency delivery may be necessary. Tocolytics should not be given by the emergency physician in the presence of suspected abruption.

PLACENTA PREVIA   Placenta previa, implantation of the placenta over the cervical os, accounts for 20 percent of bleeding episodes in the second half of pregnancy. Incidence is increased with multiparity and prior cesarean section. The patient presents with painless bright-red bleeding. This complication should be distinguished from the "bloody show" that is passage of a very small amount of bright-red blood mixed with mucus at the onset of labor. Disruption of the placenta by digital or speculum examination can lead to catastrophic bleeding. **Whenever placenta previa is considered within the differential diagnosis digital and speculum examination should be avoided.** The safest course is to perform an emergency abdominal ultrasound study first because ultrasound is between 93 and 98 percent accurate for diagnosis.[13]

PREMATURE LABOR AND PREMATURE RUPTURE OF MEMBRANES (PROM)   *Preterm (premature) labor* is defined as labor prior to 37 weeks' gestation,[14] whereas *premature rupture of membranes* (PROM) is rupture of membranes prior to onset of labor. Preterm labor occurs in 10 percent of deliveries and is the leading cause of perinatal death and disease, accounting for approximately 85 percent of neonatal deaths not due to lethal genetic or congenital abnormalities.

With advances in prenatal neonatal care, previable PROM includes those with membrane rupture before 23 to 24 weeks. Three major factors contribute to spontaneous or induced delivery before 34 weeks: (1) PROM, (2) spontaneous preterm labor without PROM, and (3) complications that jeopardize fetal or maternal health, mandating early delivery.

Many known factors are associated with preterm labor. More common ones include PROM, abruptio placentae, illicit drug use (particularly of cocaine and amphetamines), multiple gestations, polyhydramnios, cervical incompetence, and infection. Sexually transmitted diseases, including syphilis, gonorrhea, *Chlamydia,* and bacterial vaginosis, are two to three times more likely to be associated with preterm labor. The presence of low-grade infection is felt to be one of the most important causes of PROM because bacterial colonization can reduce the tensile strength of membranes. Of importance is the association of digital pelvic examinations and increased frequency of PROM. As a result of this finding, **cervical examinations should not be performed from 37 weeks' gestation unless the results of the examination clearly will influence clinical management.** All digital examinations during the latter portion of pregnancy performed for emergency reasons should be done using sterile gloves.

Labor is defined as regular uterine contractions resulting in progressive cervical effacement and dilatation. When a woman presents to the ED with the suspected onset of labor, the date of the last menstrual period should be ascertained and the estimated date of delivery calculated. The gestational age is the number of weeks from the first

day of the LMP. If that date is not known, gestational age can be estimated clinically (see Chap. 104). The patient should be asked about the frequency and duration of contractions, about passage of blood-stained mucus ("bloody show"), and whether there has been rupture of membranes, usually signaled by a gush of fluid or constant leakage of fluid.

In addition to the routine physical examination, the fundal height should be measured, fetal heart tones auscultated, and a sterile speculum examination performed. A pooling of fluid in the vaginal vault or leakage of clear fluid from the cervix in the absence of labor is evidence of PROM. If there is no fluid, the woman should be asked to press on the fundus or perform a Valsalva maneuver to determine whether there is leakage of fluid. Any fluid should be tested with nitrazine paper (pH > 6.5 indicates amniotic fluid) and swabbed on a glass slide to be examined for ferning, indicating amniotic fluid. The presence of blood or semen may interfere with both these tests. On visual examination, if the cervix is posterior in the vagina, thick, and closed, it is not yet ripe for labor. In this case, it may be better not to perform a digital examination, but if one must be done, use sterile technique. If, in contrast, it is midposition to anterior within the vagina, moderately effaced, and approximately 2 cm dilated, the uterus is undergoing changes preparatory to delivery. Tests for *Chlamydia,* gonorrhea, and group B streptococcus should be performed and secretions examined for bacterial vaginosis. If PROM is suspected or confirmed, digital examination should be deferred if possible or, if performed, should be done using sterile gloves.

A number of critical questions must be considered. Has PROM occurred? Is the woman in premature labor? What is the best estimate of gestational age? Is there fetal distress? Is the woman a candidate for tocolytic therapy? All women suspected of premature labor or PROM require obstetric consultation.

Viability of the fetus is possible before 23 weeks of gestation, but mortality and morbidity rates are extremely high. A number of drugs have been used to inhibit labor, but none are completely effective. Some are contraindicated, and there is potential for serious side effects (Table 106-6). Tocolysis was the third most common cause of adult respiratory distress syndrome and death in pregnant women in Jackson, Mississippi, over a 14-year period.[15] Since tocolytic drugs can delay delivery by only a few days, the purpose of tocolytic therapy is to allow time for administration of glucocorticoids to speed fetal lung maturity.[16] A typical agent and dose is betamethasone 12 mg IM q24h for 2 doses or dexamethasone 6 mg IM q6h for 4 doses and weekly thereafter. If a patient presents to an ED in preterm labor and the fetus is not mature enough to do well (prior to 34 weeks' gestation), the patient should be transported to a tertiary care facility that has a high-risk intensive care unit for mother and child.

Candidates for tocolysis are women in preterm labor between 24 and 34 to 36 weeks of gestation. Prior to 23 weeks, chances of survival of the fetus are remote and the probability of permanent disability high, but fetal viablity at earlier gestational age is increasing, so the decision to begin tocolytic therapy is complicated. At about 25 weeks, even a 2-day increase in the length of gestation can add 10 percent to the likelihood of neonatal survival. Beyond 34 to 36 weeks, the infant should be mature enough to do well without specific treatment, and the possible side effects of tocolysis are to be avoided.

There is no clear protocol for management that results in a favorable outcome.[17,18] The decision to institute tocolysis and the drugs used should be made by the obstetrician who can explain the risks and benefits to the patient (see Table 106-6). Tocolytics (Table 106-7) should not be given if abruption is suspected. The American College of Gynecology has issued a practice bulletin for the management of preterm labor.[19]

The value of antibiotics has not been elucidated clearly. Infection has been shown to be associated with both preterm labor and PROM, as well as fetal morbidity, but whether use of antibiotics can prevent these complications is not clear.[18,20] Therefore, administration of an-

TABLE 106-6   Contraindications and Potential Complications to Tocolytics

Contraindications	Maternal Effects	Fetal and Neonatal Effects
β-ADRENERGICS		
Cardiac arrhythmias	Arrhythmias, ACS, CHF, hyperglycemia, hypokalemia, antidiuresis, altered thyroid function	Fetal tachycardia, hyperglycemia, cardiac hypertrophy, cardiac ischemia
Poorly controlled thyroid disease		
Poorly controlled diabetes mellitus	Physiologic tremor, nervousness, nausea and vomiting, fever, hallucinations	Neonatal tachycardia, hypocalcemia, hyperbilirubinemia, hypotension, intraventricular hemorrhage
MAGNESIUM SULFATE		
Myasthenia gravis	Flushing, lethargy, headache, muscle weakness, diplopia, dry mouth, CHF, cardiac arrest	Lethargy, hypotonia, respiratory depression, demineralization*
CALCIUM CHANNEL BLOCKERS		
Cardiac disease	Flushing, headache, dizziness, nausea, transient hypotension	None known
Caution with renal disease, avoid with magnesium		
PROSTAGLANDIN SYNTHETASE INHIBITORS		
Major renal or hepatic impairment	Nausea, dyspepsia	Constriction of DA, pulmonary impaired renal function (reversible) with oligohydramnios, intraventricular hemorrhage, hyperbilirubinemia, necrotizing enterocolitis
Active PUD		
Coagulation disorders, thrombocytopenia		
NSAID-sensitivity		

*With prolonged use.

Abbreviations: ACS = acute coronary syndrome; CHF = congestive heart failure; DA = ductus arteriosus; PUD = peptic ulcer disease.

Source: Adapted from Hearne AE, Nagey DA: *Clin Obstet Gynecol* 43(4):787, 2000.

tibiotics prior transfer should be a shared decision between the transferring and receiving physicians.

EMERGENCIES DURING THE POSTPARTUM PERIOD

Pulmonary embolus (PE) as a complication of deep venous thrombosis (DVT) is one of the most common causes of maternal death either during pregnancy or in the postpartum period. Postpartum hemorrhage and infection continue to be the most common emergencies seen during the postpartum period, but amniotic fluid embolism, while rare, is associated with high morbidity and mortality rates for both mother and fetus. **Eclampsia may persist and even present occasionally during the postpartum period.** Among those who developed eclampsia in a large cohort of over 100,000 pregnant patients, almost one third occurred more than 48 h postpartum, with some occurring up to 3 weeks post delivery.[21] Peripartum cardiomyopathy (PPC) is seen during the last month of pregnancy or within 5 months of delivery.

Thromboembolic Disease

The likelihood of venous thromboembolism in normal pregnancy and the puerperium is increased by a factor of 5 when compared with the nonpregnant woman of similar age. Normal consequences of stasis from impeded blood flow and increased clotting predispose toward the formation of thrombosis and the complication of PE. Estimates of DVT during the first postpartum month may be as high as 20 times the estimates in nonpregnant women. The increased risk of PE is greatest in the first few weeks after delivery. Added risk factors include obesity, bed rest, advanced age, prior DVT and varicose veins, trauma, and multiparity. Symptoms of DVT are similar to those in nonpregnant patients. The left leg is involved more commonly. Diagnostic testing by ultrasound is most sensitive for detecting thromboses in the thigh veins. The iliac veins must be imaged by computed tomograhpy (CT) or magnetic resonance imaging (MRI).[22] Half of PEs arise from the iliac veins. The amount of radiation from a CT scan is within acceptable radiation limits for fetal exposure,[23] and MRI may be used after the first trimester. Treatment of DVT of the

TABLE 106-7   Tocolytic Therapy Protocols

Agent	Initial Dose	Maintenance	Comment
Terbutaline	0.25 mg SC	0.25 mg SC q20min up to 3 h or until contractions stop	Hold for pulse >120 beats per min
Ritodrine	50–100 μg IV per min	Increase 50 μg per min q10min (max 350 μg per min) until contractions cease	Cease if side effects develop (see Table 106–7)
Magnesium sulfate	4–6 g IV bolus over 20 min	2–3 g per h	Monitor for side effects
Nifedipine	30 MG PO or 10 mg SL q20min × 3	10–20 mg PO or SL q4–6h	Monitor for side effects
Indomethacin	50 mg PR, or 50–100 mg PO	25–50 mg PO q6h × 48 h	
Kotorolac	60 mg IM	30 mg IM q6h × 48 h	
Sulindac	200 mg PO	200 mg PO q12h 48 h	

Abbreviations: SL = sublingual; PR = per rectum.

Source: Adapted from Hearne AE, Nagey DA: *Clin Obstet Gynecol* 43(4):787, 2000.

thigh is anticoagulation with heparin or low-molecular-weight heparin (LMWH) in standard doses.

PE should be in the differential diagnosis of any pregnant woman complaining of shortness of breath, syncope, chest pain, or shock. The threshold for ordering a CT or ventilation-perfusion scan to diagnose PE should be low. Either of these studies can be performed safely in the pregnant patient. Treatment is similar to that in nonpregnant patients, except for use of warfarin. Thrombolytics can be used.

Postpartum Hemorrhage

Postpartum hemorrhage is implicated in approximately 28 percent of pregnancy-related deaths. Since most postpartum hemorrhages occur in the first 24 h after delivery, unless the delivery takes place at home or in a free-standing birthing center, such patients are unlikely to present to the ED. However, delayed hemorrhage may be seen days to weeks postpartum.

The differential diagnosis of hemorrhage in the period immediately following delivery includes uterine atony, uterine rupture, laceration of the lower genital tract, retained placental tissue, uterine inversion, and coagulopathy. After 24 h, retained products may cause bleeding. Other causes include uterine polyps or a coagulopathy, most commonly von Willebrand disease.

Physiologic bleeding that takes place in the postpartum period may be of variable duration, not uncommonly extending for periods of up to 5 weeks after delivery. The patient should be questioned about difficulty delivering the placenta. Manual delivery of the placenta increases the risk of postpartum hemorrhage.

A careful history and physical examination should elicit the diagnosis in most cases (Table 106-8). The most common cause of bleeding within the first 24 h is uterine atony. Normally, after delivery, the uterus is firm, globular in shape, and palpable at or below the umbilicus. When uterine atony occurs, the uterine fundus is "doughy" in consistency and possibly palpable above the umbilicus. If the tone of the uterus is good but blood is seen to be coming from the cervical os, the possibility of retained products of conception or uterine rupture must be considered. Uterine rupture is more common after prior cesarean section as a result of separation of the scar. Prior uterine surgery and multiparity also can predispose to this complication. Very rarely, rupture occurs in the face of no prior risk factors. Diagnosis of the cause will allow proper treatment.

The management of postpartum hemorrhage depends on stabilization of the patient and diagnosis of the cause of bleeding (see Table 106-9). If bleeding is massive, two large-bore intravenous lines should be started, a CBC and clotting studies should be performed, and the patient should be typed and crossmatched for blood. A red-top tube should be kept by the bedside, and if a clot has not formed by 7 min, a coagulopathy, either causing the bleeding or resulting from the blood loss, may be present.

Good lighting and suction should be maintained. A speculum examination should be performed to inspect for trauma to the vaginal, vulvar, or cervical tissues. Any lacerations should be repaired after local anesthesia is provided. If a laceration is extensive, the patient should be taken immediately to the operating room.

If a mass is seen in the vaginal vault and the uterus cannot be palpated on the abdominal examination, the possibility of uterine inversion is strong. Emergency obstetric consultation is required.

If blood is seen to be coming from the cervix, the possibility of atony or retained products of conception is high. If atony is present and the uterus is large and doughy, the patient should be treated with oxytocin. It is administered by diluting 20 to 30 units in 1 L of NS or LR solution and infusing the fluid at 200 mL per h. Methylergonovine maleate, an alternative agent, can be given at a dose of 0.2 mg IM, has an onset of action of 7 min, and lasts for 2 h. This agent should not be used if hypertension or preeclampsia is present. Once bleeding is controlled, the patient can be discharged on an oral maintenance dose of 0.2 mg methylergonovine every 6 h.

If the uterus has good tone, the possibility of retained products of conception is high. An ultrasound study confirms the diagnosis.

Postpartum Infections

Pelvic infection is the most common serious complication of the puerperium. Any persistent fever over 38.0°C (100.4°F) is caused by genital tract infection until proven otherwise. Extragenital causes of fever include respiratory tract infection (more common after cesarean section), pyelonephritis, mastitis, and thrombophlebitis.

The route of delivery is the single most significant risk factor for uterine infection, with the vast majority of endometrites occurring secondary to cesarean section. Other risk factors include lower socioeconomic level, multiple gestations, younger maternal age, longer duration of labor and membrane rupture, and internal fetal monitoring. Women with these risk factors who were not given antibiotics prophylactically have been found to have a 90 percent rate of pelvic infection. Digital examination after 37 weeks' gestation also is thought to predispose to infection.

The most common pathogens are those which normally reside in the bowel and also colonize the perineum, vagina, and cervix. Both gram-positive and gram-negative aerobes, anaerobes, *Mycoplasma hominis,* and *Chlamydia trachomatis* are seen. *Gardnerella vaginalis* is isolated more often in younger women. Many infections are polymicrobial.

Signs and symptoms of postpartum endometritis are foul-smelling, profuse, bloody discharge and abdominal pain. Only scant discharge may be present, especially in patients with group A β-hemolytic streptococci. Shaking chills suggest bacteremia. Uterine and adnexal tenderness is found on bimanual examination.

Infection may be localized to the decidua and adjacent myometrium and, if this is the case, responds readily to antibiotic therapy. Complications include parametrial phlegmons; surgical, incisional, and pelvic abscesses; infected hematomas; septic pelvic thrombophlebitis; necrotizing fasciitis; and peritonitis. Necrotizing fasciitis is a feared complication with high mortality and morbidity rates. Risk factors for this complication are obesity, diabetes mellitus, and hypertension.

The mainstay of treatment is antibiotic therapy (see below), drainage of any collections of purulent material, and debridement of necrotic tissue. Routine vaginal cultures are of little clinical utility be-

TABLE 106-8   Physical Findings, Cause, and Treatment of Postpartum Hemorrhage

Finding	Cause	Treatment
Enlarged, doughy uterus	Uterine atony	Oxytocin 20–30 U/L at 200 mL per h or methylergonovine maleate 0.2 mg IM and 0.2 mg PO q6h
Globular, firm uterus	Retained products of conception	Dilatation and curettage
Inability to palpate uterus	Uterine inversion	Manual reduction
Blood in vagina but not coming from uterus	Laceration of lower genital tract	Repair in emergency department or operating room
History of cesarean section	Possible uterine rupture	Surgery
Blood does not clot in red-top tube	Coagulopathy	Fresh-frozen plasma

cause of contamination with local flora. Blood culture results are positive in a minority of patients.

Oral antibiotics can be used on an outpatient basis for mild illness, i.e., the disease is confined to the decidua and myometrium. Any patient who appears toxic or moderately ill, has had a cesarean section, or has underlying comorbid conditions should be hospitalized for parenteral therapy. There are many regimens of therapy. The combination of ampicillin and gentamicin is sufficient for 90 percent of patients. The β-lactam antimicrobials have the advantages of being safe and requiring administration of only one drug, thus being cost-effective. Cephalosporins that can be used include cefoxitin (2 g IV every 6 h), cefotetan (2 g IV every 12 h), and cefotaxime (2 g IV every 6 h). Other regimens include clindamycin (500 mg IV every 6 h) and gentamicin (4.2 mg/kg IV daily) or metronidazole (500 mg IV every 8 h) plus ampicillin and an aminoglycoside.

AMNIOTIC FLUID EMBOLUS   Mortality rates between 60 and 80 percent have been reported for amniotic fluid embolism. Neurologic morbidity rates are even higher, and few patients are without sequelae. In a national registry of patients with amniotic fluid embolus, if the amniotic fluid had meconium staining, no mother survived without a neurologic deficit.[24] If the infant is still in utero at the time of the embolus, both mortality and neurologic morbidity rates are high. The only significant relationship found thus far is fetal male sex.

Onset is sudden, with the mother displaying cardiovascular collapse. Seizure or seizure-like activity at the time of collapse is common. Patients display profound cardiovascular instability, severe hypoxemia, and if survival is long enough, DIC. Death is rapid, with many patients dying within 1 h of onset of symptoms.

Care is supportive, with use of high concentrations of oxygen and standard treatment of DIC (see Chap. 219) if the patient survives long enough. Delivery of the infant should be immediate, but infant mortality and morbidity rates remain high even with immediate delivery.[24]

PERIPARTUM CARDIOMYOPATHY   Peripartum cardiomyopathy (PPC) is the development of heart failure during or shortly after labor with no apparent cause. Most women have an underlying cause found during workup for PPC.[25] Causes include chronic hypertension, mitral stenosis, obesity, viral myocarditis, and preeclampsia. Terbutaline administration for tocolysis has been found to have an association with congestive heart failure in patients with no underlying heart disease. In a small group, no cause can be found. PPC appears to be similar to the idiopathic cardiomyopathy seen in young nonpregnant women. Biopsy shows evidence of myocarditis in up to 30 percent.

Patients present with signs and symptoms of congestive heart failure. Dyspnea, orthopnea, cough, palpitations, and chest and abdominal pain are common complaints. Massive dilated cardiac chambers are seen on chest radiograph and echocardiograph. Treatment is with

FIG. 106-1. Algorithm for medical screening of pregnant women. EMC = emergency medical condition; EMTALA = Emergency Medical Treatment and Active Labor Act. (Reproduced with permission from American College of Emergency Physicians: Providing Care under Federal Law: EMTALA. Dallas, ACEP, 2000.)

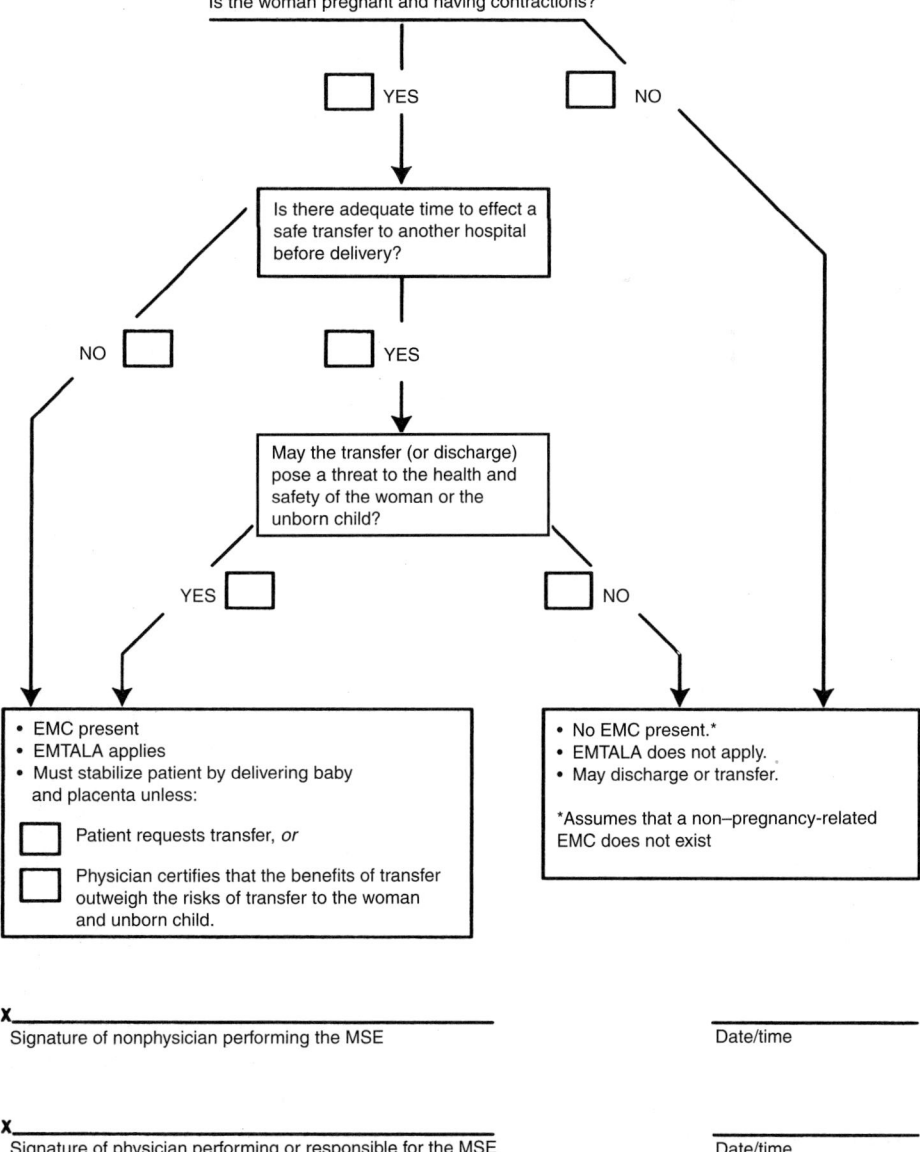

diuretics and fluid restriction. Digitalis should be used with caution because 60 percent of patients have complex ventricular arrhythmias. Afterload reduction has been used, but ACE inhibitors should be avoided if the patient is undelivered. Because of the high association of PE with PPC, anticoagulation with heparin is often recommended. If no underlying cause can be found, the prognosis is very poor, with mortality of almost 50 percent at 1 year. Many survivors demonstrate diminished contractile reserve when studied with dobutamine challenge in periods remote from pregnancy.[25]

TRANSFER OF THE PREGNANT PATIENT

There are times when a pregnant patient will require transfer to another hospital. If the emergency physician works in a hospital that does not provide obstetric services, it is highly recommended that he or she be familiar with the protocols in place for transfer and inpatient care of these patients. The Emergency Medical Treatment and Active Labor Act (EMTALA) specifically addresses the issue of the pregnant patient. All rules and regulations of EMTALA mandating care before and during transfer apply. Additionally, if a woman is having contractions, she is considered to have an emergency medical condition if there is insufficient time for transfer before delivery or the transfer may pose a threat to the health or safety of the child. In this situation, the patient may not be transferred prior to delivery unless the patient requests transfer.[26] If contractions are not present, an emergency medical condition is not automatically present, and the regular rules of providing medical care and determining the need for transfer of patients applies (Figure 106-1).

REFERENCES

1. Hoyert DL, Freedman MA, Strobino DM, et al: Annual summary of vital statistics: 2000. *Pediatrics* 108:1241, 2001.
2. State-specific maternal mortality among black and white women-United States, 1987–1996. *MMWR* 48:492, 1999.
3. Berg CJ, Atrash HK, Koonin LM, et al: Pregnancy-related mortality in the United States, 1987–1990. *Obstet Gynecol* 88:161, 1996.
4. Hoyert DL, Danel I, Tully P: Maternal mortality, United States and Canada, 1982–1997. *Birth* 27:4, 2000.
5. Cacciatore B, Tiitenen A, Stenman U, et al: Normal early pregnancy: Serum hCG levels and vaginal ultrasonography findings. *Br J Obstet Gynaecol* 97:899, 1990.
6. Sebire NJ, Rees H, Paradinas F, et al: The diagnostic implications of routine ultrasound examination in histologically confirmed early molar pregnancies. *Ultrasound Obstet Gynecol* 18:662, 2001.
7. Weigel RM, Weigel MM: Nausea and vomiting of early pregnancy and pregnancy outcome: A meta-analytical review. *Br J Obstet Gynaecol* 96:1312, 1989.
8. Sullivan CA, Johnson CA, Roach H, et al: A pilot study of intravenous ondansetron for hyperemesis gravidarum. *Am J Obstet Gynecol* 174(5):1565, 1996.
9. Brent R: Medical, social, and legal implications of treating nausea and vomiting of pregnancy. *Am J Obstet Gynecol* 186(5 pt 2):S262, 2002.
10. Zhou Y, Damsky C, Fisher SJ: Preeclampsia is associated with failure of human cytotrophoblasts to memic a vascular adhesion phenotype: One cause of defective endovascular invasion in this syndrome? *J Clin Invest* 99:2152, 1997.
11. Sibai BM: Treatment of hypertension in pregnant women. *New Engl J Med* 335:257, 1996.
12. Ajayi RA, Soothill PW, Campbell S, et al: Antenatal testing to predict outcome in pregnancies with unexplained antpartum haemorrhage. *Br J Obstet Gynaecol* 99:122, 1992.
13. Hertzberg BS, Bowie JD, Carroll BA, et al: Diagnosis of placenta previa during the third trimester: Role of transperineal sonography. *AJR* 159:83, 1992.
14. American College of Obstetricians and Gynecologists: Preterm labor. Technical bulletin 206, June 1995.
15. Perry KG, Martin RW, Blake PC, et al: Maternal outcome associated with adult respiratory distress syndrome. *Am J Obstet Gynecol* 174:391, 1996.
16. National Institutes of Health: NIH consensus development statement: Effect of corticosteroids for fetal maturation on perinatal outcomes. Washington, NIH Consensus Develpment Conference, 1994.
17. Berkman ND, Thorp JM Jr, Lohr KN, et al: Tocolytic treatment for the management of preterm labor: A review of the evidence. *Am J Obstet Gynecol* 88(6):1648, June, 2003.
18. Terzidou V, Bennett PR: Preterm labor. *Curr Opin Obstet Gynecol* 14:105, 2002.
19. ACOG, Practice Bulletin, no. 43: Management of preterm labor. *Obstet Gynecol* 101:1039, 2003.
20. Goncalves LF, Chaiworapongsa T, Romero R: Intrauterine infection and prematurity. *Ment Retard Dev Disabil Res Rev* 8:3, 2002.
21. Mattar F, Sibai BM: Eclampsia. VIII. Risk factors for material mobility. *Am J Obstet Gynecol* 182:307, 2000.
22. Spritzer CE, Evans AC, Kay HH: Magnetic resonance imaging of deep venous thrombosis in pregnant women with lower extremity edema. *Obstet Gynecol* 85:603, 1995.
23. Hall EJ: Scientific view of low-level radiation risks. *Radiographics* 11:509, 1991.
24. Clark SL, Hankins GDV, Dudley DA, et al: Amniotic fluid embolism: Analysis of the national registry. *Am J Obstet Gynecol* 172(4):1158, 1996.
25. Witlin AG, Mabie WC, Sibai BM: Peripartum cardiomyopathy: An ominous diagnosis. *Am J Obstet Gynecol* 176:182, 1997.
26. Bitterman R: Special situations: Obstetric and psychiatric patients, in Bitterman R (ed): *Providing Emergency Care under Federal Law: EMTALA.* Dallas, ACEP, 2000, pp 125–148.

EMERGENCY DELIVERY
Michael J. VanRooyen
Kimberly B. Fortner

The anxiety experienced by emergency physicians caring for a woman in active labor is not simply due to the lack of familiarity with normal deliveries but also is due to the awareness of the potential for serious and rarely fatal complications of labor. In addition, the initial management of third-trimester emergencies such as preeclampsia, eclampsia, and hemorrhage has major consequences for maternal and infant survival.

PREHOSPITAL MANAGEMENT

Precipitous delivery in the ED setting is a relatively uncommon phenomenon. With advances in prenatal care and nearly ubiquitous availability of obstetrical units in the United States, the incidence of out-of-hospital delivery has fallen to less than 1 percent of deliveries.[1] However, the desire for planned home deliveries is on the rise and sometimes results in rapid transport to the hospital for difficult deliveries. One study in Washington State found that of 7000 planned home births, 500 women were transferred emergently to the hospital for delivery.[2] Other reasons for out-of-hospital delivery may include poorly educated patients, those with no prenatal care, inadequate preparations by family members, lack of transportation options, remote locations, and premature delivery. A relatively recent and controversial practice is intentional precipitous labor, in which a women desiring to avoid hospital charges delays care until the final stages of labor.

Emergency medical system (EMS) personnel must be trained to recognize active labor and manage the precipitous delivery appropriately. Pregnancy-related complications that may occur in the prehospital setting include preeclampsia, eclampsia, maternal hemorrhage, and complications of labor such as cord prolapse, shoulder dystocia, and fetal distress. This requires an integrated approach to management of the patient in labor, including knowledge by prehospital personnel of available obstetric and neonatal units in the system's catchment area for appropriate transport.

Transport of Pregnant Patients

The need to recognize maternal and neonatal complications in the prehospital setting has become more important with the availability of transport systems for high-risk obstetrical patients to specialty centers. The development of specialty centers has led to a significant decline in neonatal mortality, particularly for infants weighing less than 1500 g at birth. High-risk maternal units have proliferated as well, and as a consequence, transport of pregnant patients for reasons of maternal bleeding, eclampsia or preeclampsia, fetal distress, multiple gestations, fetal anomalies, and other maternal health problems including traumatic injuries has increased markedly. The most common reason for transport of obstetric patients to a tertiary care center is the premature rupture of membranes.

Prehospital units transporting the actively laboring patient should be prepared by carrying sterile delivery packs and medical supplies and medications for maternal and neonatal emergencies (Table 107-1). The transport team should be trained to assist in the precipitous delivery of an infant and educated in the use of basic obstetrical supplies. Prehospital protocols should be reviewed often so that EMS personnel remain prepared for the rare and potentially catastrophic pregnancy-related event.

Emergency Department Preparedness

Whether patients deliver in the prehospital setting or immediately on arriving to the ED, every ED should be prepared for emergency delivery by preparing a basic delivery kit, along with resources for the initial care and potential resuscitation of the newborn. (Tables 107-1 and 107-2). These include an infant warmer/isolette and supplies for neonatal resuscitation (see Chap. 13). Because of the relative infrequency of ED delivery, extra care should be taken to educate physician and nursing staff through educational programs, annual in-services, and equipment orientation sessions.

EVALUATION OF THE PREGNANT PATIENT

Any pregnant woman beyond 20 weeks' gestation who arrives in the ED with signs of active labor should be evaluated carefully to determine the condition of the mother and the fetus. An important component of this is the medical and obstetrical history of the patient, including parity and estimated date of confinement (EDC). If the last menstrual period (LMP) is known and a pregnancy wheel is not available, the EDC can be calculated by adding 9 months and 7 days to the LMP (Naegle rule). Although useful for providing a rough estimate, ultrasound examination late in the third trimester is not an accurate predictor of gestational age because estimates of EDC can vary by ±3 weeks. Fundal height also provides a rapid estimate of gestational age in the patient who does not recall LMP or EDC. Fundal height is measured in centimeters (cm = weeks of gestation ± 2 weeks) from the pubic symphysis to the top of the fundus as palpated by the examiner, although this measurement can be greatly overestimated in obese patients. In addition to the obstetrical history of the patient, it is important to obtain pertinent medical information such as allergies, medications, drug and alcohol use, and prenatal care and to elicit any past history of complications with prior deliveries or precipitous labor.

TABLE 107-1   Equipment and Supplies for Emergency Delivery

Surgical scissors
Placenta basin
Rubber suction bulb
Neonatal airways
Towels
Hemostats
Cord clamps
Sterile gloves
Sterile towels and drapes
Gauze sponge (4 × 4)
Syringes (10 mL)
Needles (23 gauge)

Note: List excludes standard adult and neonatal resuscitation equipment.

TABLE 107-2   Medications for Emergency Delivery and Indications for Use

Medication	Dose	Indication
Oxytocin 10 units/mL	Infuse 2 L of 20 units/L NS solution	Give routinely for uterine contraction and hemostasis immediately post partum
Methyl ergonovine	0.2 mg IM	Control of postpartum hemorrhage
Hydralazine 20 mg/mL	5–10 mg IVP q3–5 min to treat diastolic BP >110 mm Hg	Control of hypertensive crisis (to diastolic BP 80–90 mm Hg)
Magnesium sulfate (50% solution: 5 g/10 mL)	Bolus 4–6 g IV over several minutes	First-line control of eclamptic seizures
Calcium gluconate 10% solution	10 mL IV over several minutes	Magnesium toxicity
Fosphenytoin	10 mg/kg PE loading, followed by second loading dose of 5 mg/kg 2 h later	Second-line drug for eclamptic seizures
Terbutaline sulfate 1 mg/mL	0.25 mg SC q3h	Tocolysis
Fentanyl 50 μg/mL	50 μg (1 mL) q1h	Short-acting opiate analgesic
Lidocaine 1% solution	1–10 mL locally	Local anesthetic
Prochlorperazine 10 mg/2 mL	5–10 mg IV	Nausea and vomiting
Naloxone 0.4 mg/mL	0.8–2 mg IV	Narcotic overdose

Abbreviations: IVP = intravenous push; PE = phenytoin equivalent.

Every patient presenting with signs of active labor should have immediate monitoring of maternal vital signs (particularly blood pressure) and fetal heart rate. Doppler heart tones are helpful to confirm normal fetal heart rate (120–160 beats/min). A persistently slow fetal heart rate (<120 beats/min) is an indicator of fetal distress, and emergent obstetrical consultation is necessary.

Distinguishing True versus False Labor

The confirmation of true labor as opposed to false labor is an important initial step in the management of the term or near-term pregnant patient. *False labor* is defined as uterine contractions that do not lead to cervical changes, and false labor is characterized by irregular, brief contractions usually confined to the lower abdomen. These contractions, commonly called *Braxton-Hicks contractions,* are irregular in both intensity and duration. False labor may be persistent for several days. It is treated most commonly with hydration and rest but uncommonly may require admission with supportive care.

True labor is characterized by painful, repetitive uterine contractions that increase steadily in intensity and duration and lead to progressive effacement and dilatation of the cervix. True labor pains typically begin in the fundal region and upper abdomen and radiate into the pelvis and to the lower back. True labor also leads to progressive descent of the fetus into the pelvis in preparation for delivery and cervical dilatation and effacement.

There are three stages of labor.[3] The first stage begins with the onset of regular uterine contractions and ends with full cervical dilatation. The first stage can then be divided into two phases, latent and active. The latent phase is characterized by uterine contractions that are infrequent, irregular, but moderately uncomfortable and result in gradual cervical changes. This is a preparatory phase in which the uterus is orienting to contractions and the cervix is undergoing effacement and softening. The active phase typically is accepted as starting once the cervix has dilated to 3 to 5 cm and leads to cervical dilatation at an average rate of 1.2 cm/h in nulliparas and 1.5 cm/h in parous women. The second stage of labor, from full dilatation to delivery of the infant, is usually brief and lasts an average of 20 min for parous women and 50 min for nulliparous women. The third stage of labor is from delivery of the infant to delivery of the placenta.

Physical Examination

Patients without vaginal bleeding should be evaluated with a sterile speculum examination and a bimanual examination. Patients presenting with vaginal bleeding should be evaluated with ultrasound prior to any speculum or bimanual examination to rule out placenta previa (see below). The typical method for pelvic examination is in the lithotomy position. Stirrups are not necessary, although they are helpful. Alternatively, an inverted bedpan may be employed to elevate the patient's buttocks enough to allow speculum examination. Lubricant should be avoided unless rupture of membranes has been confirmed because lubricant may produce a false-positive nitrazine test.

If spontaneous rupture of membranes (SROM) is suspected, sterile speculum examination should be performed and digital examination avoided because studies have shown an increased risk of infection after a single digital examination.[4] It is particularly important to avoid digital examinations in the preterm patient in whom prolongation of gestation is desired. Sterile speculum examination allows confirmation of SROM by three tests: verification of pooling of amniotic fluid in the vaginal vault, a positive nitrazine test, and evidence of ferning on a microscope slide. The speculum examination also provides for visualization of the cervix with estimation of dilatation with collection of cervical cultures, in particular, group B *Streptococcus, Neisseria gonorrhoeae,* and *Chlamydia* cultures.

The abdomen should be inspected and palpated to determine fundal height and evaluated for fundal tenderness. The cervix is examined to determine effacement, dilatation, and station. *Effacement* of the cervix refers to the process of thinning that occurs during labor. Effacement conventionally has been described in terms of a percentage of normal cervical length. This method often has been confusing and poorly reproduced between examiners. More recently, the preferred method is to describe the degree of effacement in terms of actual length of remaining cervix in centimeters. Cervical *dilatation* describes the diameter of the internal cervical os and is an indicator of the progression of labor. The index and middle fingers of the examining hand are used to determine the diameter; expressed in centimeters (fingertip to 10 cm). Ten centimeters indicates full dilatation. The *station* indicates the level that the fetus occupies in the pelvis, with the reference point being the maternal ischial spines, palpable on either side of the vaginal canal at about 4 and 8 o'clock. If the presenting fetal part remains above the ischial spines, the station is described as negative. Once the presenting fetal part has reached the level of the ischial spines, the station is zero, with further descent into the pelvis described as +1 or +2. A +3 station corresponds to visible scalp at the introitus, indicating a fetal position consistent with impending delivery.

Leopold maneuvers (see below) and digital examination provide information about the presentation of the child and can indicate a potential breech presentation or cord prolapse. The frequency of malpresentation at 32 weeks is up to 15 percent, whereas nonvertex presentation at term is from 4 to 7 percent. Leopold maneuvers are the palpation of the fetus through the maternal abdomen to determine fetus position and presentation. This can be used for screening for malpresentation as well as fetal weight. Sensitivity in identification of fetal malpresentation among experienced clinicians ranges from 28 to 88 percent, but specificity is usually high (94 percent).[5,6] Nahum found that estimation of fetal weight is within 15 percent of actual with these maneuvers.[7] Conversely, Leopold maneuvers are relatively unreliable in inexperienced hands.

On digital examination, vertex presentation is best confirmed with palpation of the cranial sutures. Palpation of small parts, such as feet or hands, is often indicative of malpresentation. If very thick meconium is present on the examining finger after palpation of fingertip to 1-cm dilatation, breech presentation should be ruled out immediately. If available, sonographic verification of presentation is preferred.

Care should be taken to ensure that the pregnant woman does not remain flat on her back for a prolonged period of time because compression of venous return by the gravid uterus can lead to hypotension in the mother and decreased blood supply to the fetus. After examination, the patient should be placed in the left lateral position.

Rupture of Membranes

Determining if membranes have ruptured is an important predictor of the likelihood of imminent labor, as well the potential for complications such as infection or cord prolapse.[8] SROM occurs during the course of active labor in most patients, although it may occur prior to the onset of labor in 10 percent of third-trimester patients.

The history of SROM typically involves a reported gush of clear or blood-tinged fluid; occasionally, patients recount continued leaking or dampening of their underwear on standing or with the Valsalva maneuver. At this time, screening for symptoms of infection, such as fevers, chills, flushing, and palpitations, should occur. Rupture of membranes can be confirmed by using nitrazine paper to test residual fluid in the fornix or vaginal vault while performing a sterile speculum examination. Amniotic fluid has a pH of 7.0 to 7.4 and will turn nitrazine paper a dark blue. Vaginal fluid typically has a pH of 4.5 to 5.5, and the nitrazine strip will remain yellow. False-positive tests may occur with blood, lubricant, and the presence of *Trichomonas,* semen, or cervical mucus. Another test used to confirm rupture of membranes (ROM) is ferning, or observing sodium chloride crystals on a slide as amniotic fluid dries. At the time of this pelvic examination, it is prudent to also evaluate for signs of chorioamnionitis, such as maternal fever, maternal tachycardia, fetal tachycardia, and fundal tenderness.

If membranes are intact, an amniotomy should not be performed in the ED setting because this may lead to precipitous labor and the potential for cord prolapse. It is also important to note the presence of meconium after the ROM, indicated by the presence of thick, greenish brown fluid.

Premature Rupture of Membranes

Rupture of the amnion and chorion that occur more than 1 h prior to the onset of labor is called *premature rupture of membranes* (PROM).[9] If rupture occurs prior to 37 weeks of gestation, this is termed preterm premature rupture of membranes (PPROM). Prolonged ROM occurs if delivery does not occur within 18 h of ROM. Given that this is a major cause of maternal transports, it is important to review a few details about PROM and PPROM. Possible causative factors include infection, history of PPROM, history of trauma, multiple gestations, fetal anomalies, placental abruption, and placenta previa. Conservative management of PPROM usually is employed in gestations of less than 34 weeks; obstetricians will wait for signs of chorioamnionitis or nonreassuring fetal testing before intervening. Use of tocolytics is reserved for cases where maternal transport is necessary or if a delay of delivery is needed to initiate steroids for fetal lung maturity. Mercer and colleagues showed that latency of noninfected PPROM patients can be prolonged with ampicillin and erythromycin for 7 days.[8]

Fetal Distress

Fetal distress may occur during active labor, and care must be taken to evaluate the fetal status as often as possible. Indicators of fetal distress include decelerations in fetal heart rate, defined as a persistent drop in fetal heart rate during contractions lasting greater than 30 s after a contraction. While most EDs do not have fetal monitoring devices,

Doppler heart tones should be measured after each contraction to detect the presence of decelerations. Episodic bradycardia lasting for more than 5 min is an indication for immediate cesarean section. Interventions for decelerations attempt to increase maternal blood flow or increase maternal serum oxygenation. For decelerations, maternal repositioning to the left lateral, the right lateral, and then the knee-chest position should be attempted until return of fetal heart rate to baseline is achieved. Fetal scalp stimulation also should be initiated with sterile bimanual examination. In addition, maternal oxygen by face mask can be initiated to increase oxygen supply to the fetus for late decelerations. Lastly, an injection of terbutaline can halt uterine contractions and increase blood flow to the fetus.

EMERGENCY DELIVERY

The initial step in the management of a woman in active labor is to obtain vital signs and initiate supportive therapy, including obtaining venous access and monitoring the mother and fetus if fetal monitoring is available. If the pelvic examination reveals complete cervical effacement and fetal presentation at the introitus, then delivery is imminent. It is important to realize that patients, particularly multiparous patients, can progress very rapidly. The stage of labor and the parity of the patient should be taken into account when considering transport of a laboring patient to another facility, and also when determining if the patient can be safely transported from the ED to the labor and delivery suite. For patients who are crowning, or who are fully dilated and effaced, it is generally best to have the obstetrician come to the ED, rather than risk precipitous delivery during transport.

As the cervix becomes fully dilated and effacement becomes complete, the fetus continues to descend, and the patient will experience the urge to push. Patients delivering in the emergency setting may have difficulty controlling these expulsive efforts, and they are in even greater need of assistance, reassurance, and instruction. Preoccupation with the delivery should not exclude the needs of the mother nor minimize the importance of maternal cooperation to accomplish a controlled delivery.

Determination of fetal position is best accomplished in the emergency setting by evaluation of the presenting portion of the infant. Pelvic examination should reveal evidence of the infant's position, including palpable skull sutures and fontanels or, in the case of breech delivery, the infant's buttock or extremity. Confirmation may be accomplished by personnel familiar with Leopold maneuvers.

The typical delivery position is the dorsal lithotomy position, which allows maximum visualization and control of the delivery. However, a patient laboring naturally often may prefer delivery in the knee-chest position. If this is the case, all maneuvers for delivery must be in the opposite direction, or the patient must be rotated to the dorsal lithotomy position. As time allows, the perineum may then be prepared by washing with mild soap and water and swabbing with povidone-iodine. Drapes should be placed over the patient, and gowns, masks, and gloves should be donned by medical personnel attending the patient. Obstetrical support should be notified as indicated.

The process of fetal descent during labor and delivery is described by six cardinal movements: (1) engagement, (2) flexion, (3) descent, (4) internal rotation, (5) extension, and (6) external rotation (see Figure 107-1). The following discussion describes delivery in the cephalic, occiput anterior (OA) position. As the fetus descends through the birth canal and reaches the introitus, the perineum bulges to accommodate the fetal head. Delivery can be aided by gentle digital stretching of the inferior portion of the perineum. The perineum will undergo gradual thinning and stretching to enable passage of the newborn. The use of routine episiotomy for a normal spontaneous vaginal delivery has been discouraged in recent years and has been demonstrated to increase the incidence of third- and fourth-degree lacerations occurring at the time of delivery.[10,11] If an episiotomy is necessary, it may be performed as follows: 5 to 10 mL of 1% lidocaine solution is injected with a small-gauge needle into the posterior

fourchette and perineum. While protecting the infant's head, a 2- to 3-cm midline cut is made with scissors to extend the vaginal opening. The incision must be supported with manual pressure from below, taking care not to allow the incision to extend into the rectum.

Control of the delivery of the neonate is the major challenge. As the infant's head emerges from the introitus, the perineum should be supported by placing a sterile towel along the inferior portion of the perineum with one hand and supporting the fetal head with the other hand. Mild counterpressure is exerted to prevent rapid expulsion of the fetal head, which may lead to third- or fourth-degree perineal tears. Control of the head away from the anterior structures also will reduce anterior tears near the urethra and clitoris.

As the infant's head presents, the left hand may the be used to control the fetal chin while the right remains on the crown of the head, supporting the delivery. This controlled extension of the fetal head will aid in the atraumatic delivery. The mother is then asked to breathe through contractions rather than bearing down and attempting to push the baby out rapidly. Immediately after delivery of the infant's head, the infant's nose and mouth should be suctioned. This is particularly important in infants presenting with meconium in order to prevent aspiration. A simple suction bulb will assist in routine clearing of the infant's nose and mouth. After suctioning, the neck should be palpated for the presence of a nuchal cord. Nuchal cord is a common condition, found in 25 percent of all cephalad-presenting deliveries.[12] If the cord is loose, it should be reduced over the infant's head, and the delivery may proceed as usual. If the cord is wound tightly, it may need to be clamped in the most accessible area by two close clamps and transected to allow delivery of the infant.

After clearing the airway, delivery of the body is allowed to progress. After delivery of the head, the head will restitute, or turn to one side or the other. As the head rotates, the physician's hands are placed on either side of the head, providing gentle downward traction to deliver the anterior shoulder. Care should be taken to provide only gentle traction because jerky or forceful movements may cause a brachial plexus injury. Once the anterior shoulder is visible, the physician's hand then gently guides the fetus upward, delivering the posterior shoulder and allowing the remainder of the infant to be delivered. At this point, it is very important to control the delivery of the body to prevent perineal lacerations.

A point of practical concern is the need to maintain control of the newly born infant such that inadvertent dropping does not and cannot occur. The combination of amniotic fluid, blood, and vernix results in a very slippery infant. It is useful to prepare for the delivery by placing the posterior (left) hand underneath the axilla of the infant prior to delivering the rest of the body. The anterior hand may then be used to grasp the ankles of the infant and ensure a firm grip. In obstetrical training, students often are instructed to hold the infant close to their chest "like a football." In order to promote the clearing of secretions in the neonate, it is best to hold the infant so that the head is below the heart, tilting downward with the infant's head secured in the palm of the hand.

The infant is then loosely wrapped in a towel and stimulated as it is dried. In the setting of an uncomplicated delivery, the mother may hold the child immediately while the cord is being cut, providing the child has responded well to initial stimulation and has a clear airway and good respiratory effort. The umbilical cord is double clamped 3 cm distal to its insertion at the umbilicus and transected with sterile scissors. The infant is further dried and warmed under an incubator, where postnatal care may be provided and Apgar scores calculated at 1 and 5 min after delivery. Scoring includes general color, tone, heart rate, respiratory effort, and reflexes (Table 107-3).

In the case of suspected meconium aspiration, the infant is delivered, the cord is double clamped and cut immediately, and the infant is placed in an incubator for airway assessment and possible intubation prior to stimulating the child to breathe spontaneously. Intubation allows for the trachea to be suctioned adequately prior to spontaneous breathing, thus reducing the risk of meconium aspiration. If a cyanotic

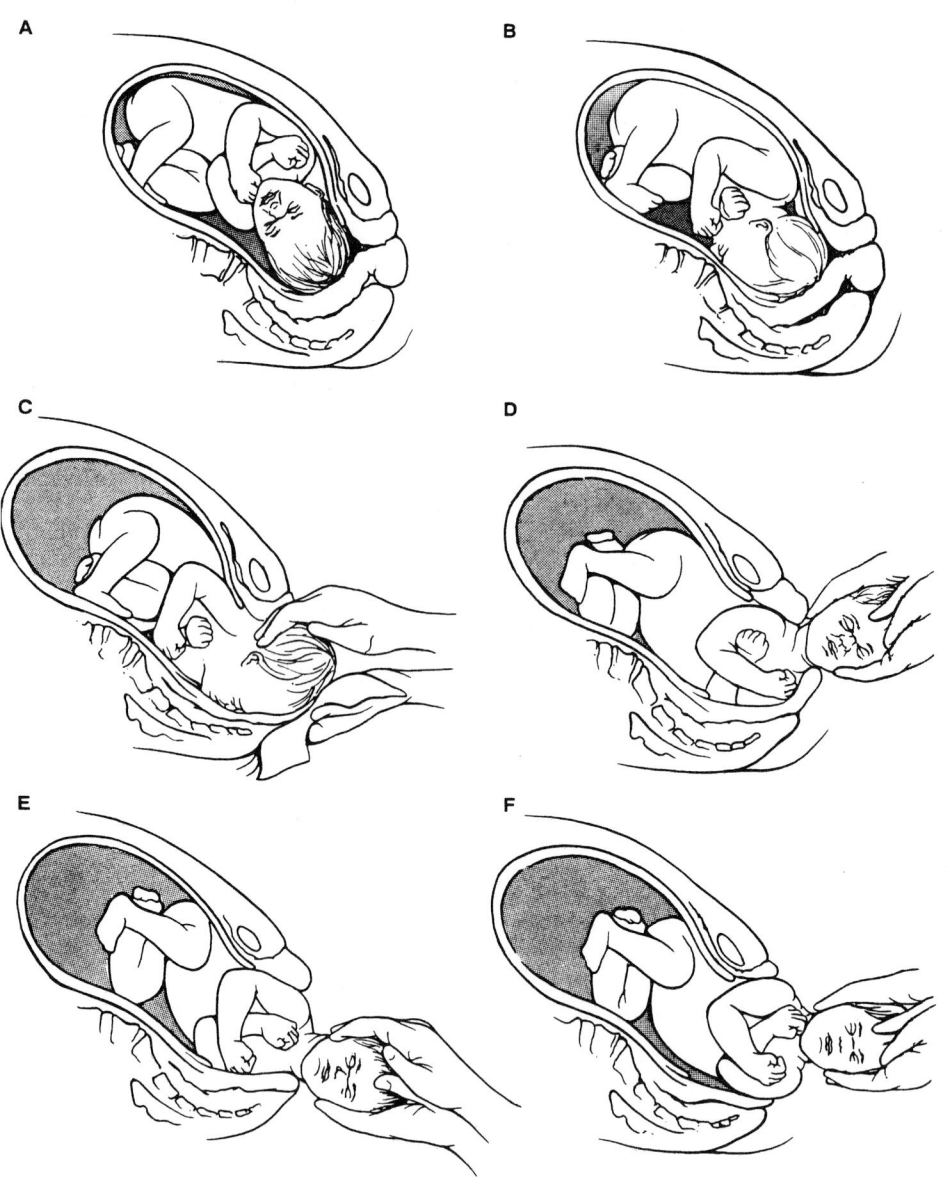

A **B** **C** **D** **E** **F**

FIG. 107-1. Movements of normal delivery. Mechanism of labor and delivery for vertex presentations. **A.** Engagement, flexion, and descent. **B.** Internal rotation. **C.** Extension and delivery of the head. After delivery of the head the infant's nose and mouth should be suctioned and the neck checked for encirclement of the umbilical cord. **D.** External rotation bringing the thorax into the anteroposterior diameter of the pelvis. **E.** Delivery of the anterior shoulder. **F.** Delivery of the posterior shoulder. Note that after delivery, the head is supported and used to gently guide delivery of the shoulder. Traction should be minimized.

or apneic child is delivered and does not respond immediately to stimulation, neonatal resuscitation is instituted (see Chap. 13).

Delivery of the Placenta

After the infant is delivered and the umbilical cord is clamped, the placenta delivers in 15 to 30 min. The placenta should be allowed to separate spontaneously, assisted with gentle traction. Aggressive traction

TABLE 107-3   APGAR Scoring for Newborns

	Sign	0 Points	1 Point	2 Points
A	Activity (muscle tone)	Absent	Arms and legs flexed	Active movement
P	Pulse	Absent	Below 100 beats/min	Above 100 beats/min
G	Grimace (reflex irritability)	No response	Grimace	Sneeze, cough, pulls away
A	Appearance (skin color)	Blue-gray, pale all over	Normal, except for extremities	Normal over entire body
R	Respiration	Absent	Slow, irregular	Good, crying

on the cord risks uterine inversion, tearing of the cord, or disruption of the placenta, which can result in severe vaginal bleeding. After removal of the placenta, the uterus should be massaged gently to promote contraction. Oxytocin (10 to 20 IV units in 1 L NS at 250 mL/h or 10 units intramuscularly) is administered to maintain uterine contraction.

Uterine atony may follow a precipitous delivery and may lead to excessive vaginal bleeding. Additional oxytocin may be administered, as well as methylergonovine 0.2 mg IM, or carboprost tromethamine, .25 mg IM. With significant postpartum hemorrhage, vigorous bimanual massage should be continued while administering contractile agents. Episiotomy or laceration repair may be delayed until an experienced obstetrician is able to close the laceration and inspect the patient for fourth-degree (rectovaginal) tears.

COMPLICATIONS OF DELIVERY

Cord Prolapse

In the event that the bimanual examination reveals palpable, pulsating cord, the examiner's hand should not be removed but rather should be used to elevate the presenting fetal part to reduce compression on the cord.[12] Immediate obstetrical assistance is necessary because a ce-

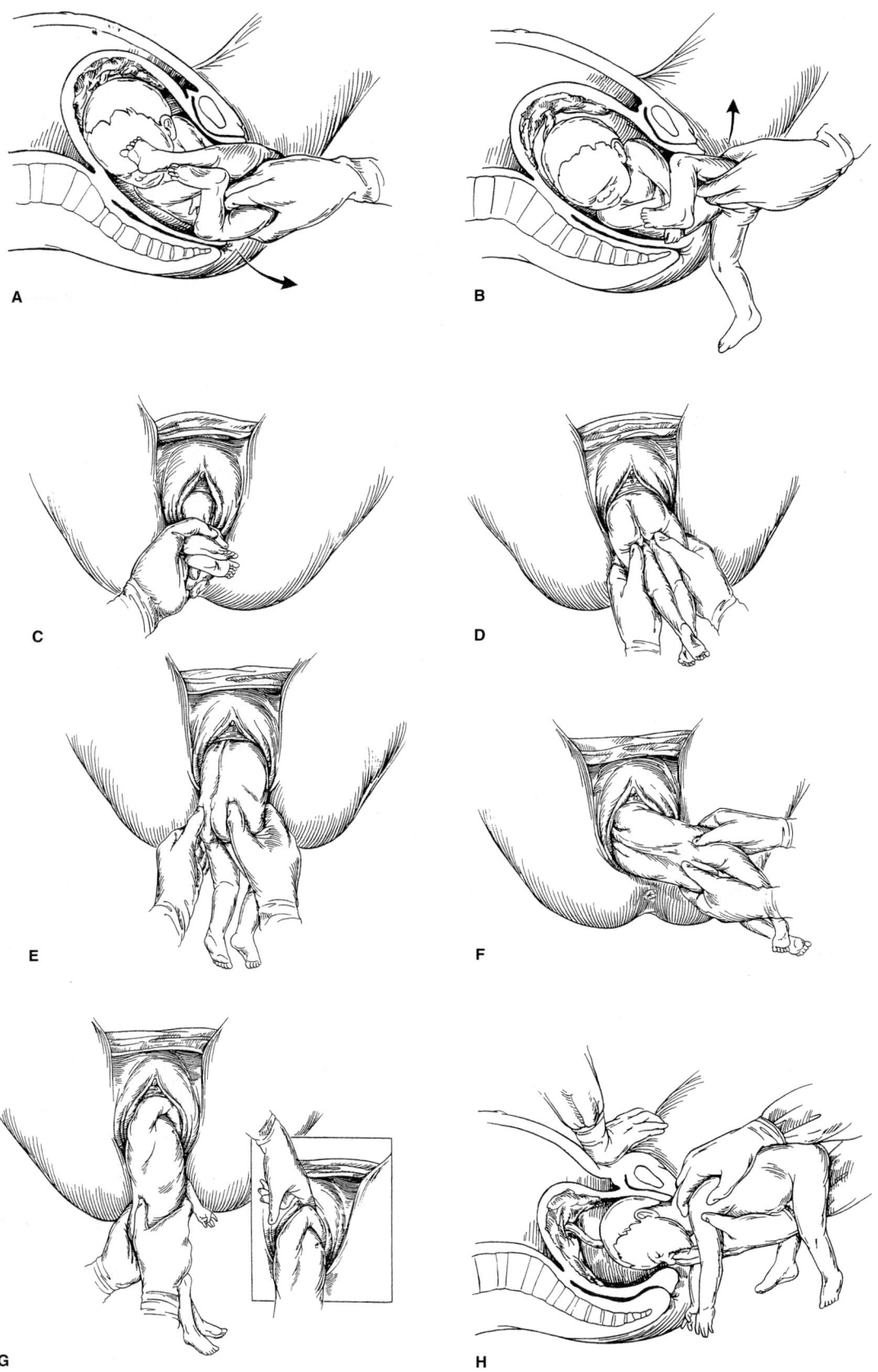

FIG. 107-2. Management of the vaginal frank breech delivery. **A.** The Pinard maneuver. The operator's hand is placed behind the fetal thigh, putting gentle pressure at the knee and allowing delivery of the leg. **B.** A similar maneuver of the opposite leg. **C.** The feet are grasped with the thumb and third finger over the lateral malleolus and the second finger is placed between the two ankles. **D.** With maternal expulsive efforts, the breech is delivered to the level of the umbilicus. The sacrum should be kept anterior. **E.** Again, with maternal expulsive efforts, the infant is delivered to the level of the clavicles, keeping the sacrum an-terior. **F.** The fetus is rotated 90° allowing visualization of the now anterior right arm. **G.** The arm is well visualized and a single digit is used to deliver it. Delivery of the opposite arm is accomplished by rotating the fetus 180° in a clockwise direction and repeating the maneuver. **H.** Delivery of the fetal vertex is accomplished by placing the operator's fingers over the maxillary processes of the fetus, keeping the body parallel to the floor. The body should never be lifted above parallel to prevent hyperextension of the neck. An assistant applies suprapubic pressure, aiding flexion of the fetal head and accomplishing delivery.

sarean section is indicated. The examiner's hand should remain in the vagina while the patient is transported and prepared for surgery in order to prevent further compression of the cord by the fetal head. No attempt should ever be made to reduce a prolapsed cord.

Shoulder Dystocia

Shoulder dystocia is the impaction of fetal shoulders at the pelvic outlet after delivery of the head. Typically, the anterior shoulder is trapped behind the pubic symphysis, leading to delay of delivery of the rest of the infant. It usually occurs in the delivery of larger infants with disproportionately large shoulders compared with the fetal head. Although rare, shoulder dystocia is a serious concern because of the risk of fetal morbidity and mortality if it is not managed promptly and appropriately. Complications of shoulder dystocia include brachial plexus injury from overaggressive traction and fetal hypoxia from impaired respirations and compression of the umbilical cord and compromised fetal circulation.

Shoulder dystocia is first recognized after delivery of the fetal head, when routine downward traction is insufficient to deliver the anterior shoulder. After delivering the infant's head, it retracts tightly against the perineum (the turtle sign).[13] If a shoulder dystocia is recognized, the physician should use the momentum from delivery of the head to deliver the anterior shoulder. After delivery of the anterior shoulder, the infant's nose and mouth can then be suctioned. If the shoulder is still impacted, call for assistance and have an assistant note the time. It is then important to position the mother in the extreme lithotomy position, with legs sharply flexed up to the abdomen (the McRobert maneuver) with the legs held by the mother or an assistant. The bladder should be drained if this has not been done already. A generous episiotomy also may facilitate delivery. Next, **an assistant should apply suprapubic pressure to disimpact the anterior shoulder from the pubic symphysis. It is important to remember never to apply fundal pressure because this will further impact the shoulder on the pelvic rim.** Pressure also can be applied to the infant's sternum to decrease shoulder diameter.

To deliver the impacted anterior shoulder, a corkscrew maneuver (Woods' maneuver) is the first manipulation attempted. The physician grasps the posterior scapula of the infant with two fingers and rotates the shoulder girdle 180 degrees in the pelvic outlet in an attempt to rotate the posterior shoulder into the anterior position and in the process deliver the shoulder. Gentle traction may then be applied as the mother pushes, and the infant is delivered through an oblique pelvic diameter. If the corkscrew maneuver fails to reduce the dystocia, the physician may then attempt to deliver the posterior shoulder. The examiner's hand is passed posteriorly in the vagina, and the infant's posterior arm is felt. The elbow is grasped and flexed, and the arm is delivered with the posterior shoulder, and the anterior shoulder usually follows.

Breech Presentation

Breech presentations occur in 3 to 4 percent of term pregnancies and are associated with a morbidity rate three to four times greater than that of cephalad presentations.[14] Breech presentations occur most frequently in premature infants, since final rotation in the pelvis may not have occurred (25 percent of pregnancies at less than 28 weeks and 7 percent of pregnancies at 32 weeks of gestation). The major concern in breech deliveries is head entrapment. In a normal cephalic delivery, the larger head dilates the cervical canal, thus ensuring that the rest of the infant follows. With breech deliveries, however, the head emerges last and may become trapped by an incompletely dilated cervix.

Breech presentation is associated with a greater incidence of fetal distress and umbilical cord prolapse. Breech presentations may be classified as frank, complete, incomplete, or footling. Frank and complete breech presentations serve as a dilating wedge nearly as well as the fetal head, and delivery may proceed in an uncomplicated fashion.

The main point for the emergency physician to remember in a breech presentation is to keep hands away and let the delivery happen spontaneously. This allows the presenting portion of the fetus to maximally dilate the introitus prior to presentation of the fetal head. It is recommended that the examiner literally refrain from touching the fetus until the umbilicus appears. At that point, the physician should place fingers medial to each thigh, pressing out laterally to deliver the legs (Figure 107-2). The fetus should then be rotated to the sacrum anterior position, and the trunk and lower half should be wrapped in a towel. When the scapulae appear, gently rotate until the right humerus can be followed down, rotated across the chest, and swept out. The fetus should then be turned in a counterclockwise position to allow delivery of the other arm. Then, keeping the infant's head flexed, the physician should place the index and middle fingers over the infant's maxillary bones (not in the infant's mouth) to help keep the head flexed. This should allow the mother to expel the fetus. It is important not to pull on the fetus because this may impact the head in the pelvis or entrap the extended fetal arm. Footling and incomplete breech positions are not considered safe for vaginal delivery because of the possibility of cord prolapse or incomplete dilatation of the cervix. In any breech delivery, obstetrical consultation should be obtained immediately.

Preterm Delivery

Preterm delivery is a major cause of precipitous childbirth and is often the cause of emergency delivery. Preterm infants also present more often in the breech position and have a greater incidence of morbidity and mortality. Carefully control the delivery to reduce the likelihood of trauma to the fragile preterm infant. Deliver the infant slowly and immediately dry and warm the infant while performing the initial assessment because the premature infant is much more likely to require resuscitation. The decision whether to initiate resuscitative efforts in the ED is often difficult because patients may deliver an extremely premature fetus of unknown gestational age. In general, even very premature deliveries (18–22 weeks) should receive initial resuscitative efforts until determination of viability is made (see Chap. 13).

REFERENCES

1. Curtin SC: Trends in the attendant, place, and timing of births, and in the use of obstetric interventions: United States, 1989–1997. *Natl Vital Stat Rep* 47:1–12, 1999.
2. Pang JW, Heffelfinger JD, Huang GJ, et al: Outcomes of planned home births in Washington State: 1989–1996. *Obstet Gynecol* 100:253, 2002.
3. Dystocia and the Augmentation of Labor. ACOG Technical Bulletin Number 218, December 1995.
4. Johnston MM, Sanchez-Ramos L, Vaughn AJ, et al: Antibiotic therapy in preterm, premature rupture of membranes: A randomized prospective double blind trial. *Am J Obstet Gynecol* 163:743, 1990.
5. Lydon-Rochelle M, Albers L, Gorwoda J, et al: Accuracy of Leopold maneuvers in screening for malpresentation: A prospective study. *Birth* 20: 132, 1993.
6. Thorp JM Jr, Jenkins T, Watson W: Utility of Leopold maneuvers in screening for malpresentation. *Obstet Gynecol* 78:394, 1991.
7. Nahum GG: Predicting fetal weight: Are Leopold's maneuvers still worth teaching to medical students and house staff? *J Reprod Med* 47: 271, 2002.
8. Mercer BM: The Preterm Prediction Study: Prediction of preterm premature rupture of membranes through clinical findings and ancillary testing. The National Institute of Child Health and Human Development Maternal-Fetal Medicine Units Network. *Am J Obstet Gynecol* 183:738, 2000.
9. Capeless EL, Mead PB: Management of preterm premature rupture of membranes: Lack of a national concensus. *Am J Obstet Gynecol* 157:11, 1987.
10. Borgatta L, Piening SL, Cohen WR: Association of episiotomy and delivery position with deep perineal laceration during spontaneous delivery in nulliparous women. *Am J Obstet Gynecol* 160:294, 1989.
11. Shiono P, Klebanoff MA, Carey JC: Midline episiotomies: More harm than good? *Obstet Gynecol* 75:765, 1990.
12. Critchlow CW, Leef TL, Benedetti TJ, et al: Risk factors and infant outcomes associated with umbilical cord prolapse: A population-based case-control study among births in Washington State. *Am J Obstet Gynecol* 170: 613, 1994.

13. Nocon JJ, McKenzie DK, Thomas LJ, et al: Shoulder dystocia: An analysis of risks and obstetric maneuvers. *Am J Obstet Gynecol* 168:1732, 1993.
14. Hearne A, Driggers R: Normal labor and delivery, operative delivery, and malpresentations. In Baakowski BJ, Hearne AE, Lambrou NC, Fox HE, Wallaih EE (eds): *The Johns Hopkins Manual of Gynecology and Obstetrics,* 2d ed. Baltimore, Johns Hopkins University Press, 2002, pp. 91, 92.

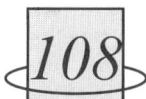

VULVOVAGINITIS
Gloria J. Kuhn

Vulvovaginitis is inflammation of the vulva and vaginal tissues. It is usually characterized by a vaginal discharge and/or vulvar itching and irritation. A vaginal odor may be present. It accounts for 10 million visits to physicians per year in the United States, and is the most common gynecologic complaint in prepubertal girls.[1]

The most common causes of acute vulvovaginitis include:

1. Infections,
2. Irritant or allergic contact,
3. Local response to a vaginal foreign body, and
4. Atrophic vaginitis.

The three most frequent infectious causes are bacterial vaginosis (BV) caused by replacement of normal flora by overgrowth of anaerobes and *Gardnerella vaginalis,* candidiasis (usually caused by *Candida albicans*) and, trichomoniasis (caused by *Trichomonas vaginalis*).[2] BV is the most common cause of vaginal discharge or malodor. Polymicrobial infection in women with vaginitis is not uncommon. Vulvovaginal candidiasis, contact vaginitis, and atrophic vaginitis may occur in virgins and after menopause, but other forms of infectious vulvovaginitis are generally found only in sexually active women.

GENERAL APPROACH TO VULVOVAGINITIS

A detailed gynecologic history should be obtained and a pelvic examination performed. Microscopic evaluation of fresh vaginal secretions using both normal saline solution (demonstrating clue cells for BV and motile *Trichomonas vaginalis* for trichomoniasis) and 10 percent potassium hydroxide (KOH) slide preparation (demonstrating yeast or pseudohyphae for candidiasis) and fishy odor in BV (whiff test) will, in most instances, provide a diagnosis (Table 108-1). Checking the pH and microscopic examination of secretions is mandatory because symptoms are nonspecific, signs on physical examination may vary, and patients may have more than one etiology causing vulvovaginitis. Culture for *T. vaginalis* is more sensitive than microscopic examination but is very infrequently performed. One of the most helpful diagnostic tools is measurement of the pH of the vaginal secretions using Nitrazine paper. A pH greater than 4.5 is typical of BV or trichomoniasis, while a pH below 4.5 represents physiologic discharge or a fungal infection.[2]

TABLE 108-1 Diagnosis of Vaginitis Based on Vaginal Secretions

Test	Finding	Diagnosis
pH	4.0–4.5	Normal
	4.0–4.5	Candidiasis
	>4.5	Bacterial vaginosis
	>4.5	Trichomoniasis
Normal saline solution	Clue cells	Bacterial vaginosis
	Motile trichomonads	Trichomoniasis
	Pseudohyphae and/or buds	Candidiasis
KOH preparation	Fishy odor (whiff test)	Bacterial vaginosis
	Pseudohyphae and/or buds	Candidiasis

Signs of vulval inflammation and minimal discharge in the absence of vaginal pathogens suggest the possibility of mechanical, chemical, allergic, or other noninfectious causes of vulvovaginitis.

All treatment recommendations are taken from the 2002 guidelines for the treatment of sexually transmitted diseases from the Centers for Disease Control and Prevention (CDC).[2]

NORMAL VULVOVAGINAL ENVIRONMENT

In females of childbearing age, estrogen causes the development of a thick vaginal epithelium with a large number of superficial cells serving a protective function and containing large stores of glycogen. Glycogen is used by the normal flora, consisting of lactobacilli and acidogenic corynebacteria, to form lactic and acetic acids. The resulting acidic environment favors the normal flora and discourages the growth of pathogenic bacteria. Lack of estrogen or a dominance of progesterone results in an atrophic condition, with loss of the protective superficial cells and their contained glycogen. This results in loss of the acidic environment. Normal vaginal secretions may vary in consistency from a thin, watery material to one that is thick, white, and opaque. The quantity may also vary from scant to a rather copious amount. This material is odorless and produces no symptoms. The normal vaginal pH varies between 4.0 and 4.5. Alkaline secretions from the cervix before and during menstruation and semen (which is alkaline) reduce acidity, predisposing to infection. Before menarche and after menopause, the vaginal pH varies between 6 and 7. Because of scant nerve endings in the vagina, the patient usually does not have symptoms until both the vagina and vulva are involved in an inflammatory or irritant process.

Factors thought to contribute to vaginitis in prepubertal females include less-protective covering of the introitus by the labia majora, low estrogen concentration, exposure to irritants such as bubble bath, poor hygiene, and specific pathogens. The role of poor hygiene and infection is disputed.[1] Infectious etiologies may be more common in adolescents.[3]

BACTERIAL VAGINOSIS

BV is a clinical syndrome that occurs when the normal H_2O_2-producing *Lactobacillus* species in the vagina are replaced by high

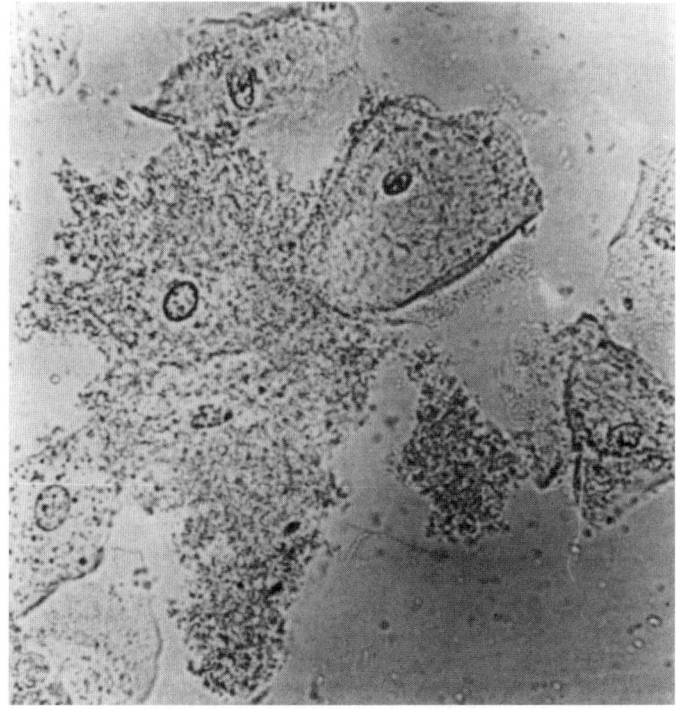

FIG. 108-1. Stippled clue cell of *G. vaginalis* vaginitis.

concentrations of anaerobic bacteria, *G. vaginalis,* and *Mycoplasma hominis.* BV is the most common cause of a malodorous discharge, but more than half of the women who meet the clinical criteria for diagnosis are asymptomatic. The cause of this microbial alteration in the normal vaginal flora is not understood. While BV is rarely seen in women who have never been sexually active, it is not clear whether the disease is the result of a sexually transmitted pathogen. However, BV is associated with having multiple sex partners.[2]

Bacterial vaginosis can be diagnosed by the use of clinical and microscopic criteria. The CDC states that for the disease to be diagnosed, three of the following signs or symptoms must be present:

1. A homogeneous, white, noninflammatory discharge that smoothly coats the vaginal walls;
2. Presence of clue cells on microscopic examination (epithelial cells coated by bacteria) (Figure 108-1);
3. pH greater than 4.5; and
4. A fishy odor to the discharge after addition of KOH (whiff test).[2]

Gram staining, which demonstrates a concentration of bacterial morphotypes characteristic of BV, is an acceptable laboratory method of diagnosing BV. Culture of *G. vaginalis* is not recommended.[2]

Research demonstrates an association between BV and adverse pregnancy outcomes because of preterm labor and premature rupture of membranes (PROM), leading to recommendations that high-risk patients (i.e., those who previously delivered a premature infant) be screened for BV during the second trimester of pregnancy.[4] BV is also associated with pelvic inflammatory disease, endometritis, and vaginal cuff cellulitis after surgical procedures.

All symptomatic patients, unless allergic to the drug, should be treated with metronidazole regardless of pregnancy status.[2] Several drug regimens are available (Table 108-2). There is no proof of teratogenicity from metronidazole in humans and this drug is recommended for pregnant patients.[2]

Treatment is not recommended for asymptomatic nonpregnant patients who are not undergoing surgery. Because of the association of BV with postsurgical infection, strong consideration should be given to prophylactic treatment of infected women prior to surgical abortion. More data are needed before recommendation for treatment of all asymptomatic infected women undergoing other surgical procedures

TABLE 108-2   Treatment Regimens for Bacterial Vaginosis

Agent	Dose
RECOMMENDED REGIMENS	
Metronidazole*	500 mg PO bid for 7 d
Clindamycin cream 2%	One full applicator intravaginally qhs for 7 d
Metronidazole gel 0.75%	One full applicator intravaginally bid for 5 d
ALTERNATIVE REGIMENS†	
Metronidazole	2 g PO in a single dose
Clindamycin	300 mg PO bid for 7 d
REGIMENS FOR PREGNANT WOMEN	
High-risk patients	
Metronidazole	250 mg PO tid for 7 d
Alternative regimens†	
Metronidazole	2 g PO in a single dose
Clindamycin	300 mg PO bid for 7 d
Low-risk symptomatic patients	
Metronidazole	250 mg PO tid for 7 d
Alternative regimens†	
Metronidazole	2 g PO in a single dose
Metronidazole gel 0.75%	One full applicator intravaginally bid for 5 d
Clindamycin	300 mg PO bid for 7 d

*Avoid alcohol during and 24 h after treatment.
†Lower efficacy.

is made. However, consideration of treatment of these patients prior to surgery seems reasonable.[2] **All pregnant women should be treated because of the negative impact this infection has on pregnancy.**[2]

Overall cure rates 4 weeks after treatment do not differ significantly between a 7-day regimen of either oral metronidazole, metronidazole vaginal gel, or clindamycin vaginal cream. Metronidazole vaginal gel has the benefit of fewer side effects (i.e., gastrointestinal disturbance and unpleasant taste) but should not be used in women who are allergic to the oral preparation. All patients on oral metronidazole should avoid alcohol during use and for 24 h after, and in some cases longer, after treatment because of the disulfiram-like reaction that can occur. The vaginal clindamycin cream appears less efficacious than the metronidazole regimens. Based on frequency of cure rates, alternative treatments to metronidazole are not as efficacious.

The use of clindamycin vaginal cream during pregnancy is not recommended because of the possibility of preterm deliveries among pregnant women treated with this medication (Table 108-2). Recurrence of symptoms is seen within 3 months in 30 percent of treated patients who initially respond. The reasons for this are unclear. Prolonged therapy for 10 to 14 days may be tried.[5]

CANDIDA VAGINITIS

Candida species are a common cause of vaginitis. There are no reliable prevalence data of vulvovaginal candidiasis (VVC) because the disease is not reportable, many women self-medicate with over-the-counter preparations, and as many as half the women given this diagnosis have other conditions. Although the actual prevalence is unknown for the above reasons, it is estimated that 75 percent of women will experience at least one infection during their childbearing years (with the highest attack rate during the third trimester of pregnancy), making it the second commonest vaginal infection. A small subpopulation of women, less than 5 percent, have repeated episodes of disease with no clinically proven factors being responsible for recurrent infection.

The organism can be isolated from up to 20 percent of asymptomatic, healthy women of childbearing age, some of whom are celibate. Therefore, this infection is not considered a sexually transmitted disease (STD), although it can be transmitted that way. At least one study, although small, has shown frequent intercourse to be a risk factor for infection.[6] Factors that favor increased rates of asymptomatic vaginal colonization include pregnancy, oral contraceptives, uncontrolled diabetes mellitus, and frequent visits to STD clinics (perhaps as a result of antimicrobial therapy). It is rare in premenarcheal girls but does occur.[3] It has a decreased incidence after menopause unless replacement estrogen is being used, emphasizing the hormonal dependence of VVC. Immunity to *Candida* infections is primarily cell mediated.

C. albicans strains account for 85 to 92 percent of those strains isolated from the vagina. *C. glabrata* and *C. tropicalis* are the commonest non-*albicans* strains and are often more resistant to conventional therapy. Candidal organisms gain access to the vaginal lumen and secretions predominantly from the adjacent perianal area. Candidal organisms must first adhere to the vaginal epithelial cells for colonization to take place, and *C. albicans* adheres in greater numbers than do other strains.

Factors that enhance the germination of *Candida* (e.g., pregnancy and estrogen therapy) tend to precipitate symptomatic vaginitis, while conditions that inhibit germination (normal flora and local mucosal cell-mediated immunity) prevent acute vaginitis in carriers of yeast. The growth of *Candida* is held in check by the normal vaginal flora, and symptoms of vaginitis usually occur only when the normal balance is upset. Conditions that inhibit growth of normal vaginal flora, particularly *Lactobacillus* species (e.g., systemic antibiotics, especially broad-spectrum agents), diminish the glycogen stores in vaginal epithelial cells (e.g., diabetes mellitus, pregnancy, oral contraceptives, and hormonal replacement therapy), or increase the pH of vaginal secretions (e.g., menstrual blood or semen), may cause increased colonization by *Candida,* which is an opportunistic organism, and cause subsequent symptomatic infection. Tight-fitting, particularly syn-

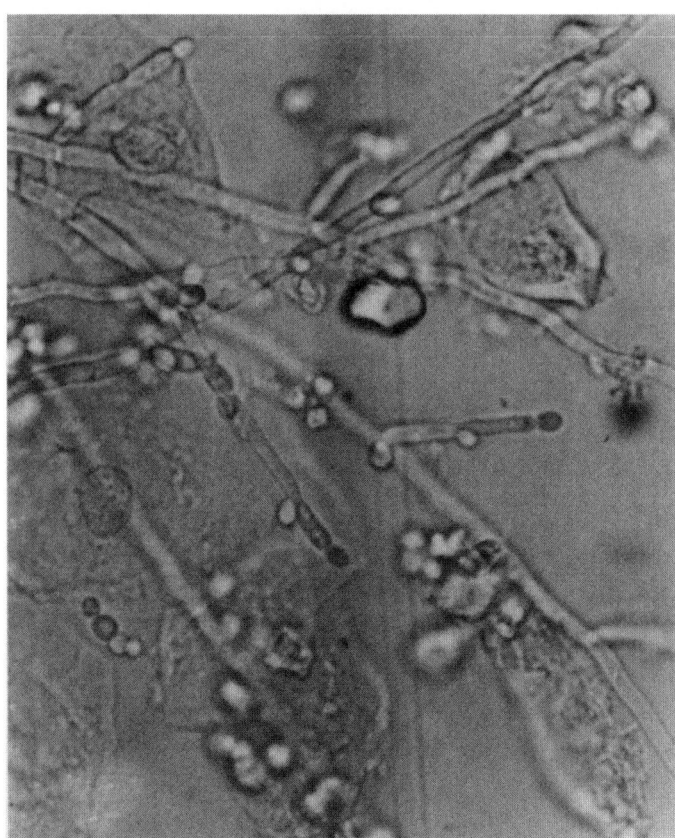

FIG. 108-2. Hyphal elements of *C. albicans* seen on high-power magnification during saline microscopy. The patient had florid candidal vaginitis.

thetic, undergarments may also contribute to the problem because of increased temperature, moisture, and local irritation.

Clinical symptoms include leukorrhea, severe vaginal pruritus (commonest symptom), external dysuria, and dyspareunia. Symptoms vary in severity, but exacerbation is frequently seen in the week prior to menses or with coitus. Odor is unusual.

Gynecologic examination may reveal vulvar erythema and edema, vaginal erythema, and, occasionally, thick "cottage-cheese" discharge, seen most often in pregnant patients. The discharge may vary from none to watery to homogeneously thick.

The diagnosis is made by finding a normal vaginal pH (4 to 4.5) and positive results on microscopic exam. Exam of a wet mount or normal saline sample of vaginal secretions will reveal yeast buds and pseudohyphae (Figure 108-2; sensitivity 40 to 60 percent). Two drops of 10 percent KOH added to the vaginal secretions dissolves the vaginal epithelial cells, leaving yeast buds and pseudohyphae intact, increasing the sensitivity (80 percent) of microscopic examination and yielding almost 100 percent specificity. Culture is almost never initiated from the ED. It is suggested for symptomatic patients with negative findings on microscopic examination. However, even this can lead to a false diagnosis as 10 to 20 percent of women usually harbor *Candida* spp. and other yeasts in the vagina.[2] Therefore, treatment of culture-positive patients is limited to those with compatible symptoms.

Most treatment regimens (see Table 108-3) are effective in relieving in excess of 80 percent of infected women.[7] The topically applied azole drugs are more effective than nystatin, with relief of symptoms in 80 to 90 percent of patients who complete treatment. Creams, lotions, sprays, vaginal tablets, suppositories, and coated tampons are all equally efficacious, and the choice of vehicle should depend on the patient's preference. The azole drugs are all available over-the-counter with treatment for 1, 3, or 7 days. Uncomplicated VVC (i.e., mild to moderate symptoms, sporadic, nonrecurrent disease in a normal host with normally susceptible

TABLE 108-3   Treatment Regimens for Vulvovaginal Candidiasis*

Agent	Formulation	Dosage Regimen
Uncomplicated VVC		
Butoconazole (Femstat)	2% Cream	5 g/d × 3 days
Clotrimazole (Lotrimin, Mycelex-G)	100 mg vaginal tablet	2 tablets/d × 3 days
Miconazole (Monistat)	200 mg vaginal suppository	1 suppository/d × 3 days
Nystatin (Mycostatin)	100,000-unit vaginal tablet	1 tablet/d × 14 days
Tioconazole (Vagistat)	6.5% ointment	5 g intravaginally × one dose
Fluconazole (Diflucan)†	150 mg oral tablet	1 tablet × one dose
Complicated VVC		
Fluconazole (Diflucan)†*	150 mg oral tablet	1 tablet on days 1 and 3
Clotrimazole (Lotrimin, Mycelex-G)	500 mg vaginal suppository or tablet	1 suppository/tablet weekly
Pregnant patients†	**Topical azole therapy only**	**Apply for 7 days**

*Not all possible regimens listed.
†Oral therapy not recommended for pregnant patients.

C. albicans) responds to all azoles, including single-dose therapy. Complicated VVC (i.e., severe symptoms, recurrent disease, abnormal host, or resistant organism such as *C. glabrata*) requires therapy lasting from 10 to 14 days with topical or oral azoles.[2,7] Other than initial burning and irritation, side effects of local agents are unusual. Oral agents occasionally cause nausea, abdominal pain, and headaches.

One-day treatment with oral fluconazole is as effective as use of topical preparations but cannot be used in pregnancy and can cause gastrointestinal intolerance, headache, and rash.[8] Ketoconazole can cause liver toxicity as well as adverse drug interactions with a variety of other medications. Oral agents are not recommended to treat candidiasis in pregnant patients. Partners should not be treated unless the woman has frequent recurrences.

Self-medication should only be advised in women with previously diagnosed VVC and recurrence of similar symptoms. If symptoms persist or recur within 2 months, the patient should be seen so that vaginal and microscopic examinations can be performed. Recurrent VVC is defined as four or more episodes per year and occurs in less than 5 percent of healthy women.[9] All possible precipitating factors, such as high blood-glucose levels, should be controlled. However, the majority of women with recurrences do not have obvious precipitating causes.

Management of women with frequent recurrences is aimed at control, rather than cure, with a long-term suppressive prophylactic regimen. Why a minority of women, many of whom have no underlying pathology, have frequent recurrences of infection with resulting morbidity is not fully understood. Current views suggest that local vaginal immune mechanisms may be responsible for frequent relapses. Diagnosis should be certain, oral contraceptives stopped, and blood glucose level checked in diabetics.

TRICHOMONAS VAGINALIS

The causative organism of trichomoniasis is a flagellated protozoan, *T. vaginalis,* that may live quiescently in paraurethral Skene's glands and from this nidus of infestation cause overt infection in the susceptible vagina. Trichomonads are frequently found in the urethra and may be recovered from urine. It is estimated that 2 to 3 million American women contract the disease annually. ***Trichomonas* is almost always a STD,** and its prevalence correlates with the overall level of sexual activity of the population studied. Recent epidemiologic surveys indicate a possible decline in prevalence. Vaginal trichomoniasis may be associated with adverse pregnancy outcomes, particularly PROM and preterm delivery.[10] Seventy percent of men having intercourse with infected women demonstrated the organism within 48 h, while 85 percent of women whose male partners were infected developed *Trichomonas* infection. There is a high prevalence of gonorrhea in women with trichomoniasis. Oral contraceptives, spermicidal agents, and barrier contraceptives are all thought to reduce transmission.

Infection ranges from asymptomatic carrier state to severe, acute inflammatory disease. A vaginal discharge is reported by 50 to 75 percent of patients. It may vary in character from the classic picture of a yellow-green frothy discharge, seen in 20 to 30 percent of patients, to a gray discharge to scant or no discharge. Other symptoms include vulvovaginal soreness and irritation (25 to 50 percent), pruritus, which may be severe (25 to 50 percent), dysuria (25 percent), and malodorous discharge (25 percent). A sense of vulvovaginal fullness may be intense or mild. As many as half of symptomatic women complain of some degree of dyspareunia. Symptoms may be more severe before, during, or after menstruation when the vaginal pH is more alkaline. Lower abdominal pain is rare and should alert the physician to the possibility of other diseases.

Just as symptoms vary in severity, so do the findings on examination. Gynecologic examination reveals the classic "strawberry cervix" secondary to diffuse punctate hemorrhages in only 2 percent of patients. Diffuse erythema is seen in 10 to 33 percent of patients.

The diagnosis is made through use of the "hanging-drop" slide test, which has a sensitivity of 80 to 90 percent in symptomatic patients. A cotton swab is used to obtain a specimen of secretions from the vaginal vault (not the endocervix) and is placed within a drop of normal saline solution on a glass slide. Microscopic examination reveals many polymorphonuclear leukocytes (PMNs) and motile, pear-shaped, flagellated

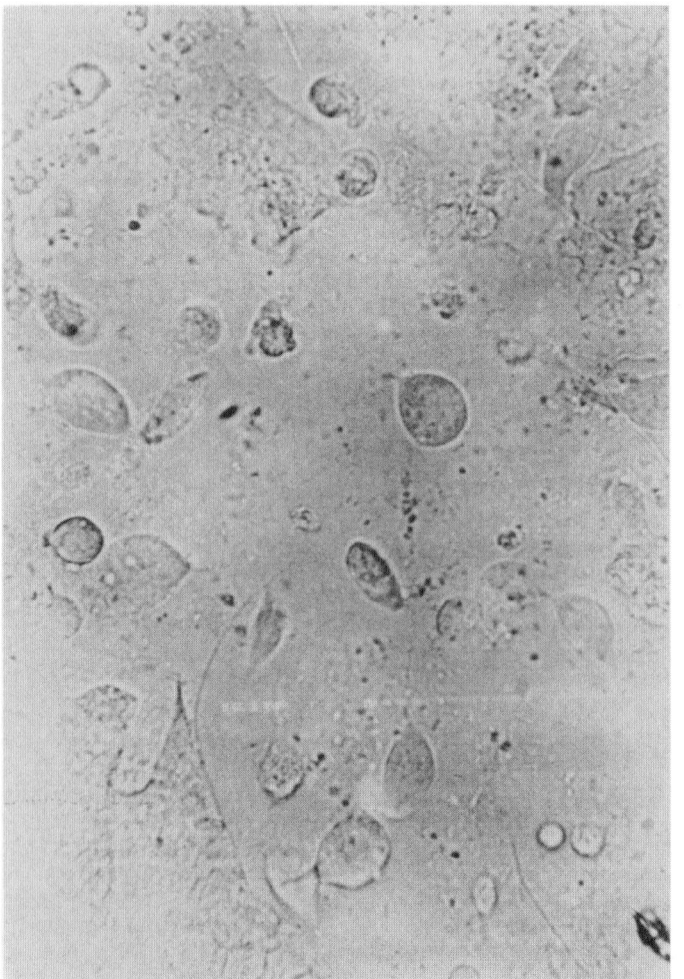

FIG. 108-3. Trichomoniasis: high-power microscopic view of secretions showing multiple trichomonads.

trichomonads, which are slightly larger than the leukocytes (Figure 108-3). As a screening test in asymptomatic individuals, the microscopic test may only be 50 to 70 percent percent sensitive, but has virtually 100 percent specificity. Cultures are approximately 95 percent sensitive and should be considered in symptomatic patients with elevated pH, PMN excess, and absence of motile trichomonads and clue cells.

T. vaginalis may survive up to 24 h in tap water, in hot tubs, in urine, on toilet seats, and in swimming pools, but the usual sequence of events begins with a large deposit of inoculum of organisms contained in the alkaline semen at time of intercourse. Because up to 25 percent of women and 90 percent of men harboring the organisms are asymptomatic, it is difficult to control spread of disease. The cornerstone of therapy remains metronidazole (Table 108-4).[2] Recurrence of disease is frequent and may necessitate more than one course of treatment. There is a 90 percent cure rate with either the single- or multiple-dose regimen. Cure rates increase to more than 90 percent when sexual partners are treated simultaneously. The single-dose treatment is preferable because of lower cost, fewer side effects, and greater patient compliance. Patients not responding may require a 7-day course of therapy. Patients who are allergic may be desensitized but there is no alternative treatment that is efficacious (CDC recommendation).

GENITAL HERPES

Genital herpes is a sexually transmitted infection caused by a deoxyribonucleic acid (DNA)-containing virus specific to human beings. Approximately 25 million individuals are infected with genital herpes in the United States. Sexual transmission can occur during asymptomatic periods. Usually, genital herpes is the most frequently encountered of the diseases causing genital ulcers in the United States,[2] and it may be one of the most frequent sexually transmitted diseases. There are two antigenic groups: herpes simplex virus 1 (HSV-1) and herpes simplex virus 2 (HSV-2). Initially, HSV-1 caused oral lesions and HSV-2 genital lesions, but this is no longer the case. Overall, 85 to 90 percent of genital herpes infections are caused by HSV-2, but some studies have found up to 30 percent are caused by HSV-1. Most cases of recurrent genital herpes are caused by HSV-2. Neonatal infection with high mortality and morbidity rates after passage through an infected birth canal has been seen. It is estimated that at least 50 million persons in the United States are infected.[2] It remains a recurrent disease with no cure at this time.

Initial presentation occurs 1 to 45 days (mean 5.8 days) after exposure. Usually, initial infection is more severe and lasts longer than do subsequent recurrences. There may be both local and systemic manifestations. The lesions begin as painful, fluid-filled vesicles or papules, which progress to well-circumscribed, occasionally coalescent, shallow-based ulcers. They then heal by reepithelialization of mucous membranes or by crusting by the epidermal surface. Symptoms peak in 8 to 10 days and decrease over the next week. Ulcers last 4 to 15 days, with total healing in 21 days. Lymphadenopathy is usually present, and when the deep inguinal nodes are involved, severe pelvic pain may result. Urethritis is usually present, causing severe dysuria, which may cause urethral spasm and urinary retention. Initial disease involves the cervix in more than 80 percent of cases. Pharyngitis and secondary spread of lesions to other body sites, usually below the waist, have been reported in up to two-thirds of patients. Systemic symptoms, such as

TABLE 108-4 Treatment Regimens for Trichomoniasis

Agent	Dose
RECOMMENDED REGIMEN	
Metronidazole	2 g PO in a single dose
ALTERNATIVE REGIMEN	
Metronidazole	500 mg PO bid for 7 d

Note: Avoid alcohol during and for at least 24 h after treatment. Metronidazole can be used in pregnant women, but is not approved for use by the US FDA until the second trimester; and only if other treatment fails.

fever, malaise, headache, and myalgias, are common. Hepatitis, aseptic meningitis, and autonomic nervous system dysfunction can occur. Aseptic meningitis has been seen more frequently with HSV-2 than with HSV-1 infection and has been reported in approximately 30 percent of patients. Sacral autonomic nervous dysfunction is rare but can result in decreased cutaneous sensation and bladder and bowel dysfunction. After the attack is over, the inactive virus resides in the sacral dorsal root ganglia. Under various stimuli, both exogenous and endogenous, the virus travels down the sensory nerve root to the lower genital area, where it replicates and becomes symptomatic.

Recurrent episodes are usually milder than the initial disease, and the patient usually does not have systemic symptoms. A recurrence may be heralded by genital tingling. Recurrent genital lesions are fewer, smaller, and more often unilateral. Lesions may be ulcerative or resemble a fissure or excoriations. Recurrences tend to occur in the same location and have the same appearance from episode to episode. Symptoms last 4 to 8 days, and the lesions have usually disappeared by 10 days. Frequency of attacks and intervals between attacks are highly variable. The average number of symptomatic recurrences is 5 to 8 per year. Asymptomatic infections, defined as culture-positive viral shedding in the absence of symptoms or lesions, have been documented.

Approximately 25 percent of initial presentations occur in women with preexisting antibody to herpes simplex virus. The initial episodes tend to be less severe. They may, in fact, represent recurrent infections in patients who had previous asymptomatic infections. Clinically, it is impossible to distinguish between HSV-1 and HSV-2 infections, but HSV-1 usually causes milder initial disease, results in recurrence less frequently, and results in milder recurrent episodes.

Diagnosis is suspected by clinical presentation and confirmed by either culture, which is the preferred virologic test according to 2002 CDC guidelines (may become positive within 2 to 3 days of inoculation), or polymerase chain reaction (PCR). Although PCR is extremely sensitive in detecting low concentrations of viral DNA, the CDC has not yet recommended it as the test of choice. The virus can be isolated from vesicle fluid and the base of a wet ulcer. Intact vesicles, if present, should be unroofed and the fluid cultured directly. Scrapings of an ulcer may be taken for a Papanicolaou (Pap) smear or Tzanck preparation. A Tzanck smear stained with either Wright or Giemsa stain is positive if multinucleated giant cells are present, which may be seen in up to 50 percent of cases, but may be falsely positive. Serologic analysis is useful in classifying the initial herpetic episode as primary or nonprimary but is usually not indicated.

Treatment is not curative. Multiple antiviral agents and regimens are available (Table 108-5). Systemic antiviral agents provide partial control of the signs and symptoms and accelerate healing of the lesions, but do not affect the frequency or severity of recurrences. Topical therapy is ineffective.[2] Patients with severe disease may need hospitalization and intravenous therapy. In recurrent episodes, treatment should be started during the prodrome or within 1 day of onset of lesions if treatment is to be beneficial. For patients with frequent recurrences (six or more episodes per year) daily suppressive therapy can be used but should be discontinued after 1 year to allow assessment of the patient's recurrent episodes. Daily suppressive therapy reduces the frequency of recurrences by at least 75 percent. Suppressive therapy does not lessen the rate of viral shedding, and therefore patients should be advised of their continued risk of infecting sexual partners.

The safety of acyclovir and valacyclovir during pregnancy has not been established, however there has been no increased risk for major birth defects in pregnant women treated with these agents as compared to the general population. In pregnant patients with life-threatening disease, such as encephalitis, pneumonitis, or hepatitis, intravenous acyclovir should be used. It should not be used for recurrent episodes or as suppressive therapy. Pregnant women treated with the drug should be reported to the Glaxo-Wellcome registry, which is kept in cooperation with the CDC (1-800-722-9292, extension 38465). Current registry findings do not indicate an increased risk for major birth defects after acyclovir treatment.[2]

Systemic analgesics may be needed. Some patients have severe dysuria when the urine comes in contact with vaginal and vulvar tis-

TABLE 108-5 Treatment of Genital Herpes

Agent (Oral Tablets or Caplets)	Dose
INITIAL EPISODE	
Acyclovir	400 mg tid for 7–10 d
Famciclovir	250 mg tid for 7–10 d
Valacyclovir	1 g bid for 7–10 d
EPISODIC RECURRENT INFECTION	
Acyclovir	400 mg tid for 5 d
Famciclovir	125 mg bid for 5 d
Valacyclovir	500 mg bid for 5 d
DAILY SUPPRESSIVE THERAPY	
Acyclovir	400 mg bid
Famciclovir	250 mg bid
Valacyclovir	1 g daily
INTRAVENOUS THERAPY FOR SEVERE INITIAL PRESENTATION	
Acyclovir	5–10 mg/kg qid for 5–7 d
PREGNANCY	
Acyclovir	If severe or IV required 5–10 mg/kg qid for 5–7 d

Note: All agents categorized class B may be used for pregnant patients.

sues. Pouring warm water over these tissues during urination may provide symptomatic relief. HSV infection is a major source of morbidity and mortality for newborns. When active lesions are present at time of delivery, cesarean section may be necessary. Every effort should be made to prevent infection during pregnancy and to treat active disease.

CONTACT VULVOVAGINITIS

Contact dermatitis results from the exposure of vulvar epithelium and vaginal mucosa to a primary chemical irritant or an allergen. In either case, characteristic local erythema and edema occur. Severe reactions may progress to ulceration and secondary infection. Common irritants and/or allergens include chemically scented douches; soaps; bubble baths; deodorants; perfumes, dyes, and scents in toilet paper, tampons, and pads; feminine hygiene products; topical vaginal antibiotics; and tight slacks, pantyhose, and synthetic underwear.

Clinically, patients report local swelling and itching or a burning sensation. The gynecologic examination reveals an erythematous and edematous vulvovaginal area. Local vesiculation and ulceration are seen more commonly with allergens or when primary irritants are used in strong concentrations. Vaginal pH changes may promote colonization and infection with *C. albicans*, thus obscuring the primary cause.

Diagnosis of contact vulvovaginitis is made by ruling out an infectious cause and by identifying the offending agent. Most cases of mild vulvovaginal contact dermatitis resolve spontaneously when the causative agent is withdrawn. For patients with severe, painful reactions, cool sitz baths and wet compresses of dilute boric acid or Burow's solution may afford relief. Topical corticosteroids, such as hydrocortisone acetate (0.5 to 2.5 percent), fluocinolone acetonide (0.01 to 0.2 percent), or triamcinolone acetonide (.025 percent), relieve symptoms over a few applications and promote healing. Creams can be applied two or three times a day. Oral histamines may be helpful if a true allergic reaction is present. Superinfection with *C. albicans*, should it occur, should be treated as previously described. In these cases Mycolog (nystatin/triamcinolone) can be used.

Vulvovaginitis in the HIV-1-Positive Woman

Presence of vulvovaginitis may predispose women to infection by the human immunodeficiency virus (HIV) virus. Women who are HIV-1-positive may have an increased incidence of vulvovaginitis and may be more likely to infect others during this period. There is evidence that disturbance of the normal vaginal flora and presence of BV may be a risk factor for acquisition of HIV infection.[2] Among HIV-1-seropositive women, the prevalence of *Candida* vulvovaginitis is reported to be as high as 62 percent.[11] Rates of colonization are similar in nonimmunocompromised HIV-positive women and HIV-negative women. When CD4[+] T-cell counts are below 200/μL rates of colonization are increased as is symptomatic vaginitis. Recurrence of disease is also more frequent in immunocompromised HIV-positive women, as compared to HIV-positive women with CD4[+] T-cell counts >200/μL and HIV-negative women.[12] Treatment of VVC infection resulted in decreased viral shedding and thus infectivity in women who have *Candida* vaginitis.[13] The optimal treatment of HIV-positive patients remains undefined; therefore, these patients should be treated with the same regimen as HIV-negative women.[7] Treatment of patients with trichomoniasis has resulted in decrease of cell-free HIV-1 in vaginal secretions which may lead to decreased infectivity.[14] Herpes genitalis is thought to be associated with an increased risk for HIV infection.[2]

VAGINAL FOREIGN BODIES

Children and adolescents may insert objects intravaginally during periods of genital exploration or sexual stimulation. In young girls, the most commonly inserted foreign bodies are rolled-up pieces of toilet paper, toys, and small household objects. In adolescents and adult women, it is often a forgotten tampon or sponge contraceptive. Foreign objects left in place for more than 48 h can cause severe localized infections due to *Escherichia coli,* anaerobes, or overgrowth of other vaginal flora. Patients present with a foul-smelling and/or bloody vaginal discharge. The only treatment necessary for vaginitis secondary to the presence of a foreign body is removal of the object.[1] In most cases, the vaginal discharge and odor will disappear without further therapy within several days.

PINWORMS

Pinworms *(Enterobius vermicularis)* may migrate from the anus to the vagina in children and cause intense pruritus that is often most intense during the night, when gravid female worms pass out from the intestinal tract to lay eggs on the perineal skin. Cellophane tape can be used to obtain material for a slide, which can be examined microscopically for the presence of ova, which are large and double-walled in appearance. The child and all family members need treatment with an antiparasitic agent, either mebendazole 100 mg PO × 1 and repeated in 2 weeks; albendazole, 400 mg PO × 1 and repeated in 2 weeks; or pyrantel pamoate 11 mg/kg PO × 1 dose with a repeat dose q 2 weeks × 2 (maximum single dose 1g). Repeat treatment 2 weeks later should be administered because mature worms seem more vulnerable to treatment than do young worms. Albendazole is contraindicated in pregnancy; mebendazole can be used with caution. Pyrantel pamoate is available without prescription.

ATROPHIC VAGINITIS

During menarche, pregnancy, and lactation, and after menopause, the vaginal epithelium lacks the stimulation of estrogen. The maturation of the vaginal and urethra mucosa depends on the presence of estrogen and can be altered by the absence of estrogen or the presence of antiestrogenic factors, such as hormones, drugs, or diseases. Menopause results in a vaginal mucosa that is attenuated, pale, and almost transparent as a result of decreased vascularity. The vagina loses its normal rugae. The squamous epithelium atrophies, the glycogen content of the cells decreases, and the vaginal pH ranges from 5.5 to 7.0. The mucosa is only three or four cells thick and is less resistant to minor trauma and infection. Marked atrophic changes can cause atrophic vaginitis. It is important to distinguish between symptomatic atrophic vaginitis,

which is rare, and an atrophic vagina that is a result of physiologic changes of menopause. When symptomatic vaginitis occurs, the vaginal epithelium is thin, inflamed, and even ulcerated. Symptoms include vaginal soreness, dyspareunia, and occasional spotting or discharge, which may be a thin, scant, yellowish or pink material. The cervix atrophies and retracts and may become flush with the apex of the vault. The upper one-third of the vagina constricts, and the entire vagina becomes shorter in length and loses its elasticity. The increased vaginal pH may permit the growth of nonacidophilic coliform organisms, bacteria not normally found in the vagina, and the disappearance of *Lactobacillus* species. This can lead to the development of a clinical vaginal infection with copious purulent discharge. Unless estrogenic replacement therapy is used, *Candida* and *Trichomonas* infections are rare. The changes seen vary widely from one patient to another.

A Papanicolaou (Pap) smear of the cervix and vagina is mandatory in the face of bleeding to rule out carcinoma. A wet preparation will show erythrocytes and increased PMNs associated with small, round epithelial cells, which are immature squamous cells that have not been exposed to sufficient estrogen.

The treatment of atrophic vaginitis consists primarily of topical vaginal estrogen. Nightly use of vaginal tablets is effective. Estradiol absorption from vaginal tablets has been found to be negligible when low dose formulations (10 to 25 μg) are used.[15] Estrogen should not be prescribed for any patient with a past history of cancer of any of the reproductive organs. Atrophic vaginitis is usually not seen in patients who are already on systemic estrogen replacement therapy. Patients should be referred for follow-up to monitor therapy and for the results of the Pap smear.

REFERENCES

1. Jaquiery A, Stylianopoulos A, Hogg G, et al: Vulvovaginitis: Clinical features, aetiology, and microbiology of the genital tract. *Arch Dis Child* 81:64, 1999.
2. Centers for Disease Control: 2002 Guidelines for treatment of sexually transmitted diseases: Recommendations and reports. *MMWR* 51(RR-06):1, 2002.
3. Koumantakis EE, Hassan EA, Deligeoroglou EK, et al: Vulvovaginitis during childhood and adolescence. *J Pediatr Adolesc Gynecol* 10:39, 1997.
4. French JI, McGregor JA, Draper D, et al: Gestational bleeding, bacterial vaginosis, and common reproductive tract infections: Risk for preterm birth and benefit of treatment. *Obstet Gynecol* 93:715, 1999.
5. Sobel JD: Vaginitis. *New Engl J Med* 337:1896, 1997.
6. Foxman B: The epidemiology of vulvovaginal candidiasis: Risk factors. *Am J Public Health* 80:329, 1990.
7. Reef SE, Levine WC, McNeil MM, et al: Treatment options for vulvovaginal candidiasis. *Clin Infect Dis* 20(suppl 1):S80, 1995.
8. Sobel JD, Brooker D, Stein GE, et al: Single oral dose fluconazole compared with conventional clotrimazole topical therapy of *Candida vaginitis.* Fluconazole Vaginitis Study Group. *Am J Obstet Gynecol* 172:1263, 1995.
9. Rodgers CA, Beardall AJ: Recurrent vulvovaginal candidiasis: Why does it occur? *Int J STD AIDS* 10:435; quiz 440, 1999.
10. Fiscella K: Racial disparities in preterm births. The role of urogenital infections. *Public Health Rep* 111:104, 1996.
11. Martin HL, Richardson BA, Nyange PM, et al: Vaginal lactobacilli, microbial flora, and risk of human immunodeficiency virus type 1 and sexually transmitted disease acquisition. *J Infect Dis* 180:1863, 1999.
12. Spinillo A, Michelone G, Cavanna C, et al: Clinical and microbiological characteristics of symptomatic vulvovaginal candidiasis in HIV-seropositive women. *Genitourin Med* 70:268, 1994.
13. Duerr A, Sierra MF, Feldman J, et al: Immune compromise and prevalence of *Candida* vulvovaginitis in human immunodeficiency virus-infected women. *Obstet Gynecol* 90:252, 1997.
14. Wang CC, McClelland RS, Reilly M, et al: The effect of treatment of vaginal infections on shedding of human immunodeficiency virus type 1. *J Infect Dis* 183:1017, 2001.
15. Notelovitz M, Funk S, Nanavati N, et al: Estradiol absorption from vaginal tablets in postmenopausal women. *Obstet Gynecol* 99:556, 2002.

PELVIC INFLAMMATORY DISEASE
Amy J. Behrman
William H. Shoff
Suzanne M. Shepherd

Pelvic inflammatory disease (PID) comprises a spectrum of infections of the female upper reproductive tract. It is a common and serious disease initiated by ascending infection from the cervix and vagina. PID may include salpingitis, endometritis, and tubo-ovarian abscess and may extend to produce pelvic peritonitis and perihepatitis. The annual rate of PID in industrialized countries has been reported to be as high as 10 to 20 per 1000 women of reproductive age, with as many as 1.5 million cases estimated to occur per year in the United States.[1] These numbers likely underestimate the true incidence because of widely variable symptoms and the relatively poor reliability of the clinical diagnosis. Long-term sequelae, including tubal factor infertility (TFI), ectopic pregnancy, and chronic pain, may occur in as many as 25 percent of patients. The annual direct costs of the acute disease and its sequelae were estimated to be $1.88 billion in 1998.[1]

Patients with PID frequently present to the ED with nonspecific complaints and findings. Early diagnosis and aggressive treatment may provide rapid clinical and microbiologic improvement, identify coexisting disease, decrease transmission, and minimize the likelihood of serious sequelae.

ETIOLOGY

Neisseria gonorrhoeae and *Chlamydia trachomatis* can be isolated in many, if not most, cases of PID, and therapy traditionally has been directed primarily against these organisms. However, newer, more sensitive, and more specific culture techniques have improved our understanding of PID significantly. Polymicrobial infection, including anaerobic and aerobic vaginal flora, clearly has been demonstrated in studies relying on cultural material from the upper reproductive tract. Earlier culdocentesis studies suggested that 80 percent of PID was polymicrobial, but there is evidence that this may represent a degree of contamination of the cul-de-sac by the procedure. Laparoscopy cultures more conservatively point to mixed infection in 30 to 40 percent of cases. Pathogenic organisms may include anaerobes, *Gardnerella vaginalis,* enteric gram-negative rods, *Haemophilus influenzae, Streptococcus agalactiae, Mycoplasma hominis,* and *Ureaplasma urealyticum. N. gonorrhoeae* and *C. trachomatis* often may be instrumental in the initial infection of the upper genital tract, whereas anaerobes, facultative anaerobes, and other bacteria are isolated increasingly as inflammation increases and abscesses form. Bacterial vaginosis also may play a role in the initiation of ascending infection, particularly after abortion or gynecologic surgery.[2,3] HIV-1 infection is associated with an increased incidence of *C. trachomatis* infection and an increased risk of progression to PID.[4] PID also may result from *M. tuberculosis* in endemic areas.[5] The microbiology of PID also reflects the predominant sexually transmitted diseases prevalent within a given population.

Pathology and Risk Factors

Most cases of PID are presumed to originate with sexually transmitted diseases (STDs) of the lower genital tract, followed by ascending infection of the upper tract. The original STD may be asymptomatic. It is estimated that 10 to 20 percent of untreated gonococcal or chlamydial cervicitis may progress to PID. The precise mechanisms by which infection and inflammation in the upper genital tract are initiated and propagated remain under investigation. Although the cervical mucus serves as a functional barrier to ascending infection much of the time, its efficacy may be decreased by hormonal changes during ovulation and by retrograde menstruation. Bacteria also may be carried by or along with sperm into the uterus and tubes. Uterine infection usually is limited to the endometrium but may be more invasive in a gravid or postpartum uterus. Tubal infection initially affects only the mucosa, but acute, complement-mediated transmural inflammation may develop rapidly and increase in intensity with repeated infection. Inflammation may extend to uninfected parametrial structures, including the bowel. If purulent material from the tubes spills into the abdomen, pelvic peritonitis may result. Infection may extend by direct or lymphatic spread beyond the pelvis to involve the hepatic capsule with acute perihepatitis and focal peritonitis (FitzHugh-Curtis syndrome).

Risk factors for PID within a sexually active population include multiple sexual partners, history of other STDs, history of sexual abuse, and frequent vaginal douching.[6–9] Younger age is associated with increased risk, possibly because of a larger zone of cervical ectopy in young women, increased cervical mucosal permeability, lower prevalence of protective chlamydial antibodies, risk-taking behavior, or a combination of these factors. Consistent barrier contraception is associated with lower risk of PID. Intrauterine device (IUD) use has been associated with a two- to ninefold increased risk for PID, but recent data indicate that the risk with current IUDs may be much less.[10] Oral contraceptive pills (OCPs) have been thought to increase the risk of endocervical infection (probably by increasing the zone of cervical ectopy) but to decrease the risk of symptomatic PID, possibly by increasing the viscosity of cervical mucus, decreasing menstrual blood flow (and hence decreasing retrograde menstruation), or modifying local immune responses. Recent data, however, suggest that OCPs may have no effect on PID incidence.[11] Bilateral tubal ligation (BTL) does not provide protection against PID, but patients with BTL may have delayed and/or milder forms of the disease.[12] Pregnancy decreases the risk of PID because the cervical os is protected by a mucous plug. However, PID can occur during the first trimester and may cause fetal loss.

In addition to host factors, genetic polymorphisms of PID pathogens may affect the likelihood that a lower tract infection will progress to frank PID. P9-Opa(b) protein expression in *N. gonorrhoeae*[13] and CHSP60 antigen expression in *C. trachomatis*[14] are recent examples of specific bacterial genes implicated in PID pathogenesis.

Complications

PID is associated with a number of serious clinical sequelae. Tubo-ovarian abscess is reported in up to one-third of women hospitalized for PID. Infection and inflammation can lead to scarring and adhesions within tubal lumens. The rate of potentially fatal ectopic pregnancy is 12 to 15 percent higher in women who have had PID. TFI is increased 12 to 50 percent in women with a past diagnosis of PID, and the incidence of TFI increases with the number and severity of past PID episodes. Asymptomatic or silent PID appears to be associated with TFI as well; 50 percent of women with TFI have no history of PID but do have scarring of the fallopian tubes and exhibit antibodies to *N. gonorrhoeae* and/or *C. trachomatis.* Chronic pelvic pain and/or dyspareunia has been reported in 18 percent of women with past histories of PID.

DIAGNOSIS

Clinical Findings

HISTORY Lower abdominal pain is the most frequent presenting complaint in PID. Other symptoms may include abnormal vaginal discharge, vaginal bleeding, postcoital bleeding, dyspareunia, irritative voiding symptoms, fever, malaise, nausea, and vomiting. PID may be minimally symptomatic or asymptomatic.[15] The differential diagnosis of these nonspecific presentations includes cervicitis, ectopic pregnancy, endometriosis, ovarian cyst, ovarian torsion, spontaneous abortion, septic abortion, cholecystitis, gastroenteritis, appendicitis, diverticulitis, pyelonephritis, and renal colic.

PHYSICAL EXAMINATION   The physical examination is usually notable for lower abdominal tenderness, cervical motion tenderness, and uterine and/or adnexal tenderness. The positive predictive value (PPV) of these findings will vary depending on the prevalence of PID in a given clinical population. However, one large multicenter trial found adnexal tenderness to be the most sensitive finding on physical examination (95 percent sensitive, $p < 0.001$).[16] Mucopurulent cervicitis is common and has a significant negative predictive value when absent.[15] Disproportionate unilateral adnexal tenderness and/or adnexal mass or fullness may indicate an ovarian abscess. Abdominal guarding and rebound tenderness will develop with peritonitis. Right upper quadrant tenderness, particularly with jaundice, may indicate FitzHugh-Curtis syndrome. Signs of other STDs should be noted and evaluated.

Laboratory Evaluation

Laboratory evaluation in the ED always should include a pregnancy test. The possibility of ectopic pregnancy or septic abortion must be considered, and concurrent pregnancy will influence PID therapy. Saline- and potassium hydroxide-treated wet preparations of vaginal secretions should be examined for leukorrhea (more than one polymorphonuclear leukocyte per epithelial cell), trichomoniasis, and clue cells. The absence of leukorrhea in saline preparations is a negative predictor for PID.[15] Endocervical swabs should be sent for culture and can be Gram stained for gonococci. DNA probes for gonorrhea and *Chlamydia* are useful and increasingly available. Quantitative culture for *Chlamydia*, the most common causal agent for PID, identifies rapidly replicating bacteria that appear to be associated with active disease,[17] but these results will not be available to the emergency physician at the time of evaluation.

Elevated white blood cell counts, sedimentation rates, and/or C-reactive protein support the diagnosis of PID. The rapid plasma reagin test for syphilis should be performed. Patients should be counseled and tested for hepatitis and HIV. HIV-infected women with PID may present more often with tubo-ovarian abscess and coinfection with *Candida* and human papillomavirus.[15] Blood cultures do not aid in the diagnosis or management of PID.[18]

Procedures

A number of procedures can be performed to improve the accuracy of PID diagnosis. These procedures are not necessary, nor are they indicated, in every case of presumptive PID. However, since PID is difficult to diagnose definitively on clinical grounds and may mimic surgical emergencies,[19] the clinician should be familiar with these modalities.

Transvaginal pelvic ultrasound may demonstrate thickened (>5 mm), fluid-filled fallopian tubes or free pelvic fluid in acute, severe PID. These findings alone are not specific enough to make a definitive diagnosis. However, pelvic abscesses may be seen as complex adnexal masses with multiple internal echoes. In the individual who appears toxic or has asymmetric pelvic findings, ED pelvic ultrasound is an important diagnostic tool for the identification of a tubo-ovarian abscess. Pelvic ultrasound also will be useful in evaluating the possibility of ectopic pregnancy in those patients in whom the differential diagnosis includes both entities. Power Doppler transvaginal sonography is reported to be extremely accurate in diagnosing PID and assessing the severity of the disease.[20]

Endometrial biopsy can be used for the histopathologic diagnosis of endometritis. Endometritis is uniformly associated with salpingitis. Specimens for culture also may be obtained but frequently will be contaminated with vaginal flora. The procedure is performed with an endometrial suction pipette/curette and is well tolerated. Endometrial biopsy is approximately 90 percent specific with similar sensitivity. However, diagnostic utility in the ED is limited because results are not immediately available.

Culdocentesis can be performed rapidly in the ED. However, its utility is also limited. The potential positive findings of leukocytes and bacteria are nonspecific and may be a product of other inflammatory processes, such as appendicitis or diverticulitis, or due to contamination with vaginal contents.

Laparoscopy is the "gold standard" for the diagnosis of PID. It is significantly more sensitive and specific than clinical criteria alone. The minimum criteria to diagnose PID laparoscopically include visible hyperemia of the tubal surface, tubal wall edema, and the presence of exudate on the tubal surface and fimbriae. Pelvic masses consistent with tubo-ovarian abscess or ectopic pregnancy also can be visualized directly. Hepatic capsule exudate and/or adhesions may be demonstrated. Material may be obtained for definitive culture without the risk of vaginal contamination. However, the procedure is invasive and expensive, requiring an operating room and anesthesia. Findings on laparoscopy do not necessarily correlate with the severity of illness because the laparoscopist can see only the surfaces of structures. Laparoscopy may fail to define up to 20 percent of cases.[21]

Diagnostic Guidelines

To expedite treatment and maximize compliance, the diagnosis of PID in ED and clinics is usually based on clinical criteria with or without laboratory evidence. The Centers for Disease Control and Prevention (CDC) regularly reviews STD research and epidemiology in order to update guidelines for diagnosis and treatment. Current guidelines[15] for PID stratify diagnostic criteria into the three groups shown in Table 109-1.

THERAPY

Treatment

Treatment of PID is aimed at relieving acute symptoms, eradicating current infection, and minimizing the risk of long-term sequelae. There is no clear role for anti-inflammatory drugs at this time, but effective analgesia should be administered. Therapy initiated in the ED must include empirical broad-spectrum antibiotics to cover the full range of likely organisms. All regimens should be effective against anaerobes, gram-negative facultative organisms, and streptococci, as well as *N. gonorrheae* and *C. trachomatis*. Long-term outcomes are improved if antibiotics are begun immediately.[15]

No published studies have effectively compared parenteral and oral antibiotic regimens or inpatient versus outpatient regimens with regard to documented elimination of endometrial and tubal infection. Many studies have demonstrated the effectiveness a variety of parenteral and

TABLE 109-1   Treatment Guidelines for PID Based on Diagnostic Criteria

Group 1: Minimum criteria. Empirical treatment indicated if no other etiology to explain findings
   Uterine or adnexal tenderness
   Cervical motion tenderness
Group 2: Additional criteria improving diagnostic specificity
   Oral temperature $>101°F$ ($38.3°C$)
   Abnormal cervical or vaginal mucopurulent secretions
   Elevated erythrocyte sedimentation rate
   Elevated C-reactive protein
   Laboratory evidence of cervical infection with *N. gonorrheae* or
      C. trachomatis (i.e., culture or DNA probe techniques)
Group 3: Specific criteria for PID based on procedures that may be appropriate for some patients
   Laparoscopic confirmation
   Transvaginal ultrasound (or MRI) showing thickened, fluid-filled tubes
      with/without free pelvic fluid or tubo-ovarian complex
   Endometrial biospy showing endometritis.

Source: Adapted from CDC.[15]

TABLE 109-2   Parenteral Treatment Regimens for PID

1. Cefotetan 2 g IV q12h *or* cefoxitin 2 g IV q6h *and* doxycycline 100 mg PO or IV q12h
2. Clindamycin 900 mg IV q8h *and* gentamicin 2 mg/kg IV loading dose followed by 1.5 mg/kg q8h
3. Ofloxacin 400 mg IV q12h *or* levofloxacin 500 mg IV q24h (prefer >18 years of age due to concerns regarding adverse effects on cartilage)[22] *with or without* metronidazole 500 mg IV q8h *or* ampicillin-sulbactam 3 g IV q6h and doxycycline 100 mg PO or IV q12h

Note: PO doxycyline has the same bioavailability as IV and avoids painful infusion. Gentamicin dosing may be every 24 h.
Source: Adapted from the CDC.[15]

oral regimes in the elimination of acute symptoms and the achievement of microbiologic cures. Currently accepted treatment regimens are summarized in Tables 109-2 and 109-3. Physicians should be familiar with current patterns of drug resistance in their patient populations.

If an IUD is present, it should be removed after antibiotics have been started.

Twenty-four hours after clinical improvement, patients with PID who require initial intravenous antibiotics can be switched to oral antibiotics, which should be continued for a total of 14 days. Oral therapy is usually doxycycline (100 mg PO bid). In the setting of tubo-ovarian abcess, oral therapy should be continued with clindamycin (450 mg PO qid) *or* metronidazole with doxycycline for better anaerobic coverage.

All patients should be reevaluated in 72 h for evidence of substantial clinical improvement (defervescence, decreased abdominal tenderness, decreased uterine, adnexal, and cervical motion tenderness) and compliance with their regimen.

Surgical Intervention

Patients who do not improve within 72 h should be reevaluated for possible laparoscopic or surgical intervention, i.e., drainage of pus loculations or tubo-ovarian abscess, or to reconsider other possible diagnoses.

The majority of tubo-ovarian abscesses (60–80 percent) will resolve with antibiotic administration alone. If patients do not respond clinically to antibiotics, laparoscopy may be useful to identify pus loculations requiring drainage, or alternative pathologies. An enlarging pelvic mass may indicate bleeding secondary to vessel erosion or a ruptured abscess. Unresolved abscesses may be drained percutaneously, laparoscopically, or surgically.

DISPOSITION

Guidelines for the admission (Table 109-4) and inpatient treatment of PID patients have evolved over the past decade (see Table 109-2). Parenteral therapy no longer requires admission in many settings, and there are no data to demonstrate that inpatient treatment is more effective than outpatient treatment in optimizing long-term clinical outcomes. Admission of adolescents and those with coexisting HIV infection should be reviewed on an individual basis.[22] Admission

TABLE 109-3   Oral/Outpatient Treatment Regimens for PID

1. Ofloxacin 400 mg PO bid for 14 days *or* levofloxacin 500 mg PO qd for 14 days (prefer >18 years of age due to concern regarding adverse effects on cartilage)[21] *with or without* Metronidazole 500 mg PO bid for 14 days
2. Ceftriaxone 250 mg IM once *or* cefoxitin 2 g IM once and probenecid 1 g PO once *and* doxycycline 100 mg PO bid for 14 days *with or without* metronidazole 500 mg PO bid for 14 days

Note: Other parenteral third-generation cephalosporins can be substituted for ceftriaxone or cefoxitin.
Source: Adapted from the CDC.[15]

TABLE 109-4   Admission Considerations

Surgical emergency cannot be excluded from the differential
Pregnancy
Failure to respond to outpatient treatment
Inability to tolerate or comply with outpatient treatment
Severe toxicity, nausea, vomiting
Tubo-ovarian abscess

Source: Adapted from the CDC.[15]

decisions in the ED are based on severity of illness, likelihood of compliance with outpatient medications, likelihood of major anaerobic infection (IUD, suspected pelvic or tubo-ovarian abscess, or history of recent uterine instrumentation), certainty of diagnosis, coexisting illness and immunosuppression, pregnancy, patient age, and other major fertility issues. A gynecologist must be consulted on all patients considered for admission, including those with coexisting pregnancy, IUD, or tubo-ovarian abscess. A surgeon should be consulted if appendicitis cannot be excluded. Abdominal computed tomographic examination with oral and intravenous contrast material is the best modality to use in this instance to clarify the situation.

PREVENTION

Uncomplicated endocervical infections with *N. gonorrheae* and *C. trachomatis* are often underdiagnosed and undertreated. One study found a 10.4 percent prevalence of unrecognized genital gonorrhea and *Chlamydia* infection in a general urban ED population.[23] Improving education, diagnosis, and empirical treatment rates for these infections, as well as for minimally symptomatic PID, should result in a lower incidence and prevalence of PID and should decrease the incidence of major long-term sequelae, such as infertility and ectopic pregnancy. In addition, routine screening for *N. gonorrheae* and *C. trachomatis* in women at risk for PID using DNA probes of cervical specimens or urine[15,24] could theoretically reduce the incidence of PID and its sequelae.

Patients discharged with PID may be noncompliant with medications, may not understand their diagnoses, and frequently do not obtain partner treatment. Patients should be educated about these issues, as well as the advisability of testing and treatment for other STDs, including syphilis and HIV. Patients should understand the use of barrier contraceptives and other "safe sex" techniques to lessen their risk of reinfection.

Finally, and perhaps most important, partner treatment is crucial to preventing repeated episodes of PID. Partners of PID patients should be treated empirically for *N. gonorrheae* and *C. trachomatis* if they have had sexual contact with the patient in the 60 days preceding the onset of her symptoms. Sexual contact should be avoided until one full course of treatment is completed for each partner.[14]

REFERENCES

1. Rein DB, Kassler WJ, Irwin KL, et al: Direct medical cost of pelvic inflammatory disease and its sequelae: Decreasing but still substantial. *Obstet Gynecol* 95:397, 2000.
2. Peipert JF, Montagno AB, Cooper AS, Sung CJ: Bacterial vaginosis as a risk factor for upper genital infection. *Am J Obstet Gynecol* 177:1184, 1997.
3. Koumans EH, Kendrick JS, CDC Bacterial Vaginosis Working Group: Preventing adverse sequelae of bacterial vaginosis: A public health program and research agenda. *Sex Transm Dis* 28:292, 2001.
4. Brunham RC, Kimani J, Bwayo J, et al: The epidemiology of *Chlamydia trachomatis* within a sexually transmitted diseases core group. *J Infect Dis* 173:950, 1996.
5. Avan BI, Fatmi Z, Rashid S: Comparison of the clinical and laparoscopic features of infertile women suffering from genital tuberculosis (TB) or pelvic inflammatory disease or endometriosis. *J Pakistan Med Assoc* 51:393, 2001.

6. Marks C, Tideman RL, Estcourt CS, et al: Assessment of risk for pelvic inflammatory disease in an urban sexual health population. *Sex Transm Infect* 76:470, 2000.

7. Ness RB, Soper DE, Holley RL, et al: Douching and endometritis: Results from the PID Evaluation and Clinical Health (PEACH) study. *Sex Transm Dis* 28:240, 2001.

8. Champion JD, Piper J, Shain R, et al: Minority women with sexually transmitted diseases, sexual abuse and risk for pelvic inflammatory disease. *Res Nurs Health* 24:38, 2001.

9. Dayal M, Barnhart RT: Noncontraceptive benefits and therapeutic uses of the oral contraceptive pill. *Semin Reprod Med* 19:295, 2001.

10. Shelton JD: Risk of clinical pelvic inflammatory disease attributable to an intrauterine device. *Lancet* 357:443; 2001.

11. Ness RB, Soper DE, Holley RL, et al: Hormonal and barrier contraception and risk of upper genital tract disease in the PID Evaluation and Clinical Health (PEACH) study. *Am J Obstet Gynecol* 185:121, 2001.

12. Levgur M, Duvivier R: Pelvic inflammatory disease after tubal sterilization: A review. *Obstet Gynecol Surv* 55:41, 2000.

13. Makepeace BL, Watt PJ, Heckels JE, et al: Interactions of *Neisseria gonorrhoeae* with mature human macrophage opacity proteins influence production of proinflammatory cytokines. *Infect Immun* 69:1909, 2001.

14. Kinnunen A, Molander P, Morrison R, et al: Chlamydial heat shock protein 60—specific T cells in inflamed salpingeal tissue. *Fertil Steril* 77:162, 2002.

15. Centers for Disease Control and Prevention: 2002 Guidelines for treatment of sexually transmitted diseases. *MMWR* 51(RR-6):1, 2002.

16. Peipert JF, Ness RB, Blume J, et al: Clinical predictors of endometritis in women with symptoms and signs of pelvic inflammatory disease. *Am J Obstet Gynecol* 184:856, 2001.

17. Geisler WM, Suchland RJ, Whittington WLH, et al: Quantitative culture of *Chlamydia trachomatis:* Relationship of inclusion-forming units produced in culture to clinical manifestations and acute inflammation in urogenital disease. *J Infect Dis* 184:1350, 2001.

18. Apuzzio JJ, Hessami S, Rodrigquez P: Blood cultures for women hospitalized with acute pelvic inflammatory disease: Are they necessary? *J Reprod Med* 46:815, 2001.

19. Cohen SB, Weisz B, Seidman DS, et al: Accuracy of the preoperative diagnosis in 100 emergency laparoscopies performed due to acute abdomen in nonpregnant women. *J Am Assoc Gynecol Laparosc* 8:92, 2001.

20. Molander P, Sjoberg J, Paavonen J, et al: Trasvaginal power Doppler findings in laparoscopically proven acute pelvic inflammatory disease. *Ultrasound Obstet Gynecol* 17:233, 2001.

21. Molander P, Finne P, Sjoberg J, et al: Observer agreement with laparoscopic diagnosis of pelvic inflammatory disease using photographs. *Obstet Gynecol* 101:875, 2003.

22. Lehmann CE, Biro FM: Drug treatment of non viral sexually transmitted diseases: Specific issues in adolescents. *Pediatr Drugs* 3(7):481, 2001.

23. Mehta SD, Rothman RE, Kelen GD, et al: Clinical aspects of the diagnosis of gonorrhea and chlamydia infection in an acute care setting. *Clin Infect Dis* 32:655, 2001.

24. Nelson HD, Helfand M: Screening for chlamydial infection. *Am J Prevent Med* 20:95, 2001.

BREAST DISORDERS
Janet Simmons Young

The most common breast problems in the ED usually involve breast pain, breast mass, nipple discharge, breast infection, or postoperative complications. Rarely is the problem emergent, but a patient's perception for the potential for cancer may contribute to increased anxiety over the presenting problem.

EPIDEMIOLOGY

Few data are available regarding the incidence of emergency presentations for general breast disorders. Approximately one in every three to four women in the United States sees a physician with a chief complaint relating to their breasts.[1] In 2001, incidence of all breast cancers exceeded 192,000 new cases, with an estimated 40,200 deaths attributable to breast cancer.[2] Therefore, while the acuity of the problem may be low, the prevalence of presenting breast disorders may be quite high.

ANATOMY AND PHYSIOLOGY

Adult Anatomy

Normal breast tissue is a circular mass of glandular tissue located on the anterior chest wall and extending from the sternocostal junction medially to the midaxillary line laterally and from the second to the sixth ribs in the midclavicular line. Sensory innervation is from a dermatomal distribution, whereas the arterial supply to the breast arises from the internal mammary, lateral thoracic, thoracodorsal, and subscapular arteries. The lymphatic drainage of the breast is primarily to the axilla, with a small portion going to internal mammary lymph nodes. Lymph flow is not regionally distributed; lymphatic drainage to either the axilla or the internal mammary chain can originate in any quadrant of the breast.

Breast Physiology

Stromal and lobular tissues continue to develop until approximately 25 years of age. The adult breast is composed of approximately 20 percent ductal tissue, whereas the remaining breast volume consists of fat and connective tissue that give the breast its characteristic texture and shape.

Cyclic variances in estrogens, progesterone, follicle-stimulating hormone (FSH), and luteinizing hormone (LH) signal stromal and glandular changes in breast physiology. Due to the effects of rising circulating progesterone and a small peak in estrogen levels, the resulting interlobular edema causes the breast swelling, engorgement, and tenderness associated with the premenstrual phase. Breast tissue volume and tenderness are at a minimum 5 to 7 days after menstruation due to the relative lack of progesterone, allowing for a more sensitive and comfortable breast examination. At the onset of menstruation, the rapid decline in estrogen and progesterone levels leads to ductal involution. In contrast, menopausal breast changes involve actual loss of glandular tissue secondary to the gradual loss of estrogen and progesterone synthesis. The resulting postmenopausal breast consists predominantly of prepectoral fat, connective tissue, mammary ducts, and minimal lobular elements.

HISTORY AND PHYSICAL EXAMINATION

A routine breast examination can be a significant source of anxiety for the patient. The history and examination should be as private, comfortable, and reassuring as possible and should be followed by a discussion in which the diagnosis and treatment strategy are both understandable and acceptable to the patient.

Patient History

The patient should be questioned about onset of any mass or pain, location of the affected area, and duration of the symptoms. Complaints that vary with menses suggest a benign cause, whereas cancers are often asymptomatic. Radiation of the pain to any other body site is particularly important when a malignancy is suspected. The presence of symptoms in the contralateral breast parenchyma is also more reassuring for a benign diagnosis. The color and consistency of a nipple discharge, if present, should be evaluated, although the color of the discharge does not differentiate a benign from a malignant process. Changes that the patient notes on breast self-examination may be significant and should be correlated with the menstrual cycle. Family history specifically inquiring about the presence of first-degree relatives with breast cancer and other risk factors (delayed childbearing after age 30, biopsy confirmation of atypical hyperplasia, or history of chest irradiation) should be obtained. However, it also must be remembered that most women who develop breast cancer have no obvious risk factors beyond the two strongest factors, namely, female gender and age. More than 50 percent of breast cancers are diagnosed in women 65 years of age or older, and women under age 30 are diagnosed with less than 1 percent of all breast cancers.[3]

Physical Examination

The breast tissue examination (Figure 110-1) is best performed with the patient supine with the ipsilateral forearm behind the head. Palpation in a rotatory clockwise or counterclockwise motion ensures evaluation of the entire breast mound. The upper outer quadrant of each breast should be examined with extra care because approximately half of breast carcinomas originate in that area, with a higher propensity for left-sided involvement.[4–6] Asymmetry in glandular consistency and nodules or thickenings should be described by their quadrant of location (upper and lower, inner and outer) and distance from the nipple-areola complex. Examination of the nipple-areola complex occurs by gentle manipulation to detect subareolar masses and latent nipple discharge. The breasts then should be compared with the patient in an upright or sitting position, with any breast asymmetry or skin dimpling noted. Subtle abnormalities in the lower quadrants may be accentuated by having the patient raise her arms above her head. The axillae should be examined to note the presence, consistency, and mobility of any palpable lymph nodes. The anterior and posterior neck as well as the supraclavicular area should be examined for lymphadenopathy.

PHYSIOLOGY AND DISORDERS OF THE LACTATING BREAST

During pregnancy, marked glandular growth occurs under the influence of estrogen, progesterone, placental lactogen, prolactin, and chorionic gonadotropin, as well as maternal cortisol and thyroid hormones. Proliferative and secretory glandular changes, which begin early in the first trimester, prepare the breast alveolar cells for milk production at parturition. However, inhibition of lactation during pregnancy is mediated by a central nervous system (CNS) dopaminergic pathway. The abrupt fall of progesterone, human placental lactogen, and estrogen that occurs at parturition leads to the glandular secretion of colostrum and the cessation of milk production inhibition. Within 3 to 4 days, milk rich in lipid, protein, carbohydrate, and immunoglobulin is produced. The nursing infant's tactile stimulation of the nipple-areola complex provides a neurogenic signal to maintain milk production that can lead to discharge for years if stimulation is maintained after weaning.

ABNORMAL LACTATION

Any inappropriate secretion of milky discharge from the breast is referred to as *galactorrhea*. Galactorrhea often results from abnormally elevated levels of prolactin, although some women will have normal prolactin levels on testing. Physiologic causes of elevated serum prolactin levels are sleep, stress, exercise, volume depletion, intercourse or orgasm, pregnancy, and breast stimulation. Abnormal stimulation of the chest wall, such as from surgery, trauma, or herpetic infection, can increase prolactin secretion. Elevated levels of prolactin can occur from inadequate inhibition of secretion or from increased production of prolactin. Any exogenous damage or disruption of the pituitary

FIG. 110-1. Positioning for the examination of the breasts. [From August, DA and Sondak, VK: Breast disease, in Greenfield LJ (ed): *Surgery: Scientific Principles and Practice.* Philadelphia, Lippincott, 1996, pp 1357–1415.]

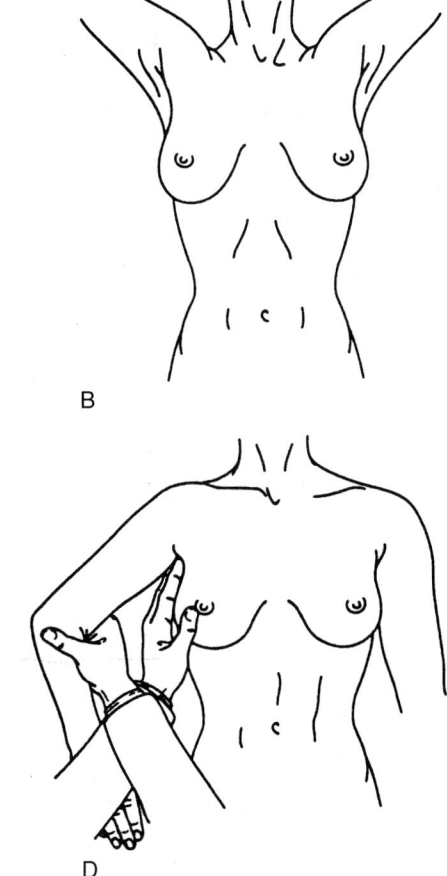

A

B

C

D

stalk or endogenous hypothalamo-pituitary signaling may result in increased prolactin secretion. Prolactinomas, benign anterior pituitary neoplasms, are distinguished by symptoms of galactorrhea, amenorrhea, hirsutism, facial acne, visual field deficits, and headaches. Other neoplastic disorders implicated in hyperprolactinemia are renal cell carcinoma, lymphoma, craniopharyngioma, bronchogenic carcinoma, and hydatidiform mole.

Multiple medications are known to interfere with dopamine-mediated inhibition of prolactin. Specifically, antidepressants such as monoamine oxidase inhibitors (MAOIs), selective serotonin reuptake inhibitors (SSRIs), and tricyclic antidepressants (TCAs) target dopamine to exert their clinical effects. The antihypertensives atenolol, methyldopa, reserpine, and verapamil, as well as the antipsychotic phenothiazines and antihistamines, are known to cause galactorrhea. Several herbs, often contained in dietary supplements, are associated with galactorrhea: anise, fennel, nettle, clover, and thistle. Fenugreek seed has even been used to induce lactation. Many illegal drugs such as amphetamines, cocaine, opioids, and marijuana can cause galactorrhea.

Consideration of systemic diseases should be given in the evaluation of galactorrhea. Chronic renal failure results in a diminished capacity to clear circulating prolactin. Hypothyroidism causes increased thyrotropin-releasing hormone (TRH), which results in increased pituitary secretion of prolactin. Hypercortisolism (Cushing disease) and acromegaly due to abnormal growth hormone secretion are both associated with galactorrhea.

Evaluation of the patient with galactorrhea should focus on a history of associated menstrual abnormalities and the presence of acne, hirsutism, infertility, or libido changes. Symptoms of increased intracranial pressure and hypothyroidism also should be investigated. All medications and dietary supplements should be reviewed with the patient.

The physical examination should include evaluations of the visual fields, breasts, skin, and thyroid gland. ED studies include a urine or serum pregnancy test, neuroimaging (computed tomography or magnetic resonance imaging), and neurosurgical consultation if there is concern for an intracranial mass. Treatment, other than the discontinuation of a suspected medication, may be deferred to the primary care physician or the follow-up specialist.

COMPLICATIONS OF LACTATION

Breast engorgement usually presents on the third to fifth postpartum day, with symptoms of painful, hard, and enlarged bilateral breasts. The pain may be accompanied by a low-grade fever. The presence of carbohydrate-rich milk during lactation facilitates bacterial overgrowth and colonization by *Candida* species in the lactiferous ducts should obstruction to flow from any of the major ducts occur. Pumping the breasts usually alleviates the pain and allows for decompression of the nipple-areola complex, facilitating effective breast-feeding. Topical antifungals, in conjuction with breast pumping, usually are effective at eradicating the fissuring and scaly rash of the nipple and areola due to *Candida albicans.*

Puerperal mastitis occurs most often after bacterial colonization secondary to areolar inflammation and glandular obstruction, creating an increased susceptibility to suppurative mastitis during nursing. Puerperal mastitis, or endemic mastitis, often occurs during the first few weeks to months postpartum, when the skin of the nipples is damaged most easily, and much later when the infant may inflict dental trauma. The patient may report fever, chills, myalgias, or flulike symptoms, and examination of the breast reveals an erythematous, localized area of pain. Puerperal mastitis is most commonly caused by *Staphylococcus aureus,* although *Eschericia coli* and *Streptococcus* spp. are also known pathogens. Treatment requires breast emptying, skin cleansing, analgesia, and antistaphylococcal penicillins or cephalosporins.[7] There is no need to interrupt breast-feeding with puerperal mastitis. However, if the infection fails to respond rapidly to antibiotics, an abscess should be suspected.

Differentiation between mastitis, usually associated with cellulitis of the overlying skin, and breast abscess, usually accompanied by palpable fluctuance, can be difficult. An abscess may present with the signs and symptoms of mastitis or may demonstrate only minimal focal induration. Ultrasound examination of the erythematous area may be helpful in diagnosis of a subcutaneous purulent collection. Interruption of breast-feeding to prevent neonatal infection and cephalosporins or clindamycin for anaerobic coverage may be required. Immediate referral for surgical drainage is necessary, although an excisional biopsy of tissue also may be performed by the surgeon to rule out an inflammatory carcinoma.[8]

INFLAMMATORY BREAST CONDITIONS

Breast Infections

The differential diagnosis of an inflammatory breast complaint includes infectious mastitis, breast abscess, periductal mastitis, ruptured breast cysts, inflammatory carcinomas, lymphosarcomas, carcinoma erysipeloides (inflammatory skin metastases from thyroid carcinoma), syphilis, tuberculosis, and Paget dermatitis.[9] ED presentations of each entity can mimic other, more benign conditions. While the classic *peau d'orange* appearance is highly suggestive for cancer, other signs such as the clarity of erythematous demarcation, the amount of tissue involved, or the presence of ulceration are not pathognomonic for any specific diagnosis. A failure to improve with antibiotics indicates the need for immediate surgical consultation and possible biopsy to exclude the presence of an inflammatory neoplasm.[10]

Acute Mastitis and Breast Abscess

Acute infections of the breast generally present with erythema, edema, tenderness, malaise, and often fever. Mastitis, or superficial cellulitis of the breast, usually is treated conservatively with antistaphylococcal antibiotics and frequent reassessment. Puerperal mastitis, which was discussed in the preceding section, is also treated with antibiotics and frequent breast emptying. Breast cellulitis, if recognized early, responds to antibiotic treatment with an antistaphylococcal penicillin (e.g., dicloxacillin 250 mg PO qid for 7 days) or first-generation cephalosporin (such as cephalexin 500 mg PO qid for 7 days). In contrast, a breast abscess presents with inflammatory skin changes, mastalgia, but may or may not exhibit induration. Abscesses require surgical drainage. Oral versus parenteral antibiotic administration is based on the extent of breast involvement and the degree of systemic illness. Periareolar abscesses often simply may be incised and drained, whereas **general anesthesia may be required for larger peri- or retroareolar abscesses.** Breast ultrasound or needle aspiration may be helpful for diagnosis. A large-bore needle, usually 16-gauge or larger, may be necessary to aspirate purulent material under local anesthesia. Aspiration permits bacterial culture and sensitivity testing and may be adequate management for very small fluid collections with limited breast involvement. While aspiration of the fluctuant mass does in fact cause microscopic tissue displacement, there is little evidence to suggest, in contrast to lung neoplasms, that breast aspiration will spread an indolent cancer significantly.[11] In either case, infections should respond rapidly to antibiotics, demonstrating at least partial resolution within 48 h. Repeat clinical evaluation is recommended at 48 to 72 h. Duration of therapy should occur for at least 2 weeks. However, management for breast abscess should include a referral for surgical evaluation for open drainage.

Occasionally, either mastitis or abscess may result in systemic toxicity. General indications for admission and immediate surgical consultation are patients with obvious sepsis or hemodynamic compromise, immunosuppressed or immunocompromised hosts (e.g., diabetics), rapidly progressive infection, or failure of outpatient antibiotic therapy. Parenteral antibiotics recommended are cefazolin 1 g IV every 8 h or nafcillin 2 g IV every 4 h. In penicillin-allergic patients, fluoroquinolones, rifampin, or vancomycin should be considered, although multiple-drug-resistant *Staphylococcus* spp. have been reported.

Periductal Mastitis (Mammary Duct Ectasia)

Periductal mastitis, also called *plasma cell mastitis* or *mammary duct ectasia,* is an uncommon benign disorder characterized by dilated or ectatic ducts with retained secretions surrounded with significant inflammation. Women over 40 years of age generally present with constant mastalgia associated with nipple retraction or discharge. In severe cases, subareolar abscesses form and can burrow through the skin at the areolar border to form mammary duct fistulas. Younger women tend to present with cellulitis or recurrent subareolar abscesses, whereas perimenopausal and postmenopausal women are more likely to present with nipple discharge and retraction, or sterile subareolar masses.

Infection should be treated, and the patient should be referred to a specialist for definitive diagnosis and treatment.

Hidradenitis Suppurtiva

Hidradenitis suppurtiva frequently presents with recurrent multiple cutaneous abscesses, sinus tracts, and scarring of the breast folds, axillae, and groin and perineum. It is a chronic inflammatory disease involving the obstruction of sweat glands associated with polymicrobial colonization, with *Staphylococcus* and *Streptococcus* spp. implicated in the pathogenesis of infection.[12] Frequently, patients present with painful sebaceous abscesses along the inferior, pendulous surface of the breast and request incisional drainage for pain relief. Incision and drainage usually are adequate therapy for a limited area of abscess formation. Antibiotics are rarely used for outpatient management of simple abscesses in immunocompetent patients, although antibiotic suppression therapy may be used by the specialist to decrease the frequency and severity of the disease. There is no cure for the disease except extensive surgical excision of the apocrine tissue, which often results in higher recurrence rates at the excisional sites.

Inflammatory Breast Cancer

Of all the potential presentations of a breast malignancy, *inflammatory breast cancer* (IBC) is the entity associated with the greatest mortality and longest delay from initial presentation to definitive diagnosis. IBC accounts for 1 to 3 percent of all breast cancers. The clinical presentation is composed of symptoms of mastalgia and breast inflammation due to tumor infiltration of dermal lymphatics that results in an inflammatory response of the breast stroma. The combination of erythema and edema results in the classic orange-peel *(peau d'orange)* appearance of the overlying skin and ultimately nipple retraction as the edema progresses. Initially, the patient presents with a clinical syndrome of breast enlargement, breast warmth, tenderness, edema, erythema, and sometimes discoloration of the overlying skin. The abscence of a palpable underlying mass or axillary lymphadenopathy does not rule out the diagnosis. The signs of inflammatory breast cancer are often indistinguishable clinically from infection. Prompt mammography and biopsy of the skin and any palpable or radiographic breast lesions are required by the follow-up physician. Similarly, the diagnosis of IBC must be considered promptly if there is not an initial good response to antibiotics or if a breast cellulitis or abscess fails to completely resolve.

Axillary Lymphadenopathy and Pain

In women with axillary adenopathy, the possibility of breast cancer metastatic to axillary nodes must be considered. This is true even if careful physical examination does not reveal a palpable breast abnormality. Referral to a breast specialist for bilateral mammograms is in-

dicated. Unless there is excellent evidence that the adenopathy may be attributed to an infectious or other benign etiology, palpable axillary nodes should prompt a referral to a breast specialist.

NONINFLAMMATORY PAINFUL BREAST DISORDERS

Mastodynia

One of the most common urgent presentations is for breast pain, also termed *mastodynia* or *mastalgia.* The discomfort usually is cyclic, waxing or waning with the menstrual cycle. Cyclic mastodynia is usually most severe in the immediate premenstrual phase and decreases or resolves completely following menstruation. The pain is bilateral and usually is most severe in the upper outer quadrants of the breast. It may be referred to the axilla, underarm, or scapula. Diagnosis relies on the history and physical examination to confirm that the pain actually originates from the breast. At times, the examination reveals tender, nodular breasts, suggesting a diagnosis of fibrocystic changes, although breast cancer must remain in the differential diagnosis. For most patients, occasional use of nonsteroidal anti-inflammatory drugs is the only therapy required. Patients with breast pain should be referred to their primary care physicians for follow-up treatment and imaging, if necessary.

Nipple Discharge

Table 110-1 lists some common causes of nipple discharge. Most discharges, even bloody, are not usually due to malignancy. In general, milky, green, gray, or black discharges that are either unilateral or bilateral and can be expressed from several ducts are not suggestive of cancer.[13] However, follow-up to the patient's primary care physician for mammography and possible fluid analysis of the discharge is always needed.

Intraductal papillomas usually present with a unilateral bloody nipple discharge in women from 20 to 40 years of age. Bleeding is secondary to increased tissue vascularity. A mass may not be palpable on examination. Other etiologies of bloody nipple discharge include mammary duct ectasia and breast cancer. Again, outpatient follow-up is required for mammogram and eventual biopsy.

Bilateral spontaneous milky nipple discharge can be indicative of an elevated serum prolactin level. Discussion of this entity can be found earlier in this chapter. Any postmenopausal nipple discharges are significant and should be referred immediately to a breast specialist.

SKIN AND NIPPLE ABNORMALITIES

Mondor Disease

Thrombophlebitis of the superficial thoracoepigastric vein, or *Mondor disease,* results in a cordlike mass in the breast, sometimes associated with skin changes such as dimpling. Without an identifiable etiology in most cases, localized trauma or an inflammatory process has been associated with Mondor disease. Breast pain is the usual presenting complaint, with examination findings of a characteristic cordlike mass in the superficial subcutaneous tissue of the breast, most commonly in the lower quadrants. Mondor disease, which can be mistaken for an inflammatory cancer, is benign and self-limited. Treatment is usually a nonsteroidal anti-inflammatory medication for symptomatic relief.

Nipple Irritation

Nipple irritation may be caused by repeated friction from clothing or sunburn. The nipples are easily protected from chronic abrasion by application of a small dab of petroleum jelly or use of protective pads

TABLE 110-1 Relationship Between Nipple Discharge and Possible Etiologies

Purulent	Infection
Milky/galactorrhea	Pregnancy
	Prolactinoma
	Pituitary adenoma
	Drugs (phenothiazines, H_2 blockers)
Serous/serosanguineous	Intraductal papilloma
	Fibrocystic changes
	Duct ectasia
	Cancer
Watery	Papilloma
	Cancer

Source: Adapted with permission from Neinstein LS: Breast disease in adolescents and young women. *Pediatr Clin North Am* 46(3):607, 1999.

inserted into the cups of a support bra. Nipple irritation, however, also may be indicative of atopic dermatitis, erosive adenomatosis, or Paget disease. Erosive adenomatosis is a benign proliferation of the lactiferous ducts presenting with eczema or an erosion of the nipple. Treatment is surgical excision, and referral to a breast specialist is needed. Paget disease, which is heralded by the appearance of a weeping, eczematoid lesion of the nipple, occurs in less than 2 percent of all breast cancers. However, Paget disease is almost always associated with an underlying breast carcinoma and usually is diagnosed in postmenopausal women. Paget disease may present with an associated palpable breast mass, often correlating with the presence of an intraductal carcinoma. Because skin edema and inflammatory changes may respond transiently to incorrectly prescribed topical treatments, there is usually a delay of 6 to 12 months in diagnosis. Urgent referral for bilateral mammography and follow-up with a breast specialist are mandatory.

FIBROCYSTIC DISEASE AND THE EVALUATION OF BREAST MASS

The most common cause for benign breast disease in premenopausal women is fibrocystic breast disease, which is a constellation of breast symptoms linked by the common pathognomonic finding of breast cysts. The nodularity and tenderness, which occur as a result of breast tissue responses to hormonal cycling, is called *fibrocystic breast disease* or *fibrocystic changes of the breast.* Fibrocystic changes do not include skin thickening, edema, discoloration, nipple retraction, or discharge. If the history and physical examination in the ED are normal, then outpatient mammography and specialist follow-up should occur if the patient is over age 40. If the patient is under age 30 and presents with a breast mass, then fibrocystic changes or a fibroadenoma are more likely, and the patient will require outpatient ultrasonography, possible needle aspiration, and referral to a breast specialist. Women with recurrent or severe symptoms, skin changes, solid masses, nipple abnormalities, or severe anxiety about the possibility of cancer should be referred to a breast specialist.

Breast cancer is rare in patients younger than 20 years of age and uncommon in women younger than 30 years of age. Risk factors for young women include inheritance of the *BRCA1* or *BRCA2* gene, a history of childhood malignancy, or a history of chest irradiation. A family history of a first-degree relative with breast cancer, increased exposure to endogenous estrogens (nulliparity or delayed childbearing until after age 30), or biopsy-confirmed breast atypical hyperplasia increases the risk for women aged 30 years and older. However, most patients diagnosed with breast cancer have only two risk factors: age greater than 50 years and female gender.[2]

Physical signs that should prompt immediate surgical referral include a palpable mass with or without the following: lymphadenopathy, skin ulceration, fixation to the chest wall, fixed axillary nodes, or the presence of ipsilateral arm edema.

Characteristics associated with a delayed diagnosis of breast cancer are nonwhite race, lower socioeconomic status, normal/false-negative mammogram, presentation with nipple lesions or axillary mass, or inadequate biopsy technique.[14,15]

BREAST TRAUMA

Blunt trauma to the breast is usually seen in association with multiple thoracic injuries and often accompanied by extensive chest wall ecchymoses, commonly referred to as a "seat belt sign." Traumatic breast injuries rarely necessitate specific therapy unless there is significant avulsion of breast tissue or an expanding hematoma, which should prompt immediate surgical intervention. The presence of a significant isolated breast injury should raise the possibility of abuse or cancer. Long-term sequelae of beast trauma include inflammatory and architectural distortions of the breast, as well as persistent microcalcification observed on mammography. Fat necrosis is the most common type of inflammatory response to breast injury, but few patients actually remember a discrete breast injury. Fat necrosis can be confused easily with carcinoma because it may present with a palpable mass and even skin dimpling and retraction. While no specific treatment is required for fat necrosis, the presence of cancer must be excluded. Any persistent mass after trauma must raise the question of underlying pathology or malignancy, and referral to a breast specialist for evaluation is required.

PERIOPERATIVE AND POSTOPERATIVE COMPLICATIONS

Hematoma

Immediate postoperative hemorrhage or expanding hematoma formation is best evaluated and treated by the operating surgeon. Emergent evaluation requires determination if the hematoma is expanding, tensely distended, or stable. Expanding hematomas, especially those occurring within the first few postoperative days, may signify the presence of continued bleeding and usually require surgical evaluation for evacuation of the hematoma or ligation of bleeding vessels. Later presentations of breast hematoma are usually managed conservatively, with analgesics, a compressive bra, and the correction of any coagulopathy. Aspiration of the hematoma generally is not effective in the ED. The presence of an infected hematoma requires inpatient management, percutaneous drainage, or open drainage and packing, and parenteral antibiotics generally are indicated.

Infection

Postoperative wound infections may be treated with an oral first-generation cephalosporin on an outpatient basis if there is no evidence of abscess, systemic signs of toxicity, or immunocompromise. Worsening signs of cellulitis or systemic response to infection, development of purulent drainage, or failure to improve after 48 h require inpatient management. Postoperative drain infections generally require drain removal and antibiotic therapy. Any fluid collections that develop subsequently usually require drainage either by repeated aspiration or by incision. The operating surgeon should be consulted for any of these complications.

REFERENCES

1. American College of Obstetrics and Gynecology: *Precis V: An Update in Obstetrics and Gynecology.* Washington, ACOG, 1994, p 75.
2. American Cancer Society: *Cancer Facts and Figures, 2002.* Atlanta, American Cancer Society (www.cancer.org, accessed March 2002).
3. Ries LAG, Eisner MP, Kosary CL, et al (eds): *SEER Cancer Statistics Review, 1973–1999.* Bethesda, MD, National Cancer Institute (http://seer.cancer.gov/csr/1973_1999, 2002; accessed December 2002).

4. McMasters KM, Wong SL, Chao C, et al: Defining the optimal surgeon experience for breast cancer sentinel lymph node biopsy: A model for implementation of new surgical techniques. *Ann Surg* 234:292, 2001.

5. Hill AD: Lessons learned from 500 cases of lymphatic mapping for breast cancer. *Ann Surg* 232:81, 2000.

6. Borgstein PJ: Functional lymphatic anatomy for sentinel node biopsy in breast cancer: Echoes from the past and the periareolar blue method. *Ann Surg* 232:203, 2000.

7. Whitaker-Worth DL: Dermatologic diseases of the breast and nipple. *J Am Acad Dermatol* 453(5 pt 1):733, 2000.

8. Scott-Connor CE, Schorr SJ: The diagnosis and management of breast problems during pregnancy and lactation. *Am J Surg* 170:401, 1995.

9. Schwartz RA: Cutaneous metastatic disease. *J Am Acad Dermatol* 33(2 pt 1):161, 1995.

10. Wrightson WR, Edwards MJ, McMasters KM: Primary squamous cell carcinomas of the breast presenting as breast abcess. *Am Surg* 65:1153, 1999.

11. Liberman L: Clinical management issues in percutaneous core breast biopsy. *Radiol Clin North Am* 38(4):791, 2000.

12. Jemec GB: The bacteriology of hidradenitis suppurtiva. *Dermatology* 193:203, 1996.

13. Gulay H: Management of nipple discharge. *J Am Coll Surg* 178:471, 1994.

14. Tartter PI: Delay in diagnosis of breast cancer. *Ann Surg* 229:91, 1999.

15. Simon MS: Racial differences in breast cancer survival: The interaction of socioeconomic status and tumor biology. *Am J Obstet Gynecol* 176:S233, 1997.

111 UROGYNECOLOGIC DISORDERS AND GYNECOLOGIC ONCOLOGY

Michael Londner

Daniela Meshkat

INCONTINENCE

The six main anatomic structures contributing to continence are:

The *detrusor muscle,* a meshwork of fibers surrounding the bladder.

The *urethra,* a 3- to 4-cm tube surrounded mainly by smooth muscle.

The *urethral sphincter,* which provides the secondary defense against urinary incontinence and about 50 percent of total urethral resistance.

Two posterior *pubourethral ligaments,* which suspend the urethra, holding it close to the pubic bone.

The *autonomic nervous system,* the parasympathetic and sympathetic nerves that supply the lower genitourinary tract. Parasympathetic fibers S_2 to S_4 cause detrusor contraction (cholinergic drugs do the same). Sympathetic fibers T_{10} to L_2 have α- and β-adrenergic components. Alpha fibers stimulate the bladder neck and urethral contraction while relaxing the detrusor muscle. Beta fibers relax the urethra and contract the detrusor muscle.

Pudendal nerves provide voluntary urethral contraction.

Continence is maintained because intraurethral pressure exceeds intravesical pressure. The levator ani and surrounding fascia and ligaments help to maintain urethral anatomy in times of abrupt changes associated in intra-abdominal pressure.

The four most common classifications of continence are:

Urinary stress incontinence
Urge incontinence
Total incontinence
Overflow incontinence

Stress urinary incontinence occurs when urine is lost involuntarily as a result of increased intra-abdominal pressure, i.e., when the intraurethral pressure is less than the intra-abdominal pressure. It is associated with multiparity, vaginal delivery, pregnancy, menopause, chronic cough (i.e., chronic obstructive pulmonary disease), or other forms of

pelvic relaxation. Symptoms include leaking of urine during cough, straining, laughing, sneezing, running, or other causes of increased intra-abdominal pressure. Stress incontinence per se is not a diagnosis that is important to establish in the ED. Of importance is the differential diagnosis, which includes infection, neurologic disease, medications, or other systemic illness as possible causes of stress urinary incontinence. A thorough history and physical examination are required, along with a comprehensive neurologic examination. Further, a full vaginal examination with inspection of all the vaginal walls is necessary. If important etiologies in the differential diagnosis are excluded, the patient can be referred safely to a consulting gynecologist. Outpatient workup includes stress testing and, if necessary, urodynamic testing. Nonoperative options include Kegel exercises, estrogen, α-adrenergic stimulants, intravaginal weights, biofeedback, transcutaneous electrical nerve stimulation (TENS), and urethral plugs. Operative management to correct the defect and restore the anatomy of the urethra is the approach used most commonly. Surgery may be laparoscopic, vaginal, abdominal, or a combination of these. The list of procedures and variations is very long, but the most common include the Marshall-Marchetti-Kranz, Burch, Pereyra, Stamey, and Raz procedures, collagen injections, and sling suspensions.

Urge incontinence occurs in the setting of detrusor muscle instability. The incidence of this entity is around 15 to 20 percent of all women with incontinence, but it increases markedly with increasing age. It is often seen in conjunction with stress urinary incontinence, when it is known as *mixed incontinence.* The precise etiology of urge incontinence is unknown, but it is seen in the presence of foreign bodies (suture inadvertently placed in the bladder), intravesical stones, menopause (hypoestrogen states), and/or infection. Symptoms include urinary urgency, frequency, nocturia, and incontinence. Observing involuntary detrusor contractions during cystometric or urodynamic studies is diagnostic. Treatment includes pharmacologic agents (e.g., anticholinergics, β-sympathomimetics, musculotrophics, tricyclic antidepressants, or dopamine agonists), bladder training, biofeedback, and functional electrical stimulation.

Total incontinence is most commonly the result of a urinary fistula. Fistulas usually occur as a result of pelvic surgery, radiation, and obstetric injuries (in underdeveloped countries). Patients present with constant, painless leaking of urine and/or recurrent infections. Placing a tampon into the vagina and instilling methylene blue or sterile milk into the bladder helps to make the diagnosis. In the event that a vesicovaginal fistula is present, the tampon will stain blue. If there is no staining, then indigo carmine is injected intravenously. If the tampon then stains blue, a ureterovaginal fistula is present. An intravenous pyelogram (IVP) should be obtained in either situation to help define the anatomy and rule out other multiple fistulas. Treatment is initiated with insertion of a diverting Foley catheter and may lead to spontaneous healing if the injury is recent. Usually, however, operative repair is required.

Overflow incontinence is a result of urinary retention from a hypotonic detrusor muscle. This is seen in the setting of neuropathy secondary to diabetes, spinal cord injuries, outflow obstruction, postoperatively, or lower motor neuron diseases (i.e., multiple sclerosis). Symptoms include postvoid bladder fullness (the "feeling" of never having an empty bladder), small quantities on micturition, and leaking. Diagnosis is made through complete history and physical examination with emphasis on the neurologic examination and determination of postvoid residual volume. Therapy is directed at treating the underlying cause and teaching intermittent self-catheterization.

PROLAPSE

The female pelvic organs, i.e., vagina, uterus, bladder, and rectum, are held in proper alignment by supporting ligaments, fascia, and the pelvic floor muscles. When any or all of these structures fail, the pelvic organs may prolapse within and occasionally protrude through the vagina. This prolapse or displacement may occur singly or more commonly in combination. Prolapse can be divided into two broad categories, uterine and vaginal.

Uterine prolapse is graded as first through third degrees:

First degree: The cervix remains within the vagina.
Second degree: The cervix protrudes beyond the introitus.
Third degree: This implies descent of the entire uterus outside the vulva, also known as *procidentia.*

This classification system is slowly being replaced with staging of all pelvic prolapses through one pelvic organ prolapse quantification (POPQ) profile, now standardized terminology.

A prolapsed, elongated, inflamed, edematous cervix may be mistaken for uterine prolapse if careful evaluation is not undertaken. Procidentia represents complete failure of all supporting structures. The vagina can prolapse without accompanying uterine prolapse, but the uterus cannot prolapse without bringing the upper vagina with it.

Vaginal prolapse is best subdivided into four basic quadrants:

Upper anterior vaginal wall: cystocele (represents weakness of the pubocervical fascia)
Lower anterior vaginal wall: urethral displacement
Upper posterior vaginal wall: enterocele (usually associated with herniation into the pouch of Douglas)
Lower posterior vaginal wall: rectocele

In addition, inversion of the vagina is known as *vault prolapse.* Most commonly, prolapse results from attenuation of pelvic fascia, ligaments, and muscles following extensive stretching during vaginal delivery. However, prolapse can occur after easy labor or in the nulliparous woman, in which case it is considered a congenital or developmental weakness of pelvic connective tissue. Virtually any cause of repeated increased intra-abdominal pressure may lead to prolapse, including chronic cough, ascites, heavy lifting, or habitual straining on defecation. These mechanisms should raise concern to search for occult malignancy, e.g., lung cancer in a person with chronic cough or colon cancer in someone straining to defecate. Atrophy of the supporting tissue plays a significant role in initiating or worsening this condition.

The degree of symptomatology is quite variable. The most common complaint is a "feeling of heaviness or fullness in the pelvis." Others may describe "something falling out." More diffuse complaints include backache, pelvic discomfort, and discomfort or straining with defecation or urination. Cystocele may present with frequency, urgency, incontinence, or ultimately, retention (especially if displacement causes kinking of the ureter), whereas rectocele may present with difficulty evacuating the rectal vault.[1] A characteristic not to be overlooked is the worsening of symptoms with prolonged standing followed by alleviation when lying down. Women may become extremely tolerant of prolapse symptoms and present with advanced complications such as infection of the prolapsed segment, decubitus ulceration, bleeding, and carcinoma of the cervix.

Diagnosis revolves around a thorough history and physical examination, including vaginal examination. Use of a Sim's speculum or separating the two halves of the standard Grave's speculum and using the posterior blade allows for adequate vaginal inspection. Depress the posterior vaginal wall, and ask the patient to bear down. This will demonstrate descent of the anterior vaginal wall in the setting of cystocele and/or urethral displacement. Reversing the speculum to elevate the anterior vaginal wall allows visualization of the intruding posterior wall during straining, demonstrative of enterocele or rectocele. A rectal examination often will help to distinguish rectocele from enterocele.

Treatment modalities are grouped into nonoperative and operative.[2] The patient's age, future fertility, degree of sexual activity, and degree of prolapse must be considered in defining a management plan. Nonoperative treatments generally are tried first if future childbearing

is desired, the degree of pathology is mild, or the patient is a poor surgical candidate. These options include Kegel (pelvic floor strengthening) exercises, pessaries, estrogen, and electrical muscle stimulation. Operative management options are used in patients failing nonoperative treatments, those with severe prolapse, and those who are symptomatic. The overall goal of surgery is to return the pelvic anatomy to as close to normal as possible. Procedures include anterior/posterior colporrhaphy, enterocele repair, hysterectomy, obliteration of the vaginal vault, urethropexies (colpocleisis), urethral sling procedures, and/or suspension of the vaginal vault.

URETHRAL SYNDROME

Urethral syndrome describes a complex of symptoms involving the lower urinary tract and including urinary frequency, urgency, dysuria, suprapubic discomfort, postvoid fullness, incontinence, and/or dyspareunia with no objective findings of urologic pathology. Grandmultiparity, delivery without episiotomy, two or more abortuses, and pelvic relaxations appear to predispose.[3] The true incidence of urethral syndrome in the United States among adult women is unknown, as is the cause. The most widely accepted etiology of this enigmatic syndrome is an inflammatory process. Other etiologies include psychogenic factors, *Chlamydia* or *Mycoplasma* infection, atrophic urethritis in the perimenopausal/postmenopausal patient, fastidious organism bacterial infection, urethral stenosis and/or spasm, allergy, neurogenic, and trauma during intercourse. The diagnosis is one of exclusion founded on a thorough history and physical examination, followed by urine microscopic examination and culture. Referral is often obtained then for dynamic cystourethroscopy and urodynamic studies. Treatment encompasses many modalities because the etiology is uncertain.[4] The first approach is often pharmacologic, with antibiotics (doxycycline) or anticholinergics, followed by instillation of dimethyl sulfoxide, periurethral injection of triamcinolone, serial urethral dilation with or without massage, cryosurgery (internal urethrotomy and urethrolysis), bladder neck reconstruction, biofeedback, and psychotherapy. Recent research has led to the use of urethral suppositories with multiple medications, including lidocaine, hydrocortisone, and topical estrogens. Lastly, supportive therapy is helpful in all patients.

GYNECOLOGIC MALIGNANCIES

The female reproductive tract cancers account for 13 percent of all cancers in women, following breast, lung, and colon cancer. Symptoms occurring as a result of natural progression of malignancy include bleeding, nausea and vomiting, obstructive uropathy, failure to thrive, and/or paraneoplastic syndromes. Treatment with surgery, chemotherapy, and radiation can cause complications. Surgical complications include bowel and urogenital tract injury, thromboembolism, and bleeding. Chemotherapy-related complications include anemia, febrile neutropenia, thrombocytopenia, neuropathy, uropathy, nausea and vomiting, extravasation injury, and stomatitis. Radiation-related complications focus mainly on injury to the gastrointestinal and genitourinary tracts.

Ovarian Cancer

Cancers of the ovary and fallopian tube are discussed together because of the rarity of fallopian tube cancer and similarity in gross and microscopic appearance, pattern of spread, and disease process. Over 25,000 women are diagnosed with ovarian cancer yearly in the United States, with about half dying from the disease. A woman with no family history has a 1 to 2 percent chance of developing ovarian cancer in her lifetime. Peak incidence occurs between the ages of 55 and 65 years, although some types occur earlier. The following risk factors have been identified: infertility, low parity, high-fat diet, lactose intolerance, history of breast or colon cancer, and a family history of site-specific ovarian cancer or its associated syndromes. Oral contraceptives seem to be protective against ovarian cancer.

Cancers of the ovary and fallopian tube come in three main histologic types: epithelial (85 percent), germ cell tumors (10 percent), and sex cord stromal tumors (5 percent). Patients often present after the disease has spread beyond the ovary, with symptoms such as abdominal pain, bloating, ascites, early satiety, weight loss, and/or respiratory distress secondary to effusion. Sertoli-Leydig tumors produce androgens, often resulting in masculinization and often occurring at age 25 years. **It is most important to recognize that a woman presenting to the ED with ascites has a gynecologic malignancy until proven otherwise.** As a first diagnostic step after pelvic examination, computed tomographic (CT) scanning can be done in the ED. Aspiration of ascitic fluid should not be done.

The single most important factor in the large death rate is the advanced stage at diagnosis. Diagnosis and staging of ovarian cancer are based on surgical evaluation. The International Federation of Gynecology and Obstetrics (FIGO) devised an extensive and universal staging classification. In summary (a simplification):

Stage I: Growth limited to one or both ovaries
Stage II: One or both ovaries with pelvic extension
Stage III: One or both ovaries with growth outside the pelvis
Stage IV: One or both ovaries with distant metastasis

Treatment of ovarian cancer may involve surgery, chemotherapy, and/or radiation therapy.

Uterine Cancer

Uterine cancer is the most common gynecologic malignancy. In 1997, 32,800 cases were diagnosed. The average age at occurrence is 58 years. Adenocarcinoma of the endometrium is the most common histologic type. Other histologic types of endometrial cancer that occur less frequently are papillary serous, clear cell, adenosquamous, and adenocanthoma. Sarcomas are malignancies of the uterine muscle. They behave very aggressively and have a worse prognosis than endometrial cancer.

Multiple risk factors have been associated with endometrioid adenocarcinoma of the uterus, such as early menses, late menopause, nulliparity, obesity, diabetes, hypertension, and unopposed estrogen use. The use of progestins has dramatically reduced the risk of endometrial cancer. Tamoxifen, an antiestrogen that competes with estrogen at its receptor site, has been shown to increase the risk of adenocarcinoma of the uterus.

The most common symptom of endometrial cancer is postmenopausal bleeding. Sarcomas, however, may present with bleeding but also with abdominal pain or prolapse of friable tissue through the cervical os.

The diagnosis of uterine cancer is made by sampling the endometrium. This may be achieved through office endometrial biopsy, a dilatation and curettage specimen, or hysteroscopy. A pathologic specimen must be obtained for proper diagnosis and further treatment planning. A sonogram that measures the endometrial stripe as greater than 5 mm in a postmenopausal woman must be evaluated.

Staging for uterine cancer is as follows (summary of staging):

Stage I: Confined to the uterine corpus
Stage II: Involvement of the cervix
Stage III: Extends to the uterine serosa, ovary, vagina, and para-aortic/pelvic lymph nodes
Stage IV: Involvement of the bladder/bowel, inguinal/intra-abdominal lymph nodes

Staging is surgical. Treatment involves surgery and also may include radiation and chemotherapy.

The vaginal cuff, vagina, and pelvis are common sites for recurrence. Patients with recurrence often present with vaginal bleeding, vaginal or pelvic masses, or uremia secondary to ureter obstruction. Pulmonary metastases are less common in recurrent uterine cancer but still need to be considered in a women presenting with respiratory symptoms and a history of uterine cancer.

Cervical Cancer

Currently, 15,800 new cases of cervical cancer are diagnosed each year. The average age at the time of diagnosis is 54 years. Risk factors include early coitus, multiple sexual partners, high-risk male partners, smoking, human papillomavirus, and HIV infection (or other immunosuppressive states). The diagnosis of cervical cancer in an HIV-positive patient is now considered an AIDS-identifying illness. Smoking increases the risk of cervical cancer in women by 3.5 times, and even passive smoke increases the risk 3-fold. Approximately 90 percent of cervical cancers are of squamous histologic type, but adenocarcinoma, which comprises 5 to 10 percent of cervical cancers, is increasing and has a worse prognosis.

The presenting signs and symptoms of cervical cancer, in decreasing order, are postmenopausal bleeding, abnormal vaginal bleeding, postcoital bleeding, vaginal discharge, pain, or leg swelling. Diagnosis must be made by cervical biopsy (not only Papanicolau smear). Often, on speculum examination, a mass or ulcerative lesion is seen on the cervix. The gynecologic consultant should be called to perform a biopsy, cone biopsy, or loop electrosurgical excision procedure (LEEP).

Staging of cervical cancer is performed clinically. Once a diagnosis is made by biopsy, a thorough physical examination must be performed, including an examination under anesthesia (cystoscopy and proctoscopy) of the parametrium, pelvic sidewalls, bladder, and rectum, and a chest x-ray. These results are combined to clinically stage the individual. The tumor tends to spread by direct extension, causing parametrial thickening, and by lymphatic spread to obturator nodes and then to pelvic and para-aortic nodes.

The staging of cervical cancer is complex, but the following is a brief overview:

Stage I: Confined strictly to the cervix
Stage II: Beyond the cervix but not to the pelvic sidewall
Stage IIA: No parametrial involvement
Stage IIB: Parametrial involvement
Stage III: Extends to the pelvic sidewall
Stage IV: Beyond the true pelvis, bladder or rectum involvement

Treatment of cervical cancer requires a team of gynecologic oncologists and radiation oncologists. In stage I to IIA cervical cancer, radical hysterectomy or radiation therapy has demonstrated similar excellent 5-year survival rates. Any persons with stage IIB or greater must be treated with radiation.

Recurrent or persistent cancer causes devastating problems for patients, their families, and clinicians. Patients have a markedly diminished 5-year survival rate when recurrence occurs. Recurrent cervical cancer can be treated palliatively or with some hope of a cure. Curable lesions are those which are easily resected, i.e., single lesions located at the vaginal apex or in the lung or lesions located centrally in the pelvis without lymph node involvement. Pelvic exenterative surgery is very extensive surgery removing the bladder, rectum, uterus (if not already done), and vagina. A colostomy is required, and a neovagina and urinary diversion are created. Patients with recurrent cervical cancers often present to the ED with vaginal bleeding, uremia secondary to ureter obstruction or invasion, deep venous thrombosis, leg swelling, or pain.

Vaginal Cancer

Vaginal cancer accounts for only 1 to 2 percent of all gynecologic malignancies. The true definition of primary vaginal cancer is that it must arise from the vagina and not be an extension or metastasis from the cervix or vulva. The main histologic type is squamous cell carcinoma. Squamous lesions usually occur in postmenopausal woman, whereas other histologic types (rhabdosarcoma, endodermal sinus tumor, adenocarcinoma, and clear cell adenocarcinoma from diethylstilbestrol) usually occur in younger women. The last diethylstilbestrol (DES) administration was around 1971, which would place these women in their forties. The mean age of occurrence for vaginal cancer is 60 to 65 years of age. Epidemiologic factors contributing to the occurrence of vaginal cancer are immunosuppression, chronic irritation (long-term pessary use or prolapse of female organs), decreased socioeconomic status, radiation for cervical cancer, hysterectomy for dysplasia, multiple sexual partners, and DES exposure. The tumor usually presents in the posterior upper third of the vagina. Abnormal vaginal bleeding is the presenting symptom most of the time. Some complain of abnormal discharge or postcoital bleeding.

Staging for vaginal cancer is summarized as follows:

Stage I: Vaginal wall involvement
Stage II: Parametrial involvement
Stage III: Pelvic wall involvement
Stage IV: Bladder/rectum or beyond pelvic involvement

Most vaginal cancers are best treated with radiation therapy.

Embryonal rhabdomyosarcomas (sarcoma botryoides) occur in children younger than 5 years of age and present with vaginal bleeding, discharge, or grapelike masses protruding from the vagina. These cancers respond very well to the chemotherapeutic regimen of vincristine, dactinomycin, and cyclophosphamide with either surgery or radiation. Complications associated with vaginal cancers are bleeding, infections, fistulas, or complications from chemotherapy, radiation, or surgery.

Vulvar Cancer

Vulvar cancer is responsible for only 1 to 4 percent of all gynecologic malignancies and less than 1 percent of all cancers. Most women diagnosed with vulvar cancer are older than 55 years of age. The most common histologic type is squamous cell carcinoma, followed by melanoma, basal cell carcinoma, adenocarcinoma, sarcoma, Bartholin gland tumors, and metastasis. Luckily, the prognosis is generally good because recognizable symptoms allow for early diagnosis. The most common presenting symptoms include a mass, pruritus, pain, or ulceration (in decreasing order of frequency). The cause for vulvar cancer is still unknown, but there have been associations of vulvar cancers with other cancers of the anogenital tract. Human papillomavirus (HPV) types 16, 18, 31, 35, and 39 all have been suggested as causative factors.

It seems that the etiology is multifactorial, and HPV alone is not the culprit. Other possibilities include immunodeficiency, vulvar dystrophy, smoking, and exposure to aniline dyes such as benzene. Multicentric lesions are seen more commonly in younger women, whereas unifocal lesions are seen most often in older women. On physical examination, the lesions may appear white, pigmented, raised, thickened, nodular, or ulcerative. A vulvar biopsy should be performed liberally in women with any suspicious lesions. Treatment depends on the stage at the time of diagnosis. More recent years have welcomed the advent of more conservative treatment modalities. The treatment of choice is surgery with adjuvant radiotherapy in more advanced stages.

Staging is summarized as follows:

Stage I: Confined to the vulva or perineum and less than 2 cm
Stage II: Confined to vulva or perineum and greater than 2 cm
Stage III: Any size lesion spread to lower urethra, vagina, or anus with unilateral positive nodes
Stage IV: Involvement of the upper urethra, bladder, rectum, or pelvic bone with positive bilateral nodes

Partial vulvectomy is the treatment of choice for patients with lesions smaller than 2 cm. The use of postoperative radiation may decrease the incidence of recurrence and improve survival in women with lesions larger than 2 cm and positive lymph nodes. The morbidity from surgery is groin wound breakdown and lymphedema from lymph node dissections. Recurrent vulvar cancer may be local or distant or involve lymph nodes. Patients often present with bleeding, lymphedema, deep venous thrombosis, or metastasis (usually to bone or lung).

Gestational Trophoblastic Disease

Gestational trophoblastic disease (GTD) is a disease of trophoblastic placental tissue. There are four forms of GTD: (1) hydatidiform mole, (2) invasive mole, (3) choriocarcinoma, (4) placental site tumors.[5]

The incidence of molar pregnancy is about 1 in 2000 pregnancies, but the incidence is much higher in Asian women. The risk of developing a second molar pregnancy is higher. Molar pregnancy is seen with a bimodal distribution. Persons younger than age 20 and older than age 40 are at greatest risk. GTD may be benign or malignant and, when malignant, can be divided into metastatic and nonmetastatic.

The benign form of this disease is hydatidiform mole, either partial or complete. Table 111-1 lists some of the major differences between partial and complete moles.

Treatment of hydatidiform mole is suction curettage or hysterectomy. Hyperthyroidism or hypertension must be stabilized prior to surgery. Follow-up is essential because dilatation and curettage alone is curative in only 80 percent of patients, leaving 20 percent at risk for persistent trophoblastic disease.

Gestational trophoblastic neoplasm (GTN) includes invasive mole and choriocarcinoma. These tumors can progress to malignancy and ultimately death if left untreated. Luckily, they are highly responsive to chemotherapy.

Invasive mole is the myometrial invasion of the hydatidiform mole. Common sites for metastasis of this cancer are the lungs and vagina. Invasive moles occur in 1 of 15,000 pregnancies, and 15 percent of hydatidiform moles result in invasive moles. Diagnosis is confirmed by consistently elevated or rising beta human chorionic gonadotropin (β-hCG) levels after a molar evacuation.

Choriocarcinoma is characterized by atypical trophoblastic hyperplasia with direct and vascular invasion into the myometrium and distant sites, most commonly the lungs, brain, liver, pelvis, or vagina. The incidence of choriocarcinoma is approximately 1 in 40,000 pregnancies. Twenty-five percent follow abortion or ectopic pregnancies, 25 percent are seen with term gestations, and the remaining 50 percent result from hydatidiform moles. Fortunately, only 2 to 3 percent of hydatidiform moles result in choriocarcinoma.

TABLE 111-1 Some Major Differences between Partial and Complete Moles

	Complete Mole	Partial Mole
Symptoms	Vaginal bleeding Uterine size > estimated gestational age Hyperemesis gravidarum Pre-eclampsia at <20 weeks gestation Hyperthyroidism Trophoblastic embolization Absent fetal heart tones	Incomplete or missed abortion Vaginal bleeding
Diagnosis	Ultrasonography reveals "snowstorm" appearance coupled with a high β-hCG level	Usually on histologic examination from tissue obtained from a missed or incomplete abortion

Symptoms of GTN are continued bleeding after dilatation and curettage for hydatidiform mole or bleeding after a pregnancy event (e.g., vaginal delivery, cesarean section, ectopic pregnancy, miscarriage, or abortion). Patients with metastasis may present with dyspnea, cough, chest pain, central nervous system abnormalities, or vaginal mass. The most common site for metastasis is the vagina, followed by the lung.

Treatment depends on the presence of metastasis. Patients with no metastatic disease who wish to preserve their fertility are treated with single-agent chemotherapy, methotrexate, or dactinomycin; otherwise, hysterectomy is the treatment of choice. This initial therapy leads to cure in 85 to 90 percent of patients. When metastatic disease is present, combination chemotherapy is given.

COMPLICATIONS OF GYNECOLOGIC MALIGNANCIES

The complications of gynecologic malignancies are related to the natural progression of disease, surgery, chemotherapy, or radiation. Any combination of these complications can occur depending on the type and stage of neoplasm and treatment modality.

The complications related to the natural progression of disease often represent the symptoms that help to diagnose the disease. These include, but are not limited to, genital tract bleeding, gastrointestinal obstruction, masses or ascites, fistulae (both genitourinary and gastrointestinal), obstructive uropathy, metastasis, lymphedema, and hypercoagulable states leading to deep venous thrombosis or pulmonary embolism.

By far the most common oncologic complication (most frequently seen with cervical or uterine cancer) **is bleeding.** It may be acute or chronic, massive or minimal, external or internal. Sources include friable tissue, tumor erosion into iliac or femoral vessels, adnexal mass rupture, or coagulopathies that develop secondary to chemotherapy or radiation. Assessment and management begin with the principles of emergency care. Then a thorough history and physical examination, including prior diagnoses and treatment, should be undertaken to find the likely source and cause of bleeding. Where externally accessible sites of bleeding occur, apply direct pressure. If this fails to control the bleeding, next use topical silver nitrate or Monsel's solution. If bleeding persists, topical absorbable hemostat material can be applied such as Gelfoam, Instat, or Surgicel. Where the vagina is the source of bleeding, vaginal packing may become necessary. Use a long strip of continuous gauze, and place a Foley catheter to prevent urinary retention. Regardless of the causes of bleeding, after stabilization, the gynecology service should be consulted.

Patients occasionally present with abdominal distention and discomfort. This often is concomitant with other complications of cancer and therefore may be accompanied by early satiety, nausea, vomiting, anorexia, weight loss, constipation or diarrhea, urinary frequency, urgency, incontinence, dyspnea, or orthopnea. As always, the first step is complete history and physical examination, including both pelvic and rectal examinations. Diagnostic testing may reveal worsening of known disease, recurrence of cancer, new cancer, torsion of a large ovary, bowel perforation, or intra-abdominal hemorrhage. Consultation with a gynecologist, gynecologic oncologist, or surgeon is indicated.

Gastrointestinal complications include obstructions and fistulae. Obstruction is common as a progressive symptom of malignancy, especially with ovarian and uterine tumors that are associated with enlarging masses or ascites. The resulting obstruction may be mechanical or due to tumor ileus from encasement of the nerve plexus leading to dysfunction of a segment of bowel. Patients often present with nausea, vomiting, early satiety, abdominal pain, distention, constipation, and/or obstipation. The normal management scheme for obstruction applies (as discussed in Chap. 79 in more depth). Surgical palliation may give temporary symptomatic relief, but recurrence rates are extremely high. Consultation with a gynecologist, gynecologic oncolo-

gist, or surgeon is indicated to discuss and provide permanent proximal decompression and supplemental nutrition.

Fistula formation occurs secondary to bowel encasement or obstruction. The fistula may drain to the abdominal wall, peritoneal cavity, vagina, uterus, or bladder. Instillation of colored medium (e.g., charcoal, food dye in tube feeds), upper gastrointestinal series, barium enema, or a fistulogram often aids diagnosis. Consultation with a gynecologist, gynecologic oncologist, or surgeon is indicated to determine the best treatment.

Urinary tract complications also include obstruction and fistula. Ureteral obstruction classically is seen in cervical cancer but also occurs with progression or recurrence of other pelvic malignancies. Radiation also may cause permanent scarring of the lumen leading to obstruction. Patients may develop acute renal failure and require percutaneous or cystoscopic emergent decompression. A vesicovaginal or ureterovaginal fistula may develop at the site of untreated cancer or recurrent cancer or after radiation therapy.

Chronic mild lymphedema of the lower extremities often follows inguinal node resection. Pedal lymphedema is seen after pelvic radiation therapy. Aside from the associated discomfort, the greatest concern is deep venous thrombosis, especially if lymphedema is unilateral. Duplex ultrasound is necessary. Lymphedema is treated supportively with elevation and support stockings.

Thromboembolic disease has long been associated with gynecologic malignancies and is discussed in Chap. 59.

Most of the side effects of chemotherapeutic agents are predictable and can be lessened with adjuvant medications. Risk factors for poor tolerance of chemotherapy are advanced age, advanced disease, poor nutritional status, or severe systemic involvement. Chemotherapeutic agents may have debilitating effects on many organ systems (Table 111-2).

The complications related to radiation are temporally divided into acute and chronic. The chronic manifestations may be further broken into gastrointestinal, genitourinary, and pulmonary. Acute findings include nausea, vomiting, diarrhea, cystitis, nephritis, pneumonitis, and myelosuppression. Gastrointestinal symptoms are often self-limiting and are controlled with supportive therapy, including antiemetics, antidiarrheals, and avoidance of high-fiber diets. Newer studies point to glutamine-rich diets, and the use of sucralfate may further reduce diarrhea. The genitourinary symptoms range from infection to hemorrhagic cystitis with extreme pain. Treatment of these symptoms includes adequate hydration, surveillance for infection, and bladder irrigation with analgesia or steroids. Resolution of myelosuppression is often spontaneous and begins after radiation has been completed.

Chronic findings are divided into gastrointestinal, genitourinary, and pulmonary. The most common complication is radiation enteritis, which presents with chronic diarrhea, malabsorption, or digestive difficulty. Other chronic gastrointestinal complications include strictures, fistulas, perforations, obstructions, and hematochezia. These findings often occur within 2 years of treatment. Management should be a collaborative effort between the oncologist, surgeon, and gastroenterologist. Emergency management includes adequate hydration and symptomatic relief. Genitourinary complications include incontinence, fistula formation, stricture formation, and hemorrhagic cystitis. Incontinence and fistulas were discussed earlier. The most severe complication of stricture formation is obstructive uropathy. This always should be considered as recurrence of disease until proven otherwise and as a result of radiation by diagnosis of exclusion. Both hemorrhagic cystitis and stricture require cystoscopy for evaluation. An oncologist and urologist should institute appropriate treatment.

Lastly, secondary malignancies may arise from radiation therapy. This results from the local nonmalignant tissue being exposed to ionizing radiation. The resulting damage to genetic material leads to mutation that is the presumed mechanism for carcinogenesis. The secondary malignancy is often observed years after the initial radiation therapy, and accuracy in predicting its occurrence is difficult at best.

TABLE 111-2 Chemotherapeutic Agents and Their Toxicities

Agent	Toxicity	Type of Cancer Treated
	ALKYLATING AGENTS	
Cyclophosphamide	Myelosuppression, cystitis, hepatitis, alopecia	Ovarian, breast, sarcoma
Ifosfamide	Myelosuppression, CNS abnormalities, bladder and rental toxicity	Ovarian, cervical
Chlorambucil	Myelosuppression, dermatitis, hepatitis, gastrointestinal dysfunction	Ovarian
Nitrogen mustard	Nausea, vomiting, myelosuppression	Ovarian, malignant effusions
Cisplatin (alkylating like)	Nephrotoxicity, tinnitus, hearing loss, myelosuppression, peripheral neuropathy, nausea, vomiting	Ovarian, cervical, germ cell
Carboplatin (alkylating like)	Neuropathy, ototoxicity, myelosuppression, nephrotoxicity	Ovarian, germ cell
	ANTIMETABOLITES	
Methotrexate	Myelosuppression, hepatitis, pneumonitis, stomatitis	Breast, ovarian, choriocarcinoma
5-Fluorouracil	Myelosuppression, alopecia, nausea, vomiting	Breast, ovarian
Hydroxyurea	Nausea, vomiting, anorexia, myelosuppression	Cervical
	PLANT ALKALOIDS	
Vinblastine	Myelosuppression, alopecia, nausea, vomiting, neurotoxicity	Germ cell, choriocarcinoma
Vincristine	Myelosuppression, alopecia, nausea, vomiting, neurotoxicity	Germ cell, cervical, sarcoma
Paclitaxel (Taxol)	Myelosuppression, alopecia, arrhythmias, hypersensitivity	Ovarian, breast
Etoposide (VP-16)	Myelosuppression, alopecia, hypotension	Germ cell, choriocarcinoma
	ANTITUMOR ANTIBIOTICS	
Bleomycin	Fever, anaphylaxis, pulmonary fibrosis, dermatitis	Cervial, germ cell, malignant effusions
Doxorubicin (Adriamycin)	Myelosuppression, alopecia, cardiotoxicity, nausea, vomiting	Ovarian, breast, uterine
Mitomycin-C	Nephrotoxicity, stomatitis, nausea, vomiting, myelosuppression	Breast, ovarian, cervical
Actinomycin-D (Dactinomycin)	Nausea, vomiting, dermatitis, myelosuppression, stomatitis	Germ cell, choriocarcinoma

REFERENCES

1. Romanzi LJ, Chaikin DC, Blaivas JG: The effect of genital prolapse on voiding. *J Urol* 161:581, 1999.
2. Cundiff GW, Addison WA: Management of pelvic organ prolapse. *Obstet Gynecol Clin North Am* 25:907, 1998.
3. Gurel H, Gurel SA, Atilla MK: Urethral syndrome and associated risk factors related to obstetrics and gynecology. *Eur J Obstet Gynecol Reprod Biol* 83:5, 1999.
4. Wesselmann U, Burnett AL, Heinberg LJ: The urogenital and rectal pain syndromes. *Pain* 73:269, 1997.
5. Newlands ES, Paradinas FJ, Fisher RA: Recent advances in gestational trophoblastic disease. *Hematol Oncol Clin North Am* 13:225, 1999.

112 COMPLICATIONS OF GYNECOLOGIC PROCEDURES
Michael A. Silverman
Karen M. Hardart

Because of convenience, cost effectiveness, and apparent safety, the number of ambulatory surgeries continues to increase. The indications appropriate for ambulatory surgery also continue to increase. These trends are accompanied by a decrease in the length of hospitalization following major gynecologic surgery. Unanticipated hospital admission after ambulatory surgery occurs in approximately 1 percent of cases and is an important measure of outcome.[1] Gynecologic outpatient surgery has been associated with an unscheduled admission rate of more than 5 percent, with postoperative emesis being the most common reason for admission.[2]

HISTORY AND PHYSICAL EXAMINATION

The most common reasons for ED visits during the postoperative period following gynecologic procedures are pain, fever, and vaginal bleeding. A focused but thorough evaluation should be performed. The history should include the surgical procedure performed (abdominal versus vaginal), the reason for it, time of symptom onset and its proximity to the surgery, complications already experienced, the patient's postsurgical history, and medications prescribed. The interval between the surgery and the onset of symptoms is very important in determining their cause. For example, most cases of early postoperative fevers (less than 24 h) are not infectious, and causes may include pulmonary atelectasis, hypersensitivity reactions to antibiotics, pyogenic reactions to tissue trauma, or hematoma formation.

Relevant examination of all appropriate systems should then be performed. It should not be assumed that the etiology of the complaint is gynecologic. Other potential explanations of the symptoms should be investigated. Postoperative pain and tenderness can be difficult to assess. Some tenderness is normal, but rebound tenderness is not. After laparoscopy, patients may have pain radiating to their shoulder for several days because of remaining CO_2 bubbles. Postoperative pain and tenderness is more concerning if associated with nausea and vomiting and a change in bowel sounds. The surgical wound should be examined, and a pelvic examination should be performed, including both a sterile speculum and a bimanual examination. The pelvic examination should be performed with caution, or even deferred in infertility patients, due to the possibility of rupturing enlarged ovarian follicles. The sterile speculum examination should visualize the cervix, or if it is absent, the vaginal cuff, and any evidence of bleeding, discharge, erythema, or cuff or labial cellulitis should be noted. Cervical cultures should be considered. Bimanual examination after a vaginal or abdominal hysterectomy should evaluate for tenderness, masses, and an intact cuff. Following hysteroscopy or dilation and curettage, cervical motion, uterine, and adnexal tenderness should be evaluated. A rectal examination should always be performed to evaluate tenderness or masses.

Laboratory studies should be directed towards the patient's complaints. A complete blood count with a manual differential count is almost always indicated. A serum β-human chorionic gonadotropin level should be obtained for all women with childbearing potential. A catheterized urine specimen, along with urine, blood, wound, and cervical (if present) cultures, should be obtained if the patient is febrile. A chemistry panel may be necessary to evaluate hepatic and renal function.

Imaging procedures are often necessary. A chest radiograph can confirm pneumonia or inappropriate air under the diaphragm. Air or insufflated CO_2 should be completely absorbed by the third postoperative day. Supine and erect abdominal series help confirm bowel obstruction. Pelvic sonogram remains the gold standard for visualizing the pelvic structures. However, a computed tomography (CT) scan may be necessary, especially if an abscess is suspected.

COMPLICATIONS OF ENDOSCOPIC PROCEDURES

Laparoscopy

Both diagnostic and therapeutic gynecologic laparoscopy are accomplished by passing a rigid endoscope through a trocar that is inserted bluntly through a small infraumbilical incision into the abdominal cavity after a Veress needle has been used to insufflate the abdomen with carbon dioxide. The pneumoperitoneum must be sufficient to displace the bowel and is maintained throughout the surgery. Additional trocars can be placed so that other accessories can be used during the surgery. Laparoscopy is almost always an ambulatory surgical procedure and is performed under general anesthesia with endotracheal intubation.

There are numerous indications for gynecologic laparoscopy, ranging from diagnosing gynecologic disorders (e.g., endometriosis or ectopic pregnancy) to performing complex gynecologic surgery. The most common surgical procedure in the United States is female sterilization. More than 60 percent of these procedures are performed laparoscopically and have a complication rate of 1.6 per 100 procedures.[3] Infertility is one of the most common indications for diagnostic laparoscopy. Laparoscopy is also used for lysis of adhesions, CO_2 laser ablation of endometriosis, uterine surgery (including myomectomy), tubal surgeries (including salpingectomy), ovarian surgery (including oophorectomy and oophorocystectomy), paraovarian cyst excision, laparoscopic vaginal hysterectomy, and retropubic urethropexy.

All of these procedures entail the same potential complications, but more complex surgeries carry considerably more risk. The incidence of major complications in the United States for laparoscopy may be as low as 0.22 percent.[4] In the last decade, the most comprehensive survey on this topic reported complications for 45,042 procedures as follows: hemorrhage 1 percent, unintended laparotomy 1 percent, blood transfusion for hemorrhage 0.45 percent, and bowel or urinary tract injury 0.41 percent. Further studies have supported these data.[5–7] Approximately half of all complications may be related to the installation of laparoscopy, though some studies show that open laparoscopy may be safer.[7,8] In 1996, the overall incidence of complications in major operative laparoscopy was reported as 10.4 percent.[9] This rate is still significantly less than the 25 to 50 percent overall complication rate of abdominal surgery, such as hysterectomy or oophorectomy through abdominal incisions, although data related to the two approaches are not directly comparable because of other factors that may mandate a traditional surgical procedure.

The major complications associated with laparoscopy are thermal injury of the bowel, perforation of a viscus, bleeding or other vascular injury, ureteral or bladder injuries, and incisional hernia or wound dehiscence.

Thermal injury is the most serious potential complication. While many significant complications of laparoscopy are recognized in the operating room under direct visualization, patients with thermal injury may not develop symptoms for several days and up to several weeks postoperatively. Various series have reported the incidence of electrothermal injuries to be in the range of 0.5 to 3.2 per 1000 cases. Patient presentations may include bilateral lower quadrant pain and tenderness, fever, elevated white blood cell count, or peritonitis. Plain radiographs may show an ileus or free air under the diaphragm. Patients with greater-than-expected pain after laparoscopy should be considered to have a bowel injury until proven otherwise. Early gynecologic consult is critical if a thermal injury is suspected.

Traumatic injury to the bowel is usually less serious than thermal injury. The small diameter Veress needle is usually the cause of a bowel perforation, which is recognized on withdrawal of the needle. A sharp trocar may cause more damage, though most surgeries are now performed with a blunt trocar. Gastric perforation may result, usually due to stomach distention from aerophagia or as a result of a difficult intubation. The large or small bowel may also be perforated. These injuries are usually noted during the operation. On rare occasions, perforation may occur through a single loop of bowel adherent to the anterior abdominal wall. Complications include peritonitis, abscess, enterocutaneous fistula, and septic shock.

Vascular injury occurs at a rate of 0.1 to 6.4 per 1000 cases. While such injuries may be immediately life-threatening, they are almost universally recognized during the operation. Patients may present with a postoperative hematoma. Local compression, if feasible, is the initial treatment. If the mass enlarges or signs of hypovolemia occur, the wound must be explored by the gynecologist.

Bladder and ureteral injuries may occur from mechanical or thermal trauma. Trocar or dissection injuries to the bladder are typically recognized intraoperatively. Thermal injuries, however, may not be initially apparent and may present with peritonitis or fistula. The diagnosis of a ureteral injury is usually delayed. Thermal injury may present up to 14 days postoperatively with abdominal or flank pain, fever, and peritonitis. There may be an elevated white blood cell count, and an intravenous pyelogram (IVP) shows extravasation of urine or an urinoma. Mechanical obstruction of the ureter from sutures or staples may be recognized intraoperatively by direct visualization, but may present up to 1 week postoperatively with fever and flank pain. An IVP or a CT scan of the abdomen and pelvis helps define the site and degree of obstruction.

Incisional hernias and dehiscence are rare complications after laparoscopy. Incisional hernias are more common when defects larger than 10 mm are made and may develop within the first postoperative week. Patients may be asymptomatic or may present with pain, mass, evisceration, or signs and symptoms of a mechanical bowel obstruction. Fever may occur if the bowel is incarcerated, and peritonitis may develop following bowel perforation. Dehiscence usually involves protrusion of the omentum, and, in rare cases, the small bowel passes through the opening. Immediate incisional repair by a gynecologist is usually sufficient; however, a laparotomy may be necessary if the bowel is incarcerated or perforation is a risk.

Wound infection after laparoscopy is uncommon and often not a serious complication. Most are minor skin infections that can be managed expectantly with oral antibiotics or with drainage. The risk of infection after laparoscopy is much lower than that after abdominal or vaginal surgery. Excluding minor skin infections, pelvic infection is reported in fewer than 1 in 1000 cases. Pelvic cellulitis and abscess can occur, and severe necrotizing fasciitis, while rare, has been reported. Most infections are probably secondary to a subacute coexisting infection present prior to the procedure or secondary to skin contamination. Broad-spectrum antibiotics typically provide a rapid response.

Hysteroscopy

Hysteroscopy is the direct visualization of the uterine cavity using a rigid or flexible fiberoptic instrument. Hysteroscopy can be done as an office procedure under intravenous sedation or in an operating room under general anesthesia, spinal or epidural anesthesia, or intravenous sedation. Hysteroscopy is done for both diagnostic and therapeutic purposes. The most common indication for hysteroscopy is abnormal vaginal bleeding. Other indications include uterine leiomyomata, intrauterine adhesions, proximal tubal obstruction, removal of intrauterine devices, müllerian anomalies, and infertility evaluation. Therapeutic applications include directed biopsies, removal of small myomata or polyps, and endometrial ablation for menorrhagia. Complications of hysteroscopy occur in less than 1 percent of cases and include fluid overload, uterine perforation with possible damage to intraabdominal organs, infection, toxic shock syndrome, anesthesia reaction, postoperative bleeding, and embolism.[10]

Fluid overload is rare but can occur from absorption of electrolyte and nonelectrolyte solutions during lengthy procedures. The entry of dextran into the circulation can lead to pulmonary edema and disseminated intravascular coagulation. For this reason, no more than 500 mL of dextran should be used during a procedure. A lack of recovery of distention medium in excess of 1000 mL also places the patient at risk for fluid overload. If fluid overload is suspected, hyponatremia is likely. Therapy to decrease the serum sodium level may prevent generalized cerebral edema, seizures, and death (see Chap. 27).

Uterine perforation is a relatively common complication. A midline uterine perforation generally does not have significant sequelae. A lateral perforation may lacerate uterine vessels and cause substantial bleeding. Most often, the perforation is noted at the time of surgery, and a laparoscopy is done to investigate for bleeding and/or damage to bowel or bladder. If the complication is not noted at the time of surgery, the patient may present with peritoneal signs if the bowel has been injured or pain and/or bleeding if the vessels were lacerated.

Infection is very rare and most commonly occurs in patients with concurrent genital tract infections. Endometritis or even toxic shock can result.

Postoperative bleeding may be uterine or cervical in origin. Cervical lacerations may be caused by forceful dilation or tears from the tenaculum. Uterine bleeding can result from resection procedures. After hemodynamic stabilization of the patient, the gynecologist can place a Foley or balloon catheter into the uterine cavity and fill it with approximately 10 to 15 mL of water or saline solution. One technique is to remove one-half the fluid from the balloon after 1 h and the other half after 2 h. If bleeding remains stopped, the patient can usually be discharged. If bleeding persists, the patient should be admitted. The catheter is reinflated and left overnight, and occasionally reexploration is required.

Embolism is the most feared complication of using CO_2 gas as a distention medium. The risks of such an occurrence are low when the principles of low flow and low pressure are followed.

COMPLICATIONS RELATED TO MAJOR ABDOMINAL SURGERY

Complications from major abdominal procedures that lead to ED visits usually occur at least 3 days postoperatively. Expected complications include, but are not confined to, wound infection and related morbidity, phlebitis (both superficial and deep), urinary tract infection, bladder and ureteral injury, ileus and bowel obstruction, pneumonia, and atelectasis.

Hysterectomy remains one of the most common major surgical procedures in the United States, with abdominal hysterectomy being performed more frequently than laparoscopic hysterectomy and vaginal hysterectomy.[11] It also carries significant morbidity, with postoperative infection rates reported between 3.9 and 50 percent for abdominal hysterectomies and 1.7 to 64 percent for laparoscopic vaginal hysterectomies. There are numerous risk factors for postoperative infections. Lower socioeconomic status is a risk factor for infection in gynecologic surgery, which may be related to inadequate nutrition or poor hygiene. Obesity also carries an increased risk of infection, possibly due to poor hygiene, altered nutrition, or increased operative time. Additional risk factors include altered immunocompetence, diabetes, lack of prophylactic antibiotics when indicated, or excessive operative blood loss.

Wound Infection

CLINICAL FEATURES Wound infections may occur early postoperatively or up to several months after the surgery. Greater than 90 percent occur within the first 2 postoperative weeks. Early infections range from mild cellulitis to those associated with fever, tachycardia, increased wound tenderness, and severe local cellulitis. As the infection progresses, the wound may be fluctuant or indurated. Wound breakdown and dehiscence can occur if treatment is not initiated rapidly. The infected incision is swollen, erythematous, edematous, and tender. There may be spontaneous purulent drainage from the wound. Initial management consists of opening the incision, probing with a sterile cotton swab to confirm an intact fascia, vigorous cleaning with saline solution, and packing with saline-soaked wet-to-dry dressings. If staples have been placed, they should be removed. Aerobic and anaerobic cultures should be obtained. The operating gynecologist should always be informed about the patient. Late-onset infections are characterized by persistent low-grade fevers and purulent drainage from the incision. Local wound care as described above is appropriate.

DISPOSITION Parenteral therapy with a penicillin-based antibiotic and aggressive local wound care are typically used for early postoperative infections, particularly when there is underlying cellulitis. Consultation with the gynecologic surgeon would be appropriate. Most patients are readmitted.

Infected Vaginal Cuff Hematoma, Cellulitis, or Abscess

CLINICAL FEATURES A vaginal cuff is formed during a hysterectomy and is composed of the contiguous retroperitoneal space immediately above the vaginal apex and the surrounding soft tissue. This cuff may become infected, leading to cellulitis, hematoma, or abscess.

Vaginal cuff cellulitis is a common complication following both abdominal and vaginal hysterectomy. Symptoms and signs usually present between postoperative days 3 and 5, and may begin in the hospital or just after discharge. Patients often complain of lower abdominal pain, pelvic pain, back pain, fever, and abnormal vaginal discharge. Induration, tenderness of the vaginal cuff, and possibly a purulent discharge or labial edema or erythema are prominent during the pelvic examination. The white blood cell count is usually elevated.

A vaginal cuff abscess usually presents early in the postoperative course. Patients complain of fever, chills, pelvic pain, and rectal pressure. On examination, lower abdominal and vaginal cuff tenderness is present. A tender fluctuant mass near the cuff may be palpable, and purulent drainage from the cuff may be seen.

Infected cuff hematomas may present later in the postoperative course, and if large, are associated with a decrease in the patient's hemoglobin and hematocrit levels. The hematoma may not be palpable on examination.

DISPOSITION Patients should be readmitted for intravenous antibiotics and possible drainage. Broad-spectrum antibiotics should be started early, with coverage for gram-negative, gram-positive, and anaerobic organisms. Most pelvic infections require similar treatment. Triple antibiotic therapy with ampicillin (2 g IV q6h), gentamicin (1.5 mg/kg load IV, then 1.0 mg/kg IV q8h) and clindamycin (900 mg IV q6h) are still appropriate. Aztreonam (1 to 2 g IV q8h) can be substituted if the patient is at risk for nephrotoxicity. Other options that are more expensive but have a more favorable profile when renal compromise is an issue include ticarcillin-clavulanate (3.1 g IV q6h) or ampicillin-sulbactam (3 g IV q4 to 6h). Abscess, septic pelvic thrombophlebitis, or drug fever should be considered in patients who do not respond. A CT scan may be necessary for diagnosis or to better define an abscess or hematoma.

Postoperative Ovarian Abscess

CLINICAL FEATURES Patients with fever and abdominal and pelvic pain shortly after discharge from the hospital may have a pelvic abscess. Such abscesses are usually ovarian in nature. A sudden increase in pain may be a signal that the abscess has ruptured. This is a surgical emergency and requires a laparotomy. If time permits or the diagnosis is in question, a CT scan can aid in identifying the size and location of the abscess.

DISPOSITION   Patients with a pelvic abscess need to be admitted. Some abscesses respond to broad-spectrum antibiotics, and others may require drainage either by an interventional radiologist or by colpotomy.

Dehiscence and Evisceration

CLINICAL FEATURES   Wound disruption is a failure of normal healing and includes the breakdown of any layers of a surgical incision. Dehiscence is disruption of all layers, including fascia and peritoneum. Evisceration occurs when there is complete breakdown of the healing processes through all levels of the abdominal wall and the omentum or bowel presents through the incision. The classic sign of impending dehiscence is the sudden outpouring of serosanguineous blood from the abdominal incision. Most often this occurs between postoperative days 5 and 8. The patient may describe a "pop" or tearing sensation. About one-third of cases of wound dehiscence are associated with evisceration. While gynecologic surgery has a lower wound disruption rate than the 1 to 3 percent reported following major abdominal surgery, the mortality rate is high, up to 35 percent or greater.[12]

DISPOSITION   When evisceration has occurred, the abdomen should be covered with moist sterile towels and supported with tape to prevent further extrusion of the gut.

The patient should be taken directly to the operating room for closure. In cases in which there is a sudden appearance of blood but no bowel, it is best to follow the same procedure because evisceration usually is imminent.

Ureteral Injury

CLINICAL FEATURES   Operative injury to the ureter results from one of three types of trauma: crushing, transection, or ligation. Each type of injury may be either partial or complete. This complication occurs more often during the performance of abdominal hysterectomy than during any other pelvic surgery. In patients who develop flank pain shortly after surgery, ureteral injury should be suspected. Patients may have fever and costovertebral angle tenderness. A urinalysis should be performed, and if obstruction is suspected, an abdominal and pelvis CT with intravenous contrast or an IVP should be obtained. If obstruction is noted, it is usually near the ureterovesical junction.

DISPOSITION   Patients should be admitted for attempted ureteral catheterization under cystoscopic guidance and possibly exploratory laparotomy. Percutaneous nephrostomy with delayed repair may also be considered.

OTHER COMPLICATIONS OF GYNECOLOGIC SURGERY

Urinary Retention

Urinary retention in a healthy female after gynecologic surgery is uncommon. However, many women experience either an inability to void or incomplete emptying of the bladder during the postoperative period. Urinary retention is usually a temporary result of pain or bladder atony resulting from anesthesia.

CLINICAL FEATURES   Inability to void is more frequent after operations such as radical hysterectomy or those that involve the urethra and bladder neck (i.e., anterior repair or any modification of the retropubic urethropexy). Most problems with voiding following any of these procedures resolve with time and without medication.

DISPOSITION   Retention can be initially relieved with insertion of a Foley catheter for 12 to 24 h. Most patients are able to void after this period. An alternative method is intermittent straight catheterization. Patients are instructed to attempt to void on a timed schedule at intervals of less than 3 h. Patients should be taught to perform self-catheterization if they are unable to void. Self-catheterization can be taught in the ED, and the patient should be reassured that voiding function will return in time. If a patient still has trouble voiding after temporary placement of a Foley catheter, the problem may be ureteral spasm, which can be treated with phenazopyridine (200 mg, tid) or oxybutynin (5 mg bid/tid).

Vesicovaginal Fistula

CLINICAL FEATURES   Vesicovaginal fistulas may occur after total abdominal hysterectomy. Patients present 10 to 14 days after surgery with a watery vaginal discharge. The diagnosis can be confirmed by inserting a cotton tampon into the vagina and then instilling methylene blue or indigo carmine dye via a transurethral catheter. If the tampon stains blue, a vesicovaginal fistula is present. If no staining occurs, a ureterovaginal fistula must be ruled out by injecting 5 mL of indigo carmine dye IV. If a ureterovaginal fistula is present, the tampon should stain blue within 20 min.

DISPOSITION   Gynecologic consultation is necessary. A Foley catheter should be inserted for prolonged drainage if a vesicovaginal fistula is present. With continuous drainage, up to 15 percent close spontaneously within 4 to 6 weeks. The remainder ultimately require surgical repair.

Osteomyelitis Pubis

CLINICAL FEATURES   Osteomyelitis pubis is a rare complication of pelvic surgery that presents 6 to 8 weeks after surgery with pain and tenderness along the symphysis pubis, especially with ambulation. Osteomyelitis pubis results from direct or contiguous seeding of the periosteum from pelvic surgery. It has been seen following certain types of bladder neck suspension. Patients have a low-grade fever, elevated sedimentation rate, and leukocytosis. Blood should be drawn for culture, since the results are sometimes positive.

DISPOSITION   Patients should be admitted for parenteral antibiotics and possibly surgical debridement.

Wound Hematoma

CLINICAL FEATURES   Hematomas are a common complication of wound closure and are more frequent in transverse than in vertical incisions. The wound itself may swell and be painful.

DISPOSITION   In general, smaller hematomas can and should be managed expectantly. If there are any signs of infection, the wound should be opened and drained. An ultrasound examination of the incision may be helpful if hematoma is suspected. The patient should be instructed to return if signs of infection develop.

Wound Seroma

CLINICAL FEATURES   Wound seromas are relatively common in gynecologic incisions. A wound seroma is a collection of serous fluid and may drain spontaneously. In general, it is the presence of drainage, not fever or pain, that prompts patients to seek emergency care.

DISPOSITION   If the wound remains intact after gentle probing, the seroma can be watched and usually disappears. If the seroma has reached a large size, drainage can be performed by aspiration and light pressure over the lymphocyst. Wound infection precautions should be given.

Postconization Bleeding

CLINICAL FEATURES High-grade squamous intraepithelial lesions of the cervix may be treated by loop electrocautery or cold-knife conization. The most common complication of these procedures is bleeding. If delayed hemorrhage occurs, it usually occurs 7 days postoperatively. Bleeding following this procedure can be rapid and severe.

DISPOSITION Visualization of the cervix is the key to controlling such bleeding. Application of Monsel solution (a commercially available ferrous subsulfate solution) is a reasonable first step if it is readily available. Monsel solution should be available from the hospital pharmacy. Direct pressure for 5 min with a large cotton-tipped swab may be effective. Alternatively, cauterization with silver nitrate may be attempted. If these maneuvers are not successful, a gynecologist should be consulted for suturing or cauterization of the bleeding arteriole. The vagina can be packed with gauze if the bleeding is severe until more definitive therapy is available. Often the patient must be taken to the operating room for repair because adequate visualization is difficult in the ED.

Septic Pelvic Thrombophlebitis

CLINICAL FEATURES Septic pelvic thrombophlebitis (SPT) is a diagnosis of exclusion complicating 0.1 to 0.5 percent of gynecologic procedures. The diagnosis is made when a patient with a postoperative fever does not respond to appropriate antibiotics in the absence of an undrained abscess or infected hematoma. Patients with SPT rarely present to the ED, since the complication typically presents in the hospital and delays discharge.

There are two forms of SPT. The classic form occurs 2 to 4 days after abdominal surgery and is characterized by fever, tachycardia, gastrointestinal distress, and unilateral abdominal pain. A palpable abdominal cord develops in 50 to 67 percent of cases. The enigmatic form complicates vaginal delivery and pelvic surgery. Patients have spiking fevers despite clinical improvement on antibiotics. Findings upon pelvic examination may be normal in patients with either form.

DISPOSITION Heparin and antibiotics for 7 to 10 days is the mainstay of treatment. Long-term anticoagulation is not needed unless septic pulmonary emboli have occurred. Antibiotics against heparinase-producing *Bacterioides* species (e.g., clindamycin 600 to 900 mg IV q8h) should be given to all patients.

Induced Abortion

There are three major methods for termination of a pregnancy: instrumental evacuation by the vaginal route, stimulation of uterine contraction, and major surgical procedures. Abortions performed surgically have complication rates of 18 to 29 percent[13,14] and can be immediate, delayed, or late. Immediate complications, less than 24 h after the abortion, include bleeding and pain. Most immediate complications are arrested at surgery, but many present within 24 h to the ED. Retained products of conception, uterine perforation, and cervical lacerations are the most common causes of immediate bleeding and pain. Delayed complications occur between 24 h and 4 weeks postabortion and include excessive bleeding, primarily due to retained products of conception, and postabortive endometritis. Late complications include postabortal amenorrhea, psychological problems including depression, and Rh isoimmunization.

If a cervical laceration is noted, treatment includes pressure followed by application of Monsel solution or use of silver nitrate sticks.

Suturing may be necessary if there is no resolution of bleeding. Uterine perforation occurs in approximately 1 to 3 per 1000 abortion procedures. Most perforations are noted at the time of surgery and are asymptomatic. However, those that go unnoticed can present with pain and/or bleeding and possibly signs of shock. The incidence of retained products of conception is 0.5 to 1.0 percent. On physical examination, the cervical os is generally open. The uterus is usually boggy, enlarged, and tender. A pelvic sonogram should be obtained to evaluate the uterine cavity for retained products. Repeat dilatation and curettage is necessary. If coexistent endometritis is present, treatment with antibiotics (as previously noted) is required for 10 to 14 days. Usual therapy includes broad-spectrum antibiotics until the patient is afebrile for 24 to 48 h.

Postabortal endometritis not associated with retained products of conception presents with a firm yet tender uterus and closed cervical os. Uncomplicated endometritis requires antibiotics, as previously discussed, and possible reaspiration based on sonographic findings. Rh_0 (D) immune globulin (300 μg IM) should be given to Rh-negative women after a spontaneous or induced abortion. If it is not prescribed within 72 h, the overall risk of sensitization in the second pregnancy is approximately 3 percent.

Brachytherapy

Brachytherapy is the treatment of malignant tumors by radioactive sources that are implanted, typically under general anesthesia, close to (intercavitary) or within (interstitial) the tumor. It may be used as adjuvant therapy following surgery or as primary therapy if the malignancy is advanced. Currently, radiation therapy is geared mainly toward cervical and uterine cancers and remains limited in ovarian cancer.

The normal tissues of the cervix and uterus can tolerate very high doses of radiation. In contrast, the sigmoid, rectosigmoid, and rectum do not, and are therefore more susceptible to radiation injury. Usually the small bowel is spared because it is in motion. Acute radiation cystitis can occur in the immediate postoperative period. Symptoms of cystitis are present but cultures are negative. Treatment is to increase oral intake and take a urinary analgesic. Chronic radiation cystitis with hematuria requires continuous bladder irrigation.

Radiation-induced soft tissue necrosis can also be a significant complication. It is thought to be due to a progressive endarteritis leading to decreased blood flow and eventually hypoxia. Often this leads to inflammation, infection, tissue breakdown, and fistula formation. The use of hyperbaric oxygen has been shown to enhance healing.

Postoperative Fatigue

Postoperative fatigue following major gynecologic surgery is quite common and often underappreciated by both the patient and physician. Sixty to ninety percent of posthysterectomy patients report postoperative fatigue to the point of interference with daily activities. Pain, sleep disturbances, and psychological factors all play a role in postoperative fatigue; however, the majority of patients have fatigue persist past resolution of postoperative pain. An average of 10 weeks is required before patients can resume normal activities. Anemia can contribute to fatigue and oral iron supplementation should be considered. In some cases, postoperative fatigue can persist for 6 to 12 months. In these chronic cases, depression and anxiety disorders should be ruled out.

Assisted Reproductive Technology

Transvaginal ultrasonographically guided aspiration of oocytes is used universally during in vitro fertilization. Previously, laparoscopic oocyte collection was used, which carried the occasional complications of laparoscopic surgery, including those related to general anesthesia. Complications related to ultrasound-guided retrieval and preparation for retrieval of oocytes are rare and include ovarian hyperstimulation syndrome, pelvic infections, intraperitoneal bleeding, and adnexal torsions.[15] However, the acute abdomen has developed hours to weeks after the procedure and has required prompt surgical intervention.

Ovarian hyperstimulation syndrome can be a life-threatening complication of induction of ovulation.[16] The incidence of the moderate-to-severe form is 1 to 2 percent. Symptoms include abdominal distention, ovarian enlargement, and weight gain in the mildest form. In the most severe form, patients have massive third-spacing of fluids into the abdominal cavity, which can lead to ascites, electrolyte imbalances, pleural effusions, and hypovolemia. Clinically, one sees increased coagulability and decreased renal perfusion. The decreased renal perfusion leads to increased salt and water reabsorption in the proximal tubule, leading to oliguria. **Abdominal and pelvic examinations are contraindicated due to extremely fragile ovaries that are at high risk of rupture or hemorrhage.** Defer examination until after discussion with the gynecologist. Patients are also at high risk for ovarian torsion because of the size of their ovaries. Electrolyte studies, renal function tests, a complete blood count, coagulation studies, and blood for type and cross-match should be obtained. An electrocardiogram to evaluate hyperkalemia should also be obtained. The gynecologist should be consulted for admission. Treatment is volume repletion.

Postembolization Syndrome

Since the mid 1990s, uterine artery embolization has become a more common approach for treating symptomatic uterine fibroids.[17] This nonsurgical approach is safe and effective and helps patients avoid myomectomy and hysterectomy. Performed by invasive radiologists, typically in collaboration with the patient's gynecologist, this procedure may be performed on an outpatient basis under conscious sedation, though many patients spend one night in the hospital for pain control. All patients who undergo the procedure experience some form of postembolization syndrome: pelvic pain and fever lasting 2 to 10 days as a result of transient myometrial and persistent fibroid ischemia. Patients may present to the ED with pain ranging from mild to severe. The emergency physician must work to control the pain as well as consider other etiologies that may cause the patient's symptoms, particularly an infectious etiology such as endometritis. Evaluation may include a complete blood count and a CT scan. Between 1 and 9 percent of patients may have symptoms of menopause after this procedure, with temporary or permanent loss of menses. While up to 10 percent of patients ultimately undergo hysterectomy, approximately 1 percent of patients undergo hysterectomy due to infection. Vaginal discharge and fibroid expulsion are other complications. Some patients may require admission for pain control and/or intravenous antibiotics.

REFERENCES

1. Fortier J, Chung F, Su J: Unanticipated admission after ambulatory surgery—A prospective study. *Can J Anaesth* 45:612, 1998.
2. Hedayati B, Fear S: Hospital admission after day-case gynecological laparoscopy. *Br J Anaesth* 83:776, 1999.
3. Jamieson DJ, Hillis SD, Duerr A, et al: Complications of interval laparoscopic tubal sterilization: Findings from the United States collaborative review of sterilization. *Obstet Gynecol* 96:997, 2000.
4. Hulka J, Peterson HB, Phillips JM, Surrey MW: Operative laparoscopy: American Association of Gynecologic Laparoscopists' 1993 membership survey. *J Am Assoc Gynecol Laparosc* 2:133, 1995.
5. Chapron C, Querlou D, Brukat MA, et al: Surgical complications of diagnostic and operative gynaecological laparoscopy: A series of 29,966 cases. *Hum Reprod* 13:867, 1998.
6. Harkki-Siren P, Kurki T: A nationwide analysis of laparoscopic complications. *Obstet Gynecol* 89:108, 1997.
7. Leonard F, Lecuru F, Rizk E, et al: Perioperative morbidity of gynecological laparoscopy. A prospective monocenter observational study. *Acta Obstet Gynecol Scand* 79:129, 2000.
8. Hasson HM, Rotman C, Rana N, et al: Open laparoscopy: 29-year experience. *Obstet Gynecol* 96:763, 2000.
9. Saidi MH, Vancaillie TG, White AJ, et al: Complications of major operative laparoscopy: A review of 452 cases. *J Reprod Med* 41:471, 1996.
10. Jansen FW, Vredevoogd CB, Ulzen KV, et al: Complications of hysteroscopy: A prospective, multicenter study. *Obstet Gynecol* 96:266, 2000.
11. Farquhar CM, Steiner CA: Hysterectomy rates in the United States. *Obstet Gynecol* 99:229, 2002.
12. Graham DJ, Stevenson JT, McHenry CR: The association of intra-abdominal infection and abdominal would dehiscence. *Am Surg* 64:660, 1998.
13. Jensen JT, Astley SJ, Morgan E, et al: Outcomes of suction curettage and miferistone abortion in the United States. A prospective comparison study. *Contraception* 59:153, 1999.
14. Autry AM, Hayes EC, Jacobson GF, et al: A comparison of medical induction and dilation and evacuation for second trimester abortion. *Am J Obstet Gynecol* 187:393, 2002.
15. Dicker D, Ashkenazi J, Feldberg D, et al: Severe abdominal complications after transvaginal ultrasonographically guided retrieval of oocytes for in-vitro fertilization and embryo transfer. *Fertil Steril* 59:1313, 1993.
16. Venn A, Henninki E, Watson I, et al: Mortality in a cohort of IVF patients. *Hum Reprod* 16:2691, 2001.
17. Goodwin SC, McLucas B, Lee M, et al: Uterine artery embolization for the treatment of uterine leiomyomata. *J Vasc Intervent Radiol* 10:1159, 1999.

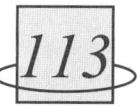

PELVIC ULTRASONOGRAPHY
Robert F. Reardon
Dietrich V. K. Jehle

Ultrasonography is a standard diagnostic tool used in the evaluation of pregnancy and female pelvic pathology.[1] Bedside pelvic ultrasound is used commonly in the ED in order to guide the evaluation of women with pelvic pain, pregnancy-related problems, and maternal trauma. The use of early pelvic ultrasound is essential for the timely diagnosis of ectopic pregnancy and placenta previa. Recent studies have demonstrated that bedside transabdominal and transvaginal ultrasound performed by emergency physicians improves early detection and decreases morbidity of patients with ectopic pregnancy.[2–5] The availability of bedside pelvic sonography decreases the ED length of stay for women with early pregnancy.[6]

This chapter describes many other indications for ED bedside pelvic sonography. Since training and experience with pelvic sonography are highly variable among emergency physicians, a cautious approach to "ruling out" serious conditions should be employed initially. For example, ordering a "formal" ultrasound to be performed in the radiology or obstetrics and gynecology department is reasonable when no intrauterine pregnancy is identified in a symptomatic pregnant patient.

IMAGING TECHNIQUES

Transabdominal imaging and transvaginal imaging are complementary studies in evaluating the female pelvis. Transabdominal sonography (TAS) gives a good overview of the pelvis but requires a full urinary bladder. The bladder acts as an acoustic window to the pelvis for transabdominal scanning. If it is empty, retrograde filling of the bladder with 300 to 500 mL of saline, with careful avoidance of introducing air, may be necessary to obtain adequate visualization. By contrast, transvaginal sonography (TVS) is best performed with an empty bladder. Transabdominal scanning of the pelvis usually is performed with lower-frequency transducers (3–5 MHz) that provide a larger field of view and deeper penetration but have poorer resolution. TVS uses a higher-frequency probe (5–8 MHz) and provides better resolution with a smaller field of view because the transducer is placed closer to the area of interest. The standard transabdominal views are sagittal, with the marker dot cephalad, and transverse, with the marker dot toward the patients right (Figures 113-1 through 113-4). The standard transvaginal views are sagittal, with the marker dot toward the ceiling, and coronal, with the marker dot toward the patient's right (Figures 113-5 through 113-8). Orientation of pelvic anatomy using the transvaginal probe is difficult initially, but identifying the uterus before searching for other pelvic structures is a good way to simplify transvaginal imaging. Keeping the marker dot of the transvaginal probe in one of only two positions, toward the ceiling or toward the patient's right, also will help to simplify transvaginal imaging. Finally, palpation of the lower abdomen during transvaginal imaging will push mobile loops of bowel out of the pelvis and allow identification of relatively fixed structures such as ovaries and adnexal masses.

SONOGRAPHIC PELVIC ANATOMY

Transabdominal versus Transvaginal Imaging

Transabdominal midline images of the pelvis in the longitudinal plane show the long axis of the uterus posterior to the distended bladder. The cervix is immediately posterior to the deepest point of the bladder. The posterior cul-de-sac (pouch of Douglas) is a potential space posterior to the uterus where free intraperitoneal fluid may be seen (Figure 113-9). When a normal (anteverted) uterus is seen, the uterus meets the vagina at an angle of 90 degrees or greater, depending on the amount of bladder distention. Retroversion of the uterus is a normal variant and can make transabdominal visualization of the uterus difficult. The position of the uterus is less important when the transvaginal probe is used.

Uterus

Normal uterine size for a nulliparous menstruating female is up to 8 cm in length and 3 to 5 cm in transverse and anteroposterior (AP) diameter. Maximal uterine size for multiparous women may be 1 to 2 cm greater in each plane. The empty uterus is a thick-walled, muscular organ with moderate echogenicity. It contains a hyperechoic midline stripe formed by the opposed surfaces of the endometrial cavity. In the nonpregnant patient, the appearance of the endometrium is variable depending on the phase of the menstrual cycle. Early in the cycle, the proliferative endometrium is thin, measuring 2 to 8 mm in width (see Figure 113-8). Late in the cycle, during the secretory phase, the endometrium generally measures 7 to 14 mm and displays increased

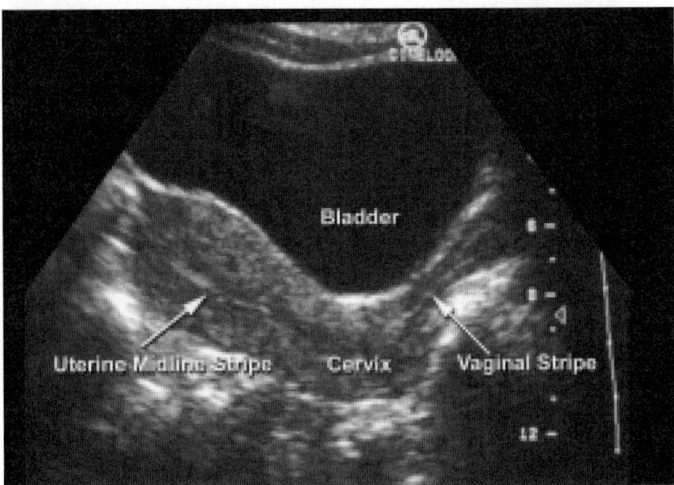

FIG. 113-2. Normal pelvic anatomy in the standard midline sagital view with TAS. The uterus and vagina are posterior to the bladder. The cervix is immediately posterior to the angle (deepest part) of the bladder.

echogenicity (see Figure 113-6). The echogenicity and size of the menstrual endometrium are variable and depend on the amount of blood and clot present within the uterus. The endometrium of the postmenopausal patient without hormone-replacement therapy is generally less than 9 mm in width. Postmenopausal women with vaginal bleeding and/or increased endometrial width need evaluation for endometrial carcinoma. A markedly thickened postpartum endometrium suggests the presence of retained products of conception (Figure 113-10).

Ovaries

The ovaries usually can be found lateral to the body of the uterus, anterior to the internal iliac vessels, and anteromedial to the external iliac vessels (Figure 113-11). There is significant variability in the position of the ovaries in women with a past history of pregnancy, and they may be found posterior or cephalad to the uterus (Figure 113-12). Also, a distended bladder may displace the ovaries cephalad. A normal ovary is about 2 by 2 by 3 cm in size and contains several small hy-

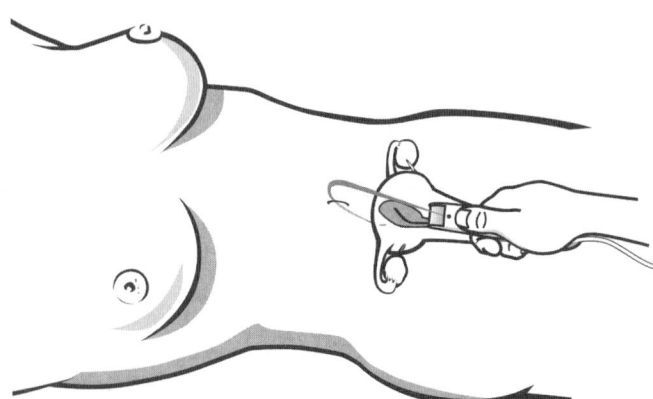

FIG. 113-1. Technique for TAS showing how to obtain the standard midline sagital view. The probe is placed just above the pubic bone with the marker dot cephalad.

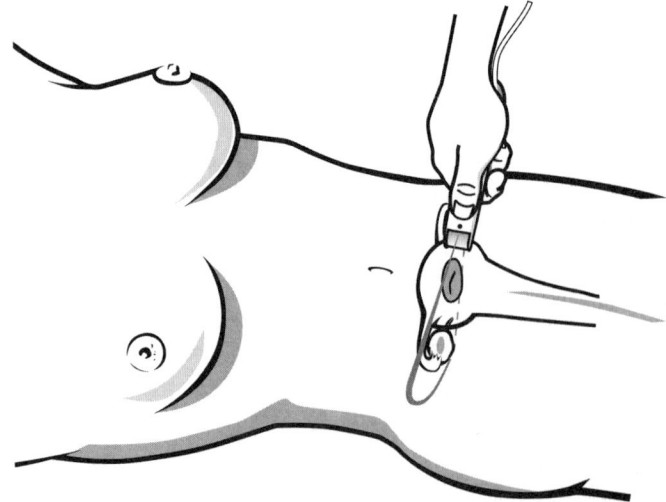

FIG. 113-3. Technique for TAS showing how to obtain the standard transverse view. The probe is placed just above the pubic bone with the marker dot toward the patient's right.

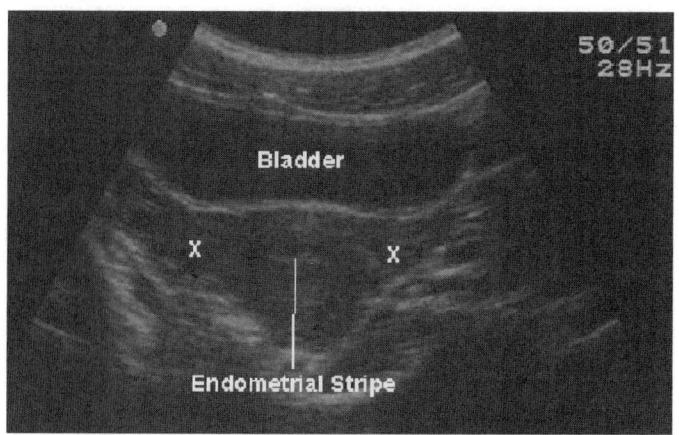

FIG. 113-4. Normal pelvic anatomy in the standard transverse view with TAS. The uterus is posterior to the middle of the bladder. The right ovary is seen on the left of the image, and the left ovary is difficult to identify.

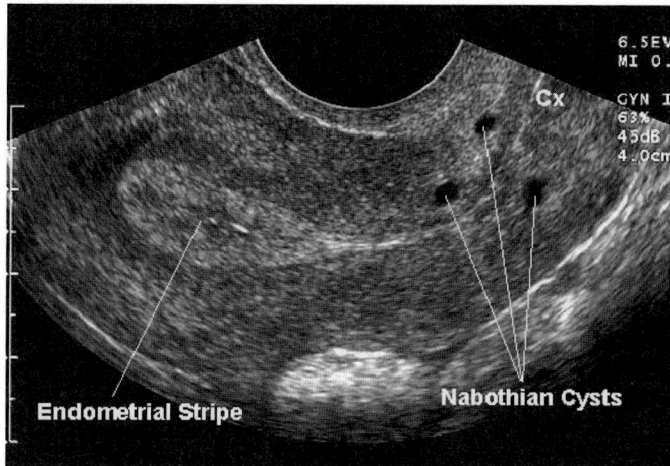

FIG. 113-6. Normal uterus in the standard midline sagital view with TVS. The endometrium is in the secretory phase, so the midline stripe is thick and prominent, and there are three Nabothian cysts in the myometrium near the cervix.

poechoic structures, which are the maturing follicles (see Figure 113-11). The sonographic appearance of the ovary changes throughout the menstrual cycle as several follicles are recruited and then a dominant follicle emerges, followed by the development of a corpus luteum.

NORMAL EARLY PREGNANCY

Ultrasound Findings

The first sonographic finding in early pregnancy is the gestational sac (Table 113-1). This is a discrete hypoechoic structure that is slightly eccentric in its location within the uterine cavity (Figure 113-13). The decidua capsularis and decidua vera are seen as two distinct hyperechoic layers surrounding the early gestational sac; this is known as the *double decidual sac sign* (Figure 113-14). The yolk sac is the next embryonic structure to be visualized. It appears as a small hyperechoic ring within the gestational sac (Figure 113-15). Finally, the embryo (fetal pole) can be seen adjacent to the yolk sac[7] (Figure 113-16). Cardiac activity usually can be observed whenever a fetal pole is present.

The normal fetal heart rate seen in early pregnancy is 112 to 136 beats per minute, slower than heart rates observed in the second and third trimesters. If the ovaries are imaged early in pregnancy, a corpus luteum cyst may be seen (see Figure 113-16). These cysts are benign and usually measure about 2 to 4 cm in diameter. Corpus luteum cysts are generally anechoic but sometimes bleed into themselves causing internal echoes.

Pregnancy Testing

The biochemical diagnosis of pregnancy may be made very early with the use of qualitative serum beta human chorionic gonadotropin (β-hCG) tests of blood and urine. Modern tests can detect serum β-hCG levels of 20 mIU/mL or lower in urine and can diagnose pregnancy within 7 to 10 days after conception, at 3 weeks of gestational age (measured from the first day of the last menstrual period). Quantitative serum β levels correlate approximately with the gestational age of the normal pregnancy. At any given gestational age, serum β-hCG titers are markedly higher when twins (or multiple gestations) are

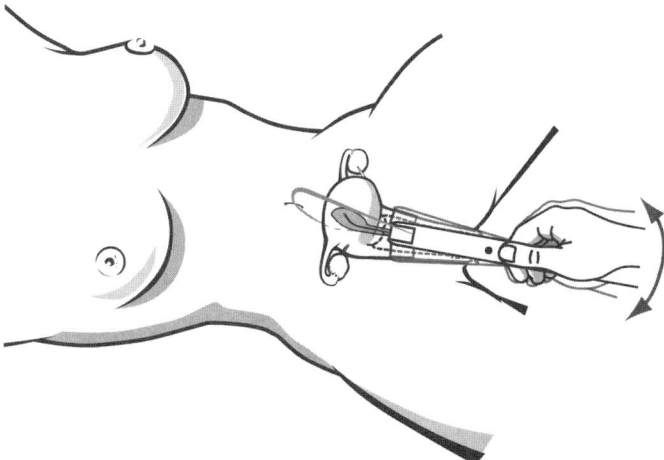

FIG. 113-5. Technique for TVS showing how to obtain the standard midline sagital view. The marker dot is toward the ceiling, and the probe handle is moved from side to side to scan the entire pelvis.

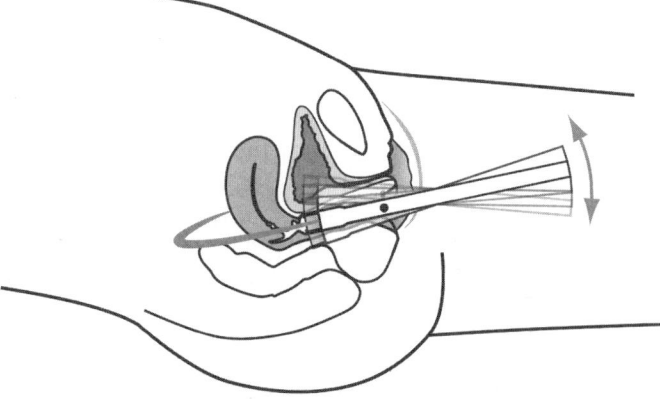

FIG. 113-7. Technique for TVS showing how to obtain the standard coronal view. This drawing is a cross section from the patient's right. The marker dot is toward the patient's right, and the handle is moved up and down to scan the entire pelvis.

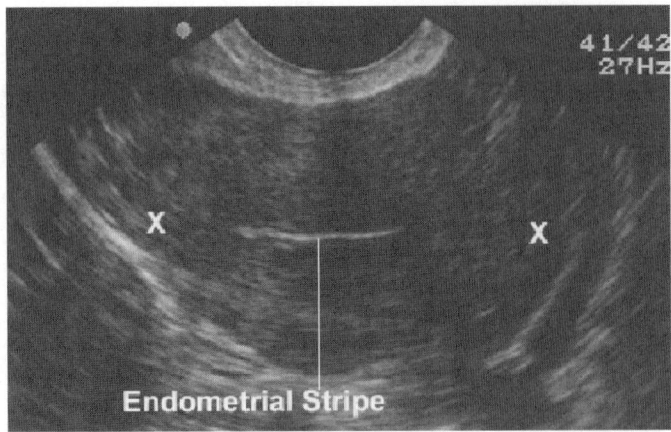

FIG. 113-8. Normal uterus in the standard coronal view with TVS. The endometrium is in the proliferative phase, so the midline stripe is thin.

present. Table 113-1 indicates the approximate gestational age at which different sonographic and serum markers appear in early pregnancy. The standards shown in the table are those of the International Reference Preparation (IRP). Some institutions may use an older standard called the Second International Standard, with values approximately one-half the IRP values.

Determining Gestational Age

When sonographic evidence of an early pregnancy is definitive, the gestational age of the pregnancy can be estimated by measurements of the gestational sac, crown-rump length, or biparietal diameter. Measurement of sonographic structures very early in pregnancy allows a better estimate of gestational age than later measurements because the growth of the embryo during the first trimester is consistent among individuals and not dependent on genetic or nutritional factors. Measurement of the mean gestational sac diameter or the crown-rump length provides the best estimate of gestational age during the first trimester. Mean sac diameter (MSD) is the average of three gestational sac measurements:

$$MSD = \frac{length + width + depth}{3}$$

Gestational age measured in days is:

$$Gestational\ age\ (days) = MSD\ (mm) + 30$$

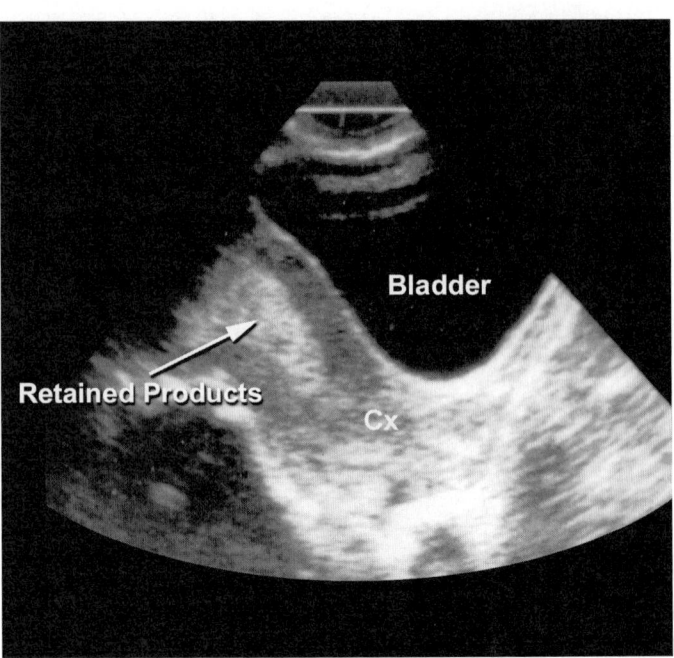

FIG. 113-10. Retained products of conception. TAS in the midline sagital view showing a very thick midline stripe due to an incomplete abortion. *(Courtesy of J. Mateer, M. B. Phelan, and the Department of Emergency Medicine, Medical College of Wisconsin.)*

If an embryo is identified, crown-rump length (CRL) can be measured easily. It is important to obtain the maximal embryo length, excluding the extremities and yoke sac.

$$Gestational\ age\ (wks) = CRL\ (cm) + 6.5$$

Both MSD and CRL give very accurate estimates of gestational age. A significant discrepancy between CRL and MSD dates suggests a failing pregnancy. After the first trimester, gestational age should be estimated by measuring the biparietal diameter (BPD) of the fetal skull. The BPD is a transverse measurement of skull diameter at the level of the thalamus. The markers are positioned at the leading edge (outside) of the near side of the skull and the leading edge (inside) of the far side of the skull. Modern ultrasound equipment is capable of calculating the gestational age automatically when any of the preceding measurements are marked on the display (Figure 113-17).

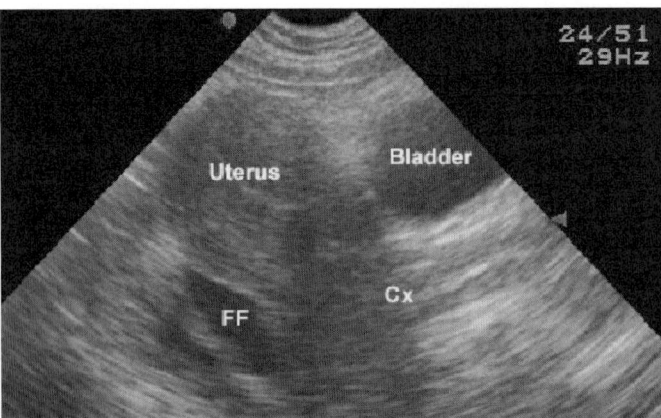

FIG. 113-9. Free pelvic fluid (FF). TAS in the midline sagital view showing anechoic free fluid *(left lower)* in the posterior cul-de-sac behind the uterus *(center)*. The hypoechoic bladder is in the right upper portion of the image (cx = cervix).

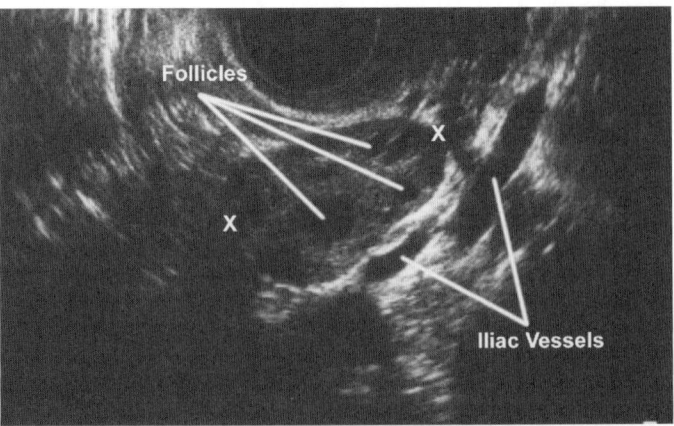

FIG. 113-11. Normal ovary. TVS showing the appearance of a normal premenopausal ovary with multiple small anechoic follicles. It is in the usual location adjacent to an iliac vessel on the right.

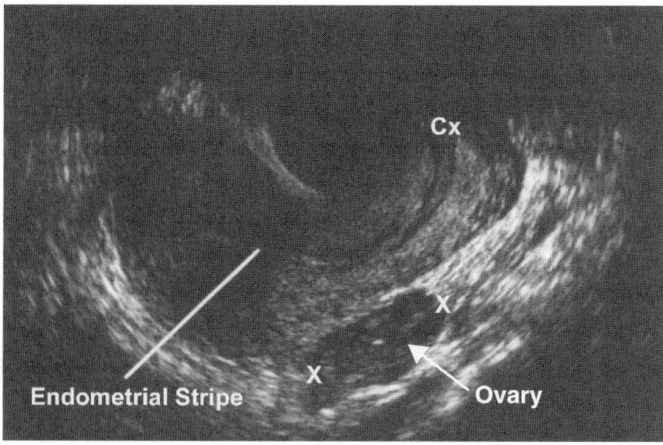

FIG. 113-12. Ovary in an unusual location. TVS in the standard mid-line sagital view showing a normal-size ovary in the posterior cul-de-sac behind the uterus. The cervix is well visualized on the right.

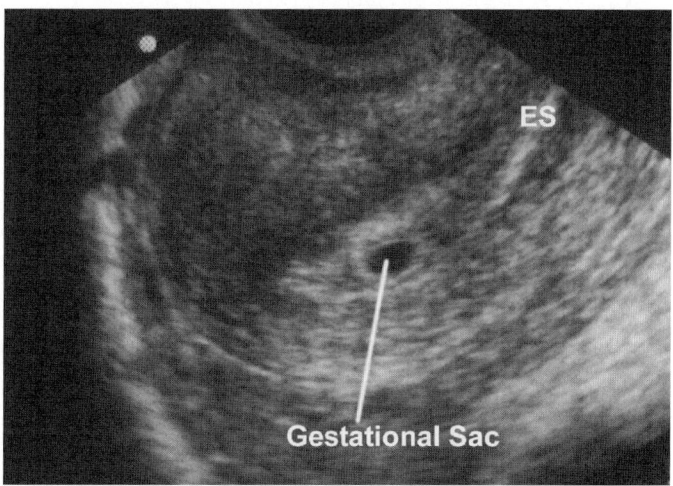

FIG. 113-13. Gestational sac. TVS showing a small anechoic gestational sac within the uterus slightly eccentric to the midline stripe (ES = endometrial stripe).

ECTOPIC PREGNANCY

Diagnosing ectopic pregnancy (EP) in a timely manner is a challenge for emergency physicians. Significant morbidity and mortality may result from a missed or delayed diagnosis. Early diagnosis of an EP may allow nonsurgical therapy with methotrexate. (See Chap. 103 for a detailed discussion of EP.) About half of all EPs are missed on first presentation to the ED.[4] Liberal use of transvaginal pelvic ultrasound decreases the rate of missed ectopic pregnancy.[3,4,7,8]

Ectopic Location

EP occurs when the fertilized ovum implants anywhere except in the endometrium of the intrauterine cavity. Approximately 95 percent of EPs occur in the fallopian tube, with the ampulla being the most common location of implantation. Other sites of implantation include the interstitial region (proximal tube), the cervix, and the abdomen. Interstitial EPs are located in the fallopian tube as it traverses the uterine wall and may appear to be inside the uterus.[9]

Initial Evaluation of Patients at Risk for EP

A detailed approach to the woman at risk for EP is discussed in Chap. 103. A protocol that includes bedside TVS allows emergency physicians to evaluate high-risk patients more quickly and effectively.[4,6] If no intrauterine pregnancy (IUP) is present, both TAS and TVS should be performed.

TABLE 113-1   Estimated Sonographic and Serum βhCG Landmarks

Gestational Age	Transabdominal Landmarks	Transvaginal Landmarks	Serum βhCG Level, IRP
4–5 weeks	± Gestational sac	Gestational sac	1000 mIU/mL
5 weeks	Gestational sac ± yolk sac	Gestational sac with yolk sac, ± fetal pole	1000–7000 mIU/mL
6 weeks	Yolk sac and fetal pole	Yolk sac and fetal pole with cardiac activity	10,000–23,000 mIU/mL

Abbreviation: IRP = International Reference Preparation.
Source: Cacciatore B, Tiitinen A, Stenman U, et al: Normal early pregnancy: Serum hCG levels and vaginal ultrasonography findings. *Br J Obstet Gynaecol* 97:899, 1990.

Ultrasound Evaluation

Patients who are at risk for an EP usually should have both a TAS and a TVS. TAS can identify an IUP after about 6 weeks of gestational age. TAS sometimes can detect masses that are too high in the pelvis to be seen by TVS (Figure 113-18). In addition, TAS can be used to estimate the amount of free intraperitoneal blood in patients with a ruptured EP. Therefore, it is prudent to scan both the pelvis and the right upper quadrant in all patients at risk for EP. Patients who have free fluid in both the pelvis and Morison pouch require an urgent obstetrics consultation and aggressive resuscitation. TVS is more sensitive and specific for evaluating early pregnancy. TVS can identify an IUP at about 5 weeks and can detect more subtle signs of EP such as tubal rings, adnexal masses, and small amounts of pelvic free fluid. ED TVS has 69 percent sensitivity and 99 percent specificity for diagnosing EP.[8] TVS can differentiate between an IUP and an EP in 75 percent of pregnant women who present with pain or bleeding. Finding a definitive IUP rules out the diagnosis of EP as long as there is just a single gestation. Patients taking fertility drugs have a significant chance of both an IUP and an EP. The presence of a yolk sac, fetal pole, or cardiac activity within an intrauterine gestational sac confirms the presence of an IUP. Visualization of a gestational sac alone is not definitive evidence of an IUP unless a double decidual sign is seen clearly. In patients with an EP, about 15 percent can be identified immediately by

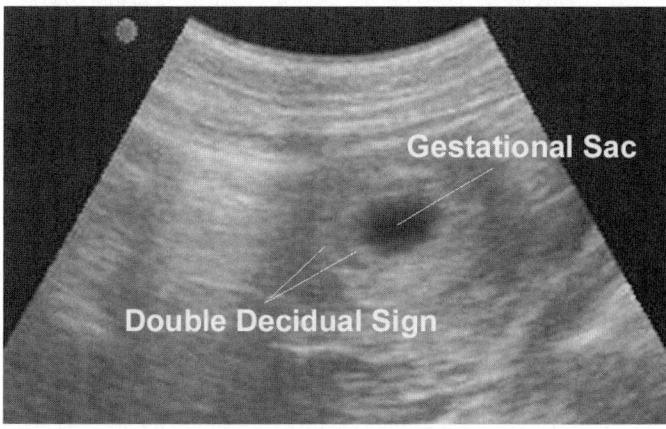

FIG. 113-14. Gestational sac and double decidual sign. TAS showing an anechoic gestational sac surrounded by two clear hyperechoic rings formed by the decidua capsularis and the decidua vera.

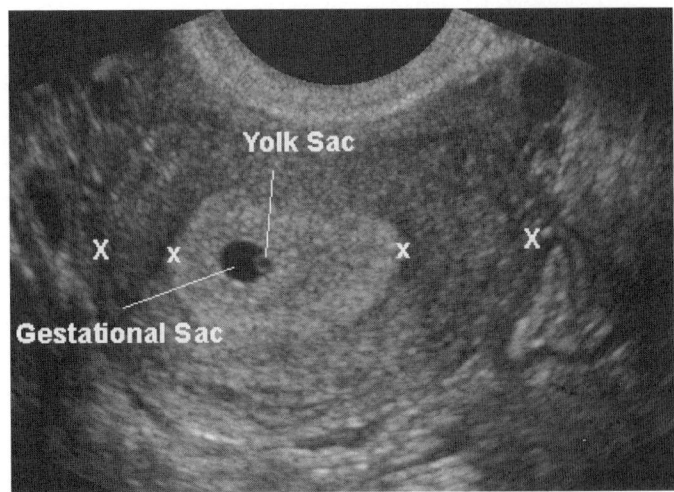

FIG. 113-15. Yolk sac. TVS showing a small discrete hyperechoic ring inside of a hypoechoic gestational sac. There is a thick hyperechoic decidual reaction surrounding the gestational sac.

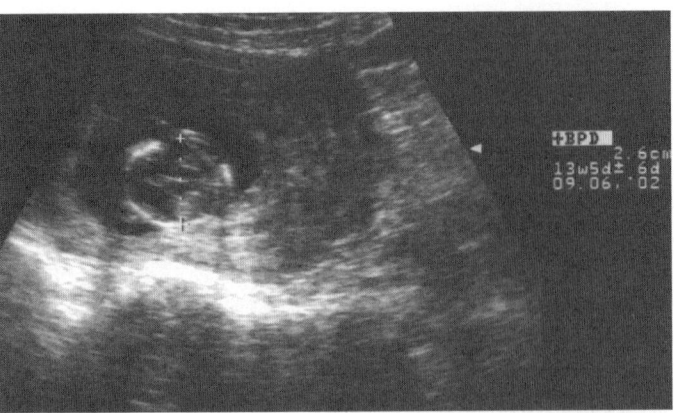

FIG. 113-17. Pregnancy dating. TAS showing how to measure the biparietal diameter (BPD) of a fetal skull *(left)* and a display of the gestational age and estimated date of confinement *(right)* that the ultrasound machine calculated automatically.

transvaginal ultrasound. Signs of an obvious EP include an extrauterine gestational sac with a yolk sac and/or fetal pole and/or cardiac activity (Figure 113-19). Finding a tubal ring in the adnexa is not definitive evidence of an EP, but it is highly suggestive (Figure 113-20). Also, an EP is strongly suspected when pelvic free fluid or a complex adnexal mass is seen[10–12] (Figures 113-21 and 113-22). TVS is very sensitive for detecting pelvic free fluid. When free pelvic fluid is seen in combination with a tubal ring or a complex adnexal mass, the diagnosis of EP is almost certain (see Figure 122-20). Identification of pelvic free fluid is easy using TVS, even for inexperienced sonographers (see Figures 113-9 and 113-21). However, identifying a tubal ring or complex mass can be more difficult because a more complete sonographic survey of the pelvis is required. Therefore, request for a "formal" pelvic ultrasound should be considered when no obvious IUP or EP is identified, especially when pelvic free fluid is seen or the risk of EP is high.

Quantitative Serum β-hCG and Discriminatory Zone

Although a quantitative β-hCG level used to be the pivotal test in rule out EP protocols, the utility of a single quantitative β-hCG level is questionable. **Transvaginal pelvic ultrasound is clearly the best initial test and indicated to rule out an EP, regardless of the β-hCG level.**[13,14]

Implications and use of the "discriminatory zone" in the evaluation of EP is discussed in Chap. 103.

Potential Errors Related to Sonography in the Diagnosis of EP

Several errors related to sonography should be avoided in evaluating a patient with a potential EP. Overreliance on the serum β-hCG level was discussed earlier. It is prudent to perform a complete sonographic survey of the pelvis if the uterus is empty, regardless of the β-hCG level. Assumption that the uterus is empty due to a very early IUP or spontaneous abortion may prove erroneous.

Misinterpretation of pelvic sonography can lead to a delayed diagnosis of EP, with disastrous results. An anechoic fluid collection without a clear double decidual reaction (pseudo-gestational sac) may be misinterpreted as an IUP. A pseudo-gestational sac is present in about 10 to 20 percent of patients who have an EP.[15] A pseudo-gestational sac is the result of endometrium that is stimulated by trophoblastic hormones and intrauterine bleeding (see Figures 113-18 and 113-23).

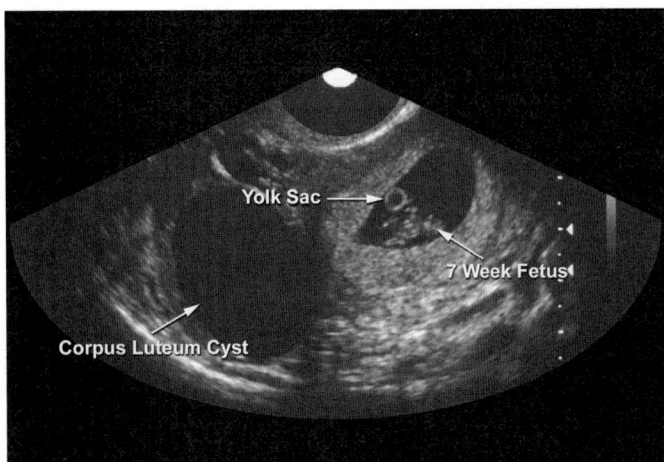

FIG. 113-16. Yolk sac and embryo. TVS showing an intrauterine pregnancy at 7 weeks' gestational age. A discrete embryo (fetal pole) is seen adjacent to the yolk sac, and a large hyopoechoic ovarian cyst (corpus luteum cyst) is seen on the left.

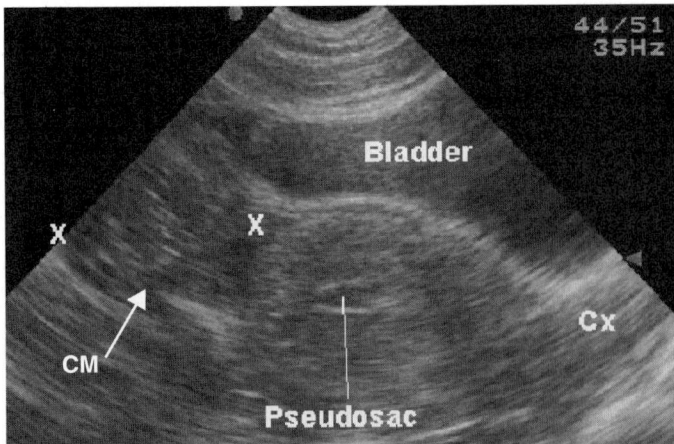

FIG. 113-18. Complex mass high in the pelvis. TAS in the standard midline sagital view showing a complex mass/ectopic pregnancy *(left)* cephalad to the uterus and a pseudo-gestational sac within the uterus *(center)* (cx = cervix; cm = complex mass).

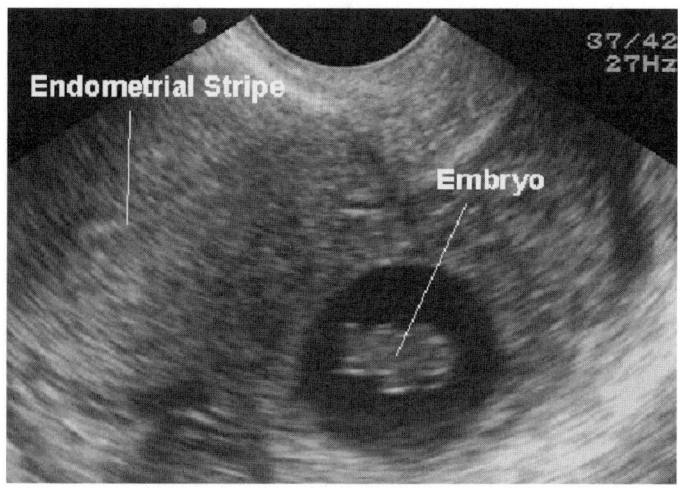

FIG. 113-19. Obvious ectopic pregnancy. TVS showing a clear embryo inside of a large gestational sac *(right)* adjacent to an empty uterus *(left)*. Cardiac activity was seen inside the embryo.

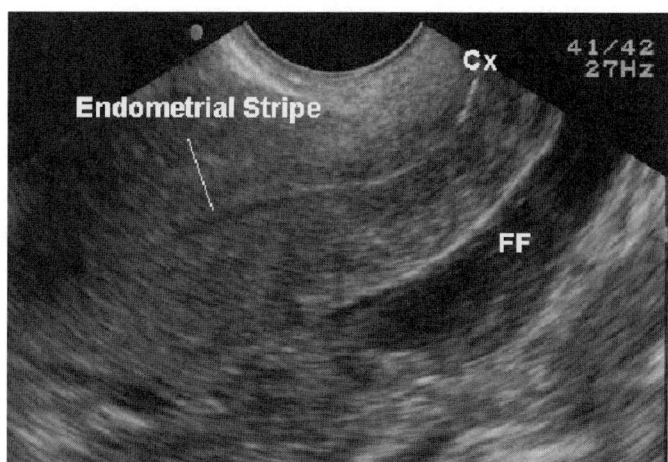

FIG. 113-21. Pelvic free fluid. TVS showing a moderate amount of free fluid (FF) in the posterior cul-de-sac (pouch of Douglas) behind an empty uterus. This was the only abnormal finding in this patient with an ectopic pregnancy.

The double decidual sac sign can be used to differentiate a true gestational sac from a pseudo-gestational sac. Failure to appreciate the presence of free pelvic fluid or the implications may be disastrous. About two-thirds of patients with an EP will have pelvic free fluid. Also, pelvic free fluid is the only abnormal sonographic finding in about 15 percent. The greater the volume of free intraperitoneal fluid, the greater is the likelihood of EP. In fact, pregnant patients with free fluid in Morison pouch have a large hemoperitoneum and almost a 100 percent chance of having an EP.[5] Not performing sonography of the right upper quadrant is a mistake because identifying free fluid in Morison pouch is very easy, even for inexperienced sonographers.

Missing a subtle adnexal mass or tubal ring is a mistake that may be difficult to avoid. Identifying such abnormalities usually requires a complete sonographic survey of the pelvis, which requires increased training and experience.

Misjudging the intrauterine or extrauterine location of a pregnancy is a serious mistake. The location of the uterus should be identified clearly before a gestational sac, yolk sac, and/or fetal pole is called an IUP or EP. A normal pregnancy should be located in the fundus of the uterus.

Interstitial pregnancies can be difficult to differentiate from an IUP and should be considered when a patient presents in shock with an apparent IUP by ultrasound.[9]

Heterotopic Pregnancy

Usually the presence of an IUP is sufficient evidence that an EP does not exist. However, in the case of patients who are taking progestational/fertility agents, this assumption should not be made. The incidence of simultaneous intrauterine and extrauterine pregnancy (heterotopic pregnancy) in the general population is now thought to be as high as 1 per 4000 pregnancies, although historically this was only reported in 1 per 30,000 pregnancies. Those taking medications to enhance fertility are at much higher risk for heterotopic pregnancy. Patients who have a history of in vitro fertilization may have an incidence as high as 1 per 100 to 200 pregnancies. For this reason, sonographic imaging of the entire pelvis should be completed even after identification of an obvious IUP in such patients.

ABNORMAL FIRST-TRIMESTER INTRAUTERINE PREGNANCY

Spontaneous Abortion

Abortion is discussed in Chap. 106. Most pregnancy losses occur early in the first trimester, and few are lost after fetal cardiac activity is

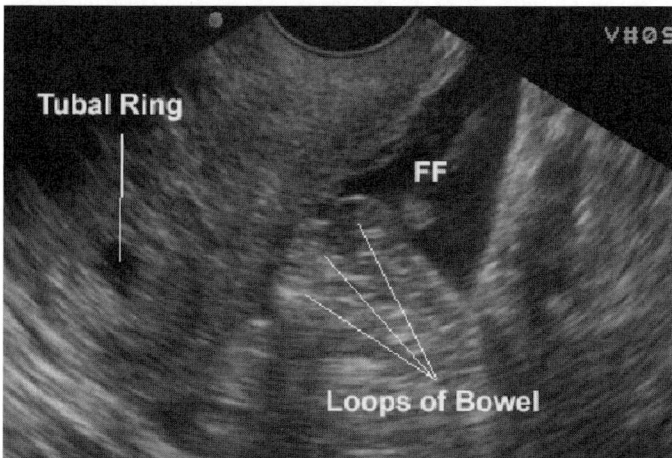

FIG. 113-20. Ectopic pregnancy. TVS showing a tubal ring *(left)* and adnexal free fluid (FF) *(right)*. Loops of bowel are clearly outlined by the hypoechoic free fluid *(center)*.

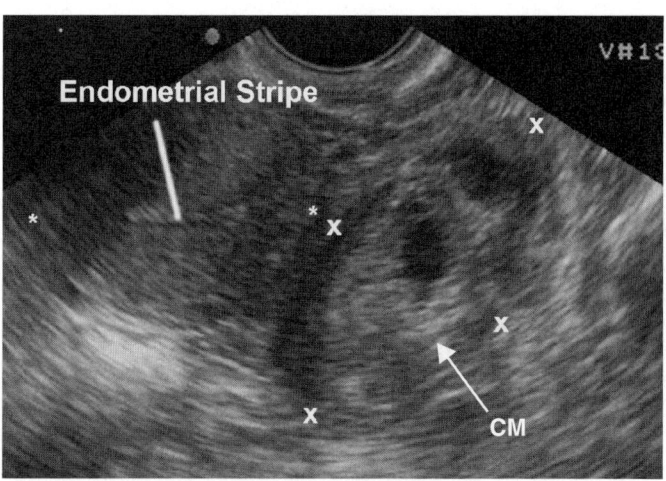

FIG. 113-22. Complex mass (CM). TVS showing a complex mass/ ectopic pregnancy *(right)* adjacent to an empty uterus *(left)*.

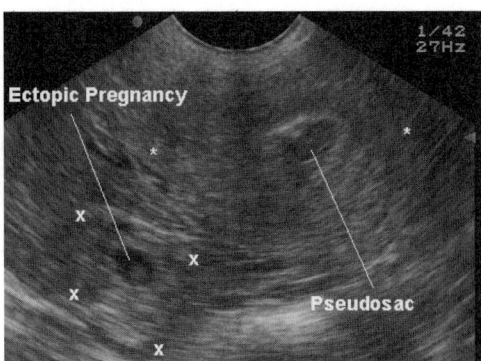

FIG. 113-23. Pseudo-gestational sac. TVS showing a fluid collection (pseudo-gestational sac) inside the uterus *(right)* and a tubal ring associated with an ectopic pregnancy *(left).*

noted sonographically.[7] After a completed abortion, an empty uterus should be visualized sonographically; thus a postpartum endometrial stripe greater than 10 mm in a symptomatic patient suggests the presence of retained products of conception (see Figure 113-10).

Threatened Abortion and Viability of an Early IUP

The pivotal step in the evaluation of a patient with first-trimester vaginal bleeding is pelvic sonography. If a live IUP is seen and there is a single gestation, expectant management is the rule.

There are several sonographic criteria that can be used to decide whether an early IUP is viable or whether early fetal demise has occurred. Major criteria are those which uniformly predict fetal demise. Inability to visualize a yolk sac or embryo in a large gestational sac is a major criterion for demise; this is referred to as a *blighted ovum* (Figure 113-24). Specifically, absence of a yolk sac when the MSD is 10 mm or greater with TVS or when the MSD is 20 mm or greater with TAS indicates certain fetal demise.[7] In addition, absence of an embryo when the MSD is 16 mm or greater with TVS or when the MSD 25 mm or greater with TAS predicts fetal demise with confidence.[7] Visualization of a grossly distorted gestational sac uniformly predicts fetal demise but is somewhat subjective (Figure 113-25). A gestational sac located in the lower portion of the uterus adjacent to the cervix is probably in the process of aborting.[7] An irregular, thin, or weakly echogenic choriodecidual reaction surrounding the gestational sac, decreased amniotic fluid volume, or a fetal heartbeat below 90 beats/min after 6 weeks' gestational age are all suggestive but not diagnostic of a failing pregnancy.

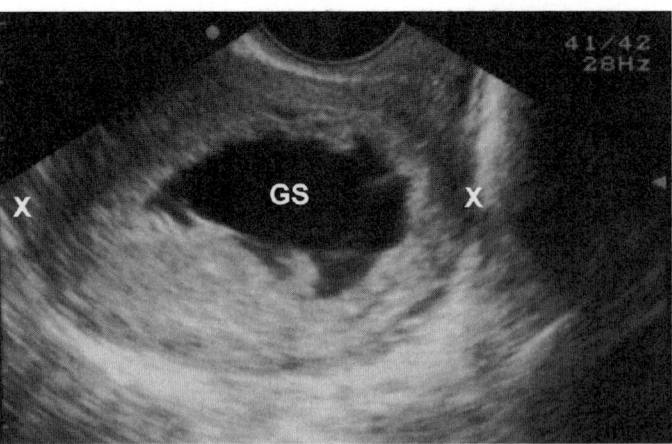

FIG. 113-25. Fetal demise. TVS showing a large gestational sac (GS) that is grossly distorted. There is some debris inside the sac but no clear yolk sac or embryo.

Subchorionic Hematoma

An intrauterine hematoma is present in about one-fourth of patients with threatened abortion. In the first trimester, blood may accumulate in the endometrial cavity between the chorionic membranes and the uterine wall; this is known as a *subchorionic hematoma* or *implantation bleed* (Figure 113-26). The presence of a subchorionic hematoma may more than double the chances of pregnancy loss in threatened abortion. The size and location are important factors in judging the significance of such bleeding. Small hematomas under the placenta are more important than larger hematomas elsewhere.

Vaginal Bleeding with No IUP

The sonographic finding of an empty uterus in a patient with vaginal bleeding and a positive pregnancy test poses a difficult diagnostic dilemma. Very early IUP or completed spontaneous abortion are possible, but 25 percent of these patients will have an EP.[16] When echogenic material is seen within the uterus, retained intrauterine products from an incomplete abortion or from partial resorption after fetal demise may be present (see Figure 113-10); this should not be confused with intrauterine blood and clots, which can occur with an

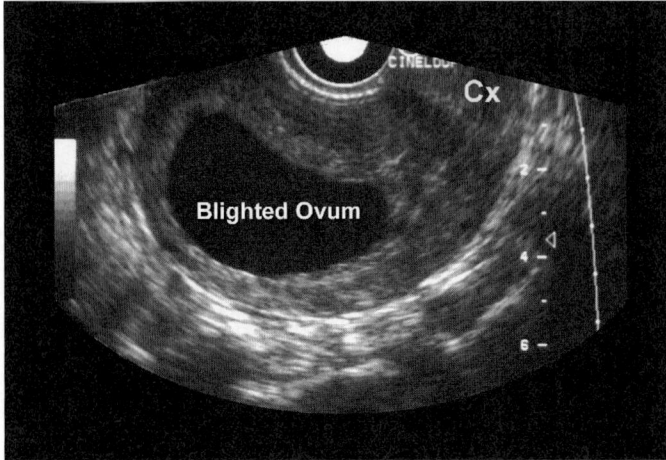

FIG. 113-24. Blighted ovum. TVS showing a large empty intrauterine gestational sac (cx = cervix).

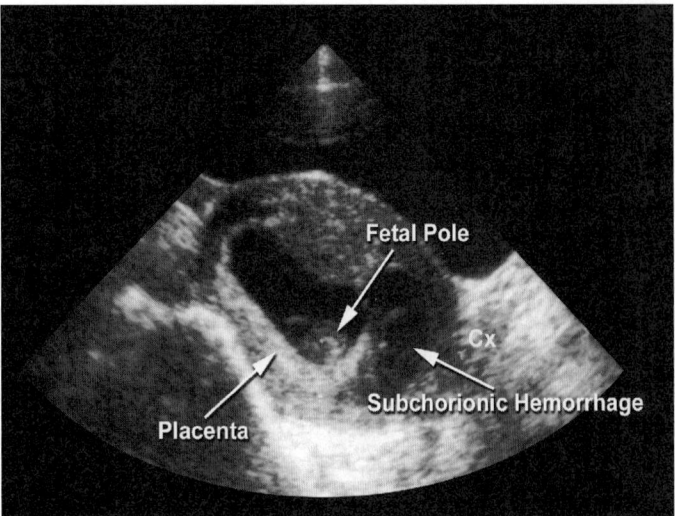

FIG. 113-26. Subchorionic hemorrhage. TAS midline sagital view showing an intrauterine pregnancy. The placenta is posterior, and the lower placental margin is displaced by an anechoic hemorrhage.

EP. Completed spontaneous abortion is confirmed only by passage of obvious products of conception or identification of chorionic villi pathologically. Serial quantitative serum β-hCG determinations may be helpful in this setting. After spontaneous abortion, serum β-hCG levels fall rapidly during the first 7 days. Close follow-up with serial sonography and serum β-hCG determinations may be needed before a final diagnosis can be ascertained.

Molar Pregnancy

Gestational trophoblastic neoplasia is a proliferative disease of the trophoblast. It is discussed in Chap. 106. Most cases (80 percent) present as a hydatidiform mole and follow a benign course. More malignant forms of the disease are invasive mole (12-15 percent) and choriocarcinoma (5-8 percent). Patients with a hydatidiform mole most commonly present with vaginal bleeding but may present with early preeclampsia or hyperemesis gravidarum. A larger than expected uterus for gestational age and a markedly elevated serum β-hCG level (>100,000 mIU/mL) are risk factors for malignant disease and are important clues to making this diagnosis. Most cases of molar pregnancy involve the entire placenta, but molar disease involving only part of the placenta or fetus also has been described. Pelvic ultrasound is the initial study of choice when a molar pregnancy is suspected.[1] A hydatidiform mole appears as an intrauterine echogenic mass with multiple small hypoechoic vesicles interspersed (Figure 113-27). It is said to have a characteristic appearance of grapes. However, the appearance of first-trimester moles may be confused with a blighted ovum or threatened abortion. A theca lutein cyst may be seen on examination of the ovaries in as many as half the cases of gestational trophoblastic disease (GTD). They are large, multiseptated ovarian cysts caused by markedly high levels of serum β-hCG. A benign mole usually resolves after evacuation of the uterus. Choriocarcinoma may metastasize to the lung, vagina, brain, or liver and is very sensitive to chemotherapy.

SECOND- AND THIRD-TRIMESTER PREGNANCY

Ultrasound evaluations of second- and third-trimester pregnancies are often done in order to evaluate fetal age and well-being when maternal problems arise. Maternal vaginal bleeding, preeclampsia, diabetes, drug abuse, and trauma all may compromise the fetus. Ultrasound can be used to quickly evaluate several important structures that may have a bearing on the final outcome of the pregnancy. Although emergency physicians are not relied on to perform routine ultrasound examinations during late pregnancy, many of the structures and abnormalities seen in late pregnancy are easily recognizable, even to those with little ultrasound training.

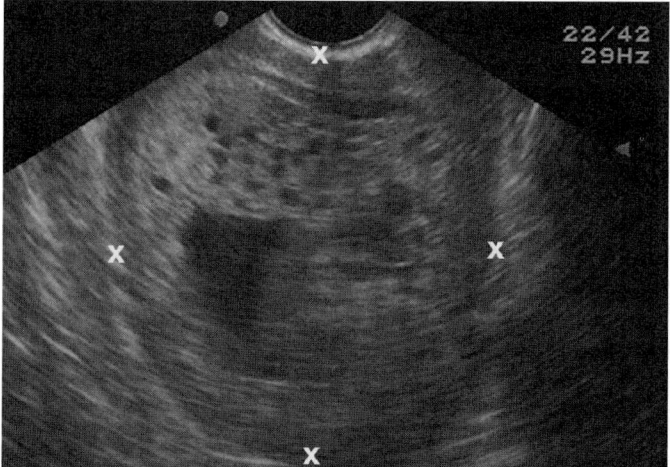

FIG. 113-27. Molar pregnancy. TVS showing a large complex intrauterine mass with cystic regions that have the characteristic appearance of grapes.

Immediate Fetal Viability

The visualization of fetal movements and fetal heart rate (normal = 120 to 160 beats/min) takes priority in the acute setting.[1] The diagnosis of fetal death is established by careful sonographic imaging of the fetal chest for at least 3 min with lack of cardiac activity. Two experienced sonographers should confirm the diagnosis.

Oligohydramnios and Polyhydramnios

The amount of amniotic fluid should be estimated. Subjective estimates of amniotic fluid volumes are best left to experienced sonographers, but extremes of polyhydramnios and oligohydramnios may be obvious to the neophyte. Amniotic fluid volume is large compared with fetal volume in normal early pregnancy; this should not be mistaken for polyhydramnios. A single measurement of the length of the deepest pocket of amniotic fluid gives a gross estimate of the volume and may be the best method of measurement for the inexperienced sonographer. A pocket more than 8 cm deep indicates polyhydramnios, and a pocket less than 1 cm deep indicates oligohydramnios. A four-quadrant index also can be used to estimate the volume of amniotic fluid. The uterus is divided into four quadrants, and the deepest pocket in each quadrant is measured. If the sum of the four measurements is less than 5 cm, oligohydramnios is present. If the sum is greater than 20 cm, polyhydramnios is present. An obstetrician should be consulted immediately when oligohydramnios is found because it is associated with fetal renal malformation, severe growth retardation, and fetal death. Polyhydramnios may be associated with fetal anomalies, preterm labor, and premature rupture of membranes, but it is generally considered less serious.

Umbilical Cord

Sonographic examination of the umbilical cord should reveal two arteries and a single larger vein. A cord that contains only one artery is associated with a 25 to 50 percent chance of fetal abnormalities. The cord vessels are best counted at the cord insertion into the fetus because the two umbilical arteries may normally fuse at the placental end of the cord.

Fetal Gender

Both male and female genitalia are easily recognizable but should be clearly identified before the gender of the fetus is revealed. Lack of visualization of the penis and scrotum without clearly identifying the female labia is not adequate, and in this case no estimate of fetal gender should be made. Errors in sonographic sex determination occur relatively frequently; thus emergency physicians should avoid forecasting gender because it adds little to emergency care.

Fetal Structures and Abnormalities

Fetal anatomy such as fetal head, chest, abdomen, and extremities can be visualized quite easily in the second and third trimesters, even for those with little ultrasound experience. Most routine fetal ultrasound examinations and detection of anomalies should be performed by physicians who specialize in fetal sonography.

COMPLICATIONS IN THE SECOND HALF OF PREGNANCY

Placenta Previa

During the evaluation of third-trimester bleeding, the greatest utility of sonography is to establish the presence or absence of placenta previa.

Since the sensitivity of sonography for the diagnosis of placental abruption is very poor, a presumptive diagnosis of placental abruption is often made after placenta previa has been ruled out. Placenta previa occurs when the blastocyte implants on the endometrium close to the cervical os and the placenta covers the os (Figure 113-28). Painless vaginal bleeding in the third trimester is the classic clinical presentation (see Chap. 106). Complete placenta previa is diagnosed when the placenta is implanted on both sides of the cervical os. A partial placenta previa covers part of the cervical os but does not bridge it. A marginal placenta previa abuts the cervical os but does not cover it. Since partial and marginal previas can both cause bleeding and ultrasound cannot distinguish between the two diagnoses, they are commonly grouped together. A low-lying placenta that does not cover or abut the cervical os may still cause bleeding but not as frequently or severely as placenta previa.

ULTRASOUND EXAMINATION FOR SUSPECTED PLACENTA PREVIA Ultrasound is highly sensitive in detecting placenta previa, but a significant number of false-positive examinations occur. Since the consequences of placenta previa are so serious, it is important not to underdiagnose the condition. The best sonographic examination for placenta previa is the standard transabdominal midline sagittal view (see Figures 113-1, 113-2, and 113-28). In order to rule out placenta previa, the cervical os must be clearly visualized and must be free of overlying placenta. Visualization of the placenta at a site distant from the os makes previa unlikely but does not rule it out because an accessory placental lobe also may be present. When the relationship between the internal cervical os and the placenta cannot be clearly established using the standard examination, other sonographic approaches may be attempted. Traction on the fetal head with the patient in the Trendelenburg position may allow an improved view of the cervical os in late pregnancy. Completely emptying the urinary bladder may improve transabdominal images of the cervical os in some cases. TVS gives better visualization of the cervix and is preferred in patients who have not had vaginal bleeding. The theoretical risk of dislodging clots and causing significant bleeding by introducing a probe into the vagina has led some clinicians to use transperineal sonography instead. Transperineal sonography is performed by placing the abdominal transducer on the perineum between the urethra and the vagina. This method has been found to be very accurate for diagnosing placenta previa.

Sonographic false-positive diagnoses of placenta previa may occur for a number of reasons. An overly distended urinary bladder may cause a low-lying placenta to appear as a previa. A myometrial contraction may mimic the placenta or push the edge of the placenta into the proximity of the cervical os. Diagnosing placenta previa at an early gestational age makes a false-positive diagnosis more likely. Many placentas that appear to cover or abut the cervical os during the second trimester are found to be a safe distance from the os on later examinations. This apparent migration of the placenta is probably due to different growth rates of the placenta and the lower uterine segment. Most previas diagnosed before 20 weeks resolve prior to delivery.

Placental Abruption

Premature separation of the placenta from the wall of the uterus is called *placental abruption* (see Chap. 106 for details). Abruption can be severe or mild, acute or chronic, and retroplacental or marginal. Abruption causes varying degrees of pain, and bleeding may be mild or absent. Sonography has very poor sensitivity for diagnosing placental abruption, and lack of sonographic evidence certainly does not rule out abruption. However, a clinical presentation suggestive of placental abruption without sonographic evidence of a placenta previa should be assumed to be an abruption until proven otherwise.

Retroplacental Hematoma

Retroplacental hematoma separates the placenta from the uterine wall centrally and is likely the result of bleeding from spiral arteries. Sonographically, it appears as a hypoechoic stripe between the placenta and underlying myometrium, but it may have variable echogenicity depending on the age of the bleeding. An acute hematoma may be isoechoic with the placenta, so it may appear as simply a thickened region of the placenta. It will become hypoechoic in 1 to 2 weeks. A retroplacental contraction may mimic a hematoma, and an old heterogeneous hematoma may look like a retroplacental fibroid. Retroplacental hematomas cause placental infarction and may result in fetal growth retardation, fetal death, and massive maternal hemorrhage. When a retroplacental hematoma is apparent sonographically, fetal mortality is directly related to the size of the hematoma.

Marginal Hematoma

Marginal hematomas occur at the edge of the placenta in the subchorionic plane. They are probably the result of bleeding from veins at the margin of the placenta. They are generally associated with less severe complications than retroplacental hematomas, but bleeding still may be severe. Some physicians have claimed that marginal hematomas are of no consequence to the fetus; however, some studies have shown that large hematoma volumes are associated with poor fetal outcomes.

TRAUMA IN PREGNANCY

When trauma occurs during pregnancy, the first priority is the stabilization of the mother. The most common cause of fetal death is maternal death. Ultrasound of the maternal abdomen should be accomplished early after significant blunt trauma.[1] The uterus is well protected within the pelvis during the first trimester of pregnancy; however, during the second and third trimesters, it is at much greater risk of injury due to its intra-abdominal position. The sonographic appearance of intraperitoneal blood may be noted in the pelvis before it is detected in the Morison pouch or elsewhere. Signs of fetal distress may be the first warning sign of occult maternal hemodynamic compromise. After initial maternal stabilization, the well-being of the fe-

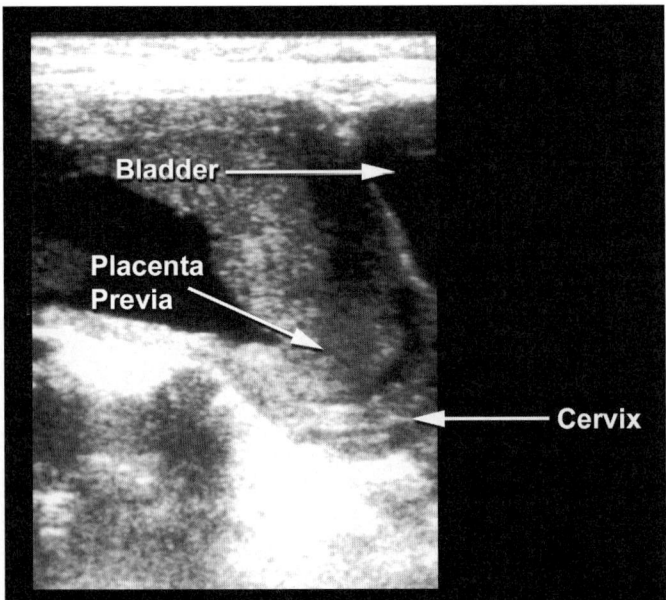

FIG. 113-28. Placenta previa. TAS midline sagital view showing the lower portion of the uterus in a third trimester pregnancy. The placenta is anterior, and the placental margin is covering the cervix.

tus should be evaluated. Placental abruption and direct fetal injury must be suspected following significant maternal trauma in the second and third trimesters.

Fetal Sonographic Evaluation

Ultrasound can be used to assist in the initial evaluation of the fetus after maternal trauma.[1] First, ultrasound can aid in making a quick estimate of gestational age. Knowledge of the gestational age is important because subsequent management decisions may be influenced by its determination. Next, immediate fetal viability can be ascertained by sonography. If the fetus is dead (no cardiac activity and no fetal movement), management of the mother will become the sole priority. Gross injury to the fetus, placenta, or uterus may be apparent on the initial ultrasound examination. Oligohydramnios following maternal trauma suggests uterine injury or premature rupture of the membranes. Large placental abruptions may be visualized, and fetal distress (fetal heartbeat above 180 or below 120 beats/min) may indicate unrecognized maternal, fetal, or placental injury. Urgent delivery of the significantly compromised fetus is indicated if the gestational age is at least 24 to 26 weeks (see Chap. 254). Traumatic uterine rupture is usually accompanied by massive bleeding and requires repair or hysterectomy regardless of gestational age. Although sonographic imaging may detect some large abruptions and gross fetal injury, cardiotocographic monitoring is a much more sensitive indicator. Fetal bradycardia, late decelerations, and loss of beat-to-beat variation are signs of distress. Fetal distress and frequent uterine contractions nearly always appear within 4 h of significant traumatic placental abruption.

PELVIC MASSES

Uterine Masses

A leiomyoma (uterine fibroid) is a benign proliferation of the smooth muscle and connective tissue of the uterus. It is the most common cause of uterine enlargement not related to pregnancy. Fibroids have a variety of sonographic appearances, ranging from hypoechoic masses with irregular uterine contours to echogenic structures with distinct calcified borders (Figure 113-29). When a fibroid degenerates, multiple small cystic spaces are visualized within the fibroid. Fibroids can be intramural, submucosal, subserosal, or pedunculated. A fibroid may outgrow its blood supply, leading to necrosis and severe pain, espe-

cially during pregnancy. Rarely, a fibroid degenerates into a uterine sarcoma. In addition, endometrial or ovarian carcinoma may invade the myometrium. Therefore, complex or cystic uterine masses require further investigation.

Cervix and Vagina

The vagina and cervix are best visualized with TAS. Visualization of the cervix with the transvaginal probe requires that the probe be withdrawn into the distal vagina. Nabothian cysts are benign growths that are seen commonly in the region of the cervix (see Figure 113-6). Gartner duct cysts are also benign and may be seen at the anterior and lateral walls of the vagina. Imperforate hymen causes primary amenorrhea, lower abdominal pain, and urinary symptoms during puberty. A tender lower abdominal mass may be palpable on physical examination, and pelvic sonography will confirm that the vagina is filled with blood; this is called *hematocolpos*. A distended urinary bladder and a blood-filled distended uterus, or *hematometra*, also may be noted. Perineal examination will reveal a bulging hymen; incision and drainage are required.

Adnexal Masses

Developing ovarian follicles may measure up to 2 cm at midcycle. Functional ovarian cysts measure greater than 2.5 cm and are well defined, thin-walled, and anechoic. Most simple ovarian cysts resolve spontaneously, and serial sonographic examinations are helpful to follow their progression. In postmenopausal patients, even well-defined anechoic ovarian cysts require further workup, especially if they are greater then 5 cm in diameter. Sonographically, polycystic ovary disease appears as bilaterally enlarged ovaries with multiple small follicles or a small number of very large follicles. In some cases, the follicles are so tiny that they cannot be seen sonographically; thus a normal appearance of the ovaries does not rule out the diagnosis.

Complex Adnexal Masses

Hemorrhagic ovarian cysts, endometriomas, tubo-ovarian abscesses, benign ovarian tumors, and malignancies all can present as a complex adnexal mass (Figure 113-30). Dermoids have the appearance of focal bright echoes inside a complex adnexal mass. Adnexal tumors that are hyperechoic, septated, and very irregular are more likely to be malignant and require further investigation. When a large complex adnexal mass and ascites are present, the likelihood of ovarian carcinoma high.

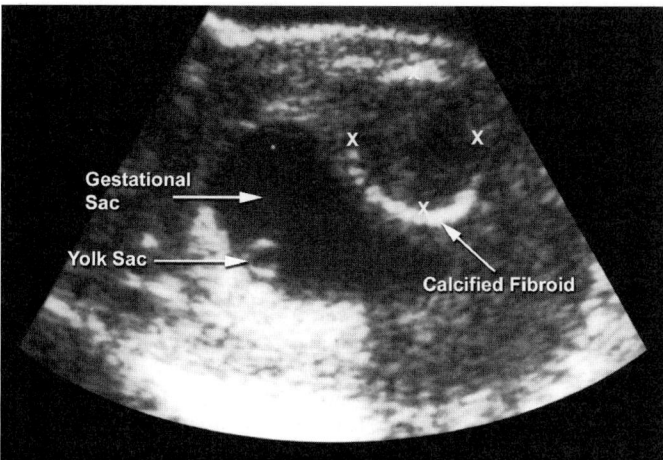

FIG. 113-29. Leiomyoma (fibroid). TAS showing a calcified mass on the anterior wall of the uterus with distal shadowing. An intrauterine gestational sac and yolk sac are seen in the uterine fundus.

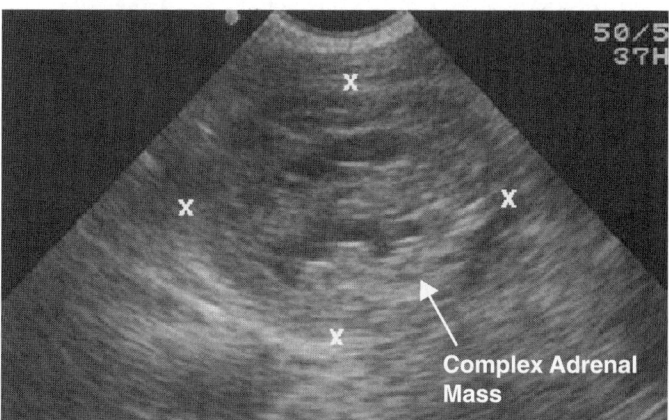

FIG. 113-30. Complex adnexal mass. TAS showing a large, well-demarcated mass with both hypoechoic and hyperechoic regions. This is a tubo-ovarian abscess, but a hemorrhagic ovarian cyst or ovarian tumor could have a similar appearance.

OTHER CONDITIONS

Pelvic Inflammatory Disease and Tubo-Ovarian Abscess

The diagnosis of pelvic inflammatory disease (PID) is usually made clinically, without the aid of ancillary studies. Ultrasound findings are unlikely to be noted early in the course of PID. In cases of severe PID, the ultrasound examination may demonstrate free fluid in the cul-de-sac or pyosalpinx. Pyosalpinx is a swollen, pus-filled fallopian tube, which appears sonographically as a distinct circular structure with low-level echoes in the lumen when imaged in cross section. Pyosalpinx may appear to be a multicystic mass if multiple loops of distended tube are lying adjacent to one another. Sonographic evidence of pyosalpinx has been shown to be specific for the diagnosis of PID. Tubo-ovarian abscess (TOA) is a complication of PID that can be diagnosed accurately using pelvic ultrasound. An abscess will appear as a complex mass with both cystic and solid components (see Figure 113-30). Percutaneous or transvaginal drainage of a TOA may be facilitated by ultrasound guidance.

Ovarian Torsion

Doppler ultrasound is used commonly for the evaluation of suspected ovarian torsion; however, the diagnostic accuracy of Doppler studies for ovarian torsion is poor. When torsion is present, the lack of internal ovarian blood flow on Doppler examination probably indicates that an ovary is beyond salvage. Also, the absence of blood flow to the ovary can be seen in a variety of cystic ovarian lesions when torsion is not present. Massive ovarian edema is an entity caused by intermittent or partial adnexal torsion. Doppler flow is present, and resolution of the edema often occurs after detorsion of the adnexa. Simple gray-scale pelvic sonography is helpful when adnexal torsion is suspected because most patients with ovarian torsion have a significantly enlarged ovary.[17] Finding normal-sized ovaries makes adnexal torsion unlikely.

REFERENCES

1. American College of Emergency Physicians: Clinical policy for the initial approach to patients presenting with a chief complaint of vaginal bleeding. *Ann Emerg Med* 29(3):435, 1997.
2. Durham B, Lane B, Burbridge L, Balasubramaniam S, et al: Pelvic ultrasound performed by emergency physicians for the detection of ectopic pregnancy in complicated first-trimester pregnancies. *Ann Emerg Med* 29(3):338, 1997.
3. Mateer JR, Aiman EJ, Brown MH, et al: Ultrasonographic examination by emergency physicians of patients at risk for ectopic pregnancy. *Acad Emerg Med* 2(10):867, 1995.
4. Mateer JR, Valley VT, Aiman EJ, et al: Outcome analysis of a protocol including bedside endovaginal sonography in patients at risk for ectopic pregnancy. *Ann Emerg Med* 27(3):283, 1996.
5. Rodgerson JD, Heegard WG, Plummer D, et al: Emergency department right upper quadrant ultrasound is associated with a reduced time to diagnosis and treatment of ruptured ectopic pregnancies. *Acad Emerg Med* 8(4):331, 2001.
6. Shih CH: Effect of emergency physician-performed pelvic sonography on length of stay in the emergency department. *Ann Emerg Med* 29(3):348, 1997; discussion 352.
7. Dart RG: Role of pelvic ultrasonography in evaluation of symptomatic first- trimester pregnancy. *Ann Emerg Med* 33(3):310, 1999.
8. Kaplan BC, Dart RG, Moskos M, et al: Ectopic pregnancy: Prospective study with improved diagnostic accuracy. *Ann Emerg Med* 28(1):10, 1996.
9. Dewitt C, Abbott J: Interstitial pregnancy: A potential for misdiagnosis of ectopic pregnancy with emergency department ultrasonography. *Ann Emerg Med* 40(1):106, 2002.
10. Cacciatore B: Can the status of tubal pregnancy be predicted with transvaginal sonography? A prospective comparison of sonographic, surgical, and serum hCG findings. *Radiology* 177(2):481, 1990.
11. Brown DL, Doubilet PM: Transvaginal sonography for diagnosing ectopic pregnancy: Positivity criteria and performance characteristics. *J Ultrasound Med* 13(4):259, 1994.
12. Nyberg DA, Hughes MP, Mack LA, et al: Extrauterine findings of ectopic pregnancy of transvaginal US: Importance of echogenic fluid. *Radiology* 178(3):823, 1991.
13. Dart RG, Kaplan B, Cox C: Transvaginal ultrasound in patients with low beta-human chorionic gonadotropin values: How often is the study diagnostic? *Ann Emerg Med* 30(2):135, 1997.
14. Counselman FL, Shawn GS, Heller RA, et al: Quantitative β-hCG levels less than 1000 mIU/mL in patients with ectopic pregnancy: Pelvic ultrasound still useful. *J Emerg Med* 16(5):699, 1988.
15. Dart R, Howard K: Subclassification of indeterminate pelvic ultrasonograms: Stratifying the risk of ectopic pregnancy. *Acad Emerg Med* 5(4):313, 1998.
16. Dart RG, Burke G, Dart L: Subclassification of indeterminate pelvic ultrasonography: Prospective evaluation of the risk of ectopic pregnancy. *Ann Emerg Med* 39(4):382, 2002.
17. Houry D, Abbott JT: Ovarian torsion: A fifteen-year review. *Ann Emerg Med* 38(2):156, 2001.

THE NORMAL CHILD
Peter Mellis

Children account for approximately 30 percent of visits in most EDs. The majority have minor or self-limited illnesses that may optimally be cared for in a nonemergent setting. However, the differentiation of critically ill pediatric patients from the larger number of less ill children with similar complaints represents one of the most important and challenging diagnostic skills for emergency physicians. The key to mastering process of identifying ill children is a knowledge of child development as applied to the emergency setting.

GENERAL PRINCIPLES OF THE DEVELOPMENTAL APPROACH

Although there are many specific aspects of the developmental approach, a few general principles are applicable to all age groups of children and their families.

Communicate with the Child

Children are best approached in a positive and gentle manner, with an awareness that the first impression sets the tone for the encounter. Review the emergency record for patient's name and age so that an introduction and a developmentally structured interaction may be planned. An awareness of the child's age-related communication skills and perspective will result in a more meaningful evaluation. Whenever possible, look at the child from his or her own eye level. Use the child's motor skills, vocabulary, and specific life experiences as reference points. Hunger, discomfort, fear of separation or pain, and feelings of loss of control should be addressed directly. Recognize that the ED is a strange and threatening environment and, whenever possible, isolate the child from the sights and sounds of other patient care experiences that may heighten the child's own anxiety. Most importantly, be honest with children regarding expectations for their experience so that trust can be established.

Communicate with the Family

Assess and treat the child in the context of his or her family, avoiding separation whenever possible. ED policy should encourage parental accompaniment of children to the clinical area. It is optimal to consider that there are two patients, child and parent(s), each with expectations that must be addressed. Caregivers have essential historical information and, in the case of infants and toddlers, are physically necessary to the performance of a meaningful physical assessment. At all ages, children watch their parents for cues with respect to how to respond to the medical staff. Parents who understand and accept the sequence of events involved in emergency care become allies in enlisting their child's cooperation. Whenever possible, parents should be encouraged to remain present during procedures and maintain visual and physical contact from a sitting position. Appropriate exceptions include parental discomfort and critical illness. Because parents are intimately familiar with their child's range of verbal and nonverbal behaviors, the examiner must take the phrase "this is not my child" as parental concern for an abnormal level of consciousness. This reliance on parental knowledge is particularly applicable to the assessment of a child with developmental delay.

Assess by Means of Observation

Every effort should be made to gain information regarding a young child before interacting with him or her directly. Infants and young children communicate a normal level of consciousness through age-appropriate motor and social responses to their environment. Observe the child's behavior from a distance, preferably without his or her awareness. This can often be accomplished while obtaining the history from the caretakers. Antipyretic therapy and satisfying hunger are often crucial to achieving this period of optimal observation. Often more is learned regarding neurologic status from a brief period of observation than from the traditional physical examination. Nonemergent, uncomfortable examination components and procedures should be performed last.

Obtain Meaningful Vital Signs

Normal ranges for heart rate, respiratory rate, and blood pressure differ significantly with age and must be interpreted in the context of a child's activity at the time (Table 114-1). Anxiety, pain, fever, and crying will increase all values, and these states should be documented, if present. Optimal vital signs are obtained without eliciting an adverse reaction to the examiner (e.g., respiratory rate taken by observing abdominal movements and heart rate auscultated through clothing). If fever is a concern, temperature should be obtained rectally in infants, toddlers, and uncooperative children, because the oral, axillary, and tympanic routes are less reliable. Temperature measured by the oral route is likely to be feasible and accurate in children by 4 to 5 years of age. Blood pressure should be measured on previously well children who are 5 years and older (school age), children with chronic disease associated with hypertension (e.g., renal disease), and all children who are critically ill. Oxygen saturation should be determined for those in respiratory distress. Weight is a pediatric vital sign, because of dosing considerations and the importance of growth as an indicator of chronic disease in children. Appropriate scales and growth charts should be available in EDs. For resuscitation purposes, bedside estimates of weight are frequently inaccurate, and length-based resuscitation resources (e.g., Broselow tapes) are recommended.

GROWTH AND DEVELOPMENTAL STAGES

The process of development is not unique to children, but the pace at which change occurs and the implications for patient care are maximal during this period of life. *Developmental stages* are described with associated age ranges, but these are best viewed as a sequence of events with significant individual variations in rate of progression. For purposes of facilitating patient care in the ED, two aspects of each developmental stage must be considered. *Physical aspects* include growth and physiologic parameters unique to a given developmental stage, a knowledge of which is essential to provide excellent care. *Neurologic aspects* include motor, language, and social and psychological milestones that affect patient assessment and responses during acute illness or injury. These milestones and their related strategies are summarized in Table 114-2. Based on a knowledge of these principles, the examiner is well equipped to proceed with a developmentally *age-specific approach.*

Early Infancy (0 to 6 Months)

PHYSICAL ASPECTS Rapid growth rate is a characteristic feature of young infants, for whom the major work is eating. After a 5 to 10 percent

TABLE 114-1   Pediatric Vital Signs (Awake and Resting)

Age	Heart Rate/min, Upper Limit	Respiratory Rate/min, Upper Limit	Blood Pressure,* Lower Limit	Weight,† kg
0–1 mo	180	60	60/40	3–4
2–12 mo	160	50	70/45	5–10
12–24 mo	140	40	75/50	10–12
2–6 y	120	30	80/55	13–25
6–12 y	110	20	90/60	25–40
>12 y	100	20	90/60	40–60

*May be estimated by
  systolic blood pressure (5th percentile) = 70 + [2 × (age in years)]
†May be estimated by
  ≤12 mo; weight (kg) = 4 + (age in months/2)
  1–12 y; weight (kg) = 10 + [2 × (age in years)]

loss over the first 3 days of life, term infants regain birth weight by 10 days of age. A 20- to 30-g per d weight gain is the best overall sign of health. Normal infants double their birth weight by 5 months. Young infants have a high ratio of surface area to body mass, with a proportionally large head, resulting in a high rate of heat loss and risk of hypothermia. The normal anterior fontanelle is slightly depressed when a child is upright. Young infants are obligate nose breathers and may experience partial airway obstruction with abnormal positioning or viral upper respiratory tract infections. Normal neonates may exhibit periodic breathing, or 5- to 10-s pauses followed by tachypnea due to immature central control of respiration. Cardiac output and minute ventilation are relatively rate dependent in early infancy. A heart rate faster than 180 beats/min and a respiratory rate faster than 60 breaths/min should be considered abnormal. Blood pressure is well maintained by compensatory mechanisms at this age, with hypotension a very late finding in shock. The pulmonary vascular bed dilates over the first 6 weeks of life, so that congenital heart lesions resulting in a left-to-right shunt, for example, ventricular septal defect, will present after this age. The primary series of immunizations, including diphtheria-pertussis-tetanus (DPT), oral poliovirus, pneumococcal conjugate vaccine (PCV), and *Haemophilus influenzae* type b (HIb), are completed by age 6 months (Table 114-3). The rotavirus vaccine had been added to the primary immunization series, but possible association with intussusception has resulted in cessation of its use.

NEUROLOGIC ASPECTS   Motor development is the major indicator of neurologic health and proceeds in a cephalocaudal fashion. Neonates demonstrate involuntary "primitive" reflexes, such as the suck, grasp, and Moro (startle) responses, which may be elicited to demonstrate muscle tone and should always be symmetric. By 1 month of age, infants can lift their heads, follow a moving object, and demonstrate a social smile. By 4 months, head control is steady, the child will reach for and grasp objects with the whole hand, a cooing response may be elicited, and rolling over has begun. During this period, normal infants learn trust from their parents and will respond positively to a gentle examiner. This is the period of least parental confidence, and many ED visits are made because of lack of knowledge and a need for reassurance.

TABLE 114-2   Developmental Stages and Emergency Department Assessment Strategy

Stage	Milestone	Strategy
Early infancy (0–6 mo)	Motor: lifts head, reaches Verbal: cooing Social: responsive smile	Observation Examine in parent's arms Direct approach
Late infancy (6–18 mo)	Motor: reaches/obtains, sits, walks Verbal: jargon, few words Social: stranger anxiety/dependence	Observation Examine in parent's arms Indirect approach
Toddler (18–36 mo)	Motor: walks well, scribbles Verbal: speaks in phrases Social: stranger anxiety/autonomy	Observation Indirect approach
Preschool (3–5 y)	Motor: runs well, colors Verbal: speaks in sentences Social: magical thinking	Indirect or direct approach Explain briefly just before procedures
School age (5–12 y)	Motor: schoolwork, sports Verbal: concrete reasoning Social: task oriented	Direct approach Explain in detail before procedures
Adolescence (12–17 y)	Motor: adult Verbal: abstract reasoning Social: autonomy, rebellion	Direct approach Confidentiality Treat as adult

TABLE 114-3   Recommended Schedule of Childhood Immunizations

Age	DTaP	IPV	HIb	PCV	MMR	HepB	VZV
Birth						HepB	
2 mo	DTaP	IPV	HIb	PCV		HebB	
4 mo	DTaP	IPV	HIb	PCV			
6 mo	DTaP	IPV*	HIb	PCV		HepB*	
12–15 mo			HIb	PCV	MMR		VZV†
15–18 mo	DTaP						
4–6 y	DTaP	IPV			MMR‡		
11–12 y	Td						

*Third dose of IPV and HepB may be given at any time at ages 6 to 18 mo.
†VZV may be given at any time at ages 12 to 18 mo.
‡Second dose of MMR may be given at any time at ages 4 to 12 y.
Abbreviations: DTaP = diphtheria-tetanus-acellular pertussis, HepB = hepatitis B (live), HIb = *Haemophilus influenzae* type b conjugate, IPV = inactivated polio virus, MMR = measles-mumps-rubella (live), PCV = pneumococcal conjugate vaccine; Td = tetanus toxoid with diphtheria adjuvant (adult), VZV = varicella zoster virus (live).
Source: American Academy of Pediatrics, Committee on Infectious Diseases: Recommended childhood immunization schedule: United States, January–December 1998. *Pediatrics* 101:154, 1998. http://www.cispimmunize.org/applicationT.cfm?filenm-/cisp/pro/pro_body.html.

AGE-SPECIFIC APPROACH   Assessment is optimally made by direct interaction with the use of a pleasant, confident tone of voice and smiling face directed toward the infant. Observation of muscle tone, spontaneous activity, eye contact, responsive smile, and recognition of parents is most important. Examination of the infant is best performed when the infant is in the parent's lap, with use of brightly colored or pleasant-sounding objects to elicit a motor response. Feeding the infant or eliciting the sucking reflex with a finger often will result in greater cooperation. Optimal examination is done in order of least to most invasive interactions, that is, observation, auscultation, and palpation, being careful to avoid uncomfortable procedures such as ear and throat examination until the remainder of the exam is complete. Parental confidence should be directly reinforced. Young infants should be carefully monitored during procedures involving sedation or abnormal positioning, because of the risk of airway compromise. The motor abilities of young infants result in a limited potential for self-inflicted accidental injury. Whenever an injury is developmentally inconsistent with the stated mechanism, the potential for child abuse must be investigated.

Late Infancy (6 to 18 Months)

PHYSICAL ASPECTS   Normal infants triple their birth weight by 1 year of age, but the rate of growth slows during this period. The primary teeth begin to erupt by 6 months of age, with an average acquisition rate of one per month. Head size, center of gravity, and ratio of body surface area to body mass remain large in comparison with those of adults. The anterior fontanelle is closed by 18 months of age. The measles-mumps-rubella vaccination is given at 12 to 15 months of age, and the varicella vaccine is given at 12 to 18 months of age. The DPT and HIb boosters are given during this same period (see Table 114-3).

NEUROLOGIC ASPECTS   The normal infant sits with minimal support, transfers objects from hand to hand, and babbles by 6 months. By 9 months of age, the infant is crawling, pulling to a standing position, and verbalizing with nonspecific jargon. By 12 months, the infant has a mature pincer-type grasp, begins to walk, and acquires specific words. The developmental combination of mobility and grasp results in increasing risk of toxic and foreign-body ingestion. Between 9 and 12 months, a strong sense of "stranger anxiety," related to fear of separation from parents, is acquired and complicates every aspect of physical assessment. Conversely, the failure of an older infant or toddler to recognize and preferentially respond to parents suggests significant disease.

AGE-SPECIFIC APPROACH   Assessment of an older infant and toddler begins with observation, preferably without the child's awareness of the examiner's presence. The child should be undressed to obtain a meaningful respiratory rate and to observe the work of breathing. Spontaneous motor activity, such as sitting and pulling up, and purposeful responses to parental overtures, such as reaching for objects and smiling, are indicators of a normal level of consciousness. The child should see the examiner approach gradually and engage his or her caretakers first. An entire examination requiring any degree of cooperation is best performed while the child is held on the parent's lap or shoulder so that perception of separation is avoided. As for younger infants, the examination proceeds from least to most invasive interactions. Procedures in this age group require adequate physical restraint. Although parental restraint is acceptable for nonpainful examination procedures, parents should not be asked to immobilize their child for invasive procedures. Caretakers should be encouraged to remain present to reassure their child during procedures, if it is their desire to do so. The high level of anxiety at this age frequently results in persistently uncooperative behavior despite adequate analgesia. Sedation for procedures may require a significantly higher per-kilogram dose of an anxiolytic or analgesic drug to achieve the desired effect.

Toddler (18 to 36 Months)

PHYSICAL ASPECTS   Decelerating growth rate and decreased appetite are seen during this period, although the head approaches its adult size. The 20 primary teeth are in place by 36 months, and dental caries are common. High center of gravity, mobility, and curiosity lead to increasing risk for head and orthopedic injuries. A toddler's open growth plates are far more likely to sustain epiphyseal fracture than ligamentous injury. Traction injuries to the arm will frequently result in subluxation of the annular ligament of the radial head (i.e., "nursemaid's elbow").

NEUROLOGIC ASPECTS   By 18 months of age, most children can walk well, feed themselves, follow simple commands, and use four to six words to indicate their desires. Stranger anxiety peaks at this age but remains important throughout the toddler period. By 24 months, most children can run, climb stairs, and speak with three-word phrases, although only 50 percent of speech is intelligible to nonfamily members. Toddlers understand far more than their spontaneous speech would indicate and learn by imitating the behavior of their family members. When given opportunity to draw, a toddler will scribble with a brief attention span. Parents consistently underestimate the mobility and problem-solving ability of a toddler, resulting in a peak risk for falls and ingestions at this age.

AGE-SPECIFIC APPROACH   An examination strategy of indirect observation followed by direct interaction in the safety of the parent's arms should be followed, as described for older infants. The examiner should encourage the parent to have the toddler walk and follow commands as an important component of the assessment for acute systemic or neurologic disease. Allow the child a favorite object, such as a doll or blanket, for comfort during the examination. Talk to the child in simple language about what you will do and offer to let the child touch or hold the examination instruments to gain their trust. Older toddlers may indicate the site of pain specifically, but many will be unable to communicate localized pain or tenderness. As described above, perform the physical assessment in order of least to most invasive examination components. As for older infants, restraint is routinely indicated for painful procedures and a higher per-kilogram dose of an anxiolytic or analgesic drug may be required. Because of likelihood of epiphyseal fracture, a young child with tenderness over the growth plate after injury should be immobilized with a splint, even if x-ray films are negative.

Preschool Age (3 to 5 Years)

PHYSICAL ASPECTS   Growth rate slows significantly during this period, and appetite decreases further. Children develop a more lean body habitus. The incidence of injuries increases with increasing activity. The preschool child is no longer restrained in a car seat and is at risk for defined injury complexes from improperly fitting lap and shoulder belts. A DPT booster is given shortly before beginning school, between the ages of 4 and 6 years (see Table 114-3).

NEUROLOGIC ASPECTS   Preschool children develop progressive autonomy in terms of mobility and self-care. Attraction to books, drawing, and coloring is common. Expressive language skills expand rapidly, and children this age are often able to identify site(s) of specific complaint. However, a strong sense of fear of pain remains, and the level of anxiety remains high in the emergency setting. Preschool children live in the present and have a limited sense of time and history, so that prior symptoms are frequently forgotten. Self-centered "magical" reasoning is the rule, so that many preschool children believe that ED care is punishment for misbehavior. This is occasionally reinforced by parents who state they will "have the doctor give you a shot," which should be discouraged.

AGE-SPECIFIC APPROACH Many preschool children may be directly approached and examined in the traditional systematic fashion. However, some will require the indirect approach described for toddlers, and the nearby presence of a parent is typically essential for cooperation. The examiner should always talk directly with the preschooler to establish rapport and confirm the general complaint. Identification of recent positive experiences such as birthdays or favorite cartoon characters is frequently helpful in gaining cooperation. However, preschool children should be expected to identify only the current complaint, and reliance on parental history should remain. Cooperation during the physical examination is likely, although less comfortable components are still best performed at the end. The performance of painful procedures requires a careful approach. It is always best to be honest regarding discomfort, but information should be given immediately before performing the procedure to minimize the effects of fantasy regarding pain and causality and delaying tactics. Comfort and distraction by the parent are frequently effective for minor procedures; however, restraint, as for toddlers, is typically necessary. Rewards such as verbal praise and a sticker for bravery often significantly enhance the memory of the experience for the child and family.

School Age (5 to 12 Years)

PHYSICAL ASPECTS The school years represent the slowest period of growth in childhood, and the body habitus is typically slender. The primary teeth are loosening and the secondary teeth erupt. The lymphatics reach maximal dimensions relative to body size by 6 years of age. There is increased physical activity, including organized sports, during this period, and injuries become common.

NEUROLOGIC ASPECTS School-age children experience rapid language growth and maturing motor ability. Concrete reasoning ability emerges with an ability to understand cause and effect. The child is increasingly aware of his or her body and develops a sense of modesty. Task-oriented behavior is common, and school and sports activity are typically the central events of the child's life. School-age children are eager to please and often reluctant to express their fears of pain and death.

AGE-SPECIFIC APPROACH The direct examination approach is typically successful for school-age children. Parental accompaniment and respect for modesty should be maintained. Historical information should be elicited from child and parent. An effort to inquire about school or extracurricular interests will enhance rapport. Change in school performance is a helpful indicator of chronic disease. Painful procedures are best preceded by explanations to both parent and child, given well in advance with honesty regarding discomfort. The child should be given some degree of choice in the manner in which the procedure is completed, such as a comfortable position, to minimize the sense of loss of control.

Adolescence (12 to 17 Years)

PHYSICAL ASPECTS The teen years mark a second period of rapid growth, beginning at age 10 in girls and age 12 in boys. Secondary sexual development begins shortly after beginning the growth spurt, with menarche starting between 10 and 16 years in girls. Sexual activity and drug use are common during adolescence, and many teens are parents themselves, complicating the differential diagnosis and issues of maturity and reliability in carrying out the follow-up plan.

NEUROLOGIC ASPECTS Abstract reasoning ability progressively develops during adolescence, paired with a self-centered world view and self-consciousness regarding appearance. Feelings of immortality and denial of the consequences of risky behavior are common. Loss of autonomy is the greatest fear of an adolescent, and mistrust of and rebellion toward authority is normal. Previously well-controlled chronic disease frequently becomes unstable as a result of these developmental issues. Psychiatric disease and suicidal behavior are increasingly recognized in this age group. The parents of teenagers are frequently angered by these changes and may project these feelings on the ED staff.

AGE-SPECIFIC APPROACH The traditional history and physical examination with respect for modesty are effective in the assessment of adolescents. The examiner should communicate to the teenager that he or she will be treated "like an adult." Choices must be allowed, such as parental presence during the examination, with proper limit setting regarding cooperative behavior. The parent's concerns must be addressed individually and, if necessary, in private. Confidentiality should be stressed, particularly as the law requires with respect to pregnancy and sexually transmitted disease.

MEDICAL CONSENT AND THE TREATMENT OF MINORS

Consent for evaluation and treatment must be obtained for medical care to be delivered in a lawful manner. State laws vary regarding the age of majority at which consent may be given by a patient, varying between 18 and 21 years of age. In the case of minor children, consent must be obtained from the legal guardian (typically a parent, unless custody has been removed) before initiation of treatment. This does not apply, however, to triage and examination, and children should be evaluated without delay to determine the nature of the illness or injury.[1] If the child is not accompanied by persons able to provide consent, the parent or guardian should be contacted by phone and witnessed consent obtained. Such attempts should be documented in the medical record. Written documentation from the parent or legal guardian granting consent may suffice in many states, but this should not obviate attempted phone contact for permission to treat. In the absence of consent, the patient should be evaluated sufficiently to determine the presence or absence of an emergent situation. In the setting of an emergency situation in which delay in treatment may threaten the life or health of the child, consent can be assumed and care initiated with ongoing attempts to locate the parent or guardian. If any doubt exists, the emergency physician and patient are best served by providing treatment with documentation of efforts to determine the presence of an emergency and obtain consent for treatment. In the absence of an emergency, further care should not be provided unless specifically permitted under state law (Table 114-4). Most states permit minors to seek treatment for child abuse, substance abuse, sexually transmitted diseases, and pregnancy-related complaints without parental consent. Most states consider a child "emancipated" and able to provide consent if a member of the armed forces, married, or self-supporting and living independently. Some states permit older minors to give consent for nonemergent care. Many states have a process for obtaining concurrent judicial review and consent. Emergency physicians are encouraged to become familiar with the specific state laws applicable to consent issues.[1] As a matter of courtesy and necessity, verbal consent should be obtained from older minors, typically at age 12 years and older.

Parental refusal of consent for care in the setting of possible life-threatening emergency or child abuse presents emergency physicians with a significant challenge. If parental consent cannot be obtained, a court order should be obtained through the appropriate local mechanism to allow the provision of necessary care for the well-being of the child.

TABLE 114-4 Consent for Treating Minors

Age of consent is typically 18 y but may vary by state. A minor should be
evaluated but not receive treatment in an emergency department without
consent obtained from a parent or legal guardian, with the following
exceptions:
- Life- or limb-threatening emergency
- State-protected right to treatment
  - Child abuse
  - Pregnancy-related complaints
  - Sexually transmitted disease
  - Substance abuse
  - Outpatient mental health (some states)
- State-defined "emancipated minor" status
  - Married
  - Member of armed forces
  - Self-supporting and living independently

REFERENCE

1. Consent for Emergency Medical Services for Children and Adolescents.
   American Academy of Pediatrics; Committee on Pediatric Emergency Medicine: Policy statement. *Pediatrics* 111(3); 703, 2003.

115 FEVER
Carol D. Berkowitz

Fever is the most common chief complaint of children presenting to
the ED and accounts for approximately 30 percent of pediatric outpatient visits. Physicians evaluating febrile children must differentiate
mildly ill from seriously ill children, a challenge that may be compounded when no focus of infection is apparent. The extent of the diagnostic workup and the institution of appropriate management, including the use of antibiotics and the need for hospitalization, must be
determined. Many factors, such as clinical assessment, physical findings, age of the patient, immunization status, and height of the fever,
influence the evaluation and management decisions.

PATHOPHYSIOLOGY

Fever is defined as a rise in deep body temperature associated with a
resetting of the body's thermostat. This thermostat is located in the
preoptic region of the anterior hypothalamus, near the floor of the third
ventricle. Exogenous fever-producing substances (pyrogens), such as
bacteria, bacterial endotoxin, antigen-antibody complexes, yeast,
viruses, and etiocholanolone, may stimulate the formation and release
of endogenous pyrogens. Endogenous pyrogens are produced by neutrophils, monocytes, hepatic Kupffer cells, splenic sinusoidal cells,
alveolar macrophages, and peritoneal lining cells and are believed to
induce the synthesis of prostaglandins in the hypothalamus. Endogenous pyrogens include interleukin 1, interleukin 6, and tumor necrosis
factor.[1] The body's thermostat is then reset at a higher setting, and the
patient, whose own temperature is below that of the body's thermostat,
experiences a chill. Peripheral vasoconstriction, shivering, central
pooling, and behavioral activity (e.g., putting on a sweater or drinking
hot tea) lead to an increase in body temperature.

CLINICAL FEATURES

The possible beneficial effects of fever have been debated for many
years. Aside from these considerations, it is important to recognize
that fever represents a symptom of some underlying disease, and one
must determine what this disease is.

An initial question is, "What degree of temperature elevation represents a fever?" One survey conducted among pediatric training programs revealed a wide variability in the temperature considered a
"fever" in infants younger than 2 months. This figure has ranged from
38°C to 39.4°C (100.4°F to 103°F). It is important to recognize that
oral temperatures are generally 0.6°C (1°F) lower than rectal temperatures and axillary temperatures are 0.6°C (1°F) lower than oral temperatures. Temperatures taken with infrared thermometers that scan
the tympanic membrane are of variable reliability and reproducibility.[2]
Body temperature normally varies from morning to evening with the
body's circadian rhythm. The degree of variation, which is greater in
young women and small children, is approximately 1.1°C (2°F).

Current practice guidelines suggest a temperature of 38°C as a sufficient fever to warrant an evaluation. The relation between height of
fever and incidence of bacteremia is discussed below. In general,
higher temperatures are associated with a higher incidence of bacteremia. The incidence of meningitis is about twice as high in children
with fevers above 41.1°C (105.9°F) than in children with fevers between 40.5°C and 41.0°C (104.9°F and 105.8°F). The incidence of
pneumonia and bacteremia is about the same in both groups.

Some studies, many of which have also been retrospective, have
produced variable results and have indicated that children with higher
temperatures have more diagnostic studies ordered but the same incidence of different diseases.

INFANTS UP TO 3 MONTHS

Diagnosis

The age of the patient influences the extent of the workup. Early studies suggested that infants younger than 3 months were at high risk for
life-threatening infection. Recent studies based on outpatients showed
that the incidence of serious bacterial infection, including bacteremia
and meningitis, is about 3 to 4 percent, although serious nonbacterial
infections (e.g., aseptic meningitis) are a frequent cause of fever in this
age group (Table 115-1).

Presentation History

The history often provides a clue to the diagnosis. When evaluating infants younger than 1 to 2 months, it is critical to review the birth history, because the etiology of the infant's infection may be birth related.
The key points to consider include the length of the gestation, the use
of antibiotics in the mother or infant, and the presence of any neonatal complications, such as fever or tachypnea. Although an organ-
specific list of inquiries may be helpful in treating older infants, it is
less useful in younger ones, because the signs and symptoms of sepsis
may be very nonspecific. For instance, vomiting and diarrhea accompany many problems, including gastroenteritis, otitis media, urinary
tract infections, and meningitis. Cough or respiratory symptoms
would be consistent with a respiratory infection. Frequency of urination is important to assess as a measure of the state of hydration.

**TABLE 115-1 Incidence of Serious Bacterial Infection
with Fever in Infants ≤3 mos of Age**

Infants up to 3 mo old with temperature of ≥38°C	3–4%
Rochester criteria for low-risk bacteremia	0.2%
Nontoxic appearance	
No soft tissue infection	
WBC	500–15,000/μL
Normal urinalysis	
Stools	<5 WBC/hpf with diarrhea

Abbreviations: hpf = high power field; WBC = white blood cell count.

Physical Examination

Infants should be undressed completely to enable a full assessment. Vital signs are important to evaluate. For instance, tachypnea may be a clue to lower respiratory tract infection. Crying and the ease of consolation should be evaluated. Inconsolable crying, or increased irritability when handled, is frequently seen in infants with meningitis. Although fullness of the anterior fontanelle may be noted in some of these infants, other signs of meningeal irritation, such as nuchal rigidity, are most often absent. A head-to-toe evaluation should be carried out to determine whether there is a focus of infection, such as an inflamed eardrum or evidence of cellulitis.

Clinical assessment of the severity of illness of young, febrile infants is, however, problematic. Young infants lack social skills, such as the social smile, and their ability to interact with examiners is limited. There is a report in the literature of an infant with group B streptococcal bacteremia who was judged by house staff and faculty to be clinically well. The absence of any diagnostic abnormalities in the medical history or on physical examination suggests the need for extensive laboratory tests to detect occult infection. These tests would include a complete blood count (CBC) and differential, erythrocyte sedimentation rate (ESR), blood culture, lumbar puncture, chest x-ray, urinalysis and culture, and a stool culture if there is a history of diarrhea, particularly if leukocytes are noted on a stool smear. Some authors also recommend a quantitative C-reactive protein as an index of serious bacterial infection.[3] Urinary tract infections may not produce symptoms other than fever, so urinalysis and culture should be included routinely in the evaluation. Urinary tract infections may be associated with bacteremia in up to 30 percent of infected infants[4] and are the most common bacterial infection in this age group.

The recognition of occult serious infection in well-appearing young, febrile infants is problematic. Most investigators agree that no single variable can correctly identify these infants. Combinations of variables are more helpful in the differentiation process. Criteria have been identified by a number of investigators but are generally referred to as the Rochester criteria for low risk for serious bacterial infection in infants younger than 3 months. **These criteria include nontoxic appearance, no soft tissue infection, white blood cell counts (WBCs) between 5000 and 15,000/μL, fewer than 1500 bands/μL, normal urinalysis, and stool with fewer than 5 WBCs/high power field in infants with diarrhea.[3] The risk of serious bacterial infection in the absence of these variables is about 0.2 percent.**

Management

The appropriate management of young febrile infants presents another area of disagreement.[5] There appears to be no "community standard of practice" regarding the need for hospitalization; some physicians hospitalize all febrile infants younger than 3 months, and others hospitalize only those younger than 1 month. Some have attributed this difference in management to a difference in bias, with physicians in practice having a bias toward wellness (the infant is basically healthy) and those working in the ED having a bias toward illness (worst-case scenario approach).[6] Because the differentiation between sick and well infants is so difficult, especially to less experienced examiners, all such febrile infants need extensive septic workups. The decision not to hospitalize a small febrile infant must be made after careful clinical and appropriate laboratory assessment and after ensuring the reliability of follow-up.

Current management strategies include the administration of ceftriaxone at a dose of 50 mg/kg to febrile infants between 1 and 3 months of age who are judged to be at low risk for serious bacterial infection when the above criteria are used.[7] A caretaker with a telephone is an additional criterion for such outpatient management. Similarly, Baskin and colleagues[8] proposed parenteral ceftriaxone and 24-h observation for inpatient management of febrile infants between 2 and 4 weeks of age and also judged to be at low risk. Infants could be discharged if cultures were negative after 24 h. In the future, the ready availability of rapid viral assays may alter the use of expectant antibiotics in this age group.[9,10]

INFANTS OF 3 TO 24 MONTHS

Diagnosis

Many of the considerations noted in the evaluation of infants younger than 3 months apply for older infants. Children between 3 and 36 months have been the focus of considerable research, because this group appears to be at higher risk for occult bacteremia (Table 115-2). These studies have sought to identify clinical and laboratory characteristics of bacteremic patients.

Clinical judgment appears to be more reliable in the assessment of older infants. Characteristics that evaluating physicians should note are willingness of patients to make eye contact, playfulness and positive response to interactions, negative response to noxious stimuli, alertness, and ease of consolation. Toxic infants will not respond appropriately.

Presentation History

The medical history and physical examination frequently will reveal the source of infection. Viral illnesses, including respiratory infections and gastroenteritis, account for most febrile illnesses and usually have system-specific symptoms, such as vomiting, diarrhea, rhinorrhea, cough, or rashes. In this age group, such symptoms are more often indicative of an organ-specific infection. Bacterial infections of the respiratory tract most notably include otitis media, pharyngitis, and pneumonia. Otitis media is generally caused by *Streptococcus pneumoniae* or nontypable *Haemophilus influenzae,* and antibiotic therapy, such as amoxicillin, should be directed at these organisms. Although pneumonia is commonly of viral etiology, it is appropriate to institute antibiotic therapy with amoxicillin or erythromycin. The physical signs of meningitis, such as nuchal rigidity and Kernig or Brudzinski signs, may be inapparent in children even up to the age of 2 years. A bulging fontanelle, vomiting, irritability that increases when the infant is held, inconsolability, or a febrile seizure may be the only signs suggestive of meningitis. Infants with aseptic meningitis generally should be hospitalized and ensured adequate long-term follow-up, because they are at greater risk for subsequent neurologic and learning disabilities.

The presence of petechiae on physical examination should alert physicians to the potential presence of a serious underlying infection.[11] Up to 20 percent of children may have bacteremia or meningitis, most frequently with *Neisseria meningitidis* or *H. influenzae.* Petechiae in association with high fever (≥40°C), ESR at or above 30 mm per h, and WBCs of at least 15,000/μL are most frequently correlated with bacteremia. The pneumonic ILL, for *i*rritability, *l*ethargy, and *l*ow capillary refill (>2 s or hypotension), has been proposed as a clue to bacteremia associated with petechiae.[12]

Bacteremic infants may or may not have an obvious focus of infection. The height of the fever is a clue to bacteremia in infants. Al-

TABLE 115-2   Incidence of Serious Bacterial Infection with Fever in Infants Aged 3–24 Months

Infants 3–24 mo old with temperature of ≥39.5°C	5% before pneumococcal vaccine
Higher risk of bacteremia	
WBC	>15,000/μL
Bands	>500/μL
ANC	>10,000/μL

Abbreviations: ANC = absolute neutrophil count; WBC = white blood cell count.

though bacteremia may be seen at lower temperatures, a temperature above 39.5°C (103.1°F) in infants aged 3 to 36 months is associated with a higher incidence of bacteremia. **Specifically, occult pneumococcal bacteremia was reported with the following prevalences: 1.2 percent with temperatures from 39.0°C to 39.4°C, 2.5 percent with temperatures from 39.5°C to 39.9°C, 3.2 percent with temperatures from 40.0°C to 40.4°C, and 4.9 percent with temperatures above 40.5°C.**[13]

Certain laboratory tests have been recommended to assist further in identifying bacteremic patients. WBC counts of at least 15,000/μL, band counts of at least 500/μL, total polymorphonuclear counts of at least 10,000/μL, and band plus polymorphonuclear counts equal to or more than 10,500/μL are associated with an increased incidence of bacteremia, although bacteremia also occurs without these findings. An absolute neutrophil count equal to or more than 10,000/μL is associated with an increased likelihood of bacteremia and is an indication for a blood culture and the initiation of expectant antibiotic therapy.[13] Other studies, such as an ESR, quantitative C-reactive protein, antigen assays, cytokine levels, and polymerase chain reaction are more expensive, not readily available, and offer no advantage over the WBC.

The incidence of bacteremia in children 3 to 24 months of age with a temperature of 39.5°C (103.1°F) or over was about 5 to 6 percent before the widespread use of the conjugated heptavalent pneumococcal vaccine. **The incidence was 12 to 15 percent in patients with WBCs of at least 15,000/μL.** An ESR at or above 30 mm per h had the same significance as WBCs of 15,000/μL or more. The organism most commonly causing bacteremia in this age group had been *S. pneumoniae*. *Haemophilus influenzae* has been rarely implicated in cases of occult bacteremia since the availability of *H. influenzae* vaccine. It is anticipated that the heptavalent pneumococcal vaccine will have a similar impact on the incidence of occult pneumococcal bacteremia, because 83 to 92 percent of *S. pneumoniae* recovered in bacteremic children involves one of the seven serotypes contained in the vaccine.[14,15] Is it important to perform a blood culture to detect occult bacteremia? Opinions differ, especially since the advent of the heptavalent pneumococcal vaccine. It is apparent that bacteremic patients do better if they receive antibiotics early in the course of the disease. Many bacteremic children do have a focus of infection and, hence, are treated anyway. In addition, in at least 25 percent of bacteremic patients with no focus of infection, the bacteremia is resolved without antibiotics. Others develop soft tissue infections, which are then appropriately managed. The ability of oral antibiotics to prevent the development of meningitis in bacteremic children is still unclear. The blood culture appears to be useful for following patients who may not be returning for periodic evaluations. Some physicians who support the continued acquisition of blood cultures have speculated on the emergence of *N. meningitidis* as the most prevalent pathogen once *H. influenzae* and *S. pneumoniae* have been eliminated through immunization. Kuppermann and colleagues cited the devastating effects of meningococcemia.[16] Conversely, as the prevalence of occult bacteremia is reduced, the rate of contaminated blood cultures will exceed that of truly positive blood cultures, thereby increasing the cost of health care without providing any benefit. The prevalence of blood cultures positive for *N. meningitidis* before *H. influenzae* and *S. pneumoniae* immunizations was 1 to 5 percent. The decision to obtain a blood culture should take into account the immunization status of the child and of other children in the community and whether the child is at high risk for an infection for any reason.

Management

Is there a role for the use of expectant antibiotics in children suspected of having occult bacteremia? Retrospective studies have shown that early antibiotics diminish the incidence of persistent bacteremia. In a prospective, randomized study comparing oral penicillin with no antibiotics, no improvement was reported in any bacteremic child who did not receive antibiotics. Other investigators reported more equivocal results.

Outpatient daily injections of ceftriaxone are being used by some physicians for children at increased risk of occult bacteremia. Controlled trials investigating the efficacy of this therapy have demonstrated a reduction in the incidence of meningitis in bacteremic children treated with ceftriaxone compared with those treated with oral or no antibiotics. Parenteral ceftriaxone should never be initiated without appropriate antecedent diagnostic studies. Treatment should be discontinued if cultures are negative. The risk from the overuse of ceftriaxone is the emergence of resistant organisms, a phenomenon that has been reported.[17,18]

Current recommendations suggest the following approach to well-appearing infants between 3 and 36 months of age: for those 2 to 3 years with a temperature below 39.5°C, no blood testing should be done, because the incidence of occult bacteremia is less than 1 percent; for those 2 to 3 years with a temperature above 39.5°C or those 3 to 24 months with a temperature above 39°C, a CBC with an automated differential count should be obtained, because the incidence of occult bacteremia is 2.6 percent. If the absolute neutrophil count is more than 10,000/μL, obtain a blood culture and initiate expectant antibiotics with ceftriaxone at a dose of 50 mg/kg given twice 24 h apart.[13] If cultures are negative after 48 h, no further treatment is needed. Any child who appears ill or toxic should be admitted to the hospital.[19] Likewise, children who are felt to be at risk for a serious bacterial infection and do not have reliable follow-up or the ability to return to the hospital should also be admitted for inpatient management.

Another dilemma surrounds the management of positive blood culture results. All patients with positive blood cultures should be recalled for repeat evaluation. If they are receiving appropriate antibiotics, are clinically well, and have been afebrile, they should be instructed to complete the course of therapy. If they are afebrile and clinically well but have never been treated with antibiotics, opinions differ regarding the need for additional blood cultures and antibiotic therapy. In general, neither is necessary unless the child has developed a specific focus of infection. However, any patient who remains febrile or does poorly even if on antibiotics should receive complete septic evaluation (CBC, blood culture, lumbar puncture, chest film, and urine culture), be hospitalized, and receive parenteral antibiotics (Figure 115-1).

OLDER FEBRILE CHILDREN

Diagnosis

Children older than 3 years are easier to evaluate. They can specify their complaints and have illnesses similar to those of younger children, in particular upper respiratory infections and gastroenteritis. The risk of bacteremia appears lower in this age group, but the incidence of streptococcal pharyngitis is higher, especially in children between the ages of 5 and 10 years and those with hyperpyrexia. Infectious mononucleosis may present with fever, tonsillar hypertrophy, and exudate, as does streptococcal pharyngitis. Marked lymphadenopathy or hepatosplenomegaly would support the diagnosis. Pneumonia in this age group may be caused by *Mycoplasma pneumoniae*. These children present with cough and fever. Rales may not be apparent early in the illness, although the chest film would show evidence of an infiltrate. Bedside cold agglutinins, if positive, provide a clue to the correct diagnosis. Children with pneumonia secondary to *mycoplasma* should be treated with a macrolide such as erythromycin at 30 to 40 mg/kg per d (maximum dose, 1 g), or azithromycin at 10 mg/kg on day 1, and then 5 mg/kg on days 2 to 5, or clarithromycin at 7.5 mg/kg every 12 h.

EMERGENCY DEPARTMENT CARE

Managing the Fever

Once the issue of fever as a symptom has been addressed, it is appropriate to determine the need for fever-reducing measures.

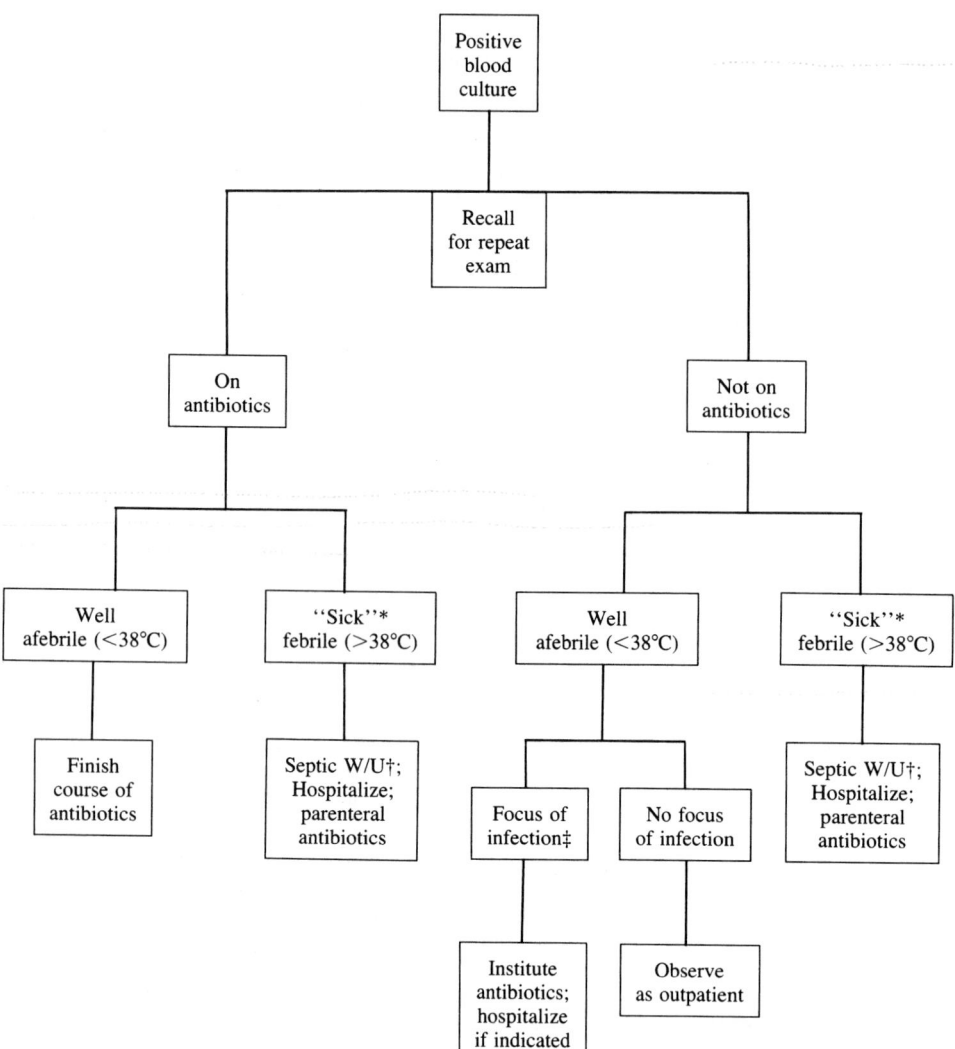

FIG. 115-1. Management of bacteremic children. *"Sick" = irritable, lethargic, anorexic, or vomiting. †Septic W/U (workup) = blood culture, lumbar puncture, chest x-ray, complete blood count, differential, urinalysis, and urine culture. ‡Focus of infection = otitis media, pneumonia, or cellulitis.

Many parents are concerned about the harmful effects of the fever; many are aware of the risk of febrile seizures. Children who are prone to febrile seizures are not benefited by antipyretics alone because the seizure frequently occurs early in the illness, often before the parents are aware that the child is ill. Aside from febrile seizures, fever is not known to produce any harmful effects in children. Many children, however, feel uncomfortable during the fever, so it is appropriate to institute measures directed at symptomatically reducing the fever.

The body loses heat in four ways: (1) radiation (60 percent), that is, heat loss from the body to the air in the surrounding environment; (2) evaporation (25 percent), that is, heat loss through the evaporation of perspiration, water, or any liquid applied to the body surface; (3) convection (10 percent), that is, heat loss when air currents blow over the skin; and (4) conduction (approximately 5 percent), that is, heat loss through contact with a solid surface. Heat loss through conduction is increased by the use of cooling blankets.

One can facilitate heat loss in children by using any combination of these measures. Unwrapping a bundled child increases heat loss through radiation, and rehydrating a dehydrated child increases the heat loss through evaporation. Sponging also helps to reduce fever by evaporation. Sponging should be done slowly and only with tepid water. Very rapid cooling by sponging can result in peripheral vascular collapse, and death among small, critically ill infants has been reported. Sponging with ice water is uncomfortable for children and results in shivering, and sponging with alcohol carries the risk of intoxication, hypoglycemia, and coma. Vigorous rubbing of the skin induces vasodilatation and improves heat loss.

Studies have shown that sponging and antipyretics used together are more effective than either modality used alone. Acetaminophen, ibuprofen, and aspirin are equally effective and appear to work centrally to block prostaglandin synthesis. Heat is lost through peripheral vasodilatation and sweating.

Drug dosage for aspirin or acetaminophen is 10 to 15 mg/kg per dose at 4-h intervals (maximum dose, 600 mg). Increasing the dose does not result in a better or more sustained effect. Administration of either drug by rectal suppository slightly delays absorption. No studies have evaluated the efficacy of alternating the two drugs at 2-h intervals to avoid the recrudescence of fever. Administration of the drugs simultaneously at the usual dosage produces a reduction in temperature that is sustained for 6 h rather than for 2 to 4 h. The dosage of ibuprofen is 5 mg/kg for fevers below 39°C (102.2°F) and 10 mg/kg for fevers above 39°C (102.2°F). Ibuprofen may be given every 6 to 8 h, with a maximum daily dose of 40 mg/kg. The key to assuring a good outcome is judicial management, follow-up, and reassessment. It is not appropriate to simply administer ceftriaxone and assume that any infection an infant may have has been appropriately treated. Emergency physicians must be certain that infants can be reevaluated to ensure that other problems have not emerged.

The use of aspirin has been curtailed after reports linking aspirin and Reye syndrome. Aspirin should not be used in children with chickenpox or with influenza-like illnesses. The effects of aspirin are cumulative, and over half of the reported overdoses involves therapeutic misuse. Other side effects of aspirin include gastrointestinal upset and hemorrhage and coagulation disturbances. Acetaminophen is also toxic if taken in inappropriate doses, but there is minimal likelihood of any cumulative effect, and children are less prone than adults to hepatotoxicity. Side effects of ibuprofen are similar to those of aspirin and include gastrointestinal ulceration, bleeding, and perforation. Platelet disturbances have been reported but are felt to be reversible with cessation of therapy.

REFERENCES

1. Kluger MJ: Fever revisited. *Pediatrics* 90:846, 1992.
2. Petersen-Smith A, Barber N, Coody D, et al: Comparison of aural infrared with traditional rectal temperatures in children from birth to age three years. *J Pediatr* 125:83, 1994.
3. Dagan R, Sofer S, Phillip M, Shachak E: Ambulatory care of febrile infants younger than 2 months of age classified as being at low risk for having bacterial infections. *J Pediatr* 112:355, 1987.
4. Hoberman A, Wald ER: Urinary tract infections in young febrile children. *Pediatr Infect Dis J* 16:11, 1997.
5. Lieu TA, Baskin MN, Schwartz S, Fleisher GR: Clinical and cost-effectiveness of outpatient strategies for management of febrile infants. *Pediatrics* 89:1135, 1992.
6. Young PC: The management of febrile infants by primary-care pediatricians in Utah: Comparison with published practice guidelines. *Pediatrics* 95:623, 1995.
7. Baskin MN, O'Rourke EJ, Fleisher GR: Outpatient treatment of febrile infants 28 to 89 days of age with intramuscular administration of ceftriaxone. *J Pediatr* 120:22, 1992.
8. Baskin MN, O'Rourke EJ, Fleisher GR: Management of febrile infants 15 to 28 days of age with parenteral ceftriaxone and 24 hours of in-patient observation. *Arch Pediatr Adolesc Med* 148:49, 1994.
9. Sharma V, Dowd MD, Slaughter AJ, et al: Effect of rapid diagnosis of influenza virus type a on the emergency department management of febrile infants and toddlers. *Arch Pediatr Adolesc Med* 156:41, 2002.
10. Byington CL, Taggart EW, Carroll KC, Hillyard DR: A polymerase chain reaction-based epidemiologic investigation of the incidence of nonpolio enteral infections in febrile and afebrile infants 90 days and younger. *Pediatrics* 103:1098, 1999.
11. Mandl KD, Stack AM, Fleisher GR: Incidence of bacteremia in infants and children with fever and petechiae. *J Pediatr* 131:398, 1997.
12. Brogan PA, Raffles A: Fever and petechiae. *Arch Dis Child* 83:506, 2000.
13. Kuppermann N: Occult bacteremia in young febrile children. *Pediatr Clin North Am* 46:1073, 1999.
14. Giebink GS: The prevention of pneumococcal disease in children. *New Engl J Med* 345:1177, 2001.
15. Lee GM, Fleisher GR, Harper MB: Management of febrile children in the age of the conjugate pneumococcal vaccine: A cost-effectiveness analysis. *Pediatrics* 108:835, 2001.
16. Kuppermann N, Malley R, Inkelis SH, et al: Clinical and hematologic features do not reliably identify children with unsuspected meningococcal disease. *Pediatrics* 103:E20, 1999.
17. Bradley JS, Scheld WN: The challenges of penicillin-resistant pneumococcal infection. *Clin Infect Dis* 24:S213, 1997.
18. Silverstein M, Bachur R, Harper MB: Clinical implications of penicillin and ceftriaxone resistance among children with pneumococcal bacteremia. *Pediatr Infect Dis J* 18:38, 1999.
19. Fleisher GR, Rosenberg N, Vinci R, et al: Intramuscular versus oral antibiotic therapy for the prevention of meningitis and other bacterial sequelae in young febrile children at risk for occult bacteremia. *J Pediatr* 124:504, 1994.

116 BACTEREMIA, SEPSIS, AND MENINGITIS IN CHILDREN
Peter Mellis

The identification and treatment of potentially life-threatening systemic infectious disease in children represents a continuing challenge for the emergency physician, most frequently in the setting of the evaluation of the febrile infant. Although most children with fever have

self-limited viral or minor focal bacterial infection, a subset will have serious bacterial disease with potential for morbidity and mortality. This chapter provides an overview of the presentation, diagnosis, and management of bacteremia, sepsis, and meningitis in pediatric patients in the ED. Although each is discussed separately, it must be kept in mind that these entities represent different points along a spectrum and may occur concurrently as a result of progression of disease.

BACTEREMIA AND SERIOUS BACTERIAL INFECTION

Pathophysiology

Children between the ages of birth and 3 years are at relatively increased risk for bloodborne bacterial disease due to immaturity of the reticuloendothelial system. The term *bacteremia* refers to the presence of a positive blood culture without reference to specific clinical symptomatology. Bacteremia may resolve spontaneously, progress to *septicemia* with clinical signs of abnormal perfusion parameters and altered mental status, or be associated with focal *serious bacterial infection* (SBI), most often involving the lung, kidney, meninges, bowel, bone, or joint. The risk of bacteremia and SBI decrease with age, with the greatest incidence in the first 3 months of life (Table 116-1). For purposes of discussion, the relative risks can be broken down into three age groupings: neonates (0 to 28 days), young infants (29 to 90 days), and children (3 to 36 months).

Neonates with fever have a 5 percent risk for bacteremia and a 15 percent incidence of SBI, predominantly due to pathogens encountered at the time of birth.[1] Bacteremia in this age group results in a fulminant septicemic process within hours to days of birth (*early-onset disease*) or a focal SBI developing weeks to months later (*late-onset disease*). Group B *Streptococcus* is by far the most common bacterial pathogen in this age group, followed by *Escherichia coli, Listeria monocytogenes,* and *Enterococcus* sp.

Infants 29 to 90 days of age are at a progressively lesser risk for late-onset infection from these neonatally acquired pathogens but are increasingly susceptible to community-acquired pathogens. This age group thus represents a transition period from neonates and those infants 3 months and older.

Children 3 months and older are susceptible to infection from community-acquired pathogens and are at relatively less risk for bacteremia and SBI in comparison with younger infants. Bacteremia in this age group is a result of SBI or may occur as a primary process and precede the development of focal serious infection. Focal SBI that may be associated with bacteremia includes meningitis, pneumonia, pyelonephritis, bacterial enteritis, facial cellulitis, septic arthritis, and osteomyelitis (Table 116-2). The reader is referred to subsequent chapters for descriptions of the pathogenesis and microbiology of these

TABLE 116-1   Age-Related Risk Groups and Causes of Bacteremia in Children

Group	Risk	Pathogens
Neonates 0–28 d	High risk	Group B *Streptococcus* *Escherichia coli* *Listeria monocytogenes* *Enterococcus* sp.
Young infants 29–90 d	Intermediate risk	Neonatal pathogens (above) Community-acquired pathogens (below)
Older infants 3–36 mo	Low risk	*Streptococcus pneumoniae* *Neisseria meningitidis* *Haemophilus influenzae* b (unimmunized) Group A *Streptococcus* *Escherichia coli* (pyelonephritis) *Salmonella* sp. (gastroenteritis) *Staphylococcus aureus* (osteomyelitis)

TABLE 116-2   Serious Bacterial Infections Associated with Bacteremia

Meningitis
Pneumonia
Pyelonephritis
Bacterial enteritis
Facial cellulitis
Septic arthritis
Osteomyelitis

infections in children. Pneumonia is most frequently viral in etiology in older infants and children, with a less than 3 percent incidence of associated bacteremia, most often due to *Streptococcus pneumoniae*. Urinary tract infection (UTI) is usually caused by *E. coli* ascending infection, with associated bacteremia most commonly noted in infants younger than 6 months. Bacterial enteritis caused by *Salmonella* sp. and facial cellulitis, septic arthritis, and osteomyelitis caused by *Staphylococcus aureus* and *S. pneumoniae* carry some risk of bacteremia in infancy. The development of generalized septicemia without a primary focus is quite rare in immunologically competent children, occurring primarily with *Neisseria meningitidis* infection.

Bacteremia may also occur in the 3- to 36-month age group without clinically recognized septicemia or focal SBI. This disease process, termed *occult bacteremia* (OB), most recently has been determined to have an incidence of 2 percent in children 3 to 36 months of age, with rectal temperatures of 39°C or higher, a well clinical appearance, and no major focal bacterial infection.[2] *Streptococcus pneumoniae* accounts for more than 80 percent of OB and carries a 5 percent risk of persistent bacteremia and a 10 percent risk of complicating SBI.[2] The recent introduction of a pneumococcal conjugated vaccine (PCV) has significantly decreased this risk. Based on clinical trials for this vaccine, the incidence of *S. pneumoniae* bacteremia and SBI are expected to decrease by up to 90 percent in fully immunized children.[3] Because the PCV is not yet universally administered, is not protective against all serotypes of *S. pneumoniae,* and definitive studies after vaccine introduction have not yet been published, this organism is expected to continue playing a significant but declining role in OB and SBI. Although *Haemophilus influenzae* type b (Hib) historically accounted for a significant proportion of complicating SBI from OB, the impact of the Hib vaccine has been dramatic in virtually eliminating this organism as a potential pathogen in adequately immunized patients.[4] Other organisms, such as *Neisseria meningitidis* and *Salmonella* sp., contribute a minority of cases of bacteremia but with a high rate of subsequent focal SBI. Although uncommon, group A *Streptococcus* has increasingly been reported as a cause of bacteremia. Primary varicella infection in immunocompetent children is a risk factor for group A *Streptococcus* bacteremia, particularly in the setting of fever persistent through the fourth day of illness.[5]

The primary issue with respect to identification and treatment of OB is the incidence of subsequent SBI. Studies conducted in the post-Hib vaccine era have demonstrated a less than 20 percent incidence of complicating SBI for those with OB. For all patients in this age group with fever but no SBI, given a 2 percent incidence of OB, this represents a less than 0.5 percent risk of complicating SBI.[2] However, no studies of complicating SBI after OB have been performed since the introduction of the pneumococcal conjugate vaccine. The present risk of OB and progression to complicating SBI in adequately immunized children is likely to be much lower.[3]

The widespread emergence of penicillin- and cephalosporin-resistant strains of *S. pneumoniae* has complicated the choice of optimal therapy for bacteremia, SBI, and meningitis in particular. Antibiotic treatment within the prior month has been demonstrated to be a risk factor for infection due to a resistant strain.[6] The emergence of poly-drug-resistant organisms in community-acquired infections has led to a national effort to reduce the use of unnecessary antibiotics.

Clinical Features

Fever, defined as a temperature greater than 38°C (>100.4°F) measured by an age-appropriate route, is a frequent presenting complaint in the ED and may be a sign of potentially serious infection in children. However, the presence and degree of fever are nonspecific for purposes of identification of bacteremia and SBI. Indeed, the absence of fever does not exclude infection, and the finding of hypothermia (temperature < 36.8°C (<98°F) may be a grave prognostic finding in the setting of sepsis.[7] Infant temperatures should be obtained by the rectal route in the ED, because the axillary and auditory canal routes are less reliable in the identification of fever. Unlike the perception of tactile fever, a history of fever measured by the parent by the rectal route carries the same significance as fever detected in the ED. To facilitate the patient's comfort and the physician's assessment of mental status, antipyretic therapy (acetaminophen 10 to 15 mg/kg or, for children 6 months or older, ibuprofen 5 to 10 mg/kg PO or PR) should be administered early in the course of ED evaluation. However, the degree of defervescence in response to antipyretic therapy is not predictive of the risk of bacteremia and SBI.

Historical risk factors for neonatally acquired bacterial infection in infants younger than 3 months include premature delivery, ruptured amniotic membranes for more than 24 h before delivery, positive prepartum maternal vaginal culture for group B *Streptococcus,* and maternal amnionitis before or after delivery. Specific symptoms suggestive of a focus of infection in this age group are rare. High fever is uncommon in this age group, and serious infection most commonly presents with low-grade fever or normal temperature. **The symptoms and signs suggestive of bacteremia and SBI in neonates and young infants most frequently produce an overall ill appearance.** Parents may report poor feeding, decreased activity, or irritability in response to attempts to console ("paradoxical irritability"). Physical examination findings suggestive of an ill appearance include poor eye contact and muscle tone, including weak suck, poor head control, and indifferent response to stimuli. Signs of respiratory distress and poor perfusion parameters are suggestive of septicemia and should be specifically sought. Although uncommon, findings suggestive of a specific focus of infection, such as otitis media, skin, soft tissue, bone, or joint inflammation, place young infants in a higher-risk group for SBI. However, due to the nonspecific nature of the signs and symptoms of illness at this age, the history and physical examination alone are unreliable screening tools for bacteremia and SBI in neonates, with marginally improved predictive value in infants 30 to 90 days old.[8]

Children 3 months and older found to have bacteremia and SBI most often are noted to have fever with rectal temperatures of 39°C or higher, although serious infection can uncommonly occur without the finding of fever. As for younger infants, the most important historical and physical findings are related to overall appearance. **Parental report of persistent lethargy or irritability with associated fever raises significant concern for SBI with associated bacteremia.** Symptoms of respiratory, gastrointestinal, soft tissue, bone, or joint inflammation should be elicited. The reader is referred to subsequent chapters for a complete description of the symptoms suggestive of focal SBI in children. Historical risk factors of importance include incomplete immunization status, prior SBI, and underlying conditions that impair immune response, such as sickle cell anemia and human immunodeficiency virus. The physical examination is performed in two phases. The first is a global assessment of the child's appearance to categorize the child as "ill" versus "well," optimally after antipyretic therapy has been administered. This assessment should specifically include mental status, evaluated by observing response to parental physical and social stimulation, and perfusion and hydration parameters. A well appearance is demonstrated by an awake, responsive infant or child with good eye contact, developmentally appropriate social interaction with family members, normal muscle tone, and vigorous cry. An ill appearance is demonstrated by lethargy or irritability, failure to respond to or be consoled by family members, weak cry, poor muscle tone, or abnormal peripheral perfusion parameters. If the examination findings are equivocal, the child should be reassessed within a short period and, if unchanged, considered "ill appearing." The performance of an overall assessment of appearance has been shown to improve the sensitivity of the history and physical examination in detecting SBI.[9] The second phase of physical examination is devoted to eliciting signs of specific SBI and minor focal infection. Signs of meningitis may be subtle and are reviewed later in this chapter. **The finding of a minor focus of infection, such as upper respiratory infection, otitis media, pharyngitis, or gastroenteritis, does not exclude the possibility of bacteremia or SBI.**

The clinical presentation of the patient at risk for OB includes age of 3 to 36 months, rectal temperature of 39°C (102°F) or higher, well appearance by the above criteria, and no other signs of infection or signs of minor focal infection only. However, only 2 percent of patients with these findings will have a positive blood culture. Further, it is impossible to distinguish well-appearing febrile children with OB from those without bacteremia by clinical features alone.[10] Conversely, a well-appearing child with an untreated rectal temperature lower than 39°C and no signs of focal SBI is at extremely low risk for bacteremia.

Diagnosis

Because of the relatively greater risk for bacteremic illness and lack of sensitivity of the clinical examination, the febrile or ill-appearing neonate, regardless of temperature, should be evaluated comprehensively for SBI by a *sepsis workup*. This workup should include complete blood count, blood culture, urinalysis and urine culture (catheterized or suprapubic technique), and cerebrospinal fluid (CSF) culture, cell count, Gram stain, and protein and glucose measurements. Respiratory symptoms or signs are indications for chest x-ray. The differential diagnosis for septic-appearing neonates includes congenital cardiac disease, metabolic disease, nonaccidental trauma, and bowel obstruction.

Infants 30 to 90 days of age are optimally evaluated by a *low-risk* versus *high-risk* stratification that combines clinical and routine laboratory assessments[11] (Table 116-3). Low-risk infants are those who were born at full term, have no underlying medical problems, and have not been treated previously with antibiotics. On physical examination, these young infants have a well appearance with no identified focus of possible bacterial infection to specifically include otitis media, skin, soft tissue, joint, or bone infection. To be considered low risk, these young infants also must have negative laboratory screening tests.

TABLE 116-3 Low-Risk Criteria for Febrile Infants 30 to 90 Days of Age

History
  Full term (≥37 wk of gestation)
  No prior infections or underlying medical problems
  No current antibiotics
Physical examination
  "Well appearance"
  No focus of infection (otitis, cellulitis, bone/joint)
Laboratory
  WBC 5000–15,000/μL with <1500 bands/μL
  Urinalysis <10 WBCs/hpf, negative for leukocyte esterase, nitrite
  Stool smear <5 WBCs/hpf (if diarrhea present)
  Normal chest x-ray (if respiratory symptoms/signs present)
Follow-up
  Reliable parents
  Home telephone and transportation

Abbreviations: hpf = high-powered field, WBC = white blood cell count.
Source: Dagan R, Powell KR, Hall CB, et al: Identification of infants unlikely to have serious bacterial infection although hospitalized for suspected sepsis. *J Pediatr* 107:855, 1985.

These are defined as white blood cell counts (WBCs) of 5000 to 15,000/μL with fewer than 1500 bands/μL, urinalysis showing fewer than 10 white blood cells per high power field, and negative findings for leukocyte esterase and nitrite, and, when diarrhea is present, a stool smear with fewer than 5 WBCs per high power field. Cultures of the blood and urine (suprapubic or catheterized) should be performed. Stool should be cultured if diarrhea is bloody or white blood cells are present, as above. A chest x-ray is indicated if there are significant respiratory findings, such as frequent cough, tachypnea, grunting respirations, rales, or wheezes. Lumbar puncture should be performed routinely in febrile infants younger than 60 days and strongly considered for those 60 to 90 days of age because of limited sensitivity of the clinical assessment at these ages for the detection of meningitis. Febrile infants 30 to 90 days of age who meet low-risk criteria have less than a 1 percent risk of bacteremia and less than a 2 percent risk of SBI. In contrast, young infants categorized as high risk with ill appearance are reported to have up to a 10 percent risk of bacteremia and a 15 percent risk of SBI.[11] Infants 30 to 90 days of age considered high risk by clinical or laboratory parameters should have a complete evaluation for sepsis, as for neonates.

The laboratory assessment of children 3 to 36 months and older should be individualized based on the overall appearance of the child, clues from the history and physical examination, and a knowledge of the incidence of bacteremia and SBI in this age group. Most importantly, an ill-appearing febrile child, regardless of age, should be stabilized and comprehensively evaluated for sepsis as just described. In contrast, the well-appearing febrile infant and child should have an directed laboratory evaluation based on clinically identified risk factors for bacteremia and associated SBI. Specifically, laboratory evaluation for pyelonephritis, pneumonia, bacterial enteritis, and bone or joint infection should be performed independently of the evaluation for bacteremia, sepsis, or meningitis.

Blood culture has limited usefulness in the outpatient management of radiographically identified pneumonia but should be considered in those patients ill enough to warrant admission. Similarly, blood cultures are indicated in febrile children 6 months or younger who have UTI and in those with clinical features of pyelonephritis requiring admission. Blood cultures are also appropriate for pediatric patients with presumed sepsis, meningitis, bacterial enteritis, facial cellulitis, septic arthritis, and osteomyelitis. All febrile patients who are immunocompromised, such as with sickle cell anemia and human immunodeficiency virus, also should have blood cultures obtained (Table 116-4). The identification of a clearly recognizable viral syndrome such as bronchiolitis or vesicular stomatitis or pharyngitis renders the yield of laboratory testing for bacteremic disease negligible.

The WBC is a nonspecific test that may assist in the identification of bacteremia and SBI but is not diagnostic and must be interpreted in the clinical context. Although the incidence of bacteremia rises with a WBC of 10,000/μL or more, there is no threshold value that distinguishes bacteremic from non-bacteremic patients or identifies patients with SBI with adequate sensitivity and specificity. A WBC of

TABLE 116-4 Indications for Blood Cultures in Children

Unexplained ill appearance, regardless of age or fever
Febrile neonates
Febrile young infants aged 30–90 d
Febrile with immune deficiency state, e.g., sickle cell disease
Sepsis
Meningitis
Pneumonia (requiring admission)
Pyelonephritis (age ≤6 mo or requiring admission)
Bacterial enteritis (age ≤24 mo)
Facial cellulitis
Septic arthritis
Osteomyelitis

5000/μL or fewer in ill-appearing infants is suggestive of overwhelming bacterial sepsis but in well-appearing infants suggests benign viral illness with transient bone marrow suppression. The choice of a WBC threshold of 15,000/μL or more for obtaining a blood culture in the setting of a well-appearing child with temperature of 39°C or higher and no or minor focus of infection represents a compromise, because this threshold will identify only 65 percent of those with OB. Moreover, only 7.5 percent of febrile, well-appearing children 3 to 36 months of age with a WBC of 15,000/μL or more will prove to be bacteremic. Decreasing the WBC threshold for obtaining a blood culture to improve sensitivity markedly decreases the specificity and predictive value of the test.[12] Other available screening tests, such as absolute neutrophil count, band count, erythrocyte sedimentation rate, and C-reactive protein, have failed to provide significantly greater sensitivity or specificity for the identification of bacteremia. Although the blood culture is the "gold standard" for the identification of bacteremia, its result usually cannot be predicted by a screening test with any degree of confidence at the time of initial ED evaluation. The pursuit of OB or finding of a minor focus of bacterial infection, such as otitis media, should not distract emergency physicians from evaluating febrile young children for symptoms or signs of focal serious bacterial infection.

Treatment

EMERGENCY   The treatment plan for febrile infants, like the diagnostic evaluation, must be stratified by patient age and directed toward the age-related and organ system-specific probable pathogens (Figures 116-1 and 116-2 and Table 116-5). Febrile neonates, after being fully evaluated for sepsis, should be stabilized with supportive care and treated with broad-spectrum IV antibiotics to cover group B *Strepto-*

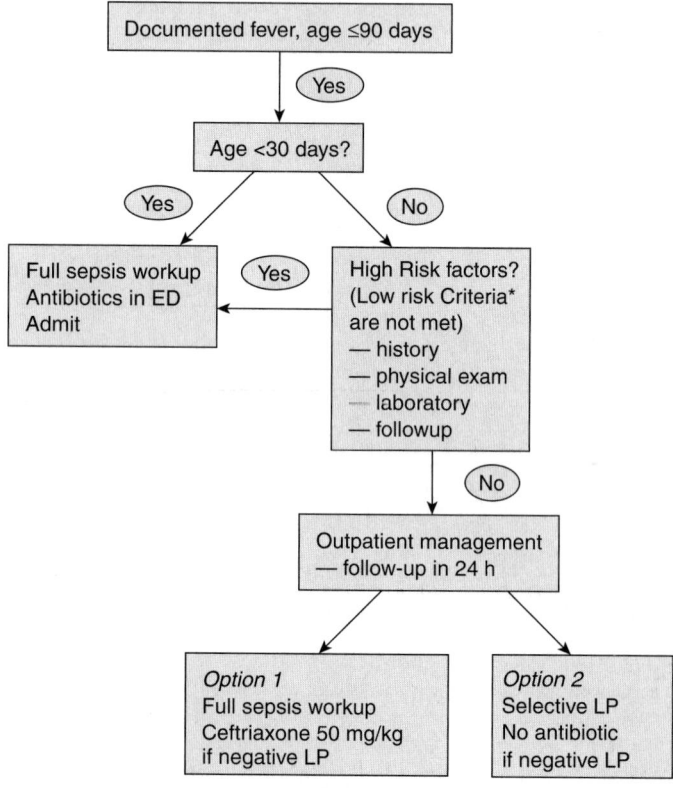

*See Table 116-3

FIG. 116-1. Management scheme for febrile infants 0 to 90 days of age.

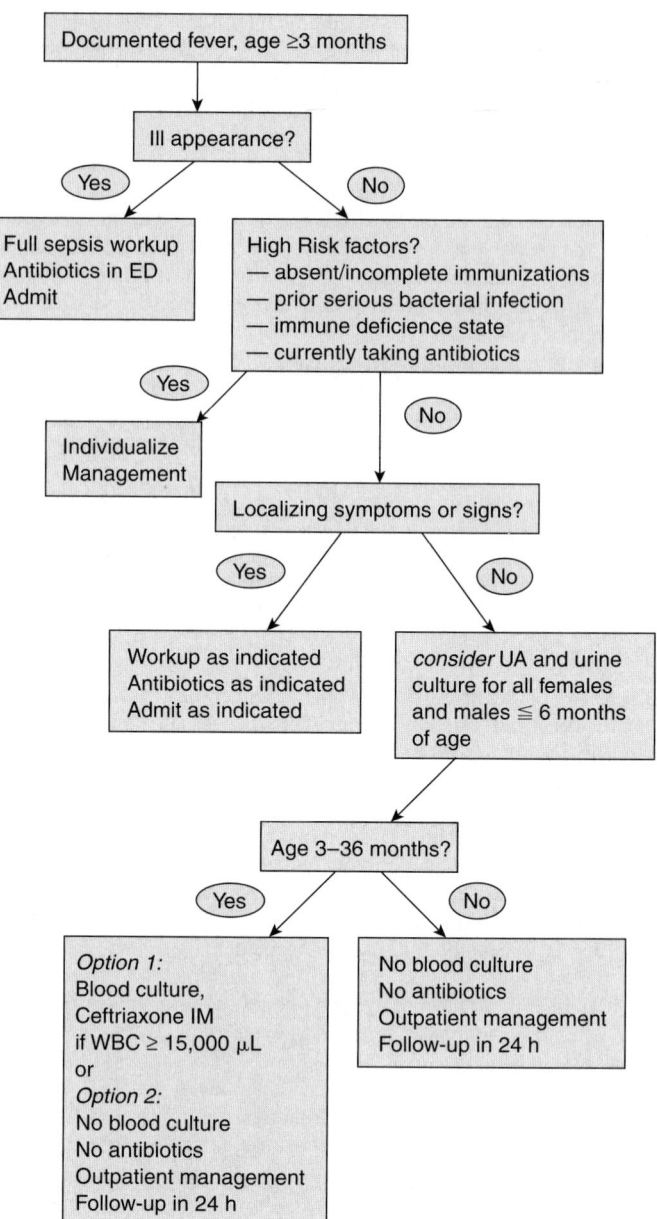

FIG. 116-2. Management scheme for febrile infants and children 3 months and older.

coccus, E. coli, L. monocytogenes, and *Enterococcus* sp. pending culture results. Optimal therapy includes ampicillin, 100 mg/kg per d, and cefotaxime or ceftriaxone, 50 mg/kg IV per d, with initial doses given in the ED before admission. Jaundiced neonates should not be treated with ceftriaxone, because this agent may displace protein-bound bilirubin.

Young infants 30 to 90 days of age considered to be high risk for SBI based on the foregoing clinical or laboratory parameters should be similarly evaluated for sepsis and treated with ampicillin and cefotaxime or ceftriaxone to cover neonatally and community-acquired pathogens. Young infants 30 to 90 days of age considered low risk for SBI based on clinical and laboratory parameters may be reasonably managed as outpatients in two ways, if follow-up is feasible based on the physician's judgment of parental reliability and availability of a home telephone and source of transportation. The more traditional and conservative approach is to perform a lumbar puncture on all such young infants to exclude bacterial and aseptic meningitis definitively and treat with ceftriaxone, 50 mg/kg per d intramuscularly, before discharge. Alternatively, it has been shown that well-appearing infants in

TABLE 116-5   Initial Intravenous Antibiotic Dosages for Bacteremia, Sepsis, and Meningitis

Age Group	Occult Bacteremia	Sepsis*	Meningitis
Neonates	Not applicable	Ampicillin, 100 mg/kg *plus* Cefotaxime, 50 mg/kg *or* Ceftriaxone, 50mg/kg	Ampicillin, 100 mg/kg *plus* Cefotaxime, 50 mg/kg *or* Ceftriaxone, 50 mg/kg
Young infants (30–90 d)	Not applicable	Ampicillin, 100 mg/kg *plus* Cefotaxime, 50 mg/kg *or* Ceftriaxone, 50 mg/kg *plus consider* Vancomycin, 15 mg/kg†	Ampicillin, 100 mg/kg *plus* Cefotaxime, 100 mg/kg *or* Ceftriaxome, 100 mg/kg *plus* Vancomycin, 15 mg/kg‡
Older infants and children	Ceftriaxone, 50 mg/kg§	Cefotaxime, 50 mg/kg *or* Ceftriaxone, 50 mg/kg *plus consider* Vancomycin, 15 mg/kg*	Cefotaxime, 100 mg/kg *or* Ceftriaxone, 100 mg/kg *plus* Vancomycin, 15 mg/kg†

*Use meningitis doses if the patient is considered too unstable for lumbar puncture in the emergency department.
†Consider addition of vancomycin in sepsis only with critical illness.
‡Add vancomycin only if there is evidence of bacterial meningitis in the cerebrospinal fluid.
§May be given IM.

this age group considered low risk may be safely managed as outpatients with selective lumbar puncture and without antibiotics, provided strict adherence to clinical, laboratory, and follow-up criteria is maintained.[13]

The treatment of febrile infants 3 to 36 months of age remains a subject of considerable controversy. As for all infants, an ill-appearing febrile child should be stabilized with supportive care and fully evaluated for sepsis, and broad-spectrum IV antibiotics such as cefotaxime or ceftriaxone should be administered in the ED. Fortunately, most penicillin- and cephalosporin-resistant strains of *S. pneumoniae* demonstrate only intermediate resistance at this time and may be adequately treated with a third-generation cephalosporin. Treatment of focal SBI presumptively identified by diagnostic testing in the ED depends on the likely pathogens and is reviewed in subsequent chapters. Treatment of meningitis is reviewed later in this chapter. The optimal treatment for children at risk for OB has not been established. Published observational retrospective studies,[14] prospective randomized trials,[15,16] and meta-analyses of pertinent prior studies[17] have concluded that expectant antibiotic treatment of patients at risk for OB results in a shorter duration of fever and a lower rate of subsequent focal SBI. However, no study has shown that oral antibiotics alter the rate of subsequent development of meningitis. Initial therapy for pediatric patients at risk for OB with ceftriaxone, 50 mg/kg IM, has been recommended because of a reported significant reduction in the incidence of subsequent culture-positive meningitis as compared with oral antibiotics or observation without therapy.[14,17] However, critical reviews of these studies have shown significant methodologic flaws that seriously undermine the conclusion that antibiotic therapy prevents subsequent SBI, in particular the failure to include partially treated meningitis as an adverse outcome. At the present time, there is no standard of care for the treatment of well-appearing febrile children 3 to 36 months of age who are at risk for OB. Independent of other diagnostic considerations, reasonable approaches for treatment of possible OB include (1) blood culture if WBC is at least 15,000/µL, followed by ceftriaxone, 50 mg/kg IM, and (2) no blood culture and antibiotic therapy only for identified bacterial infection, in either case with follow-up within 24 h. The second approach is more completely justified if the patient is known to have had two or more doses of the PCV and Hib vaccines. If antibiotic treatment for OB is chosen, emergency physicians should be wary of the efficacy of antibiotic treatment in

preventing focal SBI and the potential for delayed diagnosis for partially treated infection with altered presentation, for example, UTI or meningitis.[18]

OUTPATIENT   Follow-up within 24 h and clear instructions regarding indications for early return are the cornerstones of management of well-appearing febrile infants 3 to 36 months of age. Young infants 30 to 90 days of age may be similarly managed as outpatients if all "low-risk" clinical, laboratory and follow-up criteria are met. Communication with a patient's primary physician to facilitate such follow-up represents optimal management. In the absence of a primary physician, consideration should be given to performing such follow-up in the ED. The parents should be educated regarding the effective use of antipyretics and instructed to return with the child to the ED immediately for symptoms of ill appearance suggestive of SBI. Patients who return to the ED with the report of a positive blood culture for *S. pneumoniae* and who are afebrile and well appearing on follow-up may be managed as outpatients with repeat blood culture, oral antibiotic therapy, and follow-up in 24 h.

ADMISSION   All febrile neonates and ill-appearing infants should be admitted for observation and parenteral antibiotic treatment pending culture results. Young infants 30 to 90 days of age who fail to meet "low-risk" criteria also should be admitted and treated. Infants 3 months or older who return to the ED with (1) a report of any gram-negative organism on blood culture or (2) persistent fever or ill appearance with a report of positive blood culture for *S. pneumoniae* should have a complete evaluation for sepsis, parenteral antibiotic therapy in the ED, and admission for continued treatment.

SEPSIS

Pathophysiology

Sepsis is a life-threatening clinical syndrome defined by bacteremia with clinical evidence of invasive, systemic infection that can progress with variable rapidity to circulatory failure. Sepsis can occur in isolation or with focal bacterial disease, such as meningitis. The pathophysiology of sepsis is related to (1) colonization with a bacterial pathogen, usually nasopharyngeal, (2) invasion of the blood by encapsulated organisms and release of inflammatory mediators, and (3) host defense-response failure. This process results in systemic manifestations that are clinically detectable. Circulatory consequences may include alteration in systemic vascular tone and decreased myocardial contractility. Neurologic effects include decreased cerebral perfusion pressure and abnormal temperature homeostasis. Sepsis also may result in a microvascular angiopathy and disseminated intravascular coagulopathy involving the kidneys, lungs, skin, and central nervous system (CNS).

Host defense risk factors for sepsis include impaired splenic function (e.g., congenital absence, surgical removal, or functional impairment in sickle hemoglobinopathy) and congenital metabolic disease (e.g., galactosemia), and the rarer primary or acquired humoral and cellular immunodeficiency states. The presence of an indwelling foreign body or obstruction to drainage of a body cavity represents additional risk factors.

The likely pathogens for sepsis demonstrate an age-related distribution. In the first month of life, group B *Streptococcus* and *E. coli* dominate and can cause an explosive sepsis syndrome that may increasingly be recognized in the ED with the trend to early newborn discharge. The risk presented by these organisms falls dramatically by the third month of life. In infancy and early childhood, *N. meningitidis* predominates as the pathogen for sepsis, with life-long peak incidence during this age. *Streptococcus pneumoniae* is more likely to cause focal disease but may also result in sepsis syndrome, particularly with sickle cell disease and other causes of asplenia. In school-age children, *N. meningitidis* predominates as the cause of sepsis, but group A *Streptococcus* has increasingly been implicated. Rocky Mountain spotted fever, caused by *Rickettsia rickettsii* and acquired by tick bite in endemic areas of the United States, must not be overlooked as a possible cause of sepsis in the summer and fall seasons.

Clinical Features

The sepsis syndrome may present with a subtle or obvious, rapidly progressive clinical picture. Neurologic symptoms most frequently include altered mental status, with irritability, confusion, or lethargy. Poor feeding, lack of spontaneous motor activity, and hypotonia are common findings. Hyperpyrexia, defined as a rectal temperature higher than 41°C (106°F), may occur, although this is not specific for sepsis. Hypothermia also may occur in sepsis, particularly in infants younger than 3 months, and is a grave prognostic finding.[7] Tachypnea and retractions may reflect hypoxia, metabolic acidosis, or underlying pneumonia. Early septic shock is accompanied by subtle findings of resting tachycardia, widened pulse pressure, warm distal extremities, and brisk capillary refill. Subsequently, classic signs of hemodynamic compensation occur, including weak distal pulses, delayed capillary refill, and cool extremities. Ultimately, these are followed by signs of decompensation with decreased sensorium and hypotension. Cutaneous findings may include petechiae, which may progress to coalescent purpura over hours to days.

Diagnosis

Sepsis represents a *clinical* diagnosis of exclusion in the ED, pending the results of cultures and treatment, because of the potential for rapid progression of disease. Obvious septic shock rarely presents a problem of diagnosis but rather of management. In more subtle cases, the combination of altered mental status and abnormal vital signs should suggest to the emergency physician the possibility of sepsis. Because of the characteristically nonspecific presentation, febrile or ill-appearing neonates should be considered septic until proven otherwise.

No laboratory test is diagnostic, although a WBC greater than 20,000/μL is supportive of bacterial sepsis. However, a WBC in the "normal" range in an ill-appearing child is not reassuring. A WBC smaller than 5000/μL or a platelet count smaller than 150,000/μL is a grave prognostic sign, particularly for disease due to *N. meningitidis*.[7]

The diagnostic evaluation of septic-appearing infants in the ED should routinely include a complete blood count, electrolyte panel, blood glucose level, and urinalysis. Cultures of the blood and urine should be obtained by sterile technique. Diarrheal stool, if present, should be stained for white blood cells and cultured. A chest x-ray is indicated for signs of respiratory distress or critical illness, and arterial blood gas measurement should be considered. Liver and renal functions, coagulation studies, and fibrin split product analysis should be considered for critically ill children. Lumbar puncture should be performed to obtain CSF for culture, cell count, protein, and glucose. Lumbar puncture should be deferred if the patient has an unstable airway or a respiratory or hemodynamic status demanding resuscitation. Gram-stained smears made from CSF and petechial scrapings may provide immediate diagnostic information regarding the identity of the organism.

The differential diagnosis for a "septic-appearing" child includes infectious, cardiac, metabolic, and traumatic disease. Major focal bacterial infections, such as meningitis and pericarditis, and systemic viral disease (e.g., respiratory syncytial virus) may present with findings of fever, altered mental status, and cardiorespiratory compromise. Young infants with congenital heart disease or viral myocarditis may present in cardiogenic shock with respiratory distress and signs of poor perfusion. Toxic ingestion, diabetic ketoacidosis, and congenital metabolic disease may present with altered mental status as the major complaint. Child abuse with head or abdominal injury may present with altered mental status, temperature instability, and signs of poor perfusion without historical or cutaneous evidence of trauma.

Treatment

EMERGENCY Stabilization must take priority over completion of the diagnostic workup. Restoration of oxygenation and perfusion are the first priorities in the initial management of sepsis. An ill-appearing child should be provided high-flow oxygen and continuous monitoring of heart rate, respirations, and blood pressure, and oxygen saturation should be initiated. Attention to airway patency should continue throughout the assessment, with particular emphasis during procedures such as lumbar puncture. Secure vascular access should be obtained early, and, in the setting of signs of poor perfusion, fluid resuscitation should be done with multiple 20 mL/kg boluses of NS with serial reassessments. In such cases, an indwelling Foley catheter should be placed to ensure adequate response to fluid resuscitation by establishment of urine output of 1 to 2 mL/kg per h. In young infants in particular, hypoglycemia should be identified early by bedside testing and corrected with IV 25 percent dextrose (D25 or 25 g/100 mL) as a 0.5 g/kg bolus. Endotracheal intubation and mechanical ventilation are indicated if a patient is judged to have advanced respiratory or circulatory failure or neurologic compromise with potential for loss of airway control. Intubation also should be considered for septic-appearing patients who require interhospital transport. If serial fluid bolus therapy does not restore evidence of adequate perfusion, inotropic support with dopamine in the setting of normal blood pressure or epinephrine in hypotensive states is indicated.

Antibiotic therapy should initiated in the ED as soon as possible and should not be withheld pending lumbar puncture if the patient is too unstable for this procedure. Antibiotic selection is made according to the likely age-related pathogens (see Table 116-5). In the first 2 months of life, ampicillin, 100 mg/kg, and cefotaxime or ceftriaxone, 50 mg/kg IV, are indicated. Adequate initial therapy for children 3 months and older is cefotaxime or ceftriaxone, 50 mg/kg IV. These doses should be doubled if meningitis has not been excluded by lumbar puncture, to facilitate CSF drug delivery. Because of the widespread emergence of penicillin- and cephalosporin-resistant strains of *S. pneumoniae*, vancomycin, 15 mg/kg IV, should be considered as part of the initial therapy for critically ill, septic children, particularly in the setting of an underlying immune deficiency state.[19] In endemic areas during the summer and early fall, doxycycline, 4 mg/kg IV, should be considered for septic children with possible Rocky Mountain spotted fever. Care must be taken to monitor patients after antibiotic administration for abrupt vascular collapse due to acute bacterial lysis with release of endotoxins.

ADMISSION   All children with suspicion for bacterial sepsis should be admitted for monitoring and treatment pending culture results. Disposition decision-making for a possibly septic child must specifically include choice of the appropriate pediatric inpatient unit. A child with limited suspicion for sepsis who is alert and requires no cardiorespiratory stabilization in the ED may be admitted to a pediatric floor unit for antibiotic therapy pending culture results. A child with evidence of cardiorespiratory or neurologic compromise requiring stabilization in the ED should be admitted to a pediatric intensive care unit (PICU) because of the risk of progression of disease. If interhospital transfer to a PICU is necessary, a pediatric transport team should be used.

MENINGITIS

Pathophysiology

In most cases, bacterial meningitis occurs as a complication of a primary bacteremia. The inflammatory response to the products of bacterial multiplication may result in alteration of the permeability of the blood-brain barrier, with extension of infection and inflammation to the brain itself. The resulting brain edema, increased intracranial pressure, decreased cerebral blood flow, and vascular thrombosis produce neuronal injury. Less commonly, meningitis occurs by the hematogenous route from a distant primary focal infection, direct extension from adjacent infection, or after head injury with cribriform plate fracture. The incidence of meningitis is highest between the ages of birth and 2 years, with age-related peak risks during the neonatal period and between 3 and 8 months. Host defense factors resulting in impaired splenic function or immunodeficiency are associated with increased risk for sepsis and meningitis.

The pathogenic organisms responsible for bacterial meningitis parallel those responsible for sepsis. In the neonatal period, group B *Streptococcus* and *E. coli* predominate. In older infants and children, *S. pneumoniae* and *N. meningitidis* are the likely pathogens. Although penicillin-resistant strains of *S. pneumoniae* are increasing in frequency, there is no evidence that these organisms are more virulent.[20] Infants and children who have not received the Hib vaccine continue to be at risk for Hib meningitis.

Clinical Features

Because the presenting symptoms are subtle and overlap with those of less serious infection, a high index of suspicion for meningitis is crucial. Two modes of presentation are seen. The most frequently encountered pattern is an insidious progression of a febrile illness over several days. Less commonly, a fulminant progression to septic shock and meningitis may occur over hours, most commonly caused by group B *Streptococcus* in neonates and young infants and *N. meningitidis* in young infants and older children.

Symptoms and signs of bacterial meningitis depend on the patient's age, duration of illness, and pretreatment with antibiotics. No single complaint or physical finding is specific. However, the findings of fever associated with altered mental status constitute a reasonable basis for suspicion for meningitis. Infants typically present with nonspecific symptoms including decreased responsiveness, poor feeding, and vomiting. Although common, fever is not universally present at the time of diagnosis. Symptoms and signs of "paradoxical irritability" despite parental comforting attempts, decreased responsiveness to

age-appropriate stimuli, vomiting, hypotonia, bulging fontanelle, or respiratory distress may be seen. Older children usually will complain of headache, photophobia, nausea, and vomiting. As for infants, signs of lethargy and confusion are primary indicators for suspicion of meningitis, and fever may not be consistently present. Nuchal rigidity and the classic findings of the Kernig sign (neck pain elicited with passive knee extension) and the Brudzinski sign (involuntary lower extremity flexion elicited with passive neck flexion) are helpful only if positive. Seizures occur early in 25 percent of patients with bacterial meningitis and are typically initially generalized but may be focal.[20] Focal neurologic findings, focal or prolonged seizures, and presentation with obtundation or coma suggest an adverse outcome. Pretreatment with oral antibiotics is associated with an altered presentation characterized by less consistent findings of fever or altered level of consciousness and longer duration of symptoms before diagnosis.[18]

Diagnosis

On the basis of reasonable clinical suspicion, a lumbar puncture must be performed to make or exclude the diagnosis of meningitis. The blood WBC is not an adequate screen for meningitis. In the absence of fever, computed tomography of the brain may be necessary to exclude intracranial mass lesion before lumbar puncture. If meningitis is strongly suspected, computed tomography should not delay antibiotic therapy. The CSF should be obtained for culture and sensitivity, protein and glucose levels, cell count, and Gram stain. Cerebrospinal fluid leukocytosis with a predominance of polymorphonucleocytes, CSF protein level greater than 100 mg/mL, and CSF glucose level less than 50 percent of blood glucose level are considered positive screening test results for bacterial meningitis. *Listeria* may be associated with CSF lymphocytosis. The Gram stain has a 70 percent sensitivity for preliminary identification of the offending organism and should be reported as soon as available. Because of the emergence of penicillin-resistant strains of *S. pneumoniae,* perform CSF latex agglutination for bacterial antigens on all patients with abnormal CSF to identify high-risk patients. If prior treatment with antibiotics has occurred, the emergency physician should have a lower threshold for performing a lumbar puncture, and bacterial antigen techniques are routinely indicated, because these are often essential to diagnosis. A complete blood count, electrolyte panel, blood glucose, urinalysis, and cultures of blood and urine should be obtained before performing the lumbar puncture. Indications for deferring lumbar puncture in the ED include cardiorespiratory compromise or risk of increased intracranial pressure. In such cases, antibiotic therapy should be given in the ED, and lumbar puncture should be performed as soon as possible in the inpatient setting.

The differential diagnosis for bacterial meningitis includes the same spectrum of systemic disease as described for sepsis. *Aseptic meningitis* refers to evidence of meningeal inflammation with negative CSF cultures and is more common than bacterial meningitis. Most frequently, this is due to viral meningeal infection, but other causes, such as tuberculosis or syphilis, should be considered. Parameningeal infection or brain abscess may rarely mimic the presentation and laboratory features of meningitis. Central nervous system mass lesion, nonaccidental head injury, and toxic drug ingestion also should be considered in afebrile patients.

Treatment

EMERGENCY   As for clinically septic children, treatment for bacterial meningitis begins with stabilization of oxygenation, ventilation, and perfusion parameters. Provision of supplemental oxygen and monitoring of heart rate and oxygen saturation during and after lumbar puncture are appropriate, with careful attention to prevention of airway compromise during the procedure. Children with meningitis are often septic and may require vigorous initial isotonic fluid bolus therapy to restore systemic and CNS perfusion. However, subsequent fluid should be provided at a maintenance rate to minimize brain edema. Neurologic complications are frequent and must be treated aggressively to prevent secondary CNS injury. Seizures are treated with lorazepam, 0.1 mg/kg IV, and, if necessary, phosphenytoin, 15 mg/kg, or phenobarbital, 10 mg/kg IV, with correction of hypoglycemia or other underlying metabolic disorder. Severe respiratory distress and decreasing mental status with risk of loss of control of airway protective reflexes should prompt elective endotracheal intubation. Increased intracranial pressure is treated with mannitol, 1 g/kg IV. Hyperventilation has fallen into disfavor.

Empirical antibiotic therapy for the likely age-related pathogens should be initiated as soon as possible in the ED. Recommended antibiotic dosages are higher with meningitis, because of poor drug penetration across the blood-brain barrier and concern for the possibility of antibiotic resistance. In the first 3 months of life, ampicillin, 200 mg/kg, and cefotaxime or ceftriaxone, 100 mg/kg IV, are indicated. Children 3 months and older should receive cefotaxime or ceftriaxone, 100 mg/kg (maximum, 2 g) IV (see Table 116-5). Due to the widespread emergence of penicillin- and cephalosporin-resistant strains of *S. pneumoniae*, vancomycin, 15 mg/kg IV, also should be administered routinely as initial therapy to children older than 1 month who have presumed bacterial meningitis.[19]

Steroid therapy has been shown to decrease the incidence of neurologic complications significantly in bacterial meningitis due to Hib, if given before or at the time of initial antibiotic therapy. However, this benefit has not been demonstrated for meningitis due to *S. pneumoniae* or *N. meningitidis,* and steroid therapy may actually worsen neurologic sequelae. Current guidelines are to *consider* steroid therapy in cases of suspected bacterial meningitis, specifically dexamethasone, 0.15 mg/kg IV, before or immediately after the initial antibiotic dose to children 1 month or older (www.cispimmunize.org/applicationT. clm?filem-/cisp/pro/hib/hib_inf.html).[19,21]

Prophylaxis of contacts to eliminate carriage of organisms from the upper respiratory tract is indicated after identification of an index case of meningitis caused by organisms capable of causing epidemic disease. For Hib disease, a regimen of rifampin, 20 mg/kg (maximum, 600 mg), once per day for 4 days is indicated for (1) household members if there is a home contact younger than 4 years and (2) day-care center staff and enrollees resembling households, defined as children younger than 2 years with contact of 25 h per week or more. For *N. meningitidis* disease, a regimen of rifampin, 10 mg/kg (maximum, 600 mg), twice per day for 2 days is indicated for all household members, day-care center contacts, and medical personnel who have had direct physical exposure to the index case before antibiotic therapy. There is no indication or effective prophylaxis for *S. pneumoniae* disease.

ADMISSION   All pediatric patients with identified or presumed meningitis should be admitted for supportive care, monitoring for complications, and antibiotic therapy. As for sepsis, the disposition decision for children with meningitis also must include choice of the appropriate pediatric inpatient unit. Stable patients may be admitted to a monitored isolation bed on a pediatric floor unit for antibiotic therapy pending culture results. Children with evidence of cardiorespiratory or neurologic compromise should be admitted to a PICU, because of the risk of progression of disease. If transfer of such a patient is necessary, a pediatric transport team should be used for referral to a tertiary care center.

REFERENCES

1. Bonadio WA, Webster H, Wolfe A, et al: Correlating infectious outcome with clinical parameters of 1130 consecutive febrile infants aged zero to eight weeks. *Pediatr Emerg Care* 9:84, 1993.
2. Alpern ER, Alessandrini EA, Bell LM, et al: Occult bacteremia from a pediatric emergency department: Current prevalence, time to detection and outcome. *Pediatrics* 106:505, 2000.
3. Black SB, Shinefield HR, Hansen J, et al: Postlicensure evaluation of the effectiveness of seven valent pneumococcal conjugate vaccine. *Pediatr Infect Dis J* 20:1105, 2001.
4. Adams WG, Deaver KA, Plikaytis BD, et al: Decline of childhood *Haemophilus influenzae* type b (Hib) disease in the Hib vaccine era. *JAMA* 269:221, 1993.
5. Doctor A, Harper MB, Fleisher GR: Group A beta-hemolytic streptococcal bacteremia: Historical overview, changing incidence, and recent association with varicella. *Pediatrics* 96:428, 1995.
6. Tan TQ, Mason EO, Kaplan SL: Penicillin-resistant systemic pneumococcal infections in children: A retrospective case-control study. *Pediatrics* 92:761, 1993.
7. Wong VK, Hitchcock W, Mason WH: Meningococcal infections in children: A review of 100 cases. *Pediatr Infect Dis J* 8:224–227, 1989.
8. Baker MD, Avner JR, Bell LM: Failure of infant observation scales in detecting serious illness in febrile 4- to 8-week-old infants. *Pediatrics* 85:1040, 1990.
9. McCarthy PL, Lembo RM, Fink HD, et al: Observation, history, and physical examination in diagnosis of serious illnesses in febrile children ≤ 24 months. *J Pediatr* 110:26, 1987.
10. Teach SJ, Fleisher GR: Efficacy of an observation scale in detecting bacteremia in febrile children three to thirty-six months of age, treated as outpatients. *J Pediatr* 126:877, 1995.
11. Dagan R, Powell KR, Hall CB, et al: Identification of infants unlikely to have serious bacterial infection although hospitalized for suspected sepsis. *J Pediatr* 107:855, 1985.
12. Jaffe DM, Fleisher GR: Temperature and total white blood cell count as indicators of bacteremia. *Pediatrics* 87:670, 1991.
13. Baker MD, Bell LM, Avner JR: Outpatient management without antibiotics of fever in selected infants. *New Engl J Med* 329:1437, 1993.
14. Harper MB, Bachur R, Fleisher GR: Effect of antibiotic therapy on the outcome of outpatients with unsuspected bacteremia. *Pediatr Infect Dis J* 14:760, 1995.
15. Bass JW, Steele RW, Wittler RR, et al: Antimicrobial treatment of occult bacteremia: A multicenter cooperative study. *Pediatr Infect Dis J* 12:466, 1993.
16. Fleisher GR, Rosenberg N, Vinci R, et al: Intramuscular versus oral antibiotic therapy for the prevention of meningitis and other bacterial sequelae in young, febrile children at risk for occult bacteremia. *J Pediatr* 124:504, 1994.
17. Baraff LJ, Oslund S, Prather M: Effect of antibiotic therapy and etiologic microorganism on the risk of bacterial meningitis in children with occult bacteremia. *Pediatrics* 92:140, 1993.
18. Rothrock SG, Green SM, Wren J, et al: Pediatric bacterial meningitis: Is prior antibiotic therapy associated with an altered clinical presentation? *Ann Emerg Med* 21:146, 1992.
19. American Academy of Pediatrics, Committee on Infectious Diseases: Therapy for children with invasive pneumococcal infections. *Pediatrics* 99:289, 1997.
20. Arditi M, Mason EO, Bradley JS, et al: Three-year multicenter surveillance of pneumococcal meningitis in children: Clinical characteristics and outcome related to penicillin susceptibility and dexamethasone use. *Pediatrics* 102:1087, 1998.
21. Red Book 2001. American Academy of Pediatrics. *Haemophilus influenzae* infections, 2001.

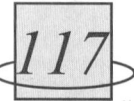

COMMON NEONATAL PROBLEMS
Tonia J. Brousseau
Niranjan Kissoon

The assessment of neonates in the ED is more difficult than that of older children and adults. Symptoms are usually vague and nonspecific. Signs are usually subtle and, even when recognized, may not be helpful in pinpointing a diagnosis. For example, respiratory distress may be due to primary respiratory or cardiac disease, generalized sepsis, abdominal pathology, or metabolic derangements. Examination of neonates is time consuming and requires special skills in the approach to the infant and the anxious parent.

The prerequisites for the proper evaluation of neonates are a great deal of patience and an appreciation of the marked variations in normal vegetative functions. Many visits are initiated because of parental concerns related to feeding patterns; weight gain; stool frequency, color, and consistency; and breathing patterns. Physicians involved in the care of neonates in the ED therefore should be knowledgeable about patterns of normal vegetative functions in neonates. Routine early discharge from the newborn nursery has increased the number of ED visits for issues that previously would have been recognized and addressed before discharge. This trend requires a more thorough knowledge of neonatal issues by the emergency physician.[1]

NORMAL VEGETATIVE FUNCTIONS

Feeding Patterns

The feeding of infants requires practical interpretation of specific nutritional needs and the widely varying limits of a normal baby's appetite and behavior regarding food. Variation in times between feedings is to be expected in the first few weeks during the establishment of a self-regulation plan. By the end of first month, more than 90 percent of infants establish a suitable and reasonably regular schedule. Most healthy bottle-fed infants want six to nine feedings every 24 h by the end of the first week of life; breast-fed infants prefer shorter intervals.[2,3]

Feedings should be considered as having progressed satisfactorily if the infant is no longer losing weight by 5 to 7 days and is gaining weight by 12 to 14 days. Parents usually need reassurance that their infant is obtaining adequate nutrition because of the wide variation in the intakes of normal infants. It is important to appreciate that infants cry for reasons other than hunger and that they need not be fed every time they cry.

Weight Gain

Although it is difficult to precisely judge the caloric intake of breast-fed infants and feeding frequency varies widely, intake is adequate if the neonate is gaining weight appropriately and appears content between feedings. Normal newborns may lose 5 to 10 percent of their birth weight during the first 3 to 7 days of life. A weight loss of up to 10 percent is acceptable if the infant's examination and behavior are normal. On average, infants gain between 20 and 30 g per d in the first 3 months of life and between 15 and 20 g per d for the next several months. It is important to weigh the infant completely undressed.

An infant's weight between 3 and 12 months of age can be calculated approximately by the following formula:

$$\frac{\text{age (months)} + 9}{2} = \text{expected weight (kg)}$$

Although plotting the infant's weight on a growth chart is preferred, this formula provides a reasonable reference of expected weight between 3 and 12 months of age in the ED.

Stool Patterns

The number, color, and consistency of bowel movements can change greatly in the same infant and across infants regardless of diet or environment. Breast-fed infants frequently will produce six or seven stools per day, whereas formula-fed infants generally produce one to two stools per day. The stools of breast-fed infants are softer than those of elemental or breast-fed infants. An excessive intake of human milk or maternal use of laxatives further increases the water content of the infant's stool. Overfeeding or use of formula that is too concentrated or too high in sugar content also can produce loose stools.[2]

Stool color has no significance unless blood is present. Occasionally, an infant may not have a bowel movement on a given day. The first stool, which consists of meconium, is usually passed within the first 24 h after birth. Transition stools, which are greenish brown, ap-

pear after initiation of milk feeding and are replaced by typical milk stools 3 to 4 days later. Infrequent bowel movements do not necessarily mean constipation, because breast-fed infants may occasionally go 5 to 7 days without a bowel movement. A history of not passing meconium in the first 48 h of life may be suggestive of Hirschsprung disease.

Breathing Patterns

The normal respiratory rate is 30 to 60 breaths/min in infants. For premature infants, the rate is higher and fluctuates more widely. Because fluctuations occur rapidly, the respiratory rate should be counted for a full minute with the infant in full resting state, preferably asleep. A rate consistently over 60 breaths/min during periods of regular breathing should be evaluated further.

Because the breathing of newborn infants is almost entirely diaphragmatic, the soft front of the thorax usually is drawn inward during inspiration while the abdomen protrudes. In a quiet infant, this paradoxical pattern has no clinical significance; however, when it changes to predominantly thoracic breathing, intra-abdominal or intrathoracic pathology should be suspected. Alternatively, an increase in abdominal breathing suggests pulmonary disease.

Newborn infants, especially those born prematurely, may exhibit periodic breathing characterized by alternating periods of a normal rate and periods of a markedly slow rate of respiration, with pauses of more times for 3 s or longer. Such alternating respiratory patterns have been observed in 30 to 95 percent of premature babies during sleep, but less frequently in term infants. Periods of apnea longer than 20 s or accompanied by bradycardia or cyanosis should be evaluated.

Sleeping Patterns

Infants are not born with the ability to sleep through the night. Instead, they awaken every 20 min to 6 h, and sleep periods are spread evenly across the day and night. By 3 months of age, most of their sleep occurs at night, and by 6 months, most infants are sleeping through the night.

Night waking is defined as waking and crying once or more between midnight and 5 am for at least 4 of 7 nights per week for at least 4 consecutive weeks. This occurs in approximately 25 percent of infants usually younger than 12 months. This prevalence rises to about 50 percent among breast-fed infants. When the child cries during the night, parents can check to ensure that there is no physical reason for the crying. Having determined that there is no physical problem, parents should ignore the crying so that the child learns to fall asleep on its own. If parents usually feed the child at that time and the child is older than approximately 6 months, the volume of the night feedings should be tapered until they are discontinued and all nourishment is given during the daytime.[3]

REASONS FOR EMERGENCY DEPARTMENT VISITS

A review of presenting complaints in our pediatric ED, a tertiary-care referral center, over a 6-month period indicated the spectrum most likely to be seen by the emergency physician (Table 117-1). Complaints in neonates are usually not single; rather, they are often symptom complexes. Such symptom complexes reflect the nonspecific nature of signs and symptoms in neonates and the similar presentation of many diseases of diverse etiology.

Crying, Irritability, and Lethargy

The symptom complex of crying, irritability, and lethargy is fairly common yet difficult to treat, even in the presence of an identifiable cause. Most neonates exhibit varying degrees and periods of crying

TABLE 117-1   **Common Presenting Complaints**

Crying, irritability, lethargy (see Table 117-2)
Gastrointestinal tract symptoms
    Feeding difficulties
    Regurgitation
    Vomiting
    Diarrhea
    Abdominal distention
    Constipation
Cardiorespiratory symptoms
    Rapid breathing
    Cough and nasal congestion
    Noisy breathing and stridor
    Apnea, periodic breathing
    Blue spells, cyanosis
Jaundice
Eye discharge, redness
Diaper rash, oral thrush
Fever and sepsis
Sudden infant death

during a 24-h period. However, infants who present with an episode of acute, inconsolable crying should be observed closely for an underlying cause (Table 117-2).

Intestinal Colic

Colic is a paroxysm of crying for 3 h per d or more for 3 days/week or more over a 3-week period and causes significant parental distress. The incidence of colic is about 13 percent, with no seasonal variation. Colic is a symptom complex consisting of the sudden onset of paroxysmal crying lasting several hours, a flushed face, circumoral pallor, tense abdomen, drawn up legs, cold feet, and clenched fists. It may begin as early as the first week of life but seldom lasts beyond 3 to 4 months of age. A careful history is important in the diagnosis of colic; findings at physical examination are normal, and laboratory tests are not required. However, when the diagnosis is unclear, a careful history, physical examination, and appropriate laboratory investigations are necessary to rule out conditions listed in Table 117-2. In doubtful situations, admission for observation or return for reassessment is reasonable.

The cause of colic is unknown. Proposed causes include excessive intake of air, insufficient intake of fluid, allergy to protein, and mater-

TABLE 117-2   **Conditions Associated with Uncontrollable Crying, Irritability, and/or Lethargy in Neonates**

Intestinal colic
Trauma
    Nonaccidental trauma
    Falls
    Open diaper pin
    Strangulation of digit or penis
    Corneal abrasion or foreign body
Infections
    Meningitis
    Sepsis
    Otitis media
    Urinary tract infection
    Gastroenteritis
    Necrotizing enterocolitis
Surgical
    Incarcerated hernia
    Anal fissure
    Intestinal malrotation/volvulus
Improper feeding practices
Cardiovascular
    Heart failure
Metabolic abnormalities

nal stress. Just as the cause remains obscure, no single treatment has been proven effective for all infants who have colic. Applying heat to the abdomen, decreasing external stimulation, and rocking the infant have been advocated as useful interventions at various times. Administration of drugs (including sedatives) rarely is beneficial or indicated. A 1-week trial of hypoallergenic formula (non-cow's milk protein) may be beneficial and is occasionally a worthwhile intervention in severe cases. Reassuring the parents that colic is a common, self-limited problem in young infants and encouraging them to share caregiving responsibilities during this time can be helpful.

The emergency physician can also be helpful by making the following suggestions:

1. Changes in care-taking styles (e.g., increased soothing activities such as carrying and rocking, feeding more frequently, and use of a pacifier and less overstimulation)
2. Changes in environment (e.g., background music or car and stroller rides)
3. Changes in feeding for refractory cases (e.g., removal of cow's milk from the diet of an infant who has visible peristalsis, persistent regurgitation, and symptoms after ingesting cow's milk protein; removal of cow's milk from the diet of the mother of a breast-fed baby; but not switching to formula from breast milk or changing formula).[4]

Abuse and Trauma

Distinguishing between accidental and nonaccidental injuries is vital. The most common accidental newborn skin lesion is a scratch.[5] By making an accurate determination, the practitioner achieves two equally important objectives: (1) protecting victims of abuse from future harm, which is often more severe than the present injuries; and (2) avoiding the damage done by unwarranted suspicion of abuse and the time-consuming investigative process that ensues.

Recognition of abuse and neglect (maltreatment) is likely only if the possibility is entertained in the differential diagnosis. The approach to the family should be supportive, empathic, and non-accusatory (see Chap. 297 for a detailed discussion).

If the diagnosis is suspected, the child should be admitted for protection, and the appropriate agencies should be notified for further investigation.

Infections

Neonatal infections are manifested by a variety of symptoms and signs, such as temperature instability, feeding difficulties, fever, jaundice, and respiratory distress. Neck rigidity and Kernig and Brudzinski signs are usually absent in neonates with meningitis. A septic neonate may present with a normal or subnormal temperature. Urinary tract infections are often associated with nonspecific signs, such as irritability, vomiting, diarrhea, or poor feeding, and diagnosis is established by urine culture rather than urinalysis. There is general consensus that all neonates (younger than 28 days) with possible sepsis should be hospitalized and given broad-spectrum antibiotic therapy pending results of appropriate cultures (e.g., urine, blood, and cerebrospinal fluid [CSF]). See Fever and Sepsis, below.

Surgical Lesions

Surgical conditions in neonates can present with a wide variety of symptoms, including respiratory distress, fever, lethargy, weight loss, poor feeding, feeding intolerance, or abdominal distention. Progression of symptoms can be helpful in decision-making but may not be easily or accurately elicited from an infant or poorly observant parent.

The surgically correctable causes of respiratory distress in newborns are less frequent and include choanal atresia, congenital lobar emphysema, micrognathia (Pierre-Robin syndrome), laryngomalacia, tracheomalacia, tracheoesophageal fistula, and vascular rings. Most of these anomalies are identified in the newborn nursery, but in the ED these diagnoses should be considered in any infant with respiratory distress. In the neonate with abdominal symptoms, the most common diagnoses include necrotizing enterocolitis and congenital anomalies, such as malrotation with midgut volvulus, duplication, gastroschisis, and omphalocele.

Malrotation usually presents in the first month of life with sudden onset of bilious vomiting. The incidence is 1 in 500 live births and 50 percent are diagnosed in the first month of life. Bilious vomiting should always be considered a surgical emergency. These symptoms should prompt an immediate surgical evaluation or consultation. Delayed presentation or surgical correction results in an increased morbidity and mortality.

Pyloric stenosis classically presents between 2 and 6 months of age and is the most common surgically correctible cause of vomiting in newborns. With more sensitive evaluation using ultrasound, it is often diagnosed and corrected in the first month of life. In fact, more than 90 percent of newborns have no electrolyte disturbances at the time of diagnosis. A volumetric evaluation is an appropriate and effective tool to use in the ED if ultrasound is not immediately available. To perform a volumetric evaluation, place an 8-French naso- or orogastric tube and attempt aspiration of gastric contents 3 to 4 h after the last feed. If less than 5 mL is obtained, pyloric stenosis is unlikely. If more than 5 mL is obtained, pyloric stenosis is more likely, and a diagnostic ultrasound should be obtained to make the diagnosis.

Incarcerated inguinal hernias and intussusception are most common after 2 months of age. Incarcerated hernia and intussusception account for most abdominal surgical emergencies in the 2-month to 1-year age group; incarcerated hernia decreases in incidence after 1 year of age.

The diagnosis of abdominal emergencies is challenging in the ED. A systematic approach helps to minimize missed diagnoses. The most common signs are irritability and crying, followed by poor feeding, vomiting, constipation, and abdominal distention. Prudent use of laboratory and imaging studies will minimize misdiagnosis. The early involvement of a surgeon in the care of all pediatric patients who have significant abdominal symptoms is recommended.[6–8]

Improper Feeding Practices

Improper feeding practices may result in an irritable infant with periods of inconsolable crying. These symptoms usually result from overfeeding without adequate burping during feedings. The infant swallows large amounts of air, resulting in bowel distention, reflux, and occasionally respiratory distress. Instruction in proper feeding practices usually alleviates the problem.

GASTROINTESTINAL TRACT SYMPTOMS

Common presenting gastrointestinal symptoms are listed in Table 117-1.

Feeding Difficulties

Most visits for feeding difficulties occur because parents perceive that the infant's food intake is inadequate. The neonate's pattern of intake is not fully established until about 1 month of age. If weight gain is satisfactory and the infant is satisfied after feedings, intake is adequate. Parents usually can provide accurate information of the intake of bottle-fed infants. Weighing breast-fed infants before and after feedings is not advised, because weights may be inaccurate. In addition, weighing may have adverse psychological effects on a mother whose infant is doing poorly.

Rarely, anatomic abnormalities may can cause difficulty in feeding and swallowing. A careful history usually pinpoints such difficulties as having started at birth. The infants appear malnourished and dehydrated. The most likely causes are esophageal obstruction (e.g., stenoses, strictures, laryngeal clefts, or cleft palate) and compression of the esophagus or trachea by a double aortic arch. Infants with a recent decrease in intake have an acute disease, usually an infection, and should prompt an urgent evaluation.

Gastroesophageal Reflux

Regurgitation of small amounts is common in neonates due to reduced lower esophageal sphincter pressure and relatively increased intragastric pressure. Parents may confuse regurgitation with vomiting. Vomiting results from forceful contraction of the diaphragm and abdominal muscles, whereas regurgitation is independent of any effort and likely represents the ultimate degree of gastrointestinal reflux. If the neonate is thriving, parents can be reassured that regurgitation is of no clinical significance and will decrease as the infant grows. Such infants usually respond well to thickening of feedings. The infant's upper body should be elevated after feedings, if thickening of feedings alone does not resolve the regurgitation. Infants who are not thriving or having respiratory symptoms should be investigated for anatomic causes of regurgitation or chronic aspiration.

Regurgitation rarely results from pathologic processes, such as intrinsic compression of the esophagus or occasionally compression of the trachea, in which case it is usually accompanied by stridor and cough. Dysphagia, irritability, anemia, and malnutrition are sequelae of chronic regurgitation with esophagitis, but this condition is rare. Investigations such as scintigraphy, pH monitoring, endoscopy, and biopsy are used to confirm the diagnosis of reflux esophagitis. These invasive tests are not done on an emergency basis.

Vomiting

Vomiting results from many causes and is rarely an isolated symptom. During the first few weeks of life, vomiting is uncommon and is often confused with regurgitation. Vomiting beginning at birth is most likely due to an anatomic abnormality, such as tracheoesophageal fistula, upper gastrointestinal obstruction, or midgut rotation. More commonly, acute vomiting may be part of the symptom complex of some diseases, especially increased intracranial pressure, and infections (e.g., sepsis, urinary tract infections, and gastroenteritis).

Projectile vomiting is usually seen in infants with pyloric stenosis and usually assumes its characteristic pattern after the second and third weeks of life. This condition usually occurs in firstborn males and is characterized by projectile vomiting at the end of feeding or shortly thereafter. The vomitus does not contain bile or blood. Examination of these infants should be done with the infant relaxed and the stomach empty. Prominent gastric waves may be seen going from the left to right. A firm olive mass may be felt by palpating under the liver edge. Malnutrition and dehydration are rarely seen because of early diagnosis.

In any infant who is vomiting, signs of dehydration should be sought. Hepatobiliary, urinary tract, and central nervous system disease can also cause vomiting. Vomiting due to inborn errors of metabolism may present with hypoglycemia and metabolic acidosis. Infants who are vomiting should be admitted for evaluation and therapy.

Necrotizing Enterocolitis

Necrotizing enterocolitis remains incompletely understood, but the cause is multifactorial. It is a result of inflammation or injury to the bowel wall that has been associated with infectious causes and hypoxic-ischemic insults. Although there is a higher incidence in premature infants, it may be seen in the term newborn. Initial symptoms may range from feeding intolerance, abdominal distention, bloody stools, and apnea or shock. The classic x-ray findings include pneumatosis intestinalis (intramural air) and hepatic portal air. Free air in the abdomen may be seen, if perforation has already occurred. Management is directed by symptomatology. A pediatric surgeon should be consulted or a transfer arranged to an appropriate facility after stabilization. Broad-spectrum antibiotics should be administered, including ampicillin, cefotaxime, and clindamycin to cover gram-positive, gram-negative, and anaerobic organisms.

Blood in the Diaper

Blood in the diaper or stool can be a difficult complaint to evaluate in the ED. In the first 2 to 3 days of life, blood in the diaper is most commonly due to swallowed maternal blood. This possibility may be confirmed by the Kleihauer-Betke or Apt-Downey test (see Chap. 254), which differentiates fetal from maternal hemoglobin in the stool. After the first few days of life, most causes are idiopathic, but coagulopathies, necrotizing enterocolitis, anal fissures, allergic or infectious colitis, and congenital defects should be considered. Visualization of a bleeding anal fissure on examination may be helpful, but not visualizing a fissure does not confirm or exclude the diagnosis. Cow's milk allergy is an IgE-mediated disorder causing changes in the bowel mucosa that result in bloody stools. Eosinophils may be present in the stool, and the diagnosis may be confirmed by resolution of the problem after cow's milk is removed from the diet. For unresponsive or severe cases, biopsy may be needed to make a diagnosis. A careful history and thorough examination of the infant, with focus on the abdomen and rectum, may be helpful. Blood in the stool should be confirmed by a guaiac test for occult blood. A single event in a newborn that has no other findings may be observed as an outpatient. Persistent symptoms or other findings should be evaluated on an inpatient basis with appropriate subspecialty care.

Diarrhea and Dehydration

Diarrhea refers to stools that are abnormally frequent and liquid. The modifier *abnormal* is critical because stools can normally be frequent and liquid in young children. In the United States, rotavirus predominantly affects infants between ages 3 to 15 months. The peak incidence is in the winter months, and rotavirus accounts for as many as 50 percent of the cases of acute diarrhea in winter. Enteric adenoviruses (serotypes 40 and 41) are the second most common viral pathogen in infants. In summer, most cases of diarrhea are caused by bacteria (including *Escherichia coli*, *Salmonella*, and *Shigella*). Parasitic causes of diarrhea are rare in neonates.

A history of bloody diarrhea strongly suggests a bacterial pathogen. A suspicion or diagnosis of Salmonella gastroenteritis in a newborn should prompt a full sepsis evaluation and admission for antibiotic therapy. The history should assess the infant's state of hydration and possible causative agents. Information regarding oral intake, frequency and volume of stools, general appearance of the infant, mental status, and frequency of urination can help in assessing hydration. The parent should be asked about fever, antibiotic therapy, and exposure to infant day-care centers or other children and adults with diarrheal illness.

All children with diarrhea should be carefully weighed unclothed for comparison with previous weight and to provide a baseline for monitoring subsequent weights during the course of the disease. In an infant, the normal extracellular fluid volume is 25 percent of body weight; therefore, a loss of 8 percent of body weight as extracellular fluid would result in severe dehydration. The actual weight loss is usually greater than 8 percent because of concomitant loss of cellular water. A neonate with gastrointestinal losses may prompt further evaluation and should be considered for admission, because loss of seemingly small volumes of stool may cause significant dehydration.

The physical examination should begin with a general assessment, with particular attention to the state of hydration (Table 117-3). Mucous membranes should be evaluated for moistness. The appearance of the anterior fontanel and eyes should be assessed. Skin hydration and turgor may provide a sense of the degree of dehydration. The finding of doughy and tented skin is associated with hypernatremic dehydration. The child's mental status with regard to interaction with the examiner and the parent may reflect the severity of the illness and dehydration.

Temperature, pulse, and blood pressure also may provide information concerning the degree of illness. The rest of the physical examination should focus on signs of concurrent viral illness, such as upper respiratory tract infections and abdominal findings. A rectal examination is often useful in obtaining a stool sample for detection of occult blood, culture, examination for leukocytes, measurement of pH, and detection of reducing substances. It can also rule out anal fissures as the cause of bloody stools.

Serum electrolyte levels, in particular sodium and bicarbonate, should be assessed in any neonate with diarrhea and dehydration. A markedly elevated serum urea nitrogen with a relatively normal creatinine may indicate recent or rapid dehydration. Serum creatinine values tend to be low in infants and young children, and a creatinine value of 1 mg/dL may represent a doubling in the normal value. The rest of the evaluation should include a stool sample for the above-mentioned tests and a urine sample for culture and analysis.

Most newborns should be admitted to the hospital for rehydration. The loss of even seemingly small volumes of stool may cause severe

TABLE 117-3   Clinical Assessment of Severity of Dehydration

Signs and Symptoms	Mild Dehydration	Moderate Dehydration	Severe Dehydration
Body weight loss, %	3–5	6–9	≥10
General appearance and condition, infants and young children	Thirsty, alert, restless	Thirty; restless or lethargic but irritable to touch or drowsy	Drowsy; limp, cold, sweaty, cyanotic extremities; may be comatose
Radial pulse	Normal rate and strength	Rapid and weak	Rapid, feeble, sometimes impalpable
Respiration	Normal	Deep, may be rapid	Deep and rapid
Anterior fontanel	Normal	Sunken	Very sunken
Systolic blood pressure	Normal	Normal or low	Low, may be unrecordable
Skin elasticity	Pinch retracts immediately	Pinch retracts slowly	Pinch retracts very slowly
Eyes	Normal	Sunken	Grossly sunken
Tears	Present	Absent or reduced	Absent
Mucous membranes	Moist	Dry	Very dry
Urine flow	Normal	Reduced amount and dark	Anuria, severe oliguria
Capillary refill	Normal	±2 s	>3 s
Estimated fluid deficit, mL/kg	30–50	60–90	≥100

dehydration in the neonate. Oral hydration may be attempted in the hospital, depending on personnel and cardiovascular stability of the patient. Oral rehydration should be attempted in children who are less than 5 percent dehydrated. If the infant is breast fed, rehydration should be continued and an oral electrolyte and glucose solution supplement should be given until diarrhea subsides. An age-appropriate diet should be resumed after initial feedings, with oral rehydration solutions as tolerated. A lactose-free or elemental formula should not be substituted unless stools are positive for reducing substances. The total fluid intake of oral electrolyte solution and regular diet should be approximately 150 mL/kg per d.[9,10]

However, if there are any indications of significant peripheral vascular compromise or shock, or if vomiting is persistent, or if there is more than 5 percent dehydration, intravenous hydration is recommended (see Chap. 132).

Abdominal Distention

Abdominal distention may be normal in neonates and is usually due to lax abdominal musculature and relatively large intra-abdominal organs. It may also be accentuated by excessive gas within the bowel. If the infant is comfortable and feeding well and the abdomen is soft, there is no need for concern. Abdominal distention may also occur in association with bowel obstruction, constipation, necrotizing enterocolitis, or ileus due to sepsis or gastroenteritis. Congenital organomegaly (e.g., hepatomegaly, splenomegaly, or renal enlargement) undetected in the perinatal period also may present as abdominal distention.

Constipation

Infrequent bowel movements in neonates do not necessarily mean that the infant is constipated. Infants occasionally may go without a bowel movement for 5 to 7 days and then pass a normal stool. However, if the infant has never passed stools, especially if there has not been a stool in the first 48 h of life, the possibility of intestinal stenosis or atresia, Hirschsprung disease, or meconium ileus or plug should be considered.

Constipation occurring after birth but within the first month of life suggests Hirschsprung disease, hypothyroidism, or anal stenosis. The diagnosis of Hirschsprung disease is supported by absence of feces on rectal examination and an abrupt change in bowel luminal size on barium enema, and is confirmed by a rectal biopsy demonstrating absence of ganglion cells. Infants with hypothyroidism present with feeding problems, a weak or hoarse cry, hypothermia, hypotonia, and peripheral edema. The child should be admitted for further evaluation and treatment. Hypothyroidism is part of the routine newborn metabolic screening but varies from state to state. Emergency physicians should be familiar with the diseases that are screened for in their state and how they may obtain the results.

CARDIORESPIRATORY SYMPTOMS

Neonates are prone to respiratory problems for a variety of reasons. Anatomic predisposing factors are a barrel-shaped chest, a flattened diaphragm, limitation of diaphragmatic movement by abdominal compression, smaller airway diameter, and higher closing volumes. The high compliance of the chest wall, low compliance of the lungs, and less fatigue-resistant fibers in the diaphragm and intercostal muscles are other significant contributory factors. Cardiorespiratory symptoms are also more common in neonates, because structural and functional abnormalities of the airway and heart are more likely to present early in life. A cardiorespiratory arrest should be considered due to respiratory pathology until proven otherwise.

Cardiorespiratory symptoms in neonates are nonspecific and may be due to primary organ failure (cardiovascular or respiratory) or secondary to a variety of systemic diseases, such as sepsis, metabolic acidosis, abdominal pathology, and severe meningitis. Regardless of the cause, the assessment and stabilization of the cardiac and respiratory systems are priorities and should be accomplished before or concurrently with establishing a diagnosis.

Rapid Breathing

Rapid breathing can be due to minor problems, such as abdominal distention, or to life-threatening illnesses, such as sepsis. **Rapid breathing or grunting should always be considered a medical emergency.** Physical examination should include observation for grunting during feeding. Admission for investigations, monitoring, and therapy should be considered in all but the mildest cases. When a cause cannot be identified on initial presentation, a full sepsis workup (full blood count, blood culture, urinalysis, chest x-ray, and CSF examination) should be done, and broad-spectrum antibiotics should be administered (Table 117-4).

Pneumonia

The lungs are the most common sites of infection in neonates, with group B *Streptococcus* being the most common cause of lower respiratory infection. The infection is most likely acquired in utero from a contaminated amniotic fluid environment. Affected infants frequently develop fulminant illness within hours of birth. Other common bacterial pathogens in newborns and infants include *Streptococcus pneumoniae* and *Haemophilus influenzae* serotype B. Chlamydial pneumonia usually occurs after 3 weeks of age and is accompanied by conjunctivitis in 50 percent of cases. Infants with bacterial and viral pneumonia may present with fussiness, stuffy nose, decreased appetite, abrupt onset of high fever, nasal flaring, grunting, retraction, tachypnea, and tachycardia.

Patients with chlamydial pneumonia are usually afebrile, tachypneic, and have a prominent "staccato" cough. Wheezing is uncommon, but the chest x-ray may demonstrate hyperinflation with bilateral interstitial infiltrates. The definitive diagnosis is by a nasopharyngeal swab for culture, but the peripheral blood count may reveal an eosinophilia.

Respiratory syncytial virus (RSV), adenovirus, and parainfluenza virus can also cause pneumonia in otherwise well infants.

TABLE 117-4 Causes of Rapid Breathing in Neonates

Pneumonia
  Bacterial
  Viral
  Chlamydia
  Aspiration
Bronchiolitis
Illness in other organ systems
  Septicemia
  Central nervous system (e.g., meningitis)
  Abdomen (e.g., distention, gastroenteritis)
  Metabolic acidosis
Congenital diseases
  Repiratory disease
    Delayed presentation of diaphragmatic hernia
    Tracheoesophageal fistula
    Lobar emphysema
    Tracheal stenosis, webs
  Heart disease
    Cardiac failure (e.g., hypoplastic left heart, critical coarctation of aorta, aortic stenosis, patent ductus arteriosus)
    Cyanotic disease (e.g., transposition of great arteries)
    Vascular ring
  Neuromuscular disease
    Infant botulism
    Muscle weakness

In addition to pneumonia, infections with *Bordetella pertussis* may cause paroxysms of cough accompanied by cyanosis in an otherwise well-appearing infant. The cough is not accompanied by the characteristic whoop in neonates. Pertussis always must be considered in infants who have severe, paroxysmal cough and post-tussive vomiting. Apnea also may be the only presenting symptom. Because many adults are susceptible to infection with pertussis, such an infection should be considered if the caretaker also has a persistent cough. Infants younger than 6 months who are suspected of having pertussis should be admitted to the hospital. Pertussis is diagnosed through culture of the nasopharynx, but because special culture medium is required, the laboratory should be consulted about proper technique when this culture is required. A lymphocytosis of the peripheral blood count is nonspecific but may support the diagnosis.

The approach to the febrile neonate with suspected bacterial pneumonia should include a full evaluation for sepsis (blood and urine cultures, chest radiographs, and complete blood count). The blood culture results are typically negative, but obtaining two culture samples instead of one during the initial evaluation may increase the diagnostic yield fourfold. A lumbar puncture should be done if there are no contraindications.

Infants who have fever and pneumonia should be hospitalized and receive parenteral antibiotics. The most common organisms include group B *Streptococcus*, *Listeria*, and *Haemophilus influenzae*. A premature infant who has recently been in the neonate intensive care unit may have a nosocomial cause such as *Staphylococcus aureus* or *Pseudomonas aeruginosa*. Chlamydial or *B. pertussis* pneumonia should be treated with erythromycin or sulfamethoxazole. Infants with pneumonia who are afebrile may be treated as outpatients when a viral pathogen is suspected. Inability to eat, respiratory distress, and hypoxemia are criteria for hospitalization. Outpatients should be seen daily until symptoms resolve.[11]

Bronchiolitis

Bronchiolitis is an acute lower respiratory tract illness in early life preceded by signs and symptoms of an upper respiratory infection or apnea. Bronchiolitis is a highly seasonal disease, comparatively few cases are seen during the summer months, and activity peaks during winter months. Serious cases of bronchiolitis occur most commonly in infants younger than 1 year and in those who are premature (<34 weeks of gestational age) or have an underlying medical problem. The greatest risk of a complicated course is in the first 3 months of life. Bronchiolitis is seen more commonly in families of low socioeconomic status or infants who have not been breast fed.

Respiratory syncytial virus is the most common cause, accounting for more than 60 to 90 percent of bronchiolitis cases. Transmission is by direct contact with nasal secretions of infected individuals much more frequently than by aerosol spread. Shedding of the virus can be documented 1 to 2 days before symptoms occur and for 1 to 2 weeks thereafter. Those exposed are probably not contagious for the entire period of time but should be considered contagious 24 to 48 h before the onset of symptoms and for several days thereafter.

Many other viral agents also can cause bronchiolitis, although the illness is milder. The parainfluenza viruses are the second most common cause of bronchiolitis and are responsible for autumn and spring epidemics, usually before and after RSV outbreaks. Influenza type A virus, adenovirus, rhinovirus, and *Mycoplasma pneumoniae* also can precipitate bronchiolitis.

Acute bronchiolitis presents in infancy with serous nasal discharge accompanied by sneezing. These symptoms are followed by diminished appetite, cough, dyspnea, irritability, and, commonly, periods of apnea. **Apnea is more common in neonates and preterm infants younger than 34 weeks of gestational age and usually presents within the first 3 days of illness.** Physical examination reveals a rapid respiratory rate (>60 breaths/min), cyanosis, air hunger, wheezing,

hyperinflation, intercostal and subcostal retractions, and a palpable liver and/or spleen due to hyperinflation of the lungs. Fever is usually low grade or absent, except in the presence of otitis media, when a temperature as high as 40°C may be present. Chest x-rays usually show hyperinflation with patchy atelectasis.

The diagnosis of bronchiolitis is usually made clinically. There is no need to send nasopharyngeal washings for diagnosis unless the infant is younger than 2 months, when washings may obviate a sepsis evaluation. A wheezing infant with a history of the aforementioned symptoms for several days, particularly during the peak season for RSV, can be assumed to have bronchiolitis. Immunofluorescence or enzyme-linked immunosorbent assays performed on respiratory secretions are very sensitive and specific for detection of RSV. Other diagnostic tests, such as blood gas analysis or cell counts, are directed by clinical assessment but are rarely necessary.

Most cases of bronchiolitis are mild and can be managed without hospitalization. Infants usually recover without β-adrenergic agents or other medications used for relief of wheezing. The decision to hospitalize an infant with bronchiolitis should be based on a number of clinical criteria in addition to other considerations, such as reliability of parents and the likelihood of obtaining acceptable follow-up. **Infants who are born prematurely, have underlying heart or lung disease, are younger than 3 months, or have low initial oxygen saturation (<92 percent) are at greater risk to develop progressive or life-threatening illness.** In addition, infants who are not feeding well or are dehydrated should be hospitalized.

Infants for whom hospitalization is being considered may receive a course of a nebulized β-adrenergic agent (albuterol 0.1 to 0.15 mg/kg per dose, up to 5 mg). The drug should be continued only if the infant shows improvement. Racemic epinephrine has demonstrated more consistent beneficial results than β-adrenergic agents and warrants a trial in sicker patients. The continued use of such agents in the absence of an initial beneficial response is not routinely recommended. It is not possible to predict which individuals with bronchiolitis may respond to β-adrenergic agents. The use of corticosteroids is not useful in the treatment or outcome of bronchiolitis. The use of antibiotics generally does not affect the clinical course of bronchiolitis, but the presence of a high fever or severe course of illness may be an indication for temporary antibiotic coverage.[12,13]

ILLNESS INVOLVING OTHER ORGAN SYSTEMS

The search for pathologic conditions in other organ systems is mandatory, because the presence of respiratory symptoms does not preclude pathology in another organ. For example, generalized sepsis, meningitis, gastroenteritis, and metabolic acidosis may present with respiratory distress as the predominant symptom.

CONGENITAL DISEASES

Respiratory Disease

Occasionally an H-type tracheoesophageal fistula may present in the first month of life or later with recurrent pneumonia, respiratory distress after feedings, and problems in clearing mucus. Tracheal stenosis may present initially with noisy breathing or a high-pitched cry and tremendous respiratory difficulty even after mild upper respiratory infections. Similarly, neonates with chronic respiratory insufficiency, such as bronchopulmonary dysplasia, may present as respiratory failure even after mild upper respiratory infections.

Heart Disease

Rapid breathing due to cardiac disease is usually not associated with significant retractions and use of accessory muscles. As a general rule, a well-developed neonate who presents with unexplained cyanosis and tachypnea should be suspected of having congenital cardiac disease. In neonates with transposition of the great arteries and ventricular septal defect or critical coarctation of the aorta, congestive cardiac failure may be the presenting feature. Infants with underlying cardiac disease may present to the ED in the first few weeks of life after the ductus arteriosus closes. Emergency physicians should be familiar with the simple but potentially life-saving administration of prostaglandins. Prostaglandin E_1 is started at 0.05 to 0.1 μg/kg per min and titrated according to improvement of partial pressure of oxygen. Signs of heart failure may be very subtle but are life threatening and require emergency referral[14] (see Chap. 120).

Neuromuscular Disease

Any form of muscle weakness may be associated with shallow breathing and a compensatory increase in respiratory rate. Infantile botulism is a possible cause and usually preceded by constipation, and the infant may have a poor cry and feeding difficulties. Ocular palsy, apnea and weakness or hypotonia, and lethargy are later symptoms. Other causes of hypotonic neuromuscular diseases include Down syndrome, hypoxic-ischemic encephalopathy, spinal cord lesions such as myelomeningocele, and peripheral nerve diseases such as myasthenia gravis, metabolic disorders, and myotonic dystrophy.

Cough and Nasal Congestion

Cough may be a prominent feature of most of the primary respiratory conditions listed in Table 117-4. It also may be the initial presentation of a variety of congenital anomalies, including cleft palate, laryngeal tracheomalacia, laryngotracheal cleft, tracheal webs, tracheoesophageal fistula, tracheal hemangiomas, and vascular rings. Although congenital malformation resulting in cough and nasal congestion is more likely to occur in neonates, in most instances, cough is due to a viral upper respiratory infection and may be associated with sneezing and nasal congestion. It also may be a prominent feature of bronchiolitis and chlamydial and pertussis infections. Treatment of the underlying condition is required. Cough suppressants should be avoided in neonates. The focus should be the diagnosis of the etiology, not suppressing the cough. Over-the-counter cough medications usually are not effective and may contain ingredients that increase mucus production or cause drowsiness or irritability. Nasal congestion is best treated with instillation of saline drops and suction, when necessary.

Noisy Breathing and Stridor

Noisy breathing is a common presenting complaint in neonates and is usually benign. Stridor is usually due to congenital anomalies (e.g., webs, cysts, atresia, stenosis, clefts, or hemangiomas) anywhere from the nose to the trachea and bronchi. Infants who were intubated in the neonatal period may develop subglottic stenosis. Infection (e.g., croup, epiglottitis, and abscess) as a cause of stridor in neonates is rare. Stridor worsening with cry or increased activity suggests laryngomalacia or subglottic hemangioma; stridor and feeding difficulties suggest vascular ring, laryngeal cleft, or tracheoesophageal fistula; stridor with hoarseness or weak cry suggests vocal cord paralysis. Laryngomalacia is the most common cause of stridor in the neonate. It is characterized by noisy, crowing, inspiratory sounds, which usually decrease during the first year of life. When the diagnosis is in doubt, the infant should be admitted for evaluation.

Apnea and Periodic Breathing

Periodic breathing, which may occur in normal neonates, should be differentiated from apnea. However, periodic breathing may precede apnea, and both may occur in the same patient. Apnea is a cessation of respiration for 20 s or bradycardia and cyanosis. It signifies critical illness and warrants prompt investigation and admission for monitoring and therapy.

Apnea may be precipitated by any of the disease conditions listed in Table 117-4 and usually indicates respiratory muscle fatigue and impending respiratory arrest. Resuscitation, including airway support and ventilation, should be followed by a thorough search for the inciting condition. If no obvious cause is found, the neonate should be assumed to be septic or have meningitis. Cultures should be obtained and broad-spectrum antibiotics started.[15]

Cyanosis

An infant with cyanosis usually presents a diagnostic challenge, because such findings may be due to many disorders. If cyanosis is associated with rapid but unlabored breathing, the most likely cause is cyanotic congenital heart disease with a right-to-left shunt. Methemoglobinemia, although rare, may mimic cyanotic heart disease and could be easily diagnosed by ordering an arterial blood gas with a co-oximeter. Irregular or shallow breathing may be associated with sepsis, meningitis, cerebral edema, or intracranial hemorrhage and also may be accompanied by cyanosis. If breathing is labored (e.g., grunting or retractions), pulmonary disease (e.g., pneumonia or bronchiolitis) is likely. All infants with cyanosis should be admitted for monitoring and further investigation.

Jaundice (Hyperbilirubinemia)

Jaundice (Table 117-5) may appear at different times during the neonatal period and may require a complete diagnostic evaluation. This is the most common reason for re-evaluation and admission as a result of earlier discharge from the newborn nursery. Jaundice during the first 24 h rarely presents to the ED. The most common causes of jaundice seen in the ED are physiologic jaundice, jaundice due to sepsis, or breast-milk jaundice. Occasionally, infants with hemolysis due to autoimmune disease may present to the ED.

Physiologic jaundice is due to the hemolysis of fetal red blood cells. It is characterized by bilirubin rising at a rate of less than 5 mg/dL per 24 h, with a peak of 5 to 6 mg/dL during the second to the fourth days of life, and a decrease to less than 2 mg/dL by 5 to 7 days. Septic infants with hyperbilirubinemia may have an increase in bilirubin by greater than the acceptable 5 mg/dL per 24-h period, and other features of sepsis, such as vomiting, abdominal distention, respiratory distress, and poor feeding. Jaundice associated with breast feeding is thought to be due to the presence of substances that inhibit

TABLE 117-5   Causes of Jaundice in Neonates

<24 h	ABO, Rh incompatibility
	Sepsis
	Congenital infections (e.g., rubella, toxoplasmosis, cytomegalovirus infection)
	Excessive bruising from birth trauma (cephalhematoma or intramuscular hematoma)
2–3 d	Physiologic
3 d to 1 wk	Septicemia
	Syphilis, toxoplasmosis, cytomegalovirus infection
>1 wk	Septicemia, congenital atresia of bile ducts, serum hepatitis
	Congenital hemolytic anemias (sickle cell anemia, spherocytosis)
	Hemolytic anemia due to drugs (e.g., in glucose-6-phosphate dehydrogenase deficiency)
	Rubella, herpetic hepatitis
	Hypothyroidism
	Breast-milk jaundice

glucuronyl transferase in breast milk; it may start as early as the third to fourth day and reaches a peak of 10 to 27 mg/dL by the third week of life. Although cessation of breast feeding will result in a rapid decline of bilirubin over 2 to 3 days, it is not routinely recommended. Breast feeding jaundice is unlikely to cause kernicterus and usually can be treated with phototherapy, when necessary.

A proper history and physical examination provide clues to the causes of jaundice. A well-looking child who is gaining weight and feeding well is unlikely to be septic. Laboratory evaluation should include a full blood count to test for anemia, a smear for hemolysis, direct and total bilirubin determinations, a reticulocyte count, and a Coombs test. Admission to the hospital, appropriate cultures, and antibiotics are ordered for neonates who are unwell and have any of the signs or symptoms listed in Table 117-5. In all cases, arrangements should be made for monitoring of bilirubin and hemoglobin levels. Whereas most well infants can be monitored and receive phototherapy as outpatients, infants who have anemia or have bilirubin levels approaching exchange transfusion levels should be admitted. The American Academy of Pediatrics recommends initiation of phototherapy based on age. **Infants 25 to 48 h old with bilirubin levels of at least 15 mg/dL, 49 to 72 h old with levels of least 18 mg/dL, or older than 72 h with levels of at least 20 mg/dL should receive phototherapy. These recommendations are for healthy newborns, not ill-appearing or premature newborns.**[16]

Eye Discharge, Redness, and Conjunctivitis

Neonates with red eyes most likely have conjunctivitis. Neonatal conjunctivitis occurs in 1.6 to 12 percent of newborns during the first month of life. The chemical irritation from antimicrobial prophylaxis against bacterial infection is the most frequent cause occurring in the first 24 h of life, followed by *Chlamydia trachomatis* infection. Other important pathogens in this setting are *H. influenzae* and *Streptococcus pneumoniae*. *Neisseria gonorrhoeae* is no longer a major cause of neonatal conjunctivitis in the United States, because of the use of neonatal ocular prophylaxis. The failure rate of antimicrobial prophylaxis is 1 percent. However, because *N. gonorrhoeae* can damage the eye severely, it is important to always test for this pathogen as the possible cause of neonatal conjunctivitis. Viruses rarely cause isolated neonatal conjunctivitis as an isolated problem. They usually cause conjunctivitis as part of a generalized viral syndrome affecting many organs. For example, herpes simplex virus causes neonatal keratoconjunctivitis as part of a generalized viremia, with infection at other sites such as skin or mucous membranes, or with disseminated disease. The finding of vesicles anywhere on the body in association with neonatal conjunctivitis suggests herpes simplex infection. This finding warrants a full sepsis evaluation with CSF cultures for herpes simplex virus and treatment with acyclovir.

An important consideration in the evaluation of neonatal conjunctivitis is the time of onset. Chemical conjunctivitis due to ocular prophylaxis usually occurs on the first day of life. Gonococcal conjunctivitis generally has its peak time of onset between 3 and 5 days after birth. By the end of the first week of life and throughout the first month of life, *Chlamydia* becomes the most frequent cause of conjunctivitis. These times of onset presume rupture of amniotic membrane at or near the time of delivery. However, the conjunctiva can be inoculated before birth by an ascending bacterial infection.

Chlamydial conjunctivitis can vary in severity, ranging from mild to severe hyperemia with a thick mucopurulent discharge and pseudomembrane formation. Gonococcal conjunctivitis can present as a typical bacterial conjunctivitis. However, in its full-blown form, it presents as hyperacute conjunctivitis with profuse discharge. There often is severe edema of both lids. In marked contrast to other forms of bacterial conjunctivitis, *N. gonorrhoeae* has the capacity to invade superficial layers of the conjunctiva, causing ulceration of the cornea. If it is not treated, it can result in permanent loss of vision from corneal complications.

A Gram stain and culture should always be obtained in instances of neonatal conjunctivitis to look for *N. gonorrhoeae*. Because isolation of *C. trachomatis* requires specialized tissue cultures, proper technique should be used in collecting culture specimens (e.g., Dacron swabs) and specimens for antigen detection.

Gonococcal ophthalmia neonatorum is treated best with ceftriaxone (25 to 50 mg/kg per d IV or IM, not to exceed 125 mg) given once or as a single dose of cefotaxime (100 mg/kg IV or IM). Disseminated disease should be suspected until CSF cultures are negative. Admission is necessary, and ophthalmology consultation should be sought. Cefotaxime is recommended for hyperbilirubinemic infants. Infants with gonococcal ophthalmia should have their eyes irrigated with saline solution immediately and at frequent intervals until the discharge is eliminated. Topical antibiotic treatment alone is inadequate and unnecessary when systemic antibiotic treatment is given.

Chlamydial conjunctivitis and pneumonia in young infants are treated with oral erythromycin (50 mg/kg per d in four divided doses, for 14 days). Oral sulfonamides may be used after the immediate neonatal period for infants who do not tolerate erythromycin. Topical treatment of conjunctivitis is ineffective and unnecessary. Because the efficacy of erythromycin therapy is approximately 80 percent, a second course is sometimes required. A specific diagnosis of *C. trachomatis* infection in an infant should prompt the treatment of the mother and her sexual partners.

The neonate with a red eye and irritability also may have a corneal irritation or abrasion, usually due to an eyelash or scratch from a fingernail. Fluorescein evaluation with Wood's lamp or a slit lamp is helpful. Acute glaucoma, although rare, also presents as a red, teary eye. In these instances, the cornea may be stained or cloudy, the anterior chamber may be shallow, and the intraocular pressure may be increased. Prompt ophthalmologic referral of all suspected cases of glaucoma is needed. Infectious causes should be treated (Table 117-6) and follow-up care ensured.[17–19]

Diaper Rash and Oral Thrush

Candidal diaper dermatitis is an erythematous plaque with a scalloped border and a sharply demarcated edge that is studded by satellite lesions. It usually occurs in the moist, occluded diaper area and intertriginous zones and usually results from the action of organisms harbored in the gastrointestinal tract. Treatment consists of a topical anti-candidal agent with each diaper change or four times daily. Protection of the area with zinc oxide paste overlying the cream will prevent friction, and local treatment with nystatin cream will prevent spread of the infection. An oral course of fluconazole is warranted in a candidal diaper rash that is unresponsive to topical therapy (see Table 117-6). More serious conditions such as *S. aureus* superinfection require oral antibiotics. Staphylococcal scalded skin syndrome or toxic epidermal necrolysis should be considered in the more severe or atypical presentations. These conditions require prompt recognition, treatment, and admission.

Oral candidal lesions are white and flaky and may involve the tongue, lips, gingiva, and mucous membranes. These lesions are common in normal newborns, debilitated infants, and those on antibiotics. Oral lesions may affect oral intake, because of pain and discomfort. Treatment of ill infants consists of treating the underlying pathology, topical oral mucosa antifungal therapy, or oral fluconazole (Diflucan) and an anesthetic gel before feeding. Cool liquids may prevent discomfort and pain.[20,21]

Fever and Sepsis

Fever is most commonly due to acute infections. Fever is present when an infant's rectal temperature is 38°C (100.4°F) or higher as measured by a caretaker or a health care professional. Although the height of the temperature in infants older than 4 weeks suggests a bacterial etiology,

TABLE 117-6   Antibiotic Therapy for Neonatal Infections

Indication	Organisms	Antibiotic

Sepsis and meningitis	Group B *Streptococcus*
	 Escherichia coli
	 Listeria
		Ampicillin, 200–300 mg/kg per d, div q6h IV, *and*
		   Cefotaxime 200 mg/kg per d div q6h IV
		   or Ceftriaxone 100 mg/kg per d
		   Gentamycin 2.5 mg/kg per d IV for infants younger than 7 d or div q12h IV
		   for infants older than 7 d

Pneumonia	Group B *Streptococcus* *Listeria* *Chlamydia trachomatis* *Bordetella pertussis*	Same as for sepsis Same as for sepsis Erythromycin 40–50 mg/kg per d div q6h PO for 14 d Erythromycin 40–50 mg/kg per d div q6h PO for 14 d *or* Azithromycin 10–12 mg/kg per d PO for 7 d
Conjunctivitis	*Chlamydia trachomatis* *Neisseria gonorrhoeae*	Same as chlamydia pneumonia Ceftriaxone 25–50 mg/kg per d IV or IM *or* Cefotaxime 100 mg/kg per d IV or IM (in hyperbilirubinemia)

Necrotizing enterocolitis	Associated with *Escherichia coli,*
	   Pseudomonas, and
	   Staphylococcus epidermidis
		Ticarcillin 300 mg/kg per d div q6h IV or IM
		   and
		 Gentamycin 2.5 mg/kg per d IV for infants younger than 7 d or div q12h IV
		   for infants older than 7 d

Oral thrush	*Candida albicans*	Oral nystatin suspension 100,000 U 1–2 drops to each side of mouth q4–6h
		   after feedings for 7–14 d
		   or
		 Fluconazole 10 mg/kg PO loading and then 3–6 mg/kg per d for 14 d

Dermatitis	*Candida albicans*	Nystatin cream 100,000 U/g to affected area q4–6h *or* Fluconazole 10 mg/kg PO loading and then 3–6 mg/kg per d for 14 d

there is no such correlation between height of fever and possible bacterial etiology in neonates. The risk of bacterial infection rises with the height of the temperature in infants older than 4 weeks (about 3 percent with fever above 39.4°C, 6 percent with fever above 40°C, 13 percent with fever above 40.5°C, and 26 percent with fever above 41.1°C).[22,23]

Recognizing neonatal bacterial sepsis early is a difficult task. Neonates have about twice the risk of serious bacterial infection as do infants 4 to 8 weeks of age. Neonatal sepsis tends to appear as an "early-onset" or a "late-onset" syndrome, with some overlap. Early-onset disease is seen in the first few days of life, tends to be fulminant, and is usually associated with maternal or perinatal risk factors, such as maternal fever, prolonged rupture of membranes, and fetal distress. Late-onset disease usually occurs after 1 week of age, tends to develop more gradually, and is less likely to be associated with risk factors. Septic shock and neutropenia are more common with early-onset syndrome, and meningitis is more common in late-onset disease.

Clinical signs of either type of sepsis are not specific (Table 117-7). Septic infants may exhibit any of a variety of symptoms, including lethargy, poor feeding, vomiting, temperature instability (hypothermia more often than hyperthermia), unexplained apnea, respiratory distress, seizures (with or without meningitis), cyanosis, tachycardia, bleeding diathesis, and hypotension.

The bacterial causes of neonatal sepsis tend to reflect the organisms that colonize the female genital tract and nasal mucosae of caregivers. In general, the two groups of pathogens most frequently encountered are gram-positive cocci, such as β-hemolytic streptococci, and enteric organisms, such as *E. coli* and *Klebsiella* species, and *H. influenzae*. *Listeria monocytogenes* also causes sepsis and meningitis in neonates. Viral infections comprise another common cause of fever and are most likely due to enteroviruses (coxsackievirus and echovirus) acquired at the time of delivery or RSV and influenza A virus acquired postnatally.

When a neonate is thought to be septic, microscopic analysis of CSF, blood, and urine, and cerebrospinal cultures should be obtained.

All neonates should be admitted, and intravenous antibiotics should be started. Initial treatment of a neonate with suspected bacterial septicemia or meningitis entails a combination of ampicillin and an aminoglycoside. An alternative regimen of ampicillin and cefotaxime or ceftazidime is active against gram-negative bacilli and can be used in cases when gram-negative meningitis is strongly suspected. An infant with a maternal history of herpes or suspicious CSF findings (predominance of lymphocytes and erythrocytes in a nontraumatic lumbar puncture) or ill appearance should also receive intravenous acyclovir.

Febrile infants 4 to 8 weeks of age who satisfy the following criteria are at low risk and may be candidates for outpatient management:

1. No focus of bacterial infection (middle ear, skin, soft tissue, bone, or joint) on physical examination
2. Term, well appearing (alert, active, and with good muscle tone), well hydrated, and tolerating oral fluids adequately, and no respiratory distress (respiratory rate <60 breaths/min, no grunting respiration or retractions)
3. Total white blood cell counts fewer than 10/μL for CSF, fewer than 15,000/μL for complete blood count, fewer than 10 cells/high power field for urinalysis, and negative results for bacteriuria, leukocytes, esterase, and nitrite
4. No pulmonary infiltrates on chest radiograph
5. Reliable caretaker ensuring close outpatient follow-up

The decision to administer ceftriaxone empirically pending culture results in newborns younger than 28 days or infants who do not meet low-risk criteria is routine, because potentially serious complications, such as bacteremia and septicemia, and seeding of central nervous system can result. *Streptococcus pneumoniae* is the most common cause of occult bacteremia. Routine use of the pneumococcal vaccine polyvalent, Pneumovax (intramuscular or subcutaneous injection), or the pneumococcal 7-valent conjugate vaccine, Prevnar (intramuscular injection only), has been instituted and may decrease the risk of occult bacteremia, but data are not yet available to change our current standards

TABLE 117-7   Signs and Symptoms of Neonatal Sepsis

Temperature instability
Central nervous system dysfunction
Respiratory distress
Feeding disturbance
Jaundice
Rashes
Fever, hypothermia
Lethargy, irritability, seizures
Apnea, tachypnea, grunting
Vomiting, poor feeding, gastric distention, diarrhea

for empiric treatment. Therefore, the therapeutic benefit of administering ceftriaxone pending culture results decreases risk and outweighs cost considerations. Thorough and frequent reevaluations of these infants are essential to monitor changes in the clinical course and culture results.[22–24]

NEONATAL SEIZURES

Recognition of seizures in the newborn period is important, because their management and implications are different than at any other age. Seizures usually indicate a severe underlying problem that is rarely idiopathic. Newborns are more likely to present with subtle manifestations, such as eye deviation, tongue thrusting, eyelid fluttering, apnea, or pedaling movements rather than generalized activity. Neonatal seizures are discussed in detail in Chap. 125.

REFERENCES

1. Maisels JM, Kring E: Length of stay, jaundice, and hospital readmission. *Pediatrics* 101:995, 1998.
2. Schmitt BD: The first week at home with your new baby. *Contemp Pediatr* 10:77, 1993.
3. Blum NJ, Carey WB: Sleep problems among infants and young children. *Pediatr Rev* 17:87, 1996.
4. Lucassen PLBJ, Assendelft WJJ, Gubbels JW, et al: Effectiveness of treatments for infantile colic: systemic review. *BMJ* 316:1563, 1998.
5. Labbe J, Caouette G: Recent skin injuries in normal children. *Pediatrics* 108:271, 2001.
6. Mandell GA, Wolfson PJ, Adkins ES, et al: Cost-effective imaging approach to the nonbilious vomiting infant. *Pediatrics* 103:1198, 1999.
7. Konstantinos P, Chen EA, Luks FI, et al: The changing presentation of pyloric stenosis. *Am J Emerg Med* 17:67, 1999.
8. Pollock ES: Pediatric abdominal surgical emergencies. *Pediatr Ann* 25:448, 1996.
9. Gastanaduy A, Begue RE: Acute gastroenteritis. *Clin Pediatr* 38:1, 1999.
10. Armon K, Stephenson T, Macfaul R, et al: An evidence and consensus based guideline for acute diarrhoea management. *Arch Dis Child* 85:132, 2001.
11. McIntosh K: Community-acquired pneumonia in children. *New Engl J Med* 346:429, 2002.
12. Schlesinger C, Koss MN: Bronchiolitis update 2001. *Curr Opin Pulmon Med* 8:112, 2002.
13. Wright RB, Pomerantz WJ, Luria JW: New approaches to respiratory infections in children: Bronchiolitis and croup. *Emerg Med Clin North Am* 20:93, 2002.
14. Rossi AF: Pediatric cardiac intensive care, in Chang AC, Hanley FL, Wernovsky G, Wessel DL (eds): *Cardiac Diagnostic Evaluation.* Baltimore, Williams & Wilkins, 1998, p. 37.
15. Carroll JL, Marcus CL, Loughlin GM: Disordered control of breathing in infants and children. *Pediatr Rev* 14:51, 1993.
16. Dennery PA, Seidman DS, Stevenson DK: Neonatal hyperbilirubinemia. *New Engl J Med* 344:581, 2001.
17. Gonococcal infections, in *Report of the Committee on Infectious Diseases, American Academy of Pediatrics,* 24th ed. Elk Grove Village, American Academy of Pediatrics, 1997, p. 212.
18. *Chlamydia trachomatis,* in *Report of the Committee on Infectious Diseases, American Academy of Pediatrics,* 24th ed. Elk Grove Village, American Academy of Pediatrics, 1997, p. 170.
19. Wagner RS: Eye infection and abnormalities: Issues for the pediatrician. *Contemp Pediatr* 14:137, 1997.
20. Hoppe JE: Treatment of oropharyngeal candidiasis and candidal diaper dermatitis in neonates and infants: Review and reappraisal. *Pediatr Infect Dis J* 16:885, 1997.
21. Lazaks EL, Lane AT: Diaper dermatitis. *Pediatr Clin North Am* 47:909, 2000.
22. Avner JR: Occult bacteremia: How great the risk? *Contemp Pediatr* 14:53, 1997.
23. Baraff LJ: Management of fever without source in infants and children. *Ann Emerg Med* 36:602, 2000.
24. Avner JR, Baker MD: Management of fever in infants and children. *Emerg Med Clin North Am* 20:49, 2002.

THE NICU GRADUATE
Daniel G. Batton

Graduates of the neonatal intensive care unit (NICU) may be frequent visitors to the ED and often require rehospitalization during the year following discharge.[1–3] Most NICU graduates are low-birth weight infants who may have a variety of complications related to prematurity. **These infants should be evaluated based on their *corrected gestational age,* not their chronologic age.** For example, a 32-week-gestation premature infant who is 8 weeks old should be evaluated as a term infant.

Premature infants are usually discharged from the hospital at a corrected gestational age of 33 to 38 weeks, although a few infants will be well beyond 40 weeks. The normal respiratory rate at this age is 30 to 40 breaths/min, but an infant with bronchopulmonary dysplasia usually breathes 60 to 70 times per min. The heart rate ranges from 120 to 160 beats/min while awake and is considerably lower during quiet sleep. Most laboratory values are similar to adult values, although the hematocrit can be as low as 20 to 25 percent following discharge because of physiologic anemia. By 3 to 4 months corrected age the hematocrit should have increased significantly from this nadir. When caring for NICU graduates, attention must be paid not only to the presenting signs and symptoms of the acute illness, but also to general problems related to prematurity.

GENERAL CONSIDERATIONS

Cold Stress

Following hospital discharge, premature infants remain susceptible to cold stress when exposed to lower environmental temperatures, primarily because of decreased subcutaneous tissue.[4] Infants who are cold-stressed are not capable of responding by shivering, but instead attempt to maintain body temperature by increasing the metabolism of brown fat, which results in heat production. However, this process increases oxygen consumption and can lead to hypoglycemia. If this compensatory increase in metabolic rate is insufficient to overcome the low environmental temperature, then body temperature will fall. A normal body temperature, however, does not eliminate the possibility of cold stress, since body temperature may be maintained at considerable metabolic expense. The best way to avoid cold stress is for the ED to provide an adequate environmental temperature for the infant who is being evaluated. If the room temperature cannot be adjusted appropriately, a heat lamp should be available. Commercial heat lamps with automatic timers are available and can be adjusted to provide varying amounts of heat. Such lamps should be standard equipment in EDs that treat infants and children.

Hypoglycemia

Premature infants are at risk of developing hypoglycemia with an acute illness. This risk may be due in part to increased glucose consumption, cold stress, poor enteral intake during the illness, or suboptimal glycogen stores.[4] Since hypoglycemia can have serious consequences, **glucose testing is necessary for all premature infants presenting with an acute illness.** If the blood sugar is less than 45 mg percent, intravenous glucose therapy (D10W at 100 mL/kg per d) may be required.

Hypertension

Longitudinal studies of convalescing premature infants have demonstrated that systemic hypertension may develop in as many as 9 percent.[5] The possible causes include thromboembolic renal artery occlusion following umbilical artery catheterization, and bronchopulmonary dysplasia.[6] Although the normal range is age dependent, a systolic blood pressure greater than 120 mm Hg or a diastolic pressure greater than 75 mm Hg warrants consideration of systemic hypertension.[7]

Fractures

Because of decreased bone mineralization (osteopenia), fractures of the long bones and ribs are not uncommon in premature infants during their initial hospitalization. Usually by the time of hospital discharge, bone mineralization has improved to such an extent that new fractures are uncommon, but evidence of healing fractures on x-ray examination may still be present. This fact should be kept in mind if fractures are incidentally noted on an x-ray, to avoid possible misinterpretation as a sign of child abuse. Comparison of current x-rays with previous films may help to clarify the issue.

Failure to Thrive

The establishment of consistent weight gain with oral feedings is a standard criterion for hospital discharge for most premature infants. However, this does not ensure that adequate weight gain will continue following discharge. Failure to thrive may occur either because of an ongoing chronic disease (e.g., bronchopulmonary dysplasia, malabsorption, or central nervous system disease) or because of dysfunctional parenting. NICU graduates should be consuming at least 150 mL/kg per d of a standard formula if not breast feeding and should be consistently gaining approximately 20 to 30 g/d. If appropriate growth curves[8] are unavailable, a comparison of the current weight with the discharge weight (which parents usually remember) allows for a quick evaluation of this problem. Any infant with failure to thrive requires a thorough diagnostic evaluation and often hospitalization for accurate documentation of caloric intake. Prematurity itself is not an adequate explanation for postdischarge failure to thrive.

Immunizations

The recommendation by the American Academy of Pediatrics is to immunize premature infants on the same schedule as normal full-term infants in most cases.[9] However, because of prolonged hospitalization and complicated follow-up, it is possible that immunizations might be missed. Inquiry about the immunization status may uncover such a situation. Although it may not be desirable to immunize an infant during an acute illness, appropriate recommendations for follow-up should be made.

ACUTE RESPIRATORY DETERIORATION IN INFANTS WITH BRONCHOPULMONARY DYSPLASIA

Although acute respiratory deterioration can occur in any NICU graduate, this discussion focuses on those infants with ongoing pulmonary disease, such as bronchopulmonary dysplasia (BPD). BPD is usually a sequela of prematurity, hyaline membrane disease, and mechanical ventilation, although it may be associated with other conditions.[10] Features of BPD include tachypnea, hypercarbia, suboptimal oxygenation, and sometimes reactive airway disease. In more severe cases, pulmonary hypertension, pulmonary edema, and cor pulmonale are prominent. The cornerstones of therapy for BPD are oxygen and nutrition. It is essential to take a medication history, since some infants will be treated with chronic diuretics, bronchodilators, or systemic steroids, although their value remains poorly defined.

Acute respiratory deterioration in patients with BPD is usually manifested by an increase in respiratory rate and effort, a decrease in oxygenation, and poor feeding. The most common causes of acute respiratory deterioration in infants with BPD are listed in Table 118-1. A careful history can usually delineate the likely etiology. For example, a history of an upper respiratory infection or fever suggests an infectious cause, which is the most common reason for an acute respiratory deterioration in a patient with BPD. Although many viruses and bacteria can be responsible for such infections, **respiratory syncytial virus (RSV) infection is particularly common in premature infants with BPD.[2,11] Infants with BPD can quickly deteriorate during an RSV infection due to acute bronchospasm and airway obstruction from increased secretions.** Such infants usually require rehospitalization for close observation since many worsen to the point of requiring mechanical ventilation. Although the current recommendation of RSV immunoglobulin prophylaxis for premature infants may decrease the frequency of RSV infection requiring hospitalization,[12–14] this is likely to remain an important cause of acute respiratory deterioration in NICU graduates, particularly for those with underlying BPD.

Sudden respiratory deterioration in a patient with BPD is usually due to aspiration, either from gastroesophageal reflux or to a poorly coordinated suck/swallow reflex. Exposure to cigarette smoke or other environmental pollutants may also precipitate acute bronchospasm. Congestive heart failure is usually accompanied by the development of peripheral edema and excessive weight gain. Dehydration is an important cause of acute respiratory deterioration, since many infants have an altered myocardial compliance (Starling curve shifted to the right), making cardiac output more dependent on end-diastolic filling. Therefore, if an infant becomes dehydrated secondary to vomiting and diarrhea or to aggressive diuretic therapy, cardiac output will decrease and secondary respiratory deterioration will follow. When evaluating and treating an infant with BPD who acutely deteriorates, there is often a temptation to initiate or increase the use of diuretics. However, if the infant is already volume depleted, diuretics will make the infant worse. Anemia may also exacerbate respiratory distress in an infant with BPD and is suggested by the presence of pallor. Infants who are not on adequate iron supplementation could have iron deficiency anemia. Acute cor pulmonale can develop secondary to hypoxemia from any of the above-mentioned causes, and deterioration can be very rapid. Effective treatment of acute cor pulmonale in infants with BPD includes treatment of the hypoxemia and its underlying cause.

TABLE 118-1   Causes of Acute Respiratory Deterioration in Infants with BPD

Respiratory infection
Sepsis
Aspiration
   Gastroesophageal reflux
   Incoordinate sucking or swallowing
Bronchospasm
Pulmonary edema or congestive heart failure
Dehydration
   Gastroenteritis
   Diuretic therapy
Anemia

The usual evaluation of an infant with BPD who has acute respiratory deterioration includes a complete blood count, arterial blood gas determination, appropriate cultures, and a chest x-ray. Since the chest x-ray can be difficult to interpret because of chronic abnormalities, it is essential to compare the current x-ray with previous films to identify acute changes. The interpretation of blood gases can also be difficult as these infants often have a compensated respiratory acidosis with P_{CO_2} values from 50 to 70 mm Hg. If a worsening respiratory acidosis is accompanied with hypochloremia, overaggressive diuretic use may be responsible. Infants who become hypochloremic from diuretics will retain bicarbonate and have a secondary increase in P_{CO_2} since they have a limited ability to compensate.

Therapy for acute respiratory deterioration should be directed toward the specific cause, but oxygenation is the cornerstone of treatment. Although BPD infants often have chronic CO_2 retention, there is no evidence that respiratory drive is decreased with oxygen administration. Therefore, oxygen should be used liberally while definitive diagnosis and treatment are contemplated. Specific therapies for BPD have recently been extensively reviewed.[11] Care in an ED often centers on the treatment of acute bronchospasm. Although bronchospasm may be a prominent feature, the treatment of acute respiratory deterioration in an infant with BPD is not the same as that for a child with asthma. The majority of infants with BPD who need acute bronchodilator therapy require hospitalization and observation because of the potential to require mechanical ventilation.

APNEA AND HOME APNEA MONITORS

Most infants resolve apnea of prematurity before discharge and do not require apnea monitoring at home.[15] However, home monitoring is sometimes utilized for premature infants with severe apnea or if apnea persists beyond 38 weeks' gestational age.[16,17] Infants may be brought to the ED because of an apneic episode or because the parents are not sure of the significance of an alarm. Studies have demonstrated that the majority of alarms at home are not associated with a change in cardiorespiratory status and probably represent monitor malfunction, such as that caused by loose leads.[16] However, caution must be exercised before attributing an alarm to a mechanical problem with the monitor. All episodes associated with cyanosis or bradycardia, directly observed episodes of apnea (of sufficient duration, i.e., >15 s), and any episode requiring intervention, such as stimulation or mouth-to-mouth resuscitation, should be thoroughly evaluated and usually require admission. A recurrence of apnea in a premature infant who was discharged apnea-free warrants admission and a thorough search for the cause. The differential diagnosis (Table 118-2) includes respiratory infection (especially with RSV or pertussis), sepsis, gastroesophageal reflux and aspiration, aspiration during feedings, anemia, and metabolic problems such as hypoglycemia. Other more unusual causes include seizures, cardiac dysrhythmias or heart failure, and posthemorrhagic hydrocephalus. Therapy is directed toward the specific cause.

TABLE 118-2   Most Common Causes of Apnea and Bradycardia at Home in NICU Graduates

Respiratory infection (RSV or pertussis)
Sepsis
Gastroesophageal reflux and aspiration
Aspiration with feedings
Anemia
Hypoglycemia
Seizures
Cardiac arrhythmias
Posthemorrhagic hydrocephalus

POSTHEMORRHAGIC HYDROCEPHALUS

Premature infants who have had an intraventricular hemorrhage may develop posthemorrhagic hydrocephalus in the newborn period.[18] Hydrocephalus can progress during the initial hospitalization, in which case the infant is usually discharged with a ventriculoperitoneal shunt in place. Hydrocephalus may also develop gradually following discharge. Such infants may present to an ED because of progressive hydrocephalus if unshunted, or shunt obstruction and/or infection. Infants with infection usually have nonspecific signs, such as poor feeding, lethargy, irritability, fever, and vomiting, similar to those of any other child with central nervous system infection. An infant with an obstructed shunt most often has a tense fontanel and a history of vomiting, although the infant usually does not appear particularly ill. A comparison of the current head circumference with the head circumference at discharge (if available) is helpful in evaluating for progressive hydrocephalus. A imaging study such as a computed tomography scan or cranial ultrasound may be necessary to fully evaluate the size of the ventricles. Empiric antibiotic therapy should be utilized whenever a shunt infection is suspected, pending culture results. Shunt infections usually require removal of the foreign body, although successful treatment without removal has been reported for *Staphylococcus epidermidis* infections. For both shunt infections and hydrocephalus, neurosurgical consultation is required.

THE EXPECTED HOME DEATH

Some infants are discharged from the NICU with lethal conditions for which further medical intervention is not indicated, and the parents are expecting the child to die at home. In many cases the parents are instructed to take the infant to the ED to be pronounced dead by a physician. The parents should be given a letter at the time of the original hospital discharge by their physicians delineating the infant's problems to provide guidance to the emergency physician facing such a situation. This is a very traumatic time for the parents. A futile resuscitation effort is not appropriate and can prolong the parents' agony. It is very important to request autopsy permission in such cases to completely delineate the infant's problems and to provide optimal counseling for future pregnancies.

REFERENCES

1. Mutch L, Newdick M, Lodwick A, et al: Secular changes in rehospitalization of very low birth weight infants. *Pediatrics* 78:164, 1986.
2. Cunningham CK, McMillian JA, Gross SJ: Rehospitalization for respiratory illness in infants of less than 32 weeks' gestation. *Pediatrics* 88:527, 1991.
3. Yüksel B, Greenough A: Birth weight and hospital readmission of infants born prematurely. *Arch Pediatr Adolesc Med* 148:384, 1994.
4. Klaus MH, Martin RJ, Fanaroff AA (eds): *Care of the High-Risk Neonate*, 5th ed. Philadelphia: Saunders, 2001.
5. Sheftel DN, Hustead V, Friedman A: Hypertension screening in the follow-up of premature infants. *Pediatrics* 71:763, 1983.
6. Abman SH, Bradley AW, Lum GM: Systemic hypertension in infants with bronchopulmonary dysplasia. *J Pediatr* 104:928, 1984.
7. Tan KL: Clinical and laboratory observations: Blood pressure in very low birth weight infants in the first 70 days life. *J Pediatr* 112:266, 1988.
8. Ballard, RA: *Pediatric Care of the ICN Graduate*. Philadelphia: Saunders, 2000.
9. American Academy of Pediatrics: *2000 Redbook: Report of the Committee on Infectious Diseases*, 25th ed. Elk Grove Village, IL: American Academy of Pediatrics, 2000, p. 54.
10. Rush MD, Hazinski TA: Current therapy of bronchopulmonary dysplasia. *Clin Perinatol* 19:563, 1992.
11. Groothuis JR, Gutierrez KM, Lauer BA: Respiratory syncytial virus infection in children with bronchopulmonary dysplasia. *Pediatrics* 82:199, 1988.

12. Groothuis JR, Simoes E, Hemming VG, et al: Respiratory syncytial virus (RSV) infection in preterm infants and the protective effects of RSV immune globulin (RSVIG). *Pediatrics* 95:463, 1995.

13. American Academy of Pediatrics Committee on Infectious Diseases, Committee on Fetus and Newborn: Respiratory syncytial virus immune globulin intravenous: Indications for use. *Pediatrics* 99:645, 1997.

14. American Academy of Pediatrics Committee on Infectious Diseases, Committee on Fetus and Newborn: Prevention of respiratory syncytial infections: Indications for the use of palivizumab and update on the use of RSV-IGIV (RE9839). *Pediatrics* 102:1211, 1998.

15. Miller MJ, Martin RJ: Apnea of prematurity. *Clin Perinatol* 19:789, 1992.

16. Spitzer AR, Givson E: Home monitoring. *Clin Perinatol* 19:907, 1992.

17. Consensus statement: National Institutes of Health Consensus Development Conference on Infantile Apnea and Home Monitoring, Sept. 29 to Oct. 1, 1986. *Pediatrics* 79:292, 1987.

18. Volpe JJ: *Neurology of the Newborn,* 4th ed. Philadelphia: Saunders, 2001.

SIDS (SUDDEN INFANT DEATH SYNDROME) AND ALTE (APPARENT LIFE-THREATENING EVENT)

Carol D. Berkowitz

Sudden death may affect persons of any age, but it is especially devastating when it affects previously healthy individuals. In the past, between 5000 and 10,000 infants (1 to 2 per 1000 live births) succumbed yearly to sudden infant death syndrome (SIDS), also known as *crib death.* With recent changes related to infant position during sleep, the number of deaths has decreased to about 3000 and the rate to about 0.8 deaths per 1000 infants.

The term *sudden infant death syndrome* was officially designated in 1963 to describe a syndrome of unexpected death in infants younger than 1 year for which no pathologic cause could be determined by a thorough postmortem examination. The syndrome has been a leading cause of death of infants between 1 month and 1 year of age.

An understanding of SIDS is essential for emergency physicians so that they can recognize the syndrome, initiate resuscitation, manage infants who have experienced an apparent life-threatening event (ALTE; previously termed *near-miss SIDS*), and counsel the family of the victim.

PATHOPHYSIOLOGY

More than 70 different theories for SIDS have been proposed, including suffocation from sleeping with a parent, milk allergy, and thymic enlargement (status thymicolymphaticus). The main disturbance in some victims appears to be with the infant's ventilatory response, and SIDS and infantile apnea appear related, although the exact nature of this relation is uncertain. There are multiple causes of infantile apnea for which the final pathway involves respiratory muscle fatigue. Death is due to respiratory rather than to cardiac arrest, and some potential SIDS victims may be successfully resuscitated with ventilation alone. Dysrhythmias probably occur only as a terminal event, and syndromes such as prolonged QT interval or Wolff-Parkinson-White syndrome are rare associations.[1] Prospective studies monitoring normal infants showed no antecedent dysrhythmias in infants who eventually succumbed to SIDS. Conversely, approximately 2 percent of premature and low-birth-weight infants experienced bradycardia (fewer than 50 breaths/min) without apnea 1 week after discharge.

Information implicating ventilation disturbances and hypoxemia has been obtained from two sources: autopsies of infants who succumbed to SIDS, and studies of those who experienced an ALTE but survived. The ALTE group comprises infants who were found limp, cyanotic, pale, and lifeless, showed no respiratory effort, but who were successfully resuscitated.

Autopsies of some SIDS victims showed pathologic changes initially felt to be indicative of longstanding hypoxemia. These changes included smooth muscle thickening in small pulmonary arteries, right ventricular hypertrophy, hematopoiesis in the liver, increase in peri-adrenal brown fat, adrenal medullary hyperplasia, and abnormalities of the carotid body. Markers now reported with regularity include brainstem gliosis and increased neuronal apoptosis in the brainstem and hippocampus.

Recently, much attention has been given to SIDS and sleeping in the prone position.[2,3] Epidemiologic studies indicated that the incidence of SIDS is lower in countries where infants sleep supine or in the side-down position, and that a reduction in the incidence of SIDS follows a reduction in prone sleeping. Concern about aspiration in infants sleeping in the supine position are unfounded. Two mechanisms linking SIDS to prone sleeping are noted. With prone sleeping, infants will assume a face-down position, particularly in response to a cold stimulus on the face. This may result in upper airway obstruction. However, upper airway obstruction has not been observed in clinical trials; rather, infants were found to rebreathe expired air and experience hypercarbia.[4] Because of these observations related to the prone position, the American Academy of Pediatrics now recommends a supine or side-sleeping position for normal infants.

The link between child abuse, SIDS, and ALTE has also received renewed interest.[5] Familial cases of SIDS raise the possibility of abuse. Some investigators reported that 10 percent of SIDS cases are due to abuse. Some children with ALTE have been purposefully asphyxiated, and in some cases the complaints have simply been fabricated. These problems are referred to as *Munchausen syndrome by proxy.* The use of in-hospital covert video-surveillance cameras has sometimes facilitated substantiating this diagnosis. Child abuse is the diagnosed cause of death in about 2000 cases a year. The presence of bruises, long-bone fractures, rib fractures, internal hemorrhages, evidence of physical neglect, or trauma around the nares suggests abuse. Rib fractures in infants are not induced by cardiopulmonary resuscitation. A history inconsistent with the usual events surrounding a SIDS death also may raise the suspicion of abuse. In addition, some infants with abusive head trauma may present with nonspecific symptoms including apnea.[6] Appropriate diagnostic studies should be initiated to establish the correct diagnosis. An interesting report on death-scene investigations found circumstantial evidence of accidental death in 23 of 26 infants studied.[7] It is beyond the scope of emergency physicians to conduct such investigations. However, more and more communities have extensive databases that are filled in when SIDS is suspected. In addition, Child Death Review Boards are convened to ensure the full evaluation of sudden and unexpected death among children. It is important, however, to be aware of the possible role of accidental or intentional trauma in some SIDS victims.

SIDS and Apnea

Four groups of infants who appear at increased risk of SIDS have been identified: (1) term infants who have had an ALTE, (2) premature infants of low birth weight, (3) siblings of infants who have succumbed to SIDS, and (4) infants of substance-abusing mothers.[8]

Studies of infants with ALTE may reveal (1) hypoventilation (partial pressure of carbon dioxide > 45 mm Hg) and chronic hypoxemia, (2) a depressed ventilatory response to CO_2 breathing, (3) prolonged sleep apnea (>15 s, associated with cyanosis or pallor), (4) bouts of frequent short apnea, (5) increased periodic breathing (characterized by repeated 3-s pauses in breathing followed by normal breathing for shorter than 20 s with bradycardia), (6) obstructive apnea, and (7) mixed obstructive and central apnea.

Southall[9] described three separate components associated with respiratory abnormalities in infants.

First, there is central apnea, in which immaturity, tumor, head injury, infection, or congenital malformation leads to primary failure of respiratory center control. In addition, peripheral chemoreceptors act abnormally, particularly in response to hypercarbia and hypoxia. The dive reflex may contribute to apnea on a central basis. Young monkeys receiving a cold or wet stimulus to the face in the area of the trigeminal nerve stop breathing. This situation may be analogous to a young infant lying in a regurgitated feeding. Alternatively, this stimulus may lead to a face-down sleeping position and airway obstruction.

Airway obstruction is a second component. Obstructive apnea may occur in response to nasal occlusion, as with an upper respiratory infection, and is noted with tonsillar enlargement, hypotonia of the hypopharynx, or glossoptosis. It is a contributing factor in about 5 percent of ALTE episodes. It is detected by the presence of increased chest wall movement, with bradycardia and decreased partial pressure of oxygen (by surface oximeter). It is a contributing component to SIDS in infants with upper respiratory infection.

The third and most significant component is expiratory apnea. Prolonged expiratory apnea is associated with sudden atelectasis. Ventilation perfusion inequalities, hypoxia, and sudden cyanosis occur within 5 to 10 s. There is a rapid loss of consciousness. These episodes may occur even in the face of nasotracheal intubation. In older children, they may occur with crying, as cyanotic breath-holding spells.

Acute hypoxic episodes are felt to occur in 80 percent of SIDS cases.

EPIDEMIOLOGIC FACTORS

The diagnosis of SIDS is confirmed by autopsy, but many clinical and epidemiologic features characterize the syndrome. Although the overall incidence is now about 0.8 per 1000 live births, there is variation among different ethnic groups, with an incidence of 0.51 per 1000 among Asian Americans and 5.93 per 1000 among Native Americans. Some of the current ethnic variability in the incidence of SIDS may be related to compliance of caregivers' placing infants in the supine position. Victims range in age from 1 month to 1 year, with peaks at 2 months 2 weeks and at 4 months. The infant frequently has been premature or small for gestational age. Although initial reports suggested a higher incidence of SIDS among premature infants with bronchopulmonary dysplasia, this association has not been confirmed by more recent studies.

The syndrome is rare in the first month of life, probably because the neonate has a better anaerobic capacity for survival, and with a gasp may be able to raise his or her arterial partial pressure of oxygen over 20 mm Hg and continue breathing. Of the infants who are otherwise healthy, 30 to 50 percent have some acute infection, usually of the upper respiratory tract, at the time of the event. Infection with respiratory syncytial virus has been associated with apnea, particularly in premature infants and those with an antecedent history of apnea. Otitis media and gastroenteritis also have been associated with SIDS. Infected infants tend to be older than noninfected infants, and males outnumber females in the infected group by 2:1. The sex ratio is equal in the noninfected group. There is a disproportionate number of babies from the lower socioeconomic group, although this is true for deaths in infancy from all causes. Mothers frequently are younger than 20 years and unwed, smoke, use drugs, and have made few prenatal and postpartum visits. Prenatal and postnatal maternal smoking increase the incidence of SIDS. Sudden infant death syndrome is more likely to occur during the winter months and when the infant is asleep.

A disproportionate number of infants succumbs to SIDS while with a babysitter.[10] Many of these infants have been found in the prone position. For some infants, this is the first time they have been placed in the prone position, and investigators have proposed that these infants have poor strength and tone in their neck muscles. Further, some infants may have acquired an upper respiratory infection in day-care centers, a phenomenon that is well described for that setting.

The issue of the relation between co-sleeping and SIDS is controversial.[11,12] Several studies have reported an increased incidence of co-sleeping or sleeping on an inappropriate surface among SIDS victims.

Parental intoxication or substance abuse appears to be a related factor. In one study, only 1 of 40 children who had died from SIDS while co-sleeping had been supine on an appropriate surface at the time of death.

CLINICAL FEATURES

A number of scenarios may confront physicians in the ED. These scenarios mirror the range of problems that may be broadly categorized under the heading of SIDS or of ALTE (Table 119-1).

Some infants appear completely well at the time they are examined, and the parents may relate a history of cessation of respiration. The physician must then determine whether the event represented an episode of apnea, was severe enough to be life threatening, or represented a different disorder.

The sequence of events before the episode may be a clue to the cause (Table 119-2). If the infant stiffened or exhibited clonic movements, the cessation of respiration may have been postictal apnea after a seizure. With a seizure, an infant is frequently awake before becoming apneic. Gastroesophageal reflux may lead to apnea and also may occur in awake infants after a feeding. A history of an upper respiratory infection followed by paroxysmal cough with an apneic episode suggests pertussis. Hypoglycemia also may be associated with apnea, with or without a seizure. The differential diagnosis also includes infection (sepsis or meningitis) and cardiomyopathy. Infantile botulism may be the cause in 5 to 10 percent of SIDS victims.

The evaluation of healthy-appearing infants with a history of apnea is problematic. Occasionally, parents may have misinterpreted acrocyanosis, postprandial regurgitation, or skin color change with stooling as an episode of apnea. The parents should be carefully questioned about what they did to revive the baby, for example, stimulation or mouth-to-mouth resuscitation. No resuscitative efforts suggest a benign event. Conversely, the need for mouth-to-mouth resuscitation indicates a more serious event. The finding of irregular respiration or poor muscle tone on physical examination would assist in the diagnosis of an ALTE.

Some infants who have experienced an ALTE have not been fully resuscitated in the field. They should receive the benefit of vigorous cardiopulmonary resuscitation, unless signs of irreversible death (livedo reticularis, blood pH of 6, or boxcar venous pooling in the fundi) are apparent. Frequently the heart will resume beating after prolonged arrest. The infant heart is a remarkably resistant organ and may be revived after irreversible brain damage.

DIAGNOSIS

The evaluation of an infant who has experienced an ALTE should include a complete medical history, particularly of the event itself, and

TABLE 119-1   Risks for SIDS and ALTE

SIDS risks
   Term infants with an episode of ALTE
   Premature low-birth-weight infants
   Siblings of an infant who died of SIDS
   Infants of substance-abusing mothers
ALTE risks
   Respiratory center immaturity
      Hypoventilation and chronic hypoxemia
      Depressed ventilatory response to CO_2
      >15 s of sleep apnea, with cyanosis or pallor
      Increased periodic breathing: 3-s pauses, apnea >20 s, and
         bradycardia
      Prolonged expiratory apnea
   Obstructive apnea
      Apnea related to upper respiratory infection

Abbreviations: ALTE = apparent life-threatening event, SIDS = sudden infant death syndrome.

TABLE 119-2   Conditions That May Present as an Apparent Life-Threatening Event

Cardiac arrhythmias/anomalies
Child abuse
Gastroesophageal reflux
Infantile botulism
Inborn errors of metabolism
Intracranial hemmorhage
Pertussis
Respiratory syncytial virus infection
Seizure
Sepsis

take into account the perinatal and epidemiologic factors associated with SIDS and ALTE. A history of other infant deaths in the family should be obtained because of the familial incidence of SIDS. Familial cases of SIDS suggest the possibility of child abuse or of inborn errors of metabolism, such as disorders of fatty acid metabolism.[13] Autopsy results in a small subset of infants who succumbed to SIDS showed findings such as microvesicular steatosis of the liver, a sign of a disorder of fatty acid metabolism. Sometimes, sudden unexpected death has occurred in other siblings within these affected families. Initial reports suggested that siblings of SIDS victims are at increased risk (about 10-fold) for subsequent SIDS. More recent studies showed at most a twofold increase in the incidence of SIDS among SIDS siblings.

The physical examination should be complete, with special emphasis on the neurologic evaluation and the presence of any injuries. The initial laboratory assessment should include a complete blood cell count; determination of levels of serum electrolytes, blood sugar, calcium, phosphate, and magnesium; and a 12-lead electrocardiogram. A septic workup, including blood culture, cerebrospinal fluid analysis, urine culture, and chest x-ray, is indicated in most cases, although studies have shown a negligible yield in the absence of associated findings such as fever. Nasopharyngeal washings for respiratory syncytial virus or other viral assays are indicated if there are signs of an upper respiratory infection. In an infant with an ALTE, the stool should be sent for clostridial culture and botulinum toxin testing, especially if hypotonia is present. Other studies should be done when suggested by the history and physical examination; these include determination of serum ammonia, urinary organic acids, sleep and awake electroencephalograms, skull x-rays, barium swallow, and computed tomography.

TREATMENT

Initial treatment in the ED involves continued resuscitation of the infant, if necessary, and stabilization. In general, all ALTE victims and infants with a history of apnea and/or cyanosis should be admitted to the hospital. The evaluation of these infants is designed to rule out treatable causes of apnea and to determine whether, in the absence of these other causes, the infant is at risk for SIDS, an event reported in 20 to 100 percent of infants with an ALTE.

Apnea should be monitored in the hospital. Most hospitals can obtain pneumograms, which provide evidence of abnormalities related to periodic breathing or episodes of apnea. Polysomnography measures the amount of air flowing in at the mouth and nose and can detect obstructive apnea; the test is complicated and generally done in a sleep laboratory. Certain tertiary care centers are equipped to evaluate responses to CO_2 breathing and diminished inspiratory oxygen.

HOME MONITORING

Two major treatment modalities are recommended for infants who have experienced an ALTE or are at risk for SIDS. Xanthine derivatives such as caffeine and theophylline are used frequently in treating apnea of prematurity because of their central excitatory effect. Their use is asso-

ciated with the normalization of the respiratory pattern in more than 80 percent of such children. Their efficacy in the prevention of SIDS is unclear. A pragmatic approach to the use of xanthine derivatives would be to limit them to infants with abnormal pneumograms. Reversal of these abnormalities with either medication would be an indication for its use. Theophylline is given at 6 mg/kg per d and caffeine at 5 to 7.5 mg/kg per d, and a serum level of 5 to 15 mg/mL should be maintained.

Home apnea monitoring is the second modality that can be offered. Three groups were defined in a National Institutes of Health Consensus Statement in 1986 as being candidates for home monitoring. The first group consists of term infants with unexplained apnea of infancy, usually manifested by a life-threatening episode and/or abnormal pneumogram. The absence of an abnormal pneumogram does not preclude home monitoring. The second group consists of preterm infants who have continued to manifest apnea beyond term (i.e., after 40 weeks postconception). The third group consists of subsequent siblings of two or more SIDS victims, but not of one SIDS victim. Twins of SIDS victims were reported to have a 20-fold increase in their risk for SIDS. More recent studies suggested their chance is the same as for non-twin siblings. Additional candidates for home monitoring include infants with bronchopulmonary dysplasia, especially if oxygen dependent, and infants who require tracheostomy for airway support.

Home-monitoring devices usually measure chest wall movement and heart rate. The detection of bradycardia is particularly important in infants with an obstructive component, because chest wall movement is not diminished with obstructive apnea. Parents must be instructed in equipment maintenance, interpretation of the alarm, and cardiopulmonary resuscitation. Home monitoring does not mean simply supplying a family with a mechanical device. It involves the development of a medical team to support the family, interpret any episodes of apnea, and decide when home monitoring can be discontinued. Technicians who are available 24 h a day to maintain the equipment are also required.

Emergency physicians are frequently consulted about monitor alarms. Infants are brought to the ED because of alarm triggering. Physicians must be able to differentiate a false alarm from a true episode. The need for vigorous stimulation or mouth-to-mouth resuscitation suggests a serious episode. If there is concern about equipment malfunction, technical assistance should be obtained from the monitoring company.

The use of home monitors has increased dramatically in recent years. The estimated cost of monitoring (including initial assessment) ranges from $3000 to $5000 per infant, with monthly rental and maintenance costs ranging from $150 to $300. Although parental anxiety is frequently reduced, the reduction in the incidence of subsequent SIDS in monitored infants is questioned. Reports found a mortality rate as high as 50 percent among infants on home monitoring. In many cases, technical errors and parental noncompliance contributed to the infant's demise. Some infants, however, simply failed to respond to aggressive cardiopulmonary resuscitation.

The decision to discontinue monitoring is usually made by an infant's primary physician. In general, most infants remain on a monitor for 6 to 8 months. Criteria for discontinuing the monitor include 2 to 3 months with no episodes requiring stimulation or resuscitation, 3 months without apnea of 20 s or longer, no apnea associated with an upper respiratory infection or immunization, and an improvement in any neurologic problem for which the monitoring was instituted (e.g., apnea associated with seizures).

THE SIDS VICTIM

The management of a nonresuscitative SIDS infant and the infant's family is equally challenging for a physician. The emergency physician is confronted by the distraught mother who had fed her infant several hours earlier, went to check the sleeping infant, and found the baby cold, blue, and lifeless. Frequently, valiant albeit unsuccessful efforts are carried out in the ED, or the infant is revived briefly, only to succumb after several hours in the intensive care unit.

The major responsibility of the physician is then to notify, counsel, and educate the family. In most jurisdictions, victims of sudden and unexplained deaths must be referred to the coroner's office, where an autopsy is performed at the coroner's discretion. Some jurisdictions have infant death teams that fully evaluate the circumstances surrounding the unexpected death of young infants. If the physician believes the infant is a victim of SIDS, the family should be so advised but told that the final confirmation awaits the autopsy report. The emergency physician should assure the family about their lack of responsibility for the infant's death and assuage their feelings of guilt. The physician should then serve as a facilitator by maintaining contact with the family to advise them of the autopsy results. The hospital chaplain or social worker may provide additional support, but the physician's empathy is especially supportive to the family. Most communities have organizations for parents of SIDS victims, and information about these organizations can be obtained from the SIDS Alliance, 10500 Little Patuxent Parkway, Suite 420, Columbia, MD 21044, 1-800-221-SIDS. Parents also may be referred to Web sites such as http://www.sidsfamilies.com.

REFERENCES

1. Schwartz PJ, Strambla-Badiale M, Segantini A, et al: Prolongation of the QT interval and the sudden infant death syndrome. *New Engl J Med* 338:1709, 1998.
2. Ponsonby AL, Dwyer T, Gibbons LE, et al: Factors potentiating the risk of sudden infant death syndrome associated with the prone position. *New Engl J Med* 329:377, 1993.
3. American Academy of Pediatrics, Task Force on Infant Sleeping Position and SIDS: Infant sleep position and sudden infant death syndrome (SIDS) in the United States: Joint Commentary from the American Academy of Pediatrics and selected agencies of the federal government. *Pediatrics* 93:820, 1994.
4. Chiodini BA, Thach BT: Impaired ventilation in infants sleeping face down: Potential significance for sudden infant death syndrome. *J Pediatr* 123:686, 1993.
5. Reece RM: Fatal child abuse and sudden infant death syndrome: A critical diagnostic decision. *Pediatrics* 91:423, 1993.
6. Jenny C, Hymel KP, Ritzen A, et al: Analysis of missed cases of abusive head trauma. *JAMA* 281:621, 1999.
7. Bass M, Kravath RE, Glass L: Death-scene investigation in sudden infant death syndrome. *New Engl J Med* 315:100, 1986.
8. Carroll JL, Loughlin GM: Sudden infant death syndrome. *Pediatr Rev* 14:83, 1993.
9. Southall DP: Role of apnea in the sudden infant death syndrome: A personal view. *Pediatrics* 80:73, 1988.
10. Moon RY, Patel KM, Shaefer SJ: Sudden infant death syndrome in child care settings. *Pediatrics* 106:295, 2000.
11. Gessner BD, Ives GC, Perham-Hester KA: Association between sudden infant death syndrome and prone sleep position, bed sharing and sleeping outside an infant crib in Alaska. *Pediatrics* 108:923, 2001.
12. Kemp JS, Unger B, Wilkins D, et al: Unsafe sleep practice and an analysis of bedsharing among infants dying suddenly and unexpectedly: Results of a four-year, population-based, death scene investigation study of sudden infant death syndrome and related deaths. *Pediatrics* 106:e41, 2000.
13. Boles RG, Buck EA, Blitzer MG, et al: Retrospective biochemical screening of fatty acid oxidation disorders in postmortem livers of 418 cases of sudden death in the first year of life. *J Pediatr* 132:924, 1998.

120 PEDIATRIC HEART DISEASE
C. James Corrall

Pediatric cardiovascular disorders are decidedly uncommon in emergency medicine. The combination of the low incidence and the age-related differences in clinical presentation make timely recognition, sta-

bilization, and appropriate tertiary referral a challenge. In the ED, problems may range from an asymptomatic discovery of a murmur to the life-threatening presentation of a cyanotic infant in cardiogenic shock.

Congenital heart disease is usually classified based on physiology (presence or absence of cyanosis, with or without persistent fetal circulation) or on the nature of the anatomic defect (shunt, obstruction, transposition, or complex). Most pediatric heart disease is congenital, but acquired conditions also occur and include complications secondary to rheumatic fever, Kawasaki disease, and severe chronic anemias, as well as myocarditis, pericarditis, endocarditis, and the tachydysrhythmias.

Pediatric heart disease can also be classified by clinical presentation. The six common clinical presentations to primary care physicians are cyanosis, congestive heart failure, pathologic murmur in asymptomatic patients, abnormal pulses, hypertension, and syncope. Table 120-1 lists the most common lesions in each category. While this is informative in the formation of a broad differential diagnosis in very ill pediatric patients, it is perhaps best to classify heart disease according to the clinical presentation in the ED. Most often, this presentation is in children with previously undiagnosed heart disease and to a lesser degree in those with previously diagnosed heart disease or reparative surgery for the same.

Children with previously undiagnosed heart disease can be broadly classified into three categories: unstable, stable but symptomatic, and stable and asymptomatic. Unstable infants usually require immediate and decisive stabilization and aggressive management before diagnostic studies or tertiary referral can be made. Pediatric cardiology consultation should be emergently sought from the regional tertiary care center before pharmacologic intervention, if at all possible. Stable and symptomatic infants require less-aggressive measures, so there is time to focus on physiologic derangement and correction of abnormalities of oxygenation and metabolism and time for tertiary referral. A baseline electrocardiogram (ECG) and chest radiograph are indicated in such infants, particularly when a murmur appears to be pathologic (grade 3 or louder, holosystolic or diastolic in timing, and/or radiating away from the heart). Stable but asymptomatic infants can easily be referred routinely based on findings on general examination. Such infants can be electively evaluated without specific testing in the ED. Recent, well-publicized cases of pediatric sudden death from unrecognized pediatric heart disease are rare, but such infants arrive in extremis at the ED. This represents a final presentation type of pediatric heart disease that is tragic because such infants cannot often be resuscitated, even by physicians with expertise in pediatric heart disease.

Children with known heart disease arrive at the ED for treatment of routine illnesses, as well as for problems related to their unique disease. Rarely, they arrive with acute life-threatening cardiovascular complica-

TABLE 120-1   Clinical Presentation of Pediatric Heart Disease

Cyanosis	TGA, TOF, TA, Tat, TAVR
Congestive heart failure	See Table 115-3
Murmur/symptomatic patient	Shunts: VSD, PDA, ASD
	Obstructions
	Valvular incompetence
Abnormal pulses	
Bounding	PDA, AI, AVM
Decreased with prolonged amplitude	Coarctation, HPLV
Hypertension	Coarctation
Syncope (see Chap. 131)	
Cyanotic	TOF
Acyanotic	Critical AS

Abbreviations: AI = aortic insufficiency; AS = aortic stenosis; ASD = atrial septal defect; AVM = arteriovenous malformation; HPLV = hypoplastic left ventricle; PDA = patent ductus arteriosus; TA = truncus arteriosus; Tat = tricuspid atresia; TAVR = total anomalous venous return; TGA = transposition of the great arteries; TOF = tetralogy of Fallot; VSD = ventricular septal defect.

tions. Once the knowledge of preexisting heart disease is known, the physician can anticipate complications related to the unique disease, such as hemoconcentration caused by polycythemia, bacterial endocarditis, or embolism. Only infrequently do such infants have abnormal immune systems, and most handle routine pediatric illnesses well.

CARDIOVASCULAR PHYSIOLOGY

It is important to understand the interplay between normal cardiovascular dynamics in pediatric patients and the age-related changes that occur during transition to the extrauterine environment. This understanding is necessary in order to recognize the signs and symptoms of pediatric heart disease and to plan therapy appropriate to the physiologic derangement.

Perhaps the most dramatic change that occurs at birth is the transition from fetal to postnatal circulation. Immediately following birth, flow through the umbilical arteries ceases and the venous flow through the cord slows and then stops. These vascular changes are mediated by the rapid increase in partial pressure of arterial oxygen (PaO_2) that occurs during lung inflation. Following lung expansion, pulmonary vascular resistance falls and pulmonary blood flow increases. The pulmonary vascular resistance will continue to fall with increases in blood flow over the next 30 to 45 days of extrauterine life. The ductus arteriosus also closes with the rise in PaO_2, and blood shunted through a patent foramen ovale ceases. In time, these shunt channels permanently close but, until then, may reopen under conditions of decreased partial pressure of oxygen (PO_2) or other stresses.[1]

Because neonates and small children have limited ability to increase stroke volume because of the relatively noncompliant ventricular walls, they rely on changes in heart rate to adjust the cardiac output. Thus, sinus tachycardia is usually the first response to stress in infants and children and is mediated by the intrinsic pacemaker in the sinoatrial node and by various adrenergic, hormonal, and neural mediators.

Preload is the amount of blood that the heart receives to distribute to the body. Decreasing the amount of blood flowing into the heart lowers the cardiac output. Preload can be reduced by pharmacologic means such as by the use of intravenous nitrates or by blood loss. Similarly, increasing the amount of blood into the heart will increase the cardiac output in accordance with Starling forces, until the point of maximum compliance of the ventricular wall. At this point, cardiac output decreases dramatically and congestive heart failure occurs.

Afterload is the resistance to blood flow out of the heart. Afterload may be increased anatomically in neonates by an obstructive lesion, such as aortic stenosis or critical coarctation of the aorta. Afterload depends on the size of the ventricle and its compliance or elasticity. The compliance in the neonatal heart is limited, so afterload reaches critical values early. Afterload also depends on the amount of arteriolar resistance in the case of pediatric hypertension unrelated to obstructive lesions in the proximity of the heart and great vessels. Treatment of afterload problems is directed at arterial vasoconstriction or vasodilatation.

Contractility or *inotropy,* which is the ability of the cardiac muscle to pump blood out of the heart, refers to the force or power of the contraction and determines the amount of work that the heart can perform. Increasing the cardiac contractility increases the stroke volume and hence the cardiac output. Cardiac contractility is normally regulated by neural or humoral mechanisms. It may be altered pharmacologically by such medications as digoxin or dobutamine.

Cardiac rate or *chronotropy* is the ability of the heart muscle to pump blood out of the heart per fixed unit of contraction. In the typical circumstance, chronotropy and inotropy cannot be differentiated with regard to therapeutic maneuvers. Typically, both the cardiac rate and the relatively fixed contractility of the neonatal heart contribute to the overall cardiac output, with the former contributing more of the output. In pediatric hearts older than 4 to 5 years, there is a more balanced contribution to cardiac output, with the contractility playing a much more prominent role.

THERAPEUTIC PRINCIPLES

All of the medical management provided to children with heart disease is directed toward increasing cardiac output in low-output states by alteration of the heart rate, preload, afterload, or inherent contractility. As mentioned previously, some of these parameters may be rather fixed due to the inherent limitations of the neonatal ventricular noncompliance.

Heart rate is the most malleable of the cardiac physiologic parameters. Symptomatic bradycardias of all types are treated with oxygenation, atropine and, in severe cases, with epinephrine and/or isoproterenol followed by transthoracic pacemaker and transvenous pacemaker usage. Symptomatic tachycardia must be differentiated into sinus, supraventricular, or ventricular before specific therapy can be initiated.

Preload disorders are common in children and are most frequently caused by shock states with resultant hypovolemia that causes the decreased preload. Hypovolemia may be a result of increased loss of total body water, such as occurs in excessive diarrhea or vomiting, or it may be a relative loss of volume because of maldistribution. In the latter circumstance, distributive forms of shock such as in sepsis, neurogenic spinal shock, or anaphylaxis produce relative hypovolemia secondary to increased vasodilation and decreased venous return to the heart. In congestive heart failure, preload is markedly increased when the left atrial pressure becomes elevated. The resulting Starling forces produce pulmonary edema and its resultant hypoxemia. The hypoxemia reduces contractility, further increasing the left atrial pressure and accentuating the increased preload state. Treatment of such a state requires diuretics and vasodilation to reduce preload.

Adequate oxygen delivery is necessary for the myocardium during the diastolic filling phase. The oxygen supply depends on the PO_2 of the blood, the hemoglobin concentration, and the coronary perfusion pressure. Hypoxemia results from deoxygenated venous blood entering the systemic circulation by vascular shunts that may be present at any location. Hypoxemia caused by most vascular shunts responds poorly to increasing ambient inspired oxygen. In contrast, most respiratory causes of hypoxemia respond to increasing oxygen.

Anemia profoundly decreases the amount of oxygen available to the tissues by decreasing the amount of oxygen bound to hemoglobin per unit of cardiac output. Transfusions of 10 mL packed red cells per kg will raise the hemoglobin approximately 1.5 g/dL and provide improved oxygen-carrying capacity to the tissues. In special circumstances, other competing agents, such as methemoglobinemia and carboxyhemoglobinemia, with increased affinity for oxygen must be excluded.

Myocardial perfusion can only occur during the relaxation phase provided during diastole. The perfusion is markedly impaired under conditions of low cardiac output. Because the coronary perfusion pressure is the difference between the diastolic pressure minus the coronary sinus venous pressure, it follows that any situation that lowers diastolic pressure to 30 to 40 mm Hg can lead to poor coronary perfusion, myocardial ischemia, and subsequent ECG changes reflecting injury. Treatment of low diastolic pressure includes infusion with α-adrenergic agents such as phenylephrine, norepinephrine, and epinephrine to raise the diastolic pressure and coronary artery perfusion. Other factors are also important to augment perfusion, but are not as amenable to therapy by emergency physicians.

Severe acidosis adversely affects myocardial contractility and may be persistent after hypovolemia has been corrected. Sodium bicarbonate may rapidly improve contractility in such situations. If acidosis is caused by respiratory failure, airway control with endotracheal intubation and mechanical ventilation is useful to correct the hypercapnia and to decrease the metabolic demand generated by trying to overcome respiratory failure. Temperature control is also important because elevations cause an increase in oxygen consumption, causing a marginal cardiovascular system to fail. Ideally, a neutral thermal environment should be maintained to avoid such stress. Hypoglycemia frequently occurs during stressful events, and neonates are less able to respond because of decreased glycogen stores and minimal fat necessary for gluconeogenesis. Low serum glucose of less than 40 mg/dL should be corrected with an infusion of either D25 or D10 solution. Electrolyte disturbances can interfere with both inotropic and chronotropic responses to decreased cardiac output. Appropriate monitoring of concentrations of potassium, calcium, magnesium, sodium, chloride, phosphate, and bicarbonate is prudent. Finally, attempts must be made to minimize stress in ill neonates. Alleviation of external stressors such as tubing manipulation or skin care should be minimized to increase oxygen availability by decreasing agitation. Phlebotomy should be minimized, and parents should be present to console the child.

ASSESSMENT OF CHILDREN SUSPECTED OF HAVING HEART DISEASE

Children with heart disease may present with symptoms unrelated to the underlying disease, and careful neurologic, pulmonary, and cardiac assessment must be performed to determine the stability of patients and the need for supportive care. From a cardiovascular perspective, this assessment determines whether the cardiac output is low, normal, or hyperdynamic. Concurrent conditions often exist, making definition of physical findings challenging. For instance, the symptoms and signs of increasing pulmonary venous pressure and the signs of a viral upper respiratory tract infection appear similar. What appears to be a feeding disorder with easy fatigue during routine feeds may represent congestive heart failure, particularly if diaphoresis is present with labored breathing.

The physical examination of children with significant congenital heart disease is often not as dramatic as the diagnosis of congestive heart failure in adolescents. In the author's experience, unrecognized congenital heart disease in small infants is often not diagnosed until the second or third visit to the emergency department for the same illness. Most often, that illness is misdiagnosed as a viral upper respiratory illness or a feeding intolerance.

When a child with known cardiac problems presents to the ED, the historical information that must be obtained by the emergency physician is problem focused and directed toward known complications of the congenital defect. A detailed history of medications administered and recent changes in dosages and timing of administration are important in such children. New illnesses, particularly of the upper respiratory tract, should be identified. Simple common pediatric illnesses such as croup, pneumonia, or bronchiolitis may cause sudden decompensation in a child with limited cardiac reserve. These illnesses may be difficult or impossible to differentiate clinically from an exacerbation of known cardiac disease. The symptoms and signs of increased right heart failure and critical pulmonary venous pressure states and respiratory illness often overlap and are indistinguishable without echocardiography.

Exertional dyspnea is often present, but overlooked, in older children with cardiac disease. In infants, feeding intolerance is the most reliable marker of exercise tolerance. Historical evidence of slow feeding, increased tachypnea with feeding, persistent staccato cough with feeding, and diaphoresis at midfeeding all suggest borderline cardiac reserve.

In small infants, tachypnea is often the first sign manifested, followed by rales that are more typical of congestive heart failure. Hepatomegaly usually develops late and is more marked than splenomegaly. In small infants, edema is usually generalized and not associated with jugular venous distention. Accurate blood pressure measurement in infants requires an appropriately sized cuff (approximating two-thirds of the extremity). Blood pressure should be measured in both upper and lower extremities. Cardiac murmurs should be graded according to location, timing in the cardiac cycle, and loudness. There may be significant cardiac pathology in the absence of murmur and, conversely, a very loud murmur may be innocent. The

pediatric-sized stethoscope bell and diaphragm should be used to discern the exact location of murmurs. Heart sounds should also be assessed particularly for fixed splitting of the second heart sound.

Focused cardiac examination must address the difference between pathologic and innocent cardiac murmurs. In one study of newborns 1 to 5 days with a murmur, 86 percent had structural heart defects.[2] Usually, innocent flow murmurs are of low intensity and do not radiate. They are brief in the cardiac cycle and usually systolic in timing. They are never holosystolic and are usually accentuated by head position or Valsalva maneuver.[3]

The Still murmur, which is the most common innocent murmur, is usually early systolic in timing, located at the apex or the lower left sternal border, and is often confused with the murmur of a ventricular septal defect (VSD). It usually does not radiate to the back like the murmur of a VSD. Pulmonary systolic ejection murmur, which is equivalent to the Still murmur, is extremely harsh and is usually heard loudest in the second and third intercostal spaces on the left. A unique murmur, often heard in neonates, is that of peripheral pulmonic stenosis. This murmur is usually of low intensity, is usually heard in both axillae and the back, and usually vanishes by 3 to 6 months of age. It is often misdiagnosed as a congenital lesion in sick infants and results in inadvertent administration of cardiotonic medication. Significant cardiac murmurs are usually holosystolic, continuous or diastolic in timing and usually associated with radiation.[3,4]

Laboratory studies are usually not initially helpful in acutely ill, hemodynamically unstable patients, but may be of some benefit in more stable pediatric patients. Such studies are usually confined to chest radiograph, ECG and, in some centers, bedside emergency ultrasonography.

Chest radiographic studies are essential in assessing the size and shape of the heart, and in evaluating pulmonary blood flow. The chest radiograph also provides some information about the position of the aortic arch, which should be normally left sided. In the normal left-sided aortic arch, there is rightward displacement of the esophagus and trachea to the right. An abnormal right position of the aortic arch may be a clue to the diagnosis of the congenital cardiac lesion. Right-sided aortic arches are seen in truncus arteriosus, transposition of the great vessels, tetralogy of Fallot, tricuspid atresia, and total anomalous pulmonary venous return. The chest radiograph is critical to the assessment of pulmonary vascularity. In small left-to-right shunts, the pulmonary vascularity is normal. Pulmonary vascularity can also be normal in conditions that cause pulmonary stenosis, such as valvular pulmonic stenosis or functional pulmonic stenosis associated with tetralogy of Fallot. Increased pulmonary vascularity may be seen with any cause of left-to-right shunting or in any cause of left-sided failure, such as ischemia or outflow obstruction.

The ECG is useful to evaluate cardiac conduction and, in particular, the rhythm, electrical axis, chamber size. Such information is clearly age related and will require one to have access to a standard text of normal values of pediatric ECG voltages and criteria for ventricular hypertrophy.[5] The electrical force axis most often defines abnormal chamber diameters and usually does not suggest cardiac ischemia as in the adult population.

Hemodynamically Unstable Patients

Clinical signs of low cardiac output are manifested by signs of dysfunction of one or more organ systems. Shock is diagnosed by determination of skin perfusion and mental status appropriate for age. Additional information may be obtained by assessment of the distal pulse quality, amplitude, and duration. Pallor, cyanosis, and skin mottling are usually present. The infant's hands and feet appear cold, and there is delayed capillary refill that is very distinct from acrocyanosis present in some infants. Mental status changes appear as fluctuating signs of apathy, irritability, or failure to respond to painful stimuli or to parental presence. Body positioning is that of prostration with loss of head control and is preferred to that of upright sitting or standing. Sinus tachycardia is the first response to maintenance of cardiac output, followed by tachypnea in an attempt to correct the acidosis of poor perfusion and oxygen delivery. Hypotension occurs late, is dramatic in its onset, and can occur without warning. Laboratory studies are unhelpful because their results are usually normal.

Noncardiac causes of shock and low cardiac output states must be considered, diagnosed, and treated in tandem with delineation of the possibility of congenital heart disease. Congenital heart lesions that present with low cardiac output are usually classified as shunt dependent and must be treated definitively and quickly. Up to 1 percent of infants are born with one or more congenital heart anomalies. Many of these lesions are of trivial or mild consequence, but a significant number are severe enough to become incompatible with life once the ductus arteriosus begins to close. As this occurs, blood can no longer reach the lungs and distal circulation. These infants present in shock within the first 2 weeks of life. Both cyanotic and acyanotic lesions may present in this fashion. The former include severe coarctation of the aorta, critical aortic stenosis, and hypoplastic left ventricle. Transposition of the great vessels, pulmonary atresia, and hypoplastic right heart syndrome are examples of the latter presentation.

Shunt-dependent lesions mandate immediate surgical referral for repair or palliation of the anatomic condition. It may be necessary to stabilize and restore some function to the shunt-dependent lesion while awaiting transport to a tertiary care facility. One method of providing this care is with the use of prostaglandin infusion to reopen the shunt pharmacologically. Prostaglandin E$_1$ infusions are successful in reopening the ductus arteriosus in nearly 95 percent of such patients and may allow for less emergent repair of the underlying defect. It is infused at a rate of 0.05 to 0.1 µg/kg per min initially. If there is no improvement within several minutes, it is increased progressively in 0.2 µg/kg per min increments. The minimal effective dosage should be used, because of adverse effects that include fever, skin flushing, diarrhea, and periodic apnea. Intubation and ventilatory support are often necessary as well.

Cardiogenic shock can also occur as a result of dysfunctional myocardium and may mimic the signs and symptoms seen with shunt-dependent anatomic lesions. Such cardiomyopathies are uncommon in pediatric patients, but can be easily confused with anatomic lesions. Cardiomyopathies are usually defined into two groups in children: dilated and hypertrophied. Presentation varies from asymptomatic cardiomegaly discovered on routine chest radiograph to congestive heart failure, cardiogenic shock, or sudden death. Typically, such children self-limit their activities at home and then, during an acute febrile illness, decompensate rapidly and arrive in profound shock. The dilated cardiomyopathies more often cause congestive heart failure, whereas the hypertrophied cardiomyopathies cause sudden death. Emergent medical management includes supportive care as previously outlined in an attempt to enhance contractility. Tragically, little can be done to assist those unfortunate children who suffer sudden death.

TETRALOGY OF FALLOT   Although not in itself a cause of hemodynamic instability because of sudden loss of blood flow, tetralogy of Fallot often presents in a dramatic fashion as a consequence of hypercyanotic episodes or "tet spells" that mimic other more significant structural lesions. Tetralogy of Fallot is the most common cause of cyanotic congenital heart disease in children older than 4 years of age. Anatomically, it is characterized by obstruction of the right ventricular outflow tract, VSD, dextroposition of the aorta, and right ventricular hypertrophy. Functionally, obstruction of the right ventricular outflow tract and the presence of VSD have the greatest physiologic consequences. Because of the outflow tract obstruction, blood is forced from right to left, resulting in desaturation and compensatory polycythemia and hyperviscosity.

The other cardinal features on physical examination are a holosystolic VSD murmur in the third intercostal space at the left sternal border and a diamond-shaped systolic murmur of pulmonary stenosis in the second intercostal space at the left sternal border. The history may reveal exercise intolerance relieved by squatting. The main radiographic findings are a boot-shaped heart with decreased pulmonary vascular markings. A right-side aortic arch is present in 25 percent of tetralogies. Right ventricular hypertrophy with right axis deviation is the primary ECG abnormality.

The greatest threat to these patients is the hypercyanotic or tet spells. These episodes, dramatic in presentation, are characterized by episodes of paroxysmal dyspnea with labored respiration, increased cyanosis, and syncope. These episodes in concert with polycythemia lead to seizures, cerebrovascular accidents, and death. They occur as a consequence of the exertion of feeding, crying, or straining at stool, and last from a few minutes to hours. The rapid, deep hypernea results from an increase in cardiac output with exertion against fixed right ventricular outflow tract obstruction. The fixed obstruction causes increased shunting across the VSD and increased hypoxia, hypercarbia, and acidosis. The hypoxia and acidosis cause a decrease in systemic vascular resistance that further potentiates the shunt and stimulates the respiratory center to maintain and deepen the hypernea.[6]

Management of hypercyanotic spells consists of positioning and pharmacologic management. Infants should be placed in a knee-chest position. This positioning allows for an increase in venous return to the heart and an increase in systemic vascular resistance. Pharmacologic management includes administration of oxygen to decrease the hypoxemia, and injection of morphine sulfate SC or IM at a dosage of 0.2 mg/kg per dose. Many consider the administration of propranolol a contraindication to bypass surgery, so it should not be given without consultation. In extreme cases, phenylephrine infusion 10 µg/kg initial infusion, followed by infusion of 0.5 to 2 µg/kg per min, is used to increase the systemic vascular resistance and increase blood pressure.

Lack of recognition of the hypercyanotic episode and timely intervention could result in significant complications, including seizures, cerebral thrombosis, profound lactic acidosis, deterioration in cardiac rhythm, and subsequent death.

TRANSPOSITION OF THE GREAT VESSELS   This is the most common cyanotic defect that appears in the first week of life. Infants with this defect who are brought to the ED usually have dusky lips noted by parents or have an increased respiratory rate or feeding difficulty. While not as dramatic in presentation as a hypercyanotic spell of tetralogy of Fallot, the defect is easily missed on a single ED visit because of the lack of cardiomegaly or murmur.

Anatomically, in transposition of the great vessels, the aorta originates from the right ventricle, and the pulmonary artery originates from the left ventricle. The systemic veins drain as they usually do into the anatomically correct right atrium, and the pulmonary veins drain into the left atria. Thus, in transposition, the systemic and pulmonary blood flows are not admixed and exist in parallel unless alternative flow is established. To maintain life, mixing of blood occurs either at the level of the atria via an atrial septal defect or at the level of the ventricles by a VSD. If neither of these is present, flow must be maintained by a persistent ductus arteriosus.

Clinically, cyanosis and tachypnea appear within the first several days of life, but may be prolonged when a patent ductus arteriosus fails to close. Ironically, cardiomegaly is often absent and no murmur is noted. The chest radiograph is usually normal, but may show a narrow, small heart because of the overlapping of the abnormally positioned aorta and pulmonary artery. The ECG shows normal right-sided-force dominance. Rarely, depending on the anatomy, will frank congestive heart failure be present.

Treatment of this condition is initially palliative in the cardiac catheterization laboratory and involves the creation of a large artificial atrial septal defect by using a balloon catheter (Rashkind septoplasty). Initially, most emergency physicians who suspect this entity are justified in beginning an infusion of prostaglandin E$_1$, as previously outlined, while arranging transport to a facility capable of palliation. The definitive surgery that is performed later is the Mustard operation, in which an artificial baffle is created at the atrial level to direct systemic venous return into the left ventricle and the pulmonary return to the right ventricle. The left ventricle then pumps blood to the lungs, and the right ventricle pumps blood to the systemic circulation.[7]

LEFT VENTRICULAR OUTFLOW OBSTRUCTION SYNDROMES

No clinical presentation can match the rapidity of onset of cardiogenic shock, hypotension, and acidosis as seen in infants with this group of disorders. In these infants, systemic blood flow depends on a large contribution of shunted blood via a patent ductus arteriosus. When the ductus closes, cardiac output falls, perfusion becomes negligible, and a state of profound cardiogenic shock ensues. Such lesions are often complex, but include hypoplastic left heart syndrome, tricuspid atresia, and critical coarctation of the aorta. Other variants include transposition of the great vessels, as discussed previously, and some tetralogy of Fallot variants.[8]

Such infants present with decreased or absent perfusion, hypotension, and severe acidosis. When these infants present in the first week of life, they must be considered for an infusion of prostaglandin E_1, as outlined earlier. The infusion is begun at 0.1 μg/kg per min, preferably by a central line, although any access in such ill infants is acceptable. The dosage may be reduced as perfusion and color return. Side effects of the infusion include hypotension and mandate close observation of blood pressure. Other effects are apnea, focal seizures, and fever that may mimic sepsis. Because of the critical nature of these infants, immediate referral and transfer to a tertiary care facility are necessary.

Hemodynamically Stable, Symptomatic Patients

Some infants arrive at the ED with respiratory distress and are found on examination to have findings suggestive of congenital heart disease, usually with evidence of congestive heart failure. These infants have near-normal blood pressure and usually display normal skin perfusion, but may have cyanosis. Several congenital cardiac conditions may present in this fashion.

TRUNCUS ARTERIOSUS

This congenital anomaly is characterized by a single, large arterial trunk originating from the ventricular portion of the heart. This common vascular trunk supplies blood to both the systemic and the pulmonary circulation. A large VSD is usually present and may account for the murmur that is often heard. Because of the large amount of flow from both ventricles into the single large arterial conduit, flow to the pulmonary tree is greatly enhanced due to decreased flow resistance. This results in little or no cyanosis until pulmonary resistance increases and then cyanosis appears.

Clinically, these infants present with signs of increased pulmonary blood flow, dyspnea, and, occasionally, overt congestive heart failure. Chest x-ray demonstrates cardiomegaly and increased pulmonary vascularity or pulmonary edema. The ECG is initially normal until pulmonary vascular resistance increases and then signs of strain, left ventricular hypertrophy, or biventricular hypertrophy are evident.

VENTRICULAR SEPTAL DEFECT

This is the most common cardiac defect, and symptoms displayed depend on the size of the defect. Small defects are often found on routine physical examination. More than 60 percent of these close spontaneously in older childhood.

Moderate-sized VSDs cause elevated right ventricular pressure and subsequent increased pulmonary artery pressure. Infants with this defect present with increased cough with mild upper respiratory tract infections and may have mild increase in pulmonary vascularity and early congestive heart failure. Typically, the chest radiograph is interpreted as mild congestive heart failure, and treatment consists of furosemide and, occasionally, digoxin.

Large VSDs present with congestive heart failure early in infancy, resulting in early and severe pulmonary artery pressure that, if uncorrected, will result in pulmonary hypertension. Pulmonary hypertension will result in reversal of left-to-right shunt and cyanosis in a condition known as the Eisenmenger complex.

COARCTATION OF THE AORTA

This represents localized narrowing of the aortic lumen, most often distal to the origin of the left subclavian artery and in close proximity to the ductus arteriosus or its postnatal remnant, the ligamentum arteriosus.

In infancy, symptomatic infants present with congestive heart failure and feeding difficulty. Decreased pulse amplitude and duration are noted in the lower extremities, and hypertension is noted in the upper extremities. Cardiac examination reveals a systolic ejection murmur at the cardiac base, with interscapular radiation.

Older children present with decreased exercise tolerance and, occasionally, claudication to the lower extremities. In children older than 6 to 7 years of age, a characteristic rib notching of the inferior border of posterior ribs is evident. Such notching is bilateral and usually caused by hypertrophied collateral vessels.[9]

Hemodynamically Stable, Asymptomatic Patients

This class of patients presents to the ED for reasons that are not referable to the heart and are discovered to have findings suggestive of cardiac disease. Some of the more common cardiac defects have already been mentioned including mildly affected tetralogy of Fallot, small- to moderate-sized VSDs, and coarctation of the aorta. Several common structural defects warrant mention here.

ATRIAL SEPTAL DEFECT

Most children remain symptomatic throughout childhood until adolescence, when signs of increased pulmonary hypertension develop. Characteristically, the physical examination of such children reveals a split second heart sound that does not vary with inspiration. Often a soft systolic murmur heard at the upper left sternal border may mimic the pulmonary flow murmur mentioned earlier. Initially, the chest radiograph is normal but, with time, shows an increased size of the right atria and later the right ventricle. The ECG shows a characteristic prolongation of the PR interval and a incomplete or complete right bundle-branch block pattern. Cardiomegaly represents a late finding that is usually seen in adults.[10]

CONGENITAL AORTIC STENOSIS

This is a less dramatic form of left-sided outlet obstruction than described previously. Children with this defect usually arrive at the ED with fatigue, decreasing exercise tolerance, exertional dyspnea, or syncope. The diagnosis is suspected based on the greatly diminished pulse amplitude and duration and the characteristic murmur, which is usually systolic in timing and loud with radiation to the neck. Treatment consists of decreasing activities, particularly sports, and referral for evaluation of surgical intervention. In all circumstances, these children should refrain from any significant physical activity, as sudden death can result.

CONGESTIVE HEART FAILURE

Clinical Features

The most common cause of congestive heart failure (CHF) in children is congenital heart disease, which often masquerades as, or coexists with, pneumonia or sepsis. Pneumonia can cause a previously stable cardiac condition to decompensate, so that both problems exist simultaneously. The predominant symptoms include poor feeding, excessive diaphoresis, irritability or lethargy with feeding, weak cry, and, in severe cases, grunting and nasal flaring. Pulmonary congestion with rales, rhonchi, and wheezing may mimic common lower respiratory viral infections. Gallop rhythms may be difficult to ascertain because of the presence of tachycardia. Table 120-2 outlines the common symptoms and signs of an infant with congestive heart failure.

TABLE 120-2   Recognition of Congestive Heart Failure in Infants

	Right-Sided Failure	Left-Sided Failure	Both
Cardinal signs	Hepatomegaly	Tachypnea Dyspnea and sweating on feeding Rales	Cardiomegaly Failure to thrive Tachycardia
Unusual signs	Jugular venous distention Peripheral edema Anasarca		

Both increased pulmonary blood flow in left-to-right shunts and pulmonary edema decrease lung compliance, causing tachypnea in an attempt to maintain minute ventilation. Tachypnea is a cardinal sign of left-sided failure in infants. Unlike tachypnea caused by respiratory viruses, this tachypnea is usually effortless in children with congestive heart failure, because of lack of airway obstruction. Because feeding is the infant's primary form of exertion, dyspnea and sweating during feeding can often be elicited in the history. Peripheral edema, jugular venous distention, and rales are unusual and late signs in infants.

Hepatomegaly appears long before ascites, anasarca, or peripheral edema in right-sided failure in infants, but is usually a late sign. Hepatomegaly exists when the liver is more than 2 cm below the right costal margin in the absence of downward displacement by hyperexpanded lungs. In hepatomegaly, the liver border is rounded rather than sharp.

In congestive heart failure, the details of any murmur detected on physical examination contribute to the diagnosis. The chest radiograph may reveal cardiomegaly, increased or decreased vascular markings, or pulmonary edema. Often, as a consequence of the presence of a thymic shadow, the cardiac size is not readily apparent on routine posterior-anterior radiographs of the chest, but can be assessed on the lateral view by obliteration of the retrocardiac window by the enlarged heart. On the posterior-anterior view, the thymic shadow can be distinguished from the cardiac silhouette by the "sail sign," if present, and by the scalloped border that is produced by compression of the thymus against the rib cage. The ECG is often nonspecific, but may reveal only evidence of abnormal electrical axis, rhythm disturbances, or, more often, chamber hypertrophy.

Physiology of Congestive Heart Failure

Typically, most cases of CHF in children are caused by afterload increases in the pressure dynamics of one or both chambers of the heart. In these conditions, pressure builds in one chamber of the heart because of an obstructive lesion in the outflow tract of the affected chamber. Several of the more common entities early in the first weeks of life are the left ventricular outflow obstruction syndromes, followed by congenital aortic stenosis and moderate-to-severe coarctation of the aorta. With these lesions, the systemic circulation has inadequate perfusion, and renal flow is diminished. The combination of increased fluid retention and chamber dilatation results in cardiac failure. Treatment of afterload increases is aimed at vasodilatation with either specific load-altering medications, such as nitroprusside or nitroglycerin, or the use of furosemide, which has both a diuretic effect and a vasodilatory effect.

Less often, CHF can be related to increases in preload representing an overall volume overload without obstructive pressure consequences. Typical entities include large VSDs, and persistent patent ductus arteriosus in premature infants. Anemias of different etiologies should be considered, especially iron deficiency anemia in small cow milk-fed infants. Sickle cell anemia and thalassemia variants should also be considered. In the former group of conditions, decreasing the vascular volume with diuretics is beneficial. In addition, the use of digoxin may be beneficial prior to surgical repair. In the latter cases, transfusion is warranted along with judicious use of fluid restriction and diuresis.

Poor contractility is not usually considered a major cause of CHF in small infants, because the ventricular walls are still relatively noncompliant. In older pediatric patients, however, poor contractility becomes an issue. Kawasaki syndrome, idiopathic endocardial fibroelastosis, pulmonary hypertension associated with Eisenmenger syndrome, and toxic-metabolic causes should be considered in adolescent patients with CHF. Less-frequent inflammatory causes include myocarditis, constrictive pericarditis, and collagen vascular diseases. Treatment is geared toward increasing contractility with dobutamine or digoxin.

Differential Diagnosis

CONGENITAL ANATOMIC HEART DEFECTS   Once CHF is recognized, age-related categories simplify further differential diagnosis as outlined according to time of development in Table 120-3. In the first few minutes of life, CHF occurs from a variety of noncardiac origins such as asphyxia, acidosis, hypoglycemia, hypocalcemia, anemia, and sepsis. In critically ill premature neonates, a patent ductus arteriosus is the most common cause of CHF. Among full-term newborns, a hypoplastic left ventricle is the most common cause in the first week of life and coarctation of the aorta is the most common cause in the second week of life. Transposition of the great arteries presents within the first 3 days of life, with either cyanosis or CHF.[11]

VSDs alone do not cause CHF in the first weeks of life but, when complicated by transposition of the great arteries, truncus arteriosus, critical aortic stenosis, or coarctation can present with failure at any time during the first few weeks of life. Large, uncomplicated VSDs can present with CHF after weeks 3 to 4 of life as pulmonary artery pressure continues to fall, increasing the left-to-right shunt. Onset of failure is insidious between 1 and 3 months of age, when the left-to-right shunt increases as the pulmonary vascular resistance decreases further from the high fetal values.

Clinical assessment also involves estimation of the degree of severity of the congestive heart failure. For example, depending on the size of the defect, a VSD may present in a variety of ways, ranging from mild tachypnea to chronic compensated CHF accompanied by growth

TABLE 120-3   Differential Diagnosis of Congestive Heart Failure Based on Age of Presentation

Age	Spectrum	
1 min 1 hour	Noncardiac origin: anemia, acidosis, hypoxia, hypoglycemia, hypocalcemia, sepsis	Acquired
1 day 1 week 2 weeks 1 month	PDA in premature infants HPLV Coarctation Ventricular septal defect	Congenital
3 months 1 year 10 years	Supraventricular tachycardia Myocarditis Cardiomyopathy Severe anemia Rheumatic fever	Acquired

Abbreviations: HPLV = hypoplastic left ventricle; PDA = patent ductus arteriosus.

failure and frank pulmonary hypertension in later years. The finding on clinical examination of a small VSD is often out of proportion to the size of the VSD: a small VSD may have with a loud holosystolic murmur that is hemodynamically insignificant, and a large defect may produce no murmur initially.

In contrast to the gradual onset of heart failure with a VSD, coarctation of the aorta can present with abrupt onset of CHF precipitated by a delayed closure of the ductus arteriosus during week 2 of life. The severity of the symptoms is directly proportional to the degree of obstruction and can vary from mild tachypnea to cardiogenic shock. Milder degrees of coarctation, on the other hand, present later in life with isolated hypertension and diminished pulses in the lower extremities.

The onset of CHF after 3 months of age usually signifies acquired heart disease as opposed to congenital heart disease. The exception to this rule occurs when pneumonia, subacute bacterial endocarditis, or other complicating factors cause a previously stable congenital lesion to decompensate. Before 2 years of age, myocarditis, cardiomyopathies, and severe anemia are the most common diseases in the differential diagnosis. Rheumatic fever, once a common cause of CHF, is seen among children who are 8 to 12 years of age. Except in certain ethnic groups, it is now unusual.

MYOCARDITIS AND CARDIOMYOPATHIES   Myocarditis affects children of all ages and is the leading cause of end-stage cardiomyopathy requiring transplantation. Viral etiologies include enteroviruses (coxsackie, echovirus, and poliovirus), as well as mumps, influenza virus, and varicella-zoster. An emerging cause is HIV-associated myocarditis and chronic Epstein-Barr myocarditis. Many bacterial species have been associated with myopericarditis, but not myocarditis alone. Noninfectious causes include lupus erythematosus, toxins such as tricyclic antidepressants, and cocaine. Myocarditis is often preceded by a viral respiratory illness and needs to be differentiated from pneumonia. As with the latter diagnosis, presenting signs and symptoms are often respiratory distress, fever, tachypnea, and tachycardia. Clues that suggest myocarditis include generalized malaise, fever, and myalgias in age-appropriate children.

Cardiomyopathies are uncommon, but significant because of the high mortality and severe disability that they produce. They are usually classified into two groups: either dilated or hypertrophic. The dilated cardiomyopathies display impaired cardiac contractility and ventricular dilation. Most cases are idiopathic or viral in etiology. Most infants who arrive at the ED have respiratory symptoms, and a chest radiograph reveals an enlarged heart and vascular congestion. In a small percentage of these infants, acute cardiovascular collapse can result from severe CHF or dysrhythmia. Infants become acutely symptomatic when their disease is accentuated by intercurrent febrile illness. The hypertrophic cardiomyopathies display thickened myocardium and very plastic immobile contractile state.

Chest radiographs show cloudy lung fields either from inflammation or pulmonary edema. ECG may reveal ST-T segment changes that are generalized to all leads or rhythm disturbances. Evidence of ectopy signals severe diffuse disease and a high risk of sudden death. Cardiomegaly with poor distal pulses and prolonged capillary refill, however, distinguish it from common pneumonia. Once cardiomegaly is discovered, admission and echocardiogram are warranted. The latter will show a dilated, poorly contracting left ventricle with a low ejection fraction with or without a pericardial effusion. In dilated cardiomyopathies, both ventricles are usually affected and substantial dilatation is apparent at diagnosis.

At this point, the cause of myocarditis must be further delineated in a hospital, and endomyocardial biopsy may be warranted to do so. Parents must be thoroughly versed in cardiopulmonary resuscitation and be aware that a lethal dysrhythmia could cause sudden death. Infants are best kept comfortable in an upright position in an infant seat.

Oxygen is administered in a nonthreatening fashion appropriate for age, and a neutral thermal environment is established. If CHF is apparent, a diuretic is administered. Severe CHF is initially treated with inotropic infusions (for example, dopamine hydrochloride or dobutamine) along with fluid restriction, diuresis, and supplemental oxygen. Intubation and mechanical ventilation often become necessary during the hospital phase of the illness. Treatment is directed to the underlying cause in addition to the supportive therapy outlined earlier.

PERICARDITIS   Usually, this presents as cardiomegaly that is discovered incidentally on chest radiograph. Clinical signs, such as chest pain, muffled heart sounds, and a friction rub, may be present. In older patients and adolescents, classic pleuritic or positional chest pain, abdominal pain, and tachycardia may be seen. An echocardiogram is performed on an urgent basis to distinguish a pericardial effusion from dilated or hypertrophic myocarditis. The most common etiology is in association with coxsackie viral myocarditis. Bacterial pericarditis from *Haemophilus influenzae* is rare today and was uncommon even before the availability of *H. influenzae* type B conjugated vaccines. Typically, most cases of bacterial pericarditis present with profound toxicity and muffled heart sounds and jugular venous distention. If not appropriately drained in addition to antibiotic treatment, constrictive pericarditis will result in tamponade. Pericarditis that accompanies rheumatic fever, lupus erythematosus, or chronic renal failure is usually secondary and does not produce the main symptomatology. Because diagnostic pericardiocentesis can be complicated by hemorrhage, cardiac tamponade, and arrest, it is usually deferred to a pediatric cardiologist or intensivist for drainage. Pericardiocentesis with an 18-gauge over-the-needle catheter is indicated in the ED if an infant with large heart becomes rapidly unstable with loss of pulse. As in adults, the needle is placed in the sub-xiphoid region and aimed toward the left shoulder.

Typically, uncomplicated pericarditis responds to a prolonged course of anti-inflammatory medication and decreased activity or bed rest. Most cases are self-limited and require specialty consultation only for the initial evaluation.

COR PULMONALE   If an infant presents in pure right-sided CHF, the primary problem is most likely to be pulmonary in origin. Hepatomegaly and anasarca may be present, but most often, in early stages, lid edema is the first noticeable sign. Moreover, the lid edema is likely to be appreciated by the parents more than by the physician and must be specifically searched for on examination. Often it will have to be elicited by asking "Do your child's eyes look puffy?" If the underlying problem is bronchopulmonary dysplasia resulting from prematurity and infantile respiratory distress syndrome, the infant may already be on appropriate home oxygenation and diuretic therapy. Upper airway obstruction from hypertrophied adenoidal and tonsillar tissue can produce cor pulmonale, presenting as edema or anasarca. The clinical features of airway obstruction, however, are subtle; a careful history will reveal continuous mouth breathing while awake and sleeping, with or without snoring. Sleep studies and tonsillectomy are indicated. Cor pulmonale from upper airway obstruction in infants usually responds to diuresis and oxygen alone, without the need for digoxin.

Treatment

The degree and severity of CHF dictate the initial treatment. Infants who present with mild tachypnea, hepatomegaly, and cardiomegaly simply need to be seated upright in a comfortable position and kept in a neutral thermal environment to minimize preload and to avoid metabolic stress. If the work of breathing is appreciably increased by an increased pulmonary blood flow, 1 to 2 mg/kg furosemide parenterally is indicated. If pulmonary edema is present, then the hypoxemia can usually be corrected by fluid restriction, diuresis, and an increase in ambient oxygen.

Severe degrees of CHF can present with signs of low cardiac output or cardiogenic shock. Aggressive management is often necessary in secondary derangement, including respiratory insufficiency, acute renal failure, lactic acidosis, disseminated intravascular coagulation, hypoglycemia, and hypocalcemia.

For definitive diagnosis and treatment of congenital lesions presenting in CHF, cardiac catheterization followed by surgical intervention is often necessary. Stabilization and improvement of left ventricular function can often first be accomplished with inotropic agents. Digoxin is used in milder forms of CHF. Initial digitalization is performed IV, giving one-half the daily dosage followed by one-fourth of the daily dosage IV at 6- to 8-h intervals. Maintenance dioxin consists of one-eighth the daily dosage given IV or PO at 12-h intervals. For full-term infants up to 2 years of age, the dosage is 0.03 to 0.05 mg/kg per d. Hence, 0.02 mg/kg would be the appropriate first digitalizing dose to be given in the ED.

At some point, congestive heart failure progresses to cardiogenic shock, in which distal pulses are absent and end-organ perfusion is threatened. In such situations, continuous infusions of inotropic agents such as dopamine or dobutamine are indicated instead of digoxin. The initial starting range is 5 to 10 μg/kg per min. The "rule of six" simplifies the necessary calculations. A total of 6 mg/kg of body weight of either dopamine or dobutamine is placed in a microdrip chamber and filled to 100 mL with D5W or NS; 1 mL per h equals 1 μg/kg per min, so it is administered via a pump initially at 5 mL per h (5 μg/kg per min). Prior to starting a continuous inotropic infusion such as this, the acid-base status should be checked by arterial blood gas analysis. Any abnormality should be corrected with 1 to 2 mEq/kg of sodium bicarbonate as needed and cautious volume expansion with 10 mL/kg of NS if necessary.

If inotropic support is inadequate, the use of combination therapy with vasodilatory therapy is warranted. The combination of dopamine and nitroprusside has been used extensively in situations of low cardiac output and low ejection fraction states. Another combination is nitroglycerin, which is readily available to even the smallest EDs.

When pharmacologic management is unsuccessful, other measures must be considered. Typically, most emergency physicians will be able to support ventilation with endotracheal intubation and positive end-expiratory pressure. Further care after tertiary referral includes balloon-assist counterpulsation devices or membrane oxygenation until definitive surgical care of the underlying cardiac defect can be undertaken.

DYSRHYTHMIAS

In general, children are able to tolerate higher rates without the usual ischemic phenomenon often present in adults. The treatment in children is usually directed at the underlying structural aspect of the intracardiac conduction system and less at prevention of cardiac ischemia related to rate.

Dysrhythmias can occur in the absence of underlying structural heart disease or metabolic condition. Many conditions that occur in the adult population—such as hypoxia, electrolyte imbalance, collagen vascular diseases, and overzealous use of sympathomimetic agents—rarely occur in children. Because much of the prognosis with regard to the reoccurrence of a dysrhythmia depends on the nature of any underlying structural cardiac defect, cardiologic evaluation is needed for all first-time occurrences of dysrhythmias.

Recognition of dysrhythmia is age dependent, and dysrhythmia often masquerades as other cardiac entities. In small infants, poor feeding and irritability may be the only signs of illness, with signs of poor cardiac output at higher rates evident later as edema and poor capillary refill. Older children may have more specific symptoms because of their increased ability to verbalize. In such instances, more classic adult symptoms of palpitations may be elicited, as well as syncope due to increased rate.

Slow Cardiac Rates

FIRST- AND SECOND-DEGREE ATRIOVENTRICULAR BLOCKS   First-degree atrioventricular (AV) block is seen frequently and has no real serious consequence unless it occurs in the presence of another cardiac anomaly such as an atrial septal defect. Second-degree AV block requires a more thorough evaluation. Mobitz type I second-degree AV block can be a normal variant. Mobitz type II, however, is always of significance and always requires an evaluation and prolonged monitoring.

COMPLETE ATRIOVENTRICULAR BLOCKS   Complete AV block can occur and can be either congenital or acquired. Congenital complete AV block is associated with congenital heart disease or may occur independently. In the former, the prognosis is extremely guarded until the underlying defect is corrected. Often the associated congenital defect is so severe (common AV canal) that it is uncorrectable. In the latter condition, AV block occurs during gestation and is usually secondary to maternal connective tissue disease with autoimmune destruction of the AV tracts in infants. The diagnosis is usually suspected prenatally, and treatment is instituted during gestation. Postnatal therapy includes transthoracic pacemaker and transvenous pacemaker use. Acquired AV block can occur without cause in older children, occur as a manifestation of inflammatory diseases of the myocardium, or occur postpartum in adolescent patients. In this category, syncope is usually the initial presenting complaint, and prompt recognition and referral are mandatory. Treatment is with an implantable pacemaker to prevent sudden death.

Fast Cardiac Rates

SINUS TACHYCARDIA   Although usually a benign event, the differentiation from the more significant supraventricular tachycardia (SVT) is difficult. Typically, ventricular rates in excess of 230 beats/min are highly unusual and should be presumed to be the latter entity. The rate in SVT is usually fixed, with little variability with manipulation of the infant. Vagal maneuvers may be attempted to try to slow the cardiac rate. If slowing can be accomplished, P waves may be visible. The presence of P waves during slowing supports the diagnosis of sinus tachycardia. Other causes of sustained high-rate sinus tachycardia must be sought, including diarrheal dehydration, febrile illness, hyperthyroidism, sepsis, and drug effect from substance abuse or iatrogenic medication administration.

SUPRAVENTRICULAR TACHYCARDIA   This is the most common dysrhythmia in the pediatric age range. In infants, SVT presents with a 4- to 24-h history of poor feeding, tachypnea, pallor, and lethargy. In older children, palpitations and chest pain can be prominent in the symptomatology. Physical examination reveals weak pulses and a tachycardia that can be too rapid to be counted accurately. Depending on the time since onset of SVT, other physical signs can vary from CHF to cardiogenic shock with pending arrest. Low cardiac output is secondary to inadequate ventricular diastolic filling time.

Most children younger than 3 or 4 months of age will have no easily identifiable cause for the tachycardia. Children older than 4 months often have underlying structural defects or precipitators, such as fever or exposure to sympathomimetic cold remedies. Older children and adolescents are more likely to have accessory pathways. Recurrence rates for accessory pathway disease are as high as 90 percent, and recognition allows for more directed therapy at the AV node.

An ECG rhythm strip shows an unvarying ventricular rate between 220 and 360 beats/min, as opposed to a range of 150 to 200 beats/min in adults with SVT. The QRS complexes are narrow and regular. P waves are absent or abnormal. Any wide-complex rhythm that is seen is considered ventricular in origin, because SVT with aberration is usually extremely rare in children.

SVT must be distinguished from sinus tachycardia, which is the most common tachyarrhythmia in children. In sinus tachycardia, P waves are present. The normal range for heart rate in newborns is 120 to 200 beats/min. In children younger than age 5 years, it is not unusual to find a sinus tachycardia up to a rate of 200 beats/min caused by fever, stress, or hypovolemia. The latter requires prompt recognition and adequate volume expansion.[12]

Initial management of *unstable* patients with narrow or wide complex tachycardia consists of immediate synchronized cardioversion at 0.5 J/kg with increases in power output to 2 J/kg as needed. Cardioversion should be undertaken at the lowest possible output in children on digoxin. There is a greater risk of subsequent ventricular fibrillation in such patients, so prophylactic lidocaine hydrochloride should be administered in a dose of 1 mg/kg before cardioversion. If cardioversion is unsuccessful, overdrive pacing is indicated. Once cardioversion is completed, suppressive therapy with digoxin is required.

Intravenous adenosine (0.1 mg/kg followed by 0.3 mg/kg boluses every 1 to 2 min until tachycardia resolves) is the drug of choice for both wide and narrow complex supraventricular tachycardia.[13] Because the half-life of adenosine is a matter of seconds, it is administered as a rapid bolus via a peripheral IV line. Two syringes can be timed in delivery of the medication: the first syringe contains the adenosine, and the second contains 5 to 10 mL of saline flush. Both syringes can be sequentially emptied in less than 5 s. A brief (3 to 10 s) period of asystole is sometimes seen before return of a normal sinus rhythm. If necessary, the dosage can be doubled, tripled, or quadrupled to convert the rhythm (maximum dosage, 12 mg).[13]

Vagal maneuvers to convert SVT can be attempted, but are usually not successful until after the first dose of digoxin. The diving reflex, which is elicited by submersing the face in ice water, usually produces the greatest vagal tone. An alternative to submersion is to place the ice water in a plastic bag that can be lowered briefly on the infant's face.

Digoxin has been the time-honored standard of medical management of SVT in infants. Because it takes 4 to 6 h before the rhythm converts, however, it is used more for chronic management than for acute conversion. The dosage is the same as that previously listed for CHF.

Verapamil should not be used in neonates and children <5 years of age because it can result in electromechanical dissociation.[13] The dose of verapamil in older children is 0.1 mg/kg bolus, with preparation for any associated hypotension with calcium chloride at 10 mg/kg ready at the bedside. If verapamil fails or is contraindicated, then chemical cardioversion with either propranolol, procainamide, or flecainide may be attempted.[14] Propranolol administration prolongs conduction at the AV node in both antegrade and retrograde fashion and thus is extremely useful in Wolff-Parkinson-White syndrome. It is administered at a dosage of 0.1 mg/kg per dose every 6 h. Procainamide blocks only retrograde conduction and may be beneficial if the rhythm appears to be ventricular in origin. It is administered as a 5- to 15-mg/kg bolus over 20 to 30 min.[14]

ATRIAL FLUTTER This is associated with congenital heart disease approximately 90 percent of the time. The atrial rates generated typically range from 200 to 300 beats/min in practice, but rates as high as 500 beats/min have been reported. With such high rates, the flutter waves are often difficult to visualize unless vagal maneuvers result in slowing long enough to capture the flutter waves. Conduction to the ventricles is variable and can be as high as 1:1 to a more usual 3:1 or 4:1 block.

In stable patients, control of rate is a first priority and can usually be accomplished by the use of digitalization to slow the ventricular response. The ultimate goal of therapy is to eliminate the flutter waves and to decrease the conducted response of the atria. If digoxin alone is effective, procainamide can be given. Combination therapy is usually never appropriate for emergency physicians to undertake, because slowed junctional bradycardia or asystole may occur.[15]

ATRIAL FIBRILLATION Unlike adult atrial fibrillation, which is usually secondary to ischemic heart disease or pulmonary disease with chamber dilatation, childhood disease is secondary to rheumatic heart disease or dilated cardiomyopathy. Atrial fibrillation in children usually manifests as an irregular rhythm with variable conduction. Rate control is rarely problematic unless rates are in excess of 200 beats/min. In unstable patients, immediate cardioversion is usually successful at energy levels of 0.5 J/kg. Overdrive pacing is useful for those that do not convert.

Unlike adult cardioversion, anticoagulation is never necessary prior to the termination of atrial fibrillation. Medical therapy with digoxin is rarely effective, and not enough experience is available with newer agents such as diltiazem[16] or ibutilide. Even in stable patients, cardioversion is usually required. Rarely, electrophysiologic studies are warranted and ablation of the focus is required.[17]

VENTRICULAR TACHYCARDIA This is usually seen in the presence of underlying congenital heart disease. Intentional or inadvertent drug overdose should also be suspected. Occasionally, ventricular tachycardia may be idiopathic and discovered on routine examination in asymptomatic children. In the latter case, complete investigation should include a search for myocarditis, cardiomyopathy, or the prolonged QT syndrome.

Despite the poor prognosis that this rhythm holds in adults, stable asymptomatic children are usually left untreated if the heart is normal. Symptomatic children who present with syncope or chest pain require further study, but treatment should not be instituted by emergency physicians until after these studies are performed.

If patients are unstable in any way, synchronized cardioversion should be performed at an energy of 1 to 2 J/kg. If stability for transfer is uncertain, medical management with lidocaine hydrochloride is warranted. The dosage is usually a 1 mg/kg loading dose followed by a 0.5 mg/kg reload in 20 to 30 min, and then a maintenance infusion of 0.01 to 0.04 mg/kg per min infusion. Procainamide can also be used, but must be given over 30 to 60 min at a dose of 15 mg/kg IV. Other considerations include phenytoin, propranolol, or amiodarone.[18,19]

VENTRICULAR FIBRILLATION The initial energy for defibrillation is 2 J/kg and can be doubled, if necessary. Hypoxia and acidosis should be corrected to increase the success of defibrillation. A trial of amiodarone given as a 5 mg/kg infusion over 5 to 20 min followed by defibrillation may be warranted. If defibrillation is successful a continuous infusion of 5 to 15 μg/kg per min is warranted. Failure to respond after an initial infusion of amiodarone followed by three defibrillation attempts and a second 2 mg/kg bolus infusion usually indicates that the heart is unresuscitatable.[19]

ANTICIPATING PROBLEMS IN CHILDREN WITH CONGENITAL HEART DISEASE

Children with congenital heart disease are brought to the ED for routine accident care, as well as for childhood illnesses. Some childhood illnesses may predispose patients to acute cardiovascular complications. A significant number of these children are treated with digoxin, diuretics, and anticoagulants that can make care of acute problems difficult. Special problems must be anticipated and complications of therapy for other conditions avoided.

Hypoxemic Spells

Most ED procedures involve fear and apprehension, as well as pain in the preparation of wounds and fracture splint placement or reduction.

Infants with uncorrected tetralogy of Fallot can have hypoxemic episodes when total oxygen demand during painful procedures exceeds that which the restricted pulmonary blood flow can support. Strain also increases the right-to-left shunt through a VSD, as well as the reduced pulmonary blood flow. As described previously, loss of consciousness can result. Pediatric consultation should be obtained, if at all possible, before attempting conscious sedation.

Surgical Shunt Dysfunction

Because of palliative shunt procedures performed in the neonatal period prior to definitive operative repair of complex congenital heart disease, shunts can malfunction. Typically, infants in such a situation are in acute distress with increasing cyanosis. Although not as dramatic as with ductus-dependent lesions, symptoms develop when the shunt flow narrows to less than 50 percent of usual. Ordinarily, a continuous murmur is heard over the side of the shunt. Diminution or disappearance of the murmur suggests occlusion of the shunt. Typically, emergency physicians can do nothing for these infants. Palliative therapy with 100 percent oxygen is used, and transfer to a tertiary center is expedited. The use of thrombolytic therapy has been tried, but should be used by only pediatric cardiologists by direct shunt instillation or systemically. In all cases, possible replacement of the shunt or definitive surgical repair might be the only option.

Pulmonary Hypertensive Crisis

Many children with congenital heart disease have increased pulmonary artery pressure, particularly those with large VSDs. With painful procedures, these patients can experience pulmonary vasospasm. In such conditions, cyanosis and lethargy can develop and can mimic the hypercyanotic episodes of tetralogy of Fallot. Treatment is directed toward alkalinization with IV sodium bicarbonate and 100 percent oxygen to facilitate pulmonary vasodilation. Anxiolysis and analgesia are useful.

Diuretic Complications

Diuretics may be inadequate for the weight of the child because of normal growth and present as CHF. Conversely, during times of excess extraneous losses such as diarrhea or vomiting, dehydration can occur with subsequent hemoconcentration that could compromise cardiac function or shunt integrity. Careful monitoring of potassium levels is imperative during such losses.

Digoxin Toxicity

Because of the narrow therapeutic window between treatment and toxicity, digoxin toxicity can easily develop. In infants, toxicity is manifested most often by bradycardia and occasionally by other dysrhythmias. The usual adult patterns of atrial and ventricular tachycardia are not seen, except in adolescents. It is always good practice to monitor digoxin concentrations expectantly during any visit where blood will be drawn.

Usually, increased serum concentrations can be managed by withholding dosages of digoxin. Rarely, pharmacologic intervention is required for bradycardias. Ventricular dysrhythmias are managed medically with lidocaine or phenytoin. For severely intoxicated children, the use of digoxin immune globulin (Digibind) is indicated and will reverse toxicity rapidly. Usually, the dosage can be calculated readily based on the amount of digoxin elevation in nanograms above normal (see Chap. 174). A 1-ng increase in digoxin is assumed to reflect a burden of 1 mg digoxin. Each vial of digoxin-specific antibody binds 0.4 mg digoxin. Therefore, a digoxin level that is 5 ng above expected would require 12.5 vials of digoxin-specific antibody. Care should be taken to avoid volume overload.

Anticoagulation Problems

Some children with congenital heart disease are on anticoagulant therapy to prevent shunt occlusion or thrombosis of surgically implanted valves or grafts. The risk of serious bleeding is small with routine ED visits, but must be considered for any elective repair of fractures or lacerations. Prothrombin time and the international normalized ratio (INR) must be monitored. Reversal of anticoagulation with the administration of either vitamin K or fresh-frozen plasma should be undertaken only after consultation with a pediatric cardiologist.

Anemia and Polycythemia with Cyanotic Congenital Heart Disease

Children with this problem require an increase in hemoglobin concentration to compensate for hypoxemia. Children develop tachycardia, feeding difficulty, or congestive heart failure when hemoglobin concentrations fall to normal. Often, anemia will be compensated for by polycythemia, which will cause increased viscosity and the potential for cerebrovascular complications. Iron supplementation is important for prevention of anemia. When polycythemia occurs, therapeutic phlebotomy may be warranted.

Viral Infections with Congenital Heart Disease

Although few normal children have problems with common viral pathogens such as influenza virus, parainfluenza virus, or respiratory syncytial virus, children with congenital heart disease are at unique risk for major sequelae. Distinguishing minor early infections with these agents and differentiating them from the symptoms of congestive heart failure is a challenge, even for seasoned clinicians. Children with lesions that increase pulmonary blood flow are far more at risk because of pooling of alveolar secretions. The pooled secretions allow for stasis and secondary bacterial overgrowth. Dramatic increases in mortality and morbidity are evident among affected infants. No effective therapy is available for parainfluenza and influenza virus, and prophylaxis against influenza B with amantadine analogues is not approved for small children. Hospitalization and specific treatment of infants affected by respiratory syncytial virus has been difficult to justify because of conflicting studies regarding efficacy of the antivirals and ribavirin and the expense of respiratory syncytial virus-specific immune globulin. Most infants will benefit from admission for bronchodilator therapy, but the prophylactic use of antibiotics to prevent secondary bacterial pneumonia is not justified. Admission may help sort out the distinction between congestive heart failure and underlying pulmonary infection.[20]

Subacute Bacterial Endocarditis

Children with congenital heart disease are at great risk of developing endocarditis. Transient bacteremia produced by iatrogenic procedures such as dental work or gastrointestinal or urologic manipulation can lead to localized colonization and infection. Although the thrust of most primary care providers is toward prevention of this disease, cases still occur. Typically, the usual presentation is of unexplained fever in children with known congenital heart disease. Appropriate evaluation includes multiple blood cultures, urine culture and analysis, and complete blood count. Parenteral or oral antibiotics should be administered in consultation with a pediatric cardiologist familiar with the child's history. In cases of known source of infection, such as otitis media or pneumonia, multiple blood cultures should be obtained, and appropriate therapy should be directed at the site of primary infection.

Acutely ill children with high fever mandate hospitalization, multiple blood cultures, and echocardiographic study of the heart. Usually, treatment is instituted following the obtainment of cultures and is directed toward the most common pathogens. Established diagnosis is followed by 4 to 6 weeks of intravenous antibiotic therapy.[21]

ENDOCARDITIS PROPHYLAXIS PRIOR TO PROCEDURES

Prophylactic treatment is recommended for patients with congenital heart malformations and rheumatic fever with valvular disease who are undergoing surgical or dental procedures and instrumentation involving mucosal surfaces. The administration of the medication should be timed such that an effective serum level will be present during the 15 min after the mucosal manipulation, when the transient bacteremia occurs. Amoxicillin 50 mg/kg (maximum, 2 g) is given 1 h before the procedure and 25 mg/kg (maximum, 1.5 g) 6 h later. For patients with valvular disease, 2 mg/kg gentamicin is given IV or IM 30 min before the procedure and 8 h later, in addition to the amoxicillin. Erythromycin 20 mg/kg PO (maximum, 800 mg erythromycin ethylsuccinate or 1 g stearate) can be given 2 h before the procedure, with half the dose given 6 h later.

The indications for prophylaxis and treatment options are well outlined in the American Heart Association guidelines for prophylaxis of endocarditis. Cases of endocarditis can occur despite appropriate prophylaxis. Vigilance in performing appropriate blood cultures is warranted in any children with symptoms suggestive of endocarditis.[22]

EVALUATION OF FEVER IN INFANTS WITH HEART DISEASE

Infants and children with known heart disease are prone to the same illnesses as other children. When they are brought to the ED for treatment of febrile illnesses, they are most likely to be hemodynamically stable and capable of handling the illness. Any signs of congestive heart failure are indications for an admission. Otherwise, blood cultures should be obtained, as well as a complete blood count, as would be performed for any infant between the ages of 6 months and 24 months. Although occult bacteremia has the same probability for occurrence in a child with congenital heart disease, concern for bacterial endocarditis must be greater. Oral or parenteral antibiotics should be administered with great care if presumptively treating early bacteremia or subacute bacterial endocarditis. It is more prudent to arrange admission, repeated cultures, and expectant therapy for such infants than to begin antibiotic therapy blindly simply because of the presence of congenital heart disease. A follow-up visit is mandatory in 12 to 24 h for any children who are discharged home without hospital admission.

EVALUATION OF INFANTS WITH CARDIAC TRANSPLANTATION

Increasingly, infants with complex congenital heart disease are surviving and undergo cardiac or cardiopulmonary transplantation. Many of these special infants are being returned to their homes of origin after a period of intensive recovery close to the transplant hospital. As a result, these infants are often instructed to seek care in EDs far removed from the transplant hospital for "evaluation." Many emergency medicine practitioners have had no experience with infants of this complexity and are unsure of what the evaluation will entail.

Most patients are sufficiently stable and beyond the period of acute rejection of the cardiac or cardiopulmonary transplant, but may rarely present with acute, life-threatening deterioration. Allograft rejection is the leading cause of severe hemodynamic compromise in the pediatric heart or heart-lung transplant recipient. Most patients are maintained on a complex immunosuppressive regimen to suppress the immune system at multiple sites. Therapeutic monitoring of the immunosuppressive regimen is usually beyond the scope of most hospitals, but may be collected and forwarded to the transplant hospital after appropriate telephone consultation and transfer arrangements are made.

These patients are extremely ill and require careful optimization of cardiac output. All the parameters that define cardiac output (heart rate, preload, contractility, and afterload) that were previously discussed require pharmacologic manipulation to stabilize the circulation until the rejection can be reversed. Careful administration of volume, diuretics, inotropic, and afterload-reducing agents are required for stabilization prior to transfer to the transplant hospital. Corticosteroids are paramount in treatment for both cellular and vascular rejection, but should only be undertaken by direction of the transplant hospital and is probably not warranted acutely unless used to treat acute secondary adrenal insufficiency.[23]

Fortunately, most cardiac transplant recipients more commonly seek ED care for complaints that are not acutely life-threatening. The most common complaints are related to the respiratory tract, and the most common diagnoses are related to infectious processes. Fever is the presenting complaint in 25 percent of the visits, which result in positive blood cultures in approximately 10 percent of cases. By reason of severe immunocompromise, infections from opportunistic organisms and bacteremia must be considered. Surprisingly, most infections are similar to those in the nontransplanted child.[24,25] In one series drawn from an ED experience at a transplant hospital, admission was required for approximately 30 percent of the ED visits.[24] No pediatric heart transplant recipients should be considered for discharge unless consultation with the transplant hospital occurs. In all but the most unusual of circumstances, these children require transfer to the transplant hospital for more definitive care after stabilization.

REFERENCES

1. Moss AJ, Adams FH, Emmanouilides GC (eds): *Moss & Adam's Heart Disease in Infants, Children and Adolescents: Including the Fetus and Young Adult,* 5th ed. Baltimore, Williams and Wilkins, 1995, p. 1725.
2. Rein AJ, Omokhodion SI, Nir A: Significance of a cardiac murmur as the sole clinical sign in the newborn. *Clin Ped* 39:511, 2000.
3. Rosenthal A: How to distinguish between innocent and pathologic murmurs in childhood. *Pediatr Clin North Am* 31:1229, 1984.
4. McNamara DG: Value and limitation of auscultation in the management of congenital heart disease. *Pediatr Clin North Am* 37:93, 1990.
5. Myung K, Park MK, Gunteroth W (eds): *How to Read Pediatric ECGs.* St. Louis, CV Mosby, 1992.
6. Van Roenkens CN, Zuckerman AL: Emergency management of hypercyanotic crises in tetralogy of Fallot. *Ann Emerg Med* 25:256, 1995.
7. Kirklin JW, Colvin EV, McConnell ME, et al: Complete transposition of the great arteries: Treatment in the current era. *Pediatr Clin North Am* 37:171, 1990.
8. Starnes VA, Griffin ML, Pitlick PT, et al: Current approach to hypoplastic left heart syndrome: Palliation, transplantation or both? *J Thorac Cardiovasc Surg* 104:189, 1992.
9. Bernstein D: The cardiovascular system: Acyanotic congenital heart disease: Coarctation of the aorta, in Behrman RE, Kliegman RM, Arvin AM (eds): *Nelson Textbook of Pediatrics,* 15th ed. Philadelphia, WB Saunders, 1996, pp 1301–1304.
10. Makoney L, Truesdell SC, Krzmarzick TR, et al: Atrial septal defects that present in infancy. *Am J Dis Child* 140:1115, 1986.
11. Park, MK: *Pediatric Cardiology Handbook,* 3rd ed, St. Louis, Mosby, 2002.
12. Binder LS, Boeche R, Atkinson D: Evaluation and management of supraventricular tachycardia in children. *Ann Emerg Med* 20:51, 1991.
13. Paul T, Bertram H, Bokenkemp R, et al: Supravertricular tachycardia in infants, children, and adolescents: Diagnosis, pharmacological, and interventional therapy. *Paediatr Drugs* 2:171, 2000.
14. Jaeggi ET: Update on the diagnosis and treatment of supraventricular tachycardia in children. *Rev Med Suisse Romande* 121:213, 2001.
15. Garson PC, Garson A Jr, Biuk-Boelkens M, Hesslein PS: Atrial flutter in the young: A collaborative study of 380 cases. *J Am Coll Cardiol* 6:871, 1985.
16. Freed MD: Advances in the diagnosis and therapy of syncope and palpitations in children. *Curr Opin Pediatr* 6:368, 1994.
17. Pass RH, Liberman L, Al-Fayaddah M, et al: Continuous intravenous diltiazem infusion for short-term ventricular rate control in children. *Am J Cardiol* 86:559, 2000.
18. Gow R: Ventricular arrhythmias in infants and children. *Curr Opin Pediatr* 2:963, 1990.

19. Celiker A, Ceviz N, Ozme S: Effectiveness and safety of intravenous amiodarone in drug-resistant tachyarrhythmias of children. *Acta Pediatr Jpn* 40:567, 1998.

20. Antiarrhythmic Agents. Amidorone, in McEvoy GK (ed): AHFS Drug Information 2003, p 1512–1517. American Society of Health System Pharmacists, Bethesda, MD.

21. Saiman L, Prince A, Gersony WM: Pediatric infective endocarditis in the modern era. *J Pediatr* 122:847, 1993.

22. Dajani AS, Bisno AL, Chung KJ, et al: Prevention of bacterial endocarditis: Recommendations by the American Heart Association. *JAMA* 277:1794, 1997.

23. Costello JM, Pahl E: Prevention and treatment of severe hemodynamic compromise in pediatric heart transplant patients. *Pediatr Drugs* 4:705, 2002.

24. Chinnock R, Sherwin T, Robie S, et al: Emergency department presentation and management of pediatric heart transplant recipients. *Pediatr Emerg Care* 11:355, 1995.

25. Stovall S, Ainley K Frazier E, et al: Invasive pneumococcal infection in pediatric heart transplant patients. *J Heart Lung Transplant* 20:231, 2001.

121 OTITIS AND PHARYNGITIS IN CHILDREN

Kimberly S. Quayle

Susan Fuchs

David M. Jaffe

OTITIS MEDIA

Otitis media, or inflammation of the middle ear, is one of the most common pediatric diagnoses. Each year there are 25 to 30 million office visits, with direct costs of more than $5 billion a year.[1] Acute otitis media (AOM; acute suppurative, purulent, or bacterial) is associated with signs and symptoms of inflammation of the middle ear, such as otalgia, otorrhea, fever, irritability, anorexia, or vomiting.[1] Otitis media with effusion (OME; secretory, nonsuppurative, serous, or mucoid) is a relatively asymptomatic collection of fluid in the middle ear. The duration (not the severity) of OME can be divided into acute (<3 weeks), subacute (3 weeks to 3 months), and chronic (>3 months). The most important distinction between OME and AOM is that the signs and symptoms of acute infection (otalgia, otorrhea, and fever) are lacking in OME, but hearing loss may be present in both conditions.[1]

Acute Otitis Media

Infants and young children are at greatest risk for the development of otitis media, with the peak incidence occurring between 6 and 18 months.[2] In fact, in the United States, up to 50 percent of children will have had at least one episode of AOM by age 1.[1] The incidence is higher in males, Native Americans, Alaskan and Canadian Eskimos, and children who attend day care, are exposed to tobacco smoke, have a cleft palate or other craniofacial anomaly (e.g., Down syndrome), sleep in a prone position, use a pacifier, have older siblings or parents with a history of ear infections, had their first episode of AOM at younger than 6 months, or have congenital or acquired immunodeficiency.[1,2] The incidence is lower in breast-fed infants.[1]

Middle ear effusion may persist for weeks to months after an episode of AOM. Antibiotic therapy generally sterilizes the effusion but does not clear it from the middle ear space. After the first episode of AOM, 70 percent of children still have a middle ear effusion at 2 weeks, 40 percent at 1 month, 20 percent at 2 months, and 10 percent at 3 months.[3]

ETIOLOGY   Bacteria are the most common cause of AOM and can be isolated in a pure culture from the middle ear exudate in 60 to 75 percent of cases. These organisms colonize the nasopharynx and enter the middle ear via the eustachian tube. *Streptococcus pneumoniae* and *Haemophilus influenzae* are the most common pathogens (*S. pneumoniae,* 40 to 50 percent, and most common serotypes are 19, 23, 6, 14, 3, and 18; *H. influenzae,* 30 to 40 percent, primarily nontypable strains), and *Moraxella catarrhalis* is the third most common organism (10 to 15 percent).[1,4] Of importance is a major change in the increased prevalence of β-lactamase-producing *M. catarrhalis* (almost 100 percent) and *H. influenzae* (35 to 40 percent), which affects antibiotic therapy decisions.[1] *Streptococcus pyogenes* (group A) and *Staphylococcus aureus* each are found in 2 percent of cultures.[4] *Chlamydia pneumoniae* also may be a causative organism, especially in those younger than 6 months. However, in infants 6 weeks or younger, gram-negative enteric bacilli and *S. aureus* account for 10 to 20 percent of isolates.[5] Although viruses are rarely recovered from middle ear effusions, recent studies have shown an increased risk of OME after an upper respiratory tract infection due to rhinovirus, respiratory syncytial virus, adenovirus, and influenza virus A or B.

PATHOPHYSIOLOGY   Abnormal function of the eustachian tube appears to be the dominant factor in the pathogenesis of middle ear disease. Two types of tube dysfunction may result in otitis media: obstruction and abnormal patency. Obstruction can result from persistent collapse of the eustachian tube due to increased tubal compliance, an inadequate active opening mechanism, or both. Infants and younger children are susceptible to eustachian tube obstruction, because the cartilage that supports the eustachian tube is less stiff than in adults. In addition, an upper respiratory tract infection or allergies can obstruct the eustachian tube and decrease its function. The obstructed eustachian tube prevents equilibration of air pressure between the middle ear and the atmosphere and creates conditions favorable to the development of purulent or sterile effusions. The other type of dysfunction is abnormal patency, which may allow reflux of nasopharyngeal secretions.[5]

CLINICAL FEATURES   Classic signs and symptoms of AOM include ear pain (otalgia), otorrhea, and fever; however, ear pulling and irritability may be the only clues in an infant. The most important diagnostic tool is the pneumatic otoscopic examination. Before adequate visualization of the external canal and tympanic membrane (TM) can be achieved, cerumen must be removed from the canal by blunt curettage or by irrigation with warm water.[5] The presence or absence of discharge and the position or contour (normal, bulging, retracted), color (pink, grey, red, yellow), and degree of translucency (translucent, opaque, non-opaque) and mobility (normal, increased, decreased, absent) of the TM must be assessed.[6] The light reflex is of no diagnostic value. The normal eardrum is translucent and pearly gray but may become reddened with crying. The eardrum should be freely mobile in response to positive and negative pressure by the pneumatoscope; however, retracted TMs have reduced mobility. The TM of AOM is usually opaque, pale yellow, red, and sometimes bulging, and bony landmarks (long and short process of the malleus) are not easily discernible. However, the most significant sign is the loss of or decrease in mobility of the TM, which implies the presence of a middle ear effusion.[6]

Tympanometry is a noninvasive diagnostic technique used to determine the compliance of the TM and the middle ear. A fixed tone at a given intensity is delivered through a probe snugly placed in the external ear canal as the air pressure in the canal is changed from positive to negative. The tympanogram is a recording of the acoustic compliance of the middle ear, and patterns obtained are useful in distinguishing a normal ear from one with an effusion.[6] Spectral gradient acoustic reflectometry is a technique that in the uncooperative infant or child is easier to perform than tympanometry, because the instrument does not need to seal the auditory canal. It assesses the response of the TM to a sound stimulus, and a microprocessor analyzes the data into spectral gradient angles that indicate the likelihood of a middle ear effusion.[5] However, it cannot be used to distinguish the presence of an effusion due to AOM from that caused by OME.[6]

Aspiration of the middle ear is the most definitive method of verifying the presence and type of middle ear effusion and infecting organism; however, its use for this purpose in the ED setting is rarely practical. It may be beneficial in (1) children with overwhelming sepsis, (2) immunologically deficient children, (3) neonates, (4) children with persistent symptoms of AOM after more than 48 to 72 h on antimicrobial therapy, or (5) otitis media with confirmed or potential suppurative complications.[5,6] Diagnostic tympanocentesis may be performed by inserting an 2.5- to 3-in. 18-gauge spinal needle or catheter over a needle attached to a syringe through the anterior inferior or posterior inferior quadrant of the TM. The aspirate should be cultured in blood culture broth, on blood and chocolate agar plates, and sent for Gram stain.[6] When therapeutic drainage is required, a myringotomy should be performed. The incision should be made in the lower half of the TM and should be large enough to allow adequate drainage and aeration of the middle ear. Myringotomy may relieve unusually severe otalgia at initial examination or at any time during the course of the disease. In addition, it should be performed when a suppurative complication (e.g., meningitis, facial paralysis, or mastoiditis) is present.[5,6]

TREATMENT   Selection of the appropriate antibiotic is based on several factors: (1) knowledge of the likely etiologic agent or recovery of a specific pathogen from middle ear fluid, (2) the efficacy of certain antibiotics against the organism responsible for AOM, (3) antibiotic penetration into middle ear fluid, (4) a history of drug allergy, (5) compliance issues, (6) drug side effects, and (7) treatment failure or success of previous drug regimens for that child.[1] There are also patient factors that influence therapy, including age, attendance at day care, and the use of antibiotics within the past 3 months.[1,4]

Despite the approval of 16 antibiotics by the US Food and Drug Administration (FDA) for the treatment of AOM (see Table 121-1 for doses and frequency) and the changing antibiotic susceptibility patterns that have emerged over the past few years, amoxicillin remains the drug of choice. However, due to the prevalence of drug-resistant *S. pneumoniae* (DRSP) (Table 121-2), a Centers for Disease Control and Prevention (CDC) working group has developed a new management scheme.[4] **There are now two doses of amoxicillin (Amoxil): the standard dose (40 to 45 mg/kg per d) and the high dose (80 to 90 mg/kg per d).** The recommendation to use a high dose is based on the fact that amoxicillin has the longest time above the MIC90 against DRSP than any of the other antibiotics.[4] The high-dose amoxicillin is recommended as first-line treatment for those patients with a high risk of DRSP. These patients include children younger 2 years, those in day care, and those who have used antibiotics within the previous 3 months. Although this high dose is not approved by the FDA, it was felt that amoxicillin had a long safety record and a history of efficacy in treating AOM.[4]

Other potential choices include high-dose amoxicillin-clavulanate (Augmentin; 80 to 90 mg/kg per d of the amoxicillin component with 6.4 mg/kg per d of clavulanate, which requires the new 7:1 formulation) or cefuroxime axetil (Ceftin; 30 mg/kg per d). For those children not in the high-risk group, first-line treatment options include standard- or high-dose amoxicillin.[4]

If after 3 days the infant or child still has evidence of AOM (clinical failure including persistence of signs and symptoms such as ear pain, fever, or TM findings consistent with AOM), it is necessary to provide coverage against β-lactamase-producing *H. influenzae* and *M. catarrhalis* and penicillin-resistant *S. pneumoniae*. Antibiotics that are appropriate are based on the initial agents used but include high-dose amoxicillin-clavulanate, cefuroxime axetil, and intramuscular ceftriaxone (Rocephin) for the low-risk group. For the high-risk group, intramuscular ceftriaxone, clindamycin, and tympanocentesis are options.[4] The caveats are as follows. (1) Whereas the FDA has approved a single dose of intramuscular ceftriaxone for penicillin-susceptible strains, the CDC working group has recommended treatment on 3 consecutive days for those in whom high-dose amoxicillin was unsuccessful, because one dose may be insufficient in curing AOM due to

TABLE 121-1   Treatment Options for Acute Otitis Media

Generic Name (Trade Name)	Oral Dose Unless Otherwise Noted	Frequency*
Amoxicillin (Amoxil)	40–45 mg/kg per d, standard dose 80–90 mg/kg per d, high dose	tid
Amoxicillin–clavulanate (Augmentin)	40–45 mg/kg per d, standard dose 80–90 mg/kg per d, high dose, but limit clavulanate to 6.4 mg/kg per d	4:1 formula tid, 7:1 formula bid
Trimethoprim–sulfasoxazole (TMP-SMX; Bactrim, Septra)	TMP, 8–12 mg/kg per d SMZ, 40–60 mg/kg per d	bid
Erythromycin and sulfasoxazole (Pediazole, Eryzole)	40–50 mg/kg per d of erythromycin	qid or tid
Second-generation cephalosporins		
Cefaclor (Ceclor)	40 mg/kg per d	tid or bid
Cefuroxime axetil (Ceftin)	30 mg/kg per d	bid
Cefprozil (Cefzil)	30 mg/kg per d	bid
Cephalexin (Keflex, Keftab)	25–50 mg/kg per d	qid or tid
Loracarbef (Lorabid)	30 mg/kg per d	bid
Third-generation cephalosporins		
Cefixime (Suprax)	8 mg/kg per d	qd or bid
Ceftibuten (Cedax)	9 mg/kg per d	qd
Cefpodoxime (Vantin)	10 mg/kg per d	qd or bid
Cefdinir (Omnicef)	14 mg/kg per d	qd or bid
Ceftriaxone (Rocephin)	50 mg/kg per d, IM only	qd for 1–3 d
Macrolides		
Azithromycin (Zithromax)	10 mg/kg per d on day 1, then 5 mg/kg per d for 4 d	qd
Clarithromycin (Biaxin)	15 mg/kg per d	bid

*Prescription duration is 10 days, unless otherwise noted. Please see text for discussion of appropriate patients for 5–7 versus 10 days of therapy.

TABLE 121-2   High-Risk Features for Otitis Media Due to Drug-Resistant *Streptococcus pneumoniae*

Antibiotics within past 3 mo
Day-care attendance
Age <2 y

penicillin-resistant *S. pneumoniae*.[4] (2) The use of clindamycin may be appropriate for those exposed to recent antibiotics, but it is important to realize that clindamycin is not active against *H. influenzae* or *M. catarrhalis* and, hence, should be given as the sole agent in culture-confirmed *S. pneumoniae* otitis media.[4] (3) Since the report of the CDC working group, another cephalosporin, cefdinir (Omnicef), has been approved for AOM. Because its spectrum of activity is similar to that of cefuroxime axetil and it has a better taste, it may be another appropriate choice.[7] (4) The use of diagnostic tympanocentesis is another option to guide the choice of therapy.[4]

If the child is not found to have a treatment failure on day 3, but rather returns for a re-check between days 10 and 28 and is found to still have AOM (not just a middle ear effusion), then the treatment options include high-dose amoxicillin-clavulanate, cefuroxime axetil, or intramuscular ceftriaxone for the low-risk group and high-dose amoxicillin-clavulanate, cefuroxime, intramuscular ceftriaxone, or tympanocentesis for the high-risk-group, after taking into account the caveats listed above[4] (Figure 121-1).

Although there are many other β-lactamase agents effective and approved for the treatment of AOM [including cefaclor (Ceclor), cefixime (Suprax), ceftibuten (Cedax), cefproxil (Cefzil), cefpodoxime (Vantin), loracarbef (Lorabid), azithromycin (Zithromax), and clarithromycin (Biaxin)], the CDC working group did not include them due to lack of clinical efficacy.[4] Cefproxil has less β-lactamase stability than do cefuroxime, cefdinir, and cepodoxime. Cefaclor, loracarbef, cefixime, and ceftibuten have inadequate activity against penicillin-resistant *S. pneumoniae*.[1,4]

Some of the traditionally used first- and second-line antibiotics, including trimethoprim-sulfamethoxazole [TMP-SMZ (Bactrim or Septra)] and erythromycin and sulfasoxazole (Pediazole), are not in the algorithm, because resistance to TMP-SMZ is more common than resistance to penicillin and 10 percent of isolates are resistant to erythromycin. Therefore, patients who have already failed high-dose amoxicillin are likely to fail to respond to these drugs.[4] In addition, pneumococci that are resistant to erythromycin are also resistant to the newer macrolides, azithromycin and clarithromycin, and they are not as effective against *H. influenzae* as the β-lactams[4] (see Figure 121-1).

Patients who are allergic to β-lactam agents should not be given cephalosporins, so alternatives such as clindamycin, erythromycin and sulfamethoxazole in combination, TMP-SMZ, clarithromycin, or azithromycin are recommended.[1]

In infants 6 weeks or younger, several factors should be taken into account (Table 121-3). If the infant is younger than 2 weeks (or is older but has remained in a newborn nursery for a prolonged period), group B *Streptococcus, S. aureus,* and gram-negative bacilli are the most likely pathogens. A child of this age warrants a full septic workup (complete blood count, blood culture, urinalysis, urine culture, lumbar puncture with cerebrospinal fluid analysis and culture, and possibly a chest radiograph) and admission for parenteral antibiotics (ampicillin plus gentamicin, cefotaxime, or ceftriaxone). For infants between 2 and 6 weeks of age who have been discharged for more than 2 weeks from a nursery, *S. pneumoniae* and *H. influenzae* are the most likely culprits.[5] Although a full septic workup is warranted, decisions about admission and treatment options are based on the results of these tests, the appearance of the infant, availability of close follow-up, and prevailing policies.

In the numerous trials of antibiotics in the treatment of otitis media, adverse reactions requiring the discontinuation of the drug have occurred in fewer than 5 percent of patients. With ampicillin, amoxi-

cillin, and amoxicillin-clavulanate, diarrhea is the most common side effect, followed by rash. Trimethoprim-sulfasoxazole can also cause diarrhea and skin rash (including Stevens-Johnson syndrome), but the major concern is the development of neutropenia and thrombocytopenia. In addition, a patient with glucose 6-phosphate dehydrogenase deficiency should not receive sulfonamides. Erythromycin often causes gastrointestinal symptoms, including abdominal cramps, nausea, vomiting, and diarrhea. Aside from possible cross-sensitivity in patients with penicillin allergy, cefaclor can cause a serum sickness-like reaction consisting of a rash, arthralgia or arthritis, and fever.[1]

DURATION OF THERAPY   Although the CDC working group did not address the issue of duration of therapy, recent data support the use of a 5- to 7-day course of antibiotics in older children (>2 years) with mild AOM. For children younger than 2 years, any patient with perforation of the TM, those with underlying medical problems, those at higher risk of treatment failure, and those with chronic or recurrent otitis media should receive a full 10 days of treatment (except for azithromycin, which is given for 5 days).[3,8]

ADDITIONAL THERAPY   Antipyretics and analgesics may be helpful in alleviating some of the acute symptoms. A topical analgesic [antipyrine, benzocaine, and glycerin (Auralgan)] instilled into the external ear canal often provides some relief from otalgia, but it should not be used when a TM perforation is present. Decongestants, antihistamines, or glucocorticoids have no demonstrable role in the treatment of AOM. With appropriate antimicrobial therapy, most children with AOM are significantly improved within 48 to 72 h. Persistent or recurrent pain or fever after 48 to 72 h indicates a need for reexamination of the child and the possible selection of another antimicrobial agent. Reasons for response failure include a resistant organism, noncompliance, and host-related structural or immunologic abnormalities.

Standard practice has been that children with an uncomplicated course should be reexamined within 10 to 14 days of the completion of antibiotic therapy. Studies have demonstrated that this visit may be delayed to 3 to 6 weeks in certain cases. However, in view of the fact that an emergency physician is not usually providing long-term follow-up care for such patients, telephone contact with the patient's physician to arrange for a follow-up visit is recommended.

Recurrent Acute Otitis Media

Many children have repeated episodes of AOM. Recurrent AOM is defined as three or more episodes of AOM in 6 months or four episodes in 12 months, with at least one episode within the past 6 months[3,9] (Table 121-4). Some children develop symptoms and a new ear effusion, often associated with an upper respiratory tract infection, after a previous effusion has resolved, whereas others develop symptoms of AOM with no documented resolution of a previous effusion. There is a correlation between such "otitis-prone" children and the onset of AOM before 1 year of age. Other risk factors include day-care attendance and genetic susceptibility: a sibling or parent with a history of severe or recurrent AOM. The key factor is distinguishing AOM from OME via pneumatic otoscopy and even tympanocentesis.[9] Due to the risk of long-term sequelae, such as hearing loss and speech impairment, prevention of further episodes is desirable.[9] A more thorough physical examination and laboratory x-ray studies should be performed to rule out sinusitis, allergies, immune deficiencies (C3 and C5 deficiencies), submucous cleft palate, or a tumor of the nasopharynx. If none of these is present, the preferred method of prevention for this particular group of patients is prophylaxis with antibiotics: amoxicillin, 20 mg/kg per d at bedtime, or sulfasoxazole, 75 mg/kg in one or two divided doses, for 3 to 6 months, with rechecks every 1 to 2 months. Prophylaxis is especially important during the fall and winter, when respiratory tract infections tend to occur; for children younger than 2 years; and for those in day care. Although there is concern that

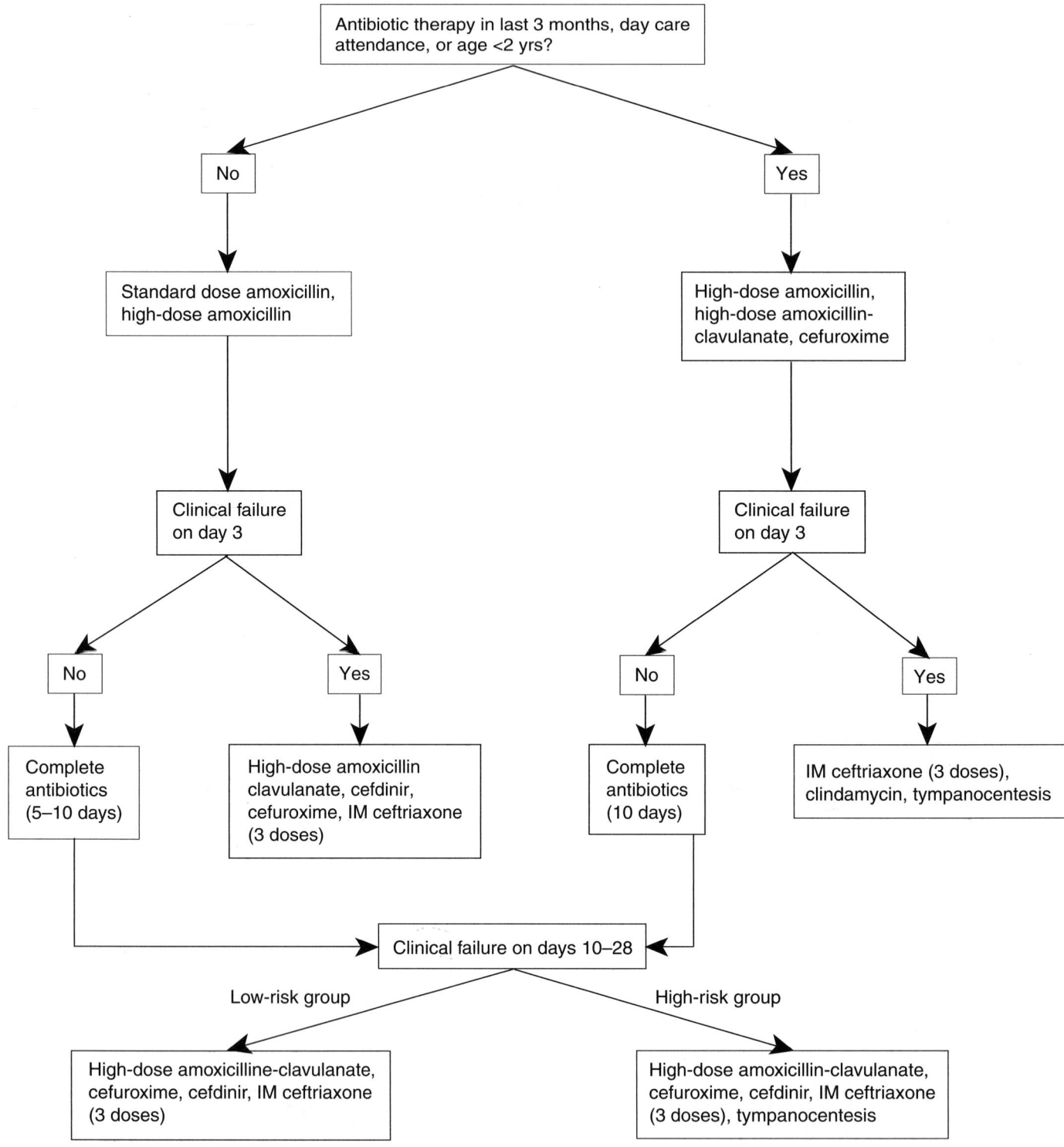

Algorithm modified and adapted from references 1,4,7,8

FIG. 121-1. Algorithm for drug therapy for acute otitis media. IM = intramuscularly. (Modified and adapted from McCracken GH Jr: Diagnosis and management of acute otitis media in the urgent care setting. *Ann Emerg Med* 39:413, 2002; Dowell SF, Butler JC, Giebink GS, et al: Acute otitis media: Management and surveillance in an era of pneumococcal resistance—a report from the drug-resistant *Streptococcus pneumoniae* therapeutic working group. *Pediatr Infect Dis J* 18:1, 1999; Klein JO, McCracken GH Jr: Summary: Role of a new oral cephalosporin, cefdinir, for therapy of infections in infants and children. *Pediatr Infect Dis J* 19:S181, 2000; Kozyrskyj AL, Hildes-Ripstein GE, Longstaffe SEA, et al: Treatment of acute otitis media with a shortened course of antibiotics. *JAMA* 279:1736, 1998.)

TABLE 121-3   Otitis Media Neonates

Age	Organisms	Workup
<2 wk or prolonged care in a nursery	Group B *Streptococcus, Staphylococcus aureus,* gram-negative bacilli	Full septic workup including lumbar puncture
2–6 wk or discharged ≥2 wk from a nursery	*Streptococcus pneumonia, Haemophilus influenzae*	Full septic workup, lumbar puncture is usual

the use of prophylaxis results in increased nasopharyngeal carriage of resistant pneumococci in this population, the benefits must be weighed against the risks and other options.[3]

Myringotomy with tympanostomy tube insertion is the next step for children who fail antibiotic prophylaxis, although some physicians might have chosen myringotomy instead of antibiotic prophylaxis. Adenoidectomy is recommended at the time of myringotomy tube placement for children with severe nasal obstruction.[5]

Persistent Acute Otitis Media

Persistent AOM is defined as the persistence of AOM within 3 days of initiating therapy or the recurrence of signs and symptoms within a few days of completing a 10-day course of antibiotics. This condition may be caused by the same pathogen (relapse) or a new bacterial species (reinfection).[5] The treatment of this problem is covered in the algorithm for AOM (see Figure 121-1). If the child still has AOM after two courses of treatment, tympanocentesis for culture and identification of the organism should be performed, although this is not always feasible. A search for a suppurative complication of otitis media (e.g., mastoiditis) or a concurrent infection (e.g., meningitis) should be performed at this time.

Chronic Suppurative Otitis Media

The persistence (>6 weeks) of a chronic inflammation of the middle ear and mastoid in the presence of a perforated or non-intact TM is known as chronic suppurative otitis media (CSOM). Purulent ear discharge may or may not be present.[10] It is thought to be a sequela of partly treated or untreated AOM or recurrent AOM. The organisms responsible for infection depend on the patient's age. In young children who develop AOM and then have a perforation or those with a tympanostomy tube, the common organisms are those that cause AOM, including *S. pneumoniae, H. influenzae,* and *M. catarrhalis.* In older children or in those with water contamination of the middle ear, *Pseudomonas aeruginosa* and *S. aureus* are the most common causative organisms, although anaerobes have also been cultured.[10] It is thought that the organisms gain access to the middle ear through the perforated TM and become pathogens in the middle ear. A thorough examination is imperative, because chronic ear drainage can be a manifestation of a cholesteatoma (which requires surgery). In the absence of a cholesteatoma, the following steps result in a more rapid improvement in ear drainage and a decreased need for tympanomastoid surgery. (1) Meticulous daily cleaning and aspiration of the external and middle ear followed by instillation of ear drops. Polymyxin B, neomycin, and hydrocortisone (Cortisporin, Pediotic suspension), topical tobramycin and dexamethasone (TobraDex), or gentamicin ophthalmic drops (Garamycin) are falling out of favor, because they may be ototoxic. Ofloxacin (Floxin otic) is FDA approved for use in CSOM in children older than 12 years and for cases of AOM in children older

than 1 year with tympanostomy tubes. Ofloxacin (Floxin otic) is currently the only FDA-approved drug for children with non-intact TMs. Ciprofloxacin with hydrocortisone (Cipro HC) is FDA approved for children and adults for the treatment of otitis externa and with an intact TM, not for CSOM. Alternatives to antibiotics include the use of ototopical antiseptic agents such as acetic acid and aluminum subacetate (Burow's solution), acetic acid (2%) otic (VoSoL), or acetic acid (2%) in aqueous aluminum acetate otic solution (Otic Domeboro).[5,10] (2) Oral antibiotics (amoxicillin-clavulanate) in addition to otic drops can be prescribed, if the organism is thought to be *P. aeruginosa,* although this is unlikely to be effective. For adults and children older than 18 years, oral ciprofloxacin is another alternative.[10] (3) If ototopical drops with or without oral antibiotics is not successful, the next step is the use of parenterally administered broad-spectrum, antipseudomonal antibiotics [ticarcillin, ticarcillin-clavulanate (Timentin), piperacillin, or ceftazidime (Fortaz, Tazicef, or Tazidime)] on an inpatient or an outpatient basis.[5,10]

Complications and Sequelae of Otitis Media

The complications and sequelae of otitis media predominantly involve the middle ear and adjacent structures within the temporal bone, but in rare instances intracranial complications may occur. The aural or intratemporal complications and sequelae include hearing loss, perforation or retraction pocket of the TM, tympanosclerosis, adhesive otitis media, ossicular discontinuity and fixation, CSOM, cholesteatoma, mastoiditis, petrositis, labyrinthitis, and facial paralysis.[11] Suppuration in the middle ear, mastoid, or both may extend into the intracranial cavity, producing the following intracranial complications: meningitis, extradural abscess, subdural empyema, focal encephalitis, brain abscess, lateral (sigmoid) sinus thrombosis, and otitic hydrocephalus.[11] These complications are uncommon except in neglected cases.[11]

Prevention of Acute Otitis Media

Because *Pneumococcus* is the most common bacterial pathogen in AOM, the use of a vaccine could decrease the incidence of AOM. A heptavalent pneumococcal conjugate vaccine is now available in the United States. It contains separate conjugates for serotypes 4, 6B, 9V, 14, 18C, 19F, and 23F. Large-scale evaluations of this vaccine in northern California and Finland have demonstrated a reduction in all AOM cases by 6 to 8.9 percent and culture-proven pneumococcal cases by 34 percent.[12] The routine use of this vaccine (recommended to be given at ages 2, 4, and 6 months, with a booster at age 2 years) could reduce the number of visits for otitis in the United States by 1 million![12]

Otitis Media with Effusion

Otitis media with effusion is defined as a collection of fluid in the middle ear, without acute clinical signs and symptoms, which often follows an episode of AOM.[13] Hearing loss is by far the most prevalent complication and morbid outcome of OME. The extent of hearing loss depends on the volume of the effusion rather on than the physical properties of the effusion, and OME is associated with a mild to moderate conductive hearing loss of 20 dB or more. Audiometry is of limited value as a diagnostic method for the identification of OME, but it

TABLE 121-4   Recurrent Acute Otitis Media

≥3 episodes in 6 mo
or
≥4 episodes in 12 mo, with 1 in past 6 mo

can be helpful in the evaluation of the effect of middle ear disease on hearing. The relation between persistent or episodic conductive hearing loss and impairment in the cognitive linguistic and speech development of children has been reported. However, the degree and duration of the hearing loss required to produce such deficits have not been defined.[13]

Other factors that should be considered in addition to hearing loss when deciding whether to treat OME include (1) occurrence in young infants, because they are unable to communicate their symptoms and may have suppurative disease; (2) an associated acute purulent upper respiratory infection; (3) permanent conductive or sensorineural hearing loss; (4) vertigo; (5) alterations in the TM (severe atelectasis and/or a deep retraction pocket in the posterosuperior quadrant or the pars flaccida); (6) middle ear changes, such as adhesive otitis or ossicular involvement; (7) persistence of the effusion for more than 3 months (chronic OME); (8) occurrence of episodes so close together that the child has OME for 6 of 12 months; (9) the presence of craniofacial abnormalities; and (10) impaired or deficient immunologic status.[13] A thorough search for an underlying cause (e.g., sinusitis, allergy, submucous cleft, or tumor) should be attempted before treatment is begun.

There are several management options for children 1 to 3 years of age with OME that persists for less than 3 months: observation (no treatment) or treatment with an antibiotic for 10 to 14 days.[13] Because most episodes of OME clear spontaneously and because of the concern for antibiotic resistance, the no-treatment option is currently preferred.[13] However, if antibiotic therapy is chosen, because bacteria that cause OME are similar to those found in AOM, the antibiotics used are the same: amoxicillin, amoxicillin-clavulanate, TMP/SMX, cefaclor, erythromycin, and sulfasoxazole.[13]

For children with OME of 3 months' duration and a hearing loss of 20 dB or more, the Agency for Health Care Policy and Research recommends referral to an otolaryngologist for myringotomy with tympanostomy tube placement as another option (in addition to the options described above).[13] However, many reserve myringotomy and tube placement for patients who have failed an antibiotic trial.

The other nonsurgical methods available, including the use of decongestants, antihistamines, and immunotherapy, have not been shown to be effective in clinical trials.[13] The addition of an oral corticosteroid (prednisone, 1 mg/kg per d in two doses for 7 days) to the use of oral antibiotics for 14 to 21 days remains controversial. Steroids should not be used in a susceptible child who has been exposed to Varicella in the past month, due to a risk of disseminated disease.

Myringotomy with tympanostomy tube placement improves the conductive hearing loss for longer periods than does myringotomy alone.[5] Tympanostomy tubes remain in place from a few weeks to several years, with an average of 6 months. Possible complications of myringotomy tubes are scarring (tympanosclerosis), localized atrophy, persistent perforation, and the rare development of a cholesteatoma.[5] For children 4 years or older who have recurrent chronic OME and who have had one or more myringotomy and tympanostomy tube operations in the past, adenoidectomy is a reasonable option.[11] The presence of upper airway obstruction, recurrent acute or chronic adenoiditis, or both is another indication to consider adenoidectomy.[5]

OTITIS EXTERNA

External otitis (OE) is any inflammatory condition of the auricle, external ear canal, or outer surface of the TM. It can be caused by infection, inflammatory dermatoses, trauma, or combinations of the three.

Pathophysiology

The flora of the normal ear canal are the same as those of normal skin. They include *Staphylococcus epidermidis*, *Corynebacterium* species, and α-hemolytic streptococcus.[14] Compromise of any of the protective features of the ear canal (e.g., shape, cerumen, or acidic pH) can lead to OE due to colonization and invasion by pathogenic organisms, especially *P. aeruginosa, S. aureus,* and fungi.[14] Causes include (1) high environmental temperature and humidity, (2) hyperhydration and maceration of epithelial tissue in the canal, (3) absorption of moisture by the stratum corneum, (4) lack of cerumen through blocked gland ducts and/or mechanical removal (scratching), (5) obstruction of gland ducts by edema and keratin debris, (6) invasion by exogenous or endogenous organisms through breaks in the damaged epithelial surface, and (7) trauma.[14]

Clinical Features

The mildest form of acute inflammatory OE is characterized by itching or a sense of fullness in the ear. As it progresses, increasing pain, itching, redness, edema, tenderness of the canal, and cheesy or purulent discharge occur. Inward pressure on the tragus or pulling the auricle up and back usually results in discomfort. If the TM can be visualized, it is often red, thick, and covered with the flat vesicles or areas of desquamating epithelium.[14] In the severe stage, pain is intense and can be caused by any movement of the jaw or the ear. There is often disseminated infection, with the presence of enlarged and tender lymph nodes. Further anterior spread of the infection affects the parotid gland and subcutaneous tissue. Posterior spread involves the mastoid, and medial spread involves cranial nerves IX through XII, with possible osteomyelitis of the skull.[14]

When there is acute localized OE (furunculosis), although pain, itching, and signs of infection, such as erythema, are present, a localized abscess is often seen. The organism responsible is usually *S. aureus*.[14] When OE is caused by fungi (otomycosis), most commonly *Aspergillus niger,* there is intense itching. Otomycosis is more common in those with underlying immune disorders and diabetes mellitus.[14]

Diagnosis

The hardest part of the diagnosis is to distinguish between OE and otitis media. Ideally, clinical inspection of the TM with a pneumatic otoscope helps establish the diagnosis; however, the TM of a child with OE may be as red and distorted as that of a child with otitis media, although mobility of the TM is normal or slightly decreased in OE. In addition, visualization of the TM may be difficult, because of edema of the canal in OE. Tympanometry can be helpful if the canal is clear, and a tight seal for the earpiece can be formed without too much discomfort. Parotitis, periauricular adenitis, mastoiditis, dental pain, and temporomandibular joint dysfunction should be considered when the discomfort is poorly localized and the ear canal and TM appear normal. In addition, pain can be referred from pharyngitis or tonsillitis, but such pain is often made worse by swallowing or eating. Foreign bodies in the ear also can cause OE.[14]

Treatment

A thorough and atraumatic cleaning of the ear canal is the most important part of therapy. For mild infections, dry mopping with a small tuft of cotton attached to a wire applicator is sufficient and may be curative. If the canal is inflamed, edematous, and occluded by debris, cleaning can be done with gentle suctioning: a soft plastic infant feeding tube (with an opening at the tip) can be used.

Mild OE can be treated with cleaning and acidifying agents alone. Acetic acid eardrops are the easiest and least expensive way to eliminate the infecting agent. A 2% solution is effective and available commercially in aqueous (Otic Domeboro) or alcohol-based (VoSoL or Orlex) solutions. These drops should be used three to four times a day for at least 1 week.[14]

Moderate OE should be treated with cleaning and antibiotic drops. If the canal cannot be cleaned sufficiently, an Oto-Wick can be placed in the canal to act as a passage for the use of drops. It can be left in place for 2 to 3 days, at which point reexamination and removal can be performed. Antibiotic preparations containing neomycin and polymyxin B (Cortisporin Otic, Otocort, and Pediotic) have been reported to cause ototoxicity.[14] Cortisporin is available as a solution and a suspension. The solution contains an acidifying agent, so it may cause more burning or stinging that the suspension. Another option is the use of Cortisporin ophthalmic suspension, which is free of acid and alcohol. Consequently, fluoroquinolone otic drops such as ofloxacin (Floxin otic) or ciprofloxacin with hydrocortisone (Cipro HC otic) are now preferred.[14] Floxin otic is approved for use with a non-intact TM. Cipro HC otic is approved for use with an intact TM. Although fluoroquinolones are not approved for children younger than 18 years via the oral route, otic fluoroquinolone drops can be used in children older than 1 year. Fluoroquinolone drops are used twice a day, as opposed to the polymyxin/neomycin drops, which must be used three to four times a day.[14] Otic chloramphenicol (Chloromycetin) should be avoided because of the risk of aplastic anemia.

Children who fail to respond within 48 h of treatment should be reexamined. If the ear is not clear and dry, other causes, such as cellulitis, abscess, CSOM, cholesteatoma, sensitization to the antibiotic, local dermatoses, or even noncompliance, should be excluded.[14] In some cases, oral antibiotics active against *S. aureus* (e.g., dicloxacillin or cephalexin) may be required. Oral ciprofloxacin, an effective antipseudomonal drug, is not approved for children younger than 18 years.

Patients with progressive, unresponsive, or severe infection may require parenteral (intravenous) therapy. Cultures of canal secretions should be taken, and a combination of an aminoglycoside (gentamicin or tobramycin) and an antipseudomonal penicillin (ticarcillin or piperacillin) should be started. If the clinical findings and course of the illness suggest an infection due to *S. aureus,* a penicillinase-resistant antibiotic [nafcillin, oxacillin, vancomycin, or ampicillin-sulbactam (Unasyn) for those older than 1 year] also should be given.[14]

The basic treatment of otomycosis is similar to that for acute bacterial OE, with cleaning followed by 2% acetic acid or M-cresyl acetate (25%) preparations. Patients who do not respond can be treated with topical antifungal medications, including suspensions of miconazole, nystatin, clotrimazole, or amphotericin B. Glucocorticoids are present in many topical otic preparations, but their value is unproven. Topical benzocaine and lidocaine may be useful to reduce the itching, but they are inadequate for the relief of moderate to severe pain, for which oral analgesics may be required.[14]

Prevention of Otitis Externa

Swimming should be prohibited during the course of treatment. Even after therapy, earplug use is suggested. If there is no perforation of the TM, irrigation with 2% acetic acid in Burow's solution (Otic Domeboro) or other acidic solutions, to return the pH to an acidic level, is helpful. Acidified isopropyl alcohol (equal parts vinegar and alcohol) or hydrogen peroxide also can be used, followed by drying with suction, compressed air, or a hair dryer set on low, 1 ft. from the ear for 1 min. The use of cotton swabs to clean the ears should be strongly discouraged,[14] because injury to the TM or ear canal can result.

PHARYNGITIS

Pharyngitis, infection of the pharynx and the tonsils, is a very common pediatric problem. Despite physicians' longstanding familiarity with pharyngitis, there remains wide variability in approach. Controversies and new developments pertain to (1) selection of patients for throat culture and antibiotic treatment, (2) use of rapid diagnostic tests for group A β-hemolytic *Streptococcus* (GABHS), (3) increased incidence of serious systemic streptococcal disease, and (4) occurrence of bacteriologic and clinical failure with penicillin treatment of GABHS.

Non-Streptococcal Pharyngitis

ETIOLOGY   Most cases of acute pharyngitis in children are caused by viral infections. Examples include adenovirus, Epstein-Barr virus (EBV; see below), influenza virus, parainfluenza virus, rhinovirus, herpes simplex virus, and enterovirus. Although many of these viruses cause symptoms in addition to sore throat and fever, such as cough, coryza, conjunctivitis, or mucosal ulcerations, some viral infections can be clinically difficult to distinguish from GABHS.

Mycoplasma and *Chlamydia* have been suggested as uncommon causes of pharyngitis in adults and adolescents; however, neither organism appears to be an important cause of pharyngitis in children.[15] Many organisms, viral, bacterial, fungal, and even protozoal, have been associated with pharyngitis; however, only a relatively few are of practical significance to the emergency evaluation of pharyngitis in the immunocompetent child. Recent studies have suggested that *Arcanobacterium haemoliticum* (formerly *Corynebacterium haemoliticum*) might be a cause of non-GABHS tonsillopharyngitis with or without a scarlatiniform rash. Erythromycin is the treatment of choice when this organism is identified.[15] Among bacterial pathogens, GABHS is clearly the most important, accounting for 15 to 30 percent of all pharyngeal infections in school-age children. GABHS pharyngitis is unusual in children younger than 3 years, and rheumatic fever is rare in this age group.[16]

DIAGNOSIS AND TREATMENT   The few non-GABHS organisms that occasionally require specific diagnosis are *Corynebacterium diphtheriae, Neisseria gonorrhoeae,* EBV, and human immunodeficiency virus (HIV) type 1. Despite the many etiologic possibilities, in school-age children the diagnostic task is most often reduced to distinguishing GABHS, which requires specific antibiotic therapy, from non-streptococcal pharyngitis.

Diphtheria is a rare but serious cause of pharyngitis in developed countries. Immunization in infancy has been effective in nearly eliminating diphtheria in childhood, but it can occur in crowded conditions where there are socioeconomic barriers to immunization. Morbidity occurs because of infectious and toxic reactions. Infectious invasion and spread occur with enough tissue necrosis to produce a pseudomembrane that can progress to cause airway obstruction. The *C. diphtheriae* bacteria also produce an exotoxin that can cause widespread organ damage, including myocarditis and cardiac dysrhythmia, neuritis with bulbar and peripheral paralysis, nephritis, and hepatitis. Diagnosis must be clinical to expedite effective therapy; however, the bacteria can be grown on Loeffler medium. Treatment is directed at killing the bacteria and neutralizing the exotoxin. Therefore, antibiotic (penicillin or erythromycin) and horse serum antitoxin must be given.

Neisseria gonorrhoeae is an infrequent but important cause of pharyngitis in sexually active adolescents. Gonococcal pharyngitis in younger children strongly suggests child sexual abuse. Gonococcal pharyngitis may be asymptomatic or cause very mild symptoms with occasional exudative tonsillitis and/or cervical lymphadenopathy. Pharyngeal throat swabs should be plated on Thayer-Martin medium to recover the organism. Rectal and vaginal or urethral cultures and serum to test for syphilis and hepatitis B should be obtained whenever gonorrhea is suspected or documented. Gonococcal pharyngitis in children and adolescents should be treated with ceftriaxone (125 mg IM once). Children who cannot tolerate ceftriaxone may be treated with a 5-day regimen of TMP/SMX. Children 9 years or older also should receive oral doxycycline (100 mg twice daily for 7 days) for presumptive *Chlamydia* infection. Children 8 years or younger should receive erythromycin, 40 mg/kg per d in divided doses. Azithromycin (20 mg/kg, 1 g maximum) PO in a single dose is an alternative treatment for *Chlamydia* in all age groups.[17]

Epstein-Barr virus is a herpesvirus that is a common cause of infection in childhood and adolescence. Although EBV has been associated with a variety of clinical syndromes, most children infected with

EBV are asymptomatic or have only mild, nonspecific symptoms. Epstein-Barr virus can cause isolated tonsillopharyngitis and pharyngitis as a manifestation of infectious mononucleosis (IM). Clinically, the classic IM syndrome begins with malaise, fatigue, and sore throat. Fever and adenopathy are the most common signs. Splenomegaly and hepatomegaly are also present in the majority of infected children, whereas skin rash, enanthem, eyelid edema, and jaundice occur much less commonly. Pharyngitis occurs in nearly all children with IM. The appearance of the throat can resemble that of bacterial GABHS disease. Dual infection with EBV and GABHS has been documented. Classic IM is much less common in children younger than 2 years, when EBV tends to cause a nonspecific febrile illness. However, IM has been reported recently to occur in toddlers more commonly than was once thought. These younger children most often have a syndrome characterized by fever, tonsillitis, lymphadenopathy, and hepatosplenomegaly.

The laboratory can be helpful in establishing the diagnosis of IM. There is an increase in the proportion and the absolute number of atypical lymphocytes in the peripheral blood smear (generally ≥50 percent lymphocytes and ≥10 percent atypical lymphocytes). Liver transaminase levels show moderate elevation (in general, aspartate aminotransferase < 600 U/dL). The heterophil antibody is present (and can be demonstrated by rapid slide test methods) in more than 90 percent of children older than 5 years with IM but in only 75 percent between the ages of 2 and 4 years, and in fewer than 30 percent younger than 2 years. Serologic testing specific for EBV can provide information as to the likelihood of acute, postacute, old quiescent, and reactivation-type infections. These determinations are made on the basis of the presence of specific patterns of IgM and IgG responses to viral capsid antigen and IgG responses to EBV early antigen and the EBV nuclear antigen.

Infectious mononucleosis is generally a benign, self-limited, but somewhat prolonged illness. In general, treatment involves nonspecific supportive modalities (fluids, acetaminophen, and rest). Fatal complications are rare. Death can be caused by neurologic complications (e.g., meningoencephalitis or Guillain-Barré syndrome), splenic rupture and hemorrhage, and bacterial and fungal sepsis. Immunocompromised children may have unusual susceptibility to fulminant EBV infection. Airway obstruction secondary to tonsillar hypertrophy also can occur. This complication responds rapidly to glucocorticoid administration (dexamethasone, 1 to 10 mg/kg maximum and then 0.5 mg/kg every 6 h) and rarely requires intubation. Airway obstruction is the only complication for which the use of steroids is widely accepted.

Human immunodeficiency virus type 1 is a recently recognized cause of acute pharyngitis.[15] Primary retroviral infection can produce an IM-like illness with fever, sore throat, and lymphadenopathy that can last for a few days or a few weeks. Findings such as gastrointestinal symptoms or mucocutaneous lesions occur more commonly with acute HIV infection and are very unusual with IM caused by EBV. Primary HIV infections should be considered in high-risk populations.

Streptococcal Pharyngitis

Pharyngitis caused by GABHS is the most common treatable cause of pharyngitis in children. The peak months of infection are January to May, but, because of the high frequency of occurrence in school-age children, the beginning of school in the fall is also associated with GABHS pharyngitis in many areas. The peak ages are 4 to 11 years, with GABHS infection being uncommon before age 3 years.

DIAGNOSIS   No set of symptoms or signs is completely specific for GABHS (Table 121-5). Nonetheless, there are findings that are typically, but not exclusively, associated with GABHS. In general, the infected child experiences sudden onset of sore throat and fever. The tonsils and pharynx appear markedly red and have a moderate to large amount of exudate. The soft palate and uvula are also red and may have petechiae. The anterior cervical lymph nodes are enlarged and

TABLE 121-5   Characteristic Signs of Streptococcal Pharyngitis

Erythema of tonsils and pharynx
Exudate of tonsils and pharynx
Erythema and edema of uvula
Petechiae of the soft palate
Enlarged, tender anterior cervical lymph nodes
Scarlatiniform rash

tender. The presence of a scarlatiniform rash and pharyngitis is virtually diagnostic of GABHS. Headache, vomiting, abdominal pain, meningismus, and torticollis also can occur. These are of little diagnostic importance but must be recognized as possibly attributable to GABHS. The presence of significant coughing, rhinorrhea, or ulcerations suggest an alternative diagnosis.

There is general agreement that clinical diagnosis alone would result in an unacceptably high rate of misdiagnosis.

The mainstay of laboratory diagnosis is still the throat culture, although rapid antigen-detection techniques are gaining popularity in pediatric offices and EDs. The tonsil or posterior pharyngeal wall should be swabbed vigorously. In many centers, the swab is sent to the laboratory in appropriate culture medium for further handling. The sample is plated on a blood agar culture medium with neomycin and nalidixic acid added. Colonies that show β-hemolysis are identified as group A by bacitracin disk tests, fluorescent antibody staining, or latex agglutination. The rate of false-negative results from single throat culture is about 10 percent. Recovery rates are maximized by good swabbing technique, multiple cultures (rarely actually performed), and incubation in a carbon dioxide-enriched environment. Positive cultures may indicate an acute GABHS infection or the carrier state. Rates of GABHS carriage change with the season but have been reported to be as high as 15 percent. There is imperfect correlation between the amount of growth (generally reported on a scale of 1+ to 4+) and the likelihood of true infection. Chronic carriers of GABHS are not at increased risk for developing true GABHS pharyngitis or suppurative and nonsuppurative (e.g., rheumatic fever and nephritis) sequelae, nor do they pose an increased risk for disease transmission.

Incubation of throat cultures takes 24 to 48 h, during which time management must occur with uncertainty as to the diagnosis. Antigen-detection procedures are often available in EDs and practitioners' offices. The tests involve extraction of group A carbohydrate antigen from a throat swab and then combining the antigen with a latex agglutination, coagglutination, or enzyme-linked immunosorbent assay. More recently, a chemiluminescent DNA probe test and optical immunoassay have become commercially available. The nonculture tests take 10 to 30 min to perform and are generally more expensive per test than direct plate culturing. Sensitivity under controlled laboratory conditions when using the culture as the gold standard ranges from 85 to 90 percent, and specificity ranges from 98 to 100 percent. Unfortunately, when measured in the field under less well-controlled circumstances, sensitivity of the latex agglutination test has been as low as 50 percent.[18] In other words, the false-positive rate is low, but the false-negative rate may be unacceptably high. The newer optical immunoassay tests are nearly as sensitive as blood agar plate culture and more sensitive than other rapid tests for GABHS; however sensitivities for these tests have varied from 79 to 95 percent when performed in office or ED settings.[18,19] Any ED or office planning to use a rapid diagnostic test must assess the performance of the test on site. A safe and commonly used approach is to obtain swabs for throat culture and rapid test simultaneously. Children with positive rapid test results are treated for GABHS. If the results are negative, the throat culture is processed and the children are managed according to an acceptable strategy while awaiting throat culture results. An important role of the rapid tests is to decrease the indiscriminate use of antibiotics in children with sore throats, most of whom do not have streptococcal pharyngitis.

TREATMENT The objectives of treatment for GABHS are (1) to prevent rheumatic fever, (2) to prevent suppurative complications (e.g., peritonsillar abscess and cellulitis, suppurative cervical lymphadenitis, and retropharyngeal abscess), and (3) to hasten clinical recovery. Group A β-hemolytic *Streptococcus* is highly sensitive to penicillin, and there has been no evidence of development of resistance in vitro despite decades of use. A single dose of intramuscular penicillin G benzathine (600,000 units if the patient weighs 27 kg or less, and 1.2 million units if the patient weighs more than 27 kg) is effective but causes significant local discomfort in more than 50 percent of recipients. A preparation containing penicillin G benzathine, 900,000 units, and penicillin G procaine, 300,000 units (CR Bicillin 900/300, introduced in 1976), is effective for children who weigh 64 kg or less and significantly reduces the magnitude and frequency of local reactions. Oral penicillin V is a popular alternative. A regimen of 250 to 500 mg two times daily for 10 days effectively eradicates infection and prevents rheumatic fever.[16,20] Amoxicillin suspension (at the same dosage as penicillin) is a more palatable alternative for children unable to swallow pills. Variable levels of compliance have been reported. Improvements in compliance can be achieved with careful parent education at the time of discharge. If compliance or follow-up are problematic, the intramuscular route should be used. Alternatives to penicillin for children with penicillin allergy include erythromycin or cephalosporins (Table 121-6). Treatment with antimicrobials, such as azithromycin, cefuroxime, cefdinir, cefixime, and cefpodoxime, for 5 days has been reported to eradicate *Streptococcus* as effectively as the traditional 10-day courses; however, the cost of medication and the effects on antimicrobial resistance also must be considered.[21]

Research also has clearly demonstrated the beneficial effects of early antibiotic therapy on reduction of signs and symptoms of GABHS pharyngitis.[15] In addition, because it is recommended that children with GABHS receive antibiotics for 24 h before returning to school or day care, early treatment benefits the children and their parents, especially parents who work outside the home. Based on these considerations, many strategies for testing and treatment have been proposed, ranging from treating all children with pharyngitis with antibiotics to withholding antibiotics from all pending culture results. Cost-effectiveness studies employing decision-analysis methods have compared some of these strategies.[22,23] The best strategy for a given institution depends on the local prevalence of GABHS, the availability and accuracy of rapid antigen testing, and the ability to follow up successfully in untreated children found to have positive culture results. A widely accepted strategy that incorporates the latest technology is to perform rapid antigen testing on all children with pharyngitis and to treat all with positive results. In addition, children with classic clinical findings or a scarlatiniform rash should be treated regardless of the result of rapid testing. Those with a negative rapid test result and equivocal or atypical clinical features for GABHS should have a throat culture performed, but treatment may be withheld pending culture results. Positive culture results indicate the need for treatment. It is not necessary to reculture to test for eradication of GABHS in asymptomatic children. Children with recurrent or persistent symptoms and those with previously documented rheumatic fever do require reculturing. Children with persistent positive culture results in this context can be treated with a different antibiotic such as amoxicillin-clavulanate, a cephalosporin, or clindamycin.[20] The asymptomatic carrier state need not be treated except in certain circumstances. These exceptions include a family history of rheumatic fever, an outbreak of rheumatic fever or glomerulonephritis, or multiple documented symptomatic episodes of streptococcal pharyngitis occurring within a family or closed community. Clindamycin, amoxicillin-clavulanate, or a combination of penicillin and rifampin have been shown to be effective in eradicating GABHS in carriers.[17]

COMPLICATIONS An increased number of apparent treatment failures with penicillin has been reported.[21] Group A β-hemolytic *Streptococcus* remains susceptible to penicillin in vitro. Alternative explanations for these findings may involve children who are carriers of GABHS and develop a viral pharyngitis, patients who reacquire the organism from a family member or another close contact, or patients who are noncompliant with the prescribed penicillin. Other proposed mechanisms include development of GABHS penicillin tolerance and the production of β-lactamase from other normal pharyngeal flora. The evidence does not support the diminished efficacy of penicillin therapy for GABHS pharyngitis. Reports of the proposed therapeutic failures have prompted many recent studies comparing the efficacy of penicillin with that of other antibiotics. In general, penicillin remains the recommended antibiotic of choice based on past experience, cost, and historically successful prevention of rheumatic fever.[16,20,21]

The overall incidence of rheumatic fever has been declining in the developed countries and is now less than 1 per 100,000 in the continental United States. A number of scattered outbreaks of acute rheumatic fever were reported in the United States during the latter part of the 1980s. There is ample justification for adherence to the American Heart Association's recommendations that one of the above-mentioned antibiotic regimens for documented GABHS pharyngitis must be provided. Antibiotic treatment begun within 9 days of the onset of infection is effective in preventing rheumatic fever.

Post-streptococcal glomerulonephritis is a nonsuppurative complication of GABHS disease that is not preventable with antibiotic therapy. Its occurrence is related to infection with nephritogenic strains of streptococci.

Indications for tonsillectomy remain uncertain and controversial. For children with many recurrent episodes of pharyngitis, tonsillectomy reduces the incidence of pharyngitis. The decision regarding tonsillectomy for such children should be individualized to account for various considerations of risks, benefits, and quality of life, including the quality of available anesthetic and surgical services, impact of recurrent illness versus surgery on the child and parents, school performance, and comparative costs to the family.

Recent outbreaks of pharyngitis caused by group G and C streptococci have been reported, often associated with contaminated food sources.[15] Although the acute clinical syndromes associated with these organisms are identical to those of GABHS pharyngitis, they are unlikely to cause preventable nonsuppurative sequelae. However, rare cases of acute glomerulonephritis after infection with group G *Streptococci* have been described.

A recent resurgence of invasive GABHS infections has been noted.[22] Serious illnesses include septicemia, toxic shock-like syndrome, pneumonia, cellulitis, lymphangitis, and necrotizing fasciitis.

TABLE 121-6 Antibiotic Choices for Group A Streptococcal Infections

Drugs	Dosage
Penicillin V*	250–500 mg bid PO for 10 d
Amoxicillin†	250–500 mg bid PO for 10 d
CR Bicillin 900/300‡	1.2 million units, IM, single dose
Benzathine penicillin G#	1.2 million units, IM, single dose
If allergic to penicillin§	
Erythromycin ethyl succinate	40 mg/kg per d PO bid for 10 d
Azithromycin	12 mg/kg per d for 5 d

*250 mg for children, 500 mg for adolescents and adults.
†Amoxicillin suspension is a better tasting alternative if the child is unable to swallow pills.
‡For patients ≤64 kg (140 lb).
#For patients >64 kg (140 lb).
§Cephalosporins also may be considered for penicillin-allergic patients.
Sources: Bisno AL: Acute pharyngitis. *New Engl J Med* 344:205, 2001; Dajani A, Taubert K, Ferrieri P, et al: Treatment of acute streptococcal pharyngitis and prevention of rheumatic fever: A statement of health professional. *Pediatrics* 96:758, 1995.

Such systemic infections may produce an extraordinarily virulent syndrome progressing rapidly to shock and death. Data suggest an appearance of new serotypes of GABHS but also an increased strain-associated virulence, rather than virulence related to a given serotype. The pathogenetic mechanism by which these virulent strains produce severe disease is not well understood.

Symptomatic therapy for GABHS and non-streptococcal pharyngitis includes acetaminophen for analgesia. A throat spray (e.g., Chloraseptic) can be used before meals and bedtime, if further analgesia is required. Lozenges should be avoided in children younger than 5 years because of the possibility of aspiration.

REFERENCES

1. McCracken GH Jr: Diagnosis and management of acute otitis media in the urgent care setting. *Ann Emerg Med* 39:413, 2002.
2. Daly KA, Giebink GS: Clinical epidemiology of otitis media. *Pediatr Infect Dis J* 19:S31, 2000.
3. Dowell SF, Marcy SM, Phillips WR, et al: Otitis media—Principles of judicious use of antimicrobial agents. *Pediatrics* 101:165, 1998.
4. Dowell SF, Butler JC, Giebink GS, et al: Acute otitis media: Management and surveillance in an era of pneumococcal resistance—a report from the drug-resistant *Streptococcus pneumoniae* therapeutic working group. *Pediatr Infect Dis J* 18:1, 1999.
5. Bluestone CD, Klein JO: *Otitis Media in Infants and Children,* 3rd ed. Philadelphia, WB Saunders, 2001.
6. Hoberman A, Paradise JL: Acute otitis media: Diagnosis and management in the year 2000. *Pediatr Ann* 29:609, 2000.
7. Klein JO, McCracken GH Jr: Summary: Role of a new oral cephalosporin, cefdinir, for therapy of infections in infants and children. *Pediatr Infect Dis J* 19:S181, 2000.
8. Kozyrskyj AL, Hildes-Ripstein GE, Longstaffe SEA, et al: Treatment of acute otitis media with a shortened course of antibiotics. *JAMA* 279:1736, 1998.
9. Pichichero ME: Recurrent and persistent otitis media. *Pediatr Infect Dis J* 19:911, 2000.
10. Bluestone CD: Efficacy of ofloxacin and other ototopical preparations for chronic suppurative otitis media in children. *Pediatr Infect Dis J* 20:111, 2001.
11. Bluestone CD: Clinical course, complications and sequelae of acute otitis media. *Pediatr Infect Dis J* 19:S37, 2000.
12. Black S, Shinefield H: Vaccines and otitis media. *Pediatr Ann* 29:648, 2000.
13. Stool SE, Berg AO: *Clinical Practice Guideline: Otitis Media with Effusion in Young Children.* Publication 94-0622. Rockville, MD, Agency for Health Care Policy and Research, 1994.
14. Hughes E, Lee JH: Otitis externa. *Pediatr Rev* 22:191, 2001.
15. Bisno AL: Acute pharyngitis. *New Engl J Med* 344:205, 2001.
16. Dajani A, Taubert K, Ferrieri P, et al: Treatment of acute streptococcal pharyngitis and prevention of rheumatic fever: A statement for health professionals. *Pediatrics* 96:758, 1995.
17. Peter G (ed): *American Academy of Pediatrics: 2000 Red Book: Report of the Committee on Infectious Diseases,* 25th ed. Elk Grove Village, IL, American Academy of Pediatrics, 2000.
18. Corneli HM: Rapid strep tests in the emergency department: An evidence based approach. *Pediatr Emerg Care* 17:272, 2001.
19. Gerber MA, Tanz RR, Kabat W, et al: Optical immunoassay test for group A beta-hemolytic streptococcal pharyngitis: An office-based, multicenter investigation. *JAMA* 277:899, 1997.
20. Bisno AL, Gerber MA, Gwaltney JM, et al: Diagnosis and management of group A streptococcal pharyngitis: A practice guideline. *Clin Infect Dis* 25:574, 1997.
21. Pichichero ME, Casey JR, Mayes T, et al.: Penicillin failure in streptococcal tonsillopharyngitis: Causes and remedies. *Pediatr Infect Dis J* 19:917, 2000.
22. Kaplan EL: Recent epidemiology of group A streptococcal infections in North America and abroad: An overview. *Pediatrics* 97(suppl):945, 1996.
23. Webb KH: Does culture confirmation of high-sensitivity rapid streptococcal tests make sense? A medical decision analysis. *Pediatrics* 101:e2, 1998.

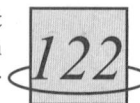

SKIN AND SOFT TISSUE INFECTIONS
Richard Malley

This chapter discusses several of the more common skin and soft tissue infections of childhood, including conjunctivitis, impetigo, sinusitis, and cellulitis. Because of its particular severity, orbital/periorbital cellulitis is highlighted in a section separate from the general discussion of cellulitis; however, the pathophysiology and clinical manifestations that are shared are not repeated.

CONJUNCTIVITIS

Definition

Conjunctivitis is an inflammation of the conjunctivae, the membranes that line the surface of the eye. This inflammation may be the result of infection, allergy, or mechanical or chemical irritation. Keratoconjunctivitis involves the cornea as well as the conjunctivae.

Etiology

The etiology of infectious conjunctivitis differs between the newborn and the older child (Table 122-1). In the newborn, pathogens that reside in the birth canal play a major role in ocular infections. *Chlamydia trachomatis* is the most frequent, but *Neisseria gonorrhoeae* poses the greatest threat to the integrity of the eye. Later in childhood, the respiratory tract pathogens predominate, particularly *Haemophilus* species. Trachoma, a recurrent chlamydial conjunctivitis seen in tropical regions, is not discussed.

Epidemiology

Conjunctivitis is the most common ocular infection of childhood. It may occur at any age. Neonates acquire most infections during passage through colonized birth canals; in older children, respiratory tract pathogens spread from person to person. Conjunctivitis is usually a sporadic disease, but epidemics of viral illness may occur.

Pathophysiology

Pathogens introduced into the conjunctival sac may proliferate and produce hyperemia and an inflammatory exudate. This exudate may be purulent, fibrinous, or serosanguineous. With certain organisms, corneal involvement (keratitis) also may occur.

TABLE 122-1 Etiology of Infectious Conjunctivitis

Frequency	Neonate	Child
Very frequent	*Chlamydia trachomatis*	Adenoviruses *Hemophilus* species
Moderately frequent	*Streptococcus pneumoniae* *Enterococcus faecalis* or *faecium* *Neisseria gonorrhoeae*	*Streptococcus pneumoniae*
Infrequent	*Hemophilus influenzae* Herpes simplex *Staphylococcus aureus*	*Neisseria gonorrhoeae* *Neisseria meningitidis* *Chlamydia trachomatis* Herpes simplex *Staphylococcus aureus* *Corynebacterium diphtheriae*

Clinical Features

Older children with conjunctivitis may complain of photophobia, ocular pain or pruritus, a sensation of a foreign body in the eye, crusting of the eyelids, or conjunctival erythema. Infants and young children are usually brought by their parents for "pink eye" or crusting. The duration of symptoms with infectious conjunctivitis is most often 2 to 4 days but may be longer in cases which are untreated or resistant to therapy.

As with any ocular complaint, the physician should perform a thorough examination of the structure and function of both eyes, including, when age appropriate, examination of visual acuity, visual fields by confrontation, extraocular muscle function, periorbital area, eyelids (with eversion), conjunctivae, cornea with fluorescein staining, pupillary reflex, anterior chamber, and fundus. Erythema and increased secretions characterize conjunctivitis. Chemosis may be seen. Intense erythema and purulent discharge are more common with an infectious rather than an allergic cause. The cornea does not stain with fluorescein in children with conjunctivitis unless an associated keratitis has developed, as with herpes simplex or adenoviruses. Most importantly, visual acuity is normal.

Fever and other systemic symptoms do not occur with isolated conjunctivitis. However, conjunctivitis may be only one manifestation of a viral upper respiratory tract infection, in which case the temperature may be elevated. Conjunctivitis may be only one manifestation of a systemic disorder, such as measles and Kawasaki disease.

Diagnosis

The diagnosis is primarily clinical. A Gram stain, which should be performed in neonates or in confusing cases, usually shows more than 5 white blood cells per oil immersion field and, in many cases, bacteria. The finding of gram-negative intracellular diplococci presumptively identifies *N. gonorrhoeae* in the first few weeks of life. Conjunctival scrapings and/or cultures may be performed in selected circumstances to diagnose *C. trachomatis* or specific viral and bacterial pathogens.

Once the diagnosis of conjunctivitis is established on the basis of diffuse injection, purulent discharge, and normal vision, infectious and noninfectious causes are next separated. *Allergic conjunctivitis* is usually distinguished by chronicity, seasonality, pruritus, and associated symptoms of allergic rhinitis; if the physician is uncertain, a Gram stain should be done (Table 122-2).

Differential Diagnosis

The differential diagnosis of the "red (or pink) eye" includes conjunctivitis, orbital/periorbital infection, foreign body, corneal abrasion, uveitis, and glaucoma. Periorbital and orbital infections cause obvious swelling and tenderness around the eye and/or loss of ocular mobility.

TABLE 122-2   Differential Diagnosis of Allergic and Infectious Conjunctivitis

	Allergic	Infectious
History		
Pruritus	Yes	No
Chronic	Yes	No
Recurrent	Yes	No
Seasonal	Yes	No
Sneezing, rhinorrhea	Yes	Variable
Examination		
Discharge	Watery	Watery or purulent
Chemosis	Present	Usually absent
Fluorescein	Negative	Negative, except keratitis
Laboratory tests		
Gram stain	Negative	White cells, bacteria

Foreign bodies should be visible on direct examination, often only following eversion of the upper eyelid. Thus the differential diagnosis usually revolves around four conditions: conjunctivitis, corneal abrasion, uveitis, and glaucoma (Table 122-3). Both uveitis and glaucoma are uncommon. The erythema in these conditions is concentrated around the limbus, and the discharge consists primarily of tears. Additionally, the vision is decreased in glaucoma, and the cornea may be cloudy. A corneal abrasion is easily identified by the uptake of fluorescein.

Complications

Conjunctivitis is generally self-limited, with the notable exceptions of herpes simplex and *N. gonorrhoeae*. The potential complications are corneal ulceration and scar formation leading to visual impairment.

Treatment

In approaching infectious conjunctivitis (Figure 122-1), the physician must decide whether the ocular disorder is one manifestation of a systemic illness such as measles, or is occurring in relative isolation. Isolated conjunctivitis may be caused by various viruses and bacteria, of which herpes simplex and *N. gonorrhoeae* are particularly severe, or by *C. trachomatis*, especially in the first 3 months of life.

Fluorescein staining always should be performed in an effort to identify the dendritic corneal ulcerations characteristic of herpetic disease. If they are identified, treatment is with acyclovir or other antiviral agents under the supervision of an ophthalmologist. Because *N. gonorrhoeae* is usually acquired during passage through the birth canal, infants younger than 1 month of age must always be tested for this pathogen with a Gram stain and culture. If gram-negative intracellular diplococci are seen on smear, a single intramuscular injection of ceftriaxone (125 mg) is indicated.

Infants older than 1 month of age and older children with an obvious clinical diagnosis of conjunctivitis do not routinely require smears or cultures. In patients younger than 3 months of age, treatment is instituted with erythromycin (50 mg/kg per d) PO for *C. trachomatis* (Table 122-4). Older children require only topical antibiotic instillation into the conjunctival sac. A child who has unusually severe disease or who fails to respond to therapy within 48 h may benefit from a laboratory investigation. Appropriate studies in the infant younger than 1 month of age includes a Gram stain and bacterial culture and either a scraping or culture for *C. trachomatis*. Older children require only a Gram stain and bacterial culture. Diagnostic tests for herpes simplex are not usually rewarding in the absence of corneal ulceration; culture for adenoviruses may be helpful in persistent or severe hemorrhagic infections to avoid unnecessary additional testing, but there is no specific treatment. All children with conjunctivitis should be reevaluated within 48 h. Failure to improve warrants further investigation and continued, careful follow-up.

IMPETIGO

Impetigo is a superficial bacterial infection of the skin confined to the epidermis. Deeper spread to the dermis leads to ecthyma. There are two varieties of impetigo: impetigo contagiosa and bullous impetigo.[1]

Impetigo is the most common skin infection seen in the pediatric ED. The prevalence is greatest in children younger than age 6 years. Impetigo may be sporadic or epidemic. Conditions favoring epidemic spread include warm weather, overcrowding, and poor hygiene. Bullous impetigo is less common than impetigo contagiosa.

Pathophysiology

Group A β-hemolytic streptococcus (GABHS) or *Staphylococcus aureus* often are the primary infecting agents and therapy should cover

TABLE 122-3   Differential Diagnosis of the "Red Eye"

	Conjunctivitis	Corneal Abrasion	Uveitis	Glaucoma
History	URI	Trauma, contact lens	JRA, sarcoid, trauma	Prematurity, Marfan syndrome, homocystinuria
Visual acuity	Normal	Normal or decreased	Normal or decreased	Decreased
Ocular examination				
External	Watery or purulent discharge	Watery discharge	Watery discharge	Watery discharge
Cornea	Usually normal; staining if keratitis	Staining	Normal or band keratopathy	Cloudy, staining
Anterior chamber	Normal	Normal	Cells, hypopyon, hyphema	Normal or shallow
Pupil	Normal	Normal	Small	Fixed
Intraocular pressure	Normal	Normal	Variable	Increased

Abbreviations: JRA = juvenile rheumatoid arthritis; URI = upper respiratory infection.

both organisms. In particular, in bullous impetigo, the primary pathogen is *S. aureus.*[1]

The intact epidermis forms a relatively impervious barrier to bacteria. The development of impetigo follows a breach in the integument; this may be an obvious abrasion or an inconspicuous insect bite. Bacteria then invade the skin and elaborate toxins, such as streptolysins, which promote local spread.

Clinical Features

The chief complaint of children with impetigo is most often that of sores on the body. There are no associated systemic manifestations such as fever or malaise. Regional lymph nodes may be minimally enlarged.

The typical lesion of impetigo contagiosa begins as an erythematous papule. Small vesicles may follow transiently, but rapid progression to crusted lesions occurs. These crusts, which are initially honey-colored and fine in consistency, may appear on any area of the body; between the upper lip and the nose is a very characteristic site. The lesions enlarge over days to weeks, and the crusts become thicker. Erythema is mild. No induration is present.

In bullous impetigo, the characteristic skin lesions are superficial bullae filled with purulent material. The bullae range in size from 0.5 to 3 cm and have minimal, if any, surrounding erythema.

The diagnosis of impetigo is clinical, and laboratory tests are not needed. Where the diagnosis is uncertain, Gram stain of the lesions is

helpful, showing abundant polymorphonuclear leukocytes and gram-positive bacteria. Local culture may be obtained from patients whose disease does not respond to standard therapy.

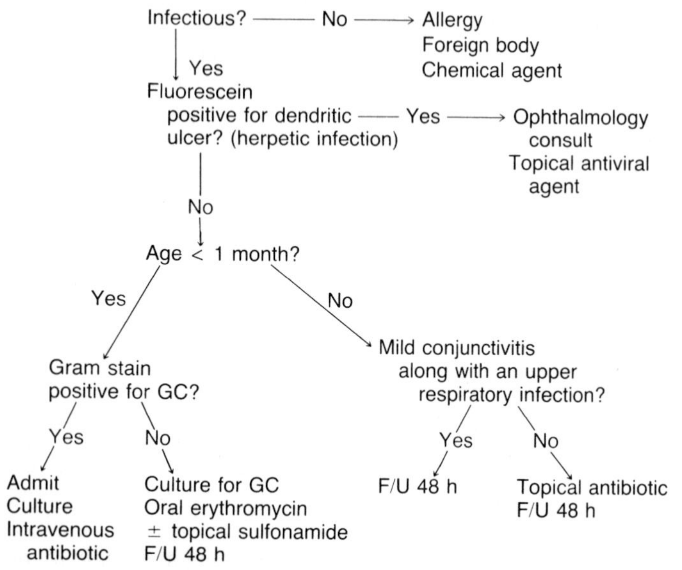

Several dermatologic disorders may resemble either impetigo contagiosa or bullous impetigo. These include tinea corporis, nummular eczema, small burns or abrasions, allergic contact dermatitis, eczema herpeticum (with underlying atopic dermatitis), and scalded skin syndrome.

Impetigo may spread locally or, in the case of streptococcal infections, lead to remote, nonsuppurative sequelae. Occasionally, impetigo may progress to cellulitis or lead to lymphadenitis in the regional nodes. The attack rate for acute poststreptococcal glomerulonephritis has been as high as 1 percent in certain epidemics; however, the disease is unusual following sporadic skin infections.

Treatment

The treatment of impetigo is oral antibiotic therapy or an appropriate topical antibiotic for limited eruptions. A first-generation oral cephalosporin such as cephalexin (50 mg/kg per d) provides effective oral therapy. Mupirocin is the only topical agent with proven efficacy. Combination topical and systemic therapy is unnecessary. Vigorous scrubbing, in addition to topical or systemic antibiotic agents, offers no advantage; routine cleanliness is sufficient.

Antibiotic therapy hastens the resolution of impetigo and limits suppurative complications. Although the incidence of glomerulonephritis may be reduced, it has not been possible to demonstrate this effect with certainty in clinical studies because of the low incidence of this disease.

FIG. 122-1. Approach to the child with an isolated, infectious conjunctivitis. F/U = follow-up; GC = gonorrhea culture.

TABLE 122-4   Treatment of Conjunctivitis by Pathogen

Viruses	
Herpes simplex	Trifluridine, vidarabine, or acyclovir, topically (neonates may also have systemic infection)
Other	Supportive
Chlamydia	
Chlamydia trachomatis	Erythromycin, 50 mg/kg per d PO, for 14 d
Bacteria	
Neisseria gonorrhoeae	Child: ceftriaxone 125 mg IM or IV Adult: ceftriaxone 250 mg IM or IV
Neisseria meningitidis	Child: penicillin, 50,000 units/kg per d, IV, for 7 d Adult: penicillin, 10 million units per d, IV, for 5 d
Hemophilus influenzae, *Streptococcus pneumoniae,* and others	Topical antibiotic ointments: sulfonamide erythromycin, etc.

SINUSITIS

Sinusitis is an inflammation of the paranasal sinuses: maxillary, ethmoid, frontal, or sphenoid. This inflammation may be on the basis of infection or allergy; it may be acute, subacute, or chronic.

The major pathogens in acute bacterial sinusitis in childhood are *Streptococcus pneumoniae, Moraxella catarrhalis,* and nontypeable *Haemophilus influenzae.*[2] The incidence of *H. influenzae* type B (Hib) sinusitis in children has likely declined with Hib vaccination, but other nontypeable *H. influenzae* are still important causative pathogens. Other potential etiologic agents found in a minority of infections include group A streptococcus, group C streptococcus, β-hemolytic streptococcus, and *Peptostreptococcus.* Similar clinical investigations in adults have been in general agreement, finding nontypeable *H. influenzae* and *S. pneumoniae* in 60 to 70 percent of the cases. Although *S. aureus* and anaerobic organisms are isolated occasionally, they rarely play a role in acute infections in childhood. Severe sinusitis is not a common illness in children, but mild or subacute disease may occur more frequently.

Pathophysiology

The ethmoid and maxillary sinuses are present at birth, but the frontal and sphenoid sinuses do not become aerated until 6 or 7 years of age. The sinuses are lined primarily by ciliated columnar epithelium and connect with the nasopharynx via narrow ostia. Normally, the epithelium is coated by a double layer of mucus: a viscid gel layer superficially and a more fluid layer underneath. Resistance to infection depends on the patency of the ostia, the function of the ciliary mechanism, and the quality of the secretions.

Obstruction of the ostia results either from mucosal swelling or, less commonly, mechanical obstruction. By far the most frequent offenders are viral upper respiratory infection and allergic inflammation. Less-common causes include cystic fibrosis, trauma, choanal atresia, deviated septum, polyps, foreign body, and tumor.

Factors that impair normal mucociliary function include viral infections, cold or dry air, certain chemicals or drugs, and, rarely, inborn errors of motility. Alterations of the mucus occur in asthma and cystic fibrosis.

The bacteria that cause sinusitis often colonize the nasopharynx of healthy children. Disruptions in one or more of the barriers described above allow these organisms to ascend through the ostia and multiply within the sinuses.

Clinical Features

The spectrum of sinusitis has not been completely defined as it relates to clinical manifestations. However, there are two major types of infection, which can usually be distinguished on clinical grounds: acute, severe sinusitis, and mild, subacute sinusitis (Table 122-5).

Acute, severe infections of the sinuses are infrequent during childhood. Symptoms are headache and bilateral nasal mucopurulent discharge. Findings include fever, localized swelling and/or erythema, and facial tenderness.

The diagnosis of sinusitis in young children is usually made on clinical grounds without any laboratory or radiographic studies. In older children and adolescents, transillumination of the maxillary or frontal sinuses may provide assistance.

Standard radiographs or preferably CT if available, should be obtained in patients with an uncertain clinical diagnosis and in cases of severe sinusitis. The most diagnostic findings for purulence are an air-fluid level or complete opacification, although it is important to remember that certain sinuses (such as frontal) are not usually aerated in young children. Mucosal thickening greater than 4 mm is usually indicative of infection but may accompany viral upper respiratory disease, particularly in the first year of life. A normal radiograph suggests, but does not prove, that a sinus is free of disease.

TABLE 122-5 Severity of Signs and Symptoms in Children with Sinusitis

	Acute, Severe Disease	Mild, Subacute Disease
Headache	+++	++
Fever	+++	+
Facial tenderness	++	—
Facial swelling	++	—
Nasal discharge	+++	++++

Ultimate confirmation of infection within the paranasal sinuses rests with demonstration of organisms by Gram stain and quantitative culture of aspirated secretions. Aspiration is not routinely indicated but can be performed in selected cases of maxillary sinusitis by an otolaryngologist. Appropriate circumstances for aspiration include (1) life-threatening complications, (2) immunosuppressive conditions, (3) clinical unresponsiveness, and (4) unusually severe disease. The presence of organisms on Gram stain and a count of at least 104 colony-forming units point to bacterial infection.[3]

Differential Diagnosis

Nasal congestion lasting 3 to 7 days often accompanies viral upper respiratory infections, and should not be diagnosed as acute sinusitis and does not need treatment with antibiotics.

Other causes of facial swelling include superficial infection (cellulitis), trauma, cold injury, and allergic edema. Facial pain may be neurogenic, odontogenic, or related to the temporomandibular joint. Unilateral nasal discharge suggests a nasal foreign body.

Complications

The proximity of the paranasal sinuses to the brain sets the scene for the occurrence of life-threatening complications from sinusitis; however, the use of antibiotics has reduced the incidence of such complications. Infection may spread from the sinuses to surrounding structures through the diploic veins, which have no valves, or by erosion through bone.

The most commonly encountered complications are periorbital cellulitis and orbital cellulitis/abscess. Periorbital infection causes swelling around the eye, while intraorbital accumulation of pus may be recognized on the basis of proptosis and decreased ocular motion. Infection may also produce osteomyelitis of the surrounding bone; in the frontal region this is referred to as Pott puffy tumor. Less-common complications of intracranial extension are epidural, subdural, or brain abscess; meningitis; and cavernous sinus thrombosis. Meningitis rarely follows sinusitis; it more commonly occurs after bacteremia. Suspicion of an intracranial complication requires neuroimaging. Brain abscess and subdural empyema are demonstrated by contrast head CT scan, and cavernous sinus thrombosis or epidural empyema may only be visualized by magnetic resonance imaging (MRI).

Treatment

Sinusitis requires therapy with antibiotics (Table 122-6). Mild, subacute infections respond well to oral therapy for 10 to 14 days. Amoxicillin (80 mg/kg per d) remains the first-choice antimicrobial. Failure to improve with amoxicillin therapy suggests infection with pathogens that are often resistant to this drug, such as *M. catarrhalis* or *H. influenzae,* or perhaps with penicillin-resistant *S. pneumoniae.* A second course of treatment with newer oral second- and third-generation cephalosporins such as cefprozil or cefpodoxime, or amoxicillin-clavulanic acid should

TABLE 122-6 Antibiotic Therapy for Sinusitis

	Acute, Severe Sinusitis	Mild, Subacute Sinusitis
Initial	Ceftriaxone, 75 mg/kg per d IV *or* Ampicillin-sulbactam, 200 mg/kg of ampicillin per d IV	Amoxicillin, 80 mg/kg per d PO
Persistent	Antibiotics as above plus surgical drainage	Cefprozil, 30 mg/kg per d PO *or* Amoxicillin-Clavulanate 40 mg/kg per d PO
Penicillin allergic	Ceftriaxone, 75 mg/kg per d IV *or* Clindamycin, 40 mg/kg per d IV	Clindamycin, 10–30 mg/kg per d PO divided every 6–8 h

TABLE 122-7 Etiology of Cellulitis

	Most Likely	Less Likely
IMMUNOCOMPETENT HOST		
Trunk/extremity	S. aureus Streptococcus pyogenes	H. influenzae
Face (periorbital/ buccal); unimmunized	H. influenzae	S. aureus S. pneumoniae
Face (periorbital/ buccal); immunized	S. aureus S. pneumoniae	H. influenzae
Any site/animal bite	S. aureus	Pasteurella multocida
Any site/human bite	Anaerobic organisms	S. aureus
IMMUNOCOMPROMISED HOST		
Any site	S. aureus, gram-negative rods	Anaerobic organisms

then be instituted; aspiration for culture may be useful for those patients in whom the infection still persists after a second course of therapy.

Acute, severe sinusitis may result in life-threatening complications and requires intravenous antibiotic therapy directed at *S. pneumoniae* (possibly penicillin-resistant), amoxicillin-resistant *H. influenzae,* and, less commonly, *S. aureus.* Ceftriaxone (50 to 100 mg/kg per d) represents a single-drug regimen effective for this disease; ampicillin-sulbactam (200 mg/kg per d) is a good alternative for the nonallergic patient. Failure of severe disease to respond promptly to antibiotic therapy or the occurrence of complications indicates the need for surgical consultation in regard to drainage procedures.

CELLULITIS

Cellulitis is an infection of the skin and subcutaneous tissues. It extends below the dermis, differentiating it from impetigo, but does not involve muscle (pyogenic myositis) or bone (osteomyelitis). Any region of the body may be involved, but two divisions are important in regard to predicting the most likely pathogens: (1) the trunk and extremities and (2) the face (buccal and periorbital cellulitis).

Children of any age may develop cellulitis, but, as noted above, disease caused by *H. influenzae* has become rare, affecting mainly infants younger than age 6 months.

The organisms that play an important role in the immunocompetent host under normal circumstances include *S. aureus, S. pyogenes* (group A β-hemolytic streptococcus), and *H. influenzae* (Table 122-7). In general, *S. aureus* is the most common and *H. influenzae* the least common among the three major pathogens, particularly in children immunized against *H. influenzae* type B.[4] However, in certain anatomic locations, particularly for young or unimmunized children, *H. influenzae* remains an important consideration. Additionally, unusual organisms may cause cellulitis in immunocompromised hosts or following their introduction in special types of wounds (see Table 122-7).

Pathophysiology

Cellulitis may occur either when a pathogen is directly inoculated into the subcutaneous tissue or following an episode of bacteremia. The majority of infections involve local invasion after a breach in the integument. The organisms responsible are usually *S. aureus* and *S. pyogenes.* In contradistinction, *H. influenzae* type B disseminates hematogenously.

Clinical Features

The child with cellulitis manifests a local inflammatory response at the site of the infection, including erythema, edema, warmth, and tenderness. There may be a history of a preceding wound or a complaint related to loss of function, such as limp with an infection of a lower extremity. Fever is unusual except in infections caused by *H. influenzae* type B (Table 122-8).

Inspection of the area of cellulitis usually shows intense erythema. A violaceous hue suggests *H. influenzae,* but has been reported with other pathogens, including *S. pneumoniae.* Red streaks may radiate proximally along the course of the lymphatic drainage, and the regional nodes may enlarge.

The diagnosis of cellulitis is made by inspection. Laboratory studies including a WBC count, blood culture, and aspirate culture are obtained for specific indications: immunocompromise, fever, severe local infection, facial involvement, and failure to respond to therapy.

The WBC count is normal in most cases of infection caused by *S. aureus* or *S. pyogenes,* which are locally invasive. On the other hand, cellulitis caused by *H. influenzae* type B results from bacteremia and is usually accompanied by a WBC count >15,000/μL.

The blood culture is usually negative in infections caused by *S. aureus* and *S. pyogenes.* On the other hand, *H. influenzae* type B, as a rule, causes a bacteremic infection.

Aspirate cultures are best obtained close to the center of an infected lesion, as the periphery may consist primarily of edema fluid devoid of organisms. The needle should be sufficiently large to permit the evacuation of purulent material—22 gauge for the face and 19 gauge for the trunk and extremities. Using a 5- or 10-mL syringe prefilled with

TABLE 122-8 Usual Clinical and Laboratory Features of Children with Cellulitis

Characteristic	H. influenzae	S. aureus
Age	<3 years	Any
Fever	Yes	No
Color of lesion	Violaceous	Erythematous
Location	Cheek, periorbital	Trunk, extremity
Preceding wound	No	Yes
WBC count	>15,000/μL	<15,000/μL
Bacteremia	Yes	No

Abbreviation: WBC = white blood cell count.

1 mL of sterile, nonbacteriostatic saline, the needle is directed into the subcutaneous tissue to a depth of approximately 0.5 to 1.0 cm, and aspiration is attempted. If there is no return, the saline is injected and reaspirated. The material obtained is used for culture and Gram stain.

Differential Diagnosis

Cellulitis must be differentiated from other causes of erythema and edema, including trauma and allergic reaction. Allergic edema is not tender and usually only mildly erythematous. Traumatic lesions may be easily distinguished when there is a history of injury and absence of fever. Cold injury, especially on the cheeks ("popsicle panniculitis"), may be confused with cellulitis.

Complications

Cellulitis caused by *S. aureus* and *S. pyogenes* may at times spread locally or involve the regional lymph nodes; distant foci occur only rarely. Bacteremic *H. influenzae* type B infections (which are exceedingly rare since the advent of universal conjugate vaccination in the United States) are more likely to spread hematogenously, involving the central nervous system, epiglottis, joints, or pericardium.

Treatment

The treatment of cellulitis is the administration of systemic antibiotic therapy. Although most patients respond rapidly to oral antistaphylococcal agents, the clinician must identify those individuals who require broad-spectrum or IV administered drugs. Obviously, signs of sepsis are indicative of hematogenous dissemination and demand treatment as an inpatient. Additionally, children younger than 6 months of age and those with impaired immunity are unable to contain local bacterial infections and will benefit from intravenous therapy.

Among otherwise healthy children older than 6 months of age, only those who are clinically ill appearing, or in whom bacteremic disease is suspected, need to be admitted to the hospital. Prior to the advent of the *Haemophilus* vaccine, physicians could identify patients at risk for invasive *H. influenzae* type B disease fairly reliably on the basis of anatomic location, presence of fever, and a WBC count greater than $15,000/\mu L$. Although the incidence of this disease has dropped considerably, it is important to remember that young infants and underimmunized children are still at some risk of being infected with this organism.

The usual therapy for patients discharged from the ED is an antistaphylococcal antibiotic, such as dicloxacillin or cephalexin. Broadspectrum therapy is recommended presumptively for patients who are immunocompromised or suspected to have bacteremia, pending a definitive isolate (Table 122-9).

PERIORBITAL/ORBITAL CELLULITIS

Cellulitis as previously defined may involve the tissues anterior to the orbital septum (periorbital cellulitis) or within the orbit (orbital cellulitis).

Children younger than age 3 years are more likely to become bacteremic than are those who are older; thus, they experience the highest incidence of periorbital disease. Orbital cellulitis may occur at any age.

S. aureus, S. pneumoniae, and *H. influenzae* are the principal etiologic agents, although the incidence of *Haemophilus influenzae* type B disease has declined significantly since the advent of universal immunization.[4] Orbital infections are most often caused by *S. aureus.*

Pathophysiology

Organisms reach the periorbital area either hematogenously or by direct extension from the ethmoid sinus. In the case of orbital disease, contiguous spread is most common.

TABLE 122-9   Initial Antibiotic Therapy for Cellulitis

	Drug	Dose
Presumptive immunocompetent		
Extremity or buccal/periorbital Afebrile	Dicloxacillin	50–100 mg/kg per d PO
	or Cephalexin	50–100 mg/kg per d PO
Febrile/leukocytosis	Ampicillin-sulbactam	200 mg/kg as ampicillin/ per d IV
	or Ceftriaxone	75 mg/kg per d IV
Immunocompromised		
Any site	Oxacillin	150 mg/kg per d IV
	or Cefazolin	100 mg/kg per d IV
	and Gentamicin	5–7.5 mg/kg per d IV
	or Tobramycin	5–7.5 mg/kg per d IV
Specific organism		
Streptococcus pyogenes	Penicillin	100,000 units/kg per d PO or IV
Staphylococcus aureus	Dicloxacillin	50–100 mg/kg per d PO
	or Oxacillin	150 mg/kg per d IV
Haemophilus influenzae Ampicillin-sensitive	Ampicillin	200 mg/kg per d IV
Ampicillin-resistant	Ceftriaxone	75 mg/kg per d IV

Clinical Features

Orbital and periorbital cellulitis cause the periorbital area to appear red and swollen. The periorbital edema is usually more prominent with preseptal infections. Proptosis or limitation of extraocular muscle function indicates orbital involvement. Fever is more common with periorbital cellulitis.

Periorbital and orbital cellulitis are distinguished from noninfectious disorders on the basis of the clinical findings and the WBC count. Leukocytosis occurs frequently with cellulitis, more often with bacteremic preseptal infections. A blood culture is often positive.

CT is performed when orbital involvement is likely. An inflammatory mass is easily demonstrated when present using this modality.

Differential Diagnosis

As for cellulitis in other regions, allergic and traumatic causes for edema must be considered. Additionally, tumors and metabolic disease may cause swelling, discoloration, and/or proptosis. Thyrotoxicosis usually occurs in adolescents. The most likely tumor is metastatic neuroblastoma. Pseudotumor occurs rarely.

Complications

Periorbital cellulitis may serve as a focus for metastatic bacterial disease; of particular concern is the occurrence of meningitis. Orbital cellulitis may evolve into a subperiosteal abscess; this condition threatens the integrity of the eye and should be considered a surgical emergency. Intracranial extension may occur rarely.

Treatment

Admission and treatment with intravenous antibiotics is the rule. Blood cultures should always be done, and an aspirate culture is indicated for any ill child. In a child younger than 6 months of age, strong consideration of a lumbar puncture is indicated whenever infection with *H. influenzae* type B is suspected. Beyond 6 months of age, in the immunized child, although the possibility of meningitis remains, a decision regarding a lumbar puncture can be based on the clinical status and examination of the patient. Presumptive therapy of periorbital or orbital cellulitis is directed against *S. aureus,* pneumococcus (both penicillin-sensitive and resistant) and *H. influenzae* (see Table 122-9). Although medical management may be sufficient in some cases,[5] surgical drainage is often necessary with abscess formation or sinusitis.

REFERENCES

1. Sadick NS: Current aspects of bacterial infections of the skin. *Derm Clin* 15:341, 1997.
2. Nash D, Wald E: Sinusitis. *Pediatr Rev* 22:111, 2001.
3. American Academy of Pediatrics, Subcommittee on Management of Sinusitis and Committee on Quality Improvement. *Pediatrics* 108(3):798, Sept. 2001.
4. Schwartz GR, Wright SW: Changing bacteriology of periorbital cellulitis. *Ann Emerg Med* 28:617, 1996.
5. Starkey CR, Steele RW: Medical management of orbital cellulitis. *Pediatr Infect Dis J* 20:1002, 2001.

123 VIRAL AND BACTERIAL PNEUMONIA IN CHILDREN

Kathleen Brown
Willie Gilford, Jr.

The diagnosis and management of pediatric pneumonia cases can present unique challenges to the emergency physician. However, having a heightened sense of awareness toward certain presenting signs and symptoms from the child or parent and the appropriate ED workup and management can serve to dismantle these challenges. Pneumonia is defined pathologically as an inflammation of lower tract lung tissue. Clinically, pneumonia is defined by the presence of pulmonary infiltrates on a chest radiograph, usually associated with a combination of clinical signs, such as cough, fever, chest pain, tachypnea, and a variety of abnormal auscultatory findings. This chapter does not discuss in detail the entities associated with the diagnosis of pneumonia, such as interstitial processes, foreign body aspiration, chemical inflammation, *Mycobacterium tuberculosis,* and certain protozoan infections (e.g., *Pneumocystis carinii*). Instead, this chapter focuses on viral and bacterial pneumonias, which are most commonly implicated as the causes of pneumonia.

EPIDEMIOLOGY

Pneumonia develops more often in early childhood than at any other age. The incidence of pneumonia in children decreases as a function of age. In North America it has been estimated at 40 per 1000 in preschool children and approximately 9 per 1000 in 10-year-olds.[1,2] Infectious causes often display seasonal variation. Parainfluenza occurs predominantly in the fall, respiratory syncytial virus (RSV) in the winter, and influenza in the spring. Bacterial pneumonia is more common in the winter, when indoor crowding promotes respiratory transmission of microbes. Several risk factors increase the incidence or severity of pneumonia: prematurity, malnutrition, low socioeconomic status, passive exposure to smoke, and attendance at day-care centers. The mortality rate of childhood pneumonia is less than 1 percent in industrialized nations, but pneumonia accounts for up to 5 million deaths annually in children younger than 5 years in developing countries.[3]

PATHOPHYSIOLOGY

Most pneumonias are acquired through aspiration of infective particles into the lower respiratory tract. There are many protective mechanisms preventing infection with aerosolized infective particles. Aerosolized particles are filtered in the nasal cavities or entrapped and cleared by the normal mucus and ciliated epithelium of the upper respiratory tract. Aspiration is further prevented by laryngeal reflexes and coughing. In the lower respiratory tract, alveolar macrophages and various immune mechanisms prevent further invasion by infectious agents. These defense mechanisms include the ingestion and killing of bacteria by macrophages, the activation of complement and antibodies that neutralize bacteria, and the transportation of particles from the lung by lymphatic drainage. Abnormalities in any of these protective mechanisms predispose patients to acquired pneumonia. Anatomic abnormalities of the respiratory tract, immune deficiencies, neuromuscular weakness, airway abnormalities that predispose the child to aspiration, and alterations in the quantity or quality of mucus secretion (e.g., cystic fibrosis) also predispose patients to acquired pneumonia. Passively acquired maternal antibodies may further prevent respiratory tract infection by pneumococcal and *Haemophilus influenzae* infections.

Suppression of the normal respiratory physiologic and anatomic defenses may occur secondary to a preceding viral infection of the upper respiratory tract. Coexistence of viral and bacterial pathogens in children has been demonstrated in 50 percent or more of cases.[4,5] Bacteria that cause pneumonia include many of the same organisms that colonize the child's upper airway. In addition, organisms that are transmitted person to person by airborne droplet spread may cause pneumonia. Less commonly, bacterial and certain viral (e.g., herpes simplex virus, varicella, rubella, rubeola, and Epstein-Barr virus) microbes may cause pneumonia through hematogenous or contiguous spread. Parenchymal invasion by bacteria results in an acute inflammatory response that includes exudation of fluid, deposition of fibrin, and infiltration of the alveoli with fluids, polymorphonuclear leukocytes, and, soon, macrophages. Accumulation of excess alveolar fluid creates the characteristic consolidation seen on chest radiograms. Viral agents, mycoplasma, and chlamydia typically cause inflammation characterized by a predominately mononuclear infiltrate involving submucosal and interstitial tissues.

ETIOLOGY

The specific etiologic agent of pneumonia can be determined in about one-third to two-thirds of cases based on results, when available, of cultures, antigen detection, and serologic techniques.[4–11] The predominant pathogens that cause pneumonia in pediatric patients are a function of the patient's age, the presence of underlying disease, the vaccination status, and attendance in day care. Because clustering of cases of pneumonia due to a particular microbe are common, it is helpful to be aware of recent local outbreaks. When an etiologic agent is not identified, the best predictor of the agent is age. The most common etiologic agents causing pneumonia according to age groups are listed in Table 123-1 and discussed below.

Newborns: Birth to 1 Month

The newborn age group is the only developmental period when bacterial infections are more common than viral agents as the leading cause of pneumonia. Most infections in this age group are caused by aspiration of the maternal genital organisms present during labor and delivery. The predominant pathogen is group B *Streptococcus,* followed by *Escherichia coli, Klebsiella* species, and other gram-negative enteric bacilli from the Enterobacteriaceae family. Other, less commonly encountered organisms include nontypeable *H. influenzae,* other streptococci (group A and β-hemolytic species), enterococci, *Listeria monocytogenes, Bordetella pertussis,* and anaerobic bacteria.[11]

Infants: 1 to 24 Months

During the first 2 years of life, viruses are the most common etiologic agent of pneumonia. Respiratory syncytial virus, parainfluenza virus, influenza virus, and adenovirus account for most lower respiratory tract infections, including pneumonia, in this age group.[1,2,4,7] There

TABLE 123-1 Etiologic Agents and Empirical Antimicrobial Therapy for Pediatric Pneumonia in Otherwise Healthy Children*

Age Group	Frequent Pathogens (in Order of Frequency)	Patients in Hospital	Outpatients
Newborn	Group B *Streptococci* Gram-negative bacilli *Listeria monocytogenes* Herpes simplex Cytomegalovirus Rubella	Ampicillin *plus* Cefotaxime *or* Gentamicin	Not recommended
1–3 mo	*Chlamydia trachomatis* Respiratory syncytial virus Other respiratory viruses	Afebrile pneumonitis: erythromycin *or* clarithromycin Febrile pneumonia: cefuroxime	Initial outpatient management not recommended
3–12 mo	Respiratory syncytial virus Other respiratory viruses *Streptococcus pneumoniae* *Haemophilus influenzae* (type b,† nontypeable) *C. trachomatis* *Mycoplasma pneumoniae*	Ampicillin *or* cefuroxime	Amoxicillin *or* Erythromycin *or* Clarithromycin
2–5 y	Respiratory viruses *S. pneumoniae* *H. influenzae* type b† *M. pneumoniae* *Chlamydia pneumoniae*	Same as for 3–12 mo	Same as for 3–12 mo
5–18 y	*M. pneumoniae* *S. pneumoniae* *C. pneumoniae* *H. influenzae* type b† Influenza viruses A and B Adenoviruses Other respiratory viruses	Erythromycin or clarithromycin‡ With or without cefuroxime or ampicillin	Erythromycin or clarithromycin‡

*Duration of antibiotic treatment: outpatients, 7 to 10 days; hospitalized, 10 to 14 days.
†*Haemophilus influenzae* type b is uncommon where there is universal *H. influenzae* type b immunization.
‡Azithromycin can be substituted for clarithromycin with equal safety and efficacy for treating *M. pneumoniae*.
Source: Adapted with permission from Jadavji T, Lau B, Lebel MH, et al: A practical guide for the diagnosis and treatment of pediatric pneumonia. *CMAJ,* 156(suppl):S703, 1997.

are at least 14 other viral agents isolated in children with pneumonia, which include rhinoviruses, enteroviruses, coronavirus, measles, varicella, rubella, herpes simplex virus, and Epstein-Barr virus.[7,8,12] Bacterial pneumonia due to *Streptococcus pneumoniae, Streptococcus pyogenes, Staphylococcus aureus,* and *H. influenzae* should be considered in infants and toddlers who are severely ill, have rapid onset and progression of symptoms, or have lobar or diffuse infiltrates, large effusions, or abscesses on radiograph.[13]

Very young infants (1 to 3 months) may present with what is often referred to as *afebrile pneumonitis,* or atypical pneumonia. This syndrome is typified by cough, tachypnea, and sometimes progressive respiratory distress in the absence of fever. **Apneic episodes can occur with RSV, chlamydia, and pertussis.** There is often radiographic evidence of bilateral diffuse pulmonic infiltrates with air trapping. The viruses listed above are the most common etiologic agents.[14] *Chlamydia trachomatis* often is identified in this scenario.[10,14] *Ureaplasma urealyticum, Mycoplasma hominis, P. carinii,* and *B. pertussis* also have been implicated in this syndrome, but the extent of their role is not as well defined.[10,15]

Preschool: 2 to 5 Years

As age advances, the overall incidence of pneumonia decreases, but the relative frequency of bacterial pathogens, in particular *S. pneumoniae,* as etiologic agents increases. Nevertheless, respiratory viruses, in particular influenza viruses A and B and adenovirus, remain the most common cause of pneumonia in this age group. The most common bacterial pathogen encountered is *S. pneumoniae.* In the recent past, *H. influen-*

zae type b was encountered nearly as frequently; however, since implementation of widespread immunization against this agent, its incidence as an agent of invasive disease is thought to be much less.[16,17] However, non-type b *H. influenzae,* which is not protected against by the vaccine, may be an increasingly common agent of bacterial pneumonia.[18] Other bacteria that are isolated less commonly include *S. aureus,* group A *Streptococcus,* and *Moraxella catarrhalis. Mycoplasma pneumoniae* has been found more frequently in this age group in recent studies.[19,20]

School Age and Adolescence

Once children reach school age, *M. pneumoniae* is the most frequent bacterial cause of pneumonia.[1,20,21] The peak incidence is between 10 and 15 years of age.[22] *S. pneumoniae* remains a common pathogen in this age group.[1] *Chlamydia pneumoniae* is estimated to be the cause of up to 19 percent of pneumonias in school-aged and adolescent patients.[9,10,19,20] These infections are usually mild or asymptomatic.[20] *S. aureus* pneumonia can occur at any age but tends to be most frequent in older children.[23] Respiratory viruses, especially adenovirus, also can cause pneumonia in this age group.

All Ages: Special Considerations

The most common etiologic agents causing severe pneumonia (requiring admission to an intensive care unit) in all age groups beyond the neonatal period include *S. pneumoniae, S. aureus,* group A *Streptococcus, H. influenzae* type b, adenovirus, and *M. pneumoniae. Staphylococcus aureus* is notorious for causing rapidly progressive disease, often with pulmonic abscesses. A resurgence of virulent group A *Streptococci* has been associated with sporadic cases of invasive disease, including necrotizing fasciitis with pneumonia and empyema in children.[24] Increased severity of *M. pneumoniae* infections in children with sickle cell disease has been described.

Gram-negative bacilli, including *Pseudomonas,* should be considered in patients who have recently been hospitalized. Anaerobic infections should be considered in children with neurologic or anatomic defects that predispose them to aspiration. Unusual causes of bacterial pneumonia in children include *Mycobacterium tuberculosis, Legionella pneumophila, Chlamydia psittaci, Francisella tularensis,* and rickettsial infections. Children with progressive or unresponsive pneumonia should be evaluated for evidence of these microorganisms. An immunocompromised host is susceptible to all of these infections and to opportunistic infections, such as *Pneumocystis carinii,* cytomegalovirus, and fungal diseases.

CLINICAL FEATURES

Clinical findings in a child with pneumonia are highly variable and depend on the specific respiratory pathogen, age, the severity of the disease, and any underlying illnesses. Tachypnea is the most frequent sign of pneumonia in children and may be an otherwise isolated finding. The best physical examination finding for ruling out pneumonia in an infant or child is the absence of tachypnea.[25] However, tachypnea is a nonspecific symptom and may occur secondary to fever, anxiety, metabolic disease, cardiac disease, or other respiratory problems. Fever can increase an infant's respiratory rate by 10 breaths/min for each degree centigrade of elevation.[26] Respiratory rates should be counted past 1 min. Several studies have shown that rates counted over a shorter period tend to overestimate the rate.[27]

Auscultation of the lungs may reveal localized rales, wheezing, and decreased air entry in the affected area. However, auscultatory findings may not be reliable in children. When a group of pediatricians was asked to examine children with lower respiratory tract symptoms, there was only fair agreement about most auscultatory findings.[28] In younger children, decreased breath sounds, rather than rales, are often heard, because the involved areas tend to be ventilated poorly. Observable findings, such as respiratory rate and work of breathing, are more reliable.[25] Signs of increased work of breathing may include retractions, chest indrawing in infants, or paradoxical (seesaw) breathing. Grunting respirations are frequently present, particularly in infants with pneumonia.[29] Abdominal distention and pain may be present secondary to a paralytic ileus or diaphragmatic irritation in lower lobe pneumonias.[30]

The clinical presentation may be suggestive of the etiologic agent (Table 123–2). Two classic presentations have been described for pneumonia: typical pneumonia and atypical pneumonia. Typical pneumonia is characterized by abrupt onset of fever, chills, pleuritic chest pain, and productive cough. Associated physical examination findings include high-grade fever, localized findings on chest examination, and a toxic appearance. Atypical pneumonia is characterized by gradual onset (over days) of headache, malaise, nonproductive cough, and low-grade fever. Associated physical examination findings may include wheezing, prolonged expiration, rhinitis, conjunctivitis, pharyngitis, and rash. The typical pattern is generally thought to be associated with a bacterial pathogen, and the atypical pattern is thought to be more characteristic of a viral infection; however, significant overlap exists, and identification of a causal agent based on clinical presentation is not always reliable.[31]

Typical clinical presentations have been described for some specific pathogens. Pneumonia due to *S. aureus* is notorious for being particularly rapid in the progression of clinical findings. Patients with *B. pertussis* pneumonia typically develop prodromal symptoms, including mild cough, conjunctivitis, and coryza, which lasts 1 to 2 weeks. A severe, paroxysmal cough often associated with emesis and

TABLE 123-2 Antibiotic Dosages for Pneumonia

Antibiotic	Dosage
Amoxicillin	40 mg/kg daily in 3 divided doses PO
Ampicillin	150 mg/kg daily in 4 divided doses IV, IM
Azithromycin	10 mg/kg daily, then 5 mg/kg daily PO
Cefotaxime	150 mg/kg daily in 3 divided doses IV, IM
Ceftazidime	50 mg/kg daily in 3 divided doses IV, IM
Cefuroxime	150 mg/kg daily in 3 divided doses, IV, IM
Clarithromycin	15 mg/kg daily in 2 divided doses PO
Erythromycin	40 mg/kg daily in 4 divided doses PO, IV
Gentamicin	2.5 mg/kg daily in 3 divided doses IV, IM

dehydration, because coughing prevents eating and drinking, is characteristic of the catarrhal phase of pertussis infections. The inspiratory whoop is generally present only in older children. A history of maternal pelvic or conjunctival chlamydial infection is present in up to 50 percent of cases in which the infant develops *C. trachomatis* pneumonia. An infant with a chlamydial infection is usually afebrile, has a distinct staccato cough (i.e., short, abrupt onset), and diffuse rales on auscultation. Such infants rarely appear systemically ill. Chlamydial pneumonia in adolescents is usually insidious in onset and often includes complaints of sore throat and dysphagia. Mycoplasmal infections generally present with the gradual onset of malaise, fever, and headache. A hacking, nonproductive cough usually begins 3 to 5 days after the onset of illness and is present in up to 98 percent of children. Mycoplasmal infection may produce pharyngitis, and rales are present in approximately 75 percent of patients. A variable rash, which may be papular, vesicular, urticarial, or erythema-multiforme-like, is present in about 10 percent of patients with *M. pneumoniae.*

The age of the patient also may affect the clinical presentation. Pneumonia often occurs in association with a sepsis syndrome in neonates.[11,22] Infants frequently lack the classic symptoms and present with a variety of nonspecific findings. Nonspecific symptoms and signs of pneumonia in infants include fever without a localizing source, apnea, poor feeding, abdominal pain, vomiting or diarrhea, hypothermia, grunting, bradycardia, lethargy, and shock. Sputum production is uncommon in non-tracheostomized children younger than 8 years.

The severity of pneumonia may be judged by clinical features. More severe pneumonia is associated with deterioration of the patient's mental status, the use of accessory muscles, and the presence of retractions, nasal flaring, splinting, and cyanosis. Infants with poor feeding and lethargy may have more severe disease. A patient with a history of immunosuppressive therapy, a history of primary immune deficiencies, or a history suggestive of an immune deficiency may have more severe pneumonia, often caused by unusual pathogens. Children with underlying illnesses, such as congenital heart disease, chronic pulmonary disease, or sickle cell disease, are often more severely compromised by pneumonia.

DIAGNOSIS

Initially it is important to differentiate pneumonia from noninfectious pulmonary conditions, such as congestive heart failure, atelectasis, primary and metastatic tumors, and congenital abnormalities, such as pulmonary hypoplasia or congenital lobar emphysema. The wide variety of conditions that may simulate pneumonia include radiologic imaging problems (e.g., poor inspiration or a prominent thymus), recurrent or acute aspiration, atelectasis, tumors, collagen vascular disorders, allergic alveolitis, chronic pulmonary diseases (e.g., cystic fibrosis or asthma), and congenital abnormalities (e.g., pulmonary sequestration). A thorough history and physical examination usually help to exclude many of these conditions.

Radiographs

The chest radiograph is considered the pragmatic reference standard for making the diagnosis.[25] The finding of consolidation on radiograph is thought to be a reliable sign of pneumonia.[32] Differentiating the various microbiologic causes of pneumonia is often more difficult. Typical patterns of clinical presentation and epidemiologic data on incidence have been described above but often overlap. Radiographically, viral pneumonias tend to appear as diffuse interstitial infiltrates, frequently with hyperinflation, peribronchial thickening, and areas of atelectasis. Bacterial pneumonias tend to have lobar or segmental consolidation. Pneumatocele formation and a combination of pneumothorax and empyema are highly suggestive of *S. aureus* infection. However, bacterial pneumonias with perihilar interstitial and nodular patterns on radiographs have been reported.[33,34] *C. trachomatis* infections usually lead to hyperexpansion and diffuse alveolar or perihilar interstitial infiltrates.

Radiographic patterns in *M. pneumoniae* infections are variable and nonspecific.[35] Lower lobe, streaky or patchy infiltrates are the most common, but many other patterns are possible, including lobar infiltrates in 10 to 25 percent of cases. Viral pneumonias also can cause lobar or segmental consolidations.[34] Several studies have investigated the accuracy of the chest radiograph in differentiating viral from bacterial disease. A recent review of these studies found sensitivities ranging from 42 to 80 percent and specificities of 42 to 100 percent.[25]

Laboratory Studies

The white blood cell count is usually elevated, with a left shift in bacterial pneumonia, especially early in the illness.[36] Typically, viral, chlamydial, and pertussis pneumonias produce lymphocytosis. However, it is not unusual for viral pneumonia to initially provoke a significant polymorphonuclear cell response. In patients with mycoplasmal pneumonia, the total white blood cell count and differential cell count are usually normal, but the erythrocyte sedimentation rate may be elevated. Chlamydial infections or parasitic infections often produce eosinophilia.

Blood culture results are rarely (5 to 10 percent) positive in children with pneumonia, even when it is proven to be bacterial.[4,8,22] Blood cultures should be obtained in infants who have high fever, appear ill, or require hospitalization. Sputum cultures also may help in identifying the causative organism but are difficult to obtain from nontracheostomized children, in particular those younger than 8 years.

Cultures of the nasopharynx and throat for viral pathogens, chlamydia, pertussis, and mycoplasma often reveal the causative agent in patients with pneumonia caused by these organisms. Bacterial cultures of these regions have no diagnostic value due to mixed oral flora. Fluorescent antibody tests for *C. trachomatis* and *B. pertussis* are preferable to culture in some settings. Rapid viral antigen tests exist for a number of organisms, including RSV and influenza. Bacterial antigen testing is available in some centers but has poor sensitivity and specificity in diagnosing the cause of pneumonia.[4,23] Serologic testing can be done for viruses, mycoplasma, parasites, and fungi in persistent or puzzling cases. Skin testing for tuberculosis also should be considered in patients not responding to traditional therapy or with apical, cavitary pneumonia.

More invasive diagnostic procedures, such as obtaining endotracheal cultures, percutaneous lung aspiration, bronchoalveolar lavage, or open lung biopsy, may be necessary in patients with severe disease that is unresponsive to empiric therapy. Results of tests for cold agglutinins are positive in 72 to 92 percent of patients with *M. pneumoniae* infection. Cold agglutinin test results also may be positive in viral infections and are less consistently positive in young children. To perform

the bedside test for cold agglutinins, place several drops of blood in a blue-stopper coagulation profile tube and place it in ice water for 15 to 30 s. The presence of floccular agglutination is considered a positive result, and the agglutination should disappear after rewarming.

TREATMENT

All patients with actual or suspected pneumonia should have oxygen saturation determined with pulse oximetry.[37] There is no evidence-based pulse oximetry threshold for the administration of oxygen, or for admission to the hospital. For previously healthy, otherwise well young children with pneumonia who live at sea level, surveyed emergency physicans selected a median pulse oximetry threshold of 93 percent for admission.[38] In this survey 99.5 percent of emergency physicians practicing at sea level would have admitted a child with an oximetry value <90%. Physicians practicing at significant elevation may select lower oximetry values as the threshold for the admission of supplemental oxygen, as children at elevation have lower baseline oximetry values.[38,39] Children with oxygen saturation levels >90% may require supplemental oxygen and admission in the presence of other factors such as age <3 months; toxic appearance; oxygen desaturation with crying, feeding, or exercise; the presence of grunting with respiration; and comorbidities such as pre-existing lung disease, prematurity, or dehydration; actual or potential ventilatory insufficiency from muscular or spinal disorders; or shock.

In patients requiring hospital admission for suspected bacterial pneumonia, intravenous antibiotics should be administered in the ED. Empiric coverage, whether outpatient or inpatient, should be guided by the age of the patient and the epidemiologic data discussed above. Tables 123-1 to 123-4 list likely organisms and suggested antibiotic therapies. In newborns, ampicillin (150 mg/kg daily) in combination with an aminoglycoside (gentamicin 2.5 mg/kg per dose) or a third-generation cephalosporin (cefotaxime 150 mg/kg daily) is preferred. The ampicillin provides coverage against *Listeria* and enterococcal species. For infants with pneumonitis syndrome or afebrile pneumonia, erythromycin (40 mg/kg daily in four divided doses) is the drug of choice. In children 3 months to 5 years of age, ampicillin (150 mg/kg daily in four divided doses) or cefuroxime (150 mg/kg daily in three divided doses) alone is usually sufficient. In children who are unresponsive to this therapy or who have a suggestive clinical presentation, mycoplasma and chlamydial infections should be considered. Appropriate coverage for these infections includes erythromycin (40 mg/kg daily in four divided doses) or clarithromycin (15 mg/kg daily in two divided doses). In children older than 5 years, erythromycin or clarithromycin alone is usually sufficient. In severely ill hospitalized children in this age group, the addition of cefuroxime should be considered. In all age groups, if resistant *S. pneumoniae* is suspected, vancomycin should be added.

Children with fulminant viral pneumonia, such as an immunocompromised patient with varicella, may require treatment with acyclovir. In RSV pneumonia, ribavirin therapy should be considered for selected high-risk children, such as those with significant underlying cardiopulmonary or oncologic diseases and those with severe RSV

TABLE 123-3   Agents for Treating Unusual Pneumonias

Cause	Drug
Varicella pneumonia	Acyclovir
Respiratory syncytial virus	Ribavirin, if high risk
Human immunodeficiency virus with interstitial pneumonia	Prednisone and zidovudine
Cytomegalovirus pneumonia	Ganciclovir and γ-globulin
Gram-negative pneumonias	Ceftazidime

TABLE 123-4   Typical Features for Some Pneumonia Pathogens

Organism	Features
Staphylococcus aureus	Very rapid progression
Bordetella pertussis	1–2 wk of cough, coryza, conjunctivitis Cough with emesis and dehydration Whooping cough in older children Lymphocytosis on complete blood cell count
Chlamydia trachomatis	Neonatal: maternal pelvic or conjunctival infection Infant: staccato cough, nontoxic appearance Adolescent: sore throat, dysphagia Lymphocytosis or eosinophilia on complete blood cell count
Mycoplasma	Gradual onset of fever, malaise, headache Hacking nonproductive cough with pharyngitis Positive for cold agglutinins

pneumonia. Lymphocytic interstitial pneumonia in children with human immunodeficiency virus should include a combination of prednisone and zidovudine. Patients with bone marrow and solid organ transplantation and cytomegalovirus pneumonia may require ganciclovir and γ-globulin. Ceftazidime or ceftriaxone should eradicate nosocomial pneumonia in most cases, but ceftazidime has improved efficacy against *Pseudomonas aeruginosa*. Children with cystic fibrosis often develop acute infectious exacerbations secondary to *Pseudomonas* and *S. aureus,* often with reduced antimicrobial resistance to standard antibiotics.

Most children with uncomplicated pneumonia can be treated as outpatients. If a bacterial cause is suspected, the patient should be placed on an appropriate antibiotic. The choice of oral antibiotic should be based on the considerations discussed above with regard to the most likely etiologic organisms based on the age and clinical presentation of the patient. For outpatient treatment, amoxicillin (40 mg/kg daily in three divided doses) is preferred for children between 3 months and 5 years. Alternatively, daily intramuscular ceftriaxone may be used.[40] After age 5 years and in penicillin-allergic children, erythromycin (40 mg/kg daily in four divided doses) or tetracycline (in children older than 9 years) is the preferred initial agent. Recent data have indicated similar cure rates, fewer side effects, and reduced termination of therapy with clarithromycin compared with erythromycin.[41,42] Azithromycin also has been shown to have a cure rate equal to that of erythromycin in children with community-acquired pneumonia.[43] Both drugs are significantly more expensive than erythromycin or tetracycline.

If viral pneumonia is suspected, no specific antibiotic therapy is warranted. Symptomatic treatment should include fever control and hydration. Patients with viral pneumonia often have a mixture of airway and air-space disease. If the patient has prominent airway disease (bronchiolitis-like) symptoms, bronchodilator therapy should be considered.

All patients discharged with a diagnosis of pneumonia should have routine follow-up with a primary care provider within 1 to 2 days. The duration of therapy depends on the clinical response, predisposing host factors, and suppurative complications. Ten days of antimicrobial treatment should suffice for most uncomplicated cases.

Disposition

ADMISSION CRITERIA   Children with hypoxia should be admitted to the hospital. There is no evidence-based definition of hypoxia, but physicians often choose a pulse oximetry threshold of <90–93% for admission. Other factors include age <3 months; toxic appearance; respiratory distress; a history of apnea or cyanosis; impaired immune function; oxygen desaturation with crying, feeding, or exercise; the presence of grunting with respiration; the presence of pre-existing lung disease; prematurity; dehydration; the potential for ventilatory insufficiency; lack of response to oral antibiotics; or inability to provide close outpatient followup. **The presence of underlying disease and the ability of the caregivers should also be considered.** The finding of a pleural effusion or pneumatocele or findings suggestive of a bacterial infection in a child younger than 1 year suggest a pathogen other than *S. pneumoniae* (in particular *H. influenzae* type b or *S. aureus*). Because such infections can progress rapidly and are not well tolerated, hospitalization is generally required. Infants with suspected *B. pertussis* or *M. tuberculosis* should be admitted. Children with moderate or severe complications from pneumonia should be hospitalized. Indications for admitting patients with RSV pneumonia are the same as those for RSV bronchiolitis.

COMPLICATIONS   Most viral pneumonias will resolve spontaneously without specific therapy. Complications are similar to those for bronchiolitis and include dehydration, bronchiolitis obliterans, and apnea. Apnea is commonly seen in very young infants with RSV, chlamydial, or pertussis infection. Pleural effusions can occur with viral pneumonias but are not common.

Uncomplicated bacterial pneumonia usually responds rapidly to antibiotic therapy. A delay in improvement or a worsening condition after therapy has begun should prompt an evaluation for possible complications. Complications of bacterial pneumonia include pleural effusions, empyemas, pneumothorax, pneumatoceles, dehydration, and development of additional infectious foci. Pneumococcal pneumonias are accompanied by pleural effusions in about 10 percent of cases. Pneumonia due to *H. influenzae* type b is complicated by pleural effusions in 25 to 75 percent of cases. Other foci of infection are frequently seen with *H. influenzae* type b and can include meningitis, septic arthritis, epiglottitis, soft tissue infections, and otitis media. Pneumonias secondary to *S. aureus* have a high rate of complications, including empyemas (80 percent) and pneumatoceles (40 percent). Mycoplasma pneumonia is only rarely complicated by pleural effusions, meningitis, encephalitis, arthritis, and hemolytic anemia. Whenever pneumonia is complicated or prolonged, roentgenographic follow-up is recommended to assure complete resolution, which may take 4 to 6 weeks or longer.

PREVENTION   Administration of the *H. influenzae* type b vaccine has nearly eliminated disease caused by this agent. A heptavalent pneumococcal (Prevnar) vaccine was approved recently for use in infants and toddlers and is expected to cause a similar reduction in pediatric pneumococcal infections.[44–46] Thus, because of the significance of such interventions, the emergency physician should inquire about immunization status and refer to a primary care physician if the patient is unimmunized.

DISCHARGE INSTRUCTIONS   All children discharged from the ED with a diagnosis of pneumonia should receive specific advice on the dosage and scheduling of medications and the signs of worsening respiratory distress. Children who become unable to ingest adequate amounts of fluid or prescribed antibiotics should be instructed to return for further care. All children discharged with the diagnosis of pneumonia should have follow-up scheduled with the primary care provider within 48 h.

ACKNOWLEDGMENT

The authors would like to acknowledge the contribution of Dr. Thomas Terndrup for his work on the prior edition of this chapter.

REFERENCES

1. Murphy TF, Henderson FW, Clyde WA Jr, et al: Pneumonia: An eleven-year study in a pediatric practice. *Am J Epidemiol* 113:12, 1981.
2. Wright AL, Taussig LM, Ray CG, et al: The Tucson Children's Respiratory Study: II. Lower respiratory tract illness in the first year of life. *Am J Epidemiol* 129:1232, 1989.
3. Grant JP: *The State of the World's Children, 1990: UNICEF.* Oxford, Oxford University Press, 1990.
4. Turner RB, Lande AE, Chase D, et al: Pneumonia in pediatric outpatients: Cause and clinical manifestations. *J Pediatr* 111:194, 1987.
5. Hietala J, Uhari M, Tuokko H, Leinonen M: Mixed bacterial and viral infections are common in children. *Pediatr Infect Dis J* 8:683, 1989.
6. McCracken GH Jr: Diagnosis and management of pneumonia in children. *Pediatr Infect Dis J* 19:924, 2000.
7. Paisley JW, Lauer BA, Mcintosh K, et al: Pathogens associated with acute lower respiratory tract infection in young children. *Pediatr Infect Dis J* 3:14, 1984.
8. Nohynek H, Eskola J, Laine E, et al: The causes of hospital-treated acute lower respiratory tract infection in children. *Am J Dis Child* 145:618, 1991.
9. Ruuskamen O, Nohynek H, Zeigler T, et al: Pneumonia in childhood: Etiology and response to antimicrobial therapy. *Eur J Clin Microbiol Infect Dis* 11:217, 1992.
10. Davies HD, Matlow A, Petric M, Glazier Rwang EEL: Prospective comparative study of viral, bacterial and atypical organisms identified in pneumonia and bronchiolitis in hospitalized Canadian infants. *Pediatr Infect Dis J* 15:371, 1996.
11. Bohin S, Field DJ: The epidemiology of neonatal respiratory distress. *Early Hum Dev* 37:73, 1994.
12. Boyer KM, Cherry JD: Nonbacterial pneumonia, in Feigin RD, Cherry JD (eds): *Textbook of Pediatric Infectious Diseases,* 3rd ed. Philadelphia, Saunders, 1992.
13. Jadavji T, Law B, Lebel MH, et al: A practical guide for the diagnosis and treatment of pediatric pneumonia. *CMAJ* 156(suppl):703S, 1997.
14. DeMuri GP: Afebrile pneumonia in infants. *Prim Care* 23:849, 1996.
15. Matlow AG, Richardson SE, Quinn PA, Wang EEL: Isolation of *Ureaplasma urealyticum* from neonatal respiratory tract specimens in a pediatric institution. *Pediatr Infect Dis J* 15:371, 1996.
16. Lee GM, Harper MB: Risk of bacteremia for febrile young children in the post-*Haemophilus influenzae* type B era. *Arch Pediatr Adolesc Med* 152:624, 1998.
17. Bower C, Condon R, Payne J, et al: Measuring the impact of conjugate vaccines on invasive *Haemophilus influenzae* type B infection in Western Australia. *Aust N Z J Public Health* 22:67, 1998.
18. Urwin G, Krohn JA, Deaver-Robinson K, et al: Invasive disease due to *Haemophilus influenzae* serotype F: Clinical and epidemiologic characteristics in the *H. influenzae* serotype B vaccine era. The *Haemophilus influenzae* Study Group. *Clin Infect Dis* 22:1077, 1996.
19. Block S, Hedrick J, Hammerschlag MR, Cassell GH, et al: *Mycoplasma pneumoniae* and *Chlamydia pneumoniae* in pediatric community-acquired pneumonia: Comparative efficacy and safety of clarithromycin vs erythromycin ethylsuccinate. *Pediatr Infect Dis J* 14:189, 1995.
20. Hammerschlag MR: Atypical pneumonias in children. *Adv Pediatr Infect Dis* 10:1, 1995.
21. Broughton RA: Infections due to *Mycoplasma pneumoniae* in childhood. *Pediatr Infect Dis* 5:71, 1986.
22. Schidlow DV, Callahan CW: Pneumonia. *Pediatr Rev* 17:300, 1996.
23. Schutze GE, Jacobs RF: Management of community acquired bacterial pneumonia in hospitalized children. *Pediatr Infect Dis J* 11:160, 1992.
24. Novotny W, Faden H, Mosovich L: Emergence of invasive group A streptococcal disease among young children. *Clin Pediatr* 31:696, 1992.
25. Margolis P, Gadomoski A: Does this infant have pneumonia? *JAMA* 279:308, 1998.
26. Gadomoski A, Permutt T, Stanton B: Correcting respiratory rate for the presence of fever. *J Clin Epidemiol* 47:1043, 1994.
27. Taylor JA, Del Beccaro M, Done S, et al: Establishing clinically relevant standards for tachypnea in febrile children less than 2 years. *Arch Pediatr Adolesc Med* 149:283, 1995.
28. Margolis P, Ferkol T, Marsocci S, et al: Accuracy of the clinical exam in detecting hypoxemia in infants with respiratory illness. *J Pediatr* 124:552, 1994.
29. Poole S, Chetham M, Anderson M: Grunting respirations in infants and children. *Pediatr Emerg Care* 11:158, 1995.

30. Kanegaye JT, Harley JR: Pneumonia in unexpected locations: An occult cause of pediatric abdominal pain. *J Emerg Med* 13:773, 1995.
31. Fang GD, Fine M, Orloff J, et al: New and emerging etiologies for community-acquired pneumonia with implications for therapy. *Medicine* 69:307, 1990.
32. Davies HD, Wang EE, Manson D, et al: Reliability of the chest radiograph in the diagnosis of lower respiratory infections in young children. *Pediatr Infect Dis J* 15:600, 1996.
33. Simpson W, Hacking P, Court S, Gardner P: The radiologic findings in respiratory syncytial virus infections in children: II. *Pediatr Radiol* 2:155, 1974.
34. Wildin S, Chonmaitree T, Swisschuk L: Roentgenographic features of common viral respiratory tract infections. *Am J Dis Child* 142:43, 1988.
35. John SD, Ramanathan J, Swischuk LE: Spectrum of clinical and radiographic findings in pediatric mycoplasma pneumonia. *Radiographics* 21:121, 2001.
36. Triga MG, Syrogiannopoulos GA, Thoma KD, et al: Correlation of leukocyte count and erythrocyte sedimentation rate with the day of illness in presumed bacterial pneumonia. *J Infect* 36:63, 1998.
37. Mower WR, Sachs C, Nicklin EL, Baraff LJ: Pulse oximetry as a fifth pediatric vital sign. *Pediatrics* 99:681, 1997.
38. Brown L, Dannenberg B: Pulse oximetry in discharge decision-making: A survey of emergency physicians. *Can J Emerg Med* 4:388, 2002.
39. Beebe SA, Heery LB, Magarian S, Culberson J: Pulse oximetry at moderate altitude: Healthy children and children with upper respiratory infection. *Clin Pediatr* 33:329, 1994.
40. Dagan R, Philip M, Watemberg NM, et al: Outpatient treatment of serious community-acquired pediatric infections using once-daily intramuscular ceftriaxone. *Pediatr Infect Dis J* 6:1080, 1987.
41. Block S, Hedrick J, Hammerschlag MR, et al: *Mycoplasma pneumoniae* and *Chlamydia pneumoniae* in pediatric community-acquired pneumonia: Comparative efficacy and safety of clarithromycin vs. erythromycin ethylsuccinate. *Pediatr Infect Dis J* 14:471, 1995.
42. Chein SM, Pichotta P, Siepman N, et al: Treatment of community-acquired pneumonia: A multicenter, double-blind randomized study comparing clarithromycin with erythromycin. *Chest* 103:697, 1993.
43. Roord JJ, Wolf BH, Gossens MM, et al: Prospective, open randomized study comparing efficacies and safeties of a 3-day course of azithromycin and a 10-day course of erythromycin in children with community-acquired acute lower respiratory tract infections. *Antimicrob Agents Chemother* 40:2765, 1996.
44. Selman S, Hayes D, Perin LA, Hayes WS: Pneumococcal conjugate vaccine for young children. *Manag Care* 9:49, 2000.
45. Scheifele D, Halperin S, Pelletier L, Talbot J: Invasive pneumococcal infections in Canadian children, 1991–1998: Implications for new vaccination strategies. Canadian Paediatric Society/Laboratory Centre for Disease Control Immunization Monitoring Program, Active (IMPACT). *Clin Infect Dis* 31:58, 2000.
46. Tan TQ: Update on pneumococcal infections of the respiratory tract. *Semin Respir Infect* 17:3, 2002.

PEDIATRIC ASTHMA AND BRONCHIOLITIS

Maybelle Kou

Thom Mayer

ASTHMA

Asthma is a chronic disease of the tracheobronchial tree characterized by airway obstruction, inflammation, and hyperresponsiveness. Triggers for cytokine-mediated inflammation and hyperresponsiveness are well known and can be as innocuous as changes in barometric pressure. The cascade of events leading to mucous plugging, airway edema, and obstruction is generally reversible with appropriate, aggressive therapy. Adequate and timely treatment is paramount to the care of children with asthma.

The National Institutes of Health (NIH) 1997 Expert Panel Report 2 (EPR-2), *Guidelines for the Diagnosis and Management of Asthma,*[1] is a publication with which all physicians should be familiar. It provides treatment algorithms for use in the acute-care setting and clear guidelines to outpatient management (see Figure 68-1). However, most institutions will need to tailor these protocols to meet regional, local, and individual hospital needs.

Epidemiology

Asthma affects 4.8 million children younger than 18 years of age.[2] The prevalence of asthma has increased in all age groups by 40 percent in the last decade. In 1995, there were about 570,000 ED visits for asthma in children aged 0 to 14 years,[3] with an admission rate of nearly 70 per 10,000. An investigation of over 113,000 pediatric asthma admissions from 1986 to 1993 revealed that although the number of discharges paralleled the general increase in population, the percentage of patients with adverse outcomes [mainly intubation but also the need for CPR] as well as death almost tripled.[4] Between 1993 and 1995, there were 170 deaths due to asthma in the age group from 0 to 14 years.[5]

Specific risk factors associated with the development of asthma in children include low birth weight, family history of asthma, urban household, low-income household, and race (children of African-American, Asian, and Hispanic descent).[6–8] These factors also have an influence on when hospitalization might be required during exacerbation. Most children presenting with asthma do so before age 8, with male predominance in the prepubertal age group. During adolescence, this ratio equalizes.

Risk factors that contribute to the deaths of children with asthma include socioeconomic background, limited access to health care, improper medication administration, and unrecognized severe disease. Extreme lability of disease, nocturnal asthma, and history of respiratory failure with previous intubation also have contributed to these deaths.

Pathophysiology

Bronchial hyperreactivity appears to have a genetic basis; however, the difficulty in distinguishing atopy from asthma has resulted in limited studies of this area. Nonetheless, asthma is classified as extrinsic IgE-mediated, intrinsic (infection-induced), and mixed (both IgE- and infection-induced). Since environmental factors are strongly implicated in the initiation of bronchial hyperreactivity, it should come as no surprise that 66 to 75 percent of asthmatic children are "allergic," many with serum IgE elevation. Concurrent sinusitis and bronchospasm secondary to chronic postnasal drip may be present. Whereas allergens and irritants are the most common and preventable triggers of asthma in children older than 2 years of age, viral respiratory infections are felt to be predisposing in those below age 2. Respiratory syncytial virus is one of many viruses that can cause wheezing; this is discussed below under "Bronchiolitis" (Table 124-1).

Sympathetic β_2-receptors cause bronchodilation, and parasympathetics govern bronchoconstriction. IgE-mediated inflammation is a contributor in the pathogenesis of an asthma attack. Mast cells release histamine, leading to the formation of arachidonic acid metabolites and the inflammatory cytokine cascade. Asthma is a two-stage process: (1) bronchoconstriction due to histamine and leukotriene release (early stage) and (2) airway mucosal edema with mucous plugging (late phase). Since resolution depends largely on the degree of mucosal inflammation, an asthma attack may persist from days to weeks.

Bronchospasm, mucosal edema, and mucous plugging cause variable and reversible airflow obstruction with subsequent air trapping and impaired oxygen exchange. While increased lung volumes and pulmonary overdistention may help maintain airway patency, the resulting tidal volume approaches the volume of the pulmonary dead

TABLE 124-1   Asthma Triggers

Trigger	Countermeasures
Environmental Air pollution Temperature extremes High humidity	Keep indoors during high-ozone days
Tobacco smoke	Adults stop smoking
Allergens Animal dander/feces Molds Pollen	Minimize carpets, down/feather bedding; control animal dander
Exercise	Pretreat before exercise
Viral respiratory infections	Simple infection control measures when others are ill
Rhinitis/sinusitis	Treat postnasal drip and sinusitis
Gastroesophageal reflux	Use preventive medications

space and results in alveolar hypoventilation. Ventilation-perfusion mismatch in areas of atelectasis contributes to hypoxia.

In the early stages of a severe exacerbation, compensatory hyperventilation may cause a fall in $Paco_2$ and even a respiratory alkalosis. More severe obstruction and inadequate alveolar ventilation ultimately result in marked CO_2 retention, respiratory acidosis, and respiratory failure. *Pseudonormalization* of $Paco_2$ is therefore ominous: The apparently "normal" $Paco_2$ of 40 mm Hg coupled with altered mental status is a clear sign of respiratory failure. The acidosis that results from hypoxia and hypercapnea leads to pulmonary vasoconstriction, pulmonary hypertension, and right-sided heart strain.

PEDIATRIC ANATOMIC DIFFERENCES   The child with asthma is at higher risk of respiratory failure than an adult due to these anatomic differences:

1. Increased compliance of the infant rib cage and immature diaphragm results in paradoxical respiration, and inward displacement of the ribs during inspiration contributes to increased work of breathing and respiratory muscle fatigue.
2. Young lung tissue lacks elastic recoil and is more prone to atelectasis, resulting in ventilation-perfusion mismatch.
3. Airway walls are relatively thicker and result in greater narrowing with bronchoconstriction.

Thus, if expiration is hampered by obstruction, complete collapse of alveoli and lung segments may occur.

Evaluation

To avoid delays in treatment, a brief physical examination should be performed before a detailed history is obtained. Treatment with inhaled β_2-agonists should not be withheld while the initial evaluation is in progress, even if the patient is in the triage area owing to lack of availability of a treatment room. Examination of vital signs should include respiratory rate, pulse, blood pressure, temperature, and pulse oximetry (Sao_2). A room-air oxygen saturation of <90–93 percent in an infant or child should prompt supplementary oxygen administration, and concern for need for admission (see Chap. 123). Supplemental oxygen should be administered immediately to a child in respiratory distress, without delay, to obtain pulse oximetry on room air. Oximetry may be inaccurate in states of poor perfusion.

After initial stabilization, perform a complete examination. The child's chest must be visible for complete examination. Inspection and auscultation should be performed to assess ventilation, accessory muscle use, and work of breathing. The severity of disease may be underestimated in the "silent" or "quiet wheezer," in whom the expiratory phase usually is prolonged and wheezing is absent due to extreme air trapping.

The tripod position is a significant indicator of distress: The child sits forward, hands over knees, on the edge of the bed. The nostrils should be inspected for presence or absence of nasal flaring, foreign bodies, and concurrent sinusitis. Hallmark "musical" polyphonic inspiratory and expiratory wheezes may not always be present on lung examination and are not prognostic of severity of disease. Extremities should be inspected to assess cyanosis and clubbing. Insensible fluid losses may result in delayed capillary refill and poor skin turgor. Pulsus paradoxus in severe exacerbation is usually 20 to 40 mm Hg and may be reflected by significant jugular venous distention, which is otherwise difficult to appreciate in the pediatric examination.

A thorough series of questions can aid the physician in assessing risk factors and comorbidities and in formulating an educational and discharge plan. A history of asthma may be denied because pediatricians who are reluctant to give the diagnosis of asthma use *reactive airway disease* as alternative nomenclature. History of precipitating factors (see Table 124-1), medications and home care, previous hospitalizations, intubation, and tracheostomy should be determined, and medical records should be reviewed. History of prematurity, bronchopulmonary dysplasia (BPD), supplemental oxygen requirement, and neonatal intensive care unit admissions should be determined.

Often such information is not volunteered. In adolescents, inquire about the use of inhalants, tobacco, drugs of abuse, and over-the-counter purchases of bronchodilators that their parents may not be aware they have been using. History of aspiration or choking, as well as possible ingestion, should be included for all ages. Family history of asthma and allergy also can give a sense of whether or not the parent or caretaker will be able to continue treatment once the ED visit terminates.

The NIH–EPR-2 (Table 124-2) is a consensus document for assessing severity of an acute asthma episode. Table 124-3 provides guidelines for assessing the general severity of the condition.

Peak expiratory flow rate (PEFR) should be determined to monitor response to acute treatment and also for the ongoing assessment and management of asthma.[1] Forced expiratory volume in 1 s (FEV_1) is estimated by measuring PEFR and correlates with the degree of airway obstruction; PEFR is already decreased by 25 percent once wheezing is detected by stethoscope (Table 124-4). PEFR values in liters per minute are based on the child's height. A PEFR of less than 50 percent indicates severe obstruction, and less than 25 percent indicates possible hypercarbia. In the ED, PEFR is an excellent tool to evaluate mild asthma or for reevaluating patients after treatment, especially those who know their "personal best" score. Pre- and posttreatment values should be obtained when possible.

TABLE 124-2   Classifying Severity of Asthma Exacerbations*

	Mild	Moderate	Severe	Respiratory Arrest Imminent
Symptoms				
Breathless	While walking	While talking (infant—softer, shorter cry; difficulty feeding)	While at rest (infant—stops feeding)	
	Can lie down	Prefers sitting	Sits upright	
Talks in	Sentences	Phrases	Words	
Alertness	May be agitated	Usually agitated	Usually agitated	Drowsy or confused
Signs				
Respiratory rate	Increased	Increased	Often >30/mn	

Guide to rates of breathing in awake children:

Age	Normal rate
<2 months	<60/min
2–12 months	<50/min
1–5 years	<40/min
6–8 years	<30/min

	Mild	Moderate	Severe	Respiratory Arrest Imminent
Use of accessory muscles; suprasternal retractions	Usually not	Commonly	Usually	Paradoxical thoraco-abdominal movement
Wheeze	Moderate, often only end expiratory	Loud; throughout exhalation	Usually loud; throughout inhalation and exhalation	Absence of wheeze
Pulse/min	<100	100–120	>120	Bradycardia

Guide to normal pulse rates in children:

Age	Normal rate
2–12 months	<160/min
1–2 years	<120/min
2–8 years	<110/min

	Mild	Moderate	Severe	Respiratory Arrest Imminent
Pulsus paradoxus	Absent <10 mm Hg	May be present 10–25 mm Hg	Often present 20–40 mm Hg (child)	Absent

Source: Expert Panel Report 2: Guidelines for the Diagnosis and Management of Asthma, 1997. National Institutes of Health Publication No. 98-4051. Bethesda, MD: NIH, 1997.

TABLE 124-3   Classification of Asthma Severity: Clinical Features Before Treatment

	Days with Symptoms	Nights with Symptoms	PEFR or FEV$_1$*	PEFR Variability
Step 4 Severe Persistent	Continual	Frequent	≤60%	>30%
Step 3 Moderate Persistent	Daily	≥5/month	>60%–<80%	>30%
Step 2 Mild Persistent	3–6/week	3–4/month	≥80%	20–30%
Step 1 Mild Intermittent	≤2/week	≤2/month	≥80%	<20%

*Percent predicted values for forced expiratory volume in 1 second (FEV$_1$) and percent of personal best for peak expiratory flow rate (PEFR) (relevant for children 6 years old or older who can use these devices).

Notes: Patients should be assigned to the most severe step in which *any* feature occurs. Clinical features for individual patients may overlap across steps. An individual's classification may change over time.

Patients at any level of severity of chronic asthma can have mild, moderate, or severe exacerbations of asthma. Some patients with intermittent asthma experience severe and life-threatening exacerbations separated by long periods of normal lung function and no symptoms.

Patients with two or more asthma exacerbations per week (i.e., progressively worsening symptoms that may last hours or days) tend to have moderate-to-severe persistent asthma.

Source: NIH Guidelines.[1]

The use of PEFR meters in children younger than age 5 is limited by patient cooperation. In older children, the ability to perform deep inspiration and forced expiration may not be feasible during an acute exacerbation.

Arterial blood gas analysis should be obtained to determine Paco$_2$ in children with impending respiratory failure, if the patient is hypoventilating, if PEFR is less than 30 percent of predicted, or if the patient is not responding as expected to treatment. It also may be helpful in differentiating intensive care unit from regular floor admission.

TABLE 124-4   Predicted Average Peak Expiratory Flow for Normal Children and Adolescents, Male and Female

Height, in.	L/min	Height, in.	L/min
43	147	56	320
44	160	57	334
45	173	58	347
46	187	59	360
47	200	60	373
48	214	61	387
49	227	62	400
50	240	63	413
51	254	64	427
52	267	65	440
53	280	66	454
54	293	67	467
55	307		

Source: From Polger G, Promedhat V: *Pulmonary Function Testing in Children: Techniques and Standards.* Philadelphia: Saunders, 1971, with permission.

Complete blood count and chemistries are usually unnecessary unless there is a concurrent febrile illness or coexisting disease. Chronic steroid use can cause leukocytosis and elevated band count. Chronic use or abuse of albuterol can cause hypokalemia. If the child is taking theophylline, a level should be obtained.

Chest x-ray is not recommended routinely but should be performed in new-onset asthma, for severe episodes requiring admission, or if pneumonia, pneumothorax, foreign body, or pneumomediastinum are in the differential diagnosis. Findings typical of asthma are hyperinflation, flattened diaphragm, increased anteroposterior diameter, peribronchial cuffing, and atelectasis.

Differential Diagnosis

NEW-ONSET ASTHMA   In the new-onset "wheezer," upper and lower respiratory and nonrespiratory causes must be differentiated (Table 124-5).

INFECTION   Fever and focal wheezing implicate infectious etiologies such as pneumonia or bronchiolitis. Nocturnal wheezing, nocturnal cough, and poor exercise tolerance may be clues of more chronic illness. Sinusitis can exacerbate asthma symptoms; a history of nasal congestion and nocturnal cough or snoring should be treated with at least a 2-week course of antibiotics and nasal steroids. Recurrent attacks, failure to thrive, and a history of sinusitis and chronic ear infections should raise suspicion of cystic fibrosis as an etiology.

CARDIAC LESIONS: CONGENITAL AND ACQUIRED   Infants with a history of bronchopulmonary dyplasia (BPD) may present with mild illness with rapid deterioration. Prolonged mechanical ventilation in the neonatal period causes smooth muscle hypertrophy and pulmonary hypertension, leading to cardiac disease. It may be necessary to distinguish pulmonary edema as a cause of wheezing; usually a history of diuretic use will aid in the diagnosis. Congenital heart lesions causing congestive heart failure, often exacerbated by concurrent viral infections, also can present with wheezing that can be mistaken for asthma. Chap. 120 presents a detailed discussion of pediatric heart disease.

TABLE 124-5   Differential Diagnosis of Asthma

Bronchopulmonary dysplasia (BPD)
Cystic fibrosis
Bronchiectasis
Pneumonia
  Bacterial
  Viral
Varicella
Pneumonitis
Gastroesophageal reflux disease
  Aspiration pneumonia
Anatomic defects of the airway
  Tracheoesophageal fistula
  Tracheomalacia
  Bronchial stenosis
  Bronchogenic cyst
  Pulmonary sequestration
Vocal cord dysfunction
Cardiovascular disorders
  Congestive heart failure
  Tricuspid atresia and transposition
  Vascular ring
Miscellaneous
  Foreign-body aspiration
  Anaphylaxis
  Hyperventilation syndrome
Salicylate ingestion
β-blocker ingestion

UPPER AIRWAY OBSTRUCTION/FOREIGN-BODY ASPIRATION

Wheezing from croup, tracheomalacia, epiglottitis, retropharyngeal abscess, upper airway foreign body, or vocal cord dysfunction can be misdiagnosed as asthma. In these situations, wheezing is loudest over the trachea, and wheezes heard in the lungs are transmitted from the upper airway. Chap. 133 presents a detailed review of upper respiratory emergencies.

GASTROESOPHAGEAL REFLUX DISEASE (GERD) A history of postprandial wheezing or coughing is indicative of GERD with microaspiration of liquid into the tracheobronchial tree. Severe GERD has been implicated in apnea and sudden infant death syndrome. Recurrent microaspiration can result in wheezing, fever, and pneumonia. Suspicion of GERD as a cause for wheezing requires further evaluation (see Chap. 117) and specific treatment.

Treatment

β_2-RECEPTOR AGONISTS β_2-Receptors are widely distributed on bronchial smooth muscle and airway epithelial cells. β_2-Receptor agonists activate adenylate cyclase, increase cyclic adenosine monophosphate (cAMP) levels, cause bronchial smooth muscle relaxation due to increased binding of intracellular calcium to the endoplasmic reticulum, and decrease myoplasmic calcium.

Albuterol (Canadian name, salbutamol; do not confuse with the long-acting salmeterol, which is contraindicated in an acute episode) is the treatment of choice. Dosage is listed in Table 124-6. Continuous aerosolized therapy with albuterol is a safe,[9] fast, and effective way to deliver medication directly to the lung capillary beds and may be associated with a reduction in hospital admission.[10] Continuous cardiac monitoring is employed with continuous albuterol infusions.

Tachycardia and jitteriness are common side effects (more so with oral medication than with inhaled medication), and rarely, dysrhythmias have been reported. During an acute attack, use of a β_2-receptor agonist may cause transient drops in Po_2 due to pulmonary vasodilatation and ventilation-perfusion mismatch.[11]

Levalbuterol (Xopenex), the R-isomer of albuterol, results in less tachycardia than racemic albuterol. It is not currently used for acute exacerbations but is used as home nebulization therapy for asthma, although there are limited data demonstrating that its benefits outweigh standard albuterol treatment. It is more expensive than albuterol.

Salmeterol (Serevent), a long-acting β_2-agonist that reduces the need for prn albuterol dosing, is not indicated for use in acute exacerbations. It is also available in combination with fluticasone (Advair) as maintenance therapy.

Tachyphylaxis has been documented with chronic and improper use of β_2-agonists[12] and appears to be related to saturation of β_2-receptors from frequent dosing intervals and/or decreased downregulation of the number of β_2-receptors on leukocytes of asthmatic pa-

TABLE 124-6 Albuterol Dosage Guidelines

Dosage for adolescents: 2.5–5.0 mg q20min $\times$ 3 doses
  or
  10–15 mg per h by continuous nebulization with at least 25% oxygen

Dosage for children: 2.5–5.0 mg q20min $\times$ 3 doses

  or

  0.5 mg/kg per h by continuous nebulization with at least 25% oxygen

Dosage for infants/neonates: 0.05–0.15 mg/kg per dose, q20min $\times$ 3 doses

  2.5 mg albuterol is prepared as 0.5 mL of 0.5% albuterol diluted with NS to a final volume of 3 mL

  or

  2.5 mg albuterol is contained in 3 mL of commercially available 0.083% albuterol solution

Source: Clinical Pharmacology 2000 *http://cpip.gsm.com* (July 2002 update).

tients. When this occurs, increasing doses of β_2-agonists prove to be ineffective. Efficacy is preserved as long as the medication is used as needed and not overused or abused. Overuse of such medications as aerosolized epinephrine (available over the counter as Primatene Mist) has been implicated in the deaths of asthmatics from tachyphylaxis and cardiac dysrhythmias. Such over-the-counter preparations have no place in asthma management, even in mild asthma.

METERED-DOSE INHALER (MDI) Although the literature has stated that MDI therapy is just as effective as nebulizer treatment in children older than 6 years of age, patient cooperation limits its effectiveness in the emergency setting. Failure to improve with home MDI use occurs in children due to tachypnea, inability to take a breath and hold it, and inability to form a seal around the chamber mouthpiece, at which point nebulized medication becomes a necessity.

SUBCUTANEOUS EPINEPHRINE If a patient is unresponsive to the preceding therapy or respiratory distress increases, subcutaneous epinephrine should be administered while intravenous line placement is attempted. Give 0.01 mL/kg aqueous epinephrine 1:1000 to a maximum of 0.3 mL. This may be repeated every 20 to 30 min for a total of three doses.

TERBUTALINE More β_2-specific than epinephrine, terbutaline can be given SC in place of epinephrine as 0.01 mL/kg of a 1 mg/mL solution up to 0.25 mL. Nebulized terbutaline has no advantage over albuterol.

Terbutaline is the only intravenous β_2-agonist available in the United States (intravenous albuterol is available in Europe and Canada). Its use could be considered in older children who have not responded to conventional therapy. Adverse effects include myocardial ischemia and tachyarrhythmias, so continuous cardiac monitoring and intensive care admission are needed when the drug is given. Intravenously, terbutaline is given as 0.05 to 0.1 μg/kg per min.

CORTICOSTEROIDS Glucocorticoids inhibit the secretion of inflammatory leukotrienes and prostaglandins and prevent and reverse the increase in vascular permeability that leads to airway edema. They also cause an increase in density of β_2-receptors on leukocyte cell membranes and reverse tolerance to β_2-agonists.

Early administration during the course of an acute exacerbation is recommended for all patients unless (1) the PEF is greater than 50 percent *and* there is an immediate response to the first treatment or (2) when exercise-induced attacks occur in a previously well child. If the parent has already administered a dose at home, the dose can be repeated in the ED. Orally, prednisone or prednisolone is administered as 2 mg/kg. Prednisolone formulations are as follows: Pediapred 5 mg/5 mL, Prelone 15 mg/5 mL, and Orapred 15 mg/5 mL, the latter of which is reportedly more palatable. Intravenous methylprednisolone is available as Solumedrol, given as a single 2 mg/kg dose.

There is no real advantage to the administration of intravenous over oral glucocorticoids in the acute setting.[13] If a child has vomited oral medicines or is already intubated, then intravenous administration is preferred. Intramuscular administration is also an option.

While the early administration of steroids in the ED may not actually change the need for admission,[14–22] we believe that steroids treat inflammation and reduce relapse attacks and therefore should be administered as early as possible in the acute attack to prevent prolonged hospitalization.

INTRAVENOUS FLUIDS Most children presenting in status asthmaticus will be dehydrated because of increased insensible losses. Administer a bolus of fluid [20 mL/kg of NS] to aid in thinning secretions and repleting lost volume, especially in patients for whom admission seems inevitable.

ANTICHOLINERGIC THERAPY Anticholinergics are thought to prevent bronchoconstriction induced by cyclic guanosine monophosphate. Nebulized ipratropium bromide (Atrovent) may provide an additive benefit when used with albuterol,[23,24] for acute asthma. It can be mixed with albuterol solution for combined administration by nebulizer. Ipratropium is a safe drug with few side effects and may be given to patients of all ages. An MDI in combination with albuterol (Combivent) is at this time indicated for adult use only.

The dosage of nebulized ipratroprium bromide is as follows:

Adolescents >14 years of age: 500 µg in an initial nebulization
Children up to 14 years of age: 125–250 µg in an initial nebulization
Neonates: 25 µg/kg in an initial nebulization

MAGNESIUM SULFATE   The exact mechanism of action of magnesium is unknown but may resemble the tocolytic effects of magnesium sulfate on uterine smooth muscle. Patients who receive intravenous magnesium show improvement in short-term pulmonary function without adverse effects, such as low blood pressure.[25,26] Magnesium sulfate may be given as 25 to 50 mg/kg IV over 20 min; this may be repeated once to a serum magnesium level of 4 mg/dL. The maximum dose for children is 2 g. Nebulized administration is not recommended.

HELIOX   Heliox is generally available as 80:20 or 60:40 mixtures of helium and oxygen. The 60:40 mixture should be used in order to administer supplemental oxygen. If available, it may be initiated in the ED. It is recommended for the asthmatic who does not improve with conventional treatment but in whom intubation is not imminent.[27] The lower density and high diffusivity of the gas allow easier passage through turbulent obstructed airways. The peak flow rate increases, while airway resistance and work of breathing decrease. It is possible to continue to administer β$_2$-agonists during Heliox treatment.

OTHER THERAPIES   Theophylline is a competitive phosphodiesterase inhibitor that was thought to aid bronchodilation by increasing cAMP. It is no longer used routinely because it has no benefits over β$_2$-agonists for treatment, has an extremely narrow therapeutic-to-toxic ratio, has adverse central nervous system and cardiac side effects, and has multiple drug interactions. It is reserved for patients who clearly respond to it or for those who remain refractory to other modes of treatment. Aminophylline 6 mg/kg (85 percent theophylline) is given in 25 to 50 mL of NaCl IV over 20 min. If the patient is already taking theophylline but the level is subtherapeutic, a loading dose can be given [mg = (desired level − measured level)/2 × kg].

Agents for Adjunctive Ambulatory Treatment

Inhaled glucocorticoids improve long-term control of asthma, minimize the use of rescue medication, and have minimal side effects compared with systemic glucocorticoids. Table 124-7 lists doses of commonly used agents.

Cromolyn sodium has long been used to inhibit mast-cell degranulation and histamine release. It is not recommended in acute attacks.

Nedocromil (Tilade) works similarly; however, it may be effective only if strict compliance is maintained. A primary feature is that it reduces the cough component of asthma; it is also considered to be "steroid sparing."

Leukotriene receptor inhibitors (LTRIs) are increasingly popular agents for use in the outpatient prophylactic management of asthma. These medications do not supersede steroid use in acute attacks. They are classified as 5-lipoxygenase inhibitors or 5-lipoxygenase-activating protein inhibitors, of which montelukast is approved for pediatric use; zafirlukast may be used in children aged 12 years and older. Currently, only limited data are available, but the initial response is encouraging and suggests less need for medication and chronic steroid use. Although initial studies have revealed a relatively good safety profile, zafirlukast has been linked to several adult cases of Churg-Strauss syndrome[28] (granulomatous necrotizing vasculitis).

TABLE 124-7   Discharge Treatment Dosage Guidelines

Sympathomimetic agents: adrenergic agonists
  Short-acting β$_2$-agonists
    Albuterol (= salbutamol)
    Nebulizer solution (5 mg/mL) 0.05 mg/kg (min 1.25, max 2.5 mg) in
      2 to 3 mL of NS q4–6h
    Or premixed 2.5 mg/3 mL of NS q4–6h
    MDI (*Proventil HFA, Ventolin,* generic) 90 µg per puff
      1–2 puffs q3–4h
    Suspension 2 mg/5 mL, 0.1 mg/kg per dose, q6–8h
  Long-acting β$_2$-agonists
    Albuterol extended-release tablets (Repetabs, Volmax)
      0.1–0.2 mg/kg q12h
    Salmeterol (*Serevent*) 21 µg per puff q12h
Anticholinergic agents
  Ipratropium bromide (*Atrovent*)
    Nebulizer (0.25 mg/mL) 0.25–0.5 mg q6h
    MDI (18 µg per puff) 1–2 puffs q6h
Treatment of inflammation
  Glucocorticoids
    Prednisone (5-, 10-, and 20-mg tablets) 1–2 mg/kg PO qd
    Prednisolone (*Prelone, Pediapred*)
      (5 mg/5 mL, 15 mg/5 mL) 1–2 mg/kg PO qd
      "Burst dose" max 60 mg per d × 3–10 days
    Inhaled steroid preparations
      Beclomethasone
        Vanceril DS (84 µg per puff) 2 puffs bid
        Beclovent (42 µg per puff) 4 puffs bid
      Triamcinolone (*Azmacort*) (100 µg/puff) 2 puffs bid
      Flunisolide (*Aerobid*) (250 µg per puff) 2 puffs bid
      Budesonide (*Pulmicort Turbuhaler*) (100, 200, and 400 µg per puff)
        200–400 µg bid
      Fluticasone (*Flovent*) (44, 10, and 220 µg per puff) 2 puffs bid
Unclassified anti-inflammatory agents
  Cromolyn sodium (*Intal*)
    MDI (800 µg per puff) 2–4 puffs bid
    Neb (10 mg/mL) 20 mL qid
  Nedocromil (*Tilade*)
    MDI (1.75 mg per puff) 2 puffs qid
  Leukotriene receptor inhibitors
    5-Lipoxygenase inhibitors
      Zileuton (*Zyflo*) 600 mg qid (not for children age 12 and under)
    5-Lipoxygenase-activating protein inhibitors
      Zafirlukast (*Accolate*) 20 mg bid (children age 12 and up)
      Montelukast (*Singulair*) 5 mg qd (children age 6 and up)
        10 mg qd (ages 12 and up)

Interleukin 4-receptor medications are not currently approved for pediatric use.

Complications of Moderate and Severe Asthma Exacerbation

Respiratory failure may occur even if treatment is in progress, mainly from muscle fatigue. Atelectasis is common and may be responsible for the overdiagnosis of pneumonia in pediatric asthmatic patients. While pneumomediastinum is rare, children may present with vague chest pains for which a radiograph can reveal the diagnosis. Most can be managed on an outpatient basis, provided that they can be seen again within 24 h or can return to the ED quickly if respiratory distress develops. Generally, mediastinal air will resorb over 2 to 3 days. A large pneumomediastinum and/or pneumothorax requiring chest tube thoracostomy will require admission for close monitoring and observation.

Reassessment and Disposition

Treatment algorithms greatly simplify the decision of whether or not a child should be admitted. Disposition can be made after 2 to 4 h of therapy for patients who remain stable (Table 124-8). A child who does not respond after 2 h of continuous treatment whose $Paco_2$ is greater than 40 mm Hg should be admitted to an intensive care unit for continuous therapy. Children with oxygen requirements, refractory asthma, and/or dyspnea on exertion may be admitted to the floor. If parents of children with newly diagnosed asthma do not feel comfortable taking care of their children even with adequate teaching, admission may be warranted (this also applies to patients with mild attacks requiring nebulization but with limited resources and inability to obtain nebulizers on weekends and at night).

An intubated patient or patient requiring continuous nebulization should be transported to a facility with pediatric intensivist capability by advanced life support (ALS) providers with pediatric airway experience.

Discharge Instructions and Ambulatory Treatment

Children responding well to conventional therapy may be discharged after 2 to 4 h of treatment. A short ED observation period is recommended for patients with an incomplete response but acceptable PEFR. Detailed discharge instructions should outline medication administration, inhaler use, and follow-up (see Table 124-7). No child should be discharged without an MDI and spacer, and prescriptions for oral glucocorticoids are generally recommended unless the attack was extremely mild (resolved with minimal treatment) or exercise-induced. A tapered dose generally is not needed for "burst dose" (3- to 10-day) therapy[29] because the side effect of adrenal suppression with prolonged use is unlikely to occur. Of the two most common forms of methylprednisolone, Pediapred is reported to taste better than Prelone; however, its lower concentration requires that three times the volume of Prelone be given for the same dose. Orapred may be prescribed instead of Prelone but is not widely available.

A courtesy call to the private pediatrician of the child who has been treated for asthma in the ED should be made because it facilitates continuity of care for the child and ensures follow-up. All children should be referred to their pediatrician for follow-up within 24 h.

BRONCHIOLITIS

Bronchiolitis, or inflammation of the bronchioles, is the term applied to the clinical syndrome of wheezing, chest retractions, and tachypnea in children younger than age 2 years; it causes more significant illness in infants younger than 6 months of age.

Epidemiology

Peak prevalence is from late October to May. The peak age of incidence in urban populations is 2 months and results in hospitalizations lasting 5 to 7 days. Disease in older children is usually milder.

Pathophysiology

Respiratory syncytial virus (RSV) causes 50 to 70 percent of clinically significant bronchiolitis. Non-RSV bronchiolitis is caused by influen-

zavirus, parinfluenzavirus, echovirus, and rhinovirus. *Mycoplasma pneumoniae* and *Chlamydia trachomatis* also produce symptoms. Adenovirus causes a particularly destructive form, bronchiolitis obliterans, observed in native Canadian Eskimo populations.

The highly infectious RSV is transmitted by direct contact with large droplets of secretions and self-inoculation by contaminated hands via the eyes and nose. No significant transmission occurs by small-particle aerosol. RSV-infected secretions remain infectious on countertops for more than 6 h. Strict attention to hand washing and use of masks and gloves can prevent transmission. RSV is shed from the respiratory tract of symptomatic and asymptomatic patients for up to 9 days. Immunocompromised patients may continue to shed for up to 6 weeks. Immunity to the virus is variable owing to antigenic diversity, so reinfection does occur. No vaccine has yet been developed.

Mucous plugging results from necrosis of the respiratory epithelium and destruction of ciliated epithelial cells. This and submucosal edema lead to peripheral airway narrowing and variable obstruction, with areas of patchy atelectasis or overdistention in lung segments. Progressive disease causes severe pneumonia, with extensive destruction of respiratory epithelium, parenchymal necrosis, and formation of hyaline membranes. Bronchiolar regeneration occurs within 3 to 4 days; however, cilia may take as long as 15 days to regenerate.

Increased airway resistance and decreased compliance result in increased work of breathing. Like the infant with lower airway obstruction, the infant with bronchiolitis breathes at higher lung volumes due to uneven resistance within the lung. Alteration of gas exchange results from the patchy atelectasis and airway obstruction.

Clinical Features

Symptoms can vary from minimal rhinorrhea to bronchiolitis or pneumonia and respiratory failure. Severe illness and apnea are more likely to occur in children with a history of prematurity, cystic fibrosis, congenital heart disease, or immunocompromise.

Infection begins with nasal discharge, pharyngitis, and cough. Fever accompanies the first few days of illness, with temperatures as high as 40°C (104°F). The parent brings the child to the ED because of wheezing, increased respiratory symptoms, nasal congestion, and difficulty feeding. Symptoms reach a peak at 3 to 5 days, generally resolving in 2 weeks with normalization of pulmonary function. Resulting wheezing can persist for weeks to months.

Physical findings include tachypnea greater than 50 to 60 breaths/min, tachycardia, mild conjunctivitis, chest retractions, prolonged expiration with hyperresonant chest, wheezes throughout, and hypoxemia. The most reliable clinical finding that correlates with hypoxemia is tachypnea, which signifies serious impairment of gas exchange. The hypoxemic child with bronchiolitis may not show cyanosis. The severity of wheezing or intercostal retractions also will not correlate with the severity of hypoxemia. Respiratory rate must be followed, but this may be difficult because variation occurs with fever and crying. Abnormal pulse oximetry is a predictor of severe disease, and most children with saturations of <90–93 percent will need admission.

YOUNG INFANTS AND APNEA The mechanism inducing RSV-related apnea in young infants is not completely understood but may be related to hypoxemia and upper airway obstruction.[30] Infants at highest risk are younger than 6 weeks old and have a history of prematurity, apnea of prematurity, and low O_2 saturation on admission. It is difficult to predict apneic events. The severity of wheezing and retractions does not correlate with frequency of apnea, and most infants younger than 1 month of age will have atypical disease and may present without wheezing and retractions. Apneic infants may require intubation during the course of the illness, sometimes requiring mechanical ventilation for up to a week or more. After extubation, these infants are not at higher risk of apnea and may be discharged without apnea monitors.

TABLE 124-8   Admission Criteria

Respiratory failure requiring intubation
Status asthmaticus:
  Persistent retractions, tachypnea
  Oxygen requirement after 2 h of therapy
Return ED visit within 24 h
Limited home resources
Pneumothorax
Complete lobar atelectasis
Large pneumomediastinum
Underlying cardiopulmonary disease

Children with underlying diseases such as bronchopulmonary dysplasia, cystic fibrosis, immunodeficiency, or congenital heart defects are at increased risk of severe RSV infection. Care must be taken in treating infants with a history of BPD because many will have a tendency toward chronic CO_2 retention. Since hypoxemia remains the major respiratory stimulus in this population, supplemental oxygen may cause further CO_2 retention; therefore, saturations of 94 to 95 percent are acceptable standards in such patients.

Numerous retrospective analyses and observations note that children with bronchiolitis as infants frequently develop asthma later on.[31]

Diagnosis

The diagnosis of bronchiolitis is suggested by clinical presentation, patient age, and history of RSV exposure or community epidemic. Immunofluorescence assays currently available are extremely sensitive but not necessary for all patients. We feel that a confirmatory test for RSV is unnecessary unless admission is being considered and then only for bed-placement purposes as deemed by individual hospitals. Since the prevalence of RSV during an epidemic is so high, routine testing is costly and is best reserved for children with predisposing medical conditions or complicated disease courses.

Complete blood counts and chemistries may not be helpful in diagnosis. The white blood cell count can be normal or elevated with a left shift. An elevated band count may be present. Chemistries should be obtained if there is poor feeding or evidence of dehydration. Chest radiography to rule out pneumonia is indicated for children with concurrent cardiopulmonary illness or those who are ill-appearing and hypoxemic and may reveal patchy atelectasis, segmental atelectasis, hyperinflation, and peribronchial thickening. The history should include questioning about possible ingestion; salicylate ingestion may present with respiratory distress and mixed metabolic acidosis and respiratory alkalosis, and β-blocker ingestions can exacerbate wheezing.

Emergency Department Management

GENERAL CARE   During RSV epidemics, the emergency physician will be exposed to a broad spectrum of patients at varying stages of disease and must be able to identify those who need admission and those who are at risk for apnea. Most cases of bronchiolitis are treated on an outpatient basis, for which follow-up in 24 h with a private pediatrician is essential. Infants in respiratory failure will require emergent intubation and admission to the intensive care unit.

Children with suspected respiratory compromise should be monitored carefully, including continuous pulse oximetry and cardiac monitor. Treatment is mainly supportive, the most important therapy being supplemental humidified oxygen. At concentrations of 28 to 40 percent, arterial hypoxemia is improved in most infants.

Increased insensible fluid loss occurs from increased work of breathing and can cause significant dehydration that warrants a 20 mL/kg NS bolus. Patients with poor fluid intake due to congestion also may require intravenous hydration and admission (especially if parents are unable to feed the child owing to uncontrollable secretions). Beyond initial resuscitation, fluid replacement should not exceed maintenance due to the potential for the development of pulmonary edema in some of these children.

Fever should be controlled with acetaminophen or ibuprofen. A 9-year prospective study of 565 children with documented RSV infection showed that the risk of secondary bacterial infection was low; subsequent secondary bacterial infections were seen more frequently in the group treated with antibiotics. Studies have failed to show any utility in obtaining blood cultures in children with fever attributable to RSV. Infants with high temperatures and documented RSV therefore are unlikely to require workup for occult bacteremia *unless they appear septic.* A complete blood count should be drawn from children *who appear toxic* and have a temperature above 38.5°C (101.3°F) to rule out intercurrent infections. Antibiotics should be reserved for concurrent otitis media or other identifiable bacterial infections.

RACEMIC EPINEPHRINE   Racemic epinephrine is an effective treatment for the wheezing of bronchiolitis. Nebulized racemic epinephrine has been compared with albuterol and found to reduce hospitalizations in children with bronchiolitis,[32] improving symptom scores of respiratory rate, wheezing, and retractions at 15 min compared with nebulized saline.[33] The exact mechanism of its action in bronchiolitis is unknown. It can be used safely in hospitalized children up to every 2 h as a 0.1% solution (0.5 mL in 3.5 mL of NS). If used in the ED, we recommend an observation period of 4 h before a disposition decision is made. Generally, infants and children showing minimal response or deterioration after a single treatment will require hospitalization.

ALBUTEROL AND IPRATROPIUM   Unless there is a history of asthma, there is a limited role for bronchodilator therapy in the treatment of bronchiolitis. A trial of bronchodilator therapy, however, is an optional and reasonable treatment and can be aborted if the child fails to show a response. Many studies of oral and nebulized albuterol alone show that it fails to improve oxygen saturation or to reduce the length of hospitalizations,[34–36] leading some authors to question the benefit of such therapy. Ipatropium also does not affect the natural course of the disease,[37] although anecdotes suggest that it may have a role in drying up secretions.

HELIOX   Heliox may be considered for children with severe obstructive symptoms and works for the same reasons as in asthma. A recent study[38] showed that its use increased SaO_2 in children when compared with oxygen alone. Its can be a useful bridge in reducing the need for intubation in certain populations of infected children.

Other Treatment Modalities

GLUCOCORTICOIDS   Controlled studies have failed to demonstrate any proven benefit to the use of glucocorticoids, including studies on oral prednisolone and dexamethasone.[39] We do not recommend the use of glucocorticoids unless there is a history of asthma; however, these drugs have been helpful in infants with a history of BPD. Initial reports on budesonide, a smaller molecule that has been studied widely in Europe and Australia, suggest a benefit. In a Finnish study[40] of 100 patients, budesonide was seen to reduce the number of hospital admissions and subsequent wheezing episodes as compared with controls. A more recent study on nebulized budesonide[41] stated that its effects in preventing postbronchiolitic wheezing were unremarkable. It is currently being introduced in the United States in a MDI form, and more studies need to be performed before it can be recommended routinely.

RIBAVIRIN   Ribavirin is a guanosine-resembling synthetic nucleoside analogue generally used as inpatient therapy. When delivered as a small-particle aerosol, it has produced improvement in oxygenation. It is thought to work by decreasing viral protein synthesis. Candidates for such treatment are those with immunodeficiency, cystic fibrosis, congenital heart disease, and severe illnesses of infancy. Since the introduction of intravenous immunoglobin, the use of ribavirin appears to be less frequent.

RESPIGAM RSV IMMUNE GLOBULIN INTRAVENOUS (HUMAN)   RespiGam has been in use for the past few years as outpatient passive immunization for infants at risk for severe RSV disease. The treatment involves monthly intravenous infusions of immunoglobulin during

RSV season. It is recommended for infants with documented BPD and for those with a gestational age of less than 35 weeks (at the discretion of the physician). The PREVENT study[42] demonstrated a reduction in the incidence and duration of RSV hospitalization and severity of illness.

PALIVIZUMAB (SYNAGIS)   Palivizumab is the first monoclonal antibody that can be given by intramuscular injection to provide protection against infection (protein binding neutralizes the virus). Like RespiGam, it is administered monthly to patients at highest risk and is desirable for children in whom vascular access is a challenge. The Impact-RSV trial showed a 55 percent reduction in hospitalizations in a group of 1500 patients, with few adverse effects.

Disposition

Parents should be educated on the natural course of RSV infection and how to identify markers of respiratory distress. Infants with visible moderate to severe respiratory distress, hypoxia, apneic spells, or dehydration should be admitted to the intensive care unit. Infants without wheezing but with sustained tachypnea (RR >60 breaths/min) also should be admitted, preferably to a step-down unit. Hospitalization should be considered in all infants with a history of BPD, congenital heart disease, and immunocompromise. Infants and children with resting oxygen saturations of less than 93 percent should be evaluated carefully for possible admission.

Those with mild disease who are taking fluids well and whose parents are capable of taking care of them may be released with good follow-up instructions. Home health visits and nebulizers may be instituted if deemed necessary. Parents should be instructed on how to perform aggressive nasal suctioning and evaluate respiratory distress. Albuterol in syrup form also may be initiated, but only for children who respond to nebulized albuterol in the ED. Use of vapor solutions available over the counter should be discouraged, and parents who smoke cigarettes should be cautioned that tobacco smoke worsens the illness. Decongestants and antihistamines are of questionable benefit; their use in infants younger than 6 months of age is not recommended.

REFERENCES

1. Expert Panel Report 2: *Guidelines for the Diagnosis and Management of Asthma*, 1997. National Institutes of Health Publication No. 98-4051. Bethesda, MD, NIH, 1997.
2. Surveillance for asthma—United States, 1960–1995. *MMWR* 47:6, 1998.
3. Surveillance for asthma—United States, 1960–1995. *MMWR* 47:14, 1998.
4. Calmes D, Leake BD, Carlisle DM: Adverse outcomes among children hospitalized with asthma in California. *Pediatrics* 101:845, 1998.
5. Surveillance for asthma—United States, 1960–1995. *MMWR* 47:7, 1998.
6. Surveillance for asthma—United States, 1960–1995. *MMWR* 47:16, 1998.
7. Goodman DC, Stukel TA, Chang CH: Trends in pediatric asthma hospitalization rates: Regional and socioeconomic differences. *Pediatrics* 101:208, 1998.
8. McFadden ER, Gilbert IA: Asthma. *New Engl J Med* 327:1928, 1992.
9. Katz RW, Kelly HW, Crowley MR, et al: Safety of continuous nebulized albuterol for bronchospasm in infants and children. *Pediatrics* 92:666, 1993.
10. Buck M: Administration of albuterol by continuous nebulization. *AACN Clin Iss* 6:279, 1995.
11. Williams JR, Bothner JP, Swanton RD: Delivery of albuterol in a pediatric emergency department. *Pediatr Emerg Care* 12:263, 1996.
12. Suissa S, Ernst P, Boivin JF, et al: A cohort analysis of excess mortality in asthma and use of inhaled beta-agonists. *Am J Respir Crit Care Med* 149:604, 1994.
13. Barnett PL, Caputo GL, Baskin M, Kuppermann J: Intravenous versus oral corticosteroids in management of acute asthma in children. *Ann Emerg Med* 29:212, 1997.
14. Tal A, Levy N, Bearman JE: Methylprednisolone therapy for acute asthma in infants and toddlers: A controlled clinical trial. *Pediatrics* 86:350, 1990.
15. Scarfone RJ, Fuchs SM, Nager AL, et al: Controlled clinical trial of oral prednisone in emergency department treatment of children with acute asthma. *Pediatrics* 92:513, 1993.
16. Rodrigo C, Rodrigo O: Early administration of hydrocortisone in emergency room treatment of acute asthma. *Respir Med* 88:755, 1994.
17. Wolfson DH, Nypaver MM, Blaser M, et al: A controlled trial of methylprednisolone in early ED treatment of acute asthma in children. *Pediatr Emerg Care* 10:335, 1994.
18. Lin RY, Resola GR, Westfal RE, et al: Early parenteral corticosteroids administration in acute asthma. *Am J Emerg Med* 15:621, 1997.
19. Dales RE, Schweitzer I, Kerr P, et al: Risk factors for recurrent emergency department visits for asthma. *Thorax* 50:520, 1995.
20. Laitinen LA, Laitinen A: Remodeling of asthmatic airways by glucocorticosteroids. *J Allergy Clin Immunol* 97:153, 1996.
21. deBlic J, Delacourt C, Le Bourgeois M, et al: Efficacy of nebulized budesonide in treatment of severe infantile asthma: A double blind study. *J Allergy Clin Immunol* 98:14, 1996.
22. Sung L, Osmond MH, Klassen TP: Randomized, controlled of inhaled budesonide as an adjunct to oral prednisone in acute asthma. *Acad Emerg Med* 5:209, 1998.
23. Schuh S, Johnson DW, Callahan S, et al: Efficacy of frequent nebulized ipatropium bromide added to frequent high dose albuterol therapy in severe childhood asthma. *J Pediatr* 126:639, 1995.
24. Qureshi F, Pestian J, Davis P, Zaritsky A: Effective nebulized ipratropium on the hospitalization rates of children with asthma. *New Engl J Med* 8:1030, 1998.
25. Ciarallo L, Sauer AH, Shannon MW: IV Mg therapy for moderate to severe pediatric asthma: Results of a randomized, placebo-controlled trial. *J Pediatr* 129:809, 1996.
26. Devi PR, Kumar L, Singhi SC, et al: IV MgSO4 in acute severe asthma not responding to conventional therapy. *Indian Pediatr* 34:389, 1997.
27. Kudukis TM, Manthous CA, Schmidt GA, et al: Inhaled Heliox revisited: Effect of inhaled helium oxygen mixture during treatment of status asthmaticus in children. *J Pediatr* 130:217, 1997.
28. Holloway J, Ferriss J, Groff J, et al: Churg-Strauss syndrome associated with zafirlukast. *J Am Osteopath Assoc* 98:275, 1998.
29. Cydulka RK, Emerman CL: A pilot study of steroid therapy after emergency department treatment of acute asthma: Is a taper needed? *J Emerg Med* 16:15, 1998.
30. Church NR, Anas NG, Hall CB, Brooks JG: RSV-related apnea in infants: Demographics and outcome. *Am J Dis Child* 138:247, 1984.
31. Korrpi M, Kuikka L, Reijomen T, et al: Bronchial asthma and hyperreactivity after early childhood bronchiolitis or pneumonia: An 8-year follow up study. *Arch Pediatr Adolesc Med* 148:1079, 1994.
32. Menon K, Sutcliffe T, Klassen TP: A randomized trial comparing the efficacy of epinephrine with salbutamol in the treatment of acute bronchiolitis. *J Pediatr* 126:1004, 1995.
33. Reijnonen T, Korppi M, Pitkakangas S, et al: The clinical efficacy of nebulized racemic epinephrine and albuterol in acute bronchiolitis. *Arch Pediatr Adolesc Med* 149:686, 1995.
34. Dobson JV, Stephens-Groff SM, McMahon SR, et al: The use of albuterol in hospitalized infants with bronchiolitis. *Pediatrics* 101(3 pt 1):361, 1998.
35. Lugo RA, Salyer JW, Dean JM: Albuterol in acute bronchiolitis-continued therapy despite poor response? *Pharmacotherapy* 18:198, 1998.
36. Cengizlier R, Saraclar Y, Adalioglu G, Tuncer A: Effect of oral and inhaled salbutamol in infants with bronchiolitis. *Acta Paediatr Jpn* 39:61, 1997.
37. Chowdury D, al Howasi M, Khalil M, et al: The role of bronchodilators in the management of bronchiolitis: A clinical trial. *Ann Trop Paediatr* 15:77, 1995.
38. Hollman G, Shen G, Zeng L, et al: Helium-oxygen improves clinical asthma scores in children with acute bronchiolitis. *Crit Care Med* 26:1731, 1998.
39. Klassen TP, Sutcliffe T, Watters LK, et al: Dexamethasone in salbutamol-treated inpatients with acute bronchiolitis: A randomized controlled trial. *J Pediatr* 130:191, 1997.
40. Reijnonen T, Korppi M, Kuikka L, et al: Anti-inflammatory therapy reduces wheezing after bronchiolitis. *Arch Pediatr Adolesc Med* 150:512, 1996.
41. Richter H, Seddon P: Early nebulized budesonide in treatment of bronchiolitis and prevention of post-bronchiolitis wheezing. *J Pediatr* 132:849, 1998.
42. The PREVENT Study Group: Reduction of RSV Hospitalization Among Premature Infants and Infants with Bronchopulmonary Dysplasia Using RSV Immune Globulin prophylaxis. *Pediatrics* 99:93, 1997.

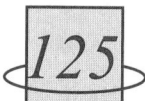

125 SEIZURES AND STATUS EPILEPTICUS IN CHILDREN
Michael A. Nigro

In children aged 0 to 9 years, the prevalence of seizures is 4.4 cases per 1000, and in those 10 to 19 years, the prevalence is 6.6 cases per 1000. Simple febrile convulsions constitute a separate category, with an incidence of 3 to 4 percent in children.

These numbers alone do not reveal the most important features of the seizure phenomenon: the increased morbidity and mortality rates that are a direct result of seizures, their cause, or their treatment. The overall mortality rate is two to three times higher in epileptic than in nonepileptic patients. The earlier the onset of seizures and the more deprived the social environment, the higher the morbidity and mortality rates are.

This chapter reviews pediatric seizures in the following clinical categories:

1. The first seizure
2. Breakthrough seizures in a known epileptic
3. Febrile seizures
4. Neonatal seizures
5. Infantile spasms
6. Seizures associated with head trauma
7. Status epilepticus

Emergency care should include (1) safely stopping the seizure, (2) identifying and immediately correcting treatable or reversible causes, and (3) initiating appropriate diagnostic studies and determining whether admission is needed or whether outpatient follow-up is appropriate. The differences in the treatment of children are distinctive enough so that, unless the physician is experienced in pediatric management or able to readily obtain pediatric or neurologic consultation, the child should be transferred to a pediatric facility.

ETIOLOGY

A *seizure* is an episodic alteration in motor activity, behavior, sensation, or autonomic function. It represents an abrupt change in brain function. The term *epilepsy* indicates recurring seizures without a simple discernible and reversible cause.

Physiologically, a seizure is an abnormal, sudden, and excessive electrical discharge of neurons (gray matter) that propagates down the neuronal processes (white matter) to affect end organs in a clinically measurable fashion. The International Classification of Epileptic Seizures is still accepted as the contemporary standard[1] (Table 125-1).

Seizures are also categorized by presumed cause: *primary, idiopathic,* or *secondary;* due to prior neurologic insult; or some underlying metabolic, structural, inflammatory, or systemic disorder. Diagnosis, treatment, and disposition strategies depend on the clinical status of the patient and the underlying cause.

Idiopathic seizures account for about 25 to 50 percent of children seen with seizures, depending on the study cited. Secondary seizures occur for a wide variety of reasons (e.g., inflammatory, structural, metabolic, or secondary to general illness). In such cases, correction of the primary problem is necessary. Thus, the primary goal of seizure evaluation is to uncover disorders that are readily identifiable and reversible.

Correcting the metabolic abnormality treats seizures due to hypoglycemia, hypocalcemia, and electrolyte imbalance. Seizures can be a complication of disorders such as systemic lupus erythematosus, sickle cell anemia, leukemia, arteriovenous malformations, or neoplasms. Seizures have been reported in children after topical application of *N,N*-diethyl-*m*-toluamide, and lindane (Kwell). Toxic ingestions of substances such as camphor, theophylline, isoniazid, tricyclic antidepressants, oral and parenteral meperidine, cyclosporine,

TABLE 125-1   International Classification of Epileptic Seizures

Partial seizures (seizures beginning focally)
　Partial seizures with elementary symptomatology (generally without impairment of consciousness)
　　With motor symptoms (includes Jacksonian seizures)
　　With special sensory or somatosensory symptoms
　　With autonomic symptoms
　　Compound forms
　Partial seizures with complex symptomatology (generally with impairment of consciousness)
　　With impairment of consciousness only
　　With cognitive symptomatology
　　With affective symptomatology
　　With "psychosensory" symptomatology
　　With "psychomotor" symptomatology
　　Compound forms
　Partial seizures secondary generalized
Generalized seizures (bilaterally symmetric without localized onset)
　Absences (petit mal)
　Bilateral massive epileptic myoclonus
　Infantile spasms
　Clonic seizures
　Tonic seizures
　Tonic–clonic seizures (grand mal)
　Atonic seizures
　Akinetic seizures
Unclassified epileptic seizures

Source: Reprinted with permission from Gestaut H: Clinical and electroencephalographic classification of epileptic seizures. *Epilepsia* 11:102, 1970.

methylphenidate, lead, and mercury can cause seizures. Viral and bacterial meningitis, viral encephalitis, brain abscess, and more uncommon problems such as cat-scratch fever and mycoplasma-related encephalopathy may present with seizures. In a child with a ventriculoperitoneal shunt, seizures can arise from associated cerebral abnormalities or shunt malfunction. Unfortunately, one must always be alert to nonaccidental trauma (shaken baby syndrome) as a cause of new onset seizures.

ELECTROENCEPHALOGRAPHY

Electroencephalographic (EEG) recording on an emergent basis is important to diagnose nonconvulsive status epilepticus. In this condition, the patient seems to be seizure free but is unresponsive. The EEG demonstrates subclinical status epilepticus. In a child who unexpectedly remains comatose or in a neonate in whom clinical seizures may be difficult to detect, immediate and continuous EEG monitoring may more effectively direct aggressive antiepileptic drug (AED) treatment.

NEUROIMAGING IN EPILEPSY

The choice of central nervous system (CNS) imaging depends in part on the circumstances and the age of the patient:

1. For neonates and young infants, cerebral ultrasound is a quick and relatively reliable method to identify intraventricular and parenchymal hemorrhage, periventricular leukomalacia, major malformations, cerebral edema, and hydrocephalus.
2. Computed tomography (CT) is needed to evaluate seizures associated with head trauma or mass lesions.
3. Magnetic resonance imaging (MRI) is preferred for evaluating migrational defects, mesial temporal sclerosis, acute parainfectious disseminated encephalomyelitis, stroke, and neoplasm.
4. Magnetic resonance angiography is best for defining vascular abnormalities, stroke, and stroke-like events.
5. Transcranial Doppler sonography can be helpful in determining impending cerebrovascular occlusive disease of sickle cell anemia.

NEWER ANTIEPILEPTIC DRUGS

Newer AEDs are generally indicated in the management of seizures as add-on drugs, although there are currently numerous studies determining their value for initial and monotherapy.

Gabapentin

Gabapentin (Neurontin) is a novel AED with ill-defined mechanism of action, although it appears to increase the effect of γ-aminobutyric acid (GABA), the major cerebral inhibitor. It has no drug interactions, is not metabolized, and is not protein bound. It is excreted solely by the kidneys. The short half-life of 5 to 6 h and the limited intestinal absorption capability require frequent dosing of three to four times a day. Dosage is 20 to 60 mg/kg per d, and maximal dosage can be reached in several days. Side effects are mild, self-limiting, and usually consist of vertigo, lightheadedness, and infrequently, behavioral changes. Rarely, myoclonic seizures have been provoked soon after initiating the drug. Antiepileptic drug levels are not useful in determining therapeutic and toxic effects.

Lamotrigine

Lamotrigine (Lamictal) probably acts on voltage-sensitive sodium channels and excitatory amino acid neurotransmitters. **Two very important features of lamotrigine include the adverse effect of rash, which can progress to Stevens-Johnson syndrome, and drug interactions.** The incidence of serious rash has been reduced by lower dosing regimens. The half-life of lamotrigine is reduced by 50 percent when administered with enzyme inducers, such as phenytoin, carbamazepine, and phenobarbital, and is doubled when used in conjunction with valproate. The combination with valproate has been associated with most adverse reactions.

Lamotrigine is indicated in the treatment of partial and generalized epilepsy, including absence, drop, and myoclonic seizures. When administered with enzyme inducers, the dose begins at 2 mg/kg per d and is increased over 8 to 12 weeks to a maximum of 15 mg/kg per d. When used with valproate (Depakote), it should be started at 0.2 mg/kg every other day, increased by 0.2 mg/kg per d to 1 mg/kg per d, and over the next 8 to 12 weeks increased to a maximum of 5 mg/kg per d. When changes are made in reducing or introducing co-medication, the lamotrigine dose will have to be modified in most instances. Given as monotherapy, the half-life is 25 to 30 h. It has minimal protein binding. Blood levels do not reflect toxic or therapeutic effects. There is no reported significant hepatic or hematologic side effect.

Topiramate

Topiramate (Topamax) became available in 1997. It acts on the GABAergic system, sodium channels, and glutamate receptors by preventing the propagation of the seizure from its focus. The half-life is 19 to 23 h, so the drug can be given twice a day. Eighty-five percent of the drug is eliminated unchanged through the kidneys, and 15 percent is metabolized by the hepatic P-450 system. It is indicated in the treatment of partial seizures and is being evaluated as monotherapy. In children, the drug is begun slowly at 1 mg/kg per d and over 8 to 12 weeks is gradually increased to a maximum of 10 mg/kg per d or 400 mg/d, if necessary. In infants the dose is increased to 20 mg/kg per d in view of greater drug clearance. The major side effect limiting dosage and rate of incrementing dosage is the effect on memory and name recall.

Tiagabine

Tiagabine (Gabitril) is a GABA reuptake inhibitor, which inhibits epileptic excitatory activity. With a relatively short half-life of 5 to 8 h, the drug can be administered three times a day. Absorption is slower and the drug more easily tolerated when given with meals.

Metabolism is via the P-450 mechanism and, as a result, the half-life is significantly reduced by co-administration with enzyme inducers, such as carbamazepine, phenytoin, and phenobarbital. The maximum effective dose in children at this time is estimated to be 1 mg/kg per d. This dose should be started at 0.1 mg/kg per d and gradually increased over the next 6 to 10 weeks. Because of high protein binding, free levels of co-administered AEDs should be monitored (phenytoin, carbamazepine, and valproate). Most common side effects are sedation, behavioral changes, and activation of myoclonic seizures.

Oxcarbazepine

Oxcarbazepine (Trileptal) is a 10-keto analogue of carbamazepine. Its active metabolite is a monohydroxy derivative that has a half-life of 10 h, allowing for a twice-daily dosing. It is begun at 10 mg/kg per d and increased to a maximum of 60 mg/kg per d or to tolerance and seizure control. It is approved for use as adjunctive treatment of partial epilepsies. It can be used in combination with any of the existing AEDs, including carbamazepine. Unlike carbamazepine, it has no epoxide metabolites and is not affected by erythromycin. It does interact with anovulatory agents in a manner similar to that of carbamazepine by decreasing their effect at low doses, and hence warrants a caution to sexually active teens.

Depacon

Depacon is the intravenous preparation of valproate. It is usually administered intravenously when the oral maintenance dose cannot be tolerated. Dosage is the usual maintenance dose administered IV over 15 min. The loading dose is 10 to 30 mg/kg IV over 15 min.

Extended-Release Agents

Carbatrol and Tegretol XR are extended-release forms of carbamazepine that permit bid dosing.

Fosphenytoin

Fosphenytoin (Cerebyx) is a prodrug of phenytoin that contains a disodium phosphate ester that is cleaved during hydrolysis, yielding a molecule of phenytoin. Phosphatases are ubiquitous and present in newborns, so fosphenytoin can be used at any age. It is water soluble and can be given intravenously and intramuscularly without soft tissue injury. A 1 mg phenytoin equivalent (PE) is the therapeutic equivalent of 1 mg of phenytoin. Fosphenytoin can be infused at 3 mg PE/kg per min, with therapeutic free phenytoin levels achieved by 7 to 8 min after infusion and 30 min after intramuscular use. Rapid infusion in alert patients may produce perineal pruritus.

Zonisamide

Zonisamide (Zonegran) is a sulfonamide indicated as adjunctive therapy for partial seizures in adults. Studies are currently underway in the United States to determine the safety and effectiveness in children, but zonisamide is used extensively in Japan in the pediatric population. Oligohidrosis and hyperthermia have been described in children as a complication of the drug. It is also contraindicated in patients with hypersensitivity to sulfonamides. Zonisamide has a long half-life of 60 to 80 h, and enzyme-inducing drugs (i.e., carbamazepine, phenytoin, and phenobarbital) increase drug clearance. Dosage begins at 1 mg/kg per d and is increased every 2 weeks at a rate of 1 to 2 mg/kg per d until seizure cessation, or a maximum of 12 mg/kg per d.

Levetiracetam

Levetiracetam (Keppra) is a novel AED indicated for adjunctive therapy for the treatment of partial seizures in adults, and studies are currently investigating the safety and effectiveness in children. Levetiracetam is not protein bound, and there have been no significant drug interactions reported with other AEDs. In adults the plasma half-life is 6 to 8 h, and 66 percent of the dose is renally excreted unchanged. In children the clearance is 40 percent higher than in adults. Dosage is initiated at 10 mg/kg per d and increased by 10 to 20 mg/kg per d every 2 weeks to a target dose of 40 to 60 mg/kg per d.

ADDITIONAL ADVANCES IN EPILEPSY TREATMENT

Vagus Nerve Stimulation

The Cyberonics vagus nerve stimulator (NeuroCybernetic Prosthesis System) is programmed to deliver a stimulus at a specific intensity and frequency for a specific interval (e.g., 15 s every 3 min). Although the mechanism of action is uncertain, electrical stimulus of the left vagus nerve can significantly reduce seizure frequency. Common side effects include hoarseness and difficulty swallowing during stimulation. Problems with instrumentation are unlikely to warrant an ED visit. If a patient is experiencing significant discomfort upon activation of the vagus nerve stimulator, the stimulator can be temporarily turned off by taping a magnet over the subcutaneous pacemaker.

Ketogenic Diet

Ketones are an alternative energy source for cerebral metabolism. By severely restricting glucose and increasing fat intake, ketosis can be maintained and seizure control improved. There are several concerns about an ED visit that warrant mention. **It is necessary to maintain ketosis; as a result, glucose infusions should be avoided, if possible, and prescriptions given should have no measurable carbohydrate content. Renal calculi and pancreatitis are two complications of the ketogenic diet.**

THE FIRST SEIZURE

Immediate anticonvulsant treatment is not needed unless the child is in status epilepticus or seizures recur in the ED[2] (Tables 125-2 to 125-4). Instead, the emergency physician can concentrate on defining the cause and determining the appropriate disposition.

History

For a first seizure, the history should be directed to the identification of risk factors for underlying neurologic or metabolic abnormality and risk factors for neurologic morbidity from seizure. **Risk factors include a family or sibling history of seizures, presence of underlying neurologic abnormality, and a history of trauma, focal seizure, or seizure lasting longer than 2 min.**

Examination and Evaluation

On physical examination, vital signs and careful physical and neurologic examinations are needed. Physical examination should assess for underlying metabolic or neurologic abnormalities, including evidence of trauma, abnormal head size, abnormal facies or body habitus suggestive of genetic abnormality, petechiae, café-au-lait spots, or adenoma sebaceum. Clinical evaluation for sources of infection, including ears, mastoids, soft tissue, chest, gastrointestinal tract, and urine, should be done. Neurologic examination must be thorough to detect any abnormality such as meningismus, distended fontanelle, cranial nerve abnormalities, or focal weakness.

Suggested laboratory studies are outlined in Table 125-2. Head CT scan is generally obtained and necessary in the ED if there are focal neurologic signs on examination, if the seizure was described as focal by the caregivers, or if there is suspicion of trauma or abuse. Fever and

TABLE 125-2   Evaluation for Neonatal Seizure, First Seizure, or Status Epilepticus (SE)

Clinical assessment
   History
   Physical examination
   Neurologic examination
Laboratory tests/procedures
   Stat bedside glucose
   CBC
   Na, K, Cl, CO_2, calcium, magnesium
   BUN, creatinine
   Urinalysis
   Consider depending on age and presentation:
      Toxicology screen
      Urine and serum amino acid screen
      Serum ammonia
      Liver function tests
      Arterial blood gases for SE or persistent altered mental status
      PCR for herpes, cytomegalovirus, and others
      EEG if nonconvulsive status suspected
      EEG for neonates
      Lumbar puncture if meningitis suspected
Imaging studies
   Head CT for trauma, altered mental status
   MRI for suspected dysplastic disorders
   Chest x-ray
   Skeletal survey if abuse suspected

Abbreviations: BUN = blood urea nitrogen; CBC = complete blood count; CT = computed tomography; EEG = electroencephalogram; MRI = magnetic resonance imaging; PCR = polymerase chain reaction.

suspicion of meningitis requires appropriate intravenous antibiotics (see Chap. 116) followed by CT (depending on clinical evaluation) and lumbar puncture. In the patient with trauma or persistent altered mental status after a first seizure, head CT should be obtained. If the child is fully recovered with no deficit, an MRI is preferred, because CNS dysplasias are not readily identifiable by CT.

Disposition

A child with a first focal seizure or any suspected or proven underlying neurologic or systemic abnormality should be admitted and neurologic consultation obtained. Children with a brief, non-focal first seizure, normal recovery, normal neurologic examination, and normal laboratory and radiologic results in the ED can be discharged after neurologic consultation and after arrangements have been made for follow-up.

In general, the EEG can be done on an outpatient basis. Antiepileptic drugs may or may not be started in the ED, depending on the recommendation of the consultant.

BREAKTHROUGH SEIZURES IN KNOWN EPILEPTICS

When seizures recur in known epileptics, something has occurred to alter the balance of the excitation-inhibition complex, causing the seizure threshold to be lowered. Complete seizure control is not always possible. A child with mental retardation, cerebral palsy, and complex partial seizures with or without secondary generalization is most likely to have recurring seizures. Tonic-clonic (grand mal) seizures are the most dramatic and often lead to emergency treatment. The usual causes of seizure breakthrough are lowered anticonvulsant blood levels, change in habits, complicating factors of epilepsy management, and progression of the underlying cause. Superimposed head trauma also may precipitate seizures (see discussion on head trauma and seizures, below). An unprovoked episode of seizures may occur in a well child with adequate levels of anticonvulsants.

TABLE 125-3   Initial and Maintenance Doses in the First Seizure (Nonstatus Partial and Tonic, Clonic, and Tonic–Clonic Seizures of Childhood

Drug	Route	Initial Dose, mg/kg per d	Maintenance Dose, mg/kg per d	Therapeutic Level Total	Free	Half-Life, h
Phenytoin (Dilantin)*	PO/PR	8	4–8	10–22	1.0–2.2	24
Fosphenytoin (Cerebyx)	IV/IM	15–20 mg PE	4–8 mg PE	10–22	1.0–2.2	18
Carbamazepine (Tegretol, Carbatrol)	PO/PR	10	10–40	6–12	1.8–2.2	14†
Valproate (Depakote, Depakene)	PO/PR	10	20–60	50–130	10–25	10
Valproate (Depacon)	IV	10	20–60	50–130	10–25	10
Primidone (Mysoline)	PO/PR	5	10–20	5–12	NA	12
Ethosuximide (Zarontin)	PO/PR	20	20–30	50–100	NA	30
Gabapentin (Neurontin)	PO	20	20–60	NA	NA	6
Lamotrigine (Lamictal)‡	PO	0.2–1.0 mg	5–15	NA	NA	12–60
Topiramate (Topamax)	PO	1.0	8–20	NA	NA	14–23
Tiagabine (Gabitril)	PO	0.1	1	NA	NA	7
Clonazepam (Klonopin)	PO	0.05	0.1–0.3	NA	NA	18–50
Acetazolamide (Diamox)	PO	10	10	NA	NA	24–42
Felbamate (Felbatol)#	PO	15	45	NA	NA	19
Oxcarbazepine	PO	10	40–60	NA	NA	10
Zonisamide	PO	1.0	12	NA	NA	60–80
Levetiracetam	PO	10	40–60	NA	NA	6–8

*Higher free phenytoin levels when administered with valproate.
†With chronic use.
‡Requires 6 to 8 weeks to achieve maintenance dose. Coadministration with valproate requires very low dosage initially, whereas coadministration with an enzyme inducer requires higher initial dosage.
#Not recommended for routine use.
Abbreviations: NA = not applicable; PE = phenytoin equivalent.

Evaluation

LOWERED ANTICONVULSANT BLOOD LEVELS

Due to Noncompliance   This is a common cause, most often in a preteen or teen who has been given the responsibility for self-medication. Noncompliance is seen more often with three times per d and daily dosing.

Related to Intercurrent Infection   Anticonvulsant levels fall during acute infections (viral or bacterial), with or without fever. Quite often, a child's seizure recurrence is an indication of the infection before the acute problem is evident (e.g., varicella or otitis media).

Interaction of Different Drugs   An example of this kind of interaction is the reduction of the phenytoin level by the induction of parahydroxylation when barbiturates are used concomitantly (see Problems of Anticonvulsant Use).

CHANGE IN HABITS

1. Altered sleep patterns because of trips, holidays, or parties.
2. A job, examinations, or an emotional stress may lead to seizures in active teens. If a pattern develops, knowledge of the pattern is quite helpful in defining treatment.
3. Alcohol use can lower the seizure threshold and increase noncompliance.
4. The use of illicit drugs or prescription drugs that lower the threshold. Examples are neuroleptic agents, lindane (Kwell), theophylline, phencyclidine, lysergic acid diethylamide, cyclosporine, isoniazid,

meperidine, tricyclic antidepressants, stimulants, and certain anesthetic agents (e.g., Ethrane).

COMPLICATING FACTORS OF EPILEPSY MANAGEMENT

1. Toxic levels of drugs. An example is phenytoin intoxication, which can increase seizure frequency. Carbamazepine and other AEDs in therapeutic dosage have been found to infrequently increase seizures. Tiagabine and gabapentin may increase myoclonic seizures.
2. The use of phenytoin in some myoclonic epilepsies.
3. Anticonvulsant-induced osteomalacia with hypocalcemia (rickets). This uncommon problem may increase the seizure frequency and typically occurs after 5 to 7 years of use.
4. Downregulation of benzodiazepine receptor sites with decreasing antiepileptic response (e.g., clonazepam and nitrazepam).
5. Carbamazepine and oxcarbazepine induced hyponatremia.

PROGRESSION OF THE UNDERLYING CAUSE   Examples are subacute focal (Rasmussen) encephalitis, neoplasm, arteriovenous malformation, and degenerative disease (ceroid lipofuscinosis and Huttenlocher-Alpers). Blume and coworkers found that 16 of 38 children undergoing cerebral resection for intractable seizures unexpectedly had cerebral tumors.[3]

When a child known to have epilepsy presents with recurring seizures, several steps may minimize the treatment time and disclose the reason for the breakthrough. The physician should first assess the airway and obtain vital signs. If the patient is febrile, a source of infection should be sought. Next, if the patient is having seizures at the time, the physician should test for the levels of anticonvulsants

TABLE 125-4   Doses for Status Epilepticus in Children

Drug	Recommended Loading Dose	Route	Repeat	Rate	Maximum Dose
Diazepam intravenous	0.2 mg/kg	IV	3 times	1 mg per min	5 mg, 0–2 y 10 mg, ≥2 y
Diazepam IV preparation for rectal administration	0.5 mg/kg	Rectal	0.25 mg/kg in 10 min	Bolus	Switch agents if 2nd dose ineffective
Diazepam gel for rectal administration (Diastat)	0–5 y 0.5 mg/kg 6–11 y 0.3 mg/kg >12 y 0.2 mg/kg	Rectal	No	Bolus	One dose. Switch agents if one dose ineffective
Lorazepam	0.1 mg/kg	IV	4 times	>2 min	0.4 mg/kg
Midazolam	0.2 mg/kg	IV	1 time	>2 min	0.4 mg/kg
Midazolam infusion		IV	Continuous	0.04–0.05 mg/kg per h	Until seizure cessation
Phenobarbital	20.0 mg/kg	IV	0	1 mg/kg per min	400 mg
Fosphenytoin	20.0 mg PE/kg	IV	0	3 mg PE/kg per min	Until effective therapeutic level reached
Clonazepam	0.3 mg/kg	NG	1 time		10 mg
Depacon	10–30 mg/kg	IV	0	Over 15 min	IV preparation of valproate
Pentobarbital	5 mg/kg	IV	Continuous	0.5–3.0 mg/kg per h	Until 3–6 s burst suppression
Propofol	1 mg/kg	IV	Continuous	3–7 mg/kg per h	No better than phenobarbital
Lidocaine	2.0 mg/kg	IV	0	5–10 mg/kg per h	Rarely effective

Abbreviation: PE = phenytoin equivalent.

(phenobarbital, phenytoin, valproic acid, or carbamazepine), electrolytes, calcium, and glucose, obtain a complete blood cell count with a differential count, and establish an intravenous line.

Treatment

Once these procedures have been completed, anticonvulsant management is initiated. Assume the anticonvulsant levels are low and give a partial loading dose. If the patient is compliant, give the daily dose of phenobarbital or phenytoin PO, if the patient is able to swallow, or IV, if not. If the patient is known to be noncompliant or if the levels of the anticonvulsant are significantly below the therapeutic range, give double the daily dose (e.g., in a child on 60 mg of phenobarbital, give 120 mg initially and repeat the dose if the seizures recur despite levels in the low therapeutic range).

If the anticonvulsant levels are within a high therapeutic range and the child is well without an obvious source of infection or other cause of breakthrough, then one can decide whether another anticonvulsant is necessary. One may decide to wait and see whether there is a trend toward increased seizure frequency, which would warrant additional medication, or whether this is a solitary episode, which would warrant observation, monitoring of drug levels, and follow-up. If the levels are within the high therapeutic range and seizures recur, additional anticonvulsants are warranted in appropriate loading doses (see Table 125-3). **Neurologic consultation should be obtained before adding another medication.**

Recurring or frequent tonic, tonic and clonic, or clonic seizures warrant loading doses that produce therapeutic levels safely and rapidly. Phenobarbital or fosphenytoin can be administered IM and IV, and Depacon (valproate) can be given intravenously. Rectal administration of liquid preparations of valproate, phenobarbital, phenytoin, primidone, and carbamazepine can result in therapeutic levels within 4 h. Using large enough doses of primidone, carbamazepine, topiramate, and tiagabine most likely will result in significant CNS toxicity and a greater likelihood of sedation, ataxia, and confusion. Because of

the greater risk of serious rash, lamotrigine should not be given in an emergency situation for immediate seizure control. Rapid loading with levetiracetam and zonisamide has not been carefully evaluated.

Seizures that begin with focal features, partial or complex partial (temporal lobe, psychomotor), may appear less dramatic and typically warrant a slower modification of drug therapy unless the seizures are prolonged or postictal Todd paralysis occurs. If a patient requires additional drugs, phenobarbital, phenytoin, and valproate can be used interchangeably without producing uncomfortable side effects.

Patients with petit mal (generalized absence) epilepsy rarely are brought to the ED, because the seizures are not alarming to the parents. If some injury occurs because of the absence spells, or if the parent is unusually concerned and brings the child for emergency treatment, determining the blood levels of anticonvulsants is most useful. Addition of another anticonvulsant can be initiated, e.g., lamotrigine (Lamictal), ethosuximide (Zarontin), valproate (Depakote), clonazepam (Klonopin), or acetazolamide (Diamox).

Disposition

Most often, epileptic patients with breakthrough seizure can be sent home, and the pediatrician or neurologist can modify the drug regimen. After the initial evaluation, modification of drug therapy, and treatment for any superimposed problems, the emergency physician should (1) arrange for follow-up, (2) emphasize the need for compliance, and (3) provide treatment for infection or other precipitating factors.

FEBRILE SEIZURE

Febrile seizure is a unique and common form of seizure in childhood. Although various types occur (tonic, tonic and clonic, and clonic), the characteristics of a simple febrile seizure distinguish it from other symptomatic and idiopathic seizure disorders. **A febrile seizure is a**

seizure associated with fever, but without evidence of intracranial infection or defined cause, usually occurring between 6 months and 5 years of age.[4,5] Typically, these seizures are generalized and last less than 15 min, and there is no postictal focal neurologic deficit. The EEG usually does not demonstrate paroxysmal (epileptic) activity, and there often is a family history of similar seizures. A rapid rise in temperature, usually above 38.8°C (101.8°F), occurs at the onset of the illness and, on occasion, recurs several times in the course of the illness. Three to four percent of young children experience febrile seizures; of these, 30 to 40 percent have recurrences, especially when the first seizure occurs when a child is younger than 1 year. The mortality from simple febrile seizures is extremely low.

Evaluation

The first febrile seizure warrants the most concern, because the benign nature of the illness has not yet been established. The initial evaluation is directed toward identifying the cause of fever and excluding serious causes, such as meningitis, encephalitis, bacterial sepsis, toxic exposure, or underlying neurologic abnormality. Any febrile illness, such as upper respiratory infection, gastroenteritis, or urinary tract infection, can be associated with a febrile seizure. Glucose test strip should be determined, but the need for other laboratory studies generally depends on the patient's clinical condition. Lumbar puncture is needed whenever intracranial infection appears likely. A child older than 18 months who is clinically nontoxic, has normal mental status, has not received prior antibiotics, and demonstrates no clinical concern for meningitis does not need lumbar puncture.

Treatment

Therapy for the cause of the fever is the main goal. Fever should be reduced with acetaminophen, 10 to 15 mg/kg PO or PR at 4-h intervals, to a total dose of 600 mg. The dose of ibuprofen is 10 mg/kg every 6 to 8 h, to a total dose of 40 mg/kg (see Chap. 115). Tepid sponging with water, never with alcohol, provides an additive response to antipyretics. A simple febrile seizure does not warrant treatment with AEDs, because of the good prognosis in untreated children and the high incidence of adverse drug effects.[6]

If a child exhibits repetitive seizures with this or prior febrile seizures, then phenobarbital can be administered with a loading dose of 15 mg/kg IV followed by 4 to 6 mg/kg per d to attain therapeutic levels of 15 to 50 μg/mL. The drug is continued until the child improves.

Chronic AED prophylaxis with phenobarbital or valproate is limited to children with (1) complex febrile seizures (prolonged or focal), (2) a preexisting neurologic deficit (e.g., cerebral palsy), (3) onset before age 6 months, (4) repeated seizures in the same illness, (5) prior nonfebrile seizures, and (6) more than three febrile seizures within 6 months. PR or PO administered diazepam also has been used successfully to prevent seizures when given at the onset of a febrile illness.[6,7] The dose of oral diazepam is 0.2 to 0.5 mg/kg given every 8 h during the febrile illness. However, about 40 percent experience side effects such as lethargy, ataxia, and irritability.

Disposition

Children with a simple febrile seizure do not need admission. Follow-up with the pediatrician or family physician should be arranged. Admit the ill child without an easily treatable problem, one in whom recurrent seizures have occurred within several hours or 1 day, or one with a complex febrile seizure.

NEONATAL SEIZURES

Seizures in neonates are difficult to identify. All neonates experiencing seizures should be considered to be at serious risk from the under-lying disorder, the effect of unremitting seizures, and increased risk for epilepsy. Prompt, effective anticonvulsant therapy and other specific therapies lessen the impact of short-term detrimental effect on long-term neurologic functioning. In many instances, the seizure itself is less important for its immediate effects than for its indication of significant underlying disease (e.g., infection, metabolic disorder, or CNS malformation) that ultimately will have more effect on morbidity and mortality.

Multifocal or fragmentary seizures occur more commonly at this age, and clonic or tonic movements independently affect the limbs simultaneously or fleetingly. Autonomic dysfunction may be the only manifestation of neonatal seizures, with the infant exhibiting pupillary changes, apnea, and cardiac irregularity. The difference in seizure presentation is due to the lack of arborization of the immature brain, which prevents rapid propagation of electrical epileptic activity, and to the particular disorders to which newborns are subject (e.g., hypoxic ischemic encephalopathy, metabolic conditions such as inborn errors of urea cycle and amino acid metabolism, and dysplastic conditions). Unilateral (partial or focal) seizures may be associated with structural lesions, and permanent neurologic deficit may be associated with them.

Non-CNS causes of neonatal seizures include sepsis, cardiac disease, hypoxia or apnea, hypoglycemia, electrolyte abnormalities such as hypocalcemia, and complex hereditary metabolic disorders. Infectious CNS causes include viral or bacterial meningitis or encephalitis (such as *Listeria*, herpes, toxoplasmosis, cytomegalovirus, or rubella) and perinatal CNS hemorrhage. Examples of dysplastic CNS disorders are Cornelia de Lange syndrome, Sturge-Weber syndrome, and tuberous sclerosis.

Evaluation

While ensuring the airway, oxygenation, and circulation, obtain a history to identify perinatal risk factors for seizures. Verify gestational age of the infant and determine whether there was premature rupture of the membranes, delivery complications, and maternal perinatal infection. Determine feeding patterns, because urea cycle defects with hyperammonemia, maple syrup urine disease, and methylmalonic acidemia usually become evident days or weeks after feedings with protein are initiated. The infant with nonketotic hyperglycinemia may exhibit seizures immediately after birth. Table 125-2 lists laboratory studies needed for the evaluation of neonatal seizures.

Most will require lumbar puncture to detect viral or bacterial meningitis. Cerebral imaging is needed to identify cerebral hemorrhage and structural abnormalities. Ultrasound may be sufficient for diagnosis in some cases, but MRI is the best study for migrational defects of the CNS (e.g., lissencephaly, heterotopia, and agenesis of the corpus callosum).

Treatment

Treatment principles in the management of neonatal seizures are as follows:

1. Identify and correct treatable causes (hypocalcemia, hypoglycemia, and electrolyte imbalance).
2. Identify and treat associated problems such as sepsis, hyperbilirubinemia, and acidosis.
3. Initiate anticonvulsant therapy with appropriate loading doses and carefully observe blood levels to adjust the maintenance dosage (Table 125-5).

Ensure adequate ventilation and oxygenation. Obtain bedside glucose determination and administer glucose as 5 mL/kg of D10W if hypoglycemia is present (see Chap. 129). For active seizures, phenobarbital is the treatment of choice, and fosphenytoin is a good alternative. Pyridoxine is sometimes given empirically for refractory seizures.

TABLE 125-5   Drug Regimen for Neonatal Seizures

5 mL/kg D10W given to infants with proven hypoglycemia or when highly suspect because of circumstances

Calcium gluconate (10%) 200–500 mg/kg per d divided in 4 doses (in proven hypocalcemic infants)

Magnesium sulfate 25–50 mg/kg IV or IM. Repeat q4–6h for 3–4 doses if necessary to normalize magnesium

Phenobarbital 20 mg/kg at rate of 1 mg/kg per min, then 3–4 mg/kg per d

Fosphenytoin 20 mg PE/kg at rate of 3 mg/kg per min, then 4–8 mg PE/kg per d in 2 divided doses IV or PO. Phenytoin maintenance 8–12 mg/kg per d in 2 divided doses to maintain a free level of 1.0–2.2

Lorazepam 0.10 mg/kg over 2 min. Repeat twice at 10-min intervals if necessary

Midazolam 0.2 mg/kg over 2 min. Repeat once if necessary. If refractory seizures use midazolam continuous infusion at 0.04–0.5 mg/kg per h

Pentobarbital as an alternative to continuous midazolam infusion. Initial pentobarbital dose is 5 mg/kg bolus followed by continuous infusion of 0.5–3.0 mg/kg per h to maintain electroencephalographic burst suppression at 3- to 6-s intervals

Abbreviations: D10W = 10% dextrose in water; PE = phenytoin equivalent.

Several factors influence drug treatment in neonates: (1) variations in the metabolic half-lives of drugs, (2) hypoxia, tissue acidosis, and renal or hepatic dysfunction increase anticonvulsant half-lives requiring lower dosing and less frequent administration, and (3) greater difficulty in identifying the end point of seizure control in neonates. Consequently, blood levels of seizure medications must be monitored during treatment.

PHENOBARBITAL   The drug of choice is phenobarbital, 10 to 20 mg/kg IV, administered at a rate of 1 mg/kg per min. Blood levels of phenobarbital of 16 to 40 μg/mL are necessary to achieve seizure control in most cases. Levels of 40 to 80 μg/mL have been maintained in resistant cases with inconsistent benefit. Dosages of 3 to 4 mg/kg per d maintain mid to high therapeutic levels and prevent toxicity. In infants younger than 7 days, the half-life of phenobarbital is 100 h; after 28 days of continuous therapy, the half-life is reduced to 60 to 70 h.

FOSPHENYTOIN   Fosphenytoin is the second drug of choice and is well tolerated in neonates. The loading dose of fosphenytoin is 15 to 20 mg PE/kg administered at a rate of 3 mg PE/kg per min, with intravenous maintenance of 4 to 8 mg PE/kg per d. Free phenytoin levels up to 2.2 μg/mL may be necessary for adequate seizure control.

PYRIDOXINE AND BIOTIN   Pyridoxine (vitamin B₆), 100 mg per d, is empirically used when no reasonable cause for seizures has been identified and the seizures remain uncontrolled. Seizure reduction rather than EEG improvement is the best indication of B₆ response. Biotin, 10 mg per d, is the long-term replacement therapy for biotinidase deficiency.

OTHER AGENTS   In poorly responsive neonatal seizure, it is reasonable to consider newer agents (e.g., topiramate) given more quickly then usual, so that a full dose is achieved in 5 to 10 days.

In status epilepticus of neonates, diazepam or lorazepam must be used with caution, because its half-life may be prolonged, and respiratory depression superimposed on an immature and possibly compromised respiratory apparatus should be anticipated. Diazepam may exaggerate hyperbilirubinemia by uncoupling the bilirubin-albumin complex and should be used with caution in jaundiced babies.

INFANTILE SPASMS

Infantile spasms are a unique form of seizures. The onset is typically between 3 and 9 months of age but may begin as late as 18 months.

Concurrently, the child exhibits regression in development. The spasms are very brief, lasting a split second, often with flexion or extension of the head and trunk. They occur singly or repeatedly in bursts of 5 to 20 spasms at a time, usually several times per day and more often upon arousal from sleep or with sudden auditory or physical stimulation. The EEG is abnormal in virtually every case. Mental retardation in patients with this disorder is as high as 85 percent. Parents are often frustrated because medical professionals fail to recognize these spasms as seizures.

There are many causes of infantile spasm, including migrational defects, prior CNS trauma, hypoxia, neurocutaneous disorders, and infectious and metabolic disorders. The idiopathic type is the most alarming, because it affects children with no prior neurologic disorder and no etiology is identified. Differential diagnosis includes benign myoclonus, dyskinesia due to gastroesophageal reflux, and tics.

Evaluation

Once infantile spasms are recognized, prompt neurologic referral is recommended. Basic assessment includes electrolytes, calcium, glucose, complete blood count, creatinine, and lumbar puncture. The lumbar puncture is warranted to identify the rare syndrome of glucose transporter defect, which is a potentially treatable cause of infantile spasms. If the cerebrospinal fluid glucose is less than 60 percent of blood glucose, this disorder should be strongly suspected. Magnetic resonance imaging is the preferred neuroimaging study and can be done electively.

Treatment

Although adrenocorticotropic hormone is still considered the most effective agent for infantile spasms, the frequency and severity of side effects warrant the use of newer, less toxic AEDs, especially topiramate, which can be increased much more rapidly in this situation, with dosages as high as 30 to 40 mg/kg, to achieve cessation of spasms. Clonazepam, valproate, and vigabatrin (in cases of tuberous sclerosis) are alternatives.[7]

HEAD TRAUMA AND SEIZURES

Head trauma can result in three types of seizures: immediate seizures, early posttraumatic seizures, and late posttraumatic seizures.

Immediate Posttraumatic Seizures

Immediate seizures result from impact and presumably are due to traumatic depolarization of neurons. The risk of recurring seizures in these patients is minimal unless there are more serious prognostic factors such as prolonged coma and penetrating head injury. Emergency treatment is the identification and correction of depressed skull fracture, intracerebral hemorrhage, or hematoma; and the reduction of cerebral edema, oxygenation, ventilation, and correction of shock, and the careful administration of anticonvulsants. Fosphenytoin is the drug of choice, given at 20 mg/kg PE at a rate of 3 mg per min (see Table 125-4). It is helpful for the neurosurgeon or neurologist to avoid the use of sedative anticonvulsants (barbiturates or diazepam), if possible. Long-term management of immediate posttraumatic seizures remains controversial. In a patient who recovers rapidly, chronic anticonvulsant use usually is not indicated. An exception would be a patient with a seizure history or a family history of epilepsy.

Early Posttraumatic Seizures

Early posttraumatic seizures occur within the first week after trauma, and epilepsy results in 20 to 25 percent of these patients. These seizures are presumed to result from the focal effects of contusions or lacerations and associated hypoperfusion, which causes ischemia and related metabolic changes. Evaluation includes assessment for intracerebral hemorrhage or hematoma, or associated metabolic abnormalities such as hyponatremia. Treatment of choice is intravenous loading of fosphenytoin (see Table 125-4) and referral to neurosurgery or neurology, as clinically appropriate. Long-term anticonvulsant therapy is generally recommended.

Late Posttraumatic Seizures

Late posttraumatic seizures occur after 1 week and may be seen as late as 10 years after the trauma. Structural changes, such as atrophy with gliosis and permanent local vascular changes, altered dendrite branching, and presumably modified neurotransmitter function, account for the development and permanence of these seizures. Of these seizures, 40 percent are focal or partial seizures and 50 percent are temporal lobe seizures, indicating the predilection for traumatic injury and known epileptogenic properties of this structure. The risk of recurring seizures in this group is reported to be as high as 70 percent, and long-term anticonvulsant therapy is necessary. Patients at greater risk for chronic posttraumatic seizures include those with depressed skull fractures, posttraumatic amnesia more than 24 h after the trauma, dural penetration, acute intracranial hemorrhage, early posttraumatic epilepsy, and a foreign body in a cerebral wound. The more severe the seizure and the later the onset, the less likely remission will occur.

Emergency management of late posttraumatic seizures consists of airway and circulation stabilization, administration of anticonvulsants, with intravenous fosphenytoin being the preferred agent (see Table 125-4), and imaging to identify neurosurgically correctable lesions. Long-term anticonvulsant therapy is needed.

STATUS EPILEPTICUS

Status epilepticus (SE) is a state of continuous seizures lasting at least 30 min. As a practical measure, seizures are usually treated as SE if they persist longer than 10 min. Classification of status seizures is listed in Table 125-6. In absence (petitmal) SE, the child appears dazed and may exhibit repetitive eye blinking.

Epilepsia partialis continua is a serious neurologic condition, although it does not appear life threatening at first. The patient exhibits repeated continuous or minimally interrupted clonic jerking of one side of the body and usually one part of an extremity for days, weeks, or months. It is typically due to encephalitis or cerebrovascular accident or associated with heterotopias and indicates a relatively poor prognosis. Initial management is similar to that of SE.

About 5 to 10 percent of children with epilepsy experience one bout of SE. The longer it persists, the greater the morbidity and the mortality rates and the more difficult it is to control the seizures. In patients

TABLE 125-6 Classifications of Status Seizures

Primary generalized convulsive status grand mal (continuous and noncontinuous)
   Tonic–clonic status
   Myoclonic status
   Clonic–tonic status
Secondary generalized convulsive status (continuous and noncontinuous)
   Tonic–clonic status with partial onset
   Tonic status
Simple partial status
   Partial motor status including epilepsia partialis continua
   Partial sensory status
   Partial status with vegetative or autonomic symptoms
   Partial status with cognitive symptoms
   Partial status with affective symptoms
Complex partial status
Absence (petit mal) status

with no neurologic sequelae, the mean duration of SE is 1 h 30 min. The mean duration of status grand mal in patients who die is 13 h.

Experimental models in animals have demonstrated permanent cell damage in the hippocampus, amygdala, cerebellum, thalamus, and middle cerebral cortical layers after 60 min of seizure activity. Even with artificial ventilation and correction of existing metabolic derangements, most changes still occur. Cell death results from the increased metabolic demands and the exhaustion of the continuously firing neurons. In addition, secondary effects exaggerate the adverse effects. The cerebral partial pressure of oxygen and amounts of cytochrome A and cytochrome A3 reductase decrease enhance the risk of cell damage. Increases in calcium, arachidonic acid, arachidonic diglycerol, prostaglandin, and leukotriene levels in the neurons exaggerate or cause cerebral edema or cell death. Increased levels of cyclic adenosine monophosphate and increased release of prolactin, growth hormone, adrenocorticotropic hormone, cortisol, insulin, glycogen, epinephrine, and norepinephrine may contribute to the progression of cell damage, with loss of physiologic responsiveness.

Later secondary effects include lactic acidosis, elevated cerebrospinal fluid pressure, hyperglycemia followed later by hypoglycemia, dysautonomia with hyperthermia, diaphoresis, dehydration, hypertension followed by hypotension, and eventually shock. In addition, excessive muscle activity leads to rhabdomyolysis, myoglobinuria, and renal failure. Neuropathologic studies have indicated that nucleovacuolation and ischemic nerve cell damage lead to neuronal dissolution.

Evaluation and Treatment

To obtain the most effective and rapid cessation of SE, the following evaluation and therapeutic goals must be reached[8,9]:

1. Specific delineation of the type and subtype of SE so that appropriate treatment can be chosen. For example, tonic-clonic generalized SE is very responsive to diazepam or phenytoin; noncontinuous clonic or tonic-clonic seizures may be refractory to diazepam.
2. Identification and treatment of the reversible precipitating cause of SE (e.g., cerebral infection, trauma, electrolyte disturbance, brain abscess, hypoglycemia, or sickle cell crisis).
3. Rapid cessation of SE to prevent secondary effects that prolong the seizures and cause irreversible neuronal damage.
4. Full support of medical systems to prevent complications of the seizures or the treatment (e.g., respiratory depression, dysrhythmia, aspiration pneumonia, shock, and myoglobulinuria).

The end point of therapy is cessation of the clinical seizures, with return of normal function. When a patient fails to arouse, the possibility of nonconvulsive status must be entertained, and then the end point is improvement in the EEG abnormality.

BENZODIAZEPINES   Lorazepam, a rapid acting benzodiazepine, is the drug of choice in SE.[10] Benzodiazepines are effective in SE via several mechanisms: (1) agonist binding at the benzodiazepine receptor increases GABA for its receptor and GABA acts as a receptor for a longer period, and (2) benzodiazepines block sustained high-frequency discharges of epileptic neurons. Benzodiazepines are effective, because they have high lipophilicity, rapid brain penetration, and brain receptor binding. Benzodiazepines are effective for prehospital control of seizures.[11,12]

Lorazepam is preferred over other benzodiazepines, because it has a longer duration of action, although it has a slightly longer onset of action than diazepam. The dose of lorazepam is 0.1 mg/kg IV given over 2 min and repeated for a maximum of 8 mg.

To maintain the seizure-free state, a long-term AED is started simultaneously with phenobarbital 20 mg/kg, at 1 mg/kg per min. Alternatively, fosphenytoin 20 mg PE/kg at 3 mg/kg per min, can be used.

Diazepam was the benzodiazepine used initially in the modern era of epilepsy management and can be used in addition to or instead of lorazepam. The dose of diazepam is 0.2 to 0.5 mg/kg IV, given at a rate of 1 mg per min and repeated as needed, to a maximum of 2.6 mg/kg. Most patients stop seizing with one or two bolus doses.

Midazolam is a very rapid-acting benzodiazepine and is rapidly absorbed intramuscularly. When given intramuscularly, seizure control occurs within 2 to 3 min of injection. It has been used by intravenous, intramuscular, nasal, and rectal routes in the treatment of SE.[13–17] Midazolam has a distribution half-life of 1.5 to 3.5 h. The initial dosage is a 0.2 mg/kg bolus, which can be repeated in 15 min. Because of its short half-life, it is used as a continuous infusion at 0.05 to 0.4 mg/kg per h to treat continuous unresponsive seizures. In one study,[17] more rapid cessation of seizures occurred with midazolam (7.8 to 4.1 vs. 11.2 to 3.6 min) than with intravenous diazepam. This result was attributed to the ease of administration of the intramuscular midazolam as compared with the time needed for intravenous site acquisition with the diazepam.

The following steps should be followed when treating continuous tonic-clonic SE (see Table 125-4):

1. Assess basic functions immediately and maintain blood pressure, airway, and pulse.
2. Obtain blood to be tested for levels of anticonvulsants, electrolytes, serum urea nitrogen, calcium, and glucose and for a complete blood cell count with differential while inserting an intravenous catheter for fluid administration.
3. If hypoglycemia is present, administer 5 mL/kg of D10W.
4. Administer lorazepam, 0.1 mg/kg IV, and repeat up to a total dose of 8 mg or early signs of respiratory depression; or administer diazepam, 0.2 mg/kg IV over 2 min, and repeat in 15 and 30 min, if necessary, to a total dose of 2.6 mg/kg.
5. Administer fosphenytoin, 20 mg PE/kg IV at 3 mg/kg per min, as the benzodiazepine is being infused.
6. Administer phenobarbital, 20 mg/kg IV at 1 mg/kg per min, if fosphenytoin is ineffective.
7. If seizures persist, give additional phenobarbital 10 mg/kg, to reach levels of 60 μg/mL.
8. If seizures continue, administer pentobarbital, under intensive care monitoring, 2 mg/kg bolus, followed by maintenance of 1 to 2 mg/kg per h, to effect 3 to 6 s of EEG burst suppression.
9. In noncontinuous SE, administer continuous midazolam at a dose of 0.04 to 0.05 mg/kg per h despite step 8.

LIDOCAINE   Lidocaine also may be useful in the management of seizures in children in whom other drugs have failed.[18] The loading dose is a 2 mg/kg IV bolus followed by an intravenous infusion of 5 to 10 mg/kg per h.

PROPOFOL   Propofol may be useful for seizures not responding to benzodiazepines or fosphenytoin,[15,16,19,20] but further study is needed before it can be recommended as a standard agent for SE in children. The meta-analyses by Classen and associates reported an average loading dose of 1 mg/kg and infusion rates of 2.94 mg/kg per h (±2.00) minimum to 6.98 mg/kg per h (±5.34) maximum.[16] There was no apparent superiority of propofol to pentobarbital in the studies they reviewed for the meta-analyses. The use of propofol has been advocated in adults with refractory SE,[10] but its prolonged use in children with refractory SE was associated with progressive severe metabolic acidosis and rhabdomyolysis, which the authors concluded was due to propofol.[19]

Noncontinuous SE can be more difficult to treat, because the end point is more elusive. Rapidly acting drugs such as diazepam and lorazepam are less effective, and a more sustained effect is necessary. Noncontinuous SE often is not responsive to appropriate therapeutic levels of phenytoin and phenobarbital. Midazolam can be given as a continuous infusion of 0.04 to 0.05 mg/kg per h. Alternatively, large doses (0.2 to 0.6 mg/kg) of clonazepam via nasogastric tube may be used to produce the desired effect of cessation of noncontinuous seizures, and the anticonvulsant effect can be maintained by additional drugs (phenytoin or phenobarbital) and clonazepam (0.1 to 0.3 mg/kg per d).

DIFFERENTIAL DIAGNOSIS OF SEIZURES

The differential diagnosis of seizures must consider many disorders that can produce loss of consciousness, unusual movements, impaired awareness, or bizarre behavior. Many of these disorders are age specific.

In newborns, jitteriness or hyperexcitability appears as high-amplitude tremulousness easily brought about by passive movement of the extremities or jarring of the crib. Drug-withdrawn infants are irritable and tremulous and may have diaphoresis, vomiting, and diarrhea, but they may also have seizures. Sepsis, hypoglycemia, and hypocalcemia may produce nonepileptic paroxysmal activity in addition to seizures. Hyperekplexia, or startle disease, mimics tonic and clonic seizures, is very responsive to clonazepam, and if left untreated has a significant risk for sudden neonatal or infant death. Seizures are part of the differential diagnosis of near-miss sudden infant death syndrome (see Chap. 119). In older infants, cyanotic and pallid breath-holding spells can occur after an abrupt trauma (a fall or a minor spanking) or a verbal reprimand. Bradycardia and a brief tonic nonepileptic seizure often occur. The prolonged QT syndrome and neurocardiogenic syncope may cause nonepileptic seizures or syncopal episodes (Chap. 131). Drug intoxication manifested by hyperkinesis, impaired awareness, or altered behavior (hallucinations) is usually accidental at this age. In adolescence, phencyclidine intoxication mimics complex partial seizures and may result in seizures with more severe overdoses.

Congenital heart disease can produce paroxysmal events at all ages. Abrupt mental status changes may occur in patients with disorders such as pulmonary hypertension, acquired cardiomyopathy, aortic stenosis, or tetralogy of Fallot (see Chap. 131).

Hyperkinetic movement disorders can be difficult to differentiate from complex partial seizures. Sydenham chorea is now rare, and drug-induced chorea (ethosuximide, carbamazepine, or diphenhydramine hydrochloride) and lupus-induced chorea are likewise very uncommon. Tourette syndrome is seen more frequently, but rarely does the child appear acutely ill. Kinesogenic chorea is a movement disorder brought on by action and mimics simple motor partial seizures. Intermittent focal dystonia can affect one limb and last from seconds to hours.

Pseudoseizures represent a particular problem because the "seizures" appear to represent a significant threat to the patient's safety, and vigorous anticonvulsant therapy is often initiated. Unfortunately, pseudoseizures often occur in patients with documented epilepsy. Secondary gain should become evident in these cases. The "seizures" are atypical in that the patient may waken fully in the interictal phase and require repeated large doses of anticonvulsants even to the point of protracted drug-induced depression. Another form of pseudoseizures consists of those described by the parent and never observed by other witnesses (Munchausen by proxy). In this case, the parent receives much attention, and psychiatric, psychologic, and social services inputs are essential.

Neurologic referral, or even hospitalization, is needed to treat pseudoseizure, prevent recurrences, provide family education, and avoid inappropriate treatment.

PROBLEMS OF ANTICONVULSANT USE

Unwanted features of anticonvulsants may be seen soon after the drug is initiated or may develop weeks, months, or years later. These problems may turn up during evaluation for other illnesses (e.g., macrocytic anemia) or be the basis for emergency treatment.

Immediate side effects often subside in time. Lethargy is usually dose related and subsides with chronic use and can occur with the oldest AED (phenobarbital) and the newest AEDs (topiramate and tiagabine). Irritability and changes in cognition can persist and be significant but are unrelated to drug levels (all drugs). Rashes may occur within days or weeks of initiation of therapy but must be differentiated from concurrent viral exanthem. Pruritic and/or morbilliform rashes usually require cessation of medication. Stevens-Johnson syndrome, with bullous skin lesions affecting mucous membranes, is a serious potential reaction. There is a risk of serious sequelae: blindness, esophageal stenosis, or loss of life.

With valproic acid use, hepatic failure may occur within days or up to 2 years after first use. The drug reaction results in behavior alteration, increasing lethargy, and vomiting. Levels of liver enzymes may be minimally to markedly elevated, and hyperammonemia with or without symptoms of hepatic failure may be found. Immediate cessation of valproate, hospitalization, and observation are necessary when symptomatic hepatic reaction is evident. In asymptomatic patients with enzyme level elevations, a reduction of the dosage and careful observation are warranted. Gastrointestinal side effects are common with initial use of valproic acid and may be so severe that more serious hepatic problems are considered. These side effects can be avoided by taking the drug with meals, by avoiding carbonated beverages and citric juices, and by using the enteric-coated form or sprinkles. Pancreatitis secondary to valproate use may occur with initial and chronic use and has been associated with fatalities.

Toxicity due to overdosage at any time can produce some readily identifiable symptoms and signs. Phenytoin toxicity occurs when serum levels exceed 25 µg/mL in most patients (>20 µg/mL in some patients). Nausea, dysarthria, diplopia, and ataxia are seen early, with progression to impaired levels of consciousness and decerebrate posturing. Virtually all anticonvulsants produce ataxia and lethargy with significant overdosage. Cardiopulmonary monitoring during high-dose drug use in SE should be employed, because cardiac dysrhythmia, hypotension, or respiratory depression can occur. The use of fosphenytoin has eliminated the problem of venous and subcutaneous extravasation-related phenytoin side effects. Chronic phenytoin use can result in folate deficiency with macrocytic anemia, acquired osteomalacia (increased vitamin D turnover), neutropenia (often transient), peripheral neuropathy, lupus-like syndromes, and myasthenic weakness.

Valproate-induced thrombocytopenia is a significant side effect warranting lowering or discontinuation of the drug, if platelet levels are significantly lowered or bleeding is evident. Lower carnitine levels due to valproate metabolism may be a contributing factor of valproate hepatotoxicity.

Drug interactions may be quite dramatic. Valproate and aspirin use can result in a bleeding diathesis. Antihistamines used in conjunction with barbiturates can be very sedating, warranting smaller doses of the antihistamine. When erythromycin is used, particular care must be exercised, because the carbamazepine levels may rise to toxic levels rapidly. Toxicity is greater when carbamazepine and lithium are used together, even though blood levels may be in the therapeutic range. Total phenytoin levels are typically reduced when valproic acid and tiagabine are also used, but free phenytoin usually remains therapeutic, and it is essential to measure free phenytoin. When barbiturates are used concomitantly with phenytoin, increased parahydroxylation can enhance metabolism of phenytoin, so that therapeutic levels fall, resulting in seizure breakthrough. Hyperbilirubinemia and hypoalbuminemia can affect anticonvulsant binding and blood levels.

Movement disorder (e.g., chorea) can result after several weeks or months of use of ethosuximide and carbamazepine. The movements may be profound and usually respond to the reduction or discontinuation of the drug and, if necessary, the use of diphenhydramine (Benadryl), 12.5 to 25 mg IV. Clonazepam and diazepam can cause acute bladder dysfunction with urinary retention.

Zonisamide has the unique complication of anhidrosis, and therefore a child may present with heat stroke. Topiramate and felbamate

are associated with weight loss, and topiramate is also associated with renal calculi.

Many problems of dose-related toxicity can be avoided by maintaining therapeutic blood levels. This is applicable for valproic acid, phenytoin, phenobarbital, and carbamazepine but has not been substantiated in new AEDs. Blood level determinations should be done randomly to determine compliance at times of increased seizure frequency or when signs of toxicity develop. In some patients, side effects develop at therapeutic levels. Idiosyncratic effects cannot be predicted, but families must be made aware that significant side effects can develop with little warning, and evaluation by a physician is recommended before a drug is dismissed. Obtaining the patient's history, consulting with the primary physician or consultant, and reviewing readily available drug information in the package insert or pharmacology databases make emergency evaluation and treatment of anticonvulsant drug reactions simpler.

ERRORS IN EMERGENCY MANAGEMENT OF SEIZURES

After a patient arrives for treatment, the initial assessment may be incomplete, resulting in inappropriate or inadequate therapy. Not identifying treatable infections, electrolyte imbalance, child abuse, and accidental trauma can lead to rapidly progressive deterioration and demise or may make seizure control difficult. By not ascertaining anticonvulsant levels in a patient with epilepsy, the physician loses an opportunity to determine whether the anticonvulsant is ineffective or simply at too low a level.

If the emergency physician communicates with the primary physician, unnecessary studies and drugs that were ineffective or produced some side effects can be avoided. In addition, it is important to consult with the patient's physician when prescribing non-anticonvulsants that might interfere with anticonvulsants or produce unwanted side effects.

In the aggressive treatment of seizures (SE and recurring breakthrough seizures), inadequate loading doses or improper drug selection may prolong the seizure and worsen the prognosis. Excessive dosage can result in respiratory depression or hypotension and, in rare instances, can exacerbate the seizures. If nonepileptic paroxysmal disorders are not recognized, the patient is put at the additional risk of unnecessary medication and inadequate treatment of the real disorder.

Emergency physicians cannot deal with all the problems facing patients with epilepsy. Follow-up care by the primary physicians or appropriate consultants ensures better compliance and, one hopes, lessens emergency situations in the future.

REFERENCES

1. Gestaut H: Clinical and electroencephalographic classification of epileptic seizures. *Epilepsia* 11:102, 1970.
2. Pellock JH: Management of acute seizure episodes. *Epilepsia* 39:328, 1998.
3. Blume WT, Girvin JP, Kaufmann JC: Childhood brain tumors presenting as chronic uncontrolled focal seizure disorders. *Ann Neurol* 12:538, 1982.
4. American Academy of Pediatrics, Provisional Committee on Quality Improvement, Subcommittee on Febrile Seizures: Practice parameter: The neurodiagnostic evaluation of the child with a first simple febrile seizure. *Pediatrics* 997:769, 1996.
5. Baumann RJ, Duffner PK: Treatment of children with simple febrile seizures: The AAP practice parameter. *Pediatr Neurol* 23:11, 2000.
6. Farwell JR, Lee YJ, Hertz DG, et al: Phenobarbital for febrile seizures: Effects on intelligence and on seizure recurrence. *New Engl J Med* 322:364, 1990.
7. Rosman NP, Colton T, Labazzo J, et al: A controlled trial of diazepam administered during febrile illnesses to prevent recurrence of febrile seizures. *New Engl J Med* 329:79, 1993.
8. Gross TV, Shinnar S: Convulsive status epilepticus in children. *Epilepsia* 34(suppl) 11:12, 1993.
9. Lowenstein DH, Alldredge BK: Status epilepticus. *New Engl J Med* 338:970, 1998.

10. Treiman DM, Meyers PD, Walton NY, et al: A comparison of four treatments for generalized convulsive status epilepticus. *New Engl J Med* 339:792, 1998.

11. Dieckmann RA: Rectal diazepam for prehospital pediatric status epilepticus. *Ann Emerg Med* 23:216, 1994.

12. Dreifuss FE, Rosman NP, Cloyd JC, et al: A comparison of rectal diazepam gel and placebo for acute repetitive seizures. *New Engl J Med* 338:1869, 1998.

13. Shorvon SD: The use of clonazepam, midazolam, and nitrazepam in epilepsy. *Epilepsia* 39:S15, 1998.

14. Rivera R, Segnini M, Baltodano A, et al: Midazolam in the treatment of status epilepticus in children. *Crit Care Med* 21:955, 1993.

15. Prasad A, Worrall BB, Bertram EH, et al: Propofol and midazolam in the treatment of refractory status epilepticus. *Epilepsia* 42:380, 2001.

16. Classen J, Hirsch LJ, Emerson RG, et al: Treatment of refractory status epilepticus with pentobarbital, propofol, or midazolam: A systematic review. *Epilepsia* 43:146, 2002.

17. Chamberlain JM, Altieri MA, Futterman C, et al: A prospective, randomized study comparing intramuscular midazolam with intravenous diazepam for the treatment of seizures in children. *Pediatr Emerg Care* 13:92, 1997.

18. Walker IA, Slovis CM: Lidocaine in the treatment of status epilepticus. *Acad Emerg Med* 4:918, 1997.

19. Hanna JP, Ramundo ML: Rhabdomyolysis and hypoxia associated with prolonged propofol infusion in children. *Neurology* 80:301, 1998.

20. Kuisma M, Roine RO: Propofol in prehospital treatment of convulsive status epilepticus. *Epilepsia* 36:1241, 1995.

126 VOMITING AND DIARRHEA IN CHILDREN
Christopher M. Holmes
Summer A. Smith

Emergency physicians frequently see children who present with vomiting and/or diarrhea as their chief complaint. A careful history and physical examination will usually sort out those children with life-threatening manifestations of their illness from those who are less urgently ill. The most common cause of vomiting, diarrhea, and dehydration is acute viral gastroenteritis. This chapter will primarily address the differential diagnosis, etiology, diagnosis, and management of acute viral gastroenteritis.

VOMITING AND DIARRHEA

Vomiting is a coordinated reflex process that results in the forceful evacuation of stomach contents. The most common cause of acute vomiting is usually a self-limited viral illness. However, more serious and potentially life-threatening illnesses may present primarily with vomiting, and are presented in Table 126-1. The management of these illnesses is beyond the intent and scope of this chapter.

Diarrhea is best defined as an excessive loss of electrolytes and fluid in the stool. Generally, young infants produce about 5 g/kg of stool a day with the amount increasing to 200 g per d by adulthood. The small bowel absorbs the vast majority of water in the gastrointestinal tract. Illnesses that interfere with absorption of water in the small intestine or secretion of water tend to produce voluminous diarrhea. In contrast, colonic processes such as dysentery produce frequent small-volume bloody stools.

Causes of diarrhea are legion, but the most common etiology of diarrhea in children is infectious. Noninflammatory infectious diarrhea is caused by viruses and parasites that localize to the proximal small bowel, or by toxin-producing bacteria. Infectious diarrhea is typically profuse and watery and commonly associated with nausea and vomiting. Fever is less likely. Clinicians frequently use the name gastroenteritis, but the stomach is generally not involved.

Other causes of acute diarrhea are uncommon, but must be consid-

TABLE 126-1 Differential Diagnosis of Vomiting

Infection
  Viral
  Bacterial
  Meningitis
  Sepsis
  Appendicitis
  Otitis media
  Urinary tract infection
  Cholecystitis
  Hepatitis
  Other infections
Intestinal obstruction
  Pyloric stenosis
  Malrotation
  Volvulus
  Incarcerated hernia
  Intussusception
Toxic ingestion
  Contaminated food poisoning
Metabolic disorder
  Diabetic ketoacidosis
  Inborn error of metabolism
Pregnancy
Pancreatitis
Trauma
  Abdominal trauma
  Head injury/increased intracranial pressure
Munchausen by proxy

ered. This includes poisoning due to anticholinesterase insecticides, organophosphates, and carbamates. These liquids may look like milk to a child if they are placed in inappropriate containers such as plastic milk jugs. Diarrhea due to these agents is accompanied by profuse sweating, lacrimation, hypersalivation, and abdominal cramps. Vomiting and diarrhea may also be a nonspecific presentation for other infectious diseases such as otitis media, urinary tract infection, or more serious conditions including intussusception, malrotation, increased intracranial pressure, and metabolic acidosis.

EPIDEMIOLOGY

In the United States, children younger than 3 years of age have 1.3 to 2.3 episodes of diarrhea each year. The prevalence is higher in children attending day-care centers. Up to one-fifth of all acute care outpatient visits to hospitals are by families with infants or children affected by acute gastroenteritis, and 9 percent of all hospitalizations of children younger than 5 years of age are for diarrhea.[1] Most enteric infections are self-limited, but excessive loss of water and electrolytes resulting in clinical dehydration may occur in 10 percent and is life-threatening in 1 percent.[2] Pathogenic viruses, bacteria, or parasites may be isolated from nearly 50 percent of children with diarrhea. Viral infection is the most common cause of acute diarrhea. Bacterial pathogens may be isolated in only 1 to 4 percent of cases. Specific pathogens, diagnostic aids, and treatment are outlined in Table 126-2. While identifying the specific viral or bacterial agent may be a challenging academic exercise, it is often not practical or necessary in the ED.

PATHOPHYSIOLOGY

Diarrhea can be caused by a variety of mechanisms including tissue invasion or toxin production (see Table 126-2). Destruction of intestinal villi results in decreased absorption of water, nutrients and electrolytes, resulting in watery diarrhea or dysentery. Enteric infections with *E. coli* may be used to illustrate the different mechanisms of diarrhea. Enteroinvasive *E. coli* (EIEC) directly invades the gut epithelium causing inflammation, which results in leukocyte infiltration and

TABLE 126-2   Clinical Features, Diagnostic Aids, and Treatment of Diarrhea

Agent	Clinical Features/Historical Clues	Diagnostic Aids	Treatment
Viral			**Rehydration**
Rotavirus	Watery diarrhea, winter, most common agent	Enzyme immunoassay available but of little help in acute management	
Enteric adenovirus	Watery diarrhea, ± concurrent respiratory symptoms		
Norwalk	Watery diarrhea, epidemic gastroenteritis, with associated fever, headache, myalgias		
Bacterial			**Rehydration *plus***
Campylobacter jejuni	Fever, abdominal pain, watery or bloody diarrhea, may mimic appendicitis, animal reservoir	Fecal WBC, stool culture	Erythromycin ethylsuccinate (EES) 50 mg/kg per d divided qid
Shigella	Fever, abdominal pain, headache, mucoid diarrhea, possible seizure, toxic megacolon, small inoculum, very contagious	Fecal WBC, stool culture, swab culture	TMP-SMX (Bactrim) 8/40 mg/kg per d divided bid *or* Ampicillin 50–100 mg/kg per d divided qid
Salmonella	Fever, dysentery, animal reservoir, large inoculum	Fecal WBC, stool culture	Antibiotics prolong carrier state and indicated only if complicated (septic, hemoglobinopathy); TMP-SMX 8/40 mg/kg per d divided bid* *or* ceftriaxone *or* cefotaxime
Escherichia coli			
Enterotoxigenic (ETEC)	Watery diarrhea, cholera-like enterotoxin	Stool culture, ELISA	TMP-SMX 8/40 mg/kg per d divided bid
Enterohemorrhagic (EHEC)	Dysentery, serotype O157:H7 associated with HUS	Fecal WBC, stool culture, PCR, serotype with HUS, check CBC, BUN, creatinine	Supportive care, no antibiotics
Enteroinvasive (EIEC)	Dysentery, *Shigella*-like	Fecal WBC, stool culture	TMP-SMX 8/40 mg/kg per d divided bid
Vibrio cholerae	Rice-water diarrhea, enterotoxin		TMP-SMX 8/40 mg/kg per d divided bid
Yersinia enterocolitica	Fever, vomiting, diarrhea, abdominal pain, may mimic appendicitis, animal reservoir	Stool culture, serology	Ceftriaxone (Rocephin) 50 mg/kg per d (controversial)
Clostridium difficile	Recent antibiotic use	Fecal WBC, stool culture, toxin assay	Metronidazole (Flagyl) 15-40 mg/kg per d divided tid, discontinue other antibiotics
Staphylococcus aureus	Food poisoning, toxin mediated	History	No antibiotics
Parasitic			**Rehydration *plus***
Giardia lamblia	Diarrhea, flatulance, mountain streams, day care	Stool ova and parasite	Metronidazole 15-40 mg/kg per d divided tid
Entamoeba histolytica	Bloody mucoid stools, hepatic abscess	Serologic test	Metronidazole 15-40 mg/kg per d divided tid

*Increasing resistance.
Abbreviatons: BUN = blood urea nitrogen; CBC = complete blood count; ELISA = enzyme-linked immunosorbent assay; HUS = hemolytic uremic syndrome; PCR = polymerase chain reaction; TMP-SMX = trimethoprim-sulfamethoxazole; WBC = white blood cell count.

fecal leukocytes on stool examination. Alternatively, diarrhea may be a result of toxin production. Enterotoxins alter cell function without causing cell death. Enterotoxigenic *E. coli* (ETEC) adheres to mucosal epithelium and elaborates an enterotoxin. The heat labile toxin, which is similar to the toxin produced by *V. cholerae,* increases cyclic adenosine monophosphate, which in turn promotes secretion of electrolytes and fluids into the intestinal lumen.

Enterohemorrhagic *E. coli* (EHEC) produces shiga-like cytotoxin, which differs from enterotoxin, and inhibits protein synthesis, ultimately causing cell death. Infection with enteropathogenic *E. coli* (EPEC) differs from the other forms of *E. coli* infection. It does not produce traditional *E. coli* enterotoxins, nor is it invasive. The organism attaches to the mucosa and destroys microvilli, interrupting absorption. Viruses and parasites cause diarrhea by a variety of mechanisms similar to those discussed above.

CLINICAL FEATURES

A careful assessment of the child's state of hydration is essential, although clinical assessment of dehydration is difficult. The most accurate and objective method is to compare the child's weight when well versus the weight while ill. The value of a history is somewhat limited by the lack of objectiveness on the part of the caregiver, but can be helpful by providing information on what fluids and foods have been offered. A history of last urine output should be obtained, but this may not be obvious in infants and toddlers who are having frequent watery stools. Dehydration may be assessed on the basis of the physical examination, along with the vital signs. Combinations of physical signs, including ill general appearance, vital signs, capillary refill >2 s, dry mucous membranes, and absent tears, are good objective predictors of the degree of dehydration (Table 126-3). The presence of two or more signs predicts 5 percent dehydration, whereas three or more signs predicts 10 percent dehydration.[3] Severe dehydration accompanied by lethargy, hypotension, and delayed capillary refill requires immediate ad-

TABLE 126-3   Clinical Signs of Dehydration

Two or more predict 5% dehydration
Three or more predict 10% dehydration
   Ill general appearance
   Capillary refill >2 s
   Dry mucous membranes
   Absent tears

Source: From Gorelick et al,[3] with permission.

ministration of parenteral fluids. Capillary refill may be affected by conditions other than dehydration, but is generally an excellent indicator of dehydration until proven otherwise.[4] Guidelines for assessing dehydration are listed in Chap. 132.

DIAGNOSIS

The approach to the child with vomiting and/or diarrhea has two main functions. First, the clinician must seek out those conditions that are life-threatening, and swiftly intervene. Anticipation and aggressive fluid resuscitation may be necessary to prevent shock or further deterioration. Historical and clinical information may be incomplete while interventions are occurring. The second purpose of the assessment is to determine the degree of dehydration and proceed with appropriate rehydration.

The less acutely ill child should have a careful history and physical examination performed with selective laboratory and radiologic evaluation. Various cultures and immunoassays of stool for the presence of enteric pathogens are now well established in most hospital laboratories. Routine stool culture for bacterial pathogens now includes *C. jejuni, Y. enterocolitica,* and *Aeromonas* in addition to *Salmonella* and *Shigella.* Subculturing for *E. coli* serotypes or stool assays for *C. difficile* toxin activity are readily available. Enzyme immunoassays are also available to test stool for the presence of rotavirus, enteric adenovirus, and astrovirus.

Most children present with a nonspecific gastroenteritis and not dysentery. The clinician must assess the likelihood of defining a treatable etiology, and as a consequence, the indication for doing a stool culture. The presence of fecal leukocytes and/or positive guaiac testing has been used as a screening tool to identify children at increased risk for invasive bacterial enteric infection. Fecal leukocyte testing has poor sensitivity and guaiac testing has poor specificity.[5] The most prudent approach is that of combining these tests with the clinical findings. If the child is febrile, has abrupt onset of diarrhea occurring more than four times a day, or blood in the stool, the illness is more likely to be caused by a bacterial pathogen and stool cultures are indicated.[6] The likelihood of identifying bacterial pathogens is increased if the patient's stool or accompanying exudates contains polymorphonuclear leukocytes.

Anaerobic stool cultures and assay of stool for *C. difficile* toxin activity should be obtained in children who have been receiving antibiotics and develop bloody diarrhea. A history of hiking or camping should prompt examination for ova and parasites. In addition, a swab of mucus or bloody exudates from the stool should be placed in transport medium and sent to the laboratory for culture of *Shigella* species. *Shigella* is a fastidious pathogen and is more likely to be recovered from a swab than from a fresh stool specimen. In cases of persistent or recurrent diarrhea, especially with weight loss or day care center exposure or in immunocompromised children, stool samples should be collected in fixative and examined for *G. lamblia, E. histolytica,* and *Cryptosporidium.* Depending on geographic location or travel history, serologic testing for *E. histolytica* infection may be indicated.

MEASUREMENT OF ELECTROLYTES AND BLOOD GLUCOSE

Dehydration caused by diarrhea is usually isotonic and measurement of serum electrolytes is not always necessary. However, it is most important to be aware of the physical findings of hypernatremic dehydration such as hyperirritability, sunken eyeballs and fontanelle, parched mucous membranes, and thickened, doughy skin. If hypernatremia is suspected, or if dehydration is moderate to severe, measurement of electrolytes is mandatory. Infants and children who have hypernatremic dehydration have special requirements for rehydration after initial fluid resuscitation and require hospitalization.

Children receiving IV therapy are generally ill enough that electrolytes and blood glucose levels should be checked initially. Protracted vomiting and/or diarrhea associated with concomitant fasting may increase the risk of hypoglycemia. Younger infants, those born small for gestational age, and children with underlying metabolic disease are at higher risk of developing hypoglycemia. Bedside measurement of blood glucose may help in managing these infants. However, several studies have shown that other laboratory findings are generally neither helpful in acute management, nor predictive of ultimate disposition and should be used selectively.[7] Laboratory testing should not replace clinical reassessment.

EMERGENCY DEPARTMENT TREATMENT

After other life-threatening diseases have been ruled out, the management of acute gastroenteritis is then directed at preventing or treating the underlying dehydration. The American Academy of Pediatrics (AAP) has published guidelines (summarized in Figure 126-1) for management of acute diarrhea and vomiting in children aged 1 month to 5 years. The AAP practice guidelines evolved in part from the recognition that practitioners in the United States often do not use oral rehydration therapy (ORT) even though there are several oral rehydration solutions (ORS) available in the United States.[8] ORT is less expensive than intravenous fluid therapy, is generally readily accepted by dehydrated children, and generally rehydrates more than 90 percent of dehydrated children with lower complication rates.[9]

ORT capitalizes on the fact that glucose-coupled sodium and water absorption remains sufficiently intact during most infections, despite significant impairment of NaCl uptake. Glucose-electrolyte solutions such as Pedialyte are readily available in the United States. The glucose concentration of these solutions does not exceed the sodium concentration in millimolar units by more than 2:1. The ideal composition of ORS is a matter of controversy and heated debate. The World Health Organization solution developed almost 30 years ago has an osmolality of about 310 mOsm/L. Newer hypoosmolar solutions such as Pedialyte, with an osmolality of about 250 mOsm/L, have proven to be equally safe, and may result in lower stool volumes and reduced duration of diarrhea.[9,10] In contrast, other clear fluids often used as replacements, such as soft drinks, juices, sports drinks, and jello water, are largely carbohydrate based. These fluids are typically deficient in NaCl, and have osmolalities ranging from 510 to 1225 mOsm/L. The use of these highly osmolar sugar-based solutions to treat acute diarrhea will predictably amplify net small intestinal fluid secretion and increase diarrhea.

Vomiting is not a contraindication to continuing ORT, although parents sometimes may not be willing to continue their efforts in the face of continued emesis. The key to success in a vomiting child is to give small volumes of ORS, often starting with 5 mL at a time given every 2 or 3 min. ORS may also be given in frozen form as a popsicle. ORT is labor-intensive, and parents may be unavailable or unwilling to give this a try.

If rehydration measures are successful, reinstatement of food should begin as soon as possible. The once common management of diarrhea and vomiting by starvation is never appropriate. Recent studies have shown that the introduction of full-strength formula or unrestricted diet immediately following rehydration is associated with decreased duration of diarrhea, positive nitrogen balance, and increased weight gain. Breast-feeding should be routinely continued in infants with acute gastroenteritis. Infants who have been receiving formula feedings and who are not dehydrated may rapidly return to their feeding. There is no need to give dilute formula. The bananas, rice, applesauce, toast (BRAT) diet widely recommended by practitioners does not provide adequate energy, fat, or protein. Instead, consumption of complex carbohydrates, lean meats, yogurt, fruits, and vegetables should be encouraged. Fatty foods and foods high in simple sugars like juices and soft drinks should be avoided. Finally, there is little evidence to support a lactose-free diet.[11]

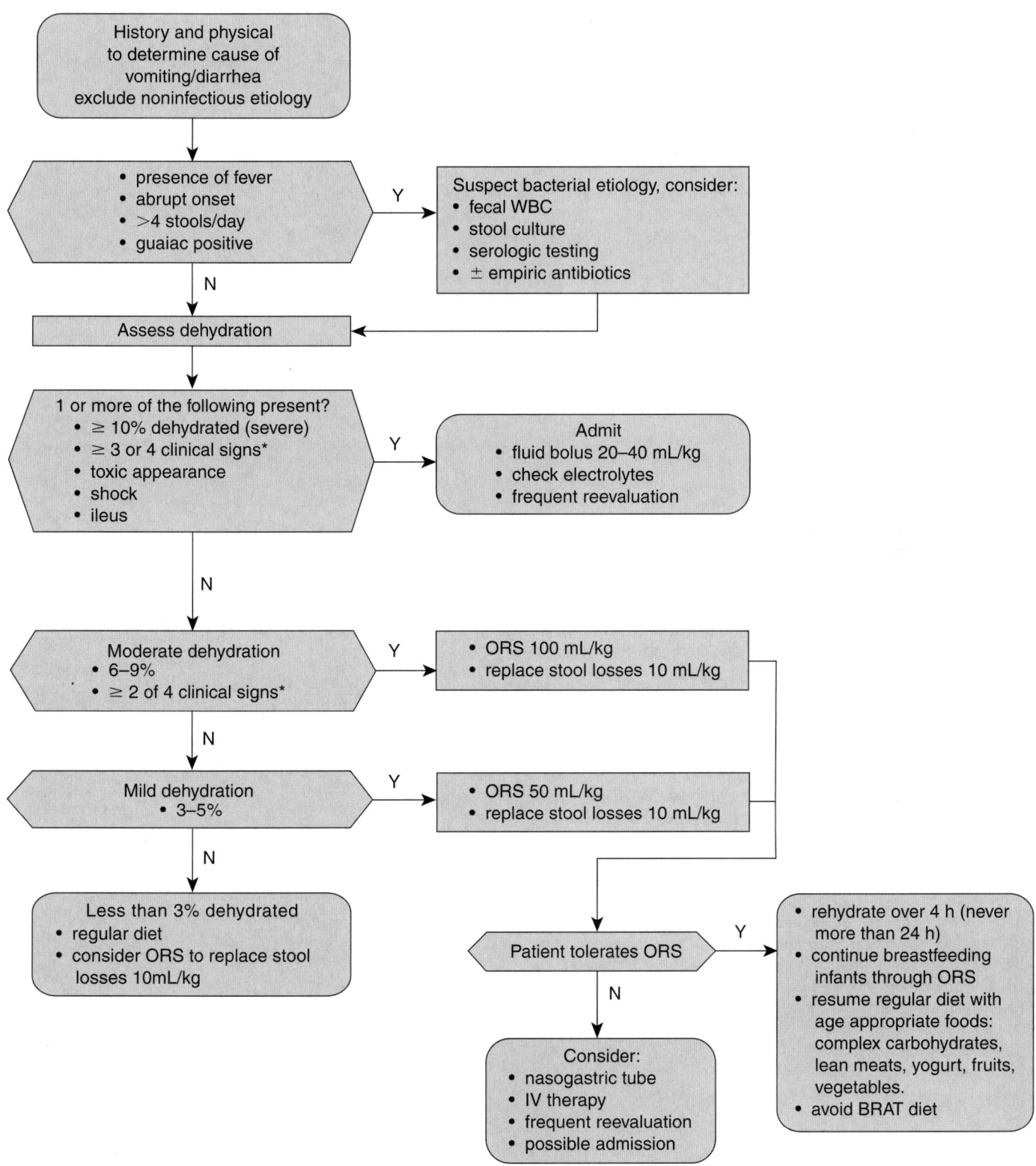

*Clinical signs of dehydration see Table 126-3. BRAT = bananas, rice, applesauce, toast; ORS = oral rehydration solution like Pedialyte; WBC = white blood cell.

FIG. 126-1. Guidelines for management of vomiting and diarrhea in children. (Adapted with permission from American Academy of Pediatrics, Provisional Committee on Quality Improvement, Subcommittee on Acute Gastroenteritis Practice Parameter: The management of acute gastroenteritis in young children. Pediatrics 97:424, 1996.)

Specific Therapy

REHYDRATION   The treatment of a child with diarrhea is directed by the degree of dehydration. If there is no dehydration, continued age-appropriate feedings are encouraged. ORT may be given in 10 mL/kg amounts to replace ongoing stool looses. Mild dehydration (3 to 5 percent) should be corrected by giving 50 mL/kg ORT plus replacement of continuing losses during a 4-h period. The continuing losses from stool and emesis are replaced by giving an additional 10 mL/kg for each stool. Age-appropriate feeding should continue after the dehydration is corrected, and as the child so desires. Moderate dehydration (6 to 9 percent) is corrected by giving 100 mL/kg ORT plus replacement over a 4-h period. Ongoing losses are corrected as above. Reassessment should occur hourly, and thus may be best accomplished in a supervised setting such as the ED or physician's office. If oral therapy fails, and intravenous access is difficult, placement of a nasogastric tube to provide ORS may be successful.

Clinical studies strongly support the use of ORT, yet the clinician must know how and when to use intravenous fluid therapy. A severely dehydrated infant or child presents with a medical emergency. Intravenous fluids should be given in 20 mL/kg increments, with immediate reassessment for continued fluids. Children in shock should receive at least 60 mL/kg in the first hour with frequent reassessments. Electrolytes and blood glucose determinations should be performed, and plans for hospitalization implemented.

Parents may request medications to treat the symptoms of diarrhea and vomiting, but their use is controversial and mostly not recommended. As a general rule, pharmacologic agents such as antiemetics, anticholinergics, opiates, and adsorbents are not suggested for use because of the self-limited nature of the vomiting and its tendency to improve as the dehydration is corrected. Side effects may be augmented in infants and children in the presence of diarrheal disease.[12] Additionally, most are not approved for use in children less than 2 years of age. The European Society for Paediatric Gastroenterology, Hepatology and Nutrition issued nine pillars of good treatment of acute gastroenteritis listed in Table 126-4.[13]

DYSENTERY   Antibiotic therapy does not affect the clinical outcome in most cases of acute diarrhea and may be contraindicated in some infections. Patients with uncomplicated *Salmonella* gastroenteritis should not be given antibiotics unless they appear septic or are bacteremic, have a hemoglobinopathy, or have an underlying chronic gastrointestinal disorder. However, infants less than 6 months of age are an exception and are generally treated with antibiotics because of their overall risk of bacteremia or suppurative disease. If the child has had diarrhea lasting longer than 10 to 14 days, has a significant fever or systemic complaints, and has inflammatory cells or blood in the stool, then empiric antimicrobial treatment may be indicated after sending a stool sample for bacterial culture. Empiric therapy should provide coverage for the usual dysenteric agents such as *Shigella, Salmonella,* and *Campylobacter.* Ampicillin or trimethoprim-sulfamethoxazole is a reasonable choice. Debilitated patients, children with an underlying gas-

trointestinal disorder, immunocompromised children, and children with severe bloody diarrhea should be treated with oral antibiotics.[14]

Children who have been receiving antibiotics and develop bloody diarrhea may have antibiotic-associated colitis. Most cases of antibiotic-associated colitis caused by *C. difficile* resolve spontaneously when antibiotics are discontinued. Infants and children with protracted diarrhea that has not improved after discontinuing antibiotics may benefit from receiving metronidazole. Cholestyramine, an anion exchange resin that adsorbs *C. difficile* toxins, may be beneficial in mild disease, but because of its limited efficacy and potential binding of antibiotics, it may not be indicated in the emergent setting.

Infants and children with bloody diarrhea may have a gastrointestinal infection due to *E. coli* O157:H7 and are at risk of developing hemolytic uremic syndrome (HUS).[15] The source most frequently identified in outbreaks has been exposure to undercooked ground meat or poultry, eggs, or unpasteurized milk. Person-to-person transmission, especially in child day care centers, is also a well-recognized risk factor for childhood HUS. The risk is highest for children under 5 years of age who are infected with *E. coli* O157:H7 and the incidence may approach 13 percent. Although antibiotic therapy may not impact outcome, these patients should be admitted for supportive care.

DISPOSITION

All infants and children who appear toxic should be admitted. Patients with 10 percent dehydration, intractable vomiting, or altered consciousness should be given an infusion of NS or LR, regardless of the serum osmolality, and admitted. Any child who presents with acute bloody diarrhea and laboratory evidence of hemolytic anemia, thrombocytopenia, and/or elevated serum creatinine should be admitted. Infants who are less ill but whose families may not be able to follow the guidelines for administering ORS should also be admitted.

Infants who are malnourished and have acute diarrhea require special attention. They more often need to be admitted to the hospital as they may develop metabolic acidosis accompanied by an increase in the anion gap and renal dysfunction. This is in contrast to most well-nourished infants, who develop hyperchloremic acidosis due to fecal loses of bicarbonate. The latter group of infants can be expected to improve with oral therapy.

Infants under 1 year of age pose a more difficult problem because of the risk of rapid dehydration and hypoglycemia. Signs of sepsis in this age group may be nonspecific. The threshold for hospital admission should be lowered in any infant who fails to make eye contact or to respond to a parent's voice. Although bilious vomiting may develop in older infants and children who acquire viral gastroenteritis, bilious vomiting in an infant under 2 years of age is a sign of intestinal obstruction until proven otherwise.

Most cases of acute gastroenteritis do not require consultation. In cases of suspected intestinal obstruction, appendicitis, or intussusception, surgical consultation is indicated. Many surgeons prefer consultation prior to radiologic confirmation of intussusception. Ingestion of toxins often requires consultation with a poison control center or toxicologist. In cases in which abuse or neglect is suspected, social service and the primary care physician should be involved. Chronic diarrhea or chronic vomiting should be discussed with the child's primary care provider to determine whether consultation is indicated.

DISCHARGE INSTRUCTIONS

Infants and children who are not dehydrated or who have responded well to oral or intravenous hydration may be discharged with instructions to take ORS and age-appropriate feedings. The family should be instructed to return to the ED or to their own physician if the child becomes unable or unwilling to drink the ORS, begins to vomit, has increased emesis, develops bilious emesis, or shows signs of

TABLE 126-4   Nine Pillars of Treatment of Acute Gastroenteritis

Use of ORS for dehydration
Hypotonic solution
Fast oral rehydration over 3–4 h
Rapid realimentation with normal feeding (including solids) thereafter
Use of special formula is unjustified
Use of diluted formula is unjustified
Continuation of breast-feeding at all times
Supplementation with ORS for ongoing losses
No unnecessary medication

Source: From Hoekstra et al,[13] with permission.

dehydration, such as decreasing urine output or decreased tearing, or if there is a decrease in the child's level of activity or state of alertness. Infants and small children should be reevaluated within 24 h, especially if they continue to have diarrhea. The family should be instructed to telephone their primary care provider and he or she should decide if a visit is necessary. If the family does not have a primary care physician, then the family should contact the ED.

REFERENCES

1. Cicrello HG, Glass RI: Current concepts of the epidemiology of diarrheal diseases. *Pediatr Infect Dis* 5:163, 1994.
2. Glass RJ, Lew JF, Gangorosa RE, et al: Estimate of morbidity and mortality rates for diarrheal diseases in American children. *J Pediatr* 118(Suppl):527, 1991.
3. Gorelick MH, Shaw KN, Murphy KO: Validity and reliability of clinical signs in the diagnosis of dehydration in children. *Pediatrics* 99:e6, 1997.
4. Gorelick MH, Shaw KN, Murphy KO, et al: Effect of fever on capillary refill time. *Pediatr Emerg Care* 13:305, 1997.
5. Hiricho L, Campos M, Rivera J, et al: Fecal screening tests in the approach to acute infectious diarrhea: A scientific overview. *Pediatr Infect Dis J* 15: 486, 1996.
6. DeWitt TC, Humphrey KF, McCarthy P: Clinical predictors of acute bacterial diarrhea in young children. *Pediatrics* 76:551, 1985.
7. Teach SJ, Yates EW, Feld LG: Laboratory predictors of fluid deficit in acutely dehydrated children. *Clin Pediatr* 36:395-400, 1997.
8. American Academy of Pediatrics, Provisional Committee on Quality Improvement, Subcommittee on Acute Gastroenteritis Practice Parameter: The management of acute gastroenteritis in young children. *Pediatrics* 97:424, 1996.
9. Santosham M, Daum RS, Dillman L, et al: Oral rehydration therapy of infantile diarrhea: A controlled study of well-nourished children hospitalized in the United States and Panama. *New Engl J Med* 306:1070, 1982.
10. Guarino A, Albano F, Guandalini S: Oral rehydration: Toward a real solution. *J Pediatr Gastroenterol Nutr* 33(Suppl 2) S2–S12, 2001.
11. Brown KH, Peerson JM, Fontaine O: Use of nonhuman milks in the dietary management of young children with acute diarrhea: A meta-analysis of clinical trials. *Pediatrics* 93:17, 1994.
12. World Health Organization: *The Rational Use of Drugs in the Management of Acute Diarrheoea in Children.* Geneva: World Health Organization, 1990.
13. Hoekstra JH, European Society of Paediatric Gastroenterology, Hepatology, and Nutrition: Acute gastroenteritis in industrialized countries: Compliance with guidelines for treatment. *J Pediatr Gastroenterol Nutr* 33:S31, 2001.
14. Richards L, Claeson M, Pierce N: Management of acute diarrhea in children: Lessons learned. *Pediatr Infect Dis J* 12:5, 1993.
15. Rowe PC, Orrbine E, Lior H, et al: Risk of hemolytic uremic syndrome after sporadic *Escherichia coli* O157:H7 infection: Results of a Canadian collaborative study. *J Pediatr* 132:777, 1998.

PEDIATRIC ABDOMINAL EMERGENCIES
Robert W. Schafermeyer

Evaluation of abdominal emergencies in children can present a diagnostic challenge. Some diseases are common to both adults and children while others are age specific, such as congenital anomalies, volvulus, malrotation, and Hirschsprung disease. One must understand the differential diagnoses of the presenting symptoms, recognize the clinical manifestations of the more common and life-threatening diseases, and be sensitive in approaching infants and children. Chap. 117 also discusses abdominal pain in neonates.

One can classify abdominal disease processes in several ways. Is the child febrile or afebrile? Does the disease appear to be obstructive or nonobstructive, abdominal, or extraabdominal in nature? Is it due to a local or a systemic process? Does the child appear healthy and happy or sick and septic?

The child's age influences the presenting signs and symptoms significantly. The spectrum of pathologic gastrointestinal (GI) conditions of a 2-day-old infant is vastly different from that of a 2-week-old, and both are quite different from that of a 2-year-old.

HISTORY

An infant or young child cannot give a complete history, but if the child is verbal, try to get the historical information from the child; then obtain the history from the parent or caregiver. Find out the accurate chronology of events, whether fever has been a part of the illness, the quality and location of pain, feeding and bowel habits, and the quality and quantity of vomiting and bowel losses. Inquire whether blood has been present in vomitus or stools. Ask about weight changes. A history of prematurity, necrotizing enterocolitis, congenital anomalies, inborn errors of metabolism, cystic fibrosis, intussusception, or sickle cell anemia are all associated with abdominal complications.

Unfortunately, because some children are either too young or too frightened to speak for themselves or have not been under continuous observation, one may miss trauma as a cause of an abdominal emergency. Such trauma may be accidental or secondary to abuse. Always keep trauma in the differential diagnosis when evaluating pediatric patients presenting with what appears to be an abdominal emergency.

EVALUATION

Children vary greatly in their ability to cooperate with a physical examination. Take a few moments to gain the confidence of the child before any painful examination or procedures are performed. Allowing the child to rest or be on the caregiver's lap may help. Remove clothing to avoid missing an incarcerated hernia, petechiae, visible masses, or peristalsis. Look first and then feel. Consider some non-touch maneuvers and observations such as the child's responses during coughing, walking, climbing onto the table, or jumping up and down.

The child can be invited to self-palpate or palpate with the physician. Start in the least painful areas. Also, evaluate extraabdominal areas such as the pharynx, mucous membranes, neck, lung fields, inguinal regions, femoral triangles, testes, and scrotum. Failure to do so may result in delayed or missed diagnoses. The rectal examination and guaiac test may provide important clues to the diagnosis. The diagnosis of Hirschsprung disease, volvulus, or intussusception may be missed without them.

The more important studies include a urinalysis, a complete blood count and differential, and a test of the stool for occult blood. Other tests, ultrasound, and x-ray evaluation should be guided by history, physical examination, how ill the child appears, and the differential diagnoses. Electrolyte and lipase determination, a pregnancy test, and chest and abdominal x-rays may be useful in certain cases. Computed tomography and ultrasonography are also helpful in the evaluation of stable patients with acute pain.[1]

Once the history, physical examination, and laboratory studies are completed, one should develop a list of differential diagnoses. If a child is critically ill, resuscitation and evaluation must be simultaneous. Early surgical consultation is essential for a child with an acute abdomen. If the child is ill but stable and the findings are equivocal, admit the patient for observation and reassessment.

KEY SYMPTOMS

The important GI signs and symptoms are pain, vomiting, diarrhea, constipation, upper or lower GI bleeding, jaundice, and masses.

Pain

Abdominal pain can be a manifestation of a variety of disease states not necessarily related to the intestinal tract.[2,3] The origin of the pain may be extraabdominal, such as one might see in a 3- to 6-year-old with tonsillitis or pneumonia. Therefore a careful general physical examination is necessary. One should distinguish between two types of pain: peritoneal and obstructive:

1. Peritoneal pain tends to be exacerbated by motion and thus keeps patients relatively immobile, for example as in appendicitis.
2. Obstructive pain is usually spasmodic and associated with restlessness and motion, for example as with intussusception.

In the very young (up to 2 years of age), pain is usually described by the caregiver in general terms, such as fussiness, irritability, and inconsolableness. With severe peritoneal pain, the caregiver may state that the child is very irritable or lethargic or seems to be grunting as if in pain. Peritonitis or pain from intussusception may present as lethargy or an altered level of consciousness.

Between 2 and 6 years of age, pain of GI origin is usually referred to the periumbilical region, and diagnosis requires correlation of the patient's observations and the physician's visual and tactile evaluation. Youngsters with pain of peritoneal origin walk with obvious discomfort and prefer to lie still. In contrast, youngsters with obstructive pain may be unable to remain still on the examining table. The etiologies of pain vary significantly with age (Table 127-1). Every emergency physician must be familiar with and recognize the life-threatening causes of pain (Table 127-2). The clinician must provide appropriate supportive therapy while completing the diagnostic evaluation and/or consultation.

TABLE 127-1   Etiology of Pain

Under 2 years	6–11 Years
Appendicitis	Appendicitis
Colic (first 4 months)	Diabetic ketoacidosis
Congenital anomalies	Functional pain
Gastroenteritis	Gastroenteritis
Incarcerated hernia	Henoch-Schölein purpura
Intussusception	Incarcerated hernia
Malabsorption (gaseous distention)	Inflammatory bowel disease
Malrotation	Obstruction
Obstruction	Peptic ulcer disease
Sickle cell pain crises	Pneumonia
Toxins (lead, arsenic)	Renal stones
Trauma	Sickle cell syndrome
Urinary tract infection	Streptococcal pharyngitis
Volvulus	Torsion of ovary or testicle
	Toxins (lead, arsenic)
	Trauma
	Urinary tract infection
2–5 Years	**Over 11 Years**
Appendicitis	Appendicitis
Diabetic ketoacidosis	Cholecystitis
Gastroenteritis	Diabetic ketoacidosis
Hemolytic uremic syndrome	Dysmenorrhea
Henoch-Schönlein purpura	Ectopic pregnancy
Incarcerated hernia	Functional pain
Intussusception	Gastroenteritis
Malabsorption (gaseus distention)	Incarcerated hernia
Obstruction	Inflammatory bowel disease
Pneumonia	Obstruction
Sickle cell pain crises	Pancreatitis
Toxins (lead, arsenic)	Peptic ulcer disease
Trauma	Pneumonia
Urinary tract infection	Pregnancy
Volvulus	Renal stones
	Sickle cell syndrome
	Torsion of ovary or testicle
	Toxins (lead, arsenic)
	Trauma
	Urinary tract infection

TABLE 127-2   Life-Threatening Causes of Pain

Appendicitis	Peptic ulcer disease: complications
Congenital anomalies (malrotation, intestinal atresia or stenosis, imperforate anus, inta-abdominal bands, etc.)	Pneumonia
	Sepsis
	Toxins (lead, arsenic, mushrooms, spider bite)
Diabetic ketoacidosis	Trauma
Ectopic pregnancy	Volvulus
Hemolytic uremic syndrome	
Incarcerated hernia	
Intussusception	

Vomiting

Vomiting is a common childhood problem and may be a specific or nonspecific manifestation of a benign process or a serious, life-threatening illness or injury. Vomiting or regurgitation may be a manifestation of a relatively minor problem (e.g., a nervous parent, poor feeding habits, or gastroesophageal reflux), or it may be a sign of a more serious illness. Bilious vomiting is always a serious manifestation in an infant or child. Vomiting may be a sign of obstructive or nonobstructive GI diseases, or of infections or metabolic disorders (Table 127-3).

Vomiting (bilious or not) is a classic symptom of mechanical intestinal obstruction in children. In the early phases of illness, before a child has developed electrolyte abnormalities (e.g., in a child with pyloric stenosis) or before a child has gangrenous bowel (e.g., intestinal volvulus), the child's general condition may appear to be good. The child may be hungry immediately after vomiting and even eat vigorously. One must not ignore the possibility of a serious underlying in-

TABLE 127-3   Causes of Vomiting

Newborn (0–2 Months)	Infant (2 Months to 2 Years)
Congenital adrenal hyperplasia	Appendicitis
Congenital anomalies	Congenital adrenal hyperplasia
Food poisoning	Diabetic ketoacidosis
Gastroenteritis	Foreign body
Gastroesophageal reflux	Gastroenteritis
Hirschsprung disease	Head trauma
Hydrocephalus	Hirschsprung disease
Inborn errors of metabolism	Hydrocephalus
Incarcerated hernia	Incarcerated hernia
Kernicterus (newborn)	Intussusception
Malrotation	Malrotation
Meconium ileus	Meningitis
Meningitis	Metabolic acidosis
Necrotizing enterocolitis	Neurologic diseases (meningitis, encephalitis, Reye syndrome, brain tumor)
Obstruction: anatomic causes	
Obstruction: renal system	
Pneumonia	Obstruction
Pyloric stenosis	Pneumonia
Sepsis	Pyloric stenosis
Toxins	Sepsis
Urinary tract infection	Toxins
Volvulus	Urinary tract infection
	Volvulus

Over 2 Years and Adolescents	
Appendicitis	Neurologic diseases
Diabetic ketoacidosis	Pancreatitis
Foreign body	Peritonitis
Gastroenteritis	Pneumonia
Head trauma	Pregnancy
Hirschsprung's disease	Sepsis
Incarcerated hernia	Toxins
Meningitis	Trauma
Metabolic acidosis	Urinary tract infection

traabdominal pathologic condition merely because a vomiting child appears to be systemically well.

Evaluate the child's circulatory and volume status and administer boluses of NS at 20 mL/kg for any child in shock or dehydrated. A one-time dose of an antiemetic may be given safely to children over 6 months of age. Children with shock or severe dehydration will need consultation. For young children who appear systemically well, 30 mL of clear liquids or infant rehydration solution can be provided at 15- to 30-min intervals.

Diarrhea

Diarrhea is an increased number of watery stools over a defined period of time. An infant may have a formed or semi-formed stool after each feeding and this could be normal. Several mechanisms can cause diarrhea in the child, including osmotic, secretory, and transit disorders. Viral and bacterial pathogens cause the majority of episodes of diarrhea. Some tumors, such as neuroblastomas, secrete hormones that can increase stool water content.

When the presenting symptom is diarrhea, one must quantify the number and volume of stools, consistency, and the presence of blood. Ascertain the norm for the child, since there is great individual variability in frequency and type of stools. Associated symptoms or the presence of diarrheal illness in other members of the family may help in establishing the diagnosis. Assess for and treat dehydration and electrolyte imbalance. Diarrhea may represent fluid expelled around an anatomic obstructive mass, such as an impaction, or functional obstruction, as in Hirschsprung disease (absence of parasympathetic ganglia cells in the muscle layers of the colon). Bloody diarrhea may be infectious or a manifestation of a systemic disease (e.g., hemolytic uremic syndrome; Table 127-4).

Treatment of diarrhea will vary depending on the cause. A suspicion of Hirschsprung or Crohn disease warrants surgical consultation. Malabsorption, hemolytic uremic syndrome, cystic fibrosis, or persistent diarrhea with weight loss and failure to thrive warrants pediatric consultation. Other causes may only require rehydration solution for 24 h and avoiding fatty or high-carbohydrate foods for a couple of days. Stool cultures are warranted in children with bloody diarrhea, diarrhea for more than 5 days, or toxic appearance, or to track an epidemic form of illness.

Constipation

Constipation is infrequent, dry, hard stools that may result from defects in filling or emptying the rectum and may be a sign of either a pathologic or functional process (Table 127–5). Eventually, watery stool works its way around the impaction and causes diarrhea. **Thus the rectal examination is very important in the evaluation of both constipation and diarrhea.**

Causes of constipation are quite different in infants and older children. In infancy, one must consider causes such as maternal drugs, congenital GI anomalies, cystic fibrosis, Hirschsprung disease, poor intake, and anal fissure. Note the abdominal shape and girth, the presence of bowel sounds and masses, and check the anal area. Check rectal tone, examine for an anal fissure, and check the stool for occult blood. If a bowel obstruction is suspected, surgical consultation is nec-

TABLE 127-4   Causes of Diarrhea

Anatomic: Hirschsprung disease
Dietary: allergy, malabsorption, overfeeding
Infectious: bacterial, parasitic, toxic, viral
Inflammatory: Crohn disease, hemolytic uremic syndrome, ulcerative colitis
Malabsorption: cystic fibrosis, enzyme deficiencies, celiac disease
Systemic: endocrinopathy, immunodeficiencies
Obstructive: fecal impaction

TABLE 127-5   Acute and Chronic Constipation

NONORGANIC	
Miscellaneous	Drugs
Anorexia nervosa	Anticholinergics
Functional	Antihistamines
Limited fluid intake	Diuretics
Minimal bulk diet	Opiates
Prolonged immobilization	Vincristine
Psychogenic	

ORGANIC	
Gastrointestinal	Metabolic
Anal fissure	Dehydration
Anal stricture/stenosis	Hypercalcemia
Cystic fibrosis	Hypokalemia
Hirschsprung disease	Hypothyroidism
Obstruction	Renal tubular acidosis
Tumor	Neuromuscular
Volvulus	Amyotonia congenita
Infectious	Cerebral palsy
Infantile botulism	Myotonic dystrophy
	Spina bifida
	Spinal cord disease or injury
	Tumor

essary. If no systemic cause or serious illness is suspected, dark thick molasses or corn syrup can be added to the diet. Finally, if the child is listless or hypotonic, one should consider infantile botulism.

In older children, one should not automatically think that the cause is functional. Constipation is seen in children who are anorexic or who have cerebral palsy, neuromuscular disease, dehydration, hypercalcemia, hypokalemia, hypothyroidism, or depression, or who have ingested drugs such as diuretics, antihistamines, anticholinergics, or narcotics. A thorough history and physical examination, including a rectal exam, are necessary. An empty rectal vault does not rule out constipation. If there are signs of bowel obstruction, tumor, or serious illness, one should consult an appropriate specialist.

Acute constipation is treated by increased oral fluids and possibly a stool softener or milk of magnesia. Chronic constipation is treated in three separate steps, and follow-up with a primary care specialist is important. The steps are clean-out, maintenance, and behavior modification.

Upper and Lower Gastrointestinal Bleeding

There are many causes of upper and lower GI bleeding, and the type of disorder is somewhat age dependent (Table 127-6). It is frequently difficult to determine the cause of minimal to moderate GI bleeding. Repeated episodes of bleeding require GI studies, endoscopic evaluation, and Meckel isotope scanning.

Bleeding in the neonate may be a sign of necrotizing enterocolitis, GI duplication, infection, milk allergy, or sepsis, or it may be nothing more than an anal fissure. GI bleeding in the healthy appearing newborn, either vomited or per rectum, may be the result of swallowed maternal blood (see Chap. 117). Small amounts of fresh blood in the diaper may result from an anal fissure. Milk allergy is an IgE-mediated disorder characterized by diffuse mucosal hyperemia. Bleeding can be mild or severe. Coagulopathies can cause GI bleeding in the newborn. The presence of small to moderate amounts of blood in the stool of an infant, particularly if associated with vomiting, should lead to consideration of malrotation of the midgut.

If the infant or child has bloody diarrhea, considerations include infectious colitis or inflammatory bowel disease.[4] If the child has colicky abdominal pain, consider intussusception. If bleeding is painless, Meckel diverticulum should be suspected. Major painless upper GI bleeding in infants or children is most commonly the result of bleeding

TABLE 127-6   Causes of Gastrointestinal (GI) Bleeding

Under 2 Months	2 Months to 2 Years	Over 2 Years
UPPER GI BLEEDING		
Bleeding diathesis	Bleeding diathesis	Esophageal varices
Swallowed maternal blood	Foreign body	Foreign body
Vascular malformation	Gastroenteritis	Gastroenteritis
	Vascular malformation	Mallory-Weiss tear
	Mallory-Weiss tear	Peptic ulcer disease
		Vascular malformation
		Varices
		Gastritis
LOWER GI BLEEDING		
Congenital duplications	Anal fissure	Colitis
Intussusception	Congenital duplication	Gastroenteritis
Meckel diverticulum	Gastroenteritis	Hemolytic uremic syndrome
Necrotizing enterocolitis	Hemolytic uremic syndrome	Henoch-Schönlein purpura
Swallowed maternal blood	Henoch-Schönlein purpura	Inflammatory bowel disease
Vascular malformation	Inflammatory bowel disease	Meckel diverticulum
Volvulus	Meckel diverticulum	Polyps
	Milk allergy	
	Polyps; benign, familial	

varices secondary to portal hypertension, which can be due to hepatitis, or congenital diseases such as cystic fibrosis, α_1 antitrypsin deficiency, glycogen storage disease, or Wilson disease. If rectal examination identifies a severe, large fissure or rectal tear, one should consider possible abuse. Treatment for fissures includes stool softeners and sitz bath.

In the older child, consider GI polyps, internal hemorrhoids, severe gastroenteritis, Henoch-Schönlein purpura, hemolytic uremic syndrome, or an anal fissure. In adolescents, one must consider stress ulceration, peptic ulcer disease, and inflammatory bowel disease.

Treatment

The child with upper or lower gastrointestinal hemorrhage must have a rapid assessment of hemodynamic status and receive aggressive treatment of hypovolemia with intravenous fluids and/or packed red blood cells. Signs of hemodynamic instability in the child include tachycardia, tachypnea, unstable vital signs, pallor, poor capillary refill, altered mental status or ongoing blood loss. Fluid should be administered until the child is hemodynamically stable and packed red blood cells should be given to children with significant hemorrhage. Fresh frozen plasma may be needed if the child also has liver disease.

Both gastrointestinal and nongastrointestinal sources of bleeding should be considered. The oropharynx should be evaluated for signs of bleeding. A nasogastric tube should be placed in all patients with a significant history of hematemesis or if the examination reveals melena. If the aspirate reveals active bleeding, then gastric lavage should be started with room temperature normal saline. A pediatric surgeon, gastroenterologist, or pediatrician should be consulted.

Jaundice

Jaundice can be an ominous sign, since it represents hepatic dysfunction. It might represent sepsis, congenital infection [TORCHS (toxoplasmosis, rubella, cytomegalovirus, herpes simplex, syphilis)], or postnatal viral hepatitis. It might represent a minor or a major ABO or Rh factor incompatibility, with the possibility of kernicterus or death. It may represent the first signs of cystic fibrosis, galactosemia, or

other hepatic enzyme deficiencies, or it could be the harbinger of an anatomic problem such as biliary atresia, a choledochal cyst, or even pyloric stenosis. All icteric patients should be evaluated promptly and consultation strongly considered (Table 127-7).

Masses

The presence of a mass could be the first sign of a congenital anomaly or a tumor (e.g., Wilms tumor or neuroblastoma). It could be a pyloric "olive" or an intussusception mass if associated with vomiting or a guaiac-positive stool. If a child has an acute surgical abdomen or intestinal obstruction, resuscitation and prompt surgical consultation is necessary. Otherwise, emergency evaluation should be followed by pediatric consultation and admission (Table 127-8).

DIAGNOSIS AND MANAGEMENT OF SELECTED DISORDERS

Gastrointestinal Emergencies in Infants in the First Year of Life

MALROTATION WITH AND WITHOUT VOLVULUS   Volvulus is a major life-threatening complication of malrotation.[5] The complications of malrotation occur most commonly in the first year of life, although malrotation can give rise to symptoms at any time in a person's life. The vast majority of cases occur within the first month of life. It is the most urgent of GI emergencies in infants and children because of consequent gangrene of the entire midgut. The time interval from the first symptom to the development of total midgut gangrene may be only a few hours.

Pathophysiology   During gestation, at approximately 6 weeks of age, the elongating intestines prolapse into the yolk sac. Upon reentry at 10 weeks, the midgut undergoes a 270° counterclockwise turn around the superior mesenteric artery. Usually the duodenum and the cecum become fixed by peritoneal bands, and the small intestine has a broad mesenteric attachment along its base. Abnormal rotation and inadequate fixation can occur during gestation. Incomplete rotation or malrotation can leave the cecum high in the abdomen, with its peritoneal attachments crossing the duodenum in an obstructing manner. The mesentery fails to fan out, and the midgut is suspended and its entire vascular supply travels along a narrow pedicle.

Clinical Features   The presenting symptoms are usually vomiting, ultimately becoming bilious, with or without abdominal distention, and streaks of blood may be seen in the stool. Infants with symptoms

TABLE 127-7   Causes of Jaundice

Unconjugated	Conjugated
ABO or Rh incompatibility	Anatomic defect: biliary, hepatic
Autoimmune hemolytic anemia	Hemolytic uremic syndrome
Hepatic: Crigler-Najjar syndrome, Gilbert disease	Hepatic abscess
	Hepatitis: congenital, acquired
Hypothyroidism	Hepatitis: TORCHS
Sepsis	Inflammatory bowel disease
Sickle cell anemia	Metabolic: cystic fibrosis,
G6PD deficiency	galactosemia, etc.
	Sepsis
	Sickle cell anemia
	Toxins
	Urinary tract infections
	Wilson disease

Abbreviation: TORCHS = toxoplasmosis, rubella, cytomegalovirus, herpes simplex, syphilis.

TABLE 127-8   Causes of Abdominal Masses

Hepatomegaly
Splenomegaly
Gastrointestinal duplication
Neuroblastoma
Presacral teratoma
Ovarian tumor
Wilms' tumor
Pyloric stenosis
Intussusception mass
Constipation (fecal mass)

of obstruction or bilious vomiting must receive prompt surgical consultation and active resuscitation. The most dramatic presentation in newborns is the sudden onset of an acute abdomen and shock, with a rigid and discolored abdomen associated with bilious or bloody vomiting and bloody stools, indicating the presence of gangrenous bowel. On physical examination, such infants may appear pale, have grunting respirations, and approximately one-third of such infants may appear jaundiced.

In older children, the pain is usually constant, not colicky. This symptom complex usually occurs in previously healthy children. However, there may have been minor episodes of vomiting or abdominal discomfort in the past. A child suspected of harboring a malrotation with possible midgut volvulus should have flat and upright abdominal x-rays. The presence of a loop of bowel overriding the liver is suggestive of the diagnosis. Occasionally, an upper GI examination may reveal an abnormal location of the ligament of Treitz.

Intussusception, duodenal stenosis, or atresia can produce a clinical picture similar to midgut volvulus.

Treatment   An infant with symptoms of obstruction or bilious vomiting must receive prompt surgical consultation, active resuscitation, and hospital admission. Start intravenous fluid immediately, and place a nasogastric tube. Send blood for type and cross-match. An elevation of the white blood cell count may suggest early gut necrosis. Electrolytes and venous blood gases may identify sodium or potassium abnormalities or ongoing acidosis. Any child with vomiting or bloody stools who is identified as having an incompletely rotated bowel requires urgent laparotomy to prevent the development of midgut volvulus and total midgut gangrene.

INCARCERATED HERNIA

Clinical Features   An incarcerated hernia will not be detected unless the infant or child is totally undressed at the time of examination. The symptoms can include irritability, poor feeding, vomiting, and an inguinal or scrotal mass. The differential diagnosis of an inguinal or scrotal mass most frequently includes hydrocele of the cord or the scrotum, undescended testicle, torsion of the testicle, torsion of the appendix testis, inguinal lymphadenopathy, inguinal node abscess, orchitis, and inguinal or scrotal trauma. The incidence of incarceration of inguinal hernias is highest in the first year of life. In both boys and girls, the incarcerated sac may contain small or large bowel. In girls, an ovary may be present in the sac.

Treatment   In most instances, it is possible to achieve manual reduction of the incarcerated hernia without the use of sedation if it has been present for only a short time. The infant should be placed in Trendelenburg position and, once the child is quiet, a gentle milking of the hernia contents toward the inguinal rings should be attempted. One may provide sedation with a short-acting agent such as midazolam or fentanyl (see Chap. 134). The few patients who do not respond to these maneuvers must undergo surgical reduction. Once the hernia is reduced, follow-up should be arranged with the pediatric surgeon within

24 to 48 h for surgical repair on an elective basis. If it was a difficult reduction, the child may need admission on the recommendation of the pediatric surgeon.

INTESTINAL OBSTRUCTION

Clinical Features   Intestinal obstruction presents in infants and young children in the classic manner, with symptoms of pain (manifested by irritability), vomiting, abdominal distention, and later, absence or diminution of bowel movements. The differential diagnosis of intestinal obstruction in newborns and infants includes intestinal atresia or stenosis, meconium ileus (newborns only), incarcerated inguinal hernia, intussusception, malrotation, malrotation with volvulus, volvulus around a congenital intraabdominal band, duplication cysts of the intestinal tract, imperforate anus, and Hirschsprung disease.

Diagnosis and Treatment   Flat and upright films of the abdomen show dilated loops of bowel with air-fluid levels (Figure 127-1). Such

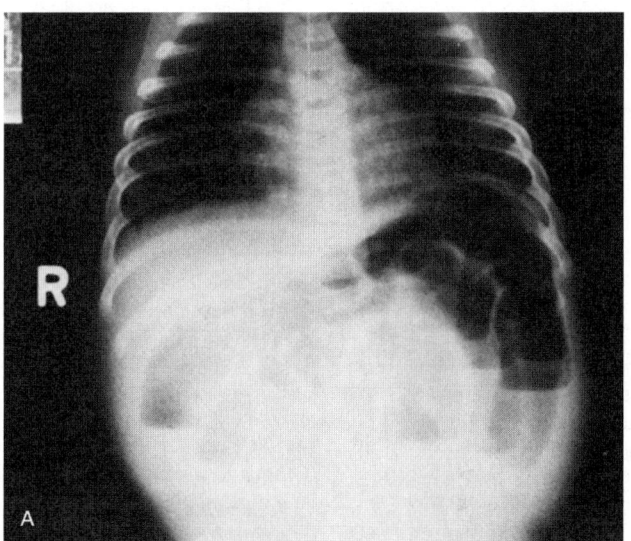

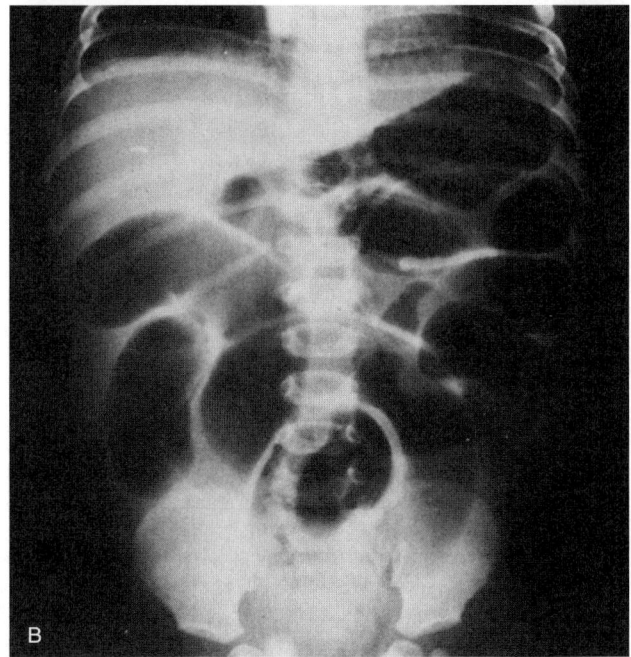

FIG. 127-1. Mechanical intestinal obstruction. **A.** Upright film. **B.** Flat film.

an appearance on the plain x-ray film warrants a barium enema examination with a Hirschsprung catheter, which helps to differentiate between Hirschsprung disease, malrotation, and colonic stenosis, and separates lower large bowel obstruction from upper small bowel obstruction.

Once intestinal obstruction is diagnosed, prepare the patient for surgical intervention by having an intravenous line started and a nasogastric tube placed; the child should be admitted.

PYLORIC STENOSIS

Consider pyloric stenosis in the infant with a history of nonbilious projectile vomiting. The disorder affects approximately 1 in 150 male and 1 in 750 female patients. It occurs more frequently in first-born males, and a familial incidence is noted in approximately 50 percent of patients. It is caused by diffuse hypertrophy and hypoplasia of the smooth muscle that narrows the antrum of the stomach to a small channel that can be easily obstructed.

Clinical Features Onset is rare before the age of 1 week, and the disorder usually begins in the second or third week of life. It seldom develops after the third month of life. Initially, the infant may only regurgitate small amounts of milk, making it difficult to distinguish the cause of vomiting from simple regurgitation, gastric reflux, or milk intolerance. Vomiting usually becomes projectile within a week of onset of symptoms, and the vomitus is never bile stained, although it may occasionally have streaks of blood. Vomiting occurs just after or near the end of feeding, and afterward the infant will refeed hungrily unless the child has become malnourished or dehydrated.

Vomiting eventually becomes projectile. Constipation may be noted because the infant is not retaining enough formula and becomes dehydrated.

Physical examination usually demonstrates a hungry infant who has failed to gain weight over the past several weeks or has lost weight. Jaundice occurs in 1 to 2 percent of cases. If one undresses and then feeds the infant, peristaltic waves can sometimes be seen passing from left to right across the upper abdomen, just prior to an episode of vomiting. Palpation of a pyloric tumor-the "olive"-is pathognomonic. The olive usually is felt near the lateral margin of the right rectus muscle just below the liver edge. Palpation of the olive is very dependent on the amount of hypertrophy of the pylorus and the skill of the clinician.

In advanced cases, the physical examination will reveal dehydration and lethargy. The child may appear moribund, with sunken eyes, decreased elasticity of the skin, and loss of subcutaneous tissue.

Diagnosis If the olive is palpated, further studies are not necessary. If no olive is palpated, abdominal ultrasonography is recommended. Accuracy depends on the use of a high-resolution machine and an experienced sonographer. Although false positives are rare, false negatives can occur in up to 20 percent of cases, often due to bowel gas interference. If the diagnosis is strongly suspected and the findings on ultrasonography are normal, an upper GI series can be performed. This usually demonstrates delayed gastric emptying and indentation of the antrum by the pyloric olive. The pyloric channel is narrowed and appears stringlike. If pyloric stenosis is not noted, the radiographer can evaluate the infant for gastroesophageal reflux. The major risk from the upper GI series is the potential for aspiration.

Treatment Once the diagnosis of pyloric stenosis is confirmed or is strongly suspected, surgical consultation should be obtained. Surgery is the treatment of choice, and the procedure is very safe. Oral intake should be restricted and an intravenous line started. Dehydration and electrolyte abnormalities must be corrected before surgery. Much of the reduced morbidity and mortality from surgery for this disease can be attributed to improved preoperative status. Extensive and protracted vomiting in pyloric stenosis may lead to hypokalemia, hyponatremia, and hypochloremic metabolic alkalosis. Fluid and electrolyte replacement is discussed in Chap. 132.

INTUSSUSCEPTION

Intussusception occurs when a portion of the alimentary tract is telescoped into another segment. It is the most common cause of intestinal obstruction between 3 months and 6 years of age and is rare under 3 months of age. The male:female ratio is 4:1.

Pathophysiology The cause of most intussusception remains unknown. A seasonal incidence seems to follow peak viral illness seasons. In some patients, recognizable causes for intussusception are found, such as Meckel diverticulum, intestinal polyp, duplication, lymphosarcoma, or as a complication of Henoch-Schönlein purpura, but these are rarely found in infants under 2 years of age. Rarely, tumors or foreign bodies may cause intussusception. Prior to 2000, the rotavirus vaccine was associated with an increased incidence of intussusception and was withdrawn from the market. Ileocolic intussusception is the most common type. The upper portion of the bowel invaginates into the lower portion, bringing the mesentery with it. Constriction of the mesentery obstructs venous return with engorgement of the intussusceptum. With edema and bleeding, there may be bloody stools, with mucus giving rise to the characteristic "currant jelly" stool.

Clinical Features The classic patient is a robust, 6- to 18-month-old infant without prior difficulty. Suddenly, the child appears to be in pain. The youngster may be playing quietly in the playpen and suddenly stop playing, begin to cry, and even roll around in discomfort. Just as suddenly, the pain ceases, and the child appears to be as happy and content as before the onset of pain. Episodes of the painful attacks may recur at intervals that become shorter and shorter and with increasing duration. Some children become very still, listless, and pale, and appear to be in a shocklike state due to the visceral pain. Vomiting is rare in the first few hours, but usually develops after 6 to 12 h. The classic "currant jelly" stool associated with intussusception is a late manifestation of the disease complex and is present even then in only 50 percent of cases.[6] Its absence should not delay evaluation for intussusception in the patient. However, a positive stool guaiac test is present in almost every case.

Fever can occur and even rise to 41°C (106°F). Respirations may be shallow and grunting in nature.

Apathy or lethargy may be the only presenting sign of intussusception in up to 10 percent of cases. Because of this, some infants will receive a lumbar puncture and other diagnostic studies, thus delaying the diagnosis and management of the child's illness.[7,8,9]

Examination between attacks may reveal the often-described sausage-shaped tumor mass of intussuscepted bowel in the right side of the abdomen. If this mass is felt in the epigastrium, the long axis is usually horizontal. At least one-third of patients do not have a palpable mass, but the absence of a mass must not delay further investigation. An ileoileal intussusception may have a less typical presentation, with symptoms and signs suggestive of intestinal obstruction.

Diagnosis and Treatment The presumptive diagnosis of intussusception is made based on the history. The apparent well being of a child in the absence of clinical findings should not mislead the physician. An x-ray examination of the abdomen may show a mass or filling defect in the right upper quadrant of the abdomen (Figure 127-2), but can be normal in 30 percent. An air contrast enema is diagnostic and is frequently curative.[7] Air insufflation is preferred over barium enema because it enables better control over colonic pressure used for the reduction,[10] and if perforation should inadvertently occur, there is no spillage of barium into the peritoneum. The pediatric surgeon should be consulted before diagnostic procedures, so that prompt surgery can be done if reduction is unsuccessful or if there is a complication.

After successful reduction, the child is generally admitted for observation for complications of reduction and because of a 5 to 10 percent recurrence rate, usually within the first 24 to 48 h following re-

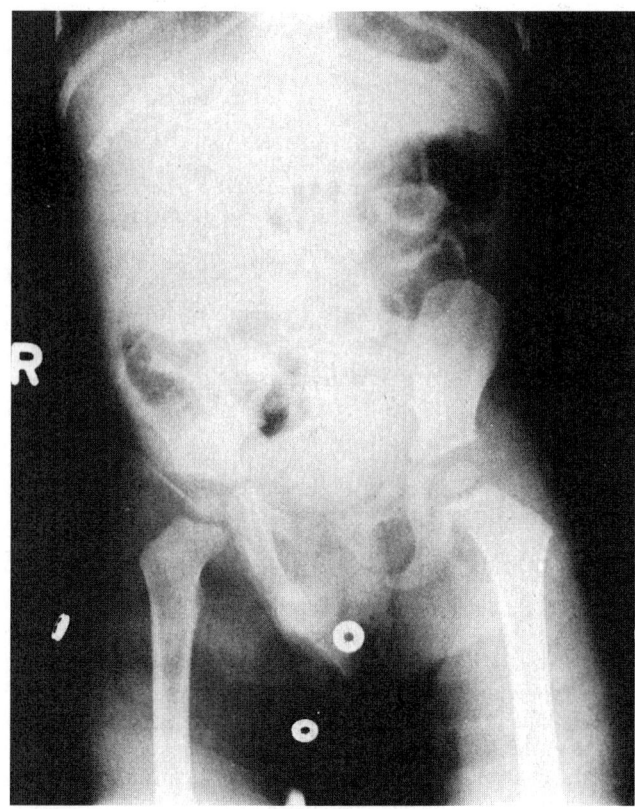

FIG. 127-2. Intussusception. Plain film with loss of bowel pattern in the right upper quadrant.

duction. A second attempt at air reduction can then be considered and is usually successful. If another episode of intussusception occurs, then surgical reduction is necessary.

Gastrointestinal Emergencies in Children 2 Years and Older

APPENDICITIS

Clinical Features Appendicitis can occur in children younger than age two, but the presentation is usually one of peritonitis or sepsis because of the delay in diagnosis.[11] The most common symptoms in children under two are vomiting, pain, diarrhea, and fever. Other clinical features that might confuse the diagnosis include irritability, grunting respiration, cough, and hip pain.[12] The child under two usually has a fever and diffuse abdominal tenderness, with localized right lower quadrant tenderness noted in less than 50 percent. One-third to one-half of the patients may have abdominal distention or abdominal rigidity. Due to the difficulty of making the diagnosis of appendicitis in children under 2 years of age, the appendix is often perforated by the time of surgery.

Over age two, appendicitis becomes a more important part of the differential diagnosis of abdominal pain. The symptoms of appendicitis may not progress in the classic fashion in young children. The usual progression involves early anorexia followed by the development of mild to moderate periumbilical pain, then vomiting and migration of the pain to the right lower quadrant of the abdomen. While adult studies indicate that pain usually precedes vomiting, the sequence may not be followed in young children. Vomiting may be the first symptom noted by the parents.[12] The typical sequence is absent in approximately one-third of children with appendicitis. Physical examination findings also vary based on the time course of the disease and the time of patient presentation.

On physical examination, tenderness may be localized to the right lower quadrant or may involve the entire abdomen. Bowel sounds are unreliable in determining the presence or absence of appendicitis. Walking, climbing onto the stretcher, or jumping up and down all cause pain. Guarding or rebound tenderness may be unreliable early in the time course of appendicitis. These signs are present more frequently in cases of a perforated appendix.[12] The following signs and symptoms make the diagnosis of acute appendicitis more difficult:

1. The temperature may be normal.
2. The white blood cell count may be normal.
3. The child may not be anorexic and may actually request food.
4. The heavily built child may manifest minimal right lower quadrant tenderness.
5. Appendicitis can follow an episode of gastroenteritis. Intensification of pain in the presence of a history of gastroenteritis should suggest an acutely inflamed appendix secondary to gastroenteritis.[13]
6. Appendicitis has been identified in children younger than 2 years of age. Incidence of perforation in this age group is much higher because of the difficulty of making a diagnosis and the confusion with gastroenteritis.

The white blood cell count has insufficient sensitivity or specificity to confirm or eliminate the consideration of appendicitis. A urinalysis may help evaluate whether the child is suffering from pyelonephritis. However, if the urine has a few white cells, the child may still have appendicitis rather than a UTI.

Ultrasonography (US) is a subject of interest in identifying patients with appendicitis. It is, however, operator dependent and has missed not only inflamed but also ruptured appendices. Increased experience with the use of ultrasound to evaluate children with abdominal pain has improved sensitivity from 76 to 93 percent and specificity from 88 to 98 percent. Non-visualization of the appendix on abdominal ultrasonography is strongly associated with false-negative ultrasound studies.[12,14,15]

Computed tomography (CT) has better sensitivity and specificity than ultrasonography in most studies in children, whether contrast is used PO or PR. CT can also identify other causes of pain. Sensitivities are reported from 95 to 97 percent and specificities from 87 to 100 percent. These two modalities are useful in the indeterminate or atypical case.[16–19] CT scans using oral and colonic contrast with small 5-mm cuts starting just above the cecum and extending distally had the highest sensitivity.[12] There is some concern that CT scans may be less accurate in younger children due to a relative lack of body fat, that make it difficult to differentiate an inflamed appendix from surrounding tissue or bowel.[20]

Treatment Once the diagnosis of appendicitis is strongly considered or confirmed, surgical consultation should be obtained and the child should be admitted to the hospital. The child should receive any appropriate supportive therapy. If the child is febrile, rectal acetaminophen may be given. The child should not receive any oral fluids or food. Start an intravenous line and administer fluid boluses, particularly if the child shows signs of sepsis or shock. Closely monitor the child's vital signs and give pain medication parenterally as appropriate.

If the diagnosis is possible but not probable, surgical consultation should be considered and the child reexamined until either resolution of the illness or a need for laparotomy is determined.

If a perforated appendix is suspected or the child appears septic, resuscitate the patient in the usual fashion by providing oxygen, ensuring adequate ventilation, and treating hypovolemia and shock. Administer broad-spectrum antibiotics such as ampicillin/sulbactam, piperacillin/tazobactam, cefoxitin, or cefotetan.

With the high potential for misdiagnosis and the difficulty of diagnosing appendicitis in children, one must rely on the history, physical exam, and clinical suspicion. No single test or combination of clinical and laboratory features is 100 percent reliable. Ultrasonography and contrast CT may reduce the rates of misdiagnosis. Understanding the spectrum of the clinical illness and the variation of signs and symptoms in children of different ages will enhance the physician's ability to manage children with acute abdominal pain.

MECKEL DIVERTICULUM   A Meckel diverticulum can cause a variety of signs and symptoms, such as bleeding, peritonitis, intussusception, and intestinal obstruction. The presence of gastric mucosa in the diverticulum may give rise to an ulcer in the adjacent ileum, which may cause symptoms such as painless rectal bleeding. Bleeding is brisk and usually bright red. The ulcer may perforate and cause peritonitis. Isotope scanning reveals the presence of a Meckel diverticulum containing gastric mucosa in up to 50 percent of cases. A scan with normal findings does not eliminate the diagnosis.

Acute inflammation in a Meckel diverticulum may simulate acute appendicitis or may initiate intussusception. Finally, the vitello-intestinal remnant attaching the apex of a Meckel diverticulum to the intraabdominal umbilical region may be the focus around which volvulus of the small bowel or an internal hernia develops, each of these giving rise to intestinal obstruction. Surgical consultation is necessary.

HENOCH-SCHÖNLEIN PURPURA AND HEMOLYTIC UREMIC SYNDROME   Henoch-Schönlein purpura (HSP) and hemolytic uremic syndrome (HUS) can cause abdominal pain and GI bleeding.

In HSP, some children may present with joint pain, abdominal pain, or seizure. Usually there is a petechial or purpuric rash on the buttocks and lower extremities. Many children have guaiac-positive stools, but rarely present with hematochezia unless there is associated intussusception. Treatment is usually symptomatic and on an outpatient basis unless the child appears ill or has a complication of the disease, such as renal failure, intestinal perforation, or a rare complication, testicular torsion.

In HUS, there is usually a history of a gastroenteritis with or without bloody diarrhea, up to 2 weeks before onset of illness. Toxigenic strains of *Escherichia coli* have been implicated as a possible link to HUS. Low-grade fever, pallor, hematuria, and hematochezia occur. The central nervous system can be involved. Hypertension occurs in up to 50 percent and seizures in up to 40 percent of cases. Acute bowel perforation, toxic megacolon, intussusception, renal failure, and pancreatitis can occur.

COLON POLYPS   Single polyps or multiple or classic familial polyposis may give rise to painless hematochezia. Single polyps are usually benign (juvenile), with no propensity for malignant degeneration. Frequently, the parent describes what is obviously a prolapsed polyp, easily palpated on rectal examination. It is rare for bleeding originating from a polyp to be life-threatening. Familial polyposis is rare and is a premalignant syndrome. The child should be referred to a pediatric surgeon.

PANCREATITIS   Pancreatitis is not common in childhood. The most common cause is abdominal trauma. It can also occur as an idiopathic or postviral process (after mumps, influenza, coxsackie, etc.) or be due to drugs or toxins. Systemic diseases such as cystic fibrosis, systemic lupus erythematosus, and α_1 antitrypsin deficiency can cause pancreatitis.[21]

Clinical findings include central abdominal pain, vomiting, and sometimes fever. The abdomen may be distended and is tender to palpation. Patients should receive fluids to correct dehydration and any hypovolemia and receive appropriate pain management. Most will need admission for intravenous hydration, pain management, and diagnostic studies.

Intraabdominal Masses

Every child should have a careful abdominal examination because intraabdominal masses grow silently at first until they cause obstruction,

bleeding, or hemorrhage into the tumor or until a parent sees a mass protruding in the abdomen. The child should be supine with his or her head turned toward the parent, and one should carefully palpate all quadrants of the abdomen. If a mass is palpated, the child should be referred to a pediatric surgeon and diagnostic imaging studies obtained. A careful rectal examination, especially if the child has constipation or a gait abnormality, must be done to check for a presacral teratoma and for ovarian masses. Both of these tumors can show calcifications on plain film x-rays in approximately 50 percent of cases.

Neuroblastomas can arise from adrenal glands or along the sympathetic chain. They often cross to the midline, and the best cure rate is obtained in children under 1 year of age. Computed tomography is the best way to evaluate this tumor. Wilms tumor is an intrarenal tumor initially and should be considered in children with hematuria. US and CT help define this tumor. Bone scan is also needed. Rhabdomyosarcoma occurs in the pelvis or anywhere there is striated muscle, and it is highly malignant.

In girls over the age of menarche, one must consider pregnancy, and if there is lower quadrant pain, one must consider ectopic pregnancy. One should obtain a serum pregnancy test and consider the use of ultrasonography.

Portal Hypertension

Portal hypertension is rare in children in the United States, but is one of the common causes of major upper GI hemorrhage. Extrahepatic portal thrombosis, parenchymal liver disease associated with fibrocystic disease, and biliary cirrhosis in youngsters with congenital biliary atresia surviving as a result of portal enterostomy are examples of conditions that can result in portal hypertension and esophagogastric varices. Other causes include a history of hepatitis, congenital diseases such as α_1 antitrypsin deficiency, glycogen storage diseases, and Wilson disease.

Massive hematemesis is the usual initial manifestation, along with hematochezia in children, whereas ascites is more common as the presenting sign in infants. A nasogastric tube can be placed to empty the stomach and to monitor for continued bleeding, and blood transfusions given as indicated. Correct any coagulation abnormalities. Emergency consultation with a surgeon, pediatric surgeon, or a pediatric gastroenterologist is necessary.

REFERENCES

1. Johnson GT, Johnson P, Fishman EK: CT evaluation of the acute abdomen: Bowel pathology spectrum of disease. *Crit Rev Diagn Imaging* 37:163, 1996.
2. Moir CR: Abdominal pain in infants and children. *Mayo Clin Proc* 71:984, 1996.
3. Mason JD: The evaluation of acute abdominal pain in children. *Emerg Med Clin North Am* 14:629, 1996.
4. Vinton NE: Gastrointestinal bleeding in infancy and childhood. *Gastroenterol Clin North Am* 23:93, 1994.
5. Andrassy RJ, Mahour GH: Malrotation of the midgut in infants and children. *Arch Surg* 116:158, 1981.
6. Yamamoto LG, Morita SY, Boychuk RB, et al: Stool appearance in intussusception: Assessing the value of the term "currant jelly." *Am J Emerg Med* 15:292, 1997.
7. Winslow BT, Westfall JM, Nicholas RA: Intussusception [review]. *Am Fam Physician* 54:213, 220, 1996.
8. Conway EE Jr: Central nervous system findings and intussusception: How are they related? *Pediatr Emerg Care* 9:15, 1993.
9. Harrington L, Connolly B, Hu X, et al: Ultrasonographic and clinical predictors of intussusception. *J Pediatr* 132:836–839, 1998.
10. Kirks DR: Air intussusception reduction: "The winds of change." *Pediatr Radiol* 25:89, 1985.
11. Puri P, O'Donnell B: Appendicitis in infancy. *J Pediatr Surg* 13:173, 1978.
12. Rothrock SG, Pagane J: Acute appendicitis in children: Emergency diagnosis and management. *Ann Emerg Med* 36:39–50, 2000.

13. Horwitz JR, Gursoy M, Jaksic T, et al: Importance of diarrhea as a presenting symptom of appendicitis in very young children. *Am J Surg* 173:80, 1997.

14. Gupta H, Dupuy DE: Advances in imaging of the acute abdomen [review]. *Surg Clin North Am* 77:1245, 1997.

15. Emil S, Mikhail P, Laberge JM, et al: Clinical versus sonographic evaluation of acute appendicitis in children: A comparison of patient characteristics and outcomes. *J Pediatr Surg* 36:780–783, 2001.

16. Dilley A, Wesson D, Munden M, et al: The impact of ultrasound examinations on the management of children with suspected appendicitis: A 3-year analysis. *J Pediatr Surg* 36:303–308, 2001.

17. Lowe LH, Penney MW, Stein SM, et al: Unenhanced limited CT of the abdomen in the diagnosis of appendicitis in children: Comparison with sonography. *AJR* 176:31–35, 2001.

18. Teo EL, Tan KP, Lam SL, et al: Ultrasonography and computed tomography in a clinical algorithm for the evaluation of suspected acute appendicitis in children. *Singapore Med J* 41:387–392, 2000.

19. Sivit CJ, Applegate KE, Stallion A, et al: Imaging evaluation of suspected appendicitis in a pediatric population: Effectiveness of sonography versus CT. *AJR* 175:977–980, 2000.

20. Friedland JA, Siegel MJ: CT appearance of acute appendicitis in childhood. *AJR Am J Roentgenol* 168:439–442, 1997.

21. Weizman Z: Acute pancreatitis in childhood: Research of pathogenesis and clinical implications [review]. *Can J Gastroenterol* 11:249, 1997.

DIABETIC KETOACIDOSIS
Frederick Place
Thom Mayer

EPIDEMIOLOGY

Diabetes can be subclassified into several different forms. Of the two major categories, type I or juvenile-onset diabetes, characterized by an abrupt and frequently complete decline in insulin production, most commonly begins in childhood. Type II or adult-onset diabetes, marked by increasing insulin resistance and most commonly found in obese adults, is being seen with increasing frequency in overweight adolescents with a strong genetic tendency. Type I diabetes (no longer called insulin-deficient diabetes mellitus) is the most common pediatric endocrine disorder with an estimated prevalence of 1 in 400. As many as 27 percent to 40 percent of new-onset diabetics present in diabetic ketoacidosis (DKA).[1,2] In known diabetics, DKA is much less common and tends to be clustered in a small subset of patients, with 5 percent of diabetic children accounting for nearly 60 percent of DKA episodes.[3] DKA is the leading cause of mortality in diabetics younger than age 24 years and cerebral edema is the leading cause of mortality in DKA.[4]

PATHOPHYSIOLOGY

The fundamental cause of DKA is an absolute or relative insulin deficiency resulting in the inability of cells to take up and utilize glucose. Counterregulatory hormones (catecholamines, cortisol, growth hormone, glucagon) are elevated, driving many of the physiologic disturbances. These hormones increase glucose production by promoting glycogenolysis, gluconeogenesis, lipolysis, ketogenesis, and further decrease glucose utilization by antagonizing insulin.

As the serum glucose exceeds the renal absorption threshold, an obligatory osmotic diuresis ensues resulting in the classic symptoms of polyuria and polydipsia. If not recognized early, this can lead to profound dehydration and electrolyte disturbances. Acidosis stems from the complex metabolic derangements induced by insulin deficiency and unopposed glucagon. The cellular milieu of the body is essentially in a state of functional starvation, unable to utilize the excess glucose. Decreased lipid uptake by adipose tissue and increased lipolysis results in an overabundance of circulating free fatty acids, which are converted by the liver into the ketoacids acetoacetate and β-hydroxybutyrate.

Despite this profound shift in substrate production, ketoacid utilization and renal elimination are both impaired, resulting in a high anion gap metabolic acidosis. In certain patients, the acid base status may be more complex. Persistent vomiting and severe volume depletion may result in a superimposed metabolic alkalosis and may mask the severity of the acidosis with a relatively normal pH. Severe dehydration and poor perfusion causing a lactic acidosis will result in a superimposed nonanion gap acidosis. Alternatively, a patient who remains relatively well hydrated will lose sodium with ketoanions in the urine while retaining chloride and demonstrate a significant nonanion gap acidosis.

CLINICAL FEATURES

Polyuria, polydipsia, and polyphagia constitute the classic triad leading to the diagnosis of diabetes. Other common insidious symptoms include weight loss, secondary eneuresis, anorexia, vague abdominal discomfort, visual changes, and genital candidiasis in the toilet-trained child. The diagnosis is established by demonstrating hyperglycemia and glucosuria in the absence of other causes such as steroid therapy, Cushing syndrome, pheochromocytoma, hyperthyroidism, or other rare disorders.

Uncontrolled diabetes will present to the emergency physician along an entire spectrum from simple hyperglycemia without ketonuria to diabetic ketosis (hyperglycemia with ketonuria) to full-blown DKA. DKA is generally defined as a metabolic acidosis (pH <7.25 to 7.30 or serum bicarbonate <15 mEq/L) with hyperglycemia (serum glucose >300 mg/dL) and ketonemia >1:2 serum dilution.[5,6] A vigorous search for precipitants should be undertaken. The most common cause of DKA in known diabetic children and adolescents is poor compliance. Other precipitants include intercurrent viral illness and focal infections such as urinary tract infection or gastroenteritis. Type I diabetics experience DKA much more commonly than do type II diabetics, but it is not uncommon for the latter to develop DKA under moderately severe physiologic stressors.

In the known diabetic, the diagnosis of DKA is relatively straightforward. Patients complain of polydipsia and polyuria (if not dehydrated), diffuse nonfocal abdominal pain often associated with vomiting, and generalized malaise, in addition to any focal complaints related to a precipitating trigger.

Physical findings in DKA are related to dehydration and the concomitant acidosis. Patients appear dehydrated, tachycardic, and hypotensive. Respiratory compensation for the acidosis is noted in the deep Kussmaul respirations and should not be misinterpreted as hyperventilation, even when associated paresthesias are present. Acetoacetate is converted to acetone and is responsible for the classic breath odor of nail polish. The level of consciousness may range from alert to somnolent to comatose. In a child with DKA and a depressed level of consciousness, cerebral edema should be strongly considered.

Abdominal pain and vomiting often accompany DKA. Care should be taken to distinguish nonspecific abdominal pain or gastroenteritis from more serious intra-abdominal disorders such as acute appendicitis. Focal abdominal tenderness, failure of pain to resolve with fluid therapy, or associated fever suggest an underlying intra-abdominal process.

An elevated glucose in the presence of ketonemia/ketonuria and acidosis almost always indicates DKA. However, other rare conditions possess similar clinical characteristics. Any condition resulting in prolonged vomiting or excessive fasting can result in ketoacidosis, but the glucose is not elevated. In the adolescent patient without known diabetes, toxic ingestions of ethylene glycol, isopropyl alcohol, or salicylates should be considered.

CEREBRAL EDEMA

Cerebral edema is the most dreaded complication of pediatric DKA. Mortality rates have been reported from 40 to 90 percent and only 14 to 57 percent of children who develop the disorder are left neurologically normal.[4,7] Cerebral edema more commonly develops in children younger than 5 years and is rare in persons older than 20 years.[7] It is likely that all patients in severe DKA have some degree of subclinical cerebral edema,[8] but the specific risk factors associated with overt, life-threatening cerebral edema are young age, severe hyperosmolality, hyponatremia, and severe acidosis.[5,7] Failure of the serum sodium to rise commensurately with the fall in glucose during therapy may be an important contributor.[9] Newer studies refute the belief that overaggressive fluid resuscitation per se is a significant risk factor.[1,5] Nevertheless, caution and restraint is prudent, particularly in the extremely hyperosmolal patient (i.e., greater than 340 mOsm/L). Recently, it has been proposed that cerebral edema is caused not by rapid changes in osmolality but rather by cerebral ischemia induced by the combination of severe dehydration and hypocarbia.[5]

While rarely noted at presentation, cerebral edema typically manifests itself 6 to 12 h after the onset of therapy (Figure 128-1). Interestingly, many patients appear to be improving clinically and biochemically prior to deterioration from cerebral edema. Premonitory symptoms occur in as few as 50 percent of individuals and include severe headache, declining mental status, seizures, and papillary edema. Unfortunately, respiratory arrest may be the first sign of cerebral edema. Early aggressive intervention based on the clinical evaluation, often before confirmatory CT findings, is vital to prevent respiratory arrest, herniation, and death.[7,10] Once respiratory arrest has occurred, meaningful recovery is unlikely to occur.[7]

Standard treatment for cerebral edema is mannitol (1mg/kg intravenous bolus) and definitive airway management if necessary. Fluid administration should be kept to the minimum possible to retain a functioning intravenous catheter. Alternately, a "heparin lock" alone can be placed in the established catheter allowing immediate intravenous access for administration of medications and other therapeutic interventions as they become necessary. If the patient appears more clinically stable and is still in the ED, half of normal maintainence fluids can be given until the child reaches the pediatric intensive care unit (Table 128-1). Hyperventilation reduces cerebral blood flow and may worsen cerebral ischemia. Dexamethasone is likewise ineffective. In the patient with clinically apparent cerebral edema that is not well supported by CT findings, consideration should be given to cerebral venous sinus thrombosis, a finding often missed on plain noncontrast head CT, and which requires contrast CT or MRI.

INITIAL LABORATORY EVALUATION

Routine blood studies should include a complete blood count (CBC); serum glucose; electrolyte panel including calcium and phosphate; venous blood gas (VBG), serum phosphate, and urinalysis (Table 128- 2). Hyperglycemia, metabolic acidosis, and ketones on urinalysis confirm the diagnosis of DKA. Other laboratory studies, such as serum ketones, blood cultures, hepatic enzymes, magnesium, serum osmolality, and lipase are at the clinician's discretion. A venous blood gas (VBG) should replace the arterial sample for assessing the degree of acidosis and hypocarbia, avoiding an additional painful procedure (or procedures). The pH from a VBG is only 0.03 less than that from an arterial blood gas (ABG) and is an accurate reflection of the acid-base status.[11]

Care should be taken in interpreting laboratory results as several factitious abnormalities may be seen in DKA. An increased white blood count is often seen in DKA and should be interpreted in context with physical findings and diagnostic studies for infection. Elevated salivary amylase in DKA confounds the diagnosis of pancreatitis and lipase is a more accurate test. Depending upon the type of laboratory analysis for creatinine, serum ketones may result in a factitious elevation in the serum creatinine.

The serum glucose is usually above 350 mg/dL, but a glucose less than 300 mg/dL is still consistent with DKA. Euglycemic DKA may occur in the young, well-hydrated diabetic who is compliant with the insulin regimen, but has relative insulin deficiency caused by an intercurrent illness. However, even in the absence of hyperglycemia, insulin is needed.

Change in the serum potassium is the most critical electrolyte disturbance in DKA. Potassium depletion may be both profound and not reflected in initial laboratory values. The average potassium deficit is 3 to 5 mEq/kg (150 to 250 mEq potassium deficit in a 50-kg adolescent) and the initial serum level is often normal or high. Potassium depletion is a result of insulin deficiency (which normally drives potassium into cells), acidemia (which causes the redistribution of potassium out of the cells in exchange for hydrogen), volume contraction, and tissue catabolism. These processes all provide increased potassium available for urinary excretion. Within this context, initial hypokalemia signifies a severe deficit and a potentially dangerous situation.

The bicarbonate concentration is invariably low. A high anion gap acidosis from the ketonemia is usually noted. In simple DKA, the bicarbonate should fall to the extent that the anion gap rises. A fall in the bicarbonate level *less* than expected for a given rise in the anion gap in the vomiting patient indicates the presence of an accompanying metabolic alkalosis. Conversely, a fall in the bicarbonate level *greater*

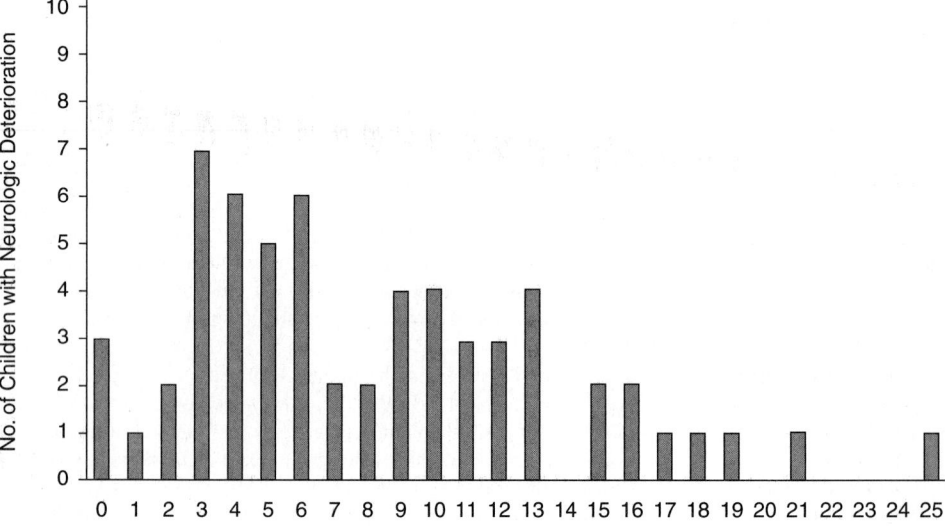

FIG. 128-1. Time between the initiation of therapy and neurologic deterioration in children with diabetic ketoacidosis and cerebral edema.

TABLE 128-1 Management of Cerebral Edema

High risk
    Younger than 5 years of age
    Severe acidosis
    Severe hyperosmolality
    Failure of serum sodium to rise
Prevention
    Judicious fluid management
    Early *clinical* recognition
Treatment
    Mannitol
    Fluid restriction
    Appropriate airway management

than expected for the rise in the anion indicates a concomitant nonanion gap acidosis. This is frequently seen in well-hydrated patients who are still able to excrete the ketoanions while retaining chloride or in severely dehydrated patients with accompanying lactic acidosis.

The serum osmolality is increased in DKA and its rise correlates with the decrease in the level of consciousness at presentation. Osmolality greater than 340 mOsm/L often results in a stuporous or comatose patient while a serum osmolality of less than 300 mOsm/L should prompt reconsideration of the cause of the decreased arousal. It is generally believed that the development of cerebral edema is correlated with the rate of decline in the serum osmolality, and it is critical that patients with high serum osmolality have their fluid deficits corrected less rapidly.

Sodium deficits average 5 to 10 mEq/kg, but the serum sodium may be normal because of excessive free water loss. More typically, it is factitiously low because of hyperglycemia and a corrected value may be arrived at by using the formula *corrected sodium = 1.6 × (serum glucose − 100)/100 + measured serum sodium.*

β-Hydroxybutyrate (3-HB) is the major ketoacid produced. But unlike acetoacetate, it does not react with the nitroprusside used in urine and serum ketone assays, so measured ketone levels may appear low for the degree of acidosis and do not reflect the true extent of ketonemia. This fact also explains the paradoxical rise in measured ketones with therapy: 3-HB is converted to acetoacetate, which reacts more strongly with the assay. Using bedside ketone testing to monitor recovery is further complicated by the persistence of urine ketones after clearance of serum ketones.[12]

TREATMENT

Intensive monitoring and meticulous care of the DKA patient improves outcome, but management varies greatly between specialties. Emergency physicians more aggressively hydrate and bolus with insulin than do pediatric intensivists and endocrinologists, despite emerging data suggesting increased risk of complications.[13]

TABLE 128-2 Laboratory Evaluation in DKA

INITIAL LABORATORY

Essential	Optional
Glucose	Magnesium
Electrolyte panel	Calcium
Venous blood gas	Serum osmolality
Phosphate	Serum ketones
Urinary ketones	CBC
	Lactate

EVERY HOUR

Bedside serum glucose measurement

EVERY TWO HOURS

Electrolyte panel, venous blood gas

Attention should be directed toward three related but independently addressed problems: perfusion status, electrolyte disturbances, and hyperglycemia and ketonemia (Table 128-3). The initial focus should always be on volume status and vital signs. Next, electrolyte disturbances should be addressed and insulin therapy begun. Other problems such as associated infections should obviously be addressed concurrently.

Fluid Resuscitation

The immediate priority is to stabilize hemodynamics and begin volume resuscitation. The average fluid deficit is 10 percent of body weight, but is often greater. An initial 20 mL/kg bolus of NS should be given to the patient clearly in shock and repeated if needed. Once vital signs have stabilized, it is important to resist the desire to correct the fluid deficit too rapidly, especially if there is a high calculated osmolality (i.e., >340 mOsm/L). The fluid deficit should be corrected slowly as in other severe dehydration states, especially in the context of a high osmolar state. Traditionally, this has meant a 50 percent deficit replacement in the first 8 h with the rest over the next 16 to 24 h. However, many institutions are now even less aggressive, replacing the deficit evenly over 24 to 48 h. This moderated approach helps avoid overhydration, pulmonary complications, and possibly cerebral edema.

Electrolyte Replacement

SODIUM Sodium depletion from vomiting and urinary losses rarely causes a problem by itself and is most often related to the extent of dehydration. The main concern with sodium lies in its correction. It has been fairly convincingly demonstrated that the failure of serum sodium to rise in the treatment of DKA is associated with the development of cerebral edema. Typical protocols recommend 0.45 percent sodium chloride correction at 1.5 times maintenance for empiric replacement therapy, but in an attempt to decrease the risk of cerebral edema, some newer protocols have advocated sodium concentrations of 0.66 to 0.8 percent sodium chloride (e.g., 125 mEq Na$^+$/L) and calculated fluid replacements to tighten control over biochemical parameters.[1,10] This approach is effective in ensuring a steady rise in the sodium concentration.[9]

POTASSIUM Potassium should be withheld until hyperkalemia (i.e., potassium >6.0 mEq/L) is excluded and the patient is urinating. Because the electrocardiogram may be normal in the face of hyperkalemia it can be falsely reassuring, thus the serum potassium level must be monitored. Potassium deficits are often large, and both initial

TABLE 128-3 Management of DKA in Children

1. 10–20 mL/kg NS bolus until hemodynamically stable*
2. Then begin 0.45% NS at 1.5 times maintainance in the ED†
3. If K$^+$ is <5.5 mEq/L and patient is urinating, add 30 mEq potassium per liter (half as KCL and half as Kphosphate). If initial K$^+$ is 2.5–3.5 mEq/L, add 40 mEq K$^+$/L; consider adding more if the K$^+$ is <2.5 mEq/L.
4. Begin regular insulin at 0.1 units/kg per h after intravenous fluid bolus (if done) is complete. Adjust dose to maintain glucose decline at 50–100 mg/dL per h. Do not decrease insulin infusion to less than 0.05 units/kg per h.
5. Add dextrose to intravenous fluids when BS is <200–250 mg/dL.
6. Follow serum electrolytes every 2 h; follow serum glucose every hour.

*Bolus therapy is not done to correct dehydration but only to restore hemodynamic stability.
†Alternatively, one can calculate fluid deficit and correct 50% over the first 12–16 h. Some authorities recommend a higher calculated sodium concentration of between 0.45% and 0.9% NS.
Abbreviations: BS = blood sugar; K = potassium; KCL = potassium chloride; NS = normal saline.

rehydration and insulin therapy can cause a precipitous decline in potassium levels due to redistribution.

Initial hypokalemia (i.e., <3.0 mEq/L) indicates a profound deficit and therapy should be aggressive. The recommended rates of potassium replacement vary widely but in general, maintenance fluids should contain between 30 and 40 mEq K^+/L. Consider higher doses for children with demonstrated hypokalemia. Serum potassium should be monitored at minimum every 2 h.

OTHER ELECTROLYTES   Phosphate depletion is well described in DKA but the value of intravenous replacement has never been proven. Many authorities recommend half of the potassium replacement in the form of potassium phosphate. In the absence of replacement, one should monitor for symptomatic hypophosphatemia (serum phosphate <1 mmol/L, muscular weakness, rhabdomyolysis, respiratory depression). The same rule applies to magnesium replacement. Hypocalcemia, when present, is likely secondary to overaggressive phosphate replacement.

Hyperglycemia and Insulin Therapy

Fluid resuscitation will reduce serum glucose levels somewhat. After the patient is hemodynamically stable, a low-dose insulin infusion should be started. The goal of insulin therapy is to evenly reverse the ketonemia and acidosis. High dose insulin therapy does not improve the rate of recovery, but it does place the patient at greater risk of hypoglycemia and hypokalemia, and a loading bolus of 0.1 units/kg, once common, is no longer considered beneficial.

The insulin infusion dose is 0.1 units regular insulin/kg per h. As a rule of thumb, serum glucose should decrease approximately 50 to 100 mg/dL per h in a slow, controlled fashion to prevent intracerebral osmole shifts. If improvement of the pH is too slow (<0.03 pH units per h), the rate can be doubled.[10] Generally, glucose corrects faster than the ketoacidosis and dextrose will need to be added to the intravenous fluids when the blood glucose dips below 250 mg/dL, with the goal of maintaining a serum glucose of 150 to 300 mg/dL until resolution of the ketoacidosis. The patient with euglycemic DKA will need the addition of glucose at the initiation of therapy. If the blood sugar continues to decline, additional glucose should be added before considering adjustment of the insulin drip. If the child is at the maximum glucose concentration available (or maximum tolerable concentration if peripheral access only), then the administration of insulin can be temporarily held for 10 to 15 min before restarting the insulin drip at a lower rate. In general, this should not be below 0.05 units/kg per h. The short half-life of intravenous insulin (5 to 10 min) along with the continued administration of glucose will correct transient hypoglycemia. Continued insulin administration is the mainstay of therapy and should be continued, allowing for reversal of the ketoacidosis. Serum potassium should be meticulously monitored, as insulin will begin driving potassium back into the cells.

The insulin infusion should not be transitioned to subcutaneous administration until a pH >7.30 and a bicarbonate >16 mEq/L has been reached and serum ketones have disappeared. At that point, subcutaneous insulin may be administered and the infusion stopped 30 to 60 min later.[10]

INSULIN PUMP   Rarely, a child with an insulin pump will present in DKA. As the majority of cases of DKA are related to inadequate insulin delivery, this would imply a malfunctioning pump. Alternatively, the pump may be functioning correctly but the child is suffering from an intercurrent illness with increased and unmet insulin needs. Either way, the pump should be shut off and the child should be treated like any other insulin dependent diabetic in DKA.

Acidosis and Bicarbonate Therapy

The routine use of bicarbonate in the treatment of DKA is not recommended because it has never been shown to improve outcome, and it has been associated with a fourfold increase in the development of cerebral edema.[5] In addition, the use of bicarbonate therapy can lead to volume overload, accelerated hypokalemia, hypernatremia, and paradoxical central nervous system acidosis.[14] Bicarbonate administration should be limited to critically ill patients with a pH <7.0 and hemodynamic compromise (unresponsive to fluid resuscitation) from depressed cardiac contractility and poor perfusion. If necessary, depending on the pH and the patient's clinical condition, bicarbonate may be administered slowly at 0.5 to 2.0 mEq/kg over 1 to 2 h. Correction should never exceed a pH of 7.1 or a serum bicarbonate of 10 mEq/L.

Disposition of Children in DKA

Most patients in DKA require admission to the intensive care unit, even when stable, because of intensive monitoring needs. Furthermore, many hospitals restrict the use of insulin infusions to intensive care settings. Known diabetics with a pH above 7.35 and a bicarbonate above 20 mEq/L with a known and resolving precipitant for DKA, a good clinical appearance, a solid social situation, and close follow-up with their primary physician may be discharged home.[15] As many as 69 percent of patients with a starting pH >7.20 or a serum bicarbonate greater than 10 mEq/L will correct their acidosis within 6 h.[6]

HYPERGLYCEMIA WITHOUT KETOACIDOSIS

New-Onset Hyperglycemia

Many children with new-onset diabetes present with classic symptoms of diabetes such as polydipsia, polyuria, and malaise, and they are identified before significant ketoacidosis develops. They are frequently sent from the outpatient physician's office for management and admission. ED management is less intensive and should be done in coordination with the child's endocrinologist. In general, children with hyperglycemia but no DKA are only mildly dehydrated, may or may not have urinary ketones, and the serum pH is over 7.3. The speed at which such children will descend toward actual DKA is largely a function of hydration status and age. Infants and very young children will progress more rapidly because of their inability to independently access fluids and their increased metabolic rate. With appropriate attention paid to hydration status and timely insulin administration, DKA is very unlikely to develop in the hospital in the absence of serious underlying illness.

ED management should be restricted to drawing baseline laboratory studies, providing fluids PO or IV, depending on the need, and possibly administering the first dose of insulin. An acceptable initial dose is 0.1 units/kg of subcutaneous regular insulin. Whether or not new-onset diabetic children are particularly sensitive to insulin is a matter of debate. Still, serum glucose should be monitored closely, every hour after insulin is administered. Children should be admitted in order to provide education about their disease and to establish their daily insulin requirements. The latter are generally in the range of 0.5 to 1.0 units/kg per day in divided doses: two-thirds in the morning and one-third in the evening.

Known Diabetics with Hyperglycemia

For the known diabetic who presents with hyperglycemia with or without an intercurrent illness or injury, management should focus on the primary reason for the ED visit. An additional dose of 10 percent of the child's normal daily insulin dose can be administered as subcutaneous regular insulin for simple hyperglycemia.

If the child has an intercurrent illness, more specific management guidelines may vary between endocrinologists and also depend on whether or not urinary ketones are present. An acceptable approach if the child has an intercurrent illness and no urinary ketones is to administer an additional 5 percent of the daily insulin dose every 4 to 6 h until the condition resolves. If the child has urinary ketones, one should administer 10 percent of the daily dose every 4 to 6 h until the ketonuria resolves, and then decrease to 5 percent, as noted above.

Glargine Insulin (Lantus)

Occasionally, a child will present with hyperglycemia without DKA after missing one or more doses of insulin glargine. Glargine is a long-lasting once-daily insulin preparation that has no peak effect. Generally, glargine is given at approximately 50 percent of the daily insulin requirement, the rest as a short-acting preparation, so that missing a single dose of glargine is not equivalent to missing all insulin doses for the day.

If the child is off schedule for insulin glargine and does not have DKA, a single injection of neutral protamine Hagedorn (NPH) insulin can be given, followed by resumption of the regular dosing schedule.

If the child is off schedule for insulin glargine and is in DKA, treatment is no different from treating DKA as described above.

REFERENCES

1. Felner EI, White PC: Improving management of diabetic ketoacidosis in children. *Pediatrics* 108:735, 2001.
2. Smith CP, Firth D, Bennett S, et al: Ketoacidosis occurring in newly diagnosed and established diabetic children. *Acta Paediatr* 87:537, 1998.
3. Rewers A, Chase HP, Mackenzie T, et al: Predictors of acute complications in children with type 1 diabetes. *JAMA* 287:2511, 2002.
4. Edge JA, Ford-Adams ME, Dunger DB: Causes of death in children with insulin dependent diabetes 1990–96. *Arch Dis Child* 81:318, 1999.
5. Glaser N, Barnett P, McCaslin I, et al: Risk factors for cerebral edema in children with diabetic ketoacidosis. *New Engl J Med* 344:264, 2001.
6. Linares MY, Schunk JE, Lindsay R: Laboratory presentation in diabetic ketoacidosis and duration of therapy. *Pediatr Emerg Care* 12:347, 1996.
7. Rosenbloom AL: Intracerebral crises during treatment of diabetic ketoacidosis. *Diabetes Care* 13:22, 1990.
8. Hoffman WH, Steinhart CM, El Gammal T, et al: Cranial CT in children and adolescents with diabetic ketoacidosis. *AJNR Am J Neuroradiol* 9:733, 1988.
9. Harris GD, Fiordalisi I, Harris WL, et al: Minimizing the risk of brain herniation during treatment of diabetic ketoacidemia: A retrospective and prospective study. *J Pediatr* 117:22, 1990.
10. Harris GD, Fiordalisi I: Physiologic management of diabetic ketoacidemia: A 5-year prospective pediatric experience in 231 episodes. *Arch Pediatr Adolesc Med* 148:1046, 1994.
11. Kelly A, Kyle E, McAlpine R: Venous pCO$_2$ and pH can be used to screen for significant hypercarbia in emergency patients with acute respiratory disease. *J Emerg Med* 22:15, 2002.
12. Laffel L: Sick-day management in type I diabetes. *Endocrinol Metab Clin North Am* 29:707, 2000.
13. Glaser NS, Kuppermann N, Yee CKJ, et al: Variation in the management of pediatric diabetic ketoacidosis by specialty training. *Arch Pediatr Adolesc Med* 151:1125, 1997.
14. Green SM, Rothrock SG, Ho JD, et al: Failure of adjunctive bicarbonate to improve outcome in severe pediatric diabetic ketoacidosis. *Ann Emerg Med* 31:41, 1998.
15. Bonadio WA: Pediatric diabetic ketoacidosis: Pathophysiology and potential for outpatient management of selected children. *Pediatr Emerg Care* 8:287, 1992.

HYPOGLYCEMIA
Randolph Cordle

Emergency physicians must recognize the sometimes subtle and other times stunning effects that hypoglycemia can cause, because prompt diagnosis and treatment may spare an otherwise normal child severe brain damage or even death. This is especially true in the first year of life when the diagnosis is difficult to make based on clinical findings alone (Table 129-1).

DEMOGRAPHICS

Most agree that a blood glucose lower than 40 mg/dL is abnormal at any age. Normally the whole blood concentration of glucose is 10 to

TABLE 129-1 Causes of Hypoglycemia in Children

Perinatal
  Transient
    Small for gestational age
    Infant of diabetic mother
    Erythroblastosis fetalis
    Polycythemia
    Infection*†
    Adrenal hemorrhage or
      glucocorticoid suppression*†
    Pre- or postmature infant
    Fetal alcohol syndrome
    Nesidioblastosis
    Fetal distress from any cause
    Congenital heart disease*
    Hypothermia*†
    Umbilical artery catheter displaced
    Exchange transfusion*†
    Cessation of high levels of IV glucose*†
    Hypoglycemia-inducing drug use by the mother
    Maternal toxemia of pregnancy
    Idiopathic*
Infancy
  Those marked* above and
  Substrate-related
    Starvation
    Idiopathic ketotic hypoglycemia
  Endocrine
    Hypopituitarism†
    Glucagon deficiency
    Glucocorticoid deficiency†
    Hypothyroidism
    Adrenocorticotropin deficiency†
    Growth-hormone deficiency†
  Inborn errors of metabolism
    Types I, III, and VI glycogen storage disease
    Hereditary fructose intolerance†
    Acyl-CoA dehydrogenase deficiency†
    Carnitine deficiency†
    HMG-CoA lyase deficiency
  Amino acid metabolic abnormality
    Propionic acidemia
    Methylmalonic aciduria
    Tyrosinemia
    Others
  Hyperinsulinism
    Islet cell adenoma†
    Functional β-cell secretory defect†
    Factitious insulin use
    Beckwith-Wiedemann syndrome†
    Nesidioblastosis†
    Islet cell hyperplasia†
    Factitious sulfonylureas use†
Childhood
  Those marked † above and
  Idiopathic ketotic hypoglycemia
  Drug-induced, especially salicylates
  Large nonpancreatic tumors; neuroblastoma
  Toxin-induced (alcohol, akee fruit)
  Fulminant hepatic disease
  Factitious disorders
  Idiopathic

*Perinatal and infant hypoglycemia.
†Perinatal, infant, and childhood hypoglycemia.
Abbreviations: CoA = coenzyme A; HMG = hydroxymethylglutaryl.

15 percent less than that found in the serum or plasma. This is due to dilution effects caused by the red blood cells in whole blood that contain little glucose. Therefore, acceptable serum or plasma glucose levels would be greater than 45 mg/dL. Values slightly above this level may still be a concern in symptomatic patients.

Pediatric hypoglycemia is relatively rare with a reported prevalence of only 6.54 in 100,000 children presenting to a pediatric ED.[1] Of these, 58 percent had a diagnosis of idiopathic ketotic hypoglycemia (IKH), and 10 percent were found to have insulin-dependent diabetes mellitus.

PATHOPHYSIOLOGY

Normally a highly sophisticated regulatory system maintains glucose concentrations within a very narrow range. This is a steady-state system, not an equilibrium, so the rate of production does not equal the rate of use at any given moment. Relative to body weight, glucose production and use are much higher in children than in adults. This difference is due to children's higher basal metabolic rate, use of glucose for growth and development, and greater activity.

All tissues can use glucose for energy metabolism. Tissues such as the heart, other muscles, and the kidneys can use other substrates quite efficiently; however, the brain, red blood cells, lymphocytes, and platelets are nearly totally dependent on glucose for their metabolism. In the fasted adult model, up to 80 percent of the glucose produced by glycogenolysis and gluconeogenesis is used for brain metabolism.[2] Nearly all the rest is used by the formed elements of blood. An adequate quantity of glucose for the brain's metabolism depends on its degree of use and the plasma glucose level.

The brain is a proportionately much larger organ in children than in adults. More than 80 percent of the fasted child's glucose use occurs by the brain. In fact, glucose use correlates better with brain weight than with body weight. In the postabsorptive state, the glucose requirement of small children is up to two and half times that of the adult, or about 5 to 7 mg/kg per min. After fasting, this requirement drops to 4 mg/kg per min, a value still much higher than that in the fasted adult. In children younger than 2 years, during the fasting state, nearly all the endogenously produced glucose is required and used by the brain. When inadequate quantities of glucose are available, development and growth stop, so that all sources of endogenous energy can be used strictly for the maintenance of brain metabolism.

During periods of inadequate glucose supply to the brain, alternative sources of energy such as ketones and Krebs cycle intermediates will be used. In adults, up to two-thirds of the brain's energy requirements, for short periods, can be supplied with these substances. However, ketones are not immediately available when acute changes in blood glucose occur, because their production occurs slowly over hours. Neonates and children with free fatty acid abnormalities, carnitine deficiency, and ketone-production-limiting hyperinsulinemias are at particular risk for devastating neuroglycopenia, because they lack the ability to effectively produce or use ketones as an alternative energy source.

Carrier-mediated transport is responsible, not only for shuttling glucose through the blood-brain barrier but also for moving it from the cerebrospinal fluid (CSF) into the extracellular space, where it can be used by the individual cells of the brain. A limiting factor in the movement of glucose from the plasma to the brain is the turnover rate of this carrier system. When the plasma glucose concentration and brain glucose use are normal, this carrier-mediated system maintains a three-fold surplus of glucose in the brain. This buffer allows for normal fluctuations of plasma glucose over time. The CSF glucose concentration is maintained at about 65 percent of that found in the blood, whereas that of the brain's extracellular fluid is maintained at about one-third the CSF glucose concentration. In general, CSF and brain extracellular glucose concentrations remain nearly constant. When the plasma glucose level drops to about 30 mg/dL, the supply to the brain cells becomes dangerously low. If not rapidly corrected, the extracellular glucose concentration may approach zero and neuronal metabolism will fail. Fortunately, acute changes in the plasma glucose concentration do not immediately affect that of the CSF and brain. Changes here lag behind those in the plasma by a few hours. As the plasma glucose concentration decreases, systemic changes occur, usually leading to a re-

supply of exogenously or endogenously produced glucose. If not, neuroglycopenia will occur. Peak CSF glucose levels do not occur until 2 h after intravenous dextrose is given. Equilibrium of glucose across the CSF, brain extracellular space, and plasma is typically not achieved for about 4 h. Assuming ongoing carbohydrate provision, plasma equilibrium occurs more quickly. Hence, when neuroglycopenic patients are given exogenous glucose, it often takes a few hours for their mental status to return to normal.

Although alternative fuel sources may temporarily maintain cerebral metabolism, the rapid return to glucose use is necessary for multiple reasons. Glucose is necessary for brain growth and development, the production of membrane lipids and structural proteins, and myelination. Prolonged or repetitive hypoglycemia may cause seizures, permanent neurologic deficits, mental retardation, or death.

Intermediary Metabolism

An elevated glucose concentration causes the release of insulin and suppression of glucagon and glucocorticoid secretion. The elevated insulin level also leads to the suppression of ketogenesis, gluconeogenesis, lipolysis, and glycogenolysis. Simultaneously, it induces glycogen production in the liver and muscle from glucose, protein production from amino acids, and fat production from lipids. Fats are also produced from endogenous lipids formed from surplus amino acids and glucose in the liver. Standard texts in endocrinology and metabolism should be reviewed for a complete discussion of intermediate metabolism. A brief discussion is provided in this chapter.

Glycogenolysis, Ketogenesis, and Gluconeogenesis

In the early fasting state, the remaining free glucose is used rapidly for energy. Thereafter, insulin levels drop as glucagon and epinephrine levels increase, thereby inducing glycogenolysis. Assuming that normal glycogen stores are present, children may be able to maintain a normal plasma glucose concentration for 4 to 6 h, only half the time seen in adults. This occurs because children produce and use more glucose per kilogram of body weight than adults, and they have smaller glycogen stores.

In the late fasting state, children become dependent on gluconeogenesis and ketogenesis. Low levels of insulin and elevated levels of growth hormone, cortisol, epinephrine, and glucagon stimulate lipolysis to provide glycerol for gluconeogenesis and free fatty acids for ketogenesis.

Gluconeogenesis is an energy consumptive reversal of glycolysis. It provides a mechanism for the production of glycogen in most organs of the body and glucose in the liver from pyruvate. During times of starvation, the majority of glucose formed in the liver enters the blood stream to meet the energy demands of glucose-dependent tissues of the blood, renal medulla, testes, and brain. In general, amino acids from skeletal muscle make up the substrates of gluconeogenesis. These substrates lose their ammonia group and donate their carbon backbone to the production of pyruvate. Eighteen of our 20 amino acids can be used as carbon donors in this process, although alanine plays a leading role due to its predominance in skeletal muscle. A quantitative deficiency in the mobilization of these precursors is thought to be the cause of IKH.

Alcohol leads to hypoglycemia by blocking gluconeogenesis in two important ways. Ethanol metabolism by alcohol dehydrogenase consumes oxidized nicotinamide adenine dinucleotide and produces reduced nicotinamide adenine dinucleotide and hydrogen ions. Elevated levels of reduced nicotinamide adenine dinucleotide push the pyruvate ⇌ lactate and oxaloacetate ⇌ malate reactions toward the consumption of pyruvate and oxaloacetate, thus depriving gluconeogenesis of two very important substrates.

Ketogenesis may play a vital role in providing glucose to the brain during the fasted state. By providing for the energy needs of the heart, kidneys, muscles, and other tissues, ketogenesis allows a higher percentage of endogenously produced glucose to be used by the brain.

Triglyceride metabolism is another source of ketones, but ketone production depends on the presence of fatty acetyl coenzyme A (CoA) and carnitine in hepatocytes. Therefore, defects in fatty acetyl-CoA or in carnitine cause non-ketotic hypoglycemia and the accumulation of abnormal fatty acid metabolites in the liver. Clinical examples of such non-ketotic hypoglycemic disorders include carnitine deficiency and Jamaican vomiting illness. In the past, treatment for non-ketotic hypoglycemic disorders included frequent feedings to prevent development of the fasting state. Carnitine deficiency may be treated by adding carnitine to the diet. Jamaican vomiting illness is caused by the toxin hypoglycin, found in the unripe akee fruit. Hypoglycin metabolites lead to esterification of carnitine and coenzyme A, preventing ketone production. Hypoglycin also suppresses gluconeogenesis.

Counter-regulatory chemicals also play a role in this system. When the glucose concentration approaches 70 mg/dL, glucagon and epinephrine levels begin to rise. By the time the glucose level reaches 55 mg/dL, an intense counter-regulatory chemical response is apparent. In children with insulin-dependent diabetes or chronic hyperinsulinemia, the epinephrine response may be blunted and may not occur until the glucose concentration is about 35 mg/dL. Under conditions of even normal glucose use, there may not be time for endogenous mechanisms to prevent severe hypoglycemia. β-Blockers often blunt the counter-regulatory catecholamine response to hypoglycemia, resulting in hypoglycemia without the classic catecholamine-induced clinical signs and symptoms. Instead, patients may develop predominantly neuroglycopenic symptoms and signs, such as seizure, "stroke," or coma. The release of glucagon is normally stimulated by hypoglycemia and elevated levels of growth hormone, epinephrine, and cortisol. However, calcium-channel blockers, β-antagonists, and anticholinergic drugs suppress its release. Therefore, these drugs may predispose individuals to hypoglycemia (Table 129-2).

CLINICAL FEATURES

Classically, hypoglycemic patients present with neuroglycopenic or excessive adrenergic signs and symptoms (Table 129-3). In general, the more rapid the decrease in glucose concentration, the more adrenergic-type symptoms will be noted. Variability and crossover in symptoms is the rule, however, and not the exception. Neonates and young children may present with poor feeding, jitteriness, emesis, ravenous hunger, lethargy, altered personality, repetitive colic-like symptoms, hypotonia, or hypothermia. In other cases, they unfortunately present after an apparent life-threatening event, seizure, or cardiac arrest. As children grow older, they begin to present more like adults, with signs of adrenergic excess followed by neuroglycopenia. If treatment is not forthcoming, the adrenergic symptoms may abate, leaving only the neuroglycopenic ones. In some cases, as with type I glycogen storage disease, patients may have no obvious symptoms despite an incredibly low blood glucose concentration. Children with unexplained catastrophic presentations such as coma, severe hypothermia, and cardiorespiratory arrest should have bedside glucose testing performed immediately, and, if clinically indicated, a specimen should be sent for

TABLE 129-2 Drugs Related to Hypoglycemia in Infants and Children

Ethanol	Sulfonylureas	Salicylates
Insulin	Phenformin/	Sulfisoxazole
β-blockers	metformin	Ethylenediaminetetraacetic
Bishydroxycoumarin	Oxytetracycline	acid
warfarin	Phenylbutazone	Manganese
Propoxyphene	Chlorpromazine	Diphenhydramine
Indomethacin	Para-aminobenzoic	Haloperidol
	acid	

TABLE 129-3 Clinical Signs of Hypoglycemia

Adrenergic Excess	Neuroglycopenia
Anxiety	Confusion
Tachycardia	Ataxia
Perspiration	Headache
Nausea	Depressed consciousness
Tremors	Blurred vision
Pallor	Lightheadedness
Chest pain	Focal neurologic deficits
Weakness	Seizures
Abdominal pain	Strabismus
Hunger	Staring
Irritability	Paresthesias

formal laboratory evaluation. Empirically treating patients after cardiac arrest with glucose may worsen neurologic outcomes, because hyperglycemia is detrimental in cases of cerebral edema and anoxia. Therefore, whenever possible, bedside testing and historical data surrounding the event should guide therapy in this population. Hypoglycemia should be suspected in all moderately to severely injured or ill children. The underlying disease process often will mask the symptoms of hypoglycemia. Children with increased physiologic stress require periodic reevaluation for hypoglycemia, because they are often unable to maintain sufficient glucose influx to meet their increased needs. This is especially true in patients whose illness, injury, or treatment prevents them from being able to express their needs.

Idiopathic Ketotic Hypoglycemia

The most common cause of hypoglycemia in non-insulin-dependent children older than 1 year is IKH. It is more a physiologic aberration than a true pathologic syndrome.[1,3] It usually presents in children younger than 18 months after a period of fasting. Often this is seen on holidays and weekends, when parents sleep late, thereby inadvertently extending the child's usual nighttime fasting period. It is also more common during illnesses preventing normal food intake. These children return to normal after a glucose load and have no suspicious findings in their history or physical examinations.[1] Historically, IKH was thought to occur because affected children were small for their age, but that idea has been called into question by more recent findings.[1,3] Currently, alanine, by far the most important amino acid in gluconeogenesis, is thought to play a major role in this disorder.[2,4] Haymond and colleagues found lower serum alanine concentrations in these patients than in age-matched control groups during fasting.[3] Giving gluconeogenic precursors during periods of fasting prevents hypoglycemia, lending further support to the theory outlined above. Children with IKH present with expected ketonemia and ketonuria. If not tested for early, the ketones may be missed, because they dissipate rapidly with correction of the hypoglycemia. If assayed, insulin normally will be suppressed to no more than 5 to 10 μ units/mL, and cortisol and growth hormone normally will be elevated during the hypoglycemic period. Abnormally elevated insulin levels should call the diagnosis into question.

DIFFERENTIAL DIAGNOSIS

The differential diagnosis of hypoglycemia differs in different age groups. Some disorders are seen only transiently in neonates, whereas others may start in the neonatal period but extend throughout childhood. Still others are not usually seen until after the neonatal period. For example, some inborn errors of metabolism always present in early infancy, whereas others may not be clinically apparent until the child is a few years old. Table 129-1 lists some causes of hypoglycemia in childhood. A full discussion of each cause is beyond the scope of this chapter. Suspicion of many of these disorders should prompt a discussion with and referral to an expert in metabolic diseases.

Many drugs (see Table 129-2) may predispose children to hypoglycemia. Some have more supporting evidence and occur more frequently than others. Aside from insulin and possibly sulfonylurea-type medications, ethanol is by far the most common cause of drug-induced hypoglycemia in children. Ethanol inhibits gluconeogenesis. Hypoglycemia after the ingestion of alcohol may occur in adults but is far more likely in children, because of their higher relative glucose use and much lower relative quantities of glycogen. Children become more quickly dependent on gluconeogenesis than do adults. This effect on liver metabolism is often seen at alcohol levels too low to cause clinical intoxication. Therefore, any child with a history of alcohol ingestion should be closely monitored for hypoglycemia and given glucose orally or parenterally. In nonintoxicated patients, this may be accomplished by feeding. Intoxicated-appearing patients should always be evaluated for hypoglycemia at presentation and every few hours thereafter, if they are unable to eat. In young children who will not be able to eat for more than 4 h, maintenance fluids containing dextrose should be given.

Rapid bedside glucometers have evolved over the years. Qualitative reagent strips, based on nonspecific reduction reactions or enzymatic reactions, were replaced by more quantitative systems. Spectrophotometers used to read subtle enzymatic induced color-indicator changes proportional to the concentration of a more specific substrate, glucose, then took over the market. These systems are still in use but require more expertise and training to avoid user error. Therefore, in most institutions, they have been replaced by more user-friendly and possibly more precise amperometric systems. Enzymatic reactions with glucose lead to loss of electrons that are quantified and correlated with a priori set normal parameters to give a glucose concentration. These systems are calibrated for use on whole blood only. Their algorithms calculate results based on relatively normal whole-blood constituent concentrations. For example, patients who have very high hematocrits may have erroneously low results. Conversely, low hematocrits may produce spuriously high results. Spuriously low results also may be found in capillary samples from patients in shock or with decreased peripheral perfusion. False low results also may be found in patients with hyperglycemic and hyperosmolar conditions or severe dehydration. The correlation between one popular (Precision PCX) monitor using electrochemical detection and laboratory instrumentation was better in adults than in neonates (correlation coefficient, 0.984 vs. 0.889). The definitive diagnosis and workup should be based on the chemical analysis and not just on the bedside screening in all age groups, especially neonates. In symptomatic patients, treatment should begin based on the bedside test result. Treatment can be altered, if necessary, upon return of the chemical analysis.

EVALUATION

Evaluation is quite complex in some cases and controversial in others. In all cases, a detailed history should be obtained and a meticulous physical examination should be performed. Inquiry regarding prior episodes of hypoglycemia should occur. Detailed data regarding family, birth, development, and past medical history are needed. History of childhood death from an unknown cause in a first- or second-degree relative should be sought. Potential access to insulin, sulfonylureas, β-blockers, salicylates, or other toxins should be determined. Physical examination should include a head-to-toe survey for signs of other serious illness and findings more specifically related to hypoglycemia. Hypopituitarism may be associated with midline defects such as abnormal incisors, palatal defects, cleft-lip defects, midface abnormalities, or abnormal palpebral fissures. Hyperpigmentation, undescended testes, severe dehydration, and micropenis may be associated with ab-

normalities arising from the adrenal or pituitary glands. Children with short stature or less than expected recent growth should be evaluated for growth hormone abnormalities.[1,3] Height, weight, and head circumference should be plotted on a standardized growth chart. Tanner stage should be determined. The fundi should be evaluated for signs of optic nerve hypoplasia associated with hypopituitarism. Each patient should have a thorough examination of the abdomen. Large masses such as those from neuroblastoma and, more importantly, hepatomegaly associated with most hypoglycemia causing glycogen storage, fatty acid oxidation, and other metabolic abnormalities should be sought.

The goal is to diagnose hypoglycemia and any other clinically important associated disease processes. Physicians should then institute appropriate therapy. Concurrently, they must differentiate between ketotic and nonketotic hypoglycemia and, based on this information, make decisions regarding the potential need for further studies. In questionable cases, it is practical to collect an extra set of blood tubes and an additional urine specimen for later use, if deemed necessary. Many study results are valuable only if they are based on samples obtained when the child is hypoglycemic. This being said, children should not be allowed to remain hypoglycemic for any significant period before treatment. Overzealous or time-consuming attempts at laboratory collection should be avoided.

Prehospital protocols for hypoglycemic children should include the collection of appropriate blood specimens before treatment whenever possible. Prehospital laboratory specimens should not be discarded except at the discretion of the consultant or admitting physician. They should be placed on ice to prevent ongoing metabolism.

Most children who present to the ED, however, probably do not need extensive laboratory evaluation. Infants and especially neonates should be evaluated thoroughly on first presentation unless the cause of hypoglycemia is clear. Developmentally normal children older than 1 year who have normal head circumference and growth, make a complete recovery after receiving glucose, have normal electrolytes, and present with findings consistent with IKH do not usually need a detailed investigation. Patients with hepatomegaly, other signs of illness, significant acidemia, hyperpigmentation, or other clinically significant physical findings require a complete evaluation at presentation. In patients for whom a full workup is deferred, appropriate tubes of blood and a urine specimen may be collected and held by the laboratory. Close follow-up should be arranged, and the patient's primary care physician should be made aware of the child's visit and findings. Should hypoglycemia recur or the child's clinical situation change, the held specimens may be extremely valuable. See Figure 129-1 for a general approach to the laboratory evaluation of these patients. Variance from this approach is not only acceptable but expected based on the specifics of the individual clinical situation.

SPECIAL ISSUES AFFECTING DIAGNOSIS

Mentally challenged children can be especially difficult to evaluate. Often they have dysautonomia and feeding difficulties. A low threshold for blood glucose evaluation is appropriate in these patients, especially if the caretakers note a change in baseline behavior or mental status.

Most children who present with self-harming thoughts, suicidal threats, or true suicide attempts should have their glucose checked as part of their medical clearance. This is especially true of diabetic children and those with access to a relative's oral hypoglycemic agents. Inpatient monitoring of glucose may be necessary if overdose of an oral hypoglycemic agent is suspected. Management of such overdoses is often complex and is beyond the scope of this chapter.

In patients thought to have a factitiously depressed glucose associated with an elevated insulin level, the C-peptide level should be determined. If exogenous insulin is the cause, the C-peptide level will be inappropriately suppressed, and typically the insulin level in these

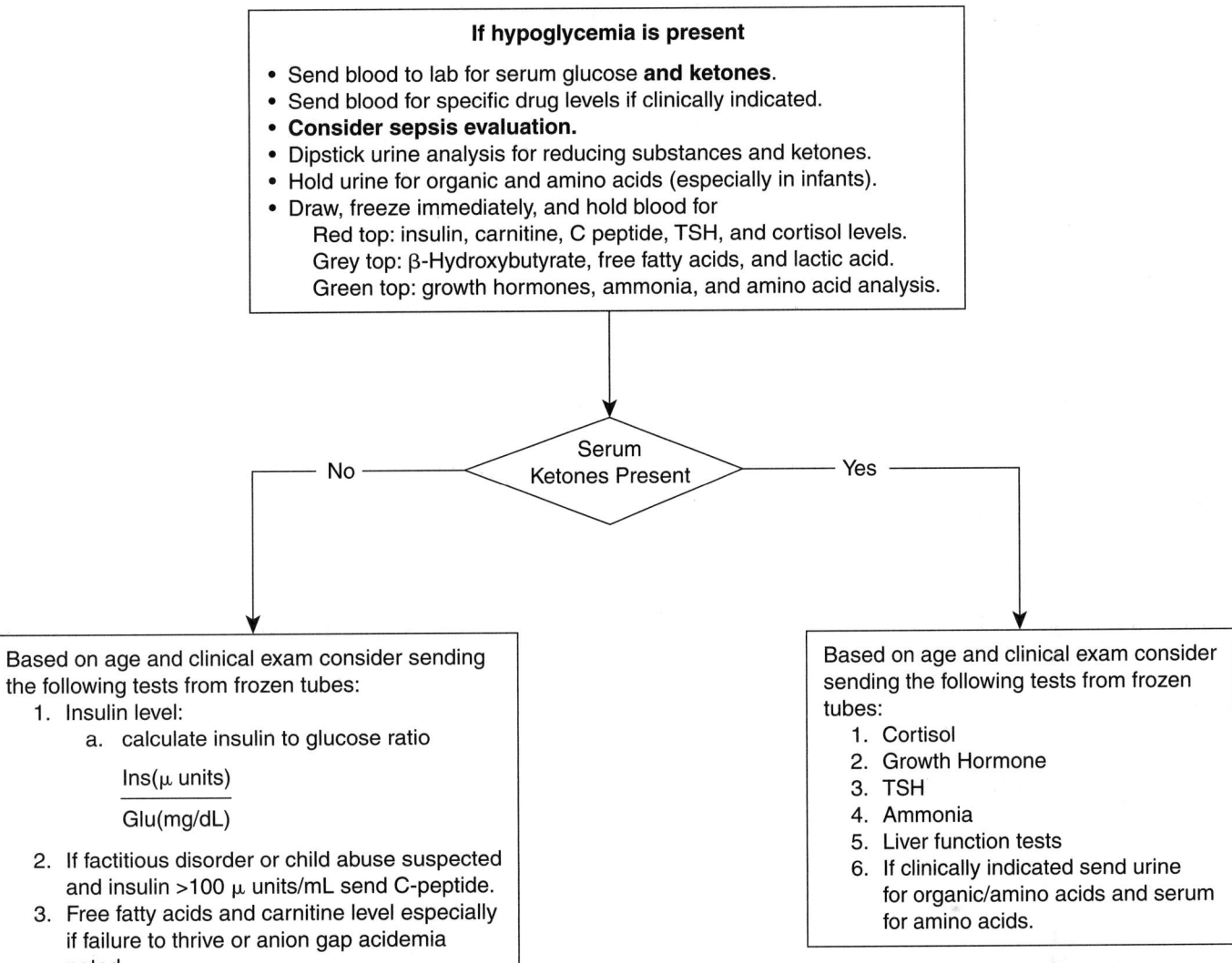

If hypoglycemia is present

- Send blood to lab for serum glucose **and ketones**.
- Send blood for specific drug levels if clinically indicated.
- **Consider sepsis evaluation.**
- Dipstick urine analysis for reducing substances and ketones.
- Hold urine for organic and amino acids (especially in infants).
- Draw, freeze immediately, and hold blood for
    Red top: insulin, carnitine, C peptide, TSH, and cortisol levels.
    Grey top: β-Hydroxybutyrate, free fatty acids, and lactic acid.
    Green top: growth hormones, ammonia, and amino acid analysis.

Serum Ketones Present — No / Yes

No branch:

Based on age and clinical exam consider sending the following tests from frozen tubes:
1. Insulin level:
    a. calculate insulin to glucose ratio

    $$\frac{Ins(\mu\ units)}{Glu(mg/dL)}$$

2. If factitious disorder or child abuse suspected and insulin >100 μ units/mL send C-peptide.
3. Free fatty acids and carnitine level especially if failure to thrive or anion gap acidemia noted.
4. Consider glucose-6-phosphatase deficiency and hereditary fructose intolerance in differential: if possible assure appropriate specific tests, urine for organic and amino acids, and serum amino acids ordered.

Yes branch:

Based on age and clinical exam consider sending the following tests from frozen tubes:
1. Cortisol
2. Growth Hormone
3. TSH
4. Ammonia
5. Liver function tests
6. If clinically indicated send urine for organic/amino acids and serum for amino acids.

FIG. 129-1. General approach to the laboratory evaluation of hypoglycemia. TSH = thyroid-stimulating hormone.

cases will be very high. Normally C-peptide is produced in equimolar quantities during the processing of proinsulin to insulin; therefore, its levels should follow those of insulin itself. In cases of insulinoma, for example, insulin and C-peptide levels will be high.[5,6]

Patients found to have hypoglycemia and non-glucose-reducing substances in their urine should have galactosemia ruled out. The dipstick urine test will be negative for glucose, but the laboratory evaluation for reducing substances will be positive in this case. This disease usually presents during infancy with failure to thrive, vomiting, hepatomegaly, and jaundice.

TREATMENT

Whenever possible, if the clinical condition allows, children should be treated with oral glucose loading. Clearly this should not occur in children unable to protect their airway. Common methods include orange juice with 2 tsp of sugar added per glass, maple syrup, honey (in older children), and, in mild cases, non-diet soda. Sucrose and fructose should not be given to any child suspected of having hereditary fruc-

tose intolerance. Lactose should not be given to children suspected of having galactosemia.

Once the glucose concentration is back to the normal range, children should be given a meal containing complex carbohydrates, proteins, and fats, with the presumption that inborn errors of metabolism have been ruled out. Children thought to have an inborn error should have consultation with a metabolic disease expert before feeding a normal diet to potentially prevent the additional buildup of substrate, due to an enzymatic defect and/or abnormally produced products of metabolism. Dextrose should be given until clarification of these issues is obtained through further testing and/or consultation.

When oral treatment is not an option, the intravenous route should be used (Table 129-4). If an intravenous line cannot be obtained, an intraosseous line should be considered. Glucose given through a nasogastric tube also can be lifesaving.

Intravenous boluses of 0.5 g/kg are most commonly used. This is equivalent to 5 mL/kg D10W, 2 mL/kg D25W, or 1 mL/kg D50W. If no clinical response is seen within 5 min, this dosing should be repeated and a bedside glucose checked. If the glucose remains below

TABLE 129-4   Treatment of Hypoglycemia

Oral (preferred); consider NG tube if IV access is poor in child unable to swallow
  Orange juice with 2 tsp sugar/8 oz.
  2–4 honey packets (not infants)

Parenteral	
IV bolus glucose	Maintenance
Infants	
5 mL/kg D10NS*	4 mL/kg per h D10 in appropriate electrolyte-containing fluid
Child	
2 mL/kg D25NS†	3 mL/kg per h D10 in appropriate electrolyte-containing fluid
Glucagon (if neither route above available) (dilute in sterile water)‡	
(Max dose 1 mg)	
Infant 50 μg/kg IV, IM, or SC	
Child 30 μg/kg IV, IM, or SC	

*D10 = 100 mg dextrose/mL NaCl.
†D25 = 250 mg dextrose/mL NaCl.
‡See text.
Abbreviation: NG = nasogastric.

50 mg/dL and three boluses have been given, the clinician should consider using one of the alternative agents listed below. The proper choice should be based on the clinical and historical findings.

Boluses in neonates should be given with D10W. Infants should receive D10W whenever possible, although D25W is acceptable. In older children, D25W may be used. D25W and especially D50W are very hyperosmolar and may cause phlebitis or tissue necrosis, if they extravasate. Even without extravasation, patients commonly complain of pain at the injection site for 1 to 2 weeks. The risk of extravasation is increased when smaller veins, such as those found in infants, are used. In addition, hyperosmolar loading in premature neonates is associated with an increased risk of intracranial germinal matrix hemorrhage and subsequent periventricular leukomalacia. The use of D25W and D50W also may lead to an increased incidence of rebound hypoglycemia due to endogenous insulin release. When time allows, diluting 50 or 25 to D10W with NS or half NS will decrease the risk of pain, phlebitis, and necrosis at the injection site by decreasing the osmolarity. This practice also prevents the administration of large volumes of free water when multiple boluses are required, as would occur if sterile water were used as the diluent. Because many of these patients are also dehydrated, this amount of electrolyte-containing solution is certainly not excessive and probably somewhat therapeutic.

Once the patient's glucose is brought into the normal range, maintenance fluids should be started. The amount of glucose required for maintenance of euglycemia varies with age, underlying glucose use, and the patient's insulin level. Neonates typically require D10 whereas older infants and children usually only require D5 in their maintenance fluids. Nonelectrolyte-containing dextrose solutions should never be used for multiple boluses or maintenance fluids. This practice can cause water intoxication, hyponatremia, intractable seizures, and death. Typically, D10NS or D10/.45NS (77 mEq/L Na+) will be appropriate. Changes can be made once the serum sodium is known.

Likewise, potassium may be added once urine output is established and the current serum concentration is known. Knowing the current serum potassium concentration before adding it to maintenance fluids is especially important in patients with potential mineralocorticoid deficiency, such as those with 21-hydroxylase deficiency.

Patients who are hyperinsulinemic often require dextrose maintenance rates of 10 to 12 mg/kg per min. In some cases, 25 mg/kg dextrose per min will be needed. The clinician will need to use more concentrated dextrose-containing electrolyte solutions in these cases. A central line should be considered if greater than D12.5 containing maintenance fluid is required.

Glucagon is an effective treatment for hypoglycemia only if the patient has intact glycogen stores.[3] Its use should be considered, especially in the prehospital arena, when an intravenous line cannot be placed. Controversy surrounds the use of glucagon in cases of sulfonylurea overdose and hyperinsulinemia. Glucagon stimulates insulin release; therefore, at least theoretically, giving it to these patients could worsen hypoglycemia. Typical glucagon dosing is 1 mg in adults, 30 μg/kg in children, and 50 μg/kg in infants. The maximum single dose is 1 mg for hypoglycemia, although higher doses are used for other indications. It may be given SC, IM, or IV. If no intravenous line is available, the intramuscular route is probably best. One exception is in small neonates who may not have adequate muscle mass. The new recombinant form of glucagon is packaged with a diluent containing glycerin, sterile water, and hydrochloric acid. In contrast to the phenol-containing diluent found in older forms of glucagon, the recombinant glucagon diluent may be used in all age groups. If a 50 percent rise in serum glucose concentration is not seen within 30 min, the clinician should suspect previous depletion of glycogen stores, an abnormality in fatty acid oxidation, or type I glycogen storage disease. Less commonly, glycogen storage disease types III, VI, and IX can present in this fashion.

In refractory cases, especially those associated with adrenal insufficiency, steroids may be useful. Hydrocortisone succinate is a good choice owing to its effective glucocorticoid and additional mineralocorticoid effects. Most adrenally suppressed patients also will have associated mineralocorticoid depression. In these cases, a steroid such as hydrocortisone must be used instead of one such as dexamethasone, which has almost no mineralocorticoid activity. The dose of hydrocortisone succinate is 1 to 2 mg/kg IV every 6 h. The minimum dose is 25 mg and the maximum dose is 100 mg.

Hyperinsulinemic patients also may be given diazoxide to inhibit insulin release and activity.[4] Octreotide may be a better choice; it is not associated with the rare hypotensive effects of diazoxide. Octreotide dosing for this potential indication is controversial. Diazoxide is given IV at 3 to 5 mg/kg for neonates and 1 to 3 mg/kg for children every 8 h. Diazoxide should be given over at least 30 min to prevent severe hypotension. In children who are able to eat, feedings every 3 to 4 h often will suffice. If given only simple carbohydrates, hyperinsulinemic children will develop postprandial hyperglycemia with subsequent rebound hypoglycemia secondary to stimulation of insulin secretion. Therefore, their diets should consist of complex carbohydrates, proteins, and fats. Raw cornstarch feedings at night usually maintain safe glucose levels and are not typically associated with the rebound phenomenon discussed above. Starches are absorbed slowly, leading to a lower but more continuous supply of glucose.[7] Children with endogenous hyperinsulinemia due to insulinomas often require nearly total pancreatectomy.

Idiopathic ketotic hypoglycemia is best treated by prevention. Prevention efforts should include avoidance of prolonged fasts, provision of frequent high-carbohydrate and high-protein meals, and monitoring for urine ketones during periods of decreased oral intake, such as illness.[3,7] If ketones are detected, the patient should be given additional carbohydrate- and protein-containing foods and/or be brought to medical attention at once.

REFERENCES

1. Pershad J, Monroe K, Atchison J: Childhood hypoglycemia in an urban emergency department: Epidemiology and a diagnostic approach to the problem. *Pediatr Emerg Care* 14:268, 1998.
2. Pagliara AS, Karl IE, Haymond M, et al: Hypoglycemia in infancy and childhood: Part I. *J Pediatr* 82:365, 1973.
3. Haymond MW, Pagliara AS: Ketotic hypoglycemia. *Clin Endocrinol Metab* 12:447, 1983.

4. Pagliara AS, Karl IE, Haymond M, et al: Hypoglycemia in infancy and childhood. Part II. *J Pediatr* 82:558, 1973.

5. Lebowitz MR, Blumenthal SA: The molar ratio of insulin to C-peptide: An aid to the diagnosis of hypoglycemia due to surreptitious (or inadvertent) insulin administration. *Arch Intern Med* 153:650, 1993.

6. Sheehy TW: Case report: Factitious hypoglycemia in diabetic patients. *Am J Med Sci* 304:298, 1992.

7. Chen YT, Cornblath M, Sidbury JB: Cornstarch therapy in type I glycogen storage disease. *New Engl J Med* 310:171, 1984.

130 ALTERED MENTAL STATUS AND HEADACHE IN CHILDREN

Nancy Pook

Natalie Cullen

Jonathan I. Singer

ALTERED MENTAL STATUS

Altered mental status (AMS) in a child is the failure to respond to the external environment in a manner appropriate to the child's developmental level, despite verbal or physical stimulation.[1] Alteration in mental status consists of impairment of awareness and arousal, the two components of consciousness. Patients with AMS require simultaneous stabilization, diagnosis, and treatment. The objectives of treatment are to sustain life and prevent irreversible central nervous system damage. Once the patient is resuscitated, the next objective is to establish the cause of AMS and stop disease progression.

Pathophysiology

There is a spectrum of alterations of mental status, ranging from confusion or delirium (disorders in perception) to lethargy, stupor, and coma (states of decreased awareness). A lethargic child has decreased awareness of self and the environment. In an emergency setting, this translates to decreased eye contact with family members and nursing and physician personnel. A stuporous child has decreased eye contact, decreased motor activity, and unintelligible vocalization. Stuporous patients can be aroused with vigorous noxious stimulation. Comatose patients are unresponsive and cannot be aroused by verbal or physical stimulation, such as phlebotomy, arterial catheterization, or lumbar puncture.[2,3]

Irrespective of the cause, AMS is indicative of depression of the cerebral cortex or localized abnormalities of the ascending reticular activating system. Both cerebral cortices must be affected to cause AMS. Classic causes of bilateral cortical impairment are toxic and metabolic states that deprive the brain of normal substrates. Altered mental status also can be produced through dysfunction of the reticular activating system that is housed in the brainstem and midbrain. This system connects cranial nerve nuclei and extends from the brainstem to the thalamus. It governs respirations, cardiovascular functions, many aspects of homeostasis, and daily wake and sleep cycles. Any abrupt interruption or selective destruction of the reticular activating system may result in AMS.[1]

The pathologic conditions that affect awareness and arousal can be described by three broad pathologic categories: supratentorial mass lesion, subtentorial mass lesion, and metabolic encephalopathy.[4]

Supratentorial mass lesions cause AMS by compressing the brainstem and/or diencephalon. Signs and symptoms of this type of lesion include focal motor abnormalities that are often present from the onset of the altered level of consciousness. The progression of neurologic dysfunction is from rostral to caudal, with sequential failure of midbrain, pontine, and medullary functions. Compromise by supratentorial lesions causes slow nystagmus toward and fast nystagmus from a cold stimulus during caloric testing.

Subtentorial mass lesions lead to reticular activating system dysfunction, in which prompt loss of consciousness is generally the rule. There is a discrete level of dysfunction. Cranial nerve abnormalities are frequently found due to the highly packed neurologically eloquent anatomy. Abnormal respiratory patterns such as Cheyne-Stokes respiration, neurogenic hyperventilation, and ataxic breathing are common. With brainstem injury, asymmetric and/or fixed pupils are found. No eye movements occur despite cold stimuli to both auditory canals.

Metabolic encephalopathy usually causes depressed consciousness before depressed motor signs, which, when present, are typically symmetric. Respiratory function is involved relatively early, and abnormalities are often secondary to acid-base imbalance. Pupillary reflexes are generally preserved. Pupils may be sluggish, but the movement is intact and symmetric. Exceptions occur with profound anoxia and the influence of cholinergics, anticholinergics, opiates, and barbiturates.

Clinical Features

One individual should act as historian to perform a methodical and comprehensive interview. The key questions that must be explored concern prodromal events leading to the change in consciousness, recent illnesses, the likelihood of an infectious exposure or exposure to intoxicants, and the likelihood of trauma, including abuse.[5] The historian should make inquiries regarding antecedent fever, headache, head tilt, abdominal pain, vomiting, diarrhea, gait disturbance, seizures, drug ingestion, palpitations, weakness, hematuria, weight loss, and rash. For infants and young children with AMS, developmental milestones should be pursued. The medical, immunization, and family histories are important in children of all ages. The clinician should be alert for any inappropriate responses or inconsistencies and delays in seeking care that may arouse the suspicion of child abuse.

One should proceed with a general examination only after cardiac and cerebral resuscitation. The objectives of the examination are to identify occult infection, trauma, toxicity, or metabolic disease.[3,4] The neurologic examination should document the child's response to sensory input, motor activity, pupillary reactivity, oculovestibular reflexes, and respiratory pattern. Although several coma scales have been published, the most simplified and functional in an emergency setting is the AVPU scale. This is a descriptive tool in which *A* means "alert," *V* means "responsive to verbal stimuli," *P* means "responsive to painful stimuli," and *U* means "unresponsive."

After a targeted history and a focused examination, the treating physician should anticipate and observe changes in the patient's status that may indicate improvement or deterioration. An additional task of the physician who attends the patient is to make an operational, if not specific, diagnosis of AMS.

Diagnosis

The differential diagnosis for AMS in children is diverse and differs slightly from that for adult patients.[1,3] The familiar mnemonic AEIOU TIPS (alcohol, encephalopathy, insulin, opiates, uremia, trauma, infection, poisoning, and seizure) remains a useful tool for organizing the diagnostic possibilities (Table 130-1).

ALCOHOL   In younger pediatric patients, alcohol ingestion is typically accidental; intentional ingestion is more likely in adolescents. Altered mental status may occur with serum levels below 100 mg/dL. Hypoglycemia may occur concurrently.

ACID-BASE AND METABOLIC DISORDERS   Children with diabetes may present in ketoacidosis. The classic presentation includes weight loss, polyuria, polydipsia, polyphagia, weakness, vomiting, abdominal discomfort, Kussmaul respirations, a fruity acetone breath, and AMS. Patients with diabetic ketoacidosis and many other pediatric disease states associated with a loss of circulating volume may develop inadequate

TABLE 130-1 AEIOU TIPS: A Mnemonic for Pediatric Altered Mental Status

A Alcohol
Acid-base and metabolic
  disorders
  Diabetes mellitus
  Dehydration
  Hypercapnia
  Hepatic failure
  Hypoxia
  Inborn errors of metabolism
Arrhythmia and cardiogenic
  causes
  Ventricular fibrillation
  Stokes-Adams attack
  Aortic stenosis
	O Opiates
	
	U Uremia
	  Chronic renal failure
	  Hemolytic uremic syndrome
	
	T Trauma
	  General trauma with
	  hypovolemia
	  Head injury
	  Mass lesion
	  Cerebral edema
	  Cerebrovascular accident
	  Electric shock
	  Decompression sickness
	  Tumor
	  Thermal

E Encephalopathy
  Hypertensive
  Reye syndrome
  Hemorrhagic shock and
    encephalopathy syndrome
  Postimmunization
  HIV disease
 	
Endocrinopathy
  Addison disease
  Congenital adrenal
    hyperplasia
  Thyrotoxicity
  Cushing syndrome
  Pheochromocytoma
  Hepatic porphyrias
 	
Electrolytes
  Na^+, Ca^{2+}, Mg^{2+}, PO_4^-
	I Infection
	  Meningitis
	  Encephalitis
	  Brain abscess
	  Visceral larva migrans
	  Severe systemic infection
	
	Intracerebral vascular disorders
	  Subarachnoid hemorrhage
	  Venous thrombosis
	  Arterial thrombosis
	  Intracerebral and intraven-
	    tricular hemorrhages
	  Cerebral emboli
	  Acute infantile hemiplegia
	  Acute confusional migraine
	  Moyamoya malformation

I Insulin
  Hypoglycemia
  Ketotic hypoglycemia
  Hyperglycemia
  Intussusception
	P Poisoning
	  Psychogenic
	
	S Seizure
	  Shunt malfunction

Source: Adapted from McCabe J, Singer J, Augustine J, Roth R: Intussusception: A supplement to the mnemonic for coma. *Pediatr Emerg Care* 3:118, 1987.

perfusion. Patients with hypotonic or hypertonic dehydration may develop AMS with and without seizures. Poorly perfused patients or patients with inadequate air exchange have insufficient oxygen delivery to the brain and exhibit insomnia, somnolence, and confusion. Patients who develop hypercapnia as a result of primary lung disease or neurologic dysfunction also may present with AMS. Those with hepatic failure present with nausea, fatigue, and behavioral alterations and may rapidly become obtunded. Patients with inborn errors of metabolism typically present early in life with poor feeding, recurrent vomiting, seizures, metabolic acidosis, lethargy, stupor, and AMS.

ARRHYTHMIA AND OTHER CARDIOGENIC CAUSES Ventricular fibrillation causes unconsciousness by diminished oxygen delivery to the brain. In a Stokes-Adams attack, heart block leads to loss of consciousness. Critical aortic stenosis leads to unconsciousness through decreased cardiac output.

ENCEPHALOPATHY Hypertensive encephalopathy may occur in pediatric patients at diastolic pressures of 100 to 110 mm Hg. Reye syndrome follows a viral illness, such as influenza or varicella. Patients are afebrile and anicteric and develop pernicious vomiting. Con-

fusion and delirium may lead to increasing obtundation. Hemorrhagic shock and encephalopathy syndrome is a symptom complex of unknown cause that affects previously healthy infants. The common features include a mild prodromal, nonspecific illness of several days' duration followed by the onset of profuse, watery diarrhea that becomes bloody, and seizures. Patients present poorly perfused, with profound metabolic acidosis and evidence of disseminated intravascular coagulation. Laboratory evidence of hepatic, renal, pancreatic, and myocardial dysfunction is common.

ENDOCRINOPATHY Altered mental status is a rare presentation of these disorders. Patients with Addison disease present with nausea, vomiting, abdominal pain, weakness, malaise, hypotension, and mental status changes, including psychosis. Presumptive evidence is provided by finding hyperpigmentation, depressed sodium and blood sugar levels, an elevated potassium level, and a variably increased calcium level. Infants with congenital adrenal hyperplasia may present in an acute salt-losing, volume-depleted hypotensive crisis or with virilization, characterized by ambiguous genitalia and cortisol insufficiency also manifested as hypoglycemia. Thyrotoxic infants may present with ventricular dysrhythmia. Patients also may exhibit symptoms similar to those of adults, including goiter, irritability, exophthalmos, hyperthermia, high-output congestive heart failure, mania, delirium, psychosis, and, later, apathy and decreasing levels of consciousness. Patients with pheochromocytoma may present with hypertensive encephalopathy.

ELECTROLYTES Hyponatremic children become symptomatic with plasma levels around 120 mEq/L. Manifestations include anorexia, headache, nausea, vomiting, irritability, weakness, cramps, disorientation, seizures, and AMS. Hypernatremic individuals develop muscle weakness, irritability, seizures, and AMS. Disorders of calcium, magnesium, and phosphorus present with neuromuscular signs, including weakness, tetany, seizures, and apathy.

INSULIN Hypoglycemia may be an end product of an endocrinopathy (e.g., adrenal insufficiency, hyperthyroidism, or hypopituitarism) or the result of an exogenous substance, such as ethanol, salicylate, oral hypoglycemics, or insulin. Hypoglycemia may result from a common stress pathway of decreased gluconeogenesis, as seen during sepsis or Reye syndrome. Adrenergic signs of palpitations, hunger, and sweating are seen at levels below 60 mg/dL. Irritability, confusion, seizures, and coma occur at levels of 40 mg/dL or lower. Infants and children are prone to develop ketotic hypoglycemia with fasting, especially with infections in early infancy. Altered mental status from hyperglycemia is rare in children. The most common cause of hyperosmolar central nervous system dysfunction is diabetic ketoacidosis.

INTUSSUSCEPTION Intussusception is readily diagnosed in the small percentage of younger children who present with a classic constellation of abdominal pain, vomiting, abdominal mass, and rectal bleeding. Altered mental status may be the initial symptom and dominant concern of the physician and the parent caring for a child with intussusception. Altered mental status remains until the bowel obstruction is reduced.[6]

OPIATES Children who have ingested opiates may present with miosis, absent bowel sounds, and lethargy. Common opiates that may be present in the household include dextromethorphan, diphenoxylate and atropine (Lomotil), and loperamide (Imodium). Ingestion of clonidine also may cause signs and symptoms similar to opiate intoxication. Abuse and neglect should always be suspected in children with opiate intoxication.

UREMIA In children with chronic renal failure, neurologic dysfunction may develop secondary to stroke, hypertension, or metabolic derangements. Encephalopathy occurs in over one-third of patients with chronic renal failure and is manifested by headache, irritability, cognitive derangement, and seizures. Hemolytic uremic syndrome is the most common cause of acute renal failure in childhood. It is characterized by oliguria, microangiopathic hemolytic anemia, and thrombocytopenia with purpura. Diverse etiologies may precipitate the disorder. The most common include a prodromal *Escherichia coli* enteritis or an invasive *Streptococcus pneumoniae* infection.

TRAUMA   Trauma may occur at the cellular or global level. In the context of multisystem trauma, a hypovolemic state may create insufficient cerebral perfusion. Such hypovolemic states may be created by other "traumatic" insults, such as primary peritonitis or ruptured appendicitis with hypovolemia. Children may have transient loss of consciousness after closed-head injury. Occasionally, a seizure may occur immediately after closed-head injury, resulting in AMS from the postictal state. The signs and symptoms of acute epidural hematoma are typically posttraumatic loss of consciousness followed by a lucid interval and then rapid progression of AMS. Acute epidural hematoma also can present with a gradual loss of consciousness associated with ipsilateral pupillary dilatation. As in adults, subdural hematomas may be acute, subacute, or chronic. Most children with subdural hematomas have external signs of trauma. The exceptions are abused infants, typically younger than 6 months who may present without external signs of injury. Abused children who are shaken typically present with a history of vomiting, seizures, and changes in respiratory pattern associated with AMS. Retinal hemorrhages or a tense fontanel may suggest the diagnosis. Children with blunt head trauma are more inclined than adults to develop diffuse cerebral swelling, increased intracranial pressure, and AMS without extracerebral or intracerebral collections of blood.

TUMOR   Primary brain tumor, or metastatic or meningeal leukemic infiltration, may alter the metabolism of the brain. Intracerebral tumors commonly produce focal neurologic dysfunction, whereas posterior fossa tumors typically block the ventricular system and create signs and symptoms suggestive of hydrocephalus. Supratentorial and infratentorial tumors may present abruptly with AMS, fever, or meningismus after an intratumor hemorrhage.[7]

THERMAL   Extremes of body temperature also may lead to central nervous system dysfunction. Progressive hypothermia leads to insidious AMS. Patients who develop body-core temperatures higher than 41°C (105.8°F) develop headache, weakness, and dizziness followed by confusion, euphoria, combativeness, and AMS. Posturing, seizures, hemiparesis, and pupillary changes may be present.[8]

INFECTION   Infection is more common as a cause of AMS in children than in adults. The incidence of bacterial meningitis and septicemia is highest in early infancy and considerably higher throughout childhood than in adulthood. Bacterial meningitis should be high on the differential diagnostic list in a pediatric patient with AMS. Unless there are contraindications to lumbar puncture, examination of cerebrospinal fluid (CSF) should be considered in lethargic, febrile pediatric patients (Table 130-2). Patients with encephalitis have fever and headache and may have signs of meningeal irritation or neurologic deficits. Herpes viruses, arbovirus, rotavirus, and Epstein-Barr virus are among the most common viral agents associated with encephalitis. Encephalitis may occur in the course of mycoplasmal illness, shigellosis, Lyme disease, or cat-scratch disease. Visceral larva migrans may produce encephalopathy in the young.

A brain abscess may create signs and symptoms suggestive of encephalitis. Patients with a brain abscess present with fever and

TABLE 130-2   Procedure: Lumbar Puncture

Relevant anatomy: CSF is produced by the choroid plexus and circulates around the brain and spinal cord within the subarachnoid space. A spinal needle traverses the skin, subcutaneous tissue, supraspinal ligament, interspinal ligament, ligamentum flavum, dura, and arachnoid before entering the subarachnoid space surrounding nerve roots that form the cauda equina in the lumbar region.

Indications: The primary indication for emergent lumbar puncture is the possibility of central nervous system infection. It is also indicated for suspected spontaneous subarachnoid hemorrhage.

Contraindications: Absolute contraindications include the presence of infection in tissues near the puncture site and increased intracranial pressure secondary to a space-occupying lesion. The presence of coagulopathy or lumbosacral deformity is a relative contraindication.

Possible complications: Common complications include localized back pain, residual paraspinal muscle spasm, and headache. Rare but debilitating events include subarachnoid bleeding, subdural bleeding, entrapped nerve through dural tear, paresis, pyogenic spondylitis, vertebral infection, meningitis, implantation of epidermal tissue with delayed epidermoid tumor. The most serious complication is cardiorespiratory arrest, which can result from a vasovagal phenomenon, malpositioning of the child's neck in flexion, or cerebral herniation.

Equipment needed: Necessary equipment consists of a lumbar puncture kit with spinal needle. A 22-gauge $1\frac{1}{2}$-in. needle is used for children <6 y. A 22-gauge $2\frac{1}{2}$-in. needle is required for children 6–12 y, and a 21-gauge $3\frac{1}{2}$-in. needle is used in children >12 y. A manometer with a three-way stopcock is used to measure CSF pressure. Consider use of a cardiorespiratory monitor and oxygen saturation measuring device.

Patient positioning: An assistant is generally required to ensure proper positioning of the patient. The classic posture for lumbar puncture is lateral recumbent with spine flexed and knees drawn upward to the chest, with shoulders and back perpendicular to the table. An alternative for a small infant is sitting with the thighs flexed toward the abdomen. It is critical to avoid flexion of the neck.

Steps of procedure:

To prevent oxygen desaturation in the young, consider delivering 5 L oxygen/min through a tight-fitting face mask for several minutes before needle insertion.

The back may be cleaned with povidone-iodine surgical scrub, or povidone-iodine solution may be allowed to air dry on the skin. Sterile draping is optional in infants and best avoided to maximize landmark exposure and proper positioning. Local anesthesia with 1% xylocaine should be administered to all children, irrespective of age.

The intersection of a line joining the superior portion of the iliac crest and the spine meets at the spinous process of L4. Optimal insertion is at the L3–L4 interspace but may be performed one space above or below.

The spinal needle is inserted into the chosen site with the stylet in place through the epidermis and dermis. Then the stylet may optionally be removed for the remainder of the procedure. The clinician may not feel an increasing resistance and "pop" into the subarachnoid space in younger children.

Manometry may be performed as indicated in cooperative children who have lumbar puncture performed in the lateral decubitus position. Classic, relaxed pressure is 5–15 cm H_2O, but normal values may range as high as 20–28 cm H_2O.

If the tap is bloody, one may replace the stylet and leave the needle in place. Insert a second spinal needle one interspace cephalad and collect fluid for analysis. Finally, withdraw both needles. This process minimizes red blood cell contamination in the collected fluid.

Place a bandage over the insertion site.

Analysis: Necessary CSF studies include bacterial culture and gram stain from tube 1, protein and glucose from tube 2, and cell count and differential from tube 3. Tube 4 may be sent for viral or fungal cultures or for latex agglutination in specific circumstances.

Abbreviation: CSF = cerebrospinal fluid.

headache that precede changes in presentation and consciousness. Affected patients also may present with generalized or focal seizure activity. Patients at risk for brain abscess include those with sinusitis, cyanotic congenital heart disease, immunodeficiency, and intravenous drug abuse.

Any systemic infection associated with vasculitis or vasodepressant toxins with shock may lead to AMS secondary to cerebral hypoperfusion.

INTRACEREBRAL VASCULAR DISORDERS Cerebrovascular events are uncommon in children, but subarachnoid hemorrhage from arteriovenous malformations or a ruptured berry aneurysm may cause focal neurologic deficits followed by status epilepticus and coma. Nuchal rigidity is an inconstant finding. Venous thrombosis may follow severe dehydration or a pyogenic infection of the paranasal sinuses, mastoid, or middle ear. Periorbital edema with cranial nerve abnormalities is a clue. Arterial thrombosis is uncommon in children, except in those with homocystinuria. Children with homocystinuria have a marfanoid appearance, dislocated lenses, and mental retardation. Intracerebral and intraventricular hemorrhages may follow birth asphyxia or trauma in neonates, but in older children they may signify a congenital or acquired coagulopathy. Signs of subacute bacterial endocarditis include splinter hemorrhages, splenomegaly, microscopic hematuria, and AMS caused by cerebral emboli. Acute infantile hemiplegia presents with an acute seizure followed by hemiparesis and coma. Acute confusional migraine may be associated with profound alterations in consciousness. Children with sickle cell anemia can develop cerebral thrombosis, status epilepticus, and coma.

POISONING Drugs may be transferred to a fetus transplacentally. Infants and children may receive drugs through neglect, abuse, or accident. Drugs may be used as a suicide gesture in adolescents. Altered mental status may be caused by exogenous intoxicants, such as ethanol, ethylene glycol, methyl alcohol, paraldehyde, salicylates, and anticholinergics, including antihistamines, cholinergics, opiates, carbamazepine, clonidine, sedative-hypnotics, amphetamines, cocaine, cannabis, nicotine, carbon monoxide, hydrocarbons, and multiple psychotropics within the categories of selective serotonin reuptake inhibitors, mood stabilizers, and antipsychotics.[9] Ingestion of household and beauty products also may cause AMS.

PSYCHOGENIC Psychogenic unresponsiveness is rare in children. It is characterized by decreased responsiveness but otherwise normal findings on neurologic examination, including normal oculovestibular reflexes. Psychogenic unresponsiveness may occur as a conversion reaction, an adjustment reaction, a panic state, or a manifestation of malingering.

SEIZURE Generalized tonic-clonic major motor seizures and absence status epilepsy are associated with prolonged unresponsiveness in pediatric patients.[10] A prolonged post-ictal phase in a febrile child with seizure suggests intracranial infection.

Diagnostic Adjuncts

Ancillary procedures for diagnosis of AMS include analysis of blood, gastric fluid, urine, and CSF (see Table 130-2); electrocardiography; roentgenography; ultrasonography; and computed tomography (CT).[11] Diagnostic tests should be guided by the clinical situation. Rapid estimation of the blood glucose level with a glucose oxidase strip is a universally accepted evaluation in pediatric patients with AMS. Confirmation by laboratory analysis of venous blood is recommended. Electrolyte determinations, liver function studies, and renal function studies may provide additional information regarding the state of hydration, suspected endocrine and metabolic derangements, and liver and kidney function. If the history is consistent with a toxic ingestion

or a toxidrome is identified, serum or urine toxicology screening is in order. The white blood cell count and differential blood cell count as independent evaluations are rarely helpful, except perhaps in management decisions regarding highly febrile children younger than 2 years. A blood culture should be obtained whenever serious bacterial infection is suspected.

An arterial blood gas or capillary blood gas analysis with pulse oximetric analysis may provide useful information in cases of trauma, respiratory distress, or suspected acid-base imbalance.

Shock or hypotension and hypoxia should be corrected before lumbar puncture, and empiric antibiotics should be given before lumbar puncture if bacterial meningitis is suspected. Lumbar puncture with CSF examination is necessary as soon as the patient is stabilized (see Chap. 116).

A 12-lead electrocardiogram should be obtained if there are pathologic auscultatory findings or a rhythm disturbance is found while monitoring the patient. An electrocardiogram may further guide therapy in cases of tricyclic antidepressant overdose.

Radiologic evaluation should be directed by the clinical scenario. Cervical spine immobilization is the first step in management of the head or multiple system trauma patient. This is followed by cervical spine radiography and/or CT of the cervical spine and head. A chest x-ray may be used to confirm or clarify examination findings and to document endotracheal tube placement. Abdominal films are indicated for the acute ingestion of radiopaque material, if suspected, or if the patient exhibits signs and symptoms of an acute abdomen, including possible intussusception. Abdominal ultrasound studies may be useful to screen cases of intussusception with an atypical presentation. A CT scan of the head may be obtained for suspected increased intracranial pressure, vascular disorder, or mass lesion.

Other studies for specific instances are blood ammonia, serum osmolality, blood alcohol level, thyroid function tests, blood lead level, or skeletal survey for suspected abuse. A portable electroencephalogram may diagnose non-motor status epilepticus.

Treatment

The first priorities in AMS are stabilization and reversal of acutely life-threatening conditions before specific diagnostic maneuvers, such as lumbar puncture, are undertaken.[5] Airway, breathing, and circulation must be assured. For suspected cervical injury, spinal immobilization is mandatory, and the airway is opened with the jaw-thrust maneuver.

Hypoxia must be corrected, and continuous pulse oximetric monitoring should be established. There is no contraindication to providing oxygen to pediatric patients. Oxygen is obviously indicated for patients with signs of hypoxemia or hypoperfusion, but hypercapnia must be avoided. Bag-valve-mask ventilation may reverse hypercapnia, but endotracheal intubation is necessary to protect the patient from aspiration.

Fluid resuscitation is necessary in hypotensive comatose patients, because cerebral perfusion depends on adequate mean arterial pressure. A fluid bolus of 20 mL/kg of isotonic crystalloid should be given quickly. Poorly perfused patients should be reassessed and boluses repeated up to a total of 60 mL/kg, as necessary. Thereafter, pressors should be used. In hemodynamically stable patients with suspected head injury, encephalitis, or meningitis, the intravenous fluids should be reduced to an hourly rate that provides two-thirds of the calculated maintenance volume. Empiric therapy may be initiated with 2 mL/kg of a solution of D25W IV if hypoglycemia is strongly suspected. Alternatively, the blood glucose level may be rapidly estimated by means of a glucose oxidase stick, and glucose-containing fluids may be given for hypoglycemia.

If there is clinical suspicion of opiate or clonidine overdose, a narcotic antagonist may be administered. The recommended dose for naloxone is 0.01 to 0.1 mg/kg IV every 2 min, until the desired effect is achieved, or a total dose of 2 mg. Any dose, if successful, may be repeated as necessary to maintain narcotic reversal. Flumazenil (Mazicon), a benzodiazepine antagonist, may be used for pure benzodiazepine ingestion in an otherwise healthy child. The dose is 0.01 mg/kg IV, with cardiac monitoring established.

Seizures should be aborted, if present. Benzodiazepines are typically first-line drugs. The longer-acting anticonvulsants, such as phenytoin or phenobarbital, also may be needed.

Acid-base balance should be restored with hydration and compensatory ventilation. Sodium bicarbonate should be used sparingly and only in circumstances in which the arterial pH is 7.0 or lower.

Core body temperature should be controlled. Maintaining euthermia is critical to minimizing metabolic demands. A child's increased relative body surface area hastens radiant heat loss. Heat loss may be minimized with the use of a heating lamp during resuscitative procedures.

Septic-appearing patients and those suspected of having intracranial infection should receive empiric intravenous antibiotics as quickly as possible. Antibiotics may be given before lumbar puncture.

Disposition

All patients with AMS should receive continuing care in an area that can provide physiologic monitoring and repeated physical examination. In general, this requires admission to an intensive care unit or transfer to a tertiary care center with pediatric intensive care capabilities. Only those patients with transient, reversible causes of AMS may be treated, monitored in the ED, and discharged after observation. Patients who are discharged (e.g., those with a closed head injury or simple febrile seizure) should receive disease-specific discharge instructions. Patients who are evaluated for AMS and discharged home should have a repeat evaluation within 24 h of discharge.

HEADACHE

Headache refers to any head pain including pain in the face, neck, and ears but is generally used to describe pain perceived in the scalp and cranium. A headache may occur in childhood as an acute process over a finite period or may occur repeatedly over an extended time frame. Those who sustain repeat, chronic headaches may have altered school performance, behavioral disturbances, and disproportionate over-reporting of all types of pain.[12]

Up to 2 percent of visits to the ED are for the chief complaint of headache,[13] but it is an associated symptom in a great proportion of visits.[14] The vast majority of children who are evaluated in an emergency setting have a benign cause for headache. In one series of 696 children with headache, 6.6 percent had emergent or urgent conditions causing headache, 80 percent of which were due to viral meningitis.[15] In another study of 150 children aged 2 to 18 years who presented to an ED with acute severe headache, the leading causes of headache were upper respiratory tract infection with fever in 57 percent, migraine in 18 percent, viral meningitis in 9 percent, and undetermined in 7 percent.[16] Two qualities associated with serious underlying disease were occipital location of headache and inability of the child to describe the quality of head pain. All patients with neurosurgical conditions had clear and objective neurologic signs.[16]

Pathophysiology

The pathogenesis for headache is complicated and often unclear. The brain and most of the overlying meninges have no pain receptors and thus are not sensitive to pain.[17] Also insensate is the cranium itself, dura, ependymal lining, and choroid plexus.[15,16] Pain may be perceived from any structure between the epidermis of the scalp and the periosteum of the skull. Extracranial pain may arise from cervical nerve roots, cranial nerves, or extracranial arteries traversing muscles or skin. Intracranial pain may arise from venous sinuses, large veins, dura around large veins, or dural arteries and arteries around the base of the brain. Irritation of cranial nerves may lead to pain at specific areas within the head and neck region. As an example, the ophthalmic branch of the trigeminal nerve innervates the supratentorial vessels, pia, arachnoid meninges, and the skull periosteum. Irritation may result in pain radiating to the forehead, eyes, and temples. The pain nociceptors in the posterior fossa (inferior to the tentorium, cranial nerve roots, and cranial nerves VII, IX, and X) refer pain to the occiput, ear, and retroauricular areas.[18] The posterior fossa is also innervated by glossopharyngeal and vagus nerves and thus may refer pain to the throat.[17]

Clinical Features

There are several common classification schemes for headaches. The most frequent approach divides headaches into two general categories, primary and secondary. Primary headaches are physiologic or functional, and secondary headaches have an anatomic basis. Primary headaches are often recurrent and are accompanied by a normal physical examination. Examples include migraine headache, tension headache, chronic daily headache, and headache associated with depression or fatigue. Secondary headaches are due to anatomic problems, such as intracranial mass, vascular malformation, or meningeal inflammation; craniofacial problems such as sinusitis, dental abscess, or otitis; or systemic disorders such as lupus cerebritis. Secondary or anatomic causes of headache have the greatest potential for morbidity or mortality. The appropriate acquisition of historical information, physical examination, and laboratory or radiologic data is necessary to identify the serious causes for headache (Tables 130-3 and 130-4).

HISTORY The child, parents, and caretakers should be asked about the characteristic features of the headache, such as quality, precipitants, timing, duration, location, associated symptoms, and family and personal medical histories. A detailed history may uncover historical features suggesting secondary headache (see Table 130-3).

Age at Presentation The complex migraine syndromes (acute confusional, abdominal, or basilar artery) may have their onset before age 4 years. Classic or common migraine is unlikely before age 6 years.[19] Incapacitating headache associated with vomiting in a child younger than 7 years should lead to consideration of an intracranial mass lesion. Other predictors for a space-occupying lesion in children younger than 7 years include absence of visual aura and absence of family history of migraine.[20]

Quality of Headache Children may be able to express the quality of head pain. The inability of a child to describe the quality of head pain does not preclude a serious underlying process.[21] Herpes zoster can cause stabbing pain or uncomfortable hyperesthesias. Boring pain may be seen with sinusitis. Aching pain occurs with tension headache, encephalitis, or

TABLE 130-3 Historical Features Suggesting Secondary Headache

Acute onset
Worst ever
Posttraumatic
Awakens from sleep
With fever
Aggravated by: sneezing, coughing, Valsalva, lying down
Morning vomiting
Altered mental status
Change in behavior
Change in pattern
Toxic exposure
Positive family history for migraines or subarachnoid hemorrhage

TABLE 130-4 Physical Findings Suggesting Secondary Headache

Altered mental status
Septic or toxic appearance
Fever >104°C in infants and children or >38°C in neonates
Hypertension or hypotension
Diaphoresis
Facial herpes zoster
Petechiae
Café-au-lait spots
Hydrocephalus
Ptosis
Visual field defect
Retinal hemorrhage or optic disc distortion
Asymmetry of motor or sensory responses
Thyromegaly
Nuchal rigidity
Head tilt

meningitis. Throbbing headache is associated with migraine, hypertension, or intracerebral hemorrhage.

Headache Precipitants Fever is the most common precipitant of headache in children.[16] The intensity of headache with fever is variable and not related to the severity of the fever. Acute, posttraumatic headache is a common pediatric event. Occasionally, a posttraumatic event may lead to chronic headaches precipitated by exertional activities. Classic adult precipitants for migraine also occur in children. Chocolate, aged cheeses, monosodium glutamate, menses, or emotional distress may precipitate migraine headaches.[18] Hypoxemia associated with an underlying medical condition, such as asthma, or created by toxic exposure (such as carbon monoxide or drug-induced methemoglobinemia) may initiate headache. Medications, such as vitamin A, oral contraceptives, tetracycline, or steroids, may induce acute or chronic headaches. Bifrontal "ice cream" headache may be induced by cold food on the palate. Headache exacerbated by chewing or teeth clenching suggests temporomandibular joint dysfunction. Prolonged reading-induced headache suggests ocular imbalance or accommodative error.

Timing of Headache Patients with obstructive hydrocephalus, pseudotumor cerebri, or brain tumor will experience headaches after lying down. They may awaken at night from sleep or experience headache upon arising in the morning.

Onset and Duration of Headache The duration of headache is not a particularly specific or sensitive feature. However, an acute event associated with fever suggests infection or inflammation, often within the craniofacial region. When the tempo of headache is hyperacute and intense at onset, subarachnoid hemorrhage is suspected. Subacute tempos suggest cluster headache, tumor, neuralgias, or migraine.

Location of Headache Occipital location is often associated with a serious underlying condition.[21] Adverse drug effect, hypertension, and basilar artery migraine tend to create occipital headaches. Pain at the vertex is seen with sphenoid sinusitis. Periauricular or temporal pain is seen with temporomandibular joint and dental pathology. Retroorbital pain is associated with meningitis, dural sinus thrombosis, ethmoid, and maxillary and frontal sinusitis. Migraine involves frontal or temporal hemicrania in adolescence but may be bifrontal or generalized in younger children. Tension headache has the greatest variance in location: headache may be generalized, frontal, occipital, or posterior cervical.

Manipulations and Avoidance During an acute headache, patients with migraine prefer the silence and darkness. They reduce their speech and seek sleep as a means of relief. As they rest, migraine patients may be noted to rhythmically rub the maximal area of pain. Migraineurs' behaviors contrast most with cluster headache patients. The latter have increased activity, pacing, rocking, or head butting. Patients with increased intracranial pressure will avoid the Valsalva maneuver. Pain intensifies with defecation, coughing, or sneezing. Children with brain tumors avoid placing their heads in a position that increases intracranial pressure. This lends to intermittent, unexplained head tilt. The emotional turmoil and chronicity of tension headaches leads to the highest degree of school absenteeism.

Associated Symptoms Associated symptoms are valuable refinements for a preliminary diagnosis and may be necessary to attain a headache classification. As an example, classic migraine or complicated migraine headache must be associated with motor, sensory, or visual disturbances. Migraineurs may see flashing lights (photopsia), bright wavy lines (teichopsia), or shimmering zigzag (scintillating scotoma). With confusional migraine, there may be visual size distortion (metamorphopsia) and distortions of space or time with sensory hallucinations. Hemiplegic migraine may be associated with paresthesias, transient hemiparesis, or aphasia. Blindness for half the visual field (hemianopsia) or other restricted visual fields is transient with migraine headache. Visual field defects or dimming of vision that are permanent suggest pseudotumor cerebri. Personality change, altered school performance, and rapid fluctuations in consciousness suggest brain tumor. Effortless, nonprojectile vomiting not associated with nausea strongly suggests brain tumor. Vomiting may occur at any time of the day, although the episodes tend to cluster in the morning. In the case of brain tumor, vomiting without systemic complaints or abdominal pain may last from days to weeks, resolve spontaneously, and then recur weeks to months later.[7] In contrast, vomiting associated with migraine headache is coupled with anorexia, nausea, and occasionally abdominal pain.[22] A headache with seizure suggests subarachnoid hemorrhage or tumor. Neck rigidity or syncope may be associated symptoms with subarachnoid hemorrhage.

Family History Children with migraine headache have a positive family history of migraine in up to 90 percent of cases. About 7 percent of children with cluster headache have a family history of similar headaches. Children whose parents have sustained subarachnoid hemorrhage have a four times greater risk of subarachnoid hemorrhage than do the general population. A family history of hypertension, diabetes, or atherosclerotic heart disease may predispose the child to medical conditions that may be associated with headache. Depressive states are occasionally hereditary. However, psychological or psychiatric disorders in parents, when combined with a dysfunctional environment, may predispose to tension headaches in the children.

Medical History Without a history of headache, it may be difficult to provisionally diagnose migraine headache, even with a classic history. Conversely, patients previously diagnosed with migraine, tension headache, fatigue headache, or depressive headache are not excluded from a more ominous diagnosis. A change in the existing headache pattern is the key. A recent inadequately treated infection may lead to bacterial dissemination. Complicated sinusitis, brain abscess, or venous thrombosis of the lateral or cavernous sinus may result from an inadequately treated parameningeal focus. Intracranial infection is more likely in children with immune deficiency. If there is a medical history of meningitis, recurrence may result from an anatomic congenital defect or immunologic impairment. Shunt malfunction or infection may cause the headache. Coagulopathy, such as hemophilia, predisposes the child to spontaneous intracerebral hemorrhage.

PHYSICAL EXAMINATION The general appearance and affect of the pediatric patient and interaction of the patient with any accompanying adult should be assessed during the acquisition of the history of present illness. The search for systemic disease, craniofacial problems, or intracranial pathology is facilitated by analysis of vital signs, a focused head and neck examination, and a detailed neurologic examination (see Table 130-4).

Vital Signs Hypertension or hypotension associated with headache is significant. Any child with encephalopathy or seizures and a diastolic pressure greater than 110 mm Hg suggests a hypertensive emergency. Hypertension as the primary cause of headache should be considered when a child's blood pressure is greater than the 99th percentile for any given age or greater than 15 mm Hg above the 95th percentile. Blood pressures two standard deviations below the mean, particularly if associated with clinical signs of poor perfusion, suggest systemic infection, profound metabolic derangement, or occult trauma. Increased respiratory rate suggests metabolic derangement, hypoxia, or, rarely, increased central neurogenic drive. Resting increased heart rate in the absence of fever may reflect sympathetic response to pain. Tachycardia may result from fever. Temperature elevation with headache suggests infection, which may be localized to the central nervous system. Subarachnoid hemorrhage also can cause fever.

Head and Neck Soft tissue swelling of the scalp may be noted after cranial trauma. Tender scalp muscles suggest a muscular contraction headache. The presence of a machine-like cranial bruit indicates arteriovenous malformation. Periorbital edema, if combined with sinus percussion tenderness, suggests sinusitis. Eyelid edema without palpable tenderness over the sinuses suggests cluster headache. Lacrimation, nasal congestion, and rhinorrhea may be seen with sinusitis or cluster headache. Ptosis, sixth nerve palsy, and mydriasis may be seen with ophthalmoplegic migraine. Papilledema reflects increased intracranial pressure. Retinal hemorrhages in a child without a hemorrhagic diathesis suggests abusive head injury. Meningeal irritation suggests subarachnoid hemorrhage or intracranial infection. Dental caries with gingival erythema, induration, or mass suggest apical abscess. Malocclusive bite, palpable tenderness, and mandibular crepitance suggest temporomandibular joint dysfunction.

NEUROLOGIC EXAMINATION Transient neurologic findings such as somnolence, visual aura, aphasia, or hemiparesis can be seen with various migraine syndromes. Fixed neurologic abnormalities such as AMS, visual field defect, or any focal finding suggest a space-occupying intracranial lesion. Patients with neurologic conditions will have clear and objective neurologic signs.[21]

Diagnostic Adjuncts

Diagnostic procedures of potential utility for headache patients include phlebotomy for complete blood cell count, erythrocyte sedimentation rate, blood sugar, basic metabolic panel, carboxyhemoglobin measurement, lead level, blood culture, and thyroid function testing. Lumbar puncture is of obvious diagnostic utility for suspected intracranial infection, subarachnoid hemorrhage, and pseudotumor cerebri. Useful imaging studies include noncontrast and contrast head CT and magnetic resonance imaging of the brain.

There are no evidence-based studies to guide the clinician in the selection of various diagnostic investigations for headache. However, **there are several scenarios with a high percentage of positive findings, including first headache; worst headache; change in pattern of a chronic headache; headache associated with seizure, fever, or meningeal signs; AMS; or focal neurologic abnormality.**[20,23–25]

Treatment

Headache management includes treatment of the underlying condition, relief of pain, modification of precipitating factors, and insuring continuity of care.

Treatment of the underlying condition can range from welcomed reassurance to a wide variety of therapeutic agents (such as oxygen, antibiotics, etc.) or therapeutic procedures (such as lumbar puncture for pseudotumor cerebri). Narcotic or non-narcotic analgesics should be given that are appropriate for the disease process and the perceived degree of pain.

Treatment options for common and classic migraine in children have not been well studied. There are no straightforward regimens that are uniformly successful. Acetaminophen is rarely helpful. Naproxen or ketorolac can be effective. Promethazine, prochlorperazine, metoclopramide, hydroxyzine, and ondansetron may reduce nausea and vomiting and induce sedation. Dihydroergotamine can be used in children older than 6 years if all other drugs have failed to provide acute headache relief. Ergotamines should not be given to children with basilar or hemiplegic migraine, because it may further reduce blood flow to the ischemic areas of the brain.

Potential precipitating factors should be addressed. For example, education can be provided for dietary avoidance for migraine. Situation modifications can be suggested for relief of tension headache. Patients with posttraumatic headache may temporarily benefit from exercise restriction. Continuity of care with the primary care physician should be arranged to ensure effective therapy, including prophylactic regimens such as β-blockers, cyclic antidepressants, or anticonvulsants for migraine.

Disposition

All patients with emergent causes of headache, such as subarachnoid hemorrhage, acute bacterial meningitis, severe hypertension, or intracranial mass lesion from tumor, hematoma, or abscess, require admission for definitive care. Any patient with intractable pain should be considered for admission.

REFERENCES

1. Rubenstein JS: Initial management of coma and altered consciousness in the pediatric patient. *Pediatr Rev* 15:204, 1994.
2. Alguire PC: Rapid evaluation of comatose patients. *Postgrad Med* 87:223, 1990.
3. Cantor RM: The unconscious child: Emergency evaluation and management. *Int Pediatr* 4:9, 1989.
4. James HE: Emergency management of acute coma in children. *Am Fam Phys* 48:473, 1993.
5. Strange GR (ed): Altered level of consciousness, in *APLS: The Pediatric Emergency Medicine Course,* 3rd ed. Elk Grove Village, IL, AAP/ACEP, 2000.
6. Singer J: Altered consciousness as an early manifestation of intussusception. *Pediatrics* 64:93, 1979.
7. Singer JI: Erroneous diagnosis within the cranial vault. *Pediatr Emerg Care* 8:297, 1992.
8. Brady WJ, Esterowitz D, Genco M: Life-threatening syndromes presenting with altered mentation and muscular rigidity. *Emerg Med Rep* 20:51, 1999.
9. Jacobs ES, Dickstein DP, Liebelt EL: Novel psychotropic medications in children: new toxicities to master. *Pediatr Emerg Care* 17:226, 2001.
10. Benson PJ, Klein EJ: New-onset absence status epilepsy presenting as altered mental status in a pediatric patient. *Ann Emerg Med* 37:402, 2001.
11. Cantor RM, Santamaria JP (eds): Altered level of consciousness, in *ACEP's Pediatric Emergency Guide,* 3rd ed. Dallas, ACEP, 1997.
12. Anttila P, Metsahonkala L, Mikkelsson M, et al: Comorbidity of other pains in schoolchildren with migraine or nonmigrainous headache. *J Pediatr* 138:176, 2001.
13. Svenson J, Cowen D, Rogers A: Headache in the emergency department: Importance of history in identifying secondary etiologies. *J Emerg Med* 15:617, 1997.
14. Field AG, Wang E: Evaluation of the patient with nontraumatic headache: An evidence based approach. *Emerg Med Clin North Am* 17:127, ix, 1999.
15. Burton LJ, Quinn B, Pratt-Cheney JL, et al: Headache etiology in a pediatric emergency department. *Pediatr Emerg Care* 13:1, 1997.

16. Lewis DW, Qureshi F. Acute headache in children and adolescents presenting to the emergency department. *Headache* 40:200, 2000.

17. Rosenblum RK, Fisher PG: A guide to children with acute and chronic headaches. *J Pediatr Health Care* 15:229, 2001.

18. Linder SL, Winner P: Pediatric headache. *Med Clin North Am* 85:1037, 2001.

19. Welborn CA: Pediatric migraine. *Emerg Med Clin North Am* 15:625, 1997.

20. Medina LS, Kuntz KM, Pomeroy S: Children with headache suspected of having a brain tumor: A cost-effectiveness analysis of diagnostic strategies. *Pediatrics* 108:255, 2001.

21. Rothner AD: Pathophysiology of recurrent headaches in children and adolescents. *Pediatr Ann* 24:458, 1995.

22. Linder SL, Winner P. Pediatric headache. *Med Clin North Am* 85:1037, 2001.

23. Bulloch B, Tenenbein M: Emergency department management of pediatric migraine. *Pediatr Emerg Care* 16:196, 2000.

24. Molofsky WJ: Headaches in children. *Pediatr Ann* 27:614, 1998.

25. Annequin D, Tourniaire B, Massiou H: Migraine and headache in childhood and adolescence. *Pediatr Clin North Am* 47:617, 2000.

131 SYNCOPE AND SUDDEN DEATH
William E. Hauda II
Thom Mayer

Although syncope is usually benign, it may be a symptom of serious cardiac disease and can predispose individuals to sudden death. The sudden death of a child may be due to cardiac, neurologic, or respiratory illnesses or trauma. This chapter discusses syncope and sudden death due to cardiovascular causes, although the other causes of sudden death are mentioned briefly.

EPIDEMIOLOGY

Syncope

Syncope is very common in adolescence and less common in younger children. Between 20 and 50 percent of adolescents experience at least one episode of syncope.[1] Syncope is a presenting symptom of 0.05 percent of pediatric visits[2] and 6 percent of hospital admissions.[1] Only 25 percent of patients referred to a cardiology or neurology specialty clinic for the evaluation of syncope are eventually diagnosed with a serious illness.[3] The most common cause of benign syncope is neurally mediated syncope.[2] Therefore, prior syncopal events are not always associated with an increased risk of future sudden death.[4]

Sudden Death

A distinction must be made between sudden unexpected death and sudden cardiac death, because the first includes many causes, such as a seizure, asthma, or toxic ingestion. Sudden cardiac death includes just those causes that directly relate to cardiovascular dysfunction. The rate of sudden unexpected death in children is 2.3 percent of all deaths, or 1.3 cases per 100,000 patient years.[5] Sudden cardiac death encompasses approximately one-third of these deaths, or about 600 deaths per year in the United States. Excluding trauma, sudden cardiac death is the most common cause of sports-related death in young athletes.[6] The sports most frequently associated with sudden death are basketball, football, and track events. The greatest risk for sudden cardiac death is among patients with congenital or acquired structural cardiac disease, including postoperative congenital heart disease. The most frequent causes of sudden cardiac death in children are acute myocarditis, cardiomyopathy, cyanotic and noncyanotic congenital heart disease, valvular heart disease, congenital complete heart block, Wolff-Parkinson-White syndrome, long QT syndrome (LQTS), Mar-fan syndrome, coronary artery disease, and anomalous coronary arteries.[7] Hypertrophic cardiomyopathy is the most common cause of sudden cardiac death in adolescents without known cardiac disease.[7]

PATHOPHYSIOLOGY

Syncope is the temporary loss of consciousness from reversible disruption of cerebral functioning and usually refers to inadequate cardiac output and cerebral hypoperfusion, resulting in a temporary loss of consciousness.

Vascular syncope occurs when a stimulus causes venous pooling in the legs, leading to a decrease in ventricular preload and a compensatory increase in heart rate and myocardial contractility. After fainting, return of consciousness occurs while lying on the floor, because gravity no longer contributes to venous pooling of blood. Neurally mediated syncope (NMS), or reflex syncope, occurs when receptors in the atria, ventricles, and pulmonary arteries sense a decrease in venous return, and an efferent brainstem response via the vagal nerve causes bradycardia, hypotension, or both. This reflex is also called the *Bezold-Jarisch reflex*. Because the pathophysiology of NMS is related to abnormal circulatory control, this form of syncope is often grouped with other forms of vascular syncope, such as orthostasis and hypovolemia.

Cardiac syncope occurs when there is an interruption of cardiac output from an intrinsic cardiac problem. These causes are divided into tachydysrhythmia, bradydysrhythmia, outflow obstruction, and myocardial dysfunction.

Any event that causes sufficient cerebral hypoperfusion can lead to sudden death. The most common causes are seizures, cardiac diseases, and metabolic diseases. Little is known about the most common dysrhythmias that cause sudden death in children, because such cardiopulmonary arrests often are note witnessed. In children, bradycardic or asystolic arrests are thought to be most common, especially in children younger than 1 year, but ventricular fibrillation is also seen in older children.[8] Overall in children, however, the incidence of ventricular fibrillation as the presenting cardiac dysrhythmia is much lower than that in adults.[8]

CLINICAL FEATURES

Syncope is characterized by a sudden onset of falling with a brief episode of loss of consciousness. Other associated symptoms or signs are usually related to the etiology for the syncopal event. Two-thirds of children experience a prodrome of lightheadedness or dizziness before the event,[3] whereas vertigo is much less common. Involuntary motor movements occur with all types of syncopal events but are more common with seizures.[3] Stokes-Adams syndrome is defined as cardiac syncope associated with very brief tonic or clonic motor activity. This is different from the longer duration tonic and clonic motor movement characteristic of a generalized seizure. Factors related to more serious causes of syncope are outlined in Table 131-1. Events that may mimic syncope in children are listed in Table 131-2.

Sudden cardiac death is usually an unexpected, unwitnessed, terminal event. When resuscitation is rapidly started in patients who have a witnessed arrest, the likelihood of survival is much greater, approaching 25 percent. Witnesses may be able to describe prodromal symptoms to aid in determining the cause of the event.[9]

TABLE 131-1   Risk Factors for a Serious Cause of Syncope

Exertion preceding the event
History of cardiac disease in the patient
Family history of sudden death, deafness, or cardiac disease
Recurrent episodes
Recumbent episode
Prolonged loss of consciousness
Associated chest pain or palpitations
Medications that can alter cardiac conduction

TABLE 131-2 Events Easily Mistaken for Syncope

Condition	Distinguishing Characteristics
Basilar migraine	Headache, rare loss of consciousness, other neurologic symptoms
Seizure	Loss of consciousness simultaneous with motor event, prolonged postictal phase
Vertigo	Rotation or spinning sensation, no loss of consciousness
Hyperventilation	Inciting event, paresthesias or carpopedal spasm, tachypnea
Hysteria	No loss of consciousness, indifference to event
Hypoglycemia	Confusion progressing to loss of consciousness, requires glucose administration to terminate
Breath-holding spell	Crying before event, child 6–18 mo old

Source: Braden DS, Gaymes CH: The diagnosis and management of syncope in children and adolescents. *Pediatr Ann* 26:422, 1997.

DIAGNOSIS

No clinical or historical features reliably distinguish vasovagal syncope from other causes.[3] The patient's history of the event and observations of witnesses present during the event are crucial to identifying the likely causes for the syncopal event. Certain historical features and a careful history and physical examination will increase an emergency physician's suspicion of a potentially serious cause (see Table 131-1). Particular attention should be directed to the cardiovascular examination, including palpation of the cardiac impulse, auscultation of the heart, and evaluation of the peripheral pulses. Orthostatic measurements will identify volume depletion or autonomic dysfunction. The physical examination will often be completely normal. An electrocardiogram (ECG) should be obtained for almost all children and usually will be normal.[3] Children who have an unmistakable episode of vasovagal syncope do not need an ECG. Other laboratory studies are directed by the nature of the history and physical examination but are not routinely helpful in identifying the cause of syncope.

Many of the diseases that cause syncope also cause sudden death in children. A syncopal event can be the presenting symptom of these more serious illnesses. Up to 25 percent of children who die suddenly have a history of at least one prior syncopal event.[5] However, because syncope is a very common event, a syncopal event by itself is not associated with an increased risk of sudden death unless certain features are present (see Table 131-1).[4] The two most common causes of sudden cardiac death among children who do not have known cardiac disease are hypertrophic cardiomyopathy and myocarditis.[5] Primary rhythm disturbances undoubtedly are underrepresented due to the inherent difficulty in identifying these causes after death.

In contrast, among athletes who have died suddenly, only 10 percent had previously experienced at least one episode of syncope.[9] Even with a standard sports screening evaluation, fewer than 5 percent of athletes who subsequently die are suspected of having cardiac disease.[9] The two most common cardiac lesions associated with sudden death among athletes are hypertrophic cardiomyopathy and aberrant coronary arteries.[9] Other coronary artery abnormalities, Marfan syndrome (ruptured aortic aneurysm), valvular heart disease, myocarditis, and dilated cardiomyopathy are less common.

History

The most crucial step in evaluating a child with a syncopal or near death event is a careful medical history. Interview any family members, friends, or witnesses who were with the child just before the event. The events leading up to the incident should be described in detail, as should any apparent change in the child's behavior or symptoms. Pay particular attention to details such as the intake of medications, drugs, fluids, and food. Note the position the child was in when syncope occurred, because recumbent positioning is less consistent with NMS or other forms of vascular syncope. **A history of syncope during exertion or exercise increases the likelihood of the more serious etiologies.** The prodromal symptoms often will aide in identifying the cause of the event. The sequence and timing of motor movements, level of consciousness, and postural positioning will help to differentiate primary seizures from NMS or other true causes of syncope. A history of previous syncopal events should be sought. Any known medical problems should be considered, especially known cardiac diseases, diabetes, seizures, medication or drug use, or psychiatric or psychological problems. Ask about a family history of structural cardiac disease, dysrhythmias, sudden death, migraines, or seizures. Statements by the witnesses that the patient appeared dead and required cardiopulmonary resuscitation must be evaluated carefully. The duration of pulselessness and the degree of intervention required should be carefully recounted by the witnesses. Anytime that cardiopulmonary resuscitation has been performed, even if by an inexperienced lay person, the event should be considered a resuscitated sudden death and evaluated comprehensively.

Physical Examination

Complete cardiovascular, neurologic, and pulmonary examinations are crucial, but the findings are normal in the vast majority of children with syncope, regardless of the seriousness of the etiology. Neurologic examination should include deep tendon reflex, gait, and coordination testing. The cardiovascular examination includes assessment of blood pressure, resting heart rate, oxygen saturation, and respiratory rate. Pulse quality should be assessed in all extremities. Blood pressure and heart rate also should be measured during positional changes (orthostatic vital signs). Auscultation should be performed to identify any murmurs, abnormalities in rhythm, and variations or abnormalities in heart sounds. Any abnormalities in the cardiovascular assessment require an indepth cardiac evaluation.

Laboratory Assessment

An ECG is recommended for nearly every patient, except those with an unmistakable vasovagal episode.[10] Abnormalities on the ECG may not correlate with the syncopal event, and some patients with an arrhythmic cause of syncope will have normal ECGs.[3] Other laboratory tests should be guided by clinical suspicion (e.g., a hemoglobin measurement for a patient with possible anemia or a glucose measurement for a patient with diabetes). Routine laboratory studies are not needed in a child with a clear episode of vasovagal syncope. However, patients with an atypical presentation or worrisome associated symptoms should have a serum chemistry panel, hematocrit, thyroid function tests, chest radiograph, and ECG in the ED. Hyperthyroidism predisposes patients to supraventricular tachycardias (SVTs), so thyroid function tests must be obtained with any child in whom an SVT is considered. In adolescents, a serum alcohol level and urine drug screen should be considered due to the possibility of illicit drug use (most commonly cocaine and amphetamines).

An echocardiogram should be obtained for patients with known or suspected cardiac disease. A patient with abnormal heart sounds, cardiac murmurs, evidence of cardiac chamber enlargement or repolarization abnormalities on ECG, or other features that suggest myocardial dysfunction requires a prompt echocardiogram. If an echocardiogram cannot be obtained in the ED, then an inpatient evaluation must be performed.

The clinical utility of other tests, such as stress tests, tilt-table tests, electrophysiologic studies, and cardiac catheterization, usually is directed by the pediatric cardiologist and is beyond the scope of this chapter.

Patients resuscitated from sudden death must have a complete evaluation unless a clear cause for the arrest is apparent. The diagnostic possibilities are extensive, so laboratory and radiographic studies should be directed by clinical and historical information. All such patients should have a serum chemistry panel, myocardial band enzymes of creatine phosphokinase (CPK-MB), complete blood cell count, serum alcohol level, urine drug screen, thyroid function tests, chest radiograph, and ECG in the ED. Look for complications resulting from the arrest, such as hypothermia, acidosis, rhabdomyolysis, and cerebral edema or hypoxia. The inpatient evaluation can include an echocardiogram, cardiac catheterization, stress test, and electrophysiologic testing as directed by the pediatric cardiologist.

SPECIFIC CONDITIONS

Neurally Mediated Syncope

This category comprises vasovagal syncope, vasodepressor syncope, neurocardiogenic syncope, reflex syncope, and simple faint. Three clinical patterns of NMS occur: vasodepressor syncope (due to vasodilation), cardioinhibitory syncope (due to vagal stimulation), and mixed syncope (due to both). Any disorder that causes vasodilatation, vagal stimulation, or both can result in syncope. Neurally mediated syncope is the most common cause of syncope in children[2] and usually is preceded by a sensation of warmth, nausea, lightheadedness, and a visual grayout or tunneling of vision.[10] This type of syncope frequently lasts less than 1 min.[3] Common precipitating factors include prolonged recumbence just before standing or prolonged standing, sight of blood or disfiguring injury (e.g., fractures or soft tissue injuries), emotional upset, mild physical trauma or pain, physical exertion, and hot or crowded conditions. Other contributing factors that are less common include hypovolemia, anemia, dehydration, and pregnancy. Neurally mediated syncope also can occur with swallowing, urination, defecation, and coughing; breath-holding spells are a variant of this form of syncope. Medications that alter vascular tone or heart rate may contribute to the development of syncope, including β-blockers, calcium-channel blockers, and diuretics. Surreptitious use of diuretics is common among athletes, such as wrestlers, who must maintain weight restrictions.

Identifying NMS as the cause of syncope can be difficult in an ED. Because NMS is related to a wide range of clinical states and physiologically is mediated by inadequate compensatory mechanisms to maintain blood pressure and cardiac output, the distinction between syncope, NMS, and other causes of orthostatic syncope is often blurred. However, NMS and other orthostatic causes of syncope are generally considered to be benign illnesses.

ORTHOSTATIC SYNCOPE Patients typically will complain of lightheadedness and weakness after standing for a period ranging from seconds to minutes. Factors that predispose children to orthostatic syncope include anemia, dehydration, and medications, especially calcium-channel blockers and angiotensin-converting enzyme inhibitors.[2] A drop of greater than 20 mm Hg in blood pressure with an increase in heart rate of more than 20 beats/min while checking vital signs with the child in the supine to standing position is often considered diagnostic of orthostatic hypotension.

SITUATIONAL SYNCOPE Urination, defecation, coughing, and swallowing have been described as causing syncope. The pathophysiology probably is related to an exaggerated Valsalva response causing cardioinhibitory syncope. Stretching, neck extension, external neck pressure, and hair grooming also have been described as causing syncope, presumably due to carotid sinus hypersensitivity or abnormal Valsalva responses.

FAMILIAL DYSAUTONOMIA Abnormalities in heart rate and blood pressure control can be inherited as a primary disorder, such as the Riley-Day syndrome. This disorder results from abnormal development of the sensory and autonomic ganglia, perhaps due to a lack of nerve growth factor during embryogenesis. Manifestations include failure to thrive, developmental delay, temperature instability, abnormal sweating, absent lacrimation, breath-holding spells, and seizures.

Cardiac Dysrhythmias

Outpatient continuous portable ECG monitoring (Holter monitoring) identifies the cause of syncope in only 3 percent of pediatric patients.[3] A cardiac dysrhythmia should be suspected if the syncope is associated with an intense sympathetic stimulus, such as fright, anger, surprise, or physical exertion.[11] The event usually will start and end abruptly, in contrast to nonarrhythmogenic causes such as hypoglycemia or seizures, which are more gradual. Associated symptoms may include palpitations or irregularities of heartbeat.

LONG QT SYNDROME This disorder may be inherited or acquired and is characterized by a prolonged QT interval on the ECG. Although the incidence of inherited LQTS is rare (1 in 5000 births), LQTS is associated with hypertrophic cardiomyopathy and thus accounts for up to half of the cases of sudden cardiac death.[12] Classically, a patient with LQTS should have a corrected QT interval that is longer than 0.44 s on the ECG.[11] Other abnormalities on the ECG associated with LQTS include torsade de pointes, T-wave alternans, notched T waves in three leads, and prominent U waves. Patients with a LQTS may have a normal ECG in the ED.[3] These patients may be diagnosed by a history of LQTS in a family member (familial LQTS), stress testing (exertional LQTS), or Holter monitoring (intermittent LQTS). The history also should include any recent use of medications that can prolong the QT interval (Table 131-3). The 10-year mortality rate can be reduced from 70 to 4 percent by appropriate treatment.[12] Genetic studies to date have identified four genetic loci associated with LQTS, all of which encode proteins involved in sodium and potassium transport. Two congenital syndromes not associated with structural heart disease are also recognized: Romano-Ward syndrome is an autosomal dominant heterozygous condition not associated with deafness, whereas Jervell-Lange-Nielsen syndrome is the homozygous disease associated with deafness.

WOLFF-PARKINSON-WHITE SYNDROME Wolff-Parkinson-White syndrome is characterized by antegrade conduction through an accessory pathway causing a reentrant SVT. Symptoms are manifested when conduction down the accessory pathway occurs at very rapid rates, leading to a reentrant SVT. An ECG may show the characteristic delta wave, but it may be normal. Although Wolff-Parkinson-White syndrome occurs in only 0.1 percent of the general population, it is more common in patients with Ebstein malformation, corrected transposition of the great arteries (levo-TGA), and hypertrophic cardiomyopathy. The risks of sudden death and syncope are greatest in patients who have atrial dysrhythmias such as atrial fibrillation and atrial flutter. Patients at greatest risk for death are those who conduct antegrade over the accessory pathway, allowing 1:1 conduction of an atrial dysrhythmia. Atrial fibrillation and atrial flutter are rare before adolescence.

ATRIOVENTRICULAR BLOCK This condition is most common in children with congenital heart disease but also occurs as a rare congenital disorder. Atrioventricular (AV) block is most common after heart surgery but also occurs with acquired heart disease, such as hypertrophic cardiomyopathy and myocarditis, and muscular dystrophy. Acquired AV block occurs in 87 percent of children with carditis associated with Lyme disease.[13] Congenital AV block was first described

TABLE 131-3 Medications That Prolong the QT Interval

Macrolide antibiotics
    Erythromycin (many trade names)
    Clarithromycin (Biaxin)
    Azithromycin (Zithromax)
Tricyclic antidepressants
    Imipramine (Tofranil)
    Amitriptyline (Elavil)
    Amoxapine (Asendin)
    Desipramine (Norpramin)
    Nortriptyline (Pamelor)
    Others
Phenothiazines
    Thioridazine (Mellaril)
    Pimozide (Orap)
Antifungals
    Fluconazole (Diflucan)
    Ketoconazole (Nizoral)
Gastrointestinal prokinetics
    Cisapride (Propulsid)
Antihistamines
    Astemizole (Hismanal)
    Terfenadine (Seldane)
    Diphenhydramine (Benadryl)
Epinephrine
    Local anesthetics used by dentist or physician
Trimethoprim
    Trimethoprim-sulfamethoxazole (Bactrim)
Antiarrhythmics
    Class IA
        Quinidine (many trade names)
        Procainamide (Pronestyl)
        Disopyramide (Norpace)
    Class IC
        Ecainide (Enkaid)
        Flecainide (Tambocor)
Anti-nausea
    Dolasetron (Anzemet)
Appetite Suppressant
    Phentermine (Adipex, Fastin)
Quinolone Antibiotics
    Moxifloxacin (Avelox)

by Morquio in 1901, and although the risk of death is highest in infants, asymptomatic children may also die in adolescence.[14] Congenital AV block is also associated with mothers who have connective tissue disease. Syncope from a high-degree AV block not related to positional changes or exertion is called a *Stokes-Adams attack.* Prophylactic pacemaker insertion is routinely performed in children with acquired or congenital AV block.

SICK SINUS SYNDROME Sick sinus syndrome is also known as *tachycardia-bradycardia syndrome.* Isolated sinus node dysfunction rarely causes syncope; a syncopal event is more likely to be due to a reentrant atrial tachycardia. Most commonly, these dysrhythmias are associated with prior heart surgery, especially the Mustard or Senning operation for transposition of the great vessels and the Fontan operation. Syncope and sudden death can occur after pacemaker placement, because the pacemaker will prevent bradycardia but not tachycardia.

SUPRAVENTRICULAR TACHYCARDIA Any cause of SVT can lead to syncope while recumbent if the heart rate is high enough to inhibit cardiac filling or if coincident vasomotor abnormalities occur.[15] Wolff-Parkinson-White syndrome and atrial fibrillation are the most common causes, but primary SVT can also occur. Episodes of SVT are associated with congenital heart disease, including Ebstein anomaly and levo-TGA.

PACEMAKER MALFUNCTION Although pacemakers are not common in childhood, any child with a pacemaker who has syncope or presyncope should be presumed to have a pacemaker malfunction. Syncope can be caused in several ways: lack of pacemaker output (low battery, broken lead, or malfunction), noncapture of myocardium (exit block or lead fracture), retrograde AV conduction (reflex vasodilatation from enhanced jugular venous pulsations with a ventricular pacemaker), and pacemaker-mediated tachycardia (sensed atrial tachycardia or retrograde P waves with an atrial sensing pacemaker).

Structural Cardiac Disease

HYPERTROPHIC CARDIOMYOPATHY Also known as *idiopathic hypertrophic subaortic stenosis,* this disease is a dynamic and a fixed subvalvular obstruction. Exertional syncope is a common presentation, but infants may present with congestive heart failure and cyanosis. Any child with exertional related syncope must have this diagnosis considered. Onset of symptoms in early childhood is associated with a greater risk of mortality; the 10-year mortality rate is 50 percent for children diagnosed before 14 years of age.[16] Syncopal events appear to be related to myocardial ischemia and/or ventricular tachycardia, probably as an LQTS. An echocardiogram is necessary to exclude or confirm this diagnosis and should be done in the ED or on the inpatient ward. Most investigators recommend implantable cardiac defibrillators in children with hypertrophic cardiomyopathy.

DILATED CARDIOMYOPATHY This disorder is unusual in children but can occur by three general mechanisms: idiopathic, with congenital heart disease, or after myocarditis. Syncope and death are thought to be caused by ventricular dysrhythmias or severe myocardial dysfunction.

ARRHYTHMOGENIC RIGHT VENTRICULAR DYSPLASIA This disorder is rare in the United States but is a common cause of adolescent death in Italy. Presentation is more common in older adolescents or adults. Patients usually present with congestive heart failure, cardiomegaly, and syncope or sudden death from an dysrhythmia. Electrocardiographic abnormalities include left bundle branch block and T-wave inversion, but some patients may have a normal ECG. Even the echocardiogram, cardiac catheterization, and myocardial biopsy can be nondiagnostic.

CONGENITAL CYANOTIC AND NONCYANOTIC HEART DISEASE Hypercyanotic spells may progress to syncope in tetralogy of Fallot, tricuspid atresia, TGA, and Eisenmenger syndrome. Children with structural heart disease are also prone to ventricular dysrhythmias and AV block.

VALVULAR DISEASES Several valvular lesions are associated with syncope and sudden death. In general, the degree of valve dysfunction correlates with the risk of sudden death. *Aortic stenosis* is usually due to a congenital defect, often associated with a bicuspid valve, although unicommissural or severely dysplastic valves also occur. Other associated cardiac anomalies, in particular coarctation of the aorta, also occur. Most patients are identified by the presence of a murmur. Exertional syncope is due to reduced cerebral blood flow and is commonly associated with chest pain, dyspnea on exertion, and poor exercise tolerance. *Mitral valve prolapse* (MVP) itself is probably not associated with an increased risk of sudden death.[17] A child with MVP and syncope requires a more intensive diagnostic workup. Adults with MVP and significant mitral regurgitation have more frequent dysrhythmias, but this has not been shown in children. *Ebstein malformation of the tricuspid valve* is an uncommon disorder. Sudden death is thought to be due to the development of supraventricular or ventricular dysrhythmias.

PULMONARY HYPERTENSION Primary pulmonary hypertension (without structural heart disease) is uncommon but can present in adolescence. It is often associated with dyspnea on exertion, shortness of breath, exercise intolerance, and syncope. Eisenmenger syndrome is acquired pulmonary hypertension due to a cardiac shunt. High blood flow to the pulmonary circulation from a left-to-right shunt leads to a reactive increase in pulmonary resistance. After months to years, the development of pulmonary hypertension causes the shunt to reverse to a right-to-left shunt, and cyanosis becomes apparent. One-half of patients with pulmonary hypertension develops syncope. Physical findings include an increased ventricular impulse, a loud second heart sound, and cyanosis, which is particularly prominent in patients with Eisenmenger syndrome. Syncope and sudden death in these patients usually are related to a dysrhythmia.

CORONARY ARTERY ABNORMALITIES Many of these patients present with sudden death during exercise or have a history of exercise-induced syncope. Abnormalities of coronary artery origin include the left main artery arising from the right sinus of Valsalva or, less frequently, the right artery arising from the left sinus. In both cases, the aberrant artery often passes between the aorta and the pulmonary artery, thus placing it at risk for extrinsic compression, especially during physical exertion. Other abnormalities include myocardial overbridging, coronary artery fistulae, coronary artery spasm, coronary ostial stenosis, coronary artery aneurysms, and stenosis from Kawasaki disease.

Noncardiovascular Causes

SEIZURES Although not truly syncope, a seizure may appear to be a syncopal event even to the medical professional. Seizures often have little or no prodrome and are associated with a loss of consciousness. Seizures usually have a prolonged recovery phase (postictal phase), which most syncopal events lack. Other findings commonly associated with a seizure include onset while supine, convulsions immediately with loss of consciousness, and a warm, flushed, or cyanotic skin color. Many patients who are diagnosed with a syncopal event in the ED are later found to have a seizure disorder.[2] Adding to the confusion, up to 71 percent of syncopal events may have associated behavior that could be called a seizure. Unfortunately, electroencephalographic monitoring is frequently normal even in patients who have experienced a seizure.

BREATH HOLDING Breath-holding spells are probably related to NMS. Typically, the children are 6 to 18 months old and have an intense emotional trigger that causes crying and then a breath hold during expiration.[18] The children then become cyanotic or pale and lose consciousness from the progressive cerebral hypoperfusion. Myoclonic activity or seizure activity may occur. The episode is usually short, requires no specific intervention, and rapidly resolves with gasping respirations and progressive loss of cyanosis or pallor. Up to 20 percent of children with breath-holding spells develop NMS in later life.[18]

ATYPICAL MIGRAINE Basilar artery migraines may be associated with syncope due to poor cerebral circulation during vasospasm. Most patients with this disorder also will have headache, a family history of migraines, symptoms referable to the posterior cerebral circulation (visual changes, dysarthria, tinnitus, vertigo, or ataxia), and a normal heart rate and blood pressure during the event.

HYPERVENTILATION Severe hypocapnia can cause syncope by intense cerebral vasospasm that leads to cerebral hypoperfusion. Typically, there is also a history of dyspnea, chest tightness, lightheadedness, tunnel vision, carpopedal spasm, or paresthesias.

HYSTERIA Hysterical syncope is an event that occurs without neurologic or cardiovascular changes but otherwise has the visual appearance of syncope. Often these events occur in front of an audience, are independent of posture, and rarely result in injury. Patients frequently will fall gracefully and without injury to the floor. The patient may even describe the event, often in an indifferent or unconcerned manner, clearly indicating that consciousness was not lost.

HYPOGLYCEMIA Syncope due to hypoglycemia is more commonly of a gradual onset and is associated with diaphoresis, tachycardia, hunger, and generalized weakness. Unconsciousness resolves with glucose administration but does not usually resolve with recumbency. A history of disorders of glucose production (enzyme or storage deficiencies) or glucose use (diabetes) is usually present.

TREATMENT

Syncope

Most children with syncope will be fully recovered by the time they arrive at the ED.[2,3] Continued altered level of consciousness should prompt an evaluation for causes other than syncope. Treatment should be tailored to current symptoms. Signs of compromised oxygenation, ventilation, or circulation should be addressed immediately. A cardiac monitor should be applied to the patient while gathering the history and physical findings to document any transient dysrhythmias. Vascular access and blood for laboratory studies should be obtained for all children except those in whom a simple vasovagal event explains the symptoms.

Treatment is targeted to specific identified etiologies for the syncopal event. Ongoing cardiac dysrhythmias or seizures should be managed as appropriate. Most patients, however, will have no treatable dysrhythmias in the ED.

Sudden Death

A child who survives an out-of-hospital cardiac arrest must be rapidly stabilized, and any identified conditions must be quickly treated. In general, the principles of pediatric advanced life support are followed (see Chap. 14). Unstable ventricular or supraventricular rhythms should be treated immediately with a cardioverter using direct-current countershocks in a synchronized or unsynchronized fashion. Wide QRS-complex tachydysrhythmias should not be treated with class 1A agents such as procainamide and quinidine if LQTS is suspected, because these medications act by also prolonging the QT interval. Class IB drugs, such as phenytoin or amiodarone, should be used instead.

Treatment in the ED is directed at identifying the probable cause for the arrest so that future events can be prevented. The possible etiologies are extensive, so laboratory and radiographic studies are directed by clinical and historical information. All patients should have a serum chemistry panel, complete blood cell count, serum alcohol level, urine drug screen, thyroid function tests, chest radiograph, and ECG in the ED. The inpatient evaluation can include an echocardiogram, cardiac catheterization, stress test, and electrophysiologic testing.

DISPOSITION

Syncope

A child who had a syncopal event can present a challenging disposition decision. When the cause of syncope is not readily apparent from the ED evaluation, multiple additional tests are frequently performed but rarely provide further diagnostic information.[19] Unfortunately, few studies have examined the most effective evaluation in the ED and the hospital.

Obviously, any child with a dysrhythmia documented by prehospital providers or on the ECG in the ED must be admitted. Children who have any of the risk factors listed in Table 131-1 also should be admitted in consultation with a pediatric cardiologist. Patients with a normal ECG but a history suspicious for dysrhythmia are candidates for outpatient ambulatory cardiac monitoring. Identified causes of syncope should be treated as appropriate in the ED, and admission to the hospital should be directed by the need for further evaluation or therapy. All children admitted for a syncope evaluation should be placed on a cardiorespiratory monitor in the hospital.

If, after appropriately thorough history, physical, and laboratory evaluations, a clear precipitating cause for the syncope cannot be identified in the ED, the child may be discharged to home with close follow-up by the child's primary physician or a cardiologist. Because NMS accounts for up to 50 percent of the cases of syncope in children, most pediatric patients without cardiac risk factors or exercise-induced symptoms may be safely evaluated as outpatients.[19] Many of these children will have additional tests as outpatients, including portable rhythm monitoring, tilt-table testing, and stress testing, although the cost effectiveness of this approach remains in doubt.[19]

Sudden Death

After stabilization, children who have suffered a sudden cardiac arrest should be transferred to a pediatric intensive care unit that is capable of managing cardiac disorders. These children must be transferred with a crew capable of treating cardiac arrest from any dysrhythmia. In general, this should be done with a dedicated pediatric critical care transport team and consultation with the receiving pediatric intensivist.

REFERENCES

1. Manolis AS: Evaluation of patients with syncope: Focus of age-related differences. *Am Coll Cardiol Curr J Rev* 3:13, 1994.
2. Pratt JL, Fleisher GR: Syncope in children and adolescents. *Pediatr Emerg Care* 5:80, 1989.
3. McHarg ML, Shinnar S, Rascoff H, Walsh CA: Syncope in childhood. *Pediatr Cardiol* 18:36, 1997.
4. Driscoll DJ, Jacobsen SJ, Porter CJ, Wollan PC: Syncope in children and adolescents. *J Am Coll Cardiol* 29:1039, 1997.
5. Driscoll DJ, Edwards WD: Sudden unexpected death in children and adolescents. *J Am Coll Cardiol* 5:118B, 1985.
6. Maron BJ, Epstein SE, Roberts WC: Causes of sudden death in competitive athletes. *J Am Coll Cardiol* 7:204, 1986.
7. Klitzner TS: Sudden cardiac death in children. *Circulation* 82:629, 1990.
8. Walsh CK, Krongrad E: Terminal cardiac electrical activity in pediatric patients. *Am J Cardiol* 51:557, 1983.
9. Maron BJ, Shirani J, Poliac LC, et al: Sudden death in young competitive athletes. *JAMA* 276:199, 1996.
10. Gutgesell HP, Barst RJ, Humes RA, et al: Common cardiovascular problems in the young: Part I. *Am Fam Phys* 56:1825, 1997.
11. Moss A, Schwartz PJ, Crampton RS, et al: The long QT syndrome: Prospective longitudinal study of 328 families. *Circulation* 84:1136, 1991.
12. Jancin B: Long QT syndrome tracked to a genetic cause. *Pediatr News* 30:8, 1996.
13. McAlister HG, Klementowicz PR, Andrews C, et al: Lyme carditis: An important cause of reversible heart block. *Ann Intern Med* 110:339, 1989.
14. Michaelson M, Jonzon A, Riesenfeld T: Isolated congenital complete atrioventricular block in adult life. *Circulation* 92:442, 1995.
15. Leitch J, Klein G, Yee R, et al: Syncope associated with supraventricular tachycardia. *Circulation* 85:1064, 1992.
16. McKenna WJ, Franklin RCG, Nikoyannopoulos P, et al: Arrhythmia and prognosis in infants, children, and adolescents with hypertrophic cardiomyopathy. *J Am Coll Cardiol* 11:146, 1988.
17. Bisset GS, Schwartz DC, Meyer RA, et al: Clinical spectrum and long-term follow-up of isolated mitral valve prolapse in 119 children. *Circulation* 62:423, 1980.
18. Lombroso CT, Lerman P: Breath holding spells. *Pediatrics* 39:563, 1967.
19. Gordon TA, Moodie DS, Passalacqua M, et al: A retrospective analysis of the cost-effective workup of syncope in children. *Cleveland Clin Q* 54:391, 1987.

132 FLUID AND ELECTROLYTE THERAPY
William Ahrens

INTRODUCTION

Fluid and electrolyte abnormalities are among the most common problems confronting physicians who care for children. This is primarily due to the high incidence of gastroenteritis in the pediatric population, and the vulnerability of children to the loss of water and solutes. In poor countries, diarrheal diseases are common causes of infant death. In the United States, they often result in prolonged ED stays and hospitalization. Electrolyte abnormalities are most commonly secondary to fluid imbalances.

FLUID REQUIREMENTS

The key to managing fluids in infants and children is the realization that there are vast differences in the maintenance requirement of water in the first 2 years versus the rest of life. This reflects a direct correlation between caloric expenditure, reflected by the basal metabolic rate, and the requirement for free water. Rapidly growing infants have an extremely high basal metabolic rate and require an enormous number of calories relative to their body weight. They therefore require a correspondingly enormous amount of water. The daily turnover of free water in infants is up to 3 to 4 times that of adults. This includes increased insensible losses from the skin and respiratory tract, which are usually electrolyte free. Urine accounts for approximately 50 percent of daily fluid requirements and is the predominant cause of sensible losses; because infants have a decreased ability to concentrate urine, they lose a relatively large amount of free water through their kidneys in order to excrete solutes. In addition, a larger percentage of young infants' total body water is contained in the extravascular space in comparison with older children and adults. This puts them at greater risk for cardiovascular compromise when confronted with sudden fluid losses.[1,2]

Caloric expenditure and therefore fluid requirements can be estimated from body surface area, which is huge in infants in comparison to adults. However, in the ED, weight is a sufficiently accurate and more easily obtained method of calculating fluid requirements. The fundamental formula is:

For the first 10 kg: 100 mL/kg per d
For the second 10 kg: 50 mL/kg per d
For more than 20 kg: 20 mL/kg per d

For example,

1. A 10-kg baby requires 100 mL × 10 kg, or a total of 1000 mL per d.
2. A 20-kg baby requires 100 mL × 10 kg = 1000 mL + (50 mL × 10 kg) = 500 mL, for a total of 1500 mL per d.
3. A 40-kg baby requires 100 mL × 10 kg = 1000 mL + (50 mL × 10 kg) = 500 mL + (20 mL × 20 kg) = 400 mL, for a total of 1900 mL per d.

Hypermetabolic states increase the need for free water. The most common of these are fever (which increases the free water requirement by approximately 12 percent per degree of elevation in temperature centigrade above normal), and increased sweating.

Electrolyte requirements remain constant throughout childhood and can be estimated by body weight. All infant formulas contain sufficient electrolytes to satisfy these, as do Ricelyte and Pedialyte. The requirement for sodium is 2 to 3 mEq/kg per d and for potassium is 2 mEq/kg per d (Table 132-1).[1,2]

ISOTONIC DEHYDRATION

Isotonic dehydration occurs when there is a proportionately equal loss of sodium and water; the serum sodium thus remains within the normal

TABLE 132-1   Maintenance Requirements for Fluid and Electrolytes, Based on Body Weight

Body weight	0–10 kg	10–20 kg	>20 kg
Total water volume	100 mL/kg	1000 mL + 50 mL/kg for each kg >10 kg	1500 mL + 20 mL/kg for each kg >20 kg
Sodium	3 mEq/kg	3 mEq/kg	3 mEq/kg
Potassium	2 mEq/kg	2 mEq/kg	2 mEq/kg
Chloride	5 mEq/kg	5 mEq/kg	5 mEq/kg

range of 130 to 145 mEq/L. It most often results from diarrheal illness and is the most common fluid and electrolyte problem encountered in pediatrics. Fluid is initially lost from the extracellular space. Intracellular fluid then shifts into the vascular tree, which protects circulating blood volume at the expense of intracellular dehydration.

The clinical manifestations of isotonic dehydration depend on the absolute volume deficit, the rate at which fluid is lost, and the age of the patient. When fluid is lost over a relatively long period, a large deficit may be well tolerated and clinical manifestations can be rather subtle, even though up to 40 percent of intracellular fluid may be lost. This most commonly occurs in patients with protracted diarrheal illnesses. In contrast, sudden massive loss of fluid such as occurs in cholera-associated or rotavirus diarrhea can be fatal if not treated aggressively, because most of the volume is lost from the extracellular space and there is insufficient time for intracellular fluid to shift into the vascular tree. This is especially true in young infants, because a relatively large percentage of their total body water is contained in the extracellular space. Rapid fluid loss can result in cardiovascular collapse, whereas older children will remain well compensated.

EVALUATION

The most accurate way to estimate the degree of dehydration is calculating weight loss, which in acute situations amounts to free water deficit. However, this information is rarely available. In practice, estimating the degree of dehydration depends on integrating multiple factors. Patients usually have a history of vomiting and diarrhea. It is useful to quantitate the approximate number of stools and to determine whether the patient is able to tolerate any oral feedings without vomiting. Parents are asked what liquids the child has been given, since excess free water can cause hyponatremia, and homemade remedies may contain excess sodium. A history of decreased urine output implies significant fluid loss, but may be difficult to quantitate when associated with significant diarrhea.

Physical examination has been demonstrated to provide a reliable estimation of the degree of dehydration[2] (Table 132-2). Hypotension

indicates hypovolemic shock. The patient's mental status is important: normal mental status usually implies mild dehydration, whereas irritability signifies at least moderate fluid loss. Lethargy implies severe volume loss and/or an electrolyte abnormality, especially hypernatremia. Decreased skin turgor and sunken eyes and fontanel imply moderate to severe fluid loss and usually occur when intracellular fluid has had time to diffuse into the intravascular space. In these patients, vital signs may be only slightly abnormal and not indicative of the degree of dehydration.

It is important to realize that assessing the degree of dehydration in very young infants is notoriously difficult, and fluid losses are often underestimated.[1–3]

LABORATORY FINDINGS

In isotonic dehydration, the sodium level is within the normal range. The potassium level is usually normal or slightly decreased. The serum bicarbonate level is often decreased: in mild dehydration it is usually in the range of 15 to 20 mEq/L, whereas in more severe cases it falls below 10 mEq/L. A low serum bicarbonate level reflects stool losses, the presence of ketones from "starvation," and in severe dehydration, lactic acidosis. The blood urea nitrogen level usually rises with increasingly severe fluid losses. Urine specific gravity also rises in significant dehydration and may reach 1.030. In young infants, a decreased ability to concentrate urine may result in a falsely low specific gravity. In infants and children with mild to moderate dehydration, it is usually unnecessary to evaluate serum electrolytes. In neonates and young infants it is prudent to evaluate serum electrolytes if there is a history of significant fluid losses.[4]

MANAGEMENT

The management of dehydrated children depends on the degree of fluid loss, as well as a patient's ability to tolerate oral liquids (Table 132-3). Mildly dehydrated patients (<5 percent) who tolerate oral fluids can usually be discharged home on clear liquids with close follow-

TABLE 132-2   Estimation of Dehydration

Extent of Dehydration	Mild	Moderate	Severe
Weight loss†			
Infants	5%	10%	15%
Adolescents	3%	4–6%	7–9%
Pulse	Normal	Slightly increased	Very increased
Blood pressure	Normal	Normal to orthostatic, >10 mm Hg change	Orthostatic to shock
Behavior	Normal	Irritable, more thirsty	Hyperirritable to lethargic
Thirst	Slight	Moderate	Intense
Mucous membranes*	Normal	Dry	Parched
Tears	Present	Decreased	Absent, sunken eyes
Anterior fontanelle	Normal	Normal to sunken	Sunken
External jugular vein	Visible when supine	Not visible except with supraclavicular pressure	Not visible even with supraclavicular pressure
Skin* (less useful in children >2 years of age)	Capillary refill <2 s	Slowed capillary refill, 2–4 s (decreased turgor)	Very delayed capillary refill (>4 s) and tenting; skin cool, acrocyanotic, or mottled*
Urine specific gravity	>1.020	>1.020; oliguria	Oliguria or anuria

*These signs are less prominent in patients who have hypernatremia.
†A 3-month-old has about 70% total body water; a 15-year-old has about 60%.

TABLE 132-3 Dehydration in Children

Dehydration that occurs gradually is much better tolerated in infants and children than a sudden large loss of fluid.

Mental status is an important indicator of hydration status.

In mild or moderate dehydration electrolytes are almost always normal.

In moderately dehydrated infants and children it is safe to predicate therapy by calculating a deficit of 10%.

In patients in whom intravenous access is difficult, it is reasonable to attempt hydration using a nasogastric tube.

up. A "next-day hydration check" is especially desirable in infants less than 4 to 5 months of age. Moderately dehydrated patients generally require intravenous therapy, although oral rehydration is an option. Severely dehydrated patients require aggressive resuscitation. Boluses of 20 mL/kg of NS or LR solution are given until improved mental status, vital signs, and peripheral perfusion indicate stable intravascular volume. In patients in shock this may require 60 to 80 mL/kg. Isotonic crystalloid is utilized because it will stay in the intravascular space. Fluid replacement then consists of replacing 50 percent of the estimated volume deficit in the first 8 h, and the remainder of the deficit in the next 16 h. It is important to remember that maintenance fluids must be added to the deficit replacement; failure to do so will result in inadequate replenishment of volume. Some patients may require additional fluids to replace ongoing losses, such as can occur with profound diarrhea. For practical purposes, it is safe to assume a 10 percent deficit in healthy infants and children who appear dehydrated.

For example, a 12-kg infant is estimated to be 10 percent dehydrated. After a 20-mL/kg bolus of NS, she is alert and perfusion is adequate. Fluid orders can then consist of:

1. Maintenance is 100 mL/kg × 10 kg/24 h = 1000 mL + (50 mL/kg × 2 kg/24 h) = 100 mL, for a total of 1100 mL/24 h or 46 mL per h.
2. Deficit = 10 percent of body weight (1.2 kg) = 1200 mL; replace 600 mL over the first 8 h or 75 mL per h; replace 600 mL over the next 16 h or 38 mL per h.

Thus, for the first 8 h, maintenance + deficit = 121 mL per h; for the next 16 h, maintenance + deficit = 84 mL per h.

Appropriate rehydrating solutions in infants are D5 .25NS or D5 .45NS. In infants, D5 .20NS is utilized for maintenance rehydration in isotonic dehydration. In children, D5 .45NS can be used for maintenance rehydration in isotonic dehydration. Glucose is added to the solution to minimize further catabolism. After the patient has urinated, potassium can be added at a maximum concentration of 40 mEq/L. Most patients will begin to tolerate oral feeding with clear liquids within 24 h. All severely dehydrated patients are admitted to the hospital.

Patients who are moderately dehydrated can be managed in a number of ways. Some patients can be aggressively rehydrated with NS over a period of 2 to 4 h in the ED and safely discharged. Resuscitation consists of 40 to 50 mL/kg. Rapid nasogastric rehydration in lieu of intravenous therapy has also been shown to be a viable option in dehydrated infants. This may be preferable to both clinicians and parents when confronted with an infant or child in whom intravenous access is difficult to obtain. It may also be considered in more severely dehydrated infants in whom intravenous access is difficult, but in whom an intraosseous line seems inappropriately invasive. A more detailed discussion of oral rehydration follows below.

The success of rapid rehydration may be correlated with an initial serum bicarbonate level of greater than 13 mEq/L, but further study is needed to clarify this. Extreme caution should be exercised in using rapid rehydration in neonates and young infants, since the underlying gastroenteritis is likely to continue and these patients are at relatively high risk of cardiovascular compromise. If they are discharged, follow-up must be expedient and absolutely certain. Patients with persistent profuse diarrhea and those with intractable vomiting are candidates for

admission. Fluid management is then the same as for severely dehydrated patients, with 50 percent of the deficit replaced in the first 8 h and the remaining 50 percent replaced over the next 16 h. Oral rehydration is also an option and is discussed further below.[5–8]

HYPERNATREMIC DEHYDRATION

Hypernatremia is defined as a serum sodium greater than 150 mEq/L. Hypernatremic dehydration occurs when there is a relatively greater loss of free water than sodium. It often occurs when patients with gastroenteritis are treated with salt-rich solutions. The predominant clinical problems related to hypernatremic dehydration result from the increase in serum osmolarity. As sodium rises and osmolarity increases, fluid is drawn from the interstitial and intracellular spaces into the vascular tree. This protects circulating blood volume and peripheral perfusion and can result in deceptively normal vital signs, despite severe dehydration. Loss of intracellular fluid causes doughy, tenting skin. Faced with osmotic disequilibrium, brain cells create charged molecules in an effort to preserve intracellular volume and electrical neutrality. Despite this, mental status changes are common, including irritability, lethargy, and seizures.

The most essential aspect of managing hypernatremic dehydration involves replacing lost free water in such a way that the serum sodium falls no more than 10 to 15 mEq/L per d. A more rapid decrease in serum osmolarity can result in the influx of water into brain cells, resulting in cerebral edema. In patients in whom perfusion is inadequate, a 10- to 20-mL/kg bolus of NS is administered. The management of hypernatremic dehydration is predominantly based on clinical experience, and there is no universal agreement on the optimal subsequent hydrating solution to be used, but D5 .45NS will be adequate in the majority of cases and is probably less risky than the more hypotonic D5 .25NS. It is most important that rehydration be spread out over 48 to 72 h, rather than the 24 h used for isotonic dehydration. Frequent monitoring of serum sodium during the resuscitation is necessary. In cases of severe hypernatremia (Na^+ >165 mEq/L), it is reasonable to consult a pediatric intensivist or nephrologist after the patient is stabilized. Even with optimal management, patients with severe hypernatremia are at risk for neurologic sequelae. The essence of resuscitation of hypernatremic dehydration is a slow correction of serum sodium in order to minimize the possibility of sudden changes in brain cell osmolarity.

DIABETES INSIPIDUS

Diabetes insipidus, which is most commonly caused by a deficiency of the antidiuretic hormone (ADH) arginine vasopressin, usually occurs secondary to damage to the neurohypophysial unit and commonly occurs after severe head trauma, central nervous system infections, and suprasellar tumors, especially craniopharyngiomas. An extremely rare form of diabetes insipidus is characterized by a failure of the renal tubules to respond to vasopressin and is referred to as *nephrogenic;* it is a congenital disorder.

Clinically, diabetes insipidus is characterized by polyuria that can be massive. Most patients also manifest polydipsia. The excessive loss of free water can result in hypernatremia. The patient's urine is usually extremely dilute, with a specific gravity of less than 1.005 and an osmolality of 50 to 200 mOsm/L. Diagnosis can be made by water deprivation testing or by serum assay of vasopressin.

Diabetes insipidus is treated with desmopressin (DDAVP), an analogue of vasopressin. The dose is individualized, and consultation with a pediatric endocrinologist is advisable.[1]

HYPONATREMIC DEHYDRATION

Hyponatremia is defined as a serum sodium level of less than 130 mEq/L. There are many causes of hyponatremia, which are usually categorized on the basis of whether total body water is increased, decreased, or normal. Hyponatremic dehydration most commonly occurs when a parent replaces acute fluid losses from vomiting and diarrhea with water. Much less common causes of hyponatremic dehydration include adrenal insufficiency states, third-space losses from ascites or pancreatitis, and diuretic use.

In severe cases of hyponatremic dehydration, shock can result. However, the most common clinical manifestations of symptomatic hyponatremia involve the central nervous system. Although a gradual reduction in serum sodium is usually well tolerated, a sudden decrease can result in irritability, lethargy, and seizures. Seizures are most common with a serum sodium level of less than 120 mEq/L, but are more dependent on the rate of fall than the absolute value of serum sodium. Hyponatremia should be considered in infants who have a first-time seizure not associated with a fever, especially if there is a history of vomiting and diarrhea.

The management of hyponatremic dehydration associated with cardiovascular instability consists of the infusion of NS in 20-mL/kg boluses until the patient is stable. Many patients with gastroenteritis who suffer hyponatremic-induced convulsions will stop seizing following the administration of a bolus of NS alone. Subsequent management is aimed at restoring both the volume and sodium deficits. The standard formula used in correcting serum sodium is:

$$(\text{Na desired} - \text{Na measured}) \times 0.6 \times \text{kg body weight}$$

in which 0.6 reflects the fractional distribution of sodium. To prevent overcorrection, the desired sodium level is usually 125 mEq/L, which corrects osmolarity sufficiently to prevent further seizures. In stable patients with acute hyponatremia, volume resuscitation and sodium correction can be carried out over 24 h, as there is no physiologic advantage to raising the serum sodium rapidly. In patients with profound hyponatremia or persistent seizures, it may be necessary to infuse 3% saline at a dose up to 12 mEq/kg; in clinical practice this is rarely necessary. In patients with chronic severe hyponatremia, rapid correction of serum sodium has resulted in central pontine demyelinization.[9]

HYPONATREMIA WITH INCREASED TOTAL BODY WATER

Causes of hyponatremia associated with increased total body water include acute water intoxication, the syndrome of inappropriate secretion of antidiuretic hormone (SIADH), edema-forming states including nephrotic syndrome, cirrhosis, and congestive heart failure.

Acute water intoxication can result in a profound rapid decrease in serum sodium. It is often psychogenic, but can occur in young infants who are accidentally given large amounts of free water. If seizures occur, treatment with 3% saline may be necessary. In most cases, fluid restriction suffices to lower serum sodium.

In SIADH, antidiuretic hormone (ADH) is secreted without an appropriate physiologic reason, and this stimulates the resorption of free water, causing a dilutional hyponatremia. SIADH occurs in a variety of disease states, including meningitis and following head trauma. In the ED a frequent cause of SIADH is meningitis. The most important laboratory finding in SIADH is a urine osmolarity greater than serum osmolarity. Hypouricemia is also usually present. The fundamental treatment is fluid restriction.

In nephrosis and cirrhosis, hyponatremia is usually mild and chronic. Even though total body water is increased, intravascular volume may be low due to third-spacing. Treatment usually consists of diuresis, with a combination of albumin followed by a diuretic. These patients are best managed in consultation with a pediatric nephrologist.

ORAL REHYDRATION

It has been repeatedly demonstrated that oral rehydration is as effective as intravenous therapy in treating infants with mild to moderate dehydration. It has had an enormous impact in developing countries, where prepackaged electrolyte solutions are available in lieu of infinitely more expensive intravenous solutions. Although time constraints may limit oral therapy in EDs in the United States, emergency physicians who do work in international medicine must be familiar with its use.

Water and electrolyte solutions created for treating dehydrated patients differ from maintenance solutes, primarily in their composition of electrolytes. Rehydration solutions contain 60 to 90 mEq/L sodium and 2 to 2.5 percent glucose, compared with maintenance solutions, which contain approximately 45 to 50 mEq/L sodium (Table 132-4). The higher sodium content is thought to facilitate the absorption of water in the small intestine. Some controversy exists regarding the propensity of the World Health Organization's rehydrating formula, containing 90 mEq/L sodium, to cause hypernatremia. In dehydrated patients, this appears to be rare, but reformulated oral rehydrating solutions containing 50 to 60 mEq/L sodium are preferred by some. Studies continue to investigate the optimum sodium content of oral rehydration solutions, as well as the optimum composition of sugars. Current evidence indicates that reduced osmolarity formulas limit the duration of diarrhea. In practice, maintenance solutions can be effectively used if rehydrating solutions are unavailable.

Fluid replacement is accomplished by administering 50 mL/kg over 4 h to mildly dehydrated patients and 100 mL/kg to patients with moderate dehydration. Vomiting can be reduced by administering the fluid slowly. This can be done by using a teaspoon or eyedropper. Ongoing losses from continuing diarrhea are also replaced. Once adequate hydration is reestablished, supplemental feeding should be encouraged. This is especially important in malnourished infants.

Severe dehydration, persistent vomiting, continuing severe diarrhea, or significant hypernatremia may preclude the use of oral rehydration when intravenous therapy is available. However, if necessary, the vast majority of these patients can be salvaged by persistent administration of small quantities of oral fluids.[10,11]

TABLE 132-4 Composition of Commercial Oral Hydration Solutions

	Na⁺ (mEq/L)	K⁺ (mEq/L)	Cl⁻ (mEq/L)	Base (mEq/L)	Carbohydrate (% Weight for Volume)
Maintenance solutions					
Resol (Wyeth)*	50	20	50	Citrate, 34	2% Glucose
Ricelyte (Mead Johnson)	50	25	45	Citrate, 34	3% Rice syrup solids
Pedialyte (Ross)	45	20	35	Citrate, 30	2.5% Glucose
Rehydrate solutions					
Rehydralite (Ross)	75	20	65	Citrate, 30	2.5% Glucose
World Health Organization formulation (for use in cholera)	90	20	80	HOC_3^-, 30	2% Glucose

*Includes calcium, 4 mEq/L; magnesium, 4 mEq/L; phosphate, 5 mEq/L.

SPECIFIC SITUATIONS

Pyloric Stenosis

The protracted vomiting that characterizes pyloric stenosis can result in significant losses of hydrogen ion, chloride, potassium, and occasionally, sodium. This leads to the characteristic hypochloremic metabolic alkalosis. Fluid replacement must take into account potentially severe losses of chloride and potassium. Appropriate replacement can be accomplished with NS with 40 mEq/L potassium. Serum electrolytes should be monitored during therapy.[1]

Adrenogenital Syndrome

The most common cause of adrenogenital syndrome in children is congenital adrenal hyperplasia secondary to deficiency of 21-hydroxylase. Defective steroidogenesis results in a deficiency of cortisol and an overproduction of intermediary metabolites. Affected infant boys appear normal, whereas infant girls have ambiguous genitalia. Adrenal insufficiency can also occur in patients who have been on long-term treatment with steroids.

Patients can present with vomiting, lethargy, and failure to thrive. Profound volume deficit can lead to shock. Glucocorticoid deficiency can result in hypoglycemia, and mineralocorticoid deficiency causes hyponatremia and hyperkalemia. Metabolic acidosis may be present.

Initial resuscitation is with NS until adequate perfusion is reestablished. Hypoglycemia is treated with intravenous glucose. In infants, D25 in a dose of 2 to 4 mL/kg is usually adequate. In older children and adolescents, D50 in a dose of 1 to 2 mL/kg is appropriate. Neonates are best treated with D10 at 1 to 2 mL/kg to avoid rapid shifts in osmolarity. Treatment also consists of initiating glucocorticoid therapy with hydrocortisone at a dose of 50 mg/m² per dose IV every 6 h. Mineralocorticoid therapy is not necessary during the acute adrenal crisis.[1]

Cystic Fibrosis

Patients with cystic fibrosis have an elevated concentration of sodium and chloride in sweat. During hot weather or strenuous exercise, affected children can suffer severe salt depletion and corresponding electrolyte abnormalities. Intercurrent pulmonary infection may be present. Profound chloride loss is compensated for by a rise in serum bicarbonate, resulting in a metabolic alkalosis. Hyponatremia is present, and serum potassium is decreased. Patients can present with lethargy and signs of hypoperfusion. Treatment is with NS, with supplemental potassium.[1]

Hypokalemia

Potassium is the predominant intracellular cation. Hypokalemia occurs when the serum potassium falls below 3.4 mEq/L, and most commonly occurs secondary to profuse vomiting with or without diarrhea. Therapy with loop diuretics can also cause hypokalemia. In diabetic ketoacidosis, profound hypokalemia can result from osmotic diuresis, although in the face of the hydrogen-potassium shift that accompanies acidemia, serum levels may be normal or falsely elevated. Uncommon causes of hypokalemia are renal tubular acidosis and familial hypokalemia-induced paralysis.

Severe potassium depletion can result in skeletal muscle weakness, ileus, and cardiac conduction disturbances. A prominent electrocardiographic (ECG) manifestation is the U wave. Clinical manifestations generally reflect the rate of fall of serum potassium rather than the absolute level.

In most cases, hypokalemia occurs slowly, and it is difficult to determine whole body stores based on the serum level. In general, oral replacement over several days is adequate. Dehydration must be corrected. If intravenous therapy is necessary, 0.2 to 0.3 mEq[K⁺]/kg per h is adequate. In extremely urgent situations, such as hypokalemia-induced respiratory insufficiency, 1 mEq[K⁺]/kg per h can be administered, with continuous ECG monitoring. This is usually done through a central line. In diabetic ketoacidosis, potassium repletion should begin early in the course of therapy, since diuresis-induced depletion can result in profound hypokalemia as acidosis is corrected and serum potassium shifts into cells.[1]

Hyperkalemia

Hyperkalemia is defined as a serum potassium level greater than 5.5 mEq/L. In infants and children, hyperkalemia is most commonly due to hemolysis that occurs during blood drawing and does not reflect serum levels. Causes of true hyperkalemia include renal failure, rhabdomyolysis, the use of potassium-sparing diuretics, and adrenal corticoid insufficiency. Metabolic acidosis can result in hyperkalemia due to the hydrogen-potassium shift.

Cardiac conduction delay is the most common manifestation of hyperkalemia and is potentially life-threatening. Peaked T waves are the first manifestation, followed by prolonged PR interval and then widening of the QRS complex, an ominous finding that can precede ventricular dysrhythmias and asystole. Any patient with ECG changes requires emergent therapy to reverse cardiac conduction toxicity. Asymptomatic patients with normal ECGs usually do well with therapy to enhance potassium excretion. Most commonly, this occurs in patients with renal failure who have sustained a gradual rise in serum potassium.

Treatment of symptomatic hyperkalemia is directed at immediately antagonizing its deleterious effects on cardiac conduction and at enhancing potassium excretion (Table 132-5).

Sodium polystyrene sulfonate is a resin that exchanges sodium for potassium at a 1:1 ratio and therefore enhances potassium excretion. It can be administered orally or by enema. A dose of 1 g/kg will lower serum potassium by up to 1.2 mEq/L. When it is administered orally, it is usually given with a cathartic to enhance transit time through the gastrointestinal tract. Hypernatremia or volume overload are potential complications. In patients with hyperkalemia secondary to renal failure, dialysis is usually necessary. In patients with hyperkalemia secondary to metabolic acidosis, normalization of serum pH usually restores serum potassium to normal levels.[1]

Disorders of Calcium

Normally, 99 percent of total body calcium is contained in bone. Normal serum levels are maintained by a complex interaction between dietary intake, absorption from the GI tract and resorption from bone, and renal excretion. Serum calcium is inversely proportional to serum phosphorus. The active form of vitamin D stimulates absorption of calcium and phosphorus from the GI tract; its formation depends on exposure to sunlight and healthy kidneys. Parathyroid hormone increases calcium resorption from bone in response to hypocalcemia and increases phosphorus excretion. Calcitonin decreases calcium resorption from bone in response to hypercalcemia.

TABLE 132-5   Treatment of Hyperkalemia

1. Calcium gluconate 10%* 100 mg/kg IV given at rate not to exceed 100 mg per min; onset of action, minutes; duration, 60 min
2. Sodium bicarbonate 1–2 mEq/kg IV; onset of action, minutes; duration, hours
3. Regular insulin 0.1 units/kg IV, with D25W, 0.5 g/kg IV over 30 min. Check glucose every 30 min. Onset, 30 min
4. Sodium polystyrene sulfonate 1–2 g/kg PO, NG, or PR
5. Albuterol inhalation, 0.5% solution; onset of action, minutes

*10% calcium gluconate contains 100 mg/mL.

In the serum, 45 to 50 percent of serum calcium exists in the ionized or free form; most of the remainder is bound to albumin. pH affects the proportion of calcium that is ionized and therefore bioavailable. Acidosis increases and alkalosis decreases the fraction of ionized calcium.

HYPOCALCEMIA This can result from hypoparathyroidism or end-organ resistance to parathyroid hormone. True hypoparathyroidism can be idiopathic, follow thyroid surgery, and can be associated with magnesium deficiency. End-organ resistance to parathyroid hormone is most commonly associated with vitamin D deficiency. The most common causes of this are dietary deficiency and chronic renal failure. Young infants fed cow's milk, which is high in phosphate, can develop significant hypocalcemia. A common cause of hypocalcemia is hyperventilation; the decreased P_{CO_2} results in an acute respiratory alkalosis that rapidly decreases ionized calcium.

Clinical manifestations of hypocalcemia include muscle weakness, vomiting, and irritability. Infants may simply appear "jittery." In severe cases, tetany, laryngospasm, carpopedal spasm, and seizures can occur. Carpopedal spasm is especially common in patients with hyperventilation syndrome. The most characteristic ECG abnormality is a prolonged QT interval.

Laboratory evaluation of hypocalcemia of unknown etiology includes total serum and ionized calcium, phosphate, total protein and albumin, measurement of parathyroid hormone, and blood urea nitrogen and creatinine.

Intravenous calcium is the treatment of choice for symptomatic hypocalcemia. Calcium gluconate 10% is administered in a dose of 100 mg/kg at a rate not to exceed 100 mg per min, with continuous ECG monitoring. Further management depends on determining the etiology of hypocalcemia.[1]

HYPERCALCEMIA This exists when serum calcium exceeds 11 mg/dL and most often results from increased bone resorption. Probably the most common cause in children is malignancy involving the lymphoreticular system. Less common causes include vitamin D intoxication and hypervitaminosis A.

Clinical manifestations of hypercalcemia include fatigue, irritability, anorexia and vomiting, and constipation. Affected patients may be clinically dehydrated and complain of polyuria. An ECG may reveal bradycardia and a shortened QT interval.

The laboratory evaluation of hypercalcemia includes evaluation of total serum and ionized calcium levels, a complete blood count, and evaluation of total protein and albumin and alkaline phosphatase. An evaluation of the vitamin D level may also be indicated, depending on the patient's medical history.

The treatment of hypercalcemia depends on the etiology. In the acute scenario, patients with functioning kidneys can be treated by aggressive intravenous hydration followed by furosemide, which will enhance calcium excretion.[1]

REFERENCES

1. Adelman RD, Solhaug MJ: Pathophysiology of body fluids and fluid therapy, in Behrman RE, Kliegman RM, Jenson HB (eds): *Nelson Textbook of Pediatrics*. 16th ed. Philadelphia: Saunders, 2000, pp. 197-227.
2. Roberts KB: Fluid and electrolytes: Parenteral therapy. *Pediatr Rev* 22:380, 2001.
3. Gorelick MH, Shaw KN, Murphy KO: Validity and reliability of clinical signs in the diagnosis of dehydration in children. *Pediatrics* 99:1, 1997.
4. Teach SJ, Yates EW, Feld LG: Laboratory predictors of fluid deficit in acutely dehydrated children. *Clin Pediatr* 36:395, 1997.
5. Luten RC: Rapid rehydration in pediatric patients. *Ann Emerg Med* 28:353, 1996.
6. Reid SR, Bonadio WA: Outpatient rapid intravenous rehydration to correct dehydration and resolve vomiting in children with acute gastroenteritis. *Ann Emerg Med* 28:318, 1996.
7. Mackenzie A, Barnes G: Randomized controlled trial comparing oral and intravenous rehydration therapy in children with diarrhea. *BMJ* 303:393, 1991.
8. Nagar AL, Wang VJ: Comparison of nasogastric and intravenous methods of rehydration in pediatric patients with acute dehydration. *Pediatrics* 109:566, 2002.
9. Androgue HJ, Madias NE: Hyponatremia. *New Engl J Med* 342:1581, 2000.
10. Sarker SA, Mahalanabis D, Alam NH, et al: Reduced osmolarity oral rehydration solution for persistent diarrhea in infants: A randomized controlled clinical trial. *J Pediatr* 138:532, 2001.
11. Cohen MB, Mezoff AG, Laney DW Jr, et al: Use of a single solution for oral rehydration and maintenance therapy of infants with diarrhea and mild to moderate dehydration. *Pediatrics* 95:639, 1995.

UPPER RESPIRATORY EMERGENCIES
Randolph Cordle

STRIDOR

The physical sign common to all causes of upper respiratory tract (URT) obstruction is stridor.

Stridor is due to Venturi effects created by somewhat linear airflow through a semicollapsible tube, the airway. During inhalation the relative pressure in the center of the airway becomes greater than that at its edges. This pressure differential leads to partial collapse of the airway walls. During expiration, the previously collapsed areas reopen due to the relative increase in air pressure. Forced expiration or expiration against a partially closed glottis may cause expiratory stridor even in patients with a normal airway. Physiologic airway support increases with caudal progression through the major airways. Therefore, less inspiratory collapse is found in the trachea compared with the supraglottic airway.

Both inspiratory and expiratory stridor are associated with obstruction at the supraglottic, glottic, and subglottic levels, as well as the trachea and primary bronchi. Supraglottic obstructions cause inspiratory stridor, with marked inspiratory and expiratory variation, while obstruction at the glottic and subglottic areas commonly cause both inspiratory and expiratory stridor of lesser magnitude. Finally, obstructions at the level of the trachea and primary bronchi may be associated with inspiratory or expiratory stridor, although usually of a much lesser degree. Although the posterior walls of the trachea and bronchi are somewhat collapsible, relatively good support is provided by the horseshoe-shaped cartilage within its walls. In premature infants and infants with tracheomalacia, these supports are not well formed and inspiratory and expiratory stridor may be impressive.

Expiratory stridor, or wheeze, is common in distal airways, since intrathoracic pressure may become much greater than atmospheric pressure during expiration. The pressure differential creates high flow through the semicollapsible bronchi, resulting in wheezes. This information can be clinically useful while evaluating a wheezing child. Commonly, gentle pressure over the chest wall or midabdomen during expiration will increase the intrathoracic pressure and exacerbate wheezing, thus making the patient's bronchoconstriction obvious. This maneuver may also assist in detecting inspiratory stridor because the child will follow this forced expiration with a much deeper inspiration than at rest. Patients with marked variation in the pattern of stridor should be considered to have a foreign body in the airway until proven otherwise. The quality of the pitch is not clinically useful for diagnosis. The age of the patient will narrow the differential diagnosis considerably (Table 133-1).

Stridor in Children below 6 Months of Age

An infant under 6 months of age with a long duration of symptoms (weeks to months) typically has a *congenital* cause of stridor, with the

TABLE 133-1 Common Causes of Stridor

Children <6 months of age
  Laryngotracheomalacia: chronic, resolves by age 2
  Vocal cord paresis or paralysis
  Arnold-Chiari malformation
Children >6 months of age: acute
  Viral croup
  Epiglottitis
  Retropharyngeal abscess
  Foreign body aspiration

major causes being laryngomalacia, tracheomalacia, and vocal cord paresis or paralysis.

Laryngomalacia accounts for 60 percent of all neonatal laryngeal problems. It is due to a developmentally weak larynx. Collapse occurs with each inspiration at the epiglottis, aryepiglottic folds, and arytenoids. Generally, the stridor worsens with crying and agitation. It often improves with neck extension and when in the prone position. This is a self-limited disorder resolving by 2 years of age in over 90 percent of cases. Symptom exacerbations may occur with upper respiratory infections or increased work of breathing due to any cause. It only rarely is associated with respiratory distress, failure to thrive, apnea, or feeding problems. Definitive diagnosis is by fiberoptic laryngoscopy. Rarely, tracheotomy or epiglottoplasty may be needed. In many cases the tracheal support structures are similarly affected, leading to the diagnosis of laryngotracheomalacia. Less commonly, the larynx will be adequately supported while the trachea is not, leading to a diagnosis of tracheomalacia.

The next most common cause of neonatal stridor is vocal cord paralysis or paresis. Most infants will have a history of birth trauma, shoulder dystocia, macrosomia, forceps delivery, an abnormal cry, or other intrathoracic anomaly. Diagnosis is typically by flexible fiberoptic laryngoscopy with visualization of the cords during speech or crying. In emergent respiratory failure, endotracheal intubation can be quite difficult in a child with bilateral vocal cord paralysis. Placing the bevel of the endotracheal tube parallel to the small remaining glottic opening and rotating the endotracheal tube one-quarter turn while applying gentle pressure may assist in passing the tube. Force should not be used, as this may damage the laryngeal structures. Needle cricothyroidotomy and subsequent tracheotomy may be required to secure the airway. It is unlikely that the laryngeal mask airway (LMA) would be helpful in this case. Use of the LMA is contraindicated in abnormal or obstructed airways because the path of least resistance to flow will likely be around the mask and not into the airway. Retrograde intubation may be difficult as well, owing to the size of the structures and potential difficulty in passing the wire from the trachea into the hypopharynx.

Arnold-Chiari (Chiari II) malformation should be considered in children with trisomy 21, myelomeningocele, hydrocephalus, sacral dimple, sacral epidermal abnormality, or other neurologic abnormalities who present with stridor. Chiari II malformations are likely due to failure of the fetal neural folds to fully close. The developing ventricular system fails to fill with CSF and distend properly due to continual drainage through this opening in the developing spinal cord. The posterior fossa subsequently develops too small to contain the developing brainstem, cerebellum, and associated structures. As the brainstem and cerebellum develop, they partially herniate both towards the tentorium and through the enlarged foramen magnum into the spinal canal. Chiari II, but not Chiari I, malformations are usually associated with other CNS abnormalities. Compression of the cerebellar tonsils, pons, medulla, and upper cervical spinal cord can lead to difficulty swallowing, arm weakness, facial weakness, nystagmus, inability to look upward, apnea, and stridor. Recognizing this cause of stridor is important diagnostically and therapeutically, as inline stabilization must be maintained if intubation is required to prevent further compression of vital CNS structures and death. Urgent neurosurgical consultation and likely decompression are also required.

Stridor in Children above 6 Months of Age

The patient above 6 months of age with a relatively short duration of symptoms (hours to days) characteristically has an acquired cause of stridor. Causes are either inflammatory, such as croup or epiglottitis, or noninflammatory, such as foreign-body aspiration. The remainder of the chapter discusses the most common acquired causes of stridor: epiglottitis, peritonsillar abscess, viral croup, foreign-body aspiration, retropharyngeal abscess, and bacterial tracheitis (Table 133-2).

EPIGLOTTITIS

Clinical Features

Since the introduction of the *Haemophilus influenzae* vaccine, the incidence and demographics of this disease have changed remarkably. Currently *H. influenzae* is thought to be responsible for less than 25 percent of cases. Now, gram-positive organisms such as *Streptococcus pyogenes, Staphylococcus aureus,* and *Streptococcus pneumoniae* are responsible for most cases in immunized children. In immunocompromised children, herpes simplex, *Candida,* and varicella must also be considered.

Prior to the introduction of the *Haemophilus* vaccine, the median age of this disease was 3 years, with 25 percent occurring in children under age 2. Although epiglottitis can occur at any age, its median age of presentation has shifted to older children and adults.

The classic symptoms are an abrupt onset over several hours of high fever, sore throat, stridor, dysphagia, and drooling. Some cases may develop over 1 to 2 days. Physical examination reveals a toxic-appearing, apprehensive child with an ashen-gray color. The child often sits in a tripod position, or the "sniffing" position, with the neck slightly extended and the chin forward. As opposed to the child with croup, there is no cough. The voice may be muffled, but supraglottic foreign bodies, peritonsillar abscess, and retropharyngeal abscess may present similarly. If inflammatory changes extend beyond the epiglottis to include the vocal cords, voice pitch will be altered as well.

Older children and adults may have much more subtle presentations. In fact, some older children will complain of only a severe sore throat. Stridor may or may not be present. The diagnosis is suggested by severe sore throat, the finding of a relatively normal-appearing oropharynx, and striking tenderness with gentle movement of the hyoid.

Diagnosis

The ideal approach to the diagnosis of epiglottitis varies depending on the practice environment. Each institution should have a written "Suspected Epiglottitis Management Protocol." The steps necessary in all protocols include:

1. Immediate recognition and triage to a resuscitation area
2. Continuous monitoring by someone trained in the management of the difficult airway
3. Rapid consultation with appropriate colleagues
4. Consideration and risk-benefit analysis of patient transfer with appropriate personnel present during the transfer
5. Bedside radiology without disturbing patient or, if moved to the x-ray suite, constant monitoring by a physician with appropriate airway equipment and skills

Lateral neck radiographs are usually unnecessary in patients with the classic presentation for epiglottitis. When the diagnosis is uncertain, radiographs should be taken with the neck extended during inspiration using soft tissue technique. The child typically holds his or her head in the

TABLE 133-2   Common Acquired Causes of Stridor

	Viral Group	Bacterial Tracheitis	Epiglottitis	Peritonsillar Abscess	Retropharyngeal Abscess	Foreign-Body Aspiration
Etiology	Parainfluenza viruses Occasionally RSV Influenza	*Staphylococcus aureus* (most) *Streptococcus pneumoniae* *Haemophilus influenzae*	*Streptococcus pneumoniae* *Haemophilus influenzae*	*Streptococcus pyogenes* *Staphylococcus aureus*	Polymicrobial *Streptococcus pyogenes* *Staphylococcus aureus* Beta-lactamase producers Gram-negative rods Oral anaerobes	Variable Peanuts Sunflower seeds Balloons/other toys Hot dogs Raisins/grapes
Age	6 mo–3 y Peak 1–2 y	3 mo–13 y Majority <3 y	All ages Classically 1–7 Median now 7	10–18 y (most) 6 mo–5 y (rare)	6 mo–4 y Peak <1 y Rare >4 y	Any 6 mo–5 y most common 80% <3 y About $\frac{2}{3}$ deaths <1 y
Onset	1–5 days	2–7 day viral upper respiratory infection Suddenly worse over 8–12 h	Rapid, hours	Antecedent pharyngitis	Insidious over 2–3 days after an upper respiratory infection or local trauma	Immediate or delayed possible
Position effect	None	None	Worse supine Prefer erect	Worse supine	Almost opisthotonic May improve in sniffing position	Usually none Location-dependent
Stridor	Inspiratory and expiratory	Inspiratory and expiratory	Inspiratory	Uncommon	Inspiratory when severe	Location-dependent
Cough	Seal-like bark	Usually Possible thick sputum	No	No	No	Often transient or positional
Voice change	Hoarse Not muffled	Usually normal Possibly raspy	Muffled "Hot potato"	Muffled "Hot potato"	Often muffled "Hot potato"	Location-dependent Primarily if at or above glottis
Drool	No	Rare	Yes	Often	Yes	Rare—often if esophageal
Dysphagia	No	No	Yes	Yes	Yes	Rare—typically if esophageal
Radiologic appearance	Subglottic narrowing "steeple" Distended hypopharynx	Subglottic narrowing Ragged tracheal air shadow Tracheal foreign bodies	Enlarged epiglottis Vallecular space loss Supraglottic ballooning	May see enlarged tonsillar soft tissue	Thickened bulging pretracheal soft tissue	Often normal Possible radiopaque density Ball-valve effect Segmented atelectasis Air contrast effect may be seen

sniffing position and has prolonged inspiration already, making it quite easy to obtain radiographs. Lateral neck radiographs are not required if the patient is already intubated, as often the typical findings for epiglottitis will not be seen in such cases. False-positive findings may occur if the radiograph is taken during expiration or with the head flexed. False-negative radiographic evaluations do occur, and if suspicion for the diagnosis still exists despite normal-appearing films, direct visualization of the epiglottis is necessary to exclude the diagnosis.

In evaluating lateral neck radiographs, the epiglottis, vallecula, hypopharynx, tracheal air column, arytenoids, and retropharyngeal or prevertebral space should be assessed. The epiglottis is normally tall and thin, projecting up into the hypopharynx (Figure 133-1). Normally there is a poorly delineated space between the epiglottis and the anterior aspect of the hypopharynx. In epiglottitis, the epiglottis is swollen and appears squat and flat, like a thumbprint at the base of the hypopharynx (Figure 133-2). Commonly, the vallecular airspace is obscured. Another common finding is ballooning of the hypopharynx just above the area of the larynx. This is illustrated by the different sizes of the hypopharynx in Figures 133-1 and 133-2. While not spe-

cific for epiglottitis, this distention does indicate significant obstruction of the upper respiratory tract. The retropharyngeal space is normally 3 to 4 mm wide. Commonly it is stated that it should be less than the width of the adjacent vertebral body. The tracheal air column should be of uniform width and smooth, without densities on its internal walls.

In some scenarios, gentle direct visualization can be attempted. Most proponents of this practice would agree that it should be performed only at sites where experts in pediatric airway management are present with appropriate equipment to maintain the airway by whatever means necessary. Typically this is done in the following stepwise manner. In his or her position of comfort, the child is asked to open their mouth wide. If the epiglottis is not seen, the child is asked to stick their tongue out, with a tongue blade used to depress the anterior aspect of the tongue in the hope of visualizing the epiglottis. Having the child inspire slowly the entire time the tongue blade is in their mouth will prevent gagging. If the epiglottis is still not seen, as is common, fiberoptic laryngoscopy by an operator skilled in the technique, and with the ability to intubate over the scope, is the safest next step.

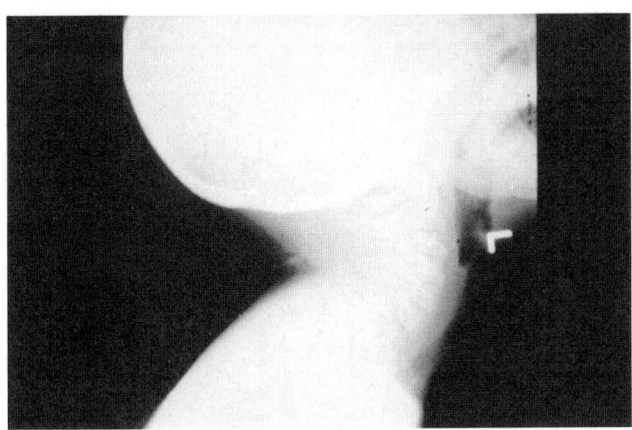

FIG. 133-1. A normal lateral neck x-ray. Open arrow points to epiglottis.

Airway Management

Should the child develop respiratory fatigue or if airway obstruction or apnea occurs before the airway has been secured, bag-valve-mask ventilation can be effective. Securing the pop-off valve may be necessary to provide adequate inspiratory pressures.

Patients with epiglottitis who are initially seen in an office, clinic, or ED without pediatric or ear-nose-throat (ENT) subspecialty support should be transported to a referral center by ground or air, whichever is more appropriate, accompanied by personnel who can manage the airway. Oxygen should be given as needed. Nebulized racemic epinephrine should be considered to decrease airway edema. The child should be kept seated upright. Heliox can also be a temporizing measure until consultants arrive (see discussion of croup, below). The referral center should be alerted as soon as possible, so that decisions concerning intubation or tracheostomy can be made in concert with consultants, and so that support personnel can be mobilized as needed. Patients usually are intubated by the most skilled individual available as soon as the diagnosis is made. Sedation, paralytics, and vagolytics are used as indicated. In a child who is able to maintain an airway, the decision to administer paralytics must be accompanied by the absolute certainty that intubation will be successful. To reduce the incidence of postextubation stridor, a tube one size smaller than usual should be used. Tube sizes above and below this size should be immediately available. The correct tube size will have a slight leak on auscultation at end inspiration. Evaluation of returned volume, ETCO$_2$ monitoring,

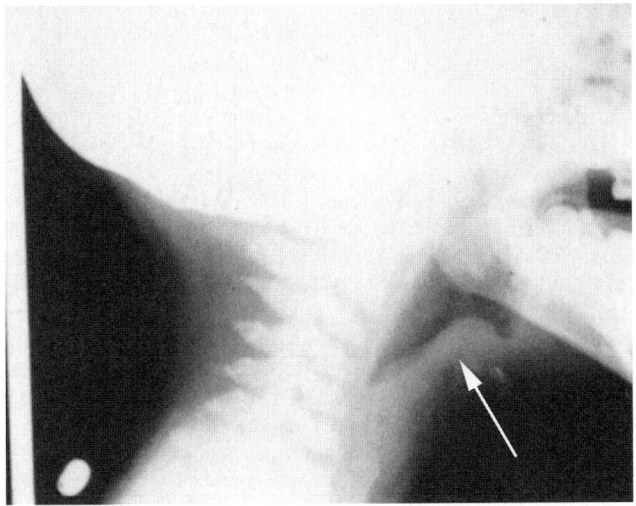

FIG. 133-2. Lateral neck view of a child with epiglottitis.

and chest wall motion will provide far more valuable information on adequacy of ventilation than does the tidal volume set on the ventilator due to leakage of air around the tube, especially as the swelling dissipates. The tube should be secured immediately, with as little patient movement as possible afterward to minimize the likelihood of tube dislodgement.

Supportive Therapy

A second- or third-generation cephalosporin such as cefuroxime, cefotaxime, or ceftriaxone is generally administered to ensure adequate coverage of *H. influenzae*. With the increasing incidence of *S. pneumoniae* as a cause for epiglottitis and the marked increase in resistance of this organism to cephalosporins, one may empirically give vancomycin also. Some recommend adding nafcillin instead, based on the increasing incidence of gram-positive cocci, including *S. aureus*, as etiologic agents. Blood cultures are positive in 80 to 90 percent of patients. Cultures of the epiglottis itself are much less sensitive. Typically oral antibiotics are continued for 7 to 10 days after the patient is extubated.

VIRAL CROUP

Viral croup (laryngotracheitis or laryngotracheobronchitis) is responsible for most cases of stridor after the neonatal period. Children 6 months to 3 years of age are most commonly affected, with a peak incidence between 1 and 2 years of age. Croup is relatively uncommon after age 6. This is due to the much greater effect of a small amount of mucosal edema and inflammation in the airway of a small child versus that of an older child. As little as 1 mm of airway edema in an infant may cause a decrease in cross-sectional area of 50 to 60 percent. This leads to increased resistance and work of breathing. In the adult airway, 1 mm of edema is nearly inconsequential. The incidence of true croup is thought to be equal in males and females, but many authors believe that moderate to severe cases are twice as common in males. Most cases occur in the late fall or early winter.

Acute viral croup is thought to be on a continuum with spasmodic croup. Prospectively it is very difficult or impossible to differentiate them. Retrospectively, spasmodic croup is seen more commonly in atopic children, has no seasonal variation, usually has almost complete symptom resolution within 6 h, is not characteristically associated with fever, and is often recurrent. Both spasmodic croup and acute viral croup have characteristic nocturnal exacerbations.

Etiology

Practically all cases are viral. Parainfluenza virus types I, II, and III are most common, but sometimes indistinguishable syndromes can be caused by influenza A or B, respiratory syncytial virus (RSV), rhinoviruses, adenoviruses, and even measles virus. Cases caused by adenovirus may be associated with hemorrhagic cystitis and conjunctivitis. Measles pneumonitis should be considered in atypical cases and, if suspected, treated aggressively. In nonimmunized or immunosuppressed adults, measles pneumonitis may prove fatal. The incubation period for parainfluenza virus is 2 to 6 days, and virus is usually shed for about 2 weeks. In cases caused by RSV, the shedding may continue for a much longer period and symptoms may take months to clear completely. In children over the age of 5, *Mycoplasma pneumoniae* infection has also been associated with a crouplike syndrome.

Signs and Symptoms

There is typically a 1- to 5-day prodrome consisting of cough, coryza, and occasionally other upper respiratory infection-type symptoms. This is followed by a 3- to 4-day period of barking cough. The cough is typically worse in the late evening and at night and may occur strictly during these times. Children may or may not have a low-grade fever during the illness. The typical duration of symptoms ranges from 3 to 7 days regardless of the treatment. Typically the third and fourth days are the worst, and then the child starts to improve. Children who do not follow this general course should be reevaluated.

Viral croup is classically associated with biphasic stridor, although often the inspiratory component is much greater than the expiratory component. Stridor is unaffected by position but increases with crying or agitation. Intercostal retractions and tachypnea are common signs. The voice is often hoarse but not muffled. If inflammation extends from the trachea to the more distal bronchi, wheezing or crackles may be present.

Diagnosis

Croup is a clinical diagnosis. Generally laboratory tests are unnecessary. The white count is typically normal or demonstrates a slight lymphocytosis. Blood cultures or nasopharyngeal washings are not clinically useful, since knowing the exact etiologic agent does not change management.

Radiographs are needed only if other causes of stridor are being considered, or in atypical or prolonged cases. A lateral neck film and posteroanterior (PA) chest radiograph should be obtained as appropriate. The aryepiglottic area is normal. The lateral neck radiograph may demonstrate slightly ill-defined tracheal air shadows, narrowing on inspiration greater than that on expiration, and slight distention of the hypopharynx. Typically, fixed subglottic obstructions—such as papillomas, foreign bodies, hemangiomas, and subglottic stenoses—cause narrowing of the airway that does not change with the phase of respiration. Many of the latter noncroup causes also cause asymmetry in appearance, whereas croup causes symmetrical changes in the air column. The PA chest x-ray is most useful to rule out radiopaque foreign body. In cases of croup, the normally squared shoulders of the subglottic tracheal air shadow will appear more like a steeple, pencil tip, nail, or hourglass.

General Treatment

Pulse oximetry should be measured and supplemental humidified oxygen given. Children with croup should not be sedated except in the course of a rapid-sequence intubation. Antibiotics are not indicated for patients with a confident diagnosis of croup. Antipyretics should be given for fever to decrease minute ventilation and work of breathing. The least invasive route possible should be used to provide hydration to replace insensible water losses from respiratory distress and fever. Urine output, or the number of wet diapers, should be monitored and intravenous hydration provided only if necessary.

Exposure to humidified air, either cold night air or moist air from a shower, has been reported useful by parents for years, but humidification in croup tents has been shown not to be effective. Mild humidification may calm and soothe the child while possibly causing some mucosal vasoconstriction. Croup tents should not be used. In addition to lack of efficacy, they lead to increased anxiety, separation from parents, decreased ability of staff to monitor the child, and difficulty in maintaining oxygen provision at adequate levels.

In general, calculating a croup score (Table 133-3)[1] is more useful as a research tool than as an adjunct to clinical practice. Its primary role is to provide a semiobjective scale by which to classify patients for comparative studies. Its usefulness as a tool for clinical decision making with individual patients is much less clear. The score, if calculated, should only be used as one piece of data in the decision-making process. For example, a child with severe retractions and markedly decreased air entry may have a score of only 5, but would be considered at high risk by most clinicians and treated aggressively. Generally, healthy-appearing children with stridor only when agitated do not re-

TABLE 133-3   Modified Westley Croup Score*

Clinical Indicators	Score
Inspiratory	
None	0
At rest, with stethoscope	1
At rest, no stethoscope required to hear	2
Level of consciousness	
Normal	0
Altered	5
Air entry	
Normal	0
Decreased	1
Severely decreased	2
Cyanosis	
None	0
Agitated	4
Resting	5
Retractions	
None	0
Mild	1
Moderate	2
Severe	3
	Total =

*Note: Multiple variations of this are used in the literature. When discussing scores, one must know which scale is being used. Score 8 or greater indicates respiratory failure.
Source: Adapted from Super DM, Cartelli NA, Brooks LJ, et al: A prospective randomized double-blind study to evaluate the effect of dexamethasone in acute laryngotracheitis. *J Pediatr* 115:323, 1989, with permission.

quire treatment with epinephrine. Children with stridor at rest or who appear in distress should receive epinephrine as discussed below. All children receiving catecholamines should receive steroids as well. The use of steroids, as discussed below, is generally agreed upon in moderate to severe episodes of croup. In mild croup, controversy exists regarding the absolute need of steroid treatment, but there is increasing evidence of efficacy in this population as well. The use of steroids in the mildest cases may vary between reasonable clinicians. Further research using clinically important endpoints should clarify their use in this population.

Epinephrine

Racemic epinephrine, a nearly equimolar mixture of the two isomers (D and L) of epinephrine, is a mainstay of moderate to severe croup treatment. The majority of its activity is due to the L-isomer. The D-isomer is only about 30 percent as active as the L-isomer. The drug is quite effective when nebulized. Positive effects can be seen in as little as 10 min, with maximal effects seen at about 1 h. In most cases its therapeutic effects are practically gone by 2 h. Nebulized epinephrine decreases airway edema by vasoconstriction of the boggy mucosal vessels. It does not alter the natural course of disease, but does improve ventilation. Use of racemic epinephrine decreases the number of children with croup requiring intubation, intensive care unit admission, and admission to the hospital in general.

L-epinephrine, a pure isomer, is used as an advanced cardiac life support (ACLS) drug in a 1:1000 concentration. It is at least as effective and safe as racemic epinephrine (Table 133-4). Although some forms contain sulfur dioxide, a known respiratory irritant, this has not caused significant problems in this patient group. Both racemic and

TABLE 133-4   Epinephrine for Stridor

Drug	Concentration	Accurate Dosing*	Quick Dosing
L-Epinephrine	1 : 1000 1 mL = 1 mg	0.5 mL/kg (max 5 mL)	2.5 mL <1 y 5 mL >1 y
Racemic epinephrine	2.25%	0.05 mL/kg (max 0.5 mL)	0.25 mL <6 mo 0.5 mL >6 mo

*Diluted if necessary with normal saline to make 3–5 mL total volume.

L-epinephrine are relatively contraindicated and may worsen the obstruction seen in patients with severe left ventricular outflow obstruction (idiopathic hypertrophic subaortic stenosis, subvalvular aortic stenosis, etc.). When the drug is used in these patients, very close monitoring is indicated.

Ledwith's group monitored patients for 3 h after epinephrine nebulization and found that 38 percent of the patients who had a recurrence requiring admission did so between the second and third hour.[2] Prendergast et al. also demonstrated that there was an upward trend in the croup score between the second and third hours in those patients ultimately requiring admission.[3] The current recommendation for moderate to severe croup is to administer nebulized epinephrine with early steroids (see below) and monitor these patients in the ED for at least 3 h before considering discharge (Table 133-5).

Dexamethasone

Steroids should be given within 1 h of presentation, and early effects of steroid use may be seen at $\frac{1}{2}$ to 2 h. Most likely this is due to vasoconstriction of the edematous mucosa. Steroid effects on immune modulation and protein synthesis occur later and may be responsible for their longer-term clinical benefits. Certainly any child receiving nebulized epinephrine should also receive steroids.

Dexamethasone, a fluorinated derivative of prednisolone, has antiinflammatory effects about 25 times greater than those of hydrocortisone at equal doses. It has minimal to no mineralocorticoid effect. Its half-life is about 2 days (range 36 to 72 h). Peak effects are seen in 2 h with persistent effects over the next 1 to 2 weeks. Early studies used 0.6 mg/kg of dexamethasone IM. This was the standard to which alternative dosages and interventions were compared. It was then shown[4] that doses greater than 0.3 mg/kg of dexamethasone IM were clearly beneficial, but doses less than this had marginal benefit. Subsequent studies demonstrated that oral dexamethasone was as effective as intramuscular dexamethasone at the same dosages. Studies, primarily from the adult asthma literature, have demonstrated near bioequivalence of intravenous and oral steroids. Giving steroids orally has become standard practice for asthma and croup.[5] Geelhoed's group demonstrated that 0.15 mg/kg, 0.3 mg/kg, and 0.6 mg/kg of oral dexamethasone have essentially equivalent effectiveness.[6] This author

TABLE 133-5   Discharge Criteria for Croup

At least 3 h since last epinephrine
Nontoxic appearance
Able to take fluids well
Not clinically dehydrated (labs not necessary)
Room-air oxygen saturation greater than 90%
Age greater than 6–12 months*
Weather conditions allow rapid return to ED for worsening
Parents have a phone and no social issues for concern
Caretaker seems able to recognize change in child's clinical status
Relatively short transit time from home to hospital

*Controversial.
Source: Adapted from Kunkel NC, Baker D: Use of racemic epinephrine, dexamethasone, and mist in the outpatient management of croup. *Pediatr Emerg Care* 12:156, 1996.

personally uses 0.3 mg/kg of dexamethasone PO. Although 0.15 mg/kg is likely equivalent, giving the higher dose allows a buffer zone for a little bit of medicine being spit out. The greatest problem with giving oral steroids is vomiting and the bitter taste. Various steroid preparations are available (Table 133-6). Using crushed dexamethasone tablets or giving the medication in small aliquots over the first 30 min is said to reduce the number of children who vomit. This author typically gives the 10 mg/mL IV formulation PO. This makes the volume nearly inconsequential (20-kg child = 0.6 mL), the taste nearly irrelevant, and the incidence of vomiting near zero, a major benefit for our nursing colleagues.

More recent studies have investigated the use of nebulized steroids. If steroids could be selectively deposited at the area of inflammation, they could have a greater effect on the disease process with fewer side effects. Johnson's study using dexamethasone resulted in benefits that were not clinically significant, and two children in the study developed bacterial tracheitis with associated neutropenia.[7] Nebulized dexamethasone is not recommended. Multiple other studies using budesonide have had more encouraging results. Limited data suggests nebulized budesonide may have efficacy similar to epinephrine in moderate cases. Some will try a nebulized dose of budesonide in these cases as it allows for earlier discharge when effective. Whether or not an oral dexamethasone dose should be given as well in these cases is controversial and open to further research. A few conclusions can be drawn. Nebulized budesonide is effective, but has lower efficacy in most studies than dexamethasone given orally or IM.[8] Results are mixed regarding an additive effect of nebulized budesonide with oral dexamethasone. One of Klassen's studies demonstrated a number needed to treat (NNT) of four for nebulized budesonide in addition to oral dexamethasone. The outcome measure in this study was a two-point decrease in Westley croup score during a 4-h treatment period.[8,9] Although still controversial, it may be reasonable to give a dose of nebulized budesonide in addition to oral dexamethasone in moderate to severe presentations of croup where this potential effect could be clinically useful.

A child with resting stridor, increased P_{CO_2}, decreased P_{O_2}, impaired mental status, cyanosis, age less than 1 year (some say 6 months), or a croup score above 8 (see Table 133-3) should be considered in early respiratory failure and managed aggressively to prevent progression to respiratory arrest.

Fortunately, if treated aggressively, less than 1 percent of admitted patients will need intubation. Intubation should be performed whenever clinically indicated by the most experienced operator available. Based loosely on the available literature and on personal experience, this author strongly considers elective intubation in the following situations.

1. A croup score above 8 without rapid improvement
2. Two catecholamine nebulizations required within 1 h and patient fatiguing or getting worse
3. Hourly nebulizations required beyond the second hour
4. Acute mental status changes associated with respiratory distress
5. Worsening respiratory failure despite ongoing treatment
6. Severe croup in a child with neonatal lung disease
7. Moderately severe to severe croup in a child who needs transfer (especially if by helicopter)

TABLE 133-6   Steroids for Croup

Steroid	Concentration	Dose	Route	Informaton
Dexamethasone	0.25, 0.5, 1, 1.5, 2, 4, 6 mg tablets	0.3 mg/kg	PO	Crush in juice, acetaminophen elixir, or applesauce
	4, 10, 20, 24, mg/mL	0.3 mg/kg	IV	Erratic GI absorption
	8, 16 mg/mL	0.3 mg/kg	IM	Minimize volume
	0.5 mg/5 mL elixir	0.3 mg/kg	PO	May contain 5% alcohol Taste varies by brand
	0.1 or 1 mg/mL oral solution	0.3 mg/kg	PO	May contain 30% alcohol
	10 mg/mL IV solution	0.3 mg/kg	PO	No need to dilute
Budesonide	2 mg/4 mL	2 mg	Nebulized	Not available in U.S.
Prednisolone	5 mg/5 mL syrup	1 mg/kg	PO	Pediapred 5% alcohol
	15 mg/5 mL syrup	1 mg/kg	PO	Prelone
	15 mg/5 mL	1 mg/kg	PO	Orapred; great taste and less volume
Prednisone	1, 2.5, 5, 10, 20, 50 mg tablets	1 mg/kg	PO	
	1 or 5 mg/mL syrup	1 mg/kg	PO	Poor taste

In children with a less than 40 percent oxygen requirement, a trial of heliox should be given before intubation whenever feasible (see below).

The cricoid cartilage is normally the narrowest part of the young child's airway and will be especially narrow in croup owing to mucosal inflammation of the trachea. Subglottic stenosis after extubation can be minimized by using a tube that is 0.5 to 1.0 mm smaller than would typically be used. Never force a tube through the cricoid ring. Be sure a slight air leak is present after intubation.

Fiberoptic laryngoscopy should be considered in atypical or recurrent presentations of a crouplike syndrome. It may also be indicated in children who fail to respond to standard therapy and occasionally in the very young to rule out laryngomalacia and other congenital causes of stridor.

Heliox

Helium is much less dense than either oxygen or nitrogen. Replacing nitrogen with helium decreases airway resistance. Heliox will improve ventilation in patients with nearly all types of upper airway obstruction. In fact, Weber's group[10] compared heliox to racemic epinephrine in a small number of patients with moderate to severe croup and demonstrated similar reductions in modified Taussig croup scores in the first and subsequent 3 h. Heliox may also restore laminar flow, improving ventilation and ventilation/perfusion matching. The work of breathing also decreases. Carbon dioxide diffuses much faster through a helium-oxygen mixture than it does through a nitrogen-oxygen mixture. This may make ventilation more effective. One easily forgotten point is that oxygen and helium gas cannot occupy the same space. Due to the rule of partial pressures, if the helium concentration is increased, the oxygen concentration must decrease. Helium has therapeutic effects only when its concentration makes up 60 to 80 percent of the inspired gas. Therefore an individual who requires greater than 35 to 40 percent oxygen cannot use this modality. The flow of oxygen and helium must be high enough to exceed the patient's minute ventilation to prevent entrainment of room air and increased dead-space ventilation.

The indications for the use of heliox are still somewhat controversial. Most would agree that children not requiring high-flow oxygen should be given a trial of heliox for poor ventilation secondary to partial upper airway obstruction. At a minimum this may serve as a temporizing measure and allow for a more controlled intubation. Following intubation, helium may be given through the ventilator circuit as a mixture with oxygen. Volume and flow readings from the ventilator will be inaccurate if helium is used, since ventilators are calibrated for use with a nitrogen-oxygen mixture.

BACTERIAL TRACHEITIS

Bacterial tracheitis, also known as membranous croup or membranous laryngotracheobronchitis, is rare. It is generally caused by bacterial superinfection of an antecedent viral upper respiratory infection. It is most commonly seen in children less than 3 years of age, with a median age of incidence of $4\frac{1}{2}$ years. Nearly all reported cases have arisen in children between 3 months and 13 years of age. Typically, 2 to 7 days of a crouplike syndrome is followed by worsening symptoms and the development of a toxic appearance over a period of several hours. Children appear septic or similar in appearance to those with epiglottitis with a few important differences. As a rule, children with bacterial tracheitis have severe inspiratory and expiratory stridor, cough with occasional thick sputum production, a raspy or hoarse voice, and no dysphagia. They may also complain of a gnawing or burning substernal chest discomfort.

The history, physical exam, laboratory, and radiologic findings may help diagnose less obvious cases in well-appearing patients. Most patients will have a markedly elevated white count with an impressive left shift. Blood cultures are typically negative. Anteroposterior (AP) and lateral neck radiographs usually demonstrate subglottic narrowing of the trachea. Irregular densities may be seen within the trachea and its borders may appear ragged and indistinct.

Management is similar to that of epiglottitis. Ideally, these patients should go to the operating room for sedation, intubation, and bronchoscopy. Culture and Gram stain of the mucopurulent secretions should be obtained at this time. Gram-stain findings may help guide antibiotic therapy. In less severe cases without respiratory distress, bronchoscopy may be performed without immediate intubation. This is the exception to the rule, however, as greater than 85 percent of cases will require intubation.

Antibiotics effective against *S. aureus, S. pneumoniae,* and beta lactamase-producing gram-negative organisms such as *H. influenzae* and *Moraxella catarrhalis* should be given empirically. Vancomycin and a third-generation cephalosporin, such as cefotaxime or ceftriaxone, are commonly used.

FOREIGN-BODY ASPIRATION

Demographics

The peak incidence of foreign body aspiration is in the 1- to 3-year-old age group. At least 90 percent of cases are seen in children under age 4 and it has been reported in infants as young as 3 months. In children younger than 6 months, foreign-body aspiration is often secondary to a feeding given by a well-meaning sibling.

The most commonly aspirated foreign bodies fall into two groups: foods and toys. The most dangerous objects are those that are cylindrical or small, smooth, and round. Commonly aspirated foods include peanuts, sunflower seeds, raisins, grapes, hot dogs, and small sausages.

In 1979, the federal government instituted the Consumer Product Safety Act, which has decreased the incidence of toy aspiration. However, watchdog groups warn that most toys are not properly evaluated for safety prior to marketing. Anticipatory guidance should include recommendations that consumers directly inspect toys and follow all warning labels.

Although small, round metal objects typically do not cause tissue reactions, vegetable matter does. Aspirated vegetable matter commonly causes an intense pneumonitis and subsequent pneumonia and/or suppurative bronchitis. Aspirated vegetable matter is often difficult to remove if not found early. It swells with the absorption of moisture from the surrounding lung, and if left long enough, seeds may even sprout.

At presentation, many patients with foreign-body aspiration may be completely asymptomatic with a normal physical exam. Some data suggest that the majority will present with or will have previously had symptoms consistent with but not specific for foreign body aspiration. The study of Laks and Barzilay demonstrated fever in 36 percent, wheeze in 35 percent, crackles in 38 percent, and tachypnea in 45 percent of patients at presentation.[11] Although the location of the aspirated foreign body does play a role in determining the symptoms and signs seen on presentation, there is overlap between groups. Classic dogma is that laryngotracheal foreign bodies cause stridor, whereas bronchial foreign bodies cause wheezing. Studies have shown, however, that about 30 percent of laryngotracheal foreign bodies and up to 10 percent of bronchial foreign bodies will demonstrate wheezing and stridor, respectively. More importantly, a significant proportion will have no cough, wheeze, or stridor. It is true that the majority of patients presenting with severe immediate-onset stridor or cardiac arrest after aspiration will be found to have a laryngotracheal foreign body. Patients with alternating wheezing and stridor may have a mobile foreign body. Other signs and symptoms of foreign-body aspiration may include cough, history of a choking episode, history of persistent or recurrent pneumonia, apnea, pharyngeal pain, or persistent symptoms of croup or asthma remaining after adequate treatment for 5 to 7 days. Foreign-body aspiration should be considered in all children given a diagnosis of unilateral wheezing. Upper esophageal foreign bodies may impinge upon the posterior aspect of the trachea, leading to signs and symptoms of airway obstruction. Commonly the patient will present with stridor. Contrary to most cases of airway aspiration, patients with an esophageal foreign body typically will have dysphagia.

Diagnosis

A high index of suspicion is required to diagnose this disorder. Foreign-body aspiration should always at least be considered in a young child with respiratory symptoms, regardless of the duration of symptoms, since many children may present more than 24 h after foreign body aspiration. If the clinical scenario clearly indicates the presence of a foreign body or airway obstruction, a protocol for obstructed airway should be implemented immediately (see Chap. 14). When the diagnosis is considered in a stable child, plain radiographs may be helpful if positive. Clinicians should never rule out foreign-body aspiration based only on plain radiographs, as they may be entirely normal in up to one-third of foreign-body aspiration cases. Most aspirated foreign bodies are not radiopaque.

Nonradiopaque foreign bodies at the laryngeal or tracheal locations may be identified by looking for telltale air contrast of the foreign body in relation to the surrounding normal soft tissues. Computed tomography (CT) may be helpful. In most cases, however, additional radiologic procedures are not ideal, and laryngoscopy and rigid bronchoscopy are indicated.

In cases of complete obstruction, segmental atelectasis may be seen on plain radiographs. In other cases, intermittent or partial obstruction occurs, creating a ball-valve effect (Figure 133-3). In these cases, additional radiographs or fluoroscopy may be helpful. Partial obstruction, most commonly of the right mainstem bronchus, may cause obstructive emphysema of the involved lung by allowing air past the obstruction on inhalation, but preventing its passage on exhalation. In cooperative, stable children, inspiratory and expiratory PA chest radiographs to search for hyperinflation of the involved lung with contralateral mediastinal shift and decreased excursion of the ipsilateral diaphragm may be indicated. Forced expiration by having a parent gently push on the child's lower abdomen during expiration may increase the sensitivity, but this has not been adequately studied. In young or uncooperative children, the ball-valve phenomenon may best be demonstrated by fluoroscopy. Bilateral decubitus PA chest radiographs may also be used, but are less sensitive than fluoroscopy. The obstructed side will remain fully inflated with the ipsilateral diaphragm inferiorly displaced when the involved side is down. When the unobstructed side is down, it will show the normal findings of diaphragmatic elevation, rib splinting, and decreased relative volume compared to the other side (Figures 133-4 and 133-5). Foreign-body aspiration is definitively diagnosed preoperatively in only about half of cases. Clinically suspected foreign-body aspiration should ultimately be ruled out by bronchoscopy.

Esophageal foreign bodies may sometimes cause stridor. Esophageal foreign bodies more commonly are radiopaque, and are therefore more easily seen on plain radiography. In general, narrow, flat foreign bodies such as coins will be oriented in the coronal plane if they are in the esophagus. The tracheal cartilages with the exception of the cricoid ring are incomplete and horseshoe-shaped, with the opening directed posterior. These anatomic characteristics cause most narrow, flat radiopaque tracheal foreign bodies to be sagittally oriented on radiography, but certainly exceptions to these generalities do occur. Radiolucent foreign bodies in the esophagus may be suspected in many cases due to an air-fluid level or soft tissue changes in the area just cephalad to the obstruction. Older children may complain of something stuck in the throat. Discussion of esophageal foreign-body management is found in Chap. 76.

Treatment

If a child who is presumed to have aspirated a foreign body has severe signs and symptoms but is maintaining the airway, and is alert and able to speak, the predetermined obstructed airway protocol should be instituted. If local personnel are not able to remove the foreign body, a transport team experienced in the management of the difficult pediatric airway should be summoned to the patient's location. Ideally, the transport team will have a physician member trained and experienced

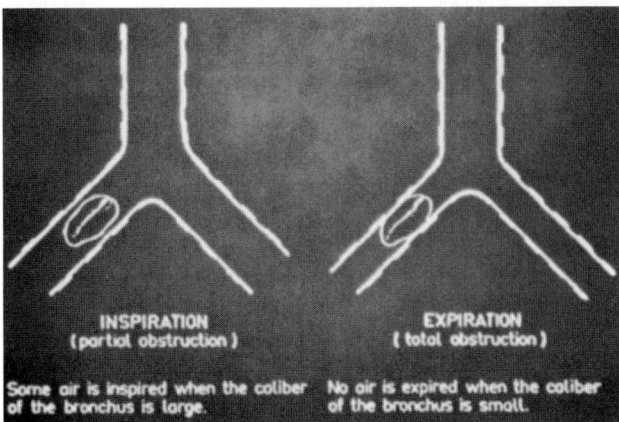

FIG. 133-3. Inspiratory and expiratory films in foreign-body aspiration.

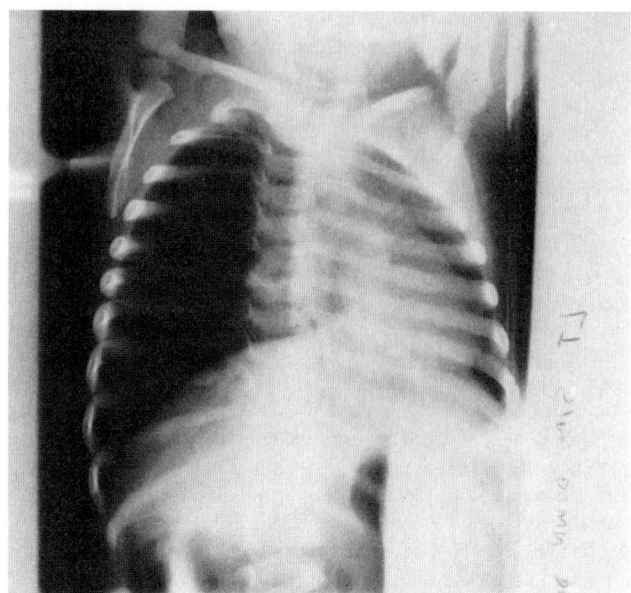

FIG. 133-4. Normal decubitus film with left side down.

in the removal of foreign bodies and in the management of the diffi-cult pediatric airway. In general, the foreign body should be removed. If this is not possible, as in the case of a supralaryngeal foreign body, the child should be electively intubated prior to transport. Exceptions may occur based on clinical circumstances. Racemic epinephrine or heliox may be an alternative.

The outcome of patients with laryngotracheal foreign-body aspira-tion and sudden collapse or cardiopulmonary arrest primarily depends on appropriate bystander basic life support and emergency medical system response. Basic pediatric CPR and foreign-body removal are discussed in Chap. 14, and pediatric airway management is dis-cussed in Chap. 15. The management of swallowed foreign bodies is discussed in Chap. 76.

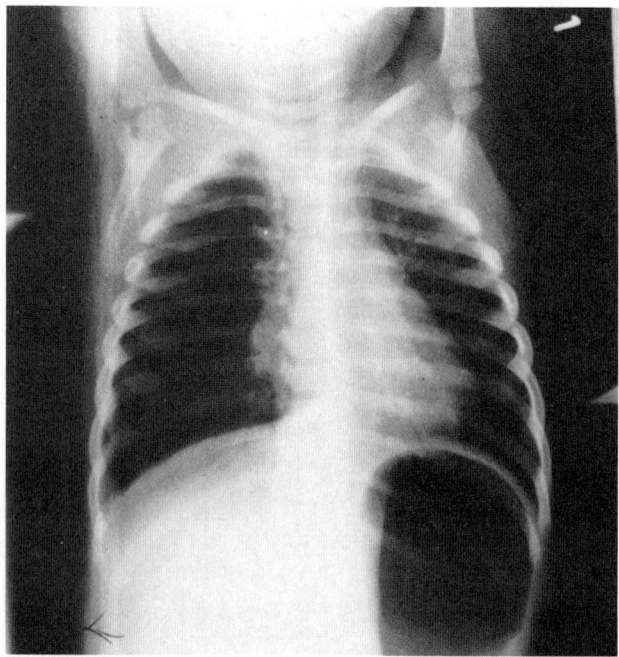

FIG. 133-5. Decubitus film, right side down, with foreign-body aspi-ration on the right side.

PERITONSILLAR ABSCESS

Peritonsillar abscess in children most commonly presents in adoles-cents with an antecedent sore throat. Often there is a period of im-provement prior to the onset of progressively worsening symptoms. Peritonsillar abscess may rarely occur in the younger child. Most com-monly, patients appear acutely ill with fevers, chills, dysphagia, tris-mus, drooling, or a muffled or "hot potato" voice. When present, tris-mus is thought to be due to secondary inflammation of the neighboring pterygoid muscles. There may be ipsilateral ear pain and torticollis. Torticollis may represent an attempt to relax the ipsilateral sternocleidomastoid muscle so as to decrease pressure on the periton-sillar space.

The peritonsillar space includes the superior aspect of the tonsil and the area lateral to the adenoids to the area of the pyriform sinus. Once a tonsillar infection has escaped the boundary of the tonsillar capsule, purulent material may flow relatively freely throughout this area. These anatomic relationships are important to remember, as they help to explain the classic physical findings of this disease process.

Careful visualization of the oral cavity is a must to reliably rule out this infection. The majority of cases will involve the superior aspect of the peritonsillar space, which can lead to discovery with meticulous examination. This may be nearly impossible in the young child with trismus. Diagnosis in this case is more challenging. In this instance, some have recommended CT scanning of the oropharyngeal and cer-vical soft tissues, while others believe that this practice may be dan-gerous as the child could acutely obstruct the airway. One possible al-ternative is an ultrasound examination at the bedside.[12–17] The literature on this topic is controversial and the reported accuracy likely dependent on the operator's experience, inclusion and exclusion crite-ria used in the study, and the pretest likelihood of abscess (or preva-lence of disease in those included). Ultrasound may be useful for lo-calization purposes when an abscess is seen.

Typically, however, bilateral tonsillar erythema and exudate will be noted on exam. The uvula and anterior pillar of the tonsil on the af-fected side may be displaced away from the involved tonsil. The in-volved tonsil is, as a rule, anteriorly and medially displaced. Cervical adenopathy is often present but does not differentiate this process from the much more common causes of pharyngitis.

When uvular deviation, marked soft palate displacement, severe trismus, airway compromise, or localized areas of fluctuance are noted, the diagnosis of peritonsillar abscess can be made with confi-dence and no imaging study is required. In less obvious cases with minimal or no trismus, no localized areas of fluctuance, and no dis-placement of pharyngeal structures, differentiating peritonsillar ab-scess from peritonsillar cellulitis is difficult. If a child appears toxic, the diagnosis should certainly be considered peritonsillar abscess un-til proven otherwise. In younger children, imaging may be required to help differentiate these processes (see above). In nontoxic-appearing adolescents with good follow-up, involved parents, and findings most consistent with peritonsillar cellulitis, a trial of antibiotics may be the best choice for initial treatment. Penicillin, a macrolide, or clin-damycin are most commonly used.

The definitive treatment of peritonsillar abscess has changed sig-nificantly over the last decade. Previously, most cases were taken to the operating room for incision and drainage. Today, the majority of cases are treated as outpatients with needle aspiration, antibiotics, and pain control. Clearly, definitive follow-up is a must. The local proto-col and individual physician comfort should dictate who performs the peritonsillar abscess aspiration. Very young and uncooperative chil-dren may be better served with formal incision and drainage in the op-erating room. Some have used ketamine successfully to accomplish this safely in the emergency department. The patient must be under control during needle aspiration to prevent injury to the jugular vein and carotid artery. In general, a single episode of peritonsillar abscess is not an indication for tonsillectomy.

RETROPHARYNGEAL ABSCESS

Demographics

Retropharyngeal abscess, although relatively rare, is the second most commonly seen deep neck space infection. The usual age range is 6 months to 4 years, with the peak incidence in infants. Retropharyngeal abscess is quite rare after age 4 because repeated upper respiratory-type infections have obliterated the retropharyngeal lymph nodes by this age in most children. Most cases of retropharyngeal abscess evolve insidiously over a few days following a relatively minor upper respiratory infection. Localized trauma to the posterior pharyngeal wall is another cause. This most commonly occurs in children who fall with a stick or similar object in their mouths.

Anatomic Relationships

Two major cervical lymph node chains enter the retropharyngeal space. They drain lymph not only from the nasopharynx but also the adenoids and the posterior paranasal sinuses. The retropharyngeal space is the potential space located between the posterior pharyngeal wall (more properly the buccopharyngeal fascia) and the prevertebral fascia. It extends from the base of the skull to the level of T1 or T2 in the area of the posterior mediastinum. It is the only deep neck space that extends the entire length of the neck. Anatomists believe that it may actually be in continuity with the prevertebral space, which extends to the level of the psoas muscle. For this reason or due to erosion through the prevertebral fascia, infections in the retropharyngeal space are known to have extended this entire length.

Signs and Symptoms

The symptoms most commonly found in patients with a retropharyngeal abscess are, individually, not specific, but, together, point toward the correct diagnosis. Although not commonly recognized in preverbal children, older children will complain of sore throat. Most have a history of high fever. Other symptoms include dysphagia, decreased oral intake, and stiff neck.

In general, children with retropharyngeal abscess appear quite ill. Signs of retropharyngeal abscess include muffled voice, persistently hyperextended neck, inspiratory stridor, meningismus, and, if partial airway obstruction is present, respiratory distress and tachypnea. Ipsilateral cervical adenopathy has also been described but is not specific. Often a unilateral or bilateral retropharyngeal mass can be visualized during examination of the oropharynx. Unilateral masses are typically easier to detect than bilateral ones. Although palpation will commonly demonstrate fluctuance, this practice is dangerous and unnecessary. Laboratory testing is neither sensitive nor specific for retropharyngeal abscess.

Classic teaching is that a lateral neck radiograph should be obtained when one suspects this infection. This radiograph should be taken during inspiration with the neck extended so as to limit false-positive results. Diagnostic criteria for this radiograph are controversial (Figure 133-6). Most would agree that the normal prevertebral soft tissue should be no wider at the second cervical vertebra than the diameter of the vertebral body at the same level. Radiographs showing slightly wider prevertebral soft tissues at this level without obvious bulging have a low specificity for retropharyngeal abscess. If the criterion for a positive test is considered two times the diameter of the vertebral body at the same level, the sensitivity is about 90 percent, but the specificity is still not very good unless air-fluid levels are seen within the retropharyngeal soft tissues. Still others have suggested using values of 7-mm prevertebral soft tissue width at C2 and 14-mm prevertebral soft tissue width at C6 as the criteria for the presence of a retropharyngeal abscess. The sensitivity and specificity of these criteria would seem to be quite dependent on the age and position of the

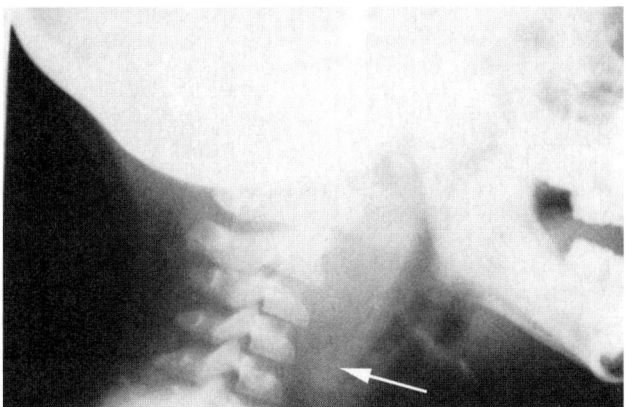

FIG. 133-6. Lateral neck view of a child with retropharyngeal abscess and widened retropharyngeal space.

patient. Others have found no correlation between the findings on lateral neck radiographs and CT scans in patients who clinically appear to have a retropharyngeal abscess. Therefore, definitive diagnosis should be based on CT scan results whenever possible. CT scan differentiates cellulitis from abscess and helps with surgical planning by demonstrating the degree of extension that has occurred. It can also be used to clarify equivocal x-ray findings. CT's sensitivity for retropharyngeal abscess is thought to be near 100 percent. Unstable patients should be intubated before going to the CT scan suite. A physician accustomed to managing the difficult pediatric airway and appropriate equipment should accompany stable patients. Risks and benefits of sedation must be seriously considered in non-intubated patients.

Treatment

After the airway has been stabilized, the patient should receive analgesia and in most cases be prepared for surgery. Retropharyngeal cellulitis and very small localized abscesses may do well with antibiotics alone. All other cases should undergo an incision and drainage procedure. These decisions should be made in consultation with an otolaryngologist.

Most retropharyngeal abscesses are found to contain mixed flora when cultured. Common organisms include *S. aureus, S. pyogenes, S. viridans,* and beta lactamase-producing gram-negative rods such as *Klebsiella.* Oral anaerobes such as *Peptostreptococcus* species, *Fusobacterium* species, and *Bacteroides* species are also frequently seen. Antibiotic choice is controversial. Single-agent therapy with ampicillin/sulbactam may be best. Others use clindamycin and/or nafcillin with a third-generation cephalosporin. Some believe that high-dose penicillin G is most appropriate. In patients who are not allergic to penicillin, ampicillin/sulbactam provides the broadest coverage of the potential etiologic agents. Penicillin-allergic patients who are not known to be allergic to cephalosporins may achieve the best results with clindamycin and a third-generation cephalosporin.

Most patients do quite well, but complications do occur. Airway obstruction from sudden rupture of the abscess cavity can be rapidly fatal. Aspiration pneumonia and empyema have been described. Abscess extension throughout the neck can cause airway obstruction and infection can extend into the mediastinum. Erosion into the carotid artery and internal jugular vein thrombosis have been reported. Extension to the retroperitoneum, involving the psoas muscle, has been reported.

We acknowledge the previous contributions of Nicholas Relich to this chapter.

REFERENCES

1. Westley CR, Cotton EK, Brooks JG: Nebulized racemic epinephrine by IPPB for the treatment of croup: *Am J Dis Child* 132:484, 1978.

2. Ledwith CA, Shea LM, Mauro RD: Safety and efficacy of nebulized racemic epinephrine in conjunction with oral dexamethasone and mist in the outpatient treatment of croup. *Ann Emerg Med* 25:331, 1995.

3. Prendergast M, Jones JS, Hartman D: Racemic epinephrine in the treatment of laryngotracheitis: Can we identify children for outpatient therapy? *Am J Emerg Med* 12:613, 1994.

4. Rittichier KK, Ledwith CA: Outpatient treatment of moderate croup with dexamethasone: intramuscular versus oral dosing. *Pediatrics* 106:1344, 2000.

5. Klassen TP, Rowe PC: Outpatient management of croup. *Curr Opin Pediatr* 8:449, 1996.

6. Geelhoed GC, Macdonald WPG: Oral and inhaled steroids in croup: A randomized, placebo-controlled trial. *Pediatr Pulmonol* 20:355, 1995.

7. Johnson DW, Schuh S, Koren G, et al: Outpatient treatment of croup with nebulized dexamethasone. *Arch Pediatr Adolesc Med* 150:349, 1996.

8. Klassen TP, Craig WR, Moher D, et al: Nebulized budesonide and oral dexamethasone for treatment of croup: A randomized controlled trial. *JAMA* 279:1629, 1998.

9. Klassen TP, Watters LK, Feldman ME, et al: The efficacy of nebulized budesonide in dexamethasone-treated outpatients with croup. *Pediatrics* 97:463, 1996.

10. Weber JE, Chudnofsky CR, Younger JG, et al: A randomized comparison of helium-oxygen mixture (Heliox) and racemic epinephrine for the treatment of moderate to severe croup. *Pediatrics* 107:E96, 2001.

11. Laks Y, Barzilay Z: Foreign body aspiration in childhood. *Pediatr Emerg Care* 4:102, 1988.

12. Miziara ID, Koishi HU, Zonata AI, et al: The use of ultrasound evaluation in the diagnosis of peritonsillar abscess. *Rev Laryngol Otol Rhinol (Bord)* 122:201, 2001.

13. Scott PM, Loftus WK, Kew J, et al: Diagnosis of peritonsillar infections: A prospective study of ultrasound, computerized tomography, and clinical diagnosis. *J Laryngol Otol* 113:229, 1999.

14. Kew J, Ahuja A, Loftus WK, et al: Peritonsillar abscess appearance on intra-oral ultrasonography. *Clin Radiol* 53:143, 1998.

15. Strong EB, Woodward PJ, Johnson LP, et al: Intraoral ultrasound evaluation of peritonsillar abscess. *Laryngoscope* 105:779, 1995.

16. Ahmed K, Jones AS, Shah K, et al: The role of ultrasound in the management of peritonsillar abscess. *J Laryngol Otol* 108:610, 1994.

17. Buckley AR, Moss EH, Biokmanis A: Diagnosis of peritonsillar abscess; value of intraoral sonography. *AM J Roentgenol* 162:961, 1994.

134 ACUTE PAIN MANAGEMENT AND PROCEDURAL SEDATION IN CHILDREN

Michael N. Johnston
Erica L. Liebelt

Appropriate and safe treatment of pain and anxiety in children is an integral component of an EDs clinical practice. Children are reported to be less adequately treated for pain in the emergency department compared to adults. However, national mandates for hospitals to assess and treat pain adequately have brought about increasing awareness and education to health care providers about this important entity.[1] Indeed, some experts believe that this heightened awareness of pain should be deemed the "fifth vital sign." Furthermore, many of the myths and misperceptions that have contributed to inadequate pain management in children have disappeared in recent years due to the emergence of more scientific evidence, expertise, and education in this area.

Children presenting to the emergency department experience numerous types of acute pain—the most common being that resulting from illness, injury, or from necessary medical procedures. Pediatric pain experience, perception, and expression are determined by many factors, including the nature of the illness, injury, or procedure, developmental level, emotional and cognitive state, personal concerns, the meaning of pain, family attitudes, culture, and the environment. Anything that is painful for an adult is likely to be painful for a child, and it is the responsibility of the emergency medicine physician to recognize, assess, and treat all types of pain.

PAIN ASSESSMENT

Because the ED is a common setting where children in a multitude of different scenarios experience pain, it is extremely important that physicians, nurses, and other health care professionals be familiar with the basic concepts and tools of pain assessment. One comprehensive general approach to pain assessment in children is QUESTT, which includes several assessment strategies providing both qualitative and quantitative information about pain (Table 134-1).[2]

Question the child for a description and location of the pain, using age- and culturally-appropriate and familiar language. A variety of familiar and age-appropriate words such as "owie," "boo boo," or "hurt" may be necessary to describe pain when questioning a child. Toddlers as well as some older children who have difficulty understanding pain scales can usually locate pain by pointing to the affected part.

Use a pain rating scale to provide a quantitative measure of pain intensity. Scales differ in their developmental appropriateness, i.e., the child's ability to grasp numeracy, abstract thought, and pictorial appreciation (Figures 134-1, 134-2, 134-3, and 134-4).

Evaluate behavior and physiologic responses to pain, such as facial expression. This is particularly useful in nonverbal children.

Secure parents' and caregivers' involvement. They know their child best. Parents should be encouraged to participate in their child's pain assessment and management.

Take the cause of pain into account. Because of the nature of emergency medicine, the emergency physician is perhaps most cognizant of the numerous and different types of pain that a child experiences. The nature of the pathology or type of procedure permits anticipation of the type, duration, and intensity of pain. For example, pain caused by a single venipuncture is short in duration as opposed to the persistent pain caused by a migraine headache.

Take action. Ensure that all appropriate modalities are enlisted to treat the specific disorder and the pain, with ongoing assessment and documentation of pain until it is resolved. A child who presents to the ED without a parent or guardian to consent should have severe pain managed without delay. Every institution should have policies that outline the procedures to follow in such cases.

Numerous measures and scales for assessing children's pain have been developed in the last 20 years, and these can be classified as physiologic, behavioral, or self-report, depending on the nature of the response that is measured.[3] Tools specific to an age group or developmental stage should be selected. Children who are developmentally delayed, emotionally disturbed, or non-English speaking require special assessment. Pain severity in infants must be inferred from physiologic and behavioral responses, but for the toddler and older child, subjective measures can be included. Finally, pain measurement should be repeated and improvement assessed until pain has abated.

Objective or Nonself-Report Pain Assessment (Physiologic and Behavioral Scales)

Physiologic changes from pain include tachycardia, tachypnea, crying, sweating, blood pressure elevation, decreased oxygen saturation, pupil

TABLE 134-1   QUESTT Approach for Pain Assessment in Children

Question the child.
Use pain rating scales.
Evaluate behavior and physiological changes.
Secure parents' involvement.
Take cause of pain into account.
Take action and evaluate results.

Source: Data from Baker CM, Wong DL,[2] with permission.

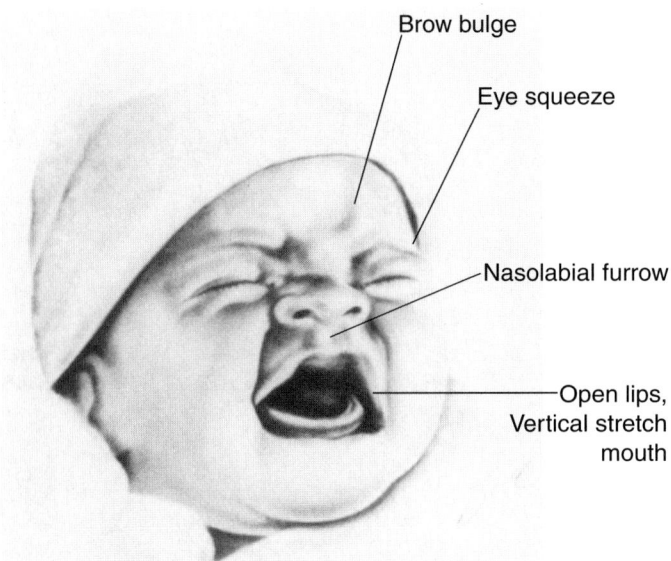

FIG. 134-1. Neonate's facial reaction to painful stimulus. (Reprinted and modified with permission from Grunau RVE, Craig KD, et al: Facial activity as a measure of neonatal pain expression. *Adv Pain Res Ther* 15:147, 1990.)

dilation, flushing or pallor, nausea, and muscle tension. No single physiologic change has been shown to correlate directly with a child's pain experience. These parameters can be muted in persistent pain and can be confounded by fear, anxiety, or fever.

The observation of children's physical behaviors when they experience pain is another method of assessing and measuring their pain. Specific behaviors associated with pain include withdrawal of the painful part, pulling ears, or refusing to use a body part. Facial expression has been demonstrated to be one of the most consistent behavioral indicators of pain. Description of the presence of a brow bulge, eye squeeze, nasolabial furrow, open lips, vertical stretch mouth, horizontal stretch mouth, lip purse, taut tongue, and chin quiver can provide an assessment of infant pain expression (see Figure 134-1).[4]

A number of objective numeric scores have been developed and validated for the assessment of pain intensity for infants and nonverbal toddlers. The CRIES scale was developed for the assessment of postoperative pain in neonates and infants at 32 to 60 weeks of gestation. This scale takes into account cry quality, need for oxygen, changes in heart rate and blood pressure, expression, and state of sleepiness.[5] Another example is The Children's Hospital of Eastern Ontario Pain Scale (CHEOPS), which assesses pain by describing six behaviors—crying, facial expression, verbal expression, torso position, touch behavior, and leg position—on a 13-point scale that ranges from 4 (no pain) to 13 (worst pain).[6] This scale is reliable in children under 5 years of age.

The primary limitation of behavioral scales is that they are indirect measures of children's pain. Children's distress behaviors are not nec-

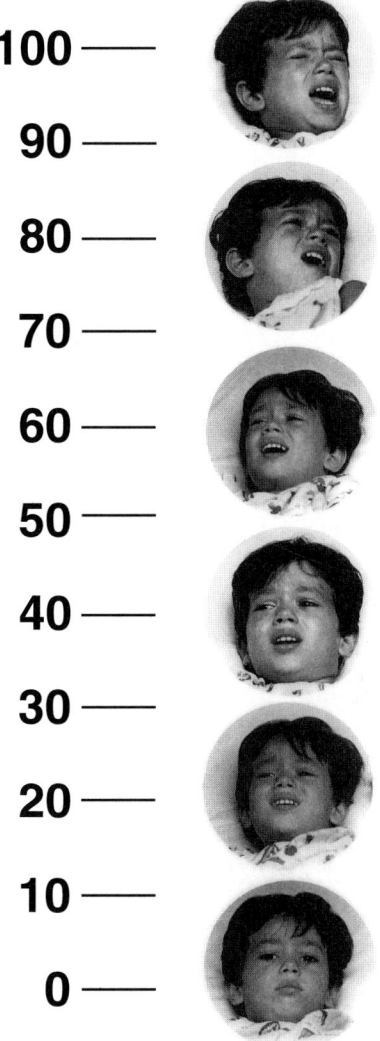

FIG. 134-3. Oucher pain scale. [The Hispanic version of the OUCHER was developed and copyrighted by Antonia M. Villarrael, PhD, RN (University of Pennsylvania) and Mary J. Denyes, PhD, RN (Wayne State University) in 1990. Reprinted with permission.]

essarily direct expressions of the intensity or quality of their pain experiences.

Subjective (Self-Report) Pain Assessment

Self-report pain measures are the gold standard for assessing children's pain. A child's self-report of pain provides direct information about many different aspects of the pain, including the sensory characteristics, the affective component, and other cognitive, behavioral, and emotional factors. Numerous creative and developmentally appropriate pain intensity rating scales have been developed and validated for children. Self-reports can be used reliably for developmentally normal children over the age of 4 years.

Facial expression scales are popular pain assessment tools because they are simple to use, and most children can readily identify with facial expressions of actual children or of cartoon drawings. The Wong-Baker FACES pain scale, which can be used for children age 3 years and up, demonstrates six cartoon facial expressions from "no hurt" to a tearful face representing "the worst hurt you could imagine" (see Figure 134-2).[7] It is useful in the ED setting because the scale is compact and can be purchased in the form of a pin or badge that can be pinned to a coat, making it always available. The OUCHER pain scale

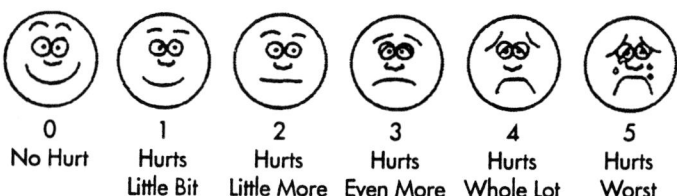

FIG. 134-2. FACES pain scale. (From Wong DL, Hockenberry-Eaton M, Wilson D, et al: *Whaley and Wong's Nursing Care of Infants and Children,* 6th ed. St. Louis, MO: Mosby, 1999, p. 1153. Copyright © Mosby. Reprinted with permission.)

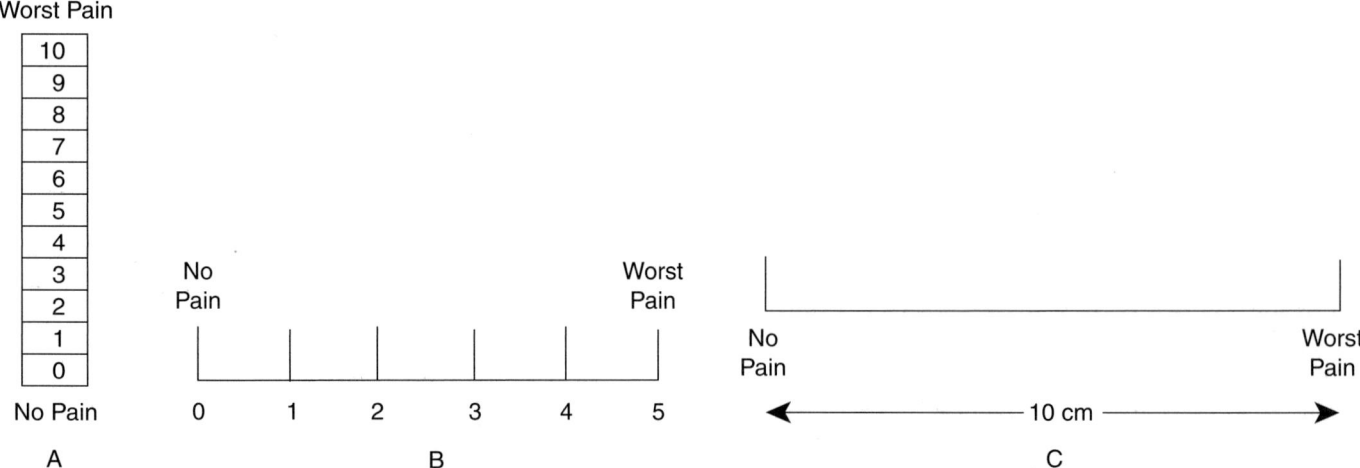

FIG. 134-4. **A.** Pain thermometer. **B.** Numeric rating scale. **C.** Visual analog scale.

is a photographic serial representation of children demonstrating the facial appearance of increasing intensity of pain along a vertical numeric scale ranging from 0 to 100 (see Figure 134-3).[8] There are a number of versions of this assessment tool depicting different ethnic and racial groups.

Numeric scales can be used with children 5 years of age and older, provided that they can count and have a concept of the relative magnitude of numbers (see Figure 134-4). The pain thermometer or pain ladder are examples of such scales. They also have the advantage of not requiring special photographic images. Visual analogue scales (VAS) are simple, versatile, and well-validated scales that are probably best used for the sequential evaluation of pain. A VAS usually consists of a 10-cm horizontal line with endpoints marked as "no pain" and "worst pain possible." The child is asked to place a mark on the line that best describes his or her amount of pain. Then, the distance from the "no pain" end to the mark is recorded. Sequential measurements with a ruler may make this cumbersome for routine assessment in the ED. The colored analogue scale or CAS is similar to a mechanical VAS and was developed specifically for assessing pain in children.[9] Children adjust the position of the slider, and the numbers corresponding to different slider positions are on the back of the scale. Unlike traditional VAS and numeric scales, the CAS varies in three dimensions—color, width, and length—so children can more easily understand that different scale positions reflect different values in pain intensity.

School-aged children and adolescents can use verbal numerical rating scales similar to those used by adults. Children are asked to rate the intensity of pain on a scale of 0 (no pain) to 10 (worst pain). This tool is simple to use, easy to record, and can easily be used for sequential evaluation of pain and response to pain relief interventions.

PAIN TREATMENT

Nonpharmacologic Modalities

Cognitive behavioral and physical techniques are useful nonpharmacologic adjuncts to pediatric acute pain management. Several simple age- and development-specific interventions can significantly decrease a child's anxiety and pain perception. Cognitive behavioral modalities include reassurance and explanation, relaxation, distraction, music, psychoprophylaxis, biofeedback, and guided imagery. Guided imagery can be used with children as young as 3 or 4 years, who have a rich fantasy world and can be encouraged to imagine their favorite place or activity. Environmental alterations such as dimmed lights, a quiet room, or stereo headphones may relieve anxiety. Distraction techniques such as storytelling, singing, and playing games

are effective. Hypnosis has also been shown to be helpful in relieving pain, but may not be practical in a busy emergency department. General strategies for nonpharmacologic pain relief techniques according to age and developmental stage are outlined in Table 134-2. Physical techniques include kinesthetic or tactile stimulation, application of heat and cold, and massage, as well as the more complex modalities of transcutaneous electrical nerve stimulation (TENS), acupuncture, acupressure, and electro-acupressure. Medical play demonstrating to the child what is going to happen is also useful for preschool and school-age children. Open and honest discussion with adolescents about procedures is imperative.

Pharmacologic Modalities

The choice of a pharmacologic agent for a pediatric patient's pain management should consider the nature of the procedure, the duration of the procedure, and the most appropriate route of administration. This choice should be made in conjunction with the use of nonpharmacologic techniques. Pharmacologic analgesic therapy can be categorized into systemic (opioid and nonopioid analgesics) or nonsystemic (local anesthetic agents with topical, local, or regional administration). Avoidance of painful intramuscular and subcutaneous injections when possible is particularly important when treating children. Furthermore, absorption may be erratic and less predictable than with intravenous administration. The intravenous route is recommended for titration of opioid medications. Noninvasive topical or mucosal techniques for the delivery of systemic pharmacologic agents should be used where appropriate.

Suggested systemic medications, dosages, routes of administration, and comments for nonopioid analgesics are outlined in Tables 134-3 and 134-4 and for opioids in Table 134-5. Nonsystemic analgesic medications and techniques for administration, such as local anesthetics, topical anesthetics, and regional anesthetics are discussed in detail in Chap. 37.

Systemic Pharmacologic Agents

ACETAMINOPHEN   Acetaminophen is a commonly-used analgesic and antipyretic that is useful for mild pain and as an adjunct for moderate pain in combination with some opioids. Its analgesic properties do not differ significantly from those of aspirin, but it has a safer profile in the pediatric population. Acetaminophen is a weak inhibitor of prostaglandin biosynthesis and thus possesses only very weak antiinflammatory effects. Acetaminophen is rapidly absorbed from the gastrointestinal tract and onset of action is within 20 to 40 min with a

TABLE 134-2   Selected Nonpharmacologic Pain Management Techniques for Different Ages

Age	Techniques
Infant (0–12 months)	Tactile stimulation: rocking, swaddling, stroking Sucking a pacifier Distraction with bubbles, toys
Toddler (1–3 years)	Tactile stimulation: holding, patting, stroking Distraction with books, puppets, music, action rhymes Parental presence Medical play with a doll and/or equipment before procedure Guided imagery Comfort from blanket or toy from home
Preschooler (4–5 years)	Comfort from blanket or toy from home Medical play with a doll and/or equipment from procedure Guided imagery to remember and play out a superhero story or cartoon character Distraction with music, storytelling, singing a song, reciting nursery rhymes, remembering a movie Reward after procedure with discussion of this prior to procedure
School-age (6–12 years)	Procedural rehearsal and preparation Verbal reward along with toy or other incentive Guided imagery used prior to and during the procedure Breathing and muscle relaxation Thought stopping and positive self-talk during the procedure Parental presence Distraction by listening to music, watching television, or playing video game
Adolescent (>13 years)	Discuss openly issues involving pain Allow teen to choose useful techniques Guided imagery Distraction with music, TV, video games

peak effect in 2 h. The plasma half-life is 1.25 to 3 h, but may be increased by liver disease and following overdose. Acetaminophen is primarily metabolized by the liver through conjugation with a small amount metabolized by the cytochrome P450 enzyme system.

Recent reports about children developing fulminant hepatic liver failure from acetaminophen use emphasize the importance of educating caregivers about appropriate dosing, using the proper measuring device for each acetaminophen formulation, and the appropriate dosing intervals. Most of the reported cases of liver toxicity were due to inappropriate use of acetaminophen in supratherapeutic doses for ex-

tended periods of time, or in children who had underlying risk factors for developing toxicity. Thus it is also important to obtain a detailed history about other medical problems and other medications the child is consuming that may make the child more susceptible to the toxic effects of acetaminophen, even in therapeutic doses. Table 134-3 lists the doses and different formulations for acetaminophen.

TABLE 134-3   Pediatric Dosing Units and Formulations of Acetaminophen

Dose	Max Dose
Oral: 10–15 mg/kg q4h Rectal: 25–40 mg/kg first dose, then 20 mg/kg q6h†	75 mg/kg per d to a total of 4 g/d

Formulation	Mg of Acetaminophen per Dosing Unit
Infant drops (solution, suspension)*	80 mg per 0.8 mL (1 dropperful)
Suspension liquid or elixir*	160 mg per 5 mL (1 teaspoon)
Chewable tablets	80 mg or 160 mg per tablet
Caplets	160, 325, 500, 650 mg per caplet
Tablets	160, 325, 500 mg per tablet
Tablets (extended release)	625 mg per tablet
Suppositories	80, 120, 325, 650 mg per suppository

*The dosing devices that come with the product should be used with that product only.
†*Source:* Birmingham PK, Tobin MJ, Fisher DM, et al: Initial and subsequent dosing of rectal acetaminophen in children: A 24-hour pharmacokinetic study of new dose recommendations. *Anesthesiology* 94:385, 2001.

TABLE 134-4   Pediatric Dosages for Nonsteroidal Anti-Inflammatory Drugs (NSAIDS)

Drugs	Dose (mg/kg per dose)	Comments
Enteral NSAIDS		
Aspirin	Oral: 10–15 mg/kg q4h Rectal: As above	GI irritation Platelet dysfunction Reye syndrome in children Max dose: 4 g/d or 2.5 g/m^2

Ibuprofen
Drops:
  50 mg/1.25 mL
Suspension:
  100 mg/5 mL
Chewables:
  50 mg, 100 mg
Tablets:
  100 mg, 200 mg
	Oral: 7–10 mg/kg q6–8h	GI irritation, bleeding
		Renal insufficiency
		Max dose: 40 mg/kg per d or 2.4 g/d

Naproxen Suspension: 125 mg/5 mL Tablet: 200, 235, 375, 500 mg	Oral: 5–7 mg/kg q8–12h	GI irritation Max dose: 1.5 g/d or 15 mg/kg
Parenteral NSAIDS		
Ketorolac	IV/IM: 0.5–1.0 mg/kg q6h	Max single dose: 30 mg IV, 60 mg IM Max daily total dose: 120 mg/d

TABLE 134-5   Pediatric Dosages for Opioid Analgesics

Drug	Dose Enteral	Dose Parenteral	Duration of Action	Toxicity/Adverse Reactions
Opioids				
Morphine	Oral: 0.3–0.5 mg/kg q4–6h Onset: 15–30 min	IV: 0.05–0.1 mg/kg Onset: 5–10 min IM/SC: 0.1–0.2 mg/kg Onset: 15–30 min	2–4 h	Respiratory depression (esp. with IV push) Hypotension Nausea, vomiting Pruritus
Codeine	Oral: 1–2 mg/kg q4h Onset: 30–60 min	IM: 0.5–1 mg/kg	4 h	Nausea Use with caution in renal failure Not recommended for IV use
Hydromorphone	Oral: 0.03 mg/kg q4–6h Onset: 15–30 min	IV: 0.015 mg/kg Onset: 15 min	2–4 h	Less pruritus than morphine
Meperidine	NA*	IV/IM: 1–2 mg/kg Onset: IV 5–10 min IM 10–15 min	2–3 h	Respiratory depression (esp. with IV push) Hypotension Seizures Avoid with MAO inhibitors
Oxycodone	Oral: 0.1 mg/kg q4h Onset: 10–15 min	NA	3 h	Less nauseating than codeine
Fentanyl	NA	IV: 1–3 μg/kg Onset: 1–2 min	30–60 min	Respiratory depression (esp. with IV push) Chest wall rigidity (see text for treatment) Use $\frac{1}{3}$ dose in children <6 months old
Opioid Antagonist				
Naloxone	NA	IV/IM/IO/ETT: 0.001–0.01 mg/kg	30–40 min	Duration of action is shorter than agonists Potential for hypertension, pulmonary edema, and seizures, particularly in opioid-dependent patients

Abbreviation: NA = not applicable.

ASPIRIN   Aspirin is one of the oldest medications for treating minor pain, but it fell out of favor with the pediatric population with the emergence of acetaminophen in the 1970s. It has the advantage of possessing analgesic, anti-inflammatory, and antipyretic properties. Disadvantages include gastrointestinal irritation, nausea, and inhibition of platelets that can lead to bleeding. Moreover, it may induce bronchospasm in some asthmatic patients. There is a strong association between Reye syndrome and the use of aspirin in children with influenza and varicella. Thus the FDA advises that it not be used in children with these diseases. Dehydrated patients may be more susceptible to salicylate toxicity, even in therapeutic doses. For the management of acute pain, nonsteroidal anti-inflammatory drugs (NSAIDs) are a better choice because they are more potent than aspirin with fewer side effects.

NSAIDs   Nonsteroidal anti-inflammatory drugs (NSAIDs) have become the most commonly used nonopioid medications for treating a wide variety of conditions associated with acute pain in the emergency department, including minor trauma, dysmenorrhea, and headache. Ibuprofen (Advil, Motrin) has anti-inflammatory, analgesic, and antipyretic properties. The analgesic effect is related to inhibition of prostaglandin synthesis through inhibition of cyclooxygenase. It can be used in children over 6 months of age as an alternative to acetaminophen. **NSAIDs should not be given to children with aspirin sensitivity and vice versa, because of cross-sensitivity of aspirin and NSAIDs.** The most frequent adverse effects involve gastrointestinal (GI) tract irritation and renal dysfunction. Renal failure has been reported. Dehydrated patients are at higher risk for renal failure. There is a rare association with aseptic meningitis and severe hepatic reactions. Safety and efficacy have been established for children over 6 months of age. Ibuprofen, like acetaminophen, comes in multiple formulations and caregivers should be instructed on the appropriate dose and time intervals (see Table 134-4). There is no evidence to support the practice of alternating acetaminophen and ibuprofen for superior analgesia. This practice may lead to confusion about dosing and inadvertent overdose.

Ketorolac (Toradol) is an anti-inflammatory, antipyretic, and potent analgesic agent with similar actions and side effect profile to other NSAIDs, with slightly less GI irritation when given intravenously or intramuscularly than oral NSAIDs. Overall, ketorolac has a lower incidence of side effects and longer duration of action than morphine. It acts peripherally, does not affect opiate receptors, and does not cause respiratory depression. Ketorolac is the only intravenous NSAID approved by the FDA. It may be used in combination with opioids, resulting in an opioid-sparing effect. Thus smaller opioid dosages may provide adequate pain relief. It should not be admixed in the same syringe as opiates or hydroxyzine due to incompatibilities. Ketorolac also has good oral bioavailability, but has not been shown to be more efficacious than less expensive NSAID oral preparations. There is limited data on its use in children less than 16 years of age. In addition to GI irritation and platelet effects, ketorolac has been reported to adversely affect renal function, particularly in the dehydrated patient. Additionally, an increased risk of renal failure in patients on diuretics has been reported. Because ketorolac is highly protein-bound, it should be used cautiously in the presence of other protein-bound drugs such as warfarin. Interactions with renal clearance of lithium resulting in increased lithium levels have been reported. There is potential for cumulative adverse effects if ketorolac is combined with aspirin or other NSAIDs. There have been reports of bronchospasm and anaphylactoid reactions in adults. Duration of ketorolac therapy should not exceed 5 days. The efficacy and safety of the new COX-2 inhibitors, celecoxib and rofecoxib, have not been evaluated in children less than 18 years of age.

OPIOIDS   Opioid medications remain the mainstay of analgesic pharmacotherapy for severe pain. Opioids include the phenanthrene derivatives (e.g., morphine, codeine, hydrocodone, hydromorphone, oxycodone, and oxymorphone), the phenylpiperidine derivatives (e.g., meperidine and fentanyl) and the diphenylheptane derivatives (propoxyphene and methadone). **The three classes do not share allergic cross-sensitivity, so a patient with allergy to one class can be**

given an agent from another class. It is important to realize that there is a continuum between systemic analgesia and sedation with opioids. Close clinical and physiologic monitoring is essential with opioid use in the ED patient, as is an understanding of the relationship between level of pain, opioid dose, and conscious state. Opioids in general have analgesic effects at lower doses than those required for sedation.

Opioids are probably used too infrequently and in inadequate doses because of inexperience and unfounded fears of addiction. Most of the opioids can be given orally, intravenously, rectally, sublingually, subcutaneously, or intramuscularly (see Table 134-5). In the ED, the intravenous route is best for the rapid delivery and expeditious control of acute pain. Side effects with these drugs include respiratory depression, nausea, vomiting, pruritus, urticaria, and hypotension.

Adverse cardiorespiratory complications associated with opioid use may depend on the child's age and medical conditions. Infants <3 months of age, premature infants, history of apnea, airway compromise (large tonsils, abnormal airway anatomy), cardiorespiratory disease, hemodynamic instability, obtundation, neuromuscular disease, renal or liver disease, or intracranial hypertension are examples of medical conditions associated with an increased risk of cardiorespiratory complications following opioid administration. The presence of a risk factor does not preclude the use of an opioid analgesic. These children may be safely treated by titrating the medication to effect (which may entail reducing the standard dose by 50 percent) and continuous monitoring with high nursing surveillance.

Morphine remains the gold standard opioid for the management of moderate to severe acute pain. Its oral bioavailability is poor. Infants less than 3 months old are particularly sensitive to its respiratory depressant effects. Morphine induces histamine release and should not be used in children with asthma and in children who are hypovolemic.

Hydromorphone (Dilaudid) is a hydrogenated ketone of morphine and is five to seven times more potent. It is well absorbed following oral, rectal, or parenteral administration. It has a more rapid onset and a shorter duration of action than morphine when given orally. It may produce less sedation, pruritus, and nausea than morphine.

Meperidine (Demerol) is a synthetic derivative of morphine and is one-tenth as potent an analgesic per milligram of drug. Onset and duration of action are shorter than morphine, and meperidine has slightly better oral bioavailability. Normeperidine (6-*N*-desmethylmeperidine) is a toxic meperidine metabolite excreted by the kidney. Normeperidine is a cerebral irritant that can cause effects ranging from dysphoria and irritability to convulsions. Because of the unique toxic metabolite, meperidine is contraindicated in patients with impaired renal function. This metabolite will also accumulate in patients with normal renal function receiving prolonged therapy (e.g., sickle cell vasoocclusive crisis and burn patients). Dangerous drug-drug interactions contraindicate its use in patients on monoamine oxidase inhibitor (MAOI) drugs. Therefore meperidine should be reserved for otherwise healthy children who have demonstrated an unusual reaction or allergic response during treatment with other opioids, such as morphine or hydromorphone.

Fentanyl is a short-acting synthetic opioid, 80 to 100 times as potent as morphine. When administered intravenously it has a rapid onset of action of less than 1 min and a short duration of action (30 to 45 min) due to its high lipid solubility and rapid redistribution. The major ED role for fentanyl is as an analgesic component for short, painful procedures. In infants, it is less of a cardiovascular and respiratory depressant than morphine, and causes less histamine release, but the respiratory depressant effect may lag behind the analgesic effect. Fentanyl is associated with skeletal and thoracic muscle rigidity, especially following rapid intravenous administration. This may cause chest wall rigidity and laryngospasm (glottic rigidity), as well as generalized muscular rigidity. This effect is more likely to occur with high-bolus dosing (5 μg/kg), but can occur with lower dosing (1 to 2 μg/kg) given as a rapid bolus. Small infants, less than 6 months of age, are at greater risk. The management for chest wall rigidity includes: naloxone 0.001 to 0.01 mg/kg or neuromuscular blockade

(succinylcholine 2 mg/kg, or rocuronium 0.6 to 1.0 mg/kg, or pancuronium 0.1 mg/kg), and mechanical ventilation with 100 percent oxygen. Given the high potency of fentanyl, exercise caution to avoid inadvertently flushing a residual bolus of the drug remaining in the intravenous line.

Codeine is readily absorbed from the gastrointestinal tract, and a very useful agent in the ED for adjunct oral pain therapy with acetaminophen. Codeine is usually given orally because it maintains two-thirds of its effectiveness in oral form when compared to parenteral use. It is valuable for moderate pain associated with severe otitis media, dental abscess, or stomatitis. At therapeutic doses, the analgesic effect reaches a peak within 2 h and persists between 4 and 6 h. The plasma concentration does not correlate with brain concentration or relief of pain. Codeine crosses the blood-brain barrier, is found in fetal tissue and breast milk, but is not bound to plasma proteins. The plasma half-life is about 2.9 h. The elimination of codeine is primarily by the kidneys, and about 90 percent of an oral dose is excreted by the kidneys within 24 h of dosing. It can cause extreme nausea and many patients state they are "allergic" to codeine because of the nausea and vomiting.

Hydrocodone (Hycodan) is an oral analgesic that is more potent than codeine with less associated nausea and vomiting. Oxycodone (Roxicodone) is 10 times more potent than codeine and retains about 50 percent of its efficacy when given orally. It is often combined with aspirin (Percodan) or acetaminophen (Percocet, Tylox). Sustained release oxycodone (Oxycontin) has become a popular drug of abuse/street drug. There is no indication for its routine use in the treatment of acute pain in children.

Documented clinical experience is insufficient to establish the safety and an appropriate dosing regimen for propoxyphene in children. Thus it is not recommended for use in pediatric patients.

Nonsystemic Pharmacologic Agents

Nonsystemic topical, local, and regional anesthetic techniques are of great value in the management of painful conditions or procedures in the pediatric ED patient and may minimize the need for opioids and sedatives. The amide and ester local anesthetic medications (lidocaine, bupivacaine, prilocaine, and procaine) and refrigerant agents are the most commonly used nonsystemic agents. Techniques range from topical applications such as lidocaine, epinephrine, and tetracaine (LET) and eutectic mixture of local anesthetics (EMLA), to ethyl chloride, local infiltration of local anesthetics, peripheral nerve block, hematoma block, and intravenous Bier block. The general discussion of these agents as well as specific comments regarding their use in children is found in Chap. 37.

PROCEDURAL SEDATION AND ANALGESIA

Terms and Definitions

Historically, "conscious sedation" was defined as a medically controlled state of depressed consciousness that allows protective reflexes to be maintained, retains the patient's ability to maintain a patent airway independently and continuously, and permits appropriate responses by the patient to physical stimulation or verbal command. Unfortunately, the term "conscious sedation" rapidly became a term that was universally applied to almost every sedation event in the outpatient setting, despite the fact that most sedation events in the ED do not meet this focused definition. The American College of Emergency Physicians in 1998 recommended the term "procedural sedation and analgesia" (PSA) be adopted and published a newer definition of sedation that more clearly reflected how sedation techniques are applied in the ED. This clinical policy defined PSA as "techniques of administering sedatives or dissociative agents with or without analgesia to induce a state that allows the patient to tolerate unpleasant procedures while maintaining cardiorespiratory function. Procedural sedation and analgesia is intended to result in a depressed level of consciousness, but one that allows the patient to maintain airway control independently and, specifically, the drugs, doses, and techniques used are not likely to produce a loss of protective airway reflexes."[10] The Joint Commission on Accreditation of Healthcare Organizations (JCAHO) revised its standards for sedation practices in 2001, dropping the term "conscious sedation" and providing additional definitions for levels of sedation.[11] A universal set of terms and definitions for PSA has recently been proposed (Figure 134-5).[12]

Goals

The goals of pediatric PSA are to minimize pain, fear, and anxiety, maintain patient safety, control behavior, provide amnesia, and return the patient to a state safe for discharge. Factors involved in the selection of the sedation regimen include the specific procedure being performed, duration of the procedure, the developmental age and physical condition of the child, and physician experience with the agents. A checklist of requirements for procedural sedation in children is shown in Table 134-6.

In the ED environment, PSA should only be performed by physicians appropriately skilled in airway and resuscitation management, and only for patients considered to be ASA class E, I, or II, or selected class III, after appropriate consultation (Table 134-7). The American Academy of Pediatrics (AAP) and the American Society of Anesthesiologists (ASA) have published guidelines for monitoring and management of pediatric patients during and after sedation for diagnostic and therapeutic procedures.[13,14] Significant features of these documents are discussed below and should be incorporated into the ED's sedation policy.

Patient Evaluation

The first step is assessment of the patient for sedation in the emergency department. The history should identify any abnormalities of the major organ systems and airway, including current upper respiratory tract infection, fever, and dehydration; previous adverse experience with sedation, analgesia, or anesthesia; any neurologic disorder or impairment; medications and allergies; and time and nature of the patient's last oral intake. Focused physical examination should include baseline vital signs and oxygen saturation, and evaluation of cardiorespiratory status and the oropharynx and airway.

Appropriate candidates for sedation protocols in the ED are healthy patients or patients with mild systemic disease (see Table 134-7). Children with severe systemic disease (ASA III or IV); infants <3 months of age; premature infants <60 weeks postconceptual weeks of age; and children with underlying respiratory or airway disease, neurologic conditions, CNS injury, multiple trauma, or liver or kidney disease are at increased risk for sedation complications and require consultation with an anesthesiologist. For nonemergent sedation, fasting for 2 h from clear liquids and 8 h for solids and nonclear liquids is recommended. However, this length of fasting is often not possible in the busy ED environment. Children requiring urgent or emergent sedation despite recent oral intake should not receive deep sedation to avoid depression of protective airway reflexes that may result in aspiration. Procedures should be delayed, if possible, to facilitate gastric emptying that may decrease the risk of regurgitation and aspiration. Overall, noncompliance with AAP/ASA fasting guidelines for elective sedation is not a contraindication to PSA in the pediatric ED. The potential risk of aspiration appears to be low in most urgent and emergent sedations. However, physicians should always bear in mind the timing of the last oral intake and balance the risks of sedation with the urgency of the needed procedure and planned sedation depth. Routine use of agents such as ranitidine to raise gastric pH or metoclopramide to stimulate gastric emptying is not recommended or supported by current literature. Informed consent should be obtained from the child's

---

Procedural Sedation and Analgesia Definitions and Terminology*

General

PSA: A technique of administering sedatives, analgesics, and/or dissociative agents to induce a state that allows the patient to tolerate unpleasant procedures while maintaining cardiorespiratory function. PSA is intended to result in a depressed level of consciousness but one that allows the patient to maintain airway control independently and continuously. Specifically, the drugs, doses, and techniques used are not likely to produce a loss of protective airway reflexes.

Current Sedation State Terminology

Minimal sedation (anxiolysis): A drug-induced state during which patients respond normally to verbal commands. Although cognitive function and coordination may be impaired, ventilatory and cardiovascular functions are unaffected.

Moderate sedation (formerly "conscious sedation"): A drug-induced depression of consciousness during which patients respond purposefully to verbal commands, either alone or accompanied by light tactile stimulation. Reflex withdrawal from a painful stimulus is not considered a purposeful response. No interventions are required to maintain a patent airway, and spontaneous ventilation is adequate. Cardiovascular function is usually maintained.

Dissociative sedation: A trance-like cataleptic state induced by the dissociative agent ketamine and characterized by profound analgesia and amnesia, with retention of protective airway reflexes, spontaneous respirations, and cardiovascular stability.

Deep sedation: A drug-induced depression of consciousness during which patients cannot be easily aroused but respond purposefully after repeated or painful stimulation. The ability to independently maintain ventilatory function may be impaired. Patients may require assistance in maintaining a patent airway and spontaneous ventilation may be inadequate. Cardiovascular function is usually maintained.

General anesthesia: A drug-induced loss of consciousness during which patients are not arousable, even by painful stimulation. The ability to independently maintain ventilatory function is often impaired. Patients often require assistance in maintaining a patent airway, and positive pressure ventilation may be required because of depressed spontaneous ventilation or drug-induced depression of neuromuscular function. Cardiovascular function may be impaired.

*Adapted from Green SM, Krauss B: Procedural sedation terminology: Moving beyond "conscious sedation." *Ann Emerg Med* 39:433, 2002.

FIG. 134-5. Procedural sedation and analgesia definitions and terminology.

TABLE 134-6   Checklist for Procedural Sedation in Children

__Standardized documents
  __History and physical exam including
    __ASA physical status class I and II
    __Airway evaluation
  __Informed consent
  __Standard chart for records before, during, and after sedation
__Fasting guidelines
  __Last oral intake
    __Solids
    __Liquids
__Personnel
  __Qualifications, training, and duties
    __Physician
    __Nurses
__Monitoring equipment
  __Pulse oximetry
  __Continuous electrocardiogram and respiratory monitoring
  __Blood pressure
__Resuscitation equipment and emergency drugs
  __Suction
  __O_2 and O_2 delivery system
  __Airway equipment
  __Resuscitation drugs
  __Reversal drugs
  __Equipment for venous access
__Recovery area and discharge criteria
  __Personnel
  __Equipment
__Outcome Monitor
  __Standard quality improvement form for Procedural Sedation
    __Indication
    __Drugs used
    __Complications
    __Outcome

Abbreviation: ASA = American Society of Anesthesiologists.

parent or legal guardian with explanations about the procedure, sedation and analgesia plan, and associated risks. All information can be documented on a sedation assessment and monitoring record.

Equipment and Monitoring

The ED must be appropriately equipped for administering sedation to children of all ages and sizes. An oxygen source capable of delivering >90 percent oxygen and positive-pressure ventilation, appropriate size masks, and functioning suction apparatus with Yankauer-tip catheters must be at the child's bedside. Appropriately-sized laryngoscopes, endotracheal tubes, intravenous catheters, and emergency medications must be readily available. Airway management and breathing equipment must be checked before each sedation procedure.

The child should be attached to a cardiac monitor and pulse oximeter. During the procedure, one person whose sole responsibility is monitoring the patient, a registered nurse with basic life support and pediatric advanced life support (PALS) training, or a physician who is not performing the procedure, must be present. Continuous quantita-

TABLE 134-7   American Society of Anesthesiologists Physical Status Classification System

I	Healthy, no underlying organic disease
II	Mild or moderate systemic disease that does not interfere with daily routines
III	Organic disease with definite functional impairment
IV	Severe disease that is life-threatening
V	Moribund
E (suffix)	A procedure undertaken as an emergency

tive monitoring of oxygen saturation (pulse oximetry) and heart rate, and intermittent monitoring of respiratory rate and blood pressure should be recorded at 5- to 10-min intervals. Level of consciousness (response to verbal commands/tactile stimuli) and pulmonary ventilation (observing chest wall excursion and/or auscultation of breath sounds and/or capnography) should also be monitored. Limited studies on end-tidal CO_2 ($ETCO_2$) monitoring during procedural sedation have shown that significant increases in $ETCO_2$ may occur without clinical recognition of hypoventilation. Thus capnography may become an important component of the sedation monitoring armamentarium. All drugs and doses administered must be clearly documented, with special attention to calculation of single and cumulative doses in milligrams per kilogram. After the procedure the child must be observed and monitored in an area with suitable equipment and vital signs recorded every 15 min. Pulse oximetry should be maintained until the patient is fully alert. Observation should be continued until all discharge criteria are met (Table 134-8). Appropriate discharge instructions with follow-up should be conveyed to the child's caretaker.

SEDATION AGENTS AND TECHNIQUES

Indications for sedating infants and children in the emergency department include diagnostic imaging procedures (CT or MRI scans), as an adjunct to analgesia, and anesthesia for painful diagnostic and therapeutic procedures. Table 134-9 lists common pharmacologic options for sedation. Nonpharmacologic techniques should also be considered when preparing to sedate children and should not be forgotten in the midst of a busy emergency department. As previously discussed, parental involvement, verbal preparation, relaxation, tactile stimulation, guided imagery, and distraction techniques are all effective. Manual restraint (sheets or papoose boards) may be required as an adjunct to the nonpharmacologic and pharmacologic approach to procedures for infants and toddlers. Parents should not be asked to provide or be responsible for the restraint of the child, but rather should be encouraged to provide comfort.

An ideal pharmacologic agent for sedation is one that is effective, has rapid onset, is easily titratable with a predictable duration of action, is quickly eliminated or reversible, has no adverse effects, and is easy and painless to administer. Although no ideal agent exists, there are several good drugs and regimens that when administered appropriately can provide safe and adequate analgesia and/or anesthesia. Sedatives can be administered by a variety of routes including intravenous, intramuscular, oral, rectal, sublingual, transmucosal, and intranasal; each route has advantages and disadvantages. Intravenous administration allows the most precise titration of drug to the desired effect; intramuscular administration is usually painful and not titratable (ketamine being the exception). Oral and transmucosal routes are more readily accepted by children than nasal or rectal routes. Despite the options for administration routes, side effects can occur with any route of administration.

Specific Agents

BENZODIAZEPINES   Benzodiazepines provide anxiolysis and amnesia but not anesthesia. They can be used alone as a sedative, or in

TABLE 134-8   Recommended Discharge Criteria

Patient is alert and oriented; infants and those with initially abnormal mental status are at their baseline level of functioning
Vital signs are stable and within age-appropriate limits, including pain level
Protective reflexes are intact (gag, cough, swallow)
Patient does not have protracted nausea and vomiting
Patient is able to ambulate at the preprocedural level
Patient is discharged in the company of a responsible adult
Written instructions given for postsedation diet, medications, activities, and contact phone number in case of emergency

TABLE 134-9 Sedative Drugs for the Pediatric Patient

Drug	Route/Dose	Duration of Action	Contraindication
Benzodiazepines			
Midazolam (Versed)	IV: 0.05–0.1 mg/kg (single max dose 2 mg) Subsequent incremental doses at 3-min intervals to desired effect or up to a total of 0.2 mg/kg IM: 0.3 mg/kg PO: 0.5–0.75 mg/kg (max dose 15 mg) Nasal: 0.3–0.5 mg/kg (max dose 5 mg) PR: 0.5 mg/kg (max dose 15 mg)	30–45 min	Uncontrolled pain CNS depression Shock Hypersensitivity to benzodiazepines
Diazepam (Valium)	IV: 0.1–0.2 mg/kg (max dose 10 mg) PO: 0.2–0.3 mg/kg PR: 0.5 mg/kg	2–6 h	
Barbiturate			
Pentobarbital (Nembutal)	IV/IM: 4–6 mg/kg (max dose 150 mg) PR: <4 y 3–6 mg/kg >4 y 1.5–3.0 mg/kg	2–4 h	CNS depression Hypersensitivity to barbiturates Hepatic impairment Porphyria
Nitrous oxide	50% N_2O/50% O_2 via inhalation	3–5 min after ceasing inhalation	Previous narcotic/sedative within 4 h Impaired mental status Increased ICP or head trauma Intoxication Nausea/vomiting Pregnancy Pneumothorax Bowel obstruction
Ketamine (Ketalar)	IV: 1–2 mg/kg Administer atropine (0.01 mg/kg) concurrently, consider co-administration of midazolam 0.05 mg/kg (max 2 mg) IM: 4–5 mg/kg (combine atropine in the same syringe), consider coadministration of midazolam 0.05 mg/kg (max 2 mg) PO/PR: 10 mg/kg (administer with atropine 0.02 mg/kg) consider coadministration of midazolam 0.5 mg/kg (max 15 mg)	IV: 20–60 min IM: 30–90 min PO/PR: 60–120 min	Age ≤3 months History of airway instability/tracheal stenosis URI/asthma exacerbation Cardiovascular disease/hypertension Increased ICP states (head trauma, hydrocephalus, brain tumor) Poorly controlled seizure disorder Glaucoma or acute globe injury Psychosis, porphyria, thyroid disorder
	REVERSAL AGENTS		
Naloxone (Narcan)	IV/IM: 0.01–0.1 mg/kg per dose (max single dose 2 mg) Repeat to desired effect every 2 m	20–45 min	Use smaller doses 0.001 mg/kg in children dependent on opioids
Flumazenil (Romazicon)	IV/IM: 0.01 mg/kg per dose (max initial dose 0.2 mg) Repeat at 60-s intervals to desired effect or maximum of 0.05 mg/kg or 1.0 mg	20–45 min	Chronic benzodiazepine therapy for seizures Concomitant use of medications that have the potential to cause seizures (tricyclic antidepressants, theophylline, buproprion, isoniazid) Hypersensitivity to benzodiazepines

Abbreviations: ICP = intracranial pressure; URI = upper respiratory infection.

conjunction with a narcotic or local anesthetic for a painful procedure. Midazolam (Versed) is a short-acting benzodiazepine that has an onset of action within 5 min and a duration of action of 30 to 45 min. Midazolam is safe and effective for use in the ED in children undergoing laceration repair, fracture reduction, and other painful procedures. Adverse effects include respiratory depression and paradoxical inconsolability. Anecdotally, this latter effect appears to happen with increased frequency in children with attention deficit hyperactivity disorder, and is reversible with flumazenil.

Diazepam (Valium) is a longer-acting benzodiazepine that has been used extensively as a sedative for children and has amnestic properties. Diazepam can be used for extended diagnostic procedures and for muscle relaxation for orthopedic reductions. It has been largely replaced by midazolam.

SEDATIVE/HYPNOTICS Chloral hydrate is a pure sedative/hypnotic with no analgesic properties that has been used primarily for sedation of infants and young children requiring painless diagnostic procedures.[15] The time to sedation is relatively long (45 to 60 min) and its effects can last several hours because of its active metabolite, trichloroethanol, making it an impractical agent for use in the ED. Adverse effects include nausea, vomiting, and paradoxical delirium/excitement, which are not reversible. Serious adverse effects including airway obstruction and death have been reported with chloral hydrate use. It is not recommended for use in the busy ED environment.

The short-acting barbiturates can provide rapid onset of sedation for painless procedures such as computed tomography and magnetic resonance imaging studies in children with no preexisting central nervous system depression.[16] Again, they have no analgesic or amnestic properties. Intravenous pentobarbital has an onset of action within 30 s and children are usually appropriately sedated within 5 min. Its duration of action is 30 to 60 min, making it a better choice for children undergoing emergent procedures. Respiratory and central nervous system (CNS) depression can occur that can be exacerbated in the presence of other depressants such as opioids and benzodiazepines; patients must be closely monitored.

Methohexital is an ultra short-acting barbiturate similar to thiopental. It has been given rectally at doses of 20 to 25 mg/kg for induction of anesthesia in the past. More recently, intravenous use has been reported for sedation during painful procedures and radiologic imaging studies.[16,17] The average intravenous dose is 1 mg/kg. Care must be taken as methohexital can cause myoclonus and may induce seizures in patients with temporal lobe epilepsy. Again, respiratory and CNS depression can occur, especially when given concurrently with other depressants such as opioids and benzodiazepines. More experience is needed before this agent can be recommended for routine use.

Etomidate is an ultra short-acting sedative hypnotic when given intravenously. It is routinely used in many EDs for rapid sequence intubation. As a newer agent for PSA, there are few published studies in children.[18,19] It has minimal hemodynamic effects on patients; myocardial oxygen consumption is unchanged. Reported adverse effects are pain on injection, nausea, vomiting, myoclonus, and short-term adrenal suppression (more commonly seen with long-term use). It has no analgesic properties and therefore must be coadministered with an analgesic for painful procedures. Limited evidence suggests doses of 0.1 to 0.2 mg/kg given as an IV bolus. Again, respiratory and CNS depression can occur, especially when given concurrently with other depressants such as opioids and benzodiazepines. More experience is needed before this agent can be recommended for routine use in children.

NARCOTICS   A discussion of individual narcotics is found in the preceding analgesia and pain management section. Narcotics can be administered intravenously in conjunction with an anxiolytic such as a benzodiazepine for sedation for painful procedures.

NITROUS OXIDE   Limited studies in children have shown nitrous oxide (N_2O) to be an effective and safe sedative/analgesic either alone or in combination with a local anesthetic for laceration repair, orthopedic procedures, and other minor surgical procedures.[20,21] It offers many advantages over other pharmacologic agents for use in the outpatient setting and ED. It provides analgesia, anxiolysis, and sedation without the need for intravenous line placement, has a low incidence of complications and adverse effects, and can result in shorter ED lengths of stay due to rapid recovery. Nitrous oxide interacts with the endogenous opioid system to confer analgesia and appears to blunt the patient's reaction to pain. It produces a sense of euphoria, relief from anxiety, and an almost detached attitude toward pain and the patient's surroundings.

In the outpatient setting, nitrous oxide should be delivered as a fixed-ratio mixture of nitrous oxide to oxygen, usually 50 percent N_2O to 50 percent oxygen (oxygen concentration must be a minimum of 30 percent) by a self-administered demand-valve apparatus with a scavenger device. This mode of administration protects against equipment failure and/or human error, which may result in too high a concentration of nitrous oxide. The gas is routinely delivered by an inspiratory effort of the patient, minimizing the risk of loss of consciousness and protective reflexes because the mask will fall off when the patient is sedated. The gas/oxygen mixture can be inhaled through a face mask, mouthpiece, or nasal hood in which a flavored lip balm lining or concentrated "child-friendly" scent can be applied to disguise the odor of the gas. For younger children unable to hold their own mask, the physician or parent can assist in the delivery of the mixture by placing the mask lightly on the child's face.

Nitrous oxide has a rapid onset of action of 3 to 5 min and a short duration of action on withdrawal of 3 to 5 min. The gas is not metabolized, and is eliminated by the lungs unchanged. Short-term use has no significant effects on other organs. The most commonly reported side effects are nausea and vomiting. Diffusional hypoxia is another potential concern since nitrous oxide rapidly diffuses out of the blood and into the alveoli, where it can displace oxygen and cause hypoxia. This theoretical concern has not been supported by clinical evidence. Nevertheless, supplemental oxygen should be administered throughout the recovery phase. Nitrous oxide use in the ED also has the potential for abuse, environmental contamination, and potential teratogenic effects, especially with chronic exposure. The use of nitrous oxide is contraindicated in patients with pneumothoraces, bowel obstruction, middle ear effusions, and patients undergoing procedures using balloon-tipped catheters because of its rapid diffusion into gas-collecting areas of the body, which could cause acute expansion, overdistension, and perforation. It also should be avoided in patients with head injuries, psychiatric diseases, or drug intoxication. Because of nitrous oxide's opioid agonist properties, it may result in deep sedation or general anesthesia if combined with a sedative or opioid. Thus extreme caution should be exercised when administering it to a patient with recent administration of either of these medications.

KETAMINE   Ketamine is a unique sedative analgesic that has been studied extensively in children undergoing outpatient procedures.[22–24] PSA using ketamine should be referred to as dissociative sedation, reflecting its unique properties.[25] A derivative of phencyclidine, ketamine produces a dissociative effect resulting in a trancelike cataleptic state, providing a combination of sedation, amnesia, and analgesia. Spontaneous respirations and pharyngeal muscular tone are maintained, as well as protective airway reflexes of coughing and swallowing. Ketamine has very few negative inotropic effects, making it a reasonable option for acutely ill patients. Its sympathomimetic actions may produce mild to moderate increases in heart rate, blood pressure, and cardiac output. However, in the catecholamine-depleted child, use of ketamine may result in hypotension due to unopposed direct vasodilatory effects. It also is a good option for the difficult-to-control child with mental retardation or behavioral disorder, in whom initial intravenous access can be difficult to obtain. Clinical effects from intravenous and intramuscular ketamine occur within several minutes and last about 30 min. It has also been shown to be effective when administered by the transmucosal, oral, and rectal routes. Because ketamine stimulates salivary and tracheobronchial secretions, it should be administered concurrently with an anticholinergic drug, either atropine or glycopyrrolate. Both agents may be combined in a single intramuscular injection. Hallucinatory emergence reactions have been reported with ketamine, although less frequently in children less than 10 years of age. Whether a benzodiazepine should always be given with ketamine is controversial. Recent studies suggest that the administration of midazolam with ketamine does not reduce the overall incidence of emergence reactions in children, but may decrease the incidence of vomiting in children less than 10 years old.[26,27] This combination may prolong the patient's recovery time because benzodiazepines will inhibit ketamine's metabolism. Ketamine can also cause increased intracranial and intraocular pressure because of increased cerebral blood flow. Other adverse effects are nystagmus, random limb movement, ataxia (may last up to 24 h), and vomiting. Ketamine has the potential for causing laryngospasm and thus should not be used in patients with upper respiratory or pulmonary infections or who have increased salivary secretions. If laryngospasm occurs, the child should be ventilated with a bag-valve-mask. Paralysis and emergent intubation must be performed if this is unsuccessful. Contraindications to ketamine's use are age ≤3 months; history of airway instability or tracheal stenosis; procedures involving stimulation of the posterior pharynx; cardiovascular disease including congestive heart failure and hypertension; head injury associated with loss of consciousness, altered mental status, central nervous system masses, abnormalities, or hydrocephalus; poorly controlled seizure disorder; glaucoma; acute globe injury; or psychosis.

Other Agents

Propofol is an ultra short-acting intravenous anesthetic marketed in the United States as Diprivan. It has been reported as a safe and effective nonanesthetic sedative for adults undergoing fracture reduction, reduction of joint dislocations, minor surgical procedures (incision and drainage of abscesses), cardioversion, and chest tube placement in the ED.[28] It has been used in the ICU setting in pediatric patients.[29] Propofol has been used in children in the ED for difficult fracture reduction, incarcerated inguinal hernia reductions, laceration repair, foreign body removal, and cardioversion.[30,31] Propofol's onset of action occurs within seconds and its duration of action is extremely short, requiring continuous infusion for maintenance of clinical effects. After discontinuation of the drug in sedative doses, patients are usually awake and responsive within minutes. It does not possess any analgesic properties in sedative doses and must be used in conjunction with narcotics for painful procedures. Propofol has potent dose-related respiratory depressant effects, may quickly result in deep sedation, and may produce hypotension. More experience is needed before it can be recommended for routine use in children in the ED.

In the past, the "DPT cocktail," consisting of Demerol (meperidine), Phenergan (promethazine), and Thorazine (chlorpromazine), was a popular sedative/analgesic choice for children in the emergency department. Unfortunately, the intramuscular route does not allow for titration of effects and its onset of action is variable. The wide range of doses used and combination of three sedatives adds to confusion and potential for serious respiratory depression. In addition, the efficacy of this "cocktail" can be variable, while its duration of action can be several hours, making it a poor choice for sedation in the ED.[32]

Reversal Agents

Naloxone is an opioid antagonist that should be readily available for reversal of respiratory depression, apnea, and severe hypotension. It can be administered in incremental doses of 0.01 to 0.1 mg/kg (maximum single dose 2 mg) to the desired reversal of life-threatening effects, because it would not be desirable to reverse all of the analgesia in a patient undergoing a painful procedure. Naloxone's duration of action is short (approximately 45 min); thus reversal of toxic effects of longer-acting opioids such as morphine, or large doses of short-acting opioids such as fentanyl, may require additional doses.

Flumazenil is a benzodiazepine antagonist that reverses the central nervous system depression, and to some degree the respiratory depression, secondary to inadvertent excess sedation. Incremental doses of 0.01 to 0.02 mg/kg (maximum single dose 0.2 mg) every 1 to 2 min can be titrated to the desired reversal effect. Respiratory depression and hypoventilation should be managed with standard airway management techniques and assisted ventilation if necessary. Flumazenil has also been shown to reverse the paradoxical delirium secondary to midazolam.[33] In the setting of a polypharmaceutical overdose, flumazenil should not be administered. It should not be used in patients on chronic benzodiazepine therapy or on tricyclic antidepressant medications because of the risk of seizures. Flumazenil's duration of action is about 40 to 60 min. Because the duration and degree of reversal depends on the plasma concentrations of benzodiazepine as well as the amount of flumazenil given, the sedative and respiratory depressive effects of the benzodiazepine may last longer than the antagonism produced by flumazenil. Both drugs should be readily available and appropriate doses calculated prior to initiation of the procedure.

REFERENCES

1. Committee on Psychosocial Aspects of Child and Family Health, American Academy of Pediatrics: The assessment and management of acute pain in infants, children, and adolescents. *Pediatrics* 108:793, 2001.
2. Baker CM, Wong DL: Q.U.E.S.T: A process of pain assessment in children. *Orthop Nurs* 6:8, 1987.
3. Liebelt E: Assessing children's pain in the emergency department. *Clin Pediatr Emerg Med* 1:260, 2000.
4. Grunau RVE, Craig KD: Pain expression in neonates: Facial action and cry. *Pain* 28:395, 1987.
5. Krechel SW, Bildner J: CRIES: a new neonatal postoperative pain measurement score. Initial testing of validity and reliability. *Paediatr Anaesth* 5:53, 1995.
6. McGrath PJ, Johnson G, Goodman JT, et al: CHEOPS: A behavioral scale for rating postoperative pain in children. *Adv Pain Res Ther* 9:395, 1985.
7. Wong DL, Hockenberry-Eaton M, Wilson D, et al: *Wong's Essentials of Pediatric Nursing,* 6th ed. St. Louis, MO: Mosby, 2001.
8. Beyer J, Aradine C: Content validity of an instrument to measure young children's perceptions of the intensity of their pain. *J Pediatr Nurs* 1:386, 1986.
9. Tyler DC, Tu A, Douthit J, et al: Toward validation of pain measurement tools for children: a pilot study. *Pain* 52:301, 1993.
10. American College of Emergency Physicians: Clinical policy for procedural sedation and analgesia in the emergency department. *Ann Emerg Med* 31:663, 1998.
11. Joint Commission on Accreditation of Healthcare Organizations: 2001 sedation and anesthesia care standards. Available at: http://www.jcaho.org/accredited+organizations/hospitals/standards/revisions/2001/sedation+and+anesthesia+care.htm. Accessed June 20, 2002.
12. Green SM, Krauss B: Procedural sedation terminology: Moving beyond "conscious sedation." *Ann Emerg Med* 39:433, 2002.
13. Committee on Drugs, American Academy of Pediatrics: Guidelines for monitoring and management of pediatric patients during and after sedation for diagnostic and therapeutic procedures. *Pediatrics* 89:1110, 1992.
14. American Society of Anesthesiologists: Practice guidelines for sedation and analgesia by nonanesthesiologists. *Anesthesiology* 96:1004, 2002.
15. Binder LS, Leake LA: Chloral hydrate for emergent pediatric procedural sedation: A new look at an old drug. *Am J Emerg Med* 9:530, 1991.
16. Pomeranz ES, Chudnofsky CR, Deegan TJ, et al: Rectal methohexital sedation for computed tomography imaging of stable pediatric emergency department patients. *Pediatrics* 105:1110, 2000.
17. Sedik H: Use of intravenous methohexital as a sedative in pediatric emergency departments. *Arch Pediatr Adolesc Med* 155:665, 2001.
18. Ruth WJ, Burton JH, Bock AJ: Intravenous etomidate for procedural sedation in emergency department patients. *Acad Emerg Med* 8:13, 2001.
19. Dickinson R, Singer AJ, Carrion W: Etomidate for pediatric sedation prior to fracture reduction. *Acad Emerg Med* 8:74, 2001.
20. Burton JH, Auble TE, Gillman MA: Effectiveness of 50% nitrous oxide/50% oxygen during laceration repair in children. *Acad Emerg Med* 5:112, 1998.
21. Gamis AS, Knapp JF, Mathias S: Nitrous oxide analgesia in a pediatric emergency department. *Ann Emerg Med* 18:177, 1989.
22. Green SM, Rothrock SG, Lynch EEL, et al: Intramuscular ketamine for pediatric sedation in the emergency department: Safety profile in 1,022 cases. *Ann Emerg Med* 31:688, 1998.
23. Green SM, Rothrock SG, Harris T, et al: Intravenous ketamine for pediatric sedation in the emergency department: Safety profile with 156 cases. *Acad Emerg Med* 5:971, 1998.
24. Green SM, Hummel CB, Wittlake WA, et al: What is the optimal dose of intramuscular ketamine for pediatric sedation? *Acad Emerg Med* 6:21, 1999.
25. Green SM, Krauss B: The semantics of ketamine. *Ann Emerg Med* 36:480, 2000.
26. Wathen JE, Roback MG, Mackenzie T, et al: Does midazolam alter the clinical effects of intravenous ketamine sedation in children? A double-blind, randomized, controlled emergency department trial. *Ann Emerg Med* 36:579, 2000.
27. Sherwin TS, Green SM, Khan A, et al: Does adjunctive midazolam reduce recovery agitation after ketamine sedation for pediatric procedures? A randomized, double-blind, placebo controlled trial. *Ann Emerg Med* 35:229, 2000.

28. Swanson ER, Seaberg DC, Mathias S: The use of propofol for sedation in the emergency department. *Acad Emerg Med* 3:234, 1995.
29. Hertzog JH, Campbell JK, Dalton HJ, et al: Propofol anesthesia for invasive procedures in ambulatory and hospitalized children: Experience in the pediatric intensive care unit. *Pediatrics* 103:e30, 1999.
30. Havel CJ Jr, Strait RT, Hennes H: A clinical trial of propofol versus midazolam for procedural sedation in a pediatric emergency department. *Acad Emerg Med* 6:989, 1999.
31. Skokan EG, Pribble C, Bassett KE, et al: Use of propofol sedation in a pediatric emergency department: A prospective study. *Clin Pediatr* 40:663, 2001.
32. American Academy of Pediatrics Co: Reappraisal of lytic cocktail/demerol, phenergan, and thorazine (DPT) for the sedation of children. *Pediatrics* 95:598, 1995.
33. Shannon M, Albers G, Burkhart K, et al: Safety and efficacy of flumazenil in the reversal of benzodiazepine-induced conscious sedation. *J Pediatr* 131:582, 1997.

135 PEDIATRIC EXANTHEMS

Michael S. Weinstock
Alexander M. Rosenau

Rashes represent skin signs that are useful in making the diagnosis of a variety of infectious and noninfectious illnesses. Rashes with diverse etiologies can look alike. An assessment of the signs and symptoms preceding or presenting along with the exanthem augment an accurate history in determining the diagnosis. Useful historical data includes prior immunizations, potential human or animal contacts, and recent environmental exposure.

Concerns for bioterrorism make it necessary for the emergency physician to recognize rare disorders such as cutaneous anthrax and variola, which are discussed below.

Another important concern for emergency medicine is the evaluation of rashes in large numbers of U.S. schoolchildren. Epidemics of nonspecific rashes in schoolchildren have been reported in 27 states and Canada since October 2001,[1] affecting up to 47 percent of children in some schools. The rashes are variously described as pruritic and erythematous, involving primarily the cheeks and arms, or as migratory urticaria. There are no associated systemic symptoms, and the rash is self-limited. Parvovirus B19 has been suspected as the cause in some cases, but the cause has not been determined in the vast majority of reported epidemics. The Centers for Disease Control and Prevention (CDC) recommends that epidemic-type rashes in schoolchildren be reported to the local health department. Information gathering should include (1) collect uniform information from patients so that rashes in schools can be differentiated from other types of rashes; (2) determine if family members or non-school contacts are affected; (3) provide follow-up to ensure that rashes have resolved; and (4) evaluate any associated systemic signs and symptoms.

The various etiologic agents and associated exanthems are noted in Tables 135-1, 135-2, and 135-3. Further discussion of cutaneous disorders is found in Section 21 and in general texts of dermatology.[2,3]

BACTERIAL

Bullous Impetigo

Bullous impetigo, or staphylococcal impetigo, is a local skin infection caused by phage group II staphylococci. The staphylococci produce an epidermolytic toxin that acts locally to cause separation of the skin at the granular layer, giving rise to bullae. The infection occurs primarily in newborn infants and young children. The characteristic skin lesions of bullous impetigo are superficial, flaccid, thin-walled bullae that oc-

cur most often on the extremities but can occur anywhere. They range in size from 0.5 to 3 cm. They can arise from normal skin or may have a thin, red halo. The bullae are filled with a clear, pale-to-yellow fluid and rupture easily, leaving a moist, denuded base that dries rapidly with a shiny coating. Extensive areas of skin may be involved if left untreated.

The clinical appearance of the lesions usually makes diagnosis easy. However, single lesions or extensive involvement may not be as typical. Staphylococci cultured from the fluid of aspirated bullae will establish the diagnosis.

Systemic antistaphylococcal antibiotics, usually oral, along with local wound cleansing and topical antibiotics (such as Neosporin) are effective in eradicating the infection. Prognosis for complete recovery is good.

Impetigo Contagiosum

Impetigo is a superficial pyoderma caused by infection with staphylococci, although group A β-hemolytic streptococci may also be cultured. It is a common skin infection, primarily affecting young children, especially in warm, humid conditions. Impetigo can arise at the site of insect bites or superficial cutaneous trauma; sometimes there is no apparent predisposing skin lesion. Fever and systemic signs are uncommon.

The skin lesions start as small erythematous macules and papules. These develop into discrete, thin-walled vesicles, which become pustular and quickly rupture (Figure 135-1). As the vesicles rupture, a yellow fluid forms an exudate, which dries to form a stratified golden yellow crust that accumulates. The crusts can be readily removed, leaving a smooth, red surface. The crusts can spread the infection to other parts of the body. Initially the lesions are discrete, but they may enlarge and become confluent. Local adenopathy may be present. The infection occurs most frequently on the face, neck, and extremities.

The diagnosis of impetigo can be readily made on the basis of the typical clinical appearance. Cultures are generally not necessary. Systemic antibiotic therapy must be combined with wound scrubbing and cleansing and application of Neosporin or mupirocin ointment for optimal results. Effective antibiotics include oral antibiotics such as

TABLE 135-1   Different Causes of Exanthems

Vesiculopustules	*Maculopapules*
Drug eruption	Drug eruption
Herpes simplex	Secondary lues
Variola	Scarlet fever
Vaccinia	Echovirus 9, 16
Varicella	Coxsackie A5, A9, A16, B5
Generalized zoster	Reovirus 2
Rickettsialpox	Erythema infectiosum
Coxsackie A and B	Gianotti-Crosti syndrome
Reovirus 2	Rubella
Mycoplasma pneumonia	Rubeola
Echovirus 4	Hepatitis
Contagious ecthyma (orf)	Infectious mononucleosis
	Arbovirus (dengue)
	Rickettsioses
Urticaria	*Petechiae*
Varicella (urticaria around vesicle)	Drug eruption
Coxsackie A5, A9	Bacterial endocarditis
Infectious hepatitis	Echovirus
Mononucleosis	Coxsackie A5, A9
Mycoplasma pneumoniae	Mononucleosis
Hepatitis	Rubella
	Thrombocytopenia with many acute infectons

Source: From Burnett JW, Crutcher WA, in Moschella SL, Hurley HJ (eds): *Dermatology.* Philadelphia: Saunders, 1985, with permission.

TABLE 135-2 Selected Seasonal Rashes

Summer	Fall	Winter	Spring
Enteroviruses	Enteroviruses	Varicella	Rickettsia
Rickettsia	Rickettsia		Rubella
	Pityriasis rosea		Varicella
			Pityriasis rosea

erythromycin, clindamycin, cephalosporins, amoxicillin-clavulanate and dicloxacillin.

Erysipelas

Erysipelas, or St. Anthony's fire, is cellulitis and lymphangitis of the skin caused by group A β-hemolytic streptococci. It is frequently accompanied by fever, chills, malaise, headache, and vomiting.

The rash is characterized by local redness, heat, swelling, and a raised, indurated border. There is marked involvement of the superficial dermal lymphatics. The rash starts as an erythematous plaque that rapidly enlarges by peripheral extension. At first, it is scarlet, hot, brawny, swollen, and tender. The edge is raised and sharply demarcated. The rash can vary in appearance from a transient hyperemia to intense inflammation, vesiculation, and bulla formation. The face is the most frequent site. A skin wound, fissure, or ulcer may act as a portal of entry.

Diagnosis is made on clinical grounds, although aspiration of the leading edge of the lesion will frequently demonstrate streptococci. A brief course of parenteral penicillin is usually warranted because of the rapid advancement of the infection, the acutely toxic state of the patient, and the possibility of suppurative complications. Rapid clinical response is usually obtained. Macrolide antibiotics may be used in patients unable to take penicillin.

Mycoplasma Infections

Mycoplasma pneumoniae infections are a common cause of pneumonia, upper respiratory infections, and bronchitis in children between 5 and 19 years of age. The most frequent presenting clinical findings in children and adults are fever, cough, sore throat, malaise, headache, chills, and rash. An erythematous maculopapular rash, the most frequent presentation, is located on the trunk and may be discrete or confluent. However, the most frequently reported exanthem is consistent with erythema multiforme and Stevens-Johnson syndrome, with lesions occurring primarily on the trunk, legs, and arms. The rash occurs most commonly during the febrile period. An enanthem of generalized ulcerative stomatitis or pharyngitis-tonsillitis associated with the exanthem is common. The diagnosis can be confirmed by the use of either serum cold agglutinins or several specific antibody tests.

Mycoplasma responds to several antimicrobials, including erythromycin, azithromycin, fluoroquinolones, and doxycycline. Infection with *M. pneumoniae* should be suspected in patients with pneumonia and a rash.

Scarlet Fever

Scarlet fever is an acute febrile illness, primarily affecting young children, caused by group A β-hemolytic streptococci. Recently group C streptococci have been implicated as well. Clinical manifestations include acute onset with fever, sore throat, headache, vomiting, and abdominal pain followed by a distinctive exanthem in 1 to 2 days.

There are both an exanthem and an enanthem associated with scarlet fever. They are caused by an erythrogenic toxin elaborated by the streptococcal organism. The tonsils and pharynx are red and covered with exudate, although occasionally pharyngeal findings are minimal. The tongue has a white coating through which red and hypertrophied papillae project, creating the appearance of a "white strawberry tongue." The white coating disappears by day 4 or 5, and the tongue acquires a bright-red appearance, the "red strawberry tongue." Bright-red or hemorrhagic spots may be seen on the soft palate or anterior pillars of the tonsillar fossae.

The exanthem of scarlet fever begins 1 or 2 days after the onset of the illness. It starts on the neck, axillae, and groin, spreading to the trunk and extremities. The rash is red and finely punctate, consisting of 1- to 2-mm papules that give the rash a characteristic rough, sandpaper feel. It is sometimes easier to identify the rash by palpation. The rash blanches with pressure. Linear petechial eruptions, Pastia's lines, are often present in the antecubital and axillary folds. There is facial flushing with circumoral pallor. A brawny desquamation occurs at 2 weeks, yielding fine flakes of dry skin.

The diagnosis of scarlet fever is readily made on clinical grounds. Throat swabs usually culture group A β-hemolytic streptococci, al-

TABLE 135-3 Disease Descriptions

	Season	Rash	Fever	Vesicles
Coxsackie hand, foot, and mouth	Summer Fall	Palm Sole Buttock Mouth Tongue Gingiva Soft palate Buccal	Yes	4–8 mm vesicle
Coxsackie herpangina	Summer Fall	Posterior pharynx Tonsil Uvula Soft palate Faucial pillars	Yes	2 mm pharynx vesicles 2–4 mm ulcers (crater)
Herpes labialis	Anytime	Gingiva Lip Hard palate	Yes/No	Vesicles
Herpetic gingivostomatitis	Anytime	Anterior two-thirds of oral cavity, including alveola of gingiva. *Note:* coxsackie lesions favor the posterior pharynx	Yes	Vesicles

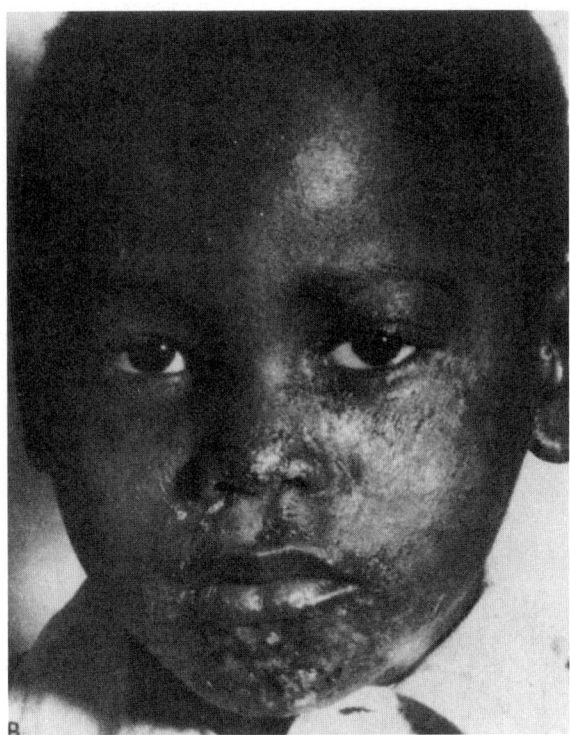

FIG. 135-1. Impetigo contagiosum. [Reproduced with permission from Marples RR, Leyden JL: Bacterial infections, section I, fundamental cutaneous microbiology, in SL Moschella, HJ Hurley (eds): *Dermatology.* Philadelphia, PA: Saunders, 1985, pp. 590.]

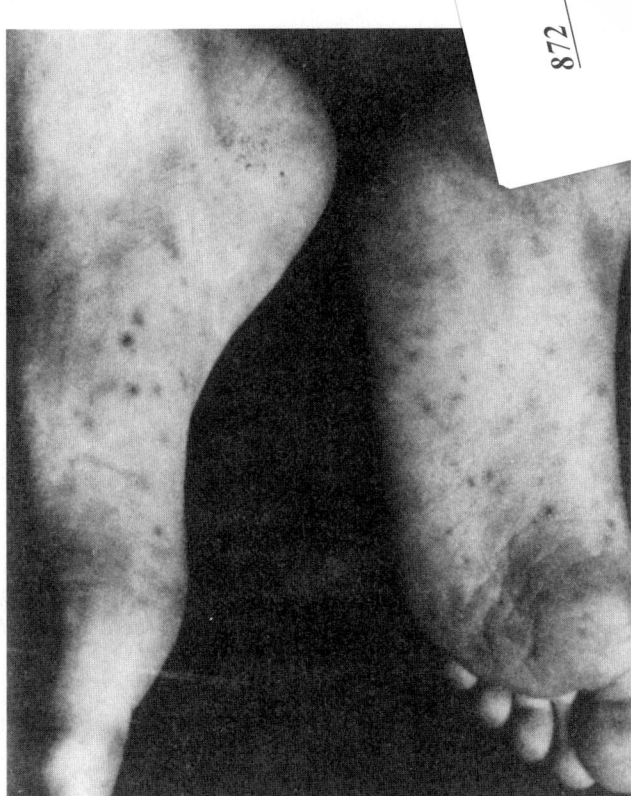

FIG. 135-2. Rocky Mountain spotted fever. [Reproduced with permission from Burnett JW, Crutcher WA: Viral and rickettsial infections, in SL Moschella, HJ Hurley (eds): *Dermatology.* Philadelphia, PA: Saunders, 1985, pp. 673.]

though group C may be cultured as well. Treatment with antibiotics is necessary to reduce the incidence of rheumatic fever and nephritis, and will probably ameliorate the course of the disease. Penicillin is the antibiotic of choice, or use one of the macrolides for those who are penicillin-allergic.

RICKETTSIAL

Rocky Mountain Spotted Fever

Rocky Mountain spotted fever (RMSF) is an infectious disease caused by *Rickettsia rickettsii,* which is transmitted by ticks. The prominent clinical manifestations of RMSF can be directly related to the primary pathologic lesion in the endothelial cells lining small blood vessels where the organism multiplies. Rash, headache, mental confusion, terminal heart failure, and shock are manifestations of the generalized vasculitis.

The incubation period is from 2 to 12 days with either a sudden or gradual onset of symptoms. Peak severity usually occurs within 1 to 2 weeks. Headache, fever, toxicity, rash, and myalgia are the major clinical features. The rash (Figure 135-2), a pathognomonic feature of the disease, usually appears on the second or third day. The initial lesions first appear on the wrist and ankles, spreading rapidly to the extremities and trunk. These lesions also are found on the palms and soles of the patient. Initially lesions are small, erythematous macules that blanch on pressure. They rapidly become maculopapular and petechial.

Laboratory diagnostic confirmation is difficult during the early phase of the disease, frequently mandating treatment based on clinical criteria. Serologic tests are used to confirm the diagnosis of RMSF. Some laboratory data may be helpful in establishing the presumptive diagnosis early, such as hyponatremia, leukopenia, and thrombocytopenia.

Specific therapy consists of doxycycline or chloramphenicol. In seriously ill children over the age of 8, doxycycline is given at a dose of 2 to 4 mg/kg per d, divided in two doses. Chloramphenicol 100 mg/kg per d, in four divided doses, up to 3 g, is an alternative. Treatment can be terminated 2 or 3 days after fever returns to normal for 24 h. The mortality of RMSF in the United States has held steady for a decade at 3 to 6 percent of identified cases despite treatment.

VIRUSES

Enteroviruses

Enteroviruses are an exceedingly common cause of illness and exanthem in young children. Enteroviruses are small, single-stranded RNA viruses belonging to the picornavirus group and consist of polioviruses and nonpolioviruses (coxsackievirus and echovirus). There are many types of coxsackieviruses and echoviruses that have been associated with illnesses. They usually occur in epidemics and are most prevalent in the summer and early fall. Transmission usually occurs by the fecal-oral route and possibly by the respiratory route.

The clinical manifestations of infection with coxsackieviruses and echoviruses are extensive. The spectrum of disease includes nonspecific febrile illness, upper respiratory infection, parotitis, croup, bronchitis, pneumonia, bronchiolitis, vomiting, diarrhea, abdominal pain, hepatitis, pancreatitis, conjunctivitis, pericarditis, myocarditis, orchitis, nephritis, arthritis, meningitis, and encephalitis.

Similarly, the associated skin manifestations include an array of exanthems. Diffuse macular eruptions, morbilliform erythema, vesicular lesions, petechial and purpural eruptions, rubelliform rash, roseola-like rash, and scarlatiniform eruptions have been reported.

Strict clinical-virologic associations have been difficult to demonstrate. A single clinical syndrome can be associated with many types coxsackieviruses and echoviruses. On the other hand, some types of coxsackieviruses and echoviruses have been associated with multiple illnesses and exanthems.

Hand, foot, and mouth disease is an acute infectious illness, caused by enteroviruses, that primarily affects children. Initial manifestations include fever, anorexia, malaise, and sore mouth. Oral lesions appear 1 to 2 days later and cutaneous lesions shortly thereafter. The oral lesions begin as vesicles on an erythematous base, which ulcerate. The vesicles are usually 4 to 8 mm in size, and are very painful. They are located on the buccal mucosa, tongue, soft palate, and gingiva. The exanthem starts as red papules that change to gray vesicles about 3 to 7 mm in size. They are found on the palms and soles, but may occur on the dorsum of the feet and hands and on the buttocks as well. They may be oval, linear, or crescentic and may run parallel to skin lines. They heal in 7 to 10 days.

Herpangina is a febrile disease of children that is associated with many types of coxsackieviruses and echoviruses. The onset is acute with fever to 40°C (104°F), headache, sore throat, dysphagia, anorexia, and occasionally stiff neck. In the pharynx, there are one or more yellowish-white 2-mm vesicles with hyperemic borders. They are located in the posterior pharynx on the tonsils, uvula, soft palate, and anterior faucial pillars. The vesicles usually ulcerate, leaving a shallow, gray-yellow crater 2 to 4 mm in size. The lesions persist for 5 to 10 days.

Boston exanthem is caused by echovirus 16. It is an acute illness with fever, anorexia, pharyngitis, and lymphadenopathy. An enanthem similar to herpangina may be present. The exanthem begins as small, discrete, pink macules that develop into papules. It appears on the face and chest, spreads centrifugally, and may involve the palms and soles. As in roseola, the rash may appear with defervescence of the fever.

Infection due to echovirus 9 is common and produces a typical enteroviral illness. Clinical manifestations include fever, headache, nausea, vomiting, abdominal pain, cough, coryza, pharyngitis, and nuchal rigidity. The exanthem is rubelliform, a maculopapular rash beginning on the face and neck, then extending to the trunk and feet and sometimes the palms and soles. Occasionally, there are lesions on the buccal mucosa and soft palate that resemble Koplik spots. Petechiae may occur. The appearance of this rash and the presence of nuchal rigidity makes this illness occasionally mimic meningococcemia. The exanthem persists for about 5 days.

Infection with coxsackievirus A9 is a common cause of exanthem. It is an acute febrile illness with a discrete erythematous maculopapular rash that begins on the face and neck and extends to the trunk and extremities. Aseptic meningitis may occur. The rash may also be vesicular or urticarial.

The clinical differentiation of enteroviral disease is difficult. Since there is no specific therapy for enteroviral infection, it is more important to consider bacterial diseases in the differential diagnosis in order to exclude treatable causes of sepsis, meningitis, myocarditis, and pneumonia. Symptomatic therapy for enteroviral infections includes adequate hydration, antipyretics, and viscous lidocaine gel for painful oral lesions.

Herpes Virus (Figures 135-3 and 135-4)

Herpes simplex infection is characterized by umbilicated vesicles that become pustules. Lesions occur at the mouth, lips, gingiva, and fingertips. Treatment with oral antiviral therapy is effective for primary infections. Acyclovir, valacyclovir, or famciclovir can be used.

Erythema Infectiosum

Erythema infectiosum (fifth disease) is an acute, febrile illness with a unique exanthem. Outbreaks of erythema infectiosum occur primarily in the spring. During epidemics, the attack rate is highest in children 5 to 15 years of age, but all age groups can be affected. The illness is caused by infection with human parvovirus, a single-stranded DNA virus.

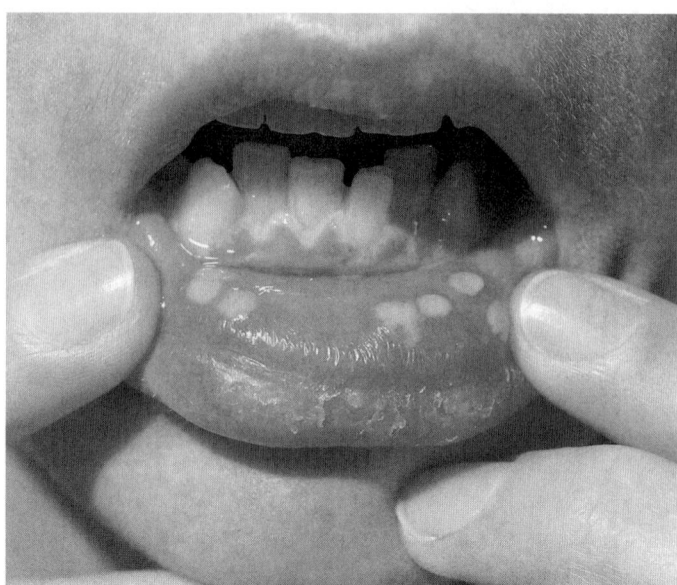

FIG. 135-3. Herpes simplex virus infection: primary gingivostomatitis. (Reproduced with permission from Fitzpatick TB, Johnson RA, Wolff K: *Fitzpatrick's Color Atlas & Synopsis of Clinical Dermatology,* 4th ed. New York, NY: McGraw-Hill, 2001, p. 787.)

The abrupt appearance of the rash is frequently the first manifestation of erythema infectiosum. It begins with a characteristic fiery red rash on the cheeks. The rash is a diffuse erythema of closely grouped tiny papules on an erythematous base. The edges are slightly raised. The erythema is most intense below the eyes and extends over the cheeks in a pattern reminiscent of butterfly wings; it is sometimes re-

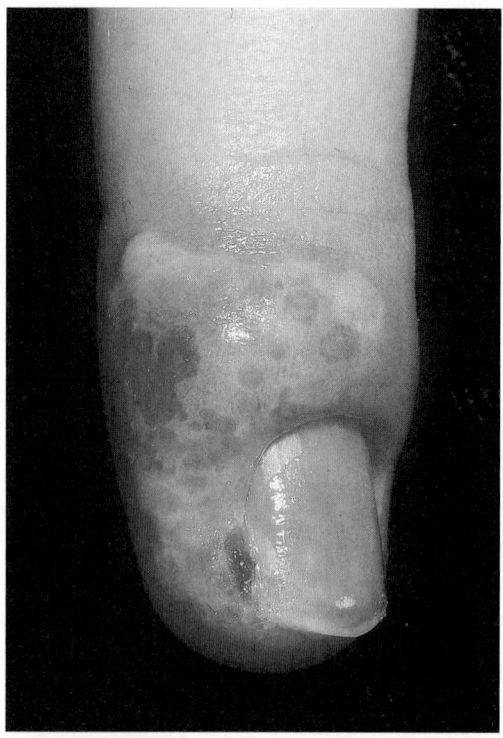

FIG. 135-4. Herpes simplex virus infection: herpetic whitlow. (Reproduced from Fitzpatick TB, Johnson RA, Wolff K: *Fitzpatrick's Color Atlas & Synopsis of Clinical Dermatology,* 4th ed. New York, NY: McGraw-Hill, 2001, p. 789.)

ferred to as a *slapped-cheek appearance.* There is circumoral pallor as well as sparing of the eyelids and chin. The facial rash fades after 4 to 5 days. Approximately 1 to 2 days after the appearance of the facial rash, a nonpruritic macular erythema or erythematous maculopapular rash occurs on the trunk and limbs. It is at first localized to the deltoid areas, trunk, and forearms, but usually extends to involve a large area. This stage of the exanthem may last 1 week. A distinctive aspect of the rash is that it fades with central clearing, giving a reticulated or lacy appearance. The palms and soles are rarely affected.

The exanthem may recur in the ensuing 3 weeks, sometimes briefly. The intensity of the recurrent exanthem varies and may be related to exposure to environmental factors such as sunlight, hot baths, and perhaps, physical exertion or emotional upset. Associated symptoms frequently occur and may include fever, malaise, headache, sore throat, cough, coryza, nausea, vomiting, diarrhea, and myalgia. Arthralgias and arthritis can occur, but usually only in adults. These symptoms may occur before or after the onset of the rash.

There is no specific treatment for human parvovirus infection. Symptomatic therapy is all that is required. Recovery is usually complete.

Measles

Prior to a nationwide immunization program in 1965, measles was an expected disease of childhood. It is a highly contagious, endemic myxovirus infection. It is a winter-spring disease in temperate climates, but it occurs throughout the world.

After exposure, the incubation period for the disease is about 10 days. The prodromal period lasts approximately 3 days and is characterized by upper respiratory symptoms. The onset of clinical measles is characterized by general malaise, systemic toxicity, fever, coryza, conjunctivitis, photophobia, and cough.

The exanthem develops about the fourteenth day following exposure. The rash first appears behind the ears and at the hairline of the forehead. It spreads in a centrifugal pattern from the head to the feet. It is initially erythematous and maculopapular but rapidly progresses to confluence, especially on the face. Initially the rash is red and blanches on pressure. As it fades, it takes on a copper-to-brownish hue. With healing there may be some fine desquamation. The rash generally lasts 7 days.

Koplik spots are an associated pathognomonic enanthem. The lesions are white, 1-mm discrete spots that first appear on the buccal mucosa opposite the lower molars and then spread to involve the entire buccal mucosa. The treatment of measles is supportive.

Infectious Mononucleosis

The diagnosis of infectious mononucleosis can be entertained in those children, adolescents, and young adults who present with fever, sore throat, malaise, and fatigue accompanied by tonsillopharyngitis and lymphadenopathy. The Epstein-Barr virus (EBV) is the etiologic agent of this illness. The age of initial (primary) infection varies and appears to depend upon socioeconomic status. The mononucleosis symptom complex is associated with the primary infection. A 2- to 5-day prodromal period of malaise and fatigue with or without fever may precede the full onset of the syndrome. The adenopathy is usually confined to the anterior and posterior cervical chain but may be generalized. There is a 5-percent incidence of a generalized erythematous maculopapular rash associated with an enanthem consisting of petechiae on the soft palate. The incidence of the rash increases to almost 100 percent in those patients taking ampicillin or its congeners. The treatment for infectious mononucleosis is supportive.

Rubella

Rubella (German measles) was once a common childhood disease that had its highest incidence during the spring. The incubation period is 12 to 25 days following exposure with a 1- to 5-day prodrome of fever, malaise, headache, and sore throat.

The exanthem varies and is sometimes difficult to identify. It may present as a short-lived blush, or it may have the more common 2- to 3-day course. The exanthem begins as irregular pink macules and papules on the face spreading to the neck, trunk, and arms in a centrifugal distribution. It coalesces on the face as the eruption reaches the lower extremities and then clears in the same fashion. As enanthem of pinpoint petechiae involving the soft palate (Forschheimer spots) may accompany the rash but is nonspecific.

Lymphadenopathy is a clinical manifestation of rubella, with the enlargement characteristically in the suboccipital and posterior auricular nodes. The clinical diagnosis of the individual case is often difficult, but the epidemic nature of the illness, along with the seasonal variation and high expression rate of the exanthem, help in establishing the diagnosis. A history of inadequate immunizations may assist in the diagnosis. There is no specific therapy.

Varicella

Varicella, or chickenpox, is a result of infection with varicella-zoster virus, a herpes virus.[4] In normal children it is characterized by a pruritic generalized vesicular exanthem with mild systemic manifestations. Cases generally occur in late winter and early spring. The incidence of varicella has declined dramatically in surveillance areas with significant vaccine coverage. It is highly contagious in the prodromal and vesicular stage. Varicella most frequently occurs in children less than 10 years old, but it may occur at any age.

The exanthem starts on the trunk or scalp and first appears as faint red macules. Within 24 h, the rash acquires the typical vesicular appearance of varicella. The rash consists of teardrop vesicles on an erythematous base, which then dry and crust over (Figure 135-5). Successive fresh crops may appear for a few days. The extent of the rash may be minimal, but usually it will spread centrifugally and become widespread. Palms and soles are spared. Vesicles may occur on mucous membranes and proceed to rupture and form shallow ulcers. Low-grade fever, malaise, and headache are frequently present but are usually mild. The diagnosis of varicella is usually made clinically on the basis of its distinctive rash. A Tzanck smear of the vesicle contents will demonstrate varicella giant cells with inclusion bodies.

Complications of varicella can occur, including encephalitis, pneumonia, nephritis, and infection of the vesicles with staphylococci or streptococci. Neonates born to mothers with perinatal varicella infection may develop serious illness.

Uncomplicated varicella requires no specific therapy. Acetaminophen may be used as needed, but aspirin should be avoided as it may predispose to the development of Reye syndrome. Oral antihistamines may be useful to reduce itching. Most importantly, lesions should be cleansed regularly to prevent secondary infection. In the absence of central nervous system complications, the prognosis is excellent. Routine use of acyclovir for uncomplicated varicella infections in children is not recommended. While limited data are available on pediatric use, no unusual toxicity or problems have been noted.

Immunocompromised patients with varicella require aggressive treatment with antiviral drugs such as acyclovir. The dose of acyclovir is 80 mg/kg per d in four divided doses up to 800 mg/dose. Administration of varicella zoster immune globulin (VZIG) should be considered for immunocompromised patients exposed to individuals with varicella.

With the advent of significant vaccine coverage, surveillance and public health reporting are important for outbreak management.

Variola

Due to an international effort to isolate and eradicate variola, smallpox is now a historical disease. The virus is known to exist only in two

Chickenpox
(varicella)

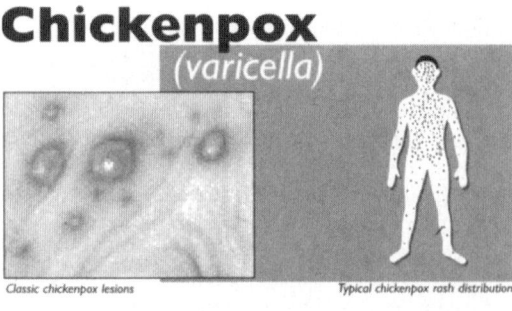

Classic chickenpox lesions · Typical chickenpox rash distribution

IMAGES OF CHICKENPOX (VARICELLA)

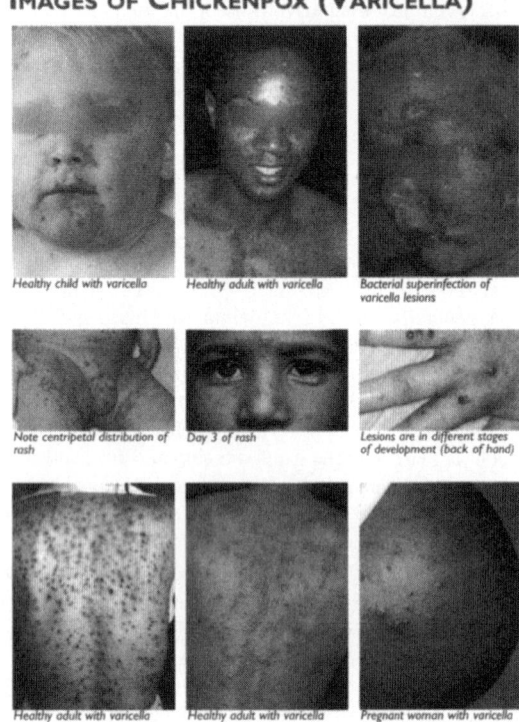

Healthy child with varicella · Healthy adult with varicella · Bacterial superinfection of varicella lesions

Note centripetal distribution of rash · Day 3 of rash · Lesions are in different stages of development (back of hand)

Healthy adult with varicella · Healthy adult with varicella · Pregnant woman with varicella

FIG. 135-5. Varicella. [Reproduced from the Centers for Disease Control (CDC). www.bt.cdc.gov/agent/smallpox/diagnosis/pdf/spox-poster-full.pdf]

Smallpox
(variola)

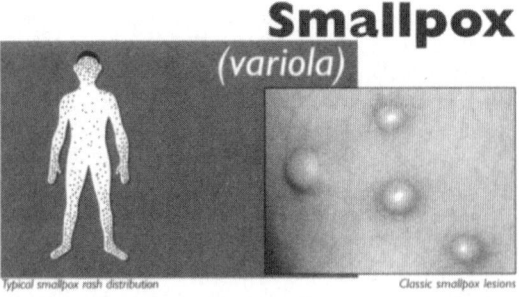

Typical smallpox rash distribution · Classic smallpox lesions

IMAGES OF SMALLPOX

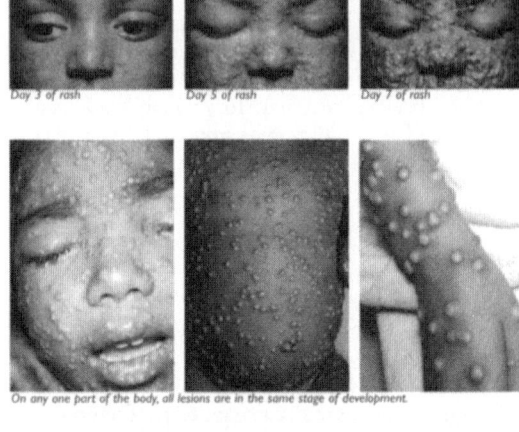

Day 3 of rash · Day 5 of rash · Day 7 of rash

On any one part of the body, all lesions are in the same stage of development.

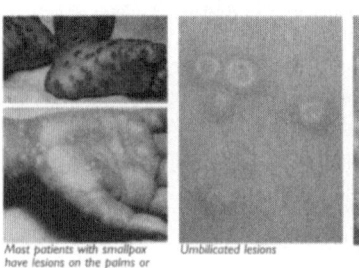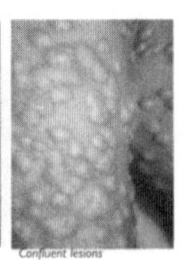

Most patients with smallpox have lesions on the palms or soles · Umbilicated lesions · Confluent lesions

FIG. 135-6. (PLATE 1). Smallpox. [Reproduced from the Centers for Disease Control (CDC). www.bt.cdc.gov/agent/smallpox/diagnosis/pdf/spox-poster-full.pdf]

laboratories worldwide, one in the former Soviet Union and one in the U.S..

With the breakup of the former Soviet Union in the early 1990s, concern regarding biological agent proliferation surfaced. The reach of international terrorism has heightened awareness of the use of nuclear, biological, and chemical threats, including smallpox, as weapons of terror.

Variola or smallpox (Figure 135-6, **Plate 1**) is a highly transmissible poxvirus with a mortality rate that can exceed 30 percent. Transmission is by droplet (from oropharynx, person to person) or through contact with virus from infected persons. An incubation period of 2 weeks allows for known contacts to be successfully immunized through vaccination.

The rash associated with smallpox is quite striking. With careful examination it is easily differentiated from the exanthem of varicella (chickenpox). Varicella causes superficial lesions that occur in crops. The lesions proceed through a cycle of papule, vesicle, pustule, and scab formation, so many different stages of the lesions are present simultaneously. The greatest density of lesions occurs on the trunk with chickenpox.

By contrast, smallpox causes deep lesions of greatest density on the face and extremities, and all lesions present are in the same stage.

These lesions begin as a maculopapular rash: first affecting the mouth and face, then proceeding to the trunk and legs. Vesicles form within 2 days, and then become pustules. Smallpox is associated with high fever, headache, backache, and the previously described rash. A high percentage of untreated patients die on the sixth day. Among those who survive, the rash forms scabs and crusts by the eighth day.

Smallpox identified in the ED requires activation of the institutional response plan including immediate isolation and consultation with public health and hospital authorities.

Anthrax

Although cutaneous anthrax (Figure 135-7, **Plate 2**) is not uncommon among the farmers of southwestern Texas, the recent threat of bioterrorism and the appearance of virulent strains of both inhalation and cutaneous anthrax has heightened the need for early recognition and continued surveillance.

Spores of *Bacillus anthracis* can be introduced subcutaneously. The clinical manifestations are usually very striking. Most develop lesions on exposed surfaces of the body such as the face, neck, arms, and hands. The lesion usually starts as a small, painless often pruritic

FIG. 135-7. (PLATE 2). Cutaneous anthrax in a 9-year-old girl. [Reproduced with permission from DOIA (Dermatology Online Atlas) University Erlangen, Department of Dermatology, Nürnberg, Germany, www.dermis.net/index_e. htm.]

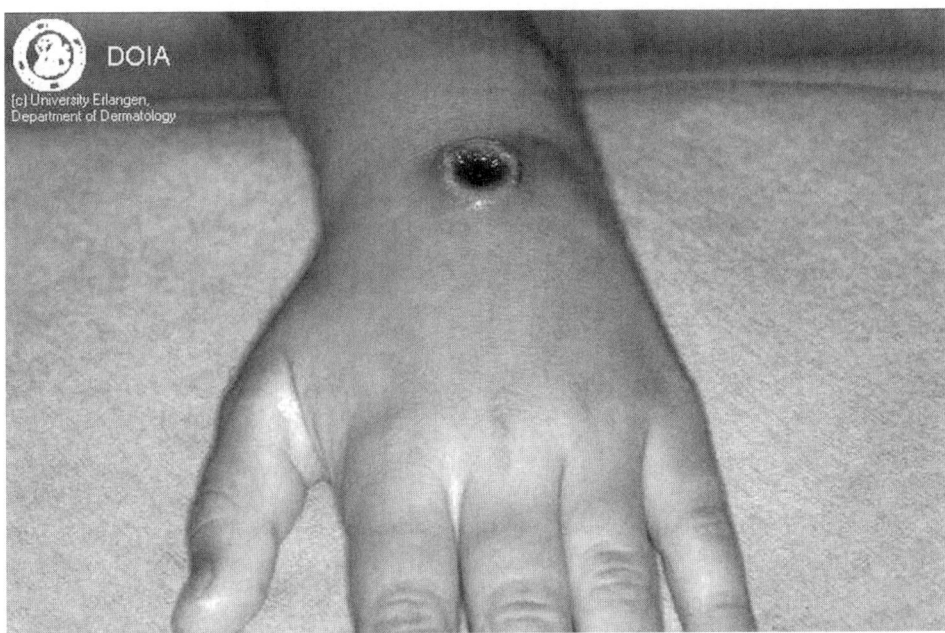

papule. It progresses rapidly (usually over 2 to 3 days) with initial enlargement of the papule followed by vesiculation and rapid ulceration with eschar formation. Regional adenopathy is often present. The differential diagnosis includes brown recluse spider bite, necrotic herpes simplex, tularemia, accidental vaccinia, and ecthyma.

Gram stain of the vesicular fluid demonstrates sporulating grampositive rods. Clinically, the presence of edema out of proportion to the size of the lesion, the absence of pain, and the rarity of polymorphonuclear leukocytes on Gram stain make the diagnosis of cutaneous anthrax relatively easy to make. Untreated, the fatality rate can be as high as 20 percent.

B. anthracis is highly susceptible to many antibiotics. For cutaneous anthrax, penicillin has been used historically, but ciprofloxacin or doxycycline are now recommended (www.cdc.gov/ncidod/EID/vol8no2/01-0521.htm).

Roseola Infantum

Roseola infantum, or exanthem subitum, is a common acute febrile illness of childhood. There appears to be no seasonal preponderance to its occurrence. The most likely etiologic agent has been identified as the human herpesvirus 6, although other viruses have been associated with a roseola-like illness.

Roseola is characterized by a febrile period of 3 to 5 days, defervescence, and the appearance of a rash for 1 or 2 days. Primarily, young children are affected, with most patients being between 6 months and 3 years of age. The illness begins abruptly with high fever, sometimes as high as 40.6°C (105.1°F). The child is usually alert and active but may be irritable, especially with very high fever. Associated symptoms are usually mild and may include cough, coryza, anorexia, and abdominal discomfort. Lymphadenopathy may be present. Febrile convulsions may occur. The fever persists for 3 to 5 days, and most often returns to normal by crisis. The child rapidly becomes well.

The exanthem in roseola usually coincides with defervescence of the fever, but it may follow a short afebrile interlude. The rash is an erythematous macular or maculopapular eruption that consists of discrete, rose or pale-pink lesions 2 to 5 mm in size. It is most prominent on the neck, trunk, and buttocks, but the face and proximal extremities may also be involved. The lesions blanch with pressure. There is no mucous membrane involvement. The rash lasts 1 to 2 days but may fade rapidly, usually without desquamation.

There is no specific treatment for roseola. Acetaminophen is useful for fever control and convulsions should be treated vigorously. Recovery is usually complete.

ETIOLOGY UNCLEAR

Erythema Nodosum

Erythema nodosum is an inflammatory exanthem of unknown etiology. It is probably an inflammatory reaction to a stimulus. In the past, erythema nodosum was most closely associated with streptococcal infections, tuberculosis, and sarcoid, although fungal infections, *Yersinia* infections, vasculitis, inflammatory bowel disease, and leukemia are also known to stimulate the syndrome. Now it is more commonly associated with drugs, especially oral contraceptives. Persons of any age can be affected. Constitutional symptoms may be present at the onset, including fever, malaise, myalgias, and arthralgias.

Erythema nodosum presents a distinctive clinical appearance. Bilateral, very tender nodules develop symmetrically. They usually occur on the shins, but can occur on the arms, thighs, calves, and buttocks. The nodules are 1 to 5 cm in diameter, and individual lesions may coalesce to form sizable areas of induration. The skin over the nodules is red, smooth, and shiny. No ulceration occurs. After a week or two, the color of the lesions changes from red to blue and may achieve a dull, purple, bruised appearance. The eruption lasts several weeks.

The diagnosis of erythema nodosum is usually readily made on clinical grounds. A thorough history and physical, and perhaps laboratory evaluation must be performed to exclude an underlying cause. There is no known therapy to alter the course of the disease. Nonsteroidal antiinflammatory drugs may provide relief from the sometimes significant pain associated with these lesions.

Kawasaki Disease (Mucocutaneous Lymph Node Syndrome)

Kawasaki disease, or mucocutaneous lymph node syndrome (MLNS) is a disease of unclear etiology found predominantly in children under 9 years of age.[5,6]

The diagnosis of this disorder is based on a constellation of clinical findings. The patient must exhibit a prolonged fever associated with at least four of the following: (1) conjunctivitis, (2) rash,

(3) lymphadenopathy, (4) changes in the oropharynx consisting of injection of the pharynx and lips with prominent papillae of the tongue (strawberry tongue), and (5) extremity erythema and edema.

The rash has been described as erythematous, morbilliform, urticarial, scarlatiniform, or erythema multiforme-like. It has a predilection for the perineum. Additional supportive evidence which may help in the presumptive diagnosis includes leukocytosis, elevation of acute-phase reactants, elevated liver function tests, arthritis, arthralgia, and irritability.

In the second phase, there is usually a sharp rise in the platelet count, desquamation of the fingers and/or toes, and the most serious complication, the development of coronary artery aneurysm. A small percentage (1 to 2 percent) of patients with coronary artery aneurysm develop sudden cardiac failure, resulting in death from myocardial infarction with coronary artery thrombosis.

The differential diagnosis includes drug allergy, toxic epidermal necrolysis, staphylococcal toxin-mediated syndromes, erythema multiforme, and scarlet fever. The etiologic speculations include a hyperimmune response to a variety of infections, a viral syndrome, an allergic or toxic response to pollutants, drugs, or toxic agents, and a possibility of a rickettsial disease.

Treatment of Kawasaki disease continues to evolve. Intravenous gamma globulin (IVIG, intravenous immunoglobulin) is now routinely recommended. Aspirin remains an important component of the therapy for Kawasaki disease. Steroids, while somewhat controversial, are assuming an increasingly important role, especially in those cases refractory to IVIG. Bed rest, supportive therapy, and frequent monitoring are mainstays of treatment.

Pityriasis Rosea

Pityriasis rosea is a mild inflammatory exanthem of unknown cause. The available evidence suggests a viral etiology. Pityriasis rosea affects all age groups but occurs most commonly in patients 10 to 35 years old. It tends to occur in spring and fall but not in epidemics. Pityriasis rosea is not contagious. A pityriasis rosea-like eruption has been associated with some drugs and viruses. Occasionally there are prodromal symptoms including malaise, headache, sore throat, fatigue, and arthralgia.

The rash of pityriasis rosea evolves over a period of several weeks. It begins with a "herald patch," a solitary, erythematous lesion with a raised edematous border most frequently occurring on the chest or back. It is 2 to 6 cm in diameter. About 1 or 2 weeks later, there is a widespread, symmetrical eruption of pink- or salmon-colored maculopapular lesions. The patches are oval and are covered with dry epidermis which desquamates to form a ring of scale at the periphery. The lesions are 0.5 to 1.5 cm in diameter and are at first discrete, but can become confluent. The long axes of the patches frequently run parallel to lines of skin tension, giving rise to the "Christmas tree" pattern seen on the back. The eruption is generalized and chiefly affects the trunk, although it can occur anywhere. The lesions can be localized. Mucous membranes can be involved with plaques, hemorrhagic punctate spots, or ulcers. Successive crops of skin lesions can occur, and the entire illness can last 3 to 8 weeks. Healing is complete, without sequelae or evidence of organ involvement.

The diagnosis of pityriasis rosea is made by the clinical appearance. It can be confused with viral exanthem, drug eruptions, syphilis, and seborrheic dermatitis. Potassium hydroxide preparation of skin scrapings will serve to distinguish pityriasis rosea from tinea corporis. A serologic test for syphilis must be done to exclude that diagnosis.

Therapy is directed at alleviating symptoms. There is some early evidence indicating that treatment with erythromycin may speed the resolution of this exanthem. Further studies may be useful in this regard. The rash is sometimes very itchy. Oatmeal baths and oral antihistamines will provide temporary relief. Emollients will help dryness and irritation. Secondary infection must be prevented with thorough cleansing.

REFERENCES

1. Update: Rashes among schoolchildren. *MMWR* 51:524, 2002.
2. Knoop K, Stack L, Storrow A (eds): *Atlas of Emergency Medicine,* 2nd ed. New York: McGraw Hill, 2002.
3. Freedberg IM, Eisen AZ, Wolff K, et al (eds): *Fitzpatrick's Dermatology in General Medicine,* 6th ed. New York: McGraw-Hill, 2003.
4. Seward J, Watson B, Peterson C, et al: Varicella disease after introduction of varicella vaccine in the United States, 1995-2000. *JAMA* 287:606, 2002.
5. Brogan P, Bose A, Burgner D, et al: Kawasaki disease: An evidence based approach to diagnosis, treatment, and proposals for future research. *Arch Dis Child* 86:286, 2002.
6. Fukunishi M, Kikkawa M, Hamana H, et al: Prediction of non-responsiveness to intravenous high dose gamma globulin therapy in patients with Kawasaki disease at onset. *J Pediatrics* 137:172, 2000.

136

MUSCULOSKELETAL DISORDERS IN CHILDREN
Courtney Hopkins-Mann
David Leader
Donna Moro-Sutherland
Richard A. Christoph

GENERAL PRINCIPLES

The anatomy of the pediatric musculoskeletal system is unique and reflects the active growth and development that occurs during childhood. Fracture classification, treatment approach, and types of complications are directly related to this unique anatomy. Perhaps the most helpful way to divide pediatric musculoskeletal injuries is into those occurring before and those occurring after fusion of the physes. In general, both injury patterns and treatment approaches in children in whom closure of the physes has already occurred is similar to those of the adult. Therefore, the major focus of this discussion is directed at injuries occurring in the prepubescent child. In addition, diseases specific to the pediatric population that cause non-traumatic musculoskeletal complaints will also be covered.

The long bones of children consist of discrete anatomic areas. The physis is an area of growth cartilage and may occur at one (e.g., the phalanges) or both (e.g., the tibia and the femur) ends of a long bone. The area of bone between a physis and the adjacent joint is termed the epiphysis. An apophysis is an area of bone between a physis and is a point for muscle or ligament attachment. The midshaft of a long bone is referred to as the diaphysis. The metaphysis of a long bone represents the area between the diaphysis and the physis (see Figure 267-6).

The long bones of children are generally less dense and more porous than the long bones of adults. The resulting increased compliance contributes to the tendency of pediatric long bones to respond to mechanical stress by bowing and buckling, rather than fracturing through and through, as is seen in adult fracture patterns. The periosteum of the diaphysis and the metaphysis is thicker in children and is continuous from the metaphysis to the epiphysis, surrounding and protecting the mechanically weaker physis. The weakness of the physis is in part related to the reduced oxygen tension found in the hypertrophic zone of the physis. This hypertrophic zone is the location of frequent fractures within the physis. The physis is also sensitive to alterations in the blood supply to this hypertrophic zone as well as to nutritional, hormonal, and mechanical influences, and physeal injuries can result in growth disturbance.

The growth of the musculoskeletal system and its response to injury are also influenced by the growth of muscle and connective tissue. The ligaments of children are stronger and more compliant than in adults, and tolerate mechanical forces better than the weaker physis.

Therefore, apophyseal detachments or epiphyseal fractures are much more common than ligamentous injuries during childhood.

FRACTURE PATTERNS

Fractures Involving the Physis

The weakest layer of the physis is the hypertrophic cell zone. This area is particularly susceptible to shearing, bending, and tension stresses, and represents the layer of the physis that is most consistently fractured. Consequently, the reserve and proliferative cartilage cells in the first two zones of the injured physis usually remain with the epiphysis. This is important because the predominant circulatory support of the cells in these two reproductive zones of the physis arises through the epiphyseal vasculature and thus is more likely to be spared in the event of physeal injury.

Compression forces alone may also affect bone growth. This is particularly true when compression forces are applied to the epiphyseal side of the physis. The injury to bone growth caused by compression results from interruption of the epiphyseal circulation to the reproductive cells of the physis.

Perhaps the easiest way to divide pediatric orthopedic injuries is into those occurring in children who are skeletally immature with open physes, and those whose physes have closed. The type of injury in the skeletally immature child is usually described with relation to the physis. The Salter and Harris classification system (see Figure 267-7) is based on the relationship of the fracture line to the physis and the prognosis for growth disturbance.

Salter-Harris Type I Fracture

Type I physeal injuries occur when the epiphysis separates from the metaphysis. The cleavage is through the hypertrophic cell zone of the physis, with the reproductive cells of the physis remaining with the epiphysis. There are no associated fragments of bone as the thick periosteal attachments surrounding the physis remain intact. The epiphysis may, however, somewhat displace from the metaphysis. Type I injuries have a low incidence of growth disturbances.

The diagnosis of a Salter-Harris type I injury must be suspected clinically in a child who presents with point tenderness over a physis after trauma. Radiographic findings are typically subtle and soft tissue swelling or a joint effusion may be the only abnormality. Epiphyseal displacement can usually be appreciated on x-rays in one or more views; however, in the absence of epiphyseal displacement, the diagnosis is usually a clinical one.

Treatment of most type I fractures consists of immobilization of the suspected fracture using an appropriate splint, cold compresses, and elevation to limit swelling. Referral to an orthopedic surgeon for follow up evaluation allows for monitoring for bone growth disturbances, which is essential.

Salter-Harris Type II Fracture

In a type II injury, the fracture line extends a variable distance along the hypertrophic cell zone of the physis and then out through a piece of metaphyseal bone. The periosteum overlying the metaphyseal fragment remains intact, whereas the periosteum on the opposite side of the fracture is torn away from the diaphysis while remaining adherent to the epiphysis. Growth is preserved since the reproductive layers of the physis maintain their position with the epiphysis and the epiphyseal circulation. Diagnosis is made radiographically by noting a triangular-shaped fragment of metaphysis that is not associated with discernible injury to the epiphysis.

Treatment of a type II fracture consists of closed reduction of any displacement followed by immobilization in a splint, ice, elevation, analgesia, and orthopedic follow up.

Salter-Harris Type III Fracture

Type III physeal injuries are intraarticular. The fracture line extends intraarticularly from the epiphysis, through the hypertrophic zone of the physis, with the cleavage plane continuing along the physis to the periphery. The prognosis for subsequent bone growth relates to the preservation of circulation to the epiphyseal bone fragment; however, the prognosis is usually quite favorable.

The diagnosis of a type III injury is made radiographically and is based on the appearance of an epiphyseal fragment, not associated with an apparent metaphyseal fracture. There may or may not be an associated periosteal injury. Occasionally, additional imaging with CT or MRI is used to better evaluate the extent of fracture and articular surface involvement. Treatment is usually open reduction to ensure proper alignment of the articular surface.

Salter-Harris Type IV Fracture

In type IV injuries, the fracture line originates at the articular surface and extends through the epiphysis, the entire thickness of the physis, and continues through the metaphysis. The risk of growth disturbance with this type of fracture is significant and reduction must be precise.

The diagnosis of a type IV injury is made radiographically upon identification of epiphyseal and metaphyseal fragments. Treatment is open surgical reduction and internal fixation.

Salter-Harris Type V Fracture

Type V injuries typically involve the knee or ankle and are the result of a profound compressive force transmitted to the physis, resulting in crushing of the chondrocytes in both the reserve and proliferative zones. Displacement of the epiphysis is usually only minimal despite the significant damage to the physis.

The diagnosis of a type V injury may be difficult initially leading to a lack of appreciation of the seriousness of the injury. An initial diagnosis of a sprain or a type I physeal fracture may prove incorrect in view of subsequent development of premature growth arrest during follow up. Radiographs may appear normal or may demonstrate focal narrowing of the physeal plate. There is also typically a joint effusion. The history will point to a type V injury, however, as a significant mechanism has usually been sustained. Treatment consists of casting and orthopedic monitoring in anticipation of bone growth arrest.

Torus Fractures

The porus nature and resulting compliance of the metaphyses of pediatric long bones, coupled with the relative thickness of the periosteum in this area, confer unique fracture characteristics in children. Compressive forces often result in a bulging or buckling of the periosteum rather than a more complete fracture line. Cortical, or *torus*, fractures are so named to describe prominence or bulging of the bony cortex, usually involving the metaphysis.

A simple torus fracture will not produce a visible deformity to the shape of the extremity; however, there is typically soft tissue swelling and point tenderness over the bony injury. In children who are not obese, the torus fracture is occasionally palpable as a ridge over the metaphyseal area of the long bone.

Radiographically, the torus fracture may be subtle. The contour of the metaphyseal flare should be carefully inspected. Any asymmetry, bulging, or deviation of the cortical margin indicates a torus fracture. Soft tissue swelling is also usually evident. Torus fractures are not typically associated with severe angulation, displacement, or rotational abnormalities, so reduction is rarely necessary. The extremity is splinted in a position of function with orthopedic follow up within 1 week.

Greenstick Fractures

Stress and force may be applied to the porous, compliant bones of children in such a way as to create an incomplete cortical fracture. A *greenstick* fracture is characterized by cortical disruption and periosteal tearing on the convex side of the bone, with an intact periosteum on the concave side of the fracture. Greenstick fractures are more stable and somewhat less painful than complete fractures, since the area of intact periosteum limits bony displacement.

The need for reduction is determined by the degree of angulation of the fracture, the age of the child, and the anatomic location of the injury.

Plastic Deformities (Bowing or Bending Fractures)

Plastic deformities, also referred to as bowing or bending fractures, are almost exclusively limited to the forearm and lower leg long bones. Usually, this type of injury is noted in combination with a completed fracture of the other bone of the forearm or lower leg. The cortex of the diaphysis of the long bone is deformed, but the periosteum along the entire diaphysis is preserved. These injuries result from the compliance and porosity of the child's bones, with the associated tendency to deform or bend rather than fracture in the traditional sense.

The diagnosis of a plastic deformity fracture is made radiographically. Proper interpretation of the radiographs requires an awareness of the normal shape of the long bones involved, since fracture lines and disruptions in the periosteum will be absent. Comparison films of the uninvolved extremity may be useful in determining the degree of deformity.

Prompt orthopedic consultation is required for any plastic deformities as proper reduction and realignment is essential. Reduction usually involves completion of the fracture with restoration of proper alignment.

Fractures from Child Abuse

See Chap. 297 for complete discussion of child abuse.

UPPER EXTREMITY INJURIES

Fractures of the Clavicle

Clavicle fractures occur during two distinct time frames: the newborn period and childhood. Fractures of the clavicle in the newborn usually result from birth injury (Figure 136-1). Risk factors include high birth weight and shoulder dystocia. The infant may demonstrate upper extremity palsy secondary to a brachial plexus injury or may have "pseudoparalysis" of the extremity secondary to pain. Although many clavicle fractures are detected at birth, the diagnosis may be delayed especially if the fracture is nondisplaced. An ED visit may be made when the newborn is not moving one arm during the first week of life, or when a parent notices a small "lump" or callus at the clavicle during the first 2 to 3 weeks of life. Most clavicle fractures in the newborn do not need specific treatment. Pain control and careful handling of the baby are usually all that are required.

Clavicle fractures outside of the newborn period usually result from accidental injury in a mobile child. However, clavicle fractures in children younger than 2 years old should raise the possibility of abuse. The most common mechanism of injury is either a fall onto an outstretched hand or onto the lateral side of the shoulder. The clavicle may fracture in three general sites: the diaphysis, the medial end, or the lateral end. Fractures of the diaphysis usually occur in the middle third of the clavicle and are the most common of all clavicle fractures. Treatment is an arm sling, as tolerated by the child. Even displaced and overlapping fractures tend to heal well with simple immobilization in a simple sling for 3 to 4 weeks. Complete healing and remodeling can take more than 1 year, and a small callus will become palpable in most cases if the fracture was displaced. Routine follow up with the primary care physician is sufficient.

Fractures at the medial end of the clavicle are uncommon. Given the strong ligamentous attachment of the clavicle to the sternum, injuries to this area are usually epiphyseal disruptions. Clinical presentation and treatment depend on the direction of the displacement. When the displacement is anterior, there is usually tenderness, and a palpable protrusion of the distal end of the clavicle. Open reduction and fixation is generally needed. If the displacement is posterior, compression of the trachea and esophagus can lead to complaints of dysphagia and respiratory difficulty. Treatment of a posterior displacement is urgent reduction.

Fractures of the distal end of the clavicle are also uncommon in children and again more likely to be epiphyseal disruptions. Injuries to the distal end of the clavicle are more likely to result from direct trauma to the area. Generally, these types of fractures can be managed by a conservative sling if they are minimally displaced. However, surgical reduction may be needed for more displaced fractures to provide for optimal healing and function of the shoulder.

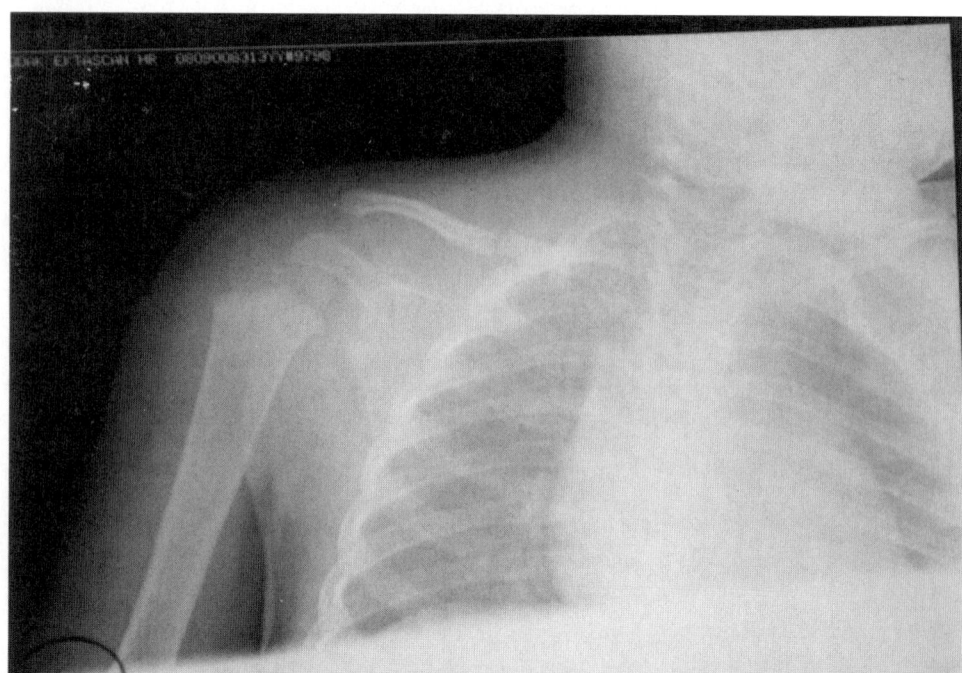

FIG. 136-1. Nondisplaced clavicle fracture in an infant.

Fractures of the Humerus

Fractures of the humerus can be divided into three groups: fractures of the proximal humerus, humeral diaphysis, and supracondylar fractures. Supracondylar fractures are discussed as part of the elbow.

Fractures of the proximal humerus may occur at the physis or the proximal humeral metaphysis, and they have an extraordinary ability to repair themselves. Physeal fractures occur more commonly in adolescents because this area becomes relatively weak during this time because of rapid growth. Fractures of the proximal humeral metaphysis are more common in preadolescents. Treatment depends on both the age of the child and the degree of displacement. Orthopedic consultation is needed to determine the best approach. In general, the younger child can tolerate a greater degree of displacement. For slightly displaced fractures, treatment is conservative with immobilization in a sling and orthopedic follow up. Fractures displaced >30 degrees often need closed reduction and immobilization.

Fractures of the humeral diaphysis are uncommon in children. Direct trauma can cause a transverse fracture and violent rotation can cause a spiral fracture. The possibility of abuse must be considered in small children presenting with fractures of the diaphysis of the humerus because of the significant force required for fractures in this area. Potential for healing is again good and treatment is usually conservative with immobilization in a long arm plaster splint and orthopedic follow up. Closed reduction may be required for displaced fractures. Transverse fractures tend to be more unstable than spiral fractures. One complication with respect to fractures of the humeral diaphysis is radial nerve injury. The fracture fragment may injury the nerve as it runs in the radial groove. Documentation of radial nerve function is therefore extremely important and should also be noted after any reduction attempt.

Pediatric Elbow

Compared to other fractures, elbow fractures in children are commonly missed in the ED. Radiologic diagnosis of these injuries are extremely challenging because of the large cartilaginous component of the elbow. A thorough understanding of the anatomy of the immature elbow helps to reduce the risk of misdiagnosis. Familiarity with proper alignment, angulation, various stages of development of ossification centers, and quality of fat pads will aid the emergency physician in correctly diagnosing an elbow fracture.

ORDERING RADIOGRAPHS   True lateral and anteroposterior (AP) radiographs of the elbow are needed. There are three key points to consider in the interpretation of every radiograph of the pediatric elbow. In a true lateral radiograph, the anterior humeral line should bisect the capitellum in the middle third. If the capitellum falls posterior to the line, one needs to consider an extension-type supracondylar fracture as the most likely diagnosis. Other diagnoses to consider include lateral condyle fractures or, rarely, a transphyseal fracture. The radius should point to the capitellum in all views. If not, lateral condyle fracture, radial neck fracture, Monteggia fracture, or elbow dislocation must be considered in the evaluation. A sensitive indicator of angulation of the distal humerus in the frontal plane is the Baumann angle. The normal angle is 9 to 26 degrees. It is commonly abnormal in supracondylar fractures.[1,2]

Lateral radiographs are used to evaluate for subtle effusions when an occult fracture is suspected. The normal anterior fat pad is seen as a drop of oil hugging the distal humerus anteriorly. No posterior fat pad should be appreciated. The quality of the anterior fat pad may be the only hint that a fracture is present. The anterior fat pad may be unappreciated due to soft tissue swelling, grainy in appearance, or the classic "sail sign" may be seen, which clues the physician to hunt further for a fracture line in either the humerus, radius, or olecranon. When a posterior fat pad is visualized, it usually suggests a hemarthrosis secondary to an intraarticular injury. If a fracture is not apparent, oblique views can be obtained, which may detect a subtle fracture. If no fracture line is present, it is an occult supracondylar fracture until proven otherwise.

OSSIFICATION CENTERS   There are six ossification centers apparent in the pediatric elbow and are seen at varying ages. It is important to become familiar with the orientation of the ossification centers around the elbow as they may be confused for a fracture. The mnemonic used over the years is CRITOE [capitellum, radial head, internal (medial) epicondyle, trochlea, olecranon, external (lateral) epicondyle]. See Table 136-1.

ELBOW INJURIES   Elbow injuries are divided into supracondylar fractures, lateral condylar fractures, medial epicondylar fractures, distal humeral physeal fractures, olecranon fractures, radial head and neck fractures, elbow dislocations, and radial head subluxation.

Supracondylar Fractures   Supracondylar fractures are the most common fractures in children under 8 years old. The majority of supracondylar fractures occur in children from 3 to 10 years of age, with the peak incidence occurring between ages 5 and 7. The extension type is by far the most common, accounting for 90 to 98 percent of cases. It is caused by a fall on an outstretched hand (FOOSH) with the elbow hyperextended. The flexion-type fracture is a rare occurrence resulting from falling on a flexed elbow. The complications from this type of injury, though uncommon, can be significant if the injury is missed or treatment is delayed. Complications range from transient neuropraxia to Volkmann ischemic contracture.

Classification of the types of supracondylar fractures is based on the extent of fracture fragment displacement. Type I fractures have minimal or no displacement. Type II fractures are displaced with a variable amount of angulation, but the posterior cortex of the humerus is intact. Type III fractures are completely displaced with no cortical contact. The distal fragment may be posteromedially (IIIa) rotated and, as such, can impinge against the radial nerve or be posterolaterally (IIIb) rotated. In posterolaterally displaced fractures, the brachial artery and median nerve are at risk for injury. There is a higher incidence of compartment syndrome with IIIb supracondylar fractures.[1,3] If a pulseless, pale, cold hand is present, an orthopedic surgeon should be urgently consulted and the limb elevated. Traction and reduction are indicated if the hand is cool, pale, and pulseless. The simple absence of a pulse in an otherwise viable hand is a contraindication to manipulation in the ED.

The level of displacement and the prereduction physical examination dictates treatment of pediatric supracondylar fractures. Type I supracondylar fractures are inherently stable. The goal of therapy is comfort and immobilization. The arm is placed in a double sugar-tong splint or a long-arm posterior splint with the elbow at 90 degrees and the forearm in pronation or neutral rotation for 3 weeks. Orthopedic follow-up should be within 48 h. Type II and type III fractures need orthopedic consultation in the ED for definitive management.

LATERAL CONDYLAR FRACTURES   Lateral condyle fractures account for approximately 10 percent of elbow fractures in children, and are usually Salter-Harris type IV. The mechanism of injury is varus

TABLE 136-1   Sequence of Appearance of Ossification Centers of the Elbow

Ossification Center	Age of Appearance
Capitellum	3 mo–2 y
Radial Head	4–5 y
Medial epicondyle (**I**)	4–6 y
Trochlea	8–10 y
Olecranon	8–10 y
Lateral epicondyle (**E**)	10–12 y

stress on an extended elbow with the forearm in supination. Swelling and tenderness are usually limited to the lateral elbow, and neurovascular injury is uncommon. Diagnosis can be made with standard AP and lateral views, however, an oblique view should be obtained if clinical suspicion is high, as this is often the best view for evaluating the extent of the fracture and displacement. Treatment is based on amount of displacement and articular congruence. Nonunion, malunion, osteonecrosis, cubitus valgus, and tardy ulnar nerve palsy are well-described complications, so orthopedic consultation is needed to determine the best treatment approach.

MEDIAL EPICONDYLAR FRACTURES   Fractures of the medial epicondyle tend to occur in older children, between the ages of 10 and 14 years. They are not true Salter-Harris injuries, as the apophysis rather than the physis is involved. Simple fractures of the medial epicondyle are extraarticular injuries with limited soft tissue involvement, but nearly half of injuries are associated with elbow dislocation. Fractures are classified by the amount of displacement and associated extremity injuries, and orthopedic consultation is needed to determine the best approach.

DISTAL HUMERAL PHYSEAL FRACTURES   Most injuries occur in children younger than 2.5 years old. Recognition is both difficult and important, especially in infants, in whom this particular injury is often the result of child abuse. This injury is felt to result from a twisting mechanism that shears off the distal epiphysis.

OLECRANON FRACTURES   Olecranon fractures generally result from a fall onto the elbow. Orthopedic consultation is best to guide treatment. If the fracture is displaced less than 5 mm, it should be immobilized in the most stable position, usually 45 degrees of elbow flexion, for 3 to 6 weeks. Open reduction and internal fixation are indicated for unstable fractures. Olecranon fractures occur in association with fractures of the radial head and neck. A "simple" olecranon fracture may be part of a Monteggia lesion, so radial head position should be evaluated carefully.

RADIAL HEAD AND NECK FRACTURES   Fractures of the radial head and neck are uncommon in children. The radial neck is fractured more frequently than the radial head, and most radial neck fractures occur through the metaphysis. The most common mechanism is a fall. Orthopedic consultation should be obtained to guide treatment. Open reduction is indicated when angulation is more than 60 degrees or displacement is more than 50 percent.

ELBOW DISLOCATION   Elbow dislocations occur most frequently in males (70 percent), usually from a fall on the outstretched hand. The most common type of dislocation is posterior, usually accompanied by some lateral displacement. The radiographs need to be thoroughly scrutinized to rule out the presence of associated fractures, particularly of the medial epicondyle and radial neck. Neurologic injury is associated with approximately 10 percent of elbow dislocations. Ulnar neuropathy is the most common and is usually associated with medial epicondyle entrapment. Radial nerve abnormalities are rare. Median nerve damage is the most problematic. It may be caused by kinking of the nerve inside the joint, coursing behind the medial epicondyle, or entrapment in an epicondyle fracture. Arterial injuries with elbow dislocation are rare, and most reported cases occurred with an open injury. In the presence of neurovascular compromise, an urgent orthopedic consultation is warranted. Postreduction films must be obtained to verify reduction and to rule out any associated fractures. Acute management involves immobilization of the reduced elbow in a posterior mold after closed reduction followed by protected motion in 5 to 7 days. The major long-term complication is stiffness. Long-term results are generally excellent in the absence of prolonged immobilization.

RADIAL HEAD SUBLUXATION (NURSEMAID'S ELBOW)   The peak incidence of radial head subluxation is 2 to 3 years of age, with a range from 6 months to 7 years. Girls are seen more commonly than boys. Left-sided injury is more common, presumably because most caretakers are right-handed. The usual mechanism of injury is sudden longitudinal traction on the arm with the elbow extended, such as occurs when a child is pulled up by the arm. The annular ligament of the radius displaces into the radiocapitellar articulation. The clinical examination reveals a toddler who will not move the affected arm, but is otherwise not in any distress. The arm is kept in an adducted, semiflexed, and prone position. On palpation there is no significant point tenderness or swelling. There may be some discomfort on palpation of the radial head on the affected side. Attempts at pronation and supination of the forearm are painful. Radiographs are not necessary if the clinical suspicion of radial head subluxation is high. There are two maneuvers for reduction, the supination technique, and the hyperpronation technique. The supination technique (Figure 136-2) is performed by holding the child's elbow at 90 degrees with one hand, then firmly supinating the wrist, and finally by flexing the elbow so that the wrist is directed to the ipsilateral shoulder. The hyperpronation technique[4] (Figure 136-3) is reported to be more successful, and it can be used primarily, or as a backup technique when supination fails. The hyperpronation technique is performed by holding the child's elbow at 90 degrees in one hand, then firmly pronating the wrist. Full arm function should return within 30 min, and if it does not, the alternative technique can be applied, or an alternative diagnosis should be considered. An arm sling may be offered until all pain resolves, but is usually not necessary.

Forearm Injuries

Forearm injuries heal well with few complications if appropriately managed. Clinical and radiographic assessment should include the forearm and the joints above and below the primary injury, because there is a high rate of associated fractures or dislocations at those joints. In general, the potential for remodeling is better with more distal injuries. Proximal injuries of the midshaft can be problematic and occasionally require open fixation.

Fractures of the radial and ulnar shafts usually result from a fall onto an outstretched hand. The majority of shaft fractures involve the distal third of the forearm. Clinically, there is point body tenderness, swelling, and obvious deformity. Although all forearm fractures need orthopedic follow-up, the patient's age and degree of deformity determine the need for immediate referral and reduction. Any fracture with rotational deformity or more than 10 degrees of angulation in any plane, requires consultation with an orthopedist to determine the need for reduction. Recognition of a bowing type fracture is also essential because failure to correct the bowing may lead to permanent deformity and disability. However, detection of a bowing fracture may prove difficult, although comparison views may help. As with incomplete yet angulated greenstick fractures, bowing fractures may require completion of the break to establish proper realignment.

Isolated fractures of the ulna are extremely rare. Typically, the same force causes either a fracture or dislocation of the radius. The combination of an ulnar fracture with a dislocation of the radial head is called a *Monteggia fracture.* Clinically, there may be tenderness about the elbow; however, even without significant clinical findings, films of the elbow are essential with fractures of the ulna to evaluate for possible dislocations. Any suspected Monteggia fracture-dislocation requires immediate evaluation by an orthopedist. The *Galeazzi fracture* is a radial shaft fracture with an associated dislocation of the distal radioulnar joint. Although this injury is uncommon, immediate orthopedic consultation is again warranted.

Fractures of the distal radius and ulna are very common. Their propensity to heal with proper management is excellent. Clinically, the child has point tenderness over the distal forearm, frequently associ-

FIG. 136-2. Supination technique. Hold the elbow at 90 degrees, then firmly supinate the wrist and flex the forearm toward the ipsilateral shoulder.

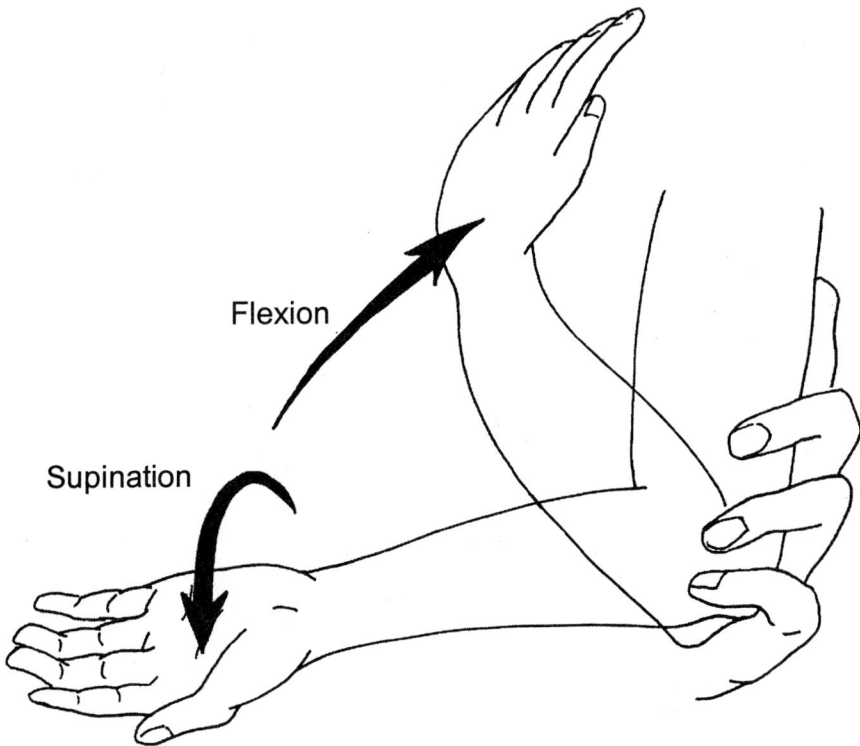

ated with localized swelling. Torus or buckle type fractures are extremely common and are occasionally overlooked given their radiographically subtle nature. Once identified, these types of fractures are well managed in a volar or sugar tong splint with orthopedic follow up in 1 week.

Greenstick or complete fractures with more than 10 degrees of angulation in any plane require consultation with an orthopedist to determine whether reduction is necessary. Otherwise, immobilization in a splint with follow up within the week is adequate treatment. Greenstick and complete fractures of the distal radius and ulna have a tendency to become further displaced if not appropriately immobilized; so placing the child in a sugar tong splint is preferred over a simple volar splint.

Salter-Harris types I and II injuries of the distal radius physis are very common and growth disturbance is rare. Any child with point tenderness or swelling over the physis should be immobilized and have orthopedic follow up arranged. For Salter-Harris types III, IV, and V injuries, immediate orthopedic consultation is necessary.

FIG. 136-3. Hyperpronation technique. Hold the elbow at 90 degrees, then firmly pronate the wrist.

Wrist Injuries

Fractures of the carpal bones are quite rare in children. The scaphoid may be fractured in older adolescents with the typical mechanism being that of a fall to an outstretched hand. There is typically snuff box tenderness and pain with longitudinal compression of the thumb. However, unlike adults, nonunion is less common. Any suspected fracture of the scaphoid should be immobilized in a thumb spica splint and orthopedic followup provided even in the absence of radiographic findings.

Phalangeal Fractures

The most common injury is that to the distal phalanx resulting from a crush injury, typically seen when the child catches his or her hand in a door. Any distal phalanx "tuft" fracture should be immobilized and if there is an associated nail bed injury, the fracture is considered "open" and the child should be sent home on a course of antibiotics and orthopedic follow up arranged in 1 week.

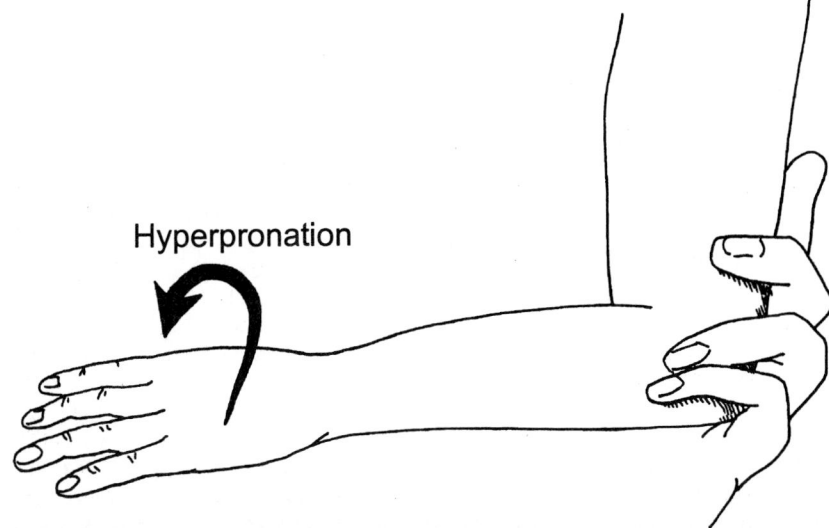

Fractures of the phalangeal shaft should be examined for displacement, rotational deformity, and tendinous disruption. Significantly displaced or rotated fractures need to be reduced and immediate consultation with an orthopedist is warranted to determine the type of reduction.

LOWER EXTREMITY INJURIES

Pelvic Fractures

The infrequent nature of pediatric pelvic fractures is largely related to the relative cartilaginous pliability of the immature pediatric pelvis as compared to the adult pelvis. Therefore, pediatric pelvic fractures usually result from a tremendous force.[5] The exception is the avulsion-type injury, which usually results from sudden muscle contractions associated with athletic injuries.

The most common mechanism for non-avulsion-type pelvic fractures is pedestrian versus motor vehicle collisions. The incidence of associated injuries is extremely high and include injuries to the genitourinary system, abdomen, chest, and central nervous system. After the child is stabilized, there should be a careful evaluation for associated injuries. Multisystem injury must be assumed in a child with a pelvic fracture, and transfer to a facility equipped to manage the pediatric multiple trauma patient is warranted. In children, life-threatening hemorrhage usually results from injury to other body areas rather than from injury to the pelvic vessels.

Avulsion-type injuries of the pelvis result from sudden contraction of musculature attached to the pelvis and typically occur during athletic activities. These injuries are usually seen in the adolescent after secondary ossification centers develop. Therefore, avulsion injuries are unusual before 8 years of age. Clinically the child will complain of sudden pain and have point tenderness and possibly swelling over the fracture site. Nearly all avulsion fractures can be managed conservatively with rest, limitation of activity until symptoms resolve, and orthopedic follow up.

Hip Injuries

Although fractures of the proximal end of the femur are quite rare in children, trauma can result in a epiphyseal disruption or a fracture of the head, neck, trochanteric, or subtrochanteric region of the femur. Treatment is almost always urgent surgical reduction and stabilization, and immediate orthopedic consultation is indicated. Proximal fractures involving the femoral head or neck have a high risk of complications such as avascular necrosis and growth arrest, unlike those involving the trochanteric or subtrochanteric regions. Treatment is dependent on both age and degree of displacement, with older children more likely to be treated operatively.

Traumatic dislocations of the hip are also rare in the pediatric population and are best divided into those occurring in the older adolescent and those occurring in the skeletally immature child. As with adults, most dislocations in adolescents are posterior and result from significant trauma. The mechanisms of injury are also similar to those of adults. The exception is the dislocation occurring in the immature hip, in children younger than 10 years of age, which can occur with minimal low-energy trauma. Treatment for pediatric hip dislocations is urgent closed reduction. Immediate orthopedic consultation is indicated as any significant delay in reduction is associated with a higher incidence of complications. The amount of time the hip is dislocated is a risk factor for avascular necrosis of the femoral head: there is a 20 times higher risk if reduction is delayed more than 6 h.[6]

Fractures of the Femoral Shaft

The femur is second bone to ossify in the fetus and the largest of the long bones in the body. The strength of the femur continues to increase in later childhood and therefore significant force is usually required to fracture the femoral shaft. Pediatric femur fractures occur more commonly in boys and seem to follow a bimodal distribution with peaks during late-toddler age and mid-teenage years.

The most common mechanisms of injury are falls, pedestrian versus automobile incidents, and motor vehicle collisions. Child abuse should be considered in children who are not yet walking.

The clinical findings in a child with a femur fracture are obvious. There is typically tenderness and swelling over the fracture site. The child may hold the leg externally rotated and likely refuse to bear weight. Shortening of the extremity may also be noticed. Given the high degree of traumatic force needed to produce the fracture, the child should receive a through evaluation for associated trauma. Evidence of hemodynamic instability such as hypotension is usually not related to an isolated femur fracture in a young child and should prompt a search for other injuries.[7]

All femoral shaft fractures require immediate orthopedic consultation. Treatment depends on the child's age, size, degree of malalignment, and reliability of follow up. Management is controversial and institution dependent; however, current trends favor early closed reduction and immobilization in a hip spica cast for closed femur fractures in children weighing less than 40 pounds or who are younger than 5 years of age. Operative repair with flexible nails and plates is gaining popularity in the 7- to 12-year age group.

Slipped Capital Femoral Epiphysis

Slipped capital femoral epiphysis (SCFE) is a disorder of childhood during which there is chronic slipping of the femoral epiphysis of the hip. The morbidity can be significant with complications commonly including avascular necrosis and premature closure of the physis. SCFE is the most common cause of hip disability in adolescents. Etiology is multifactorial and any child may develop SCFE during a growth spurt; however, most children are obese adolescents whose hips are exposed to repetitive minimal trauma. Boys are affected three times more commonly than girls and present at an average age of 14 to 16 years old. Girls typically present earlier, at around 11 to 13 years of age, with occurrence after menarche being rare. Hormonal and genetic factors also appear to play a role in the development of SCFE. Associations are seen in children with juvenile chronic arthritis, certain human leukocyte antigen (HLA) types, endocrinopathies, renal failure, and previous radiation or chemotherapy (Figure 136-4).

The slippage may be chronic, acute, or acute on chronic. Although most children will have some degree of chronic slipping, acute worsening of displacement may occur after minimal trauma. Clinically, the child presents with pain at the hip or referred to the thigh or knee. The pain may be vague and chronic in nature. Any adolescent with chronic pain in the groin, hip, thigh, or knee area deserves bilateral hip radiographs to evaluate for SCFE. Any delay in diagnosis can lead to significant disability, and given the incidence of referred pain to the knee, a high index of suspicion for SCFE needs to be maintained to prevent misdiagnosis and treatment delays.

Radiographically, epiphyseal slippage may be detected by examining the anatomic relationship of the femoral neck to the femoral head (Figure 136-5). Several techniques of measuring the presence or degree of slip have been suggested; however, subtle cases can challenge or even evade the best radiologists on plain radiographs. Therefore, any child with pain history suspicious for SCFE should receive orthopedic consultation in the ED. Once the diagnosis is made, management includes strict non-weight-bearing and definitive operative management.

The differential diagnosis includes a traumatic transphyseal fracture of the proximal femur. Although the location of the abnormality may be the same on radiographic evaluation, the conditions may usually be differentiated based on the clinical history and radiographic evidence of preexisting femoral abnormalities. SCFE has a typically in-

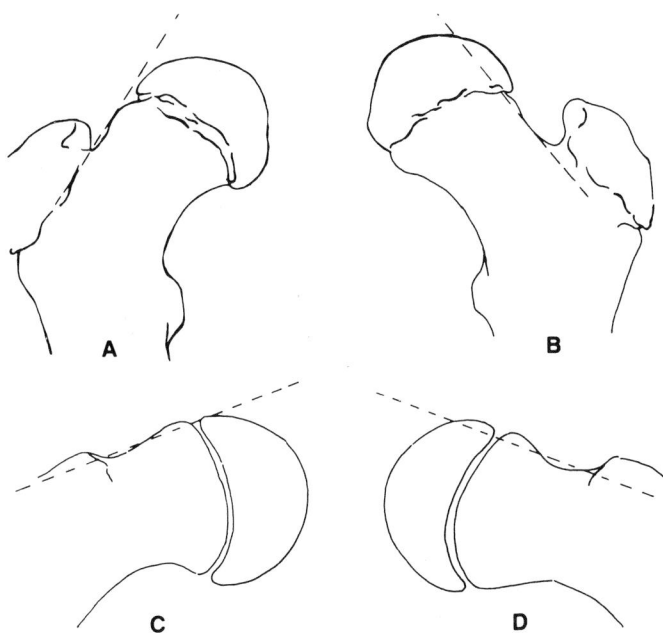

FIG. 136-4. A line drawn along the lateral (superior) aspect of the femoral neck fails to transect the lateral quarter of the femoral head in medical SCFE, seen in **A** and **C**. The normal anatomic relationship is illustrated in **B** and **D**.

sidious onset, a history of preceding intermittent hip pain, and precipitating trauma is minimal. In contrast, significant and acute trauma is necessary to fracture the femoral physis in a healthy hip.

KNEE INJURIES

Compared to the adult, ligamentous injuries to the pediatric knee are much less common than are fractures. The Ottawa knee rules (see Table 274-1) have been validated for children ≥2 years of age and can help determine the need for radiographs.[8]

Fractures through the *distal femoral physis* are uncommon yet carry a significant complication rate. The popliteal artery lies close to the distal femoral metaphysis and may be injured along with the peroneal nerve with traumatic distal femoral physeal separations. Growth arrest may also occur secondary to permanent physeal damage. Al-

though Salter-Harris type I injuries may not be appreciated on x-rays, any child suspected of having a significant injury should receive orthopedic follow up. Any displaced distal femoral physeal disruption needs immediate orthopedic evaluation for reduction (Figure 136-6).

Patellar injuries in children are usually dislocations. In fact, *patellar dislocation* is one of the most common causes of a traumatic hemarthrosis in children. The typical mechanism is one of pivoting the knee on a fixed lower leg. Often reduction has already occurred at the scene although a history of the "knee popped out of place" can usually be obtained. If the patient presents with the patella still dislocated, the displaced patella is usually sitting laterally and the knee held in flexion. Reduction need not be delayed for x-rays and is easily accomplished by gently extending the knee while another provider helps "lift" the patella into place. Although the patella does not actually need to be moved into place, the second provider can help prevent a traumatic reduction resulting in additional fractures. The child should receive x-rays after the reduction to assess for any fractures, which are most typically seen at either the lateral femoral condyle or the medial margin of the patella. Immobilization in a knee immobilizer and orthopedic follow up are indicated. Most patients improve with conservative management and rehabilitation; however, some children are predisposed to chronic dislocations and may eventually need realignment of their extensor mechanism.

Fractures of the *patella* are uncommon in children and occur from either direct traumatic force or more commonly in the adolescent participating in sporting events. Unique to children is the "sleeve" fracture of the patella where the distal patellar "sleeve" is avulsed from the body of the patella. The typical mechanism of an avulsion "sleeve" fracture is that of forceful contraction of the quadriceps against a fixed

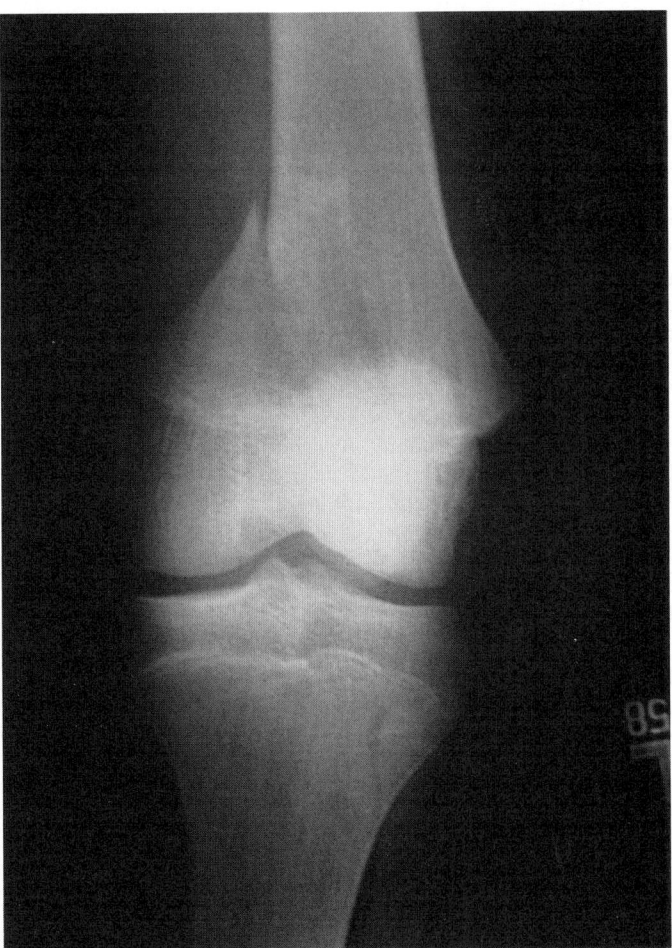

FIG. 136-6. Distal femur fracture.

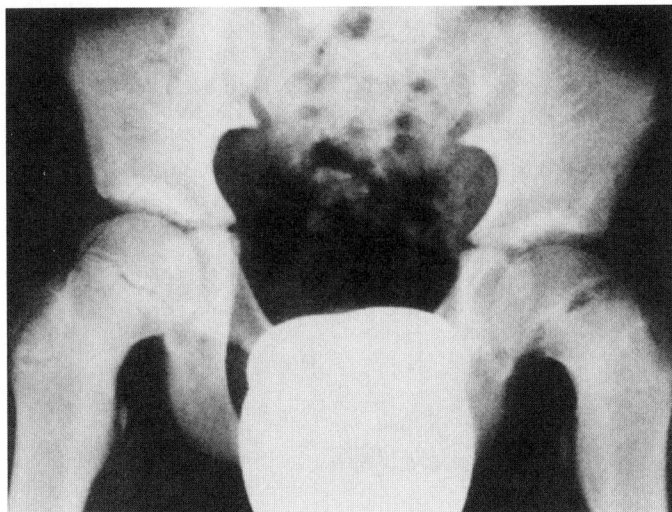

Right   Left

FIG. 136-5. AP radiograph illustrating a medical SCFE involving the left hip.

lower leg. Consultation with an orthopedist is advised to determine the appropriate treatment which depends on the degree of displacement.

Proximal tibial injuries include injuries to the *tibial spine, tibial tuberosity, and proximal tibial physis.* Mechanically speaking, an avulsion fracture of the tibial spine is the equivalent of an anterior cruciate ligament (ACL) rupture in an adult. The ACL inserts on the tibial eminence and this ligament and its insertion are much stronger than the epiphyseal bone in children. Nondisplaced fractures may be managed conservatively with immobilization and orthopedic follow up. However, any displaced fractures need reduction and immediate orthopedic consultation.

Tibial tuberosity fractures are typically avulsion-type and occur most commonly from strong contraction of the quadriceps against a fixed leg. Again, these injuries are most likely sports related. They may be classified as type I, II, or III, depending on the location of the fracture line. Type I injuries are characterized by a fracture through the small distal portion of the tibial tuberosity. Type II fractures occur after the coalescence of the secondary ossification centers of the tuberosity to the metaphysis. The fracture splits the epiphysis of the tuberosity from the epiphysis of the proximal tibia. Type III injuries involve a fracture into the joint and are at risk for developing compartment syndrome. Types I and II fractures are usually treated with immobilization. Displaced type II and type III injuries need reduction and fixation and require immediate orthopedic consultation.

Fractures of the *proximal tibial physis* are relatively uncommon and most are Salter-Harris type I. As with distal femoral physeal fractures, vascular injury to the popliteal artery is a concern and documentation of intact pulses is especially important.

Fractures of the Tibia and Fibula

Most fractures of the tibia and fibula occur at the shaft. If the fracture is minimally displaced and there is no evidence of compartment syndrome, the leg can be immobilized in a long leg posterior splint and orthopedic follow up arranged. However, if there is more than 10 degrees of angulation in any plane, reduction is recommended and immediate orthopedic consultation is indicated.

Of particular interest in the child is the *toddler's fracture,* which refers to an isolated spiral fracture of the distal tibia in a toddler. The typical mechanism is external rotation of the foot with the knee flexed, such as may occur in a child's walker. Parents may notice that the child is limping or refusing to bear weight after seemingly insignificant or occasionally unrecalled history of trauma. Clinically, there appears to be pain with palpation and rotation of the distal tibia, although swelling may be minimal or absent. Radiographically, a fracture line may be noticed at the distal third of the tibial shaft; however, initial standard x-rays may be normal with nondisplaced fractures. The addition of oblique views may show a fracture line when standard views are negative. Immobilization and follow up with a bone scan or repeat x-rays in a week is suggested when a toddler's fracture is clinically suspected and initial radiographs are negative. The child should be immobilized in a long leg splint and given orthopedic follow up for definitive casting and to ensure that proper alignment is maintained during the healing process.

Ankle Injuries

Ankle injuries in children include both ligamentous disruptions as well as fractures. Ligamentous injuries are uncommon before physeal closure because of the generally stronger nature of ligaments when compared to the strength of open physes. Ankle sprains in older children with closed physes are graded and treated as they are in adults.

Fractures of the pediatric ankle may involve the distal tibia, the fibula, or both. A thorough evaluation and appropriate treatment are extremely important because any articular surface disruption in this joint can have long-term complications despite a seemingly benign initial presentation. Additional imaging techniques such as CT and MRI are frequently used to help define the extent of fracture involvement. Treatment goals are to restore maximum function and prevent complications such as growth arrest, osteoarthritis, and chronic pain.

The most common fractures of the distal fibula are Salter-Harris types I and II, which account for approximately 90 percent of isolated distal fibula fractures. Clinically, findings with a Salter-Harris I fracture may be subtle; however, typically there is tenderness at the growth plate and soft tissue swelling is common. Isolated Salter-Harris I fractures of the distal fibula can be distinguished from a lateral ligamentous ankle sprain by the presence of point tenderness over the physis. Plain radiographs only show soft tissue swelling at the lateral fibula. In general, any type I or II fracture that is nondisplaced may be managed by immobilization and orthopedic follow up.

The most common fractures of the distal tibia are also Salter-Harris types I and II. In general, these fractures may be managed with closed reduction if any displacement is present, followed by immobilization. Salter-Harris III fractures account for approximately 25 percent of distal tibia fractures and typically require open reduction of any displacement. The Tillaux fracture is a Salter-Harris type III fracture of the anterolateral portion of the distal tibia. The location of the Tillaux fracture is a result of the order in which the distal tibial physis closes. Closure occurs centrally, then medially, and finally laterally making the anterolateral portion most vulnerable. Therefore, this type of fracture is typically seen in a child who is nearing skeletal maturity. Treatment is surgical reduction.

Salter-Harris IV fractures include the triplane fracture, which involves fractures in the sagittal, coronal, and transverse planes resulting in multiple fracture fragments. The management is surgical reduction.

Foot and Phalanx Injuries

In early childhood, the pliability and lack of ossification of the foot make fractures in this area rare. As ossification increases with age, fractures become more common; however, significant injuries are still unusual. The foot may be divided into the hindfoot (calcaneus and talus), the midfoot (navicular, cuboid, second and third cuneiforms), and the metatarsals and phalanges. Fractures of the mid- and hindfoot are rare; however, when they occur, they usually result from a fall. Recognition of fractures in these areas may be difficult and CT and MRI may be necessary to identify and define these fractures. Fractures of the metatarsals and phalanges are relatively common in children and typically result from a direct blow from a falling object. They typically heal without sequelae. Crush injury to the foot may cause vascular compromise and compartment syndrome.

Most nondisplaced fractures of the metatarsals and phalanges may be managed by immobilization and follow up with an orthopedist. Significantly displaced fractures of the metatarsals and phalanges as well as those of the great toe that have intraarticular involvement may require fixation, although this can typically be done on an outpatient basis.

SELECTED NONTRAUMATIC MUSCULOSKELETAL DISORDERS OF CHILDHOOD

Acute Septic Arthritis

Septic arthritis occurs in all age groups, but especially in children younger than 3 years of age. The reported incidence of septic arthritis varies from 2 to 5 per 100,000 per year in the general population to 28 to 38 per 100,000 per year in patients with rheumatoid arthritis. The knee is the most commonly involved joint, followed in frequency by the hip and the elbow. Any joint can be infected, and infection of more than one joint can occur.

Bacteria are the usual pathogens in acute skeletal and joint infections. Bacteria may access the joint hematogenously, by direct extension from adjacent osteomyelitis or from inoculation as in arthrocentesis or femoral venipuncture. Of these routes, hematogenous spread is the most common. The etiologic organisms encountered in septic arthritis vary with the age of the child (Table 136-2).

Even though septic infections of joints in children are uncommon, they are important because of their potential to cause permanent disability. The normal joint has several protective components. Healthy synovial cells possess significant phagocytic activity, and synovial fluid normally possesses significant bactericidal activity. In patients with bacteremia and hematogenous spread, a large number of bacteria are delivered into the vascular synovial membranes. If infection occurs, polymorphonuclear leukocyte (PMN) infiltration, vascular congestion, and lining cell proliferation occur. Early on, increased secretion of synovial fluid occurs and may be serosanguineous, cloudy, or suppurative with PMN counts ranging from 500 to 200,000 and exceeding 50,000/μL after the earliest stages. Synovial fluid glucose concentration is decreased, and the protein content is elevated. If this progresses and bacterial proliferation occurs, a persistent purulent effusion develops, accompanied by the clinical findings of a swollen, tender joint. Eventually proteolytic enzymes released by PMN, as well as direct pressure, lead to cartilage and bone destruction.

Children with septic arthritis are frequently misdiagnosed on their initial visit because the earliest signs and symptoms are subtle. This is particularly true of neonates, who characteristically do not appear ill and in half of cases do not have fever. Older infants, toddlers, and children usually have fever and localizing signs. Infants may have only pseudoparalysis of an extremity or apparent pain on movement of the affected extremity. The child with hip or knee septic arthritis will limp or not walk at all. The child maintains the infected hip in flexion, abduction, or internal rotation. On physical examination, the manifestations are those of any localized infection (i.e., erythema, swelling, tenderness, and pain). Older children will appear ill, often with high fever [40 to 40.5°C (104 to 105°F)], with apprehension, and irritability.

Plain film radiographs are frequently nondiagnostic early in the course of infection, but should be obtained to help identify osteomyelitis, fracture, or another process in the differential diagnosis.

Widening of the joint space with joint effusion and distention are late findings. Fat lines are displaced early in the septic arthritis because of capsular distention. Views of the contralateral side may be useful for comparison. Ultrasonography may be useful to document the presence of a joint effusion, and can aid in needle aspiration. CT and MRI both provide improved soft tissue resolution, and can aid in the diagnosis.

The differential considerations are listed in Table 136-3.

If septic arthritis is suspected, a CBC, blood cultures, erythrocyte sedimentation rate (ESR), C-reactive protein (CRP), and throat cultures should be obtained. About half will have WBC counts of less than 15,000 cells/μL. In approximately 90 percent of cases the ESR is high, with mean values ranging from 68 to 82 mm/h. The ESR is nonspecific and may be elevated in the presence of other infectious or immunologic conditions. The CRP may be useful as values greater than 20 mg/L have high predictive values for septic arthritis.

Joint fluid should be aspirated and sent for cell count, Gram stain, glucose, and culture. Isolation of an organism from the joint fluid is the primary criterion for the diagnosis of septic arthritis. Organisms that may be seen on the smear may not grow in culture, because of the bacteriostatic effect of joint fluid. In approximately one third of cases, a specific pathogen is not identified. If obtained, blood cultures are positive in less than half, and they are the only source from which the causative agent is isolated in about 10 percent.

Concurrent infections at other sites have been reported and may help define the pathogen (e.g., urine gram-negative bacilli; skin/wound *S. aureus;* urethra, cervix, rectum, and pharynx *N. gonorrhea).* Obtaining cultures from these sites should be dictated by the age of the child and the clinical circumstances.

The management of acute septic arthritis consists of prompt joint drainage to remove bacterial products and infectious debris, and antibiotic administration. Table 136-4 lists antibiotic therapy. The prognosis

TABLE 136-3 Differential Considerations for the Acutely Inflamed Pediatric Joint

Trauma
Septic arthritis
Acute rheumatic fever
Post-streptococcal reactive arthritis
Gonococcal arthritis
Lyme disease
Sickle cell crisis
Henoch-Schönlein purpura
Legg-Calvé-Perthes disease
Slipped capital femoral epiphysis
Reactions and toxic synovitis
Osteomyelitis
Juvenile rheumatic arthritis
Transient synovitis
Hemophilia
Osgood-Schlatter disease

TABLE 136-2 Causes of Suppurative Arthritis in Children in Decreasing Incidence

Newborn (0–2 Months)	Infant (2–36 Months)	Child (>36 Months)
Staphylococcus aureus	Staph. aureus	Staph. aureus
Group B Streptococcus	Streptococcus species	Streptococcus species
Gram-negative bacilli	Gram-negative bacilli	Gram-negative bacilli
Neisseria gonorrhoeae	H. influenza	N. gonorrhoeae
Haemophilus influenzae	Unknown or unidentified	
Candida albicans*		

*Hospital acquired.

TABLE 136-4 Initial Antibiotic Therapy of Acute Suppurative Arthritis in Children

Age	Suspected Organism	Antibiotics
Newborn (0–2 months)	Staphylococcus aureus	Methicillin or nafcillin*
	Group B Streptococcus	Ampicillin, and cefotaxime or ceftriaxone
	Gram-negative bacilli	Cefotaxime/ceftriaxone
	Neisseria gonorrhoeae	Cefotaxime/ceftriaxone
	Unknown	Methicillin or nafcillin* and cefotaxime or ceftriaxone
Infant (2–36 months)	S. aureus	Methicillin or nafcillin*
	Streptococcus species	Clindamycin/cefotaxime/ceftriaxone
	Gram-negative bacilli	Cefotaxime/ceftriaxone
	Haemophilus influenzae	Cefuroxime or cefotaxime/ceftriaxone
	Unknown	Methicillin or nafcillin* and cefotaxime or ceftriaxone
Child (>36 months)	S. aureus	Methicillin or nafcillin*
	Streptococcus species	Clindamycin/cefotaxime/ceftriaxone
	Gram-negative bacilli	Cefotaxime/ceftriaxone
	N. gonorrhoeae	Cefotaxime/ceftriaxone
	Unknown	Methicillin or nafcillin* and cefotaxime or ceftriaxone

*Vancomycin, if methicillinase-resistant S. aureus is suspected. PCN allergic patient: clindamycin + chloramphenicol.

depends on the length of time between symptom onset and treatment. More than 4 days increases the likelihood of orthopedic complications, and infants have less-favorable outcomes, possibly because of delays in diagnosis.

Henoch-Schönlein Purpura

Henoch-Schönlein purpura (HSP) is a small-vessel vasculitis characterized by purpura, arthritis, abdominal pain, and hematuria. It is the most common cause of nonthrombocytopenic purpura in children. The specific pathogenesis of HSP is unknown, but the vasculitis involves primarily small vessels and is mediated by immune complexes through IgA and the alternate complement pathways. The cause of HSP is also unknown, but HSP typically follows an upper respiratory infection. A variety of infectious and noninfectious stimuli appear to precipitate the immunologic mechanisms of the vasculitis.

The hallmark of the disease is the rash, beginning as pinkish maculopapules that initially blanch on pressure and progress to petechiae or purpura that are characterized as palpable. This rash has a propensity for the lower trunk, buttocks, perineum, and lower extremities (see Chap. 135). The lesions tend to occur in crops lasting from 3 to 10 days, and may appear at intervals that vary from a few days to several months. In addition, the vasculitis includes involvement of the glomeruli, with the subsequent development of hematuria and with the potential for long-term renal sequelae. Renal involvement occurs in 25 to 50 percent of children, and hepatosplenomegaly and lymphadenopathy may be found during active disease.

Edema and damage to the vasculature of the gastrointestinal (GI) tract may also lead to intermittent abdominal pain that is often colicky in nature. More than half of patients develop occult heme-positive stools, diarrhea (with or without blood) or hematemesis. A small proportion of children with severe abdominal colic caused by Henoch-Schönlein purpura experience massive gastrointestinal hemorrhage or intussusception.

Arthritis may be present in more than two-thirds of children with HSP, and is usually localized to the knees and ankles often with associated edema. The effusions are serous, not hemorrhagic in nature, and resolve after a few day without residual deformity or articular damage.

The clinical diagnosis is usually clear in those children manifesting all or several of the characteristics of the disorder. Making the diagnosis is often more difficult if acute arthritis is the only symptom. The role of the ED is establishing the diagnosis or maintaining a high index of suspicion. The diagnostic evaluation is also influenced by the need to exclude other causes of vasculitis. Otherwise, the care is entirely supportive. Routine laboratory test are neither specific or diagnostic. Affected children often have a moderate thrombocytosis and leukocytosis. The erythrocyte sedimentation rate (ESR) may be elevated. Consideration of specific laboratory or imaging studies is influenced by specific symptoms. In a child presenting exclusively with hematuria and abdominal pain, a urinalysis, urine culture, kidneys, ureters, and bladder (KUB) radiogram, CBC, and chemistry profile to assess renal function may be required. Intussusception in HSP is usually ileo-ileal in location, and barium enema may be used for both identification and nonsurgical reduction. Renal involvement is manifested by red blood cells, white blood cells, casts, or albumin in the urine. In summary, when the entire clinical picture presents itself, the extent of the diagnostic workup is much reduced.

Symptomatic treatment, including adequate hydration, bland diet, and pain control with acetaminophen, is provided for self-limited complaints of arthritis, edema, fever, and malaise. Avoidance of competitive activities and keeping the lower extremities elevated intermittently may decrease local edema. If there is significant edema of the scrotum, elevation of the scrotum and local cooling may decrease discomfort.

Admission to the hospital may be required when the diagnosis is in doubt, for observation and control of abdominal pain, for monitoring of renal function, or for fluid hydration in cases of recurrent emesis. Children with extremely mild symptoms can be safely discharged and observed as outpatients, with close follow-up with their primary care provider. Intestinal complications (e.g., hemorrhage, obstruction, and intussusception) may be life threatening and managed with corticosteroids and, when necessary, air enema reduction or surgical reduction or resection of the intussusception. Therapy with oral or intravenous corticosteroids is associated with improvement of GI and CNS complications, and high doses may be helpful in advanced renal involvement. Steroid use should be directed by the admitting pediatrician.

The major complications of HSP are renal involvement and development of nephrotic syndrome or bowel perforation. The overall prognosis is excellent for this relatively common, self-limited disease. Chronic renal disease becomes more common in older children. Less than 1 percent of patients with HSP develop persistent renal disease, and fewer than 0.1 percent develops serious renal disease.

Juvenile Rheumatoid Arthritis

Juvenile rheumatoid arthritis (JRA) is one of the most common rheumatic diseases of children and is a major cause of chronic disability. It is characterized by an idiopathic noninfectious synovitis of the peripheral joints, and arthritis with associated soft tissue swelling and effusion. The peak age of onset is between 1 and 3 years, and a second peak occurs in the early teen years. Although the etiology is unknown, an autoimmune response in reaction to exposure to certain viruses is suspected. JRA has three principal types of onset: (1) oligoarthritis (pauciarticular disease); (2) polyarthritis; and (3) systemic-onset disease.

Oligoarthritis (pauciarticular disease) is the most common form of JRA in children. It usually affects the joints of the lower extremities, such as knees and ankles, and typically a single large joint such as the knee. Permanent joint damage is uncommon.

Polyarticular disease occurs in approximately a third of cases, and is characterized by involvement of both large and small joints. As many as 20 to 40 separate joints are often affected, but the involvement of 5 or more joints is the criterion for this classification. There is a female preponderance. Polyarticular disease often resembles the usual presentation of adult rheumatoid arthritis. Rheumatoid nodules over the elbow extensor surfaces and Achilles tendon portend a more severe course. Long-term morbidity is related to progressive joint destruction, particularly of the hips and knees. Cervical spine involvement is common with an increased risk of atlantoaxial subluxation. Rheumatoid factor (RF) serology may be positive or negative, and antinuclear antibody (ANA) titers are positive in 25 percent of RF-negative patients, and in 75 percent of RF-positive patients.

Systemic JRA is associated with high fevers and chills, characteristically with spikes to at least 39°C (102.2°F) for a minimum of 2 weeks. There is also an accompanying characteristic faint erythematous macular coalescing rash on the trunk, palms, and soles. In addition to arthritis, patients with systemic-onset disease often have hepatosplenomegaly, lymphadenopathy, and a serositis, such as pleuritis or pericardial effusion. The arthritis in this form may progress to permanent joint damage. Serology for RF and ANA are negative in this form of JRA.

Laboratory evaluation is not highly specific for JRA. Arthrocentesis may be necessary to exclude acute suppurative arthritis, especially in pauciarticular presentations. Hematologic abnormalities often reflect the degree of systemic or articular inflammation, with elevated white blood cells and platelet counts. The ESR usually mirrors these findings, along with elevation of the CRP, serum globulins, and serum immunoglobulins. However, it is not unusual for the ESR to be normal in some children with JRA. ANAs are present in at least 40 to 85 percent of all children with pauciarticular or polyarticular JRA, but are unusual in children with systemic-onset disease. Early in the course of JRA, radiographs demonstrate only soft tissue swelling and synovial effusions. The findings of bone and cartilage destruction occur later.

The diagnosis of JRA will likely not be made in the ED, and the ED focus should be primarily to exclude other diagnostic considerations.

Hospital admission is recommended for those children in who the diagnosis is in doubt or who are treated empirically for suspected acute suppurative arthritis while synovial fluid cultures are pending.

The initial therapy for patients with an established diagnosis include aspirin or other nonsteroidal anti-inflammatory drug (NSAID). Corticosteroids are used when the diagnosis is certain and for overwhelming systemic illness, including pericarditis, myocarditis, or iridocyclitis unresponsive to other therapy.

A pediatric rheumatologist should direct other management strategies including intraarticular glucocorticoid injections, and use of methotrexate (which has generally replaced gold therapy), chloroquine, anticytokine therapy, or cytotoxic drugs.

Kawasaki Disease

Kawasaki disease (also called mucocutaneous lymph node syndrome) is an acute febrile vasculitis of childhood, involving small and medium size arteries, and characteristic involvement of the coronary arteries. It is an acute, self-limiting disease of unknown etiology.

The disease is recognized worldwide. In the United States, the peak incidence is in children 18 to 24 months of age, with 80 percent occurring in children younger than 4 years of age and 95 percent of cases occurring in children younger than 10 years of age. Males are affected more often than females (1.5:1), and children of Asian descent are at increased risk.

The diagnosis is based entirely on clinical findings. Table 136-5 lists the diagnostic clinical criteria, and the disorder is also discussed in Chap. 135. Fever is commonly the first finding of the acute phase. The fever is high, often exceeding 40°C (104°F), and prolonged, lasting from 1 to 2 weeks in untreated patients. Bulbar conjunctivitis is nonpurulent and bilateral, and has onset shortly after the appearance of fever. Changes involving the oropharynx are prominent during the acute febrile period, and include erythema and cracking of the lips and erythema of the buccal mucosa and posterior pharynx. The tongue may have a strawberry appearance due to prominent lingual papillae. The rash is quite variable and may appear morbilliform, maculopapular, or scarlatiniform. Most commonly the rash is a raised deep-red, plaquelike eruption. It may even present a fine pustular eruption, and vesicular rashes are rare. In infants, this rash may be most prominent on the perineum. Cervical adenopathy is another early symptom, and nodes are usually unilateral, nonsuppurative, and measure >1.5 cm in size. Changes to the peripheral extremities occur as induration of the dorsum of the hands and feet with erythema over the palms and soles. The palms and soles can become quite painful. A wide variety of associated findings can be present in Kawasaki disease, as listed in Table 136-6. Irritability is profound in Kawasaki disease, and aseptic meningitis frequently is found.

The acute febrile phase of the disease lasts about 10 days, during which most of the diagnostic criteria (see Table 136-5) are likely to be present. The subacute phase of the disease (from days 11 through 21)

TABLE 136-5   Diagnostic Criteria for Kawasaki Disease

Fever of at least 5 days' duration (100%)
Presence of at least four of the following five conditions:
1. Bilateral conjunctivitis (85%)
2. Changes of the lips and oral mucosa (90%)
   Dry, red, fissured lips
   Strawberry tongue
   Oropharyngeal edema
3. Changes of the extremities (75%)
   Erythema of palms and soles
   Edema of hands and feet
   Periungual desquamation
4. Polymorphous rash (80%)
5. Cervical lymphadenopathy (70%)
Illness not explained by other known disease process

TABLE 136-6   Associated Features of Kawasaki Disease

Cardiovascular system	Genitourinary system
Coronary artery aneurysms	Urethritis with sterile pyuria
Myocarditis-pericarditis	Proteinuria
Mitral or aortic insufficiency	Pulmonary system
Dysrhythmias	Pneumonitis
Peripheral ischemia	Cough, coryza
Central nervous system	Gastrointestinal system
Irritability	Hydrops of the gall bladder
Aseptic meningitis	Hepatitis
Anterior uveitis	Nausea, vomiting, diarrhea
Sensorineural hearing loss	Abdominal pain
Hematologic system	
Thrombocytosis (subacute phase)	
Anemia	

usually is associated with a decrease in fever, rash, and lymphadenopathy. Conjunctival injection and irritability may persist. Arthralgias and arthritis occur in many children at this time, as well as the dramatic desquamation of the fingers and toes. Thrombocytosis is an important finding in Kawasaki disease and this usually occurs during the subacute phase. At this time the platelet count is generally over 650,000/μL and may exceed 1 million. It is during this phase when the patient is at greatest risk for development of coronary artery thrombosis. The convalescent phase begins about day 21, when all clinical and associated signs and symptoms have disappeared, and continues until the ESR and platelet count return to normal in 6 to 10 weeks.

Cardiovascular manifestations of the disease comprise the major complications of Kawasaki disease. An acute carditis develops in 50 percent of patients, with patients developing myocarditis with symptoms of tachycardia and gallop rhythms indicating mild to severe congestive heart failure. Less-frequently occurring manifestations of carditis include pericarditis, conduction disturbances, and valvular insufficiencies. Patients with Kawasaki disease have approximately a 20 percent risk of developing coronary aneurysms without treatment. Patients younger than 1 year of age have an even greater risk. The risk of coronary aneurysm is reduced to 4 to 5 percent following treatment. Most aneurysms develop after the acute phase between days 15 to 45 of the illness. Untreated, the coronary artery aneurysms are quite prone to thrombosis during the subacute phase because of the hypercoagulable state created by the thrombocytosis. Myocardial infarction and dysrhythmia are the most common causes of sudden death and occur in 1 to 2 percent of patients, usually in the third to fourth week.

The laboratory findings are nonspecific in patients with Kawasaki disease. The CBC often shows an elevated WBC count with a left shift. A mild nonhemolytic anemia may be present. A remarkable thrombocytosis appearing during the second week of the illness, and other secondary laboratory abnormalities consistent with a diffuse systemic vasculitis may be present.

The differential diagnosis is extensive because of the nonspecific nature of its clinical features. The emergency department role is primarily that of establishing the diagnosis. Treatment is admission for administration of intravenous gamma globulin (IVGG), aspirin therapy, and cardiac evaluation. The use of IVGG has substantially decreased the morbidity and mortality associated with the disease. If used in the first 10 days of the illness, IVGG reduces the incidence of coronary artery aneurysms to 3 to 4 percent. It also is effective in promoting resolution of established aneurysms. IVGG is administered as a single dose of 2 g/kg infused over 8 to 12 h with specific protocols to monitor the patient. Aspirin therapy is started at 100 mg/kg per d divided in four doses and continued until the fever has resolved. Low-dose aspirin at 3 to 5 mg/kg per d (maximum, 40 to 80 mg per d) is then continued for 2 to 3 months or until the platelet count has normalized. Patients exhibiting coronary aneurysms despite IVGG therapy should receive aspirin for at least 1 year following the resolution of the aneurysm. A cardiologist should be involved in the evaluation and follow-up of any patient with Kawasaki syndrome. Repeat echocardiograms are usually performed 14 days and 6 to 8 weeks after onset of the illness, or more frequently if there is evidence of cardiac involvement.

Children suspected of having Kawasaki disease who do not fulfill diagnostic criteria may have "atypical" Kawasaki disease. This atypical presentation may be seen more commonly in the younger child. If the emergency physician suspects a child may have an atypical presentation, consultation with a pediatric infectious disease or rheumatology specialist is warranted.

Legg-Calvé-Perthes Disease

Legg-Calvé-Perthes disease (LCPD) is a hip disorder that generally has onset between the ages of 4 and 9 years in 80 percent of patients, with a range of occurrence from 2 to 13 years. It is the most well-known form of avascular necrosis of the femoral head. Males outnumber females by a ratio of 4:1, and it is bilateral in 10 percent of cases. Most children with the disorder are short, with average or above average weight. They often have delayed skeletal maturation.

The exact cause is unknown, although the pathophysiology is vascular occlusion. LCPD begins with repeated episodes of ischemia of the femoral head, leading to infarction and necrosis. This avascular necrosis of the femoral head is then complicated by a subchondral stress fracture. A process of reossification and remodeling (resorption) takes place and may take from 2 to 4 years. Resultant collapse and flattening of the femoral head may occur, with subsequent potential for subluxation. The outcome is a painful hip joint associated with a restricted range of motion, muscle spasms, and contractures of the soft tissues.

The onset of symptoms in LCPD is usually insidious. Presentation as an acute emergency is rare. Mild hip pain and limp have been present for weeks to months before making the diagnosis. Initially, pain is mild to none and is often referred to the anteromedial thigh or knee. Physical findings include decreased hip abduction and internal rotation. Sometimes the initial presentation is associated with trauma. Proximal thigh atrophy, and in advanced cases, limb shortening may also be noted.

Radiographically, LCPD progresses and is divided into four stages: initial, fragmentation, reossification, and healed. In the initial stage (1 to 3 months), the capital femoral epiphysis fails to grow because of the lack of blood supply. This results in the radiograph of the hip demonstrating only widening of the cartilage space of the affected hip and a smaller size of the ossific nucleus of the femoral head (Figure 136-7). The second radiographic sign is the appearance of the sub-

chondral stress fracture line in the femoral head (Caffey sign). The third radiologic finding is increased radiopacity of the femoral head caused by new bone deposited on avascular trabeculae. Subsequently, calcification of the necrotic marrow occurs, with resultant crushing of the avascular trabeculae in the dome of the epiphysis. Further distortions of the femoral head evolve during the healing process, along with subluxation and extrusion of the femoral head from the acetabulum.

Diagnosis of LCPD demands a high index of suspicion, because initial radiographs often are normal. Bone scan and MRI are helpful early on to make the diagnosis. The technetium-99m bone scan demonstrates markedly reduced uptake of nuclide within the affected femoral head. These findings precede apparent plain film abnormalities, with possibility to diagnose LCPD months earlier than the x-ray alone. Likewise, MRI also provides superior resolution and sensitivity, with areas of low signal intensity reflecting necrotic regions within the femoral head.

The differential diagnosis includes toxic synovitis, acute rheumatic fever, tuberculosis arthritis, tumors such as eosinophilic granuloma, osteoid osteoma, and osteoblastoma, and lymphoma. Patients diagnosed with LCP disease should be made non-weight bearing and referred to a pediatric orthopedist for management. Current treatment focuses on maintaining containment of the femoral head through the use of splints or occasionally surgery. Factors related to a poorer prognosis include older age at clinical onset, extensive capital femoral epiphyseal involvement, premature epiphyseal closure, and reduced range of hip motion.

Osgood-Schlatter Disease

This very common syndrome is an apophysitis of the tibial tubercle resulting from repeated normal stresses or overuse. These repetitive stresses imposed by the patellar tendon on its site of insertion results in a series of micro-avulsions of the ossification center and the underlying cartilage. An inflammatory process is established, with resultant patellar tendonitis and a remarkable prominence, induration, and tenderness of the tibial tuberosity. No evidence of avascular necrosis of the tibial tubercle is present. Patients are usually between 10 and 15 years of age at time of onset; it more commonly occurs in running or jumping athletes. Boys are affected more often than girls, and most cases are bilateral, although symptoms are commonly asymmetric.

Signs and symptoms of Osgood-Schlatter disease are chronic, intermittent pain and tenderness over the anterior aspect of the knee and the tibial tuberosity. Pain is aggravated by activates such as running, kneeling, squatting, and climbing stairs, and improves with rest. On examination, there is a prominence and soft tissue swelling over the tibial tubercle. Tenderness and thickening of the patellar tendon may be present. The remainder of the knee examination usually is normal, and there is no knee effusion.

While radiographs are not essential, they usually are obtained. Radiographic findings of soft tissue swelling and irregularities of the tibial tubercle are nonspecific. The irregularity of the ossification of the tibial tubercle is normal in this age group. A lateral knee radiograph is best for demonstrating abnormalities, which may show prominence of the tibial tuberosity, calcification in the tibial tubercle region, or separate ossicles from the anterior border of the tubercle.

The disease is self-limited, and most patients respond to conservative care that consists of rest and avoidance of the offending activity. This is perhaps the most difficult instruction to enforce in young athletes. To ensure compliance, a brief period of immobilization or non-weight bearing may be necessary. Flexibility exercises to stretch the quadriceps and hamstrings to alleviate stress on the tubercle and avoid recurrences are helpful. Applying ice after activity may decrease swelling and pain. NSAIDs may be used but have not been shown to decrease the course of disease. A neoprene sleeve on the knee reduces patellar mobility with resultant reduction of forces on the tubercle. Corticosteroid injections into the patellar tendon or para-apophyseal

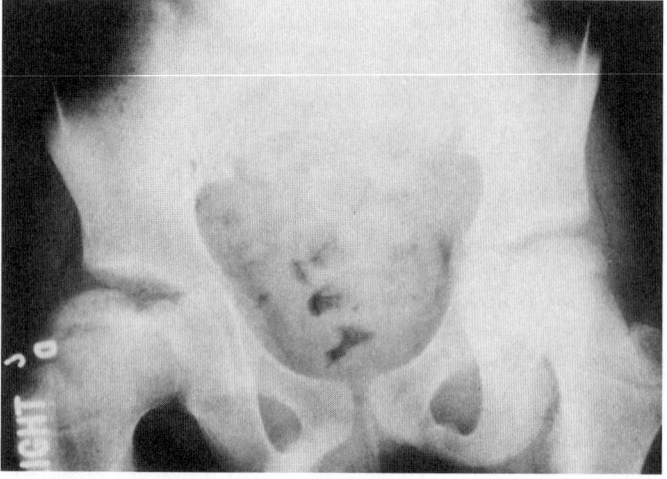

FIG. 136-7. Legg-Calvé-Perthes disease. The right hip illustrates joint-space widening, reduced size of the ossific nucleus of the femoral head, and increased opacification of the femoral head.

soft tissues should not be administered. Other than the presence of an ossicle that causes pain with kneeling, there are no long-term disabilities or problems associated with this condition.

Poststreptococcal Reactive Arthritis

Because of increased group A β-hemolytic infections, the incidence of poststreptococcal reactive arthritis (PSRA) is also increasing. PSRA is a poorly understood clinical syndrome in which arthritis of one or more joints occurs following a group A streptococcal infection of the pharynx. Like acute rheumatic fever (ARF), PSRA is a reactive arthritis characterized by a streptococcal infection, a symptom-free interval, and subsequent aseptic inflammation of one or more joints. Other major criteria of ARF are absent in PSRA. It is not certain whether PSRA represents a mild or early form of ARF, or whether it is an entirely separate entity.

In addition to group A β-hemolytic streptococci, primary infections with *Salmonella, Staphylococcus,* and other groups of *Streptococcus* are reportedly associated with reactive arthritis. Unlike ARF, reactive arthritis is not associated with carditis or other major criteria, and is a milder illness. PSRA also begins sooner (approximately 10 days) after streptococcal infection than does ARF (approximately 21 days). The arthritis in PSRA is generally more severe and prolonged and unusually resistant to treatment with salicylates, in contrast to the migratory salicylate-sensitive arthritis generally associated with ARF.

The differentiation between ARF and PSRA is clinical. The arthritis of ARF is classically a migratory polyarthritis, while the arthritis of PSRA is described as a nonmigratory mono- or oligoarthritis. ARF poststreptococcal nonsuppurative sequelae are more commonly observed in younger patients (mean age 12 ± 4 years). The typical patient with reactive arthritis is older, but it may occur in children as young as 4 years of age. Erythema nodosum and erythema multiforme are frequently associated with PSRA, while encountered only infrequently in cases of ARF.

To establish the diagnosis of PSRA, antecedent infection with group A streptococcus must be established, either by culture of the bacterium from the throat or by demonstration of an elevation or a fourfold rise in anti-streptolysin O (ASO) or anti-DNase B titer. If group A streptococcus is recovered from the throat, specific antibacterial therapy should be given. The diagnosis of PSRA should be made only after careful historical and clinical evaluation for nonsuppurative complications or other causes of polyarthritis. The issue of antibiotic prophylaxis as recommended for ARF is controversial with PSRA, but may be considered on a short-term basis. If, after further evaluation, there is no evidence of carditis or chorea, prophylaxis may be discontinued. Treatment of PSRA is nonsteroidal anti-inflammatory medications.

Acute Rheumatic Fever

ARF primarily affects children of school age. The incidence of ARF has steadily fallen in developed countries over the past 50 years. However, a resurgence in cases of group A β-hemolytic streptococcal infections over the past 10 years has increased concerns about ARF and other nonsuppurative sequelae of streptococcal infections. Outbreaks of ARF are regularly reported in North America. It is preceded by infection with certain strains of group A β-hemolytic *Streptococcus* (mucoid types 3, 5, and 18). Different layers of the cell wall of the streptococcal organism appear to stimulate antibody production to variable host tissues. The hallmark histologic feature of rheumatic fever is the Aschoff body, found in the connective tissue and created by edematous, fragmented collagen fibers. The connective tissue of the heart, joints, central nervous system, and subcutaneous tissues and skin are targeted by the immune reaction. The carditis is an endomyocarditis, with valvulitis primarily involving the mitral and aortic valves. The arthritis is characterized by synovial edema and periarticular swelling with joint effusions.

The child develops the disorder 2 to 6 weeks following a streptococcal pharyngitis. While nonspecific symptoms of systemic illness predominate early on, physical examination eventually reveals evidence of arthritis, carditis, choreiform movements, erythema marginatum, or subcutaneous nodules, individually or in combination. Table 136-7 illustrates Jones criteria for establishing a diagnosis of acute rheumatic fever. Either two major criteria or one major and two minor criteria plus evidence of an antecedent streptococcal infection are necessary to establish the diagnosis.

Arthritis occurs in 60 to 75 percent of initial attacks and is characterized as a migratory, fleeting polyarticular arthritis primarily affecting the large joints. The carditis occurs in a third of new cases and may be mild or severe. Its presence is heralded by any combination of a new cardiac murmur, tachycardia, a gallop rhythm, a pericardial friction rub, congestive heart failure, or a hyperactive precordium. Sydenham chorea occurs in 10 percent of cases and may have its initial appearance months following a streptococcal infection. Chorea may be the sole manifestation of acute rheumatic fever. The skin rash of acute rheumatic fever (erythema marginatum) is described as serpiginous and persists only for several days. It usually coexists with the presence of carditis in some form. Subcutaneous nodules are more rare and are located on the extensor surfaces of the wrists, elbows, and knees. The greatest morbidity and mortality is associated with the development of carditis.

Diagnostic studies are used to clarify the associated antecedent infection by group A streptococcus (a pharyngeal swab for culture, antistreptolysin titers, or streptozyme titers), or are employed to identify and assess the presence and extent of carditis. An electrocardiogram is obtained to assess for conduction delays or hypertrophy. A chest x-ray serves to identify cardiac dilatation or pulmonary vascular congestion or edema. Echocardiography is used to identify evidence of valvulitis or valvular insufficiency and also to exclude other diagnostic considerations.

The differential diagnosis includes JRA, septic arthritis, Kawasaki disease, viral or other forms of cardiomyopathy, leukemias, and other forms of vasculitis, including drug reactions. Rarely, tumors of the central nervous system require differentiation from ARF when the child's sole clinical manifestation is chorea.

Treatment of ARF in the emergency department is directed primarily toward the management of complicating features of carditis. In the absence of cardiac or hemodynamic instability (and such is the rule), early consultation with a pediatric cardiologist is recommended, and admission to the hospital is generally advised in the early stages until the diagnosis is confirmed. Arthritis is managed with high-dose aspirin therapy (75 to 100 mg/kg per d) to achieve a serum salicylate level of 20 to 30 mg/dL. The aspirin dose is reduced after approximately 1 week to 50 mg/kg per d for an additional 4 to 6 weeks. Significant carditis or congestive heart failure is managed with prednisone, 1 to 2 mg/kg per d. This is continued for 2 weeks following the resolution of symptoms and the return of the ESR to normal. The

TABLE 136-7   Revised Jones Criteria for the Diagnosis of Acute Rheumatic Fever

Major	Minor
Carditis	Fever
New or changing murmurs	Arthralgia
Cardiomegaly, congestive heart failure	History of previous attack of ARF
	Elevated ESR, C-reactive protein
Pericarditis	Prolonged PR interval on electrocardiogram
Migratory polyarthritis	
Chorea	Rising titer of antistreptococcal antibodies
Erythema marginatum	
Subcutaneous nodules	

Note: Diagnosis is likely when two major criteria or one major and two minor criteria are met. Group A *Streptococcus* may be documented by a history of scarlet fever, isolation of group A *Streptococcus* from throat culture, or rising titers of antistreptococcal antibodies.

duration of glucocorticoid therapy requires a subsequent taper of the steroids over a 4- to 6-week period. Chorea can be managed with haloperidol, 0.01 to 0.03 mg/kg per d in four divided doses. All children with ARF are treated with penicillin, even if the cultures for group A *Streptococcus* are negative. The dose of benzathine penicillin is 600,000 units IM if <27 kg, and 1.2 million units IM if ≥27 kg. Benzathine penicillin G can be administered in a single dosage of 1.2 million units. Penicillin V administered PO is also effective. Erythromycin may be substituted for the penicillin-allergic patient. All therapy, if pursued, is administered for 10 days.

Long-term prophylactic therapy against group A *Streptococcus* is begun upon completion of the acute phase of therapy. Acceptable prophylactic regimens include benzathine penicillin G, 1.2 million units administered IM every month, or daily oral penicillin V or sulfadiazine. Five years of prophylactic antibiotics for those children without cardiac involvement is recommended. Patients with manifestations of carditis are placed on life-long prophylaxis.

Transient Synovitis of the Hip

Toxic or transient synovitis is a benign, self-limiting inflammatory process of the hip. It afflicts males more than females and is the most common cause of acute hip pain in children less than 10 years of age. The peak incidence is between ages 3 and 6 years, but has been reported from 9 months to adolescence. It is eight times more frequent than septic arthritis of any joint. The etiology is unknown and believed to be a post-viral illness sequelae most often, but trauma, bacterial infection, and postvaccine or drug-mediated reactions have also been cited as possible causes. Arthralgia and arthritis are secondary to a transient inflammation and hypertrophy of the synovial membrane.

Symptoms are characterized by an abrupt onset of unilateral hip pain, limp, and restricted hip motion (preferentially held in abduction and external rotation). The child may complain of pain in the anteromedial or anterolateral thigh and knee. Although children complain of discomfort with movement of the limb, it generally remains possible to put the hip through a full range of motion. This is in contrast to the septic hip in which pain and spasms are more severe, and range of motion is decreased. The child is nontoxic appearing, and other signs of systemic illness are absent. There can be either no fever, or a low grade temperature elevation. The mean WBC and ESR are significantly lower than in septic arthritis, but they cannot be used to distinguish between transient synovitis and septic arthritis and septic arthritis in individual patients. Patients at risk for septic arthritis usually have temperature >38.5°C (101.3°F), an ESR >20, leukocytosis, severe pain, tenderness on palpation, spasm, and refusal to walk.

Radiographs of the hip may be normal or may demonstrate an effusion, and are obtained to exclude pathologic osseous conditions. There are no bone changes associated with transient synovitis. Ultrasound is more sensitive than plain films at detecting joint effusions, although accuracy is decreased in patients younger than 1 year of age. Reports of an effusion of the hip by ultrasound in toxic synovitis vary from 50 percent to 95 percent.

The differential diagnosis includes slipped capital femoral epiphysis and other hip fractures, Legg-Calvé-Perthes disease, and septic arthritis of the hip. Less-common causes include acute rheumatic fever, juvenile rheumatoid arthritis, and, rarely, tuberculosis of the hip.

Joint aspiration is only necessary if septic arthritis is in the differential diagnosis. When obtained, synovial fluid is sterile, and clearly transudative with negative organisms on Gram stain. If the peripheral WBC and ESR are substantially elevated and a hip effusion is noted on radiograph or ultrasound, a diagnostic arthrocentesis should be performed to exclude a septic joint. Synovial fluid should be sent for Gram stain, aerobic and anaerobic cultures, and acid-fast bacilli with culture. If an infection is demonstrated, an orthopedic consultation should be obtained with consideration for open irrigation of the hip in the operating room and admission for intravenous antibiotics.

Rest and non-weight bearing until the pain resolves for a usual period of 3 to 7 days, followed by limited activity for 1 to 2 weeks, are the treatments of choice. Nonsteroidal anti-inflammatory medications are the first-line therapy for pain. The duration of pain is typically 3 to 4 days, but may last as long as 2 weeks. Exacerbations of symptoms can occur if the child resumes normal activity too early.

There is no evidence of serious sequelae resulting from toxic synovitis. As long as the diagnosis is certain, reevaluation by the primary care physician can be arranged within 2 weeks.

REFERENCES

1. Skaggs D, Pershad J: Pediatric elbow trauma. *Ped Emerg Care* 13(6):425, 1997.
2. Skaggs DL: Elbow fractures in children: Diagnosis and management. *J Am Acad Orthop Surg* 5(6):303, 1997.
3. Wu J, Perron AD, Miller MD, et al: Orthopedic pitfalls in the ED: Pediatric supracondylar humerus fractures. *Am J Emerg Med* 20(6):544, 2002.
4. Macias CG, Bothner J, Wiebe R: A comparison of supination/flexion to hyperpronation in the reduction of radial head subluxations. *Pediatrics* 102(1):110, 1998.
5. Grisoni N, Connor S, Marsh E, et al: Pelvic fractures in a pediatric level I trauma center. *J Orthop Trauma* 16(7):458, 2002.
6. Mehlman CT, Hubbard GW, Crawford AH, et al: Traumatic hip dislocation in children. Long-term followup of 42 patients. *Clin Orthop* (376):68, 2000.
7. Sanders JO, Browne RH, Mooney JF, et al: Treatment of femoral fractures in children by pediatric orthopedist: Results of a 1998 survey. *J Pediatr Orthop* 21(4):436, 2001.
8. Bulloch B, Neto G, Plint A, et al: Validation of the Ottawa Knee Rule in children: A multicenter study. *Ann Emerg Med* 42(1):48, 2003.

SICKLE CELL DISEASE

Peter J. Paganussi
Thom Mayer
Maybelle Kou

Sickle cell disease (SCD) is among the most common pediatric genetic conditions encountered in emergency medicine (especially in urban settings) and is found primarily in people of African, Mediterranean, Indian, or Middle Eastern heritage.

In the United States about 8 percent of the African-American population carries the hemoglobin (HgbS) gene and about 0.15 percent (approximately 1/500) are homozygous (HgbSS).[1] These individuals have a predominance of "sickled" hemoglobin, thus resulting in symptomatic SCD. Patients with this hemoglobinopathy have both sickle (A_2) and fetal hemoglobin. The most frequently encountered heterozygous sickle genotypes are HgbSA (sickle cell trait), Hgb-β thalassemia (sickle β thalassemia), and HgbSC (sickle cell-hemoglobin SCD). These less common variants of the homozygous disorder have similar, but far less severe, clinical manifestations. While patients with sickle cell trait have a normal life expectancy, those with SCD have a significant mortality rate, with 20 to 30 percent of all deaths from SCD occurring before 5 years of age and a mean age at death of 14 years.[2] Current survival has been greatly improved as a result of more aggressive infection prophylaxis and advances in therapy. Nonetheless, the highest mortality occurs in children between 1 and 3 years of age, with sepsis being the leading cause of death.[3]

Clinical effects of the disorder can begin in infancy but usually are not seen until 5 to 6 months of age, because high levels of fetal hemoglobin are present following birth, and the β-Hgb subunit is not predominant until about 3 months of age. SCD is characterized by abnormal sickle-shaped cells that are less deformable than normal red blood cells. Aggregation of these less pliant, abnormally-shaped cells leads to obstruction and thrombosis of small vessels, resulting in ischemia and tissue infarction, leading to end-organ dysfunction.

This chapter discusses sickle cell disease in children. Chapter 221 reviews sickle cell disease in adults.

PATHOPHYSIOLOGY

The genetic abnormality responsible for the disease is caused by a single amino acid substitution of valine for glutamic acid in the β subunit of the hemoglobin molecule. The resultant hemolytic anemia is caused by the abnormal properties of HgbS. Affected red blood cells undergo repeated cycles of sickling and unsickling, with the HgbS strands polymerizing abnormally in response to deoxygenation. Without an attached O_2 molecule, they tend to coalesce and stretch into long monofilaments, thereby resulting in the distorted sickle shape of the red cell membrane. These irreversibly sickled cells diminish blood viscosity, causing hemolysis and obstructing the microcirculation of end-organ tissues. Capillary obstruction deprives tissues of oxygen and metabolic nutrition. It has long been presumed that the resultant hypoxia and ischemia cause the pathologic and clinical features of the disease. This entire process is felt to be self-perpetuating and sustains continued sickling. Others have recently proposed that plasma proteins, endothelial cells, and other genetically driven mechanisms play a major role in this complex process. A few investigators have even questioned whether vasoocclusion exists at all, theorizing that tissue ischemia and infarction result from shunting of blood away from end-organ vascular beds rather than occlusion by deformed, sickled cells.[4]

CLINICAL PRESENTATION AND DIAGNOSIS

Patients with SCD classically present with signs and symptoms classified by the type of crisis they manifest: vasoocclusive, hematologic, or infectious (Table 137-1). The National Heart, Lung, and Blood Institute has recently published treatment guidelines on the management of sickle cell patients, which summarize the current understanding of this disease.[5]

Vasoocclusive Crises

Vasoocclusive crises are the classic "sickle crises" characterized by painful events, often involving the back, chest, extremities, or abdomen, but which may also involve the central nervous, renal, or genitourinary systems. They are the most common reason for ED visits by children with SCD.[6] These vasoocclusive events account for more morbidity and hospitalizations than any other set of complications. The episodes are highly variable from patient to patient, with many patients reporting no crises at all, whereas others experience them on a regular basis, varying in location, duration, and severity. Typical sickle cell patients average about four severe attacks per year, with few patients reporting crises daily.

TABLE 137-1   Types of Sickle Cell Crises

Vasoocclusive crises
  Musculoskeletal
    Long bones
    Lumbosacral
    Dactylitis
  Abdominal pain
    Generalized
    Right-upper-quadrant syndrome
  Acute chest syndrome
  Central nervous system crisis
  Renal crises
  Priapism
Hematologic crises
  Acute splenic sequestration
  Aplastic crises
Infectious crises

Some of these vasoocclusive crises seem to have triggers, that include stress (emotional or physical), cold water immersion/exposure (especially as associated with shivering postexposure), dehydration, high altitudes/hypoxia, or infection (bacterial or viral, with the latter being the most common trigger in children under the age of 10 years).

Most vasoocclusive crises occur without any obvious cause. They result from the classic mechanism of sludging of sickled red blood cells into the microcirculation, resulting in tissue hypoxia and infarction. The associated pain may recur in the same location(s), but it can be anywhere in the body. Young children tend to have pain in the limbs, whereas adolescents more commonly complain of abdominal pain. *Musculoskeletal* crises are the most common vasoocclusive crises followed by *abdominal pain*. With musculoskeletal pain, the location can be anywhere, but mostly involves the long bones, i.e., the femur, tibia, and humerus. Lumbosacral pain is also commonly reported. Often there are no demonstrative physical findings, but point tenderness may be found in the painful locations. Inguinal pain with difficulty in weight bearing and walking should raise the suspicion of avascular necrosis of the femoral head. Radiographs and/or a bone scan will aid in the diagnosis.

Infants may present with *sickle dactylitis,* also known as hand and foot syndrome. This occurs secondary to ischemia and infarction in the bone marrow of the extremities. Nutrient arteries that supply the metacarpals and the metatarsals become occluded and cause avascular necrosis. Clinically one sees swelling and pain of the hands and feet, often with an accompanying low-grade fever (i.e., less than 38.6°C or 101.5°F). One or all four extremities may be involved. Dactylitis is usually seen in children under the age of 2 years and is rare after the age of 5.

Abdominal pain is the next most common type of vasoocclusive crisis seen in children with SCD and is characterized by its abrupt onset, lack of localization, and recurrence. Patients often complain of diffuse, generalized abdominal pain, typically in the absence of significant peritoneal signs. Bowel sounds usually remain present and auscultate normally during these attacks. It can be extremely difficult to differentiate whether the pain is caused by vasoocclusive crisis or by a more common type of surgically correctable condition. While peritoneal signs are often absent in crisis, abdominal guarding and rebound tenderness may be present to cloud the diagnosis. Mesenteric infarction as well as splenic and hepatic infarction are the most likely causes of the pain, but the differential also should include pancreatitis, hepatitis, appendicitis, perforated viscus, and pelvic inflammatory disease or other gynecologic pathology. It is important to determine if the abdominal pain in SCD patients has substantially changed in character, quality, duration, severity, and associated symptoms. If such changes are present, infection or other related diagnoses should be explored.

Because of the rapid turnover of red blood cells, bilirubin gallstones commonly form. This can result in biliary colic and/or cholecystitis with a secondary gallstone ileus [right-upper-quadrant (RUQ) syndrome]. Any sickle cell patient in crisis with RUQ pain should be carefully evaluated for this possibility. Approximately 75 percent of sickle patients have demonstrable bilirubin gallstones; fortunately only about 10 percent become symptomatic.

RUQ syndrome is characterized by the sudden onset of RUQ pain, anorexia, extreme hyperbilirubinemia (greater than 50 mg/dL), and progressive hepatomegaly. RUQ syndrome is usually benign and self-limiting in the pediatric patient population. It is felt to result from intrahepatic cholestasis and is usually reversible with intravenous fluids and other supportive measures. However, in a small number of adult patients, this syndrome can progress to liver failure. With all of the aforementioned conditions, ultrasound examination and/or computed tomography (CT) of the abdomen and pelvis may be useful. Prompt surgical consultation is initiated in patients in whom the diagnosis cannot be clarified.

Infections can cause vasoocclusive crises; therefore, determining the presence of an infectious process is critical. Painful crises are often associated with a low-grade fever and leukocytosis, but any temperature above 38.4°C (101.1°F) (or an absolute band count greater than 300 cells per cubic millimeter) is more likely to represent an infectious etiology than tissue ischemia.

General Treatment of Vasoocclusive Crises

Regardless of the end-organ involved, acute pain management, assuring adequate hydration, and provision of supplemental oxygen in appropriate settings are all essential features of the treatment of SCD.

ACUTE PAIN MANAGEMENT By definition, the patient in acute pain in the ED has exhausted the therapeutic options used at home and indicates the need for aggressive pain control, which will nearly always need to be provided by the parenteral route. Selection of the agent, route, and dose should be based on consideration of: (1) effective agents used at home; (2) drugs, dosages, and side effects providing relief in previous episodes; and (3) timing of medications recently taken by the patient. SCD patients or their family members are the best source for determining which medications (and at what dose) have been most effective in previous episodes. When available, consultation with a patient's physician can be invaluable in providing information and coordinating treatment. The patient's pain should be quantitated using a numerical scale or a modified Wong-Baker scale in younger children (see Chap. 134).[7] Pain relief should be assessed frequently (no less than every 15 to 30 min) with a goal of 50 to 60 percent pain relief from previous intervals (Table 137-2). Intravenous morphine sulfate, usually at a dose of 0.1 to 0.15 mg/kg, or hydromorphone (0.02 to 0.05 mg/kg) may be given initially, followed by one-quarter to one-half the loading dose at subsequent reevaluation intervals. Pain intensity, pain relief, mood, and sedation level should be assessed and documented at each reassessment interval. Patient-controlled anesthesia pumps may also be used as well.

HYDRATION THERAPY Hydrational status of all SCD patients should be assessed clinically and by use of blood chemistries, blood count, and urine specific gravity. Fluid overload should be avoided by using D5 ¼NS or ½NS. Fluid replacement should not exceed 1.5 times maintenance levels (2250 mL/m^2 per d), except in cases in which SCD patients are hypotensive, in which case fluid boluses of 10 to 20 mL/kg of RL or NS may be needed initially.

Other Vasoocclusive Events

Acute chest syndrome, the second most common reason for hospitalization in a SCD patient, is an acute illness characterized by fever and development or worsening of respiratory symptoms, accompanied by a new pulmonary infiltrate on chest radiograph.[5] However, chest radiographic changes typically are delayed by hours to days, which may make the diagnosis of acute chest syndrome somewhat more difficult. Patients often present with pleuritic chest pain, cough, dyspnea, hypoxia, and leukocytosis. Two multicenter studies [the Multicenter Acute Chest Syndrome Study (MACSS)[8,9] and the Cooperative Study of Sickle Cell Disease (CSSCD)[10]] have delineated the nature of pulmonary end-organ pathology, which includes acute chest syndrome, pulmonary infarction, pneumonia, reactive airway disease, and fat embolism syndrome. Diagnostic workup of acute chest syndrome includes chest radiograph, pulse oximetry and/or arterial blood gases,

CBC, and reticulocyte count. Treatment is guided by the severity of the disease, but always includes hydration, pain control, and oxygen therapy (Table 137-3).

***Stroke or CNS crises* (Table 137-4) occur in 5 to 10 percent of children (15 to 25 percent in all age categories) with SCD, and may be characterized by acute onset of hemiparesis, seizures, headaches, transient ischemic attacks, dizziness/vertigo, sensory hearing loss, cranial nerve palsies, paresthesias, and inexplicable coma.** These crises tend to be painless but are abrupt in onset. Cerebral infarction is more common in children, while cerebral hemorrhage is more typical in adults. The overall rate of subarachnoid hemorrhage (SAH) is increased in sickle disease patients.[11] Computed tomography (CT) scan, lumbar puncture, and magnetic resonance imaging (MRI) are all helpful for diagnosis.

Renal vasoocclusive events are common but generally asymptomatic. Symptoms of renal infarction may include flank pain, renal colic, and costovertebral angle tenderness to percussion or palpation. Gross or microscopic hematuria may be evident, and some patients may actually pass renal tissue in their urine secondary to papillary necrosis. Monitoring of baseline renal function (i.e., BUN and creatinine) is always recommended in SCD patients.

Priapism consists of a painful, sustained erection of the penis in the absence of sexual stimulation and is the result of the accumulation of sickled cells in the corpora cavernosa. Severe and prolonged attacks can cause impotence. This occurs in up to 30 percent of males with SCD; surgical decompression is usually required in such prolonged attacks (Table 137-5).[12]

Newer approaches to priapism include oral administration of α-adrenergic agonists (terbutaline and pseudoephedrine) or intrapenile injection of vasodilators such as hydralazine, and/or needle aspiration of the corpora cavernosa.

Hematologic Crises

The hallmarks of these crises are an acute drop in serum hemoglobin levels and clinical symptoms of generalized weakness and malaise, fatigue, shortness of breath or exertional dyspnea, progressive congestive heart failure, and/or shock. There are two types of hematologic crisis—splenic sequestration and aplastic crisis (Table 137-6).

TABLE 137-3   Treatment of Acute Chest Syndrome

Oxygen Therapy
Assessment
   Continuous pulse oximetry
   Baseline arterial blood gases
   Calculation of the alveolar-arterial (A-a) gradient
Treatment
   Moderately hypoxic patients
      P_{AO_2} 70–80 mm Hg
      SaO_2 92–95 percent
      Oxygen 2–4 L/min
      Pain control
   Severely Hypoxic Patients
      P_{AO_2} <70 mm Hg
      SaO_2 <90 percent
      Worsening A-a gradient
      10% Drop from baseline status
      Ventilatory support
      Transfusion therapy
Antibiotic Therapy (febrile or severely ill patients)
   Intravenous broad-spectrum coverage
      Macrolide or quinolone (to cover atypical pneumonia)
      Cephalosporin
Pain Control (see Table 137–2)
Hydration
   D5¼NS or D5½NS (see Chap. 132)

TABLE 137-2   Pain Medication Guidelines for SCD in Children

Intravenous route (avoid intramuscular)
Morphine sulfate 0.1–0.15 mg/kg IV
Hydromorphone 0.02–0.05 mg/kg IV
One-quarter to one-half the loading dose at 15- to 30-min intervals
Medication titrated to pain relief, pain intensity, mood, and sedation

TABLE 137-4   Treatment of CNS Crises

Acute Ischemic Stroke
   Thrombolytic therapy (guided by current indications and contraindications, the most important of which is age <18 years)
   Hydration
      Monitor by blood count, chemistries, and urine specific gravity
      D5 ¼NS or D5 ½NS as indicated clinically and by lab studies
      Replacement not to exceed 1.5 times maintenance (maintenance = 2250 mL/M^2 per d)
   Exchange transfusion
      Avoids increased blood viscosity of normal transfusion
      Must be titrated to avoid hypotension (which could lower cerebral perfusion further)
   Seizure control
      Seizures should be treated
      Prophylactic treatment or corticosteroids are not recommended
   Maintain normoglycemia
   Treat hypothermia
Transient Ischemic Attacks (TIAs)
   Exchange transfusion if the patient has significant large vessel disease on TCD, CT, MRI
   Antiplatelet therapy (aspirin, clopidogrel, dipyridamole/aspirin)
   TCD screening for asymptomatic patients; chronic transfusion for those with confirmed abnormalities
Subarachnoid hemorrhage
   Neuro/pediatric ICU monitoring
   Exchange transfusion with a goal of <30% HbS
   Nimodipine (guided by empiric results)

Abbreviation: TCD = transcranial Doppler.

ACUTE SPLENIC SEQUESTRATION   This occurs primarily in infants and young children and is the second most common cause of death in children with SCD under the age of 5 years. The spleen enlarges, accompanied by a decline in hemoglobin concentration; hence patients present with splenomegaly and hypovolemic shock. These symptoms may occur suddenly or insidiously, and repeated episodes are common, as a result of sickled cells blocking splenic outflow and drainage, thus causing pooling of both peripheral blood and sickled cells in the spleen. These crises are often preceded by a viral infection, often with parvovirus B19, although rhinoviruses and echoviruses have also recently been implicated.[13]

Splenic sequestration crises are often divided into major and minor types. In major sequestration, the spleen enlarges rapidly and the serum hemoglobin levels drop to less than 6 g/dL, or to 3 g/dL from that particular patient's baseline. A minor episode is more insidious and leads to progressive splenomegaly, with hemoglobin levels generally greater than 6 g/dL. Reticulocyte counts tend to be higher than normal, reflecting the compensatory increase in bone marrow activity. Management includes transfusion of packed RBCs and exchange transfusions. Ultimately splenectomy may become necessary.

APLASTIC CRISIS   Among the most life-threatening of all complications related to SCD, this complication occurs when bone marrow erythropoiesis slows or completely ceases, resulting in erythroid aplasia. It is characterized by fatigue, dyspnea, increased headache and severe anemia (with hematocrit levels of 10 percent or lower, hemoglobin levels of 1 to 3 g/dL or less, and reticulocyte counts as low

TABLE 137-5   Treatment of Priapism

Analgesia
IV hydration
Urologic consultation
Oral α-adrenergic agents (terbutaline or pseudoephedrine)
Intrapenile injection of hydralazine
Needle aspiration of corpora cavernosa
Exchange transfusion (if not relieved in 2–3 h)

TABLE 137-6   Comparison of Findings in Sequestration and Aplastic Crises in Sickle Cell Disease

	Sequestration Crisis	Aplastic Crisis
Onset	Sudden	Gradual
Pallor	Present	Present
Jaundice	Normal	Normal
Abdominal pain	Present	Absent
Hemoglobin level	Very low	Low or very low
Reticulocytes	Unchanged or increased	Decreased
Marrow erythroid activity	Unchanged or increased	Decreased

as 0.5 percent).[14] White blood cell (WBC) counts and platelet counts tend to remain stable despite the lack of erythropoiesis. Many of these crises are precipitated by human parvovirus B19, although folic acid deficiency and bone marrow suppressive/toxic drugs such as phenylbutazone have also been implicated.[15] Fortunately these crises tend to occur only once in the lifetime of a patient with SCD and are usually self-limiting. RBC transfusions are usually necessary secondary to the severe anemia. This helps to avoid any secondary cardiopulmonary complications.

Infections/Infectious Crises

Children with SCD are markedly more at risk for development of serious infection, particularly sepsis from encapsulated organisms, both because of splenic malfunction and the inability to form specific IgG antibodies to polysaccharide antigens. Indeed, *Streptococcus pneumoniae* sepsis is the most common cause of death in children with SCD.[16] Two primary prevention strategies have been undertaken to reduce this risk: vaccination and prophylactic penicillin therapy.

Current standard practice in children with SCD is to administer 23-valent polysaccharide *S. pneumoniae* vaccine at 24 months of age.[17] While the antigen response in SCD patients is markedly less than in normal patients, there still appears to be some benefit to vacination.[18] The use of prophylactic penicillin is the single most important advance in preventing *S. pneumoniae* sepsis in SCD patients, preventing 80 percent of such episodes (Table 137-7). The widespread use of *Haemophilus influenzae* vaccine has dramatically reduced the incidence of infection by this organism.

Acute bone pain is a common presenting complaint in SCD and there is substantial overlap in the clinical, radiologic, and laboratory findings of marrow ischemia, osteomyelitis, and septic arthritis. Current NHLBI recommendations suggest an unambiguous bacterial diagnosis be confirmed and blood, subperiosteal, or joint fluid cultures be obtained prior to antibiotic therapy, which should include coverage for *Salmonella*.[5]

Fever without a known source should be treated as a serious illness in children with SCD (Table 137-8). Parents and children should be

TABLE 137-7   Prophylactic Penicillin Therapy

Newborns to 36 months
   Penicillin VK 125 mg PO twice daily
3 years to 5 years
   Penicillin VK 250 mg PO twice daily
>5 years
   Alternate therapies include:
      Discontinuing therapy
      Continuing penicillin VK 250 mg twice daily
      Immediate treatment of febrile episodes ("just-in-time" therapy)

TABLE 137-8   Treatment of Fever of Unknown Origin

Toxic-appearing children or those with T >40°C
Immediate parenteral antibiotics while work-up proceeds
Admission and close observation
Lumbar puncture
Non-toxic appearing children or T <40°C
Parenteral antibiotics if:
Abnormal oxygen saturation or chest x-ray
Peripheral WBC count >30,000 or <5000
History of sepsis
Hemoglobin <5 g/dL
Platelet count <100,000/μL
Antibiotic coverage
Coverage for encapsulated organisms (e.g., ceftriaxone 75 mg/kg)

instructed that any temperature over 38.5°C (101.3°F) is a serious emergency, the diagnostic work-up of which should include CBC, chest radiograph, UA, pulse oximetry, and cultures of blood, urine, and throat.[19] Therapy in such children is summarized below.

Only those children who have remained clinically stable for three or more hours after their first antibiotic dose, and who have close follow-up arranged within 24 h should be considered for outpatient treatment. These children should receive parenteral antibiotics followed by oral therapy with broad-spectrum agents (e.g., ceftriaxone 75 mg/kg followed by cefixime 8 mg/kg loading dose, followed by 4 mg/kg q12h).[20]

Transfusion Therapy

Blood transfusions are often necessary in children undergoing splenic sequestration crisis and severe aplastic crisis. In addition, transfusions may be needed in the management of cerebrovascular accident (CVA), priapism, or as perioperative management prior to surgery. Naturally, transfusion carries risk: alloimmunization, HIV infection, hepatitis, volume overload, and iron toxicity (secondary to repeated transfusions). Transfusion can also markedly decrease erythropoiesis.

The decision to institute transfusion therapy can be difficult. In general, if the patient is stable and laboratory values indicate a serum hemoglobin ≥6 g/dL and a high reticulocyte count >20 percent or >250,000/μL, transfusion therapy can be avoided. However, if patients show evidence of heart failure, hypotension resistant to intravenous fluid bolus, dyspnea resistant to oxygen therapy, or marked fatigue, transfusion may be necessary, in which case a hematologist should be consulted. In cases of acute deterioration requiring immediate restoration of oxygen-carrying capacity, an initial infusion of 10 mL/kg of packed RBCs can be started while exchange transfusion is arranged.

Other Therapies for SCD

Increased concentrations of hemoglobin F inhibit sickle hemoglobin polymerization and sickling of red cells, thereby improving the clinical course of the disease in some patients. The most common agent used to increase HgbF concentrations is hydroxyurea, which can decrease hospitalizations and crises.[21] Hydroxyurea is not used to treat acute crises.

DISPOSITION

Disposition depends upon ED findings, observation, and response to initial therapy. The following is a list of guidelines to aid ED physicians in determining which children with SCD require hospitalization:

1. Temperature greater than or equal to 38.5°C (101.3°F), WBC counts greater than 30,000/μL, or left shift and/or other hematologic parameters greatly altered from baseline values
2. Any signs of respiratory distress, hypoxia, and/or lobar infiltrate on chest x-ray

3. Any new CNS findings or presence of neurologic crisis
4. Splenic sequestration or aplastic crisis
5. Acute abdomen on physical exam
6. Prolonged priapism
7. Any type of vasoocclusive crisis that does not respond to intravenous hydration and analgesia (usually after about 4 to 6 h of therapy)
8. Inability to maintain adequate oral hydration
9. Patients in whom the diagnosis remains uncertain
10. Follow-up (i.e., telephone contact, return visit, etc.) is uncertain or unlikely because of distance, inconvenience, or poor compliance

If patients with vasoocclusive crisis are discharged home, they should be advised to maintain adequate oral hydration, take pain medication (a 2- to 3-day supply should be provided), and return immediately if fever over 38°C/100.4°F occurs, the pattern of pain worsens or changes, or vomiting begins. All patients treated and released from the ED should be reevaluated in 24 to 48 h by their private pediatrician, physician, or hematologist (generally 24 h for children and 24 to 48 h for adults).

Variants of Sickle Cell Disease

SICKLE CELL TRAIT (SCT)   This is the carrier state of SCD and the most frequently encountered sickle cell variant. It is erroneous to consider this a mild form of SCD. Hematologically these patients are normal. Their RBCs have a normal lifespan; therefore there is no demonstrable anemia. The peripheral smear should not reveal sickled cells except in the presence of extreme hypoxia.

Clinically these patients have minimal complications, with the kidney being the most commonly affected organ. Hematuria is found in about 1 percent of patients with SCT and is most likely due to papillary necrosis following microinfarcts in the renal medullary tissue. Severe hypoxia and/or exposure to high altitudes can cause splenic infarction and CNS complications; there is also an increased incidence of sudden death in these patients during physical exertion or training. This is thought to be secondary to increased sickling under these extreme conditions. In general, the vast majority of these patients are asymptomatic and lead normal lives with a normal life expectancy.

SICKLE CELL HEMOGLOBIN-SC DISEASE   This heterozygous variant results when the gene for HgbS is inherited from one parent and the gene for HgbC is inherited from the other parent. These patients can have a mild to moderate anemia and usually a mild reticulocytosis. Their peripheral smear reveals an abundance of target cells and a few sickle-shaped cells. Additionally HgbC may be seen precipitated as rhomboid crystals in the RBCs. Splenomegaly is the major feature of HgbSC disease and persists into adulthood in about 60 percent of patients.

Patients with HgbSC disease can have painful crises and organ infarcts; they are also at higher-than-normal risk for bacterial infections. Avascular necrosis of the femoral head, ocular complications or visual loss, and renal medullary infarcts have all been reported in these patients. Women with SC disease have an increased incidence of complications during pregnancy. Overall, while some patients have complications as profound as those with SCD, most patients with HgbSC disease have few clinical complications.

SICKLE CELL BETA-THALASSEMIA DISEASE   Also a heterozygous sickle cell variant, this occurs when the gene for sickle hemoglobin is inherited from one parent and the gene for β-thalassemia is inherited from the other. The clinical severity of the disease, frequency of complications, and the degree of the resultant anemia depends on the type of β-thalassemia gene inherited. Approximately 80 to 90 percent of affected individuals have a β-thalassemia gene that allows for the production of some normal beta chains; thus some normal HgbA is produced. These patients in general do quite well; they have a mild hemolytic anemia (with near normal Hgb levels), suffer few painful crises, and sustain minimal end-organ damage. The remaining 10 to

20 percent of patients inherit a β-thalassemia gene that produces no beta chains; therefore they have no normal hemoglobin. These individuals have a severe hemolytic anemia and vasoocclusive symptoms similar to those seen with SCD. Splenomegaly is found in 70 percent of patients with this variant.

REFERENCES

1. Davis H, Schoendorf KC, Gergen PJ, et al: National trends in the mortality of children with sickle cell disease-1968 through 1992. *Am J Public Health* 87:1317, 1997.
2. Leikin SL, Gallagher D, Kinney TR, et al: Mortality in children and adolescents with sickle cell disease. Cooperative study of sickle cell disease. *Pediatrics* 84:500, 1989.
3. Gill FM, Sleeper LA, Weiner SJ, et al: Clinical events in the first decade in a cohort of infants with sickle cell disease. Cooperative study of sickle cell disease. *Blood* 86:776, 1995.
4. Buchanon GR: Newer concepts in the management of sickle cell disease. *Pediatrics* 100:1, 1995.
5. National Heart, Lung, and Blood Institute: The Management of Sickle Cell Disease, National Institutes of Health, Publication 02-2112. NHLBI: Bethesda, MD, 2002.
6. Pollack CV, Jr: Emergencies in sickle cell disease. *Emerg Med Clin North Am* 11:365, 1993.
7. Wong DL, Baker CM: Pain in children: Comparison of assessment scales. *Pediatr Nurs* 14:9, 1998.
8. Vichinsky EP, Neumayr LD, Earles AN, et al: Causes and outcomes of the acute chest syndrome in sickle cell disease. *New Engl J Med* 342:1855, 2000.
9. Vichinsky EP, Styles LA, Colangelo LH, et al: Acute chest syndrome in sickle cell disease: Clinical presentation and course. *Blood* 89:1787, 1997.
10. Oheme-Frempong K, Weiner SJ, Sleeper LA, et al: The Cooperative Study of Sickle Cell Disease: Cerebrovascular accidents in sickle cell disease: Rates and risk factors. *Blood* 91:288, 1998.
11. Powers DL: Management of cerebral vasculopathy in children with sickle cell disease. *Br J Haematol* 108:666, 2000.
12. Mantadakis E, Cavender JD, Rogers ZR, et al: Prevalence of priapism in children and adolescents with sickle cell anemia. *Am J Pediatr Hematol Oncol* 21:518, 1999.
13. Malloh AA, Quadah A: Acute splenic sequestration together with aplastic crisis caused by human parvovirus B19 in patients with sickle cell disease. *J Pediatr* 122:593, 1993.
14. Rao SP, Miller ST, Cohen BJ: Transient aplastic crisis in patients with sickle cell disease. *Am J Dis Child* 146:1328, 1992.
15. Serjeant GR, Serjeant BE, Thomas PW, et al: Human parvovirus infection in homozygous sickle cell disease. *Lancet* 341:1237, 1993.
16. Zarkowsky HS, Gallagher D, Gill FM, et al: Bacteremia in sickle hemoglobinopathies. *J Pediatr* 109:579, 1986.
17. Bjornson AB, Falletta JM, Verto-OI, et al: Serotype-specific immunoglobulin G antibody responses to pneumococcal polysaccharide vaccine in children with sickle cell anemia. *J Pediatr* 129:828, 1996.
18. Gaston MH, Verter JI, Woods G, et al: Prophylaxis with oral penicillin in children with sickle cell anemia: A randomized trial. *New Engl J Med* 314:1593, 1986.
19. Platt OS: The febrile child with sickle cell disease: A pediatrician's quandary. *J Pediatr* 130:693, 1997.
20. Williams LL, Williams JA, Harris SC, et al: Outpatient therapy with ceftriaxone and oral cefixime for selected febrile children with sickle cell disease. *J Pediatr Hematol Oncol* 18:257, 1996.
21. Davies S, Olujohungbe A: Hydroxyurea for sickle cell disease. Cochrane Database of Systematic Reviews (2): CD002202, 2001.

EVALUATING THE CHILD WITH SPECIAL HEALTH CARE NEEDS

Douglas R. Trocinski
Donna Moro-Sutherland

In the United States, more than 12 million children have special health care needs. Children with special health care needs are those who have or are at increased risk for chronic physical, developmental, behavioral, or emotional conditions and who require health and related services of a type or amount beyond that required by children in general (Table 138-1).[1]

A 1994 survey suggested that 18 percent of U.S. children fit the definition of having special health care needs (Table 138-2). Prevalence increases with age, with school-age children being twice as likely as toddlers to require additional services. Children from families with lower income and less advanced education and living in urban centers make up most of this population.[2] Since the landmark ruling allowing the care of Katie Beckett, a ventilator-dependent child, to be managed at home, technologic innovations and progressive parental advocacy have increased the feasibility of non-hospital-based care for this expanding pediatric population.[3]

Many children with special care needs now receive in-home care and participate in activities that assist them to integrate into the community. This patient population often requires special equipment and assistance to perform their daily activities and a specialized and focused approach to medical management. Special equipment may include apnea monitors, tracheostomies, feeding tubes and pumps, central venous lines or percutaneous intravenous catheters and pumps, ventilators, internal pacemakers or defibrillators, colostomies, oxygen, nebulizers, or ventricular peritoneal shunts.[4] Providing care to these patients may be particularly stressful if information about their problems and needs is unavailable. All resources, including family, primary care pediatricians, specialists, and home health nurses, should be sought to facilitate care in times of need.

Formulation of an emergency care plan has been advocated by the Emergency Medical Services for Children program through its Children with Special Health Care Needs Task Force and the American Academy of Pediatrics' Committee on Children with Disabilities. Essential components of a program of providing care plans include: use of a standardized form; a method of identifying at-risk children; completion of a data set by the child's physicians and other health care professionals; education of families, other caregivers, and health care professionals in the use of the emergency plan; regular updates of the information; 24-h access to the information by authorized emergency health care professionals; and maintenance of patient confidentiality. Emergency hospital and prehospital care is believed to be negatively affected by a frequent lack of accurate, timely information about the children's special needs and particular histories.[5]

> If the child is at risk for future medical emergencies, the child and family should participate in developing a written emergency care plan. Copies of this plan should be kept in easily accessible places at the child's home and any other location where the child regularly spends time. The plan should include provisions for any special training that will be needed by emergency medical personnel, family members, or other persons who may be called on to provide emergency care for the child.[5]

TABLE 138-1 What to Keep in Mind When Treating Children with Special Needs

Some patients have baseline vital signs outside the normal range for the child's age
Vital signs may be controlled by the child's medical device, i.e., ventilator or pacemaker
Weight may be significantly higher or lower than expected for the child's actual age
Standard prehospital quick reference charts or a Broselow tape may prove inaccurate for these patients
Difficulty tolerating respiratory distress or shock
Consider urgent any medical or traumatic event the child experiences
Expect and prepare for potential rapid patient deterioration
Many have a sensitivity or allergy to latex
Localized reaction or anaphylaxis could develop
Be proactive
Have latex-free items on hand
Ask about medications given before or during transport

Source: Smith E, Adirim TA, Singh T: Special kids special care. Emergency management of children with special health-care needs. *JEMS* 25:83, 2000.

TABLE 138-2 Congenital or Developmental Disorders and Associated Medical Conditions

Chromosomal disorders
  Down syndrome (trisomy 21 syndrome)
    Seizure disorder (12–15%); cataracts (15%); serous otitis media (50–70%); deafness (75%); congenital heart disease (50%): ASD, VSD, AV canal, PDA, tetralogy of Fallot, pulmonary hypertension; gastrointestinal atresias (12%); Hirschsprung disease (1%); constipation, fecal impaction from medications or hypothyroidism; thyroid disease (15%); diabetes mellitus; leukemia (1%); atlantoaxial instability (14–22%); acquired hip dislocation (6%); and psychiatric disorders (22%)
  Fragile X syndrome
    Recurrent serous otitis media (60% in males), strabismus (30–56% in males), seizures (14–50% in males), autism (16% in males), self-abusive, and mitral valve prolapse (22–77% in males)
  Trisomy 18
    Congenital heart disease (99%): VSD, ASD, and PDA
  Cri-du-chat syndrome (partial deletion 5p-)
    Catlike cry in infancy, microcephaly, and downward slant of the palpebral fissures
  Turner syndrome (XO syndrome)
    Short stature in females, horseshoe kidney, heart disease (bicuspid aortic valve in 30%, coarctation aorta in 10%, valvular aortic stenosis, mitral valve prolapse, aortic dissection later in life, and hypertension
  Noonan syndrome
    Webbing of the neck, pectus excavatum, cryptorchidism, and pulmonic stenosis
Disorders with facial defects as major feature
  Pierre Robin syndrome
    Micrognathia, glossoptosis, and cleft soft palate; primary defect: early mandibular hypoplasia
  Waardenburg syndrome
    Lateral displacement of medial canthi, partial albinism, and deafness
    Occasional associations: VSD, Hirschsprung disease, esophageal atresia, and anal atresia
  Treacher Collins syndrome
    Malar hypoplasia with downward slanting palpebral fissures, defect of lower lid, and malformation of the external ear
Disorders with limb defects as major feature
  Holt-Oram syndrome
    Upper limb defect, cardiac anomaly (ASD, VSD, arrhythmia), and narrow shoulders
  Fanconi pancytopenia syndrome
    Radial hypoplasia, hyperpigmentation, pancytopenia, and renal anomaly
  Radial aplasia thrombocytopenia (TAR syndrome)
Inherited metabolic disorders
  Phenylketonuria (autosomal recessive)
    Light pigmentation, eczema (33%), poor coordination, seizures (25%), and autistic behavior
  Hunter syndrome (X-linked recessive)
    Developmental lag after age 6–12 mo, coarse facies, growth deficiency, stiff joints by age 2–4 y, clear corneas, and hepatosplenomegaly
  Hurler syndrome (autosomal recessive)
    Developmental lag after age 6–10 mo, coarse facies, stiff joints, mental deficiency, cloudy corneas by age 1–2 y, hepatosplenomegaly, and rhinitis
  Lesch-Nyhan syndrome (X-linked recessive)
    Spasticity, choreoathetosis, self-mutilation, autistic behavior, and growth deficiency
Connective tissue disorders
  Marfan syndrome
    Arachnodactyly with hyperextensibility, lens subluxation, and aortic dilatation
  Ehlers-Danlos syndrome
    Hyperextensibility of joints, hyperextensibility of skin, and poor wound healing with thin scar
  Osteogenesis imperfecta congenita
    Short, broad, long bones; multiple fractures; and blue sclera
Hamartoses
  Sturge-Weber sequence
    Flat facial hemangiomata and meningeal hemangiomata with seizures
  Tuberous sclerosis syndrome
    Hamartomatous skin nodules (thumb print macules), seizures, angiomyolipomata (45–81%), phakomata, and bone lesions
  Neurofibromatosis syndrome
    Multiple neurofibromata, café-au-lait spots, presence or absence of bone lesions, seizures and/or EEG changes in 20%, cerebrovascular compromise, and headaches
  Peutz-Jeghers syndrome
    Mucocutaneous pigmentation, intestinal polyposis, 35% of patients have extraintestinal malignancies
Environmental agents (toxins)
  Fetal alcohol syndrome
    Vision problems (94%), recurrent serous otitis (93%), hearing loss (66%), heart defects (29–41%), renal hypoplasia, duplication of the kidney and collecting system, and bladder diverticula (10%)
    Other environmental exposures include fetal hydantoin syndrome, fetal trimethadione syndrome, fetal valproate syndrome, fetal warfarin syndrome, and retinoic acid embryopathy
Trauma
  Traumatic brain injury
    Visual and hearing disturbances; cranial nerve damage; spasticity, incoordination, ataxia, and feeding disorders; GERD
  Cerebral palsy
    Seizures (33%), strabismus (50%), hearing loss (10%), hip dislocation, scoliosis, contractures, gait disorder, GERD (8–10%), chronic aspiration and recurrent RAD, pulmonary fibrosis and bronchiectasis

(continued)

TABLE 138-2   Congenital or Developmental Disorders and Associated Medical Conditions *(Continued)*

Miscellaneous

Angelman syndrome (happy puppet syndrome)

Puppet-like gait, paroxysms of laughter, and characteristic features; seizures vary from major motor to akinetic, beginning usually at age 18–24 mo

Beckwith-Wiedemann syndrome

Macroglossia, omphalocele, macrosomia, and ear creases; neonatal polycythemia and hypoglycemia in early infancy; associated with Wilms' tumor

CHARGE syndrome

*C*oloboma, *h*eart disease (tetralogy of Fallot, PDA, double-outlet right ventricle with an atrioventricular canal, VSD, ASD, and right-sided aortic arch), *a*tresia choanae, *r*etarded growth and development and/or CNS anomalies, *g*enital anomalies and/or hypogonadism, and *e*ar anomalies and/or deafness

Prader-Willi syndrome

Mental retardation, hypotonia, hypogonadism, obesity, hyperphagia, gastric perforation, hypoventilation, obstructive sleep apnea, cor pulmonale, NIIDM, scoliosis, strabismus, inability to vomit, decreased sensitivity to pain, seizure disorder, hypoxia, right-sided heart failure, and pulmonary hypertension

Rett syndrome

Hyperventilation, breath holding, air swallowing, bruxism, ataxia, muscle wasting, poor circulation, scoliosis, seizures, and intermittent flushing

Vater syndrome

Vertebral defects and VSD, imperforate anus, tracheoesophageal fistula, renal anomalies, and single umbilical artery

Williams syndrome

Elfin-like syndrome, cardiovascular disease, supravalvular aortic stenosis, pulmonic stenosis, coarctation of the aorta, strabismus, joint contractures, hypertension, urethral stenosis, vesicoureteral reflux, constipation, ulcers, and hypercalcemia

Abbreviations: ASD = autistic spectrum disorder; AV = atrioventricular; CNS = central nervous system; EEG = electroencephalogram; GERD = gastroesophageal reflux disease; NIDDM = non–insulin-dependent diabetes mellitus; PDA = patent ductus arteriosus; RAD = reactive airway disease; TAR = thrombocytopenia–absent radius; VSD = ventricular septal defect.

Sources: Grossman SA, Richards CF, Anglin D, Hutson HR: Caring for the patient with mental retardation in the emergency department. *Ann Emerg Med* 35:69, 2000; Jones KL: *Smith's Recognizable Patterns of Human Malformation,* 5th ed. Philadelphia, WB Saunders, 1996.

Emphasis on each child as an individual and the importance of the parents and caregivers as valuable resources for the prehospital and emergency room providers should not be overlooked. The emergency information set or passport should improve the emergency care of children with special health care needs.

GENERAL MANAGEMENT

Emergency management of a child with special health care needs should focus on two points: management of the child's ABCs and using the most valuable resource, the child's caregiver. These long-term caregivers know the child's baseline status and are familiar with the medications and supportive equipment the child requires. The child's "go-bag" is a valuable resource containing specialized, individualized medical equipment, such as extra tracheostomy tubes, appropriate size suction catheters, equipment necessary to change a tracheostomy tube, syringes and adapters necessary to decompress a feeding catheter, a bag-valve-mask resuscitator, and needles necessary to access central lines.[4]

Cerebral Palsy

The term *cerebral palsy* describes a collection of nonprogressive disorders of movement and posture originating from an injury sustained by the developing brain within the first 3 to 5 years of life. This relatively common disorder has a prevalence of approximately 2 per 1000 individuals and may be associated with other central nervous system sequelae, including seizures, cognitive impairments, and sensory, communication, and behavioral abnormalities. It may be classified by motor abnormality (spastic, dyskinetic, ataxic, hypotonic, and mixed), distribution (diplegia, hemiplegia, quadriplegia, etc.), and degree of involvement. Although most children sustain their injuries in the prenatal or perinatal period, many etiologies over many different developmental periods have been suggested. Prenatal injury may occur from teratogen exposure, genetic syndromes, intrauterine infections, brain malformations, or fetal placenta unit malfunctions. The perinatal period may be complicated by preeclampsia, complications of labor and delivery, sepsis or central nervous system infection, asphyxia, or prematurity. The young child may develop cerebral palsy by way of meningitis, traumatic brain injury, or toxic exposures. Approximately 25 percent of all cases have no obvious source of injury.[6]

Cerebral palsy patients often present to the ED as a result of the many varied medical problems directly and indirectly associated with this disorder. Seizures may affect up to two-thirds of children with cerebral palsy, predominating in the spastic subtypes. The nature and complexity of the seizure syndromes may differ considerably between patients but, as with most epileptic syndromes, is generally consistent within the individual. The initial evaluation and management generally follow accepted tenets of seizure interventions, including protecting the airway, protecting the patient from injury, and treating the acute episode with anticonvulsants. However, the seizure history may be quite complex, and adequate seizure control may require multiple medications, necessitating attention to potential drug interactions and consultation with the primary neurologist when therapeutic adjustments are required.[6] See Chap. 125 for a detailed discussion of seizure management in children.

Oral motor dysfunction and gastroesophageal reflux often lead to a multitude of respiratory symptoms, including aspiration, wheezing, pneumonia, and chronic congestion. Evaluation of acute respiratory complaints must include a thorough history of past respiratory function to delineate underlying pulmonary abnormalities associated with prematurity, reactive airway disease, or tracheomalacia. Physical examination should include response to repositioning the child with poor head control to improve airway mechanics and decrease pooling of saliva, evaluation of air movement, accessory muscle use, nasal flaring, and retractions. The clinician also should entertain the possibility of a foreign body aspiration in light of the presentation and cognitive level of function of the individual patient. Ancillary tests, including x-ray evaluation, blood gas analysis, and gastroesophageal reflux investigation, may be completed as indicated by the clinical situation. Impaired respiratory function determined to be secondary to a reactive airway process should be treated with bronchodilators and steroids, as indicated. However, poor response to bronchodilator therapy should prompt consideration of an aspiration etiology and other treatment options. Admission is warranted for secondary pneumonia, persistent respiratory compromise, or removal of a foreign body in consultation with the appropriate primary physician.

Gastrointestinal complaints may include dehydration, feeding tube complications (discussed later in this chapter), and constipation. Dehydration may be the result of oral motor dysfunction or an infectious process. Children with severe involvement, growth retardation (in particular below the 5th percentile), or marginal reserves may dehydrate in response to relatively minimal vomiting and diarrhea. In addition to the clinical signs of dry mucous membranes, tachycardia, and physical sequelae of dehydration, close involvement with the family with regard to weight loss, baseline level of functioning, and ability to orally hydrate will help the emergency physician anticipate the need for rehydration therapy and admission. Intravenous access may be difficult in these children and may require the use of central or intraosseous access in addition to tube feeds, if available. Constipation, stemming from increased tone, impairment of sphincter relaxation, and limited fluid and fiber intake, may present as pain, change in bowel habits, anorexia, or overflow diarrhea. Acute therapy may include judicious use of enemas, suppositories, or dietary adjustments. Mineral oil should be avoided in children with aspiration histories to avoid pulmonary complications and impaired fat-soluble vitamin absorption. Fleets enemas should not be used chronically to avoid electrolyte abnormalities. Often, these children have home programs in place for chronic constipation and will require the involvement of their gastroenterologist or pediatrician for acute management and disposition.

The child with cerebral palsy may develop pain or cutaneous complications from orthopedic braces. The risk of orthopedic injuries is increased secondary to disuse and nutritionally induced osteopenia. Although fractures may occur from therapy, falls from beds or wheel chairs, or accidental injury, there must be a high index of suspicion for inflicted injury, particularly in displaced fractures. Orthopedic injuries may have subtle clinical findings and should be suspected in the irritable, severely impaired, or nonverbal child. Treatment should be completed in consultation with an orthopedic surgeon and may include hospitalization, casting, or soft wraps on the child with limited mobility.

Meningomyelocele and Neural Tube Defects

Neural tube defects, resulting from the failure of the neural tube to spontaneously close in the early embryonic stage of development, account for most congenital abnormalities of the central nervous system. The etiology of neural tube defects is thought to be multifactorial, but folic acid deficiency has been associated and supplementation is currently recommended as early as possible in pregnancy. The most severe form of neural tube defect, occurring with an incidence approaching 1 in 1000 live births, is the meningomyelocele, which includes involvement of the spinal cord, meninges, and vertebral column. Complex medical problems result from the impairment of sensory and motor control of voluntary and autonomic activities at or below the site of the lesion. The spectrum of medical complications includes neurogenic bowel and bladder dysfunction, contractures, scoliosis, hydrocephalus, Chiari II malformation, tethering of the spinal cord, spinal cord syrinx, vesicoureteral reflux, recurrent urinary tract infections, constipation, growth failure, latex allergy, gastroesophageal reflux, respiratory compromise, seizures, vision impairment, osteoporosis, and cognitive impairment, among others.

Hydrocephalus, requiring early shunt placement, is present in 75 percent or more of patients with meningomyelocele. Symptoms suggestive of shunt malfunction include altered mental status, irritability, nausea and vomiting, vision disturbances, neck pain, headache, seizures, or swelling along the shunt path. The presentation of shunt malfunction may, in some cases, be vague, necessitating reliance on parents and other primary care givers for information regarding symptoms of past malfunction, baseline neurologic functioning, and determination of the severity of the presenting symptoms, as discussed in detail later in this chapter.

Chiari II malformation is present in many children with meningomyelocele and consists of malformation of the cerebellum, hindbrain, and brainstem. Infants may present with apnea, vocal cord paralysis, stridor, oral motor dysfunction, vision disturbances, upper extremity weakness, and incoordination, whereas the older child most often presents with vision dysfunction, motor incoordination, headache, and hand weakness. These symptoms may result from even minor cervical hyperflexion and extension injuries. New-onset stridor in the child

with meningomyelocele should be aggressively evaluated for Chiari II malformation by magnetic resonance imaging of the craniocervical junction and closely monitored for the progression of stridor to complete airway obstruction. If respiratory function is not severely compromised and the history is found to be static, outpatient disposition may be considered in consultation with subspecialists caring for the child. Aggressive immobilization and evaluation for upper cervical spine injury should be completed for the child with Chiari II malformation involved with any deceleration mechanism secondary to the instability of the craniocervical junction and increased likelihood of injury.

Urinary tract complaints include recurrent urinary tract infection, urinary retention or incontinence, complications of straight catheterization, or complications of urologic surgery. Children may be receiving medications or prophylactic antibiotics to enhance continence and minimize damage to the upper urinary tract. Because bacterial colonization of the urine is common, only children with symptomatic infection should receive broad-spectrum antibiotic coverage. Formation of a false channel during self-catheterization is suspected with difficult catheter passage, pain, or urethral bleeding. Recatheterization should not be attempted in the ED for these symptoms for fear of compounding the underlying injury. Rather, urologic consultation should be obtained. Long-term indwelling catheterization predisposes the patient to the development of latex allergy.

The insensate areas distal to the neural tube defect are susceptible to burns and pressure sore development. Local wound care, padding, frequent repositioning, and discontinuing of bracing may be required for superficial wound healing. Careful evaluation is required to differentiate cellulitis, abscess, or osteomyelitis. Deep infections and osteomyelitis may require admission, surgical intervention, and long-term antibiotic therapy.

Autism

Autism describes a heterogeneous disorder of brain development that affects behavior; impairs social interaction, language, and communication skills; and, often, features repetitive motor activities. The term *autistic spectrum disorder* is used to encompass the wide variety of clinical expressions, severity, and level of functioning. Autistic spectrum disorder has a prevalence of 2 per 1000 (autistic disorder approximates 1 in 1000), with recent evidence suggesting that these numbers are increasing with improved and earlier detection.[7] In general, most children with autism do not have associated medical disorders and will have emergency medical needs similar to those of age-matched, developmentally normal children. Exceptions include, but are not limited to, an association of autism in children with tuberous sclerosis and rare coincidence of autism with Williams syndrome and neurofibromatosis. Although the medical problems may not be unusual, interactions with autistic children may be difficult secondary to sensory defensiveness, unusual social behaviors, and potentially aggressive self-protective responses to medical procedures and examinations. Parents and primary care givers can inform the physician of the most effective means of communication for each patient. Judicious use of sedation for painful or difficult procedures should be employed with specific attention to patient safety and potential medication interactions.

Mental Retardation and Developmental Delay

Mental retardation occurs in approximately 2.5 percent of the population and is classically defined by cognitive impairment and decreased adaptive behaviors resulting from injury, disease, or abnormality occurring before the age of 18 years. Mental retardation is associated with disorders, such as Down syndrome, Rett syndrome, Williams syndrome, fragile X, and fetal alcohol syndrome, but has no such associations in the majority of patients. The intellectual impairment and associated behavior difficulties create challenges for medical care providers. Mentally retarded children are often difficult to approach, have impaired social and communication skills, and may become aggressive or combative when confronted by new or painful stimuli. As with the autistic child, the parent or primary care giver is an essential source of information for effective interaction strategies. In addition, all potential sources of information should be investigated to complete a history clouded by a decreased level of intellectual function. The various medical problems found in these patients can be specific to the underlying syndrome but generally can be approached in ways similar to those with developmentally normal children. Medication profiles should be reviewed to prevent drug interactions and to identify potential drug side effects.

Down Syndrome

Down syndrome is a relatively common genetic disorder, most often resulting from a trisomy of chromosome 21, occurring in slightly more than 1 in 1000 live births. The syndrome is characterized by developmental delay, mental retardation, congenital heart defects, gastrointestinal system abnormalities, increased risk of upper respiratory and ear infections, and atlanto-occipital instability. Congenital heart defects affect 40 to 60 percent and include atrioventricular canal defects, ventricular and atrial septal defects, tetralogy of Fallot, and patent ductus arteriosus. These defects generally are detected in early infancy, but pulmonary hypertension and congestive heart failure may develop with time if treatment is not successful. Common gastrointestinal tract abnormalities include esophageal atresia, tracheoesophageal fistula, pyloric stenosis, duodenal atresia, Meckel diverticulum, Hirschsprung disease, and imperforate anus. Feeding difficulties in the infant with Down syndrome therefore should prompt further investigation and immediate surgical intervention, if indicated. There is also an increased risk of gastroesophageal reflux, which responds to standard therapy. Midfacial malformations affect the normal functioning of eustachian tubes, leading to recurrent and chronic infections of the ear, sinuses, and upper respiratory tract. Deceleration injuries raise the possibility of atlantoaxial subluxation or dislocation.

Spinal Cord Injury

More than 1000 new cases of traumatic spinal cord injury occur each year in children as a result of motor vehicle accidents, athletic activities, falls, inflicted trauma, and birth trauma. Spinal cord injuries may result in complications similar to those described for meningomyelocele but also may include pain, heterotopic bone ossification, hypercalcemia, renal calculi, and autonomic dysreflexia. Upper thoracic and cervical injuries also may lead to respiratory insufficiency secondary to phrenic nerve impairment or weakness of abdominal and chest wall musculature.

Autonomic dysreflexia is a serious, potentially life-threatening complication of cord injuries proximal to the mid-thoracic level. It consists of paroxysmal sympathetic and parasympathetic hyperactivity initiated by stimuli below the level of the lesion, such as bladder overdistention, fecal impaction, or fracture. The symptoms of autonomic dysreflexia are sweating, flushing, pounding headache, hypertension, bradycardia, and piloerection. The primary intervention is to determine and eliminate the offending stimulus through bladder emptying, disimpaction with local anesthesia, discontinuation of painful procedures, or repositioning. If elevated blood pressure does not respond to repositioning or stimulus reduction, standard treatment of a hypertensive emergency should be instituted.

Chronic dysesthesias or paresthesias become more frequent as the child reaches adolescence. Pain management should consist of analgesics and other pain-control strategies in concert with the primary physician. Prolonged narcotic use should be avoided.

Heterotopic bone formation may present with pain, heat, swelling, and restricted movement, most commonly in the hips, knees, elbows, or shoulders. Underlying fracture, infection, or skin breakdown should be excluded.

Spinal cord–injured patients of any age are at increased risk for psychiatric and emotional difficulties related to loss of function and body image. Depression, anxiety, uncontrolled anger, or temper tantrums usually can be handled in the outpatient setting, but hospitalization may be required for suicidal ideation or extreme behavioral and emotional difficulties.

TECHNOLOGY-DEPENDENT CHILDREN

Definition: one who needs both a medical device to compensate for the loss of a vital body function and substantial and ongoing nursing care to avert death or further disability.[8]

Examples of technology-dependent children include those who require ventilator support or who have pacemakers, tracheostomies, gastrostomy tubes, or central venous catheters.[8,9] The primary care physician and home health nurse should be contacted early in the evaluation process to avoid unnecessary tests and admissions and to simplify care.

Tracheostomy Care

Complications related to tracheostomy tubes include decannulation, obstruction, tube reinsertion into a false passage, pneumomediastinum, and pneumothorax. Granuloma or stricture formation at the stoma or where the tip of the tube meets the tracheal wall can lead to localized bleeding with manipulation of the cannula. Erosion into the innominate artery is a rare occurrence usually related to an inferiorly placed tracheostomy stoma. Infections related to tracheostomy care include tracheitis, pneumonia, and asthma. See Chap. 244 for further discussion of airway devices.

Mechanical Ventilation

Ventilator-related complications, such as pneumothorax, are managed according to accepted standard principles. Bag ventilation is necessary in the case of ventilator failure.

Complications of Feeding Tubes

The special needs child with a nasogastric tube may develop sinusitis, nasal and esophageal irritation, tube dislodgement or clogging, or pulmonary aspiration. Gastrostomy tubes can be associated with gastroesophageal reflux, peristomal wound infection, peritonitis, gastric perforation or hemorrhage, gastrocolic fistula, gastric ulceration, and gastric outlet obstruction. Complications of gastrojejunostomy tubes include diarrhea, tube migration, small bowel perforation, and intussusception. Stomal complications include dermatitis, allergic hypersensitivity, granulation, cellulitis, and fungal infections.

Complications of parenteral feeding include catheter obstruction or occlusion, air embolism, catheter breakage, catheter displacement, or catheter-related infection. Other complications include cholestasis that may lead to irreversible liver disease or metabolic bone disease.

Cerebrospinal Fluid Shunts

Complications related to ventricular peritoneal shunts include mechanical malfunction, overdrainage, and infection. Approximately 75 percent of patients with ventricular peritoneal shunts experience a shunt malfunction in their lifetime. Signs and symptoms of ventricular peritoneal shunt obstruction include headache, visual disturbances, vomiting, lethargy, irritability, papilledema, bulging fontanelle or enlarged head, engorged head veins, and Macewen sign (cracked-pot sound during skull percussion). Neurologic findings may include increased deep tendon reflexes or lower extremity tone, positive Babinski sign, lateral (6th) or upward (4th) gaze (sunsetting), and respiratory compromise. Seizures are generally accompanied by other signs and symptoms and are seldom, if ever, the only sign of shunt malfunction.

Shunt infections are characterized by nonspecific signs and symptoms, including change in sensorium, fever, irritability, shunt malfunction, vomiting, or abdominal pain. Antibiotics should be selected to treat gram-positive (most commonly, coagulase-negative *Staphylococcus*, *Staphylococcus aureus,* and *Streptococcus* species) and gram-negative (*Escherichia coli, Enterococcus* species, and *Haemophilus influenzae*) species. Infections most commonly occur within a few months of shunt placement, many within the first few weeks, and they generally decrease in frequency with time.

Shunt malfunction evaluation should include shunt series (plain radiographs of the skull, neck, chest, and abdomen) and head computed tomography to assess ventricular size and shunt positioning. Increased cerebral ventricle size, particularly when compared with previous studies, is indicative of shunt malfunction. However, malfunction may be present with unchanged ventricular size, due to a loss of surrounding tissue compliance. If shunt malfunction or infection is suspected, neurosurgical consultation should be obtained for further evaluation, including shunt aspiration, admission, and monitoring.

Urinary Diversions

Urinary diversions seen with the special needs child include vesicostomies, ureterostomies, ileal loop conduits, and bladder augmentations. Complications with vesicostomies include prolapse and stomal stenosis; ureterostomies leading to stenosis; ileal loop conduits leading to prolapse, peristomal hernia, or stenosis; bladder ruptures and perforations; and small bowel obstruction. Most complications should be managed in consultation with the child's attending urologist.

REFERENCES

1. McPherson M, Arango P, Fox H, et al: A new definition of children with special care needs. *Pediatrics* 102:137, 1998.
2. Gausche M, Seidel J: Out of hospital care of pediatric patients. *Pediatr Clin North Am* 46:1305, 1999.
3. Spaite DW, Karriker KJ, Seng M, et al: Training paramedics: Emergency care for children with special health care needs. *Prehosp Emerg Care* 4:178, 2000.
4. Smith E, Adirim TA, Singh T: Special kids special care. Emergency management of children with special health-care needs. *JEMS* 25:83, 2000.
5. Committee on Pediatric Emergency Medicine: American Academy of Pediatrics. Emergency preparedness for children with special health care needs. *Pediatrics* 104:e53, 1999.
6. Eicher PS, Batshaw ML: Cerebral palsy. *Pediatr Clin North Am* 40:537, 1993.
7. Sandler AD, Brazdziunas D, Cooley WC, et al: The pediatrician's role in the diagnosis and management of autistic spectrum disorder in children. *Pediatrics* 107:1221, 2001.
8. Haffner JC, Schurman SJ: The technology-dependent child. *Pediatr Clin North Am* 48:751, 2001.
9. Fein JA, Cronan K, Posner JC: Approach to the care of the technology-dependent child, in Fleisher R, Ludwig S (eds): *Textbook of Pediatric Emergency Medicine,* vol 127, 4th ed. Philadelphia, Lippincott Williams & Wilkins, 2000, pp. 1645–1665.

139 UROLOGIC AND GYNECOLOGIC PROBLEMS IN CHILDREN
Samy Saad
Olly Duckett

BOYS

Scrotal Pain and Swelling

Scrotal swelling must be categorized clinically into either an emergent or benign disease process. The most important condition to identify is testicular torsion. Common causes of scrotal swelling include testicular torsion, epididymitis, torsion of the appendix testes, varicoceles, hernias, hydroceles, and trauma. Less common causes of scrotal

swelling include Henoch-Schönlein purpura, orchitis, tuberculosis, and rarely in children, tumors.

HISTORY AND PHYSICAL EXAMINATION *Age* is a factor in diagnosis. Testicular torsion is most common in neonates and postpubertal boys. Appendiceal torsion and Henoch-Schönlein purpura are more common in school-aged males (prepubertal). Epididymitis more often presents in adolescents and adults. Hydroceles are often found in the first 2 years of life, whereas varicoceles are uncommon before the age of 10.

Time course of symptoms is important in establishing diagnosis. Abrupt onset of symptoms within minutes to hours raises the suspicion of torsion. Intermittent, acute pain associated with scrotal swelling suggests intermittent torsion with spontaneous detorsion. More gradual onset of symptoms over 1 to 3 days is more indicative of epididymitis or appendiceal torsion. Hernias and hydroceles often are reported as a gradual onset of swelling over a prolonged period of time, frequently with variations in the amount of swelling. A history of swelling that progresses toward the end of the day or with prolonged ambulation suggests a communicating hydrocele or hernia. Ask about any history of *genital trauma* because children and adolescents often are reluctant to disclose such episodes.

Determining the *severity and location* of symptoms can aid in diagnosis. The pain of testicular torsion is severe from the onset and can radiate to the abdomen and be associated with nausea and vomiting. Urinary symptoms such as frequency, urgency, and dysuria suggest epididymitis. Painless scrotal swelling suggests more benign etiologies such as hernias, hydroceles, or varicoceles.

The *physical examination* includes inspection and palpation of the phallus, scrotum, testicles, epididymis, and inguinal region. The position of the testes in the scrotum should be evaluated-one testicle riding higher in the scrotum than the other or a transverse lie of the testicles indicating a bell-clapper deformity is associated with testicular torsion. The inguinal canal should be evaluated for hernias or communicating hydroceles. Assess the degree of swelling, redness, or thickening of the scrotum. In both epididymitis and testicular torsion, the affected hemiscrotum typically displays significant erythema and swelling after 24 h. The abdomen should be examined in all those with genital complaints, and the genitals should be examined in all those with abdominal complaints, because the differential diagnoses of pain in both areas overlap.[1]

The normal testicle should be examined first. The testicle is examined by gently grasping the testicle between the thumb and forefinger. Evaluate the epididymis similarly. The epididymis should be felt at the posterosuperior aspect of the testicle. A swollen, tender testicle is indicative of torsion, but the epididymis is usually more tender than the testicle in epididymitis. Tenderness limited to the upper pole of the testicle indicates torsion of the appendix. The pathognomonic blue-dot sign, a bluish discoloration at the superior pole of the testis indicates a torsed appendage. This bluish discoloration represents the necrotic torsed appendage and is often visible through the skin at the upper pole. Late in the course of epididymitis and appendiceal torsion, loss of testicular landmarks occurs and makes it very difficult to differentiate these entities from testicular torsion.

The cremasteric reflex should be assessed by stroking or pinching the inner aspect of the thigh and watching for unilateral elevation of the testicle. An intact cremasteric reflex lowers the probability of testicular torsion. Normal boys between 30 months and 12 years of age should have an intact cremasteric reflex. The cremasteric reflex may be difficult to assess if there is severe scrotal edema.

ANCILLARY STUDIES Laboratory evaluation should include a routine urinalysis. Blood work is not routinely indicated except in patients with fever or other systemic symptoms. Pyuria suggests a urinary tract infection, and in younger patients the urinary tract may be the source of epididymitis, but a small number of children with torsion may have pyuria.

All boys with acute testicular pain and swelling should be referred for immediate imaging to rule out testicular torsion. *Color Doppler imaging* has a sensitivity of over 95 percent for the diagnosis of torsion, is noninvasive, and is readily available and so is the preferred study. Absent or decreased flow in one testis indicates testicular torsion. The accuracy of nuclear scanning is similar to that of Doppler imaging. Its disadvantages include the lack of routine availability, delay in instituting the study, and inability to display scrotal anatomy. In nuclear scanning, little or no isotope reaches the testis in testicular torsion, whereas uptake is normal or increased in patients with epididymitis.

Testicular Torsion

Testicular torsion is the twisting of the spermatic cord and its contents within the tunica vaginalis causing decrease or absence of blood flow to the affected testicle. Testicular salvage is usually possible when duration of symptoms is less than 12 h, but the rates decrease significantly after 12 h, approaching zero after 24 h of symptoms. Ideally, surgical repair should be undertaken within 6 h of symptoms. The history is usually abrupt onset of testicular pain, followed by scrotal swelling and edema, often with associated nausea, vomiting, and lower abdominal pain. There may be a history of a sudden movement, position change, or genital trauma precipitating the event. A history of similar painful episodes with spontaneous resolution may represent previous episodes of torsion/detorsion. The classic signs of torsion are an enlarged, exquisitely tender testicle that rides higher in the scrotum than the normal testicle and usually has a transverse lie. Rarely, there may be a palpable mass in the spermatic cord where the blood vessels have twisted. In most cases the cremasteric reflex is absent in the affected testicle. The scrotal wall is usually erythematous and edematous. In cases of prolonged symptoms, the scrotum may be too edematous to evaluate cremasteric reflex or to accurately examine the testicular structures. As the process of torsion becomes more chronic, the testicle becomes fixed to the overlying, often thickened scrotal wall.[2]

Adolescence is the most common age for testicular torsion, but torsion may affect children of all ages (Table 139-1). Roughly 10 percent of cases of testicular infarction are caused by *neonatal torsion*. This entity differs from pubertal torsion in that in neonatal torsion the peritoneal attachments are inadequate or absent, and the testis, epididymis, and tunica vaginalis twist as a unit. This type of torsion is known as *extravaginal torsion*. Neonatal torsion occurs in utero or in the first 10 days of life. If torsion occurred in utero, the testis is not salvageable. However, if the child develops scrotal swelling with a history of a normal scrotum at birth, immediate pediatric surgical consultation may salvage the testis.[3]

When the diagnosis of torsion is considered, a pediatric surgeon or urologist should be consulted immediately. At that time, a decision of surgical exploration versus imaging must be made. This decision most often is based on the experience of the surgeon and duration of symp-

toms. Treatment of testicular torsion is surgical exploration. At the time of exploration, if the affected testicle is nonviable after being detorsed, it should be removed. The contralateral healthy testicle should be fixed or pexed to prevent future torsion. As a temporizing measure, the emergency physician may attempt to *manually detorse* the testicle by elevating the affected testicle toward the inguinal ring and rotating the epididymis medially (see Chap. 95). Manual detorsion is unsuccessful most of the time and should be abandoned if the patient experiences any further discomfort. Relief of pain indicates correct detorsion and may allow for some blood return to the testicle. Surgical consultation remains necessary despite relief of pain.

Torsion of the Appendix

Torsion of the appendix testis or appendix epididymis may present with similar symptoms as testicular torsion but has a more gradual onset and is managed quite differently. **The most common age of presentation is between 7 and 12 years, although it can occur at any age.** The pain is typically less intense than the pain of testicular torsion. The scrotum is usually normal or mildly erythematous. The testes are equal in size, and early on, the tenderness is localized to the superior pole of the testicle. Commonly, there will be a bluish discoloration of the overlying skin giving the pathognomonic blue-dot sign at the superior aspect of the affected testicle. Imaging reveals normal blood flow to the testicle. Treatment includes scrotal elevation, bed rest, and analgesia with nonsteroidal anti-inflammatory drugs. Inflammation usually resolves within 1 week.[3]

Epididymitis

Epididymitis is rarely seen in *prepubertal* children, but when present, urologic evaluation, including renal/bladder sonogram and a voiding cystourethrogram, is warranted to rule out associated genitourinary abnormalities. Before puberty, coliform bacteria (*Escherichia coli*) and other urinary pathogens predominate. *Chlamydia trachomatis* and *Neisseria gonorrhoeae* are the most common infectious organisms in *sexually active adolescents*.[3]

Symptoms include fever, chills, and urinary symptoms (e.g., dysuria, frequency, urgency, and urethral discharge). Symptoms also may begin with flank pain that gradually spreads to the epididymis and scrotum. The epididymis becomes tender and edematous. The testicle is not tender unless the infection is complicated by epididymoorchitis. The overlying hemiscrotum is usually red, swollen, and tender. Prehn's sign (elevation of the scrotum above the pubis) relieves pain in epididymitis but not in torsion. However, this sign is not reliable in children. Urinalysis and urine cultures should be obtained, and while pyuria suggests epididymitis, pyuria also can be present with testicular torsion. The most frequent misdiagnosis of testicular torsion is epididymitis. Consequently, if there is any question about the accuracy of the diagnosis of epididymitis, imaging studies are indicated (see above).

Treatment in prepubertal boys is trimethoprim-sulfisoxazole 10 mg/kg per 24 h, divided twice a day, for 7 to 10 days. In sexually active adolescents, treatment for sexually transmitted pathogens is indicated (see Chap. 141). Analgesia and scrotal elevation may help with symptoms. Hospitalization is warranted if the patient has constitutional symptoms (i.e., fever, vomiting, or chills) or epididymoorchitis. In some cases of untreated epididymitis or orchitis, abscess formation develops and requires surgical intervention.[4]

Hernia

Hernia is a defect in the abdominal wall, usually in the area of the inguinal ring. The hernia sac most commonly contains ileum, but it may contain omentum. In girls, an ovary or fallopian tube may be encountered within the hernia sac. The chief complaint is usually that of an intermittent mass in the scrotal area. The mass is usually painless,

TABLE 139-1   Differential Diagnosis of Scrotal Pain and Swelling

	Testicular Torsion	Appendiceal Torsion	Epididymitis
Age	All ages	Prepuberty	Prepuberty with UTI, adolescence
Onset	Abrupt or intermittent	1–3 days	1–3 days
Severity	Painful	Painful	Moderate pain
Other	Horizontal lie	Blue dot sign	Tender epididymis, testis normal

although some patients do report mild discomfort. Inability to reduce the hernia and severe pain are indications of incarceration and require emergency surgical consultation. Reducible hernias should be referred for elective surgical correction (see Chap. 80). Parents should be instructed to observe for signs or incarceration or strangulation while awaiting repair.[5]

Hydrocele

A hydrocele is a fluid-filled remnant of the processus vaginalis that surrounds the testis. Hydrocoele is noted most often in infancy and is more prevalent in premature boys. By 12 to 18 months of age, the processus vaginalis obliterates, and the hydrocele resorbs. Persistence beyond 2 years of age usually requires surgical repair.[6]

It can be very difficult to differentiate hydrocoele from hernia, and hydrocoele also can coexist with hernia. The examiner must be able to palpate above the mass and palpate normal cord to exclude any associated hernia. Both hernias and hydrocoeles can be reduced or compressed, and both can transilluminate. Referral to a specialist is often needed to distinguish between the two and to exclude other causes such as lymph nodes, varicocele, spermatocele, epididymal cyst, or tumor.[5]

Varicocele

Varicocele is a painless scrotal swelling that is due to dilatation and elongation of the veins of the pampiniform plexus. Varicocele is more common on the left side because the left spermatic vein drains into the left renal vein, whereas the right one drains into the inferior vena cava. The examination should be performed in the erect position. Varicocele presents as a vermiform mass of dilated veins superior and posterior to the testis. The mass tends to increase in size with the Valsalva maneuver. Right-sided varicocele or any varicocele at a young age should prompt a search for pelvic or abdominal pathology. If left untreated, testicular atrophy may occur. Urologic referral for surgical repair is necessary if the varicocele is painful, bilateral, or of significant size. Uncomplicated varicocele requires no surgery.[7]

Disorders of the Foreskin

PHIMOSIS   Phimosis is a condition in which the foreskin cannot be retracted over the glans penis. In congenital (physiologic) phimosis, males have a tight foreskin with the inner prepuce adhered to the glans penis at birth. This phimosis resolves spontaneously but may remain present for several years. Most physiologic phimosis resolves by 3 to 5 years of age such that the glans can be fully exposed. Acquired phimosis is a condition in which a previously retractable foreskin is no longer retractable. Acquired phimosis occurs as a result of poor hygiene, poorly performed circumcision, repetitive forceful retraction of the foreskin, or balanitis, which leads to scar formation and formation of tight opening of the foreskin.[8] Phimosis (congenital or acquired) is not a reason for circumcision as long as there is no urinary obstruction, pain, or hematuria, only reassurance and proper hygiene are recommended. One of the few indications for treatment is persistent ballooning of the foreskin during voiding. Daily cleaning without forceful retraction of the foreskin is the only treatment necessary for phimosis. Some studies have demonstrated success with topical steroid cream for acquired phimosis. Many parents seek medical attention for their sons who have been circumcised in the newborn period and have a secondary phimosis. The treatment is revision of the circumcision under general anesthesia. Referral to a pediatric urologist also is warranted if there is any urinary obstruction, pain, recurrent infection, or hematuria.[1]

PARAPHIMOSIS   Paraphimosis is a true urologic emergency. Paraphimosis is the inability to bring the foreskin back over the glans pe-

nis once the foreskin has been retracted. If the foreskin remains retracted for a prolonged time, it may form a constricting ring that will cause venous congestion, with progressive swelling of the glans penis and foreskin. Arterial occlusion secondary to edema and swelling can lead to gangrene of the glans penis. Paraphimosis occurs only in uncircumcised or partially circumcised males and occurs most commonly after forceful retraction of the foreskin without timely reduction, such as after urethral catheterization or penile examination. Poor hygiene may predispose to acquired phimosis, which can lead to paraphimosis from tight fibrotic tissue.[9]

Patients usually present with pain, erythema, and swelling of the shaft skin and glans penis. Partial or complete urinary retention may occur in infants and children. On examination, there is a constricting band just proximal to the glans penis. The rest of the penile shaft appears normal. Paraphimosis should be reduced as soon as possible with the aid of conscious sedation or penile block using lidocaine hydrochloride without epinephrine. The most common technique for foreskin reduction is to hold a gauze sponge with the index and third fingers of each hand proximal to the foreskin and use the thumbs to push the glans back into the foreskin. It may take a minute or two of constant pressure before the glans slips through the paraphimotic ring. Ice and pressure may help to reduce the swelling before reduction. If manual reduction is unsuccessful, emergent urologic consultation is necessary.[3]

Invasive procedures should be done by a urologist or pediatric surgeon but, if gangrene is imminent, must be done by the emergency physician. Options include a dorsal incision at the level of the constricting ring that will release the foreskin. Single or multiple punctures of the foreskin using a 21-gauge needle to drain some of the edema from the edematous foreskin followed by manual reduction is another commonly employed technique. Injection of hyaluronidase into the edematous foreskin is effective in decreasing the swelling and permits the foreskin to be reduced. Following emergency reduction, referral to a urologist is necessary for eventual circumcision to avoid recurrence of the condition.

BALANITIS/POSTHITIS   Balanitis is an infection of the glans penis, and posthitis is an infection of the foreskin. Poor hygiene predisposes to these infections. *Candida albicans* can be causative in prepubertal children, and sexually transmitted organisms can be causative pathogens in sexually active adolescents or victims of sexual abuse. On examination, the foreskin, glans penis, or both are swollen, tender, and red. Management includes oral and topical antistaphylococcal/antistreptococcal antibiotics, warm baths, and good local hygiene.[1]

Disorders of the Penile Shaft

PRIAPISM   Priapism is a prolonged, frequently painful erection of the penis without any sexual stimulation or desire. Priapism is divided into low flow (ischemic) and high flow (arterial) based on the status of penile arterial blood flow. Low-flow priapism is more frequent than the high-flow type. *Low-flow priapism* is a true urologic emergency that requires rapid intervention to prevent long-term complications such as corporal fibrosis and erectile dysfunction. It results from decreased penile venous outflow. Common causes are sickle-cell disease (the most common etiology in children), tumor infiltration (leukemia), medications, illicit drugs (marijuana), and idiopathic. *High-flow priapism* is caused by increased arterial blood flow; it is usually caused by arterial-cavernosal shunt formation secondary to a groin or straddle injury. This type of priapism does not cause ischemia and therefore is not a true emergency condition because the patient is at low risk for permanent complications.[10]

Diagnosis and management depend largely on the patient's history and physical examination. Penile examination during the acute state is helpful in differentiating between the two types. Low-flow priapism usually involves the corpus cavernosum but spares the glans and corpus spongiosum; therefore, the penile shaft will be painful and hard, while the glans penis is soft. In high-flow priapism, the whole penis is partially rigid and painless. Management is the same in both types of priapism. Urologic consultation should be initiated at the time of presentation. In sickle-cell priapism, the combination of hydration, pain control, and partial or complete exchange transfusion is successful in up to 80 percent of the patients. The aim of transfusion is to achieve a target hemoglobin S concentration of 30 percent or less. If supportive measures fail, aspiration of the corpus cavernosum followed by injection of phenylephrine or epinephrine may be effective.[11]

HAIR TOURNIQUET   Young boys occasionally present to the ED with acute strangulation injury of the penis. The causative agent is usually a hair or a thread. The child may present with a chief complaint of penile swelling, redness, or pain. Occasionally, the parents will report urinary retention or inconsolable crying in an infant or nonverbal child. The physician should perform a genital examination in the inconsolable infant. On physical examination, the physician often will find an edematous, erythematous, tender penis with a circumferential constriction. Often the hair or thread will not be visible, even with thorough examination. The extent of damage is directly related to the duration of strangulation. Complication includes urethrocutaneous fistula and gangrene of the glans penis. Cutting the hair or applying a hair-removal agent such as Nair may relieve constriction. If this does not work or removal of the hair or the constricting agent is not certain, immediate urologic evaluation should be initiated.

ZIPPER INJURY   The skin of the penis or scrotum can get caught in the movable part or between the teeth of a zipper. Gentle manipulation, after local infiltration with 1% lidocaine, is the most successful way to release the entrapment. Release of the skin can be achieved by cutting the median bar of the movable part of the zipper with a bone-cutting plier. If all procedures fail, removal under general anesthesia or circumcision by the urologist may be required.

MEATAL STENOSIS   Meatal stenosis is a benign condition of circumcised boys, usually after toilet training. It is usually caused by frequent meatal inflammation from prolonged exposure to the moist environment of the diaper (ammoniacal dermatitis). Other etiologies include balanitis, recurrent catheterization, or complication of reconstructive surgery of the penis. The delicate meatal edge becomes adherent to itself in a side-to-side fashion secondary to inflammation and loss of the superficial epithelial lining. The adhesion usually occurs from the ventral side toward the dorsal side. Boys usually complain of difficulty controlling urinary stream, burning, or blood spotting in the underwear. Patient may demonstrate a prolonged voiding time during observation. There is a characteristic dorsal deflection of the stream due to a ventral lip of scar tissue as a result of fusion of the meatal edges. Treatment is urethral meatomy by a pediatric urologist.[1,8]

GIRLS

Evaluation and examination of the female child with gynecologic complaints provokes anxiety in parents, patients, and physicians. The physician must understand the different anatomy and illnesses seen in prepubertal children as compared with adolescents (Table 139-2). Prepubertal females lack secondary sex characteristics, and the labial and vaginal tissue is thinner and more atrophic due to lack of estrogen stimulation. The age of menarche in North American females is 12.5 years, with a lower limit of 10 years of age.

A thorough history will determine the extent of the gynecologic examination. The child should be informed that the parent or caretaker approves the examination. The physician should explain everything that will happen during the examination and why the examination is necessary. The child needs to have as much control over the examina-

TABLE 139-2   Sexual Maturity Ratings (SMRs, Tanner Stages) in Girls

SMR Stages	Pubic Hair	Breast	Age, Years
I	None	None	
II	Sparse, slightly pigmented over mons or labia	Breast and papilla elevated, areola diameter increased	10–13
III	Dark, increased amount, coarse on mons	Breast and areola enlarged	12–14
IV	Adult in character confined to mons	Mounding of areola above plane of breast	12–14
V	Adult feminine triangle	Mature, nipple projects	14–17

tion as feasible. Forcible restraint is contraindicated. An examination under sedation or anesthesia is indicated for agitated or uncooperative patients whose symptoms require complete pelvic examination.

The parent or caretaker should be present during the physical examination. The physician should leave the room as the girl disrobes and prepares for the examination, giving the caretaker time to explain and comfort the child. The best position for examination of the external genitalia is the frog-legged position, where the child lies supine with the feet together and the knees spread apart. The vestibule and hymen can be visualized by gently pressing the labial pads downward and laterally. The patient can be examined in the caretaker's lap in the frog-legged position. The prone knee-chest position is another option that allows for good visualization of the lower half of the vaginal vault and the anal area. Magnification of the genitalia may be achieved with an otoscope with the earpiece removed or a culposcope, if available.[12]

Labial Adhesions

Labial adhesions are a midline fusion of the labia minora (Figure 139-1). Adhesions can occur secondary to labial irritation, abrasions, or trauma, following which epithelialization occurs. The etiology of the irritation may be irritants such as harsh soap, bubble bath, or diaper rash. Trauma of the labia minora from sexual abuse may predispose to adhesions. These adhesions may be thin or dense, partial or complete. Labial adhesions may be asymptomatic and only diagnosed on routine physical examination or may be observed by the caregiver. Rarely, urethral obstruction may occur, resulting in urinary tract infection or

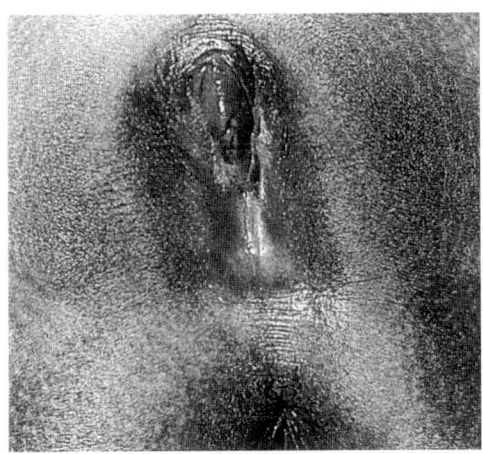

FIG. 139-1. Labial adhesions. Agglutination and adhesion of the labia minora, as a result of healing after inflammation, produce the appearance of a smooth flat surface overlying the introitus, divided centrally by a thin lucent line. *(Courtesy Dr. D. Lloyd.)*

voiding symptoms.[3] The adhesions usually resolve spontaneously during puberty. Management includes good hygiene and application of estrogen cream to the adhesion area twice a day for 2 to 3 weeks (reversible secondary sexual changes can occur as a side effect). Separation of the adhesions can be achieved by traction following the application of topical anesthetic or under general anesthesia if the child is uncooperative. After separation of the adhesions, lubrication of the vulva and good hygiene are advised to prevent recurrences.[8]

Precocious Puberty and Menarche

Precocious puberty is the appearance of physical signs of sexual development in children prior to age 9. It is usually idiopathic in origin but can be associated with endocrine or neurologic disorders.[13] Specialist referral is needed. Premature menarche is cyclic vaginal bleeding in prepubertal girls in the absence of pubertal development. It is a diagnosis of exclusion after other serious causes of vaginal bleeding have been eliminated.

Ovarian Torsion

Ovarian torsion results from twisting of the ovary at its pedicle. An ovarian mass or cyst predisposes to ovarian torsion. Complete ovarian torsion compromises the vascular supply and, if untreated, will lead to ischemia and atrophy of the ovary. The child usually presents with lower abdominal pain, nausea, and vomiting. A tender pelvic mass may or may not be palpable. Diagnosis is difficult because of the nonspecific symptoms and findings. Sonography may demonstrate an edematous ovary with prominent follicles. However, Doppler flow is not always absent in torsion. Patients with suspected ovarian torsion need urgent surgical evaluation.

Vaginal Obstruction

Vaginal obstruction can be due to imperforate hymen or transverse vaginal septum (Figure 139-2).[14] Girls with vaginal obstruction may be missed until the age of menarche, at which time the symptoms of failure to menstruate, cyclic abdominal pain, abdominal mass, or urine retention develop. Imperforate hymen usually presents as a bulging, shiny, blue- to purple-colored mass seen at the genital area. The urethral meatus is distinct from the mass. Girls with imperforate hymen require evaluation for associated vaginal, urethral, anorectal, and spinal abnormalities. Transverse vaginal septa may occur in the lower, middle, or upper vagina. Most of the septa are in the upper vagina. Treatment is surgical repair.

Urethral Prolapse

Urethral prolapse occurs primarily in young African-American females. The mucosa of the distal urethra prolapses and forms a circular mass surrounding the urethral meatus. The child usually presents with blood spotting in the underwear, dysuria, obstructive voiding symptoms, or a mass. On physical examination, a doughnut-shaped mass that is usually friable and hyperemic protrudes from the urethral opening. The examiner should locate the vaginal opening posterior to the prolapsed urethra. Differential diagnosis includes periurethral abscess, prolapsed urethral polyp, ectopic ureter, prolapsed ectopic ureterocele, papilloma, condyloma accuminata, and sarcoma botryoides. Specialty referral is needed for proper diagnosis and treatment.[3]

Vaginal Foreign Bodies

Foreign bodies should be considered when a child presents with vaginal bleeding, foul-smelling discharge, or irritation. Symptoms may persist for long periods and usually are not resolved by antibiotics or proper hygiene unless the foreign body is removed. Toilet paper is the

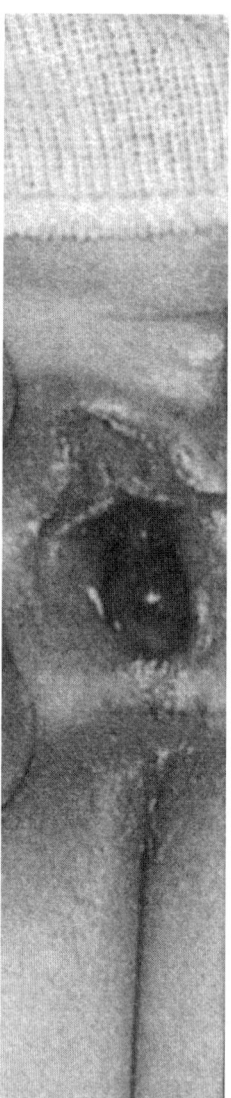

FIG. 139-2. Imperforate hymen with neonatal hematocolpos. A dark purplish bulge at the introitus was noted by the mother during a diaper change.

most common foreign body in the prepubertal girl. Other objects, including toy parts, coin, erasers, beads, and nuts, have been reported. Examination of the girl in the knee-chest position is usually helpful to visualize the vaginal vault and possibly the foreign body. If the foreign body is observed, removal may be successful with a forceps, cotton-tipped swab, or gentle vaginal irrigation with warm NS. If all these methods fail, examination and removal under conscious sedation or anesthesia should be considered. The complications of retained foreign bodies include vaginitis, rectovaginal or vesicovaginal fistula formation, endometritis, or salpingitis.[14]

Vaginitis

Vaginitis is the most common cause of pruritus vulvae and vaginal bleeding in children. Prepubertal girls are prone to bacterial vaginitis because of their thin, atrophic, and more alkaline vaginal mucosa. Wiping from back to front after urination or a bowel movement, bubble baths, tight clothing, or perfumed soap can predispose to vaginitis. *Bacterial vulvovaginitis* frequently presents with copious yellow-green vaginal discharge, pruritus, bleeding, or erythema.[8,15] The most common bacteria are respiratory or enteric pathogens such as group A beta-hemolytic streptococci, *Haemophilus influenzae, Staphylococcus aureus, Shigella,* and *E coli. Gardnerella* and *Trichomonas* are rare in prepubertal girls because these pathogens prefer a more estrogenized vagina. Management is usually achieved by following proper hygiene and taking the appropriate antibiotics.[16]

Candida vaginitis is less common in prepubertal girls than in older females because of the alkaline pH of the vagina. Predisposing factors are depressed cellular immunity, poor perineal ventilation, recent antibiotic intake, diabetes mellitus, pregnancy, and the use of oral contraceptives. The patient usually presents with nonodorous discharge, pruritus, dysuria, and vulvar erythema. The classic thick, white, cheesy discharge is present in only a few patients. In young girls and infants, an erythematous perineal rash and satellite lesions are common. Inspection of the lower third of the vagina may reveal thick discharge and whitish plaques adherent to the vaginal mucosa. Microscopic examination of the discharge (see Chap. 108) usually confirms the presence of yeast buds or hyphae. In infants and young children, the topical application of antifungal medications such as clotrimazole (Lotrimin) or nystatin (Mycostatin) cream four times daily for 7 to 10 days is usually effective.[17]

Genital Trauma

Accidental genital trauma is commonly the result of falls, bicycle, or straddle injuries. Other sports-related injuries such as those common to water sports and horseback riding also can cause genital trauma. Sexual assault or abuse also should be in the differential diagnosis.[18] The most common injuries are hematomas or lacerations of the labia majora. These injuries may be associated with injuries to the vagina, rectum, urethra, or perineum. Urethral injuries may cause urinary retention; the patient must be able to void before leaving the emergency department. In girls with penetrating trauma, the length of the penetrating object should be estimated to determine if it could penetrate the pelvic floor. Examination includes a careful evaluation of the urethra, external genitalia, vulva, vagina, and rectum. Patients with lesions that are actively bleeding, lacerations that extend beyond superficial layers, any rectal bleeding, positive stool guiac examination, or hematomas need emergency evaluation by a gynecologist. Since the perineal/vulvar area is extremely vascular, lesions that continue to bleed also need gynecologic consultation. Small hematomas can be observed in the ED until the physician feels comfortable that the hematoma is not expanding. Discharge instructions include strict bed rest for 12 to 24 h (may ambulate for bathroom and meals).

Vaginal Bleeding

Vaginal bleeding is common in early puberty. The most common cause is irregular or delayed periods due to the lack of regular ovulation. These anovulatory periods are most common during the first 2 years after menarche. Stress, excessive weight loss, and intense exercise regimens can all cause abnormal menstrual bleeding. Pregnancy should be considered. Medications and systemic disorders such as hypothyroidism, hyperthyroidism, hyperprolactinemia, Cushing disease, liver disease, or renal failure may all lead to increased or irregular vaginal bleeding. Excessive bleeding since menarche should prompt an evaluation for coagulopathies such as von Willebrand disease, platelet abnormalities, or factor deficiencies. Polycystic ovary disease (PCO) is a common cause of vaginal bleeding due to increased unopposed estrogen. Patients with PCO display physical characteristics such as hirsutism, increased acne, and obesity. Other considerations include a vaginal foreign body, trauma, or vaginal neoplasms.

Dysfunctional Uterine Bleeding

The overwhelming majority (95 percent) of vaginal bleeding in adolescents is dysfunctional uterine bleeding (DUB). DUB is a diagnosis of exclusion, and the differential diagnosis includes all the causes of

vaginal bleeding mentioned earlier.[19,20] The possibility of pregnancy always must be considered in pubertal children. For further discussion of DUB, refer to Chap. 101.

REFERENCES

1. Lundquist ST, Stack LB: Genitourinary emergencies: Diseases of the foreskin, penis and urethra. *Emerg Med Clin North Am* 19(3):529, 2001.
2. Pillai SB, Besner GE: Pediatric testicular problems. *Pediatr Clin North Am* 45(4):813, 1998.
3. Sheldon CA: Pediatric genitourinary examination. *Pediatr Clin North Am* 48(6):1339, 2001.
4. Marcozzi D, Suner S: Non-traumatic acute scrotum. *Emerg Med Clin North Am* 19(3):547, 2001.
5. Garrett JE, Cartwright PC, Snow BW, et al: Cystic testicular lesions in the pediatric population. *J Urol* 163(3):928, 2000.
6. Kaplan GW: Scrotal swelling in children. *Pediatr Rev* 21(9):311, 2000.
7. Kass EJ: Adolescent varicocele. *Pediatr Clin North Am* 48(6):1559, 2001.
8. Brown MR, Cartwright PC, Snow BW, et al: Common office problems in pediatric urology and gynecology. *Pediatr Clin North Am* 44(5):1091, 1997.
9. Choe JM: Paraphimosis: Current treatment options. *Am Fam Physician* 62(12):2623, 2000.
10. Harmon WJ, Nehra A: Priapism: Diagnosis and management. *Mayo Clinic Proc* 72(4):350, 1997.
11. Pautler SE, Brock GE: Erectile dysfunction: Priapism from priapus to the present time. *Urol Clin North Am* 28(2):391, 2001.
12. Hairston L: Physical examination of the prepubertal girl. *Clin Obstet Gynecol* 40(1):127, 1997
13. Root AW: Precocious puberty. *Pediatr Rev* 21(1):10, 2000
14. Meglio GD: Genital foreign bodies. *Pediatr Rev* 19(1):34, 1998.
15. Acquavella AP, Braverman P: Adolescent gynecology in the office setting. *Pediatr Clin North Am* 46(3):489, 1999.
16. Schroeder B: Vulvar disorder in adolescent. *Obstet Gynecol Clin North Am* 27(1):34, 2000.
17. Paek SC, Merritt DF, Mallory SB, et al: Pruritus vulvae in prepubertal children. *J Am Acad Dermatol* 44(5):795, 2001.
18. Kairys SW, Alexander RC[JKM5], et al: Guidelines for evaluation of sexual abuse of children. *Pediatrics* 103(1):186, 1999.
19. Bravender T, Emans SJ: Dysfunction uterine bleeding. *Pediatr Clin North Am* 46(3):545, 1999.
20. Mitan LA, Slap GB: Adolescent menstrual disorders. *Med Clin North Am* 84(4):851, 2000.

PEDIATRIC URINARY TRACT INFECTIONS

Michael F. Altieri

Mary Camarca

Thom Mayer

EPIDEMIOLOGY

Urinary tract infections (UTIs) are an important cause of febrile illnesses in infants and children in the United States. UTI occurs in 4 to 7 percent of febrile infants.[1] Symptomatic UTIs occur in approximately 2 percent of children from 1 to 5 years of age and in up to 3 to 5 percent of school-aged girls.[2] Since the presenting signs and symptoms are often nonspecific, especially in younger infants, the index of suspicion of UTI should be high. The incidence of UTI varies greatly with age, gender, historical factors such as prematurity, and history of previous UTI. Proper initial evaluation, interpretation of laboratory data, treatment, and follow-up are essential to avoid renal scarring. The American Academy of Pediatrics recommendations for UTI are contained in this chapter.[3]

PATHOPHYSIOLOGY

In the neonatal period, UTI originates via hematogenous spread resulting in bacterial seeding of the renal parenchyma. After the neonatal period, bacteria gain access to the urinary tract via perineal and periurethral colonization, with subsequent retrograde contamination of the lower urinary tract structures. Virulence of the pathogen, host immunity, and structural and functional aspects of the urinary tract all play important roles in the development of UTI. Much is known about structural and functional factors contributing to the risk of UTI. Congenital urinary tract anomalies, vesicoureteral reflux, and urolithiasis are associated with a higher incidence of UTI.[3-6] However, it is now clear that pyelonephritis in the absence of vesicoureteral reflux is far more common than previously thought. Behavioral and functional factors, such as poor hygiene, voluntary urinary retention, and constipation, have been associated with increased risk of UTI.[7,8]

There are several host factors that increase susceptibility to bacteriuria and UTI. These are listed in Table 140-1.

It has also recently been shown that circumcision in males decreases the rate of positive urine cultures. Therefore, circumcision could possibly be considered as part of UTI therapy.[9,10]

Renal stones in children vary with geographic region. Stones are more common in Asia and the Middle East than in the United States, and are more often bladder stones. In the United States, stones are more common in the southeast and occur more frequently in white children with a relatively even incidence distribution between boys and girls. Stones are most often found in the renal pelvis and ureter. Stone formation is more common in children with congenital malformation of the urinary tract, chronic UTI, and metabolic disorders.[11] Although bacteriuria and UTI may complicate renal stones, sterile pyuria may also be found.[12] One study found UTI associated with 47 percent of patients with renal stones.[13] Certain urease-producing bacteria, most commonly *Proteus*, may lead to stone formation (struvite stones). These stones are the result of crystallization of magnesium and phosphorus in an alkaline urine. Antibiotics alone are unsuccessful in treating struvite stones since the causative bacteria are encased within the stone.[14] Treatment includes stone removal and subsequent urine sterilization with appropriate antibiotics.

CLINICAL FEATURES

Other than fever, few symptoms are consistently found in infants and children diagnosed with UTI. Neonates may present with jaundice, poor feeding, irritability, and lethargy. Older infants and young children commonly present with gastrointestinal complaints, such as abdominal pain, vomiting, and change in appetite. The classic signs of dysuria, urinary frequency, urgency, or hesitancy are more likely to be present in older children and adolescents. The clinical signs and symptoms of UTI also vary with the primary site of infection along the urinary tract. The symptoms of dysuria, frequency, and urgency are more often associated with lower tract (uncomplicated) infections, such as

TABLE 140-1 Host Factors Affecting Bacteriuria

Age
Colonization
  Fecal
  Periurethral
  Preputial
Gender
Genetics (uroepithelial receptors)
Genitourinary abnormalities
  Neurogenic bladder
  Pregnancy
  Vesicoureteral reflux
Iatrogenic factors
  Antibiotic use
  Catheterization
Native immunity
Sexual activity

Source: From Chon et al.[21]

cystitis and urethritis. More systemic symptoms, such as fever, chills, vomiting, and dehydration, suggest upper tract (complicated) infection. However, pyelonephritis often occurs in the absence of such symptoms. Since the signs and symptoms of UTI are nonspecific, the diagnosis should be considered in all febrile neonates and children. Furthermore, UTIs may be associated with bacteremia. Ginsburg and McCracken noted an inverse relationship between age and bacteremia in young infants: 31 percent in neonates, 21 percent in children aged 1 to 2 months, 14 percent in children aged 2 to 3 months, and 5.5 percent in children older than 3 months.[10] Follow-up diagnostic studies are often needed to distinguish between lower and upper tract disease and to identify potential long-term sequelae.[15,16]

DIAGNOSIS

Gram-negative enteric bacteria are the most commonly isolated organisms in UTI. While P-fimbriated *Escherichia coli* accounts for the vast majority of infections, *Klebsiella, Proteus,* and *Enterobacter* species are also important pathogens. *Enterococcus* species, *Staphylococcus aureus,* and group B streptococci are the most frequently isolated gram-positive organisms and are more likely to be causative organisms in the neonatal period. Coagulase-negative staphylococcal UTI occurs in teens and young adults. *Chlamydia trachomatis* infection of the urinary tract should be suspected in children and adolescents who present with microhematuria.[17] The diagnosis of a urogenital chlamydial infection can be made by inoculating cell cultures with urethral smears or by utilizing polymerase chain reaction tests (PCR) for *Chlamydia*. Direct immunofluorescence testing can also be used. Adenovirus may cause acute cystitis, occurs more commonly in young boys, and is clinically indistinguishable in many cases from bacterial disease.

While urine culture is the gold standard for the diagnosis of UTIs in children, emergency physicians must rely on clinical data and urinalysis pending the results of urine culture to subsequently confirm the diagnosis.

With a child who is not toilet-trained, a specimen for urinalysis and culture should be obtained through catheterization or suprapubic sampling. Bagged urine specimens are not acceptable because of the high degree of contamination. Urine specimens from older children with voiding control should be obtained from a cleanly voided midstream clean catch. Parents should be instructed on the proper technique for avoiding contamination of specimens. Periurethral contamination of specimens can be avoided by having girls sit backward (facing the rear of the toilet). This position favors labial retraction and better exposure of the urethral meatus. Because bacterial contaminants grow rapidly at room temperature, a urine specimen that cannot be cultured immediately should be kept on ice or at a temperature of 4°C (39.2°F) until culturing can be accomplished.

Urine chemical test strips are screening tests for the detection of leukocyte esterase and urinary nitrites. Esterases are released into the urine after the breakdown of white blood cells, providing presumptive evidence of infection. Neonates and infants may have false-negative leukocyte esterase because their leukocyte response may be limited. Nitrates are converted to nitrites by gram-negative urinary pathogens, so infections from gram-positive organisms would be expected to provide negative test strips. **In most studies, the sensitivities of a positive test result for urinary leukocyte esterase or nitrite compared to a positive urine culture result are less than 50 percent, so a negative urine test strip does not rule out a UTI.** Hematuria, proteinuria, and pyuria are commonly associated with UTIs, but are nonspecific findings and can occur in the absence of infection.

Microscopic urinalysis improves diagnostic sensitivity and specificity. **The combined presence of pyuria (more than five white blood cells per high-power field) and bacteriuria on urine microanalysis improves the sensitivity to approximately 65 percent, with a positive predictive value of about 81 percent.**

Urine culture must be obtained in all cases in which UTI is suspected, regardless of the results of test strip or microscopic urinalysis. A guide to interpreting urine culture results based on the various methods of obtaining urine samples is contained in Table 140-2.

TREATMENT

Table 140-3 summarizes the approach to management of children with UTI. Inpatient management should be instituted for any child less than 3 months of age with a febrile UTI. Older infants and children who have significant dehydration or appear toxic; have urinary stents or other urinary foreign bodies or renal insufficiency; and those who are immunocompromised should be considered for inpatient management. In addition, if a child's compliance and follow-up are questionable, inpatient treatment should be considered.

Children older than 3 months with febrile UTIs who appear nontoxic and only mildly dehydrated and who do not have persistent vomiting may be rehydrated in the ED. These children may initially receive intravenous antibiotic therapy and may then be discharged home on a course of oral antibiotics. Prior to discharge, they should demonstrate adequate oral intake and retention of fluids and have arrangements made for follow-up care within 48 h. Specific antibiotics and their dosing for both inpatient and outpatient therapy are contained in Table 140-4, but therapy should be guided with an understanding of the antibiotic resistance patterns in the hospital and community. As noted in Table 140-4, there has been an increasing use of third-generation cephalosporins. There is now increasing development of bacterial resistance to third-generation cephalosporin drugs. Cefepime and other fourth-generation cephalosporins have remained active against these organisms. Cefepime has been shown to be very effective in children with UTIs from the age of 1 month upwards. It is administered at a dose of 50 mg/kg per dose IV q8 to 12h.[18] Instructions should be given to the caregiver regarding the need for follow-up of culture results.

DIAGNOSTIC IMAGING

The most appropriate radiologic studies for the follow-up of children with UTIs have been debated,[19] and various algorithms have been proposed.[15,16,20] Although imaging studies for UTIs are rarely indicated as part of the diagnostic work-up in the ED (except in cases in which there is a palpable mass), it is important to arrange follow-up for all children with febrile UTIs. The following is a reasonable approach to diagnostic to diagnostic imaging. First, the goals of radiologic imaging are to (1) identify existing upper tract disease capable of causing cortical scarring so that appropriate antibiotic therapy can be instituted, (2) identify treatable lesions of the genitourinary system, and (3) guide an approach to prevent further renal scarring and subsequent impairment of renal function.

TABLE 140-2 Interpretation of Positive Urine Culture Results

Method of Collection	Quantitative Culture: UTI Present
Suprapubic aspiration	Growth of urinary pathogens in any number (exception of up to $2–3 \times 10^3$ coagulase-negative staphylococci)
Catheterization	Febrile infants or children with $\geq 5 \times 10^4$ CFU/mL of single pathogen
Midstream clean void	Symptomatic patients with $\geq 10^5$ CFU/mL of a single urinary pathogen
Midstream clean void	Asymptomatic patients with two specimens on different days with $>10^5$ CFU/mL of the same organism

Abbreviation: CFU = cell-forming units.
Source: Adapted from Hellerstein,[20] with permission.

TABLE 140-3 Management of Urinary Tract Infections

Age Range and Clinical Status	Management
<3 months Febrile UTI	Hospitalize; IV antibiotics for 4–5 d with good clinical response, discharge when tolerating oral medication and diet; 10 d of therapeutic doses of medication and then suppressive medication
>3 months through adolescence Acute pyelonephritis, ill or dehydrated, or with comorbidities	Hospitalize; IV antibiotics until afebrile 24–36 h and able to take oral medication and fluids; discharge on 10-d course of oral medication If renal scarring on RCS, IV therapy may be extended to 7 d
>3 months through adolescence Acute pyelonephritis, but not ill or dehydrated, no comorbidities	IM or IV antibiotic; start oral medication at therapeutic doses after 12–18 h; contact physician after 24 h if unable to take oral medication or adequate fluids; contact physician at 48 h for adjustment in medication and to schedule F/U urine and imaging studies
Infancy to adolescence Acute cystitis	5–7 d of therapeutic doses of oral antibiotic for UTI; urinalysis and culture after 4–5 d Sitz baths and/or analgesia for symptomatic relief
Adolescence Acute cystitis	Single IM or IV dose of ceftriaxone or aminoglycoside; single oral dose of trimethoprim-sulfamethoxazole; 3-d oral regimen with trimethoprim-sulfamethoxazole or nitrofurantoin; F/U urinalysis and culture after 4–5 d

Abbreviations: F/U = follow-up; RCS = renal cortical scan.
Source: Adapted from Hellerstein,[20] with permission.

In the past, indications for imaging of pediatric patients with UTI included neonates, females with recurrent UTI (two or more episodes), and males of any age with UTI. However, one of the recent recommendations from the AAP Committee on Quality Improvement Subcommittee on Urinary Tract Infection states that:

> infants and young children two months to two years of age with UTI who do not demonstrate the expected clinical response within two days of antimicrobial therapy should undergo ultrasonography promptly and either voiding cystoureterogram (VCUG) or radionuclide cystography (RNC) should be performed at the earliest convenient time. Infants and young children who have the expected response to antimicrobials should have a sonogram and either VCUG or RNC performed at the earliest convenient time.[3]

Acutely febrile and/or toxic children with UTI as the documented or presumed source of fever should have a renal cortical scan (RCS) to assess for renal involvement. If renal scarring and/or active infection is present, the patient should have intravenous antibiotic therapy extended by 7 to 10 days to reduce scarring and eliminate infection. If the RCS results are negative, males should have a voiding cystourethrogram (VCUG) and females an isotope cystogram (IC) to assess for vesicoureteral reflux. In afebrile children, the VCUG for males and IC for females should initially be assessed, followed by RCS if the results are positive. Renal sonography may be done at the time of RCS, VCUG, or IC to assess for dilatation of the collection system, although its utility has recently been questioned.[22]

While such radiologic imaging is not necessarily coordinated by the ED, it is important for emergency physicians to be aware of the necessity of follow-up and the reasons for imaging so that it can be coordinated with the patient's inpatient physician or primary care provider.

TABLE 140-4 Common Antimicrobial Drugs Used in Pediatric Urinary Tract Infections

Drug	Dosage and Interval
Parenteral Therapy	
Ampicillin	100 mg/kg per d q12h (<1 week) q6–8 h (>1 week)
Cefriaxone	75 mg/kg per d
Cefotaxime	150 mg/kg per d q6–8h
Gentamicin	5 mg/kg per d q12h (<1 week) 7.5 mg/kg per d q8h (>1 week)
Cefepime	150 mg/kg per d q8–12h
Oral Therapy	
Amoxicillin	20–40 mg/kg per d q8h
Augmentin (amoxicillin-elavulanate)	50 mg/kg per d q8h
Trimethoprim-sulfamethoxazole (TMP-SMX)	8–12 mg/kg per d TMP, 30–60 mg/kg per d SMX q12h
Cephalexin	25–50 mg/kg per d q6h
Cefixime	8 mg/kg per d q12h

REFERENCES

1. Hoberman A, Chao H-P, Keller DM, et al: Prevalence of urinary tract infections in febrile infants. *J Pediatr* 23:17, 1993.
2. Gonzalez R: Urinary tract infections, in Behrman R, Klieman R, Arvin A, et al, (eds): *Nelson's Textbook of Pediatrics,* 16th ed. Philadelphia, Saunders, 2002.
3. American Academy of Pediatrics Committee on Quality Improvements. Subcommittee on Urinary Tract Infection: Practice parameter: The diagnosis, treatment, and evaluation of the initial urinary tract infection in febrile infants and young children. *Pediatrics* 103:843, 1999.
4. Bock GH: Urinary tract infections, in Hockerman R (ed): *Primary Pediatric Care,* 3d ed. St. Louis, Mosby-Year Book, 1997, pp. 1640–1644.
5. Gearhart P, Herzberg G, Jeffs RD, et al: Childhood urolithiasis: Experiences and advances. *Pediatrics* 87:445, 1991.
6. Smellie JM, Normand ICS, Katz G: Children with urinary tract infection: A comparison of those with and those without vesicoureteric reflux. *Kidney Int* 20:717, 1981.
7. Smellie JM, Normand ICS: Urinary tract infections in children. *Postgrad Med* 61:895, 1985.
8. Bethyn AJ, Jenkins HR, Roberts R, et al: Radiologic evidence of constipation in urinary tract infection. *Am J Dis Child* 73:534, 1995.
9. Nayir A: Circumcision for the prevention of significant bacteriuria in boys. *Pediatr Nephrol* 16:1129–1139, 2001.
10. Ginsburg CM, McCracken GH: Urinary tract infections in young infants. *Pediatrics* 69(4):409, 1982.
11. Gearhart JP, Hersberg GZ, Jeffs RD: Childhood urolithiasis: Experiences and advances. *Pediatrics* 87:445, 1991.
12. Skoog SJ, Scherz HC: Office pediatric urology, in Gillenwater JY, Grayhack JT, Howards SS, et al (eds): *Adult and Pediatric Urology.* Baltimore, Lippincott Williams & Wilkins, 2002, pp. 2696–2703.
13. Stapleton FB: Clinical approach to children and urolithiasis. *Semin Nephrol* 16:389, 1996.
14. Milliner DS, Murphy ME: Urolithiasis in pediatric patients. *Mayo Clinic Proc* 68:241, 1993.
15. Conway J, Cohn R: Evolving role of nuclear medicine for diagnosis and management of urinary tract infections. *J Pediatr* 124:87, 1994.
16. Goldraich N, Goldraich I: Update on dimercaptosuccinic acid renal scanning in children with urinary tract infection. *Pediatr Nephrol* 9:221, 1995.
17. Meglic A, Cavic M, Hren-Vencelj H, et al: Chlamydial infection of the urinary tract in children and adolescents with hematuria. *Pediatr Nephrol* 15:132–133, 2000.
18. Arrieta AC, Bradley JS: Empiric use of cefepime in the treatment of serious urinary tract infections in children. *Pediatr Infect Dis J* 20:350–355, 2001.
19. Dick PT, Feldman W: Routine diagnostic imaging for childhood urinary tract infection: A systematic overview. *J Pediatr* 128:15, 1996.
20. Hellerstein S: Urinary tract infections: Old and new concepts. *Pediatr Clin North Am* 42:1433, 1995.
21. Chon CH, Lai FC, Dairiki-Shortllife LM, et al: Pediatric urinary tract infections. *Pediatr Clin North Am* 48:(6):1441, 2001.
22. Hoberman A, Charron M, Hickey RW, et al: Imaging studies after a first febrile urinary tract infection in young children. *NEJM* 348(5):195, 2003.

141 SEXUALLY TRANSMITTED DISEASES
Joel Kravitz
Susan B. Promes

Sexually transmitted diseases (STDs) are encountered commonly in ED and urgent care settings. About 50 million people in the United States are infected with genital herpes simplex virus (HSV), an estimated 600,000 gonococcal infections are diagnosed each year, and up to 4 million cases of chlamydial infection were estimated to be diagnosed in the United States in 1993.[1]

Infection with some of the STDs discussed in this chapter increase the likelihood of acquiring HIV and/or hepatitis B, and these disorders are discussed in Chaps. 144 and 86, respectively. Thus diagnosis of an STD suggests the need for HIV and hepatitis counseling and testing.

Diagnosis and treatment of the STDs consists of three principles: protecting the health and future fertility of the patient, protecting the health of the patient's sexual contacts, and providing a "gateway" into the health care system for future screening and education with an emphasis on prevention. Prevention methods for STDs include male latex condoms, female condoms, contraceptive sponges, and diaphragms.[2] Vaginal spermicides are not protective against gonorrhea, chlamydia, or HIV.[2] *The Morbidity and Mortality Weekly Report* (http://www.cdc.gov/mmwr/) of the Centers for Disease Control and Prevention (CDC) is an excellent source of updates given the frequent changes in STD treatment guidelines and development of new antibiotics.[2]

DIAGNOSIS

The most important aspect of STD diagnosis is maintaining a high level of awareness. In one inner-city ED, half the patients with a urinary tract infection (UTI) had one or more positive STD cultures.[3] The signs and symptoms of an STD may be obvious, such as a genital lesion or vaginal discharge, or less specific, such as dysuria or lower abdominal pain. Obtaining a through sexual history will help determine the risk of STD, HIV, or hepatitis and also will direct the extent of the physical examination and laboratory testing. Special populations with a high morbidity risk from STDs include pregnant women, sexually active adolescents, and homosexual men.[2] When evaluating for potential STDs, pregnancy status should be determined, and questions should be asked about sexual assault, domestic violence, and sexual practices.

Careful examination of the genital area, including a speculum examination in female patients, is important. In males, retracting the foreskin and carefully examining between skin folds, particularly in obese patients, is an important part of the physical examination. Vaginal or urethral cultures or polymerase chain reaction (PCR) assays for gonorrhea and chlamydia should be obtained. Viral and bacterial cultures for disorders such as HSV infection or lymphogranuloma venereum should be obtained if clinically indicated.

STDs Presenting with Urethritis, Cervicitis, and/or Discharge

CHLAMYDIAL INFECTIONS *Chlamydia trachomatis* is one of the causes of nongonococcal urethritis. It commonly coexists with gonorrhea infection. The prevalence of chlamydial infection ranges from 3 to 5 percent in the general population to 15 to 20 percent among individuals attending STD clinics.[1,4] In men, chlamydial infection is often asymptomatic but can cause urethritis, epididymitis, proctitis, or Reiter's syndrome (urethritis, conjunctivitis, and rash). In women, mild, asymptomatic cervicitis is the most common presentation. Symptoms, when present, usually include vaginal discharge and dysuria. The discharge may be mucopurulent when *Neisseria gonorrhoeae* is a coinfectant. Urethral chlamydial infection should be considered in the differential diagnosis of sterile pyuria. Complications in women include pelvic inflammatory disease (PID) and infertility.

Diagnosis The yield from culture is low. Indirect detection methods such as direct immunofluorescence, enzyme-linked immunosorbent assays (ELISAs), and DNA probes are available. The sensitivity range for all of them is 70 to 95 percent.[2] The CDC has recommended that a nucleic acid amplification test (NAAT) such as Amplicor, Abbot LCx, BD ProbeTEC, or Gen-Probe APTIMA be used as a screening tool for *C. trachomatis* infections due to their high sensitivity.[5]

Treatment Treatment is with azithromycin 1 g PO in a single dose or doxycycline 100 mg PO bid for 7 days. Both regimens are equally efficacious.[2] Table 141-1 lists alternative treatment options. Sexual partners should be referred for testing and treatment if there has been sexual contact in the last 60 days. In pregnant women, azithromycin is safe, and cultures should be repeated 3 weeks later. To minimize transmission, patients should be counseled to avoid sexual contact for 7 days, regardless of 1- or 7-day treatment regimens.

GONOCOCCAL INFECTIONS *N. gonorrhoeae* is a gram-negative diplococcus. Like its frequent coinfectant, *C. trachomatis*, asymptomatic gonococcal infection is believed to be the most common presentation, particularly in women. Subclinical gonorrheal infections coupled with poor detection methods yield complications ranging from ectopic pregnancy (9 percent) to chronic pelvic pain (20 percent) to acute PID (10 to 40 percent).[1,4,6] Women tend to present with nonspecific lower abdominal discomfort and mucopurulent cervicitis after a 7- to 14-day incubation period. In contrast, 80 to 90 percent of men develop symptoms within 2 weeks. Dysuria and purulent penile discharge are the most common presenting symptoms for men, but presentations also can include acute epididymitis and prostatitis. Rectal infection with micropurulent anal discharge and pain occurs in 30 to 50 percent of women with gonococcal cervicitis and can be the only site of infection in homosexual men. *N. gonorrhoeae* also can be isolated from the pharynx but rarely causes pharyngitis. Disseminated gonococcal infection occurs in approximately 2 percent of untreated primary gonorrhea. Disseminated gonococcemia is characterized by petechial or pustular (acral) skin lesions on an erythematous base (50–70 percent), asymmetric arthralgias, tenosynovitis or septic arthritis (30–40 percent), and fever or general malaise (80 percent).

Diagnosis Cervical or urethral culture on a selective medium is the standard for diagnosis, having a sensitivity of 80 to 90 percent. If the transport and storage conditions are not conducive to maintaining the viability of the endocervical or urethral swab specimen, the CDC recommends that a NAAT be performed on endocervical or urethral swab specimens or a NAAT be performed on the urine as a screening tool for gonorrhea infections.[5] A Gram stain of a urethral smear showing intracellular gram-negative diplococci is sensitive and specific in men but much less useful in women. Diagnosis of disseminated gonococcal infection is more difficult, with only 20 to 50 percent of blood, lesion,

TABLE 141-1 Antimicrobial Therapy for STDs

Disease	First-Line Treatment	Alternate(s)
Chlamydia	Azithromycin 1 g PO single dose *or* Doxycycline 100 mg PO bid × 7 d	Erythromycin 500 mg PO qid × 7 d *or* Ofloxacin 300 mg PO bid × 7 d *or* Levofloxacin 500 mg PO qd × 7 d
Gonorrhea	Cefixime 400 mg PO single dose *or* Ceftriaxone 125 mg IM single dose *or* Ciprofloxacin 500 mg PO single dose *or* Ofloxacin 400 mg PO single dose *or* Levofloxacin 250 mg PO single dose	Spectinomycin 2 g IM single dose *or* Norfloxacin 800 mg PO single dose *or* Gatifloxacin 400 mg PO single dose
Trichomoniasis	Metronidazole 2 g PO single dose	Metronidazole 500 mg PO bid × 7 d
Bacterial vaginosis	Metronidazole 500 mg PO bid × 7 d *or* Metronidazole vaginal gel 0.75% qd for 5 d	Clindamycin 2% cream intravaginally qhs × 7 d
Syphilis (primary, secondary, early tertiary)	Benzathine penicillin G 2.4 million units IM in a single dose	Doxycycline 100 mg PO bid × 14 d
Syphilis (latent, tertiary)	Benzathine penicillin G 2.4 million units IM weekly × 3 weeks	
HSV (primary)	Acyclovir 400 mg PO tid × 7–10 d *or* Famciclovir 250 mg PO tid × 7–10 d *or* Valacyclovir 1 g PO bid × 7–10 d	Acyclovir 200 mg PO 5 times a day × 7–10 d
HSV (recurrent)	Acyclovir 400 mg PO tid × 5 d *or* Famciclovir 125 mg PO bid × 5 d *or* Valacyclovir 500 mg PO bid × 5 d	Acyclovir 800 mg PO bid × 5 days *or* Valacyclovir 1 g PO qd × 5 days
Chancroid	Azithromycin 1 g PO single dose *or* Ceftriaxone 250 mg IM single dose *or* Ciprofloxacin 500 mg PO bid × 3 d	Erythromycin base 500 mg PO qid × 7 d
Lymphogranuloma venereum	Doxycycline 100 mg PO bid × 3 weeks	Erythromycin base 500 mg PO qid × 3 weeks
Donovanosis	Doxycycline 100 mg PO bid × 3 weeks *or* TMP-SMX DS PO bid × 3 weeks	Ciprofloxacin 750 mg PO bid × 3 weeks *or* Azithromycin 1 g PO weekly × 3 weeks *or* Erythromycin base 500 mg PO qid × 3 weeks

Source: Adapted from the Centers for Disease Control and Prevention: Sexually transmitted diseases treatment guidelines—2002. *MMWR* 51(RR-6), 2002.

and joint cultures being positive. Obtaining cervical, rectal, and pharyngeal samples may improve the chance of a culture-proven diagnosis.

Treatment Ceftriaxone 125 mg IM, cefixime 400 mg PO, ciprofloxacin 500 mg PO, ofloxacin 400 mg PO, or levofloxacin 250 mg PO, all in single doses, are all acceptable treatments (see Table 141-1). Patients also should be treated for presumed chlamydial infection. Although penicillin may be effective, over the years some strains of *N. gonorrhoeae* have grown resistant to this antibiotic. Areas of Asia and the West Coast of the United States (i.e., California and Hawaii) are seeing an emergence of quinolone-resistant *N. gonorrhoeae* (QRNG).[2,7] The CDC currently recommends avoiding quinolones for infections that may have been acquired in Asia, the Pacific, or California.[2] Pregnant women should be treated with a cephalosporin or, if allergic, 2 g spectinomycin IM in a single dose. Instructions to sexual contacts are the same as with chlamydial infections. PID or disseminated disease is usually treated with higher doses of ceftriaxone. Gonococcemia requires hospitalization for antibiotics (cefotaxime 1g q8h, levofloxacin 500 mg

PO daily) and evaluation for possible endocarditis and meningitis. Patients with gonococcal arthritis also may require orthopedic surgical drainage and irrigation. Decisions to admit patients are based on their overall clinical picture as well as their ability to follow up on an outpatient basis.

NONGONOCOCCAL URETHRITIS (NGU) NGU is diagnosed when the *N. gonorrhoeae* diplococci are not seen on urethral smears. While the causative agent is most commonly *C. trachomatis* (30 to 50 percent), the prevalence of *Chlamydia* infection is lower in older men. Other agents include *Ureaplasma urealyticum* (20 to 25 percent), *Mycoplasma genitalum,* and *Trichomonas,* with 20 to 30 percent being idiopathic in etiology. Specific tests for *U. urealyticum* and *M. genitalum* are not indicated. Treatment is as for chlamydial infection.

TRICHOMONAL INFECTIONS *Trichomonas vaginalis* is a flagellated protozoan that causes urogenital infections in men and women. The World Health Organization (WHO) estimates that 180 million cases occur annually worldwide. The prevalence is less than 1 percent in women overall but up to 15 percent in those attending STD clinics. Because of the organism's ability to phagocytize viral particles, *T. vaginalis* has been proposed to increase the host's susceptibility to viral infections such as HIV and HSV. Incubation ranges from 3 to 28 days. Disease is characterized most commonly by vulvar irritation and a malodorous, yellow-green discharge. Lower abdominal pain can be present occasionally. In men, the disease is often asymptomatic, but it can cause urethritis. In women, trichomoniasis in pregnancy has been associated with premature rupture of the membranes, preterm delivery, and low birth weight.

Diagnosis   Microscopic examination of wet preparations of cervical smears or spun urine samples that reveal the classic motile parasites is diagnostic, although sensitivity is 60 to 70 percent. Culture is the most sensitive test available.

Treatment   Metronidazole 2 g PO in a single dose is the usual treatment, or alternatively, 500 mg PO bid for 7 days. Avoidance of alcohol while on this treatment should be stressed because of the disulfiram-like reaction that can occur. Sexual partners should be treated due to the high likelihood of retransmission. Metronidazole gel is available, but treatment efficacy is less than 50 percent compared with oral preparations. With respect to pregnant patients, data do not indicate that treatment of asymptomatic infection prevents adverse outcomes; several studies, including a Medicaid cohort study, a large case-control study, and two meta-analyses, suggest that use of metronidazole in pregnancy has not demonstrated a consistent association with teratogenic or mutagenic effects above the baseline population rate.[3] Oral metronidazole is still considered a class C drug by many sources, and many clinicians avoid oral treatment in the first trimester, although the CDC guidelines state that pregnant women may be treated with a single 2-g dose of metronidazole.

STDs with Genital Ulcers

Disorders characterized by genital ulcers are syphilis, herpes virus, chancroid, lymphogranuloma venereum, and granuloma inguinale. Characteristics of the lesions and their accompanying signs and symptoms are provided in Table 141-2.

SYPHILIS   *Treponema pallidum,* a spirochete, is the causative agent of syphilis as well as yaws and pinta. The organism enters the body through mucous membranes or nonintact skin. It remains very sensitive to penicillin; thus diagnosis rather than treatment is the main difficulty in controlling this disease. Unfortunately, the last 7 years has seen a marked increase in syphilis thought to be secondary to behavior associated with drug use.[1,2,8]

Syphilis consists of three phases: primary, secondary, and tertiary or latent syphilis.

Primary. The initial stage of infection is characterized by a painless chancre with indurated borders on the penis, vulva, or other areas with sexual contact. The incubation period is about 21 days, with lesions then disappearing after 3 to 6 weeks. There are no constitutional symptoms, and a lesion may even be absent with primary disease.

Secondary. This stage, which occurs 3 to 6 weeks after the end of the primary stage, includes nonspecific symptoms such as sore throat, malaise, fever, and headaches. Rash and lymphadenopathy are the most common symptoms. The rash often starts on the trunk and flexor surfaces of the extremities, spreading to the palms and soles. It takes on many forms but is often dull red-pink and papular (resembling pityriasis rosacea). Like primary syphilis, secondary syphilis also resolves spontaneously.

Tertiary (latent). This syndrome is seen in about one-third of patients who have had latent secondary syphilis. Involvement of the nervous and cardiovascular systems is characteristic of this stage, which occurs 3 to 20 years after the initial infection. Granulomatous lesions (gummas) are widespread. Specific manifestations include meningitis, dementia, neuropathy (tabes dorsalis), and thoracic aneurysm.

Diagnosis   Dark-field microscopy can identify treponemes in scrapings from primary lesions as well as from secondary lesions. Several serologic tests are also available, including nontreponemal tests (RPR, VDRL) and specific treponemal antibody tests (fluorescent treponemal antibody absorption, or FTA-ABS). Nontreponemal tests are positive about 14 days after the appearance of the chancre and falsely positive in 1 to 2 percent of the population. Nontreponemal antibodies can persist in some patients for years after treatment (the *serofast reaction*). FTA-ABS tests are slightly more sensitive and specific but more difficult to perform.

Treatment   The treatment of primary and secondary syphilis is benzathine penicillin G 2.4 million units IM in a single dose. Doxycycline 100 mg PO bid for 2 weeks may be used for penicillin-allergic individuals. Treatment of tertiary or latent syphilis is 2.4 million units of benzathine penicillin G IM given 1 week apart for 3 weeks.

TABLE 141-2   Clinical Features of Genital Ulcers

Disease	Clinical Diagnosis	Painful Ulcers	Inguinal Adenopathy	Comment
Syphilis	Indurated, relatively clean base; heals spontaneously	No	Firm, rubbery nodes; tender	Primary (chancre); secondary (rash, mucocutaneous lesions, lymphadenopathy); tertiary (cardiac, ophthalmic, auditory, CNS lesions)
Herpes simplex infection	Multiple, small, grouped vesicles coalesce and form shallow ulcers; vulvovaginitis	Yes	Tender bilateral adenopathy	Cytologic detection insensitive; false-negative culture common; type-specific serologic test
Chancroid	Multiple, painful, irregular, purulent ulcers	Yes	Painful, suppurative, inguinal lymph nodes	Cofactor for HIV transmission; 10% have HSV or syphilis
Lymphogranuloma venereum	Small and shallow ulcer, associated proctocolitis with fistulas and strictures	No	Tender lymph nodes	Caused by *C. trachomatis* L1, L2, L3
Granuloma inguinale	Painless, beefy red, bleeding ulcers	No	No	Endemic in Africa, Australia, India, New Guinea; rare in U.S.

Source: Adapted from Centers for Disease Control and Prevention: Sexually transmitted diseases treatment guidelines—2002. *MMWR* 51(RR-6), 2002.

HERPES SIMPLEX INFECTIONS   HSV type 1 or type 2 can cause genital herpes infections by infection of mucosal surfaces or nonintact skin. Many herpes infections are transmitted by those with undiagnosed or asymptomatic infections. Genital infections are caused more commonly by HSV type 2 (HSV-2).

Infections can be asymptomatic. When symptomatic, infections present as painful vesiculopustular lesions on an erythematous base. The painful lesions occur 7 to 10 days after contact with an infected individual, often preceded by 1 to 2 days of a tingling or burning sensation at the site. Primary infections sometimes can be associated with profuse, watery vaginal discharge. Lesions ulcerate after 3 to 5 days, at which time infectivity is at its highest. It is important to note that infections can be asymptomatic. Systemic symptoms are seen in 70 percent of primary infections and include fever and chills, headache, myalgias, and tender inguinal adenopathy. Dysuria is common and may progress to urinary retention secondary to severe pain. Complete healing usually occurs within 3 weeks, and viral shedding persists for 10 to 12 days after the onset of the rash. Recurrent infections due to the latent virus occur in 60 to 90 percent of patients. These are usually milder and of shorter duration, and systemic symptoms are less common.

Diagnosis   Diagnosis of the classic lesions is often made on clinical grounds. A Tzanck smear may be taken of the lesions to demonstrate large intranuclear inclusions, although this is less sensitive than direct culture. Viral cultures can be done, but sensitivity drops as the lesions heal. PCR is available in some laboratories for detection of HSV in spinal fluid, but its role in genital herpes detection is not yet clear.

Treatment   For a first clinical episode, treatment is with acyclovir 400 mg PO tid for 7 to 10 days, or acyclovir 200 mg PO five times a day for 7 to 10 days, or famciclovir 250 mg PO tid for 7 to 10 days, or valacyclovir 1 g PO bid for 7 to 10 days. Treatment duration can be extended if the lesions persist. For treatment of proctitis or oral infections, higher doses are used (acyclovir 400 mg five times a day for 7 to 10 days). Acyclovir at 5 to 10 mg/kg may be given IV every 8 h for 5 to 7 days to patients requiring hospitalization. Famcyclovir and valacyclovir have high oral bioavailability. Episodic recurrent infection should be treated for 5 days with acyclovir 400 mg PO tid, or acyclovir 800 mg PO bid, or famciclovir 125 mg PO bid, or valacyclovir 500 mg PO bid. Effectiveness requires beginning treatment either at the onset of the prodrome or within 1 day of the onset of the lesions. Suppressive therapy is available for people with more than six episodes per year; this reduces but does not eliminate viral shedding.

CHANCROID   *Haemophilus ducreyi* is a pleomorphic gram-negative bacillus that causes painful genital ulcers and lymphadenitis. Though more common in developing countries, it has seen a resurgence in recent years in the United States. Chancroid, when present, is a clue to search for other infections; 10 percent of infected patients in the United States are coinfected with HSV or *T. pallidum* (this number is higher in developing countries), and chancroid is a cofactor for HIV transmission (more so than other ulcerative diseases, for as yet unknown reasons).

After an incubation period of 4 to 10 days, a papule, often painful, on an erythematous base appears at the site of infection. One to two days later, the lesion becomes eroded, ulcerated, and often pustular (not vesicular, like HSV). The ulcers are usually 1 to 2 cm in diameter with sharp, undermined margins and are very painful. The friable base of the ulcer is covered with yellow-gray necrotic exudates. Multiple lesions may be present in up to 50 percent of patients (more so in women), and "kissing lesions" (infection of adjacent skin areas due to autoinoculation) are seen. Half of patients develop acute, painful inguinal lymphadenopathy 1 to 2 weeks after primary infection. If untreated, the lymph nodes necrose and suppurate, leaving an abscess or periadenitis involving the overlying skin and forming a bubo. Constitutional symptoms are rare with this STD.

Diagnosis   Diagnosis can be made on clinical grounds, but other diseases (such as syphilis) need to be excluded. A swab of a lesion or pus from a suppurative lymph node (bubo) can be cultured but requires special media and is met with only limited success.

Treatment   Azithromycin 1 g PO in a single dose, or ceftriaxone 250 mg IM in a single dose, or ciprofloxacin 500 mg PO bid for 3 days, or erythromycin base 500 mg PO qid for 7 days are all effective (see Table 141-2). Symptoms improve in about 3 days, and lesions are visibly improved within a week. Larger ulcers may require 2 to 3 weeks to heal. Partners should be treated if they have had sexual contact in the last 10 days, regardless of symptoms.

LYMPHOGRANULOMA VENEREUM (LGV)   Specific serotypes of *C. trachomatis* cause this disease, known in other countries as *struma, tropical bubo,* or *Nicolas-Favre-Durand disease.* Although endemic in other parts of the world, LGV is seen only sporadically in the United States. The primary lesion can take on many forms and can be confused with other STDs (see Table 141-2).

The painless primary chancre is almost never noticed and lasts only 2 to 3 days. Generally, 1 to 3 weeks (rarely as long as 6 months) following the initial lesion, inguinal lymphadenopathy is noted. The lymphadenopathy is unilateral in 60 percent of patients. Often the overlying skin has a purplish hue. It progresses to suppurative lymphadenopathy, resulting in either spontaneous abscess rupture or firm inguinal masses. Scarring of these masses can give linear depressions parallel to the inguinal ligament, forming the so-called groove sign. LGV infections can have associated systemic symptoms of fever, chills, arthralgias, erythema nodosum, and rarely, meningoencephalitis.

Diagnosis   Serologic tests and culture are the mainstays of diagnosis. Complement fixation titers for LGV greater than 1:64 are also consistent with LGV infection.

Treatment   Doxycycline 100 mg PO bid for 21 days is the usual regimen. Buboes may require drainage. Mild untreated cases will resolve spontaneously in 8 to 12 weeks. Table 141-1 gives alternative treatments.

DONOVANOSIS   Granuloma inguinale, also called *donovanosis,* is caused by *Calymmatobacterium granulomatis,* a gram-negative intracellular bacterium. It is rare in the United States but is endemic in India, southern Africa, and Pacific nations.

After a variable incubation period of 2 weeks to 6 months, donovanosis begins as subcutaneous nodules on the penis or labia/vulvar area. The nodules then progress to the more classic painless, ulcerative lesions that are highly vascular, explaining both the appearance (beefy red) and their tendency to bleed easily. There is no significant lymphadenopathy.

Diagnosis   *C. granulomatis* is difficult to culture, and diagnosis often requires visualization of Donovan bodies on tissue biopsy.

Treatment   Doxycycline 100 mg PO bid or TMP-SMX DS PO bid, both for 3 weeks, will stop progression of the lesions, although longer treatment may be needed to allow complete healing of the ulcers. Ciprofloxacin and azithromycin are alternatives.

GENITAL WARTS   Human papillomaviruses (HPVs) are DNA viruses that cause genital warts by direct transmission. Visible genital warts generally are due to HPV type 6 or type 11, whereas other genotypes have been associated with the development of cervical cancer. The flesh-colored papules or cauliflower-like projections usually appear after an incubation period of 1 to 8 months and may coalesce to form condylomata acuminata. In women, they are seen on the external genitalia, are often painless, and often enlarge during pregnancy. Infected males often complain of nonhealing penile lesions, occasionally with pruritus and urethral discharge. Perianal condylomata have been seen in up to 80 percent of women with vulvar condylomata and are seen frequently in homosexual males.

Diagnosis PCR is the most sensitive method for detecting subclinical cases. Soaking of the genital area with dilute acetic acid for 3 min can differentiate between normal skin (shiny white) and areas of neoplasia (dull gray-white) to detect subclinical infections. For the most part, diagnosis is clinical, with care to exclude other STDs.

Treatment Treatment decisions are based on the size and number of lesions, the amount of discomfort they are causing, and patient preferences. Recommended treatment is podofilox 0.5% solution or gel applied with a cotton swab or a finger to the visible warts twice a day for 3 days, followed by 4 days of no therapy, with the cycle repeated up to four times. Also recommended is imiquimod 5% cream applied at bedtime three times a week for up to 16 weeks. The treatment area should be washed 6 to 10 h after treatment with imiquimod. Most patients experience a local inflammatory reaction after treatment. Cryotherapy or trichloroacetic acid (TCA) in a physician's office is used with failure of patient-applied methods.

STDS IN SPECIAL POPULATIONS

STD Treatment during Pregnancy

Pregnant patients with STDs should be referred to the physician providing their prenatal care. Penicillin, ceftriaxone, azithromycin, cefixime, metronidazole, and acyclovir are felt to be safe for use during pregnancy.

Sexual Assault Prophylaxis

Sexual assault is discussed in detail in Chap. 298, but a review of prophylactic regimens follows in this chapter as well.

Once all appropriate forensic investigations and cultures have been taken, prophylaxis in the form of single doses of ceftriaxone 125 mg IM, metronidazole 2 g PO, and azithromycin 1g PO should be given, with adjustments as needed for allergy and pregnancy. Hepatitis B vaccination (and the subsequent complete three-shot course), without HBIG, should be given to those unimmunized. Postexposure therapy with zidovudine has shown a decreased risk for HIV infection in health care workers exposed to blood, but these studies cannot be extrapolated to the sexual assault patient. While the CDC does not endorse a particular recommendation on HIV prophylaxis, the decision should be made on a case-by-case basis. The assault survivor should be reevaluated in 72 h to further discuss this risk. Repeat evaluation for STDs should be done in 1 to 2 weeks to make sure that infection has been eradicated.

GENERAL RECOMMENDATIONS FOR STD TREATMENT AND FOLLOW-UP

When treating patients for STDs in the ED, it is important to remember that many STDs occur together, follow-up and compliance are poor, and lack of treatment can contribute to infertility. For these reasons, a standardized approach is suggested for patients with suspected STDs. This should include:

1. Treating even when an STD is only suspected, especially for gonorrhea and chlamydia, with emphasis on single-dose treatments that are administered in the ED
2. Ascertaining pregnancy status and consulting obstetrics if the patient is pregnant
3. Obtaining a serologic test for syphilis

4. Reporting appropriate diseases to the state health department
5. Providing counseling for STD prevention and HIV testing
6. Advising partner(s) to seek treatment
7. Arranging for appropriate follow-up
8. Documenting treatment, counseling, and follow-up on the medical record

REFERENCES

1. Borchardt KA, Noble MA: *Sexually Transmitted Diseases.* Boca Raton, FL, CRC Press, 1997.
2. Centers for Disease Control and Prevention: 2002 Guidelines for treatment of sexually transmitted diseases. *MMWR* 47:May 10, 2002.
3. Berg E, Benson D, Haraszkiewicz P, et al: High prevalence of sexually transmitted diseases in women with urinary infections. *Acad Emerg Med* 3(11):1030, 1996.
4. Adimora AA, Hamilton H, Holmes KK, et al: *Sexually Transmitted Diseases: Companion Handbook.* New York, McGraw-Hill, 1994.
5. Centers for Disease Control and Prevention. "Screening Tests to Detect *Chlamydia trachomatis* and *Neisseria gonorrhea* Infections—2002." *MMWR* 51(RR15); 1–27, October 18, 2002.
6. Scientific American Medicine SAM-CD: *Sexually Transmitted Diseases.* New York, Scientific American, December 1998.
7. Hooper DC: New uses for new and old quinolones and the challenge of resistance. *Clin Infect Dis* 30:243, 2000.
8. Aral SO: Sexually transmitted diseases: Magnitude, determinants and consequences. *Int J STDs AIDS* 12:211, 2001.

TOXIC SHOCK SYNDROME AND STREPTOCOCCAL TOXIC SHOCK SYNDROME
Shawna J. Perry
Ashley E. Booth

TOXIC SHOCK SYNDROME

Toxic shock syndrome (TSS) is a severe, life-threatening syndrome characterized by high fever, profound hypotension, diffuse erythroderma, mucous membrane hyperemia, pharyngitis, diarrhea, and constitutional symptoms. It can progress rapidly to multisystem dysfunction with severe electrolyte disturbances, renal failure, and shock. It was first described in 1978 by Todd in seven children with *Staphylococcus aureus* infections. In 1981, however, a nationwide epidemic of TSS associated with extended tampon use was widely recognized among otherwise healthy young women.[1] The incidence of TSS has dropped precipitously over the past 20 years, with the majority of cases unrelated to menses and crossing all segments of society. A similar but more menacing TSS-like syndrome, streptococcal toxic shock syndrome (STSS), has emerged over the last decade. It is associated with invasive and noninvasive streptococcal infections and has a rapidly progressive course and a very high case-fatality rate.

The case definition for TSS by the Centers for Disease Control and Prevention (CDC) is given in Table 142-1. In the absence of a definitive laboratory marker, the strict application of the case definition is warranted but undoubtedly excludes the less severe (subclinical) cases.[2]

Epidemiology

CDC surveillance of TSS from 1979 through 1996 reported 5296 definite and probable cases (Figure 142-1). TSS was initially a disease of young, healthy, menstruating women; 50 percent of cases reported in 1986 and 1987 were found in this group. Tampon use increased the

TABLE 142-1 Case Definition of Toxic Shock Syndrome

An illness with the following chinical manifestations:

Fever: temperature ≥102.0°F (≥38.9°C)

Rash: diffuse macular erythroderma

Desquamation: 1–2 weeks after onset of illness, particularly on the palms and soles

Hypotension: systolic blood pressure ≤90 mm HG for adults or less than fifth percentile by age for children aged <16 years; orthostatic drop in diastolic blood pressure greater than or equal to 15 mm Hg from lying to sitting, orthostatic syncope, or orthostatic dizziness

Multisystem involvement (three or more of the following)

Gastrointestinal: vomiting or diarrhea at onset of illness

Muscular: severe myalgia or creatine phosphokinase level at least twice the upper limit of normal

Mucous membrane: vaginal, oropharyngeal, or conjunctival hyperemia

Renal: blood urea nitrogen or creatinine at least twice the upper limit of normal for laboratory or urinary sediment with pyuria (greater than or equal to 5 leukocytes per high-power field) in the absence of urinary tract infection

Hepatic: total bilirubin, alanine aminotransferase enzyme, or asparate aminotransferase enzyme levels at least twice the upper limit of normal for laboratory

Hematologic: platelets less than 100,000/mL

Central nervous system: disorientation or alterations in consciousness without focal neurologic signs when fever and hypotension are absent

Laboratory criteria: negative results on the following tests, if obtained:

Blood, throat, or cerebrospinal fluid cultures (blood culture may be positive for *Staphylococcus aureus*)

Rise in titer to Rocky Mountain spotted fever, leptospirosis, or measles.

Case classification:

Probable: a case in which five of the six clinical findings described above are present

Confirmed: a case in which all six of the clinical findings described above are present, including desquamation, unless the patient dies before desquamation occurs

---

risk of TSS in susceptible females 33 times. Only 135 cases of TSS were reported in the year 2000, of which 3 cases occurred in men and 2 fatalities were from menstrual-related cases of TSS (MRTSS).[3] The decline in cases is presumably due to changes in the composition of tampons, general public awareness of the risks of tampon use, and increased medical awareness and detection. Tampons are now composed of cotton and rayon. Since 1990, the U.S. Food and Drug Administration (FDA) has required a limit on tampon absorbency into one of four ranges (junior, regular, super, and super-plus) corresponding to the level of flow. Tampons should be changed every 4 to 8 h, and patients with a history of MRTSS should not use tampons.

Although the use of contraceptive sponges and diaphragms places the individual at risk, occurring in 12 percent of non-menstrual-related TSS (NMTSS), their exact contribution to the development of TSS is unclear. The proportion of NMTSS cases has increased since 1980 primarily because of the decrease in the number of menstruation-related cases. The absolute number of cases of NMTSS has remained relatively constant, however, with 41 percent of TSS cases being NMTSS.[3] There is an increasing incidence of NMTSS in males. Men constitute one-tenth of patients with TSS, with a mortality rate 3.3 times that of MRTSS in women. Nonsurgical skin lesions are associated most frequently with NMTSS in children 2 years of age or younger.

The means by which *S. aureus* enters the host in TSS are numerous and have been well documented in a wide variety of clinical settings. *S. aureus* has been isolated from the vaginas of 98 percent of women with TSS, compared with an 8 to 10 percent carrier rate in control subjects. It is presumed that women who develop menstrual TSS are colonized with *S. aureus* before the onset of menstruation. TSS also has been reported following influenza and influenza-like illnesses and is associated with a significant mortality rate (43 percent). Nasal packing (nasal tampons) is also associated with TSS, with 20 to 40 percent of the adult population carrying *S. aureus* in the nasal vestibule. The recent increase in body art and piercing has introduced another pathway for infection.[4]

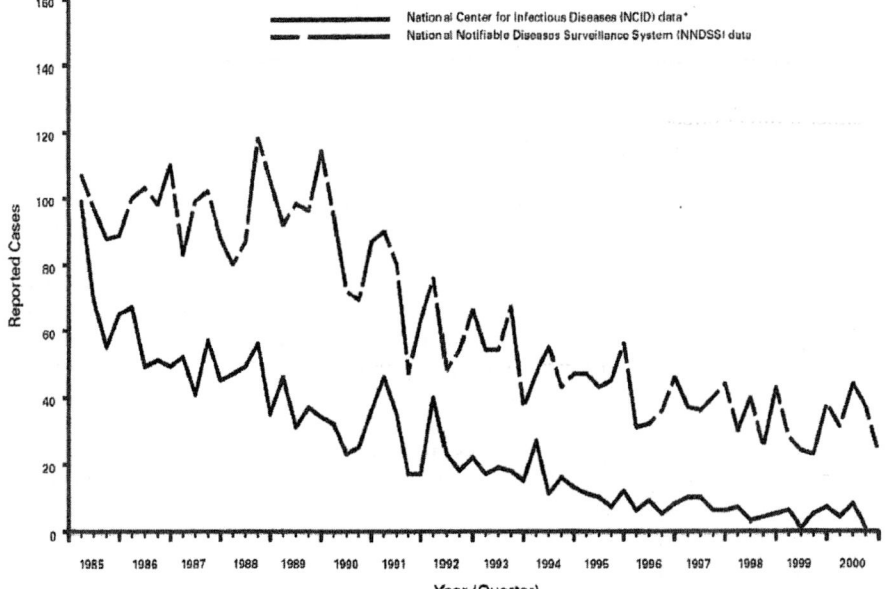

Summary of Notifiable Diseases --- United States, 2000

TOXIC-SHOCK SYNDROME (TSS). Reported cases by quarter — United States, 1985–2000

National Center for Infectious Diseases (NCID) data*
National Notifiable Diseases Surveillance System (NNDSS) data

* Includes cases meeting the CDC definition for confirmed and probable cases of staphylococcal TSS. Data for 4th quarter 2000 are not yet available.

In 2000, a total of 13 cases of staphylococcal TSS were reported to NCID. Of those cases, six persons (46%) had menstrual TSS as of July 11, 2001.

FIG. 142-1. Toxic shock syndrome by quarter in the United States, 1981–2000.

Pathophysiology

Most cases of TSS have been associated directly with colonization or infection with *S. aureus*. An exotoxin, toxic shock syndrome toxin (TSST-1), has been implicated as a significant factor in the production of symptoms associated with TSS either through direct toxic effects on the host or through stimulation of secondary mediators in response to TSST-1. The biologic properties of TSST-1 include the ability to (1) induce fever directly on the hypothalamus or indirectly via interleukin 1 (IL-1) and tumor necrosis factor (TNF) production, (2) promote T-lymphocyte "superantigenization" and overstimulation, (3) induce interferon production, (4) enhance delayed hypersensitivity, (5) suppress neutrophil migration and immunoglobulin secretion, and (6) enhance host susceptibility to endotoxins.

Ninety percent of MRTSS are caused by *S. aureus* strains that produce TSST-1, which is present in less than half of NMTSS cases. Enterotoxins B and C have been identified from isolates of NMTSS and have a biochemical structure almost identical to that of TSST-1. This explains the similarity in clinical manifestations of MRTSS and NMTSS. NMTSS may be mediated by unidentified precursors and toxins or by-products of TSST-1.[5]

The amount of TSST-1 produced by toxigenic strains of *S. aureus* in MRTSS is enhanced by certain vaginal conditions: temperature of 39 to 40°C (102.2–104°C F), a neutral pH, a P_{O_2} of greater than 5 percent, and supplemental CO_2. These conditions can be met with the change in vaginal pH from acidic to neutral during menses and an increase in O_2 and CO_2 content of the vagina with the introduction of tampons or intravaginal devices. Other influences include synthetic fibers in tampon composition and a synergistic relationship between *S. aureus* and *Escherichia coli*.[6]

The most impressive aspect of the pathophysiology is the massive vasodilatation and rapid movement of the serum proteins and fluids from the intravascular to the extravascular space. Hypotension is accounted for by (1) decreased vasomotor tone, causing pooling of blood in the periphery and decreasing venous return, (2) nonhydrostatic leakage of fluid into the interstitium, causing decreased intravascular volume and generalized nonpitting edema, primarily of the head and neck, (3) depressed cardiac function, including decreased wall motion and decreased shortening fraction, and (4) total-body water deficits secondary to vomiting, diarrhea, and fever.

Hypoalbuminemia, hypoferrinemia, and proteolysis caused by IL-1 are consistent with the peripheral edema, anemia, and rhabdomyolysis seen in TSS. TNF induces profound acidosis, shock, and multisystem organ failure in animal models similar to the effects of TSS. The multisystem organ failure may be a reflection of either a direct effect of the toxin on tissues or the rapid onset of hypotension and decreased perfusion. Low convalescent titers to TSST-1 and enterotoxins B and C are found in the majority of patients with TSS for up to 1 year after infection.[5]

Clinical Features

TSS should be considered in any unexplained febrile illness associated with erythroderma, hypotension, and diffuse organ pathology. Diagnostic criteria for TSS are listed in Table 142-1. Patients with MRTSS usually present between the third and fifth day of menses. The median time to onset of illness in postoperative NMTSS is 2 postoperative days. There appears to be a spectrum of severity of TSS. Mild cases of TSS may be excluded from the CDC case definition. *Mild TSS* generally is characterized by fever and chills, myalgias, abdominal pain, sore throat, nausea, vomiting, and diarrhea. Hypotension is usually not present, and the illness is self-limited. *Severe TSS* is an acute-onset multisystem disease with symptoms, signs, and laboratory abnormalities reflecting multiple-organ involvement. Headache is the most common complaint. Some patients may experience a prodrome consisting of malaise, myalgias, headache, nausea, vomiting, and diarrhea. Sudden onset of fever and chills occurs approximately 1 to 4 days prior to presentation. Diffuse myalgias, particularly in the proximal aspects of the extremities, abdomen, and back, are reported by virtually all patients; arthralgias are also common. Profuse, watery diarrhea and repeated vomiting are reported by 90 to 98 percent of patients. Orthostatic light-headedness or syncope may be present. Patients may complain of sore throat, headache, paresthesias, photophobia, abdominal pain, or cough.

Physical examination reveals hypotension or an orthostatic decrease in systolic pressure of 15 mm Hg in all patients. In general, victims of TSS appear acutely ill. The initial state usually lasts about 24 to 48 h; the patient may be obtunded, disoriented, oliguric, and hypotensive. There may be nonpitting edema of the face and extremities. Other prominent signs may include profound muscle weakness and tenderness or abdominal tenderness. Diarrhea is usually watery and profuse, frequently with associated incontinence. One-half to three-quarters of patients have pharyngitis, with a strawberry red tongue; conjunctival hyperemia and vaginitis are also seen. Tender, edematous external genitalia, diffuse vaginal hyperemia, "strawberry" cervix, scant purulent cervical discharge, and bilateral adnexal tenderness are seen in 25 to 35 percent of patients with MRTSS.

The rash of TSS is a diffuse, blanching erythroderma, classically described as painless "sunburn," that fades within 3 days of its appearance and is followed by full-thickness desquamation, especially of the palms and soles, during convalescence. This CDC criterion is missed most often because it may be subtle or difficult to detect in darkly pigmented patients. Variations include patchy erythroderma and localized maculopustular eruptions. In all cases, a fine, generalized desquamation of the skin, with peeling over the soles, fingers, toes, and palms, occurs from 6 to 14 days after the onset of illness. Most severely ill patients experience loss of hair and nails 2 to 3 months later.

Specific focal neurologic findings occur rarely. Patients present with varying degrees of altered consciousness. Approximately 75 percent of patients have nonfocal neurologic abnormalities without signs of meningeal irritation. Confusion, disorientation, agitation, hysteria, somnolence, and seizures have been reported, consistent with a toxic encephalopathy from cerebral edema. If the clinical picture is unclear, a computed tomographic (CT) scan and lumbar puncture should be performed. Figure 142-2 illustrates the temporal relationships of the major manifestations of TSS.

Abnormal laboratory values reflect the multisystem involvement in TSS. Leukocytosis, lymphocytopenia, and mild anemia with peripheral smears consistent with microangiopathic hemolytic anemia may be present. Azotemia, myoglobinuria, and abnormal urinary sediment (sterile pyuria and red blood cell casts) are seen as acute renal failure develops. Liver function abnormalities and hyperbilirubinemia are seen in approximately 3 percent of patients with clinical evidence of coagulopathy. Metabolic acidosis secondary to hypotension is also seen. Electrolyte abnormalities, including hypocalcemia, hypophosphatemia, hyponatremia, and hypokalemia, are common. Hypocalcemia is out of proportion to the degree of hypoalbuminemia and may be difficult to correct if there is a concomitant decrease in the serum magnesium level.

Acute renal failure secondary to acute tubular necrosis is a complication of TSS. It appears to be secondary to prerenal deficits, renal ischemia caused by hypotension, rhabdomyolysis, and possibly direct damage from TSST-1 mediators. Ventricular arrhythmias, bundle-branch block, first-degree heart block, and T-wave and ST-T-wave changes have been reported. Echocardiography of patients with TSS shows wall motion abnormalities and decreased shortening fraction, suggestive of toxic cardiomyopathy. Adult respiratory distress syndrome (ARDS) with refractory hypotension represents the ultimate end-organ damage secondary to TSS.

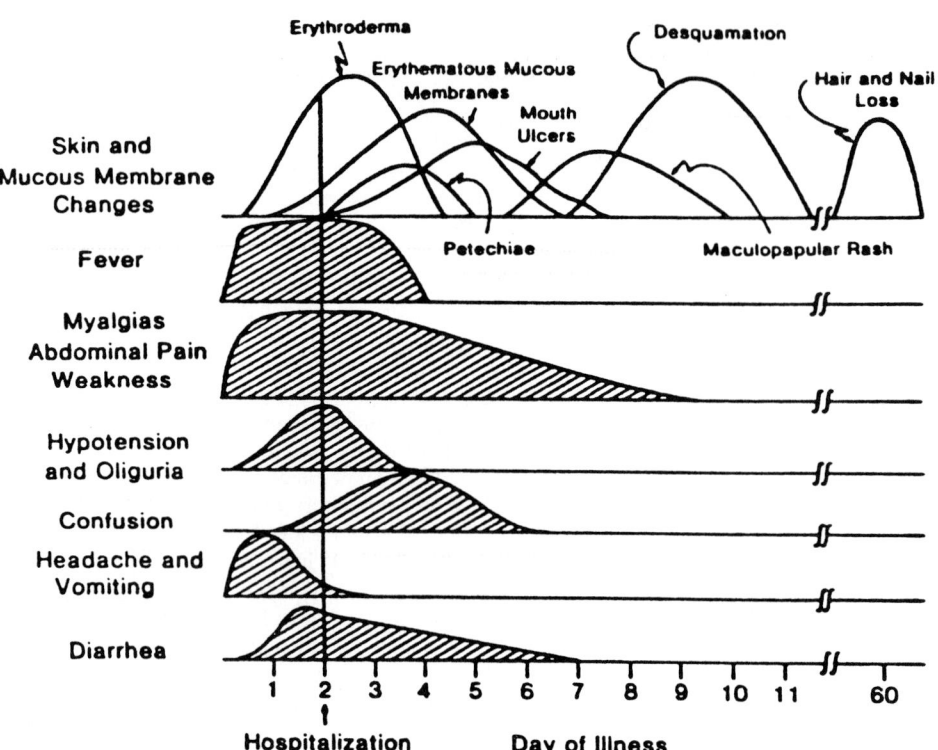

FIG. 142-2. Composite drawing of major systemic, skin, and mucous membrane manifestations of toxic shock syndrome. (From Chesney PJ, David JP, Purdy WK, et al: Clinical manifestations of toxic shock syndrome. *JAMA* 246:741, 1981, with permission.)

Differential Diagnosis

Other systemic illnesses characterized by fever, rash, diarrhea, myalgias, and multisystem involvement resemble TSS (Table 142-2). Kawasaki disease (see Chap. 135) is characterized by fever, conjunctival hyperemia, and erythema of the mucous membranes with desquamation. It is primarily a disease of children. Staphylococcal scalded-skin syndrome (SSSS; see Chap. 246) is seen most commonly in children younger than 5 years of age and is characterized by fever, generalized painful erythroderma, and conjunctivitis. Staphylococcal scarlet fever is so similar to TSS, with full-thickness desquamation, that only pathologic specimens or serologic evidence of the exfoliatin toxin will differentiate the two entities. In streptococcal scarlet fever, the "sandpaper" rash is distinct from the macular "sunburn" rash of TSS.

Rocky Mountain spotted fever (see Chaps. 135 and 248) has a presentation similar to that of TSS, but the rash is usually petechial and delayed in onset. Toxic epidermal necrolysis (see Chap. 246) resembles SSSS and occurs primarily in adults. Erythema multiforme (see Chap. 246) can be associated with fever, pharyngeal erythema, and toxemia. The rash is multiform, with symmetric involvement of the lower extremities.

Septic shock (see Chap. 32) always must be considered in the differential diagnosis of TSS. In general, the appearance of a rash and the laboratory abnormalities associated with TSS will aid in distinguishing these two entities.

TABLE 142-2   Differential Diagnosis of Toxic Shock Syndrome

Acute pyelonephritis	Acute viral syndrome
Septic shock	Leptospirosis
Acute rheumatic fever	Systemic lupus erythematosus
Streptococcal scarlet fever	Rocky Mountain spotted fever
Staphylococcal scarlet fever	Tick typhus
Staphylococcal scalded skin syndrome	Gastroenteritis
Legionnaire disease	Kawasaki disease
Pelvic inflammatory disease	Reye syndrome
Hemolytic uremic syndrome	Toxic epidermal necrolysis
	Erythema multiforme

Treatment

The most important aspect of initial treatment is the aggressive management of circulatory shock. Continuous monitoring of the heart rate, respiratory rate, blood pressure, oxygen saturation, urinary output, and central venous pressure is essential. Pulmonary capillary wedge pressure monitoring also may be needed in severe cases. During the first 24 h, patients may require 4 to 20 L of crystalloid and fresh-frozen plasma. There have been reports of patients requiring up to 20 L of fluid in the first 24 h of hospitalization. A dopamine infusion beginning at 5 to 20 μg/kg per min may be used if volume correction fails to restore normal arterial pressure. Large amounts of IV fluid and pressors to treat refractory hypotension can result in the rapid onset of pulmonary edema. ARDS may then complicate TSS and require mechanical ventilation with positive end-expiratory pressure.

Evaluation must include arterial blood gas analysis, a complete blood count with peripheral smear, serum electrolyte determinations including magnesium and calcium, coagulation studies, urinalysis, and chest radiograph. Patients with abnormal coagulation profiles and evidence of bleeding require colloid replacement, fresh-frozen plasma, or transfusions. Thrombocytopenia may require platelet transfusions. An electrocardiogram and echocardiogram also may be indicated.

A focus of infection should be sought aggressively and treated promptly. Cultures of all potentially infected sites and blood should be obtained prior to initiating antibiotic therapy. Foreign bodies such as tampons or nasal packing should be removed. Early consultation with a surgeon or a gynecologist is recommended if drainage or debridement of infectious sites is warranted.

Although antimicrobial agents have not been shown to affect the outcome of the acute illness, they are recommended and are given to most patients to eradicate the focus of toxin-producing staphylococci as well as to decrease the recurrence rate. Antibiotic selection should include an antistaphylococcal penicillin or cephalosporin with β-lactamase stability. Nafcillin or oxacillin in doses of 2 g IV every 4 h provides adequate antimicrobial coverage. Cefazolin 2 g IV every 6 h, also provides adequate coverage, but the first-generation cephalosporins are less β-lactamase-stable than the antistaphylococcal penicillins. In penicillin-allergic patients, clindamycin, vancomycin, and first-generation cephalosporins can be used. Vancomycin may be used if methicillin-resistant strains are encountered. Although data on the optimal duration of antimicrobial therapy are not available, it seems prudent to administer parenteral antibiotics for at least 3 days or until the patient improves clinically. Oral antistaphylococcal antibiotics (dicloxacillin or clindamycin in penicillin-allergic patients) then should be administered for an additional 10 to 14 days. Methylprednisolone and IV immunoglobulin have shown improvement in some cases of TSS.[7,8]

Most patients become afebrile and normotensive within 48 h of hospitalization. Initial laboratory abnormalities resolve within 1 to 2 weeks, although full anemia correction occurs in 4 to 6 weeks.

Numerous sequelae of TSS have been reported and include late onset of maculopapular rash, decreased renal function, reversible loss of hair and nails, prolonged neuromuscular abnormalities, and cyanotic extremities. Neurologic deficits are common, with 50 percent of patients exhibiting residual memory deficits, decreased ability to concentrate, and diffuse electroencephalographic abnormalities.

The mechanism responsible for these sequelae is not yet clear; it has been suggested that they are due to either the delayed effects of the toxin or circulating immune complexes or are drug-mediated.

Patients not treated with β-lactamase-stable antimicrobial drugs can have recurrence of the disease.[7] Most recurrent episodes of MRTSS in women are seen by the second month following the initial episode and happen on the same day of menses as the prior attack, although some have recurred in less than 1 month and some more than 1 year later. In the majority of patients having recurrence, convalescent antibody titers are low and nonprotective. The initial episode is the most severe, although deaths have resulted from recurrences of initially mild cases of TSS.

STREPTOCOCCAL TOXIC SHOCK SYNDROME

The decline in the incidence of TSS in the late 1980s was followed closely by the emergence of an even more serious illness. Initially classified as streptococcal toxic shock-like syndromes (TSLS) by the CDC, a consensus definition was formulated in 1993. It was identical to the case definition for TSS except that TSLS develops in association with a severe soft tissue infection, and culture results from a normally sterile site must be positive for *Streptococcus pyogenes* [group A streptococcus (GAS)]. The current case definition, as published in 1997, is shown in Table 142-3.[9]

STSS is defined as any group A streptococcal infection associated with invasive soft tissue infection, the early onset of shock, and organ failure. Similar in presentation to TSS, STSS has a higher mortality rate, may occur in patients of all ages, and occurs in most countries of the world. Labeled the "flesh-eating bacteria," the most serious GAS soft tissue infections associated with STSS are streptococcal necrotizing fasciitis and streptococcal myositis.

STSS associated with GAS invasive infections, in contrast to previous reports of GAS bacteremia, most commonly affects individuals between the ages of 20 and 50 *without* predisposing illnesses.[10] There is regional variability in the populations at risk for developing STSS and necrotizing fasciitis from GAS infections. Extremes of age, diabetes, alcoholism, drug abuse, treatment with nonsteroidal anti-inflammatory drugs (NSAIDs), and immunodeficiency appear to be risk factors for GAS invasive infections.[11–13] STSS rarely develops from symptomatic pharyngitis.

It is estimated that in the United States each year there are 2000 to 3000 cases of STSS and 500 to 1500 cases of necrotizing fasciitis.[9] The mortality rate is very high for STSS, at 30 to 80 percent.[12] In patients with STSS, 70 percent of the soft tissue infections progress to necrotizing fasciitis or myositis requiring surgical intervention. The morbidity rate of STSS is 65 to 80 percent with surgical intervention to control the infection.[11–14] The mortality rate for streptococcal

TABLE 142-3   Case Definition of Streptococcal Toxic Shock Syndrome

An illness with the following clinical manifestations occurring within the first 48 h of hospitalization or, for a nosocomial case, within the first 48 h of illness:

Hypotension defined by a systolic blood pressure less than or equal to 90 mm Hg for adults or less than the fifth percentile by age for children aged less than 16 years

Multiorgan involvement characterized by two or more of the following:

Renal impairment: creatinine greater than or equal to 2 mg/dL (≥177 μ/L) for adults or greater than or equal to twice the upper limit of normal for age; in patients with preexisting renal disease, a greater than twofold elevation over the baseline level

Coagulopathy: platelets less than or equal to 100,000/mL (≤100 × 106/L) or disseminated intravascular coagulation, defined by prolonged clotting times, low fibrinogen level, and the presence of fibrin degradation products

Liver involvement: alanine aminotransferase, aspartate aminotransferase, or total bilirubin levels greater than or equal to twice the upper limit of normal for the patient's age; in patients with preexisting liver disease, a greater than twofold increase over the baseline level

Acute respiratory distress syndrome: defined by acute onset of diffuse pulmonary infiltrates and hypoxemia in the absence of cardiac failure or by evidence of diffuse capillary leak manifested by acute onset of generalized edema, or pleural or peritoneal effusions with hypoalbuminemia

A generalized erythematous macular rash that may desquamate

Soft tissue necrosis, including necrotizing fasciitis or myositis, or gangrene

Laboratory criteria for diagnosis

Isolation of group A streptococcus

Case classification

Probable: a case that meets the clinical case definition in the absence of another identified etiology for the illness and with isolation of group A streptococcus from a nonsterile site

Confirmed: a case that meets the clinical case definition and with isolation of group A streptococcus from a normally sterile site (e.g., blood or cerebrospinal fluid or, less commonly, joint, pleural, or pericardial fluid)

myositis is 85 to 100 percent, and up to 60 percent for necrotizing fasciitis even with aggressive treatment.[12,13] The rate of recurrence is unknown.

Epidemiology

Although severe invasive infections caused by *S. pyogenes* (GAS) have been reported with increasing frequency during the past decade, it is not entirely clear whether these reports reflect an actual increase in the incidence of disease or increased awareness. The latter is likely due to the dramatic nature of the infections and the coining of the phrase "flesh-eating bacteria" by the tabloid press to describe invasive necrotizing infections caused by GAS. It is believed that there has been a true recent increase in the GAS virulence properties that may account for the changes in clinical diseases caused by GAS. Few population-based studies exist on its prevalence. Reports on the incidence range from 1 to 5 per 100,000.[13] STSS may be underdiagnosed when associated with GAS invasive infections, since 90 percent of patients are in shock or develop shock within 4 to 6 h of admission. Prospective population-based surveillance studies from Canada from 1991 through 1995 demonstrated an incidence of STSS associated with necrotizing fasciitis of 13 to 46 percent.[11,14] There also have been recent reports of TSLS caused by non-group A streptococcal infection, specifically groups B, C, and G. In 1998, a documented group B streptococcal necrotizing fasciitis and TSLS was reported in three patients with significant underlying disease; the authors postulated that group B streptococcus has acquired an increased ability to cause fasciitis and may be the cause of a new clinical syndrome in adults.[15–17]

Pathophysiology

The resurgence of GAS invasive infections appears to be the result of the production of more virulent exotoxins from the M-type isolates of GAS. Streptococcal pyogenic exotoxins (SPEs) are produced by 90 percent of GAS isolates.[17] Multiple exotoxins (SPEs A, B, C, F, G, H, I, and J) have been identified.[8] SPE A, also known as the *scarlet fever toxin,* is the most powerful and most frequently found SPE in STSS. It has a molecular structure similar to that of enterotoxin B of NMTSS. The SPEs A and B display features similar to those of TSS-mediated exotoxins, including pyrogenicity, superactivation of T cells, and synthesis of TNF, IL-1, and IL-6.[17] These powerful cytokines can induce severe acidosis, shock, and multisystem organ failure, as in TSS. The effects of the "superantigens" SPE A and SPE B are hypothesized to be similar to yet more profound than those of TSST-1, with greater induction of TNF, IL-1, IL-6, and other cytokines, thereby causing more severe signs and symptoms.[17] The patients suspected of being most at risk for developing STSS are those without immunity to M-type 1 SPE A– or B–producing strains of GAS. SPE C has been found in fewer GAS isolates, and its role in STSS is not clear.

The portal of entry for streptococci include the vagina, pharynx, mucosa, and skin in 50 percent of cases of STSS but is not identifiable in most patients.[13] Most commonly, infection begins at a site of minor local trauma, usually without disruption of the skin. Cases have developed from burns, lacerations, abrasions, hematomas, minor nonpenetrating muscle injuries, surgical and orthopedic procedures, and recent infections with varicella or influenza.[12,13]

Clinical Features

Pain is the most common initial symptom of STSS, usually of abrupt onset, severe, and preceding local tenderness or physical findings.[12] Eighty percent of patients have signs of soft tissue infection; this progresses to necrotizing fasciitis or myositis in 70 percent of patients. Although most commonly affecting the extremities, the location of the pain may suggest an intra-abdominal process, such as peritonitis or pelvic inflammatory disease, or other conditions, such as pneumonia or pericarditis. Up to 20 percent of patients may experience a prodromal influenza-like episode including fever, chills, myalgias, and diarrhea. Fever is the most common early sign. Confusion is present in 55 percent of patients, and coma or combativeness also may occur. Other early signs and symptoms of STSS may include dizziness, diffuse rash, and abdominal pain. The initial diagnosis of STSS may be difficult, if not impossible, to distinguish from TSS. If necrotizing fasciitis is present, fever, severe pain, swelling, and redness at the site of the wound are seen. Myositis is an uncommon complication of invasive GAS infection with a very high fatality rate. The most common symptom is severe pain; swelling and erythema may be the only early physical findings. Muscle compartment syndromes may develop rapidly.

On physical examination, fever is the most common presenting sign, followed closely by shock. Shock is apparent at presentation or develops within 4 to 8 h of admission in virtually all patients with STSS. It may be refractory to treatment or require massive volume replacement. The development at the site of the soft tissue infection of vesicles and bullae with progression to violaceous or blue discoloration is considered an ominous sign of necrotizing fasciitis or myositis. ARDS develops in 55 percent of patients, usually following the onset of hypotension; intubation is required in the majority of cases. A diffuse erythematous rash is much less prevalent in STSS (10 percent), but if it does occur, there is desquamation.

Laboratory evaluation shows mild elevation in the white blood cell count (13,000/L) with a profound bandemia as high as 40 to 50 percent. Liver function test values may be two times normal; decreased platelet levels and disseminated intravascular coagulopathy may be seen. Renal dysfunction persists or progresses in all patients; dialysis is required commonly. Creatinine kinase levels become elevated if the

soft tissue infection becomes necrotizing. Blood cultures are positive for GAS in 60 percent of patients, and more than 90 percent of patients with STSS have positive tissue culture results with a known site of infection.[11] One recent report suggests that magnetic resonance imaging may be useful in the early diagnosis of GAS necrotizing fasciitis.[18] Definitive diagnosis of STSS is made by positive GAS culture results from a normally sterile site in addition to the clinical and laboratory parameters defined in the case definition (see Table 142-3).

Diagnosis

The differential diagnosis is the same as for TSS (see Table 142-2) with the significant addition of invasive and noninvasive GAS infections, necrotizing fasciitis, myositis, and serious infections caused by *Clostridium perfringens, C. septicum,* and mixed organisms, such as anaerobic and aerobic bacteria. Although pain usually involves an extremity, symptoms also may suggest peritonitis, pelvic inflammatory disease, pneumonia, or pericarditis.

Treatment

The initial treatment of STSS is similar to that of TSS, with aggressive management of shock and early use of vasopressors (see "Treatment" under "Toxic Shock Syndrome"). Antibiotic therapy should be initiated immediately in the ED to treat STSS and the associated infection if present: intravenous penicillin G 24 million U/d in divided doses, and clindamycin 900 mg IV every 8 h.[12] Erythromycin 1.0 g IV every 6 h should be used in penicillin-allergic patients or the combination of ceftriaxone 2 g IV every 24 h and clindamycin 900 mg IV every 8 h. Intravenous immunoglobulins (IVIGs) have been observed to improve 30-day survival rates as an adjunctive therapy for patients with STSS, perhaps by neutralizing bacterial exotoxins associated with STSS.[8,19] The recommended dose of IVIGs is 2 g/kg with a repeat dose in 48 h should the patient remain unstable. IgA deficiency is an absolute contraindication to the use of IVIGs.[19]

Although antibiotics are important, prompt and aggressive exploration and debridement of suspected deep-seated *S. pyogenes* infection sites are mandatory. If STSS is suspected, immediate surgical consultation is indicated because 70 percent of patients with STSS require debridement, fasciotomy, or amputation.

Disposition

All patients suspected of having STSS should be admitted to an intensive care unit with emergent surgical debridement if warranted. Early surgical consultation on these patients is needed.

REFERENCES

1. Todd J: Toxic-shock syndrome associated with phage group-1 staphylococci. *Lancet* 2:1116, 1978.
2. Centers for Disease Control: Case definition for toxic shock syndrome. *MMWR* 46:30, 1997.
3. Chesney PJ: Toxic shock syndrome: Management and long-term sequelae. *Ann Intern Med* 96:84, 1982.
4. Tweeten SS: Infectious complications of body piercing. *Clin Infect Dis* 26:735,1998.
5. Chance TD: Toxic shock syndrome: Role of the environment, the host and the microorganism. *Br J Biomed Sci* 53:284, 1996.
6. Berkley SF: The relationship of tampon characteristics to menstrual toxic shock syndrome. *JAMA* 258:917, 1987.
7. Todd J: Corticosteroid therapy for patients with toxic shock syndrome. *JAMA* 252:3399, 1984.
8. Schleivert P: Use of intravenous immunoglobins in the treatment of staphylococcal and streptococcal toxic shock syndromes and related illnesses. *J Allergy Clin Immunol* 108:107, 2001.

9. Centers for Disease Control: Case definitions for infectious conditions under public surveillance. *MMWR* 46:34, 1997.

10. Stevens DL: Streptococcal toxic-shock syndrome: Spectrum of disease, pathogenesis, and new concepts in treatment. *Emerg Infect Dis* 1(3):1, 1995.

11. Davies HD: Invasive group A streptococcal infections in Ontario, Canada. *New Engl J Med* 335:547, 1996.

12. Kaul R: Population-based surveillance for group A streptococcal necrotizing fasciitis: Clinical features, prognostic indicators, and microbiologic analysis of seventy-seven cases, Ontario Group A Streptococcal Study. *Am J Med* 103:18, 1997.

13. Stevens D: Invasive streptococcal infections (Review Article). *J Infect Chemother* 7:69, 2001.

14. Gardam MA: Group B streptococcal necrotizing fasciitis and streptococcal toxic shock-like syndrome in adults. *Arch Intern Med* 158:1704, 1998.

15. Hirose Y: Toxic shock-like syndrome caused by non-group A beta-hemolytic streptococci. *Arch Intern Med* 157:1891, 1997.

16. Stevens DL: Severe streptococcal infections associated with a toxic shock-like syndrome and scarlet fever toxin A. *New Engl J Med* 321:1, 1989.

17. Hackett SP: Superantigens associated with staphylococcal and streptococcal toxic shock syndrome are potent inducers of tumor necrosis factor synthesis. *J Infect Dis* 168:232, 1993.

18. Drake DB, Woods JA, Bill TJ: Magnetic resonance imaging in the early diagnosis of group A beta streptococcal necrotizing fasciitis: A case report. *J Emerg Med* 16:403, 1998.

19. Kaul R, McGeer A, Norrby-Teglund A, et al: Intravenous immunoglobulins therapy for streptococcal toxic shock syndrome: A comparative observational study. *Clin Infect Dis* 28:800, 1999.

143

COMMON VIRAL INFECTIONS: INFLUENZAVIRUSES AND HERPESVIRUSES

Robert A. Brownstein

Viral illnesses are among the most common reasons for ED visits. Although some may be trivial, such as the common cold, others are life-threatening, and still others cause chronic diseases and contribute to the development of certain malignancies. Effective therapies for some viruses are now available, with more drugs and vaccines in development. Influenzaviruses and the herpesvirus family are discussed in this chapter.

INFLUENZA A AND B

Influenzaviruses are single-stranded RNA viruses of the orthomyxovirus family. There are three types—A, B, and C—as determined by their genetic material. Type C does not cause significant human disease and does not warrant further discussion. The virions have surface glycoproteins that contain either hemagglutinin or neuraminidase activity. Different subtypes of influenza (i.e., influenza A-H1N1 versus influenza A-H2N2) have large differences between the hemagglutinin (H) or neuraminidase (N) molecules, whereas different strains of the same subtype have minor differences in the H or N molecules.

Antigenic drift is caused by minor mutations in the RNA genome of either the H or N molecule causing a change in antigenicity. Influenza A has much more frequent drift than B, and H more than N, so that the H molecules of influenza A show virtually annual changes, accounting for decreased antigenicity and facilitating annual epidemics.

Antigenic shift occurs by genetic reassortment within a host infected by two different influenzaviruses, producing a new virus with little or no antigenic similarity to the old viruses. The population lacks immunity against the new virus but has high levels of immunity against the old virus, giving the new virus a competitive advantage. This type of shift has occurred three times with hemagglutinin and twice with neuraminidase in this century (thus we have H1, H2, and H3 and N1 and N2). Antigenic shifts are responsible for the flu pandemics, such as in 1918.

Epidemiology

Flu occurs worldwide—in the winter months in the northern and southern hemispheres and sporadically year round in the tropics. In the United States, flu generally occurs from November to April. Droplets generated by coughing spread influenza. During epidemics, attack rates are in the 20 to 30 percent range and may be as high as 50 percent during pandemics.[1] The Centers for Disease Control and Prevention (CDC) and local health departments track influenza activity monthly. Influenza A attack rates are higher for children than for adults, but the disease carries a higher mortality rate in adults, especially the elderly. Influenza B produces a similar illness with high attack rates for children and lower attack rates for adults, probably because of preexisting immunity due to a lower rate of antigenic drift.

After exposure, the incubation period is usually about 2 days. Viral shedding (contagiousness) starts approximately 24 h before the onset of symptoms, rises to peak levels within 48 h, and then declines over the next 3 to 7 days. In young children, viral shedding is prolonged.

Pathophysiology

Following exposure, the virus enters the columnar cells of the respiratory tract epithelium. Host defenses include mucociliary clearance, nonspecific proteins, and if present, specific immunoglobulin A (IgA) molecules. The invaded epithelial cells release large numbers of virions before cell death; thus large numbers of virions are available for spread with respiratory secretions. Influenza viral particles are rarely found outside the respiratory tract.

Clinical Features

Classic flu symptoms include fever of 38.6° to 39.8°C (101°–103°F), with chills or rigor, headache, myalgia, and generalized malaise. Respiratory symptoms include dry cough, rhinorrhea, and sore throat, frequently with bilateral tender, enlarged cervical lymph nodes. The onset of symptoms typically is rapid and dramatic; many patients recall the exact time of onset. Ocular symptoms include eye pain, light sensitivity, tearing, and pain with lateral gaze. Myalgias and arthralgias, but not arthritis, are extremely common. The myalgias often affect back muscles in adults and calf muscles in children. Almost half of affected children have gastrointestinal symptoms, but these are unusual in adults. The elderly usually do not have classic symptoms and may have only fever, malaise, confusion, and nasal congestion.

The fever generally lasts 2 to 4 days, followed by rapid recovery from most of the systemic symptoms. Cough, fatigue, and occasionally depression may last for several weeks.

Diagnosis

Traditionally, diagnosis has been through the use of viral cultures or serologic tests, which do not yield results for several days. These tests are not useful in individual patients except to confirm diagnosis after recovery from acute illness, but they do provide useful epidemiologic data. Some studies have shown that a clinical diagnosis of flu during a known outbreak has an accuracy of approximately 85 percent,[2,3] but bacteremia also should be considered in patients with rigor and myalgias. New rapid antigen tests are available that may change the approach to flulike illnesses. These tests enable rapid diagnosis and institution of antiviral agents and may decrease the empirical use of antibiotics. Commercially available tests require less than $\frac{1}{2}$ h to perform and have sensitivities of 57 to 81 percent, with specificities of 93 to 100 percent.[4]

Complications

The complications of acute influenza infection include primary influenza pneumonitis, secondary bacterial pneumonia, croup, exacerbation of chronic obstructive pulmonary disease, and Reye syndrome. Other rare complications include Guillain-Barré syndrome, myocarditis, and pericarditis.

Primary influenza pneumonitis occurs most commonly in those with preexisting cardiac or pulmonary disease, but in large outbreaks it has occurred in previously healthy adults. The initial symptoms are typical flulike symptoms with progression to cough and dyspnea. There is significant hypoxia. Radiologic findings are bilateral infiltrates similar to acute respiratory distress syndrome (ARDS). Bacterial cultures and Gram stains are negative, and antibiotics do not help. Treatment is primarily supportive. Most clinicians support the use of anti-influenza agents, but there are no good studies demonstrating efficacy. The mortality rate of influenza pneumonitis remains high.

Secondary pneumonia is similar clinically to pneumonia occurring without antecedent flu. This complication presents 1 to 2 weeks after the flu, with a brief well period in between. Secondary pneumonia is most common in the elderly and in those with diabetes mellitus or cardiopulmonary disease. Treatment is initially with broad-spectrum antibiotics and pulmonary support, with narrowing of antibiotic coverage when culture results become available.

Reye syndrome has been associated with influenza B and varicella-zoster infections and with the use of aspirin. It occurs primarily in children between the ages of 2 and 16 years and begins with vomiting and progresses to altered mental status or coma. There is hepatomegaly due to fatty infiltration of the liver. There are elevated levels of liver enzymes, elevated ammonia levels, and an elevated prothrombin time. Hypoglycemia is common. The case-fatality rate is from 10 to 40 percent. The American Academy of Pediatrics has recommended that aspirin not be used for fevers caused by influenza or varicella.[5]

Treatment

Amantadine and rimantadine are currently approved for the treatment of influenza A. Neither has activity against influenza B. For maximal effectiveness, both need to be started within 48 h of onset of symptoms and can reduce the duration of systemic symptoms by 1 to 2 days. The dose is 100 mg bid for 5 days for both drugs. Amantadine is cleared renally, and the dose needs to be adjusted in the elderly and in patients with renal insufficiency. The recommended dose for persons older than age 65 is 100 mg daily. Amantadine causes an increase in seizure activity in patients with a preexisting seizure disorder. Rimantadine is cleared hepatically, and a 50 percent dose reduction is recommended in patients with severe liver dysfunction. Rimantadine has a significantly lower incidence of central nervous system (CNS) side effects than does amantadine. Neither drug should be used during pregnancy. Both amantadine and rimantadine can be used in children older than 1 year of age, although only rimantadine is officially approved for prophylaxis in children. Amantadine costs approximately $10 for a course of therapy versus about $25 for a course of rimantadine in adults.

Oseltamivir and zanamivir (Tamiflu and Relenza) are neuraminidase inhibitors that are active against both influenza A and B. Both have been shown to reduce systemic symptoms of influenza if started in the first 48 h after onset of clinical illness. Both reduce the duration of illness by about 1 day. Zanamivir is an inhaled medicine, dosed twice a day for 5 days, for about $55 for a course of treatment. Zanamivir can cause bronchospasm and should not be given to patients with underlying pulmonary disease. Oseltamivir is dosed at 75 mg twice a day PO for 5 days for around $65. Nausea is reported frequently with oseltamivir and can be decreased by taking the drug with food.

Prophylaxis

The flu vaccine is formulated annually and contains two strains of influenza A and one of influenza B. It is 70 to 90 percent effective in preventing illness in those under age 65. For patients over age 65 and not in chronic care facilities, it is 30 to 70 percent effective in preventing hospitalizations due to flu and pneumonia. For those in chronic care facilities, it is 50 to 60 percent effective in preventing hospitalizations due to flu and pneumonia and approximately 80 percent effective in preventing excess deaths due to flu and pneumonia.[6] The vaccine is recommended for all persons over age 65; for residents of chronic care facilities; for adults and children with chronic cardiopulmonary disease; for persons with diabetes mellitus and other chronic metabolic diseases, renal disease, or hemoglobinopathies; and for the immunosuppressed and health care workers. Children and teenagers who require aspirin therapy should be immunized because of the risk of Reye syndrome. Women who will be pregnant during flu season should be immunized. The vaccine is safe for pregnant and lactating women. A whole-virus vaccine is used in adults, whereas a split-virus vaccine is used in children younger than age 12. The only contraindication to immunization is known allergy to egg protein or other vaccine components.

All four anti-influenza medicines are effective in preventing flu, with efficacy rates of 75 to 90 percent when used at the same doses as for treatment but for a prolonged duration (zanamivir is not approved by the Food and Drug Administration for prophylaxis). Consideration should be given to instituting chemoprophylaxis in a chronic care facility where flu has been definitively diagnosed, regardless of vaccination status of patients, because there is added benefit for patients with both vaccine and chemoprophylaxis. The medicines should be given for at least 14 days and then until the outbreak has subsided for a full week. For those at high risk who cannot be vaccinated, a 6- to 8-week course of chemoprophylaxis during peak flu season is indicated. Postexposure prophylaxis consists of immunization followed by 14 days of chemoprophylaxis.

HERPESVIRUSES

The herpesviruses are a ubiquitous class of enveloped DNA viruses that cause an expanding list of human illness. The herpesviruses all have the ability to dwell in the host as a lifelong latent infection and may cause clinical disease at a time distant from the primary infection. Some have been shown to be carcinogenic. Each herpesvirus has distinguishing clinical characteristics and will be discussed individually. Human herpesviruses 6 and 7, which cause roseola, and human herpesvirus 8, implicated in Kaposi sarcoma, are not discussed in this chapter. As a class, the herpesviruses are transmitted by close contact, since they are unable to survive in the environment and are unable to penetrate intact skin. The varicella-zoster virus (VZV) can be spread via aerosolized particles as well as by close contact. Most transmission of the herpes simplex virus (HSV) and of Epstein-Barr virus (EBV) occurs during asymptomatic shedding. Viruses discussed below are HSV, VZV, EBV, and cytomegalovirus (CMV).

HERPES SIMPLEX VIRUSES 1 AND 2

Epidemiology

HSV has been found in all populations throughout the world. Transmission is via contact of infected secretions (saliva or genital) with mucous membranes or with open skin. There is serologic evidence of exposure to HSV-1 in most persons by the time of puberty, and the rates are higher among lower socioeconomic classes. HSV-2 is spread primarily sexually, and its rates are variable among different adult populations, depending on sexual behavior.

Pathophysiology

After exposure, the virus replicates locally in the epithelial cells, causing lysis of the infected cells and producing an inflammatory response. This response results in the characteristic rash of HSV, which is indistinguishable from the rash of VZV. The rash consists of small, thin-walled vesicles on an erythematous base. Continued replication results in viremia in immunocompromised hosts but rarely in normal hosts. Following primary infection, the virus becomes latent in a sensory nerve ganglion.

Clinical Features

ORAL HSV HSV-1 primarily causes oral lesions but may cause genital infection. HSV-2 causes identical lesions, primarily genital, but may cause oral lesions. The primary oral infection of HSV-1 is often mild or asymptomatic. In children under age 5, it may present as a pharyngitis or gingivostomatitis associated with fever and cervical lymphadenopathy. The lesions are distributed throughout the mouth, unlike the limited posterior involvement of herpangina. Admission of the young may be necessary due to poor oral intake and dehydration. In teenagers and young adults, there simply may be a posterior pharyngitis or tonsillitis. The primary lesions generally last 1 to 2 weeks. The diagnosis is largely clinical. Viral cultures take days to weeks to be performed and thus are of little use in an ED setting. The use of intravenous acyclovir at a dose of 5 mg/kg has been recommended for severe gingivostomatitis that requires admission and intravenous hydration.[7] Oral acyclovir has been shown to shorten the duration of symptoms in children if begun within the first 72 h of symptoms. No treatment other than oral hygiene is required for mild or moderate disease.

Recurrent oral lesions occur in 60 to 90 percent of infected individuals, are usually milder, and generally occur on the lower lip at the outer vermilion border, but considerable variation exists, with individuals usually having recurrences at the same site as prior recurrences. The recurrences often are triggered by local trauma, sunburn, or stress. The outbreaks frequently are preceded by prodromal symptoms of local adenopathy and pain or tingling. The lesions usually follow the prodrome within the first 48 h and may last for up to 10 days, but they are usually crusted over by 48 h. Treatment of recurrent oral herpes labialis with oral acyclovir 400 mg five times per day in adults shortens duration of symptoms. Topical acyclovir is ineffective. Topical pencyclovir applied every 2 h for 4 days shortens duration of symptoms.[8] In patients with severe or frequent recurrences, prophylaxis with oral acyclovir can reduce outbreaks by 50 to 75 percent.[7]

GENITAL HSV HSV-1 and 2 cause identical genital infections, with HSV-2 causing the majority. These are also covered in Chap. 141 on sexually transmitted diseases. A few items of importance are presented here. Recurrent genital lesions carry a small threat of intrauterine infection in pregnant patients, as does primary genital HSV (1 or 2), and initiation of oral acyclovir and consultation with an obstetrician or perinatologist and follow-up within 72 h are recommended. Cesarean section is recommended for all women with active lesions present when labor commences, whether primary or recurrent.[9] Primary lesions carry a higher risk of transmission to the neonate.[10]

OCULAR HSV HSV infections of the eye can lead to corneal blindness and usually are caused by HSV-1. An ulcerative keratitis is the most common manifestation. Herpetic vesicles can be seen on the conjunctiva or on the lid margin as a blepharitis. There is a regional adenopathy. Fluorescein staining may show a diagnostic dendritic ulceration of the cornea. Due to the threat of permanent vision loss, consultation with an ophthalmologist is mandatory, and antiviral therapy should be begun immediately. Superficial keratitis usually heals completely in several weeks. Recurrent ocular infections may involve the deeper structures, with a high risk of visual loss, and if deeper structures are involved, immediate consultation with an ophthalmologist and the administration of intravenous acyclovir are appropriate. Following acute treatment, long-term treatment with acyclovir can reduce recurrences of ocular HSV.[11]

ENCEPHALITIS Herpes simplex encephalitis, which is usually caused by HSV-1, is rare but is one of the most common types of viral encephalitis. The mechanism of entry into the CNS is not known definitely but is believed to be along neural routes. The temporal lobes are the major targets. Temporal abnormalities seen by computed tomography (CT), magnetic resonance imaging (MRI), or electroencephalography increase the likelihood of HSV encephalitis if present.

Clinically, there may be a preceding viral-like illness, or the onset may be sudden. There may be no cutaneous manifestation of an HSV infection. There may be headache, fever, and altered mental status, indicated by speech disturbances or focal seizures. Temporal lobe seizures may present as olfactory hallucinations. The cerebrospinal fluid (CSF) findings are nonspecific, showing an elevated white blood cell count with mononuclear predominance. Cultures usually are negative for HSV. Immediate diagnosis is not possible, and if a suspicion of HSV encephalitis exists, empirical treatment should be initiated as soon as possible. The test of choice for diagnosis is the CSF detection of HSV DNA by polymerase chain reaction (PCR). The sensitivity is 90 to 95 percent, with a specificity of greater than 95 percent.[12] The PCR results can be available in 8 to 12 h if it is done on site. There are reports of false-negative results early in the course of disease.[13] The traditional "gold standard" for diagnosis has been a brain biopsy, with sensitivity and specificity of 96 and 99 percent, respectively; however, the biopsy method has a 3 percent surgical complication rate and a significant delay in obtaining the biopsy specimen and the results. For untreated persons, the mortality rate is close to 70 percent. Treatment should be initiated in the ED if the diagnosis is suspected. Treatment is with intravenous acyclovir at 10 mg/kg every 8 h.

BELL PALSY HSV may affect the peripheral branches of the cranial nerves. HSV-1 is a frequent cause of Bell palsy, which has been described classically as an idiopathic palsy of the peripheral branch of cranial nerve VII (CN VII). It occurs equally among men and women and occurs most frequently in the middle aged and has been reported in children. CN VII controls the facial muscles and the stapedius muscle, taste sensation of the anterior two-thirds of the tongue, and lacrimal gland secretory function. Clinical features include facial hemiplegia or hemiparesis, taste disturbance in greater than 50 percent of the patients, decreased blinking, variably dry eyes or increased tearing, jaw or face pain, and numbness of the face and/or neck in 60 percent of patients. The diagnosis is made by definite findings of peripheral nerve VII involvement and exclusion of other treatable causes. The motor control of the muscles of the forehead are from bilateral motor cortices to the CN VII motor nuclei, so central CN VII lesions spare the forehead but cause unilateral weakness of the lower face. A peripheral lesion results in paralysis of the forehead, along with the face. Attempting to close the eye on the affected side results in an upward gaze (Bell phenomenon). Paralysis of the stapedius muscle results in hyperacusis on the affected side.

Ruling out of other conditions is important in making the diagnosis. The results of a detailed examination of the cranial nerves should be normal except for the aforementioned findings associated with CN VII. The findings on examination of the ear, tympanic membrane, mastoid, and parotid gland should be normal in order to make a diagnosis of Bell palsy. A CN VII palsy in association with otitis media, mastoiditis, or parotitis is a potential ear, nose, and throat (ENT) emergency and should prompt immediate consultation. The presence of vesicles on the tympanic membrane or in the ear canal is diagnostic of the Ramsay Hunt syndrome and is discussed in the section on VZV. A history of chronic ear infections, prior ear surgery or tumor, or recent head trauma excludes a diagnosis of Bell palsy. If the presentation and examination are consistent with Bell palsy, imaging of the CNS (CT or MRI) is not indicated, but if there are atypical features, recent trauma, or doubt, then imaging is recommended along with ENT consultation. The differential diagnosis includes stroke, tumor, atypical Guillain-Barré syndrome, and Lyme disease, especially if in endemic areas and if bilateral.

Treatment with prednisone for anti-inflammatory effect at 60 mg PO daily or 1 mg/kg per d for 5 days and then tapered over the next 5 days, along with acyclovir 400 mg five times per day for 10 days, has been recommended by some.[14] Other groups have reviewed the data and found them to be inconclusive[15] or trending toward favoring treatment, but without sufficient evidence to make recommendations.[16] Follow-up is with either ENT or neurology as an outpatient. The prognosis is generally good for total recovery, but patients with total paralysis are at increased risk of long-term or permanent paralysis and should be seen in follow-up within 2 to 3 days, and patients with incomplete paralysis should be instructed to return if the weakness becomes total paralysis. Among patients with incomplete paralysis, 6 percent will have residual weakness at 1 year. Among the patients with complete paralysis, 84 percent had total or good recovery at 1 year, with 16 percent having poor to fair recovery.[17]

Eye care is important in preventing damage due to impaired blinking and decreased tearing. Artificial tears should be used frequently during the day at any sign of dryness or every 2 h. At night, a lubricating ointment with or without an eye patch should be used. Care of the eye is the most important therapeutic intervention that can be made by emergency physicians.

HERPETIC WHITLOW   Herpetic whitlow is a primary or recurrent HSV infection of the finger. HSV-1 is seen in children who autoinnoculate their fingers during an episode of oral herpes. HSV-1 is also seen in health care workers who are exposed to infected oral secretions. HSV-2 is more common among adults due to digital/genital contact in the community. The disease is usually limited to a single digit. Herpetic whitlow frequently is painful and accompanied by axillary adenopathy. Vesicles, which may be recognizable early in the course of the disease, coalesce and may appear to contain pus but actually contain necrotic epithelial cells causing the purulent appearance. Healing occurs spontaneously over 2 to 3 weeks if local wound care and pain control are used. Whitlow may be misdiagnosed as a paronychia and incised, which may delay healing or allow a secondary infection to occur. When incised, no purulent material will be expressed. For patients with frequent painful recurrences, suppressive therapy with acyclovir may be effective.[7]

IMMUNOCOMPROMISE   Immunocompromised patients are at increased risk of disseminated or severe typical and atypical HSV disease, usually resulting from reactivation of latent virus. HSV infection in immunocompromised patients may cause esophagitis, proctitis, colitis, and pneumonitis, as well as encephalitis. Definitive diagnosis is difficult without a biopsy of the affected tissue because these patients generally all have latent HSV and frequently are shedding HSV in their secretions. Any evidence of disseminated or CNS disease mandates admission and intravenous acyclovir. The decision to admit or treat an immunocompromised patient with mucocutaneous HSV on an outpatient basis is based on severity of disease, reliability of the patient, and ability of the patient to stay hydrated. Each decision is made on a case-by-case basis, in conjunction with the patient's primary care provider. Additionally, patients with large areas of skin involvement by burns or eczema are at risk of severe or fatal HSV infection, although most commonly resolution will occur without treatment. Consultation and consideration for admission for these patients are recommended.

HERPES ZOSTER: CHICKENPOX

Epidemiology

Herpes zoster virus (VZV, human herpesvirus 3) is the cause of chickenpox as a primary infection, which may reactivate later in life as zoster (shingles). Prior to the use of the varicella vaccine, 90 percent of primary infection occurred among children 10 years of age or younger, with the majority of these in children younger than age 3. Only approximately 10 percent of individuals over age 15 remain susceptible to VZV. Chickenpox is endemic, occurring year round, but there are annual epidemics in late winter and early spring. After exposure, attack rates are close to 80 percent among susceptible household contacts. The route of spread is presumed to be respiratory. Patients are infectious for approximately 48 h before the appearance of the rash until the vesicles are crusted over.

Pathophysiology

After exposure, viral replication occurs at an unknown site, followed by a viremia. Viral replication in the skin results in degenerative changes in epithelial cells, leading to multinucleated giant cells in vesicles. The rash usually appears 14 to 15 days after exposure. The rash then fades, and the virus becomes latent in a dorsal root ganglion.

Clinical Features

Chickenpox in children is discussed in Chap. 135. Dermatologic features are similar in adults and children. However, the mortality rate among adults is about 15 times that in children, or 30 per 100,000. The disease process is more prolonged and severe in adults than in children. The most serious complications are encephalitis, cerebellar ataxia, and pneumonitis. The typical prodrome of 1 to 2 days of low-grade fever and malaise is followed by the appearance of clear vesicles with an erythematous base on the face and trunk. Vesicular fluid quickly becomes turbid due to the accumulation of cellular debris. As the lesions continue to age, they scab over. The rash spreads centripetally to involve the extremities. Over the next several days, new lesions appear in crops. A hallmark of chickenpox is the presence of lesions in various stages. Accompanying the rash is fever, malaise, pruritus, and anorexia. Varicella encephalitis is characterized by an altered level of consciousness, fever, vomiting, headaches, and seizures. Cerebellar ataxia is characterized by ataxia, vomiting, tremor, and altered speech, with complete resolution within a month. A serious potential complication in children is Reye syndrome, so even in adults, aspirin-containing products should be avoided. Varicella pneumonitis presents with cough, tachypnea, and dyspnea approximately 4 days after the onset of illness. Chest x-rays reveal a diffuse pneumonitis. Women in the second or third trimester of pregnancy are at higher risk of severe pneumonitis. Women in the immediate perinatal period are at increased risk of severe disease, as are neonates. Chickenpox during pregnancy can cause fetal anomalies.[5]

Treatment

Oral acyclovir is recommended for patients older than age 12 and those with chronic illnesses or on chronic salicylate therapy. For adults, the dosage of acyclovir is 800 mg PO qid for 5 days. For maximal benefit, acyclovir should be started within 24 h of development of the rash. All patients with varicella encephalitis or pneumonitis should be admitted for intravenous acyclovir. Treatment of pregnant or peripartum women who develop chickenpox should be discussed with an obstetrician or perinatologist because some physicians will elect to admit for intravenous acyclovir. Neonates who develop chickenpox or whose mothers develop postpartum chickenpox should be admitted for intravenous acyclovir. Immunocompromised patients tend to have more severe disease and should be admitted for intravenous acyclovir.

Varicella-zoster immune globulin (VZIG) is available to confer passive immunity to exposed susceptible adults or immunocompromised children and pregnant women. VZIG also should be given to any neonate with chickenpox or whose mother developed chickenpox within 5 days before delivery or 48 h after delivery.[5]

Varicella vaccine is now recommended for children who are 1 year of age or older. It is also recommended for adults with either a reliable history of never having chickenpox or with serologic evidence of susceptibility. The vaccine is a live attenuated cell-free vaccine. Because it is a live vaccine, it is contraindicated in immunocompromised patients, household contacts of immunocompromised patients, and pregnant or lactating women.

HERPES ZOSTER: SHINGLES

Herpes zoster (shingles) is the reactivation of latent VZV infection. There is a lifetime incidence of almost 20 percent, with the majority of cases being among the elderly. It occurs only in people who have had chickenpox. After a single occurrence in an immunocompetent host, there is a 4 percent likelihood of a second occurrence.

The lesions of shingles are identical to those of chickenpox but are limited to a single dermatome in distribution. Thoracic and lumbar dermatomes are most common. The cranial nerves may be affected as well, with the potential complications of herpes zoster ophthalmicus (HZO) and Ramsay Hunt syndrome. What triggers the reactivation is unknown. The disease begins with a prodrome of pain in the affected area for 1 to 3 days, followed by the outbreak of a maculopapular rash that quickly progresses to a vesicular rash. The course of the disease is usually around 2 weeks, but it may persist for a full month.

HZO is due to involvement of the ophthalmic branch of CN V and is a vision-threatening condition. The Hutchinson sign (lesions on the tip of the nose) may be seen before ocular involvement is recognized, but its absence does not rule out HZO.[18] Ocular involvement can be seen in the presence of only a slight rash on the forehead. HZO induces a keratitis and may be followed by involvement of deeper structures. There is usually facial pain, regional adenopathy, and occasionally, a red eye preceding the appearance of the rash. A dendriform corneal ulcer often can be identified with fluorescein staining. The presence of a skin rash helps differentiate HZO from ocular HSV. HZO or suspected HZO mandates an ophthalmologic consultation due to the threat to vision.

CN VII also can be affected. Involvement of the maxillary or mandibular branches can result in intraoral lesions. Involvement of the geniculate ganglion of CN VII results in Ramsay Hunt syndrome, which presents clinically as a facial palsy resembling Bell palsy with a unilateral motor weakness, loss of taste on the anterior two-thirds of the tongue, and vesicles in the ear canal or on the tympanic membrane (the only sites of CN VII cutaneous innervation). Ramsay Hunt syndrome also has been described as a cause of altered mental status in the elderly.[19] This is treated in the same fashion as Bell palsy. Immunocompromised patients should be admitted for intravenous acyclovir.

The most common complication of shingles is postherpetic neuralgia (PHN). This is uncommon in younger patients but increases in frequency with age. The pain at times may be so severe as to be debilitating. Occasionally, the anterior horn cells become involved, causing a transient local weakness or paralysis, with these patients being particularly prone to severe pain. PHN occurs in 10 to 20 percent of all patients after an episode of acute zoster but in up to 70 percent of patients aged 70 years or older. It generally resolves in 1 to 2 months but may last greater than a year in some patients.

The treatment of zoster in the normal host is aimed at decreasing the risk of PHN, since the antivirals have a clinically small but statis-

tically significant effect on the duration of the acute disease. Treatment should begin as soon as possible and within 72 h of onset of disease for maximal benefit. The present literature shows that all three currently available antiherpes agents are more effective than placebo at reducing the duration of PHN but not at reducing its incidence.[20–22] Corticosteroids have not been shown to be effective but have been shown to improve quality-of-life indices in affected elderly, and a 21-day taper beginning at 60 mg PO daily should be considered in patients older than age 50 if no contraindications exist.[23]

Initial treatment of patients with PHN is typically systemic analgesia, often narcotics. Patients should be referred back to their primary care provider because first-line agents often fail, and a trial of amitriptyline or carbamazepine may be tried as second-line therapy.

Immunocompromised patients have an increased risk of disseminated disease. This can be recognized clinically by evidence of the rash involving more than a single dermatome or crossing the midline. Disseminated disease may occur in patients with skin lesions limited to a single dermatome. Patients with disseminated disease may develop pneumonitis, hepatitis, meningoencephalitis, or other organ system involvement and should be admitted for intravenous acyclovir. Immunocompromised patients with shingles without evidence of dissemination can be treated as outpatients with oral acyclovir at the standard dosing, with instructions to return if the rash spreads or if they develop respiratory symptoms, headaches, or other signs of organ system disease. Close follow-up with their primary care provider is recommended.

EPSTEIN-BARR VIRUS: INFECTIOUS MONONUCLEOSIS

Human herpesvirus 4, known as Epstein-Barr virus (EBV), is the primary cause of the infectious mononucleosis syndrome. EBV is found in humans throughout the world. Serologic testing reveals that 90 to 95 percent of the adult population has developed antibodies to EBV.[24] Approximately half the population will seroconvert as young children, with a second peak occurring during the teen and young-adult years.

EBV is spread by close contact between an individual shedding the virus and a susceptible individual. EBV is not able to survive outside the human host for any significant amount of time, and spread via fomites has not been demonstrated. Transmission among teenagers is often via the exchange of saliva during kissing. Adults may shed EBV asymptomatically for up to 18 months after clinical recovery, and EBV may be demonstrated in the throats of up to 20 percent of all adults. In immunocompromised persons, up to 50 percent may demonstrate EBV.

After infection, there is a 1- to 2-month incubation period during which viral replication occurs in B lymphocytes in the reticuloendothelial system. The presence of EBV induces the production of specific anti-EBV antibodies, as well as the production of the heterophil antibodies. Heterophil antibodies react with antigens on the red blood cells of sheep, horses, and cows. Heterophil antibodies are not specific for EBV and can be produced by infection with CMV or toxoplasmosis, as well as other infections. Heterophil antibodies are rarely produced in infants.

Following asymptomatic incubation, EBV can produce a wide array of illnesses. Classic infectious mononucleosis is manifested by fever, exudative pharyngitis, lymphadenopathy, splenomegaly, and an atypical lymphocytosis. Infants and young children frequently have asymptomatic infections. A prodrome of malaise, fatigue, and fever may be present for several days before the onset of the symptoms in classic mononucleosis. An elevated liver transaminase level is found uniformly in mononucleosis. Hepatomegaly and jaundice are unusual in children and young adults but common in older adults. A severe sore throat is a common presenting complaint, and the appearance may be of a severe bilateral exudative tonsillitis/pharyngitis. Bilateral tender cervical adenopathy is virtually universal. At some point in the illness, approximately half of patients will have palpable splenomegaly. Splenomegaly is most prominent during week 2 of illness and then resolves over the next 1 to 2 weeks. The majority of patients have an uncomplicated course and recover fully. Chronic fatigue syndrome is not caused by EBV infection.

Generally, the treatment is supportive in the absence of complications. If ampicillin is given to a patient with EBV to treat a possible strep throat infection, there is an approximately 95 percent incidence of rash due to transient production of EBV-induced antibodies against ampicillin. Acyclovir has in vitro effects on EBV replication, but in vivo clinical studies have failed to show any clinically significant effect.[25]

Complications of EBV infections are uncommon and usually do not result in long-term morbidity. The upper airway in approximately 3 percent of children may be obstructed by severe tonsillitis/pharyngitis. Management includes ENT consultation for airway control, if required. Prednisone 1 to 2 mg/kg per d should be given to patients with airway compromise. Humidified oxygen and a nasopharyngeal airway are also helpful. Tonsillectomy is usually not necessary and should be reserved for patients who fail to respond to conservative measures. If endotracheal intubation is required, a prolonged period of intubation should be anticipated due to the extent of edema.

The spleen may rupture spontaneously or secondary to minor trauma. The incidence of splenic rupture is believed to be 0.1 to 0.5 percent of patients with EBV. It occurs most commonly during week 2 or 3 of illness. Presenting complaints may be abdominal pain, left scapular pain, or hypotension. Abdominal pain is unusual in infectious mononucleosis and should prompt consideration of splenic rupture. Patients with EBV should be instructed to avoid contact sports and strenuous activity for 4 weeks following the onset of clinical disease. Patients with splenic rupture should be admitted to a surgical service.

Hematologic complications include autoimmune hemolytic anemia and thrombocytopenia. Corticosteroids will benefit some patients with hematologic complications and should be initiated in the ED for those admitted with severe anemia or severe thrombocytopenia. Refractory severe thrombocytopenia may be treated with splenectomy.

Neurologic complications of EBV are quite rare but may include encephalitis, meningitis, cranial nerve palsies, and the Guillain-Barré syndrome. The CSF usually contains atypical lymphocytes. Recovery is usually complete.

In immunocompromised patients, EBV may be a cause of B-cell lymphomas and other lymphoproliferative syndromes. EBV has been implicated as a causal agent in African Burkitt lymphoma and in nasopharyngeal carcinomas. Death may be caused by overwhelming EBV infection in patients with Duncan disease (an X-linked recessive disorder), which is clinically silent until EBV infection. Patients with HIV may develop hairy leukoplakia that will respond to acyclovir therapy.

The diagnosis of EBV is based on clinical findings and nonspecific laboratory tests. Confirmatory EBV-specific antibody testing is available, but same-day results generally are not available, so these tests have little value in the setting of the ED. The complete blood count is usually moderately elevated, with elevated percentages of lymphocytes and monocytes. Atypical lymphocytes usually are found and may be up to 30 percent of the white blood cells.

The heterophil antibodies are produced in 80 to 90 percent of patients older than age 4. More than 50 percent of children younger than age 4 will not have detectable heterophil antibodies.[26] Commercially available tests for heterophil antibodies (Monospot, Mono-plus, Mono-latex, and Mono-lex) have a sensitivity of 78 to 83 percent, with a specificity of 98 to 100 percent.[27] False-negative results may occur more frequently during the first week of illness. Patients with classic symptoms of infectious mononucleosis, atypical lymphocytes, and a positive heterophil antibody test generally require no further testing to confirm the diagnosis. Patients with classic symptoms who have a negative heterophil antibody test should have repeat heterophil testing performed in a week, and if they are still negative, specific EBV antibody testing may be indicated. Viral capsid antigen (VCA) antibodies of the IgG and IgM classes are present in high titers during acute disease, with IgG persisting for life and IgM persisting for 4 to 8 weeks. The presence of IgM antibodies to VCA is a sensitive and specific indicator of acute EBV infection. Antibodies to Epstein-Barr nuclear antigen develop 4 to 6 weeks after the onset of clinical illness and persist for life; their presence is evidence against acute EBV infection. Other illnesses that may present with a similar clinical picture but with negative EBV tests include CMV mononucleosis, acute toxoplasmosis, primary HIV infection, and strep throat.

CYTOMEGALOVIRUS

Cytomegalovirus (CMV, or human herpesvirus 5) is another ubiquitous virus with worldwide distribution. It is, like the other members of the herpesvirus family, capable of causing a primary illness and then existing in a latent state in the human host indefinitely with the ability to reactivate at a later time. It is present in approximately 1 percent of newborns and in 40 to 100 percent of adults, depending on geographic location, socioeconomic status, attendance at day care, and sexual behavior. There are two peaks of seroconversion, the first in the perinatal period and the second during young adulthood, presumably related to sexual activity. CMV is not spread easily by casual contact but requires repeated or prolonged intimate contact for transmission. It is found in milk, saliva, urine, semen, and cervical secretions. CMV is also transmitted by blood transfusions containing viable leukocytes, as well as solid organs or bone marrow during transplantation.

CMV is one of the TORCH agents [*t*oxoplasmosis, *o*ther (viruses), *r*ubella, *C*MV, and *h*erpes (simplex viruses)] and is capable of causing intrauterine infection. Fewer than 25 percent of neonates with intrauterine CMV will display symptoms. Those at highest risk are those whose mother acquires primary disease during the first half of the pregnancy. A seropositive mother's antibodies to CMV appear to provide the fetus some protection. Classic intrauterine CMV (congenital cytomegalic inclusion disease) involves multiple organs, including jaundice, hepatosplenomegaly, microcephaly, petechiae, and inner ear problems, as well as CNS defects. Children who are asymptomatic at birth still may have hearing loss that results in lower IQ scores and learning disabilities later in life.

In contrast to intrauterine infection, perinatal infection (presumably acquired from the cervix of the mother during birth or from breast milk) is usually asymptomatic and has no long-term consequences.

In healthy immunocompetent children and adults, CMV infection is also usually asymptomatic. When CMV does cause disease in this setting, it is typically an illness resembling EBV infectious mononucleosis. Typical presenting complaints include fever, chills, myalgia, and headache. Clinical features include a prolonged fever (1-5 weeks), an atypical lymphocytosis, lymphadenopathy, splenomegaly, and mild elevations of the liver transaminase levels. Pharyngitis and tonsillitis usually are not present. There are rarely complications or long-term health consequences. The diagnosis of CMV mononucleosis should be considered in individuals who have a mononucleosis-type illness but are heterophil-antibody negative. The complications of CMV in immunocompetent patients include the Guillain-Barré syndrome, viral pneumonitis, hepatitis, hemolytic anemia, and thrombocytopenia.

In patients with HIV, CMV can cause illness with significant morbidity. Symptomatic infections generally do not occur in patients who are simply HIV-positive, but they do occur in those with more advanced disease, such as AIDS-related complex (ARC) or AIDS. The most common illness is CMV retinitis, which occurs in more than 10 percent of AIDS patients. Typical complaints are of floaters or decreased vision. Careful funduscopic examination may reveal characteristic retinal hemorrhages and exudates. Progression to blindness will occur without chronic suppressive therapy with intravenous ganciclovir or foscarnet. CMV may cause gastrointestinal disease as either esophagitis or colitis. Additionally, CMV can cause an adrenalitis resulting in adrenal insufficiency.

CMV causes significant morbidity and mortality in transplant patients. It can infect numerous different organs, causing colitis, hepatitis, pneumonia, and CNS disease. The most serious infection is CMV pneumonia, which is most common in recipients of bone marrow transplants. The CMV seen in transplant patients may represent primary infection after exposure from the transplanted tissue or transfused blood products or reactivation of latent infection. The primary infections tend to be more severe. CMV infections occur 4 to 8 weeks after transplantation typically, and CMV should be included in the differential diagnosis for patients presenting with a febrile illness within the first 3 months after transplantation. CMV also may contribute to rejection of the transplanted organ.

The diagnosis of CMV is difficult because most people are seropositive. The presence of IgM antibodies is helpful but not very sensitive or specific because of false-negative results during some acute infections and their persistence beyond acute infection in others. To make a definitive diagnosis based on serologies, a conversion from seronegative to seropositive or an acute rise in antibody titer should be seen, and this will require samples from before the illness and during the illness. Another method of diagnosis is by viral culture, which, using the "shell" method, takes only 48 h. Children can shed virus in their urine and respiratory secretions for extended periods following infection, but in healthy adults, virus usually is not shed in the urine or respiratory tract except during acute illness. Healthy adults may shed virus in semen and cervical secretions. In immunocompromised individuals, a biopsy of the organ suspected to be infected with CMV is the preferred method of diagnosis because of the prevalence of false-positive cultures in immunocompromised patients. Biopsy specimens of infected organs will show characteristic CMV inclusion bodies. In the ED, definitive diagnosis is not available, and suspicion of CMV should be based on clinical grounds such as presentation and time from transplantation. A review of transplant records may yield clues, such as the recipient and donor CMV status prior to transplantation. The disposition of the patient depends on the clinical setting, not on the diagnosis of CMV, and should be discussed with the patient's primary care provider.

CMV is treated with either ganciclovir or foscarnet. Ganciclovir is approved for therapy of CMV retinitis in AIDS patients and for prevention of CMV in transplant patients. It is also used for treating CMV infections in other organ systems. In AIDS-associated CMV retinitis, ganciclovir is given initially at higher doses for 2 to 3 weeks, followed by lifetime suppressive therapy. For other CMV infections, ganciclovir is given for a period of 2 to 3 weeks and then stopped. Foscarnet is used for resistant CMV infections or for patients unable to take ganciclovir. Neither medication cures patients of CMV but instead suppresses the acute disease process.

REFERENCES

1. Monto AS, Kioumehr F: The Tecumseh Study of Respiratory Illness: IX. Occurrence of influenza in the community. *Am J Epidemiol* 102:553, 1975.
2. Knight V, Fedson D, Baldini J, et al: Amantadine therapy of epidemic influenza. *Infect Immun* 1:200, 1970.
3. VanVoris LP, Betts RF, Roth FK, et al: Successful treatment of naturally occurring influenza A/USSR/77 H1N1. *JAMA* 245:1128, 1981.
4. Anonymous: Rapid diagnostic tests for influenza. *Med Lett Drugs Ther* 41:121, 1999.
5. American Academy of Pediatrics Committee on Infectious Diseases: *The Red Book: Report of the Committee on Infectious Diseases,* 24th ed. Elk Grove Village, IL, American Academy of Pediatrics, 1997.
6. Advisory Committee on Immunization Practices: Recommendations of the Advisory Committee on Immunization Practices: Prevention and control of influenza. *MMWR* 46:1, 1997.
7. Kesson AM: Position paper of the Pediatric Special Interest Group of the Australian Society for Infectious Diseases: Use of acyclovir in herpes simplex virus infections. *J Paediatr Child Health* 34:9, 1998.
8. Spruance SL, Rea TL, Thomig C, et al: Penciclovir cream for the treatment of herpes simplex labialis: A randomized, multicenter, double-blind, placebo-controlled trial. *JAMA* 277:1374, 1997.
9. Gibbs RS, Amstey MS, Sweet RL, et al: Management of genital herpes infection in pregnancy. *Obstet Gynecol* 71:779, 1988.
10. Brown ZA, Bendetti J, Ashley R: Neonatal herpes simplex virus infection in relation to asymptomatic shedding at the time of labor. *New Engl J Med* 324:1227, 1991.
11. Herpetic Eye Disease Study Group: Acyclovir for the prevention of recurrent herpes simplex virus eye disease. *New Engl J Med* 339:300, 1998.
12. Cinque P, Cleator GM, Weber T, et al for the EU Concerted Action on Virus Meningitis and Encephalitis: The role of laboratory investigation in the diagnosis and management of patients with suspected herpes simplex encephalitis: A consensus report. *J Neurol Neurosurg Psychiatry* 61:339, 1996.
13. Weil AA, Glaser CA, Amad Z, Forghani B: Patients with suspected herpes simplex encephalitis: Rethinking an initial negative polymerase chain reaction result. *Clin Infect Dis* 34:1154, 2002.
14. Adour KK, Ruboyianes JM, VanDoertsen PG, et al: Bell's palsy treatment with acyclovir and prednisone compared with prednisone alone: A double blind, randomized, controlled trial. *Ann Otol Rhinol Laryngol* 105:371, 1996.
15. Sipe J, Dunn L: Aciclovir for Bell's palsy (idiopathic facial paralysis). *Cochrane Database Syst Rev* 2: 2001.
16. Grogan PM, Gronseth GS: Practice parameter: Steroids, acyclovir, and surgery for Bell's palsy (an evidence-based review): Report of the Quality Standards Subcommittee of the American Academy of Neurology. *Neurology* 56:830, 2001.
17. Peitersen E: The natural history of Bell's palsy. *Am J Otolaryngol* 4:107, 1982.
18. Marsh RJ: Herpes zoster ophthalmicus. *J R Soc Med* 90:670, 1997.
19. Rahimi AR: Ramsay Hunt syndrome. *Geriatrics* 53:93, 1998.
20. Jackson JL, Gibbons R, Meyer G, Inouye L: The effect of treating herpes zoster with oral acyclovir in preventing postherpetic neuralgia. *Arch Intern Med* 157:909, 1997.
21. Tyring S, Barbarash RA, Nahlik JE, et al and the Collaborative Famciclovir Herpes Zoster Study Group: Famciclovir for the treatment of acute herpes zoster: Effects on acute disease and postherpetic neuralgia. *Ann Intern Med* 123:89, 1995.
22. Beutner KR, Friedman DJ, Forszpaniak C, et al: Valaciclovir compared with acyclovir for improved therapy for herpes zoster in immunocompetent adults. *Antimicrob Agents Chemother* 39:1546, 1995.
23. Whitley RJ, Weiss H, Gnann JW Jr, et al and the NIAID Collaborative Antiviral Study Group: Acyclovir with and without prednisone for the treatment of herpes zoster. *Ann Intern Med* 125:376, 1996.
24. Pereira MS, Blake JM, Macrae AD: Epstein-Barr virus antibodies at different ages. *Br Med J* 4:526, 1969.
25. Van der Horst C, Joncal J, Ahronheim G, et al: Lack of effect of peroral acyclovir for the treatment of acute infectious mononucleosis. *J Infect Dis* 164:788, 1991.
26. Sumaya CV, Ench Y: Epstein-Barr virus infectious mononucleosis in children: II. Heterophil antibody and viral specific responses. *Pediatrics* 75:1011, 1985.
27. Gerber MA, Shapiro ED, Ryan RW, Bell GL: Evaluations of enzyme-linked immunosorbent assay procedure for determining specific Epstein-Barr virus serology and of rapid test kits for diagnosis of infectious mononucleosis. *J Clin Microbiol* 34: 3240, 1996.

HIV INFECTION AND AIDS

Richard E. Rothman
Catherine A. Marco
Gabor D. Kelen

Patients with HIV present at various stages of infection, with a wide spectrum of illnesses involving virtually every organ system.

EPIDEMIOLOGY

As of December 2001, approximately 21.8 million individuals have died from HIV-related illnesses throughout the world, and an estimated 40 million people are living with HIV/AIDS. The epidemic has disproportionately affected the poorest countries due to lack of resources for implementing effective preventive programs and inadequate access to therapies known to delay progression of HIV-related diseases. HIV prevalence is greatest in sub-Saharan Africa with 28.5 million people infected. The epidemic is fastest growing in central Asia and eastern Europe, with 250,000 new infections reported in 2001. The Joint United Nations Program on AIDS (UNAIDS) predicts that by 2020, HIV will be responsible for more than one-third of all infectious disease-related deaths worldwide.[1]

In the United States, the Centers for Disease Control and Prevention (CDC) estimate that 900,000 people are currently living with HIV and that approximately 40,000 new HIV infections occur each year. As of June 2001, 460,000 deaths from HIV/AIDS have been reported.[2] Although mortality from HIV infection dropped by more than 70 percent from 1996 to 1999 (largely attributable to highly active antiretroviral therapy), rates of decline have slowed more recently. Factors likely responsible for this slowing include delayed test seeking in certain populations, limited access to health care, and limitations of new therapies.

Risk factors associated with HIV infection include homosexuality or bisexuality, injection drug use, heterosexual exposure, receipt of a blood transfusion prior to 1985, and vertical and horizontal maternal-neonatal transmission. Changes in the distribution of AIDS cases in adults/adolescents by mechanism of transmission since the start the HIV epidemic are shown in Table 144-1.[3] In homosexual and bisexual men, rates of newly acquired HIV, HIV progression to AIDS, and AIDS-related deaths have all declined (largely due to access to antiretroviral therapy and, in part, to effective prevention strategies). Similarly, substantial declines in perinatal transmission have occurred, primarily attributable to increased use of zidovudine (AZT) in pregnant women. Meanwhile, rates of new HIV infection have continued to rise among young, disadvantaged minority populations (many of whom use the ED for both primary and emergency care). During the past several years, the highest percentages of increase in reported AIDS cases have occurred among women and minority populations. These changes are principally due to an increase in HIV prevalence among injection drug users and their women partners. AIDS remains the leading cause of death among black males aged 25 to 44 and is the third leading cause of death among black women of the same age group.

Increasing use of ED services by HIV-infected persons is due in part to changes in the demographic distribution of HIV cases and AIDS-related illnesses. Seroprevalence studies in one inner-city ED reflect these trends, with rates of HIV infection among unselected adult patients rising from 6 to 11.4 percent over a 4-year period.[4]

PATHOPHYSIOLOGY

HIV is a cytopathic retrovirus of the lentivirus family that kills infected cells. The virus is extremely labile and is neutralized easily by heat and common disinfecting agents such as 50% ethanol, 35% isopropyl alcohol, 0.3% hydrogen peroxide, Lysol, or a 1:10 solution of household bleach. There are two major subtypes of HIV, HIV-1 and HIV-2. HIV-1 is the predominant subtype worldwide and is the cause of AIDS. HIV-2 causes a similar immune syndrome but is restricted primarily to western Africa and seen rarely in the United States.

The HIV virion is composed of a central RNA molecule and a reverse-transcriptase protein surrounded by a core protein encased by a lipid-bilayer envelope. Following infection, HIV selectively attacks host cells involved in immune function, primarily $CD4^+$ T-cell counts. Within the host cell, HIV-encoded RNA is reverse-transcribed into DNA by the enzyme reverse transcriptase. The viral genome then becomes permanently integrated into the host's genome, where it may lie dormant or be actively transcribed and translated to produce virally encoded proteins and new HIV virions. As a result of infection, immunologic abnormalities eventually occur, including lymphopenia, qualitative $CD4^+$ T-cell function defects, and autoimmune phenomena. Profound defects in cellular immunity ultimately result in a variety of opportunistic infections and neoplasms.

HIV has been isolated from saliva, urine, cerebrospinal fluid (CSF), pus, brain, tears, alveolar fluid, synovial fluid, and amniotic fluid. Transmission of HIV has been shown to occur via semen, vaginal secretions, blood or blood products, breast milk, and transplacental transmission in utero. Transmission has never been documented to occur by casual contact. There is only one documented case of transmission from health care provider to patient in the United States involving an infected dentist in Florida who transmitted the virus to six patients.

NATURAL HISTORY/CLINICAL STAGES OF HIV INFECTION

Symptoms of acute HIV infection are reported to occur in 50 to 90 percent of patients.[5] The diagnosis is missed in up to 75 percent of cases due to nonspecific presentation (resemblance to a flulike or mononucleosis-like syndrome) and a low index of suspicion. Symptoms of acute HIV syndrome usually develop 2 to 4 weeks develop after exposure and last for less than 14 days. The most common presentations of acute HIV infection are fever (>90 percent), fatigue (70–90 percent), pharyngitis (>70 percent), rash (40–80 percent), headache (30–70 percent), and lymphadenopathy (40–70 percent); other commonly reported symptoms include weight loss, headache, and diarrhea.[6,7] Benefits and implications of early disease detection are discussed below (see "Diagnosis").

Seroconversion reflects detectable antibody response to HIV and usually occurs 3 to 8 weeks after infection, although delays of up to 11 months have been reported. This is followed by a long period of asymptomatic infection during which patients generally have no find-

TABLE 144-1   Trends in Distribution of AIDS Cases by Mechanism of Transmission in Adults/Adolescents (% Cases Shown)

Primary Risk Factors*	1985	1990	1995	2000	Cumulative Total
Male homosexual contact	78	58	42	32	46
IDU	15	23	26	20	25
Male homosexuality + IDU	—	6	5	4	6
Heterosexual contact	0	6	11	16	11
Transfusion recipient	1	2	1	1	1
Hemophilia/ coagulation disorder	1	6	1	0	1
Other/no risk reported†	5	6	15	27	9

*Perinatal transmission not included here.

†*Primarily* refers to persons whose mode of exposure was not reported and who have not been followed up to determine their mode of exposure and a smaller number of persons who are not reported with one of the exposures listed above after follow-up; includes 34 persons who were exposed to HIV-infected blood or body fluids in health care, laboratory, or household settings.

Abbreviation: IDU = injection drug use.

Source: Modified from CDC HIV/AIDS Surveillance Reports (1985–present).

ings on physical examination except for possible persistent generalized lymphadenopathy, characterized by enlarged lymph nodes involving at least two noncontiguous sites other than inguinal nodes. The mean incubation time from exposure to the development of AIDS in untreated patients is estimated at 8.23 years for adults and 1.97 years for children under age 5. Virologic studies of patients during this period suggest that a steady state of HIV replication and $CD4^+$ T-cell death and replacement exists until increased levels of HIV replication occur. Variables most predictive of disease stage are viral burden and $CD4^+$ T-cell counts, with a steeper decline in $CD4^+$ T-cell count and a higher viral burden associated with rapid progression and poor outcome.[8]

Early symptomatic infection is characterized by conditions that are more common and more severe in the presence of HIV infection but, by definition, are not AIDS-indicator conditions. Examples include thrush, persistent vulvovaginal candidiasis, peripheral neuropathy, cervical dysplasia, recurrent herpes zoster infection, and idiopathic thrombocytopenic purpura. These conditions occur with increased frequency as the $CD4^+$ T-cell count drops below 500 cells/µL. As the $CD4^+$ T-cell count drops below 200 cells/µL, frequency of opportunistic infections increases dramatically. AIDS is defined by the CDC as the appearance of any indicator condition (Table 144-2) or a $CD4^+$ T-cell count of less than 200 cells/µL. Median survival time after the $CD4^+$ T-cell count has fallen to less than 200 cell/µL is 3.7 years; median survival after an AIDS-defining complication is 1.3 years. Late symptomatic or advanced HIV infection exists in patients with a $CD4^+$ T-cell count of less than 50 cells/µL or clinical evidence of end-stage disease, including disseminated *Mycobacterium avium* complex or disseminated cytomegalovirus (CMV). Immune reconstitution with potent antiretroviral therapies and effective prophylaxis significantly delay the time to onset of opportunistic infections and death, even in patients with AIDS-defining conditions.

DIAGNOSIS

HIV infection may be diagnosed using a number of methods: detection of viral-specific antigen, identification of HIV nucleic acid, isolation of the virus by culture, and detection of antibodies to HIV. The standard and most common method is detection of antibodies to the virus. Testing involves sequential use of an enzyme-linked immunosorbent

TABLE 144-2   Indicator Conditions for Case Definitions of AIDS

Esophageal candidiasis
Cryptococcosis
Cryptosporidiosis
Cytomegalovirus retinitis
Herpes simplex virus
Kaposi's sarcoma
Brain lymphoma
Mycobacterium avium complex
P. carinii pneumonia
Progressive multifocal leukoencephalopathy
Brain toxoplasmosis
HIV encephalopathy
HIV wasting syndrome
Disseminated histoplasmosis
Isosporiasis
Disseminated *M. tuberculosis* disease
Recurrent *Salmonella* septicemia

Added in 1993:

$CD4^+$ T-cell count <200 cells/µL
Pulmonary tuberculosis
Recurrent bacterial pneumonia
Invasive cervical cancer

assay (ELISA) and a Western blot (WB) assay. ELISA is approximately 99 percent specific and 98.5 percent sensitive; WB is nearly 100 sensitive and specific if performed under ideal laboratory conditions. Criteria for positive results are a repeatedly positive ELISA followed by a positive WB. ELISA detects the binding of specific serum antibodies to HIV antigens that are adherent to a microtiter plate. WB detects HIV antibodies to discrete viral antigens that are electrophoretically separated and transferred to nitrocellulose paper. A positive WB requires detection of at least two gene products. Reasons for indeterminate tests are not well understood but may be indicative or early seroconversion.

Diagnosis of acute-stage HIV infection cannot be made with standard serologic tests because seroconversion usually has not yet occurred. Methods for earlier detection of HIV-1 include techniques to detect DNA, RNA, or HIV antigens. None of these assays is considered more accurate than routine serology, but they should be considered in patients suspected to be in the window period who present with an acute retroviral syndrome. Sensitivity of the various tests differs with stage of disease and test technique but generally is reported as greater than 99 percent for DNA polymerase chain reaction (PCR), 95 percent for quantitative HIV RNA or viral load, 95 to 100 percent for viral culture of peripheral blood mononuclear cells (PBMCs), and up to 100 percent for the most recent p24 antigen detection assays (which are used for screening blood donors). Real-time nucleic acid tests also may hold promise for screening acute HIV infection in ED patients as these tests become more sensitive, specific, and feasible.

Although acute HIV infection is missed in up to 75 percent of all cases, the benefits of early recognition generally are considered to outweigh the risks and costs of offering testing to patients in whom suspicion for acute HIV infection exists. For the individual patient, potential benefits include early and aggressive antiretroviral therapy, which can lead to immune reconstitution, prevention of viral mutation and drug resistance, slowing of disease progression, and improved long-term prognosis. Additional health outcomes may be realized due to the recognized public health benefits (i.e., decreased disease transmission) associated with modification of high-risk behavior in those found to be HIV-positive.[6,9] For patients in whom acute HIV infection is suspected but is not confirmed (i.e., those with a high-risk profile presenting with fever of unknown origin and/or a syndrome suspicious for acute seroconversion), counseling and urgent referral to outpatient follow-up for appropriate testing should be initiated in the ED.

There are two other rapid HIV tests with which the ED physician should be familiar. The single-use diagnostic system (SUDS) is used to screen rapidly for antibodies to HIV-1 in plasma or serum. SUDS tests are used in most hospital laboratories in cases of occupational exposure. Reported sensitive and specificity are greater than 99 percent, but the tests require performance by well-trained laboratory technicians. OraSure manufactures both a saliva-based and finger-stick blood-based assay for rapid HIV testing. Sensitivity and specificity are comparable with standard serology, and advantages include availability of results in less than 20 min and minimal training required for performance. The blood-based test has been approved recently by the Food and Drug Administration (FDA).

Knowledge of recent $CD4^+$ T-cell counts and HIV viremia load can be extremely helpful in placing patients' ED presentation in an appropriate context. $CD4^+$ T-cell counts of less than 200 cells/µL and a viral load of greater than 50,000 is associated with increased risk of progression to AIDS-defining illnesses and often are used as indicators for initiation of antiretroviral therapy. When this information is unavailable or the stage of disease is unknown, the total lymphocyte count may be used to approximate the $CD4^+$ T-cell count, since a total lymphocyte count of less than 1000 cells/µL has been shown to be strongly predictive of a $CD4^+$ T-cell count of less than 200 cells/µL.

Testing for HIV in the ED generally has been considered to be of limited utility, except in situations where health care workers are exposed to patients' blood or in cases of sexual assault.[10] Although HIV screening in the ED remains controversial, both primary data and systematic review of the literature support the value of EDs offering HIV screening to either high-risk patients (i.e., those with identifiable risk factors) or high-risk populations (i.e., those in whom HIV seroprevalance is at least 1 percent).[11,12] Benefits of recognition may be particularly important with acute seroconversion, where early initiation of therapy may lead to improved outcomes and decreased transmission of disease. Time limitations, cost, difficulty with follow-up, and confidentiality frequently are cited as reasons for not testing. The development of rapid, easy-to-use diagnostic testing methods that offer immediate results likely will stimulate further investigation and possibly CDC or other national support for ED-based HIV screening programs in the near future.

CLINICAL FEATURES AND TREATMENT

The spectrum of disease caused by HIV infection varies greatly. Many patients with asymptomatic infection may come to the ED for complaints unrelated to HIV disease.[13] Other patients may have involvement of virtually any organ system, commonly with multiple interrelated problems. The protean manifestations of HIV and the complex array of related opportunistic infections can make ED evaluation and diagnosis of HIV-positive patients difficult.

Evaluation of HIV-infected patients should be carried out with the same priority-based logical approach used for all ED patients, with attention to concerns particular to this population. Attempts to develop specialized triage guidelines for HIV-positive patients have as yet been unsuccessful.[14] Patients with unstable vital signs require attention to the ABCs and rapid stabilization. Universal precautions (in some hospitals termed *standard precautions*) must be used in all cases. The history and physical examination should focus on identifying the clinical stage of disease in order to direct attention to the most likely complications. History gathering must include a thorough review of past and current medications and previous infections and attention to the activities of daily living. Physical findings that might assist with staging include the presence of thrush, evidence of temporal wasting, or dementia. Diagnostic and therapeutic maneuvers are directed toward recognition of organ system involvement, assessment of the severity of disease, and institution of symptomatic and specific therapy. An overview of the more common HIV-related presentations and treatment follows. For the most up-to-date information, as well as more details on drug dosing, the reader is referred to the CDC Web site (www.cdc.gov.hiv) or an annually updated guide to care of the HIV-positive patient, which provides an excellent clinical resource tool.[15]

Constitutional Symptoms and Febrile Illnesses

Systemic symptoms, such as fever, weight loss, and malaise, are common in HIV-infected patients and account for the majority of HIV-related presentations.[13,14] In the ED, systemic infection and malignancy must be excluded. Appropriate laboratory investigation may include electrolyte determinations, complete blood count, blood cultures (aerobic, anaerobic, and fungal), urinalysis and culture, liver function tests, chest radiograph, and serologic testing for syphilis, cryptococcosis, toxoplasmosis, CMV infection, and coccidiomycosis. Lumbar puncture may be considered if there are neurologic signs or symptoms or unexplained fever.

When evaluating fever in patients with later-stage HIV and AIDS, it is important to remember that this population may not manifest the typical signs and laboratory findings associated with systemic infection. Clinical impression therefore is critical in determining appropriate disposition. Ill-appearing patients should receive fluid resuscitation and empirical antibiotics in the ED and then be admitted for further evaluation and management. Outpatient evaluation and treatment are indicated only when all the following conditions are met: The source of the fever does not dictate admission, appropriate laboratory

studies have been initiated, the patient is able to function adequately at home (e.g., can maintain sufficient oral intake), and timely medical follow-up can be arranged.

In HIV-positive patients without obvious localizing signs or symptoms, sources of fever vary by stage of disease. Patients with $CD4^+$ T-cell counts greater than 500 cells/μL generally have causes of fever similar to nonimmunocomprised patients, whereas those with $CD4^+$ T-cell counts between 200 and 500 cells/μL are most likely to have early bacterial respiratory infections.[16] For patients with $CD4^+$ T-cell counts less than 200 cells/μL, most common causes of fever without obvious localizing findings are early *Pneumocystis carinii* pneumonia (PCP), central-line infection, *M. avium* complex, *M. tuberculosis,* CMV, drug fever, and sinusitis. Less common causes include endocarditis, lymphoma, *Histoplasma capsulatum* and *Cryptococcus neoformans.* Fever caused by HIV infection alone tends to occur in the afternoon or evening and generally is responsive to antipyretics.

Prior to the widespread use of highly active antiretroviral therapy, disseminated *M. avium* complex (MAC) was the most common opportunistic bacterial infection in AIDS patients, causing disseminated disease in up to 50 percent of patients at some time during their illness. MAC occurs predominantly in patients with $CD4^+$ T-cell counts of 100 cells/μL or less. Persistent fever and night sweats are typical. Associated symptoms include weight loss, diarrhea, malaise, and anorexia. Dissemination to the bone marrow, liver, and spleen result in anemia and elevated alkaline phosphatase levels. Diagnosis may be made by acid-fast stain of stool or other body fluids or by blood culture. Cultures using the lysis-centrifugation method are more sensitive for MAC (and histoplasmosis) and should be ordered in patients with late-stage disease and fever of unknown origin. Treatment for MAC, which reduces bacteremia and improves symptoms (but does not eradicate disease), is with clarithromycin combined with ethambutol and rifabutin.

With increased use of highly active antiretroviral therapy, a more focal and invasive form of MAC has emerged called *immune reconstitution illness to MAC*.[17] Typical presentation is lymphadenitis, with symptoms commonly starting weeks to months after starting highly active antiretroviral therapy; pathogenesis may be cytokine-mediated and attributable to restoration of a pathogen-specific immune response to infection. Current treatment guidelines advise continuing antiretroviral therapy and starting antimicrobials; steroids may be beneficial. Immune reconstitution illness also has been seen with a group of other infections including tuberculosis, CMV, *Cryptococcus,* hepatitis, herpes zoster, and progressive multifocal leukoencephalopathy (PML).

CMV is the most common cause of serious opportunistic viral disease in HIV-infected patients. Disseminated disease commonly involves the gastrointestinal, pulmonary, and CNS systems. The most important manifestation is retinitis (see below). Treatment is with foscarnet or ganciclovir; oral ganciclovir can be used for prophylaxis.

Fever in injection drug users (IDUs) always should raise concern for infective endocarditis, which often has a nonspecific presentation in the ED (see Chap. 145). While previous studies have failed to identify reliable clinical or laboratory predictors of this disease, recent developments indicate that expedited approaches to ruling out infective endocarditis in febrile IDUs may be forthcoming[18] and ultimately may include molecular diagnostic assays such as PCR.[19] Current standard of care, however, is to admit all febrile IDUs and await the results of blood cultures and echocardiography due to the significant morbidity and mortality rates of missed endocarditis and the difficulties associated with outpatient follow-up in this population.

The most common noninfectious causes of fever are neoplasm and drug fever. Non-Hodgkin lymphomas are the most frequently occurring neoplasm and typically present as high-grade, rapidly growing mass lesions. New CNS symptoms, particularly a change in mental status in the presence of fever, should be evaluated with neuroimaging. Definitive diagnosis requires biopsy. Radiotherapy and chemotherapy are effective treatment regimens. Drug fever may be secondary to intravenous drug abuse or adverse drug reactions (see below).

Neurologic Complications

CNS disease occurs in 90 percent of patients with AIDS, and 10 to 20 percent of HIV-infected patients present initially with CNS symptoms. Neurologic disease is caused by a variety of opportunistic infections and neoplasms, as well as by the direct and indirect effects of HIV infection on the CNS. Common presenting symptoms indicative of CNS pathology include seizures, altered mental status, headache, meningismus, and focal neurologic deficits. The most common causes of neurologic symptoms include AIDS dementia, *Toxoplasma gondii,* and *C. neoformans.* Since the widespread use of highly active antiretroviral therapy, rates of CNS infections and malignancy have declined significantly, whereas rates of AIDS dementia remain unchanged.

ED evaluation should include a complete neurologic examination and, when appropriate, computed tomography (CT) and lumbar puncture (LP). In general, CT should precede LP. Fever, meningismus, altered mental status, or headache are independent predictors of space-occupying lesions.[20,21]

Although there are no uniform consensus guidelines on workup of HIV-positive patients with headache, the following approach is recommended.[21] Evaluation of HIV-positive patients with headache should proceed as in the non-HIV-infected population; neuroimaging and LP are indicated for those in whom an alternative explanation is not found or for those who have a clear indication for workup (e.g., worst headache of life). For those with CD4[+] T-cell counts of less than 200 cells/μL, a more aggressive approach is advocated.[21] Headache in combination with altered mental status, seizures, or focal findings requires emergent imaging; LP should be performed if imaging is unrevealing. Isolated headaches that are protracted or changed in quality (even in the absence of other neurologic findings) also should prompt immediate neuroimaging.[20]

Non-contrast-enhanced CT is an appropriate initial imaging study in the ED in HIV-infected patients with neurologic deficits because the addition of contrast material has been shown to be of marginal value in patients with completely normal non-contrast-enhanced CT scans.[22,23] In patients in whom clinical suspicion for central nervous system (CNS) pathology is high but the CT scan is equivocal or negative, contrast-enhanced CT scanning or magnetic resonance imaging (MRI) should be arranged in the ED. Specific CSF studies that may be of value include opening and closing pressures, cell count, glucose, protein, Gram stain, India ink stain, bacterial culture, viral culture, fungal culture, toxoplasmosis and cryptococcosis antigen, and coccidioidomycosis titer. If possible, excess CSF should be held for additional testing if the diagnosis remains unclear after initial workup. Even if the ED evaluation is unrevealing, all patients with new or changed neurologic signs or symptoms should be admitted to the hospital for further workup.

AIDS DEMENTIA

AIDS dementia complex (also referred to as HIV encephalopathy or subacute encephalitis) is a progressive process commonly heralded by subtle impairment of recent memory and other cognitive deficits caused by direct HIV infection; it occurs in 10 to 15 percent of HIV-positive patients. In the early stages, diagnosis can be confused with depression, anxiety disorders, or substance abuse. Later phases of the illness are characterized by obvious changes in mental status and more severe disturbances, including aphasia and motor abnormalities. Patient with an established diagnosis of AIDS dementia who present to the ED with progressive signs or symptoms warrant further emergent workup to rule out other systemic or CNS processes. A CT scan in AIDS dementia typically shows cortical atrophy and ventricular enlargement. AIDS dementia is associated with elevated protein levels in the CSF in 50 to 70 percent of cases.

TOXOPLASMOSIS

Toxoplasmosis is the most common cause of focal encephalitis in patients with AIDS. Symptoms may include headache, fever, focal neurologic deficits, altered mental status, and seizures. Serologic tests are not useful in making or excluding the diagnosis because antibody to *T. gondii* is prevalent in the general population. The presence of antibody to *T. gondii* in the CSF is helpful if present, although there is a high rate of false-negative results. On a non-contrast-enhanced CT scan, toxoplasmosis typically appears as multiple subcortical lesions with a predilection for the basal ganglia.

In general, only a non-contrast-enhanced CT scan is indicated in the ED, with follow-up studies to further delineate the lesion done in the inpatient setting. With contrast enhancement, toxoplasmosis lesions are ring-enhancing, with surrounding areas of edema. MRI is slightly more sensitive than contrast-enhanced CT scan in detecting the extent and number of lesions with toxoplasmosis. Other causes in the differential diagnosis of ring-enhancing lesions on contrast-enhanced CT include lymphoma, fungal infection, and cerebral tuberculosis. In the ED, it is often not possible to differentiate these causes based on initial imaging studies, but general patterns in the appearance of lesions, based on underlying pathology, have been described. Toxoplasmosis tends to have a greater number of lesions with a predilection for the basal ganglia and corticomedullary regions, whereas lymphoma is characterized more often by singular lesions, typically in the periventricular white matter or corpus callosum. Tuberculosis is distinguished by a characteristic inflammatory appearance on CT, with a thick, isodense exudate filling the basal cisterns

Patients with suspected toxoplasmosis should be admitted and treated with pyrimethamine (100- to 200-mg load, then 50-100 mg per d) and sulfadiazine (4-8 g per d), with folinic acid added (10 mg per d) to reduce hematologic toxicity. Steroids (Decadron 4 mg IV q6h) are beneficial for significant edema or mass effect. Failure to improve suggests an alternative diagnosis, which may require biopsy. For patients responsive to toxoplasmosis therapy, chronic suppressive therapy with pyrimethamine, sulfadiazine, and folinic acid is usually indicated after initial treatment. Oral TMP-SMX, one DS tab qd is recommended for prophylaxis in patients with positive toxoplasmosis serologic test results and CD4[+] T-cell counts of less than 100 cells/μL.

CRYPTOCOCCOSIS

Cryptococcal CNS infection may be seen in up to 10 percent of AIDS patients, although, as with toxoplasmosis, the incidence has declined recently due to use of highly active antiretroviral therapy. Infection can produce either focal cerebral lesions or diffuse meningoencephalitis. The most common presenting signs are fever and headache, followed by nausea, altered mentation, and focal neurologic deficits. Presentation may be subtle, and meningismus is uncommon. Neuroimaging studies are usually normal. Diagnosis relies on identifying organisms in CSF by cryptococcal antigen (nearly 100 percent sensitive and specific), culture (95–100 percent sensitive), or staining with India ink (60–80 percent sensitive). Serum cryptococcal antigen is also useful but has slightly lower sensitivity (approximately 95 percent). Elevated intracranial pressure is associated with cryptococcal meningitis, and an opening pressure of greater than 25 cm H_2O should prompt drainage of fluid until pressure is less than 20 cm H_2O or 50 percent of opening pressure. Patient with CNS cryptococcosis shall be admitted for antibiotic therapy; preferred treatment is intravenous amphotericin B 0.7 mg/kg per d with oral flucytosine 100 mg/kg per d for 14 days. Sixty percent of patients may be expected to respond to therapy, and side effects are frequent, most notably bone marrow suppression. Initial therapy should be followed by 8 to 10 weeks of oral fluconazole. Lifelong maintenance therapy with fluconazole (200 mg per d) is indicated for patients but may be discontinued if immune reconstitution is shown.

OTHER NEUROLOGIC DISORDERS

Other, less common CNS infections that should be considered in the presence of neurologic symptoms include bacterial meningitis, histoplasmosis (usually disseminated), CMV infection, PML, herpes simplex virus (HSV) infection, neurosyphilis, and tuberculosis. Noninfectious CNS processes include CNS lymphoma (typically manifested as a subacute neurologic deterioration over several months with a single ring-enhancing lesion on CT), cerebrovascular accidents, and metabolic encephalopathies.

The most common disorder of the peripheral nervous system occurring in up to 50 percent of HIV-infected patients is HIV neuropathy, characterized by painful sensory symptoms in the feet. Although HIV infection itself is the most common culprit, HIV therapies also should be considered as a possible cause, and changing treatment regimens may be helpful. Symptomatic relief with pain-modifying agents such as nortriptyline should be used judiciously because of their potential for causing delirium in patients with concurrent HIV dementia. Narcotic analgesia may be helpful in severe cases.

Ophthalmologic Manifestations

Seventy-five percent of patients with AIDS develop ocular complications. Although a wide range of ophthalmic diseases occurs, recognition of a few is most critical. The most common ophthalmic finding in patients with AIDS is retinal microvasculopathy, which is characterized by retinal cotton-wool spots identical in appearance to those of diabetes or hypertension. Retinal microaneurysms are also seen, primarily in the periphery. These lesions are believed to be incidental and do not cause visual disturbances. The diagnostic dilemma is to distinguish these findings from early CMV infection, and ophthalmologic consultation is recommended.

CMV retinitis is the most frequent and serious ocular opportunistic infection and the leading cause of blindness in AIDS patients. In the highly active antiretroviral therapy era, the incidence of CMV infection has been reduced due in large part to immune reconstitution associated with the therapy.[16] Presentation of CMV retinitis is variable. It may be asymptomatic early on but later causes changes in visual acuity, visual field cuts, photophobia, scotoma, or eye redness or pain. Findings on indirect ophthalmoscopy are characteristic, with fluffy white perivascular lesions and areas of hemorrhage within them. First-line treatment is intraocular ganciclovir implant with oral ganciclovir 1.0 to 1.5 g PO tid; alternative first-line therapy is ganciclovir 5 mg/kg IV bid for 14 to 21 days. Visual loss and blindness occur in all cases without early detection and prompt treatment. Even with treatment, there are frequent relapses and progression of disease, with 10 percent of affected patients ultimately going blind.

Herpes zoster ophthalmicus usually presents with paresthesia and discomfort in the distribution of cranial nerve V_1, followed by the appearance of the typical zoster skin rash. Ocular complications include conjunctivitis, episcleritis, iritis, keratitis, secondary glaucoma, and rarely, retinitis.[24,25] Early recognition and treatment are essential to prevent ocular damage. Preferred treatment is intravenous ayclovir (30–36 mg/kg per d) for at least 7 days. The role of maintenance therapy is unclear.

A number of lesions can affect the areas around the eye in HIV patients, most notably Kaposi sarcoma and molluscum contagiosum. Patients with such lesions may be referred to an ophthalmologist for local excision or cryotherapy.

Pulmonary Complications

Pulmonary complications occur frequently in HIV-positive patients at both early and later stages of immunosuppression. Presenting complaints frequently are nonspecific and include cough, hemoptysis, shortness of breath, and chest pain. ED evaluation should be directed toward determining the likely diagnosis because early treatment has a significant impact on morbidity and mortality rates. Appreciation of the epidemiologic characteristics and common findings associated with various pathogens can assist the emergency physician in arriving at an appropriate differential and working diagnosis, leading to sound treatment and disposition decisions.

The most common causes of pulmonary abnormalities in HIV-infected patients include community-acquired bacterial pneumonia, PCP, *M. tuberculosis* (MTB) infection, CMV infection, *C. neoformans* infection, *H. capsulatum* infection, and neoplasms. In addition to the history and physical examination, evaluation of patients with pulmonary complaints may be assisted by pulse oximetric analysis, arterial blood gas determination, sputum culture, Gram staining, acid-fast staining, blood culture, and chest x-ray. Pulmonary radiographic findings are helpful in determining likely causes (Table 144-3). Admission should be considered for patients with new-onset pulmonary symptoms, especially those with hypoxia. Decisions regarding patients with known pulmonary involvement are based on comparison with baseline status, the effectiveness of ongoing or previous treatment, and the individual's ability to obtain outpatient follow-up. Of note, the widely used Patient Pneumonia Outcome Research Team (PORT) criteria[26] for guiding hospitalization decisions in patients with community-acquired pneumonia did not include HIV-positive patients in their derivation and therefore cannot be applied; further study to address this gap is will be important. Specific symptoms are discussed below with selected common causes.

Despite substantial decreases in the incidence of PCP due to effective prophylaxis and the increased use of highly active antiretroviral therapy, it continues to be the most common opportunistic infection among AIDS patients.[27] Approximately 70 percent of HIV-infected patients will acquire PCP at some time during their illness, and PCP is often the initial opportunistic infection that establishes the diagnosis of AIDS. This disease is the most frequent serious complication of HIV infection in the United States and the most common identifiable cause of death in patients with AIDS. The classic presenting symptoms of PCP are fever, cough (typically nonproductive), and shortness of breath (progressing from being present only with exertion to being present at rest).

Symptoms are often insidious and accompanied by fatigue. Chest x-rays most often show diffuse interstitial infiltrates (see Table 144-3). Although typical radiographic findings occur in up to 80 percent of

TABLE 144-3   Chest Radiographic Abnormalities: Differential Diagnosis in the AIDS Patient

Finding	Etiologies
Diffuse interstitial infiltration	PCP
	CMV
	MTB
	MAI
	Histoplasmosis
	Coccidioidomycosis
	Lymphoid interstitial pneumonitis
Focal consolidation	Bacterial pneumonia
	M. pneumoniae
	P. carinii
	MTB
	MAI
Nodular lesions	Kaposi sarcoma
	MTB
	MAI
	Fungal lesions
	Toxoplasmosis
Cavitary lesions	PCP
	MTB
	Bacterial infection
	Fungal infection
Adenopathy	Kaposi sarcoma
	Lymphoma
	MTB
	Cryptococcosis

patients, negative x-rays are reported in 15 to 20 percent of patients with PCP.[28] In patients with nondiagnostic x-ray findings and signs and symptoms suggestive of PCP, further testing should be pursued. The lactate dehydrogenase (LDH) level is elevated in patients with PCP, but the test for LDH has relatively low sensitivity and specificity, making its use in the ED impractical. Arterial blood gas analysis usually demonstrates hypoxemia and an increase in the alveolar-arterial (A-a) gradient. Early PCP should be suspected if a patient demonstrates a decrease in pulse oximetric values with exercise. Presumptive diagnosis of PCP is often assumed in the emergency department if there is hypoxia without any other explanation. Inpatient diagnostic testing may include bronchoscopy with lavage, biopsy, and culture or examination of induced sputum by indirect immunofluorescence using monoclonal antibodies.

Initial therapy for PCP is TMP-SMX (TMP 15 mg/kg per d and SMX 75 mg/kg per d) either PO or IV for 3 weeks in two or three divided doses (typical oral dosage 2 DS tablets tid). Adverse reactions (most commonly rash, fever, and neutropenia) occur in up to 65 percent of AIDS patients. Pentamidine isothionate 4 mg/kg per d is one of a number of effective alternative agents. Steroid therapy should be instituted for patients with a Pao_2 of less than 70 mm Hg or an alveolar-arterial gradient of greater than 35.[29] The usual regimen is oral prednisone 40 mg bid for 5 days, then 40 mg daily for 5 days, and then 20 mg daily for an additional 11 days. Seventy percent of patients will have reinfection within 18 months. Prophylactic therapy is an important step in preventing reinfection and also has been shown to reduce the risk of developing bacterial pneumonia; oral TMP-SMX 1 DS tablet daily is the preferred agent. Prophylaxis is also recommended in all patients with CD4[+] T-cell counts below 200 cells/μL. Repeat infections may be less responsive to therapy.

The incidence of MTB is increasing, particularly among the homeless, institutionalized, immigrant, and intravenous drug using populations. Reactivation of prior infection is common, and there is a much greater risk of direct progression of disease from recently acquired infection. The incidence of tuberculosis (TB) in the AIDS population is estimated to be 200 to 500 times that in the general population.[30] Prevalence studies demonstrate significant regional variations, attributed to both the demographic characteristics of the populations and the efficacy of local public health control measures. Clinical manifestations of TB in HIV infection vary significantly according to the severity of immunosuppression. Whereas PCP does not occur until the CD4[+] T-cell count is approximately 200 cells/μL, TB frequently occurs in patients with CD4[+] T-cell counts of 200 to 500 cells/μL. Classic pulmonary manifestations include cough with hemoptysis, night sweats, prolonged fevers, weight loss, and anorexia. With worsening immunosuppression, atypical and extrapulmonary manifestations are more common. Frequent sites of dissemination are peripheral lymph nodes, bone marrow, and the urogenital system. Classic upper lobe involvement and cavitary lesions are less common, particularly among late-stage AIDS patients.[30] Negative purified protein derivative (PPD) TB test results are frequent among AIDS patients due to immunosuppression. Definitive diagnosis may be made by stain and culture of sputum, although in some cases bronchoscopy with biopsy may be required. In the ED, physicians should maintain a high index of suspicion for TB among HIV-infected patients with pulmonary symptoms due to the high rates of person-to-person transmission. Immediate isolation should be instituted until the diagnosis is ruled out. Specific procedures for ruling out TB vary by region and site and have been found to be inadequate in some EDs.[31] Any patient identified as high risk based on clinical presentation should be placed in isolation, with the decision for further isolation based on results of chest x-ray and detailed historical and clinical information. Current treatment guidelines recommend a four-drug initial empirical therapy (see Table 144-4). Multidrug-resistant TB remains an issue of concern and should increase the awareness of the need for early isolation. All HIV-infected patients with positive PPD test results should receive prophylaxis with isoniazid plus pyridoximine for 1 year or rifampin plus pyrazinamide for 2 months.

Bacterial pneumonias are the most common pulmonary infections in HIV-infected patients. Common pathogens include *Streptococcus pneumoniae*, *Haemophilus influenzae*, and *Staphylococcus aureus*. Productive cough, leukocytosis, and the presence of a focal infiltrate suggest bacterial pneumonia, especially in those with earlier-stage disease. The response to empirical therapy tends to be good; a specific diagnosis can be established by Gram staining and culture.

Patients with severe immunosuppression are predisposed to disseminated fungal infections such as *C. neoformans* and *Aspergillus fumigatus*. Other noninfectious disorders of the lung seen in HIV-infected patients include neoplasms (e.g., Kaposi sarcoma) and lymphocytic interstitial pneumonitis. CMV or MAC infections are unlikely unless the CD4[+] T-cell count drops below 50 cells/μL.

Cardiovascular Manifestations

Cardiovascular manifestations of HIV infection are changing in the era of highly active antiretroviral therapy. Common in late-stage disease and often difficult to diagnose in the ED (in part because they mimic more generalized or systematic symptoms such as fever and malaise), these complications may be related to opportunistic infections, structural defects, or drug toxicity. HIV-associated cardiovascular conditions include cardiomyopathy, infective endocarditis (injection drug users), pericardial effusion, congestive heart failure (CHF), coronary artery disease (CAD), arrhythmias, and HIV-associated pulmonary hypertension.[32] Following standard ED workup for these conditions, consultation with a cardiologist and infectious disease specialist may be indicated.

Gastrointestinal Complications

Gastrointestinal manifestations of HIV infection are common. Approximately 50 percent of AIDS patients will present with gastrointestinal complaints at some time during their illness. The most frequent presenting symptoms include odynophagia, abdominal pain, bleeding, and diarrhea. ED evaluation should focus on recognizing the severity of symptoms and obtaining appropriate initial diagnostic studies. Therapy should include volume and electrolyte repletion and initiation of antibiotic therapy when appropriate. Disposition should be based on the duration of symptoms, the clinical appearance of the patient, and the response to ED therapy.

ORAL/ESOPHAGEAL MANIFESTATIONS Oral lesions are common in HIV-infected patients, frequently contributing to malnutrition. The appearance of oral lesions in HIV patients may serve as a potential clinical marker for viral load and degree of immunodeficiency.[33] Oral candidiasis or thrush affects more than 80 percent of AIDS patients. The tongue and buccal mucosa are commonly involved, and the plaques characteristically can be easily scraped from an erythematous base. Differentiation from hairy leukoplakia (usually manifested as adherent, white, thickened lesions on the lateral tongue borders) may be challenging, but microscopic examination on potassium hydroxide smear can be used to confirm the diagnosis. The development of oral candidiasis is a poor prognostic sign and is predictive of progression to AIDS. Most oral lesions can be managed symptomatically on an outpatient basis. Clotrimazole or nystatin suspension or troches (five times daily) are the preferred treatment. Refractory or recurrent disease can be managed with oral fluconazole. Amphotericin B is reserved for severe cases.

Other causes of painful oral and perioral lesions include oral hairy leukoplakia, HSV infection, and Kaposi sarcoma. HSV infection usually can be recognized by typical vesicular lesions, with diagnosis confirmed by identifying multinucleated giant cells from scrapings or by culture. Both HSV infection and hairy leukoplakia are responsive to oral acyclovir. Oral Kaposi sarcoma appears as a nontender, well-circumscribed, slightly raised violaceous lesion. Diagnosis requires biopsy; topical treatments may be palliative.

Esophageal involvement may occur with *Candida,* HSV, and CMV. Complaints of odynophagia or dysphagia are usually indicative of esophagitis and may be extremely debilitating. Disease typically occurs in patients who have oral thrush and CD4$^+$ T-cell counts of less than 100 cells/μL. Treatment of esophagitis in the ED is usually presumptive. Endoscopy, histologic staining, culture, and biopsy are reserved for patients who fail to respond or have atypical presentations. Presumptive treatment for *Candida,* which accounts for 50 to 70 percent of cases, is with oral fluconazole (100–400 mg per d for 2–3 weeks) or oral ketoconazole (200–400 mg per d for 2–3 weeks). Intravenous caspofungin or intravenous amphotericin B may be used for oral treatment failures.[34] Relapses are common, and intravenous amphotericin B may be required occasionally. Treatment failures endoscopically discovered to be caused by CMV and HSV are treated with gancyclovir and acylovir, respectively.

DIARRHEA Diarrhea is the most frequent gastrointestinal complaint and is estimated to occur in 50 to 90 percent of AIDS patients. Causes include bacteria (*Shigella, Salmonella,* enteroadherent *Escherichia coli, Entamoeba histolytica, Campylobacter, M. avium intracellulare, Clostridium difficile,* and others), parasites (*Giardia lamblia, Cryptosporidium, Isospora belli,* and others), viruses (CMV, HSV, HIV, and others), and fungi (*H. capsulatum, C. neoformans,* and others). In 20 to 30 percent of cases, a pathogen is never found. Diarrhea is also a known side effect of protease inhibitors, most notably nelfinavir and ritonavir.

ED evaluation of patients with diarrhea should include microscopic examination of stool for leukocytes, ova, and parasites and acid-fast staining and bacterial culture of stool. Clinical clues regarding the cause of diarrheal illnesses may be provided by patient history and confirmed by supplementary testing. Results usually are not available during the ED visit. Bacterial pathogens generally follow a more acute and fulminant course, whereas parasitic infections are more frequently indolent. If bacterial infection is suspected, empirical treatment with ciprofloxacin, which covers the common bacterial pathogens, can be started. *Cryptosporidium* and *Isospora* infections are common parasitic causes and are associated with profuse watery diarrhea. Both can be identified by a modified acid-fast stain. *I. belli* infection is usually responsive to TMP-SMZ, but relapse is common. *Cryptosporidiosis* tends to be difficult to treat.[35]

In patients with end-stage disease, the most common pathogens are CMV and *M. avium intracellulare;* both diagnoses usually require biopsy. Prolonged antimicrobial therapy is indicated for treatment. Resistance and relapse are frequent for both entities. About 15 percent of patients with late-stage AIDS suffer from severe, high-volume watery diarrhea with no pathogen identified even after thorough investigation. The presumed diagnosis is AIDS-related enteropathy. Patients often require admission for correction of electrolyte abnormalities and rehydration. Octreotide, the somatostatin analogue, may be helpful in some cases.

ED management should be directed toward repletion of fluid and electrolytes. Patients who appear nontoxic and can tolerate liquids can be referred for outpatient follow-up of test results. Patients with severe diarrhea who do not require antibiotics may benefit from symptomatic therapy, such as attapulgite (Kaopectate), psyllium (Metamucil), and if necessary, diphenoxylate hydrochloride with atropine (Lomotil).

OTHER GASTROINTESTINAL MANIFESTATIONS Hepatomegaly occurs in approximately 50 percent of AIDS patients. Elevation of the alkaline phosphatase level is seen frequently. Jaundice is rare. Coinfection with hepatitis B and hepatitis C is common, especially among injection drug users. Opportunistic infections with CMV, *Cryptosporidium, M. avium intracellulare,* and MTB also may cause signs of hepatitis.

Anorectal disease is common in AIDS patients. Proctitis is characterized by painful defecation, rectal discharge, and tenesmus. Common causative organisms include *Neisseria gonorrhoeae, Chlamydia trachomatis,* syphilis, and HSV. Proctocolitis includes the same symptoms in the presence of diarrhea, and multiple bacterial organisms may be responsible (most commonly *Shigella, Campylobacter,* and *E. histolytica*). Diagnostic evaluation should include anoscopy, with microscopic examination, Gram stain, and culture of pus and/or stool.

Renal Manifestations

Renal insufficiency among AIDS patients may be secondary to prerenal azotemia, drug nephrotoxicity, or HIV-associated nephropathy, which may cause chronic renal insufficiency due to focal and segmental glomerulosclerosis. Renal tubular acidosis is common and may explain a finding of hyperchloremic metabolic acidosis. Management decisions should be made in conjunction with nephrology.

Cutaneous Manifestations

Generalized cutaneous conditions, such as xerosis (dry skin), seborrheic eczema, and pruritus, are common and may be manifested prior to development of opportunistic infections. Treatment is with emollients and, if necessary, mild topical steroids. Pruritus may respond to oatmeal baths and antihistamines. Other infections, including *S. aureus* (manifested as bullous impetigo, ecthyma, or folliculitis), *Pseudomonas aeruginosa* (which may present with chronic ulcerations and macerations), and syphilis, are seen frequently and should be treated with standard therapies. Several specific dermatologic conditions are discussed in more detail below.

Kaposi sarcoma (KS) appears more often in homosexual men than in other risk groups. Clinically, it consists of painless, raised brown-black or purple papules and nodules that do not blanch. Common sites are the face, chest, genitals, and oral cavity; however, widespread dissemination involving internal organs may occur. Since cutaneous KS is not generally associated with significant rates of morbidity or mortality, therapy is indicated only for extensive, painful, or cosmetically disfiguring lesions. Cryotherapy or radiation can be used for localized disease; widespread disease may be responsive to chemotherapy with vincristine, vinblastine, or doxyrubicin.

HSV infections are common and may be localized or systemic. In patients with significant immunosuppression, infection may become progressive, manifested as chronic ulcerative mucocutaneous lesions. Diagnosis and treatment are the same as for other patients with HSV infection (see Chap. 143). Recommended regimens are described in Table 144-4. Intravenous therapy with an antiviral agent (acyclovir 5–10 mg/kg per d, famciclovir 250 mg PO tid, or valacyclovir 1 g bid) is needed for extensive disease.

Reactivation of varicella-zoster virus is more common in patients with HIV infection and AIDS than in the general population. The clinical course is prolonged, and complications are more frequent. In HIV-positive patients, oral acyclovir 800 mg five times a day, oral famciclovir 500 mg tid for 7 days, or oral valacyclovir 1 g tid for 7 days is usually sufficient. However, in patients with disseminated disease or ophthalmic zoster, admission is indicated for intravenous acyclovir.

Intertriginous infections with either *Candida* or *Trichophyton* are seen frequently in HIV-positive patients and can be diagnosed by microscopic examination of potassium hydroxide preparations of lesion scrapings. Treatment includes topical imidazole creams, such as clotrimazole, miconazole, or ketoconazole.

Scabies occurs in about 20 percent of HIV-infected patients, but classic intertriginous lesions are less common. Any patient with a scaly, persistent pruritic eruption should be treated with permethrin 5 percent cream, ivermectin, or crotamiton. Norwegian scabies is a particularly invasive variant of scabies and poses a challenging treatment difficulty. Norwegian scabies may be seen in immunosuppressed

TABLE 144-4   Treatment Recommendations for Common HIV-Related Infections

Organ System	Infection	Therapy
Systemic	MAI	Clarithromycin 500 mg PO bid *and* Ethambutol 15 m/kg per d PO ± Rifabutin 300 mg/kg per d PO
	CMV	Ganciclovir, 5 mg/kg IV bid × 2 weeks, then 5 mg/kg per d *or* Foscarnet 90 mg/kg q12h × 3 weeks, then 90 mg/kg per d
Pulmonary	*P. carinii*	TMP-SMX 15–20 mg TMP/kg per d *and* 75–100 mg SMX/kg per d, PO or IV × 3 weeks *or* Pentamidine 4 mg/kg per d, IV or IM, × 3 weeks
	*M. tuberculosis**	Isoniazid 5 mg/kg per d PO *and* Rifampin 10 mg/kg per d PO *and* Pyrazinamide 15–30 mg/kg per d PO *and* Streptomycin 15 mg/kg per d IM
CNS	Toxoplasmosis†	Pyrimethamine 50–100 mg/kg per d PO × 6–8 weeks *and* Sulfadiazine 4–8 mg/kg per d × 6–8 weeks *and* Folinic acid 10 mg per d PO × 6–8 weeks
	Cryptococcosis‡	Amphotericin B 0.7 mg/kg per d IV × 2 weeks *and* Flucystosine 100 mg/kg per d IV × 2 weeks *then* Fluconazole 400 mg per d PO × 8–10 weeks
Ophthalmologic	CMV#	Ganciclovir implant *and* Ganciclovir 1.0–1.5 g PO tid *or* Ganciclovir 5 mg/kg IV bid × 2–3 weeks
GI	Candidiasis	Clotrimazole, 10 mg, 5×/d troches *or* Nystatin 500 K units 5×/d, gargle
	Thrush (*Candida*)	
	Esophagitis (primarily *Candida*)	Fluconazole, 100–400 mg per d, PO
	Salmonellosis	Ciprofloxacin, 500 mg bid PO (2–4 wks); maintenance therapy required
	Cryptosporidiosis	No known effective cure; best results with HAART§
Cutaneous	HSV	Acyclovir, 200 mg PO 5×/d × 7 d *or* Famciclovir 125 mg PO bid × 7 d *or* Valacyclovir 1 g PO bid × 7 d *or* for *severe disease* Acyclovir 5–10 mg/kg q8h IV × 7 d
	Herpes zoster	Acyclovir 800 mg PO 5×/day × 7–10 d *or* Famciclovir 500 mg PO tid × 7–10 d *or* Valacyclovir 1 g PO tid × 7–10 days *or* for *ocular* or *disseminated disease* Acyclovir 5–10 mg/kg q8h × 5–7 d
	Candida or *tricophyton*	Topical clotrimazole bid or tid × 3 weeks *or* Topical miconazole bid or tid × 3 weeks *or* Topical ketoconazole bid or tid × 3 weeks

*Specific drug regimen must be adjusted if on HAART.
†Maintainance therapy required.
‡Maintainance therapy required, may discontinue if CD4 >150 for >16 weeks.
#Maintainance therapy required until CD4$^+$ T-cell count >150.
§HAART: highly active antiretroviral therapy.

patients, and patients typically exhibit extensive hyperkeratosis and crusting of the hands, feet, and scalp. Pruritus is less impressive than is seen in typical scabies. Extensive mite proliferation and high contagion are common. Treatment failures and secondary infection also are common.

Human papillomavirus infections occur with increased frequency in immunocompromised patients. Treatment is cosmetic or symptomatic and may include cryotherapy, topical therapy, or laser therapy. Other dermatologic conditions that occur with increased frequency among HIV-infected patients include psoriasis, atopic dermatitis, and alopecia. Referral for dermatologic consultation is appropriate.

Psychiatric Disorders

Epidemiologic studies of patients infected with HIV and AIDS show a high lifetime prevalence of psychiatric disorders compared with the general population. Persons at highest risk for HIV infection (i.e., injected drug users and homosexual men) frequently suffer from mood disturbances prior to contracting HIV. Infection with HIV produces brain injury and is associated with a variety of CNS and metabolic disturbances that can produce psychiatric symptoms. HIV infection is also a significant psychosocial stressor, leading to social isolation, poverty, and hopelessness.

Evaluation of psychiatric symptoms in the ED should focus on an aggressive search for underlying organic causes of the acute presentation.[36] Delirium suggests the presence of a primary physiologic disease; the workup should include laboratory studies, neuroimaging, and LP. The differential diagnosis includes CNS and toxic-metabolic derangements. Frequently, a period of observation may be required if a patient is found to be intoxicated or experiencing withdrawal symptoms.

AIDS psychosis is poorly understood. Patients may present with psychiatric symptoms, such as hallucinations, delusions, or other abnormal behavioral changes. The cause is unclear, and treatment has been identical to that for other psychoses. Acute episodes require admission.

Depression occurs in 20 percent of patients, most commonly in those with lower CD4$^+$ T-cell counts.[37] Depressive illnesses are often responsive to hospitalization and psychosocial intervention. Antidepressant therapy may be considered if symptoms of depression continue longer than 2 weeks. However, due to the increased propensity to develop medication side effects, close patient monitoring is required. Patients with suicidal ideation usually require inpatient psychiatric management.

An increased incidence of mania is observed in both the early and late stages of HIV infection. Late-stage mania is closely associated with dementia and carries a poor prognosis. Management of HIV-positive patients with psychiatric complaints must include attention to violent behavior and suicidality. Assessment and stabilization may require physical restraints and acute pharmacologic intervention. Neuroleptics and benzodiazepines may be used in combination. Haloperidol and diazepam are used frequently. Droperidol has a more rapid onset and shorter half-life than haloperidol but can cause torsades de pointes and sudden death, particularly in patients with prolonged QT$_c$ syndromes. Lorazepam offers improved intramuscular absorption over diazepam. Medications should be used judiciously due to frequent polypharmacy.

Sexually Transmitted Diseases

Sexually transmitted diseases (STDs) are epidemiologically associated with HIV infection. Diseases that cause genital ulcers, such as herpes, chancroid, and syphilis, are believed to provide vascular portals of entry for HIV. Prevalence studies demonstrate a three- to fivefold increased odds ratio of HIV seropositivity in patients with genital ulcers.[38] A similarly increased risk of HIV infection has been recently found among patients with gonorrhea and chlamydial infections.

These studies, along with recent ED-based prevalence surveys, have led to a recommendation for increased surveillance of STDs as a means of controlling HIV transmission.[39] All patients with symptoms suggestive of an STD should be tested for gonorrhea, chlamydia, and syphilis. Primary (chancre) and secondary (rash, mucocutaneous lesions, and adenopathy) syphilis should be treated with a single intramuscular dose of benzathine penicillin, 2.4 million units. For latent syphilis or unknown duration of secondary syphilis, three weekly injections are recommended. Any patient with known or suspected syphilis should be evaluated for the possibility of neurosyphilis, which is known to have an increased incidence in the HIV-infected population. Therapy for other STDs is based on current CDC guidelines (see Chap. 141).

Immunizations of HIV-Infected Patients

According to the U.S. Public Health Service Immunizations Practices Advisory Committee, HIV-infected persons should not receive live virus or live bacteria vaccines. The one exception to this is the measles-mumps-rubella (MMR) vaccine, which is indicated in all HIV-positive patients prior to onset of severe immunsuppression. In those with severe immunosuppression, MMR vaccination should be withheld due to increased risk of complications and decreased likelihood of benefit.

Killed vaccines pose no danger to immunosuppressed patients.[40] Since symptomatic HIV-infected persons have a suboptimal response to vaccines, all single-dose vaccines are advised to be given as early as possible in the course of HIV infection. Table 144-5 summarizes the CDC recommendations for common immunizations. Pneumococcal vaccine is recommended for all patients over 2 years of age because the risk for invasive pneumococcal infection is 50 to 100 times greater than in the general population. Tetanus-diphtheria vaccine is recommended as a booster every 10 years for those who have completed primary series. Hepatitis B vaccine is recommended for all high-risk individuals, including injected drug users, sexually active homosexual men, and sexually active men and women with STDs or more than one sexual partner in the past 6 months. Patients should be referred to a primary care provider for routine immunization.

Antiretroviral Therapy (ART)

The most notable recent advance in the management of HIV is the advent of highly active antiretroviral therapy (HAART) in 1996. Since then, sharp declines in AIDS incidence occurred through 1999 (although they have leveled off recently), and numbers of deaths among

TABLE 144-5   Immunization Recommendations for HIV-Infected Patients

Vaccine	Asymptomatic	Symptomatic
DPT (to age 7)	Yes	Yes
Td	Yes	Yes
OPV (oral polio vaccine)	No	No
IPV (inactivated polio vaccine)	Yes	Yes
MMR (measles-mumps-rubella)	Yes	No*
Haemophilus B (Hib) flu (HbCV)	No (although not contraindicated)	Yes
Pneumococcal	Yes	Yes
Influenza (inactivated)	No (although not contraindicated)	Yes
Hepatitis B	Yes	Yes

*Severely immunocompromised children should not receive MMR.
Source: Bartlett JG: *Medical Management of HIV Infection.* Baltimore, Johns Hopkins University, Division of Infectious Diseases, 2002; and Centers for Disease Control and Prevention: Standard for pediatric immunization practices: Recommended by the National Vaccine Advisory Committee. *MMWR* 42:1, 1993.

persons with AIDS have declined steadily.[3,41] Explanations for the slowing of the decline in AIDS incidence include poor patient compliance with treatment regimens, costs, adverse side effects, and development of drug-resistant strains of HIV.

The fundamental goal of HIV therapeutics is long-term management of a chronic infection. Specific treatment recommendations are evolving constantly based on both advances in drug modalities and increasing information from clinical trials on response to therapy. General therapeutic goals, which remain constant, include (1) clinical: prolongation of life and improved quality of life; (2) virologic: greatest possible reduction in viral load to halt disease progression and prevent/reduce resistant variants; (3) immunologic: immune reconstitution, both quantitative (CD4$^+$ T-cell count) and qualitative (pathogen-specific immune response); and (4) therapeutic: rational sequencing of drug to attain virologic goals while reducing side effects and maintaining therapeutic options.

The emergency physician should be familiar with general classes of antiretroviral drugs, principles for initiating therapy, and common adverse reactions. Three main classes of drugs that independently interrupt the normal HIV life cycle include the nucleoside reverse-transcriptase inhibitors (NRTIs), the nonnucleoside reverse-transcriptase inhibitors (NNRTIs), and the protease inhibitors (PIs). Mechanisms of action and example of agents in each class are as follows: (1) NRTIs interfere with the action of reverse transcriptase [e.g., AZT (Retrovir)]; (2) NNRTIs bind to reverse transcriptase and block RNA- and DNA-dependent DNA polymerase activity [e.g., efavirenz (Sustiva)]; and (3) PIs block HIV protease, a key enzyme in establishing HIV infectivity [e.g. Indinavir (IDV)]. Eighteen antiretroviral drugs are currently approved by the FDA. A complete list and up-to-date guide for their use can be found on the CDC Web site (www.cdc.gov/hiv/pubs/mmwr). Initial preferred treatment regimens include 2 NRTIs + 1 PI; 2 NRTIs + 2 PIs or 2 NRTIs and 1 NNRTI. Factors that are considered in initiation include likelihood of adherence, potential for long-term side effects, potential for drug interaction, and preservation of future treatment options.

The optimal time to initiate therapy and the best drugs to use are still being evaluated. Treatment should be offered to all patients with symptoms ascribed to HIV infection. For the asymptomatic patient, treatment should be offered to those with CD4$^+$ T-cell counts below 350 cells/μL at any viral load and at higher CD4$^+$ T-cell counts (>350 cells/μL) with higher viral loads (>55,000 copies/mL).[42]

Education and counseling also constitute an integral part of ART therapy. For these reasons, decisions regarding initiation of and changes in ART always should be made in consultation with the primary care physician and an infectious disease consultant.

PRECAUTIONS FOR HEALTH CARE WORKERS

Health care workers are often exposed to the blood and body fluids of HIV-infected patients or patients at high risk of harboring the HIV virus. ED-based studies have demonstrated that substantial numbers of patients continue to have unsuspected HIV infection and that HIV seropositivity cannot be predicted accurately, even with the aid of risk factors assessment. Universal precautions should be practiced, and all contacts with blood or body fluids should be considered potentially infectious. Universal precautions include gloves, gown, mask, and eye protection for any situation with the potential for exposure by splash, spray, touch, puncture, or immersion. These measures are also indicated for all ED procedures, including examination of bleeding patients, chest tube placement, central line placement, suturing, wound care, and LP.[43]

The risk of acquiring HIV through occupational exposure is low. The likelihood of contracting AIDS after a parenteral exposure has been estimated at 0.32 percent; for mucocutaneous exposure, risk is approximately 0.09 percent. HIV transmission through nonintact skin has been documented, but the estimated risk is considerably lower than for mucocutaneous exposure. Approximately 80 percent of documented occupational exposure cases have resulted from hollow-bore

needle-stick injuries. As of June 2000, the CDC had documented 56 cases of HIV seroconversion temporally associated with an occupational exposure and an additional 138 cases of possible occupationally related seroconversion (i.e., seroconversion after a specific exposure was not clearly documented but was suspected by history).

Postexposure Prophylaxis

OCCUPATIONAL   Guidelines for postexposure prophylaxis (PEP) of health care workers following an occupational exposure are based on a case-control study of needle-stick injuries from an HIV-infected source (which included 33 patients who seroconverted and 739 control subjects). This study reported that AZT prophylaxis was associated with a 79 percent reduction in disease transmission.[44] Risks for seroconversion include (1) deep injury, (2) visible blood on the device, (3) needle placement in a vein or an artery, and (4) a source with late-stage HIV infection. The most recent PEP recommendations were released in 2001 and advise treatment based on exposure category and risk of the source; decisions should be made in consultation with an infectious disease specialist.[45]

PEP should be initiated as quickly as possible, preferably within 1 to 2 h. The interval after which there is no benefit for starting PEP is not known, although animal studies suggest little benefit if PEP is started 24 to 36 h after exposure. For these reasons, the decision should not delay initiation of PEP because modifications can be made after treatment has started. Decisions about PEP are based on assessments of type of exposure (superficial, deep, cutaneous, mucosal, hollow-bore needle, etc.) and exposure risk category (risk of HIV-infected material from the source). Treatment regimens vary by type of exposure. CDC guidelines recommend two basic alternatives: a basic regimen, which consists of two-drug therapy, often consisting of AZT and lamivudine (3TC), and an expanded regimen, which adds a third drug, such as indinavir (Crixivan) or nelfinavir (Viracept). Typically, the expanded regimen is recommended for high-risk exposures (defined as large-bore needle, visible injury, visible blood in device, or needle from patient artery/vein) and/or high-risk source (defined as symptomatic HIV, AIDS, acute seroconversion, or high viral load). Appropriate testing and treatment for other, more highly infectious agents such as hepatitis should be initiated as well. PEP treatment duration is 4 weeks. Gastrointestinal and constitutional side effects can be considerable; those who start treatment thus should be counseled and referred for timely follow-up.

NONOCCUPATIONAL   Management of patients with possible sexual, injected drug use, or other nonoccupational exposure to HIV has become relevant because the U.S. Public Health Service issued a recommendation for the use of antiretroviral drugs to reduce the risk of acquisition of HIV following occupational exposure. The CDC has withheld making definitive statements regarding PEP for nonoccupational exposures because of the lack of available data regarding the use of antiretroviral agents in this setting. Recommendations may be forthcoming shortly as experience and data accumulate.

Patient adherence, the lack of data on the long-term effects of antiretroviral treatments, drug resistance, and a possible increase in high-risk behaviors have all been cited as reasons against offering PEP for nonoccupational exposures. However, further evaluation of PEP in patients with nonoccupational exposure to HIV infection may prove beneficial from both a clinical and a public health perspective.

Since the ED is often the initial site for evaluation and treatment of patients who have had these high-risk contacts, it is important for emergency physicians to develop a rationale approach. In ED patients with high-risk exposure, clinical workup should include a thorough history of the exposure and past high-risk behaviors, baseline laboratory and HIV testing, and consultation with a specialist.[46,47] PEP must be considered on a case-by-case basis and generally should be restricted to situations in which the risk of infection is high, the intervention can be initiated promptly (<36 h), adherence to the regimen is likely, and the individual is most likely to maintain risk-reduction behavior over time.[48] Advantages of therapy also must be balanced carefully with the risk of medication side effects. All sexual assault victim should be counseled about the risk and benefits of treatment.

In the ED, when the physician is faced with a case in which PEP is being considered, the assistance of experts should be sought. Risks and benefits of therapy should be considered in consultation with an infectious disease specialist and the patient's primary care provider. The CDC has a 24-h telephone hotline for physicians designed to assist with appropriate decision making regarding PEP (PEP Hotline: 1-888-448-4911).

DRUG REACTIONS

When managing HIV-positive and AIDS patients, emergency physicians must take into consideration the various drug interactions, reactions, and toxicities that can be causative of the clinical presentation of an HIV or AIDS patient. Current highly active antiretroviral therapies include a standard three-drug regimen that may cause a range of changes in metabolic or physiologic functions and also may be toxic. These interactions may be compounded by antibiotic prophylaxis being taken to fight against opportunistic infections. Drug reactions and interactions in seropositive patients should be considered when other diagnoses have been ruled out in specific presentation.

Drug interactions may be categorized as pharmacokinetic interactions [changes in level(s) of one or more drugs] or pharmacodynamic interactions (changes in effect, therapeutic response, or side effect of one or more drugs).[49] As antiretroviral drugs and combination therapies continue to be widely used and further developed, the possible drug reactions and interactions also will become more complex.

Review of current reference sources and consultation with a hospital pharmacologist and an infectious disease specialist are indicated when drug reactions are suspected.

ETHICAL CONSIDERATIONS

Many ethical considerations are involved in testing and treatment of HIV-infected patients. Confidentiality regarding HIV-related diagnoses is paramount to providing appropriate care for ED patients.[50] Treatment without discrimination, as with all disease states, should be initiated in all patients unless they specifically request otherwise.

Resuscitation of patients with advanced AIDS may be controversial, but decision making is no different than for patients with other debilitating conditions. Since ED physicians often have limited information about individual patients, their wishes, and the state of their disease, it is recommended that appropriate therapy and resuscitative measures be undertaken unless advance directives are available. Care should be taken that the label *HIV* or *AIDS* does not bias the judgment that resuscitative efforts are futile. Contact with a patient's primary care physician and family early during the ED stay helps in decision making about care.

DISPOSITION

Consultation with an infectious disease specialist and sometimes others with expertise in HIV infection is often necessary to provide proper therapy and disposition. Disposition decisions, as for all patients, are based on the need for definite inpatient evaluation or management and determination of the patient's ability to function as an outpatient (with special consideration regarding oral intake, ambulation, and availability of appropriate medical follow-up).

REFERENCES

1. Joint United Nations Program on HIV/AIDS: AIDS Epidemic Update. Available at www.unaids.org; accessed October 2002.
2. Centers for Disease Control and Prevention: A Glance at the HIV Epidemic. Available at www.cdc.gov/hiv/pubs/facts.htm; accessed October 2002.
3. Centers for Disease Control and Prevention: HIV/AIDS Surveillance Report. Available at www.cdc.gov/nchstp/hiv aids/stats/hasrlink.html; accessed October 2002.
4. Kelen GD, Hexter DA, Hansen KN, et al: Trends in human immunodeficiency virus (HIV) infection among a patient population of an inner-city emergency department: Implications for emergency department based screening programs for HIV infection. *Clin Infect Dis* 21:867, 1995.
5. Schacker T, Collier AC, Hughes J, et al: Clinical and epidemiologic features of primary HIV infection. *Ann Intern Med* 125:257, 1996.
6. Perlmutter BL: How to recognize and treat acute HIV syndrome. *Am Fam Phys* 60(2):535, 1999.
7. Kahn JO, Walker BD: Acute human immunodeficiency virus type 1 infection. *New Engl J Med* 339:33, 1998.
8. O'Brien WA, Hartigan PM, Martin D, et al: Changes in plasma HIV-1 RNA and CD4-lymphocyte counts and the risk of progression to AIDS. *New Engl J Med* 334:42, 1996.
9. Pilcher CD, McPherson JT, Leone PA, et al: Real-time, universal screening for acute HIV infection in a routine HIV counseling and testing population. *JAMA* 288:216, 2002.
10. Kelen GD, Digiovanna T, Bisson L, et al: Human immunodeficiency virus infection in emergency department patients: Epidemiology, clinical presentations and risk to health care workers: The Johns Hopkins experience. *JAMA* 262:516, 1989.
11. Kelen GD, Shahan JB, Quinn TL: HIV screening and counseling: Experience with rapid and standard serologic testing. *Ann Emerg Med* 33(2):147, 1999.
12. Rothman RE, Ketlogetswe K, Dolan T, Kelen GD: Should emergency departments conduct routine HIV screening? A systematic review. *Acad Emerg Med* 10(3):278, 2003.
13. Kelen GD, Johnson G, Digiovanna TA, et al: Profile of patients with human immunodeficiency virus infection presenting to an inner-city emergency department: Preliminary report. *Ann Emerg Med* 19(9):963, 1990.
14. Haukoos JS, Witt MD, Zeumer CM, et al: Emergency department triage of patients infected with HIV. *Acad Emerg Med* 9(9):880, 2002.
15. Bartlett JG, Gallant JE: 2001-2002 Medical Management of HIV Infection. The Johns Hopkins University School of Medicine, 2002 (http://hopkins-aids.edu).
16. Moylett EH: HIV: Clinical manifestations. *J Allergy Clin Immunol* 110(1):3, 2002.
17. Shelburne SA 3d, Hamill RJ, Rodriguez-Barradas MC, et al: Immune reconstitution inflammatory syndrome: Emergence of a unique syndrome during highly active antiretroviral therapy. *Medicine* 81(3):213, 2002.
18. Majmudar MD, Kelen GD, Rothman RE: Defining new criteria for the diagnosis of infective endocarditis (IE) in febrile intravenous drug users (IDUs). *Acad Emerg Med* 7(5):561, 2000.
19. Rothman RE, Majmudar MD, Kelen GD, et al: Detection of bacteremia in emergency department patients at risk for infective endocarditis using universal 16S rRNA primers in a decontaminated polymerase chain reaction assay. *J Infect Dis* 186:1677, 2002.
20. Rothman RE, Keyl PM, McArthur JC, et al: A decision guideline for emergency department utilization of noncontrast head computed tomography in HIV-infected patients. *Acad Emerg Med* 6:1010, 1999.
21. Graham CB, Wippold FJ, Pilgram TK, et al: Screening CT determined by CD4 count in HIV-positive patients presenting with headache. *Am J Neuroradiol* 21:451, 2000.
22. Berger JR, Nath A: A careful neurologic examination should precede neuroimaging studies in HIV-infected patients with headache. *Am J Neuroradiol* 21:441, 2000.
23. Barber CJ, Rowlands PC, McCarty M, et al: Clinical utility of cranial CT in HIV-positive and AIDS patients with neurological disease. *Clin Radiol* 42(3):164, 1990.
24. Greenwood J, Graham EM: The ocular complications of HIV and AIDS. *Int J STD AIDS* 8:358, 1997.
25. Baven ER, Wison P, Atkins M, et al: Natural history of untreated CMV retinitis. *Lancet* 346:1671, 1995.
26. Fine MJ, Auble TE, Yealy DM, et al: A prediction rule to identify low-risk patients with community-acquired pneumonia. *New Engl J Med* 336:243, 1997.
27. Wolff AJ, O'Donnell AE: Pulmonary manifestations of HIV infection in the era of highly active antiretroviral therapy. *Chest* 120(6):1888, 2001.
28. Huang L, Stanell JD: AIDS and the lung. *Med Clin North Am* 80:4, 1996.

29. NIH-UC Expert Panel for Corticosteroids as Adjunctive Therapy for *Pneumocystis* Pneumonia: Consensus statement for use of corticosteroids as adjunctive therapy for *Pneumocystis* pneumonia in AIDS. *New Engl J Med* 323:1500, 1990.

30. Markowitz N, Hansen NI, Hopewell PC, et al: Incidence of tuberculosis in the United States among HIV-infected persons. *Ann Intern Med* 126:123, 1997.

31. Moran GJ, McCabe F, Morgan TM, et al: Delayed recognition and infection control for tuberculosis in the emergency department. *Ann Emerg Med* 26:290, 1995.

32. Barbaro G, Fisher SD, Giancaspro G, et al: HIV-associated cardiovascular complications: A new challenge for emergency physicians. *Am J Emerg Med* 19(7):566, 2001.

33. Patton LL: Sensitivity, specificity, and positive predictive value of oral opportunistic infections in adults with HIV/AIDS as markers of immune suppression and viral burden. *Oral Surg Oral Med Oral Pathol* 90(2):182, 2000.

34. Mora-Duarte J, Betts R, Rotstein C, et al: Comparison of caspofungin and amphotericin B for invasive candidiasis. *New Engl J Med* 347:2020, 2002.

35. Neild PJ, Nelson MR. Management of HIV-related diarrhoea. *Int J STD AIDS* 8:286, 1997.

36. Lyketsos CG, Fishman M, Treisman G: Psychiatric issues and emergencies in HIV infection. *Emerg Med Clin North Am* 13:163, 1995.

37. Lyketsos CG, Hoover DR, Guccione M, et al: Depressive symptoms as predictors of medical outcomes in HIV infection. *JAMA* 270:2563, 1993.

38. Dickerson MC, Johnston J, Delea TE, et al: The causal role for genital ulcer disease as a risk factor for transmission of human immunodeficiency virus. *Sex Transm Dis* 23:429, 1996.

39. Yearly DM, Greene TJ, Hobbs GD: Underrecognition of cervical *Neiserria gonorrhoeae* and *Chlamydia trachomatis* infections in the emergency department. *Acad Emerg Med* 4:962, 1997.

40. Centers for Disease Control and Prevention: Standard for pediatric immunization practices: Recommended by the National Vaccine Advisory Committee. *MMWR* 42:1, 1993.

41. Andrews L: Progress in HIV therapeutics and the challenges of adherence to antiretroviral therapy. *Infect Dis Clin North Am* 14(4):901, 2000.

42. Carpenter C, Cooper DA, Fischl MA, et al: Antiretroviral therapy in adults: Updated recommendations of the International AIDS Society—USA Panel. *JAMA* 283:381, 2000.

43. Kelen GD, Hansen KN, Green GB, et al: Determinants of emergency department procedure- and condition-specific universal (barrier) precaution requirements for optimal provider protection. *Ann Emerg Med* 25:743, 1995.

44. Cardo DM, Culver DH, Ciesielski CA, et al: A case-control study of HIV seroconversion in health care workers after percutaneous exposure: Centers for Disease Control and Prevention Needlestick Surveillance Group. *New Engl J Med* 337:1485, 1997.

45. Centers for Disease Control and Prevention: Updated U.S. Public Health Service Guidelines for the management of occupational exposures of HBV, HCV and HIV and recommendations for postexposure prophylaxis. *MMWR* 29:501, 2001.

46. Merchant RC: Nonoccupational HIV postexposure prophylaxis: A new role for the emergency department. *Ann Emerg Med* 36(4):366, 2000.

47. Moran GJ: Pharmacologic management of HIV/STD exposure. *Emerg Med Clin North Am* 18:4, 2000.

48. Katz MH, Gerberding JL: The care of persons with recent sexual exposure to HIV. *Ann Intern Med* 128:312, 1998.

49. Hovanessian HC: New developments in the treatment of HIV disease: An overview. *Ann Emerg Med* 33(5):546, 1999.

50. Parsa M, Walsh M: Ethics seminars: HIV testing, consent, and physician responsibilities. *Acad Emerg Med* 8:1197, 2001.

145 INFECTIVE ENDOCARDITIS

Richard E. Rothman

Samuel Yang

Catherine A. Marco

The majority of patients with infective endocarditis (IE) have an identifiable predisposing cardiac abnormality or risk factor for disease. Clinical presentation is often nonspecific and can be highly variable, as the disease can affect nearly every organ system and have either an indolent or fulminant course. Diagnosis relies on a set of explicit criteria, which include findings from blood culture, echocardiography, and several days of inpatient observation. Unrecognized disease is associated with a wide range of complications and mortality approaching 100 percent.

EPIDEMIOLOGY

In developed countries, the incidence of IE ranges from 2.4 to 11.9 cases per 100,000 patient-years.[1-4] Incidence is higher in urban versus rural populations, likely reflecting the impact of injection drug use (IDU). Currently just over 25 percent of cases occur in patients less than 30 years of age; approximately 50 percent occur in patients aged 31 to 60; and slightly less than 25 percent occur in those greater than 60 years of age. Factors contributing to the age distribution include decreased incidence of rheumatic heart disease, increased prevalence of degenerative valvular disease (due to aging), and increasing use of invasive medical procedures, including hemodialysis, intravenous catheters, and intracardiac devices. The disease is uncommon among children, where it is associated primarily with structural congenital heart disease, rheumatic heart disease, or nosocomial catheter-related bacteremia. IE affects men more commonly than women in a ratio of 1.7:1. The aortic valve is most commonly affected, followed in decreasing frequency by the mitral, tricuspid, and pulmonic valves. Significant variation in mortality occurs based on organism, presence of complications, and treatment modality (medical versus surgical).

The majority of cases of IE occur either in those with a predisposing identifiable cardiac structural abnormality (congenital or acquired) or a recognized risk factor for disease [including IDU, indwelling catheters, poor dental hygiene, or infection with human immunodeficiency virus (HIV)]. Recent reviews of IE cases in two suburban hospitals in North America showed distribution of cases of IE as follows: native valve related IE (NVE), 59 to 70 percent, IDU, 11 to 16 percent, and prosthetic valve IE (PVE), 14 to 30 percent.[5,6] Studies in inner-city populations, however, find IDUs to account for up to 40 percent of cases.[7]

For NVE in the developed world, mitral valve prolapse is now the most commonly recognized predisposing cardiac lesion for IE. Incidence in this population is 100 per 100,000 patient years. Other commonly recognized underlying structural defects found in those with IE include congenital defects (most commonly bicuspid aortic valve), degenerative cardiac lesions (particularly calcific aortic stenosis), and rheumatic heart disease. In developing countries, rheumatic heart disease remains the leading underlying risk factor for IE. For NVE, left-sided disease predominates and mortality ranges from 16 to 27 percent. Risk factors associated with mortality for patients with left-sided native valve endocarditis include comorbidity, abnormal mental status, congestive heart failure, bacterial etiology other than *Streptococcus viridans* and *Staphylococcus aureus,* and medical therapy without valve surgery.[8]

Although the exact incidence is difficult to determine, estimated risk for IE in IDUs is 2 to 5 percent per year. Mean age of disease is 30 years. When IE occurs in IDUs it has a predilection for the right side, with tricuspid valve involvement occurring in the vast majority of cases. Morality (<10 percent) is lower than that seen in NVE. Other features of IDU-related IE include increased susceptibility to recurrence (approximately 40 percent) and increased mortality (56 percent) in those with concurrent HIV and evidence of immunosuppression (as measured by a CD4$^+$ T-cell count of less than 200).[7,9]

Prosthetic valve endocarditis (PVE) occurs in 3 to 6 percent of prosthetic valve recipients. Risk for IE is greatest during the initial 6 months after valve surgery and thereafter declines to a lower risk at 0.2 to 0.4 percent per year. No significant difference in risk for IE exists between those with mechanic versus bioprosthetic valves. Cases with onset within 60 days after surgery are called *early PVE* and are usually acquired in the hospital. Cases occurring beyond 60 days post-surgery are called *late PVE* and are usually community acquired. Mortality rates are highest for those with early (30 to 80 percent) versus late PVE (20 to 40 percent) and are largely attributable to the greater virulence of the causative organisms involved.[10]

PATHOPHYSIOLOGY

The normal endothelium is resistant to infection and thrombus formation unless it is injured by high pressure gradients and turbulent flow states. These abnormal hemodynamic states occur most commonly in those with preexisting valvular or congenital cardiac defects. Turbulent blood flow then strikes against the endocardium, ultimately leading to denuding of the endothelium. In IDUs, endothelial damage likely occurs by a different mechanism, as a result of repetitive bombardment with particulate matter (i.e., talc) present in injected material, or as a result of ischemia brought on by vasospasm from the injected drug. Cocaine is known to be particularly associated with increased rates of IE.[11,12] The resultant endothelial damage promotes deposition of platelets and fibrin, which form sterile vegetations called nonbacterial thrombotic endocarditis (NBTE). NBTE can also arise as a result of hypercoagulable states, such as in patients with malignancy (marantic endocarditis) or systemic lupus erythematosus (Libman-Sacks endocarditis), and in areas surrounding foreign bodies, such as intracardiac catheter or prosthetic valves.

In the setting of preexistent NBTE, transient bacteremia may result in colonization of vegetations and ultimately conversion of NBTE to IE. Transient bacteremia can occur from trauma to the skin or mucosal surfaces of the oropharynx or gastrointestinal or genitourinary tracts (all of which are normally laden with endogenous flora). Even in the absence of trauma, however, spontaneous bacteremia can occur in patients with severe periodontal disease or other localized infections. In cases of bacteremia, the bacterial load usually does not exceed 10 organisms per milliliter of blood, and the bloodstream is usually sterilized in less than 30 min. In the presence of NBTE, however, this time interval is believed to be sufficient for bacteria to adhere to the vegetation and transform it into an infected lesion.

The coexistence of bacteremia and NBTE does not uniformly result in IE. In order to cause IE, the infecting organism must be able to adhere to the NBTE on the endothelium. Different organisms vary in this ability based on their intrinsic cellular factors. Furthermore, although NBTE is generally believed to be present in those who develop IE, it not an absolute prerequisite, and highly invasive organisms (e.g., *S. aureus*) can directly invade the endocardium.[11] Adherent organisms stimulate further deposition of platelets and fibrin, leading to sequestration into a "protected site," into which phagocytic cells have difficulty penetrating. Metabolically inactive and nongrowing organisms,

common in IE, also provide relative protection from the bactericidal effects of antibiotics. As the disease progresses, the vegetation continuously fragments, shedding surface organisms into the circulation and resulting in sustained bacteremia.

MICROBIOLOGY

A wide range of bacteria and fungi, as well as *Rickettsia* and *Chlamydia* species can cause endocarditis. Bacteria are the predominant cause overall, with only a small number of species responsible for the majority of cases. Causative microorganisms vary based on the specific conditions (i.e., native versus prosthetic valve) and risk factors (injection drug use) that predispose patients to IE (Table 145-1). *Staphylococcus aureus* is the single most common cause.[13]

Native Valve Endocarditis (Non IDU)

Among non-IDUs with NVE, streptococcus is responsible for more than 50 percent of cases, followed by staphylococci and enterococci.[14] Infection occurs most frequently in those with preexisting valvular abnormalities. Disease course with streptococci-associated IE tends to be indolent.

Staphylococci-associated IE occurs both in patients with previously normal valves and those with known valvular abnormalities. Most are caused by coagulase-positive organisms *(S. aureus)* which cause rapid destruction of valves, multiple distal abscesses, myocardial abscesses, conduction defects, and pericarditis.

Patients with enterococcal endocarditis generally have underlying valvular disease and multiple predisposing abnormalities, most commonly diabetes mellitus. Enterococcal NVE may occur following manipulation of the genitourinary or lower gastrointestinal tract.

Negative culture can occur in approximately 5 percent of patients with IE and in one-third to one-half of these cases cultures are negative because of prior antibiotic exposure.[15] The remainder of cases are caused by infection with fastidious organisms, such as the HACEK group (*Haemophilus, Actinobacillus, Cardiobacterium, Eikenella,* and *Kingella*), *Bartonella* species, or *Coxiella burnetii.* In patients who meet diagnostic criteria for culture-negative IE, the clinician should advise the laboratory of the suspected diagnosis, to allow initiation of specialized testing to recover these fastidious organisms, which is critical for appropriate antimicrobial therapy.

IDU-Associated IE

Skin flora and contaminated injection devices are the most frequent sources of microorganisms involved in IDU-associated IE. *S. aureus* accounts for more than 50 percent of cases, followed in decreasing fre-

TABLE 145-1   Microbiology of Infective Endocarditis

	NATIVE VALVE ENDOCARDITIS (% CASES)			PROSTHETIC VALVE ENDOCARDITIS (% CASES)	
	Nonaddict	IV Drug Addict		Early (<60 d)	Late (>60 d)
Streptococci	55	12	*S. epidermidis*	33	29
Enterococci	5	8	*S. aureus*	15	10
S. aureus	20	57	Streptococci	8	30
S. epidermidis	5	3	Enterococci	2	6
Gram-negative rods	6	7	Gram-negative rods	17	10
Fungus	1	5	Fungi	10	5
Polymicrobial	3	3	Diphtheroids	8	3
Culture negative	5	5	Others	2	2
			Culture negative	5	5

Source: Adapted from Bansal.[14]

quency by streptococcal species (including enterococci), gram-negative bacilli (predominantly *Pseudomonas* and *Serratia* species), and fungi (5 percent, mostly *Candida* species). *S. viridans* is a relatively infrequent cause of IDU-associated IE. Polymicrobial infective endocarditis, although relatively uncommon, is seen most often in association with IDU.

Prosthetic Valve Endocarditis

Microorganisms involved in early PVE most often reflect contamination during the perioperative period, with *S. epidermidis* being the most frequently isolated organism. Early PVE is often associated with valve dysfunction and has a fulminant clinical course. Late PVE has similar bacteriology and clinical manifestations as native valve endocarditis, with streptococcus accounting for 30 percent of cases; disease course tends to be less fulminant. *Aspergillus* and *Candida albicans* account for the majority of cases of mycotic PVE, and are associated with large vegetations and embolic complications.

CLINICAL FEATURES

Classically, the clinical course of IE has been categorized as either acute or subacute. Acute IE is characterized by rapid onset, with high fevers and rigors, hemodynamic deterioration, and death within days to weeks if left untreated. Typically, acute IE has been associated with highly virulent organisms such as *S. aureus*. Subacute IE is characterized by an indolent course with progressive constitutional signs and symptoms and gradual deterioration. Patients often have symptoms for several weeks prior to diagnosis; progression of disease is more insidious and complications may take months to develop. Subacute IE has been generally associated with relatively avirulent organisms such as viridans streptococci. While it is important to be familiar with these traditional distinctions, these terms are less widely utilized today as correlation of disease course with its infecting pathogen has been found to be variable, certain pathogens have been found to cause either form of disease, and classic presentations are rarely encountered. IE can thus better be understood as a continuum, with an understanding of clinical conditions as they relate to the pathophysiologic process and the organ systems that are affected.

Bacteremia

Early bacteremia produces signs and symptoms that are often nonspecific and protean (Table 145-2), usually beginning within 2 weeks of the precipitating infection. The patient with IE often presents to the ED early in the course of the disease, with vague constitutional complaints such as fever, chills, nausea, vomiting, fatigue, and malaise. Fever (>38°C) is present in almost all patients with IE (>90 percent overall, and >98 percent in those with IDU-associated IE). It may be absent, however, in elderly persons or patients with a history of antibiotic or antipyretic use, severe congestive heart failure, or renal failure. Since prevalence of IE among febrile IDUs is extremely high (10 to 15 percent), and it has been well demonstrated that clinical findings are insufficient to reliably exclude the diagnosis of IE in this population, all febrile IDUs should be admitted to evaluate for bacteremia and IE.[16–18] Unexplained fever in a patient with a prosthetic valve should also prompt careful evaluation for PVE, as should prolonged unexplained constitutional symptoms in patients at risk (see section on diagnosis). As the level of bacteremia increases, sepsis ultimately occurs with the usual features of hemodynamic compromise.

Cardiac

Cardiac findings in patients with IE are common and due to local invasion. Heart murmurs are useful if present and are most often regurgitant in nature due to destruction of the valves or adjacent structures

TABLE 145-2 Clinical Features of Infective Endocarditis

Symptoms	Percent	Signs	Percent
Fever	80	Fever	90
Chills	40	Heart murmur	85
Weakness	40	New murmur	3–5
Dyspnea	40	Changing murmur	5–10
Anorexia	25	Skin manifestations	18–50
Cough	25	Osler nodes	10–23
Malaise	25	Splinter hemorrhages	15
Skin lesions	20	Petechiae	20–40
Nausea/vomiting	20	Janeway lesions	<10
Headache	20	Splenomegaly	20–57
Stroke	20	Embolic phenomena	>50
Chest pain	15	Septic complications	20
Abdominal pain	15	Mycotic aneurysm	20
Mental status change	10–15	Renal failure	10
Back pain	10	Retinal lesions	2–10

Source: Adapted from Bayer A, Scheld WM: Endocarditis and intravascular infections, in Mandell GL, Bennett JE, Dolin R (eds): *Principles and Practice of Infectious Diseases.* Philadelphia: Churchill Livingstone, 2000, p. 866.

by enlarging vegetations. While murmurs are reportedly present in up to 85 percent of cases of IE, they may be difficult to detect in the ED. In patients with right-sided IE, less than 50 percent have murmurs detectable on admission.

Acute or progressive congestive heart failure, now the leading cause of death in patients with IE, occurs in up to 70 percent of patients. Causes of CHF include distortion or perforation of valvular leaflets, rupture of the chordae tendineae or papillary muscles, or perforation of cardiac chambers (a devastating but rare complication). Valvular abscesses and pericarditis are caused by local extension of infection into valve rings or the pericardium, respectively. Other important cardiac complications include heart blocks and arrhythmias that result from extension of infection through the interventricular septum to the conduction system.

Embolic

The extracardiac manifestations of IE are usually the result of arterial embolization of fragments of the friable vegetation, and are second to CHF as the leading cause of complications of IE. Embolization to any major artery may occur. Infarcts or abscesses of remote tissues may occur, depending on whether emboli are bland or septic.

Central nervous system complications occur in 20 to 40 percent of cases of IE. Most common is embolic stroke. The middle cerebral artery is affected most frequently, and hemiplegia is a common presentation. Mycotic aneurysms of the cerebral circulation are also relatively frequent. Rupture of the aneurysm results in subarachnoid hemorrhage. Retinal artery emboli may cause acute monocular blindness. Pulmonary complications are most common in IDUs, who are predisposed to right-sided disease, typically involving the tricuspid valve. Clinical manifestations include pulmonary infarction, pneumonia, empyema, or pleural effusion. Coronary artery emboli usually arise from the aortic valve, and may cause acute myocardial infarction, or myocarditis with arrhythmias. Embolic splenic infarction may cause left upper quadrant abdominal pain with radiation to the left shoulder. Patients with suspicious presentations should have an abdominal CT performed. Splenomegaly occurs in up to 60 percent of cases of IE and is usually suggestive of indolent disease. Renal emboli may present with flank pain or hematuria. Emboli lodging in the mesenteric arteries may result in acute abdominal pain and guaiac-positive stool, while those involving arteries of the extremities may produce acute limb ischemia.

Circulating Immune Complexes

The persistent bacteremia of IE stimulates the host humoral and cellular immune systems. This results in circulating immune complexes, which have been detected in virtually all patients. A variety of classic cutaneous and peripheral manifestations have been described in IE as a result of local immune-mediated vasculitis or microemboli. Although common (occurring in greater than 50 percent of cases), they are not specific for IE, and may be seen in other disease states including systemic lupus erythematosus, hemolytic anemia, and gonococcal infections. Petechiae are initially red, nonblanching lesions that become brown after several days and are found in 20 to 40 percent of patients. They occur most frequently on the conjunctivae, buccal mucosa, and extremities. Splinter or subungual hemorrhages appear as linear dark streaks under the fingernails or toenails; they occur in approximately 15 percent of cases, but may also be caused by local nail trauma. Osler's nodes are small, tender subcutaneous nodules that develop on the pads of the fingers or toes. They are found in up to 25 percent of cases, but usually disappear within hours or days. Janeway lesions are small hemorrhagic painless plaques located on the palms or soles. Roth spots are oval retinal hemorrhages with pale centers located near the optic disc. Digital clubbing is an infrequent finding and usually found only in those with longstanding disease. Immune complex deposition may also occur along the glomerular basement membrane, resulting in the development of focal or diffuse glomerulonephritis. Renal insufficiency and azotemia are resulting complications.

DIAGNOSIS

From the standpoint of the emergency physician, diagnosis of infective endocarditis still requires hospitalization, as results from the cornerstone components of the current diagnostic criteria (culture, echocardiography, and clinical observation) require time to accrue. Studies that have attempted to establish prediction rules for identification of patients with IE in acute care settings have failed.[17] All patients in whom the suspicion for IE exists (see below) should therefore be admitted and evaluated using the diagnostic criteria described below.[16-18]

Diagnostic Criteria

The Duke criteria are now the most widely utilized scheme for diagnosing IE.[19] Application of the criteria requires gathering critical diagnostic data (i.e., blood culture results, echocardiographic and clinical findings, and determination of the presence of recognized risk factors for disease) which compromise major or minor Criteria (Table 145-3). As a second step, specific combinations of these criteria are used to assign a final diagnostic category of definite, possible, or rejected IE (Table 145-4). Sensitivity of the Duke criteria is about 90 percent, although investigations continue in an attempt to improve specificity.[20]

Pilot studies provide promising data indicating that immediate echocardiography combined with 24-h blood culture results may provide comparable sensitivity and specificity relative to the Duke criteria for the evaluation of febrile IDUs.[21] However, these studies are ongoing and will require validation. Current recommendations are to admit all patients in whom IE is suspected for formal evaluation.

Differential Diagnosis and Consideration of IE

The differential diagnosis is extremely broad and includes viral illnesses, HIV-related fevers, acute rheumatic fever, systemic complications of collagen vascular disorders, drug reactions, and many other disorders. Endocarditis should be considered in all patients with known risk factors and/or unexplained febrile illnesses. General recommendations regarding decision making are: (1) all febrile IDUs with fever should be admitted because of the high incidence of disease (up to 15 percent) and noncompliance with outpatient follow-up; (2) patients with a cardiac prosthesis and fever (or persistent malaise, vasculitis, or new murmur) should be hospitalized due to increased risk of IE and the high morbidity and mortality associated with prosthetic valve infections; (3) patients with a new murmur or change in murmur with evidence of vasculitis or embolization should be admitted. Explicit admission guidelines are less clear for others, but the diagnosis

TABLE 145-3   Definitions of Major and Minor Criteria Used in the Duke Criteria*

Major criteria
Positive blood culture for IE
  Typical microorganism consistent with IE from two separate blood cultures* as noted below:
    Streptoccocus bovis, Viridans streptococci, HACEK group, *or*
    Community-acquired *Staphyloccocus aureus* or enterococci in the absence of a primary focus, *or*
  Microorganisms consistent with IE from persistently positive blood cultures defined as:
    At least two positive cultures of blood samples drawn >12 h apart, *or*
    All of three or a majority of four or more separate blood cultures (with first and last sample drawn at least 12 h apart)
Evidence of echocardiographic involvement
  Positive echocardiogram for IE defined as:
    Oscillating intracardiac mass on valve or supporting structures, in the path of regurgitant jets, or on implanted material in the absence of
      an alternative anatomic explanation, *or*
    Abscess, *or*
    New partial dehiscence of prosthetic valve
  New valvular regurgitation (worsening or changing of preexisting murmur not sufficient)
Minor criteria
Predisposition: predisposing heart condition or injection drug use
Fever: temperature >38°C
Vascular phenomena: major arterial emboli, septic pulmonary conjunctival hemorrhages, and Janeway lesions
Immunologic phhenomena: glomerulonephritis, Osler nodes, Roth spots, and rheumatoid fever
Microbiologic evidence: positive blood culture but does not meet a major criterion as noted in Table 145-4* or serologic evidence of active infection
  with organism consistent with IE
Echocardiographic findings: consistent with IE but do not meet a major criterion as noted in Table 145-4

*Excludes single positive cultures for coagulase-negative staphylococci and organisms that do not cause IE.
Abbreviations: HACEK = *Haemophilus, Actinobacillus, Cardiobacterium, Eikenella, and Kingella;* IE = infective endocarditis.
Source: From Durack et al.[19]

TABLE 145-4   Definitions of Infective Endocarditis According to the Duke Criteria

Definite infective endocarditis
    Pathologic criteria
        Microorganisms demonstrated by culture or histologic examination of a vegetation or in a vegetation that has embolized, or in an intracardiac abscess, *or*
        Pathologic lesions: vegetation or intracardiac abscess present, confirmed by histology showing active endocarditis
    Clinical criteria, using specific definitions listed in Table 145-2
        Two major criteria, *or*
        One major and three minor criteria, *or*
        Five minor criteria.
Possible infective endocarditis
    Findings consistent with infective endocarditis, that fall short of "definite," but not "rejected."
Rejected
    1. Firm alternate diagnosis for manifestations of endocarditis, *or*
    2. Resolution of manifestations of endocarditis, with antibiotic therapy for 4 d or less, *or*
    3. No pathologic evidence of infective endocarditis at surgery or autopsy after antibiotic therapy for 4 d

must be strongly considered in patients with any other known cardiac risk factor presenting with unexplained febrile illness or systemic complaints, as well as any patient with a prolonged (>2 weeks) unexplained fever.

Evaluation of Bacteremia (Culture and PCR)

All patients with suspected IE should have blood cultures drawn in the ED prior to initiation of antibiotic therapy. Blood cultures should be drawn from three separate sites. Since low-grade bacteremia is known to be common in patients with IE, it is recommended that a minimum of 10 mL of blood be used for each bottle. Additional sets of blood cultures have been shown to be useful in patients already receiving antibiotics. It is recommended that there be at least 1 h between the first and last blood culture. However, for those patients who are ill-appearing or have any evidence of systemic complications, antibiotics should not be withheld to await retrieval of delayed sets of cultures.

Polymerase chain reaction (PCR) techniques are currently under evaluation for the more rapid diagnosis of infective endocarditis.[22,23]

Other Diagnostic Tests

An ECG should be done in all patients with suspected IE. Although usually nonspecific, important conduction abnormalities may be uncovered that indicate extension of the infection. Prolonged PR interval, new left bundle-branch block, or new right bundle-branch block with left anterior hemiblock suggest spread of infection from the aortic valve into the conduction system. Junctional tachycardia, Wenckebach block, or complete heart block in the setting of suspected IE indicate likely extension of infection from the mitral annulus into the AV node or proximal bundle of His. If these are uncovered, cardiology and cardiothoracic surgery should be consulted, as urgent or emergent surgery may be indicated. Chest radiographs should be obtained as they may reveal other complications, such as pulmonic emboli in patients with right-sided valvular involvement or congestive heart failure in those with left-sided IE.

There are no definitive laboratory tests that can be used to make the diagnosis of IE in the acute care setting. Laboratory abnormalities that are strongly associated with IE but are relatively nonspecific include anemia (70 to 90 percent of cases), elevated erythrocyte sedimentation rate, (>90 percent of cases), and hematuria.

Echocardiography

Echocardiography should be performed on all patients in whom the diagnosis of IE is under consideration for the following reasons: (1) echocardiographic abnormalities comprise one of the two major criteria required for definitive diagnosis of IE; (2) evaluation of the cardiac valve and its surrounding structures provides critical information regarding valvular function and associated complications, data which

are important for guiding management decisions. Most hospitals defer imaging to the inpatient unit since all patients with suspected IE should be admitted. However, for any patient with evidence of significant cardiovascular compromise, imaging should be obtained emergently.

Transthoracic two-dimensional (2-D) echocardiography (TTE) is rapid and noninvasive and should be the first choice of imaging for those with native valves in whom good quality images can be obtained. Specificity for vegetations is excellent (98 percent). However, sensitivity varies according to population. It is highest among IDUs (88 to 94 percent), who more often have larger vegetations, a preponderance of right-sided lesions, and a favorable acoustic precordial window characteristic of younger patients. For those with chest wall deformities, obesity, or chronic obstructive pulmonary disease (COPD), sensitivity is diminished. Transesophageal echocardiography (TEE) is invasive, requiring more time and skill than TTE. Sensitivity and specificity (for any valvular abnormalities) are significantly higher than for TTE, due to improved image resolution. TEE is recommended in the following patient populations with suspected IE: (1) patients with prosthetic valves; (2) those in whom inadequate images are likely to be obtained with TTE as described above; and (3) those with intermediate or high clinical probability of IE (an assessment which is difficult to make and usually not feasible in the ED). While rarely indicated in the ED, TEE is of particular value for assessment of the complications associated with IE, such as myocardial abscess and perivalvular extension.

TREATMENT AND PROPHYLAXIS

Initial Stabilization

Patients with endocarditis may present with respiratory compromise due to decreased cardiac output (secondary to valvular defects), diminished pulmonary capacity (due to pulmonary emboli), altered mental status, or acidosis (related to CNS emboli and/or sepsis). In such cases rapid airway stabilization, including endotracheal intubation, is indicated.

Valvular rupture may present with acute cardiac decompensation. Rupture of left-sided valves more commonly results in cardiac decompensation, and should be managed with afterload reduction. Intraaortic balloon counterpulsation (IABP) may be indicated for the emergent management of unstable mitral valve rupture. However, the use of IABP is contraindicated for aortic valve rupture.

Neurologic complications, including stroke, should be managed with standard protocols, in addition to definitive therapy for endocarditis.

Empiric Treatment of Suspected Endocarditis of Native Valves

Empiric antibiotic therapy should be initiated promptly for suspected acute endocarditis. There is not complete agreement in the literature

TABLE 145-5 Empiric Therapy of Suspected Bacterial Endocarditis*

Patient Characteristics	Recommended Agents	Initial Dose
Uncomplicated history	Ceftriaxone	1–2 g IV
	or nafcillin	2 g IV
	plus gentamycin	1–3 mg/kg IV
Injection drug use, congenital heart disease, hospital-acquired, suspected MRSA, or already on oral antibiotics	Nafcillin	2 g IV
	plus gentamycin	1–3 mg/kg IV
	plus vancomycin	15 mg/kg IV
Prosthetic heart valve	Vancomycin	15 mg/kg IV
	plus gentamycin	1–3 mg/kg IV
	plus rifampin	300 mg PO

*Because of controversy in the literature regarding the optimal regimen for empiric treatment, antibiotic selection should be based on patient characteristics, local resistance patterns, and current authoritative recommendations.

regarding specific antibiotic selection. Antibiotic selection should be based on patient characteristics and local resistance patterns. Table 145-5 lists some sample empiric treatment regimens based on current recommendations.[24–26] Although some authors recommend awaiting culture results prior to antibiotic therapy for patients with subacute bacterial endocarditis,[27] we recommend prompt ED initiation of antibiotic therapy for all patients suspected of endocarditis. For patients with suspected native valve infection, empiric antibiotic therapy may include a penicillinase-resistant penicillin or a cephalosporin *and* an aminoglycoside. For patients with complications (including injection drug use, congenital heart disease, those who develop endocarditis while taking oral antibiotics, nosocomial infections, or those with suspected methicillin-resistant *S. aureus*), vancomycin should be added to the treatment regimen.

Empiric Treatment of Suspected Endocarditis of Artificial Valves

For patients with suspected artificial valve endocarditis, empiric therapy should include vancomycin, an aminoglycoside, and rifampin.

Definitive Antibiotic Treatment of Endocarditis

Definitive antibiotic treatment should be based on culture and sensitivity results. Selection of the most appropriate antibiotics and treatment duration should be undertaken in consultation with the primary care physician, and if appropriate, an infectious disease consultant. Most patients will require 4 to 6 weeks of antibiotic therapy. Certain

patients may be managed successfully with outpatient parenteral antibiotic therapy following definitive diagnosis of certain pathogens.[28]

Surgical Treatment

Surgical management of endocarditis may be indicated in patients with severe valvular dysfunction, such as acute congestive heart failure or impaired hemodynamic status. The presence of large vegetations does not necessarily indicate a need for surgical intervention. Surgical intervention may also be indicated in patients with relapsing prosthetic valve endocarditis, major embolic complications, fungal endocarditis, new conduction defects or arrhythmias resultant from infection, or persistent bacteremia after appropriate antibiotic therapy. Prompt surgical consultation is indicated in patients who may be surgical candidates.[29,30]

Anticoagulation

Anticoagulation for native valve endocarditis has not been shown to be beneficial.[9] Additionally, anticoagulation may significantly increase the risk of intracranial hemorrhage. Patients with prosthetic valves who are treated at baseline with anticoagulants may be cautiously maintained on established regimens, with particular caution for central nervous system complications.

Prophylaxis

Antibiotic prophylaxis against endocarditis should be administered for patients with risk factors for endocarditis, including prosthetic heart valves, congenital cardiac malformations, acquired valvular dysfunction, hypertrophic cardiomyopathy, mitral valve prolapse with documented regurgitation, or a history of endocarditis. Prophylaxis is not routinely indicated for patients with mitral valve prolapse without regurgitation, pacemakers, physiologic murmurs, prior coronary artery bypass surgery or angioplasty, or previous surgical repair of atrial septal defect, ventricular septal defect, or patent ductus arteriosus.

Although there is some controversy regarding which procedures warrant endocarditis prophylaxis, current recommendations include dental work (including cleaning), bronchoscopy, cystoscopy, urethral instrumentation, and endoscopic retrograde cholangiopancreatography. Prophylaxis is not indicated for local injections, laceration suturing, intravenous line placement, blood drawing, endotracheal intubation, endoscopy, vaginal delivery, urethral catheterization, or uterine dilation and curettage.

Current recommendations for endocarditis prophylaxis include stratification into high-, moderate-, and low-risk populations.[31–33] A simplified strategy is listed in Table 145-6.

TABLE 145-6 Prophylaxis Against Endocarditis for High-Risk Patients

Procedure	Antibiotic Agent	Dose
Dental/oral/respiratory/esophageal procedures	Amoxicillin	2 g PO, 1 h before procedure
	or Ampicillin	2 g IM or IV, 30 min before procedure
	or Clindamycin	600 mg PO, 1 h before procedure, or 600 mg IV, 30 min before procedure
	or Azithromycin	500 mg PO, 1 h before procedure
Genitourinary/gastrointestinal procedures	Ampicillin	2 g IM or IV, 30 min before procedure
	plus Gentamycin	1.5 mg/kg IM or IV, 30 min before procedure
	plus Ampicillin	1 g IV or IV, 6 h after procedure
	or Amoxicillin	1 g PO, 6 h after procedure
	Alternative regimen: Vancomycin	1 g IV over 1–2 h, completed 30 min before procedure
	plus Gentamycin	1.5 mg/kg IV or IM, within 30 min of procedure

REFERENCES

1. Cabel CH, Abrutyn E: Progress toward a global understanding of infective endocarditis. Early lessons from the International Collaboration on Endocarditis investigation. *Infect Dis Clin North Am* 16:255, 2002.
2. Berlin JA, Abrutyn E, Strom BL, et al: Incidence of infective endocarditis in the Delaware Valley, 1988–1990. *Am J Cardiol* 76:933, 1995.
3. Hogevik H, Olaison L, Andersson R, et al: Epidemiologic aspects of infective endocarditis in an urban population: A 5-year prospective study. *Medicine* 74:324, 1995.
4. Hoen B, Alla F, Selton-Suty C: Changing profile of infective endocarditis. *JAMA* 288:75, 2002.
5. Watanakunakorn C, Burkert T: IE at a large community teaching hospital 1980: A review of 210 episodes. *Medicine* 72:90, 1993.
6. Sandre RM, Shafran SD: IE: Review of 135 cases over 9 years. *Clin Infect Dis* 22:27, 1996.
7. Miro JM, Rio A, Mestres CA: Infective endocarditis in intravenous drug abusers and HIV-1 infected patients. *Infect Dis Clin North Am.* 16:273, 2002.
8. Hasbun R, Bikram HR, Barakat LA, et al: Complicated left-sided native valve endocarditis in adults: Risk classification for mortality. *JAMA* 289:1933, 2003.
9. Pulverenti J, Kerns E, Benson C, et al: IE in injection drug users: Importance of human immunodeficiency virus serostatus and degree of immunosuppression. *Clin Infect Dis* 22:40, 1996.
10. Vongpatanasin W, Hillis L, Lange R: Prosthetic heart valves. *New Engl J Med* 335:407, 1996.
11. Frontera JA, Gradon JD: Right-side endocarditis in injection drug users: Review of proposed mechanisms of pathogenesis. *Clin Infect Dis* 30: 374, 2000.
12. Brown PD, Levine DP: Infective endocarditis in the injection drug user. *Infect Dis Clin North Am* 16:645, 2002.
13. Mylonakis E, Calderwood SB: Infective endocarditis in adults. *New Engl J Med* 345:1318, 2001.
14. Bansal RC: Infective endocarditis. *Med Clin North Am* 79:1205, 1995.
15. Barnes PD, Crook DWM: Culture negative endocarditis. *J Infect* 35:209, 1997.
16. Samet JH, Shevitz A, Flower J, et al: Hospitalization decision in febrile intravenous drug users. *Am J Med* 89:53, 1990.
17. Young GP, Hedges JR, Dixon L, et al: Inability to validate a predictive score for IE in febrile intravenous drug users. *J Emerg Med* 11:1, 1993.
18. Weisse AB, Heller DR, Schimenti RJ, et al: The febrile parenteral drug users: A prospective study in 121 patients. *Am J Med* 94:274, 1993.
19. Durack DT, Lukes AS, Bright DK: New criteria for diagnosis of infective endocarditis: utilization of specific echocardiographic findings. Duke Endocarditis Service. *Am J Med* 96:200, 1994.
20. Li JS, Sexton DJ, Mick N, et al: Proposed modifications to the Duke criteria for the diagnosis of infective endocarditis. *Clin Infect Dis* 30:633, 2000.
21. Majmudar MD, Kelen GD, Rothman RE: Defining new criteria for the diagnosis of infective endocarditis (IE) in febrile intravenous drug users (IDUs): A new gold standard for the acute care setting? *Acad Emerg Med* 7:561, 2000.
22. Libsy G, Gutschik E, Durack DT: Molecular methods for diagnosis of infective endocarditis. *Infect Dis Clin North Am* 16:393, 2002.
23. Rothman RE, Majmudar MD, Kelen GD, et al: Detection of bacteremia in emergency department patients at risk for infective endocarditis using universal 16S rRNA primers in a decontaminated polymerase chain reaction assay. *J Infect Dis* 186:1677, 2002.
24. Wilson WR, Karchmer AW, Dajani AS, et al: Antibiotic treatment of adults with infective endocarditis due to streptococci, enterococci, staphylococci, and HACEK microorganisms. *JAMA* 274:1706, 1995.
25. Slovis SM, Roberts RR: Infectious endocarditis, in Harwood-Nuss A, Wolfson AB (eds): *The Clinical Practice of Emergency Medicine.* Philadelphia, Lippincott Williams & Wilkins, 2001, pp. 710–716.
26. Alestig K, Hogevik H, Olaison L: Infective endocarditis: A diagnostic and therapeutic challenge for the new millennium. *Scand J Infect Dis* 32: 343, 2000.
27. Eykyn SJ: Endocarditis; basics. *Heart* 86:476, 2001.
28. Andrews MM, von Reyn CF: Patient selection criteria and management guidelines for outpatient parenteral antibiotic therapy for native valve infective endocarditis. *Clin Infect Dis* 33:203, 2001.
29. Chamoun AJ, Conti V, Lenihan DJ: Native valve infective endocarditis: What is the optimal timing for surgery? *Am J Med Sci* 320:255, 2000.
30. Ferguson E, Reardon MF, Letsou GV: The surgical management of bacterial valvular endocarditis. *Curr Opin Cardiol* 15:82, 2000.
31. Dajani AS, Taubert KA, Wilson W, et al: Prevention of bacterial endocarditis: Recommendations by the American Heart Association. *JAMA* 277:1794, 1997.
32. http:www.americanheart.org/ and http://216.185.112.5/presenter.jhtml?identifier=1745, accessed 11/21/02.
33. Osmon DR: Antimicrobial prophylaxis in adults. *Mayo Clin Proc* 75:98, 2000.

TETANUS
Donna L. Carden

EPIDEMIOLOGY

Tetanus is an uncommon disease in the United States but continues to have a substantial global health impact. The worldwide incidence of tetanus approaches 1 million cases per year. Tetanus is associated with a mortality rate of 20 to 50 percent and at least half of these deaths occur in neonates. The prevalence of tetanus is highest in developing countries where it is among the ten most frequent causes of death and an important cause of infant mortality.[1]

The institution of widespread immunization programs for children, routine boosters in adults, mechanization of agriculture, and use of chemical fertilizers rather than animal manure has resulted in a decline in the average annual incidence of tetanus in the United States to fewer than 50 cases per year.[2] In the United States, the majority of tetanus occurs in temperate areas, such as Texas, California, and Florida,[2] and is associated with a mortality rate of approximately 11 percent. Most patients who develop tetanus have an inadequate immunization history.[2] Only 27 percent of Americans older than age 70 years have adequate immunity to tetanus.[3]

The majority of patients diagnosed with tetanus who sought medical care for their initial injury did not receive adequate tetanus prophylaxis.[2] Heroin abusers, especially those who inject themselves subcutaneously, are at increased risk of contracting tetanus.[4]

PATHOPHYSIOLOGY

Tetanus is an acute, often fatal disease caused by wound contamination with *Clostridium tetani,* a motile, nonencapsulated anaerobic grampositive rod. *C. tetani* exists in either a vegetative or a spore-forming state. The spores are ubiquitous in soil and in animal feces and are extremely resistant to destruction, surviving on environmental surfaces for years. *C. tetani* is usually introduced into a wound in the spore-forming, noninvasive state but can germinate into a toxin-producing, vegetative form if tissue oxygen tension is reduced. Factors such as the presence of crushed, devitalized tissue, a foreign body, or the development of infection, favor the growth of the vegetative, toxin-producing form of *C. tetani.*[5]

Once converted into the vegetative form, *C. tetani* produces two exotoxins: tetanolysin, which appears to be clinically insignificant, and tetanospasmin, a powerful neurotoxin that is responsible for the clinical manifestations of tetanus. Although the infection caused by *C. tetani* remains localized to the site of injury, tetanospasmin reaches the nervous system by hematogenous spread of the exotoxin to peripheral nerves and by retrograde intraneuronal transport. Blood-borne tetanospasmin does not cross the blood-brain barrier, but retrograde intraneuronal transport of the exotoxin enables tetanospasmin to gain access to the central nervous system.[1]

Tetanospasmin acts on the motor end plates of skeletal muscle, in the spinal cord, in the brain, and in the sympathetic nervous system.

This extremely potent exotoxin prevents the release of the inhibitory neurotransmitters glycine and γ-aminobutyric acid (GABA) from presynaptic nerve terminals, releasing the nervous system from its normal inhibitory control. Loss of inhibition may also affect the preganglionic sympathetic neurons resulting in sympathetic overactivity and high circulating catecholamine levels.[6]

CLINICAL FEATURES

The exotoxin tetanospasmin is responsible for the clinical manifestations of generalized muscular rigidity, violent muscular contractions, and instability of the autonomic nervous system. Wounds that become infected with toxin-producing *C. tetani* are most often puncture wounds,[2] but vary widely in severity from deep lacerations to minor abrasions.[2,5] However, a wound cannot be identified in up to 10 percent of patients with tetanus. Tetanus can also develop after surgical procedures, otitis media, and abortion, and can develop in neonates through infection of the umbilical stump and in drug abusers.

The incubation period ranges from less than 24 h to more than 1 month. The shorter the incubation period, the more severe the disease and the worse the prognosis for recovery.[1]

Clinical tetanus can be categorized into four forms: local, generalized, cephalic, and neonatal. The different categories of clinical tetanus depend on what population of neurons are involved.

Local tetanus is manifested by rigidity of muscles in proximity to the site of injury and usually resolves completely after weeks to months. Local tetanus may progress to the generalized form of the disease.

Generalized tetanus is the most common form of the disease.[2] The most frequent presenting complaints of patients with generalized tetanus are pain and stiffness in the masseter muscles (lockjaw).[7] Nerves with short axons are affected initially; therefore, symptoms appear first in the facial muscles, with progression to the neck, trunk, and extremities.[7] The transition from muscle stiffness to rigidity leads to the development of trismus and the resultant characteristic facial expression: risus sardonicus (sardonic smile) (Figure 146-1). Reflex convulsive spasms and tonic muscle contractions are responsible for the development of dysphasia, opisthotonos (Figure 146-2), flexing of the arms, clenching of the fists, and extension of the lower extremities. Patients are conscious and alert unless laryngospasm or contraction of respiratory muscles results in respiratory compromise.

Disturbances of the autonomic nervous system, generally a hypersympathetic state, occur during the second week of clinical tetanus and

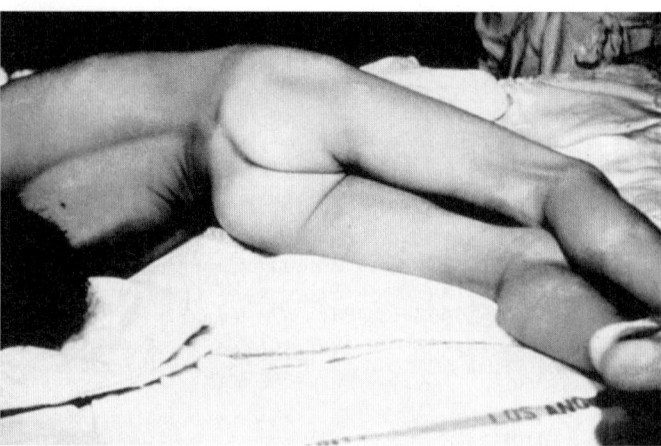

FIG. 146-2. *Opisthotonos* of tetanus. (Photograph reproduced with permission from the Immunization Action Coalition, St. Paul, MN.)

present as tachycardia, labile hypertension, profuse sweating, hyperpyrexia, and increased urinary excretion of catecholamines.[8] The autonomic complications of generalized tetanus are difficult to manage and contribute significantly to morbidity and mortality.

Cephalic tetanus follows injuries to the head or occasionally otitis media and results in dysfunction of the cranial nerves, most commonly the seventh. It has a poor prognosis.

Neonatal tetanus is responsible for more than 400,000 deaths worldwide per year. It develops in children born to inadequately immunized mothers, frequently after unsterile treatment of the umbilical cord stump. Infants with neonatal tetanus present with weakness, irritability, and an inability to suck during the second week of life.[1]

DIAGNOSIS

Tetanus is diagnosed solely on the basis of clinical evidence. Most patients who develop the disease have an unknown or inadequate immunization history.[2] There are no laboratory tests to diagnose tetanus, although serum antitoxin titers of >0.01 IU/mL are usually protective and may be helpful retrospectively. Wound culture is of limited value, because *C. tetani* may be cultured from wounds in the absence of clinical disease and may not be recovered in patients with documented tetanus.[5]

Table 146-1 presents the differential diagnosis of tetanus. Strychnine poisoning most closely mimics the clinical picture of generalized tetanus.

TREATMENT

Patients with tetanus should be managed in an intensive care unit. Respiratory compromise requires immediate neuromuscular blockade and orotracheal intubation. Environmental stimuli must be minimized to prevent the precipitation of reflex convulsive spasms.

The initial wound should be identified and dèbrided to improve the oxidation-reduction potential of the infected tissue and to prevent further toxin production.

TABLE 146-1   Differential Diagnosis of Tetanus

Strychnine poisoning
Dystonic reaction (phenothiazines, metoclopramide)
Hypocalcemic tetany
Peritonsillar abscess
Peritonitis
Meningeal irritation (bacterial meningitis, subarachnoid hemorrhage)
Rabies
Temporomandibular joint disease

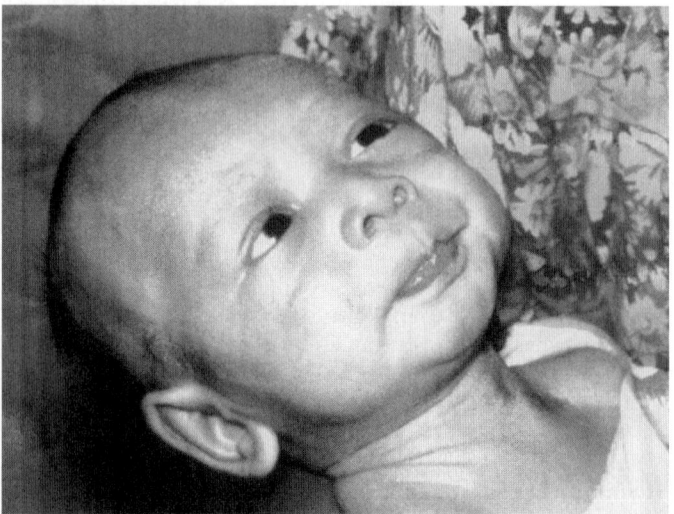

FIG. 146-1. *Risus sardonicus* (sardonic smile) of tetanus. (Photograph reproduced with permission from the Immunization Action Coalition, St. Paul, MN.)

Tetanus Immunoglobulin

Human tetanus immunoglobulin (TIG) neutralizes circulating tetanospasmin and toxin in the wound but not toxin that is already fixed in the nervous system. Even though TIG does not ameliorate the clinical symptoms of tetanus, it significantly reduces mortality.[9] Although the optimal dose of TIG is unknown, 3000 to 6000 units is the usual recommended dose, administered IM opposite the site of tetanus toxoid administration. **It should be given before wound debridement, because exotoxin may be released during wound manipulation.** Repeated doses of TIG are unnecessary, because the half-life of the antitoxin is 28 days.[7]

Antibiotics

Antibiotics are of questionable utility but are traditionally administered. Parenterally administered metronidazole is the antibiotic of choice.[10] Penicillin, a centrally acting GABAA antagonist may potentiate the effects of tetanospasmin, thus its use should be avoided.[1]

Muscle Relaxants

Tetanospasmin prevents neurotransmitter release at inhibitory interneurons, and therapy of tetanus is aimed at restoring normal inhibition. The benzodiazepines are centrally acting inhibitory agents that have been used extensively for this purpose. However, the large intravenous doses of benzodiazepines required in tetanus may result in metabolic acidosis secondary to the propylene glycol vehicle. Thus, the water-soluble agent, midazolam, is the preferred agent for producing muscle relaxation in patients with tetanus.[7] Other drugs, such as baclofen, a specific GABAB agonist, have been used to treat tetanus-induced muscle spasms.[11]

Neuromuscular Blockade

To control ventilation and muscular spasms as well as to prevent fractures and rhabdomyolysis, prolonged neuromuscular blockade may be required in the treatment of tetanus. Succinylcholine is recommended for emergency airway control, while vecuronium is the neuromuscular blocking agent of choice for prolonged blockade because of minimal cardiovascular side effects.[12] Concomitant sedation with narcotics, barbiturates, or benzodiazepines is mandatory.

Treatment of Autonomic Dysfunction

Labetalol, the combined α- and β-adrenergic blocking agent, is useful in treating the manifestations of sympathetic hyperactivity of tetanus.

Short-acting β-blockers such as esmolol may be advantageous in cases where β-blockade alone is associated with severe hypertension from unopposed α-adrenergic stimulation. Adrenergic-blocking drugs, although effective in the treatment of the autonomic dysfunction of tetanus, may precipitate myocardial depression or sudden death if sympathetic activity transiently diminishes.[13,14]

Magnesium sulfate inhibits the release of epinephrine and norepinephrine from the adrenal glands and adrenergic nerve terminals, eliminating the source of catecholamine excess in tetanus.[15] Morphine sulfate reduces sympathetic α-adrenergic tone and central sympathetic efferent discharge and produces peripheral arteriolar and venous dilatation.[7]

Clonidine, a central α-receptor agonist, has also been used to manage tetanus-induced cardiovascular instability. Continuous epidural block with bupivacaine has been suggested but may be difficult to administer and manage.

Active Immunization

Patients who recover from tetanus must undergo active immunization, because the disease does not confer immunity. Adsorbed tetanus toxoid (0.5 mL) should be administered IM at the time of presentation and at 6 weeks and 6 months after injury. Tetanus-diphtheria (Td) should be administered to patients older than 7 years of age,[16] and diphtheria-pertussis-tetanus (DPT) should be administered to patients younger than 7 years of age.[17] Tetanus immunization should be administered to unimmunized or inadequately immunized pregnant women. Table 146-2 summarizes the guidelines for active tetanus immunization and Table 146-3 summarizes the management of tetanus.

Adverse reactions following tetanus immunization include local adverse events such as erythema, induration, and pain at the injection site. Local reactions are common and usually self-limited. Exaggerated local reactions occur occasionally following tetanus toxoid and involve extensive pain and swelling of the entire extremity. Exaggerated local reactions occur most often in adults with high serum tetanus antitoxin levels who have received frequent doses of tetanus toxoid. These patients should not receive tetanus toxoid more frequently than every 10 years. Severe systemic reactions to tetanus immunization include generalized urticaria, anaphylaxis, or neurologic complications, including peripheral neuropathy and Guillain-Barré syndrome. A severe allergic reaction including acute respiratory distress or cardiovascular collapse following a previous dose of tetanus toxoid is a contraindication to further immunization. A moderate or severe acute illness is also a reason to defer routine immunization although a minor illness is not. If tetanus toxoid is contraindicated, passive immunization with TIG against tetanus should be considered.[18]

TABLE 146-2   Summary Guide to Tetanus Prophylaxis in Wound Management

History of Adsorbed Tetanus Toxoid (Doses)	CLEAN, MINOR WOUNDS		ALL OTHER WOUNDS*	
	Td† 0.5 mL IM	TIG, 250 U IM	Td† 0.5 mL IM	TIG, 250 U IM
Unknown or less than three	Yes‡	No	Yes	Yes
Three or more§	No¶	No	Yes**	No

*For example, wounds >6 h old, contaminated with soil, saliva, feces, or dirt; puncture or crush wounds; avulsions; wounds from missiles, burns, or frostbite.
†DPT for children <7 years of age (DT if pertussis vaccine is contraindicated); Td for persons >7 years of age.
‡The primary immunization series should be completed. Three doses total are required, with the second dose given at least 4 weeks after the first and the third dose 6 months later.
§If only three doses of fluid toxoid have been received, then a fourth dose of *absorbed* toxoid should be given.
¶Yes, if routine immunization schedule has lapsed in a child <7 years of age or if >10 years since last dose.
**Yes, if routine immunization schedule has lapsed in a child <7 years of age or if >5 years since last dose. Boosters more frequent than every 5 years may predispose to side effects.
Abbreviations: DPT = diphtheria-pertussis-tetanus; DT = diphtheria-tetanus toxoids; Td = tetanus-diphtheria; TIG = tetanus immunoglobulin.
Source: Adapted from the American College of Emergency Physicians,[16,17] with permission.

TABLE 146-3   Treatment of Tetanus

Respiratory management	Succinylcholine for emergency intubation; vecuronium for prolonged neuromuscular blockade
Immunotherapy	TIG ≥ 500 U IM as a single dose *and*
	Tetanus toxoid (DPT or Td depending on age), 0.5 mL IM at presentation, and 6 weeks and 6 months after presentation
Antibiotic therapy	Metronidazole, 500 mg IV every 6 h
Muscle relaxation	Midazolam, 5–15 mg/h continuous IV infusion *or*
	Lorazepam, 2 mg IV to effect *or*
	Diazepam, 5 mg IV every 1–3 h to effect
Neuromuscular blockade	Vecuronium, 6–8 mg per h IV
Management of autonomic dysfunction	Labetalol, 0.25–1.0 mg per min continuous IV infusion *or*
	Magnesium sulfate, 70 mg/kg IV loading, then 1–4 g per h continuous infusion to maintain blood level of 2.5–4 mmol/L
	Morphine sulfate, 0.5–1.0 mg/kg per h
	Clonidine, 300 μg every 8 h by nasogastric tube

REFERENCES

1. Bleck TP: *Clostridium tetani* (tetanus), in Mandell GL, Bennett JG, Dolin R, et al (eds): *Principles and Practice of Infectious Diseases,* 5th ed. New York, Churchill Livingstone, 2000, pp. 2537–2543.

2. Bardenheier B, Prevots DR, Khetsurian N, et al: Tetanus: Surveillance—United States, 1995–1997. *MMWR* 47(SS-2):1, 1998.

3. Gergen PJ, McQuillan GM, Kiely M, et al: A population-based serologic survey of immunity to tetanus in the United States. *New Engl J Med* 332: 761, 1995.

4. Centers for Disease Control and Prevention: Tetanus among injecting-drug-users-California, 1997. *MMWR* 47:149, 1998.

5. Kefer MP: Tetanus. *Am J Emerg Med* 10:445, 1992.

6. Mellanby J, Green J: How does tetanus toxin act? *Neuroscience* 6:281, 1981.

7. Ernst ME, Klepser ME, Fouts M, et al: Tetanus: Pathophysiology and management. *Ann Pharmacother* 31:1507, 1997.

8. Wright DK, Lalloo UG, Nayiager S, et al: Autonomic nervous system dysfunction in severe tetanus: Current perspectives. *Crit Care Med* 17:371, 1989.

9. Blake PA, Feldman TM, Buchanan TM, et al: Serologic therapy of tetanus in the United States, 1965–1971. *JAMA* 235:42, 1976.

10. Ahmadsyah I, Salim A: Treatment of tetanus: An open study to compare the efficacy of procaine penicillin and metronidazole. *Br Med J* 291:648, 1985.

11. Muller H, Borner U, Zierski J, et al: Intrathecal baclofen for treatment of tetanus-induced spasticity. *Anesthesiology* 66:76, 1987.

12. Powles AB, Ganta R: Use of vecuronium in the management of tetanus. *Anaesthesia* 40:879, 1985.

13. Buchanan N, Smit L, Cane RD, De Andrade M: Sympathetic overactivity in tetanus: Fatality associated with propranolol. *Br Med J* 2:254, 1978.

14. Southern PA, Blaise GA: Treatment of tetanus-induced autonomic nervous system dysfunction with continuous epidural blockade. *Crit Care Med* 14:251, 1986.

15. James MF, Manson ED: The use of magnesium sulfate infusions in the management of very severe tetanus. *Intensive Care Med* 11:5, 1985.

16. American College of Emergency Physicians, Scientific Review Committee: Tetanus immunization recommendations for persons seven years of age and older. *Ann Emerg Med* 15:1111, 1986.

17. American College of Emergency Physicians, Scientific Review Committee: Tetanus immunization recommendations for persons less than seven years old. *Ann Emerg Med* 16:1181, 1987.

18. Plotkin SA, Orenstein, WA (eds): *Vaccines,* 3rd ed. Philadelphia: WB Saunders, 1999.

147 RABIES

David J. Weber
David A. Wohl
William A. Rutala

More than 2.5 billion people are at risk of rabies in over 100 countries.[1] Rabies ranks number 10 worldwide as a cause of mortality and causes an estimated 50,000 to 60,000 deaths annually, despite the availability of effective vaccines for postexposure treatment.[1] In addition, millions of persons, primarily in developing countries, undergo costly postexposure treatment.[2] In the United States, rabies continues to be endemic in many wild animals. Although human rabies is rare in the United States, postexposure rabies prophylaxis is likely provided to more than 35,000 persons per year.[2] Prevention efforts in the United States are estimated to cost between $230 million and $1 billion.[2]

This chapter briefly reviews the microbiology, epidemiology, clinical presentation, and treatment of rabies. Because animal bites and scratches are commonly seen by primary care and emergency medical physicians, the postexposure management of persons potentially exposed to a rabid animal is reviewed in detail. Comprehensive reviews of rabies have been published in the medical literature.[3–6] Current information is available on the rabies homepage produced by the Centers for Disease Control and Prevention (www.cdc/gov).[7]

MICROBIOLOGY

Rabies virus is the prototype member of the genus Lyssavirus, of the family Rhabdoviridae, order Mononegavirales.[6] Members of this order have a single-stranded, negative-sense, nonsegmented RNA genome that is tightly encapsulated into ribonucleocapsid structures. Members of the family Rhabdoviridae are grouped on the basis of their conical or bullet shape as visualized by electron microscopy. Their host range includes vertebrates (primarily mammals and fish), invertebrates (primarily arthropods), and plants. The Rhabdoviridae that infect animals and humans are divided into two genera, the Lyssavirus (Greek *Lyssa,* frenzy) and Vesiculovirus (Latin *vesicula,* little bladder).[3] Vesiculoviruses (e.g., vesicular stomatitis virus) cause disease in cattle, swine, horses, and a variety of other vertebrates.[3] Humans occasionally develop infection, which is most commonly characterized by a nonfatal, nonspecific influenza-like viral syndrome.

The rabies group of lyssaviruses is comprised of at least seven serotypes or genotypes: classic rabies virus, Lagos bat virus, Mokola virus, Duvenhage virus, European bat lyssavirus 1, European bat lyssavirus 2, and Australian bat virus.[4–6] Rarely lyssaviruses other than rabies cause human disease (<10 total cases described worldwide).

PATHOPHYSIOLOGY

Once introduced, the initial infection and multiplication occur within local monocytes for the first 48 to 96 h. Subsequently, the virus spreads across the motor end-plate, and ascends and replicates along peripheral nervous axoplasm to the dorsal root ganglia, the spinal cord, and the central nervous system (CNS). Following CNS replication in the gray matter, the virus spreads outward by peripheral nerves to virtually all tissues and organ systems. Viral infection of the salivary glands engenders infectivity of saliva; the infectivity of other body fluids is less well established.

Histologically, rabies is similar to other forms of encephalitis: diffuse and extensive monocellular infiltration with focal hemorrhage and demyelination, predominantly in perivascular areas in the gray matter of the CNS, basal ganglia, and the spinal cord. Negri bodies, where CNS viral replication occurs, are the characteristic histologic finding for rabies. They are eosinophilic intracellular lesions found within cerebral neurons and are highly specific for rabies. Negri bodies are encountered in about 75 percent of proven animal rabies; thus although their presence is pathognomonic for rabies, their absence does not exclude rabies as a diagnostic possibility.

EPIDEMIOLOGY

Rabies is primarily a disease of animals.[3] The epidemiology of human rabies is a reflection of both the distribution of the disease in animals and the degree of human contact with these animals.[3] In those parts of the world where canine rabies has been controlled [i.e., the United States (Table 147-1), Canada, and Europe], dogs account for less than 5 percent of the cases in animals. Where canine rabies has not been controlled (i.e., most developing countries of Asia, Africa, Latin America, and South America), dogs account for 90 percent or more of reported cases in animals. The major wildlife vectors of rabies are: dogs (major vector of rabies throughout the world, particularly Asia, Latin America, and Africa); foxes (Europe, the Arctic, and North America); raccoons (eastern United States); skunks (midwestern United States, western Canada); coyotes (Asia, Africa, and North America); mongooses (yellow mongoose in Asia and Africa; Indian mongoose in the Caribbean islands); and bats (vampire bats from northern Mexico to Argentina, insectivorous bats in North America and Europe). In 2000, 49 states, the District of Columbia, and Puerto Rico reported 7369 cases of rabies in animals, a 4.3 percent increase from the number of cases reported in 1999.[8] Wild animals accounted for 93 percent of the reported cases: raccoons (37.7 percent); skunks (30.2 percent); bats (16.8 percent); foxes (6.2 percent); and other wild animals including beavers, otters, bobcats, rodents, and lagomorphs (rabbits, hares, and picas) (2.2 percent). Rabid domestic animals included cats (3.4 percent); cattle (1.1 percent); dogs (1.6 percent); horses, donkeys, and mules (0.71 percent); sheep, goats, and camels (0.15 percent); and other animals such as ferrets (0.06 percent). **The following animals very rarely have been found to be rabid and hence their bite almost never requires postexposure prophylaxis for rabies: squirrels, hamsters, guinea pigs, gerbils, chipmunks, rats, mice, domesticated rabbits, and other small rodents.**

Animal reservoirs for rabies are found worldwide with the exception of some islands (e.g., Hawaii, Great Britain), Australia, and Antarctica. Rabies infections of mammalian species occur in geographically discrete outbreaks. Disease transmission within an outbreak is primarily intraspecific and involves a single, distinctive rabies variant.

Transmission of rabies virus usually begins when the contaminated saliva of an infected host is passed to a susceptible host. The most common mode of rabies viral transmission is through the bite of a rabid animal. Other routes of documented transmission have included contamination of mucous membranes (i.e., eyes, nose, mouth), aerosol transmission during spelunking in bat-infested caves or while working in the laboratory with rabies virus, corneal transplants, and iatrogenic infection through improperly inactivated vaccine.

TABLE 147-1 Geographic Boundaries of North American Reservoirs for Rabies

1. An expanding reservoir of raccoon rabies that now encompasses the entire East coast from Maine to Florida.
2. A longstanding reservoir in red and arctic foxes in Alaska, that has spread to include foxes across Canada as far east as Ontario, Quebec, and the upper parts of the northern New England states.
3. Three separate variants that infect striped skunks in longstanding reservoirs in California, the north central states, and the south central states.
4. Two different variants in gray foxes in small but longstanding reservoirs in Arizona and Texas.
5. A small reservoir of coyotes in southern Texas.

The risk of developing rabies following an animal bite or scratch by a rabid animal depends on whether a bite or scratch occurred, the number of bites, the depth of the bites, and the location of the wounds (Table 147-2).

The epidemiology of human rabies in the United States between 1946 and 2000 has been well described in a series of reports from the CDC.[8–11] In the United States, deaths in humans caused by rabies totaled 99 in the 1950s, 15 in the 1960s, 23 in the 1970s, 10 in the 1980s, and 32 from 1990 through 2000. The median age of patients reported from 1980 through 1996 was 27 (range: 4 to 82 years of age) and 20 (63 percent) were male. Cases were reported from 20 states; 7 cases (22 percent) were reported from California and 6 from Texas. Eleven patients were exposed to rabies in eight foreign countries. The onset of illness occurred in all months and with no apparent seasonal pattern.

Of the 32 patients that died of rabies between 1980 and 1996, a definite history of animal exposure was identified in only 7 (22 percent); 6 resulted from a dog bite received in a foreign country and 1 was from a bat bite received in the United States. Contact with an animal was identified in 12 persons; 8 with a bat, 2 with a dog, 1 with a cow, and 1 with a cat. For the remaining 13 patients, a potential source of animal exposure was not identified. Of the 10 deaths from 1997 through 2000, 9 persons had a bat variant isolated (only 1 had a history of a bite by a bat) and 1 person acquired disease from a dog bite in Ghana.

Current epidemiologic patterns of rabies in the United States have been summarized as follows:[10] The annual reports of rabies in wildlife far exceed those of rabies in domestic animals; rabies variants in bats are associated with a disproportionate number of infections in humans (~90 percent), although bats constitute only about 15 percent of all reported rabies cases in animals annually; most other cases of human rabies diagnosed in the United States are attributable to infections acquired in areas of enzootic canine rabies outside the United States; most persons with a case of rabies that originated in the United States have no history of an animal bite; and rabies is diagnosed after death in more than one-third of the latter group. During the past half century, the number of humans dying of rabies has dramatically decreased to an average of 2 to 3 per year. Although the number of deaths is low, most deaths occur because individuals are unaware that they have been exposed to and infected with rabies virus, and therefore they do not seek effective postexposure prophylaxis.[12] Molecular epidemiologic studies have linked most of these cryptic rabies exposures to rabies virus variants associated with insectivorous bats. As a result of this data, the Centers for Disease Control has altered its recommendations for postexposure prophylaxis (see below).

PREEXPOSURE PROPHYLAXIS

Preexposure prophylaxis with rabies vaccine is highly recommended for persons whose recreational or occupational activities place them at risk for acquiring rabies (Tables 147-3 and 147-4).[13] Although the initial rabies preexposure vaccine regimen is similar, the need for booster doses, the timing of booster doses, and the need and timing of serologic tests to confirm immunity differ based on the degree of individual risk for exposure to rabies. Emergency medicine health care providers should refer persons at risk for rabies who have not received

TABLE 147-2 Risk of Rabies in Absence of Postexposure Prophylaxis Following Exposure to a Rabid Animal

Multiple severe bites around the face: 80–100%
Single bite: 15–40%
Superficial bite(s) on the extremity: 5–10%
Contamination of open wound by saliva: ~0.1%
Transmission via fomites (e.g., tree branch): theoretical (no cases reported)
Indirect transmission (e.g, raccoon saliva on a dog): theoretical (no cases reported)

TABLE 147-3 Rabies Preexposure Prophylaxis Schedule—United States, 1999

Type of Immunization	Route	Regimen
Primary	Intramuscular	HDCV, PCEC, or RVA; 1.0 mL (deltoid area), one each on days 0,* 7, and 21 or 28
	Intradermal	HDCV; 0.1 mL, one each on days 0,* 7, and 21 or 28
Booster	Intramuscular	HDCV, PCEC or RVA; 1.0 mL (deltoid area), one each on day 0* only
	Intradermal	HDCV, 0.1 mL, day 0* only

* Day 0 is the day the first dose of vaccine is administered.
Abbreviations: HDCV = human diploid cell vaccine; PCEC = purified chick embryo cell vaccine; RVA = rabies vaccine adsorbed.
Source: Adapted from Centers for Disease Control and Prevention.

preexposure prophylaxis to their local physician or health department for appropriate immunization.

Preexposure vaccination does not eliminate the need for additional therapy after a rabies exposure, but simplifies postexposure prophylaxis by eliminating the need for human rabies immune globulin (HRIG) and by decreasing the number of doses of vaccine required (see below).

POSTEXPOSURE PROPHYLAXIS

Postexposure prophylaxis is indicated for persons possibly exposed to a rabid animal (Figure 147-1). All persons presenting with an animal bite or scratch should be evaluated for the presence of a life-threatening condition, such as arterial laceration, pneumothorax, or respiratory compromise.[14] Appropriate emergency care for animal bites should be provided.[14] Key aspects include tetanus prophylaxis, wound cleansing, measures to prevent bacterial infection, and evaluation for rabies prophylaxis. Cleansing of the wound with a 20 percent solution of soap and water is an essential first step in rabies prevention. In experimental animals, simple wound cleansing has been shown to markedly reduce the likelihood of rabies.

All persons bitten or scratched by an animal, whether domestic or wild, should be evaluated for the need to initiate rabies postexposure prophylaxis. The decision to initiate rabies postexposure prophylaxis should be based on the following:[7] geographic location of the incident; the type of animal that was involved; and how the exposure occurred (i.e., provoked or unprovoked), the vaccination status of the animal, and whether the animal can be safely captured and tested for rabies (Table 147-5). Excellent guidelines are often available from the local health department. For the purpose of rabies postexposure prophylaxis, a bite exposure is defined as any penetration of the skin by the teeth of an animal. Bites to the face and hands carry the highest risk, but the site of the bite should not influence the decision to begin therapy.[13] Scratches, abrasions, open wounds, or mucous membranes contaminated with saliva or other potentially infectious material (such as brain tissue) from a rabid animal constitute nonbite exposures. If the material containing the virus is dry, the virus can be considered noninfectious. A fully vaccinated dog or cat is unlikely to become infected with rabies, although rare cases have been reported among animals that had received only a single dose of vaccine. No documented vaccine failures have occurred among dogs or cats that had received two vaccinations.

Other contact by itself, such as petting a rabid animal and contact with blood, urine, or feces (e.g., guano) of a rabid animal, does not constitute an exposure and is not an indication for prophylaxis.[13] However, local health departments may vary in their recommendations for salivary exposure.

Bats are increasingly implicated as an important wildlife reservoir for variants of rabies virus transmitted to humans. Minor bites by bats and awakening in a room with a bat have been associated with the development of rabies. For this reason, the CDC recommends the following actions where bat-human contact has occurred.[15] In all cases in which bat-human contact has occurred or is suspected, the bat should be collected and tested for rabies. If the bat is unavailable, the need for postexposure prophylaxis should be assessed by public health officials. Postexposure prophylaxis should be considered after direct contact between a human and a bat, unless the exposed person is certain a bite, scratch, or mucous membrane exposure did not occur. Postexposure prophylaxis may be considered for persons who were in the same room as a bat and who might be unaware that a bite or direct contact had occurred (e.g., when a sleeping person awakens to find a bat in the

TABLE 147-4 Rabies Preexposure Prophylaxis Guide

Risk Category	Nature of Risk	Typical Population	Preexposure Recommendations
Continuous	Virus present continuously, often in high concentrations; specific exposures likely to go unrecognized; bite, nonbite, or aerosol exposure	Rabies research laboratory workers,* rabies biologics production workers	Primary course Serologic testing every 6 months; booster immunization if antibody titer is below acceptable level†
Frequent	Exposure usually episodic with source recognized, but exposure also might be unrecognized; bite, nonbite, or aerosol exposure	Rabies diagnostic lab workers,* spelunkers, veterinarians and staff, and animal-control and wildlife workers in rabies-enzootic areas.	Primary course Serologic testing every 2 years; booster immunization if antibody titer is below acceptable level†
Infrequent (greater than population at large)	Exposure nearly always episodic with source recognized; bite or nonbite exposure	Veterinarians and animal-control and wildlife workers in areas with low rabies rates, veterinary students, travelers visiting areas where rabies is enzootic and immediate access to appropriate medical care including biologics is limited	Primary course; no serologic testing or booster immunization
Rare (population at large)	Exposure always episodic with source recognized; bite or nonbite exposure	U.S. population at large, including persons in rabies-enzootic areas	No immunization necessary

*Judgment of relative risk and extra monitoring of immunization status of laboratory workers is the responsibility of the laboratory supervisor.
†Minimum acceptable antibody level is complete virus neutralization at 1:5 serum dilution by the rapid fluorescent focus inhibition test. A booster dose should be administered if the titer falls below this level.
Source: Adapted from Centers for Disease Control and Prevention.[13]

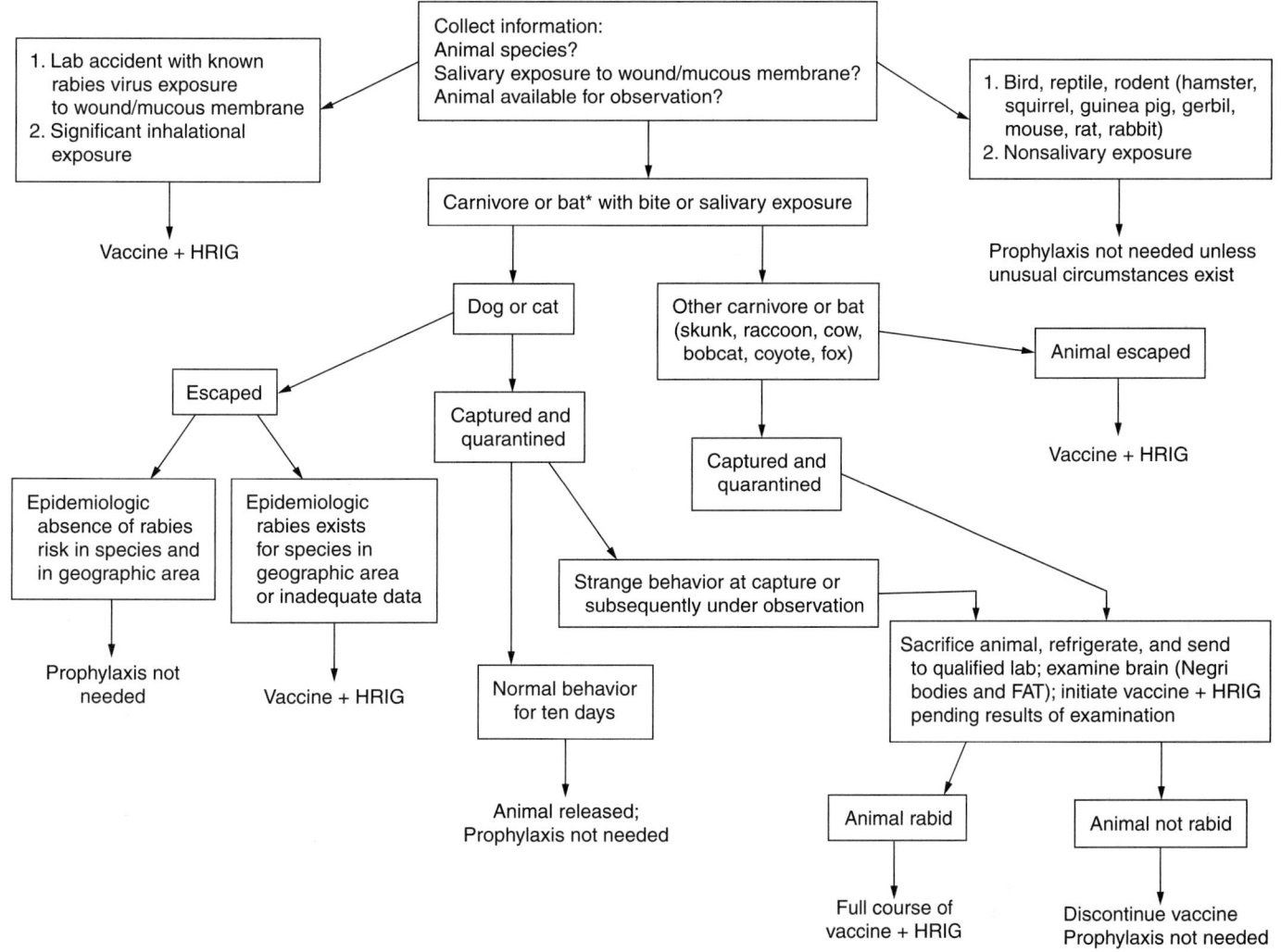

FIG. 147-1. Clinical guidelines for administration of postexposure prophylaxis. DFA = direct fluorescent antibody test; HRIG = human rabies immune globulin. (Adapted from Mann JR: Rabies risk: Systemic evaluation and management of animal bites. *Compr Ther* 7:53, 1981. Used with permission.)

room or an adult witnesses a bat in a room with an unattended child, mentally disabled person, or intoxicated person). Seeing a bat does not constitute an exposure.

The CDC recommends that a healthy dog, cat, or ferret that bites a person should be confined and observed for 10 days.[13] Such animals should be evaluated by a veterinarian at the first sign of illness during confinement. Any illness in the animal should be immediately reported to the local health department. If signs suggestive of rabies develop, the animal should be euthanized, its head removed, and the head shipped under refrigeration (not frozen) for examination of the brain by a qualified laboratory designated by the local or state health department. Any stray or unwanted dog, cat, or ferret that bites a person may be euthanized immediately and the head submitted for rabies examination. Animals other than dogs, cats, or ferrets that might have exposed a person to rabies should be immediately reported to the local health department. Prior vaccination of an animal does not preclude the necessity of euthanasia and testing if the period of virus shedding is unknown for that species.

There are anecdotal reports of person-to-person transmission of rabies.[16] Fluids from the upper and lower respiratory tracts of humans frequently test positive for rabies virus. Despite the lack of proven health care-associated transmission, ~30 percent of health care workers who have had contact with a human case of rabies have received postexposure prophylaxis. Given the mechanism of disease transmis-

sion and concern among health care workers, contact isolation precautions should be used for patients with known or suspected rabies, and health care workers who care for such patients should wear either masks and eye protection or face shields.[16] Health care workers with nonintact skin or mucous membrane exposure to infective saliva should receive postexposure prophylaxis.

In the United States, postexposure prophylaxis consists of a regimen of one dose of HRIG and five doses of rabies vaccine over a 28-day period (Table 147-6). Human rabies immune globulin and the first dose of rabies vaccine should be given as soon as possible after exposure, preferably within 24 h. Four formulations of three inactivated rabies vaccines are available in the United States, including human diploid cell vaccine (HDCV) (produced in human diploid cells; Imovax, Pasteur Merieux Connaught), rabies vaccine adsorbed (RVA) (produced in fetal rhesus diploid lung cells; Rabies Vaccine Adsorbed, SmithKline Beecham), and purified chick embryo cell culture vaccine (PCEC) (produced in chick embryo cells; RabAvert, Chiron). All currently used vaccines are produced in cell culture and are significantly less toxic than older vaccines that were produced in neural tissue. Side effects, including mild erythema, swelling, and pain at the injection site, have been reported among 30 to 74 percent of vaccine recipients. Systemic reactions, such as headache, nausea, abdominal pain, muscle aches, and dizziness, have been reported among 5 to 40 percent of recipients. Serum-sickness-like reactions (type III hypersensitivity) have

TABLE 147-5   Rabies Postexposure Prophylaxis Guide

Animal Type	Evaluation and Disposition of Animal	Postexposure Prophylaxis Recommendations
Dogs, cats, and ferrets	Healthy and available for 10 days of observations	Persons should not begin prophylaxis unless animal develops clinical signs of rabies*
	Rabid or suspected rabid	Immediate immunization
	Unknown (e.g., escaped)	Consult public health officials
Skunks, raccoons, foxes, and most other carnivores; bats	Regard as rabid unless animal proven negative by laboratory tests†	Consider immediate immunization
Livestock, small rodents, lagomorphs (rabbits and hares), large rodents, (woodchucks and beavers), and other mammals	Consider individually	Consult public health officials; bites of squirrels, hamsters, guinea pigs, gerbils, chipmunks, mice, rats, domesticated rabbits, and other small rodents, almost never require antirabies postexposure prophylaxis

*During the 10-day observation period, begin postexposure prophylaxis at the first sign of rabies in a dog, cat, or ferret that has bitten someone. If the animal exhibits clinical signs of rabies, it should be euthanized immediately and tested.
†The animal should be euthanized and tested as soon as possible. Holding for observation is not recommended. Discontinue vaccine if immunofluorescence test results of the animal are negative.
Source: Adapted from Centers for Disease Control and Prevention.[13]

been noted among approximately 6 percent of persons receiving booster doses of HDCV, 2 to 21 days after administration of the booster dose. Such reactions have not been life threatening and have not been reported with the RVA or PCEC vaccines. Anaphylaxis and neurologic symptoms have only rarely been associated with the current rabies vaccines. Severe egg allergy is a contraindication to the use of the PCEC vaccine. Once initiated, rabies prophylaxis should not be interrupted or discontinued because of local or mild systemic adverse reactions to rabies vaccine.[13] Usually such reactions can be successfully managed with anti-inflammatory and antipyretic agents. When a person with a history of serious hypersensitivity to rabies vaccine must be revaccinated, antihistamines may be given. Epinephrine should be readily available to counteract anaphylactic reactions, and the person should be observed carefully immediately after vaccination.

HRIG is administered only once (i.e., at the beginning of antirabies prophylaxis) to provide immediate antibodies until the patient responds to rabies vaccine by producing antibodies. Failure to use HRIG has led to rabies, despite appropriate postexposure prophylaxis with HDCV. If HRIG was not given when vaccination was begun, it can be given through the seventh day after administration of the vaccine.[13] Beyond the seventh day, HRIG is not indicated because an antibody response is presumed to have occurred. The CDC recommends that as much as possible of the full dose be infiltrated around the wound. HRIG should never be administered in the same syringe or into the same anatomical site as the vaccine. Even if the wound has to be sutured, it should be infiltrated locally with HRIG. This practice is safe and does not create an additional risk of infection. However, caution is needed when injecting into a tissue compartment, such as the finger pulp, because excessive HRIG can increase compartment pressure and lead to necrosis.[17]

The CDC recommendations for postexposure prophylaxis should be followed *EXACTLY.* Although no postexposure prophylaxis vaccine failures have been reported in the United States since the licensing of HDCV in 1980, 13 persons outside the United States have contracted rabies after postexposure prophylaxis with tissue culture-derived vaccine.[3] Each of these cases involved deviation from the recommended protocol; wounds were not cleansed, passive immunization with HRIG was not provided, or rabies vaccine was injected into the gluteal rather than the deltoid area.

In order to reduce costs and because HRIG may not be available in other countries, postexposure regimens using intradermal administration of vaccine have been studied and approved by the World Health Organization and HRIG is advised only for the highest risk exposures.

However, in the United States, only regimens recommended by the CDC should be used because of their proven efficacy.

POSTEXPOSURE PROPHYLAXIS IN SPECIAL CIRCUMSTANCES

Prior Rabies Immunization

If exposed to rabies, persons previously vaccinated should receive two intramuscular doses (1 mL each) of vaccine, one immediately and one 3 days later.[13] "Previously vaccinated" refers to persons who have received one of the recommended preexposure or postexposure prophylaxis regimens of HDCV, RVA, or PCEC, or those who have received another vaccine and had a documented rabies antibody titer. HRIG is unnecessary and should not be given in these cases because an anamnestic antibody response will follow the administration of a booster regardless of the prebooster antibody titer.

Immunocompromised Persons

Immunization of immunocompromised persons presents special challenges. First, vaccines may represent a danger to the immunocompromised person. Second, the immune response of immunocompromised persons to vaccination may not be as good as that of immunocompetent persons; higher doses or additional immunizations may be required, although even with these modifications, the immune response may be suboptimal. The Advisory Committee on Immunization Practices (ACIP) considers these persons severely immunocompromised: congenital immunodeficiency; human immunodeficiency virus (HIV) infection; leukemia or lymphoma; aplastic anemia; generalized malignancy; or therapy with alkylating agents, antimetabolites, radiation, or large amounts of corticosteroids.[18]

Because rabies vaccine is formulated with inactivated virus, it does not represent a danger to immunocompromised persons and may be administered to such persons using the standard recommended doses and schedule (see Table 147-6). Furthermore, the recommendations for the use of HRIG are the same in immunocompromised and immunocompetent persons. However, corticosteroids, other immunosuppressive agents, and immunosuppressive illnesses can interfere with the development of active immunity and predispose the patient to developing rabies if exposed. Immunosuppressive agents should not be administered during postexposure prophylaxis, unless essential for the

TABLE 147-6   Rabie Postexposure Prophylaxis Schedule—United States, 1999

Immunization Status	Treatment	Regimen*
Not previously immunized	Wound cleansing	All postexposure prophylaxis should begin with immediate thorough cleansing of all wounds with soap and water; if available, a virucidal agent such as povidone-iodine solution should be used to irrigate the wounds
	HRIG	Administer 20 IU/kg body weight. If anatomically feasible, *the full dose* should be infiltrated around the wound(s) and any remaining volume should be administered IM at an anatomical site distant from vaccine administration; also, HRIG should not be administered in the same syringe as vaccine; because HRIG might partially suppress active production of antibody, no more than the recommended dose should be given
	Vaccine	HDCV, RVA, or PCEC 1.0 mL (deltoid area†), one each on days 0,‡ 3, 7, 14, and 28
Previously immunized#	Wound cleansing	All postexposure treatment should begin with immediate thorough cleansing of all wounds with soap and water; if available, a virucidal agent such as a povidone-iodine solution should be used to irrigate the wounds
	HRIG	HRIG should *not* be administered
	Vaccine	HDCV, RVA, or PCEC 1.0 mL (deltoid area†), one each on days 0‡ and 3

*These regimens are appropriate to all age groups, including children.
†The deltoid area is the only acceptable site of vaccination for adults and older children. For younger children, the outer aspect of the thigh may be used. Vaccine should never be administered in the gluteal area.
‡Day 0 is the day the first dose of vaccine is administered.
#Any persons with a history of preexposure prophylaxis with HDCV, RVA, or PCEC; prior postexposure prophylaxis with HDCV, RVA, or PCEC; or previous immunization with any other type of rabies vaccine and a documented history of antibody response to the prior immunization.
Abbreviations: HDCV = human diploid cell vaccine; HRIG = human rabies immuneglobulin; PCEC = purified chick embryo cell vaccine; RVA = rabies vaccine adsorbed.
Source: Adapted from Centers for Disease Control and Prevention.[13]

treatment of other conditions. When rabies postexposure prophylaxis is administered to persons receiving steroids or other immunosuppressive therapy, it is especially important that serum be tested for rabies antibody to ensure that an adequate response has developed.[13] To test the adequacy of the immune response, serum collected 2 to 4 weeks after the postexposure prophylaxis should completely neutralize challenge virus at a 1:5 serum dilution by rapid fluorescent focus inhibition test (RFFIT).[13]

Travelers

Preexposure prophylaxis is recommended for international travelers based on the local incidence of rabies in the countries to be visited, the availability of appropriate antirabies biologics, and the intended activity.[19] Such persons include veterinarians, animal handlers, field biologists, spelunkers, and certain laboratory workers. Chloroquine phosphate (and possibly other structurally-related antimalarials such as mefloquine, which is administered for malaria chemoprophylaxis) may interfere with the antibody response to HDCV. Always immunize persons receiving antimalarial chemoprophylaxis by the intramuscular route.

Between 1980 and 2000, seven persons died in the United States from rabies after having been bitten by a dog while visiting a foreign country. In that same period, three U.S. citizens died in foreign countries from exposure that occurred in the foreign country. For this reason, all persons who have returned from abroad should be questioned regarding whether they received an animal bite or scratch in an area with endemic rabies. Persons bitten or scratched by an animal in an area with endemic rabies should receive appropriate postexposure prophylaxis if the injury has occurred within the known incubation period (which may extend up to 5 years).

U.S. citizens and residents who are exposed to rabies while traveling in countries where rabies is endemic may sometimes receive postexposure prophylaxis with regimens or biologics that are not used in the United States. If postexposure prophylaxis is begun outside the United States using a non-FDA-approved regimen or biologic of nerve tissue origin, it may be necessary to provide additional treatment when the patient reaches the United States.[13] State and local health departments should be contacted for specific advice in such cases. The ma-

jor modification used abroad, usually in an attempt to reduce cost, is the substitution of various schedules for intradermal injection or the use of non-FDA-approved vaccines.

Pregnancy

Adverse pregnancy outcomes or fetal abnormalities have not been associated with rabies vaccination. Because of the potential consequences of inadequately treated rabies exposure, and because adverse events have not been associated with rabies postexposure prophylaxis during pregnancy, pregnancy is not considered a contraindication to rabies postexposure prophylaxis or HRIG.[13] If there is substantial risk of exposure to rabies, preexposure prophylaxis may also be indicated during pregnancy.

Children

The risk of rabies and the management of postexposure prophylaxis in children have been reviewed.[17] In infants and children, the dose of rabies vaccine for preexposure and postexposure prophylaxis is the same as that recommended for adults (see Table 147-6). The dose of HRIG for postexposure prophylaxis is based on body weight. For small children with multiple bites, the calculated dosage of HRIG may be insufficient to infiltrate all wounds. However, sterile saline can be used to dilute the volume twofold or threefold to permit thorough infiltration.[17]

CLINICAL DISEASE

Rabies virus causes acute encephalitis in all warm-blooded hosts, including humans, and the outcome is almost always fatal. While patients with rabies may manifest a variety of clinical symptoms and signs, the disease tends to follow a characteristic course (Table 147-7).

Rabies infection is most commonly initiated by the bite of a rabid animal. Most commonly, the incubation period ranges from 20 to 90 days.[3] However, incubation periods have been reported as short as 4 days and as long as 19 years. Incubation periods exceeding 1 year have been well documented in the literature. For patients who died from rabies in the United States between 1980 and 1996 and for whom a definite animal bite occurred, the median incubation period was 85 days

TABLE 147-7 Natural History of Clinical Rabies in Humans

Clinical Stage	Defining Event	Usual Duration	Common Symptoms and Signs*
Incubation period	Exposure	20 to 90 days	None
Prodrome	First symptom	2 to 10 days	Pain or paresthesia at site of bite Malaise, lethargy Headache Fever Nausea, vomiting, anorexia Anxiety, agitation, depression
Acute neurologic phase	First neurologic sign	2 to 7 days	Anxiety, agitation, depression Hyperventilation, hypoxia Aphasia, incoordination Paresis, paralysis Hydrophobia, pharyngeal spasms Confusion, delirium, hallucinations Marked hyperactivity
Coma	Onset of coma	0 to 14 days	Coma Hypotension, hypoventilation, apnea Pituitary dysfunction Cardiac arrhythmia, cardiac arrest
Recovery	Death or initiation of recovery	Months	Pneumothorax Intravascular thrombosis Secondary infections

*Not every symptom or sign may be present in each case.

(range: 53 to 150 days).[10] The incubation period has been reported to be shorter when the site of bite is on the head than when it is on an extremity.[3]

During the prodromal period, the symptoms and signs of rabies are often nonspecific. They include fever, sore throat, chills, malaise, anorexia, headache, nausea, vomiting, dyspnea, cough, and weakness. Early in the course some patients may report symptoms suggestive of rabies such as limb pain, limb weakness, and paresthesias at or near the presumed exposure site. Nonspecific neurologic symptoms may be reported including apprehension, anxiety, agitation, irritability, depression, and psychiatric disturbances.

The prodrome merges into the acute neurologic phase, which begins when the patient develops objective signs of central nervous system disease. Two major forms of acute neurologic disorder have been described: furious and paralytic. Furious rabies is noted in about 80 percent of patients and is characterized by hyperactivity, disorientation, hallucinations, and bizarre behavior. Periods of hyperactivity may alternate with periods of calm. Signs of autonomic dysfunction are frequently present and include hyperthermia, tachycardia, hypertension, and excessive salivation. About 50 percent of patients have classic hydrophobia in which attempts at drinking fluids result in severe spasms of the pharynx, larynx, and diaphragm. Paralytic rabies is noted in about 20 percent of patients and is characterized by paralysis, which may be maximal in the extremity that was bitten, diffuse, and symmetrical, or it may ascend in a pattern similar to Guillain-Barré syndrome. Accompanying signs may include fever and nuchal rigidity.

Coma almost always occurs within 10 days of the onset of symptoms. In the series reported by Noah and colleagues, the median duration of illness was 19 days (range: 7 to 28 days).[10] All patients in the series died. Death occurs from a variety of complications including pituitary dysfunction, seizures, respiratory dysfunction with progressive hypoxia, cardiac dysfunction with dysrhythmias and arrest, autonomic dysfunction, renal failure, and secondary bacterial infections.

Rarely have patients recovered from rabies, but in all such cases the patient had received either postexposure or preexposure prophylaxis with duck embryo vaccine or suckling mouse brain vaccine before the onset of symptoms. Despite intensive therapy, no persons without postexposure prophylaxis have survived in the United States since 1980.

DIAGNOSIS AND TREATMENT

Rabies should be included in the differential diagnosis of any acute encephalitis. The diagnosis of rabies is frequently made postmortem. This occurs because of the rarity of the disease, the increasing number of persons without an obvious exposure, and clinical confusion with other disorders. Important clues to diagnosis include a history of an animal bite and the development of the pathognomonic signs of hydrophobia and aerophobia. Tetanus should not be confused with rabies, because in tetanus the mental status is usually normal and the cerebrospinal fluid is normal. Other diseases that may be confused with rabies include poliomyelitis, Guillain-Barré syndrome, transverse myelitis, postvaccinial encephalomyelitis, intracranial mass lesions, cerebrovascular accidents, poisoning with atropine-like compounds, and other forms of viral encephalitis.[20]

During the incubation period of rabies, no diagnostic test is available for animals or humans that will indicate infection. Routine laboratory tests are of limited value for the diagnosis of rabies. Specific tests are required to diagnose rabies. Because no single test is uniformly informative, a battery of tests is commonly recommended. Useful laboratory specimens include serum, cerebrospinal fluid, saliva, and tissue, such as skin from highly innervated locations (e.g., nuchal skin biopsy).[4] The appearance of antibodies to specific viral antigens, either via serum binding or neutralization tests, is diagnostic in a patient with encephalitis and no history of previous immunization. Rabies virus has been isolated antemortem by animal inoculation or cell-culture passage from human saliva, brain tissue, cerebrospinal fluid, urine, and tracheal secretions. These samples can be probed for viral nucleic acid. Viral antigen can be detected by the direct fluorescent antibody (DFA) test on brain biopsy material, corneal touch impressions, or a full-thickness nuchal skin biopsy from the hairy nape of the neck. Early in the course of illness, the most reliable diagnostic test is a nuchal skin biopsy with immunofluorescent rabies antibody staining. Once clinical symptoms develop, a brain biopsy is universally positive when properly stained, but the invasive nature of this test precludes routine use. Tests to detect serum antibodies are useful, but while serum antibody may be present as early as day 5 of clinical illness, it may be absent after 10 to 14 days or more. Recently, nested polymerase chain reaction of RNA (RT-PCR) extracted from saliva has been shown to be a useful adjunct in rabies diagnosis, especially as a confirmatory test.

No specific therapy exists to treat rabies. Treatment is directed at the clinical complications of the disease. Although rabies is not treatable, every attempt should made at rapid diagnosis as it justifies public health measures to limit contacts with the patient and permits reconstruction of a history in which others may have been exposed to the same infective source.[4]

REFERENCES

1. Haupt W: Rabies-the risk of exposure and current trends in prevention of human cases. *Vaccine* 17:1742, 1999.
2. Rupprecht CE, Smith JE, Fekadu M, et al: The ascension of wildlife rabies: A cause for health concern or intervention? *Emerg Infect Dis* 1:107, 1995.
3. Fishbein DB, Robinson LE: Current concepts: Rabies. *N Engl J Med* 329:1632, 1993.
4. Rupprecht CE, Hanlon CA, Hemachudha T: Rabies re-examined. *Lancet Infect Dis* 2:327, 2002.
5. Plotkin SA: Rabies. *Clin Infect Dis* 30:4, 2000.
6. Smith JS: New aspects of rabies with emphasis on epidemiology, diagnosis, and prevention of the disease in the United States. *Clin Microbiol Rev* 9:166, 1996.
7. Centers for Disease Control and Prevention: Rabies home page at http://www.cdc/gov/ncidod/dvrd/rabies.
8. Krebs JW, Mondu AM, Rupprecht CE, Childs JE: Rabies surveillance in the United States during 2000. *JAMA* 219:1687, 2001.
9. Anderson LJ, Nicholson KG, Tauxe RV, et al: Human rabies in the United States, 1960 to 1979: Epidemiology, diagnosis, and prevention. *Ann Intern Med* 100:728, 1984.
10. Noah DL, Drenzek CL, Smith JS, et al: Epidemiology of human rabies in the United States, 1980 to 1996. *Ann Intern Med* 128:922, 1998.
11. Krebs JW, Smith JS, Rupprecht CE, Childs JE: Mammalian reservoirs and epidemiology of rabies diagnosed in human beings in the United States, 1981-1998. *Ann N Y Acad Sci* 916:345, 2000.
12. Messenger SL, Smith JS, Rupprecht CE: Emerging epidemiology of bat-associated cryptic cases of rabies in humans in the United States. *Clin Infect Dis* 35:738, 2002.
13. Centers for Disease Control and Prevention: Human rabies prevention—United States, 1999. Recommendations of the Advisory Committee on Immunization Practices (ACIP). *MMWR* 48(RR-1):1, 1999.
14. Weber DJ, Hansen AR: Infections resulting from animal bites. *Infect Dis Clin North Am* 5:663, 1991.
15. Centers for Disease Control and Prevention: Human rabies-California, Georgia, Minnesota, New York, and Wisconsin, 2000. *MMWR* 49:1111, 2000.
16. Weber DJ, Rutala WA: Risks and prevention of nosocomial transmission of rare zoonotic diseases. *Clin Infect Dis* 32:446, 2001.
17. Lang J, Plotkin SA: Rabies risk and immunoprophylaxis in children. *Adv Pediatr Infect Dis* 13:219, 1998.
18. Centers for Disease Control and Prevention: Recommendations of the Advisory Committee on Immunization Practices (ACIP): Use of vaccines and immune globulin in persons with altered immunocompetence. *MMWR* 42(RR-4):1, 1993.
19. Centers for Disease Control and Prevention: Health information for international travelers, 1999-2000. McLean, VA, International Medical Publishing, 2000.
20. Whitley RJ, Gnann JW: Viral encephalitis: familiar infections and emerging pathogens. *Lancet* 359:507, 2002.

MALARIA
Jeffrey D. Band

With the increase in international travel and the continued shift of travel to tropical locales, it is not surprising that physicians are seeing more patients with infectious diseases acquired in the tropics. Malaria, a protozoan disease transmitted by the bite of the *Anopheles* mosquito,

remains one of the most significant of these. Four species of the genus *Plasmodium* infect humans: *P. vivax, P. ovale, P. malariae,* and *P. falciparum.* Annually, over 250 million persons develop malaria, and more than 2.5 million persons die.[1] The incidence of malaria has been increasing in recent years despite aggressive worldwide attempts at control. Not only is the mosquito vector becoming less susceptible to a variety of insecticides, but *P. falciparum*—the parasite responsible for the most deadly form of malaria—is becoming increasingly resistant to antimalarial medications.

Malaria, especially disease due to *P. falciparum,* represents a medical emergency in any nonimmune host. Its early manifestations are largely nonspecific and can mimic other infectious diseases. Failure to diagnose infection rapidly can be disastrous. Likewise, failure to use specific antimalarial agents to which the individual strain is susceptible can result in early death. A diagnosis of malaria must be considered in any person returning from the tropics with an unexplained febrile illness. Questions regarding recent travel should become routine in emergency departments.

EPIDEMIOLOGY

Malaria transmission occurs in large areas of Central and South America, the Caribbean, sub-Saharan Africa, the Indian subcontinent, Southeast Asia, the Middle East, and Oceania. Certain species may predominate in a given geographic area.[2] For example, *P. vivax* is more common in the Indian subcontinent and in Central America, whereas *P. falciparum* is the most prevalent form in Africa, Haiti, and New Guinea.

The risk of contracting malaria, which varies considerably between regions, is largely dependent on the intensity of transmission in both urban and rural areas and, for travelers, on the itinerary and time and type of travel. In 1999 and 2000, the Centers for Disease Control and Prevention (CDC) reported 2942 cases of malaria, including 1660 cases among U.S. civilians, 735 cases among foreign civilians, and 101 cases occurring in U.S. military personnel. Cases occurring among U.S. citizens traveling abroad have increased to the highest levels observed in more than 30 years.[3] Of the more than 1402 total cases in 2000, 783 (56 percent) were acquired in Africa (two-thirds from countries in sub-Sahara or West Africa), 238 (17 percent) in Asia (primarily from the Indian subcontinent), 230 (16 percent) in the Caribbean and Central America, 22 (2 percent) in Oceania, and only 57 (4 percent) in South America. *P. vivax* accounted for 42 percent of all cases, and *P. falciparum* accounted for another 49 percent. Mixed infections were uncommon, representing less than 1 percent of all cases. Thus more than half of all cases of malaria, including the majority of cases due to *P. falciparum,* were acquired from travels in sub-Saharan Africa. Yet, for every traveler to sub-Saharan Africa, at least 10 travelers visit potential malarious areas of Asia and South America each year. Clearly, the intensity of exposure appears to be much higher in sub-Saharan Africa. Four patients became infected in the United States in 2000; two through congenital transmission and two through locally acquired transmission via possible needle-stick injuries while caring for infected patients. Six deaths attributable to malaria were reported during 2000.

Resistance of *P. falciparum* to chloroquine continues to spread[4] (Table 148-1). In addition, strains of *P. falciparum* are resistant to other chemotherapeutic agents, including pyrimethamine-sulfadoxine, quinine, mefloquine, doxycycline, and new agents such as halofantrine and artesunate (the latter two agents are not available in the United States). Recently, strains of *P. vivax* have been isolated from patients who have failed chloroquine therapy.[5] Prior to 1990, no strains of *P. vivax, P. ovale,* or *P. malariae* were resistant to chloroquine.

PATHOPHYSIOLOGY

The organism is transmitted primarily by the bite of an infected female anopheline mosquito. This vector is found most frequently in tropical and subtropical regions below 2500 m (8200 ft) above sea level. Plasmodial

TABLE 148-1   Geographic Distribution of Malaria, Including Resistant Strains

Geographic Region	Areas with Malaria	Countries with Chloroquine-Resistant *P. falciparum* (CRPF)	Countries with Fansidar-Resistant *P. falciparum*
Central America	All countries	None	None
Caribbean	Dominican Republic and Haiti	None	None
South America			
Temperate	Argentina	None	None
Tropical	All countries	All countries except Paraguay	Interior Amazon Basin
East Asia	China	China	South China
Eastern South Asia	All countries except Brunei and Singapore	All infected areas	Infected areas except Philippines
Middle South Asia	All countries	All countries	Afghanistan and Bhutan
Western South Asia and Middle East	Iraq, Oman, Saudi Arabia, Syria, Turkey, and United Arab Emirates	All countries except Syria and Turkey	None
Northern Africa	All countries except Tunisia	None	None
Sub-Saharan Africa	All countries except Reunion and Seychelles	Widespread	Widespread
Southern Africa	All countries except Lesotho and Saint Helena	Widespread	Occasional
Oceania	Limited to Papua New Guinea, Solomon Islands, and Vanuatu (small foci elsewhere)	Widespread	Widespread

sporozoites are injected into the host's bloodstream during the mosquito's blood meal and are carried via the bloodstream to the liver. The hepatic parenchymal cells are invaded, and asexual reproduction of the parasite begins (pre-erythrocytic schizogony or exoerythrocytic stage). As thousands of daughter merozoites are formed (amplification cycle), the parenchymal liver cell ruptures, releasing daughter merozoites back into the circulation, where they rapidly invade erythrocytes (erythrocytic stage). In *P. vivax* and *P. ovale* infection, a portion of the intrahepatic forms are not released, remain dormant for months, and can later activate and cause clinical relapses.

The clinical manifestations of malaria first appear during the erythrocytic stage. Once merozoites enter this stage, they never reinvade the liver. Merozoites mature within the erythrocyte and take on various morphologic forms, including the early ring forms, trophozoites, and schizonts (which represent a mass of new merozoites). Eventually, the target erythrocyte lyses, and new merozoites invade uninfected red blood cells, continuing the infection and causing clinical manifestations. Lysogeny may become regular, occurring at 2- to 3-day intervals in established and untreated infections, producing the classic periodicity of symptoms.

After several cycles, a proportion of the merozoites develop into sexual forms (gametocytes). On ingestion by another feeding anopheline mosquito, male and female gametocytes undergo sexual reproduction and become infective sporozoites ready for their next host.

Each species of *Plasmodium* has specific characteristics, including typical morphologic forms and selective red blood cell tropism (Table 148-2). Many of these characteristics are responsible for important pathophysiologic consequences.

Malaria also may be transmitted by direct transfusion of infected blood or passed transplacentally from mother to fetus. In these cases, an exoerythrocytic phase is absent.

Disease ensues after an incubation period ranging from 8 days in the nonimmune and unprotected host to several weeks or more. Both incomplete suppression by partially active chemoprophylaxis and incomplete immunity can markedly prolong the incubation period to months or even years. For U.S. residents who developed malaria asso-

TABLE 148-2   Characteristics of Malaria-Causing *Plasmodium* Species

	P. falciparum	*P. vivax*	*P. ovale*	*P. malariae*
Incubation period	8–25 d	8–27 d	9–17 d	15–30 d
Asexual erythrocytic cycle	48 h	48 h	48 h	72 h
Relapse	No	Yes	Yes	No
Red blood cell (RBC) preference	Reticulocytes (but can infect RBCs of all ages)	Reticulocytes	Reticulocytes	Older cells
Morphologic characteristics				
Degree of parasitemia	High (multiple rings per RBC)	Low	Low	Low
Ring forms and early trophozoites	Ring forms predominate; threadlike cytoplasm with double-chromatic dots	Ameboid cytoplasm	Compact cytoplasm	Compact cytoplasm
Mature trophozoites	Rarely seen	Observed	Observed	Observed
Schizonts	Rarely seen	Observed	Observed	Observed
Gametocytes	Banana shaped	Round	Round	Round

ciated with travels abroad during 2000, disease became evident within 1 month after arrival home in 80 percent of *P. falciparum* cases but in only 40 percent of *P. vivax cases.* Only 1 percent of persons became ill more than 1 year after returning to the United States.[3] Only the asexual intraerythrocytic parasite is responsible for the symptoms and pathophysiologic consequences. The hallmark of malaria is the recurring febrile paroxysm that corresponds to hemolysis of infected erythrocytes and release of antigenic products with activation of macrophages and production of proinflammatory cytokines.

Hemolysis can be high with *P. falciparum* infection because parasitemia can be overwhelming and erythrocytes of all ages are susceptible. Parasitized erythrocytes lose flexibility and are removed in the microcirculation, with resulting obstruction and tissue anoxia of the lungs, kidneys, brain, and other vital organs. Noncardiac pulmonary edema, renal failure, and cerebral malaria may result. Sequestration accounts for the paucity of observed mature parasites in the peripheral smear of patients infected with *P. falciparum.*

In addition to prolonged high fever, hemolysis, and in the case of infection with *P. falciparum,* obstruction to capillary flow, immunologic sequelae also may occur, resulting in glomerulonephritis, nephrotic syndrome, thrombocytopenia, and polyclonal antibody stimulation. Lastly, hypersplenism with resulting pancytopenia may occur, especially in cases of prolonged, untreated malaria.

CLINICAL FEATURES

Typically, patients develop a prodrome of malaise, myalgia, headache, and low-grade fevers, often accompanied by chills.[6] In some patients, headache, chest pains, cough, abdominal pain, arthralgias, or diarrhea may be prominent. The early manifestations are quite nonspecific and can be confused easily with a viral syndrome, influenza, hepatitis, and other less severe self-limited clinical entities. Illness usually progresses to severe chills followed by high-grade fevers accompanied by tachycardia, nausea, orthostatic dizziness, and extreme weakness. After several hours, the fever abates, and the patient becomes diaphoretic and exhausted. Over time, the paroxysms of malaria—chills and fever followed by diaphoresis—may occur at nearly regular intervals that correspond to the length of the asexual erythrocytic cycles (see Table 148-2). The classic paroxysms of malaria are often lacking in malaria due to *P. falciparum* or in persons who received some form of chemoprophylaxis.

The findings on physical examination are also not specific for malaria. Most patients appear acutely ill with high fevers, tachycardia, and tachypnea. Splenomegaly and tender abdomen are present commonly in advanced infection. The liver may or may not be enlarged. Features quite atypical for malaria include lymphadenopathy and a maculopapular skin rash.

Laboratory features include normochromic normocytic anemia with findings suggestive of hemolysis, a normal or mildly depressed total leukocyte count, thrombocytopenia, an elevated erythrocyte sedimentation rate, elevated lactose dehydrogenase, and mild abnormalities in liver and renal functions. Other laboratory abnormalities include hyponatremia, hypoglycemia, and a biologic false-positive VDRL.

Complications of malaria can occur rapidly in untreated infection, especially when the agent is *P. falciparum.*[7] Infections caused by any species of *Plasmodium* can result in hemolysis, splenic enlargement, and occasionally, splenic rupture. An immune-mediated glomerulonephritis is also common to all forms but tends to occur most often in *P. malariae* infection. With the ability to cause high parasitemia levels and sequestration with capillary sludging, *P. falciparum* infection can be fatal. Cerebral malaria—characterized by somnolence, coma, delirium, and seizures—is associated with mortality rates in excess of 20 percent. Reversible causes of encephalopathy must be excluded. The cerebrospinal fluid is usually normal, except for a slightly elevated opening pressure and protein concentration. A mild pleocytosis also may be present. Other life-threatening complications associated with *P. falciparum* infection include respiratory failure due to noncardiogenic acute pulmonary edema (similar to adult respiratory distress syndrome), renal failure (acute tubular necrosis), and severe metabolic abnormalities, including lactic acidosis and profound hypoglycemia. Any target organ is susceptible to the effects of severe tissue hypoxia from the cytoadherence between the parasitized erythrocyte and the vascular endothelium of the host.

The very young, the elderly, and pregnant women are at greatest risk for complications due to *P. falciparum.* In addition to these host factors, additional risk factors for fatal malaria include an immunocompromised state, asplenia, failure to take appropriate chemoprophylaxis, refusal of or delay in seeking medical care, and misdiagnosis.[8]

DIAGNOSIS

The definitive diagnosis is established by the visualization of parasites on Giemsa-stained thick and thin blood smears. In early infection, especially infection due to *P. falciparum,* in which parasitized erythrocytes are sequestered from the bloodstream, parasitemia may be undetectable. Also, parasitemia fluctuates over time; it generally is highest during chills and as the fever is on the rise. High fevers are schizonticidal. In highly suspicious cases, failure to detect parasitemia is not an indication to withhold therapy. Delay in the diagnosis and treatment of malaria can have disastrous results. If parasitemia is not seen in the stained thin smear, a thick smear that concentrates blood cells may provide the diagnosis (Table 148-3). Extreme care in the preparation of slides is important because debris may result in false-positive smears. If parasites are not visualized, repeated smears should be obtained at least twice daily for 2 to 3 days to exclude malaria completely, although the first smear is positive in greater than 90 percent of cases.[9] Newer molecular probes for rapid diagnosis and speciation of the invading pathogen are available or in development, but each of these tests has major limitations when compared with an experienced light microscopist.[10] The two major questions to be answered by the blood smear are the degree of parasitemia present (correlates with prognosis) and whether *P. falciparum* is responsible for infection. Most patients with *P. falciparum* infection should be managed in the hospital setting, as should any patient with more than 3 percent parasitemia. Clues to the diagnosis of *P. falciparum* infection include the presence of small ring forms with double-chromatin knobs within the erythrocyte, multiply infected rings in individual red blood cells, a paucity of trophozoites and schizonts on smear, the pathognomonic crescent-shaped (banana-shaped) gametocyte, and parasitemia exceeding 4 percent. Repeated smears should be obtained daily to assess the efficacy of drug treatment.

TREATMENT

Therapeutic decisions are based on the severity of the illness, the agent, and whether the patient may be infected with chloroquine-resistant *P. falciparum.*[2,9] If *P. falciparum* infection can be excluded,

---

TABLE 148-3   Guidelines for Preparing Malaria Smears

Use scrupulously clean slides; manufacturers' precleaned slides may have residual debris.

Obtain a large drop of blood from the patient's finger by using a blood lancet.

Place the cleaned surface of the slide against the drop of blood; with a quick circular motion, make a film the size of a dime. Do not mix excessively or distortion will result. The thick smear should be of such depth that newsprint would be barely legible. (Let the smear air dry for 30 to 60 min.)

Obtain a small drop of blood from the patient's finger, and with a second clean slide, spread the blood gently over the slide. Air dry the thin film, fix it with methyl alcohol, and stain it with Giemsa stain.

If the thin smear is negative, examine the thick smear. Once air dried, the thick film should not be fixed prior to staining with Giemsa.

most persons can be managed in the ambulatory setting. Close follow-up, including repeated smears, is necessary. Patients with significant hemolysis or those who have underlying severe chronic medical problems that can be aggravated by high fevers or hemolysis are best hospitalized. Infected infants and pregnant women are also best managed in the hospital.

Chloroquine is the drug of choice for treatment of infection due to *P. vivax, P. ovale,* and *P. malariae.* Table 148-4 summarizes the treatment regimens for malaria. With treatment, the parasite load should decrease significantly within the first 24 to 48 h. No asexual forms of the parasite should be detectable 3 to 4 days after treatment is completed. Gametocytes, the sexual forms that do not cause disease in the human host, may persist for several weeks after treatment and are not an indicator of treatment failure. Chloroquine has no effect on the exoerythrocytic parasites, which may be dormant in the liver with infection due to *P. vivax* and *P. ovale.* Unless terminal treatment is administered with primaquine, clinical relapses commonly occur. Primaquine should not be used in patients with glucose-6-phosphate dehydrogenase deficiency because primaquine may induce massive hemolysis of erythrocytes. Table 148-5 summarizes the commonly described adverse effects and precautions or contraindications of the an-

timalarial medications. Despite treatment with both chloroquine and primaquine, infection or relapse may persist.

Treatment of *P. falciparum* infection is generally best managed in a hospital setting, particularly if the level of parasitemia exceeds 3 percent. Unless one is certain that the patient could not have chloroquine-resistant *falciparum* infection (based on geographic exposure; see Table 148-1), it is best to assume that the infecting strain is resistant to chloroquine and to initiate treatment with a combination of quinine and doxycycline with or without pyrimethamine-sulfadoxine. Clindamycin can be substituted for doxycycline in patients in whom doxycycline is contraindicated. Mefloquine is also a very effective therapy for chloroquine-resistant *P. falciparum* (and the asexual erythrocyte stages of the other *Plasmodium* species) either alone or combined with doxycycline. It should not be used if it had been prescribed for chemoprophylaxis. Atovaquone-proguanil, a recently approved fixed-dose medication (Malarone) agent, is also highly effective, with cure rates exceeding 95 percent.[11] It is generally well tolerated and offers another excellent option in treatment. It should not be prescribed for therapy if used as chemoprophylaxis with suspected failure. It may be more effective than mefloquine.

Persons presenting with complications caused by *P. falciparum* or with high parasitemia but unable to tolerate oral medications due to

TABLE 148-4   Treatment Regimens for Malaria

Clinical Setting	Drug	Dosage Guidelines	
		Adults	Children
Uncomplicated infection with *P. vivax, P. ovale, P. malariae,* and chloroquine-sensitive *P. falciparum*	Chloroquine phosphate *plus*	1-g load (600-mg base), then 500 mg (300-mg base) in 6 h, then 500 mg (300-mg base) per day for 2 d (total dose 2.5 g)	10-mg/kg base to maximum of 600 mg load, then 5-mg/kg base in 6 h and 5-mg/kg base per day for 2 d
	Primaquine phosphate*	26.3-mg load (15-mg base) per day for 14 d on completion of chloroquine therapy	0.3-mg/kg base for 14 d on completion of chloroquine therapy
Uncomplicated infection with chloroquine-resistant *P. falciparum*	(a) Quinine sulfate *plus*	650 mg PO tid for 3–7 d	8.3 mg/kg PO tid for 3–7 d
	Doxycycline†	100 mg PO bid for 7 d	Contraindicated in children < 8 years of age†
	Plus or minus Pyrimethamine-sulfadoxine (fansidar)‡	3 tablets (75 mg/1500 mg) PO × 1 dose	Over 2 months old >50 kg 3 tabs 30–50 kg 2 tabs 15–29 kg 1 tab 10–14 kg $\frac{1}{2}$ tab 4–9 kg $\frac{1}{4}$ tab
	or (b) Mefloquine *plus* doxycycline§ *or*	750 mg PO initially followed by 500 mg in 6–8 h See above	10–15 mg/kg base followed by 5–10 mg/kg base in 6–8 h See above
	(c) Atovaquone-proguanil (Malarone)	4 adult-strength (250/100) tabs daily × 3 d	>40 kg, adult dose 31–40 kg, 3 adult tablets × 3 d 21–30 kg, 2 adult tablets × 3 d 11–20 kg, 1 adult tablet × 3 d
Complicated infection with chloroquine-resistant *P. falciparum*	Quinidine gluconate	10-mg/kg load over 2 h (maximum 600 mg), then 0.02 mg/kg per min continuous infusion until patient is stabilized and able to tolerate PO therapy (see above)	Same as adults¶
	plus Doxycycline†	100 mg IV q12h until tolerating PO therapy (see above)	Contraindicated in children < 8 years of age†

*Terminal treatment for *P. vivax* and *P. ovale* only.
†Clindamycin is an alternate to doxycycline at dose of 10 mg/kg (max 900 mg) every 8 h for 3–7 days.
‡Optional; of unlikely value if acquisition is with fansidar resistance.
§Optional; many experts feel comfortable with mefloquine alone.
¶Consult an expert in pediatric infectious disease immediately for guidance.

TABLE 148-5   Adverse Effects, Precautions, and Contraindications of Antimalarial Drugs

Drug	Minor Toxicity	Major Toxicity	Precautions/Contraindications
Chloroquine	Nausea/vomiting, diarrhea, pruritus, postural hypotension, rash, fever, headache, dizziness	Rare; hypotension and shock after parenteral therapy; retinopathy after prolonged use	Avoid in patients with severe psoriasis and some types of porphyria
Quinine or quinidine	Cinchonism (nausea and vomiting, headache, tinnitus, dizziness, visual disturbance)	Hypotension, cardiac dysrhythmias, hypoglycemia, Coombs-positive hemolysis, abortions, neuromuscular paralysis (myasthenia)	Contraindicated in cardiac disease; cautiously in pregnancy, myasthenia gravis
Fansidar (pyrimethamine-sulfadoxine)	GI disturbances, phototoxicity, headaches, dizziness, skin rash	Fatal cutaneous eruptions reported, agranulocytosis	Contraindicated during pregnancy and in infants or if the patient is allergic to sulfonamides or pyrimethamine
Mefloquine	Nausea/vomiting, cramps, diarrhea, anorexia; dizziness, headaches, nightmares, and bradycardia	Rare unless underlying heart disease with bradycardia or the patient is on selected cardiotoxic medications (dysrhythmias, arrest); acute toxic confusional states may occur, as can seizures	Precaution during pregnancy and in children weighing < 10 kg; avoid if the patient is receiving quinidine; avoid if the patient has heart conduction disturbance or if underlying seizure or major neuropsychiatric disorders.
Doxycycline	GI disturbances, phototoxicity, vaginal candidiasis	Rare; esophageal ulcerations if not taken with fluids	Contraindicated during pregnancy, in children < 8 years of age; may depress prothrombin time in patients receiving anticoagulants
Atovaquone-proguanil (Malarone)	Nausea, vomiting, cramps, oral ulcers, headaches, dizziness	Rare serious allergic reactions and alopecia reported.	Contraindicated in pregnancy and in children < 11 kg (no safety data).
Primaquine*	Nausea, vomiting, diarrhea, cramps, methemoglobulinemia	Massive hemolysis in patients with G6PD deficiency, exacerbation of systemic lupus erythematosus or rheumatoid arthritis	Contraindicated in G6PD deficiency, pregnancy

*Terminal treatment for *P. vivax* and *P. ovale* infections only.
Abbreviations: G6PD = glucose-6-phosphate dehydrogenase; GI = gastrointestinal.

vomiting should receive intravenous medications. Supportive care is critical for these patients and includes close hemodynamic monitoring, use of judicious fluid replacement, correction of significant metabolic abnormalities, and additional support as needed (e.g., dialysis, mechanical ventilation, and so on). Exchange transfusions have been lifesaving in some patients with parasitemia in excess of 10 percent,[12] although a recent meta-analysis suggested that exchange transfusion showed no significant benefit in survival when compared with antimalarial chemotherapy alone.[13] Glucocorticoids have not been shown to be of benefit in the treatment of cerebral malaria and should not be used.[14] Quinidine is the intravenous drug of choice due not only to its widespread availability but also to its enhanced activity against *P. falciparum*. Parenteral quinine is available only from the CDC. Its use should be reserved for individuals developing significant cardiotoxicity while receiving intravenous quinidine.

Quinine and quinidine are potent inducers of insulin release and may cause severe hypoglycemia. Sudden changes in orientation, sweating, tremor, tachycardia, or anxiety should prompt measurement of plasma glucose concentration. Cinchona alkaloids are myocardial depressants, so cardiac monitoring is needed during administration. Terminal treatment with primaquine is not needed in patients with *P. falciparum* malaria due to the absence of dormant asexual forms in the liver. Newer artemisinin compounds (e.g., artemisinin, artemether, and artesunate) are active against quinine-resistant strains of *P. falciparum*.[15] These agents are not yet available in the United States and have been used either alone or in combination with mefloquine or benflumetol in a fixed-dose tablet (coaretemether).

PREVENTION

Malaria is largely preventable through the use of personal protective measures and appropriate chemoprophylaxis. Recent studies confirmed that travelers to malarious areas frequently do not use anti-mosquito measures or take antimalarial drugs.[8,16] Of the 825 U.S. civilians who acquired malaria abroad during 2000, 635 (77 percent) reported that they had not followed a chemoprophylactic drug regimen recommended by CDC for the area to which they had traveled.[3] Between dusk and dawn, travelers should remain in well-screened areas, use mosquito nets if needed, and wear long-sleeved, light-colored clothing. A pyrethrum-containing insect spray should be used during evening hours and before retiring to bed. Permethrin can be sprayed on clothing for additional protection, and an insect repellent containing *N,N*-diethyl-*m*-toluamide (DEET) in concentrations no higher than 35 percent should be applied to exposed skin. Newer formulations of DEET exist with polymer encapsulation and sustained-release properties that provide long-acting protection at lower concentrations. These are especially useful for children, in whom lower concentrations of DEET are recommended, and for persons with intense, prolonged exposures.[17]

Appropriate chemoprophylaxis depends on where one will be traveling. If potential exposure to infected mosquitoes is likely, prophylaxis is warranted even if such exposure will be brief. Table 148-6 summarizes the chemotherapeutic agents of choice.[2,4,18] Recommendations can be obtained by calling the CDC 24-h malaria hotline (888-232-3228) or by accessing the CDC's Internet site at *http://www.cdc.gov/travel*, which provides up-to-date information on resistance patterns in countries. Failure to take appropriate chemoprophylaxis has been identified as a significant risk factor for fatal infection.[19] Studies exploring other chemoprophylactic options, such as proguanil combined with dapsone, primaquine and related newer analogues (tafenoquine), and monotherapy with daily azithromycin, appear promising.

Last, even with the religious use of antimosquito measures and chemoprophylaxis, malaria can be contracted or can recur. For reasons discussed earlier, malaria must be considered whenever fever occurs in someone who has traveled to a malarious area or who has received

TABLE 148-6 Recommendations for Chemoprophylactic Regimens for Prevention of Malaria*

Drug	Adult Dose	Pediatric Dose
TRAVEL TO AREA WHERE CRPF HAS NOT BEEN REPORTED		
Primary drugs		
Chloroquine phosphate	500 mg (300-mg base) PO, 1 per week (before, during, and for 4 weeks after last exposure)	8.3 mg/kg (5-mg/kg base) PO, 1 per week up to adult dose
Hydroxychloroquine	400 mg (300-mg base) PO, 1 per week (before, during, and for 4 weeks after last exposure)	6.6 mg/kg (4-mg/kg base) PO, every day up to adult dose
Second-line drugs		
Doxycycline	100 mg PO every day (2 days before, during, and for 4 weeks after last exposure)	>8 years of age: 2 mg/kg PO every day up to adult dose
Atovaquone-proguanil (Malarone)	250 mg/100 mg PO every day (2 days before, during, and for 1 week after last exposure)	62.5 mg/25 mg >40 kg 1 adult tab/d 31–40 kg 3 ped tabs/d 21–30 kg 2 ped tabs/d 11–20 kg 1 ped tab/d
TRAVEL TO AREAS WHERE CRPF HAS BEEN REPORTED		
Primary drugs		
Mefloquine	250 mg (228-mg base) PO, 1 per week (before, during, and for 4 weeks after last exposure)	>45 kg 1 tab/week 31–45 kg $\frac{3}{4}$ tab/week 20–30 kg $\frac{1}{2}$ tab/week 12–19 kg $\frac{1}{4}$ tab/week 5–11 kg 5 mg/kg base/week
Atovaquone-proguanil	See above	See above
Doxycycline†	See above	See above
Secondary drugs		
Primaquine	30 mg PO every day (2 days before, during, and for 1 week after last exposure)	0.5 mg/kg per d up to adult dose
TRAVEL TO AREAS WHERE MDRPF HAS BEEN REPORTED		
Primary drugs		
Doxycycline	See above	See above
Atovaquone-proguanil	See above	See above
Secondary drugs		
Primaquine	See above	See above
Artemisinin derivations	Investigational	Investigational

*For prolonged exposure in areas with *P. vivax* or *P. ovale,* primaquine (see Table 148-5) should be added at completion of prophylaxis.
†Doxycycline is the preferred first-line agent for travels to rural Thailand (border areas along Cambodia and Burma) due to prevalence of mefloquine resistance. Atovaquone-proguanil (Malarone) recently has demonstrated comparable efficacy in this area and is an alternative to doxycycline.
Abbreviations: CRPF = chloroquine-resistant *P. falciparum;* MDRPF = multiple-drug-resistant *P. falciparum.*

"successful" therapy in the past. Vaccines directed against various antigens of the malaria parasite are currently in trials, but the findings thus far have not been overwhelmingly encouraging and quite preliminary.[20]

REFERENCES

1. World Health Organization (WHO): Expert Committee on Malaria, 20th Report. *WHO Technical Report Service* 892:1, 2000.
2. Centers for Disease Control and Prevention: *Health Information for International Travel 2000–2001.* Atlanta, US Department of Health and Human Services, 2002.
3. Centers for Disease Control and Prevention: CDC surveillance summaries: Malaria surveillance—United States, 2000. *MMWR* 51:9, 2002.
4. World Health Organization (WHO): *International Travel and Health, 2002.* Geneva, WHO, 2002.
5. Than M, Kyaw MP, Soe AY, et al: Development of resistance to chloroquine by *Plasmodium vivax* in Myanmar. *Trans R Soc Trop Med Hyg* 89:307, 1995.
6. Svenson JE, MacLean JD, Gyorkos TW, et al: Imported malaria: Clinical presentation and examination of symptomatic travelers. *Arch Intern Med* 155:861, 1995.
7. Warrell DA, Molyneaux ME, Beales PF: Severe and complicated malaria. *Trans R Soc Trop Med Hyg* 84(suppl):1, 1990.
8. Dorsey G, Ghandhi M, Oxygi JH, et al: Difficulties in the prevention, diagnosis and treatment of imported malaria. *Arch Intern Med* 160:2505, 2000.
9. White NJ: The treatment of malaria. *N Engl J Med* 335:800, 1996.
10. Moody A: Rapid diagnostic tests for malaria parasites. *Clin Microbiol Rev* 15:66, 2002.
11. Looareesuwan S, Churley JD, Canfield CJ, et al: Malarone (atovaquone and proguanil hydrochloride): A review of its clinical development for treatment of malaria. Malarone Clinical Trials Study Group. *Am J Trop Med Hyg* 60:533, 1999.
12. Phillips P, Nantel S, Benny WB: Exchange transfusion as an adjunct to the treatment of severe falciparum malaria: Case report and review. *Rev Infect Dis* 12:1100, 1990.
13. Riddle MS, Jackson SL, Sanders JW, et al: Exchange transfusion as an adjunct therapy in severe *Plasmodium falciparum* malaria: A meta-analysis. *Clin Infect Dis* 34: 1192, 2002.
14. Hoffman SL, Rustama D, Punjabi NH, et al: High-dose dexamethasone in quinine-treated patients with cerebral malaria: A double-blind placebo-controlled trial. *J Infect Dis* 158:325, 1988.
15. Pittler MH, Ernst E: Artemether for severe malaria: A meta-analysis of randomized clinical trials. *Clin Infect Dis* 28:597, 1999.
16. Lobel HO, Kozarsky PE: Update on prevention of malaria for travelers. *JAMA* 278:1767, 1997.
17. Fradin MS: Mosquitoes and mosquito repellents: A clinician's guide. *Ann Intern Med* 128:931, 1998.
18. Conner BA: Expert recommendations for antimalarial prophylaxis. *J Travel Med* 8:557; 2001.
19. Centers for Disease Control and Prevention: Malaria deaths following inappropriate malaria chemoprophylaxis—United States, 2001. *MMWR* 50: 597, 2001.
20. Hoffman SL, Goh LM, Luke TC, et al: Protection of humans against malaria by immunization with radiation-attenuated *Plasmodium falciparum* sporozoites. *J Infect Dis* 185:1155, 2002.

INFECTIONS FROM HELMINTHS
Harold H. Osborn

Parasitic diseases outrank cancer as a leading cause of death globally.[1] Parasitic infections can be acquired by consuming infected food or water, walking barefoot on contaminated soil, and from insect bites. Parasitic diseases are becoming increasingly encountered in industrialized nations. Immigration and travel are major factors in this recent trend. Tourism has replaced agriculture as the biggest industry in the world, with over 50 million people traveling from the developed to the underdeveloped world each year.[2] Over 650 million people crossed international borders in 1999, and that number will rise to over 1 billion annually by the year 2010.[3]

According to the World Health Organization (WHO), worldwide 3.5 billion people harbor intestinal parasites, of which 450 million are symptomatic, and the number of those infected is increasing in all WHO regions.[4] There are 1.3 billion cases (24 percent prevalence) of *Ascaris* and 902 million cases (17 percent prevalence) of *Trichuris* around the globe (Table 149-1). Malaria is by far the most important parasite in the world today, infecting 270 million people annually with between 1.5 and 2.7 million deaths per year.[5]

Parasitic disease is an important cause of morbidity and mortality in the U.S. due to several factors: the persistence of endemic parasites; immigration to the U.S. of infected individuals from Asia, Africa, and Latin America; increased travel by Americans, particularly to the underdeveloped parts of the world; and the rise of parasitic infections among immunosuppressed patients, especially those afflicted with HIV.[6]

Cryptosporidium and *Giardia* are important pathogens causing traveler's diarrhea, and have also become major causes of diarrhea in immunocompetent individuals in the U.S.[7] Person-to-person spread of these parasites has led to diarrheal illness in day-care centers and other institutions, and contamination of municipal water supplies has led to major outbreaks. In 1993, over 400,000 people in Milwaukee, Wisconsin became ill after *Cryptosporidium* contaminated the drinking water, and 54 people died as a result.[8] About 10 to 15 percent of the chronic diarrhea and wasting in AIDS patients is due to infection with *Cryptosporidium parvum.* Recently, surveys of water throughout the United States indicated that 50 percent of rivers and lakes may be contaminated with *Cryptosporidium.*[9] This parasite cannot be contained by chlorination, iodination, or ozonation of the water; it must be eliminated by filtration. Outbreaks of diarrhea in the summer of 1996 due to the consumption of strawberries contaminated with *Cyclospora,* a coccidian, further highlight the challenge of emerging parasitic diseases in the United States.

TABLE 149-1 Prevalence of Specific Parasitic Diseases Worldwide

Organism	No. of Cases
Ascaris	1.3 billion
Filaria	120 million
Leishmania	12 million
Onchocerca	18 million
Paragonimus	20 million
Schistosoma	200 million
Taenia saginata	45 million
Taenia solium	3 million
Trichuris	902 million
Trypanasoma brucei	(African trypanosomiasis) 55 million
Trypanasoma cruzi	(American trypanosomiasis) 18 million

The agents that cause parasitic diseases belong to three major groups: helminths (worms), protozoa, and arthropods. The multicellular helminths include nematodes (roundworms), cestodes (flatworms), and trematodes (flukes). There are about 20 species of helminths that are natural parasites of man, but many others cause zoonoses (infections of animals which also infect man). The protozoa are single-celled organisms that cause a variety of diseases ranging from malaria to amebiasis. Arthropods are classified as ectoparasites, and are medically important as obligate intermediate hosts and as mechanical vectors in many diseases. This chapter concentrates on diseases caused by helminths. Malaria is discussed in Chap. 148, and parasitic diseases organized by syndromes are also discussed in Chap. 206. Diseases in immunocompromised hosts (e.g., HIV patients) are discussed in Chap. 144.

HISTORY

The recognition of parasitic disease begins with the elicitation of a careful history. Specifically, the clinician should inquire about travel to or immigration from high-risk areas. Parasites flourish in warm, moist climates, in locations where sanitation is poor, and in places where many people have low socioeconomic status and inadequate nutrition. Children are infected with parasites more frequently than adults because of their oral behavior, poor hygiene, and limited ability to ward off arthropod vectors.

Parasitic disease should be considered in any patient with unexplained fever, abdominal pain, diarrhea, skin ulcers, rash, or eosinophilia. The history should include dates of travel or immigration, destination or country of origin, living conditions, and activities. Travel to or from certain specific areas of the world may implicate particular parasitic agents. Hmong tribesmen, who came to this country from Indochina in large numbers after the Vietnam War, often harbor *Paragonimus westermani* (lung fluke), whereas visitors to Russia or the Rocky Mountains may return with *Giardia.* The history should also include questions about sexual orientation and contacts, drug use, and past illnesses, as well as a complete review of systems. The use of pretravel medications, including antimalarial and antidiarrheal agents, should also be elicited.

The presence of risk factors can provide a clue to specific parasitic diseases (Table 149-2). Cases of acute Chagas disease (trypanosomiasis) and babesiosis following blood transfusions have been described in the United States and Canada. Institutionalized patients may suffer from amebiasis and can become infected with *Hymenolepsis nana* (the most common tapeworm in the United States) or *Giardia.* Immunocompromised hosts (including those on steroids or antineoplastic agents) are susceptible to infection by *Strongyloides, Toxoplasma, Cryptosporidium,* and *Pneumocystis carinii* and can develop a life-threatening hyperinfection syndrome with *Strongyloides stercoralis.* It is interesting to note that patients with AIDS, while susceptible to *Toxoplasma, Cryptosporidium, Pneumocystis, Isospora, Microsporidium,* and *Cyclospora,* are not any more susceptible to *Amoeba* and *Strongyloides* than immunocompetent individuals. Finally, the consumption of raw food has been associated with a variety of parasitic diseases, including fish, pork, and beef tapeworm.

PATHOPHYSIOLOGY

Parasites differ in their pathogenicity and in their capacity to produce invasive or systemic disease. The subclass Coccidia, for example, includes both *Toxoplasma* and *Isospora.* However, *Isospora* is unable to invade the intestinal mucosa and thus produces only enterocolitis, whereas *Toxoplasma* crosses the intestine and produces severe systemic illness.

Sometimes various forms of the same parasite differ in their ability to cause illness. The adult form of *Trichinella spiralis* remains in the intestine, while the larval form crosses and migrates to striated and cardiac muscle. Amebiasis can be manifested as both an intestinal and

TABLE 149-2   Risk Factors for Parasitic Disease

Risk Factor	Parasite
Blood transfusion	*Plasmodium* species, *Trypanosoma, Babesia, Toxoplasma*
Intravenous drug use	*Plasmodium* species
Homosexuality	*Entamoeba* (also seen after colonic irrigation therapy), *Giardia, Cryptosporidium*
Immunocompromised host	*Toxoplasma, Pneumocystis, Strongyloides, Cryptosporidium, Microsporidium, Isospora,* and *Cyclospora*
Hypogammaglobulinemia	*Giardia, Cryptosporidium*
Institutionalization	*Hymenolepsis nana, Entamoeba histolytica, Giardia*
Day-care centers	*Giardia, Cryptosporidium*
Livestock workers	*Cryptosporidium*
Pica	*Toxocara* (visceral larva migrans), hookworm (*Necator americanus*)
Consumption of raw food	
Sushi, sashimi, gefilte fish	*Diphyllobothrium, Anisakis*
Pork	*Taenia solium, Trichinella, Sarcocystis*
Beef	*Taenia saginata, Toxoplasma, Sarcocystis*

visceral infection. Pathogenicity may vary among strains within a genus. Infection with *Entamoeba* can result in an asymptomatic cyst carrier state or hepatic abscesses, depending on the strain involved.

Finally, organisms differ in their virulence. The infectious dose of *Giardia* and *Cryptosporidium* is on the order of 10^1 to 10^3 organisms. By contrast, the infectious dose of *Vibrio cholerae* and *Salmonella* is 10^5 to 10^8 organisms. This may be an important factor in the genesis of outbreaks in institutions and day-care centers.

CLINICAL FEATURES

Unfortunately, symptoms may be nonspecific, and the latency period between exposure and symptom appearance may be years. Symptoms can be acute or chronic, specific or vague. Parasitic disease can present with relatively common complaints, such as headache, fever, cough, and malaise, or with acute, life-threatening complications, such as seizures, hemoptysis, melena, and intestinal obstruction. A differential diagnosis can be attempted on the basis of history and knowledge of typical symptoms associated with various parasitic agents (Table 149-3).

DIAGNOSIS

Although viruses and bacteria are generally the most common causes of infectious diarrhea, parasites constitute a significant cause as well.

The majority of diarrhea-inducing infections are noninflammatory, usually arising in the upper small bowel from the action of an enterotoxin (e.g., *V. cholerae* or enterotoxigenic *Escherichia coli*) or other processes that alter the absorptive function of the villous tip (e.g., *Cryptosporidium, Giardia,* rotavirus, and Norwalk-like virus). In contrast, inflammatory diarrhea, which often presents as dysentery (bloody stools), arises in the colon from an invasive process, sometimes mediated by a cytotoxin (e.g., *Salmonella, Shigella, Campylobacter, Clostridium difficile,* and *Amoeba*).

If diarrhea has persisted for more than a few days, is bloody in nature, or is accompanied by substantial fever, dehydration, or weight loss, the patient should be evaluated more closely. Diarrheal illness that lasts 10 days or longer, occurs in those with risk factors (see Table 149-2), or persists in those without evidence of a bacterial infection should prompt a vigorous search for parasites.

TABLE 149-3   Symptoms of Parasitic Disease

Symptom	Possible Cause
Abdominal pain	*Ascaris, Clonorchis, Diphyllobothrium, Entamoeba, Fasciola, Giardia,* hookworm, *Hymenolepsis, Schistosoma, Taenia, Trichuris*
Anemia	*Babesia, Diphyllobothrium,* hookworm, *Leishmania donovani, Plasmodium* species, *Trichuris*
Asthma	*Ascaris, Strongyloides, Toxocara*
Conjunctivitis and keratitis	Filariae (*Onchocerca volvulus*), Taenia, *Trichinella, Trypanosoma*
Diarrhea	*Dientamoeba, Entamoeba, Fasciola, Fasciolopsis, Giardia,* hookworm, *Hymenolepsis, L. donovani, Palantidium, Schistosoma, Strongyloides, Taenia, Trichinella, Trichuris*
Edema	*Fasciolopsis,* filariae (*Wuchereria bancrofti*), *Trichinella, Trypanosoma*
Eosinophilia	*Ascaris, Dracunculus, Fasciola,* filariae (*W. bancrofti, Brugia malayi*), fluke (*Paragonimus westermani, Chlonorchis sinensis, Fasciolopsis leuski*), *Hymnenolepsis,* hookworm, *Schistosoma, Strongyloides, Taenia, Toxocara, Trichinella, Trichuris*
Fever	*Ascaris, Babesia, Entamoeba, Fasciola,* filariae (*W. bancrofti*), fluke (*C. sinensis*), *Giardia, L. donovani, Plasmodium* species, *Toxocara, Trichi, Trichuris, Trypanosoma*
Hematuria	*Schistosoma*
Hemoptysis	*Ascaris, Echinococcus, Paragonimus*
Hepatomegaly	Fluke (*C. sinensis, Opisthorchis viverrini, Fasciola*), *L. donovani, Plasmodium* species, tapeworm (*Echinococcus*), *Schistosoma, Toxocara, Trypanosoma*
Intestinal obstruction	*Ascaris, Diphyllobothrium,* fluke (*Fasciolopsis buski*), *Strongyloides, Taenia*
Jaundice	Fluke (*C. sinensis, O. viverrini*), *Plasmodium* species
Meningitis	*Acanthamoeba,* malaria (*Plasmodium falciparum*), *Naegleria,* primary amebic meningoencephalitis, *Toxocara, Trichinella, Trypanosoma*
Myocardial disease	*Taenia, Trichinella, Trypanosoma (T. cruzi)*
Nausea and vomiting	*Ascaris, Entamoeba, Giardia, Leishmania, Taenia, Trichinella, Trichuris*
Pneumonia	*Ascaris,* filariae (*W. bancrofti, B. malayi*), fluke (*P. westermani*), *Strongyloides, Trichinella*
Pruritus	*Dientamoeba, Enterobius,* filariae (*O. volvulus*), *Trichuris*
Seizures	*Hymenolepsis, Trichinella, Paragonimus,* tapeworm (*Echinococcus, Cysticercus*)
Skin ulcers	*Dracunculus,* hookworm, *L. donovani, Trypanosoma*
Splenomegaly	*Babesia, Toxoplasma, Plasmodium*
Urticaria	*Ascaris, Dracunculus, Fasciola, Strongyloides, Trichinella*

Examination of a stool sample for fecal leukocytes is neither sensitive nor specific for inflammatory causes.[10]

Examination of a stool specimen for ova and parasites has traditionally been the method of choice for detecting intestinal parasites, including the cysts and trophozoites of protozoa and the larvae, eggs, and adults of helminths. Three specimens collected on different days are examined. The stool must be free of substances such as bismuth, barium, nonabsorbable antidiarrheal agents, and mineral oil.[11] Antimicrobial agents should be stopped at least 1 week prior to the stool collection. Fresh specimens are best, and specimens over an hour old should be preserved with formalin or polyvinyl alcohol. Multiple stool examinations are particularly important when dealing with formed stool, which usually contains fewer parasites than do diarrheal specimens.

Occasionally *Giardia, Cryptosporidium,* and the larvae of *Strongyloides* may be detected by examining a duodenal aspirate or by having the patient swallow a string attached to a gelatin capsule (Entero-test). However, detection of *Giardia* by examination of several stool specimens is just as effective as examination of duodenal contents.

Special procedures for removing parasites include the following: warm water concentration through a filter for *Strongyloides* (Baermann test), sticky tape swab of the perianal area for *Enterobius,* and passage of urine through a nucleopore filter for *Schistosoma haematobium.* Use of special stains such as an acid-fast stain to detect *Cryptosporidium, Isospora,* and *Cyclospora,* and a modified trichrome stain for microsporidia may be helpful.

The enzyme-linked immunosorbent assay (ELISA) technique can be used to make a serologic diagnosis of parasitic infection. Immunoassay tests have been used to detect antigens of *Giardia* and *Cryptosporidia* in particular in the stool. Immunodiagnostic assays are more sensitive and cost effective than the standard examination for ova and parasites.[12] The increased accuracy and availability of these tests have obviated the need for the standard examination for ova and parasites and the invasive duodenal fluid examination in the diagnosis of *Giardia* and *Cryptosporidium parvum.* Many experts now recommend immunoassay screening for these two most common parasitic pathogens first if parasitic disease is suspected. Microscopic examinations of the stool that are costly, time-consuming, and require a skilled technician should be reserved for patients with persistent symptoms and laboratory exclusion of the common enteric pathogens.

Malaria-causing plasmodia, *Babesia,* microfilaria of *Wuchereria* and *Brugia,* and the trypanosomes that cause Chagas disease can be detected by Giemsa-stained thick and thin films of peripheral blood.

Finally, organisms that affect the central nervous system (e.g., *P. falciparum,* which causes cerebral malaria, and *Acanthamoeba* or *Naegleria,* which cause amoebic meningoencephalitis) can be detected by culture or microscopic examination of centrifuged cerebrospinal fluid. *Pneumocystis* is detected by characteristic findings on chest x-ray, elevated lactate dehydrogenase (LDH) levels, and evidence of hypoxemia, and is confirmed by lung biopsy with special stains, while *Toxoplasma* is detected by characteristic findings on computed tomography (CT) scan in association with elevated serum antibody levels, and is rarely confirmed by brain biopsy.

HELMINTHS

Nematodes (Roundworms)

Nematodes are cylindrical, unsegmented, elongated white worms. Their mode of entry into the human host varies from ingestion of eggs (*Ascaris* and *Enterobius*) to penetration of the skin (*Necator, Ancylostoma,* and *Strongyloides*) to inoculation by insect bite *(Wuchereria).*

ASCARIS *Ascaris lumbricoides* has a worldwide distribution, and its lifespan if left untreated is 2 to 7 years. Larval invasion follows the ingestion of *Ascaris* eggs, and during this stage the parasite migrates through the lungs. Clinical disease is due to pulmonary hypersensitivity or intestinal complications. Patients may have fever, cough, dyspnea, hemoptysis, and eosinophilia. Obstruction of the common bile duct and the intestine have been described. The chest x-ray may reveal eosinophilic pneumonitis (Loeffler syndrome). The diagnosis is made by finding eggs, or occasionally an adult worm, in the stool. Serologic tests, including bentonite flocculation, ELISA, and indirect hemagglutination, may be helpful. Treatment is with mebendazole, albendazole, or pyrantel pamoate. Intestinal obstruction may necessitate surgery, especially in children.

ENTEROBIUS (PINWORM) Adult *Enterobius* (pinworm) resides in the cecum, appendix, ileum, and ascending colon after its eggs are in-

gested. The gravid female migrates to the anus, especially at night, where it causes intense pruritus. Autoinfection with hand-to-mouth transmission is possible after scratching. A host of problems from vaginitis to enuresis have been attributed to *Enterobius* infection, without good evidence. It is most prevalent in temperate climates during the winter and fall. The diagnosis is confirmed with a cellophane tape swab of the anus. All family members should be examined. Treatment is with pyrantel pamoate, albendazole, or mebendazole, and should be repeated after 2 weeks.

NECATOR (HOOKWORM) *Necator americanus* prevails in the southern United States and is often seen in immigrants from warmer climates. Infection is associated with the use of human feces as fertilizer and the lack of shoes and latrines. Because each worm can withdraw 0.03 to 0.2 mL of blood a day, infection often leads to chronic anemia. Pica and geophagy are often seen in infected children. Patients may have cough, low-grade fever, abdominal pain, diarrhea, weakness, weight loss, heme-positive stools, and eosinophilia. The diagnosis is made by finding ova in the stool. In mild infections, multiple stool specimens or concentration techniques may be necessary. The parasite burden may be estimated using the Beaver stool or Kato slide smear method. Infections with less than 2100 eggs per gram of feces (<50 adult worms) are usually not hematologically significant, whereas infections with over 11,000 eggs per gram results in significant anemia. Hookworm is best treated with mebendazole, albendazole, or pyrantel pamoate.

STRONGYLOIDES (THREADWORMS) Adult threadworms reside in the mucosa of the small intestine. Because entry of the parasite is through the skin, penetration can lead to allergic manifestations, pruritus, and an erythematous rash. Migration throughout the lungs can produce cough, dyspnea, and pneumonia. The intestinal phase is manifested by abdominal pain, diarrhea with mucus and blood, and eosinophilia. Autoinfection can occur due to internal production of infective larvae. Larval migration in the skin produces larva currens. Fatalities may occur due to hyperinfection in elderly and immunocompromised patients (e.g., patients with leprosy, nephrotic syndrome, hepatic disease, or lymphoproliferative disorders and those on steroids). The diagnosis is confirmed by finding larvae in the stool. Occasionally, use of a formalin ether concentration method or duodenal aspiration may be necessary. Various stages of the parasite may be found in the sputum. An ELISA test is also available. An upper gastrointestinal series may reveal a deformed duodenal bulb, and *Strongyloides* may be confused with ulcer disease. Treatment is with thiabendazole or ivermectin.

TRICHURIS TRICHIURA (WHIPWORM) Like *Ascaris, Trichuris trichiura* is found in rural communities in the southern United States. The infection is most often acquired in childhood because the ova are deposited in the soil where children play and defecate freely. The adult worm resides in the cecum. Patients complain of anorexia, insomnia, abdominal pain (including pain in the right upper quadrant), fever, flatulence, bloody diarrhea, weight loss, and pruritus, and may have eosinophilia and microcytic hypochromic anemia. *Trichuris* can result in colitis or rectal prolapse in children. The diagnosis is made with the finding of ova in the stool. Mebendazole or albendazole are the drugs of choice for treatment.

TRICHINELLA SPIRALIS Trichinosis is common in Mexico and the United States and results from the consumption of infected pork, and less commonly, bear and walrus meat. In the early stages of infection with *Trichinella spiralis,* the patient may present with acute myocarditis, nonsuppurative meningitis, bronchopneumonia, or catarrhal enteritis. The primary lesions are in striated muscle. Clinical symptoms depend on the site of invasion. Patients may present with nausea and vomiting, diarrhea, fever, urticaria, periorbital edema, (pathognomonic) splinter hemorrhages, myalgia, muscle spasm, stiff neck, headache, and psychiatric disturbances. Laboratory manifestations of trichinosis include leukocytosis, eosinophilia, elevated creatine phosphokinase, and electrocardiographic changes. The diagnosis can be confirmed with latex agglutination, skin test, and a bentonite flocculation test. Biopsy of tender muscle may be helpful after the fourth week. Since *T. spiralis* encysts in striated muscle, stool examination is not helpful after the initial gastrointestinal phase in making the diagnosis. The differential diagnosis includes staphylococcal and *Salmonella* food poisoning, shigellosis, and amebiasis. Albendazole or mebendazole are indicated for treatment of the intestinal phase, but may be ineffective after encystment. Steroids are indicated for severe infections, such as CNS disease and myocarditis, but are not advocated routinely because their use can increase the number of circulating larvae. Most cases are mild and never come to medical attention.

Trematodes (Flukes)

Trematodes are leaflike, symmetrical flatworms lacking a body cavity but possessing a ventral sucker to hold their position. They live in intermediate hosts such as snails, crabs, and fish, and shed their eggs from the human host in the feces (*Schistosoma, Clonorchis,* and *Fasciola*), urine *(Schistosoma haematobium),* or sputum *(Paragonimus).*

SCHISTOSOMA Schistosomes penetrate the skin, creating a papular pruritic rash. The adult form resides in the venous system. Symptoms of acute disease-fever, lymphadenopathy, and hepatosplenomegaly (so-called Katayama fever)—are rarely seen. More typically, patients present in the chronic stage with granulomas in the liver (portal hypertension) and bladder (obstructive hydroureter). Patients may present with diarrhea, abdominal pain, melena, hepatosplenomegaly, hematemesis, and in the late stages, ascites and liver failure. With *S. haematobium,* dysuria and hematuria may be found. The diagnosis is suggested by a positive immunofluorescent antibody test result and confirmed by finding eggs in the feces or on rectal biopsy. Treatment is with praziquantel.

Cestodes (Flatworms)

The cestodes are flatworms commonly referred to as tapeworms. They have a scolex, or head, equipped with suckers, or hooks. Cestodes grow by segmentation, extending proglottides from the neck.

TAENIA *Taenia solium* (pork tapeworm) is occasionally encountered in the United States in immigrants or visitors from Central America and the Middle East. *Taenia saginata* (beef tapeworm) is seen more often, especially in those who consume raw beef (e.g., steak tartare). Adult worms live in the small intestine. Infected patients can be asymptomatic or present with nausea and vomiting, headache, abdominal pain, pruritus, constipation, diarrhea, and intestinal obstruction. The larval stage of *T. solium* can cause clinical disease (cysticercosis), which can be serious and sometimes fatal. *Taenia* cysts may be found in subcutaneous tissue, the eye, the brain, and the heart, and cause seizures and hydrocephalus. Radiographs of the soft tissues may reveal curvilinear calcifications indicative of cysts, and cysts can be seen in the meninges and brain parenchyma on CT scanning. The diagnosis is made by finding gravid proglottids in the stool. An ELISA or hemagglutination reaction may be helpful, but results of both can be falsely negative if the cysts are calcified. Treatment of the adult (intestinal) stage is with praziquantel. The larval (tissue) stage is treated with albendazole.

DIPHYLLOBOTHRIUM *Diphyllobothrium* (fish tapeworm) has been reported in the Pacific northwest, Minnesota, Michigan, and other areas where raw fish (e.g., sushi and sashimi) and gefilte fish are consumed. *Diphyllobothrium* can compete with the host for vitamin B_{12}, and thus patients can present with pernicious anemia. Treatment is the same as for *Taenia.*

TREATMENT

The geographic spread and emerging drug resistance of parasites have created challenges for successful treatment. A number of reports have recently highlighted persistent shedding of schistosome eggs despite multiple treatments with praziquantel, the drug of choice.[13] Successful treatment of malaria has been compromised by strains of *P. falciparum* that are resistant to chloroquine which now have a global distribution. Pockets of malaria resistant to sulfadoxine-pyrimethamine have been found throughout Africa. Mefloquine, a fluoroquinolone, has historically been available for the treatment of multidrug resistant *P. falciparum.* Now, however, monotherapy with mefloquine is associated with over 50 percent failure rates in some areas.[14] Strains of *Leishmania* resistant to antimonial compounds have also been reported.

In many cases international pharmaceutical companies have stopped manufacturing drugs of proven efficacy and have curtailed the research and development of new drugs and vaccines due to financial considerations. Eflornithine, a medication used for trypanosomiasis, is prohibitively expensive and is no longer manufactured. Drugs for schistosomiasis (oxaminiquine and metrifonate) are expensive and in very short supply.

The treatment of parasites is complex and constantly changing[15] (Table 149-4). Patients with potentially life-threatening infections

TABLE 149-4   Commonly Used Antiparasitic Drugs

Drug	First-Line Agent	Alternative Agent	Side Effects
Albendazole (Zental)	*Trichinella, Echinococcus granulosus, Cysticercus, Ascaria,* cutaneous larva migrans, *Enterobius, Gnathostoma, Trichuris,* hookworm (*Ascaris duodenale, Necator americanus), Microsporidium*	*Capillaria, Trichostrongylus,* visceral larva migrans	Diarrhea, abdominal pain
Amphotericin B (Fungizone)	Amebic meningoencephalitis *(Naegleria)*	*Leishmania (L. braziliensis, L. mexicana)*	Fever, headache, anorexia, nausea, diarrhea, muscle and joint pain, azotemia, anemia, renal tubular acidosis (RTA), leukopenia
Atovaquone (Mepron)	*Babesia*		Headache, dizziness, nausea, vomiting, anemia, neutropenia, hyperglycemia
Bithionol (Bithin)	Fluke *(Fasciola hepatica)*		Photosensitivity, nausea and vomiting, urticaria
Chloroquine	*Plasmodium* species (except resistant *P. falciparum)*		Pruritus, vomiting, headache, confusion, skin eruptions, myalgias, blurred vision
Clindamycin (Cleocin)	*Babesia,* chloroquine-resistant *P. falciparum*		C. difficile diarrhea

(continued)

TABLE 149-4   Commonly Used Antiparasitic Drugs *(Continued)*

Drug	First-Line Agent	Alternative Agent	Side Effects
Diethylcarbamazine (Hetrazan)	Filariae (*Wuchereria bancrofti, Loa loa*, tropical pulmonary eosinophilia), visceral larva migrans		Allergic reactions, GI symptoms
Fumagillin	*Microsporidia*		Thrombocytopenia
Iodoquinol (Yodoxin)	*Entamoeba (Entamoeba histolytica), Dientamoeba*	*Balantidium*	Rash, acne, enlarged thyroid, nausea, diarrhea, anal pruritus; rarely: optic atrophy, peripheral neuropathy
Ivermectin (Mectizan)	Filariae *(Onchocerca volvulus), Strongyloides*, cutaneous larva migrans		Fever, pruritus, tender nodes, bone and joint pain, headache
Lindane (Kwell)		Lice, scabies	Eczema, conjunctivitis, aplastic anemia
Mebendazole (Vermox)	*Angiostrongylus, Ascaria, Capillaria, Enterobius*, filariae *(Mansonella perstans) Trichuris*, hookworm, *Trichinella*	*Leishmania*, visceral larva migrans	Diarrhea, abdominal pain, agranulocytosis
Mefloquine (Lariam)		Chloroquine-resistant *P. falciparum*	Vertigo, nausea, nightmares, headache
Meglumine (Glucantime)	*Leishmania*		Joint and muscle pain, nausea
Metronidazole (Flagyl)	*Entamoeba (E. histolytica, E. polecki), Dracunculus, Trichomonas, Blastocystis, Giardia*	*Balantidium*	Nausea, headache, dry mouth, reaction with alcohol; rarely: seizures, ataxia, leukopenia, pancreatitis
Niclosamide (Niclocide)	Fluke *(Fasciolopsis buski)*, tapeworm *(Diphyllobothrium, Taenia, Dipylidium)*	Tapeworm *(Hymenolepis)*	Nausea, abdominal pain
Nifurtimox (Lampit)	*Trypanosoma (T. cruzi)*		Anorexia, vomiting, sleep disorder, tremors
Nitoazoxanide (Cryptaz[16], Alinia)	*Cryptosporidia*		Hypertension, headache, abdominal pain
Paromomycin (Humatin)	*Entamoeba, Dientamoeba, Cryptosporidium*	*E. histolytica, Giardia Leishmania*	GI disturbance; rarely: eighth nerve and renal damage
Pentamidine isethionate (Pentam)	*P. carinii*	*Trypanosoma (T. brucei), Leishmania*	Hypotension, hypoglycemia, vomiting, blood dyscrasia, renal damage, GI disturbance
Praziquantel (Biltricide)	Fluke, *Schistosoma*, tapeworm *(Hymenolepis, Cysticercus)*; tapeworm *(Diphyllobothrium latum, Taenia, Dipylidium, Hymenolepis nana, Cysticercus cellulosae)*		Malaise, headache, dizziness, abdominal upset, fever, eosinophilia
Primaquine phosphate	*P. vivax, P. orale* (prevention of relapse only)		G6PD hemolysis, neutropenia, GI disturbances
Pyrantel pamoate (Antiminth)	*Ascaria, Enterrobius*, hookworm, *Trichostrongylus, Moniliformis*		GI disturbances, headache, dizziness, rash, fever
Pyrimethamine (Daraprim)	Chloroquine-resistant *P. falciparum, Toxoplasma*		Blood dyscrasias, folate deficiency; rarely: rash, vomiting, seizures, shock
Quinacrine (Atabrine)		*Giardia*	Dizziness, headache, vomiting, diarrhea, yellow skin, toxic psychosis, insomnia, rash, blood dyscrasias
Quinine sulfate (Quinamm)	*Babesia*, chloroquine-resistant *P. falciparum*		Cinchonism, hemolytic, anemia, blood dyscrasias, photosensitivity, hypoglycemia, arrhythmias, hypotension
Sodium stibogluconate (Pentostam)	*Leishmania*		Muscle pain, joint stiffness, nausea, diarrhea, rash, pruritus, liver and heart damage, bradycardia; rarely: hemolytic anemia, sudden death
Spiramycin (Rovamycin)		*Toxoplasma*	GI symptoms
Suramin sodium (Germanin)	*Trypanosoma* (African)		Vomiting, pruritus, urticaria, paresthesias, neuropathy
Tetracycline (Achromycin)	*Dientamoeba*		Nausea, vomiting, metallic taste, discolored teeth in children

(continued)

TABLE 149-4   Commonly Used Antiparasitic Drugs *(Continued)*

Drug	First-Line Agent	Alternative Agent	Side Effects
Thiabendazole (Mintezol)	*Angiostrongylus, Strongyloides,* visceral larva migrans, cutaneous larva migrans	*Capillaria, Dracunculus, Trichostrongylus*	Nausea, vertigo, rash, leukopenia, hallucinations, erythema multiforme, Stevens-Johnson syndrome, rarely: shock, seizures
Tinidazole (Fasigyn)	*Amoeba (E. histolytica), Trichomonas*	*Giardia*	Colitis
Trimethoprim-sulfamethoxazole (Septra, Bactrim)	*Isospora, Pneumocystis carinii, Cyclospora*		Allergic reactions

Source: Adapted from Drugs for parasitic infections, *Med Lett* April 1, 2002, p. 1, with permission. Available at: www.medletter.com.

(e.g., cerebral malaria, *Pneumocystis* pneumonia, amebic meningoencephalitis, or CNS toxoplasmosis) should be started on antiparasitic treatment immediately in the emergency department and rapidly admitted to the hospital. Patients who are dehydrated from gastrointestinal losses or fever should receive intravenous hydration. Those who can take fluids orally can be rehydrated by mouth.

Patients with diarrhea who appear severely ill, toxic, or dehydrated; those who cannot tolerate anything by mouth; and those with organ system involvement (e.g., lung, blood, or CNS) should be admitted for intravenous hydration, further diagnostic evaluation, and antiparasitic drug treatment as indicated. Patients who do not require hospitalization can be treated with antiparasitic agents if a specific diagnosis has been made and should be referred for follow-up. Those who can tolerate oral fluids can be reliably rehydrated with the WHO oral rehydration solution. Such a solution can be prepared by adding 3.5 g sodium chloride (or three-quarters teaspoon of table salt), 2.5 g sodium bicarbonate (or 2.9 g sodium citrate or 1 teaspoon of baking soda), 1.5 g potassium chloride (or 1 cup of orange juice or two bananas), and 20 g glucose (or 40 g sucrose or 4 tablespoons of sugar) to a liter (1.05 quart) of clean water. This makes a solution of approximately 90 mmol sodium, 20 mmol potassium, 80 mmol chloride, 30 mmol bicarbonate, and 111 mmol glucose per liter.

REFERENCES

1. Northrop-Clewes CA, Shaw C: Parasites. *Br Med Bull* 56:193, 2000.
2. World Health Organization: *The World Health Report 1996: Fighting Disease, Fostering Development.* Geneva, World Health Organization, 1996.
3. World Tourism Organization (WTO) News, available at: http://www.world-tourism.org/newslett/aprjun00/results.htm, second quarter 2000.
4. World Health Organization, Division of Control of Tropical Disease: Intestinal Parasites Control, available at: http://www.who.int/crd/html/intest.html, 1998.
5. Campbell CC: Malaria: An emerging and reemerging global plague. *FEMS Immunol Med Microbiol* 18:32, 1997.
6. James SL: Emerging parasitic infections. *FEMS Immunol Med Microbiol* 18:313, 1997.
7. Wittner M, Tanowitz HB: Intestinal parasites in returned travelers. *Med Clin North Am* 76:1433, 1992.
8. Mackenzie MD: A massive outbreak in Milwaukee of *Cryptosporidium* infection transmitted through the public water supply. *N Engl J Med* 331:161, 1994.
9. Widmer G, Carraway M, Tzipori S: Waterborne *Cryptosporidium*: A perspective from the USA. *Parisitol Today* 12:286, 1996.
10. Huicho L, Sanchez D, Contraras M, et al: Occult blood and fecal leukocytes as screening tests in childhood infectious diarrhea: An old problem revisited. *Pediatr Infect Dis J* 12:474, 1993.
11. Rosenblatt JE: Laboratory diagnosis of parasitic infections. *Mayo Clin Proc* 69:779, 1994.
12. Morris AJ, Murray PR, Reller RB: Contemporary testing for enteric pathogens. *J Clin Microbiol* 34:1776, 1996.
13. Stephenson I, Wiselka M: Drug treatment of tropical parasitic infections. *Drugs* 60:985, 2000.
14. Nosten F, Luxemburger C, Kuile FO, et al: Treatment of resistant *P. falciparum* malaria with three day artesunate-mefloquine combination. *J Infect Dis* 170:971, 1994.
15. The Medical Letter: Drugs for parasitic infections. The Medical Letter Inc., April 1, 2002.
16. The Medical Letter: Nitazoxanide (Alinia)—A new anti-protozoal agent. The Medical Letter Inc., April 14, 2003.

150

FOOD-BORNE AND WATER-BORNE DISEASES
William T. Anderson

The spectrum of food-borne and water-borne disease is changing with the emergence of new pathogens, reemergence of old pathogens and the increase in antibiotic resistance among these agents. The globalization of the food economy and explosion in international travel have facilitated the transmission of disease between continents.[1] Single outbreaks of food-borne or water-borne illnesses are capable of causing sickness in hundreds of thousands of people. Food or water may act as a vehicle for transmission of actively growing organisms or as a transfer medium for nonreplicating viruses, toxins, protozoa, bacteria, or chemical agents.

Food-borne illness is the occurrence of two or more cases of a similar illness resulting from the ingestion of a common food.[2]

Water-borne illness is defined by the Centers for Disease Control and Prevention (CDC) as an illness that occurs after consumption or use of water intended for drinking or as illness associated with recreational water such as swimming pools, whirlpools, hot tubs, spas, water parks, and naturally occurring fresh and marine surface waters.[3]

EPIDEMIOLOGY: FOOD-BORNE DISEASE

Food-borne diseases are estimated to cause approximately 76 million illnesses, 325,000 hospitalizations, and 5000 deaths in the United States each year. The majority of these illnesses are caused by unknown or unidentified pathogens.[4] Three pathogens, *Salmonella, Listeria,* and *Toxoplasma* cause 1500 deaths each year, more than 75 percent of all deaths caused by known pathogens.[4] Newly recognized pathogens include *Campylobacter jejuni, Escherichia coli* O157:H7, *Listeria monocytogenes,* and *Cyclospora cayetanensis.*[4] A growing list of foods previously thought to be safe have been identified as new vehicles for transmission. *E. coli* O157:H7, generally associated with undercooked beef or unpasteurized dairy products, is now linked with items such as fruits, salad vegetables, yogurt, water, and acidic foods.

International trade has allowed people to come into contact with previously unfamiliar pathogens that are native to remote parts of the world.[5] Bacteria, viruses, parasites, and chemical contamination at the site of processing can be disseminated to a multitude of locations thousands of miles away. Low-dose contamination at a central processing site can cause widespread outbreaks.[5] Consolidation of the food industry has led to a larger market share and greater geographic distribution of products from a single supplier or distributor.[5] This increases the risk of larger outbreaks of disease. In 1994, a nationwide outbreak of over 224,000 cases of *Salmonella enteritidis* from one distributor occurred when ice cream premix was transported in tanker trucks that had not been completely sanitized after transporting nonpasteurized liquid eggs.[6]

The eating habits of the U.S. population have changed, with a greater emphasis on incorporating fruits and vegetables into the diet.[1] To meet this increased demand, the volume of imported fresh fruits and vegetables has escalated. Imports can account for more than 75 percent of fruits and vegetables available at local grocery stores.[1] Outbreaks of food-borne illness have occurred recently in produce such as fresh squeezed orange juice, raspberries, frozen strawberries, sliced tomatoes, and lettuce.[5]

Also, a larger percentage of meals are consumed outside the home.[5] Nearly 44 percent of food-borne outbreaks in the United States from 1993 to 1997 occurred in cafeterias, restaurants, or delicatessens.[2] Many restaurants rely on transient personnel who have inadequate knowledge of safe food-handling techniques.[7] In the home, there has been a decline in basic food preparation skills. Many adults who prepare meals do not routinely wash their hands after handling raw meat or poultry.[7]

The number and the percentage of people with increased vulnerability to illness have changed. A demographic shift to an older population base[8] and patients with compromised immunity secondary to AIDS, immunosuppressants, chemotherapy, or chronic illnesses also represent an expanding segment of the population with heightened susceptibility to food-borne illness.[5,8]

Travelers are at an increased risk of food-borne illnesses secondary to exposure to new, previously unseen pathogens, increased exposure through meals at hotels and restaurants, and unpredictable standards for public health cleanliness and water-supply systems.[9] The relative risk of food-borne infection with viruses, bacteria, or parasites varies by country, but ranges from 20 to 50 percent for all travelers.[1] Enterotoxigenic *E. coli* is recognized as the major cause of traveler's diarrhea, but other strains of *E. coli* are also associated with travel, including enterohemorrhagic and enteroinvasive *E. coli*.[9] The prevalence of *Salmonella typhi* necessitates typhoid immunization for travelers to many countries.[9] *Salmonella enteritidis* outbreaks have occurred due to contaminated meals on airlines and railways.[9] Other pathogens associated with international travel include *Brucella*, hepatitis A,[9] *Vibrio, Shigella, Campylobacter, Giardia lamblia,* and *Cryptosporidium*.[10]

Food industry influences have contributed to the emergence of new pathogens in food-borne disease. The routine use of antibiotics to promote growth in food animals in North America and Europe for more than 50 years has facilitated an increase in antibiotic-resistant strains of *Salmonella* and *Campylobacter jejuni. Salmonella* contamination was found in 20 percent of supermarket ground meat samples. Of these isolates, 84 percent were resistant to at least one antimicrobial, including ceftriaxone, the drug of choice in treating *Salmonella* infection in children.[4,11] The disposal of the more than 1 billion tons of manure and associated pathogens that are an annual by-product of the farming industry can contribute to the contamination of fruits and vegetables at harvest.[5]

National and international surveillance systems provide only rough estimates of the incidence of disease. Cholera is the only food-borne disease that must be reported internationally.[12] Many governments are reluctant to provide information on food-borne diseases, particularly if a country's economy is based on tourism or food exports.[12] International surveillance systems and laboratories have insufficient resources for accurate reporting.[12] Globally, only 1 to 10 percent of incidents of food-borne illnesses are reported.[12] Some countries have estimated that food-borne illnesses may be 300 to 350 times more common than reported.[12]

EPIDEMIOLOGY: WATER-BORNE DISEASE

United States public water systems are regulated under the Safe Water Drinking Act and the Surface Water Treatment Rule.[3] These regulations require water utilities to disinfect surface water and groundwater, and use parameters such as turbidity, coliform counts, and the presence of human enteric viruses, *Cryptosporidium parvum* and *Giardia lamblia* cysts as target organisms to assess efficacy of treatment.[3]

The CDC identified 39 outbreaks of water-borne disease in the United States associated with drinking water that caused illness in 2068 people from 1999 to 2000.[3] Most outbreaks of water-borne illness remain unrecognized when they do not cause an acute serious illness, involve few people, have long incubation periods, or involve private, noncommunity water systems.[3] A 1994 outbreak of cryptosporidiosis, the largest water-borne disease outbreak ever reported in the United States, accounted for 403,000 total cases of which 4400 people were hospitalized. The outbreak was traced to a community water system. Surface water from Lake Michigan had been filtered and chlorinated, but a deterioration in the water quality and the decreased effectiveness of the coagulation-filtration process led to inadequate removal of *Cryptosporidium parvum* oocysts. The treated water had met all state and federal quality standards that were then in effect. The outbreak was recognized by widespread absenteeism among employees of hospitals, students, and schoolteachers; a shortage of antidiarrheal drugs citywide; and a marked increase in the number of emergency department visits.[13]

PATHOPHYSIOLOGY

Normal physiologic defense mechanisms that exist to prevent disease from food- and water-borne pathogens include gastric acid, the normal flora of the gastrointestinal tract, intestinal motility, and mucous glycoproteins of the intestinal mucus. The effectiveness of each of these barriers can be altered by age, concomitant infections, chronic illnesses, medications, and the pathogen itself.

A gastric pH of 3 or less is generally found in most healthy adults and can effectively kill most food-borne pathogens.[14] A reduction in acidity can occur secondary to antacids, H_2 blockers, and proton-pump inhibitors. Chronic underlying medical conditions such as diabetes mellitus, pernicious anemia, and gastric surgery also reduce gastric pH. Hypochlorhydria has also been demonstrated in *Helicobacter pylori* infections.[14]

Nonpathogenic indigenous intestinal bacteria inhibit colonization of pathogens by direct competition for nutrients and by the production of fatty acids or chemicals that are bactericidal. Alterations of intestinal flora commonly occur after antibiotic use, as well as secondary to radiation therapy, chemotherapy, and abdominal surgery.[14] Recent antibiotic use lowers resistance to *Salmonella* infections and has been implicated as a risk factor for infection with *E. coli* O157:H7.[14]

The normal motility of the intestinal tract provides an important defense mechanism by minimizing the contact between the mucosal surface and potential pathogens. Bowel stasis permits multiplication and overgrowth of food-borne or water-borne pathogens and contributes to retrograde migration from the colon to the small intestine. Antiperistaltic agents, narcotics, and previous radiation therapy theoretically can prolong gut transit time and increase pathogen infectivity.[14]

The most common cause of bacterial food-borne illnesses in the United States is *Campylobacter* followed in order by *Salmonella, Shigella,* and *E. coli*.[15] Infectivity of bacteria occurs by a variety of methods. Protein toxins are produced by *Vibrio cholerae* and enterotoxic *E. coli*. These toxins alter fluid and electrolyte movement across the mucosal surface, producing large volumes of fluid in excess of the absorptive capacity of the colon, causing excessive diarrhea and rapid dehydration. *E. coli* can adhere to the mucosal surface via surface pili or fimbria that bind to intestinal epithelial cell receptors. *Shigella, Salmonella,* enteroinvasive *E. coli, Campylobacter,* and *Vibrio parahaemolyticus* can invade the mucosal cells directly, causing cellular death. Cytotoxins, such as the Shiga toxin of *Shigella dysenteriae* or Shiga-like toxins produced by enterohemorrhagic *E. coli* O157:H7, enteropathogenic *E. coli,* and *V. parahaemolyticus* cause cellular membrane disruption and cell lysis.[16]

Food-borne viruses are usually transmitted person to person by the fecal-oral route and are infectious in very low doses. Viruses do not multiply or produce toxins, and food items simply act as transfer media. Testing for viral etiologies of diarrheal disease is rarely done, leading to underreporting of viral food-borne outbreaks. Viral gastroenteritis, caused by Norwalk viruses, astroviruses, rotaviruses, and enteric adenoviruses are the most common form of food-borne disease with an estimated annual incidence in the United States of 23,000,000 illnesses.[4,10]

Simultaneous infection with more than one viral pathogen is common. Viral contamination can occur at the source, after harvesting, or during food preparation. Bivalve mollusk (oysters, clams, and mussels) contamination usually occurs at the source in polluted shallow coastal waters. The application of raw sewage or sludge to fruit and vegetable crops is another source of primary viral contamination. Viral contaminants remain active when they are inadequately cooked or consumed raw, particularly in oysters.[17]

Viral contamination from infected food handlers is largely associated with cold food items that require much handling during preparation, such as salads and sandwiches, ice, or ready-to-eat foods.[10]

Water-borne transmission of virus is an effective mechanism of infectivity. Outbreaks have been associated with contamination of private wells, small water systems, and community water systems.[3] Seasonal outbreaks of Norwalk gastroenteritis have been associated with swimming in lakes and pools.

Hepatitis A is the only reportable food-borne viral disease, and the true incidence of illness is underreported. Hepatitis A outbreaks are likely to be recognized weeks after contaminated food has been consumed and samples are unavailable for testing. Most infections are the result of consumption of infected bivalves, but outbreaks associated with infected raw produce have occurred.[10]

Viruses can be eliminated at any step along the food-handling process. Heating is an effective means of inactivating hepatitis A virus particles in mollusks, and their exposure to temperatures of 85° to 90°C for at least 90 s is recommended.[17] Viruses are a small target for ionizing radiation. Enteric viruses are often acid resistant, and hepatitis A virus is quite resistant to drying. Viruses in water or on surfaces can be inactivated by chlorine, ozone, or ultraviolet light.[17]

DIAGNOSIS AND TREATMENT

Symptoms associated with food-borne illness are very common and often nonspecific except for syndromes associated with particular chemical agents such as ciguatera toxin, organophosphates, or histamine (scombroid). Obtaining a complete history of an acute diarrheal illness is important. In a presumed food-borne illness, determining the exact time of exposure can help direct the evaluation to particular causative agents, although significant overlap exists between syndromes of food-borne illness (Table 150-1).[10] Extending a history beyond 3 or 4 days will provide only limited benefit in identifying pathogens such as hepatitis A, *Cryptosporidium,* and *Salmonella* with prolonged incubation periods.

A history of two or more people within a household becoming ill simultaneously may indicate a food-borne etiology. If additional cases occur within 24 to 36 h, non-food-borne sources such as viruses are more likely. Patients should be questioned about inadequate food-handling practices at home, such as preparation of food several hours prior to consumption, insufficient cooking or reheating of food, cross contamination between raw and cooked foods on common preparation surfaces, or people with poor personal hygiene handling the food.[18]

Patients should be questioned about other activities associated with an increased risk of food-borne disease, such as frequent restaurant meals, exposure to day care centers, consumption of street-vended food or raw seafood, overseas travel, and camping with the ingestion of lake or stream water.

Host factors that reduce resistance and immunocompetence should be identified. The recent use of antibiotics and medications that reduce gastric acidity, such as H_2 blockers, proton-pump inhibitors, and

TABLE 150-1   Etiologic Agents for Foodborne Diseases and Usual Incubation Periods

1–6 h
  Norwalk viruses
  Astrovirus, calcivirus
  Staphylococcus aureus
  Bacillus cerus vomiting toxin
  Ciguatoxin
  Scombroid toxins
  Paralytic or neurotoxic shellfish poisoning
  Puffer fish, tetrodotoxin
  Heavy metals
  Monosodium glutamates
  Short-acting mushroom toxins
6–24 h
  Bacillus cereus diarrheal toxin
  Clostridium perfringens
  Vibrio parahaemolyticus
  Long-acting mushroom toxins
24–48 h
  Nontyphoidal Salmonella
  Enterotoxigenic *E. coli* (ETEC)
  Clostridium botulinum
  Trichinella spp. intestinal phase
2–6 d
  Shigella
  Campylobacter
  Escherichia coli O157:H7
  Vibrio cholerae
  Streptococcus group A
  Yersinia enterocolitica
6–14 d
  Cryptosporidium parvum
  Salmonella typhi
  Cyclospora
  Giardia lamblia
>14 d
  Hepatitis A
  Brucella
  Listeria monocytogenes invasive disease
  Trichinella spp. systemic phase

Source: From Centers for Disease Control and Prevention (CDC): Diagnosis and Management of Foodborne Illness: A primer for physicians. *MMWR* 50:RR-2, 2001.

antacids, should be identified. Identify patients with AIDS or other immunocompromised conditions.

Children younger than age 5 and adults older than age 65 have the highest attack rate for infection with *E. coli* and are at the greatest risk for hemolytic-uremic syndrome.[14] Residents of chronic care facilities are at increased risk for illness and death because of their close proximity, increased frequency of fecal incontinence, and a general debilitated state with multiple concurrent illnesses.[14]

A recent history of swimming in pools, water parks, lakes, and other recreational water facilities is important and should raise suspicion for cryptosporidiosis, although other pathogens such as enterohemorrhagic *E. coli* have been linked to water park outbreaks.[3]

Physical examination should be directed at identifying toxic or dehydrated patients, identifying the presence of blood in the stool, and excluding other diarrheal illnesses.

A variety of diagnostic tests are available for confirmation of pathogens in suspected outbreaks. The majority of patients will have a self-limited illness that resolves by the time culture results are available. Stool cultures are indicated if the patient is febrile, has bloody diarrhea, has severe abdominal pain, if the illness is clinically severe or persistent, or if the patient has significant historical risk factors for food-borne illness.[10] Routine testing of all patients with infectious diarrhea for ova and parasites and stool cultures is not cost effective. Stool cultures should minimally include the more frequent causes of food-borne illnesses: *Campylobacter, Salmonella,* and *Shigella.* The frequency of *E. coli* O157:H7 food-borne illness has increased, but only 50 percent of laboratories routinely culture for it.[15] Cultures for other organisms should be based on prevalence rates in the community or an increased index of suspicion based on history and physical examination. Testing for some pathogens such as *E. coli* O157:H7 and *Vibrio* spp. may need to be specifically requested.

When fecal leukocytes are present, the culture yield is higher for bacterial pathogens, but the absence of fecal leukocytes does not exclude a bacterial etiology. The Gram stain can identify *Campylobacter,* one of the most common causes of gastroenteritis, with a sensitivity of 66 to 99 percent, and still has a role in the diagnosis of diarrheal disease.[19] Blood cultures should be obtained when bacteremia or systemic infection are suspected.[10]

Emergency physicians should be cognizant of which pathogens are, and equally as important, are *not* routinely cultured for in their laboratories. Optimal sensitivity of the stool culture test requires more than a single specimen, but samples should preferably be obtained in the emergency department, especially if testing for ova and parasites is required. Multiple specimens yield optimal results. Rectal swabs are not adequate for specimen collection.

Direct antigen detection tests and molecular biology techniques are available for rapid identification of certain viral, bacterial, and parasitic agents in clinical specimens.[10] Rapid diagnostic tests for the presence of Shiga toxin have become available for use in clinical laboratories.[10] Microbiologic and chemical laboratory testing of vomitus and implicated food items is warranted in an outbreak, but not routinely.

Public health authorities usually become aware of and initiate investigations of potential food-borne or water-borne outbreaks when there is an increase in the frequency of pathogens reported to them by hospitals or a cluster of suspicious cases. Chap. 153 outlines reportable communicable diseases. Variations of this reporting structure do occur.

Many episodes of acute gastroenteritis secondary to food-borne agents are self-limited and require only fluid replacement and supportive care. Parenteral rehydration is indicated for patients who cannot tolerate oral fluids or if they cannot adequately orally replace fluids lost with copious diarrhea. Because many antidiarrheal agents have potentially serious adverse effects in infants and young children, their routine use is not recommended in this age group.[10] Antimicrobial therapy should be based on severity of illness, likelihood of resolution with supportive care, detection of the organism in clinical specimens, and antimicrobial susceptibility tests.[10] Details of treatment after diagnosis are listed in Table 150-2.[10] Ciprofloxacin 500 mg PO bid × 3–5 days or 1 gm PO × 1 dose, or TMP-SMX DS, PO bid × 3–5 days, is the preferred initial ED treatment for suspected bacterial infectious diarrhea. The use of antibiotics to treat *E. coli* O157:H7 may increase the risk of hemolytic-uremic syndrome.[16]

TABLE 150-2   Bacterial Food-Borne Illnesses

Organism	Incubation Period	Signs and Symptoms	Illness Duration	Food Source	Lab Testing	Treatment*
Bacillus anthracis	2 d–weeks	Nausea, vomiting, bloody diarrhea, abdominal pain	Weeks	Contaminated meat	Blood	Penicillin, ciprofloxacin
Bacillus cereus (diarrheal toxin)	10–16 h	Watery diarrhea, nausea, cramps	24–28 h	Meat, stew, gravy, vanilla sauce	None	Supportive only
Bacillus cereus (enterotoxin)	1–6 h	Sudden fever, nausea, vomiting, may have diarrhea	24 h	Rice, meats	None	Supportive only
Brucella spp.	7–21 d	Fever, chills, headache, myalgias, arthralgias, bloody diarrhea	Weeks	Raw milk, goat cheese, meats	Blood, serology	Rifampin and doxycycline
Campylobacter	2–5 d	Bloody or watery diarrhea, cramps, fever	2–10 d	Poultry, milk, water	Special stool culture	Erythromycin or ciprofloxacin*
Clostridium botulinum (adults, children)	12–72 h	Vomiting, diarrhea, diplopia, dysphagia, descending muscle weakness	Variable, can end in death	Improperly canned foods, fermented fish, bottled garlic, herb-infused oils, baked potatoes in foil, foods kept in a warm oven for hours	Stool, serum, and food assayed for toxin at CDC or state laboratories	Botulinum antitoxin
Clostridium botulinum (infants)	3–30 d	Lethargy, poor feeding, hypotonia	Variable	Honey, home-canned foods	As above	Botulinum immune globulin
Clostridium perfringens	8–16 h	Watery diarrhea, nausea, cramps	24–48 h	Meat, poultry, gravy, dried or precooked foods	Quantitative culture of stool	Supportive only
Enterohemorrhagic *E. coli*	1–8 d	Bloody diarrhea, abdominal pain, vomiting	5–10 d	Meat, unpasteurized milk, raw fruit and vegetables, salami, contaminated water, salad dressings	Specific stool culture	Supportive only
Enterotoxigenic *E. coli*	1–3 d	Watery diarrhea, vomiting, cramps	3–10 d	Fecal contamination of water or food	Specific stool culture	Ciprofloxacin* or TMP-SMX
Enterohemorrhagic *E. coli*	1–8 d	Bloody diarrhea, abdominal pain, vomiting	5–10 d	Meat, unpasteurized milk, raw fruit and vegetables, salami, contaminated water, salad dressings	Specific stool culture	Supportive only

(continued)

TABLE 150-2 Bacterial Food-Borne Illnesses *(Continued)*

Organism	Incubation Period	Signs and Symptoms	Illness Duration	Food Source	Lab Testing	Treatment*
Enterotoxigenic *E. coli*	1–3 d	Watery diarrhea, vomiting, cramps	3–10 d	Fecal contamination of water or food	Specific stool culture	Ciprofloxacin* or TMP-SMX*
Listeria monocytogenes	9–48 h for GI, 2–6 weeks for invasive disease	Fever, myalgias, nausea, diarrhea in pregnant women, flu-like illness Can lead to premature delivery Elderly or immunocompromised can have sepsis or meningitis	Variable	Soft cheese, unpasteurized milk, deli meats, and hot dogs	Blood or CSF culture	IV ampicillin, or TMP-SMX
Salmonella spp.	1–3 d	Diarrhea, fever, cramps, vomiting *S. typhi* and *paratyphi* cause chills, myalgias, headache, with rare diarrhea	4–7 d	Eggs, poultry, unpasteurized milk or juice, cheese, raw fruits and vegetables, street vendors, fecal water contamination	Stool cultures	Ciprofloxacillin* or TMP-SMX*
Shigella spp.	24–48 h	Bloody diarrhea, fever, cramps	4–7 d	Fecal food or water contamination person-person spread by fecal-oral contamination	Stool culture	TMP-SMX if susceptible
S. aureus	1–6 h	Sudden severe nausea, vomiting, diarrhea	24–48 h	Unrefrigerated meats, potato and egg salad, cream pastries	None	Supportive only
Vibrio cholerae	24–72 h	Severe watery diarrhea and vomiting	3–7 d, death from dehydration	Contaminated water, fish, shellfish, street vendors	Specific stool culture	Ciprofloxacin in adults, TMP-SMX in children
Vibrio vulnificus	1–7 d	Vomiting, diarrhea, abdominal pain, sepsis, wound infections, liver disease and elderly can have skin bullae	2–8 d, death can result	Raw shellfish and fish, open wounds exposed to seawater	Specific wound or blood cultures	Doxycycline or ceftazidime
Yersinia spp.	24–48 h	Mimics appendicitis, can have rash	1–3 weeks	Undercooked pork, unpasteurized milk, contaminated water	Specific stool or blood culture	Ciprofloxacin,* doxycycline,* ceftriaxone,* or gentamycin*

*Antibiotics for severe cases only.
Abbreviation: TMP-SMX = trimethoprim-sulfamethoxide.
Source: Adapted from CDC, Diagnosis and management of foodborne illness: A primer for physicians. *MMWR* 50(No RR-2):1, 2001.[10]

CHRONIC SEQUELAE

Chronic secondary complications of food-borne illness occur in about 2 to 3 percent of patients.[20] If the host and pathogen have common surface antigens, host recognition of the foreign antigen can initiate an autoimmune response. A low but consistent incidence (0.2 to 2.4 percent) of seronegative reactive arthritis has been noted following outbreaks of *Salmonella typhimurium, Shigella flexneri,* and *Campylobacter jejuni.*[20,21] Superantigens—protein virulence factors that can elicit extreme immune responses in the host—have been isolated from several food-borne bacteria. These are thought to be associated with multiple autoimmune disorders, such as rheumatoid arthritis, multiple sclerosis, Graves disease, and psoriasis.[20] A link between *Campylobacter* and Guillain-Barré syndrome has been suspected for over a decade. It is estimated that possibly 40 percent of Guillain-Barré cases are secondary to primary infection, with *Campylobacter* usually developing 7 to 21 days after resolution of gastrointestinal symptoms.[20,21] Hemolytic-uremic syndrome (HUS), characterized by acute renal failure, thrombocytopenia, and microangiopathic hemolytic anemia, develops in some patients, particularly children, following acute colitis with *E. coli* O157:H7. HUS is caused by toxin-mediated damage to the glomerular epithelial cells and possibly the tubular epithelial cells and is the leading cause of acute renal failure in children.[20,21] Other organisms that have been linked to HUS include other strains of *E. coli, Citrobacter,* *Campylobacter, Shigella, Salmonella,* and *Yersinia.*[21] Adults with *E. coli* O157:H7 infection may develop HUS or thrombotic thrombocytopenic purpura (TTP), a microangiopathic disorder that resembles HUS but is accompanied by neurologic abnormalities.[10] Many of the acute symptoms of ciguatera poisoning can persist as a waxing and waning chronic symptom complex that is often misdiagnosed as chronic fatigue syndrome, brain tumor, or multiple sclerosis.[21]

PREVENTION AND SURVEILLANCE

Traditional Surveillance

Effective food-borne disease surveillance is critical to determine the frequency of cases, identify newly emerging pathogens, and isolate factors that contribute to disease transmission.[8] Traditional surveillance systems for food-borne illnesses rely on clinical microbiology laboratories reporting identified pathogens or suspected outbreaks to state health departments, which then report them to the CDC.[22] This type of passive surveillance requires a person with a diarrheal illness to seek care from a physician who then in turn obtains a stool culture. The current underreporting of food-borne illnesses is a direct consequence of this interdependent chain of events in which elimination of even one step results in a case not being identified.[22]

FoodNet

FoodNet is a collaborative project of participating data collection sites in the CDC, U.S. Department of Agriculture, and the Food and Drug Administration (FDA) that became operational in 1995. It employs an active surveillance strategy for diarrheal illnesses and food-borne illnesses in sentinel populations monitored at over 300 clinical laboratories throughout the United States[22] with a surveillance population of approximately 33.1 million people.[15] FoodNet investigators actively contact these laboratories for confirmed cases of *Salmonella, Shigella, Campylobacter, E. coli* O157:H7, *Listeria, Yersinia, Vibrio, Cyclospora,* and *Cryptosporidium.* They have built a comprehensive database of food-borne illness in these regions.[23] Physician practice patterns for ordering stool specimens have also been monitored. Population surveys allow an approximation of the number of patients with diarrheal illness who seek medical care.[23] This information is centrally based at the CDC and facilitates timely recognition and response to food-borne outbreaks.

PulseNet

PulseNet, completed in May 1998, is a national computer network of public heath laboratories that perform DNA fingerprinting on two bacteria: *E. coli* O157:H7 and *Salmonella typhimurium.* Using a standardized methodology for pulsed-field gel electrophoresis (PFGE), designated network laboratories in the United States can rapidly determine whether food-borne illnesses in multiple locations are linked to a common pathogen and food source. The state or local health department enters bacterial PFGE patterns into a centralized national electronic database. Matching patterns from different locations during a defined time period will trigger an alert to a possible multilocation food-borne-illness outbreak.[23]

Prevention

The current system for ensuring food safety is complex, with authority divided between federal, state, and local governments. Currently in the United States, the FDA inspects food-processing plants, and along with the U.S. Department of Agriculture, regulates the interstate commerce of these foods. Final delivery destinations, such as restaurants, supermarkets, and cafeterias, are regulated by local health departments. The movement of food from the farm or water sources follows a predictable process-specific pathway. Contamination can occur at one or more points in the process.

Hazard Analysis and Critical Control Points (HACCP) is an applied methodology mandated for the meat and poultry industries in 1998. HACCP identifies vulnerable points in food production, such as sensitive ingredients, human interactions, and critical processing steps that are at high risk of contamination. It requires cooperation between government regulatory agencies and the food industry and replaces simple inspection of a final product. Industry-wide solutions can be implemented once contamination points are identified.[1,7,8,24] HACCP directives do not extend to the home, food service, or retail establishments.

Emergency physicians should advise infected patients of the potential risks they pose to family members or others, particularly if they are food handlers or health care workers.[17] A small number of factors in food handling are responsible for a large percentage of food-borne disease.[18] The most important steps that can be taken in the home to prevent food-borne disease are thorough cooking and eating cooked food promptly. Educate patients that food from animal sources such as meat, dairy, and eggs should be either pasteurized or completely cooked and not eaten undercooked or raw. Cross contamination from the juices or drippings from raw meat, poultry, eggs, or shellfish with other foods must be avoided by washing hands or common preparation surfaces with soap and water. Prepared food should not be left for extended periods of time at temperatures that will promote bacterial growth.[18] The World Health Organization has established rules for the preparation of safe food in the home that can be accessed via the Internet at http://www.who.int/fsf/gldnrls.htm.[18]

REFERENCES

1. Kaferstein Y, Motarjemi Y, Bettcher D: Foodborne disease control: A transnational challenge. *Emerg Infect Dis* 3:503, 1997.
2. Centers for Disease Control and Prevention (CDC): Surveillance summaries: Surveillance for foodborne-disease outbreaks: United States, 1993–1997. *MMWR* 49:SS-01, 2000.
3. Centers for Disease Control and Prevention (CDC): Surveillance summaries: Surveillance for waterborne disease outbreaks: United States, 1999–2000, *MMWR* 51:SS-8, 2002.
4. Mead PS, Slutsker L, Deitz V, et al: Food-related illness and death in the United States. *Emerg Infect Dis* 5:607, 1999.
5. Altekruse S, Cohen M, Swerdlow D: Perspective: Emerging foodborne diseases. *Emerg Infect Dis* 3:285, 1997.
6. Hennessy T, Hedberg C, Slutsker L, et al: A national outbreak of *Salmonella enteritidis* infections from ice cream. *N Engl J Med* 334:1281, 1996.
7. Collins J: Impact of changing consumer lifestyles on the emergence/re-emergence of foodborne pathogens. *Emerg Infect Dis* 3:471, 1997.
8. Altekruse S, Swerdlow D: The changing epidemiology of foodborne diseases. *Am J Med Sci* 311:23, 1996.
9. Cartwright R, Chahed M: Foodborne disease in travelers. *World Health Stat Q* 50:102, 1997.
10. Centers for Disease Control and Prevention: Diagnosis and management of foodborne illness: A primer for physicians. *MMWR* 50(No. RR-2):1, 2001.
11. White DG, Zhao S, Sudler R, et al: The isolation of antibiotic resistant *Salmonella* from retail ground meats. *N Engl J Med* 345:1147, 2001.
12. Motarjemi Y, Kaferstein F: Global estimation of foodborne illness. *World Health Stat Q* 50:5, 1997.
13. Centers for Disease Control and Prevention (CDC): Surveillance summaries: Surveillance for waterborne disease outbreaks: United States, 1993–1994. *MMWR* 45:SS-1, 1996.
14. Klontz K, Adler W, Potter M: Age-dependent resistance factors in the pathogenesis of foodborne infectious disease. *Aging Clin Exp Res* 9:320, 1997.
15. Preliminary FoodNet data on the incidence of foodborne illnesses—selected sites, United States, 2000. *MMWR* 50:13, 2001.
16. Wong CS, Jelacic S, Habeed RL, et al: The risk of hemolytic-uremic syndrome after antibiotic treatment of *Escherichia coli* O157:H7 infections. *N Engl J Med* 342:1930, 2000.
17. Cliver D: Virus transmission via food. *World Health Stat Q* 50:90, 1997.
18. World Health Organization (WHO): The WHO Golden Rules for Safe Food Preparation. Geneva: WHO, http://www.who.ch/programmes/fsf/gldnrls.htm.
19. Hines J, Nachamkin I: Effective use of the clinical microbiology laboratory for diagnosing diarrheal diseases. *Clin Infect Dis* 23:1292, 1996.
20. Bunning K, Lindsay J, Archer D: Chronic health effects of microbial food-borne disease. *World Health Stat Q* 50:51, 1997.
21. Lindsay J: Chronic sequelae of foodborne diseases. *Emerg Infect Dis* 3:443, 1997.
22. FoodNet Working Group: Foodborne Diseases Active Surveillance Network (FoodNet). *Emerg Infect Dis* 3:581, 1997.
23. Slutsker L, Altekruse S, Swerdlow D: Foodborne diseases, emerging pathogens and trends. *Infect Dis Clin North Am* 12:199, 1998.
24. Tauxe R: Emerging foodborne diseases: An evolving public health challenge. *Emerg Infect Dis* 3:425, 1997.

ZOONOTIC INFECTIONS
John T. Meredith

The World Health Organization classifies zoonotic infections as those diseases and infections that are naturally transmitted between vertebrate animals and humans.[1] This broad class of diseases includes more than 200 specific diseases and syndromes covering an extremely variable range of clinical syndromes and medical therapy.[2] Zoonotic infections can be transmitted to humans by direct contact with an infected animal or infected animal product, by ingestion of contaminated water or food products, by inhalation, and through arthropod vectors.

In North America, an estimated 4 million people are infected annually.[3] Zoonotic infections represent a significant public health problem in underdeveloped regions dependent economically on agricultural animals. The growth and mobility of the world's population has resulted in the appearance of new zoonotic infections and the reemergence of previously eliminated ones. More than 50 percent of the newly identified infectious agents since 1976 are associated with animals.[4] Thus diversity of presentation, human mobility, and zoonotic reemergence make the diagnosis and management of zoonotic infections a challenge for emergency physicians.

RISK ASSESSMENT

A zoonotic infection should be considered part of the differential diagnosis of any undifferentiated infectious syndrome: fever, headache, myalgias, malaise, and weakness. However, diagnosis is difficult. Determining risk factors for acquiring a zoonotic infection can help focus the differential diagnosis.

Specific avocations and occupations that involve animal contact[5] and certain medical comorbidities carry an increased risk (Table 151-1).[6] The type of animal exposure is an important factor. Dressing, skinning, or handling an animal's skin; a history of animal bite or scratch; and ingestion of animal or dairy products all carry an associated risk of zoonotic infection. Recent travel and history of habitation, particularly in an underdeveloped country or rural area, are additional risk factors. Zoonoses can occur at any time of the year, but in the United States, most zoonoses show an increased incidence in the spring and summer.

Zoonoses that can present as an undifferentiated febrile illness or sepsis are listed in Table 151-2. The table lists only some of the more common zoonotic diseases.

TICK-BORNE ZOONOTIC INFECTIONS

More zoonotic diseases are transmitted by ticks than by any other vector.[7] In the United States more than 15,000 cases are diagnosed each year.[8,9] Tick-borne diseases should be considered in the differential diagnosis of nonspecific febrile illnesses, especially if there is associated rash. Many patients do not recall a history of a tick bite.[8] Tick-borne zoonoses have a geographic distribution (Table 151-3) and seasonal variation, with the highest U.S. incidence in spring and summer.

Tick Removal

The most effective way to remove an embedded tick is a three-step approach. First, viscous lidocaine is applied to kill the tick and anesthetize the bite site. Second, careful and gentle traction is applied to the tick's head with fine forceps. Third, all parts of the tick need to be removed. Residual tick body parts can stimulate a granulomatous reaction and persistent infection.

Techniques to avoid include the use of a burning match or any action resulting in crushing the tick. These attempts can cause infection by tick regurgitation into the wound site, and often result in incomplete tick removal.

Rocky Mountain Spotted Fever

The causative organism of Rocky Mountain spotted fever (RMSF) is *Rickettsia rickettsii,* a pleomorphic, obligate intracellular organism, and the vector is the *Dermacentor* tick. Deer, rodents, horses, cattle, cats, and dogs are zoonotic hosts.[10] The classic clinical picture of RMSF is the triad of fever, rash, and tick exposure, but only about half of the patients can recall a tick bite. Other signs and symptoms include malaise, myalgias, lymphadenopathy, abdominal pain, nausea, vomiting, diarrhea, hepatosplenomegaly, headache, conjunctivitis, confusion, meningismus, renal failure, respiratory failure, and myocarditis.

The rash of RMSF occurs on days 1 to 15 of the illness but is absent in about 20 percent of patients.[11,12] The characteristic maculopapular rash begins on the hands, feet, wrists, and ankles, and then spreads centripetally up the trunk (see Chap. 248 for more detailed discussion). Laboratory abnormalities are usually nonspecific, but the combination of neutropenia, thrombocytopenia, elevated liver function studies, and hyponatremia suggests RMSF, especially in advanced disease. Diagnosis can be confirmed with a rise in antibody titer between acute and convalescent serum, skin biopsy with immunofluorescent testing,[12,13] or culture, although none of these are useful for ED diagnosis. Preferred treatment is doxycycline 100 mg PO bid for 7 days, or for 2 days after temperature normalizes. While chloramphenicol is still an alternative, it can cause serious toxicity, including myelosuppression. It is contraindicated in children <2 years of age, pregnancy and breast-feeding, G6PD deficiency, porphyria, and those with hepatic or renal disease.

Lyme Disease

Lyme disease is the most common vector-borne zoonotic infection in the United States, with approximately 15,000 cases reported annually.[14] The responsible organism is *Borrelia burgdorferi,* a spirochete, and the vector is the *Ixodes* deer tick. Lyme disease is most prevalent in the Northeast, but all continental 48 states have reported it.[14] The overall risk of Lyme disease after a deer tick bite is relatively low, approximately 3 percent in highly endemic areas. However, the risk of infection is proportional to the length of time the tick feeds on the host. There is almost no risk if duration of attachment is <72 h, and about 25 percent risk of infection if the tick has been attached for 72 h or more.[15]

The disease has three stages. The initial stage of illness is often characterized by erythema migrans. Erythema migrans is an erythematous plaque with central clearing. It is the most common clinical manifestation associated with *B. burgdorferi* infection, occurring in about 60 to 80 percent of cases.[8] It develops within 2 to 20 days at the site of the tick bite and is a result of a vasculitis. It may persist for

TABLE 151-1   Risk Factors for Zoonotic Infection

Risk Category	Examples
Agricultural workers	Farmers, cattle ranchers, sheep ranchers, and migrant workers
Animal processing workers	Slaughterhouse workers, animal-hide processors, and workers in any manufacturing plant that deals with animal products or by-products
Outdoor enthusiasts	Forestry workers, lumbermen, surveyors, park rangers, hunters, spelunkers, fishermen, and those who regularly engage in outdoor recreational activities
Pet owners	Those with a dog, cat, bird, rodent, rabbit, reptile, or fish
Professionals	Veterinarians, animal researchers, and animal handlers
Immunocompromised patients	Those with congenital immunodeficiencies, diabetes mellitus, alcoholism, renal failure, liver failure, cancer, splenectomy, or HIV

TABLE 151-2 Systemic Zoonotic Infections

Agent	Animal Reservoir	Physical Findings	Diagnostic Tests	Treatment
Aeromonas spp.	Fish, reptiles	Nonspecific fever, severe crepitant cellulitis with systemic toxicity		Fluoroquinolones, TMP-SMX, cephalosporin (third or fourth generation), or Amox/Clav
Brucella canis	Dog	Nonspecific fever	Serologic testing, blood culture	Doxycycline plus gentamicin or rifampin
Capnocytophaga	Dogs and cats	Fever, sepsis, and endocarditis from infected bite	Culture of bite wound	Amoxicillin-clavulanate, or clindamycin plus either a fluoroquinolone or TMP-SMX
Chlamydia psittaci	Birds	Fever, pneumonia, endocarditis, sepsis	Serologic testing and sputum culture	Tetracycline or erythromycin
Coxiella burnetii (Q fever)	Cats, livestock animals, ticks	Fever, pneumonia, hepatitis, meningitis, endocarditis	Serologic testing	Azithromycin, doxycycline, or a fluoroquinolone
Ehrlichia spp.	Tick	Nonspecific fever, sepsis, meningitis, hepatitis	Serologic testing, peripheral blood smear, immunocytologic testing, PCR testing	Doxycycline
Leptospira spp.	Birds, dogs, rodents	Fever, pneumonia, conjunctivitis, lymphadenopathy	Darkfield microscopic examination of body fluids serologic testing	Penicillin G IV; doxycycline IV or PO, or ampicillin IV
Francisella spp. (tularemia)	Rabbits, cats, wild animals	Fever, sepsis, meningitis, pneumonia, hepatitis, rash	Serologic testing	Tobramycin or gentamicin plus chloramphenicol for meningitis
Rickettsia rickettsii	Ticks	Fever, diarrhea	Stool culture	Doxycycline or chloramphenicol
Salmonella enterica	Dogs, cats (rarely), reptiles (turtles)	Fever, sepsis, cellulitis, meningitis, endocarditis, septic arthritis	Blood culture	Ciprofloxacin or ceftriaxone
Streptococcus inae cellulitis	Livestock	Fever, pneumonia, meningitis, lymphadenopathy	Blood culture	Erythromycin, vancomycin, or TMP-SMX
Yersinia pestis	Dogs, cats, rodents		Blood culture, culture of suspected sites	Gentamicin, streptomycin, doxycycline, or chloramphenicol

Abbreviations: Amox/Clav = amoxicillin clavulanate; TMP-SMX = trimethoprim-sulfamethoxazole.

up to 1 month and recur in the secondary stage of Lyme disease.[15] Untreated erythema migrans resolves spontaneously in 3 to 4 weeks.

The secondary stage of illness develops with the dissemination of the *Borrelia* spirochete and occurs within a few days to 6 months of the initial infection. This stage is characterized by fever, adenopathy, neuropathies, cardiac abnormalities, arthritic problems, and multiple annular dermatologic lesions. The multiple annular lesions occur in up to 50 percent of the patients infected, and are the most characteristic component of the secondary stage of illness.

The most common neurologic symptom in the secondary stage of illness is the development of cranial neuritis, most often unilateral or bilateral facial nerve palsy. This palsy can also occur concomitantly with the initial rash of erythema migrans. Neuroborreliosis occurs in 15 percent of the untreated cases, and can consist of periodic headache, neck stiffness, difficulty in mentation, cerebellar ataxia, myelitis, encephalitis, motor or sensory radiculoneuritis, mononeuritis multiplex, and facial palsy.[14] Asymmetric oligoarticular arthritis of the large joints, with a particular predilection for the knees, is another complication. Brief attacks of asymmetrical oligoarticular arthritis are commonplace in the untreated patient in the secondary stage of illness. These attacks are characteristically separated by months of remission.[16] Cardiac abnormalities occur in up to 8 percent of patients and present as varying degrees of atrioventricular block, sometimes requiring the insertion of a temporary pacemaker for stabilization. Additionally, myopericarditis may also be a manifestation on initial presentation.

The tertiary stage of illness occurs years after the initial infection and can be characterized by chronic arthritis, myocarditis, subacute encephalopathy, axonal polyneuropathy, and leukoencephalopathy.[14]

Diagnosis is principally clinical, though confirmation may be obtained by either polymerase chain reaction testing, polyvalent fluorescence immunoassay, or Western immunoblot testing.[14] *Borrelia burgdorferi* has been cultured with difficulty. Of special note, the advanced, chronic neurologic forms of Lyme disease can persist for more than 10 years.[16]

Treatment of primary stage and to some degree the secondary stage of Lyme disease can be accomplished with several antimicrobial agents: doxycycline, amoxicillin, cefuroxime, ceftriaxone, or erythromycin. When only the initial rash of erythema migrans is present, the response to therapy is excellent. The duration of antimicrobial therapy in the primary stage of illness is 14 to 21 days. The more advanced secondary stage of illness requires longer duration of therapy, up to 28 days. However, there is a controversy in the treatment of the tertiary stage of illness.[14,16] Intravenous antibiotics, ceftriaxone or penicillin, are recommended for the tertiary stage of Lyme disease, with duration of therapy extending from 28 to 60 days. But this late phase of illness may not respond to aggressive antimicrobial therapy.

A vaccine was commercially available, but was withdrawn from the market in February 2002.[17] Vaccination was felt to be the best prevention against Lyme disease. As the tick feeds on an immunized host, antibodies are ingested, destroying spirochetes in the gut of the engorging tick prior to transmission to the host.

However, there was little demand for the vaccine, and it was expensive. Optimal protection required immunization at 0, 1, and 12 months, one booster immunization every 1 to 3 years. There was concern that immunization would lead recipients to disregard physical precautions against tick-borne diseases in general.

TABLE 151-3   Tick-Borne Zoonotic Infections

Disease	Vector	Animal Reservoir	Clinical Features	Antibiotic Treatment	Geographic Distribution
Babesiosis	*Ixodes dammini, I. scapularis,* and *I. pacificus*	Cattle, horses, dogs, cats, rodents, deer	Fatigue, malaise, anorexia, nausea, headache, sweats, rigors, abdominal pain, emotional lability, depression, dark urine, hepatomegaly, fever, petechiae, ecchymosis, occasional rash, and occasionally pulmonary edema	For the seriously ill, atovaquone and azithromycin, or quinine plus clindamycin	Coastal areas of MA, RI, and NY; also in MD, VA, MN, WI, GA, WA, and Mexico
Colorado tick fever	*Dermacentor andersoni*	Deer, marmots, porcupines	Fever, chills, headache, myalgias, nausea, vomiting photophobia, abdominal pain, and occasional sore throat; also may have conjunctivitis, lymphadenopathy, hepatosplenomegaly, stiff neck, retroorbital pain, weakness, and lethargy	Supportive care	Western and northwestern US and southwestern Canada
Human granulocytic ehrlichiosis	*Ixodes scapularis*	Dogs, deer, other mammals	Fevers, chills, malaise, headache, nausea, muscle aches, cough, sore throat, and pulmonary infiltrates (especially in children)	Doxycycline or tetracycline	Japan, Malaysia, and the Eastern, northeastern, and northcentral US
Human monocytic ehrlichiosis	*Amblyomma americanum* (Lone Star tick) and *D. variabilis*	Dogs, deer, other mammals	Fevers, chills, malaise, headache, nausea, muscle aches, cough, sore throat, and pulmonary infiltrates (especially in children)	Doxycycline or tetracycline	Japan, Malaysia, and southern US
Lyme disease (*Borrelia burgdorferi*)	*Ixodes dammini*	Deer, sheep, deer mice	Erythema migrans, meningitis, encephalitis, neuropathy, and joint and heart symptoms	Doxycycline, amoxicillin, cefuroxime, erythromycin, ceftriaxone, or cefotaxime	Atlantic central and northcentral US
Rocky Mountain spotted fever (*Rickettsia rickettsii*)	*Dermacentor andersoni* (wood tick) and *D. variabilis* (dog tick)	North American mammals	Petechiae, purpura, pulmonary infiltrates, jaundice, myocarditis, hepatosplenomegaly, meningitis, encephalitis, and lymphadenopathy	Doxycycline or chloramphenicol	Most of the continental US, although more prevalent in the southeast and southcentral US
Relapsing fever (*Borrelia* spp.)	*Ornithodoros* spp.	Human body lice, wild rodents, humans	Fever, chills, headache, myalgias, and arthralgias; pain, nausea, vomiting, and hypotension	Erythromycin or doxycycline	Worldwide
Tularemia (*Francisella tularensis*)	*Dermacentor* spp. and *Amblyomma* spp.	Rabbits, deer, dogs	Pneumonia, regional lymphadenopathy and headache, cough, myalgias, arthralgias, nausea, vomiting, ulceration at inoculation site, and ocular findings	Tobramycin or gentamycin, and chloramphenicol for meningitis	US (except Hawaii) and Canada

Routine prophylactic treatment is not recommended, since only approximately 3 percent of the bites transmit the disease, and because prophylactic antibiotic administration may depress the immune response to the disease.[18] Recommended considerations for prophylactic treatment include treating patients bitten by deer ticks in areas where Lyme disease is highly endemic, the nymphal deer tick is at least partially engorged with blood, and/or when the deer tick has been feeding for more than 72 h.[18]

A single 200-mg dose of doxycycline given within 72 h of the deer tick bite is effective in preventing Lyme disease.[19] It is important to note that nearly one-third of those treated with single dose doxycycline will develop nausea and vomiting.[19]

Relapsing Fever

Relapsing fever is caused by *Borrelia* spirochetes. *Ornithodoros* ticks are the vectors, and the principal zoonotic reservoirs are wild rodents.[20,21] Often the initial presentation is that of a rash or pruritic eschar at the site of a tick bite. An average incubation period of 7 days precedes the onset of fever, chills, cephalgia, myalgia, arthralgia, abdominal pain, and general malaise. Characteristically, the febrile episodes are interspersed with afebrile periods. Leukocytosis, thrombocytopenia, and an elevated erythrocyte sedimentation rate are the typical laboratory findings. Diagnosis is confirmed with the appearance of spirochetes on Wright- or Giemsa-stained peripheral blood smears. Treatment is with doxycycline or erythromycin (doxycycline 100 mg PO bid for 10 days or erythromycin 500 mg qid for 10 days).[20,22]

Colorado Tick Fever

Colorado tick fever is caused by an RNA virus. The principal vector is the tick of the species *Dermacentor,* and the zoonotic reservoirs are deer, marmots, and porcupines. The disease is endemic to the western mountainous regions of the United States, but only about 300 cases are reported annually. The incubation period is 3 to 7 days, and the onset of illness is characterized by fever, chills, headache, myalgias, and photophobia. There may be a macular or petechial rash. Complications are rare. Diagnosis is most often based on clinical findings and geography. The virus can be isolated from blood or cerebrospinal fluid (CSF) by inoculating suckling mice.[23] Treatment is supportive.

Tularemia

Tularemia, which has been characterized as "a plague-like disease of rodents,"[24] is caused by a gram-negative, nonmotile coccobacillus, *Francisella tularensis.* The zoonotic vectors are ticks of the *Dermacentor* spp. and the *Amblyomma* spp., and the principal zoonotic reservoirs are rabbits, hares, and deer.[9] Tularemia can be contracted through tick bites or through open wounds while dressing an infected zoonotic host. The clinical presentation depends on the method of inoculation, and the clinical forms are called ulceroglandular, glandular, typhoidal, pneumonic, and oropharyngeal. The ulceroglandular form is the most common. It is characterized by an ulcer at the site of the tick bite, and painful regional adenopathy. The glandular form consists of painful adenopathy without ulcerations. The typhoidal form consists of fever, chills, cephalgia, and abdominal pain. The ocular-oropharyngeal form and pneumonic form are the result of deposition into the eyes or inhalation of the *F. tularensis* bacterium. Laboratory findings are nonspecific, and the diagnosis can be determined by culture and enzyme-linked immunosorbent assay (ELISA).[24,25]

Treatment is with tobramycin (5 mg/kg IV divided in 3 doses for 7–14 d) or gentamicin (5 mg/kg per d in three divided doses for 7 to 14 d). Chloramphenicol and ciprofloxacin are also effective in treating tularemia. A live attenuated vaccine is available for research workers and laboratory personnel.[24]

Babesiosis

Babesiosis is a malaria-like disease transmitted by ticks with the etiologic agents being protozoan parasites: *Babesia microti* and *Babesia equi.*[26] The major zoonotic reservoirs are domesticated mammals, rodents, and deer. *Ixodes* ticks function as the principal vector. Blood transfusions have been implicated in the transmission of babesiosis.[26] Clinically, the presentation is generalized malaise, anorexia, fever, and chills that can progress to intermittent sweats, myalgia, headache, and hemolytic anemia. Splenectomy and immunosuppression are risk factors. Laboratory tests can provide evidence of hemolysis, liver dysfunction, anemia, thrombocytopenia, and renal failure. Interestingly, approximately 20 percent of patients with babesiosis have a concurrent infection with Lyme disease.[9] Diagnosis is made by finding intraerythrocytic ring forms on a Giemsa-stained peripheral blood smear, though false-negative results can occur when the level of parasitism is low.

Treatment is with atovaquone (750 mg PO q12h) plus azithromycin (500 mg PO on day 1, then 250 mg/d) both for 7 days. Clindamycin plus quinine is an alternative regimen.

Ehrlichiosis

Ehrlichiosis is a zoonotic disease with two principal presentations: *human granulocytic ehrlichiosis* and *human monocytic ehrlichiosis.* The etiologic agent, *Ehrlichia chaffeensis,* that is responsible for the granulocytic form is similar in ribosomal RNA gene-sequence to *Ehrlichia phagocytophila* and *Ehrlichia equi.*[9,27,28] The predominant form in the United States is the monocytic form caused by *Ehrlichia chaffeensis.* The *Ehrlichia* bacteria are gram-negative pleomorphic coccobacilli that infect circulating leukocytes.[27] The zoonotic reservoirs are thought to be deer, dogs, and other mammals, with the vectors being *Ixodes* spp. and *Amblyomma* spp. ticks. Approximately 90 percent of patients have a tick bite history in the 3 weeks prior to the onset of symptoms.[9,27] Characteristic clinical presentation is that of a febrile illness with cephalgia, malaise, nausea, vomiting, abdominal pain, anorexia, and myalgia. In 20 percent of the cases, a maculopapular or petechial rash is present that only infrequently involves the soles and palms occurs during the initial phase of illness. In contrast, over 80 percent of patients infected with Rocky Mountain spotted fever develop a maculopapular rash.[9] With disease progression, a minority of patients go on to develop severe complications of renal failure, respiratory failure, and encephalitis. The acute phase of illness lasts less than 4 weeks, with the majority of patients recovering and preceding on to a convalescent phase. Laboratory studies can demonstrate leukocytopenia, thrombocytopenia, and liver dysfunction at 1 week from the onset of acute symptoms. Diagnosis is based on seroprevalence studies using an indirect immunofluorescent antibody test.[9,27] The diagnosis is made by either a fourfold rise or a decrease in antibody titer between the acute phase and convalescent phase of illness. Treatment is with doxycycline, 100 mg PO bid for 7 to 14 days.[27]

ZOONOTIC ENCEPHALITIS

Zoonotic encephalitis is most often an arboviral infection transmitted hematologically by an arthropod vector and animal host. Often the vector is a mosquito or tick and the animal host is a small animal or bird. The one exception is rabies (see Chap. 147), which follows peripheral nerve tracts after inoculation from an infected animal's bite. Additionally, encephalitis may be seen in the nonviral zoonotic infections of *Bartonella henselae, Brucella canis,* borreliosis, *Coxiella burnetii, Ehrlichia* spp., listeriosis, leptospirosis, Lyme disease, RMSF, psittacosis, and toxoplasmosis.[9,29,30]

The clinical presentation is a prodromal illness with malaise, myalgia, fever, and occasionally parotitis. This prodromal phase advances to a sudden decline in mental status associated with headache and fever. However, there are no specific signs and symptoms that determine the exact etiology and causative organism of encephalitis. The CSF is often abnormal, showing a slightly elevated opening pressure, normal to slightly elevated protein concentration, normal glucose levels, and predominance of lymphocytes. The electroencephalogram is abnormal with diffuse bilateral slowing interrupted by occasional spike activity. CSF viral cultures are frequently sterile, and the infectious agent is rarely isolated from the CSF.[29–32] ELISA of serum can be used to detect most arboviral infections causing encephalitis. Computed axial tomography is often negative with no evidence of focal findings or abnormalities. Magnetic resonance imaging often does reveal evidence of encephalitis by the imaging of cerebral swelling. If the CT scan were negative, following up with an MRI scan would be the prudent course of investigation. Treatment is supportive and directed toward decreasing elevated intracranial pressure.

West Nile Virus Encephalitis

The West Nile virus was first isolated in the West Nile District of Uganda in 1937, and since then was commonly found in vertebrates in Africa, Eastern Europe, West Asia, and the Middle East.[33] It is a member of the Japanese encephalitis serocomplex of the Flaviviridae family of viruses.[34] In 1999 it was detected in the western hemisphere.

The mode of transmission involves mosquitoes, primarily of the *Culex* species, that feed on infected birds, which serve as the natural reservoir for the virus. Over 110 species of birds have been identified as being infected by the West Nile virus in the United States. Most of these birds are crows, ravens, and jays.[34]

Infected mosquitoes transmit the virus to humans and other animals when taking a blood meal.

There is an incubation period of 3 to 15 days after an infected bite. About 20 percent of those bitten develop fever and a flu-like illness, "West Nile fever." The classic presentation for West Nile fever is that of a mild dengue-like illness of sudden onset with fever, lymphadenopathy, headache, abdominal pain, vomiting, rash, conjunctivitis, eye pain, and anorexia. Duration is typically 3 to 6 days.[34]

Meningoencephalitis occurs in approximately 1 in 150 patients that become infected and is more common than meningitis. Risk factors for the development of meningoencephalitis are immunocompromised host (HIV, TB, or malaria), or advanced age. Complaints of weakness out of proportion to physical examination findings are common and myoclonus is nearly a universal finding. Interestingly, complete flaccid paralysis may occur and can be confused with Guillain-Barré syndrome. Other neurologic findings include parkinsonian-like signs, ataxia, extrapyramidal signs, cranial nerve abnormalities, myelitis, optic neuritis, and seizures. Treatment for West Nile virus is supportive.[34]

Laboratory findings for West Nile virus infection are limited to a total leukocyte count that is either normal or slightly elevated. Hyponatremia has been occasionally associated with patients with encephalitis. Cerebrospinal fluid demonstrates mostly lymphocytes, protein elevation, and a normal glucose. Computed tomography of the brain shows no evidence of acute disease, though with progressive meningoencephalitis cerebral edema may be noted.

Diagnosis is made by identifying West Nile virus (WNV)-specific IgM antibody in serum or CSF specimens. IgM-specific antibody is an acute-phase identifier that can persist in serum for up to 12 months postinfection. IgG WNV-specific antibody is found in the convalescent phase in both serum and CSF. As of this writing, PCR testing is still in an experimental stage.[34]

Methods to reduce the exposure risk for West Nile virus include use of mosquito repellents, clothing with long sleeves and long pants, and avoiding the outdoors during dawn and dusk. The insect repellent recommended is DEET (N,N-diethyl-m-toluamide and related compounds). Personal insect repellents should not be used on infants under 6 months of age. Use of mesh covers on strollers is recommended for this age group, along with protective clothing.[34]

ZOONOTIC MENINGITIS

Zoonotic meningitis can be caused by brucellosis, listeriosis, plague, salmonellosis, tularemia, leptospirosis, Lyme disease, ehrlichiosis, Q fever, RMSF, and psittacosis. CSF is almost always abnormal, showing a slightly elevated opening pressure, normal to slightly elevated protein concentration, normal glucose levels, and predominance of lymphocytes. Treatment is directed toward the specific organism cultured from the CSF. However, empiric antibiotic coverage should be administered immediately in any presumptive case of meningitis in an effort to reduce mortality and morbidity.[31] See Chap. 235 for specific empiric recommendations.

RESPIRATORY ZOONOTIC INFECTIONS

Respiratory zoonotic infections can be divided into upper (pharyngitis) and lower respiratory infections (pneumonia).

Upper Respiratory Zoonotic Infections

Recurrent culture-proven streptococcal pharyngitis in a household member can have a zoonotic source—often the household pet.[35,36] For complete eradication of this form of streptococcal pharyngitis from a family, the family pet, in addition to family members, may require a course of antistreptococcal antimicrobial therapy. Prolonged exudative pharyngitis raises the suspicion of a zoonotic origin or atypical pharyngitis, particularly if the exudative pharyngitis includes systemic symptoms and leukocytosis, and is refractory to standard antistreptococcal therapy. In this case, it is pertinent to inquire about animal exposure. Dogs and domesticated farm animals can be the source of *Streptococcus* spp., *Corynebacterium ulcerans, Yersinia* spp., and viral vesicular stomatitis. All of these zoonoses can present as an exudative pharyngitis.[5] Nondomesticated animals can be a source of exudative pharyngitis as a result of *Bordetella* spp., *Francisella tularensis, Streptobacillus moniliformis,* and *Yersinia pestis.*[5] Both pet birds and wild birds carry *Chlamydia psittaci,* which can cause an atypical exudative pharyngitis in humans.

Lower Respiratory Zoonotic Infections

Zoonotic pneumonia presents as an atypical, community-acquired pneumonia with systemic symptoms. Most often the presentation consists of productive or nonproductive cough, fever, chills, headache, myalgias, and a nonspecific rash. Symptoms can progress very rapidly. Zoonotic pneumonia should be considered in any case of gramnegative community-acquired pneumonia and in any case of atypical pneumonia with systemic symptoms (Table 151-4).[36]

A detailed history provides the data necessary for the consideration of zoonotic pneumonia. Inquiries about animal exposure, occupation, and recent travel are warranted for patients with an atypical pneumonia. Particular attention should be paid to slaughterhouse workers and those individuals exposed to ticks, birds, and other fowl. Additionally, a history of outdoor activity, recreational history, and food-contact history should be obtained.[37]

Inhalation anthrax (Bacillus anthracis) is acquired most often from handling unsterilized, imported animal hides or imported raw wool, and is generally fatal. Inhalation anthrax is a mediastinitis without alveolar involvement, and is not a true pneumonia. Initial symptoms are flulike in character and progress to respiratory failure in 3 to 4 days, with marked mediastinal and hilar edema. Treatment is with either ciprofloxacin (400 mg IV q12h) or with doxycycline (100 mg IV q12h), plus clindamycin (900 mg IV q8h) and/or rifampin (300 mg IV q12h). Treatment may be needed for 60 days.

Brucellosis (Brucella spp.) occurs most often in slaughterhouse workers exposed to aerosols containing *Brucella* bacteria. The con-

TABLE 151-4 Zoonotic Pneumonias

Disease	Organism	Reservoirs	Treatment
Inhalation anthrax	*B. anthracis*	Imported animal hides, raw wool, sick domestic animals	Ciprofloxacin, clindamycin, and rifampin
Brucellosis	*Brucella* spp.	Food animals and product handling, ingestion, inhalation	Doxycycline plus rifampin or gentamicin, or TMP-SMX plus gentamicin
Psittacosis, ornithosis	*C. psittaci*	Bird exposure—pet and pet shop, veterinarians, turkey farms	Macrolides, or a fluoroquinolone, or doxycycline
Q fever	*C. burnetii*	Inhaled endospores from animal-contaminated soil; cat afterbirth, ticks	Tobramycin, doxycycline, erythromycin, or a fluoroquinolone
Tularemia	*F. tularensis*	Aerosol from dead birds, animals; bacteremic spread from bubo; ticks and biting flies	Gentamicin, or chloramphenicol for meningitis
Leptospirosis	*L. interrogans*	Domestic and wild animals, contaminated water, veterinarians, farmers	Doxycycline, ampicillin, amoxicillin, or penicillin
Pasteurellosis	*P. multocida*	Underlying respiratory disease; contact with cat, dog in home	Doxycycline, penicillin, third-generation cephalosporin, or Amox/Clav
Melioidosis	*P. pseudomallei*	Penetrating injury in endemic area in rodent-contaminated soil or water	Ceftazidime plus TMP-SMX; chloramphenicol or doxycycline
Rocky Mountain spotted fever	*R. rickettsii*	Tick-associated, typical rash	Doxycycline or chloramphenicol
Toxoplasmosis	*T. gondii*	Contact with domestic food animals and pets, ingestion of cysts, pneumonia in immunocompromised persons	Pyrimethamine plus sulfadiazine and folinic acid
Plague	*Y. pestis*	Contact with mammals and fleas; veterinarians; outdoor activities in endemic area; cats	Gentamicin, streptomycin, doxycycline, or ciprofloxacin
Viral pneumonias			
Hantavirus pulmonary syndrome	Bunyaviridae	Rodent feces, urine, and saliva	Ventilator oxygenation or ribavirin
Influenza pneumonia	Influenza A	Aquatic fowl, pigs, horses, marine mammals	Supportive care; amantadine or rimantadine

Abbreviations: Amox/Clav = amoxicillin clavulanate; TMP-SMX = trimethoprim-sulfamethoxazole.

sumption of unpasteurized dairy products is another way of acquiring brucellosis. Often the presentation is one of an upper respiratory infection with a cough, hoarseness of voice, and wheezing. Typically, peritracheal and hilar lymph node enlargement is seen on x-ray. Pulmonary infiltrates or consolidation are uncommon. With longstanding resolution, calcified granulomas and lymph nodes are characteristic findings.[38] Doxycycline (100 mg PO bid for up to 6 weeks) combined with gentamicin (2 mg/kg IV q8h) or rifampin (10 mg/kg per d up to 600 mg/d) is effective therapy.[38,39]

Psittacosis is also known as parrot fever, parrot disease, or ornithosis, and is caused by *Chlamydia psittaci,* an organism common to most birds and domesticated fowl. Human acquisition is from the inhalation of dust from dried bird feces, feather dust, or aerosolized avian respiratory secretions. Psittacosis is characterized by an incubation period of 5 to 14 days followed by abrupt onset of fever, chills, cephalgia, myalgia, and generalized malaise. Pneumonia is atypical, with a nonproductive cough and lobar or interstitial infiltrates on chest radiograph. Extrapulmonary manifestations involving the heart, central nervous system, liver, and kidney are common.[40,41] Macrolides (azithromycin, clarithromycin, or erthyromycin for 7–14 d) are the drugs of choice for treatment, with doxycycline (100 mg PO bid for 7–14 d) as an alternative.

Q fever (Coxiella burnetii) is the only rickettsial infection acquired by aerosol inhalation rather than by an arthropod vector. Q fever is common among domesticated farm animals in the United States and is shed in urine, afterbirth products, and feces. Feedlots are often contaminated with *C. burnetii,* which is highly resistant to environmental degradation. The disease is often self-limiting, with variable pulmonary manifestations and extrapulmonary findings. In addition to pulmonary infiltrates, pericarditis, myocarditis, and endocarditis, granulomatous hepatitis can occur.[42] Treatment is with doxycycline

(100 mg PO bid for 10 to 14 d), with erythromycin (250 mg PO qid for 10 to 14 d) as an alternative.

Pasteurellosis (Pasteurella multocida) is endemic to the normal oral flora of cats and most dogs. Often associated with necrotizing cellulitis from bite wounds, bronchitis, bronchopneumonia, and suppurative pleural effusion can occur as a result of pulmonary infection.[43] Treatment is with amoxicillin-clavulanate (500 mg/125 mg PO tid for 10 to 14 d), tetracycline (doxycycline 100 mg PO bid for 10 to 14 d), penicillin (penicillin V 500 mg PO qid for 10 d), or a third-generation cephalosporin.

Rocky Mountain spotted fever (Rickettsia rickettsii), a rickettsial infection carried by an arthropod vector, can result in a pulmonary capillary vasculitis with associated bronchiolitis.[9] Often a nonproductive cough is present. The chest radiographic findings vary from a normal radiograph to one that shows diffuse interstitial infiltrates and pleural effusions. A secondary bacterial pneumonia is commonly associated with this rickettsial pneumonia. Recommended treatment is with docycline.[44]

Plague (Yersinia pestis) is endemic to the United States and is most often found in rock squirrels and ground rodents of the Southwest. Cats can also be carriers of plague. The principal vector is the rodent flea. Humans and household pets can become infected when bitten by an infected flea. Often an eschar is found at the site of the flea bite, followed by the development of a bubo, an enlarged, suppurative, proximal lymph node. Sepsis and pneumonia from hematologic spread then follow the bubo formation. The pneumonic form is highly contagious and rapidly fatal if not aggressively treated. Additionally, the pulmonary plague can be disseminated from one person to another through aerosolization of respiratory secretions.[45] Treatment is with gentamicin (2 mg/kg IV loading dose followed by 1.7 mg/kg IV tid for 10–14 d), streptomycin (1 g IM bid for 10–14 d), or doxycycline or ciprofloxacin.

Influenza viruses cause zoonotic pneumonia. Influenza types A, B, and C infect humans, but zoonotic infections are limited to influenza type A.[46] Migrating aquatic fowl are thought to be the natural animal reservoir for influenza type A. Horses and marine mammals can also serve as reservoirs for this zoonotic virus. Influenza can be transmitted between certain species, such as between pigs and humans.[46] Antigenic drift of the viral surface proteins hemagglutinin and neuraminidase in conjunction with a zoonotic reservoir accounts for the frequent human pandemics of influenza. Treatment and prevention of influenza and influenza pneumonia are discussed in Chap. 143.

Hantavirus, identified in 1977, is a viral zoonosis. The recognized etiologic agent in North America is the Sin Nombre virus, which belongs to the Bunyaviridae family of viruses. To date, at least 10 distinctive serotypes have been identified, each with a specific rodent vector, geographic distribution, and clinical manifestation.[47,48] The deer mouse *(Peromyscus maniculatus)* is the primary vector in the United States.[47,48] Infected rodents excrete hantavirus in feces, urine, and saliva. Human infection occurs with the inhalation of dried, particulate feces, contact with urine, or by a rodent bite. The majority of hantavirus serotypes have a predilection for the kidney, and the most common worldwide presentation is that of acute renal failure with concurrent thrombocytopenia, ocular abnormalities, and flulike symptoms. In the United States, the presentation of this zoonosis is that of hantavirus pulmonary syndrome,[47,48] which consists of an initial flulike prodromal illness of 3 to 4 days' duration, rapidly followed by pulmonary edema, hypoxia, hypotension, tachycardia, and metabolic acidosis. Dizziness, nausea, vomiting, absence of cough, and thrombocytopenia are common and may help to differentiate hantavirus pulmonary syndrome from acute respiratory distress syndrome, bacterial pneumonia, and influenza pneumonia.[2] Hantavirus pulmonary syndrome carries a very high mortality rate of 50 to 70 percent. Diagnosis is with an immunofluorescent or immunoblot assay. Treatment consists of supportive care with attention to adequate oxygenation and possibly the use of an inhalation solution of ribavirin.[47,48]

GASTROINTESTINAL ZOONOTIC INFECTIONS

Many of the parasitic, bacterial, and viral organisms responsible for gastroenteritis share a zoonotic source in addition to a human source. In the evaluation of patients with suspected gastroenteritis, information regarding travel history and animal exposure is extremely important. Occupational exposure to cattle, horses, poultry, sheep, swine, or reptiles, and even exposure to a household pet can be significant in determining a zoonotic origin. Dogs in particular are well known to have a 40 percent carriage rate for *Giardia lamblia* and a 30 percent carriage rate for the bacterial enteropathogens *Salmonella* spp. and *Yersinia* spp.[49]

Zoonotic gastroenteritis often presents with fever, headache, and abdominal pain, often localizing to the right lower quadrant. Patients may have diarrhea or constipation. Laboratory findings may consist of electrolyte and acid-base abnormalities if diarrhea is severe. Leukocytosis may be seen if an interstitial invasion has occurred, and eosinophilia is often a finding with intestinal parasitic infestation. Most cases of zoonotic gastroenteritis are self-limiting and require only fluid hydration. However, specific pathogens may require specific therapy (Table 151-5).

DERMATOLOGIC ZOONOTIC INFECTIONS

Dermatologic findings are common in zoonotic infections, as the dermis is often the site of inoculation and may display focal findings. The common dermatologic infections of impetigo, ecthyma, and cellulitis can be transmitted zoonotically, as can human infestations with mites and lice. The dermatophytoses *Tinea verrucosum* and *Microsporum canis* account for the majority of zoonotic dermatophyte infections, with *M. canis* accounting for 15 percent of all human dermatophy-

TABLE 151-5 Gastrointestinal Zoonotic Infections

Zoonoses	Animal Reservoir	Antibiotic Therapy
Brucellosis	Dogs and farm animals	Rifampin plus doxycycline, or TMP-SMX plus gentamicin
Campylobacter spp.	Dogs, cats, farm animals, poultry, unpasteurized milk	Erythromycin, fluoroquinolones
Giardia lamblia	Beavers, dogs, cats, farm animals	Metronidazole, tinidazole, quinacrine
Salmonella spp.	Reptiles (turtles), aquatic animals, dogs, cats, and humans *(S. typhi)*	Fluoroquinolones or TMP-SMX
Tularemia	Rabbits, cats, wild animals	Tobramycin, gentamicin, or doxycycline
Yersinia entercolitica	Dogs and cats	Fluoroquinolone, TMP-SMX, or third-generation cephalosporin
Vibrio cholerae	Shellfish	Doxycycline, ciprofloxacin, TMP-SMX (strain 0139 resistant to TMP-SMX)

Abbreviation: TMP-SMX = trimethoprim-sulfamethoxazole.

toses.[50] Chancriform lesions (ulcerations at the site of inoculation) can result from zoonotic infection of bacterial, mycobacterial, fungal, or viral etiology.

The most significant bacterial chancriform zoonotic lesions are *Bacillus anthracis* (anthrax), *Bartonella henselae* (cat-scratch disease), *Erysipelothrix rhusiopathiae* (erysipeloid), *Francisella tularensis* (tularemia), *Listeria monocytogenes* (listeriosis), *Mycobacterium marinum,* and *Pseudomonas mallei* (glanders).[5,50,51] The vast majority of these chancriform zoonotic infections occur in livestock workers, cattle ranchers, veterinarians, stable workers, horse trainers, slaughterhouse workers, poultry workers, and farmers. Significant zoonotic fungal chancriform infection is principally from *Blastomyces dermatitidis* (cutaneous blastomycosis) and *Sporothrix schenckii* (sporotrichosis). Dog and cat owners, along with veterinarians, are most at risk of contracting these two fungal zoonoses.[50,51] All of the chancriform zoonotic infections most commonly appear at the site of inoculation, often the hands or forearms.

Zoonotic dermatoses of viral etiology include *Vaccinia* spp. (cowpox), *Paravaccinia* spp. (pseudocowpox), and bovine papular stomatitis. These cutaneous viral zoonoses often occur on the hands and forearms of patients who work closely with cattle, sheep, goats, or horses.

Systemic zoonoses can be accompanied by dermatologic findings, usually a generalized maculopapular rash, which is common in bartonellosis, lymphocytic choriomeningitis, Colorado tick fever, leptospirosis, psittacosis, and rickettsial infections. However, the maculopapular rash associated with most zoonotic infections is nonspecific and does not facilitate the diagnosis. Those zoonotic infections with specific dermatologic findings that can aid in diagnosis are infections from *Aeromonas* spp., Lyme disease, RMSF, *Vibrio* spp., and viral hemorrhagic fevers (Table 151-6).[5,9]

Of special note is cutaneous anthrax (Figure 135-7), also known as woolsorter's disease. Cutaneous anthrax accounts for 95 percent of all anthrax infections seen by physicians. This variant is most common in Third World nations dependent on livestock, and agriculture-based societies. With disruption of the dermal layer of the skin, anthrax spores are deposited, and within 1 to 5 days a pruritic macule becomes visible at the inoculum site. The hands and fingers are the most commonly infected areas of the body, but arms, lower legs, and feet can also be involved. The macule evolves into an ulcerative site with multiple

TABLE 151-6 Specific Zoonotic Dermatologic Findings

Zoonoses	Characteristic Rash
Aeromonas spp.	Crepitant cellulitis with systemic toxicity
Lyme disease	Erythema migrans at the focus of the tick bite
Rocky Mountain spotted fever	Maculopapular rash on soles and palms with centripetal spread, advance characteristic of petechial hemorrhage and necrosis
Viral hemorrhagic fever	Petechial and purpuric rash

vesicles. These vesicles are serosanguineous and contain the anthrax bacillus. Gram stain or culture of the vesicular fluid is often diagnostic. The ulcer eventually progresses to a painless black eschar and falls off within 2 weeks. Antibiotic coverage is the same as for pulmonary or systemic anthrax, but it does not alter the progression of cutaneous anthrax. But antibiotic therapy does inhibit the progression from cutaneous to systemic anthrax.

ZOONOSES ACQUIRED FROM HOUSEHOLD PETS

There are more than 30 significant human diseases acquired from household pets.[52] Dogs and cats are the two most common household pets in North America and account for the majority of these zoonotic infections. Small rodents, pet birds, reptiles, and aquarium fish account for only a fraction of the zoonotic infections in the United States (Table 151-7).[51,53] Although pet owners often have close contact with their pets, pet-acquired zoonoses are rare and not often recognized. Yet these infections have a very diverse etiology and encompass parasitic, bacterial, rickettsial, and fungal infections.

Up to 50 percent of dogs are infected with at least one intestinal parasite, and 15 percent of adult dogs actively excrete *Toxocara canis*, the source of *toxocariasis* and visceral larva migrans.[49] Despite its prevalence in dogs, human toxocariasis is infrequently diagnosed, probably because infection is often subclinical. Typically, the only indication of infection is eosinophilia. Children may display fever, cough, and nonspecific rash, as well as an inability to gain weight. Rarely, pulmonary infiltrates, hepatosplenomegaly, and seizures may occur. Diagnosis is by either biopsy of infected tissue or by ELISA. Treatment in the symptomatic patient consists of albendazole (400 mg bid for ≥5 d) or Mebendazole, (100–200 mg PO bid for ≥5 d). Corticosteroids can be used to control the allergic component.

Other intestinal parasites that may be transmitted to humans from household pets include *Ancylostoma caninum* (cutaneous larva migrans), *Echinococcus granulosus* (echinococcosis), and *Dipylidium*

caninum (dipylidiasis or dog and cat tapeworm).[49] Cutaneous larva migrans is often a self-limiting, pruritic, erythematous serpiginous rash caused as the larva migrates through the skin, and is often acquired from fecally contaminated soil. Topical or oral thiabendazole is effective therapy for shortening the disease course.[50,51]

Though dogs and other carnivores are the definitive hosts for *E. granulosus, echinococcosis* is most common in areas of cattle and sheep ranching. This zoonosis involves multiple organ systems: liver, lung, muscle, bone, kidney, and brain. Typically, there is a unilocular cyst containing multiple larvae that enlarge over time. Diagnosis and treatment usually occur at the time of surgical resection. Aspiration of the cyst is contraindicated, because leakage of the cystic fluid can spread the infection and cause an anaphylactic reaction.

Dipylidiasis, caused by a tapeworm common to both dogs and cats, is found worldwide. Human infection is rare; however, when infection does occur, it is often in children and presents with the nonspecific symptoms of diarrhea and pruritus ani. Occasionally, the cucumber-shaped proglottides are seen moving in the child's stool. Treatment is with praziquantel (5–10 mg/kg PO single dose), or niclosamide (2 mg PO single dose).

Cats are the host of the intracellular protozoan *Toxoplasma gondii,* which causes *toxoplasmosis.* Human toxoplasmosis can occur in three ways: by ingestion of uncooked or raw meat, especially pork or mutton containing the *Toxoplasma* cysts; by ingestion of the oocysts from cat and wild-animal feces; and transplacentally.[49,52] Transplacental transmission can result in congenital abnormalities of retinochoroiditis, hydrocephalus, hepatosplenomegaly, and thrombocytopenia in 10 percent of the children infected. The majority of children transplacentally infected with toxoplasmosis display no significant abnormalities. Nevertheless, pregnant women should limit their contact to only indoor cats and avoid contact with cat feces. The encysted trophozoite can become reactivated in a previously infected host if the host becomes immunocompromised.[54]

Bacterial zoonoses from household pets include, but are not limited to, brucellosis, leptospirosis, salmonellosis, and campylobacteriosis. *Brucellosis (Brucella canis)* is an uncommon infection in humans and is most often acquired from dogs. Pigs, cattle, and goats are less frequent transmitters. The typical human course for brucellosis is self-limited, with fever, headache, myalgias, and nonspecific laboratory findings. Doxycycline plus rifampin or gentamycin is the standard therapy in treating human brucellosis, or alternatively, TMP/SMX plus gentamycin.

Leptospirosis (Leptospira canicola) infects almost all mammals, but dogs are the principal vector for humans. Humans become infected through exposure to body fluids, particularly urine, of an infected animal. The acute phase of leptospirosis is characterized by headache,

TABLE 151-7 Pet-Associated Zoonotic Infections

Dog	Cat	Bird	Rodent	Fish and Reptiles
Anthrax	Anthrax	Cryptococcosis	Leptospirosis	Erysipeloid
Brucellosis	Campylobacteriosis	Erysipeloid	Listeriosis	*Mycobacterium marinum*
Campylobacterosis	Cryptosporidiosis	Listeriosis	Lymphocytic choriomeningitis	Salmonellosis
Crytosporidiosis	Histoplasmosis	*Mycobacterium*	Murine typhus	Vibriosis
Dirofilariasis	Pasteurellosis	Ornithosis *(C. psittaci)*	Plague	
Echinococcosis	Plague	Salmonellosis	Rat-bite fever *(S. moniliformis)*	
Histoplasmosis	Q Fever	Tularemia	Salmonellosis	
Leptospirosis	Rabies	Viral encephalitis	Tularemia	
Pasteurellosis	Salmonellosis		Yersiniosis	
Rabies	Toxocariasis			
Rocky Mountain spotted fever	Tularemia			
Salmonellosis				
Toxocariasis				
Tularemia				
Yersiniosis				

malaise, myalgias, and fever. Nonspecific rash, meningitis, uveitis, myositis, and leptospiruria follow the acute phase. Doxycycline (100 mg PO bid for 10 to 14 d) or high-dose penicillin (penicillin G 20 to 24 million units IV qd for 10 to 14 d) are the mainstays of treatment for leptospirosis.[35,51]

Campylobacteriosis (Campylobacter jejuni) is a major cause of infectious diarrhea in humans. This zoonotic infection also occurs in dogs, cats, pigs, poultry, cattle, and horses. Human infection from a pet is uncommon, but the presence of a puppy or kitten with a diarrheal illness in the house and human contacts experiencing diarrhea should raise the suspicion of pet-acquired campylobacteriosis. Though the disease is often self-limiting, treatment with erythromycin can facilitate resolution in protracted cases.[49]

Nontyphoidal salmonellosis is typically a self-limiting gastrointestinal illness prevalent among dogs. Human transmission is rare. Diarrhea in any pet should alert the pet owner to use increased personal hygiene and to dispose of the pet's feces properly.[35,52]

The ticks and fleas inhabiting dogs and cats can transmit the zoonotic infections of tularemia, plague, and Rocky Mountain spotted fever. Transmission is often by cat bite, tick bite, or scratch. Dogs do not directly transmit tularemia, but do serve as carriers of the ticks that can transmit this zoonosis.

Plague *(Yersinia pestis)* is endemic in the rodent population of the southwestern United States. Dogs and cats can also be sources of this zoonosis. Transmission occurs when bitten by fleas inhabiting an infected rodent, dog, or cat or by eating infected rodents. Plague has three forms: bubonic or suppurative lymphadenopathy (the most common), the pneumonic form, and the septicemic form. Because of the aggressive nature of *Y. pestis,* treatment should not be delayed.

Rocky Mountain spotted fever *(Rickettsia rickettsii)* is a tick-transmitted, systemic zoonosis, with the tick *Dermacentor* as principal vector and reservoir. Animal reservoirs consist of rodents, rabbits, and infrequently, dogs. Zoonotic fungal infections are occasionally acquired by humans. The most common of these infections is a dermatophytosis from *Microsporum canis.* It is estimated that up to 30 percent of human dermatophytoses have a zoonotic origin.[50] Treatment is with topical ketoconazole or other imidazole antifungals.

ZOONOTIC INFECTIONS AND IMMUNOCOMPROMISED PATIENTS

Immunocompromised patients deserve special consideration and encompass a very large group: patients with congenital immunodeficiencies, diabetes mellitus, chronic renal failure, or liver failure; splenectomized patients; chronic alcoholics; cancer patients; and HIV-positive patients. Of all of these patients, those undergoing chemotherapy and those with AIDS have the greatest risk of acquiring a zoonotic infection.[55] It is estimated that 30 to 40 percent of immunocompromised patients may own pets.[54] *Salmonella* and *Campylobacter* are the two most common infections acquired by immunocompromised patients from their pets,[55] but the overall risk of transmission of *Salmonella* and *Campylobacter* from contact with pets is low. Additionally, *Mycobacterium marinum* from aquatic pets, and *Bartonella* from cats, are also commonly acquired by immunocompromised patients. Other acquired zoonotic infections that immunocompromised patients are susceptible to include *Toxoplasma gondii, Cryptosporidium, Giardia, Rhodococcus equi,* and *Bordetella bronchiseptica* (Table 151-8). With the exception of *Bartonella* (cat-scratch disease), most of these zoonotic infections are acquired by immunocompromised patients from sources other than exposure to animals.[54] These sources are principally from contaminated food or water. Nevertheless, it is important for emergency physicians to inquire about animal exposure and zoonotic risk factors when evaluating immunocompromised patients. Consultation with an infectious disease specialist and a veterinarian may be warranted in evaluating immunocompromised patients in the ED.

TABLE 151-8 Zoonotic Infections Among Immunocompromised Patients

Infection	Source	Clinical Findings	Antibiotic Treatment
Cat-scratch disease *Bartonella henselae*	Cats	Pyogenic granulomas, regional lymphadenopathy, and fever	Erythromycin or doxycycline
Bordetella *Bordetella bronchiseptica*	Dogs	Fever, pharyngitis, and cough	Erythromycin or TMP/SMX
Campylobacter *Campylobacter* spp.	Dogs, cats	Gastroenteritis and diarrhea	Erythromycin, ciprofloxacin, or azithromycin
Cryptococcus *Cryptococcus neoformans*	Bird droppings and cats	Flulike symptoms early, photophobia, headache, cranial nerve symptoms, and meningeal irritation later	Amphotericin B, fluconazole
Cryptosporidium	Dogs	Diarrhea	Nitazoxanide[56]
Giardia *Giardia lamblia*	Dogs, cats	Gastroenteritis and diarrhea	Metronidazole, tinidazole, albendazole, quinacrine
Listeria *Listeria monocytogenes*	Livestock, and dairy products	Sepsis and meningitis	Ampicillin, high-dose penicillin, or TMP/SMX
Mycobacterium			
M. avium	Pet birds	Pneumonia and gastroenteritis	Clarithromycin plus ethambutol
M. marinum	Fish	Cutaneous granulomas, skin ulcerations at distal extremities	Clarithromycin, doxycycline, TMP/SMX, or rifampin and ethambutol
Rhodococcus *Rhodococcus equi*	Farm animals	Pneumonia and cavitating lung lesions	Vancomycin, erythromycin, or imipenem plus rifampin
Salmonella *Salmonella* spp.	Dogs, cats, reptiles, and farm animals	Gastroenteritis, diarrhea, and sepsis	Ciprofloxacin, ceftriaxone, azithromycin, or TMP/SMX
Toxoplasmosis *Toxoplasma* gondii	Cats	Pneumonia, brain abscesses, encephalitis, and ocular disease	Pyrimethamine, plus sulfadiazine and folinic acid

Abbreviation: TMP/SMX = trimethoprim-sulfamethoxazole.

REFERENCES

1. World Health Organization (WHO): Zoonoses Technical Report Series, 1959. Geneva, WHO, 1959.
2. Hart CA, Trees AJ, Duerden BI: Zoonoses: Proceedings of the third Liverpool Tropical School Bayer symposium on microbial diseases held on 3 February 1996. *J Med Microbiol* 46:4, 1997.
3. Simpson GL: Vector borne and animal associated infections, in Brillman CJ, Quenzer RW (eds): *Infectious Diseases in Emergency Medicine,* 2d ed. Philadelphia, Lippincott-Raven, 1998, p. 209.
4. Institute of Medicine: *Emerging Infections: Microbial Threats to Health in the United States.* Washington, National Academy Press, 1992.
5. Weinberg AN, Weber DJ: Animal associated human infections. *Infect Dis Clin North Am* 5:xi, 1991.
6. Walker DH, Barbour AG, Oliver JH, et al: Emerging bacterial zoonotic and vector-borne diseases: Ecological and epidemiological factors. *JAMA* 275:463, 1996.
7. Centers for Disease Control: Lyme disease: United States, 1987 and 1988. *MMWR* 38:668, 1989.
8. Doan-Wiggins L: Tick-borne diseases. *Emerg Med Clin North Am* 9:303, 1991.
9. Spach DH, Liles WC, Campbell GL, et al: Tick-borne diseases in the United States. *N Engl J Med* 329:936, 1993.
10. Centers for Disease Control: Rocky Mountain spotted fever: United States, 1990. *MMWR* 40:451, 1991.
11. Kirkland KK, Sexton DJ: Therapeutic delay in Rocky Mountain spotted fever. *Clin Infect Dis* 12:1118, 1995.
12. Woodward TE: Rocky Mountain spotted fever: Epidemiological and early clinical signs are keys to treatment and reduced mortality. *J Infect Dis* 150:465, 1984.
13. Walker DH: Rocky Mountain spotted fever: A seasonal alert. *Clin Infect Dis* 12:1111, 1995.
14. Steere AC: Lyme disease. *N Engl J Med* 345:115, 2001.
15. Wright SW, Trott AT: North America tick-borne diseases. *Ann Emerg Med* 17:964, 1988.
16. Shadick NA, Phillips CB, Logigian EL, et al: The long-term clinical outcomes of Lyme disease: A population-based retrospective cohort study. *Ann Intern Med* 121:560, 1994.
17. Hayes EB, Piesman DSc: How can we prevent lyme disease. *NEJM* 348:24, 2424, June 12, 2003.
18. Shapiro ED: Doxycycline for tick bites: Not for everyone. *N Engl J Med* 345:133, 2001.
19. Nadelman RB, Nowakowski J, Fish D, et al: Prophylaxis with single-dose doxycycline for the prevention of Lyme disease after an *Ixodes scapularis* tick bite. *N Engl J Med* 345:79, 2001.
20. Fihn S, Larson EB: Tick-borne relapsing fever in the Pacific Northwest: An underdiagnosed illness? *West J Med* 133:203, 1980.
21. Horton JM, Blaser MJ: The spectrum of relapsing fever in the Rocky Mountains. *Arch Intern Med* 145:871, 1985.
22. Mandell GL, Bennett JE, and Dolin R (eds): Mandell, Douglas & Bennett's: *Principles & Practice of Infectious Diseases,* 5th ed. 2000, Churchill-Livingstone, Edinburgh, 2000.
23. Emmons RW: An overview of Colorado tick fever. *Prog Clin Biol Res* 178:47, 1985.
24. McCoy GW, Chapin CW: Further observation of a plague-like disease of rodents with a preliminary note on the causative bacteria. *J Infect Dis* 10:61, 1912.
25. Evans ME, Gregory DW, Schaffner W, et al: Tularemia: A 30-year experience with 88 cases. *Medicine (Baltimore)* 64:251, 1985.
26. Boustani MR, Gelfand JA: Babesiosis. *Clin Infect Dis* 22:611, 1996.
27. Bakken JS, Krueth J, Wilson-Nordskog C, et al: Human granulocytic ehrlichiosis (HGE): Clinical and laboratory characteristics of 41 patients from Minnesota and Wisconsin. *JAMA* 275:199, 1995.
28. Dawson JE: Human ehrlichiosis in the United States, in Reminton JS, Swartz MN (eds): *Current Clinical Topics in Infectious Diseases.* Cambridge, MA, Blackwell Science, 1996, p. 164.
29. Whitley RJ, Cobbs CG, Alford CA, et al: Diseases that mimic herpes simplex encephalitis: Diagnosis, presentation, and outcome. *JAMA* 262:234, 1989.
30. Rennels MB: Arthropod-borne virus infections of the central nervous system. *Neurol Clin* 2:241, 1984.
31. Johnson RT, Mims CA: Pathogenesis of viral infections of the nervous system. *N Engl J Med* 278:23, 1968.
32. Kennard C, Swash M: Acute viral encephalitis: Its diagnosis and outcome. *Brain* 104:129, 1981.
33. Smithburn KC, Hughes TP, Burke AW, et al: A neurotropic virus isolated from the blood of a native of Uganda. *Am J Trop Med* 20:471, 1940.
34. Petersen LR, Marfin AA: West Nile virus: A primer for the clinician. *Ann Intern Med* 137:173, 2002.
35. Goldstein EJC: Household pets and human infections. *Infect Dis Clin North Am* 5:1177, 1991.
36. Weinberg AN: Respiratory infections transmitted from animals. *Infect Dis Clin North Am* 5:649, 1991.
37. Brachman PS: Inhalation anthrax. *Ann NY Acad Sci* 353:83, 1980.
38. Greer AE: Pulmonary brucellosis. *Dis Chest* 29:508, 1956.
39. Fox MD, Kaufman AF: Centers for Disease Control: Brucellosis in the United States, 1965–1974. *J Infect Dis* 136:312, 1977.
40. Centers for Disease Control: Compendium of measures to control *Chlamydia psittaci* infection among humans (psittacosis) and pet birds (avian chlamydiosis), 1998. *MMWR* 47:1, 1998.
41. Grayston JT, Thom DH: The chlamydial pneumonias. *Curr Clin Top Infect Dis* 11:1, 1991.
42. Sawyer LA, Fishbein DB, McDade JE: Q fever: Current concepts. *Rev Infect Dis* 9:935, 1987.
43. Weber DT, Wolfson JS, Swartz MN, et al: *Pasteurella multocida* infections: Report of 34 cases and review of the literature. *Medicine (Baltimore)* 63:133, 1984.
44. Byrd RP, Vasquez J, Roy TM: Respiratory manifestations of tick-borne diseases in the southeastern United States. *South Med J* 90:1, 1997.
45. Perry RD, Fetherston JD: *Yersinia pestis:* Etiologic agent of plague. *Clin Microbiol Rev* 10:35, 1997.
46. Webster RG, Sharp GB, Claas EC: Interspecies transmission of influenza viruses. *Am J Respir Crit Care Med* 152:525, 1995.
47. Centers for Disease Control: Hantavirus pulmonary syndrome: Colorado and New Mexico, 1998. *MMWR* 47:249, 1998.
48. Duchin JS, Koster FT, Peters CJ, et al: Hantavirus pulmonary syndrome: Clinical description of seventeen patients with a newly recognized disease. *N Engl J Med* 330:949, 1994.
49. Bauer D: The capacity of dogs to serve as reservoirs for gastrointestinal disease in children. *Ir Med J* 87:184, 1994.
50. Scott DW, Horn RT Jr: Zoonotic dermatoses of dogs and cats. *Vet Clin North Am* 17:117, 1987.
51. Elliot DL, Tolle SW, Goldberg L, et al: Pet-associated illness. *N Engl J Med* 16:985, 1985.
52. Tan JS: Human zoonotic infections transmitted by dogs and cats. *Arch Intern Med* 157:1933, 1997.
53. Chomel BB: Zoonoses of house pets other than dogs, cats, and birds. *Pediatr Infect Dis J* 11:479, 1992.
54. Glaser CA, Angulo J, Rooney JA: Animal-associated opportunistic infections among persons infected with the human immunodeficiency virus. *Clin Infect Dis* 18:14, 1994.
55. Angulo FJ, Glaser CA, Juranek DD, et al: Caring for pets of immunocompromised persons. *J Am Vet Med Assoc* 205:1711, 1994.
56. Nitazoxanide (Alinia)—A new anti-protozoal agent. *Med Lett* 54:29, April 14, 2003.

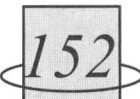

SOFT TISSUE INFECTIONS
Steven G. Folstad

NECROTIZING SOFT TISSUE INFECTIONS

Although these individual infectious entities are often discussed separately, necrotizing soft tissue infections actually represent a spectrum of illness differentiated primarily by the depth of soft tissue involvement. The similar feature in all of these infections is, as the name implies, some extent of tissue necrosis. The spectrum of these illnesses extends from localized infection involving only the subcutaneous tissue, as is the case in necrotizing cellulitis, through extensive soft tissue fascial plane involvement and sepsis, as in necrotizing fasciitis, to the deep myonecrosis and sepsis seen with gas gangrene. These necrotizing infections are most commonly polymicrobial in nature, and involve mixed aerobic and anaerobic organisms. There are a few specific bacteria, such as the *Clostridium* species and group A *Streptococcus* that can produce a single organism infection. With each of these infections soft tissue gas production may or may not be present.

Due to the rapid progression of illness and the high mortality rate associated with the more invasive of these infections, early recognition and aggressive treatment are essential. A keen eye for the early subtle signs and symptoms that differentiate these from the much less severe forms of cellulitis is required to lessen the high morbidity and mortality seen with these infections.

Gas Gangrene (Clostridial Myonecrosis)

Clostridial myonecrosis is a rapidly progressive and serious life- and limb-threatening deep subcutaneous tissue infection caused by several of the spore-forming clostridial species of organism. It is the deepest of the necrotizing soft tissue infections. Severe myonecrosis with gas production and sepsis are the hallmarks of this disease.

EPIDEMIOLOGY *Clostridium* species are ubiquitous organisms found throughout our environment. There are approximately 1000 cases of gas gangrene reported to the Centers for Disease Control and Prevention (CDC) each year in the United States.[1] The incidence of disease secondary to these organisms is decreasing, presumably due to better wound management and more effective antibiotic therapy. For example, the incidence of gas gangrene in battle-related injuries was 5 percent during World War I; this dropped to 0.2 percent during the Korean War, and to 0.01 percent during the war in Vietnam.

PATHOPHYSIOLOGY There have been seven *Clostridium* species identified as causing gas gangrene. *Clostridium perfringens* is attributed to 80 to 95 percent of cases, with *C. septicum* being the second most common etiology.[2] The clostridial organisms are large, gram-positive, spore-forming anaerobic bacilli normally found in the soil, gastrointestinal tract, and female genitourinary tract. They produce over ten exotoxins that are responsible for the cellular destruction as well as the rapid progression and systemic toxicity of the disease. The exotoxin that is considered to be the most significant is the α-toxin. This toxin has direct cardiodepressant activity. It also hydrolyzes cell membranes, causes tissue necrosis, inactivates leukocytes, and hemolyzes erythrocytes. Secondary toxic effects may be caused by the release of myoglobin, creatine phosphokinase (CPK), and potassium from tissue breakdown.

There are two potential mechanisms for infection with clostridial organisms. The most common is through direct inoculation from an open wound. Similarly to tetanus, clostridial species thrive best in contaminated wounds with crushed or ischemic edges that tend to offer a favorable anaerobic environment. Uterine myonecrosis due to clostridial infection has also been documented following cesarean section delivery. This is most likely due to the significant incidence of clostridial colonization in the female genitourinary tract. The second mechanism for infection is by hematogenous spread, particularly in the immunocompromised. Almost a third of cases of "spontaneous gas gangrene" are caused by *C. septicum*, with an even higher incidence in cases related to malignancies.

CLINICAL FEATURES The incubation period is usually less than 3 days. The most common presenting complaints in early gas gangrene are pain out of proportion to physical findings, as well as a sensation of "heaviness" of the affected part. On examination, the area may demonstrate a brawny edema with crepitance. Crepitance is a later finding, however, and its absence does not rule out the diagnosis. The skin will develop a bronze or brownish discoloration with a malodorous serosanguineous discharge, and bullae may be present. Systemic manifestations include a low-grade fever with tachycardia out of pro-

portion to the fever. The patient may be confused or irritable and have a rapid deterioration of the sensorium. Laboratory evaluation may reveal any or all of the following: metabolic acidosis, leukocytosis, anemia, thrombocytopenia, coagulopathy, myoglobinemia and myoglobinuria, and liver or kidney dysfunction. Gram stain of the bullae often shows pleomorphic gram-positive bacilli with or without spores, red blood cells, but very few white blood cells. Radiologic studies may demonstrate gas within the involved muscle and surrounding soft tissue, and when the infection involves the trunk, possibly gas within the peritoneal or retroperitoneal space.

Surgical exploration is also helpful in the diagnosis. In the early stages, the muscles are edematous and pale but still bleed when cut; in later stages, the muscles lose contractility and on dissection appear beefy red without bleeding and gas bubbles may be evident between the tissues.

The differential diagnosis of clostridial myonecrosis must encompass other gas-forming infections, including necrotizing fasciitis, streptococcal myositis, and clostridial or nonclostridial anaerobic cellulitis. The crepitance of infection should be differentiated from other causes of subcutaneous emphysema such as pneumothorax, pneumomediastinum, and fractured larynx or trachea. The edema and pallor, with loss of distal pulses, seen in an affected extremity should be differentiated from vascular thrombosis conditions such as phlegmasia cerulea dolens.

TREATMENT Treatment consists of four main phases:

1. *Resuscitation* should begin in the ED immediately upon making a presumptive diagnosis. Aggressive fluid resuscitation using crystalloid, plasma, and packed cells is usually needed to replace red blood cells lost due to hemolysis and to correct hypotension due to shock. Volume status should be closely monitored using urine output and central venous pressure readings. Avoid the use of vasoconstrictors when possible due to the possibility of decreasing perfusion to already ischemic muscle.
2. *Antibiotic therapy* using penicillin G, 24 million units IV per d in divided doses plus clindamycin, 900 mg q8h IV, is recommended. Ceftriaxone or erythromycin are alternative choices. Sodium penicillin is recommended over potassium penicillin to reduce the risk of worsening hyperkalemia in patients with hemolysis and tissue necrosis. Mixed infections with other anaerobes, gram-negative rods, and staphylococci are common. Therefore, multiple-antibiotic therapy using aminoglycosides, penicillinase-resistant penicillins, or vancomycin is recommended. Tetanus prophylaxis should be given as indicated.
3. *Surgical debridement* is a mainstay of therapy and may include fasciotomy, debridement, or amputation. Early removal of the infected tissue by surgical debridement is most important. The borders for debridement are guided by the appearance of the muscle.
4. *Hyperbaric oxygen (HBO) therapy* should be initiated as soon as possible after surgical debridement. Although there are no prospective human studies, retrospective data suggest a twofold reduction in mortality in patients receiving concomitant HBO therapy.[3] Typical HBO therapy consists of 100 percent oxygen at 3 atm of pressure for 90 min immediately following surgery, with three dives in the first 24 h followed by two dives a day for 4 or 5 days.

Wound care at the time of initial evaluation and treatment is the most important factor in preventing clostridial infections. Debridement of crushed or dead tissue and copious irrigation prior to wound closure will help prevent the development of an environment favorable to clostridial growth. Amoxicillin/clavulanate, imipenem, meropenem, or ampicillin/sulbactam may be beneficial.

Gas Gangrene (Nonclostridial Myonecrosis)

Most cases of nonclostridial myonecrosis are caused by mixed infections involving both aerobic and anaerobic organisms. The clinical presentation, evaluation, and treatment of nonclostridial myonecrosis is very similar to that caused by the clostridial species, and only the differences seen with the nonclostridial infections will be discussed here.

A recent Japanese study examined the treatment outcome of a small group of patients with nonclostridial myonecrosis.[4] Each patient had a mixed infection with an average of 5.1 different species of organisms being isolated. The range of organisms per patient was 2 to 10. Both aerobic and anaerobic organisms were found in all cases. The most common bacteria were: *Enterococcus* (100 percent); *Staphylococcus* (71 percent); α-Streptococci (57 percent); *E. coli, Klebsiella,* and *Proteus* (each at 43 percent); and *Bacteroides* (43 percent). Other less common bacteria included *Peptostreptococcus, Bacillus, Citrobacter, Enterobacter,* and *Morganella* (each at 14 percent). *Clostridium* was also isolated in 29 percent of these mixed infections.

The pain associated with the onset of infection was not as pronounced as with typical clostridial infection, and the authors felt that this led to a delay in presentation (2 to 10 days after symptom onset), and contributed to their significant mortality rate of 43 percent.

Broad-spectrum antibiotic coverage is of the utmost importance due to the mixed nature of the organisms involved with these infections. Coverage for aerobic gram-positive and gram-negative organisms as well as anaerobes is necessary. The most commonly recommended drugs are: ampicillin/sulbactam, ticarcillin/clavulanate, piperacillin/tazobactam, imipenem, or meropenem. Vancomycin, a fluoroquinolone, and clindamycin can be used in penicillin-allergic patients. Fluoroquinolones should be added for freshwater infections. Early surgical debridement and HBO therapy are recommended as for clostridial infections.

Streptococcal Myositis

This is an extremely rare muscle infection caused by an invasive form of group A *Streptococcus*. Clinically, it is difficult to distinguish from other forms of myonecrosis, except there is typically no gas production. It is a very virulent infection that has a high rate of bacteremia, and subsequent toxic shock syndrome (see Chap. 142). The case mortality rate is reported to be in the 80 to 100 percent range. There will be further discussion of group A streptococcal infections later in this chapter.

Necrotizing Fasciitis (Polymicrobial Infection)

Necrotizing fasciitis is characterized by widespread necrosis involving the subcutaneous tissue and fascia. The infection does not spread through the fascial layer into the underlying muscle, as it does with the clostridial and nonclostridial myonecrosis infections. It is an infectious process that has been recognized for centuries, but was brought to the world's attention in the mid-1990s when the tabloid press began reporting about an outbreak of "flesh-eating bacteria."

As with gas gangrene, there is a mixed-organism form of this infection, which is the most common, and a single-organism form, which is typically caused by group A *Streptococcus*. The presentation, evaluation, and treatment of these two forms of infection are very similar, and a discussion of the differences of the group A *Streptococcus* infection will follow in a separate section.

EPIDEMIOLOGY   There are 10 to 20 cases of invasive group A streptococcal infection per 100,000 population, and about 27 cases per 10,000 hospital admissions.[5]

Those with underlying illnesses such as diabetes and peripheral vascular disease are at higher risk. Smoking and intravenous drug use are also significant predisposing factors.

A majority of cases involve the lower extremities, with the upper extremities, perineum, trunk, head and neck, and buttocks following in decreasing order of incidence.

PATHOPHYSIOLOGY   The majority of cases of necrotizing fasciitis are mixed aerobic and anaerobic. Common pathogens include: the gram-positive α, β, *and* γ streptococci, *Staphylococcus aureus,* the gram-negative *E. coli, Pseudomonas* spp., *Enterobacter, Klebsiella,* and *Proteus,* and the anaerobic bacteria *Bacteroides, Clostridium,* and *Peptostreptococcus.* Most patients are infected with several strains of bacteria. One study of 182 patients with positive cultures showed a mean of 4.4 organisms per patient, and up to 6 organisms per wound culture.[6]

The exact pathogenesis of this infection is not clear, but there seems to be a symbiotic relationship between the different bacteria that acts to promote the overall infection. The facultative gram-negative organisms lower the oxygen-reduction potential of the tissue, which promotes an environment for anaerobic organism growth. The anaerobic organisms impede phagocyte function in the host immune response, which favors aerobic bacterial growth.

The mechanism for the wide spread of fascial plane necrosis appears to be secondary to a vasculitis and thrombosis of regional blood vessels. Bacterial tissue toxins cause inflammation in the walls of larger regional blood vessels, which eventually leads to thrombosis in the vessel lumen, as well as ischemia of the skin, subcutaneous fat, and fascia that the vessel supplies. This ischemic tissue environment promotes the spread of bacterial growth, propagating the process occurring in regional blood vessels, resulting in rapid spread of the infection.

The most common mechanisms for infection are soft tissue trauma and surgery, with insults such as intravenous injection, surgical incision, abscess, insect bite, and ulcer. Diabetes and underlying malignancy are predetermining risk factors for spontaneous infection.

The overall mortality rate is usually reported in the 25 to 50 percent range. Bacteremia is reported in 25 to 30 percent of cases, and is a strong predictor of mortality. Other patient factors that have been shown to affect mortality are age less than 1 year or greater than 60; intravenous drug use; comorbid conditions, especially cancer, chronic renal disease, and congestive heart failure; certain characteristics of the clinical course such as positive blood culture, trunk or perineal involvement, infection related to peripheral vascular disease, and delayed time to diagnosis or treatment.

CLINICAL FEATURES   The primary presenting complaint in patients with necrotizing fasciitis is pain well out of proportion to the physical findings. The skin appears erythematous and possibly edematous. Discoloration, vesicles, and crepitus are typically later findings. A low-grade fever and tachycardia are common. Early on, the sensorium is typically clear. Necrotizing fasciitis infections can progress with alarming rapidity, within hours.

DIAGNOSIS   CBC with differential, and chemistry including liver enzymes, coagulation studies, arterial blood gas, and possibly serum lactate should be obtained. Aerobic and anaerobic culture specimens should be obtained of the blood, and if possible of the infected area. Bedside soft tissue biopsies sent for rapid frozen section can be helpful in making an early diagnosis.[7] The tissue biopsy specimen needs to extend down to the level of the deep fascial plane.

The "finger test" is another bedside diagnostic aid that may help in making an early diagnosis. This test is performed in the following manner: After local anesthesia, a 2-cm incision is made in the suspected area of tissue down to the deep fascial plane. A lack of bleeding or the presence of a foul, cloudy fluid is a very suggestive sign. A finger is then placed in the incision, just superior to the deep fascia, and pushed forward. If the finger dissects the soft tissue away from the fascia without difficulty, the test is considered positive, and indicative of necrotizing fasciitis. In healthy tissue the subcutaneous fat adheres strongly to the deep fascia.

Very early surgical consultation is indicated in all suspected cases of necrotizing fasciitis.

TREATMENT   The treatment of necrotizing fasciitis is similar to that of gas gangrene, and should be considered to consist of four phases: (1) *aggressive fluid and blood resuscitation, and avoidance of vasopressors;* (2) *antibiotic therapy* similar to that for nonclostridial myonecrosis should be empirically given-imipenem or meropenem, or vancomycin, clindamycin and a fluoroquinolone in penicillin-allergic patients; (3) *surgical debridement* is again the mainstay of therapy; (4) *hyperbaric oxygen (HBO)* therapy can be instituted following surgical debridement.

Necrotizing Fasciitis (Group A *Streptococcus*)

As with gas gangrene, the basic presentation, evaluation, and treatment for group A streptococcal (GAS) necrotizing fasciitis is very similar to that of the polymicrobial type, and only the differences will be discussed here.

The overall incidence is reportedly 10 to 20 cases per 100,000 population.[8] Most series report an overall mortality rate of 20 to 60 percent for invasive GAS infections, supposedly due to more virulent strains of bacteria.

Concomitant *Varicella* infection, especially in children, and NSAID use increase the risk for invasive GAS infection. *Varicella* lesions are presumed to be a portal of entry for the GAS bacteria into the host. It is unclear if the use of NSAIDs predisposes certain patients to invasive GAS infection, or if it acts to mask the early symptoms of disease.

Clinically, patients with GAS necrotizing fasciitis present very similarly to those with the polymicrobial form of infection; however, there is usually no gas formation in the soft tissue. Patients tend to have a more rapid progression of illness and are more prone to bacteremia and subsequent development of toxic shock syndrome (TSS) (see Chap. 142). Necrotizing fasciitis secondary to GAS is a subsegment of the overall spectrum of invasive GAS infections. The most severe end of this spectrum is TSS, and it is estimated that 50 percent of patients with GAS TSS had necrotizing fasciitis as the initiating infection.

Treatment should initially begin with a broad-spectrum antibiotic regimen as discussed above, but it can be changed to a combination of penicillin and clindamycin when cultures identify an isolated GAS infection. Penicillin alone often fails in severe GAS infections. Clindamycin has a synergistic effect with penicillin and improves treatment success greatly. Some of the mechanisms of clindamycin efficacy include: suppression of bacterial toxin synthesis, promotion of phagocytosis of the bacterium by inhibiting M protein synthesis, suppression of synthesis of penicillin-binding proteins, and a prolonged postantibiotic effect in comparison to penicillin.

HBO therapy is of minimal benefit with infections involving aerobic organisms.

Necrotizing Cellulitis

Necrotizing cellulitis is the most superficial form of necrotizing soft tissue infection, with the involved tissue being limited to the skin and subcutaneous fat. This is often determined at the time of surgery, or from a superficial tissue biopsy sent for rapid frozen section. Other synonyms for the disorder are crepitant cellulitis and synergistic necrotizing cellulitis.

PATHOPHYSIOLOGY   This infection is also typically associated with a preceding soft tissue trauma or surgery, but can occur spontaneously, usually in patients with an underlying malignancy or diabetes. The invading bacteria cause direct local tissue necrosis and vasculitis, which lead to edema and eventual thrombosis. This is similar to that seen with necrotizing fasciitis, but involves only the more superficial vessels.

Clostridial species are common pathogens, with *Clostridium perfringens* being the most commonly found in the setting of trauma or surgery, and *Clostridium septicum* more commonly found in the setting of malignancy and spontaneous infection. Clostridial infection is typically associated with significant gas production in the subcutaneous tissue.

Nonclostridial necrotizing cellulitis is caused by a variety of other anaerobic bacteria, similar species as those previously discussed for the deeper soft tissue infections. Infection may be caused by a single organism, but is most commonly polymicrobial. There is usually less gas production than that seen with clostridial infection, and there may be no gas at all.

CLINICAL FEATURES   Pain and erythema at the site of infection are the most common presenting complaints. The pain is often severe, but not typically to the degree of that seen with the deeper necrotizing infections. There may be an ecchymotic or frankly necrotic center to the infected area. Vesicles or blebs may also be present. The presence of crepitance is strongly suggestive of a necrotizing infection. Systemic symptoms are typically mild or absent due to the more localized nature of the infection.

TREATMENT   Surgical debridement of the local skin and subcutaneous fat is required, but extensive soft tissue removal is not needed. Surgical debridement is typically curative; however, administration of broad-spectrum antibiotics, similar to those used in the deeper infections should be started early, and continued until significant improvement is seen in the patient's clinical condition.

CELLULITIS

Cellulitis is a local soft tissue inflammatory reaction secondary to bacterial invasion of the skin. The classic symptoms of cellulitis have been attributed previously to bacterial invasion and subsequent proliferation within the local tissues; however, there is some evidence that suggests that the majority of symptoms may instead be secondary to a complex set of immune and inflammatory reactions triggered by cells within the skin itself.[9]

Epidemiology

Cellulitis is presumed to selectively affect the elderly, the immunocompromised, and those with peripheral vascular disease. Epidemiologic data on prevalence and incidence of disease has typically been difficult to obtain and interpret. One study of over 300,000 patient visits over a 1-year period[10] identified almost 4000 cases of cellulitis, or 1.3 percent of all patient visits. Patient characteristics demonstrated a slight male predominance (61 percent); a mean age of 46 years; a vast majority of infections involving either the lower or upper extremities (48 and 41 percent respectively); and interestingly, in this study predisposing medical conditions such as diabetes, peripheral vascular disease, cancer, and alcohol abuse were each seen in less than 5 percent of patients.

Pathophysiology

Cellulitis is a local inflammation of the skin characterized by pain, induration, warmth, and erythema. It is caused by invasion of the tissues by bacteria, most commonly staphylococci or streptococci in adults and *Haemophilus influenzae* in children. In diabetic patients, additional consideration needs to be given to Enterobacteriaceae and rarely clostridia. Lymphangitis and lymphadenopathy are seen occasionally in previously healthy patients, but purely local inflammation is much more common. Systemic involvement with fever, leukocytosis, and bacteremia is seen most typically in patients with underlying immunosuppressive disorders.

Efforts at isolating causative organisms from infected tissue have had a very poor yield. Needle aspiration of the leading edge of an area of cellulitis produces organisms in less than 10 percent of cultures, and even punch biopsy from the same area yields organisms in only about 20 percent of cultures. Only areas with suppuration or abscess formation have significantly higher yields. Although bacterial invasion is what triggers the inflammation, the organisms are largely cleared from the site within the first 12 h, and the infiltration of lymphoid and reticular cells and their products is what produces the majority of symptoms. Cells such as Langerhans cells and keratinocytes release the cytokines interleukin-1 and tumor necrosis factor that enhance infiltration of the skin by circulating lymphocytes and macrophages. The net effect of this is much more rapid clearing of bacteria, but at the price of a significantly greater inflammatory response.

Clinical Features

Patients with cellulitis typically present with localized tenderness, warmth, induration, and erythema. Specific note should be made on physical examination of evidence of lymphangitis or lymphadenitis; although uncommon, these may suggest more serious infection. The presence of high fever and chills suggests bacteremia, especially in patients with underlying medical disorders. Recurrent attacks can lead to impairment of lymphatic drainage, permanent swelling, dermal fibrosis, and epidermal thickening. These chronic changes are known as *elephantiasis nostra* and predispose patients to further attacks of cellulitis.

In otherwise healthy patients, the clinical presentation is sufficient for diagnosing cellulitis. In patients with underlying disease or signs of bacteremia, blood cultures and leukocyte counts are indicated. Local means of isolating the organism are controversial, but in the case of a toxic-appearing patient, they may be worthwhile. Differentiating deep venous thrombosis from cellulitis in the lower extremities is often difficult and may require Doppler studies or venogram.

Treatment

Simple cellulitis in otherwise healthy adult patients can be treated on an outpatient basis with dicloxacillin (500 mg PO q6h), a macrolide (erythromycin ethylsuccinate 500 mg PO q6h, azithromycin 500 mg PO initial dose, then 250 mg PO qd × 4 d, clarithromycin 500 mg PO q12h), or amoxicillin-clavulanate (875/125 mg PO q12h), with all treatments lasting for 10 days except for azithromycin. The exception to this is cellulitis involving the head or neck, for which most patients should be admitted for intravenous antibiotics. Appropriate intravenous antibiotics include parenteral first-generation cephalosporins (cefazolin 1 g IV q6h) and penicillinase-resistant penicillins (nafcillin or oxacillin 2 g IV q4h). In diabetics, a parenteral second- or third-generation cephalosporin (ceftriaxone 1 to 2 g IV qd) should be used, or imipenem (500 mg IV q6h), meropenem (0.5 to 1 g IV q8h), or trovafloxacin (200 to 300 mg IV qd) in severe cases.[11] A once-daily treatment with cefazolin (2 g IV) plus probenacid (1 g PO) has recently been shown to be as efficacious as a once-daily dose of ceftriaxone (1 g IV), and much more cost effective.[12] This may be a viable option for patients who have access to home health services or an outpatient treatment center.

Disposition

Patients with evidence of bacteremia and those with underlying diseases such as diabetes mellitus, alcoholism, or other immunosuppressive disorders should be admitted for intravenous antibiotics. Empirical therapy may be started with the antibiotics listed earlier and changed as indicated by culture results.

Follow-up intervals depend on initial presentation, but generally within 2 or 3 days is sufficient to evaluate the success of treatment.

ERYSIPELAS

Epidemiology

Previously, erysipelas involved the face more frequently, but now it is primarily an infection of the lower extremities.

Pathophysiology

Erysipelas is a superficial cellulitis with lymphatic involvement that is caused primarily by group A *Streptococcus*. Atypical infections most commonly seen with other groups of streptococci are also noted. Infection is typically achieved through a portal of entry into the skin, with traumatic wounds, ulcers, and infected dermatoses of the lower extremities being the most common sites. Lymphedema and injury at the site of entry were the most common risk factors in one recent study (odds ratio 71.2 and 23.8 respectively).[13] Toe-web intertrigo had the highest population attributable risk, and proper diagnosis and treatment of toe-web intertrigo could prevent up to 60 percent of cases of lower extremity erysipelas. Leg edema, venous insufficiency, and obesity were also risk factors for infection (odds ratio 2.5, 2.9, and 2). Most often erysipelas occurs proximal to the portal of entry into the skin.

Clinical Features

The onset of symptoms is usually abrupt, with a sudden onset of high fever, chills, malaise, and nausea representing the prodromal phase. Over the next 1 to 2 days a small area of erythema with a burning sensation develops. As the infection continues, a red, shiny, hot plaque forms. The plaque has a tense, painful induration that is sharply demarcated from the surrounding normal tissue. Lymphatic inflammatory changes, known as *toxic striations,* and local lymphadenopathy are common. Purpura, bullae, and small areas of necrosis also are seen. The presence of bullae suggests a more serious form of infection, often requiring longer treatment courses and hospital admissions.[14] Systemic symptoms continue until antibiotic therapy is initiated. On resolution of the infection, desquamation of the site typically occurs.

The diagnosis is based primarily on physical findings. Leukocytosis with an increase in the neutrophil count is common. Performing a needle aspiration of the infection site is rarely successful at isolating an organism, but swabbing the portal of entry, when identifiable, may have a higher success rate. Blood cultures are positive in only around 5 percent of patients, and so are not helpful. Serologic testing to determine ASO and anti-DNase B titers may be more specific but is of little use in the ED.

The differential diagnosis includes other forms of local cellulitis. Some believe that necrotizing fasciitis is a complication of erysipelas infections and should be considered in all cases.

Treatment

Penicillin G (1 to 2 million units IV q6h) may be used in nondiabetic patients for initial treatment due to the high incidence of streptococcal infection. Penicillinase-resistant penicillins (nafcillin or oxacillin 2 g IV q4h), parenteral second- or third-generation cephalosporins (ceftriaxone 1 to 2 g IV qd), or amoxicillin-clavulanate (875/125 mg PO q12h) should be used in diabetic patients and those with facial disease. Imipenem (500 mg IV q6h) is recommended in severe cases. Erythromycin, cephalosporins, or a macrolide should be used in patients with penicillin allergy. Essentially all patients with erysipelas should be admitted to the hospital for intravenous antibiotics.

CUTANEOUS ABSCESSES

The development of cutaneous abscesses most often is caused by a breakdown in the skin's normal protective barrier, followed by contamination with local resident bacterial flora. In most cases, involving otherwise immunocompetent patients, appropriate surgical incision and drainage are the only treatment required.

Epidemiology

Cutaneous abscesses are a common ED presentation, representing 1 to 2 percent of presenting complaints. There has been little recent investigation into the bacteriology or recommended treatment of simple cutaneous abscesses. This is probably secondary to the excellent outcome with simple incision and drainage procedures regardless of the location or etiology.

Pathophysiology

Intact, healthy skin usually acts as an excellent barrier to bacterial invasion. Cutaneous factors such as constant desquamation of the epidermis, continually shedding bacteria, and the lower pH of 3 to 5 of the skin also contribute to the skin's protective function. Host cellular and humoral defenses further protect invading bacteria from developing subsequent infection. When favorable host factors are lacking, or in cases of overwhelming bacterial contamination, a break in the skin's integrity either superficially (abrasion, laceration, or thermal injury) or from deep inoculation (laceration, puncture, or bite) may lead to colonization and subsequent infection. Infection typically starts as a local superficial cellulitis. Many organisms that colonize normal skin can cause necrosis and liquefaction with subsequent accumulation of leukocytes and cellular debris. Loculation and subsequent walling off of these products of infection lead to abscess formation. As the infection progresses and the area of liquefaction increases, the abscess wall thins and ruptures spontaneously, draining either cutaneously or into an adjoining tissue compartment.

The bacterial etiology of soft tissue abscesses often can be predicted by knowledge of the normal flora colonizing specific areas of the body. Environmental factors such as temperature, humidity, and the general hygiene of a patient play a role in the likelihood of infection, but only by increasing the number of bacteria colonizing the skin. In abscesses involving the scalp, trunk, and extremities, staphylococcal species are the most common infecting organism. *Staphylococcus aureus,* the least common of the staphylococcal species isolated on normal skin, is the most common species causing infection. *S. epidermidis* and *S. hominis* are also seen frequently. Streptococci commonly colonize the oral and nasal mucosa and can be seen in abscesses involving the adjoining soft tissues. The intertriginous and perineal areas often are colonized by the gram-negative aerobes *Escherichia coli, Proteus mirabilis,* and *Klebsiella* species. Abscesses involving the axillae are most often infected with *P. mirabilis* for reasons that are not clear. Abscesses in the perirectal and genital areas are most commonly mixed anaerobic and aerobic in nature, with *Bacteroides* species being the most common anaerobe.

In abscesses secondary to foreign bodies, *S. aureus* is the most commonly isolated species. Bite injuries, especially by cats, are at risk for infection with *Pasteurella multocida,* but also can involve *S. aureus,* as well as *Streptococcus viridans* and *Eikenella corrodens.* Human bites are less likely to involve *P. multocida,* but have a high incidence of involvement with the anaerobe *Bacteroides fragilis* and the gram-positive *Corynebacterium jeikeium,* as well as the usual staphylococcal and streptococcal organisms. In infections associated with intravenous drug abuse, mixed infections prevail, with anaerobic bacteria predominating. The most common anaerobic organisms are *Peptostreptococcus* species, with *Staphylococcus* and *Streptococcus* species being the predominating aerobic organisms. Interestingly, a significantly higher percentage of anaerobic infections have been noted in patients injecting cocaine. This has been attributed to the relative anaerobic environment created by the vasoconstrictive effect of the cocaine.

Clinical Features

Patients present with an area of swelling, tenderness, and erythema. Inspection of the area may reveal fluctuance, induration, or active drainage. Lymphadenitis, localized lymphadenopathy, or fever may indicate systemic involvement of the infection, but in otherwise healthy patients, cutaneous abscesses tend to remain localized. A careful history should be obtained, with special attention given to underlying immunocompromising illnesses, steroid or other immunosuppressive drug use, and alcoholism. Close inspection of the area for evidence of predisposing injury or foreign body is important. Radiography may be indicated to evaluate for certain radiopaque foreign bodies, and ultrasound may be useful in identifying nonradiopaque objects. Ultrasound can accurately identify many small foreign objects or at least a small fluid collection representing surrounding abscess. The limiting factor in the use of ultrasound is that because of the superficial location of most of these objects, a very high-frequency ultrasound transducer is required (7.5 to 10 MHz). Specific abscesses that may be encountered in the ED are discussed below.

BARTHOLIN GLAND ABSCESSES   Bartholin gland abscesses are discussed in Chap. 108.

PARONYCHIA AND FELONS   Paronychia and felons are discussed in Chap. 285.

HIDRADENITIS SUPPURATIVA   Hidradenitis suppurativa is a recurrent, chronic infection that is a disorder of the terminal follicular epithelium within apocrine gland-bearing skin.[15] The blockage of the apocrine glands is secondary to an adjacent folliculitis. The folliculitis, and secondary blockage of the surrounding apocrine glands by keratinous material, leads to inflammation, local cellulitis, and subsequent abscess formation. Multiple areas of infection develop and coalesce to form chronic draining fistulous tracts. These tracts tend to occur in the axilla, groin, and perianal regions, where the apocrine sweat glands predominate. Hidradenitis suppurativa is more common in women and blacks, and there appears to be a genetic factor involved in its development. Obesity, shaving, and mechanical irritation have been considered risk factors, but study data have never supported this. The onset of symptoms almost universally occurs after the onset of puberty, and a relationship between androgens and hidradenitis suppurativa has been closely considered. Androgen administration has been shown to worsen symptoms; however, antiandrogen therapy has shown mixed results at best.

The causative organism is usually *Staphylococcus,* but *Streptococcus* also can be involved. In the groin, gram-negative organisms and anaerobes also may be seen. Patients often will present with multiple lesions in different stages of development and healing, but with an acute exacerbation in one or a few areas. ED treatment is directed primarily at incision and drainage of the acute infection with referral to a surgeon for further definitive treatment. Oral antibiotics should be considered in patients with significant areas of cellulitis or systemic symptoms.

Patients with longstanding disease are at risk of developing an aggressive form of squamous cell carcinoma that is associated with local invasion, recurrence after excision, distant metastasis, and high mortality.

INFECTED SEBACEOUS CYSTS   Sebaceous glands occur diffusely throughout the body. Blockage of the duct of a sebaceous gland may lead to development of a glandular cyst that may exist for a long period of time without becoming infected. Once bacterial invasion occurs, abscess formation is common. Patients typically present with an erythematous, tender cutaneous nodule that is commonly fluctuant. Simple incision and drainage are the appropriate ED treatment. The cyst always contains a capsule that must be removed to prevent further infection. This is usually best done at a later follow-up visit when the initial inflammation has improved or resolved. Occasionally the wall of the sac can be grasped with a forceps and removed at the time of drainage.

PERIRECTAL ABSCESSES   These are discussed in Chap. 82.

PILONIDAL ABSCESSES Pilonidal abscesses are located along the superior gluteal fold. It is thought that a pilonidal sinus forms along the gluteal fold possibly at the time of embryogenesis, although others believe it to be secondary to local soft tissue trauma. These sinuses are lined with squamous epithelium and hair. It is blockage of the sinus tract with hair and other keratinous material that leads to bacterial invasion and infection. The causative organisms typically are normal skin flora, with *Staphylococcus* species being the most common. Contamination with peritoneal and fecal organisms is also possible. Patients tend to develop symptoms in their late teens and early twenties, and without definitive surgical treatment, they tend to have recurrent infections, sometimes developing a chronic draining fistulous tract. Patients typically present to the ED with a tender, swollen, and fluctuant nodule located along the superior gluteal fold. Systemic symptoms are rare. The appropriate initial treatment includes incision and drainage using care to remove all excess hair and debris from the abscess cavity. The cavity should be packed with iodoform gauze, and the patient should return in 2 to 3 days for advancement of the packing. Antibiotics generally are not needed. Surgical referral is recommended for more definitive treatment. This now typically consists of wide surgical excision, and healing by secondary intention.

STAPHYLOCOCCAL SOFT TISSUE ABSCESSES *Staphylococcus* species are ubiquitous throughout the skin and have a particular affinity for hair follicles, where infection is common. Inflammation of a hair follicle caused by bacterial invasion is known as *folliculitis* and is best treated noninvasively with warm soaks. A deeper invasion into the soft tissue surrounding a hair follicle can lead to a localized abscess formation called a *furuncle* (boil). These are most commonly found on the face, neck, back, axilla, inner thighs, and other areas exposed to friction. Unless severe, warm compresses usually are adequate to promote spontaneous drainage. In the thick skin on the back, neck, lateral thighs, and buttocks, several furuncles may coalesce to form a large area of infection containing many interconnected sinus tracts and abscesses. This is known as a *carbuncle* and often requires wide surgical excision for complete resolution. Carbuncles are seen much more commonly in diabetics and may demonstrate signs of systemic involvement.

Diagnosis Most simple cutaneous abscesses in otherwise healthy patients are local infections without need for further evaluation. Clinical presentation of a tender, swollen, often erythematous nodule strongly suggests infection. A palpable area of fluctuance is typically enough for the diagnosis of abscess. Notice should be made of the admitting vital signs, with particular attention to temperature and heart rate. Fever or tachycardia suggests systemic involvement of the infection and may indicate the need for further laboratory testing. In patients with diabetes, alcoholism, and other immunocompromising conditions, the threshold for further diagnostic studies should be lower. A complete blood count and in certain situations (such as possible osteomyelitis) an erythrocyte sedimentation rate usually are all that are needed to evaluate for possible systemic involvement. Diabetic patients routinely should have their blood glucose checked.

In simple abscesses involving otherwise healthy patients, a routine culture and sensitivity is not needed. If it is felt that antibiotic treatment is indicated, the causative organisms usually can be predicted by the general location of the abscess. If further certainty is required, a Gram stain of the abscess aspirate most often will lend the required information, and results can be obtained while the patient is still in the ED. Gram-positive cocci in clusters suggest infection with *S. aureus*, whereas many different organisms suggest a mixed anaerobic and aerobic infection. In patients in whom possible deep or chronic infection may complicate the course, early wound cultures with sensitivities may prove useful. Immunocompromised patients demonstrating systemic signs of infection also should have blood cultures drawn. In patients in whom foreign body involvement is a potential issue, plain radiographs or possibly ultrasound should be used to assist in identification.

Treatment Incision and drainage is the only treatment necessary in most cases of superficial and localized abscesses. Often it is difficult to determine clinically if an area of fluctuance is present within an area of induration and swelling. Needle aspiration of the most likely area of induration often can help in the diagnosis. When pus is encountered with aspiration, incision and drainage should be performed. When no pus is located, a trial of antibiotic therapy and warm compresses is appropriate initially. Patients should have a follow-up evaluation in 48 to 72 h to identify the need for incision and drainage.

Consideration must be given to the best location for abscess drainage. Abscesses well suited to ED treatment are those that are superficial, well localized, and not in close proximity to nerves or vascular structures. Fluctuant masses should be examined for pulsations or bruits if near vascular structures. Patient comfort is also an important consideration. Infiltration of a local anesthetic most often gives poor pain relief. The lower pH of infected tissue typically greatly reduces the effectiveness of a local anesthetic. Injecting additional fluid into an already swollen and tender area also increases pain. Regional or field blocks can be effective. Some may require systemic sedation and analgesia, and those in whom adequate analgesia cannot be obtained in the ED should be taken to the operating room for appropriate surgical drainage.

Before the procedure, consent should be obtained and complications explained. Complications are few with superficial abscesses, but include residual local numbness, the risk of injury to deeper nerves and blood vessels, and poor or delayed wound healing, especially in those with diabetes or peripheral vascular disease. Some estimate should be made of the residual scarring that may be anticipated, especially in areas of cosmetic significance.

The patient should be positioned to ensure appropriate access to the abscess and in the most comfortable position possible. The area should be prepared with povidone-iodine solution and draped in a sterile fashion. After appropriate anesthesia, the abscess should be opened widely over the area of greatest fluctuance, using a no. 11 or 15 scalpel blade to ensure adequate drainage. As much pus as possible should be expressed by gentle compression. Hemostats are then used to break up any loculated areas within the abscess cavity. The cavity is irrigated with saline and packed loosely with gauze tape to hold it open to promote drainage while the infection resolves. The packing should be left in place long enough for the cavity to heal from the inside out, preventing recollection of the abscess. Patients are discharged with instructions for warm compresses or soaks three to four times a day. A follow-up visit should be scheduled in 2 to 3 days for recheck and advancement or replacement of the packing. Wounds that continue to actively drain at the time of follow-up should have the packing replaced. Replacing the packing performs some degree of debridement of the abscess cavity, as well as providing fresh packing for absorption of pus and debris. Wounds that are not actively draining can have the packing replaced and advanced as needed to allow for internal healing while keeping the incision open to promote drainage.

The use of antibiotics in patients with cutaneous abscesses is somewhat controversial. The risk of systemic infection following local incision and drainage appears to be low. An ED study demonstrated that in 50 afebrile patients in whom blood cultures were drawn 2 and 10 min after incision and drainage of cutaneous abscesses, none of the cultures was found to be positive.[16] There are no good data suggesting that antibiotic treatment following incision and drainage speeds infection resolution in otherwise healthy patients. Generally, it is felt that in patients without underlying immunocompromising conditions or signs of systemic infection, antibiotics are not indicated following incision and drainage of superficial cutaneous abscesses. With a lack of hard scientific data pointing to clear-cut guidelines for antibiotic therapy, clinical judgment needs to be exercised. In patients with diabetes, alcoholism, or other underlying immunocompromising illnesses, or in those on immunosuppressant medications such as steroids or chemotherapeutics, the threshold for antibiotic use should be much lower. Furthermore, patients who present with signs of systemic disease such as fever and chills and those with cellulitis extending beyond the abscess borders also should be considered for antibiotic therapy. Abscesses involving the hands or face should be treated more aggressively with antibiotics because of the higher morbidity associated with prolonged infection or complications. The specific antibiotic used should be chosen according to the most likely pathogen involved. This can be somewhat predicted by the location of the infection. Duration of therapy should be directed to some degree by the severity of infection but typically should continue for 5 to 7 days.

Of separate concern are patients with underlying structural heart disease at risk for bacterial endocarditis. Certain structural cardiac conditions lead to a higher incidence of bacterial endocarditis. Furthermore, the severity of disease and morbidity are increased in patients with certain underlying cardiac diseases who develop bacterial endocarditis. The American Heart Association publishes guidelines for patients it considers at increased risk for developing bacterial endocarditis.[17] Table 152-1 outlines the cardiac conditions considered to be at high and moderate risk based on predicted outcomes if endocarditis does occur. Note that several types of patients frequently encountered in the ED, namely patients after coronary artery bypass grafting, those with pacemakers, and those with mitral valve prolapse without valvular regurgitation, are not recommended for endocarditis prophylaxis. Despite the apparent low risk of transient bacteremia following incision and drainage of a simple cutaneous abscess, the American Heart Association recommends prophylactic antibiotics for those patients in the high- and moderate-risk categories prior to the procedure. No mention is made of postprocedure treatment. The antibiotic selected should be directed at the most likely organism causing the abscess. Suggested antibiotic treatment by organism for soft tissue infections is shown in Table 152-2,[11] and should be used for preprocedure prophylaxis for endocarditis. An intravenous or intramuscular antistaphylococcal penicillin, clindamycin, or first-generation cephalosporin is appropriate for patients not able to take oral medications. In patients with known methicillin-resistant *S. aureus* infection, vancomycin is recommended for prophylaxis.

SPOROTRICHOSIS

Sporotrichosis is a mycotic infection caused by the fungus *Sporothrix schenckii,* commonly found on plants and vegetation and in soil. Infection is caused by traumatic inoculation and usually remains within the local soft tissues and lymphatics. Disseminated forms, although more rare, do occur.

TABLE 152-1   Cardiac Conditions at Risk for Endocarditis

Endocarditis prophylaxis recommended:
  High-risk category:
    Prosthetic cardiac valves
    Previous bacterial endocarditis
    Complex cyanotic heart disease (e.g., single ventricle, transposition of the great vessels, tetralogy of Fallot)
    Surgically constructed systemic pulmonary stunts or conduits
  Moderate-risk category:
    Most other congenital cardiac malformations
    Acquired valvular dysfunction (e.g., rheumatic heart disease)
    Hypertrophic cardiomyopathy
    Mitral valve prolapse with valvular regurgitation and/or thickened leaflets
Endocarditis prophylaxis not recommended:
  Negligible-risk category (no greater risk than general population):
    Isolated secundum atrial septal defect
    Surgical repair of ASD, VSD, or PDA
    Previous coronary artery bypass grafting
    Mitral valve prolapse without valvular regurgitation
    Physiologic, functional, or innocent heart murmur
    Cardiac pacemakers

Abbreviations: ASD = atrial septal defect; VSD = ventricular septal defect; PDA = patent ductus arteriosus.

TABLE 152-2   Oral Antibiotic Recommendations for Common Skin Infections

Staphylococcus and Streptococcus Species

Common infections:
  Cellulitis; erysipelas (typically *Streptococcus*); sebaceous cyst abscesses; abscesses secondary to foreign bodies; hidradenitis suppurativa; pilonidal abscesses; folliculitis, boils, and carbuncles (typically *Staphylococcus*)
Antibiotic recommendations:
  Cloxacillin or dicloxacillin, 250–500 mg q6h
  Cephalexin 250–500 mg q6h (high resistance rate with *Staphylococcus*)
  Clindamycin 150–450 mg q6h
  Amoxicillin-clavulanate 875/125 mg q12h
  Erythromycin 250–500 mg q6h
  Clarithromycin 500 mg q12h
  Azithromycin 500 mg first day, then 250 mg qd × 4 d

Escherichia, Proteus, and *Klebsiella* Species

Common infections:
  Cutaneous abscesses involving the axilla, perineum, and groin; Bartholin gland abscesses; perirectal abscesses, hidradenitis suppurativa involving the groin; pilonidal abscesses
Antibiotic recommendations:
  Trimethoprim-sulfamethoxazole 160/800 mg q12h
  Amoxicillin-clavulanate 875/125 mg q12h
  Ciprofloxacin 500–750 mg q12h
  Ofloxacin 200–400 mg q12h
  Levofloxacin 250–500 mg qd

Bacteroides Species

Common infections:
  Cutaneous abscesses involving the groin and perineum; human bites; abscesses secondary to IV cocaine use; Bartholin's gland abscesses; hidradenitis suppurativa involving the groin and perineum, perirectal abscesses, pilonidal abscesses
Antibiotic recommendations:
  Clindamycin 150–450 mg q6h
  Metronidazole 500 mg q6h
  Amoxicillin-clavulanate 875/125 mg q12h

Pasturella multocida

Common infections:
  Animal bites, especially cats
Antibiotic recommendations:
  Penicillin V 250–500 mg q6h
  Doxycycline 100 mg q12h
  Amoxicillin-clavulanate 875/125 mg q12h
  Trimethoprim-sulfamethoxazole 160/800 mg q12h

Epidemiology

The organism responsible for sporotrichosis occurs worldwide and is found most commonly in soil, sphagnum moss, and decaying vegetable matter. Inoculation into the host most commonly occurs from a spine or barb on a plant puncturing the skin during handling. It is a common disease among florists, gardeners, and agricultural workers. Transmission from infected animals, especially cats, has been documented, and veterinarians and animal handlers are also at increased risk. The largest outbreak of sporotrichosis in the United States involved 15 states and 84 persons, all of whom handled conifer seedlings shipped in sphagnum moss contaminated with *S. schenckii.*[18]

Pathophysiology

S. schenckii is a thermally dimorphic fungus that changes from its mycelial form to its yeast form on entering a body-temperature environment. Local infection occurs in most cases, with disease limited to cutaneous or lymphocutaneous areas. Osteoarticular involvement including osteomyelitis, septic arthritis, bursitis, and tenosynovitis occurs and may be related to a local cutaneous infection or secondary to hematogenous spread. Systemic forms, including pulmonary and meningeal, are much more rare.

Clinical Features

The incubation period averages 3 weeks from the time of initial inoculation, but varies from a few days to several weeks. After the fungus enters the body through a break in the skin, three types of localized infections may occur. The *fixed cutaneous* type is characterized by lesions restricted to the site of inoculation and may appear as a crusted ulcer or verrucous plaque. *Local cutaneous* type infections also remain local but present as a subcutaneous nodule or pustule. The surrounding skin becomes erythematous and may ulcerate, resulting in a chancre. Local lymphadenitis is common. The *lymphocutaneous* type is the third and most common type. It is characterized by an initial painless nodule or papule at the site of inoculation that later develops subcutaneous nodules with clear skip areas along local lymphatic channels. The local reactions in all three types of infections tend to be relatively painless but show no signs of improvement without treatment.

Patients occasionally develop extracutaneous illness from what is most probably hematogenous spread. It is not clear what the exact pathogenesis of infection is since most cases do not involve the cutaneous form of the infection at the same time. Most cases of extracutaneous sporotrichosis involve the skeletal system. An indolent form of monarticular arthritis is the most common symptom. Osteomyelitis, tenosynovitis, and carpal tunnel syndrome are occasionally seen as well. Multiarticular arthritis is usually only seen in patients with underlying immunocompromising illness. Rarely patients will develop pulmonary involvement, which typically occurs in elderly alcoholic males, and clinically resembles tuberculosis. Chronic lymphocytic meningitis can be a delayed complication of sporotrichosis infection, and should be considered in patients with chronic meningeal symptoms.

Diagnosis

History and physical findings are the keys to diagnosis. Histopathologic stains are of little help because the organisms are scarce in tissues. Fungal cultures are the best way to isolate the fungus, and tissue biopsy cultures often are diagnostic. Routine laboratory tests are nonspecific, but an increased white blood cell count, eosinophil count, and erythrocyte sedimentation rate may be noted. The differential diagnosis includes tuberculosis, tularemia, cat-scratch disease, leishmaniasis, staphylococcal lymphangitis, and nocardiosis.

Treatment

Itraconazole (100 to 200 mg qd for 3 to 6 months) is the treatment of choice for localized and systemic infections.[19] Fluconazole is less effective than itraconazole and should be reserved for those few patients not tolerating itraconazole. Ketoconazole has shown even poorer results than fluconazole. Intravenous amphotericin B is effective, but adverse reactions usually limit its use to disseminated forms.

REFERENCES

1. Gas Gangrene. Medline Plus, http://www.nlm.nih.gov/medlineplus/ency/article/000620.htm.
2. Corey E: Nontraumatic gas gangrene: Case report and review of emergency therapeutics. *J Emerg Med* 9:431, 1991.
3. Stephens M: Gas gangrene: Potential for hyperbaric oxygen therapy. *Postgrad Med* 99:217, 1996.
4. Takahira N, Shindo M, Tanaka K, et al: Treatment outcome of nonclostridial gas gangrene at a level I trauma center. *J Orthop Trauma* 16:12, 2002.
5. Childers B, Potynondy L, Nachreiner R, et al: Necrotizing fasciitis: A fourteen-year retrospective study of 163 consecutive patients. *Am Surg* 68:109, 2002.
6. Elliott D, Kufera J, Myers R, et al: The microbiology of necrotizing soft tissue infections. *Am J Surg* 179:361, 2000.
7. Majeski J, Majeski E: Necrotizing fasciitis: Improved survival with early recognition by tissue biopsy and aggressive surgical treatment. *South Med J* 90:1065, 1997.
8. Stevens D: Streptococcal toxic shock syndrome: Spectrum of disease, pathogenesis, and new concepts in treatment. http://www.cdc.gov/ncidod/EID/vol/no3/downstev.htm. *EID* 1(3):69, 1995.
9. Sachs M: Cutaneous cellulitis. *Arch Dermatol* 127:493, 1991.
10. Dong S, Kelly K, Oland R, et al: ED management of cellulitis: A review of five urban centers. *Am J Emerg Med* 19:535, 2001.
11. Gilbert D, Moellering R, Sande M: *The Sanford Guide to Antimicrobial Therapy,* 33rd ed. Hyde Park, VT, Antimicrobial Therapy, Inc., 2003.
12. Grayson M, McDonald M, Gibson K, et al: Once-daily intravenous cefazolin plus oral probenacid is equivalent to once-daily intravenous ceftriaxone plus oral placebo for the treatment of moderate-to-severe cellulitis in adults. *Clin Infect Dis* 34:1440, 2002.
13. Dupuy A, Benchikhi H, Roujeau J, et al: Risk factors for erysipelas of the leg (cellulitis): Case-control study. *BJM* 318:1591, 1999.
14. Guberman D, Gilead L, Zlotogorski A, et al: Bullous erysipelas: A retrospective study of 26 patients. *Am Acad Dermatol* 41(5 Pt 1):733, 1999.
15. Brown T, Rosen T, Orengo I, et al: Hidradenitis suppurativa. *South Med J* 91:1107, 1998.
16. Bobrow B, Pollack C, Gamble S, et al: Incision and drainage of cutaneous abscesses is not associated with bacteremia in afebrile adults. *Ann Emerg Med* 29:404, 1997.
17. Danjani A, Taubet K, Wilson W, et al: Prevention of bacterial endocarditis: Recommendations by the American Heart Association. *JAMA* 277:1794, 1997.
18. Dixon D, Salkin I, Duncan R, et al: Isolation and characterization of *Sporothrix schenckii* from clinical and environmental sources associated with the largest U.S. epidemic of sporotrichosis. *J Clin Microbiol* 29:1106, 1991.
19. Stalkup J, Bell K, Rosen T: Disseminated cutaneous sporotrichosis treated with itraconazole. *Cutis* 69:371, 2002.

REPORTABLE INFECTIOUS DISEASES
Jane H. Brice

J. Brent Myers

The Centers for Disease Control and Prevention (CDC) in Atlanta publishes a list of notifiable infectious diseases that is updated and revised routinely. The most recent update as of this writing (2002) includes 54 nationally notifiable diseases and is summarized in Table 153-1.[1] The requirement to report these diseases is mandated by state or territory laws and regulations, and therefore, the list differs for each state or territory.

The reliability of the national reporting system rests on health care providers, laboratories, and other public health personnel, as is emphasized by the CDC: "The usefulness of public health surveillance data depends on its uniformity, simplicity, and timeliness."[2] Without consistent and timely notification, it becomes very difficult to monitor trends in disease patterns, to detect unusual occurrences or pockets of disease, and to assess the effectiveness of public health interventions to eradicate or contain disease. In effort to improve the consistency and timeliness of notification, the CDC has established a nationwide, computerized system that collects and analyzes data on a weekly basis.[3] Data reported by the 50 states, the District of Columbia, and the U.S. territories are summarized in the *Morbidity and Mortality Weekly Report,* which can be accessed online at www.cdc.gov/mmwr.

In an effort to ensure uniformity, the CDC maintains a revised case definition for all notifiable diseases. What follows is a summary of the

TABLE 153-1 Nationally Reportable Communicable Diseases

Acquired immunodeficiency syndrome (AIDS)	Malaria
	Measles
Anthrax	Meningococcal disease
Botulism	Mumps
Brucellosis	Pertussis
Chancroid	Plague
Chlamydia trachomatis genital infections	Poliomyelitis, paralytic
	Psittacosis
Cholera	Q fever
Coccidioidomycosis	Rabies, animal
Cryptosporidiosis	Rabies, human
Cyclosporaisis	Rocky Mountain spotted fever
Diphtheria	Rubella
Ehrlichiosis	Rubella, congenital syndrome
Encephalitis or meningitis, arboviral	Salmonellosis
Escherichia coli O157:H7	Shigellosis
Giardiasis	Streptococcal disease, invasive, group A
Gonorrhea	
Haemophilus influenzae invasive disease	*Streptococcus pneumoniae,* drug-resistant invasive disease
Hansen's disease (leprosy)	Streptococcal toxic shock syndrome
Hantavirus pulmonary syndrome	Syphilis
Hemolytic-uremic syndrome, post-diarrheal	Syphilis, congenital
	Tetanus
Hepatitis A	Toxic shock syndrome
Hepatitis B	Trichinosis
Hepatitis C/non-A, non-B	Tuberculosis
HIV infection, pediatric	Tularemia
Legionellosis	Typhoid fever
Listeriosis	Varicella (deaths only)
Lyme disease	Yellow fever

case definitions for each of the specified nationally notifiable diseases. Unless otherwise noted, these case definitions were obtained from the 1997 *Morbidity and Mortality Weekly Report (MMWR)* update on reportable diseases.[2] These case definitions establish uniform notification criteria and are subject to revision. For the most up-to-date information, go to http://www.cdc.gov/epo/dphsi/casedef/index.htm.

ACQUIRED IMMUNODEFICIENCY SYNDROME (AIDS)

AIDS is a chronic illness with varying manifestations; for patients 13 years of age or older, reporting is required if the patient demonstrates (1) a CD4$^+$ T-cell count of less than 200/μL, (2) a CD4$^+$ T-cell percentage of total lymphocyte of less than 14 percent, or (3) any of the following: pulmonary tuberculosis, recurrent pneumonia, invasive cervical cancer, or 23 other clinical conditions discussed elsewhere in this text (Chap. 144) and via the *Morbidity and Mortality Weekly Reports.*[4–6] For patients less than 13 years of age, a revised system has been developed to include a child's infection status, immunologic status, and clinical status. Infection status is discussed in the HIV section (below). The immunologic status is based on age-appropriate CD4$^+$ T-cell counts. The clinical status includes the asymptomatic, the moderately symptomatic, and the severely symptomatic, with this latter category including the majority of the traditional AIDS-defining illnesses.[5]

ANTHRAX

Anthrax is an acute illness with one of several distinct clinical presentations. The cutaneous form is characterized by a skin lesion evolving over 2 to 6 days from a papule to a vesicle to a depressed black eschar. The inhalation form presents with a brief upper respiratory infection followed by hypoxia and dyspnea. On chest radiography, there will be evidence of mediastinal widening from adenopathy. The intestinal

form is distinguished by severe abdominal pain and cramping followed by fever and sepsis. Finally, in the oropharyngeal form, a mucosal lesion in the oral cavity develops along with cervical adenopathy, edema, and fever.

The laboratory diagnosis is made by (1) isolation of *Bacillus anthracis* from a clinical specimen, (2) anthrax electrophoretic immunotransblot (EITB) reaction to the protective antigen and/or lethal factor bands in at least one serum specimen obtained after onset of symptoms, or (3) demonstration of *B. anthracis* through immunofluorescence.

BOTULISM

Foodborne An acute illness of varying severity, foodborne botulism is manifested by diplopia, blurred vision, bulbar weakness, or symmetric paralysis that may be of rapid onset. Laboratory confirmation of this illness consists of demonstration of botulinum toxin in serum or stool or in food the subject recently consumed. A positive *Clostridium botulinum* culture from stool also serves as confirmation of the diagnosis.

Infant A constellation of symptoms in an infant under 1 year of age including constipation, poor feeding, and failure to thrive followed by progressive weakness, impaired respiration, and death should suggest infant botulism. Laboratory confirmation of the diagnosis is made in the same manner as described for foodborne botulism.

Wound The symptoms for wound botulism mirror those found in the foodborne form. The laboratory diagnosis is made by finding botulinum toxin in serum or obtaining a positive culture from the wound.

BRUCELLOSIS

Infection with *Brucella* may be either of acute or insidious onset. Brucellosis is characterized by fever, night sweats, undue fatigue, anorexia, weight loss, headache, and arthralgias. The laboratory diagnosis may be made in several ways: (1) culture positive from a clinical specimen, (2) at least a fourfold increase in *Brucella* agglutination titers between the acute and convalescent phases in serum taken at least 2 weeks apart and studied in the same laboratory, or (3) positive immunofluorescence of *Brucella* in a clinical specimen.

CHANCROID

Chancroid is a sexually transmitted disease caused by the organism *Haemophilus ducreyi*. It is manifested by a painful genital ulcer with inflamed inguinal lymph nodes. Isolation of the organism from a clinical specimen confirms the diagnosis.

CHLAMYDIA TRACHOMATIS GENITAL INFECTIONS

Genital infection with *Chlamydia trachomatis* is sexually transmitted and may present in several different manners. There may be evidence of urethritis, epididymitis, cervicitis, or acute salpingitis, or the infection may be completely asymptomatic. It is therefore essential to test for *Chlamydia* whenever there is a suspicion of infection or when there is evidence of other sexually transmitted infection. *Chlamydia* also may cause conjunctivitis or pneumonia in newborns through perinatal transmission. Finally, *Chlamydia* causes lymphogranuloma venerum, which is discussed below. The diagnosis of *Chlamydia* is confirmed through either a positive culture or detection of the antigen or nucleic acid on immunofluorescence.

CHOLERA

Cholera infection is manifested by a diarrheal illness of varying severity. The presence of vomiting does not exclude the diagnosis. Isolation of the toxigenic *Vibrio cholerae* O1 or O139 from stool or emesis confirms the diagnosis. Serologic evidence of recent infection also may confirm a recent illness caused by cholera. The CDC requests notification for cholera only if the one of the two *Vibrio* serotypes listed above is isolated; there is no need to notify the CDC for other serotypes.

COCCIDIOIDMYCOSIS

Infection with the fungus *Coccidioides immitis* may manifest in an acute or chronic illness and may, in some persons, be maintained in an asymptomatic state. This fungus is endemic in the southwestern United States. Those demonstrating symptoms usually complain of an influenza-like febrile respiratory illness. The disease may disseminate in approximately 0.5 percent of patients.

Coccidioidomycosis should be considered in those with one or more of the following: (1) influenza-like signs and symptoms (i.e., fever, cough, chest pain, myalgia, arthralgia, and headache), (2) pneumonia or other pulmonary lesion on chest radiograph, (3) erythema nodosum or erythema multiforme rash, (4) involvement of bones, joints, or skin by dissemination, (5) meningitis, and/or (6) involvement of viscera or lymph nodes.

Laboratory confirmation is made through (1) culture, histopathology, or molecular evidence of *C. immitis,* (2) serologic tests including detection of IgM by immunodiffusion, enzyme immunoassay, latex agglutination, or tube precipitation or detection of rising titer of IgG by immunodiffusion, enzyme immunoassay, or complement fixation, or (3) coccidioidal skin-test conversion after onset of symptoms.

CRYPTOSPORIDIOSIS

Diarrhea, abdominal cramps, loss of appetite, low-grade fever, and nausea and vomiting are the cluster of signs and symptoms associated with cryptosporidiosis. The infection may be asymptomatic in some persons. The illness also can be prolonged and life-threatening in immunocompromised patients. It is caused by the protozoa *Cryptosporidium parvum.*

In the laboratory, the diagnosis is confirmed by detection of oocysts in stool, demonstration of *Cryptosporidium* in intestinal fluid or small bowel biopsy specimens, detection of *Cryptosporidium* antigen in stool by specific immunodiagnostic testing, use of polymerase chain reaction (PCR) techniques where routinely available, or demonstration of reproductive stages in tissue preparations.[1]

CYCLOSPORAISIS

Cyclosporaisis is an intestinal illness caused by the protozoa *Cyclospora cayetanensis.* Symptoms include watery diarrhea, weight loss, increased flatus, nausea, fatigue, and perhaps vomiting. Other symptoms may include anorexia, abdominal bloating/cramping, and low-grade fever. Asymptomatic and relapsing infections can occur. Laboratory confirmation is accomplished by one of four methods: (1) detection of oocysts in stool by microscopic examination, (2) detection of *Cyclospora* in intestinal fluid or bowel biopsy specimens, (3) demonstration of sporulation, or (4) detection of DNA by PCR in stool, duodenal/jejunal aspirates, or small bowel biopsy specimens.[1]

DIPHTHERIA

Diphtheria is characterized by upper respiratory symptoms, including sore throat, low-grade fever, and an adherent membrane to tonsils, pharynx, and/or the nose. There is a cutaneous form of diphtheria that does not need to be reported to the CDC. Isolation of *Corynebacterium diphtheriae* from clinical specimens or a histopathologic diagnosis of diphtheria confirms the illness.

EHRLICHIOSIS

Ehrlichiosis is a tick-borne illness characterized by acute onset of a flulike illness with fever, headache, myalgias, and malaise. In addition, some cases may demonstrate nausea, vomiting, or rash. Laboratory abnormalities may include thrombocytopenia, leukopenia, and/or elevated liver enzymes. Intracytoplasmic bacterial aggregates (morulae) may be visible in the leukocytes of some patients. Three categories of ehrlichiosis should be reported and are described below.

HME   A variant of the disease caused by *Ehrlichia chaffeensis.* Laboratory confirmation is achieved by demonstration of a fourfold increase in antibody titer to *E. chaffeensis* by immunofluorescence assay (IFA) in paired serum samples, positive PCR with demonstration of *E. chaffeensis* DNA, identification of morulae in leukocytes with a positive IFA titer to *E. chaffeensis* antigen, immunostaining of *E. chaffeensis* antigen in biopsy or autopsy specimen, or culture of *E. chaffeensis* from a clinical specimen.

HGE   A variant of the disease caused by *E. phagocytophila.* The laboratory mechanisms described for *E. chaffeensis* detection and confirmation are the same procedures used for *E. phagocytophila.*

Ehrlichiosis, Human, Other, or Unspecified Agent   This variant of the disease is confirmed in the laboratory by either a fourfold change in antibody titer to more than one *Ehrlichia* species by IFA in paired samples in which a dominant reactivity cannot be established or by the identification of an *Ehrlichia* species other than *E. chaffeensis* or *E. phagocytophila* by PCR, immunostaining, or culture.[1]

ENCEPHALITIS OR MENINGITIS, ARBOVIRAL

Arboviral central nervous system (CNS) infections range in severity from febrile headache to encephalitis; these illnesses are often indistinguishable from other viral CNS infections. Arboviral meningitis is characterized by fever, headache, stiff neck, and pleocytosis. Arboviral encephalitis is characterized by a febrile illness associated with any of the following neurologic signs and symptoms: headache, confusion, altered sensorium, nausea and vomiting, meningismus, cranial nerve palsy, paresis or paralysis, sensory deficit, altered reflexes, seizures, abnormal movements, or coma. The diagnosis is made based on laboratory detection of (1) a fourfold or greater rise in serum antibody titer, (2) isolation of virus or finding of viral antigen or genomic sequences in tissue, blood, cerebral spinal fluid (CSF), or other bodily fluids, (3) IgM antibody detected on enzyme immunoassay from serum or CSF, or (4) virus specific IgM antibodies demonstrated in serum by antibody-capture EIA and confirmed by demonstration of virus-specific IgG antibodies in the same or later specimen by another serologic assay. Eastern equine encephalitis/meningitis, western equine encephalitis/meningitis, California serogroup encephalitis/meningitis, St. Louis encephalitis/meningitis, Powassan encephalitis/meningitis, and West Nile meningitis/encephalitis are reportable to the CDC.[1]

ENTEROHEMORRHAGIC *ESCHERICHIA COLI* (EHEC)

A diarrheal disease of variable severity, *E. coli* infections have gained national prominence through several foodborne outbreaks. A recently revised CDC case definition includes not only the well-recognized *E. coli* O157:H7 but also other subtypes of *E. coli* capable of producing enterohemorrhagic illness. The diarrhea of this disease is often bloody and associated with abdominal cramping. It may be complicated by hemolytic-uremic syndrome (HUS) or thrombotic thrombocytopenic purpura (TTP). It also may be asymptomatic.

In the laboratory, isolation of *E. coli* O157:H7 or a Shiga toxin producing *E. coli* is confirmatory. A probable case is defined as one in which (1) there is isolation of *E. coli* O157 from a clinical specimen pending H7 or Shiga toxin production, (2) there is an epidemiologic link with a confirmed or probable case, (3) there is identification of a Shiga toxin from a clinically compatible case, or (4) there is definitive evidence of an elevated antibody titer to a known EHEC serotype from a clinically compatible case. The CDC should be notified concerning both confirmed and probable cases.[1]

GIARDIASIS

Caused by the protozoan *Giardia lamblia,* this intestinal illness is characterized by diarrhea, abdominal cramps, weight loss, malabsorption, and bloating. Some individuals may remain as asymptomatic carriers. Diagnosis is confirmed by demonstration of *G. lamblia* cysts in stool; *G. lamblia* trophozoites in stool, duodenal fluid, or small bowel biopsy; or *G. lamblia* antigen in stool by specific immunodiagnostic test.[1]

GONORRHEA

This sexually transmitted disease is characterized by varying manifestations, including urethritis, cervicitis, or salpingitis. It may be asymptomatic in some persons or may become disseminated. Laboratory detection of *Neisseria gonorrhoeae* in clinical specimens confirms the diagnosis. Other methods of laboratory confirmation include detection of antigen or nucleic acid in specimens or observation of gram-negative intracellular diplococci in a urethral smear obtained from a male patient.

HAEMOPHILUS INFLUENZAE INVASIVE DISEASE

Invasive diseases caused by *H. influenzae* include meningitis, bacteremia, epiglottitis, or pneumonia. Laboratory isolation of *H. influenzae* from a normally sterile site such as blood, CSF, or joint fluid is necessary to confirm the diagnosis.

HANSEN DISEASE (LEPROSY)

Hansen disease is a chronic infection with *Mycobacterium leprae* involving the skin predominantly but which can include peripheral nerves and the mucosa of the upper airway as well. There are four clinical forms of Hansen disease. Tuberculoid leprosy is characterized by one or a few well-demarcated, hypopigmented, and anesthetic skin lesions. Often these lesions have active, spreading edges and a clearing center. Peripheral nerve swelling or thickening also may be present. In the lepromatous form, a number of erythematous papules and nodules may be present or an infiltration of face, hands, and feet with lesions in a bilateral and symmetric pattern that progresses to thickening of the skin. The borderline or dimorphous form presents with skin lesions characteristic of both the tuberculoid and lepromatous forms. Finally, in the indeterminate form, early lesions, usually hypopigmented macules, are present that do not develop the more characteristic features of the tuberculoid or lepromatous forms.

Demonstration of acid-fast bacilli in skin or dermal nerves makes the diagnosis. Specimens should be obtained from a full-thickness skin biopsy of a lepromatous lesion, if possible.

HANTAVIRUS PULMONARY SYNDROME

Hantavirus pulmonary syndrome is a febrile illness characterized by bilateral interstitial pulmonary infiltrates and respiratory compromise resembling adult respiratory distress syndrome. There is typically a prodrome of fever, chills, myalgias, headache, and gastrointestinal distress. Common laboratory findings include one or more of the following: hemoconcentration, left shift in white blood cell count, neutrophilic leukocytosis, thrombocytopenia, or circulating immunoblasts.

Hantavirus should be considered in the setting of one or more of the following: (1) febrile illness [temperature greater than 38.3°C (101°F)] in a previously healthy individual with bilateral interstitial edema that may resemble adult respiratory distress syndrome radiographically and respiratory compromise requiring oxygen support developing within 72 h of hospitalization or (2) unexplained respiratory illness resulting in death and autopsy examination demonstrating noncardiogenic pulmonary edema without identifiable cause.

Detection of hantavirus-specific IgM or rising titers of IgG, detection of hantavirus-specific ribonucleic acid sequences by PCR techniques in clinical specimens, and detection of hantavirus antigen by immunohistochemistry are all acceptable laboratory methods for confirming the diagnosis.

HEMOLYTIC-UREMIC SYNDROME, POSTDIARRHEAL

HUS presents as acute onset of microangiopathic hemolytic anemia, renal injury, and low platelet count. Most cases occur within 3 weeks of an acute diarrheal illness. A low platelet count is typical early in the illness (within the first 7 days) but may have normalized by the time the patient seeks care. If the platelet count is not less than 150,000/μL within 7 days of the onset of the gastrointestinal illness, consider another diagnosis. TTP has similar features and is distinguished from HUS by the presence of fever and CNS involvement. Additionally, it may have a more gradual onset. Few cases of TTP are associated with a diarrheal illness.

In the laboratory, both of the following findings will be present: (1) anemia of acute onset with microangiopathic changes (schistocytes, burr cells, or helmet cells on smear) and (2) acute renal failure with hematuria, proteinuria, or increased creatinine levels (50 percent over the patient's baseline values, or greater than 1.0 mg/dL for a child under 13 years of age, or greater than 1.5 mg/dL for persons over 13 years of age with previously normal renal function).

HEPATITIS

Hepatitis is characterized by acute and discrete onset of symptoms and jaundice or elevated serum aminotransferase levels. At present, hepatitis A, B, C, and non-A and non-B are reportable. The laboratory diagnosis of each of the hepatitis viruses is listed below.

Hepatitis A. Detection of IgM to the hepatitis A virus (anti-HAV).
Hepatitis B. (1) Detection of IgM to hepatitis B core antigen (anti-HBc) or hepatitis B surface antigen (HBsAg) and (2) anti-HAV negative, if done.
Hepatitis C. (1) Detection of antibody against hepatitis C antigen (anti-HCV) with verification by an additional, more specific assay, (2) serum aminotransferase levels greater than 7 times the upper limit of normal, (3) anti-HAV negative, (4) anti-HBc negative (if done), and (5) HBsAg negative.
Non-A, non-B hepatitis. (1) Serum aminotransferase levels greater than 2.5 times the upper limit of normal, (2) anti-HAV negative, and (3) anti-HBc (if done) and/or HBsAg negative.
Delta hepatitis. (1) HBsAg or anti-HBc positive and (2) detection of antibodies to hepatitis delta virus (not a reportable disease).

Persons with chronic hepatitis, those who are hepatitis B surface antigen positive, or those who are anti-hepatitis C virus positive should not be reported unless they have acute illness compatible with viral hepatitis at the time of the laboratory finding.[1]

PERINATAL HEPATITIS B

In infants aged 1 to 24 months, infection with hepatitis B may range from an asymptomatic state to fulminant hepatitis. On laboratory investigation, the infant will be HBsAg positive.

HIV INFECTION

Adults, Adolescents, and Children 18 Months of Age and Older
HIV cases are reportable if they meet the following criteria: (1) Positive result on a screening test for HIV antibody (e.g., repeatedly positive enzyme immunoassay) followed by a positive result on a confirmatory test for HIV antibody (e.g., Western blot), (2) positive report on any one of the virologic tests: HIV nucleic acid detection (e.g., PCR), HIV p24 antigen test (including neutralization), or HIV isolation in viral culture), or (3) clinical criteria meeting the definition of AIDS (see AIDS section above). If the actual laboratory results are not available, a signed note from the patient's physician documenting the laboratory results used to fulfill the preceding criteria is acceptable.

Children Less than 18 Months of Age A definitive diagnosis is confirmed if two of the virologic tests mentioned above are positive. The diagnosis is reported as presumptive if only one of the virologic tests is positive. These virologic tests must be obtained at two different times; cord blood may not be used for testing. As with adults, adequate physician documentation of laboratory results is acceptable if the actual laboratory results are not available.[7]

LEGIONELLOSIS

Infection with *Legionella* causes two distinct illnesses: (1) legionnaires' disease, manifested by fever, myalgia, cough, and pneumonia, and (2) Pontiac fever, which is a milder illness without pneumonia. Laboratory confirmation of *Legionella* infection can be made by any of the following methods: (1) isolation of *Legionella* from respiratory secretions, lung tissue, pleural fluid, or other normally sterile site, (2) demonstration of fourfold or greater rise in reciprocal immunofluorescence antibody titer to greater than or equal to 128 against *L. pneumophila* serogroup 1 between paired acute and convalescent serum specimens, (3) detection of *L. pneumophila* serogroup 1 in respiratory secretions, lung tissue, or pleural fluid by direct fluorescent antibody testing, or (4) detection of *L. pneumophila* serogroup 1 antigen in urine by radioimmunoassay or enzyme-linked immunosorbent assay.

LISTERIOSIS

Invasive disease associated with *Listeria monocytogenes* is characterized by meningitis and/or bacteremia. In pregnant females, infection may result in miscarriage or stillbirth. Confirmation is achieved by isolation of *L. monocytogenes* from a normally sterile site or, in the setting of childbirth, from fetal or placental tissue.[1]

LYME DISEASE

This tick-borne illness presents with systemic manifestations, including those of the dermatologic, rheumatologic, neurologic, and cardiac systems. The best clinical marker is erythema migrans, the initial skin lesion that occurs in 60 to 80 percent of patients. Other acute symptoms include fatigue, fever, headache, mildly stiff neck, arthralgias, and myalgias. Late manifestations are variable and are best discussed by system:

Musculoskeletal. Recurrent brief and intermittent episodes (over weeks or months) of objective joint swelling in one or several joints, sometimes followed by chronic arthritis.
Central nervous system. Any of the following (alone or in combination): lymphocytic meningitis, cranial neuritis (particularly facial palsy that occasionally is bilateral), radiculopathy, or rarely, encephalomyelitis.
Cardiovascular. Acute onset of high-grade (second- or third-degree) atrioventricular (AV) block that resolves in days to weeks and sometimes is associated with myocarditis (note that palpitations, bradycardia, bundle-branch block, or myocarditis alone is not enough).

Isolation of the organism *Borrelia burgdorferi* from a clinical specimen or demonstration of antibody (IgM or IgG) against *B. burgdorferi* in serum or CSF confirms the diagnosis. A two-test approach (enzyme-linked immunosorbent assay followed by Western blot) is recommended.

MALARIA

Malaria is caused by infection with one of the *Plasmodium* species. Most patients have fever. Other complaints include headache, chills, sweats, myalgias, nausea, vomiting, diarrhea, or cough. Untreated infection by *P. falciparum* can lead to coma, renal failure, pulmonary edema, and death. In the laboratory, malaria parasites can be seen on blood smear.

MEASLES (RUBEOLA)

Measles is an illness characterized by all the following (1) generalized rash lasting more than 3 days, (2) temperature greater than or equal to 38.3°C (101°F), and (3) cough, coryza, or conjunctivitis. The laboratory diagnosis can be made by any of the following: (1) positive serologic tests for measles IgM, (2) significant rise in measles antibody levels by any standard serologic assay, or (3) isolation of measles virus from clinical specimens.

MENINGOCOCCAL DISEASE

Meningococcal disease is most commonly evident as meningitis and/or meningococcemia. It may progress rapidly to purpura fulminans, shock, and death. Isolation of *Neisseria meningitidis* from a normally sterile site such as blood or CSF confirms the diagnosis.

MUMPS

An illness with acute onset, mumps is characterized by unilateral or bilateral tender, self-limited swelling of parotid or other salivary gland for 2 or more days without other cause. The laboratory diagnosis is evident by (1) isolating mumps virus from a clinical specimen, (2) a significant rise between acute and convalescent titers in serum mumps IgG, or (3) finding mumps IgM in serum.

PERTUSSIS

Pertussis is an illness with cough lasting for 2 weeks or longer without other cause and with one of the following: (1) paroxysms of cough, (2) inspiratory whoop, or (3) posttussive vomiting. The laboratory confirmation is found in isolation of *Bordetella pertussis* from clinical specimens or a positive PCR for *B. pertussis*.

PLAGUE

An illness characterized by fever, chills, headache, malaise, prostration, and leukocytosis, plague manifests predominantly in one of the following clinical forms: (1) bubonic plague, manifested by regional lymphadenitis, (2) septicemic plague, in which there is septicemia without evident bubo, (3) pneumonic plague, where pneumonia results from either inhalation of infectious droplets (primary pneumonic plague) or hematologic spread from bubonic or septicemic cases (secondary pneumonic plague), or (4) pharyngeal plague, in which there is pharyngitis and cervical lymphadenitis resulting from exposure to larger infectious droplets or ingestion of infected tissues.
Presumptive laboratory diagnosis is made by (1) an increase in serum antibody titers to *Yersinia pestis* fraction 1 antigen without plague vaccination or (2) detection of fraction 1 antigen by fluorescent assay. Confirmatory laboratory diagnosis is produced by (1) isolation of *Y. pestis* in clinical specimens or (2) a fourfold or greater rise in serum antibody titer to *Y. pestis* fraction 1 antigen.

POLIOMYELITIS, PARALYTIC

Paralytic poliomyelitis is an illness of acute onset characterized by flaccid paralysis of one or more limbs. Deep tendon reflexes are absent or diminished. There are no accompanying sensory or cognitive losses; there should be no other apparent cause for the findings. Laboratory testing only serves to classify the case into categories set up by the CDC. The clinical case definition is sufficient for reporting.

PSITTACOSIS

Psittacosis is a disease found among bird handlers that presents with fever, chills, headache, photophobia, cough, and myalgia. In the laboratory, any of the following methods will confirm the diagnosis: (1) isolation of *Chlamydia psittaci* from respiratory secretions, (2) a fourfold or greater increase in antibodies against *C. psittaci* by complement fixation or microimmunofluorescence (MIF) to a reciprocal titer of at least 32 between paired acute and convalescent serum samples, or (3) detection of serum IgM to *C. psittaci* by MIF to a reciprocal titer of at least 16.

Q FEVER

The acute infection with *Coxiella burnetti* is characterized by fever, myalgias, malaise, and retrobulbar headache. More severe cases may result in hepatitis, pneumonia, and meningoencephalitis. Chronic infections may result in potentially fatal endocarditis (especially in those with preexisting vavular disease) and the chronic fatigue syndrome. In addition, asymptomatic infections have been reported. Diagnosis is confirmed by (1) at least a fourfold change in antibody titer to *C. burnetti* phase II or phase I antibody titer in paired serum specimens, ideally taken 3 to 6 weeks apart, (2) isolation of *C. burnetti* from a specimen by culture, or (3) demonstration of *C. burnetti* in a clinical specimen by antigen or nucleic acid testing.[1]

RABIES, ANIMAL

The laboratory diagnosis of animal rabies is the only necessary item for reporting. The diagnosis usually is made by a positive direct fluorescent antibody test (preferably performed on CNS tissue) or by isolation of rabies virus in cell culture or in a laboratory animal.

RABIES, HUMAN

In humans, rabies is an acute encephalomyelitis that almost always progresses to coma and death within 10 days of the first symptom. Laboratory confirmation of the illness can be made in any of the following manners (although the CDC strongly recommends confirming the diagnosis by *all* the suggested methods): (1) direct fluorescent antibody of viral antigen in clinical specimen (preferably the brain or the nerves surrounding hair follicles in the nape of the neck), (2) isolation in cell culture or in a laboratory animal of rabies virus from saliva, CSF, or CNS tissue, or (3) identification of a rabies neutralizing antibody titer of greater than 5 in the serum or CSF of an unvaccinated person.

ROCKY MOUNTAIN SPOTTED FEVER

This is a tick-borne illness of acute onset characterized by headache, myalgia, fever, and petechial rash that appears on the palms and soles in two-thirds of patients. Laboratory diagnosis may be made by one of several methods: (1) a fourfold or greater rise in antibody titer to *Rickettsia rickettsii* antigen by immunofluorescence antibody, complement fixation, latex agglutination, microagglutination, or indirect hemagglutination antibody test in acute and convalescent specimens taken 4 weeks apart, (2) positive PCR to *R. rickettsii,* (3) positive immunofluorescence of skin lesion (biopsy) or organ tissue (autopsy), or (4) isolation of *R. rickettsii* from a clinical specimen.

RUBELLA (GERMAN MEASLES)

Rubella is characterized by all of the following: (1) acute onset of generalized maculopapular rash, (2) temperature greater than 37.2°C (99°F), if measured, and (3) arthralgia/arthritis, lymphadenopathy, or conjunctivitis. Laboratory confirmation is obtained by (1) isolation of rubella virus, (2) significant rise in serum rubella IgG titers between the acute and convalescent phases by any standard serologic assay, or (3) positive serologic test for rubella IgM. It should be noted that rubella IgM tests are occasionally falsely positive in persons with other viral illnesses such as Epstein-Barr virus, cytomegalovirus, or parvovirus infection or in the presence of rheumatoid factor.

RUBELLA, CONGENITAL SYNDROME

The congenital syndrome of rubella is an illness of infancy resulting from rubella virus infection in utero. Infants present with signs and symptoms from the following categories: (1) cataracts/congenital glaucoma, congenital heart disease, hearing loss, and pigmentary retinopathy or (2) purpura, splenomegaly, jaundice, microcephaly, mental retardation, meningoencephalitis, and radiolucent bone disease. Deafness is the most common deficit. Laboratory detection is undertaken by any of the following methods: (1) isolation of rubella virus, (2) demonstration of rubella-specific IgM, (3) infant rubella antibody levels persistently high for longer than expected from passive maternal antibody transfer (infant antibodies should decrease by a twofold dilution each month of life), or (4) a positive PCR for rubella virus.[7]

SALMONELLOSIS

Infection with *Salmonella* causes diarrhea, abdominal pain, and occasionally, nausea and vomiting of variable severity. Infections may be asymptomatic or may cause extraintestinal disease. Isolation of *Salmonella* from a clinical specimen confirms the diagnosis.

SHIGELLOSIS

Shigellosis presents with diarrhea, nausea, abdominal cramping, and tenesmus of varying severity; alternatively, asymptomatic infections may occur. Isolation of *Shigella* from a clinical specimen confirms the diagnosis.

STREPTOCOCCAL DISEASE, INVASIVE, GROUP A

Invasive group A streptococcal disease is associated with any of several clinical syndromes, including (1) pneumonia, (2) bacteremia associated with cutaneous infection (cellulitis, erysipelas, or infection of a surgical or nonsurgical wound), (3) deep soft tissue infection (myositis or necrotizing fasciitis), (4) meningitis, (5) peritonitis, (6) osteomyelitis, (7) septic arthritis, (8) postpartum sepsis (puerperal fever), (9) neonatal sepsis, or (10) nonfocal bacteremia. Laboratory isolation of group A streptococci *(Streptococcus pyogenes)* by culture from a normally sterile site makes the diagnosis.

STREPTOCOCCAL TOXIC SHOCK SYNDROME

Streptococcal toxic shock syndrome (STSS) is a severe, rapidly progressive illness associated with either invasive or noninvasive group A streptococcal infection. This syndrome may occur with infection at any site but is associated most often with a cutaneous lesion. To be considered as STSS, all the following manifestations must be present within 48 h of hospitalization:

1. *Hypotension.* Systolic blood pressure less than 90 mm Hg for adults or less than the fifth percentile by age for children under 16 years of age.

2. *Multiorgan involvement* with two or more of the following:
   a. *Renal.* Creatinine greater than 2 mg/dL for adults, or twice the upper limit of normal for age, or twice the baseline value for persons with underlying renal dysfunction.
   b. *Coagulopathy.* Platelets less than 100,000/μL or disseminated intravascular coagulopathy.
   c. *Hepatic.* Total bilirubin, alanine aminotransferase, or aspartate aminotransferase twice the upper limit of normal for age or twice normal baseline values for those persons with underlying liver disease.
   d. *Respiratory.* Adult respiratory distress syndrome.
   e. *Dermatologic.* Generalized erythematous macular rash that may desquamate.
   f. *Musculoskeletal.* Soft tissue necrosis including necrotizing fasciitis, myositis, or gangrene.

The laboratory diagnosis is made by isolating group A *Streptococcus* in a normally sterile site.

STREPTOCOCCUS PNEUMONIAE DRUG-RESISTANT INVASIVE DISEASE

Drug-resistant, invasive *S. pneumoniae* is associated with many clinical syndromes depending on the site of infection. Isolation of the organism from a normally sterile site and finding a "nonsusceptible" isolate form the crux of the diagnosis.[1]

STREPTOCOCCUS PNEUMONIAE, INVASIVE, CHILDREN < 5 YEARS OF AGE

Invasive *S. pneumoniae* is associated with many clinical syndromes depending on the site of infection. Isolation of the organism from a normally sterile site confirms the diagnosis.[1]

SYPHILIS

The manifestations of syphilitic illness vary with the time period between infection and detection. Primary syphilis is recognized by the one or more chancres, usually on the genitalia. Secondary syphilis is identified by the presence of localized or diffuse mucocutaneous lesions. The primary chancre may still be present. Laboratory diagnosis for primary or secondary syphilis rests on demonstrating *Treponema pallidum* by dark-field microscopy, direct fluorescent antibody (DFA-TP), or equivalent method.

Latent syphilis has no clinical symptoms. The early latent period occurs in those infected within the previous 12 months, and the late latent period occurs in those infected for greater than 1 year. Persons in whom the period of infection cannot be documented and in whom there are no clinical symptoms are referred to as being latent of unknown duration. Laboratory diagnosis of latent syphilis can be made in one of the following ways: (1) no past diagnosis of syphilis and a reactive nontreponemal test (VDRL or RPR) and a reactive treponemal test (FTA-ABS or MHA-TP) or (2) history of syphilis therapy and current test titer with fourfold increase from last nontreponemal test titer.

Neurosyphilis is evident by the presence of CNS findings in the setting of a reactive serologic test for syphilis and a reactive VDRL in CSF. Late syphilis with clinical manifestations other than neurosyphilis is manifested by inflammatory lesions of the cardiovascular system, bone, and skin. Rarely, lesions of the upper or lower respiratory tracts, mouth, eye, abdominal organs, reproductive organs, lymph nodes, or skeletal muscles occur. Evidence of late syphilis is seen after more than 15 years of untreated infection.

Syphilitic stillbirth is fetal death after at least a 20-week gestation or in a fetus weighing greater than 500 g in which the mother had untreated or inadequately treated syphilis at delivery. This should be reported as congenital syphilis.

SYPHILIS, CONGENITAL

Infection in utero with *T. pallidum* causes an illness of varying severity in children. Those under 2 years of age may present with hepatosplenomegaly, rash, condyloma lata, snuffles, jaundice (nonviral hepatitis), pseudoparalysis, anemia, or edema from nephrotic syndrome and/or malnutrition. Older children may have the stigmata of syphilis: interstitial keratitis, nerve deafness, anterior bowing of the shins, frontal bossing, mulberry molars, Hutchinson teeth, saddle nose, rhagades, or Clutton joints.

Identification of *T. pallidum* by dark-field microscopy, fluorescent antibody, or other specific stains in specimens from lesions, placenta, cord blood, or autopsy material confirms the diagnosis.

TETANUS

Tetanus has an acute onset and is characterized by hypertonia and/or painful muscular contractions typically of the muscles of the neck and jaw without other cause. Since there are no serologic tests available to confirm the suspicion of tetanus, a clinically compatible case is sufficient for diagnosis.

TOXIC SHOCK SYNDROME

Toxic shock syndrome is an illness manifested by:

1. Temperature greater than or equal to 38.8°C (102°F)
2. Diffuse macular erythroderma
3. Desquamation, particularly affecting the palms and soles, 1 to 2 weeks following onset of illness
4. Hypotension, as defined by:
   a. Systolic blood pressure less than or equal to 90 mm Hg for adults or less than the fifth percentile by age for those persons under 16 years of age
   b. Orthostatic decrease in diastolic blood pressure greater than or equal to 15 mm Hg from lying to sitting
   c. Orthostatic syncope or dizziness
5. Multisystem involvement (three or more):
   a. *Gastrointestinal.* Vomiting or diarrhea at outset
   b. *Muscular.* Severe myalgia or creatinine phosphokinase twice the upper limit of normal
   c. *Mucous membranes.* Vaginal, oropharyngeal, or conjunctival hyperemia
   d. *Renal.* Blood urea nitrogen or creatinine twice the upper limit of normal or urinary sediment with pyuria in the absence of urinary tract infection
   e. *Hepatic.* Total bilirubin, alanine transferase, or aspartate transferase twice the upper limit of normal
   f. *Hematologic.* Platelets less than 100,000/μL
   g. *Central nervous system.* Disorientation or alteration in consciousness without focal neurologic signs when fever and hypotension are absent

Although the diagnosis is primarily a clinical one, laboratory evaluation should include no rise in Rocky Mountain spotted fever, leptospirosis, or measles titers, if obtained, and negative blood, throat, and CSF cultures. Blood culture positive for *S. aureus* is not inconsistent with the diagnosis of toxic shock syndrome.

TRICHINOSIS

Trichinosis presents with variable manifestations. Most commonly a person will complain of fever, myalgia, and periorbital edema. Eosinophilia may be present on white blood cell differential. Trichinosis is caused by ingestion of *Trichinella* larvae in meat most commonly. On laboratory evaluation, *Trichinella* larvae may be found in tissue obtained by muscle biopsy, or the serologic test for *Trichinella* will be positive.

TUBERCULOSIS

Tuberculosis is a chronic infection characterized pathologically by formation of granulomas. Caused by *Mycobacterium tuberculosis,* the most common site of infection is the lungs, although other organs may be involved. The following criteria must be met for a reportable case of tuberculosis: (1) a positive tuberculin skin test, (2) other signs and symptoms compatible with tuberculosis (abnormal chest radiograph or clinical evidence of current disease), (3) treatment with two or more antituberculosis medications, and (4) completed diagnostic evaluation. Laboratory confirmation can be made by any of the following methods: (1) isolation of *M. tuberculosis* from a clinical specimen, (2) detection of *M. tuberculosis* from a clinical specimen by nucleic acid amplification test, or (3) acid-fast bacilli in a clinical specimen when culture has not or cannot be obtained.

TULAREMIA

Seven clinical forms characterize infection with *Francisella tularensis:* (1) ulceroglandular: cutaneous ulcer with regional lymphadenopathy; (2) glandular: regional lymphadenopathy without an ulcer; (3) ocularglandular: conjunctivitis with preauricular lymphadenopathy; (4) oropharyngeal: tonsillitis, stomatitis, or pharyngitis and cervical lymphadenopathy, (5) intestinal: intestinal pain, vomiting, and diarrhea; (6) pneumonic: primary pleuropulmonary disease; or (7) thyroidal: febrile illness without early localizing signs and symptoms. The presumptive laboratory diagnosis is made by detection of serum antibody titers to the organism in an individual with no history of *F. tularensis* vaccination or by detection of *F. tularensis* in a clinical specimen by fluorescent assay. Confirmatory laboratory testing is accomplished by the isolation of *F. tularensis* in a clinical specimen or by detection of a fourfold or greater change in serum antibody titer to *F. tularensis* antigen.[1]

TYPHOID FEVER

The insidious onset of fever, headache, malaise, anorexia, relative bradycardia, constipation or diarrhea, and cough are characteristic of typhoid fever. Caused by the bacteria *Salmonella typhi,* typhoid fever may be relatively mild or even asymptomatic. Isolation of *S. typhi* in blood, stool, or other clinical specimen seals the diagnosis.

VARICELLA (CHICKENPOX, DEATHS ONLY)

Varicella is an illness characterized by the acute onset of diffuse maculopapulovesicular rash with no other apparent cause. Laboratory confirmation is achieved by (1) isolation of varicella virus from a clinical specimen, (2) positive direct fluorescent antibody (DFA) for the virus, (3) detection of nucleic acid by PCR, or (4) significant rise in serum IgG antibody level as detected by any standard serology. Laboratory confirmation is only recommended in the event of fatal cases or other special circumstances.

A case is considered probable if the clinical criteria are met in the absence of laboratory confirmation or epidemiologic linkage. Two epidemiologically linked probable cases are considered confirmed, as is any case meeting the laboratory confirmation requirements above.

Any case in which varicella infection contributes directly or indirectly to the patient's death should be reported. A fatal case is reported as probable if it meets the probable criteria above and as confirmed if the case meets confirmed criteria above. Nonfatal cases need not be reported.[1]

YELLOW FEVER

This mosquito-borne viral illness presents with acute onset of fever, headache, myalgias, and conjunctival injection. This is followed by brief remission and recurrence of the preceding symptoms along with hepati-

tis, albuminuria, jaundice, and in some cases, renal failure, shock, and generalized hemorrhages. Laboratory diagnosis of yellow fever is made on finding (1) a fourfold or greater rise in yellow fever titer in patients with no recent history of yellow fever vaccination and in whom cross-reaction to other flaviviruses has been excluded or (2) yellow fever virus antigen or genome in tissue, blood, or other body fluids.

REFERENCES

1. http://www.cdc.gov/epo/dphsi/phs/infdis2002.htm.
2. Centers for Disease Control and Prevention: Case definitions for infectious conditions under public health surveillance. *MMWR* 46(RR-10):1, 1997.
3. http://www.cdc.gov/epo/dphsi/netss.htm.
4. Centers for Disease Control and Prevention: 1993 Revised classification system for HIV infection and expanded surveillance case definition for AIDS among adolescents and adults. *MMWR* 41(RR-17):1, 1992.
5. Centers for Disease Control and Prevention: 1994 Revised classification system for human immunodeficiency virus infection in children less than 13 years of age. *MMWR* 43(RR-12):1, 1994.
6. Centers for Disease Control and Prevention: Revision of the CDC surveillance case definition for acquired immunodeficiency syndrome. *MMWR* 36(suppl 1):10s, 1987.
7. Centers for Disease Control and Prevention: Guidelines for national human immunodeficiency virus case surveillance, including monitoring for human immunodeficiency virus infection and acquired immunodeficiency syndrome. *MMWR* 48(RR-13):29, 1999.

154

OCCUPATIONAL EXPOSURES, INFECTION CONTROL, AND STANDARD PRECAUTIONS
Kathy J. Rinnert

This chapter examines standard precautions, routes of infectious disease exposure, and infection control practices. This discussion includes an overview of exposure management and commonly encountered occupational exposures in the ED.

OCCUPATIONAL EXPOSURES

The Centers for Disease Control and Prevention (CDC) estimates that 8 million health care workers are at risk of acquiring infections in the course of providing care for their patients.

An additional 1.2 million non-health care workers are also at risk for infectious exposure, and include those engaged in law enforcement; fire, rescue, and emergency medical services; correctional facilities; research laboratories; and the funeral industry.

The Occupational Safety and Health Administration (OSHA) defines *occupational exposure* as a "reasonably anticipated skin, eye, mucous membrane, or parenteral contact with blood or other potentially infectious materials that may result from the performance of the employee's duties."[1] Blood is defined as "human blood, blood products, or blood components."[1] *Other potentially infectious materials* (OPIM) are defined as "human body fluids, such as saliva, semen, and vaginal secretions; cerebrospinal, synovial, pleural, pericardial, peritoneal, and amniotic fluids; any body fluids visibly contaminated with blood; unfixed human tissue or organs; HIV (human immunodeficiency virus) or HBV (hepatitis B virus) containing cell or tissue cultures, culture mediums, or other solutions; and all body fluids where it is difficult or impossible to differentiate between body fluids."[1] Health care workers should treat all bodily secretions, fluids, and tissues as potentially infectious substances.

Sources of exposure for blood-borne, airborne or droplet, and contact-related pathogens are multiple and varied. Health care activities that expose medical personnel to blood-borne diseases include placement of venous access, phlebotomy, needle recapping, specimen handling, administration of injected medications, lumbar puncture, chest tube insertion, airway suctioning, placement of nasogastric and orogastric tubes, intubation, placement of urinary catheters, and hemorrhage control. Health care activities that bring workers into close physical proximity to patients or their environment expose workers to airborne or droplet-dispersed organisms. Dressing changes, wound debridement, and wound irrigation may expose health care workers to contaminated materials or infectious agents. Workplace activities that may expose health care personnel to contact-dispersed organisms or parasites include cleaning patient care areas or equipment, changing linens, caring for incontinent and diapered patients, and physical examination. A seemingly innocuous physical examination (including integument, scalp, eyes, oropharynx, respiratory tract, and wounds) is not an activity without risk, depending on the nature of the infectious agent or exposure source.

The Hospital Infection Control Practices Advisory Committee (HICPAC) of the Centers for Disease Control and Prevention has developed a listing of selected infections and conditions that may be encountered in the ED, along with recommended occupational exposure precautions.[2,3] While the geographic distribution and population incidence of most infectious diseases are well known, this does not imply that infectivity is limited to specific ethnic groups, races, or subsets of the population. As the world population becomes increasingly mobile, patients with geographically isolated diseases may migrate to regions where the disease incidence may be low or nonexistent. In addition, many infectious diseases display heterogeneous and varying symptom complexes, including prolonged latent or asymptomatic stages. Therefore providing care to an apparently healthy, asymptomatic patient does not preclude the possibility of disease infectivity and exposure. Since health care workers cannot readily identify those who are infected or risky, it is prudent to employ infection control practices and utilize personal protective equipment (PPE) during all patient care activities. It is on this premise that the concept of standard precautions is based.

Portals for infectious disease entry are percutaneous, mucous membrane (oral, ocular, nasal, or rectal), respiratory, and dermal.

Percutaneous exposures are the most commonly reported and pose the highest risk for the contraction of blood-borne disease. Needle sticks or cuts by sharp objects account for the majority of percutaneous injuries. Workplace activities that put personnel at risk for percutaneous injuries include phlebotomy, initiation of intravenous access, manipulation of access devices, suturing, and medication injection. Since the majority of these activities are nursing functions, it is not surprising that nurses are the most likely recipients of needle-stick injury.

Mucous membrane exposures are the second most commonly reported occupational exposure, and result from splatters, splashes, and sprays of blood and body fluids. Risk is entailed by such health care tasks as wound management (hemorrhage control, exploration, cleansing, irrigation, and debridement), airway suctioning, nasogastric or orogastric tube placement, intubation, and handling specimen containers of blood or body fluids.

Respiratory exposures result from the inhalation of airborne or droplet particulate materials. Health care workers risk respiratory exposure when they are confined with an expectorating, coughing, or sneezing patient for prolonged periods or in a poorly ventilated environment.

Dermal exposure involves skin contact with patients (direct contact) or environmental surfaces or objects that are contaminated with infectious materials (indirect contact). The risk of infection is increased if worker contact involves a large surface area or if the dermis is not intact (abraded, chapped, or excoriated). Drug-resistant organisms, such as methicillin-resistant *S. aureus* and vancomycin-resistant enterococci, pose additional dermal exposure risk. Transmission of these diseases may be related to contact with infected patients, medical equipment used on them, or both. Workplace activities that place the health care worker at risk include patient examination, turning or moving patients, and changing linens or wound dressings. Parasites of the integument (e.g., scabies, lice, etc.) are also agents of dermal exposure. Other dermal exposures include hypersensitivity reactions of health care workers that may occur with prolonged or repeated exposure to specific inert substances (e.g., latex).

The risk of infection in an exposed health care provider depends on the route (portal) of exposure, the concentration (number of organisms) of pathogen in the infectious material, the infectious characteristics (virility) of the pathogen, the volume (dose) of infectious material, and the immunocompetence (susceptibility) of the exposed individual. Infectious characteristics may vary as the pathogen mutates, becoming resistant to treatment agents (e.g., antibiotics, antivirals, antifungals, etc.) or the host's immune defenses. The potential for infection may be incrementally higher as the route of exposure changes; that is, percutaneous exposures have greater potential for infection than do mucous membrane exposures, respiratory exposures, or dermal exposures.

LEGISLATIVE REGULATIONS

OSHA has drafted federal regulations that prescribe safeguards to protect workers and reduce risk of exposure to blood and body fluids.[4] Updated and more detailed standards (known as the Blood Borne Pathogens Standard) were then published in Title 29 of the Code of Federal Regulations in December 1991 and amended in September 2000 by the Needlestick Safety and Prevention Act.[5,6]

The standards require health care facilities to develop programs involving five major initiatives for the mitigation of blood-borne disease transmission. These are (1) to develop a written exposure control plan, (2) to utilize engineering controls to reduce risk by removing the hazard or isolating the worker from exposure, (3) to utilize work practice controls to standardize and maximize the safety with which work tasks are performed, (4) to identify mechanisms for compliance with Title 29 standards, and (5) to communicate workplace hazards to those with potential for blood-borne disease exposures. CDC and OSHA websites should be accessed to keep abreast of future amendments and revisions of these regulations and standards.

INFECTION CONTROL

Infection control practices are designed to prevent transmission of microbial agents and to provide a wide margin of safety for health care workers. These practices include hand washing; use of PPE; cleaning, disinfecting, and sterilizing patient care equipment and environmental surfaces; decontamination and laundering of soiled uniforms, clothing, and patients' linens; disposal of needles, sharps, and infectious waste; and patient location. Infection control measures that are simple, part of the routine work environment, and uniform across all situations have the greatest likelihood of compliance.

A complete infection control program includes administrative controls, equipment engineering, work practice controls, education of the work force, and medical management.

Administrative controls are designed to organize, define, and direct infection control activities. The most important of these is the development of a written infection control (exposure) plan. This plan defines all policies, procedures, and activities related to the education, prevention, and management of infectious diseases in the work force. Jobs and specific work tasks are identified and evaluated for potential exposure to infectious diseases. Initial and recurrent training in infectious disease hazards and risk activities must be provided to all health care workers.

Equipment engineering serves to reduce employee exposure by removing the hazard or isolating the health care provider from exposure. Examples include self-sheathing needles, needleless drug administration devices, sharps containers, disposable airway equipment, syringe splash guards, and PPE. Medical safety devices may significantly mitigate occupational exposures experienced by health care personnel, and recommendations for task-specific use of these devices are shown in Table 154-1.[7]

TABLE 154-1 Task-Specific Recommendations for Use of Medical Safety Devices

Patient Care Activity	Self-Sheathing Needles	Needleless Administration Devices	Splash Guards	Sharps Containers
Wound care, lavage	No	No	Yes	No
Venipuncture	Yes	No	No	Yes
Intravenous line placement	Yes	No	No	Yes
IM, SQ, IV medication administration	Yes	Yes	No	Yes
Cricothyrotomy, needle decompression	Yes	No	No	Yes
Intubation, airway adjunct placement, suctioning	No	No	No	No†
Nasogastric or orogastric tube placement	No	No	No	No†
Specimen handling	No•	No	No	No†
Childbirth	No	No	No	No†
Resuscitation activities	Yes	Yes	No	Yes

*Utilize self-sheathing device if specimen has needle permanently attached.
†Utilize sharps container or noncrush container for contaminated hardware, devices, equipment, or specimens.
Source: Adapted from Kelen et al,[7] with permission.

PPE is "specialized clothing or equipment which does not permit blood or potentially infectious substances to pass through or reach worker clothing, skin, eyes, mouth, or other mucous membranes under normal conditions of use."[1] PPE includes such items as examination gloves, face masks, eye protection, face shields, and impervious gowns, leggings, and shoe covers. PPE may significantly mitigate occupational exposures experienced by health care personnel, and recommendations for task-specific use of PPE are shown in Table 154-2.[7]

Work practice controls modify the performance of a task to minimize exposure to blood and blood-containing body fluids and infectious materials. Work practice controls necessitate the development of policies concerning disposal of needles and sharps containers (i.e., avoid shearing, bending, recapping, or breaking); disposal of contaminated linens, clothing, and infectious waste; disinfection techniques for reusable equipment; and restriction of employee activities (e.g., avoidance of eating, drinking, smoking, and application of cosmetics) while in work areas that have a reasonable likelihood of exposure to blood and body fluids.

Education of the work force should include information about the agents of infectious disease, epidemiology, methods of disease transmission, disease signs and symptoms, risky work activities, risk reduction strategies, and postexposure management. Such education must occur at initial employment, with recurrent training provided at specified intervals. Health care providers must also be aware that utilization of PPE and engineering controls does not totally eliminate infection risk.

Medical management practices include preexposure preventive vaccinations, acute postexposure medical evaluation, infectious disease counseling, disease prophylaxis, and medical testing and referral. OSHA mandates preexposure vaccines at initial employee training and within 10 days of employment for all personnel at risk of exposure.[1] The Advisory Committee on Immunization Practices (ACIP) and the

TABLE 154-2 Task-Specific Recommendations for Use of PPE

Patient Care Activity	Disposable Gloves	Mask and Protective Eyewear	Impervious Gown
Measuring blood pressure	No*	No	No
Measuring pulse	No*	No	No
Measuring temperature	No*	No	No
Examination of bleeding patient	Yes	No†	No†
Wound management, dressing	Yes	No†	No†
Minor hemorrhage control	Yes	No†	No†
Profuse hemorrhage control	Yes	Yes	Yes
Cardiopulmonary resuscitation	Yes	No†	No†
Venipuncture	Yes	No	No
Intravenous line placement	Yes	No	No
IM, SQ, IV medication administration	Yes	No	No
Cricothyrotomy, needle decompression	Yes	Yes	No
Intubation, airway adjunct placement, suctioning	Yes	Yes	No
Childbirth	Yes	Yes	Yes
Nasogastric or orogastric tube placement	Yes	Yes	No†
Specimen handling	Yes	No	No

*Utilize gloves if task performance includes possible contact with patient's blood, secretions, or body fluids.
†Utilize mask, protective eyewear, and impervious gown if possibility of splashing or spray exists.
Source: Adapted from Kelen et al.[7]

Hospital Infection Control Practices Advisory Committee (HICPAC) make specific recommendations concerning the use of certain immunizing agents in health care personnel.[8]

MANAGEMENT OF HEALTH CARE PERSONNEL POTENTIALLY EXPOSED TO HBV, HCV, OR HIV

Once an infectious exposure has occurred, a plan for postexposure prophylaxis (PEP) medical management should be available to health care providers 24 h a day. This plan should include immediate medical assessment, risk analysis, counseling, treatment and prophylaxis, and follow-up appropriate to the type and source of the exposure.[8–11] The emergency physician, often the first to examine the exposed person and make an assessment of the relative risk of the transmission, serves an important role in managing occupational exposures.

A standardized approach to the management of exposures to blood or body fluids will ensure efficient and efficacious treatment of these incidents. An outline for general management has been developed and is shown in Table 154-3.[10]

The exposed person's medical record (the occupational exposure report) should contain specific information relative to the exposure incident. Key elements include the circumstances of exposure, medical history of the source person, and medical history of the exposed person. The CDC recommends specific data elements be included in the occupational exposure report (Table 154-4).[9]

Treatment of the exposure site is similar to standard wound care. Wounds and skin sites that have been exposed to potentially infectious materials should be washed with soap and water; mucous membranes should be flushed with water. The application of caustics (bleach), antiseptics, or disinfectants directly into the wound is not recommended.

The exposure event should be evaluated for the potential to transmit HBV, HCV, and HIV, based on the type of body substance involved and the route and severity of the exposure (Table 154-5).[9] Blood, fluid containing visible blood, or OPIM (including semen, vaginal secretions, and cerebrospinal, synovial, pleural, peritoneal, pericardial, and amniotic fluids) or tissue may transmit blood-borne viruses. Exposures to these fluids through a percutaneous injury or mucous membrane contact are situations that pose a risk for virus transmission and require further evaluation. For dermal exposure, follow-up is indicated only if it involves exposure to blood or OPIM and the skin is not intact (abraded, chapped, excoriated, open wound).

Testing to determine the HBV, HCV, and HIV infection status of an exposure source should be performed as soon as possible (Table 154-6).[9] An FDA-approved rapid HIV-antibody test should be considered. Direct viral assays (HIV p24 antigen enzyme immunoassay, HIV RNA, HCV RNA) are not recommended. If the exposure source is not

TABLE 154-3   Outline for Management of Exposures to Blood or Body Fluids

Expedite triage

Irrigate exposed areas

Obtain history regarding exposure circumstances, source patient, and vaccination history of exposed (see Table 154-4)

Obtain blood samples for laboratory studies (using consents when required) from exposed person; obtain urine pregnancy test for women of childbearing potential

Order laboratory studies from source patient, if known

Determine need for tetanus immunization

Determine need for hepatitis B PEP (see Table 154-7)

Determine need for HIV PEP (Tables 154-8 and 154-9)

Counsel exposed person regarding risk of specific blood-borne pathogens and discuss risks/benefits of available treatment options

Review dosing and side effects of recommended treatments (see Tables 154-10, 154-11, and 154-12)

Arrange follow-up through employee health clinic or other resource

Source: Moran,[10] with permission.

TABLE 154-4   Recommendations for the Contents of the Occupational Exposure Report

Date and time of exposure

Details of the procedure being performed, including where and how the exposure occurred; if related to a sharp device, the type and brand of device and how and when in the course of handling the device the exposure occurred

Details of the exposure, including the type and amount of fluid or material and the severity of the exposure (e.g., for a percutaneous exposure, depth of injury and whether fluid was injected; for a skin or mucous membrane exposure, the estimated volume of material and the condition of the skin [e.g., chapped, abraded, intact])

Details about the exposure source (e.g., whether the source material contained HBV, HCV, or HIV; if the source is HIV-infected, the stage of disease, history of antiretroviral therapy, viral load, and antiretroviral resistance information, if known)

Details about the exposed person (e.g., hepatitis B vaccination and vaccine-response status)

Details about counseling, postexposure management, and follow-up

Source: From CDC.[9]

known, epidemiologic data should be used to determine the exposure risk. Testing of needles or sharps instruments is not recommended as reliability is suspect. If the source is known to have HIV information about the state of the infection (CD4[+] T-cell count, and viral load, current and previous antiretroviral therapy) may guide the choice of an appropriate PEP regimen. If this information is not immediately known, the initiation of PEP should not be delayed, as changes in the regimen may be made on follow-up (within 72 h postexposure).[9]

Factors to consider in the management of HBV exposure include the hepatitis B surface antigen (HBsAg) status of the source and the hepatitis B vaccination and vaccine response status of the exposed person. Every unvaccinated health care worker who has been exposed to blood or body fluids should receive the hepatitis B vaccine series. Summary recommendations for the percutaneous or mucosal exposure to blood according to the HBsAg status of the exposure source and the vaccination/vaccine-response status of the exposed person is shown in Table 154-7.[9] Hepatitis B immune globulin (HBIG), when indicated, should be administered as soon as possible after the exposure (ideally within 24 h). After a period of 7 days, the effectiveness of HBIG is unknown. When hepatitis B vaccine is indicated, it should be given as soon as possible.

For occupational HCV exposures the CDC recommends anti-HCV testing of the source patient. The exposed person should be tested for

TABLE 154-5   Factors to Consider in Assessing the Need for Follow-Up of Occupational Exposures

Type of exposure

Percutaneous injury

Mucous membrane exposure

Nonintact skin exposure

Bites resulting in blood exposure to either person involved

Type and amount of fluid/tissue

Blood

Fluids containing blood

Potentially infectious fluid or tissue (semen; vaginal secretions; and cerebrospinal, synovial, pleural, peritoneal, pericardial, and amniotic fluids)

Direct contact with concentrated virus

Infectious status of source

Presence of HBsAg

Presence of HCV antibody

Presence of HIV antibody

Susceptibility of exposed person

Hepatitis B vaccine and vaccine response status

HBV, HCV, and HIV immune status

Source: From CDC.[9]

TABLE 154-6   Evaluation of Occupational Exposure Sources

Known sources

Test known sources for HBsAg, anti-HCV, and HIV antibody

   Direct virus assays for routine screening of source patients are *not* recommended

   Consider using a rapid HIV-antibody test

   If the source person is *not* infected with a blood-borne pathogen, baseline testing or further follow-up of the exposed person is *not* necessary

For sources whose infection status remains unknown (e.g., the source person refuses testing), consider medical diagnoses, clinical symptoms, and history of risk behaviors

Do not test discarded needles for blood-borne pathogens

Unknown sources

For unknown sources, evaluate the likelihood of exposure to a source at high risk for infection

   Consider likelihood of blood-borne pathogen infection among patients in the exposure setting

Source: From CDC.[9]

anti-HCV and alanine aminotransferase (ALT) at baseline and follow-up (at 4 to 6 months). Testing for HCV RNA may also be performed at 4 -to 6 weeks if earlier diagnosis of HCV is desired. All positive anti-HCV tests by enzyme immunoassay (EIA) should be confirmed by supplemental testing (i.e., recombinant immunoblot assay [RIBA]). Immunoglobulin (IG) and antivirals are not recommended for PEP after exposure to HCV-positive blood. Medical personnel exposed to HBV- or HCV-infected blood do not need to take any precautions to prevent secondary transmission during the follow-up period; however, they should not donate blood, plasma, organs, tissue, or semen.

Health care personnel potentially exposed to HIV should receive expedited evaluation (ideally in less than 1 h) and should be tested for HIV at baseline. If the source patient is HIV-negative, baseline testing or further follow-up for the exposed person is not normally necessary. Factors to consider in the management of HIV exposure include the type of exposure (percutaneous, mucous membrane, or dermal),

the volume of the exposure (small or large), and the HIV status of the source patient. The CDC provides detailed recommendations concerning PEP for percutaneous, mucous membrane, and nonintact skin exposures (Tables 154-8 and 154-9).[9] These recommendations apply to situations when a person has been exposed to a source person with HIV infection or when information suggests the likelihood that the source is HIV-infected. PEP should be initiated as soon as possible; if later testing determines the source patient to be HIV-negative, PEP should be discontinued. PEP is substantially less effective if started more than 24 to 36 h postexposure, although the interval after which no benefit is gained is not known. Therefore, PEP should be started even when the postexposure interval exceeds 36 h. In addition, the optimal duration of PEP is unknown; the CDC recommends 4 weeks.

In an effort to balance the substantial risk of PEP toxicity (over 50 percent of those who initiate PEP discontinue treatment due to side effects), and with the negligible risk of HIV infection even when exposed to HIV-positive blood, the CDC has developed two drug regimens for PEP. The basic two-drug regimen is appropriate for most HIV exposures. The expanded three-drug regimen is used for those exposures determined to be an increased risk for transmission. Recommended drug regimens and dosing information for the basic and expanded HIV PEP regimens are shown in Tables 154-10 and 154-11.[12] Since HIV PEP may cause a number of side effects (Table 154-12),[10] patients should be closely monitored at baseline and at 2 weeks with blood cell counts and renal and hepatic tests. HIV-antibody testing should be performed for at least 6 months postexposure. Exposed health care personnel should be advised to use the following measures to prevent secondary transmission during the follow-up period (6 to 12 months): exercise sexual abstinence or use condoms; refrain from donating blood, plasma, organs, tissue, or semen; and avoid breastfeeding. Exposed workers should be advised to seek medical evaluation for any acute illness which occurs during the follow-up period, as this may signal the onset of acute retroviral syndrome.

The postexposure management for occupational exposures is complex due to the variable circumstances of the exposure (route, body

TABLE 154-7   Recommended PEP for Percutaneous and Mucous Membrane Exposure to HBV

Vaccination and Antibody Response Status of Exposed Workers*	TREATMENT		
	Source HBsAg† Positive	Source HBsAg† Negative	Source Unknown or Not Available for Testing
Unvaccinated	HBIG‡ × 1 and initiate HB vaccine series#	Initiate HB vaccine series	Initiate HB vaccine series
Previously vaccinated			
Known responder§	No treatment	No treatment	No treatment
Known nonresponder**	HBIG × 1 and initiate revaccination or HBIG × 2††	No treatment	If known high-risk source, treat as if source were HBsAg positive
Antibody response unknown	Test exposed person for anti-HBs‡‡ 1. If adequate,§ no treatment is nesessary 2. If inadequate,** administer HBIG × 1 and vaccine booster	No treatment	Test exposed person for anti-HBs 1. If adequate,§ no treatment is necessary 2. If inadequate,** administer vaccine booster and recheck titer in 1–2 months

*Persons who have previously been infected with HBV are immune to reinfection and do not require postexposure prophylaxis.

†Hepatits B surface antigen.

‡Hepatitis B immune globulin; dose is 0.06 mL/kg IM.

#Hepatitis B vaccine.

§A responder is a person with adequate levels of serum antibody to HBsAg (i.e., anti-HBs ≥10 mIU/mL).

**A nonresponder is a person with inadequate response to vaccination (i.e., serum anti-HBs <10 mIU/mL).

††The option of giving one dose of HBIG and reinitiating the vaccine series is preferred for nonresponders who have not completed a second 3-dose vaccine series. For persons who previously completed a second vaccine series but failed to respond, two doses of HBIG are preferred.

‡‡Antibody to HBsAg.

Source: From CDC.[9]

TABLE 154-8 Recommended HIV Postexposure Prophylaxis for Percutaneous Injuries

	INFECTION STATUS OF SOURCE				
Exposure Type	HIV-Positive Class 1*	HIV-Positive Class 2*	Source of Unknown HIV Status†	Unknown Source‡	HIV-Negative
Less severe#	Recommend basic 2-drug PEP	Recommend expanded 3-drug PEP	Generally, no PEP warranted; however, consider basic 2-drug PEP§ for source with HIV risk factors**	Generally, no PEP warranted; however, consider basic 2-drug PEP§ in settings where exposure to HIV-infected persons is likely	No PEP warranted
More severe††	Recommend expanded 3-drug PEP	Recommend expanded 3-drug PEP	Generally, no PEP warranted; however, consider basic 2-drug PEP§ for source with HIV risk factors**	Generally; no PEP warranted; however, consider basic 2-drug PEP§ in settings where exposure to HIV-infected persons is likely	No PEP warranted

*HIV-Positive, Class 1—asymptomatic HIV infection or known low viral load (e.g., <1500 RNA copies/mL). HIV-Positive, Class 2—symptomatic HIV infection, AIDS, acute seroconversion, or known high viral load. If drug resistance is a concern, obtain expert conultation. Initiation of postexposure prophylaxis (PEP) should not be delayed pending expert consultation, and, because expert consultation alone cannot substitute for face-to-face counseling, resources should be available to provide immediate evaluation and follow-up care for all exposures.
†Source of unknown HIV status (e.g., deceased source person with no samples available for HIV testing).
‡Unknown source (e.g., a needle from a sharps disposal container).
#Less severe (e.g., solid needle and superficial injury).
§The designation "consider PEP" indicates that PEP is optional and should be based on an individualized decision between the exposed person and the treating clinician.
**If PEP is offered and taken and the source is later determined to be HIV-negative, PEP should be discontinued.
††More severe (e.g., large-bore hollow needle, deep puncture, visible blood on device, or needle used in patient's artery or vein).
Source: From CDC.[9]

TABLE 154-9 Recommended HIV Postexposure Prophylaxis for Mucous Membrane Exposures and Nonintact Skin* Exposures

	INFECTION STATUS OF SOURCE				
Exposure Type	HIV-Positive Class 1†	HIV-Positive Class 2†	Source of Unknown HIV Status‡	Unknown Source#	HIV-Negative
Small volume§	Consider basic 2-drug PEP**	Recommend basic 2-drug PEP	Generally, no PEP warranted; however, consider basic 2-drug PEP** for source with HIV risk factors††	Generally, no PEP warranted; however, consider basic 2-drug PEP** in settings where exposure to HIV-infected persons is likely	No PEP warranted
Large volume‡‡	Recommend basic 2-drug PEP	Recommend expanded 3-drug PEP	Generally, no PEP warranted; however, consider basic 2-drug PEP** for source with HIV risk factors††	Generally, no PEP warranted; however, consider basic 2-drug PEP** in settings where exposure to HIV-infected persons is likely	No PEP warranted

*For skin exposures, follow-up is indicated only if there is evidence of compromised skin integrity (e.g., dermatitis, abrasion, or open wound).
†HIV-Positive, Class 1—asymptomatic HIV infection or known low viral load (e.g., <1500 RNA copies/mL). HIV-Positive, Class 2—symptomatic HIV infection, AIDS, acute seroconversion, or known high viral load. If drug resistance is a concern, obtain expert conultation. Initiation of postexposure prophylaxis (PEP) should not be delayed pending expert consultation, and, because expert consultation alone cannot substitute for face-to-face counseling, resources should be available to provide immediate evaluation and follow-up care for all exposures.
‡Source of unknown HIV status (e.g., deceased source person with no samples available for HIV testing).
#Unknown source (e.g., splash from inappropriately disposed blood).
§Small volume (i.e., a few drops).
**The designation "consider PEP" indicates that PEP is optional and should be based on an individualized decision between the exposed person and the treating clinician.
††If PEP is offered and taken and the source is later determined to be HIV-negative, PEP should be discontinued.
‡‡Large volume (i.e., major blood splash).
Source: From CDC.[9]

TABLE 154-10   Basic HIV Postexposure Prophylaxis (PEP) Regimens

Basic Two-Drug Regimen
    Zidovudine (600 mg/d divided in 2–3 doses)
       + Lamivudine (150 mg bid)
Alternate Basic Two-Drug Regimens
    Lamivudine (150 mg bid) + Stavudine (40 mg twice daily *OR* if body
       weight <60 kg, dose 30 mg bid)
    Didanosine (400 mg daily on an empty stomach *OR* if body weight
       <60 kg, dose 125 mg bid) + Stavudine (40 mg bid *OR* if body weight
       <60 kg, dose 30 mg bid)

Source: Demangone,[12] with permission.

substance involved, volume of infectious material, etc.), health status of the exposed person (previous immunizations, comorbid conditions, immunocompetence, nature of the exposure site), health status of the source person (previous immunizations, comorbid conditions, immunocompetence, current and past therapies for infectious diseases, etc.), and recommendations for treatment and prophylaxis given the current understanding of the optimal therapies (immunomodulators, vaccinations, antibiotics/antivirals, etc.). Since CDC guidelines for managing these complex cases are constantly evolving, optimal case management can be extremely difficult.

To address these issues and facilitate care, the CDC offers three resources. The National Clinician's Post-Exposure Prophylaxis Hotline (PEPline) offers 24-h telephone consultation for physicians managing occupational exposures to blood-borne pathogens. Expert clinicians from the University of California-San Francisco and San Francisco General Hospital provide immediate, confidential, and free consultation (1-888-448-4911, www.ucsf.edu/hivcntr). The service is intended primarily for cases that represent a management challenge, such as delayed (over 24 to 36 h) reporting of exposure, unknown source, pregnancy in the exposed patient, suspected resistance of the source virus, and toxicity of the initial PEP regimen.[9] A second source of information developed and maintained by the University of California-Los Angeles, is Needlestick! (www.needlestick.mednet.ucla.edu). This interactive, Web-based, electronic medical record is intended to assist emergency physicians with the management of occupational exposures. The physician anonymously and confidentially enters relevant data and the program uses contingency tables and current CDC guidelines to provide advice regarding testing and treatment. The Hepatitis Hotline provides guidance to clinicians in regard to the acute and chronic management of hepatitis (1-888-443-7232, www.cdc.gov/hepatitis).

INFECTION PRECAUTIONS

In 1985, the CDC first introduced the concept of universal blood and body fluid precautions. The focus of these "universal" precautions centered on blood and blood-containing fluids (substances implicated in the transmission of blood-borne pathogens) with inadequate attention to infections transmitted by airborne/respiratory droplet or direct/indirect contact.

In 1996, the CDC's Hospital Infection Control Practices Advisory Committee (HICPAC) devised a new system of isolation precautions.

TABLE 154-11   Expanded HIV Postexposure Prophylaxis (PEP) Regimens

Expanded Regimen
Basic two-drug regimen plus *ONE* of following:
    Indinavir (800 mg every 8 h on an empty stomach)
    Nelfinavir (750 mg tid with food or 1250 mg bid with food)
    Efavirenz (600 mg daily, at bedtime)
    Abacavir (300 mg bid)

Source: Demangone,[12] with permission.

TABLE 154-12   Drugs Commonly Used for HIV Postexposure Prophylaxis

Drug (Trade Name)	Dosage	Primary Toxic Effects
Zidovudine (Retrovir; ZDV, AZT)	300 mg bid or 200 mg tid	Neutropenia, anemia, nausea, fatigue, malaise, headache, insommia, myositis
Lamivudine (Epivir; 3TC)	150 mg bid	Headache, abdominal pain diarrhea, rarely pancreatitis
ZDV plus 3TC (Combivir)	1 tablet bid (each tablet contains 300 mg ZDV and 150 mg 3TC)	Toxicity of ZDV and 3TC combined is approximately equal to ZDV alone
Indinavir (Crixivan; IDV)	800 mg q8h on an empty stomach	Nephrolithiasis (reduced by drinking large amounts of water), crystalluria, hematuria, nausea, headache, elevated liver function test results, hyperglycemia; many drug interactions including terfenadine, astemizole, cisapride, triazolam, midazolam, rifampin, rifabutin, ketoconazole
Nelfinavir (Viracept)	750 mg tid with food	Diarrhea, hyperglycemia; drug interactions same as indinavir

Source: Moran,[10] with permission.

The new guidelines contain two tiers of precautions: standard and transmission-based. Standard precautions assume a broad approach to health care and patient protection, by including agents transmitted by routes other than blood. Transmission-based precautions are designed for patients with documented or suspected transmissible pathogens for which additional protection beyond standard precautions is required. Transmission-based precautions are of three types: airborne, droplet, and contact. These precautions are to be utilized in addition to, not in place of, standard precautions.[2,3]

Standard Precautions

Standard precautions are exercised when caring for *all* patients, and include hand washing, gloves, mask and eye protection or face shield, gowns, handling of patient care equipment and linens, environmental controls, workplace controls, and patient location or placement.

Hand washing is performed after touching blood, body fluids, secretions, excretions, and contaminated items *even if gloves are worn*. Hands should be washed immediately after gloves are removed, between patient contacts, and when otherwise indicated to avoid the transfer of organisms to other patients or environments. It may be necessary to wash hands between procedures on the same patient to prevent cross-contamination of various body sites. Plain soap and water are recommended for routine use. Washing with an antimicrobial agent or waterless antiseptic may be utilized for control of outbreaks or hyperendemic infections.

Clean, nonsterile gloves are used when touching blood, body fluids, secretions, excretions, and contaminated items. Clean gloves should also be utilized when touching nonintact skin and mucous membranes. Gloves should be changed between tasks and procedures following contact with material that may contain a high concentration of microorganisms. Gloves should be removed and hands washed before touching noncontaminated items, environmental surfaces (phones, light switches, writing implements, etc.), or other patients.

Face masks, eye protection, and face shields that are fluid resistant are worn to protect mucous membranes of the eyes, nose, and mouth during patient care activities and the performance of procedures likely to generate splashes or sprays of blood, body fluids, secretions, excretions, and infectious materials. Masks that become significantly soiled, moistened by the user's exhaled vapor, or contaminated by fluids are immediately replaced, since loss of protective function occurs if the barrier device is completely saturated.

Clean, nonsterile gowns that are fluid resistant are used to protect the worker's skin and clothing during patient care activities and the performance of activities likely to generate splashes or sprays of blood, body fluids, secretions, and excretions. Soiled gowns should be replaced as soon as possible, since barrier protection is lost if the garment is saturated with contamination. Sleeve protectors, booties, and leggings should be used if a large volume of contamination or infectious material that is difficult to contain is anticipated.

Patient care equipment and linens soiled with blood, body fluids, secretions, and excretions should be handled so as to prevent skin and mucous membrane exposure, contamination of clothing, and transfer of microorganisms to other patients and environments. Reusable items should be cleaned and reprocessed to eliminate infectivity. Single-use items should be promptly discarded.

Environmental controls relate to hospital procedures for the decontamination of objects in patient care areas. Environmental surfaces, beds, bed rails, bedside equipment, and frequently touched surfaces should be cleaned and disinfected between patient uses.

Workplace controls (work practice controls) include proper disposal of needles, scalpels, and other sharp instruments. Workers should avoid recapping, excessive handling, and manipulation of sharp devices. Disposal should emphasize the use of self-sheathing devices, use of puncture-resistant containers, and replacement of sharps containers prior to overflowing. Patients who contaminate the environment or those who cannot assist in their own hygiene should be located in a private room if available.

Airborne Precautions

In addition to standard precautions, airborne precautions are utilized for patients known to be or suspected of being infected with microorganisms transmitted by airborne droplet nuclei. Airborne precautions also apply to small particle residue (5 μm or smaller) of evaporated droplets containing microorganisms that remain suspended in the air and can be dispersed widely by air currents over a long distance. Examples of infectious agents spread by this method are found in Table 154-13.[2]

The placement of patients in the ED requires a room with (1) monitored negative air pressure in relation to surrounding areas, (2) 6 to 12 air changes per hour, and (3) discharge of the room air to the outdoors or high-efficiency filtration of the air before it is circulated to other areas in the hospital. The door to the patient's room must be kept closed, and the patient must remain in the room. Movement and transportation of the patient should be limited. If movement is unavoidable, the patient should wear respiratory protection to avoid contamination of other areas within the hospital. Health care providers entering the room must wear respiratory protection, such as a personalized, fitted mask with efficient filters (approved particulate respirator).

Droplet Precautions

In addition to standard precautions, droplet precautions are employed for patients known to have or suspected of having serious illnesses transmitted by large particle droplets (>5 μm in size) that can be generated by the patient during talking, sneezing, or coughing or during the performance of procedures. Examples of infectious agents spread by this method are listed in Table 154-14.[2]

Patients should be placed in a private room. Special air handling and ventilation are not required, and the door may remain open. If a private room is not available, the patient may be placed in a room with other patients who have active infections with the same microorganism (i.e., cohorting). When this is not possible, maintain spatial separation of at least 3 ft between the infected patient and other patients and visitors. Patient transportation should be limited. Patients who must be moved for testing and procedures should don face masks to minimize the dispersal of droplets. Health care personnel should wear face masks when working within 3 ft of the patient.

Contact Precautions

In addition to standard precautions, contact precautions should be utilized with patients known to have or suspected of having serious illnesses easily transmitted by direct patient contact or by contact with items in the patient's environment. Examples of such infectious diseases are shown in Table 154-15.[2]

If the examination and care of a patient result in contact with infective materials and a high concentration of microorganisms (wound drainage or fecal material), changing of gloves is required. Hand washing with an antimicrobial agent or waterless antiseptic is required after removal of gloves. After glove removal and hand washing, workers should avoid contact with potentially contaminated environmental surfaces or items in the patient's room.

Upon entering the patient's room, a clean, nonsterile gown should be worn if one anticipates substantial contact with the patient or if the patient is incontinent or has diarrhea, a colostomy, an ileostomy, or wound drainage not contained by dressings. The gown should be removed prior to leaving the patient's room, and care should be taken to avoid contact with potentially contaminated environmental surfaces.

Transportation and movement should be limited. If the patient must be moved, one should ensure that contamination spread is minimized by large, bulky dressings. Bulky, absorbent, leak-proof dressings are utilized to *contain* contaminated secretions and therefore *limit* spread of disease.

Durable, multiuse medical equipment (e.g., blood pressure cuffs, stethoscopes, bedside commodes, etc.) should be dedicated to a single patient (or cohort of similarly infected patients) to avoid sharing between noninfected patients. Personnel who use personal medical equipment (e.g., stethoscopes) should thoroughly clean these items between using them on different patients if the possibility of contamination exists.

TABLE 154-14   Droplet-Spread Infectious Diseases

Invasive *Haemophilus influenzae* type B (including meningitis, pneumonia, epiglottitis, sepsis)
Invasive *Neisseria meningitidis* (including meningitis, pneumonia, sepsis)
Serious bacterial respiratory infections:
   Diphtheria (pharyngeal)
   Mycoplasma pneumonia
   Pertussis
   Pneumonic plague
   Streptococcal pharyngitis, pneumonia, scarlet fever
Serious viral infections:
   Adenovirus
   Influenza
   Mumps
   Parvovirus B19
   Rubella

Source: Modified from CDC.[2]

TABLE 154-13   Airborne-Spread Infectious Diseases

Rubeola (measles)
Varicella (including disseminated zoster)
Tuberculosis

Source: Modified from CDC.[2]

TABLE 154-15   Contact-Spread Infectious Diseases

Multidrug-resistant infections or colonization (gastrointestinal, respiratory, skin, wound sites)

Enteric infections with low infective dose or prolonged environmental survival:

   Clostridium difficile

   Enterohemorrhagic *Escherichia coli* O157:H7

   Shigella

   Hepatitis A

   Rotavirus

Respiratory syncytial virus

Parainfluenza virus

Enteroviral infections

Skin infections that are highly contagious or that may occur on dry skin:

   Diphtheria (cutaneous)

   Herpes simplex virus (neonatal or mucocutaneous)

   Impetigo

   Major, noncontained abscesses, cellulitis, decubiti

   Pediculosis

   Scabies

   Staphylococcal furunculosis

   Herpes zoster (disseminated or in an immunocompromised host)

Viral hemorrhagic conjunctivitis

Viral hemorrhagic infections (Ebola, Lassa, Marburg)

Source: Modified from CDC.[2]

COMMON OCCUPATIONAL EXPOSURES

Hepatitis

Viral hepatitis represents a group of infections that produce a large burden of disease in the United States, and is most commonly caused by one of five different viruses (known as hepatitis A, B, C, D, and E).

Hepatitis A and E are transmitted by the fecal-oral route and can cause extensive single-source outbreaks of disease. These viruses do not cause persistent infection, nor have they been identified as the causative agents of chronic viral hepatitis. In contrast, hepatitis B, C, and D are transmitted by several routes, including virus shed from mucous membranes or by percutaneous exposure. Each of these may cause persistent infection, and have been identified as etiologic agents in chronic viral hepatitis and cirrhosis. Persistent infections caused by HBV and HCV may ultimately result in the development of primary hepatocellular carcinoma. Hepatitis A and B can be prevented by vaccination.

Hepatitis A virus (HAV), a single-strand RNA picornavirus, is worldwide in its distribution, with the highest prevalence of infection in geographical regions with substandard water and sanitation. Occupationally acquired HAV is primarily contracted via the fecal-oral route, by either person-to-person contact or via ingestion of contaminated food or water. Rarely has HAV been transmitted by the transfusion of blood or blood products. Since HAV is associated with a substantial viremia that may persist for several weeks, percutaneous transmission of the virus is possible if health care workers receive a blood or body fluid exposure from a patient in the prodromal phase.

Passive immunity to HAV is conferred by intramuscular injection of immunoglobulin (IG). Preexposure administration of IG (0.02 mL/kg IM) confers protection for 1 to 2 months, while a higher dose (0.06 mL/kg IM) confers protection for 3 to 5 months. Postexposure use of IG (0.02 mL/kg IM) is more than 85 percent effective in preventing hepatitis, with greatest efficacy seen when it is administered early in the incubation period. Active immunity to HAV is conferred by two highly effective, formalin-inactivated vaccines currently licensed in the United States; Havrix (SmithKline Beecham) and Vaqta (Merck & Co., Inc.).[13] Primary vaccination consists of two doses, given at 0 and 6 to 12 months. Dosage differs depending on the age of the recipient, as well as the type and formulation of the vaccine being

administered. Both Havrix and Vaqta are licensed in two formulations, pediatric and adult. Health care personnel should always follow the manufacturer's dosage recommendations. Protective antibody levels develop in 94 to 100 percent of adults 1 month after the initial dose. All healthy persons exhibit protective levels of antibodies following the second dose.[13] Other preventive measures for health care providers include the use of standard precautions, with the addition of contact precautions when caring for patients who are incontinent or diapered. Acute postexposure medical examination, counseling, risk/benefit analysis, treatment (IG and HAV vaccine), and follow-up are required for exposed health care personnel.

HBV is a partially double-strand, circular DNA hepadnavirus with worldwide distribution. HBV is an established cause of acute and chronic hepatitis and cirrhosis, and is the cause of up to 80 percent of hepatocellular carcinomas. The virus is occupationally transmitted by parenteral or mucosal exposure to virus-containing blood or body fluids. The rate of HBV transmission to susceptible health care workers ranges from 6 to 30 percent after a single needlestick exposure to an HBV-positive patient.[9]

Passive immunity to HBV is available using HBIG, which is prepared from human plasma known to contain a high titer of antibody to the HBV surface antigen (anti-HBs). In the occupational setting, multiple doses of HBIG (0.06 mL/kg IM) initiated within 1 week following percutaneous exposure to HBsAg-positive blood provides an estimated 75 percent protection from HBV infection. Highest efficacy is found when HBIG is administered within 12 h of exposure. The efficacy of combination treatment with HBIG and the hepatitis B vaccine series has not been studied in the occupational setting. The combination of HBIG and HBV vaccine, as opposed to immunoglobulin or vaccine alone, conferred increased efficacy in the perinatal setting (70 to 75 percent vs. 85 to 95 percent), and is presumed to apply to occupational exposures as well.[9] Active immunity to HBV is conferred by two highly effective, recombinant vaccines commercially available in the United States; Engerix-B (SmithKline Beecham) and Recombivax HB (Merck & Co., Inc.). Primary vaccination consists of three doses, given on a 0-, 1-, and 6-month schedule. Dosage differs depending on the age of the recipient, as well as the type and formulation of the vaccine being administered. Both Engerix-B and Recombivax HB are licensed in two formulations, pediatric and adult. Health care personnel should always follow the manufacturer's dosage recommendations. Protective antibody levels develop in over 90 percent of healthy adults. A combined hepatitis A and B vaccine, Twinrix (SmithKline Beecham) is made of the antigenic components used in Havrix and Engerix-B. Primary vaccination consists of three doses, given on a 0-, 1-, and 6-month schedule, similar to that used for single antigen hepatitis B vaccines. The utility of this combination vaccine in the setting of occupational exposures is unknown. Other HBV preventive measures for health care providers include the use of standard precautions. Acute postexposure medical examination, counseling, risk/benefit analysis, treatment (HBIG and HBV vaccine), and follow-up are required for exposed health care personnel.

Hepatitis C virus (HCV) is an enveloped, single-strand RNA flavivirus. HCV is the most common chronic blood-borne infection in the United States and a major cause of chronic liver disease worldwide. Chronic hepatitis develops in approximately 60 to 70 percent of HCV-infected patients and may progress to cirrhosis (10 to 20 percent) and hepatocellular carcinoma (1 to 5 percent).[14] The most common and efficient route of HCV transmission is parenteral. The average incidence of anti-HCV seroconversion after unintentional needle sticks or sharps exposure from an HCV-positive source is 1.8 percent (range, 0 to 7 percent).[14]

Neither IG nor antiviral therapy (interferon or rifampin) is recommended as postexposure prophylaxis. No vaccine currently exists to prevent HCV. Preventive measures must focus on limiting exposure risk via standard precautions. Acute postexposure medical examination, counseling, and follow-up disease monitoring are required for exposed health care personnel.

Hepatitis D virus (HDV) is a single-strand, circular RNA virus. The genome of HDV is contained within an envelope provided by HBV and HBV surface proteins are required for HDV viral assembly. HDV infection can occur simultaneously with HBV infection (coinfection) or as a superinfection of patients with chronic HBV infection. Occupational transmission is primarily by parenteral contact with blood.

Prevention of HDV depends on prevention of HBV infection (immunization) and reducing exposure to blood and body fluids. No vaccine for HDV currently exists. Preventive measures for health care providers include the use of standard precautions. Acute postexposure medical examination, counseling, risk/benefit analysis, treatment (HBIG and HBV vaccine), and follow-up are required for exposed health care personnel.

Hepatitis E virus (HEV) is a nonenveloped, single-strand RNA calicivirus. HEV is the major etiologic agent of enterically transmitted non-A, non-B hepatitis worldwide. The virus is endemic and epidemic in developing countries that lack the infrastructure to ensure adequate sanitation and water purification. HEV is spread primarily by the fecal-oral route.

No vaccine for HEV currently exists. Preventive measures for health care providers include the use of standard precautions, with the addition of contact precautions when caring for patients who are incontinent. Acute postexposure medical examination, counseling, and follow-up are required for exposed health care personnel.

Human Immunodeficiency Virus

HIV is a lentivirus with an enveloped genome of two identical, single-strand RNA molecules. There are two types of human lentiviruses: HIV-1, the predominant HIV type in most parts of the world, and HIV-2, primarily found in West Africa. The capacity of HIV to recombine and generate mosaic genotypes confounds treatment efforts and vaccine development. The virus mutates at varying rates over time in various individuals, and data suggest that the host's ongoing immune response is a driving force for genetic variation.

Occupational exposure occurs with percutaneous, mucous membrane, or dermal exposure to HIV-infected blood or body fluids. The average risk of HIV transmission after a percutaneous exposure to HIV-infected blood is approximately 0.3 percent.[9] Risk of infection after percutaneous injury is increased for deep injury, injury by a device previously placed in the source patient's artery or vein, visible blood on the device causing the injury, and death of the source patient as a result of AIDS within 60 days postexposure. The risks of acquiring HIV after mucous membrane and nonintact skin exposure to HIV-infected blood are approximately 0.09 percent and less than 0.09 percent respectively.[9] Risk of infection after mucous membrane or dermal exposure is increased for large-volume exposures or those involving mucous membranes or skin which has lost its integrity. Chemoprophylaxis should be recommended to exposed workers after occupational exposures associated with highest risk for HIV transmission. The U.S. Public Health Service regularly updates and publishes guidelines relating to postexposure prophylaxis for health care workers exposed to blood-borne pathogens including HIV, HBV, and HCV. Detailed recommendations are discussed earlier in this chapter and in Tables 154-3 through 154-12.

If warranted, chemoprophylaxis should begin as soon as possible after the exposure, ideally within 1 to 2 h. Animal studies show that antivirals are less effective if initiated more than 24 to 36 h after the exposure event.[9] No vaccine currently exists to prevent HIV infection. A large consortium of public health agencies and academic institutions including the World Health Organization (WHO), Joint United Nations Program on HIV/AIDS (UNAIDS), International AIDS Vaccine Initiative (IAVI), U. S. National Institutes of Health (NIH), and the Centers for Disease Control and Prevention (CDC) have been working

to develop an HIV vaccine. A number of experimental vaccines are currently undergoing phase II and III clinical trials.[15]

HIV preventive measures for health care providers include the use of standard precautions. Acute postexposure medical examination,[9] counseling,[11] risk/benefit analysis, treatment (basic or expanded PEP regimen), and follow-up are required for exposed health care personnel.

Tuberculosis

Four subspecies of mycobacteria exist, each of which can cause tubercular disease: *Mycobacterium africanum, Mycobacterium bovis, Mycobacterium microti,* and *Mycobacterium tuberculosis. Mycobacterium tuberculosis* is the primary cause of TB in humans.

Transmission of TB occurs through inhalation of aerosolized bacilli. As few as 1 to 10 bacilli can cause infection, but only about 20 percent of exposed individuals become infected.

Preventive measures include environmental controls (rooms with negative-pressure ventilation and ultraviolet radiation) in health care settings, application of directly observed therapy, and vaccine development. Occupational exposures for health care providers can be mitigated through use of standard and airborne precautions. These measures include the routine use of National Institute for Occupational Safety and Health (NIOSH)-approved particulate filtration respirator (PFR) masks during patient encounters at risk for TB. The most effective control measure is curative treatment of patients with infectious pulmonary TB. While bacille Calmette-Guérin (BCG) vaccine is the most widely administered of all vaccines worldwide, questions regarding its efficacy and its tendency to cause a dermal hypersensitivity reaction to purified protein derivative (PPD) has precluded its use in the United States. The CDC has advocated preventive chemotherapy (antibiotics) and vaccine development for those at risk for developing active TB; however, research does not currently support these measures.[16] Routine annual or semiannual PPD testing or chest x-rays may be warranted if personnel work in high-risk environments.

Measles

Rubeola, or measles, is an acute viral illness caused by a single-strand RNA paramyxovirus. Worldwide, measles is the most common vaccine-preventable cause of death among children. Obstacles to measles eradication in the United States include increasing numbers of susceptible children and infants who are not immunized, and circulation of measles virus from other geographic regions of the world.

Transmission of measles is primarily person-to-person via large respiratory droplets. Airborne transmission via aerosolized droplet nuclei has been documented in closed areas. While isolation of patients is the mainstay of outbreak control, this mechanism is not effective in preventing subsequent cases. Primary prevention by immunization is preferred.

Measles vaccine is available in monovalent form as Attenuvax (Merck & Co., Inc.). Combination vaccines include measles-mumps-rubella (MMR) (M-M-RII, Merck & Co., Inc.) and measles-rubella (MR) (M-R-Vax, Merck & Co., Inc.). All vaccines are highly effective and are administered subcutaneously in a 2-dose schedule, with the second administration occurring at least 1 month after the initial dose. Health care personnel should always follow manufacturer's dosage recommendations. According to the ACIP, MMR is the vaccine of choice when protection against any of the three diseases is required, unless any of its component vaccines is contraindicated.

Adults who may be at increased risk for exposure to and transmission of measles (including persons who work in health care facilities) should be considered for vaccination. For postexposure prophylaxis, measles vaccine provides permanent protection and may prevent disease if given within 72 h of exposure. This route of prophylaxis is preferable to using immune globulin. Immunoglobulin (IG) may prevent or modify disease if given within 6 days of exposure. Any immunity conferred by IG is temporary.[17] Preventive measures for health care providers include use of standard and airborne precautions, as well as vaccination if immunization status is unclear.

Mumps

Mumps is an acute viral illness caused by a single-strand RNA paramyxovirus. Humans are the only known host.

Transmission of mumps occurs through airborne transmission or direct contact with infected droplet nuclei or saliva.

While isolation of patients is the mainstay of outbreak control, this mechanism is not effective in preventing subsequent cases. Primary prevention by immunization is preferred. Mumps vaccine is available in monovalent form as Mumpsvax (Merck & Co., Inc.). Combination vaccines include measles-mumps-rubella (MMR) (M-M-R II, Merck & Co., Inc.) and rubella-mumps (Biavax II, Merck Co., Inc.). All vaccines are highly effective and are administered subcutaneously in a 2-dose schedule, with the second administration occurring at least 1 month after the initial dose. Health care personnel should always follow the manufacturer's dosage recommendations. According to the ACIP, MMR is the vaccine of choice when protection against any of the three diseases is required, unless any of its component vaccines is contraindicated.

Adults who may be at increased risk for exposure to and transmission of mumps (including persons who work in health care facilities) should be considered for vaccination. For postexposure prophylaxis, neither mumps immune globulin nor IG is effective and they are not recommended for that use.[17] Mumps vaccine after exposure is not harmful and may provide protection against subsequent exposures. Preventive measures for health care providers include use of standard and droplet precautions, as well as vaccination if immunization status is unclear.

Rubella

Rubella, or German measles, is an exanthematous viral illness caused by an enveloped RNA togavirus. Some of the most important consequences of rubella are miscarriages, stillbirths, fetal anomalies, and therapeutic abortions that result when rubella infection occurs during early pregnancy.

Transmission of rubella is due to person-to-person spread via airborne transmission or droplets shed from the respiratory secretions of infected persons. While isolation of patients is the mainstay of outbreak control, this mechanism is not effective in preventing subsequent cases. Primary prevention by immunization is preferred.

Rubella vaccine is available in monovalent form as Meruvax (Merck & Co., Inc.). Combination vaccines include measles-mumps-rubella (MMR) (M-M-R II, Merck & Co., Inc.), measles-rubella (MR) (M-R-Vax, Merck & Co., Inc.), and rubella-mumps (Biavax, Merck & Co., Inc.). All vaccines are highly effective and are administered subcutaneously in a 2-dose schedule, with the second administration occurring at least 1 month after the initial dose. Health care personnel should always follow the manufacturer's dosage recommendations. According to the ACIP, MMR is the vaccine of choice when protection against any of the three diseases is required, unless any of its component vaccines is contraindicated.

Adults who may be at increased risk for exposure to and transmission of rubella (including persons who work in health care facilities) should be considered for vaccination. For postexposure prophylaxis, neither rubella vaccine nor IG is effective.[17] Vaccination after exposure is not harmful and may possibly avert later disease. Preventive measures for health care providers include use of standard and droplet precautions, as well as vaccination if immunization status is unclear.

Varicella and Herpes Zoster

Varicella zoster virus (VZV) is a double-strand DNA herpes virus. Primary infection with VZV results in varicella (chickenpox). Herpes zoster (shingles) is the result of recurrent VZV infection. Chickenpox is highly contagious and poses a serious nosocomial and occupational infection risk.

Transmission of VZV occurs person-to-person from infected respiratory tract secretions. Transmission may also occur by direct contact or inhalation of aerosols from vesicular fluid of skin lesions of acute varicella or zoster.

When administered within 96 h of exposure, varicella zoster immunoglobulin (VZIG) may modify or prevent clinical varicella its and complications. VZIG is indicated for use in susceptible individuals at risk for complications who have had significant exposure (prolonged direct contact). Of note, VZIG provides temporary protection and should be given as soon as possible after the exposure. Susceptible workers with significant exposure should be furloughed from work from days 10 to 21 postexposure. Receipt of VZIG does not change this recommendation.

Active immunity is provided by the VZV vaccine Oka (Merck & Co., Inc.). The vaccine is administered subcutaneously in a 2-dose schedule, with the second dose given 4 to 8 weeks after the initial dose. Health care personnel should always follow the manufacturer's dosage recommendations. Postexposure use of varicella vaccine may prevent infection.[18] Preventive measures for health care providers include use of standard, airborne, and contact precautions, as well as vaccination if immunization status is unclear. Medical providers who are susceptible to varicella should avoid infected patients if immune caregivers are available.

Influenza

Influenza is a highly infectious viral illness caused by a single-strand RNA orthomyxovirus. Influenza A and B are the two types of influenza virus that cause epidemic human disease. Peak influenza activity levels are found in temperate climates between late December and early March.

Influenza virus is transmitted via aerosolized or droplet transmission from the respiratory tract of infected persons. A less important mode of transmission of droplets is by direct contact.

Two measures are available to reduce the impact of influenza: immunoprophylaxis with inactivated (killed virus) vaccine, and chemoprophylaxis with influenza-specific antiviral agents. Antiviral agents for influenza are an adjunct to vaccine and are not a substitute for vaccine. A trivalent vaccine is prepared on an annual basis (typically two strains of influenza A, one strain of influenza B) representing the influenza viruses likely to circulate in the upcoming winter. Immunity following vaccination rarely exceeds 1 year. Vaccine efficacy varies depending on the age and immunocompetence of the vaccine recipient and the degree of similarity between the viruses in the vaccine and those in circulation. The vaccine is most effective if administration precedes exposure by no more than 2 to 4 months. Health care providers should receive annual vaccination, ideally in October. One dose of the vaccine is administered by the intramuscular route. Health care personnel should always follow the manufacturer's dosage recommendations. Intranasally administered, live, attenuated influenza virus vaccines (LAIVs) are under development in the United States. Monovalent, bivalent, and trivalent formulations have been studied. An application for FDA licensure is under review.

Four antiviral agents are approved for preventing or treating influenza. Dosage recommendations and duration of administration vary by age group and medical conditions. Amantadine and rimantadine are FDA approved for both prophylaxis and treatment of influenza type A in persons 1 year of age and older. Both agents come as oral formulations (tablets, capsules, and syrup). Zanamivir (available as an inhaled powder) is approved for treatment of influenza A or B in persons 7 years of age and older who have been symptomatic for no more than 2 days. Zanamivir is not approved for prophylaxis. Oseltamivir (available as a tablet), is approved for the treatment of influenza A and B in persons 1 year of age and older who have been symptomatic for no more than 2 days. This agent is approved for prophylaxis of influenza infection among persons 13 years of age and older.[19] Additional preventive measures include use of standard, airborne, and contact precautions.

Scabies

Scabies is a highly contagious, pruritic skin disorder caused by an arachnid, *Sarcoptes scabiei* var. *hominis.* The human scabies mite is endemic in many developing countries, where the prevalence ranges from 20 to 100 percent.

Human scabies is transmitted primarily by direct personal contact with infected individuals. Although less common, transmission may also occur by contact with contaminated bedding and clothing. The mite has been found to survive for 2 to 3 days on inanimate objects. The scabies mite is motionless at room temperature and lacks the ability to jump or fly from person to person.

The average person infected with scabies harbors 10 to 15 live adult female mites at any given time. Patients with crusted (Norwegian) scabies, an atypical form of scabies, harbor mite populations in the thousands to millions. This form is often seen in physically or mentally handicapped, immunocompromised, or institutionalized persons. Some sources advise testing patients who exhibit crusted scabies for HIV. Preventive measures for health care providers include use of standard and contact precautions in patients with pruritic eruptions.

Pediculosis

Pediculosis is a dermal infestation caused by a parasitic insect (louse). Infestations in various body regions (e.g., head, thorax, and groin) are caused by the head louse *(Pediculus humanus capitis),* the body louse *(Pediculus humanus corporis),* and the crab louse *(Phthirus pubis).* Adult lice are about the size of a sesame seed and can live for up to 30 days on an infested individual. Adult forms also feed on blood and may survive up to 2 days on inanimate objects.

Lice are transmitted by direct contact with infected individuals or common use of infected bedding, clothing, or combs, brushes, or headgear. Prevention of occupational exposures in health care providers includes use of standard and contact precautions.

Latex Allergy

Latex is a milky cytosol secreted by lactifer cells from the rubber tree, *Hevea brasiliensis.*[20] The cytosol contains *cis*-1,4 polyisoprene, which is immunologically inert. The manufacturing process results in the cross-linking of chains of polyisoprene, yielding a polymer that exhibits excellent tensile strength, elasticity, and barrier capacity.[20] Such desirable characteristics have lead to the use of rubber latex in the manufacture of many medical products, including gloves (for surgery, examination, and housekeeping and cleaning), intravascular devices (balloon catheters, intravenous tubing, and ports), airway devices (nasopharyngeal airways, endotracheal tubes, and oxygen masks), tourniquets, blood pressure cuffs, electrocardiogram leads, tape, and dressings.

Immune reactions to latex products may take three forms: irritant, contact dermatitis (type IV), and IgE (type I). Irritant reactions are nonimmune in nature and result in dry dermal erythema limited to the site of contact. Contact dermatitis occurs as a result of dermal exposure to chemicals used in the manufacturing of latex products. Thiurams and thiazoles are the most common chemicals to induce this type IV response. This reaction, which may extend beyond the site of contact, results in a dry dermal erythema, pruritus, weeping, and vesiculation. Such loss of skin integrity permits the access of latex proteins to the immune system and may result in an IgE-mediated response. IgE (type I) response is an immunologic reaction to protein allergens contained in latex. Clinical manifestations of such reactions include urticaria, asthma, rhinitis, angioedema, laryngeal edema, and anaphylaxis. IgE reactions may occur as a result of mucosal, dermal, contact, or inhalational exposure. Cornstarch powder, which serves as a lubricant to ease the donning of latex gloves, binds and aerosolizes protein allergens, leading to inhalation exposure.

At highest risk of developing IgE-mediated latex allergy are individuals with high exposure to latex and those who are atopic. Workers in industries that make rubber products (e.g., tire manufacturers and doll makers) and those who use rubber products (e.g., housekeepers, hairdressers, and health care workers) are at high risk of developing this allergy. While anyone can develop latex allergy, specific populations are at higher risk. Individuals likely to develop latex allergy include those with a history of multiple allergies (including dermal, respiratory, oral, or facial reactions to latex or rubber products), asthma (reactive airways disease), eczema, multiple food allergies (especially to bananas, avocados, and other tropical fruit), frequent surgical or dental procedures, multiple urogenital procedures (e.g., bladder, vaginal, and rectal), spina bifida and related conditions of spinal dysraphism, congenital urinary anomalies, or sensitivity to ethylene oxide (a sterilizing agent).

Since September 1998, the U.S. Food and Drug Administration has promulgated uniform labeling for all medical products. Many latex-free medical products exist on the market and may be substituted for currently used products. Prevention of disease in health care workers is critical and requires the use of synthetic or low-allergen powder-free gloves.[20] NIOSH and the CDC have published several documents that describe the hazards of latex allergy and suggest steps health care providers may take to protect themselves.[21] To protect themselves from latex exposure and allergy in the workplace, health care personnel may: use nonlatex gloves for workplace activities that do not involve contact with infectious materials; use synthetic or low-allergen powder-free gloves when handling infectious materials; avoid oil-based hand lotions or creams when wearing latex gloves (to prevent glove deterioration); wash hands with mild soap and dry thoroughly upon removal of latex gloves; frequently clean work areas and equipment contaminated with latex-containing dust; obtain education and training regarding latex allergy; and recognize the symptoms of latex allergy. Health care providers should be aware that hypoallergenic latex gloves do not reduce the risk of latex allergy, but do reduce reactions to chemical additives in latex.

SARS

As of this writing (May 2003), Severe Acute Respiratory Syndrome (SARS) is thought to be due to coronavirus, and is characterized as asymptomatic or mild, moderate, or severe. Clinical criteria of moderate disease are temperature of >38°C (100.4°F) and one or more findings of respiratory illness; additional criteria for severe disease include radiographic evidence of pneumonia, or respiratory distress syndrome, or autopsy findings consistent with pneumonia or respiratory distress syndrome without an identifiable cause. In addition, epidemiologic criteria for disease are travel within 10 days of onset of symptoms to an area with SARS, or close contact within 10 days of onset of symptoms of a person suspected to have SARS. As of this writing there is no diagnostic testing available outside of a research setting. Infection control guidelines consist of hand washing with soap and water or alcohol-based hand rubs for all possible contacts. Infection control of EMS vehicles with potential contamination includes the use of any EPA-registered detergent-disinfectant currently used by healthcare facilities for environmental sanitation. All surfaces and equipment should be cleaned. At ED triage, questions about SARS exposure should be asked. If positive, a surgical mask should be placed on the patient and the patient should be kept away from others in the waiting room. In the ED or EMS vehicles, full personal protective attire should be used. Health care personnel should use an N-95 filtering disposable respirator. Patients need admission for medical care, but not for infection control, unless infection control is not possible outside of a hospital setting (prison, homeless shelter, dormitory, etc.). In April, 2003, SARS was added to the list of quarantinable communicable diseases in the US. Since SARS information is changing rapidly, the CDC should be consulted for the most recent case and epidemiologic definitions, laboratory testing, travel advisories, and infection control guidelines. (http://www.cdc.gov/ncidod/sars).

REFERENCES

1. U.S. Department of Labor: Occupational Exposure to Blood-borne Pathogens: Precautions for Emergency Responders. Washington, DC, OSHA 3130, 1992.
2. Centers for Disease Control and Prevention, Hospital Infection Control Practices Advisory Committee: Guideline for isolation precautions in hospitals: I. Evolution of isolation practices. *Am J Infect Control* 24:24, 1996.
3. Centers for Disease Control and Prevention, Hospital Infection Control Practices Advisory Committee: Guideline for isolation precautions in hospitals: II. Recommendations for isolation precautions in hospitals. *Am J Infect Control* 24:32, 1996.
4. Occupational Safety and Health Act of 1970. 91st Congress, Pub. L 91-596, section 2193, December 1970, amended by Pub. L 101-553, section 3101, November 1990, amended by Pub. L 106-430, section 3067. Washington, DC, November 2000.
5. U.S. Department of Labor: Bloodborne Pathogens Standard. Title 29 CFR, part 1910.130, July 1992, revised April 2001, Washington, DC.
6. Needlestick Safety and Prevention Act. 106th Congress, Pub. L 106-430, section 3067, Washington, DC, November 2000.
7. Kelen GD, Hansen KN, Green GB, et al: Determinants of emergency department procedure- and condition-specific universal (barrier) precaution requirements for optimal provider protection. *Ann Emerg Med* 25:743, 1995.
8. Centers for Disease Control and Prevention, Immunization of Health-Care Workers: Recommendations of the Advisory Committee on Immunization Practices (ACIP) and the Hospital Infection Control Practices Advisory Committee (HICPAC). *MMWR* 46:1, 1997.
9. Centers for Disease Control and Prevention: Updated U.S. Public Health Service Guidelines for the Management of Occupational Exposures to HBV, HCV, and HIV and Recommendations for Postexposure Prophylaxis. *MMWR* 50:1, 2001.
10. Moran GJ: Emergency department management of blood and body fluid exposures. *Ann Emerg Med* 35:47, 2000.
11. Centers for Disease Control and Prevention: Updated guidelines for HIV counseling, testing, and referral. *MMWR* 50:1, 2001.
12. Demangone D: HIV: Acute Retroviral Syndrome and Occupational Exposure Guidelines. *Emerg Med Specialty Rep* Suppl. 538Z, 2002.
13. Centers for Disease Control and Prevention: Prevention of hepatitis A through active or passive immunization: Recommendations of the Advisory Committee on Immunization Practices (ACIP). *MMWR* 48:1, 1999.
14. Centers for Disease Control and Prevention: Recommendations for prevention and control of hepatitis C virus (HCV) infection and HCV-related chronic infection. *MMWR* 47:1, 1998.
15. Centers for Disease Control and Prevention, National Center for HIV, STD, & TB Prevention: Testing a Vaccine Designed to Help Curb the Devastating Toll of HIV in the Developing World. Update Atlanta, February 1999.
16. Centers for Disease Control and Prevention: Development of new vaccines for tuberculosis: Recommendations of the Advisory Council for the Elimination of Tuberculosis (ACET). *MMWR* 47:1, 1998.
17. Centers for Disease Control and Prevention: Measles, mumps, and rubella-Vaccine use and strategies for elimination of measles, rubella, and congenital rubella syndrome and control of mumps: Recommendations of the Advisory Committee on Immunization Practices (ACIP). *MMWR* 47:1, 1998.
18. Centers for Disease Control and Prevention: Prevention of varicella: Update recommendations of the Advisory Committee on Immunization Practices (ACIP). *MMWR* 48:1, 1999.
19. Centers for Disease Control and Prevention: Prevention and control of influenza: Recommendations of the Advisory Committee on Immunization Practices (ACIP). *MMWR* 51:1, 2002.
20. Kelly KJ, Walsh-Kelly CM: Latex allergy: A patient and health care system emergency. *Ann Emerg Med* 32:723, 1998.
21. Centers for Disease Control and Prevention: Preventing Allergic Reactions to Natural Rubber Latex in the Workplace. Publication 97-135. Atlanta, Department of Health and Human Services, National Institute for Occupational Safety and Health, 1997.

155 PHARMACOLOGY OF ANTIMICROBIALS, ANTIFUNGALS, AND ANTIVIRALS
Ralph H. Raasch

This chapter reviews the basic pharmacology of commonly prescribed antimicrobial agents used in the emergency department. Topics discussed are mechanisms of action, indications for use in the emergency department, contraindications, adverse drug reactions, dosage adjustments for renal or hepatic insufficiency, use in pregnancy, and important drug interactions. Additional information regarding the treatment of specific infections will be found in other chapters of this text and Principles of Drug Interactions are discussed in Chap. 157.

ANTIBACTERIAL DRUGS

Effective antibacterial drugs have the ability to either inhibit the growth of (bacteriostatic effect) or kill (bactericidal effect) bacteria. These drugs have an antibacterial effect as a result of a variety of mechanisms, including the inhibition of cell wall synthesis, inhibition of intrabacterial protein synthesis, alteration in nucleic acid metabolism, or intrabacterial enzyme inhibition (Table 155-1). The mechanism of action does not necessarily correlate with bacteriostatic or bactericidal effects, which are also highly dependent on the concentration of antibiotic to which bacteria are exposed. Drugs of choice for most infections are not based on a bacteriostatic or bactericidal effect of an agent but rather on whether the drug reaches the site of infection in adequate quantities, the spectrum of the agent, its safety, and its cost.

Mechanisms of Action

CELL WALL-ACTIVE AGENTS   Beta-lactam (penicillins, cephalosporins) and glycopeptide antibiotics (vancomycin, teicoplanin) must bind to receptors in the bacterial cell wall in order to cause an antibacterial effect. The target receptors (there are at least seven) for

TABLE 155-1   Mechanisms of Action of Antibacterial Drugs

Cell wall active agents
Penicillins
Vancomycin
Cephalosporins
Teicoplanin
Protein synthesis inhibitors
Aminoglycosides
Macrolides
Linezolid
Tetracyclines
Clindamycin
Quinupristin/dalfopristin
Nucleic acid inhibitors
Quinolones
Rifampin
Nitrofurantoin
Enzyme inhibitors
Sulfonamides
Trimethoprim

Source: From Hardman et al.[1]

penicillins and cephalosporins are collectively called *penicillin-binding proteins* (PBPs). With binding to the PBPs, autolytic enzymes within the cell wall are activated, resulting in the deterioration of the peptidoglycan component of the cell wall, cell wall weakening, and eventual cell lysis. Glycopeptide antibiotics bind to a terminal dipeptide (alanine-alanine) in the cell wall peptidoglycan and then by steric hindrance prevent the necessary cross-linking for a competent cell wall structure. At usual doses, β-lactam and glycopeptide antibiotics are bactericidal. Resistance can arise to these antibiotics due to mutations in the PBPs, leading to markedly reduced beta-lactam binding (e.g., in oxacillin-resistant *Staphylococcus aureus* or penicillin-resistant *Streptococcus pneumoniae*), or when the terminal dipeptide mutates to a lactate-alanine (e.g., vancomycin-resistant *Enterococcus faecium*) that markedly reduces the level of vancomycin binding.

PROTEIN SYNTHESIS INHIBITORS   Several classes of antibacterial drugs bind to ribosomes within bacteria, thereby blocking necessary protein synthesis. Aminoglycosides and tetracyclines bind to the 30S ribosomal subunit, whereas macrolide antibiotics and clindamycin bind to the 50S subunit. Ribosomal binding inhibits transfer RNA function, thereby decreasing the amount of protein synthesis. In order for these ribosomal binding drugs to work, they must enter the cell through the cell wall and bind in adequate concentrations to reversibly inhibit protein synthesis. Resistance mechanisms arise when there is reduced cell wall permeability, an active efflux pump that removes the antibiotic from the cell, or ribosomal binding-site mutations that decrease antibiotic affinity. All these mechanisms may result in resistance to each of the drug classes listed above.

NUCLEIC ACID INHIBITORS   Fluoroquinolone antibiotics inhibit DNA gyrase, the enzyme responsible for DNA unwinding for transcription and then recoiling during bacterial replication. These agents must reach the nucleus of the bacterial cell in order to provoke these effects; hence resistance can arise when cell wall permeability is reduced, active efflux occurs, or a DNA gyrase mutation has arisen that reduces fluoroquinolone binding. Rifampin is a broad-spectrum antimicrobial agent active against many gram-positive and gram-negative bacteria and mycobacteria. Rifampin inhibits RNA synthesis by binding to DNA-dependent RNA polymerase, thereby blocking the initiation of RNA chain formation. Nitrofurantoin is modified by bacterial metabolism to a compound that damages DNA. Susceptible bacteria rarely become resistant to nitrofurantoin.

ENZYME INHIBITORS   Sulfonamides and trimethoprim block sequential steps in the formation of folic acid. Sulfonamides inhibit dihydropteroate synthase, the enzyme that converts *para*-aminobenzoic acid (PABA) to dihydrofolic acid; then trimethoprim inhibits dihydrofolate reductase, the enzyme that converts dihydrofolic to tetrahydrofolic acid. Resistance to these drugs can arise by enzyme mutations that reduce the affinity of the sulfonamide or trimethoprim to their respective enzyme targets.[1]

Table 155-2 summarizes the classification and names of most antibiotics within each antibiotic class referred to above. Available routes of administration are also listed.[2]

Indications in the Emergency Department and Drugs of Choice

Drugs of choice for specific infections are based largely on clinical experience of effectiveness, supported by clinical trial reports and case series, with an acceptable level of adverse events. Successful effectiveness is based on the knowledge of the likely bacterial pathogen responsible for a specific infection type and the usual antimicrobial spectrum of antibiotics. Alternate drugs of choice are selected in cases of resistance to an initial drug, a history of intolerance or allergy to the drug of choice, or because of a higher risk of adverse events.

TABLE 155-2   Classification of Antibacterial Drugs with Common Trade Names

Penicillins	Cephalosporins
Natural penicillins	*First generation*
Penicillin G—IV, PO*	Cefazolin (Ancef)—IV
Penicillin V (Pen-Vee K)—PO	Cephalexin (Keflex)—PO
	Cefadroxil (Duricef)—PO
Aminopenicillins	Cephapirin (Cefadyl)—PO
Ampicillin (Omnipen)—IV, PO	
Amoxicillin (Amoxcil)—PO	*Second generation*
	Cefaclor (Ceclor)—PO
Penicillinase-resistant penicillins	Cefotetan (Cefotan)—IV
Oxacillin (Bactocill)—IV, PO	Cefoxitin (Mefoxin)—IV
Nafcillin (Unipen)—IV, PO	Cefprozil (Cefzil)—PO
Dicloxacillin (Dynapen)—PO	Cefuroxime (Zinacef)—IV
Cloxacillin (Cloxapen)—PO	Cefuroxine axetil (Ceftin)—PO
Antipseudomonal penicillins	*Third generation*
Ticarcillin (Ticar)—IV	Cefotaxine (Claforan)—IV
Piperacillin (Pipracil)—IV	Ceftriaxone (Rocephin)—IV
	Ceftazidime (Fortaz)—IV
β-lactam–β-lactamase inhibitor combination	Cefpodoxime (Vantin)—PO
Amoxicillin-clavulanic acid	Ceftibutin (Cedax)—PO
(Augmentin)—PO	
Ampicillin-sulbactam (Unasyn)—IV	*Fourth generation*
Ticarcillin-clavulanic acid	Cefepime (Maxipime)—IV
(Timentin)—IV	
Piperacillin-tazobactam (Zosyn)—IV	*Macrolides/tetracyclines*
	Erythromycin (Erythrocin)—IV, PO
Monobactams and carbapenems	Azithromycin (Zithromax)—IV, PO
Aztreonam (Azactam)—IV	Clarithromycin (Biaxin)—PO
Imipenem (Primaxin)—IV	Tetracycline (Tetracyn)—PO
Meropenem (Merrem)—IV	Minocycline (Minocin)—PO
Ertapenem (Invanz)—IV	Doxycycline (Vibramycin)—IV, PO
Aminoglycosides	*Folate Inhibitors*
Amikacin (Amikin)—IV	Trimethoprim-sulfamethoxaxole
Gentamicin (Garamycin)—IV	(Bactrim, Septra)—IV, PO
Neomycin (Mycifradin)—PO	Trimethoprim (Trimpex)—PO
Netilmicin (Netromycin)—IV	
Streptomycin—IM, IV	*Miscellaneous*
Tobramycin (Nebcin)—IV	Clindamycin (Cleocin)—IV, PO
	Vancomycin (Vancocin)—IV, PO
Fluoroquinolones	Metronidazole (Flagyl)—IV, PO
Ciprofloxacin (Cipro)—IV, PO	Linezolid (Zyvox)—IV, PO
Levofloxacin (Levaquin)—IV, PO	Nitrofurantoin (Macrodantin)—PO
Gatifloxacin (Tequin)—IV, PO	Quinupristin/dalfopristin
Moxifloxacin (Avelox)—IV, PO	(Synercid)—IV

* Usual routes of administration.
Source: From Koda–Kimble et al.[2]

Taking into account those infections most likely to be present in emergency department patients and the most likely pathogens involved in these infections, Table 155-3 summarizes drugs of choice for these infections.[2]

Antibiotic Dosage and Dosage Adjustments

Providing an antibiotic in adequate dosage is one of the requirements for successful treatment. Drug dosage usually takes into account achievable serum and tissue levels and the concentrations necessary (determined in the laboratory) to inhibit the growth of susceptible bacteria. These empirical doses are then usually evaluated in clinical trials for various indications to ensure that positive treatment outcomes occur at one or more tested doses. Thus standard dosing guidelines are available that usually will result in successful treatment, assuming that a susceptible organism is present and issues regarding drug penetration to the site of infection (i.e., abscess) are not present. In cases

TABLE 155-3 Antibiotics of Choice for Treatment of Common Adult Infections in the ED

SITE/TYPE OF INFECTION	SUSPECTED ORGANISMS	DRUG OF CHOICE	ALTERNATIVE
Respiratory			
Pharyngitis	Group A streptococci	Penicillin V	Macrolide
Bronchitis, otitis,	S. pneumoniae	amoxicillin, amox/clav,	Macrolide or doxycycline
Acute sinusitis	H. influenzae	or cefuroxime	
Epiglottitis	H. influenzae,	Ceftriaxone	Cefuroxime
	Group A streptococci		
Community-acquired pneumonia			
Normal host	S. pneumoniae, viral,	Azithromycin	Levofloxacin
	Mycoplasma		
Aspiration	Aerobes and anaerobes	Clindamycin	Cefoxitin
Alcoholic	S. pneumoniae, Klebsiella	Ceftriaxone	Levofloxacin
Urinary tract infection	E. coli and other enteric	Amoxicillin or TMP/SMX	Ciprofloxacin, cephalexin,
	Gram-negative rods		or nitrofurantoin
Sexually-transmitted infections			
Urethritis	N. gonorrhea, Chlamydia	Ceftriaxone	Ciprofloxacin
Genital ulcers	Treponema pallidum,	Penicillin G	Doxycycline
	Herpes simplex virus	Acyclovir	Valacyclovir
Skin/soft tissue			
Cellulitis	Group A streptococci,	Cephalexin	Dicloxacillin
	S. aureus		
Necrotizing Fasciitis	Polymicrobial	Imipenem or meropenem	
		Plus vancomycin	
Fresh/brackish water infections	Mixed flora, Aeromonas	TMP/SMX	Fluoroquinolone
Cat bite	Pasteurella, mixed flora	Amox/clav	Clindamycin and
			ciprofloxacin
Meningitis			
Normal host	S. pneumoniae,	Ceftriaxone and	
	N. meningitides, S. aureus	vancomycin	
Immunocompromised or >50	Listeria, H. influenzae	add Ampicillin	
Acute Abdomen (perforation)	Gram-negative rods, anaerobes,	AM/SB or Pip/TZ	Cefoxitin or cefotetan
	Enterococci		

Abbreviations: AM/SB = ampicillin/sulbactam; TMP/SMX = trimethoprim/sulfamethoxazole; Pip/TZ = piperacillin/tazobactam; amox/clav = amoxicillin/clavulanate.

Source: Adapted from Bryan, JH, Kitzis, A, Jui, J, Guide to Antibiotic Use in the Emergency Department. Emergency Medicine Residents Association, Dallas, TX, 2003.

where there may be antibiotic penetration issues, such as meningitis, endocarditis, or osteomyelitis, the highest doses recommended should be given. Dosage adjustments of many antibiotics are necessary for patients with renal disease to prevent adverse events that would occur with drug accumulation (if dosage reduction did not occur). Because the highest doses of drugs usually are given intravenously, dosage adjustments are most relevant for intravenous administration. Oral doses are typically at the "low end" of the dosage range, meaning that toxic drug accumulation is much less likely when oral doses are given in renal dysfunction. Hence little dose modification is necessary with oral dosing. Dosage modifications in liver disease are less clear because of a poorer understanding of how liver function tests measure a decrease in drug elimination characteristics or rate. Adverse events (dose-related and allergic) of antibacterial drugs will be discussed in the next section. Guidelines for dosing adjustment, primarily with intravenous therapy, are summarized in Table 155-4.[2]

Adverse Effects and Contraindications of Antibacterial Drugs

Allergic reactions and direct pharmacologic-based toxicity are the two general categories of adverse drug reactions to antibiotics. Allergic reactions are not dose-related, they are unpredictable, and they cannot be studied effectively in animal models. Reactions can vary from very mild skin rashes to life-threatening circumstances, such as toxic epi-

dermal necrolysis or anaphylactic reactions. Drug fever, hepatitis, and interstitial nephritis are also examples of allergic drug reactions. Direct dose-related toxicity is the result of the pharmacologic properties of the drug. These reactions are possible in any recipient (including animal models) if the dose or accumulated drug in the body is high enough. Dose-related adverse events typically are reversible if the antibiotic is discontinued. There is some predictability to these reactions, such as renal dysfunction caused by an aminoglycoside, if the blood level of drug is high enough for an extended period of time. It is these dose-related or pharmacologic side effects that are avoided if appropriate dose adjustments of antibiotics are made as in the dosing guidelines in Table 155-4. Certain adverse effects of antibiotics, such as pseudomembranous colitis, do not fall easily into either category; all antibiotics can cause this side effect. The common allergic and dose-related adverse effects of antibacterial drugs are summarized in Table 155-5. This table also includes the Food and Drug Administration (FDA) safety-in-pregnancy categories.[1-5]

Contraindications and Drug Interactions

There are certain important contraindications to the use of several of the antibacterial drugs. In general, a contraindication exists if the patient has a previous history of allergy to the drug being considered for use. This circumstance is most pertinent for patients with a penicillin or cephalosporin allergy, but in particular, the nature of the allergy is

TABLE 155-4   Dosage Guidelines for Selected Antibacterial Drugs in Adults

Drug	Major Route of Elimination	Maximum Daily IV Dose (g)	Dose Adjustment for Creatinine Clearance (mL/min)		
			>50	10–50	<10
Ampicillin	Renal	12	1–2 g q4–8h	1 g q6h	1 g q12h
Aztreonam	Renal	8	1–2 g q6–8h	1–2g q12h	1 g q12h
Cefazolin	Renal	8	1–2 g q8h	1 g q12h	1 g q24h
Cefotaxime	Renal	12	1–2 g q4–8h	1–2 g q12h	1 g q12h
Cefotetan	Renal	6	1–2 g q12h	1–2g q24h	1 g q24h
Ceftazidime	Renal	6	1–2 g q8h	1–2g q24h	0.5 g q24h
Ceftriaxone	Biliary	4	1–2 g q12–24 h	No adjustments	
Ciprofloxacin	Renal	1.2	0.4 g q8-12h	0.4g q12h	0.4 g q24h
Clindamycin	Biliary	4.8	0.6–0.9 g q6–8h	No adjustments	
		In hepatic failure, limit dose to 0.6 g q8h			
Imipenem	Renal	2	0.5 g q6–8h	0.5g q12h	0.5 g q24h
Metronidazole	Biliary	2	0.5 g q6–8h	No adjustments	
		In hepatic failure, limit dose to 0.5 g q12h			
Nafcillin, Oxacillin	Biliary	12	1-2 g q4-6 h	No adjustments	
Penicillin G	Renal	24 MU*	3-4 MU q4h	2MU q6h	1MU q6h
Piperacillin	Renal	18	3g q4–6h	3g q6h	2 g q6h
Tobramycin, gentamicin	Renal	7 mg/kg per dose	q24h	q36h	Do not use
Vancomycin	Renal	15 mg/kg per dose	q12–24h	q24–48h	Use levels

* Million units.
Source: From Koda–Kimble et al.[2]

important to understand when making decisions for alternate therapy. For example, a patient with a history of respiratory distress, wheezing, urticaria, or hives during a previous course of β-lactam treatment would be at significant risk for another potential life-threatening reaction upon reexposure to another β-lactam. In this case, a penicillin or cephalosporin would be strongly contraindicated. β-Lactam therapy could still be used if absolutely necessary but should be accomplished first in a desensitization protocol in the intensive care unit. On the other hand, if the patient history is a mild maculopapular rash while taking amoxicillin or other penicillin, the chances are very high that subsequent treatment with a cephalosporin would not provoke another allergic event.

Drug interactions with antibacterial drugs, fortunately, are infrequent, but several must be kept in mind. Two mechanisms for interactions predominate with these drugs. **The first mechanism is an inhibition of absorption of oral antibiotics. The best example of this interaction occurs when any of the tetracycline or fluoroquinolone antibiotics are given at the same time as divalent cations (Ca^{2+}, Mg^{2+}, Fe^{2+}).** If this occurs, the ions bind to the antibiotic and reduce markedly the amount of drug that is absorbed orally. Tetracyclines and fluoroquinolones should not be given with calcium or iron preparations or with antacids. **Second, certain antibiotics can slow the metabolism of other drugs by inhibiting several of the hepatic cytochrome P450 enzymes in the liver. In particular, ciprofloxacin, clarithromycin, and trimethoprim-sulfamethoxazole are drugs that are able to provoke this enzyme inhibition.** Summaries of these antibiotic contraindications and drug interactions are included as Tables 155-6 and 155-7, respectively.[4]

ANTIFUNGAL DRUGS

New antifungal agents for systemic infections have been developed over the last 5 years. These agents are effective for significant infec-

tions with a lower adverse-effect risk than traditional antifungal drugs (e.g., amphotericin B). The mechanism of action of antifungal agents is primarily based on actions that decrease cell wall integrity. Amphotericin B (and its lipid-based derivatives) binds to cell wall ergosterol, increasing cell wall permeability that eventually results in cell lysis. Triazole antifungals (e.g., fluconazole, itraconazole) block ergosterol synthesis by inhibition of a fungal cytochrome P450-dependent enzyme. Caspofungin is another enzyme inhibitor, in this case, the inhibition is of beta-glucan synthetase. Beta-glucan, like ergosterol, is another necessary component of the cell wall of several fungal species. Flucytosine is an antimetabolite that disrupts DNA function after conversion intracellularly to 5-fluorouracil. These agents for systemic fungal infections are summarized in Table 155-8. Multiple topical antifungal preparations are available, as summarized in Table 155-9, and are indicated for *Candida* or tinea infections.[3–5]

Of the various lipid-based amphotericin B preparations, liposomal amphotericin B (Ambisome) is becoming the preferred product primarily because of a lower rate of infusion-related reactions and perhaps a lower frequency of renal dysfunction compared with the other lipid products. Because amphotericin B has the broadest antifungal spectrum of all these systemic agents, it is the preferred drug for empirical therapy, including ED use, until further diagnostic workup determines the likely pathogen involved. All amphotericin B infusions, whether conventional (infused over 4 h) or lipid-based (infused over 2 h) can be preceded by routine premedications to diminish the frequency of infusion-related fever and chills. Acetaminophen (650 mg PO) and diphenhydramine (Benadryl, 25–50 mg PO or IV) should be given 30 min prior to the infusion. If rigors occur, meperidine (Demerol, 25–50 mg IV) likely will promote resolution of the rigor. With these premedications, a "test dose" (1 mg) infused slowly is not necessary.

In addition to the preceding infusion-related reactions, amphotericin B toxicity is related to renal dysfunction. The lipid-based products

TABLE 155-5   Antibacterial Adverse Effects

Antibiotic Class	Allergic Reactions	Dose-Related Effects
β-lactams (penicillins, cephalosporins, monobactams, carbapenems) Pregnancy category* B	Anaphylaxis, urticaria, rash, fever, serum sickness; hepatitis, nephritis, anemia, thrombocytopenia Cross-reactivity between penicillins and cephalosporins is ~5%; little cross-reactivity between cephalosporin and aztreonam or imipenem	Diarrhea (Augmentin), biliary sludging (ceftriaxone); phlebitis; seizures (imipenem, penicillin G); anti-platelet effects and hemolytic anemia; decreased vitamin K synthesis and disulfiram reaction (cefotetan); nausea, hypotension (rapid infusion of imipenem).
Aminoglycosides Pregnancy category C	Rare	Nephrotoxicity: incidence 10–15%, usually reversible Ototoxicity: incidence 1–5%, causes deafness and/or dizziness; toxicity is both dose- and duration-related
Macrolides Pregnancy category B C (clarithromycin)	Cholestatic jaundice: associated with IV erythromycin	GI toxicity: nausea, vomiting diarrhea, cramping—mostly with erythromycin
Clindamycin Pregnancy category B	Rash	Diarrhea—most common adverse effect; pseudomembranous colitis
Tetracyclines Pregnancy category D	Rash, anaphylaxis, urticaria, fever, hepatitis	Nausea, diarrhea; increase in BUN; deposits and discolors teeth and bone (avoid in pediatrics); dizziness and vertigo (minocycline)
Vancomycin Pregnancy category C	Rash (rare)	Infusion-related reactions: phlebitis, "red person syndrome" from rapid fusions—give 1 g over 60 min; oto- and nephrotoxicity is rare with current formulations
Fluoroquinolones Pregnancy category C	Rare	Nausea, vomiting, diarrhea; confusion, headache, seizures; tendonitis and tendon rupture; prolonged QT interval
Sulfonamides Pregnancy category X	Rash, Stevens-Johnson syndrome, exfoliative dermatitis (more common in AIDS); hepatitis; bone marrow suppression	Nausea, vomiting, diarrhea; crystalluria (doses taken with insufficient fluids)

*United States FDA Safety-in-Pregnancy Code: A: controlled human studies show no risk; B: no evidence of risk in humans; the chance of fetal harm is remote but remains a possibility; C: risk cannot be ruled out; well-controlled human studies are lacking, and animal studies have shown risk or are lacking; there is a chance of fetal harm if administered during pregnancy; D: positive evidence of risk; studies in humans have demonstrated fetal risk; X: contraindicated in pregnancy; the risk of fetal abnormalities outweighs the potential benefit of the drug.
Source: From Cunha BA.[3]

TABLE 155-6   Antibiotic Contraindications

Antibiotic Class	Contraindications
Penicillins	History of hypersensitivity to penicillins, cephalosporins, imipenem (carbapenems)
Cephalosporins	Hypersensitivity to cephalosporins, imipenem (carbapenems), penicillins
Fluoroquinolones	Hypersensitivity to any of the fluoroquinolones; tendonitis or tendon rupture; use of QT interval–prolonging drugs (amiodarone, procainamide)
Tetracyclines	Hypersensitivity to any of the tetracyclines
Macrolides	Hypersensitivity to any of the macrolides; treatment of meningitis (inadequate CNS penetration)
Vancomycin	Hypersensitivity to vancomycin
Clindamycin	Hypersensitivity to clindamycin; treatment of meningitis (inadequate CNS penetration)
Aminoglycosides	Previous allergic or toxic reactions to any of the aminoglycosides
Metronidazole	Hypersensitivity to metronidazole; first trimester of pregnancy
Sulfonamides	Hypersensitivity to sulfonamides or related drugs (sulfonylureas, thiazides, loop diuretics), pregnancy at term, lactation

Source: From Burnham et al.[4]

significantly reduce but do not totally eliminate the risk of renal toxicity. Consequences of the renal effects of amphotericin B are renal tubular acidosis and renal wasting of bicarbonate, potassium, and magnesium. Serum electrolyte levels should be followed closely, with aggressive supplementation of potassium and magnesium being frequently necessary. Amphotericin B is also responsible for causing frequent elevations of blood urea nitrogen (BUN) and serum creatinine, which, again, have been reduced with the use of the lipid-based products. Nevertheless, increases in creatinine are possible with any of these amphotericin products and, if present, should result in reduction of the daily dose or, preferably, infusion of the product every other day if the creatinine level rises to greater than 2.5 to 3.0 mg/dL.

Fluconazole, itraconazole, voriconazole, and caspofungin are very safe drugs and do not provoke the renal dysfunction associated with amphotericin B. Occasionally, liver function test elevations and hepatitis result from triazole therapy, so patients on prolonged courses of these drugs should be followed with liver function tests monthly. Triazoles (particularly itraconazole) can interact with other drugs metabolized by the cytochrome P450 system. In particular, warfarin, phenytoin, cyclosporine, and tacrolimus levels routinely increase in patients on these drugs who are then given itraconazole. Fluconazole is a less potent inhibitor of cytochrome P450, so significant interactions with fluconazole are less frequent. Flucytosine can cause reversible bone marrow suppression, with leukopenia and thrombocytopenia. The pregnancy category for the amphotericin products is category B, and for the triazoles, caspofungin, and flucytosine, it is category C. Finally, dose-modification issues are only relevant for fluconazole and flucytosine as follows: For creatinine clearance less than 50 mL/min, reduce

TABLE 155-7   Antibacterial Drug Interactions

Antibiotic Class	Drug Interactions
Penicillins	Oral contraceptives—failure (infrequent) Allopurinol—increased rash with ampicillin Aminoglycosides—when administered IV simultaneously, inactivation occurs Probenecid—reduced renal elimination of penicillin
Cephalosporins	Warfarin—cefotetan and cefoperazone enhance the anticoagulant effect of warfarin Antacids—may reduce the oral absorption of cefaclor, cefdinir, and cefpodoxime
Fluoroquinolones	Antacids, iron salts, sucralfate—absorption of the fluoroquinolone is reduced by chelation Theophylline—metabolism is slowed by ciprofloxacin, may cause theophylline toxicity; warfarin elimination is slowed by fluoroquinolones—follow clotting times carefully
Tetracyclines	Antacids, iron salts—bind to tetracycline and reduce oral absorption (occur least with doxycycline) Oral contraceptives—failure
Macrolides	Clarithromycin can increase levels of warfarin, cyclosporin, lovastatin, theophylline—monitor additive effects carefully
Vancomycin	Aminoglycosides—may increase risk of nephrotoxicity
Aminoglycosides	Neuromuscular blockers—may prolong respiratory depression; loop diuretics—may increase auditory toxicity
Trimethoprim-sulfamethoxazole	Warfarin—can prolong clotting times; phenytoin—increase in serum levels and possible toxicity

Source: From Burnham et al.[4]

TABLE 155-8   Antifungal Agents for Systemic Infections*

Drug	Spectrum	Usual Doses
Amphotericin B, IV	*Aspergillus,*	
Conventional (Fungizone)	*Candida,*	0.5–1.0 mg/kg per d
Lipid complex (Abelcet)	*Cryptococcus,*	5.0 mg/kg per d
Liposomal (Ambisome)	*Histoplasmosis,*	5.0 mg/kg per d
Colloidal dispersion (Amphotec)	*Mucormycosis*	5.0 mg/kg per d
Triazoles*		
Fluconazole (Diflucan), IV, PO	*Candida, Cryptococcus,*	400 mg per d
Itraconazole (Sporonox), IV, PO	*Aspergillus* (not fluconazole),	200 mg bid
Voriconazole (Vfend), IV, PO	*Histoplasmosis*	4 mg/kg bid
Caspofungin (Cancidas), IV	*Aspergillus, Candida, (not Cryptococcus)*	70 mg × 1, 50 mg qd
Flucytosine (Ancobon), PO	*Candida, Cryptococcus* (should not be used as monotherapy)	25–37.5 mg/ kg q6h

Source: From Cunha BA[3] and Burnham et al.[4]
*Triazoles and imidazoles should not be used with astemizole† or terfenadine,† because the combination can result in QT$_c$ prolongation.
†No longer available in the U.S.

TABLE 155-9   Selected Topical Antifungal Agents

Class and Products	Dosage Forms	Comments
Allylamines/benzylamines		
Butenafine (Mentax) Naftitine (Naftin) Terbinafine (Lamisil)	1% cream, gel, solution, spray	Treatment for 1–4 weeks for tinea
Imidazoles		
Clotrimazole (Lotrimin, Mycelex)	1% cream, lotion, vaginal tablets	Topical (*Candida,* tinea) apply bid; Vag. tab 100 mg × 7d or 500 mg hs × 1
Miconazole (Micatin, Monistat)	2% cream, ointment, vag. supp.	As above, except 200 mg vag. supp. × 3 d
Tioconazole (Vagistat-1)	6.5% vag. ointment	Application hs × 1
Miscellaneous (for tinea only)		
Haloprogin (Halotex)	1% cream, solution	Apply bid 2–4 weeks
Tolnaftate (Tinactin, Ting)	1% cream, solution, gel, powder, spray	Apply bid 2–6 weeks Less effective than Imidazoles

Source: From Anderson et al.[5]

fluconozole to 200 mg daily and flucytosine to 25 to 37.5 mg/kg every 12 h; for creatinine clearance less than 10 mg/min, flucytosine should be further reduced to 25 to 37.5 mg/kg every 24 h.[1–5]

ANTIVIRAL AGENTS

Recent advances in the development of antiviral agents has increased our ability to treat infections caused by herpes simplex virus (HSV I and II), varicella-zoster virus (VZV), cytomegalovirus (CMV), influenza A and B, and human immunodeficiency virus (HIV). Table 155-10 summarizes the mechanism of action of the agents used for these viral infections, except for HIV, and the antiviral spectrum of each agent.[1] Table 155-11 summarizes the antiviral mechanisms of the antiretroviral (anti-HIV) drugs, their dosing regimens, and their common adverse effects. Uses for the non-HIV antiviral agents for patients in the emergency department are summarized in Table 155-12. Adverse effects of these drugs are compiled in Table 155-13.[2,4]

Acyclovir (and penciclovir) and ganciclovir are excellent drugs for the treatment of HSV and CMV infections, respectively. When given orally, however, the absorption of these agents is less than optimal. As a result, large oral doses are necessary to achieve adequate blood and tissue levels to inhibit viral replication. Drug formulation and product development generated the three *prodrugs* valacyclovir, famciclovir, and valganciclovir. In the case of valacyclovir and valganciclovir, a valine ester has been added to acyclovir and ganciclovir, respectively, that produces enhanced absorption from the gastrointestinal tract. On reaching the liver, the valine is hydrolyzed and removed, resulting in the emergence of acyclovir or ganciclovir. Specifically, acyclovir oral absorption is about 16 percent of a dose, whereas for valacyclovir absorption increases to about 55 percent. Valganciclovir absorption is about 60 percent of an oral dose; for ganciclovir the percentage of dose absorbed in only 5 percent. This is why the dosage of the prodrugs is significantly less than the oral doses of the parent compounds.

As far an antiretroviral therapy is concerned, treatment is *always* a combination of at least three drugs using agents with different mechanisms of action. Current drugs either inhibit the enzyme responsible for the conversion of HIV RNA to a DNA copy (reverse transcriptase) for replication in human T cells or inhibit a viral protease that promotes the maturation of new HIV virions prior to their budding from host cells.

TABLE 155-10 Antiviral Agents for Systemic Herpes, Varicella, CMV, and Influenza Virus Infections

Drug	Mechanism of Action	Activity Against
Acyclovir (Zovirax), valacyclovir (Valtrex) Penciclovir, famciclovir (Famvir)	Purine nucleoside analogues; triphosphate form inhibits HSV DNA polymerase and viral DNA replication	HSV I and II, VZV
Ganciclovir (Cytovene), valganciclovir (Valcyte)	Nucleoside analogue (guanine); when phosphorylated, inhibits viral DNA polymerase	HSV I and II, VZV, CMV
Foscarnet (Foscavir)	Inorganic pyrophosphate analogue that inhibits DNA polymerase	HSV I and II, VZV, CMV
Cidofovir (Vistide)	Nucleotide analogue that inhibits viral DNA polymerase	HSV I and II, VZV, CMV
Amantadine (Symmetrel), rimantadine (Flumadine)	Inhibits uncoating of virus and uptake of nucleic acid by host cells	Influenza A
Olseltamivir (Tamiflu), zanamivir (Relenza)	Inhibitor of influenza virus neuraminidase with possible alteration in viral aggregation and release	Influenza A and B

Source: From Hardman et al.[1]

Several important comments are necessary regarding the adverse effects of the antiretroviral agents. Certain reactions may be life-threatening and thus may be important circumstances that could arise in the emergency department. First, lactic acidosis is being recognized increasingly as a significant adverse effect of therapy. The onset of the acidosis may be subacute, so patients will complain of several weeks of fatigue, anorexia, weight loss, confusion, and loss of energy. Arterial lactic acid levels may be increased two to three times, and resolution of the acidosis typically is slow, even after discontinuation of the antiretroviral drugs. Lactate levels should be checked in patients with the preceding symptoms who have been receiving antiretroviral agents, especially stavudine (d4T, Zerit) or didanosine (ddI, Videx). Second, the hypersensitivity syndrome secondary to abacavir (Ziagen) must be noted. As briefly described in Table 155-11, the syndrome is characterized by rash and other systemic complaints. The reaction is reversible with discontinuation of abacavir. However, if the patient then takes abacavir again, cardiovascular and respiratory insufficiency has been observed that can be life-threatening. Rechallenge should be done only under the supervision of a clinician very experienced in HIV care. Finally, it should be noted that there are multiple and important drug interactions between the antiretroviral drugs themselves and with drugs used for other indications. A comprehensive summary of these interactions is beyond the scope of this chapter. Excellent resources, such as the references for this chapter, can help with a listing of these drug interactions. Multiple online sources are also available and are updated frequently. These sources, in particular, include www.hivatis.org and www.pedhivaids.org.[2–5]

TABLE 155-11 Antiviral Agents for HIV Infection

Drug	Usual Dose	Adverse Events and Administration Issues
Nucleoside reverse-transcriptase inhibitors		
Zidovudine (Retrovir) (AZT, ZDV)	300 mg PO bid	Bone marrow suppression with anemia, macrocytosis; headache, nausea, vomiting; can be given with or between meals
Didanosine (Videx) (ddI)	200 mg PO bid or 400 mg qd (>60 kg) 250 mg qd (<60 kg)	Peripheral neuropathy; pancreatitis, nausea diarrhea; lactic acidosis (myalgia, fatigue, anorexia); give between meals
Zalcitabine (Hivid) (ddC)	0.75 mg PO q8h	Peripheral neuropathy; stomatitis; give between meals
Stavudine (Zerit) (d4T)	40 mg bid (>60 kg) 20 mg bid (<60 kg)	Peripheral neuropathy, hepatitis; lactic acidosis; can be given with or between meals
Lamivudine (Epivir) (3TC)	150 mg PO bid	Few adverse events: headache, nausea, pancreatitis; can give with or between meals
Abacavir (Ziagen)	300 mg PO q12h	Hypersensitivity reaction (fever, rash, nausea, abdominal pain, malaise); do not readminister abacavir; headache, lactic acidosis; can give with or between meals
Tenofovir (Viread)	300 mg qd	Nausea, diarrhea, vomiting; take with food
Nonnucleoside reverse-transcriptase inhibitors		
Nevirapine (Viramune)	200 mg PO qd × 7 d; then 200 mg bid	Rash (can be severe), hepatitis, nausea, vomiting, diarrhea; give with/without food
Delavirdine (Rescriptor)	400 mg PO q8h	Rash, nausea, headache; give with or without food
Efavirenz (Sustiva)	600 mg PO hs	Vivid dreams, headache, rash (can be severe), dizziness, light-headedness; avoid taking with high-fat meals—increases toxicity
Protease inhibitors		
Indinavir (Crixivan)	800 mg q8h or 400 mg bid with 400 mg bid ritonavir	Kidney stones; hyperbilirubinemia (indirect), nausea, vomiting, hepatitis, increased glucose and lipids; lipodystrophy; must be taken between meals
Lopinavir (Kaletra) (fixed combination with ritonavir)	3 capsules bid	Nausea, vomiting, diarrhea, hepatitis; increase in glucose and lipids; lipodystrophy; take with food
Ritonavir (Norvir)	400 mg bid in combination with other protease inhibitors	As above
Nelfinavir (Viracept)	1250 mg bid	Diarrhea (~20%); increase in lipids; lipodystrophy; take with meal or snack
Saquinavir (Fortovase)	1200 mg tid or 400 mg bid with ritonavir	Nausea, diarrhea, abdominal pain, headache; hepatitis, increases in glucose and lipids Lipodystrophy; take with food
Amprenavir (Agenerase)	1200 mg bid, or 450 mg bid with 100 mg bid ritonavir	Rash, nausea, vomiting, diarrhea, circumoral paresthesias; lipodystrophy; can be taken with or between meals

Source: From Koda-Kimble et al[2] and Burnham et al.[4]

TABLE 155-12   Antiviral Therapy (Non-HIV) in the ED

Diagnosis	Drug	Dosage	Route
Herpes encephalitis	Acyclovir	10 mg/kg q8h × 10 d (adult) 500 mg/m^2 q8h (6 mo–12 yr)	IV
Mucocutaneous Herpes (immunocompromised)	Acyclovir	5 mg/kg q8h × 7 d (adult) 250 mg/m^2 q8h (<12 yr)	IV
Varicella-zoster (immunocompromised)		Same as above for herpes encephalitis	IV
Herpes zoster (normal host)	Acyclovir, or famciclovir, or valacyclovir	800 mg 5 times/day × 7–10 d 500 mg tid × 7 d 1 g tid × 7 d	PO PO PO
Varicella (chickenpox)	Acyclovir	20 mg/kg (≤800 mg) qid (adults and children >2 yr) × 5 d	PO
Influenza A	Amantadine	100 mg bid × 10 d (adults and children >9 yr) 4.4–8.8 mg/kg per d, but <150 mg/d (children 1–9 yr)	PO
	Rimantadine	100 mg bid × 7 d (adults and children >10 yr) 5 mg/kg per d, but <150 mg/d (children 1–10 yr)	PO
	Oseltamivir	75 mg bid (adults) × 5 d	PO
	Zanamivir	10 mg (2 inhalations) bid × 5 d (adults and children >12 yr)	Inhalation

Source: From Koda-Kimble et al.[2]

TABLE 155-13   Adverse Effects of Selected Antiviral Agents

Drug	Adverse Effects
Acyclovir	IV: Phlebitis and irritation (9%); increase in BUN and creatinine (5–10%)—keep patient well hydrated; CNS toxicity (1%)—confusion, hallucinations (reversible) PO: Nausea/vomiting (7%), itching, rash (2%), hepatitis (1–2%)
Amantadine	Nausea, dizziness and insomnia (5–10%); depression, anxiety, hallucination, confusion, dry mouth, constipation, orthostatic hypotension, ataxia, peripheral edema (1–5%)
Famciclovir	Headache (6–9%), nausea (4–5%), diarrhea (1–2%)
Oseltamivir	Nausea, vomiting (9–10%), vertigo (1%)
Rimantadine	Insomnia, dizziness, headache, fatigue; nausea, vomiting, anorexia, dry mouth, abdominal pain (1–3%)
Valacyclovir	Headache (13–17%), nausea (10–16%), vomiting and diarrhea (1–7%)
Zanamivir	Bronchospasm, nasal/throat irritation, decline in respiratory function, headache, cough (1–2%)

Source: From Koda-Kimble et al.[2]

REFERENCES

1. Hardman JG, Limbird LE, Gilman AG, et al (eds): *Goodman & Gilman's The Pharmacological Basis of Therapeutics,* 10th ed. New York, McGraw-Hill, 2001.
2. Koda-Kimble MA, Young LY, Kradjian WA, et al (eds): *Handbook of Applied Therapeutics,* 7th ed. Philadelphia, Lippincott Williams & Wilkins, 2002.
3. Cunha BA: *Antibiotic Essentials.* Royal Oak, MI, Physician' Press, 2002.
4. Burnham TH, Wickersham RM, Novak KK, et al (eds): *Drug Facts and Comparisons.* St Louis, Wolters Kluwer, 2002.
5. Anderson PO, Knoben JE, Troutman WG (eds): *Handbook of Clinical Drug Data,* 10th ed. New York, McGraw-Hill, 2002.
6. McEvoy GK (ed): *AHFS Drug Information 2003.* American Society of Health-System Pharmacists, Bethesda, MD.

GENERAL MANAGEMENT OF POISONED PATIENTS

Jason B. Hack

Robert S. Hoffman

It is generally accepted that, given a large enough exposure, all chemicals have the potential to be poisons. Inadvertent exposures to chemical substances have to fulfill specific criteria in order to be considered "nontoxic" (Table 156-1). Once fulfilled, these patients can be managed with only a brief observation period prior to discharge.

A *poisoning* occurs when exposure to a substance adversely affects the function of any system within an organism. The setting of the poison exposure may be occupational, environmental, recreational, or medicinal. A poisoning may result from varied portals of entry, including inhalation, insufflation, ingestion, cutaneous and mucous membrane exposure, and injection. Historically most poisonings have occurred when substances are tasted or swallowed. Toxins may be airborne in the form of gas or vapors or in a suspension such as dust. Caustics, vesicants, or irritants may directly affect the skin, or a toxin may pass transdermally and affect internal structures. Parenteral exposure is also common through intravenous or subcutaneous injection of medications or drugs of abuse.

A poison may affect the normal activity of an organism in a variety of ways. It may inhibit or alter cellular function, change organ function, or may change uptake or transport of substances into, out of, or within the organism. The toxin may prevent the organism from obtaining or utilizing essential substrates from the environment.

In 2000, there were more than 2 million toxic exposures reported to poison centers in the United States, just over half of which involved children younger than 6 years old.[1] Some authors currently list poisoning as the third leading cause of death in the United States, and between 1985 and 1995, the incidence of toxin-related deaths is said to have increased approximately 300 percent. Although many of these exposures were referred to as "accidents," most were preventable. School counselors, primary care physicians, and emergency physicians can educate families about poisonings, potentially poisonous substances, and techniques for protecting children from their environment. Nonfood (potentially harmful) items should not be stored in food areas, and toxins should not be stored in empty food containers. Hospitals and pharmacies must work together to recognize potential drug interactions, ensure patient identification, and develop procedures to check proper dosing, warning labels, and packaging on products with potential toxicity.

Poison centers are an integral part of the management of potentially exposed patients. These centers are typically staffed with specialists trained in the management of poisoned patients, who have extensive reference material at their disposal. Poison centers have immediate access to medical toxicologists if more extensive evaluation is required. Routine consultation in cases where toxic exposure is suspected can help focus diagnosis and treatment and may reduce costs and unnecessary hospitalizations.

RESUSCITATION

Diagnosis and resuscitation proceed simultaneously. The first priorities are always the ABCs (airway, breathing, and circulation). Once the airway and respiratory status is secured, abnormalities of blood pressure, pulse, rectal temperature, oxygen saturation and hypoglycemia must be corrected. Although the proper use of antidotes (Table 156-2) is essential in the treatment of poisoned patients, only in very rare incidences (such as cyanide poisoning) would the administration of an antidote take precedence over completing the primary evaluation and normal attempts to stabilize the ABCs.

Patients may be unresponsive or have an altered mental status for many reasons. Four possible etiologies (hypoxia, opioid intoxication, hypoglycemia, and Wernicke's encephalopathy) are readily treated by the administration of specific antidotes. Within the first few minutes after the patient's arrival, the administration of empiric antidotes (the "coma cocktail"), including supplemental oxygen, naloxone, 50 mL D50W for adults and 1 g/kg glucose for children, and 100 mg thiamine in adults should be considered after taking into account the medical history, vital signs, and laboratory data immediately available. These treatments are simple, inexpensive, and generally without undue risk of an adverse reaction when used appropriately.

In unresponsive children thiamine is generally not administered empirically. However, 1 g/kg of glucose (2 mL/kg of D50W for adults, 4 mL/kg of D25W or 10 mL/kg of D10W for children) is often administered when serum glucose cannot be rapidly ascertained or hypoglycemia is confirmed. Naloxone (0.01 mg/kg titrated to effect) may be given, particularly in older children where unintentional or intentional opioid exposure cannot be excluded. Intentional poisoning of children as a form of child abuse does occur.

The suggestion that the administration of thiamine should precede the administration of D50W to prevent the precipitation of acute Wernicke's encephalopathy is unfounded.[2] The most important management issue with both D50W and thiamine is that both should be given in a timely manner in the emergency department so that these often occult diagnoses are added to the differential diagnosis and are treated promptly.

Although opioid intoxication often presents with the classic triad of central nervous system (CNS) depression, miosis, and respiratory depression, only respiratory status is useful as an indicator of a patient response to naloxone.[3] Many toxins, though, produce miosis or CNS depression, and some opioids classically leave pupil size unaltered, making these findings less useful in isolation.

Naloxone, administered in a dose of 0.1 to 2.0 mg IV in adults and children is a competitive opioid antagonist that can be administered IV or IM, and is appropriate to use for a hypoventilating but nonintubated, opioid-intoxicated patient. Extremity restraints for the patient should be considered before administering the drug. Naloxone may completely reverse the symptoms observed, restoring effective ventilations and mental status for 20 to 60 min, so patients should be observed for 2 to 3 h afterward. The risks include the precipitation of an acute opioid withdrawal syndrome. Although acute withdrawal is never life-threatening in adults, vomiting from withdrawal can result in aspiration. Thus, the reflexive administration of large doses of naloxone should be discouraged. Patients who become resedated may require additional naloxone doses administered either in intermittent boluses or via a continuous infusion. The latter is achieved by the administration of two-thirds the dose of the naloxone that fully aroused the patient in the initial bolus, but infused over an hour with the dose adjusted to the patient's ventilatory status.

EMERGENCY DEPARTMENT DIAGNOSIS

History

As much detailed information as possible must be obtained about the exposure. Ask about the number of exposed persons, the type of exposure, amount or dose, and route of exposure. In addition, the

TABLE 156-1   Criteria for Nontoxic Ingestions

Only one substance is involved in the exposure.

The substance must be absolutely identified.

The substance's product label must not contain any consumer product safety commission signal words indicating a potential hazard of toxicity.

The exposure must have been unintentional.

The route of exposure must be known.

An approximate amount of the substance involved in the exposure must be known.

The exposed individual must be free of symptoms for the extent of the observation period.

Follow-up consultation must be easily available or a responsible parent or guardian must be present.

Note: All of the listed criteria must be fulfilled in order for an ingestion to be classified as nontoxic.

Source: Adapted from Mofenson HC, Grensher J, Caraccio TR: Ingestions considered nontoxic. *Emerg Med Clin North Am* 2:159, 1984, and Mofenson HC, Grensher J: The nontoxic ingestion. *Pediatr Clin North Am* 17:583, 1970.

patient's intent must be determined. Underlying motivation, potential for secondary gain, and perceived risk of arrest all may affect the history elicited from the patient. Corroborating information should be obtained from the patient's private physician, witnesses, or emergency medical technicians. Ask about the environment in which the patient was found, empty pill bottles or containers nearby, smells or unusual materials in the home, the occupation or hobbies of the patient, or the presence of a suicide note.

Toxicologic Physical Examination

Undress the patient completely for a comprehensive physical examination. Check the patient's clothing for objects still retained in the pockets or substances hidden on the patient's body (waistbands, groin, or between skin folds). Care must be taken when searching belongings, particularly pockets, because health care providers have been stuck by uncapped needles or lacerated by sharp objects.

Assess the general appearance of the patient. The presence of agitation, confusion, or obtundation should be noted. Examine the skin for cyanosis or flushing, excessive diaphoresis or dryness, signs of injury or injection, ulcers, or bullae. Bruising may be a clue for trauma, duration of unconsciousness, or coagulopathy. Examine the eyes for pupil size, reactivity, nystagmus, dysconjugate gaze, or excessive lacrimation. Hypersalivation or excessive dryness should be noted upon examination of the oropharynx. The chest examination should include careful evaluation of the lungs to assess for bronchorrhea, or wheezing, and the heart must be assessed for its rhythm, rate, and regularity. Bowel sounds, urinary retention, and abdominal tenderness or rigidity must also be noted. The extremities must be evaluated for tremor or fasciculation. Cranial nerves, reflexes, resting muscle tone, coordination, cognition, and the ability to ambulate all must be assessed.

Toxidromes

Toxidromes are grouped, physiologically based abnormalities of vital signs, general appearance, skin, eyes, mucous membranes, lungs, heart, abdomen, and neurologic examination that are known to occur with specific classes of substances and typically are helpful in establishing a diagnosis when the exposure is not well defined (Table 156-3). Similarly, certain clinical findings may help narrow the etiologic possibilities (Tables 156-4 and 156-5).

Toxicologic Screen

In the acute care setting, the utility of toxicologic screening tests of blood and/or urine in many circumstances is very limited, and does not contribute significantly to the evaluation, management or outcome of

patients. Most toxicology screens are enzyme-multiplied immunoassay tests (EMITs), which are used to evaluate the presence of markers for commonly available substances including marijuana, opioids, cocaine, amphetamines, tricyclic antidepressants (TCAs), barbiturates, and benzodiazepines. Interpretation of test results often leads to confusion.

Positive results may occur with many substances because they persist in body fluids for days to weeks, depending on the chronicity of use. Thus, "falsely" positive results may not be related to the acute symptoms. Furthermore, positive results may occur from substances that cross-react with the assay (e.g., chlorpromazine, propranolol, pseudoephedrine, and selegiline for amphetamines; chlorpromazine, cyclobenzaprine, thioridazine, diphenhydramine, and cyproheptadine for TCAs). Negative results may be due to sampling error (e.g., very dilute urine after hydration) or from assay specificity (e.g., opioid screens do not detect methadone and meperidine; amphetamine screens do not detect MDMA; benzodiazepine screens do not detect rohypnol).

Patients may require emergent interventions before the tests return. Often basic supportive measures alone can successfully manage many commonly encountered ingestions or intoxications. The diagnosis of less frequently encountered exposures is usually dependent upon specialized testing that is not obtainable in a timely manner.

Toxicologic screens may have a place in the evaluation of children. The unexpected return of a positive result for a controlled or illegal substance should prompt further evaluation of the child's home environment and may require hospital admission for the child's protection. If the test result is replicated with a confirmatory study, authorities must be notified.

GENERAL DECONTAMINATION

The general approach to most toxic exposures involves the removal of the patient from the substance and the substance from the patient. Toxins outside the body must be washed away. Toxins within the body must be either bound within the gut lumen to make them unavailable for absorption or have their elimination enhanced from the gut, the blood, or the tissues.

Gross Decontamination

Decontamination is generally achieved by undressing patients completely and washing them thoroughly with copious amounts of water. Patients requiring assistance should be attended to by properly gowned staff in an isolated area. The towels used to dry patients and patient clothing, shoes, socks, watches, and jewelry should be handled as hazardous waste. Gross decontamination should occur prior to the patient's entry into the ED or other areas in the hospital. In mass casualty exposures, this will typically occur at a staging area adjacent to the ED (see Chap. 6).

Eyes

Ocular exposures should be treated immediately by copious irrigation (usually 2 L) with NS. Ophthalmic anesthetic such as 0.5% tetracaine may be necessary to relieve blepharospasm. Lid retractors may be required for adequate irrigation. Alkalies require specific considerations. Unlike acids which can be washed off, alkalies penetrate deep into tissues. Lengthy continuous irrigation (possibly 1 or even 2 h) may be required, until the tears in the conjunctival sac have stabilized at <8.0. The pH of normal tears is slightly acidic. The pH of NS solution is 5.6. Equilibration of 10 min or longer may be required for accurate pH determination. Ophthalmologic consultation is recommended.

Gastrointestinal Decontamination

Each of the methods used to decontaminate the gastrointestinal (GI) tract have potential benefits and risks that must be considered prior to

TABLE 156-2   Common Antidotes: Doses and Indications

Antidote	DOSE Pediatrics	Adult	Poison
***N*-acetylcysteine**	140 mg/kg PO load, followed by 70 mg/kg PO q4h for 18 total doses		Acetaminophen
Activated charcoal	1 g/kg PO		Most ingested poisons
Antivenom Fab	4–6 vials IV initially over 1 h may be repeated. 2 vials every 6 h for 18 h		Envenomation by *Crotalidae*
Calcium gluconate 10% (9 mg/mL elemental calcium)	0.6–0.8 mL/kg IV	10–30 mL IV	Hypermagnesemia, hypocalcemia (ethylene glycol, hydrofluoric acid), calcium channel antagonists, black widow spider venom)
Calcium chloride 10% (27.2 mg/mL elemental calcium)	0.2–0.25 mL/kg IV	10 mL IV	
Cyanide antidote kit Amyl nitrate	Not typically used	1 ampule in oxygen chamber of ambu-bag 30 s on/30 s off	Cyanide poisoning
Sodium nitrite	0.33 mL/kg IV (3% solution)	10 mL (3% solution)	Hydrogen sulfide (use only sodium nitrate)
Thiosulfate	Thiosulfate: 1.65 mL/kg IV	Thiosulfate: 12.5 g IV	
Deferoxamine	90 mg/kg IM (1 g max) or 15 mg/kg per h IV (1 g max)	2 g IM or 15 mg/kg per h (6–8 g/d max)	Iron
Dextrose	1 g/kg IV		Hypoglycemia
Digoxin Fab Acute	10–20 vials IV		Digoxin and cardiac glycosides
Chronic	1–2 vials IV	3–6 vials IV	
Ethanol 10% for IV administration	10 mL/kg over 30 min, then 1.5 mL/h*		Ethylene glycol, methanol
Folic acid/leucovorin	1–2 mg/kg q 4–6h IV		Methanol, methotrexate (only leucovorin)
Fomepizole	15 mg/kg IV, then 10 mg/kg q12h		Methanol, ethylene glycol, disulfiram
Glucagon	50 μg/kg	1–10 mg IV	Calcium channel blocker, β-blocker
Methylene blue	1–2 mg/kg Neonates: 0.3–1 mg/kg	1–2 mg/kg	Oxidizing chemicals (e.g., nitrites, benzocaine, sulfonamides)
Octreotide	1 μg/kg q6h SC	50–100 μg SC q6h	Refractory hypoglycemia after oral hypoglycemic agent ingestion
Naloxone	As much as is needed. Typical starting dose 0.4 mg–10 mg IV		Opioid, clonidine
Physostigmine	0.02 mg/kg IV	1–2 mg IV	Anticholinergic substances (not tricyclic antidepressants)
Pralidoxime (2-PAM)	20–40 mg/kg IV	1–2 g IV	Cholinergic substances
Protamine	1 mg neutralizes 100 U of administered heparin; administered over 15 min 0.6 mg/kg	25–50 mg IV: empiric	Heparin
Pyridoxine	Gram for gram ingestion if amount of isoniazid is known 70 mg/kg IV	5 g IV	Isoniazid, *Gyromitra esculenta,* rocket fuel
Sodium bicarbonate	1–2 mEq/kg IV bolus followed by 2 mEq/kg per h		Sodium channel blockers, alkalinization of urine or serum
Thiamine	100 mg IV		Ethylene glycol, Wernicke syndrome, "wet" beri-beri
Vitamin K₁	2–5 mg/d PO	25–50 mg TID	Anticoagulants
Whole-bowel irrigation	0.5 L/h PO	1.5–2 L/h PO	Multiple indications

*This is an approximation. Dose should be titrated to level (see Chap. 166).

TABLE 156-3   Toxidromes

Toxidrome	Representative Agent(s)	Most Common Findings	Additional Signs and Symptoms	Potential Interventions
Opioid	Heroin Morphine	CNS depression, miosis, respiratory depression	Hypothermia, bradycardia. Death may result from respiratory arrest, acute lung injury	Ventilation or naloxone
Sympathomimetic	Cocaine Amphetamine	Psychomotor agitation, mydriasis, diaphoresis, tachycardia, hypertension, hyperthermia	Seizures, rhabdomyolysis, myocardial infarction Death may result from seizures, cardiac arrest, hyperthermia	Cooling, sedation with benzodiazepines, hydration
Cholinergic	Organophosphate insecticides Carbamate insecticides	Salivation, lacrimation, diaphoresis, nausea, vomiting, urination, defecation, muscle fasciculations, weakness, bronchorrhea	Bradycardia, miosis/mydriasis, seizures, respiratory failure, paralysis Death may result from respiratory arrest from paralysis, bronchorrhea, or seizures	Airway protection and ventilation, atropine, pralidoxime
Anticholinergic	Scopolamine Atropine	Altered mental status, mydriasis, dry/flushed skin, urinary retention, decreased bowel sounds, hyperthermia, dry mucous membranes	Seizures, dysrhythmias, rhabdomyolysis Death may result from hyperthermia and dysrhythmias	Physostigmine (if appropriate), sedation with benzodiazepines, cooling, supportive management
Salicylates	Aspirin Oil of wintergreen	Altered mental status, respiratory alkalosis, metabolic acidosis, tinnitus, hyperpnea, tachycardia, diaphoresis, nausea, vomiting	Low-grade fever, ketonuria Death may result from acute lung injury	MDAC, alkalinization of the urine with potassium repletion, hemodialysis, hydration
Hypoglycemia	Sulfonylureas Insulin	Altered mental status, diaphoresis, tachycardia, hypertension	Paralysis, slurring of speech, bizarre behavior, seizures Death may result from seizures, altered behavior	Glucose containing solution intravenously, and oral feedings if able, frequent capillary blood for glucose measurement, octreotide
Serotonin syndrome	Meperidine or dextromethorphan and MAOI; SSRI and TCA; SSRI/TCA/MAOI and amphetamines; SSRI alone	Altered mental status, increased muscle tone, hyperreflexia, hyperthermia	Intermittent whole-body tremor Death may result from hyperthermia	Cooling, sedation with benzodiazepines, supportive management, theoretical benefit—cyproheptadine

Abbreviations: CNS = central nervous system; MDAC = multidose activated charcoal; MAOI = monoamine oxidase inhibitor; SSRI = selective serotonin reuptake inhibitor; TCA = tricyclic antidepressant.

their use. The three general methods of decontamination involve removal of the toxin from the stomach via the mouth, binding it inside the gut lumen, or mechanically flushing it through the GI tract. The toxin ingested, the time course, the patient's clinical status, and the skills of the physician at the bedside determine the choice of method(s) used. GI decontamination must never be initiated as a punitive action.

GASTRIC EMPTYING

Emesis

Emesis can be achieved by administration of syrup of ipecac. Syrup of ipecac is a plant-derived compound composed of two alkaloidal substances—emetine and cephaeline—that work both peripherally on the stomach and centrally on the chemotactic trigger zone to induce vomiting. Dosing of syrup of ipecac is 15 mL for children 1 to 12 years of age, and 30 mL for adults, usually followed by sips of water. The dose may repeated only once if vomiting does not occur within 30 min. Approximately 90 percent of patients vomit within 20 min after the first dose, and up to 97 percent vomit after a second dose. A typical patient vomits less than three to five times, and symptoms usually resolve within 2 h.

The ingested toxin should be suspected as the etiology if protracted vomiting occurs. Contraindications to the administration of syrup of ipecac include ingestions that have the potential to alter mental status; active or prior vomiting; caustic ingestion; a toxin with more pulmonary than GI toxicity (e.g., hydrocarbons); and ingestions of toxins that have the potential for inducing seizures. Rare complications of syrup of ipecac include aspiration, Boerhaave syndrome, Mallory-Weiss tear, and intractable vomiting.

Indications for in-hospital use of syrup of ipecac are extremely limited. Most patients reach the hospital beyond the time frame when the toxin would still be expected to remain in the stomach, because either the toxin has been absorbed or has passed through the pylorus. Also, even when syrup of ipecac is given with activated charcoal less than 60 min after ingestion, it has not been demonstrated to alter outcome when compared to treatment with activated charcoal and a cathartic alone. Ipecac's administration also delays the time to administration of oral antidotes such as *N*-acetylcysteine by 1 to 6.5 h.

Possible rare hospital indications for its use include very recent ingestions of substances not expected to compromise the airway or lead to altered mental status, hemodynamic derangement, or seizure; a recent ingestion of a pill that is known not to fit into the holes of the appropriately sized orogastric tube; or a substance known not to adsorb to activated charcoal (see the following sections).

TABLE 156-4 Agents that May Alter Presenting Signs or Symptoms*

Drugs	Seizures	Change in Blood Pressure	Change in Ventilation	Change in Heart Rate	Temperature Change
Alcohol withdrawal	✓	↑	↑	↑	↑
Amphetamines	✓	↑	↑	↑	↑
Anticholinergic	✓	↑	↑	↑	↑
Baclofen	✓	↓	↓	↑	↓
Caffeine	✓	↑	↑	↑	
Camphor	✓				
Cocaine	✓	↑	↑	↑	↑
Gyrometria exculenta (mushroom)	✓				
Isoniazid	✓				
Lithium	✓				
Methaqualone	✓	↑	↓	↑	
Serotonin syndrome	✓	↑	↑	↑	↑
Theophylline	✓	↑	↑	↑	
Tricyclic antidepressants	✓	↑	↓	↑	
β-Blockers	✓	↓		↓	
Calcium-channel blockers		↓		↓	
Clonidine		↓	↓	↓	↓
Ethanol		↓	↓	↑	↓
Phenothiazines		↓	↓	↑	
Opioids		↓	↓	↓	↓
Organophosphates	✓	↓	↓	↓	
Meprobamate		↓	↓		
Monoamine oxidase inhibitor overdose	✓	↑	↑	↑	↓
Phencyclidine		↑	↓	↑	↑
Sedative hypnotic withdrawal	✓	↑	↑		↑
Phenylpropanolamine		↑	↑	↑	
Barbiturates		↓	↓	↓	↓
Ethchlorvynol		↓	↓	↓	
Glutethamide		↓	↓		
Salicylates		↓	↑	↑	↑
Nicotine	✓	↑	↑	↑	
Hydrocarbons		↓	↑	↑	
Toxic alcohols	✓	↓	↑	↑	
Iron	✓	↓	↑	↑	

*Listed are the most common or most classically seen with the agent.

Although debated by many authors, syrup of ipecac may still be indicated, especially when it can be given in the home immediately after an ingestion of a known toxin that does not have the previously listed contraindications while it still is expected to be in the stomach. This may be especially true in remote locations where transport times to definitive health care may be prolonged.

Orogastric Lavage

The principal method of gastric emptying in the emergency department is orogastric lavage, which is performed with the patient lying in the left lateral decubitus position. A 36- to 40-French tube is used for adults and a 22- to 24-French tube for children. The tube is inserted after careful measurement of the length from the chin to the xiphoid process. Correct positioning must be assessed by insufflation of air to ensure accurate placement in the stomach. Lavage with room-temperature water is commonly continued until the effluent becomes clear. Before the tube is removed, activated charcoal should be instilled in a dose of 1 g/kg, if indicated. The contraindications to lavage include pills that are known not to fit into the holes of the orogastric lavage hose, nontoxic ingestions, non-life-threatening ingestions, caustic ingestions, any patient whose airway integrity is not assured, or toxic ingestions that are more damaging to the lungs than to the GI tract. Complications include insertion of the tube into the trachea, aspiration, esophageal or gastric perforation, decreased oxygenation during the procedure,[4] and inability to withdraw the tube once inserted (knot formation).

Although the perceived benefits of orogastric lavage are the immediate return of small pills or pill fragments, and a reduction in the amount of substance available for further intoxication, studies typically

TABLE 156-5   Odors and Skin Findings

ODORS

Almonds	Cyanide
Eggs	Hydrogen sulfide, mercaptans
Fish	Zinc sulfide
Garlic	Organic phosphorus compounds
Freshly mown hay	Phosgene
Geraniums	Lewisite
Swimming pool	Chlorine gas
Mothballs	Camphor, naphthalene, *P*-dichlorobenzene
Violets	Turpentine
Wintergreen	Methyl salicylate
Peanuts	Vacor

SKIN FINDINGS

Cyanosis	Anything causing deoxyhemoglobin or methemoglobin
Yellowing of skin	Excessive consumption of vegetables containing carotene (e.g., carrots, squash), local coloration from cigarettes, dinitrophenol, picric acid
Flushing	Anticholinergic medications, scombroid, ethanol in patients aldehyde dehydrogenase deficient, rectal foreign body, disulfiram, niacin, nitrates
Gray	Metallic silver or gold
Eschar formation	Radioactive material, anthrax, brown recluse spider venom
Bullae	Barbiturates, chemotherapeutic agents
Red skin	Vancomycin, carbon monoxide, boric acid
Transverse lines across nails	Sign of major systemic insult (e.g., arsenic, chemotherapy)

demonstrate drug removal ranging from only 35 to 56 percent. Of three large studies that evaluated the clinical efficacy of orogastric lavage,[5,6] only two showed any benefit from the procedure, and only if it was initiated in patients within 1 h of the ingestion. Indications for this procedure are generally limited to recent ingestion of a life-threatening toxin that requires ventilatory support because of depressed mental status, or risk of seizures.

TOXIN ADSORPTION IN THE GUT

Activated Charcoal

The most appropriate agent to decontaminate the GI tract is activated charcoal, which is produced by pyrolysis of carbonaceous materials and "activation" by steam cleaning to increase its surface area. Activated charcoal works by adsorbing the toxin within the gut lumen, making the toxin less available for absorption into the tissues. It also enhances elimination by establishing a free-drug concentration gradient favoring movement into the GI lumen to enhance elimination ("GI dialysis"),[7] and it can also bind substances excreted in the bile, interrupting enterohepatic circulation. The benefits of this technique include its capability to decontaminate the gut without requiring invasive procedures, its rapid administration, and its proven safety in both adults and children.

Activated charcoal is typically given in a slurry of water or juice by mouth or through a nasogastric tube, in an activated charcoal-drug dose of 10:1 (thought to be the smallest dose of activated charcoal that can be given without reducing its efficacy)[8] or in 1 g/kg, whichever is larger. In adults, the first dose of activated charcoal is often given with a cathartic to reduce GI transit time. Sorbitol and magnesium citrate solution are the most commonly used cathartics (see "Cathartics" below).

Activated charcoal should not be given if esophageal or gastric perforation are suspected, or if emergency endoscopy might be needed (as in caustic ingestion). Complications that are exceedingly rare, include aspiration and intraluminal impaction in patients with abnormal gut motility.

Clear indications for administration of activated charcoal are ingestion of any drug known to adsorb to it or after an unknown ingestion by patients with protected airways. There is no indication for activated charcoal in isolated ingestion of substances known not to adsorb to activated charcoal (such as iron, lithium, or lead).

Multiple-Dose Activated Charcoal

One dose of activated charcoal is usually sufficient to achieve a therapeutic effect. Multiple-dose activated charcoal, however, is indicated in specific instances, such as after ingestion of very large doses; substances that form bezoars in the GI tract; potentially injurious toxins that slow gut function; toxins that are released slowly into the gut lumen; and those with enterohepatic, enteroenteric circulation. Multiple-dose activated charcoal is usually given as follows: the first dose is up to 1 g/kg body weight, which is then followed by subsequent doses of 0.25 to 0.50 g/kg. Repeated doses of activated charcoal should be given in intervals ranging from 1 to 4 h. Although intubated patients having ingested life-threatening toxins who have decreased gut motility can receive multiple doses, the stomach must be suctioned just prior to the administration of the next dose of activated charcoal to minimize gastric distention.

To prevent excessive fluid loss and electrolyte imbalance, only the first dose of activated charcoal should be given with a cathartic, and only if the toxin itself is not expected to cause diarrhea.

Multiple-dose activated charcoal is contraindicated in patients with non-life-threatening ingestions that result in decreased gut motility, because of increased risks of aspiration from gastric distention, and impaction of charcoal within the gut.

Cathartics

Often, activated charcoal is administered with an osmotic cathartic, such as 70% sorbitol (1 g/kg), or a 10% solution of magnesium citrate (in a dose of 250 mL for adults and 4 mL/kg for children). Cathartics have been repeatedly shown to decrease the transit time for the passage of the activated charcoal (and presumably the adsorbed toxin) through the GI tract.[9,10] Although most studies fail to show a benefit of administering a cathartic alone,[11,12] several studies suggest that there is a decrease in peak serum plasma concentrations and area under the curve, when the cathartic is administered with activated charcoal.[12–14] No definitive clinical human data, however, suggest that the addition of a cathartic to a dose of activated charcoal either limits the toxin's bioavailability or changes the patient's clinical outcome.

Indications for use of cathartics generally mirror those for the administration of activated charcoal. When multiple-dose activated charcoal is used, only the first dose is accompanied by a cathartic, to limit complications. Complications of cathartic administration include nausea and abdominal pain, severe volume depletion, electrolyte imbalances and fluid shifts, and hypermagnesemia in patients with renal compromise.

Contraindications for cathartic use are: ingestion of a substance that will result in diarrhea; children younger than age 5; patients with renal failure (magnesium-containing cathartics are contraindicated); intestinal obstruction; or ingestion of any caustic material.

Whole-Bowel Irrigation

Whole-bowel irrigation is the installation of large volumes of polyethylene glycol in an osmotically balanced electrolyte solution that causes neither fluid nor electrolyte shifts. This technique is accomplished in adults by the installation of 2 L/h polyethylene glycol solution either by mouth or through a nasogastric tube. In children, the volume administered is 50 to 250 mL/kg per h or as much polyethylene glycol solution as can be tolerated. The end point is clear rectal effluent.

When done properly, this technique produces a rapid catharsis by mechanically forcing ingested substances through the bowel at a rapid rate.

Contraindications include: patients with preceding diarrhea; ingestions that are expected to result in significant diarrhea (except for heavy metals, as these substances do not adsorb well to activated charcoal); and patients with absent bowel sounds or with obstruction. Complications include bloating, cramping, and rectal irritation from frequent bowel movements. Close nursing care is needed to maintain patient cleanliness.

Controlled studies clearly demonstrating improvement in clinical outcome after this procedure are lacking, but many authors describe limited symptomatology following potentially toxic doses of substances known not to adsorb to activated charcoal.[15] Table 156-6 lists common indications for whole-bowel irrigation.

Frequently, an antiemetic is required to prevent the nausea and vomiting that results from gastric distention with large volumes of whole-bowel irrigation solution. Care must be taken to avoid phenothiazine derived antiemetics that may slow gut function. Generally, either metoclopramide or ondansetron are used for this purpose.

ENHANCED ELIMINATION

Alkalinization

Urinary alkalinization is beneficial in the treatment of certain ingestions. The urinary pH is manipulated to exploit physiologic properties of specific toxins. Only nonionized substances are free to move passively across membranes. Ionized particles must remain in the fluid-filled compartments in which they were formed. Weak acids are mostly uncharged at physiologic pH, but become charged in alkaline environments. After intravenous administration, bicarbonate becomes concentrated in the urine resulting in significant elevation of urinary pH (if the patient has a normal serum potassium). By significantly raising the urinary pH with intravenous sodium bicarbonate, toxins that are weak acids are converted from their nonionized form to their ionized form and are therefore held within the urinary collection system. This "ion trapping" keeps the toxin within the renal tubules, thereby enhancing its excretion out of the body in the urine. This creates an imbalance in the concentration gradient of the toxin between the blood and the urinary collection system, drawing more toxin into the renal tubular lumen. The ideal toxin that can be eliminated by this technique is one with substantial urinary excretion and with a pK_a less than the serum pH (Table 156-7).

Urinary alkalinization is typically achieved by the administration of an intravenous bolus of 1 to 2 mEq/kg sodium bicarbonate, followed by either intermittent boluses of sodium bicarbonate or a continuous intravenous infusion to achieve a urinary pH of 7.5 to 8.0. Serum pH should not be allowed to rise above 7.5 to 7.55. Pronounced hypokalemia may result from this technique and must be corrected aggressively. Hypokalemia induces the kidneys to reabsorb potassium and excrete hydrogen ions, inhibiting the production of alkaline urine. This may result in relatively acidic urine when compared to the serum pH.

The benefit of urinary alkalinization is a decrease in toxin serum half-life from increased urinary excretion. The risks include volume

TABLE 156-6   Conditions in Which Whole-Bowel Irrigation May be Helpful

Heavy metals
Body packers
Iron
Lithium
Sustained or delayed release formulations
Potential for bezoar formation

TABLE 156-7   Modalities That May Enhance Elimination for Certain Substances

Drugs	Agents Where Urinary Alkalinization is Commonly Considered	Agents Where Hemodialysis is Commonly Considered
2-4-D (herbicide)	✓	
Phenobarbital	✓	
Chlorpropamide	✓	
Salicylates	✓	✓
Methanol	✓	✓
Ethylene glycol		✓
Lithium		✓
Theophylline*		✓
Amanita (mushrooms)*		✓

*Indicates also removed by hemoperfusion.

overload (congestive heart failure, pulmonary edema), pH shifts, and hypokalemia. Therefore, contraindications to this procedure include patients who cannot tolerate the volume or sodium load, are hypokalemic, have renal insufficiency, and ingestion of a toxin that does not respond to alkalinization.

Acidification of Urine

Acidification of urine can somewhat enhance elimination of amphetamines, phencyclidine, and some other drugs. However, the risks, particularly in relation to rhabdomyolysis, far outweigh any benefits.

Forced Diuresis

Forced diuresis has never been shown to be effective for any ingestion. Given the potential of harm, this technique should not be used.

Hemodialysis/Hemoperfusion

Hemodialysis is generally reserved for specific toxins that must be both potentially life-threatening and amenable to removal by this method (see Table 156-7). The benefits include the ability to remove toxins that are already absorbed from the gut lumen, removal of substances that do not adhere to activated charcoal, and the ability to remove both the parent compound and the active toxic metabolites. Hemodialysis is much less effective when the toxin ingested has a large volume of distribution (>1 L/kg), has a large molecular weight (more than 500 Da), or is highly protein bound.

Hemodialysis is rarely absolutely contraindicated, but relative contraindications include hemodynamic instability, very small children, and patients with poor vascular access or profound bleeding diatheses. Risks of hemodialysis are typically minimal in experienced centers, but they include large fluid shifts, electrolyte imbalances, infection and bleeding at the catheter site, and intracranial hemorrhage. Exchange transfusion should be considered in small children who cannot receive hemodialysis because of technical limitations.

Hemoperfusion, which is also used for decontamination of a patient's systemic circulation, involves placing a filter filled with activated charcoal into the circuit of the hemodialysis machine. This filtration alleviates the constraints of protein binding and molecular size, both of which limit the utility of hemodialysis. Toxins that can be removed by this method must adsorb well to activated charcoal and have a small volume of distribution. While potentially useful for phenobarbital, phenytoin, and ethchlorvynol, in practice, it is only commonly recommended for theophylline overdoses.

REFERENCES

1. Litovitz T, Klein-Schwartz W, White S, et al: 2000 Annual Report of the American Association of Poison Control Centers Toxic Exposure Surveillance System. *Ann Emerg Med* 19:337, 2001.
2. Hack JB, Hoffman RS: Thiamine before glucose to prevent Wernicke encephalopathy: Examining the conventional wisdom. *JAMA* 279:583, 1998.
3. Hoffman JR, Schringer DL, Votey SR, Luo JS: The empiric use of naloxone in patients with altered mental status: A reappraisal. *Ann Emerg Med* 20:246, 1991.
4. Thompson AM, Robins JB, Prescott LF: Changes in cardiorespiratory function during gastric lavage for drug overdose. *Hum Toxicol* 6:215, 1987.
5. Merigian KS, Woodward M, Hedges JR, et al: Prospective evaluation of gastric emptying in the self-poisoned patient. *Am J Emerg Med* 8:479, 1990.
6. Pond SM, Lewis-Driver DJ, Williams GM, et al: Gastric emptying in acute overdose: A prospective randomized controlled trial. *Med J Aust* 163:345, 1995.
7. Levy G: Gastrointestinal clearance of drugs with activated charcoal. *New Engl J Med* 307:676, 1982.
8. Olkkola K: Effect of charcoal-drug ratio on antidotal efficacy of oral activated charcoal in man. *Br J Clin Pharmacol* 19:767, 1985.
9. Krenzelok EP, Keller R, Stewart RD: Gastrointestinal transit times of cathartics combined with charcoal. *Ann Emerg Med* 14:1152, 1985.
10. Harchelroad F, Cottington E, Krenzelok EP: Gastrointestinal transit times of a charcoal/sorbitol slurry in overdose patients. *J Toxicol Clin Toxicol* 27:91, 1989.
11. Minton NA, Henry JA: Prevention of drug absorption in simulated theophylline overdose. *J Toxicol Clin Toxicol* 33:43, 1995.
12. Al-Shareef AH, Buss DC, Allen EM, Routledge PA: The effects of charcoal and sorbitol (alone and in combination) on plasma theophylline concentrations after a sustained-release formulation. *Hum Exp Toxicol* 9:179, 1990.
13. Picchioni AL, Chin L, Gillespie T: Evaluation of activated charcoal-sorbitol suspension as an antidote. *J Toxicol Clin Toxicol* 19:433, 1982.
14. Goldberg MJ, Spector R, Park GD, et al: The effect of sorbitol and activated charcoal on serum theophylline concentrations after slow-release theophylline. *Clin Pharmacol Ther* 41:108, 1987.
15. Roberge RJ, Martin TG: Whole-bowel irrigation in an acute oral lead intoxication. *Am J Emerg Med* 10:577, 1992.

PRINCIPLES OF DRUG INTERACTIONS
George Delgado, Jr.
Jamie Pilarowski

The use of medications to treat disease is not without peril. Clinicians are required to assess the risks and benefits of drug therapy before implementing such treatment. For a clinician to treat certain conditions, it may be necessary to use multiple medications. Using multiple medications can increase the risk of drug interactions through an increase or decrease in efficacy or toxicity due to one agent or multiple agents. Although a drug interaction can be predicted at times, drug interactions may not consistently result in the same clinically observable outcome and may vary due to dosing, differences between agents in a certain class, concomitant disease states of a patient, and duration of administration.

The mechanisms of these drug interactions are pharmacokinetic and pharmacodynamic in nature. Pharmacokinetic mechanisms of drug interactions can occur in one of the four different phases of the body's processing of medication: absorption, distribution, metabolism, and elimination. Some interactions that involve absorption include:

1. Prevention of absorption through binding of the medication in the gut [e.g., ciprofloxacin (Cipro) and antacids]
2. Increased absorption by inhibition of gut lining metabolism [e.g., felodipine (Plendil) and grapefruit juice]
3. Changes in absorption capacity by alteration of gut flora (e.g., ampicillin and oral contraceptives)

4. Changes in gut pH or motility [e.g. ranitidine (Zantac) and ketoconazole (Nizoral)]

Distribution interactions usually involve drugs that are normally highly protein bound. Increased concentrations of a highly bound agent can occur by displacement from its binding site by another agent. For example, sulfonylureas and warfarin (Coumadin), which are over 90 percent protein bound, when given together may increase the international normalized ratio (INR) and increase the risk of bleeding. Metabolism interactions can occur when a medication decreases or increases the metabolism of another agent. Of particular importance are those medications that are metabolized by the cytochrome P450 (P450) enzyme family. There are two mechanisms for P450-mediated interactions, induction and inhibition. An induction interaction is the result of decreased degradation or increased synthesis of P450 enzymes, thereby accelerating the conversion of active medication to its inactive metabolites. For instance, nafcillin administered with warfarin induces metabolic enzymes that increase the metabolism of warfarin, resulting in a decreased anticoagulant effect. An inhibition interaction, which can refer to competition of substrates (drugs) for a site or enzyme inactivation, results in a decreased rate of drug metabolism, leading to a prolonged half-life and a potential for increased pharmacodynamic effects. For example, the concomitant use of metronidazole (Flagyl) and warfarin decreases warfarin metabolism, resulting in an increase in anticoagulant effect. Agents commonly associated with interactions with other agents are presented.

ANTICOAGULANTS

Concurrent administration of warfarin with agents such as alcohol, macrolides, sulfonamides, azole antifungals, and amiodarone (Cordarone) may significantly increase the anticoagulation activity. Some nonsteroidal anti-inflammatory drugs (NSAIDs), such as phenylbutazone and naproxen, have been reported to displace warfarin from plasma proteins, whereas others do not appear to have effects. Selective cyclooxygenase 2 (Cox-2) inhibitors may slightly elevate prothrombin times. Chronic alcohol ingestion, nafcillin, barbiturates, and rifampin may significantly decrease the anticoagulation activity.[1]

ANTIMICROBIAL AGENTS

Although most drug interactions are sources of concern, some are predictable and can be used to enhance the effect of some antimicrobials.[2] In fact, the interaction of probenecid in combination with penicillins or cephalosporins has been used to decrease the need for multiple doses of shorter-acting antibiotics by inhibiting their elimination.

Some of the more troubling adverse effects of drug interactions concern antimicrobials that induce or inhibit hepatic or renal metabolism of other drugs. The agents most commonly associated with these types of drug interactions are rifampin, erythromycin, isoniazid, and the azole antifungals. For example, rifampin, an inducer of the hepatic P450 system, increases clearance of many medications and therefore reduces efficacy. Medications that have been shown to interact with rifampin include digoxin, calcium channel blockers, amiodarone, 3-hydroxy-3-methylglutaryl coenzyme A reductase inhibitors, azole antifungals, corticosteroids, and theophylline.

ANTIRETROVIRAL AGENTS

The increasing complexity of highly active antiretroviral therapy (HAART) for treating human immunodeficiency virus infection warrants special attention for drug interactions. The most common drug interactions occur with the use of a nonnucleoside reverse transcriptase inhibitor or a protease inhibitor, which are metabolized primarily by the P450 system and inhibit or induce the metabolism of other agents that use the P450 system. This interaction can be quite problematic because of the typical HAART regimen consisting of two nucleoside reverse transcriptase inhibitors in addition to a nonnucleoside reverse transcriptase inhibitor or a protease inhibitor. For example, a HAART regimen that includes ritonavir (Norvir; a strong inhibitor of cytochrome P4503A4) and used concomitantly with certain 3-hydroxy-3-methylglutaryl coenzyme A reductase inhibitors can significantly increase the risk of rhabdomyolysis.[3,4]

THEOPHYLLINE

Theophylline is still used in children and on occasion in adults to provide preventative and symptomatic relief of bronchospasm in patients with chronic asthma, bronchitis, and emphysema. Interventions are discussed in detail in Chap. 173. When adding a macrolide or fluoroquinolone, caution must be used because the interaction may result in an increase in theophylline levels.

CARDIOVASCULAR DRUGS

Antihypertensives such as metoprolol succinate (Lopressor), propranolol hydrochloride (Inderal), and verapamil (Calan and Isoptin) exhibit decreased bioavailability secondary to induction by medications such as rifampin and phenobarbital (Luminal), which are strong inducers of the P450 system.[5] The end result of this interaction is the lowering of these agents below therapeutic levels. Cimetidine (Tagamet), a P450 inducer, may produce the opposite effect. Another significant inhibition interaction can be seen with the azole antifungal agents and the dihydropyridine calcium channel blockers, such as amlodipine (Norvasc) and felodipine. This combination inhibits the metabolism of calcium channel blockers and should be avoided. Certain calcium channel blockers also have been shown to increase other drug levels through a decreased clearance. For example, diltiazem (Cardizem), nifedipine (Procardia and Adalat), and verapamil can decrease the clearance of theophylline by more than 25 percent. Another example is the coadministration of cyclosporine with diltiazem or verapamil, which can result in a lower maintenance dose for cyclosporine. Verapamil is also responsible for increasing the bioavailability of simvastatin (Zocor). The dose of simvastatin should be reduced if the combination of the two cannot be avoided.

Digoxin, due to its narrow therapeutic index and kinetic profile, should be taken into consideration when discussing drug-to-drug interactions. Digoxin's long half-life, large volume of distribution, fairly extensive tissue binding, and high percentage of renal excretion (>80 percent) combined with its narrow therapeutic index set the path for numerous interactions. Some of the most clinically relevant drug interactions include amiodarone, spironolactone (Aldactone), and verapamil, which decrease digoxin clearance and increase serum digoxin levels. In addition, serum digoxin levels rise with quinidine coadministration through a decrease in digoxin clearance and displacement of digoxin from binding sites in tissue. Diuretics also may play a role in interactions by potassium and magnesium depletion, which may increase the risk of digoxin side effects, such as arrhythmias. β-blockers, such as carvedilol (Coreg), have been shown to increase the bioavailability of digoxin when given in combination.

QT PROLONGATION

Various individual or classes of drugs, electrolyte imbalances, and some congenital syndromes prolong the QT interval, which itself potentiates the development of torsades de pointes. Some of these drugs may cause QT prolongation alone or in combination with other drugs that have the same potential. For example, quinidine, ibutilide (Corvert), amiodarone, and haloperidol (Haldol) can cause QT prolongation and or torsades de pointes on their own, but other drugs, such as the azole antifungals, when used in combination with agents known to prolong QT intervals may further increase the risk of developing this arrhythmia.

HERBAL MEDICINE

With the overwhelming increase in the number of patients consuming herbal and dietary supplements in addition to their prescription medications, it is important to consider the potential for interactions between them.[6–8] Because herbal products are not strictly regulated and tested by the Food and Drug Administration, the data regarding these interactions are limited. The data that do exist are from case reports or from other countries. Table 157-1 lists a summary of some of the important herbal and drug interactions. The Natural Medicines Comprehensive Database (http://www.naturaldatabase.com) and the NIH Office of Dietary Supplements, IBIDS Consumer Database (http://www.dietary-supplements.info.nih.gov) are other sources of information.

ANTIEPILEPTIC DRUGS

Epilepsy is a chronic disease state in which patients may require years of treatment with antiepileptic drugs. Some epileptic patients will require treatment with more than one antiepileptic drug to maintain seizure control. Further, concomitant disease states may require the administration of other drug therapies, thus increasing the potential for interactions.[9,10]

Many of the older antiepileptic drugs are metabolized by the P450 system and are inducers or inhibitors of these enzymes. Carbamazepine (Tegretol), phenobarbital, phenytoin, and primidone (Mysoline) are inducers, whereas valproic acid (Depakene) is an inhibitor. In addition, some of these older agents may be more highly protein bound (i.e., phenytoin and valproic acid), which can have an effect on drug interactions. Most of the newer antiepileptic drugs undergo minimal or no metabolism by the P450 system, so many possible drug interactions can be avoided. In addition, many of the newer agents do not induce or inhibit enzymes involved in the metabolism of other drugs.

One clinically significant drug interaction that is important to keep in mind with coadministration of antiepileptic drugs is the reduction of contraceptive efficacy via increased metabolism and clearance of oral contraceptive drugs. Antiepileptic drugs implicated in this type of interaction include carbamazepine, phenytoin, phenobarbital, oxcarbazepine (Trileptal), and felbamate (Felbatol). Not all of the newer antiepileptic drugs are known to contribute to this interaction, but caution should be advised and the patient counseled on alternative methods of birth control.

Other drugs that are susceptible to increased metabolism via enzyme induction by phenytoin, carbamazepine, phenobarbital, and primidone are theophylline, warfarin, digoxin, cyclosporine, antiretroviral agents, and griseofulvin. The induction caused by these antiepileptic drugs could decrease the efficacy of these drugs and potentially cause treatment failure.

Valproic acid, an enzyme inhibitor, may increase plasma concentrations of phenytoin, carbamazepine, phenobarbital, and lamotrigine (Lamictal), thus putting the patient at risk of supratherapeutic levels if used in combination without dosage adjustment and monitoring.

PSYCHOTROPICS

There are several antidepressant and antipsychotic medications in use today, but only some of the more important interactions with these agents are discussed. One of the most impressive and significant interactions concern a specific class of antidepressants known as the monoamine oxidase inhibitors. These agents [phenelzine (Nardil), selegiline (Eldepryl), and tranylcypromine (Parnate)] are not as commonly prescribed today due to newer agents that have a better safety profile. Monoamine oxidase inhibitors have a rare but potentially fatal interaction when taken with specific foods high in tyramine content and with certain drugs. A marked pressor effect is seen and may develop into hypertensive crisis with subsequent cerebral vascular accident and death. Symptoms include headache, stiff neck, nausea,

TABLE 157-1 Herbal Interactions

Herbal Medication	Potential Interaction	Effect/Possible Mechanism
Coenzyme Q	Warfarin	Decreased INR (coenzyme Q contains vitamin K derivatives)
Danshen	Warfarin	Increased INR (decreased warfarin clearance/increased bioavailability; also, danshen may contain coumarin derivatives); hemorrhage reported
Dong Quai	Caffeine; theophylline	Exaggerated sympathomimetic activity
	Antiplatelet drugs; warfarin	Increased INR/increased bleeding tendency (platelet inhibition; dong quai contains coumarin derivatives)
Feverfew	Antiplatelet drugs (NSAIDs, ticlopidine, clopidogrel, dipyridamole); warfarin	Inhibition of platelet aggregation (increased risk of bleeding)
	Anti-serotonin migraine drugs (e.g., sumatriptan)	Inhibition of serotonin release (increased risk of serotonin syndrome–like picture)
Garlic	Warfarin	Increased INR (potential fibrinolytic/antiplatelet activity of garlic); hemorrhage reported
	Antihyperglycemic agents	Hypoglycemia (additive effect on glucose levels)
Ginger	Antiplatelet drugs; warfarin	Platelet inhibition
	Antihypertensives	Variable effects (may cause loss of BP control in patients on antihypertensives)
Ginkgo	Antiplatelet drugs; warfarin; aspirin; rofecoxib	Antiplatelet activity/increased bleeding tendency (CNS hemorrhage reported with warfarin)
	Trazodone	Increased production of one of the active metabolites of trazodone (potential for trazodone toxicity including coma)
Ginseng	Warfarin	Decreased INR (increased warfarin metabolism)
	Antihypertensive agents	Increase or decrease in blood pressure
	Antihyperglycemic agents	Hypoglycemia (additive effect of glucose levels)
Kava	Antiplatelet drugs; warfarin	Increased risk of bleeding (platelet inhibition)
	Benzodiazepines	Increased anxiolytic properties (additive effect)
St. John's wort	Tricyclic antidepressants, theophylline, indinavir, monoamine oxidase inhibitors, cyclosporin, oral contraceptives, warfarin, alprazolam, simvastatin, tacrolimus	Decreased levels of mentioned agents (enzyme induction by St. John's wort)
	Digoxin	Decreased digoxin levels (increased P-glycoprotein activity)
	SSRI	Increased serotonin effects
Yohimbine	Clonidine, tricyclic antidepressants	Hypertension (α_2 antagonism)

Abbreviations: CNS = central nervous system; INR = international normalized ratio; NSAIDs = nonsteroidal anti-inflammatory drugs; SSRI = serotonin selective reuptake inhibitor.

vomiting, diaphoresis, and an abrupt increase in blood pressure. Some of the common medications that must be restricted in patients on monoamine oxidase inhibitors include meperidine (Demerol), dextromethorphan, asthma inhalants, carbamazepine, decongestants (topical and systemic), and agents with sympathomimetic activity (see Chap. 160).

Another psychotropic agent with the potential for drug interactions is haloperidol. Haloperidol, a phenothiazine antipsychotic agent, is metabolized by the P450 system (primarily 2D6 and 3A4). Carbamazepine and other inducers may decrease plasma concentrations of haloperidol, chlorpromazine (Thorazine), clozapine (Clozaril), and risperidone (Risperdal), whereas valproic acid may inhibit metabolism of certain psychotropic agents.[10,11]

The most common and troubling drug interactions with lithium include NSAIDs, angiotensin converting enzyme inhibitors, and diuretics. The NSAIDs and angiotensin converting enzyme inhibitors decrease lithium clearance and increase lithium concentrations, whereas diuretics can produce either effect depending on the class of the diuretic (i.e., where the diuretic works in the renal system). For example, loop and thiazide diuretics increase lithium concentrations by increasing lithium reabsorption. Conversely, carbonic anhydrase inhibitors and osmotic diuretics can increase lithium excretion. Caffeine and theophylline also can increase lithium excretion.

CONCLUSION

One of the many challenges of medicine is choosing the most appropriate medication, which may be complicated further by the use of multiple agents and comorbid conditions that may alter the pharmacodynamics and pharmacokinetics of these medications. A few of the significant drug interactions are reviewed in this chapter. As more drugs gain approval and the popularity of herbal supplements continues to grow, so will the potential for interactions. Awareness of the general pharmacokinetic properties of a given class of medication may help to avoid a potentially fatal drug interaction.

REFERENCES

1. Wittkowsky AK: Drug interactions update: Drugs, herbs and oral anticoagulation. *J Thromb Thrombolysis* 12:67, 2001.
2. Gregg CR: Drug interactions and anti-infective therapies. *Am J Med* 106:227, 1999.
3. Rainey PM: HIV drug interactions: The good, the bad, and the other. *Ther Drug Monit* 24:26, 2002.
4. Williams D, Feely J: Pharmacokinetic-pharmacodynamic drug interactions with HMG-CoA reductase inhibitors. *Clin Pharmacokinet* 41:343, 2002.

5. Flockhart DA, Tanus-Santos JE: Implications of cytochrome P450 interactions when prescribing medication for hypertension. *Arch Intern Med* 162:405, 2002.
6. DeSmet PA: Herbal remedies. *New Engl J Med* 347:2046, 2002.
7. Valli G, Giardina EV: Benefits, adverse effects and drug interactions of herbal therapies with cardiovascular effects. *J Am Coll Cardiol* 39:1083, 2002.
8. Izzo AA, Ernst E: Interactions between herbal medicines and prescribed drugs. A systematic review. *Drugs* 61:2163, 2001.
9. Patsalos PN, Froscher W, Pisani F, et al: The importance of drug interactions in epilepsy therapy. *Epilepsia* 43:365, 2002.
10. Hachad H, Ragueneau-Majlessi I, Levy RH: New epileptic drugs: Review on drug interactions. *Ther Drug Monit* 24:91, 2002.
11. Spina E, Perucca E: Clinical significance of pharmacokinetic interactions between antiepileptic and psychotropic drugs. *Epilepsia* 43(suppl 2):37, 2002.

158 TRICYCLIC ANTIDEPRESSANTS
Kirk C. Mills

EPIDEMIOLOGY

Although their popularity has decreased in recent years, tricyclic antidepressants (TCAs) remain a frequent cause of drug exposure and overdose, in most cases requiring emergent medical care. Approximately 1 in every 30 adult exposures to a pharmaceutical medication involves a TCA.[1] The 2001 Annual Report of the American Association of Poison Control Centers Toxic Exposure Surveillance System demonstrates that TCAs are associated with more drug-related deaths than any other class of prescription medication.[1] Over the past decade there have been an average annual reporting of 18,000 exposures and 110 associated deaths related to TCAs. The relatively low exposure-to-death ratio of TCAs underscores their low therapeutic index and potential for severe toxicity resulting in death. Most reported TCA exposures occur in young adults, with approximately 60 percent of all exposures believed to be intentional.

TCAs are used primarily for the treatment of major depression. In addition, they are prescribed frequently for other psychiatric and medical conditions such as obsessive-compulsive disorder, attention-deficit disorder, panic and phobia disorders, anxiety disorders, eating disorders, chronic pain syndromes, peripheral neuropathies, nocturnal enuresis, migraine headache prophylaxis, and selected drug-withdrawal therapy. Pediatric and adolescent use has increased significantly over the past few years. There are currently eight different TCAs available in the United States (Table 158-1), but many more varieties are available in other countries. The five most commonly reported TCAs involved in drug exposures include amitriptyline (40 percent), imipramine (17 percent), doxepin (14 percent), nortriptyline (12 percent), and desipramine (6 percent). Two related antidepressants, maprotiline and amoxapine, have minor structural differences when compared with traditional TCAs but have similar toxicity in overdose and thus will be included in this chapter. Cyclobenzaprine (Flexeril) is a muscle relaxant that is almost structurally identical to amitriptyline but lacks antidepressant activity. It tends to have less cardiotoxicity than amitriptyline but still can produce significant central nervous system (CNS) sedation and antimuscarinic toxicity in overdose.[2] Therapeutic doses of TCAs are highly variable. Initially, lower doses are used, followed by gradual increases until the desired therapeutic response is achieved. In addition, this process allows most patients to become acclimated to the typical TCA-induced adverse effects such as CNS sedation and dry mucous membranes.

TCA-related drug toxicity is not just limited to cases of drug overdose (Table 158-2). There are at least seven different possible mechanisms for developing TCA-related drug toxicity while taking therapeutic doses. First, mild to moderate toxicity will develop commonly if unacclimated individuals are started on higher therapeutic doses. Second, toxicity can result when TCAs are combined with other medications having similar pharmacologic actions (e.g., antihistamines, antipsychotics). Third, a subset of the population consists of slow metabolizers of TCAs, and as such, these people will develop higher plasma TCA levels for any given dose. Fourth, many drugs have the potential to inhibit the metabolism of TCAs, resulting in elevated TCA plasma levels. Fifth, some TCAs are available as mixed-drug formulations combined with either benzodiazepines or antipsychotic agents, having the potential for additional drug toxicity. Sixth, patients with certain medical conditions such as underlying heart problems or seizure disorders are more susceptible to TCA toxicity at therapeutic doses. Seventh, TCAs have the potential to produce serotonin syndrome, especially in combination with other serotonergic medications (see Chap. 159).

TABLE 158-1 Tricyclic Antidepressants

Generic Name	Trade Name(s)	Formulations (mg)	Adult Daily Dose (mg)	Active Metabolites
Amitriptyline	Elavil	10, 25, 50, 75, 100, 150	75–300	Nortriptyline
Amoxapine*	Asendin	25, 50, 100, 150	50–300	7-Hydroxyamoxapine 8-Hydroxyamoxapine
Clomipramine	Anafranil	25, 50, 75	50–200	Desmethylclomipramine
Cyclobenzaprine*	Flexeril	10-mg tablet	20–40	None
Desipramine	Norpramin Pertofrane	10, 25, 50, 75, 100, 150	75–200	None
Doxepin	Adapin, Sinequan	10, 25, 50, 75, 100, 150 Oral solution 10 mg/mL	75–300	Desmethyldoxepin
Imipramine	Tofranil	10, 25, 50	75–200	Desipramine
Maprotiline*	Ludiomil	25, 50, 75	75–150	Desmethylmaprotiline
Nortriptyline	Pamelor, Aventyl	10, 25, 50, 75 Oral solution 2 mg/mL	75–150	None
Protriptyline	Vivactil	5, 10	15–40	None
Trimipramine	Surmontil	25, 50, 100	75–200	Desmethyltrimipramine

*See text for clarification.

TABLE 158-2 Mechanisms for TCA Drug Toxicity at Therapeutic Doses

Development of serotonin syndrome
Drug interactions with medications that inhibit hepatic metabolism (P450 system)
Drug interactions with medications sharing similar pharmacologic actions
Elevated levels of TCAs due to genetically slow hepatic metabolism
Patients with preexisting cardiovascular or CNS disease
Some combination TCA medications contain other active ingredients (e.g., antipsychotics)
Unacclimated individuals starting on high therapeutic doses

PATHOPHYSIOLOGY

TCAs have a distinct chemical structure consisting of three aromatic rings: a central seven-member ring, two outer benzene rings, and an aminopropyl side chain connected to the central ring. There are only minor structural differences among the TCAs, usually on the central aromatic ring or aminopropyl side chain. Amoxapine is unique in that it has an aromatic side chain. Maprotiline has an ethylene bridge across a six-member center ring, giving it a tetracyclic chemical structure. It is not surprising that other chemicals that share the same basic tricyclic chemical structure as the TCAs, such as carbamazepine and phenothiazines, would manifest similar toxicity in overdose.

TCAs are nonselective agents that exhibit a multitude of pharmacologic effects (Table 158-3) and have considerable variation in potency. There are subtle and potentially clinically significant pharmacologic differences among the TCAs at therapeutic plasma levels. However, these differences become less important at the higher plasma levels typically seen in overdose. Only a few of their pharmacologic actions are believed to have a direct therapeutic effect, such as inhibition of amine reuptake (norepinephrine, serotonin) and antagonism of postsynaptic serotonin receptors (5-HT$_2$). Thus the remaining pharmacologic actions are essentially without therapeutic benefit but significantly contribute to TCA-related adverse effects and overdose toxicity. Most clinical findings seen in TCA overdose can be explained by the following seven pharmacologic actions, listed in descending order of general potency.

Antihistaminic Effects

TCAs are potent inhibitors of peripheral and central postsynaptic histamine receptors. Doxepin is a prime example, but its nonspecific pharmacologic activity makes it impractical to use for treatment of seasonal allergies or other allergic conditions. Antagonism of central histamine receptors leads primarily to CNS sedation and may contribute significantly to the development of coma frequently seen in TCA overdose.

Antimuscarinic Effects

TCAs are competitive inhibitors of acetylcholine at central and peripheral muscarinic receptors but do not antagonize acetylcholine at nicotinic receptors. This action, commonly referred to as being *anticholinergic*, is imprecise and inaccurate. Central antimuscarinic symptoms vary from agitation to delirium, confusion, amnesia, hallucinations, slurred speech, ataxia, sedation, and coma. Peripheral antimuscarinic symptoms include dilated pupils, blurred vision, tachycardia, hyperthermia, hypertension, decreased oral and bronchial secretions, dry skin, ileus, urinary retention, increased muscle tone, and tremor. Antimuscarinic symptoms are especially common when TCAs are combined with other medications that also have antimuscarinic activity. Examples include antihistamines, antipsychotics, antiparkinsonian drugs, antispasmodics, and some muscle relaxants.

TABLE 158-3 Pharmacologic Profile of Tricyclic Antidepressants

Pharmacologic Activity	Potency	Clinical Presentation	Treatment
Antagonism of postsynaptic histamine receptors	++ to ++++	Sedation	Supportive care alone
Antagonism of postsynaptic muscarinic receptors	++ to ++++	Sedation, coma, agitation, confusion, hallucinations, seizures, mydriasis, dry mucous membranes, dry skin, tachycardia, mild hypertension, hyperthermia, ileus, urinary retention, tremor	Supportive care alone (physostigmine contraindicated)
Antagonism of postsynaptic α-adrenergic receptors	++ to ++++	Sedation, miosis, orthostatic hypotension, reflex tachycardia	Intravenous fluids Norepinephrine
Inhibition of norepinephrine reuptake	+ to ++++	Agitation, mydriasis, diaphoresis, tachycardia, early hypertension	Supportive care alone
Inhibition of serotonin reuptake	+ to ++++	Sedation, mydriasis, myoclonus, hyperreflexia (see serotonin syndrome)	Supportive care alone Consider cyproheptadine for treatment of serotonin syndrome
Inhibition of voltage-gated sodium channels	+ to ++++	Impaired conduction, wide QRS, other conduction abnormalities; impaired cardiac contractility; wide complex sinus tachycardia, ventricular ectopy Hypotension	Sodium bicarbonate Hyperventilation Hypertonic saline Intravenous fluids Sodium bicarbonate Hypertonic saline
Inhibition of voltage-gated potassium channels	+ to +++	Prolongation of QT interval, ventricular ectopy, torsades de pointes	Magnesium sulfate Cardiac overdrive pacing
Antagonism of postsynaptic serotonin (5-HT) receptors	+ to ++	None, possible therapeutic benefit	None
Antagonism of postsynaptic GABA-A receptors	+ to ++	Seizures	Benzodiazepines Phenobarbital or propofol
Antagonism of postsynaptic dopamine receptors	+ to ++	Extrapyramidal symptoms ranging from dystonic reactions to neuroleptic malignant syndrome	Supportive care

Physostigmine is an inhibitor of acetylcholinesterase activity and potentially can reverse antimuscarinic symptoms. Historically, it was used to reverse TCA-induced antimuscarinic symptoms, but its use is often associated with life-threatening complications. Although antimuscarinic symptoms are a common finding in TCA overdose, they are not directly responsible for TCA-related deaths. Therefore, antimuscarinic symptoms are an important clinical marker of TCA toxicity, but they do not require specific therapy other than supportive care alone. Physostigmine has no role in the current management of TCA overdose in the ED.

Inhibition of α-Adrenergic Receptors

Inhibition of postsynaptic central and peripheral α-adrenergic receptors is a characteristic action of most TCAs. They do not inhibit β-adrenergic receptors. TCAs have a much greater affinity for $α_1$- than $α_2$-adrenergic receptors. Inhibition of $α_1$ receptors produces CNS sedation, orthostatic hypotension, and pupillary constriction. This action frequently offsets antimuscarinic-induced pupillary dilatation. Thus patients with TCA toxicity can present with constricted, dilated, or midpoint-sized pupils. Orthostatic hypotension is often associated with reflex tachycardia. The antihypertensive effect of clonidine can be negated by TCAs because of their ability to block the binding of clonidine to $α_2$ receptors.

Inhibition of Amine Uptake

Inhibition of amine reuptake is believed to be the most important mechanism by which TCAs are efficacious in treating depression. TCAs are potent inhibitors of norepinephrine (NE) and serotonin (5-HT) reuptake but have little affinity for inhibition of dopamine (DA) reuptake.[3] Inhibition of neurotransmitter reuptake leads to increased synaptic levels and subsequent augmentation of the neurotransmitter response. Inhibition of NE reuptake is thought to produce the early sympathomimetic effects occasionally seen in some TCA overdoses and may contribute to the development of cardiac dysrhythmias. Serotonin syndrome results from increased 5-HT brainstem activity and has been produced by TCAs that are particularly potent 5-HT uptake inhibitors such as clomipramine and amitriptyline. In general, TCAs must be used in combination with other serotonergic agents to produce serotonin syndrome. Myoclonus and hyperreflexia often are attributed to increased serotonin activity.

Sodium Channel Blockade

TCA-induced cardiotoxicity is the single most important factor contributing to patient mortality. Life-threatening cardiotoxicity results from TCA-induced inhibition of sodium influx through voltage-dependent sodium channels. Inhibition of fast sodium channels in His-Purkinje cells leads to delayed depolarization and conduction abnormalities.[4] Impaired sodium entry into myocardial tissue leads to decreased contractility. Sodium channel blockade is often referred to synonymously as *membrane stabilizing, quinidine-like,* or *local anesthetic effect.* Sodium channel blockade results in a prolongation of phase 0 of the action potential, which becomes more pronounced with rapid heart rates, hyponatremia, and acidosis. This effect expresses itself on the electrocardiograph (ECG) as prolongation of PR and QRS intervals and right-axis deviation (RAD). The RAD is most pronounced in the terminal 40 ms of limb leads, as demonstrated on ECG by a terminal R wave in lead aVR and an S wave in lead I. Rapid influx of sodium is necessary for the release of intracellular calcium stores and subsequent myocardial contractility. Some of the negative chronotropic effect of sodium channel blockade can be attenuated by the sinus tachycardia secondary to antimuscarinic activity. Bradycardia is particularly worrisome when accompanied by QRS complex widening because it indicates profound sodium channel blockade. Lo-

cal changes in electrical conduction can predispose to ventricular dysrhythmias by establishing reentry loops. In summary, severe sodium channel blockade culminates in depressed myocardial contractility, various types of heart blocks, hypotension, cardiac ectopy, widening of the QRS complex, and RAD of the terminal 40 ms.

Sodium channel blockade can be overcome in part by serum alkalinization (pH 7.50–7.55) and increasing the serum sodium concentration. In humans, intravenous sodium bicarbonate ($NaHCO_3$) is thought to be more effective than either hyperventilation (alkalinizes blood) or sodium chloride (increases [Na^+]) in treating TCA cardiotoxicity. One explanation for the greater effectiveness of $NaHCO_3$ is that it produces both alkalemia and increased serum [Na^+]. The mechanism by which blood alkalinization partially reverses sodium channel blockade remains unknown. Previously, it was believed to be related to enhancement of plasma TCA serum protein binding. Alkalinization probably decreases the overall inhibition to sodium ion influx. Recent animal data suggest that hypertonic saline (7.5% saline) may be more efficacious than $NaHCO_3$ or hyperventilation in reversing TCA cardiotoxicity.[5] Whether this finding also will be applicable to humans is currently unknown. Hypertonic saline is believed to act primarily by increasing the extracellular sodium concentration gradient, thus favoring the inward movement of sodium ions.

Potassium Channel Antagonist

TCAs block myocardial potassium channels and inhibit the efflux of potassium ion during repolarization. This effect is seen on ECG as QT interval prolongation, which is more pronounced at slower heart rates. Many TCA overdose patients develop sinus tachycardia, which is partially protective against severe QT_c interval prolongation. Torsades de pointes is a life-threatening complication of severe QT interval prolongation, but it is seen rarely in TCA overdoses.[6]

GABA-A Receptor Antagonist

Generalized seizures occur commonly in the setting of TCA overdoses. Possible mechanisms for these seizures include TCA-induced γ-aminobutyric acid receptor A (GABA-A) antagonism, neuronal sodium channel blockade, central antimuscarinic activity, and effects on biogenic amines. The exact etiology of these seizures remains speculative, but TCA-induced antagonism of the GABA-A receptors may represent the most important mechanism. All drugs that inhibit GABA-A neurotransmission are associated with seizures. Benzodiazepines and barbiturates are potent GABA-A agonists and are considered the anticonvulsants of choice in treating TCA-induced seizures. Propofol (Diprivan) is a short-acting intravenous anesthetic with anticonvulsant activity. It should be considered for patients with resistive seizures, especially in the setting of hypotension.

PHARMACOKINETICS

All TCAs share similar pharmacokinetic properties. They are highly lipophilic and readily cross the blood-brain barrier, and peak plasma levels occur between 2 and 6 h after ingestion at therapeutic doses. Gastrointestinal absorption can be prolonged because of their antimuscarinic effect on gut motility. Bioavailability is only 30 to 70 percent because of extensive first-pass hepatic metabolism. They are highly protein bound to $α_1$ acid glycoproteins. Their apparent volume of distribution is extremely large and ranges from 10 to 50 L/kg. Tissue TCA levels are commonly 10 to 100 times greater than plasma levels. Only 1 to 2 percent of the total-body burden of TCAs is found in the blood. These pharmacokinetic properties explain why attempts at removing TCAs by hemodialysis, hemoperfusion, peritoneal dialysis, or forced diuresis generally are unproductive.

TCAs are eliminated almost entirely by hepatic oxidation, which consists of N-demethylation of the amine side-chain groups and hydroxylation of ring structures. The removal of a methyl group from the tertiary amine side chain usually produces an active metabolite designated by the desmethyl prefix (see Table 158-1). These active metabolites often will have different pharmacologic activities when compared with the parent compounds. Amoxapine and maprotiline both have active metabolites. Although secondary amines such as desipramine, nortriptyline, and protriptyline are effective antidepressants, their metabolites generally are considered inactive. Clinical toxicity from tertiary TCAs usually lasts longer than that from secondary TCAs alone because of the production of active metabolites. Some TCAs undergo enterohepatic circulation prior to their eventual oxidation, conjugation, and renal elimination, but this does not significantly contribute to their toxicity.

The average elimination half-life of TCAs is approximately 24 h (range 6–36 h) at therapeutic doses, but this can increase to 72 h after overdose. Inhibition of TCA metabolism by other drugs that use the same hepatic enzymes can prolong the half-life of TCAs. This carries the risk of elevating TCA plasma levels and producing clinical TCA toxicity at therapeutic doses. Approximately 7 percent of the U.S. population are genetically slow metabolizers of TCAs. This predisposes them to develop higher plasma levels at any given daily TCA dose.

TOXICITY

Therapeutic doses for TCAs are highly variable and are determined by many factors but range from 1 to 5 mg/kg per d (see Table 152-1). Any dose greater than this has the potential to produce TCA toxicity. Life-threatening symptoms usually occur with ingestions of greater than 10 mg/kg in adults. Pediatric patients are particularly susceptible to the antimuscarinic activity of TCAs. Other patients at higher risk for TCA toxicity include patients who have coingested cardiotoxic or CNS-depressive medications, geriatric patients, and patients with heart disease. Desipramine is the most potent sodium channel blocker among the TCAs.[7] It has twice the fatality rate of other TCAs. Some TCAs, especially desipramine, are able to precipitate severe cardiotoxicity (e.g., wide QRS complex, hypotension) without producing significant antimuscarinic symptoms. TCA-related fatalities are commonly associated with ingestions of greater than 1 g. Most TCA overdose fatalities occur within the initial hours after ingestion, often before the patient reaches the hospital. Fatalities more than 24 h after ingestion are unusual with appropriate medical therapy.

While quantitative plasma TCA levels are very helpful in monitoring chronic drug therapy, results are rarely available to emergency physicians during the time of patient evaluation and therefore have negligible impact on patient care. Some studies have shown that patients with a combined plasma level of parent TCA and metabolite of greater than 1000 ng/mL are at greater risk for developing seizures and cardiotoxicity. However, the severity of clinical toxicity does not always correlate with the extent of plasma TCA elevation. Patients can develop severe toxicity at plasma levels less than 1000 ng/mL.[8,9] Conversely, patients with plasma TCA levels much greater than 1000 ng/mL may not develop seizures or ventricular dysrhythmias. Serious toxicity rarely develops at therapeutic levels alone (<300 ng/mL). When this occurs, other causes should be entertained to explain the patient's condition. As always, the most important thing is to treat the patient and not the drug level.

An interesting but confounding characteristic of TCAs is their ability to undergo significant postmortem drug redistribution.[10] Plasma levels can increase by as much as 10- to 50-fold after death as tissue binding sites release TCAs back to the blood. This is a time-dependent process. The diagnostic accuracy of postmortem TCA levels is inversely proportional to the time they were obtained after death. The relevance of TCA postmortem drug redistribution to emergency physicians relates to ED deaths of patients taking TCAs therapeutically.

CLINICAL FEATURES

The clinical presentation of TCA toxicity varies tremendously from mild antimuscarinic symptoms to severe cardiotoxicity secondary to sodium channel blockade. In up to 70 percent of TCA poisonings, coingested drugs also are involved, and the additional toxicity from these coingestants should be considered when evaluating these patients. Antimuscarinic symptoms commonly serve as markers for TCA toxicity (e.g., dry mouth and axillae, sinus tachycardia), but they alone are rarely responsible for patient fatalities. Moreover, antimuscarinic symptoms are not uniformly present in TCA toxicity. As an example, sinus tachycardia is the most frequent dysrhythmia noted in TCA toxicity, but it is only present in approximately 70 percent of symptomatic patients. Altered mental status is the most common symptom reported following TCA exposure.

Mild to moderate TCA toxicity may present as drowsiness, confusion, slurred speech, ataxia, dry mucous membranes and axillae, sinus tachycardia, urinary retention, myoclonus, and hyperreflexia. Antimuscarinic syndrome classically is associated with decreased bowel tones and ileus. However, bowel function is fairly resistant to inhibition, and the presence of active bowel tones does not rule out the possibility of antimuscarinic syndrome. Mild hypertension is observed occasionally and rarely requires treatment. Nontolerant individuals occasionally develop coma and respiratory depression after relatively small overdoses without obvious peripheral antimuscarinic effects and without QRS complex widening. Overflow urinary incontinence may be mistaken for normal micturition in pediatric (diaper-dependent) patients.

Serious toxicity is almost always seen within 6 h of major TCA ingestion and consists of the following symptoms: coma, cardiac conduction delays, supraventricular tachycardia, hypotension, respiratory depression, premature ventricular beats, ventricular tachycardia, and seizures.[8] Secondary complications from serious toxicity include aspiration pneumonia, anoxic encephalopathy, hyperthermia, and rhabdomyolysis. Pulmonary edema is a well-recognized complication of TCA overdose. Seizures usually are generalized and brief in duration. The exception to this rule is seen in amoxapine and maprotiline overdoses. These agents can cause status epilepticus. Amoxapine seizures commonly occur without corresponding QRS complex widening.

DIAGNOSIS

TCA toxicity should be suspected in all patients with a positive serum TCA drug screen in conjunction with corresponding clinical toxicity and/or characteristic ECG abnormalities. Most cases ultimately will prove to be associated with elevated quantitative TCA plasma levels. However, these are not routinely available to the emergency physicians, nor do they have an impact on ED care. Conversely, qualitative TCA drug tests are available in most hospitals and have a rapid turnaround time, but they cannot differentiate between therapeutic and toxic levels. False-positive qualitative serum TCA drug screen results can occur with diphenhydramine, carbamazepine, cyclobenzaprine, cyproheptadine, and phenothiazines. Some of these medications also can produce typical TCA ECG abnormalities and similar clinical toxicity. False-negative serum TCA drug tests are extremely unusual. They should be repeated with a new specimen if there is a high clinical suspicion for TCA exposure. Urine drug testing may be helpful in identifying other toxicologic causes for the patient's condition. The differential diagnosis of TCA toxicity encompasses those drugs which can mimic any one of the three criteria used in making the diagnosis (Table 158-4). However, the quintessential point for emergency physicians is that the initial treatment for all these medications is identical and should not be delayed until definitive drug test results become available.

ECG abnormalities are seen commonly with TCA toxicity and generally are useful in identifying patients at increased risk for seizures and ventricular dysrhythmias. The classic TCA electrocardiogram is

TABLE 158-4   Differential Diagnosis of Tricyclic Antidepressant Toxicity

Drug	False-Positive Serum Drug Screen	Wide QRS/Right Axis Deviation	Antimuscarinic Activity	Point of Differentiation
Carbamazepine	Possible	At levels greater than 20 μg/mL	Yes	History of seizure disorder Elevated serum carbamazepine level
Cyclobenzaprine	Possible	Very unlikely but theoretically possible	Yes	History of cyclobenzaprine use for muscle pain or back problems
Diphenhydramine	Possible	At moderate to high doses	Yes	History of over-the-counter drug use, allergies, or insomnia
Phenothiazines	Possible	Yes, dose dependent	Yes	History of psychotic disorder treated with antipsychotic medication
Class IA antiarrhythmics	No	Yes	Yes	History of heart problems History of leg cramps (quinine)
Class IC antiarrhythmics	No	Yes	No	History of heart problems
Propranolol	No	Seen at moderate to high doses	No	Bradycardia almost always seen Positive response to glucagon
Propoxyphene	No	Often seen in overdose	No	Opiate toxidrome Reversal with naloxone (may require large doses)
Cocaine	No	At high doses	No	Sympathomimetic presentation Positive urine cocaine drug screen
Lithium	No	At elevated serum levels	No	History of bipolar disorder Elevated serum lithium level
Hyperkalemia	No	At increased serum levels	No	Elevated serum $[K^+]$

shown in Figure 158-1, consisting of sinus tachycardia, RAD of the terminal 40 ms (lead aVR), and prolongation of the PR, QRS, and QT intervals. This classic ECG pattern is seen frequently in moderate to severe TCA toxicity, but its absence does not eliminate the possibility of TCA toxicity during the first 6 h after ingestion. Typical ECG findings resolve over the next few days. Moderate prolongation of the QT interval is noted frequently, even at therapeutic TCA doses. Nonspecific ST-segment and T-wave abnormalities are observed commonly in TCA overdose. Less common ECG abnormalities include right bundle branch block and high-degree atrioventricular blocks.

Life-threatening complications can occur in the absence of significant ECG abnormalities.[9] However, these complications are more likely in the presence of a widened QRS complex greater than 100 ms and/or RAD of the terminal 40 ms of greater than 120 degrees. The risk of seizures increases as the QRS complex exceeds 100 ms, and ventricular dysrhythmias are more likely if QRS complex prolongation exceeds 160 ms. RAD is demonstrated commonly as a positive terminal R wave in lead aVR and a negative S wave in lead I (Figure 158-2). Widening of the QRS complex and positive deflection of the terminal QRS complex in lead aVR are equally helpful in identifying patients at risk for serious toxicity.[11] They usually occur together but can occur in exclusion of each other. The development of RAD of the terminal 40 ms and/or QRS complex widening appears to be less predictable of TCA-induced cardiotoxicity in young children.[12] Pediatric electrocardiograms tend to have a wider range of acceptable variant features, and this complicates the ECG identification of TCA toxicity. **ECG abnormalities universally develop within 6 h of ingestion** and typically resolve over 36 to 48 h.[13] The identification of either **QRS complex widening of greater than 100 ms or terminal RAD greater than 120 degrees warrants NaHCO$_3$ therapy** and admission to a monitored hospital bed. Unfortunately, up to 10 percent of the population will have a prolonged QRS complex of more than 100 ms or terminal RAD without exposure to sodium channel blocking drugs. Therefore, these ECG abnormalities in isolation are not 100 percent specific for TCA tox-

icity. Many patients on TCA therapy do not have prior electrocardiograms available for comparison. Thus any observed ECG abnormalities must be assumed attributable to TCA exposure until proven otherwise.

TREATMENT

All patients should be evaluated immediately for alterations of consciousness, hemodynamic instability, and respiratory impairment. Every patient requires an intravenous line, continuous ED cardiac monitoring, and an electrocardiogram. Serial electrocardiograms will be required in most patients. Suggested laboratory studies include determinations of serum electrolyte, creatinine, and glucose levels. A quantitative serum acetaminophen determination is recommended in all overdose patients. Most symptomatic patients will require arterial blood gas measurement. Patients with antimuscarinic symptoms may require a urinary catheter to prevent urinary retention and a nasogastric tube if bowel sounds are absent. Patients who are asymptomatic initially may deteriorate rapidly and therefore should be monitored closely for several hours. Emergency physicians should report all TCA exposures to a regional poison control center.

Gastrointestinal Decontamination

Although the best method of gastrointestinal decontamination in TCA ingestions remains undefined, a few generalizations are still possible.[14] Syrup of ipecac cannot be recommended. Activated charcoal (AC) has been shown to bind TCAs effectively and to decrease their absorption. Therefore, all patients should receive 1 g/kg of AC. Whether gastric lavage and AC is better than AC alone remains unproven. Studies have shown that the gastric lavage is most effective when it is performed within the first few hours after ingestion. Most emergency physicians opt to perform gastric lavage and give AC to patients who present relatively early after TCA ingestion. The proper method of performing gastric lavage in alert patients is to place the

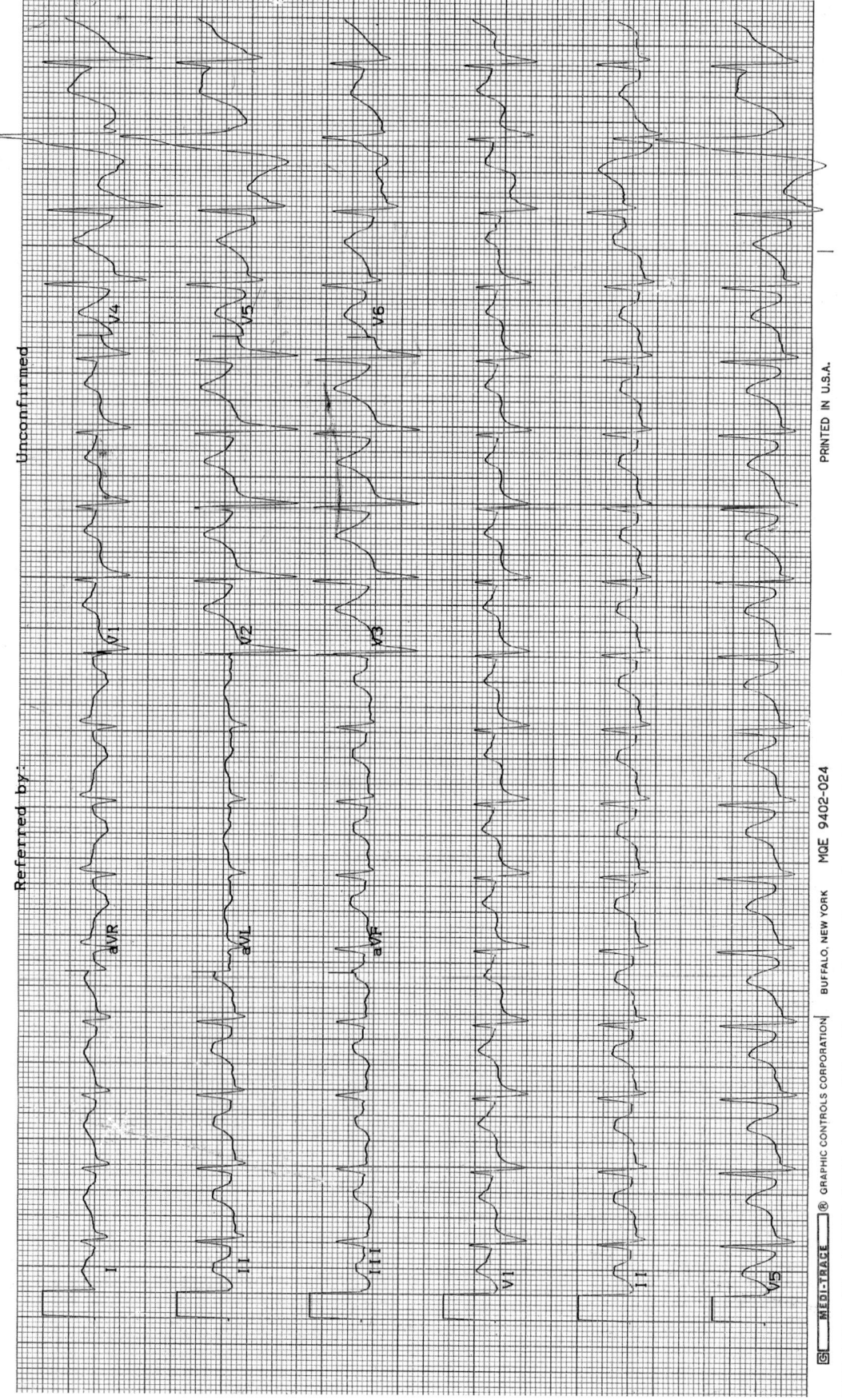

FIG. 158-1. Classic TCA ECG abnormalities. Sinus tachycardia and prolonged PR, QRS, and QT intervals. Also, right axis deviation (RAD) of terminal 40 ms.

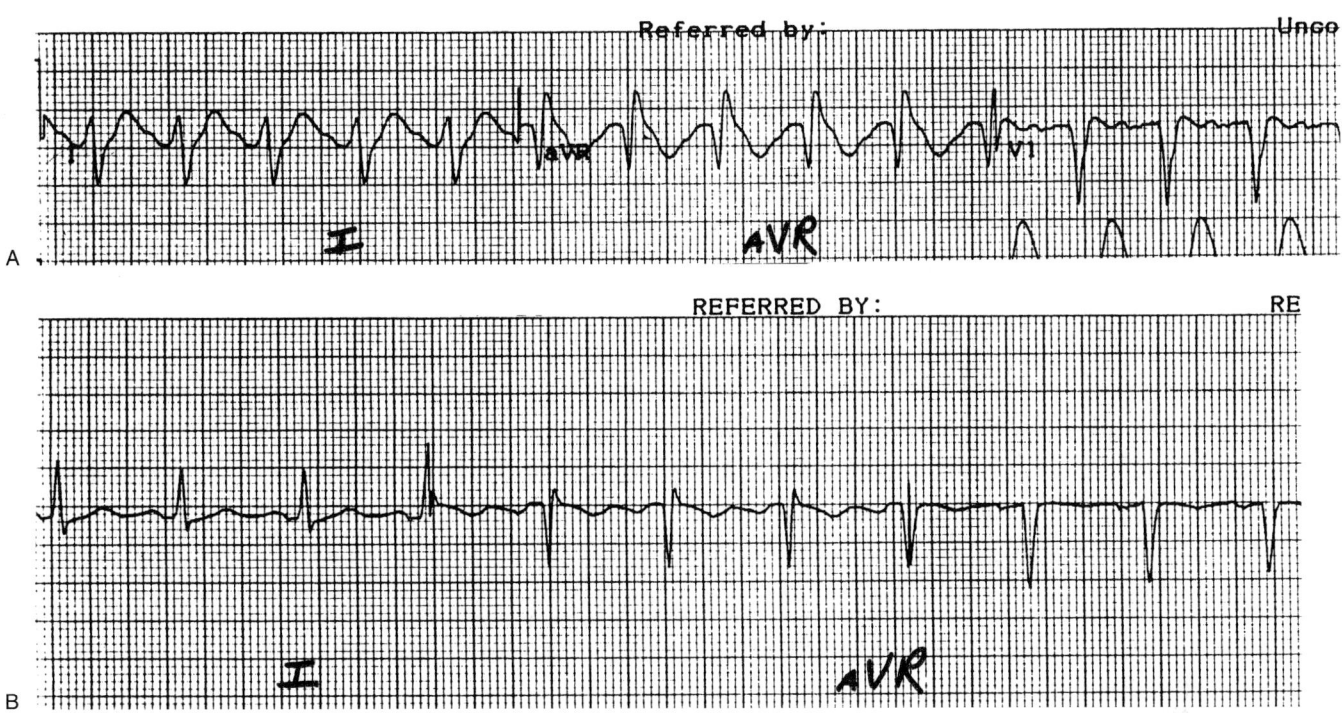

FIG. 158-2. A. An example of terminal 40 ms RAD during TCA toxicity. Note the large R wave in lead aVR and S wave in lead I. **B.** The same patient after complete resolution of TCA toxicity. Note the decrease in the R wave height in lead aVR and the S wave in lead I.

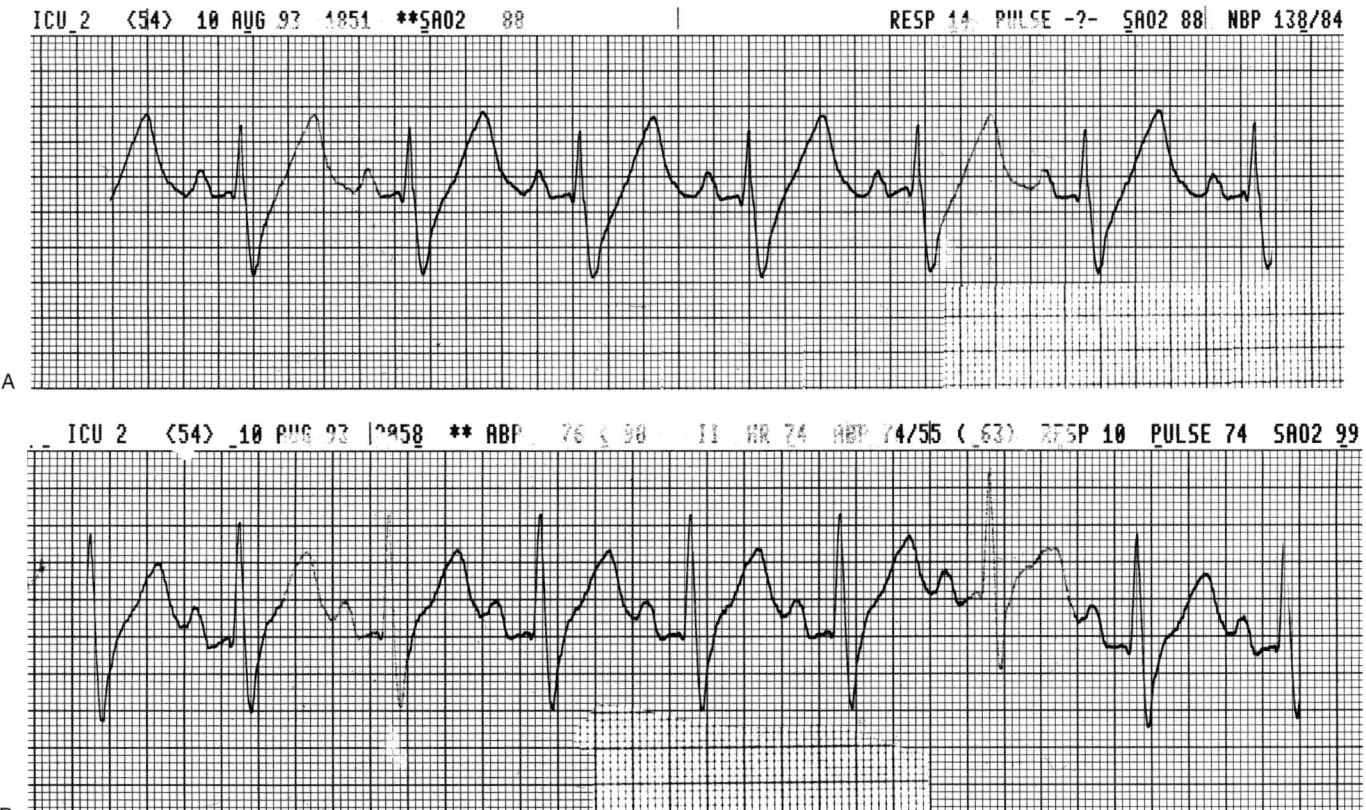

FIG. 158-3. A. Cardiac rhythm strip of a patient with a wide QRS complex recorded 3 h after ingesting amitriptyline. **B.** Narrowing of the QRS complex in same patient after receiving an intravenous bolus of sodium bicarbonate.

patient in the left lateral decubitus position to prevent pulmonary aspiration. Obtunded patients require endotracheal intubation prior to performing gastric lavage. Asymptomatic patients with reliable histories of minimal TCA ingestions can be treated with AC alone and observed for toxicity. Some authors have recommended giving repeat doses of AC to enhance TCA elimination, but these recommendations should be viewed cautiously in the setting of decreased intestinal motility.

Sodium Bicarbonate Therapy

Indications for NaHCO₃ therapy include QRS complex widening greater than 100 ms, hypotension refractory to fluid hydration, terminal RAD in aVR of greater than 3 mm, and ventricular dysrhythmias. Sodium bicarbonate has been shown to improve conduction, increase contractility, and suppress ventricular ectopy. It is given as an initial bolus of 1 to 2 mEq/kg, which can be repeated until patient improvement is noted or until blood pH equals 7.50 to 7.55 (Figure 158-3). Alkalinization beyond this point can be deleterious and therefore is discouraged. Continuous infusions of NaHCO₃ usually are administered as 3 ampules (50 mEq/50 mL) placed in 1 L of D5W or 2 ampules added to D5½NS (slightly hypertonic with NaHCO₃ added) solution and run at a rate of 2 to 3 mL/kg per h. Adjustments in the intravenous rate are made based on blood pH measurements, serum sodium level, and clinical response to therapy. Hypokalemia is an expected complication of NaHCO₃ therapy. Intravenous potassium supplementation usually is required, and serum potassium levels should be measured frequently.

Altered Level of Consciousness

Patients with altered level of consciousness require a trial of intravenous dextrose, thiamine, naloxone, and oxygen to rule out reversible causes of CNS depression. Antagonism of postsynaptic muscarinic, histamine, and α-adrenergic receptors contributes to the development of altered mentation in TCA overdoses. Coma from TCA toxicity typically is rapid in onset. Unresponsive patients may have unrecognized head or neck trauma. Flumazenil should not be given to patients suspected of having mixed-drug overdoses involving TCAs and benzodiazepines because this may precipitate generalized seizures. There is a very high incidence of pulmonary aspiration among TCA overdose patients who present comatose to the ED. Agitation is observed commonly prior to the onset of coma, as well as in previously comatose patients as they awaken. Agitation is best controlled with reassurance, decreased environmental stimulation, and benzodiazepines. As mentioned previously, physostigmine should not be administered to patients taking TCAs.

Seizures

Most seizures occur within the first 3 h following ingestion. Typically, these seizures are generalized and brief in duration. Multiple seizures are reported in approximately 10 to 30 percent of TCA overdoses. Focal seizures are atypical and require further neurologic evaluation. Seizures are especially common with maprotiline and amoxapine ingestions and require aggressive management because status epilepticus is frequently associated with these two particular antidepressants. Benzodiazepines (e.g., diazepam, lorazepam) are the anticonvulsants of choice to stop existing seizure activity. Barbiturates (e.g., phenobarbital) are indicated to treat seizures resistant to benzodiazepines. The initial intravenous dose of phenobarbital is 15 mg/kg, but this can be increased in patients with continued seizure activity and adequate blood pressure. Hypotension is a major side effect. Endotracheal intubation and respiratory support will be required when benzodiazepines are combined with barbiturates or propofol. **Phenytoin is an ineffective anticonvulsant for stopping TCA-induced seizures. Physostigmine and NaHCO₃ do not stop TCA-induced seizures.** If seizures continue despite adequate dosing with benzodiazepines and phenobar-

bital, consideration should be given to paralyzing the patient with a neuromuscular blocking agent. This will stop the physical manifestations of the seizure and its secondary effects, which include metabolic acidosis, hyperthermia, rhabdomyolysis, and renal failure. It does not stop brain seizure activity. Therefore, following the induction of muscle paralysis, these patients require electroencephalographic (EEG) monitoring and continued anticonvulsant therapy.

Hypotension

Hypotension should be treated initially with isotonic crystalloid fluids in increments of 10 mL/kg. In the setting of impaired cardiac contractility, pulmonary edema can develop if excessive fluids are administered. Hypotension that does improve with appropriate fluid challenges should be treated with NaHCO₃ (regardless of QRS complex width). Vasopressors should be used when hypotension is unresponsive to fluids and sodium bicarbonate therapy. The most effective vasopressor is norepinephrine (1 μg/min titrated to effect up to 30 μg/min) because it directly competes with TCAs at α-adrenergic receptors. Dopamine is less effective than norepinephrine in reversing TCA-induced hypotension.[15] In many cases, dopamine administration actually will cause a lowering in systolic blood pressure due to its β-adrenergic and dopaminergic actions that promote vasodilation. If used, it should be adjusted at the upper range of the dose (12–20 μg/kg per min). A pulmonary artery catheter should be placed in patients whose hypotension is refractory to fluid, NaHCO₃, and vasopressor therapy. Mechanical irritation of the heart during pulmonary artery catheter placement may precipitate life-threatening conduction abnormalities and ventricular dysrhythmias. Hypotension induced by TCAs represents a potentially reversible cause of cardiovascular collapse. Mechanical support of the circulation with cardiopulmonary bypass, overdrive pacing, or aortic balloon pump assistance may be warranted in patients with refractory hypotension, although no studies document their effectiveness.

Dysrhythmias

TCAs frequently alter cardiac rate, conduction, and contractility. Asymptomatic patients with sinus tachycardia, isolated PR and QT interval prolongation, or first-degree atrioventricular (AV) block do not require specific pharmacologic therapy. Conduction blocks greater than first-degree AV block are worrisome because they can progress rapidly to complete heart block secondary to impaired infranodal conduction. Most patients with QRS complex prolongation greater than 100 ms should be treated with NaHCO₃ therapy, although this is somewhat controversial. This recommendation is made despite the absence of randomized, controlled human trials demonstrating NaHCO₃ therapy benefits in otherwise asymptomatic patients with QRS complex prolongation.[16] Nonetheless, the early use of sodium bicarbonate in the setting of sodium channel blockade has become a common practice for treating QRS complex widening. Hyperventilation represents a reasonable alternative to sodium bicarbonate therapy in the setting of renal failure, pulmonary edema, or cerebral edema.

Ventricular dysrhythmias should be treated immediately with sodium bicarbonate administration. Lidocaine is the second agent of choice in treating ventricular dysrhythmias. Excessive lidocaine administration is capable of producing seizures. Bretylium generally is considered a third-line drug for ventricular dysrhythmias. Synchronized cardioversion is appropriate in patients with unstable dysrhythmias. Torsade de pointes should be treated initially with 2 g of IV magnesium sulfate. Efforts should be made to rule out other causes of torsades de pointes. Overdrive pacing frequently is required to prevent a recurrence of this dysrhythmia. IV isoproterenol may be of some benefit in treating recurrent torsade de pointes when overdrive pacing is not available. **The following medications are contraindicated in the treatment of TCA-induced dysrhythmias: all class IA and IC antiarrhythmic agents, β-blockers, calcium channel blockers, and all class III antiarrhythmic agents.**

DISPOSITION

Patients who remain asymptomatic 6 h after ingestion do not require hospital admission for toxicologic reasons. They may still require hospital admission because of other coexisting medical or psychiatric conditions. Psychiatric evaluation is warranted for intentional drug ingestions. All symptomatic patients require hospital admission to a monitored bed. Patients demonstrating signs of moderate to severe toxicity should be admitted to an intensive care unit. Hospitalized patients can be cleared medically after 12 to 24 h of being asymptomatic—including a normal or baseline electrocardiogram, normal mental status, and resolution of all antimuscarinic symptoms.

REFERENCES

1. Litovitz TI, Klein-Schwartz W, Rodgers GC, et al: 2001 Annual report of the American Association of Poison Control Centers Toxic Exposure Surveillance System. *Am J Emerg Med* 20:391, 2002.
2. Spiller HA, Winter ML, Mann KV, et al: Five-year multicenter retrospective review of cyclobenzaprine toxicity. *J Emerg Med* 13:781, 1995.
3. Buckley NA, McManus PR: Can the fatal toxicity of antidepressant drugs be predicted with pharmacological and toxicological data? *Drug Saf* 18:369, 1998.
4. Kolecki PF, Curry SC: Poisoning by sodium channel blocking agents. *Crit Care Clin* 13:829, 1997.
5. McCabe JL, Cobaugh DJ, Menegazzi JJ, et al: Experimental tricyclic antidepressant toxicity: A randomized, controlled comparison of hypertonic saline solution, sodium bicarbonate, and hyperventilation. *Ann Emerg Med* 32:329, 1998.
6. Phillips S, Brent J, Kulig K, et al: Fluoxetine versus tricyclic antidepressants: A prospective multicenter study of antidepressant drug overdoses. The Antidepressant Study Group. *J Emerg Med* 15:439, 1997.
7. Preskorn SH: Pharmacokinetics of antidepressants: Why and how they are relevant to treatment. *J Clin Psychiatry* 54(suppl 9):14, 1993.
8. Hulten B-A, Adams R, Askenasi R: Predicting severity of tricyclic antidepressant overdose. *Clin Toxicol* 30:161, 1992.
9. Caravati EM, Bossart PJ: Demographic and electrocardiographic factors associated with severe tricyclic antidepressant toxicity. *Clin Toxicol* 29:31, 1991.
10. Hilberg T, Bugge A, Beylich K-M: An animal model of postmortem amitriptyline redistribution. *J Forens Sci* 38:81, 1993.
11. Liebelt EL, Francis PD, Woolf AD: ECG lead aVR versus QRS interval in predicting seizures and arrhythmias in acute tricyclic antidepressant toxicity. *Ann Emerg Med* 26:195, 1995.
12. Berkovitch M, Matsui D, Folgelman R, et al: Assessment of the terminal 40-millisecond QRS vector in children with a history of tricyclic antidepressant ingestion. *Pediatr Emerg Care* 11:75, 1995.
13. Liebelt EL, Ulrich A, Francis PD, et al: Serial electrocardiogram changes in acute tricyclic antidepressant overdoses. *Crit Care Med* 25:1721, 1997.
14. Bosse GM, Barefoot JA, Pfeifer MP, et al: Comparison of three methods of gut decontamination in tricyclic antidepressant overdose. *J Emerg Med* 13:203, 1995.
15. Tran PT, Panacek EA, Rhee KJ, et al: Response to dopamine vs norepinephrine in tricyclic antidepressant-induced hypotension. *Acad Emerg Med* 4:864, 1997.
16. Hoffman JR, Votey SR, Bayer M, et al: Effect of hypertonic sodium bicarbonate in the treatment of moderate-to-severe cyclic antidepressant overdose. *Am J Emerg Med* 11:336, 1993.

159

NEWER ANTIDEPRESSANTS AND SEROTONIN SYNDROME
Kirk C. Mills

The newer antidepressants are commonly referred to as *atypical, heterocyclic,* or *second-generation antidepressants*. These terms distinguish them from the more traditional monoamine oxidase inhibitors (MAOIs) and tricyclic antidepressants (TCAs). This distinction is important because newer antidepressants are more selective in their pharmacologic activity and have drastically different toxicologic behavior than MAOIs and TCAs. As a group, the newer antidepressants are the most popular form of psychopharmacologic therapy for the treatment of major depression. They are also commonly prescribed in the treatment of many other psychiatric disorders such obsessive-compulsive disorder, panic disorders, and eating disorders. The newer antidepressants are being used increasingly in older children and adolescent patients. However, fluvoxamine (Luvox) and sertraline (Zoloft) are the only newer antidepressants that are approved by the Food and Drug Administration (FDA) for pediatric use. Over the past decade, the American Association of Poison Control Centers Toxic Exposure Surveillance System has reported annual increases in drug exposures to newer antidepressant agents.[1] Fortunately, the newer antidepressants produce less severe toxicity in overdose and are associated with fewer fatalities than either MAOIs or TCAs. For some of the newer antidepressants, very little overdose information is available to base treatment recommendations. Importantly, all antidepressants, especially the MAOIs and selective serotonin reuptake inhibitors (SSRIs), have the potential to produce the serotonin syndrome, a recently recognized drug-induced disorder.

GENERAL PRINCIPLES OF NEWER ANTIDEPRESSANTS

The newer antidepressants are a heterogeneous group of drugs that differ significantly in chemical structure, mechanism of action, pharmacokinetic characteristics, and adverse effect profile. Nonetheless, they also share many important similarities that are summarized in the following eight points. These points are not repeated for each individual drug.

1. Most newer agents do not significantly inhibit cardiac sodium, calcium, or potassium ion channels. Therefore, they do not demonstrate the same cardiotoxicity or electrocardiographic conduction abnormalities typically seen with TCAs. Exceptions to this rule are citalopram and to a much lesser extent fluoxetine and venlafaxine.
2. These agents do not inhibit monoamine oxidase activity and are not associated with tyramine-like reactions. The use of indirect sympathomimetics is not contraindicated.
3. These agents have negligible affinity for acetylcholine, dopamine, γ-aminobutyric acid (GABA), glutamate, or β-adrenergic receptors. Although their exact mechanism of action remains poorly understood, it is traditionally attributed to inhibition of neurotransmitter reuptake (except mirtazapine).
4. Newer antidepressants (except bupropion) appear to have a much higher safety margin than the MAOIs and TCAs. Nonetheless, they can still cause fatalities, especially at very high doses or when combined with other drugs. There is extremely limited human data on the "typical" presentation or optimal management. Therefore, current management recommendations may require modification as more information becomes available. Emergency physicians should routinely contact a regional poison control center (PCC) to report exposures. Also, consultation with a medical toxicologist is available through most regional PCCs.
5. Attempts at enhancing the elimination of newer antidepressants via hemodialysis, hemoperfusion, forced diuresis, or multiple-dose activated charcoal are unlikely to be successful and therefore are not recommended. Whole-bowel irrigation does not offer any advantage over single-dose activated charcoal in providing gastrointestinal decontamination to patients exposed to newer antidepressants.
6. The newer antidepressants are not detected by routine hospital serum and urine drug screens. Certain specialty laboratories do have the capability to measure parent drug and metabolite plasma levels, but this information is only useful for the confirmation of suspected drug overdose. Specific levels are not immediately available, nor do they affect patient management. Postmortem drug redistribution is likely to occur with the newer antidepressants, affecting forensic investigation.

7. The newer antidepressants are metabolized primarily by hepatic enzyme systems (cytochrome P450 pathways). Drug interactions can be expected when two medications that share the same metabolic pathway are given together. In addition, hepatic dysfunction can lead to elevated drug levels and subsequent drug toxicity.

8. All the newer antidepressants carry warnings against combination with MAOIs because the two can precipitate serotonin syndrome. Although the manufacturers' contraindications do not specify other serotonergic medications, risks and benefits should be carefully assessed before combining these as well.

TRAZODONE

Trazodone hydrochloride (Desyrel) was released in the United States in 1982 for the treatment of endogenous depression. During the past decade, the frequency of reported trazodone exposures has increased markedly, but the fatality rate remains quite low (1 in 1200 exposures). This is approximately seven to ten times less than the fatality rate for MAOI or TCA exposures. The average daily therapeutic dose for trazodone is between 150 and 400 mg, with a maximum dose of up to 600 mg restricted to psychiatric inpatients. Trazodone is available as 50-, 100-, and 150-mg tablets. There is a low potential for trazodone abuse, and a distinct withdrawal syndrome has not been observed with its abrupt discontinuation. Trazodone is a category C risk in pregnancy.

Trazodone is a triazolopyridine derivative that is structurally unrelated to other antidepressants. Its antidepressant action is believed to be due to a combination of serotonin [5-hydroxytryptamine (5-HT)] reuptake inhibition and antagonism of postsynaptic 5-HT$_2$ receptors.[2] Trazodone is a moderately potent nonselective α-adrenergic receptor blocker with at least five times greater affinity for α$_1$- than α$_2$-adrenergic receptors. Consequently, trazodone is frequently associated with orthostatic hypotension, which is maximal within the first 6 h of use and can be minimized by taking the medication at bedtime. Sedation, which is a common side effect of trazodone therapy, is believed to be secondary to inhibition of central α-adrenergic and histamine receptors.

Trazodone is absorbed rapidly and completely, with peak plasma levels occurring between 1 and 2 h following oral administration. It is highly protein bound and has a moderate volume of distribution (1.2 L/kg). Trazodone primarily undergoes hepatic oxidation by the cytochrome P450 isoenzyme system. It has one active metabolite, *m*-chlorophenylpiperazine (*m*-CPP), which has a complex pharmacologic profile, such as inhibition of 5-HT uptake, stimulation and inhibition of multiple postsynaptic serotonin receptors, and interactions with other neurotransmitter systems. The overall contribution of *m*-CPP to the therapeutic and toxic effects of trazodone is currently under investigation. The half-life of trazodone ranges from 5 to 9 h at therapeutic doses but can increase up to 13 h in overdose.

The adverse-effect profile for trazodone is very favorable when compared with other antidepressants except for its association with priapism. Trazodone is one of the most common causes of drug-induced priapism. The estimated incidence of priapism ranges from 1 in 1000 to 1 in 10,000 patients. Any patient with a history of increased frequency, duration, or inappropriate penile or clitoral engorgement should discontinue trazodone therapy immediately. Human volunteer and laboratory animal studies have proven that trazodone is far less cardiotoxic than TCAs. Therapeutic use of trazodone has been reported occasionally to be arrhythmogenic, especially in patients with underlying cardiac risk factors such as conduction abnormalities or ischemic heart disease. Examples of cardiac rhythm abnormalities reported in association with trazodone therapy include sinus arrest, sinus bradycardia, various atrioventricular blocks, complete heart block, atrial fibrillation, and ventricular dysrhythmias (premature ventricular beats or torsade de pointes). The most frequently reported dose-related adverse effects are drowsiness, dizziness, dry mouth, nausea and vomiting, and orthostatic hypotension. There have been rare case reports of patients experiencing reversible liver enzyme elevation, jaundice, and abnormal liver histology in association with trazodone therapy.

Acute Overdose Toxicity

There is no established toxic dose for trazodone. **As a general guideline, serious toxicity in an average adult is not expected with ingestions of less than 2 g. This safety margin is reduced significantly when other medications are coingested with trazodone.** The most common symptom of acute trazodone poisoning is central nervous system (CNS) depression. Other CNS-related symptoms include ataxia, dizziness, coma, and seizures. Trazodone rarely produces coma or seizures when it is the only drug ingested. Pupils are usually of normal size and remain reactive to light. Infrequently, patients may complain of muscle weakness. Trazodone-induced CNS symptoms show marked improvement within 6 to 12 h after ingestion and are almost always resolved by 24 h. Orthostatic hypotension is the most frequently reported cardiovascular abnormality noted in trazodone overdose and usually responds to fluid administration. Mild abnormalities of sinus rhythm, such as sinus bradycardia and tachycardia, are encountered frequently. The most common electrocardiographic abnormality is moderate prolongation of the QT$_c$ interval. Polymorphic ventricular tachycardia (torsade de pointes) has been reported in rare cases. Commonly reported gastrointestinal complaints include nausea, vomiting, and nonspecific abdominal pain. Respiratory depression is observed infrequently with pure trazodone overdoses. Priapism has been reported following an acute overdose of 3.5 g.

Treatment

An intravenous line should be started and cardiac monitoring initiated on all patients. In pure trazodone ingestions, significant neurologic and cardiac toxicity is not expected, and supportive care is usually the only treatment required. Specific antidotal therapy is not available. Gastrointestinal decontamination can be applied selectively in patients in whom the dose ingested can be calculated accurately. Ingestion of 2 g requires only 1 g/kg of activated charcoal as long as trazodone is ingested as a single agent and the patient does not have any underlying cardiac or neurologic risk factors. Gastric lavage is probably unnecessary. Ingestions of more than 2 g of trazodone or coingestions have a higher incidence of coma, seizures, and respiratory arrest. In these patients, early gastric lavage followed by administration of activated charcoal is indicated. Hypotension should be treated initially with isotonic intravenous fluid administration. If the use of a vasopressor becomes necessary, direct-acting vasopressors (e.g., norepinephrine) are recommended. Drugs with β-adrenergic receptor activity (e.g., dopamine) theoretically can potentiate the hypotension in the presence of trazodone-induced α-adrenergic receptor antagonism. Patients who have remained asymptomatic for at least 6 h can be discharged safely from the emergency department, assuming that any necessary psychiatric evaluation has been completed or arranged. All intentional trazodone ingestions should be evaluated properly for the presence of other drugs (e.g., acetaminophen). Patients with neurologic and/or cardiac symptoms persisting longer than 6 h after ingestion will require hospital admission to a monitored bed. In addition, patients with coingestants associated with delayed toxicity will require prolonged observation or formal hospital admission.

NEFAZODONE

Nefazodone (Serzone), was approved in 1995 for the treatment of depression. It is both structurally and functionally related to trazodone. Nefazodone inhibits serotonin reuptake and also antagonizes postsynaptic 5-HT$_2$ receptors.[3] It has little affinity for other receptors except slight antagonism of postsynaptic α_1 receptors. Nefazodone is available in 50-, 100-, 150-, 200-, and 250-mg tablets. The recommended effective dose for nefazodone is between 300 and 600 mg/d. Although nefazodone is absorbed rapidly, it has a bioavailability of only 20 percent due to extensive first-pass hepatic metabolism. Peak levels occur within 1 h, and its elimination half-life ranges from 2 to 6 h. It is 99 percent protein-bound, with a relatively small volume of distribution. It has three active metabolites: hydroxynefazodone, desethylhydroxynefazodone, and *m*-CPP. The hydroxynefazodone metabolite is pharmacologically equivalent to the parent compound. The *m*-CPP metabolite is noteworthy only because it is also produced by trazodone. Nefazodone can inhibit the metabolism of terfenadine, astemizole, cisapride, and pimozide, which in turn can lead to life-threatening prolongation of the QT interval (torsade de pointes). Certain benzodiazepines such as alprazolam and triazolam have markedly increased CNS effects in the presence of nefazodone. Carbamazepine inhibits the metabolism of nefazodone by up to 75 percent. Overall, nefazodone has a favorable adverse-effect profile. Compared with placebo, however, nefazodone has a higher incidence of headache, dizziness, drowsiness, asthenia, tremor, dry mouth, nausea, constipation, and blurred vision. It also predisposes patients to postural hypotension and priapism but not to the same degree as trazodone. Nefazodone has a category C rating in pregnancy.

Treatment

Experience with nefazodone in overdose is extremely limited. Unpublished premarketing data suggest that nefazodone is relatively safe in overdose. The most common symptoms reported include nausea, vomiting, and somnolence. There were no fatalities with pure nefazodone ingestions ranging from 1000 to 11,200 mg. Based on its pharmacokinetic profile, the onset of nefazodone toxicity would be expected to occur within the first 6 h following an overdose. At present, management of nefazodone overdoses should follow the aforementioned guidelines for trazodone.

BUPROPION

Bupropion (Wellbutrin) has been available in the United States since 1989 for the treatment of major depression. The actual incidence and severity of bupropion exposures are unknown. However, since bupropion has been approved recently for the treatment of smoking cessation (Zyban), the potential for bupropion poisoning is considerable. The same pharmaceutical company manufactures bupropion under two trade names: Wellbutrin and Zyban. For smoking cessation, Zyban (150 mg) is administered either once or twice daily for no more than 12 consecutive weeks. The maximum daily dose of Zyban is 300 mg. Wellbutrin comes in a variety of doses and formulations, including sustained-release tablets (100 and 150 mg) and regular-release tablets (75 and 100 mg). The recommended starting dose of Wellbutrin is 100 mg given twice daily, gradually increasing up to 300 mg/d. The incidence of seizures increases drastically at doses of greater than 450 mg/d, and higher doses therefore are prohibited. The combination of the two bupropion preparations is obviously contraindicated. Other contraindications include patients with bulimia, anorexia nervosa, epilepsy, or taking MAOIs. Bupropion is a category B drug in pregnancy. The information in this section is derived from studies using only the Wellbutrin form of bupropion. It is assumed that this information is equally applicable to Zyban exposures.

Bupropion has a monocyclic phenylaminoketone chemical structure that resembles those of the phenylethylamines (e.g., amphetamine).[4] However, bupropion does not produce stimulant effects or drug-addictive behavior at therapeutic doses. The therapeutic mechanism of action for bupropion is poorly understood but currently attributed to a weak ability to inhibit neuronal reuptake of serotonin, norepinephrine, and dopamine. It does not directly stimulate postsynaptic receptors. Bupropion is absorbed rapidly after oral administration and undergoes extensive first-pass hepatic metabolism. It is highly protein-bound, has an extremely large volume of distribution, and readily crosses the blood-brain barrier. Peak plasma levels occur within 2 h for regular-release tablets and within 3 h for sustained-release preparations. Its elimination half-life ranges between 14 and 20 h. Bupropion has one important metabolite, hydroxybupropion, that is less potent than bupropion, preferentially inhibits norepinephrine reuptake, and may contribute to seizure development.

Bupropion antidepressant therapy is well tolerated. It does not produce CNS depression, orthostatic hypotension, or cardiovascular changes or impair sexual function at therapeutic doses. The most commonly reported adverse effects are of mild severity and include dry mouth, dizziness, agitation, nausea, headache, constipation, tremor, anxiety, confusion, blurred vision, and increased motor activity. Seizures have been reported with therapeutic doses, but are rare. The drug should be discontinued and the patient should receive emergency department evaluation for a first seizure. Bupropion has been reported to infrequently produce catatonia, hallucinations, psychosis, and paranoia that probably are related to its dopaminergic activity. Rarely, angioedema and urticaria, including plaque-like lesions on the palms, have been described. Skin allergy becomes evident within the first few weeks of therapy. The drug must be stopped; if not, the rash can progress to angioedema or Stevens-Johnson syndrome.

Abrupt discontinuation of bupropion has not been associated with any withdrawal symptoms but may pose a slight theoretical risk of precipitating neuroleptic malignant syndrome because bupropion is considered a dopamine agonist. Bupropion is relatively free of significant drug interactions. In general, bupropion should not be combined with SSRIs, lithium, MAOIs, TCAs, dopaminergic drugs (e.g., levodopa), or drugs that are known to lower patient seizure threshold (e.g., phenothiazines).

Acute Overdose Toxicity

Bupropion differs from other new antidepressants in that it has a low toxic-to-therapeutic ratio. Toxicity can occur at doses equal to or just slightly greater than the maximum therapeutic dose of 450 mg/d. As a general rule, significant toxicity is not expected in pure bupropion overdose with adult ingestions of less than 450 mg. The largest case series of bupropion overdoses reported that symptomatic patients ingested a mean of 2310 mg, and the lowest symptomatic dose was 200 mg.[5] Patients who remained asymptomatic ingested a mean of 1325 mg, and the largest asymptomatic dose was 4000 mg. The most commonly reported symptoms in pure bupropion overdose include sinus tachycardia (43 percent), lethargy (41 percent), tremor (24 percent), generalized seizures (21 percent), confusion (14 percent), and vomiting (14 percent). Mild hyperthermia is reported occasionally. Sinus tachycardia is the most common electrocardiographic abnormality. An isolated case of moderate QT-interval prolongation has been reported in conjunction with a massive bupropion overdose. Otherwise, bupropion does not produce myocardial conduction abnormalities. Hypotension is unexpected in pure bupropion overdoses but has been reported in mixed-drug overdoses. Hypertension is usually of only mild to moderate severity. Coma and cardiac arrest have been reported in severe bupropion overdoses. The hallmark of bupropion toxicity is generalized seizures. The actual incidence of seizures is unknown but probably is greater than the estimated 21 percent obtained by retrospective studies. There is no correlation between the development of seizures and the presence of other symptoms such as sinus tachycardia. Therefore, **seizures can develop in otherwise asymptomatic patients.** Seizures usually occur within the first 1 to 4 h after ingestion of regular-release bupropion. The average time of seizure onset is

3.7 h, but they may be delayed for up to 8 h. Recent case reports suggest that sustained-release preparations may predispose patients to seizures up to 14 h after exposure. Laboratory study findings are usually normal except for rare cases of mild hypokalemia.

Treatment

Possible early onset of generalized seizures should be anticipated in all cases of bupropion ingestion. A peripheral intravenous line should be established and cardiac monitoring initiated in all patients. Rapid gastrointestinal decontamination is recommended using gastric lavage and administration of 1 g/kg of activated charcoal. Syrup of ipecac is contraindicated due to risk of seizures. Significant cardiotoxicity is not expected except in mixed-drug overdoses. Sinus tachycardia is rarely of hemodynamic significance. Seizures that last longer than 5 min, are focal in nature, or repetitive should be treated aggressively with benzodiazepines. Diphenylhydantoin (phenytoin) is generally less effective than benzodiazepines or phenobarbital in stopping drug-induced seizures but was reportedly effective in stopping seizure activity in one case of bupropion-induced status epilepticus. Hospital admission is recommended for all patients with seizures, sinus tachycardia, or lethargy. Asymptomatic patients having ingested only regular-release bupropion should be observed for 8h before discharge. In many cases, a psychiatric evaluation also may be necessary. Patients ingesting more than 450 mg of sustained-release bupropion require longer periods of monitoring, probably for 24h, although consensus guidelines have not yet been established.

MIRTAZAPINE

Mirtazapine (Remeron), a tetracyclic compound structurally unrelated to other currently available antidepressants, has been available in the United States since 1996.[6] In contrast to all other atypical antidepressants, mirtazapine does not inhibit neuronal amine uptake. Instead, it blocks central presynaptic α_2-adrenergic receptors and postsynaptic serotonin receptors, subtypes 5-HT$_2$ and 5-HT$_3$. This has the net therapeutic effect of increasing central norepinephrine and serotonin (5-HT$_1$) neurotransmission. Mirtazapine has a high affinity to block histamine (H$_1$) receptors and a moderate affinity to block muscarinic receptors. Mirtazapine is commonly associated with somnolence (antihistamine effect) and less often associated with weight gain and increased appetite. It is supplied as 15-, 30-, and 45-mg tablets, with an average daily dose range of between 15 and 45 mg. It is rated category C in pregnancy. Mirtazapine has a similar pharmacokinetic profile as other atypical antidepressants. It is absorbed rapidly and completely following oral administration. Bioavailability is approximately 50 percent due to significant first-pass hepatic metabolism. Peak levels occur within 2 h after ingestion. Mirtazapine is metabolized by the hepatic oxidase enzyme system (cytochrome P450) with only minor active metabolites. The elimination half-life for mirtazapine averages 26 h for males and 37 h for females. The difference in mirtazapine half-life between men and women is attributed to decreased cytochrome P450 metabolism in females. Mirtazapine is highly protein-bound (85 percent) and has a large volume of distribution (5 L/kg). Plasma levels are unlikely to be affected by attempts at extracorporeal removal. Postmarketing surveillance identified a rare incidence of agranulocytosis associated with mirtazapine.

Acute Overdose Toxicity

Mirtazapine appears to be associated with limited toxicity in overdose. Very few cases of mirtazapine overdose have been reported in the medical literature. The most common signs and symptoms were sedation, confusion, sinus tachycardia, and mild hypertension.[7] Doses up to 1350 mg have been tolerated without significant sequelae. The risk of coma and respiratory depression is greatest at larger doses or when combined with other CNS-depressant drugs. Vital-sign abnormalities are rarely of clinical significance and have not required specific treatment.

Treatment

Treatment guidelines have not been established for mirtazapine overdoses. Based on the currently available data, the following recommendations seem logical but may require modification as experience with mirtazapine increases. For this reason, PCC consultation is strongly encouraged for most cases involving the use of mirtazapine. Fortunately, mirtazapine toxicity usually resolves over 24 h with supportive care alone. Single-dose activated charcoal is the gastrointestinal decontamination method of choice. Gastric lavage may be warranted in selected patients presenting early after large overdoses or with significant coingestants. Syrup of ipecac is contraindicated, and whole-bowel lavage is unnecessary. Symptomatic patients should be admitted to a monitored bed, but significant cardiac toxicity is unlikely. Electrocardiographic abnormalities other than sinus tachycardia have not been reported. Asymptomatic patients can be medically cleared after 8 h of observation.

SELECTIVE SEROTONIN REUPTAKE INHIBITORS

SSRIs represent a structurally heterogeneous group of drugs that share a selective affinity to inhibit presynaptic serotonin reuptake without significantly affecting norepinephrine or dopamine reuptake. The increase in synaptic serotonin levels may not entirely explain their therapeutic effects.[8] As with most antidepressant agents, acute alterations in biogenic amine levels do not correlate with immediate clinical response to drug therapy. Secondary receptor and cellular compensatory mechanisms currently are believed to play an important role in their mechanism of action. SSRIs are essentially devoid of direct presynaptic or postsynaptic receptor interactions. Thus they are associated with very few unwanted pharmacologic actions, in contrast with TCAs.

SSRIs represent the most common form of pharmacotherapy for depression in the United States. They are also the most frequent class of antidepressants reported in drug overdoses. Fatalities are uncommon, with an average of only 1 death in every 1000 drug exposures. There are currently five SSRIs available in the United States: fluoxetine (Prozac, released in 1988), sertraline (Zoloft, released in 1991), paroxetine (Paxil, released in 1993), fluvoxamine (Luvox, released in 1994), and citalopram (Celexa, released in 1998). There are slight potency differences between SSRIs, but their clinical efficacy appears to be comparable. The following represents the suggested average daily dose and maximum daily dose for SSRIs: fluoxetine (average 20–80 mg, maximum 80 mg), paroxetine (average 20–50 mg, maximum 50 mg), citalopram (average 20–40 mg, maximum 60 mg), sertraline (average 50–200 mg, maximum 200 mg), and fluvoxamine (average 50–300 mg, maximum 300 mg). In pregnancy, all SSRIs have a category C rating for teratogenic risk.

The SSRIs have similar pharmacokinetic profiles, including rapid and complete oral absorption, peak plasma levels occurring 4 to 8 h after ingestion (citalopram, 2 to 4 h), significant first-pass hepatic metabolism, a high degree of protein binding (except citalopram), and a large volume of distribution. Fluoxetine is the only SSRI with a clinically significant active metabolite, norfluoxetine, that is equally potent as fluoxetine. The half-lives of fluoxetine and norfluoxetine are 2 to 4 days and 7 to 14 days, respectively. The effects of fluoxetine may last for up to 5 weeks because of the prolonged period necessary to allow for norfluoxetine metabolism. Sertraline and paroxetine have similar half-lives of approximately 24 h. The half-life of citalopram is estimated at 33 h, whereas fluvoxamine has the shortest half-life at 15 h. The SSRIs are metabolized almost entirely by the hepatic cytochrome P450 isoenzyme system. It is becoming increasingly recognized that the SSRIs can inhibit the metabolism of other drugs dependent on the cytochrome P450 isoenzyme system.[9] Clinically significant drug interactions are most likely to occur with drugs that have a low therapeutic index, e.g., TCAs, antipsychotics, anticonvulsants, benzodiazepines, opiates, theophylline, warfarin, terfenadine, astemizole, pimozide, and cisapride. SSRIs are contraindicated in combination with MAOIs. A 2-week abstinence ("washout") period for most SSRIs and a 5-week abstinence period for fluoxetine are needed before prescribing MAOIs. The administration of other serotonergic agents in combination with SSRIs also should be avoided whenever possible.

The most serious drug-related adverse effect of SSRI psychopharmacotherapy is the potential to produce serotonin syndrome (see below). Other CNS-related adverse effects include headache, sedation, insomnia, dizziness, weakness or fatigue, tremor, and nervousness. Seizures are very uncommon but have been reported with all SSRIs. Serotonin has varying effects on the dopaminergic system. In many cases, extrapyramidal-related symptoms such as dystonic reactions, akathisia, dyskinesia, hypokinesia, and parkinsonian symptoms have been reported in association with SSRI therapy.[10] Consequently, SSRIs should be used cautiously with antipsychotic agents because SSRIs can potentiate antidopaminergic activity. Gastrointestinal complaints such as nausea, diarrhea, constipation, vomiting, and anorexia are reported commonly by patients taking SSRIs. Other adverse effects less commonly reported include dry mouth, increased sweating, blurred vision, hyponatremia, and hypoglycemia. Hyponatremia is believed to be secondary to inappropriate secretion of antidiuretic hormone [syndrome of inappropriate secretion of antidiuretic hormone (SIADH)]. Sexual dysfunction (e.g., anorgasmia) is a relatively common SSRI-related adverse effect and is reversible with drug discontinuation. Priapism has been reported but is extremely rare. A withdrawal syndrome consisting of nonspecific neurologic, psychiatric, and gastrointestinal symptoms has been described in conjuncture with abrupt SSRI discontinuation. It is less likely to occur with fluoxetine because it has a long-acting metabolite.

Acute Overdose Toxicity

Despite the tremendous popularity of SSRIs, there is limited information on their toxicity in overdose. The greatest amount of human overdose experience has been with fluoxetine.[11] The information from case series involving the other SSRIs is consistent with the information accumulated on fluoxetine.[12–15] However, important differences may exist between the different SSRIs that will become evident only with greater exposure of patients to individual SSRIs. Fortunately, all of the SSRIs are characterized by a high therapeutic-to-toxic ratio, and fatalities are uncommon with pure SSRI overdoses. Approximately 50 percent of all adult patients and 75 percent of pediatric patients remain asymptomatic following SSRI overdose. The most common symptoms seen in SSRI overdose include nausea, vomiting, sedation, tremor, and sinus tachycardia. These symptoms are almost identical to the adverse-effect profile of SSRIs except for sinus tachycardia, which is more common in overdose and rarely reported as an adverse effect. Less frequently observed symptoms include mydriasis, seizures, diarrhea, agitation, hallucinations, hypertension, and hypotension. Sertraline may produce mild CNS stimulation in pediatric patients.[13] Sinus bradycardia was observed more frequently in fluvoxamine overdoses than with other SSRIs. Citalopram produced QRS widening in approximately one-third of cases when more than 600 mg was ingested.[15] In another case series, prolongation of the QT interval has been reported in association with significant citalopram ingestions. Other SSRIs have been reported rarely to produce similar electrocardiographic abnormalities. It most cases, the electrocardiographic abnormalities gradually resolve over 24 h. Tachycardia, mild hypotension, and lethargy are seen more commonly when SSRIs are combined with ethanol. Mixed-drug ingestions can produce a wide variety of additional symptoms depending on the coingestant toxicity. Serotonin syndrome can occur as a consequence of acute SSRI overdose. The results of laboratory tests are usually normal in SSRI overdoses. As mentioned previously, SSRI therapy

has been associated with drug-induced SIADH secretion, which may result in symptomatic hyponatremia.

Treatment

Patients who intentionally overdose with SSRI require establishment of a peripheral intravenous line and cardiac monitoring. Overall, pure SSRI overdoses are associated with limited toxicity except for the infrequent development of life-threatening complications such as generalized seizures and serotonin syndrome. The optimal method of gastrointestinal decontamination in SSRI poisoning remains undetermined. Based on the high therapeutic index and unlikelihood of serious toxicity, single-dose activated charcoal (1 g/kg) is logical for most ingestions, and gastric lavage is probably unnecessary in the majority of SSRI overdoses. However, gastric lavage may have greater utility in the setting of mixed-drug overdoses or if extremely large doses of SSRIs have been ingested recently. Due to the potential for seizures and CNS sedation, syrup of ipecac is contraindicated in adult intentional ingestions.

All patients should be observed for at least 6 h, during which supportive care is generally all that is required. Psychiatric evaluation is warranted for intentional ingestions. Hospital admission is recommended for all patients who remain tachycardic or lethargic 6 h after ingestion. Patients at higher risk for complications include those with underlying seizure disorders, symptoms of serotonin syndrome, or mixed-drug overdoses that have the potential for additional or delayed toxicity. Sodium bicarbonate therapy is indicated in cases of SSRI-induced QRS prolongation, primarily seen after citalopram ingestions of greater than 600 mg, and is administered in an identical manner as described in Chap. 158. Other SSRIs have been associated only rarely with QRS widening. Benzodiazepines are recommended as initial anticonvulsant therapy. Barbiturates are probably equally effective as benzodiazepines but are more sedating. There have been rare reports of delayed seizures, up to 16 h after ingestion. Delayed onset of serotonin syndrome or extrapyramidal reactions are theoretical possibilities that should be considered in all patients.

VENLAFAXINE

Venlafaxine (Effexor) is a bicyclic compound that is structurally different from other antidepressants. It was released in 1994 for the treatment of depression. In contrast to the SSRIs, venlafaxine is a nonselective inhibitor of serotonin, norepinephrine, and dopamine reuptake.[16] Whether this nonselectivity offers any advantage over SSRIs, bupropion, trazodone, nefazodone, or mirtazapine is currently unknown. Venlafaxine has no significant direct effect on presynaptic or postsynaptic neurotransmitter receptors and does not inhibit MAO activity. It is available in 25-, 37.5-, 50-, 75-, and 100-mg tablets. The recommended starting dose is 75 mg/d, which can be increased gradually up to a maximum daily dose of 225 mg. It has a category C rating in pregnancy.

Peak levels occur 2 h after ingestion. It is poorly protein-bound (27 percent), and it has volume of distribution of 6 to 7 L/kg and a half-life of approximately 5 h. The majority of venlafaxine undergoes hepatic cytochrome P450 oxidation, but it is a weak inhibitor of cytochrome P450 enzyme activity. To date, no significant pharmacokinetic drug interactions have been reported. It has one active metabolite, O-desmethylvenlafaxine, that is pharmacologically similar to its parent drug, except for a longer half-life of 11 h. The adverse-effect profile for venlafaxine is similar to that for SSRIs. The only notable exception is the occurrence of mild to moderate hypertension when doses exceed 225 mg/d, which is probably secondary to inhibition of norepinephrine reuptake. Venlafaxine has the same potential as other serotonin agonists to produce serotonin syndrome. Therefore, it should not be combined with MAOIs or other serotonin agonists. Because of its shorter half-life, venlafaxine requires only a 1-week abstinence period before initiating MAOI therapy. However, a 2-week abstinence period is still required after MAOI discontinuation before starting venlafaxine therapy.

Acute Overdose Toxicity

Information regarding venlafaxine toxicity in overdose is limited to isolated case reports. Unfortunately, most of these cases also include significant coingestants, confounding the interpretation of "pure" venlafaxine toxicity. Sympathetic nervous system stimulation, via inhibition of norepinephrine reuptake, predisposes patients to tachycardia, hypertension, diaphoresis, tremor, and mydriasis. These symptoms are seen frequently in venlafaxine overdoses. Severe hypotension, requiring vasopressors, was reported in one case. Otherwise, most vital-sign abnormalities are of moderate severity and do not require specific pharmacologic therapy. CNS sedation is also reported commonly and occasionally progresses to coma requiring endotracheal intubation and ventilatory support. Generalized seizures are reported frequently and tend to occur early after ingestion. Electrocardiographic abnormalities include sinus tachycardia, QRS widening, and QT_c-interval prolongation. In most cases, symptoms completely resolve gradually over 36 h with supportive care alone.

Treatment

There are no established guidelines for treating venlafaxine overdoses. All patients require at least 6 h of observation. Venlafaxine toxicity is often precipitous and should be anticipated in all intentional overdoses. Patients require establishment of a peripheral intravenous line and cardiac monitoring. Venlafaxine appears to have greater toxicity in overdose than SSRIs and probably deserves more aggressive gastric decontamination. Gastric lavage should be strongly considered for most intentional ingestions with early presentation. Accidental ingestions can be treated with single-dose activated charcoal alone. Benzodiazepines are the anticonvulsants of choice. Hypertension and sinus tachycardia rarely require specific pharmacologic therapy. β-blockers have the theoretical disadvantage of allowing unopposed α-adrenergic receptor stimulation. Sodium bicarbonate therapy should be considered invenlafaxine overdoses associated with QRS widening of greater than 100 ms. All symptomatic patients should be admitted to a monitored bed.

SEROTONIN SYNDROME

Serotonin syndrome is a rare but important idiosyncratic drug-induced complication of antidepressant therapy.[17] It can be produced by any drug or, more commonly, by a combination of drugs that increase central serotonin neurotransmission (Table 159-1). The stimulation of specific postsynaptic serotonin receptors ($5-HT_{1A}$ and $5-HT_2$) is required for full expression of this syndrome. Drugs (such as ondansetron) that block serotonin postsynaptic receptors are incapable of inducing this syndrome. Most cases occur at therapeutic levels, with fewer than 13 percent of cases being associated with drug overdose. Serotonin syndrome is characterized by alterations in cognition and behavior, autonomic nervous system function, and neuromuscular activity. The degree of abnormality in any one area is highly variable. Serotonin syndrome usually occurs either relatively soon after the dose of a potent serotonin agonist (MAOI or SSRI) has been increased or shortly after a second serotonergic agent (e.g., dextromethorphan) has been added. The importance of serotonin syndrome in emergency practice is twofold. First, the diagnosis of serotonin syndrome is very challenging due to its nonspecific symptomatology. Mild cases of serotonin syndrome frequently are attributed to other psychiatric and medical disorders. Severe cases are often misdiagnosed as neuroleptic malignant syndrome. Second, **without proper recognition of patients at risk for serotonin syndrome, emergency physicians may**

TABLE 159-1 Serotonergic Potential of Various Drugs

Extreme Potency	Moderate Potency	Low Potency	None
Amitriptyline	Amphetamine	Amantadine	Acetaminophen
Citalopram	Buspirone	Bromocriptine	Granisetron
Clomipramine	Cocaine	Bupropion	Metoclopramide
Dexfenfluramine	Desipramine	Carbamazepine	Morphine
Dextromethorphan	Doxepin	Cisapride	NSAIDs
Fenfluramine	Levodopa	Codeine	Ondansetron
Fluoxetine	LSD	Pentazocine	Salicylates
Fluvoxamine	Mescaline	Pergolide	
Imipramine	Mirtazapine	Reserpine	
Isocarboxazid	Nefazodone		
L-Tryptophan	Nortriptyline		
5-Hydroxytryptophan (5-HTP)‡	St. John's wort‡		
Lithium	Sumatriptan		
MDMA	Trazodone		
Meperidine			
Moclobemide*			
Pargyline†			
Paroxetine			
Phenelzine			
Selegiline			
Sertraline			
Tramadol			
Tranylcypromine			
Venlafaxine			

*Not available in the United States.
†No longer manufactured in the United States.
‡Over-the-counter herbal product.
Note: The serotonergic potential of the drugs listed was determined by both objective and subjective criteria and can be influenced by different doses and formulations.
Abbreviations: LSD = lysergic acid diethylamide; MDMA = 3,4-methylenedioxymethamphetamine; NSAIDs = nonsteroidal anti-inflammatory drugs.

inadvertently precipitate serotonin syndrome by administering serotonergic agents (e.g., meperidine). Therefore, emergency physicians should exercise the same drug-interaction precautions in treating patients taking newer antidepressants as those listed in Chap. 160.

The true incidence and severity of serotonin syndrome are unknown. Prospective studies on serotonin syndrome tend to overestimate its incidence and underestimate its severity. Conversely, case reports often are associated with incomplete documentation and tend to overestimate the severity and underestimate the incidence of serotonin syndrome. The most commonly reported signs and symptoms associated with serotonin syndrome are listed in Table 159-2. Interestingly, muscle rigidity, when present, is especially prominent in the lower extremities. This finding can serve as a valuable clinical marker for serotonin syndrome. Patients with ataxia should be examined carefully for lower extremity hypertonia. Unilateral muscle rigidity or focal neurologic findings have not been reported. Seizures are always generalized and usually short-lived. Hyperthermia is usually of moderate severity, but temperatures greater than 41°C (106°F) have been reported. Hypertension is twice as common as hypotension and is associated with a more favorable prognosis.

TABLE 159-2   Clinical Presentation of Serotonin Syndrome*

Cognitive-Behavioral	%	Autonomic Dysfunction	%	Neuromuscular Dysfunction	%
Confusion/disorientation	54	Hyperthermia	46	Myoclonus	57
Agitation	35	Diaphoresis	46	Hyperreflexia	55
Coma	28	Sinus tachycardia	41	Muscle rigidity	49
Anxiety	16	Hypertension	33	Tremor	49
Hypomania	15	Tachypnea	28	Hyperactivity	43
Lethargy	15	Dilated pupils	26	Ataxia	38
Seizures	14	Unreactive pupils	18	Shivering	25
Insomnia	10	Flushed skin	14	Babinski sign	14
Hallucinations	6	Hypotension	14	Nystagmus	13
Dizziness	6	Diarrhea	12	Teeth chattering	6
		Abdominal cramps	5	Opisthotonus	6
		Salivation	5	Trismus	6

*Percentages are based on a retrospective study of 127 cases of serotonin syndrome.
Source: Adapted from Mills,[17] with permission.

There are no confirmatory laboratory tests for serotonin syndrome. Therefore, the diagnosis of serotonin syndrome is based entirely on clinical suspicion and exclusion of other psychiatric and medical conditions. Serum chemistry tests, drug levels, cerebrospinal fluid analysis, and brain computed tomographic scan results are usually within normal limits. The differential diagnosis for serotonin syndrome is identical to those conditions listed in Table 160-3.

The initial treatment of serotonin syndrome includes discontinuing all serotonergic drugs and providing appropriate supportive care. All patients with serotonin syndrome should be admitted to the hospital until their symptoms have resolved completely. More severely ill patients require admission to an intensive care unit. Approximately 25 percent of patients require endotracheal intubation and ventilatory support. Most patients will show dramatic improvement within 24 h of symptom onset. However, fatalities have been reported. There is an estimated 11 percent mortality rate associated with serotonin syndrome.

At present, there are no accepted guidelines for the use of serotonin antagonists in the treatment of serotonin syndrome. Isolated human case reports suggest that cyproheptadine, methysergide, and propran-olol have the potential to be effective antiserotonergic agents. Benzodiazepines are nonspecific serotonin antagonists and can be used to decrease patient discomfort and promote muscle relaxation. Cyproheptadine (Periactin) appears to be the most effective antiserotonergic agent in humans.[17,18] It should be on most hospital formularies. The initial dose is 4 to 8 mg PO. This dose can be repeated in 2 h if no response is noted to the initial dose. Cyproheptadine therapy should be discontinued if no response is noted after 16 mg has been administered. Patients who respond to cyproheptadine are usually given 4 mg every 6 h for 48 h to prevent recurrences. The use of dopamine agonists (e.g., bromocriptine) has no accepted role in managing patients with serotonin syndrome. Dantrolene (0.5–2.5 mg/kg IV every 6 h, maximum 10 mg/kg per 24 h or 50 to 100 mg bid PO) is a nonspecific muscle relaxant that is used occasionally in serotonin syndrome, but it should be restricted primarily to the treatment of malignant hyperthermia. Patients with muscle rigidity, seizures, or hyperthermia should be monitored closely for rhabdomyolysis and/or metabolic acidosis. Once a patient recovers from serotonin syndrome, it is best to avoid future exposure to serotonergic drugs (see Table 159-1), although the risk of recurrence is unknown.

REFERENCES

1. Litovitz TI, Klein-Schwartz W, Rodgers GC, et al: 2001 Annual report of the American Association of Poison Control Centers Toxic Exposure Surveillance System. *Am J Emerg Med* 20:391, 2002.

2. Haria M, Fitton A, McTavich D: Trazodone: A review of its pharmacology, therapeutic use in depression, and therapeutic potential in other disorders. *Drugs Aging* 4:331, 1994.

3. Cyr M, Brown CS: Nefazodone: Its place among antidepressants. *Ann Pharmacother* 30:1006, 1996.

4. Goodnick PJ: Pharmacokinetics of second-generation antidepressants: Bupropion. *Psychopharmacol Bull* 27:513, 1991.

5. Spiller HA, Ramoska EA, Krenzelok EP: Bupropion overdose: A 3-year multicenter retrospective analysis. *Am J Emerg Med* 12:43, 1994.

6. Puzantian T: Mirtazapine, an antidepressant. *Am J Health System Pharm* 55:44, 1998.

7. Bremmer JD, Wingard P, Walshe TA: Safety of mirtazapine in overdose. *J Clin Psychiatry* 59:233, 1998.

8. Mourilhe P, Stokes PE: Risks and benefits of selective serotonin reuptake inhibitors in the treatment of depression. *Drug Saf* 18:57, 1998.

9. Mitchell PB: Drug interactions of clinical significance with selective serotonin reuptake inhibitors. *Drug Saf* 17:390, 1997.

10. Caley CF: Extrapyramidal reactions and the selective serotonin-reuptake inhibitors. *Ann Pharmacother* 31:1481, 1997.

11. Borys DJ, Setzer SC, Ling LJ, et al: Acute fluoxetine overdose: A report of 234 cases. *Am J Emerg Med* 10:115, 1992.

12. Klein-Schwartz W, Anderson B: Analysis of sertraline-only overdoses. *Am J Emerg Med* 14:456, 1996.

13. Lau GT, Horowitz BZ: Sertraline overdose. *Acad Emerg Med* 3:132, 1996.

14. Myers L, Krenzelok EP: Paroxetine (Paxil) overdose: A pediatric focus. *Vet Hum Toxicol* 39:86, 1997.

15. Personne M, Sjoberg G, Persson H: Citalopram overdose: Review of cases treated in Swedish Hospitals. *Clin Toxicol* 35:237, 1997.

16. Ellingrod VL, Perry PJ: Venlafaxine: A heterocyclic antidepressant. *Am J Hosp Pharm* 51:3033, 1994.

17. Mills KC: Serotonin syndrome: A clinical update. *Crit Care Clin* 13:763, 1997.

18. Graudins A, Stearman A, Chan B: Treatment of the serotonin syndrome with cyproheptadine. *J Emerg Med* 16:615, 1998.

160 MONOAMINE OXIDASE INHIBITORS
Kirk C. Mills

EPIDEMIOLOGY

Monoamine oxidase inhibitors (MAOIs) have been in clinical use for almost 50 years; they were the first effective agents in the treatment of major depression. However, because of their inherent toxicity and the development of safer antidepressants, MAOIs are generally now reserved for atypical or refractory cases. Despite their declining popularity, there were still 200,000 MAOI prescriptions filled in the United States during 2000 (personal communication, GlaxoSmithKline). Emergency physicians should recognize that MAOIs have a low therapeutic index, generally cause severe toxicity in overdose, predispose to tyramine reactions, and can produce serotonin syndrome in combination with other serotonergic agents. There are only three antidepressant MAOIs available in the United States: phenelzine (Nardil), tranylcypromine (Parnate), and isocarboxazid (Marplan). The American Association of Poison Control Centers Toxic Exposure Surveillance System recorded approximately 6000 exposures to MAOIs during the past decade.[1] Of these exposures, 80 percent occurred in adults, 60 percent were intentional ingestions, and 75 percent of patients developed symptoms. There were also 58 reported MAOI-related deaths during the same 10-year period, averaging 1 death for every 100 exposures. However, the mortality may increase up to 33 percent following intentional MAOI overdose, as reported in one case series.[2] In contrast, trazodone (an atypical antidepressant) averages 1 death for every 1200 exposures. This disparity underscores the greater toxicity of MAOIs when compared with newer antidepressant agents.

The only federally approved indication for MAOI antidepressant therapy is for the treatment of nonendogenous depression (i.e., atypical depression or depression refractory to other antidepressants). Other conditions that have shown positive responses to MAOI antidepressant therapy include social phobia disorders, panic disorders, posttraumatic stress syndrome, obsessive-compulsive disorder, bulimia, and narcolepsy. MAOIs are not approved for use in children younger than 16 years of age. Several newer MAOI antidepressants with improved safety and tolerability have been developed, but they are available only outside the United States. The most popular of the newer more selective MAOIs is moclobemide (Aurorix), and it is widely available in Canada and Europe. Surprisingly, it can be purchased in the United States over the Internet without a prescription.

St. John's wort *(Hypericum perforatum)* is a popular over-the-counter herbal treatment for depression. It contains many active ingredients, some of which have the ability to inhibit monoamine oxidase and block serotonin reuptake.[3] A specific history of herbal supplement use should be sought because most patients do not consider St. John's wort a "drug." Although generally safe, St. John's wort still should be viewed with caution because even mild MAOI activity may become more clinically significant in overdose or with certain drug interactions.

Selegiline (Eldepryl) is a MAOI that is devoid of antidepressant activity but is used as an adjunct in the treatment of Parkinson disease.[4] However, at increasing doses, it has activity similar to that of traditional MAOI antidepressants (see below). Some drugs have MAOI activity as an unrelated pharmacologic action such as procarbazine (Matulane), a chemotherapeutic agent for severe Hodgkin lymphoma, and furazolidone (Furoxone), a synthetic nitrofuran with antimicrobial and antiprotozoan activity. Patients taking these medications may be predisposed to MAOI-related drug interactions. Although the information in this chapter has relevance to all drugs with MAOI activity, it focuses primarily on phenelzine, tranylcypromine, isocarboxazid, and selegiline toxicity.

PATHOPHYSIOLOGY

Monoamine oxidase (MAO) is an intracellular enzyme bound to the outer mitochondrial membrane.[5] It has been identified in most human cells. A notable exception is erythrocytes, which do not contain mitochondria. MAO removes amine groups from both endogenous and exogenous biogenic amines. This oxidative deamination process is the primary mechanism by which endogenous biogenic amines such as norepinephrine (NE), dopamine (DA), and 5-hydroxytryptamine

(serotonin or 5-HT) become inactivated. A second important function of MAO is to decrease the systemic availability of absorbed dietary biogenic amines (e.g., tyramine) via hepatic and intestinal metabolism. Therefore, inhibition of MAO leads to the accumulation of neurotransmitters in presynaptic nerve terminals (both centrally and peripherally) and allows for increased systemic availability of dietary amines. Monoamine oxidase has a negligible role in metabolizing circulating catecholamines, which are either secreted endogenously (e.g., by the adrenal gland) or administered intravenously (e.g., epinephrine). This function is accomplished by the enzyme catechol-*O*-methyl transferase (COMT), which is located extraneuronally and is not affected by MAOIs.

MAO is actually two separate isoenzymes, designated MAO-A and MAO-B. Each isoenzyme has its own relative preference for different neurotransmitters, dietary amines, and MAOIs. These substrate preferences are entirely dose-dependent and can be overcome at higher substrate concentrations or MAOI doses (e.g., selegiline). For example, MAO-A has a 1000 times greater affinity for serotonin than MAO-B, but the ability of MAO-B to metabolize serotonin increases at higher serotonin concentrations. Norepinephrine is metabolized primarily by MAO-A, whereas MAO-A and MAO-B have equal ability to metabolize dopamine and tyramine. Overall, the human brain contains more MAO-B than MAO-A, with MAO-B predominance increasing with advancing age. Dopamine neurons appear to lack MAO-B activity and have limited MAO-A activity.[6] Significant MAO-B activity has been detected in surrounding astrocytes and glial cells. Thus dopamine inactivation may depend on astrocyte and glial cell metabolism. Interestingly, MAO-B is the exclusive isoenzyme found in serotonergic neurons. This paradox may be explained by simple conservation of energy, where the MAO-B isoenzyme has a lower affinity for 5-HT and allows for more 5-HT to become recycled. It also allows for increased metabolism of nonserotonin bioamines, thus keeping the neuron free of false neurotransmitters. Intestinal MAO activity is mostly secondary to MAO-A, whereas approximately equal proportions of both isoenzymes are found in the liver. This dual representation of both isoenzymes in the liver affords greater protection against a tyramine reaction.

MAOIs share structural similarities with endogenous amines (e.g., NE, 5-HT, DA), and this allows them to act as potential substrates for MAO. The antidepressant activity of phenelzine, tranylcypromine, and isocarboxazid generally has been attributed to their ability to increase NE and 5-HT neurotransmission by increasing presynaptic concentrations of serotonin and norepinephrine. The actual mechanism by which they exert their therapeutic effects remains unproved but is probably related to delayed postsynaptic receptor modifications (e.g., downregulation). Other potential mechanisms of action include indirect release of neurotransmitters and inhibition of neurotransmitter reuptake. MAOIs also inhibit other enzyme systems (e.g., pyridoxal phosphokinase, diamine oxidase, etc.), but this finding is of uncertain clinical significance. At therapeutic doses (10 mg per d), selegiline has limited effects on NE and 5-HT metabolism. The therapeutic benefit of selegiline in Parkinson disease is thought to be related to increased striatal dopamine neurotransmission and protection against neuronal damage from oxidative stress.[4,6] However, at doses greater than 30 mg per d, selegiline is capable of increasing presynaptic NE and 5-HT concentrations and thus has the potential to produce drug-related toxicity similar to that of phenelzine and tranylcypromine.

All the currently available MAOI antidepressants are irreversible and nonselective (MAO-A, MAO-B) in their enzyme inhibition. MAOIs form irreversible covalent bonds with the MAO enzymes, and this renders the enzyme permanently inactive. Once an irreversible MAOI has been discontinued, it takes approximately 2 weeks before new enzyme synthesis has returned MAO activity to 50 percent of normal. MAOIs do not affect enzyme production. Reversible MAOIs competitively inhibit MAO activity. Thus new enzyme synthesis is not necessary to restore MAO activity, and MAO activity will return gradually to normal over a period of hours as the drug-enzyme complex spontaneously dissociates. Examples of reversible MAOIs include moclobemide, toloxatone, brofaromine, cimoxatone, and befloxatone. These agents are currently not available in the United States.

All MAOIs are absorbed rapidly and completely from the gastrointestinal tract.[7] They have relatively low bioavailability because of a large first-pass effect of hepatic metabolism. Their dependence on hepatic metabolism predisposes them to potential drug interactions with other drugs requiring hepatic oxidation. Peak drug levels usually occur within 1 to 3 h of ingestion. They have relatively large volumes of distribution (1–5 L/kg) and are highly protein-bound. Elimination half-life averages between 2 and 3 h. It is important to recognize that clinical toxicity is usually delayed well after most of the MAOI has already been metabolized. Thus blood MAOI levels do not correlate with clinical toxicity. Selegiline has many active metabolites, such as desmethylselegiline, amphetamine, and methamphetamine. Tranylcypromine has long been suspected of having amphetamine as a metabolite, but this has rarely been detected. Phenelzine metabolism results in multiple active metabolites such as B-phenylethylamine, which also serves as a substrate for MAO-B. The pharmacokinetic profile of most MAOIs suggests that attempts at extracorporeal removal (e.g., hemodialysis) or administering repeat doses of activated charcoal would be unsuccessful in significantly reducing MAOI plasma levels.

TYRAMINE REACTION

Tyramine is an exogenous dietary amine that normally is metabolized by intestinal and hepatic MAO enzymes.[8] In patients taking a nonselective MAOI, a greater amount of tyramine is able to reach the systemic circulation. Tranylcypromine is associated more frequently with tyramine reactions than phenelzine or isocarboxazid. Selegiline (MAO-B selective) is unlikely to produce a tyramine reaction if taken at therapeutic doses. Tyramine is classified as an indirect sympathomimetic and is structurally similar to amphetamine. Like most indirect sympathomimetics, tyramine enters the presynaptic neuron through amine uptake pumps. Once inside the neuron, indirect sympathomimetics are capable of releasing presynaptic stores of norepinephrine and to a lesser degree serotonin and dopamine. Tyramine also can displace epinephrine from the adrenal gland. This action produces the "cheese" reaction (aged cheese contains a large amount of tyramine). In similar fashion, broad (fava) beans contain large quantities of dopamine.

Tyramine is found in over 70 foods and beverages, and any one of these sources may trigger such a reaction.[9] It has been reported that less than 30 percent of patients comply with a MAOI-restrictive diet. In addition, approximately 4 to 8 percent of compliant patients will experience a tyramine reaction during their course of therapy. Nonetheless, newer guidelines call for avoiding only a few high-risk food groups such as meat or fish that is not fresh, sauerkraut, aged meats and cheeses, alcohol (Chianti wine and vermouth), pickled fish (herring), concentrated yeast extracts, and broad beans.

The tyramine reaction is typically of rapid onset, occurring within 15 to 90 min of ingestion of the dietary amine. The severity of this reaction is highly variable and partially related to the total amount of tyramine ingested. The hallmark symptom of the tyramine reaction is a severe occipital or temporal headache. Other associated symptoms include hypertension, diaphoresis, mydriasis, neck stiffness, pallor, neuromuscular excitation, palpitations, and/or chest pain. Most symptoms resolve gradually over 6 h without specific therapy, but fatalities have been reported rarely, usually due to intracranial hemorrhage or myocardial infarction. Therefore, an electrocardiogram should be obtained on all patients with tyramine-associated chest pain. Focal neurologic findings or a persistent, severe headache warrants investigation with a computed tomographic (CT) scan of the head.

In cases of severe hypertension, the drug of choice remains phentolamine, which is given IV in 2.5- to 5-mg doses every 5 to 15 min

until the blood pressure is controlled. The half-life of phentolamine is approximately 20 min, and its duration of action less than 1 h. Nitroprusside is another rapidly acting direct vasodilator that is always administered as a continuous infusion (1–4 μg/kg per min). In cases of moderate hypertension, nifedipine and prazosin have been reported to be effective. Newer recommendations for the treatment of accelerated chronic hypertension discourage the use of nifedipine due to concerns of excessive blood pressure reduction. These concerns may not apply to the acute hypertension seen in tyramine reactions. β-Adrenergic blockers should be considered contraindicated due to unopposed α-receptor stimulation. Hospital admission should be strongly considered for patients whose symptoms do not resolve completely within 6 h of onset. Patients who are asymptomatic after 4 h of observation can be discharged safely home.

DRUG INTERACTIONS

Chronic MAOI drug therapy predisposes to many potentially significant drug interactions (Table 160-1). However, documentation of human MAOI-drug interactions is often limited to single case reports or case series. Controlled human studies are impractical due to the life-threatening nature of these reactions. Animal studies often have limited applicability to human toxicity. Most important, emergency physicians should never administer medications to patients taking MAOIs unless absolutely necessary. Drug compatibility with MAOIs always should be confirmed prior to drug administration.

TABLE 160-1 Drugs Contraindicated with MAOIs*

Indirect Sympathomimetics	Miscellaneous Drugs
Benzphetamine	β-Blockers
Bretylium	Bupropion
Cocaine	Buspirone
Dexfenfluramine	Caffeine
Diethylpropion	Carbamazepine
Dopamine	Cyclobenzaprine
Ephedrine	Dextromethorphan
Fenfluramine	Disulfiram
Guanethidine	Ergot alkaloids
Isometheptene	Fentanyl
Mephentermine	Furazolidone
Metaraminol	Ketamine
Methamphetamine	Levodopa (L-dopa)
3,4-Methylenedioxymethamphetamine (MDMA)	Lithium
Methyldopa	Meperidine
Methylphenidate	Mirtazapine
Pemoline	Oral hypoglycemic agents
Phentermine	Phenothiazines
Phencyclidine	Procarbazine
Phenylpropanolamine	St. John's wort
Propylhexedrine	Sumatriptan
Pseudoephedrine	Theophylline
Reserpine	Tramadol
Ritodrine	Tricyclic antidepressants
Tyramine	

*See additional list of drugs causing serotonin syndrome in Chap. 159, on newer antidepressants, Table 159-1.

Drug interactions involving MAOIs can be grouped into three categories: pharmacodynamic, pharmacokinetic, and idiosyncratic. The most common pharmacodynamic reaction involves indirect-acting sympathomimetics. They have the potential to produce a hyperadrenergic condition similar to the tyramine reaction (see above) and can be found in over-the-counter preparations, drugs of abuse, and some prescription products. Pharmacokinetic drug interactions have been noted with MAOIs because they are metabolized through the cytochrome oxidase enzyme system and thus can inhibit the metabolism of other drugs. The potentiation of opiate and sedative-hypnotic drugs is an example of this type of enzyme inhibition. Tranylcypromine and phenelzine have been shown to increase insulin release and predispose to hypoglycemia, especially in patients taking oral sulfonylurea agents. Insulin dosage also may warrant reduction. Serotonin syndrome (see Chap. 159) is a rare, potentially life-threatening idiosyncratic reaction. It occurs most commonly when MAOIs are combined with other serotonergic agents. However, specific emphasis pertaining to emergency physicians is placed on the avoidance of using meperidine,[10] dextromethorphan, or tramadol in combination with MAOIs. Even after a patient discontinues MAOI therapy, it still takes 2 weeks before 50 percent of MAO enzyme activity returns. Consequently, there always should be at least a 2-week abstinence period between the time of MAOI discontinuation and the time that any contraindicated drug is administered. This recommendation is particularly important to prevent the development of serotonin syndrome.

It is also important to note which medications are generally considered safe in patients on MAOIs (Table 160-2). Aspirin, acetaminophen, ibuprofen, and morphine have been used in combination with MAOIs without complications. Morphine should be given in decreased doses due to impaired morphine metabolism and enhanced opiate effects. Direct-acting sympathomimetic agents (e.g., norepinephrine) can be used with caution, employing the lowest possible effective dose. Direct sympathomimetics do not rely on the release of neurotransmitters for their activity, and they are inactivated by the enzyme COMT, which is unaffected by MAOIs.

TABLE 160-2   Drugs Considered Safe with MAOIs*

Direct sympathomimetics
Albuterol aerosol
Dobutamine
Epinephrine
Isoproterenol
Methoxamine
Norepinephrine
Terbutaline
Miscellaneous drugs
Acetaminophen
Aspirin
Barbiturates
Benzodiazepines
Calcium channel blockers
Cephalosporins
Corticosteroids
Granisetron
Inhalation anesthetics
Lidocaine
Morphine
Nitroglycerin
Nitroprusside
Nonsteroidal anti-inflammatory drugs
Ondansetron
Penicillins
Phentolamine
Procainamide
Tropisetron

*Always use the lowest effective dose.

CLINICAL FEATURES (ACUTE OVERDOSE)

MAOIs have a dangerously low toxic-to-therapeutic ratio. Ingestions of greater than 2 to 3 mg/kg of body weight can be life-threatening, and doses of less than 2 mg/kg still may produce mild to moderate toxicity. The lethal-dose MAOI toxicity is reported to be between 4 and 6 mg/kg.[11] Deaths have been reported in adults with as little as 170 mg of tranylcypromine and 375 mg of phenelzine. Selegiline overdoses have not been reported but should be assumed to produce toxicity similar to that of the traditional MAOI antidepressants until determined otherwise. The average therapeutic dose of tranylcypromine ranges from 20 to 40 mg per d, with a maximum dose of 60 mg per d. It is available as a small, round, red 10-mg tablet. Therapeutic doses of phenelzine range between 45 and 75 mg per d, with a maximum of 90 mg per d. The drug comes as a small, round, orange 15-mg tablet. Isocarboxazid is manufactured as a 10-mg tablet with therapeutic doses ranging between 10 and 60 mg per d. Selegiline has a standard dose of 10 mg per d and comes as an aqua 5-mg capsule.

An important clinical aspect of MAOI is that **symptoms of overdose are characteristically delayed** between 6 and 12 h after ingestion but can be delayed as long as 24 h. The delayed onset of toxicity is believed to be secondary to the gradual accumulation of NE and 5-HT in the brain and in peripheral sympathetic neurons. Symptoms of MAOI overdose are most consistent with a hyperadrenergic state secondary to excessive stimulation of α- and β-adrenergic receptors, but symptoms related to excessive serotonin receptor activity are also seen. Patients on chronic MAOI therapy may show earlier signs of toxicity due to preexisting enzyme inhibition. In severe cases, the hyperadrenergic state can be followed rapidly by hypotension and central nervous system depression resembling a sympatholytic condition. Toxicity usually persists for 1 to 4 days after ingestion.

The signs and symptoms of MAOI toxicity are often nonspecific. Even in its most severe form, it can resemble numerous other conditions (see below). Most clinical overdose information has come from single case reports or case series, with tremendous variation in presentation. Hence there is no "typical" presentation to MAOI toxicity, nor is there an orderly progression of symptoms. The clinician should anticipate the appearance of life-threatening symptoms in all MAOI overdose patients. The initial symptoms of MAOI overdose are reported to include headache, agitation, irritability, nausea, palpitations, and tremor. The earliest signs of MAOI toxicity include sinus tachycardia, hyperreflexia, hyperactivity, fasciculations, mydriasis, hyperventilation, nystagmus, and generalized flushing. In cases of moderate toxicity, opisthotonus, muscle rigidity, diaphoresis, chest pain, hypertension, diarrhea, hallucinations, combativeness, confusion, marked hyperthermia, and trismus may become evident. A peculiar ocular finding described as "Ping-Pong gaze" has been observed with some cases of MAOI toxicity and refers to bilateral wandering horizontal eye movements. The mechanism of this gaze disorder is unknown. In all cases, it resolves gradually as the patient improves. Severe toxicity is accompanied by bradycardia, cardiac arrest, hypoxia, papilledema, hypotension, seizures, coma, and worsening hyperthermia. Hypotension is an ominous finding that commonly remains resistant to therapeutic attempts at correction. Fetal demise, cerebral edema, pulmonary edema, and intracranial hemorrhage all have been reported in association with MAOI overdoses. The most common electrocardiographic abnormality seen in MAOI toxicity is sinus tachycardia, but T-wave abnormalities are not uncommon. Deaths usually are secondary to multiple-organ failure.

DIAGNOSIS

There are no confirmatory laboratory or drug tests. MAOI overdose remains a clinical diagnosis based solely on the history of excessive MAOI ingestion. Plasma MAOI levels and drug screens cannot be relied on to assist in making the diagnosis of MAOI toxicity for two reasons. First, all commonly used drug screens are qualitatively unable to detect MAOIs. Second, specific quantitative plasma MAOI levels are not available routinely in most hospitals, nor do they correlate with observed clinical toxicity. Selegiline is likely to produce amphetamine metabolites, which can be detected on most urine drug screens. Tranylcypromine has the potential to produce amphetamine metabolites, but these have been detected rarely. The best use of laboratory tests is to assist in the differential diagnosis of MAOI toxicity and to identify possible complications of MAOI overdose, which include hypoxia, rhabdomyolysis, renal failure, hyperkalemia, metabolic acidosis, hemolysis, and disseminated intravascular coagulation. Leukocytosis and thrombocytopenia are seen commonly with MAOI toxicity.

The differential diagnosis of an MAOI overdose includes all drugs and medical conditions capable of producing a hyperadrenergic state, altered mental status, and/or muscle rigidity. As evidenced by the extensive number of conditions listed in Table 160-3, the differential diagnosis of unknown MAOI ingestion is extremely challenging. In addition, MAOI toxicity also can be associated with a sympatholytic presentation, thus broadening the differential possibilities even further. In reality, without a history of exposure to MAOIs, it is highly unlikely that the correct diagnosis will be made in the ED, since no confirmatory tests are available.

An interesting diagnostic dilemma exists when a patient on chronic MAOI therapy presents with elevated blood pressure. At therapeutic doses, hypertension can result from tyramine reactions, spontaneous hypertensive crisis, and serotonin syndrome. Tyramine reactions are likely to occur in close relation to food or drug ingestions containing indirect sympathomimetics. Spontaneous hypertensive crisis is a rare condition, usually occurring in relation to recent MAOI dosing.[12] Serotonin syndrome occurs most commonly shortly after exposure to other serotonergic agents and usually is associated with significant cognitive-behavioral and neuromuscular abnormalities.

TABLE 160-3 Differential Diagnosis of Monoamine Oxidase Inhibitor Overdose

Intoxications	Medical conditions	Adverse drug reactions
Amphetamines	Heat stroke	Dystonic reactions
Antimuscarinics	Hypoglycemia	Malignant
Cathinone	Hyperthyroidism	hyperthermia
Clonidine (early)	Pheochromocytoma	Serotonin syndrome
Cocaine		Tyramine reaction
Lysergic acid		Spontaneous
diethylamide		hypertensive crisis
(LSD)		Neuroleptic malignant
Methylphenidate		syndrome
MDMA*		
Nicotine (early)		
Phencyclidine		
Phenylpropanolamine		
Strychnine		
Theophylline		
Tricyclic		
antidepressants		
(early)		
Withdrawal states	Infectious diseases	Psychiatric
Ethanol	Encephalitis	Lethal catatonia
(delirium	Meningitis	
tremens)	Rabies	
Sedative-	Sepsis	
hypnotics	Tetanus	
Clonidine		
β-Blockers		

*3,4-Methylenedioxymethamphetamine.

TREATMENT

General Care

All potential MAOI overdose patients require immediate attention, establishment of at least one preferably large-base peripheral intravenous line, cardiac monitoring, supplemental oxygen, and gastric decontamination. General laboratory tests should be ordered on all patients, with particular emphasis on identifying early hyperkalemia, metabolic acidosis, and rhabdomyolysis. There are no known antidotes for MAOI toxicity. ED management therefore is directed toward supportive care and early treatment of complications. Onset of toxicity is usually gradual and delayed, sometimes up to 24 h after ingestion. However, the abrupt development of seizures, coma, respiratory insufficiency, hyperadrenergic storm, and cardiovascular collapse is entirely possible. Greater toxicity for any given dose of MAOI is predicted in the setting of significant underlying medical problems, pediatric patients, geriatric patients, or coingested drugs.

The best method of gastric decontamination in the setting of MAOI overdose has never been studied. Therefore, the following recommendations are general guidelines based on the pharmacokinetic profile of MAOIs as well as results of human case reports. **Syrup of ipecac is contraindicated.** Activated charcoal should be administered as a single dose of 1 g/kg as soon as possible. Multiple-dose administration of activated charcoal is not expected to be advantageous. Gastric lavage is recommended in all significant ingestions and should be performed within the first 2 h of ingestion to maximize drug removal. Since MAOIs are absorbed rapidly, delayed gastric lavage or whole-bowel irrigation is unlikely to be of any clinical benefit. Hemodialysis, hemoperfusion, and peritoneal dialysis have no established role in the treatment of MAOI poisoning. Urinary acidification is not recommended because it is ineffective at enhancing MAOI elimination and predisposes to acute renal failure secondary to myoglobin precipitation within renal tubules.

Management of Specific Conditions

HYPERTENSION   The acutely hypertensive patient should be treated only with short-acting intravenous antihypertensive agents because of the potential to develop precipitous hypotension. In most cases, an intraarterial catheter is required for accurate blood pressure monitoring. The traditional antihypertensive agents of choice are phentolamine and nitroprusside. Phentolamine is a nonspecific α-adrenergic receptor blocker usually administered in 2.5- to 5.0-mg boluses every 10 to 15 min until blood pressure elevation is controlled. It also can be given as a continuous infusion (0.2–0.5 mg per min) for maintenance therapy. Phentolamine use is commonly associated with reflex tachycardia. Nitroprusside is as effective as phentolamine. It is given as a continuous infusion with an initial rate of 1 μg/kg per min and then titrated according to blood pressure response. Prolonged high doses of nitroprusside can predispose to cyanide toxicity, but this potential complication is rarely noted in the ED. The addition of thiosulfate to nitroprusside infusions eliminates the possibility of cyanide toxicity. Nitroglycerin is indicated for the relief of anginal chest pain and in patients with signs of myocardial ischemia. Fenoldopam is a recently approved short-acting parenteral antihypertensive agent.[13] Its mechanism of action is secondary to peripheral dopamine (D_1) receptor stimulation. It reportedly does not cross the blood-brain barrier. Fenoldopam is administered as a titratable infusion with a suggested starting dose of 0.05 to 0.1 μg/kg per min. Intravenous diltiazem is expected to be an effective antihypertensive agent, but its long duration of action makes it less desirable than the previously mentioned shorter-acting agents. β-Blockers pose a theoretical risk of increasing the blood pressure through unopposed vasoconstriction and would appear to be contraindicated. Despite this concern, β-blockers have been used occasionally to treat hyperadrenergic symptoms in MAOI overdose without serious complications. At best, β-blockers should be used with great caution in the setting of MAOI toxicity. Labetalol is a β-blocker with slight α-receptor blocking ability. The theoretical benefit of its α-blocking capacity must be balanced against its β-blocking activity, which is seven times greater.

HYPOTENSION   Hypotension carries a poor prognosis in MAOI overdose. Isotonic intravenous fluid boluses of 10 to 20 mL/kg are the initial treatment of hypotension. When vasopressors are required, it is important to avoid all indirect-acting agents (see Table 160-1). Norepinephrine is the vasopressor of choice, with epinephrine as the second choice. MAOI patients usually demonstrate an increased sensitivity to vasopressors, and lower initial doses are recommended.

DYSRHYTHMIAS   Sinus tachycardia rarely calls for specific drug therapy unless it is producing cardiac ischemia. Lidocaine and procainamide are the most effective antiarrhythmics in treating MAOI-induced ventricular dysrhythmias. Bradycardia may degrade quickly into asystole in the later stages of the overdose and requires pacemaker placement. Pharmacologic treatment of bradycardia includes atropine, isoproterenol, and dobutamine. Bretylium should be avoided due to its indirect sympathomimetic activity.

SEIZURES   Benzodiazepines are the anticonvulsants of choice in treating MAOI-induced seizures. Barbiturates are as effective as benzodiazepines but may cause hypotension, especially at higher doses. Phenytoin is generally ineffective in stopping drug-induced seizures. General anesthesia and/or muscle paralysis may be necessary in cases of status epilepticus to prevent the metabolic acidosis, hyperthermia, and rhabdomyolysis that commonly accompany persistent seizure activity. Muscle paralysis is best accomplished using nondepolarizing neuromuscular blocking agents. The action of succinylcholine may be enhanced by MAOIs. Pancuronium is probably less desirable than other nondepolarizing agents (e.g., vecuronium) because of its propensity to produce elevations in heart rate and blood pressure. Electroencephalographic monitoring is required when muscle paralysis is used to control the peripheral manifestations of seizure activity. See Chap. 232 for details of treating seizures.

HYPERTHERMIA   Antipyretics generally are ineffective at lowering drug-induced fever. Benzodiazepines are useful first-line agents by reducing muscle hyperactivity and thus decreasing secondary heat production. Increasing evaporative and conductive heat loss is essential for the successful treatment of hyperthermia. This is best accomplished by using cool mist spray, evaporative fans, and ice baths. Hyperthermia is often resilient in the setting of persistent muscle rigidity. Muscle paralysis (nondepolarizing agents) should be considered when diffuse rigidity is refractory to benzodiazepine therapy. Dantrolene has been used successfully as a muscle relaxant in resistant cases of muscle rigidity. The intravenous dose of dantrolene ranges from 0.5 to 2.5 mg/kg every 6 h. Dantrolene should be used only when other measures have failed to relieve muscle rigidity. Older reports of MAOI-induced hyperthermia cited successful treatment with phenothiazines (chlorpromazine). However, these agents are not currently recommended owing to their potential to lower the seizure threshold, worsen hypotension, and produce extrapyramidal reactions.

ADMISSION CRITERIA

All intentional MAOI overdoses and accidental exposures of greater than 1.0 mg/kg require admission to an intensive care unit. Accidental exposures of less than 1.0 mg/kg still require hospital admission but are unlikely to develop life-threatening complications. Therefore, these patients can be admitted to a less acutely monitored bed. Asymptomatic patients should be monitored for at least 24 h before medical clearance. Vital-sign abnormalities should be recognized early and treated appropriately. Dietary and medication restrictions should be followed meticulously during the hospitalization. All patients should be instructed to avoid contraindicated foods and medications for a minimum of 2 weeks. Consultation with a medical toxicologist through the nearest regional poison control center is strongly recommended. Patients who require transfer to hospitals with intensive care units should be transferred as soon as possible to avoid the problems anticipated with delayed onset of toxicity. All patients being transferred should be accompanied by medical personnel capable of performing advanced cardiac life support and endotracheal intubation. It is important to remember that **even a single MAOI pill may produce life-threatening drug interactions** such as serotonin syndrome under the right circumstances.

REFERENCES

1. Litovitz TI, Klein-Schwartz W, Rodgers GC, et al: 2001 Annual report of the American Association of Poison Control Centers Toxic Exposure Surveillance System. *Am J Emerg Med* 20:391, 2002.
2. Meredith TJ, Vale JA: Poisoning due to psychotropic agents. *Adverse Drug React Acute Poisoning Rev* 4:83, 1985.
3. Thiede HM, Walper A: Inhibition of MAO and COMT by *Hypericum* extracts and hypericin. *J Geriatr Psychiatry Neurol* 7(suppl 1):S54, 1994.
4. Youdim MBH, Finberg JPM: Pharmacological actions of l-deprenyl (selegiline) and other selective monoamine oxidase B inhibitors. *Clin Pharmacol Ther* 56:725, 1994.
5. Boulton AA, Eisenhofer G: Catecholamine metabolism: From molecular understanding to clinical diagnosis and treatment. *Adv Pharmacol* 42:273, 1998.
6. Youdim MBH, Riederer P: Dopamine metabolism and neurotransmission in primate brain in relationship to monoamine oxidase A and B inhibition. *J Neural Transm Gen Sect* 91:181, 1993.
7. Mallinger AG, Smith ES: Pharmacokinetics of monoamine oxidase inhibitors. *Psychopharmacol Bull* 27:493, 1991.
8. Brown C, Taniguchi G, Yip K: The monoamine oxidase inhibitor-tyramine interaction. *J Clin Pharmacol* 29:529, 1989.
9. Shulman KI, Walker SE, MacKenzie S, et al: Dietary restriction, tyramine, and the use of monoamine oxidase inhibitors. *J Clin Psychopharmacol* 9:397, 1989.
10. Stack CG, Rogers P, Linter SPK: Monoamine oxidase inhibitors and anesthesia. *Br J Anaesth* 60:222, 1988.
11. Linden CH, Rumack BH, Strehlke C: Monoamine oxidase inhibitor overdose. *Ann Emerg Med* 13:1137, 1984.
12. Lavin MR, Mendelowitz A, Kronig MH: Spontaneous hypertensive reactions with monoamine oxidase inhibitors. *Biol Psychiatry* 34:146, 1993.
13. Post JB IV, Frishman WH: Fenoldopam: A new dopamine agonist for the treatment of hypertensive urgencies and emergencies. *J Clin Pharmacol* 38:2, 1998.

ANTIPSYCHOTICS
Richard A. Harrigan
William J. Brady

A group of antipsychotic drugs, classically termed *neuroleptics,* have been in use since the 1950s for the treatment of schizophrenia and other related psychoses (Table 161-1). Although they have revolutionized the treatment of these disorders, these agents are known to cause myriad adverse effects, both in therapeutic and toxicologic situations. A propensity to affect neurologic function led to the term *neuroleptic,* which is less appropriate today in light of the development of newer agents for the treatment of schizophrenia that are less likely to cause these effects; thus, these agents are now usually classified as *antipsychotic* agents (see Table 161-1). In addition to the treatment of various psychoses, however, these drugs also are used for nonpsychiatric con-

TABLE 161-1 Pharmacologic Classification of Typical and Atypical Antipsychotic Agents

Class	Generic Name	Brand Name
TYPICAL ANTIPSYCHOTICS		
Phenothiazines		
Aliphatic	Chlorpromazine	Thorazine
	Triflupromazine	Vesprin
Piperazine	Fluphenazine	Prolixin
	Perphenazine	Trilafon
	Prochlorperazine	Compazine
	Trifluoperazine	Stelazine
Piperidine	Thioridazine	Mellaril
	Mesoridazine	Serentil
Thioxanthenes	Thiothixene	Navane
Butyrophenones	Haloperidol	Haldol
Diphenylbutylpiperidines	Pimozide	Orap
Dihydroindolones	Molindone	Moban
Dibenzazepines		
Dibenzoxazepine	Loxapine	Loxitane
ATYPICAL ANTIPSYCHOTICS		
Dibenzazepines		
Dibenzodiazepine	Clozapine	Clozaril
Thienobenzodiazepine	Olanzapine	Zyprexa
Dibenzothiazepine	Quetiapine	Seroquel
Benzisoxazoles	Risperidone	Risperdal
Benzisothiazol piperazine derivative	Ziprasidone	Geodon

ditions, such as chemical restraint of agitated or violent patients; control of nausea and emesis; pain and nausea relief in various headache syndromes; suppression of hiccups; and control of various involuntary motor disorders, including Tourette syndrome, Huntington chorea, and various disorders of the basal ganglia.

Conventional, or *typical,* antipsychotics are a diverse group of older agents that gained widespread acceptance for the control of the positive symptoms (e.g., hallucinations, delusions, and disordered thought) of schizophrenia and related psychoses. These agents cause numerous adverse effects, however, and do little if anything to ameliorate the cognitive dysfunction and negative symptoms (e.g., withdrawal, flat affect, and loss of drive) that are also characteristic of the disease. Thus, a newer class of *atypical* antipsychotic drugs has emerged, featuring improved clinical efficacy and a different side-effect and toxicologic profile. Despite the numerous adverse effects seen with antipsychotic agents, their therapeutic index is high, and lethal ingestion is rare. The most recent Toxic Exposure Surveillance System summary of fatal exposures from the American Association of Poison Control Centers lists only 23 reported deaths with an antipsychotic agent as the principal agent ingested; in only 6 of those cases was the antipsychotic the sole agent involved.[1]

PHARMACOLOGY

The *typical antipsychotics* share a similarity in pharmacotherapeutic and adverse-effect profiles. They are all dopamine receptor antagonists; this blockade in the limbic system is thought to be primarily responsible for the antipsychotic activity of these agents. Dopaminergic antagonism in the basal ganglia also occurs, causing disinhibition of cholinergic neurons; this, in turn, may lead to various involuntary movement disorders, termed *extrapyramidal side effects,* as discussed below. In addition to blocking dopaminergic receptors, typical anti-

psychotics also block, to varying degrees, α-adrenergic (principally α₁), muscarinic, and histaminic receptors. Alpha₁-adrenergic antagonism leads to orthostatic hypotension and reflex tachycardia because of peripheral vasodilatation. Anticholinergic activity at muscarinic sites leads to hyperthermia, tachycardia, pupillary dilatation, dry mouth, urinary retention, and constipation. Histamine blockade results in central nervous system sedation. Generally speaking, drugs of higher potency (i.e., low milligram-per-day dosage) tend to cause significant dopaminergic antagonism and thus are more likely to cause extrapyramidal effects; examples include haloperidol, fluphenazine, and thiothixene. Drugs of lower potency (i.e., high milligram-per-day dosage) are less likely to cause extrapyramidal effects, but are more likely to cause sedation and orthostatic hypotension, because of strong antihistaminic and anticholinergic/muscarinic effects. Examples of lower-potency drugs include chlorpromazine and thioridazine. It should be emphasized, however, that all typical antipsychotics could cause some degree of extrapyramidal symptoms, sedation, orthostatic hypotension, and various anticholinergic effects.

The newer *atypical antipsychotics,* in addition to featuring varying degrees of antagonistic activity at dopaminergic, α-adrenergic, histaminic, and cholinergic/muscarinic receptor sites, block serotonergic sites with varying affinity. These drugs exhibit greater clinical efficacy in that they also improve negative symptomatology and cognitive dysfunction, and they are less likely to cause extrapyramidal effects and thus are more attractive than the typical antipsychotics. There is evidence that these newer agents also are effective in treatment-resistant patients who are so labeled due to treatment failures with the typical antipsychotic agents.

The pharmacokinetics of all antipsychotic agents are similar, given well-controlled, therapeutic situations. Bioavailability is erratic and peak plasma levels occur 2 to 6 h after oral administration, although clinical effects are seen within the first 30 to 60 min. Of the new atypical antipsychotics, only ziprasidone is currently available in injectable form. Protein binding, lipophilicity, and volume of distribution are uniformly high for all antipsychotics, rendering dialysis an ineffective means of treating toxicity. Elimination is by hepatic metabolism—both hepatic microsomal enzyme oxidation and enterohepatic circulation—followed by renal excretion, to varying degrees. The newer atypical antipsychotics all carry warnings regarding use in patients with concomitant hepatic disease. Only quetiapine and ziprasidone do not carry such precautions in renal disease, because of trivial excretion of unchanged drug by the kidney. Plasma-level monitoring can establish compliance, but is not generally recommended with the antipsychotics, in either therapeutic or toxicologic assessment situations.

ADVERSE EFFECTS

Extrapyramidal Disorders

Although these dopaminergic receptor-mediated side effects can be seen with any antipsychotic agent, they are classically associated, and most frequently seen, with the typical agents, especially those of higher potency. However, any of the following conditions can occur with all antipsychotic drugs, as well as with other structurally similar agents that are not classified as antipsychotics, such as droperidol, promethazine, metoclopramide, and prochlorperazine.

Dystonic reactions are involuntary muscle contractions that may affect the muscles of the neck (torticollis), jaw (trismus), trunk (opisthotonos), tongue, or those surrounding the eye (oculogyric crisis). Laryngospasm, although rare, may also occur, and threaten the airway. Dystonia may involve an isolated muscle group or, more frequently, a combination of the above. Affected patients commonly exhibit evidence of adrenergic hyperactivity, including diaphoresis, tachycardia, tachypnea, and hypertension, and are often in obvious pain and quite anxious.[2] A history of therapeutic (including long-acting depot preparations of some antipsychotics such as fluphenazine and haloperidol) and illicit drug use is key; dystonic reactions have been reported with a variety of agents, including tricyclics, "street Valium" (haloperidol), and cocaine.[2] Acute treatment includes administration of diphenhydramine 25 to 50 mg IM or IV; the latter route provides the most rapid relief, usually within 10 min. If symptoms are not relieved, the dose may be repeated in 15 to 30 min, or an alternative agent can be used, such as benztropine (Cogentin) 1 to 2 mg, optimally via either parenteral route. Benzodiazepines may serve as adjunctive therapy and are especially useful when cocaine is the offending agent. **Because of the prolonged effects of the dystonia-inducing agent, oral therapy with either diphenhydramine or benztropine should be continued for 2 to 5 days.[2]**

Akathisia is a condition in which patients demonstrate motor restlessness with corresponding anxiety; it can be mistaken for a worsening of the underlying psychiatric disorder. This assumption may lead to a dose increase of the offending agent, thus making the symptoms worse. Administration of diphenhydramine or related agents may be diagnostic and therapeutic; a reduction in dose of the antipsychotic, or a switch to a less potent agent, is a possible long-term solution. *Bradykinesia,* or drug-induced parkinsonism, is another extrapyramidal side effect of this drug class and should be treated in a similar fashion.

Tardive Dyskinesia

This involuntary movement disorder is idiosyncratically associated with chronic therapy, and classically—although not exclusively—with the typical antipsychotic agents. Symptoms include involuntary, repetitive, choreoathetoid movements of the face, mouth, and tongue, and may be mild or severe and debilitating; uncommonly, the limbs and trunk are also affected. Elderly patients, especially those with diabetes mellitus and organic brain disorders, seem to be at increased risk. The overall incidence is approximately 5 percent per year of exposure to the offending agent. The pathophysiology of tardive dyskinesia is unclear. Traditionally, it has been attributed to an emerging supersensitivity of dopaminergic receptors in the striatum under chronic blockade by the antipsychotic agent. Alternate theories also implicate other neurotransmitters, whereas others invoke the possibility of direct neurotoxicity resulting in free radical production. The new atypical antipsychotics are believed to be much less likely to cause this syndrome, although this is not yet clear. A number of drugs and treatment modification strategies have been advanced as therapeutic options for tardive dyskinesia; there are no emergency management issues other than recognizing the syndrome.[3]

Neuroleptic Malignant Syndrome

This syndrome is an idiosyncratic, rare, and potentially fatal reaction most commonly associated with the use of antipsychotic drugs, although other drug classes also have been implicated. Clinical features include hyperthermia, muscle rigidity, autonomic instability, and alteration in mental status. Neuroleptic malignant syndrome (NMS) may occur at any time during therapy with the causative agent or may present when dopamine agonist therapy is discontinued. Risk factors include age (young or middle-aged adults are most commonly affected); a concomitant condition of exhaustion, dehydration, or a general debilitated state; and a history of NMS. Typically, patients present with high fever, from 39°C (102.2°F) to 42°C (107.6°F), but onset of hyperthermia may be delayed.[4] Manifestations of autonomic dysfunction include tachycardia, labile hypertension, pallor, vasoconstriction, and diaphoresis.[5] A "lead-pipe" rigidity of the musculature is almost universal, while other manifestations of motor dysfunction also may occur, including tremors, myoclonus, dystonia, dyskinesia, dysphagia, dysarthria, and opisthotonos. Alteration in mental status ranges from confusion and agitation to stupor or coma.[4] Characteristic laboratory findings include leukocytosis, myoglobinuria, and elevation of crea-

tine phosphokinase. Metabolic acidosis, renal insufficiency, electrolyte abnormalities, and elevated hepatic transaminases may also occur. The differential diagnosis includes meningoencephalitis, tetanus, rabies, collagen vascular disease, malignant hyperthermia, lethal catatonia, heatstroke, thyroid storm, pheochromocytoma, strychnine poisoning, and toxicity from a variety of drugs, including anticholinergic poisoning and the serotonin syndrome. Perhaps the two syndromes most difficult to distinguish from NMS are malignant hyperthermia and lethal catatonia, as all three feature fever and muscle rigidity. Malignant hyperthermia is associated with causative exposure to certain anesthetic agents, whereas lethal catatonia, a type of heat exhaustion, follows a period of manic hyperactivity and does not feature autonomic instability.

The cornerstone of treatment of NMS is supportive care, with rapid cooling, fluid and electrolyte repletion, and critical care monitoring all being paramount. Intubation should be considered, and aggressive muscle relaxation should be pursued with intravenous benzodiazepines (e.g., lorazepam 2 mg IV, diazepam 5 mg IV. The offending pharmacologic agent should be discontinued, or the previously withdrawn dopamine agonist should be restarted.[4,5] Dantrolene (1 mg/kg to 2.5 mg/kg IV initially; titrate to effect, max 10 mg/kg cumulative), a nonspecific skeletal muscle relaxer that is employed in the treatment of malignant hyperthermia, also has been used with good results, especially in cases wherein muscle rigidity is a predominant feature.[5] Specific therapy for NMS has been advocated, some of which is based on the presumed pathophysiology of the syndrome, which is central dopamine depletion.[4,5] Bromocriptine, carbidopa/levodopa, and amantadine have been used with equivalent success, both alone and in combination.[5] Centrally acting dopa-mine agonists may be most important in the treatment of significant hyperthermia and mental status alteration, and vasodilators such as minoxidil (2.5 mg PO) and nitroprusside (start at 0.3 mg/kg per min) should be considered when vasoconstriction is a problem. Ag-gressive therapy has led to a reduction in mortality from NMS.

Selected Miscellaneous Adverse Effects

In addition to the various dopamine-related side effects just described (extrapyramidal disorders, tardive dyskinesia, and NMS), the antipsychotics may cause a variety of other untoward effects, some of which are highlighted here. All antipsychotics may cause sedation and impair mental capacity to some degree; patients should be cautioned regarding activities requiring mental alertness, such as driving and operating heavy machinery. Photosensitivity may occur with the typical antipsychotics, especially the phenothiazines; it is not characteristic of the atypical agents, with the exception of risperidone. To varying degrees, all may lower the seizure threshold. Both typical and atypical agents are pregnancy category C, with the exception of clozapine, which is category B; none of these agents are recommended in breast-feeding women. Clozapine therapy carries the risk of agranulocytosis and is reserved for use in severely ill schizophrenics who have failed conventional treatment regimens; weekly monitoring of the leukocyte count is indicated. Weight gain, hyperglycemia, and hyperlipidemia are variably associated with the atypical antipsychotics, with the apparent exception of ziprasidone. This agent does have a propensity to increase the QT interval on the electrocardiogram, however, and thus it is not recommended for use with other drugs that lengthen the QT interval or in uncorrected conditions predisposing to QT prolongation (e.g., hypokalemia, hypomagnesemia).[6]

ACUTE OVERDOSE

Clinical Features

In general, overdose with these drugs features an exaggerated version of the response that is expected, based on knowledge of the aforementioned adverse effects. Central nervous system depression, ranging from mild sedation to deep coma, frequently occurs and is attributable to anticholinergic and antihistaminic effects. Some degree of sedation is generally seen with overdose of any antipsychotic drug, but has been found to occur more frequently with chlorpromazine.[7] Seizures may be seen, as well as dysfunction in temperature regulation.[7,8] Anticholinergic and extrapyramidal effects may occur as with nontoxic ingestion and tend to vary with the potency of the drug: low-potency compounds tend to cause anticholinergic effects, and high-potency agents tend to cause extrapyramidal disorders.[2]

Cardiovascular effects may be seen as alterations in heart rate, blood pressure, and cardiac conduction. Tachycardia can be attributed both to anticholinergic effects and to a reflex response to vasodilatation. Hypotension is caused by both α_1-adrenergic blockade and a direct depressant effect on the myocardium. Atrioventricular and intraventricular conduction disturbances may also occur, as well as other electrophysiologic effects, ranging from asymptomatic prolongation of the QT interval to fatal ventricular dysrhythmia.[6–8] **The piperidine phenothiazines (e.g., thioridazine) are the antipsychotic drugs with the highest potential for serious dysrhythmia: they may behave like type Ia antidysrhythmics in overdose, possibly causing wide-complex tachycardia and torsade de pointes.**[6–8] Prolongation of the QT interval, torsade de pointes, and sudden death are all well-documented to have occurred with haloperidol, yet the frequency of occurrence is significantly less than with thioridazine.[6] Although not an antipsychotic, droperidol, a butyrophenone-derivative similar to haloperidol, deserves mention here because of its utility both as an antiemetic and in the chemical control of the agitated patient. Droperidol received a Food and Drug Administration (FDA)-prompted drug warning advisory in December 2001, citing the risk of QT prolongation and torsade de pointes. It was accompanied by a recommendation that droperidol use be restricted to clinical situations wherein other agents fail, and then only if the corrected QT interval is <440 msec in males and <450 msec in females; the scientific rationale behind this was recently reviewed and questioned in the emergency medicine literature.[9]

Clinical experience with overdose involving the newer atypical agents is relatively sparse, but emerging. Clozapine, with its profound anticholinergic effects, causes central nervous system depression and seizures, but appears to be unlikely to cause cardiac conduction disturbances or agranulocytosis. Risperidone principally causes neurologic (lethargy, spasms, and dystonia), cardiovascular (tachycardia, QT prolongation, and wide-complex tachycardia), and electrolyte disturbances. **In massive overdose risperidone is also associated with miotic pupils and a wider variety of dysrhythmias, including supraventricular tachycardias and bradycardia.** In most cases, risperidone overdose is well-tolerated.[10,11] Olanzapine poisoning causes central nervous system depression—at times profound and requiring intubation for airway protection—and miosis.[12] Quetiapine overdose may lead to alterations in neurologic (depressed sensorium) and cardiovascular (hypotension and tachycardia) status, and in one case of massive overdose, it was associated with significant prolongation of the QT interval.[13] Ziprasidone, the newest atypical antipsychotic agent, is contraindicated in cases of known or suspected QT-interval prolongation but has limited overdose data available; thus far, mild sedation and some prolongation of the QT interval have been observed without serious neurologic or cardiovascular complications.[14,15]

Treatment

Supportive care and decontamination of the gastrointestinal tract are the key principles of treatment (Table 161-2). Patency of the airway and assurance of adequate ventilation are paramount, especially in light of the fact that these agents may cause profound alterations in level of consciousness. Oxygen and naloxone should be administered to all patients with altered mental status, and blood glucose should be

TABLE 161-2 Care of the Acute Ingestion

Airway, breathing, IV access, and cardiac monitor
Altered mental status
  Naloxone 0.4 mg to 2.0 mg IV; titrate to effect (usual maximum 10 mg)
  Dextrose 25 g (50 mL) of D50 solution IV (if rapid glucose
    determination suggests low blood sugar, or if is unavailable) and
    repeat ×1 if no response.
Hypotension
  Crystalloid infusion
  Norepinephrine 4 mg/500 mL D5W; begin at 2–4 μg/min; titrate to effect
Ventricular dysrhythmias
  Sodium bicarbonate, 1–2 mEq/kg IV bolus; if infusion necessary,
    100–150 mEq/L D5W, titrate over 4–6 h with target arterial pH
    approximately 7.50
  Lidocaine 1.0–1.5 mg/kg IV bolus; maintenance infusion of 2 g/250 mL
    D5W at 1–4 mg/min
Torsade de pointes
  Magnesium sulfate 2–4 g IV
  Overdrive pacing
  Isoproterenol 2 mg/250 mL D5W at 5 μg/min
Gastrointestinal decontamination
  Activated charcoal 1–2 g/kg PO
  If patient is intubated, orogastric lavage using >34 French tube, followed
    by activated charcoal
Seizures
  Benzodiazepines
    Lorazepam 2–4 mg IV (2 mg per min); may repeat if necessary
      (consider airway protection)
    Diazepam 5–10 mg IV (5 mg per min); may repeat if necessary
      (consider airway protection)
  Phenobarbital up to 20 mg/kg IV at maximum 50 mg per min
  Fosphenytoin 15–18 mg/kg PE IV at maximum 150 mg PE per min

rapidly assessed at the bedside. Crystalloid intravenous fluids should be given for hypotension. If further therapy is needed, vasopressors with β-adrenergic activity theoretically should be avoided (e.g., dopamine, epinephrine, and isoproterenol), because the α-adrenergic blockade seen with the antipsychotic agents results in unopposed β-adrenergic agonism, causing vasodilatation and worsening hypotension.

Continuous cardiac monitoring and a 12-lead electrocardiogram are cardinal management features. The QT interval should be determined and monitored. Ventricular dysrhythmias should be managed with type Ib antidysrhythmic agents (e.g., lidocaine), avoiding class Ia agents (e.g., quinidine, disopyramide, and procainamide), which may worsen cardiac toxicity. Wide-complex tachycardias should be treated with intravenous sodium bicarbonate due to the potential for blockade of fast sodium channels with certain agents, especially thioridazine.[7,8] Torsade de pointes, if it occurs, should be managed with cardiac pacing, isoproterenol, or magnesium infusion.[7,16]

Gastrointestinal decontamination should be instituted as soon as the patient is stabilized; in most cases, PO administered activated charcoal (1 g/kg) will suffice. Gastric lavage should be considered in patients who present to the ED very soon after a life-threatening ingestion. Multidose activated charcoal is theoretically indicated because of the partial metabolism by enterohepatic circulation. High protein binding and a large volume of distribution, general characteristics of this drug class, render hemodialysis and forced diuresis ineffective management techniques.

In addition to stabilization of the airway and cardiovascular status and attention to gastrointestinal decontamination, other therapy may be given as needed. Intravenous benzodiazepines, phenobarbital, and phenytoin should be considered for control of seizures. Electrolyte disturbances have been reported sporadically; serum chemistries should be obtained in serious ingestions, especially to exclude other causes of altered mental status and dysrhythmia, which may occur. Specific drug levels are not readily available and are not helpful in the acute management of these patients. Acute extrapyramidal disorders should be treated as described above.

Disposition

Patients with alteration in mental status, which usually includes a depressed level of consciousness, and patients with evidence of cardiotoxicity are best managed in the intensive care unit. Thioridazine has been shown to cause serious dysrhythmias both early in the clinical course and after a significant delay; patients ingesting this agent warrant electrocardiographic monitoring for at least 24 h, even if asymptomatic.[7,8] Patients should receive appropriate psychiatric evaluation after ED assessment and treatment if they are asymptomatic, have a physical examination and electrocardiogram without evidence of lingering toxicity (e.g., no QT-interval prolongation), and are not believed to have ingested a piperidine phenothiazine. If psychiatric evaluation is not warranted, they may be discharged from the ED.

REFERENCES

 1. Litovitz TL, Klein-Schwartz W, White S, et al: 2000 Annual report of the American Association of Poison Control Centers Toxic Exposure Surveillance System. *Am J Emerg Med* 19:337, 2001.
 2. Fines RE, Brady WJ, DeBehnke DJ: Cocaine-associated dystonic reaction. *Am J Emerg Med* 15:513, 1997.
 3. Egan MF, Apud J, Wyatt RJ: Treatment of tardive dyskinesia. *Schizophr Bull* 23:583, 1997.
 4. Lev R, Clark RF: Neuroleptic malignant syndrome presenting without fever: Case report and review of the literature. *J Emerg Med* 12:49, 1994.
 5. Schneider SM: Neuroleptic malignant syndrome: Controversies in treatment. *Am J Emerg Med* 9:360, 1991.
 6. Glassman AH, Bigger JT Jr: Antipsychotic drugs: Prolonged QT interval, torsade de pointes, and sudden death. *Am J Psychiatry* 158:1774, 2001.
 7. Buckley NA, Whyte IM, Dawson AH: Cardiotoxicity more common in thioridazine overdose than with other neuroleptics. *J Toxicol Clin Toxicol* 33:199, 1995.
 8. LeBlaye I, Donatini B, Hall M, Krupp P: Acute overdosage with thioridazine: A review of the available clinical exposure. *Vet Hum Toxicol* 35: 147, 1993.
 9. Horowitz BZ, Bizovi K, Moreno R: Droperidol—behind the black box warning [editorial]. *Acad Emerg Med* 9:615, 2002.
10. Acri AA, Henretig FM: Effects of risperidone in overdose. *Am J Emerg Med* 16:498, 1998.
11. Duenas-Laita A, Castro-Villamor MA, Martin-Escudero JC, Perez-Castrillon JL: New clinical manifestations of acute risperidone poisoning. *J Toxicol Clin Toxicol* 37:893,1999.
12. O'Malley GF, Seifert S, Heard K, et al: Olanzapine overdose mimicking opioid intoxication. *Ann Emerg Med* 34:279, 1999.
13. Hustey FM: Acute quetiapine poisoning. *J Emerg Med* 17:995, 1999.
14. Burton S, Heslop K, Harrison K, Barnes M: Ziprasidone overdose. *Am J Psychiatry* 157:835, 2000.
15. House M: Overdose of ziprasidone. *Am J Psychiatry* 159:1061, 2002.
16. Vukmir RB: Torsade de pointes: A review. *Am J Emerg Med* 9:250, 1991.

LITHIUM
Sandra M. Schneider
Daniel J. Cobaugh

EPIDEMIOLOGY

Apart from treatment of bipolar disorder, many other medical and psychiatric uses for lithium have been suggested, including impulsive/aggressive behavior, neutropenia, alcohol dependence, cluster and migraine headaches, and hypothyroidism. Lithium toxicity may result from accidental or intentional overdose or from an alteration in lithium

clearance. The true incidence of toxicity and subsequent medical outcomes are not known because there is no mandatory reporting requirement for toxic exposures in the United States.

It has been estimated that up to 75 to 90 percent of patients who are chronically treated with lithium will develop toxicity some time in their therapy. For the year 2001, the American Association of Poison Control Centers has reported over 4,607 potential toxic exposures to lithium. Of these, 253 were in children. There were 44 that resulted in death.[1]

PATHOPHYSIOLOGY

Lithium is thought to cause toxicity through several mechanisms. It has the ability to compete with other similar-molecular-weight ions, including sodium, potassium, magnesium, and calcium, displacing them from both intracellular and bone sites. Competition with and displacement of other ions can result in lithium retention and subsequent toxicity. Therefore, activities, medical conditions, and medications that affect water and electrolyte balance can contribute to lithium toxicity. Loss of salt, water, or both leads to an increase in proximal reabsorption of lithium and a rise in lithium level. Inhibition of arginine vasopressin and the resulting hydro-osmotic effects also have been attributed to lithium. Some of the toxic effects of lithium may be due to inhibition of 3-glycogen synthase kinase (GSK) that is present in high quantities in brain and is involved in cell proliferation and differentiation.[2]

It is also thought that lithium, through adenylate cyclase inhibition, causes decreases in intracellular cyclic adenosine monophosphate (cAMP). Decreases in cyclic guanosine monophosphate (cGMP) also may occur. It has been suggested that lithium may increase inositol monophosphate (IMP) and reduce free inositol through inhibition of IMP. Activated inositol may interact with G proteins to form intracellular messengers that enhance intracellular calcium release and activate protein kinase C.[3] Lithium is also thought to interfere with the release and reuptake of the neurotransmitter norepinephrine at the nerve terminal site. Lithium may enhance serotonin release from the hippocampus. Lithium has been implicated in the serotonin syndrome when combined with other medications that alter serotonin. It also may have a protective effect against apoptosis and promote growth and regeneration of axons.[4] Finally, risk of lithium toxicity exists when it is combined with a variety of medications. Most often toxicity involves a drug-drug interaction with lithium. A number of these potential drug interactions are listed in Table 162-1. Herbal diuretics may in-

TABLE 162-1   Drug Interactions with Lithium

Major	
Haloperidol	

Moderate	
ACE inhibitors	NSAIDs
Anorexiants	Phenytoin
Benzodiazepines	Tetracyclines
Caffeine	Theophyllines
Calcium antagonists	Thiazide diuretics
Carbamazepine	Urea
Clozapine	Urinary alkalizers
Fluoxetine	Succinylcholine
Iodide salts	Nondepolarizing muscle
Loop diuretics	paralytics
Methyldopa	Phenothiazines
Metronidazole	Tricyclic antidepressants

Minor	
Carbonic anhydrase inhibitors	Sympathomimetics, parenteral

Abbreviations: ACE = angiotensin-converting enzyme; NSAIDs = nonsteroidal anti-inflammatory drugs.

crease toxicity.[5] In addition, the use of succinylcholine and vecuronium in patients taking lithium may result in a prolonged neuromuscular blockade.

The pharmacokinetics of lithium also play a vital role in toxicity. The absorption of lithium is rapid and complete following oral administration. There is delayed uptake and elimination in the brain, recently confirmed by magnetic resonance imaging (MRI).[6] The difference in the concentration in the brain and serum may vary two- to threefold.[6] **Serum levels do not predict central nervous system (CNS) levels.** Delayed absorption may occur with sustained-release products and following ingestion of a large number of pills. Toxic effects ap-pear later and last longer. Lithium has a volume of distribution of 0.79 L/kg, which is similar to that of body water. Lithium distribution to and from the CNS is slower, resulting in CNS symptoms that do not correlate with serum levels. Sustained toxic effects, even after hemodialysis, can be due to the slow distribution in the CNS. Lithium is not bound to plasma proteins. The half-life of lithium is reported to be approximately 29 h. There is no appreciable hepatic metabolism, and it is excreted primarily unchanged in the urine. The presence or development of renal insufficiency is an important factor in the development of lithium toxicity. Sodium and water loss due to heat and exercise may lead to lithium retention. The elderly are prone to toxicity due to a decreased volume of distribution and reduced renal clearance.

CLINICAL EFFECTS

Adverse effects are common with lithium, occurring in 35 to 90 percent of treated patients.[7] The most common adverse effects (Table 162-2) are hand tremor, polyuria due to loss of urinary concentration ability, and rash. Hand tremor occurs in up to 65 percent of patients at some time,[8] and worsening of a baseline tremor is an important signal of developing toxicity. Decreasing the intake of caffeine or adding a beta blocker may improve the tremor, but often a decrease in dose is necessary.[7] Neurologic side effects include memory loss, decreased mental concentration, and fatigue. Ataxia and dysarthria can develop and often will improve with cessation of therapy. Long-term lithium treatment can lead to electroencephalographic changes, including diffuse slowing, an increase in theta and delta waves, and a decrease in alpha activity.

A decrease in urinary concentrating ability occurs in most patients but is largely asymptomatic. Up to 12 percent of patients will develop nephrogenic diabetes insipidus.[9] In some patients, incomplete distal renal tubular acidosis develops (defect in urine acidification without academia).

Gastrointestinal (GI) side effects, including nausea, vomiting, and diarrhea, are common at initiation of treatment and generally are transient. They can be decreased by giving the dose with food or dividing the dose over the day. GI symptoms that develop during the course of treatment may signal toxicity. Cardiovascular changes develop in part because lithium interferes with the sodium-potassium pump, leading to intracellular hypokalemia. This results in electrocardiographic findings of U waves, flattened or inverted T waves, and ST-segment depression. Bradycardia, QT_c prolongation, bundle-branch block, and junctional dysrhythmias have been reported. Cardiac effects occur in 20 to 30 percent of patients. Other less common side effects include syncope due to sinus node dysfunction, induced hypothyroidism, and a folliculitis that occurs mainly in the spring.

Lithium toxicity may result from acute intentional overdose, from chronic exposure, or as a result of a change in lithium clearance (e.g., medications, dehydration, or salt depletion). Toxicity developing in patients taking chronic lithium therapy may be due to a change in the daily dose of medication or physiologic changes impairing elimination of the drug. Renal failure or intravascular volume depletion is a precipitating cause in nearly all cases of chronic toxicity.[9] Other factors known to precipitate lithium toxicity are listed in Table 162-3.

TABLE 162-2   Side Effects with Chronic Lithium Therapy

Neurologic
  Fine tremor*
  Fatigue*
  Poor memory
  Loss of concentration
  Dysphoria
  Muscle weakness
  Decreased reaction time
  Lack of spontaneity
  Worsening of dementia
  Truncal ataxia
  Ataxic gait
  Dysarthria
  Extrapyramidal symptoms (cogwheeling)
Renal
  Polyuria*
  Atrophy of nephron
  Decreased ability to concentrate urine
  Nephrogenic diabetes insipidus
  Inhibition of antidiuretic hormone
  Incomplete distal renal tubular acidosis
Cardiovascular*
  T-wave flattening or inversion
  U waves
  Prolonged QT interval
  Sinus bradycardia
  Sinoatrial block
  First-degree atrioventricular block
Endocrine
  Increased thyroid-stimulating hormone and decreased T4 and T3
    (hypothyroid effect)
  Euthyroid goiter
  Increased calcium and parathyroid hormone
  Increased magnesium
  Weight gain
  Increased glucose
Gastrointestinal
  Anorexia*
  Nausea and vomiting*
  Diarrhea*
  Abdominal pain
Dermatological
  Maculopapular rash*
  Psoriasis
  Acne
  Folliculitis
  Edema of hands and feet
  Alopecia
Miscellaneous
  Eye burning, itching, and tearing
  Increased white blood cell count

*Common.

Patients with acute overdose may have elevated serum concentrations with limited signs of toxicity. Acute ingestions classically cause more GI toxicity and less CNS toxicity. After ingestion, there is delay in transport of lithium into the intracellular compartment and across the blood-brain barrier. With time, equilibration occurs, and toxicity develops. Neurologic symptoms often develop as GI symptoms are abating. Levels in patients with an acute ingestion do not correlate well with either symptoms or prognosis.

Patients with chronic exposure have lower serum concentrations and higher cellular levels and classically display earlier and greater neurologic changes. Levels in such patients correlate better with prognosis and toxicity. Acute-on-chronic ingestions have aspects of both profiles of ingestion. As in most toxicities, the best guideline for therapy is the patient's condition, not the serum concentration of the implicated agent.

TABLE 162-3   Factors Precipitating the Development of Lithium Toxicity (Excluding Drug Interactions)

Renal failure
Volume depletion
Hyperthermia/neuroleptic malignant syndrome
Infection
Congestive heart failure
Diabetes mellitus
Preexisting cerebral pathology (white matter infarct, frontal meningioma, HIV)
Gastroenteritis
Surgery
Cirrhosis
Decreased sodium intake

Recognizing lithium toxicity may be challenging, particularly in patients with chronic overdose. Table 162-4 lists a common grading system for toxicity. Patients commonly present with muscle fasciculations, ataxia, agitation or lethargy, and muscle weakness. At times, it may be difficult to distinguish between lithium toxicity and organic delirium. Although most patients present with slowing of their cognitive function, cases of lithium toxicity presenting as mania have been reported. As toxicity worsens, confusion, lethargy, stupor, and finally, coma develop. Rarely, extrapyramidal signs develop. Proximal muscle weakness, extensor plantar response, and auditory, visual, and tactile hallucinations have been reported. The electroencephalogram shows diffuse slowing and disorganization, with frontal intermittent rhythmic delta activity in severe cases.

In addition to neurologic changes, renal dysfunction is common. Lithium at therapeutic doses has been implicated in nephrogenic diabetes insipidus as well as in decreased creatinine clearance, oliguria, and albuminemia. There appears to be a relationship between these effects on renal function and lithium serum concentration. Due to diabetes insipidus, patients complain of polyuria and polydipsia. Fluid losses may exacerbate toxicity. Acute renal failure may develop, particularly in patients with preexisting renal impairment, advanced age, diabetes, hypertension, or dehydration.

GI symptoms are common in both acute and chronic toxicity. Patients present with gastroenteritis, nausea, vomiting, diarrhea, bloating, or generalized abdominal pain. Leukocytosis can occur. Cardiac abnormalities are more common in acute toxicity, with hypotension, conduction abnormalities, and ventricular dysrhythmias. Electrocardiographic changes with transient ST-segment depression and T-wave inversion are seen in some patients. As indicted earlier, QT_c prolongation, conduction abnormalities, and bradycardia are seen. Less common effects include hyperthermia, hypothermia, peripheral neuropathy, and severe leukopenia.

Up to 10 percent of patients die, generally of respiratory failure or cardiovascular collapse. Most patients who recover will have no long-term sequelae. Chronic renal failure occasionally develops. Permanent cerebellar damage may develop and progress over several weeks following the toxic episode.[10] These patients have truncal ataxia, ataxic gait, scanning speech, and diffuse incoordination. Short-term memory loss, dementia, and a tremor of the hands and head accompany the cerebellar signs. Most patients improve over several months, but symptoms are permanent in some patients. Permanent seizure disorder has been reported.

TREATMENT

As in all toxicities, initial stabilization of patients must include protection of the airway, ventilatory support, and hemodynamic support. Intravenous access, cardiac monitoring (including a 12-lead electrocardiogram), and laboratory analysis of blood and urine, including renal function, fluid/electrolytes, calcium, magnesium, complete blood count, urine specific gravity, and drug concentration for lithium, acetaminophen, and other possible ingestants, should be obtained. A complete medical history, including an assessment of baseline neurologic function, must be documented. It is also necessary to search for precipitating factors such as volume depletion or electrolyte imbalance. A complete listing of medications (prescription, over-the-counter, and herbal agents) taken in the preceding week should be obtained. The neurologic examination should be focused on the issues discussed above.

Seizures should be treated with intravenous benzodiazepines (see Chap. 232). Refractory seizures may require phenobarbital or general anesthesia. **Phenytoin decreases renal excretion of lithium** and often is ineffective in drug-induced seizures.

GI decontamination is difficult in lithium toxicity. Often these patients present with chronic toxicity, and there is no role for gastric decontamination. Activated charcoal is ineffective at adsorbing lithium at gastric pH.[11] Its use is not contraindicated, however, because it may be effective in cases of polydrug toxicity. Gastric lavage or ipecac is as effective in lithium overdose as in other drug overdoses, and if it is done early after ingestion, some drug can be removed. Since lithium tablets are often quite large, small-bore tubing may be ineffective in removing the drug. Whole-bowel irrigation (polyethylene glycol, 2 L/h in adults and 500 mL/h in children) is helpful, especially in cases where sustained-release lithium products have been ingested. Whole-bowel irrigation initiated in the first hour can remove 60 percent of the drug.[12]

Aggressive hydration with normal saline is important. Nearly all patients with significant toxicity have some sodium and volume deficit. Sodium and water depletion interferes with lithium elimination, and this increases and prolongs toxicity. In fact, in volume-depletion states, lithium may be resorbed preferentially by the kidney in an attempt to counter sodium loss. Volume repletion reestablishes normal elimination kinetics. Forced diuresis does not enhance lithium elimination once fluid losses have been replaced. In fact, loop and thiazide diuretics can be dangerous because they further sodium and water loss.[13]

Although nearly all toxicologists agree that hemodialysis should be used for severely toxic patients, the threshold for initiating this treatment is still debated. Patients with levels greater than 3.5 mEq/L (4.0 mEq/L in acute ingestion), patients with little change in their lithium level of 1.5 to 3.5 mEq/L after 6 h of hydration, or patients with sustained levels of more than 1.0 mEq/L after 36 h will benefit from hemodialysis.[14] In addition, patients with renal failure, those with rapidly increasing levels, or those who have ingested sustained-

TABLE 162-4   Grading of Lithium Toxicity

Level	Clinical Features	Treatment
Grade 1	1.5–2.5 mEq/L: nausea, vomiting, tremor, hyperreflexia, ataxia, agitation, muscular weakness	Hydration, Kayexalate
Grade 2	2.5–3.5 mEq/L: stupor, rigidity, hypertonia, hypotension	Hydration, Kayexalate, possible dialysis
Grade 3	>3.5 mEq/L: coma, seizures, myoclonus, collapse	Hemodialysis

Note: Levels are valid in chronic ingestions only.

release preparations should be considered for treatment. However, a recent study of the outcome of patients meeting these criteria, treated with and without dialysis, showed no major difference, suggesting that these criteria may be conservative.[15] Addition of bicarbonate to the dialysate has been shown to lead to greater intracellular extraction of lithium.[16]

The goal of hemodialysis is to reduce the serum lithium level to less than 1 mEq/L. Because of the cellular concentration of lithium, an increase in serum levels following termination of dialysis is common.[16] Drug levels must be monitored for up to 8 h following dialysis. If levels rise to greater than 1 mEq/L, hemodialysis should be reinstituted. Use of either high-volume continuous venovenous hemofiltration (HV-CVVH) or hemodialysis followed by continuous venovenous hemofiltration (CVVHD) may prevent a rebound in level.[17,18,19] Peritoneal dialysis and charcoal hemoperfusion have been used but are less effective than hemodialysis (Table 162-5). Because of the intracellular concentration of lithium in the CNS, neurologic symptoms may persist and even worsen during treatment.

In less severe toxicity, sodium polystyrene sulfonate (SPS, or Kayexalate; 15 g PO qid or 30 g PR) may be useful in decreasing serum half-life of lithium.[20] Approximately 75 percent of lithium is bound to SPS in vitro compared with less than 25 percent when activated charcoal is used. Although experience with SPS is limited, it may be useful for mild to moderate toxicity. Because SPS is an exchange resin, large electrolyte shifts may occur during its use, and the electrolyte level must be monitored and derangements treated aggressively.

Treatments mentioned in anecdotal case reports, such as sodium bicarbonate and acetazolamide (both in urinary alkalinization) and aminophylline, cannot be recommended at this time. Among treatments found to be ineffective or harmful are water loading, diuretics (furosemide, thiazide, ethacrynic acid, or spironolactone), and ammonium chloride.

DISPOSITION

Admission decisions must be weighed by the presence and persistence of factors predisposing the patient to toxicity, the acuity of the toxicity, and the circumstances that led to the toxicity. Acute ingestions must be treated as already described, and patients should be monitored for 4 to 6 h, even if asymptomatic, and receive psychiatric consultation. **Any patient with *acute* ingestion of a sustained-release preparation should be admitted.** Patients with levels of greater than 1.5 mEq need admission.

Patients with grade 1 *chronic* toxicity without additional risk factors may be managed with hydration for 4 to 6 h. Once levels return to the normal range (less than 1.5 mEq), there is clinical improvement, and usually, after psychiatric evaluation, the patient may be discharged. Repeat values obtained within 24 h by home health services can be considered. Patients with grade 2 or 3 chronic toxicity require admission.

TABLE 162-5   Comparison of Half-Life of Lithium with Treatment

Therapy	Serum Half-Life, h	Clearance, mL/min
No treatment	14–54	15
Saline		15
Peritoneal dialysis		10–15
Hemodialysis	4–6	50
Sodium polystyrene sulfonate	12	
Charcoal hemoperfusion		20

REFERENCES

1. Litovitz TL, Klein-Schwartz W, Rodgers GC Jr, et al: 2001 Annual report of the American Association of Poison Control Centers Toxic Exposure Surveillance System. *Am J Emerg Med* 20:391, 2002.
2. Shaldubina A, Agam G, Belmaker BH: The mechanism of lithium action: State of the art, ten years later. *Prog Neuropsychopharmacol Biol Psychiatry* 25:855, 2001.
3. Kofman O, Belmaker RH: Biochemical behavior and clinical studies of inositol in lithium treatment and depression. *Biol Psychiatry* 34:839, 1989.
4. Chen RW, Chuang DM: Long-term lithium treatment suppresses p53 and Bax expression but increases Bcl-2 expression. *J Biol Chem* 274:6039, 1999.
5. Pyevich D, Bogenschutz MP: Herbal diuretics and lithium toxicity. *Am J Psychiatry* 158:1329, 2001.
6. Kilts CD: In vivo imaging of the pharmacodynamics and pharmacokinetics of lithium. *J Clin Psychiatry* 61(suppl 9):41, 2000.
7. Dunner D: Optimizing lithium treatment. *J Clin Psychiatry* 61(suppl 9):76, 2000.
8. Gelenberg AJ, Jefferson JW: Lithium tremor. *J Clin Psychiatry* 56:283, 1995.
9. Bendz H, Aurell M, Balldin J, et al: Kidney damage in long-term lithium patients: A cross-sectional study of patients with 15 years or more on lithium. *Nephrol Dial Transplant* 9:1250, 1994.
10. Manto M, Godaux E, Jacquy J, Hildebrand JG: Analysis of cerebellar dysmetria associated with lithium intoxication. *Neurol Res* 18:416, 1996.
11. Favin FD, Klein-Schwartz W, Oderda GM, Rose SR: In vitro study of lithium carbonate adsorption by activated charcoal. *Clin Toxicol* 26:443, 1988.
12. Smith SW, Ling LH, Halstenson CE: Whole bowel irrigation as treatment for acute lithium overdose. *Ann Emerg Med* 20:536, 1991.
13. Finley PR, Warner MD, Peabody CA: Clinical relevance of drug interactions with lithium. *Clin Pharmacokinet* 29:172, 1995.
14. Jaeger A, Sauder P, Kopferschmitt J, et al: When should dialysis be performed in lithium poisoning? A kinetic study in 14 cases of lithium poisoning. *Clin Toxicol* 31:429, 1993.
15. Bailey B, McGuigan M: Comparision of patients hemodialyzed for lithium poisoning and those for whom dialysis was recommended by PCC but not done: What lesson can we learn? *Clin Nephrol* 54:388, 2000.
16. Szerlip HM, Heeger P, Feldman GM: Comparison between acetate and bicarbonate dialysis for the treatment of lithium intoxication. *Am J Nephrol* 12:116, 1992.
17. Jacobsen D, Aasen G, Grederichsen P, Eisenga B: Lithium intoxication: Pharmacokinetics during and after terminated hemodialysis in acute intoxications. *Clin Toxicol* 25:81, 1987.
18. van Bommel EFH, Kalmeijer MD, Ponssen HH: Treatment of life-threatening lithium toxicity with high-volume continuous venovenous hemofiltration. *Am J Nephrol* 20:408, 2000.
19. Meyer RJ, Flynn JT, Brophy PD, et al: Hemodialysis followed by continuous hemofiltration for treatment of lithium intoxication in children. *Am J Kidney Dis* 37:1044, 2001.
20. Roberge RJ, Martin TM, Schneider SM: Use of sodium polystyrene sulfonate in a lithium overdose. *Ann Emerg Med* 22:1911, 1993.

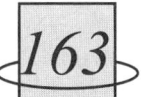

BARBITURATES
Raquel M. Schears

Barbiturates have been in common clinical use for a century. These agents possess sedative properties, which are used to reduce anxiety, and hypnotic properties, which are used to induce sleep, hence their informal classification as sedative-hypnotics. The therapeutic efficacy of these agents in the emergency department is best illustrated in their use as anticonvulsants in the treatment of seizure disorders, for conscious sedation to facilitate procedures, and as induction agents in rapid-sequence intubation.[1] There are also recent case series reports of administering barbiturates to treat severe withdrawal from alcohol and γ-hydroxybutyrate (GHB), resistant to benzodiazepine therapy.[2] The prophylactic use of barbiturates as antihypertensives in the management of elevated intracranial pressure (ICP) has been abandoned for lack of supporting evidence.[3,4] Currently, inducing "barbiturate coma" is considered a last resort for intractable ICP elevations after all medical and surgical treatment has failed.[5] Also recently challenged is the efficacy of prescribing barbiturate-containing combination analgesics available in the United States and Canada, for the treatment of migraine headache and other chronic pain disorders. The United Kingdom, France, Germany, and Australia have removed these agents from the market because of their high liability of physical dependence and abuse, coupled with their potential risk of lethal overdosage and lack of outcome-based benefit.[6]

Barbiturate abuse, both prescription and illicit, peaked in the 1970s. The availability, as measured by sales and by the accidental death rate, was significantly correlated with their use for suicide. During the last two decades, the number of toxic exposures involving barbiturates and the incidence of overall barbiturate-related deaths have declined dramatically. This trend has been attributed to the advent and popularity of safer sedative-hypnotics such as the benzodiazepines and other major tranquilizers, rescheduling of barbiturates to class II, III, and IV drugs, and improvements in supportive care in overdose settings. Since 1990, there have been U.S. reports of increasing illicit barbiturate use among adolescent populations. Reasons for this include youth misperceptions that barbiturates are harmless, and even helpful when taken in combination with cocaine and methamphetamines to mitigate unpleasant stimulant extremes. By 1998, forensic data from mass suicide rituals and state-required reporting by Oregon physicians prescribing medications to assist in their patients' suicide, continued to underscore both the predictable lethality and strategic preference for prescription barbiturates used in intentional overdose.[7] The *2000 Annual Report of the American Association of Poison Control Centers* documented that barbiturates were involved in 4484 reported poisonings, with half of these recorded as intentional overdoses, which resulted in 16 fatalities.[8] Although children were involved in 1138 of the total reported barbiturate poisonings, none died from their explosure.[8] Overall (in adults and children), barbiturates consistently rank among the top 5 toxic agents in overdosage, associated with major complications and fatalities.

PHARMACOLOGY

The parent compound, barbituric acid (2,4,6-trioxohexahydropyrimidine), itself has no central depressant activity. R group substitutions, primarily at position 5, give these compounds their sedative-hypnotic properties. Substituting sulfur for the oxygen at position 2 creates a thiobarbiturate, which is more lipid soluble than an oxybarbiturate (Figure 163-1). High lipid solubility allows an agent to rapidly transit the blood-brain barrier and confers a shorter duration of action and greater degree of hypnotic activity. By convention, barbiturates have been classified according to their duration of action (Table 163-1).

Long-acting barbiturates tend to be weaker acids (lower pK_a values), less lipid soluble, and less protein bound than shorter-acting barbiturates. This translates to a delayed onset of action, decreased volume of distribution, and longer duration of action when compared

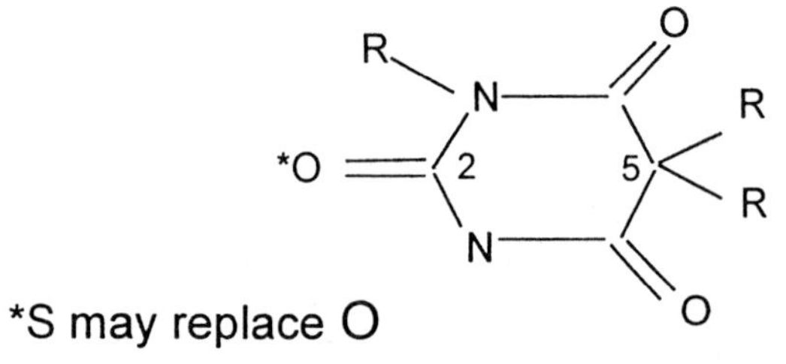

*S may replace O

FIG. 163-1. Chemical structure of barbituric acid.

with short-, ultrashort-, and intermediate-acting compounds. Furthermore, tissue permeability of long-acting barbiturates is uniquely affected by body fluid pH changes. Only nonionized drug is membrane permeable. Phenobarbital has a pK_a of 7.24 and is 95 percent ionized at pH 7.4. Ionization will increase in a basic medium, and permeability will decrease. (Conversely, an acidic medium will facilitate phenobarbital permeability by maintaining more drug in a nonionized state.) Alkaline diuresis takes advantage of this equilibrium and forces the remaining 5 percent of the drug into an ionized form. Thus, the charged drug is trapped under basic conditions for renal elimination. Unfortunately, ion-trapping as a drug elimination strategy only works for long-acting barbiturates.

Short-, ultrashort-, and intermediate-acting barbiturates are not affected by body pH changes. Secobarbital, for example, has a pK_a of 7.9 and is 98 percent nonionized at pH 7.4. Rate of barbiturate delivery to the membrane determines tissue permeability with these classes. These compounds are stronger acids (higher pK_a values), more lipid soluble, and more protein bound, enabling a more rapid onset of action, greater volume of distribution, and shorter duration of action compared with the long-acting barbiturates.

Bulk absorption of barbiturates occurs in the stomach and small intestine, where most of the drug exists in a nonionized state. Overall, barbiturates readily diffuse into the body tissues and cross the blood-brain barrier, with highest concentrations occurring in the brain, liver, kidney, and adipose tissue. Barbiturates are excreted in breast milk and easily cross the placenta. Fetal blood barbiturate concentrations closely reflect maternal plasma levels. Interestingly, in utero exposure to phenobarbital has been significantly linked to a distinctive pattern of physical abnormalities in infants,[9] and in separate reports, with verbal intelligence deficits in adult men.[10] Tolerance develops with chronic barbiturate use, and higher doses are required to produce the same effects. Most barbiturates are metabolized in the liver to inactive by-products. Hepatic biotransformation occurs primarily through routes involving the cytochrome P450 microsomal enzyme system. All barbiturates are capable of inducing the activity of this enzyme system, which affects many other drug actions. For example, patients with chronic barbiturate use will have an increased rate of metabolism of oral contraceptives, anticoagulants, and corticosteroids when taken concurrently. Depending on the degree of hepatic biotransformation, variable amounts of barbiturates are excreted unchanged in the urine. Barbital and phenobarbital are less protein bound and thus most dependent on the renal excretion pathway. Elimination half-life of barbiturates can be greatly accelerated in infants and children and very prolonged in the elderly and in patients with liver or renal disease. The main action of barbiturates is to depress activity in nerve and muscle tissues. In the central nervous system (CNS) this is accomplished by enhancing the action of the primary inhibitory neurotransmitter γ-aminobutyric acid (GABA) at the postsynaptic membrane. Additionally, barbiturates may act by inhibiting calcium-mediated excitatory neurotransmitter release at the presynaptic junction.

CLINICAL FEATURES

Mild to moderate barbiturate intoxication closely resembles the drug "high" produced by alcohol. Drowsiness, disinhibition, ataxia, slurred speech, and mental confusion are common features that escalate with increasing dose. The progressive CNS depression seen with *severe* barbiturate intoxication predictably manifests as a range from stupor to coma to complete neurologic unresponsiveness. Scales gauging the depth of coma are useful in describing patient presentation and monitoring interval changes in the level of consciousness during treatment in overdose settings.[11] The most common vital sign abnormalities seen in overdose are hypothermia, respiratory depression, and hypotension. The abnormal temperature control and respiratory depression are centrally mediated phenomena, whereas hypotension is primarily a result of increased vascular capacitance and venous pooling. The end prod-

TABLE 163-1   Selected Properties and Classification of Commonly Used Barbiturates

	Long Acting*		Intermediate Acting*		Short Acting*		Ultrashort Acting*	
Generic name	Barbital†	Phenobarbital†	Amobarbital	Amobarbital plus secobarbital	Pentobarbital	Secobarbital	Thiopental	Methohexital
Trade name	Veronal	Luminal	Amytal	Tuinal	Nembutal	Seconal	Pentothal	Brevital
Street name‡	Carbutol	Purple hearts, goof balls, phennies	Blue heavens, downers	Gorilla pills, F-66's, rainbows, double trouble	Yellow jackets, Abbotts, Mexican yellows	Reds, red devils/birds, lilly, pinks, pink ladies.	ND	ND
pK_a	7.4	7.24	7.75	7.85	7.96	7.90	7.6	7.9
Major route of detoxification	Renal (33%)	Renal (30%)	Hepatic	Hepatic	Hepatic	Hepatic	Hepatic	Hepatic
Plasma protein binding (%)	5	20	ND	ND	35	44	80	73
Volume of distribution V_D (L/kg)	ND	0.7	1.05	1.0	1.0	1.5	1.4–6.7	1.1
Hypnotic dose (mg)	300–500	100–200	50–200	100	50–100	100–200	50–100	50–120 IV
Duration of action (h)	>6	>6	3–6	3–6	<3	<3	0.3	0.3
Plasma half-life (h)	ND	24–96	14–42	16–40	21–42	20–28	6–46	1–2
Fatal dose (g)§	10	5	ND	ND	30	30	ND	ND

Abbreviation: ND = no data.

*This classification scheme is a convention only; it preceded the discovery that the elimination half-lives do not conform to the apparent duration of action.

†Only drugs responsive to alkaline diuresis.

‡Barbituates possessing street names are relatively common drugs of abuse.

§In nontolerant individuals.

Source: Adapted with permission from Lee D: Sedative-hypnotic agents, in Goldfrank LR, Howland MA (eds): *Goldfrank's Toxicologic Emergencies,* 7th ed. New York, NY: McGraw-Hill Companies, 2001, p. 932.

uct of these derangements can be a patient who is cold, apneic, and in shock. Pulse rate is not diagnostic; pupil size, light reactivity, nystagmus, and deep tendon reflexes are variable. Gastrointestinal tract motility is slowed, resulting in delayed gastric emptying and ileus. Skin bullae, referred to as "barbiturate blisters," are uncommon and may indicate nothing more than the effects of local skin pressure.[11] Even when it is known that a barbiturate was ingested, it is prudent to consider coingestions and alternate explanations for the observed symptom complex.

Early deaths in barbiturate overdose result from cardiovascular collapse and respiratory arrest. Most common complications are hypoglycemia, followed by the delayed pulmonary problems of aspiration pneumonia, noncardiogenic pulmonary edema, and adult respiratory distress syndrome. Current mortality rates range between 1 and 3 percent and are more often the result of multiple organ system failure. Lethal dose is uncertain, but severe poisoning can be assumed if more than 10 times the hypnotic dose has been ingested in a single exposure.[11]

The Oregon reporting data on physician-assisted suicide indicated all 27 patients who received prescriptions of either secobarbital (≥9 g) or phenobarbital (6 g), achieved their death wish. The median interval between ingestion to unconsciousness was 10 min (range, 1 to 30 min), and the mean interval between ingestion and death was 30 min (range, 4 min to 26 h).[7]

Laboratory evaluation in barbiturate overdose should include determination of glucose levels, blood chemistries, complete blood count, arterial blood gas measurement (if indicated), toxicology screen, chest radiograph, and an electrocardiogram. Barbiturate serum levels are useful in establishing the diagnosis of a comatose patient and should be obtained and used to distinguish long- from short-acting agents because treatment approaches differ. As a rule of thumb, patients presenting with a serum concentration of more than 10 mg/dL

for a long-acting barbiturate, more than 7 mg/dL for an intermediate-acting barbiturate, and more than 3 mg/dL for a short-acting barbiturate, left untreated, have a greater risk of death from the exposure.[11] These measurements are not reliable in predicting clinical course in overdose because they do not reflect brain barbiturate concentrations and may underestimate the clinical condition of a patient in the setting of polydrug exposure. Such levels are also invalid in chronic barbiturate abusers who have developed physiologic tolerance and in patients with renal or hepatic disease who have decreased clearance.[11]

TREATMENT

In barbiturate overdose, reaching a treatment center predicts favorable outcome largely because supportive management alone is effective over a broad range of serum concentrations.

Airway Assessment and Stabilization

Airway assessment and stabilization are the first management priorities. Intubation in severe sedative-hypnotic overdose is often required and should precede any attempt at gastrointestinal evacuation. Standard monitoring of vital signs, cardiac electrical activity, pulse oximetry, intravenous access, and supplemental oxygen therapy should be initiated on ED arrival.

Volume Expansion

Volume expansion is the mainstay of circulatory support in barbiturate-induced shock. In the absence of cardiac failure, rapid infusion of 1 to 2 L of isotonic intravenous fluid is indicated; administration of bolus therapy, e.g., 200-mL aliquots, is prudent in the elderly, those with cardiac decompensation, or in the setting of known renal impairment.

If fluid resuscitation fails to correct hypotension, vasopressors such as dopamine and norepinephrine should be initiated.

Gastric Emptying

Gastric lavage should not be considered unless a patient has ingested a potentially life-threatening amount of barbiturates *and* the procedure can be undertaken within 60 min of ingestion.[12]

Lavage is not superior to activated charcoal alone. Given the CNS depression associated with this overdose, the induction of emesis should be avoided. The patient should be intubated for airway protection prior to performing lavage when it is indicated. Oral activated charcoal augments drug extraction by adsorbing drugs from the gastrointestinal tract. Multiple-dose activated charcoal (MDAC) is beneficial in reducing serum phenobarbital concentrations; however, no significant difference in clinical outcome has yet been demonstrated. Still, most studies suggest that activated charcoal is at least as effective as gastric lavage and may be better, given its immediate functional effectiveness. The current toxicology Position Statement is to consider MDAC only if a patient has ingested a life-threatening amount of phenobarbital.[13] Loading dose of activated charcoal is 50 to 100 g. Concurrent administration of cathartic agents remains unproven and is not recommended; standard MDAC is 20 to 50 g every 4 h.

Forced Diuresis

Forced diuresis with fluid loading and diuretic therapy is most effective for phenobarbital. Intravenous furosemide should be titrated to effect a urinary flow of 4 to 6 mL/kg per h. Diuresis is contraindicated in the setting of hypotension or shock. Iatrogenic congestive heart failure and fluid overload preclude the usefulness of this therapy for other barbiturates that have limited renal excretion.[11]

Urinary Alkalinization

Urinary alkalinization (see Chap. 156) will promote the excretion of long-acting barbiturates (e.g., phenobarbital) only. **Alkalinizing the urine is not effective for shorter-acting barbiturates** because these drugs are primarily metabolized by the liver with negligible renal excretion, exist as stronger acids, and are often more protein bound. The utility of this strategy requires that the drug be appreciably excreted in the urine and that more of it can be trapped in its ionized form in the tubular fluid under basic conditions, to facilitate increased renal excretion. The 5- to 10-fold increase in basal renal excretion rate for phenobarbital, is accomplished by giving a 1 to 2 mEq/kg sodium bicarbonate bolus IV, followed by 50 to 100 mEq in 500 mL of D5W. The drip rate is considered sufficient when an arterial pH of 7.45 to 7.50, urinary pH of 8.0, and urinary output of 2 mL/kg per h is maintained. Serum potassium must remain at least 4 mEq/L to achieve continuous urinary alkalinization. Adequacy of therapy should be monitored every 2 to 4 h.

Hemodialysis and Hemoperfusion

Hemodialysis and hemoperfusion are techniques that are used to maximize barbiturate elimination; these techniques are reserved for patients who are deteriorating despite institution of aggressive supportive care. Effectiveness of these modalities was previously limited by drug characteristics and technical difficulties. However, recent reports of high-efficiency hemodialysis, which uses high blood flow rates, demonstrate a rapid fall in phenobarbital levels linked to dramatic improvement in clinical condition.[14]

Further research into this modality must be undertaken before it can be recommended as the preferred mode of extracorporeal therapy for refractory phenobarbital intoxication.

DISPOSITION

Mild to moderate barbiturate intoxication responds well to general supportive care and including a single dose of activated charcoal. Frequent reassessment of neurologic status and vital sign parameters indicating improvement over 6 to 8 h allow eventual patient transfer to psychiatric services. Severe overdose will require intensive care unit admission, ongoing medical stabilization (MDAC only for lethal phenobarbital ingestion), and delayed psychiatric intervention. Early poison center contact and specialty service consultation is recommended.

BARBITURATE ABSTINENCE SYNDROME

Barbiturates are notorious for their rapid development of tolerance, high liability for physical dependence and abuse, and multiple drug interactions. Abrupt discontinuation of barbiturates in a chronically dependent user will produce minor withdrawal symptoms within 24 h and major life-threatening symptoms within 2 to 8 days. The severity of the withdrawal reflects the degree of physical dependence and drug half-life. Cessation of short-acting barbiturates results in more severe abstinence symptoms than stopping long-acting barbiturates. This is consistent with the clinical observation that the brain has more time to adapt to declining drug concentrations that are gradual. Clinical manifestations of abstinence mimic those described for alcohol withdrawal. *Minor symptoms* include anxiety, restlessness, depression, insomnia, anorexia, nausea, vomiting, muscle twitching, abdominal cramping, and sweating. *Major symptoms* include psychosis, hallucinations, delirium, generalized seizures, hyperthermia, and cardiovascular collapse.

Priorities in the treatment of major abstinence symptoms are cardiovascular stabilization and seizure control. Intravenous benzodiazepines usually are effective in treating seizures, although intravenous barbiturates may be required. Due to the mortality associated with sedative-hypnotic abstinence, gradual in-hospital withdrawal of the addicting agent is recommended.

REFERENCES

1. Lerman B, Yoshida D, Levitt MA: A prospective evaluation of the safety and efficacy of methohexital in the emergency department. *Am J Emerg Med* 14:351, 1996.
2. Sivilotti M, Burns MJ, Aaron CK, et al: Pentobarbital for severe gamma-butyrolactone withdrawal. *Ann Emerg Med* 38:660, 2001.
3. Biros MH, Heegaard W: Prehospital and resuscitative care of the head-injured patient. *Curr Opin Crit Care* 7:444, 2001.
4. Anonymous: The Brain Trauma Foundation. The Joint Section on Neurotrauma and Critical Care. Use of barbiturates in the control of intracranial hypertension. *J Neurotrauma* 17:527, 2000.
5. Allen CH, Ward JD: An evidence-based approach to management of increased intracranial pressure. *Crit Care Clin* 14:485, 1998.
6. Sellers EM, Hoornweg K, Busto UE, et al: Risk of drug dependence and abuse posed by barbiturate containing analgesics. *Can J Clin Pharmacol* 6:18, 1999.
7. Sullivan AD, Hedberg K, Fleming DW: Legalized physician-assisted suicide in Oregon-the second year. *New Engl J Med* 342:598, 2000.
8. Litovitz TL, Klein-Schwartz W, White S, et al: 2000 Annual report of the American Association of Poison Control Centers Toxic Exposure Surveillance System. *Am J Emerg Med* 19:337, 2001.
9. Holmes, LB, Harvey EA, Coull BA, et al: The teratogenicity of anticonvulsant drugs. *New Engl J Med* 344:1132, 2001.
10. Reinisch JM, Sanders SA, Mortensen EL, et al: In utero exposure to phenobarbital and intelligence deficits in men. *JAMA* 274:1518, 1995.
11. McCarron MM, Schulze BW, Walberg CB, et al: Short-acting barbiturate overdosage: Correlation of intoxication score with serum barbiturate concentration. *JAMA* 248:55, 1982.
12. Anonymous: Position statement: Gastric lavage. American Academy of Clinical Toxicology; European Association of Poisons Centres and Clinical Toxicologists. *Clin Toxicol* 35:711, 1997.

13. Anonymous: Position statement and practice guidelines on the use of multi-dose activated charcoal in the treatment of acute poisoning. American Academy of Clinical Toxicology; European Association of Poisons Centres and Clinical Toxicologists. *J Toxicol Clin Toxicol* 37:731, 1999.
14. Palmer BF: Effectiveness of hemodialysis in the extracorporeal therapy of phenobarbital overdose. *Am J Kidney Dis* 36:640, 2000.

BENZODIAZEPINES
George M. Bosse

Benzodiazepines are pharmacologic agents commonly used for the treatment of anxiety, insomnia, seizures, and alcohol withdrawal. They also are used in conscious sedation as well as general anesthesia. Table 164-1 lists common generic benzodiazepines currently approved for use in the United States.

Benzodiazepines are frequently agents of accidental and intentional overdose. In the 2000 Annual Report of the American Association of Poison Control Centers Toxic Exposure Surveillance System, benzodiazepines accounted for 49,849 exposures, both as single agents and in combination with other drugs.[1] Although the ingestion of benzodiazepines alone appears to result in relatively few deaths, increased rates of morbidity and mortality do result from mixed overdose. Parenteral administration of benzodiazepines may also result in significant complications, particularly respiratory depression and hypotension.

PHARMACOLOGY

A specific benzodiazepine receptor has been identified in the central nervous system (CNS).[2] Specific peripheral receptor sites also have been identified, but the predominant clinical effects of benzodiazepines are mediated through the CNS receptors. Although the receptor has not been fully characterized, research supports the existence of a neuronal cell-surface protein complex containing a benzodiazepine receptor, a γ-aminobutyric acid (GABA) receptor, and a chloride channel. GABA is an inhibitory neurotransmitter. Effects of stimulation of GABA pathways include sedation, anxiolysis, and striated muscle relaxation. Stimulation of the benzodiazepine receptor appears to increase the sensitivity of the GABA-receptor complex to stimulation by GABA. The enhancement of GABA transmission by the administration of benzodiazepines is thought to occur either by increasing the affinity of the GABA receptor for its ligand or by improving coupling between the GABA receptor and its associated chloride channel. Increased GABA output leads to inhibitory effects throughout the neuroaxis and the resulting typical clinical effects of benzodiazepines. The presence of an endogenous ligand for the benzodiazepine receptor has been proposed, but such a ligand has not been identified conclusively.

In general, benzodiazepines are well absorbed from the gastrointestinal tract. The onset of action after oral ingestion is limited more by the rate of absorption from the gastrointestinal tract than by the relatively rapid passage from the bloodstream into the brain. With the exception of lorazepam and midazolam, intramuscular injection of benzodiazepines results in unpredictable absorption.

Benzodiazepines are all relatively lipid-soluble, with some variation among the agents. Increased lipid solubility is associated with more rapid diffusion across the blood-brain barrier. After single doses, the more highly lipophilic benzodiazepines have a shorter onset of action but also a shorter duration of activity. This short duration of activity occurs because of rapid egress of the drug from the brain and bloodstream into inactive tissue storage sites. For this reason, the half-life may not be a good indicator of the duration of action in an acute ingestion. For example, diazepam is a derivative with a long elimination half-life but a relatively short duration of action.

Benzodiazepine derivatives undergo metabolism by hepatic biotransformation through either oxidation or conjugation. Several derivatives are metabolized by both oxidative and conjugative processes. Oxidation often produces active metabolites that prolong the biologic half-life of the parent compounds. Oxidation is more susceptible to impairment by such factors as disease states (e.g., chronic liver disease), demographic characteristics (e.g., old age), and concurrent treatment with drugs that impair oxidizing capacity (e.g., cimetidine, estrogen, isoniazid, ethanol, and phenytoin). Conjugation is a rapid process that produces inactive metabolites. Examples of agents that undergo conjugation primarily include oxazepam, lorazepam, and temazepam. Administration of benzodiazepines that undergo conjugation may be safer in susceptible groups. Other approved agents in the United States undergo both oxidation and conjugation.

Selection of a benzodiazepine for use by a physician depends on the clinical properties of the particular derivative. Although individual drugs are marketed for specific conditions, there is considerable overlap of activity. For this reason, some hospital formulary committees have limited the number of available agents.

CLINICAL FEATURES

Isolated benzodiazepine overdose is notable for the relative lack of significant rates of morbidity and mortality.[3] Most reported cases of serious toxicity have occurred in the setting of coingestion of other agents or with parenteral administration. Death due solely to benzodiazepine overdose is rare in otherwise healthy individuals. However, deaths in seemingly isolated overdoses have been reported and appear to be more likely with short-acting derivatives, such as triazolam, alprazolam, and temazepam.

The clinical presentation of benzodiazepine intoxication is nonspecific. Clinical assessment also may be difficult because of the frequent coingestion of other agents. Except for additive effects, drug interactions of benzodiazepines with other sedative-hypnotics are unusual.

TABLE 164-1 Benzodiazepines Approved for Use in the United States

Generic Name	Brand Name	Half-Life, h*	Metabolite Characteristics†
Alprazolam	Xanax	6–26	Inactive
Clorazepate dipotassium	Tranxene	1.1–2.9	Active
Chlordiazepoxide	Librium	5–30	Active
Clonazepam	Klonopin	39	Inactive
Diazepam	Valium	20–70	Active
Estazolam	Prosom	10–24	Inactive
Flurazepam	Dalmane	2–3	Active
Lorazepam	Ativan	9–19	Inactive
Midazolam	Versed	2–5	Inactive
Oxazepam	Serax	5.4–9.8	Inactive
Quazepam	Doral	25–41	Active
Temazepam	Restoril	10–16	Inactive
Triazolam	Halcion	1.6–5.4	Inactive

*Elimination of half-life of parent compound.
†Some of the derivatives listed as having inactive metabolites actually are converted to active compounds. However, rapid metabolism results in no appreciable accumulation of active intermediates.

The nonspecific presentation of benzodiazepine toxicity is similar to that of other sedative-hypnotics. However, other agents can have at least a few distinguishing features. Chloral hydrate is known to precipitate cardiac dysrhythmias. Ethchlorvynol can produce prolonged coma and may be suspected by the presence of a vinyl-like odor. Glutethimide may give rise to fluctuating levels of CNS impairment and anticholinergic signs. Barbiturates are more likely than benzodiazepines to produce coma and depressant myocardial effects.

The predominant manifestations of benzodiazepines are neurologic. CNS effects include drowsiness, dizziness, slurred speech, confusion, ataxia, and general incoordination and impairment of intellectual function. Coma, particularly if prolonged, is atypical and should prompt suspicion of intoxication with other agents or a non-toxin-related medical condition. The elderly are more prone to manifest the CNS effects of benzodiazepines.

Paradoxical reactions, including excitement, anxiety, aggression, hostile behavior, rage, and delirium, have been reported but are quite uncommon. Although unclear, the etiology of such effects is probably not idiosyncratic. Benzodiazepines may have a disinhibiting effect, which, in the presence of various extrinsic factors, can lead to such actions as aggressive or hostile behavior. Other effects that have been reported and that have unclear etiologies include headache, nausea, vomiting, chest pain, joint pain, diarrhea, and incontinence.

Uncommonly, respiratory depression and hypotension may occur, generally with either parenteral administration or in the presence of coingestants. Intravenous administration is more likely to cause serious cardiorespiratory effects with rapid administration of large doses. In addition, the elderly and those with underlying cardiorespiratory disease are more susceptible to adverse effects of intravenous administration. The use of propylene glycol as a diluent in parenteral preparations of diazepam also has been implicated as a factor in cardiorespiratory arrest.

Extrapyramidal reactions have been associated with the use of benzodiazepines. Various allergic, hepatotoxic, and hematologic reactions also have been reported, but they are infrequent. In general, benzodiazepines have no long-term organ-system toxicity other than that which can be ascribed to indirect effects from CNS or cardiorespiratory depression.

Laboratory data in benzodiazepine ingestion are of limited value. Determination of serum benzodiazepine levels is not indicated routinely because they do not correlate well with the clinical state. Qualitative testing may be helpful, but the laboratory may not test routinely for all available derivatives. Familiarity with laboratory capabilities at a given institution is essential.

TREATMENT

Benzodiazepines often are ingested with other agents, and the history frequently is inaccurate. Therefore, in patients with depressed or altered mental status, administration of concentrated dextrose, thiamine, and naloxone (see Chap. 156) should be considered. Induction of emesis should be avoided in benzodiazepine overdose because CNS depression may ensue. Gastric lavage is safer and is recommended if the amount ingested is large or in coingestions with toxic agents. Activated charcoal binds benzodiazepines effectively and should be administered in most situations. Elimination enhancement by forced diuresis, hemodialysis, or hemoperfusion is not effective, and most patients do not manifest toxicity serious enough to warrant consideration of such measures. The patient should be monitored closely for CNS and respiratory depression.

Indications for observation or hospital admission include significant alterations in mental status, respiratory depression, and hypotension. If CNS depression persists or is profound, other agents or conditions must be considered. Unfortunately, there is insufficient literature to recommend a specific duration of appropriate emergency department observation.

Flumazenil is a unique selective antagonist of the central effects of benzodiazepines,[4] although there have been inconclusive claims that it may be effective in other drug overdose. Potential clinical applications include the management of benzodiazepine overdose and reversal of benzodiazepine-induced conscious sedation. Its use in benzodiazepine toxicity may obviate the need for tracheal intubation and respiratory support. As a diagnostic aid in obscure alterations of mental status, flumazenil may reduce the need for expensive and invasive procedures, such as computed tomography or lumbar puncture.

However, flumazenil has limited utility in the emergency department.[5] It is useful mainly in reversing the effects of benzodiazepines administered for diagnostic and therapeutic procedures. Even in such cases, management is usually accomplished safely and easily by allowing the effects of the benzodiazepine to subside without antidotal administration. The plasma elimination half-life of flumazenil is approximately 1 h. Its duration of action is variable and depends on the dose of flumazenil and the benzodiazepine administered. **Recurrent benzodiazepine toxicity may result once the effects of flumazenil have worn off.** This is less likely for an agent with a short duration of action, such as midazolam. The dose of flumazenil is 0.2 mg IV every minute to response or to a total of 3 mg.

Several considerations should limit the empirical administration of flumazenil to a poisoned patient (see Table 165–3). Generalized seizures have occurred in patients given flumazenil after coingestions of benzodiazepines and seizure-inducing agents, particularly cyclic antidepressants.[6,7] Seizure activity after flumazenil administration also has occurred in patients physically dependent on benzodiazepines and in patients receiving benzodiazepines for control of a seizure disorder. The putative explanation for this convulsive activity is either the reversal of the cerebroprotective and anticonvulsive effects of benzodiazepines or the precipitation of a benzodiazepine withdrawal syndrome. Another reason to avoid empirical administration of flumazenil in overdose patients is that the history is often unreliable or unavailable. **Flumazenil is also contraindicated in patients with a suspected elevation of intracranial pressure, such as in severe head injury.** This contraindication is due to its effects on cerebral hemodynamics. In all cases of benzodiazepine toxicity, supportive care is the cornerstone of treatment.

BENZODIAZEPINE ABUSE AND WITHDRAWAL

Genuine physiologic addiction to benzodiazepines may occur, particularly with prolonged use and high doses.[3,8] However, the abuse potential of benzodiazepines appears to be low in comparison with that of agents such as alcohol, cocaine, opiates, and barbiturates.[9,10] Benzodiazepine abuse usually occurs in individuals with a history of abuse of other psychoactive drugs. Primary drug abuse with benzodiazepines alone is not common.

Benzodiazepine withdrawal may occur on abrupt discontinuation and is more likely in patients with prolonged use and high doses. Because of the long biologic half-life of several derivatives, withdrawal manifestations may not occur for several days to over 1 week after the benzodiazepine has been discontinued. Unfortunately, it is often difficult to distinguish between withdrawal and underlying symptoms for which the drugs were prescribed initially.

Reported withdrawal manifestations include anxiety, irritability, insomnia, nausea, vomiting, tremor, sweating, and anorexia. Serious manifestations, including confusion, disorientation, psychosis, and seizures, also have been reported. For patients with an acute organic brain syndrome, a history of possible benzodiazepine withdrawal always should be pursued. Withdrawal reactions may be avoided by dose tapering. Treatment of withdrawal reactions may be accomplished by drug substitution or by reintroduction of a benzodiazepine and subsequent tapering.

REFERENCES

1. Litovitz TL, Klein-Schwartz W, White S, et al: 2000 Annual Report of the American Association of Poison Control Centers Toxic Exposure Surveillance System. *Am J Emerg Med* 19:337, 2001.
2. Mohler H, Okada T: Benzodiazepine receptor: Demonstration in the central nervous system. *Science* 198:849, 1977.
3. Guadreault P, Guay J, Thivierge RL, Verdy I: Benzodiazepine poisoning: Clinical and pharmacologic considerations and treatment. *Drug Safety* 6:247, 1991.
4. Votey SR, Bosse GM, Bayer MJ, Hoffman JR: Flumazenil: A new benzodiazepine antagonist. *Ann Emerg Med* 20:181, 1991.
5. Goldfrank LR: Flumazenil: A pharmacologic antidote with limited medical toxicology utility, or an antidote in search of an overdose. *Acad Emerg Med* 4:935, 1997
6. Spivey WH, Roberts JR, Derlet RW: A clinical trial of escalating doses of flumazenil for reversal of suspected benzodiazepine overdose in the emergency department. *Ann Emerg Med* 22:1813, 1993.
7. Spivey WH: Flumazenil and seizures: An analysis of 43 cases. *Clin Ther* 14:292, 1992.
8. Marriott S, Tyrer P: Benzodiazepine dependence: Avoidance and withdrawal. *Drug Safety* 9:93, 1993.
9. Warneke LB: Benzodiazepines: Abuse and new use. *Can J Psychiatry* 36:194, 1991.
10. Woods JH, Katz JL, Winger G: Use and abuse of benzodiazepines: Issues relevant to prescribing. *JAMA* 260:3476, 1988.

NONBENZODIAZEPINE HYPNOSEDATIVES
Raquel M. Schears

The term *nonbenzodiazepine hypnosedative* is currently used to refer to a diverse group of agents that share the ability to promote sleep and allay anxiety, categorically exclusive of the benzodiazepines. Several of these chemical entities, such as etchlorvynol, meprobamate, glutethimide, and methaqualone, are rarely subscribed for clinical use, yet ingestions continue to be reported.[1] Newer agents such as buspirone, zaleplon, and zolpidem are commonly prescribed, making toxicity and overdose characteristics important to recognize (Tables 165-1 and 165-2). EM physicians encounter the effects of these agents in patients presenting with symptoms of intentional overdose, recreational misuse, alleged assault, withdrawal syndromes, or during major trauma evaluations when detected on drug screen.

In the U.S., some chemical compounds exist that possess secondary hypnosedative properties, but were primarily labeled as nonfood,

TABLE 165-1 Reported Toxic Exposures and Associated Fatalities of Nonbenzodiazepine Hypnosedatives in 2001

Substance	No. of Exposures	Deaths
Buspirone	2726	3
Chloral hydrate	238	4
Etchlorvynol	22	0
Glutethimide	3	0
Meprobamate	167	3
Carisoprodol	6991	20
Methaqualone	24	0
γHB and γHB-related drugs (γHB/γBL/BD)	1916	6

Source: From Litovitz et al.[1]

nondrug products. This initial designation allowed these agents to be marketed as untested dietary supplements or industrial solvents, without a legitimate clinical purpose. Lacking prior proof of safety and efficacy, the human hazards posed by such entities tend to be revealed and responded to gradually as morbidity patterns and evidence of lethality mounts. Relevant in this context are γ-hydroxybutyrate (γHB), and its precursors γ-hydroxybutrolactone (γBL) and 1,4-butanediol (BD), which convert to γHB in vivo. These drugs are creating novel public health issues and dangerous toxicity in acute ingestion and abrupt withdrawal. Despite increasing FDA regulations since 1990, whereby γHB manufacture and sales were banned, up until recently (March, 2000) when γHB was designated a Federal Schedule I Controlled Substance enforced by the DEA, these compounds continue to be easily accessible and widely abused.[2] Statistics on raves, circuit parties, and bodybuilder club cultures indicate these drugs are increasingly prevalent in intentional misuse and overdose.[3,4] γHB and its congeners are further indicted as agents used in drug-facilitated sexual assault (γSA), episodes of polydrug abuse among consenting gay and bisexual men prompting high-risk sexual behavior, and have been linked to driving impairment as single-agent exposures in forensic reports.[4-6] Curtailing illicit and licit use of γHB and related compounds is proving more difficult than previously anticipated. These observations create an imperative for EM physicians to be well versed in the presentation and management of γHB-related emergencies.

Agents in this chapter share certain pharmacologic and clinical similarities. These drugs tend to be highly lipophilic and concentrate in the central nervous system (CNS), causing variable degrees of CNS depression with gradual redistribution and eventual hepatic degradation. Clinically, mild intoxication manifests as sedation and incoordination, which progresses to lethargy, worsening ataxia, and deepening coma in overdose. It is recognized that reaching a treatment center predicts a favorable outcome in all types of overdose, including those seen with the nonbenzodiazepine hypnosedatives. In fact, declining mortality associated with these agents over broad dose ranges is attributed mostly to improvements in standard supportive care. Therefore general treatment guidelines take precedence in management of all these agents in overdose (see Chap. 156). Departures from general clinical presentation or management in overdose unique to a specific agent are covered in the discussion specific to the agent below.

γ-HYDROXYBUTYRATE (γHB) AND γHB-RELATED COMPOUNDS: γ-HYDROXYBUTROLACTONE (γBL) AND 1,4- BUTANEDIOL (BD)

γHB is an endogenous metabolite of γ-aminobutyric acid (γABA), the major inhibitory neurotransmitter in the CNS. γHB functions as a putative neurotransmitter or neuromodulator itself, capable of inducing profound CNS depression. It produces a biphasic dopamine response and triggers the release of endogenous opiate-like substances. γHB centrally mediates sleep cycles, emotional control, and retention of memory. It also functions in glucose metabolism, temperature regulation, and blood flow. Ingestion of γHB results in rapid gastrointestinal (GI) absorption, with peak plasma concentrations and coincident clinical effects occurring within 30 to 60 min. γHB quickly crosses the blood-brain barrier, concentrating in the CNS, kidney, heart, and muscle tissue. The average drug half-life is 30 min. γHB is metabolized in the liver and then almost completely oxidized to carbon dioxide and water by the lungs and expired. Less than 2 percent of γHB is eliminated unchanged in the urine, and this occurs so rapidly that after 12 h it is undetectable. Exposed adults can experience comatose states typically lasting 1 to 2 h, with spontaneous recovery of consciousness usually within 4 hours.

γHB was developed as an anesthetic more than 40 years ago. It had escaped clinical use in the United States until late 2002, when Orphan

TABLE 165-2   Selected Properties and Characteristic Overdose Features of Nonbenzodiazepine Hypnosedative Drugs

Drug Class	Azapirones	Alcohols	Carbinols	Piperidinediones	Carbamated Propandiol
Generic name	Buspirone	Chloral hydrate*	Ethchlorvynol*	Glutethimide*	Meprobamate* (‡carisoprodol)
Trade name	Buspar	Noctec	Placidyl	Doriden	Miltown, Equanil (Soma, Rela)
Street name	ND	(+Ethanol: knockout drops, Mickey Finn)	Pickles, jelly beans, Mr. Green Jeans	(+Codeine: sets, hits, packs, loads, threes and eights, four doors)	(Soma ± Tylenol with codeine Soma Do, Soma Coma)
Detoxification	Hepatic, fecal 30%	Hepatic, renal 10%	Hepatic, renal 10%	Hepatic	Hepatic, renal 10%
Plasma protein binding (%)	95	35–40	50–60	47–59	20
V_d (L/kg)	433	0.6–1.6	3–4	2.7	0.75
Hypnotic dose (mg)§	15–30	500–1000	500–1000	250–500	400
Plasma half-life (h)**	2–3 (M)	8 (M)	10–20	12 (M)	6–16
Fatal dose (g)	ND	5–10	10	10–20	12
Lethal bleed level (mg/dL)	ND	25	15	3–10	20
Overdose clues	Drowsiness Dysphoria Miosis	Breath odor: pear Ventricular dysrhythmias GI bleeding	Breath odor: vinyl Prolonged coma Hypothermia ARDS	Anticholinergic symptoms Fluctuating, prolonged coma	Gastric concretions Severe hypotension Fluctuating, prolonged coma
Extracorporeal methods	ND	HP > HD	HP > HD	HP	HP > HD

(continued)

*Agent causes significant life-threatening abstinence syndrome requiring hospital admission.
†Legal synthesis in USA terminated 1984.
‡Prodrug metabolizes to DEA controlled schedule drug in the respective drug class category.
#Due to the fluctuating legal status of GHB, Orphan Medical (1-888-8ORPHAN) maintains the current legislative status of GHB by state.
§All agents have both sedative and hypnotic properties; maximum adult hypnotic dose listed can be given in divided doses to that total dose/day for sedative purposes.

Medical began marketing it as Xyrem (sodium oxybate), a schedule III controlled substance. Currently it is the only FDA-approved form of γHB available for the treatment of cataplexy associated with narcolepsy. All use of the medication is tracked through an industry-sponsored registry (see Table 165-2). It is hoped that by monitoring physician prescription practices and patient consumption, tight control over American distribution will be ensured. In Europe, γHB has long been used to manage alcohol and narcotic withdrawal and treat narcolepsy.

Unregulated sales of γHB in the United States began in the 1980s when it was first sold to bodybuilders as a health food product allegedly capable of "fat-burning" metabolic powers during sleep. In the 1990s it was marketed to ravers as "liquid ecstasy" for its purported euphoric effects when used during all-night dance parties. Drug-facilitated sexual assault also surfaced in connection with γHB, fluni-trazepam, and most recently γHB congeners, during the last 5 years. Very small quantities of these drugs are required to cause rapid onset of disinhibition, passivity, loss of will to resist, relaxation of muscles, and lasting antegrade amnesia. γHB is an odorless, colorless, and nearly tasteless liquid, powder, or capsule.[7] Concerns regarding such illicit use, compounded by the growing popularity of γHB, prompted passage of a 1996 federal law, the Drug-Induced Rape Prevention and Punishment Act, which sets prison terms of up to 20 years for anyone convicted of using any controlled substance with the intent to commit a violent crime, including sexual assault. Also within the last few years, γHB-related agents have become increasingly recognized as prevalent drugs of abuse for their aphrodisiac effects, and a corre-

sponding public health problem has developed among consenting gay and bisexual men who frequent "circuit parties." These are ticketed multiday gatherings with an estimated annual attendance in the United States in the hundreds of thousands. In a recent survey of circuit party participants (N = 295), nearly all respondents reported use of drugs during the party weekends, including ecstasy (75 percent), ketamine (58 percent), crystal methamphetamine (36 percent), γHB or γBL (25 percent), and Viagra (12 percent). Two-thirds of the men reported having sex (oral or anal), 49 percent reported having anal sex, and 28 percent reported having unprotected anal sex during the 3-day period. An association was found between the use of drugs and risky sexual behavior.[4]

γHB can be ordered from other countries via the Internet, is relatively inexpensive and easy to synthesize from its related compounds. A common method of synthesizing illicit γHB is to react liquid γBL with an equal volume of water in the presence of a base to open its ring structure. On a volume basis, the potency of γBL is twice that of γHB prepared by this method. Consumers of these agents may not recognize these potency differences, leading to dosing errors and serious side effects. Also, the direct sale of "natural" dietary supplements containing the newer-generation γHB precursors, γBL and BD, are the subject of several FDA health risk warnings, partial manufacturer recalls, and extensive Internet marketing strategies which assure consumer anonymity, flexible supply, and continued demand. γBL is sold in herbal products (unregulated) and is a component of acetone-free nail polish removers and cyanoacrylate glue. It has greater bioavailability and faster onset of action (20 min) than γHB on an equimolar

TABLE 165-2   Selected Properties and Characteristic Overdose Features of Nonbenzodiazepine Hypnosedative Drugs *(Continued)*

Quinazolines	Pyrazolopyrimidin	Imidazopyridines	Neurotransmitter
Methaqualone*	Zaleplon	Zolpidem	Gamma hydroxybutyrate* (GHB)# GHB-related compounds: ‡Gamma-hydroxybutyrolactone ‡1,4 Butanediol
Qualude, Parest, Mequin, Sopor†	Sonata	Ambien, Stilnox, Niotal, Bikalm	Xyrem
Quads, ludes, soapers, mandies, love-drug, wall banger	ND	ND	Grievous Bodily Harm, Georgia Home Boy, Liquid Ecstasy, Liquid X, or E, GHB, GBH, Soap, Scoop, Easy Lay, Salty Water, Cherry Menth, Organic Qualude, Xen "Party Drug"
Hepatic	Hepatic	Hepatic	Hepatic
80–90	60%	92	ND
5.8–6.0	1.4	.54	.4–.58
150–300	10	20	3000
19	1	2–5	0.3
8	ND	ND	ND
10–15	ND	ND	14–290
Hyperacusis Hypertonicity, seizures Bleeding diathesis	Drowsiness Headache	Somnolence Vomiting	GCS score: 4–6 (median) Athletic physique, seizure-like activity, apnea Sudden unexplained, reversible coma Extreme combativeness with stimulation
HP	ND	ND	ND

**Half-life given at therapeutic dose; generally half-life in overdose is considerably longer. M = active metabolites. Fatal dose is an estimate complicated by history of tolerance, coingestion, and patient reliability. Extracorporeal methods: HP = hemoperfusion, HD = hemodialysis, > denotes preferred method; ND = no data; V_d = volume of distribution; ARDS = acute respiratory distress syndrome.
Source: Adapted from Lee D: Sedative-hypnotic agents, in Goldfrank LR, Howland MA (eds): *Goldfrank's Toxicologic Emergencies,* 7th ed. New York, NY: McGraw-Hill, 2001, p. 932, with permission.

basis. Usually these substances are considered alternatives to "ecstasy" or methamphetamine and are often coingested with alcohol, which in the case of BD potentiates toxicity. BD competes with ethanol, the preferred substrate of alcohol dehydrogenase (ADH) in vivo. This competitive inhibition of ADH delays onset of BD metabolism and may consequently mask symptoms for up to 8 h in patients with concurrent exposure. Historical clues to γHB intoxication are very similar from case to case and commonly involve this scenario: patient reports going out drinking, and either develops a sudden sense of extreme drunkenness after just one or two drinks, or experiences an abrupt onset of uncharacteristic aggressive behavior, followed by sudden drowsiness, dizziness, euphoria, or coma with rapid reawakening and amnesia.[2,3]

Clinical Features of Toxicity

The toxic effects of γHB and γHB-related compounds target the CNS, cardiovascular system, and respiratory system, but spare hepatorenal function. Symptoms include labile level of consciousness (agitation, combativeness, somnolence, coma, sudden reawakening emergence), variable neuromuscular movement (hypotonia, tremor, myoclonus, seizure-like activity), vomiting, hypothermia, bradycardia, respiratory depression, apnea, and death. Solid evidence that γHB and γHB-related compounds alone cause lethal outcome in overdose exists. Since 1992, the DEA has documented 9600 adverse γHB reactions or overdoses in 46 states, and identified 71 γHB-related fatalities, the majority of which occurred after 1996. In 15 of these deaths, a γHB-related compound was the sole drug isolated in forensic analysis.[2,7] Over the last 10 years, ED encounters for γHB-related poisonings are up 100-fold, and at least 30 cases of γHB DFSA have been clearly documented (data from NIDA and NIH National Symposium, Bethesda, MD, 6/27/2000). The burden of additional toxicity risk contributed by websites claiming the hazards of these drugs are exaggerated is not known. However, casual attitudes of friends attending γHB overdose victims have been linked to fatal delays in obtaining emergency medical treatment.[2,3]

Clinical effects are dose-related. Low doses produce euphoria, nystagmus, ataxia, and dizziness; moderate doses produce sedation; and high doses produce coma, respiratory depression, apnea, and rarely, death. Under controlled conditions, 10 mg/kg results in amnesia, hypotonia, and ataxia; 30 mg/kg induces euphoria, drowsiness, and dizziness. Doses of 50 mg/kg produce unconsciousness. Doses above 50 mg/kg cause bradycardia, respiratory depression, and seizure-like activity. Since most γHB is "home brewed," dose purity and strength are uncertain, and anywhere between one-half teaspoon and 4 tablespoons have been reported to elicit adverse effects. Mixed in alcoholic beverages, the two sedatives are synergistic. Likely clinical features in the ED include: Glasgow coma scale (GCS) scores as low as 3 to 5, may be followed by emergence delirium and vomiting, which appears inversely related to initial GCS score; i.e., 85 percent of the vomiting reported in exposure case series had GCS scores of 8 or less.[8] Mild bradycardia, moderate bradypnea with Cheyne-Stokes respirations, and seizure-like activity have also been noted. Urinary and fecal incontinence are commonly seen with γBL and BD overdose. Episodes of marked agitation on stimulation (intubation, sternal rub) are the hallmark of γHB intoxication, along with findings of only mild respiratory acidosis despite periods of prolonged apnea and hypoxia.

Treatment

No standard treatment protocol or antidote exist for γHB intoxication. However, several supportive measures are recommended, which begin with the ABCs of resuscitation. Aspiration precautions are advised because of the potential for sudden changes in mental status. Furthermore, airway protection via rapid sequence intubation (RSI) followed by assisted ventilation may be the best strategy in managing both the profound CNS and respiratory depression seen in serious γHB intoxication. (Because γHB functions as an anesthetic induction agent, RSI can proceed with paralytic agents alone.) Secondly, improper manufacture of γHB using recipes obtained via the Internet often results in mixtures of γBL and sodium hydroxide or lye, which can lead to caustic alkaline burns of the esophagus and lungs with aspiration.

Neither naloxone nor flumazenil has been effective in reversing unconsciousness induced by γHB, and the use of physostigmine to reverse coma may be dangerous and lacks supportive evidence. In other overdose settings in which bradycardia complicates presentation, physostigmine administration has caused asystole and cardiac arrest. The bradycardia seen in γHB intoxication is attributed to central vagal activity, and responds to atropine if simple stimulation fails to suffice. Routine cardiovascular monitoring, establishment of intravenous access, and laboratory testing for electrolyte balance, blood glucose level, and arterial blood gas measurement are considered good management. Drug screening is costly and of little value in most patients presenting with γHB overdose. γHB is only detectable in the urine for 6 to 12 h after ingestion, resulting in many false-negative results.

Both charcoal and lavage are of limited value for single γHB ingestion due to the small amount of drug ingested and its rapid absorption.[9] Patients with symptoms of mild intoxication who improve rapidly (after 6 h or less of observation) and clear completely can be discharged from the ED. All others should be admitted for observation. Serious GHB and GHB precursor intoxication, complicated by coingestion of alcohol or other CNS depressants, often will require emergent airway stabilization and cardiovascular support. Because of the altered hepatic metabolism seen **in patients taking BD concurrently with alcohol, it is recommended that these patients be observed until their blood alcohol concentrations are not detectable.** The role of gastric decontamination for coingestants also lacks proven efficacy if more than 1 h has elapsed since ingestion, or if less than life-threatening amounts were taken.[10] Extracorporeal elimination methods have not been evaluated in GHB overdose.

Drug Facilitated Sexual Assault

When a patient presents to the ED seeking treatment for alleged drug-facilitated sexual assault, the best recommendation is compassionate advocacy and a complete evaluation. Currently, this is accomplished through supporting the psychological state of the victim and collecting evidence of the alleged crime. Many ED jurisdictions in the U.S. utilize sexual assault nurse examiners (SANE), specifically trained in this sensitive role. The presence of a clinical symptom pattern consistent with drug-facilitated sexual assault and a history of drug ingestion within 72 h are indications for toxicologic screenings. Both blood and urine specimens should be obtained. (Minimum collection: single gray topped tube for blood, refrigerate; 100 mL of urine.) Specimens should be submitted for testing according to strict chain-of-custody procedures, which will be critical if the case is prosecuted. Drug screening requires patient consent, and SANE must inform the patient what drugs will be included in the screen. Any documentable use of recreational or prescription drug use by the victim should be recorded in the medical record prior to the findings of positive results of the drug screen if negative impact on the victim's credibility is to be minimized. A complete toxicologic screen can cost upwards of $800. Currently, the strategy of many SANE programs has been to turn over the biological specimens collected with the rape kit to the appropriate law enforcement authorities. Thus the screening costs are passed on to the investigating agency. If a report is not generated regarding the incident, but the victim wants a toxicologic screen, the victim should be informed of the cost and financial burden.[11]

A previously free nationwide urine testing program developed to assess the incidence of drug use in sexual assault cases recently reported the findings on ethanol, γHB, flunitrazepam, and nine other drug classes (amphetamines, barbiturates, benzodiazepines, cannabinoids, cocaine, methaqualone, opiates, phencyclidine, and propoxyphene). Of the 1179 samples, 468 were negative for all substances tested. There were no samples identified as positive for phencyclidine or methaqualone. Of the remainder (711 samples) 35 percent of the drug-positive samples contained multiple drugs. The drug found in the majority of the positive specimens was ethanol, followed by cannabinoids, cocaine, benzodiazepines, amphetamines, and γHB. Although many drugs appear to be associated with the crime of sexual assault, the prevalence of γHB and related compounds is of special concern because of the lack of routine screening tests available to detect these drugs.[5]

Detection of γHB and γHB-related drugs requires targeted analysis such as gas chromatography-mass spectrometry. Currently, forensic laboratory screening of biological specimens for γHB can be facilitated through contacting the National Medical Services Laboratory in Willow Grove, PA at 1-800-522-6671 or go to www.nmslab.com, for further information.

Withdrawal

Sharply contrasting with overdose, there are numerous recent small case series documenting the existence of tolerance and dependence liability with chronic γHB use.[12] γHB dependence is characterized by multiple daily doses taken around the clock (every 1 to 3 h) for months to years, often with a history of multiple unsuccessful attempts to self-taper. Furthermore, high-frequency users appear to be at the greatest risk for developing manifestations of severe delirium and psychosis as part of an acute life-threatening withdrawal syndrome that occurs rarely with abrupt discontinuation of γHB use. The spectrum of acute withdrawal is similar to that seen with other hypnosedatives, including benzodiazepines, barbiturates, and alcohol, suggesting a common mechanism. Usually patients report only 6 to 8 h of abstinence before the onset of craving and symptoms that consistently include a triad of anxiety, tremor, and insomnia. Several other historical associations have been documented, including the presence of emotional lability, prior diagnosis of nonpsychotic psychiatric disorders, and/or substance abuse in the majority of patients suffering from γHB withdrawal symptoms. Presentation to the ED is often delayed until more severe symptoms of agitation and vivid hallucinations are experienced. The observed withdrawal syndrome can last 5 to 15 days. Severe withdrawal is characterized by mild autonomic instability, and progressive psychosis and delirium, which develop within 2 days of last use. Patients require ICU monitoring for the degree of physical and chemical restraint needed to maintain sedation, control CNS symptoms, and prevent injury. Patients often suffer complications of pulmonary edema, hyperthermia, and rhabdomyolysis, and are at high risk for γHB relapse on hospital discharge. The critical need for psychiatric assessment and treatment for chemical dependence is best anticipated from the ED and incorporated into the treatment of acute withdrawal.[12]

The treatment of γHB withdrawal is also evolving. Although there are no prospective studies, it seems that the similarity of γHB withdrawal to that of benzodiazepines, ethanol, and other hypnosedatives, place a GABA agonist as first-line treatment in the ED. Huge intravenous doses of benzodiazepines (diazepam 100 mg/24 h; 2.5 g/4 d) initiated early for sedation purposes and to decrease severity and duration of symptoms has been described. Barbiturates (pentobarbital 1 to 2 mg/kg IV every 30 to 60 min with slow taper over 5 to 6 d) are considered alternatives for cases refractory to benzodiazepines. Chloral hydrate, 1 gm PO is another option. Other agents, such as IV propofol or fentanyl, can be given in an ICU setting under the direction of a toxicologist.

Low-dose antipsychotics (haloperidol and risperidone) have also been used successfully. However, administering antipsychotics may adversely affect thermoregulation, precipitate acute dystonic reactions, and lower the seizure threshold. For these reasons, the current best strategy is to avoid these agents in the management of acute γHB withdrawal.

BUSPIRONE

Buspirone, introduced in 1984, is a prototype anxiolytic drug from the azapirone family. The agent is not chemically or pharmacologically related to the other hypnosedatives, although its efficacy profile is comparable with that of the benzodiazepines. Clinical indications for buspirone use are not fully delineated; however, it appears most useful in the treatment of conditions such as chronic anxiety, especially in the elderly, and mixed anxiety-depression states. It does not affect γABA or benzodiazepine receptors, and therefore produces less sedation, euphoria, psychomotor impairment, and ethanol potentiation. It does affect CNS serotonergic, dopaminergic, and noradrenergic neurotransmission, but the mechanisms are not fully understood. Buspirone appears to have several merits when compared to the hypnosedatives, including a virtual absence of abuse potential, a wide margin of therapeutic safety, and no documented delayed toxicity or withdrawal reactions with abrupt discontinuation of chronic use.[13]

Buspirone is rapidly absorbed, highly protein-bound, and widely distributed to the tissues. Metabolism occurs in the liver, with at least one active metabolite generated. Fecal elimination accounts for 20 to 40 percent of drug clearance. Experience in overdose may be limited by the drug's wide margin of safety. Patients have taken up to 3 g (which is 150 times the average anxiolytic dose) in overdose without lasting ill effects. Most common clinical symptoms in overdose are nonspecific drowsiness and dysphoria. Rarely, hypotension, bradycardia, seizures, GI upset, dystonia, and priapism have also been described. Spontaneous acute hypertensive reactions have developed in patients taking buspirone and monoamine oxidase inhibitors concurrently. No other adverse drug interactions or unexpected toxicities have emerged with buspirone use.[13] Treatment in overdose is supportive. Serum levels are not useful clinically, and extracorporeal methods of elimination enhancement have not been evaluated.

CHLORAL HYDRATE

Introduced in 1869, chloral hydrate (a schedule III drug with recognized abuse potential) is the oldest hypnosedative agent, and was used as a popular sedative in clinical medicine until the advent of barbiturates largely supplanted its use in the early 1900s. Chloral hydrate is still used effectively for promoting sedation in children because in therapeutic doses it does not depress respiratory drive or circulatory function. Drawbacks include its narrow margin of safety, minimal analgesic activity, and propensity to develop tolerance and physical dependence. Withdrawal symptoms mimic those of alcohol abstinence. Toxic doses produce severe CNS and respiratory and cardiovascular depression. Ethanol potentiates the sedative effects of chloral hydrate when taken in combination. This observation led to the street use of the two substances for malicious intent, as in slipping someone a "Micky Finn" or "knockout drops."

Chloral hydrate absorption occurs rapidly and completely from the GI tract. It is a well-known mucous membrane irritant, especially when taken in quantity or undiluted. It functions as a CNS depressant via an unknown mechanism of action. Toxic doses also depress myocardial contractility, shorten the refractory period, and sensitize the myocardium to catecholamines. These factors create the substrate for resistant ventricular dysrhythmias that are the leading cause of mortality in overdose.[14] Chloral hydrate is lipid-soluble and easily transits all cell membranes. Volume of distribution and protein-binding properties are moderate. Metabolism occurs in the liver via alcohol dehydrogenase and results in the generation of a longer-acting active metabolite, trichloroethanol ($t_{1/2}$ = 4 to 12 h), thought responsible for most of the drug's sedative action and toxic effects in overdose. Neither the parent drug nor the metabolite induces hepatic enzyme activity.

Clinical clues to the ingestion of chloral hydrate are a pearlike breath odor, hypotension, cardiac dysrhythmias, and GI bleeding. Because chloral hydrate is radiopaque and can cause intestinal perforation, abdominal x-rays may help narrow the differential diagnosis and guide decontamination. Electrocardiogram (ECG) often shows a shortened QT interval indicative of the decreased refractory period seen in chloral hydrate overdose. Persistent ventricular dysrhythmias commonly signal terminal events, because they are resistant to standard antidysrhythmic therapy. Propranolol, a β-adrenergic antagonist, is considered the drug of choice in treating dysrhythmias associated with chloral hydrate overdose. Consider overdrive pacing in the management of persistent fatal dysrhythmias. Avoid β-adrenergic drugs such as epinephrine, isoproterenol, and dopamine, which are capable of potentiating dysrhythmias in the catecholamine-sensitized myocardium. If hypotension does not respond to volume loading, an α-acting pressor such as norepinephrine is first-line therapy. Serum levels are rarely helpful in guiding clinical management. Barring evidence of intestinal perforation, gastric lavage and activated charcoal can be administered for ingestions presenting to the ED within an hour, once the airway has been controlled. Hemodialysis and hemoperfusion have been shown to be beneficial in severe overdose.

ETHCHLORVYNOL

Ethchlorvynol, a schedule IV drug, was marketed initially in 1955 as an alternative to barbiturates, possessing a more rapid onset and shorter duration of action. However, the drug's high abuse potential, coupled with its tendency toward tolerance, physical dependence, and life-threatening withdrawal, overshadowed any claim of superior efficacy. The drug is available as a liquid-filled capsule, allowing both intravenous and oral abuse.

Ethchlorvynol is absorbed rapidly from the GI tract. It is highly lipophilic, concentrates in the CNS, and possesses a large volume of distribution. Its biphasic distribution is characterized by an initial period of adipose tissue deposition after ingestion (3 to 5 h), with sedative effects that disappear only to resurface later (7 to 10 h), when the drug redistributes from fat stores. Ethchlorvynol is moderately protein-bound and metabolized in the liver, but does not induce microsomal enzymes. It also crosses the placenta and causes neonatal withdrawal symptoms. Mechanisms of CNS sedative action and hepatic degradation are unknown. Ethanol potentiates its CNS depressant effects.

Distinguishing clinical clues in oral and intravenous overdose are a vinyl-like breath odor (although the patient may report a mintlike taste in the mouth), dyspnea, and dry cough. CNS effects include nystagmus, lethargy, and extremely prolonged coma. Isoelectric electroencephalographic (EEG) tracings have been reported, but do not preclude full recovery. Hemodynamic instability progresses from an initial bradycardia to severe hypotension and hypothermia. Noncardiogenic pulmonary edema can be seen in massive ingestions, although it is more characteristic of intravenous overdose. Polydrug exposures that potentiate CNS depression can result in acute respiratory arrest and cardiovascular collapse. Successful treatment of ethchlorvynol overdose centers on the usual attention to supportive care and general decontamination. Serum levels of ethchlorvynol are not helpful in guiding management except to confirm diagnosis or trigger use of an extracorporeal elimination method in refractory cases. Charcoal hemoperfusion is superior to hemodialysis because of the drug's degree of protein binding and redistribution characteristics. Forced diuresis is not recommended because the risks of inducing pulmonary edema outweigh the minimal benefit gained from strategic enhancement of renal elimination.

GLUTETHIMIDE

Glutethimide was introduced in 1954 as a safe, nonaddicting hypnosedative drug substitute for barbiturates. However, its clinical usefulness was quickly eclipsed by recognition of its potential adverse effects, which closely resembled those of barbiturates. Similarities include its ability to induce prolonged coma, addiction, tolerance, and severe withdrawal. In large overdose, several complications (e.g., cerebral and pulmonary edema, hypotension, seizures, and sudden apnea) make treatment of this schedule II substance more difficult. Illicit abuse involves the street belief that taking combinations of codeine and glutethimide produce a similar but longer-acting euphoria than can be obtained with intravenous heroin use. Side effects with chronic use include "hangover," headaches, blurred vision, rash, bone marrow suppression, hypocalcemia, and osteomalacia.

Poor water solubility causes glutethimide to be slowly and erratically absorbed from the GI tract. However, coingestion of alcohol markedly enhances drug dissolution and absorption. The drug is lipophilic and initially concentrates in the CNS and adipose tissue, with eventual redistribution. Drug half-lives up to 40 h have been observed in overdose. Glutethimide has a large volume of distribution, is moderately protein-bound, and is capable of inducing hepatic microsomal enzymes. Hepatic degradation results in several active metabolites that may play a role in the prolonged fluctuating coma seen in overdose.[15] Glutethemide crosses the placenta, and fetal blood concentrations equal those of the mother. Minimal amounts of unchanged drug are excreted in breast milk.

Clinical manifestations of glutethimide overdose mirror those seen with barbiturate toxicity with two exceptions. Anticholinergic symptoms are prominent, and the unique fluctuating nature of the prolonged coma complicates management. Mydriasis, dry mucous membranes, tenacious secretions, tachycardia, hypertension, ileus, urinary retention, hyperpyrexia, delirium, seizures, and agitation may be observed.

Serum levels of one of the active metabolites, 4-HG, may correlate better with toxicity than do levels of the parent compound. As with ethchlorvynol, complete clinical recovery is possible despite an isoelectric EEG if the patient has been spared the insults of cerebral hypoxia and/or ischemia. Coingestion of other CNS depressants, prolonged coma, and age over 60 years, predict negative outcomes in glutethimide overdose.[15]

Late gastric lavage (12 h after ingestion) has been shown to be beneficial in obtunded patients because of the drug's anticholinergic effect of delaying gastric emptying. In asymptomatic patients presenting 4 h or more after ingestion, the poor water solubility of glutethimide limits the effectiveness of lavage. Activated charcoal is recommended in all patients, but the utility of multiple-dose activated charcoal (MDAC) remains unproven. The use of physostigmine to reverse anticholinergic CNS toxicity is not recommended. Forced diuresis is not effective and can precipitate the development of pulmonary edema. Improvement in clinical outcomes for the elderly and those patients with severe intoxications (serum glutethimide levels >40 mg/L) has been documented using extracorporeal techniques to increase drug clearance. Hemoperfusion is the preferred method, but efficacy remains controversial, limiting its application to overdose patients not responding to supportive measures alone. Given the potential for delayed, erratic absorption and characteristic fluctuating mental status,

admission and prolonged observation of patients with significant exposures is indicated.

MEPROBAMATE

Meprobamate has been in clinical use since 1955 as an anxiolytic hypnosedative; this remains its only approved use in the U.S. Meprobamate is classified as a schedule IV drug because of known potential for inducing tolerance and dependence. Several combination products remain available even though the abuse potential of meprobamate probably surpasses that of the benzodiazepines, which are the currently favored, considerably safer, prescription alternative for anxiolysis. Thus toxic exposures continue to be reported, with intentional overdose commonly implicated as the rationale. More significantly, carisoprodol (Soma), a widely prescribed, noncontrolled skeletal muscle relaxant whose active metabolite is meprobamate, is clearly emerging as a street drug of abuse. Often carisoprodol is combined with acetaminophen and codeine. The combination is known as "Soma-Do" and "Soma-Coma." According to the 2001 Annual Report of the American Association of Poison Control Centers, exposures and fatalities attributable to carisoprodol vastly outnumbered those reported for meprobamate (see Table 165-1). It has also recently been shown that physicians groups commonly prescribing carisoprodol are not sufficiently aware of either its abuse potential or that it is metabolized to a controlled substance.[16]

Absorption of meprobamate occurs in the small intestine. The compound is poorly water soluble, stable in acidic environments, and able to decrease gastric motility. These characteristics lend themselves to the development of gastric concretions. Meprobamate has a large volume of distribution, is poorly protein bound, and is metabolized primarily in the liver, where it can induce microsomal enzymes. Approximately 10 percent of the drug is excreted unchanged in the urine. Meprobamate crosses the placenta, and fetal blood levels approximate those of the mother. It is also excreted in breast milk. Meprobamate depresses the CNS by reducing sensory transmission, particularly in the thalamus. In overdose, meprobamate also concentrates in myocardial tissue, causing direct cardiotoxicity, manifesting as depressed contractility and hypotension, often in the absence of respiratory depression.

Clinical features of meprobamate toxicity are similar to those of the other hypnosedatives. CNS symptoms range in mild exposures from nystagmus and dysarthria to ataxia, confusion, and deep coma in overdose. In contrast to barbiturates, hypotension may be an early sign of toxicity occurring in lesser stages of coma. Prolonged and fluctuating coma is due to continued drug absorption from concretions. Hypotension is the hallmark of serious meprobamate overdose. Also, seizures, cardiac dysrhythmias, and pulmonary edema have been reported rarely. Abstinence syndromes reflecting the degree of physical dependence and tolerance develop quickly, usually within 1 to 2 days of drug discontinuation, and can be severe.

Utility of serum levels of meprobamate is limited but confirmative of ingestion. It may guide the need for extracorporeal removal. The treatment approach after stabilization of the airway and circulation centers on gastric decontamination given meprobamate's propensity to form concretions. Single- and multiple-dose activated charcoal MDAC appear to be safe and effective in increasing the clearance of meprobamate, although solid clinical outcome data are lacking.[17] Delayed gastric lavage and whole-bowel irrigation using a polyethylene glycol solution until rectal effluent is clear is advocated but not well studied. According to some anecdotal reports, gastrostomy and endoscopic removal of concretions have been successful. Hemoperfusion is the preferred extracorporeal method to enhance drug elimination when usual intensive supportive measures fail or serum levels dictate. Forced diuresis is not advised because the limited benefit of increasing the amount of drug cleared renally must be balanced against the greater risk of inducing pulmonary edema. Management of hypotension should include the early use of vasopressors and inotropes to avoid fluid overload.

METHAQUALONE

One of the more ubiquitous hypnosedative barbiturate substitutes, methaqualone was introduced in 1965 and withdrawn from the U.S. market in 1984 because promotions of safety and nonaddictiveness proved false. High abuse potential owed to methaqualone's popularity as a street aphrodisiac. The college pastime of "luding out," slang for a standard combination of 300 mg methaqualone ingested with wine, was used for attainment of characteristic deep relaxation, disinhibition, and euphoria.[18] In the 1980s the drug was used more often to mitigate the unpleasant side effects of popular stimulants as a "cocaine downer." Even though clandestine manufacture continues abroad, supporting drug smuggled into the United States, actual reports of toxicity and mortality are becoming rare. Cessation of legal synthesis and readily available benzodiazepine alternatives explain this trend.

The drug is a CNS depressant like all the other hypnosedatives, but its mechanism of action is more of a mystery. In contrast to other hypnosedatives, which depress muscle tone and reflexes, methaqualone increases muscle tone and motor activity by selectively depressing polysynaptic spinal reflexes at high dose. Methaqualone is rapidly absorbed from the GI tract, is highly lipophilic, and concentrates in the brain, adipose tissue, and liver. It exists as a weak base with a large volume of distribution and is highly protein bound. The majority of its metabolism occurs in the liver; no active metabolites are generated, and microsomal enzymes are moderately induced.

Clinically, hypertonicity, clonus, hyperreflexia, and muscle twitching are unique features in overdose. Additionally, the usual hypnosedative symptom profile of lethargy, ataxia, dysarthria, seizures, and coma at escalating dose is observed. Hyperacusis is also reported and may be a helpful diagnostic clue to ingestion. More often the drug-induced dissociative "high," poor judgment, and coincident impulsive behavior, result in death due to trauma, as opposed to fatalities resulting from direct toxic effects in overdose.[18] Cardiopulmonary symptoms include hypotension due to decreased myocardial contractility and respiratory depression. However, such symptoms occur less commonly than with other hypnosedatives, even in comatose patients. Coingestion of other CNS depressants can lead to severe respiratory depression and sudden apnea. Pulmonary edema can be seen as a result of increased capillary permeability, a risk common to most hypnosedative agents.

GI distress and hemorrhage have been noted in methaqualone overdose. Drug-induced inhibition of platelet aggregation, prolonged prothrombin and partial thromboplastin times, and decreased factors V and VII are causative. As with other hypnosedative agents, decontamination and supportive care remain the mainstays of therapy. Specific management considerations for methaqualone overdose include early use of benzodiazepines to control hypertonicity and seizures, along with administration of blood products (i.e., platelets, vitamin K, fresh-frozen plasma) in the setting of hemorrhage. Charcoal hemoperfusion is more effective than hemodialysis in clearing methaqualone, but is reserved for patients who fail to respond to maximal supportive therapy or whose serum methaqualone levels are greater than 10 to 15 mg/dL. Severe abstinence symptoms occur in chronic users when this drug is stopped abruptly and require hospital admission for gradual withdrawal.

ZALEPLON AND ZOLPIDEM

In 2000, zaleplon, a pyrazolopyrimidine derivative, became the newest available nonbenzodiazepine hypnosedative drug developed to combat insomnia. It is marketed for its rapid absorption and onset, as well as its significant presystemic metabolism ($t_{1/2} = 1$ h). Zaleplon has inactive metabolites that are primarily renally excreted. The comparative

efficacy of zaleplon and zolpidem has not been formally established. However, zaleplon does not produce the cognitive impairment, next-day sedation, amnesia, or rebound insomnia after discontinuation of nightly use that is seen with zolpidem and benzodiazepine derivatives. There have been no case reports of fatal acute overdose with zaleplon as a single substance, and evidence for pharmacologic tolerance or withdrawal is lacking. The abuse potential of zaleplon is comparable to that seen with triazolam in healthy volunteers with a history of drug abuse (i.e., considerably less than alcohol, cocaine, opiates, and barbiturates).[19]

Zolpidem is the other short-acting hypnosedative agent introduced in 1988 for the treatment of jet lag, anxiety, and insomnia. It is an imidazopyridine derivative, structurally different from benzodiazepines and other hypnosedatives. It binds preferentially to one of the benzodiazepine receptor subtypes (omega-1, benzodiazepine-1) in the CNS. Zolpidem is rapidly absorbed, has an onset of action within 30 min, and is effective for up to 6 h. It is metabolized in the liver to inactive metabolites that are excreted in the urine and feces. The advantage of zolpidem over the benzodiazepines had been the absence of reported addiction, tolerance, or withdrawal symptoms in most patients. Also, it had been extensively marketed to the elderly as a safer alternative to the benzodiazepines, which were shown to increase fall and fracture risk. However, recent studies indicate that these risks remain for older persons taking zolipem.[20] Also, the potential for abuse, previously believed to be limited by the presence of adverse effects of the drug at higher doses, has begun to surface. Still, to date only fifteen cases of abuse or dependence have been noted in the literature.[21] Apparently the drug is chronically abused for its psychomotor stimulant action, and tolerance and withdrawal effects can result, including rebound insomnia and seizures on abrupt discontinuation. Recently the WHO Expert Committee on Drug Dependence recommendations listed zolpidem, diazepam, and γHB for international control.[22] Experience in acute overdose is limited, but there are a few case reports of coma and rapidly remitting respiratory failure attributed to zolpidem alone.

Signs of acute zolpidem overdose in larger series commonly include drowsiness, vomiting, and rarely coma with respiratory depression. These symptoms escalate with dose and are complicated by coingestion of other psychotropic drugs and ethanol. In most cases, symptoms of intoxication remit rapidly, and therapy is usually limited to general supportive measures. Treatment is not aided by obtaining serum drug levels; the utility of MDAC and extracorporeal elimination enhancement methods has not been evaluated in overdose.

Anecdotally, flumazenil has been effective in reversing the CNS and respiratory actions of zolpidem.[23] The recommended initial dose is 0.2 mg intravenously given over 30 s. If no improvement in consciousness is observed within 30 s, an additional dose of 0.3 mg may be administered over 30 s. This dosing regimen (0.2 mg followed by 0.3 mg) can be repeated one more time, to a total dose of 1 mg, at an interval of 1 min if adequate consciousness is not obtained. Flumazenil at a total dose of 1 mg or less IV leaves 50 percent of the benzodiazepine receptors unoccupied, and therefore should limit the risk of acute withdrawal so long as this dose is not exceeded. Flumazenil is best avoided in multidrug exposures seen in the majority of adult overdose presenting to the ED, for fear of precipitating seizures. Contraindications to the use of flumazenil are shown in Table 165-3. In the event of a flumazenil-induced seizure, a therapeutic dose of benzodiazepine should be effective.

TABLE 165-3 Contraindications to Flumazenil

Suspected TCA overdose
Co-ingestion of seizure inducing agents
Known seizure disorder
Suspected or known physical dependence to benzodiazepines
Overdose of unknown agents
Suspected increased intracranial pressure

REFERENCES

1. Litovitz TL, Klein-Schwartz W, Rodgers GC Jr, et al: 2001 Annual Report of the American Association of Poison Control Centers Toxic Exposure Surveillance System. *Am J Emerg Med* 20:391, 2002.

2. Zvosec DL, Smith SW, McCutcheon JR, et al: Adverse events, including death, associated with the use of 1,4-butanediol. *New Engl J Med* 344:87, 2001.

3. Weir E: Raves: A review of the culture, the drugs and the prevention of harm. *Can Med Assoc J* 162:1843, 2000.

4. Mansergh G, Colfax GN, Marks G, et al: The circuit party men's health survey: Findings and implications for gay and bisexual men. *Am J Public Health* 91:953, 2001.

5. ElSohly MA, Salamone SJ: Prevalence of drugs used in cases of alleged sexual assault. *J Analytical Toxicol* 23:141, 1999.

6. Couper FJ, Logan BK: GHB and driving impairment. *J Forensic Sci* 46:919, 2001.

7. Miotto K, Darakjian J, Basch J, et al: Gamma-hydroxybutyric acid: Patterns of use, effects and withdrawal. *Am J Addict* 10:232, 2001.

8. Chin RL, Sporer KA, Cullison B, et al: Clinical course of gamma-hydroxybutyrate overdose. *Ann Emerg Med* 31:716, 1998.

9. Anonymous: Position statement: gastric lavage. American Academy of Clinical Toxicology; European Association of Poisons Centres and Clinical Toxicologists. *Clin Toxicol* 35:711, 1997.

10. Anonymous: Position statement and practice guidelines on the use of multi-dose activated charcoal in the treatment of acute poisoning. American Academy of Clinical Toxicology; European Association of Poisons Centres and Clinical Toxicologists. *J Toxicol Clin Toxicol* 37:731, 1999.

11. Ledray LE: The clinical care and documentation for victims of drug-facilitated sexual assault. *J Emerg Nurs* 27:301, 2001.

12. Dyer JE, Roth B, Hyma BA: Gamma-hydroxybutyrate withdrawal syndrome. *Ann Emerg Med* 37:147, 2001.

13. Pecknold JC: A risk-benefit assessment of buspirone in the treatment of anxiety disorders. *Drug Safety* 16:118, 1997.

14. Gaulier JM, Merle G, Lacassie E, et al: Fatal intoxications with chloral hydrate. *J Forensic Sci* 46:1507, 2001.

15. Hansen AR, Kennedy KA, Ambre JJ, et al: Glutethimide poisoning: A metabolite contributes to morbidity and mortality. *New Engl J Med* 292:250, 1975.

16. Reeves RR, Carter OS, Pinkofsky HB, et al: Carisoprodol (soma): Abuse potential and physician unawareness. *J Addict Dis* 18:51, 1999.

17. Hassan E: Treatment of meprobamate overdose with repeated oral doses of activated charcoal. *Ann Emerg Med* 15:73, 1986.

18. Wetli CV: Changing patterns of methaqualone abuse: A survey of 246 fatalities. *JAMA* 249:621, 1983.

19. Rush CR, Frey JM, Griffiths RR: Zaleplon and triazolam in humans: Acute behavioral effects and abuse potential. *Psychopharmacology* 145:39, 1999.

20. Wang PS, Bohn RL, Glynn RJ, et al: Zolpidem use and hip fractures in older people. *J Am Geriatr Soc* 49:1685, 2001.

21. Soyka M, Bottlender R, Moller HJ: Epidemiological evidence for a low abuse potential of zolpidem. *Pharmacopsychiatry* 33:138, 2000.

22. World Health Organization: WHO Expert Committee on Drug Dependence. Thirty-second report. *World Health Organization Technical Report Series* 903:I–V, 1, 2001.

23. Lheureux P, Debailleul G, DeWitte O, et al: Zolpidem intoxication mimicking narcotic overdose: Response to flumazenil. *Hum Exp Toxicol* 9:105, 1990.

ALCOHOLS
William A. Berk
Wilma V. Henderson

ETHANOL

Ethanol is unique among drugs of potential abuse. It is legal and culturally acceptable in most societies—and therefore ubiquitous. While potentially acutely and chronically toxic, it confers health benefits when used moderately. Finally, most medical morbidity associated with acute intoxication is the result not of direct drug effect, but of secondary injuries.

Ethanol is the most frequently used and abused intoxicant in the United States[1] and most other societies, including those where it is proscribed. Nearly three-quarters of adult Americans consume at least one alcoholic drink each year. Beer ranks as the fourth most popular beverage in terms of volume consumed, after soft drinks, milk, and coffee. Adult consumption of beverages containing ethanol peaked in 1980–1981 at 2.77 gallons per person of pure ethanol, but by 1997 this had declined to 2.2 gallons.[1]

Distilled spirits typically contain ethanol volumes of 40 to 50 percent (80 to 100 proof), although brands with volumes of 75 percent or more exist. Wines have an ethanol volume of 10 to 20 percent, while beers range from 2 to 6 percent. One drink is considered to be 0.5 oz or 15 g of alcohol, which is equivalent to 12 oz (355 mL) of beer, 5 oz (148 mL) of wine, or 1.5 oz (44 mL) of 80 proof spirits. Ethanol is also a constituent of mouthwashes (up to 75 percent volume), colognes (40 to 60 percent), and medicinal preparations (0.4 to 65 percent).

Though the statistics that show that the cost to society of alcohol abuse can be numbing, a few are worthy of mention here. Ethanol use in the U.S. cost $185 billion in 1998 and contributes to approximately 100,000 deaths per year,[1] dwarfing the value of any potential health benefits that might accrue from its use. Forty per cent of motor vehicle fatalities (15,000/year) are related to alcohol use. One-quarter of the victims of interpersonal trauma report alcohol use by their assailants,[2] and alcohol abuse as reported by the injured woman is the strongest predictor for acute injury related to domestic violence.[3] The prevalence and lifelong risk of alcohol abuse or dependence are 7 and 13 percent, respectively.[4]

Data from the 1995 National Hospital Ambulatory Medical Care Survey indicates that 2.7 percent of all ED visits are related to alcohol use.[5] Ethanol has been detected in the blood of 15 to 40 percent of ED patients, depending on locale. However, despite its prevalence, emergency physicians and inpatient specialists fail to recognize 50 percent of patients with ethanol dependence. The formal diagnosis of alcoholism has rested on instruments such as the CAGE and the Michigan Alcohol Screening Test. In the clinical setting, pointed questioning, when appropriate, about quantity of ethanol intake, medical complications usually caused by drinking, and whether the patient or others has ever felt he or she had a drinking problem will usually uncover such problems. It is increasingly clear that the ED-based interventions can be quite effective in treatment of alcoholism and its consequences.[6,7]

Pathophysiology

Ethanol is a central nervous system depressant which inhibits neuronal activity. Alcohol intoxication is associated with the depression of the excitatory neurotransmitter glutamate and alcohol increases the inhibitory activity of the neurotransmitters γ-aminobutyric acid (GABA) and glycine. Alcohol may also affect phosphorylation of proteins involved in ligand-gated channels that provide signaling functions. Changes in the number and sensitivity of these receptors that occur with chronic alcohol use appear to underlie at least some components of the alcohol withdrawal syndrome. The clinically observed cross-tolerance that exists between ethanol and other sedative-hypnotic agents, including benzodiazepines and barbiturates, appears related to the similar affects that these agents have on brain chemistry.

Ethanol absorption occurs in the mouth and esophagus to a small extent, in the stomach and large bowel to a moderate extent, but chiefly in the proximal portion of the small bowel. Approximately 2 to 10 percent of ethanol may be excreted by the lungs, in urine, or in sweat, the proportion being dependent on blood concentration. The remainder is metabolized to acetaldehyde in the liver by one of two pathways. In the cell, cytosol alcohol dehydrogenase with nicotinamide adenine dinucleotide as a cofactor produces acetaldehyde, which in turn is metabolized by aldehyde dehydrogenase. The second pathway, which is clinically significant at high blood ethanol concentrations and has increased activity with repeated exposures to ethanol, is a microsomal alcohol oxidizing system. Gender-related differences in the metabolism of ethanol explain the considerably higher blood ethanol levels in women versus men after similar dosing on a gram-per-kilogram basis. Women have a smaller volume of distribution (0.6 L/kg) for ethanol than men (0.7 L/kg) and have decreased first-pass metabolism of ethanol because their gastric walls contain less alcohol dehydrogenase than do those of men.[8]

Clinical Features

Symptoms and signs of ethanol intoxication include slurred speech, nystagmus, disinhibited behavior, central nervous system depression including coma, and decreased motor coordination and control. A lowering of blood pressure or even hypotension with resultant reflex tachycardia are common secondary to a decrease in total peripheral resistance or as a result of volume loss. Changes in posture may result in syncope.[9] However, when hypotension is present, other causes must be considered.

Because of the phenomenon of tolerance, blood alcohol levels correlate poorly with degree of intoxication. While death from respiratory depression may occur in unhabituated individuals at concentrations of 400 to 500 mg/dL, it is not uncommon for some alcoholics to appear minimally intoxicated at blood concentrations as high as 400 mg/dL.[10] Although most states have adopted 80 or 100 mg/dL as the legal definition of intoxication for the purposes of driving a motor vehicle, there is considerable evidence to suggest that impairment may be seen with levels as low as 5 mg/dL, especially in unhabituated individuals.

A mild lactic acidosis may be seen. However, **significant acidosis should never be attributed to alcohol intoxication,** and should prompt an aggressive search for another cause. In the presence of volume depletion, a mild contraction alkalosis may be noted, as may prerenal azotemia.

Treatment

Management of acute ethanol intoxication consists of attending to associated injuries or medical illness and observation until clinical sobriety is attained. A careful examination should be performed to evaluate for complicating injuries or medical conditions. Ethanol levels are not necessarily required for mild or moderate intoxication when no other abnormality is suspected. It is appropriate in all patients with depressed level of consciousness or altered mental status. The most appropriate fluid is D5NS. This fluid addresses volume issues as well as glycogen depletion.

Hypoglycemia should be excluded by a bedside glucose determination. In the event of severe depression of mental status, causes other than alcohol ingestion must be considered, especially subdural hematoma, which can occur in the absence of external signs of trauma.

Fluid administration does not hasten alcohol elimination;[11] therefore intravenous access for fluid administration alone is unnecessary in uncomplicated cases of mild to moderate intoxication unless clinical signs of volume depletion are present. Any alcoholic with CNS depression, even if apparently attributable to intoxication, should receive thiamine. Folate and other vitamins are indicated only if there are clinical signs or laboratory confirmation of deficiency. Ethanol does not bind to activated charcoal, which should be administered only if other substances have been ingested that are adsorbable. Careful and serial observation is crucial, as in the vast majority of uncomplicated cases rapid improvement occurs over a few hours. **Mental status that fails to improve and any deterioration should be considered secondary to other causes** and evaluated aggressively. Respiratory depression may result in carbon dioxide retention, which on rare occasion may require intubation. Unhabituated patients eliminate ethanol from the bloodstream at a rate of 15 to 20 mg/dL per h, while alcoholics average 25 to 35 mg/dL per h.

Alcoholics should be questioned about concomitant drug use. In the past, ethylene glycol or methanol was occasionally substituted for or combined with ethanol. Today cocaine has clearly become the most common concomitant drug used by alcoholics. The attraction of abusing these drugs together may relate to the formation of a metabolite, cocaethylene, which although less potent than cocaine, has a half-life that is 3 to 5 times longer.[12] The risk of sudden death among users of both drugs simultaneously may be as high as 20 times that with cocaine alone.

Ethanol is the most common cause of an osmolar gap (see Chap. 27) (Table 166-1). The concomitant presence of an anion-gap (AG) metabolic acidosis may help characterize the presence of a coingestant. Methanol and ethylene glycol poisoning are associated with significant widened AG-type acidosis. The metabolic derangements ascribed to alcohol toxicity are readily reversed by volume repletion.

A long-running debate continues about whether alcohol ingestion complicates the care of the injured patient. Some feel that it does, either by increasing trauma severity through mechanical means (some have proposed decreased tone in the abdominal musculature), or through its toxic effects in combination with trauma to injured organs, particularly the brain. However, most studies have found that expenditures for diagnostic studies and morbidity are similar in intoxicated and sober trauma victims when controlling for severity of trauma.

Disposition

Morbidity and mortality in association with acute intoxication are predominantly the result of injuries, often motor vehicle collisions related to ethanol-induced deficits in judgment or physical capabilities. Patients with acute ethanol intoxication alone rarely require hospital admission. However, questions frequently arise over alcoholics who appear clinically sober while still having considerable blood ethanol concentrations. Medical judgment of mental competence should not be confused with any particular blood alcohol concentration level. Patients whose intoxication has resolved to the extent that they do not constitute a danger to themselves or others, *and* who will not be responsible for their own transportation, may be discharged on their own recognizance or preferably in the company of responsible friends or relatives who can assist them and take some responsibility for their care. Patients who are to drive themselves home should have ethanol levels close to zero, not merely below a given state's legal level for driving, as there is the theoretical potential for psychometric disability at very low levels, and the potential liability for the emergency physician is unfortunately huge.

ISOPROPANOL

Isopropanol, also known as isopropyl alcohol and 2-propanol, is commonly found in the home as rubbing alcohol. It is also used widely in

TABLE 166-1   Substances that Contribute to the Osmolar Gap

Substance	Molecular Weight	mOsm/L at 100 mg/dL	Correction Factor
Ethanol	46	22	4.6
Isopropanol	60	17	6.0
Methanol	32	31	3.2
Ethylene glycol	62	16	6.2

Note: To estimate concentration of an alcohol in mg/dL, use the following formula: (osmolar gap − 10) × correction factor. This estimation is only valid if the alcohol is the only unmeasured abnormal contributor to osmolarity. Measured osmolality, if higher than predicted by the known concentration(s) of the measured alcohol(s), implies the presence of another osmotically active substance.

industry as a solvent and disinfectant and is a component of a variety of skin and hair products, jewelry cleaners, detergents, paint thinners, and antifreeze. Poisoning usually results from ingestion, but may also occur after inhalation or dermal exposure in poorly ventilated areas—for example, during alcohol sponge bathing. Toxicity occurring after administration of an isopropanol enema has also been reported. Its principal metabolite, acetone, does not cause the eye, kidney, cardiac, or metabolic toxicity caused by the metabolites of methanol and ethylene glycol.

Isopropanol is approximately twice as potent as ethanol in causing central nervous system depression and its duration is two to four times that of ethanol. As a result it is on occasion utilized as a substitute intoxicant by alcoholics as well as in suicide attempts. After ethanol, it is the second most commonly ingested alcohol. Though more toxic than ethanol, it is considerably less so than methanol or ethylene glycol.

Pathophysiology

Isopropanol is a clear, volatile liquid with a bitter, burning taste and an aromatic odor. It is rapidly absorbed after being ingested, with 80 percent of an oral dose being absorbed after 30 min and complete absorption within 2 h. The substance has a volume of distribution of 0.6 to 0.7 L/kg. Small and clinically insignificant amounts are resecreted by the salivary glands and stomach.

The kidneys excrete 20 to 50 percent of an absorbed dose unchanged. However, the major pathway for the metabolism of isopropanol is in the liver (50 to 80 percent), where it is oxidized to acetone by alcohol dehydrogenase (Figure 166-1). Acetone is excreted primarily by the kidneys, with some excretion through the lungs. However, similar to ETOH but unlike methanol and ethylene glycol, significant acidosis ascribable solely to isopropanol or its metabolites does not occur. A hallmark of isopropanol toxicity is ketonemia and ketonuria, but without elevated blood glucose or glycosuria. This feature (i.e., presence of ketones) helps differentiate isopropanol ingestion from poisoning with ethylene glycol or methanol.

Isopropanol most closely follows concentration-dependent (first-order) kinetics. The half-life of isopropanol in the absence of ethanol is 6 to 7 h, while the half-life of acetone is 22 to 28 h. The long half-life of acetone may be the cause of the prolonged symptomatology often associated with isopropanol poisoning. Ethanol administration has not been used clinically to inhibit isopropanol metabolism to acetone.

The toxic dose of 70 percent isopropanol is approximately 1 mL/kg, with the lethal dose in an adult approximately 2 to 4 mL/kg. As little as 0.5 mL/kg may cause symptoms, but survival has been reported following ingestions of up to 1 L. Children are especially susceptible to toxic effects and may develop symptoms with as little as three swallows of 70 percent isopropanol.

Clinical Features

The clinical features of isopropanol intoxication are similar to those seen with ethanol intoxication except that the duration of symptoms and signs is longer and central nervous system depression may be more profound because of the formation of acetone. Onset of symptoms occurs within 30 to 60 min, with peak effects in a few hours. Nystagmus is usually present. Severe poisoning is marked by early onset of coma, respiratory depression, and hypotension.

Massive ingestion may cause hypotension secondary to peripheral vasodilatation, with contributions possible from hemorrhagic gastritis. Serious dysrhythmias are rare.

Hemorrhagic gastritis secondary to gastric irritation appears early and is a striking feature of isopropanol ingestions, resulting in nausea, vomiting, abdominal pain, and upper gastrointestinal hemorrhage.

Hypoglycemia may occur secondary to depressed gluconeogenesis. Less common complications include hepatic dysfunction, acute tubular necrosis, myoglobinuria, hemolytic anemia, rhabdomyolysis, and myopathy.

Isopropanol poisoning should be suspected when the fruity odor of acetone or smell of rubbing alcohol is present on the breath. Patients will have ketonuria and ketonemia without glycosuria or hyperglycemia, in the presence of an elevated osmolar gap. A spurious increase in serum creatinine as a result of acetone may sometimes be seen. Generally there is no abnormal anion gap, although this may be seen as a result of hypotension and related lactic acidosis. The use of alcohol screening panels helps detect unsuspected isopropanolism.

Although isopropanol levels of 50 mg/dL are associated with mild intoxication in individuals who are not habituated to ethanol, alcoholic patients may be considerably more resistant to the central nervous system effects of isopropanol.

Treatment

If there is suspicion of isopropanol poisoning, intravenous access should be established. If indicated, there should be bedside testing for blood glucose, and administration of thiamine and naloxone. Patients should be monitored for central nervous system or respiratory depression. Because of the rapid absorption of isopropanol, there is no utility to performing gastric lavage. Activated charcoal binds isopropanol poorly and is not necessary in the absence of ingestion of adsorbable substances. Laboratory studies are guided by the results of examination and clinical condition. Serum electrolytes, CBC, glucose, and acetone should generally be obtained. Blood type and screen may be appropriate in anticipation of the possibility of significant gastric hemorrhage.

In severely obtunded patients, airway management may require intubation and ventilatory support. Hypotension usually responds to intravenous fluids. In severe cases, support with vasopressors may be required. Patients with severe hemorrhagic gastritis may require blood transfusion. If a significant acidosis is present, vigorous investigation for another cause must be made. Hemodialysis is indicated when hypotension is refractory to conventional therapy, results in hemodynamic instability, or when the predicted peak isopropanol level is greater than 400 mg/dL. Hemodialysis is effective in eliminating both isopropanol and acetone. Peritoneal dialysis is less effective than hemodialysis.

Disposition

Patients with lethargy or prolonged central nervous system depression should be admitted to the hospital. Those who remain asymptomatic

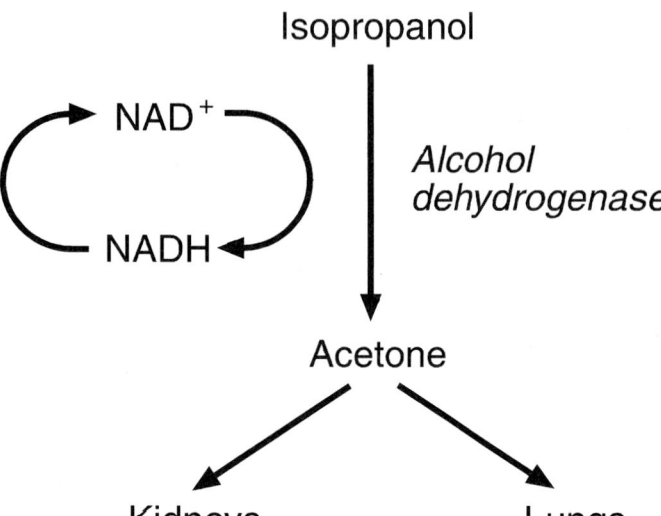

FIG. 166-1. Metabolic pathway of isopropanol.

for 6 to 8 h may be discharged or referred for substance abuse counseling or psychiatric evaluation.

METHANOL

Methanol—also referred to as methyl alcohol, wood spirits, or wood alcohol—is used widely in commercial, industrial, and marine solvents. A product of wood distillation, it is a component of many paint removers, varnishes, shellacs, windshield washing fluids, and antifreeze formulations. Methanol poisoning has resulted from the consumption of contaminated whiskey, accidental ingestion by desperate alcoholics, or intentional ingestion during suicide attempts. Methanol is also present in measurable but small amounts in wine and distilled spirits, accounting for the fact that low levels may be detectable in the blood after binge drinking. Methanol's toxicity is due to the formation of two toxic metabolites, formaldehyde and formic acid. Therapeutic strategies are therefore based on prevention of the formation of these metabolites or their removal from the body.

Pathophysiology

Methanol is a colorless, volatile liquid with a distinctive odor. It is well absorbed from the gastrointestinal tract, with peak levels attained 30 to 90 min after ingestion. Most incidents of toxicity occur after oral ingestion, but significant absorption may also occur through the lungs or skin. The serum half-life after mild toxicity is 14 to 20 h. With severe toxicity, this increases to 24 to 30 h. Methanol has a volume of distribution of 0.6 to 0.7 L/kg.

Following ingestion, highest concentrations are found in the kidney, liver, and gastrointestinal tract, but high levels are also found in the vitreous humor and optic nerve. Most methanol—90 to 95 percent—is eliminated by the liver, while renal excretion accounts for 2 to 5 percent; pulmonary excretion is minimal. In overdose situations, elimination follows saturation (zero-order) kinetics.

Toxicity from methanol poisoning results from the metabolism by hepatic alcohol dehydrogenase of methanol to formaldehyde and formic acid (Figure 166-2). The accumulation of formic acid is associated with the onset of clinical symptoms. Lactate is produced from formate-induced inhibition of mitochondrial respiration, as a result of tissue hypoxia, and to a lesser extent as a result of a decrease in the intracellular NAD^+/NADH ratio caused by the oxidation of methanol and thus stimulation of anaerobic glycolysis and lactate production. Formaldehyde production in the retina causes optic papillitis and retinal edema, in severe cases resulting in blindness. Since folate is a cofactor in the breakdown of formic acid to carbon dioxide and water, alcoholics who are folate-deficient may be especially susceptible to methanol toxicity due to increased accumulation of formic acid.

The amount of methanol required to cause toxicity varies; death has been reported after ingestion of a dose as small as 15 mL of a 40 percent solution. Although 30 mL of a 40 percent solution is considered the minimal lethal dose, amounts as large as 500 to 600 mL have been ingested with survival reported.

Clinical Features

The symptoms of methanol poisoning may not appear for up to 12 to 18 h after ingestion because of the time it takes for methanol to be metabolized to its toxic metabolites. The delay in symptoms may be even longer if ethanol has been ingested and is competing with methanol for metabolism by alcohol dehydrogenase. The cardinal clinical manifestations of methanol poisoning are central nervous system depression similar to that of ethanol, visual disturbances, abdominal pain, nausea and vomiting, and wide-anion-gap metabolic acidosis. As with isopropanol, the early phase of elation commonly seen in ethanol intoxication is absent.

On arrival at the hospital, the victim may be confused or, in severe cases, comatose. There may be complaints of headache or vertigo, and seizures may occur. Visual disturbances are seen in approximately 50 percent of patients. These include diplopia, blurred vision, decreased visual acuity, photophobia, descriptions of "looking into a snow field," constricted visual fields, and blindness. The clinician may find nystagmus, fixed and dilated pupils, retinal edema, and optic atrophy or hyperemia of the optic disk. Computed tomography of the brain may reveal basal ganglia infarcts consistent with the parkinsonian syndrome, which has been reported after methanol poisoning. Methanol is a potent mucosal irritant and causes severe abdominal pain as well as nausea and vomiting in over one-half of cases; pancreatitis has also been commonly reported. However, serious ingestions may occur without gastrointestinal symptoms. Although an increased osmolar gap is usually present with serious methanol ingestion, **methanol poisoning with a normal osmolar gap can be seen.** This is due to completed conversion of methanol to its toxic metabolites.

Hypotension and bradycardia are late findings and suggest a poor prognosis. Outcome is best correlated with the severity of the acidosis rather than serum methanol concentration.

Diagnosis of methanol poisoning rests on history, the presence of the characteristic clinical features outlined above, and the presence of a wide-anion-gap metabolic acidosis and osmolar gap. While confirmation of a tentative diagnosis depends on identification of the substance in the bloodstream, treatment should be initiated based on compatible clinical presentation to avoid morbidity resulting from delay. In any case, serum methanol determinations at many institutions depend on outside laboratories and may not be available for several hours. However, if the ethanol level is known, the methanol level can be estimated from the osmolar gap (see Table 166-1).

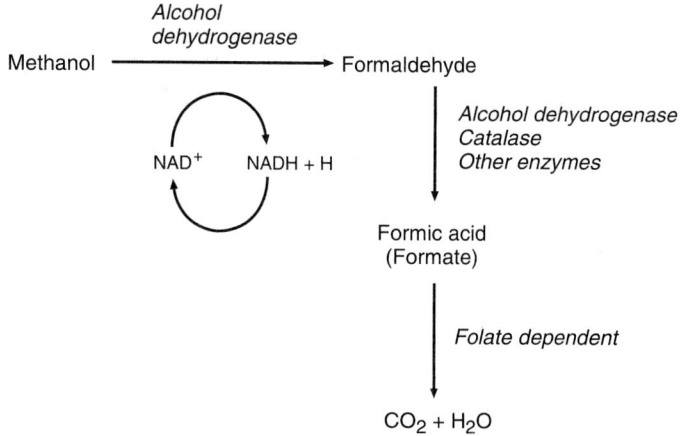

FIG. 166-2. Metabolism of methanol in the liver.

Normal methanol blood concentration from endogenous sources is 0.05 mg/dL. Asymptomatic individuals usually have peak levels below 20 mg/dL, while levels above 50 mg/dL indicate serious poisoning. Central nervous system symptoms usually appear when levels rise above 20 mg/dL, eye problems are associated with levels greater than 50 mg/dL, and the risk of fatality rises with levels greater than 150 to 200 mg/dL.

The differential diagnosis should include other potential causes of a wide-anion-gap metabolic acidosis—i.e., ethylene glycol, diabetic ketoacidosis, paraldehyde, isoniazid, salicylates, iron, lactic acidosis, phenformin, uremia, carbon monoxide, cyanide, alcoholic ketoacidosis, and toluene.

Treatment

Intravenous access should be established, with immediate bedside testing for blood glucose and administration of thiamine and naloxone if indicated. The general measures involved in treatment are 1) supportive care, 2) correction of acidosis, 3) administration of fomepizole or ethanol to decrease conversion to toxic metabolites, and 4) dialysis to eliminate the methanol. Unless the patient presents immediately after the ingestion, gastric aspiration or lavage is unlikely to be of benefit. Activated charcoal is ineffective in the absence of ingestion of other, adsorbable substances. Serum electrolytes, CBC, glucose, and ethanol level (if there is any possibility of coingestion of this substance), in addition to a methanol level are generally needed as a minimum. Care should be taken to maintain an adequate airway with intubation if necessary for proper airway protection and ventilatory support. Sodium bicarbonate should be administered with the goal of maintaining a near normal pH, since correction of metabolic acidosis moderates some of the toxic effects of methanol poisoning, including visual impairment.

Prevention of metabolism of methanol to its toxic metabolites by competitive inhibition of alcohol dehydrogenase is a mainstay of methanol ingestion management. Ethanol has to a great extent been supplanted by a pharmacologically superior agent, fomepizole (also referred to as 4-methylpyrazole).[13,14] A competitive inhibitor of alcohol dehydrogenase, fomepizole has an affinity for the enzyme that is 8000 times that of ethanol.[15] In addition, it does not produce central nervous system depression or metabolic toxicity, and it does not require the monitoring of levels and dosage adjustments. Fomepizole is administered in a loading dose of 15 mg/kg, followed by doses of 10 mg/kg every 12 h for four doses. Each dose is given by slow intravenous infusion over 30 min. More frequent dosing (q4h) is required during hemodialysis because fomepizole is removed during the procedure.

Ethanol, the traditional initial treatment of methanol intoxication, competitively inhibits the metabolism of methanol by alcohol dehydrogenase. Ethanol's affinity for the enzyme is 10 to 20 times that of methanol, and its presence largely inhibits the formation of the toxic metabolites. Blood ethanol level should be maintained between 100 and 150 mg/dL to completely inhibit formation of toxic metabolites. Blood concentrations below 100 mg/dL are considerably less effective and therefore increase the risk of severe toxicity. Ethanol may be administered IV, PO, or by nasogastric tube.

Oral administration uses 20 to 30% concentration usually by nasogastric tube. Higher concentrations can lead to gastritis. Also, oral loading presents significant risks should alterations in mental status ensue.

Intravenous administration is preferred, though it may result in superficial thrombophlebitis. The intravenous solution should contain 10 percent ethanol in D5W. If the recommended solution of 10 percent ethanol in D5W is utilized, the loading dose is 10 mL/kg and maintenance is 1.5 mL/kg per h. When intravenous ethanol is not immediately available, oral therapy can be initiated with commercial distilled spirits. To calculate the ethanol content of distilled spirits, the following formula may be used:

$$\text{ethanol (g)} = \text{volume of beverage (mL)} \times 0.9 \times (\text{proof}/200)$$

Ethanol levels should be assayed on a frequent basis, with the dose adjusted to maintain a concentration of 100 to 150 mg/dL. If dialysis is initiated, a higher maintenance infusion starting at 0.24 g/kg per h will be necessary, as ethanol is dialyzable. As hypoglycemia may occur with ethanol administration, especially in children, blood glucose levels should be monitored closely.

Indications for treatment and doses of fomepizole and ethanol are shown in Table 166-2.

Fomepizole should be considered the drug of choice when inhibition of alcohol dehydrogenase is desired. Ethanol is indicated in the presence of known fomepizole allergy or when fomepizole is not readily available. Case reports suggest that fomepizole is safe to use in children, who are especially susceptible to some of the side effects of ethanol.[16] Fomepizole is expensive: the current cost of the loading dose alone is greater than $1000, compared with just a few dollars for ethanol. Although there is no formal study of the cost effectiveness of fomepizole, it seems likely that much if not all of its cost would be offset by savings in intensive care monitoring, laboratory tests, and nursing manpower. **Use of fomepizole or alcohol does not alter the indications for dialysis.**

Folate is a cofactor for the conversion of formic acid to carbon dioxide. It is especially important to provide supplements to alcoholic patients

TABLE 166-2 Indications and Treatment for Methanol and Ethylene Glycol Poisoning

Agent	Indications for Treatment	Treatment
Methanol	Methanol >20 mg/dL Ingestion ≥0.4 mg/kg History, symptoms suggestive of poisoning	Ethanol Loading dose: 10% ethanol in D5W at 10 mL/kg over 30 min* Infusion: 10% ethanol in D5W at 1.5 mL/kg per h to maintain ethanol level at 100–150 mg/dL† *or* Fomepizole 15 mg/kg over 30 min, then 10 mg/kg q12h × 4 doses *and* Folinic acid 1 mg/kg IV (max 50 mg) q4h NaHCO₃ 1 mEq/kg IV for severe acidosis
Ethylene glycol (EG)	EG >20 mg/dL Suspicion of ingestion Suspicion and anion gap acidosis	Ethanol Loading dose: 10% ethanol in D5W at 10 mL/kg over 30 min* Infusion: 10% ethanol in D5W at 1.5 mL/kg per h to maintain ethanol level at 100–150 mg/dL† *or* Fomepizole 15 mg/kg over 30 min, then 10 mg/kg q12h‡ × 4 doses *and* Thiamine 100 mg IV Pyridoxine 100 mg IV 10% Calcium gluconate 10 mL IV for hypocalcemia NaHCO₃ 1 mEq/kg IV for severe acidosis

*A 100-kg person will require 1 L of fluid.
†If ethanol <100 mg/dL, reload using following formula: Desired ETOH concentration in mg/dL—actual concentration in mg/dL × 0.6 L/kg × kg.
‡During dialysis dosage must be altered. Consult hospital pharmacist or poison control center.

who may be folate deficient. Administration of folic acid 50 mg IV every 4 h for several days to all patients is recommended.

Indications for dialysis are shown in Table 166-3. These indications are the same for patients treated with fomepizole. Hemodialysis is considerably more effective than peritoneal dialysis, but peritoneal dialysis may be utilized if hemodialysis is unavailable. Dialysis eliminates both the parent compound and its toxic metabolites. Dialysis and fomepizole or ethanol are continued until levels are zero and acidosis has resolved.

Disposition

Disposition decisions are based on criteria identical to those used for ethylene glycol poisoning (see below). It should be emphasized that **asymptomatic patients with a history of any possible methanol ingestion should be admitted** and treatment initiated, even if no acidosis is evident.

ETHYLENE GLYCOL

Ethylene glycol has many commercial uses as a coolant (antifreeze), preservative, and glycerine substitute; it has also been used in lacquers, cosmetics, polishes, and detergents. It accounted for 4938 poison exposures and 16 deaths in the United States as reported to poison control centers in 2001.[17] It may be ingested as an alcohol substitute by alcoholics, in suicide attempts, and accidentally by children. Ethylene glycol's toxicity is the result of the formation of two toxic metabolites, formaldehyde and formic acid. As with methanol, therapeutic strategies are based on prevention of formation of these metabolites or their removal from the body.

Pathophysiology

Ethylene glycol is a colorless, odorless, sweet-tasting substance. It is highly water-soluble and rapidly absorbed when ingested orally, but not when exposure is via the lungs or skin. Peak blood levels occur within 1 to 4 h of an ingestion. The volume of distribution is 0.83 L/kg and the plasma half-life is 3 to 5 h. Ethylene glycol is metabolized in the liver and kidneys to toxic metabolites—aldehydes, glycolate, oxalate, and lactate—which in turn cause toxicity to the lungs, heart, and kidneys. These metabolites also cause the metabolic acidosis associated with ethylene glycol poisoning.

Ethylene glycol is metabolized to glycoaldehyde by alcohol dehydrogenase (Figure 166-3). This conversion involves the reduction of NAD^+ to NADH, which causes inhibition of the citric acid cycle and formation of lactic acid. Glycoaldehyde is further metabolized to glycolic acid and to glyoxylic acid, which in turn are converted to several new compounds. Pyridoxal phosphate is a cofactor in the conversion of glyoxylic acid to glycine, which is nontoxic, while thiamine pyrophosphate is the cofactor in the conversion of glyoxylic acid to another nontoxic compound called α-hydroxy-β-ketoadipate. A deficiency of either pyridoxal phosphate or thiamine may shift the metabolism of ethylene glycol to the production of toxic metabolites.

Glyoxylic acid is also metabolized to formic acid and oxalic acid. Glycolic acid contributes to the metabolic acidosis observed in ethylene glycol poisoning. Oxalate crystalluria is a striking feature caused by calcium oxalate salt deposition, but occurs in the urine in only about 50 percent of cases.

The potentially lethal dose in adults is 2 mL/kg, although survival has been reported after ingestions ranging from 240 to 2000 mL.

TABLE 166-3 Indications for Dialysis with Methanol Poisoning

Signs of visual or central nervous system dysfunction
Peak methanol levels >20 mg/dL
pH <7.15
History of ingesting >30 mL

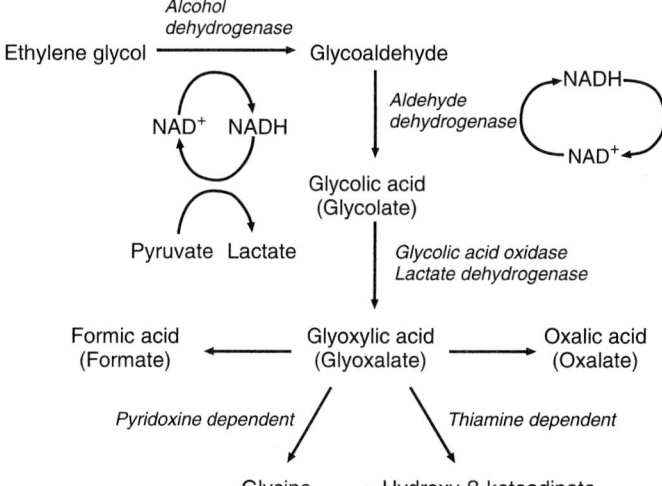

FIG. 166-3. Metabolic pathway of ethylene glycol.

Clinical Features

Ethylene glycol poisoning often exhibits three distinct clinical phases, the severity and progression of which depends on the amount ingested. The initial phase is characterized by central nervous system depression, usually within 1 to 12 h after ingestion. Patients may appear inebriated, with slurred speech and ataxia but without the odor of ethanol on their breath. Hallucinations, coma, seizures, and death may also occur during this initial phase. These central nervous system symptoms correlate with peak glycoaldehyde production. The optic fundus is usually normal, differentiating the syndrome from methanol poisoning, although nystagmus and ophthalmoplegia may be observed. Lumbar puncture may demonstrate elevated CSF pressure and protein and a few polymorphonuclear cells.

The second, cardiopulmonary phase develops 12 to 24 h after ingestion. Tachycardia, mild hypertension, and tachypnea are the most common symptoms; congestive heart failure, acute respiratory distress syndrome, cardiomegaly, and circulatory collapse are also observed. Myositis has also been reported less commonly during this phase.

The third phase, marked by nephrotoxicity, occurs 24 to 72 h after ingestion. Early symptoms consist of flank pain and costovertebral angle tenderness. Oliguric renal failure and acute tubular necrosis ensue. Complete anuria may occur, but most patients recover without renal damage if they receive appropriate therapy. Nephrotoxicity is caused by aldehyde metabolites and oxalic acid. Two forms of urinary calcium oxalate crystals may be identified on microscopic evaluation of the urine. The dihydrate form (octahedral crystals) shows tent-shaped crystals, and the monohydrate form (monoclinic crystals) shows crystals that are dumbbell- or prism-shaped. The monohydrate form was at one time felt to represent a salt of hippurate, explaining previous reports of hippurate crystals in the urine.

Hypocalcemia may develop secondary to precipitation of calcium as calcium oxalate and may be severe enough to cause tetany and prolongation of the QT interval. Elevated serum creatine phosphokinase levels may accompany and explain the generalized myalgias experienced by some patients.

Ethylene glycol intoxication should be considered when a patient presents with inebriation and no ethanol scent on the breath, a wide-anion-gap metabolic acidosis with osmolar gap, and calcium oxalate crystalluria. The mechanisms of anion-gap metabolic acidosis and osmolar gap are similar to those observed with methanol.

Tentative diagnosis and initiation of treatment should be based on history and characteristic clinical presentation. As with methanol poisoning, confirmation of a tentative diagnosis depends on identification of the substance in the bloodstream, but treatment should be initiated based on compatible clinical presentation to avoid morbidity resulting from delay. Serum levels greater than 20 mg/dL are likely to result in toxicity. Survival has been reported with levels up to 650 mg/dL, while fatality has been associated with levels >98 mg/dL.

Leukocytosis is common and should not be considered a manifestation of infection unless clinical signs are present. One-third of patients may have hypocalcemia, with shortening of the QT interval present on the electrocardiogram. Serious intoxication has been reported in the absence of an osmolar gap or calcium oxalate crystalluria. The mechanism for the absence of an osmolar gap is based on the same explanation as given for methanol (above).

As with methanol, the differential diagnosis should include other potential causes of a wide-anion-gap metabolic acidosis.

Treatment

The management of ethylene glycol poisoning is similar to that of methanol poisoning. Indications for gastric emptying and guidelines for administration of sodium bicarbonate are the same as those given for methanol, above. If the patient is hypocalcemic, 10 mL of calcium gluconate 10 percent should be given IV. Pyridoxine 100 mg and thiamine 100 mg IM or IV should be administered daily to facilitate metabolism of ethylene glycol by nontoxic pathways. Magnesium has also been shown to be a cofactor in the metabolism of toxic metabolites and should be given if patients are hypomagnesemic, as is often the case with alcoholics.

Laboratory tests that may be useful in evaluating patients suspected of ethylene glycol ingestion include complete blood count; serum electrolytes; acetone; alcohol toxicology panel with ethanol, isopropanol, and methanol determinations; electrolytes; blood urea nitrogen; creatinine; salicylate level; arterial blood gases; urinalysis; serum ethylene glycol level; calcium; creatine phosphokinase (CPK); and magnesium levels. Lactate levels should also be determined if the reason for the severe acidosis is unclear.

Competitive inhibition of alcohol dehydrogenase's breakdown of ethylene glycol with fomepizole or ethanol should be initiated in the ED when overdose is suspected or confirmed. Fomepizole (see above) has supplanted ethanol as the initial treatment of choice.[18] Dosing is the same for ethylene glycol as for methanol. Ethanol's affinity for alcohol dehydrogenase is 100 times that of ethylene glycol, resulting in a prolongation of the half-life of ethylene glycol to 17 h. Indications for treatment and doses of fomepizole or ethanol are shown in Table 166-2.

Oral and intravenous dosing guidelines for ethanol are identical to those outlined for methanol, above. Due to ease of administration, greater affinity for alcohol dehydrogenase, and a superior side-effect profile, fomepizole is the drug of choice unless it is not readily available or there is a history of allergy to fomepizole. Fomepizole has been well tolerated by children in case reports,[19] though the overall magnitude of clinical experience is considerably less than for adults.

Indications for dialysis are shown in Table 166-4. Although there are reports of patients with normal renal function who met other standard criteria for hemodialysis who were treated effectively and safely with fomepizole alone,[15] we feel that use of the agent should not change the indications for hemodialysis. As for methanol, fomepizole or ethanol administration and dialysis should be continued until serum blood levels of whichever substance has been ingested are zero and acidosis has resolved.

TABLE 166-4 Indications for Dialysis with Ethylene Glycol Poisoning

The triad of history, clinical presentation, and laboratory results consistent with ethylene glycol poisoning are present
Ethylene glycol >20 mg/dL
Signs of nephrotoxicity
Metabolic acidosis is present

As with methanol, hemodialysis has been shown to be considerably more effective, but peritoneal dialysis may be used if hemodialysis is unavailable.

Disposition

Any patient with the serious signs and symptoms associated with ethylene glycol or methanol intoxication, or a history of significant ingestion even in absence of symptoms, should be admitted to an intensive care setting. Suicidal patients should receive a psychiatric evaluation when their condition improves and prior to discharge from any facility.

Patients seen at facilities unable to provide hemodialysis or intensive care should be transferred if sufficiently stable as soon as possible to institutions capable of providing such care. Because the symptoms of ethylene glycol and methanol intoxication may be delayed, patients who have ingested these substances should be admitted to the hospital for observation and laboratory testing even if they are initially asymptomatic.

REFERENCES

1. Secretary of Health and Human Services: Tenth Special Report to the U.S. Congress on Alcohol and Health. Washington, DC, U.S. Department of Health and Human Services, 2000.
2. Whiteman PJ, Hoffman RS, Goldfrank LR: Alcoholism in the emergency department: An epidemiologic study. *Acad Emerg Med* 7:14, 2000.
3. Kyriacou DN, McCabe F, Anglin D, et al. Emergency department-based study of risk factors for acute injury from domestic violence against women. *Ann Emerg Med* 31:502, 1998.
4. Grant BF: Prevalence and correlates of alcohol use and DSM-IV alcohol dependence in the United States: Results of the National Longitudinal Alcohol Epidemiologic Survey. *J Stud Alcohol* 464:464, 1997.
5. Li G, Keyl PM, Rothman R, et al: Epidemiology of alcohol-related emergency department visits. *Acad Emerg Med* 5:788, 1998.
6. D'Onofrio G, Bernstein E, Bernstein J, et al: Patients with alcohol problems in the emergency department, Part 2: Intervention and Referral. *Acad Emerg Med* 5:1210, 1998.
7. Gentilello LM, Rivara FP, Donovan DM, et al: Alcohol interventions in a trauma center as a means of reducing the risk of injury recurrence. *Ann Surg* 230:473, 1999.
8. Frezza M, Di Padova C, et al: The role of decreased gastric alcohol dehydrogenase activity and first-pass metabolism. *New Engl J Med* 322:95, 1990.
9. Narkiewicz K, Cooley RL, Somers VK: Alcohol potentiates orthostatic hypotension: Implications for alcohol-related syncope. *Circulation* 398:398, 2000.
10. Sullivan JB, Hauptman M, Bronstein AC: Lack of observable intoxication in humans with high blood alcohol concentrations. *J Forensic Sci* 32:1660, 1987.
11. Li J, Mills T, Erato R: Intravenous saline has no effect on blood ethanol clearance. *J Emerg Med* 17:1, 1999.
12. Farre M, de la Torre R, Gonzalez ML, et al: Cocaine and alcohol interactions in humans: Neuroendocrine effects and cocaethylene metabolism. *J Pharmacol Exp Ther* 283:164, 1997.
13. Brent J, McMartin KE, Phillips S, et al: Methylpyrazole for Toxic Alcohols Study Group. Fomepizole for the treatment of methanol poisoning. *New Engl J Med* 344:424, 2001.
14. Megarbane B, Borron SW, Trout H, et al: Treatment of acute methanol poisoning with fomepizole. *Intensive Care Med* 27:1370, 2001.
15. Sivilottti MLA, Burns MJ, McMartin KE, et al: Toxicokinetics of ethylene glycol during fomepizole therapy: Implications for management. *Ann Emerg Med* 36:11, 2000.
16. Brown MJ, Shannon MW, Woolf A: Childhood methanol ingestion treated with fomepizole and hemodialysis. *Pediatrics* 108:E77, 2001.
17. American Association of Poison Control Centers: Toxic Exposure Surveillance System (TESS) 2001 Annual Report. Washington, DC, AAPCC, 2001.
18. Brent J, McMartin K, Phillips S, et al: Fomepizole for the treatment of ethylene glycol poisoning. Methylpyrazole for Toxic Alcohols Study Group. *New Engl J Med* 340:832, 1999.

19. Benitez JG, Swanson-Biearman B, Krenzelok EP: Nystagmus secondary to fomepizole administration in a pediatric patient. *J Toxicol Clin Toxicol* 238:795, 2000.

OPIOIDS
Suzanne Doyon

Opioids refer to all agonist, antagonist, endogenous, and exogenous substances that possess morphine-like activity. In the United States, the most commonly abused opioids are heroin and methadone. In 2001, heroin-related visits occurred in 0.1 percent of all ED encounters and in 13 percent to 14 percent of ED encounters involving substances of abuse in the United States. That same year, mentions of prescription opioid analgesics, including methadone, also constituted 0.1 percent of all ED encounters. ED mentions of hydrocodone (Vicodin) and oxycodone (Percocet, OxyContin) have almost doubled since 1999, while mentions of codeine have significantly decreased.[1]

PHARMACOLOGY

Opioids modulate nociception in the terminals of afferent nerves in the central nervous system (CNS) and peripheral nervous system (PNS) and the gastrointestinal tract. They are agonists at the μ, κ, and σ receptors in these tissues. Importantly, the International Union of Pharmacology has adopted a new nomenclature for opioid receptors. The μ is now called OP3, κ, OP2, and σ, OP1, reflecting the chronologic order of discovery. Although there are similarities between these receptor types, such as linkage to a G-protein, they vary largely and are considered nonuniform. Furthermore, individual receptors have specific and different distribution throughout the CNS and PNS.[2] The orphanin, sigma, and epsilon receptors are no longer considered opioid receptors because they lack sensitivity to naloxone or are not found in humans.[3]

Importantly, binding of a drug to a receptor is not limited to one receptor type. Specificity and affinity of a drug for opioid receptors is variable. For example, tramadol possesses 1/6000 the affinity of morphine at the OP3 receptor site.

Stimulation of the OP3 receptors, further subdivided into subtypes a and b, results in analgesia, respiratory depression, cough suppression, and, occasionally, euphoria.[3] For example, most of the analgesic effect of morphine is mediated via OP3a stimulation. All currently available opioids have some activity at the OP3b receptor and result in

some degree of respiratory compromise. Stimulation of OP2 receptors results in spinal analgesia, miosis, and diuresis. The clinical role of OP1 receptors is largely unknown.[3]

Interestingly, there is a lot of interplay between opioid receptors and other receptors. For example, *N*-methyl-D-aspartate (NMDA) receptor blockade enhances the analgesic effect of morphine. Another example of receptor interplay is the localized release of dopamine in the mesolimbic pathway (often referred to as the "pleasure pathway") common to almost all OP3 and OP1 opioids. The end result is a variable feeling of euphoria. Heroin and fentanyl, two exquisitely lipophilic opioids that have high affinity for the OP3 and OP1 receptors, are euphoria-inducing. A third example of receptor interplay is the induction of mast cell histamine release by morphine and meperidine.[3]

PHARMACOKINETICS

A detailed discussion of the absorption, distribution, and elimination of opioids is beyond the scope of this chapter. However, knowledge of duration of action and elimination half-life is useful and is provided in Table 167-1. Most opioids are more effective given parenterally than orally. This phenomenon is due to variable but significant first pass effect. Opioids with good oral potency are codeine, oxycodone, levorphanol, and methadone. The metabolism of codeine, morphine, propoxyphene, oxycodone, meperidine, and methadone is mostly hepatic. The hepatic metabolites may be pharmacologically active. Concurrent use or abuse of benzodiazepines, barbiturates, and alcohol is common. Coingestants, like antiretroviral agents, can inhibit the hepatic metabolism, especially the metabolism of methadone. Further discussion of opioid pharmacology is found in Chaps. 36 and 38.

CLINICAL FEATURES

The opioid intoxication toxidrome encompasses a wide variety of signs and symptoms. Opioids cause respiratory depression, mental status changes, analgesia, miosis, orthostatic hypotension, nausea and vomiting (especially if opioid-naïve), histamine release resulting in localized urticaria and bronchospasm, decreased gastrointestinal (GI) motility, and urinary retention secondary to increased vesical sphincter tone. The depression of the mental status can be variable but may be extremely profound. The respiratory depression may also be variable. One should look for shallow respirations, cyanosis, bradypnea, hypercarbia, and hypoxia. Miosis is not universally present. In fact, normal or even enlarged pupils have been documented secondary to exposure to meperidine, morphine, propoxyphene, pentazocine, and diphenoxylate. Mydriasis can also result from coingestants or may signal severe cerebral hypoxia.

TABLE 167-1   Classification and Characteristics of Major Opioid Agonists

	Analgesic Dose Equivalent to 10 mg of Morphine (mg)	Analgesic Duration of Action (h)	Elimination Half-Life (h)
Natural			
Codeine	120	4–5	2.2–3.6
Morphine	10	4–5	1.4–2.4
Semisynthetic			
Heroin	5	4–5	0.5
Hydromorphone (Dilaudid)	1.3	4–5	2–3
Oxycodone (Percodan, OxyContin)	10	4–5	—
Oxymorphone (Numorphan)	1	4–6	2–3
Hydrocodone (Vicodin)	10	4–6	3.5–4.5
Synthetic			
Diphenoxylate (Lomotil)	2.5	—	—
Fentanyl (Sublimaze)	0.125	1	1.5–6.0
Meperidine (Demerol)	75	2–4	2.4–4.0
Methadone (Dolophine)	65	4–5	24–48
Propoxyphene (Darvon)	240	4–6	6–12

DIAGNOSIS

The diagnoses of opioid overdose or withdrawal remain clinical. The classic triad of coma, miosis, and respiratory depression strongly suggests opioid intoxication, chronic or acute. Studies attempted to determine clinical criteria predictive of the presence of opioid overdose. The criteria of respirations ≤12 breaths/min, presence of miosis, and circumstantial evidence of opioid use (drug paraphernalia, needle marks, presence of a tourniquet, bystander corroboration) were highly sensitive in predicting response to naloxone (92 percent), hence establishing the diagnosis of exposure to opioids.[4] Unfortunately, in this study, only a respiratory rate was used as a measure of respiratory depression, not an assessment of depth or quality of respirations, nor a pulse oximetry or blood gas measurement. A detailed review suggests examination of the urine for opioids may aid in the diagnosis of opioid intoxication but the results have a high false negative rate and are not immediately available to the clinician.[4]

The diagnosis of opioid withdrawal is established when a constellation of withdrawal symptoms are temporally related to the abrupt cessation of a licit or illicit opioid, or both.

Differential Diagnosis

The differential diagnosis of opioid overdose includes the effects of other agents such as clonidine, organophosphates and carbamates, phenothiazines, sedative-hypnotic agents, and carbon monoxide. Clonidine overdoses are characterized by periods of apnea that respond to tactile or auditory stimulation. Organophosphate and carbamate overdoses cause muscle fasciculations, profuse vomiting and diarrhea, and sweating. Phenothiazines cause CNS depression and miosis from decreased adrenergic tone. Olanzapine and risperidone overdoses are associated with profound CNS depression and miosis. γ-Hydroxybutyrate is also associated with profound CNS depression, bradypnea, and, occasionally, miosis. Sedative-hypnotic agent and carbon monoxide cause profound CNS depression but are not usually associated with miosis. Hypoglycemia, hypoxia, CNS infections, postictal states, and pontine hemorrhages should also be considered in the differential diagnosis.

The differential diagnosis of withdrawal includes drugs and toxins that promote an adrenergic state, other drug withdrawals, and other conditions such as hyperthyroidism. Most patients will volunteer the diagnosis of opiate withdrawal in their history.

TREATMENT

Proper airway management is crucial to proper treatment of opioid intoxicated individuals. Bag-valve-mask support may be needed initially to help maintain adequate oxygenation. It may be followed by the administration of naloxone, endotracheal intubation, or both.

Naloxone was introduced in 1976. It is a pure antagonist at all OP receptors, with particular affinity for the OP3 receptor. Naloxone competitively binds to the OP receptors preventing the binding of any other agonist, partial agonist, or mixed agonist-antagonist, but without producing any effect, positive or negative, on the receptor proper. Naloxone can fully reverse the opioid-induced respiratory depression, mental status changes, miosis, and analgesia. Administration of naloxone to opioid-naïve individuals results in little or no effect, even when large, supratherapeutic doses are used. Opioid antagonists, such as naloxone and the longer-acting naltrexone, have been studied in the treatment of acute spinal cord injury, cocaine and ethanol dependence, acute overdoses of ethanol, clonidine, and valproic acid with mixed results.

Naloxone can be administered intravenously, intratracheally, intramuscularly, subcutaneously, intralingually, and occasionally, in the erectile tissue of the penis. The intravenous route is preferred. Onset of action after intravenous injection is extremely rapid, in the order of

1 to 2 min. The duration of action of naloxone is 20 to 60 min, shorter that that of most opioids. Its elimination half-life is 60 to 90 min.

The reversal effects of a dose of naloxone is variable and is largely dependent on the dose of opioid. A very small dose, for example 0.05 mg IV, is recommended in an opioid-dependent individual who presents with CNS depression but with minimal respiratory depression. Naloxone 0.4 mg IV is recommended in the non-opioid-dependent individual who presents with CNS depression but with minimal respiratory depression. This dose, however, may induce withdrawal in the opioid-dependent individual. Escalating doses (titration) of naloxone 0.05 to 0.4 mg IV can be administered until desired effect. Incremental dosing of naloxone will avoid the acute precipitation of opioid withdrawal. A full 2.0 mg IV should be administered to the patient presenting with significant respiratory depression, regardless of drug use history. In the latter cases, repeated doses of 2 mg IV every 3 min are recommended, until a maximum of 10 mg IV has been reached or respiratory depression is reversed. Exposures to propoxyphene, fentanyl, pentazocine, or dextromethorphan, and sustained-release preparation of oxycodone may require these larger-than-ordinary doses.

Recent literature recommends the same dose ranges in the pediatric patient. However, there is one exception to this recommendation, naloxone 0.01 mg/kg IV is still recommended to treat CNS and respiratory depression in the neonate in the immediate postpartum period.[5]

The therapeutic dose of naloxone varies somewhat from the diagnostic dose. Reversal of opioid toxicity with naloxone will last 20 to 60 min. Repeated intravenous boluses or naloxone infusions are occasionally required in order to support respirations. This is especially true for long-acting opioids such as propoxyphene, methadone, or Levo-alpha-acetylmethadol (LAAM), or for sustained-release preparations. A continuous infusion should only be considered if the patient has responded to the naloxone bolus and requires multiple subsequent boluses. To calculate the infusion rate and dose, the initial bolus dose that was successful in reversing the respiratory depression, i.e., the "wake-up dose," is determined. Administer two-thirds of the wake-up dose per hour by intravenous infusion. For example, two-thirds of a 1-mg dose is approximately 0.6 mg. Multiplying that dose by a factor of 10 equals 6 mg. Mix 6 mg of naloxone in 1 L of D5W and run at 100 mL/h. Adjustments in infusion rates may be required if the patient develops respiratory depression (rebolus and increase infusion rates) or withdrawal symptoms (decrease infusion rates). It is recommended that patients maintained on naloxone infusions be admitted to a monitored unit.[5]

Naloxone has a remarkably safe profile. The most common adverse effects associated with naloxone (anxiety, nausea, vomiting, diarrhea, abdominal cramps, piloerection, yawning, and rhinorrhea) are related to the precipitation of the opioid withdrawal syndrome. Again, the precipitation of opioid withdrawal can be minimized by careful naloxone dosing.[5–8]

Endotracheal intubation is a therapeutic option in some cases of opioid overdoses with severe respiratory depression unresponsive to naloxone, where adequate ventilation cannot be achieved by bag-valve-mask.[9] Endotracheal intubation offers the advantage of protecting the airway, easy access for suctioning, alternate route of administration for naloxone, and total airway control. Rapid sequence intubation, omitting the administration of anesthetic/ sedative agents, is the preferred technique. In experienced hands, endotracheal intubation is not associated with many complications.

For ingested opioids, gastric decontamination may be worthwhile. Syrup of ipecac and gastric lavage are not recommended because of the potential risk of aspiration of stomach contents in patients with altered mental status. Activated charcoal should be administered if large amounts of opioids have been ingested with 1 h of presentation to the ED. This time frame can be extended under special circumstances. Fifty grams of activated charcoal PO, followed by a cathartic such as sorbitol 0.5 to 1.0 g PO are standard doses. Delayed and multiple doses of activated charcoal may be useful in diphenoxylate hydrochloride-atropine sulfate (Lomotil) overdoses and in cases of large ingestions of sustained-release preparations.

An acetaminophen level should be obtained in cases of propoxyphene, oxycodone, hydrocodone, tramadol, and codeine overdose, as well as any intentional suicidal ingestion.

The optimal observation period after an opioid intoxication has not been defined for most opioids. Although some authors report a 0 percent incidence of recurrence of toxicity, a more recent, larger, and better-designed study including exposures to a multitude of different opioids reported a 30 percent incidence of recurrence of toxicity.[10] Therefore, an observation period of 4 to 6 h in the ED is recommended for most cases of opioid intoxication. Except in certain cases illustrated below, it is acceptable to discharge the opioid-intoxicated patient after this reasonable period of observation, especially if the patient has demonstrated complete resolution of all symptoms and signs. The moderate to severely intoxicated patient with an exposure to a long-acting opioid like propoxyphene, methadone, or LAAM, or after an ingestion of a sustained release preparations usually requires a 24- to 48-h hospital admission.[8] A psychiatric evaluation is needed for all exposures with suicidal intent.

SPECIAL CONSIDERATIONS

Meperidine

Meperidine and its metabolite, normeperidine, are proconvulsive agents. Normeperidine is reported to have twice the convulsant activity of meperidine. This explains why meperidine overdoses may cause seizures in the absence of hypoxia.[8] Normeperidine is largely renally excreted and will accumulate in cases where renal function is diminished: chronic renal failure, cancer, elderly, and sickle cell patients. Orally administered meperidine is more likely to lead to an accumulation of the toxic metabolite than is parenterally administered meperidine because of a large first-pass effect. Therefore, patients with underlying renal dysfunction who receive oral meperidine, especially repeated doses, are at increased risk of developing toxic seizures. Seizures are quite variable in pattern, from multifocal myoclonus to generalized tonic-clonic seizures. Patients with meperidine-induced seizures are observed for 24 to 48 h in the hospital and should receive a full seizure diagnostic evaluation. Seizures are best treated with small amounts of benzodiazepines only and avoidance of meperidine.

Serotonin Syndrome

The combination of meperidine or dextromethorphan with monoamine oxidase inhibitors (MAOIs) can result in an increase in the amount of serotonin in the neuronal terminals in the CNS. The serotonin syndrome is characterized by disorientation, severe hyperthermia, hypo-/hypertension, and muscle rigidity. Deaths have been reported. Treatment involves the administration of benzodiazepines, aggressive cooling methods, and the avoidance of naloxone.

Propoxyphene

Propoxyphene and its metabolite, norpropoxyphene, are cardiotoxic and neurotoxic. Propoxyphene overdoses have been associated with intraventricular conduction disturbances, heart block, prolonged QT interval, and ventricular bigeminy. Both propoxyphene and norpropoxyphene block fast sodium channels in myocardial tissue. Seizures have also been documented secondary to propoxyphene overdoses. Naloxone cannot reverse either of these independently occurring effects. For propoxyphene overdose, place the patient on a cardiac monitor. If, after 6 h, the patient is asymptomatic and the electrocardiogram (ECG) is normal, the patient can be referred to psychiatry or

discharged. Symptomatic patients or those with an abnormal ECG should be admitted and monitored for 24 to 48 h. The administration of sodium bicarbonate, 1 mEq/kg IV, may reverse the cardiotoxic effects of propoxyphene, by overcoming the sodium channel blockade and restoring sodium channel function.

Mixed Agonist-Antagonists

The mixed agonist-antagonists include pentazocine (Talwin), butorphanol (Stadol), and nalbuphine (Nubain). These agents have variable but mostly antagonist activity at the OP3 receptor. They may cause significant naloxone-responsive respiratory depression in overdose. Mixed agonists-antagonists usually precipitate withdrawal when taken in excess by an opioid-dependent individual, hence reducing the potential for abuse.

Diphenoxylate Hydrochloride-Atropine Sulfate (Lomotil)

Diphenoxylate hydrochloride-atropine sulfate is a frequently prescribed antidiarrheal agent. The medication is manufactured in a pill form containing a combination of diphenoxylate hydrochloride 2.5 mg and atropine sulfate 0.025 mg (Lomotil). It is a schedule IV drug. Initially, an anticholinergic toxidrome dominates the clinical picture, with flushing, tachycardia, hyperthermia, hallucinations, dry mucous membranes, and urinary retention. These signs and symptoms regress as the patient enters the second phase of intoxication, which is characterized by a predominantly opioid-like picture caused by the effects of diphenoxylate hydrochloride. There are two important caveats to remember when treating a patient intoxicated with this mixed ingestion. First, children younger than 6 years of age can be particularly sensitive to diphenoxylate hydrochloride. Second, absorption can be delayed up to 6 to 12 h in some cases. Current recommendations are that all children younger than age 6 years be admitted to the hospital and closely observed for 24 h because signs of respiratory depression may be delayed and severe. Multiple-dose activated charcoal is recommended in all cases of moderate to severe Lomotil intoxication. Adults appear to be somewhat resistant to the toxic effects of Lomotil but should still be observed in the ED for 6 h.

Tramadol

Tramadol (Ultram, Ultracet) overdoses are associated with agitation, hypertension, respiratory depression, seizures, and death, especially at doses exceeding 500 mg orally in an adult. Treatment remains supportive. Naloxone is ineffective in reversing seizures. Withdrawal to tramadol is expected in long-term tolerant individuals. It is treated the same way as other opioid-withdrawal syndromes.

Oxycodone

Oxycodone has become a very popular street drug of abuse. Sustained-release oxycodone preparations (OxyContin) are readily available in the United States. Large overdoses have resulted in life-threatening toxicity and death.[8] Crushing the tablet will destroy the drug-delivery mechanism and make the drug immediately available. Ingestion, insufflation, or injection of crushed oxycodone is common and is associated with a large number of deaths in the United States. Large OxyContin overdoses may be resistant to even large doses of naloxone.[8]

Acute Lung Injury

Special mention must be made of opioid-induced acute lung injury (previously known as noncardiogenic pulmonary edema), a rare complication associated with toxicity from some drugs, including opioids. Acute lung injury can occur immediately or be delayed up to 24 h following heroin or methadone abuse and should be suspected in any patient who develops tachypnea, rales, or decreased oxygen saturation with a normal cardiac silhouette on x-ray. An older study reported a 48 percent incidence among heroin abusers.[10] However, street heroin in the United States was less potent (i.e., lower concentration) at the time of the study than currently, and adulterants may have played a role in pulmonary toxicity. The pathophysiology is poorly understood, but some degree of direct capillary injury is present. Treatment includes positive oxygenation, intubation, and use of end-expiratory pressure. Monitoring with Swan-Ganz catheterization is recommended. Naloxone, diuretics, and digoxin are usually not indicated.

Mixed Drugs

The administration of naloxone as an antidote for heroin-cocaine (Speedball) and heroin-scopolamine (Polo, Homicide, Sting, etc.) mixtures may "unmask" the underlying cocaine or scopolamine intoxication. Cocaine has a relatively short duration of action but the same is not true of scopolamine. Unmasked scopolamine overdoses often require control with benzodiazepines. Physostigmine can be given to reverse scopolamine toxicity, but should only be given by experienced physicians familiar with the use of this antidote.[11]

Body Stuffers/Packers

Retained drug packets pose special challenges to the clinician. Current literature supports the use of a polyethylene glycol solution (GoLYTELY) administered by nasogastric tube at a rate of 2 L/h in adult patients, until the rectal effluent is clear. Multiple dose activated charcoal is also recommended. Large doses of naloxone may be required to reverse the respiratory depression associated with the leakage or breakage of the packets.

Contaminants

Intravenous heroin continues to contain many adulterants, including strychnine, quinine, lactose, and talc. The actual role of many adulterants in the etiology of medical illnesses attributable to intravenous drug usage remains largely unknown. An exception to this statement must be made in the case of 1-methyl-4-phenyl-1,2,3,6-tetrahydropyridine (MPTP). A meperidine analog was synthesized in the 1980s that contained a contaminant called MPTP. When used IV, it caused a severe form of movement disorder similar to Parkinson disease. MPTP is metabolized by monoamine oxidase B in the substantia nigra to mercaptopyrazidepyrimidine (MPP), which is directly neurotoxic.[12]

Medical Complications

Chap. 306 discusses Medical complications from intravenous drug use.

OPIOID WITHDRAWAL

Downregulation of endogenous endorphins, dynorphins, and opioid receptors occurs from chronic usage. Abrupt cessation of opioid use does not allow time for upregulation of receptors and results in increased neuronal firing and withdrawal.

Opioid withdrawal usually starts with feelings of anxiety, insomnia, yawning, lacrimation, diaphoresis, rhinorrhea, and diffuse myalgias. It then progresses to piloerection, mydriasis, nausea, profuse vomiting, diarrhea, and abdominal cramping. Opioid withdrawal reactions are very uncomfortable but are not of themselves life-threatening. Vomiting and aspiration of gastric contents can cause pneumonitis and vomiting and diarrhea can cause dehydration and electrolyte disturbances. Onset of withdrawal is usually within 12 h of last heroin usage and within 30 h of last methadone exposure. It can be precipitated by the administration of antagonists such as naloxone or the longer-acting naltrexone or the administration of partial agonists such as buprenorphine. Symptoms of opioid withdrawal can be rendered more tolerable by the administration of the central α_2-agonist clonidine, antiemetics, and antidiarrheal agents. Clonidine may be used at a dose of 5 μg/kg PO if the blood pressure is above 90 mm Hg systolic.

The management of opioid-dependent individuals hospitalized for medical or surgical reasons remains controversial. It is generally agreed upon that detoxification from opioids during the acute course of a medical illness is usually unsuccessful. Alleviation of withdrawal symptoms should be the goal of therapy. Daily administration of a verified dose of methadone PO (or half the verified dose IM if the patient's status is NPO) is recommended to inhibit withdrawal symptoms and reduce craving. This applies only to individuals who are actively enrolled in a methadone maintenance program and in whom the dose can be verified. The habitual user who is not on methadone maintenance therapy can receive methadone 20 mg PO or 10 mg IM. These dosages should inhibit withdrawal symptoms but not induce euphoria. **No methadone should be administered to the habitual user until the appearance of withdrawal symptoms.** Buprenorphine (Buprenex) is a partial agonist that is, in its parenteral form, Food and Drug Administration approved for the treatment of pain. Suprenorphine (Suboxone) in its oral form is approved for the treatment of opioid detoxification and for opioid maintenance. It is not currently approved for the treatment of opioid withdrawal. However, some authors have demonstrated that buprenorphine 0.3 to 1.2 mg IV or IM every 6 h can safely be administered to medically ill opioid-dependent patients experiencing withdrawal.[13] The practice of administering buprenorphine before discharging a patient, or in an outpatient nondrug treatment setting, is strongly discouraged. If buprenorphine is administered before the onset of objective signs of withdrawal, it will precipitate withdrawal in the opioid-dependent individual who recently used an opioid.

REFERENCES

1. Substance Abuse and Mental Health Services Administration Office of Applied Studies: *Emergency Department Trends from the Drug Abuse Warning Network, Final Estimates 1994–2001,* DAWN Series D-21, DHHS Publication No (SMA) 02-3635, Rockville, MD, 2002.
2. Stein C: The control of pain in peripheral tissues by opioids. *New Engl J Med* 332 (25):1685, 1995.
3. Dhawan BN, Cesselin F, Raghubir R, et al. Internation Union of Pharamcology XII. Classification of opioid receptors. *Pharmacol Rev* 48:567, 1996.
4. Hoffman JR, Schriger DL, Luo J: The empiric use of naloxone in patients with altered mental status: A reappraisal. *Ann Emerg Med* 20(3):246, 1991.
5. Moore PA, Rumack BH, Conner CS, et al: Naloxone underdosage after narcotic poisoning. *Am J Dis Child* 134:156, 1981.
6. Goldfrank LR, Weisman RS: A dosing nomogram for continuous infusion intravenous naloxone. *Ann Emerg Med* 15(5):566, 1986.
7. Schug SA, Zech D, Grond S: Adverse effects of systemic opioid analgesics. *Drug Saf* 7(3):200, 1992.
8. Schneir AB, Vadeboncoeur TF, Offerman SR, Barry JD, Williams SR, Clark RF: Massive OxyContin ingestion refractory to naloxone. *Ann Emerg Med* 40:425, 2002.
9. Smith DA, Leake L, Loffin JR, Yealy DM: Is admission after intravenous heroin overdose necessary? *Ann Emerg Med* 21:1326, 1992.
10. Duberstein JL, Kaufman DM: A clinical study of an epidemic of heroin intoxication and heroin induced pulmonary edema. *Am J Med* 51:704, 1971.
11. Perrone JM, Hamilton RH, Nelson L, et al: Scopolamine poisoning among heroin users—New York City, Philadelphia, and Baltimore 1995 and 1996. *MMWR* 45:392, 1996.
12. Burns RS, Lewitt PA, Ebert MH, et al: The clinical syndrome of striatal dopamine deficiency: Parkinsonism induced by MPTP. *New Engl J Med* 312:1418, 1985.
13. Welsh CJ, Meenakshi S, Cohen A, Boyles L, Bennett M, Weintraub E: The use of intravenous buprenorphine in the treatment of opioid withdrawal in medially ill hospitalized patients. *Am J Addict* 11:135, 2002.

168

COCAINE, AMPHETAMINES, CAFFEINE, AND NICOTINE
Jeanmarie Perrone
Robert S. Hoffman

COCAINE AND AMPHETAMINES

The life-threatening nature of cocaine toxicity is common knowledge as a result of the many reports of actors, musicians, and athletes who have died from the drug. These drugs produce toxicity by activating the sympathetic nervous system. Although cocaine abuse is the most commonly reported cause of serious stimulant toxicity, amphetamines and other substances that resemble cocaine also produce unique toxic complications. The regional prevalence of each of these drugs of abuse may help the clinician discern which agent is present in a patient with sympathomimetic findings.

Epidemiology

Cocaine abuse is a major problem in the United States, especially in urban areas, although any assessment of prevalence is limited. The 2000 National Household Survey on Drug Abuse reported that 1.2 million Americans were current cocaine users.[1] This represents 0.5 percent of the population aged 12 years and older. The estimated number of persons using crack cocaine in the year 2000 was 265,000.[2] Cocaine use is highest among young persons aged 18 to 25 years and appears to be increasing in this age group. In 1998, it was estimated that there are more than half a million new cocaine users each year.[2]

ED visits by cocaine-abusing patients have tripled since 1988. Fatal injuries (homicides, suicides, falls, and overdoses) following cocaine use are a leading cause of death among young adults in New York City, and probably in many other urban environments as well.[3] A 3-year study demonstrated cocaine metabolites in 26 percent, and free cocaine in 18 percent, of all patients with fatal injuries. Methamphetamine use is reported as a frequent cause of drug-related ED visits in the western United States, and its use is increasing in other regions.

Cocaine

Cocaine is the naturally occurring alkaloidal extract of *Erythroxylum coca*, a plant indigenous to South America. The water-soluble hydrochloride salt is absorbed across all mucosal surfaces, including the oral, nasal, gastrointestinal, and vaginal epithelium; thus cocaine can be applied topically, swallowed, or injected intravenously. Although the hydrochloride form is most often insufflated (snorted) or injected intravenously, ether extraction yields crack cocaine, a form that is stable to pyrolysis and can be smoked, producing the popping sound that characterizes its name. The onset and duration of action vary with the route of administration. When cocaine is insufflated nasally, the peak effect occurs within 30 min and the duration of effect is 1 to 3 h. The delayed and prolonged effect is a result of vasoconstrictive properties that limit mucosal absorption. A portion of insufflated cocaine is swallowed and thus absorbed from the stomach as well. Gastrointestinal absorption is also delayed by vasoconstriction, producing a peak effect at 90 min and a duration of effect as long as 3 h. Both the intravenous and the inhalational routes produce a rapid peak effect (within 30 s to 2 min), with a duration of effect of 15 to 30 min. This rapidly intense onset but brief duration of drug effect is theorized to explain why more crime and increased risk of human immunodeficiency virus (HIV) infection is associated with this highly addictive drug; more frequent use is required to maintain the "high." Each use increases the risk. Cocaine is primarily metabolized to ecgonine methyl ester by plasma cholinesterase. Relative deficiency of this enzyme may predispose affected patients to life-threatening toxicity.[4] Benzoylecgonine is the other major metabolite excreted in the urine and is the one routinely tested by most urine toxicology screens.

Cocaine is both a local anesthetic and a central nervous system (CNS) stimulant. Like other local anesthetics, cocaine inhibits conduction of nerve impulses by blocking fast sodium channels in the cell membrane. Cocaine also has quinidine-like effects on conduction causing QRS widening and QT_c prolongation. Thus, in large doses, cocaine may exert a direct toxic effect on the myocardium resulting in negative inotropy, wide-complex dysrhythmia, bradycardia, and hypotension. Central effects are mediated through activation of the sympathetic nervous system via enhanced effects of excitatory amino acids and blockade of presynaptic reuptake of norepinephrine, dopamine, and serotonin. The resultant excess of neurotransmitters at postsynaptic receptor sites leads to sympathetic activation, producing the characteristic physical findings of mydriasis, tachycardia, hypertension, and diaphoresis, and predisposing the user to dysrhythmias, seizures, and hyperthermia. Cocaine use produces a euphoria associated with enhanced alertness and a general sense of well-being. It is thought that the psychological addiction, drug craving, and withdrawal effects are mediated through interference with dopamine and serotonin balance in the central nervous system. Subsequent dopamine depletion at the nerve terminals may account for the dysphoria and depression associated with long-term abuse. Many of the ED visits attributed to cocaine are for the depression associated with chronic abuse.

Amphetamines

Amphetamines comprise a broad class of structurally similar derivatives of phenylethylamine. The derivative methamphetamine, also known as "ice," is abused by ingestion, intravenous injection, inhalation, or insufflation. Methylphenidate (Ritalin), widely prescribed for attention deficit disorder, has become a popular drug of abuse by insufflation of crushed tablets. As with cocaine, amphetamine's absorption and peak effects occur rapidly with inhalation, insufflation, and intravenous injection. However, the effects of some amphetamines such as methamphetamine (MDA) and methylenedioxymethamphetamine (MDMA) may persist for 12 h.

Amphetamines enhance the release and block the reuptake of catecholamines and may also directly stimulate catecholamine receptors. Some amphetamine metabolites inhibit monoamine oxidase, thus also increasing cytoplasmic concentrations of norepinephrine. Certain amphetamine derivatives can also induce release of serotonin and affect central serotonin receptors. These serotonergic effects account for the hallucinogenic properties of some amphetamine derivatives such as MDMA and methylenedioxyethamphetamine (MDEA or mescaline). Dopamine receptor activity may contribute to the withdrawal phenomenon. Mortality from amphetamine toxicity, like that from cocaine, is a result of hyperthermia, dysrhythmias, seizures, hypertension (intracranial hemorrhage or infarction), and encephalopathy.

The stimulants ephedrine and phenylpropanolamine produce toxic syndromes similar to those caused by cocaine and amphetamines, although there are some distinguishing features. Phenylpropanolamine, previously available in many over-the-counter diet aids and decongestants, was withdrawn from the market in December 2000, because of the increased risk of intracranial hemorrhage associated with its use.[5] It is primarily a peripheral α-adrenergic agonist that causes significant vasoconstriction resulting in hypertension and, often, a marked reflex bradycardia. Although less-commonly available now, overdose from supplies in the home may lead to hypertensive encephalopathy or cerebrovascular accident.

Ephedrine is a plant-derived indirect-acting sympathomimetic with both α- and β-adrenergic activity caused by the release of dopamine and norepinephrine from neuronal stores. It is widely available as a "natural" stimulant in health food supplements promoted for dieting, energy, and to stay alert. Significant cardiovascular and neurologic toxicity, psychosis and severe hypertension have been reported, including several deaths.[6]

CLINICAL FEATURES

Cardiac

Cocaine induces dysrhythmias, myocarditis, cardiomyopathy, and myocardial ischemia and infarction. Other vascular complications include aortic rupture and aortic and coronary artery dissection. Even at relatively low doses, cocaine induces vasoconstriction in coronary arteries,[7] one of the proposed mechanisms of cocaine-induced myocardial ischemia and infarction. Coronary vasoconstriction is exacerbated by β-adrenergic blockade and antagonized by phentolamine, suggesting that it is mediated through the stimulation of α-adrenergic receptors.[7,8] This effect is even further potentiated by cigarette smoking. Myocardial ischemia has also been demonstrated in chronic abusers undergoing cocaine withdrawal. It is thought that cocaine withdrawal is a dopamine-depleted state, resulting in intermittent coronary spasm. Animal data demonstrate increased platelet aggregation and thrombogenesis, accelerated atherosclerosis, direct myocardial toxicity, and increased myocardial oxygen demand.

A profile of the patient at risk for myocardial ischemia can be elucidated from a compilation of 91 case reports of patients with cocaine-induced myocardial infarction and a prospective evaluation of patients with cocaine-associated chest pain.[9,10] The average patient with cocaine-associated myocardial infarction was young and male (mean age 32.8 years, range 18 to 52; male:female ratio, 7:1) and most (83 to 89%) were cigarette smokers and regular cocaine users. Two-thirds of patients presented within 3 h of cocaine use, and all routes of cocaine administration were reported. Of the patients with follow-up cardiac catheterization, coronary artery disease was present in 31%. Electrocardiographic (ECG) abnormalities were variably present, and both Q-wave and non-Q-wave infarctions occurred. Many studies have reported myocardial infarction in patients with atypical histories and unremarkable ECGs.

Myocardial ischemia and infarction and aortic dissection are also reported in association with ephedrine, phenylpropanolamine, or amphetamine use. Additionally, reports of mitral and aortic valve abnormalities associated with use of the amphetamine combination phentermine-fenfluramine prompted a voluntary recall of these drugs. Cardiopulmonary toxicity from other amphetamine diet aids has also been reported.

Central Nervous System

A vast array of neurologic syndromes is described in association with cocaine abuse, most commonly seizures, intracranial infarctions, and hemorrhages. Pathology results from the hyperadrenergic tone, inducing severe transient hypertension, hemorrhage, or focal vasospasm and, sometimes, exacerbation of underlying abnormalities of cerebral blood vessels. In a dog model, lethal doses of intravenous cocaine initially induced seizures, lactic acidosis, hyperthermia, and death.[11] Progression of toxicity could be prevented by sedation and cooling. In this animal model, diazepam was an optimal sedative because it prevented hyperthermia and seizures and improved survival.

Although coronary vasospasm has been well documented in humans exposed to cocaine, a recent study using magnetic resonance angiography also demonstrated cerebral vasoconstriction following cocaine administration.[12] Other CNS manifestations reported include spinal cord infarctions, cerebral vasculitis, and intracranial abscesses. Acute dystonic reactions following cocaine use and withdrawal are also reported. Choreoathetosis and other repetitive movements (termed "crack dancing") are associated with cocaine and amphetamine intoxication, and all seem to be related to dopamine dysregulation. An interesting syndrome termed "cocaine washout" occurs in patients following a prolonged crack binge. Patients have a depressed level of consciousness but can be aroused to normal with stimulation. Resolution of lethargy can take up to 24 h. Unilateral blindness occurs

secondary to central retinal artery occlusion and bilateral blindness from diffuse vasospasm. A syndrome of corneal abrasions and ulcerations secondary to smoke and irritation is known as "crack eye." Keratitis caused by methamphetamine use is described as well.

Amphetamines, phenylpropanolamine, and ephedrine are also associated with intracranial hemorrhages, infarctions, encephalopathy, and seizures. Amphetamines also cause a CNS vasculitis resulting in focal neurologic deficits. A profound paranoid psychosis occurs with chronic amphetamine abuse and withdrawal.

Pulmonary

Respiratory effects of cocaine use have become more prevalent with the epidemic of crack cocaine smoking. Pulmonary hemorrhage, barotrauma, pneumonitis, asthma, and pulmonary edema are described. Pneumomediastinum, pneumothorax, and pneumopericardium result from barotrauma secondary to the Valsalva maneuver performed following inhalation or insufflation in an attempt to enhance drug effect. Pneumonitis, asthma, and bronchiolitis may be immunologic phenomena or the result of the numerous adulterants known to be present in cocaine. A recent case control study in an urban ED examined the association between bronchospasm and cocaine use. The authors demonstrated a higher incidence of recent cocaine use in patients presenting with new-onset bronchospasm as compared with age- and sex-matched urban ED patients.[13] Another study demonstrated bronchoconstriction following the inhalation of crack but not following intravenous injection of cocaine.[14] This suggests that such bronchospasm may be a result of local airway irritation. Acute lung injury may be catecholamine-mediated, in view of a similar syndrome described in patients with adrenergic excess from pheochromocytoma and intracranial hemorrhage. Upper airway irritation and a presumed thermal uvulitis occurs in patients smoking crack cocaine.

Gastrointestinal

Patients who are thought to have swallowed poorly packaged cocaine following police pursuit are called "body stuffers." Such patients are often brought to the hospital by police and may or may not show signs of cocaine intoxication. In contrast, the "body packer" swallows a large number of well-sealed packages of cocaine in order to smuggle drugs into this country. Because of the large quantities of relatively pure drug contained in these packages, toxicity and death can occur if even a single bag ruptures.

Cocaine-induced mesenteric vasospasm may contribute to the many reported cases of intestinal ischemia, bowel necrosis, ischemic colitis, and splenic infarctions. In addition, gastrointestinal bleeding and perforation occur in association with cocaine use.

Renal

Traumatic and nontraumatic rhabdomyolysis occurs secondary to cocaine or amphetamine use. In an early series of cocaine-induced rhabdomyolysis, one-third of patients developed acute renal failure and half of those died.[15] Risks for developing rhabdomyolysis include altered mental status, seizures, dysrhythmias, and hemodynamic instability including cardiac arrest.[15] **Patients whose initial serum creatine phosphokinase (CPK) is less than 1000 U/L with normal creatinine, white blood cell count, and only one or no risks in addition to cocaine itself, are unlikely to develop complications[12]** and need not necessarily be admitted for this alone. In addition to renal failure resulting from rhabdomyolysis, stimulants may further exacerbate renal injury through hyperthermia, vasoconstriction, hypotension, and hypovolemia. Clinicians must be aware of this potential late complication and augment fluid resuscitation to maintain a urine output of 1 to 3 mL/kg per h. Renal infarction has been described following intravenous cocaine use.

The Pregnant Patient

Cocaine is a potent vasoconstrictor that alters uteroplacental blood flow. An increased incidence of spontaneous abortions,[16] abruptio placentae, fetal prematurity, and intrauterine growth retardation results from cocaine abuse in pregnancy.[17] Both spontaneous abortions and abruptio placentae appear to occur from placental vasoconstriction and increased uterine contractility, with concomitant maternal hypertension. Intoxication of a breast-fed infant secondary to maternal cocaine use has been reported as well. Methamphetamine abuse during pregnancy has similar detrimental effects on fetal growth.

DIAGNOSIS

The cocaine- or amphetamine-intoxicated patient can often be identified initially by vital signs. Adrenergic stimulation may produce tachycardia, tachypnea, hypertension, and sometimes hyperthermia. The patient's mental status can range from normal to paranoid or severely agitated to coma. Organ-system involvement may be suspected from symptoms such as chest pain, palpitations, dyspnea, headache, or focal neurologic complaints. The patient may be postictal or may present with seizures. Other physical findings may include mydriasis and diaphoresis. In the absence of an adequate history, it may be difficult to distinguish this presentation from other conditions of catecholamine excess, such as withdrawal from alcohol or sedative-hypnotics. Metabolic (lactic) acidosis may be present following seizures or as a result of vasoconstriction and hypoperfusion. As with all intoxicated patients, occult trauma and hypoglycemia must be excluded.

Concomitant use of alcohol and other drugs frequently alters the clinical presentation. For example, a patient ingesting both opioids and stimulants may present with a decreased level of consciousness and few if any other revealing findings. When the opioid is reversed with naloxone, the stimulant effects are unmasked, often with impressive findings.

Laboratory Evaluation

Any patient with significant agitation or elevated temperature should have a chemistry panel and creatine phosphokinase (CPK) obtained to screen for a metabolic acidosis, renal failure, or rhabdomyolysis. Hyponatremia, often with altered mental status, occasionally occurs following the use of hallucinogenic amphetamines (e.g., MDMA). Cardiac markers including myocardial band enzymes of creatine phosphokinase (CPK-MB) or troponin are appropriate to screen for cardiac injury. A urine test strip positive for hemoglobin with only few or no red blood cells by microscopy suggests rhabdomyolysis. Obtain baseline coagulation and liver function studies in patients with hyperthermia, because these values increase dramatically in the first 24 h. Most patients with altered mental status who do not awaken with glucose or naloxone should undergo computed tomography of the head, because associated neurovascular injuries are common. A chest radiograph and ECG are fundamental to the evaluation. Laboratory confirmation of cocaine or amphetamine use is readily available but must be interpreted with caution. Because urine drug screening for the cocaine metabolite benzoylecgonine is sensitive to 200 to 300 ng/mL, cocaine use within the past 24 to 72 h will typically be detected, depending on dose and chronicity of cocaine use. Cocaine can be detected in chronic users by more sensitive techniques (radioimmunoassay, gas chromatography) for up to 2 weeks after last use of the drug, so a positive drug screen requires clinical correlation. Most of the rapid screening tests for cocaine are fairly specific for cocaine metabolites and exhibit little cross-reactivity. However, amphetamine immunoassays cross-react with interfering substances and other phenylethylamine compounds, so they are not very specific. In addition, excessive use of certain nasal inhalers that contain stimulant-class drugs may cross-react with immunoassay methods and yield false-positive tests.

TREATMENT

The basic protocol specific to stimulants outlined in Chap. 156 should be followed. Charcoal should be given. Intravenous access should be obtained and supplemental oxygen delivered to those with potential cardiac or CNS ischemia. **The cornerstone of therapy is adequate sedation and monitoring of vital signs.** The patient with hypertension and tachycardia will often respond to treatment with benzodiazepines, which decrease central sympathetic outflow. Lorazepam 2 mg or diazepam 5 mg can be administered intravenously and titrated with repeated doses to decrease the autonomic excess and CNS stimulation. Haloperidol, droperidol, and chlorpromazine should be avoided as these lower the seizure threshold and may contribute to hyperthermia or dysrhythmias. A core temperature should be measured. Hyperthermia is potentially lethal and patients must be cooled rapidly to decrease subsequent morbidity and mortality. Application of ice packs, and coolmist spray to the skin and fans to increase heat loss by convection and evaporation may decrease temperature adequately. See Chap. 193 Heat Emergencies, for further discussion of management of hyperthermia. Aggressive fluid resuscitation is critical to maintain urine output.

Seizures may be treated with benzodiazepines as well (see Chap. 232); however, in status epilepticus, phenobarbital loading or neuromuscular blockade may be necessary to control motor activity and prevent hyperthermia, acidosis, and rhabdomyolysis. Computed tomography is recommended in all cases of stimulant-induced seizures because the finding of intracranial pathology creating a seizure focus is common.

The patient complaining of chest pain should be evaluated for possible myocardial ischemia, as well as for the common pulmonary etiologies already discussed. Patients suspected of acute coronary syndrome should be managed by standard protocol with nitrates, morphine, benzodiazepines and aspirin (see Chap. 51).[18–20] **β-Adrenergic antagonist therapy is absolutely contraindicated** because unopposed stimulation of α-adrenergic receptors may worsen coronary and peripheral vasoconstriction, hypertension, and possibly ischemia.[18,19] This recommendation is also emphasized in the most recent *Advanced Cardiac Life Support Guidelines*. Although labetalol (a mixed α- and β-adrenergic antagonist) has been suggested by some authors, labetalol increases seizures and mortality in an animal model of cocaine toxicity and does not decrease cocaine-induced coronary vasoconstriction in humans. Consultation may be helpful before administering thrombolytic therapy in cocaine-associated myocardial infarction. Despite the increased incidence of coronary atherosclerosis, thrombolytic agents should not be used when severe hypertension is present or vasospasm or coronary artery dissection are suspected.[21,22] Emergent catheterization, when available, is a safer diagnostic and therapeutic alternative.

Wide-complex tachydysrhythmias and QRS prolongation secondary to the quinidine-like effects of cocaine may be treated by alkalinizing the serum to a pH of 7.45 to 7.5 with sodium bicarbonate. Although lidocaine has been used safely in this setting, some animal studies and theoretical evidence suggest that lidocaine may potentiate cocaine neurotoxicity and should be used with caution in patients with dysrhythmias who are not responsive to sodium bicarbonate.

Severe hypertension not responding to sedation may require treatment with nitroprusside infusion or phentolamine (phentolamine starting dose: 2.5 to 5 mg IV). Blood pressure may be lowered aggressively if the patient is not suspected to have chronic hypertensive disease. Treatment for refractory hypertension would be similar to that for hypertensive emergencies of any etiology (see Chap. 57).

The treatment of patients with cardiovascular or neurologic sequelae of amphetamine or other stimulant use is comparable to that outlined for cocaine. Acidification of the urine to increase amphetamine excretion was previously recommended but should not be done because of the increased risk of renal tubular precipitation of myoglobin in the presence of rhabdomyolysis. Dialysis has no value.

The management of an asymptomatic cocaine "body packer" brought in by police or customs officials constitutes a dilemma for the emergency physician. If the patient shows no signs of toxicity, we recommend a dose of activated charcoal followed by whole-bowel irrigation with polyethylene glycol electrolyte lavage solution (GoLYTELY or Colyte) to gently hasten elimination of the potentially lethal packets. If the patient begins to show signs of intoxication, such as agitation, hypertension, or tachycardia, benzodiazepines should be administered while immediate surgical consultation for emergent laparotomy and packet removal is made. Neither upper nor lower endoscopy should be routinely attempted because both routes are associated with packet rupture. Following passage of the "last" packet, a radiologic imaging procedure (a barium-enhanced upper gastrointestinal series with small bowel follow-through or abdominal computed tomography with contrast) should be performed to ensure that the gut has been purged of all containers. In contrast to "body packers," "body stuffers" (people who ingest poorly packaged drugs while trying to avoid arrest) are more likely to be seen in the ED. These patients can be given a dose of activated charcoal, sedated (if indicated), and given supportive care if intoxicated, because the toxicity should be shorter-lived and often involves smaller amounts of drug.

Drug Interactions

There are a few potential drug interactions to be aware of in the treatment of the stimulant-poisoned patient. Because cocaine is metabolized by plasma cholinesterase, coadministration of other drugs such as succinylcholine and mivacurium, which are metabolized by plasma cholinesterase, may have a prolonged duration of effect as a result of decreased metabolism.

Both lidocaine and cocaine are local anesthetics and act as sodium-channel antagonists. It is thought that neurotoxic effects from both occur by similar mechanisms. Despite some theoretical risk of treating cocaine-induced dysrhythmias with lidocaine, it has been used safely to date in patients with cocaine-associated myocardial infarction.

Monoamine oxidase inhibitors block the degradation of catecholamines and lead to increased levels of presynaptic catecholamines. Amphetamines are indirect-acting sympathomimetic amines and weak inhibitors of monoamine oxidase as well. Thus, patients taking monoamine oxidase inhibitors who subsequently use amphetamines or phenylpropanolamine (and to a lesser extent cocaine) may precipitate an acute syndrome of excessive catecholamine release, resulting in severe hypertension, tachycardia, hyperthermia, agitation, tremors, and possible severe neurotoxicity.

Withdrawal

Cocaine withdrawal is characterized by irritability, paranoid ideation, and delayed depression. Symptoms are generally milder than for amphetamines. Psychological addiction may be particularly strong. Amphetamine withdrawal is characterized by drowsiness, lethargy, hunger, tremor, and chills. There is considerable potential for long-term depression and suicide.

DISPOSITION

Patient disposition depends on initial patient presentation, response to therapy, the stimulant involved, and expected duration of effect. Patients who present with adrenergic excess following recent cocaine use and who respond to sedation may be expected to improve completely during a period of observation in the ED secondary to the relatively limited duration of cocaine effect. In contrast, amphetamines have a longer duration of effect and may be expected to produce more prolonged toxicity, necessitating hospital admission or prolonged observation in some cases. Patients demonstrating resolution of toxicity and clear sensorium in the absence of focal complaints or end-organ dam-

age should be advised of the medical risks of their drug abuse and referred to appropriate detoxification, counseling, and social support services. In general, patients with significantly increased creatine phosphokinase levels, hyperthermia, myoglobinuria, or ECG changes consistent with myocardial ischemia should be hospitalized in an intensive care setting.

Disposition of patients who present with cocaine-associated chest pain is discussed in Chap. 51.

CAFFEINE

Caffeine is probably the most commonly used drug in the world. Its ubiquitous presence in coffee, tea, soda, and other drinks allows both for unperceived use and addiction. In addition, the use of large doses of caffeine in products designed to reduce weight or enhance arousal gives rise to the potential for substantial overdose and toxicity (Table 168-1). Although clearly an underestimation of true exposures and toxicity, U.S. poison centers received more than 5000 calls in 2001, including 1 fatality.[23]

Pharmacologically, caffeine (1,3,7-trimethylxanthine) is best described as a methylxanthine, and as such, has properties very similar to theophylline (1,3-dimethylxanthine) and theobromine (3,7-dimethylxanthine) (see Chap. 173). Although caffeine can be administered IV, IM, SC, and PR, the most common route of absorption is PO. Whether in a pill or a liquid, it is rapidly and completely absorbed within approximately 30 to 60 min, depending on the presence of food. Once absorbed, caffeine's mechanism of effect is similar to theophylline, and includes β-adrenergic stimulation (largely through the release of endogenous epinephrine and norepinephrine) adenosine antagonism, and in overdose, phosphodiesterase inhibition.

There is no clearly defined toxic dose. At low doses (approximately 200 mg in adults), the literature is clearly supportive of caffeine's ability to enhance arousal and performance both of cognitive and psychomotor skills.[24] However, at higher doses (about 1 g) toxicity is indistinguishable from theophylline toxicity with severe gastrointestinal symptoms as the first manifestation. This is followed by tachycardia, tachypnea, agitation, and electrolyte abnormalities such as hypokalemia and hyperglycemia. As levels increase, seizures, dysrhythmias, and cardiovascular instability may occur. Ingestions of 100 to 150 mg/kg or blood levels of 100 μg/mL are consistent with life-threatening toxicity.

Treatment begins with basic supportive care. Volume depletion results from vomiting, tachypnea, diuresis, and vasodilation. Therefore, patients with good cardiovascular function should be aggressively resuscitated with NS. Antiemetics, such as metoclopramide (5 to 10 mg IV or IM), will ease gastrointestinal symptoms and facilitate the administration of activated charcoal, which both prevents absorption and

TABLE 168-1   Caffeine Content of Various Products

Product	Caffeine Content, mg
No Doz Maximum, Vivarin	200
Espresso coffee	120
Regular coffee	103
No Doz	100
Jolt Cola	72
Aspirin-free Excedrin	65
Excedrin ES	65
Instant coffee	57
Black tea	53
Most sodas	35–55

enhances elimination. Seizures are best treated with benzodiazepines, followed by barbiturates or propofol (see Chap. 232). Phenytoin is ineffective in theophylline-induced seizures and by analogy should not be used for caffeine toxicity. For life-threatening toxicity such as recurrent seizures, ventricular dysrhythmias or cardiovascular instability hemodialysis or charcoal hemoperfusion is indicated.

NICOTINE

Nicotine is available in all tobacco products (cigarettes, cigars, pipe tobacco, snuff, and chewing tobacco), in smoking cessation products (gums, sprays, and patches), and in liquid form for use as a pesticide. Consequently, like caffeine, nicotine is pervasive in modern society with nearly one fourth of Americans smoking regularly. Although not specifically used or abused as a stimulant, on a pharmacologic level, nicotine is exactly that.

Nicotine is most commonly absorbed through the pulmonary system, but also demonstrates excellent transdermal, transmucosal (oral or nasal), and gastrointestinal absorption. The rate of absorption is highly dependent on the route of administration. For example, following inhalation, CNS levels are achieved in less than 10 s, whereas gastrointestinal absorption is delayed because of poor absorption in the acid stomach.

Once absorbed, nicotine binds to the nicotinic subset of muscarinic receptors in the autonomic, central nervous, and muscular systems. At typical doses used by smokers, an electroencephalogram (EEG) can demonstrate CNS stimulation of the reticular activating system.[25] Clinically, this corresponds to improved memory and attention.[25] As levels increase, nausea, vomiting, salivation, and tremor are common. Hypertension, tachycardia, and seizures may follow. Ultimately, overstimulation of receptors leads to blockade, with coma, hyporeflexia, muscle fasciculations, weakness, and paralysis resulting.[26]

A typical cigarette may contain 13 to 30 mg of nicotine. Although it is generally accepted that a child who ingests more than one cigarette is likely to become symptomatic, life-threatening toxicity would only be expected with exposures to concentrated forms of nicotine such as the pesticides or smoking cessation products.[27] Nicotine levels can be obtained, and levels greater than 50 ng/mL are predictive of severe toxicity. However, levels are not available emergently.

Management begins with decontamination. Gastric emptying is rarely required, as most patients will have spontaneous emesis. Activated charcoal may help prevent absorption of remaining drug, but is typically difficult to administer because of consequential nausea and vomiting. Dermal decontamination with soap and water may be beneficial following topical exposures. Subsequent therapy is completely supportive, as there is no antidote. Benzodiazepines may be used for seizures and endotracheal intubation and mechanical ventilation may be required if significant neuromuscular weakness develops. Fortunately, because nicotine has a very short half-life (on the order of 1 to 4 h in nonsmokers) symptoms typical resolve rapidly.

REFERENCES

1. Office of Applied Studies: *Summary of Findings from the 2000 National Household Survey on Drug Abuse.* Rockville, MD, Substance Abuse and Mental Health Services Administration, October, 2001, http://www.samhsa.gov/oas/drugs.htm#Cocaine.
2. The National Clearinghouse for Alcohol and Drug Information: "Trends in initiation of drug use" Cocaine and Crack Cocaine. http://www.health.org/govstudy/bkd332/8trends.htm.
3. Marzuk PM, Tardiff K, Leon AC, et al: Fatal injuries after cocaine use as a leading cause of death among young adults in New York City. *New Engl J Med* 332:1753, 1995.
4. Hoffman RS, Henry GC, Howland MA, et al: Association between life-threatening cocaine toxicity and plasma cholinesterase activity. *Ann Emerg Med* 21:247, 1992.
5. Kernan WN, Viscoli C, Brass LM, et al: Phenylpropanolamine and the risk of hemorrhagic stroke. *New Engl J Med* 343:1826, 2000.
6. Haller CA, Benowitz NL: Adverse cardiovascular and central nervous system events associated with dietary supplements containing ephedra alkaloids. *New Engl J Med* 343:1833, 2000.
7. Lange RA, Cigarroa RG, Yancy CW, et al: Cocaine-induced coronary artery vasoconstriction. *New Engl J Med* 321:1557, 1989.
8. Lange RA, Cigarroa RG, Flores ED, et al: Potentiation of cocaine-induced coronary vasoconstriction by beta-adrenergic blockade. *Ann Intern Med* 112:897, 1990.
9. Hollander JE, Hoffman RS: Cocaine-induced myocardial infarction: An analysis and review of the literature. *J Emerg Med* 10:169, 1992.
10. Hollander JE, Hoffman RS, Gennis P, et al: Prospective multicenter evaluation of cocaine associated chest pain. *Acad Emerg Med* 1:330, 1994.
11. Catravas JD, Waters IW: Acute cocaine intoxication in the conscious dog: Studies on the mechanism of lethality. *J Pharmacol Exp Ther* 217:350, 1981.
12. Kaufman MJ, Levin JM, Ross MH, et al: Cocaine-induced cerebral vasoconstriction detected in humans with magnetic resonance angiography. *JAMA* 279:376,1998.
13. Osborn HH, Tang M, Bradley K, et al: New onset bronchospasm or recrudescence of asthma associated with cocaine abuse. *Acad Emerg Med* 4:689, 1997.
14. Tashkin DP, Kleerup EC, Koyal SN, et al: Acute effects of inhaled and intravenous cocaine on airway dynamics. *Chest* 110:904, 1996.
15. Brody SL, Wrenn KD, Wilber MM, Slovis CM: Predicting the severity of cocaine associated rhabdomyolysis. *Ann Emerg Med* 19:1137, 1990.
16. Ness RB, Grisso JA, Hirschinger N, et al: Cocaine and tobacco use and the risk of spontaneous abortion. *New Engl J Med* 340:333, 1999.
17. Plessinger MA, Woods JR: Cocaine in pregnancy: Recent data on maternal and fetal risks. *Obstet Gynecol Clin North Am* 25:99, 1998.
18. Hollander JE: The management of cocaine-associated myocardial ischemia. *New Engl J Med* 333:1267, 1995.
19. Lange, RA, Hillis DL: Medical progress: Cardiovascular complications of cocaine use. *New Engl J Med* 345:351, 2001.
20. Weber JE, Shofer FS, Larkin GL, et al: Validation of a brief observation period for patients with cocaine-associated chest pain. *New Engl J Med* 348:510, 2003.
21. Hollander JE, Burstein JL, Hoffman RS, et al: Cocaine-associated myocardial infarction: Clinical safety of thrombolytic therapy. *Chest* 107:1237, 1995.
22. Hollander JE, Wilson LD, Leo PJ, Shih RD: Complications from the use of thrombolytic agents in patients with cocaine associated chest pain. *J Emerg Med* 14:731, 1996.
23. Litovitz TL, Klein-Schwartz W, Rodgers GC Jr, et al: 2001 Annual report of the American Association of Poison Control Centers Toxic Exposure Surveillance System. *Am J Emerg Med* 20:391, 2002.
24. Bryant CA, Farmer A, Tiplady B, et al: Psychomotor performance: investigating the dose-response relationship for caffeine and theophylline in elderly volunteers. *Eur J Clin Pharmacol* 54:309, 1998.
25. Griesar WS, Zajdel DP, Oken BS: Nicotine effects on alertness and spatial attention in non-smokers. *Nicotine Tob Res* 4:185, 2002.
26. Saxena K, Scheman A: Suicide plan by nicotine poisoning: A review of nicotine toxicity. *Vet Hum Toxicol* 27:495, 1985.
27. Smolinske SC, Spoerke DG, Spiller SK, et al: Cigarette and nicotine chewing gum toxicity in children. *Hum Toxicol* 7:27, 1988.

169 HALLUCINOGENS
Karen N. Hansen
Katherine M. Prybys

INTRODUCTION

Over the centuries, humans have purposefully ingested naturally occurring mind-altering substances, such as psilocybin-containing mushrooms and peyote cactus, to achieve mystical or religious enlightenment. Modern interest in hallucinogenic drugs dates from Albert Hofmann's 1943 discovery of the properties of lysergic acid diethylamide (LSD) through inadvertent exposure.

The popularity of hallucinogens (Table 169-1) as recreational drugs peaked in the 1960s, but has undergone a resurgence among

TABLE 169-1 Characteristics of Hallucinogens

Drug	Chemical Classification	Mechanism of Action	Typical Dose	Duration of Action	Clinical Features	Complications	Specific Treatment
LSD	Indole alkylamine	5-HT$_2$ agonist	50–300 μg	8–12 h	Mydriasis Sympathomimetic symptoms Nausea Muscle tension	Persistent psychosis Hallucinogen persisting perception disorder	Supportive Benzodiazepines
Psilocybin	Indole alkylamine	5-HT$_2$ agonist	5–100 mushrooms, 4–6 mg of psilocybin	4–6 h	Mydriasis Sympathomimetic symptoms Nausea	Seizures (rare) Hyperthermia (rare)	Supportive Benzodiazepines
Mescaline	Phenylethylamine	5-HT$_2$ agonist	3–12 "buttons," 200–500 mg of mescaline	6–12 h	Mydriasis Abdominal pain Vomiting Dizziness Sympathomimetic symptoms	Rare	Supportive Benzodiazepines
MDMA ("Ectasy")	Phenylethylamine	5-HT release	50–200 mg	4–6 h	Mydriasis Sympathomimetic symptoms Bruxism Jaw tension Ataxia	Arrhythmias Hypertension Seizures Hyperthermia Rhabdomyolysis DIC Chronic neuropsychiatric problems	Benzodiazepines Hydration Active cooling
Phencyclidine (PCP)	Piperadine derivative	Glutamate antagonist at NMDA receptor	1–9 mg	4–6 h	Miosis or midsized pupils Nystagmus Hypertension Sympathomimetic, anticholinergic, and cholinergic symptoms	Coma Seizures Hyperthermia Rhabdomyolysis Hypertension Hypoglycemia	Benzodiazepines Hydration Active cooling Multiple doses of activated charcoal Alkalinize urine (for rhabdomyolysis)
Marijuana	Cannabinoid	Binds cannabinoid receptor	5–15 mg of THC	2–4 h	Tachycardia Conjunctival injection Impaired motor coordination	Rare	Supportive Benzodiazepines

Abbreviations: DIC = disseminated intravascular coagulation; NMDA = N-methyl-D-aspartate; THC = tetrahydrocannabinol.

adolescents and young adults which started in the early 1990s.[1] According to data from the Monitoring the Future study,[2] use of LSD within the U.S. has declined over the past few years, while marijuana and MDMA ("ecstasy" or "Adam") have become increasingly popular. In 2001, 6.6 percent of high school seniors reported using LSD within the previous 30 days, and 10.9 percent had used it at least once in their life.[2] In the same year, 37 percent of high school seniors reported recent use of marijuana, and a remarkable 49 percent admitted trying it at some time in their life.[2] Of particular concern is the increasing popularity of the psychoactive amphetamine derivative MDMA. In 2000, 11 percent of high school seniors reported recent use of MDMA.[2] According to a large national survey, the percentage of college students reporting use of MDMA within the previous year increased 69 percent (from 2.8 to 4.7 percent) between 1997 and 1999.[3] Encouragingly, use of phencyclidine (PCP) has declined. In 2000, only 0.1 percent of Americans over age 12 reported using PCP during the previous year, and only 2.6 percent reported ever trying it.[4]

The term *psychedelic* is sometimes preferred to *hallucinogen.* Many of the drugs within this group rarely produce true hallucinations, which are sensory perceptions occurring in the absence of any external stimulus. Perceptual alterations based on some environmental cue are termed *illusions,* and are far more common. These effects may involve any sensory modality, but are most often visual. Users may also experience distortions of body image, and a distorted sense of the passage of time. Alterations in mood and heightened suggestibility are common.

The classic hallucinogens include agents from the indole alkylamine (LSD, psilocybin), and phenylethylamine (mescaline and others) chemical families. These drugs share a common proposed mechanism of action, and are capable of producing the profound psychological effects and sensory distortions characteristic of the psychedelic "trip." In addition to classic hallucinogens, a number of other drugs, such as MDMA ("ecstasy"), PCP, and marijuana possess the ability to alter sensory perceptions, and can be placed within the broader category of hallucinogens.

LSD

LSD (lysergic acid diethylamide) can be chemically synthesized or obtained by hydrolysis of ergot alkaloids from the fungus *Claviceps purpurea.* It is the most potent hallucinogenic compound known. Evidence suggests that the psychedelic effects of LSD are mediated through serotonergic (5HT) systems, and that LSD acts as an agonist at $5HT_2$ receptors.

The typical LSD dose of 50 to 300 μg is most commonly delivered through ingestion of a small square of dried "blotter" paper saturated with a solution of the compound. Blotter acid is often imprinted with fanciful designs or cartoons, which may serve as trademarks for the manufacturer. Other forms of LSD include "microdots" (tiny tablets), "windowpane" (gelatin sheets), impregnated sugar cubes, and liquid LSD. LSD is relatively inexpensive; a dose typically costs less than $15.

LSD is rapidly absorbed following ingestion. Onset of psychedelic effects occurs after about 30 min, peak effects occur within the first 4 h, and the total duration of an LSD "trip" is between 8 and 12 h. The serum half-life of LSD is approximately 3 h.[5] Physiologic effects of LSD usually precede psychedelic effects, and are dominated by sympathomimetic symptoms. These include marked mydriasis, and mild elevations of pulse, blood pressure, and temperature. Facial flushing, mild gastric distress, piloerection, bruxism, increased muscle tension, and hyperreflexia may be seen. Severe or life-threatening complications are extremely uncommon. Seizures have been reported rarely. Massive overdose of LSD may produce coma, respiratory arrest, hyperthermia, and coagulopathy.[6]

The psychedelic effects of LSD may be perceived as pleasurable or horrifying, depending on the user's prevailing mood and expectations ("set"), and external environmental factors ("setting"). Acute adverse psychological effects ("bad trip") include panic attacks, extreme paranoia, acute psychotic reactions, and depressive reactions. Potential physical trauma as a consequence of dangerous or impulsive behavior is a serious hazard. Occasional suicides have been reported. Prolonged and sometimes permanent psychosis following LSD use has been well described, and affects up to almost 5 percent of users.[7] The term "flashback" has been replaced by *hallucinogen persisting perception disorder,*[7,8] a debilitating malady in which patients experience chronic perceptual distortions reminiscent of the drug-induced state, often accompanied by anxiety or panic.

Patients who present to the ED due to effects of LSD are conscious and alert and will usually be able to give a history of the drug ingestion. Diagnosis is based on a history of use and the presence of sympathomimetic signs. Sensitive assays have been developed for the detection of LSD, but are not usually available or necessary in the emergent clinical setting. Routine toxicology screens available in most EDs will not usually detect LSD, but may be indicated if other intoxicants are suspected. If the history is clear, and in the absence of medical complications or possible coingestants, observation in a safe, quiet environment is appropriate. Reassurance and emotional support are generally the only interventions required to manage a patient experiencing a "bad trip." Oral or parenteral benzodiazepines may be given if the patient is extremely agitated or exhibiting significant sympathomimetic stimulation. Haloperidol may be used as a second choice if additional sedation is required, but may have a small theoretical risk of lowering the seizure threshold. Patients who are lucid and medically stable may be released into the custody of family or friends. Patients with paranoid or psychotic symptoms lasting longer than 8 to 12 h may require hospital admission. Rare patients with medical complications due to massive overdose may require hospital admission, but can be expected to recover quickly with supportive management.[6]

PSILOCYBIN

Psilocybin and the related compound psilocin are hallucinogens of the indole alkylamine class, and are structurally related to LSD. Psilocybin and psilocin are believed to act as 5-HT_2 agonists in a manner similar to LSD. They occur naturally in mushrooms of the *Psilocybe* genus, most notably *P. semilanceata* (liberty cap) and *P. cubensis.* Psilocybin-containing mushrooms grow naturally in many areas of the U.S. and Europe, and kits containing spores and the ingredients necessary for propagation are advertised in drug-oriented publications. Hallucinogenic mushrooms purchased on the street are often nonpsychoactive mushrooms which have been adulterated with LSD or PCP.[9] Psilocybin-containing mushrooms may be dried or cooked without losing potency. Because mushroom size and the concentration of psychoactive compounds vary, there is little correlation between the number of mushrooms ingested and hallucinogenic effect. A user may ingest as few as 5 or as many as 100 mushrooms for a single "dose."

Symptom onset occurs about 30 min after ingestion of psilocybin-containing mushrooms, and the total duration of hallucinogenic effects is about 4 to 6 h. The hallucinogenic effects are similar to, but less powerful than, those produced by LSD. Other common effects include mydriasis, mild tachycardia, hyperreflexia, and nausea and vomiting. Serious medical side effects are extremely rare, but seizures and hyperthermia have occurred, and the death of a small child has been reported.

ED management of patients presenting with isolated hallucinogenic mushroom ingestion is largely supportive. Routine drug screens will not detect psilocybin or psilocin. However, a drug screen may be indicated if there is a possibility that the mushrooms ingested were adulterated with PCP. If the patient's symptoms are not consistent with psilocybin, the possibility that the mushrooms ingested were of another more toxic variety should be considered (see Chap. 204).

MESCALINE

Mescaline (3,4,5-trimethoxyphenylethylamine) is the hallucinogenic alkaloid found in the Mexican peyote cactus *Lophophora williamsii*, a small spineless cactus that grows throughout the southwestern U.S. and northern Mexico. Mescaline is a member of the phenylethylamine class of hallucinogens, and is structurally related to amphetamines. Like LSD, mescaline is believed to act as an 5-HT$_2$ agonist,[10] but mescaline is a much weaker hallucinogen than LSD.

The small 8-mm crowns of the peyote cactus are dried and sold as peyote "buttons," each containing approximately 45 mg of mescaline. A typical dose of 200 to 500 mg will require 3 to 12 of these "buttons." Mescaline can be extracted from peyote or chemically synthesized, but these methods are expensive. Pills or capsules sold on the street as "mescaline" are unlikely to be genuine,[9] and may instead contain LSD or PCP.

Peyote is bitter tasting, and causes significant uncomfortable physical side effects within an hour of ingestion. Initial signs and symptoms, which often include nausea and vomiting, abdominal discomfort, diaphoresis, dizziness, nystagmus, ataxia, and headache, generally resolve in about 2 h. Adrenergic stimulation causes mydriasis and mild elevations in pulse, blood pressure, and temperature. Hallucinogenic effects very similar to those produced by LSD begin several hours after ingestion and persist for 6 to 12 h. Death due to aberrant behavior while under the influence of the drug can occur, but reports of significant morbidity or mortality due to physiological effects of mescaline are absent from the literature. Patients presenting to the ED due to peyote ingestion can usually be managed supportively. Routine drug screens do not detect mescaline.

MDMA

MDMA (3,4-methylenedioxymethamphetamine, "ecstasy" or "Adam") is a synthetic phenylethylamine derivative, structurally related to both amphetamines and mescaline. MDA (3,4-methylenedioxyamphetamine) and MDEA (3,4-methylenedioxyethamphetamine, "Eve") are related compounds with similar properties. MDMA is believed to act as an indirect monoamine agonist by causing release and inhibiting reuptake of 5-HT and dopamine.[11]

MDMA is usually ingested in doses of 50 to 200 mg. Tablets are typically round and white, and are often imprinted with logos such as birds, butterflies, lightning bolts, or four-leaf clovers. At the turn of the century, the street price for a dose is approximately $20 to $30. The drug is colorless and tasteless, and has become notorious as a "date rape" drug. Acute effects last about 4 to 6 h. MDMA rarely causes actual hallucinations, but can produce sensory effects such as alterations in the intensity of colors or sensation of textures. Users often report feelings of euphoria, enhanced sociability, verbosity, and heightened sexual interest. Common physical manifestations of MDMA include sympathomimetic effects, particularly mydriasis and mild elevations of pulse and blood pressure, as well as nausea, jaw tension, bruxism, dry mouth, muscle aches, and ataxia.

The increase in popularity of MDMA has been accompanied by an increase in reports of serious complications and death related to its use. Fatal arrhythmias and death due to cardiac effects have been reported in patients with and without underlying cardiac disease.[12] Severe hypertension and intracranial hemorrhage have been reported.[12] A pattern of toxicity manifested by hyperthermia, seizures, disseminated intravascular coagulation (DIC), rhabdomyolysis, and renal failure is well recognized.[13] This pattern shares many features of the serotonin syndrome.[14] Acute liver damage has occurred, not always attributable to hyperthermia. Hyponatremia, due to excessive water consumption or possibly inappropriate antidiuretic hormone secretion,[14] has been reported.

Serious concerns have arisen regarding the possibility of persistent neurotoxic effects from MDMA use. Mounting evidence indicates that repeated use of MDMA may result in neurotoxic injury to serotonin axon terminals and long-term functional consequences.[15] MDMA has been shown to cause significant reductions in both the number of serotonin transporters in the brain and levels of serotonin metabolites in the cerebrospinal fluid.[15] A corresponding dramatic loss of serotonergic neurons was observed on examination of brain tissue from primates even 1 year after drug administration. Significant dopaminergic toxicity has also been found in a recent study using nonhuman primates.[16] Neuropsychiatric studies performed on chronic MDMA users demonstrate long-lasting cognitive impairment and mood dysfunction, including memory impairment, diminished learning ability, and depression. More human clinical studies are necessary to definitively establish a link between MDMA use and permanent neurologic damage.

Patients presenting to the ED with complications due to MDMA should receive activated charcoal if the ingestion was recent. Arrhythmias are managed with standard therapy. Hypertension and tachycardia will often respond to treatment with benzodiazepines. Rapid intravenous titration with very high doses of benzodiazepines may be required to control symptoms. If hypertension is severe, phentolamine or nitroprusside can be used. β-Blockers such as propranolol should be avoided due to the risk of unopposed alpha stimulation.[17] Hyperthermia should be managed aggressively with active cooling measures. Patients with temperatures exceeding 40°C (104°F) have increased morbidity and mortality, and may require rapid sequence intubation and paralysis using a nondepolarizing neuromuscular blocking agent. The use of dantrolene or specific serotonin antagonists[13] has been suggested, but no prospective clinical studies support use of these agents in treatment of MDMA toxicity.

PHENCYCLIDINE

Phencyclidine (PCP) is a synthetic piperadine derivative. It is a dissociative anesthetic agent structurally related to ketamine. PCP is unlike the classic hallucinogens in that it causes clouding of the sensorium rather than heightened sensory awareness. PCP is believed to act as a glutamate antagonist at the NMDA (N-methyl-D-aspartate) receptor.[18]

PCP can be easily and inexpensively synthesized. Powdered drug ("angel dust") is most often combined with tobacco, marijuana, or other vegetable matter and smoked, but PCP can be ingested orally, sniffed intranasally, or injected intravenously. Unfortunately PCP is often sold as another drug, or used to adulterate another drug, and thus may be unknowingly ingested.[9] The onset of action depends on the mode of administration, and is about 5 min if PCP is smoked. Acute effects generally last 4 to 6 h, but can persist much longer.

Because of the remarkable variability of clinical effects, recognition of PCP intoxication can be challenging. Patients may present with CNS stimulation or depression, and may be physically violent, catatonic, or comatose. A combination of cholinergic, anticholinergic, and sympathomimetic effects may be present. Many patients have taken a combination of drugs, compounding the clinical picture.[19] In a series of 1000 PCP-intoxicated patients, nystagmus and hypertension were the most common findings, each occurring in 57 percent of patients.[19] Hypertension was generally mild. Other prevalent manifestations were: acute brain syndrome (37 percent); violent (35 percent), agitated (34 percent), or bizarre (29 percent) behavior; hallucinations or delusions (19 percent); and tachycardia (30 percent).[19] Diaphoresis, muscle rigidity, dystonic reactions, ataxia, and a decreased response to painful stimuli have also been described. Pupil size is variable; unlike classic hallucinogens, widely dilated pupils are not common.[19]

Medical complications due to PCP use occur frequently. Coma has been seen in 10.6 percent,[20] and seizures in 3.1 percent[19] of PCP-intoxicated patients. Elevated serum creatine kinase (CK), due to increased muscle activity and/or a possible direct toxic effect of PCP, was found in 70 percent of patients in one study.[19] Rhabdomyolysis may occur, sometimes resulting in renal failure requiring dialysis.[20] Hypoglycemia,[19] hypertension causing intracerebral hemorrhage,[21] and hyperthermia causing hepatic necrosis have also been reported. In addition, significant traumatic injury and even death may occur as a result of the violent or aberrant behavior characteristic of PCP use.

The ED evaluation of a patient with known or suspected PCP intoxication should include examination for occult trauma and evaluation for the possibility of hypoglycemia or rhabdomyolysis. A urine dipstick positive for occult blood when no red blood cells are seen on microscopic examination suggests myoglobinuria, and should prompt the physician to obtain a total CK level to screen for rhabdomyolysis. Results of toxicologic screening for PCP can be misleading. Tests can be falsely negative; also, chronic PCP users may test positive for weeks following their last use,[22] so a positive test does not necessarily indicate acute PCP intoxication.

PCP is secreted into the stomach, so administration of multiple doses of activated charcoal could theoretically facilitate drug removal. In reality, patients intoxicated with PCP are often uncooperative or combative, and it may be impractical or impossible to administer this form of therapy. If possible, activated charcoal should be administered to patients known to have large or recent ingestions of PCP.

Violence and agitation are common features of PCP intoxication, and sedation and/or physical restraints are frequently required to prevent patients from harming themselves and to protect ED personnel. Pharmaceutical intervention is preferable to physical measures because the muscular activity caused by a patient fighting against restraints may contribute to the development of rhabdomyolysis. Parenteral benzodiazepines are recommended, but haloperidol can also be used.

Management of patients with PCP intoxication is generally supportive, but patients with severe CNS toxicity or who have specific medical complications require appropriate intervention. They should be evaluated for other causes of altered consciousness, including hypoglycemia and trauma. Seizures should be treated with benzodiazepines, and patients in status epilepticus may require endotracheal intubation and neuromuscular blockade. Hyperthermia is treated with rapid cooling measures, and if severe, endotracheal intubation with neuromuscular blockade should be considered. Hypertension usually responds to sedation, but severe hypertension can be treated with nitroprusside. Treatment of rhabdomyolysis includes aggressive hydration. Use of intravenous sodium bicarbonate to alkalinize the urine is controversial but may help prevent acute tubular necrosis (see Chap. 279).

Patients with significant medical complications due to PCP, such as rhabdomyolysis, seizures, hyperthermia, or severe hypertension, require hospital admission. Patients exhibiting only minor clinical features of PCP intoxication (lethargy, bizarre behavior, violent behavior, or agitation) can often be discharged if improved following a period of observation.[20]

MARIJUANA

Dried leaves and flowers from the hemp plant *Cannabis sativa* is called marijuana, and dried resin from the flower tops of this plant is known as hashish. The psychoactive ingredient of marijuana is Δ^9-tetrahydrocannabinol (Δ^9-THC). Δ^9-THC binds to a specific brain receptor for which an endogenous ligand has been discovered.[23]

Marijuana is most often smoked, but can be ingested. Symptoms persist for 2 to 4 h, or longer if ingested. Drowsiness, euphoria, heightened sensory awareness, paranoia, distortions of time and space, and feelings of unreality are described. Hallucinations do not normally occur at usual doses. Common physiologic effects of marijuana are mild tachycardia, injected conjunctiva, bronchodilation, orthostatic hypotension, and impaired motor coordination. Although significant medical complications occur rarely if at all, users may experience panic reactions, or even brief toxic psychoses due to Δ^9-THC.

Acute psychiatric symptoms due to marijuana use can usually be managed with reassurance alone, but benzodiazepines can be used if

medication is warranted. **Urine tests are unreliable indicators of acute marijuana intoxication because it is detectable for days after use in novice users, and for weeks after the last use in chronic users.[24]**

OTHER HALLUCINOGENS

Several drugs with hallucinogenic properties are enjoying increasing popularity due to information disseminated on the Internet. Numerous websites promote the use of psychoactive drugs that are "natural" and legal, such as *Salvia divinorum* and toad venom. *S. divinorum* is a plant in the mint family that can be chewed, smoked, or made into tea. The active ingredient, salvinorin A, is a potent κ opioid agonist,[25] and can cause profound hallucinations. It is currently legal in the U.S. and can be purchased through Internet sites. Possible adverse medical effects are largely unknown.

Bufotenin and related compounds are indolalkylamines with hallucinogenic properties that are present in venom from toads of the *Bufo* genus. Toads are "milked," or venom can be ingested through the practice of "toad-licking"; dried toad skins are also sold and smoked. Unfortunately toad venom may also contain toxic cardioactive steroids with digoxin-like properties, and can cause severe toxic reactions and death.[26] Digoxin-specific Fab fragments may be lifesaving for critically ill patients exposed to toad venom.[26]

Seeds of the Morning glory plant (*Ipomoea violacea, Ipomoea tricolor,* and others) contain lysergic acid amide (ergine), a compound closely related to LSD. They are sometimes intentionally ingested for the hallucinogenic effects. Several hundred seeds may be taken as a "dose." Physical and psychologic manifestations closely resemble effects of LSD, and patients can be managed similarly.

Accidental or intentional ingestion of large amounts of nutmeg can cause delirium with hallucinations. Nutmeg is the dried seed from the tropical *Myristica fragrans* tree. The hallucinogenic properties of nutmeg may be due to a component, myristicin, but the mechanism is not well understood. Ingestion of 1 to 3 nutmegs or 5 to 15 g of the ground spice produces psychologic effects which begin in 3 to 6 h and last for 6 to 24 h. Uncomfortable physical symptoms are prominent, and may include tachycardia, flushing, dry mouth, nausea, and abdominal pain. Signs and symptoms may resemble anticholinergic poisoning, but pupils are usually small or midsized. Management is generally supportive.

Jimson weed (*Datura stramonium*) and Angel's trumpet (*Datura candida*) are plants which grow naturally in the U.S., and contain the anticholinergic alkaloids atropine, scopolamine, and hycoscyamine. Seeds or other parts of the plant can be ingested or smoked, and cause the anticholinergic toxic syndrome. Delirium, hallucinations, and seizures can occur, along with other classic anticholinergic effects such as mydriasis, tachycardia, dry mouth and skin, blurred vision, urinary retention, and hyperthermia. Gastric emptying can be delayed, so gastric decontamination is an important part of the management of such patients. Whole bowel irrigation is recommended for patients who have ingested a large number of seeds. Medications with anticholinergic properties, such as phenothiazines, should be avoided. Physostigmine is effective treatment for severe anticholinergic symptoms.

Ketamine and dextromethorphan are chemically related to PCP, and have hallucinogenic properties. Like PCP, they are believed to act at the NMDA receptor. Ketamine, called "vitamin K" or "special K," is usually taken in powdered form, mixed in a drink, or snorted. Effects can be similar to those of PCP. Dextromethorphan is legal and readily available in over-the-counter cough suppressants, and has become increasingly popular among adolescent drug users. A large quantity must be ingested for the user to experience hallucinogenic effects. Dextromethorphan-containing preparations often include other ingredients such as acetaminophen, so the potential for toxic coingestion should be considered in any patient who has consumed a hallucinogenic dose of dextromethorphan.

DIFFERENTIAL DIAGNOSIS

Among the many conditions that may mimic hallucinogen intoxication are alcohol or benzodiazepine withdrawal, anticholinergic poisoning, thyrotoxicosis, central nervous system (CNS) infections, structural CNS lesions, and acute psychosis. Hypoglycemia should be considered in all patients with altered mental status. Numerous prescription and nonprescription medications can also cause hallucinations. Hallucinogens are usually taken intentionally, so in most cases a history of what was taken and the mode of administration will be available. However, the identity of street drugs is often misrepresented; the possibility that the substance used was adulterated or substituted by another more toxic drug, particularly PCP, should be considered. Drug testing is of limited utility since routinely available drug screens will not detect many hallucinogens. In addition, a positive test for PCP or marijuana can be misleading, as it may be indicative of use days or even weeks prior to testing.

GENERAL MANAGEMENT

The initial ED management of a patient presenting with hallucinations, bizarre behavior, or altered thought processes should be concentrated on assessing the patient's general medical condition and stabilizing the airway, breathing, and circulation as appropriate. Hypoxia and hypoglycemia should be recognized and treated promptly.

Most hallucinogens are rapidly absorbed. Patients experiencing adverse effects due to hallucinogen use do not usually present to the ED until several hours after the drug was administered. Therefore gastric decontamination is of limited utility in most cases of hallucinogen intoxication. Administration of oral activated charcoal is indicated for recent ingestions. Hemodialysis is not indicated, as it does not effectively remove hallucinogens from the body.

In many cases, calm reassurance in a supportive environment will sufficiently soothe the violent patient. In other cases, pharmacologic intervention, and possibly physical restraints, may be necessary in order to ensure the safety of the patient and the ED staff and to facilitate evaluation and treatment of the patient. Benzodiazepines are considered the mainstay of treatment. Diazepam 5 to 10 mg PO or IV, or lorazepam 1 to 2 mg PO, IM, or IV can be given depending on the severity of symptoms and the clinical situation. Repeated doses can be given as needed, provided the patient is monitored for the possibility of respiratory depression. Phenothiazines should not be used. Use of haloperidol, a butyrophenone, may be considered when a second sedating agent is required. However, haloperidol lowers the seizure threshold, has anticholinergic properties, and can cause dystonic reactions. Haloperidol's theoretical risk of reduction of the seizure threshold is often cited, but rarely experienced in practice. It should be avoided if the patient is exhibiting significant anticholinergic symptoms. Haloperidol can be administered intramuscularly or intravenously in 5-mg increments. Physical restraints are sometimes necessary, but their use should be minimized and avoided if possible. Physical restraints may cause injury, may exacerbate paranoia and agitation, and may contribute to the development of rhabdomyolysis in patients who struggle against them.

The management of patients with hallucinogen intoxication is largely supportive, but medical complications can occur and should be treated appropriately. Tachycardia and hypertension often respond to sedation with benzodiazepines alone. Significant arrhythmias are treated using standard protocols. Severe hypertension can be treated with nitroprusside. The dose of a nitroprusside infusion starts at 0.5 μg/kg per min, and can be titrated to a maximum of 10 μg/kg per min as needed. Propranolol should probably be avoided because many of the hallucinogens cause significant adrenergic stimulation, and use of a β-blocker may lead to paradoxical hypertension due to unopposed alpha stimulation.[17] Rapid cooling measures should be initiated for patients with significant hyperthermia. Treatment of severe hyperthermia may require neuromuscular paralysis and endotracheal intubation. Seizures are treated with benzodiazepines and standard anticonvulsants. Patients with rhabdomyolysis require aggressive hydration and intravenous sodium bicarbonate to achieve a urinary pH of 6.5 to 8.

DISPOSITION

Most patients seen in the ED due to adverse reactions from hallucinogen use can be discharged into the custody of family or friends if they are lucid and medically stable after a period of observation. Patients with persistent psychotic symptoms or other significant psychiatric disturbance require psychiatric evaluation and possible hospital admission. Patients with significant medical complications of hallucinogen use, such as severe hypertension, hyperthermia, seizures, or rhabdomyolysis, should be admitted to the hospital for continued treatment and observation.

REFERENCES

1. Golub A, Johnson BD, Sifaneck SJ, et al: Is the U.S. experiencing an incipient epidemic of hallucinogen use? *Subst Use Misuse* 36:1699, 2001.
2. Johnston L, O'Malley P, Bachman J: Monitoring the Future national results on adolescent drug use: Overview of key findings, 2001, in NIH Publication No. 02-5105. Bethesda, MD, National Institute on Drug Abuse, 2002.
3. Strote J, Lee JE, Wechsler H: Increasing MDMA use among college students: Results of a national survey. *J Adolesc Health* 30:64, 2002.
4. Substance Abuse and Mental Health Administration: Summary of findings from the 2000 National Household Survey on Drug Abuse, in NHSDA Series H-13, DHHS Publication No.(SMA)01-3549. Rockville, MD, Office of Applied Studies, Department of Health and Human Services, 2001.
5. Aghajanian G, Bing O: Persistence of lysergic acid diethylamide in the plasma of human subjects. *Clin Pharmacol Ther* 5:611, 1964.
6. Klock JC, Boerner U, Becker CE: Coma, hyperthermia, and bleeding associated with massive LSD overdose: A report of eight cases. *Clin Toxicol* 8:191, 1975.
7. Abraham HD, Aldridge AM: Adverse consequences of lysergic acid diethylamide. *Addiction* 88:1327, 1993.
8. American Psychiatric Association: *Diagnostic and Statistical Manual of Mental Disorders.* Washington, DC, American Psychiatric Association, 1994.
9. Renfroe CL, Messinger TA: Street drug analysis: An eleven year perspective on illicit drug alteration. *Semin Adolesc Med* 1:247, 1985.
10. Davis M: Mescaline: Excitatory effects on acoustic startle are blocked by serotonin2 antagonists. *Psychopharmacology (Berl)* 93:286, 1987.
11. Johnson MP, Hoffman AJ, Nichols DE: Effects of the enantomers of MDA, MDMA, and related analogues on [3H]serotonin and [3H]dopamine release from superfused rat brain slices. *Eur J Pharmacol* 132:269, 1986.
12. Dowling GP, McDonough ET, Bost RO: 'Eve' and 'ecstasy': A report of five deaths associated with the use of MDEA and MDMA. *JAMA* 257:1615, 1987.
13. Satchell SC, Connaughton M: Inappropriate antidiuretic hormone secretion and extreme rises in serum creatinine kinase following MDMA ingestion. *Br J Hosp Med* 51:495, 1994.
14. Mueller PD, Korey WS: Death by "ecstasy": The serotonin syndrome? *Ann Emerg Med* 32:377, 1998.
15. McCann UD, Eligulashvili V, Ricaurte GA: (+/−)3,4-Methylenedioxymethamphetamine ("Ecstasy")-induced serotonin neurotoxicity: Clinical studies. *Neuropsychobiology* 42:11, 2000.
16. Ricaurte GA, Yuan J, Hatzidimitrou BJ, et al: Severe dopaminergic neurotoxicity in primates after recreational dose regimen of MDMA ("ecstasy"). *Science* 297:2260, 2002.
17. Romaska E, Sacchetti AD: Propranolol-induced hypertension in treatment of cocaine intoxication. *Ann Emerg Med* 14:1112, 1985.
18. Javitt DC, Zukin SR: Recent advances in the phencyclidine model of schizophrenia. *Am J Psychiatry* 148:1301, 1991.
19. McCarron MM, Schulze BW, Thompson GA, et al: Acute phencyclidine intoxication: Incidence of clinical findings in 1,000 cases. *Ann Emerg Med* 10:237, 1981.
20. McCarron MM, Schulze BW, Thompson GA, et al: Acute phencyclidine intoxication: Clinical patterns, complications, and treatment. *Ann Emerg Med* 10:290, 1981.

21. Eastman JW, Cohen SN: Hypertensive crisis and death associated with phencyclidine poisoning. *JAMA* 231:1270, 1975.

22. Simpson GM, Khajawall AM, Alatore E, et al: Urinary phencyclidine excretion in chronic abusers. *J Toxicol Clin Toxicol* 19:1051, 1982.

23. Devane WA, Hanus L, Breuer A, et al: Isolation and structure of a brain constituent that binds to the cannabanoid receptor. *Science* 258:1946, 1992.

24. Dackis CA, Pottash ALC, Annitto W, et al: Persistence of urinary marijuana levels after supervised abstinence. *Am J Psychiatry* 139:1196, 1982.

25. Roth BL, Baner K, Westkaemper R, et al: Salvinorin A: A potent naturally occurring nonnitrogenous *k* opioid selective agonist. *Proc Natl Acad Sci USA* 99:11934, 2002.

26. Brubacher JR, Padinjarekuttu PR, Banina T, et al: Treatment of toad venom poisoning with digoxin-specific Fab fragments. *Chest* 110:1282, 1996.

170 SALICYLATES
Luke Yip

EPIDEMIOLOGY

The widespread availability of aspirin [acetylsalicylic acid (ASA)] in prescription and over-the-counter (OTC) preparations, confusion between product names and brand names, and the ease with which incremental chronic dosing can cause toxicity make salicylism a common and sometimes fatal occurrence. Data from the American Association of Poison Control Centers Toxic Exposures Surveillance System showed that in 2000, aspirin was implicated in 20,892 exposures, with 12,658 cases (61 percent) treated in a health care facility; 45 deaths (0.2 percent of cases) were attributed to salicylate toxicity.[1]

Many people use OTC medications without realizing that they may contain significant amounts of salicylate. For example, Pepto Bismol (261 mg salicylate per 30 mL) will deliver large amounts of salicylate in patients who misuse the product. Children may become salicylate-toxic from extensive application of keratolytic agents or other agents containing oil of wintergreen (methyl salicylate). **One milliliter of a 98% methyl salicylate solution contains 1400 mg of salicylate. Liniments and products used in hot vaporizers have high concentrations of methyl salicylate, and an ingestion of 5 to 10 mL can be lethal for an infant or a toddler.**

PATHOPHYSIOLOGY

Absorption of salicylate may be delayed or erratic depending on the product. After ingestion of large amounts of non-enteric-coated ASA, absorption from the gastrointestinal (GI) tract may be slowed because of the inhibitory effect of ASA on gastric emptying and the impaired dissolution of tablets in gastric fluids at high concentrations. Peak serum salicylate levels may not be reached for 18 to 24 h, although toxic levels usually are evident within 6 h. Methyl salicylate is a liquid that produces peak levels earlier, whereas peak levels following enteric-coated or sustained-release ASA overdose have been reported to occur 60 h after ingestion.[2] Some formulations of ASA may coalesce to form a gelatinous gastric mass after an intentional overdose, and this mass becomes a source for continued absorption.

After absorption, ASA is hydrolyzed to salicylic acid (salicylate) and is distributed throughout body tissues. Salicylate is responsible for both the therapeutic and the toxic effects of ASA. The severity of toxicity depends on the cellular salicylate concentration. At higher salicylate concentrations, a lesser percentage of the drug is protein bound, and more free drug is available to diffuse into tissues. The pK_a of salicylate is 3.0, and at physiologic pH (7.40), almost all salicylate molecules are ionized. If the systemic pH decreases, the change in equilibrium will form a greater portion of nonionized molecules. This is an important concept because nonionized molecules will cross cellular membranes, such as the blood-brain barrier. Thus, for a given serum salicylate concentration, brain salicylate concentrations will be substantially higher in the presence of acidemia.[3] Although the precise mechanism remains to be determined, the concentration of salicylate in the brain is correlated directly with mortality rate.[3]

The ionized state of salicylate can be used to enhance its elimination. If the urine pH is above 8.0, more salicylate molecules in the urine will be ionized compared with the renal tubular cell pH of 7.4, and reabsorption across the urinary tubule will be reduced.[4]

Acute salicylate overdose may produce nausea and vomiting as a result of local gastric irritation and stimulation of the chemoreceptor trigger zone. Vomiting may result in volume depletion, which reduces renal perfusion and urine flow, adversely affecting renal salicylate elimination and contributing to acid-base and electrolyte disturbances.

Salicylate initially increases respiratory rate through a direct stimulatory effect on the medullary respiratory center in the central nervous system (CNS),[5] but very high salicylate concentrations depress respiration, a finding usually seen later in the course. Salicylate also stimulates skeletal muscle metabolism, which causes an increase in oxygen consumption and carbon dioxide production.[5] The clinical manifestation of the initial respiratory center stimulation (the dominant component) and the increase in carbon dioxide production cause an increased respiratory rate, resulting in respiratory alkalosis.[5] Initially, this will counter the enduring metabolic acidosis. If ventilatory compensation fails to keep pace with increased carbon dioxide production, respiratory acidosis will develop and will compound the metabolic acidosis. The loss of the respiratory buffering effect is detrimental because the kidneys, even under ideal conditions, cannot react with sufficient rapidity to counter the acidosis meaningfully. Also, the critical alkalemia seen early when respiratory alkalosis predominates causes the kidneys to increase bicarbonate and potassium excretion. The urinary bicarbonate loss eventually will decrease the body's bicarbonate stores and impair compensation for the metabolic acidosis of salicylism.

Salicylate enhances lipolysis, uncouples oxidative phosphorylation, and inhibits various Krebs cycle enzymes involved in energy production and amino acid metabolism, resulting in (1) increased catabolism that leads to increased carbon dioxide production, (2) increased heat production, (3) increased glycolysis and peripheral demand for glucose, and (4) production of metabolic intermediaries (i.e., organic acids, lactate, pyruvate, and keto acids) that contribute to the metabolic acidosis of salicylate toxicity.[6] Overall, the acid-base disturbance associated with salicylate poisoning is mixed and includes respiratory alkalosis, metabolic alkalosis (due to volume contraction), and wide anion-gap metabolic acidosis.

Salicylate-induced noncardiogenic pulmonary edema has been observed in humans and studied in animals. Salicylate toxicity causes increased pulmonary vascular permeability, whereas pulmonary vascular pressures and cardiac performance are unaffected. This vascular injury also may involve the kidneys. Proteinuria is a prominent early finding in salicylate toxicity, starting at a serum salicylate concentration of greater than 30 mg/dL, and it is related directly to salicylate concentrations.

Salicylate also affects both central and peripheral glucose homeostasis. Salicylate causes mobilization of glycogen stores, resulting in hyperglycemia. However, salicylate is also a potent inhibitor of gluconeogenesis. Therefore, normoglycemia, hyperglycemia, or hypoglycemia may occur in salicylate toxicity. The brain involves a unique problem with glucose delivery. Animal studies demonstrate that toxic doses of salicylate produce a profound decrease in brain glucose concentration despite normal serum glucose levels.[7] This finding suggests that the supply of glucose to the brain in salicylate poisoning may be inadequate, even though serum glucose levels are normal.

Antiplatelet activity is a well-known effect of ASA, but hemorrhage is a rare complication of acute, single, massive overdose of salicylate. *Chronic* administration of large doses of salicylate may cause significant hypoprothrombinemia when the serum salicylate concentration exceeds 60 mg/dL.[8]

Salicylate ototoxicity is characterized by a reversible sensorineuronal hearing loss that is not idiosyncratic; it is related to serum salicylate concentrations.[9] When serum salicylate concentrations exceed 40 mg/dL, hearing loss reaches its maximum of 40 dB.[9]

CLINICAL FEATURES AND DIAGNOSIS

Clinical manifestations of salicylism depend on the dose of salicylate ingested, duration of exposure, and age of the patient. In general, acute ingestion of less than 150 mg/kg may produce "mild" toxicity, with nausea, vomiting, and GI irritation, but significant toxicity is not expected. Acute ingestion of 150 to 300 mg/kg may produce "mild to moderate" toxicity, with vomiting, hyperpnea, diaphoresis, tinnitus, and acid-base disturbances. Acute ingestion of more than 300 mg/kg may produce "severe" toxicity.

Intoxication in Children

Acute pediatric salicylate intoxication is characterized by a known history of ingestion and onset of symptoms within a few hours of ingestion. Patients usually present soon after the ingestion. Symptoms are usually mild and the intoxication well tolerated.[10] When the duration of salicylate intoxication is between 12 to 24 h, metabolic acidosis and acidemia (pH < 7.35) occur primarily in children younger than age 4, and nearly all children younger than age 1 have acidosis.[11] The acid-base disturbance in older children (age 4 or older) changes to a mixed disturbance with respiratory alkalosis and increased anion-gap metabolic acidosis; alkalemia (pH > 7.45) tends to be observed.

Chronic or "therapeutic" (repeated dose) pediatric salicylate poisonings generally are more serious and are associated with a higher mortality than acute salicylism.[10,12] Often, several days elapse between the initial salicylate administration and the onset of symptoms.[12] There is frequently a coincidental illness that prompted salicylate administration, and children usually appear more ill than those with acute intoxication. The presenting signs are hyperventilation, volume depletion, acidosis, severe hypokalemia, and CNS disturbances.[10] Chronic salicylism is often mistaken for an infectious process. Young children are prone to develop hyperpyrexia, which indicates a worse prognosis.[12] Renal failure may be a significant complication, but pulmonary edema is unusual in the pediatric population.[12] The delay in diagnosis may account for the more severe clinical picture with "therapeutic" salicylism.

Intoxication in Adults

Acute salicylate intoxication in adults is usually due to intentional ingestion, most often occurs in young women, and the patient frequently has a psychiatric or drug overdose history. The typical clinical presentation includes nausea, vomiting, tinnitus, sweating, and hyperventilation, which are reported to occur when the serum salicylate concentration is above 30 mg/dL.[13] However, tinnitus may develop when the serum salicylate concentration exceeds 19.6 mg/dL.[13] Most patients have a mixed acid-base disturbance of respiratory alkalosis and metabolic acidosis.[14] However, when patients also have ingested sedative drugs that impair the hyperpneic response associated with salicylate toxicity, their acid-base profile is altered. Respiratory acidosis, rather than respiratory alkalosis, is more likely to occur.[14] Patients with mixed ingestions have a normal anion-gap metabolic acidosis 40 percent of the time compared with patients who have a larger mean anion gap when salicylate was ingested alone.[14] Therefore, salicylate intoxication in adults who present with a normal anion-gap metabolic acidosis should raise the suspicion that a coingestion including a CNS depressant has occurred. **A normal anion gap does not rule out salicylate toxicity in patients with an unknown ingestion.**

The complex triple-mixed acid-base disturbance of increased anion-gap acidosis, metabolic alkalosis, and respiratory alkalosis may not be seen frequently in salicylate toxicity, but when it is noted, the differential diagnosis is limited. The only other single entity that leads to increased anion-gap acidosis seen with the other two components is sepsis (lactic acidosis, contraction metabolic alkalosis, and respiratory alkalosis). The main contribution to the metabolic acidosis in sepsis is lactate. In contrast, any lactic acidosis associated with salicylate poisoning should be mild unless there is significant hypotension and impaired tissue perfusion. The presence of significant lactic acidosis should prompt a search for an alternate etiology (see Chap. 25).

Uncommon features of acute adult salicylism include fever, neurologic dysfunction, renal failure, adult respiratory distress syndrome (ARDS), noncardiogenic pulmonary edema, and hypoglycemia. Each of these uncommon manifestations indicates more severe poisoning, with associated greater morbidity and mortality rates. Hyperpyrexia appears to be an adverse prognostic indicator, and death is usually preceded by a predominant metabolic acidosis and neurologic deficits.[14] Other rare complications may include rhabdomyolysis, gastric perforation, and GI hemorrhage. Risk factors for death from acute salicylate toxicity include unconsciousness on presentation, fever, severe acidosis, seizures, cardiac dysrhythmias, and advanced age. The development of respiratory acidosis is usually a premorbid event.

The diagnosis of chronic salicylate intoxication (chronic excessive dosing) in adults is different, particularly in the elderly. These patients are more likely to have underlying medical conditions that they are treating with salicylates. Signs and symptoms of chronic intoxication include hyperventilation, tremor, papilledema, agitation, paranoia, bizarre behavior, memory deficits, confusion, and stupor.[15] Neurologic abnormalities are much more common in chronic salicylate poisoning and often mislead physicians. Chronic salicylism should be considered in any patient with unexplained CNS dysfunction, especially in the presence of a mixed acid-base disturbance, tachypnea or dyspnea, unexplained noncardiogenic pulmonary edema, or nonfocal neurologic or behavioral abnormalities. Adults with chronic salicylate toxicity have a higher morbidity rate, including pulmonary edema, seizures, and renal failure, as well as higher mortality rate. The distinction between acute and chronic salicylate toxicity may not always be clear. A patient may present many hours after an acute severe salicylate overdose, when altered mental status, acidosis, elevated prothrombin time, and serious toxicity with a "therapeutic" serum salicylate concentration are signs consistent with a chronically poisoned patient. Significant toxicity may be evident despite declining or "therapeutic" serum salicylate concentrations. In these situations, the patient's clinical status is most important when assessing the severity of toxicity.

Chronic salicylism may develop in patients taking carbonic anhydrase inhibitors for treatment of glaucoma.[16] The normal anion-gap (hyperchloremic) metabolic acidosis produced by carbonic anhydrase inhibitors increases the volume of distribution for salicylate and facilitates its entry into the CNS, causing toxicity at a "therapeutic" serum salicylate concentration.

SPECIFIC ISSUES

The Done nomogram was created to assist in clarifying the level of salicylate intoxication that should prompt intervention: ". . . this [nomogram] provides only a rough guide to a single criterion of severity in previously well patients. . . . it obviously does not supplant clinical judgment."[17] Although widely taught and used for over 40 years, the Done nomogram typically is misunderstood and often is misused. Thus it is strongly recommended that the patient's clinical condition and early course, rather than the nomogram, guide clinical management. The nomogram was based primarily on previously healthy pediatric patients with acute single salicylate ingestion.[17] The patients' presentations were graded clinically. The initial serum salicylate concentration was extrapolated based on toxicokinetic data. The clinical grade was then correlated with the extrapolated initial salicylate concentration. The potential usefulness of the nomogram is to assist in predicting the degree of toxicity after an acute single ingestion of ASA in patients who have not been taking salicylate recently. The nomogram is *not* useful when:

salicylate has been ingested over several hours or days,
the preparation is an enteric-coated or a sustained-release tablet,
the compound is oil of wintergreen, which is absorbed rapidly,
the patient has renal insufficiency or failure,
the time of ingestion is unknown or uncertain,
the patient is acidemic, or
a salicylate level drawn before 6 h after ingestion returns nontoxic.

In such situations, the degree of toxicity is determined by serial evaluation of a patient's clinical condition and serial salicylate levels. Evolution of a "nontoxic" salicylate level into severe salicylate intoxication has surprised many physicians. Failure to anticipate worsening intoxication is generally due to reliance on a single salicylate level, without regard for the formulation used or the time of ingestion. If the level was drawn before 6 h, it may underestimate the severity. It is prudent in most patients to obtain serial serum salicylate levels every 1 to 2 h until the levels are declining and the patient's clinical status stabilizes. Acidemia must alter estimation of the severity of the intoxication. Due to its limitations and deceptive utility, **use of the Done nomogram is not recommended,** and for this reason, a description of its use is not provided in this text.

The presence of salicylate may be determined with the ferric chloride test, which uses several drops of 10% ferric chloride added to 1 mL of urine. A purple color will be seen in the presence of salicylic acid, acetoacetic acid, or phenylpyruvic acid. This test is very sensitive to small quantities of salicylic acid, and a positive test result does not indicate salicylate poisoning or toxicity. False-negative results have not been reported. However, false-positive results may occur when a small quantity of urine that has been used for test-strip analysis with the N-Multistix or Bili Labstix is then used for ferric chloride testing. Presumably, some impregnated chemical from the dipstick dissolves in the urine and causes a false-positive reaction. Another bedside test for salicylic acid uses the Ames Phenistix, which turns brown when either salicylic acid or phenothiazines are present in the urine or serum. Adding one drop of 20 N sulfuric acid to the strip bleaches out the color in the case of phenothiazines but not in the case of salicylic acid. The color change is often difficult to interpret. Both the ferric chloride and Ames Phenistix tests are qualitative tests. All positive urine results must be confirmed with serum salicylate level. There are severe limitations associated with bedside detection techniques for salicylic acid, and I do not advocate their use in the clinical setting.

Assessing the condition of patients who have ingested enteric-coated or a sustained-release ASA preparation is difficult. These products are formulated to remain intact in the acidic gastric environment but to dissolve in the alkaline intestinal fluids. Drug release is therefore primarily a function of gastric emptying, and peak levels may not be apparent until 10 to 60 h after ingestion.[2] Another problem with enteric-coated and sustained-release tablets is their large size, which makes them difficult to remove from the stomach even through a no. 40 French gastric lavage tube. A plain radiograph of the abdomen has been recommended for enteric-coated medications, but not all are radiopaque.[18] Thus a positive radiograph can confirm that pills are present, but a negative radiograph does not rule out enteric-coated or sustained-release ASA tablets in the GI tract. If a potentially lethal number of enteric-coated or sustained-release tablets has been ingested, the patient should be observed for at least 24 h and serial serum salicylate levels obtained until a declining level is ensured.[2]

Many standard texts assert that urinary alkalinization is impossible until hypokalemia has been corrected.[11] The kidneys will attempt to excrete hydrogen ion in order to retain potassium, leading to paradox-

ical aciduria despite alkalemia. However, there seem to be little or no clinical data specifically regarding the role of potassium replacement in alkalinization of urine during salicylate intoxication. In one human study, no correlation was found between serum potassium levels and urinary pH, and the patients' urines remained acidic despite alkalemia and normokalemia.[19] Although it is important to administer supplemental potassium to hypokalemic patients, do not delay the administration of sodium bicarbonate until normokalemia is achieved. Potassium and sodium bicarbonate should be administered simultaneously.

When aggressive management for ARDS with endotracheal intubation, mechanical ventilation, and sedation becomes necessary, hyperventilation must be maintained, or acute deterioration may occur as a result of iatrogenic respiratory acidosis, causing a rapid shift of salicylate into the CNS.

TREATMENT

There is no specific antidote for salicylate toxicity. The main goals of therapy are immediate resuscitation; maintenance of airway, breathing, and circulation; correction of volume depletion and metabolic derangements; GI decontamination; and reduction in body salicylate burden. The first step is to determine that clinically significant salicylate toxicity exists. This decision is made based on serial clinical assessment of the patient and serial serum salicylate concentrations. Essential laboratory tests include serum salicylate levels, electrolytes, glucose, blood urea nitrogen, and creatinine. Arterial blood gases, chest and abdominal radiograph, electrocardiogram, complete blood count, serum calcium level, and urinalysis with urine pH determination should be obtained as clinically indicated.

Reducing a patient's salicylate burden involves minimizing further absorption of salicylate from the GI tract and hastening elimination of salicylate already absorbed. Salicylate absorption is effectively reduced by the administration of activated charcoal (AC) both for regular and for sustained-release forms.[20] AC 1 to 2 g/kg should be administered to patients who have ingested potentially toxic amounts of salicylate. In contrast, no convincing data support the use of repeated or multiple doses of AC. Evidence supports the use of whole-bowel irrigation as a more effective means of GI decontamination when dealing with enteric-coated or sustained-release ASA in the GI tract.[21]

Patients with severe salicylate intoxication are usually volume depleted and have acid-base disturbances that require general supportive and specific measures to enhance elimination. Careful assessment of a patient's volume and electrolyte status is important, particularly in the elderly and in patients with a history of cardiac disease. Fluid replacement of volume deficits should be undertaken while preparations are made for other measures. Potassium (40 mEq/L) should be supplemented in the NS (may require central line administration) after adequate urine output has been established. Note that correction of acidemia might further exacerbate hypokalemia due to a shift of potassium into cells.

Urinary salicylate clearance is directly proportional to urine flow rate, but more important, it is logarithmically proportional to urine pH.[19] Urine alkalinization is more effective than forced diuresis or forced alkaline diuresis, and it avoids the potential complication of fluid overload that may result from forced diuresis, especially in those with marginal cardiac reserve or cardiac performance.[19]

Opinions differ on the approach to initial fluid resuscitation and alkalinization of the urine. In practice, often both hydration and urine alkalinization are initiated simultaneously. My approach has been to volume replete patients with NS with a target urine output of 1 to 2 mL/kg per h. Concurrently, in a second intravenous line, administer an intravenous bolus of sodium bicarbonate (1 to 2 mEq/kg), followed by a continuous infusion of D5W, to which 3 ampules (either 44 or 50 mEq/ampule) of sodium bicarbonate have been added, starting at 1.5 to 2.0 times the maintenance rate and then adjusted to maintain the urine pH above 7.5. Except for the fluids used for hydration, all intravenous fluids administered should contain a minimum of 50 g/L of glucose (D5W) because hypoglycemia has been implicated in the pathophysiology of salicylate CNS injury.[7] When hypoglycemia or neurologic symptoms are present, a minimum of 100 g/L glucose (D10W) has been suggested. It is important to diligently monitor the patient's clinical course. The patient's urine pH and serum salicylate concentration, as well as volume, acid-base and electrolyte status, and cardiopulmonary and neurologic status, should be evaluated at least every hour.

Patients with salicylate-induced (noncardiogenic) pulmonary edema should be managed as are patients with ARDS from other causes. Pulmonary edema begins to improve concomitantly with the lowering of serum salicylate levels. This would suggest that aggressive efforts toward rapid elimination by hemodialysis may be beneficial in this subset of patients. In addition, early hemodialysis enables removal of salicylate without the volume challenge that accompanies sodium bicarbonate administration, and it avoids the possibility of aggravating pulmonary edema.

Hemorrhagic complications are seen rarely in single massive salicylate overdoses. Chronic administration of large doses does cause significant hypoprothrombinemia when serum salicylate concentration exceeds 60 mg/dL.[8] However, hemorrhage, even under this scenario, is seen rarely in clinical practice or in animal experiments. When bleeding does occur, it rarely appears to be a contributing factor in mortality from salicylate toxicity. Patients with clinically significant bleeding should be treated with fresh-frozen plasma. Observations in animals and humans indicate that administering large doses of vitamin K after the development of hypoprothrombinemia has little or no effect on the plasma prothrombin time when serum salicylate concentration is high. After discontinuing salicylate, the prothrombin time rapidly returns to normal.

Hemodialysis is considered the extracorporeal technique of choice for the treatment of serious salicylate toxicity because hemodialysis can correct acid-base and electrolyte abnormalities while rapidly reducing the body salicylate burden.[22] Indications for hemodialysis include:

clinical deterioration or failure of improvement despite intensive supportive care and an alkaline diuresis,
lack of success in establishing an alkaline urine,
renal insufficiency or renal failure,
severe acid-base disturbance,
altered mental status, and
patients with ARDS.

Serum salicylate concentration may be helpful but should not be the sole determinant in the decision to initiate hemodialysis. A level of 100 mg/dL after an acute ingestion in a healthy patient may not require hemodialysis, whereas a patient with a level of 30 mg/dL in a chronic ingestion may be moribund. One should err on the side of hemodialysis in patients who are elderly, have chronically ingested ASA, have altered mental status, have acidemia, or have a severe underlying disease (e.g., coronary artery disease or chronic obstructive pulmonary disease).

In significant ingestions, serum salicylate levels should be monitored at least every 2 h until a peak has been reached and then every 4 to 6 h until the peak falls into the nontoxic range. In severe ingestions, serum salicylate levels should be determined hourly, and clinical decisions should be based on the trend of the serum salicylate levels as well as the patient's clinical status.

DISPOSITION

A patient may be discharged following adequate GI decontamination if there is progressive clinical improvement, no significant acid-base disturbance, and a documented serial decline in serum salicylate lev-

els toward the therapeutic range. If there is any doubt, the patient should be admitted to an intensive care setting. Although the determination of serial salicylate levels offers valuable information regarding the effectiveness of the treatment implemented, it is a poor substitute for clinical evaluation of a patient. Management decisions are never based solely on a particular salicylate level. Early consultation with a clinical toxicologist is prudent.

REFERENCES

1. Litovitz TL, Klein-Schwartz W, White S, et al: 2000 Annual report of the American Association of Poison Control Centers Toxic Exposure Surveillance System. *Am J Emerg Med* 19:337, 2001.
2. Wortzman DJ, Grunfeld A: Delayed absorption following enteric-coated aspirin overdose. *Ann Emerg Med* 16:434, 1987.
3. Hill JB: Salicylate intoxication. *New Engl J Med* 288:1110, 1973.
4. Smith PK, Gleason HL, Stoll CG, et al: Studies on the pharmacology of salicylates. *J Pharmacol Exp Ther* 87:237, 1946.
5. Tenny SM, Miller RM: The respiratory and circulatory actions of salicylate. *Am J Med* 19:498, 1955.
6. Schwartz R, Landy G: Organic acid excretion in salicylate intoxication. *J Pediatr* 66:658, 1965.
7. Thurston JH, Pollock PG, Warren SK, et al: Reduced brain glucose with normal plasma glucose in salicylate poisoning. *J Clin Invest* 49:2139, 1970.
8. Clausen FW, Jager BV: The relation of the plasma salicylate level to the degree of hypoprothrombinemia. *J Lab Clin Med* 31:428, 1946.
9. Myers EN, Bernstein JM, Fostiropolous G: Salicylate ototoxicity: A clinical study. *New Engl J Med* 11:587, 1965.
10. Gaudreault P, Temple AR, Lovejoy FH: The relative severity of acute versus chronic salicylate poisoning in children: A clinical comparison. *Pediatrics* 70:566, 1982.
11. Done AK: Treatment of salicylate poisoning: Review of personal and published experiences. *Clin Toxicol* 1:451, 1968.
12. Snodgrass W: Salicylate toxicity following therapeutic doses in young children. *Clin Toxicol* 18:247, 1981.
13. Mongan E, Kelly P, Nies K, et al: Tinnitus as an indication of therapeutic serum salicylate levels. *JAMA* 226:142, 1973.
14. Gabow PA, Anderson RJ, Potts DE, et al: Acid-base disturbances in the salicylate-intoxicated adult. *Arch Intern Med* 138:1481, 1978.
15. Greer HD III, Ward HP, Corbin KB: Chronic salicylate intoxication in adults. *JAMA* 193:555, 1965.
16. Anderson CJ, Kaufman PL, Sturm RJ: Toxicity of combined therapy with carbonic anhydrase inhibitors and aspirin. *Am J Ophthalmol* 86:516, 1978.
17. Done AK: Significance of measurements of salicylate in blood in cases of acute ingestion. *Pediatrics* 26:800, 1960.
18. Savitt DL, Hawkins HH, Roberts JR: The radiopacity of ingested medications. *Ann Emerg Med* 16:331, 1987.
19. Prescott LF, Balali-Mood M, Critchley JAJH: Diuresis or urinary alkalinisation for salicylate poisoning? *Br Med J* 285:1382, 1982.
20. Levy G, Tsuchiya T: Effect of activated charcoal on aspirin absorption in man. *Clin Pharmacol Ther* 13:317, 1972.
21. Kirshenbaum LA, Mathews SC, Sitar DS, et al: Whole-bowel irrigation versus activated charcoal in sorbitol for the ingestion of modified-release pharmaceuticals. *Clin Pharmacol Ther* 46:264, 1989.
22. Jacobsen D, Wiik-Larsen E, Bredesen JE: Haemodialysis or haemoperfusion in severe salicylate poisoning? *Hum Toxicol* 7:161, 1988.

ACETAMINOPHEN
Oliver L. Hung
Lewis S. Nelson

Acetaminophen (*N*-acetyl-*p*-aminophenol, paracetamol, or APAP) is the most popular over-the-counter analgesic used in the United States, and is one of the most commonly reported toxic exposures reported to poison centers nationwide. Poisonings often occur because of the erroneous belief that this medication is benign or because the victim was unaware that it was an ingredient in the ingested preparation. According to the Toxic Exposure Surveillance System in 2000, acetaminophen accounted for 5 percent of all toxic exposures, but also accounted for 23 percent of reported fatalities.[1]

PHARMACOLOGY

The recommended dosing of acetaminophen is 650 to 1000 mg every 4 to 6 h up to 4 g a day in adults and 10 to 15 mg/kg every 4 to 6 h in children. After ingestion, acetaminophen is rapidly absorbed from the gastrointestinal tract. In therapeutic doses, peak serum levels are usually achieved within 30 min to 2 h. Even in overdose, peak serum levels are usually achieved within 2 h. However, delayed absorption of acetaminophen is reported following overdoses of preparations in which acetaminophen is combined with propoxyphene (e.g., Darvocet) or diphenhydramine (e.g., Tylenol PM), as well as those with altered release kinetics (e.g., Tylenol Arthritis Pain Extended Relief).

Acetaminophen is primarily metabolized by the liver through sulfation (20 to 46 percent) and glucuronidation (40 to 67 percent). A small percentage (<5 percent) of acetaminophen undergoes direct renal elimination. A small percentage is also oxidized by cytochrome P450 (CYP2E1, CYP1A2, and CYP3A4) to a reactive metabolite

NAPQI (*N*-acetyl-*p*-benzoquinoneimine), which is quickly detoxified by hepatic glutathione to a nontoxic acetaminophen-mercaptate compound that is renally eliminated (Figure 171-1).

However, following acetaminophen overdose, hepatic metabolism through glucuronidation and sulfation is easily saturated. A larger proportion of acetaminophen is therefore metabolized by cytochrome P450 to NAPQI, depleting glutathione. When hepatic stores of glutathione decrease to less than 30 percent of normal, NAPQI binds to other hepatic macromolecules and hepatic necrosis ensues (Figure 171-2).[2] Within the hepatic lobule, cytochrome P450 is concentrated within hepatocytes surrounding the terminal hepatic vein and least concentrated within hepatocytes surrounding the portal triad. As a result, acetaminophen-induced hepatic injury develops in the characteristic pattern of centrilobular necrosis.

Although the clinical manifestations of acetaminophen toxicity are classically delayed, hepatic injury actually occurs very early. In an animal model of acetaminophen hepatic toxicity, early signs of hepatocyte injury occurred within 12 h of exposure.[3] This was based on microscopic evidence as well as immunofluorescent staining of NAPQI-hepatic protein adducts (3-Cys-A) within hepatocytes. Hepatocyte changes progressed until day 2, when cell lysis occurred, releasing hepatic enzymes, such as transaminases, and NAPQI-hepatic protein adducts into the circulation where they were detected in the

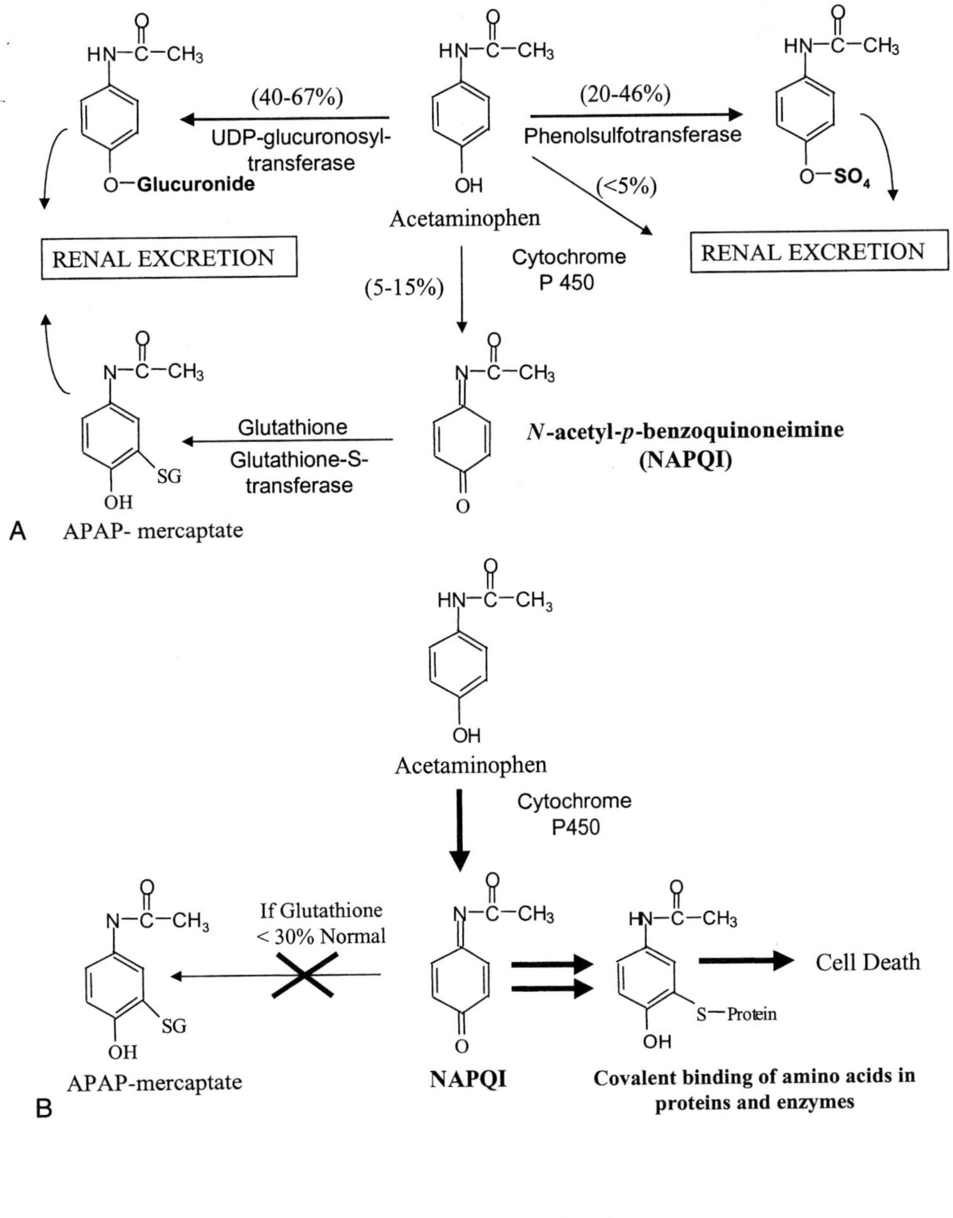

FIG. 171-1. A and **B.** Acetaminophen [*N*-acetyl-*p*-aminophenol (APAP)] metabolism.

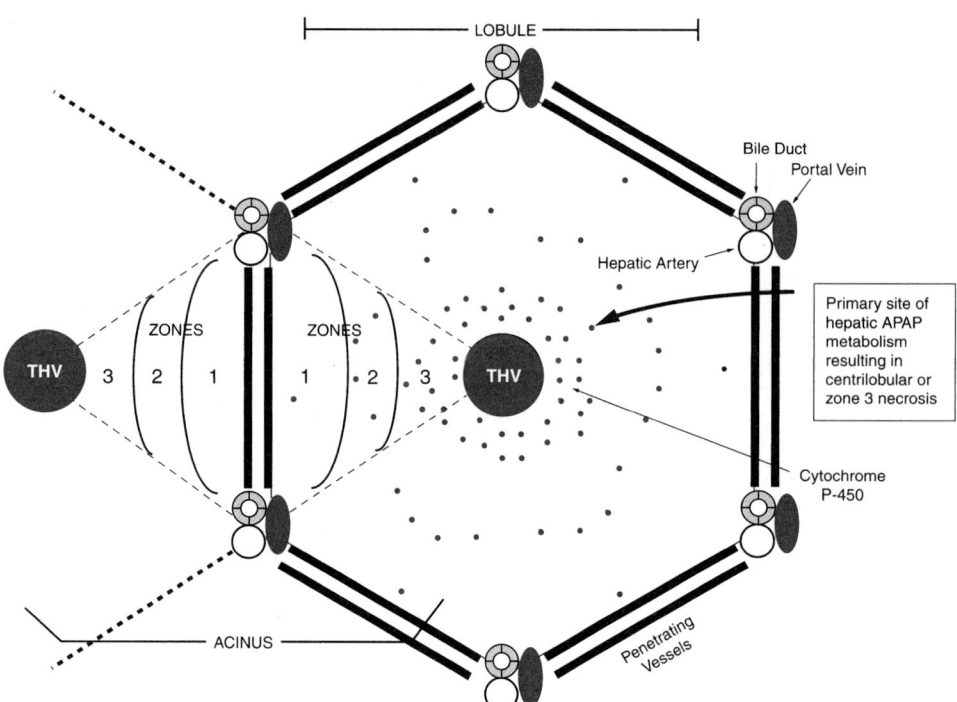

FIG. 171-2. Hepatic architecture. Although morphologically the liver is described by the lobule, it is better described functionally by the acinus. The acinus includes the tissue located between adjacent portal triads and it contains zones of differing metabolic function. Zone 3, located closest to the hepatic vein, contains the greatest concentration of cytochrome P450, accounting for the pathologic finding of centrilobular necrosis in patients with acetaminophen hepatotoxicity. THV = terminal hepatic vein.

serum. This corresponds generally to the development of overt clinical toxicity in humans.

CLINICAL PRESENTATION

The clinical presentation of human acetaminophen toxicity can be approximately divided into four stages. During the first 24 h after exposure (stage 1), patients often have minimal signs and symptoms of toxicity. Some may have minor, nonspecific signs and symptoms such as anorexia, nausea, vomiting, pallor, and malaise. By days 2 to 3 (stage 2), clinical signs of hepatotoxicity that may be discerned in hepatotoxic patients include right upper quadrant abdominal pain and tenderness, and abnormal laboratory tests, such as elevated serum aspartate aminotransferase (AST), alanine aminotransferase (ALT), and bilirubin. Even without treatment, most of these patients will recover without sequelae. By days 3 to 4 (stage 3), however, the conditions of some patients will progress to fulminant hepatic failure. Characteristic findings include metabolic acidosis, coagulopathy, renal failure, encephalopathy, and recurrent gastrointestinal (GI) symptoms. Those patients who survive the complications of fulminant hepatic failure will begin to recover over the next week (stage 4), with complete resolution of hepatic dysfunction in survivors.

Patients with insufficient glutathione stores (e.g., alcoholics and AIDS patients) and patients with induced cytochrome P450 enzymatic activity (e.g., alcoholics and those taking concurrent anticonvulsant or antituberculous medications) may be at greater risk for developing acetaminophen-induced hepatotoxicity following overdose.[4,5] In contrast, children, because of their greater ability to metabolize acetaminophen through hepatic sulfation, may be at decreased risk for developing hepatotoxicity following a moderate overdose when compared to adults.[6,7]

Acetaminophen may also cause acute, extrahepatic toxic effects, presumably because of the presence of cytochrome P450 present in other organs. Ingestion of massive doses of acetaminophen (4-h acetaminophen level >800 μg/mL) is associated with the acute development of altered sensorium (coma, agitation) and a metabolic (lactic) acidosis.[8] Lactic acidosis can occur with extremely high levels of APAP in the absence of both liver failure or hypotension. Acetaminophen overdose is also infrequently associated with the development

of isolated renal insufficiency. In rare cases, cardiac toxicity and pancreatitis may occur.

DIAGNOSIS

A toxic exposure to acetaminophen is suggested when greater than 140 mg/kg is ingested in a single dose or when greater than 7.5 g is ingested within a 24-h period. The confirmation of acute acetaminophen poisoning depends solely on obtaining a serum acetaminophen level and estimating the time since ingestion. Unlike other types of poisoning, the initial clinical findings are nonspecific and delayed in onset; thus the reliance on laboratory evaluation. An acetaminophen level should be obtained for all patients presenting to the ED with a presumed intentional overdose of any type. In one study, 1 in 500 patients presenting to the ED after an overdose who denied ingesting acetaminophen was determined by laboratory testing to have a potentially toxic acetaminophen level.[9] Empirical testing of all patients with intentional overdoses may be cost-effective. The cost of treating a single patient for complications of acetaminophen-induced hepatotoxicity is commonly estimated to outweigh the cost of laboratory testing for 500 patients who prove to have nontoxic acet-aminophen levels.

The implication of a measured acetaminophen level is determined by plotting it on the Rumack-Matthew nomogram[10] (Figure 171-3). This nomogram was empirically based on a retrospective analysis of previous acetaminophen overdose patients and their clinical outcomes. The original nomogram line was based on a 4-h acetaminophen level of 200 μg/mL, but was subsequently modified in the United States by the Food and Drug Administration (FDA) to increase the safety margin by moving the line to a 4-h acetaminophen level of 150 μg/mL. More importantly, the nomogram only applies to an acetaminophen level obtained after 4 h postingestion and before 24 h postingestion. It cannot be applied to acetaminophen levels obtained outside this 20-h window.

Obtaining multiple acetaminophen levels following acute overdose is rarely indicated in the absence of hepatotoxicity. An initial level below the nomogram line may rarely "cross the line" in patients who ingest acetaminophen preparations known to have prolonged absorption kinetics (see "Pharmacology" above). However, the clinical significance of crossing the line in this fashion is unknown. Similarly, be-

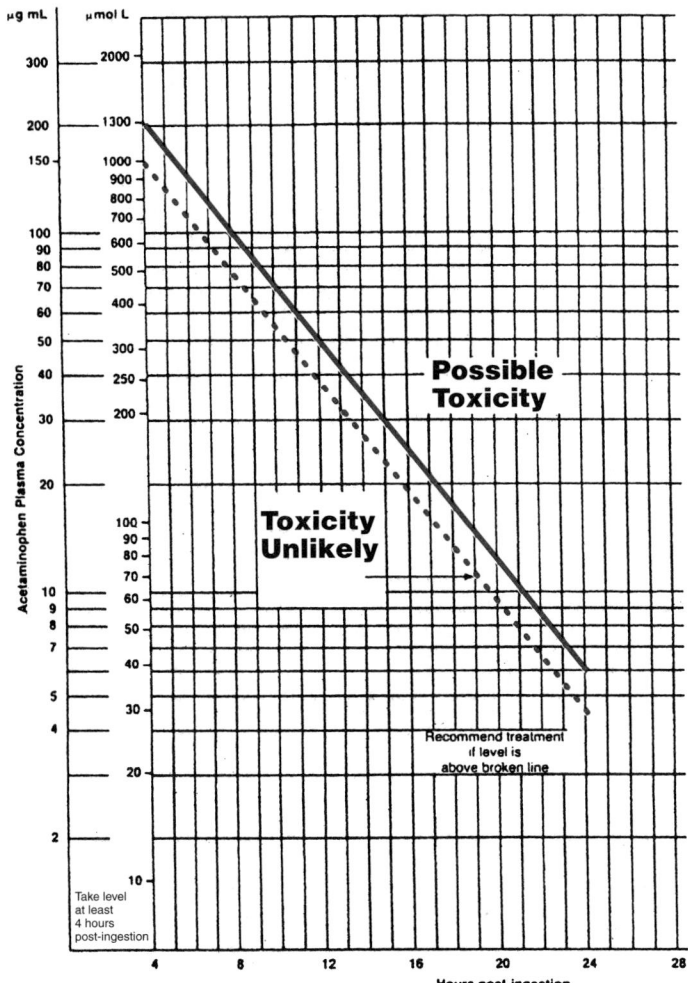

FIG. 171-3. Rumack-Matthew nomogram. (Reproduced with permission from Rumack BH, Matthew H: Acetaminophen poisoning and toxicity. *Pediatrics* 55:871, 1975.)

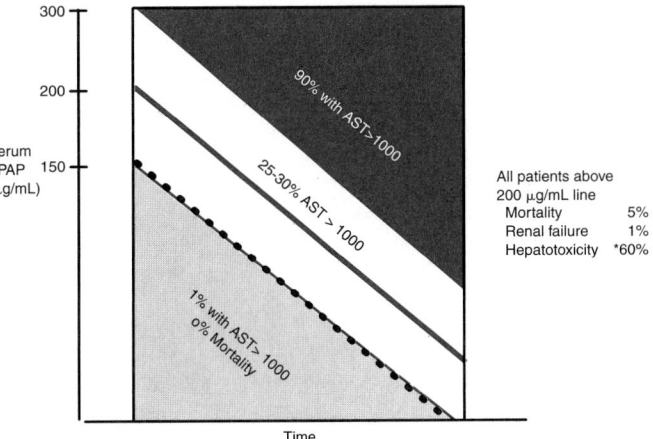

FIG. 171-4. Outcome of acetaminophen poisoned patients without *N*-acetylcysteine; such therapy initiated prior to 8 h postingestion reduces adverse outcomes to that expected if the acetaminophen level was below the nomogram line. APAP = *N*-acetyl-*p*-aminophenol (acetaminophen); AST = aspartate aminotransferase.* Defined as AST >1000. (Adapted with permission from Smilkstein MJ, Knapp GL, Kulig KW, et al: Efficacy of oral *N*-acetylcysteine in the treatment of acetaminophen overdose. *New Engl J Med* 319:1557, 1988.)

the antidote. In addition, more aggressive forms of decontamination, such as orogastric lavage or whole-bowel irrigation with polyethylene glycol are unnecessary because of the rapid gastrointestinal absorption of acetaminophen and the great success of treating acetaminophen poisoning with NAC. However, aggressive gastrointestinal decontamination should be considered in cases of polydrug overdose in which a coingestant is likely to be life-threatening (e.g., a tricyclic antidepressant or a sustained-release calcium-channel blocker).

The mainstay for the prevention or treatment of acetaminophen toxicity is the administration of NAC. Although its mechanisms of action are not fully understood, NAC is thought to have two important beneficial effects. In early acetaminophen poisoning (less than 8 h after ingestion), NAC averts toxicity by preventing the binding of

cause the nomogram was constructed and verified by using only a single serum level, the clinical implications of a level initially above the line that falls below it on repeat analysis are unknown.

Based on data obtained before the widespread use of antidotal therapy, patients with serum acetaminophen levels above the original 200 μg/mL nomogram were observed to have a 60 percent risk of developing hepatotoxicity (defined as AST >1000 IU/mL), a 1 percent risk of renal failure, and a 5 percent risk of mortality.[11] In addition, patients with extremely high serum acetaminophen levels (above a parallel line coinciding with a 300 μg/mL 4-h level) were observed to have a greater risk (90 percent) of developing hepatotoxicity (Figure 171-4). The safety level below the U.S. nomogram line (4-h level corresponding to 150 μg/mL) was confirmed in a prospective study involving 11,195 patients.[12] The risk of hepatotoxicity in patients with acetaminophen levels below the nomogram was 1 percent. No patients received antidotal therapy, and all recovered without any complications (Figure 171-5).

TREATMENT

Treatment for acetaminophen toxicity consists of GI decontamination, the timely use of the antidote, *N*-acetylcysteine (NAC), and supportive care. For most cases of acetaminophen poisoning, adequate GI decontamination consists of the early administration of activated charcoal orally or through nasogastric tube. Inducing emesis by administering syrup of ipecac is undesirable because it delays the administration of

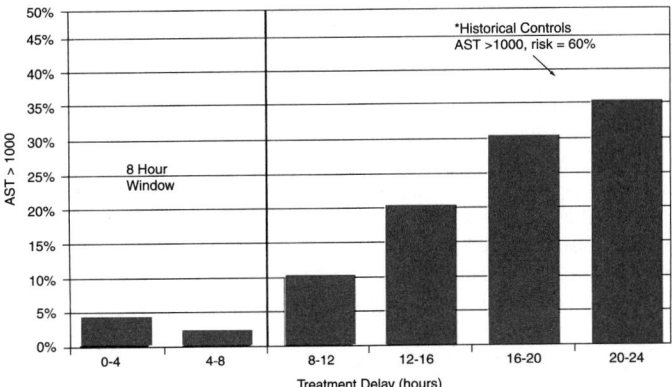

FIG. 171-5. The effect of the delay to the initiation of antidotal therapy on patients presenting with an initial acetaminophen level above the nomogram line. Initiation of *N*-acetylcysteine therapy prior to 8 h postingestion nearly prevents the development of hepatotoxicity, defined as an AST >1000. Although the benefit of *N*-acetylcysteine is less pronounced when initiated more than 8 h postingestion, without antidotal therapy 60 percent of the patients in this group, based on historical controls, are expected to develop hepatotoxicity. AST = aspartate aminotransferase. (Adapted with permission from Smilkstein MJ, Knapp GL, Kulig KW, et al: Efficacy of oral *N*-acetylcysteine in the treatment of acetaminophen overdose. *New Engl J Med* 319:1557, 1988.)

NAPQI to hepatic macromolecules. NAC may do this by acting as a glutathione precursor or substitute, a sulfate precursor, or it may directly reduce NAPQI back to acetaminophen. In established acetaminophen toxicity, or greater than 24 h after acetaminophen ingestion, NAC diminishes hepatic necrosis by acting as an antioxidant, decreasing neutrophil infiltration, improving microcirculatory blood flow, or increasing tissue oxygen delivery and extraction.

The standard 72-h oral NAC regimen used in the United States is a loading dose of 140 mg/kg followed by maintenance doses of 70 mg/kg every 4 h for 17 additional doses. If treatment is initiated within 8 h of acetaminophen ingestion, NAC is nearly 100 percent effective in preventing the development of hepatotoxicity.[12] The longer the initiation of NAC therapy is delayed beyond 8 h after ingestion, the greater the risk of developing hepatotoxicity. **Even by 24 h after acetaminophen ingestion, however, NAC treatment is associated with a lower risk of hepatotoxicity than occurred in historical controls[11]** (see Figure 171-5).

The major complications of oral NAC therapy are nausea and vomiting, due in part to its foul rotten egg odor and taste. To hide these disagreeable characteristics, the standard 10 or 20 percent NAC solution should be diluted to a 5 percent concentration in a chilled beverage, such as fruit juice or a soft drink, prior to administration. NAC's disagreeable odor may be further minimized by having the patient sip the drink through a straw from a covered cup or by administering the dose by nasogastric tube. Some patients with persistent nausea and vomiting may require concomitant antiemetic treatment with agents such as intravenous metoclopramide (Reglan), 0.1 mg/kg up to 1.0 mg/kg, ondansetron (Zofran), 0.15 mg/kg, or granisetron (Kytril), 0.01 mg/kg.

Intravenous NAC regimens are routinely used in other countries and are being used successfully with increasing frequency in certain parts of the United States. Intravenous NAC is better tolerated by most patients, and the only major limitation is the development of rate-related anaphylactoid reactions that are easily treated.[13] Intravenous NAC therapy is as effective as oral therapy for patients with early acetaminophen poisoning,[14,15] although its efficacy in patients presenting more than 10 h postingestion is less clear. At this time, the clinical experience with intravenous NAC in the United States remains too limited to recommend it as a routine replacement in most regions for the traditional oral NAC regimen. However, intravenous administration of NAC may be required to treat patients with refractory vomiting and in patients with contraindications to oral therapy (e.g., caustic ingestions). In addition, intravenous NAC may be preferable to oral NAC for the treatment of acetaminophen-induced fulminant hepatic failure,[16] because oral NAC has not been adequately studied in this setting. Currently, there is no intravenous NAC formulation available in the United States. If it is to be used, the oral NAC preparation, which is sterile, can be administered intravenously. The recommended dose varies by locale, but administering a dose identical to that given in the oral regimen is reasonable without other expert guidance. Although not an FDA-approved route of administration, there is sufficient support in both the literature and clinical practice to allow its use.

Clinical experience suggests that patients with poor glutathione reserves, such as alcoholics and the chronically ill, have similar excellent clinical outcomes when the standard treatment guidelines are applied to their care. As such, there is no need to alter the use of the acetaminophen treatment nomogram or modify the dosing of *N*-acetylcysteine for these patients.

In many clinical situations, NAC therapy is often started in close temporal proximity to the administration of activated charcoal. **Although NAC is adsorbed by activated charcoal, there is no evidence that activated charcoal inhibits the clinical effectiveness of NAC.**[17] This loss is likely unimportant in most situations because the current dosing of NAC is probably excessive. This may explain why NAC appears to be equally effective in preventing hepatotoxicity following even very large acetaminophen overdoses. Separating the first dose of NAC and activated charcoal by 1 to 2 h when possible is a rea-

sonable (but not necessary) method to minimize potential NAC and activated charcoal interaction.

Finally, the weight of evidence suggests that NAC therapy is both safe and efficacious during pregnancy and that the approach to treating a pregnant patient following an acetaminophen overdose should remain the same. Although an ovine model demonstrated that NAC is unable to cross the placenta, there are data in humans establishing that it does.[18] Still, NAC treatment has never been associated with fetal malformations in humans, but fetal demise and malformations have been described following delayed NAC treatment in first-trimester pregnant women after acetaminophen overdose.[19]

TREATMENT GUIDELINES

Treatment guidelines for acetaminophen poisoning are based on the time to presentation to the ED after ingestion: acetaminophen ingestions less than 4 h prior to presentation; acetaminophen ingestions greater than 4 h but less than 24 h ago; and acetaminophen ingestions of unknown time or greater than 24 h prior to presentation (Figure 171-6). No further acetaminophen serum measurements are necessary once the need for NAC therapy has been determined. Treatment with NAC should continue for the full 72-h course (18 doses).

For patients who present to the ED within 4 h and who are determined to likely have a significant overdose of their acetaminophen ingestion, treatment begins with GI decontamination (usually activated charcoal) and awaiting the determination of a 4-h postingestion acetaminophen level. If the hospital laboratory can report an acetaminophen level within 8 h postingestion, the clinician should wait for the serum acetaminophen level and plot it on the nomogram to determine whether NAC therapy is necessary. If the hospital laboratory cannot determine the acetaminophen level within 8 h, the clinician should empirically administer the first dose of NAC (within 8 h of acetamin-

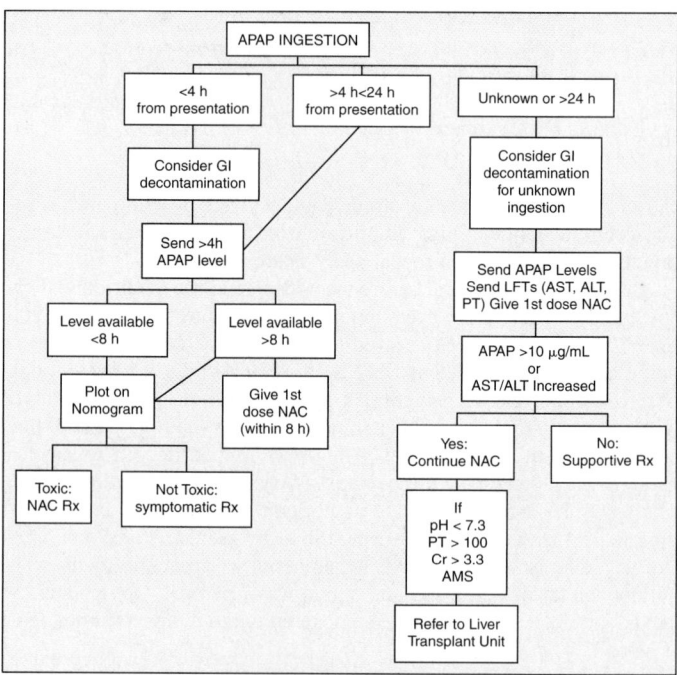

FIG. 171-6. Treatment guidelines for acetaminophen ingestion. All times noted are postingestion. Because the details of individual cases vary considerably, strongly consider calling the regional Poison Control Center (1.800.222.1222) for more specific or comprehensive assistance. ALT = alanine aminotransferase; AMS = altered mental status; APAP = *N*-acetyl-*p*-aminophenol (acetaminophen); AST = aspartate aminotransferase; LFTs = liver function tests, NAC = *N*-acetylcysteine; PT = prothrombin time; Rx = treatment.

ophen ingestion) without waiting for the measurement. Subsequently, when the acetaminophen level is determined, the need for additional NAC therapy should be determined with the use of the nomogram.

For patients who present longer than 4 h but less than 24 h following acetaminophen ingestion, the serum acetaminophen level should be determined by the laboratory as soon as possible. GI decontamination may be performed, particularly for suspected coingestants, but it may have limited effectiveness because of the delay in presentation. Similarly, if the hospital laboratory can determine the acetaminophen level within 8 h postingestion, the clinician should await the acetaminophen level and plot it on the nomogram to determine if NAC therapy is necessary. Otherwise, the first dose of NAC (within 8 h of acetaminophen ingestion, if possible) should be empirically administered. When the acetaminophen level is determined, it should be plotted on the nomogram to determine if additional NAC therapy is necessary.

Finally, for patients in whom the time of acetaminophen ingestion remains unknown or is >24 h, the clinician should consider whether GI decontamination is required. A serum acetaminophen level and liver function tests (AST, ALT) should be determined. In addition, the first dose of NAC therapy should be administered as soon as possible. In this scenario, a detectable acetaminophen level (greater than 10 μg/ml) suggests that the patient may be at risk for developing hepatotoxicity. Similarly, elevated AST and ALT enzymes suggests the possibility of ongoing hepatic toxicity. Therefore, continued NAC therapy is indicated if the acetaminophen level is measurable or if the serum AST or ALT is elevated. If APAP <10 μg/mL and the AST/ALT are not elevated, then NAC can be discontinued.

Standard supportive therapy should be initiated early for intravenous access, and a 12-lead electrocardiogram interpretation obtained to exclude cardiac toxins (e.g., cyclic antidepressants, digoxin, β-blockers, calcium channel blockers). Hypoxemia, hypoglycemia, and opiates should be quickly considered and excluded for all patients presenting with altered sensorium. All patients requiring NAC therapy should be admitted to the hospital until the completion of the therapy. In general, admission to a hospital floor bed is adequate unless the patient is hemodynamically unstable or the patient is suicidal and 24-h direct observation cannot be arranged. Patients who are not at risk for developing acetaminophen-induced hepatotoxicity (e.g., acetaminophen level below the nomogram, unmeasurable acetaminophen level with normal hepatic transaminase levels) should be observed in the ED for a minimum of a 4- to 6-h period to exclude potentially toxic coingestants. Psychiatric evaluation should be considered for patients with intentional acetaminophen overdoses.

FULMINANT HEPATIC FAILURE

Unfortunately, a small percentage of patients who overdose with acetaminophen will develop fulminant hepatic failure. The mortality rate for patients without NAC therapy is estimated at 58 to 80 percent. Most fatalities occur on days 3 to 5 after overdose and are attributed to hepatic complications such as cerebral edema, hemorrhage, shock, adult respiratory distress syndrome (ARDS), sepsis, and multiorgan failure. Patients who eventually survive from fulminant hepatic failure generally begin to show evidence of recovery by days 5 to 7. Eventually, all survivors will develop complete hepatic regeneration without any persistence of hepatic impairment.

NAC is beneficial in the treatment of acetaminophen-induced fulminant hepatic failure. When compared to controls, NAC therapy was associated with increased survival (48 vs 20 percent), decreased cerebral edema (40 vs 68 percent), and decreased vasopressor requirements (40 vs 80 percent).[16] NAC also appears to be beneficial in the treatment of other forms of hepatic failure, too, including viral hepatitis and alcoholic cirrhosis.[20]

Prognostic indicators exist to determine those patients with the highest risk of mortality from acetaminophen-induced fulminant hepatic failure. As a result, they also serve as early predictors of patients

who may subsequently require liver transplantation. A variety of laboratory and clinical markers are used including serum pH, prothrombin time (PT), serum creatinine, and mental status evaluation. The presence of a metabolic acidosis, pH <7.3, despite fluid and hemodynamic resuscitation, or a combination of coagulopathy (PT >100), renal insufficiency (creatinine >3.3 mg/dL), and grade III or IV encephalopathy is extremely useful in predicting poor outcome.[21]

Treatment for acetaminophen-induced fulminant hepatic failure includes NAC therapy, correction of coagulopathy and acidosis, monitoring for and aggressive treatment of cerebral edema, and early patient referral to a liver transplant center. Unlike the treatment of early acetaminophen toxicity, NAC therapy should be continued past the 72-h standard regimen until the patient recovers, receives a liver transplant, or dies. Because all clinical studies supporting the use of NAC for fulminant hepatic failure used the intravenous administration of NAC, intravenous NAC therapy may be preferable to oral NAC for the treatment of fulminant hepatic failure. Intravenous NAC should be administered at the same dosage as oral NAC. Because of the risk of anaphylactoid reaction, intravenous NAC infusions should be administered slowly and adjusted based on repeated blood pressure measurements to prevent hypotension.

SPECIAL CONSIDERATIONS: MULTIPLE-DOSE ACETAMINOPHEN INGESTIONS AND EXTENDED-RELEASE TYLENOL

Multiple closely-spaced acetaminophen ingestions and Tylenol Arthritis Pain Extended Relief ingestions represent two unique aspects of acetaminophen poisoning because the Rumack-Matthew nomogram cannot be readily applied. Tylenol Arthritis Pain Extended Relief (formerly Tylenol Extended Relief) is a formulation (McNeil Pharmaceuticals) that consists of a bi-layered formulation containing a total of 650 mg of acetaminophen. Theoretically, both of these situations could result in less toxicity than a single ingestion of the same total dose of acetaminophen because the time intervals between serum peaks may allow the liver to regenerate its supply of glutathione. Because there is little clinical data concerning both of these scenarios, treatment guidelines remain conservative.

The situation in which multiple ingestions of acetaminophen over a period of time occur cannot be interpreted on the nomogram because a single time of ingestion cannot be determined. One way to resolve this is to assume that a single ingestion occurred at the earliest possible time stated by the patient. An acetaminophen level is plotted on the Rumack-Matthew nomogram based on this artificial time, and treatment decisions are made accordingly. For example, if patient ingests 5 doses of 50 mg/kg of acetaminophen over a 4-h period beginning 8 h ago, a single acetaminophen ingestion is assumed to have occurred 8 h ago and the serum level is plotted on the nomogram.

Because of the uncertainty of potential toxicity of Tylenol Arthritis Pain Extended Relief, it is commonly recommended to obtain a second acetaminophen level 4 to 6 h later in those situations in which the first measured level (4 to 8 h postingestion) is elevated but below the nomogram line.[22] A full course of NAC therapy should be instituted (or continued if already started) if the second acetaminophen level is above the nomogram line. If the initial level is above the nomogram line, standard therapy should be administered and there is no need to obtain a second level.

REFERENCES

1. Litovitz TL, Klein-Schwartz W, White S, et al: 2000 Annual report of the American Association of Poison Control Centers Toxic Exposure Surveillance System. *Am J Emerg Med* 19:337, 2000.
2. Mitchell JR, Jollow DJ, Potter WZ, et al: Acetaminophen-induced hepatic necrosis. I. Role of drug metabolism. *J Pharmacol Exp Ther* 187:211, 1973.

3. Roberts DW, Bucci TJ, Benson RW, et al: Immunohistochemical localization and quantification of the 3-(cystein-S-yl)-acetaminophen protein adduct in acetaminophen hepatotoxicity. *Am J Pathol* 138:359, 1991.

4. Brackett CC, Bloch JD: Phenytoin as a possible cause of acetaminophen hepatotoxicity: Case report and review of the literature. *Pharmacotherapy* 20:229, 2000.

5. Bray GP, Harrison PM, O'Grady JG, et al: Long-term anticonvulsant therapy worsens outcome in paracetamol-induced fulminant hepatic failure. *Hum Exp Toxicol* 11:265, 1992.

6. Mohler CR, Nordt SP, Williams SR, et al: Prospective evaluation of mild to moderate pediatric acetaminophen exposures. *Ann Emerg Med* 35: 239, 2000.

7. James LP, Wells E, Beard RH, Farrar HC: Predictors of outcome after acetaminophen poisoning in children and adolescents. *J Pediatr* 140:522, 2002.

8. Roth B, Woo O, Blanc P: Early metabolic acidosis and coma after acetaminophen ingestion. *Ann Emerg Med* 33:452, 1999.

9. Ashbourne JF, Olson KR, Khayam-Bashi H: Value of rapid screening for acetaminophen in all patients with intentional drug overdose. *Ann Emerg Med* 18:1035, 1989.

10. Rumack BH, Matthew H: Acetaminophen poisoning and toxicity. *Pediatrics* 55:871, 1975.

11. Prescott LF: Paracetamol overdosage. *Drugs* 25:290, 1983.

12. Smilkstein MJ, Knapp GL, Kulig KW, et al: Efficacy of oral *N*-acetylcysteine in the treatment of acetaminophen overdose. *New Engl J Med* 319:1557, 1988.

13. Bailey B, McGuigan MA: Management of anaphylactoid reactions to intravenous *N*-acetylcysteine. *Ann Emerg Med* 31:710, 1998.

14. Yip L, Dart RC, Hurlbut KM: Intravenous administration of oral *N*-acetylcysteine. *Crit Care Med* 26:40, 1998.

15. Perry HE, Shannon MW: Efficacy of oral versus intravenous *N*-acetylcysteine in acetaminophen overdose: Results of an open-label, clinical trial. *J Pediatr* 132:149, 1998.

16. Keays R, Harrison PM, Wendon JA, et al: Intravenous acetylcysteine in paracetamol induced fulminant hepatic failure: A prospective controlled trial. *BMJ* 303:1026–1029, 1991.

17. Spiller HA, Krenzelok, EP, Grande GA, et al: A prospective evaluation of the effect of activated charcoal before oral *N*-acetylcysteine in acetaminophen overdose. *Ann Emerg Med* 23:519, 1994.

18. Horowitz RS, Dart RC, Jarvie DR, et al: Placental transfer of *N*-acetylcysteine following human maternal acetaminophen toxicity. *J Toxicol Clin Toxicol* 35:447, 1997.

19. Riggs BS, Bronstein AC, Kulig K, et al: Acute acetaminophen overdose during pregnancy. *Obstet Gynecol* 74;247, 1989.

20. Harrison PM, Wendon JA, Gimson AES, et al: Improvement by acetylcysteine of hemodynamics and oxygen transport in fulminant hepatic failure. *New Engl J Med* 324:1852, 1991.

21. O'Grady JG, Alexander GJM, Hayllar KM, et al: Early indicators of prognosis in fulminant hepatic failure. *Gastroenterology* 87:439, 1988.

22. Cetaruk EW, Dart RC, Hurlbut KM, et al: Tylenol Extended Relief overdose. *Ann Emerg Med* 30:104, 1997.

172 NONSTEROIDAL ANTI-INFLAMMATORY DRUGS

G. Richard Bruno

Wallace A. Carter

Nonsteroidal anti-inflammatory drugs (NSAIDs) are among the most widely used and prescribed drugs in the United States. They are effective antipyretics, nonnarcotic analgesics, and anti-inflammatory agents. There are between 35 and 70 million NSAID prescriptions written in the United States each year, and several agents are now available over the counter.[1] The world market for NSAIDs is reported to be a $6 billion per year industry. Given the tremendous use and easy availability of NSAIDs, they are relatively safe agents with respect to acute ingestion and overdose. The American Association of Poison Control Centers (AAPCC) reports 290,031 NSAID exposures resulting in 997 major outcomes (life-threatening signs and symptoms or

significant residual disability) and 38 deaths between 1997 and 2000. These cumulative data compare favorably to aspirin and acetaminophen, with fewer major outcomes and deaths per exposure (Table 172-1). The morbidity from NSAIDs in acute overdose is far overshadowed by complications of NSAIDs at therapeutic doses. It is estimated that NSAID-related gastrointestinal (GI) bleeding accounts for 16,500 deaths and 103,000 hospitalizations annually in the United States.[2] NSAIDs have also been reported to account for a substantial proportion of drug-induced renal failures.

PHARMACODYNAMICS

Overview

NSAIDs are structurally varied compounds with common therapeutic effects (Table 172-2). NSAIDs inhibit the enzyme cyclooxygenase (Cox), which is responsible for the production of prostaglandins from arachidonic acid. NSAIDs mediate inflammation through inhibition of prostaglandin production, but may also inhibit neutrophils via nonprostaglandin mechanisms. NSAIDs work as antipyretics through inhibition of prostaglandin E_2 (PGE_2) in the hypothalamus. NSAIDs appear to attenuate prostaglandin-mediated hyperalgesia and local pain-fiber stimulus.

Cyclooxygenase

There are at least two forms of cyclooxygenase: Cox-1 and Cox-2. Cox-1 is found predominantly in blood vessels, stomach, and kidneys at steady levels. Cox-2 is not usually found at significant levels in human tissue with the exception of possibly the brain and kidneys; rather, production of Cox-2 is induced by local inflammatory mediators.

There exist three general types of cyclooxygenase inhibitors: nonselective, partially selective, and selective (see Table 172-2). The vast majority of NSAIDs nonselectively inhibit both Cox-1 and Cox-2. It is the inhibition of Cox-1 that is believed to be responsible for many of the unwanted GI side effects of NSAIDs. There was a good deal of effort put forth to find more selective agents that would preferentially inhibit Cox-2. The partially selective agents (etodolac and meloxicam) are selective for Cox-2 at low doses, but become nonselective at higher doses. Recently, selective inhibitors of Cox-2 have been introduced with much anticipation and also some controversy. The new selective compounds do not appear to be more effective mediators of inflammation or analgesics, but they do appear to cause fewer GI side effects due to the lack of Cox-1 effects. The controversy surrounding these agents is the relative value of their GI sparing effects and less frequent dosing versus their significantly higher cost.

PHARMACOKINETICS

All NSAIDs are rapidly absorbed from the GI tract and are highly protein bound in the plasma. Most NSAIDs undergo at least partial me-

TABLE 172-1 Major Outcomes and Deaths

Cumulative AAPCC Data, 1997–2000	NSAIDs	Acetaminophen	Aspirin
Number of exposures	290,031	269,143	62,076
Major outcomes*	997	2,678	827
Deaths	35	287	175

*Major outcomes are defined as signs or symptoms that are life threatening or result in significant disability.

Abbreviations: AAPCC = American Association of Poison Control Centers; NSAIDs = nonsteroidal anti-inflammatory drugs.

TABLE 172-2   Classes of Nonsteroidal Agents Available in the United States

Nonselective NSAIDs
Salicylates
   Aspirin
   Salsalate (Salflex, Disalcid)
   Diflusinal (Dolobid)
Acetic acids
   Tolmetin (Tolectin)
   Ketorolac (Toradol)
   Diclofenac (Voltaren)
   Indomethacin (Indocin)
   Sulindac (Clinoril)
   Nabumetone (Relafen)
   Mefenamic acid (Ponstel)
   Meclofenamate (Meclomen)
Propionic acids
   Ibuprofen (Advil, Motrin, Nuprin)
   Naproxen (Naprosyn, Aleve)
   Ketoprofen (Orudis)
   Fenoprofen (Nalfon)
   Flurbiprofen (Ansaid)
   Oxaprozin (Daypro)
Pyrazolones
   Phenylbutazone
Oxicams
   Piroxicam (Feldene)
Partially selective Cox-2 inhibitors
   Etodolac (Lodin)
   Meloxicam (Mobic)
Selective Cox-2 inhibitors
   Valdecoxib (Bextra)
   Celecoxib (Celebrex)
   Rofecoxib (Vioxx)

tabolism in the liver via glucuronic acid conjugation or oxidation in the microsomal enzyme system before elimination in the urine or feces. Plasma half-lives of NSAIDs range from 2 to 4 h for ibuprofen to longer than 50 h for the long-acting agents piroxicam and phenylbutazone. The new selective Cox-2 inhibitors have a plasma half life of approximately 15 h.

SIGNIFICANT DRUG-DRUG INTERACTIONS

Warfarin

Warfarin and NSAIDs have important interactions. Two NSAIDs (phenylbutazone and naproxen) have been reported to displace warfarin from plasma proteins, leading to increased warfarin levels in serum and elevated prothrombin times. The selective Cox-2 inhibitors at therapeutic doses have also been reported to slightly elevate prothrombin times. Phenylbutazone has been shown to decrease elimination of warfarin. Other NSAIDs have not been reported to change warfarin protein binding or elimination, but the use of nonselective NSAIDs is not recommended in warfarin users because they inhibit platelet aggregation, significantly increasing the risk for bleeding.

Diuretics and Other Antihypertension Agents

NSAIDs may decrease the effectiveness of some antihypertensives, including diuretics, α-adrenergic blockers, angiotensin-converting enzyme inhibitors, and β-adrenergic blockers. The blood pressure change when both NSAIDs and antihypertensives are used ranges from little effect to hypertensive urgencies. Inhibition of prostaglandin synthesis is believed to be central to the attenuation of antihypertensive effects. Lower prostaglandin levels result in decreased renal sodium clearance, water retention, changes in vascular tone, and alter-

ations in the renin-angiotensin system, all which may attenuate the effectiveness of antihypertensive agents.[3]

Decreased Renal Clearance of Drugs

NSAIDs may also decrease the renal clearance and elimination of certain drugs. **NSAID use inhibits renal clearance of lithium and leads to elevated serum lithium levels. Methotrexate elimination is also decreased with coadministration of NSAIDs and has resulted in fatal toxicity.**

CLINICAL PRESENTATION OF TOXICITY

Toxicity of NSAIDs at Therapeutic Doses

NSAIDs are relatively safe drugs that have a number of well-documented side effects at therapeutic doses. Morbidity and death from renal insufficiency and GI bleeding with chronic NSAID use far overshadow those of acute NSAID overdose. Other organ systems that may show toxicity at therapeutic doses include the central nervous system (CNS), and the cardiovascular, respiratory, hepatic, and dermatologic systems. It is generally believed that indomethacin and the long-acting agents phenylbutazone and piroxicam are responsible for a greater proportion of side effects, and that the propionic acid agents such as ibuprofen are responsible for fewer side effects.

Central Nervous System

Toxic CNS side effects of NSAIDs are far less frequent than GI or renal toxicity; however, various CNS effects include headache, cognitive difficulties, behavioral change, and aseptic meningitis. Acute psychosis has been reported with indomethacin and sulindac use and is hypothesized to result from the structural similarity of these NSAIDs to serotonin.

One of the most interesting side effects of NSAID use is aseptic meningitis. The literature reports cases in which patients repeatedly present with symptoms of headache, fever, neck stiffness, and fever within hours of taking NSAIDs. Cerebrospinal fluid analysis in these patients reveals elevated white blood cell and protein levels, and normal or decreased glucose levels. Symptoms resolve after NSAID use is stopped and can be elicited with repeat NSAID challenges. This phenomenon is most often seen with patients who have underlying autoimmune diseases, such as systemic lupus erythematosus. The phenomenon is thought to be a hypersensitivity reaction. Infectious meningitis must be excluded before the diagnosis of NSAID-induced aseptic meningitis is entertained.[4]

Pulmonary System

NSAIDs have been responsible for various adverse pulmonary reactions, including hypersensitivity pneumonitis, bronchospasm in asthmatics, and pulmonary edema. Patients with NSAID-related hypersensitivity pneumonitis present with symptoms of fever, cough, shortness of breath, pulmonary infiltrates on chest x-ray, leukocytosis, and often peripheral eosinophilia. Cessation of NSAID use results in the resolution of symptoms, whereas readministration causes a recurrence of symptoms. NSAIDs implicated in hypersensitivity pneumonitis include naproxen, diflunisal, piroxicam, sulindac, and diclofenac. The mechanism of NSAID-mediated pneumonitis is believed to be an immune-mediated hypersensitivity reaction.

NSAID-induced bronchospasm is a well-described phenomenon in patients with reactive airway disease. The spectrum of hypersensitivity reaction varies from rhinitis to severe bronchospasm with laryngeal edema. Patients with underlying reactive airway disease and nasal polyps appear to be at greater risk for these complications. Aspirin is most often involved in hypersensitivity reactions. Aspirin-induced bronchospasm occurs in 8 to 20 percent of all asthmatics and in 14 to 23 percent of asthmatics with nasal polyps.[5] **Cross-sensitivity between aspirin and other NSAIDs is believed to be as high as 90 percent.** The mechanism of hypersensitivity to NSAIDs in asthmatics does not appear to be IgE mediated anaphylaxis; rather, it is an anaphylactoid reaction resulting from excessive leukotriene production.[6]

Gastrointestinal System

Gastrointestinal adverse effects result in the greatest morbidity from the therapeutic use of NSAIDs. These undesired effects range from dyspepsia to life-threatening bleeding from gastric or duodenal ulcerations. At therapeutic doses, nonselective NSAID inhibition of cytoprotective gastric prostaglandins (PGI_2 and PGE_2) increases the risk of gastric erosion, gastritis, and GI bleeding. There is a two- to five-fold increased risk of perforation or hemorrhage in NSAID users over the non-NSAID-using population. Data suggest that the risk for life-threatening bleeding is between 1.3 and 4 percent per year among NSAID users. It is estimated that NSAID-related GI bleeding contributes to 16,500 deaths and 103,000 hospitalizations annually in the United States.[2] Patients specifically at risk for GI bleeding include those who are elderly, those with a previous history of ulcers, those on high doses of NSAIDs, and those on corticosteroids.[7]

This significant risk for GI-related morbidity from the nonselective NSAIDs lead to the development of the newer selective Cox-2 inhibitors. These agents have been shown in multiple studies to have significantly reduced rates of gastric erosions and bleeding at therapeutic doses compared to nonselective NSAIDs.[8]

Liver

Both selective and nonselective NSAIDs may cause a spectrum of hepatic dysfunction, from asymptomatic elevation of transaminases to fulminant hepatic failure. NSAIDs that have caused idiosyncratic fulminant hepatic failure include diclofenac, bromfenac, ibuprofen, sulindac, naproxen, phenylbutazone, and oxaprozin. Hepatic toxicity can occur at any time during NSAID administration and is most common in patients with underlying liver disease, in the elderly, and in patients with preexisting autoimmune diseases.

Kidneys

The inhibition of prostaglandin synthesis by NSAIDs has specific effects on the kidneys. It appears that many of the renal effects of NSAIDs are mediated through Cox-2 inhibition.[9] These effects range from mild changes in fluid and electrolyte homeostasis to acute renal insufficiency. NSAIDs promote sodium and water retention by attenuating prostaglandin-mediated inhibition of chloride reabsorption. NSAIDs may lead to hyperkalemia, either by increased potassium reabsorption secondary to decreased sodium concentration at the distal tubule, or by decreased secretion of renin. There is at least one report in the literature of cardiac arrest secondary to NSAID-induced hyperkalemia.[10]

Prostaglandins have a vasodilatory effect on the renal vasculature. The most important of these renal vasodilatory prostaglandins are PGI_2 and PGE_2. Prostaglandin-mediated vasodilatation is probably of little importance in euvolemic patients with normally functioning kidneys. However, prostaglandins appear to attenuate the vasoconstricting effects of the renin-angiotensin system and sympathetic nervous system during times of stress, during periods of decreased intravascular volume (sepsis, hemorrhage, and diuretic therapy), and in disease states that predispose patients to sodium retention (congestive heart failure, cirrhosis, and nephrotic syndrome).[11] The lack of these va-

sodilatory prostaglandins due to Cox inhibition by NSAIDs may put stressed kidneys at risk for azotemia and renal insufficiency. Similar precautions must be used when using both nonselective and selective Cox-2 inhibitors in patients predisposed to intravascular volume depletion, preexisting renal insufficiency, diabetes, and the aforementioned comorbid states.

Hematologic System

Nonselective NSAIDs inhibit platelet formation of thromboxane A_2, a potent stimulator of platelet aggregation. This leads to qualitative platelet deficiencies. The new Cox-2 inhibitors have far fewer antiplatelet effects than traditional NSAIDs. This may explain why there may be an increase in cardiac and neurovascular events in patients taking the Cox-2 inhibitor rofecoxib versus the nonselective Cox-1 inhibitor naproxen.[1]

Most NSAIDs decrease platelet aggregation only when significant concentrations of the drug are present. Increased bleeding tendencies secondary to NSAIDs are not widely reported in the literature. However, patients taking aspirin are at risk for increased bleeding during surgery, and patients maintained on coumadin are advised to avoid all NSAIDs.

NSAIDs may cause other blood disorders. Bone marrow suppression is a rare but reported hematologic complication with use of NSAIDs. Aplastic anemia has been reported with almost all classes of NSAIDs, but phenylbutazone, indomethacin, and diclofenac are responsible for most cases.[12] NSAID use has also resulted in agranulocytosis, red cell aplasia, thrombocytopenia, and hemolytic anemia.

Skin

NSAIDs account for approximately 10 percent of cutaneous drug reactions.[13] Agents most frequently involved in dermatologic complications include phenylbutazone, piroxicam, and benoxaprofen.[14] Drug reactions to NSAIDs range from benign maculopapular rashes to the severe Stevens-Johnson syndrome and toxic epidermal necrolysis. NSAIDs are some of the most often-implicated drugs in cases of toxic epidermal necrolysis, accounting for up to one-third of drug-related cases in one series.[15] NSAIDs of all types (oral and topical) can cause photosensitivity reactions, including increased sensitivity to sun exposure (phototoxic) and true photoallergic reactions. Piroxicam and ketoprofen are the NSAIDs most frequently involved in photoallergic reactions. One NSAID of the oxicam family, isoxicam, was removed from the U.S. market after fatal skin reactions.

Pregnancy

Prostaglandins are found in high concentration in the term uterus and have a stimulatory effect on normal labor. NSAIDs inhibit uterine motility through Cox-mediated inhibition of prostaglandin synthesis. Indomethacin is sufficiently effective at slowing uterine contractions that it has been used to treat preterm labor. Although NSAIDs are not believed to be teratogenic in humans, they do cross the placenta later in pregnancy. **One of the most significant effects of fetal exposure to NSAIDs is premature constriction of the ductus arteriosus, which may result in pulmonary hypertension.** Other reported effects of in utero exposure to NSAIDs include oligohydramnios, renal dysfunction, necrotizing enterocolitis, and CNS hemorrhage.

NSAID-induced inhibition of platelet aggregation may place the fetus and the mother at increased risk for bleeding. Mothers who take NSAIDs during the latter part of pregnancy appear to be at risk for increased peripartum hemorrhage. **The safest recommendation is to avoid NSAID use during pregnancy, especially during the third trimester.**

ACUTE OVERDOSE

Most patients with acute overdoses suffer little morbidity, but patients with significant overdoses may present with CNS, metabolic, hemodynamic, GI, or renal dysfunction.[16] It is generally accepted that patients taking NSAIDs of the pyrazolone (phenylbutazone and oxyphenylbutazone) and the fenamic acid (mefenamic acid) families may present with the most severe clinical symptoms. It does not appear that NSAID metabolism is changed after acute overdose, and symptoms of acute overdose are usually apparent within 4 h of ingestion. There is little data about acute overdose of the relatively new Cox-2 inhibitors, but they are assumed to have similar safety profiles as the traditional NSAIDs.

Central Nervous System

CNS manifestation of acute NSAID overdose is usually minimal, but patients with significant overdose may present with altered mental status. Other CNS manifestations of acute overdose have included diplopia, nystagmus, and headache. Seizures have been reported after large overdoses and appear to be of special concern after ingestion of mefenamic acid.

Cardiovascular System

Acute NSAID overdose has resulted in hypotension and bradydysrhythmia. NSAIDs are not known to be primary causes of dysrhythmias, but fluid and electrolyte abnormalities may place patients at risk. Cardiovascular dysfunction is responsive to conventional critical care management.

Electrolytes

Electrolyte and acid-base abnormalities have been reported in acute NSAID overdoses. Alterations in serum electrolytes may occur secondary to decreased prostaglandin synthesis or from NSAID-induced renal failure. Sodium and water retention may lead to volume overload in patients having preexisting renal failure, cirrhosis, or congestive heart failure. Hyperkalemia, hypocalcemia, and hypomagnesemia have been reported in NSAID overdoses complicated by acute renal failure.[17]

Increased anion-gap acidosis has been observed with large overdoses of the propionic acid NSAIDs ibuprofen and naproxen. Prostaglandin inhibition is not directly responsible for the anion-gap acidosis; rather, acidosis is likely to be related to lactic acidosis. Case reports of large overdoses suggest that the acidosis may be related to large quantities of these mildly acidic NSAIDs and their metabolites in serum.[18] However, these studies neither measured nor considered lactate as the possible mechanism. Concurrent lactic acidosis in the setting of NSAID-induced seizures may worsen the acidosis in some cases.

Gastrointestinal-Hepatic System

Patients presenting after acute NSAID overdose may have abdominal pain, nausea, and vomiting. Life-threatening GI hemorrhage is not a typical finding after acute overdoses. Overdose may also result in hepatic injury, as witnessed by elevated transaminase levels and cholestasis.

Renal Failure

Acute renal failure is rare after NSAID overdose, but NSAID overdose may place a stressed renal system at risk for failure. Clinical presentation may include hematuria, elevations in blood urea nitrogen/creatine, and oliguria. The mechanism of renal insufficiency in acute overdose is believed to be renal vascular changes secondary to Cox-mediated prostaglandin inhibition. Patients with underlying renal insufficiency appear to be at greatest risk for acute renal failure. Most patients have recovery of renal function, but the need for long-term dialysis has been reported.

TREATMENT

Most patients who present with NSAID overdose will be asymptomatic. Patients who present with symptomatic ingestions (altered mental status, seizure, electrolyte disturbances, anion-gap acidosis, or renal insufficiencies) should be treated with supportive care using emergency medicine and toxicology principles. Airway management should be initiated in obtunded or apneic patients, hypotension should be managed with fluid boluses or vasopressor agents when refractory, and seizures should be treated initially with intravenous benzodiazepines.

Patients who present as hemodynamically stable with a report of acute ingestion should have a directed history and physical examination with attention focused on mental status, GI symptoms, and any signs of renal dysfunction (Figure 172-1). The history should include amount and type NSAID ingested and questions about coingestants. Ibuprofen is the most common NSAID encountered in acute ingestion, and it is generally accepted that an ingestion of less than 100 mg/kg is unlikely to result in toxicity and that greater than 400 mg/kg places the patient at greatest risk for toxicity. Most authorities believe that patients with acute ingestions will show symptoms within 4 h.

Laboratory Evaluation

Laboratory evaluation of patients with acute ingestions should focus on acid-base status, electrolyte level, and renal function. Hepatic profile, complete blood count, coagulation profile, and aspirin and acetaminophen levels should also be sent. Evaluation of drug levels for specific NSAIDs are not indicated. **A nomogram for ibuprofen intoxication does exist but is not clinically useful.** NSAID levels do not correlate well with observed toxicity or outcomes.[19]

Decontamination and Enhanced Elimination

Gastric decontamination should be initiated in all patients with suspected NSAID overdoses. Activated charcoal with the cathartic sorbitol should be given orally or through a nasogastric tube. Repeated doses of activated charcoal without sorbitol are indicated in symptomatic patients. Dialysis and charcoal hemoperfusion are not effective in enhancing elimination, because NSAIDs are highly protein bound. Manipulation of serum and urine pH through alkalinization is not helpful in enhancing elimination.

DISPOSITION OF PATIENTS WITH ACUTE OVERDOSES

Most patients with asymptomatic NSAID ingestions can be safely discharged after screening for coingestants and a 4- to 6-h period of observation. Any patient with symptomatic overdose (altered mental status, abnormal vital signs, electrolyte abnormalities, or acute renal failure) should be admitted for observation and supportive care. The psychosocial situation within which the overdose occurred requires careful evaluation.

Prognosis

The majority of NSAID overdoses will not cause significant sequelae. Even patients with major symptoms have a good prognosis if they overcome the initial insult (see Table 172-1).

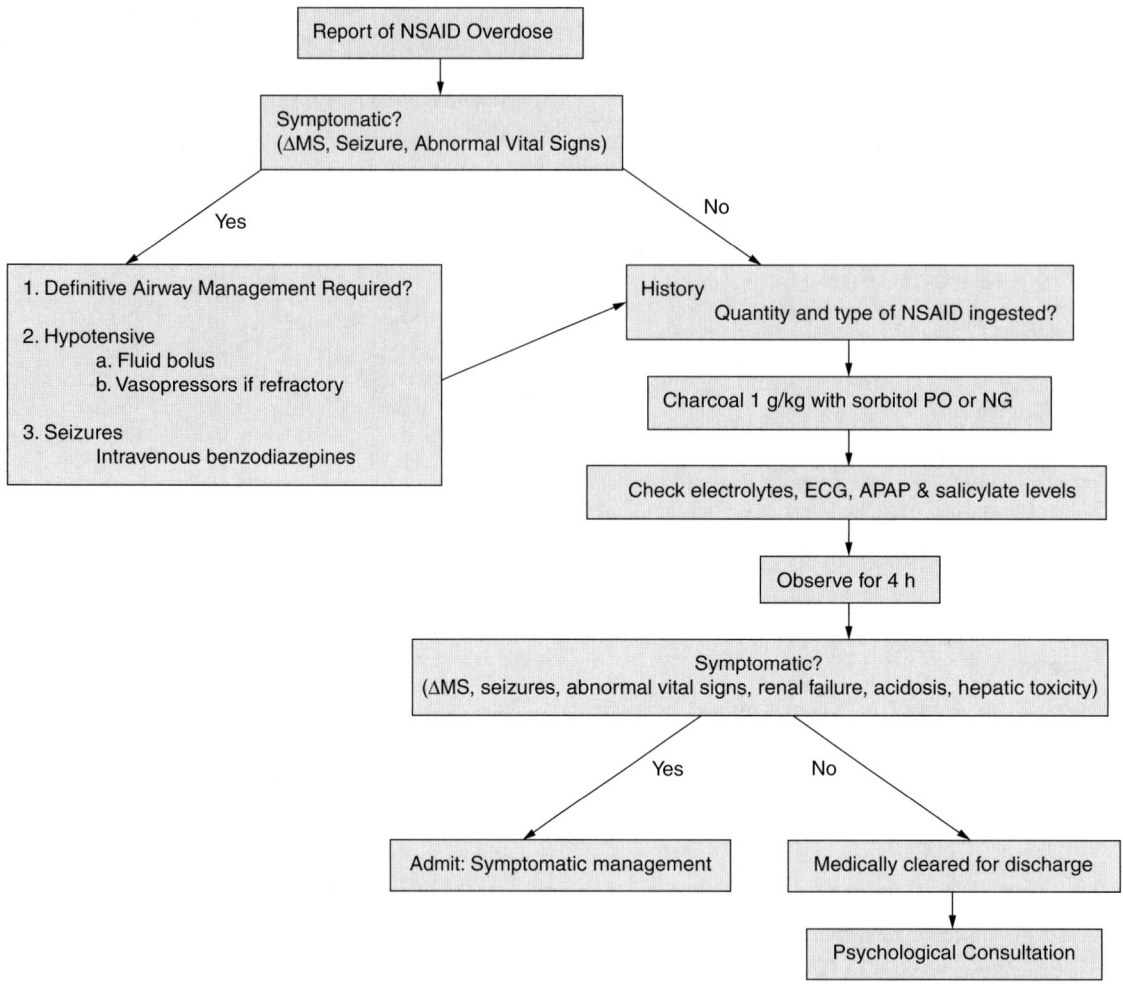

FIG. 172-1. Approach to treatment of acute NSAID overdose. APAP = acetaminophen.

REFERENCES

1. Singh G, Ramey DR, Morfeld D, et al: Comparative toxicity of non-steroidal anti-inflammatory agents. *Pharmacol Ther* 62:175, 1994.
2. Singh G, Triadafilopoulus G: Epidemiology of NSAID-induced GI complications. *J Rheumatol* 26(Suppl):18, 1999.
3. Houston MC: Nonsteroidal anti-inflammatory drugs and antihypertensives. *Am J Med* 90(5A):42S, 1991.
4. Hoppmann RA, Peden JG, Ober SK: Central nervous system side effects of nonsteroidal anti-inflammatory drugs. *Arch Intern Med* 151:1309, 1991.
5. Camu F, Lauwers MH, Vanlersberghe C: Side effects of NSAIDs and dosing recommendations for ketorolac. *Acta Anaesthesiol Belg* 47:143, 1996.
6. Babu K, Salvi S: Aspirin and Asthma. *Chest* 118:1470, 2000.
7. Hawkey CJ: Gastrointestinal safety of Cox-2 specific inhibitors. *Gastroenterol Clin* 30:921, 2001.
8. Langman MJ, Jensen DM, Watson DJ, et al: Adverse upper gastrointestinal effects of rofecoxib compared with NSAIDs. *JAMA* 282:1929, 1999.
9. Komers R, Anderson S, Epstein M: Renal and vascular effects of selective cyclooxygenase-2 inhibitors. *Am J Kidney Dis* 38:1145, 2001.
10. Kharasch MS, Johnson KM, Strange GR: Cardiac arrest secondary to indomethacin-induced renal failure: A case report. *J Emerg Med* 8:51, 1990.
11. Kleinknecht D: Interstitial nephritis, the nephrotic syndrome, and chronic renal failure secondary to nonsteroidal anti-inflammatory drugs. *Semin Nephrol* 15:228, 1995.
12. Storti E, Molinari E: Blood disorders secondary to the use of non-steroidal anti-inflammatory drugs. *Haematologica (Pavia)* 73:239, 1988.
13. Roujeau JC, Stern RS: Severe adverse cutaneous reactions to drugs. *New Engl J Med* 331:1272, 1994.
14. Alhava E: Reported adverse drug reactions and consumption of nonsteroidal anti-inflammatory drugs. *Pharmacol Toxicol* 75(Suppl 2):37, 1994.
15. Roujeau JC, Kelly JP, Naldi L, et al: Medication use and the risk of Stevens-Johnson syndrome or toxic epidermal necrolysis. *New Engl J Med* 333:1600, 1995.
16. Hall AH, Smolinske SC, Conrad FL, et al: Ibuprofen overdose: 126 cases. *Ann Emerg Med* 15:1308, 1986.
17. Al-Harbi NN, Somnuek D, Lirenman DS: Hypocalcemia and hypomagnesemia after ibuprofen overdose. *Ann Pharm Fr* 31:432, 1997.
18. Martinez R, Smith DW, Frankel LR: Severe metabolic acidosis after acute naproxen sodium ingestion. *Ann Emerg Med* 18:1102, 1989.
19. McElwee NE, Veltri JC, Bradford DC, et al: A prospective, population-based study of acute ibuprofen overdose: Complications are rare and routine serum levels not warranted. *Ann Emerg Med* 19:657, 1990.

THEOPHYLLINE
Heather Marshall
Charles L. Emerman

Theophylline use is complicated by its narrow therapeutic window, with a metabolism that depends on the patient's coincident medical problems and use of other medications. The *2000 Annual Report of the American Association of Poison Control Centers Toxic Exposure Surveillance System* reported 1146 exposures to aminophylline or theophylline, resulting in 18 deaths.[1] This represents a decrease in the number of exposures from 5 years ago, but a similar number of fatalities and incidents with major toxicity. Most theophylline exposures are unintentional overdoses occurring in adults. A theophylline level greater than 20 μg/mL (110 μmol/L) is generally considered in the toxic range, although side effects may be seen at lower levels and some patients may remain asymptomatic at higher levels.[2] Recent changes in the U.S. Food and Drug Administration dosing guidelines are aimed at reducing the likelihood of developing toxic levels. Life-threatening toxicity from theophylline poisoning can result in significant cardiac, neurologic, and metabolic abnormalities. Several modalities are available for treating theophylline toxicity, but indications for their use in patients without life-threatening symptoms is controversial.

PHARMACOLOGY

Theophylline and related products (Table 173-1) have a complex mechanism of action that has not been entirely elucidated. Although traditional teaching is that theophylline acts by inhibiting the action of phosphodiesterase, the concentration required for effective in vivo inhibition far exceeds the concentration usually produced by clinical dosages. Others have suggested that theophylline may act by affecting the binding of cyclic adenosine monophosphate, cyclic glucose monophosphate phosphodiesterase inhibition, prostaglandin antagonism, modification of intracellular calcium, stimulation of catecholamine release, or adenosine antagonism. In addition to its bronchodilatory effect, theophylline affects both the immune and inflammatory mechanisms.[3] Crossover studies have found that theophylline blunts the late asthmatic response.[4] Theophylline is readily absorbed after oral administration, with peak levels occurring 90 to 120 min after ingestion. Oral absorption is enhanced by fasting or ingestion of large volumes of fluid and is decreased following ingestion of certain foods. Enteric-coated tablets and sustained-released preparations reach peak plasma levels between 6 and 8 h. The newer, once-daily preparations have an erratic absorption rate, particularly after eating, which may lead to drug "dumping" (rapid absorption) and elevated theophylline levels. Peak levels are reached within 30 min after intravenous administration of aminophylline. The absorption of IM and PR administered drug is erratic and unpredictable. Consequently, these routes should not be used.

Theophylline is approximately 60 percent protein bound, with less binding in neonates and patients with cirrhosis. The volume of distribution ranges from 0.3 to 0.7 L/kg, with an average of 0.5 L/kg. Theophylline is primarily (85 to 90 percent) eliminated by the hepatic cytochrome P450 system, and the remaining 10 to 15 percent is eliminated by urinary excretion. Metabolism generally follows first-order elimination. The half-life is 4 to 8 h in young, healthy, nonsmoking adults, and shorter in children and smokers. Most bronchodilation occurs by serum concentrations of 15 μg/mL, leading to recommendations to lower the target for dosing from 20 μg/mL. The use of aminophylline in the management of acute asthma is controversial. Several reviews conclude that **intravenous administration of aminophylline is not effective in adults for the management of acute exacerbations of chronic obstructive pulmonary disease (COPD) or asthma.[3,5,6] There may, however be some utility to its use in children with acute asthma.[7]** Theophylline products may be useful for outpatient management, particularly for patients who cannot or will not use inhalers, patients with prominent nighttime symptoms, or those who have maximized or cannot tolerate other asthma controlling agents such as long acting β-agonists or corticosteroids. A number of factors affect theophylline's half-life, including cigarette use, diet, cardiac and liver disease, and medications that interfere with the cytochrome P450 pathway (Table 173-2). The effect of fluoroquinolone antibiotics is variable, with levofloxacin causing little change in theophylline clearance. Passive smoke exposure increases theophylline

TABLE 173-1   Theophylline Content of Related Drugs

Drug	Theophylline Content (%)
Aminophylline	80–85
Oxtriphylline	65
Dyphylline	50

TABLE 173-2   Factors Affecting Theophylline Half-Life

Decreased Half-Life	Increased Half-Life
DRUGS	
Carbamazepine	Cimetidine
Phenobarbital	Allopurinol
Phenytoin	Zileuton
	Ticlopidine
	Interferon
	Methotrexate
	Estrogens
ANTIBIOTICS	
Sulfinpyrazone	Erythromycin
	Clarithromycin
	Quinolones
	Thiabendazole
ANTIDYSRHYTHMICS	
	Mexiletine
	Propranolol
	Verapamil
	Tocainide
	Propafenone
CONDITIONS AND OTHER FACTORS	
Smoking	Cirrhosis
Charcoal-broiled foods	Congestive heart failure
Children	Pneumonia
Hyperthyroidism	Severe chronic obstructive pulmonary disease
St. John's wort	Viral illness in children
	Obesity
	Neonates

clearance, as does the use of St. John's wort. Theophylline acts as an adenosine antagonist. It markedly inhibits the coronary vasodilating effects of adenosine and may interfere with the usefulness of pharmacologic stress tests. Theophylline has been reported to reverse adenosine-induced bronchoconstriction. Few studies have examined the effects of theophylline on the therapeutic use of adenosine to reverse supraventricular tachycardia. One study reported on the successful conversion from supraventricular tachycardia in two patients with therapeutic theophylline levels. A few case reports describe the use of adenosine in theophylline-induced arrhythmias, but experience on which to base recommendations is inadequate. Aminophylline has been reported to reverse toxicity caused by overdose of multiple antihypertensive agents. There are some reports that aminophylline reduces the incidence of contrast-induced nephropathy, although other reports do not confirm this.[8,9]

TOXIC EFFECTS

Theophylline has a range of toxic effects from minor gastrointestinal symptoms to life-threatening dysrhythmias. Although it is commonly thought that symptom severity is serum-level dependent, in fact, life-threatening adverse effects may occur with little warning and before minor symptoms are evident. Many patients with elevated levels are asymptomatic and the type of symptom is not predictive of the theophylline level.[10]

Cardiovascular

Even at therapeutic levels (10 to 20 μg/mL), theophylline can cause cardiac side effects. Sinus tachycardia may occur after administration, and increased atrial automaticity, with premature atrial contractions, atrial tachycardia, multifocal atrial tachycardia, atrial fibrillation, and atrial flutter, occurs more frequently with levels above 20 μg/mL. Ventricular dysrhythmias with premature ventricular contractions and self-limited runs of ventricular tachycardia may also occur. Sustained ventricular tachycardia may occur in older patients with chronic overdose at levels of approximately 40 to 60 µg/mL. Younger patients with acute intentional overdose may tolerate levels above 100 µg/mL without developing life-threatening cardiac effects. Patients with a history of dysrhythmias may experience a recurrence of dysrhythmias with levels less than 40 µg/mL. Patients who are reported to poison control centers are more likely to have cardiac complications than any other serious manifestation of toxicity.[11] Hypotension has also been associated with acute ingestion but may also occur with chronic overmedication.

Neurologic

Even with therapeutic levels, theophylline use can be associated with agitation, headache, irritability, sleeplessness, tremors, and muscular twitching. Seizures, including both generalized tonic–clonic and focal motor, have been reported in patients with therapeutic levels. Patients with a history of epilepsy are particularly susceptible to aminophylline-induced seizures. Animal data indicates that chronic cocaine use may increase the susceptibility to theophylline induced seizures. There are human case reports of nonconvulsive status epilepticus with bizarre posturing associated with cocaine use. The incidence of seizures increases as toxic levels increase.[12] Status epilepticus resistant to treatment can occur as the level rises above 25 µg/mL. When seizures occur at only mildly elevated levels, there are usually underlying neurologic deficits. The occurrence of seizures does not appear to correlate with prognosis. Theophylline toxicity is also associated with hallucinations and psychosis.

Metabolic

Theophylline produces a dose-dependent increase in circulating catecholamines. There is a concomitant increase in glucose, free fatty acid, insulin levels, and white blood cell count. Hypokalemia may occur, with the fall in serum potassium level inversely related to the theophylline concentration. Hypokalemia appears to be a particular problem in patients with acute overdose or acute overdose superimposed on chronic use. Administration of a β-agonist may also be associated with hypokalemia and, with the hypokalemia produced by theophylline overdose, may lead to cardiac dysrhythmias. Lactic acidosis may also be present.

Gastrointestinal

Theophylline has a direct central nervous system effect, leading to nausea and vomiting (the most frequent and usually the earliest symptom). In addition, theophylline increases gastric acid secretion. Nausea and vomiting can be seen with therapeutic levels, although the incidence of nausea and vomiting increases markedly with levels above 15 µg/mL. Approximately 25 percent of patients with levels greater than 20 µg/mL have nausea or vomiting. Gastrointestinal bleeding, with epigastric pain, may also occur. Esophageal reflux has also been reported.

TREATMENT

Gastric emptying with gastric lavage may be considered for patients who have a potentially toxic ingestion occurring within the previous 1 to 2 h. Gastric lavage is probably not indicated for patients whose dose is calculated to have raised their levels to less than 30 µg/mL (approximately 10 mg/kg), unless coingestion of other medications is suspected. Ipecac may complicate the use of other therapies for enhancing the elimination of theophylline and, given the seizure potentiation, probably should be avoided. In addition, vomiting is usually a prominent symptom in theophylline toxicity.

Theophylline undergoes hepatobiliary enteric circulation leading to recommendations for multiple-dose oral-activated charcoal administration. Treatment begins with activated charcoal administered in a dose of 1 g/kg. The use of repeated doses (1 g/kg, up to 50 g) of activated charcoal at 2- to 4-h intervals significantly decreases the half-life of theophylline. Charcoal may also be administered as a continuous nasogastric infusion at rates of 0.25 to 0.5 g/kg per h. Cathartics can enhance the passage of ingested theophylline through the gastrointestinal tract. Some investigators have found magnesium citrate not to be effective in lowering the theophylline level. However, there have been reports of magnesium toxicity after the use of magnesium cathartics and thus sorbitol may be a better choice. A 70 percent sorbitol solution (100 mL) is used in combination with activated charcoal for patients with potentially toxic ingestions. Caution should be used since cathartics may cause fluid and electrolyte imbalances.

The treatment of theophylline toxicity is often hindered by the gastrointestinal disturbances produced by toxic levels. Antiemetic therapies noted to be effective in controlling theophylline-induced emesis are ranitidine (50 mg IV) or metoclopramide (high-dose, 0.5 to 1.0 mg/kg). Ondansetron has also been shown to be efficacious.[13] The control of nausea and vomiting permits the use of repeated doses of activated charcoal to enhance drug elimination.

There are reports of successful use of whole-bowel irrigation with polyethylene glycol solution, although one study showed no additional benefit over activated charcoal.[14] The use of whole-bowel irrigation as an adjunct therapy to activated charcoal remains controversial.

Recent prospective studies, however, indicate that hemoperfusion is associated with a higher complication rate without any significant increase in clinical efficacy over hemodialysis.[15] The clearance rate induced by hemodialysis is approximately 200 mL/kg per h. Charcoal hemoperfusion with resin or charcoal filters produces extraction ratios above 0.85, with clearance rates of up to 300 mL/kg per h. Recent case reports also show the use of continuous venovenous hemofiltration as an effective alternative to hemoperfusion, especially because it is available in most hospitals and because it is well tolerated in the hemodynamically unstable patient.[16] The guidelines for extracorporeal drug removal (hemoperfusion/hemodialysis) remain controversial (Table 173-3). In the view of some investigators, hemoperfusion or hemodialysis is not absolutely indicated at any theophylline level in the absence of life-threatening symptoms, such as status epilepticus or resistant ventricular dysrhythmias. Others have felt that patients with increased half-lives, advanced age, or theophylline levels above 80 µg/mL may be candidates for early hemoperfusion or hemodialysis as a preventive intervention. Young, healthy patients with an acute ingestion may be able to tolerate levels over 100 µg/mL without adverse incident. The decision to use hemoperfusion or hemodialysis should be made considering the potential for life-threatening toxicity.

Hypotension or cardiac arrhythmias are another indication of severe theophylline toxicity requiring aggressive supportive care. If the hypotension is refractory to fluids and conventional vasopressor ther-

TABLE 173-3 Indications for Hemoperfusion/Hemodialysis

Clinical Conditions	Recommendation
Life-threatening toxicity (i.e., seizures tachydysrhythmias) not responsive to other therapy	Indicated
Acute overdose with level ≥100 µg/mL	Possibly indicated
Chronic overdose with level ≥60 µg/mL	Possibly indicated
Elderly patient with known prolonged theophylline half-life, severe liver or severe cardiac disease, or level ≥40 µg/mL	Controversial
Theophylline level ≤30 µg/mL	Not indicated

apy, α-adrenergic agents such as phenylephrine may be considered. β-Blocker therapy, particularly with propranolol, also reverses the theophylline-induced vasodilation, thereby improving hypotension and tachyarrhythmias. β-Blockers should be administered cautiously in low doses and monitored for adverse effect. Alternatively, esmolol, an agent with cardioselectivity and a short duration of action, has been successfully used.[17]

In addition to being treated with β-blockade, cardiac arrhythmias may be treated with other antiarrhythmics. Verapamil has been effective in animal studies. The use of digoxin, lidocaine, and phenytoin has been reported for treatment of ventricular dysrhythmias (see Chaps. 28 and 29). Adenosine is effective in the treatment of theophylline-induced supraventricular arrhythmias, although it has been associated with bronchospasm. The contributory effect of hypokalemia should be considered in treating patients with resistant ventricular dysrhythmias, and correction of serum electrolyte abnormalities may be effective in terminating recurrent dysrhythmias.

Seizures may be difficult to control with standard anticonvulsant therapy. Benzodiazepines (diazepam, 10 mg IV, or lorazepam) remain the first-line anticonvulsants of choice and may require high doses. Second-line therapy is with a barbiturate such as phenobarbital. The airway should be protected in patients with theophylline-induced status epilepticus, especially following the administration of oral activated charcoal. Patients with status epilepticus resistant to traditional therapy may require general anesthesia with electroencephalographic monitoring and more aggressive measures to lower the serum theophylline level.

INDICATIONS FOR TREATMENT AND ADMISSION

Although theophylline toxicity can lead to life-threatening side effects, elevated theophylline levels are common and most patients tolerate them with only minor toxic manifestations.[18] Serum theophylline concentrations do not correlate well with severity of toxicity in chronic exposures. However, serum levels for acute exposures are more valuable in predicting toxicity and clinical course. No well-conducted studies have demonstrated that prophylactic use of antiarrhythmics or antiepileptics decreases morbidity or mortality rates. Similarly, while hemodialysis, hemoperfusion, and oral activated charcoal therapy enhance theophylline clearance, there is no compelling evidence that their use lowers morbidity or mortality rates for patients with only mild toxic symptoms or minimally elevated levels.

Ventricular dysrhythmias or seizures may occur in patients before the manifestation of other minor toxic effects, leading some authors to advocate aggressive therapy. Older patients with concomitant medical problems are more susceptible to life-threatening theophylline toxicity following chronic overmedication than are younger patients with an acute overdose.[19] The prophylactic use of hemoperfusion has been reported to decrease rates of major morbidity in elderly patients.

In general, patients with a history of seizures or ventricular dysrhythmias should be monitored until their theophylline level returns to normal. Patients with levels below 25 μg/mL and minor symptoms do not require specific therapy other than discontinuation or modification of theophylline administration. Such patients generally do not require hospitalization. Patients with levels above 30 μg/mL should be treated with oral activated charcoal (repeated) and monitored for toxic side effects. Hemoperfusion or hemodialysis use is controversial but may be indicated for older patients with levels above 40 μg/mL, especially with chronic intoxications or for younger patients with acute intentional overdose with levels above 100 μg/mL.

PREVENTION

Theophylline toxicity is only rarely a result of intentional overdose. Patients being started on certain medications, in particular cimetidine and macrolide or fluoroquinolone antibiotics, should have their the-

ophylline dose decreased by approximately 25 percent, with monitoring of the effect on levels. Aminophylline infusions should be started using standard guidelines with close monitoring of serum levels. Because the history of outpatient theophylline use has been found to be a poor guide to the serum concentration, loading doses of aminophylline should be calculated using the initial theophylline level. The initial dose of oral theophylline should not exceed 900 mg/d. Starting patients at a much lower dose (400 mg/d) helps to avoid the nausea and vomiting frequently accompanying initial theophylline use. Levels should be determined in order to monitor therapy.

The presence or absence of mild side effects is not a good predictor of drug levels.[10] Patients should be cautioned not to alter their medication regimen without physician guidance.

REFERENCES

1. Litovitz T, Klein-Schwartz W, Rodgers GC, et al: 2001 Annual report of the American Association of Poison Control Centers Toxic Exposure Surveillance System. *Am J Emerg Med* 20:391, 2002.
2. Bertino JS, Walker JW: Reassessment of theophylline toxicity: Serum concentrations, clinical course, and treatment. *Arch Intern Med* 147:757, 1987.
3. Weinberger M, Hendeles L: Theophylline in asthma. *New Engl J Med* 334: 1380, 1996.
4. Jarjour NN, Lacouture PG, Busse WW: Theophylline inhibits the late asthmatic response to nighttime antigen challenge in patients with mild atopic asthma. *Ann Allergy Asthma Immunol* 81:231, 1998.
5. Parameswaran K, Belda J Rowe BH: Addition of intravenous aminophylline to beta₂-agonists in adults with acute asthma (Cochrane Review). In: *The Cochrane Library,* Issue 1, 2002. Oxford: Update Software.
6. Barr RG, Rowe BH, Camargo Jr, CA. Methyl-xanthines for exacerbations of chronic obstructive pulmonary disease (Cochrane Review). In: *The Cochrane Library,* Issue 1, 2002. Oxford: Update Software.
7. Mitra A, Bassler D, Ducharme FM: Intravenous aminophylline for acute severe asthma in children over 2 years using inhaled bronchodilators (Cochrane Review). In: *The Cochrane Library,* Issue 1, 2002. Oxford: Update Software.
8. Huber W, Jeschke B, Page M et al: Reduced incidence of radiocontrast-induced nephropathy in ICU patients under theophylline prophylaxis: A prospective comparison to series of patients at similar risk. *Intensive Care Med* 27:1200, 2001.
9. Shammas NW, Kapalis MJ, Harris M, et al: Aminophylline does not protect against radiocontrast nephropathy in patients undergoing percutaneous angiographic procedures. *J Invasive Cardiol* 13:738, 2001.
10. Melamed J, Beaucher WN: Minor symptoms are not predictive of elevated theophylline levels in adults on chronic therapy. *Ann Allergy Asthma Immunol* 75:516, 1995.
11. Shannon M: Life-threatening events after theophylline overdose: A 10-year prospective analysis. *Arch Intern Med* 159:989, 1999.
12. Sesler CN: Theophylline toxicity: Clinical features of 116 consecutive cases. *Am J Med* 88:567, 1990.
13. Roberts JR, Carney S, Bolyle SM, Lee D: Ondansetron quells drug-resistant emesis in theophylline poisoning. *Am J Emerg Med* 11:609, 1993.
14. Burkhart K, Euerz R, Donovan J: Whole-bowel irrigation as adjunctive treatment for sustained-release theophylline overdose. *Ann Emerg Med* 11:1774, 1993.
15. Shannon M: Comparative efficacy of hemodialysis and hemoperfusion in severe theophylline intoxication. *Acad Emerg Med* 4:674, 1997.
16. Henderson JH, McKenzie CA, Hilton PJ, Leach RM: Continuous venovenous hemofiltration for the treatment of theophylline toxicity. *Thorax* 56:242, 2001.
17. Seneff M, Scott J, Friedman B, Smith M: Acute theophylline toxicity and the use of esmolol to reverse cardiovascular instability. *Ann Emerg Med* 19:67, 1990.
18. Emerman CL, Devlin C, Connors AF: Risk of toxicity in patients with elevated theophylline levels. *Ann Emerg Med* 19:643, 1990.
19. Shannon M: Predictors or major toxicity after theophylline overdose. *Ann Intern Med* 119:1161, 1993.

DIGITALIS GLYCOSIDES
William Dribben
Mark A. Kirk

EPIDEMIOLOGY

For centuries, digitalis glycosides have been recognized for their medicinal benefits and potential toxicity. Digitalis preparations are used most commonly in the treatment of supraventricular tachydysrhythmias and congestive heart failure. In addition to their availability as pharmaceuticals, cardiac glycosides are also found in plants such as foxglove, oleander, and lily of the valley. It is important that physicians recognize digitalis toxicity because potentially fatal cardiac dysrhythmias can be reversed with prompt administration of a highly specific antidote, digoxin-specific Fab fragments.[1] According to the American Association of Poison Control Centers (AAPCC), 2977 exposures to cardiac glycosides were reported in 2001. Of these exposures, 652 (22 percent) patients demonstrated moderate or major morbidity, with 13 (0.4 percent) deaths.[2] Even though digitalis use has declined due to newer modes of therapy for supraventricular tachydysrhythmias and congestive heart failure, reported exposures and morbidity and mortality have remained constant over the past 10 years.

PHARMACOLOGY AND PATHOPHYSIOLOGY

Digoxin is currently the most widely used digitalis preparation. It is absorbed rapidly from the gastrointestinal tract and is eliminated primarily through renal excretion. It has a volume of distribution of 6 L/kg. The half-life of a therapeutic dose is 36 to 48 h.

Digitalis has a narrow therapeutic-toxic margin. Toxicity results from an exaggeration of its therapeutic actions. Digitalis binds to a specific receptor site on the cardiac cell membrane, inactivating the $Na^+K^+ATPase$ pump.[3] This pump concentrates sodium extracellularly and potassium intracellularly to maintain the electrochemical membrane potential vital to conduction tissues. When $Na^+K^+ATPase$ is inhibited, the sodium-calcium exchanger removes accumulated intracellular sodium in exchange for calcium. This exchange increases sarcoplasmic calcium and is the mechanism thought to be responsible for the positive inotropic effect of digitalis. Inhibition of the $Na^+K^+ATPase$ pump also results in an increase in extracellular potassium.[3] Other potential mechanisms accounting for increased cytosolic calcium resulting in increased inotropic and/or toxic effects may be due to actions directly at calcium channels on the sarcoplasmic reticulum or via activation of the ryanodine receptor.[4] Digitalis increases vagal tone and decreases conduction through the atrioventricular (AV) node. In toxic doses, these effects result in various bradydysrhythmias. Automaticity is increased due to slowing of conduction in the electrical system along with a shortened refractory period in the myocardium. Intracellular calcium overload can create delayed afterdepolarizations, causing electrical oscillations in cell membranes that give rise to triggered dysrhythmias.[5]

CLINICAL FEATURES

Determine if toxicity is due to an accidental ingestion, massive intentional ingestion, or chronic toxicity from therapeutic use of digitalis. If the ingestion is intentional, historical information may be inaccurate or incomplete, and coingestants should be suspected. The time of ingestion is extremely helpful in interpreting laboratory information. Because various plants contain digitalis glycosides and cause similar toxicity to medicinal forms, an attempt should be made to accurately identify any ingested plants.

Preexisting medical conditions and current medications may identify risk factors that potentiate digitalis toxicity. Increased susceptibil-

ity is seen in patients who are elderly, have coexisting diseases (e.g., heart disease, renal dysfunction, hepatic dysfunction, hypothyroidism, and chronic obstructive pulmonary disease), electrolyte disturbances (e.g., hypokalemia, hypomagnesemia, and hypercalcemia), and hypoxia.[6] Drug interactions, most notably class IA antidysrhythmics, calcium channel blockers, and β-blockers, potentiate digitalis toxicity.

Cardiac dysrhythmias in digitalis toxicity are nonspecific and may be life-threatening. Suspect digitalis toxicity in patients with any dysrhythmia or junctional escape rhythms and AV block. The most common dysrhythmia is frequent premature ventricular beats, especially in a diseased heart. Bidirectional ventricular tachycardia, a tachycardia with an alternating axis and QRS complex, is rare but relatively specific for digitalis toxicity[7] (see Chap. 28 for examples of dysrhythmias).

In addition to cardiac manifestations, gastrointestinal distress, dizziness, headache, weakness, syncope, and seizures may occur. Reported psychiatric symptoms include confusion, disorientation, delirium, and hallucinations. Any elderly patient taking digitalis who presents with mental status changes should be evaluated for toxicity. Patients with toxicity have reported seeing yellow-green halos around objects.[8]

DIAGNOSIS

The history, physical examination, and laboratory studies provide important clues, with no single element that excludes or confirms the diagnosis.

Laboratory Evaluation

Serum potassium and digoxin levels will assist in providing information necessary to make adequate therapeutic decisions. Acute poisoning of the $Na^+K^+ATPase$ pump may result in markedly elevated serum potassium levels.[3] A high incidence of hyperkalemia has been noted in patients with severe acute poisoning. The serum potassium level may be a better indicator of end-organ toxicity and a better prognostic indicator than the serum digoxin level in the acutely poisoned patient. Hyperkalemia is less common in chronically poisoned patients. Potassium status may be less predictive in patients with renal insufficiency or volume depletion or in those who are receiving diuretic therapy.

Accepted therapeutic digoxin levels are 0.5 to 2.0 ng/μL. In most laboratories, the serum digoxin level is not part of the routine toxicologic screen and must be specifically requested. Serum digoxin levels in both acute and chronic toxicity should be interpreted in the overall clinical context and not relied on as the sole indicator of the presence or absence of toxicity. In acute exposures, digoxin is absorbed into the plasma compartment and then redistributed slowly into the tissue compartment. Hence high digoxin levels are not always associated with clinical signs and symptoms of poisoning. Serum levels are most reliable when obtained 6 h after ingestion, when distribution is complete. In patients with clinical evidence of chronic digitalis toxicity, a "therapeutic" level does not exclude toxicity, especially when predisposing factors are present. Conversely, levels above the upper limits of normal do not always cause symptoms. Given the preceding limitations, it is still most common that the higher the serum level, the greater is the likelihood of toxicity.[9]

A positive serum assay is diagnostic of acute ingestion if the patient has not received digitalis glycosides therapeutically. The rare exception is in the presence of a digoxin-like immunoreactive substance that has been detected in neonates and patients with renal insufficiency or hepatic dysfunction. In addition, naturally occurring digitalis glycosides from plants and animals may cross-react with the digoxin assay. The degree of cross-reactivity is unknown, and no correlation has been established between serum levels of these glycosides and toxicity.

Additional laboratory evaluation includes a determination of adequate oxygenation, renal and hepatic function, and electrolyte determinations in addition to potassium. Continuous electrocardiographic monitoring is essential to detect dysrhythmias.

Differences in the Presentation of Acute and Chronic Toxicity

A distinct clinical presentation exists for both acute and chronic digitalis glycoside toxicity (Table 174-1). Acute poisoning most often results from accidental or intentional ingestion. There may be an asymptomatic period of several hours prior to development of symptoms. Gastrointestinal symptoms are often the earliest manifestation of toxicity. In the early period of toxicity, increased central vagal tone produces cardiac dysrhythmias that are typically bradydysrhythmias or supraventricular dysrhythmias with AV block; however, life-threatening ventricular dysrhythmias may develop at any stage in an acute massive ingestion.[7] Acute toxicity correlates most closely with hyperkalemia and correlates poorly with the serum digoxin level.[10]

Chronic toxicity occurs most typically in the elderly cardiac patient taking digoxin and diuretics. Signs and symptoms may mimic more common illnesses such as influenza and gastroenteritis. An altered mental status or psychiatric symptoms may not be recognized as signs of digitalis toxicity. Almost any cardiac dysrhythmia may be seen, but ventricular dysrhythmias occur more frequently in chronic than in acute poisonings.[7] The serum digoxin level is not an accurate predictor of toxicity, and the serum potassium level is usually decreased or normal, but may even be elevated in the setting of renal failure.

Differential Diagnosis

Other toxins causing bradydysrhythmias include calcium channel blocker and β-blocker overdoses, class IA antidysrhythmics (procainamide and quinidine) overdoses, clonidine overdoses, organophosphate insecticide poisoning, and cardiotoxic plants (e.g., rhododendron, monkshood, tobacco, false hellebore, and yew berry). Sinus node disease also can mimic digitalis toxicity.

Factors Enhancing Toxicity

A number of factors increase susceptibility to digitalis toxicity. True end-organ sensitivity is seen with myocardial disease or ischemia and metabolic or electrolyte abnormalities. **Hypokalemia, hypomagnesemia, and hypercalcemia all predispose to increased toxicity.**[3] The elderly are more susceptible to toxicity. Decreased renal function, hepatic disease, hypothyroidism, chronic obstructive pulmonary disease,

TABLE 174-1   Clinical Presentation of Digitalis Toxicity

Acute toxicity	
Clinical history	Intentional or accidental ingestion
GI effects	Nausea and vomiting
CNS effects	Headache, dizziness, confusion, coma
Cardiac effects	Predominately supraventricular tachydysrythmias with AV block, bradydysrythmias
Electrolyte abnormalities	Hyperkalemia
Digoxin level	Marked elevation
Chronic toxicity	
Clinical history	Typically in elderly cardiac patients taking diuretics; may have renal insufficiency
GI effects	Nausea, vomiting, diarrhea, abdominal pain
CNS effects	Fatigue, weakness, confusion, delirium, coma
Cardiac effects	Almost any ventricular or supraventricular dysrhythmia can occur; ventricular dysrhythmias are common
Electrolyte abnormalities	Normal or decreased serum potassium, hypomagnesemia
Digoxin level	Minimally elevated or "therapeutic" range

TABLE 174-2   Treatment of Digitalis Glycoside Poisoning

Asymptomatic patients
  Obtain accurate history
  Continuous cardiac monitoring
  Intravenous access
  Gastrointestinal decontamination:
    Activated charcoal (1 g/kg)
  Frequent reevaluation
  Fab fragments at bedside (Calculate dose; Table 174-3)
Symptomatic patients
  ABCs
    Intravenous access
    Continuous cardiac monitoring
  Treat altered mental status
    Oxygen
    Glucose (if indicated)
    Naloxone (if indicated)
  Dysrhythmias
    Bradydysrhythmias
      Atropine (0.5–2.0 mg IV)
      Pacemaker (external or transvenous)
      Fab fragments (IV infusion)
    Ventricular dysrhythmias
      Fab fragments (IV infusion or bolus)
      Magnesium sulfate (2–4 g IV)
      Lidocaine (1 mg/kg) or
        fosphenytoin (15 mg PE/kg) infuse at 150 mg PE/min
      Electrocardioversion (10–25 J; last resort)
  Cardiac arrest
    CPR
    ACLS protocols
    Fab fragments (IV bolus; give 5–10 vials if amount ingested is unknown)
Electrolyte abnormalities
  Hyperkalemia
    Avoid calcium chloride or calcium gluconate
    Glucose-insulin (See Chap. 27)
    Sodium bicarbonate (See Chap. 27)
    Fab fragments (IV infusion or bolus)
    Potassium resin binder (See Chap. 27)
    Hemodialysis
  Hypomagnesemia
    Evaluate renal status prior to replacement
    Magnesium sulfate (2–4 g IV)
Gastrointestinal decontamination
  Activated charcoal (1 g/kg; then 0.5 g/kg q4–6 h)

and drug interactions all can augment toxic effects.[6] Drug interactions potentially resulting in digitalis toxicity include quinidine, procainamide, β-blockers, calcium channel blockers, amiodarone, spironolactone, indomethacin, clarithromycin, and erythromycin.

EMERGENCY DEPARTMENT CARE

Management of any poisoned patient includes general supportive care, treatment of specific complications of toxicity, prevention of further drug absorption, enhanced drug elimination, antidote administration, and safe disposition (Table 174-2). Patients with intentional or accidental ingestions may present with no symptoms. Still, life-threatening complications of toxicity should be anticipated. Management of the asymptomatic patient should focus on preventing drug absorption and closely monitoring for the development of toxicity. Continuous cardiac monitoring, intravenous access, and frequent reevaluations should be provided for any patient with a potentially toxic ingestion of digitalis. Toxicity may not develop for several hours after an acute ingestion; therefore, extended observation (12 h) is required for anyone with a confirmed ingestion.[9] Admission to the intensive care unit and frequent reassessment are required for any patient developing signs of toxicity.

Treatment of Life-Threatening Conditions

For the patient with life-threatening dysrhythmias, ensure a patent airway, adequate ventilation, and effective circulation. Rapidly correct conditions such as hypoxia, hypoglycemia, hypovolemia, and electrolyte abnormalities.

Conventional and antidote therapies are available to treat digitalis-induced dysrhythmias. Atropine and cardiac pacing (external and transvenous) have been used successfully in treating bradydysrhythmias. Both phenytoin and lidocaine depress ventricular automaticity and increase the fibrillation threshold. Because of phenytoin's ability to accelerate conduction at the AV node, it has been considered the antidysrhythmic of choice by some for digitalis-induced ventricular dysrhythmias. Bretylium has effectively suppressed dysrhythmias in the clinical setting, although in a digitalis-toxic animal model it was found to enhance dysrhythmias.[11] Class IA antidysrhythmics, such as quinidine and procainamide, are contraindicated because they depress AV nodal conduction, which in turn may enhance digitalis-induced cardiac toxicity. Intravenous magnesium has been reported to counteract ventricular irritability in digitalis toxicity.[12] Electrocardioversion may induce intractable ventricular fibrillation and should be considered only as a last resort. If necessary, use a low setting (10–25 J), and prepare to treat resulting ventricular fibrillation. In severe toxicity, conventional treatment may be unsuccessful. When available, digoxin-specific Fab fragments are the treatment of choice for dysrhythmias that are life-threatening and do not respond immediately to conventional therapy.[13]

Hyperkalemia secondary to acute exposures also may be life-threatening and needs immediate treatment. Treatment includes intravenous administration of glucose, insulin, and sodium bicarbonate and enteral administration of a potassium-binding resin (see Chap. 27).[13] Calcium chloride or calcium gluconate administration in the face of digitalis-induced hyperkalemia may promote cardiac toxicity and should be avoided. If digitalis-induced hyperkalemia is not corrected rapidly by conventional therapy, then Fab fragments are indicated for reversal (see below).[13]

Gastrointestinal Decontamination and Enhanced Elimination

Ipecac clearly has no role in the emergency department management of digitalis glycoside poisoning. After initial stabilization, administer activated charcoal to prevent further drug absorption.[14] Gastric lavage is not recommended as asystole has been reported in a digoxin-toxic patient, presumably from vagal stimulation during lavage. If lavage is contemplated, pretreatment with atropine prior to performing gastric lavage has been suggested. Cathartics, forced diuresis, hemodialysis, or hemoperfusion have no role in enhancing elimination of digitalis.

Digoxin-Specific Fab Antibody Therapy

Digoxin-specific Fab antibody fragments (Digibind, GlaxoSmith-Kline; DigiFab, Savage Laboratories) are derived from ovine IgG antibodies to digoxin. Fab fragments distribute widely throughout tissues and remove digitalis from tissue binding sites[13] as well as the plasma. According to AAPCC data from 2001, 314 patients received antidotal therapy with digoxin-specific Fab antibody fragments.[2] In a series of 150 severely poisoned patients, 90 percent showed reversal or significant improvement in life-threatening dysrhythmias and hyperkalemia after Fab fragment administration.[13] In most cases, clinical improvement in cardiac rhythm occurs within 1 h of antidote administration. Patients developing cardiac arrest prior to Fab administration had a 50 percent survival, which is significantly improved from survival by treatment with conventional therapies.[13] Fab fragments also have been reported to be beneficial in treating digitoxin and oleander poison-

ings.[15] Although Digibind was used in most of the studies regarding the effectiveness and safety of Fab fragments, in 2001, the Food and Drug Administration (FDA) approved DigiFab for use in cardiac glycoside poisoning.[16] Indications for digitalis-specific Fab fragments are ventricular dysrhythmias, hemodynamically significant bradydysrhythmias unresponsive to standard therapy, and hyperkalemia in excess of 5.5 mEq/L[13] associated with a toxic digitalis level or a presumptive diagnosis of overdose. Elevated serum digoxin levels should not be the sole indication for Fab fragment administration. DigiFab is indicated for the same conditions as Digibind and has similar pharmacokinetic and pharmacodynamic properties.[16]

Fab fragment administration has resulted in few adverse effects.[13] Cardiogenic shock has been reported in patients dependent on digoxin for inotropic support.[17] In addition, ventricular response to atrial fibrillation may be increased. Hypokalemia may develop rapidly as digitalis toxicity is reversed. Only mild, acute hypersensitivity reactions including rash, flushing, and facial swelling have been reported. No incidences of serum sickness or anaphylaxis have been observed, even in patients with repeated administration.[17] Skin testing has not proven to be useful in predicting allergic responses and may delay urgently needed treatment.[18] Failures to Fab fragment therapy have been attributed to inadequate dosing, moribund state prior to administration, and incorrect diagnosis of digitalis toxicity.[17]

The Fab fragment dosage is based on an estimation of total-body load of digoxin.[13] This can be determined from the serum digoxin level or based on the estimated dose ingested (Table 174-3). Clinical series have reported that an average of 200 to 480 mg (5–12 vials) were required to effectively treat severely digitalis-toxic patients.[13] When the ingested dose is unknown, 5 to 10 vials are recommended as initial treatment in life-threatening situations. Fab fragments are administered IV through a 0.22-μm filter over 30 min, except in a cardiac arrest, where it may be given as a bolus.

The serum digoxin level has no correlation with clinical toxicity following Fab administration because most laboratories use assays that measure both bound and unbound digoxin, although there are some laboratories that measure only free digoxin levels. Minutes after Fab fragment administration, the free digoxin level falls to zero, but the total serum digoxin level (bound to Fab fragments) increases 10- to 20-fold.[13] The Fab-digoxin complex is eliminated by renal excretion.[19] In

TABLE 174-3   Calculating Digoxin-Specific Fab Fragment Dosage

Calculate total-body load:

  Based on history of amount ingested:

    Total body load = amount ingested (mg) $\times$ 0.80 (bioavailability)

  Based on serum digoxin concentration:

  Total body load

$$= \frac{\text{serum digoxin level (ng/mL)} \times 5.6 \text{ L/kg} \times \text{patient's weight (kg)}}{1000}$$

Calculate number of vials of digoxin-specific Fab fragments needed to neutralize the calculated total-body load:

  It is assumed that an equimolar dose of Fab fragments is required for neutralization; one vial (40 mg) of Fab fragments binds 0.6 mg of digoxin.

$$\text{Number of Digibind vials required} = \frac{\text{total-body load}}{0.6}$$

$$\text{Number of DigiFab vials required} = \frac{\text{total-body load}}{0.5}$$

A simple and accurate variation of the above calculations:

$$\text{Number of vials of Fab} = \frac{\text{serum digoxin level (ng/mL)} \times \text{patient's weight (kg)}}{100}$$

the case of renal failure, the complex may persist in the circulation for prolonged periods. Recurrent toxicity can occur up to 10 days after Fab fragment administration in patients with renal failure. Hemodialysis does not enhance the elimination of the digoxin-Fab complex,[19] although plasma exchange may be of benefit.[20]

DISPOSITION

Patients with signs of toxicity or a history of a large ingested dose, especially if coexisting risk factors increase susceptibility to digitalis toxicity, should be admitted to a monitored unit. Contacting the local poison center and medical toxicologist can facilitate difficult management and treatment decisions regarding when to administer Fab fragments. Any patient receiving Fab fragments requires intensive care unit observation for at least 24 h. All suspected suicidal patients should have a psychiatric evaluation prior to discharge. Accidental exposures with no signs of toxicity after 12 h can be discharged home.

REFERENCES

1. Woolf AD, Wenger T, Smith TW, et al: The use of digoxin-specific Fab fragments for severe digitalis intoxication in children. *New Engl J Med* 326:1739, 1992.
2. Litovitz TL, Klein-Schwartz W, Rodgers GC, et al: 2001 Annual Report of the American Association of Poison Control Centers Toxic Exposure Surveillance System. *Am J Emerg Med* 20:391, 2002.
3. Smith TW: Digitalis: Mechanisms of action and clinical use. *New Engl J Med* 318:358, 1988.
4. Sagawa T, Sagawa K, Kelly JE, et al: Activation of cardiac ryanodine receptors by cardiac glycosides. *Am J Physiol Heart Circ Physiol* 282:1118 2001.
5. Rosen MR: Cellular electrophysiology of digitalis toxicity. *J Am Coll Cardiol* 5:22A, 1985.
6. Wofford JL, Ettinger WH: Risk factors and manifestations of digoxin toxicity in the elderly. *Am J Emerg Med* 9:11, 1991.
7. Moorman JR, Pritchett EL: The arrhythmias of digitalis intoxication. *Arch Intern Med* 145:1289, 1985.
8. Piltz JR, Wertenbaker C, Lance SE, et al: Digoxin toxicity: Recognizing the varied visual presentations. *J Clin Neuro-ophthalmol* 13:275, 1993.
9. Seltzer A: Role of serum digoxin assay in patient management. *J Am Coll Cardiol* 5:106A, 1985.
10. Bismuth C, Gaultier M, Conso F, et al: Hyperkalemia in acute digitalis poisoning: Prognostic significance and therapeutic implications. *Clin Toxicol* 6:153, 1973.
11. Vincent JL, Dufaye P, Berre J, et al: Bretylium in severe ventricular arrhythmias associated with digitalis intoxication. *Am J Emerg Med* 2:504, 1984.
12. French JH, Thomas RG, Siskind AP, et al: Magnesium therapy in massive digoxin intoxication. *Ann Emerg Med* 13:562, 1984.
13. Antman EM, Wenger TL, Butler VP, et al: Treatment of 150 cases of life-threatening digitalis intoxication with digoxin-specific Fab antibody fragments: Final report of a multicenter study. *Circulation* 81:1744, 1990.
14. Lalonde RL, Deshpande R, Hamilton PP, et al: Acceleration of digoxin clearance by activated charcoal. *Clin Pharmacol Ther* 37:367, 1985.
15. Shumaik GM, Wu AW, Ping AC: Oleander poisoning: Treatment with digoxin-specific Fab antibody fragments. *Ann Emerg Med* 17:732, 1988.
16. Thompson CA: FDA approves digoxin-toxicity remedy. *Am J Health-Syst Pharm* 58:2021, 2001.
17. Hickey AR, Wenger TL, Carpenter VP, et al: Digoxin immune Fab therapy in the management of digitalis intoxication: Safety and efficacy results of an observational surveillance study. *J Am Coll Cardiol* 17:590, 1991.
18. Kirpatrick CHG, Digibind Study Advisory Panel: Allergic histories and reactions of patients treated with digoxin immune Fab (ovine) antibody. *Am J Emer Med* 9(suppl 1):7 1991.
19. Clinton GD, McIntyre WJ, Zannikos PN, et al: Free and total serum digoxin concentrations in a renal failure patient after treatment with digoxin immune Fab. *Clin Pharm* 8:441, 1989.
20. Zdunek M, Mitra A, Mokrzycki MH: Plasma exchange for the removal of digoxin-specific antibody fragments in renal failure: Timing is important for maximizing clearance. *Am J Kidney Dis* 36:177, 2000.

β-BLOCKER TOXICITY
Teresa M. Carlin

β-Blockers are commonly prescribed drugs in clinical practice. They have a multitude of therapeutic indications that include the treatment of myocardial infarction, angina, arrhythmias, obstructive cardiomyopathy, diastolic dysfunction, migraine headaches, thyrotoxicosis, anxiety, tremor, glaucoma, and hypertension. Accidental and intentional ingestions are not uncommon presentations in the ED. According to the American Association of Poison Control Centers, during 2001, there were over 12,000 exposures to β'''blockers.[1] Of these, three quarters were unintentional and more than a quarter were among children less than 6 years of age. Almost 20 percent resulted in serious toxicity and there were 39 deaths.

PHYSIOLOGY

The β-receptor is a glycoprotein within the cell membrane coupled to an intracellular second messenger, cyclic adenosine monophosphate (cAMP), by a regulatory protein called the *G protein*. When catecholamines bind to beta receptors, the G protein undergoes a conformational change that activates adenyl cyclase. Adenyl cyclase catalyzes the formation of cAMP. cAMP stimulates protein kinase, which phosphorylates calcium channels, leading to calcium entry into cells. Additional calcium is released into the cytosol from cellular storage organelles. The expression of this reaction depends on which beta receptor is activated.[2]

At least three types of β-adrenergic receptors exist. The β_1 subunit is located in the myocardium, kidney, and eye, while the β_2 subunit is found in smooth muscle, skeletal muscle, the liver, pancreas, and adipose tissue. The β_3 subunit is located in adipose tissue. β_1 activation promotes cardiac inotropy and chronotropy. Additionally, it causes the kidney to release renin and the eye to produce aqueous humor. Stimulation of the β_2-receptors causes smooth muscle relaxation, which results in vasodilatation, brochodilation, and uterine relaxation. β_2 activation also increases metabolic substrate availability needed for stress by stimulating lipolysis and glycogenolysis. The β_3 subunit alters lipid metabolism.[2]

PHARMOCOLOGY AND PATHOPHYSIOLOGY

β-Blockade blunts the production of cAMP via β-receptor stimulation. If the β_1 subunit is preferentially antagonized, the effect is negative inotropy and negative chronotropy, the hallmark of β-blocker toxicity. Vasoconstriction, bronchospasm, and hypoglycemia may occur when the β_2-receptor is blocked.

Other mechanisms may contribute to β-blocker toxicity. Membrane-stabilizing activity of several beta blockers causes cardiovascular depression, similar to quinidine, and is associated with QRS complex widening.[3]

The pharmacologic properties of various β-blockers influence their spectrum of toxicity[3] (Table 175-1). These properties include cardioselectivity (β_1 antagonist activity), membrane-stabilizing activity, lipid solubility, and partial agonist activity. For example, lipid-soluble agents such as propranolol rapidly cross the blood-brain barrier and achieve high concentrations in brain tissue. Additionally, propranolol has a membrane-stabilizing activity similar to quinidine. These properties may contribute to the central nervous system (CNS) manifestations of propranolol overdose, namely, depression of mental status and seizures.[3,4] Membrane-stabilizing activity makes drugs such as propranolol potentially more cardiotoxic. Since propranolol is not cardioselective, it is theoretically more likely to present with β_2 effects such as wheezing than a cardioselective drug such as atenolol. Cardioselective

TABLE 175-1 β-Blocker Pharmacologic Profile

Agent	Beta-Selective	Partial Agonist	Membrane-Stabilizing Activity	Lipophilic
Acebutolol	Yes	Yes	Yes	Weak
Atenolol	Yes	No	No	Weak
Esmolol	Yes	No	No	Weak
Labetolol	No	No	No	Moderate
Metoprolol	Yes	No	Weak	Moderate
Nadolol	No	No	No	Weak
Oxprenolol	No	Yes	Yes	Moderate
Pindolol	No	Yes	Yes	Moderate
Propranolol	No	No	Yes	High
Sotalol	No	No	No	Weak
Timolol	No	No	No	Weak

Source: Adapted from Frishman WH, Jacob H, Eisenberg E: *Am Heart J* 98:

β-blockers, however, may lose specificity for the $β_1$-receptor at toxic doses. Several β-blockers have partial agonist activity, and thus weak stimulation of the beta receptor occurs concurrently with blockade. Bradycardia is initially less pronounced with these agents. Experimental evidence implicates calcium and potassium homeostasis as a contributing mechanism of toxicity.[5]

Clinically relevant pharmacokinetic characteristics include drug formulation (regular versus sustained release), rate of drug absorption, lipid solubility, and volume of distribution (Vd). Absorption of normal-release β-blockers occurs rapidly, with peak effects in 1 to 4 h. For this reason, toxic symptoms begin soon after ingestion. The high degree of protein binding, the large Vd, and the lipid solubility predict that extracorporeal drug removal will not be useful for most β-blockers. Hemodialysis may be effective for atenolol, nadolol, and sotalol because these agents have lower binding, are hydrophilic, and have Vd values similar to that of water.

CLINICAL PRESENTATION

Patients who ingest β-blockers manifest a spectrum of clinical presentations ranging from minimal symptoms to profound bradycardia and hypotension, the hallmark of toxicity (Table 175-2). Conduction abnormalities, dysrhythmias, and cardiogenic shock also occur. Wide-complex bradyarrhythmias are seen rarely. Symptoms typically develop within 2 to 4 h of acute ingestion.[6] Sudden deterioration with cardiovascular collapse may occur.[7] Most individuals ultimately requiring treatment for cardiovascular depression after exposure with propranolol, metoprolol, or atenolol develop symptoms by 6 h after ingestion.[4,6] Sotalol is an exception to this rule. Sotalol, unlike other β-blockers, is classified as a Vaughan Williams class III antiarrhythmic. Class III antiarrhythmic drugs cause a prolonged QT interval, which may degenerate into a ventricular dysrhythmia for as long as the QT interval remains abnormal. Premature ventricular contractions, bigeminy, ventricular tachycardia, ventricular fibrillation, and torsades de pointes have been reported. It is unclear whether other β-blockers, particularly sustained-released preparations, can present with delayed toxicity.[6] There is no report in the literature of delayed onset of symptoms (e.g., outside a 6-h window) with sustained-released products.

Slowing of the heart rate due to sinus node suppression or conduction abnormalities occurs in all significant β-blocker intoxications except overdoses of β-blockers with partial agonist activity. In fact, ingestion of β-blockers with partial agonist activity such as pindolol may present with hypertension and tachycardia.[3,4] QRS complex

widening is associated with the membrane-stabilizing activity of some β-blockers, such as propranolol.

The single most important predictive factor associated with cardiovascular morbidity in β-blocker exposure may be the coingestion of another cardioactive drug, such as calcium channel blockers and tricyclic antidepressants.[8] In the absence of a coingestion, the most important predictive factor is whether the β-blocker possesses membrane-stabilizing activity.[8] Examples of β-blockers that possess membrane-stabilizing activity include propranolol, acebutolol, and pindolol. Atenolol, sotalol, timolol do not possess membrane-stabilizing activity. Metoprolol has membrane-stabilizing effects only at high doses[3,8] (see Table 175-1).

The CNS is another target of β-blocker toxicity. CNS manifestations include depressed mental status, coma, psychosis, and seizures. These symptoms may occur secondary to poor perfusion or direct neuronal toxicity. It is postulated that the more lipophilic β-blockers such as propranolol cause greater CNS and cardiac toxicity compared with less lipophilic agents.[4] Studies suggest a significant association between a QRS complex duration of greater than 100 ms and seizure activity. However, a normal QRS complex does not exclude the risk of seizure.[4] Status seizures are rare but may be refractory to treatment.

Noncardioselective β-blockers may antagonize the $β_2$ subunit. Bronchospasm with wheezing and metabolic derangements such as hypoglycemia have been reported but are infrequent occurrences. Case reports suggest that hypoglycemia in children may have a delayed presentation.[9,10] Rare complications of poisoning include esophageal spasm, mesenteric ischemia, and acute renal failure.

DIAGNOSIS

A limited number of other medications, chemicals, and natural toxins potentially result in bradycardia and hypotension. Common drugs include calcium channel antagonists, centrally acting alpha agonists, and digoxin. Many plants (e.g., oleander, digitalis, and rhododendron) contain cardiac glycosides that may cause symptoms following ingestion of plant parts or consumption of teas brewed from the plant. Chinese medicinal preparations and aphrodisiacs often contain animal-derived cardiac glycosides (e.g., bufotoxin) that may cause bradycardia and hypotension. Such chemicals as organophosphate insecticides, cyanide, or hydrogen sulfide cause bradycardia.

The diagnosis of β-blocker toxicity is made on clinical grounds. Drug levels correlate poorly with clinical presentations.[11] However, specific drug levels, if available, may help confirm an exposure. A 12-lead electrocardiogram and continuous rhythm monitoring are essential in evaluation and ongoing assessment. Laboratory testing is directed at supportive monitoring of renal function, glucose level, oxygenation, and acid-base status. Radiographs to detect β-blocker pills

TABLE 175-2 Common Symptoms of β-Blocker Toxicity

Cardiac
  Asymptomatic
  Hypotension
  Bradycardia
  Cardiac conduction delays and blocks
  Cardiovascular shock
  Asystole
CNS
  Depressed mental status
  Psychosis
  Seizures
Metabolic
  Hypoglycemia
Pulmonary
  Respiratory depression
  Apnea
  Bronchospasm

in the gastrointestinal tract are not useful because these drugs are not radiopaque.[12]

TREATMENT

Standard approach to poisoning should be initiated (see Chap. 156). For serious cases, treatment begins by establishing adequate airway patency, ventilation, and oxygenation. Multiple intravenous access sites, as well as central venous access, may be required.

The goal of specific cardiovascular drug therapy is to restore perfusion to critical organ systems by improving myocardial contractility, increasing heart rate, or both. Current therapy (Table 175-3) is derived from reports of case studies and includes glucagon, adrenergic agonists, atropine, and phosphodiesterase inhibitors. Overall, these therapies have met with variable success.

Syrup of ipecac should never be used to decontaminate the gastrointestinal tract after β-blocker overdose. Enhanced vagal tone associated with vomiting may be detrimental after β-blocker exposure because of its association with cardiovascular collapse.[13] Additionally, β-blocker-intoxicated patients may experience a rapid decline in mental status, which increases the risk of aspiration during vomiting.

Gastrointestinal decontamination with 1.0 g/kg plain activated charcoal should be initiated unless oral intake is contraindicated. Gastric lavage may be beneficial prior to instillation of charcoal if it can be accomplished within 1 to 2 h of ingestion.

Glucagon is a first-line agent in the treatment of acute β-blocker overdose. Glucagon is thought to activate myocardial adenyl cyclase by a mechanism independent of β-receptor stimulation. Adenyl cyclase generates cAMP, which causes positive inotropic and chronotropic effects.[14] An intravenous bolus of glucagon achieves maximum serum concentration within 1 min and has a half-life of 6.6 min. Therefore, a bolus dose of glucagon should be followed by a continuous infusion. The bolus dose of glucagon is .05 to .15 mg/kg (3–10 mg for the average 70-kg adult) followed by a continuous infusion of 1 to 10 mg per h. There is no defined maximum therapeutic dose. Of note, the positive inotropic and chronotropic effects of glucagon may not be maintained for a prolonged period due to possible tachyphylaxis. How long the myocardial effects will last over time is not known.[14]

Nausea and vomiting are commonly reported side effects of high-dose glucagon therapy that may be related to esophageal sphincter relaxation. Patients should be monitored during therapy for hypoglycemia and hypokalemia secondary to reflex release of insulin. The

TABLE 175-3   Treatment Algorithm for Cardiovascular Effects of β-Blocker Ingestions

Standard initial interventions*
Fluid bolus (NS)
Atropine trial for symptomatic bradycardia
Glucagon
    Bolus: .05–.15 mg/kg (3–10 mg for average size adult) followed by
        infusion: 1–5 mg per h (repeat bolus as necessary)
Epinephrine
    Infusion: 1 μg/kg per min and titrate to effect (doses up to
        30–100 μg per min have been used successfully)
Isoproterenol
    Infusion: 2 μg per min and titrate to effect (doses up to
        160-200 μg per min have been used successfully)
Consider other inotropic drugs
    Dopamine infusion: 5 μg/kg per min and titrate to 20 μg/kg per min
    Norepinephrine infusion: 0.5 μg per min and titrate to 4.0 μg per min
Amrinone
    Bolus: 0.75 mg/kg over 2 min followed by infusion: 5 μg/kg per min
        and titrate
Cardiac pacing for refractory bradycardia
Intra-aortic balloon pump for refractory shock

* ABC's, two large bore IVs, cardiac monitor, glucose check, activated charcoal.

manufacturer uses a glycerin diluent with a phenol preservative. Excessive phenol exposure can cause thrombophlebitis, seizures, hypotension, or dysrhythmias. To avoid these unwanted effects, **the supplied diluent should be discarded and the glucagon reconstituted with NS** solution to a concentration not to exceed 1 mg/mL.[14,15] The dose needed to treat β-blocker overdose could exceed the amount available at a hospital pharmacy.[16]

β-Adrenergic receptor agonists (catecholamines) are used routinely for β-blocker toxicity. However, results have been variable. The most effective therapy may be glucagon followed by epinephrine. Isoproterenol and dopamine may be the least effective.[17] Clinical improvement has been noted with isoproterenol used in high doses (160–200 μg per min).[18] Canine models of propranolol overdose also support the use of high-dose catecholamines such as isoproterenol and dopamine.[19]

Phosphodiesterase inhibitors also have been used to treat β-blocker toxicity. In theory, drugs such as amrinone inhibit the ability of phosphodiesterase to break down cAMP, thereby facilitating maintenance of intracellular calcium levels. In original models, amrinone demonstrated positive inotropic effects without increasing myocardial oxygen demands in propranolol-induced heart failure.[20] However, in other animal studies, amrinone and milrinone increased cardiac output but had no appreciable effect on heart rate. When administered with glucagon, neither amrinone nor milrinone provided any additional benefit over glucagon.[21] Thus phosphodiesterase inhibitors have no advantage over glucagon. However, if glucagon is not available, phosphodiesterase inhibitors can be reasonable alternatives. The dosage of amrinone used in adults is an initial bolus of 0.75 mg/kg over 2 min, followed by a continuous infusion of 5 to 10 μg/kg per min. Atropine is unlikely to be effective in the management of β-blocker-induced bradycardia and hypotension.

Canine studies and case reports suggest that calcium chloride therapy may improve the depressed hemodynamic status, mainly by positive inotropic action.[22–25] Serum calcium improves transport of extracellular calcium into the cell and release of calcium from intracellular storage organelles, which supports myofibril contraction and promotes positive inotropy.[22–25]

Insulin may prove to be a novel therapy in β-blocker toxicity. In a canine model, high-dose insulin-dextrose therapy improved survival in severe overdoses when compared with glucagon or epinephrine. Further trials are needed to confirm beneficial effects in humans before therapy can be recommended routinely.[24,26]

Treatment of ventricular dysrhythmias due to sotalol requires pharmacologic measures different from those required for other β-blockers. Isoproterenol, lidocaine, and overdrive pacing have been used successfully. Magnesium also may be of benefit.[27]

Extrinsic pacing may be required to maintain heart rate.[28] However, electrical capture is not always successful, and if capture does occur, blood pressure is not always restored.[17] Cardiac pacing may be most beneficial in treating torsades de pointes associated with sotalol.[27] Occasionally, extreme means of resuscitation, including extracorporeal circulation and aortic balloon pump, have been successful.[29,30] Intra-aortic balloon pump should be considered when glucagon and high-dose catecholamines fail to reverse drug-induced cardiogenic shock.[30] Based on previously described pharmacokinetic properties, hemodialysis would not be expected to effectively remove lipophilic β-blocker drugs that have a large volume of distribution or extensive protein binding. Hemodialysis may be useful for atenolol, nadolol, and sotalol overdose because these drugs have a lower volume of distribution and less protein binding than do other β-blockers.

DISPOSITION

Patients who develop altered mental status, bradycardia, conduction delays, or hypotension should be managed in the intensive care unit. Patients with cardioactive coingestants or with ingestions of sustained-released β-blocker formulations probably warrant inpatient monitoring because the risk of delayed toxicity is unclear.[8]

Patients with probable β-blocker overdoses who remain asymptomatic and demonstrate no signs of hemodynamic instability for 6 h after ingestion appear to be at little risk of subsequent deterioration.[6,8] Sotalol deserves special consideration because it has class III antiarrhythmic activity and has a long half-life. One group of authors suggests that the need for observation of a sotalol ingestion beyond 6 h depends on the QT_c interval.[6,8]

REFERENCES

1. Litovitz TL, Klein-Schwartz, Rodgers GC Jr, et al: 2001 Annual report of the American Association of Poison Control Centers Toxic Exposure Surveillance System. *Am J Emerg Med* 20:391, 2002.
2. Kerns W, Kline J, Ford M: Beta-blocker and calcium blocker toxicity. *Emerg Med Clin North Am* 12:365, 1994.
3. Frishman W, Jacob H, Eisenberg E, Ribner H: Clinical pharmacology of the new β-adrenergic blocking drugs: 8. Self-poisoning with β-adrenergic blocking agents: Recognition and management. *Am Heart J* 98:798, 1979.
4. Reith D, Dawson A, Epid D, et al: Relative toxicity of β-blockers in overdose. *Clin Toxicol* 34:273, 1996.
5. Kerns W, Ransom M, Tomaszewski C, et al: The effects of extracellular ions on beta-blocker cardiotoxicity. *Toxicol Appl Pharmacol* 137:1, 1996.
6. Love J. β-Blocker toxicity after overdose: When do symptoms develop in adults? *J Emerg Med* 12:799, 1994.
7. Salzberg MR, Gallagher EJ: Propranolol overdose. *Ann Emerg Med* 9:26, 1980.
8. Love JN, Howell JM, Litovitz TL, Klein-Schwartz W: Acute beta-blocker overdose: Factors associated with the development of cardiovascular morbidity. *Clin Toxicol* 38:275, 2000.
9. Smith RC, Wilkinson J, Hull RL: Glucagon for propranolol overdose. *JAMA* 254:2412, 1985.
10. Hesse B, Pedersen JT: Hypoglycemia after propranolol in children. *Acta Med Scand* 81:344, 1986.
11. Love J. β-Blocker toxicity: A clinical diagnosis. *Am J Emerg Med* 12:356, 1994.
12. Savitt DL, Hawkins HH, Roberts JR: The radiopacity of ingested medications. *Ann Emerg Med* 16:331, 1987.
13. Soni N, Baines D, Pearson I: Cardiovascular collapse and propranolol overdose. *Med J Aust* 10:629, 1983.
14. White CM: A review of potential cardiovascular uses of intravenous glucagon administration. *J Clin Pharmacol* 39:442, 1999.
15. Mofenson HC, Caraccio TR, Laudano J: Glucagon for propranolol overdose. *JAMA* 255:2025, 1986.
16. Love JN, Tandy TK: β-Adrenoreceptor antagonist toxicity: A survey of glucagon availability. *Ann Emerg Med* 22:267, 1993.
17. Weinstein RS: Recognition and management of poisoning with β-adrenergic blocking agents. *Ann Emerg Med* 13:1123, 1984.
18. Agura ED, Wexler LF: Massive propranolol overdose. *Am J Med* 80:55, 1986.
19. Avery GJ II, Spotnitz HM, Rose EA, et al: Pharmacologic antagonism of β-adrenergic blockade in dogs: I. Hemodynamic effects of isoproterenol, dopamine, and epinephrine in acute propranolol administration. *J Thorac Cardiovasc Surg* 77:267, 1979.
20. Alousi AA, Canter JM, Fort DJ: The beneficial effect of amrinone on acute drug-induced heart failure in the anesthetized dog. *Cardiovasc Res* 19:483, 1985.
21. Love JN, Leasure JA, Mundt DJ: A comparison of combined amrinone and glucagon therapy to glucagon alone for cardiovascular depression associated with propranolol toxicity in a canine model. *Am J Emerg Med* 11:360, 1993.
22. Love JN, Hanfling D, Howell JM: Hemodynamic effects of calcium chloride in a canine model of acute propranolol intoxication. *Ann Emerg Med* 28:1, 1996.
23. Pertoldi F, D'Orlando L, Mercante WP: Electromechanical dissociation 48 hours after overdose: Usefulness of calcium chloride. *Ann Emerg Med* 31:777, 1998.
24. Albertson TE, Dawson A, de Latorre F, et al: TOX-ACLS: Toxicologic-oriented advanced cardiac life support. *Ann Emerg Med* 37:S78, 2001.
25. Brimacombe J, Scully M, Swainton R: Propranolol overdose: A dramatic response to calcium chloride. *Med J Aust* 155:267, 1991.
26. Kerns W II, Schroeder D, Williams C, et al: Insulin improves survival in a canine model of acute beta-blocker toxicity. *Ann Emerg Med* 29:748, 1997.
27. Leatham EW, Holt DW, McKenna WJ: Class III antiarrythmics in overdose: Presenting features and management principles. *Drug Saf* 9:450, 1993.
28. Kenyon CJ, Aldinger GE, Joshipura P, et al: Successful resuscitation using external cardiac pacing in β-adrenergic antagonist-induced bradysystolic arrest. *Ann Emerg Med* 17:711, 1988.
29. McVey FK, Corke CF: Extracorporeal circulation in the management of massive propranolol oversdose. *Anaethesia* 46:744, 1991.
30. Lane AS, Woodward AC, and Godman MR: Massive propranolol overdose poorly responsive to pharmacologic therapy: Use of the intra-aortic balloon pump. *Ann Emerg Med* 16:1381, 1987.

176   CALCIUM CHANNEL BLOCKERS
Kennon Heard
Jeffrey A. Kline

EPIDEMIOLOGY

Emergency physicians are familiar with the use of calcium channel blockers (CCBs) for the treatment of hypertension, angina pectoris, and for control of ventricular rate in supraventricular dysrhythmias. Less common uses include prophylactic treatment of migraine headaches, treatment of arterial vasospasm from Raynaud disease, treatment of esophageal spasm, and treatment of pulmonary hypertension.[1] For the last 5 years, CCBs have accounted for more poisoning deaths than any other cardiovascular drug, and are the second most common cause of prescription drug poisoning death. More than 4500 cases of CCB poisoning are treated in health care facilities annually.[2]

PHARMACOLOGY AND PATHOPHYSIOLOGY

Intracellular calcium is the primary stimulus for smooth and cardiac muscle contraction and for impulse formation in sinoatrial pacemaker cells. At therapeutic concentrations, CCBs bind to the α subunit of the L-type calcium channel, causing the channel to favor the closed state, thereby decreasing calcium entry during phase II depolarization. At very high concentrations, some CCBs (notably, verapamil) may occupy the channel canal and completely block calcium entry through the L-channel. The result is profound smooth muscle relaxation, weakened cardiac contraction, blunted cardiac automaticity, and intracardiac conduction delay.[1] Clinically, these effects are recognized as hypotension and bradycardia. Animal data suggest that verapamil overdose also impairs myocardial carbohydrate intake, which contributes to the negative cardiac inotropy.[3]

Table 176-1 reviews the therapeutic effects of three major CCB classes that are widely used in the clinical setting: the phenylalkylamines (verapamil), the benzothiazepines (diltiazem), and the dihydropyridines (nifedipine and most newer agents). Verapamil is the most potent negative inotrope of all CCBs, causing at least equal depression of heart contraction compared with smooth muscle dilatation at any concentration.[4] This cardiotoxic effect may be one reason that verapamil overdose causes more deaths than all other CCBs combined. Dihydropyridines bind more selectively to vascular smooth muscle calcium channels compared with cardiac calcium channels, and therefore relax smooth muscle at concentrations that produce almost no negative inotropy. Dihydropyridines have been structurally modified to make them more lipid soluble in an effort to prolong their durations of action. These modified dihydropyridines are known as *second-generation dihydropyridines*. They cause more gradual smooth-muscle relaxation, producing less reflex baroreceptor activation and less reflex tachycardia than is observed with first-generation dihydropyridines.

The older agents—verapamil, nifedipine, and diltiazem—all have relatively short serum half-lives. Consequently, sustained-release formulations have been developed for all of these agents. As sustained-

TABLE 176-1   Relative Negative Inotropic Effect versus Vascular Smooth Muscle Relaxing Effect of Calcium Channel Antagonists in Humans

Class	Trade Name	Vascular Selectivity*
Phenylalkylamines:		
Verapamil	Calan, Verelan, Isoptin	1.0
Benzothiazepines:		
Diltiazem	Cardizem, Dilacor	1.0
Dihydropyridines:		
Nifedipine	Procardia, Adalat	0.1
Amlodipine	Norvasc	0.1
Nicardipine	Cardene	0.01
Isradipine	DynaCirc	0.01
Felodipine	Plendil	0.01
Nisoldipine	Baymycard (in U.K.)	0.0001

*Ratio of percent negative inotropy to percent vasodilation at $10^{-7}\,M$.
Note: An index number closer to 1.0 indicates that the drug causes an equal degree of reduction in cardiac function compared with vasodilation.

TABLE 176-2   Single Ingestion Toxicity from Calcium Channel Blockers

Agent	Lowest Dose	Mean Toxic Dose
Verapamil	720 mg	16 mg/kg
Diltiazem	420 mg	5.7 mg/kg
Nifedipine	50 mg	8 mg/kg

Source: Adapted from Romoska EA et al.[5]

release formulations prolong drug absorption, onset of symptoms may be delayed and toxicity may be prolonged. Several of the second-generation dihydropyridines have prolonged duration of action, and therefore are generally not formulated as sustained-release products. While clinical data on overdose of these agents is limited, pharmacokinetic data suggest that delayed onset of toxicity is less likely. As newer formulations are released frequently, it is often helpful to contact a Regional Poison Control Center for help in determining if a given product is formulated as a sustained-release preparation.

CLINICAL FEATURES

Calcium channel blocker poisoning is associated with many clinical effects. The most prominent and life-threatening effects are an extension of the therapeutic effects on the cardiovascular system. Patients with moderate verapamil or diltiazem poisoning often have sinus bradycardia, varying degrees of atrioventricular block, and hypotension.[5] Mild or moderate dihydropyridine overdoses usually cause peripheral vasodilatation with resultant hypotension and reflex tachycardia.[5] In severe overdose, any of these agents may cause complete heart block, depressed myocardial contractility, and vasodilatation that ultimately results in cardiovascular collapse.

Hyperglycemia and lactic acidosis are also common manifestations of severe overdoses. These effects are caused by antagonism of calcium channels on pancreatic β cells, leading to decreased serum insulin levels, decreased myocardial glucose metabolism and increased anaerobic metabolism resulting from circulatory impairment associated with negative inotropy and vasodilation produced by the drug. The net effect is a metabolic profile similar to diabetic ketoacidosis. Hypokalemia may also be observed.

Pulmonary and central nervous system effects are generally secondary to decreased myocardial function and impaired organ perfusion. Cardiogenic pulmonary edema is sometimes observed in severe overdoses, especially if large volumes of crystalloid are infused during resuscitation. Noncardiogenic pulmonary edema has also been reported.[6] Seizures, delirium, and coma have been reported, and are presumed to be secondary to cerebral hypoperfusion. Alteration in consciousness in patients with adequate mean arterial pressure should not be attributed to CCB toxicity, and should prompt an evaluation for other causes.

DIAGNOSIS

From a large series of CCB overdoses, the lowest dose that produced toxicity in adults is shown in Table 176-2. A history of ingestion that

is near these doses should be considered potentially toxic. Doses in excess of the mean toxic dose (see Table 176-2) should be expected to produce toxicity.[5]

Many clinicians now prescribe verapamil, diltiazem, nifedipine, and some of the second-generation dihydropyridines as extended-release preparations. Compared with standard-release preparations, extended-release preparations have delayed and prolonged toxicity. Therefore, it is important to determine the exact formulation of the ingested agent to guide management decisions. If the history cannot identify the exact formulation, the clinician should assume it is sustained release and modify treatment in a conservative way. Further critical history should include the possibility of coingestants. The time of ingestion should be determined. **The onset of symptoms can be delayed as much as 12 h with significant overdose.** Thus, the conclusion that toxic manifestations will not occur should not be based solely on a questionable remote time of ingestion.

The physical examination of a patient with CCB poisoning is frequently unremarkable other than cardiovascular findings of a slow heart rate relative to the arterial blood pressure. Following dihydropyridine ingestion, patients will usually have systemic vasodilatation leading to flushed skin, tachycardia and mild to moderate hypotension. Peripheral edema is commonly seen as a side effect of chronic nifedipine therapy.

Toxicity from diltiazem or verapamil will frequently cause profound bradycardia and hypotension. Systemic hypoperfusion may cause secondary findings such as alteration in mental status, signs of pulmonary edema, or decreased urine output.

Electrocardiographic findings include sinus bradycardia, varying degrees of heart block, and slowing of intraventricular conduction. Reflex tachycardia is commonly seen with mild to moderate ingestion of dihydropyridines. Junctional rhythms and ventricular escape rhythms are frequently noted in severe overdoses with verapamil or diltiazem.

No laboratory findings are critical to the acute management of CCB toxicity. Hyperglycemia is often noted following CCB ingestion, differentiating CCB toxicity from β-blocker toxicity that may cause hypoglycemia. Lactic acidosis will manifest as an elevated anion gap and low serum bicarbonate. Hypokalemia is also noted in severe overdoses. Serum calcium levels are usually normal. Ionized serum calcium levels may be followed when calcium chloride is administered as therapy, but the optimum serum calcium level for patients with severe CCB poisoning is not known. Finally, a screening serum acetaminophen level should be performed for patients that present following suicidal overdose.

DIFFERENTIAL DIAGNOSIS

Table 176-3 shows the critical differential diagnosis for bradycardia, heart block, and hypotension. Hypothermia should be detected during vital sign assessment. Myocardial infarction may be evident on the initial or subsequent electrocardiogram. Hyperkalemia should be suspected in patients with renal failure.

Differentiation of CCB toxicity from cardiac glycoside toxicity is difficult but critical. These drugs may be used for the same indications, and patients are frequently taking both. While calcium salts are standard therapy for CCB poisoning, they may case cardiovascular

TABLE 176-3 Differential Diagnosis

Hypothermia
Acute coronary syndrome
Hyperkalemia
Cardiac glycoside toxicity
β-Blocker toxicity
Types 1a, 1c antidysrhythmic toxicity
Central α-adrenergic agonist (e.g., clonidine) toxicity

collapse when given to a patient with digoxin poisoning. Unfortunately, patient acuity may not allow serum digoxin measurement, and treatment decisions must be made on clinical impression. In general, patients with chronic digoxin poisoning will have more ventricular ectopy than patients with CCB toxicity. However, as the main manifestation of acute cardiac glycoside poisoning is heart block and bradycardia, bedside differentiation may be difficult. **If the diagnosis of acute digoxin poisoning cannot be excluded, administration of digoxin Fab should precede calcium administration.** Alternatively, other treatments for CCB toxicity should be initiated.

β-Adrenergic antagonist toxicity may be clinically indistinguishable from CCB toxicity. In general, β-blocker toxicity is not as severe and patients tend to have hypoglycemia and normal to elevated serum potassium concentrations. However, these findings are not consistent enough to have diagnostic value. Fortunately, the treatment for these two poisonings is similar. Calcium, β-adrenergic agonists, glucagon, and pacing are considered useful therapy for both.

MANAGEMENT

Decreased level of consciousness following CCB ingestion is a result of cerebral hypoperfusion or coingestion. During the initial resuscitation, patients with altered mental status should be considered for treatment with an opiate antagonist and have a serum glucose level determination. Early airway management should be implemented in patients with any degree of mental status impairment or hemodynamic instability. Decontamination with the associated risk of aspiration will be required for all but the most trivial ingestions. Endotracheal intubation may minimize this risk. In addition to the vomiting associated with decontamination, glucagon often will precipitate vomiting. Finally, early airway management will allow the physician to concentrate on treating the often-precipitous cardiovascular collapse without having to perform a "crash airway."

Following airway management, patients will generally require cardiovascular stabilization. Therapies directed at improving heart rate should be directed at increasing end-organ perfusion rather than restoring a specific heart rate. For example, some patients with heart rates in the 30 to 40 beats/min range will maintain adequate blood pressure and perfusion, and therefore will only require monitoring rather than a specific intervention. Conversely, patients may respond to cardiac pacing with an increase in heart rate to 90 to 100 beats/min but no improvement in blood pressure or perfusion. These patients obviously require additional therapy to increase myocardial function.

Therapies directed specifically at increasing heart rate include several medications and cardiac pacing. Atropine alone is rarely effective for CCB-induced bradycardia, but administration is commonly recommended. Isoproterenol may be useful (2 to 10 μg/min intravenous infusion) to increase heart rate, but peripheral vasodilation may worsen hypotension. Calcium salts may improve both heart rate and blood pressure, but the response is variable. External and transvenous pacing may be attempted, and are often successful at restoring an acceptable rate, but blood pressure frequently will improve minimally or not at all. However, pacing is indicated for patients with severe bradycardia (heart rate <30).

In general, it is reasonable to administer crystalloid during the initial resuscitation of a hypotensive CCB-poisoned patient. However, overaggressive fluid administration may worsen pulmonary edema.

Therefore, consider pulmonary artery catheterization prior to continued fluid resuscitation beyond 2 L.

Specific treatments of the hemodynamic effects of CCB toxicity are well described, but the therapies are untested in controlled human trials. The recommendations given below are based on animal data and human case reports/series. Case reports often document the use of multiple therapies simultaneously. Severely toxic patients responding to calcium (repeated boluses or infusions), multiple adrenergic agonists, and glucagon have been documented. Given the complexity of managing these cases, pulmonary artery catheterization should be considered in patients requiring more than one vasopressor.

Calcium Salts

Administration of calcium salts improves blood pressure in animal models and in human case reports.[7–9] Effects on heart rate are variable. Calcium chloride is preferred to calcium gluconate as it provides triple the amount of calcium on a weight-to-weight basis. However, calcium chloride must be administered through secure intravenous access as extravasation may result in tissue necrosis. Calcium chloride is usually given as a 1 to 3 gm intravenous bolus. The effects of calcium administration may be transient, and repeat dosing is commonly required, and continuous infusions of 2 to 6 g/h may also be used. Serum calcium levels may become markedly elevated, which may lead to reluctance toward subsequent dosing. However, for patients who do not respond to other therapies, it is reasonable to continue calcium administration even when serum calcium levels are markedly elevated. Animal studies of severe verapamil toxicity report response to an infusion of 5 mg/kg per min of calcium chloride. One human case report documents survival following administration of 30 g of calcium chloride over 12 h resulting in a serum calcium level of 5.94 mmol/L (23 mg/dL).[7]

Adrenergic Agents

Patients who do not respond to calcium administration or who require repeated doses are usually given adrenergic agonists. While animal data suggest that other therapies may offer improved metabolic function and improved survival in severe poisonings, adrenergic agonists have several advantages over more specific therapies. Physicians and nurses are familiar with these agents. Therapy can be initiated quickly and most patients will respond favorably. This prevents a period of nontreatment while the supplies for more esoteric therapies are gathered. Given the availability of these therapies and the familiarity of clinicians with their use, adrenergic agonists should be considered the first line of treatment for persistent hypotension following CCB ingestion. Cases of CCB poisoning responding to dopamine, epinephrine, and norepinephrine have been reported.[10] When standard doses are inadequate, it is reasonable to use high doses titrated to a systolic blood pressure of >90 mm Hg, although addition of another agent (such as insulin/glucose or glucagon) should also be considered. Phosphodiesterase inhibitors such as amrinone and milrinone have also been reported to improve blood pressure in animal studies and human case reports.[11,12] Figure 176-1 outlines the authors' suggested choices and dosing of β-adrenergic agents.

Insulin

Over the last 5 years, hyperinsulin/euglycemia (HIE) has emerged as a promising new treatment for the myocardial suppression associated with CCB poisoning. Several well-designed animal studies have demonstrated improved cardiac metabolic and mechanical function and improved survival when HIE is compared to glucagon, epinephrine, or placebo for treatment of verapamil poisoning.[3,13] Several human case reports have also suggested that HIE therapy improves perfusion in cases of CCB poisoning unresponsive to other therapies.[14,15] Unlike glucagon, insulin is readily available and inexpensive. Finally, the main adverse effect is hypoglycemia, a condition that may be eas-

FIG. 176-1. Proposed protocol for treatment of moderate to severe CCB poisoning.

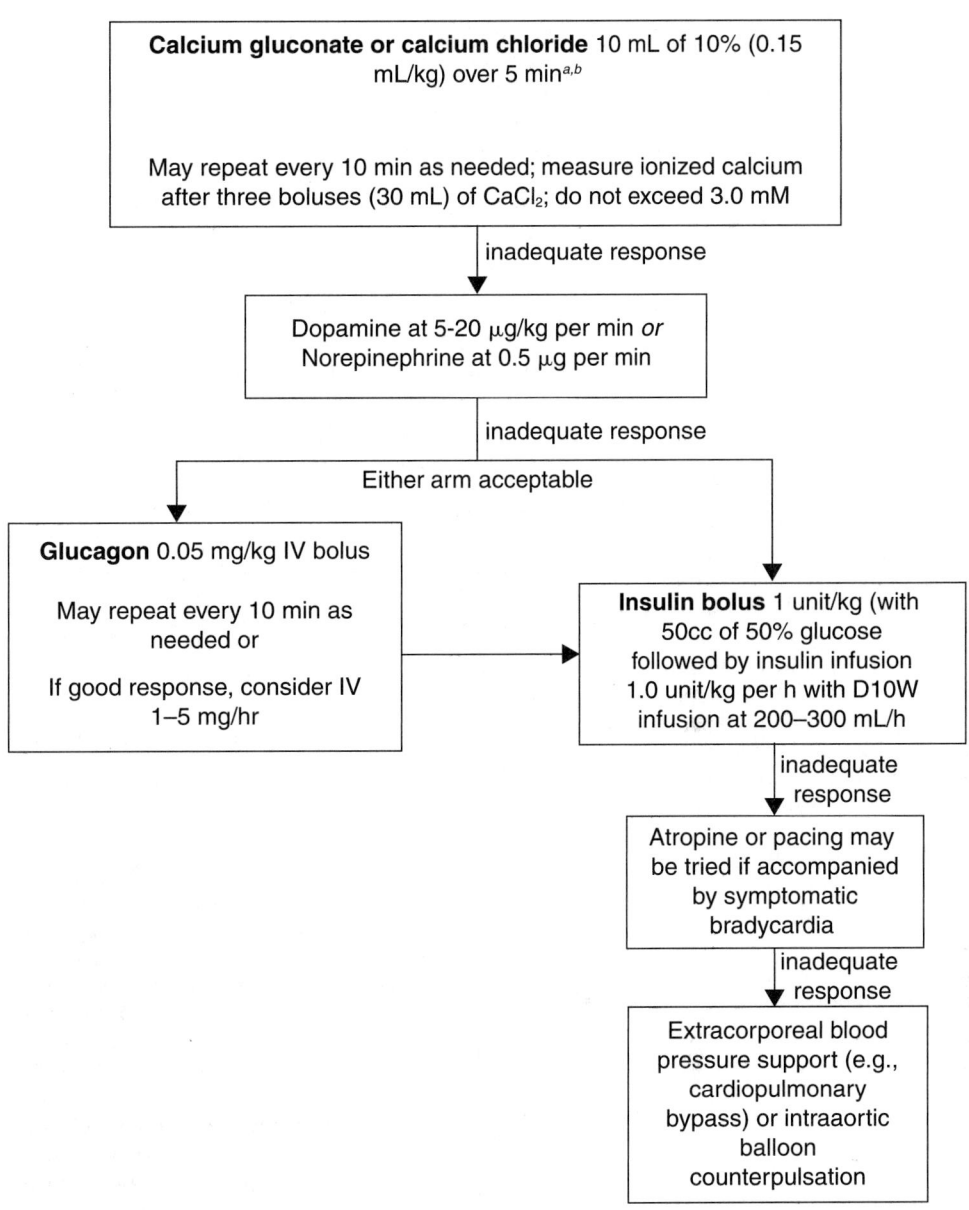

Calcium gluconate or calcium chloride 10 mL of 10% (0.15 mL/kg) over 5 min[a,b]

May repeat every 10 min as needed; measure ionized calcium after three boluses (30 mL) of CaCl₂; do not exceed 3.0 mM

↓ inadequate response

Dopamine at 5-20 μg/kg per min *or* Norepinephrine at 0.5 μg per min

↓ inadequate response

Either arm acceptable

Glucagon 0.05 mg/kg IV bolus

May repeat every 10 min as needed or

If good response, consider IV 1–5 mg/hr

Insulin bolus 1 unit/kg (with 50cc of 50% glucose followed by insulin infusion 1.0 unit/kg per h with D10W infusion at 200–300 mL/h

↓ inadequate response

Atropine or pacing may be tried if accompanied by symptomatic bradycardia

↓ inadequate response

Extracorporeal blood pressure support (e.g., cardiopulmonary bypass) or intraaortic balloon counterpulsation

[a] Calcium chloride provides three times as much free calcium as calcium gluconate.
[b] Use with caution if digoxin toxicity is possible.

ily detected with appropriate monitoring and responds rapidly to treatment. While failures are not unknown, most reports document a therapeutic response within 15 to 30 min. Current insulin dosing recommendations vary between 0.1 and 1 unit/kg. One anecdotal report noted a rapid response following a tenfold dosing error that resulted in administration of 1000 units of insulin to a patient that had failed to respond to dopamine, norepinephrine, glucagon, and calcium therapy. The patient's blood pressure increased dramatically within 15 min and the patient was off all vasopressors within 5 h, and no supplemental glucose was required. Given the success of HIE in animal models and recent clinical reports, HIE should be considered as a second line to vasopressors, and on a level with glucagon. Table 176-4 provides a suggested protocol for HIE.

Glucagon

Glucagon has been considered the treatment of choice for moderate to severe CCB toxicity. Glucagon improves blood pressure in animal models, and several case reports have also noted improvement in hemodynamics following glucagon therapy.[16,17] However, failures of therapy have also been reported.[15] The current recommended dose in adults is 0.05 mg/kg as a bolus. A response is usually seen within 15 min. If there is no response, doses should be repeated every 10 min up to 0.15 mg/kg. Patients that respond should be started on an infusion of 0.075 to 0.15 mg/kg per h. Similar dosing may be used for pediatric patients. Glucagon should be reconstituted using saline rather than the provided diluent, as this diluent contains phenol, which may cause toxicity when administered in high doses. The main adverse effects of glucagon are vomiting and hyperglycemia. Therefore, endotracheal intubation should be strongly considered prior to initiation of glucagon therapy. Finally, supplies of glucagon are often limited. Hospital glucagon supplies are often rapidly depleted and it may be necessary to contact other institutions for additional supplies. When these factors are considered, it is likely that HIE will replace glucagon as standard treatment for CCB toxicity in the near future.

Patients who do not respond to the above therapies may benefit from extraordinary measures. Hemodynamic support devices, such as intraaortic balloon pumps, left ventricular assist devices, and even extracorporeal circulatory devices, may provide adequate blood pressure to allow clearance of the drug and resolution of symptoms.[18]

TABLE 176-4   Suggested Protocol for Insulin Therapy of Severe Calcium Channel Blocker Overdose

Administer 50 mL of 50% glucose IV.

Administer insulin, 1 unit/kg IV bolus.

Begin insulin infusion at 0.5–1 unit/kg per h and D10W at 200–300 mL per h (adult) or 15–20 mL/kg per h (pediatric).

Monitor serum glucose every 20 min. Titrate glucose infusion rate to maintain serum glucose between 150 and 300 mg/dL.

Once infusion rates have been stable for 60 min, glucose monitoring may be decreased to hourly.

Monitor serum potassium and start intravenous potassium infusion if serum potassium is below 3.5 mEq/L.

Abbreviation: D50 = glucose 50% (0.5 g/mL) in water.

DECONTAMINATION

While routine gastric lavage has fallen out favor with many toxicologists, CCB overdoses are often life-threatening and may not respond to therapy. Given these considerations, the authors recommend gastric lavage for any patient that presents within 60 min of a potentially life-threatening CCB ingestion, and for any patient who requires intubation following CCB ingestion.

Calcium channel blockers are well bound to charcoal, and should be administered to adults following any potentially significant ingestion. In addition, charcoal should be routinely administered following accidental ingestion of verapamil in children, as life-threatening toxicity has been reported following ingestion of a single tablet.

Whole-bowel irrigation (WBI) is frequently advocated for ingestion of sustained-release calcium channel blockers. While prospective data are lacking, anecdotal case reports note that a large amount of medication may be recovered. Given the potential for severe toxicity, WBI should be strongly considered for patients who present following large ingestions of sustained-release products.

DISPOSITION

In general, patients will show manifestations of toxicity within 6 h of ingestion of non–sustained-release products. Patients who are asymptomatic, who have received charcoal decontamination, and who have normal vital signs following a 6-h observation period can be discharged after appropriate psychiatric evaluation. Toxicity may be delayed for up to 12 h following ingestion of sustained-release products.[19] In general, patients that ingest potentially toxic doses of sustained-release products should be admitted to a monitored setting for at least 24 h.

REFERENCES

1. Abernethy DR, Schwartz JB: Calcium antagonist drugs. *New Engl J Med* 341:1447, 1999.
2. Litovitz TL, Klein-Schwartz W, Rodgers GC: 2001 Annual report of the American Association of Poison Control Centers Toxic Exposure Surveillance System. *Am J Emerg Med* 20:391, 2002.
3. Kline JA, Leonova E, Raymond RM: Beneficial myocardial metabolic effects of insulin during verapamil toxicity in the anesthetized canine. *Crit Care Med* 23(7):1251, 1995.
4. Morel N, Buryi V, Feron O, et al: The action of calcium channel blockers on recombinant L-type calcium channel alpha1-subunits. *Br J Pharmacol* 125(5):1005, 1998.
5. Ramoska EA, Spiller HA, Winter M, Borys D: A one-year evaluation of calcium channel blocker overdoses: Toxicity and treatment. *Ann Emerg Med* 22(2):196, 1993.
6. Brass BJ, Winchester-Penny S, Lipper BL: Massive verapamil overdose complicated by noncardiogenic pulmonary edema. *Am J Emerg Med* 14(5):459, 1996.
7. Buckley N, Dawson AH, Howarth D, Whyte IM: Slow-release verapamil poisoning. Use of polyethylene glycol whole-bowel lavage and high-dose calcium. *Med J Aust* 158(3):202, 1993.
8. Hariman RJ, Mangiardi LM, McAllister RG Jr, et al: Reversal of the cardiovascular effects of verapamil by calcium and sodium: Differences between electrophysiologic and hemodynamic responses. *Circulation* 59(4): 797, 1979.
9. Henry M, Kay MM, Viccellio P: Cardiogenic shock associated with calcium-channel and beta blockers: Reversal with intravenous calcium chloride. *Am J Emerg Med* 3(4):334, 1985.
10. Erickson FC, Ling LJ, Grande GA, Anderson DL: Diltiazem overdose: Case report and review. *J Emerg Med* 9(5):357, 1991.
11. Goenen M, Col J, Compere A, Bonte J: Treatment of severe verapamil poisoning with combined amrinone-isoproterenol therapy. *Am J Cardiol* 58(11):1142, 1986.
12. Koury SI, Stone CK, Thomas SH: Amrinone as an antidote in experimental verapamil overdose. *Acad Emerg Med* 3(8):762, 1996.
13. Kline JA, Tomaszewski CA, Schroeder JD, Raymond RM: Insulin is a superior antidote for cardiovascular toxicity induced by verapamil in the anesthetized canine. *J Pharmacol Exp Ther* 267(2):744, 1993.
14. Boyer EW, Shannon M: Treatment of calcium-channel-blocker intoxication with insulin infusion. *New Engl J Med* 344(22):1721, 2001.
15. Yuan TH, Kerns WP 2nd, Tomaszewski CA, et al: Insulin-glucose as adjunctive therapy for severe calcium channel antagonist poisoning. *J Toxicol Clin Toxicol* 37(4):463, 1999.
16. Stone CK, May WA, Carroll R: Treatment of verapamil overdose with glucagon in dogs. *Ann Emerg Med* 25(3):369, 1995.
17. Walter FG, Frye G, Mullen JT, et al: Amelioration of nifedipine poisoning associated with glucagon therapy. *Ann Emerg Med* 22(7):1234, 1993.
18. Hendren WG, Schieber RS, Garrettson LK: Extracorporeal bypass for the treatment of verapamil poisoning. *Ann Emerg Med* 18(9):984, 1989.
19. Tom PA, Morrow CT, Kelen GD: Delayed hypotension after overdose of sustained release verapamil. *J Emerg Med* 12(5):621, 1994.

177 ANTIHYPERTENSIVE AGENT TOXICITY

Arjun Chanmugam

Keith Thomasset

Hypertension is one of the most common diseases in the United States, affecting almost 24 percent of the population.[1] Medications used to control hypertension are among the most commonly prescribed drugs. As a result, the potential for overdose, inadvertent or intentional, is quite high. In 2001, according to the Toxic Exposure Surveillance System, cardiovascular drugs, including antihypertensive medications, accounted for nearly 4 percent of all adult toxic exposures.[2] There are many classes of antihypertensive medications available for use, with new agents introduced into the market frequently.

The initial management of patients with an acute overdose of antihypertensive medication remains relatively uniform. Airway, breathing, and circulation remain the initial priorities. Thus, oxygen, cardiac monitoring, and intravenous access remain the key initial interventions. If mental status changes are present, glucose and naloxone should also be considered as initial interventions. If no contraindications are present, antihypertensive-induced hypotension should be treated initially with volume expansion, using NS or an equivalent crystalloid solution (such as LR solution). In most adults, initial fluid therapy should consist of bolus challenges of 500 mL or 10 to 20 mL/kg over 10 to 15 min. If hypotension persists despite fluid challenges, the use of a vasopressor may be warranted. In most cases, dopamine is the vasopressor of choice, with infusion rates started at 2 to 5 μg/kg per min and increased as appropriate.

Supportive measures and appropriate monitoring should be instituted as early as possible. The use of activated charcoal is indicated in most overdose situations, but gastric decontamination should be considered only in appropriate patients (discussed below). The management of patients with antihypertensive poisonings rarely relies on serum levels of medications but instead depends on symptoms. However, a key to managing these patients is to determine the medication involved and to target interventions specific for that class of antihypertensive agent (Table 177-1). In the following discussion, antihypertensive toxicology is divided into sections based on the class of medications. β-Blockers, monoamine oxidase inhibitors, and calcium-channel blockers are discussed in separate chapters.

DIURETICS

Diuretics are among the most commonly prescribed of all antihypertensives because they are recommended as a first-line medication in the treatment of hypertension.[1] Diuretics can be subdivided into several groups based on their mechanism of action.

Thiazide and Loop Diuretics

Thiazide and loop diuretics are two classes of diuretics commonly used. The classic thiazide diuretic is hydrochlorothiazide, which can be used as single-drug therapy or as part of a multidrug regimen. Combination products are becoming more common in the treatment of hypertension, and hydrochlorothiazide is often used as a component of these fixed-combination medications. In general, toxicity associated with thiazide diuretics is rare.

The pharmacologic action of thiazide diuretics (e.g., chlorthalidone, hydrochlorothiazide, and metolazone) is a result of their ability to inhibit reabsorption of sodium and chloride at the distal convoluted tubule. This results in a greater excretion of water and other essential electrolytes, including potassium and bicarbonate. At higher doses,

TABLE 177-1 Common Antihypertensive Medications

Agent	Mechanism of Action	Therapeutic Range	Oral LD$_{50}$	Dialysis	Maximum Tolerated Exposure	Therapeutic Interventions and Comments
Hydrochlorothiazide	Inhibits reabsortion of Na$^+$ and Cl$^-$ in the distal convoluted tubule of the kidney	12.5–100mg qd (in divided doses)	10 g/kg in mice/rats	Partially	1 g	IV fluids, correct electrolytes, vasopressor if necessary
Furosemide	Decreases reabsorption of Na$^+$ and Cl$^-$ in the loop of Henle	20–600 mg qd	1000 mg/kg in rats/dogs	No	Not established	IV fluids, correct electrolytes, vasopressor if necessary
Spironolactone	Specific antagonist of aldosterone	25–400 mg qd		Yes	Not established	IV fluids, correct electrolytes
Triamterene	Inhibits the reabsorption of sodium ions in exchange for potassium and hydrogen ions at the distal tubule	100–150 mg bid	380 mg/kg in mice	Yes	Not established	IV fluids, correct electrolytes, vasopressor if necessary
Acetazolamide	Inhibits carbonic anhydrase in the kidney	Up to 1000 mg qd in divided doses	No deaths reported	Possibly	Not established	IV fluids, correct electrolytes, pH, vasopressor if necessary
Mannitol	Osmotic diuresis	0.5–2 g/kg	Not known	Yes	Not established	IV fluids, correct electrolytes, vasopressor if necessary
Clonidine	Central α$_2$-adrenergic agonist	0.1–2.4 mg/d	465 mg/kg	No	11.25 mg	IV fluids, vasopressor, naloxone, tolazoline
Captopril	Angiotensin-converting enzyme inhibition	6.25–150 mg qd	No deaths reported	Yes	7.5 g	IV fluids, vasopressor, naloxone
Enalapril	Angiotensin-converting enzyme inhibition	5–40 mg qd	2000 mg/kg in mice/rats	Yes	300 mg	IV fluids, vasopressor, naloxone
Lisinopril	Angiotensin-converting enzyme inhibitor	2.5–80 mg qd	Not well established	Yes	400 mg	IV fluids, vasopressors (dopamine), naloxone
Losartan	Angiotensin-receptor inhibitor	12.5–100 mg qd	2000 mg/kg in rats	No	Not well established	IV fluids, vasopressors (dopamine)
Valsartan	Angiotensin-receptor inhibitor	80–320 mg qd	Not well established	No	Not well established	IV fluids, vasopressors (dopamine)
Candesartan	Angiotensin-receptor inhibitor	2–32 mg in one or two divided doses daily	Not well established	No	Not well established	IV fluids, vasopressors (dopamine)
Methyldopa	Central inhibition of α-adrenergic receptors, false neurotransmission, and/or reduction of plasma rennin activity	250–3000 mg qd	>1.5 g/kg in mice/rats	Yes	Not established	IV fluids, vasopressor

(continued)

TABLE 177-1 Common Antihypertensive Medications *(Continued)*

Agent	Mechanism of Action	Therapeutic Range	Oral LD$_{50}$	Dialysis	Maximum Tolerated Exposure	Therapeutic Interventions and Comments
Hydralazine	Direct relaxation of arteriolar smooth muscle	10–50 mg qid	173 mg/kg in rats	No	Not established	IV fluids; vasopressor therapy should be avoided secondary to potential dysrhythmias
Minoxidil	Direct peripheral vasodilation	5–100 mg qd in divided doses	1321–3492 mg/kg in rats	Partially	Not established	IV fluids; vasopressor therapy should be avoided secondary to potential dysrhythmias
Sodium nitroprusside	Relaxation of arteriolar and venous smooth muscles	0.5+10 µg/kg per min	—	Yes, for thiocyanate toxicity	Unknown	Prolonged use can result in cyanide and/or thiocyanate toxicity; for cyanide toxicity, treat with cyanide antidote kit (see Chap. 188)
Prazosin	Competitive blockade of α$_1$-adrenergic receptors	1–20 mg qd in divided doses	Not known	No	200 mg	IV fluids, vasopressor
Doxazosin	Arteriolar dilator, competitive blockade of postsynaptic α$_1$-adrenergic receptors	1–16 mg qd	1000 mg/kg in mice and rats	No	70 mg	IV fluids, vasopressors (dopamine)
Terazosin	Arteriolar dilator, competitive blockade of postsynaptic α$_1$-adrenergic receptors	1–20 mg in one or two divided doses daily	Not well established	No	Not well established	IV fluids, vasopressors (dopamine)
Fenoldopam	Postsynaptic dopamine 1 receptor agonist	0.1–1.6 µg/kg per min	Not established	Yes	Not established	IV fluids, vasopressors

thiazide diuretics can function similar to carbonic anhydrous inhibitors. Calcium regulation is also affected by thiazide diuretics by two separate mechanisms: 1) inhibition of vitamin D synthesis and thus, decreased calcium absorption from the gastrointestinal tract; 2) increased renal absorption of calcium. The net result, however, is calcium retention and possibly hypercalcemia.

Loop diuretics include drugs such as furosemide, bumetanide, ethacrynic acid, and torsemide. These agents act on the ascending limb of the loop of Henle to decrease reabsorption of sodium, chloride, and water. They act similarly to the thiazide diuretics in that they alter the regulation of other essential electrolytes, particularly potassium and calcium. Unlike thiazide diuretics, the loop diuretics increase the excretion of calcium. Loop diuretics also increase venous capacitance and are used in acute situations with elevated cardiac filling pressures.

The toxicity associated with thiazide and loop diuretics involves two basic processes: volume contraction and electrolyte derangements. Findings associated with intravascular volume depletion include hypotension (sometimes only orthostatic hypotension), tachycardia, and altered mental status. Common electrolyte derangements include hyponatremia, hypokalemia, hypocalcemia (loop diuretics), hypomagnesemia, hyperuricemia (thiazide diuretics), and hypochlor-emic metabolic alkalosis. Occasionally, an increased anion gap without acidosis is noted because of concentration of unmeasured anions in the serum. Other adverse reactions from thiazide and loop diuretics may include rash, pruritis, hearing loss, leukopenia, and thrombocytopenia.

Normal saline administration is the preferred therapy for hypovolemia, hyponatremia, and alkalosis. The use of vasopressors is rarely indicated for hypotension. Potassium replacement should be instituted early, although renal function should be assessed and monitored during therapy to avoid inducing iatrogenic hyperkalemia in acute or chronic renal failure. In general, if comorbid conditions are not present, most asymptomatic individuals can be medically cleared after therapy and observation. Poisonings sufficient to cause significant electrolyte abnormalities are likely to be associated with total body deficits of various elements and may require prolonged therapy.

Potassium-Sparing Diuretics

The most common medications of this subclass are spironolactone, triamterene, and amiloride. Spironolactone, a competitive inhibitor of aldosterone, acts to allow potassium retention while inducing sodium and water excretion. Triamterene has direct effects on the renal tubule to inhibit sodium exchange for potassium and hydrogen. Amiloride's mechanism of action, also independent of aldosterone, is to promote potassium retention in exchange of sodium and water. Volume depletion, hyperkalemia, hyponatremia, and hypochloremia are common manifestations of toxicity for this class of medication. Treatment for potassium-sparing diuretic toxicity is directed at maintaining intravascular volume, repleting sodium, and reversing the hyperkalemia. Hypotension is best initially treated with intravenous fluids, usually normal saline. If hypotension is persistent, a vasopressor such as dopamine is warranted. The most serious manifestations of hyperkalemia include neurologic and cardiovascular dysfunction. Treatment of hyperkalemia should remain a priority, and can be serious enough to warrant dialysis.

Carbonic Anhydrase Inhibitors

The prototype for this subclass of diuretic is acetazolamide, which is a nonbacteriostatic sulfonamide whose adverse reactions include severe allergic reaction and Stevens–Johnson syndrome. The primary action of this class of diuretic is to inhibit carbonic anhydrase in the kidney to prevent the reversible reaction of carbon dioxide and water to form carbonic acid. This results in loss of bicarbonate ions in the urine, along with sodium, potassium, and water. Overdose with this class of medication can lead to volume depletion and electrolyte disturbances, as well as non–anion-gap metabolic acidosis. Treatment is directed at reversing volume depletion, monitoring electrolytes, and restoring normal pH balance.

Osmotic Agents

Osmotic agents, such as mannitol, are not absorbed by the nephron. Rather, they induce diuresis by raising the osmolarity of the glomerular filtrate, thereby attracting more water in the tubules to increase urine volume. The main effect of osmotic agents is to decrease intravascular volume, but toxicity can result in pulmonary edema, anaphylaxis, and acute renal failure. Overdoses can cause profound volume loss, accompanied by electrolyte imbalances. Treatment is aimed at repleting the intravascular volume and correcting any electrolyte imbalances. Other adverse reactions—such as pulmonary congestion, acidosis, electrolyte loss, dryness of mouth, thirst, marked diuresis, urinary retention, edema, headache, blurred vision, convulsions, nausea, vomiting, rhinitis, skin necrosis, thrombophlebitis, chills, dizziness, urticaria, dehydration, fever, and angina-like chest pains—have been reported during or following mannitol infusion.

CENTRALLY ACTING ANTIHYPERTENSIVE AGENTS

A number of centrally acting antihypertensive agents are available for use. Examples include clonidine, guanabenz, guanfacine, and methyldopa. Clonidine is the most used agent in this class and has long been a favorite for the acute management of hypertension. Two forms of clonidine are commonly prescribed, an oral version and a transdermal patch. Clonidine has gained prominence in recent years because of its ability to mitigate opiate and alcohol withdrawal symptoms. Although it has not been approved by the Food and Drug Administration for this use, clonidine has been used in clinical practice for the treatment of narcotic withdrawal for almost two decades.[3] With the advent of the clonidine patch in 1986, drug delivery could be reliably maintained for 7 days at a variety of doses, which increased its attractiveness for prescribers. However, plasma concentrations of clonidine remain high enough to maintain a hypotensive effect for approximately 8 h after the removal of the patch. Regardless of the route of administration, clonidine's most common adverse effects are dry mouth and drowsiness.

Clonidine

Clonidine is an imidazoline whose principle site of action is on the α_2 receptors in the lower brainstem. Stimulation of the central α_2 receptor decreases norepinephrine release in the central nervous system (CNS), resulting in a lower heart rate and blood pressure. Although clonidine acts as a central α_2-adrenergic receptor agonist, it has other effects. For example, it reduces noradrenergic output in the locus ceruleus, which is stimulated by the cessation of narcotic use, thereby mitigating the symptoms of opioid withdrawal. At higher doses, clonidine can act as a partial peripheral α-agonist, resulting in a paradoxical increase in blood pressure and heart rate. However, this effect is relatively short-lived and the antihypertensive effects usually predominate.

Clonidine exposure appears particularly prevalent in children. During a recent 6-year period there were over 10,000 clonidine exposures in children (<19 years), with a majority among those less than 6 years. Most were of little to no consequence, but about 10 percent were moderate to serious. There was only one death.[4]

The primary symptoms associated with clonidine toxicity include hypotension and bradycardia, which can lead to cardiac ischemia and congestive heart failure. Mental status changes range from agitation and hallucinations to sedation and coma. Respiratory depression and recurrent apnea can occur, especially in children. The other symptoms of clonidine toxicity include seizures, diarrhea, hypothermia, and miosis.

Treatment of clonidine overdoses is centered on maintaining adequate blood pressures. In the acute phase of toxicity, a brief episode of blood pressure elevation may occur. This paradoxical hypertensive response is due to peripheral α_1-adrenergic receptor stimulation but usually evolves rapidly into hypotension as central α_2-agonist stimulation predominates. Treatment is rarely indicated for transient blood pressure elevation, but if aggressive intervention is warranted, nitroprusside is the drug of choice because of its rapid onset and dissipation. The peak effects of clonidine usually occur in 1 to 3 h. Intravenous fluids are usually adequate for the treatment of hypotension, but in cases of persistent hypotension, a dopamine infusion beginning at a midlevel dose rate of 2 to 5 μg/kg per min can be initiated.

The other serious cardiovascular condition caused by clonidine toxicity—sinus bradycardia—must be monitored closely. Symptomatic bradycardia should be treated with repeated doses of atropine sulfate. The other toxic effects of clonidine occur less commonly but may be serious. Respiratory depression is rare, but recurrent apnea, especially in children, may require intubation. Seizures require supportive measures and usually respond to standard anticonvulsant therapy. Hypothermia associated with clonidine toxicity also responds to standard interventions.

In cases of severe refractory hypotension or CNS depression, the use of naloxone has been suggested, although its mechanism of action is not well understood. Tolazoline 10 mg IV titrated every 15 min to a maximum of 40 mg, is only recommended after intravenous fluids, dopamine, atropine, and naloxone have failed to reverse the cardiovascular effects of clonidine.[5] There is also a single case report of clonidine toxicity being successfully treated with yohimbine, a CNS α_2-adrenergic antagonist.[6]

Clonidine's range of toxicity has not been well established. Severe toxicity has been reported in children at doses as low as 0.1 mg, whereas adults have survived with levels exceeding 15 mg. Symptoms of clonidine toxicity can persist for up to 72 h, so admission should be considered for any patient suspected of clonidine overdose.

Similar to clonidine, the following agents also exert their effects by decreasing norepinephrine release from the distal nerve terminals in the CNS. The additional agents should also be considered in this group include guanabenz, guanethidine, guanfacine, and methyldopa. Reserpine is also a centrally acting agent that exerts its action by depleting norepinephrine and other catecholamine stores in the central nervous system. Overdoses of these medications results in effects similar to the α_2-adrenergic receptor agonists, which include hypotension, symptomatic bradycardia, dry mouth, and potential mental status changes.

Hypotension should be treated with intravenous crystalloid; if necessary, vasopressors such as norepinephrine or dopamine should be considered. Bradycardia can be treated with atropine. Methyldopa can be dialyzed, but there is no clear evidence that dialysis of the other agents is beneficial. A rebound hypertensive condition, similar to that of clonidine withdrawal, may occur with the abrupt cessation of any centrally acting antihypertensive medication.

PERIPHERAL α_1-ADRENERGIC RECEPTOR ANTAGONISTS

Agents in this class exert their hypotensive effects by antagonism of peripheral α_1-adrenergic receptors. The result is a decrease in systemic vascular resistance. Agents in this class can be administered PO and IV. The oral agents include doxazosin, prazosin and terazosin. Intravenous agents used in this class include phenoxybenzamine and phentolamine. Reported toxicity associated with this drug class is relatively uncommon. A first-dose phenomenon has been reported with the use of these agents that results in an unanticipated sudden hypotensive episode, potentially leading to syncope. Inadvertent hypotension generally occurs within 30 to 60 min after the first dose has been given and is usually preceded by tachycardia. The first-dose phenomenon usually occurs in individuals with impaired hepatic function or congestive heart failure.

Other toxic symptoms include headache, vertigo, paresthesias, gastrointestinal discomfort, and weakness. Case reports have indicated that priapism, pulmonary edema, and acidosis can also occur as a result of overdose with these agents. However, the most common manifestation of α_1-adrenergic receptor antagonist overdose remains hypotension and tachycardia. Treatment is supportive with intravenous fluids, careful monitoring, and vasopressors, if necessary.

DIRECT VASODILATORS

Hydralazine

Hydralazine, a smooth muscle vasodilator whose mechanism of action is poorly understood, is available both in tablet form and in parenteral form. Acute toxicity with hydralazine is uncommon, and no fatalities as a result of acute poisoning have been reported. Chronic use does lead to a hydralazine-induced systemic lupus erythematosus syndrome, but this generally occurs in individuals who have slow hepatic acetylation. Treatment is supportive; the hypotension associated with hydralazine responds well to intravenous fluids. Vasopressors should be used with caution in order to avoid precipitating dysrhythmias. If a vasopressor is necessary, dopamine should be used judiciously. Symptomatic tachycardia can be cautiously treated with β-blockers.

Minoxidil

Minoxidil is a direct-acting peripheral vasodilator that lowers systolic and diastolic blood pressure without much affect on the CNS. It also has the advantage of not interfering with vasomotor reflexes and therefore does not induce orthostatic hypotension.

In tablet form, minoxidil is usually reserved for the treatment of severe or refractory hypertension, and reported toxicity has been rare. A common side effect of minoxidil is hirsutism. In 1988, a 2 percent topical solution of minoxidil was approved for the treatment of baldness. At least one case report exists involving ingestion of the topical solution. Regardless of the preparation, the most common symptoms of toxicity include hypotension and tachycardia.[7] In patients with renal failure, fluid retention, and pericardial effusion have been reported. Treatment is supportive and includes intravenous fluids. If the hypotension is persistent, dopamine or phenylephrine should be considered. Vasopressors with β-adrenergic activity, such as epinephrine, should be avoided because of the potential for excessive cardiac stimulation. β-Blockers can be used for symptomatic tachycardia.

Sodium Nitroprusside

This is the drug of choice for most true hypertensive emergencies. It is a rapidly absorbed and rapidly dissipated drug whose principle action is to lower blood pressure by relaxing smooth muscle in arteries and veins. Sodium nitroprusside causes toxicity by three primary mechanisms: 1) the most common adverse effect is direct vasodilation resulting in hypotension and dysrhythmias; 2) thiocyanate toxicity occurs infrequently, resulting in tinnitus, altered mental status changes, nausea, and abdominal pain; 3) in rare cases, cyanide toxicity can occur, resulting in coma, metabolic acidosis, or respiratory arrest. In very rare cases, and in susceptible patients, methemoglobinemia can occur, which, if levels reach greater than 15 percent, can result in symptomatic cellular hypoxia. Toxicity associated with sodium nitroprusside is usually related to prolonged administration or occurs in patients with renal or hepatic failure.

Nitroprusside reacts with hemoglobin to form cyanomethemoglobin and cyanide. Methemoglobin is derived from hemoglobin and will bind cyanide until the intraerythrocyte methemoglobin has been saturated. Thiosulfate will react with the remaining cyanide to form thiocyanate, which is excreted in the urine. A limiting factor in cyanide metabolism is the amount of thiosulfate in the body, and that limit is usually achieved at a nitroprusside infusion rate of 5 μg/kg per min.

The direct vasodilatation effects of nitroprusside can result in excessive hypotension, resulting in mental status changes and dysrhythmias. Thiocyanate toxicity causes anorexia, fatigue, and mental status changes, including psychosis, weakness, seizures, tinnitus, and hyperreflexia. Cyanide toxicity is often associated with the odor of almonds on breath and can result in acidosis, tachycardia, mental status changes, and death.

Excessive hypotension secondary to nitroprusside administration can be avoided by careful monitoring using an arterial line and frequent clinical evaluations. In general, blood pressure reduction should not exceed a 25 percent reduction in mean arterial pressure. Should hypotension occur, stopping the infusion is usually effective since the half-life of nitroprusside is only a few minutes.

Thiocyanate toxicity can be minimized by avoiding prolonged administration of nitroprusside and by limiting drug use in patients with renal insufficiency. If necessary, thiocyanate can be removed by dialysis. Cyanide toxicity can be avoided by the coadministration of sodium thiosulfate or by limiting the administration of nitroprusside. Details of the treatment of cyanide toxicity are discussed in Chap. 188.

DOPAMINE AGONISTS

Fenoldopam is an agent used in the management of acute severe hypertension. It is used as a nitroprusside alternative in patients with renal dysfunction, negating the risk of cyanide/thiocyanate toxicity.[8] Lack of experience and the associated expense of this agent have resulted in minimal use to date. This agent exerts its effects by agonism of the dopamine 1 receptor. The result is peripheral vasodilation and a reduction in blood pressure. Toxicity with fenoldopam is theorized to result in hypotension. These effects of fenoldopam are short lived based on its relatively short half-life (5 to 10 min). Treatment involves discontinuation of the agent and the administration of intravenous crystalloid. If hypotension persists, vasopressor therapy with agents such as dopamine or norepinephrine is warranted.

ANGIOTENSIN-CONVERTING ENZYME INHIBITORS

Angiotensin-converting enzyme inhibitors (ACEIs) come in two basic forms: an active drug form, best represented by captopril, and a prodrug form, represented by enalapril. Recently, enalaprilat, the active form of enalapril, became available for intravenous use. However, there are many ACEIs available today, and all work to inhibit the conversion of the prohormone angiotensin I to the potent endogenous vasoconstrictor angiotensin II. Besides being a vasoconstrictor, angiotensin II stimulates aldosterone release to increase sodium and water retention. Aside from these two effects, ACEIs have other mechanisms of action to decrease total peripheral resistance without increasing heart rate or cardiac output. For example, by inhibiting ACE (also known as bradykininase), the degradation of the vasodilator peptide bradykinin is prevented.

Adverse effects of ACEIs include hypotension, angioedema, rash, anaphylactoid reactions, cough, drug fever, proteinuria, glomerulopathy, neutropenia, and agranulocytosis. With overdoses of ACEIs, the most important concern is hypotension, which can be profound. The preferred therapy to reverse the hypotension is the administration of normal saline (NS), and, if necessary, vasopressors, such as intermediate- or high-dose dopamine, can be added. Although ACEIs are dialyzable, peritoneal dialysis and hemodialysis are not recommended at this time. Naloxone has been reported to be useful in reversing the hypotension induced by captopril, although its mechanism is unclear.[9] The mechanism is theorized to involve the ACEIs ability to inhibit the metabolism of enkephalins and potentiate their opioid effect, including a decrease in blood pressure.[10]

ANGIOTENSIN II RECEPTOR ANTAGONISTS

This class of agents exerts its antihypertensive effects via inhibition of the angiotensin II receptor. Common agents in this class include, but are not limited to, losartan, valsartan, and candesartan. Experience with toxic effects of these agents appears to be limited in humans to date. Symptoms experienced are primarily extensions of the agents' therapeutic effects and are similar to those of ACE inhibition. Hypotension and reflex tachycardia are the commonly seen effects of these agents. Bradycardia may be seen as a result of excess vagal stimulation. Hyperkalemia can also be seen in patients receiving these agents. Supportive measures, including intravenous NS, adequate monitoring (including electrolytes–potassium). Close observation is indicated for anyone who may have ingested an overdose of an angiotensin II receptor antagonist.

REFERENCES

1. Joint National Committee on Detection, Evaluation, and Treatment of High Blood Pressure: The sixth report of the Joint National Committee on Detection, Evaluation, and Treatment of High Blood Pressure. *Arch Intern Med* 157:2413, 1997.
2. Litovitz TL, Klein-Schwartz W, Rodgers GC Jr, et al: 2001 Annual report of the American Association of Poison Control Centers Toxic Exposure Surveillance System. *Am J Emerg Med* 20(5):391, 2002.
3. Center for Substance Abuse Treatment: *Treatment Improvement Protocol Series January 1, 1995.* Washington, DC: US Department of Health and Human Services, Public Health Service, 1995.
4. Klein-Schwartz W: Trends and toxic effects from pediatric clonidine exposures. *Arch Pediatr Adolesc Med* 56:392, 2002.
5. Conner CS, Watanabe AS: Clonidine overdose: A review. *Am J Hosp Pharm* 36:906, 1979.
6. Roberge RJ: Yohimbine as an antidote for clonidine overdose. *Am J Emerg Med* 14:678, 1996.
7. Poff SW, Rose SR: Minoxidil overdose with ECG changes: Case report and review. *J Emerg Med* 10:53, 1992.
8. Post JB 4th, Frishman WH: Fenoldopam: A new dopamine agonist for the treatment of hypertensive urgencies and emergencies. *J Clin Pharmacol* 38(1):2, 1998.
9. Varon J, Duncan SR: Naloxone reversal of hypotension due to captopril overdose. *Ann Emerg Med* 20:1125, 1991.
10. Millar JA, Sturani A, Rubin PC, Reid JL: Attenuation of the antihypertensive effect of captopril by the opioid receptor antagonist naloxone. *Clin Exp Pharmacol Physiol* 10:253, 1983.

PHENYTOIN AND FOSPHENYTOIN TOXICITY
Harold H. Osborn

Phenytoin (3-hydroxymethyl-5,5-diphenylhydantoin) is a primary anticonvulsant for all types of epilepsy except absence. It is useful in the treatment of status epilepticus in conjunction with other more rapidly acting anticonvulsants.[1] Phenytoin has been used prophylactically in a variety of clinical settings characterized by acute symptomatic seizures (head trauma, alcohol withdrawal, and drug overdose) but thus far has proven useful only in the setting of head trauma and then only in the immediate posttraumatic period. Phenytoin has been employed in the management of chronic pain syndromes. Historically, it has also been used as an antidysrhythmic agent, especially in the set-

ting of digoxin toxicity, but it is no longer considered a first-line agent. Morbidity or mortality is unusual after intentional phenytoin overdose if good supportive care is provided. Most phenytoin-related deaths have been caused by rapid intravenous administration or hypersensitivity reactions.

Data with regard to exposures from the American Association of Poison Control Centers are almost certainly underestimates. Major toxicity is more likely to be reported from adverse parenteral events, and minor drug reactions are more common with oral preparations. Nevertheless, in 2001, 3941 exposures were reported, 53 percent of which were unintentional, 35 percent were intentional, 8 percent were adverse reactions, and the rest were "other." Among these exposures, 23 percent were considered inconsequential, 24 percent were considered minor, 13 percent were considered moderate, and fewer than 3 percent were considered major. Only six deaths were reported.[2]

MECHANISM OF ACTION

Phenytoin exerts its anticonvulsant effect by blocking voltage-sensitive and frequency-dependent sodium channels in the neurons. Phenytoin stabilizes sodium channels in an inactive state, and this inhibitory effect, similar to the action of local anesthetics, depends on the voltage and frequency of firing of the neuron. Phenytoin has no effect on the amplitude or duration of the action potential. Rather, it limits the ability of the neuron to fire trains of action potentials at high frequency by delaying recovery. In this fashion, it suppresses repetitive neuronal activity and prevents the spread of a seizure focus. At higher concentrations, phenytoin delays activation of outward potassium currents in nerves and prolongs the neuronal refractory period. It also may exert an anticonvulsant effect by influencing calcium channels or γ-aminobutyric acid receptors (GABA), although this has not been fully established.

PATHOPHYSIOLOGY

The toxic effects of phenytoin vary with route administration, duration of exposure, and dosage used. Of these determinants of toxicity, the most important is the route of administration. The intravenous administration of phenytoin carries the greatest risk, in large part due to the other constituents of the parenteral vehicle (see "Effects of Propylene Glycol and Ethanol Diluents"). The most serious reactions after intravenous administration are cardiovascular (bradycardia, hypotension, and asystole), although tissue necrosis and sloughing after extravasation have been described.[3] Major cardiac toxicity occurs only after parenteral administration; in general, oral overdose does not lead to cardiovascular morbidity.[4] It is more common in the elderly and those with underlying cardiac disease but has been described in young healthy patients.

Many of the side effects of the oral preparation are dose related and are predictable at higher plasma concentrations. Nevertheless, different individuals have different tolerance profiles, and adverse effects can be evident in some at seemingly therapeutic doses, whereas others may only display untoward effects well beyond the therapeutic range. Early toxicity is manifested by vestibular, ocular, or cerebellar signs: nystagmus, dysdiadochokinesia, and ataxia. At higher levels, central nervous system (CNS) depression and other cognitive effects (confusion, dizziness, and loss of concentration and memory) are seen. Only two areas of the brain normally exhibit spontaneous neuronal burst discharge: the hippocampus and the cerebellum. The ability of phenytoin to suppress these areas may result in impaired memory and balance, respectively. Paradoxically, very high levels of phenytoin may be associated with seizures, although this is, at best, a rare occurrence. Acute oral overdose is usually manifested by nystagmus, nausea and vomiting, ataxia, dysarthria, choreoathetosis, opisthotonos, and CNS depression or excitation.[5] Deaths from oral ingestion of phenytoin are extremely rare and occur in association with the ingestion of other substances. The chronic administration of phenytoin is associated with numerous side effects that involve a variety of organ systems. Many of these effects depend on dose and duration, but some are idiosyncratic. Hypersensitivity reactions to phenytoin usually occur within the first few months of therapy and include fever, skin rashes, blood dyscrasia, and, rarely, hepatitis. Deaths due to Stevens-Johnson syndrome have occurred, and anyone with this syndrome should never receive phenytoin again.

PHARMACOKINETICS

Phenytoin is a weak acid with a pK_a of 8.3. Thus, in the acid milieu of the stomach and even at physiologic pH, its aqueous solubility is limited. The parenteral form of phenytoin is adjusted to pH 12 to keep the drug in solution, but it is very irritating to the tissues, and intramuscular injection results in local precipitation of phenytoin with erratic absorption and therefore is not recommended. Absorption after oral ingestion is slow, variable, and often incomplete, especially after an overdose. Consequently, it may be necessary to obtain serial levels in suspected overdose to determine peak levels. Significant differences in bioavailability exist among different phenytoin preparations. Peak levels typically occur from 3 to 12 h after a *single* oral dose.

After absorption, phenytoin is distributed throughout the body, with a volume of distribution of 0.6 to 0.8 L/kg. Brain tissue concentrations equal those in plasma within about 10 min of intravenous infusion and correlate with therapeutic effects, whereas cerebrospinal fluid and myocardium equilibrate within 30 to 60 min. At steady state, concentrations are higher in neural tissue than in the serum. Within the CNS, concentrations are higher in the brainstem and cerebellum than in the cerebral cortex.

PROTEIN BINDING AND FREE PHENYTOIN FRACTIONS

Phenytoin is extensively (90 percent) bound to plasma proteins, especially albumin. The free, unbound, form is the biologically active moiety responsible for the drug's clinical effect and toxicity. The free phenytoin fraction normally constitutes 10 percent of the plasma level. The unbound fraction of the drug is greater in the following groups of patients: neonates; the elderly; pregnant women; individuals with uremia, hypoalbuminemia (cirrhosis, nephrosis, malnutrition, burns, trauma, or cystic fibrosis), and hyperbilirubinemia; and individuals taking drugs that displace phenytoin from binding sites (salicylate, valproate, phenylbutazone, tolbutamide, and sulfisoxazole).

Although patients with decreased protein binding may have higher levels of free phenytoin and a greater biologic effect, they may have lower levels of total phenytoin, because more of the drug is available for metabolism. Theoretically, such patients may become toxic with total phenytoin levels in the therapeutic range. Patients who exhibit toxic signs in the therapeutic range and those with decreased protein binding should have free phenytoin levels measured.

Phenytoin concentrations are most commonly measured by an enzyme-mediated immunoassay technique, which is specific and sensitive to less than 1 μg/mL. If available, free phenytoin concentrations are more useful to predict toxicity. Corrected serum phenytoin levels can be calculated in hypoproteinemic patients with a known serum albumin level. To calculate the phenytoin concentration (C_{normal}) that would be present if a patient's serum albumin were normal, the following equation is used:

$$C_{normal} = \frac{C_{measured} \times 4.4}{albumin\ concentration}$$

where the phenytoin concentration is in micrograms per milliliter and the albumin concentration is in grams per deciliter.

METABOLISM

After absorption and distribution, only 4 to 5 percent of phenytoin is excreted unchanged in the urine. The remainder is metabolized by hepatic microsomal enzymes. The drug is primarily hydroxylated to a series of inactive compounds. The major metabolite (60 to 70 percent) is the parahydroxyphenyl derivative. It is processed by glucuronidase, secreted in the bile, reabsorbed, and subsequently excreted in the urine. Phenytoin is not appreciably removed by hemodialysis or hemoperfusion. The metabolism of phenytoin is capacity limited (dose dependent). At plasma concentrations below 10 μg/mL, elimination is first order (a fixed percentage of drug metabolized per unit of time). However, at higher concentrations, including those in the therapeutic range (10 to 20 μg/mL), the metabolic pathways may become saturated, and the elimination may change to zero-order kinetics (a fixed amount metabolized per unit of time). This change in kinetics can markedly prolong the half-life of phenytoin, which is normally 6 to 24 h. An understanding of capacity-limited kinetics is essential to the proper dosing of phenytoin, the avoidance of side effects with chronic therapy, and the management of overdoses. At higher levels in the therapeutic range, any increase in the daily dose may result in a disproportionate increase in the plasma level. Thus, incremental doses should be limited to 30 mg at a time, and levels should be carefully monitored when it is necessary to raise phenytoin doses above 300 mg (about 5 mg/kg) per day.

Because the half-life of phenytoin is 24 h or less, once-a-day regimens may result in erratic levels and become problematic for patients requiring tight seizure control. Only one phenytoin preparation (Phenytoin Kapseals) is approved by the Food and Drug Administration for once-a-day use. Concomitant use of drugs that inhibit or enhance hepatic microsomal activity may result in an increase or decrease of phenytoin level, respectively. Phenytoin also affects the metabolism of various other agents (Table 178-1).

EFFECTS OF PROPYLENE GLYCOL AND ETHANOL DILUENTS

The acute cardiovascular toxicity seen with intravenous phenytoin infusion has frequently been ascribed to its diluent. The vehicle for the older parenteral formulation of phenytoin (Dilantin) is 40 percent propylene glycol and 10 percent ethanol, adjusted to a pH of 12 with sodium hydroxide. The glycol component has been shown to cause coma, seizures, circulatory collapse, ventricular dysrhythmias, atrioventricular node depression, and hypotension in human and animals.[6] Propylene glycol is a strong myocardial depressant and vasodilator and increases vagal tone. Other toxic effects of propylene glycol include hyperosmolality, hemolysis, and lactate-associated metabolic acidosis. Louis and Kutt compared the acute toxicities of intravenous phenytoin and propylene glycol alone and in combination in a feline model.[7] Phenytoin alone did cause hypotension but did not cause significant electrocardiographic effects; rather, it partly reversed the toxic effects that occurred when propylene glycol was given.[7] Acute toxic effects of propylene glycol are also strongly related to the rate of infusion. This is further evidence for its role in intravenous phenytoin toxicity, a phenomenon that is almost always related to infusion rate. The ethanol diluent fraction of parenteral phenytoin also may precipitate a reaction in patients taking disulfiram. The glycol preparation is still available in the United States (although the original manufacturer no longer makes it). With intravenous infusion pumps controlling the rate of administration, use of cardiac and blood pressure monitors, and dilution with normal saline, adverse effects are not as common, and phenytoin is less expensive than the alternative (see "Fosphenytoin" below).

The limitations of this parenteral form of phenytoin (incomplete aqueous solubility, irritating nature of the vehicle, and tendency to precipitate in intravenous solutions) have prompted a search for a more suit-

TABLE 178-1 Phenytoin and Drug Interactions

Phenytoin *increases* serum levels of
　Zidovudine
　Oral anticoagulants
　Primidone
Phenytoin *increases* toxicity of
　Acetaminophen
　Acetazolamide
Phenytoin *decreases* serum levels of
　Amiodarone
　Carbamazepine
　Levodopa
　Methadone
　Contraceptives
　Glucocorticoids
　Cyclosporine
　Disopyramide
　Mexiletine
　Doxycycline
　Furosemide
　Quinidine
　Theophylline
　Valproic acid
　Ethanol (chronic)
Phenytoin levels are *increased* by
　Amiodarone
　Oral anticoagulants
　Chloramphenicol
　Isoniazid
　Cimetidine
　Disulfiram
　Trimethoprim
　Fluconazole
　Phenylbutazone*
　Sulfonamides*
　Valproic acid*
　High-dose salicylate*
　Tolbutamide*
Phenytoin levels are *decreased* by
　Antineoplastic drugs
　Diazoxide
　Folic acid
　Rifampin
　Sucralfate
　Theophylline
　Phenobarbital
　Diazepam
　Ethanol
　Calcium

*These drugs displace phenytoin from its protein-binding sites, thus increasing the free phenytoin fraction, although the total phenytoin level may *decrease.*

able preparation. Recently, a prodrug of phenytoin, *fosphenytoin,* has been synthesized that is more soluble and less irritating to the tissues.

FOSPHENYTOIN

Fosphenytoin is the disodium phosphate ester of phenytoin. It is freely soluble in aqueous solutions and is formulated with Tris buffer only at a pH of 8.8. Fosphenytoin is a pro-drug and is converted to phenytoin by phosphatases in the blood and various organs. **For simplicity, the concentration and dose of fosphenytoin are expressed in phenytoin equivalents (150 mg fosphenytoin = 100 mg phenytoin).** The conversion half-life is 10 to 15 min.[8] Fosphenytoin is tolerated IV and IM, and patients can be successfully loaded within 30 min with one or more intramuscular injections without significant side effects.[9]

Given IV, fosphenytoin can cause pruritus and hypotension. Due to the time delay while conversion takes place, it is not clear whether fos-

phenytoin administered IV can result in therapeutic levels more quickly and with fewer side effects than intravenous phenytoin. Blood pressure and cardiac monitoring are recommended when loading with fosphenytoin IV but not IM. The adverse and toxic effects of fosphenytoin are the same as with phenytoin, except that the effects of glycol and ethanol are not present with fosphenytoin. The ability to administer fosphenytoin intramuscularly offers a clear advantage over phenytoin and is especially useful in the prehospital and non-acute care settings and in those patients lacking venous access.

In clinical trials fosphenytoin administered IV has caused hypotension in 8 percent of subjects. Borderline heart block has been observed, and bradycardia, seizures, and asystole have been reported in a patient given 225 mg IV who had undiagnosed mitral valve prolapse.[10,11] Negative inotropic effects have been documented in a guinea pig left atrium model. Phlebitis and pain at the injection site are much less common than with phenytoin. Paresthesias have been reported in 21 percent of epileptic patients treated with fosphenytoin.[12]

SERUM LEVELS AND RANGE OF TOXICITY

Therapeutic phenytoin levels are described as being 10 to 20 μg/mL (40 to 80 mmol), with a free phenytoin level of 1 to 2 μg/mL.[13] Although 50 percent of seizure patients achieve reduction of seizure frequency with amounts below these levels, some patients require levels above 20 μg/mL for adequate seizure control. The therapeutic range for phenytoin is rather narrow. However, some patients have a greater propensity for side effects than others. Individual variation in toxicity is a function of baseline neurologic status, individual response to the drug, and free drug fraction. Patients with underlying brain disease are predisposed to toxicity and may become toxic at low levels. Long-term therapy must be individualized and based on clinical response, drug levels, and signs of toxicity. In general, toxicity correlates fairly well with increasing plasma levels (Table 178-2), but this is not a universal tenet, because some patients tolerate levels above 40 μg/mL quite well. Nystagmus usually appears first at a phenytoin level of 20 μg/mL but may occur at lower or higher levels. Almost all patients with phenytoin-induced seizures will have levels well above 30 μg/mL. Signs of toxicity occur at free phenytoin levels of 2.0 μg/mL and are consistently severe above 5.0 μg/mL.

CLINICAL FEATURES

Central Nervous System Toxicity

As toxic phenytoin levels are reached, inhibitory cortical and excitatory cerebellar and vestibular effects begin to occur. The usual initial sign of toxicity is nystagmus, which is seen first on forced lateral gaze and then becomes spontaneous. Vertical, bidirectional, or alternating nystagmus may occur with severe intoxication. A decreased level of consciousness is common with initial sedation, lethargy, ataxic gait,

TABLE 178-2 Correlation of Plasma Phenytoin Level and Side Effects

Plasma Level (μg/mL)	Side Effects
<10	Usually none
10–20	Occasional mild nystagmus
20–30	Nystagmus
30–40	Ataxia, slurred speech, nausea and vomiting
40–50	Lethargy, confusion
>50	Coma, seizures

and dysarthria progressing to confusion, coma, and even apnea in a large overdose. Chronically impaired cognitive function or acute encephalopathy may occur. Nystagmus may disappear at levels sufficient to cause coma, and complete ophthalmoplegia and loss of corneal reflexes may occur. Therefore, absence of nystagmus does not exclude severe phenytoin toxicity. Nystagmus then returns as serum drug levels decrease and coma lightens.

Phenytoin-induced seizures are usually brief and usually generalized. They are quite rare and almost always are preceded by other signs of toxicity, especially in acute overdose.[14] Cerebellar stimulation and alterations in dopaminergic and serotonergic activities may be responsible for acute dystonias and movement disorders, such as opisthotonos and choreoathetosis. Depressed or hyperactive deep tendon reflexes, clonus, and extensor toe responses also may be elicited. Some signs of neurologic toxicity may outlast the presence of drug by months, especially mild peripheral neuropathy or acute reversible cerebellar degeneration with ataxia.

Cardiovascular Toxicity

Cardiac toxicity after oral phenytoin overdose in an otherwise healthy patient has not been reported and, if observed, requires assessment for other causes (e.g., hypoxia and other drugs). Cardiovascular complications have been almost entirely limited to cases of intravenous administration. Complications include hypotension with decreased peripheral vascular resistance, bradycardia, conduction delays progressing to complete atrioventricular nodal block, ventricular tachycardia, primary ventricular fibrillation, and asystole. Electrocardiographic changes include increased PR interval, widened QRS interval, and altered ST segments and T waves. Bradycardia, hypotension, and syncope in healthy volunteers have been reported even after small undiluted intravenous doses. Some of these complications can be attributed to rapid intravenous administration of the preparation containing propylene glycol and are avoidable with cautious administration (Table 178-3). Even slowly administered intravenous phenytoin ($\leq$25 mg/min) has been reported to cause cardiac arrest in critically ill patients receiving dopamine infusions to support blood pressure.

Fosphenytoin lacks propylene glycol but nevertheless has been associated with cardiovascular toxicity. Thus, we have come full circle in our understanding of phenytoin toxicity. Having first attributed all the toxic cardiovascular effects to phenytoin and then to the vehicle, we now realize that phenytoin, fosphenytoin, and propylene glycol can cause significant cardiovascular toxicity.

Vascular and Soft Tissue Toxicity

Intramuscular injection of phenytoin results in localized crystallization of the drug and hematoma, sterile abscess, and myonecrosis at the injection site. Complications after intravenous infusion have included skin and soft tissue necrosis requiring skin grafting, compartment syndrome, gangrene, amputation, and death. Delayed bluish discoloration of the affected extremity (the "purple glove syndrome") followed by erythema, edema, vesicles, bullae, and local tissue ischemia also have been described.[15] The propylene glycol diluent, strong alkalinity of the intravenous solution, administration of the preparation undiluted, and crystallization of the drug contribute to tissue toxicity. Fosphenytoin, in contrast, is better tolerated when given IV or IM.

Hypersensitivity Reactions

Hypersensitivity reactions usually occur within 1 to 6 weeks of beginning phenytoin therapy and can include fever, systemic lupus erythematosus, erythema multiforme, toxic epidermal neurolysis, Stevens-Johnson syndrome, hepatitis, rhabdomyolysis, acute interstitial pneumonitis, lymphadenopathy, leukopenia, disseminated intravascular coagulation, and renal failure. One should always ask about a history of previous hypersensitivity reactions before deciding to restart phenytoin in the ED setting.

Miscellaneous Effects

Other side effects from phenytoin include gingival hyperplasia, hirsutism, hypocalcemia, megaloblastic anemia responsive to folate administration, pseudolymphoma, and hemorrhagic disease of the newborn responsive to vitamin K (Table 178-4). Gingival hyperplasia is so common, its absence should suggest poor compliance. Another clinically significant effect in some patients is hyperglycemia, felt to be secondary to inhibition of insulin release, which can lead to diabetic

---

TABLE 178-3   Guidelines for Safe Phenytoin or Fosphenytoin Loading

Intravenous
   Loading dose is 18 mg/kg phenytoin or fosphenytoin in PE*
   Mix total dose of phenytoin in 150–200 mL of NS (keep concentration $\leq$6.7 mg/mL); mix fosphenytoin in NS (keep concentration 1.5–25 mg PE/mL)
   Administer phenytoin through Millipore filter by using an infusion pump
   Rate of administration should not exceed 25 mg/min of phenytoin or 150 mg/min PE fosphenytoin (less in patients with cardiovascular disease)
   Monitor the blood pressure and cardiac rhythm continually during the infusion
   In the event of complications, immediately stop the infusion and administer isotonic crystalloid and other treatment as indicated
Intramuscular
   Administer 15 mg/kg fosphenytoin PE preparation in one or multiple intramuscular sites
Oral†
   Loading dose is 20 mg/kg
   Phenytoin tablets or suspension may be used
   Patient must be conscious with an intact gag reflex and not actively seizing or vomiting
   Administer the total amount in one dose

*PE = phenytoin equivalents (150 mg fosphenytoin = 100 mg phenytoin)
†Unlike intravenous loading, not all patients orally loaded will reach a therapeutic level.

TABLE 178-4   Toxicity of Phenytoin

Central nervous system
   Dizziness, tremor (intention), visual disturbance, horizontal and vertical nystagmus, diplopia, miosis or mydriasis, ophthalmoplegia, abnormal gait (bradykinesia, truncal ataxia), choreoathetoid movements, vomiting, dysphagia, respiratory distress, irritability, agitation, confusion, hallucinations, fatigue coma, death (rare), encephalopathy, pseudodegenerative disease, dysarthria, meningeal irritation with pleocytosis, seizures (rare)
Peripheral nervous system
   Peripheral neuropathy, urinary incontinence
Hypersensitivity reactions
   Eosinophilia, rash, pseudolymphoma (diffuse lymphadenopathy), systemic lupus erythematosus, pancytopenia, hepatitis, pneumonitis
Gastrointestinal
   Nausea and vomiting, hepatotoxicity
Skin
   Hirsutism, acne, rashes (including Stevens-Johnson syndrome)
Other
   Fetal hydantoin syndrome, gingival hyperplasia, coarsening of facial features, hemorrhagic disease of the newborn, hyperglycemia, hypocalcemia
Parenteral preparations
   May cause hypotension, bradycardia, conduction disturbances, myocardial depression, ventricular fibrillation, asystole, and sloughing of tissues

ketoacidosis or nonketotic hyperosmolar coma in diabetics. The teratogenic fetal hydantoin syndrome is well described, so oral phenytoin therapy in a pregnant patient should never be initiated or continued by an emergency physician without consultation and close follow-up from an attending neurologist and obstetrician.

DIFFERENTIAL DIAGNOSIS

Intoxication with almost any CNS active or sedative hypnotic drug, especially ethanol, carbamazepine, benzodiazepines, barbiturates, and lithium, may mimic early phenytoin intoxication. Disease states resembling phenytoin toxicity include hypoglycemia, Wernicke's encephalopathy, and posterior fossa hemorrhage or tumor. Although seizures may be caused by phenytoin at toxic levels, other epileptogenic drug overdoses and seizures due to trauma, drug and alcohol withdrawal, and infection should be considered first.

TREATMENT

Initial general treatment of severe oral phenytoin overdose, including intravenous access and airway management, is similar to that for other ingested drugs. Acidosis (respiratory or metabolic) should be corrected to decrease the active free phenytoin fraction. Multiple doses of oral activated charcoal (1 g/kg) within the first 24 h may be of benefit, given the known poor solubility and resultant extended absorptive phase of oral phenytoin in overdose.[16] Hemodialysis and hemoperfusion are of no clinical benefit in phenytoin poisoning. Seizures may be treated with intravenous benzodiazepines or phenobarbital, with the caution that seizures are not common in phenytoin overdose and other causes must be ruled out. Cardiovascular toxicity is extremely rare in oral overdose and should suggest other etiologies.

Cardiac monitoring after oral ingestion is unnecessary. Atropine and temporary cardiac pacing may be used for symptomatic bradydysrhythmia associated with intravenous phenytoin. Hypotension that occurs during intravenous administration of phenytoin or fosphenytoin usually responds to discontinuation of the infusion and the administration of isotonic crystalloid. Hospital admission and appropriate orthopedic or plastic surgery consultation should be obtained for patients with any significant extravasation of intravenous phenytoin or other signs of local vascular or tissue toxicity after infusion. To minimize complications due to infusion, intravenous phenytoin and fosphenytoin should be administered under close observation, with constant cardiac and blood pressure monitoring. The infused solution should be given slowly ($\leq$25 mg phenytoin, or $\leq$150 mg fosphenytoin phenytoin equivalents/min) through a large, well-positioned catheter. Phenytoin should never be administered intravenously without first diluting it in normal saline.

ADMISSION CONSIDERATIONS

Patients with serious complications after an oral ingestion (seizures, coma, altered mental status, ataxia, etc.) should be admitted for further evaluation and treatment. Others with only mild symptoms may be treated with activated charcoal in the ED and discharged after their levels have returned to normal, provided they are not actively suicidal. Prolonged observation and frequent assessment of levels are not practical in many EDs. Thus, patients with continuing symptoms may need to be admitted or their case followed in an observation unit. Given the long and erratic absorption phase of phenytoin after oral overdose, the decision to discharge or medically clear a patient for psychiatric evaluation cannot be based on one serum level. Patients with symptomatic chronic intoxication should be admitted for observation unless signs are minimal, adequate care can be obtained at home, and patients are 8 to 12 h from their last therapeutic dose. Phenytoin therapy should be stopped in all cases, and, if toxicity continues to resolve, a serum level may be reassessed in 2 to 3 days to guide resumption of therapy.

Patients with significant or persistent complications after the intravenous administration of phenytoin or fosphenytoin should be admitted. Those with transient effects need not be.

REFERENCES

1. Working Group on Status Epilepticus: Treatment of convulsive status. *JAMA* 270:854, 1993.
2. Litovitz TL, Klein-Schwarz W, Rodgers GC, et al: 2001 Annual report of the American Association of Poison Control Centers Toxic Exposure Surveillance System. *Am J Emerg Med* 20:391, 2001.
3. Earnest MP, Mark JA, Drury LR: Complications of intravenous phenytoin for acute treatment of seizures. *JAMA* 249:762, 1983.
4. Wyte CD, Berk WA: Severe oral phenytoin overdose does not cause cardiovascular morbidity. *Ann Emerg Med* 20:508, 1991.
5. Mellick LB, Morgan JA, Mellick GA: Presentations of acute phenytoin overdose. *Am J Emerg Med* 7:61, 1989.
6. Gross DR, Kitzman JV, Adams HR: Cardiovascular effects of intravenous administration of propylene glycol in calves. *Am J Vet Res* 40:783, 1979.
7. Louis S, Kutt H: The cardiocirculatory changes caused by intravenous Dilantin and its solvent. *Am Heart J* 74:523, 1967.
8. Eldon MA, Loewen GR, Voigtman RE: Pharmacokinetics and tolerance of fosphenytoin and phenytoin administered intravenously to healthy subjects. *Can J Neurol Sci* 20(suppl):180, 1993.
9. Dean JC, Smith KR: Safety, tolerance, and pharmacokinetics of intramuscular fosphenytoin in neurosurgery patients. *Epilepsia* 34(suppl 6):111, 1993.
10. Gerber N, Mays DC, Donn KH, et al: Safety, tolerance, and pharmacokinetics of IV doses of the phosphate ester of hydroxymethyl diphenylhydantoin, a new prodrug of phenytoin. *J Clin Pharmacol* 28:1023, 1988.
11. Leppik IE, Boucher R, Wilder BJ, et al: Phenytoin prodrug, pre-clinical and clinical studies. *Epilepsia* 30(suppl 2):S22, 1989.
12. Leppik IE, Boucher BA, Wilder BJ, et al: Pharmacokinetics and safety of a phenytoin prodrug given IV or IM in patients. *Neurology* 40:456, 1990.
13. McNamara JO: Drugs effective in the therapy of epilepsies, in Hardman JG, Limbird LE (eds): *Goodman and Gilman's the Pharmacological Basis of Therapeutics,* 10th ed. New York, McGraw-Hill, 2001, p. 521.
14. Osorio I, Burnstein TH, Pemler B: Phenytoin induced seizures: A paradoxical effect at toxic concentrations in epileptic patients. *Epilepsia* 30:230, 1989.
15. Hanna DR: Purple glove syndrome: A complication of intravenous phenytoin. *J Neurosci Nurs* 24:340, 1992.
16. Howard CE, Roberts S, Ely DS: Use of multiple-dose activated charcoal in phenytoin toxicity. *Ann Pharmacother* 28:201, 1994.

IRON
Joseph G. Rella
Lewis S. Nelson

INTRODUCTION

There were approximately 30,000 calls related to iron supplement ingestion made to U.S. poison control centers in 2000.[1] Iron is widely available, particularly in homes with small children, and for this reason many of the exposures involve children younger than age 6 years. Fortunately, most children remain asymptomatic or develop only minimal toxicity. Alternatively, children with large overdoses, or adults with intentional overdose, risk dying without aggressive supportive and antidotal therapy. Recent changes in the available iron formulations, as well as in current supplemental iron dispensing practices, may reduce the incidence and consequences of iron poisoning.

PHYSIOLOGY

A 70-kg (154-lb) male has a total body iron store of about 4 g, two-thirds of which is incorporated into hemoglobin. The remainder is found in other iron-containing molecules such as myoglobin, cytochromes, and other enzymes and cofactors, or stored as ferritin. Because excess iron is toxic, the body uses several mechanisms to maintain appropriate iron availability while preventing toxicity. These mechanisms include serum protein binding, intracellular storage, and, most importantly, regulation of gastrointestinal (GI) absorption.

The oral bioavailability of inorganic iron is less than 10 percent and ferrous iron (Fe^{2+}) is better absorbed than ferric (Fe^{3+}). Most dietary iron is in the ferric form, and this is reduced to ferrous by a brush border ferrireductase. Chelated iron, most readily found in heme, is best absorbed, suggesting one beneficial effect of eating meat. Fe^{2+} is transported into enterocytes by a membrane proton-coupled metal transporter called DMT1. Once absorbed, iron is bound by poorly understood chaperone molecules that sequester the iron in ferritin. In times of iron need, the body produces transferrin, which moves iron from the enterocytes into the body. Alternatively, the stored iron in the intestinal cell is eventually eliminated when the mucosal cell is sloughed. This is the principal mechanism for limiting absorption, and failure of this mechanism occurs in iron overdose.

Transferrin, the carrier protein that binds Fe^{3+}, is the major mechanism for safe iron transport through the body. The total iron-binding capacity (TIBC) primarily measures the amount of serum transferrin. The TIBC is generally two to three times the normal serum iron concentration. Ferritin is a large intracellular storage protein that can reversibly bind as many as 4500 molecules of iron. When an iron deficit exists, iron is transported from ferritin and the GI tract to the liver, spleen, and bone marrow, where it is incorporated into appropriate molecules.[2,3] It is noteworthy that, under normal conditions, unbound iron, or free iron, does not exist within the body.

PATHOPHYSIOLOGY

Iron is a potent catalyst for the production of oxidants such as free radicals. Through this mechanism, iron is a direct GI irritant and causes vomiting, diarrhea, abdominal pain, mucosal ulceration, and bleeding soon after a significant ingestion. As the mucosal surface is injured, iron passes unimpeded into the blood. When the ability of transferrin to combine with iron is exhausted, free iron becomes available. Free iron enters the mitochondria where it inhibits oxidative phosphorylation resulting in metabolic (lactic) acidosis. Iron also participates in the production of toxic hydroxyl free radicals and subsequent membrane lipid peroxidation of various organ systems. Clinical effects of free iron include coagulopathy through inhibition of serum proteases,[4] hepatotoxicity, myocardial and vascular dysfunction,[5] and encephalopathy.

Chelated sources of supplemental iron, such as Ferrochel, are less toxic in overdose because the ligand sterically limits the iron from participating in redox reactions.[6] Similarly, carbonyl iron is a nonionic iron molecule that does not participate in redox reactions.

TOXIC DOSE

It is the amount of ingested elemental iron that determines a patient's potential for experiencing toxicity. The fraction of elemental iron in various preparations ranges from 12 to 33 percent. Ferrous sulfate, the most commonly available form, contains 20 percent elemental iron (e.g., a 325-mg tablet of ferrous sulfate contains 65 mg of elemental iron). Pediatric multivitamins typically contain 10 to 18 mg of elemental iron per tablet. Toxic effects are reported following oral doses as low as 10 and 20 mg/kg elemental iron.

In general, moderate toxicity occurs at doses of 20 to 60 mg/kg of elemental iron, and severe toxicity can be expected following ingestion of greater than 60 mg/kg elemental iron.[7]

LABORATORY ASSESSMENT

Serum iron levels used to determine toxicity and to direct management must be used with caution. In general, serum iron levels between 300

and 500 µg/dL correlate with significant GI toxicity and mild systemic toxicity, and serum iron levels between 500 and 1000 µg/dL correlate with moderate systemic toxicity. Levels greater than 1000 µg/dL are associated with significant morbidity. However, **low levels do not necessarily mean absence of toxicity.** Serum levels may be low because of variable times to peak level following ingestions of different iron preparations,[8,9] and deferoxamine can artificially lower serum iron levels.

Leukocytosis and hyperglycemia have also been examined for their ability to predict iron toxicity. One early study found that a white blood cell (WBC) count of greater than 15,000/µL with glucose level of greater than 150 mg/dL correlated with an iron level of more than 300 µg/dL.[10] This study, however, assumed that a serum iron level of greater than 300 µg/dL denoted toxicity, which is not always true. Subsequent studies were unable to validate the association between these laboratory values and also did not correlate these laboratory values with clinical illness.[11,12]

TIBC has little value in the assessment of iron-poisoned patients. It becomes falsely elevated in the presence of elevated serum iron levels or deferoxamine.[13] Additionally, the relationship of the TIBC to the serum iron level is not useful, because in conditions of chronic iron overload (e.g., thalassemia and hemochromatosis), significant organ pathology occurs despite a TIBC that exceeds the serum iron level.

Radiopaque iron tablets are visible on x-ray and can guide GI decontamination when visualized. However, many iron preparations are not routinely detected, including pediatric chewable and liquid preparations, and negative radiographs do not exclude iron ingestion.[12]

CLINICAL FEATURES

Although five stages of toxicity are traditionally described, more practically, acute iron toxicity manifests in two clinical stages: local GI toxicity and systemic toxicity.

Abdominal pain, vomiting, and diarrhea characterize *stage 1* of iron poisoning. Iron is directly irritating and corrosive to the GI tract and typically induces vomiting within the first few hours following ingestion. The absence of GI symptoms within 6 h of ingestion essentially excludes a diagnosis of significant iron ingestion. Vomiting is the clinical sign most consistently associated with acute iron toxicity.[10–12] Patients with symptoms of gastric irritation may either recover over several hours or progress to the development of systemic toxicity.

Stage 2, or the "latent" stage, of iron poisoning does not always occur. Manifesting within the 6- to 24-h period following ingestion, GI symptoms may resolve, so a patient may have few, if any, symptoms, which may falsely reassure a physician. However, this is not a truly quiescent phase. Patients who have significant toxicity will have ongoing clinical illness and progressive systemic deterioration because of volume loss and worsening metabolic acidosis, despite the absence of GI symptoms. Alternatively, the resolution of GI findings may signal the end of mild poisoning, and in such a scenario, patients should have normal vital signs, a normal physical examination, and normal laboratory studies.

Systemic toxicity characterizes *stage 3* of iron toxicity. During this stage, intracellular iron disrupts cellular metabolism with resultant shock and lactic acidosis. Iron-induced coagulopathy may worsen bleeding and hypovolemia. The coagulopathy may be biphasic, with prolonged prothrombin time and partial thromboplastin time within the first 24 h that appear reversible with chelation therapy as free iron initially interferes with the activity of factors in the coagulation cascade.[4] Later, as iron poisoning causes hepatic injury, factor production decreases, potentially worsening the coagulopathy. During this stage renal failure, cardiomyopathy, and failure of other critical organ systems may also occur.

Stage 4, the hepatic stage of iron poisoning, develops 2 to 5 days following ingestion. It results from iron uptake by the reticuloendothelial system with local lipid peroxidation and manifests as elevation of aminotransferases and may progress to hepatic failure.

Stage 5 of iron poisoning refers to delayed sequelae, including gastric outlet obstruction secondary to the corrosive effects of iron on the pyloric mucosa. These changes are rare and occur 4 to 6 weeks after ingestion.

TREATMENT

Evaluation and Supportive Care

Iron poisoning is a clinical diagnosis. Patients who arrive at an ED asymptomatic, who have not ingested a toxic amount, with normal findings on physical examination, and who remain so for 6 h following ingestion, do not require specific medical treatment for iron poisoning. Patients who vomit once or twice from the gastric irritant effects of iron, but who are otherwise asymptomatic, can also be observed and may require no specific treatment. Patients who are symptomatic should first be stabilized with attention to airway, breathing, and circulation, after which GI decontamination and chelation therapy with deferoxamine may proceed (Table 179-1). Dialysis is not effective in clearing iron. Antiemetics such as metoclopramide (10 mg IV in adults; 0.1 mg/kg in pediatric patients) or ondansetron (4 mg IV over 2 to 5 min, or IM in adults; 0.1 mg/kg to a maximum of 4 mg in pediatric patients ages 2 to 12 years) should be used for repetitive vomiting.

Patients with persistent vomiting and abnormal vital signs or other signs of poor perfusion or shock should be aggressively fluid resuscitated and treated with deferoxamine. Coagulopathy should be treated with parenteral vitamin K_1 (5 to 25 mg SC) and fresh-frozen plasma (10 to 25 mL/kg in adults; 10 mL/kg in pediatric patients). Significant blood loss may require transfusion.

Laboratory tests should include complete blood cell count and determination of serum electrolyte levels, renal and liver function studies, coagulation parameters, and serum glucose and serum iron levels, with the understanding that the importance of these values may be limited.

Arterial blood gas (ABG) and serum lactate determination is usually unnecessary in mild cases because determination of serum electrolytes (anion gap evaluation) will yield all the important information. However, in the moderately to severely toxic patient, or in those with respiratory compromise, ABG determination, often more rapidly available, will yield vital information regarding the patient's acid–base status. Blood typing, screening, and cross-matching should be requested from the blood bank in anticipation of potential need.

Gastrointestinal Decontamination

In general, syrup of ipecac is not used, because it may obscure the initial signs of clinical toxicity and it is not thought to be more effective at gastric emptying than is iron-induced vomiting. **Activated charcoal does not adsorb significant amounts of iron, and its use is not recommended.** Furthermore, it may complicate endoscopy, should that be necessary. Cathartics should not be used. Orogastric lavage may not be effective if the ingested tablets are large or if several hours have elapsed since ingestion, but it may be useful within 60 min after ingestion. There are no data to support the efficacy of sodium bicarbonate or phosphosoda to form insoluble iron salts. Pills located on radiograph may indicate a potential for progressive toxicity and may guide decontamination.

Whole-bowel irrigation with a polyethylene glycol solution has demonstrated efficacy in children with large iron ingestions. Administration of 250 to 500 mL/h in children, and 2 L/h in adults, by nasogastric tube may clear the GI tract of iron pills before absorption can occur. Endoscopy has been used to remove large iron loads but may not be practical where there are large numbers of pills requiring multiple endoscope insertions. Gastrotomy may rarely be an option in profoundly ill patients where other measures are unsuccessful or impractical.[14]

Deferoxamine

Deferoxamine is a specific chelating agent derived from *Streptomyces pilosus;* it has been used to treat iron toxicity since the 1960s. Deferoxamine binds primarily to free iron and secondarily to iron from ferritin, hemosiderin, and non–protein-bound ferric salts, as well as to intracytoplasmic and mitochondrial free iron, to form the complex ferrioxamine, which is renally excreted. It is safely administered to children and pregnant women. Complete complexation of ingested iron is not the goal of therapy. Indeed, only a small fraction of the total amount of ingested iron is found in the urine following chelation. Deferoxamine administration may prove clinically effective by removing a critical amount of intracellular iron from its target, thus restoring cellular function.

Patients without hypotension or dehydration are treated with intramuscular administration of deferoxamine 90 mg/kg up to 1 g in children and 2 g in adults. The dose may be repeated every 4 to 6 h as clinically indicated (see below). This route of administration, however, can become difficult because of the volume of injected material required when used in children.

In patients with severe iron poisoning in whom fluid loss and hypovolemia are significant, and who require aggressive fluid resuscitation, deferoxamine should be administered intravenously. Intramuscular deferoxamine is not reliably absorbed in hypotensive patients. Rate-related hypotension is the limiting factor in intravenous administration, and it is recommended to begin the infusion slowly (5 mg/kg per h). A second intravenous access may be required so as not to impede volume resuscitation.

Deferoxamine can be increased to 15 mg/kg per h within the first hour of treatment, as tolerated. In fact, much higher doses have been used safely. However, it is generally not recommended to exceed a total daily dose of 6 to 8 g, although there are no specific data supporting this limit in acutely iron-poisoned patients. Administering deferoxamine at this rate will achieve a total of 6 g in about 6 h in an average-sized adult. Once this amount is reached, it is prudent to decrease the rate of deferoxamine administration, because of several associated risks. Adverse effects may include mucormycosis infection,[15] renal insufficiency,[16] pulmonary toxicity,[17] and sepsis from *Yersinia enterocolitica,* which may be related to duration of therapy.

The determination of the efficacy and duration of deferoxamine therapy involves acquisition of serial urine samples. As ferrioxamine is excreted, the urine color changes to what is classically called vin rose, but may actually appear brown or rusty. Theoretically, the disappearance of the vin rose means that a patient no longer has significant toxicity. It is important to obtain a urine sample prior to initiating treatment because patients who are hypovolemic will likely produce concentrated urine, which may also be somewhat dark and may be confused with the vin rose appearance. False-negatives, color-change latency, and difficulty visualizing a color change can limit the utility of this test.

There is some controversy surrounding the duration of deferoxamine therapy. Recommended end points range from clinical recovery and normal iron levels, to measurement of iron-to-creatinine ratios,[18] to clinical recovery with normal iron level in conjunction with normal urine color.[7] Because measured iron levels are artificially depressed by the presence of deferoxamine and urine color change can be unreliable, and because iron toxicity is a clinical diagnosis, clinical recovery of the patient is probably the most important factor in terminating therapy. For patients who continue to exhibit severe iron toxicity after 24 h of deferoxamine therapy, the therapy should continue carefully at a decreased dose, for reasons mentioned earlier.

Previously advocated was the *deferoxamine challenge test,* a *half-dose* of 50 mg/kg intramuscular injection of deferoxamine followed by examination of urine samples for change in color that would indicate the presence of chelated free iron and therefore confirm iron toxicity. More recently, a *first dose* of 90 mg/kg IM has been used, also using

TABLE 179-1 Treatment of Iron Ingestion

Gastrointestinal decontamination
  No ipecac, no activated charcoal
  Consider gastric lavage in first hour
  Consider whole-bowel irrigation
  Consider endoscopy to remove pills
Local gastric irritation only
  Fluid resuscitation
  Antiemetics
    Metoclopramide 0.1 mg/kg IV in children, 10 mg IV in adults
      or
    Ondansetron 0.1 mg/kg IV to a maximum of 4 mg in children, 4 mg IV
      over 2–5 min in adults
Mild systemic toxicity
  Fluid and metabolic resuscitation
  Deferoxamine 90 mg/kg IM or IV (up to 1 g in children) q4–6 h as
    clinically indicated, not to exceed total daily dose of 6 g
Moderate or severe systemic toxicity
  Fluid and metabolic resuscitation
  Deferoxamine 90 mg/kg IV at a rate of 5 mg/kg per h, can increase to rate
    of 15 mg/kg per h if there is no rate-related hypotension; not to exceed
    total daily dose of 6 g

change in urine color to verify toxicity. There may be several problems with this management strategy. Single-dose deferoxamine can be unreliable in eliciting a visible color change in urine, especially if a pre-deferoxamine urine sample was not obtained, and should not be the sole factor in deciding toxicity.[7]

REFERENCES

1. Litovitz T, Klein-Schwartz W, White S, et al: 2000 Annual report of the American Association of Poison Control Centers Toxic Exposure Surveillance System. *Am J Emerg Med* 19:337, 2001.
2. Schneider BD, Leibold EA: Regulation of mammalian iron hemostasis. *Curr Opin Clin Nutr Metab Care* 3:267, 2000.
3. Andrews NC: Iron metabolism: Iron deficiency and iron overload. *Annu Rev Genomics Hum Genet* 1:75, 2000.
4. Tenenbein M, Israels SJ: Early coagulopathy in severe iron poisoning. *J Pediatr* 113:695, 1988.
5. Tenenbein M, Kopelow ML, deSa DJ: Myocardial failure and shock in iron poisoning. *Hum Toxicol* 7:281, 1988.
6. Jeppsen RB: Toxicology and safety of Ferrochel and other iron amino acid chelates. *Arch Latinoam Nutr* 51 (Suppl):26, 2001.
7. Schauben JL, Augenstein WL, Cox J, Sato R: Iron poisoning: Report of three cases and a review of therapeutic intervention. *J Emerg Med* 8:309, 1990.
8. Burkhart KK, Kulig KW, Hammond KB, et al: The rise in the total iron-binding capacity after iron overdose. *Ann Emerg Med* 20:532, 1991.
9. Ling LJ, Hornfeldt CS, Winter JP: Absorption of iron after experimental overdose of chewable vitamins. *Am J Emerg Med* 9:24, 1991.
10. Lacouture PG, Wason S, Temple AR, et al: Emergency assessment of severity in iron overdose by clinical and laboratory methods. *J Pediatr* 99:89, 1981.
11. Chyka PA, Butler AY: Assessment of acute iron poisoning by laboratory and clinical observations. *Am J Emerg Med* 11:99, 1993.
12. Palatnick W, Tenenbein M: Leukocytosis, hyperglycemia, vomiting, and positive x-rays are not indicators of severity of iron poisoning. *Am J Emerg Med* 14:454, 1996.
13. Bentur Y, St Louis P, Klein J, Koren G: Misinterpretation of iron-binding capacity in the presence of deferoxamine. *J Pediatr* 118:139, 1991.
14. Foxford R, Goldfrank LR: Gastrotomy: A surgical approach to iron overdose. *Ann Emerg Med* 14:1223, 1985.
15. Daly AL, Velazquez LA, Bradley SF, Kauffman CA: Mucormycosis: Association with deferoxamine therapy. *Am J Med* 87:468, 1989.
16. Koren G, Bentur Y, Strong D, et al: Acute changes in renal function associated with deferoxamine therapy. *Am J Dis Child* 143:1077, 1989.
17. Tenenbein M, Kowalski S, Sienko A, et al: Pulmonary toxic effects of continuous desferrioxamine administration in acute iron poisoning. *Lancet* 339:699, 1992.
18. Yatscoff RW, Wayne EA, Tenenbein M: An objective criterion for the cessation of deferoxamine therapy in the acutely iron poisoned patient. *Clin Toxicol* 29:1, 1991.

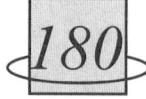

180 HYDROCARBONS AND VOLATILE SUBSTANCES
Paul M. Wax
Michael B. Beuhler

INTRODUCTION

Hydrocarbons are a diverse group of organic compounds consisting primarily of carbon and hydrogen atoms arranged in various aliphatic and aromatic configurations. Products containing hydrocarbons are found in many household and occupational settings. Examples include fuels, lighter fluids, lamp oil, paints, paint removers, pesticides, medications, cleaning and polishing agents, spot removers, degreasers, lubricants, and solvents. Volatile liquid chemicals or gases are substances sometimes abused for their euphoric effects. Examples of commonly abused volatiles include many hydrocarbon-containing substances such as glue (which contains toluene), propellants (e.g., butane, trichloroethylene, Freon), and gasoline. Other volatile chemicals not generally classified as hydrocarbons, such as nitrites (e.g., isobutyl nitrite) and nitrous oxide, are also subject to abuse. Hydrocarbon and volatile substance exposure may cause life-threatening toxicity and, in some cases, sudden death.

Classification

Most hydrocarbons are produced from petroleum distillation, which results in predominantly aliphatic (open-chain) mixtures of hydrocarbons of different chain lengths. Gasoline, for instance, consists of approximately 80 percent saturated and unsaturated aliphatic hydrocarbons of chain length C_4 to C_{10} and 20 percent aromatic hydrocarbons. Chain length and branching determines the phase of the hydrocarbon at room temperature. Short-chain aliphatic compounds, such as methane, propane, or butane, are gases; long-chain aliphatic compounds, such as waxes, are solids. Intermediate-chain (C_5 to C_{15}) aliphatic compounds are in liquid form and account for most hydrocarbon exposures seen in the ED (Table 180-1). Pulmonary toxicity secondary to aspiration is the most common complication from ingesting liquid aliphatic hydrocarbons.

The wood distillates (e.g., turpentine and pine oil) are derived from pine, consist mainly of cyclic terpene derivatives, and comprise another class of hydrocarbons. Gastrointestinal (GI) absorption of wood distillates tends to be greater than that of aliphatic petroleum distillates, increasing the risk for central nervous system (CNS) depression.

Aromatic hydrocarbons (containing a benzene ring; Table 180-2) and halogenated hydrocarbons (aliphatics with at least one substituted

TABLE 180-1 Substances that Predominantly Contain Aliphatics

Substance	Commercial Use
Gasoline	Motor fuel
Kerosene	Stove and lamp fuel
Mineral seal oil	Furniture polish
Naphtha (petroleum ether)	Lighter fluid
Diesel oil	Lubricant
N-hexane	Plastic cement, rubber cement
Methane, butane, propane	Fuel

TABLE 180-2 Common Aromatic Hydrocarbons

Substance	Commercial Use
Benzene	Chemical intermediate, gasoline (small amount; average 0.8%)
Toluene	Airplane glue, plastic cement, acrylic paint
Xylene	Solvent, cleaning agent, degreaser

halogen group; Table 180-3) are widely used industrial solvents. Freon is the trade name for a group of halogenated hydrocarbons that contain fluoride. Although many of these chlorofluorocarbons (CFCs) are thought to cause atmospheric ozone changes and are being replaced by more environmentally friendly compounds, Freon may still be found as a refrigerant gas and component of fire extinguishing systems. Inhalational exposure is the usual route of toxicity for aromatic and halogenated hydrocarbons, although ingestion of these chemicals may also be problematic. Substance abusers and workers in certain occupational settings are most often affected. Such exposures may result in significant systemic toxicity. Along with their potent CNS effects, specific cardiovascular, hepatic, renal, and hematologic toxicity are attributed to aromatic and halogenated hydrocarbons.

Finally, some compounds have toxicity related to an additive, such as lead in gasoline (greatly decreased in the United States) and pesticides in a hydrocarbon base. With these, **the toxic additive usually dictates the clinical approach.**

Epidemiology

Exposures to hydrocarbons and volatiles most commonly occur in one of two settings: ingestion or inhalation. Hydrocarbon ingestions account for approximately 3 to 10 percent of all unintentional childhood poisonings in the United States. Ingestions of gasoline, kerosene, lighter fluid, mineral seal oil, and turpentine are most frequent. In less-developed countries kerosene ingestion accounts for 33 to 59 percent of unintentional childhood poisonings.[1] It is estimated that 3.5 to 10 percent of young people have experimented with volatile substance inhalation to produce inebriation.

Most hydrocarbon exposures have a benign clinical course. The 2001 American Association of Poison Control Centers Toxic Exposure Surveillance System revealed that 79,608 potential hydrocarbon exposures were reported to poison control centers (3.5 percent of all reported exposures). Of the 3793 (4.8 percent) persons who developed moderate to major toxicity 12 died.[2] An epidemiologic study of volatile substance abuse in the United Kingdom revealed that 605 people younger than age 18 years died from volatile substance abuse during the period 1981 to 1990.[3] The most commonly implicated volatiles were butane (39 percent), aerosols (26 percent), cleaners (16 percent), and glue (10 percent).

TABLE 180-3 Common Halogenated Hydrocarbons

Substance	Commercial Use
Carbon tetrachloride	Solvent, refrigerant, aerosol propellant
Chloroform	Solvent, chemical intermediate
Methylene chloride	Paint stripper, varnish remover, aerosol paint, degreaser
Trichloroethylene (TCE)	Spot remover, degreaser, typewriter correction fluid
Trichloroethane (TCA)	Spot remover, degreaser, typewriter correction fluid
Tetrachloroethylene (perchloroethylene)	Dry cleaning agent, degreaser

PATHOPHYSIOLOGY AND CLINICAL FEATURES

Determinants of Toxicity

The toxic potential of hydrocarbons depends on physical characteristics (volatility, viscosity, and surface tension), chemical characteristics (aliphatic, aromatic, or halogenated), presence of toxic additives (pesticides or heavy metals), route of exposure, concentration, and dose.

Viscosity, defined as the resistance to flow, and surface tension, denoting "creeping" ability, plays a major role in determining the aspiration potential. Viscosity is measured in Saybolt Universal Seconds (SUS). **Patients ingesting substances with viscosities less than 60 SUS (e.g., gasoline, kerosene, mineral seal oil, turpentine, and aromatic and halogenated hydrocarbons) are at greater risk for aspiration than are those ingesting substances with viscosities greater than 100 SUS (e.g., diesel oil, grease, mineral oil, paraffin wax, and petroleum jelly).** Low surface tension also increases the risk of aspiration. Volatility denotes the ability of a substance to vaporize. A compound with high volatility evaporates easily and usually has low viscosity and low surface tension. Inhalation of volatile agents, such as aromatic hydrocarbons, halogenated hydrocarbons, or gasoline, results in systemic absorption and the potential for significant toxicity.

Dermal exposure to hydrocarbons causes local toxicity, and occasionally leads to systemic absorption. Dermal toxicity secondary to intravenous administration of hydrocarbons has also been reported. When used intravenously, hydrocarbons may cause pulmonary toxicity by their first-pass exposure through the lungs (first capillary bed encountered).

Toxicity from hydrocarbon exposure can be divided into different clinical syndromes based on the organ system(s) predominately affected. Characteristic presentations usually affect one or more of the following systems: pulmonary, neurologic (central and/or peripheral), GI, cardiac, hepatic, renal, hematologic, or dermal.

Pulmonary Toxicity

Pulmonary complications, especially aspiration, are the most frequent adverse effects of hydrocarbon exposure. Typically, this involves the unintentional childhood ingestion of small amounts of aliphatic hydrocarbon mixtures commonly stored in the household. Aliphatic hydrocarbons have a limited GI absorption; toxicity usually results from aspiration of the low-viscosity compounds or inhalation (with resulting systemic absorption) of compounds with high volatility. Although ingestion of aromatic or halogenated hydrocarbons may also result in aspiration, GI absorption is greater. Hence, CNS and other systemic toxicity secondary to GI absorption often predominate after aromatic and halogenated hydrocarbon ingestion. High-viscosity compounds such as lubricants, mineral oil, or tar, are not aspirated readily and tend to be less toxic when ingested. Occasionally, however, aspiration occurs that results in the development of lipoid pneumonia. Deaths from hydrocarbon lipoid pneumonia have been reported.

The risk and degree of aspiration is not dependent on volume ingested. Experimentally in rats, as little as 0.2 mL instilled intratracheally has caused pneumonitis. Pulmonary toxicity does not result from GI absorption but occurs from direct aspiration of the hydrocarbon into the pulmonary tree. This occurs at the time of ingestion when the hydrocarbon migrates from the hypopharynx into the airway. There is no evidence that hydrocarbons reflux from the stomach into the airway. Spontaneous vomiting, however, does increase the risk of aspiration.[4] Pulmonary toxicity manifested as acute bilateral pneumonitis has also been reported from the inhalation of an aerosolized aliphatic hydrocarbon such as gasoline or kerosene as well as from pyrrolized fluorinated compounds.[5]

Hydrocarbon aspiration causes chemical pneumonitis by direct toxic injury to the pulmonary parenchyma and altered surfactant function. Destruction of alveolar and capillary membranes results in increased vascular permeability and edema. Early distal airway closure and alveolar collapse produces clinical bronchospasm and ventilation/perfusion mismatch. The CNS manifestations seen after ingestion of a poorly GI-absorbed aliphatic hydrocarbon are thought to be from hypoxia secondary to the hydrocarbon induced pneumonitis and/or direct CNS toxicity following the pulmonary absorption of a volatile hydrocarbon. Pneumatoceles, pneumothoraces, and/or pneumomediastinum are occasionally associated with hydrocarbon aspiration. Other complications include bacterial superinfection, acute respiratory distress syndrome, and death. Long-term pulmonary dysfunction may occur.

In one study of 950 children who ingested products containing hydrocarbons and who were brought to the hospital, 19 percent had clinical or radiographic evidence of pulmonary aspiration.[6] In another study of 184 pediatric hydrocarbon ingestions called to a poison center, 35 percent had initial symptoms, but only 3 percent had progressive pulmonary symptoms.[7]

The clinical manifestations of pulmonary aspiration are usually apparent almost immediately on ingestion. The early effects result from irritation of the oral mucosa and tracheobronchial tree. Symptoms include coughing, choking, gasping, dyspnea, and burning of the mouth. Patients with these symptoms should be assumed to have aspirated until proven otherwise. Physical examination may reveal grunting respirations, retractions, tachypnea, tachycardia, and cyanosis. An odor of the hydrocarbon may be noted on the patient's breath. An elevated temperature of 39°C (102.2°F) or greater is common and may occur upon initial presentation or be delayed for 6 to 8 h. Auscultation may be normal, or reveal wheezing and decreased or absent breath sounds. Arterial blood gas analysis may demonstrate a widened alveolar-arterial oxygen gradient or frank hypoxemia. The development of a necrotizing pneumonitis and hemorrhagic pulmonary edema usually occurs within hours in severe aspiration. Most fatalities from these complications occur within 24 to 48 h. With less-severe damage, symptoms usually subside within 2 to 5 days, except with pneumatoceles and lipoid, pneumonias whose symptoms may persist for weeks to months.

Although most patients with clinically significant aspiration have abnormal chest x-rays, the time course of radiographic changes varies and correlation with physical examination may be poor. Changes may be seen as early as 30 min after aspiration, but **the initial radiograph in the symptomatic patient may be deceptively clear.** Radiographic changes usually appear by 2 to 6 h and are almost always present by 18 to 24 h, if they are to occur. The infiltrates range in appearance from streaking to flocculent to homogeneous, and are usually located in the dependent lobes. Multilobar involvement is more common than single-lobe involvement and right-sided involvement is more common than left-sided involvement. Radiographic changes limited to bilateral perihilar regions with clear lung bases are also common, however mild radiographic changes do not automatically mean the patient will become symptomatic.

Central Nervous System Toxicity

CNS toxicity may result from either a direct toxic response to the systemic absorption of the hydrocarbon, as an indirect result of severe hypoxia secondary to aspiration, or as a result of simple asphyxiation due to either loss of ventilatory drive, or the use of a plastic bag or other device during "bagging." Systemic absorption occurs through GI absorption, the inhalation of highly volatile petroleum distillates, or by direct dermal penetration, usually by prolonged contact with chlorinated hydrocarbons. GI absorption resulting in CNS toxicity is common with ingestion of terpene containing hydrocarbons (Pine-sol), especially in the elderly.[8]

Exposure to volatile hydrocarbons may occur inadvertently or deliberately when associated with solvent abuse. Volatile solvent abuse most often occurs in teenagers and younger adults, especially from lower socioeconomic backgrounds and in particular cultures (e.g., Native Americans). These patients are described as "huffers" or "baggers" depending on whether they inhale through a rag soaked with the hydrocarbon held to the mouth or rebreathe into a plastic bag containing the hydrocarbon. The act of rebreathing to facilitate inhalation may also contribute to toxicity by producing significant hypercarbia and hypoxia. Table 180-4 lists many of the most commonly abused volatiles.

Many of the hydrocarbons that affect the CNS have a natural affinity for the lipid-rich neural tissue. They behave similarly to the inhalational anesthetic agents. Hydrocarbon intoxication may be confused with ethanol inebriation. CNS depression ranges in severity from dizziness, slurred speech, ataxia, and lethargy to obtundation, coma and apnea. These effects are usually dose-dependent. Although hydrocarbons are CNS depressants, they often have an initial excitatory effect manifested as euphoria, exhilaration, and giddiness, effects sought by those who abuse them. More severe excitatory features include tremor, agitation, and convulsions. Perceptual changes, such as confusion, hallucinations, and psychosis, may occur.

Chronic CNS sequelae may result from recurrent inhalational exposure to hydrocarbons in the workplace or with solvent abuse.[9] These sequelae are seen among house painters and solvent abusers exposed to toluene-containing substances. Recurrent headaches, cerebellar ataxia, and a chronic encephalopathy consisting of tremors, emotional lability, mental status changes, cognitive impairment, and psychomotor impairment, characterize the syndrome. These effects may be transitory or permanent. The development of encephalopathy, ataxia, tremor, chorea, and myoclonus also is associated with the habitual sniffing of leaded gasoline. In this case, symptoms are thought to be secondary to the effects of tetraethyl lead and its toxic metabolites.

Peripheral Nervous System Toxicity

Exposure to *n*-hexane, methyl *n*-butyl ketone, and other six-carbon aliphatic hydrocarbons is associated with the development of a characteristic peripheral polyneuropathy caused by demyelinization and retrograde axonal degeneration.[10] Onset of symptoms may be delayed for months to years after initial exposure. Toxicity is attributed to a metabolite, 2,5-hexanedione, produced by the cytochrome P450-mediated biotransformation of the parent compounds. This neurotoxic metabolite is thought to inhibit glutaraldehyde-3-phosphate dehydrogenase, which supplies energy for axonal transport. Long, distal nerves seem to be most vulnerable, characteristically producing foot

TABLE 180-4   Commonly Abused Volatile Substances

Product	Volatile Agent
Acrylic spray paint	Toluene
Adhesives/glue	Toluene, trichloroethylene
Aerosol propellants	Propellants and butane
Cigarette lighter refills	Butane
Degreasing agents	Trichloroethylene
Dry-cleaning agents	Tetrachloroethylene
Fire extinguishers	Bromochlorodifluoromethane
Inhalational anesthetics	Nitrous oxide, halothane
Lighter fluid	Naphtha
Nitrites (poppers)	Isobutyl nitrite, amyl nitrite
Paint stripper	Methylene chloride
Petrol	Gasoline
Plastic modeling cement	Methyl ethyl ketone, toluene
Spot removers	Trichloroethylene, trichloroethane
Typewriter correction fluid	Trichloroethane, trichloroethylene

and wrist drop with numbness and paresthesias. Unleaded gasoline sniffing has produced a similar clinical picture as well.[11]

Gastrointestinal Toxicity

Most hydrocarbons act as intestinal irritants, resulting in burning in the mouth and throat, abdominal pain, belching, nausea, vomiting, and diarrhea. Vomiting, which occurs in approximately one-third of the patients with aliphatic hydrocarbon ingestions, is particularly troublesome because of the increased risk of pulmonary aspiration. Corrosive GI injury, as well as pancreatitis, has been reported with ingestion of some chlorinated hydrocarbons.[12]

Cardiac Toxicity

Life-threatening dysrhythmias, such as ventricular tachycardia and ventricular fibrillation, may occur with systemic absorption (gastrointestinal or inhalational) of a variety of hydrocarbon compounds. Most commonly, dysrhythmias occur after exposure to halogenated hydrocarbons and aromatic hydrocarbons. Exposures to predominantly aliphatic mixtures, such as gasoline or mineral spirits, and exposure to butane have also been reported to cause dysrhythmias and sudden death.[13] The mechanism of toxicity is believed to be secondary to a sensitization of the heart to catecholamines. The term "sudden sniffing death" describes solvent abusers who die suddenly after exertion, panic, or fright. The sudden release of catecholamines in these situations is thought to induce these fatal dysrhythmias.[13] Cardiac dysrhythmias as a consequence of industrial exposure to volatile hydrocarbons have also been described. Other mechanisms for sudden death include asphyxia, respiratory depression, and vagal inhibition. The use of exogenous catecholamines, such as epinephrine, may precipitate sudden dysrhythmias and should be avoided except if required for cardiac resuscitation. Decreases in myocardial contractility and peripheral vascular resistance as well as bradycardia and atrioventricular conduction blocks have also been associated with volatile solvent abuse.

Hepatic Toxicity

Hydrocarbon-induced hepatic damage resulting from halogenated hydrocarbons is well described. Carbon tetrachloride toxicity has been used as a model for toxin-induced hepatic dysfunction. As little as 3 mL of carbon tetrachloride has been associated with the development of fatal liver injury.[14] Other halogenated hydrocarbons, such as chloroform and methylene chloride, are also associated with liver dysfunction.[12] Free-radical metabolites of these agents that cause lipid peroxidation are apparently responsible for hepatocellular destruction.

Pathologic examination reveals acute fatty degeneration of the liver with areas of centrilobular necrosis. The time-course of hepatic dysfunction with acute exposures appears similar to acetaminophen hepatotoxicity. Liver function tests may be elevated within 24 h after ingestion, with the development of liver tenderness and jaundice in 48 to 96 h. Chronic exposure to carbon tetrachloride may be associated with the development of cirrhosis and hepatomas.

Renal and Metabolic Toxicity

Solvent abuse and occupational exposure to hydrocarbons may result in renal dysfunction. Exposure to hepatotoxic halogenated hydrocarbons, such as carbon tetrachloride, trichloroethylene, and chlorinated paraffins, have caused acute renal failure, as well as centrilobular hepatic necrosis.[15] In large ingestions, occasionally unchanged renal excretion of aliphatic hydrocarbons may occur, resulting in visible hydrocarbon droplets in the urine. Hemorrhagic cystitis has also been reported for some hydrocarbon ingestions.

Renal tubular acidosis may occur in patients who abuse toluene-containing substances. Patients present with a non-anion gap metabolic acidosis, hypokalemia, and hypophosphatemia. The serum potassium may be so low (<2 mEq/L) that severe muscle weakness develops, occasionally resulting in quadriparesis. Once treatment begins, the serum potassium may significantly plummet, resulting in severe muscle weakness and occasionally apnea. Significant rhabdomyolysis may also result. Toluene toxicity may also cause a high anion gap metabolic acidosis as a result of the accumulation of hippuric acid and benzoic acid metabolites. Proteinuria and renal insufficiency can occur in patients who abuse toluene.

Hematologic Toxicity

Chronic exposure to benzene, the prototypical aromatic hydrocarbon, is associated with an increased incidence of hematologic disorders including aplastic anemia, acute myelogenous leukemia, and multiple myeloma.[16] This association has received much attention because of the extensive use of benzene in the workplace. The etiology of these blood dyscrasias is probably not benzene itself but rather a toxic metabolite. Although aplastic anemia is associated with glue sniffing, this is most likely a result of the benzene fraction of the glue, and not the toluene. Hydrocarbon-induced hemolysis has occurred following the acute ingestion of gasoline, kerosene, and tetrachloroethylene, and inhalation of mineral spirits. Consumptive coagulopathy has also been reported. Significantly delayed methemoglobinemia has been reported after exposure to hydrocarbons containing amine functional groups such as aniline ($-NH_2$), and hemolytic anemia has been reported from ingestion of naphthalene.

A peculiar complication of methylene chloride exposure is the endogenous production of carbon monoxide.[17] This is unlike ordinary carbon monoxide exposure from exogenous sources where maximum carboxyhemoglobin level occurs at the time of the exposure. **With methylene chloride exposure, carbon monoxide formation may continue after cessation of exposure caused by slow release of methylene chloride from the tissues prior to its metabolism to carbon monoxide.** When patients exposed to methylene chloride present with CNS and cardiac symptoms, impairment caused by significant carbon monoxide production must be considered.

Dermal Toxicity

Dermal exposure to hydrocarbons may also result in toxicity. Cutaneous injury is most often associated with the short-chain aliphatic, aromatic, and halogenated hydrocarbons. These agents act as primary irritants and as sensitizers. Clinically, skin findings can range from local erythema, papules, and vesicles to a generalized scarlatiniform eruption and an exfoliative dermatitis. A "huffer's rash" may be noted over the face of patients who chronically abuse the volatile hydrocarbons. Pruritus may also be present. A defatting dermatitis, similar to a chronic eczematoid dermatitis, may occur. Frostbite of the face may develop during the inhalational abuse of fluorinated agents. Cellulitis and sterile abscesses have been associated with the injection of hydrocarbons, and even a small amount of injected hydrocarbon can cause significant injury.[18] Extensive partial-thickness and full-thickness burns following immersion in hydrocarbons may also occur. Occasionally, highly permeable hydrocarbons can penetrate the skin, resulting in systemic toxicity. Exposure to heated high-viscosity, long-chain aliphatics, such as tar, asphalt, or bitumen, present a particularly challenging problem because of their association with burns and hyperthermia, and difficulty with decontamination.[19]

TREATMENT

Prehospital

Not all patients who have ingested hydrocarbons require emergency department evaluation. In a retrospective study of 211 patients with hydrocarbon ingestions called to a poison center, fewer than 1 percent required physician intervention.[7] This data suggests that patients who are asymptomatic or who quickly become asymptomatic after ingestion can be watched safely at home. This approach of home observation for asymptomatic patients can be supported when the ingestion is accidental, the ingredients are known and do not cause significant systemic toxicity when ingested, and reliable follow-up can be ensured.

All symptomatic patients and intentional exposures should be referred to the hospital for further evaluation. Patients who ingest hydrocarbons that may cause significant systemic toxicity (e.g., aromatic, halogenated hydrocarbons, or toxic additives), whether or not symptomatic, should also be referred to the hospital. Volatile substance abusers and others exposed to volatiles should have immediate cardiac monitoring and advanced life support transport, if available, because of the potential for life-threatening dysrhythmias.

Emergency Department

General principles of poison management apply to the initial approach to patients once they reach the hospital. Establishing the airway and maintaining ventilation is the critical first maneuver in any patient who presents with respiratory depression and/or significant CNS depression. The detection of a sweet odor may be associated with certain halogenated hydrocarbon exposures (especially chloroform or trichloroethylene) while a petrol odor suggests gasoline or some other petroleum derivative. Continuous cardiac monitoring should be initiated, and an electrocardiogram should be obtained. Hydrocarbon-induced dysrhythmias, if present, would generally occur shortly after the exposure, especially with inhalational use. Hypotension should be treated with aggressive fluid resuscitation. **Catecholamines, such as dopamine, norepinephrine, or epinephrine, should be avoided to prevent precipitating dysrhythmias, especially following exposure to halogenated hydrocarbons and aromatic hydrocarbons.** The administration of glucose, thiamine, and naloxone should be considered in cases of altered mental status (see Table 180-5).

The patient needs to be fully undressed to prevent ongoing contamination from hydrocarbon-soaked clothes. Dermal decontamination with soap and water, and eye decontamination with saline irrigation, should be performed. Prehospital decontamination is preferable. It is unlikely that a patient contaminated with a simple hydrocarbon will generate enough vapors to affect the staff, but it is important for staff to wear protective gloves and aprons to prevent possible secondary exposure, especially for organophosphate containing mixtures.

Useful diagnostic tests include the chest x-ray and arterial blood gas to detect pulmonary aspiration and hypoxemia. Abdominal radiographs may show evidence of chlorinated hydrocarbon ingestions, such as carbon tetrachloride, because of the radiopaque nature of these polyhalogenated substances.[18] Tests of liver and renal function should be obtained in all aromatic and halogenated hydrocarbon exposures to check for the development of hepatic and renal injury. A carboxyhemoglobin level is useful to evaluate the extent of endogenous carbon monoxide production following methylene chloride exposure. Pulse oximetry will not differentiate between oxyhemoglobin and carboxyhemoglobin. Routine drug screens are not useful for the detection of hydrocarbons, but as in all intentional ingestions, an acetaminophen level, ethanol level, anion gap, and osmolality may be helpful in assessing for the presence of other coingestants.

Gastrointestinal Decontamination

For most hydrocarbon ingestions, gastrointestinal decontamination would provide little benefit; supportive care and appropriate treatment of coexisting ingestions are all that is required. The necessity for GI decontamination depends on the type of hydrocarbon and route of exposure. The risk of systemic toxicity by intestinal absorption has to be weighed against the risks of aspiration associated with gastric empty-

TABLE 180-5   ED Management of Hydrocarbon Exposures

Find out what type of hydrocarbon and route of exposure
  Utilize MSDS (material safety data sheets) and Regional Poison Control Center as resources
Ingestion: aliphatic mixtures (gasoline, kerosene, lamp oil, etc.; see Table 180-1)
GI decontamination: usually unnecessary.
Skin decontamination: if spilled on clothes or skin, soap and water
Diagnostic: observe for evidence of aspiration and CNS symptoms (CXR, pulse oximetry)
Treatment
    If evidence of aspiration-respiratory support (oxygen, inhaled β-agonists, ventilatory support)
    No need for steroids, no need for antibiotics unless documented infection
    Disposition: admit if symptomatic, discharge home with follow-up if unintentional ingestion and asymptomatic after 6 h
Ingestion: aromatics, halogenated, other volatiles (see Tables 180-2, 180-3, 180-4)
GI decontamination: consider activated charcoal, gastric aspiration if highly toxic (e.g., CCl$_4$, chloroform, benzene)
Skin decontamination: if spilled on clothes or skin, soap and water
Diagnostic adjuncts
    Observe for evidence of aspiration and CNS symptoms (CXR, pulse oximetry)
    Continuous cardiac monitoring for dysrhythmias
    Abdominal radiographs to evaluate suspected chlorinated hydrocarbon ingestions
    Methylene chloride: check COHB level, serial levels may be necessary, O$_2$
    Toluene: check potassium, anion gap, CPK
    Benzene: follow CBC
    Potent halogenated hydrocarbons (CCL$_4$, chloroform, TCE, TCA) follow LFTs
    Nitrites and amines: check methemoglobin level
Treatment
    Oxygen
    Avoid exogenous catecholamines if possible (dopamine, norepinephrine)
    Consider β-adrenergic antagonists to treat dysrhythmias
    Consider NAC therapy for potent halogenated hydrocarbon exposure
    Consider HBO if markedly elevated COHB level from methylene chloride
    Disposition: admit symptomatic exposures or hydrocarbons with delayed toxicity (CCl$_4$)
Inhalation: aliphatic mixtures, aromatics, halogenated, other volatiles
Treat as aromatics above but no need for GI decontamination
Dermal: tar and asphalt
Immediate cooling with water
Debridement of blistered skin
Remove adherent substance with petroleum based solvent (e.g., De-Solv-It, Tween 80, Polysporin)

Abbreviations: CBC = complete blood count; CCL$_4$ = carbon tetrachloride; COHB = carboxyhemoglobin; CPK = creatine phosphokinase; CXR = chest x-ray; HBO = hyperbaric oxygen; LFT = liver function test; NAC = *N*-acetyl-L-cysteine; TCA = trichloroethane; TCE = trichloroethylene.

ing. The majority of hydrocarbon ingestions, which consist of aliphatic hydrocarbons mixtures (see Table 180-1), do not require GI decontamination. These agents have poor GI absorption and their toxicity is limited primarily to pulmonary aspiration. In the typical childhood accidental ingestion, the actual amount ingested is usually one swallow or about 5 mL. Suicidal ingestions, which involve larger amounts of hydrocarbons, frequently are associated with spontaneous emesis, and further decontamination is usually not required.

GI decontamination may be warranted when the ingested hydrocarbon is known to have good GI absorption and may cause significant systemic toxicity (e.g., toluene, chloroform, wood distillates) or an additive in the toxic agent (e.g., organophosphate pesticides are often mixed in petroleum distillates). The CHAMP mnemonic (camphor, halogenated hydrocarbons, aromatic hydrocarbons, metals, pesticides) is helpful in remembering most situations where GI decontamination should be considered. Unfortunately, little data is available that evaluates the clinical benefits of gastrointestinal decontamination in these settings. If the patient presents to the ED shortly after the ingestion of these toxic hydrocarbons, aspiration with a small nasogastric tube may be useful. In patients who present with an altered mental status, the airway should be protected with a cuffed endotracheal tube, although in smaller children younger than 8 years of age, the cuff should be kept inflated only during the period of lavage because of cuff-related injury from prolonged inflation. Ipecac-induced emesis is contraindicated as its risks appear to outweigh any potential benefits. Although activated charcoal may adsorb some hydrocarbon compounds, its use is not recommended for most hydrocarbon ingestions. Charcoal instillation may distend the stomach increasing the risk for vomiting and aspiration. The use of charcoal should only be considered if one of the CHAMP-type hydrocarbons has been ingested, and extreme caution should be exercised because of aspiration risk.

The use of cathartics to hasten GI transit and facilitate decontamination has no proven efficacy in hydrocarbon ingestions. Many patients will already have diarrhea from the hydrocarbon, and further catharsis is not required. Oil-based cathartics, which had been used in the past to thicken the ingested hydrocarbon to increase its viscosity and decrease the subsequent risk of aspiration, are contraindicated. They may actually increase GI absorption and are associated with an increased risk of lipoid pneumonia when aspirated.

Pulmonary Treatment

Nebulized oxygen is helpful in the treatment of pulmonary aspiration. Inhaled β_2-agonists may also be useful, especially in the setting of bronchospasm, but their role in the treatment of hydrocarbon pneumonitis has not been studied. Positive end-expiratory pressure (PEEP) or continuous positive-airway pressure (CPAP) may sometimes be required, but because of the potential for further injury from barotrauma, one should observe for the development of pneumatoceles or pneumothorax. In cases of severe pulmonary aspiration resulting in refractory hypoxemia, treatment with extracorporeal membrane oxygenation and high-frequency jet ventilation has proved successful.[20,21] Consensus that corticosteroids are contraindicated because they impair the cellular immune response and increase the chance of bacterial superinfection remains. Antibiotics have no proven role in prophylaxis and are usually not required except in cases of continued pulmonary deterioration because of the risk of a superimposed bacterial pneumonitis.

Other

There are few antidotes to counteract the actions of hydrocarbons. N-acetylcysteine and hyperbaric oxygen may have a role in preventing hepatic toxicity after carbon tetrachloride (and possibly chloroform) exposure, but more studies are needed. Hyperbaric oxygen therapy may be indicated for patients who develop significant carbon monoxide toxicity after exposure to methylene chloride, but has not been studied. β-blockers may be useful in the treatment of hydrocarbon-induced malignant dysrhythmias.[22] Although extracorporeal removal with hemodialysis, hemoperfusion, or peritoneal dialysis has been attempted for severe intoxications, clinically controlled evidence of efficacy is lacking. Specific antidotal treatment directed at the complications of toxic additives, such as organophosphates, pyrethrins or heavy metals, may also be needed.

The treatment of tar and asphalt injuries is a particular problem because of the difficulty in removing these substances without causing further tissue injury. Immediate prehospital cooling with cold water to limit injury is important. Debridement of blistered skin can aid in the removal of adherent substances. De-Solv-It, a surface-active petroleum-based solvent, is both nonirritating and effective in removing these agents; however, it should only be applied briefly and personal protection should be employed (gloves, eyewear).[19] Polyoxyethylene sorbitan-containing ointments, such as Polysorbate 80 or Tween 80, are also useful. Petrolatum-containing preparations, such as Neosporin (although occasionally sensitizing) or Polysporin, may also work and are readily available. It is possible to apply the ointment (not De-Solv-It) under an occlusive dressing and allow the patient to go home, having them return for follow up in 24 h after it has solubilized the tar to wash it off. It is not necessary to remove all tar during the first visit, and close follow up is recommended. In some instances, excision and skin grafting are required to treat the more significant hot tar burns.

DISPOSITION

A medical toxicologist or regional poison control center should be consulted on most symptomatic hydrocarbon exposures and asymptomatic exposures that involve halogenated, aromatic, and hydrocarbon exposures with toxic additives. Hospitalization is required for patients who have ingested aliphatic hydrocarbons who are symptomatic at the time of evaluation, and patients exposed to significant amounts of methemoglobinemia-producing hydrocarbons. After a 6-h observation period, asymptomatic patients with a normal chest x-ray may be discharged home, but follow up should be assured as delayed toxicity (18+ h) has been reported.[6,23] Similar disposition of asymptomatic patients, with abnormal chest x-rays has also been suggested if reliable follow-up can be ensured. Some physicians, however, prefer to observe these patients for 24 h in the hospital. Hospitalization is recommended for those who ingest hydrocarbons capable of producing delayed complications (e.g., halogenated hydrocarbons causing hepatic toxicity) and those with toxic additives (organophosphates and organic metal compounds). All patients taking ingestions with suicidal intent or presenting with complications of solvent abuse should have psychiatric evaluation.

REFERENCES

1. Gupta P, Singh RP, Murali MV, et al: Kerosene oil poisonings childhood menace. *Indian Pediatr* 29:979, 1992.
2. Litovitz TL, Klein-Schwartz WK, Dyer KS, et al: 2001 Annual report of the American Association of Poison Control Centers Toxic Exposure Surveillance System. *Am J Emerg Med* 20:391, 2001.
3. Esmail A, Meyer L, Pottier A, et al: Deaths from volatile substance abuse in those under 18 years: Results from a national epidemiological study. *Arch Dis Child* 69:356, 1993.
4. Press E: Cooperative kerosene poisoning study: Evaluation of gastric lavage and other factors in the treatment of accidental ingestion of petroleum distillate products. *Pediatrics* 29:648, 1962.
5. Bracco D, Favre JB: Pulmonary injury after ski wax inhalation exposure. *Ann Emerg Med* 32:616, 1998.
6. Anas N, Namasonthi V, Ginsburg CM: Criteria for hospitalizing children who have ingested products containing hydrocarbons. *JAMA* 246:840, 1981.
7. Machado B, Cross K, Snodgrass WR: Accidental hydrocarbon ingestion cases telephoned to a regional poison center. *Ann Emerg Med* 17:804, 1988.
8. Welker JA, Zaloga GP: Pine oil ingestion: A common cause of poisoning. *Chest* 226:1822, 1999.
9. Goodheart RS, Dunne JW: Petrol sniffer's encephalopathy: A study of 25 patients. *Med J Aust* 160:178, 1994.
10. Herskowitz A, Ishii N, Schaumburg H: n-Hexane neuropathy: A syndrome occurring as a result of industrial exposure. *New Engl J Med* 285:82, 1971.
11. Burns TM, Shneker BF, Juel VC: Gasoline sniffing multifocal neuropathy. *Pediatr Neurol* 25:419, 2001.
12. Chan YL, Yang CC, Deng JF, et al: Diverse manifestations of oral methylene chloride poisoning: Report of 6 cases. *Clin Toxicol* 36:497, 1999.
13. Shepherd RT: Mechanism of death associated with volatile substance abuse. *Hum Toxicol* 8:289, 1989.

14. Ruprah M, Mant TGK, Flanagan RJ: Acute carbon tetrachloride poisoning in 19 patients: Implications for diagnosis and treatment. *Lancet* 1:1027, 1985.

15. Erickson TB, Aks SE, Zabaneh R, et al: Acute renal toxicity after ingestion of lava light liquid. *Ann Emerg Med* 27:781, 1996.

16. Rinsky RA, Smith AB, Hornung R, et al: Benzene and leukemia: An epidemiologic risk assessment. *New Engl J Med* 316:1044, 1987.

17. Leikin JB, Kaufman D, Lipscomb JW, et al: Methylene chloride: Report of five exposures and two deaths. *Am J Emerg Med* 8:534, 1990.

18. Kleinschmidt K, Goto GS, Roth B: Multiple small volume subcutaneous WD-40 injections with severe local and systemic toxicity. *J Toxicol Clin Toxicol* 37:653, 1999.

19. James NK, Moss AL: Review of burns caused by bitumen and the problems of its removal. *Burns* 16:214, 1990.

20. Chyka PA: Benefits of extracorporeal membrane oxygenation for hydrocarbon pneumonitis. *J Toxicol Clin Toxicol* 34:357, 1996.

21. Bysani GK, Rucoba RJ, Noah ZL: Treatment of hydrocarbon pneumonitis: High-frequency jet ventilation as an alternative to extracorporeal membrane oxygenation. *Chest* 106:300, 1994.

22. Kobayashi H, Hobara T, Kawamoto T, et al: Effect of 1,1,1-trichloroethane inhalation on heart rate and its mechanism: A role of the autonomic nervous system. *Arch Environ Health* 42:140, 1987.

23. Kuspis DA, Mrvos R, Krenzelok EP: Extended home follow-up with symptomatic pediatric hydrocarbon ingestions. *J Toxicol Clin Toxicol* 40:669, 2002.

CAUSTICS
G. Richard Bruno
Wallace A. Carter

The American Association of Poison Control Centers (AAPCC) reports approximately 103,000 potentially caustic exposures in the United States annually (Table 181-1),[1] including dermal and ocular exposure and oral ingestions. Most exposures are unintentional, with many occurring in children younger than age 6. In 2000, there were approximately 387 exposures that resulted in significant morbidity and 20 in death. Intentional adult ingestions with suicidal intent account for a greater percentage of serious injuries than unintentional oral ingestions by curious children.

Many chemicals used in industry have caustic potential. Alkali substances used in industry include sodium hydroxide and potassium hydroxide in cleaning fluids, calcium hydroxide in concrete, lithium hydroxide in photography, and ammonium hydroxide in fertilizers (Table 181-2). Common acids used in industry include hydrochloric acid and

sulfuric acids as cleaners, hydrofluoric acid in etching and metal cleaning, chromic acid in metal plating, and formic acid in leather/textile tanning. Industrial strength cleaners and chemicals accounted for 3,129 alkali exposures and 1,519 acid exposures in the 2000 AAPCC data (see Table 181-1).[1]

Household caustics are common, and many are less-concentrated forms of industrial-strength cleansers. Alkali caustics found in the home include sodium hydroxide in drain cleaners, oven cleaners, and Clinitest tablets (see Table 181-2). Caustic ammonium compounds are found in glass, tub, and tile cleaners. Household bleach (sodium hypochlorite) is the most common alkali exposure reported in AAPCC data, accounting for more than 49,000 exposures per year.[1] Most bleach exposures are benign, but 53 patients suffered major morbidity and 3 deaths were reported in the 2000 AAPCC data. Common household acids include sulfuric acid in drain cleaners and automobile batteries, hydrochloric acid in cleaners, formic acid in airplane glue, and hydrofluoric acid in rust removers.

PATHOPHYSIOLOGY OF CAUSTIC INJURIES

Alkali

Alkali injuries can induce deep tissue injury from liquefaction necrosis. After caustic alkali exposures, proteins are rapidly denatured and lipids undergo saponification. Initially, there is direct cellular destruction from contact with the alkali. This is followed by thrombosis of local microvasculature that leads to further tissue necrosis. Solid or granular alkali caustics often injure the oropharynx and proximal esophagus. Liquid alkali ingestions are characterized by esophageal injuries. Severe intentional alkali ingestion may cause multisystem organ injuries, including gastric perforation and necrosis of abdominal viscera. Severe injuries to the pancreas, gallbladder, and small intestine after intentional ingestion have been reported.

The most common household alkali is bleach, a 3 to 6 percent sodium hypochlorite solution with a pH of approximately 11. Household liquid bleach is not corrosive to the esophagus, but ingestion may cause emesis secondary to gastric irritation or pulmonary irritation related to chlorine gas production in the stomach or when mixed with other substances.[2] Industrial-strength bleach may contain much higher concentrations of sodium hypochlorite, and ingestion may result in esophageal necrosis. Other injuries reported with bleach include pneumonitis after aspiration and sight-limiting ocular injuries.

TABLE 181-1   Epidemiology of Caustic Ingestions Reported to the American Association of Poison Control Centers, 2000

	No. Exposures	Age <6	Unintentional	Intentional	Major Outcome*	Death
Alkalis						
Chemicals	26,959	14,039	26,062	546	117	1
Rust remover	20	3	19	0	0	0
Drain cleaners	3,890	630	3,614	232	61	3
Industrial cleaners	3,129	869	2,958	100	20	0
Total alkali exposures	*33,998*	*15,541*	*32,653*	*878*	*198*	*4*
Acids						
Chemicals	14,576	2,466	14,028	373	108	10
Rust remover	315	64	303	9	4	2
Drain cleaner	1,099	106	968	27	9	1
Industrial cleaner	1,519	534	1,476	32	9	0
Total acid exposures	*17,509*	*3,170*	*16,778*	*441*	*130*	*13*
Disc batteries	1,804	1,080	1,754	43	6	0
Bleach	49,020	19,481	46,383	1,949	53	3
Total caustic exposures	*102,331*	*39,272*	*97,568*	*3,311*	*387*	*20*

*Major outcomes are defined as signs or symptoms that are life-threatening or result in significant disability.
Source: From Litovitz et al, with permission.[1]

TABLE 181-2   Common Caustic Compounds

	Found In
Alkali	
Sodium hydroxide	Industrial chemicals, Clinitest tablets, drain cleaners, oven cleaners
Potassium hydroxide	Drain cleaners, batteries
Calcium hydroxide	Cement
Ammonium hydroxide	Hair straighteners, skin peels, toilet cleaners, glass cleaners, fertilizers
Lithium hydroxide	Photographic developer, batteries
Sodium tripolyphosphate	Detergents
Sodium hypochlorite	Bleach
Acids	
Sulfuric acid	Automobile batteries, drain cleaners, explosives, fertilizer
Acetic acid	Printing and photography, disinfectants, hair neutralizer
Hydrochloric acid	Cleaning agents, metal cleaning, chemical production
Hydrofluoric acids	Rust remover, petroleum industry, glass etching, jewelry cleaners
Formic acid	Model glue, leather and textile manufacturing, tissue preservation
Chromic acid	Metal plating, photography
Nitric acid	Fertilizer, engraving, electroplating
Phosphoric acid	Rustproofing, metal cleaners, disinfectants

Solid alkali ingestions may have greater potential for proximal esophageal tract injury and less for distal injury.

Acids

Injuries by strong acids produce coagulation necrosis. Tissue destruction and cell death result in eschar formation, which is believed to protect against deeper injury. Ingested acids settle in the stomach, where gastric necrosis, perforation, and hemorrhage may result. It was previously thought that acids were esophagus-sparing, with most tissue injury concentrated in the stomach, but a study by Zargar and colleagues[3] reported a similar incidence of gastric and esophageal injury (85.4 percent gastric and 87.8 percent esophageal) after acid ingestion. Despite relatively less tissue destruction, strong acid ingestion results in a higher mortality rate than does strong alkali ingestion. This higher mortality rate after acid ingestion is hypothesized to result from complications of systemic absorption of acid (metabolic acidosis, hemolysis, and renal failure).

CLINICAL FEATURES

Patients who present after caustic ingestion may have severe pain, odynophagia, dysphonia, oral and facial burns, respiratory distress, and/or abdominal pain, and may be drooling, coughing, or vomiting. Dysphonia, stridor, and respiratory distress may indicate laryngotracheal injury, whereas dysphagia, odynophagia, epigastric pain, and vomiting may indicate esophageal and gastrointestinal (GI) injury.

Conflicting data exist on the reliability of presenting signs and symptoms to predict upper GI injuries. An early retrospective study of caustic ingestions by Gaudreault and colleagues[4] reported 12 percent of patients who presented without initial signs or symptoms of upper GI injury were subsequently found to have serious esophageal injuries of grade 2 or higher (Table 181-3). A subsequent prospective study by Gorman and coworkers found that no single symptom, or group of symptoms, had 100 percent positive or negative predictive value for esophageal injury.[5] All patients with serious esophageal injuries (grade 2 or 3) in the study by Gorman and colleagues had some initial sign or symptom (drooling, abdominal pain, etc.).

TABLE 181-3   Endoscopic Grading of Upper Gastrointestinal Caustic Injuries

Grade 0	Normal examination findings
Grade 1	Edema and hyperemia of mucosa
Grade 2a	Friability, hemorrhages, erosions, blisters, whitish membrane, exudates, and superficial ulcerations
Grade 2b	Grade 2a plus deep discrete or circumferential ulceration
Grade 3a	Small scattered necrosis
Grade 3b	Extensive necrosis

Source: From Zargar et al,[11] with permission.

MANAGEMENT

Initial Assessment

During the initial and subsequent evaluations, the ED staff should take precautions to prevent personal injury secondary to caustic exposure.

The first step is immediate airway evaluation. Patients with respiratory distress may have significant oral, pharyngeal, and/or laryngotracheal injury, and may require emergency airway management. Ideally, patients with potential airway injuries should have fiberoptic evaluation of the airway prior to intubation to determine the extent of the damage, but this may not always be possible. **Blind nasotracheal intubation is contraindicated** secondary to the potential for exacerbating airway injuries. Oral intubation with direct visualization is the first choice for definitive airway management, but surgical cricothyrotomy may be required if oral intubation is not possible. When in doubt, it is prudent to establish an airway early rather than risk greater difficulty later as secondary effects of injury, such as edema, complicate the situation.

A directed history and physical examination should be performed to determine the type and amount of caustic ingested. It should also be determined whether the ingestion was intentional or unintentional. Patients should be assessed for hemodynamic instability. Etiologies for shock in these patients include GI bleeding, complications of GI perforation, and volume depletion. Patients should be examined for peritoneal signs from hollow viscus perforation, and mediastinitis should be considered in patients complaining of chest discomfort. Carefully examine eyes and skin to detect dermal and ocular caustic exposures.

Laboratory and Ancillary Tests

Laboratory evaluation should include arterial blood gas level, electrolyte panel, hepatic profile, complete blood count, and coagulation profile. Strong acid ingestions may cause severe acid-base disorders, and an arterial line may be indicated if serial blood gas determinations are required. Obtain serum calcium and magnesium levels after hydrofluoric acid exposures. All patients should have an upright chest radiograph to detect peritoneal and mediastinal air. After intentional ingestions, an ECG should be done and aspirin and acetaminophen levels should be obtained to screen for potential coingestants.

Gastric Decontamination

Charcoal should not be given to caustic ingestions, because caustics do not bind well to activated charcoal and charcoal will impede visualization when endoscopy is performed. Ipecac should not be given because vomiting could precipitate perforation, and vomiting will result in repeat exposure of the airway and gastrointestinal mucosa to the caustic agent. The risk of inserting a nasogastric tube generally outweighs the benefits. A nasogastric tube should not be inserted in the ED for alkali ingestions because the risk of perforation is considered great. For acid injuries, a nasogastric tube may be inserted by the endoscopist to aspirate residual material.

Neutralization and Dilution

Dilution or neutralization are not recommended at this time, because the risks outweigh the benefits. Potential dangers of such therapy include vomiting, airway injury, and perforation.

Benefits of dilution or neutralization have not been clearly demonstrated in the clinical setting. However, in animal models, dilution can decrease tissue destruction.[6–8] Prior concerns that neutralization therapy (neutralization of strong bases with acids and the reverse) can produce harmful exothermic reactions have been questioned.[7,8] Still, until more clinical data are available, dilution or neutralization should not be done in the ED or the prehospital setting.

Endoscopy

Endoscopy is an important tool used to evaluate the location and severity of injury to the esophagus, stomach, and duodenum after caustic ingestion. Indications for endoscopy vary, so the endoscopist should be consulted in all cases of caustic ingestion. Some authorities recommend endoscopy in all cases of caustic ingestions, whereas others advocate endoscopy based on signs and symptoms.[9] Recent data supports the latter idea (i.e., patients with endoscopically significant lesions all had signs or symptoms of oral pharyngeal injury).[10] Currently, endoscopy is indicated in the presence of any signs or symptoms of serious injury (vomiting, drooling, dyspnea, or stridor), in the presence of oral-pharyngeal burns, and after intentional ingestions.

Zargar and colleagues[3] developed the most commonly referenced system for endoscopic staging of upper GI tract caustic injuries and prospectively demonstrated the safety of using the endoscope in caustic ingestions. Injuries are divided into four grades (see Table 181-3).[11] Patients with grade 2b and 3 injuries are at risk of long-term sequelae, including stricture formation. Patients with grade 3 lesions are at greatest risk of perforation, fistula, and hemorrhage.

Traditionally, endoscopists have terminated their examination at the first sign of severe esophageal injury (grade 2b or 3). However, a more complete examination to document all injuries to the esophagus, stomach, and duodenum may outweigh the risk of perforation. Most experts agree that **the timing of the endoscopy should be within the first several hours after ingestion** and that follow-up exams should be avoided between days 5 and 15. Other noninvasive diagnostic means to evaluate and follow caustic GI injuries include abdominal computed tomography (CT) and ultrasonography. For patients not requiring emergent laparotomy, CT may be used to screen for intraabdominal necrosis outside the GI tract or in areas not reachable with the endoscope. Sonographic evaluation, both transabdominal and endoscopic, has been advocated for evaluation and follow-up of gastric injury after caustic ingestion.[12,13]

Steroids

One of the most controversial aspects of caustic ingestion management is the use of steroids. The ability of steroids to inhibit the inflammatory response led to the hypothesis that steroids may decrease stricture formation after caustic ingestion. The largest study of steroid use in human caustic ingestions was not able to demonstrate such a benefit from steroids.[14] Opponents of steroid use believe that steroids may increase the risk of infection, perforation, and hemorrhage, but no compelling data support these assertions.[15,16]

Steroid use has never been recommended in acid ingestions, because the risk of esophageal stricture formation is believed to be lower. Recommendations vary for steroid use after alkali caustic ingestions, from not using steroids at all to using them only in endoscopic grade 2b lesions (circumferential deep ulcerated lesions). Steroids are not indicated in grade 1 and grade 2a lesions because these lesions do not form strictures and grade 3 lesions are probably best handled by surgical resection. If used, steroids should be used early for alkali inges-

tions, within the first 6 h, at a dose approximately equivalent to 2 mg/kg per 24 h of prednisolone for 3 weeks, followed by a taper.

Antibiotics

There is no good data to support use of prophylactic antibiotics after caustic ingestions. However in cases in which steroids are utilized, addition of penicillin or another antibiotic that covers oral flora appears to be prudent.

Systemic Toxicity

Morbidity or death from alkali injuries usually results from the complications of direct tissue necrosis, but acid ingestions may result in systemic toxicity from absorption of the acid in addition to local tissue destruction. Acid-base disorders, hemolysis, and renal failure may result. In cases of systemic toxicity, traditional critical care principles should be applied to optimize the patient's hemodynamics. Manipulation of serum pH with sodium bicarbonate may be required if the serum pH is consistently below 7.10 due to metabolic acidosis.

Ocular Exposures

Ocular injuries after caustic exposures can be devastating to vision. The Eye Bank Association of America reports that 300 of the 1000 corneal transplants in the United States in 1995 were secondary to eye injuries caused by chemicals.[17] Caustic alkali injuries to the eye are generally more severe than acid-related eye injuries. Alkali injuries penetrate deep into ocular tissue and continue to be destructive after superficial removal, whereas acid injuries are usually superficial. The coagulation necrosis after acid injury limits the penetration of acid into ocular tissue.

Ocular injuries should be immediately treated with copious irrigation. Patients should have continuous irrigation with at least 2 L of NS per affected eye. Nitrazine (pH) paper should be utilized to ensure that the offending acid or base is eliminated. The expected pH after irrigation should be between 7.5 and 8.0, and irrigation should continue until this pH range is achieved. A waiting period of 10 min before checking the pH will more accurately reflect the pH of the eye and not the irrigation fluid. After irrigation, all patients should have a complete eye examination, including fluorescein staining, and all except the most superficial exposures should have ED ophthalmology consultation.

Treatment of Dermal Exposures

Caustic injuries to the skin most frequently occur on the extremities. Most acid injuries, excluding hydrofluoric acid, respond well to local copious saline irrigation. Alkali dermal exposures may appear deceptively superficial, yet burn more deeply and for extended periods. Management of these injuries should include copious irrigation and local wound debridement to remove residual compound. In cases of lime exposure and other caustic powders, patients should brush off the dry compound and remove contaminated clothing before irrigating.

Portland or ready-mix cement is an alkali mixture of lime that warrants special mention. When water is added to the dry mixture, calcium, sodium, and potassium hydroxide are produced. Patients may initially present with severe pain without obvious injury, but eventually develop blisters and skin necrosis if the affected area is not irrigated early. All cutaneous caustic injuries require close follow-up or early referral to a plastic surgeon to ensure the injuries are not progressing.

Experimental Therapies

Many different therapies have been tried to decrease the toxic effects of caustic ingestions. Most experiential therapies have been aimed at preventing esophageal strictures after caustic alkali ingestion. Animal data have showed decreased stricture formation with drugs that affect collagen deposition, including interferon-α-2b, octreotide, β-aminopropionitrile, N-acetylcysteine, and D-penicillamine.[18] Pentoxifylline, a local inflammatory and microcirculation mediator, has also been used experimentally. Oral agents to coat and protect the GI tract from insult, including sucralfate, bismuth subsalicylate, and sodium polyacrylate, have been tried experimentally with some success. None of these agents have been evaluated in controlled clinical trials in humans, and more data are needed before a recommendation with respect to their use can be made.

Surgery/Stents/Dilation

Major ingestions of caustic agents may result in immediate perforation of the GI tract and require emergency surgery. The indications for emergency laparotomy include peritoneal signs or free intraperitoneal air. Esophageal perforation diagnosed by mediastinal air on plain films or by endoscopy is also an indication for emergency surgery. More controversial is the management of severe esophageal injuries, grade 2b and 3, without obvious perforation. Some authorities recommend early dilation therapy (in the first 3 weeks) with or without stenting, whereas others report good results with early surgical resection.

DISPOSITION

All patients with symptomatic caustic ingestions should be admitted to the hospital. Patients with grade 1 and 2a lesions will do well, but warrant hospitalization to ensure that symptoms do not progress. The majority of ocular injuries will require ophthalmology consultation in the ED and follow-up. Mild to moderate dermal injuries can be safely discharged after local wound irrigation, aseptic dressings, and close follow-up. The following dermal exposures may warrant admission: injuries that cross flexor or extensor surfaces, facial injuries, injuries to the perineum, partial-thickness injuries to greater than 10 to 15 percent of body surface area, all full-thickness injuries, and less severe injuries in patients at the extremes of age.

SPECIAL SITUATIONS

Disc Batteries

Disc batteries are a common, potentially caustic ingestant. Each year, there are approximately 2000 disc battery ingestions in the United States, mostly by children younger than age 6 (see Table 181-1). Batteries may contain manganese dioxide, zinc, mercuric acid, silver oxide, or lithium in an alkaline medium. Most disc batteries pass through the GI tract without incident. Batteries have the potential for alkali injury if they leak secondary to casing damage or from hydroxide production related to external current from intact batteries. Pressure necrosis may also play a role in injury if the disc battery becomes lodged in the GI tract. Heavy-metal toxicities, while a theoretical consideration in disc battery ingestion, have not been documented.[19]

Chest and abdominal radiographs should be obtained to determine the position of the battery. Batteries in the airway or esophagus should be removed by endoscopy/bronchoscopy immediately. If a battery has passed the gastroesophageal junction and appears to be in the stomach, then a follow-up film should be obtained in 24 to 48 h to ensure that the battery has passed through the pylorus. Batteries in the intestines should pass without difficulty, but checking the stools and follow-up film are used to ensure passage. See Chap. 76 for more discussion.

Hydrofluoric Acid

Hydrofluoric acid is a relatively weak acid ($pKa = 3.8$) used in industry for glass etching, metal cleaning, and petroleum processing. It may also be found in household products such as chrome wheel cleaner and rust remover. Despite being a relatively weak acid, hydrofluoric acid has great potential for causing morbidity and death. The major mechanism of injury with hydrofluoric acid is not coagulation necrosis; rather, the free fluoride ion complexes with body calcium and magnesium, resulting in cellular death. Most injuries are to the upper extremities. Patients often present with benign-appearing wounds but complain of a tremendous amount of pain. These wounds often have a slight white discoloration but may become black and necrotic as cellular damage results. Severe injuries may result in hypocalcemia, hypomagnesemia, hyperkalemia, acidosis, and ventricular dysrhythmias. Ventricular fibrillation and death have been reported with dermal exposure of between 2.5 and 22 percent of body surface area.

Treatment of minor hydrofluoric acid injuries consists of first thoroughly irrigating the affected area with water and then placing the area in a paste of calcium gluconate or benzalkonium chloride solution. The paste can be made with surgical lubricant and calcium gluconate powder (2.5 percent wt/vol) or alternately with a commercially-available preparation of benzalkonium chloride (Zephiran). The affected area is soaked in the gel, with pain relief being used as the end point for therapy. Other effective treatments include intradermal injections of 5 percent calcium gluconate or magnesium sulfate around the affected area (not to exceed 0.5 mL/cm^2). For distal upper extremity injuries that do not respond to the aforementioned treatments, intraarterial infusion of calcium gluconate has been used. It is recommended that 10 mL of 10 percent calcium gluconate diluted in 40 mL of NS be infused over 4 h or until pain resolves. The use of **calcium chloride should be avoided** for fear of skin necrosis if extravasation occurs.[20] Oral ingestion of hydrofluoric acid has a high mortality rate. NG tube placement and gastric lavage with NS are recommended. Oral magnesium or calcium should be given in hydrofluoric ingestions on a milliequivalent-for-milliequivalent basis. If the amount of hydrofluoric acid ingested is not known, then 300 mL of magnesium citrate or calcium salts should be given. In serious exposures of any type, attention should be focused on hemodynamic monitoring for dysrhythmias. Serum calcium and magnesium levels should also be followed closely. Intravenous supplementation with large amounts of calcium and magnesium may be required.

Airbag-Related Burns

Recently reported caustic injuries that ED clinicians should be aware of are chemical burns related to airbag deployment. A small amount of aerosolized sodium hydroxide and sodium carbonate is released during airbag deployment. These caustic alkalis may burn skin or enter the eye and cause significant injury in the form of a chemical keratitis. Skin injuries are usually minor, related to direct contact with aerosolized alkalis or heat from melted clothing. Skin exposure usually requires only basic burn care. Caustic ocular exposures should be managed with copious irrigation, pH testing, and ophthalmology consultation.[21]

LONG-TERM MORBIDITY

Most long-term sequelae from caustic exposure are related to injuries to the GI tract. Acid ingestions may scar the pylorus and result in gastric outlet obstruction. Caustic alkali ingestions may result in esophageal strictures, which may result in dysphagia, odynophagia, and malnutrition. Controversy exists about the appropriate treatment—long-term dilation therapy versus surgery—or strictures.[22]

Patients with caustic injuries to the esophagus are at risk for cancer of the esophagus. Increased risk for esophageal malignancy is up to 1000 times greater in patients with a history of caustic ingestion and is often seen decades after the initial ingestion and resulting esophageal injury. Some authorities advocate prophylactic esophagectomy in grade 3 lesions to decrease risk of potential future malignancy.

REFERENCES

1. Litovitz TL, Klein-Schwartz W, White S, et al: 2000 Annual report of the American Association of Poison Control Centers toxic exposure surveillance system. *Am J Emerg Med* 19:335, 2001.

2. Karnak I, Tanyel FC, Bukupamukcu N, et al: Pulmonary effects of household bleach ingestions in children. *Clin Pediatr* 35:471, 1996.

3. Zargar SA, Kochhar R, Nagi B, et al: Ingestion of corrosive acids: Spectrum of injury to the upper gastrointestinal tract and natural history. *Gastroenterology* 97:702, 1989.

4. Gaudreault P, Parent M, McGuigan M, et al: Predictability of esophageal injury from signs and symptoms: A study of caustic ingestion in 378 children. *Pediatrics* 71:767, 1983.

5. Gorman RL, Khin-Maung-Gyi MT, Klein-Schwartz W, et al: Initial symptoms as predictors of esophageal injury in alkaline corrosive ingestions. *Am J Emerg Med* 10:189, 1992.

6. Homan CS, Maitra SR, Lane B, et al: Therapeutic effects of water and milk for acute injury of the esophagus. *Ann Emerg Med* 24:14, 1994.

7. Homan CS, Singer AJ, Henry MC, et al: Thermal effects of neutralization and water dilution for acute alkali exposures in canines. *Acad Emerg Med* 4:27, 1997.

8. Homan CS, Singer AJ, Thomajan C, et al: Thermal characteristics on neutralization therapy and water dilution for strong acid ingestion: an in-vivo canine model. *Acad Emerg Med* 5:286, 1998.

9. Christesen HB: Prediction of complications following unintentional caustic ingestion in children. Is endoscopy always necessary? *Acta Paediatr Scand* 84:1177, 1995.

10. Lamireau T, Rebouissoux L, Delphine D, et al: Accidental caustic ingestion in children: Is endoscopy always mandatory? *J Pediatr Gastroenterol Nutr* 33:81, 2001.

11. Zargar SA, Kochhar R, Mehta SK: The role of fiberoptic endoscopy in the management of corrosive ingestion and modified endoscopic classification of burns. *Gastrointest Endosc* 37:165, 1991.

12. Aviram G, Kessler A, Reif S, et al: Corrosive gastritis: Sonographic findings in the acute phase and follow-up. *Pediatr Radiol* 27:805, 1997.

13. Kamijo Y, Kondo I, Soma K, et al: Alkaline esophagitis evaluated by endoscopy. *J Toxicol Clin Toxicol* 39:623, 2001.

14. Anderson KD, Rouse T, Randolph JG: A controlled trial of corticosteroids in children with corrosive injury of the esophagus. *New Engl J Med* 323:637, 1990.

15. Howell JM, Dalsey WC, Hartsell FW, et al: Steroids for the treatment of corrosive esophageal injury: A statistical analysis of past studies. *Am J Emerg Med* 10:421, 1992.

16. Oakes DD: Reconsidering the diagnosis and treatment of patients following ingestion of liquid lye. *J Clin Gastroenterol* 21:85, 1995.

17. Blais BR: Treating chemical eye injuries. *Occup Health Saf* 65:23, 1996.

18. Kaygusux I, Celik O, Ozakaya O, et al: Effects of interferon-α-2b and octreotide on healing of esophageal corrosive burns. *Laryngoscope* 111:1999, 2001.

19. Litovitz T, Schnitz BF: Ingestion of cylindrical and button batteries: An analysis of 2382 cases. *Pediatrics* 89:747, 1992.

20. Graundis A, Burns MJ, Aaron CK: Regional intravenous infusion of calcium gluconate for hydrofluoric acid burns of the upper extremities. *Ann Emerg Med* 30:604, 1997.

21. Ulrich D, Noah E, Fuchs P, et al: Burn injuries by air bag deployment. *Burns* 27:196, 2001.

22. Berkovits RN, Bos CE, Wijburg FA, et al: Caustic injury of the oesophagus: Sixteen years experience, and introduction of a new model oesophageal stent. *J Laryngol Otol* 110:1041, 1996.

INSECTICIDES, HERBICIDES, RODENTICIDES

Walter C. Robey III
William J. Meggs

Pesticides include insecticides, herbicides, and rodenticides. In the United States, over 90,000 pesticide exposures were reported to the Toxic Exposure Surveillance System (TESS) of the American Association of Poison Control Centers in 2001,[1] with 46,929 exposures to children under 6 years of age. There were 17 deaths.

Pesticide intoxication results from intentional, accidental, and occupational exposures. Because of the number of chemical compounds marketed as multiple formulations and brand names and the complex clinical syndromes that result from exposure to their active ingredients, management often necessitates using a resource such as the Poison Index or consultation with a poison center. Pesticides contain inert ingredients such as petroleum distillates that also can be toxic to humans. Pesticides have class-specific toxicities. Many have both local and systemic effects. Supportive care is of utmost importance in pesticide poisonings, but for some compounds, the use of antidotes may be lifesaving.

INSECTICIDES

Chemical insecticides are toxic to the nervous system. Toxicity may include acute, chronic, and delayed sequelae of acute exposure. The four major classes of insecticides used today are the organophosphorous compounds, carbamates, organochlorines, and pyrethrins. Another compound, N,N-diethyl-3-methylbenzamide (DEET), is marketed as a personal insect repellant. Organophosphorous and carbamate pesticides are cholinesterase inhibitors that have replaced organochlorine insecticides because of their improved effectiveness and lack of persistence in the environment and human tissues. In 2001, 47,777 insecticide exposures were reported to TESS, with 19,437 exposures to children younger than 6 years of age. Six fatalities were reported. There were 150 cases of major toxicity, 74 of which involved organophosphorous pesticides. Insecticide poisonings occur worldwide.[2]

Organophosphorous Compounds

EPIDEMIOLOGY Commonly used organophosphorous chemicals include diazinon, orthene, malathion, parathion, and chlorpyrifos. In addition to their use as insecticides, they have been used as chemical warfare agents since World War II. Recently, Sarin was used in the terrorist attack on the Tokyo subway in 1995.[3] Organophosphorous and carbamate compounds are the most common insecticides associated with systemic illness. Potency does vary, however. Highly potent compounds such as parathion are used primarily in agriculture. Those of intermediate potency include coumaphos and trichlorfon, which are used in animal care. Diazinon and chlorpyrifos were restricted recently from household use in the United States due to concerns about human neurotoxicity. Poisoning results primarily from accidental exposure in the home, in recently sprayed or fogged areas using pesticide applicators, in agriculture, in industry, and in the transport of these products. Exposure to flea-dip products has been reported in pet groomers and children. Widespread food contamination and the potential for mass toxic exposure are always a risk.[4] In addition, these chemicals are involved in intentional poisonings including homicides. Systemic absorption of organophosphates occurs by inhalation and by mucous membrane, transdermal, transconjunctival, and gastrointestinal exposure. When a patient presents with a pesticide exposure, the clinician should ask questions about first aid, prehospital intervention and decontamination, product name, manufacturer, product concentration and formulation, circumstances of exposure, amount, onset of symptoms, and patient age and medical history. In patients with Alzheimer disease, taking donepezil, tacrine, or rivastigmine can potentiate seizures and other toxic effects of organophosphorous and carbamate exposures.

PATHOPHYSIOLOGY Organophosphorous and carbamate compounds inhibit the enzyme cholinesterase in the nervous system, leading to an accumulation of the neurotransmitter acetycholine in the central nervous system (CNS), the autonomic nervous system, and at neuromuscular junctions.

Acetylcholinesterase (true, or red blood cell acetylcholinesterase) is found primarily in erythrocyte membranes, nervous tissue, and skeletal muscle. Plasma cholinesterase (pseudocholinesterase, butyrylcholinesterase) is found in the serum, liver, pancreas, heart, and brain. Inhibition of cholinesterase leads to acetylcholine accumulation at nerve synapses and neuromuscular junctions, resulting in overstimulation of acetylcholine receptors. This initial overstimulation is followed by paralysis of cholinergic synaptic transmission in the CNS, in autonomic ganglia, at parasympathetic and some sympathetic nerve endings (e.g., sweat glands), and in somatic nerves. A *cholinergic crisis* results in a central and peripheral clinical toxidrome.

Organophosphorous compounds bind irreversibly to cholinesterase, thus inactivating the enzyme through the process of phosphorylation. *Aging* is a term describing the permanent, irreversible binding of the organophosphorous compound to the cholinesterase. The time to aging is slightly variable with different agents. It can take minutes to a day or more. The interval after exposure during which administration of an antidote can reverse the process is initial. **Once aging occurs, the enzymatic activity of cholinesterase is permanently destroyed,** and new enzyme must be resynthesized over a period of weeks before clinical symptoms resolve and normal enzymatic function returns. Therapeutic agents must be given before aging occurs to be effective.

CLINICAL FEATURES   Clinical presentations depend on the specific agent involved, the quantity absorbed, and the type of exposure. Most acutely poisoned patients are symptomatic within the first 8 h and nearly all within the first 24 h. However, highly fat-soluble compounds may cause recurrent or delayed symptoms and signs on redistribution from adipose tissue. Organophosphorous agents such as malathion are associated with local irritation of the skin and respiratory tract with resulting dermatitis and wheezing, respectively, without evidence of systemic absorption. A few cases of persistent reactive airways disease independent of cholinesterase inhibition have been reported.[5]

Acute systemic organophosphorous poisoning results in a variety of clinical CNS, muscarinic, nicotinic, and somatic motor manifestations. In mild to moderate poisoning, symptoms occur in various combinations. Time to onset of symptoms is variable, most often within 8 h, but can be delayed up to 24 h for compounds requiring metabolic activation. Onset is most rapid with inhalation and least rapid with transdermal absorption; however, dermatitis or skin excoriation may hasten this. Symptoms can occur within minutes with massive ingestion.

CNS symptoms of cholinergic excess include anxiety, restlessness, emotional lability, tremor, headache, dizziness, mental confusion, delirium, hallucinations, and seizures. Coma with depression of respiratory and circulatory centers may result. Aggressive behavior has been described. Inhibition of acetylcholinesterase in the parasympathetic branch of the autonomic nervous system has been described with two pneumonics, *DUMBELS* and *SLUDGE,* plus the "killer bees," as given in Table 182-1.

Muscarinic receptor stimulation by acetylcholine leads to salivation, lacrimation, diaphoresis, urinary incontinence, diarrhea, gastrointestinal distress, emesis, and bradycardia. Bradycardia or tachycardia may occur with severe poisoning.[6] Bronchospasm and bronchorrhea resulting from acetylcholine excess can lead to hypoxia and tachycardia. Miotic pupils and blurred vision are due to cholinergic effects on the pupillary constrictors and ciliary body.

Acetylcholine is the presynaptic neurotransmitter at nicotinic receptors in the sympathetic ganglia and adrenal medulla. Overstimulation results in pallor, mydriasis, tachycardia, and hypertension. Parasympathetic stimulation usually predominates, but mixed autonomic effects are common. Nicotinic stimulation at neuromuscular junctions results in muscle fasciculations, cramps, and muscle weakness. This syndrome may progress to paralysis and areflexia. Respiratory muscle paralysis results in acute respiratory failure and death. Miosis and muscle fasciculations are considered reliable signs of toxicity.

TABLE 182-1   SLUDGE + Killer Bees and DUMBELS Pneumonics for the Muscarinic Effects of Cholinesterase Inhibition by Organophosphate and Carbamate Insecticides

S	Salivation
L	Lacrimation
U	Urinary incontinence
D	Defecation
G	GI pain
E	Emesis
	+

Killer Bees: Bradycardia, Bronchorrhea, Bronchospasm

D	Defecation
U	Urination
M	Muscle weakness
B	Bradycardia, bronchorrhea, bronchospasm
E	Emesis
L	Lacrimation
S	Salivation

An *intermediate syndrome* (IMS) may occur 1 to 4 days after an acute organophosphorous poisoning.[7] Paralysis of neck flexor muscles, muscles innervated by the cranial nerves, proximal limb, and respiratory muscles occurs, and respiratory support may be needed. Electromyography (EMG) may assist in making the diagnosis. Aggressive, early antidote therapy and supportive measures may prevent this syndrome. Symptoms usually resolve within 4 to 18 days.

Organophosphate-induced delayed neuropathy occurs 1 to 3 weeks after acute poisoning. This mixed sensorimotor syndrome is due to the inhibition of neuropathy target esterase. This may mimic Guillain-Barré syndrome.

Irreversible neurologic and neurobehavioral sequelae after acute organophosphate poisoning include neuropsychiatric deficits and paralysis.[8] More lipid-soluble organophosphates may not produce immediate symptoms of toxicity, and symptoms may persist for several weeks. Low-grade chronic organophosphorous exposures occur among farm workers, pesticide manufacturing plant workers, exterminators, and patients taking cholinergic ophthalmologic preparations. Symptoms and signs are often less dramatic and nonspecific, with varying degrees of headache, nausea, weakness, diarrhea, or fatigue and a subtle cholinergic syndrome. Neuropsychiatric effects have been described with chronic exposure and include cognitive dysfunction, impaired memory, and psychiatric illnesses such as depression.

Special Considerations   Children are at greater risk of toxicity when exposed, due to size and lower baseline levels of cholinesterase activity. Chemical warfare nerve agents such as Soman, Sarin, Tabun, and VX are organophosphorous compounds that inactivate acetylcholinesterases. They are rapid acting and extremely potent, and death can occur within minutes of inhalation or dermal exposure. Soman ages within minutes, giving little time to administer antidotes.

DIAGNOSIS   Suspicion of exposure to organophosphorous agents is based on history, the presence of a suggestive toxidrome, laboratory cholinesterase assays, and reference laboratory testing for specific compounds. Diagnosis is often difficult owing to a constellation of clinical findings that can be variable in both acute and chronic poisonings. Misdiagnoses such as flu and viral syndromes have occurred. Degree of toxicity may be based on the presence of specific signs and symptoms.

Noting a characteristic hydrocarbon or garlic-like odor may assist in diagnosis. The cholinergic toxidrome may vary depending on the predominance of muscarinic, nicotinic, and CNS manifestations of the toxin and the severity of the intoxication. An initial test dose of intravenous atropine that does not result in the expected improvement in signs and symptoms in the case of poisoning may assist in making a diagnosis (see "Treatment" below). Differential diagnosis of CNS alterations includes all nontoxic causes of mental status changes, coma, and seizures. Muscarinic manifestations may imitate asthma, exacerbation of chronic obstructive pulmonary disease, cardiogenic pulmonary edema, acute gastroenteritis, mushroom toxicity, and primary cardiac brachycardia or hypotension. Miosis may appear late, whereas the presence of mydriasis may indicate hypoxia. Ocular exposure may cause persistent miosis. Nicotinic manifestations may imitate other causes of striated muscle dysfunction and respiratory failure. Sympathomimetic toxins and other causes of sympathetic hyperactivity such as withdrawal syndromes should be considered when signs and symptoms of nicotinic stimulation predominate. Exposure to medicinal cholinergic agents used in the treatment of glaucoma, myasthenia gravis, and Alzheimer disease should be considered.

Functional assays of plasma and red blood cell (RBC) cholinesterases are helpful for diagnosis and as a guide for therapy but may not be readily available. RBC cholinesterase enzymatic activity is a more accurate indicator of synaptic cholinesterase inhibition, but plasma cholinesterase is easier to assay and more available. The degree of cholinesterase inhibition necessary to produce symptomatic illness is variable, but symptoms generally occur when the enzyme is depressed below 50 percent baseline values. In theory, cholinesterase levels should correlate with toxicity, but **false-negative results occur, with symptomatic patients having determinations in the normal range.** Standardization among laboratories is poor. There is a large individual variability in baseline measurements, and deviation from baseline may be significant when laboratory values are in the normal range.

Unless pralidoxime is given before aging occurs, plasma cholinesterase takes up to 4 to 6 weeks and RBC acetylcholinesterase as long as 90 to 120 days to return to baseline after exposure. Plasma cholinesterase **levels have little prognostic value** in patients with acute organophosphate poisoning. Levels do not correlate with the amount of atropine required or the need for mechanical ventilation.[9] When the rate of cholinesterase falls gradually, as in chronic exposure, clinical symptoms may be subtle. Plasma cholinesterase levels may be depressed in genetic variants, chronic disease states, liver dysfunction, cirrhosis, malnutrition and low serum albumin states, neoplasia, infection, and pregnancy. RBC acetylcholinesterase is affected by factors that influence the circulating life of erythrocytes such as hemoglobinopathies.

Routine laboratory test abnormalities are nondiagnostic but may include evidence of pancreatitis, hypo- or hyperglycemia, leukocytosis, and liver function abnormalities. A chest radiograph may show pulmonary edema in severe cases. The electrocardiogram may be abnormal and correlate with the degree of toxicity and outcome. Common abnormalities include ventricular dysrhythmias, torsade de pointes, and idioventricular rhythms. Heart blocks and prolongation of the QT_c interval are common.[10] EMG may identify and quantify acetylcholinesterase inhibition at neuromuscular junctions.

TREATMENT Treatment consists of airway control, intensive respiratory support, general supportive measures, decontamination, prevention of absorption, and the administration of antidotes. *Therapy should not be withheld pending determination of cholinesterase levels.*

Protective clothing must be worn to prevent secondary contamination of health care workers. Neoprene or nitrile gloves must be used instead of latex. Patients with suspected exposure must be removed from the contaminated environment. All clothes and accessories must be removed completely, placed in plastic bags, and disposed of as hazardous materials. The patient is immediately decontaminated externally with copious amounts of soap and water and possibly a second washing with dilute ethanol. Decontamination includes the scalp, hair, fingernails, skin, conjunctivae, and skin folds. Body fluids are contaminated. Abrasion or irritation of the skin should be avoided. Contaminated runoff water should be contained and disposed of as hazardous materials. Instruments can be decontaminated using chlorine bleach.

The patient is placed on 100 percent oxygen, a cardiac monitor, and pulse oximeter. A 100 percent nonrebreather mask will optimize oxygenation in the patient with excessive airway secretions and bronchospasm, and may reduce the chance of ventricular dysrhythmias during antidote therapy. Gentle suction will assist in clearing airway secretions from hypersalivation, bronchorrhea, or emesis. Coma, seizures, respiratory failure, excessive respiratory secretions, or severe bronchospasm may necessitate endotracheal intubation. **A nondepolarizing agent should be used when neuromuscular blockade is needed. Succinylcholine is metabolized by plasma cholinesterase, and therefore, prolonged paralysis may result.** An intravenous line is established, and baseline blood sampling and determination of cholinesterase levels should be done. Hypotension may necessitate initial fluid boluses of NS. Gastric lavage should be considered in recent or large ingestions. Activated charcoal is recommended for all ingestions. Protection of the airway must be ensured before lavage due to the risk of aspirating a hydrocarbon vehicle. When there is significant diarrhea due to cholinergic effects, catharsis is withheld. Hemodialysis and hemoperfusion are of no proven value.

Atropine and pralidoxime are antidotes for significant organophosphorous poisonings. Atropine, a competitive antagonist of acetylcholine at CNS and peripheral muscarinic receptors, is used to reverse muscarinic and central effects secondary to excessive parasympathetic stimulation. The dose is titrated until copious tracheobronchial secretions attenuate. Large amounts may be necessary. Pupillary dilatation is not a therapeutic end point. Atropine should not be withheld in the face of a tachycardia that may be the result of hypoxia due to secretions, respiratory muscle paralysis, or ganglionic stimulation. If secretions are present, an initial dose of 1 mg or more of atropine is given IV in the adult and 0.01 to 0.04 mg/kg in children (but never less than 0.1 mg). Intramuscular administration up to 6 mg is possible, if not ideal. Normally, this dose should produce antimuscarinic symptoms; therefore, failure to respond to a trial dose is indicative of organophosphorous poisoning. The dose may be repeated every 5 min until muscarinic symptoms subside. The dose necessary to dry secretions may be on the order of hundreds of milligrams in massive overdoses, and prolonged therapy may be necessary. Atropine infusion for as long as several weeks has been reported. Inadequate atropinization may lead to treatment failure. Alternate anticholinergic agents include high-dose diphenhydramine. Nebulized atropine or ipratropium may improve pulmonary symptoms. Ipratropium and glycopyrrolate do not cross the blood-brain barrier and are ineffective in treating CNS symptoms. Atropine does not reverse muscle weakness.

Compounds called *oximes* are used to displace organophosphates from the cholinesterases. Pralidoxime (2-PAM) is a specific antidote that restores acetylcholinesterase activity by regenerating phosphorylated acetylcholinesterase and appears to prevent toxicity by detoxifying the remaining organophosphorous molecules. Clinically, pralidoxime ameliorates muscarinic, nicotinic, and CNS symptoms. Pralidoxime reverses muscle paralysis if given early, before aging occurs. If possible, blood samples for cholinesterase levels are obtained before administration of pralidoxime, but it is important that pralidoxime be administered as soon as possible before permanent and irreversible binding, or aging, occurs. It is recommended for use even more than 24 to 48 h after exposure. Pralidoxime is more effective in acute than in chronic intoxications. The dose is 1 to 2 g for adults and 20 to 40 mg/kg up to 1 g in children, and it is infused in NS over 5 to 10 min. It also can be given by the intramuscular route. A continuous infusion of 500 mg per h in adults (5–10 mg/kg per h in children) is preferable to repeated bolus dosing if paralysis does not resolve after the initial dose or if paralysis returns. Pralidoxime should be continued for 24 to 48 h while monitoring cholinesterase levels. Combination therapy reduces atropine requirements. **Pralidoxime is not administered to asymptomatic patients or to patients with known carbamate exposures presenting with minimal symptoms.**

Response to pralidoxime therapy with a decrease in muscle weakness and fasciculations and relief of muscarinic effects with atropine usually occurs within 10 to 40 min of administration. Use of pralidoxime may prevent later subacute or chronic sequelae.

Seizures are treated with airway protection, oxygen, benzodiazepines, and antidote therapy. Use of diazepam has been described to decrease CNS effects and increase survival in animal studies of nerve gas poisoning.[11] Pulmonary edema and bronchospasm are treated with oxygen, intubation, positive-pressure ventilation, atropine, and pralidoxime. Altered heart rate is treated with supportive therapy and antidotes, and atropine should be given for both bradycardia and tachycardia secondary to bronchospasm or bronchorrhea with hypoxia. Management of dysrhythmias follows advanced cardiac life support guidelines. Succinylcholine, ester anesthetics, and β-blockers may potentiate poisoning and should be avoided.

DISPOSITION   Minimal exposures may require only decontamination and 6 to 8 h of observation in the ED. Reexposure must be avoided because sequential exposures can have cumulative toxicity. Patients returning to work should be limited from further exposure risk. All clothing, including shoes and belts, should be discarded properly as hazardous materials and not returned to the patient. Poisonings have occurred from contaminated clothes and leather. Admission to the intensive care unit is necessary for significant poisonings. Most patients respond to 2-PAM therapy with an increase in acetylcholinesterase levels within 48 h. If toxins are fat-soluble, the patient may be symptomatic for prolonged periods of time and dependent on 2-PAM.[12] During a period of weeks while awaiting resynthesis of new enzyme, supportive care and respiratory support may be needed. The end point of therapy is determined by the absence of signs and symptoms on withholding pralidoxime therapy. Following an acute exposure, the patient may have a variety of neurologic sequelae and nonspecific symptoms lasting days to months that may be lifelong. Chronic exposure may necessitate serial enzyme determinations to identify a trend. Death from organophosphorous poisoning usually occurs in 24 h in untreated patients. If there is no posthypoxic brain damage, and if the patient is treated early, symptomatic recovery occurs in 10 days. Respiratory failure secondary to paralysis of respiratory muscles, CNS depression, or bronchorrhea is the usual cause of death.

Carbamates

EPIDEMIOLOGY   N-Methyl carbamates (Sevin, Baygon, Lannate, Carbaryl, Aldicarb) are cholinesterase inhibitors that are structurally related to the organophosphorous compounds. Medicinal forms include physostigmine, pyridostigmine, and neostigmine.

PATHOPHYSIOLOGY   Carbamates transiently and reversibly inhibit the cholinesterase enzyme through carbamylation. Regeneration of enzyme activity by dissociation of the carbamyl-cholinesterase bond occurs within minutes to a few hours. This involves rapid, spontaneous hydrolysis of the carbamate-cholinesterase bond. Therefore, aging does not occur. Unlike organophosphorous poisoning, it is not necessary for new enzyme to be synthesized before normal function is restored after carbamate poisoning.

CLINICAL FEATURES   Symptoms of acute intoxication are similar to the cholinergic crisis observed with organophosphorous agents but are of shorter duration. Because carbamates do not effectively penetrate the CNS, less central toxicity is seen, and seizures do not occur. Presentation of carbamate poisoning in childhood, with a predominance of CNS depression and nicotinic effects, differs clinically from that of adults.[13]

DIAGNOSIS   Cholinesterase levels and thus enzymatic activity may return spontaneously to normal 4 to 8 h after a carbamate exposure. Measurement of cholinesterase activity generally is not useful in that it will be relatively normal because of rapid decarbamylation.

TREATMENT   Initial treatment of carbamate poisoning is the same as for organophosphorous compounds. Atropine is the antidote of choice and is administered for muscarinic symptoms. This is usually all that is necessary while waiting for the carbamylated acetylcholinesterase complex to dissociate spontaneously and recover function, usually within 24 h. Therapy usually is not needed for more than 6 to 12 h. The use of pralidoxime in carbamate poisoning is controversial. The carbamate-binding half-life to cholinesterase is approximately 30 min, and irreversible binding does not occur, therefore there is little need for pralidoxime. Human case reports and some but not all animal studies suggest that pralidoxime may potentiate the toxicity of monomethylcarbamate, the carbamate carbaryl.[14] It should be avoided in known single-agent carbaryl poisonings. Pralidoxime should be used in mixed poisonings with an organophosphorous compound and a carbamate or if the type of insecticide is unknown.

DISPOSITION   Morbidity and mortality generally are limited in carbamate poisonings because of the transient cholinesterase inhibition and rapid enzyme reactivation. Carbamates are less toxic than organophosphorous compounds, and the clinical course is more benign. Most patients recover completely within 24 h. In mild poisonings, observation suffices, and the patient may be discharged with follow-up. Moderate poisonings necessitate 24 h of observation that includes ruling out concomitant exposure to or toxicity from inactive ingredients or vehicles such as hydrocarbons.

Organochlorines

EPIDEMIOLOGY   Dichlordiphenyltrichloroethane (DDT) is the prototype insecticide of these chlorinated hydrocarbons. Chlordane and heptachlor are compounds that were used for termite and roach control. Dieldrin and adrin also were used commonly. Most have been restricted or banned in the United States because of their persistence in the environment, long half-life in the human body, and toxicity. Worldwide, chlorinated hydrocarbons continue to be used. Hexachlorocyclohexane (lindane) is a general garden organochlorine insecticide that is also used to treat scabies and head lice infestations. This compound is well absorbed by ingestion and inhalation. Dermal absorption occurs particularly if the skin is abraded or repeated applications are used. Children and the elderly can develop CNS toxicity and seizures with therapeutic use.

PATHOPHYSIOLOGY   Organochlorines are CNS stimulants that can be toxic after dermal, inhalation, and gastrointestinal exposures. The physical state, whether a liquid or a solid, and the type of vehicle affect transdermal absorption. Toxicity results from repetitive neuronal discharges following the action potential due to a decrease in membrane sodium channel permeability. Organochlorines are highly lipid-soluble and accumulate in human tissues. Most are capable of inducing the hepatic microsomal enzyme system. Therefore, therapeutic efficacy of other chemicals and drugs that use this system is reduced in the presence of organochlorines.

CLINICAL FEATURES   Neurologic symptoms predominate in acute organochlorine intoxication. Mild poisoning presents with dizziness, fatigue, malaise, headache, neurologic stimulation with hyperexcitability, irritability, and delirium, apprehension, tremulousness, myoclonus, and facial paresthesias. Fever is common. More severe exposure may result in seizures, coma, respiratory failure, and death. Seizures may occur early, without prodromal syndromes, and are usually short-lived.

Organochlorines are delivered dissolved in hydrocarbon solvents that can cause sedation, coma, and pneumonitis from aspiration. Sensitization of the myocardium to endogenous cathecholamines with cardiac dysrhythmias can occur from both organochlorines and the solvents. Chronic neurotoxic effects from low-level exposure to the organochlorine compound chlordane include deficits in tests of balance, reaction time, and verbal recall.[15]

DIAGNOSIS   History is important, and valuable information can be obtained from the package label regarding the product and vehicle involved. Differential diagnosis includes other causes of CNS stimulation and other insecticides. Laboratory evaluation generally is not helpful, but organochlorines can be detected in the serum and urine by specialty laboratories.

TREATMENT   Treatment includes administration of oxygen, with intubation indicated to treat hypoxia secondary to seizures, aspiration, and respiratory failure. Benzodiazepines are indicated for seizure control. Dysrhythmia control may be indicated, but atropine and epinephrine should be avoided because both organochlorines and organic solvents can sensitize the myocardium to endogenous catecholamines. Hyperthermia must be managed by cooling techniques. Removal of clothing and skin decontamination with soap and water are important. Avoid using oils on the skin because they promote absorption. Activated charcoal and possibly gastric lavage in large, recent ingestions are indicated. The exchange resin cholestyramine should be administered to symptomatic patients exposed to Chlordecone.

DISPOSITION   Patients may be observed for 6 h and admitted to the hospital if signs of significant toxicity develop or if ingestion involved a hydrocarbon.

Pyrethrins

EPIDEMIOLOGY   Pyrethrins are naturally occurring botanic substances found in the chrysanthemum plant. They are less toxic and considered safer than other compounds. Pyrethroids are synthetic analogues of pyrethrins. They are used commonly as aerosols in automated insect sprays in public areas; therefore, inhalation is the most common source of exposure. These agents are available as dusts and liquids in a hydrocarbon base. Both are common ingredients in over-the-counter household insecticides, pediculicides, and scabicides.

PATHOPHYSIOLOGY   Pyrethroids block the sodium channel at the neuronal cell membrane, causing repetitive neuronal discharge. There is an additional effect on γ-aminobutyric acid receptors. Other effects include increased nicotinic cholinergic transmission, norepinephrine release, and interference with sodium-calcium exchange across membranes.

CLINICAL FEATURES   These compounds are responsible for dermal, pulmonary, gastrointestinal, and neurologic findings. Allergic hypersensitivity reactions are the most common effects of pyrethrins. These manifest as dermatitis, asthma, allergic rhinitis, hypersensitivity pneumonitis, or anaphylaxis. Pyrethrin antigens are cross-antigenic with ragweed pollen. Dermal absorption is minimal, but these compounds are well absorbed from the gastrointestinal tract. Skin contact may lead to tingling and burning within 30 min of exposure that usually dissipates within 24 h. Contact dermatitis syndromes and allergic rhinitis result from both compounds. Allergic reactions including fatal asthma attacks have been reported. Upper and lower airway irritation occurs with local inhalation exposure. When absorbed, these compounds are metabolized rapidly in the liver, thus resulting in minimal systemic toxicity. Pyrethroids are responsible for occasional systemic occupational poisonings. Systemic symptoms of paresthesias, hyper-

excitability, tremors, incoordination, seizures, muscle weakness, respiratory failure, dizziness, headache, and nonspecific nausea, vomiting, diarrhea, and fatigue are seen with significant intentional ingestions. Alteration of consciousness, muscle fasciculations, pulmonary edema, and seizures may occur in severe poisonings.

DIAGNOSIS   Differential diagnosis includes allergic and neurologic diseases. Laboratory tests are of little value.

TREATMENT   Treatment includes removal from exposure; dermal, ocular, and gut decontamination; treatment of allergic manifestations; and supportive care. Hydrocarbon aspiration must be avoided.

DISPOSITION   Disposition is usually related to the severity of asthmatic and allergic manifestations. The clinical course is usually benign, and hospitalization is not necessary.

N,N-Diethyl-3-Methylbenzamide (DEET)

DEET (OFF! Skintastic, Deep Woods OFF!) is used extensively as an over-the-counter insect repellant that comes in a variety of product formulations ranging in concentrations from 5 to 100 percent. When used as directed, they have a large margin of safety. DEET is absorbed through the skin and is a neurotoxin that causes seizures in large ingestions and extensive dermal exposures of high-concentration products in small children. Skin absorption occurs within 2 h of topical application. Systemic toxicity manifests as restlessness, insomnia, altered behavior, confusion, CNS depression, slurred speech, ataxia, tremors, muscle cramps, hypertonia, and seizures occurring with or without prodrome. DEET-induced hypotension and bradycardia have been reported.[16] Treatment includes benzodiazepines for seizures, skin decontamination with soap and water, and activated charcoal for ingestions. Most patients recover with supportive care.

HERBICIDES

Herbicides are chemicals used to kill weeds. There are several classes that pose a health hazard despite their low acute toxicity in mammals. Toxicity in plants is due to inhibition of photosynthesis, respiration, protein synthesis, or growth stimulation mimicking plant hormones called *auxins*. Herbicidal formulations contain multiple ingredients such as organic solvents, surfactants, and preservatives that may have their own toxic effects. These may or may not be disclosed on the product label. There were 9378 exposures to herbicides reported by the American Association of Poison Control Centers in 2001.[1] Of these, 127 were intentional, with 2594 occurring in children younger than 6 years of age. About 2060 patients were treated in health care facilities, and 310 exposures resulted in moderate to major morbidity, including 4 deaths from paraquat.

Chlorophenoxy Herbicides

EPIDEMIOLOGY   The most commonly used compounds are 2,4-dichlorophenoxyacetic acid (2,4-D) and 4-chloro-2-methylphenoxyacetic acid (MCPA). 2,4,5-Trichlorophenoxy acetic acid (2,4,5-T) has been banned in the United States because of its contamination with 2,3,7,8,-tetrachlorodibenzo-*p*-dioxin (TCDD). The aerially applied defoliant Agent Orange used during the Vietnam War was a mixture of 2,4-D and 2,4,5-T. These compounds are effective against broadleaf plants and are used as weed killers on lawns and grain crops.

PATHOPHYSIOLOGY   The metabolic pathway or mechanism related to toxicity is unknown. Skeletal muscle toxicity can result in respiratory failure or rhabdomyolysis. Toxicity results from dermal contact, inhalation, or ingestion. Local exposure results in dermal and gastrointestinal irritation.

CLINICAL FEATURES   Local exposure leads to eye and mucous membrane irritation. After ingestion, nausea, vomiting, and diarrhea occur. Tachypnea may indicate pulmonary edema. Cardiovascular findings include hypotension, tachycardia, and dysrhythmias. Muscle toxicity manifests as muscle tenderness, fasciculations, myotonia, and rhabdomyolysis. The patient may become hyperthermic. Peripheral neuropathy has been described in the recovery phase and in chronic exposure.

DIAGNOSIS   Diagnosis is based on the history of exposure. Ancillary tests generally are nonspecific but may demonstrate a metabolic acidosis and evidence of hepatorenal dysfunction. Toxin levels are not immediately available. Myoglobinuria and an elevated creatine phosphate level indicate rhabdomyolysis. Differential diagnosis includes other causes of acute myopathy.

TREATMENT   Treatment is supportive, including decontamination measures and respiratory support for myopathic-related respiratory failure. Alkalinization is suggested but not proven to increase the elimination of these compounds. Rhabdomyolysis should be monitored and treated.

DISPOSITION   Severe toxicity and serious complications are not common. Since toxic effects usually appear within 4 to 6 h, patients with mild symptoms can be observed and discharged after that time. Significant toxicity warrants admission.

Bipyridyl Herbicides

These compounds, paraquat and diquat, are nonselective contact herbicides. Both are still used widely and are responsible for significant morbidity.

PARAQUAT

Epidemiology   Paraquat is manufactured as a liquid, granules, or an aerosol and is commonly combined with diquat and other herbicides. Most products contain a blue dye, a stenchant, and an emetic. Ingestion is responsible for the majority of paraquat deaths.[17] Deaths have been reported after transdermal exposure, ingestion, and inhalation. The inhalation of sprays is unlikely to cause systemic toxicity.

Pathophysiology   Paraquat is a severe local irritant and devastating systemic toxin. There is minimal transdermal absorption of paraquat in the absence of preexisting skin lesions that increase systemic absorption. Ingested paraquat is absorbed rapidly, particularly if the stomach is empty. Plasma concentration peaks within minutes to 2 h after ingestion. Paraquat is then distributed to most organs, with the highest concentration found in the kidneys and lungs. Acute exposure causes liver and renal necrosis that is followed within a few weeks by pulmonary fibrosis.

Paraquat actively accumulates in the alveolar cells of the lungs, where it is transformed into a reactive oxygen species, the superoxide radical. This anion is responsible for lipid peroxidation that leads to degradation of cell membranes, cell dysfunction, and death. A redox reaction results in two phases of lung injury. An initial destructive phase is characterized by loss of type I and type II alveolar cells, infiltration by inflammatory cells, and hemorrhage. These changes may be reversible. The later, proliferative phase is characterized by fibrosis in the interstitium and alveolar spaces. Paraquat and oxygen enhance each other's toxicity by sustaining the redox cycle. Myocardial injury and necrosis of the adrenal glands may occur.

Clinical Features   Paraquat's severe caustic effects produce local skin irritation and ulceration of epithelial surfaces. Severe corrosive corneal injury may result from eye exposure. Upper respiratory tract exposure may result in mucosal injury and epistaxis. Inhalation may lead to cough, dyspnea, chest pain, pulmonary edema, epitaxis, and hemoptysis. Respiratory symptoms may persist for several weeks after inhalation exposure.

Ingestion causes gastrointestinal mucosal lesions and ulcerations. An acute burning sensation of the lips or mouth may be followed by ulceration 1 to 2 days later. Buccopharyngeal, esophageal, and abdominal pain and vomiting occur. Caustic lesions of lips, oral cavity, and gastrointestinal tract can occur within a few minutes to hours. Hypovolemia occurs from gastrointestinal fluid losses and decreased oral intake. Cardiovascular collapse may occur early in intoxication. Multisystem effects then result, including gastrointestinal tract corrosion, acute tubular necrosis, and extensive pulmonary injury. Ingestion of greater than 30 mg/kg leads to pulmonary edema, congestive heart failure, and renal failure within hours. Seizures, gastrointestinal perforation and hemorrhage, and hepatic failure may occur. Massive ingestion may lead to multisystem failure with death within a few days. Clinical manifestations of renal failure and hepatocellular necrosis develop between the second and fifth days, with pulmonary fibrosis leading to refractory hypoxemia 5 days to several weeks later. Metabolic (lactic) acidosis is common as a result of pulmonary effects (hypoxemia) and multisystem failure.

Diagnosis   Early diagnosis and therapy are important. The history may be indicative of an accidental or intentional poisoning and of the route of exposure. The differential diagnosis includes exposure to other corrosive agents and herbicides. Qualitative and quantitative analyses for paraquat in urine and blood can assist in the diagnosis.[18] Nomograms have been presented for predicting survival based on plasma paraquat concentration and time of ingestion.[18,19] A 10-h level greater than 0.4 mg/L carries a high probability of death. Serial pulmonary function tests, chest radiographs, and arterial blood gas determinations, including alveolar-arterial gradient, may be used to monitor toxicity.

Chemistry abnormalities reflect multiorgan necrosis. Hypokalemia may be present. Chest radiographs may show pneumomediastinum or pneumothorax in the case of corrosive rupture of the esophagus. Radiographic abnormalities of diffuse consolidation indicating parenchymal injury on the chest radiograph may not parallel the severity of clinical symptoms. Upper gastrointestinal endoscopy should be performed to identify the extent and severity of mucosal lesions.

Treatment   The goal of early and vigorous decontamination is to prevent pulmonary toxicity. Any exposure to paraquat is a medical emergency, with hospitalization indicated even if the patient is asymptomatic. Early treatment is mainly supportive but is an important determinant of survival. An attempt should be made to prevent superoxide radical formation by using low inspired oxygen to produce a therapeutic hypoxemia with the goal of reducing pulmonary injury. The use of low oxygen mixtures (FIO_2 <21 percent) with positive-pressure ventilation reduces pulmonary toxicity in experimental models and may be of therapeutic benefit. Supplemental oxygen should be avoided except for severe respiratory failure. Clothing is removed, and the skin should be decontaminated with soap and water without causing abrasions that may increase absorption. Ocular irrigation with copious amounts of water or saline must take place. Fluid and electrolytic losses from gastrointestinal tract damage, vomiting, and cathartics need to be replaced. Maintaining intravascular volume and urine output is important in preventing prerenal failure. Pain associated with oropharyngeal lesions should be treated with opioids. Emesis is common, but gastric lavage via orogastric tube is recommended despite the risk of perforation.

Immediate gut decontamination with absorbants that bind paraquat is indicated. Activated charcoal (1–2 g/kg), diatomaceous Fuller's earth (1–2 g/kg in 15% aqueous suspension), or bentonite (1–2 g/kg in a 7% aqueous slurry) should be used and repeated every 4 h. A 70% sorbitol

2 mL/kg cathartic should be administered initially. **Charcoal hemoperfusion is known to remove paraquat and should be instituted as soon as possible** and continued for 6 to 8 h. Other proposed therapies are not of proven efficacy. Corticosteroids have been used traditionally and should be considered.

Supportive care includes airway protection, maintaining intravascular volume, monitoring of vital signs and arterial blood gases, pain relief, treatment of renal failure and complications, and treatment of infection. Maintaining renal function will assist in avoiding toxic accumulation in other tissues.

Disposition An attempt to determine prognosis should be made. The mortality rate from ingestion is as high as 75 percent.[17] Outcome is determined by the amount ingested; therefore, intentional ingestions tend to have a worse prognosis. A poor prognosis is seen when paraquat is ingested in a highly concentrated formulation[18] on an empty stomach, thus increasing absorption, and when ingestion results in upper gastrointestinal ulcerations and renal failure.[20] Ingestion of a concentrated liquid solution is usually fatal. Dilute solid formulations rarely cause death. Three categories of toxicity have been described. Ingestion of less than 20 mg/kg of paraquat ion or 28 mg/kg of paraquat dichloride produces no or only moderate gastrointestinal symptoms. Recovery is usually without sequelae. Ingestion of 20 to 40 mg/kg usually results in death 5 days to several weeks after ingestion. Early development of gastrointestinal corrosion, acute renal tubular necrosis, and symptoms of systemic toxicity predominate, with subsequent extensive pulmonary injury and pulmonary fibrosis causing death in most patients. Death may be delayed 2 to 3 weeks. Patients who ingest more than 40 mg/kg of paraquat usually die in 1 to 5 days. Mortality from multiorgan failure and corrosive gastrointestinal effects is 100 percent in this group.

If more than a mouthful (50 mg/kg) is ingested, death occurs within 72 h and is due to multiorgan failure, renal tubular necrosis, myocarditis, liver necrosis, adrenal necrosis, and corrosive lesions of the gastrointestinal tract. If less than a mouthful (20–50 mg/kg) is ingested, death may be delayed up to 70 days and usually results from pulmonary fibrosis.[21] Cardiogenic shock is the usual cause of death in patients with very high plasma concentrations. Death from lower levels is due to pulmonary fibrosis and respiratory failure.

DIQUAT Diquat has a similar structure and mechanism as paraquat but is less toxic. For identification purposes, formulations containing diquat do not contain the dye, stenching agent, or emetic added to paraquat. The lethal dose is similar to that of paraquat, but severe poisoning and death are less common. The extent of pulmonary injury and fibrosis is less due to diquat's lower affinity for pulmonary tissue. Diquat is caustic to the skin and gastrointestinal tract, and primary effects result in renal and liver necrosis. Treatment is similar to that for paraquat poisoning. Mortality approaches 50 percent despite diquat's lower toxicity.

Urea-Substituted Herbicides

Urea-substituted herbicides such as chlorimuron, diuron, fluometron, and isopturon are inhibitors of photosynthesis and have low systemic toxicity. In humans, methemoglobinuria may occur with ingestion. Treatment includes decontamination, supportive care, and treatment with methylene blue.

Organophosphorous Herbicides

In addition to their use as insecticides, some organophosphorous compounds are effective herbicides. Butiphos (Def) is used commonly as a cotton defoliate prior to mechanical harvesting. Treatment is identical to that for insecticides.

Glyphosate (Roundup) is a widely used herbicide that is often combined with other herbicides, including diquat. Severe toxicity is limited to ingestions of concentrated solutions. Surfactant in glyphosate formulations may be responsible for toxicity. Dermal absorption is poor, and excretion is primarily renal. Clinical effects include mucous membrane irritation and erosions, widespread organ dysfunction, and refractory cardiovascular collapse. Treatment options are limited to activated charcoal and supportive care.

RODENTICIDES

Epidemiology

A number of agents with distinct toxicities are used as rodenticides. They may be classified based on whether they are anticoagulants or nonanticoagulants, time of onset of signs and symptoms, and degree of toxicity. According to the American Association of Poison Control Centers, in 2001, there were 19,294 rodenticide exposures reported to TESS.[1] Long-acting superwarfarin anticoagulants accounted for 16,423 of these exposures, most of which were in children younger than 6 years of age. There were only 815 intentional exposures. A total of 6983 patients were treated at health care facilities, and there were 2 deaths, with none involving superwarfarins, which are now combined with a bittering agent. Moderate to major morbidity occurred in 171 exposures. Individuals at risk are suicide victims, attempted homicide or abuse victims, exterminators, the intoxicated, the impaired elderly, and psychiatric patients. Intentional ingestions are often associated with significant morbidity and mortality. Most unintentional exposures occur in young children and result in minimal or no toxicity.[1]

NONANTICOAGULANTS Nonanticoagulant rodenticides are listed by toxicity in Table 182-2.

High Toxicity Arsenic (Rough on Rats, Red Seal Rodenticide, Paris Green) is a heavy metal in the form of a white crystalline powder. It is no longer used because of its high toxicity. After ingestion, this compound combines with sulfhydryl groups and interferes with enzymatic reactions. Symptoms may occur as early as 1 h after ingestion, with death from cardiovascular collapse occurring within 24 h. Clinical presentation includes dysphagia, muscle cramps, nausea and vomiting, bloody diarrhea, cardiovascular collapse, altered mental status, seizures, and late peripheral neuropathies. Treatment consists of lavage, activated charcoal, catharsis, and chelation therapy using dimercaptosuccinic acid (DMSA, succimer), dimercaprol, or penicillamine.

Barium carbonate and other soluble forms such as barium chlorides, hydroxides, and sulfides are highly toxic compounds. This is a white powdery substance. Toxic mechanism is depolarization, stimulating all types of muscle and resulting in neuromuscular blockade,

TABLE 182-2 Nonanticoagulant Rodenticides

High toxicity
Arsenic
Barium
Phosphorous
PNU
Sodium monofluoroacetate
Strychnine
Thallium
Zinc phosphide
Moderate toxicity
α-Naphthylthiourea
Cholecalciferol
Low toxicity
Bromethalin
Norbormide
Red Squill

Abbreviation: PNU = N-3-Pyridylmethyl-N′-p-nitrophenylurea.

paralysis, and hypokalemia. Onset occurs within 1 to 8 h with nausea, vomiting, diarrhea, abdominal pain, dysrhythmias, respiratory failure, muscular weakness, paresthesias, and paralysis. Treatment includes orogastric lavage with sodium or magnesium sulfate added to lavage solution to convert carbonate to less toxic sulfate and potassium replacement.

Elemental or yellow phosphorus (J-O Paste, Rough on Rats, Stearn's Electric Brand Paste) is a yellow or brown, waxy, fat-soluble rat or roach paste that has a garlicky odor. It is easily mixed with molasses or peanut butter or spread on bread for rodents to eat. It ignites on contact with moisture. Skin contact causes local irritation and severe burns within minutes to hours. Toxicity is related to its ability to uncouple oxidative phosphorylation. It appears to have direct toxic effects on the myocardium, kidney, and peripheral vessels. Clinical manifestations after ingestion consist of an initial stage of oral burns, abdominal pain, hematemesis, possible "smoking" luminescent vomitus and stool, a garlicky odor, and possible early death from cardiovascular collapse. The second stage, lasting a few weeks, may be relatively asymptomatic. Finally, CNS depression with multisystem toxicity including a hepatorenal syndrome may occur.

Gastric lavage with dilute potassium permanganate solution may convert phosphorus to less toxic phosphates. Activated charcoal and sorbitol catharsis, with aggressive supportive care and monitoring, is needed. Emesis should be avoided. Early cardiac and CNS toxicity is a poor prognostic sign.

N-3-Pyridylmethyl-N'-p-nitrophenylurea (PNU, Vacor, DLP-787) was withdrawn from the market several years ago because of its ability to interfere with nicotinamide metabolism in the pancreas, destroying β cells within hours of ingestion. It still may be found as a yellow cornmeal-like compound or yellow-green powder in bait and has a peanut-like odor. Toxicity manifests within 24 h of ingestion as acute gastrointestinal symptoms including perforation, autonomic nervous system dysfunction, insulin-deficient hyperglycemia or diabetic ketoacidosis, dysrhythmias, and neuropathies. Treatment consists of lavage, activated charcoal, cathartics, and intravenous or intramuscular administration of nicotinamide (niacinamide) and insulin.

Sodium monofluoroacetate (SMFA, Ratbane 1080, Compound 1081) is a white crystalline, odorless, tasteless, water-soluble powder licensed only by commercial exterminators. It is toxic when absorbed through broken skin, ingested, or inhaled. The active component, fluoroacetate, is converted to fluorocitrate, which interferes with the Krebs cycle. Aerobic glycolysis is thus blocked. As a result, glucose metabolism, cellular respiration, and energy production are blocked, resulting in anaerobic metabolism and lactic acidosis. Fluorocitrate binding of calcium causes hypocalcemia. Onset of toxicity is usually delayed from 2 to 20 h after ingestion. This lag time results from the delay in conversion to fluorocitrate. Signs of toxicity are nausea or vomiting, apprehension, and then lactic acidosis, seizures, coma, respiratory depression, cardiac dysrhythmias, and pulmonary edema. Electrocardiographic abnormalities such as ST-T wave changes, tachycardia, premature ventricular contractions, ventricular tachycardia, and fibrillation are seen. Hyperkalemia and hypocalcemia are common. Hypotension, an elevated serum creatinine level, and decreased blood pH are prognostic indicators of death.[22]

Treatment includes activated charcoal, sorbitol cathartic, seizure and dysrhythmia control, and supportive care. Experimental regimens include glycerol monoacetate and a combination of calcium gluconate and sodium succinate and ethanol loading, which necessitates consultation with a toxicologist.

Strychnine is a highly toxic, naturally occurring alkaloid that comes from the seeds of the tree *Strychnis nux-vomica*. Strychnine is used rarely as a rodenticide. However, it may be a component of homeopathic tonics and cathartic pills. It is an odorless, colorless crystal or white, bitter-tasting powder that can be absorbed through the gastrointestinal tract or nasal mucosa. Toxicity results from its competitive antagonism of the inhibitory neurotransmitter glycine at the postsynaptic brain stem and spinal cord motor neuron. Signs and symptoms of CNS stimulation begin approximately 15 to 20 min after ingestion but can be delayed for up to 2 h after ingestion. Toxicity manifests by restlessness, muscle twitching, painful extensor spasms, opisthotonos, trismus, inability to swallow, and facial grimacing. Medullary paralysis and death can follow.

Of diagnostic importance is that **the patient remains conscious during episodes of painful muscle spasm and what appear to be "seizures"** and that there is no postictal phase. Differential diagnosis includes tetanus, neuroleptic malignant syndrome, encephalitis, seizure disorders, and INH or PCP toxicity. Ancillary testing is not useful for diagnosis.

Treatment includes aggressive airway control, a quiet environment (because any sensory stimulation or manipulation may precipitate contractures), and activated charcoal. Gastric lavage may precipitate convulsions. Benzodiazepines and pain medications are administered to control painful spasms, but barbiturates and neuromuscular blocking agents may be needed. Rhabdomyolysis may ensue and is treated. Recovery is usually complete if therapy is aggressive.

Thallium sulfate (Zelio Paste, Gizmo Mouse Killer) is a heavy metal with moderate to high acute toxicity that is used by industry, found in homeopathic remedies, and is a common poisoning responsible for suicides and homicidal deaths. It is a white, crystalline, odorless, and tasteless powder. It is a cumulative poison that distributes in almost every tissue of the body. Thallium combines with mitochondrial sulfhydryl groups, interfering with oxidative phosphorylation. It is absorbed readily through the skin, by inhalation, and through the gastrointestinal tract.

Gastrointestinal symptoms including hemorrhage develop acutely within 12 to 48 h. A latent period with constipation is then followed in 2 to 5 days by neurologic sequelae, painful lower extremity paresthesias, myalgias, muscle weakness, headache, lethargy, tremors, ataxia, delirium, seizures, and coma. Respiratory failure and dysrhythmias may cause death in severe cases. Chronic sequelae include various neurologic syndromes, neuropathies, and alopecia. Urine sediment may be abnormal, showing RBCs and protein. Liver function tests may be abnormal. Thallium can be measured in the hair, serum, and urine.

Thallium ingestion is treated by multiple doses of activated charcoal, sorbitol initially, and supportive care. Potassium chloride infusion increases renal secretion but also may facilitate entry into cells. Multiple doses of activated charcoal or Prussian blue (potassium ferric hexanocyanate) may interrupt enterohepatic circulation and increase secretion in stool.

Zinc phosphide (Celphos, Phosfume, Acme Mole and Gopher Killer) is a dark-gray, crystalline, water-insoluble powder. It has a characteristic phosphorus or rotten fish odor. Zinc and phosphine gas are released on contact with water and acid. Toxicity is due to the phosphine formed following hydrolysis in the stomach. This gas may be inhaled and absorbed secondarily. Exposure causes widespread cellular toxicity and necrosis to the gastrointestinal tract, kidney, and liver if ingested and to the lungs if inhaled. The exact mechanism is unclear, but it appears to inhibit cytochrome oxidase and the electron transport system.[23]

Onset of clinical syndromes may begin within hours to days of ingestion and may be delayed following inhalation. Nausea, vomiting, and epigastric pain may ensue within 10 to 15 min. Signs and symptoms include a phosphorous or fishy breath, black vomitus, and signs of gastrointestinal irritation or ulceration. There is myocardial toxicity, shock, and noncardiogenic pulmonary edema with nonprominent CNS manifestations such as agitation, coma, and seizures. Hepatorenal injury is common. Metabolic acidosis and hypocalcemic tetany may occur.

Treatment includes preventing gastric conversion to toxic substances by intragastric alkalinization with sodium bicarbonate, dilution with water or milk, activated charcoal, a cathartic, treatment of hypocalcemia, and supportive therapy. Those who survive 3 days usually recover.

Moderate Toxicity α-*Naphthyl-thiourea* (ANTU, Bontu Prep Rat Powder, Nott's Rat-TU) is very selective for target species, with humans being relatively resistant. This compound is a fine, blue-gray powder that is odorless, water-insoluble, and slightly bitter. The mechanism of action is unknown, but this toxin does appear to increase alveolar capillary permeability, causing pulmonary edema. Patients present clinically with dyspnea, cyanosis, cough, pleuritic chest pain, noncardiogenic pulmonary edema, and pleural effusion. Treatment is supportive and includes activated charcoal and catharsis.

Cholecalciferol (vitamin D₃, Quintox Rat and Mouse Bait, Rampage, Ortho Mouse-B Gon) is used by professional exterminators and the general public. It is a white, odorless crystalline substance. In rodents, toxic doses result in the mobilization of calcium from bones, producing hypercalcemia, osteomalacia, and systemic metastatic calcifications. No severe human toxicity or deaths have been reported. Small amounts probably are nontoxic and do not require therapy.

Signs and symptoms are those associated with vitamin D intoxication and hypercalcemia. Onset of toxicity is from hours to days. Clinically, patients present with weakness, nausea, vomiting, abdominal pain, constipation, and CNS depression. Nerve and muscle dysfunction and dysrhythmias may be seen. Serum calcium, magnesium, and electrolyte levels should be monitored. Normal levels obtained 48 h after acute ingestion probably exclude significant toxicity. Therapy after acute massive ingestion includes lavage, activated charcoal, and sorbitol. Treatment of moderate to severe hypercalcemia involves intravenous infusion of normal saline, furosemide, steroids, calcitonin, and biphosphates.

Low Toxicity *Bromethalin* (Assault, Vengeance, Rat Place Packs) is a newer agent, with the first toxic exposure described in 1996. It is a pale-yellow crystalline solid that is odorless. This compound produces neurotoxicity by uncoupling oxidative phosphorylation in the mitochondria of the CNS, thus interrupting nerve conduction Clinical experience in humans is limited, but toxicity presents as muscle tremors, myoclonic jerks, contractions of flexor muscles, ataxia, and focal motor seizures, personality changes, confusion, and coma. Treatment includes decontamination, benzodiazepines for seizures, and observation.

Norbormide or dicarboximide (Shoxin, Raticide) is a yellow cornmeal bait. There is no known human toxicity, but it causes irreversible smooth muscle vasoconstriction and resulting tissue hypoxia and ischemia in rats. Treatment is supportive and includes decontamination.

Red squill (Rat Snax, Rat's End, K-R-O-Powder and Bix Kit) is a bitter-tasting botanic cardiac glycoside derived from the plant *Urginea maritima,* or sea onion. Toxicity is related to the ability to block sodium-potassium adenosine triphosphatase and is similar to digoxin poisoning. Duration of onset is from 30 min to 6 h. Because of its potent emetic properties, patients present with nausea, protracted vomiting, diarrhea, and abdominal pain. Massive ingestion causes hyperkalemia, atrioventricular block, ventricular irritability with dysrhythmias, and death. This substance may crossreact with digoxin assays.

Treatment is similar to that for digoxin toxicity using antiarrhythmics and atropine as indicated. In severe poisoning, an infusion of of digitalis-specific antibody (Fab) is recommended. Activated charcoal should be given.

ANTICOAGULANTS

Warfarin-type (3α-*acetonylbenzyl-4-hydroxy-coumarin)* anticoagulants (Kill-Ko, Rat Busters) were the first anticoagulant rodenticides. They are commonly disguised as yellow corn meal or rolled oats. It is important to differentiate these short-acting anticoagulants from the more toxic long-acting superwarfarins. **Most one-time warfarin ingestions are insignificant accidental poisonings and do not cause any bleeding problems. Toxicity requires large amounts in a single exposure or a repetitive exposure over several days.** The toxic oral dose is estimated at greater than 5 to 20 mg per d for more than 5 days. Lipid solubility of the individual anticoagulant determines its elimination half-life. Onset of effect takes

place from 12 to 48 h after ingestion. Warfarin's biologic half-life is approximately 42 h. These anticoagulants inhibit, almost immediately, the synthesis of vitamin K₁-dependent clotting factors II, VII, IX, and X. Coagulopathy develops when the level of at least one critical coagulation factor falls to 25 percent of normal.[24] This time interval is approximately 12 to 18 h.

Therapy is not necessary for ingestion of a single mouthful of warfarin. For potentially toxic ingestion, therapy consists of activated charcoal and a cathartic, with a baseline International Normalization Ratio (INR) determination and repeated in 12 to 24 h. If the INR is greater than twice normal and the risk of bleeding exists, vitamin K₁ (phytonadione) administration is indicated. The suggested oral dose is 1 to 5 mg in children and 20 mg in adults administered two to four times daily due to its short half-life, and the INR is checked every 4 h initially and then every 24 h until stable.

Second-generation superwarfarins and the indandione derivatives were introduced when rodent resistance to warfarin began to appear. They are responsible for approximately 80 percent of human rodenticide exposures reported in the United States.[1] Their mechanisms are the same as those of the warfarins, but they are more potent, have more prolonged anticoagulant activity, and therefore have the potential to be highly toxic. Poisonings involving the indandione derivatives pindone, diphacinone, chlorphacinone, and valone have toxic and clinical characteristics similar to those of the superwarfarins.

The *superwarfarins* include the 4-hydroxy-coumarins brodifacoum, diphenacoum, coumafuryl, and bromadiolone. These are readily available over the counter as grain-based bait. **Since the biologic half-life of brodifacoum is approximately 120 days, a single ingestion may result in marked anticoagulation effects for weeks to months.** Acute intentional or repeated ingestions can cause severe bleeding. After intentional ingestions, adults often develop a coagulopathy within 24 to 48 h.

A single ingestion usually does not result in immediate toxic effects, and an ingestion may or may not be identified by history. Small children and depressed patients having an unexplained coagulopathy should elevate the index of suspicion. Clinical findings of toxicity consist of ecchymoses, hematuria, uterine or gastrointestinal bleeding, gingival hemorrhage and epistaxis, hematomas, and hemoptysis. Their onset, however, may be delayed for several days, and they may persist for several days.

If an ingestion is suspected, a baseline complete blood count, INR, and specific analysis of coagulation factors II and VII are done.

An abnormal INR or decreased factors may identify repetitive ingestions of a short-acting warfarin or patients who present hours or days after a large, single ingestion of a long-acting superwarfarin. While prothrombin time (PT) is usually monitored, large doses of warfarin can also cause prolongation of the activated partial thromboplastin time (aPTT) also. Specific **serum assays for superwarfarins are available in reference laboratories. Superwarfarins are not detected by warfarin assays.** The initial differential diagnosis in a patient with an elevated INR and PT includes disseminated intravascular coagulation, liver failure, pathologic inhibitors of coagulation, acquired vitamin K deficiency, or ingestion of a vitamin K antagonist. Warfarin abuse must be suspected when no other cause of vitamin K deficiency can be found.

Resuscitation of patients with acute hemorrhage consists of oxygen administration and repletion of volume losses with normal saline or transfusion. Fresh-frozen plasma should be used if bleeding is severe or unresponsive to vitamin therapy. Vitamin K₁ can be diluted and administered by slow intravenous infusion, at less than 1 mg per min, to minimize the risk of an anaphylactoid reaction and cardiovascular collapse. Oral absorption takes approximately 2 to 3 h. Because of the extended half-life of the anticoagulant, prolonged therapy with high doses of vitamin K₁ may be required to maintain hemostasis. Doses of vitamin K₁ should be titrated to effect. Initial doses of 1 to 5 mg in children and 20 mg in adults have been recommended, but doses up to

100 mg per d for 10 months have been reported. The INR is followed every 4 h and then every 24 h.

Treatment of acute ingestion consists of gastrointestinal decontamination. Recent ingestion of amounts greater than 0.1 mg/kg necessitates activated charcoal and a cathartic. Some recent studies suggest that there is no need for gastric decontamination or coagulation studies due to lack of significant toxicity of acute, unintentional superwarfarin ingestions in the pediatric patient.[25–27] INR determinations are recommended 24–48 h postingestion.[28] If the INR is elevated, high-dose vitamin K_1 is initiated for at least 6 weeks. Discontinuation of vitamin K_1 therapy is followed by serial INR determinations to ensure that further therapy is not needed. After initial parenteral therapy, prolonged oral administration for several months may be required as the INR normalizes.

Clinical Approach

Patient evaluation is similar to that described in Chap. 156. Identifying product name is essential for appropriate management, but actual active ingredients need to be known over the commercial name. It must be recognized that similar brand names are used for more than one agent and that some agents are no longer on the market but remain on consumers' shelves. It must be recognized that chemicals can be mistakenly termed rodenticides when obtaining a history and that ingestion may involve coingestants. Specific odors or CNS, cardiopulmonary, gastrointestinal, skeletal muscle, metabolic, or hemorrhagic manifestations or electrocardiographic and radiologic findings may suggest a specific toxin.

Disposition

Given the low frequency of individual physician experience with these types of exposures, poison center or toxicology consultation may assist in recommending a plan for managing the patient based on presentation and toxin. When a patient has been exposed to a rodenticide having a rapid effect, symptoms usually manifest within 4 to 6 h of ingestion. Patients who have ingested a highly toxic rodenticide and are symptomatic are admitted after initial ED therapy. Symptoms related to agents with delayed onset typically begin 12 h or more after exposure.

The threshold for hospital admission should be low for intentional ingestions. For asymptomatic patients who have accidentally ingested a superwarfarin, baseline INR and PTT determinations are done, follow-up is ensured, and coagulation studies are repeated at 24 and 48 h. Prevention measures should be emphasized.

REFERENCES

1. Litovitz TL, Klein-Schwartz W, Rodgers GC, et al: 2001 Annual Report of the American Association of Poison Control Centers Toxic Exposure Surveillance System. *Am J Emerg Med* 20:391, 2002.
2. Saadeh AM, Al-Ali MK, Farsakh NA: Clinical and sociodemographic features of acute carbamate and organophosphate poisoning: A study of 70 adult patients in North Jordan. *Clin Toxicol* 34:45, 1996.
3. Okumura T, Takasu N, Ishimatsu S, et al: Report of 640 victims of the Tokyo subway Sarin attack. *Ann Emerg Med* 28:129, 1996.
4. Buchholz U, Mermin J, Rios R, et al: An outbreak of food-borne illness associated with methomyl-contaminated salt. *JAMA* 288:604, 2002.
5. Deschamps D, Questel F, Baud FJ, et al: Persistent asthma after acute inhalation of organophosphate insecticide. *Lancet* 344:1712, 1994.
6. Agarwal SB: A clinical, biochemical, neurobehavioral, and sociopsychological study of 190 patients admitted to hospital as a result of acute organophosphorus poisoning. *Environ Res* 62:63, 1993.
7. Senanayake N, Karalliedde L: Neurotoxic effects of organophosphorus insecticides: An intermediate syndrome. *New Engl J Med* 316:761, 1987.
8. Steenland K, Jenkins B, Ames RG, et al: Chronic neurological sequela to organophosphate pesticide poisoning. *Am J Public Health* 84:731, 1994.
9. Nouira S, Abroug F, Elatrous S, et al: Prognostic value of serum cholinesterase in acute organophosphate poisoning. *Chest* 106:1811, 1994.
10. Chuang FR, Jang SW, Lin JL, et al: QTc prolongation indicates a poor prognosis in patients with organophosphate poisoning. *Am J Emerg Med* 14:451, 1996.
11. Murphy MR, Blick DW, Dunn MA, et al: Diazepam as a treatment for nerve gas poisoning in primates. *Aviat Space Environ Med* 64:110, 1993.
12. Merril FG, Mihn FG: Prolonged toxicity of organophosphate poisoning. *Crit Care Med* 10:550, 1982.
13. Lifshitz M, Rotenberg M, Sofer S, et al: Carbamate poisoning and oxime treatment in children: A clinical and laboratory study. *Pediatrics* 93:652, 1994.
14. Mercurio-Zuppala M, Hack J, Salvador A, Hoffman RS: Carbaryl poisoning: Two PAM or not two-PAM. *J Toxicol Clin Toxicol* 5:428, 1998.
15. Kilburn KH, Thornton JC: Protracted neurotoxicity from chlordane sprayed to kill termites. *Environ Health Perspect* 103:691, 1995.
16. Leach GJ, Russel RD, Houpt JT: Some cardiovascular effects of the insect repellant *N,N*-diethyl-*m*-toluamide (DEET). *J Toxicol Environ Health* 25:217, 1988.
17. Onyon LJ, Volans GN: The epidemiology and prevention of paraquat poisoning. *Hum Toxicol* 6:19, 1987.
18. Hart TB, Nevitt A, Whitehead A: A new statistical approach to the prognostic significance of plasma paraquat concentrations. *Lancet* 2:1222, 1984.
19. Scherrmann JM, Houze P, Bismuth C, Bourdon R: Prognostic value of plasma and urine paraquat concentrations. *Hum Toxicol* 6:91, 1987.
20. Bismuth C, Garnier R, Dally S, et al: Prognosis and treatment of paraquat poisoning: A review of 28 cases. *J Toxicol Clin Toxicol* 19:46, 1982.
21. Bismuth C, Baud FJ, Barnier R, et al: Paraquat poisoning: Biological presentation. *J Toxicol Clin Exp* 8:211, 1988.
22. Chi CH, Chen KW, Chan SH, et al: Clinical presentation and prognostic factors in sodium monofluoroacetate intoxication. *J Toxicol Clin Toxicol* 34:707, 1996.
23. Chugh SN, Aggarwal HK, Mahajan SK: Zinc phosphide intoxication symptoms. *Int J Clin Pharmacol Ther* 36:406,1998.
24. Freedman MD: Oral anticoagulants: Pharmacodynamics, clinical indications, and adverse effects. *J Clin Pharmacol* 32:196, 1992.
25. Ingals M, Lai C, Tai W, et al: A prospective study of acute, unintentional, pediatric superwarfarin ingestions managed without decontamination. *Ann Emerg Med* 40:73, 2002.
26. Shepard G, Klein-Schwartz W, Anderson BD: Acute, unintentional pediatric brodificoum ingestions. *Ped Emerg Care* 18:174, 2002.
27. Mullins ME, Brands CL, Daya MR: Unintentional pediatric superwarfarin exposures: Do we really need a prothrombin time? *Pediatrics* 105:402. 2000.
28. Smolinske SC, Scherger DL, Kearns PC, et al: Superwarfarin poisoning in children: A prospective study. *Pediatrics* 84:490, 1989.

ANTICHOLINERGIC TOXICITY
Paul M. Wax

Anticholinergic poisoning should always be considered in patients who present to the ED with unexplainable mental status changes. Significant anticholinergic toxicity is manifested by a dramatically altered sensorium, hallucinations, and, at times, severe agitation. A large number of agents, both pharmaceuticals and plants, have anticholinergic properties (Table 183-1). These include H_1-histamine receptor antagonists, phenothiazines, tricyclic antidepressants, antiparkinsonian drugs, belladonna containing alkaloids (deadly nightshade, henbane, mandrake, jimsonweed), and certain mushrooms. Atropine and scopolamine are naturally occurring alkaloids that represent prototypical anticholinergic compounds.

Presentations of anticholinergic toxicity may take many guises. Most commonly, patients present after ingesting an overdose of medications that have anticholinergic properties. Antihistamine overdose (particularly diphenhydramine) is the most common presentation. In young children, unintentional ingestion of just a few pills with anticholinergic properties, such as orphenadrine, may cause significant toxicity.[1] The therapeutic use of hyoscyamine-containing agents to

TABLE 183-1 Anticholinergic Substances

Antihistamines	**Belladonna alkaloids, synthetic cogeners**
Ethanolamines	Atropine (Hyoscyamine)
Dimenhydrinate (Dramamine)	Belladonna alkaloid mixtures
Diphenhydramine (Benadryl)	Glycopyrrolate (Robinul)
Ethylenediamines	Homatropine (Dia-Quel, Malcotran)
Tripelennamine (Pyribenzamine)	Methscopolamine bromide (Pamine)
Alkylamines	Scopolamine hydrobromide (Hyoscine)
Chlorpheniramine (Teldrin)	**Cyclic antidepressants**
Piperazines	Amitriptyline hydrochloride (Elavil, Amitril, Endep)
Astemizole (Hismanal)	Desipramine hydrochloride (Norpramin, Pertofrane)
Terfenadine (Seldane)	Doxepin hydrochloride (Sinequan, Adapin)
Loratadine (Claritin)	Imipramine hydrochloride (Tofranil, Pramine)
Cyclizine (Marezine)	Nortriptyline hydrochloride (Aventyl, Pamelor)
Meclizine (Antivert)	Protriptyline hydrochloride (Vivactil)
Phenothiazines	Trimipramine (Surmontil)
Prochlorperazine (Compazine)	Maprotiline hydrochloride (Ludiomil)
Promethazine (Phenergan)	Zimelidine hydrochloride
Antiparkinsonian drugs	Fluoxetine (Prozac)
Benztropine mesylate (Cogentin)	Amoxapine (Asendin)
Biperiden (Akineton)	**Ophthalmic products**
Ethopropazine (Parsidol)	Atropine and scopolamine solutions
Trihexyphenidyl (Artane)	Cyclopentolate hydrochloride (Cyclogyl)
Procyclidine (Kemadrin)	Tropicamide (Mydriacyl)
Antipsychotics	**OTC medications (including antihistamines and belladonna alkaloids)**
Phenothiazines	Analgesics: Excedrin PM, Percogesic
Chlorpromazine (Thorazine)	Cold remedies: Actifed, Allerest, Coricidin, Dristan, Flavihist, Romex, Sine-Off
Thioridazine (Mellaril)	Hypnotics: Compoz, Sleep-Eze, Sominex
Perphenazine (Trilafon)	Menstrual products: Pamprin, Premesyn PMS
Nonphenothiazines	**Skeletal muscle relaxants**
Clozaril (Clozapine)	Orphenadrine citrate (Norflex)
Molindone (Moban)	Cyclobenzaprine hydrochloride (Flexeril)
Loxapine (Loxitane)	**Mushrooms**
Antispasmodics	*Amanita muscaria*
Clidinium bromide (Quarzan, Librax)	*Amanita pantherina*
Dicyclomine (Bentyl)	**Other**
Methantheline bromide (Banthine)	Diphenidol (Cephadol, Vontrol)
Propantheline bromide (Pro-Banthine)	
Tridihexethyl chloride (Pathilon)	
Plants	
Deadly nightshade	
Mandrake	
Jimsonweed	

Source: Adapted from Goldfrank LR (ed): *Goldfrank's Toxicologic Emergencies,* 7th ed. New York: McGraw Hill, 2002, with permission.

treat infant colic and the topical use of diphenhydramine-containing salves has also resulted in anticholinergic toxicity.[2,3] In the elderly, therapeutic doses of certain pharmaceuticals may produce particularly bothersome anticholinergic side effects.[4] The use of multiple medications with anticholinergic properties increases the likelihood of toxicity and may manifest itself as new-onset delirium.[5]

Another setting of anticholinergic toxicity is the intentional ingestion (or smoking) of belladonna alkaloid-containing plants. Group ingestion by adolescents is not uncommon and may result in multiple delirious patients presenting simultaneously to the ED.[6] Alkaloid plants are abused for their hallucinogenic effects.[7] Inadvertent poisoning from the ingestion of belladonna-contaminated herbal teas and Chinese traditional medicines has also been reported.[8,9] In recent years, adulteration of commonly abused drugs such as heroin or cocaine with scopolamine or atropine has been increasingly observed.[10,11] Such intoxications are suggested in drug-abusing patients who present with signs of anticholinergic toxicity. Such mixed presentations can be particularly challenging to diagnose and treat. Finally, systemic anticholinergic toxicity may sometimes result from the ophthalmologic instillation of anticholinergic mydriatic agents, especially in the elderly.[12]

PHARMACOLOGIC PROPERTIES

There are two major subtypes of cholinergic receptors: muscarinic receptors and nicotinic receptors. Muscarinic receptors are found pre-

dominantly on autonomic effector cells that are innervated by postganglionic parasympathetic nerves, some ganglia, and the brain (particularly the hippocampus, cortex, and thalamus). Nicotinic receptors are found at peripheral autonomic ganglia, neuromuscular junctions, and also the brain. Acetylcholine is the neurotransmitter that modulates both receptor types.

The term *anticholinergic* generally refers to drugs and plant toxins that act as muscarinic receptor antagonists. Muscarinic receptor antagonists block the binding of acetylcholine to muscarinic receptors and cause little blockade at nicotine receptor sites. The expected clinical effects from these drugs are modulated through disturbances in the parasympathetic nervous system (the peripheral effects) and the brain (the central effects).

Drug absorption can occur after ingestion, smoking, or ocular use. The rate of absorption varies depending on the drug and the route of exposure. Because cholinergic blockade slows gastric emptying and decreases intestinal motility, absorption and peak clinical effects are often delayed.

The signs and symptoms of anticholinergic toxicity are a result of both central and peripheral cholinergic blockade. The central anticholinergic syndrome refers to clinical presentation where the central effects of muscarinic receptor antagonism predominate.

Clinical manifestations associated with anticholinergic overdose may only be partly explained by muscarinic receptor blockade. Pharmacologically, many of these agents are impure, and toxicity after overdose is secondary to multiple pharmacologic mechanisms. For example, the clinical findings associated with tricyclic antidepressant (TCA) overdose are only partly characterized by anticholinergic effects (and vary considerably among different tricyclic agents). The most life-threatening complications of TCA overdose are a result of the sodium channel–blocking effects on the heart producing wide-complex tachydysrhythmias, not the anticholinergic effects.

CLINICAL PRESENTATION

Anticholinergic toxicity is characterized by both peripheral and central clinical features. The characteristic features of patients with anticholinergic toxicity can be remembered as

> **Dry as a bone**
> **Red as a beet**
> **Hot as Hades**
> **Blind as a bat**
> **Mad as a hatter**
> **Stuffed as a pipe**

Dry skin (especially dry axillae) and dry mucous membranes (e.g., dry mouth) are the typical peripheral clinical manifestations and are a result of decreased sweat gland and salivary gland secretions. The skin may be warm and flushed (red) from vasodilatation. Other typical peripheral features of muscarinic blockade include hypoactive or absent bowel sounds secondary to decreased peristalsis and gastrointestinal (GI) motility. A palpable bladder secondary to urinary retention may sometimes be appreciated.

Sinus tachycardia is usually present with a pulse rate typically ranging from 120 to 160 beats/min. More malignant dysrhythmias are less common. Ingestions of large amounts of diphenhydramine have been associated with wide-complex tachydysrhythmias, but this complication is believed to be caused by a sodium channel effect and not an anticholinergic effect.[13]

Dilated pupils are another typical feature, although this clinical finding is not invariably observed despite the presence of other anticholinergic signs. Delay in onset of mydriasis for 12 to 24 h may occur.

The central anticholinergic syndrome is characterized by a dramatic delirium. While this delirium is usually accompanied by the peripheral manifestations discussed above, clinical presentations vary, and tachycardia without delirium or delirium without tachycardia may occur.

Delirium is common and may be confused with other conditions. Anticholinergic delirium is characterized by restlessness, irritability, disorientation, confusion, agitation, auditory and visual hallucinations, and incoherent speech. A particular characteristic feature of anticholinergic delirium is a dysarthria manifested by a staccato speech pattern and difficult-to-comprehend speech. This may be exacerbated by severe dysphasia from decreased mucus secretion. High-pitched cries may sometimes be heard.

The anticholinergic toxic patient has great difficulty attending and interacting appropriately with environmental stimuli. Lilliputian (little people) hallucinations have been described in this setting. Repetitive picking at the bed clothes or imaginary objects is also characteristic. Patients may also exhibit jerking movements of the extremities, and seizure activity may occur.

Agitation-induced hyperthermia is a worrisome complication of anticholinergic toxicity, and its development may be significantly potentiated by decreased sweating and the inability to dissipate heat. A markedly elevated body temperature may lead to multisystem organ dysfunction, resulting in liver, kidney, and brain injury, and coagulopathy. In some cases, these changes may be irreversible.

Central excitation and depression may both occur, and the term "agitated depression" is often the best way to describe this presentation. Depression is usually associated with higher doses. Depressive features include lethargy, somnolence, and coma.

Fatalities associated with anticholinergic overdose are characterized by severe agitation, status epilepticus, hyperthermia, wide-complex tachydysrhythmias (usually from sodium channel–blocker effect), and cardiovascular collapse.

LABORATORY EVALUATION

Routine laboratory evaluation, including measurement of electrolytes, glucose, and pulse oximetry, should be checked in the presence of abnormal mental status. In most cases of isolated anticholinergic toxicity, these tests should be normal. Limited urine drugs-of-abuse screening generally does not detect anticholinergic agents, although some rapid screens may pick up tricyclic antidepressants. Comprehensive urine drug screens (usually performed by thin-layer chromatography) may detect certain antihistamines and phenothiazines, although such testing does not usually detect plant alkaloids, scopolamine, and atropine. A positive drug screen for an anticholinergic agent does not necessarily imply an overdose or supertherapeutic ingestion, as an ingestion of a therapeutic dose of an anticholinergic agents may result in a positive screen.

DIFFERENTIAL DIAGNOSIS

The differential diagnosis of anticholinergic toxicity includes life-threatening presentations such as viral encephalitis, Reye syndrome, head trauma, alcohol and sedative-hypnotic withdrawal, postictal state, other intoxications, neuroleptic malignant syndrome, and an acute psychiatric disorder. The difference between anticholinergic toxicity and sympathomimetic toxicity (e.g., cocaine toxicity or delirium tremens) can be subtle as patients with anticholinergic or sympathomimetic toxicity may develop tachycardia, mydriasis, and delirium. The presence of dry skin and the absence of bowel sounds suggest anticholinergic poisoning. At times, patients presenting with acute psychiatric disorders may have an abnormal mental status suggesting anticholinergic toxicity, but true delirium and attention deficits are much more characteristic of the latter condition. On occasion, other central nervous system processes, such as viral encephalitis, may also affect cholinergic outflow and produce similar anticholinergic clinical signs not related to a toxic exposure.[14]

TREATMENT

Treatment of anticholinergic toxicity includes observation, monitoring, and good supportive care. Temperature monitoring is essential. Gastrointestinal decontamination with activated charcoal may be warranted to decrease absorption. Although the American Academy of Clinical Toxicology position statement on the administration of activated charcoal is equivocal regarding the potential benefits of charcoal administration after 1 h from ingestion, the decreased gut motility associated with anticholinergic ingestions may warrant charcoal administration beyond this 1-h window. Studies assessing charcoal efficacy in this setting have not been performed.

Intravenous sodium bicarbonate should be used to treat wide-complex tachydysrhythmias. Class Ia agents should be avoided because of their own sodium channel blockade effect.

The major therapeutic challenge in the treatment of moderate to severe anticholinergic poisoning involves obtaining adequate control of the agitated individual. Inadequate sedation may lead to worsening hyperthermia, rhabdomyolysis, and traumatic injuries. Physical restraints may be required to gain initial control. **Sedation is strongly recommended.** Prolonged use of physical restraints in the struggling and agitated patient may lead to further complications.

The intravenous administration of a benzodiazepine such as lorazepam (2.5 mg IV) is an appropriate first-line therapy to sedate the agitated patient. Pharmacologically, this approach is not specific to reverse anticholinergic delirium. Some patients may be refractory to relatively large doses of benzodiazepines. Phenothiazines should be avoided because of their anticholinergic effects.

The routine use of physostigmine to reverse anticholinergic toxicity remains controversial, and its use has resulted in significant complications. Physostigmine is a tertiary ammonium compound that is a reversible acetylcholinesterase inhibitor (mechanistically related to the carbamate insecticides) that crosses the blood-brain barrier. Acetylcholinesterase inhibition results in acetylcholine accumulation that reverses both central and peripheral anticholinergic effects. While once part of the coma cocktail, physostigmine may aggravate dysrhythmias and seizures and must be used with caution. In particular, the use of physostigmine to treat overdose of drugs with concomitant sodium channel effects such as tricyclic antidepressants may lead to bradycardia and asystole. **Patients without clear evidence of anticholinergic poisoning should not receive physostigmine,** as administration of the antidote to patients without muscarinic receptor blockade may produce cholinergic toxicity and sludge symptoms.

A recent retrospective study comparing benzodiazepines and physostigmine for the treatment of anticholinergic poisoning showed that physostigmine controlled agitation in 96 percent of patients and reversed delirium in 87 percent of patients, while benzodiazepines only controlled agitation in 24 percent of patients and was unable to reverse delirium.[15] This study also showed that the patients treated with physostigmine had fewer complications and a shorter recovery time than did patients treated with benzodiazepines. There were no differences in the incidence of side effects between the two groups.

Physostigmine can be considered in cases of severe agitation and delirium, especially in cases necessitating physical restraints for control and not responsive to benzodiazepines. The dose of physostigmine is 0.5 to 2.0 mg IV, slowly administered over 5 min. When effective, a significant decrease in agitation may be apparent within 15 to 20 min. Because of rapid elimination, repeat doses may be necessary every 30 to 60 min. Patients receiving physostigmine should always be placed on a cardiac monitor and observed for signs of cholinergic excess (salivation, lacrimation, urination, and defecation). Although physostigmine has been used diagnostically, in cases of uncertain anticholinergic poisoning, such diagnostic challenge is not recommended.

Contraindications to physostigmine include asthma, nonpharmacologically mediated intestinal or bladder obstruction, cardiac conduction disturbances, and suspected concomitant sodium channel poisoning.

DISPOSITION

Patients with mild symptoms of anticholinergic toxicity can be discharged after 6 h of observation if their symptoms have resolved. More symptomatic patients usually require admission for at least 24 h. Because the half-life of physostigmine is generally shorter than the half-life of many anticholinergic agents and the reversal effect may dissipate and result in recurrent toxicity, **admission for continued observation is warranted in patients who have received this antidote.**

REFERENCES

1. Garza MB, Osterhoudt KC, Rutstein R: Central anticholinergic syndrome from orphenadrine in a 3 year old. *Pediatr Emerg Care* 16:97, 2000.
2. Reilly JF Jr, Weisse ME: Topically induced diphenhydramine toxicity. *J Emerg Med* 8:59, 1990.
3. Myers JH, Moro-Sutherland D, Shook JE: Anticholinergic poisoning in colicky infants treated with hyoscyamine sulfate. *Am J Emerg Med* 15: 532, 1997.
4. Tune LE: Anticholinergic effects of medication in elderly patients. *J Clin Psychiatr* 62(S21):11, 2001.
5. Feinberg M: The problems of anticholinergic adverse effects in older patients. *Drugs Aging* 3:335, 1993.
6. Tiongson J, Salen P: Mass ingestion of jimsonweed by eleven teenagers. *Del Med J* 70:471, 1998.
7. Francis PD, Clarke CF: Angel trumpet lily poisoning in five adolescents: Clinical findings and management. *J Paediatr Child Health* 35:93, 1999.
8. Chan TY: Anticholinergic poisoning due to Chinese herbal medicines. *Vet Hum Toxicol* 37:156, 1995.
9. Hsu CK, Leo P, Shastry D, et al: Anticholinergic poisoning associated with herbal tea. *Arch Intern Med* 155:2245, 1995.
10. Hamilton RJ, Perrone J, Hoffman R, et al: A descriptive study of an epidemic of poisoning caused by heroin adulterated with scopolamine. *J Toxicol Clin Toxicol* 38:597, 2000.
11. Weiner AL, Bayer MJ, McKay CA Jr, et al: Anticholinergic poisoning with adulterated intranasal cocaine. *Am J Emerg Med* 16:517, 1998.
12. Barker DB, Solomon DA: The potential for mental status changes associated with systemic absorption of anticholinergic ophthalmic medications: Concerns in the elderly. *DICP* 24:847, 1990.
13. Holger JS, Harris CR, Engebretsen KM: Physostigmine, sodium bicarbonate, or hypertonic saline to treat diphenhydramine toxicity. *Vet Hum Toxicol* 44:1, 2002.
14. Perrone J, Chu J, Stecker MM: Viral encephalitis masquerading as a fulminant anticholinergic toxidrome. *J Toxicol Clin Toxicol* 35:627, 1997.
15. Burns MJ, Linden CH, Graudins A, et al: A comparison of physostigmine and benzodiazepines for the treatment of anticholinergic poisoning. *Ann Emerg Med* 35:374, 2000.

METALS AND METALLOIDS

Heather Long

Lewis S. Nelson

Acute metal and metalloid toxicity is an uncommon clinical entity that can be a cause of significant morbidity and mortality if unrecognized and inappropriately treated. Because of their effects on numerous enzymatic systems in the body, the metals and metalloids often present with protean manifestations primarily affecting four systems: neurologic, gastrointestinal, hematologic, and renal. Effects on the endocrine and reproductive systems are less clinically apparent. It is important to recognize an initial "index case" to prevent others from being poisoned when the metal source is environmental or industrial (Table 184-1).

LEAD

Epidemiology

Lead is the most common cause of chronic metal poisoning and remains a major environmental contaminant. Elevated blood levels in children ages 1 to 5 years have been linked with these community characteristics: urban dwellings, dwellings built before 1974 (especially those built before 1946), poverty, non-Hispanic black race or ethnicity, and higher population density.[1,2] Data from phase 2 of the National Health and Nutritional Survey III for children ages 1 to 5 years indicate that an estimated 890,000 children have blood lead levels of 10 μg/dL or higher; this estimate represents a substantial decline in the prevalence of elevated blood lead levels since 1976.[3] This decline is attributed to bans on lead in household paints, gasoline, plumbing systems, food and drink cans, lead abatement programs, and the promulgation of standards for industrial use of lead.[1]

Elevated lead levels may have detrimental effects on intellectual development,[4] so lead toxicity remains a significant public health problem. Inorganic and organic forms of lead produce clinical toxicity. Inorganic lead affects the central and peripheral nervous systems, hematopoietic system, kidney, gastrointestinal tract, liver, myocardium, and reproductive capacity. With organic lead intoxication, central nervous system (CNS) effects predominate.

Inorganic Lead

PHARMACOLOGY Absorption is by the respiratory and gastrointestinal tracts, whereas skin absorption is negligible. Dietary deficien-

TABLE 184-1   Sources of Heavy Metals

Heavy Metal	Source
Lead	
Inorganic	Soldering; battery burning/reclamation, bronzing; brassmaking; glassmaking; ingesting ceramic lead glaze; stripping old paint, "deleading" homes; "moonshine" whiskey; liquids in improperly glazed pottery; contaminated herbal medications; indoor shooting ranges; ingestion of paint chips, lead-laden floor dust, lead foreign bodies; lead bullets in abdomen or joint spaces
	Workers at risk: jewelers, painters, lead burners and smelters, pipe cutters, pigment makers, printers, welders, pottery makers, radiator repair personnel, battery reclamation workers, construction workers
Organic	Leaded gasoline
Arsenic	
Inorganic [arsenite (As^{3+}), arsenate (As^{5+}) elemental]	Insecticides, rodenticides, herbicides, mining, smelting/refining, homeopathic medicines, kelp
Organic	Parasitical medicines (veterinary)
Gas (arsine)	Mining smelting/refining, semiconductor industry; made by mixing acids with arsenic-containing insecticides
Mercury	
Elemental	Battery and thermometer manufacture; sphygmomanometer repair; dentistry; jewelry and lamp manufacture; photography; mercury mining; manufacture of scientific instruments
Salts	Taxidermy; fur processing; tannery work; chemical laboratories; manufacture of explosives, fireworks, disinfectants, button batteries, inks, and vinyl chloride
Organic (methylmercury, ethylmercury, phenylmercury)	Contaminated seafood; embalming; manufacture of drugs, fungicides, bactericides, handling of insecticides; pesticides, coated seeds; manufacture of chloralkali; working with wood preservatives

cies in calcium, iron, copper, and zinc may contribute to increased gastrointestinal absorption in children. Absorption also occurs when retained lead bullets or shot are in contact with body fluids, such as synovial fluid. In the body, lead distributes into the blood, soft tissues, and bone. Greater than 90 percent of the total body lead is stored in bone, where it easily exchanges with the blood. Lead can be transferred across the placenta, a process exacerbated by increased bone turnover during pregnancy. Excretion of lead occurs slowly; the biologic half-life of lead in bone has been estimated to be 30 years.

PATHOPHYSIOLOGY   In the CNS, 1) lead injures astrocytes, with secondary damage to the microvasculature and resulting disruption of the blood-brain barrier, cerebral edema, and seizures; 2) decreases cyclic adenosine monophosphate and protein phosphorylation, which contribute to memory and learning deficits; and 3) alters calcium homeostasis, which leads to spontaneous neurotransmitter release. In the peripheral nervous system, nerves undergo primary segmental demyelination, followed by secondary axonal degeneration, primarily of the motor nerves. In the hematopoietic system, lead interferes with porphyrin metabolism, which may contribute to lead-induced anemia. Coexisting iron deficiency may act synergistically with lead toxicity to produce a more profound anemia and, in children, may be more important than lead as the cause of a microcytic anemia. Hemolytic anemia also occurs as a result of inhibition of red blood cell (RBC) pyrimidine 5′-nucleotidase, an enzyme responsible for clearing cellular RNA degradation products. On a blood peripheral smear, these products produce the RBC basophilic stippling sometimes seen in lead-poisoned patients.

In the kidney, acute lead toxicity affects the proximal tubule, producing Fanconi syndrome with aminoaciduria, glycosuria, phosphaturia, and renal tubular acidosis. Chronic effects include persistence of partial Fanconi's syndrome for 13 years or longer,[5] interstitial nephritis, and increased uric acid levels due to increased tubular reabsorption of urate. Chronic lead toxicity has been linked to gout, hypertension, and chronic renal failure.

Toxic hepatitis with mildly elevated transaminases, normal bilirubin, and normal alkaline phosphatase can occur. Lead-induced adverse effects on the reproductive system include increased fetal wastage, premature membrane rupture, depressed sperm counts, abnormal or nonmotile sperm, and sterility. Chronic lead toxicity can depress free thyroxine levels without producing clinical hypothyroidism.

CLINICAL FEATURES   The common signs and symptoms of acute, chronic, and delayed toxicity are listed in Table 184-2. Young children are more susceptible than adults to the effects of lead. Encephalopathy, a major cause of morbidity and mortality, may begin dramatically with seizures and coma or develop indolently over weeks to months with decreased alertness and memory progressing to mania, delirium, and cerebral edema.[6] It has developed in infants with blood lead levels (PbB) of 70 μg/dL or lower. Gastrointestinal and hematologic manifestations occur more frequently with acute than with chronic poisoning, and the colicky abdominal pains may be associated with concurrent hemolysis. Patients may complain of a metallic taste and, with long-term exposure, have bluish-gray gingival lead lines. Lead toxicity also causes constitutional symptoms, including arthralgias, generalized

TABLE 184-2   Common Signs and Symptoms of Lead Poisoning

System	Clinical Manifestations
Central nervous system	Acute: encephalopathy, seizures, altered mental status, papilledema, optic neuritis, ataxia
	Chronic: headache, irritability, depression, fatigue, mood and behavioral changes, memory deficit, sleep disturbance
Peripheral nervous system	Paresthesias, motor weakness (classic wrist drop) depressed or absent DTRs, sensory function intact
Gastrointestinal	Abdominal pain (mostly with acute poisoning), constipation, diarrhea
Renal	Acute: Fanconi syndrome (aminoaciduria, glucosuria, phosphaturia) renal tubular acidosis
	Chronic: interstitial nephritis, renal insufficiency, hypertension, gout
Hematologic	Hypoproliferative and/or hemolytic anemia; basophilic stippling (rare and nonspecific)
Reproductive	Decreased libido, impotence, sterility, abortions, premature births, decreased or abnormal sperm production

Abbreviation: DTRs = deep tendon reflexes.

weakness, and weight loss. Delayed cognitive development can occur in infants and children whose cord and PbB levels are 10 μg/dL or higher. Adult and pediatric patients may be asymptomatic in the face of significantly elevated PbB levels.

DIAGNOSIS   History of an exposure, occupational, hobby, environmental, or related to retained lead bullets, is the most important clue to making the diagnosis. The physician should focus on symptoms, developmental and dietary histories (in children), pica, any house or daycare remodeling, previous serum iron and PbB levels, and possible lead toxicity in other family members. Occupational and hobby histories should be elicited for adults being evaluated and for children who may be exposed to lead secondarily from these adult activities.

The combination of abdominal or neurologic dysfunction with a hemolytic anemia should raise the suspicion of lead toxicity. Emergency physicians should consider the diagnosis in all children presenting with encephalopathy. Toxicity due to retained lead bullets has manifested in patients as long as several decades after being shot. Hyperthyroidism, pregnancy, fever, re-injury, or immobilization of the affected extremity can promote lead release after years of dormancy.

Laboratory studies in the ED should focus on evaluation for anemia and examination of bone radiographs in children for "lead bands" and abdominal radiographs for radiopaque material consistent with lead in the GI tract. The anemia can be normocytic or microcytic, possibly with evidence of hemolysis, such as an elevated reticulocyte count and increased serum-free hemoglobin.

Anemia and basophilic stippling occur variably, and their absence does not rule out lead toxicity. Basophilic stippling of RBCs is nonspecific for lead toxicity, because it is also found in arsenic toxicity, sideroblastic anemia, and the thalassemias. In children, radiographs of long bones, especially of the knee, may reveal horizontal, metaphyseal lead bands, which represent failure of bone remodeling rather than deposition of lead.

The definitive diagnosis rests on finding an elevated PbB, with or without symptoms. The PbB level is the best single test for evaluating lead toxicity, and levels of 10 μg/dL or higher are considered toxic. Screening levels may be performed on fingerstick capillary blood, but, because of the potential for environmental lead contamination, elevated levels always should be confirmed on a venous blood sample.[7] A calcium disodium edetate (CaNa^{2+}-EDTA) provocation test was used previously to evaluate total body lead stores and the need for chelation therapy when PbB levels were between 25 and 55 μg/dL, but it is no longer recommended. Also, with the lowering of the toxic PbB level to 10 μg/dL or lower, the erythrocyte protoporphyrin test can no longer be used to screen for lead toxicity, because of its unacceptably low sensitivity at these lower PbB levels.

DIFFERENTIAL DIAGNOSIS   The differential diagnosis of lead toxicity includes causes of encephalopathy, such as Wernicke encephalopathy, withdrawal from ethanol and other sedative-hypnotic drugs, meningitis, encephalitis, human immunodeficiency virus infection, intracerebral hemorrhage, hypoglycemia, severe fluid and electrolyte imbalances, hypoxia, arsenic, thallium, and mercury toxicity, and poisoning with cyclic antidepressants, anticholinergic drugs, ethylene glycol, or carbon monoxide. The abdominal pains can mimic sickle cell crisis or the hepatic porphyrias. Chronic lead toxicity can masquerade as depression, neurosis, hypothyroidism, polyneuritis, gout, iron deficiency anemia, and learning disability.

TREATMENT   All patients with appropriate symptoms and an elevated PbB level are classified as lead toxic and should be treated.

Severe Toxicity   Lead-induced encephalopathy rarely occurs now, but it remains a major cause of serious morbidity and mortality. In severely toxic patients, standard life-support measures should be instituted and seizures treated with benzodiazepines, phenobarbital, and general anesthesia, if necessary. If abdominal films demonstrate radiopaque flecks consistent with lead, whole-bowel irrigation with a polyethylene glycol electrolyte solution should be instituted. The solution should be administered PO at a rate of 500 to 2000 mL/h for adults and 100 to 500 mL/h for children until the abdominal radiograph is clear. It will not alter fluid or electrolyte balance in the patient. Larger lead bodies, such as fishing sinkers, may require surgical removal. IV fluid administration should be controlled carefully to avoid worsening cerebral edema. Lumbar puncture may precipitate cerebral herniation and should be performed carefully, if at all, with the removal of a small amount of cerebrospinal fluid only.

Chelation therapy (Table 184-3) should be instituted immediately (i.e., in the emergency department) before obtaining laboratory verification of the diagnosis, if lead encephalopathy is suspected.

TABLE 184-3   Chelation Therapy for Lead-Poisoned Patients: Indications, Dosing, and Side Effects*

Severity, PbB (μg/dL)	Dose	Side Effects

Encephalopathy	BAL 75 mg/m^2 IM q4h × 5 d
	and
	CaNa^{2+}-EDTA 1500 mg/m^2/d, for 5 d
	  as continuous IV infusion, or
	  as 2–4 divided IV doses per d
	  start 4 h after BAL
		BAL: hypertension, febrile reaction, painful injection, GI Sx, headache, lacrimation, rhinorrhea, hemolysis in G6PD-deficient patients
		CaNa$_2$-EDTA: renal toxicity (especially if dehydrated) dermatitis, headache, fever/chills, myalgias

Symptomatic
  PbB >100 (adults)
  PbB >70 (children)
	BAL 50–75 mg/m^2 IM q4h × 3–5 d
	and
	CaNa^{2+}-EDTA 1500 mg/m^2/d, for 5 d
	  as continuous IV infusion, or
	  as 2–4 divided IV doses per d
	  start 4 h after BAL
		As above

Mild symptoms or
  PbB 70–100 (adults)
Asymptomatic with
  PbB 45–69 (children)
	DMSA 350 mg/m^2 PO TID × 5 d, then BID × 14 d	DMSA: GI Sx, rash, pruritus, sore throat, rhinorrhea, drowsiness, paresthesias, transient elevations in AST and alkaline phosphatase, thrombocytosis, eosinophilia

Asymptomatic
  PbB <70 (adults)
  PbB <45 (children)
	Routine chelation not indicated
	Remove from source	

*Although the same agents are indicated for poisoning by other metals, see the text or call regional poison centers for specifics and dosing.

Abbreviations: AST = aspartate aminotransferase; BAL = British anti-Lewisite; CaNa^{2+}-EDTA = edetate calcium disodium; div = divided; DMSA = 2,3-dimercaptosuccinic acid, (succimer); G6PD = glucose-6-phosphate dehydrogenase; GI Sx = nausea, vomiting, diarrhea, abdominal pain; PbB = blood lead level.

For symptomatic patients without encephalopathy and for asymptomatic patients with elevated PbB levels requiring chelation, the use of British anti-Lewisite (BAL) or succimer (2,3-dimercaptosuccinic acid, DMSA) with or without CaNa^{2+}-EDTA and the dosing schedules are determined by the PbB levels, the presence or absence of symptoms, and changing practice as more experience with DMSA is obtained. A retrospective study of 45 children with lead levels of 45 μg/dL or higher treated with BAL plus EDTA or DMSA plus EDTA found comparable reductions in lead levels, with fewer side effects in the DMSA group.[8] The Centers for Disease Control and Prevention recommend immediate chelation therapy for children with blood lead levels of 70 μg/dL or higher.[7] In asymptomatic patients, the standards for determining lead toxicity and the need for treatment differ for children and adults (see Table 184-3).

In patients in whom the lead level is elevated on a capillary stick sample, it is best to await verification on blood, unless the clinical presentation strongly supports lead toxicity.

Like all chelating agents, the two oral chelating agents used to treat lead toxicity provide sulfhydryl groups to which the lead attaches. DMSA, an analogue of dimercaprol, effectively chelates lead in adults and children.[9,10] Its advantages include oral administration without increasing lead absorption from the GI tract, no serious adverse effects, and minimal chelation of essential metals. High cost is its main disadvantage. Repeat treatment may be necessary after a 2-week drug-free period. D-Penicillamine is a less effective chelating agent but is inexpensive. It has been used for outpatient therapy in asymptomatic children and adults with mild PbB elevations.

DISPOSITION Removal of the source of lead is mandatory for all patients. Patients should not be discharged to their former environments until appropriate deleading and decontamination measures have been accomplished. Family members and coworkers should be evaluated for occult lead toxicity.

A guide for hospitalization includes:

1. All children with symptoms or with a PbB level ≥70 μg/dL
2. All adults with CNS symptoms
3. All patients with suspected toxicity when returning to the environment is considered dangerous

PROGNOSIS Approximately 85 percent of patients who suffer encephalopathy develop permanent CNS damage, including seizures, mental retardation in children, and cognitive deficits in adults. Abdominal colic usually subsides within days after beginning chelation therapy, and other acute manifestations clear within 1 to 16 weeks with therapy. Lead-induced nephropathy may be partly reversible with chelation therapy.

Organic Lead

Exposure to tetraethyl lead, found in leaded gasoline, can occur with gasoline sniffing or in the occupational setting. Tetraethyl lead is metabolized to inorganic lead and triethyl lead. Triethyl lead is the primary toxic product that produces predominantly CNS toxicity. Symptoms range from behavioral changes with irritability, insomnia, restlessness, and nausea and vomiting to tremor, chorea, convulsions, and mania. Muscle, hepatic, and renal damage can occur. Anemia and elevated erythrocyte protoporphyrin levels usually are not found. Blood lead levels may be normal or elevated. Therapy consists of removal from the source, symptomatic treatment, and chelation only if the PbB level is elevated. Sequelae include dementia, mental status alterations, and persistent organic psychosis.

ARSENIC

Arsenic is a nearly tasteless, odorless metal; it is the most common cause of acute metal poisoning and the second leading source of chronic metal toxicity. Arsenicals are found in a variety of compounds and industries (see Table 184-1) and continue to be used as tools for homicides and suicides.

Elemental, inorganic and organic salts, and gaseous forms exist. Elemental and organic forms have little to no toxicity and will not be discussed further. Inorganic compounds include arsenite (As^{3+}) and arsenate (As^{5+}). These compounds are the most toxic forms, and the following discussion focuses on inorganic arsenic toxicity. Arsine, a gaseous form, has toxicopathologic mechanisms and treatment that differ from those of other arsenical compounds. It is discussed under a separate heading.

Pharmacology

Arsenic is well absorbed by the gastrointestinal, respiratory, and parenteral routes and may be absorbed through damaged skin. Owing to its water solubility, pentavalent arsenic (arsenate) is more readily absorbed through mucous membranes, for example, the gastrointestinal tract, than is trivalent arsenic (arsenite). Arsenite penetrates the skin more readily due to its increased lipid solubility. After absorption, arsenic localizes in erythrocytes and leukocytes or binds to serum proteins. Within 24 h, redistribution into the liver, kidney, spleen, lung, gastrointestinal tract, muscle, and nervous tissues occurs with subsequent integration into hair, nails, and bone. Elimination from the blood is rapid, and excretion is predominantly renal.[11] Toxicity of the various forms is partly determined by excretory rates, with the more toxic arsenite being excreted at a slower rate than arsenate or the organic arsenical compounds. Arsenic crosses the placenta and has produced teratogenicity in animals and humans.

Pathophysiology

Arsenic reversibly binds with sulfhydryl groups found in many tissues and enzyme systems. Acute exposure produces dilation and increased permeability of small blood vessels, resulting in gastrointestinal mucosal and submucosal inflammation and necrosis, cerebral edema and hemorrhage, myocardial tissue destruction, and fatty degeneration of the liver and kidneys. Subacute or chronic exposure can cause a primary peripheral axonal neuropathy with secondary demyelination.

Clinical Features

The signs and symptoms of toxicity vary with the form, amount, and concentration ingested and the rates of absorption and excretion of the various arsenical compounds. Arsenite is more toxic than arsenate. Symptoms usually occur within 30 min to several hours of ingestion. Severe gastroenteritis with nausea, vomiting, and cholera-like diarrhea is the hallmark of acute poisoning and may last several days to weeks, frequently necessitating hospitalization. Patients may complain of a metallic taste. Hypotension and tachycardia secondary to volume depletion, capillary leak, and myocardial dysfunction occur in moderate to severe cases. The electrocardiogram may demonstrate nonspecific ST-segment and T-wave changes with a prolonged QT$_c$, although these findings are more common in chronic intoxication. Ventricular tachycardia with a torsades de pointes morphology has been reported.[12] Secondary myocardial ischemia may occur, leading to an erroneous diagnosis of primary myocardial infarction. Acute encephalopathy, pulmonary edema, acute renal failure, rhabdomyolysis, and death may ensue.

Patients with subacute or chronic toxicity typically present with complaints of peripheral neuropathy, skin rash, or nonspecific malaise and weakness, often with a history of gastroenteritis occurring 1 to 6 weeks earlier. Survivors of acute poisonings can develop the same problems. The peripheral neuropathy develops in a stocking-glove distribution and is initially sensory, with motor symptoms developing later. Patients with severe poisoning can develop an ascending paralysis mimicking Guillain-Barré syndrome. The dermatologic manifestations vary. Hyperpigmentation, hyperkeratosis of the palms and soles, morbilliform rash, and epidermoid cancer have been reported. Mees lines (1- to 2-mm-wide transverse white lines in the nails) may be seen 4 to 6 weeks after an acute ingestion. Perforation of the nasal septum has been found in workers exposed occupationally to arsenic. Patients may complain of weakness, muscle aches, abdominal pain, memory loss, personality changes, periorbital and extremity edema, or decreased hearing secondary to sensorineural damage. Chronic encephalopathy with delirium, hallucinations, disorientation, agitation, and confabulation resembling Korsakoff syndrome has been reported. Chronic exposure to arsenic has been linked to the development of squamous cell and basal skin carcinomas, respiratory tract cancer, hepatic angiosarcoma, and possibly with leukemia.

Diagnosis

Without a history of known exposure to arsenic, the diagnosis must be based on the presenting signs and symptoms and a strong index of clinical suspicion. Physicians rarely encounter arsenic toxicity, and, unfortunately, criminal poisonings often go undetected. The diagnosis of **acute arsenic poisoning should be considered in any patient with hypotension of unknown etiology that was preceded by severe gastroenteritis.** The diagnosis of chronic arsenic toxicity should be considered in a patient with a peripheral neuropathy, typical skin manifestations, or recurrent bouts of unexplained gastroenteritis.

An abdominal radiograph may demonstrate intestinal radiopaque metallic flecks in cases of arsenic ingestions.[13] The complete blood cell count may reveal a normocytic, normochromic, or megaloblastic anemia and/or a thrombocytopenia. The white blood cell count may be elevated in acute toxicity and decreased in chronic toxicity. A relative eosinophilia, up to 21 percent, and basophilic stippling of the RBCs have been reported. Elevated reticulocyte counts are found in cases with a component of hemolytic anemia. The electrocardiogram often reveals a prolonged QT_c interval, especially in chronic poisoning.

Definitive diagnosis of acute poisoning depends on finding elevated arsenic levels in a 24-h urine collection. All urinary measurements of metals should be collected in metal-free containers after a 5-day seafood-free diet. Normal urinary arsenic level is below 0.05 mg/L, and total urinary arsenic excretion in an unexposed patient should not exceed 0.1 mg per d. If the baseline urinary level is within normal limits and arsenic intoxication is still suspected, hair and nail clippings should be harvested for laboratory analysis. Owing to the rapid distribution of arsenic in tissues, blood arsenic levels are unreliable. Toxicologic texts provide a detailed discussion of laboratory testing and interpretation of results in arsenic toxicity.

Arsenic toxicity should be included in the differential diagnosis for septic shock, encephalopathy, peripheral neuropathy (including Guillain-Barré syndrome), Addison disease, hypo- and hyperthyroidism, patients with the previously mentioned dermatologic manifestations, Korsakoff syndrome, persistent gastroenteritis and/or cholera-like diarrhea, porphyria, other metal toxicities such as thallium and mercury, and unexplained, prolonged malaise and weakness.

Treatment

Acute arsenical toxicity is a life-threatening illness requiring aggressive management. The first task is to ensure adequate respiratory and circulatory function. Hypotension and dysrhythmias are the chief causes of death. Hypotension, usually due to volume depletion, should be managed initially with crystalloid volume replacement. Invasive hemodynamic monitoring followed by further crystalloid and pressor therapy with dopamine or norepinephrine may be required. Overhydration should be avoided, because pulmonary and cerebral edema can occur. Cardiac monitoring should be instituted. Ventricular tachycardia and fibrillation may be treated with lidocaine, amiodarone, and

electrical defibrillation, as necessary. Isoproterenol, magnesium, and overdrive pacing therapies should be considered for torsades de pointes. Drugs that prolong the QT_c, including classes IA (procainamide, quinidine, disopyramide), IC, and III antidysrhythmics, should be avoided. Potassium, calcium, and magnesium levels should be monitored and corrected as necessary to prevent further prolongation of the QT_c and torsades de pointes dysrhythmias.

Gastric lavage with a large-bore orogastric tube should be performed in all cases of acute ingestion, and activated charcoal (1 g/kg of body weight) and a cathartic should be instilled. Activated charcoal poorly adsorbs arsenic but may be effective if coingestants were taken. Whole-bowel irrigation should be considered if abdominal radiographs reveal intestinal radiopaque materials consistent with arsenic. Seizures can be treated with benzodiazepines, phenobarbital, and general anesthesia as necessary.

Initial management of chronic toxicity should be directed toward prevention of further arsenic absorption and gastrointestinal decontamination, if appropriate. In cases of suspected homicidal intent, patients should be advised to avoid food and drinks prepared by others, and visitor contact with hospitalized patients should be monitored carefully.

Chelation therapy with BAL should be instituted immediately in all cases of known or suspected acute arsenical poisoning. British anti-Lewisite is dosed 3 to 5 mg/kg IM every 4 h for 2 days, followed by 3 to 5 mg/kg every 6 to 12 h. In severe, life-threatening toxicity, BAL therapy should be continued until the clinical condition stabilizes and DMSA, the less toxic oral chelating agent, can be substituted. In cases of suspected chronic toxicity with stable symptoms, therapy may be withheld pending diagnosis. DMSA is the preferred chelating agent in these patients.[14] It is given according to the dosing regimen for lead, but therapy may be required beyond the initial 19-day regimen. D-Penicillamine does not effectively chelate arsenic and should not be used.[15] During chelation, intermittent 24-h urinary arsenic levels should be measured and therapy continued until the urine level falls below 0.05 mg/L per d. Hemodialysis can remove small amounts of arsenic (2 to 4.5 mg) in patients with acute renal failure but is not indicated otherwise.[16]

Hospitalization Guidelines

Hospitalization should be considered in:

1. All patients with acute or life-threatening known or suspected arsenic poisoning
2. All chronically poisoned patients requiring BAL therapy
3. All patients in whom suicidal or homicidal intent is suspected

Disposition

In acute toxicity, prognosis may be influenced favorably by the rapid institution of BAL therapy. Recovery from arsenical neuropathy appears to be related more to initial severity of symptoms than to institution of chelation therapy, although, in those patients who do recover, BAL appears to significantly shorten the duration of illness. Often, neurologic recovery occurs slowly over months to years. Normalization of hematologic values can occur in the absence of any specific therapy. British anti-Lewisite has a variable effect on the dermatologic manifestations; hyperpigmentation is unresponsive to this therapy.

ARSINE

Arsine is a colorless, nonirritating gas encountered in the semiconductor industry, ore smelting, and refining processes and is produced when arsenic-containing insecticides are mixed with acids. Arsine attaches to sulfhydryl groups of hemoglobin, producing an acute hemolytic anemia with resulting jaundice, abdominal pain, and hemoglobinuria-induced acute renal failure. Acute poisonings are managed with blood transfusions, exchange transfusion to remove the non-dialyzable arsine, and hemodialysis for the acute renal failure. British anti-Lewisite therapy has no role in the management of arsine toxicity.

MERCURY

Mercury occurs in inorganic and organic forms. Inorganic compounds are divided further into elemental mercury and mercurous and mercuric salts. Organic mercurials exist as short- and long-chained alkyl and aryl compounds. The short-chained alkyls, such as methyl mercury and ethyl mercury, are more toxic to humans, with dimethylmercury being lethal in small amounts.[17] All forms of mercury are toxic but differ in the routes of absorption, constellations of clinical findings, and responses to therapy. Sources are listed in Table 184-1.

Pharmacology

Elemental mercury is absorbed primarily by inhalation of its vapor but also may be absorbed dermally. Absorption by the GI tract is usually negligible. Intramuscular injections of mercury can induce abscess and granuloma formation; delayed systemic toxicity can occur.[18] Intravenous injections have produced mercury pulmonary and systemic emboli. Elemental mercury crosses the blood-brain barrier, where it is ionized and trapped in the CNS.

Mercuric salts and organic mercury are absorbed primarily through the gastrointestinal tract, with the short-chained alkyl organic compounds being better absorbed than the aryl organic compounds. Mercuric salts are deposited in the ionized form primarily in the kidney and then in the liver and spleen. The salts do not enter the CNS in consequential amounts.

With organic mercury compounds, the highly lipid-soluble short-chained alkyls easily cross membranes, accumulating in RBCs, the CNS, liver, kidney, and the fetus. Longer-chained alkyl and the aryl compounds are biotransformed into inorganic mercuric ions in the body. Therefore, toxicity with these compounds more closely resembles inorganic mercury toxicity.

Inorganic and the aryl organic mercurials are eliminated in the urine and feces. The short-chained alkyl compounds are excreted primarily in the bile, where they undergo significant enterohepatic circulation.

Pathophysiology

Mercury binds with sulfhydryl groups, affecting a diverse number of enzyme and protein systems. Methyl mercury also inhibits choline acetyl transferase, which catalyzes the final step in the production of acetylcholine, and may produce an acetylcholine deficiency. Mercuric salts produce proximal renal tubular necrosis.

Clinical Features

The clinical effects of mercury poisoning depend on the form and, in some cases, the route of administration. In general, the neurologic, gastrointestinal, and renal systems are predominantly affected. The short-chained alkyl compounds, methyl, dimethyl, and ethyl mercury, have the most devastating effects on the CNS, followed by elemental mercury, whose primary toxicity is neurologic. Both forms of mercury produce erethism, a constellation of neuropsychiatric abnormalities, including anxiety, depression, irritability, mania, sleep disturbances, excessive shyness, and memory loss. Tremor, either intention or non-intention, is a common physical finding.[19] The short-chained alkyls produce paresthesias (early sign), ataxia, muscular rigidity or spasticity, and visual and hearing impairment and induce CNS teratogenic effects. Gastrointestinal effects of elemental and short-chained alkyl compounds are mild. In cases of severe, chronic poisoning with elemental mercury, stomatitis, gingivitis, and excessive salivation are seen. Chronic toxicity of elemental and organic forms may cause renal

glomerular and tubular damage. Acute elemental mercury inhalation can produce pneumonitis, adult respiratory distress syndrome, and progressive pulmonary fibrosis with death.

In contrast, the mercury salts have little to no effect on the CNS but produce a severe corrosive gastroenteritis with abdominal pain that may be followed rapidly by cardiovascular collapse. Renal effects are typical, including acute tubular necrosis within 24 h. Children exposed to all forms of mercury, except the short-chained alkyls, can develop acrodynia, an immune-mediated condition characterized by a generalized rash, fever, irritability, splenomegaly, and generalized hypotonia with particular weakness of the pelvic and pectoral muscles.

Swallowing mercury contained in a glass thermometer (elemental mercury) usually does not produce adverse effects, because the mercury is not absorbed from the GI tract unless the tract is damaged or contains fistulas.

Diagnosis

A thorough history, including occupational exposures, and typical physical findings, especially tremor or a constellation of signs and symptoms suggesting erethism or acrodynia, may alert the emergency physician to mercury toxicity. Ingestion of mercuric chloride can produce a rapidly fatal course and should be considered in any patient presenting with a corrosive gastroenteritis. Often, however, the diagnosis of mercury toxicity is subtle, arrived at only after many other diagnoses have been investigated.

For all forms of mercury, except short-chained alkyls, a 24-h urinary measurement of mercury should be performed after a 5-day seafood-free diet. A seafood meal (contaminated with mercury) can temporarily elevate the blood level to the toxic range until the mercury is eliminated. Most unexposed individuals will have levels of 10 to 15 μg/L or lower. A level higher than 20 μg/dL before or after therapy indicates meaningful exposure. In cases of chronic toxicity, this measurement may be falsely low. Whole-blood mercury levels are less reliable diagnostically.

Short-chained alkyl mercury compounds are excreted predominantly by the bile, rendering urinary measurements invalid. Laboratory diagnosis rests on finding elevated whole-blood mercury levels, because these compounds concentrate in erythrocytes. Whole-blood mercury levels are normally lower than 1.5 μg/dL.

Magnetic resonance imaging findings in methyl mercury toxicity from ingestion of contaminated seafood include marked atrophy of the visual cortex, cerebellar vermis and hemispheres, and the postcentral cortex.[20]

The differential diagnosis of mercury toxicity depends on the form ingested. Hypothyroidism, apathetic hyperthyroidism, metabolic encephalopathy, senile dementia, adverse effects of therapeutic drugs (such as lithium, theophylline, phenytoin), Parkinson disease, delayed neuropsychiatric sequelae of carbon monoxide poisoning, lacunar infarction, cerebellar degenerative disease or tumor, and ethanol or sedative-hypnotic drug withdrawal may produce behavioral changes or tremor similar to those caused by elemental mercury. Causes of corrosive gastroenteritis, such as iron, arsenic, phosphorus, acids, or alkalis, should be considered in the differential diagnosis for mercury salts. Many of the differential diagnoses for elemental mercury also apply to the organic mercury compounds. Cerebral palsy, intrauterine hypoxia, and teratogenic effects of therapeutic and illicit drugs and environmental contaminants should be considered when evaluating an infant thought to be affected in utero by the short-chained alkyl mercury compounds.

Treatment

General therapeutic measures include removal from exposure and supportive therapy. Ingestion of mercury salts should be treated with aggressive gastrointestinal decontamination, including gastric lavage and activated charcoal. Given the profuse diarrhea that may ensue, a cathartic may not be indicated. Neostigmine may improve motor function in methyl mercury-poisoned patients by improving acetylcholine levels.

British anti-Lewisite is the preferred chelator for mercury salts and is administered in a regimen of 5 mg/kg IM once, 2.5 mg/kg IM every 8 to 12 h for 1 day, and then 2.5 mg/kg IM every 12 to 24 h until clinical improvement occurs. Adjust the dosing regimen according to clinical response and development of adverse reactions. The BAL-mercury complex is dialyzable, and hemodialysis may be helpful in patients receiving BAL who have diminished renal function. Plasma exchange transfusion also was beneficial in a case of mercuric chloride ingestion.[21] British anti-Lewisite is contraindicated in methyl mercury poisoning owing to exacerbation of CNS symptoms. DMSA has demonstrated efficacy in binding mercury, including organic forms, and may become the treatment of choice for the short-chained alkyl compounds.[22] It is given as a second agent after gastrointestinal decontamination in cases of severe poisoning and is the chelator of choice in cases of chronic or mild toxicity. The dose of DMSA is 10 mg/kg PO every 8 h for 5 days and then every 12 h for 14 days.

Hospitalization Guidelines

1. All patients known or suspected of ingesting mercury salts
2. All patients known to have or suspected to have inhaled elemental mercury vapor with pulmonary injury
3. All patients requiring BAL therapy

Disposition

Outcome depends on the form of mercury and the severity of toxicity. Mild cases of elemental and mercury salt poisoning and very mild cases of organic mercury toxicity may result in complete recovery. Death can occur in severe cases of mercuric chloride poisoning and

TABLE 184-4   Miscellaneous Metal Poisoning: Unique Manifestations and Treatments of Patients Poisoned by Less Common Metals

Metal	Poisoning Source	Acute Clinical Manifestations*	Chronic Clinical Manifestations	Specific Treatment†
Bismuth	Antidiarrheals (bismuth subsalicylate), impregnated surgical packing paste	Abdominal pain, acute renal failure	Myoclonic encephalopathy	BAL (limited evidence)
Cadmium	Contaminated soil in cadmium-rich areas; alloys used in welding, soldering, jewelry, and batteries	Ingestion: GI symptoms Inhalation: pneumonitis, acute lung injury	Proteinuria, osteomalacia, ?lung cancer	Ingestion: DMSA (limited evidence; not generally indicated) Pneumonitis: chelation NOT indicated
Cobalt	"Hard metal dust" (tungsten–cobalt mixture), flexible magnets, drying agents	Contact dermatitis, asthma	Hard-metal lung disease (spectrum ranging from alveolitis to fibrosis), cardiomyopathy, hypothyroidism	NAC (animal studies suggest efficacy as chelator)
Copper	Leaching from copper pipes and containers; fungicide (copper sulfate); welding (copper oxide)	Ingestion: resembles iron poisoning; blue vomitus (copper salts), hepatotoxicity, hemolysis, methemoglobinemia Inhalation: metal fume fever (fever, chills, cough, dyspnea)	Hepatotoxicity (Indian childhood cirrhosis)	Chelation with intramuscular BAL if hepatic or hematologic toxicity
Chromium	Corrosion inhibitors (e.g., heating systems), pigment production	Skin irritation and ulceration, contact dermatitis; GI irritation, renal and hepatic failure	Mucous membrane irritation, perforation of nasal septum ("chrome holes") eczema, lung cancer	Topical 10% ascorbic acid for skin ulcers
Silver	Colloidal (metallic) silver used for medicinal purposes as oral solutions, aerosols, and douches; cauterizing and antiseptic agent (silver nitrate); jewelry, wire	Mucosal irritation (silver oxide and nitrate)	Argyria (skin discoloration due to silver deposition and melanocyte stimulation)	No effective chelator
Thallium	Rodenticides (use prohibited in U.S.); contaminated herbal products; medical radioisotope (miniscule dose); most poisonings related to homicide	Early: GI Sx, constipation Delayed (>24 h): painful ascending neuropathy, cardiac dysrhythmias, AMS Delayed (2 wk): alopecia	Sensorimotor neuropathy, psychosis, dermatitis, hepatotoxicity	MDAC Prussian blue: 125 mg/kg PO bid (not FDA approved)
Zinc	Smelting, electroplating, military smoke bombs, zinc lozenges, welding/galvanizing (zinc oxide)	Ingestion: resembles iron poisoning Inhalation: mucosal irritation, metal fume fever (zinc oxide)	Copper deficiency, sideroblastic anemia, neutropenia	Chelation with CaNa^{2+}-EDTA

*Metal salts typically cause early gastrointestinal irritation (nausea, vomiting, diarrhea, cramping, hemorrhage) with subsequent neurologic, renal, hematologic, and cutaneous abnormalities.

†Treatment universally involves removal of the patient from the source, topical decontamination, administration of activated charcoal (if metal ingested), and supportive care, including aggressive fluid and electrolyte repletion and hemodialysis, if required. Indications for chelation and its efficacy in treating metal toxicity vary with the specific metal. Consult with medical toxicologist or regional poison center for specific indications and drug doses.

Abbreviations: AMS = altered mental status; BAL = British anti-Lewisite; CaNa^{2+}-EDTA = calcium disodium edetate; DMSA = 2,3-dimercaptosuccinic acid; FDA = U.S. Food and Drug Administration; GI Sx = gastrointestinal symptoms which include but are not limited to nausea, vomiting, diarrhea, cramping; MDAC = multiple doses of activated charcoal; NAC = *N*-acetylcysteine.

with dimethylmercury exposure. Most patients with organic mercury poisoning are left with residual neurologic deficits.

OTHER METALS AND METAL SALTS

Table 184-4 lists some of the other more commonly encountered metals and metal salts, their associated toxicity, and treatment specifics. Treatment universally involves removal of the patient from the source, topical decontamination, administration of activated charcoal (if metal has been ingested), and supportive care, including aggressive fluid and electrolyte repletion and hemodialysis, if required. Indications for chelation and its efficacy in treating metal toxicity vary with the specific metal (see Table 184-4). Consult with a medical toxicologist or a regional poison center for specific indications and drug doses.

REFERENCES

1. Update: Blood lead levels—United States, 1991–1994. *MMWR* 46:141, 1997.
2. Lanphear BP, Roghmann KJ: Pathways of lead exposure in urban children. *Environ Res* 74:67, 1997.
3. Pirkle JL, Brody DJ, Gunter EW, et al: The decline of blood lead levels in the United States: The National Health and Nutrition Examination Surveys. *JAMA* 272:284, 1994.
4. Tong S, Baghurst P, McMichael A, et al: Lifetime exposure to environmental lead and children's intelligence at 11–13 years: The Port Pirie cohort study. *BMJ* 312:1569, 1996.
5. Loghman-Adham M: Aminoaciduria and glycosuria following severe childhood lead poisoning. *Pediatr Nephrol* 12:218, 1998.
6. al Khayat A, Menon NS, Alidina MR: Acute lead encephalopathy in early infancy: Clinical presentation and outcome. *Ann Trop Paediatr* 17:39, 1997.
7. Centers for Disease Control and Prevention: *Screening Young Children for Lead Poisoning: Guidance for State and Local Public Health Officials.* Atlanta: Centers for Disease Control and Prevention, 1997.
8. Besunder JB, Super DM, Anderson RL: Comparison of dimercaptosuccinic acid and calcium disodium ethylene diaminetetraacetic acid versus demercaptopropanol and ethylene diaminetetraacetic acid in children with lead poisoning. *J Pediatr* 130:966, 1997.
9. Graziano JH, Lolacono NJ, Moulton T: Controlled study of meso-2, 3-dimercaptosuccinic acid for the management of childhood lead intoxication. *J Pediatr* 120:133, 1992.
10. Lifshitz M, Hashkanazi R, Phillip M: The effect of 2,3-dimercaptosuccinic acid in the treatment of lead poisoning in adults. *Ann Med* 29:83, 1997.
11. McKinney JD: Metabolism and disposition of inorganic arsenic in laboratory animals and humans. *Environ Geochem Health* 14:43, 1992.
12. Beckman KJ, Bauman JL, Pimental PA, et al: Arsenic-induced torsades de pointes. *Crit Care Med* 19:290, 1991.
13. Hilfer RJ, Mandel A: Acute arsenic intoxication diagnosed by roentgenograms. *New Engl J Med* 266:663, 1962.
14. Muckter H, Liebl B, Reichl FX, et al: Are we ready to replace dimercaprol (BAL) as an arsenic antidote? *Hum Exp Toxicol* 16:460, 1997.
15. Kreppel H, Reichl FX, Forth W, Fichtl B: Lack of effectiveness of D-penicillamine in experimental arsenic poisoning. *Vet Hum Toxicol* 31:1, 1989.
16. Mathieu D, Mathieu-Nolf M, Germain-Alonso M, et al: Massive arsenic poisoning: Effect of hemodialysis and dimercaprol on arsenic kinetics. *Intens Care Med* 18:47, 1992.
17. Nierenberg DW, Nordgren RE, Chang MB, et al: Delayed cerebellar disease and death after accidental exposure to dimethylmercury. *New Engl J Med* 338:1672, 1998.
18. Dell-Omo M, Muzi G, Bernard A, et al: Long-term pulmonary and systemic toxicity following intravenous mercury injection. *Arch Toxicol* 72:59, 1997.
19. Taueg C, Sanfilippo DJ, Rowens B, et al: Acute and chronic poisoning from residential exposures to elemental mercury—Michigan 1989–1990. *J Toxicol Clin Toxicol* 30:63, 1992.
20. Korogi Y, Takahashi M, Okajima T, Eto K: MR findings of Minamata disease: Organic mercury poisoning. *J Magn Reson Imaging* 8:308, 1998.
21. Yoshida M, Satoh H, Igarashi M, et al: Acute mercury poisoning by intentional ingestion of mercuric chloride. *Tohoku J Exp Med* 182:347, 1997.
22. Roels HA, Boeckx M, Ceulemans E, et al: Urinary excretion of mercury after occupational exposure to mercury vapour and influence of the chelating agent meso-2,3-dimercaptosuccinic acid (DMSA). *Br J Indian Med* 48:247, 1991.

TOXICOLOGY OF HAZARDOUS CHEMICALS

Suzanne R. White

Col. Edward M. Eitzen, Jr.

Kelly R. Klein

INTRODUCTION

A *hazardous material* can be defined as any substance (chemical, nuclear, or biologic) that may pose a risk to health, safety, property, or the environment. There are currently over 627,000 potentially toxic chemicals and compounds listed in the most commonly used poisoning database, PoisIndex, and it is estimated that 600 new chemicals are introduced yearly into the workplace. Given the quantity (1.5 billion tons per year) and frequency of transport (500,000 shipments per day) of hazardous substances throughout the United States, it seems inevitable that the practicing emergency physician will be faced with the management of a chemically exposed or contaminated patient.[1]

The Hazardous Substances Emergency Events Surveillance (HSEES) database registered 24,359 hazardous chemical accidents during 1993–1997.[2] The number of events increased annually and is underestimated because petroleum products, which account for approximately 50 percent of hazardous materials spills, were not included. Other registries, such as the National Response Center, logged over 34,000 hazardous oil and chemical incidents during 2001 alone.[3] Eighty percent of events occur at fixed facilities, whereas 20 percent are transportation-related, and over 10 percent occur within hospitals and schools. Highest-risk industries include those involved in chemical manufacture (especially agricultural types), petroleum refining, electric light and power, and milling of pulp/paper.[4] Seventy percent of hazardous materials accidents occur Monday through Friday 6 A.M. to 6 P.M. Incidents typically result in one or two victims, usually employees (56 percent) and less frequently the general public (35 percent) and first responders (9 percent).[2] Of the 10 to 30 percent of incidents that involve victims, traumatic injury is common.[5,6] Nontraumatic injuries most commonly include respiratory and eye irritation, nausea, vomiting, headache, dizziness, or other neurologic effects. Sixty-five percent of fatalities following a hazardous materials incident result from trauma, 22 percent from burns, and 10 percent from respiratory compromise. Many deaths occur in agricultural workers. Most injuries and deaths are associated with exposures to chlorine, ammonia, nitrogen fertilizer, or hydrochloric acid. Other commonly involved chemicals include petroleum products, pesticides, corrosives, metals, and volatile organics. Unknown or unclassified chemicals constitute a full 25 percent of events.[2,7] It is important to note regarding hazardous materials victims that over 40 percent of the general public and 20 percent of employees are decontaminated at hospital emergency departments.[2]

As indicated by recent events, terrorist use of readily available hazardous substances has become a reality (see Chap. 8). Chemical disasters, whether they occur at industrial fixed-facility sites or are transportation-related or terrorist-mediated, share many features. They may involve mass casualties with serious concomitant injuries, such as trauma, burns, or smoke inhalation, that outstrip medical resources. Victims will arrive at the hospital without prior decontamination. Communication breakdown is prevalent, as is chaos among medical personnel who are unfamiliar with the agents involved, unaware of available resources, or have become contaminated secondarily. The need for emergency community and medical preparedness to mitigate the adverse consequences of such hazardous materials accidents cannot be overly stressed.

Preparedness steps for chemical disasters, and general principles of decontamination, are discussed in Chap. 8.

Following decontamination and the primary survey, a secondary survey should be carried out with attention to the identification of common hazardous materials toxidromes (Table 185-1). Table 185-2 lists some important dermally absorbed toxins that can result in systemic toxicity. Some agents result in delayed onset of symptoms and require 24 h of monitoring or more to identify complications. Some of these agents are listed in Tables 185-3 and 185-4. Patients with chemical contamination require special medical followup, depending on the nature of the contaminant. About 30 percent of those who are acutely symptomatic will have persistent symptoms at 2 weeks.[8] Victims of a hazardous materials incident may also experience posttraumatic stress disorder and psychological interventions can help prevent these delayed sequelae.

Children are uniquely sensitive to chemical exposures. The child's thinner stratum corneum results in increased skin permeability. A relatively greater surface area (approximately 2.5 times larger than that of adults on a pound-per-pound basis), greater fluid intake per body weight, and increased minute volume provide greater dermal, oral, and respiratory uptake of chemicals. Children are at greater risk than adults to develop methemoglobinemia when exposed to oxidant stresses based on low NADH methemoglobin reductase activity. Other factors rendering them more susceptible to toxins include lower oxygen-carrying capacity, owing to lower baseline hematocrits, and greater susceptibility to bronchospasm following exposure to inhaled toxins.[9] When wet, infants develop rapid hypothermia; therefore, special consideration for decontamination will need to be made with the use of warm liquids and control of ambient temperature. Finally, ocular irrigation is difficult in children. One method involves the use of a "papoose" followed by flooding the bridge of the nose with normal saline rather than the eyes directly.

This chapter discusses the pharmacology and toxicology of specific chemical agents: nerve agents (organophosphate-like substances); vesicants (blistering agents); respiratory toxins; metabolic toxins (including cyanide); riot-control agents; and incapacitating agents.

TABLE 185-1   Some Common Hazardous Materials Toxidromes

	NERVE AGENTS	VESICANTS	RESPIRATORY AGENTS
Substances	Tabun, Sarin, Soman, GF, VX	Lewisite, phosgene, nitrogen, and sulfur mustards	Phosgene, chlorine, vinyl chloride, nitrogen oxides, ammonia
Symptoms	Pinpoint pupils Eye pain Dyspnea, bronchospasm Muscle fasciculations Weakness Seizures, coma Tachycardia or bradycardia Diaphoresis Salivation Lacrimation Vomiting and diarrhea Abdominal cramps	Low doses cause vesicant response Skin erythema Skin blistering Cough and hoarseness Corneal ulcers Bronchospasm Sloughing of bronchial epithelium Phosgene: urticaria	Respiratory distress Pulmonary edema
Antidotes	Oxygen Atropine Pralidoxime (2-PAM) (See Chap. 182)	Supportive care Water irrigation BAL for Lewisite (See Chap. 179)	Possibly nebulized NaHCO3 for chlorine
	METABOLIC TOXINS	RIOT CONTROL AGENTS	INCAPACITATING AGENTS
Substances	Cyanides Hydrogen sulfide Carbon monoxide Ricin	Mace* Capsaicin (pepper spray)	BZ (3-quinucidinyl benzilate) Stimulants Potent opioids Hallucinogens Nausea producing drugs
Symptoms	Coma Seizures Death	Lacrimation Eye irritation Rhinorrhea Coughing, sneezing Bronchospasm	Non-lethal effects that prevent performance of duties
Antidotes	Cyanide kit for cyanides and hydrogen sulfide (see Chap. 188) 100% oxygen or hyperbaric oxygenation for CO (see Chap. 203)	Water irrigation Treat bronchospasm	Symptomatic treatment
	HYDROCARBONS		
Substances	Halogenated hydrocarbons Freons Aromatic hydrocarbons		
Symptoms	Confusion, lethargy Coma Cardiac dysrhythmias Freons: respiratory distress		
Antidotes	Symptomatic treatment Avoid sympathomimetic agents		

*Mace = omega-chloroacetophenone.

TABLE 185-2 Dermally Absorbed Agents Through Intact Skin Resulting in Systemic Toxicity

Acrylamide
Acrylonitrile, acetonitrile, propionitrile
Aniline
Chlordane
Dinitrophenol
Hydrocarbons: benzene, gasoline, toluene, toluene diisocyanate, xylene (all slowly absorbed)
Hydrogen cyanide, cyanide salts
Hydrogen fluoride (hydrofluoric acid)
Metals (organic mercury, thallium)
Methyl bromide
Methylene chloride (slow)
Nerve agents
Nitrates
Nitrobenzene
Pesticides
Phenol
T2 toxin (biological)
Others: may be absorbed through abraded skin

NERVE AGENTS

The *nerve agents* and are currently the most toxic chemical threats known. These organophosphates were developed by the Germans around World War II, placed in munitions, yet never employed on the battlefield. Despite the cessation of chemical synthesis for military use, precursors are commonly found in industry. Five organophosphate compounds are recognized as nerve agents: tabun (GA), sarin (GB), soman (GD), GF (believed to be obsolete), and VX. Properties of these liquids vary in terms of vapor pressure, persistence in the environment, and potency. VX is the most potent and persistent with a potentially fatal exposure involving a skin area of only 2 to 3 mm in diameter. GB is the most volatile. The nerve agents are mildly irritating to the eyes, mucous membranes and respiratory tract with odors variably described as fruity (tabun), odorless (sarin, VX), or fruity/camphorous (soman) (Table 185-5).

The nerve agents are powerful inhibitors of acetylcholinesterase (AChE), found in nerve, skeletal muscle, glands, and other tissues innervated by cholinergic neurons. Additionally, red blood cell (RBC) cholinesterase and plasma pseudocholinesterase are inhibited and serve as laboratory markers of toxicity. The ability of nerve agents to interfere with normal acetylcholine hydrolysis at cholinergic synapses causes accumulation of this neurotransmitter and greatly enhanced neurotransmission. Excess acetylcholine at brain synapses, for example, results in seizures, coma, respiratory depression, and apnea. Acetylcholine accumulation at the motor endplate causes initial fasciculations with progression to weakness and paralysis. Overstimulation of sympathetic and parasympathetic ganglia of the peripheral nervous system results in tachycardia, hypertension, diaphoresis, miosis, lacrimation, salivation, bronchorrhea, bronchospasm, bradycardia, vomiting, diarrhea, and urination.

The onset and type of symptoms are determined by both concentration and route of exposure to nerve agents. Following sarin vapor inhalation, death may occur within minutes. Similarly, VX dermal exposure may cause death within minutes if the exposure is massive, but symptoms may be delayed for up to 18 h following milder dermal exposures. Vital sign abnormalities may result from stimulation of both the sympathetic and parasympathetic ganglia. While bradycardia is expected from stimulation of the parasympathetic nervous system, 90 percent of patients exposed to nerve agents have normal heart rates or are tachycardic. Vapor exposure typically creates a triad of ocular, nasal, and respiratory symptoms. The eyes and nose are most sensitive, with miosis, conjunctival injection, pain, and rhinorrhea developing at low doses. At higher concentrations, respiratory effects such as chest tightness, dyspnea, and copious secretions ensue. Neurologic findings with severe exposures include giddiness, collapse, convulsions, fasciculations, and flaccid paralysis. The predominant cause of death is from centrally mediated respiratory depression and apnea. In contrast to vapor exposure, dermal exposure results in a unique pattern of symptom onset and progression. Miosis may not be evident initially, but localized sweating and fasciculations will be noted surrounding the exposed area. Nausea, vomiting, diarrhea, and fatigue develop with increasing dose. As with vapor exposures, the presence of respiratory and neurologic symptoms indicate severe toxicity.

Once a nerve agent release has been recognized, self-protection and patient decontamination take precedence over other medical treatment. There is an extremely high risk of secondary contamination to the medical personnel caring for exposed patients. Appropriate skin and respiratory protection should be donned by the hospital staff because these agents are readily absorbed by all routes (e.g., skin, mucous membranes, respiratory tract). Neither surgical nor high-efficiency particulate-arresting (HEPA) masks render protection from these agents. Even double latex gloves are ineffective in preventing dermal exposure, and butyl rubber gloves should be worn. Removal of patient clothing alone may provide significant decontamination in those who are ambulatory. While a 0.5 percent sodium hypochlorite solution (9:1 household bleach to water) effectively inactivates nerve agents, its use on patients is inadvisable. Copious amounts of tepid water with a mild soap should be adequate for skin decontamination in most situations. However, a considerable amount of VX may remain on the skin even after initial decontamination, necessitating several washings and awareness of the potential for secondary contamination.

Following decontamination, restoring oxygenation is the single most critical step, because most deaths are respiratory in nature. Succinylcholine, if used to facilitate intubation, may have prolonged effect because the plasma cholinesterase level is inhibited. Cardiac monitoring for dysrhythmias should be instituted. Described dysrhythmias include torsade de pointes. Specific antidote therapy with atropine and pralidoxime chloride (2-PAM) should be anticipated. Atropine blocks muscarinic receptors and reverses the parasympathetic findings of lacrimation, bronchorrhea, bronchoconstriction, salivation, and gastrointestinal spasm, along with some central nervous system (CNS) manifestations. It does not affect the motor endplate or symptoms of fasciculations or weakness. The dose is best determined by signs, symptoms, and route of exposure. In contrast to organophosphate pesticide

TABLE 185-3 Toxins with Delayed Onset of Symptoms or Requiring Prolonged Monitoring

Acrylonitrile, acetonitrile, proprionitrile	Cyanide toxicity
Aniline	Methemoglobinemia
Arsine	Hemolysis
Benzene	Bone marrow suppression and leukemia
Cadmium	Pulmonary toxicity
Chlorine	Pulmonary edema
Ethylene oxide	Pulmonary edema and neurotoxicity
Halogenated solvents	Hepatorenal toxicity
Hydrofluoric acid	Pulmonary edema, dermal burns electrolyte changes
Hydrogen sulfide	Pulmonary edema
Metals	Hepatorenal, neurotoxicity
Methanol	Neurologic, acid-base disturbance
Methyl bromide	Pulmonary edema
Methylene chloride	Carbon monoxide toxicity, dysrhythmias
Organophosphates (highly lipid soluble), or dermal exposure to nerve agents	Cholinergic toxicity
Nitrogen oxides	Pulmonary edema, methemoglobinemia
Ozone (rare)	Pulmonary edema
Paraquat	Pulmonary edema/fibrosis
Phosgene	Pulmonary edema
Phosphine	Pulmonary edema
Zinc phosphide	Pulmonary edema

TABLE 185-4 Differential Diagnosis of Agents Causing Dyspnea

Agent	Findings	Onset	Irritant?
Phosgene (CG)	Pulmonary edema	Delayed	Mild/none
Nerve agents	Increased secretions/bronchospasm	Immediate (vapor); delayed (dermal/liquid)	Mild
Vesicants:			
Mustards (H)	Coughing, hoarseness (central airways most commonly affected) Pulmonary hemorrhage/airway necrosis (rare)	Delayed	Yes
Lewisite (L)	Coughing, hoarseness (central airways most commonly affected) Pulmonary hemorrhage/airway necrosis (rare)	Immediate	Yes
Phosgene oxime (CX)	Eye, mucous membrane, upper airway irritation Pulmonary edema (with inhalation and skin application)	Immediate	Yes
Chlorine	Coughing, nausea and vomiting (low level) Pulmonary edema (high level)	Immediate Delayed	Yes
Ammonia	Coughing, hoarseness, bronchospasm	Immediate	Yes
Hydrogen sulfide	Burning eyes and mucous membranes Pulmonary edema	Immediate Delayed	Yes
Riot control agents (CS, CN, OC)	Coughing, eye and mucous membrane burning (more intense than other agents)	Immediate	Yes
Cyanide (AC, CK)	Normal lung exam	Immediate	No

poisoning, high-dose or continuous atropine therapy generally is not necessary beyond 2 to 3 h following nerve agent exposure. **The end point for dosing of atropine is drying of pulmonary secretions.** Miosis is not a useful therapeutic end point, and sinus tachycardia is not a contraindication for the use of atropine. Oximes, like 2-PAM, are effective nerve agent antidotes via their ability to reactivate AChE. They carry out a nucleophilic attack on the nerve agent phosphorylated to AChE. Subsequent liberation of the enzyme occurs along with detoxification of the nerve agent. Whereas atropine is not effective in treating neuromuscular findings such as weakness or fasciculations, oximes reverse the nicotinic, muscarinic, and CNS effects of the nerve agent. One caveat to the use of oximes is the need for administration prior to "aging" of AChE. Aging is the process whereby permanent inhibition of AChE activity occurs as a result of nerve agent alkyl group hydrolysis and covalent binding. This reaction, which occurs within

2 min of soman exposure and within 5 h of sarin exposure, provides a rationale for early 2-PAM therapy. Like atropine, 2-PAM dosing in adults is determined by route of exposure and signs and symptoms (see Table 8-2). In contrast to organophosphate pesticide exposures, long-term or continuous infusions of 2-PAM have not been required in the management of victims of nerve agent exposure.

Seizures generally are not persistent once ventilatory support, atropine, and 2-PAM therapy are instituted. If present, they should be treated aggressively with benzodiazepines, which may be neuroprotective. Military Mark I autoinjector kits contain 2 mg atropine and 600 mg 2-PAM for immediate intramuscular administration in the field. The emergency physician should be familiar with this form of these antidotes, because these kits may be stockpiled for civilian first-responder use. Symptomatic patients or those with dermal exposures should be kept under close observation for 24 h.

TABLE 185-5 Nerve Agent Symptoms, Severity, and Treatment Summary

Exposure Route	Category	Signs and Symptoms	Drug Therapy
Inhalational (vapor)	Minimal	Miosis, rhinorrhea Visual complaints	Observation Consider homatropine eye drops for intractable eye pain
	Mild	Miosis, rhinorrhea, and mild dyspnea	Atropine 2 mg* 2-PAM 600 mg†
	Moderate	Miosis, rhinorrhea, moderate to severe dyspnea, nausea, vomiting	Atropine 4 mg 2-PAM 1200 mg
	Severe	Severe dyspnea, copious secretions, nausea, vomiting, diarrhea, coma, seizures, flaccid paralysis, apnea	Atropine 6 mg 2-PAM 1800 mg
Dermal (liquid)	Mild	Localized sweating, fasciculations	Atropine 2 mg* 2-PAM 600 mg†
	Moderate	Above plus nausea, vomiting, diarrhea	Atropine 2 mg* 2-PAM 600 mg†
	Severe	Above plus respiratory or neuromuscular signs (same as "severe inhalational" above)	Atropine 6 mg 2-PAM 1800 mg

*May be given IM or IV. Pediatric dose = 0.02 mg/kg (minimum 0.1 mg). Initial doses may be repeated every 10–15 min or administered by continuous infusion at 0.02–0.08 mg/kg per h. Higher doses (5 mg in adults or 0.05 mg/kg in children) may be needed to treat severe exposures.
†2-PAM is most effective if given intravenously, although the IM route is an acceptable alternative. Adult doses begin at 600 mg. The pediatric dose is 25–50 mg/kg and may be repeated in 1 h if symptoms are worsening.
Source: Modified from Sidell FR: Nerve agents, in Sidell FR, Takafuji ET, Franz DR (eds): *Textbook of Military Medicine, Medical Aspects of Chemical and Biological Warfare.* Washington, DC, Office of the Surgeon General, United States Army, 1997, pp. 129–171.

VESICANTS

The terrorist use of vesicants, or agents that produce blisters, would overwhelm the ED with patients presenting with severe dermal conditions. The toxicology of these agents is summarized below.

The three primary vesicants are mustards, lewisite, and phosgene oxime. Mustards are the most viable threat among this group, as more than a dozen countries have mustard in their arsenals and because mustards are the easiest of the chemical agents to synthesize. During World War I, mustards caused more casualties than all other chemical agents combined. More recently, 45,000 casualties occurred following their use during the Iran-Iraq war of the 1980s. Sulfur mustards (H, HS, HD) are alkylating agents that are highly reactive and electrophilic. They induce toxicity through rapid adduct formation with peptides, proteins, ribonucleic acid (RNA), deoxyribonucleic acid (DNA), and cell membranes and disappear from extracellular fluids within a few minutes. They are oily liquids with an odor of garlic, horseradish, or mustard. The median lethal dose (LD_{50}) is approximately 1.5 teaspoons, which can result in a 25 percent body surface area (BSA) burn.

Clinical effects are somewhat dose dependent. At low doses, vesication occurs, whereas at higher doses, systemic cytotoxicity is seen. Characteristically, symptoms are delayed for 4 to 8 h. Eyes, skin, and airways are relatively equally affected. Skin findings include initial erythema that progresses to blister formation over 24 h. Warm, moist areas are affected most. Ocular findings are similarly delayed and include edema of the lid, conjunctival injection, and corneal ulceration, with the most severe exposures. Respiratory involvement manifests as a dry, barking cough and hoarseness beginning 4 to 6 h postexposure. Early tachypnea or dyspnea indicates exposure to a potentially lethal amount of mustard. In such cases, bronchospasm, bronchiolar obstruction by sloughed pseudomembranous bronchial epithelium, and hemorrhagic pulmonary edema may ensue over 1 to 2 days. Systemic absorption is seen with massive exposures and results in hematopoietic, gastrointestinal tract, and CNS involvement. Overall, the expected mortality is approximately 3 percent for those reaching medical facilities.

Lewisite

Lewisite (L) is an oily colorless liquid with the odor of geraniums. It has a potency similar to that of mustard. It was used by Japan during wartime, and known stockpiles of a Lewisite-mustard mixture are possessed by Russia. While its active ingredient, trivalent arsenic, inhibits various enzymes throughout the body and interferes with glycolysis, the mechanism for vesication is not clear. In contrast to mustard exposure, skin irritation and pain are characteristically present within 15 to 30 min of Lewisite exposure. Blister formation also occurs more quickly than that seen with mustard exposure (within 2 h). Resulting lesions have less surrounding erythema and result in more tissue destruction than those caused by mustards. Ocular pain and irritation also occur within minutes, and fortunately in most cases, reflex blepharospasm seems to prevent the severe ocular injury seen with mustard exposure. Pulmonary involvement is characterized by immediate upper airway irritation and central airway inflammation. Parenchymal involvement is rare and progression to pulmonary edema occurs only in the most severe cases. Hypotension and hemolytic anemia are seen rarely and result from systemic arsenic toxicity.

Phosgene

Phosgene oxime (CX), an agent that causes extensive tissue damage, is discussed here even though it is not a true vesicant. It is actually an urticaric with an unknown mechanism of action. Following exposure, instantaneous pain and irritation of the skin, eyes, and airways occurs. The affected skin then blanches, turns grayish, and becomes urticarial, erythematous, and edematous. Vesicle formation does not occur. Necrosis of the area may penetrate to the muscle layers and results in eschar formation. Ocular findings are similar to those described for Lewisite. Pulmonary edema is common and bronchiolitis has been described.

The diagnosis of vesicant exposure is a clinical one. Urinary thiodiglycol metabolites will confirm exposure to sulfur mustards, but this test is not widely available. Treatment begins with immediate skin and eye decontamination, ideally within 1 to 2 min of exposure. This is the only effective way of preventing tissue damage. Late decontamination is recommended, however, to prevent spread to uninvolved areas of the skin and to medical or rescue personnel. Copious soap and water decontamination is appropriate for the skin. A dilute hypochlorite solution is recommended by some for skin decontamination of the relatively water-insoluble mustards and Lewisite, but this is controversial. Water alone is the preferred decontamination solution for phosgene oxime. BAL (British anti-Lewisite, or dimercaprol) is an arsenic chelator that will prevent or greatly decrease the severity of skin and eye lesions if applied topically within minutes of Lewisite exposure, but the topical form is not widely available. Given intramuscularly, BAL reduces the mortality from systemic effects of Lewisite. There are no antidotes for mustard poisoning, although mustard scavengers, antioxidants, nicotinamide-adenine dinucleotide (NAD) precursors, polymerase inhibitor, and corticosteroids are investigational. As with thermal burns, aggressive airway, fluid, electrolyte, and pain management coupled with prevention of secondary infection with topical antibiotics and sterile dressing changes is the mainstay of therapy. In contrast to thermal burns, however, mustard burns do not trigger the same magnitude of fluid loss. All burns resulting from caustic chemicals are classified as "major" by the American Burn Association and should be referred to a burn center.

RESPIRATORY AGENTS

Gases, mists, aerosols, fumes, or dusts may be inhaled. Determinants of airborne agent toxicity include many factors such as concentration of the inhaled toxin, duration of exposure, and whether the exposure occurred in an enclosed space. Other influential factors include vapor density, allergic or nonallergic bronchospastic response, exertional state or metabolic rate of the victim, and unique host susceptibility such as the underlying reactive airways disease, history of smoking, or extreme age. Aspiration of gastric contents may cause further pulmonary insult.

Other primary determinants of injury pattern include toxin particle size and solubility in water. Agents with particle diameters greater than 10 μm or that are highly water-soluble are deposited primarily in the upper airways. Examples of water-soluble chemicals include ammonia, sulfur dioxide, and acid gases such as hydrochloric acid and sulfuric acid. Following exposure, signs of upper airway irritation develop rapidly and are accompanied by eye and mucous membrane irritation. Coughing, wheezing, or stridor may progress to upper airway obstruction in severe exposures. Those inhaled toxins of smaller particle size or lower water solubility such as phosgene, ozone, or nitrogen oxides will reach the lower respiratory tract and may result in delayed symptom onset. Gases with intermediate water solubility, such as chlorine, may cause early irritative symptoms following mild exposure or delayed pulmonary edema after massive exposure.

The presence of smoke complicates the ability to predict patterns of illness following toxin inhalation. Because it is particulate, smoke carries adherent products of combustion such as acrolein, ammonia, acids, and diisocyanates deeper into the lungs than normally would be expected. Thermal physical damage to the respiratory tract also may occur, particularly in the presence of steam. General management of the patient with toxic inhalation injury involves removal from the source, application of 100 percent oxygen, humidification for irritative symptoms, and inhaled bronchodilators for bronchospasm. A detailed examination should include inspection of the upper airway for evidence of singed nasal hair, soot in the oropharynx, facial or oropharyngeal burns, erythema or parching of the mucous membranes, stridor, hoarseness, dysphagia, cough, carbonaceous sputum, tachypnea, retractions, accessory muscle use, wheezing, rales, diaphoresis, or cyanosis. Early intubation should be considered for patients with upper airway edema. Pertinent laboratory studies include arterial blood gas analysis with carboxyhemoglobin, methemoglobin, and lactate levels; RBC cyanide levels if persistent acidosis occurs; electrocardiographic (ECG) monitoring; and chest x-ray. The role for diagnostic or therapeutic bronchoscopy in inhaled toxin exposure is controversial. Administration of sodium thiosulfate to victims of smoke inhalation with persistent acidosis suspected to have cyanide toxicity is indicated. Management of noncardiogenic pulmonary edema may involve the use of positive end-expiratory pressure or bilevel positive airway pressure (BiPAP), but diuretics generally are not indicated. The use of prophylactic steroids with antibiotics is reserved for nitrogen oxide exposures. Systemic toxicity from products of combustion such as cyanide or carbon monoxide is common and is reviewed in Chaps. 188 and 203, respectively.

Many highly toxic gases produced in large quantities in the industrial sector are potential agents for malicious use. Those with a history of previous battlefield use or stockpiling, such as phosgene, chlorine, or ammonia, are of particular concern. Their toxicology is summarized below, and in Table 185-1.

Phosgene

Phosgene (CG, carbonyl chloride, D-Stoff, or green cross) is a gas with a density four times that of air. Beyond its military application, it is found in the plastics, pharmaceutical, and textile industries. Upon release, it forms a white cloud with a characteristic odor of newly mown hay. It is relatively water insoluble and therefore has poor warning properties. Only mild initial eye, nose, throat, and upper airway irritation are expected, and these may be entirely absent. The major toxicity involves an acid burn to lower airways as phosgene reaches the alveoli and hydrolyzes to carbon dioxide and hydrochloric acid. Acylation of alveolar capillary membranes results in diffuse capillary leak and noncardiogenic pulmonary edema, which is characteristically delayed for up to 24 h. This clinical latent period is followed by onset of dyspnea and chest tightness, heralding the onset of pulmonary edema. If the exposure is massive, immediate dyspnea and mucous membrane and eye irritation may occur. The onset of dyspnea or pulmonary edema within 4 h of exposure suggests a very poor prognosis. Those who become symptomatic greater than 6 h after exposure generally survive if intensive medical care is available. Recovery occurs in 3 to 4 days with respiratory supportive care and management of noncardiogenic pulmonary edema. Because exertion is known to increase pulmonary edema from phosgene, rest is mandatory for those exposed. Furthermore, a 24-h observation period with frequent reassessments is indicated for asymptomatic patients.

Chlorine

Chlorine is also widely available in the industrial sector, in the setting of laboratories, paper manufacture, swimming pool chemical distribution, and municipal water treatment. When dispersed, this dense green-yellow gas has an acrid, pungent odor and excellent warning properties. It is of intermediate water solubility, which is consistent with the observation that moderately exposed World War I soldiers exhibited both central airway damage and pulmonary edema. Early inflammatory injury results from the formation of acids and oxidants upon contact with moist membranes. Immediate ocular and upper airway irritation along with nausea and vomiting are common following

mild exposures. More significant exposure results in coughing, hoarseness, and pulmonary edema, usually within 12 to 24 h. Permanent reactive airways disease has been described following significant chlorine gas inhalation. Care is primarily supportive with the use of humidified oxygen and bronchodilators as needed. The role of nebulized sodium bicarbonate as a neutralizing therapy is controversial.[10] Chlorine may cause dermal injury at high concentration and skin decontamination may be required.

Nitrogen Oxides

Nitrogen oxides are encountered in the form of silo gas ("silo filler disease"), as products of fire combustion, in industrial processes, or as components of military blast weapons, smokes and obscurants. These oxides have limited water solubility and generally result in mainly lower airway toxicity. Slow conversion of nitrogen oxide to nitric acid in the alveoli results in delayed alveolar injury and pulmonary edema. A triphasic illness typically is seen with initial dyspnea and flulike symptoms, transient improvement, and then worsening dyspnea, which heralds the onset of pulmonary edema 24 to 72 h after exposure. Methemoglobinemia also may occur. Bronchiolitis obliterans, a potential late complication, may be prevented by the use of steroids.

Ammonia

Ammonia, widely available as a fertilizer and industrial chemical, is a highly water-soluble, colorless, alkaline corrosive gas. It has good warning properties and rapidly reacts with wet surfaces to form ammonium hydroxide. The presence of ammonia is usually obvious based on its characteristic pungent odor and immediate induction of symptoms of mucous membrane, eye, and throat irritation. Lower airway involvement resulting in bronchospasm, pulmonary edema, and residual reactive airways disease have all been described following massive exposures, especially in those who are entrapped in enclosed spaces. Treatment is supportive with humidified oxygen and bronchodilators. Anhydrous ammonia is extremely hazardous to the eyes and can penetrate the anterior chamber within 1 min of exposure. Therefore, following ocular irrigation in symptomatic patients, evaluation for the presence of corneal burns should be considered and a careful ophthalmologic examination is warranted.

Many of the chemical warfare agents can cause dyspnea. Table 8-2 outlines the differentiating features.

Overall, treatment for respiratory agents is supportive and involves removal from the source of exposure, executing the ABCs (airway, breathing, and circulation), application of humidified oxygen, and enforced rest. Flushing of the eyes and skin should be carried out as appropriate. Copious airway secretions, hypoxia, bronchospasm and pulmonary edema should be anticipated. Antibiotics are reserved for those with positive sputum gram stains or cultures. No human studies have shown benefit from the use of steroids. Their use may be considered in those with underlying reactive airway disease or nitrogen oxide exposure (see above).

METABOLIC TOXINS

Cyanide

Cyanide (AC hydrocyanic acid, CK cyanogen chloride) is the least toxic of the lethal military agents. It was employed by the French during World War I, the Nazis in World War II, and by Iraq in the 1980s. It is a popular homicidal/suicidal agent, especially among chemists and laboratory workers. Nonmilitary incidents include a mass cult suicide of the People's Temple in Guyana, Tylenol product tampering, and the World Trade Center bombing. Cyanogen sources are natural (plants), medicinal (nitroprusside), industrial (300,000 tons produced annually), fire-related (from the combustion of organonitrogen or plastics), and commercial (solvents acetonitrile, propionitirile). The military agent AC is a volatile, nonpersistent liquid or gas with the odor of bitter almonds detectable by 40 percent of the population, whereas CK is odorless and slightly irritating to mucous membranes. Cyanide is covered in detail in Chap. 188.

Hydrogen Sulfide

Hydrogen sulfide is a colorless, flammable gas that may be encountered in industry or as a natural product of organic decomposition, such as sewer or manure gas. The ability to detect its characteristic "rotten egg" odor is lost at high concentrations or with lengthy exposures to low concentrations. Its mechanism of toxicity is similar to that of cyanide, with disruption of oxidative phosphorylation through inhibition of cytochrome oxidase aa3. Cellular asphyxia and impaired adenosine triphosphate (ATP) production promote anaerobic metabolism with lactate accumulation and metabolic acidosis. It is one of the few chemical asphyxiants that also possesses irritative properties, such that respiratory and ocular irritation are common following exposure. In high concentrations, rapid loss of consciousness, seizures, and death may occur after only a few breaths. Delayed pulmonary edema and corneal destruction should be anticipated with massive exposures. Treatment involves decontamination of the skin and eyes as appropriate. Administration of the nitrite component of the cyanide antidote kit to promote low-level methemoglobin formation may result in conversion of sulfide to less toxic sulfmethemoglobin. Other treatments include 100 percent oxygen and possibly hyperbaric oxygen therapy. Phosphine and azide exposure may cause similar clinical symptoms and metabolic derangements as cyanide. Carbon monoxide is discussed in depth in Chap. 203.

Miscellaneous Industrial Toxins

Derivatives of aniline or nitrites are the industrial chemicals most frequently associated with RBC oxidant stress. Other workplace hematologic toxins include chlorates, benzene, acetanilid, nitrogen oxides, nitrophenols, *para*-toluidine, phenols, and sulfonamides.

Ricin

Ricin is a plant cytotoxin that attacks rRNA and is a ribosome inhibiting protein. It is made from the mash by-product of castor bean processing. It is available as a powder, mist, or pellet, or can be dissolved in water or a weak acid. It is extremely stable and is unaffected by extreme heat or cold. When injected, as little as 500 μg can cause death. When ricin is injected, multi-organ failure and coagulopathies result in death within 36 h. Ingestion results in multi-organ failure and profuse gastrointestinal bleeding. Inhalation results in acute respiratory distress, followed by pulmonary edema. There is no laboratory test to confirm the diagnosis. The only treatment available is supportive care. Suspected ricin poisoning should be reported to the Agency for Toxic Substances and Disease registry (ATSDR) at 1-888-422-8737. (http://www.bt.cdc.gov/agent/ricin/faq/index.asp).

HYDROCARBONS

Certain solvents such as halogenated hydrocarbons, Freons (chlorofluorocarbons), and aromatic hydrocarbons may sensitize the myocardium to the dysrhythmic effect of catecholamines. Myocardial irritability may persist for several hours following exposure. Avoidance of physical activity or sympathomimetic drugs, other than selective β_2 agonists, for the treatment of bronchospasm is warranted. Furthermore, **direct-current countershock cannot be administered to patients soaked with flammable chemicals** until decontamination has been carried out due to fire and explosion risk. Hydrocarbon inhala-

tion also results in early stimulation, followed by confusion, lethargy, stupor, or coma. Freons cause intense respiratory symptoms, which can persist for years.[11]

RIOT CONTROL AGENTS

Riot control agents such as mace, or capsaicin (pepper spray) belong to a group of compounds that cause transient but intensely noxious effects on exposure. Although generally considered to be only briefly incapacitating, fatalities from pulmonary edema have occurred following large exposures in confined spaces. Typically, symptoms include immediate irritation of the eyes and respiratory tract, blepharospasm, lacrimation, coughing, sneezing, and rhinorrhea, followed by a burning sensation of exposed skin and mucous membranes. Nausea, vomiting, headache, and photophobia may be seen. These symptoms usually disappear within a few hours after cessation of the exposure. Burns and sensitization of the skin have been described, especially if contact with the agent is prolonged. Management includes removal of the patient from the area, copious irrigation of the eyes with normal saline, and skin decontamination with soap and water. Contact with water can briefly exacerbate skin symptoms from CS. The use of bleach solutions to decontaminate the skin is not recommended as this may increase irritation or trigger blister formation from some agents. Patients with preexisting lung disease should be observed and treated for bronchospasm.

INCAPACITATING AGENTS

Military incapacitating agents produce physiologic or mental effects that render the exposed victim unable to perform assigned duties. These agents are generally not lethal, but recovery may take several hours to days. The anticholinergic deliriant, 3-quinuclidinyl benzilate (QNB, BZ) is of military interest. BZ's clinical profile most closely represents that of atropine, with a slower onset and longer duration of action. Recognition of an anticholinergic toxidrome is key to diagnosing a BZ exposure. Expected symptoms are delirium, hallucinations, mydriasis, tachycardia, ileus, dry mucous membranes, absent axillary sweat, urinary retention, and hyperthermia. Treatment involves supportive care and sedation with benzodiazepines to prevent hyperthermia and rhabdomyolysis. In the past, physostigmine was used to reverse the action of BZ, and was associated with untoward side effects. Its use should be reserved for patients with refractory seizures or tachycardia.

Incapacitation can be produced by a variety of other chemical agents including stimulants, potent opioids, hallucinogens, or nausea-producing drugs. Their battlefield use is problematic, but covert or terrorist use is possible.

ACKNOWLEDGMENT

The views, opinions, assertions, and findings contained herein are those of the authors and should not be construed as official U.S. Department of Defense or Department of the Army positions, policies, or decisions unless so designated by other documentation.

REFERENCES

1. Couturier AM, McCuney RJ: Physicians' work in emergency response. *Occup Health Safety* 66(2):46, 1997.
2. Hazardous Substances Emergency Events Surveillance (HSEES): *Five-Year Cumulative Report 1993–1997.* Atlanta, GA, Department of Health and Human Services, Agency for Toxic Substances and Disease Registry.
3. National Response Center, 2002.
4. Burgess JL, Kovalchick DF, Harter L, et al: Hazardous materials events: An industrial comparison. *J Occup Environ Med* 42(5):546, 2000.
5. Kales SN, Polyhronpoulos GN, Castro MJ, et al: Injuries caused by hazardous materials accidents. *Ann Emerg Med* 30(5):598, 1997.

6. Hall HI, Dhara VR, Price-Green PA, Kaye WE: Surveillance for emergency events involving hazardous substances: United States, 1990–1992. *MMWR* 43(2):1, 1994.

7. Phelps AM, Morris P, Giguere M: Emergency events involving hazardous substances in North Carolina, 1993–1994. *N Carolina Med J* 59(2):120, 1998.

8. Burgess JL: Hospital preparedness of hazardous materials incidents and treatment of contaminated patients. *West J Med* 167:387, 1997.

9. *Healthy Children, Toxic Environments.* Report to the Child Health Workgroup Board of Scientific Counselors. Atlanta, GA, U.S. Department of Health and Human Services, Agency for Toxic Substances and Disease Registry, 1997, pp 2–7.

10. Vinsel PJ: Treatment of chlorine gas inhalation with nebulized sodium bicarbonate. *J Emerg Med* 8(3):327, 1990.

11. Piirila P, Espo T, Pfaffli R, et al: Prolonged respiratory symptoms caused by thermal degradation products of freon. *Scan J Work, Envir, Health* 29(1):71, 2003.

VITAMINS AND HERBALS
G. Richard Braen

Vitamins and herbal preparations, particularly those sold in health food stores, are considered by many to be innocuous, but several have tremendous potential as toxins. This chapter covers most of the available vitamins and selected herbals. Agents compounded with vitamins, such as iron, are covered in other chapters. Helpful resources include: Natural Medicines Comprehensive Database (http://www.naturaldatabase.com); NIH Office of Dietary Supplements (http://dietary-supplements.info.nih.gov); and HerbMed (www.herbmed.org).

VITAMIN A

Vitamin A has two primary preformed types: retinol (vitamin A_1 alcohol) and 3-dehydroretinol (vitamin A_2). The retinyl esters of dietary vitamin A are hydrolyzed into retinol in the gastrointestinal tract. Retinol is then absorbed into intestinal mucosal cells where it combines with a fatty acid to again become a retinyl ester. The retinyl ester then travels through the lymphatic system and bloodstream to storage sites in the liver. The liver contains approximately 95 percent of the vitamin A of the entire body.

Vitamin A forms part of the visual pigments of the retina (rhodopsin and iodopsin), is important for the formation of mucus-secreting cells of the columnar epithelium, maintains bone growth, and maintains cellular membrane stability. The daily adult recommended doses range from 4000 IU for women to 5000 IU for men.

Hypervitaminosis A generally occurs when children are given excessive amounts of a high-potency supplement. Retinol is bound to a liver protein (retinol-binding protein) and is stored in this bound form. As the liver binding and storing capacities are exceeded, blood levels of a retinyl ester loosely bound to low-density lipoproteins increase. This loosely bound vitamin is believed to be toxic to cell membranes. Members of Mawson's Antarctic expedition (1911–1913) are said to have died from hypervitaminosis A after eating the livers of their dogs to try to avoid starvation.

When the total dosage is similar, water-miscible preparations are more toxic than oily preparations because of better absorption. High doses of preformed vitamin A must be ingested for long periods before signs and symptoms of hypervitaminosis A develop. There is a high degree of variability among patients in the amounts necessary to develop hypervitaminosis. Dialysis patients can be at risk of developing a type of vitamin A toxicity in which resorption of bone causes hypercalcemia.

Symptoms of hypervitaminosis A include blurred vision, appetite loss, abnormal skin pigmentation, loss of hair, dry skin, pruritus, long-bone pain, and an increased incidence of bone fractures. Massive doses can additionally cause pseudotumor cerebri.

The treatment of hypervitaminosis A depends on the condition of the patient. Generally, when vitamin A is discontinued, the symptoms resolve over a period of time and no additional treatment is needed.[1] Chap. 27 outlines treatment of hypercalcemia. β-Carotene intoxication is very rare and does not generally cause hypervitaminosis A. In diabetics and patients with hypothyroidism, however, large doses of β-carotene can cause a yellowish discoloration of the skin, which fades once β-carotene is stopped.

VITAMIN D

Vitamin D function comes from two major compounds: calciferol (vitamin D_3) and ergocalciferol (vitamin D_2). The naturally occurring provitamin forms of each of these two compounds (7-dehydrocholesterol for D_3 and ergosterol for D_2) convert to the active forms following irradiation by ultraviolet light. Most studies in humans have been made on vitamin D_3 (cholecalciferol), which is converted in the body to 1,25-dihydroxycholecalciferol, the physiologically active form of vitamin D.

Absorption of vitamin D is aided by bile and takes place in the jejunum. From there it is transported via lymph chylomicrons to the bloodstream.[1] When it reaches the liver, it is hydroxylated to 25-hydroxycholecalciferol. From the liver, it travels to the kidney, where it is again hydroxylated to 1,25-dihydroxycholecalciferol. The major function of 1,25-dihydroxyhydrocalciferol is to elevate the plasma calcium and phosphorus levels to enable normal bone mineralization.

The average daily adult requirement of vitamin D is approximately 400 IU, and therapeutic doses sometimes exceed 5000 IU. Infants may develop hypercalcemia from doses as low as 2000 IU, but adults require much higher doses before toxicity develops. The toxicity results from the hypercalcemia and includes anorexia, nausea, abdominal pain, lethargy, weight loss, polyuria, constipation, confusion, and coma.[1] Symptoms from massive doses (1000 to 3000 IU/kg) develop in 2 to 8 days. Persistently elevated levels of calcium can cause soft tissue calcification and renal failure.

Treatment of hypervitaminosis D includes discontinuation of vitamin D, reduction of the calcium intake, and reduction of serum calcium levels.

VITAMIN E

Vitamin E activity is not limited to one compound alone. Eight different fat-soluble, naturally occurring alcohols (called tocopherols and tocotrienols) have vitamin E activity, but α-tocopherol is the most active form. Because of its ability to be rapidly oxidized, α-tocopherol protects other foods from being oxidized, and thus is termed an *antioxidant*.[2] Foods high in vitamin E include wheat germ, corn, soybean, sunflower seed, cod liver, and others.

Vitamin E is absorbed and distributed through the body just as any fat-soluble vitamin, through the intestines, and then through lymphatic chylomicrons. Between 30 and 90 percent of available vitamin E in the diet is absorbed. Normal tocopherol levels in adults range from 0.5 mg to 2.0 mg/dL. The minimum daily requirement for women is about 8 mg α-tocopherol; for men, it is 10 mg α-tocopherol. An IU is the activity of 1 mg of α-tocopherol. Vitamin E needs for children increase with increasing body weight and increase for pregnant or lactating women.

Vitamin E is felt to be nontoxic at daily doses of up to 600 IU. At doses higher than 600 IU per d, taken on a long-term basis, a metabolite of vitamin E acts as a competitive inhibitor of vitamin K-dependent γ-carboxylation, increasing the daily vitamin K requirements. Additionally, through the production of thromboxane, high levels of vitamin E inhibit platelet aggregation. People ingesting large amounts of vitamin E who are taking anticoagulants should be observed closely for bleeding tendencies, but those not taking anticoagulants rarely have coagulation difficulties, except for neonates, who are more sensitive to the effects of vitamin E. Other effects in adults who take large doses for a long period of time include nausea, fatigue, headache, weakness, and blurred vision. These symptoms resolve weeks after discontinuation of the vitamin.

VITAMIN K

Vitamin K is represented by several compounds that have antihemorrhagic activity: the parent compound called menadione; vitamin K_1, which is a naturally occurring phylloquinone from plant sources; and vitamin K_2, which is a naturally occurring menaquinone from microbial sources. High levels of dietary vitamin A inhibit the absorption of vitamin K. Vitamin E at high levels acts as a vitamin K-antagonist in its liver production of clotting factors.

Phylloquinones are absorbed from the proximal intestine through an energy-requiring process. Menadione and menaquinones are absorbed from the lower intestine and colon through a passive mechanism. Both mechanisms require the presence of bile and pancreatic juice. Between 10 and 80 percent is absorbed. Once absorbed, it is carried by the lymph chylomicrons and then transferred in the blood to β-lipoproteins. Approximately 50 percent of the vitamin comes from the diet and 50 percent from bacterial synthesis in the intestines. The total dietary requirement of vitamin K is about 2 μg/kg body weight. Because most adults ingest a diet that contains 300 to 500 μg vitamin K, deficiency states are uncommon. In contrast to the other fat-soluble vitamins, vitamin K is not stored in the body to any significant extent. Approximately 70 percent of menadione is excreted in the urine. Phylloquinone is excreted mainly in bile.

Vitamin K is required for the maintenance of normal prothrombin tines through its effect on factor II (prothrombin), factor VII (proconvertin), factor IX (Christmas factor), and factor X (Stuart-Prower factor). These factors are part of the extrinsic, intrinsic, and common pathways for blood clotting. Coumarin compounds work on the clotting-factor synthesis sites in the liver to stop prothrombin synthesis and to reduce the levels of all vitamin K-dependent clotting factors.

Megadoses of menadione can be toxic. Toxic effects include hemolytic anemia, kernicterus, and hemoglobinuria in premature infants and renal tubular degeneration, liver damage, hypoprothrombinemia, and petechial hemorrhages in adults. Large doses can also paradoxically inhibit the effects of oral anticoagulants. Treatment includes stopping vitamin K, monitoring prothrombin times, and monitoring liver function studies. Additionally, doses exceeding 500 μg daily are associated with skin rashes. Fatalities from overingestion of vitamin K are rare.

VITAMIN B$_1$ (THIAMINE)

Vitamin B_1 is converted to thiamine pyrophosphate which acts as a cofactor for several metabolic reactions, including transketolations. Measurement of erythrocyte transketolase activity is used to reflect the availability of thiamine pyrophosphate in the tissues. Food sources of thiamine include fruits, grain, meats, fish, and milk, among others. The highest levels are found in pork products (0.63 mg/serving). The average daily adult requirement is 1.5 mg.[1]

Intestinal absorption of thiamine seems to be greatest in the jejunum. An active carrier-mediated absorption process occurs at normal levels of dietary thiamine, but passive diffusion is the major means of thiamine absorption at higher levels.

Thiamine is not stored in the body to any significant extent. At low dietary levels, renal excretion decreases, whereas, at high levels of ingestion, renal excretion increases proportionately. Because of the renal excretion of thiamine, there is no toxicity to the ingestion of large doses of vitamin B_1 over prolonged periods.

VITAMIN B$_2$ (RIBOFLAVIN)

Vitamin B_2 (riboflavin) works as an antioxidant through its activity in the formation of glutathione reductase and glutathione. As a part of the group of enzymes called flavoproteins, it is involved in the metabolism of fats, proteins, and carbohydrates. It is not stored in appreciable quantities in the body and must be replenished daily. Vigorous exercise increases the daily requirement of riboflavin, and a deficiency results in cracked lips, reddened tongue, and eczema of the face and genitals. The average daily adult requirement is 1.7 mg.[1]

Riboflavin is excreted through the urine, and toxicity is rare regardless of the amount ingested. No adverse effects result from overdosage.

VITAMIN B$_3$ (NIACIN)

There are two active forms of niacin—nicotinic acid and nicotinamide—which, in conjunction with thiamine and riboflavin, have antipellagra activity. Niacin, thiamine, and riboflavin all function as a coenzyme in energy metabolism. Niacin becomes part of the coenzymes nicotinamide-adenine dinucleotide (NAD) and nicotinamide-adenine dinucleotide phosphate (NADP). NAD is required in all major metabolic pathways in which there is oxidative breakdown of amino acids, fatty acids, and other compounds. It also acts in the oxidation of ethanol.

Niacin is found in poultry, meat, and fish, with less found in plants. Niacin deficiency causes changes first in cells of the skin, nervous system, and gastrointestinal tract. Deficiency states create symptoms such as anorexia, anxiety, depression, irritability, and weakness.

Whereas doses of nicotinic acid in the range of 100 to 200 times the recommended allowance of 20 mg daily lowers serum cholesterol and β-lipoprotein, nicotinamide does not. Large doses can also deplete cardiac muscle glycogen and can cause liver toxicity. Some patients experience a frightening "niacin flush" when taking a dose of more than 100 mg. The niacin flush, caused by histamine release and vasodilation, is characterized by face, neck, and chest burning, itching, and reddening.[1] It generally resolves within an hour. Antihistamines can provide symptomatic relief. Higher doses may additionally cause nausea, abdominal cramping, diarrhea, and headache. Even higher doses (2000 mg and above) over a prolonged period can produce abnormalities of liver function, impaired glucose tolerance, hyperuricemia, and skin changes such as dryness and discoloration. Subacute and chronic symptoms resolve within days to weeks.

VITAMIN B$_6$ (PYRIDOXINE)

Vitamin B_6 is a complex of three physiologically active compounds, the most active being pyridoxine. Pyridoxine is converted to pyridoxal-5-phosphate, which is a coenzyme in the transamination of amino acids that is required for the utilization of most amino acids for energy and for the synthesis of nonessential amino acids. A deficiency in vitamin B_6 in infants results in convulsive seizures (as a consequence of a reduced synthesis of γ-aminobutyric acid), anemia (caused by impaired synthesis of heme), xanthurenic aciduria (because of reduced formation of hydroxyanthranilic acid), cystathionuria (because of decreased cleavage of cystathionine to cysteine and homoserine), and homocystinuria (because of impaired formation of cystathionine). Deficiency states can be induced through ingestion of antagonists to vitamin B_6, such as isoniazid, cycloserine, and penicillamine.

Vitamin B_6 deficiency in infants may lead to growth retardation, weight loss, hyperirritability, convulsions, and anemia. Vitamin B_6 deficiency in adults may result in depression, convulsions, seborrheic dermatitis, and cheilosis. The daily requirement is 2.2 mg/d for men and 2.0 mg/d for women, with increased requirements during pregnancy and lactation. Many animal and vegetable sources contain vitamin B_6 (especially pork and glandular meats, legumes, potatoes, oatmeal, wheat germ, and bananas), but there is considerable loss of the vitamin during cooking.

In high doses, particularly over a long period of time, vitamin B_6 excess will cause nerve damage. Most people can tolerate 20 mg/d without difficulty, but 5 g/d or more over several weeks will produce an unstable gait and numbness of the feet. This is followed by similar symptoms in the hands and arms. There may be a marked loss of position and vibration senses. After withdrawal of the vitamin, recovery occurs within several months. Some patients, however, have residual neurologic losses.

Vitamin B_6 also can cause intestinal inactivation of levodopa in patients receiving that medication for Parkinson disease. Patients should be instructed not to take the vitamin at the same time as the medication.

VITAMIN B_{12}

Vitamin B_{12} deficiency causes pernicious anemia identified by macrocytosis (high mean corpuscular volume) and intramedullary hemolysis (very high lactate dehydrogenase level). Associated neurologic problems include symmetric paresthesias of the hands and feet, and decreased position and vibratory senses. Vitamin B_{12} is a very potent vitamin (relatively small amounts are needed to treat patients with pernicious anemia) that takes several forms: cyanocobalamin (vitamin B_{12}), hydroxocobalamin (vitamin B_{12a}) aquocobalamin (vitamin B_{12b}), nitritocobalamin (vitamin B_{12c}), 5′-deoxyadenosylcobalamin (coenzyme B_{12}), and methylcobalamin (methyl B_{12}). All are complex nitrogenous compounds associated with cobalamin that participate in metabolic reactions necessary for the formation of amino acids, protein, and DNA.

Partially because of the size and complexity of the vitamin B_{12} molecules, deficiencies of this water-soluble vitamin result more from absorption problems than from dietary insufficiencies.[2] Absorption depends on the production of intrinsic factor (IF) by the parietal cells of the stomach. Vitamin B_{12}–IF complexes are formed in the stomach. The complexes pass to the ileum, where IF attaches to the intestinal epithelium, facilitating the absorption of the vitamin B_{12}. Once absorbed, the cobalamin portion of the molecule attaches to the protein transcobalamin II, which carries the B_{12} through the bloodstream to various tissues. Vitamin B_{12} is stored in the liver in such quantities that it takes several years for pernicious anemia to develop in an individual who is a strict vegetarian and ingests little B_{12} or in someone unable to produce IF. Meat, eggs, dairy products, and seafood contain vitamin B_{12}.

Health food enthusiasts believe that supplemental vitamin B_{12} will energize the body, prevent mental deterioration, and protect against cancer, toxins, and infections. Because of the rate limited fashion in which vitamin B_{12} is absorbed, there is no toxicity to the ingestion of large amounts of vitamin B_{12}. Overdosage from injection is rare and results primarily in a variety of skin changes that clear over 1 to 2 weeks.

BIOTIN

Biotin is produced in the intestines by bacterial action and is a cofactor in fatty acid synthesis. Deficiencies of biotin result in baldness and dry skin, lassitude, anorexia, depression, and hypercholesterolemia. Those taking chronic antibiotics and those on extremely low-calorie diets are at risk of developing a biotin deficiency. For such individuals, 100 to 300 μg of biotin per day are recommended. There is no known toxicity to biotin overdosage.

FOLIC ACID

Folic acid is essential for the production of DNA, RNA, and proteins. Although folic acid may reverse the megaloblastic red blood cell aspects of pernicious anemia, it will not reverse the neurologic changes associated with pernicious anemia. It is found in fresh leafy green vegetables, yeasts, and liver. Folic acid is absorbed in the small and large

intestines in the form of polyglutamates. At the brush border of the intestinal cells, excess glutamates are removed from the folate molecule, making a functioning intestinal mucosa necessary for absorption.

The adult daily recommended dosage of folic acid is 400 μg/d.[2] Dietary supplementation of 100 μg/d will reverse the red cell changes of pernicious anemia but will not reverse the neurologic effects; therefore, preparations with more than 100 μg are available only through prescription. Except for the problem with masking of the hematologic changes of pernicious anemia, there are no known adverse effects to the ingestion of large doses of folic acid.

VITAMIN C

The major form of vitamin C, 1-ascorbic acid, is a strong reducing agent that participates in hydroxylation reactions such as that necessary for the formation of collagen. Scurvy results from vitamin C deficiency and results in collagen, protein, and lipid metabolism abnormalities. Additionally, the presence of vitamin C in the intestines increases the absorption rate of iron. Those with a vitamin C deficiency will also be iron depleted.

Vitamin C, which is found primarily in fruits and vegetables,[2] is absorbed through the jejunum and ileum. The absorption rates decrease with increasing intraluminal quantities of vitamin C. For example, 90 percent of a 100-mg dose might be absorbed, whereas only 20 percent of a 10-g dose might be absorbed. The daily recommended dose for adults is 60 mg. Vitamin C levels, although high in fruits and vegetables, are reduced by heat, drying, and storage.

Large doses of vitamin C can produce attacks of gout and nephrolithiasis in individuals with these conditions. Others may develop diarrhea and abdominal cramps, which subside with discontinuation. Megadoses of vitamin C may result in false negative guaiac testing of feces, and may give falsely elevated glucose levels on dipstick testing.

TABLE 186-1   Some Generally Safe Herbal Agents

Agent	General Use	Rare Adverse Effect
Chamomile	Antispasmodic	Anaphylaxis if patient allergic to ragweed
Echinacea	To cure URIs and UTIs	Anaphylaxis if patient allergic to daisies May deplete vitamin stores
Feverfew[5]	To cure migraines	Suddenly discontinuing may precipitate migraine If chewed, can cause mouth ulcers and dermatitis
Garlic	For hypertension, colic, hyperlipidemia	Hypotension, rash, nausea, vomiting, diarrhea; death has been reported in massive doses in children
Ginko	For dementia, vertigo, Raynaud disease	May inhibit platelet aggregation and interact with warfarin May cause gastrointestinal upset
Ginseng[6]	For impotence, fatigue, ulcers, stress	May interact with warfarin Lowers blood glucose May cause insomnia, nervousness
St. John's wort	As antidepressant	Phototoxicity May interact with serotonin reuptake inhibitors; avoid tyramine-containing foods
Valerian	For sedation	Interacts with other sedating drugs May have paradoxical stimulant effect

Abbreviations: URIs = upper respiratory infections; UTIs = urinary tract infections.

HERBAL AGENTS

In 1994, the Dietary Supplement Health and Education Act (DSHEA) classified herbal medicines as "dietary supplements." Under DSHEA, herbals may not be marketed with claims of definitive therapeutic effects. Instead, manufacturers are allowed to market an herbal agent by describing its *intended effect* on the human body. For example, European controlled studies show that saw palmetto is effective for alleviating symptoms of benign prostatic hypertrophy, but in the United States, claims that saw palmetto is a treatment for benign prostatic hypertrophycannot be made, and saw palmetto is advertised as an herbal agent that can "support healthy prostate function."[3]

Herbals themselves are not controlled by the Federal Drug Administration (FDA). Instead, the FDA controls the wording of the product label, even though manufacturers and distributors are not required to notify the FDA of label claims until 30 days after the product is first marketed.

In 1997, sales of over-the-counter herbal preparations exceeded $1.5 billion in the United States. Home grown and imported herbal preparations add to the total amount of herbal agents ingested, inhaled, and rubbed on. The list is staggering. Herbal agents can be classified as generally safe, potentially toxic, and toxic. Some generally safe herbal agents are listed in Table 186-1.

Some of the moderately unsafe herbal preparations include absinthe (wormwood), black cohosh, comfrey, juniper, and lobelia. *Absinthe* (wormwood)—which is popular in Europe and is being produced there in clandestine laboratories—is a toxic liquor that contains volatile oils that produce psychosis, intellectual deterioration, ataxia, headache, vomiting, and diarrhea. Absinthe is used as a flavoring in alcoholic drinks.

Black (or blue) cohosh contains an estrogen-like compound and has been used to delay or treat menopause. It may cause nausea, vomiting, dizziness, and weakness.

Comfrey is used as a digestive stimulant in teas. It has, however, been linked to liver toxicity and hepatic carcinoma. The toxic action comes from the formation of pyrroles that act on DNA.[4]

Juniper is used as a diuretic but may also be hallucinogenic. Toxicity also includes renal toxicity, nausea, and vomiting.

Lobelia is used for asthma and as an expectorant. Other uses include smoking it as a marijuana substitute for its mild euphoric effect. The active ingredients include lobeline, atropine, and scopolamine, which can produce anticholinergic symptoms.

Some herbs that are unsafe but are commonly found on store shelves include chaparral, ephedra, nutmeg, and yohimbine.

Chaparral is derived from the leaves of the creosote bush and is used for its antioxidant effects as a potential cancer preventative. It is also thought to be effective in pain control but is also thought to be hepatotoxic.

Ephedra is used in weight loss and has been implicated in multiple toxic deaths. This herbal agent is contraindicated for patients with hypertension, diabetes, or glaucoma.

Nutmeg is used for dyspepsia, muscle aches, and arthritis. It contains terpenes, ethers, and myristicin. Myristicin can produce hallucinations (at about 2 to 4 teaspoonfuls of ground nutmeg). At various dosages, it can also produce gastrointestinal upset, agitation, coma, miosis, and hypertension.

Yohimbine is thought to be an aphrodisiac. Toxic effects include hallucinations, weakness, hypertension, and paralysis. Yohimbine, if combined with pheopropanolamine, can lead to a stroke through marked elevation of the blood pressure.

In addition to any potential toxicity to overingestion or overuse of herbals themselves, herbals may also interact with prescription medications. Herbals may have either pharmacokinetic interactions (changing a drug's absorption, distribution, metabolism or elimination) or pharmacodynamic interactions (altering a drug's effects). Much of the available literature on herb-drug interactions are anecdotal and nonreproducible. There are some herb-drug interactions that, because of larger numbers of clinical reports, animal studies and/or controlled clinical studies, can be deemed to be "likely" and should be considered by the emergency physician (Table 186-2).[7,8]

TABLE 186-2   Some Likely Herb-Drug Interactions*

Herb	Herb Used for	Drug	Effect of Interaction
Cayenne (Capsicum)	Arthritis, neuralgia, analgesic	ACE Inhibitors Theophylline SR	Increase of cough Increased absorption
Dan shen (salvia)	Reduction of lactation	Warfarin	Decreased warfarin metabolism
Ephedra	Energizer, weight loss, asthma, sinus congestion	MAOIs	MAOI intoxication
Grapefruit juice	For vitamin C effects	Amiodarone Benzodiazepines Calcium channel blockers Carbamazepine Clomipramine Ethinyl estradiol Statins Sertraline	Increased drug availability of any one of these drugs because of inhibition of intestinal cytochrome P450
Licorice in chronic, high doses	Respiratory disorders, hepatitis, inflammatory diseases, infections	Antihypertensives Diuretics Prednisolone	Decreased effect (can cause pseudohyperaldosteronism by inhibiting 11-betadehydrogenase) Increased K^+ loss, myopathy Increased drug levels
St. John's wort	Depression	Cyclosporin Digoxin Indinavir	Decreased serum levels; transplant rejection Decreased serum level Decreased serum level
Yohimbine	Erectile dysfunction, sexual potency	Clonidine Tricyclic antidepressants	Decreased effect Enhanced autonomic and central effects of yohimbe

*Based on case reports, clinical studies, and animal studies.
Abbreviations: ACE = angiotensin-converting enzyme; MAOI = monamine oxidase inhibitor; SR = sustained release.

REFERENCES

1. Cushing C, Anderson AC: Hypervitaminosis, in Viccellio P, Bania T, Brent J, et al (eds): *Emergency Toxicology,* 2d ed. New York, Lippincott-Raven, 1998, p. 607.

2. Vitamin supplements. *Med Lett* 40:75, 1998.

3. Canedy D: Real medicine or the medicine show. *New York Times* 23 July 1998, p. C1.

4. Poisoning associated with herbal teas: Arizona, Washington. *MMWR* 26: 257, 1977.

5. Perharic L, Shaw D, Murray V: Toxic effects of herbal medicines and food supplements. *Lancet* 342:180, 1993.

6. Ernst E: The risk-benefit profile of commonly used herbal therapies: Ginko, St. John's wort, ginseng, echinacea, saw palmetto, and kava. *Ann Intern Med* 136, 42, 2002.

7. Rotblatt M, Ziment I (eds): *Evidence-Based Herbal Medicine.* Philadelphia, Hanley and Belfus, 2002, p. 45.

8. De Smet, Peter AGM: Herbal remedies. *NEJM* 347(25), 2046, Dec 19, 2002.

ANTIMICROBIALS

G. Richard Bruno
Wallace A. Carter

Antimicrobial agents are estimated to account for 15 to 30 percent of the world medical drug expenditure.[1] Most adverse reactions to antibiotics occur at therapeutic doses. The most common adverse effects of antimicrobial use include hypersensitivity reactions, alterations in body microbial flora, interactions with other drugs, and cutaneous drug reactions. A thorough review of adverse effects of antimicrobials at therapeutic doses is beyond the scope of this chapter. Rather, this review focuses on the medical considerations of acute antimicrobial overdose. Data from the American Association of Poison Control Centers (AAPCC) suggest that antimicrobial exposures are a frequent source of inquiry to poison control centers but rarely result in life-threatening outcomes. In 2001, the AAPCC reported 61,215 exposures, which resulted in significant morbidity in 365 cases (0.6 percent) and 13 fatalities (less than 0.02 percent).[2] Most patients who present after antimicrobial overdose are asymptomatic. Observation and screening for coingestants are adequate before medical clearance in most cases. The poison control center should be contacted to assist in patient management and to aid in accurate statistical tracking of toxin exposures.

EVALUATION AND TREATMENT OF ANTIMICROBIAL OVERDOSE

Most antimicrobial overdoses will be asymptomatic; however, significant ingestions of agents such as isoniazid (INH), chloroquine, and quinine can result in severe toxicities. The history should include the amount and type of antimicrobial ingested. Patients should also be asked about possible coingestants. Suicide potential should be assessed.

Asymptomatic antimicrobial ingestions require minimal laboratory evaluation. As is common in all cases of possible overdose, determining acetaminophen levels and taking a 12-lead electrocardiogram should be considered as a means to screen for coingestants. Emergency medicine and critical care principles should guide laboratory evaluation in symptomatic overdoses. The electrolyte level should be determined to evaluate potential anion-gap acidosis in cases of suspected INH overdose. Methemoglobin levels should be determined in dapsone, chloroquine, and primaquine overdoses.[3] Drug levels are not helpful in the management in the acute antimicrobial overdose but may be confirmatory and are available for several antibiotics (INH, quinine, and chloroquine).

Patients who present with symptomatic ingestions (altered mental status, seizure, electrolyte disturbances, anion-gap acidosis, or renal failure) should be treated with supportive care using emergency medicine principles. Gastric decontamination should be initiated in all patients with suspected antimicrobial overdoses. Activated charcoal with the cathartic sorbitol should be given orally or through a nasogastric tube. Repeat-dose activated charcoal without sorbitol is indicated in symptomatic patients. Dialysis and charcoal hemoperfusion are effective at eliminating aminoglycosides and possibly pentamidine but are not highly effective at removing other antimicrobial agents.

SPECIFIC AGENTS IN OVERDOSE

Isoniazid

Infection with *Mycobacterium tuberculosis* (tuberculosis or TB) is common in developing countries, and has over the past decade increased in incidence in the United States. Patients being treated for active TB as well as patients taking chemoprophylaxis for positive purified protein derivative (PPD) skin tests are now commonplace in many urban emergency departments. Isoniazid (isonicotinylhydrazide or INH) is a first line drug utilized in both chemoprophylaxis and treatment of active TB. INH is also associated with high morbidity and mortality in overdose. According to AAPCC data from 2001, INH is the antimicrobial agent that accounted for the most cases of significant morbidity, almost one fourth of all major morbidity from antibiotic exposures.

INH is a hydrazide of isonicotinic acid that is bacteriostatic and whose mechanism of action is not well understood. At therapeutic doses (5 mg/kg) there are numerous side effects that may cause significant morbidity including neuropathy and hepatic injury. These side effects are separate and distinct from the clinical signs and symptoms of acute overdose.

The clinical symptoms of acute INH overdose typically present initially with nausea, mental status changes, and ataxia. These symptoms may progress to the clinical triad of seizure, coma, and metabolic acidosis. Seizures are typically seen in acute INH ingestion of more than 20 to 30 mg/kg. These seizures are generalized tonic-clonic in nature, and are often refractory to standard anticonvulsive therapy (benzodiazepines, barbiturates, etc.). The postulated mechanism for INH-induced seizures is INH depletion of vitamin B_6, which decreases activity of coenzyme pyridoxal 5-phosphate, which, in turn, impairs the synthesis of the inhibitory neurotransmitter γ-aminobutyric acid (GABA).

INH ingestion should be entertained in any patient presenting with refractory seizures.[4] Seizures are treated with pyridoxine (vitamin B_6). The dose is gram-for-gram equivalent to the amount of INH ingested. For patients who ingest an unknown quantity of INH, the recommended dose of pyridoxine is 5 g IV. The pyridoxine may be administered at a rate of approximately 1 g every 2 to 3 min.[5] Single-dose therapy of pyridoxine should be effective to stop seizures, but patients who do not receive adequate pyridoxine dosing may have repeat seizures. There are case reports of pyridoxine also helping to reverse INH-induced comas.[6] It has been documented in the literature that the large doses of pyridoxine required for therapy are often not found in hospitals.[7] For those involved in emergency medicine administration and operations it is prudent to ensure adequately stocked levels of pyridoxine in the ED and pharmacy.

The acidosis associated with large INH ingestions is believed to be a lactic acidosis secondary to seizure activity. **There is little role for sodium bicarbonate in acute INH overdose.**

Most INH-induced toxicity (i.e., seizures, obtundation, and acidosis) occur within 2 h of overdose. Patients who remain asymptomatic for 6 h after presentation are unlikely to manifest delayed IHN related symptoms and are safe for medical clearance.

Antimalarial Drugs

Antimalarials are not used in the United States as frequently as other antimicrobials; however, they are among the agents with the greatest potential for toxic effects. Common agents include quinine, chloroquine, mefloquine, and primaquine.

Quinine and chloroquine may both result in severe central nervous system (CNS) and cardiac abnormalities in acute overdose. CNS manifestation of toxicity includes obtundation, headache, and seizures. Quinine also has significant ocular toxicity in acute overdose, and blindness may result with serum levels of greater than 10 to 15 μg/mL. Possible electrolyte abnormalities include hypoglycemia with quinine and hypokalemia with chloroquine. Both drugs have cardiac effects and may lead to PR, QT, or QRS prolongation. Patients may be hypotensive, with early cardiovascular collapse. Aggressive supportive care is used for overdose.[8] A decreased mortality rate has been demonstrated in chloroquine overdose treated with early intubation, gastric lavage, deep sedation with benzodiazepines, and vasoactive pressor support with epinephrine to maintain a systolic blood pressure of 100 mm Hg.[9] Sodium bicarbonate (to adjust serum pH of 7.45 to 7.50) may be helpful in treating dysrhythmias related to the sodium-channel blockade from quinine and chloroquine, although solid data do not exist to support its use.

Penicillins and the β-Lactam Agents

Penicillins and the β-lactam agents are relatively benign in acute overdose. Confusion, agitation, myoclonic jerking, and seizures have been reported with high-dose penicillin G (more than 20 to 30 million units/d), cephalosporins, and imipenem. Encephalopathy, agitation, and absence seizures have been reported with ceftazidime. CNS effects of penicillins and β-lactam agents are believed to result from antagonism of the GABA receptor. Patients most at risk for adverse CNS effects during β-lactam therapy are those with renal failure, with underlying CNS abnormalities, or who are receiving high-dose therapy.

Therapy for β-lactam agent-related seizures are based on general emergency management principles for seizure management with first-line agents being benzodiazepines.

Aminoglycosides

Aminoglycosides are not available in oral forms, so intentional ingestions have not been reported; rather most aminoglycoside acute overdoses are iatrogenic in nature. It is presumed most of these errors occur in the order process (miscalculation of dose or wrong dose dispensed). Catastrophic aminoglycoside overdoses are rare but have been reported in neonates and hospitalized patients. Aminoglycosides have a low therapeutic to toxic ratio, with ototoxicity and nephrotoxicity common in both therapeutic use and acute overdose. All aminoglycosides have the potential to damage vestibular and cochlear sensory cells, but neomycin is by far the most ototoxic. The incidence of hearing loss related to aminoglycoside has been reported to be between 2 and 25 percent. Hearing loss correlates closely with high-dose or prolonged therapy. Nephrotoxicity results from damage to the proximal renal tubules and correlates with drug dose, therapy duration, volume status, and extremes of age.

Therapy for acute aminoglycoside overdose is typically hydration and monitoring of hearing and renal function. Hemodialysis has been used to enhance elimination of aminoglycosides but it is unclear what role it should play in acute overdose because most patients recover with only supportive care.

REFERENCES

1. Blanca M: Allergic reactions to penicillins: A changing world? *Allergy* 50:777, 1995.

2. Litovitz TL, Klein-Schwartz W, Rodgers GC, et al: 2001 Annual report of the American Association of Poison Control Centers Toxic Exposure Surveillance System. *Am J Emer Med* 20:391, 2002.

3. Sin DD, Shafran SD: Dapsone and primaquine induced methemoglobinemia in HIV infected individuals. *J Acquir Immune Defic Syndr Hum Retrovirol* 12:477, 1996.

4. Sullivan EA, Geoffroy P, Weisman R, et al: Isoniazid poisonings in New York City. *J Emerg Med* 16:57, 1998.

5. Wason S, Lacouture PG, Lovejoy FH: Single high-dose pyridoxine treatment for isoniazid overdose. *JAMA* 246:1102, 1981.

6. Brent J, Nguyen V, Kulig K, Rumack BH: Reversal of prolonged isoniazid-induced coma by pyridoxine. *Arch Intern Med* 150:1751, 1990.

7. Scharman E: Isoniazid toxicity: A survey or pyridoxine availability. *Am J Emerg Med* 12:386, 1994.

8. Clemessy JL, Taboulet P, Hoffman JR, et al: Treatment of acute chloroquine poisoning: A 5-year experience. *Crit Care Med* 24:1189, 1996.

9. Riou B, Barriot P, Rimailho A, et al: Treatment of severe chloroquine poisoning. *New Engl J Med* 318:1, 1988.

CYANIDE

Larissa I. Velez

Kathleen A. Delaney

Cyanide is a potent cellular toxin with an infamous history. It was the agent of mass suicide at Jonestown, Guyana; of murder in the Tylenol-tampering incidents; and of genocide in the gas chambers of Nazi Germany.[1,2] Cyanide is widely available. Table 188-1 lists common sources of cyanide.

SOURCES OF EXPOSURE

Acute cyanide poisoning occurs in 1) occupational settings; 2) inadvertent, suicidal, or homicidal ingestions of cyanide or chemicals metabolized to cyanide[3]; 3) patients on infusions of sodium nitroprusside[4]; 4) persons who ingest plant products that contain cyanogenic glycosides[5]; and 5) inhalation of smoke from burning plastics in closed-space fires.[6–8]

Industrial Exposures

Cyanide compounds are both precursors and incidental by-products in the production of many industrial materials. Occupational exposures are caused by inhalation of hydrogen cyanide (HCN) gas and dermatologic exposure to solutions of cyanide salts. Inadvertent ingestion of cyanide salts can occur from eating in a contaminated workplace.

Smoke Inhalation

Smoke inhalation is a common, though often unrecognized, cause of acute cyanide toxicity. Large amounts of HCN are released when

TABLE 188-1   Sources of Cyanide

Burning of: wool, nylon, silk, acrylic, polyurethane, melamine, polyacrylonitrile, polyamide plastics
Industries: fabrication of plastics, electroplating, mining, photography, precious metal reclamation, solvents, hair removal from hides
Fumigants and fertilizers
"Coyote gitter" animal traps
Chemistry laboratories
Medicinal: Laetrile,* sodium nitroprusside
Plants: seeds from *Prunus* species (apricots, cherries, plums, peaches), cassava
Illicit phencyclidine (PCP) manufacturing
Cigarette smoke
Vehicle exhausts

*No longer available in U.S., but widely available via the Internet and sold outside the United States.

natural and synthetic nitrogen-containing polymers, such as wool and vinyl, are burned. Elevated cyanide levels, often associated with elevated carbon monoxide levels, are implicated in fire-related fatalities.[6–9]

Other Exposures

Suicides and homicides account for some cases of cyanide poisoning. Persons with occupational access to cyanide salts, such as chemists and jewelers, are more at risk. Naturally occurring plant glycosides have been a cause of poisoning. Amygdalin, a cyanogenic glycoside found in high concentrations in apricot pits and bitter almonds, was the principal ingredient in Laetrile. During the 1970s, the use of Laetrile as a nontraditional cancer therapy led to numerous deaths.[5] Ingestion of acetonitrile-containing cosmetic products caused severe poisoning in several children.[3]

Chronic Exposure

Adverse physiologic effects due to chronic subacute cyanide exposure have been proposed but are poorly defined. Studies of workers chronically exposed to cyanide demonstrated a higher incidence of thyroid disease and vitamin B_{12} deficiency. Cassava, a tropical root that contains the cyanogenic glycoside *linamarin,* is a food staple in many countries. Tropical ataxic neuropathy is endemic in countries where cassava consumption is high. The combination of chronic tobacco use and a diet poor in cyanide-scavenging carotenes is epidemiologically associated with the development of optic neuropathy.[10]

BIOCHEMICAL TOXICOLOGY

The avidity with which cyanide binds to metal-containing enzymes accounts for its serious cellular toxicity. Its key physiologic effect is produced by inhibition of the iron-dependent reduction of molecular oxygen to water by cytochrome aa_3, the final step in oxidative phosphorylation.[11,12] Anaerobic reduction of pyruvate to lactate and impaired conversion of adenosine diphosphate (ADP) to adenosine triphosphate (ATP) result in severe metabolic acidosis. The biochemical bases of observed effects such as altered calcium homeostasis, the release of excitatory neurotransmitters in the central nervous system (CNS), and pulmonary and coronary arteriolar vasoconstriction remain poorly defined.[2]

CLINICAL TIME COURSE OF POISONING: ROUTES OF EXPOSURE

The time course and severity of the clinical effects of cyanide are a function of the nature of the cyanide-containing compound, the route of exposure, and the concentration of cyanide to which the patient is exposed. The onset of symptoms following inhalational exposure to HCN gas is virtually immediate. Concentrations of <50 parts per million (ppm) cause restlessness, anxiety, palpitations, dyspnea, and headache.[13] Higher levels of HCN gas cause severe dyspnea, loss of consciousness, seizures, and cardiac dysrhythmias. Coma, cardiovascular collapse, and death may occur immediately on exposure to very high levels. The median lethal dose (LD_{50}) for humans is estimated to be 200 ppm for a 30-min exposure and 600 to 700 ppm for a 5-min exposure.[13]

The onset of symptoms following ingestion of a cyanide salt occurs within minutes. Death has resulted from the ingestion of as little as 50 mg of cyanide salt in an adult, while survival has been reported in much larger ingestions when antidotes are used. The LD_{50} of the potassium or sodium salt of cyanide in an untreated adult is estimated at 140 to 250 mg.[13] Symptoms of poisoning are delayed following the ingestion of compounds that require metabolic activation to release free cyanide. Acetonitrile, a solvent sold commercially as a cosmetic nail remover, undergoes hepatic oxidative metabolism that results in

the release of HCN. The onset of symptoms of cyanide poisoning following ingestion of acetonitrile occurred at 24 h in one case.[3] Cyanide is released from amygdalin by hydrolysis in the small intestine, resulting in delayed progression of symptoms. The slow release of cyanide by the spontaneous degradation of sodium nitroprusside also results in delayed toxicity, particularly during prolonged or high-dose infusions. The rate of degradation of sodium nitroprusside is increased by exposure to sunlight.[4]

CLINICAL FEATURES

History

An occupational history may provide a clue to the possibility of cyanide poisoning, particularly in the suicidal patient. Careful identification of ingestants in asymptomatic patients will prevent the discharge of a patient who has potential for delayed toxicity from a cyanogenic compound.

Symptoms of Poisoning

Antidotal treatment may be lifesaving. It is important to recognize that rapid onset of symptoms is an important clue. Patients who are alert may hyperventilate and complain of breathlessness. These symptoms can be indistinguishable from anxiety produced by knowledge of a possible exposure. CNS and cardiovascular toxicity are prominent. The severity of effects is correlated with the degree of exposure. CNS effects range from anxiety and confusion to seizures and coma. The inability to use oxygen results in functional hypoxemia except that the patient is not cyanotic, as cyanide does not significantly alter the oxygen-carrying capacity of hemoglobin. Cyanosis does follow respiratory arrest. The cardiac effects of cyanide poisoning are similar to those of hypoxemia. Sinus tachycardia, atrial dysrhythmias, and premature ventricular contractions progress to bradycardia and asystole. Ventricular tachycardia and fibrillation are uncommon. Table 188-2 summarizes common signs and symptoms of toxicity. The typical seriously poisoned patient is comatose, hyperventilating, hypotensive, and bradycardic without cyanosis. Severe metabolic acidosis is a consistent clinical clue; indeed, the absence of metabolic acidosis precludes the diagnosis of cyanide toxicity.[1] In victims of smoke inhalation, toxic cyanide levels correlate with plasma lactate levels greater than 10 mmol/L, independent of the carbon monoxide level.[8] Decreased cellular extraction of oxygen results in increased oxygenation of venous blood and a decrease in the normal arteriovenous oxygen $[(a-v)CO_2]$ difference. Although this concept facilitates understanding of the cellular effects of cyanide, it is difficult (and impractical) to detect this underuse of oxygen in an emergency setting, as normal val-

TABLE 188-2   Signs and Symptoms of Acute Cyanide Toxicity

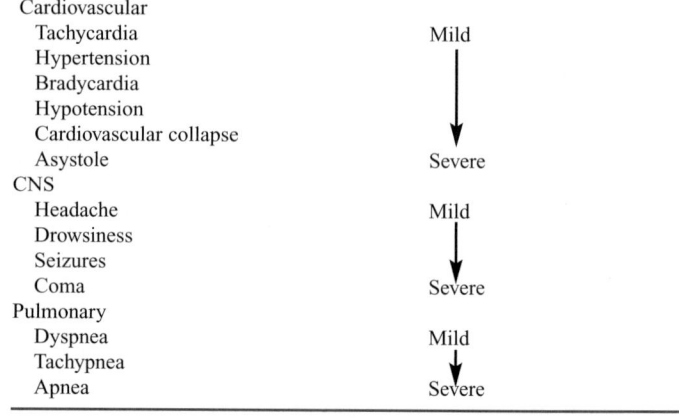

Cardiovascular	
Tachycardia	Mild
Hypertension	
Bradycardia	
Hypotension	
Cardiovascular collapse	
Asystole	Severe
CNS	
Headache	Mild
Drowsiness	
Seizures	
Coma	Severe
Pulmonary	
Dyspnea	Mild
Tachypnea	
Apnea	Severe

ues for peripheral venous oxygen saturation and the effects of oxygen therapy on these values have not been well studied. A reliable estimation of the $(a-v)CO_2$ requires that the venous sample be taken from the pulmonary artery or vena cava. A possibly useful finding related to this phenomenon is the reported "arterialization" of veins on funduscopic examination by increased venous partial pressure of oxygen.[14] A smell of bitter almonds supports the diagnosis of cyanide poisoning, but it is estimated that only 60 to 80 percent of the population can detect the characteristic almond odor of cyanide. Table 188-3 lists other anticipated laboratory abnormalities.

DIFFERENTIAL DIAGNOSIS

Cyanide poisoning should always be considered in the poisoned patient with a normal partial pressure of arterial oxygen (Pa_{O_2}) and a high anion gap metabolic acidosis because of lactate. Chap. 25 discusses the differential diagnosis of lactic acidosis and includes poisonings that accumulate lactate (iron, methemoglobin inducers, methanol, biguanides, strychnine), other cellular toxins/asphyxiants (salicylates, carbon monoxide, hydrogen sulfide, azides, arsine, phosphine, nerve agents, or other organophosphates) and seizure-causing agents (cocaine and other stimulants, theophylline, camphor, cicutoxin).

TREATMENT

The standard accepted therapy for cyanide poisoning in the United States has been well established for half a century, and is based on experimental and chemical principles developed by Chen and colleagues in 1933.[15,16] The antidotes are contained in a kit (approximately $200 per kit) now provided by Taylor Pharmaceuticals, which includes an ampule of amyl nitrite for inhalation, 10 mL of 3 percent sodium nitrite (300 mg), and 50 mL of 25 percent sodium thiosulfate (12.5 g). Table 188-4 gives the adult and pediatric doses of the three components of the kit.

Nitrites

Nitrites have significant side effects that include hypotension and the development of excessive methemoglobinemia.[11,17] **The reported death of a child from methemoglobinemia that followed aggressive treatment of a nonlethal ingestion of cyanide has led to the practice of adjusting the pediatric dose of sodium nitrite according to**

TABLE 188-3   Anticipated Laboratory Findings in Cyanide Poisoning

Test	Result	Cause
Serum electrolytes	Elevated anion gap	Lactic acidosis from anaerobic metabolism
Arterial blood gases	Metabolic acidosis Normal P_{O_2}	As above
Measured % oxygen saturation (by co-oximetry)	Normal	Hemoglobin has normal oxygen-carrying capacity
$(a-v)O_2$	Decreased	Decreased tissue oxygen use
Whole-blood cyanide level: Toxic Fatal	>0.5 μg/mL >2.5 μg/mL	Note: plasma cyanide levels are roughly 1/10 of the whole-blood cyanide levels
Fire victims COHb Lactate	Elevated >10 mmol/L	Mixed toxicity, synergistic Correlates with toxic cyanide level

TABLE 188-4   Treatment of Cyanide Poisoning

Adults
100% oxygen.
Amyl nitrite inhaler; crack vial and inhale over 30 s.*
Sodium nitrite: 10 mL IV (10-mL ampule 3% $NaNO_2$ = 300 mg).†
Sodium thiosulfate: 50 mL IV (50-mL ampule 25% $Na_2S_2O_3$ = 12.5 g).
Repeat at half dose if symptoms persist.

Children (adapted from recommendations by Berlin[17] and Isom and Johnson[19])
100% oxygen.
IV sodium nitrite and sodium thiosulfate:

Hb (g/100 mL)	3% $NaNO_2$† (mL/kg)	25% $Na_2S_2O_3$ (mL/kg)
7	0.19	1.65
8	0.22	1.65
9	0.25	1.65
10	0.27	1.65
11	0.30	1.65
12	0.33	1.65
13	0.36	1.65
14	0.39	1.65

Repeat once at half dose if symptoms persist.
Monitor methemoglobin to keep level less than 30 percent.

*Not necessary if IV is in place.
†Avoid nitrites in the presence of severe hypotension if diagnosis is unclear.

the patient's hemoglobin level, as illustrated in Table 188-4.[13,17] The amyl nitrite offers a temporizing measure when an intravenous line is not available. It does not need to be administered when sodium nitrite can be given IV.

The rationale for using nitrites was based on their capacity to form methemoglobin, which has an avid affinity for cyanide. Although the antidotal efficacy of nitrites is not disputed, their actual mechanism of action has been questioned.[12] Studies have shown that inhibition of methemoglobin synthesis by methylene blue does not affect the efficacy of the nitrites. In addition, rapid methemoglobin inducers such as 4-dimethylaminophenol (DMAP) are not more efficacious than nitrites.[2] It has also been demonstrated that the rapid clinical reversal of cyanide toxicity occurs despite the demonstration of only very small amounts of methemoglobin.[18]

Sodium Thiosulfate

Following the administration of sodium nitrite, sodium thiosulfate is infused. Sodium thiosulfate enhances the activity of the enzyme rhodanese, a mammalian enzyme that likely evolved in response to the ubiquitous presence of cyanide in nature. Rhodanese catalyzes the transfer of sulfate from sodium thiosulfate to cyanide to form thiocyanate, a less-toxic form that is excreted by the kidneys.[11,15] Studies of the cyanide LD_{50} in animals demonstrate that the therapeutic effects of sodium nitrite and sodium thiosulfate are synergistic.[11,15]

Sodium thiosulfate has very limited toxicity in comparison with nitrites and is a safer empirical therapy when the diagnosis is not clear. It may also be useful as a sole therapy for victims of inhalation injury where there is concern that the induction of methemoglobinemia in the setting of carbon monoxide exposure may further reduce oxygen carrying capacity.[7]

Oxygen

Surprisingly, the administration of 100 percent oxygen enhances the therapeutic efficacy of antidotal therapy.[11] It has been proposed that oxygen may affect the binding of cyanide to cytochrome oxidase or the ability to form methemoglobin. Animal studies of cyanide poisoning show no benefit of hyperbaric oxygen over 100 percent oxygen.[11]

Hyperbaric oxygen is useful in the management of patients with suspected cyanide poisoning who have concomitant carbon monoxide poisoning.

Other Therapies

Because of the side effects of nitrites, an effort has been made to develop equally efficacious but less toxic therapies. Dicobalt edetate (Kelocyanor), a cobalt compound with a high affinity for cyanide, is the first-line agent for the treatment of cyanide poisoning in the United Kingdom. Although highly effective as a cyanide antidote, the toxicity of dicobalt edetate is greater when cyanide is not present, limiting its use to cases where the presence of cyanide is unequivocal.[1,2,11]

Hydroxocobalamin (vitamin B_{12a}, 5 g IV; 70 mg/kg over 30 min), in combination with sodium thiosulfate, has been the antidote of choice in France since the 1970s. Because of its low toxicity and its efficacy, it is ideal in cases where the diagnosis is uncertain or in cases where the induction of methemoglobinemia may be detrimental.[8] Unfortunately, solutions of this antidote in concentrations adequate to treat cyanide poisoning are not readily available in the United States. Side effects associated with hydroxocobalamin include transient hypertension, a reddish discoloration of the skin and mucous membranes, and rare anaphylactoid reactions.[7] In practice, hydroxocobalamin is used in combination with sodium thiosulfate.

DMAP is a rapid methemoglobin-inducer developed in Germany for the treatment of cyanide poisoning. It has not been demonstrated to be more clinically efficacious than sodium nitrite. DMAP (5 mL of 5 percent solution [250 mg] IV over 1 min) is used in combination with sodium thiosulfate.

Supportive Care

Severely poisoned patients have survived with supportive care, although survival in cases of massive exposure undoubtedly has been facilitated by antidotal therapy. All patients with known or suspected cyanide poisoning should receive 100 percent oxygen by mask, be put on a cardiac monitor, and have an intravenous line in place. Hypotension should be treated with fluids and standard vasopressors (see Chap. 30). Seizures can be treated with benzodiazepines (see Chap. 232).

Decontamination

Gastric decontamination should never take priority over resuscitation of the symptomatic patient. Following resuscitation, patients with a history of ingestion may benefit from gastric decontamination with lavage and/or activated charcoal. Superactivated charcoal binds small amounts of cyanide and may be useful in decreasing the significance of an ingestion.[17] Topical exposures require copious irrigation with water.

CYANIDE AND CARBOXYHEMOGLOBIN

Patients with inhalational exposures often recover following their removal from the toxic exposure. They do not require antidotal treatment if significant recovery has occurred prior to reaching medical attention.

The decision to administer the sodium nitrite-thiosulfate antidote is straightforward when faced with a comatose, bradycardic patient with a clear history of cyanide exposure. **Hypotension is not a contraindication to sodium nitrite therapy in this setting.** A patient with mild to moderate symptoms may be observed closely for more serious signs prior to the initiation of treatment.

More difficult management decisions arise in patients with smoke inhalation who have or may have carbon monoxide exposure as well as suspected cyanide exposure, and patients who are critically ill and acidotic without any known history of cyanide exposure. It is prudent to avoid the vasodilating effects of nitrites in patients whose diagnosis is uncertain. There is a correlation between carboxyhemoglobin and cyanide levels after smoke inhalation. **The empirical administration of nitrites to patients who have elevated carboxyhemoglobin levels is relatively contraindicated because of the potential for methemoglobinemia to further decrease oxygen-carrying capacity,[7]** although a limited study failed to show clinically significant methemoglobinemia in victims of smoke inhalation who also had carbon monoxide poisoning.[6] For the victim of smoke inhalation who arrives to the ED alive and has significant unexplained lactic acidosis, the safest immediate empirical therapy that avoids the hypotensive effects of nitrites and the concerns about methemoglobin formation is the administration of sodium thiosulfate in addition to 100 percent oxygen. Hydroxocobalamin, which has orphan drug status in the United States, will be an ideal agent for both of these settings if it becomes available.[7] In critically ill, acidotic patients where the possibility of cyanide poisoning is considered, anecdotal reports support the utility of the empirical administration of sodium thiosulfate alone.

LABORATORY EVALUATION

The decision to institute antidotal treatment of cyanide poisoning must be made long before confirmatory laboratory studies can be obtained. Although cyanide levels are not closely correlated with toxicity, they can be used to confirm a clinical diagnosis in retrospect, or for forensic purposes. Whole-blood cyanide levels are the most commonly reported values.[13] Whole blood cyanide levels are normally less than 0.02 μg/mL, while potentially fatal levels are greater than 2.5 μg/mL. Because cyanide is sequestered in erythrocytes, plasma cyanide levels approximate one-tenth of the whole-blood cyanide levels.

The arterial blood gas is a rapid and useful test when cyanide poisoning is suspected. The absence of a metabolic acidosis is inconsistent with the diagnosis of acute cyanide poisoning.

As previously noted, the demonstration of a serum lactate level greater than 10 mmol/L was significantly correlated with toxic cyanide levels in victims of smoke inhalation.[8] Table 188-3 summarizes laboratory findings anticipated in cyanide poisoning.

DISPOSITION

All patients who receive antidotal therapy should be admitted. Patients who have ingested a substance that may result in delayed toxicity should also be admitted. Full recovery is anticipated in many cases of severe poisoning where treatment is initiated rapidly and cardiac arrest has not yet occurred. Recovery despite cardiac arrest also has been reported, but anoxic encephalopathy may ensue.

REFERENCES

1. Borron SW, Baud FJ: Acute cyanide poisoning: Clinical spectrum, diagnosis, and treatment. *Arh Hig Rada Toksikol* 47(3):307, 1996.
2. Beasley DGM, Glass WI: Cyanide poisoning: Pathophysiology and treatment recommendations. *Occup Med* 48(7):427, 1998.
3. Losek JD, Rock AL, Boldt RR: Cyanide poisoning from a cosmetic nail remover. *Pediatrics* 88:337, 1991.
4. Curry SC, Arnold-Capell P: Toxic effects of drugs used in the ICU: Nitroprusside, nitroglycerin, and angiotensin-converting enzyme inhibitors. *Crit Care Clin* 7:555, 1991.
5. Braico KT, Humbert JR, Terplan KL, et al: Laetrile intoxication. *New Engl J Med* 300:238, 1979.
6. Kirk MA, Gerace R, Kulig KW: Cyanide and methemoglobin kinetics in smoke inhalation victims treated with the cyanide antidote kit. *Ann Emerg Med* 22:1413, 1993.
7. Kulig K: Cyanide antidotes and fire toxicology. *New Engl J Med* 325(25):1801, 1991.
8. Baud FJ, Barriot P, Toffis V, et al: Elevated blood cyanide concentrations in victims of smoke inhalation. *New Engl J Med* 325(25):1761, 1991.
9. Silverman SH, Purdue GF, Hunt JL, et al: Cyanide toxicity in burned patients. *J Trauma* 28(2):171, 1998.

10. The Cuba Neuropathy Field Investigation Team: Epidemic optic neuropathy in Cuba-Clinical characterization and risk factors. *New Engl J Med* 333: 1176, 1995.

11. Way JL: Cyanide intoxication and its mechanism of antagonism. *Rev Pharmacol Toxicol* 24:451, 1984.

12. Baud FJ, Borron SW, Bavoux E, et al: Relation between plasma lactate and blood cyanide concentrations in acute cyanide poisoning. *BMJ* 312:26, 1996.

13. Hall AH, Rumack BH: Clinical toxicology of cyanide. *Ann Emerg Med* 15:1067, 1986.

14. Johnson RP, Mellors JW: Arterialization of venous blood gases: A clue to the diagnosis of cyanide poisoning. *J Emerg Med* 6:401, 1988.

15. Chen KK, Rose CL: Nitrite and thiosulfate therapy in cyanide poisoning. *JAMA* 149:113, 1952.

16. Chen KK, Rose CL, Clowes GHA: Methylene blue, nitrites, and sodium thiosulfate against cyanide poisoning. *Proc Soc Exp Biol Med* 31:250, 1933.

17. Berlin CM: The treatment of cyanide poisoning in children. *Pediatrics* 46:793, 1970.

18. Johnson WS, Hall AH, Rumack BH: Cyanide poisoning successfully treated without "therapeutic methemoglobin levels." *Am J Emerg Med* 7:437, 1989.

DYSHEMOGLOBINEMIAS

Sean M. Rees
Lewis S. Nelson

The dyshemoglobinemias are a constellation of disorders in which the hemoglobin molecule is functionally altered and prevented from carrying oxygen. The most clinically relevant dyshemoglobinemias are carboxyhemoglobin, methemoglobin, and sulfhemoglobin. Carboxyhemoglobin develops following carbon monoxide exposure and, because of its unique importance and prevalence, is discussed in Chap. 203. This chapter reviews methemoglobinemia and sulfhemoglobinemia. Although the exact prevalence of these disorders remains undefined, the American Association of Poison Control Centers database reports thousands of exposures to drugs and chemicals capable of producing methemoglobinemia, but, unfortunately, cases in which methemoglobinemia actually occurred are not tallied.[1]

METHEMOGLOBINEMIA

Pathophysiology

Under normal circumstances, the iron moiety within deoxyhemoglobin exists in the ferrous (Fe^{2+}) form. Iron in this oxidation state avidly interacts with compounds seeking electrons, such as oxygen, and in the process is oxidized to the ferric (Fe^{3+}) state. On exposure to a nonoxygen oxidizing agent, iron donates an electron and transforms oxidation states from Fe^{2+} to Fe^{3+}. The Fe^{3+} that remains is unreactive, and the hemoglobin that contains the Fe^{3+} is termed *methemoglobin*. Methemoglobin, therefore, is unable to bind oxygen. Under normal circumstances, a small amount of methemoglobin exists in the blood (<1 percent). A level higher than 1 percent defines methemoglobinemia. This is somewhat of a misnomer as the hemoglobin is contained within the erythrocyte and not free within the blood. The accumulation of methemoglobin is normally limited enzymatically by the rapid reduction of the ferric iron back to the ferrous form as it forms. The enzyme NADH-methemoglobin reductase (also referred to as NADH cytochrome-b_5 reductase) is primarily responsible for this reduction, in which NADH (reduced nicotinamide adenine dinucleotide) donates its electrons to cytochrome-b_5, which subsequently reduces methemoglobin to hemoglobin.[2] In this process, NAD+ (oxidized nicotinamide adenine dinucleotide) is regenerated (Figure 189-1). This pathway is responsible for reducing nearly 95 percent of the methemoglobin. A second enzymatic pathway uses NADPH and NADPH-methemoglobin reductase to effect methemoglobin reduction analogous to the NADH-linked enzyme system. This enzyme is of limited importance normally (<5 percent total reduction) because of the lack of a suitable molecule to shuttle electrons in a manner similar to cytochrome-b_5. However, this enzyme is crucial for the antidotal effect of methylene blue, which performs this function when administered exogenously (see Figure 189-1). To a very limited extent, nonenzymatic reduction systems, such as vitamin C and glutathione, may participate in the reduction of methemoglobin to hemoglobin. This limited effect of glutathione partially explains why patients with glucose-6-phosphate dehydrogenase deficiency (G6PD), who are deficient in reduced glutathione, are not at increased risk of developing methemoglobinemia.

The primary clinical effect of methemoglobin is to reduce the oxygen content of the blood. Because the hemoglobin-bound oxygen accounts for the vast majority of an individual's oxygen-carrying capacity, as the methemoglobin level rises oxygen delivery to the tissues falls. However, patients with methemoglobinemia are often more symptomatic than patients who suffer from a simple anemia that produces an equivalent reduction in oxygen-carrying capacity. This is caused by a leftward shift in the oxyhemoglobin dissociation curve, the consequence of which is a reduced release of oxygen from the erythrocyte to the tissue at a given partial pressure of oxygen (Figure 189-2).

Acquired Methemoglobinemia

Methemoglobinemia is acquired when the normal mechanisms responsible for the elimination of methemoglobin are overwhelmed by an exogenous oxidant stress, such as a drug or chemical agent (Table

FIG. 189-1. Pathophysiology of methemoglobin formation and mechanism of action of methylene blue.

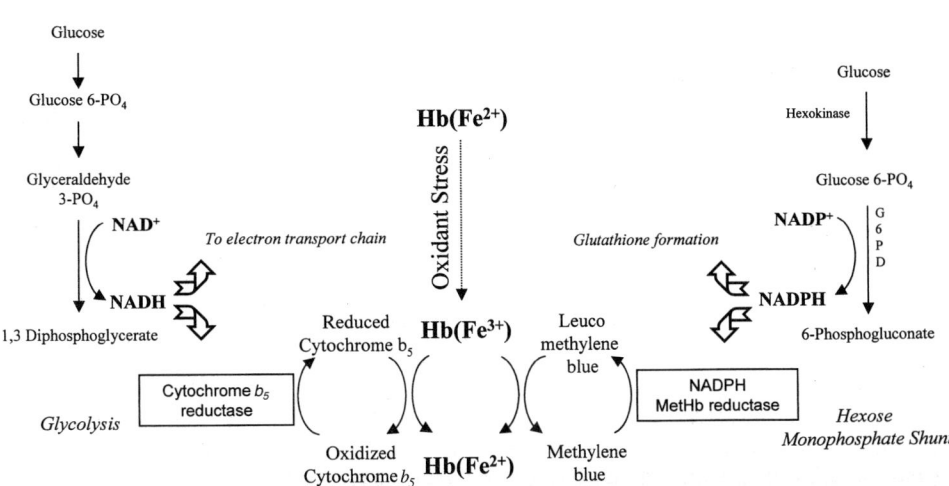

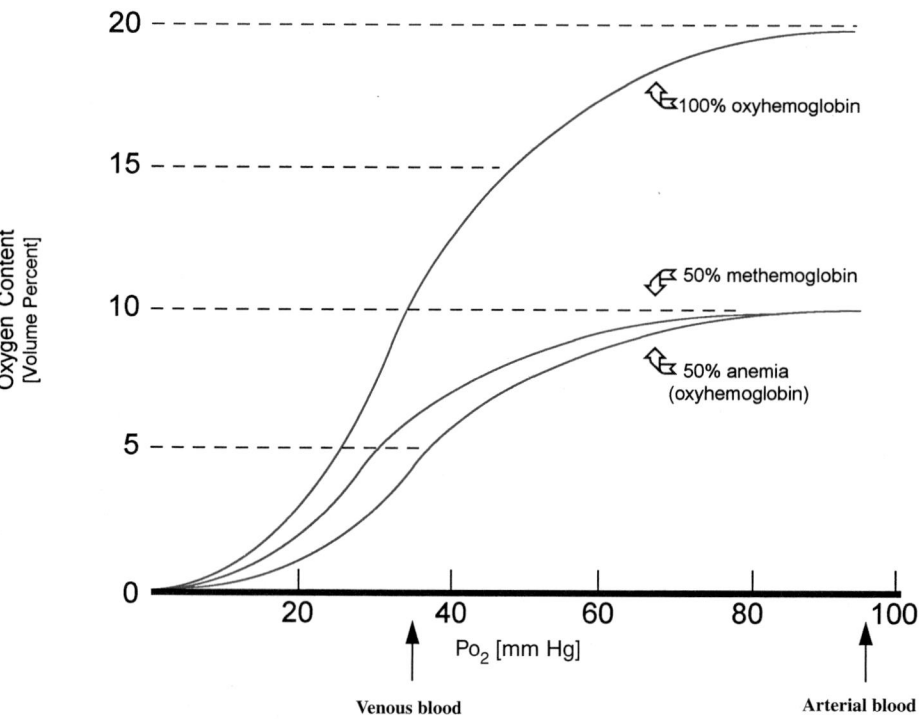

FIG. 189-2. The oxyhemoglobin dissociation curve describes the change in oxygen binding to hemoglobin as the dissolved oxygen (P_{O_2}) varies. The oxyhemoglobin dissociation curve of blood with a 50 percent reduction in erythrocytes (anemia) follows a curve similar to that of nonanemic blood, although the oxygen content is lower to start; i.e., unbinding of half of the oxygen occurs at the same P_{O_2}. The oxygen dissociation curve of blood with 50 percent methemoglobin is shifted to the left so that it is less willing to give up its oxygen despite a similar reduction in oxygen binding sites as the anemic blood.

189-1). Drugs in conventional doses rarely produce clinically significant methemoglobinemia, although subclinical methemoglobinemia may go unrecognized. Currently, most cases of drug-induced methemoglobinemia are caused by phenazopyridine (a commonly used agent for the symptomatic treatment of urinary tract infections), benzocaine (a topical anesthetic), and dapsone (an antibiotic often used in HIV-related therapy). Nitrate and nitrite salts (such as sodium nitrate) are the chemicals most often responsible for epidemic methemoglobinemia.[3] Methemoglobin induction with sodium nitrite is a therapeutic goal in the management of patients suffering from cyanide poisoning. Many of the aforementioned compounds, particularly dapsone, require metabolism to the "active" oxidant, and there may be substantial delay until toxicity is evident.

Methemoglobinemia can affect any age group and, because of undeveloped methemoglobin reduction mechanisms, the perinatal and infant age groups are more susceptible than older age groups. This explains the relatively common development of methemoglobinemia in infants given certain nitrogenous vegetables (e.g., spinach) or well-water that contains high nitrate levels. Bacteria within the gastrointestinal flora convert nitrate to the nitrite form, which is a more potent oxidant. Another common cause of acquired infantile methemoglobinemia is gastroenteritis, which is presumably caused by an increased oxidant burden originating in the gastrointestinal tract.[4]

Hereditary Methemoglobinemia

Hereditary methemoglobinemia results from either an enzymatic deficiency (i.e., NADH cytochrome-b_5 reductase) or from the presence of

an amino acid substitution within the hemoglobin molecule itself [i.e., hemoglobin M (HbM)]. Patients with NADH cytochrome-b_5 reductase deficiency develop methemoglobin levels of 20 to 40 percent, but these are easily reduced by the administration of daily oral doses of methylene blue or vitamin C. Cyanosis in these individuals begins at birth, but they remain asymptomatic and develop normally.

HbM is an abnormal form of hemoglobin in which its tertiary structure is altered and the heme iron exists in an environment favoring the ferric form. This disease only occurs in the heterozygous form, as the homozygous form is incompatible with life. Currently there is no treatment for this form of methemoglobin. As with NADH cytochrome-b_5 reductase deficiency, patients develop profound cyanosis, but tolerate the elevated methemoglobin concentrations extremely well.

Clinical Features

Patients who have normal hemoglobin concentrations do not usually develop clinically significant effects until the methemoglobin concentration rises above 20 percent of the total hemoglobin. However, patients may seek evaluation for the profound cyanosis that occurs when the methemoglobin concentration reaches about 1.5 g/dL, which is approximately 10 percent of the total hemoglobin in normal individuals. At methemoglobin concentrations between 20 and 30 percent, symptoms, including anxiety, headache, weakness, and lightheadedness develop, and patients may exhibit tachypnea and sinus tachycardia. Methemoglobin concentrations of 50 to 60 percent impair oxygen delivery to vital tissues, resulting in myocardial ischemia, dysrhythmias, depressed mental status (including coma), seizures, and lactate-associated metabolic acidosis. Levels above 70 percent are largely incompatible with life. Anemic patients may not exhibit cyanosis until the methemoglobin concentration rises dramatically above 10 percent, because it is the absolute concentration (i.e., 1.5 g/dL), not the percentage of methemoglobin, that determines cyanosis. Anemic patients may likewise suffer significant symptoms at lower methemoglobin concentrations because the relative percentage of hemoglobin in the oxidized form is greater. Patients with preexisting diseases that impair oxygen delivery to the red blood cells (e.g., chronic obstructive pulmonary disease, congestive heart failure) will also manifest symptoms

TABLE 189-1   Agents Commonly Implicated in Patients with Methemoglobinemia

Nitrates/nitrites	Dapsone
Amyl nitrite	Phenazopyridine
Isobutyl nitrite	Local anesthetics
Sodium nitrite	Benzocaine
Ammonium nitrate	Lidocaine
Silver nitrate	Prilocaine
Well water	Dibucaine
Nitroglycerin	Sulfonamides

with less significant elevations in their methemoglobin levels. On the other hand, conditions that shift the oxyhemoglobin dissociation curve to the right, such as acidosis or elevated 2,3-diphosphoglycerate, may result in somewhat better toleration of methemoglobin.

Diagnosis

The diagnosis of methemoglobinemia should be considered in all patients who present with cyanosis, and is particularly suspect in those whose cyanosis does not improve with supplemental oxygen. The blood has a characteristic "chocolate brown" color, analogous to that seen in the chocolate agar (which contains methemoglobin) used to plate gonococcus. The ability to detect this discoloration is improved when compared directly to normal blood.[5]

Pulse oximetry should be used cautiously in patients with methemoglobinemia. Because the pulse oximeter typically trends toward 80 to 85 percent in patients with methemoglobinemia, in patients with significant elevations in their methemoglobin concentrations (e.g., >20 percent), **the pulse oximeter will suggest a falsely high oxygen saturation.[6] Arterial blood gas measurement may also be initially deceptive because the partial pressure of oxygen, a measure of dissolved—not bound—oxygen, is normal.** Thus, its extrapolation to the expected oxygen saturation, as performed by the analyzer, will provide a falsely elevated result. **Definitive identification of this abnormal hemoglobin species relies on co-oximetry,** which is an in vitro spectrophotometric method that is capable of differentiating among oxy-, deoxy-, met-, and carboxyhemoglobin species. This widely available test requires only a venous specimen, although arterial blood may be used if arterial puncture is indicated for another reason. The oxygen saturation obtained from a conventional arterial blood gas analyzer will also be falsely normal, because it is calculated from the dissolved oxygen tension, which is appropriately normal.

Treatment

Patients with methemoglobinemia require optimal supportive measures to ensure oxygen delivery and the administration of appropriate antidotal therapy if indicated. In general, gastric decontamination is limited, because there often is a substantial time interval between exposure to the toxic agent and the development of methemoglobin. If a source of continuing exposure exists, decontamination is indicated, and in most stable patients, a single dose of activated charcoal is likely sufficient. Antidotal therapy with methylene blue is reserved for patients with documented methemoglobinemia or a high clinical likelihood of the disease. Highly unstable patients should receive methylene blue, and may rarely benefit from transfusion or exchange transfusion to produce an immediate enhancement of oxygen delivery.

Methylene blue serves to indirectly accelerate the enzymatic reduction of methemoglobin by NADPH-methemoglobin reductase, a normally minor enzymatic pathway. In this capacity, methylene blue is reduced to leucomethylene blue, which itself is capable of directly reducing the oxidized iron back to its oxygen carrying form (see Figure 189-1). The initial dose of methylene blue is 1 to 2 mg/kg IV (0.1 mL/kg of the 1% solution, approximately 7 mL in an adult) and its effect should be seen with 20 min. As the methemoglobin concentration falls, the most severe signs and symptoms will resolve first. Resolution of the cyanosis is a late finding, occurring only after the concentration of methemoglobin falls below 1.5 g/dL. Repeat dosing of methylene blue may be acceptable if needed, but high doses of methylene blue (>7 mg/kg) may actually induce methemoglobin formation.

Treatment failures may result if the patient is deficient in G6PD, because this enzyme is critical for the production of NADPH by the hexose monophosphate shunt (see Figure 189-1).[7] Because this group of patients does not lack NADH cytochrome-b_5 reductase, they are not at increased risk of developing methemoglobinemia, and they only lack the ability to respond to methylene blue. However, G6PD-deficient patients are at greater risk of developing hemolysis following exposure to an oxidant stress. Some oxidants, such as chlorate salts, routinely produce hemolysis even in non-G6PD-deficient patients. Importantly, hemolysis may impede a response to methylene blue, which requires an intact erythrocyte to be effective. Oxidant drugs with long serum half-lives, such as dapsone ($T_{1/2}$ ~50 h), produce prolonged oxidant stress to the red blood cell. Dapsone-exposed patients may require repetitive dosing of methylene blue. Because dapsone's hydroxylamine metabolite is responsible for its toxicity, inhibition of its formation by cytochrome P450 with cimetidine (in conventional doses) is generally recommended. In rare instances, patients may be deficient in NADPH-methemoglobin reductase, the required enzyme for methylene blue activation. Lastly, treatment failure may occur in patients with sulfhemoglobinemia, which is clinically indistinguishable from methemoglobinemia, but which is not responsive to methylene blue (see below). Patients that do not respond to methylene blue should be treated supportively. If clinically unstable, the use of blood transfusions or exchange transfusions is indicated. In the event that the newly administered red blood cell hemoglobin undergoes oxidation, it will likely respond appropriately to methylene blue. Although some additional modalities for the treatment of methemoglobinemia are being investigated, such as the use of the reducing agent N-acetylcysteine,[8] none of them are currently used clinically.

SULFHEMOGLOBINEMIA

Sulfhemoglobinemia is less common than methemoglobinemia. Although patients with sulfhemoglobinemia have a clinical presentation similar to those with methemoglobinemia, the disease process itself is substantially less concerning. Although the reduction in the patient's oxygen-carrying capacity is quantitatively similar, the patient's oxygen dissociation curve is shifted rightward, not leftward as in methemoglobinemia, favoring the release of hemoglobin-bound oxygen to the tissue. Because the pigmentation of the blood by sulfhemoglobin is substantially more intense than other colored hemoglobin species, only 0.5 g/dL of sulfhemoglobin is needed to produce a cyanosis equivalent to that produced by 1.5 g/dL of methemoglobin. At the level of the hemoglobin molecule, sulfhemoglobin occurs by oxidation of the porphyrin ring rather than the iron moiety. Many of the responsible agents are identical to those that induce methemoglobin, and the agents do not need to contain sulfur. The diagnosis is difficult to confirm. Standard co-oximetry does not differentiate sulfhemoglobin from methemoglobin because of similar spectral absorbances. The addition of cyanide to the laboratory sample differentiates the two hemoglobin species, because cyanide binds to methemoglobin and changes its spectrophotometric pattern. Thus, if the addition of cyanide to this sample fails to eliminate the methemoglobin peak, the diagnosis of sulfhemoglobinemia is confirmed. Sulfhemoglobin is not reduced by treatment with methylene blue, and generally patients require only supportive care, although transfusions may be necessary for severe toxicity.

REFERENCES

1. Litovitz TL, Klein-Schwartz W, Rodgers GC Jr, et al: 2001 Annual report of the American Association of Poison Control Centers Toxic Exposure Surveillance System. *Am J Emerg Med* 20:391, 2002.
2. Hulquist DE, Passon PG: Catalysis of methemoglobinemia reduction by erythrocyte cytochrome-b_5 reductase. *Nature* 229:252, 1971.
3. Shih RD, Marcus SM, Genese CA, et al: Methemoglobinemia attributable to nitrite contamination of potable water through boiler fluid additives—New Jersey, 1992 and 1996. *MMWR* 46:202, 1997.
4. Pollack ES, Pollack CV: Incidence of subclinical methemoglobinemia in infants with diarrhea. *Ann Emerg Med* 24:652, 1994.
5. Henretig FM, Gribetz B, Kearney T, et al: Interpretation of color change in blood with varying degree of methemoglobinemia. *J Toxicol Clin Toxicol* 26:293, 1988.

6. Barker SJ, Tremper KK, Hyatt J: Effects of methemoglobinemia on pulse oximetry and mixed venous oximetry. *Anesthesiology* 70:112, 1989.
7. Rosen PJ, Johnson C, McGehee WG, Beutler E: Failure of methylene blue treatment in toxic methemoglobinemia: Association with glucose-6-phosphate dehydrogenase deficiency. *Ann Intern Med* 75:83, 1971.
8. Wright RO, Woolf AD, Shannon MW, Magnani B: *N*-acetylcysteine reduces methemoglobin in an in vitro model of glucose-6-phosphate dehydrogenase deficiency. *Ann Emerg Med* 5:225, 1998.

HYPOGLYCEMIC AGENTS
Joseph G. Rella
Lewis S. Nelson

Diabetes mellitus is the most common endocrine disorder in the United States, and the mainstay of pharmacotherapy includes hypoglycemic agents. Poisoning by hypoglycemic agents may be the result of unintentional therapeutic misadventures, intentional self-poisoning, or homicidal intent. Many factors contribute to unintentional poisoning including prescription errors, dosing errors, and the onset of complicating metabolic factors.

It is difficult to ascertain an accurate incidence of toxicity caused by hypoglycemic agents for several reasons. Passive reporting to poison centers of overdoses is widely thought to underestimate the true number of exposures. Additionally, laboratory confirmation of actual ingestion is frequently missing from most reports, possibly contributing to a false sense of security. The *2001 Annual Report of the American Association of Poison Control Centers* recorded 7945 exposures to oral hypoglycemics, 2652 of them in children younger than 6 years of age. There were 21 reported deaths.[1]

Hypoglycemia (defined as occurrence of suggestive symptoms with serum glucose less than 50 to 60 mg/dL that responds to glucose administration) is perhaps the most common endocrine emergency. Initially, hypoglycemia precipitates a physiologic attempt to correct the deficiency in blood glucose. This response includes an autonomic nervous system–mediated release of catecholamines and glucagon, which produce the most common symptoms in hypoglycemic patients, including diaphoresis, anxiety, nausea, tremor, and palpitations.[2] However, because the brain is the only organ that uses glucose as its primary energy source, the consequential clinical findings of hypoglycemia are a result of neuroglycopenia, or insufficient glucose supply to the brain. The manifestations of neuroglycopenia are quite variable and include dizziness, decreased concentration ability, headache, diplopia, confusion, dysarthria, lethargy, coma, focal neurologic findings, and generalized seizures, including status epilepticus.[3]

In healthy persons, there are complex regulatory systems that maintain the blood glucose at a constant level. Unfortunately, certain medical conditions may impair the ability of the body to perform this task, resulting in hypoglycemia. Chronic ethanol users are at increased risk for hypoglycemia because of their diminished glycogen supply and impaired gluconeogenesis. Persons at extremes of age are also potentially at increased risk for hypoglycemia. Young children have a disproportionately higher brain requirement of glucose as well as smaller glycogen reserves. The elderly are more likely to have health problems or be using medications (e.g., β-adrenergic antagonists) that either contribute to or alter the normal counterregulatory responses to hypoglycemia.

INSULIN

Insulin is the agent most commonly associated with severe hypoglycemia in patients evaluated in the ED. The Diabetic Control and Complications Trial research group demonstrated that, although tighter glycemic control delayed the onset and progression of microvascular and neurologic complications in patients with type I diabetes, there were at least 61.2 episodes of treatment-requiring hypoglycemia per 100 patient years.[4,5] Therefore, intensive therapy directed at maintaining euglycemia increases the risk of hypoglycemia.

The pharmacokinetics of the different forms of insulin weighs heavily in management decisions. Regular insulin acts rapidly but is short-lived and produces relatively predictable hypoglycemia, whereas the long-acting insulins, such as NPH (neutral protamine Hagedorn insulin), have less-predictable kinetic characteristics. Following large subcutaneous overdose, regular insulin manifests the unpredictable kinetics characteristic of the long-acting forms of insulin (Table 190-1).

SULFONYLUREAS

Sulfonylureas represent approximately 1 percent of all prescriptions in the United States and approximately 66 percent of all oral agents prescribed for diabetes, making them a prevalent cause of hypoglycemia.[6,7] Sulfonylureas bind to adenosine triphosphate–sensitive potassium channels on pancreatic β-islet cells and induce the release of insulin by changing the cell's membrane potential.[8] First-generation sulfonylureas, such as chlorpropamide, are infrequently used because of their near-complete reliance on renal elimination and long elimination half-lives. Second-generation sulfonylureas are cleared by several routes, although they typically have half-lives that approach 24 h with therapeutic use and are expectedly longer following overdose. The second-generation agents are associated with frequent episodes of hypoglycemia, the onset of which may be both delayed (e.g., 12 to 16 h following overdose) and precipitous. Certain sulfonylureas are currently available in sustained-release formulation that results in even more unpredictable overdose kinetics and clinical effects.

BIGUANIDES

The biguanides include phenformin and metformin, both of which are derivatives of guanidine, the active component of the French lilac (*Galega officinalis*). Phenformin, withdrawn from the U.S. market in 1977 because of the high incidence of fatal lactic acidosis, was replaced by metformin in the mid-1990s for the treatment of type II diabetes. Metformin suppresses hepatic glucose output by inhibiting gluconeogenesis and stimulates insulin-mediated glucose uptake by muscle and other tissues. Unlike the sulfonylureas, it does not stimulate insulin secretion.[9] Metformin does not directly reduce blood glucose and is more appropriately termed an antihyperglycemic agent.

TABLE 190-1   Characteristics of Hypoglycemic Agents

Class/Name	Duration of Action (h)	Peak Action (h)
Insulin		
Ultrashort-acting		
Lispro (Humalog)	<6	0.5–2.5
Short-acting		
Regular (Humulin)	6–10	1–5
Semilente	12–16	Hepatic
Intermediate-acting		
Lente	16–24	6–14
NPH	16–24	6–14
Mixture*	24	bimodal
Long-acting		
PZI	24–36	8–20
Ultralente	24–28	8–20
Glargine	24+	2–20
Sulfonylureas		
First-generation		
Acetohexamide	12–24	1–2
Chlorpropamide	24–72	2–4
Tolazamide	12–24	1
Tolbutamide	6–12	1
Second/third generation		
Glipizide	10–16	.5–2
Glyburide	24	1–2
Glimepiride	16–24	2–3

*Isophane and regular insulin as 70/30 or 50/50 combinations.
Abbreviations: NPH = neutral protein Hagedorn or isophane insulin; PZI = protamine zinc insulin, no longer available in US.

Metformin is also associated with lactic acidosis that is fatal in nearly 50 percent of the cases. Lactic acidosis occurs in approximately 3 cases per 100,000 patient years of therapy, or about 10 to 20 times less frequently than with phenformin.[10] Although not completely clear, the mechanism appears to be an enhanced production and inhibited metabolism of lactic acid, with a resultant fall in serum pH and cardiovascular collapse. The risk of lactic acidosis from metformin rises with coexisting medical conditions, particularly renal insufficiency as it is cleared by the kidneys; it rarely occurs following large overdose of the drug. The association of metformin-associated lactic acidosis with the use of intravascular iodinated contrast media relates to the increased likelihood of developing renal insufficiency following the administration of radiographic contrast. In most situations, intravenous contrast medium may be administered as needed, but the patient's metformin should not be readministered until the renal function proves to be normal.[11]

α-GLUCOSIDASE INHIBITORS

There are three α-glucosidase inhibitor agents. Acarbose was the first to be marketed, followed by miglitol and voglibose. These agents, frequently used in combination with sulfonylureas, act to decrease postprandial glucose concentrations by decreasing gastrointestinal absorption of carbohydrates. Specifically, they inhibit the brush-border enzyme α-glucosidase, thereby preventing the metabolism of polysaccharides into smaller units for absorption. By themselves, α-glucosidase inhibitors do not cause hypoglycemia. Experience with α-glucosidase inhibitor overdose remains limited. However, flatulence, bloating, and malabsorption can complicate the therapeutic use of this medication and should be expected in overdose. Additionally, hepatic toxicity is reported in patients taking acarbose.[12]

THIAZOLIDINEDIONES

Although troglitazone was withdrawn from the market in 2000 secondary to reports of liver failure and death, two drugs in this class remain on the market: rosiglitazone and pioglitazone. Structurally similar to troglitazone, these agents offer the theoretical advantage over sulfonylureas of ameliorating hyperglycemia without increasing insulin secretion. These agents reduce hepatic output of glucose and increase peripheral uptake, thus enhancing the effect of endogenous insulin. Both are rapidly absorbed, undergo extensive hepatic metabolism, and are generally well tolerated. However, because of the structural similarity with troglitazone there is some concern for hepatic toxicity, although few cases of reversible hepatocellular injury are reported. Additionally, because of their ability to alter cell differentiation, the long-term consequences of the use of these agents remain undefined.[13]

BENZOIC ACID DERIVATIVES (MEGLITINIDES)

Repaglinide (Prandin, GlucoNorm) is a relatively new nonsulfonylurea insulin-releasing drug derived from benzoic acid. Its mechanism of action is thought to involve the regulation of adenosine triphosphate-sensitive potassium channels in pancreatic β-islet cells at a different site than used by sulfonylureas. Extrapancreatic activity is also likely as human trials have demonstrated reductions in overall insulin concentrations, as compared with sulfonylurea use. Repaglinide is metabolized in the liver to inactive metabolites and eliminated primarily in bile. Overdose experience with this agent is lacking.[14]

MISCELLANEOUS SOURCES OF HYPOGLYCEMIA

The ackee tree, found in Jamaica, produces a fruit that may cause hypoglycemia when eaten prior to ripening. The unripened fruit contains hypoglycins, a group of toxins that inhibit hepatic gluconeogenesis and may contribute to hypoglycemia. Epidemic ackee-associated hypoglycemia occurs during times of famine when poor nutrition and the increased eating of unripened fruit is presumably more common. Hypoglycins also produce vomiting (i.e., Jamaican vomiting sickness), central nervous system sedation, and seizures. Ackee is available in the United States in canned form, but only the unripe, fresh fruit is associated with hypoglycemia. Several medications can potentiate or have been associated with hypoglycemia (Table 190–2).

The sympathetic nervous system mediates glucose autoregulation partly through the release of epinephrine, which prevents the release of insulin and elevates blood glucose levels. This mechanism explains the role of epinephrine in the counterregulatory response to hypoglycemia. β-Adrenergic antagonists interfere with both of these effects, potentially resulting in hypoglycemia through excessive insulin release while preventing the development of the typical autonomic response to hypoglycemia.[15,16] In addition, caffeine may enhance patients' awareness of a hypoglycemic event, perhaps because of its ability to induce neuroglycopenia.[17] Low carbohydrate diets in normal individuals should not cause hypoglycemia as gluconeogenesis supplies adequate glucose.

TREATMENT

Hypoglycemia should be considered as part of the differential diagnosis for all patients with either gross or subtle alterations in their mental status. Initial management includes rapid blood glucose determination with a reagent strip or glucometer, followed by administration of 1 g/kg body weight dextrose using D50W in adults. Because approximately 3 percent of hypoglycemic patients present with a new focal neurologic deficit,[3] rapid glucose assessment prior to further care, such as computed tomography scan or thrombolytic therapy, is critical in patients with presumed cerebrovascular accidents. For children, D10W or D25W is used because the hypertonicity of the dextrose preparation may irritate or damage their smaller blood vessels.

The duration of euglycemia or hyperglycemia following intravenous dextrose administration is only about 30 min. In fact, intravenous glucose frequently induces a rebound hypoglycemia 1 to 2 h following the bolus, presumably because of pancreatic insulin release (in some type II diabetics and nondiabetics). Thus, it is critical that after the initial serum glucose correction has been made, assessment and therapy continue to prevent recurrent hypoglycemia.

Once the patient has improved following bolus therapy, D10W should be infused (1 to 2 mL/kg per h) in an attempt to maintain euglycemia. This, along with food, is generally definitive therapy for patients with insulin overdose. Failure to maintain euglycemia with even high infusion rates should prompt repeat boluses of the more concentrated dextrose solutions. Fluid overload, hypokalemia and dilutional hyponatremia and their sequelae are potential complications of large dextrose in water infusions. Feeding patients with at least 300 g of carbohydrates should allow the partial repletion of hepatic glycogen stores and help maintain euglycemia. Simple sugars in soda, chocolate, orange juice, or apple juice are probably not as useful in this effort as are carbohydrates from sandwiches or other foods.

TABLE 190-2 Drugs or Toxins Commonly Associated with Hypoglycemia

Angiotensin-converting enzyme inhibitors	Pentamidine
Acetaminophen	Phenylbutazone
Ackee	Propoxyphene
β-Adrenergic antagonists	Quinine
Chloramphenicol	Salicylates
Disopyramide	Sulfonamide
Ethanol	Streptozocin
Haloperidol	Trimethoprim-sulfamethoxazole
Monoamine oxidase inhibitors	Pyriminil
Para-aminobenzoic acid	

Glucagon should not be used as empiric therapy for hypoglycemia except in specific situations. Because the action of glucagon is to mobilize glycogen stores, those patients who are glycogen depleted (e.g., alcoholics, children, the malnourished, and the elderly) may not improve with glucagon. This may mislead the health care provider, preventing the provider from establishing the etiology of the hypoglycemia. In addition, glucagon stimulates insulin release (mechanism unclear), rendering it unsuitable as an antidote for sulfonylurea toxicity. For this reason, glucagon is better used in those patients known to have type I diabetes or in those for whom intravenous access is not easily obtained. In these patients, glucagon 1 mg IM or IV may be administered in adults and children who weigh more than 10 kg. In children who weigh less than 10 kg, 0.1 mg/kg up to a maximum dose of 1 mg may be given. Glucagon requires several minutes for effect, and intravenous administration of hypertonic dextrose should never be delayed while awaiting glucagon's effect. Because emesis is common following glucagon administration, precautions should be taken to assure airway protection. Intubation per se is not a prerequisite without other standard indications.

Diazoxide directly inhibits insulin secretion by opening potassium channels in β-islet cells. Because diazoxide may cause hypotension and sodium retention, it is rarely used today. Diazoxide may improve hypoglycemia secondary to severe oral hypoglycemic poisoning, but not that caused by insulin poisoning.[18] Diazoxide 300 mg is administered IV over 30 min and dosing may be repeated every 4 h.

Octreotide, a somatostatin analogue, inhibits insulin release by the pancreatic β-islet cells. Octreotide reverses hypoglycemia from oral hypoglycemic agents in both healthy volunteers[19] and in patients with sulfonylurea overdoses.[20] It currently has no role in the management of insulin overdose, although it is used in patients with insulinoma. The early use of octreotide should limit recurrent hypoglycemia and prevent the complications of excessive dextrose administration. Octreotide is given in a dose of 50 μg SC every 6 h.

The cornerstone of management of most poisoned patients is gastrointestinal decontamination to prevent drug absorption into the body. Several oral hypoglycemic agents have been demonstrated to effectively adsorb to activated charcoal in vitro, and there is no reason to suspect that the remainder are not similarly well adsorbed. A single dose, and perhaps several doses, of activated charcoal may be beneficial for these patients.

The use of other decontamination techniques such as emesis, gastric lavage, and whole-bowel irrigation should be considered. Emesis has not been demonstrated to produce consistent evacuation of the stomach contents and may be complicated should altered consciousness or seizure activity develop abruptly from the hypoglycemia. Gastric lavage with a large-bore tube may evacuate some (but not necessarily all) pill fragments and allow administration of activated charcoal, but is associated with aspiration, esophageal injury, and vagal complications. Whole-bowel irrigation with a polyethylene glycol–based electrolyte solution may specifically benefit patients who have ingested sustained-release preparations.

Following large subcutaneous deposition of insulin, toxicity may be reduced by removal of the reservoir. Percutaneous aspiration or excision may reduce the extent and duration of hypoglycemia, although this therapy is not commonly recommended.

The half-life of chlorpropamide may be reduced from 49 to 13 h by ion trapping through alkalinization of the urine, in a fashion analogous to treatment of salicylate toxicity.[21] However, this effect appears limited to this agent.

Metformin overdose patients generally require only gastrointestinal decontamination and expectant management. The likelihood of concomitant sulfonylurea overdose should be assessed. Metformin-associated lactic acidosis must be aggressively treated to reduce its potential mortality rate. Hemodialysis appears to be the most beneficial therapy and should be instituted early.

DISPOSITION

Patients with hypoglycemia resulting from unintentional overdose of a short- or intermediate-acting insulin may not require admission if their condition is corrected and a normal blood glucose level is maintained for 4 to 6 h prior to discharge. Those with hypoglycemia resulting from long-acting insulin or sulfonylureas should be admitted, as should those with underlying diseases such as liver or renal insufficiency or starvation. Patients with serious complications of hypoglycemia such as seizures, or those who have refractory hypoglycemia, should be closely monitored. Obviously, patients who are hypoglycemic because of an attempted suicide, attempted homicide, or abuse should be admitted as needed.

Hypoglycemia may occur in a delayed fashion after the ingestion of an oral hypoglycemic agent, particularly in children. Therefore, adults who have deliberately overdosed with oral hypoglycemics and **children who have ingested even a single pill should be admitted** for 24 h of observation, even though they may demonstrate euglycemia for many hours. Investigations of child abuse may arise from the unindicated administration of insulin to children.

REFERENCES

1. Litovitz TL, Klein-Schwartz W, Rodgers GC, et al: 2001 Annual report of the American Association of Poison Control Centers Toxic Exposure Surveillance System. *Am J Emerg Med* 20:391, 2002.
2. Service FJ: Hypoglycemic disorders. *New Engl J Med* 332:1144, 1995.
3. Malouf R, Brust JC: Hypoglycemia: Causes, neurological manifestations, and outcome. *Ann Neurol* 17:421, 1985.
4. Diabetic Control and Complications Trial (DCCT) Research Group: Hypoglycemia in the Diabetes Control and Complications Trial. *Diabetes* 46:271, 1997.
5. Davis EA, Keating B, Byrne GC, et al: Impact of improved glycaemic control on rates of hypoglycaemia in insulin-dependent diabetes mellitus. *Arch Dis Child* 78:111, 1998.
6. Bocuzzi SJ, Sung JC, Wogen J, et al: Utilization of oral hypoglycemic agents in a drug-insured U.S. population. *Diabetes Care* 24:1411, 2001.
7. Inzucchi SE: Oral antihyperglycemic therapy for type 2 diabetes: Scientific review. *JAMA* 287:360, 2002.
8. Eliasson L, Renström E, Ämmälä C, et al: PKC-dependent stimulation of exocytosis by sulfonylureas in pancreatic β cells. *Science* 271:813, 1996.
9. Bailey CJ, Turner RC: Metformin. *New Engl J Med* 334:574, 1996.
10. Crofford OB: Metformin. *New Engl J Med* 333:588, 1995.
11. McCartney MM, Gilbert FJ, Murchison LE, et al: Metformin and contrast media—A dangerous combination? *Clin Radiol* 54:29, 1999.
12. Harrigan RA, Nathan MS, Beattie P: Oral agents for the treatment of type 2 diabetes mellitus: Pharmacology, toxicity, and treatment. *Ann Emerg Med* 38:68, 2001.
13. Gale EA: Lessons from the glitazones: A story of drug development. *Lancet* 357:1870, 2001.
14. Guay DR: Repaglinide, a novel, short-acting hypoglycemic agent for type 2 diabetes mellitus. *Pharmacotherapy* 18:1195, 1998.
15. Burge MR, Schmitz-Fiorentino K, Fischette C, et al: A prospective trial of risk factors for sulfonylurea-induced hypoglycemia in type 2 diabetes mellitus. *JAMA* 279:137, 1998.
16. Boyle PJ, Kempers SF, O'Connor AM, Nagy RJ: Brain glucose uptake and unawareness of hypoglycemia in patients with insulin-dependent diabetes mellitus. *New Engl J Med* 333:1726, 1995.
17. Kerr D, Sherwin RS, Pavalkis F, et al: Effect of caffeine on the recognition of and responses to hypoglycemia in humans. *Ann Intern Med* 119:799, 1993.
18. Palatnick W, Meatherall RC, Tenenbein M: Clinical spectrum of sulfonylurea overdose and experience with diazoxide therapy. *Arch Intern Med* 151:1859, 1991.
19. Boyle PJ, Justice K, Krentz AJ, et al: Octreotide reverses hyperinsulinemia and prevents hypoglycemia induced by sulfonylurea overdoses. *J Clin Endocrinol Metab* 76:752, 1993.
20. McLaughlin SA, Crandall CS, McKinney PE: Octreotide: An antidote for sulfonylurea-induced hypoglycemia. *Ann Emerg Med* 36:133, 2000.
21. Neuvonen PJ, Kärkkäinen S: Effects of charcoal, sodium bicarbonate and ammonium chloride on chlorpropamide kinetics. *Clin Pharmacol Ther* 33:386, 1983.

FROSTBITE AND OTHER LOCALIZED COLD-RELATED INJURIES
Mark B. Rabold

Throughout history, the most celebrated and extreme reports of cold-related injuries have been in the field of military endeavor. From Hannibal's losing half his 46,000-man army crossing the Pyrenean Alps to frostbite and hypothermia to the tens of thousands of cases of trench foot during World War I, we have learned much. Perhaps the most famous cold-injury mass-casualty incident was Napoleon's retreat from Moscow during the dreadful winter of 1812–1813. Napoleon's surgeon-in-chief, Baron de Larrey, described how each evening thousands of French soldiers thawed and often inadvertently burned their frozen extremities over campfires, only to refreeze them again on the next day's march. Combined heat and cold injury coupled with refreezing and forced ambulation resulted in abysmal outcomes. In addition, thousands died from the tetanus sustained from their frostbite wounds. It was from this experience that Larrey recommended rubbing frostbitten extremities with snow. This destructive therapy was the standard of care until the 1950s and is still used occasionally by the lay public. It was not until 1956 that rapid rewarming of frozen extremities was studied by a Public Health Service medical officer in Tanana, Alaska, which laid the foundation of modern therapy.

EPIDEMIOLOGY

It is the inability to physiologically compensate for cold that produces injury.[1] However, cold itself is not the only factor in determining whether injury will occur. Duration of exposure, humidity, wind, altitude, clothing, medical conditions, behavior, and individual variability all contribute to the picture.[2,3]

Cold-induced injury may be instantaneous, as with contact frostbite after touching a cold metal bottle of fuel, or more chronic, as in chilblains. Humidity is also important because it contributes to evaporative heat loss. Wet skin is more conducive to both subcutaneous ice crystal formation and trench foot. Wind velocity and cold, the wind-chill factor, have a synergistic effect on heat loss. For example, an ambient temperature of −7°C (19.4°F), when combined with a wind of 72.5 km/h (45 mi/h), will feel equivalent to −40°C (−40°F) on a windless day. The rigors of travel at high altitude also may predispose to cold injury. Although the lower barometric pressure has not been shown to directly influence susceptibility to cold injury, a number of factors associated with high altitude travel have. The fatigue, dehydration, and hypoxia often seen in climbers or trekkers, coupled with the extreme weather conditions and remote locations, all contribute to the incidence and severity of cold-related injuries at high altitude.

Inadequate clothing is probably the most preventable cause of cold-related injuries. Constrictive clothing and boots can reduce circulation to extremities and predispose to frostbite. An exposed head and neck can account for 80 percent of body heat loss. Natural-fiber clothing, such as wool and cotton, when compared with modern synthetics, such as polypropylene, have poorer wicking ability and greater thermal conductance and moisture retention. Simply changing out of cold, wet clothes into dry ones also can be preventive. During World War I, the British decreased the number of trench foot cases from over 29,000 in 1915 to a total of less than 500 in 1916–1918 by frequent foot drying and sock changing.

Individual behavior is extremely important as well. In fact, alcohol- or drug-intoxicated persons, combined with psychiatric patients, account for the majority of frostbite cases in the United States. Impaired judgment and lack of self-preservation instincts prevent these populations from dressing adequately and making rational decisions about exposure to the cold. Alcohol consumption also increases peripheral vasodilatation and heat loss, which increases the risk for hypothermia. In addition, many of these patients smoke, which results in peripheral vasoconstriction and increases the risk of frostbite. Other examples of the precipitation of cold injury by individual behavior can be seen in case reports of significant facial frostbite by inhalation abuse of fluorinated hydrocarbons (e.g., Freon) and nitrous oxide.[4,5] There also have been case reports of full-thickness frostbite resulting from inappropriate use of dry ice as a first-aid cold pack.[6]

Certain disease states, such as atherosclerosis, arteritis, hypovolemia, diabetes, vascular injury secondary to trauma or infection, and previous cold-related injuries, may predispose to cold-related injury.[2,3,7] Military studies suggest that dark-skinned soldiers and those from warmer climatic regions are more susceptible to frostbite. Conversely, peoples indigenous to frigid climates, such as Eskimos, Tibetans, and Laplanders, are often "acclimated" to the cold and are less prone to injury.

Local cold-related injuries are classified into nonfreezing and freezing injuries.

NONFREEZING COLD INJURIES: CHILBLAINS AND TRENCH FOOT

Clinical Features

Chilblains, or pernio, is characterized by usually mild but uncomfortable inflammatory lesions of the skin of bared body areas caused by chronic intermittent exposure to damp, nonfreezing ambient temperatures with symptoms precipitated by acute exposure to cold.[8] The hands, ears, lower legs, and feet are involved most commonly. The cutaneous manifestations, which appear up to 12 h after acute exposure, include localized edema, erythema, cyanosis, plaques, nodules, and in rare cases, ulcerations, vesicles, and bullae. Patients may complain of pruritus and burning paresthesias. Rewarming may result in the formation of tender blue nodules, which may persist for several days. This is primarily a disease of women and children, and although rare in the United States, chilblains is common in the United Kingdom and other countries with a cold or temperate, damp climate. In addition, it appears that young females with Raynaud phenomenon are at greatest risk, as well as those in households with inadequate heating and lack of warm clothing.

Trench foot was given its current name after it was found frequently among World War I troops who had been confined for long periods in trenches filled with standing cold water.[9] Significant numbers of cases also were seen in the Falkland and Vietnam wars. Immersion foot describes a more severe variant of trench foot seen in downed pilots and shipwrecked sailors exposed for extended periods in life rafts in the North Atlantic Ocean. Although they are a significant problem in military operations, trench foot and immersion foot are seen rarely in the civilian population.

The pathophysiology of trench foot is multifactorial but involves direct injury to soft tissue sustained from prolonged cooling, and it is accelerated by wet conditions. The peripheral nerves seem to be the most sensitive to this form of injury. Trench foot develops slowly over hours to days and is reversible initially but will become irreversible if allowed to progress. Early symptoms progress from tingling to numbness of the affected tissues. On initial examination, the foot is pale, mottled, anesthetic, pulseless, and immobile, which initially does not change after rewarming. A hyperemic phase begins within hours after rewarming and is associated with severe burning pain and reappearance of proximal sensation. As perfusion returns to the foot over 2 to 3 days, edema and bullae form, and the hyperemia may worsen. Anesthesia frequently persists for weeks but may be permanent. In more severe cases, tissue sloughing and gangrene may develop. Hyperhidrosis and cold sensitivity are common late features and may persist for months to years. Severe cases may be associated with prolonged convalescence and permanent disability.

Treatment

Management of chilblains is supportive. The affected skin should be rewarmed, gently bandaged, and elevated. Some European studies support the use of oral nifedipine 20 mg three times daily, oral pentoxifylline 400 mg three times daily, or an oral analogue of prostaglandin E$_1$, limaprost, 20 μg three times daily as both a prophylactic and therapeutic treatment for local cold injury.[9,10] Topical corticosteroids (0.025% fluocinolone cream) and even a brief burst of oral corticosteroids, such as prednisone, have been shown to be useful. Affected areas are more prone to reinjury.

Effective prophylaxis for trench foot includes keeping warm, ensuring good boot fit, changing out of wet socks several times a day, never sleeping in wet socks and boots, and once early symptoms are identified, maximizing efforts to warm, dry, and elevate the feet. Once injury has occurred, treatment is supportive. Oral pentoxifylline 400 mg three times daily or an oral analogue of prostaglandin E$_1$, limaprost, 20 μg three times daily can be used.[9,10] Feet should be kept clean, warm, dryly bandaged, elevated, and closely monitored for early signs of infection.[9]

FREEZING COLD INJURIES: FROSTNIP AND FROSTBITE

Pathophysiology

Cutaneous vascular tone can be altered by direct heating (e.g., warming hands over a fire) and indirect heating (e.g., putting on a hat to increase core temperature) and is modulated by sympathetic adrenergic vasoconstrictive fibers. In a euthermic 70-kg male, the total basal cutaneous blood flow is 200 to 500 mL/min. However, as the skin temperature drops to 14°C (57.2°F), the flow falls to 20 to 50 mL/min. As cooling continues to 10°C (50°F), cutaneous blood flow becomes negligible, with occurrence of 5- to 10-min cycles of vasodilatation and vasoconstriction, known as the *hunter's response* (Table 191-1). For individuals who are well acclimated to the cold, such as Eskimos, the intervals between cycles are often much shorter. As the vasodilatory phases carry cooled blood back from the extremities, the core temperature begins to fall. These cycles continue until the core temperature is threatened. The body attempts to maintain thermal integrity by completely shutting down flow to the coldest extremities. This begins phase I of frostbite, and irreversible tissue damage commences.[1] As skin temperatures fall well below 0°C (32°F), ice crystals form in the extracellular space. Crystals exert an osmotic force and pull fluid from the intracellular space, resulting in cellular dehydration and hyperosmolarity. The intracellular sodium concentration may raise tenfold. As the damage continues, proteins are denatured, enzymes are destroyed, and the cellular membranes are altered. Theoretically, intracellular ice crystals then form, especially in rapid freeze and refreeze injuries, producing structural damage to the cell.

Phase II is characterized by reperfusion injury as the involved extremity is rewarmed and some initial blood flow returns. Over a period

TABLE 191-1   Frostbite Pathophysiology Summary

PREFREEZE STATE
Tissue cooling
Increased viscosity
Capillary constriction-dilatation cycle

FROZEN STATE
Extracellular ice crystal formation
Intracellular dehydration and hyperosmolarity
Fluid shifts across cell membrane
Intracellular ice crystal formation

ISCHEMIC AND VASCULAR COMPLICATIONS
Reperfusion injury
Endothelium leakage
Coagulation from vascular stasis
Leakage of destructive prostaglandins and oxygen free radicals
Vasoconstriction and arteriovenous shunting
Necrosis demarcation and gangrene

of several hours to days, the damaged endothelium-lined capillaries allow leakage of fluid into the interstitium, intracellular swelling occurs, and oxygen free radicals are generated, which furthers endothelial damage. An arachidonic acid cascade forms, which liberates prostaglandin and thromboxane. This cascade promotes vasoconstriction, platelet aggregation, and leukocyte sludging, which results in venule and arterial thrombosis and subsequent ischemia, necrosis, and dry gangrene. Profound vasoconstriction and arteriovenous shunting occur at the margin between injured and noninjured tissue. Phase II is remarkably similar to the dynamics of a burn injury.

Frostbite injury can be divided into three zones. The zone of coagulation is the most severe, usually distal, and is irreversible. The zone of hyperemia is the more superficial, typically proximal, with the least cellular damage, and generally recovers without treatment in less than 10 days. The zone of stasis is the middle ground and is characterized by severe, but possibly reversible, cell damage. It is this middle zone where treatment may have benefit.

Clinical Features

Frostbite can occur on any skin surface but generally is limited to the nose, ears, face, hands, and feet.[1,3] Frostbite has been reported in the penis and scrotum of joggers and in burn patients after prolonged treatment with ice. Also, a freezing keratitis of the cornea has been reported in snowmobilers and skiers who did not wear protective goggles.

Frostnip is on a continuum with frostbite and is a superficial freeze injury characterized by lack of extracellular ice crystal formation and absence of progressive tissue loss. The involved area appears pale from intense vasoconstriction and is associated with some discomfort. Symptoms resolve on rewarming, and tissue loss does not occur.

There has been much debate over the proper classification of the severity of frostbite.[11] One may classify frostbite into degrees of injury or into superficial and deep groups based on appearance at the time of presentation (Table 191-2). First- and second-degree injuries are classified as superficial, whereas third- and fourth-degree injuries are classified as deep. The initial clinical appearance is often deceiving, especially if some warming has not occurred. Most patients present after some warming has occurred and are in phase II of the injury.

First-degree injury is characterized by partial skin freezing, erythema, mild edema, lack of blisters, and occasional skin desquamation several days later. The patient may complain of transient stinging and burning, followed by throbbing. Prognosis is excellent.

Second-degree injury is characterized by full-thickness skin freezing, formation of substantial edema over 3 to 4 h, erythema, and formation of clear blisters rich in thromboxane and prostaglandins. The blisters form within 6 to 24 h, extend to the end of the digit, and usu-

TABLE 191-2   Classification of Cold Injury According to Severity

Classification	Symptoms
SUPERFICIAL	
First degree: partial skin freezing	Transient stinging and burning
Erythema, edema, hyperemia	Throbbing and aching possible
No blisters or necrosis	May have hyperhidrosis
Occasional skin desquamation	
(5–10 d later)	
Second degree: full-thickness injury	Numbness
Erythema, substantial edema,	Vasomotor disturbances in
vesicles with clear fluid	severe cases
Blisters that desquamate and	
form blackened eschar	
DEEP	
Third degree: full-thickness skin	Initially, no sensation
and subcutaneous freezing	Tissue feels like "block of wood"
Violaceous or hemorrhagic	Later, shooting pains, burning,
blisters	throbbing, aching
Skin necrosis	
Blue-gray discoloration	
Fourth degree: full-thickness skin,	Possible joint discomfort
subcutaneous tissue, muscle,	
tendon, and bone freezing	
Little edema	
Initially mottled, deep red, or	
cyanotic	
Eventually dry, black,	
mummified	

Source: From Britt LD, Dascombe W, Rodriquez A: *Surg Clin North Am* 71:359, 1991, with permission.

ally desquamate and form black, hard eschars over several days. The patient complains of numbness, followed later by aching and throbbing. Prognosis is good.

Third-degree injury is characterized by damage that extends into the subdermal plexus. Hemorrhagic blisters form and are associated with skin necrosis and a blue-gray discoloration of the skin. The patient may complain that the involved extremity feels like a "block of wood," followed later by burning, throbbing, and shooting pains. Prognosis is often poor.

Fourth-degree injury is characterized by extension into subcutaneous tissues, muscle, bone, and tendon. There is little edema. The skin is mottled, with nonblanching cyanosis, and eventually forms a deep, dry, black, mummified eschar. Vesicles often present late, if at all, and may be small, bloody blebs that do not extend to the digit tips. The patient may complain of a deep, aching joint pain. Prognosis is extremely poor.[3,11,12]

Treatment

FIELD MANAGEMENT   Field management of frostbite by emergency medical service personnel is simple. The hypothermia and dehydration associated with frostbite should be addressed. Wet and constrictive clothing should be removed. The involved extremities should be elevated and wrapped carefully in dry sterile gauze, with affected fingers and toes separated. Further cold injury should be avoided. In most cases, more aggressive wound management should be avoided and the patient transported to the ED. However, in some cases the patient may be several days away from evacuation, and medical services and more complex management may be indicated before arrival to the hospital (Table 191-3).

There is a correlation between the length of time tissue is frozen and the degree of cellular damage. Rapid rewarming is the single most

TABLE 191-3   Frostbite Treatment Summary

THAW
Thaw in warm-water bath (40°–42°C) for 10–30 min until extremity is pliable and erythematous
Parenteral opioid analgesics (e.g., morphine 0.1 mg/kg IV)
POSTTHAW
Debride clear blisters
Leave hemorrhagic blisters intact
Dress injured area and blisters with aloe vera cream
Tetanus immunization prophylaxis
Ibuprofen 12 mg/kg per d PO in divided doses
Consider limaprost 20 µg PO tid
Begin daily hydrotherapy

effective therapy for frostbite. However, rewarming in the field is often impractical and sometimes is dangerous. In fact, in some unusual circumstances, it is best to endeavor to keep the affected part frozen until definitive care can be administered. For instance, if the victim has frozen feet and the only avenue to evacuation is prolonged ambulation, rewarming can complicate matters significantly. The risk of refreezing the feet and causing even more severe damage is a real concern. Also, if adequate analgesia is not available, the rewarming process itself can be excessively painful. Ambulation on edematous and blistered feet may not be possible because of pain. In extreme situations such as this, it may be wise to keep the feet frozen and ambulate the patient to a location where more advanced evacuation can occur. If rewarming is attempted in the field, only clean water warmed to 40° to 42°C (104° to 107.6°F), as measured by thermometer, should be used. The use of hot, untested tap water should be avoided because the 50° to 60°C (122° to 140°F) temperatures will cause a destructive thermal injury and worsen the prognosis. Attempts to directly warm with dry air, such as campfires and heaters, should be avoided. Dry heat tends to desiccate damaged tissue, and temperature cannot be measured adequately. Adding a thermal injury to frostbite will worsen the outcome. Rubbing snow on frostbitten tissue to stimulate circulation is ineffective, destructive, and absolutely contraindicated.

Controversy surrounds management of the blisters associated with frostbite. Clear blisters are rich in tissue-injurious thromboxane and prostaglandins. Common sense suggests that blister debridement or aspiration would limit contact with these chemicals and allow direct contact with aloe vera cream to counteract their injurious effects. Also, tense blisters, which tend only to worsen when immobilization is not possible, are painful. Debridement or aspiration can bring some pain relief. When the patient is ambulating on rewarmed frostbitten feet, the associated blisters often rupture anyway. Field debridement of clear blisters is controversial, but adequate research is lacking to support or condemn this practice. Conversely, hemorrhagic blisters should not be drained in the field.

One possible complication of field aspiration or debridement is the theoretical increased risk of infection. Prophylactic use of penicillin may be wise in the field setting to combat any potential wound infection. Wounds should be cleansed daily, and if feet are involved, socks should be clean and changed at least once or twice per day. Affected digits should be covered with aloe vera cream and separated by dry, sterile cotton, and dressings should be changed daily. Pain management should begin with nonsteroidal anti-inflammatory drugs, such as ibuprofen 12 mg/kg per d PO in divided doses, to counteract the arachidonic acid cascade and should be continued even if opioid analgesics are required as well. The victim should be discouraged from smoking because it exacerbates vasoconstriction and tissue damage.[1,7,13]

EMERGENCY DEPARTMENT MANAGEMENT   When taking the patient's history, it is important to determine as many prognostic factors as possible. What was the temperature and wind velocity? How long was the extremity frozen, and if it was thawed, did any refreezing occur? Was there any self-treatment, such as rubbing with snow or use of aloe vera cream or ibuprofen? Were recreational drugs, alcohol, or tobacco involved? Are there any predisposing medical conditions?

Frostbite is often associated with systemic hypothermia and dehydration, both of which can have a negative impact on the prognosis for tissue salvage. Rehydration and general warming are important adjuncts to therapy when indicated.

Frostbitten patients often present to the ED subacutely (>24 h after injury) and with the involved extremity in a partially thawed state. This more prolonged injury and slow, partial thawing usually translate into significantly longer hospital stays and greater tissue loss. However, this should not mean that the patient is treated any less aggressively than the acute patient. The target of treatment remains minimizing tissue loss by focusing on the zone of stasis, where damaged but potentially salvageable tissue exists.

Rapid rewarming is the core of frostbite therapy and should be initiated as soon as possible. **The injured extremity should be placed in gently circulating water at a temperature of 40° to 42°C (104°–107.6°F) for approximately 10 to 30 min, until the distal extremity is pliable and erythematous.** Frostbitten faces can be thawed using moistened compresses soaked in warm water. Some patients may tolerate immersion of their ears in a bowl or pool of warmed water. Anticipate severe pain during rewarming, and treat with parenteral opiates. The patient probably will require daily hydrotherapy and physical therapy during the inpatient phase.

Blister management and the use of prophylactic antibiotics are somewhat controversial. The current consensus is that clear blisters should be debrided or at least aspirated. The blister fluid is rich in destructive thromboxane and prostaglandins. Removal limits damage from these chemicals and enables access to the underlying tissue for topical therapy. Hemorrhagic blisters should not be debrided because this often results in tissue desiccation and worse outcome. However, there is some controversy as to whether aspiration is helpful. **Both blister types should be treated with topical aloe vera cream every 6 h, which helps to combat the arachidonic acid cascade.** Affected digits should be separated with cotton and wrapped with sterile, dry gauze. Elevation of the involved extremities helps decrease edema and pain.

The role of prophylactic antibiotics is unclear. The edema associated with the first several days after injury does appear to predispose to infection. *Staphylococcus aureus, Staphylococcus epidermidis,* and β-hemolytic streptococci account for nearly half of infections, but anaerobes, *Pseudomonas,* and *Enterococcus* are important pathogens as well. Therapy with penicillin G 500,000 U IV every 6 h for 48 to 72 h is recommended in several successful protocols and seems to be beneficial. However, infection prophylaxis using topical bacitracin may be as good or better than intravenous penicillin. Silver sulfadiazine cream also has been advocated by some, but it has not been shown to be consistently beneficial. One disadvantage of using topical antibiotics is that they complicate the concurrent use of aloe vera cream. Tetanus immunization status should be assessed and appropriate vaccination administered if needed because frostbite is considered a tetanus-prone wound (see Chap. 48).

Several agents besides aloe vera cream have been advocated to battle the arachidonic acid cascade and thereby limit tissue damage. The most commonly advocated oral medication is ibuprofen 12 mg/kg per d PO in divided doses. Animal studies suggest possible future roles for oral methimazole (a thromboxane synthetase inhibitor) and topical 1% methylprednisolone acetate (a phospholipase A_2 inhibitor) in preventing the formation of arachidonic acid.

Another controversial area is the use of sympathetic blockade with either intraarterial reserpine or surgical sympathectomy to relieve vasospasm and edema. There is no role for early sympathectomy, and the controversy is beyond the scope of ED management.

Heparin and hyperbaric oxygen therapy have been studied and appear to be of little value. To date, frostbite treatment with intravenous low-molecular-weight dextran has not been studied clinically in humans, but anecdotal reports have been encouraging. Some preliminary data from a study using intraarterial recombinant tissue plasminogen activator in patients with third-degree frostbite suggest that it may hold some promise in decreasing the rate of amputation.[14] A recent limited study suggests that the oral prostaglandin E_1 analogue limaprost 20 μg three times daily may be an effective prophylactic and therapeutic vasodilator for local cold injuries at high altitudes.[10]

Early surgical intervention is not indicated in the management of frostbite. Premature surgery has been an important contributor to unnecessary tissue loss and poor results in the past. This is due primarily to the inability to assess the depth of frostbite at early stages and the fact that the blackened, mummified carapace is protective of the underlying regenerating tissue. Limited early escharotomy may be indicated if the eschar is preventing adequate range of motion or circulation. Fasciotomy is rarely, if ever, indicated. Amputation may be unavoidable, however, if wet gangrene or infection complicates recovery. It usually takes at least 3 to 4 weeks for full demarcation to occur. Most amputations and grafts occur during the third week. The mean length of hospital stay for all degrees of frostbite is reported to be from 8.5 to 33.2 days. To minimize extended hospital stays, some have advocated the early use of radionuclide angiography with bone scan at 7 to 14 days to assess tissue viability and possible early surgical debridement.[15] However, a recent case report suggests that the use of magnetic resonance imaging with magnetic resonance angiography may prove to be more helpful in the early determination of the degree of tissue damage and the eventual prognosis.[16]

Disposition

Since it is difficult to determine the extent of frostbite on initial examination, it is best to be conservative when contemplating admission.[1,3] It has been the standard of care in the past to admit all but the most isolated and superficial frostbite cases. It is important to consider the associated social factors as well. The homeless or elderly, especially when unable to care for themselves adequately, should never be discharged into subfreezing temperatures. If the frostbite is extensive and the hospital and staff are not equipped to treat the degree of severity, transfer of the patient to a tertiary hospital should be considered after initial rewarming and treatment. Patients who are discharged from the ED should be treated with topical aloe vera cream and oral ibuprofen and encouraged not to smoke. Close surgical follow-up should be arranged.

Sequelae

The sequelae of frostbite can be significant and prolonged.[3] Permanent cold sensitivity, pain, tingling, and hyperhidrosis are common. Skin color changes may occur. When deep frostbite involves bones or joints, arthritis may result. In pediatric patients, growth plate damage may result in digit shortening and radial deviation. As noted earlier, infection is a possible complication, and deep frostbite often results in amputation.

REFERENCES

1. Murphy JV, Banwell PE, Roberts AH, McGrouther DA: Frostbite: Pathogenesis and treatment. *J Trauma* 48:171, 2000.
2. Rintamaki H: Predisposing factors and prevention of frostbite. *Int J Circumpolar Health* 59:114, 2000.
3. Hassi J, Makinen TM: Frostbite: Occurrence, risk factors and consequences. *Int J Circumpolar Health* 59:92, 2000.
4. Hwang JC, Himel HN, Edlich RF: Frostbite of the face after recreational misuse of nitrous oxide. *Burns* 22:152, 1996.
5. Kurbat RS, Pollack CP: Facial injury and airway threat from inhalant abuse: A case report. *J Emerg Med* 16:167, 1998.
6. Gamble WB, Bonnecarre ER: Coffee, tea, or frostbite? Care report of inflight freezing hazard from dry ice. *Aviat Space Environ Med* 67:880, 1996.

7. Hamlet MP: Prevention and treatment of cold injury. *Int J Circumpolar Health* 59:108, 2000.

8. Carruthers R: Chilblains (perniosis). *Aust Fam Phys* 17:968, 1988.

9. Oumeish OY, Parish LC: Marching in the army: Common cutaneous disorders of the feet. *Clin Dermatol* 20:445, 2002.

10. Saito S, Shimada H: Effect of prostaglandin E₁ analogue administration on peripheral skin temperature at high altitude. *Angiology* 45:455, 1994.

11. Cauchy E, Chetaille E, Marchand V, Marsigny B: Retrospective study of 70 cases of severe frostbite: A proposed new classification scheme. *Wilderness Environ Med* 12:248, 2001.

12. Heggers JP, Robson MC, Manaualen K, et al: Experimental and clinical observations on frostbite. *Ann Emerg Med* 16:1056, 1987.

13. McCauley RL, Heggers JP, Robson MC: Frostbite: Methods to minimize tissue loss. *Postgrad Med* 88:67, 1990.

14. Skolnick AA: Early data suggest clot-dissolving drug may help save frostbite limbs from amputation. *JAMA* 267:2008, 1992.

15. Mehta RC, Wilson MA: Frostbite injury: Prediction of tissue viability with triple-phase bone scanning. *Radiology* 170:511, 1989.

16. Barker JR, Haws MJ, Brown RE, et al: Magnetic resonance imaging of severe frostbite injuries. *Ann Plast Surg* 38:275, 1997.

HYPOTHERMIA

Howard A. Bessen

EPIDEMIOLOGY

Hypothermia is defined as a core temperature of less than 35°C (95°F). While most commonly seen in cold climates, it may develop without exposure to extreme environmental conditions. Hypothermia is not uncommon in temperate regions and may even develop indoors during the summer. In the United States, an average of 700 people die from hypothermia each year. Half of those who die from hypothermia are older than 65 years of age.[1]

Individuals at the extremes of age and those with an altered sensorium for any reason are particularly susceptible to developing hypothermia. The elderly may lose their ability to sense cold, and neonates easily become hypothermic because of their large surface-area-to-volume ratio. Both groups have a limited ability to increase heat production and to conserve body heat. Individuals with an altered sensorium, if unable to carry out the appropriate behavioral responses to cold stress, may develop hypothermia despite otherwise intact thermoregulatory mechanisms.

PHYSIOLOGY OF TEMPERATURE HOMEOSTASIS

Body temperature may fall as a result of heat loss by conduction, convection, radiation, or evaporation. *Conduction* is the transfer of heat by direct contact down a temperature gradient, e.g., from a warm body to the cold environment. Since the thermal conductivity of water is approximately 30 times that of air, the body loses heat rapidly when immersed in water, producing a rapid decline in body temperature. *Convection* is the transfer of heat by the actual movement of heated material, e.g., wind disrupting the layer of warm air surrounding the body. Convective heat loss increases markedly in windy conditions. Heat also may be lost by *radiation* to the environment (primarily from noninsulated body areas) and by *evaporation of water.* Evaporation of the water contained in exhaled, water-saturated air occurs over a wide range of ambient temperatures and may be prevented by inhalation of warmed, humidified air.

Opposing the loss of body heat are the mechanisms of heat conservation and gain. In general, these are controlled by the hypothalamus; thus hypothalamic dysfunction may cause impairment in temperature homeostasis. Heat is conserved by peripheral vasoconstriction and, importantly, by behavioral responses. If behavioral responses such as putting on clothing or coming indoors from a cold environment are impaired for any reason (e.g., drug intoxication or trauma), the risk of hypothermia is increased.

Heat gain is effected by shivering and by nonshivering thermogenesis. The nonshivering component of heat production consists of an increase in metabolic rate brought about by increased output from the thyroid and adrenal glands.

ETIOLOGY

The most important causes of hypothermia are listed in Table 192-1. "Accidental" hypothermia may be divided into immersion and nonimmersion cold exposure. Exposure to cold environmental conditions may lead to hypothermia even in healthy subjects, especially in wind and rain. Inadequate clothing and physical exhaustion contribute to the loss of body heat. The high thermal conductivity of water leads to the rapid development of hypothermia during immersion. The rate of heat loss is determined by water temperature, and immersion in any water colder than 16° to 21°C (60.8° to 69.8°F) can lead to severe hypothermia.

Metabolic causes of hypothermia include various hypoendocrine states (hypothyroidism, hypoadrenalism, hypopituitarism) that lead to a decrease in metabolic rate. Hypoglycemia also may lead to hypothermia; the probable mechanism is hypothalamic dysfunction secondary to glucopenia. Other causes of hypothalamic and central nervous system (CNS) dysfunction (e.g., head trauma, tumor, stroke) may interfere with mechanisms of temperature regulation. Wernicke disease may involve the hypothalamus; this is a rare but important cause of hypothermia because it is potentially reversible with parenteral thiamine administration.

In the United States, most hypothermic patients are intoxicated with ethanol or other drugs. Ethanol is a vasodilator, and because of its anesthetic and CNS depressant effects, intoxicated subjects neither feel the cold nor respond to it appropriately. Other sedative-hypnotic and vasodilating drugs also may be implicated in the development of hypothermia, as may insulin and other hypoglycemic agents.

Sepsis may alter the hypothalamic temperature set point and is a well-known cause of hypothermia. Subnormal body temperature is a poor prognostic factor in patients with bacteremia. Severe dermal disease may impair the skin's thermoregulatory functions. Significant burns or severe exfoliative dermatitis may prevent cutaneous vasoconstriction and increase transcutaneous water loss, predisposing to the development of hypothermia. Hypothermia may develop in anyone with an acute incapacitating illness. Thus patients with severe infections, diabetic ketoacidosis, immobilizing injuries, and various other conditions may have impaired thermoregulatory function, including altered behavioral responses. Hypothermia also may be induced by resuscitation with room-temperature fluid or cold blood. This is a particular risk in patients undergoing massive volume replacement, such as trauma patients.

PATHOPHYSIOLOGY AND CLINICAL FEATURES

The response of various organ systems to lowered temperature varies widely among individuals.[2–4] In general, body temperatures from 32°

TABLE 192-1   Causes of Hypothermia: Clinical Settings

"Accidental" (environmental)
Metabolic
Hypothalamic and CNS dysfunction
Drug-induced
Sepsis
Dermal disease
Acute incapacitating illness
Iatrogenic (fluid resuscitation)

to 35°C (89.6°–95°F) constitute "mild" hypothermia. In this temperature range, the patient is in an excitation (responsive) stage, in which physiologic adjustments attempt to retain and generate heat.

When temperature drops below 32°C (89.6°F), general excitation gives way to the slowing (adynamic) stage, in which there is a progressive slowdown of bodily functions and metabolism, causing a decrease in both oxygen utilization and CO_2 production. Shivering ceases when body temperature falls below 30° to 32°C (86°–89.6°F), removing a major source of heat production.

In the initial excitation phase, heart rate, cardiac output, and blood pressure all rise. With decreasing temperature, these all decline. Cardiac output and blood pressure may be markedly depressed by the negative inotropic and chronotropic effects of hypothermia and further depressed by concomitant hypovolemia. Hypothermia causes characteristic electrocardiographic (ECG) changes and may induce life-threatening dysrhythmias[5] (Table 192-2). The Osborn (J) wave, a slow, positive deflection at the end of the QRS complex, is characteristic, though not pathognomonic, of hypothermia (Figure 192-1).

Patients are at risk for dysrhythmias at body temperatures below 30°C (86°F); the risk rises as body temperature decreases. Although various dysrhythmias may occur at any time, the typical sequence is a progression from sinus bradycardia to atrial fibrillation with a slow ventricular response, to ventricular fibrillation, and ultimately, to asystole. The hypothermic myocardium is extremely irritable, and ventricular fibrillation may be induced by a variety of manipulations and interventions that stimulate the heart, including rough handling of the patient.[3,6]

Pulmonary effects include initial tachypnea, followed by a progressive decrease in respiratory rate and tidal volume. Cold-induced bronchorrhea, along with a depression of cough and gag reflexes, makes aspiration pneumonia a common complication.

Much attention has been paid to the temperature correction of arterial blood gases in the hypothermic patient. Since the blood gas analyzer warms the blood to 37°C (98.6°F), thus increasing the partial pressure of dissolved gas, the machine will report a higher P_{O_2} and P_{CO_2} and lower pH than the actual values at the patient's body temperature. Correction factors and nomograms are available to determine the actual values in the patient's body; however, the optimal or normal values in hypothermia are not known. The simplest solution is to use the uncorrected values as if the patient were normothermic; studies suggest that this approach is the most physiologically sound. P_{CO_2} is often quite low secondary to depressed metabolism and decreased CO_2 production, and iatrogenic hyperventilation may lead to marked respiratory alkalosis.

Hypothermia causes a leftward shift of the oxyhemoglobin dissociation curve, potentially impairing oxygen release to tissues. Patients may have minimal oxygen reserves despite diminished oxygen requirements, warranting the administration of supplemental oxygen.

The CNS is affected by hypothermia, with a progressive depression of consciousness with decreasing temperature. Mild incoordination is followed by confusion, lethargy, and coma; pupils may be dilated and unreactive. These changes are associated with a decrease in cerebral blood flow. An even greater decrease in cerebral oxygen requirements may protect the brain against anoxic or ischemic damage.

TABLE 192-2   ECG Changes in Hypothermia

T-wave inversions
PR, QRS, QT prolongation
Muscle tremor artifact
Osborn (J) wave
Dysrhythmias:
  Sinus bradycardia
  Atrial fibrillation or flutter
  Nodal rhythms
  AV block
  PVCs
  Ventricular fibrillation
  Asystole

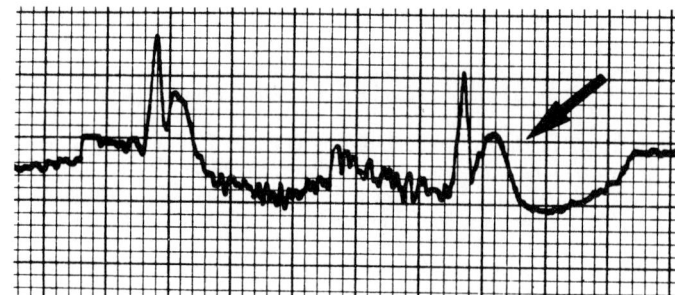

FIG. 192-1. Rhythm strip from patient with temperature of 25°C (77°F) showing atrial fibrillation with a slow ventricular response, muscle tremor artifact, and Osborn (J) wave *(arrow)*.

Hypothermia impairs renal concentrating abilities and induces a cold diuresis, leading to significant volume losses. Because of this concentrating defect, urine flow and specific gravity are unreliable indicators of intravascular volume and circulatory status. The immobile hypothermic patient is prone to rhabdomyolysis, and acute renal failure may occur because of myoglobinuria and renal hypoperfusion. Intravascular volume is also lost due to a plasma shift to the extravascular space.

The combination of hemoconcentration, cold-induced increase in blood viscosity, and poor circulation may lead to intravascular thrombosis and subsequent embolic complications. Disseminated intravascular coagulation may occur because of release of tissue thromboplastins into the bloodstream, especially when circulation is restored during rewarming. Because cold inhibits both platelet function and the enzymatic reactions of the coagulation cascade, hypothermic patients are prone to bleeding. The coagulopathy may be evident clinically but not detected with routine coagulation tests, which are performed at 37°C (98.6°F).

Endocrine function is fairly well preserved at low body temperatures. Plasma cortisol and thyroid hormone levels are usually normal or elevated unless the patient has a preexisting deficiency. Glucose levels may be normal, low, or elevated. Although hyperglycemia is common due to decreased insulin release as well as decreased glucose utilization, hypoglycemia may occur in a significant percentage of patients.

Acid-base disturbances are common in hypothermia but follow no uniform pattern. Acidosis may occur due to severe respiratory depression and CO_2 retention, as well as due to lactic acid production from shivering and poor tissue perfusion. Alkalosis may result from diminished CO_2 production with low metabolic rates, from iatrogenic hyperventilation, or sodium bicarbonate administration.

Pancreatitis (not only hyperamylasemia but true pancreatic necrosis) may occur in hypothermia. Hepatic function is depressed by cold, and drugs normally metabolized, conjugated, or detoxified by the liver may accumulate rapidly to toxic levels. Finally, local cold injury and frostbite may occur in the hypothermic patient.

DIAGNOSIS

The diagnosis of hypothermia is often not obvious, especially in patients without exposure to profoundly cold environments. Since some standard clinical thermometers record only to 34.4°C (94°F), low-reading thermometers are required to accurately measure the temperature of hypothermic patients. Electronic thermometers with flexible probes can be used to continuously monitor rectal, bladder, or esophageal temperatures.

TREATMENT

Treatment includes both general supportive measures and specific rewarming techniques. Therapy begins with careful, gentle handling because manipulation can precipitate ventricular fibrillation in the irritable hypothermic myocardium. Pulses may be difficult to detect in the profoundly hypothermic patient, and chest compressions may cause ventricular fibrillation. To avoid inappropriate chest compressions, the patient who is unmonitored or in a "nonarrested rhythm" (a rhythm other than ventricular fibrillation or asystole, such as sinus bradycardia or atrial fibrillation) should be examined carefully for respiratory activity and pulses. If no respiration is seen, ventilation should be initiated. Then 30 to 60 s should be spent attempting to palpate a pulse. If no pulses are detected, CPR should be initiated.[7,8]

Oxygen and intravenous fluids should be warmed, and patients should have constant monitoring of their core temperature, cardiac rhythm, and oxygen saturation. Pulse oximetry is usually accurate in hypothermic patients, although unreliable data may be obtained with profound vasoconstriction or a very low cardiac output. If central venous lines are placed, care should be taken to avoid entering and irritating the heart. In general, indications for endotracheal intubation are the same as in the normothermic patient. Concern has been raised regarding induction of dysrhythmias during intubation; however, there is a very low complication rate with careful intubation after oxygenation.[9]

Although dysrhythmias in the hypothermic patient may represent an immediate threat to life, most rhythm disturbances (e.g., sinus bradycardia, atrial fibrillation or flutter) require no therapy and revert spontaneously with rewarming. In addition, the activity of antiarrhythmic and cardioactive drugs is unpredictable in hypothermia, and the hypothermic heart is relatively resistant to atropine, pacing, and countershock. Ventricular fibrillation may be refractory to therapy until the patient is rewarmed. The American Heart Association's 2000 guidelines suggest initial defibrillation attempts with up to three shocks. If this is unsuccessful, CPR should be instituted and rapid rewarming begun. Defibrillation should be reattempted when the core temperature reaches 30°C (86°F).[7]

Drug Therapy

Because many hypothermic patients are thiamine-depleted alcoholics (and because Wernicke disease may cause hypothermia), patients should be given intravenous thiamine 50 mg. Between 50 and 100 mL of 50% glucose should be administered if a test-strip serum glucose measurement is low or if a rapid test is unavailable.

Administration of antibiotics, steroids, and thyroid hormone must be individualized. Serious, often occult infections may either precipitate or complicate hypothermia, and a thorough search for infection is indicated. Empirical antibiotic therapy is appropriate when a noninfectious cause of hypothermia cannot be identified.[10] Routine steroid therapy generally is not indicated, but hydrocortisone (100 mg) should be given to the patient with a history of adrenal suppression or insufficiency preceding the hypothermic episode, as well as to the patient with myxedema coma.

Hypothermia and hypothyroidism share many clinical features. While most patients with myxedema coma are hypothermic, only a small minority of hypothermic patients are hypothyroid; thyroid hormone levels are most often normal or elevated.[10] Thyroxine in large doses is necessary for the patient in myxedema coma but potentially could cause dysrhythmias or cardiac ischemia in other hypothermic patients. Therefore, thyroid hormone replacement is indicated only in patients with a known history of hypothyroidism, a thyroidectomy scar, or other strong clinical evidence of myxedema coma.

Rewarming Techniques

Many modalities are available for rewarming; the choice of method is a matter of controversy (Table 192-3). There are no prospective, controlled studies comparing rewarming methods in humans, and each method has advantages and disadvantages.

TABLE 192-3   Rewarming Techniques

Passive rewarming:
    Removal from cold environment
    Insulation
Active external rewarming:
    Warm water immersion
    Heating blankets set at 40°C
    Radiant heat
    Forced air
Active core rewarming at 40°C:
    Inhalation rewarming
    Heated IV fluids
    GI tract lavage
    Bladder lavage
    Peritoneal lavage
    Pleural lavage
    Extracorporeal rewarming
    Mediastinal lavage via thoracotomy

Passive rewarming allows patients to rewarm on their own, using endogenous heat produced by metabolism. Since patients often become hypothermic over a period of hours to days, slow, passive rewarming is physiologically sound, avoiding rapid changes in cardiovascular status and the complications associated with active rewarming methods.[11] Patients must have intact thermoregulatory mechanisms and be capable of metabolic heat production for successful passive rewarming. With severe hypothermia or hypothermia secondary to an underlying illness, patients may fail to rewarm passively; active rewarming is then indicated. In addition, since temperature rises slowly with passive rewarming, it is inappropriate for patients with cardiovascular compromise.

Active external rewarming (application of exogenous heat to the body surface) is often very effective in raising body temperature. Warm water immersion affords rapid rewarming but makes resuscitation and monitoring difficult and is impractical for use in the ED. Rewarming with heated air forced through slits in commercially available plastic or paper blankets (e.g., Bair-Hugger, Augustine Medical, Eden Prairie, MN) appears very promising; this method has been used successfully in moderately to severely hypothermic patients.[12,13]

External rewarming does have disadvantages. It may be ineffective with poor perfusion of the periphery, especially in patients in cardiac arrest. Application of external heat may cause peripheral vasodilation and venous pooling, leading to relative hypovolemia and hypotension (rewarming shock). Washout of lactic acid from the peripheral tissues may lead to rewarming acidosis, and an increase in metabolic demands of the periphery before the hypothermic heart can provide adequate tissue perfusion may lead to further tissue hypoxia and acidosis.

The core temperature may continue to decline after rewarming has begun. This *core temperature afterdrop* has been ascribed to the return of cold blood to the core induced by external warming and peripheral vasodilation. This may occur, but afterdrop also can be explained by the continued conduction of heat from the relatively warmer core to the colder peripheral tissues. The incidence and magnitude of afterdrop are unclear, as is its clinical significance.[3,6]

Active core rewarming has several theoretical advantages. Internal organs including the heart are preferentially rewarmed, decreasing myocardial irritability and returning cardiac function. Peripheral vasodilation is avoided, decreasing the incidence and magnitude of rewarming shock and acidosis. However, some internal rewarming techniques are invasive and may be unavailable or difficult to institute.

Inhalation rewarming is the administration of warmed, humidified air or oxygen by face mask or endotracheal tube. By itself, it provides a small heat gain but also minimizes heat loss from the lungs, which can account for up to 30 percent of the body's total metabolic heat production. A heater is interposed in the ventilator or face mask tubing, and the tubing must be covered with insulating material to prevent heat loss during delivery. The temperature of the gas delivered to the face mask or endotracheal tube should measure 40°C (104°F).

Intravenous fluids and blood should also be warmed to 40°C (104°F) before administration, especially in patients receiving massive volume resuscitation. Commercial fluid warmers allow the temperature of infused fluids to be controlled precisely.

Both inhalation rewarming and administration of heated fluids should be used in all patients because these are simple techniques without complications, as long as the temperature is controlled. Temperatures >50°C (122°F) can cause airway burns and intravascular hemolysis.

Gastrointestinal tract (gastric or colonic) lavage with warmed saline is technically simple, and patients can be lavaged with large volumes of warm fluid in a short time period. However, the obtunded hypothermic patient may develop pulmonary aspiration if lavaged with an unprotected airway. In a manner similar to gastrointestinal tract lavage, the bladder can be lavaged with warm saline solution using a urinary drainage catheter.

Peritoneal lavage affords relatively rapid rewarming.[14] It is widely available, may be instituted rapidly and with little technical difficulty, and has been shown to be effective in both animal studies and human applications. Potassium-free dialysis solution is warmed to 40° to 45°C (104°–113°F), instilled, and then removed; the use of two catheters (one for fluid instillation and one for removal) may increase the rewarming rate.

Pleural lavage using thoracostomy tubes has provided effective rewarming in animal studies and a few human cases.[15] Lavaging the left thoracic cavity delivers heated fluid in close proximity to the heart, potentially allowing rapid cardiac warming. Two thoracostomy tubes (for fluid inflow and outflow) generally have been employed. If this technique is chosen, care must be taken to monitor the net fluid infusion because increased intrathoracic pressure and tension hydrothorax may complicate the procedure. The risk of precipitating dysrhythmias during chest tube insertion is unknown.

Rapid internal rewarming also can be accomplished through an extracorporeal circuit.[16,17] This consists of an arteriovenous or venovenous shunt in which blood is routed to a warming device and then returned to the patient. Pump-assisted cardiopulmonary bypass using the femoral vessels for access is the most commonly used extracorporeal technique; right atrial–aortic bypass using a median sternotomy and heated hemodialysis also has been employed. Continuous arteriovenous rewarming using a countercurrent heat exchanger (a modified commercial fluid warmer) interposed between catheters placed in the femoral vessels, with flow driven by the patient's blood pressure, also has been reported.[18] This technique obviates the need for pump support and systemic heparinization but relies on the patient's circulation and is ineffective in patients with significant hypotension. Venovenous bypass is a similar technique that employs a roller pump to assist blood flow.[19]

Profoundly hypothermic patients may be rewarmed in a very short time period with these methods.[16,17] In addition to allowing rapid rewarming, pump-driven partial (femoral-femoral) or complete (right atrial–aortic) cardiopulmonary bypass provides circulatory support and oxygenation of blood, a great advantage in the management of patients in cardiac arrest or with severe cardiovascular compromise. Specialized equipment and personnel are required, however, and lack of immediate availability often precludes the use of this technique. In addition, the heparinization required for some extracorporeal techniques may cause complications in hypothermic trauma patients.

Various diathermy and radiowave techniques, although promising, have had limited use in hypothermic humans.

Finally, warm mediastinal irrigation via open thoracotomy has been used successfully in a small number of patients, although it is possible that these patients could have been resuscitated using less invasive modalities.[20] Thoracotomy has many potential complications and should be considered only in arrested patients.

Approach to Rewarming

No prospective, controlled studies comparing the various rewarming modalities have been done in humans. Therefore, firm guidelines for therapy cannot be given.

Patients with mild hypothermia, who are still in the "excitation" stage, generally improve spontaneously, as long as endogenous heat production mechanisms are functional. In addition, at temperatures above 30°C (86°F), the incidence of dysrhythmias is low, and rapid rewarming is rarely necessary.

By far the most important consideration is the patient's cardiovascular status; a secondary consideration is the presenting temperature. Some feel that patients with a stable cardiac rhythm (including sinus bradycardia and atrial fibrillation) and stable vital signs do not need rapid rewarming, even if the temperature is very low. They recommend passive rewarming and noninvasive rewarming modalities (e.g., forced-air rewarming, warm moist oxygen, and warm intravenous fluids) in this setting. Others argue that profoundly hypothermic patients, even if currently "stable," are at risk of developing life-threatening dysrhythmias. They recommend rapid rewarming until the temperature has reached 30° to 32°C (86°–89.6°F) to minimize the time period during which dysrhythmias may develop. The relative merits of each approach have not been studied.

Patients with cardiovascular insufficiency or instability, including persistent hypotension and life-threatening dysrhythmias, need to be rewarmed rapidly. Extracorporeal techniques offer many advantages but often are unavailable. If extracorporeal rewarming is not available, multiple other rewarming modalities can be used simultaneously.

PROGNOSIS

Many hypothermic patients have severe infections or other life-threatening illnesses. Patients with "uncomplicated" hypothermia (often purely due to cold exposure) have a fairly low mortality rate; patients with significant associated diseases have a much worse prognosis.[21] In terms of ultimate outcome, the underlying disease process is far more important than the initial temperature or the rewarming method chosen. Therefore, evaluation and treatment of these patients must include a search for associated diseases as well as treatment of the hypothermia itself.

If asphyxia (e.g., near-drowning) precedes the development of hypothermia, the prognosis is very poor.[22] If asphyxia has not occurred, the protective effect of hypothermia may have an important influence on prognosis. Decreased oxygen requirements can protect the brain and other organs against anoxic and ischemic damage. This means that the usual criteria indicating death or irreversibility of disease are not valid in the hypothermic patient, who may even survive prolonged cardiac arrest without neurologic sequelae.

Hypothermic patients may recover completely after presenting in a rigid, apneic state with fixed and dilated pupils. Recovery has been documented with core temperatures as low as 14.2°C (57.6°F)[23] and with cardiac arrest for 6.5 h.[24] Death in hypothermia must be defined as a failure to revive with rewarming; unless there is strong evidence that the patient is not viable, resuscitative efforts should be continued until core temperature is at least 30° to 32°C (86°–89.6°F).

DISPOSITION

Patients with mild accidental hypothermia caused purely by environmental exposure may be discharged after rewarming in the ED, provided they are asymptomatic and can return to a warm environment. Most other hypothermic patients require hospital admission, both for management of hypothermia and for evaluation and management of underlying diseases.

REFERENCES

1. Centers for Disease Control and Prevention: Hypothermia-related deaths— Utah, 2000, and United States, 1979–1998. *MMWR* 51:76, 2002.

2. Danzl DF, Pozos RF: Accidental hypothermia. *New Engl J Med* 331:1756, 1994.
3. Giesbrecht GG: Cold stress, near drowning and accidental hypothermia: A review. *Aviat Space Environ Med* 71:733, 2000.
4. Wittmers LE: Pathophysiology of cold exposure. *Minn Med* 84:30, 2001.
5. Vassallo SU, Delaney KA, Hoffman RS, et al: A prospective evaluation of the electrocardiographic manifestations of hypothermia. *Acad Emerg Med* 6:1121, 1999.
6. Lloyd EL: Accidental hypothermia. *Resuscitation* 32:111, 1996.
7. American Heart Association: Guidelines 2000 for Cardiopulmonary Resuscitation and Emergency Cardiovascular Care. Part 8: Advanced Challenges in Resuscitation. Section 3: Special Challenges in ECC. *Circulation* 102(suppl I):I-229, 2000.
8. Giesbrecht GG: Emergency treatment of hypothermia. *Emerg Med (Fremantle)* 13:9, 2001.
9. Danzl DF, Pozos RS, Auerbach PS, et al: Multicenter hypothermia survey. *Ann Emerg Med* 16:1042, 1987.
10. Muszkat M, Durst RM, Ben-Yehuda A: Factors associated with mortality among elderly patients with hypothermia. *Am J Med* 113:234, 2002.
11. Vassal T, Benoit-Gonin B, Carrat F, et al: Severe accidental hypothermia treated in an ICU: Prognosis and outcome. *Chest* 120:1998, 2001.
12. Koller R, Schnider TW, Neidhart P: Deep accidental hypothermia and cardiac arrest—Rewarming with forced air. *Acta Anaesthesiol Scand* 41:1359, 1997.
13. Steele MT, Nelson MJ, Sessler DI, et al: Forced air speeds rewarming in accidental hypothermia. *Ann Emerg Med* 27:479, 1996.
14. Otto RJ, Metzler MH: Rewarming from experimental hypothermia: Comparison of heated aerosol inhalation, peritoneal lavage, and pleural lavage. *Crit Care Med* 16:869, 1988.
15. Barr GL: Correction of hypothermia by continuous pleural perfusion. *Surgery* 103:553, 1988.
16. Walpoth BH, Walpoth-Aslan BN, Mattle HP, et al: Outcome of survivors of accidental deep hypothermia and circulatory arrest treated with extracorporeal blood warming. *New Engl J Med* 337:1500, 1997.
17. Lazar HL: The treatment of hypothermia. *New Engl J Med* 337:1545, 1997.
18. Gentilello LM, Cobean RA, Offner PJ, et al: Continuous arteriovenous rewarming: Rapid reversal of hypothermia in critically ill patients. *J Trauma* 32:316, 1992.
19. Brauer A, Wrigge H, Kersten J, et al: Severe accidental hypothermia: Rewarming strategy using a venovenous bypass system and a convective air warmer. *Intensive Care Med* 25:520, 1999.
20. Brunette DD, McVaney K: Hypothermic cardiac arrest: An 11 year review of ED management and outcome. *Am J Emerg Med* 18:418, 2000.
21. Megarbane B, Axler O, Chary I, et al: Hypothermia with indoor occurrence is associated with a worse outcome. *Intensive Care Med* 26:1843, 2000.
22. Farstad M, Andersen KS, Koller ME, et al: Rewarming from accidental hypothermia by extracorporeal circulation. A retrospective study. *Eur J Cardiothorac Surg* 20:58, 2001.
23. Dobson JA, Burgess JJ: Resuscitation of severe hypothermia by extracorporeal rewarming in a child. *J Trauma* 40:483, 1996.
24. Lexow K: Severe accidental hypothermia: Survival after 6 hours 30 minutes of cardiopulmonary resuscitation. *Arctic Med Res* 50(suppl 6):112, 1991.

HEAT EMERGENCIES

James S. Walker
David E. Hogan

Environmentally induced heat-related illnesses result when psychologic and physiologic adaptation mechanisms fail during a period of elevated heat stress. Heat-related illnesses can be trivial to life-threatening. In most circumstances, heat illnesses can be avoided through public education and preventative measures.

EPIDEMIOLOGY

Heat illnesses have been the most frequent cause of environmentally related death in the United States during the past decade—more than lightning-, tornado-, flood-, hurricane-, cold-, or winter-related fatalities.[1] Annual heat-related death rates average one per million for those 5 to 44 years of age but increase to five per million in the population older than 85 years.[2] From 1979 to 1999, 8015 heat-related fatalities were reported to the Centers for Disease Control in the United States.[2] Of these, 3829 were listed as due to "adverse weather conditions." Analysis of the 3764 weather-related deaths with known age found that 142 (4 percent) were younger than 4 years and 1068 (28 percent) were at least 75 years.[2] Heat illness is a rare but preventable cause of death in young athletes during competition. Between 1995 and 2001, 15 high school students died due to heat stroke while participating in the sport of football.

Heat-related deaths have averaged approximately 400 cases per year over the past 10 years in the United States, but the rate varies significantly according to the weather.[2] For example, fatality rates may spike to almost 200 deaths per million population during years with heat waves and droughts of substantial severity.[3] Heat waves are defined as 3 or more consecutive days of sustained temperatures above 32.2°C (90°F).[4] The number of nonfatal heat injury cases seeking medical care on a yearly basis is not known. One California study of occupational heat injuries found 1128 cases seeking medical care in a year; there were seven (0.62 percent) deaths, a 15 percent hospital admission rate, with 40 percent of workers being off work for several days after the initial medical evaluation.[5] Applying this ratio of deaths to heat-related illness cases from this study to the entire U.S. population produces an estimate of about 60,000 individuals each year who seek medical attention for heat-related illness.

The male-to-female ratio for heat illness is essentially equal, and any age can be affected. Some populations at higher risk include: the elderly (age >75 years), especially if they have chronic illness or take medications that interfere with heat loss; young children (<4 years), particularly if they have congenital nervous system disease or diarrheal illness; those with limited mobility; alcoholics; and people taking antipsychotics, major tranquilizers, anticholinergics, antiparkinsonian agents, cardiovascular medications (β-blockers, calcium channel blockers, and vasodilators), and over-the-counter sleeping aids or stimulants.[6,7] In addition, individuals with a prior history of heat stroke are at greater risk for another episode. Other risk factors for exertional heat illness include obesity, dehydration, and vigorous exertion in the heat without proper training and acclimatization. Other more rare disorders, such as congenital absence of sweat glands, progressive systemic scleroderma, hyperthyroidism, and pheochromocytoma, increase heat injury risk. The major environmental risk factor is exposure to heat stress on a constant basis without air-conditioning breaks or cooling during the night. Mortality rates for the most severe form of heat illness (heat stroke) range from 10 to 75 percent.[5] Mortality is further increased in cases with severe underlying medical conditions and in individuals who have treatment delayed for longer than 2 h after the onset of severe symptoms.

PATHOPHYSIOLOGY

Mechanisms of Heat Transfer

The body regulates heat content through four mechanisms: radiation, conduction, convection, and evaporation. Radiation and conduction are considered the dry, or sensible, methods of heat loss. Convection is usually considered a separate mechanism, but heat must first be conducted into the surrounding medium in contact with the skin (air) before it can be moved away by convection. Convection is therefore an adjunct to conduction. Evaporation represents the most efficient method of losing heat and is considered the wet, or insensible, mechanism of heat loss.

Radiation is the primary mechanism of heat loss when the environmental temperature is lower than the body temperature. Radiative loss of heat occurs through the infrared range of the electromagnetic spectrum. Infrared radiation flowing from the body into a cooler environment may account for up to 60 percent of body cooling in these conditions. When the surrounding environment is hot compared with the body, heat will be gained by radiation. Direct sunlight alone may account for a heat burden of 100 to 250 kcal/h.

Conduction of heat occurs when the kinetic energy of moving molecules of a warm surface (skin) is transferred directly to the less kinetically active molecules of a cooler surface (solid objects, water, or air). Conduction of heat energy into solid surfaces usually accounts for less than 3 percent of the total heat loss of the body. Conduction of heat into the ambient air surrounding the skin will rapidly stop as soon as that layer acquires the same temperature as the skin surface. This results in an "insulator zone" of warmed air through which little heat may be lost. Removing the warmed air next to the skin and replacing it with cooler air may increase conductive heat loss; this process is called *convection*. When conduction is coupled with convection, rates of heat energy transfer from the body may account for up to 15 percent of the total heat loss. Conduction of heat into water is 32 times more efficient than conduction into air of the same temperature. Because the specific heat of water is greater than air by a factor of several thousand, an insulator zone of warm water next to the skin cannot form to any degree.

The cooling effect of the wind on heat loss is approximately proportional to the square root of the wind velocity: a 4-km/h wind is about twice as effective as a 1-km/h wind in removing heat. Although moving the medium of the air away from the skin by convection improves heat loss by conduction, it has limits. Above 32.2°C (90°F) and 35 percent humidity, convection does not remove heat well from the body.[8] Fans alone have not been demonstrated to decrease the rate of heat stroke during periods of high environmental temperature and humidity. Populations with no home air conditioning (often in the lower socioeconomic strata) have an elevated risk of almost 50 percent for a serious heat injury when compared with populations with air conditioning.[9] Taking "heat breaks" in an air-conditioned location for periods as short as 2 h a day substantially decreases the rate of heat stroke for non-air-conditioned populations. It is clear that allowing the body to decrease the heat burden at some time during the day is critical to prevent heat illness under the above conditions.

Evaporation is the primary heat loss mechanism of the body in higher temperatures. Each gram of water evaporating from the skin and lungs removes about 0.58 kcal of heat. Even in the absence of sweating, a basal level of skin and respiratory evaporation (insensible loss) accounts for about 600 mL of water daily and 12 to 16 kcal of heat loss per hour. Evaporation accounts for over 25 percent of the heat lost in cooler settings and virtually 100 percent at high environmental temperatures. To achieve heat loss, water must be able to evaporate into the atmosphere. When the atmosphere contains high levels of humidity, evaporation is impaired and heat loss by this mechanism is decreased.

Evaporation depends on the creation of adequate amounts of sweat and adequate hydration for sweat gland secretion. Dehydration of as little as 1 percent can impair heat dissipation and physiologic responses.[10] Each 1 percent decrease in body weight from dehydration results in a core temperature increase of 0.1°C to 0.3°C (0.18°F to 0.54°F). Dehydration impairs cardiovascular and thermoregulatory functions by decreasing skin blood flow and sweating rate. During vigorous exercise, athletes will voluntarily ingest only 50 percent of their sweat loss and can rapidly dehydrate. In addition, studies on Olympic athletes indicate that highly acclimatized humans can achieve sweating rates that exceed gastric emptying rates. Such sweating rates outstrip the ability of the gastrointestinal tract to absorb water and result in dehydration and eventual hyperpyrexia. It is estimated that sweating rates faster than 1 L/h are not sustainable with oral hydration alone.

Although some clothing can reflect and reduce absorption of radiant heat, clothing may also act as an insulator causing heat gain by reducing the efficacy of convection and evaporation. Cloth traps air more efficiently close to the skin, thereby allowing the rapid development of an insulator zone of warm air, and provides increased air resistance, thereby decreasing the effectiveness of convection. Evaporation through cloth depends on the gradient of vapor pressure from the skin through the cloth and into the air.[8] Clothing that interferes with the flow of water vapor decreases evaporative efficiency. Evaporation of water from the clothing is also less effective in removing heat than evaporation directly from the skin. Wearing a hat or clothing on the trunk interferes more substantially with heat loss than covering other body areas.

Response to Heat Stress

The body tends to maintain its core temperature between 36°C and 38°C (96.8°F and 100.4°F). Native thermal regulation mechanisms begin to fail at core temperatures below 35°C (95°F) and above 40°C (104°F).[11] It is possible to maintain core temperatures of 40°C to 42°C (104°F to 107.6°F) for short periods without adverse effect. The highest documented core temperature in a survivor of heat stroke is 46.5°C (115.7°F).

Physiologic response to heat stress occurs through four primary methods: dilatation of blood vessels (particularly in the skin), increased sweat production, decreased heat production, and behavioral heat control. The primary function of heat regulation mechanisms in the human body seems to be attuned to prevention of heat loss in cold environments. It is by the release or reversal of these heat-conserving mechanisms that heat loss is achieved. As the core temperature of the body rises, the sympathetic outflow of the posterior hypothalamus (the primary heat conserving center) is inhibited, leaving unopposed the sympathetic outflow from the anterior hypothalamus. Sympathetic flow from the anterior hypothalamus results in decreased vascular tone throughout the body, particularly in the cutaneous circulation. Blood flow to the skin can increase from a basal level of 0.2 L/min to a maximum of about 8 L/min. Substantial stress may be placed on the cardiovascular system during this response, because cardiac output will increase about 3 L/min for each 1°C (1.8°F) elevation of core temperature.[9] The heart rate increases to compensate for the decrease in stroke volume from the cutaneous vascular dilation to maintain cardiac output. Any patient with underlying cardiovascular disease or a pharmacologic or physiologic impairment of these mechanisms may not be able to maintain this degree of cardiac output. Heat stress may also result in arrhythmias, myocardial ischemia, and exacerbation of congestive heart failure.

Elevated cholinergic stimulation to the skin results in increased sweat production. Elevated levels of catecholamines that occur during the heat response recruit and stimulate more sweat glands to secrete. Sharp increases in the rate of sweat production normally occur with core temperature elevations above 37°C (98.6°F).

Metabolic heat production in the body is inhibited when the core temperature rises. The major metabolic decrease in heat production is achieved when the anterior hypothalamus signals to the primary motor center in the posterior hypothalamus to inhibit shivering. Chemical thermogenesis in mammals is primarily due to the uncoupling of oxidative phosphorylation in brown fat. Because adult humans have almost no brown fat, inhibition of this mechanism is thought to have little impact on the reduction of metabolic heat production. Likewise, although increased secretion of thyrotropin-releasing hormone by the hypothalamus is seen after prolonged cold exposure, inhibition of this response in hot environments does not play a significant role in the heat response.

Behavioral control of temperature regulation is important. As individuals begin to feel hot and uncomfortable when exposed to heat stress, they may take actions to find a cool environment. Public education regarding the heat-related illness should capitalize on this response mechanism.

Acclimatization

Acclimatization is the adaptation of the body's heat stress mechanisms to increase efficiency of heat loss in a hot climate. The process does not impart a full resistance to heat illness; it only provides a maximization of the native heat removal processes. The primary methods of acclimatization occur due to changes in the onset and volume of sweating, improvement in cutaneous vascular flow and overall cardiovascular function, and alterations of the thermoregulatory set point. In most individuals, acclimatization can be achieved over 7 to 10 days.[10,11] Moderate exercise in a hot, dry environment for 60 to 100 min each day is probably the optimal approach to achieve acclimatization. Simple exposure to a hot environment for 1 to 4 h a day also may result in acclimatization within 2 weeks. Acclimatization lowers the thermal "set point" in the hypothalamus, which triggers the onset of sweating at lower core temperatures in the acclimatized human. In addition, the maximal rate of sweat production is dramatically increased to 1.5 to 3 L/h and can be sustained for longer periods. Aldosterone secretion is boosted, and sodium conservation results due to more efficient reabsorption from the sweat. Plasma volume expands, heart rate decreases for any given heat load, and exercise tolerance improves. Dilation of cutaneous blood vessels occurs at a lower core temperature to promote earlier cooling. Once removed from the hot environment, the body will deacclimate to the original physiologic parameters within 1 to 2 weeks.[10] Acclimatization protocols to decrease the frequency of heat-related illness have been developed for personnel (military, laborers, and disaster relief workers) who are preparing to deploy to hot environments.

The Path to Heat Injury

The pathway to heat injury consists of a combination of three routes: increased heat production, increased external heat gain, and decreased heat loss. Distinctions made between nonexertional (classic) and exertional heat injuries denote only the primary method by which the hyperpyrexia is achieved. Although the population characteristics, risk factors, and physiologic parameters often differ between nonexertional and exertional heat injuries, the clinical effect on the patient is ultimately the same.

Obese people are at increased risk for exertional heat illness. Adipose tissue has decreased vascularity and inhibits heat dispersal by decreasing blood flow to the skin. Obesity makes less surface area available for heat exchange, and the lower water content of adipose tissue results in the conduction of heat energy that is one third as efficient as other body tissue.

Underlying skin conditions may contribute to decreased removal of heat. Scleroderma, cystic fibrosis, eczema, psoriasis, and burns decrease sweating ability. Congenital diseases, such as ectodermal dysplasia, involving the sweat glands increase risk of heat injury. Even the presence of heat rash has been shown to decrease sweating by obstruction of sweat gland ducts with keratin debris.

Febrile illnesses with readjustment of the thermal set point above normal may contribute to the risk of heat illness. The body will use heat-conserving mechanisms to maintain the core temperature at the higher set point. Proper treatment with antipyretics such as aspirin, acetaminophen, or ibuprofen in the setting of acute febrile illnesses may decrease the risk of heat injury in individuals exposed to heat stress. However, although systemic pyrogen release has been reported due to exercise and during heat stroke, the use of antipyretics in environmental heat illness has no scientific support. Metabolic disorders, such as hyperthyroidism and pheochromocytoma, also lead to increased endogenous heat production.

Medications often interfere with heat removal mechanisms. The most notable drugs are anticholinergic agents, diuretics, phenothiazine, β-blockers, calcium channel blockers, and sympathomimetic agents.[7] Anticholinergic agents impair sweating and impair the cardiovascular response to heat. Diuretics lead to volume depletion and decreased cardiac output. Phenothiazines have anticholinergic properties and deplete central stores of dopamine that interfere with the hypothalamus thermoregulatory center. Medications, such as β-blockers or calcium channel blockers, decrease the cardiovascular response to heat and reduce peripheral blood flow and the ability to sweat. Sympathomimetics cause cutaneous vasoconstriction and inhibit sweating. Alcohol inhibits antidiuretic hormone, leading to dehydration and blunting the psychological heat avoidance response. Heroin, cocaine, and amphetamines disrupt the function of endogenous endorphins and adrenocorticotrophic hormones that are involved in heat adaptation mechanisms. Amphetamines and cocaine increase muscle activity and lead to heat production. Lysergic acid diethylamide and phencyclidine act on the central nervous system (CNS) to induce a hypermetabolic state.[7,9,10]

Classic heat injury occurs during periods of high environmental heat stress.[12,13] Physical exertion is not required, because the heat gain occurs at environmental temperatures and humidity that overwhelm the native heat loss mechanisms. Patients suffering from this form of heat illness are unable to escape from the hot environment and cannot cope with the elevated heat burden. The increase in core temperature seen in this setting is often slow, occurring over a period of hours to days. Because of this slow rise in heat burden, volume and electrolyte abnormalities have time to develop and are common. High-risk populations include the elderly, the young, and those with psychological, physiologic, and pharmacologic impairments of heat loss mechanisms.

Confinement hyperpyrexia is a special category or subtype of nonexertional hyperpyrexia and can be found in three circumstances: children left inside cars, illegal immigrants abandoned inside closed vehicles or railroad cars, and occupational heat exposure inside enclosed spaces. Between July 2000 and June 2001 in the United States, 1960 nonfatal heat injuries and 78 fatalities were reported in children after being left intentionally in motor vehicles during hot days.[14] Nonventilated vehicle compartments in a hot environment may reach temperatures of 54°C to 60°C (129.2°F to 140°F) in less than 10 min.[14] Infants have less capability than adults to deal with heat stress and, if left in motor vehicles for only a matter of minutes, may obtain a critical heat burden. The second circumstance exists along the U.S. border with Mexico. During 2000, at least 418 illegal immigrants are known to have died attempting to cross the border through the desert, with more than 50 percent of these deaths due to heat stroke, and many of these individuals were locked in closed vehicle compartments by smugglers after failed attempts to enter the United States. A particularly dangerous region is through the Tucson Sector of the border, which accounts for 22 percent of all southwest border deaths of illegal immigrants. During 2000, the U.S. Border Patrol rescued more than 846 such immigrants after smugglers had abandoned them.[15] In the third circumstance, during 2000, 21 workers died and 2554 others experienced heat-related occupational injuries due to confinement in hot environments.

Exertional heat injury usually affects individuals who are physically fit and participating in athletic events or performing jobs under conditions of high heat stress, such as the military or fighting fires. In this setting, heat production and heat gain from the environment exceed the capacity of heat removal processes. Physical exercise is the most common single source of internal heat production. Basal metabolism in an average human creates heat at approximately 50 to 60 kcal/h per square meter, or about 100 kcal/h in a 70-kg man. Heat production rapidly increases during physical activity due to skeletal muscle contraction. Strenuous exertion can increase the basal heat production rate by a factor of 20 in a short period. During vigorous competitions, athletes may create heat loads in excess of 1033 kcal/h, leading to core temperature increases of 0.3°C/min (0.54°F/min).[10] Without an efficient cooling mechanism, progressive dehydration and hyperpyrexia continue to a level of cardiovascular and metabolic failure. Avoidance of strenuous exercise during periods of high environmental heat stress, as judged by the heat index chart, coupled with acclimatization, hydration, breaks from the heat, and education, will prevent this form of heat illness.

CLINICAL FEATURES

Heat-related illnesses are generally divided into two categories: minor syndromes (heat edema, prickly heat, heat syncope, heat cramps, and heat exhaustion) and major syndromes (e.g., heatstroke). Although heat-related illnesses are clearly related to the exposure of an elevated environmental temperature, the magnitude or intensity of this heat source is only relative when the patient is a young child or an elderly adult with comorbid diseases.

Heat Edema

Heat edema is a self-limited process manifested by the mild swelling of the feet, ankles, and hands that appears within the first few days of exposure to a hot environment. Heat edema is due to the cutaneous vasodilatation and orthostatic pooling of interstitial fluid in gravity-dependent extremities. Also, an increase in the secretion of aldosterone and antidiuretic hormone in response to the heat stress contributes to the mild edema. In general, heat edema is found in elderly nonacclimatized individuals who are physically active after a period of sitting while traveling in a vehicle or airplane. Occasionally, it will occur after prolonged standing. It is commonly seen in healthy travelers just arriving from a colder climate. The edema is mild and does not impair or interfere with normal activities. Very rarely, pitting edema of the ankles may develop, but heat edema does not progress to the pretibial region.

History and physical examination are usually sufficient to exclude systemic causes of edema. ED visits for this minor heat-related syndrome are usually by elderly patients with concerns focused on the early development of congestive heart failure or deep venous thrombosis. Heat edema usually resolves spontaneously in a few days but may take up to 6 weeks. No special treatment is necessary. If a patient is insistent on treatment, elevation of the legs and the use of support hose will facilitate the removal of the interstitial fluid. Diuretics are not effective and can predispose to volume depletion, electrolyte abnormalities, or a more serious heat illness.[10]

Prickly Heat

This is a pruritic, maculopapular, erythematous rash over clothed areas of the body. Also known as *lichen tropicus, miliaria rubra,* or *heat rash,* it is an acute inflammation of the sweat ducts caused by blockage of the sweat pores by macerated stratum corneum. The ducts become dilated under pressure and ultimately rupture, producing superficial vesicles in the malpighian layer of the skin on a red base. Itching is the predominant clinical feature during this phase and is treated successfully with antihistamines. Wearing clean, light, and loose-fitting clothing and avoiding sweat-generating situations can prevent prickly heat. The use of talc or baby powder is of no benefit. Chlorhexidine in a light cream or lotion is the treatment of choice in the acute phase.

With prolonged or repeated heat exposure, a keratin plug fills the sweat duct, causing obstruction in the stratum malpighian layer. When the duct ruptures a second time, the resultant vesicle will be driven deeper into the dermis. This vesicle simulates the white papules of piloerection and is not pruritic. This is known as the *profunda stage* of prickly heat (miliaria profunda) and can readily advance into a chronic dermatitis. Infection with *Staphylococcus aureus* is a common complication and requires the use of dicloxacillin or erythromycin. The skin can be desquamated by applying 1% salicylic acid to the affected area three times a day. Caution should be used to avoid salicylate toxicity.

Heat Cramps

Heat cramps are painful, involuntary, spasmodic contractions of skeletal muscles, usually those of the calves, although they may involve the thighs and shoulders. These cramps usually occur in individuals who are sweating profusely and replace fluid losses with water or other hypotonic solutions. Heat cramps may occasionally occur during exercise or, more commonly, during a rest period after several hours of vigorous physical activity. Nonacclimatized or unconditioned individuals who are just starting manual labor in a hot environment are at high risk for developing heat cramps. Although heat cramps are self-limited and do not cause significant morbidity, the pain associated with them can readily precipitate an ED visit. In fact, the pain associated with heat cramps usually does not respond to opiates alone. In general, heat cramps are short in duration, limited to a definitive group of muscles, and do not involve enough muscle mass to cause rhabdomyolysis.

The pathogenesis of heat cramps is attributed to a relative deficiency of sodium, potassium, and fluid at the cellular level of the muscle. The production of large amounts of sweat, which has high sodium content, coupled with inadequate sodium replacement result in cellular hyponatremia. This in turn produces muscle cramps with calcium-dependent muscle relaxation. Hypokalemia from hyperventilation and volume depletion may be contributing factors.

Treatment consists of fluid and salt replacement (PO or IV) and rest in a cool environment. **For mild cases, or if an overwhelming number of patients require treatment, a 0.1 to 0.2% saline solution can be given PO. Two 10-grain (650 mg) salt tablets dissolved in a quart of water provide a 0.1% saline solution.** Many such electrolyte solution drinks (sports drinks) are commercially available and are much more palatable than 0.1% saline solution. More severe cases of heat cramps will respond to intravenous rehydration with NS. Patients with severe heat cramps may actually have hyponatremia and hypochloremia. Rarely, rhabdomyolysis occurs secondary to diffuse and protracted muscle spasm.

Heat cramps can be prevented by maintaining adequate dietary salt intake or by drinking commercial electrolyte beverages. Salt tablets by themselves should not be used because the tablets are a gastric irritant and often result in nausea and vomiting, and alone, they do not replace volume.

Heat Tetany

Heat tetany is produced by hyperventilation associated with exposure to short periods of intense heat stress. This syndrome presents as typical hyperventilation resulting in respiratory alkalosis, paresthesia of the extremities, circumoral paresthesia, and carpopedal spasm. Heat tetany can be differentiated from heat cramps by the fact there is very little pain or cramps in the muscle compartments, and paresthesias of the extremities and perioral region are more prominent. In general, concomitant heat cramps are not present. Treatment consists of removal from the heat and decreasing the respiratory rate.

Heat Syncope

Heat syncope is a variant of postural hypotension resulting from the cumulative effect of relative volume depletion, peripheral vasodilatation, and decreased vasomotor tone. It occurs most commonly in nonacclimatized individuals during the early stages of heat exposure. Accordingly, geriatric patients tend to demonstrate the highest incidence of this "minor" heat illness. It does not necessarily represent a state of significant volume depletion.

Evaluation of patients with heat syncope requires exclusion of metabolic, cardiovascular, and neurologic disorders that may produce syncope. In geriatric patients, this will commonly require a significant evaluation. Treatment consists of removal from the heat source, oral or intravenous rehydration, and rest. Many patients with heat syncope recover promptly with fluids, and hospitalization usually is not necessary. Patient education about measures to diminish the effects of venous pooling when standing are very important to prevent future syncopal episodes or injury.

Heat Exhaustion

Heat exhaustion is an acute heat-related illness that reflects significant volume depletion and may or may not have an elevated temperature. This is a syndrome characterized by nonspecific symptoms, such as weakness, malaise, lightheadedness, fatigue, dizziness, nausea, vomiting, frontal headache, and myalgias. Clinical manifestations include orthostatic hypotension, sinus tachycardia, tachypnea, diaphoresis, and syncope. The core temperature is variable and can range from normal to 40°C (104°F). In heat exhaustion, the mental status remains normal. Because of the ill-defined and nonspecific symptoms, heat exhaustion is a diagnosis of exclusion. Heat cramps and/or rhabdomyolysis may also be present on rare occasions. Physiologically, heat exhaustion is characterized by a combination of salt depletion and water depletion.

Laboratory studies almost universally will demonstrate hemoconcentration, although specific electrolyte abnormalities depend on the ratio of fluid and electrolyte losses to intake. Patients who have no fluid intake of any kind usually will have hypernatremia, whereas those who partly rehydrate with salt-containing fluids may develop isotonic hypovolemia with normal sodium and chloride levels. Serum potassium and magnesium levels are variable.

Heat exhaustion is treated with volume and electrolyte replacement and rest. Mild cases may be treated with oral electrolyte solutions. Rapid infusion of moderate amounts of intravenous fluids (1 to 2 L of saline solution) may be necessary in some patients who demonstrate significant tissue hypoperfusion. Ideally, the choice of intravenous solutions should be guided by laboratory determinations, but isotonic salt solutions may be used until specific electrolyte abnormalities are identified. In general, these patients do not require hospitalization. Patients with congestive heart failure or severe electrolyte disturbances may require admission, because of the time element needed to correct their fluid and/or electrolyte deficits.

Heat exhaustion has the potential of progressing to heatstroke. Historically, the differentiation between heat exhaustion and heatstroke consisted of anhidrosis, CNS dysfunction, and a core temperature higher than 40°C.[13] However, this distinction is suspect for the following reasons. First, the definition of "CNS dysfunction" is not standardized. Is CNS dysfunction delineated by confusion or agitation? Or does it require more severe neurologic impairment, such as delirium, seizure, or coma? Second, the presence of anhidrosis is not always clinically apparent, and patients with exertional heatstroke may still be perspiring upon arrival to the ED. Third, there is no arbitrary core temperature threshold for heatstroke. Thus, the diagnosis of heatstroke is not standardized. However, elevated hepatic enzymes is one objective tool that is really helpful in differentiating between heat exhaustion and heatstroke, especially if the patient presents with "soft" signs of CNS dysfunction, such as confusion or agitation. The only drawback is that elevated hepatic enzymes are a delayed complication of heatstroke.

Heatstroke

The classic definition of heatstroke includes the presence of a core temperature higher than 40°C, CNS dysfunction, and anhidrosis.[11–13] However, anhidrosis, or a lack of sweating, may not be present for a variety of reasons and is not considered an absolute diagnostic criterion. Subsequently, anyone with hyperpyrexia and CNS dysfunction should be considered to have a heatstroke, which is a medical emergency with multiple organ system involvement and a high mortality rate and requires immediate intervention.[11–13]

The CNS is particularly vulnerable in heatstroke, with symptoms such as irritability, confusion, bizarre behavior, combativeness, hallucinations, seizures, or coma. The cerebellum is highly sensitive to heat, and ataxia can be an early neurologic finding. Virtually any neurologic abnormality may be present in heatstroke, including plantar responses, decorticate and decerebrate posturing, hemiplegia, status epilepticus, and coma. Seizures are quite common in heatstroke and may be a complication of its treatment when cold-water immersion is used. Cerebral edema is common. Central nervous system dysfunction is universal at core temperatures higher than 42°C (107.6°F), but there is no arbitrary core temperature threshold for neurologic dysfunction in heatstroke. Neurologic injury is a function of the maximum temperature reached and the duration of exposure.[12] Patients with lower temperatures for longer periods do worse than patients with higher temperatures for shorter periods. Further, prehospital treatment may result in the patient having a normal temperature or resolution of the CNS dysfunction when evaluated in the ED.

The presence or absence of sweating has traditionally been one of the important distinctions between true heatstroke and other heat emergencies. Patients with classic heatstroke typically demonstrate marked sweating early on but eventually develop anhidrosis by the time of medical evaluation due to profound volume depletion or sweat gland dysfunction. Conversely, sweating is observed in 50 percent of patients with exertional heatstroke on initial medical assessment. Heatstroke is a total breakdown of thermoregulation. The primary cause is increased endogenous heat production.

The distinction between exertional and nonexertional heatstrokes is not clinically important, because signs, symptoms, and management are the same. The primary factor that contributes to the morbidity and mortality of heat illness is the severity of underlying or comorbid disease(s) and not the absolute height of the core temperature.[10–13]

The definitive diagnosis of heatstroke is a diagnosis of exclusion (Table 193-1). Once heatstroke is suspected, efforts to lower the body temperature should be initiated immediately by whatever means available, whether in the prehospital or ED setting. A delay in cooling contributes to the mortality rate associated with heatstroke.

TREATMENT OF HEATSTROKE

Initial Resuscitation Standard initial resuscitative measures (adequacy of airway, breathing, and circulation; initiation of high-flow oxygen; use of continuous cardiac monitoring and pulse oximetry; and intravenous access) are appropriate. An initial infusion of NS or LR solution at a rate of 250 mL/h is recommended for most patients. Glucose level should be promptly assessed with a test strip due to the high incidence of hypoglycemia in exertional heatstroke. If a patient has cardiovascular disease or is elderly, it is wise to monitor cardiac filling pressures to guide fluid therapy. This may require a central venous pressure line or a pulmonary artery catheter. A urinary drainage catheter should be inserted. Serial monitoring of the patient's core temperature is best accomplished by inserting an electronic rectal thermistor probe or a temperature probe– equipped urinary drainage catheter. Another option, especially in intubated patients, is the use of an esophageal thermometer.

TABLE 193-1 Differential Diagnosis of Heatstroke

Drug toxicity: anticholinergic toxicity, stimulant toxicity (phencyclidine, cocaine, amphetamines, ephedrine), salicylate toxicity
Drug withdrawal syndrome: ethanol withdrawal
Serotonin syndrome
Neuroleptic malignant syndrome
Generalized infections: bacterial sepsis, malaria, typhoid fever, tetanus
Central nervous system infections: meningitis, encephalitis, brain abscess
Endocrine derangements: diabetic ketoacidosis, thyroid storm
Neurologic: status epilepticus, cerebral hemorrhage

Diagnostic studies necessary to detect the end-organ sequelae of heatstroke include a complete blood cell count, comprehensive metabolic panel, coagulation profile, creatine phosphokinase, myoglobin, urinalysis, toxicology screen, electrocardiogram, and chest radiograph. A lumbar puncture and computed tomography of the head may also be indicated as part of the evaluation of altered mental status.

Cooling Techniques   Rapid reduction of the core temperature to below 40°C (104°F) is the primary goal of treatment and is accomplished by physical cooling techniques.[13] At present, there are no pharmaceutical agents that facilitate or induce the cooling process in heat stroke. Antipyretics (aspirin and acetaminophen) are not effective in reducing the temperature and can be deleterious to the patient. In clinical practice, the primary physical cooling technique that should be used allows easy patient access, is readily available, is tolerated well by the patient, and is relatively effective (Table 193-2). The two primary methods for physical cooling in the clinical setting are evaporative cooling and cold-water immersion. We feel that the primary cooling modality that best meets these criteria is evaporative cooling. Further, evaporative cooling can be used in the prehospital setting and the ED.

Evaporative cooling is performed by positioning fan(s) close to the completely undressed patient and then spraying tepid water on the patient. Inexpensive plastic spray bottles work best. We avoid covering the patient with sheets and then wetting the sheets, because this impairs evaporation of heat from the skin. Also, one person is needed to monitor and continue cooling the patient. Another effective means of providing evaporative cooling is the Makkah body-cooling unit, which is used widely in the Middle East. It is a common method of treatment for pilgrims traveling to Mecca who succumb to heatstroke. Patients are placed undressed on a modified hammock or litter and sprayed with lukewarm water (15°C; 59°F), and warm air (45°C; 113°F) is blown over them with powerful fans. The unique feature of the Makkah body-cooling unit is that it works best in patients who are vasodilated and live in a dry environment. This modality of therapy would not be ideal for patients in shock or in a humid environment.[13] Evaporative cooling by means of alcohol sponge baths is not effective

and should not be used due to the possibility of isopropyl alcohol toxicity.

Two problems associated with complications of evaporative cooling are shivering and inability of the cardiac electrodes to adhere to the skin. Shivering is treated primarily with short-acting benzodiazepines and secondarily with phenothiazines. Phenothiazines should be used with caution, because they lower the seizure threshold, can cause hypotension, and their anticholinergic properties may impair sweating. Electrodes can be applied to a patient's back.

Immersion cooling is performed by placing an undressed patient into a tub of ice water deep enough to cover the trunk and extremities. The head must be kept out of the ice water. Cardiac monitoring electrodes and temperature probes must be secured to the patient. Problems associated with immersion cooling include shivering, displacement of monitoring leads, and inability to perform defibrillation or resuscitative procedures. Also, the tub or receptacle in which the patient is placed may not be readily available. The efficiency of immersion has been documented primarily in young, healthy patients without comorbid diseases. Observations suggest that the peripheral vasoconstriction induced by the ice-water immersion may be beneficial in some patients with peripheral vascular disease or hypotension. However, this observation should not be extrapolated to all such patients, and the low peripheral resistance seen in heatstroke cannot be explained by vasodilation alone, implying that a toxin or chemical may be released by the heat-damaged tissues. Needless to say, the efficacy and safety of immersion in classic heatstroke victims or patients with significant comorbid diseases (i.e., coronary artery disease) have not been established, and there have been no controlled studies comparing the effects of these various cooling techniques on cooling times and outcome in patients with heatstroke.

Other adjuncts to evaporative cooling include ice packs to the neck, axillae, and groin. The ice packs are positioned in areas of the body where large blood vessels are relatively superficial and can facilitate the cooling process. Further, ice packs are readily available and noninvasive. Cooling blankets preclude the use of evaporative cooling and work too slowly to be considered an effective primary means of physical cooling.

Special consideration should be given for invasive cooling techniques to be used as adjuncts when the two primary means of physical cooling are not sufficient. The most rapid method of cooling a heatstroke victim is cardiopulmonary bypass. In addition, cardiopulmonary bypass has been established as an effective tool in the treatment of malignant hyperthermia. Although the availability and logistics are major drawbacks, it may be required if a patient is recalcitrant to all other measures. Cold-water gastric lavage, cold-water urinary bladder lavage, and cold-water rectal lavage are other adjunctive measures that can be performed in the ED but require some element of patient cooperation, are labor intensive, have the potential for inducing water intoxication, and are not that effective. Cold-water peritoneal lavage is yet another option but has not been validated in humans. Intravenous infusion of cold intravenous fluids should not be performed due to many complications.

Regardless of the cooling technique chosen, cooling efforts should be discontinued when the rectal temperature reaches 40°C (104°F); continued cooling below this temperature will lead to *overshoot hypothermia*.

TREATMENT OF COMPLICATIONS   Complications associated with heatstroke characteristically occur early or late (Table 193-3). In patients with a relatively intact cardiovascular system, heat stress causes a marked increase in heart rate and cardiac contractility; most patients have a high cardiac index, elevated central venous pressure, and low peripheral resistance. The low peripheral resistance is due to the vasodilatation of the vasculature in the skin. Accordingly, hypotension is a common initial finding. The tendency is to treat the hypotension with an aggressive fluid challenge ("fluids wide open");

TABLE 193-2   Comparison of Cooling Techniques

Technique	Advantages	Disadvantages
Evaporative	Simple Readily available Noninvasive Easy patient access Relatively effective	Shivering Difficult to maintain monitoring electrodes in position
Immersion	Noninvasive Relatively effective	Shivering Cumbersome Poorly tolerated Logistically difficult to access Difficult to maintain monitoring electrode and temperature probes
Ice packing	Noninvasive Readily available	Shivering Poorly tolerated
Strategic ice packs	Noninvasive Readily available Can be combined with other techniques	Shivering Poorly tolerated Medium efficiency
Cold gastric lavage	Generally available	Invasive Labor intensive Potential for water intoxication May require airway protection Limited human experience
Cold peritoneal lavage	Theoretically beneficial	Invasive Limited human experience

TABLE 193-3 Complications of Heatstroke

	Initial	Delayed
Vital signs	Hypotension Hypothermia overshoot Hyperthermic rebound	
Muscular	Shivering Rhabdomyolysis	
Neurologic	Delirium Seizures Coma	Cerebral edema
Cardiac	Heart failure	
Pulmonary	Pulmonary edema	Acute respiratory distress syndrome
Renal	Oliguria	Renal failure
Gastrointestinal	Diarrhea	Hepatic necrosis Mucosal gastrointestinal hemorrhage
Metabolic	Hypokalemia Hypernatremia	Hyperkalemia Hypocalcemia Hyperuricemia
Hematologic		Thrombocytopenia Disseminated intravascular coagulation

Source: Tek D, Olshaker JS: Heat illness. *Emerg Med Clin North Am* 10:299, 1992.

however, pulmonary edema can occur from excessive fluid administration even in young healthy individuals. A pulmonary artery catheter may be necessary in the assessment of appropriate volume replacement. Usually the blood pressure will rise in response to a cautious fluid challenge (250 mL/h), in addition to body cooling. In any age group, the presence of hypotension, decreased cardiac output, and a falling cardiac index indicates a particularly poor prognosis; the combination of a low cardiac output and an elevated central venous pressure or pulmonary artery occlusion pressure warrants the use of vasoactive catecholamines such as dopamine or dobutamine.

The fluid and electrolyte abnormalities vary with the onset and duration of the disorder, underlying disease (especially cardiovascular disease), and prior use of medications, such as diuretics.[7,10] The most important consideration with respect to fluid and electrolyte abnormalities in heatstroke is that dehydration and volume depletion may not occur in classic heatstroke but are common findings in heat exhaustion. Patients with classic heatstroke usually have a respiratory alkalosis, and those with exertional heatstroke also have a metabolic (lactic) acidosis. Accordingly, if a patient with classic heatstroke has lactic acidosis, the condition is associated with high morbidity and mortality.

Hematologic disorders may be apparent clinically and on laboratory evaluation. Findings of abnormal hemostasis include purpura, petechiae, and conjunctival, gastrointestinal, renal, or pulmonary hemorrhage. Coagulation studies may show thrombocytopenia, hypoprothrombinemia, and hypofibrinogenemia. Thermal injury to the vascular endothelium causes increased platelet aggregation, changes in capillary permeability, thermal deactivation of plasma proteins resulting in a decreased level of clotting factors, and, rarely, disseminated intravascular coagulation or fibrinolysis. All these coagulopathies tend to be a delayed complication of heatstroke, taking several days to develop.

Thermal injury to the liver is such a common finding in heatstroke that it can be used as a marker to help establish the diagnosis of heatstroke as opposed to heat exhaustion, especially if there are "soft" signs of CNS dysfunction, such as confusion or agitation. Although jaundice does not always develop, hepatic enzymes will become sig-

nificantly elevated in a delayed fashion with heatstroke. Enzyme values usually peak 24 to 72 h after the thermal insult and can be attributed to centrilobular necrosis. This in turn can have an impact on the regulation of glucose and clotting factors.[10] The liver damage is almost always reversible, with a full recovery.

Renal damage is also common in heatstroke and can be the result of direct thermal injury to the kidney, rhabdomyolysis, or volume depletion. Clinically, this will be manifested by oliguria, microscopic hematuria, proteinuria, myoglobinuria, and many granular or red cell casts.

DISPOSITION

All the minor heat illnesses except heat exhaustion can be managed totally in the ED, and then patients can be safely discharged to home care and for outpatient follow-up. Patients with heat exhaustion who are at the extremes of age and have substantial volume depletion, significant electrolyte disturbances, comorbid diseases, or heat-induced end-organ damage should be admitted to the hospital.

Heatstroke is a true medical emergency, and all patients with this diagnosis should be admitted to an area appropriate for the level of care required. Patients who are intubated, hemodynamically labile, require invasive hemodynamic monitoring, or who need continued cooling should be admitted to the intensive care unit. If the original health care facility is unable to provide the services needed for quality care, then the patient should be referred to a higher-level facility.

PREVENTION

Serious heat-related illnesses are preventable. General recommendations directed at the individual include (1) decreasing or rescheduling strenuous activity for cooler parts of the day, (2) wearing clothing that is light colored and loose fitting, (3) increasing carbohydrate intake and decreasing protein intake to decrease endogenous heat production, (4) drinking plenty of fluids even when not thirsty, (5) avoiding alcoholic beverages because they promote dehydration, (6) not using salt tablets, (7) avoiding direct exposure to the sun, and (8) taking advantage of the shade.[10,13]

The incidence of heat-related illnesses also can be significantly reduced by the institution of several public health or public education measures that (1) pay attention to environmental conditions, especially the heat index; (2) provide access to air conditioning for individuals at risk, i.e., promoting visits to malls, distributing air conditioners; (3) emphasize adequate hydration; (4) extend social service care for the chronically ill and the elderly; (5) allow for acclimatization for workers, athletes, and the military; (6) implement paced work schedules for those who need to work under adverse conditions; (7) train coaches, teachers, and youth group leaders about heat-related illnesses; (8) educate the elderly at senior citizen centers; and (9) remind parents that they should never leave their children unattended in an automobile during hot weather.[13,16] Community heath officials and governmental leaders should recognize the need to coordinate and plan the implementation of these measures in advance and not resort to crisis management.

REFERENCES

1. National Weather Service: Available at: http://www.nws.noaa.gov/om/severe_weather/heat00.pdf. Accessed September 1, 2002.
2. Centers for Disease Control and Prevention: Heat-related deaths—Four states, July–August 2001, and United States, 1979–1999. *MMWR* 51:567, 2002.
3. Centers for Disease Control and Prevention: Heat-related mortality—Chicago, July 1995. *MMWR* 44:577, 1995.
4. Centers for Disease Control and Prevention: Heat-related deaths—Los Angeles County, California, 1999–2000, and United States, 1979–1998. *MMWR* 50:623, 2001.

5. Centers for Disease Control and Prevention: Heat-related illness and deaths—United States, 1994–1995. *MMWR* 44:465, 1995.

6. Khogali M: Heat-related illnesses. *Middle East J Anesthesiol* 12:531, 1994.

7. Martinez M, Devenport L, Saussy J, Martinez J: Drug-associated heat stroke. *South Med J* 95:799, 2002.

8. Pascoe DD, Bellingar TA, McCluskey BS: Clothing and exercise: II. Influence of clothing during exercise/work in environmental extremes. *Sports Med* 18:94, 1994.

9. Aiyer M, Crnkovich DJ, Carlson RW: Recognizing hyperthermia syndromes in critically ill patients. *J Crit Illness* 9:143, 1995.

10. Tek D, Olshaker JS: Heat illness. *Emerg Med Clin North Am* 10:299, 1992.

11. Knochel JP: Heat stroke and heat stress disorders. *Dis Mon* 35:301, 1989.

12. Yaqub BA, Al-Deeb S: Heat strokes: Etiopathogenesis, neurological characteristics, treatment, and outcome. *J Neurol Sci* 156:144, 1998.

13. Bouchama A, Knochel JP: Heat stroke. *New Engl J Med* 345:1978, 2002.

14. Centers for Disease Control and Prevention: Injuries and deaths among children left unattended in or around motor vehicles—United States, July 2000–June 2001. *MMWR* 51:570, 2002.

15. US Department of Justice, Immigration and Naturalization Service: *Border Patrol Enhancing Border Safety in Tucson.* News release, July 7, 2001. Washington, DC, Office of Public Affairs, Media Services.

16. US Department of Labor: *Precautions and Quick Action Could Save Lives in Hot Summer Weather.* Trade News Release, May 28, 2002. Washington, DC, Office of Public Affairs, Department of Labor/OSHA.

194 ARTHROPOD BITES AND STINGS
Richard F. Clark
Aaron B. Schneir

The phylum Arthropoda is the largest division of the animal kingdom. Venomous bites and stings are a significant worldwide problem.[1] In the United States, the American Association of Poison Control Centers reported 85,713 cases of exposures to arthropods in 2000.[2] Just over 100 of these were listed as resulting in major or severe reactions, including severe pain, neurotoxicity, or other signs and symptoms. Fatalities among these exposures are rarely reported to poison centers, and usually result from allergic reactions to Hymenoptera stings. Clearly, these numbers are the tip of the iceberg. Toxic reactions to multiple stings by members of the order of Hymenoptera and severe systemic allergic reactions to one or more stings or bites of other insects such as deerflies, blackflies, horseflies, and kissing bugs can all present as emergency, life-threatening situations (Table 194-1).[3] Other arthropod envenomations merit review either for causing specific organ system toxicity or as infectious disease vectors. This chapter discusses the more common and serious arthropod envenomations encountered by emergency physicians.

HYMENOPTERA (WASPS, BEES, AND ANTS)

The Hymenoptera are the most important venomous insects known to humans, and more fatalities result from stings by these insects than by stings or bites from any other arthropod. There are three major subgroups or superfamilies of medical importance: (1) *Apidae,* which includes the honeybee and bumblebee; (2) *Vespidae,* which includes yellow jackets, hornets, and wasps; and (3) *Formicidae,* or ants (Figure 194-1).

Bees and Wasps (*Apidae* and *Vespidae*)

Apids, such as honeybees and bumblebees, are usually docile, stinging only when provoked. A female bee is capable of stinging only once (male bees have no stinger) because its stinger has multiple barbs that cause the sting apparatus to detach from its body, leading to evisceration and eventual death.

Africanized honeybees, or so-called killer bees, are now found in Texas, Arizona, California, and most of the temperate southeastern

TABLE 194-1 Harmful Arthropods of the United States

Class and Order	Common Name	Bite	Sting
Hexapoda (Insecta)			
Hymenoptera	Bumblebees		×
	Sweat bees		×
	Honey bees		×
	Wasps		×
	Hornets		×
	Yellow jackets		×
	Fire ants		×
	Harvester ants		×
Diptera	Mosquitoes	×	
	Deerflies	×	
	Horseflies	×	
	Stable flies	×	
	Blackflies	×	
	Biting midges	×	
Hemiptera	Bedbugs	×	
	Kissing bugs	×	
Lepidoptera	Puss caterpillars		×
	Browntail caterpillars		×
	Buck mouth caterpillars		×
Siphonaptera	Fleas	×	
Anoplura	Lice	×	
Arachnida			
Araneida	Black widow	×	
	Brown recluse	×	
	Hobo spider	×	
	Tarantula	×	
Acarina	Chiggers (mite larvae)	×	
	Ticks	×	
Scorpionida	Scorpions		×

Source: Reproduced with permission from Frazier CA: *Insect Allergy.* St. Louis, WH Green, 1987, p. 421.

and southwestern states. These bees are hybrids of African bees that escaped from laboratories in Brazil during the 1950s, which have successfully spread northward along the coasts and temperate regions of the continent. Their venom is no more toxic than that of the American counterpart, but African honeybees are very aggressive and a hive can respond to a perceived threat with more than 10 times the number of bees as a typical North American bee response. An attack from Africanized bees can lead to massive stinging resulting in multisystem damage and death from severe venom toxicity.[4] With no natural predators, it is predicted that hybrids of Africanized bees eventually will inhabit much of the southern United States.

Most of the allergic reactions reported each year from Hymenoptera occur from vespid (wasp, hornet, and yellow jacket) stings. These arthropods nest in the ground or in walls, have volatile tempers, and may be disturbed by work taking place around the nest. As with bees, only the females have adapted a stinger from the ovipositor on the posterior aspect of the abdomen. Although vespids also possess barbed stingers, they have the ability to withdraw their stingers from the victim, enabling multiple stings.

VENOM Hymenoptera venom contains several components.[5] Although histamine is one of those components and was once thought to be responsible for most of the reactions observed following envenomation, other substances have now been recognized as more important. Melittin, a known membrane-active polypeptide that can cause degranulation of basophils and mast cells, constitutes more than 50 percent of the dry weight of bee venom. Because all Hymenoptera share many of these components, cross-sensitization may occur in individuals allergic to one species. Yellow jacket venom is perhaps the most potent sensitizer.

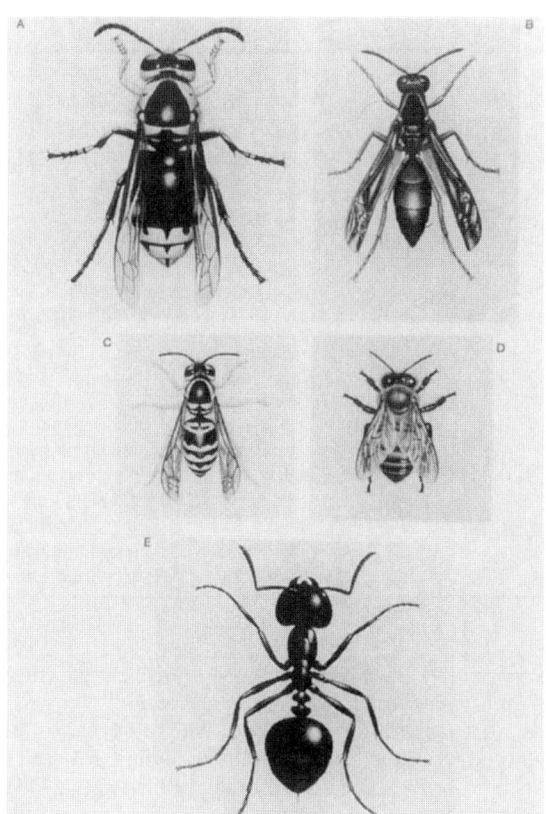

FIG. 194-1. Representative venomous Hymenoptera. **A.** Hornet *(Vespula maculata).* **B.** Wasp *(Chlorion ichneumerea).* **C.** Yellow jacket *(Vespula maculiforma).* **D.** Honeybee *(Apis mellifera).* **E.** Fire ant *(Solenopsis invicta).* (Reproduced with permission from Merck, Sharp & Dohme, Division of Merck & Co., Inc.)

CLINICAL FEATURES   The most common response to Hymenoptera venom consists of pain, slight erythema, edema, and pruritus at the sting site. In addition to this response, more significant reactions may occur.[6]

Local Reaction   A local reaction consists of an urticarial lesion contiguous with the sting site. Although there are no systemic signs or symptoms, a severe local reaction may involve one or more neighboring joints. A local reaction occurring in the mouth or throat can produce airway obstruction. Stings around the eye or on the lid may result in the development of an anterior capsule cataract, atrophy of the iris, lens abscess, perforation of the globe, glaucoma, or refractive changes. When local reactions become increasingly severe, the likelihood of future systemic reactions appears to increase and, if skin tests are positive, may warrant immunotherapy.

Toxic Reaction   When there is a history of multiple stings, such as in an Africanized bee attack, a systemic toxic reaction from venom may occur. Symptoms of a toxic reaction may resemble anaphylaxis, but there is generally a greater frequency of nausea, vomiting, and diarrhea. Light-headedness and syncope are common. There also may be headache, fever, drowsiness, involuntary muscle spasms, edema without urticaria, and occasionally convulsions. Urticaria and bronchospasm do not need to be present, although respiratory insufficiency and arrest may occur. Renal and hepatic failure also has been reported, as well as disseminated intravascular coagulation (DIC). Symptoms usually subside within 48 h, but may last for several days in severe cases. Toxic reactions are believed to occur from a direct multisystem effect of the venom.

Anaphylactic Reaction   A generalized systemic allergic or anaphylactic reaction, whether in response to a single sting or multiple stings, may range from mild to fatal, and death can occur within minutes. The majority of such reactions occur within the first 15 min, and nearly all occur within 6 h. There is no correlation between systemic reactions and the number of stings. In general, the shorter the interval between the sting and the onset of symptoms, the more severe is the reaction. Fatalities that occur within the first hour of the sting usually result from airway obstruction or hypotension. Initial symptoms usually consist of itching eyes, facial flushing, generalized urticaria, and dry cough. Symptoms may intensify rapidly with chest or throat constriction; wheezing; dyspnea; cyanosis; abdominal cramps; diarrhea; nausea; vomiting; vertigo; chills and fever; laryngeal stridor; shock; syncope; involuntary bowel or bladder action; and bloody, frothy sputum. Initial mild symptoms may progress swiftly to shock.

Generalized systemic allergic reactions to Hymenoptera venom are thought to be IgE-mediated. When an individual predisposed to allergy to bees is stung, there is usually an increase in the production of IgE antibodies, which become attached to the mast cells and basophils. This sensitizes the individual so that a subsequent sting may result in an antigen–antibody interaction releasing pharmacologically active mediators such as histamine, the slow-reacting substance of anaphylaxis (SRS-A) and eosinophil chemotactic factors of anaphylaxis (ECF-A). It is these mediators that actually cause tissue damage and systemic symptoms.

Delayed Reaction   A delayed reaction, appearing 5 to 14 days after a sting, consists of serum sickness-like signs and symptoms of fever, malaise, headache, urticaria, lymphadenopathy, and polyarthritis.[7] Frequently, the patient has forgotten about the encounter and is puzzled by the sudden appearance of symptoms. This reaction is believed to be immune complex-mediated.

Unusual Reactions   Infrequently, a reaction to Hymenoptera venom produces neurologic, cardiovascular, and urologic symptoms, with signs of encephalopathy, neuritis, vasculitis, and nephrosis. A case of Guillain-Barré syndrome has been reported as a possible consequence of a Hymenoptera sting.

Identification of the offending insect can be difficult, except for the honeybee, which predictably leaves its stinger with venom sac attached in the lesion. In general, definitive identification is unnecessary because signs and symptoms of envenomation are similar among all species of Hymenoptera. If edema persists at the sting site, secondary infection, such as cellulitis, should be considered. Severe local reactions on the foot or ankle can be misdiagnosed as gout if the insect sting is not visible.

TREATMENT   If the bee stinger is present in the wound, it should be removed. Although conventional teaching suggested scraping the stinger out to avoid squeezing remaining venom from the retained venom gland into the victim, involuntary muscle contraction of the gland continues after evisceration and the venom contents are quickly exhausted. Immediate removal is the important principle and the method of removal is irrelevant. The sting site should be washed thoroughly with soap and water to minimize the possibility of infection. For local reactions, intermittently applied ice packs at the site will diminish swelling and delay the absorption of venom while limiting edema. Oral antihistamines and analgesics may limit discomfort and pruritus. Nonsteroidal anti-inflammatory drugs (NSAIDs) can be effective in relieving pain. Standard doses of opioid analgesics also can be administered. If edema is significant, elevation and rest of the affected limb should limit swelling unless secondary infection develops, in which case antibiotics will be necessary. In local tissue reactions, there is often significant inflammatory erythema and swelling, making it difficult to distinguish from infection; as a general rule, infection is only present in a minority of cases.

TABLE 194-2   Long-Term Management for Patients with Reactions to Hymenoptera Stings

Type of Reaction	Risk of Systemic Reaction on Subsequent Stings	Should Skin Testing Be Performed	Results of Skin Testing	Recommended Treatment
Never stung	Minimal	No		None
Local reaction				
Minor local reaction: immediate pain, swelling and itching at sting site, resolves in 1 day	Minimal	No		None
Extensive local reaction: swelling develops 24–48 h after sting and resolves in 3–7 d	Less than 10 percent	No		Epinephrine syringe
Systemic reaction				
Adult (urticaria, angioedema, anaphylaxis)	High	Yes	+	Venom immunotherapy
			−	Epinephrine syringe
Child (urticaria and mild angioedema)	Low	Yes	+	Venom immunotherapy or epinephrine syringe
			−	Epinephrine syringe
Child (anaphylaxis)	Moderate	Yes	+	Venom immunotherapy
			−	Epinephrine syringe

While the initial signs and symptoms of a systemic reaction may be mild, victims can deteriorate rapidly in a matter of minutes. Treatment begins similar to that for anaphylaxis (see Chap. 34), and the most important agent to administer is epinephrine 0.3 to 0.5 mg (0.3 to 0.5 mL of 1:1000 concentration) in adults and 0.01 mg/kg in children (never more than 0.3 mg). It should be injected IM and the injection site massaged to hasten absorption. The patient should then be observed for several hours to ensure that symptoms do not intensify or relapse. Parenteral administration of standard antihistamines (diphenhydramine 25 to 50 mg IV, IM, or PO) and H_2-receptor antagonists (ranitidine 50 mg IV) is recommended. While steroids (methylprednisolone 125 mg) are of little help in combating the immediate effects, their administration tends to limit ongoing urticaria and edema and may potentiate the effects of other measures. Bronchospasm is treated with β-agonist nebulization. Hypotension may require massive crystalloid infusion, and central venous pressure monitoring may be helpful in these patients. Persistent hypotension after massive volume replacement may require dopamine. If dopamine is ineffective, an intravenous infusion of epinephrine can be used. The patient who suffers a severe systemic reaction should be admitted and monitored for potential cardiac, bleeding, renal, or neurologic complications. Antivenoms have been studied for the treatment of mass bee attacks, but are not yet commercially available.[8]

LONG-TERM MANAGEMENT AND PREVENTIVE CARE   Skin tests and radioallergosorbent tests (RASTs) are not fully reliable for determining which patients are at risk for systemic reaction during future encounters with Hymenoptera (Table 194-2).[9] Patients with negative results may have been sensitized by the skin tests themselves. **Every patient who has had a systemic reaction should be provided with an insect sting kit containing premeasured epinephrine and be carefully instructed in its use. The physician should stress that the patient must inject the epinephrine at the first sign of a systemic reaction.** Physicians should also advise their patients who are allergic to insects to wear identification (e.g., Medic Alert tags) concerning their severe allergy.

Ants *(Formicidae)*

There are five known species of fire ants *(Solenopsis)* in the United States: the native species *S. aurea, S. geminata, S. xyloni,* and at least two imported species, *S. invicta* and *S. richteri.* These two imported species entered the United States through Mobile, Alabama, in the 1930s, have now become well established throughout the Gulf Coast states, and are spreading throughout the southwest.[10] The fire ant inhabits a loose amount of dirt and breeds 9 to 10 months of the year. One mature nest can produce 200,000 ants during a 3-year period, which accounts for the rapid spread of this arthropod. The venom of the fire ant is almost entirely an insoluble alkaloid. There is potential cross-reactivity between the venoms of fire ants and other Hymenoptera, and individual stings may produce systemic toxicity in sensitized individuals.

Fire ants are characterized by their tendency to swarm when provoked and they may attack in great numbers. Most often fire ants in a swarm position themselves on their victim and sting simultaneously in response to an alarm pheromone released by one or several individuals. Immobilized or elderly patients can become rapidly covered by swarms of these ants, resulting in severe stings or death.[11] Each sting usually results in a papule that becomes a sterile pustule in 6 to 24 h (Figure 194-2). Localized necrosis, scarring, and secondary infection can result. Rarely, a systemic reaction manifested by urticaria and angioedema can occur. Fatalities within 20 min have been reported in Australia following a single sting from the jumper or red bull ant (*Myrmecia* spp.), but most fatalities had a history of prior venom al-

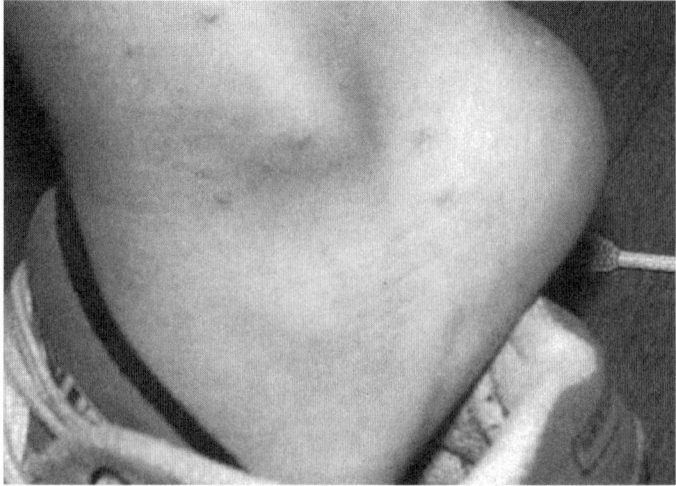

FIG. 194-2. Multiple stings from fire ants on ankle of child. Lesions are 2 days old.

lergy, all had prior cardiopulmonary disease, and none carried injectable epinephrine.[12]

Studies estimate a hypersensitivity rate to the fire ant of 16 percent in the general population, with significant crossover in those sensitized to other Hymenoptera. Treatment of fire ant stings consists of local wound care.[11] If there is evidence of systemic reaction, the usual treatment for anaphylaxis is indicated. Desensitization may be necessary in victims exhibiting potentially life-threatening reactions to these arthropods.

SPIDERS (ARANEAE)

There are more than 34,000 species of spiders worldwide, of which only a few dozen produce medically significant envenomations in humans (Tables 194-3 and 194-4). All spiders are carnivores, using venom to paralyze their prey prior to ingestion.[13] The vast majority of spiders pose little harm to humans because either their venom injecting fangs are too small to penetrate human skin, the amount of venom injected is too little to produce toxicity, or the toxins in the venom do not affect mammalian cells. Even if a reaction is elicited, it is often local and systemic toxicity is confined to a few specific species.

Necrotic Arachnidism (*Loxosceles*)

Loxosceles spiders have a worldwide distribution; their bite has the ability to produce local necrotic skin lesions and systemic toxicity.[14] Three species, *L. reclusa* (true brown recluse), *L. laeta* (corner spider), and *L. arizonica* (Arizona brown spider) produce the majority of *Loxosceles* bites in the United States. The brown recluse spider is one of the most common species found in the United States, with an endemic range in the south-central United States, from Texas to Georgia and Iowa to Louisiana. The spider has an approximately 1-cm body, a tan to brown coloration, and a violin-shaped mark on its dorsal cephalothorax. *L. reclusa* prefers warm, dry areas such as abandoned buildings, woodpiles, and cellars (Figure 194-3). The venom of the brown recluse has multiple enzymes including hyaluronidase, alkaline phosphatase, 5'-ribonucleotide phosphohydrolase and the major one responsible for necrosis, sphingomyelinase D.[13] Significant necrotic wounds are possible through neutrophil activation, platelet aggregation, and intravascular thrombosis.

TABLE 194-3   Medically Important Spiders by Geographic Location

Genus	Species	Common Name	Distribution
Loxosceles			North America, South America, Africa, Mediterranean countries
	L. reclusa	True brown recluse spider	North America (central and southeast U.S.)
	L. arizonica	Arizona brown spider	North America (southwest)
	L. rufescens		Worldwide
	L. laeta	Corner spider	South America, North America
	L. spinulosa		South Africa
	L. intermedia		Brazil
	L. gaucho		Brazil
	L. parrami	Violin spider	South Africa
Tegenaria			Europe, North America
	T. agrestis	Hobo or Northwestern brown spider	Europe, Asia (west central): native
			North America (Pacific Northwest): introduced
Latrodectus			Worldwide
	L. mactans	Black widow spider	North America
	L. bishopi	Red-legged spider	North America
	L. variolus		North America
	L. hasselti	Red-backed spider	Australia, New Zealand, Asia (southern)
	L. katipo	Katipo spider	New Zealand
	L. hesperus	Western black widow spider	North America
	L. tredecimguttatus		Mediterranean countries
	L. pallidus		Mediterranean countries, Middle East, Russia (south)
	L. indistinctus	Black button spider	Africa
	L. geometricus	Brown button spider	Worldwide
	L. rhodesiensis	Brown button spider	South Africa
Phoneutria			South America
	P. nigriventer	Brazilian armed spider	Brazil, Paraguay, Argentina, Uruguay
Atrax/Hadronyche			Australia
	A. robustus	Sydney funnel-web spider	Australia (east)
	H. formidabilis	Northern funnel-web spider	Australia (east)
	H. versutus	Australian Blue Mountains funnel-web spider	Australia (east)
	H. infensus		Australia (east)
	H. cereberus		Australia (southeast)
Cheiracanthium			Worldwide
	C. inclusum		North America
	C. mildei		Europe, eastern and central U.S.
	C. diversum		Australia, Pacific Islands, Hawaii
	C. punctorium		Europe
	C. longimanus		Australia
	C. mordax		Australia
	C. japonicum		Japan, China
	C. lawrencei (furculatum)	Sac spider	Africa

TABLE 194-4 Medically Important Spider Bites by Local Reaction and Systemic Signs

Genus	Local Reaction	Systemic Signs
Loxosceles	Initially painless Most common manifestation a mild firm erythematous lesion heals with little or no scar over several days to weeks Occasionally mild to severe pain several hours after the bite followed by erythema and blister formation within 24 h Necrotic lesion develops over the next 3 to 4 days, with eschar formation by the end of the first week	Systemic effects are rare, appear more often in children, and typically occur 24 to 72 h after the bite Nausea, vomiting, fever, chills, arthralgias, hemolysis, thrombocytopenia, hemoglobinuria, and renal failure Disseminated intravascular coagulation and death are rare
Tegenaria	Initial bite is often painless Induration may initially occur with surrounding erythema Followed by blistering, rupture, and necrosis Healing may take as long as 45 days and permanent scarring may result	Headache is the most common systemic symptom Nausea, vomiting, and fatigue can also occurr Aplastic anemia and death are rare complications
Latrodectus	Local pinprick almost always felt Immediate mild to moderate pain Pain may spread quickly to include the entire extremity Erythema appears approximately 20 to 60 min after the bite. Erythema evolves into a target lesion 1 to 2 cm in diameter	Muscle cramp-like spasms in large muscle groups Physical examination of the "cramping" extremity rarely exhibits rigidity Pain increases and becomes generalized, involving the trunk, back, and abdomen Pain lasts for 24 h or more than can be intermittent Severe hypertension may occur
Phoneutria	Severe local pain	Sympathetic stimulation: tachycardia, hypertension Parasympathetic hyperactivity: nausea, vomiting, diaphoresis, salivation Spinal cord impairment: priapism Central nervous effects: vertigo, visual changes Death from respiratory failure can be seen in 2 to 6 h
Atrax/Hadronyche	Local pain Wheal with surrounding erythema Localized sweating and piloerection	Perioral paresthesias Parasympathetic hyperactivity: nausea, vomiting, diaphoresis, salivation, lacrimation, bronchorrhea Neuromuscular stimulation: muscle fasciculation, tremors, spasms, weakness Central nervous system toxicity: altered level of consciousness Death as a result of cardiac arrest, hypotension, or pulmonary failure

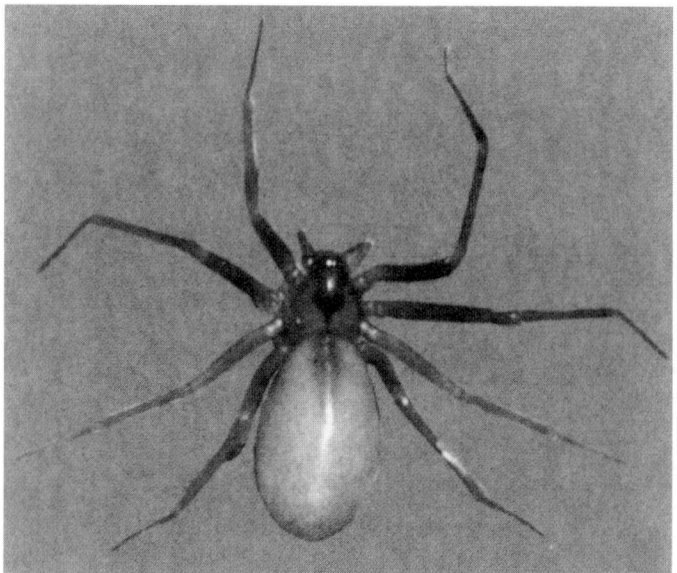

FIG. 194-3. Mature *Loxosceles reclusa*. Notice the violin or fiddle-shaped marking on the cephalothorax. [Reproduced with permission from Elston DM: What's eating you? *Loxosceles reclusa* (brown recluse spider). *Cutis* 69:94, 2002.]

CLINICAL FEATURES Bites by *Loxosceles* spiders are initially painless, often prohibiting definitive identification of the spider. The most common manifestation of a *Loxosceles* bite consists of a mild erythematous lesion that may become firm and heal with little or no scar over several days to weeks.[14] However, occasionally a more severe local reaction occurs, beginning with mild to severe pain several hours after the bite, followed by erythema and blister formation, and a bluish discoloration within the first 24 h (Figure 194-4). This lesion may become necrotic over the next 3 to 4 days, with eschar formation by the end of the first week. The necrotic, slowly healing ulcers may not reach maximum size for many weeks after envenomation, and can result in a significant cosmetic defect.

Systemic effects are rare, appear more often in children, and typically occur 24 to 72 h after the bite. Effects include nausea, vomiting, fever, chills, arthralgias, hemolysis, thrombocytopenia, hemoglobinuria, and renal failure. Disseminated intravascular coagulation and death are extraordinarily rare. Definitively diagnosing a brown recluse envenomation is difficult. The presence of a consistent clinical presentation combined with the actual spider (unusual because the bite is typically painless) or residence in an endemic area can be helpful. However, a wide variety of unrelated arthropod species and medical causes can appear similar to a *Loxosceles* envenomation. It is likely that a large number of wounds are incorrectly attributed to the bite of the brown recluse.

In patients suspected of having a bite from the brown recluse and exhibiting signs and symptoms of envenomation, a complete blood

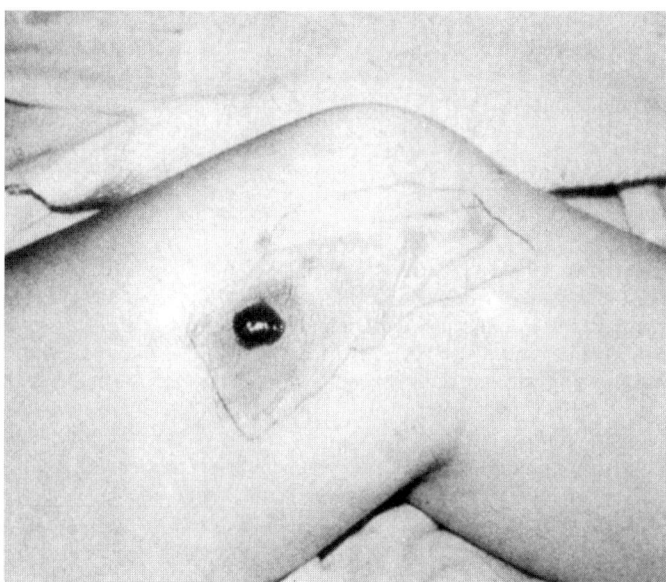

FIG. 194-4. Brown recluse spider bite approximately 12 h old.

count (CBC), basic chemistry tests, blood urea nitrogen (BUN), creatinine, and coagulation profile should be performed. Research is being done on an assay to confirm envenomation.[15] Currently, a commercial test does not exist and it remains unclear if one would be beneficial.

TREATMENT   Treatment of any possible necrotic spider bite should include the usual supportive measures. Antibiotics should be given if signs of infection are present. Analgesia may be required in some cases. Close follow-up for the patient should be arranged so that serial evaluations of the wound are performed. If ulceration does develop, surgical debridement should be delayed until clear margins are established, often 2 to 3 weeks after the bite. Patients with systemic symptoms following a brown recluse bite warrant hospitalization and close observation.

Various treatments have been advocated for brown spider bites, including hyperbaric oxygen, cyproheptadine, dapsone, steroids, and topical nitroglycerin. None of these therapies has shown clear benefit. The leukocyte inhibitor dapsone continues to be advocated by some. However, a controlled animal study failed to show benefit of dapsone, and this drug is associated with hemolysis and methemoglobinemia.[16] Antivenom could possibly be beneficial for brown recluse bites if a reliable test for envenomation can be demonstrated. However, recent research suggests diminished efficacy if antivenom administration is delayed after inoculation.[17] *Loxosceles* antivenom is not commercially available at this time.

Hobo Spider *(Tegenaria agrestis)*

A native of Europe and central Asia, the hobo or Northwestern brown spider is now found in the Pacific Northwest of the United States and Canada after its introduction through the port of Seattle in the 1930s. Because of similarity in presentation, envenomations in this area are often incorrectly attributed to the brown recluse spider, which lives elsewhere.[18] As suggested by its scientific name, the species is considered to be aggressive because of reports of biting with minor provocation. Hobo spiders are brown with gray markings, have a 7- to 14-mm body length, and a 27- to 45-mm leg span. They live in moist dark areas such as woodpiles or basements.

CLINICAL FEATURES   The clinical presentation of victims of hobo spider envenomations is similar to that of the brown recluse spider. Like brown spiders, the initial bite is often painless, delaying patient presentation until symptoms begin. Induration may initially occur with surrounding erythema, followed by blistering, rupture, and necrosis. Healing may take as long as 45 days and permanent scarring may result. Headache is the most common systemic symptom, but nausea, vomiting, and fatigue can also occur. Aplastic anemia and death are rare complications.

TREATMENT   There is no diagnostic test for hobo spider envenomation, nor is there proven treatment for local or systemic complications.[18] Surgical resection with skin grafting may be necessary but should probably not be initiated until the necrotizing process is completed.

Widow Spiders *(Latrodectus)*

Latrodectus or "widow spiders" have a worldwide distribution. In the United States, the black widow is the most well known, although of the five *Latrodectus* species found commonly in the United States, only three (*L. mactans, L. various,* and *L. hesperus*) are actually black (Figure 194-5). Other varieties may be predominantly brown *(L. geometricus)* or red *(L. bishopi).* The classic orange-red hourglass-shaped marking is noted only in *L. mactans.* Female spiders are relatively large, with a body size ranging up to 1.5 cm in length, with leg spans of 4 to 5 cm. The male spider is approximately one-third the size of the female, lighter in color, and his bite cannot penetrate human skin. Black widow spiders are found most often in woodpiles, basements, garages, and sheds. *Latrodectus* will aggressively defend her web, particularly when guarding her eggs. Most black widow bites occur between April and October and are usually seen on the hands and forearms.

The black widow spider injures its victim and its prey with a highly potent venom.[13] The most active component of the venom is α-latrotoxin, acting through a calcium-mediated mechanism leading to the release of predominantly acetylcholine and norepinephrine from nerve terminals.

CLINICAL FEATURES   Most *Latrodectus* bites are immediately felt as a pinprick sensation at the bite site, followed by increasing local pain that may spread quickly to include the entire bitten extremity. Erythema appears approximately 20 to 60 min after the bite. In the about

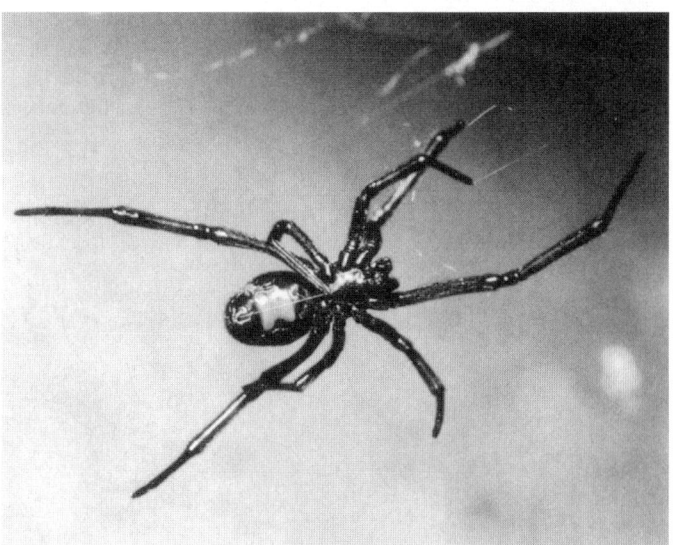

FIG. 194-5. Large female *Latrodectus mactans.* (Reproduced with permission from Stack LB: *Latrodectus mactans. New Engl J Med* 336:1649, 1997. Copyright © 1997 Massachusetts Medical Society. All rights reserved.)

two-thirds of bites, a small, <5-mm erythematous macule develops and in about one-third of cases, initial erythema evolves into a larger "target lesion" with blanched center and surrounding erythema (Figure 194-6).[19] Victims frequently complain of muscle cramplike spasms in large muscle groups, although physical examination of the "cramping" extremity rarely exhibits rigidity. The pain often increases progressively, becomes generalized, and can involve the trunk, back, and abdomen.[19] Severe abdominal wall musculature pain and cramping may be mistaken for a surgical abdomen. Approximately 60 percent of victims develop hypertension and other symptoms include headache, nausea, diarrhea, diaphoresis, photophobia, and dyspnea.[19] *Latrodectus* envenomation victims may experience severe pain for 24 h or more that can be intermittent. Rarely, pain may persist for several days.

Because an immediate pinprick sensation is almost always reported with *Latrodectus* bites, it is rare for victims not to see the offending spider. Although confirmatory testing is not available, the presence the characteristic lesion in association with severe pain and muscle spasms is virtually pathognomonic.

TREATMENT   The initial therapy is supportive care of the airway, breathing, and circulation. Cleansing of the bite site is reasonable. Pain and muscle spasms can be effectively controlled with liberal doses of opioids and benzodiazepines in approximately 70 percent of victims.[19] Although intravenous calcium gluconate has been advocated to relieve symptoms, a retrospective review of 163 patients with *Latrodectus* envenomation found this treatment to be ineffective.[19] For severe envenomations, admission is often required for continued analgesia. The most effective therapies for severe envenomation are parenteral opioids and *Latrodectus* antivenom.[19]

Administration of *Latrodectus* antivenom often causes rapid resolution of symptoms, and unlike opioids can significantly shorten the course of illness. Even in severely symptomatic cases of *Latrodectus* envenomation, patients can often be discharged from the ED after a short observation period when antivenom is administered. *Latrodectus* antivenom is produced in at least three countries with specificity for indigenous species: Red-Back Spider Antivenom (Commonwealth Serum Laboratories CSL Ltd., Australia), Button Spider Antivenom (South African Vaccine Producers Institute, South Africa), and Antivenin *Latrodectus mactans* (Merck & Co., Inc., United States). Indications, amount, and route of administration vary according to product. Antivenin *Latrodectus mactans* and Button Spider Antivenom are administered IV and Red-Back Spider Antivenom is administered by intramuscular injection. *Latrodectus* antivenom is derived from horse serum and hypersensitivity reactions are possible. One death from ana-

phylaxis has been reported after administration of Antivenin *Latrodectus mactans* in the United States; in that case, however, the antivenom was given undiluted and was IV "pushed" in a patient with asthma who had known allergies to multiple medications. Slow administration of diluted Antivenin *Latrodectus mactans* is considered safe.[20]

Armed Spiders *(Phoneutria)*

The armed spiders of South America are aggressive hunters and possess potent neurotoxic venom. Being nocturnal hunters, these spiders may enter houses during the night and hide in clothes during the day. These spiders have also been reported to hide in banana bunches during shipping and can bite workers handling these bananas at their destination. The best-known armed spider, *Phoneutria nigriventer* is large, with body size up to 3.5 cm and leg length up to 6 cm. *P. nigriventer* venom contains a mixture of potent neurotoxins that produce central nervous system, spinal cord, and autonomic effects.

CLINICAL FEATURES   The majority of *P. nigriventer* bites are reported to produce no significant symptoms. Significant envenomation produces local symptoms (severe pain) followed by sympathetic stimulation (tachycardia, hypertension), parasympathetic hyperactivity (nausea, vomiting, diaphoresis, salivation), and spinal cord impairment (priapism) and central nervous effects (vertigo, visual changes). Death from respiratory failure can be seen in 2 to 6 h, usually in children or debilitated adults. Most healthy adults will recover in 1 to 2 days.

TREATMENT   In most cases, supportive care is adequate. Local anesthetic infiltration at the bite site is useful for local pain control. A polyvalent antivenom (Instituto Butantan, Brazil) is available for cases of severe envenomation from *P. nigriventer*. Opioids are contraindicated for pain control in severe envenomation, as they appear to enhance the adverse effect of venom on respiration.

Funnel-Web Spiders *(Atrax/Hadronyche)*

Funnel-web spiders are so named because they contract a cylindrical web that extends into a recess, such as a burrow in the ground or a hole in a tree. Medically significant funnel-web spiders are found in southern and southeastern Australia, and the adjacent islands of Tasmania, Papua New Guinea, and the Solomon Islands. Funnel-web spiders of this region were originally classified into the genera *Atrax* and *Hadronyche,* but are now considered one genus. To prevent confusion, species are identified using their original genus name.

Funnel-web spiders have a shinny black body, long fangs, and females can grow up to 4 cm in body length. Females stay close to their web, but the smaller and more aggressive males tend to wander, especially during the summer following a rain. *Atrax* venom contains a potent mixture of neurotoxins with neuromotor and autonomic effects.

CLINICAL EFFECTS   *Atrax* bites may result in local reaction with immediate pain, followed by wheal formation and surrounding erythema. Later, localized sweating and piloerection have been observed. The vast majority of *Atrax* bites do not appear to result in significant envenomation or systemic toxicity. Symptoms and signs of systemic toxicity include perioral paresthesias, parasympathetic hyperactivity (nausea, vomiting, diaphoresis, salivation, lacrimation, bronchorrhea), neuromuscular stimulation (muscle fasciculation, tremors, spasms, weakness), and central nervous system toxicity (altered level of consciousness). Death following *A. robustus* envenomation has been reported as a result of cardiac arrest, hypotension, or pulmonary failure between 15 min and 3 days following a bite.

TREATMENT   To reduce venom absorption and systemic toxicity for a bite on an extremity, a compressive elastic bandage should be ap-

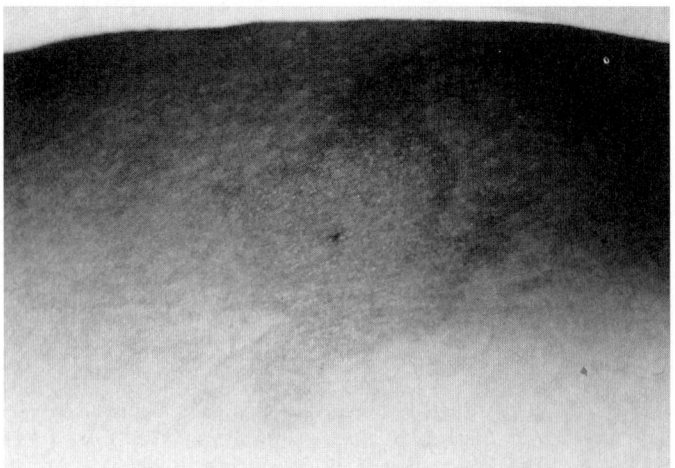

FIG. 194-6. Classic target lesion from patient bitten by a black widow spider.

plied the entire length of the limb and the extremity splinted to prevent movement. The victim should be immobilized and transported promptly to the hospital.

The specific treatment for systemic toxicity is Funnel-web Spider Antivenom (Commonwealth Serum Laboratories CSL Ltd, Australia). If the patient has signs of systemic toxicity upon arrival or develops them after the compressive elastic bandage is carefully removed, two ampules of antivenom should be administered IV every 15 min until symptoms improve; most reported cases require four vials. Supportive therapy for hypotension (intravenous fluid), bronchorrhea (atropine), tremors and agitation (benzodiazepines), and hypertension and tachycardia (β-blockers) may be necessary, but antivenom is the only therapy known to consistently improve survival.

Sac and Running Spiders *(Cheiracanthium)*

Cheiracanthium are medium-sized (7- to 15-mm body size and 30-mm leg span) house-dwelling spiders. The venom is cytotoxic and neurotoxic, but only the South African *C. lawrencei* appears capable of producing skin necrosis.

CLINICAL FEATURES   The most common symptoms are local pain, swelling, and erythema at the bite site. Mild systemic symptoms of headache, malaise, dizziness, and nausea have occasionally been reported. Skin necrosis following a *C. lawrencei* bite typically becomes apparent by the third day and heals in 7 to 10 days.

TREATMENT   Treatment is symptomatic with local wound care. Even if skin necrosis develops, healing is expected provided no secondary infection develops.

Tarantulas (*Degesiella, Aphonopelma,* and Others)

Tarantulas are large, hairy spiders belonging to the family *Theraphosidae* that have become increasingly popular as pets. The hairs found on the abdomen of most species of tarantulas in North and South America appear grossly as a velvety covering and are used defensively. When threatened, tarantulas may "flick" these hairs a short distance with their two back legs. Although North American tarantula hairs rarely penetrate human skin, the hairs have been found in some cases to imbed deeply into the conjunctiva and cornea, and can cause inflammation in all levels of the eye, from conjunctiva to retina. Patients who manifest a red eye and pain after handling a tarantula should be examined to determine if offending barbed hairs are present in the cornea or conjunctiva. Although hairs are sometimes easily seen on slit-lamp examination, they may at times be very difficult to detect. Therapy includes surgical removal of the hairs and topical steroids to control inflammation. Ophthalmia nodosa is a granulomatous, nodular reaction that can occur in cases of ocular exposure to tarantula hairs.[21] Patients may also develop a diffuse contact dermatitis from indirect hair exposure while cleaning a tarantula cage. Bites from tarantulas are typically painful, with local erythema and edema, and some patients describe local joint stiffness following nearby bites. Systemic symptoms other than fever are unusual.

Other Spiders

Wolf spiders *(Lycosa)* are small- to medium-size (3- to 5-mm body length) ground-dwelling spiders with a worldwide distribution. The venom is cytotoxic and produces local pain and occasionally induration and erythema, but no systemic symptoms. The venom is not felt to produce skin necrosis and those purported cases of *Lycosa* skin necrosis are probably either misidentification of the biting spider or a concomitant infection.

Jumping spiders (family *Salticidae*) are typically small (<15 mm), brightly colored, and very active spiders with a worldwide distribution. A bite may produce pain, swelling, pruritus, and erythema that resolves in 2 days. There are case reports of minor skin ulceration (United States) and headache and vomiting (Australia) following a jumping spider bite.

Daddy long-legged spiders (family *Pholcidae*) are common cellar and outbuilding dwellers along the Pacific coast and southwestern deserts. A repeated myth is that these spiders possess highly toxic venom, but their fangs are too short to penetrate human skin. This is false, there are no research studies on *Pholcidae* venom in mammals and no case reports of human envenomation.

SCORPIONS (SCORPIONIDAE)

Scorpions have a world-wide distribution. Highly toxic species are found in the Middle East, India, North Africa, South America, Mexico, and the Caribbean island of Trinidad. Several species of scorpions are found in the warmer parts of the southern United States. All are generally nocturnal and capable of stinging humans, but most species cause little more than localized pain similar to that following Hymenoptera stings. Cytotoxicity or inflammation does not occur from North American scorpion venom, and the exact site of the sting may not be readily apparent. In the United States, only *Centruroides exilicauda,* or the bark scorpion, found throughout Arizona, New Mexico, and parts of Texas and California, possesses venom potent enough to cause systemic toxicity.

Clinical Features

C. exilicauda venom can open neuronal sodium channels and cause prolonged and excessive depolarization. Both somatic and autonomic nerves may be affected. Systemic symptoms from the sting of this scorpion are not common but can be severe, particularly in children. Immediate onset of pain and paresthesias in the stung extremity is usually noted and may become generalized. In severe cases, cranial nerve and somatic motor dysfunction can develop, resulting in abnormal roving eye movements, blurred vision, pharyngeal muscle incoordination and drooling, occasionally leading to respiratory compromise. Excessive motor activity may present as restlessness or uncontrollable jerking of the extremities, appearing to be seizure-like activity. Nausea, vomiting, tachycardia, and severe agitation can also be present. Without antivenom treatment, symptoms can last 24 to 48 h. Cardiac dysfunction, pulmonary edema, pancreatitis, bleeding disorders, skin necrosis, and occasionally death can be seen with stings from Asian and African scorpions.

Diagnosis of a scorpion sting is clinical. Stings can be confused initially with anything that causes local pain, particularly in children. As the syndrome progresses in moderate to severe cases to include autonomic and motor findings, the diagnosis should become more apparent.

Treatment

Initial treatment is supportive with analgesics. In the United States a *Centruroides*-specific antivenom (Antivenom Production Laboratory, Arizona State University, United States) has been available only in the state of Arizona and is produced from goat-serum. Production of this antivenom has been stopped, and supplies will likely be exhausted in several years. Scorpion antivenom directed against different species have been produced for research or clinical use in more than 10 other countries. Recommendations for use and dosing of these products vary widely. Like all animal-derived antivenoms, both immediate and delayed allergic reactions including serum sickness are possible. For this reason, *Centruroides*-specific antivenom administration should be reserved for cases of severe systemic toxicity. One study outside of the United States found no benefit in routine administration of antivenom for scorpion stings.[22] Consultation with a toxicologist experienced in scorpion envenomation is recommended before using antivenom. Treatment with antivenom in cases of severe toxicity can lead to rapid resolution of symptoms; one to two vials of antivenom are usually sufficient.

TICKS (*IXODES, DERMACENTOR,* AND OTHERS)

Ticks are found throughout the world, mostly in rural areas. They are obligate, bloodsucking arthropods that are second only to mosquitoes in numbers of pathogens vectored to humans. Their bodies consist of a fused abdomen and thorax in an oval shape and vary from 1 mm or less in length to more than 1 cm when engorged with blood. Ticks attach to humans painlessly with strong jaws and cement-like adhesive.

The main concern with ticks is that they are disease vectors. Viruses, bacteria (including spirochetes and rickettsiae), and protozoa may all be transmitted by ticks. Lyme disease, Rocky Mountain spotted fever, ehrlichiosis, babesiosis, Colorado tick fever, tularemia, tick-borne relapsing fever, and tick-borne encephalitis are all tick-transmitted diseases. Lyme disease is caused by the *Borrelia burgdorferi* spirochete transmitted by the bite of *Ixodes scapularis*. Certain species of ticks have a neurotoxin and are capable of inducing tick paralysis, a symmetric ascending flaccid paralysis associated with loss of deep tendon reflexes. Most cases have been reported in children and the presentation can be nearly identical to Guillain-Barré syndrome (GBS), including progression to respiratory paralysis. A diagnosis of GBS in a child should not be considered until after a thorough search for an engorged tick. Removal of the tick leads to rapid reversal of symptoms.

Insect repellants and tight-fitting clothing can be helpful in preventing tick bites and a daily tick check is reasonable in tick-infested areas.[23] Although organic solvents, heat, and other methods have been advocated to aid in dislodging a tick so as not to leave its mouth parts beneath the skin surface and to prevent disease transmission, no technique has definitively proven superior. The generally recommended method is mechanical, and involves grasping the tick with forceps or fine-point tweezers near the point of attachment and pulling straight outward with steady, gentle traction. Transmission of pathogens is time-dependent, so prompt removal of ticks is important. Concern over the acquisition of tick-borne disease, particularly Lyme disease, has led to studies regarding the use of prophylactic antibiotics following bites. A reasonable approach is to administer a single 200-mg doxycycline oral dose to persons in Lyme disease-endemic regions who remove a partially engorged tick from their bodies.[24]

CHIGGERS (TROMBICULIDAE)

Chigger infestations result from mite larvae feeding on host skin cells. Mites are found in almost every habitat, are 0.3 to 1 mm in length, and attach themselves to host skin with mandibular structures. They tend to attach in areas where an obstacle such as tight fitting in clothing is met, such as the tops of socks, the leg bands of underwear, the waistband, or the edges of a bra. Once attached, the larvae release digestive enzymes to liquefy epidermal cells. The combination of digestive enzymes secreted by the mite and subsequent host immune response produces the "chigger bite."

Clinical Features

Although diseases such as rickettsialpox have been spread by mite vectors, the major clinical manifestation of chiggers is most often intense pruritus. The attached chigger may be seen initially as a bright red fleck on the skin, and it along with the larvae may be easily scratched off. However, the localized allergic response may last for weeks, and significant excoriation may occur at the site from intense scratching. Severe reactions may be accompanied by fever, edema, erythema multiforme-like lesions, and cellulitis (Figure 194-7).

The diagnosis of chigger infestation may be difficult as many other arthropods cause similar clinical manifestations. The history of out-

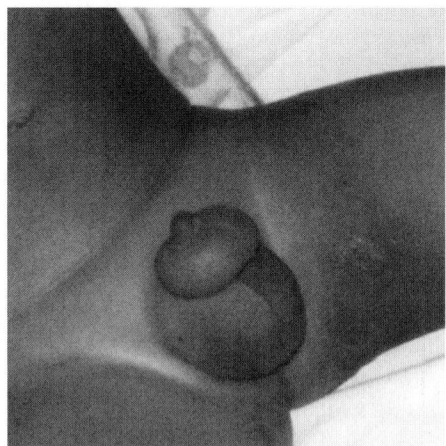

FIG. 194-7. Intense local edema from chigger bites.

door exposure combined with the presence of signs and symptoms localized to areas of snug-fitting clothing may be helpful.

Treatment

Treatment is primarily symptomatic to control the itching and consists of oral antihistamines and topical steroids. Oral steroids may be helpful in severe cases. Chiggers themselves may be killed with lindane, crotamiton, and other topical scabicides. Crotamiton may also help to relieve the pruritus. If secondary infection occurs, antibiotics are indicated.

MOSQUITOS, FLIES, FLEAS, AND LICE (DIPTERA)

Mosquitoes

Mosquitoes are aquatic-breeding arthropods found in all parts of the world. Like other members of this group, they possess one pair of wings, the second pair having evolved into smaller structures used as stabilizers.

Mosquitoes penetrate skin with a piercing motion of a bayonet-like proboscis. The actual puncturing of the skin surface causes minimal trauma and is frequently not felt by the host. A local anesthetic is injected into the wound that causes local tissue damage and local hypersensitivity. Bites can lead to both immediate and delayed reactions. An immediate skin reaction includes redness, a wheal, and itching. A delayed reaction can occur and usually consists of edema and pruritus. The immediate reaction tends to be of short duration, whereas a delayed reaction may persist for hours, days, and even weeks. Severe local reactions with skin necrosis are possible. Patients can acquire allergy to mosquito saliva constituents and develop symptoms consisting of an increasing reaction to seasonal exposures with increasingly pronounced edematous and pruritic lesions, sometimes accompanied by fever, malaise, generalized edema, severe nausea and vomiting, and necrosis with resulting scarring. Treatment is symptomatic with antihistamines (e.g., cetirizine) and NSAIDs.[25]

The greatest danger from mosquitoes in other countries is as disease vectors. Even with extensive pest control programs, arboviruses and malaria are epidemic in many parts of the world. Japanese B encephalitis, yellow fever, dengue hemorrhagic fever, and various types of equine encephalitis are among the many viruses transmitted by mosquitoes. West Nile virus–induced encephalitis is now becoming more common in the temperate regions of the United States.[26] Malaria is also encountered frequently in patients in the United States after travel, and in immigrant populations from areas where malaria is endemic. Insect repellents offer some protection from mosquito bites.[27]

Flies

Bloodsucking flies range in size from the tiny sand fly, approximately 1 to 3 mm in length, to horse flies that can be larger than 2 cm. All members stab and pierce the skin, causing some degree of pain and pruritus. Several species, such as deerflies, blackflies, horseflies, and sand flies, can produce allergic reactions, although rarely as severe as those produced by Hymenoptera venom. There is also the possibility of myiasis with fly bites, but this is rare in the United States.

The diagnosis of fly bites depends chiefly on the patient's history and a knowledge of the arthropods that frequent the area of encounter. Treatment for most local reactions to *Diptera* bites is symptomatic, whereas treatment of systemic reactions is the same as it is for Hymenoptera venom. Cold compresses may alleviate localized edema. Secondary infection from *Diptera* bites can occur, and antibiotics may be necessary in some cases. Oral antihistamines such as diphenhydramine and hydroxyzine may be helpful in relieving pruritus in these cases, but topical steroids can be used when local reactions are severe, and oral steroids are indicated when systemic hypersensitivity symptoms are present.

Fleas (Siphonaptera)

Bites of fleas, lice, and scabies produce lesions so similar that diagnosis is often difficult. Flea bites are frequently found in zigzag lines, especially on the legs and in the waist area. The lesions most often have a hemorrhagic appearing center surrounded by erythematous and urticarial patches. Flea bites are usually quite pruritic, and red spots can persist at bite sites for some time.

The main concern in the treatment of these bites is the possibility of secondary infection. Children may develop impetigo as a complication. The lesions should be washed thoroughly with soap and water. Children with flea bites should have their fingernails cut short to prevent scratching. To relieve discomfort and itching, starch baths at bedtime (about 1 kg starch to a tub full of water), local application of calamine, cool soaks, and oral or topical antihistamines might be helpful. For severe discomfort, application of a topical steroid cream or spray may be necessary. If secondary infection develops, topical or oral antibiotics may be needed.

KISSING BUGS AND BED BUGS (HEMIPTERA)

The order Hemiptera includes two blood-sucking families of arthropods with medical importance. These are *Reduviidae* (reduviid, or "kissing" bugs) and *Cimicidae* ("bedbugs" and their relatives).[28,29] Various species of kissing bugs exist predominantly in the southern United States and Central and South America. The common name "kissing bugs" derives from their habit of feeding at night on any exposed surface of a sleeping victim, commonly the face. Bedbugs are also nocturnal feeders and their distribution is worldwide. Both bugs are attracted to warm bodies and hide near beds. Bedbugs are found in nearby cracks and crevices. Both bugs are potential vectors for disease. Kissing bugs of Central and South America are vectors of Chagas' disease (trypanosomiasis), and bedbugs have been implicated as a vector for hepatitis B.

Clinical Features

Bites from both bugs are typically painless. Erythematous papules, bullae, and wheals may develop. Diagnostically, kissing bug bites can be differentiated from bedbug bites in that kissing bug bites are not in a linear formation and usually are not accompanied by telltale brown or black patterns of excrement on the bed linen, which is characteristic of bed bugs.[28] A thorough search of bedding and nearby cracks and crevices will often reveal the bugs.

Treatment

Treatment of both bites is symptomatic. Cool compresses, topical steroids, and antihistamines can be used to relieve associated pruritus. Some individuals become highly sensitive to kissing bugs and react with systemic allergic symptoms following a bite. They should be treated as previously outlined for Hymenoptera envenomation.

CATERPILLARS AND MOTHS (LEPIDOPTERA)

Lepidopterism refers to the adverse effects resulting from contact with butterflies, moths, or their caterpillars. With the exception of dermatitis from female moths of the *Hylesia* genus found in Central and South America, most symptoms are a result of contact with caterpillars.

Clinical Features

Caterpillars are the larval stage of moths and have either spines or hairs for protection. The spines can be hollow, branched, and connected to a venom gland. The spines and hairs may cause mechanical irritation, whereas the venom can produce additional symptoms. The vast majority of caterpillars are harmless to humans. Pruritus from localized "caterpillar dermatitis" and occasional diffuse urticaria are the predominant symptoms with exposures to the hairs and venom. The puss caterpillar *(Megalopyge opercularis)* is found in the southeastern United States and accounts for most of the serious envenomations in this country. After initial contact, intense local burning pain rather than pruritus is typical. A gridlike pattern of hemorrhagic papules may be seen within 2 to 3 h of these exposures and may last for several days. Regional lymphadenopathy is common, and the affected limb can swell considerably. Other symptoms include headaches, fever, hypotension, and convulsions. No deaths have been reported. Ingestion of the hickory tussock caterpillar *(Lophocampa caryae),* found in the eastern United States, has been reported with symptoms ranging from drooling to diffuse urticaria. Spines have been visualized in the oropharynx and even the esophagus in some of these patients requiring general anesthesia to help removal.[30]

Treatment

No antivenom exists for lepidopterism and treatment is symptomatic and supportive. Spines can be removed by adhesive tape. Antihistamines and steroids may be administered for pruritus. For the rare patient with hypotension, intravenous fluids and subcutaneous epinephrine should be administered.

BLISTER BEETLES (COLEOPTERA)

Although the order Coleoptera includes a large number and variety of beetles, clinically significant envenomation occurs only from blister beetles. There are approximately 1500 species of blister beetles worldwide, including 200 species in the United States. Although not naturally found in the United States, the most well known blister beetle is the "Spanish fly" *(Cantharis vesicatoria).*

Clinical Features

Blister beetles contain the highly potent vesicant cantharidin that is exuded from their joints when disturbed, or from their body when crushed. For this reason a blister beetle should be removed from the skin by blowing or flicking. Cantharidin-containing preparations are used medicinally in wart removal. Application of these substances in low concentration is without adverse effect.[31] However, higher concentrations, or contact with the beetle's venom may cause local inflammation leading to bullae formation. Severe conjunctivitis may also occur if cantharidin contacts the eyes from contaminated hands.

Owing to its lipophilicity, high concentrations of cantharidin may result in dermal absorption and systemic toxicity. Systemic toxicity also occurs following ingestion, either of the whole beetle or of cantharidin-containing preparations. Severe vomiting, hematemesis, abdominal pain, and diarrhea may occur, followed by dysuria, hematuria, oliguria, and renal failure as the toxin is concentrated in the kidneys. Death has occurred after large ingestions. Although the exact mechanism by which cantharidin produces systemic toxicity is unknown, the vesicant action may explain much of the symptoms observed. Fortunately, most preparations sold as "Spanish fly" for purported aphrodisiac properties have very low concentrations of cantharidin. It is thought that the local vascular congestion and urethral inflammation that occurs following ingestion may be interpreted by some as enhanced sexuality.

Treatment

Treatment of blister beetle toxicity is largely supportive. The skin should be irrigated thoroughly after topical exposure to remove any persistent cantharidin followed by local wound care. Symptomatic ingestions should be admitted and treated supportively.

REFERENCES

1. White J: Bites and stings from venomous animals: A global overview. *Ther Drug Monit* 22:65, 2000.
2. Litovitz TL, Klein-Schwartz W, White S, et al: 2001 Annual report of the American Association of Poison Control Centers Toxic Exposure Surveillance System. *Am J Emerg Med* 10:391, 2002.
3. Stibich AS, Carbonaro PA, Schwartz RA: Insect bite reactions: An update. *Dermatology* 202:193, 2001.
4. Diaz-Sanchez CL, Lifshitz-Guinzberg A, Ignacio-Ibarra G, et al: Survival after massive (>2000) Africanized honeybee stings. *Arch Intern Med* 158:925, 1998.
5. King TP, Spangfort MD: Structure and biology of stinging insect venom allergens. *Int Arch Allergy Immunol* 123:99, 2000.
6. Antonicelli L, Bilo MB, Bonifazi F: Epidemiology of Hymenoptera allergy. *Curr Opin Allergy Clin Immunol* 2:341, 2002.
7. Lazoglu AH, Boglioli LR, Taff ML, et al: Serum sickness reaction following multiple insect stings. *Ann Allergy Asthma Immunol* 75:522, 1995.
8. Jones RGA, Corteling RL, To HP, et al: A novel Fab-based antivenom for the treatment of mass bee attacks. *Trop Med Hyg* 61:361, 1999.
9. Hamilton RG: Diagnosis of Hymenoptera venom sensitivity. *Curr Opin Allergy Clin Immunol* 2:347, 2002.
10. Kemp SF, deShazo RD, Moffitt JE, et al: Expanding habitat of the imported fire ant *(Solenopsis invicta):* A public health concern. *J Allergy Clin Immunol* 105:683, 2000.
11. Rhoades R: Stinging ants. *Curr Opin Allergy Clin Immunol* 1:343, 2001.
12. McGain F, Winkel KD: Ant sting mortality in Australia. *Toxicon* 40:1095, 2002.
13. Rash LD, Hodgson WC: Pharmacology and biochemistry of spider venoms. *Toxicon* 40:225, 2002.
14. Sams HH, Dunnick CA, Smith ML, King LE: Necrotic arachnidism. *J Am Acad Dermatol* 44:561, 2001.
15. Krywko DM, Gomez HF: Detection of Loxosceles species venom in dermal lesions: A comparison of 4 venom recovery methods. *Ann Emerg Med* 39:475, 2002.
16. Phillips S, Kohn M, Baker D, et al: Therapy of brown spider envenomation: A controlled trial of hyperbaric oxygen, dapsone, and cyproheptadine. *Ann Emerg Med* 25:363, 1995.
17. Gomez HF, Miller MJ, Trachy JW, et al: Intradermal anti-Loxosceles Fab fragments attenuate dermatonecrotic arachnidism. *Acad Emerg Med* 6:1196, 1999.
18. Centers for Disease Control: Necrotic arachnidism—Pacific Northwest, 1988-1996. *MMWR* 45:433, 1996.
19. Clark RF, Wethern-Kestner S, Vance MV, Gerkin R: Clinical presentation and treatment of black widow spider envenomation: A review of 163 cases. *Ann Emerg Med* 21:782, 1992.
20. Clark RF: The safety and efficacy of antivenin *Latrodectus mactans. J Clin Toxicol Clin Toxicol* 39:125, 2001.
21. Belyea DA, Tuman DC, Ward TP, Babonis TR: The red eye revisited: Ophthalmia nodosa due to tarantula hairs. *South Med J* 91:565, 1998.
22. Abroug F, ElAtrous S, Nouira S, et al: Serotherapy in scorpion envenomation: A randomized controlled trial. *Lancet* 354:906, 1999.
23. Staub D, Debrunner M, Amsler L, Steffen R: Effectiveness of a repellent containing DEET and EBAAP for preventing tick bites. *Wilderness Environ Med* 13:12, 2002.
24. Wilson ME: Prevention of tick-borne diseases. *Med Clin North Am* 86:219, 2002.
25. Karppinen A, Kautiainen H, Petman L, et al: Comparison of cetirizine, ebastine and loratadine in the treatment of immediate mosquito-bite allergy. *Allergy* 57:534, 2002.
26. Petersen LR, Marfin AA: West Nile virus: A primer for the clinician. *Ann Intern Med* 137:173, 2002.
27. Fradin MA, Day JF: Comparative efficacy of insect repellents against mosquito bites. *New Engl J Med* 347:13, 2002.
28. Vetter R: Kissing bugs (Triatoma) and the skin. *Dermatol Online J* 7:6, 2001.
29. Elston DM, Stockwell S: What's eating you? Bedbugs. *Cutis* 65:262, 2000.
30. Kuspis DA, Rawlins JE, Krenzelock EP: Human exposures to stinging caterpillar: *Lophocampa caryae. Am J Emerg Med* 19:396, 2001.
31. Moed L, Shwayder TA, Chang MW: Cantharidin revisited: A blistering defense of an ancient medicine. *Arch Dermatol* 137:1357, 2001.

195

REPTILE BITES
Richard C. Dart
Frank F. S. Daly

An estimated 3 million bites and 150,000 deaths occur each year from venomous snakes in the world.[1] The American Association of Poison Control Centers reports an average of 6000 bites each year, approximately 2000 of them from venomous snakes. Because of underreporting, the true number of snake bites is possibly as high as 45,000 per year in the United States, with 7000 to 8000 from venomous snakes.[2] The major venomous snakes of the world can be divided into three groups: Viperidae (vipers), Elapidae, and Hydrophiinae (sea snakes, see Chap. 196).

Approximately 20 of the 120 snake species indigenous to North America are venomous. Most bites occur in the warm summer months, when snakes and victims are most active. In the past, it was estimated that mortality from venomous snakebite approached 25 percent. Because of the availability of antivenom and advances in emergency and critical care, mortality rates today are less than 0.5 percent; approximately 5 to 10 deaths occur per year.[3]

Except for bites by imported species, North American venomous snakebite involves the pit vipers (Crotalinae subfamily of Viperidae) or coral snakes (Elapidae family). The crotaline snakes are represented by the rattlesnakes (*Crotalus* species), pygmy rattlesnakes, and massasauga (*Sistrurus* species), and the copperheads and water moccasins (*Agkistrodon* species). Poisonous snakebites from imported exotic species are infrequent but may occur in zoo personnel as well as in amateur herpetologists. A regional poison center can provide information on snake identification, expected toxicity, and location of antivenom.

CROTALINAE (PIT VIPER) BITES

The crotaline snakes are called pit vipers because of bilateral depressions or pits located midway between and below the level of the eye and the nostril (Figure 195-1). The pit is a heat receptor that guides strikes at warm-blooded prey or predators. Crotaline snakes are also distinguished by two fangs that fold against the roof of the mouth, in contrast to the coral snakes, which have shorter, fixed, and erect fangs. Within the pit vipers, the rattle distinguishes the rattlesnake from other crotaline snakes. The mistaken belief that rattlesnakes always rattle be-

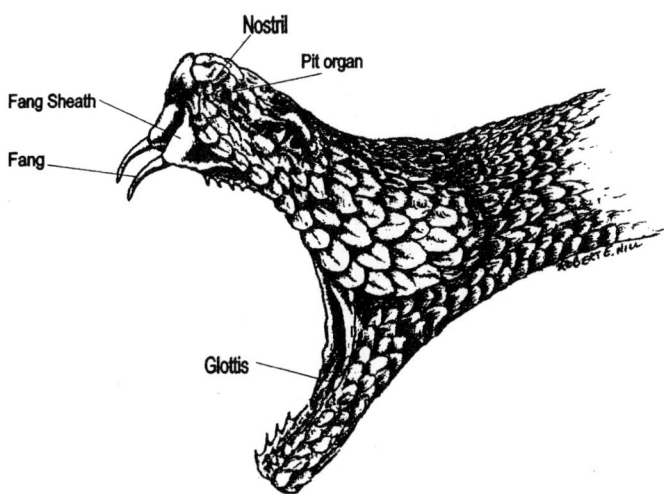

FIG. 195-1. Rattlesnake surface anatomy.

Labels in figure: Nostril, Pit organ, Fang Sheath, Fang, Glottis

fore striking has persisted for centuries. In truth, many strikes occur without a warning rattle.

Pathophysiology

Crotaline venom is a complex enzyme mixture that causes local tissue injury, systemic vascular damage, hemolysis, fibrinolysis, and neuromuscular dysfunction, resulting in a combination of local and systemic effects. Crotaline venom quickly alters blood vessel permeability, leading to loss of plasma and blood into the surrounding tissue, causing hypovolemia. Crotaline venom activates and consumes fibrinogen and platelets, causing a coagulopathy. In some species, specific venom fractions block neuromuscular transmission, leading to cranial nerve weakness (e.g., ptosis), respiratory failure, and altered sensorium.

Clinical Features

Up to 25 percent of crotaline snakebites are termed dry: venom effects do not develop. The manifestations of crotaline venom poisoning involve a complex interaction of the venom and the victim. The species and size of the snake, the age and size of the victim, the time elapsed since the bite, and characteristics of the bite (location, depth, and number, the amount of venom injected) all affect the clinical appearance. The severity of poisoning following a crotaline bite is therefore variable. An initially minimal bite may evolve into a more serious bite and require large amounts of antivenom.

The cardinal manifestations of crotaline venom poisoning are the presence of one or more fang marks, localized pain, and progressive edema extending from the bite site.[2] Other early symptoms and signs of envenomation are nausea and vomiting, weakness, oral numbness or tingling of tongue and mouth, tachycardia, dizziness, and muscle fasciculation. Envenomation may produce systemic effects with tachypnea, tachycardia, hypotension, and altered level of consciousness. In general, local swelling at the bite site becomes apparent within 15 to 30 min, but in some cases, it may not start for several hours. In severe cases, edema may progress to involve an entire limb within an hour. In less-severe cases, edema may progress over a 1- to 2-day period. Edema near an airway or in a muscle compartment may threaten life or limb without the presence of systemic effects.

Progressive ecchymosis may also occur because of leakage of blood into subcutaneous tissue. Ecchymoses may appear within minutes or hours and hemorrhagic blebs may occur within several hours. Hemoconcentration often develops as a result of fluid extravasation into subcutaneous tissue, followed by a decrease in hemoglobin over several days from blood loss secondary to coagulopathy.

Diagnosis

The diagnosis of snakebite is based on the presence of fang marks and a history consistent with exposure to a snake (e.g., walking through a field). Snake envenomation involves the presence of a snakebite plus evidence of tissue injury. Clinically, the injury may be manifest in three ways: local injury (swelling, pain, ecchymosis), coagulopathy (thrombocytopenia, elevated prothrombin time, hypofibrinogenemia), or systemic effects (e.g., oral swelling or paresthesias, metallic or rubbery taste in the mouth, hypotension, tachycardia). Abnormalities in any one of these areas indicate that venom effect is developing. The absence of any of these manifestations for a period of 8 to 12 h following the bite indicates a dry bite.

Treatment

FIRST AID   First aid measures should never substitute for definitive medical care or delay the administration of antivenom (Table 195-1). All patients bitten by a pit viper should be taken to a health care facility. **First aid treatments such as suction and incision are dangerous and should not be used.** The Coghlan's Snake Bite Kit (Coghlan's Ltd.) and similar products should not be used because they contains cups that produce little suction and seal poorly on digits. The blade in the kit, or any method of incision, can injure digital nerves, arteries, and tendons; incision is not recommended. The Sawyer Extractor (Sawyer Products) suction pump purportedly removes venom without incision; however, serious questions regarding its safety and efficacy have been raised.[4] Other useless or dangerous techniques are electric shock and ice. Electric shock treatment of the bite site is mentioned only to be condemned. This dangerous procedure is not effective and has resulted in electrical injuries. Ice-water immersion worsens the venom injury.

Tourniquets are contraindicated because they obstruct arterial flow and cause ischemia. Constriction bands may be of some use, especially when immediate medical care is not available. A constriction band is an elastic bandage or Penrose drain, rope, or piece of clothing wrapped circumferentially above the bite, applied with enough tension to restrict superficial venous and lymphatic flow while maintaining distal pulses and capillary filling. The band should be snug but loose enough to comfortably slide a finger underneath. In theory, a constriction band retards venom absorption. This should increase local tissue injury but reduce the severity of systemic effects. Anecdotal human reports and animal studies suggest that constriction band use delays venom absorption without causing increased swelling.[5] Human controlled studies are needed to better define the clinical indications for constriction band use.

EMERGENCY MANAGEMENT   In the prehospital phase, personnel should be directed to immobilize the limb, establish intravenous access in another limb, administer oxygen, and transport the victim to a medical facility. Previously placed tourniquets and constriction bands should not be removed until intravenous access is established.

As in any emergency, initial snakebite management should include advanced life support. If the patient is hypotensive, initial treatment should include rapid intravenous isotonic fluid infusion. Supplemental

TABLE 195-1   Recommended First Aid Measures

Retreat well-beyond striking range. Many victims are bitten again while trying to capture the snake.
Remain calm. Movement will increase venom absorption.
Immobilize the extremity in a neutral position below the level of the heart.
Keep physical activity minimal.
Promptly transport the victim to a medical facility regardless of whether overt signs of envenomation are quickly apparent. Signs and symptoms of snakebite may be delayed.

oxygen should be started and limb immobilization continued during transport to reduce further venom absorption. Consultation with a physician or poison center familiar with the management of snake envenomation is recommended for most cases.

Antivenom is the mainstay of therapy for poisonous snakebite.[2] Antivenom is composed of heterologous antibodies derived from the serum of animals immunized with the appropriate snake venoms. The antibodies bind and neutralize the venom molecules.

Antivenin (Crotalidae) Polyvalent is an equine-derived product, once widely used, which has been discontinued. A newer product, Polyvalent Crotalidae Immune Fab (ovine) (CroFab; FabAV) is now available in the United States. The new antivenom is produced by immunizing flocks of sheep with one of four crotaline snake venoms: Eastern diamondback *(Crotalus adamanteus),* Western diamondback *(C. atrox),* Mojave *(C. scutulatus),* or Cottonmouth *(Agkistrodon piscivorus).* The immune serum is harvested from each group and then digested with papain to produce antibody fragments (Fab and Fc). The more immunogenic Fc portion of the antibody is eliminated during purification. The four individual monospecific Fab preparations are combined to form the final antivenom product.

All crotaline bites that show evidence of progressive signs and symptoms should immediately receive antivenom. Progression is defined as worsening of local injury (e.g., pain, ecchymosis, or swelling), laboratory abnormalities (e.g., worsening platelet count, prolonged coagulation times, decreased fibrinogen), or systemic manifestations (e.g., unstable vital signs or abnormal mental status).

In clinical trials and initial clinical reports, FabAV has been effective and appears to have a better safety profile than Antivenin (Crotalidae) polyvalent.[6,7] FabAV also dissolves into solution quickly and skin testing is not required.

FabAV is administered as a larger "initial control" dose followed by three smaller maintenance doses (Figure 195-2). Initial control is defined as cessation of progression of three clinical evaluation parameters: local effects, systemic effects, and coagulopathy. The initial dose is four to six vials, which may be repeated to establish initial control of the envenomation. After initial control has been established, two-vial maintenance doses are recommended (see Figure 195-2).

Under no circumstances should antivenom be injected directly into a digit. Intramuscular injection is also not recommended because

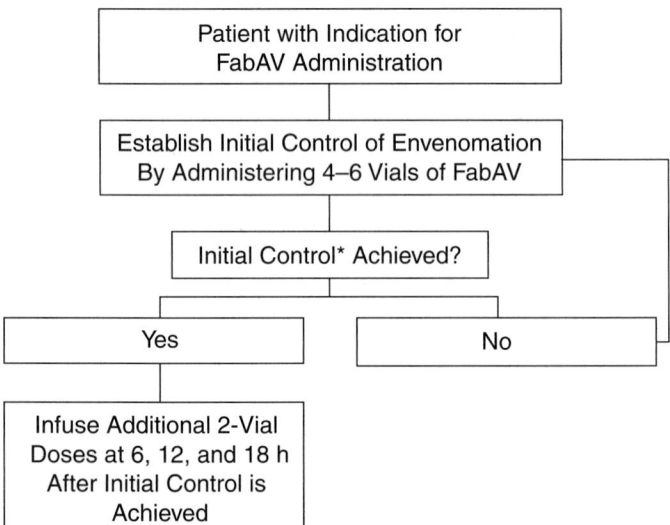

FIG. 195-2. Use of Polyvalent Crotalidae Immune Fab (ovine).

venom-induced hypovolemia may retard absorption of antivenom. Hospital pharmacies in those regions of the United States where poisonous snakes are prevalent should maintain adequate stocks of antivenom. Unfortunately, many hospitals stock insufficient amounts of antivenom, even in endemic areas.[8]

The package insert is useful as a guide for antivenom preparation. Antivenom should be administered only in a critical care facility such as an ED or intensive care unit, under direct physician supervision, and with resuscitative drugs and equipment immediately available. After reconstitution, each dose of FabAV is diluted in 250 mL of crystalloid and infused slowly for the initial 10 min, until it is evident that anaphylaxis will not occur, then the rate should be increased in a stepwise manner until the infusion is complete, usually in 1 h. The total volume, but not the number of vials, may be reduced in small children.[9]

The incidence of acute reactions to FabAV is about 14 percent.[2,7] If an acute allergic reaction occurs, the infusion should be stopped immediately and antihistamines administered (both H_1- and H_2-receptor blockers). Epinephrine infusion should be readily available and used, depending on the severity of the reaction.

It is extremely important that observation for progression of edema and systemic signs of envenomation be continued during and after antivenom infusion. Limb circumference should be measured at several sites above and below the bite, and the advancing border of edema should be outlined with a pen every 30 min. This serves as an index of the progression as well as a guide for antivenom administration. Laboratory determinations are repeated every 4 h, or after each course of antivenom therapy, whichever is more frequent. Additional doses of FabAV may be warranted if the patient's condition worsens. FabAV has been formally tested only in rattlesnake bites. Initial case reports support its efficacy in copperhead snakebite, but controlled data are needed.[10]

The value of aggressive supportive care cannot be overemphasized. Isotonic fluid resuscitation followed by vasopressor agents is appropriate for hypotension. Antivenom is the best treatment for coagulopathy, but if active bleeding occurs, blood component replacement may be necessary. Another complication of snakebite is compartment syndrome. Increased compartment pressure may occur when venom is injected or spreads into a compartment. This is often manifested by severe pain, localized to a compartment and usually resistant to opiate analgesia. Treatment of compartment syndrome is difficult (Table 195-2). The use of fasciotomy is controversial and there is no firm evidence supporting its use.

The wound area should be cleaned and the need for tetanus immunization determined. Cultures and antibiotic therapy should be initiated only if signs of infection are present. Although recommended by some authors, the data available do not support the prophylactic use of antibiotics.[11] The use of steroids is also controversial. Several studies suggest lack of efficacy or even deleterious effects. Without evidence of efficacy, steroids should be reserved for the treatment of allergic reactions or serum sickness.

TABLE 195-2 Management of Compartment Syndrome*†

Determine intracompartmental pressure.
If not elevated, continue standard management.
If signs of compartment syndrome are present and compartment pressure is >30 mm Hg:
  Elevate limb
  Administer mannitol 1–2 g/kg IV over 30 min
  Simultaneously administer *additional* antivenom, 4 to 6 vials IV over 60 min
  If elevated compartment pressure persists another 60 min, consider fasciotomy

*Elevated compartment pressure is caused by the action of the venom on the tissues; thus, the most effective treatment is to neutralize the venom, which may reduce the compartment pressure.
†This protocol delivers a high osmotic load and should not be used when contraindicated. The protocol must be completed promptly so that, if ever needed, fasciotomy may be performed as early as possible.

Delayed serum sickness develops in about 5 percent of patients after FabAV treatment. The symptoms are fever, rash, and arthralgias. Oral prednisone 60 mg/d should be started and tapered over 1 to 2 weeks.

Disposition

Patients are ready for discharge when swelling begins to resolve, the coagulopathy has been reversed, and the patient is ambulatory. During recovery, physical therapy of the bitten part (particularly the hand) is recommended after swelling has lessened and coagulopathy has resolved. Outpatient follow-up is necessary to monitor for infection and serum sickness.

It cannot be overemphasized that one can easily be deceived by a bite that initially appears innocuous. An unremarkable physical and laboratory examination at presentation does not reliably indicate an insignificant envenomation. **We recommended that physicians observe patients for at least 8 h.** Patients with severe or life-threatening bites and patients receiving antivenom should be admitted to an intensive care unit. The general ward is appropriate for patients with mild or moderate envenomations who have completed or do not require further antivenom therapy.

Patients with dry bites who have been observed for at least 8 h may be discharged. They should return if pain, swelling, or bleeding develops.

CORAL SNAKE (ELAPID) BITE

North American coral snakes include the eastern coral snake *(Micrurus fulvius fulvius)*, the Texas coral snake *(M.f. tenere)*, and the Arizona (Sonoran) coral snake *(Micruroides euryxanthus)*. The eastern coral snake is found primarily in the southeast United States. The Texas and Arizona coral snakes are found primarily in the states that bear their names. Coral snakes account for 20 to 25 bites a year.

Elapids are found throughout the world in tropical and warm climates. Medically significant groups include most venomous snakes of Australia [tiger snakes *(Notechis)*, brown snakes *(Pseudonaja)*, costal taipan *(Oxyuranus)*, dead adder *(Acanthophis)*, red-bellied black snake *(Pseudechis)*], and cobras *(Naja)*, mambas *(Dendroaspis)*, and kraits *(Bungarus)* found in Africa and southern Asia.

All coral snakes are brightly colored with black, red, and yellow rings. The red and yellow rings touch in coral snakes, but they are separated by black rings in nonpoisonous snakes, creating the well known rhyme: "Red on yellow, kill a fellow; red on black, venom lack." This rule is not always true outside of the United States.

Coral snake venom is primarily composed of neurotoxic components that do not cause marked local injury. Elapid bites produce primarily neurologic effects: tremors, salivation, dysarthria, diplopia, bulbar paralysis with ptosis, fixed and contracted pupils, dysphagia, dyspnea, and seizures. The immediate cause of death is paralysis of respiratory muscles. Signs and symptoms may be delayed up to 12 h.

The potential coral snake victim should be admitted to the hospital for observation. Coral snake venom effects may develop hours after a bite and are not easily reversed. It is suggested that three to five vials of the Antivenin *(Micrurus fulvius)* be administered to patients who have definitely been bitten because it may not be possible to prevent further effects or reverse effects that have already developed.[12] Additional coral snake antivenom is reserved for the appearance of symptoms or signs of coral snake envenomation. Because respiratory failure may result from clinical effects of the neurotoxin, baseline and serial pulmonary function parameters (such as inspiratory pressure and vital capacity), in addition to intensive care observation, may be useful. Prolonged ventilatory support may be required in severe cases. The patient must be observed closely for signs of respiratory muscle weakness and hypoventilation. Bites by the Sonoran coral snake are mild and antivenom is not usually needed.

AUSTRALIAN ELAPIDS

Approximately 3000 people are bitten by snakes each year in Australia, of whom at least 200 receive antivenom.[13] In the decade up to 1992, there was an average fatality rate of 1.8 per year, but in the years 1992 to 1994, the rate was 3.7 deaths per year (the Australian population is approximately 19 million).

Pathophysiology

The venomous snakes of Australia are members of the family Elapidae, of which the cobras are also members. The Elapidae possess a relatively unsophisticated venom delivery apparatus with nonretractile small- to medium-sized paired fangs that have grooved venom channels rather than hollow venom ducts. It is thought that the Elapidae exert voluntary control over the injection of venom, hence the occurrence of the "dry bite," without envenomation.

The venom of the Australian elapids contains several important components.[14] Neurotoxins (tiger snake, taipan, and death adder) act at the neuromuscular junction and cause paralysis. Signs usually become apparent within 2 to 4 h after the bite and may include ptosis, partial ophthalmoplegia (diplopia), dysarthria, loss of facial expression, and loss of airway control, as well as respiratory paralysis in severe cases. The procoagulant toxins (brown snake, tiger snake, taipan) act as prothrombin converters, leading to fibrinogen depletion and a consumptive coagulopathy. Intracranial hemorrhage is a recognized complication.

The brown snake can cause rapid collapse and death.[15] Brown snake venom produces severe cardiovascular depression in anesthetized dogs, and these effects may account for the sudden deaths described. Renal impairment or failure may also result from snakebite. The mechanisms are poorly understood and may include hypotension, myoglobinuria, coagulopathy, and direct renal toxicity (the brown snake). Myolysins (tiger snake, taipan, mulga snake) are structurally related to the neurotoxins but instead produce rhabdomyolysis, which may result in muscle pain, weakness, myoglobinuria, renal failure, and hyperkalemia. Local tissue destruction is uncommon with any Australian species, although mild to moderate ecchymosis and swelling may occur.

Clinical Presentation

The severity of envenomation cannot be estimated by the appearance of the bite site or initial symptoms.[16] Despite significant envenomation, patients may initially feel well and manifest no untoward clinical features. Conversely, depending on the snake involved, patients may present with myriad symptoms, including nausea, vomiting, headache, diplopia, dysphonia, progressive muscle weakness, neck stiffness, discolored urine, and seizures. Young children may not provide a history of snakebite; therefore a high index of suspicion is required in this group.

Diagnosis

Local signs after brown snake envenomation may be minimal, and unless the patient gives a history, diagnosis may be difficult. To aid in diagnosis and direct therapy, the Commonwealth Serum Laboratory Ltd. (CSL) in Australia has developed a Snake Venom Detection Kit (SVDK) to detect snake venom at the bite site or in the urine. Positive SVDK identification of venom at the bite site or in the urine is not an indication for antivenom therapy without other evidence of systemic venom effect. False-positive and false-negative results have been described for blood testing by the SVDK and so only the bite site or urine should be tested.[13]

Treatment

FIRST AID   The aim of first aid is to delay absorption of venom from the bite site until the patient is in a facility that can administer antivenom if required. The pressure-immobilization method is used for elapid bites as local soft tissue swelling is usually minimal, but this technique is not recommended for crotaline bites because the immobilization dressing causes severe pain when swelling develops.[17] All patients with elapid bites should immediately have the bitten extremity wrapped in a snug elastic bandage, applied initially over the bite site and then extending to cover the entire limb. The bandage should be applied as if to a sprained joint; if it is too loose or too tight, it will be ineffective. The limb is then splinted to prevent motion. The patient should rest until help arrives. The principle is to contain the venom within lymphatic vessels and prevent systemic absorption. Examination of lymphatic flow rates with simulated venom has demonstrated that even if the upper or lower limb is appropriately bandaged and immobilized, walking will hasten systemic envenomation.[17] Tourniquets are contraindicated because they obstruct arterial flow and add ischemic injury to venom effect. In the rare circumstance that a bite is inflicted on the trunk, firm pressure should be applied without restricting breathing.

EMERGENCY MANAGEMENT Any history suggestive of snakebite should prompt the initiation of first aid, investigation, and observation. Snakebite cases often present a number of complex clinical problems; therefore early consultation with an expert is recommended. The pressure bandage should remain in place until the patient can receive antivenom. Once in a suitable facility, objective evidence of envenomation should be sought. If signs are absent, bandages and splints should not be left on for prolonged periods. Similarly, if antivenom is indicated, the bandage should be removed once administration has commenced so that venom is available for interaction with circulating antivenom. There is no evidence that venom is inactivated by being trapped at the bite site.[13] If the patient's condition deteriorates immediately after bandage removal, the bandages may be reapplied while antivenom is given.

Antivenom should be given only in cases when there is clear clinical or laboratory evidence of systemic venom effect. Clinical indications for immediate antivenom therapy include vomiting and severe headache; neurotoxic effects such as ptosis, cranial nerve involvement, progressive muscle weakness, or diaphragmatic involvement; or evidence of coagulopathy. Pertinent investigations include complete blood count, coagulation studies, serum electrolytes, renal function, creatine kinase levels, and urine testing for hematuria or myoglobinuria.[14] Abnormal renal or coagulation studies may provide laboratory evidence of systemic venom effect before neurotoxic effects are apparent. If prothrombin or activated partial thromboplastin times are prolonged, then levels of fibrinogen and fibrin degradation products should be obtained.

In the absence of clinical or laboratory evidence of venom effect, the elastic bandage should be removed and the patient observed for 12 h. Delayed envenomation after benign presentation has been documented, but most envenomated patients will develop clinical or laboratory evidence of envenomation within 2 h of removing a bandage.[13] Therefore, coagulation studies should be repeated 2 h after bandage removal and at intervals thereafter, depending on the patient's condition.

Five antivenom products, derived from equine IgG, are produced by CSL to treat envenomation by certain groups of terrestrial Australian snakes; these are termed monovalent antivenoms.[14] A polyvalent antivenom, also equine IgG, neutralizes the venom of all five major groups of dangerous Australian snakes.

If indicated, antivenom should be given immediately in sufficient doses to improve coagulation studies. A child should receive the same dose of antivenom as an adult.[14] Pregnancy is not a contraindication to antivenom therapy. Skin testing before antivenom administration is not recommended as it may sensitize the patient to future antivenom use and delays definitive therapy.[14] If the type of snake cannot be identified, usually two appropriate monovalent antivenoms may be selected by correlating the clinical presentation with knowledge of snakes found in the geographic area. Polyvalent antivenom is used in the following circumstances: (1) monovalent antivenom is not available; (2) the SVDK is not available or has failed to identify the type of snake and the range of possible snakes would require the mixing of three or more monovalent antivenoms; (3) the patient is severely envenomated, there is insufficient time to wait for SVDK results, and the range of possible snakes would require the mixing of three or more monovalent antivenoms; or (4) stocks of appropriate monovalent antivenom have been exhausted and the patient requires further antivenom treatment.[14]

Anaphylaxis is a rare complication of antivenom therapy in Australia perhaps because of the common practice of premedication with epinephrine, antihistamines and/or corticosteroids.[18–20] Nevertheless, patients should be treated in a setting where anaphylaxis can be managed. Premedication with a subcutaneous dose of 0.3 mL of 1:1000 epinephrine (adrenaline) in an adult or 0.1 mL in a child along with a parenteral antihistamine is not used universally but recommended by some authors.[19] Although prospective data are lacking, corticosteroids may have a role in premedication and prevention of serum sickness. Most treatment protocols dictate that patients with a history of allergy to equine proteins should receive corticosteroids. In addition, a 5-day course of prednisolone may be prescribed in an attempt to reduce the incidence of serum sickness in those patients who receive large doses of antivenom.[13]

COBRA BITE

Cobras are large snakes, typically 1 to 1.5 m in length, and indigenous to most of Africa and southern Asia.[21] Cobras adapt readily to different habits and can be found around villages and inhabited areas. The bold defensive posture cobras adopt, by elevating the head and spreading the beck, is not unique to this group of snakes. Not all cobra bites result in envenomation; perhaps as much as 45 percent are dry bites. Some species of cobras have the ability to spit jets of venom toward a victim, often hitting the eyes. The incidence of cobra bite and subsequent mortality is difficult to determine because of the lack of accurate reporting systems in most of Africa and southern Asia. In rural Congo, an annual incidence of 430 cobra bites per 100,000 population has been described. In Burma and India, an annual mortality incidence between 3 and 10 per 100,000 has been reported.

Pathophysiology

Cobra venom contains a mixture of toxins. In most cobras, neurotoxins in the venom pose the greatest threat to the victim. These neurotoxins bind to postsynaptic acetylcholine receptors and produce depolarizing neuromuscular blockade. A second group of toxins are cell membrane poisons that act in a general fashion, but their chief effect is on the heart, producing arrhythmias and impaired contractility. The third group of toxins contains enzymes that break down protein and connective tissue. These necrosis-producing toxins are typical of the venom from the spitting cobras (*Naja* spp.) of Africa, China, and Sumatra.

Clinical Features

Immediate pain at the bite site is almost always present. Other symptoms and signs are variable and can include local and progressive soft tissue swelling, cranial nerve dysfunction (ptosis, diplopia, dysphagia), generalized muscle weakness followed by flaccid paralysis, and parasympathetic stimulation (salivation, bronchorrhea, nausea, vomiting). Victims who were sprayed in the eye by a spitting cobra will describe pain, tearing, and blurred vision.

Signs include impaired sensorium (drowsiness), respiratory distress, hypotension, ptosis, ophthalmoplegia, and generalized weakness or paralysis. Reaction around the bite site may develop over 48 h with local hemorrhage, bullae, and necrosis. Venom spit into the eye will produce inflammation, edema, and discharge, but no systemic symptoms or signs. Coagulopathy is rare following a cobra bite, with the exception of a bite from a spitting cobra.

Diagnosis

Because of venom potency and size of the snake, a bite resulting in envenomation will usually produce obvious symptoms. The difficulty is distinguishing cobra envenomation from bites from other snakes that possess neurotoxic venom. When possible, the snake should be killed and brought in for identification. A variety of snake venom detection assays have been developed that can identify the offending snake with reasonable accuracy from wound aspirate or urine. The availability of these kits is, unfortunately, poor in most of Africa and Asia. Standard laboratory should be obtained with local or systemic signs of envenomation: complete blood count, serum electrolytes, creatinine, and coagulation tests.

Treatment

FIRST AID   Most common first aid measures have either no proven efficacy or increase toxicity. The pressure-immobilization technique used for Australian elapids has not proven beneficial with cobra bites. The proximal lymphatic- and venous-constricting elastic-band approach used in North American crotalines is probably more reasonable, although unproven. Incisions, vacuum extractors, cooling, or ice are not beneficial. The one first aid measure beneficial is prompt and copious irrigation of the eyes having sustained a venom exposure.

EMERGENCY TREATMENT   There is no correlation between local tissue damage and systemic toxicity, so grading systems based on bite site appearance should not be used. The only proven and specific therapy for cobra envenomation is antivenom.[22] Laboratories in Africa, Asia, and Europe have developed cobra antivenom; some products are monovalent, specific for a single species, but most are polyvalent, containing antibodies against several important or common cobra species in that country or region. The animal of origin varies, as does potency and purity. All cobra antivenoms should be considered experimental agents and a high incidence of allergic reactions should be anticipated.

If the patient has evidence of systemic toxicity on arrival to the hospital, antivenom should be started before the constricting band is loosened. For patients without signs of systemic toxicity, the constricting band should be loosened only after antivenom is available. Antivenom is effective at reducing systemic toxicity but does not reduce local tissue damage and necrosis.

For patients with significant muscle weakness or paralysis, a cholinesterase-inhibiting drug, such as edrophonium or neostigmine, may produce temporary benefit until antivenom is available.[23] Respiratory failure should be treated with endotracheal intubation and ventilation.[24] Hypotension is treated with intravenous fluids initially and followed by vasopressors if there is an inadequate response. Tetanus immunization should be provided as appropriate.

DISPOSITION   Patients without signs of envenomation should still be admitted for observation for 24 h. Death from cobra envenomation typically occurs 2 to 6 h after the bite. Survival is possible without antivenom treatment provided there is good respiratory and cardiovascular supportive care.[22,24] With prompt and appropriate antivenom and supportive pulmonary care, recovery from neurotoxicity is expected, but may take up to 6 days.

GILA MONSTER BITE

Gila monsters are slow-moving lizards that inhabit the desert in the southwestern United States. They possess venom as potent as rattlesnake venom but lack the apparatus to effectively inject it. Instead of fangs, they have short, grooved teeth down which their venom flows. Therefore, envenomation requires a prolonged bite. Gila monsters bite tenaciously and may be difficult to remove from the bitten extremity.

Most bites result in local pain and swelling only, which worsens over several hours and then subsides over several more hours. Dislodged teeth often contaminate the wound. Occasionally, a more severe syndrome of systemic toxicity develops, including weakness, light-headedness, paresthesia, and diaphoresis. Severe hypertension may occur, which also resolves over several hours. There are few if any documented deaths from Gila monster bite.

First aid involves removal of the reptile from the bite site without sustaining another bite. This may require force. It helps to place the animal on a solid surface; it often loosens its grip when it is no longer suspended in midair. Otherwise, standard local wound care is sufficient, taking care to remove any teeth in the wound. The usefulness of prophylactic antibiotics is unknown and tetanus status should be updated as appropriate.

REFERENCES

1. White J: Bites and stings from venomous animals: A global overview. *Ther Drug Monit* 22:65, 2000.
2. Gold BS, Dart RC, Barish RA: Bites of venomous snakes. *New Engl J Med* 347:347, 2002.
3. Langley RL, Morrow WE: Deaths resulting from animal attacks in the United States. *Wilderness Environ Med* 8:8, 1997.
4. Bush SP, Hegewald K, Green SM, et al: Effects of a negative pressure venom extraction device (Extractor) on local tissue injury after artificial rattlesnake envenomation in a porcine model. *Wilderness Environ Med* 11:180, 2000.
5. Burgess JL, Dart RC, Egen NB, Mayersohn M: The effects of constriction bands on rattlesnake venom absorption: A pharmacokinetic study. *Ann Emerg Med* 21:1086, 1992.
6. Dart RC, McNally J: Efficacy, safety, and use of snake antivenoms in the United States. *Ann Emerg Med* 37:181, 2001.
7. Ruha A-M, Curry SC, Beuhler M: Initial postmarketing experience with Crotalidae Polyvalent Immune Fab for treatment of rattlesnake envenomation. *Ann Emerg Med* 39:609, 2002.
8. Dart RC, Stark Y, Fulton B, et al: Insufficient stocking of poisoning antidotes in hospital emergency departments. *JAMA* 276:1508, 1996.
9. Offerman SR, Bush SP, Moynihan JA, Clark RF: Crotaline Fab antivenom for the treatment of children with rattle snake envenomation. *Pediatrics* 110:968, 2002.
10. Lee C, Ryan M, Arnold T: Local manifestations of *Agkistrodon contortrix* (copperhead) envenomation treated successfully with Crotalidae polyvalent immune Fab (ovine) Crofab [abstract #214]. *J Toxicol Clin Toxicol* 39:559, 2001.
11. Tagwireyi DD, Ball DE, Nhachi CF: Routine prophylactic antibiotic use in the management of snakebite. *BMC Clin Pharmacol* 1:4, 2001. (Medline: PMID 11710972)
12. Kitchens CS, Van Mierop LHS: Envenomation by the eastern coral snake (*Micrurus fulvius fulvius*): A study of 39 victims. *JAMA* 258:1615, 1987.
13. Sutherland SK, Leonard RL: Snakebite deaths in Australia 1992-1994 and a management update. *Med J Aust* 163:616, 1995.
14. White J: *CSL Antivenom Handbook.* Melbourne, Australia, CSL Ltd, 2001.
15. Sutherland SK: Deaths from snake bite in Australia, 1981–1991. *Med J Aust* 157:740, 1992.
16. Hawdon GM, Winkel KD: Could this be snakebite? *Aust Fam Physician* 26:1386–1394, 1997.
17. Howath DM, Southee AE, Whyte IM: Lymphatic flow rates and first-aid in simulated peripheral snake or spider envenomation. *Med J Aust* 161:695, 1994.
18. Sutherland SK: Antivenom use in Australia. Premedication, adverse reactions and the use of venom detection kits. *Med J Aust* 157:734, 1992.
19. Tibballs J: Premedication for snake antivenom. *Med J Aust* 160:4, 1994.
20. White J: Envenoming and antivenom use in Australia. *Toxicon* 36:1483, 1998.
21. Davidson TM, Schafer S, Killfoil J: Cobras. *Wilderness Environ Med* 6:203, 1995.

22. Pochanugool C, Limthongkul S, Wilde H: Management of Thai cobra bites with a single bolus of antivenin. *Wilderness Environ Med* 8:20, 1997.

23. Gold BS: Neostigmine for the treatment of neurotoxicity following envenomation by the Asiatic cobra. *Ann Emerg Med* 28:87, 1996.

24. Argrawal PN, Aggarwall AN, Gupta D, et al: Management of respiratory failure in severe neuroparalytic snake envenomation. *Neurol India* 49:25, 2001.

TRAUMA AND ENVENOMATIONS FROM MARINE FAUNA

Geoffrey K. Isbister
David G. Caldicott

Despite the fact that 71 percent of the surface of the earth is covered with water and half the population of the planet lives within 125 miles of the coast, the marine environment remained largely uncharted territory until the twentieth century, when technological innovation permitted closer exploration. Today, the underwater world is increasingly important for recreation, industry, and communications, with the inevitable consequence of increased exposure to marine fauna.

The marine environment is dangerous to humans for several reasons: we can't breathe, we can't see, and swimming must be learned. The marine environment is remote to points of definitive care. Marine fauna can inflict injury through trauma (often with infection) or envenomation. Many marine animals have developed venomous systems of defense and predation. Marine toxins can be extremely potent and knowledge of these toxins lags far behind that of their land-based equivalents. Consequently, the development of marine antivenoms is still in its infancy.

EPIDEMIOLOGY

There is little information on the epidemiology of marine injuries and envenomations.[1] A notable exception is the data collected by the International Shark Attack File, maintained by the Florida Museum of Natural History, Gainesville, Florida, U.S. It contains details of more than 3000 shark attacks, and this information is available to selected marine biologists and health care professionals.[2]

One U.S. study reviewed more than 6 years of aquatic animal exposures reported to poison information centers. The commonest exposures were jellyfish stings in 31 percent, stingrays in 16 percent, venomous fish stings in 28 percent (including lionfish, catfish, and others), and gastropods in 6 percent of cases.[3] However, these percentages are likely to be biased to more severe injuries, and do not include common minor injuries such as envenomation by *Physalia* spp., sea bathers eruption, and sea urchin stings. In the United States, thousands of cases of minor jellyfish stings occur yearly from *Physalia physalis* (Portuguese Man-of-War) and *Chrysaora* species.[4]

MARINE TRAUMA

Shark Attacks

Of the many animals that live in the sea, the shark is the species best equipped to inflict severe injuries. Sharks, along with skates and rays, make up the subclass Elasmobranchii of the class Chondrichthyes ("cartilaginous fishes"), so called because their skeletons are made completely of cartilage. They are an ancient class of fish, with many living species belonging to the same genera as species that swam in the cretaceous seas 100 million years ago. They have maintained this position as top-level predators. There are 373 species of shark, up to 80 of which are currently endangered, and 32 species have been described in attacks on humans.

Any shark that can grow larger than 1.8 m (6 ft) is potentially lethal to a man, but smaller sharks, if provoked, can inflict nasty injuries.[5] Certain species appear to be disposed to attacking humans. These include the white shark *(Carcharodon carcharias),* the tiger shark *(Galeocerdo cuvier),* and several members of the *Carcharhinus* spp. There are probably between 70 and 100 shark attacks in the world each year, with between 5 and 15 deaths.[2,6,7] The mortality of shark attacks has fallen from 40 percent in the 30 years following World War II to its current rates of approximately 10 to 20 percent.[6] Death is usually a result of lack of on-scene resuscitation, hemorrhagic shock, or drowning. Despite the public perception, the risk of shark attack is extremely small when compared with almost any other injury, and one is more likely to be killed driving to a beach than by a shark attack.

Three general types of unprovoked shark attack are described: (1) The hit-and-run attack, where the victim is seized and released, or slashed on an extremity, before the victim has any time to react, and often occurs in shallow water, accounts for approximately 80 percent of shark attacks; (2) sneak attacks, or the "out-of-the-blue" attack, usually involving divers or swimmers in deeper water; and (3) bump-and-bite attacks, where the shark circles and bumps the victim prior to attacking.[5,6] These last two types tend to occur in deeper water, are multiple and sustained, involve bigger sharks, and cause the majority of deaths by shark attack.

The direct traumatic effects of a shark attack are dependent upon the severity and nature of the attack, as well as the size and species of the shark. Sharks attack the appendages of their victims (be they seals or humans), which tend to dangle lower than heads and torsos while swimming on the surface. In 70 percent of surface swimmers, the lower limb only is involved. The upper limb can be subsequently injured when patients try to fend off their attacker. Sharks are unable to chew their prey, and so sequentially strip it.[6] In more serious, concerted attacks, substantial tissue loss and extremity amputation is common.

The two major concerns regarding shark attack injuries are (1) massive tissue injury with hemorrhagic shock, and (2) an extremely high incidence of atypical microorganisms that produce wound infections. The increased survival associated with shark attack is the result of improved training of first-responders and insight into early appropriate antibiotic usage. These same principles can be applied to any major marine trauma.

Patients may be exhausted, hypothermic, and near drowned. The patient should be removed from the surf, but only as far out of the water as is necessary to commence immediate resuscitation. Injuries should be treated with the same priorities and approach like any major trauma. Plain radiographs of all injured areas should be obtained, to identify fractures or periosteal stripping, and retained foreign bodies (e.g., particles of teeth) which can remain imbedded in bone and act as a future source of sepsis. Wounds should be swabbed and sent for culture. Abrasions and small punctures can be treated with thorough irrigation and topical antibiotics, but most injuries require debridement and treatment in an operating room. Devitalized tissue should be debrided, and copious irrigation should be used in cleaning the wounds. Plastic surgical procedures and repeat surgery is often required for many months after the initial attack.

Prophylactic antibiotics are currently recommended for all shark bites.[6] The choice of antibiotics should provide coverage for *Vibrio* spp., *Staphylococcus* spp., and *Streptococcus* spp. Abdominal injuries should receive coverage effective against enteric and anaerobic organisms.

Other Major Marine Trauma

Other marine creatures have been reported in attacks on humans, but more usually in defense of territory than for feeding purposes. The great barracuda *(Sphyraena barracuda)* is the only barracuda species implicated in human attacks.[7] Attacks are generally by solitary fish and occur only in tropical climes. Moray eels, found in tropical to temperate waters, can inflict severe puncture wounds or lacerations, commonly to the hands of inquisitive divers. Other marine vertebrates known to cause traumatic injuries to humans include giant groupers, sea lions, seals, crocodiles, alligators and piranhas. Some fish (needlefish, wahoos, and triggerfish) with sharp spines and fins can inadvertently injure humans. Wounds resulting from interactions with such creatures are a combination of crush injury, abrasion, puncture, and laceration. Treatment of such injuries is analogous to that of shark bites, with an emphasis on irrigation, removal of foreign bodies (e.g., teeth), and allowing adequate wound drainage (e.g., leaving puncture wounds open).

Minor Trauma

Coral cuts are probably the most common injuries sustained underwater, usually involving the hands, forearms, elbows, and knees. The initial reactions to a coral cut are stinging pain, erythema, and pruritus. Within minutes, the break in the skin may be surrounded by an erythematous wheal, which fades over 1 to 2 h. With or without treatment, the local reaction of red, raised welts and local pruritus may progress to cellulitis with ulceration and tissue sloughing. The wounds heal slowly over 3 to 6 weeks. In extreme cases, the victim develops cellulitis with lymphangitis, reactive bursitis, local ulceration, and wound necrosis. *Coral poisoning* usually refers to systemic malaise, fever, diarrhea, and general exhaustion associated with a wound from coral.

Coral cuts should be promptly and vigorously irrigated to remove all foreign matter. Any fragments that remain can become embedded and increase the risk of infection or foreign-body granuloma. If stinging is a major symptom, there may be envenomation by nematocysts. A brief rinse with dilute acetic acid (vinegar) or papain solution may diminish the discomfort. If a coral-induced laceration is severe, it should be closed with adhesive strips, rather than sutures, if possible. Sharp debridement each day for 3 to 4 days is recommended if the wound is deep. For superficial (no fat showing) wounds, use daily saline solution or dilute povidone-iodine wet-to-dry dressing changes, or apply a topical antiseptic under a nonadherent dressing.

Bacteriology of the Marine Environment and Antibiotic Therapy

The majority of infections from marine-associated wounds are from the normal skin commensals: *Staphylococcus aureus, S. epidermidis,* α- and β-hemolytic streptococci, and certain bacilli. However, microorganisms unique to seawater or freshwater can contaminate and infect wounds.[8] The severity of these infections can be exacerbated by toxins associated with stings or bites, mechanical trauma from larger vertebrate injuries, and potential compartment syndromes from extremity injuries that penetrate deeply into tight anatomic compartments. Organisms which cause infection are referred to as marine bacteria, and halophilic, gram-negative rods cause the majority of these marine-associated infections. The most common organisms involved are *Vibrio* spp. (especially *V. vulnificus,* nontoxigenic *V. cholerae, V. alginolyticus, V. parahaemolyticus,* and *V. hollisae*) *Aeromonas* spp. [*A. hydrophila], Erysipelothrix rhusiopathiae, Photobacterium damsela, Edwardsiella tarda, Shewanella putrefaciens,* and *Mycobacterium marinum.*[8] The natural habitat of marine organisms is warmer seawater that, along with the degree of human exposure, explains the geographic distributions of wound infections.

Marine-associated infections are often diagnosed late, the history of marine exposure or injury is poorly recalled, and patients are often initially managed with inappropriate antibiotics, potentially increasing morbidity of an already virulent infection. Certain patients with underlying conditions (hepatic impairment, immunosuppression, diabetes) are susceptible to halophilic vibrio infections.[9,10] Halophilic vibrio skin infections can develop extremely rapidly, from initial con-

tact and local painful inflammation, through subepidermal bullae containing hemorrhagic fluid and vasculitis, to necrosis and small vessel thrombosis, bacteremia, and septicemia.[9,10]

The management of infected marine injuries begins with meticulous wound care, including irrigation and debridement of devitalized tissue, with particular attention to retained foreign bodies, such as teeth, vegetable matter, and spines. In all but the most superficial of injuries, debridement should take place at the soonest opportunity, in an aseptic environment, preferably an operating room. Where the patient is stable, radiographs should be obtained to identify the nature and position of foreign bodies. Quantitative wound culture prior to the appearance of clinically evident wound infection has not been shown to be useful. Similarly, the issue of prophylactic antibiotics in the treatment of most marine wounds has not been well studied.

The priority for the management of infections from marine microorganisms is recognition that they are often more serious than other common soft tissue infections. Appropriate culture techniques should be employed. Many marine microorganisms require special selective media for culture and sensitivity testing, so the clinician should alert the microbiology laboratory that a marine-acquired organism might be present. Empirical antibiotic therapy should be initiated based on the clinical condition. The need for early treatment with antibiotics is well established in definite marine infections and at risk wounds or patients.[8–10]

The choice of antibiotic is less clear. Antibiotic sensitivities vary and there is considerable discrepancy between the in vitro antibiotic susceptibility data and the clinical outcomes. Many marine wound infections are polymicrobial, and the choice of antibiotics should reflect this. Because there are no evidence-based guidelines, recommendations are tentative (Table 196-1). For all marine-acquired infections, antibiotic coverage against staphylococcal and streptococcal species is necessary, because these organisms remain the most common causes of infection. In addition, for seawater-associated infections, coverage against *Vibrio* species with a third-generation cephalosporin or fluoroquinolone should be provided (Table 196-2). For freshwater-associated infections, a fluoroquinolone, third-generation cephalosporin, trimethoprim-sulfamethoxazole, or imipenem to cover *Aeromonas* spp. is appropriate (see Table 196-2).

There are several special clinical situations of note. A patient with rapidly progressive cellulitis, myositis, or necrotizing fasciitis warrants consideration of *V. parahaemolyticus* or *V. vulnificus* infection. *V. vulnificus* can also cause primary septicemia in chronically ill individuals, particularly those with hepatic disease.[8,9] *Aeromonas hydrophila* also causes wound infections that can rapidly progress to necrotizing

TABLE 196-1 Recommendations for Antibiotic Treatment of Marine-Associated Wounds

No Antibiotics Indicated	Prophylactic/ Outpatient Antibiotics	Hospital Admission for IV Antibiotics
Healthy patient	Late wound care	Predisposing medical conditions
Prompt wound care	Large lacerations/ injuries	Long delays before definitive wound care
No foreign body	Early or local inflammation	Deep wounds; significant trauma
No bone/joint involvement		Wounds with retained foreign bodies
Small or superficial injuries		Progressive inflammatory change
		Penetration of periosteum, joint space, or body cavity
		Major injuries associated with envenomation
		Systemic illness

TABLE 196-2   Antibiotics for Marine-Associated Wound Infections

For All: Staphylococci and Streptococci Coverage	Seawater-Associated: *Vibrio* spp. Coverage	Freshwater-Associated: *Aeromonas* spp. Coverage
First-generation cephalosporin (e.g., cefazolin), *or* Penicillinase-resistant penicillin (e.g., nafcillin)	Third-generation cephalosporin (e.g., ceftazidime), *or* Fluoroquinolone (e.g., ciprofloxacin)	Fluoroquinolone (e.g., ciprofloxacin), *or* Third-generation cephalosporin (e.g., ceftazidime), *or* Trimethoprim/ Sulfamethoxazole, *or* Imipenem

myositis. *Erysipelothrix rhusiopathiae* is the infectious agent in "fish-handler's disease," and causes sharply marginated, painful, expanding plaques on the fingers or hands following cutaneous inoculation. It is sensitive to penicillin, fluoroquinolones, and the cephalosporins.[8] *Mycobacterium marinum* is an acid-fast bacillus that causes "swimming-pool granuloma" or "aquarium granuloma." Some 3 to 4 weeks following an abrasion or puncture wound, the patient develops a red papule, which progresses to a cutaneous granuloma. Because of the delay between the infecting event and presentation, patients often don't make the link, further clouding the diagnosis. It is resistant to most penicillins and is uniformly resistant to isoniazid. Clarithromycin has been recommended initially, in combination with ethambutol or rifabutin for deep-seated infections.[8] It has also been suggested that treatment with heat lamps or hot water baths may be beneficial. In common with other mycobacterial infections, therapy can be protracted. Excision is sometimes preferred.

MARINE ENVENOMATIONS

Venomous marine animals produce venom in a specialized gland, which can then be applied or injected parenterally into other organisms using a specialized venom apparatus. This is in contrast to poisonous marine animals that may have special glands that produce toxic substances, but the animal lacks a particular apparatus to deliver these substances and the poisons have to be ingested to be effective.[1,4] Venom is not a pure substance but a mixture of mainly protein and peptide toxins. The effect of a specific toxin depends on its site of action; it may be neurotoxic, hematoxic, cytotoxic, or myotoxic. The toxins in marine venoms are usually heat labile, high-molecular-weight proteins, whereas marine poisons are usually heat and gastric-acid stable metabolic byproducts of lower molecular weight.[4]

INVERTEBRATE ENVENOMATIONS

Envenoming invertebrates are found in five phyla: Cnidaria (jellyfish), Porifera (sponges), Echinodermata, Mollusca (including octopus and cone snails), and Annelida.[1,4]

Cnidaria (Coelenterate)

The phylum Cnidaria (formerly named Coelenterate) is an enormous group of about 10,000 named species, at least 100 of which are dangerous to humans.[1,4] The phylum contains four classes: Hydrozoa, Scyphozoa, Cubozoa, and Anthozoa. Cnidariae are characterized by their unique stinging apparatus, referred to as the nematocyst.[11] These structures occur in the thousands, mainly on the tentacles of the jellyfish, but also in lesser numbers on the body or bell. The nematocysts contain a minute dose of venom, in some cases highly potent venom, and a harpoon like mechanism. A physical or chemical stimulus triggers the release of the hollow, sharply pointed threadlike tube from the contained nematocyst. This process is extremely rapid (thousandths of a second), and results in the threadlike tube penetrating the skin and delivering venom SC.

HYDROZOA   The class Hydrozoa includes the hydroids, millepora (fire corals), *Physalia* species (Portuguese man-of-war and bluebottle jellyfish), limnomedusae, and Gonionemus.[1,4] The Hydrozoa class has worldwide distribution.

The feather *hydroids* are the most numerous of the hydrozoans and are plumelike animals that sting the victim when they brush against or handle it. They have nematocysts on their arms and surfaces. They occur in tropical and temperate waters, and are often attached to wrecks and wharfs. Coastal storms can break off feather hydroid branches and infest a local swimming area. Contact with hydroids generally causes only minor problems. There is an immediate sting following even a superficial brush contact, followed by itching pain, associated with the development of painful wheals and urticaria after 30 min. The welts may last for up to a week, but leave no permanent mark. With more extensive exposure, blistering and a "hemorrhagic and zosteriform" reaction can occur. These crust over after a period of days. First aid is to blot the area carefully with a dry tissue. Vinegar has been shown to inhibit nematocyst discharge in *Lytocarpus philippinus,* but studies on other species are required.[1] Pain relief can be provided with ice packs or analgesia. Itching can be treated with topical steroids.

The *Millepora* species, or fire corals, are not true corals. They resemble hard corals except they are relatively smooth. Fire corals are widely distributed in shallow tropical waters and are often mistaken for seaweed because of their innocuous appearance.[1] Tiny nematocyst-bearing tentacles protrude from numerous minute surface gastropores. The clinical effects are similar to hydroids with immediate burning or stinging pain, with rare proximal radiation. Over the course of an hour or longer, initially small mosquito-bite-size marks progress to urticarial wheals. The pain generally resolves without treatment over 1 to 2 h and in most cases, there is no further reaction. Blistering is uncommon, although occasionally lesions may become infected. First aid and treatment is similar to hydroids and minor jellyfish stings, with drying the area, ice packs and topical steroids if required.

There are at least three important *Physalia* spp., although the taxonomy remains unclear. *P. physalis* are multitentacled hydrozoan colonies, rather than single jellyfish, and include the larger, more lethal Atlantic Portuguese man-of-war, and the smaller Pacific man-of-war, although these may be separate species. The third, *P. utriculus,* a single-tentacled variety, found commonly in Australia, is often referred to as the blue bottle.[1] *Physalia* spp. have a large gas-filled float, which suspends multiple tentacles that are as long as 30 m (100 ft) in Atlantic specimens. The nematocysts occur on the tentacles, but not on the float. *Physalia* spp. are the most widely distributed jellyfish and are responsible for thousands of human envenomations in Florida, parts of Asia and Africa, Australia, and Portugal.[3,4] All species occur in swarms in shallow water and usually cause stings in the surf or are washed up on the shore. Nematocysts from fractured tentacles may remain active for months.

Stings from *Physalia* species cause immediate, intense pain that often fades over an hour, but may persist for many hours, particularly with *P. physalis*. The sting causes a characteristic linear erythematous eruption.[12] Respiratory distress and death have been reported following *P. physalis* envenomation, but not from *P. utriculus*.[13] More serious delayed effects have been reported following *P. utriculus* stings.[1]

A number of other hydrozoans are of medical importance, including the genera *Gonionemus* and *Olindias*.[1] There are at least two *Gonionemus* spp. that cause envenomation, *G. oshoro* from Japan and *G. vertens* from the eastern Russian coast. Both cause a similar clinical syndrome. There is an initial sting and erythema at the sting site. After 15 to 20 min, victims develop severe pain in muscles, joints, abdomen, chest, and back, associated with nonspecific features such as weakness, fatigue and fever. In some cases, there are respiratory symptoms. The effects resolve over 2 days. The syndrome appears to be similar to the Irukandji syndrome seen in Australia (see below). A number of *Olindias* spp. have been reported to cause stings. The most important is *O. sambaquiensis,* which occurs in coastal waters off eastern South America, including Brazil, Uruguay, and Argentina. The clinical effects are similar to other hydrozoans, with immediate pain and white welts with surrounding erythema. The pain usually lasts hours, but the marks may take weeks to resolve.

SCYPHOZOA (TRUE JELLYFISH)   The class Scyphozoa, or true jellyfish, include a number of well-known and important groups: *Cyanea* spp. (hair jellyfish), *Catastylus* spp. (blubber jellyfish), *Chrysaora quinquecirrha* (sea nettle), the *Rhizostoma, Pelagia noctiluca* (mauve stinger), and *Linuche unguiculata* (thimble jellyfish).[1,4]

Sea nettles or *Chrysaora* species are found in tropical and temperate waters. Members of the best-known species *C. quinquecirrha* are abundant in the Chesapeake Bay of North America, but also South America, the Philippines, and Japan. Envenomation from *C. quinquecirrha* are similar to those from *Physalia* species.[12] Despite possibly millions of local stings annually, there are few reports of severe signs of reactions.[1]

Cyanea species, or hair jellyfish, may grow to enormous size and occur in open and colder oceans. They have numerous hairlike tentacles with nematocysts extending for meters under the bell. The sting causes only moderate pain with a localized red reaction that may persist and appears worse than the symptoms.[1]

Catostylus mosaicus, or the common blubber jellyfish, occurs mainly in the Indo-Pacific region. However, the blubber jellyfish is unlikely to cause more than a faint prickle so is not medically significant.[1]

Pelagia noctiluca, the mauve stinger or purple jellyfish, occurs in abundance in the Mediterranean where it is a common cause of sting, and is also well known in Australia. The sting usually causes immediate intense pain and blanching, followed by urticaria and edema. The pain usually subsides but localized vesicles, blistering, edema and itchiness may last longer. Recurrence of local lesions is reported and there has been one report of a near fatal anaphylactic reaction to a sting.[1,4]

Seabather's eruption, commonly referred to by the misnomer "sea lice," is a vesicular or morbilliform pruritic dermatitis resulting from contact with the planula larvae of *Linuche unguiculata,* of the class Scyphozoa.[4] It typically occurs within 24 h after saltwater exposure. The eruption primarily involves skin surfaces covered by bathing suits, swim caps, or fins. Divers may be afflicted on the neck when floating in water churned by boat propellers that have ground floating jellyfish into fragments. Dermatitis persists for 2 to 14 days and resolves spontaneously. Other symptoms, including headache, chills, pronounced nocturnal pruritus, malaise, conjunctivitis, and urethritis, are rare.

CUBOZOA (BOX JELLYFISH)   The class Cubozoa, or box jellyfish, is divided into two important orders: Chirodropidae, including the Indo-Pacific box jellyfish *(Chironex fleckeri),* and Carybdidae, typified by *Caruka barnesi,* an Australian jellyfish that causes Irukandji syndrome.[14,15] The Indo-Pacific chirodropids have some of the most potent venoms in existence. *C. fleckeri* is sometimes described as the world's most venomous animal.[14] It is found along the northern coast of Australia and has caused at least 65 fatalities in the past century. The exact mechanism of toxicity and toxins involved in this rapid death, often within 20 min, remains unclear, but a primary cardiotoxic role is postulated.[1] Severe reactions or death can occur following skin contact with tentacles in excess of 6 to 7 m, especially in children.[14] However, the vast majority of cases are mild to moderate and cause skin welts and immediate, sometimes severe pain.[14] The toxic skin reaction may be quite intense, with rapid formation of wheals, vesicles, and a darkened reddish-brown or purple whiplike flare pattern with

stripes of 8 to 10 mm in width. In more severe stings blistering occurs and superficial necrosis develops after 12 to 18 h. On occasion, a pathognomonic crosshatched pattern may be present. Following the acute toxic reaction, a delayed hypersensitivity reaction occurs in approximately 60 percent of cases with papular urticaria at the sting sites.[14] Other important chirodropids include *Chiropsalmus quadrigatus,* which has caused deaths in the Philippines and Japan.[1] Deaths have also been reported from *Chiropsalmus quadrumanus,* which is found along the U.S. Atlantic coast.[1] The Hawaiian box jellyfish *(Carybdea alata)* produces numerous stings to beachgoers in Hawaii, although no deaths have been confirmed from this organism.[16]

Although there are numerous Carybdidae, *Carukia barnesi* has been best characterized and is responsible for the systemic envenomation referred to as the Irukandji syndrome.[1,15] The sting initially causes mild local effects with localized pain and erythema. Approximately 20 to 30 min later, severe generalized pain in the abdomen, back, chest, head, and limbs develops. The pain is usually associated with other systemic features including tachycardia, hypertension, tachyarrhythmias, sweating, piloerection, and agitation. In severe cases, pulmonary edema occurs with myocardial depression.[1,15] Other carybdids include *Carybdea* spp. and morbakka types *(Tamoya virulenta).*[1]

ANTHOZOA   The class Anthozoa is the largest class of jellyfish and includes the sea anemones, stony (true) corals, and the soft corals. Anemones are common attractive seashore creatures often found in tidal pools, where the unwary may brush up against them or inquisitively touch them. They possess tentacles loaded with nematocysts.[1] There is considerable variation in the sting of anemones, but immediate localized pain of varying severity is usual. The skin may initially blanch and then wheal formation occurs with surrounding erythema. Pain may last hours and soreness for a number of days. Severe stings may lead to vesicle formation. Systemic effects are uncommon. Treatment is symptomatic, and there is currently no evidence to support the use of any type of decontamination.

Clinical Features of Jellyfish Stings

The clinical features of Cnidaria envenomation are similar across a wide spectrum of severity. The severity depends on the venom dose, the marine species, and the victim (age and size). Mild envenomation results in bothersome acute skin reactions, with immediate stinging pain and erythema or wheal formation at the site. This usually resolves spontaneously over days to a couple of weeks, with occasional postinflammatory hyperpigmentation. Anemones, *Physalia* species, and scyphozoans may cause moderate to severe envenomations compounded by systemic symptoms. These symptoms may appear immediately or within several hours. Severe envenomation occurs most commonly with cubozoan jellyfish. Chirodropids cause severe pain from local effects and rapidly life-threatening systemic envenomation. Cubozoan jellyfish have been associated with severe systemic envenomation seen with the Irukandji syndrome, and often with only minor local effects. Severe allergic reactions have been seen with a number of jellyfish, and fatalities have been seen after *Physalia* spp. envenomation.[13]

Management of Jellyfish Stings

Therapy consists of deactivation of attached nematocysts, reversal of venom effects if possible, and symptomatic and pain relief. All victims with systemic signs or symptoms should be observed for at least 8 h, because of ongoing envenomation or delayed reactions.

FIRST AID   Deactivation of attached nematocysts is important but controversial, because of locale-dependent variations in therapy. A generally accepted method is to immediately apply a topical decontaminant, if available, to putatively inactivate undischarged nematocysts.

Freshwater rinsing is not recommended because the hypotonic solution is thought to stimulate nematocyst discharge. After decontamination, visible tentacles can be removed with forceps or a double-gloved hand.

As a decontaminant, 5% acetic acid (vinegar) is the treatment of choice to inactivate most nematocysts and is absolutely indicated in the event of a sting from *Chironex* and *Lytocarpus*. An alternative therapy for most nematocysts is isopropyl alcohol (40 to 70 percent), although it is not recommended for *Chironex*. For *Chrysaora* or *Cyanea*, a slurry of baking soda (sodium bicarbonate) is effective. Pressure immobilization bandages are not recommended for any jellyfish envenomations, including box jellyfish, despite previous suggestions.[17]

The venoms are heat labile, and despite previous advice to apply cold packs, research studies suggest heat may reduce toxicity and lethality.[16] In addition, a controlled trial of the sting from *Carybdea alata* found hot water immersion of the affected site more efficacious.[17] Some lifeguards report that a victim of a *Physalia* sting may find relief from being showered with a forceful stream of water, which implies that the mechanical removal of nematocysts may help.

TREATMENT   Symptomatic treatment is often all the treatment that is required with minor stings. Either topical anesthetics or systemic analgesia should be used. Prophylactic antibiotics are not required, but standard tetanus prophylaxis and diligent wound care should be carried out. The vast majority of jellyfish stings are not seen in EDs.

In general, only severe *Physalia* and box jellyfish stings will result in rapid decompensation. Treatment for severe *Chironex* envenomation consists of standard resuscitative measures and sheep-derived antivenom specific for *C. fleckeri* [Commonwealth Serum Laboratories (CSL) Ltd, Melbourne, Australia].[18] Pain may be severe and require opioid analgesia. Corneal envenomations can be irrigated with an isotonic solution and treated judiciously with topical steroids.

Porifera (The Sponges)

The phylum *Porifera* contains thousands of species of sponges that are composed of horny but elastic skeletons. Embedded in the connective tissue matrices are spicules of silicon dioxide or calcium carbonate. A number of sponges produce crinotoxins (slimes or surface liquids) that cause skin irritation and dermatitis referred to as stinging sponge dermatitis.[1,4] The condition is possibly worsened by embedded spicules from the sponges. There is little evidence to suggest that hypersensitivity or allergy plays a role in this dermatitis, although patch testing has produced anaphylactoid reactions.

The clinical features of sponge injuries are variable and usually referred to as stinging sponge dermatitis. Often there is no initial sensation following contact with the sponge, but after a few minutes to hours an itching or burning sensation develops. The stinging or itching sensation usually increases in intensity over 2 to 3 days, and may become almost unbearable. The effects are usually confined to the area of contact or just adjacent. There may be associated local joint stiffness, and an acute inflammatory reaction with erythema and edema develops when symptoms are severe. Untreated mild reactions subside over 3 to 7 days. Papules, vesicles and bullae may develop in some cases, followed by desquamation of the area days to weeks later. A case of erythema multiforme has been reported 10 days after initial contact. Direct eye contact or contamination of the eyes with the fingers, can cause corneal injury or iritis. Plaques and postinflammatory pigmentation may last for months and recurrent eczema and persistent arthralgias are rare complications.

The literature suggests that most sponge injuries will run their natural course, despite various first aid and medical interventions.[4] Spicules should be removed, if possible, using fine forceps, although some suggest adhesive tape. The area should be washed as soon as possible. Cold water compresses can be applied, which may reduce the

local symptoms. Although topical steroids may help to relieve secondary inflammation, they have not been found to be useful early in the treatment. Similarly topical antihistamines have also not been helpful. Pain relief with either oral or parenteral analgesia is indicated. Delayed primary therapy or inadequate decontamination may result in the persistence of bullae. Severe inflammatory reactions may be treated with systemic glucocorticoids. Severe itching may be controlled with an antihistamine.

The condition referred to as Mediterranean sponge diver disease is caused by contact with coinhabiting sea anemone on the sponge, resulting in an irritating skin rash, not as a direct result of sponge crinotoxins.

Echinodermata

The phylum Echinodermata is characterized by organisms that have penta-numerous (five parts) radial symmetry. There are two classes that contain venomous species, Asteroidea (sea stars or starfish) and Echinoidea (sea urchins). Organisms in other classes, such as Holothuroidea (sea cucumbers) contain poisons, but no venom apparatus.[1]

Sea urchins are found in all oceans. They have a globular, sometimes flattened body shape, with numerous short and long spines attached to the body shell.[4] The majority of sea urchins have solid (nontoxic) spines, and injury from these causes localized pain from cutaneous puncture or as the spines break off into the wound. The venom apparatuses of venomous sea urchins range from short sharp spines with venom glands on their tips (*Asthenosoma* spp.), to longer and hollow spines that can inject venom (*Diadema* spp.), to the triple-jawed pedicellariae (mobile grasping organs) of some other species. Contact with the venomous spines causes immediate, intense burning pain, with erythema, swelling, and often bleeding of the skin surrounding the puncture sites. The pain usually exceeds that produced by the mechanical injury, supporting the involvement of venom. The pain usually subsides over hours, but the area remains tender for a longer period of time.[1] Frequently, venomous spines break off and lodge in the victim. If a spine enters a joint, it may rapidly induce severe synovitis. Wounds from black sea urchin spines may leave a black discoloration of the skin. Secondary infection and granuloma formation from remaining spine fragments are well-described delayed effects. Systemic features have been reported, often if multiple spines are involved and may include nausea, vomiting, paresthesias, muscular paralysis, hypotension, and respiratory distress.[1] Pedicellariae can cause more severe pain and other clinical effects, predominantly neurologic.

The majority of sea stars are unlikely to cause medically significant injuries, except the crown-of-thorns sea star, *Acanthaster planci*. Crown-of-thorns sea stars are found on most reefs in the Indo-Pacific region, and have caused outbreaks in Japan and in Australia.[1] These creatures are covered with sharp, rigid spines that can passively deliver a variety of substances when they penetrate skin. This includes venom produced in special glandular tissue, mucous, bacteria and dermal tissue. Injury by the spines causes severe burning pain, often greater than expected for the mechanical injury, and lasts 1 to 2 h. Other local effects include bleeding, erythema and mild edema. In more severe cases, particularly with multiple puncture wounds the wound may become dusky or discolored. Pruritus and persisting edema can occur; perhaps as a result of allergy. Systemic effects are uncommon but may include paresthesias, nausea, vomiting, lymphadenopathy, and muscular paralysis.[1,4]

Sea cucumbers (Holothuroidea) produce a toxin that is concentrated in the tentacular organs. Direct contact may induce a contact dermatitis, which is usually mild, because the venom is diluted in seawater. The greater risk is to the corneas and conjunctivae, which may become intensely inflamed.

First aid for echinoderm wounds consists of immediate immersion in hot water to tolerance [45°C (113°F)] for 30 to 90 min or until there is significant pain relief. Prompt removal of pedicellariae and spines, especially those in intraarticular areas, is necessary but not always possible without proper imaging. Soft-tissue radiographs or magnetic resonance imaging are helpful in locating retained spines. Bolus injection of local anesthetics has also be used to remove spines to avoid surgical debridement.[19] Treatment of systemic symptoms is supportive, and analgesia may be needed. Delayed granuloma formation may require excision.

Annelida

The phylum Annelida contains the fireworms, or bristleworms, which are segmented worms covered with cactus-like bristles that can penetrate the skin.[1,4] These bristles easily detach in the skin and can be difficult to remove. Envenomation causes intense inflammation with a burning sensation and erythema. Untreated, the pain generally resolves within a few hours, but erythema may last for 2 to 3 days. Bristles should be removed with forceps or adhesive tape, and topical vinegar or isopropyl alcohol may be applied. The inflammatory response may require a course of corticosteroids.

Mollusca

The phylum Mollusca contains two envenomating classes: the gastropods (cone snails and nudibranchs) and the cephalopods (octopuses).[1,4] Cone snail shells are beautiful, univalve creatures found in shallow Indo-Pacific waters. They are predators that feed by injecting a potent mixture of neurotoxins using detachable, dart-like, radicular teeth. Stings by cone snails are rare, with few published cases in the literature. Most cases are caused by *Conus geographus* although other *Conus* spp. are implicated.[4] Most cases occur following prolonged contact with the shell, or if there is significant interference with the creature such as breaking the shell. The sting causes pain, usually similar to a bee or wasp sting. With significant envenomation, local pain is followed immediately by local numbness, which quickly spreads from the extremity to the trunk then face and throat. Partial paralysis develops within 30 min, progressing to complete voluntary muscle paralysis, respiratory failure and unconsciousness. Less-severe cases cause muscle pain, partial paralysis or ataxia, or in mild cases only local effects. Treatment is supportive and there is no specific antidote or antivenom.

The bite of the Australian blue-ringed octopus (*Hapalochlaena* spp.) causes small puncture marks. The octopus can inject tetrodotoxin, which it stores in modified venom glands. Octopus bites typically occur on the upper extremity almost always when the animal is picked up. Pain is often absent, and generalized paresthesia may be the first indication of envenomation. Further neurologic effects may develop, with flaccid paralysis progressing to ventilatory failure typical of tetrodotoxin poisoning.[4] Treatment is supportive, with mechanical ventilation as required, and full recovery is usual. No antivenom is available.

For both cone snail shell and paralytic octopus envenomations, the most commonly recommended first aid technique is pressure-immobilization, done by wrapping the limb with a lymphatic occlusive bandage and then applying a splint. The wrap is maintained until the victim is brought to a medical facility where advanced life support can be provided.

VERTEBRATE ENVENOMATIONS

The most common and important marine vertebrates to cause envenomation are stingrays, venomous fish, and sea snakes. The first two have venomous spines that cause both mechanical trauma and introduce venom into the wound as the spine sheath is ruptured upon penetration. Sea snakes have fangs and inject venom in a manner similar to terrestrial snakes.

Stingrays (Order Rajiformes)

All stingrays have a characteristic dorsoventrally flattened appearance with pectoral flaps (fins) they use for propulsion. They have a whip like tail, which houses the venomous spines.[1] When not swimming, these creatures rest on the bottom and may become buried in the sand. When an unwary human treads on a stingray, the tail reflexively whips upward and accurately thrusts the spines into the victim. This produces a puncture wound or jagged laceration and simultaneously allows the injection of venom. Most injuries occur to the lower limb from stepping on the stingray in shallow water, although injuries occur to the hands when they are caught, or divers may sustain injuries to the torso. Rarely, the spine tip breaks off and remains in the wound. Envenomation causes immediate local intense pain and variable bleeding depending on the site of injury. The pain may radiate proximally, and may last for many hours. There is often significant bleeding and the wound may be erythematous or dusky. Systemic effects have been uncommonly reported and related more to the systemic response to severe pain.

The length and size of stingray spines result in an increased risk of significant trauma and secondary infection. Morbidity and mortality can result from penetrating trauma to the trunk and internal organs, and both penetrating cardiac injuries and abdominal injuries have been reported.[1,20] The other important problem is secondary infection, mainly a concern for patients susceptible to infections, or wounds penetrating joint or tendon spaces, or wounds that are not cleaned and managed appropriately.

A number of different families of rays have been implicated in human injuries. In temperate regions, Urolophidae (stingarees) are commonly implicated, including Australia and the West coast of the United States. The family dasyatididae (stingrays, whiprays) are another important family in tropical regions, including northern Australia and the southeast coast of the United States.

Venomous Fish Stings

Venomous fish are found in tropical and, less commonly, temperate oceans, although increasing numbers are being kept in private aquariums. The important venomous fish include catfish (Siluriformes), stonefish (Synaceiidae), weeverfish (Trachinidae), and scorpion and lion fish (Scorpaenidae). The effects of the stings range in severity from severe with stonefish, to minimal from some types of catfish and other fish with nonvenomous spines.[1,20]

STONEFISH (*SYNACEIA* SPP.) Stonefish belong to the family Synanceiidae, in which there are a number of stinging fish in the genus *Synanceia,* the Australian estuarine stonefish *Synanceia trachynis, S. horrida* (Indian stonefish), and *S. verrucosa* (reef stonefish). Stonefish occur throughout tropical and warmer temperate oceans from the central Pacific, west through the Indo-Pacific to the east African coastline. Stonefish are stationary bottom-dwellers usually frequenting shallow water. They can camouflage themselves effectively, and most encounters with humans occur when they are stepped upon.

Despite the presence of myotoxic, neurotoxic and cardiotoxic components in *S. trachynis* venom, these are not important parts of the clinical effects of stonefish envenomation. Human envenomation following penetration of stonefish spine is characterized by immediate severe and increasing local pain, which may radiate proximally. The wound site usually has significant local edema and erythema.[1,20] Nonspecific systemic effects, such as sweating, nausea, hypotension, and even syncope, may occur but are more likely a result of severe pain. Despite the severe local pain and swelling, extensive tissue necrosis is not seen unless a secondary infection develops.[1]

SCORPIONFISH AND ROCKFISH (SCORPAENIDAE) Scorpion fish (Scorpaenidae) occur in all oceans of the world, but more commonly in tropical and temperate regions. At least 80 members of the family have been implicated in envenomation. Some important genera include *Pterois* spp. and *Dendrochirus* spp., the best-known species being *Pterois volitans,* the lionfish or butterfly cod. Other important ones include *Scorpaena* spp.(scorpionfish) and the bullrout *(Notesthes robusta).* They are a diverse group of fish, with differing habitats, swimming patterns, and ability to camouflage.[1] Their venom apparatus varies between species, but most have 10 to 15 dorsal spines, as well as 2 pelvic and 3 anal spines associated with venom glands. Although they are frequently large, plumelike, and ornate, the pectoral spines are not associated with venom glands.

The clinical effects are similar to stingray and stonefish envenomation, but there is usually less trauma. There is immediate and intense pain, which often radiates proximally. Untreated, the pain peaks at 60 to 90 min and persists for 4 to 6 h, but this varies considerably for different fish. There is often associated erythema and edema, and in more severe cases, there may be local discoloration and necrosis. Systemic effects are variable, but again probably relate more to the severity of pain, rather than toxin effects.

CATFISH (SILURIFORMES)   Approximately 1000 species of catfish inhabit both fresh and saltwater. Catfish have a single dorsal spine and two pectoral spines that can inflict painful wounds. The spines have venom glands within the integumentary sheath covering, which rupture and the contents are forced into the wound. Catfish also produce a crinotoxin that can be introduced into the wound during envenomation and can occasionally cause severe pain in fish handlers by merely coming in contact with the fish.[1]

Eel-tailed catfish (Plotosidae) occur in the Indo-Pacific region and live in marine, estuarine and freshwater enviroments. The striped catfish, *Plotosus lineatus,* is an important member of this family and can cause severe pain requiring hospitalization.[1,20] Other commonly reported catfish are the forktailed catfish (Ariidae), that occur worldwide and are reported to cause minor effects only. Other families have a more restricted distribution such as the family Ictaluridae, which includes the common freshwater catfish in the United States, also responsible for serious envenomations. Siluridae occur throughout Europe and Asia and cause injuries in these regions.[20]

WEEVERFISH (TRACHINIDAE)   Weeverfish (or Weaver fish) are all seawater fish and are the most venomous fish in the temperate zone. They are found in the Mediterranean and European coastal areas, and include the greater weeverfish *(Trachinus draco)* and the lesser weeverfish *(T. vipera* or *Echilchthys).* Weeverfish are bottom dwellers that sting when stepped on. The five to seven envenoming dorsal spines can penetrate a leather boot and create a substantial puncture wound. The pain from a weeverfish wound is described as being as severe as a stone fish injury, and is reported to be prone to necrosis.[1]

OTHER VENOMOUS FISH   There are a number of other groups of venomous fish. Scats (family Scatophagidae) are a less-well-known cause of envenomation. They occur in the Indo-Pacific Ocean, and there are a few reports of stings from northern Australia.[20] The most common species, the silver scat, striped butterfish or spadefish *(Selenotoca multifasciata)* causes immediate severe pain that lasts about 30 to 60 min, and has minimal local effects. Scats have become popular aquarium fish, particularly in the United States.[20] Another group of venomous fish are the family Siganidae (rabbitfish or happy moments). These fish occur in the tropical regions of the Indo-Pacific ocean. *Siganus* spp. are reported to cause severe pain that may last hours.[1]

Management of Venomous Fish and Stingray Injuries

Successful therapy for venomous fish stings requires managing both the traumatic injury and the envenomation. Treatment is directed at reversing the effects of venom, alleviating pain, and preventing infec-

tion. The wound should be irrigated immediately, and any visible pieces of the spine or integumentary sheath should be removed. Other first aid measures include control of any bleeding and hot water immersion therapy. Hot-water immersion should be done as soon as possible, using hot water to tolerance [45°C (113°F)] for 30 to 90 min or until there is pain relief. During the hot-water soak, the wound can be explored and foreign material removed.

Medical management should include first aid measures. If the pain does not respond to hot-water immersion, then oral, or more often parenteral, analgesia is required. However, local infiltration of the wound with local anesthetic without epinephrine, or a regional nerve block may be more effective.

There remains no consensus on the treatment of wounds following venomous fish stings. Once the pain is controlled the wound can be cleaned using an aseptic technique, reexplored, any foreign material removed, and débrided if there is necrotic tissue. Soft tissue radiography should be employed to visualize calcified matter. Lacerations, more often caused by stingrays, should generally be left open for delayed primary closure or sutured loosely, ensuring adequate drainage. Some authors suggest exploration and even excision of the wound to remove all foreign material.[1] Puncture wounds, usually from other venomous fish, uncommonly require exploration, but there is little evidence to support this approach.

There continues to be controversy regarding prophylactic antibiotics. The few series of venomous fish stings, and the experience of aquarium workers, is that most injuries are minor and do not require antibiotics.[20] Although some authors routinely recommend prophylactic antibiotics, the majority do not unless the wound is large or there is considerable foreign material. This is more likely in stingray wounds that have the greatest potential to cause necrosis and infection. Prevention of infection by careful cleaning of the wound and debridement, if required, are more important. A stonefish antivenom (CSL Ltd, Melbourne, Australia) is available for severe systemic reactions to stonefish and possibly other venomous fish.[1]

Sea Snakes

There are numerous species of sea snakes that are closely related to Asian and Australian elapids, all of which are venomous. They occur in the tropical and warm temperate Pacific and Indian Oceans. None are found in the Atlantic Ocean, the Caribbean, or North American coastal waters, except Hawaii. Probably the most important species is the beaked sea snake *(Enhydrina schistosa),* which has caused fatalities in southeast Asia.[4]

Most sea snakes are about 1 m (3 to 4 ft) long, although some attain lengths of up to 3 m (9 ft). They can be distinguished from land snakes by their flat tails and valvelike nostril flaps, and from eels by the presence of scales and the absence of gills and fins. Sea snakes swim in an undulating fashion and can move backward or forward in the water with equal speed. The venom apparatus consists of two to four short, hollow maxillary fangs, and a pair of associated venom glands.[1] About 20 percent of bites cause significant envenomation and up to 40 percent of these can be fatal.[4] The venom of sea snakes contains neurotoxins and myotoxins; one tends to dominate the clinical features. However, there are no toxins that affect coagulation.[1]

There is usually no pain from the bite, and it may initially go unnoticed. Symptoms typically become apparent 30 min to 4 h after the bite. The first complaint is usually because of myotoxicity, which causes muscle aches and pains, and nonspecific muscle weakness. Other symptoms include nausea, vomiting, malaise, and tachycardia. Myalgias usually occur in the neck, face, trunk, arm, and thigh. The muscle pain may become so severe that movement is limited, which is typified by trismus that develops in the jaw. Immobility secondary to pain should be distinguished from weakness or paralysis caused by neurotoxicity.[1] In some sea snakes, neurotoxicity has been reported, with ascending flaccid or spastic paralysis accompanied by ophthalmoplegia, ptosis, facial paralysis, and pupillary changes. Death is most commonly a result of ventilatory failure.

Diagnosis of a sea snake bite is based on the combination of snake identification and the presence of a puncture bite wound that was initially painless and occurred in the water. Envenomation should be suspected if the characteristic symptoms, primarily myalgias, develop. The presence of myoglobinuria and an elevated creatine kinase is also typical, indicating rhabdomyolysis. Neurotoxic symptoms are rapid in onset and usually appear within 2 to 3 h. If no symptoms develop by 6 to 8 h, envenomation is unlikely to have occurred.

First aid treatment of a sea snake bite involves pressure-immobilization of the affected limb. Supportive measures are essential, but the most effective treatment is sea snake antivenom if available. Polyvalent sea snake antivenom (CSL Ltd, Melbourne, Australia) is indicated if there is any evidence of systemic envenomation. Although tiger snake (*Notechis* spp.) antivenom and crotalid antivenom have been recommended, there is no evidence of cross-reactivity. The responses in the past to tiger snake antivenom were more likely a result of antivenom being made from animals immunized to both tiger and sea snake venom. The administration of antivenom should commence as soon as possible. Intensive supportive care and monitoring of renal, metabolic, and respiratory functions are critical.

REFERENCES

1. Williamson JA, Fenner PJ, Burnett JW, Rifkin JF (eds): *Venomous and Poisonous Marine Animals.* Sydney, Australia, University of New South Wales Press, 1996.
2. International Shark Attack File (ISAF). http://www.flmnh.ufl.edu/fish/Sharks/ISAF/ISAF.htm. 2002. (Accessed April 24, 2003.)
3. Hanley M, Tomaszewski C, Kerns W: The epidemiology of aquatic envenomations in the US: Most common symptoms and animals [abstract]. *J Toxicol Clin Toxicol* 38:512, 2000.
4. Meier J, White J: *Handbook of Clinical Toxicology of Animal Venoms and Poisons.* Boca Raton, FL, CRC Press, 1995.
5. Baldridge HD, Williams J: Shark attack: Feeding or fighting? *Mil Med* 134:130, 1969.
6. Caldicott DG, Mahajani R, Kuhn M: The anatomy of a shark attack: A case report and review of the literature. *Injury* 32:445, 2001.
7. Burgess GH, Callahan MT, Howard RJ: Sharks, alligators, barracudas, and other biting animals in Florida waters. *J Fla Med Assoc* 84:428, 1997.
8. Lehane L, Rawlin GT: Topically acquired bacterial zoonoses from fish: A review. *Med J Aust* 173:256, 2000.
9. Strom MS, Paranjpye RN: Epidemiology and pathogenesis of *Vibrio vulnificus. Microbes Infect* 2:177, 2000.
10. Upton A, Taylor S: *Vibrio vulnificus* necrotising fasciits and septicaemia. *N Z Med J* 115:108, 2002.
11. Lotan A, Fishman L, Zlotkin E: Toxin compartmentation and delivery in the Cnidaria: The nematocyst's tubule as a multiheaded poisonous arrow. *J Exp Zool* 275:444, 1996.
12. Burnett JW, Calton GJ: Jellyfish envenomation syndromes updated. *Ann Emerg Med* 16:1000, 1987.
13. Stein MR, Marraccini JV, Rothschild NE, Burnett JW: Fatal Portuguese man-o'-war *(Physalia physalis)* envenomation. *Ann Emerg Med* 18:312, 1989.
14. O'Reilly GM, Isbister GK, Lawrie PM, et al: Prospective study of jellyfish stings from tropical Australia, including the major box jellyfish *Chironex fleckeri. Med J Aust* 175:652, 2001.
15. Little M, Mulcahy RF: A year's experience of Irukandji envenomation in far north Queensland. *Med J Aust* 169:638, 1998.
16. Carrette TJ, Cullen P, Little M, et al: Temperature effects on box jellyfish venom: A possible treatment for envenomed patients? *Med J Aust* 177:654, 2002.
17. Nomura JT, Sato RL, Ahern RM, et al: A randomized paired comparison trial of cutaneous treatments for acute jellyfish *(Carybdea alata)* stings. *Am J Emerg Med* 20:624, 2002.
18. Bailey PM, Little M, Jelinek GA, Wilre JA: Jelly fish envenoming syndromes: Unknown toxic mechanisms and unproven therapies. *Med J Aust* 178:34, 2003.
19. Burnett JW: Bolus ejection: A method for removing sea urchin spines. *Ann Emerg Med* 39:94, 2002.
20. Isbister GK: Venomous fish stings in tropical northern Australia. *Am J Emerg Med* 19:561, 2001.

DYSBARISM AND COMPLICATIONS OF DIVING

Brian Snyder
Tom Neuman

Millions of recreational, commercial, and scientific dives are logged annually, and the vast majority of dives are completed without incident. However, there are physiologic effects and injuries relatively unique to the underwater environment. Generally, these effects and injuries are secondary to pressure changes on the submerged human body and the breathing of compressed gas.[1] This chapter will outline the most common diving injuries: barotrauma (otic, sinus, and pulmonary), decompression sickness ("the bends"), immersion pulmonary edema, oxygen toxicity, and nitrogen narcosis.

THE GAS LAWS

Understanding of diving injuries requires familiarity with the three relevant gas laws most pertinent to diving: Boyle's law, Dalton's law, and Henry's law.

Boyle's law states that given a constant temperature, the pressure and volume of an ideal gas are inversely related. That is, if pressure is doubled, the volume of gas is halved. This law is stated as: $P_1V_1 = P_2V_2$.

Pressure can be measured in a variety of units. The International System of Units defines pressure using the pascal (Pa). Other commonly used units of pressure include millimeters mercury (mm Hg), torr, pounds per square inch (psi), bar, or atmosphere (atm). 1 atm = 760 mm Hg = 760 torr = 14.7 psi = 1.013 bar = 101,325 Pa = 101.325 kPa. Additionally, pressure in diving settings is often described using feet of seawater (fsw) or meters of seawater (msw) (see below). In this chapter we will use atmospheres, mm Hg, and fsw for pressure units.

Because of the high density of water, a relatively small change in depth causes a great change in the pressure exerted on a body. The weight of seawater produces a change of 1 atm for each 33 ft of depth. For freshwater, pressure increases 1 atm for each 34 ft of depth. Therefore the pressure exerted on a diver at a depth of 33 ft in seawater = 1 atm for the seawater + 1 atm for the atmosphere above the water = 2 atmospheres absolute (ATA). A diver at 165 ft of seawater would experience 6 ATA of pressure (1 atm for each 33 ft of seawater = 5 atm + 1 atm for atmospheric pressure at sea level).

Thus Boyle's law dictates that as a diver descends in the water column, the volume of air-containing structures will decrease. For example, if the lungs contain volume V at the surface, a diver who descends to 33 ft of seawater holding his or her breath would have a lung volume of $1/2V$. If he or she breathes compressed air at this depth (from scuba equipment or from a surface-supplied source of gas), lung volume would return to V. If the diver then ascends to the surface without exhaling, lung volume would be $2V$ at the surface. This pressure-volume relationship governed by Boyle's law is important in the etiology of injuries due to barotrauma and produces the volume changes of bubbles in the tissues and circulation that are associated with recompression therapy.

Dalton's law states that the total pressure exerted by a mixture of gases is the sum of the partial pressures of each gas. Therefore, the partial pressure of a given component of a gas mixture will increase as the ambient pressure increases, although the proportion of gas in the mixture remains constant. The partial pressure of nitrogen in air at sea level is approximately 600 mm Hg or 0.79 ATA (the fraction of nitrogen in air, 0.79, times 760 mm Hg or 1 ATA). At a depth of 99 fsw, the partial pressure of nitrogen in air would be 4 × 600 = 2400 mm Hg (or 3.16 ATA).

Henry's law, which states that at equilibrium, the quantity of a gas in solution in a liquid is proportional to the partial pressure of the gas, along with Dalton's law explains the uptake of inert gas into tissues when breathing compressed air at depth. It is the uptake of inert gas that is intrinsic to the development of decompression sickness.

BAROTRAUMA

Barotrauma of Descent

During descent, the volume of gas in all air-containing body cavities decreases. The air space in the middle ear makes the tympanic membrane the tissue most commonly affected by this phenomenon, if active measures such as "clearing the ears" with a Valsalva or other maneuvers are not successful.[2] As the volume of gas decreases, the tympanic membrane is bent inward, causing a feeling of fullness or pain in the ear. Forcing air through the eustachian tube with a Valsalva maneuver will equalize the pressure between the middle ear and external ear canal by filling the middle ear with additional gas. Generally, divers who experience pain in an ear during descent will attempt to clear the ear and, if unsuccessful, will ascend to decrease the pressure difference and attempt equalizing again. If the diver is unsuccessful in equalizing and continues the descent, prolonged pain and injury to the tympanic membrane may result, known as barotitis or "ear squeeze."

Barotitis can range from symptoms of pain or fullness without otoscopic changes, to hemorrhage within the tympanic membrane or hemorrhage into the middle ear with hemotympanum. Ultimately, the tympanic membrane may rupture, resulting in relief of the pain, but which might also cause an influx of water into the middle ear. This in turn might cause calorically-induced vertigo and potential panic, near-drowning, or other injury. Barotitis is treated conservatively with analgesics and decongestants. If tympanic membrane rupture occurs, antibiotics can be prescribed, especially if the diving occurred in contaminated water. Divers with perforated tympanic membranes should refrain from diving until the perforation heals. Most such perforations heal without difficulty, but referral to an otolaryngologist is appropriate for individuals with larger perforations or when healing does not occur spontaneously. Divers with barotitis without perforation should refrain from diving until symptoms have resolved and the diver is again able to insufflate the middle ear.

If the external canal is occluded by cerumen or an ear plug, the inability to equalize pressure between the external canal and the tympanic membrane causes the bending of the tympanic membrane outward, producing an injury called "external ear squeeze" that produces pain and tympanic membrane hemorrhage.

If the ostia to the sinuses are occluded, air cannot enter the sinuses during descent to equalize the increasing pressure. This causes pain and mucosal edema and can lead to submucosal hemorrhage and stripping of the sinus mucosa from bone, hemorrhage (often causing bleeding from the nose into the mask), and rarely paresthesias in the infraorbital nerve distribution. Sinus barotrauma is treated with conservative measures, including decongestants and possibly antibiotics.

The inner ear is also susceptible to barotrauma, occasionally causing significant, long-term damage. If a diver attempts a forceful Valsalva maneuver to equalize the middle ear against an occluded eustachian tube, the pressure differential between the cerebrospinal fluid (CSF), transmitted through the vestibular and cochlear structures, and the middle ear air space can cause rupture of the oval or round window, fistulization of the window, tearing of Reissner membrane, or a combination of such injuries. Additionally, if the diver is able to open the eustachian tube in this situation, a rapid increase in middle ear pressure may occur. This pressure wave is transmitted to the inner ear and can also cause a similar injury. Divers with inner ear barotrauma will generally present with unilateral roaring tinnitus, sensorineural hearing loss, and profound vertigo. A "fistula test" may be positive; that is, insufflation of the tympanic membrane on the affected side causes the eyes to deviate to the contralateral side. As this injury usually occurs on descent and divers will provide a history of difficulty clearing the ears, this condition can usually be easily differentiated from other causes of vertigo, such as inner ear decompression sickness, cerebral arterial gas embolism, or alternobaric vertigo (discussed below).

Immediate complications of inner ear barotrauma are potential panic or disorientation, leading to possible drowning or a rapid ascent that predisposes the diver to pulmonary barotrauma. Divers with barotraumatic injuries to the inner ear require immediate otolaryngologic evaluation. Treatment is controversial, with some authors advocating immediate exploration, and others suggesting a trial of bed rest (head upright), medications to control vertigo, and measures to reduce CSF pressure spikes (e.g., stool softeners, no nose blowing, etc.). These authors reserve exploration for those patients whose symptoms do not respond to conservative therapy or those with severe hearing defects or significant abnormalities on an oculonystagmogram. Divers with potential inner ear barotrauma who will be treated with hyperbaric oxygen for decompression sickness or cerebral arterial gas embolism require emergent tympanostomy, as hyperbaric treatment will recreate the same pressure differentials that caused the injury, potentially causing more perilymph leakage and possibly worsening the injury.[2]

Other air-containing structures can be compressed during descent producing "squeeze" symptoms. A face squeeze occurs when air is not added to the facemask during descent, causing the face and eyes to be forced into the collapsing mask. This produces facial bruising, conjunctival injection or hemorrhage, and, rarely, changes in vision. A tooth squeeze occurs when air spaces inside a tooth—due to either decay, a filling, or abscess—become compressed during descent. A dry-suit squeeze occurs when suit folds are compressed into the underlying skin, producing local trauma manifested by painful red streaks.

Barotrauma of Ascent

During ascent the physics of gas in air-containing organs is, of course, opposite than that of descent; that is, air will expand as the pressure decreases. Air will flow through the ostia of the sinuses, and the expanding air in the middle ear will open the eustachian tube (much like during takeoff in an airplane). Should air be trapped temporarily in one middle ear cavity, the pressure differential may cause unequal vestibular impulses to the brain, resulting in vertigo (alternobaric vertigo). This is usually transient and generally requires no specific treatment.

Air also expands within the lungs. If a diver breathing compressed air ascends with a closed glottis (holds breath, coughs, vomits), most frequently seen in a rapid, panicked out-of-air ascent, the expanding air may rupture the lung. This can occur even in shallow water (e.g., a swimming pool). Pulmonary barotrauma, also called pulmonary overinflation or burst lung syndrome, can lead to pneumomediastinum. This generally only requires symptomatic treatment and may be subtle on the chest radiograph.[3] Mediastinal air can track superiorly into the neck, resulting in subcutaneous air on physical examination or air on a cervical spine radiograph. Rarely, a pulmonary overinflation injury causes pneumothorax, requiring aspiration or tube thoracostomy. If air enters the pulmonary venous circulation, embolization of the gas through the arterial system occurs. The most sensitive end organ to such embolization is the brain, and *cerebral arterial gas embolism* (CAGE) is the term applied to this condition, although the air emboli distribute to other tissues and organs.[4] Any neurologic symptom or sign in the setting of barotrauma associated with ascent should be considered to be secondary to CAGE. The symptoms, signs, and treatment of CAGE will be discussed below.

Pulmonary barotrauma (Figure 197-1) can occur without a rapid ascent or closed glottis in divers with congenital cysts, obstructive pulmonary disease, or other processes that cause air trapping. There is some debate over the safety of divers with asthma, and though the relative risk of pulmonary barotrauma may be higher (possibly as much

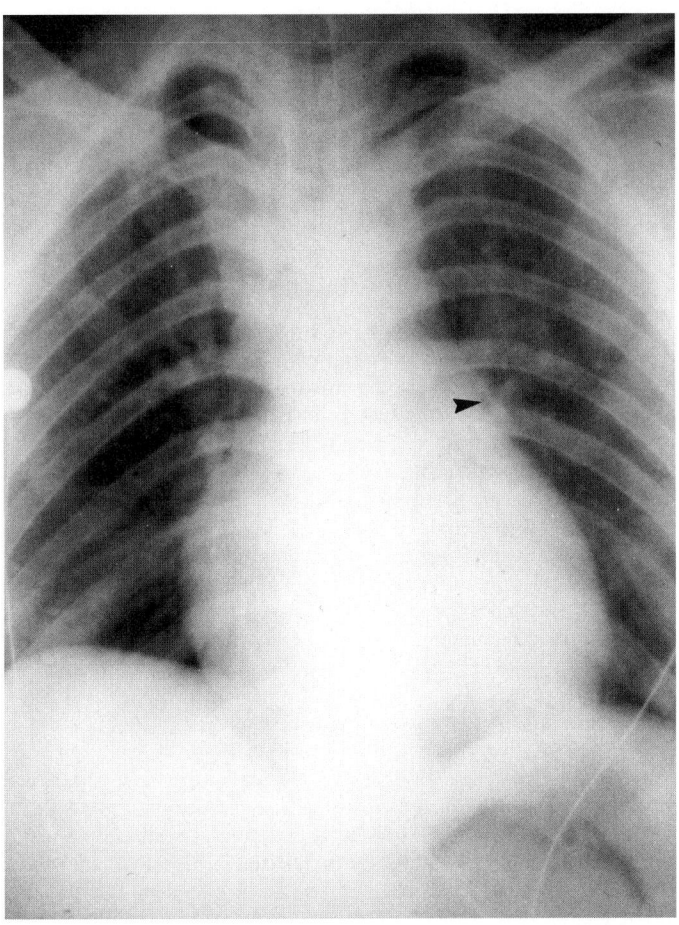

FIG. 197-1. Pulmonary barotrauma. Note the air in the mediastinum in this radiograph *(arrow)*. There is also air in the soft tissues of the neck.

as twice that of the general diving population), the absolute risk is still low because of the rarity of pulmonary barotrauma in diving (approximately 1 in 125,000 dives).[5] A physician who specializes in diving medicine should examine all divers or potential divers with asthma, and an exercise pulmonary function test (PFT) should be performed. Asthmatics can be cleared for diving if, using their usual medications, they have a normal exercise PFT, and if they understand the potential increased risk of pulmonary barotrauma.[5] Additionally, a diver who experiences a lung injury that cannot be explained by the circumstances of the dive (i.e., the diver did not have a rapid, breath-holding ascent), should be evaluated for congenital or acquired structural lung disease. These divers should probably be counseled not to dive.

An air pocket underneath a tooth may equilibrate with ambient pressure while diving, only to expand during ascent. This produces severe pain and may dislodge a filling or fracture a tooth. Swallowed air during diving may expand during ascent, producing gastric distention and abdominal cramps.

DECOMPRESSION SICKNESS AND ARTERIAL GAS EMBOLISM

Decompression Sickness

The pathophysiology of decompression sickness (DCS) is related to the obstructive and inflammatory effects of inert gas bubbles in tissues and the vascular system.[6] Besides divers breathing compressed air, DCS may also occur in caisson workers or high-altitude pilots. Bubbles may form when a body saturated with inert gas experiences a decrease in ambient pressure that causes liberation of the gas. Uptake of

inert gas occurs at different rates in different tissues and is mainly a function of blood flow.

The U.S. Navy has published dive tables to provide the limits to a dive (measured by bottom depth and time) that can be undertaken without a decompression stop ("no decompression" or "no stop" dives). Other Navy tables provide in-water decompression schedules for longer dives. A multitude of dive computers using a variety of mathematical models provide divers with relatively safe diving limits. DCS is unlikely to occur if the limits of the dive tables or dive computer are adhered to; however, adherence to such limits does not guarantee safety.

Bubbles are necessary but not sufficient to cause DCS, as bubbling occurs following many dive profiles that do not lead to DCS. Obviously, there must be a threshold at which the bubble load causes symptoms. The exact mechanism of bubble formation in DCS has yet to be determined, although preexisting gas micronuclei in circulation likely form a nidus for gas accumulation. This is inferred, as the energy required to form bubbles de novo is much higher than the energy state caused by the saturation of inert gas in tissue.[7] Bubbles may form directly in tissues or the circulation (usually the low-pressure venous circulation). Bubbles may directly obstruct blood flow, leading to direct ischemia. Additionally, the air-blood and air-endothelial interfaces initiate a variety of inflammatory and thrombotic processes, activate the endothelium leading to neutrophil adhesion and activation, and change the permeability of the endothelium, resulting in third spacing of fluid.

There is no agreed upon classification system for DCS (or "the bends" in the diving vernacular). However, the most common classification divides DCS into two main groups. Type I DCS is also called "pain-only" DCS and involves the joints, extremities, and skin ("cutis marmorata"). Lymphatic obstruction can occur in type I DCS, causing lymphedema, which usually takes days to resolve despite recompression therapy. Type II DCS (or "serious" DCS) includes neurologic DCS involving the CNS (mainly the spinal cord in compressed air divers and the brain in high-altitude decompressions), vestibular DCS ("staggers"), and cardiopulmonary DCS ("chokes"). To further complicate the nomenclature and classification of DCS, there is evidence suggesting that DCS can also occur when an arterial gas embolus causes inert gas to come out of solution after a dive profile that would otherwise not be expected to cause DCS (called type III decompression sickness).[8] As the presentation may make it difficult to discern DCS from air embolism (and in fact both can occur simultaneously), some advocate the use of the term *decompression illness* (DCI) to encompass all pathologic syndromes following a reduction in ambient pressure.

DCS in commercial and military divers, caisson workers, and aviators tends to manifest most often as joint pain. Sport divers, who usually perform multiple dives, often over a period of days, are more prone to DCS affecting the spinal cord.

Generally, the symptoms of DCS occur minutes to several hours after surfacing, but cases of DCS symptoms occurring days after diving have been reported. Symptoms from DCS occurring between dives may improve during a subsequent dive (as recompression has occurred), but get worse upon resurfacing (as the inert gas load has increased and ambient pressure has decreased). Additionally, flying with the resultant decrease in ambient pressure may precipitate or worsen DCS symptoms, and divers are generally advised to refrain from flying for at least 12 h after the last dive.[9]

Divers with type I DCS typically describe a deep pain, unrelieved but not worsened with movement. This pain can be attributed to or confused with pain caused by injury, making diagnosis problematic. The pain from type I DCS is thought to be due to distention from bubbles in ligaments or fascia, intramedullary bubbles at the ends of long bones, or the activation of stretch receptors caused by bubbles in tendons. The mechanism of simple distention of tissues is supported by the rapid improvement of symptoms with recompression. Common locations for type I DCS are knees and shoulders, and most often only a single joint is involved. Poorly localized and difficult-to-describe back pain may herald the more serious signs of spinal cord DCS.

Pulmonary DCS, generally seen only after prolonged exposures, is caused by large numbers of pulmonary artery bubbles and manifests symptoms of cough, hemoptysis, dyspnea, and substernal chest pain. Cardiovascular collapse can occur. Although now uncommon, this was the most lethal form of DCS, and was seen predominantly in aviators before the importance of oxygen prebreathing prior to high-altitude flights was recognized.

The classic description of divers with neurologic DCS (type II) begins with a sensation of truncal constriction or girdle-like pain. Often a wooly feeling begins in the feet, developing into an ascending paralysis, producing a presentation similar to a transverse myelitis. This form of DCS is usually rapid in onset and has a tendency to affect the lower cervical and thoracic regions. However, in type II DCS, neurologic deficits do not necessarily cause distinct spinal cord syndromes (i.e., an anterior or posterior spinal artery syndrome), nor will a definitive level necessarily be found, as lesions may be scattered throughout the spinal cord.[10] Autonomic involvement, with resulting incontinence and sexual dysfunction, is not uncommon. The pathophysiology of spinal cord DCS seems to be initial bubbling in the low-pressure venous plexus system that first impedes, then causes cessation of venous outflow from the cord. Decreasing venous blood flow prevents dissolved nitrogen in spinal cord tissues to egress, and in-situ bubbles within the spinal cord develop (called *autochthonous bubbles*).

An unusual initial symptom of DCS is profound fatigue. This can be difficult for the diver and clinician to differentiate from the expected fatigue resulting from the exertion of diving. Other, nonspecific symptoms such as headache, nausea, and dizziness are also frequently reported.

Vestibular decompression sickness usually occurs after deep, long dives, although it has been reported in sport divers. It manifests with vertigo, hearing loss, tinnitus, and dysequilibrium. Vestibular DCS can be differentiated from inner ear barotrauma mainly by the history, as those with barotrauma develop symptoms in the water, and generally immediately after a forced Valsalva maneuver to equalize the middle ear pressure.[4]

Arterial Gas Embolism

Arterial gas embolism (AGE) occurs when air enters the left side of the vascular system. In the setting of diving this most often occurs from pulmonary barotrauma; however, it can also occur due to a variety of complications of medical procedures, including central vascular catheterization and operations requiring cardiac bypass. Air inadvertently introduced into the venous circulation can cross from the right side of the circulation from intracardiac shunts or, presumably, pulmonary arteriovenous shunts. Air bubbles formed secondary to decompression sickness may also arterialize through these same shunts, sometimes obscuring the source of arterial bubbles. Whatever the source, when air embolizes systemically, its distribution is dependent mainly on blood flow and not gravity.

Despite its systemic nature, its most dramatic effect is on the brain. CAGE causes a variety of stroke syndromes, symptoms, and signs, depending on the part of the brain affected. In approximately 4 percent of cases, diving-related AGE from pulmonary barotrauma causes immediate apnea and cardiac arrest. The mechanism of this cardiovascular collapse is uncertain, although persons who die from AGE generally have air in the entirety of the large arteries and veins of the central vascular bed. Older hypotheses of brainstem reflexes or coronary artery air embolization to account for the cardiovascular collapse are not supported by the time course of experimental models or the clinical course of individuals who suffer from other forms of cerebrovascular accidents.

The effects of AGE secondary to pulmonary barotrauma usually occur on ascent or immediately upon surfacing. If the victim does not die immediately, the symptoms of CAGE often include loss of consciousness, seizure, disorientation, or hemiplegia. The symptoms of CAGE may spontaneously improve as the gas enters the venous cerebral circulation after a spike in blood pressure. Sometimes, by the time the patient reaches the clinician, the only signs that remain are subtle defects. In particular, parietal lobe signs and symptoms are easily overlooked. Similar to that seen in DCS, a cascade of inflammatory processes also occurs in air embolism.[4]

Treatment of Decompression Sickness and Arterial Gas Embolism

The treatment for DCS and air embolism includes administering 100% oxygen, increasing tissue perfusion with intravenous fluids, and rapid recompression. Some advocate placing patients with air embolism in the Trendelenburg position or in the left lateral decubitus position to "trap" air in the left ventricle. By the time the victim is brought onto the dive boat or the ambulance arrives, the air has usually been distributed, and the Trendelenburg position merely increases intracranial pressure, decreases cerebral perfusion, and interferes with other first aid measures. Nonetheless, some divers with AGE have collapsed when placed in a sitting or standing position. As a result, a supine position is recommended for patients with AGE. Vomiting patients should be placed in the left lateral decubitus position to prevent aspiration.

Recompression therapy with hyperbaric oxygen (HBO) treats DCS and air embolism by several mechanisms. HBO is delivered in a hyperbaric or recompression chamber. Chambers can either be *monoplace,* which are designed to treat a single patient with no inside attendant, or *multiplace,* with room for multiple patients and an inside attendant. Multiplace chambers compress the inside environment with air and provide oxygen through a mask or hood system. Some monoplace chambers are also compressed with air and provide oxygen through a mask, but most are compressed with oxygen.

The administered pressure decreases the size of bubbles, and the high partial pressure of oxygen in solution increases inert gas washout from bubbles and tissue. Mass action dictates that a gas will travel down pressure gradients; therefore nitrogen will move from bubbles with a high partial pressure of nitrogen into plasma, where it will travel to the lungs and be exhaled. Conversely, oxygen from plasma with a high partial pressure of oxygen will enter bubbles, but ultimately will diffuse into cells and be metabolized, further reducing bubble size. Additionally, HBO decreases tissue edema, increases oxygen delivery to ischemic tissues, and reduces neutrophil adhesion to the endothelium and neutrophil activation.[11]

Recompression using the United States Navy Treatment Table 6 is a commonly used method of management for DCS, employing a maximal treatment pressure of 2.8 ATA (60 fsw). Table 6 is also used for air embolism, although some advocate an initial pressurization to 6 ATA (165 fsw) to maximize bubble compression, then continuation at 2.8 ATA (the United States Navy Table 6A). Different treatment tables are utilized in other parts of the world, and there is some experience using lower treatment pressures for DCS in monoplace chambers with comparable results.[12] Some patients may benefit from repeated treatments if symptoms do not fully resolve. Recompression should occur as soon as possible, and it should not be withheld in cases with delayed presentation.[4]

Many adjuncts to standard recompression therapy have been used and studied in the treatment of DCS and CAGE.[13] For example, corticosteroids, aspirin, heparin, and lidocaine all have been advocated at some time. None have been shown to be clearly effective in humans, and heparin has been shown to be harmful in animal models. The most promising current adjunct is lidocaine in CAGE. Animal data using a model of severe air embolism show lidocaine improved somatosensory evoked potentials and cerebral blood flow.[14] Additionally, lidocaine has been shown to decrease neuropsychiatric deficits when given during anesthesia for cardiac procedures requiring bypass.[15] These operations commonly cause the entry of air into the arterial system. Dosing of lidocaine in this setting is not standardized, although typical cardiac dosing is commonly used.[16]

Divers Alert Network (Tel: 1-919-684-8111, website: www.divers-alertnetwork.org) has staff available 24 h a day to provide assistance to divers and to help clinicians treat patients with DCS or arterial gas embolism, and they can provide information and the location of the nearest recompression facility.

IMMERSION PULMONARY EDEMA

Pulmonary edema can occur while diving, and the first reported cases occurred in cold water; therefore, it was first described as "cold water" or "cold-induced" pulmonary edema. However, cases have subsequently been reported in warm water, up to 27°C (80.6°F).[17] Typical symptoms of pulmonary edema (dyspnea, chest discomfort, coughing up pink frothy secretions) occur at depth and usually improve over time or with standard treatments for pulmonary edema. This syndrome generally occurs in divers with no structural or ischemic heart disease, but evaluation for these conditions should be done. The mechanism of this condition is unknown and may be multifactorial, involving hydrostatic forces, thermal stress, and possibly increased capillary permeability. Immersion pulmonary edema is not caused by decompression and is not treated with recompression therapy. Interestingly, some divers will experience repeated episodes, while others may never experience another episode. This makes counseling of divers experiencing immersion pulmonary edema very difficult.

NITROGEN NARCOSIS

Inert gas narcosis occurs when air is breathed at a depth of 100 fsw or greater. Symptoms include loss of fine motor skills and high-order mental processes as well as behavior similar to that seen in alcohol intoxication. Symptoms increase as depth is increased beyond 100 fsw. Divers have codified this increase in symptoms as the "martini rule" (with many variations). A common description is that each 33 ft of depth (1 ATA) in excess of 100 fsw is the equivalent to drinking one martini. At depths greater than 300 fsw, unconsciousness may occur secondary to the anesthetic effect of nitrogen. At depths below 200 fsw, helium is often used in lieu of nitrogen in diving mixtures to prevent nitrogen narcosis. Symptoms of nitrogen narcosis improve upon ascent and can be worsened by fatigue, cold, and work. The effects of nitrogen narcosis are important in that divers may engage in dangerous or foolish activities during deep dives when breathing air, and the history from divers following such dives should be evaluated in this context.

OXYGEN TOXICITY

Oxygen toxicity generally affects one of two organs, the brain or lungs, depending on the partial pressure of oxygen delivered and duration of exposure. Cerebral oxygen toxicity occurs at high partial pressures with generally short exposures, whereas the clinical manifestations of pulmonary oxygen toxicity occur at lower partial pressures of oxygen but with longer exposures. Of course, pulmonary oxygen toxicity can also occur at higher partial pressures; however, the symptoms are generally not manifested, as the cerebral effects require removal from the exposure. Pulmonary oxygen toxicity can occur at partial pressures of oxygen at or below 1 ATA, as is seen in patients requiring prolonged mechanical ventilation with high fractions of inspired oxygen. Pulmonary oxygen toxicity is unusual in diving. In commercial, military, and deep diving, careful consideration is given to breathing mixtures and environmental conditions to avoid this and other complications of gas toxicity.

Cerebral oxygen toxicity most often occurs with partial pressures of oxygen greater than 1.6 ATA in the water (218 fsw while breath-

ing compressed air). Some divers may breathe "nitrox" or *oxygen-enriched air* with fractions of oxygen of 32 to 36%. Therefore cerebral oxygen toxicity can occur at lesser depths and actually is the factor that limits diving depth with nitrox. Additionally, there are oxygen rebreather systems (so-called closed circuit systems), with the diver breathing within a continuous circuit of gas that has a very high fraction of oxygen (>95%), with carbon dioxide being scrubbed out. With these systems, cerebral oxygen toxicity can occur at depths as little as 25 ft.

Cerebral oxygen toxicity manifests with twitching, nausea, paresthesias, dizziness, and seizures. A seizure may be the initial manifestation of cerebral oxygen toxicity and in the water may cause drowning. Of note, higher partial pressures of oxygen are used clinically in hyperbaric chambers (2.4 ATA, 2.8 ATA, and sometimes 3.0 ATA); however, cerebral oxygen toxicity in this setting is rare, reported in less than 1 per 1000 patients. This is because patients in hyperbaric chambers are dry, warm, and at rest, while divers are wet, often cold, and exerting themselves. Cerebral oxygen toxicity is affected by Pa_{CO_2} and cerebral blood flow and may be caused by an increase in nitric oxide production, although this is still an area of active investigation.[18]

Besides nitrogen narcosis and oxygen toxicity, other gas-related conditions important in diving medicine are toxicity from carbon monoxide and the adverse effects of elevated partial pressures of carbon dioxide. Additional issues, especially with very deep dives, include heat loss from breathing helium and the high-pressure nervous syndrome, characterized by tremor and loss of fine motor function caused by the direct effects of pressure.

REFERENCES

1. Strauss MB, Borer RC: Diving medicine: Contemporary topics and their controversies. *Am J Emerg Med* 19:232, 2001.
2. Becker GD, Parell GJ: Barotrauma of the ears and sinuses after scuba diving. *Euro Arch Otorhinolaryngol* 258:159, 2001.
3. Harker CP, Neuman TS, Olson LK, et al: The roentgenographic findings associated with air embolism in sport SCUBA divers. *J Emerg Med* 11:443, 1993.
4. Neuman TS: Arterial gas embolism and decompression sickness. *News Physiol Sci* 17:77, 2001.
5. Tetzlaff K, Muth CM, Waldhauser LK: A review of asthma and scuba diving. *J Asthma* 39:557, 2002.
6. Dutka AJ, Francis TJ: Pathophysiology of decompression sickness, in Bove AA (ed): *Bove and Davis' Diving Medicine*, 3d ed. Philadelphia, WB Saunders, 1997, pp. 159–177.
7. Doolette DJ, Mitchell SJ: The physiologic kinetics of nitrogen and the prevention of decompression sickness. *Clin Pharmacokinet* 40:1, 2001.
8. Neuman TS, Bove AA: Combined arterial gas embolism and decompression sickness following no-stop dives. *Undersea Biomed Res* 17:429, 1990.
9. Millar I: Post diving altitude exposure. *South Pacific Underwater Medicine Society Journal* 26:135, 1996.
10. Newton HB: Neurologic complications of scuba diving. *Am Fam Physician* 63:2211, 2001.
11. Martin JD, Thom SR: Vascular leukocyte sequestration in decompression sickness and prophylactic hyperbaric oxygen therapy in rats. *Aviat Space Environ Med* 73:565, 2002.
12. Li RC: The monoplace hyperbaric chamber and management of decompression sickness. *Hong Kong Med J* 7:435, 2001.
13. Catron PW, Flynn ET: Adjuvant drug therapy for decompression sickness: A review. *Undersea Biomed Res* 9:161, 1982.
14. Dutka AJ, Mink R, McDermott J, et al: Effect of lidocaine on somatosensory evoked response and cerebral blood flow after canine cerebral air embolism. *Stroke* 23:1515, 1992.
15. Mitchell SJ, Pellett O, Gorman DF: Cerebral protection by lidocaine during cardiac operations. *Ann Thorac Surg* 67:1117, 1999.
16. Mitchell SJ: Lidocaine for the treatment of decompression illness: A review of the literature. *Undersea Hyper Med* 28:165, 2001.
17. Hampson NB, Dunford RG: Pulmonary edema of scuba divers. *Undersea Hyper Med* 24:29, 1997.
18. Demchenko IT, Boso AE, O'Neill TJ, et al: Nitric oxide and cerebral blood flow responses to hyperbaric oxygen. *J Appl Physiol* 88:1381, 2000.

198

NEAR-DROWNING
Alan L. Causey
Mark A. Nichter

Submersion injuries that result in death in less than 24 h are termed *drowning*. *Near-drowning* is defined as survival longer than 24 h after a submersion event. As with other causes of accidental death, submersion injuries typically involve otherwise healthy, young individuals.

EPIDEMIOLOGY

Over the last decade more than 50,000 people have died from drowning in the U.S., and over 100,000 die each year worldwide. In the U.S., drowning is the fourth leading cause of accidental death overall, and is the second leading cause of death in those under 15 years of age. In addition, there are an estimated over 500,000 submersion events per year in the U.S. The vast majority of victims survive submersion events with outcomes ranging from minimal or transient injury to profound neurologic insult.

There are three peaks in near-drowning incidence: the first in toddlers and young children, a second in adolescents and young adults, and a third in the elderly. In addition to pools and bodies of water, infants and toddlers can drown in toilets, buckets, and bathtubs. The elderly also have an increased risk of bathtub drowning. Even in coastal areas most submersion events take place in warm, freshwater bodies of water (especially swimming pools).

Additional injuries or disorders that either precipitate or are associated with submersion events include: 1) spinal cord injuries that occur after diving into shallow water or boating mishaps, 2) hypothermia, 3) panicking, 4) syncope (e.g., due to hyperventilation prior to underwater diving), 5) seizures, and 6) other premorbid conditions (e.g., heart disease).[1,2]

PREVENTION

Submersion episodes among children less than 1 year of age are best prevented by parental vigilance during bathing. Child abuse should be considered when the victim is less than 6 months of age, or in toddlers with atypical presentations.[3] In preschool children, adult supervision in conjunction with properly installed and maintained four-sided pool fences that completely isolate the pool could prevent 50 to 90 percent of preschool-aged drownings.[4,5]

Teen and young adult drowning may be reduced by the control of alcohol and illicit drug consumption that have been implicated in 40 percent of all adult drownings and 75 percent of boating-related adult drownings.[6] The use of personal flotation devices decreases boating-related drowning. Practical experience suggests that the ability to swim is protective against teen and adult drowning, but there is little evidence to support the efficacy of swimming instructions for preventing drowning in infants and young toddlers.[7]

Drowning locations in the elderly closely parallel locations of infant and toddler drowning. Adequate pool fencing and bathtub handrails are important preventive means for the elderly population and in those patients with premorbid conditions.

PATHOPHYSIOLOGY

After submersion, the degree of pulmonary, and in particular central nervous system (CNS) insult determines the ultimate outcome. It is thought that there could be transient protection from parasympathetic activation of the diving reflex (i.e., bradycardia, apnea, peripheral vasoconstriction, and central shunting of blood flow) during submersion. However, the diving reflex may not provide significant protection in humans as was once thought. The diving reflex is strongest in young infants <6 months old, but the effects decrease with age.[8] In adults, vertical immersion (head out) and vertical submersion (head under) activates both the sympathetic and parasympathetic systems, blunting any effect of the diving reflex.[9] Physiologic stress associated with submersion undoubtedly also activates the sympathetic nervous system. Cerebral protection in cold-water submersions most likely results from rapid CNS cooling before significant cardiac dysrhythmia.

"Dry-drowning," which accounts for 10 to 20 percent of submersion injuries, occurs when there is laryngospasm, followed by hypoxia leading to loss of consciousness. More commonly, "wet drowning" occurs in which there is aspiration of water into the lungs. The effect is dilution and washout of the pulmonary surfactant with resultant diminished gas transfer across the alveoli, atelectasis, and ventilation-perfusion mismatch. In fresh-water aspiration, there is transient hemodilution, and if large enough volumes are aspirated, significant hemolysis is possible. Factors such as aspiration of contaminated foreign material, particulate matter, bacteria, vomitus, or chemical irritants can affect eventual pulmonary recovery.

Prediction of eventual outcome in near-drowning is possible using factors such as submersion time and physiologic scoring systems.[10,11] However, the utility of this prediction is debatable; the vast majority of patients who arrive at the hospital with fair cardiovascular and neurologic function survive with minimal disability, and those that arrive with unstable cardiovascular function and coma do poorly because of the hypoxic, ischemic CNS insult. Predictors are not accurate or useful for the 15 to 20 percent of near-drowning victims whose arrival condition is between these two extremes.[12]

Other end organs can also be affected from resultant hypoxemia and metabolic acidosis. Electrolyte abnormalities are seldom significant and usually transient unless there is significant renal injury from hypoxic injury, hemoglobinuria, or myoglobinuria.[12,13] Hematologic values are usually normal unless there has been massive hemolysis. Rarely, disseminated intravascular coagulation can be a complicating factor in near-drowning.

TREATMENT

Prehospital Care

Resuscitation of a submersion victim as quickly as possible optimizes outcome. This emphasizes the need to train laypersons in cardiopulmonary resuscitation (CPR), particularly swimming pool owners. After careful removal of the victim from the water (with cervical spine control/protection if there is an unknown mechanism of injury or suspicion of spinal injury), CPR should be initiated as quickly as possible.

High-flow oxygen therapy by facemask should be administered if the patient is breathing, or by positive-pressure bag-valve-mask if the patient is not breathing. For those patients who do not recover spontaneous respiratory effort, endotracheal (ET) intubation with positive-pressure ventilation should be considered, particularly if the patient remains unconscious, because of the risk of aspirating emesis.

All patients with submersion associated with amnesia for the event, loss or depressed consciousness, an observed period of apnea, or those who require a period of artificial ventilation should be transported for evaluation to an ED, even if they are asymptomatic at the scene. The patients should be warmed and monitored, and intravenous access considered (Table 198-1).

TABLE 198-1   Prehospital Care of Submersion Victims

Rapid, cautious rescue
Spinal precautions
Cardiopulmonary resuscitation
Supplemental oxygen (all patients)
Transport (all patients)

Emergency Department

Upon arrival at the ED, the treating physician should assess and secure the airway, provide oxygen, and assist ventilation as necessary. Warmed isotonic intravenous fluids should be administered and warming adjuncts (e.g., blankets, overhead warmers, warming devices) should be used. Any associated injuries should be addressed.

Patients who present to the ED with a Glasgow Coma Scale (GCS) score of ≥13 should be administered oxygen as necessary to keep their oxygen saturation (Sao$_2$) >95 percent (Table 198-2). They should be observed for 4 to 6 h, and if the pulmonary examination and room-air Sao$_2$ remain normal, they can be safely discharged home. Laboratory examination and radiographs are unnecessary, and are not predictive of discharge.[14] If, after 4 to 6 h, the patient still requires oxygen, has an abnormal pulmonary examination (rales, rhonchi, wheeze, retractions, etc.), or deteriorates in the ED, reassessment and admission or transfer to a monitored bed is needed.

Patients who present to the ED with GCS <13 should be maintained on supplemental oxygen and ventilatory support as needed. If high-flow oxygen (Fio$_2$ 40 to 60 percent) cannot maintain an adequate Pao$_2$ (>60 mm Hg in adults, >80 mm Hg in children), then the patient should be intubated and receive positive-pressure ventilation. Chest radiography and laboratory studies should be done to evaluate for pulmonary aspiration and other complications (see Table 198-2). Infrequently, childhood victims of freshwater near-drowning develop dilutional hyponatremia and seizures. In these cases, seizures are generally easily controlled with correction of the electrolyte abnormality, and residual seizure disorder is uncommon. Continuous cardiac monitoring, pulse oximetry, and frequent reassessments should be performed on all patients.

If the patient presents to the ED in cardiopulmonary arrest or asystole after a warm-water submersion event, serious thought should be given to discontinuing resuscitation efforts, as recovery without profound neurologic handicaps is rare.[15]

TABLE 198-2 Hospital Care of Submersion Victims*

	Presentation GCS ≥13	Presentation GCS <13*†
Cervical spine	Clear	Clear
Ancillary tests	Only as indicated (routine studies such as CXR are not predictive of outcome)	ABG CBC, electrolytes, glucose, PT/PTT, UA, CK, urine myoglobin, urine drug screen CXR ECG
Respiratory support	Oxygen to keep Sao$_2$ >95%	Oxygen to keep Sao$_2$ >95% Intubation and positive-pressure ventilation as needed (PEEP, CPAP)
Monitor	Oxygen saturation	Oxygen saturation Acid-base status Temperature Volume status (urine output, central venous pressure, etc.)

*Evaluate and treat any associated injuries or other conditions (e.g., hypovolemia, hypothermia, hypoglycemia, myocardial ischemia, seizures, etc.).
†Including those patients presenting with GCS ≥13 who have abnormal examinations and/or abnormal oxygen saturations after observation for 4–6 h.
Abbreviations: CBC = complete blood count; CK = creatine kinase; CPAP = continuous positive airway pressure; CXR = chest radiograph; ECG = electrocardiogram; GCS = Glasgow Coma Score; PEEP = positive end-expiratory pressure; PT = prothrombin time; PTT = partial thromboplastin time; Sao$_2$ = oxygen saturations (via pulse oximetry); UA = urinalysis.

Hospital

Hospital management of near-drowning victims is largely supportive.[16] All near-drowning victims who require emergency department resuscitation should be admitted to an intensive care unit (ICU) for continuous cardiopulmonary and frequent neurological monitoring. Most victims of significant submersion injury benefit from mechanical ventilation. Supranormal levels of positive end-expiratory pressure (PEEP) may be used to recruit fluid-filled lung units and aid oxygenation. Most victims demonstrate rapid improvement in oxygenation in the first 24 h. Victims presenting with significant aspiration pattern or severe cardiovascular collapse are predisposed to develop acute respiratory distress syndrome (ARDS). Care should be taken to avoid lung overdistension and ventilator-associated lung trauma. Bacterial pneumonia is rare and prophylactic antibiotics are not indicated.

For victims who have been resuscitated from cardiac arrest, the hemodynamic response to exogenously administered epinephrine is frequently short lived, and most will require a continuous infusion of dopamine or epinephrine in the ED or ICU. Invasive (pulmonary artery catheter) or noninvasive (echocardiogram) measures of ventricular function are often instructive. Hemodynamic recovery, when it occurs, can be expected within 48 h. Victims demonstrating no hemodynamic recovery after 48 h may slowly improve over the first week, but are more likely to have long-term neurologic damage.[12]

Results of "brain resuscitation" following significant warm-water near-drowning have been disappointing.[12,16] The degree of cerebral edema is largely determined by the duration of the anoxic or ischemic insult at the time of submersion. Efforts to control cerebral edema including the administration of mannitol, loop diuretics, hypertonic saline, fluid restriction, and mechanical hyperventilation have not shown benefit.[16] Controlled hypothermia, barbiturate "coma," and intracranial pressure monitoring have not been shown to improve outcome in pediatric near-drowning victims.[12]

Family members should be counseled about likely outcome. Using initial presentation, resuscitation, laboratory data, and serial examinations, experienced practitioners should be able to provide accurate predictions of outcomes in most cases.[17]

PROGNOSIS AND DISPOSITION

Uncomplicated

As noted above, submersion victims who are asymptomatic or mildly symptomatic can be observed for 4 to 6 h. If they continue to have a normal pulmonary examination and normal room air oxygen saturation, they can be safely discharged home. The concern for "secondary drowning" (respiratory deterioration after initial stable presentation) is unwarranted, because if deterioration is going to occur, it will do so within the 4- to 6-h observation period.[14,18,19] No data is available for long-term outcomes for these patients, but it is unlikely that there are any measurable adverse effects. Parents and patients should be advised to have close follow-up and to be evaluated for any respiratory complaints or fever.

Complicated

Since submersion time is frequently unknown or only estimated, the extent of required resuscitation is often the most objective measure of the degree of anoxic or ischemic insult. Details of initial presentation and resuscitation are frequently strong prognostic indicators.

If the submersion victim does not require cardiopulmonary resuscitation at the scene or in the ED, complete recovery within 48 h is expected. A small fraction of these patients with significant aspiration may develop severe, even life-threatening ARDS.

Victims requiring bystander CPR at the scene have a guarded prognosis. For scene-resuscitated pediatric victims, about 20 percent later die in hospital and about 5 percent are left with severe hypoxic-ischemic encephalopathy.[20] Those victims who demonstrate continuous neurologic and cardiovascular improvement after hospital admission will generally make a complete recovery. Frequently, neurologic and cardiovascular examinations are normal within 24 h of the submersion event. Victims who later die in hospital usually demonstrate deteriorating cardiovascular status. Victims who are left with severe hypoxic-ischemic encephalopathy typically have persistent abnormal cranial nerve dysfunction and coma.

Victims undergoing ED CPR have a poor prognosis. These victims have usually sustained a significant anoxic or ischemic insult to the brain and other vital organs. Complete neurologic recovery is rare, although there are anecdotal reports of neurologic recovery following ED CPR of pediatric warm-water near-drowning, possibly due to the poor descriptions of the term "CPR." In our experience of over 500 pediatric warm-water submersion victims, 75 patients required ED CPR (defined as intravenous or endotracheal epinephrine or atropine *with* chest compressions and artificial ventilation). Of these cases, 84 percent died in the hospital, and 16 percent survived with severe hypoxic-ischemic encephalopathy. Asystole, whether noted at the scene or in the emergency department, is a near-universal sign of poor prognosis in warm-water pediatric submersion injuries.

For the emergency physician, the question of whom and how vigorously to resuscitate remains unclear.[20] Though rare, complete or near-complete neurologic recovery after asystole has been reported following icy-water submersion episodes in children and adults. Consequently, victims of icy-water submersion, if removed from the water quickly, might reasonably undergo prolonged resuscitation maneuvers until CNS and cardiopulmonary viability are clear. Asystolic victims of warm-water submersion injuries with short submersion and transport times and CPR en route might reasonably undergo a vigorous resuscitation attempt.[21] CPR should be abandoned if no response is noted. Conversely, because of the poor prognosis for intact neurologic survival, emergency department resuscitation attempts might reasonably be withheld from asystolic victims of warm-water submersion with longer submersion and transport times.

ACKNOWLEDGMENT

The authors acknowledge that portions of this chapter are based upon previous work by Bruce E. Haynes.

REFERENCES

1. Watson RS, Cummings P, Quan L, et al: Cervical spine injuries among submersion victims. *J Trauma* 51:658, 2001.
2. Hwang V, Shofer FS, Durbin DR, et al: Prevalence of traumatic injuries in drowning and near-drowning in children and adolescents. *Arch Pediatr Adolesc Med* 157:50, 2003.
3. Lavelle JM, Shaw KN, Seidl T, et al: Ten-year review of pediatric bathtub near-drownings: Evaluation for child abuse and neglect. *Ann Emerg Med* 25:344, 1995.
4. Logan P, Branch CM, Sacks JJ, et al: Childhood drownings and fencing of outdoor pools in the United States, 1994. *Pediatrics* 101:e3, 1998.
5. Vincenten J, Michalsen A: Priorities for child safety in the European Union: Agenda for action. *Injury Control and Safety Promotion* 9:1, 2002.
6. Nichter MA, Everett PB: Profile of drowning victims in a coastal community. *J Florida Med Assoc* 76:253, 1989.
7. Asher KN, Rivara FP, Felix D, et al: Water safety training as a potential means of reducing risk of young children's drowning. *Inj Prev* 1:228, 1995.
8. Goksor E, Rosengren L, Wennergren G: Bradycardiac response during submersion in infant swimming. *Acta Paediatr* 91:307, 2002.
9. Schipke JD, Pelzer M: Effect of immersion, submersion, and scuba diving on heart rate variability. *Br J Sports Med* 35:174, 2001.
10. Suominen P, Baillie C, Korpela R, et al: Impact of age, submersion time and water temperature on outcome in near-drowning. *Resuscitation* 52:247, 2002.
11. Gonzalez-Luis G, Pons M, Cambra FJ, et al: Use of the pediatric risk of mortality score as predictor of death and serious neurologic damage in children after submersion. *Pediatr Emerg Care* 17:405, 2001.
12. Ibsen LM, Koch T: Submersion and asphyxial injury. *Crit Care Med* 30(Suppl):S402, 2002.
13. Orlowski JP, Szpilman D: Drowning. Rescue, resuscitation, and reanimation. *Pediatr Clin North Am* 48:627, 2001.
14. Causey AL, Tilelli JA, Swanson ME: Predicting discharge in uncomplicated near-drowning. *Am J Emerg Med* 18:9, 2000.
15. Horisberger T, Fischer E, Fanconi S: One-year survival and neurological outcome after pediatric cardiopulmonary resuscitation. *Intensive Care Med* 28:365, 2002.
16. Spack L, Gedeit R, Splaingard M, Havens PL: Failure of aggressive therapy to alter outcome in pediatric near-drowning. *Pediatr Emerg Care* 13:98, 1997.
17. Szpilman D: Near-drowning and drowning classification: A proposal to stratify mortality based on the analysis of 1,831 cases. *Chest* 112:660, 1997.
18. Pratt FD, Haynes BE: Incidence of "secondary drowning" after salt water submersion. *Ann Emerg Med* 15:1084, 1986.
19. Noonan L, Howrey R, Ginsburg CM: Freshwater submersion injuries in children: A retrospective review of seventy-five hospitalized patients. *Pediatrics* 98:368, 1996.
20. Nichter MA, Everett PB: Childhood near-drowning: Is cardiopulmonary resuscitation always indicated? *Crit Care Med* 17:993, 1989.
21. Wollenek G, Honarwar N, Golej J, et al: Cold water submersion and cardiac arrest in treatment of severe hypothermia with cardiopulmonary bypass. *Resuscitation* 52:255, 2002.

THERMAL BURNS
Lawrence R. Schwartz
Chenicheri Balakrishnan

INCIDENCE

The American Burn Association estimates there are more than 1 million burn injuries each year in the United States, generating about 700,000 ED visits and 45,000 hospitalizations.[1] Thus, the majority of burn patients are treated and discharged from the ED to be followed as outpatients. Approximately half of those hospitalized are admitted to the 125 specialized burn treatment centers, and the others are cared for in community hospitals. Fire and burn deaths account for about 4500 deaths each year.[1]

The risk of burns is highest in the 18- to 35-year-old age group. There is a male to female ratio of 2:1 for both injury and death. There is a higher incidence of scalds from hot liquids in children 1 to 5 years of age and in the elderly. The death rate in patients over 65 years of age is much higher than that in the overall burn population.[2,3]

Significant strides have been made in the overall care of the burn patient during the last two decades.[4,5] These advances are reflected in a decreased mortality rate among patients with major thermal injury; only about 4 percent of those treated in specialized burn treatment centers die from their injuries or associated complications.[6] The incidence of inpatient admissions has decreased over time owing to improvements in outpatient care both in the ED and in the burn unit. Currently, the risk of death from a major burn is associated with increased burn size, increased age, the presence of inhalation injury, and female sex.[3]

PATHOPHYSIOLOGY

Skin consists of two layers: the epidermis and the dermis. In the very young and the elderly, the skin thickness is less than that of a person in the prime of life. Skin thickness also varies significantly throughout the body. The skin is very thick in the palm of the hand and the sole of the foot. The skin on the upper part of the back is thicker than that of other parts of the body. Thus exposure to the same temperature for the same duration will lead to different depths of injury in different parts of the body.

Skin functions as a semipermeable barrier to evaporative water loss. Other functions of the skin include protection from the adversities of the environment, control of body temperature, sensation, and excretion. Partial-thickness thermal injury can result in disruption of the barrier function and contribute to free water deficits. The effect may be significant in moderate to large burns.

Thermal injury results in a spectrum of local and systemic homeostatic derangements that contribute to burn shock. These include disruption of normal cell membrane function, hormonal alterations, changes in tissue acid-base balance, hemodynamic changes, and hematologic derangement.

Fluid and electrolyte abnormalities seen in burn shock are largely the result of alterations of cell membrane potentials with intracellular influx of water and sodium and extracellular migration of potassium secondary to dysfunction of the sodium pump. In burns of greater than 60 percent of body surface area, depression of cardiac output is frequently observed with lack of response to aggressive volume resuscitation. Although disputed by others, Baxter and Shires[7] have explained this phenomenon on the basis of circulating myocardial depressants. Also, there is increased systemic vascular resistance. A significant metabolic acidosis may be present in early stages of a large burn injury.

Hematologic derangements associated with massive thermal injury consist of an increase in hematocrit with increased blood viscosity during the early phase, followed by anemia from erythrocyte extravasation and destruction. However, transfusion is not often required for patients with isolated burn injury.

Thermal injury is a progressive injury. Local effects of thermal injury include liberation of vasoactive substances, disruption of cellular function, and edema formation. The systemic response consists of responses by the neurohormonal axis and profound alterations of all organ systems. Substances implicated in these events are histamine, kinin, serotonin, arachidonic acid metabolites, and free oxygen radicals. These substances exert their primary effects at the local level and cause progression of the burn wound. Preservation of the blood supply by decreasing the inflammatory response has been attempted with pharmacologic manipulations using drugs such as nonsteroidal anti-inflammatories.[4,5]

Although many factors may influence prognosis, the severity of the burn, presence of inhalation injury, associated injuries, the patient's age, preexisting disease, and acute organ system failure are most important.[2,3] The burn's size and depth are functions of the burning agent, its temperature, and the duration of exposure. Cell damage occurs at a temperature greater than 45°C (113°F) owing to denaturation of cellular protein. The burn wound is described as having three zones: the zone of coagulation, where tissue is irreversibly destroyed with thrombosis of blood vessels; the zone of stasis, where there is stagnation of the microcirculation; and the zone of hyperemia, where there is increased blood flow. The zone of stasis can become progressively more hypoxemic and ischemic if resuscitation is not adequate. In the zone of hyperemia, there is minimal damage to the cells and spontaneous recovery is likely.

CLINICAL FEATURES

Burn Size

The size of a burn injury is quantified as the percentage of body surface area (BSA) involved.[5] One method of calculating the percentage of BSA burned is to use the Rule of Nines (Figure 199-1). This method divides the body into segments that are approximately 9 percent or multiples of 9 percent, with the perineum forming the remaining 1 percent. In infants and children, this method must be modified because of their larger heads and smaller legs.

Another method is based on the fact that the area of the back of a patient's hand is approximately 1 percent BSA. The number of "hands" that equal the area of the burn can approximate the percentage of BSA burned.

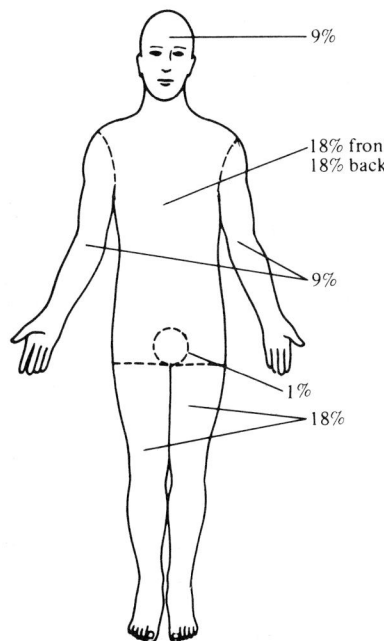

FIG. 199-1. Rule of Nines to estimate percentage of burn.

A more precise estimation of the percentage of BSA burned is obtained by using a Lund and Browder burn diagram (Figure 199-2). This allows for accurate determination of the size and depth. These charts are age-adjusted, which allows for changes in children at different ages as they grow.

Experienced burn-care nurses and physicians are reliable in estimating burn size regardless of the method used. However, it is common for inexperienced individuals to estimate burn size incorrectly when patients are first assessed in the ED.

Burn Depth

The depth of a burn has historically been described in degrees: first, second, and third. However, a classification of burn depth according to the need for surgical intervention has become the accepted approach in burn treatment centers: superficial partial-thickness, deep partial-thickness, and full-thickness burns.[4] Determination of burn depth requires judgment, using commonly seen clinical features. There is no objective method of measuring burn depth, and burn wound biopsy has not become routine practice.

A first-degree burn involves only the epidermal layer of skin. Sunburn is usually given as a common example of a first-degree burn, although sunburn is caused by ultraviolet light instead of thermal injury.[8] The burned skin is red, painful, and tender without blister formation. First-degree burns usually heal in about 7 days without scarring and require only symptomatic treatment.

Second-degree burns extend into the dermis and are divided into superficial partial-thickness and deep partial-thickness burns.

In superficial partial-thickness burns, the epidermis and the superficial (papillary layer) dermis are injured. The deeper layers of the dermis, hair follicles, and sweat and sebaceous glands are spared. Superficial partial-thickness burns are often caused by hot water. There is blistering of the skin and the exposed dermis is red and moist at the blister's base. These burns are very painful to touch. There is good perfusion of the dermis with intact capillary refill. Superficial partial-thickness burns heal in 14 to 21 days, scarring is usually minimal, and there is full return of function.

Deep partial-thickness burns extend into the deep (reticular layer) of the dermis. There is damage to hair follicles as well as sweat and sebaceous glands, but their deeper portions usually survive. Hot liquids,

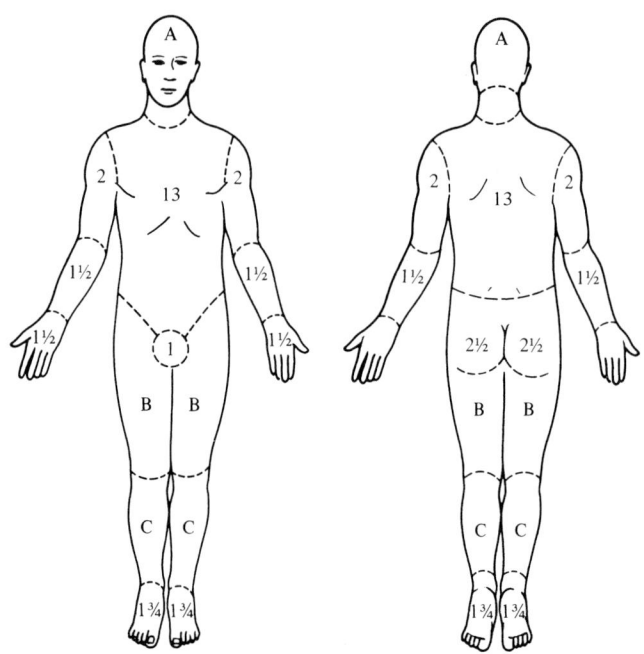

Relative Percentages of Areas Affected by Growth (Age in Years)

	0	1	5	10	15	Adult
A: half of head	9½	8½	6½	5½	4½	3½
B: half of thigh	2¾	3¼	4	4¼	4½	4¾
C: half of leg	2½	2½	2¾	3	3¼	3½

Second-degree _____ and

Third-degree _____ =

Total percent burned ____

FIG. 199-2. Lund and Browder diagram to estimate percentage of pediatric burn.

TABLE 199-1 American Burn Association Burn Unit Referral Criteria

Partial-thickness burns greater than 10% total body surface area (BSA)
Burns that involve the face, hand, feet, genitalia, perineum, or major joints
Third-degree burns in any age group
Electrical burns, including lightning injury
Chemical burns
Inhalation injury
Burn injury in patients with preexisting medical disorders that could complicate management, prolong recovery, or affect mortality
Any patients with burns and concomitant trauma (such as fractures) in which the burn injury poses the greatest risk of morbidity or mortality
Burned children in hospitals without qualified personnel or equipment for the care of children
Burn injury in patients who will require special social, emotional, or long-term rehabilitative intervention.

Source: American Burn Association, www.ameriburn.org.

Major Burns

Major burns are defined as 1) partial-thickness burns greater than 25 percent BSA in the 10- to 50-year-old age group; 2) partial-thickness burns greater than 20 percent BSA in children under 10 or adults over 50; 3) full-thickness burns of greater than 10 percent BSA in anyone; 4) burns involving the hands, face, feet, or perineum; 5) burns crossing major joints; 6) circumferential burns of an extremity; 7) burns complicated by inhalation injury; 8) electrical burns; 9) burns complicated by fractures or other trauma; 10) burns in infants and the elderly; and 11) burns in poor-risk patients. These burns typically require referral to a specialized burn treatment center.

Moderate Burns

Moderate burns are 1) partial-thickness burns of 15 to 25 percent BSA in the 10- to 50-year-old age group; 2) partial-thickness burns of 10 to 20 percent BSA in children under 10 or adults over 50; and 3) full-thickness burns of less than 10 percent BSA in anyone. Partial-thickness burns of the hands, face, feet, or perineum or circumferential burns of an extremity are excluded. These patients typically require hospitalization for burn care.

Minor Burns

Minor burns include 1) partial-thickness burns of less than 15 percent BSA in the 10- to 50-year-old age group; 2) partial-thickness burns of less than 10 percent BSA in children under 10 or adults over 50; and 3) full-thickness burns of less than 2 percent BSA in anyone, without associated injuries. These burns generally require only outpatient treatment.

Inhalation Injury

With improvements in the treatment of burn shock and sepsis, inhalation injury has emerged as the main cause of mortality in the burn patient.[2,3,6] Despite advances in respiratory support, smoke inhalation injury significantly increases mortality; half of all fire-related deaths are due to smoke inhalation. Inhalation injuries are associated with closed-space fires and conditions that decrease mentation—such as overdose, alcohol intoxication, drug abuse, and head injury. Exposure to smoke includes exposure to heat, particulate matter, and toxic gases.[10]

There is general consensus that direct thermal injury is limited to the upper airway. Thermal injuries below the vocal cords occur only in cases of steam inhalation.

Smoke contains particulate matter, usually less than 0.5 μm in size, which is formed from incomplete combustion of organic material.

steam, grease, or flame usually cause deep partial-thickness burns. The skin may be blistered and the exposed dermis is pale white to yellow in color. The burned area does not blanch; it has absent capillary refill and absent pain sensation. Deep partial-thickness burns may be difficult to distinguish from full-thickness burns. Healing takes 3 weeks to 2 months. Scarring is common; it is related to the depth of the dermal injury. Surgical debridement and skin grafting may be necessary to obtain maximum function.

Third-degree or full-thickness burns involve the entire thickness of the skin. All epidermal and dermal structures are destroyed. Full-thickness burns are usually caused by flame, hot oil, steam, or contact with hot objects. The skin is charred, pale, painless, and leathery. These injuries will not heal spontaneously, as all dermal elements are destroyed. Surgical repair and skin grafting are necessary, and there will be significant scarring.

Fourth-degree burns are those that extend through the skin to the subcutaneous fat, muscle, and even bone. These are devastating, life-threatening injuries. Amputation or extensive reconstruction is sometimes required.

SPECIFIC ISSUES

The American Burn Association has devised a classification of burns, dividing them into major, moderate, and minor, along with indications for referral to a burn unit (Table 199-1).[5,9] Children younger than 10 years of age and adults above age 50 are considered high-risk patients. Patients with underlying medical illnesses such as heart disease, diabetes, or chronic pulmonary problems are considered poor-risk.

Small particles may reach the terminal bronchioles, where they can initiate an inflammatory reaction, leading to bronchospasm and edema.

Toxic inhalants are divided into three large groups: tissue asphyxiants, pulmonary irritants, and systemic toxins.[10] The two major tissue asphyxiants are carbon monoxide and hydrogen cyanide.

Carbon monoxide poisoning is a well-known consequence of smoke inhalation injury. Severe carbon monoxide poisoning will produce brain hypoxia and coma. Comatose patients lose airway protective mechanisms, which may result in aspiration, thus further exacerbating the pulmonary injury from smoke inhalation. All patients with suspected carbon monoxide exposure should be started on 100% oxygen by non-rebreather mask and be evaluated for hyperbaric oxygen therapy (see Chap. 203).

Hydrogen cyanide is formed when nitrogen-containing polymers—such as wool, silk, polyurethane, or vinyl—are burned. Cyanide binds to and disrupts mitochondrial oxidative phosphorylation, leading to profound tissue hypoxia. Specific treatment for cyanide toxicity may be required (see Chap. 188).

Inhalation injury damages endothelial cells, produces mucosal edema of the small airways, and decreases alveolar surfactant activity, leading to bronchospasm, airflow obstruction, and atelectasis. With time, tracheal and bronchial epithelial sloughing occurs. As these patients are resuscitated with large quantities of fluid for their burn injury, pulmonary edema develops. Approximately half of intubated burn patients admitted to burn centers develop acute respiratory distress syndrome (ARDS).[11] Therefore, when inhalation injury is present, fluid resuscitation should be done carefully to avoid exacerbating pulmonary edema, and early institution of hemodynamic monitoring is recommended.

Bronchospasm may occur early, but lower airway edema is usually not clinically evident for up to 24 h. Upper airway edema, however, can occur rapidly. Although the injury is mainly to the airways, pulmonary vascular changes do occur. There is no single method capable of demonstrating the extent of inhalation injury. Diagnosis of smoke inhalation is made from the history of a fire in an enclosed space and physical signs that include facial burns, singed nasal hair, soot in the mouth or nose, hoarseness, carbonaceous sputum, and expiratory wheezing. Carboxyhemoglobin levels are useful to document prolonged exposure within an enclosed space with incomplete combustion. The chest radiograph may be normal initially; bronchoscopy and radionuclide scanning are useful in determining the full extent of injury.

Treatment of suspected inhalation injury should be instituted prior to definitive diagnosis. Humidified oxygen (100 percent) should be administered by mask. Arterial blood gases including carboxyhemoglobin levels should be obtained. In suspected cases, control of the upper airway is achieved by prompt endotracheal intubation. Indications for intubation include 1) full-thickness burns of the face or perioral region, 2) circumferential neck burns, 3) acute respiratory distress, 4) progressive hoarseness or air hunger, 5) respiratory depression or altered mental status, and 6) supraglottic edema and inflammation on bronchoscopy.

TREATMENT

The management of patients with *moderate to major* burns can be divided into three phases: 1) prehospital care, 2) ED resuscitation and stabilization, and 3) admission or transfer to a specialized burn center.

Prehospital Care

The following principles are the basis of prehospital care for burn patients: 1) stop the burning process, 2) establish the airway, 3) initiate fluid resuscitation, 4) relieve pain, 5) protect the burn wound, and 6) transport the patient to an appropriate facility.

On-site assessment of a burned patient is divided into primary and secondary surveys. In the primary survey, immediate life-threatening conditions are quickly identified and treated. Initial management of the burned patient should be the same as for any other trauma patient, with emphasis on airway, breathing, circulation, and cervical spine immobilization. During the secondary survey, a thorough head-to-toe evaluation is carried out.

The patient must be removed from the burning process and burning clothing must be immediately removed and the remainder of the clothing removed after the airway, breathing, and circulation (ABCs) are secured. All rings, watches, jewelry, and belts should be removed, as they can retain heat and produce a tourniquet-like effect on the extremity, causing ischemia. A 100 percent oxygen mask should be applied. Thought should be given to an airway that has the potential to swell rapidly, even though initial assessment may be acceptable. Prophylactic intubation should be considered in burns about the face sustained in a closed-space fire. Intravenous fluids are started with isotonic crystalloid, usually LR solution. The patient should be covered with clean sheets to protect the wound. Early cooling can reduce the depth of burn and reduce pain, but uncontrolled cooling will result in hypothermia. Analgesia can be given upon direction of the on-line medical control physician. The patient should be transported to the nearest hospital capable of caring for a burn patient or, if none is available, the nearest hospital for stabilization.

Emergency Department Management

Upon arrival at the ED, a directed history should be obtained from the patient and emergency medical services (EMS) personnel. What was the burning agent? Were chemicals involved? What was the duration of exposure? Was the fire in an open or enclosed space? If the fire was in an enclosed area, what substances were burned? Was there an explosion causing the patient to suffer a blast injury? Was there any contact with electricity? Was there any other trauma or loss of consciousness? A general history including past medical and surgical illnesses, chronic disease, allergies, medications, and tetanus immunization status should be obtained from the patient or family.

The patient's respiratory and circulatory status should be reassessed and stabilized. The adequacy of or need for cervical immobilization should also be reassessed. The patient should be examined for signs of inhalation injury, evidenced by facial burn, carbonaceous sputum, singed nasal hair, and soot in the mouth. If there is any evidence of airway compromise with swelling of the neck, burns inside the mouth, or wheezing, endotracheal intubation should be performed.

The adequacy of circulation is initially assessed by the blood pressure, pulse rate, capillary refill time, mental status, and urinary output. When possible, intravenous lines should be inserted in nonburned areas, but when this is not possible, a burned area can be used and resuscitation started according to the burn fluid-resuscitation formula.

During the secondary examination, a head-to-toe assessment, including an eye examination for corneal burns, should be done. The size of the burn and its depth should be estimated and recorded. Patients with a greater than 20 percent partial-thickness burn routinely require a nasogastric tube, as ileus frequently occurs. A urinary drainage catheter should be inserted to measure urinary output and prevent urinary retention in patients with perineal burns.

Routine laboratory tests including a complete blood count (CBC), electrolytes, blood urea nitrogen (BUN), creatinine, and glucose should be obtained. In patients with suspected inhalation injury, arterial blood gases, carboxyhemoglobin level, chest radiograph, and electrocardiogram (ECG) should be obtained. Fiberoptic bronchoscopy is indicated when there is a suspicion of inhalation injury and in intubated patients, as this is both diagnostic and therapeutic in clearing the airways. A urinalysis for myoglobin and creatine kinase (CK) levels should be done, along with an ECG in patients with electrical injury to assess muscle or cardiac injury. Additional radiographs should be taken as indicated for other suspected trauma.

The burn shock resuscitation formulas in use today are derived from laboratory studies of burn shock and resuscitation. The value of these formulas has been questioned.[12] In general, it appears that the traditional approach using crystalloid may underestimate fluid requirements when compared to resuscitation guided by cardiorespiratory monitoring. The value of early fluid resuscitation is supported by clinical experience.[12,13] However, no consensus exists on the appropriate assessment of resuscitation and its effect on outcome.[12] At this time, the formulas only provide a *guide* for fluid resuscitation that must be monitored and adjusted according to patient response.

The Baxter or Parkland formula is probably the most widely used thermal injury resuscitation regimen in North America.[4,5] This formula calls for 4 mL of LR solution multiplied by the percentage of BSA burned (second- and third-degree burns only) multiplied by the body weight in kilograms. Half of this total is given in the first 8 h after injury and the rest during the next 16 h (Table 199-2). The amounts may be large, and hemodynamic monitoring techniques are now commonly used to protect against inadvertent volume overload.

Electrical injuries, incineration burns, and associated crush injuries may produce rhabdomyolysis and myoglobinuria, leading to renal failure. Acute renal failure occurs in approximately 15 percent of patients admitted to burn centers and is associated with severe burns (mean BSA involvement 48 percent).[14] Therapy may be required to limit renal damage from myoglobinuria (see Chap. 279).

Thermal injury in the presence of concomitant multisystem trauma generally requires fluids in excess of calculated needs. Inhalation injuries have been shown to increase total fluid needs. Burn patients with preexisting cardiac or pulmonary disease require much greater attention to fluid management. Fluid resuscitation should be monitored closely by frequent assessment of the patient's vital signs, signs of cerebral and skin perfusion, and urinary output as well as hemodynamic monitoring. The urinary output should be 0.5 to 1.0 mL/kg per h.

There are several methods of calculating fluid resuscitation for infants and children. One method is to use the Parkland formula and modify it to maintain urinary output of 1 mL/kg per h. Alternatively, a pediatric maintenance rate for 24 h can be calculated plus an additional 2 to 4 mL/kg multiplied by percentage of BSA burned, with the entire amount infused over the first 24 h. In children weighing less than 25 kg, a urine output of 1.0 mL/kg per h is necessary.

It is possible for patients with major burns to receive excessive intravenous fluids during the prehospital and ED phases, particularly if two large-bore peripheral catheters are in place with fluid infusing wide open. Total fluids infused should be documented and titrated to the patient's response.

Two additions or modifications to isotonic crystalloid resuscitation have been studied: adjuvant colloid and hypertonic saline. However, neither improves patient outcome. Adjuvant colloid given along with isotonic crystalloid resuscitation has not proven beneficial and is associated with increased accumulation of water in the lungs and de-

creased glomerular filtration rate.[15] Hypertonic saline has produced an increased rate of renal failure and death.[16]

Routine tetanus toxoid prophylaxis should be administered based on the patient's immunization history. Tetanus immune globulin should be administered in patients without a history of full primary immunization. The use of systemic prophylactic antibiotics is inappropriate.

Treatment of inhalation injury includes humidified oxygen, intubation and ventilation, bronchodilators, pulmonary toilet, and hyperbaric oxygen for severe carbon monoxide poisoning.

Burns to a pregnant patient are associated with significant morbidity to mother and child. The outcome of the pregnancy is determined by the extent of the mother's injury; spontaneous termination of pregnancy is the common outcome in large-BSA burns. Fluid requirements may exceed those estimated using the formula. Fetal monitoring and early consultation with the obstetrician is recommended.

Wound Care

After evaluation and resuscitation, the burn wounds are addressed.[17] Initially in the ED, the wound is best covered with a clean, dry sheet. Later, small burns can be covered with a moist saline-soaked dressing while the patient is awaiting admission or transfer. The soothing effect of cooling on burns is most likely due to local vasoconstriction. Studies have shown that cooling stabilizes mast cells and reduces histamine release, kinin formation, and thromboxane B_2 production. In large burns, sterile drapes are better, as saline-soaked dressings applied to a large area can cause hypothermia. The admitting service should be consulted early. The use of antiseptic dressing should be avoided in the ED as the admitting service will need to assess the wound. If the patient is going to be transferred, the accepting burn unit should be contacted for specific instructions regarding burn care. Do not delay transfer for debridement of the wound. The transferring facility should utilize the regional burn center's treatment protocol.

Patients with circumferential deep burns of the limbs may develop compromise of the distal circulation. Distal pulses need to be monitored closely; a Doppler flow probe may be very helpful. If there is compromise to the circulation, escharotomy will be needed. The eschar needs to be incised on the midlateral side of the limb, allowing the fat to bulge through. This may be extended to the hand and fingers (Figure 199-3). Escharotomy may provoke substantial soft tissue bleeding.

If there are circumferential burns of the chest and neck, the eschar may cause mechanical restriction to ventilation. An escharotomy of the chest wall needs to be done to allow adequate ventilation. Incisions need to be made at the anterior axillary line from the level of the sec-

TABLE 199-2   Parkland Formula

Adults

LR 4 mL × weight (kg) × % BSA* over initial 24 h
Half over the first 8 h from the time of burn
Other half over the subsequent 16 h
Example: 70-kg adult with 40% second- and third-degree burns
4 mL × 70 kg × 40 = 11,200 mL over 24 h

Children

LR 3 mL × weight (kg) × % BSA* over initial 24 h plus
   maintenance
Half over the first 8 h from the time of burn
Other half over the subsequent 16 h

*Second- and third-degree burns only.

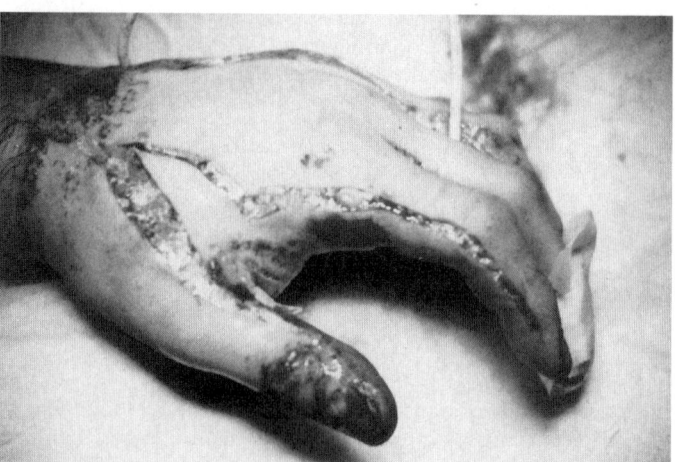

FIG. 199-3. Escharotomy of the hand.

ond rib to the level of the twelfth rib. These two incisions should be joined transversely so the chest wall can expand (Figure 199-4).

Pain Control

All burns are painful, and superficial partial-thickness burns are the most painful. Burn injury not only makes an injured area and surrounding tissue more painful, but also causes hyperalgesia, chiefly due to the A fibers. Local cooling may be soothing, but does not provide pain control.[18] Therefore pain management should be provided.

During the emergency phase, the preferred route for most medication is intravenous, because of the potential problems with absorption from the muscle and gastrointestinal tract related to decreased perfusion. Morphine is the most widely used drug for relief of pain, and relatively large doses may be required. Anxiolytic agents should be used as adjuvants in pain management.

During the acute phase and for ambulatory patients treated in the ED, opioid analgesics are required for procedural pain. Oral analgesics such as codeine, hydrocodone, oxycodone, or nonsteroidal anti-inflammatory drugs may be used for the background pain.

CARE OF MINOR BURNS IN THE EMERGENCY DEPARTMENT

The American Burn Association has defined minor burns that can be treated on an outpatient basis. To qualify as a minor burn, the injury should be isolated and not involve hands, face, feet, or perineum. The burn should not cross major joints or be circumferential. In treating a minor burn, the patient's social and medical situation should be considered. For example, an elderly patient or one with medical problems is best treated as an inpatient, even though the burn involves less than 10 percent of the BSA. The patient's reliability should be considered as an important factor for outpatient treatment. Care of minor burns requires coordination between the ED and the referral specialist who will see the patient in follow-up.[17]

As burns are painful, appropriate analgesia is required. After appropriate analgesia, the burn wound is cleaned with mild soap and water or dilute antiseptic solution. Blisters may be left intact or drained, or the overlying epithelium may be debrided; the decision depends on size and location. Large blisters or those over very mobile joints should be debrided. Small blisters on nonmobile areas should be left intact. Where compliance is questionable, patients should have the blisters debrided, because an intact or spontaneously collapsed blister may serve as a focus for wound infection. The patient's tetanus immunization status should be assessed and tetanus toxoid and/or immunoglobulin should be administered as needed.

Topical antimicrobials have an important role in reducing bacterial colonization and enhancing the rate of healing in burns.[4,5] A wide variety of topical agents are commonly used for minor burns. The most common is 1% silver sulfadiazine because it is easy to apply and has relatively little toxicity. The usual practice is to apply a thin layer of silver sulfadiazine cream to the burn and then cover it with gauze dressing. Silver sulfadiazine should not be used in patients with sulfa allergy, or on the face because of potential staining. Alternative opinions about the routine use of silver sulfadiazine have been expressed.[19]

Alternative topical agents to use in these circumstances are bacitracin or triple-antibiotic (neomycin, polymyxin B, and bacitracin zinc) ointments. Although 8.5% mafenide acetate cream and 0.2% furacin ointment are available for topical use, these should be used with caution if applied to large burns in an outpatient setting. Mafenide is a carbonic anhydrase inhibitor and can cause metabolic acidosis. Furacin is in a polyethylene glycol vehicle that can be toxic if absorbed in patients with compromised renal function. Mafenide penetrates the eschar well and has utility in treating patients with invasive infections.

Dressings are ideally changed twice daily as long as the wounds continue to weep; then they are changed daily until the burn is healed. Synthetic occlusive dressing is an alternative method of managing partial-thickness burns in outpatients. The wounds are cleansed and debrided prior to application of these dressings (e.g., Biobrane, Dow Hickam Pharmaceuticals; Tegaderm, 3M Health Care; DuoDERM, Bristol-Myers Squibb). This method is most successful for clean burns on flat surfaces. The goal is to have the dressing adhere to the wound so that it acts as artificial skin. Adherence is important, as most of the bacteria causing infection produce fibrinolytic agents. Wounds are checked at 24 to 48 h for adherence, and the dressing is left in place until spontaneous separation occurs. There is evidence that wounds treated with these synthetic occlusive dressings are better tolerated by patients, require fewer dressing changes, and heal with better appearance.[20]

Patients must be given discharge instructions that explain home burn care and symptoms and signs of infection. The patient should be advised to return to the ED immediately if there are any signs or symptoms of infection. Extremity burns should be elevated for 24 to 48 h to prevent edema. All burn wounds should be reassessed at 24 h for depth and extent of burn. The follow-up visit schedule should be clearly explained and analgesics prescribed. Deep partial-thickness, full-thickness, and mixed-thickness burns should be referred to a plastic surgeon or burn-care specialist in 2 to 4 days for reevaluation and consideration of skin grafting.

REFERENCES

1. American Burn Association: Burn incidence fact sheet. Accessed at www.ameriburn.org, January 29, 2003.
2. Ryan CM, Schoenfeld DA, Thorpe WP, et al: Objective estimates of the probability of death from burn injuries. *New Engl J Med* 338:362, 1998.
3. Muller MJ, Pegg SP, Rule MR: Determinants of death following burn injury. *Br J Surg* 88:583, 2001.
4. Sheridan RL: Burns. *Crit Care Med* 30(Suppl):S500, 2002.
5. Saffle J (ed): *Practice Guidelines for Burn Care.* Chicago, American Burn Association, 2001.
6. Saffle JR, Davis B, Williams P, American Burn Association Registry Participant Group: Recent outcomes in the treatment of burn injury in the United States: A report from the American Burn Association Patient Registry. *J Burn Care Rehabil* 16:219, 1995.
7. Baxter CR, Shires T: Physiological response to crystalloid resuscitation of severe burns. *Ann NY Acad Sci* 150:874, 1968.
8. Hendricks WM: The classification of burns. *J Am Acad Dermatol* 22:838, 1998.
9. Guidelines for the Operation of Burn Units, in Committee on Trauma, American College of Surgeons: *Resources for Optimal Care of the Injured Patient.* Chicago, American College of Surgeons, 1999. [Available from the American Burn Association website at www.ameriburn.org.]
10. Hartzell GE: Overview of combustion toxicology. *Toxicology* 115:7, 1996.
11. Dancey DR, Hayes J, Gomez M, et al: ARDS in patients with thermal injury. *Intensive Care Med* 25:1231, 1999.

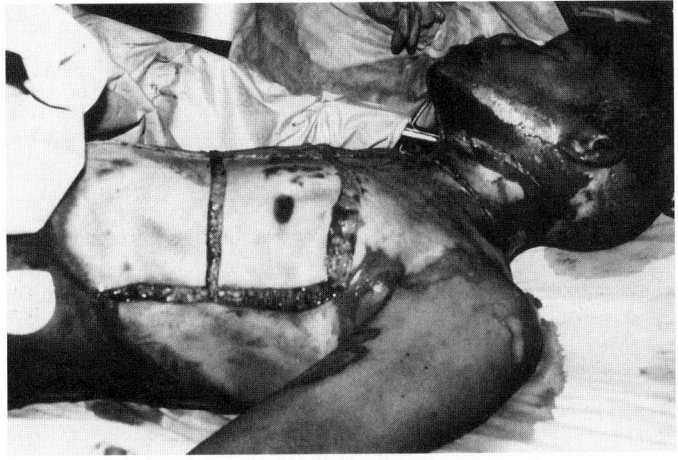

FIG. 199-4. Escharotomy of the chest wall.

12. Holm C: Resuscitation in shock associated with burns. Tradition or evidence-based medicine? *Resuscitation* 44:157, 2000.

13. Barrow RE, Jeschke MG, Herndon DN: Early fluid resuscitation improves outcomes in severely burned children. *Resuscitation* 45:91, 2000.

14. Holm C, Horbrand F, von Donnersmarck GH, et al: Acute renal failure in severely burned patients. *Burns* 25:171, 1999.

15. Gore DC, Dalton JM, Gehr TW: Colloid infusions reduce glomerular filtration in resuscitated burn victims. *J Trauma* 40:356, 1996.

16. Huang PP, Stucky FS, Dimick AR, et al: Hypertonic sodium resuscitation is associated with renal failure and death. *Ann Surg* 221:543, 1995.

17. Smith S, Duncan M, Mobley J, et al: Emergency room management of minor burn injuries: A quality management evaluation. *J Burn Care Rehabil* 18:76, 1997.

18. Werner MU, Lassen B, Pedersen JL, et al: Local cooling does not prevent hyperalgesia following burn injury in humans. *Pain* 98:297, 2002.

19. Chung JY, Herbert ME: Myth: Silver sulfadiazine is the best treatment for minor burns. *West J Med* 175:205, 2001.

20. Barret JP, Dziewulski P, Ramzy PI, et al: Biobrane versus 1% silver sulfadiazine in second-degree pediatric burns. *Plast Reconstr Surg* 105:62, 2000.

CHEMICAL BURNS

Fred P. Harchelroad, Jr
David M. Rottinghaus

More than 25,000 products are capable of producing chemical burns. Exposures occur both occupationally and during use of chemicals for activities in daily life. It is estimated that chemical burns account for 5 to 10 percent of all U.S. burn center admissions. Nonoccupational exposures number about 100,000 per year, the vast majority being minor. Deaths are rare and usually from caustic ingestion. In 2001, there were 9481 reported nonfatal chemical exposures in private industry causing days missed from work, representing about 0.5 percent of all injuries. Also, there were 96 deaths from chemical exposure in the workplace reported in 2001.[1]

Common household chemical burns are caused by lye (drain cleaners), paint removers (halogenated hydrocarbons), phenols (deodorizers, sanitizers, disinfectants), sodium hypochlorite (disinfectants, bleaches), methacrylic acid (artificial nail products), and sulfuric acid (toilet bowl cleaners). In industries, chemicals are used for cleaning, tanning, curing, extracting, preserving, soldering, and other functions. The most commonly used industrial acids are tungstic, picric, sulfosalicylic, tannic, formic, sulfuric, acetic, cresylic, trichloroacetic, chromic, hydrochloric, and hydrofluoric. Widely used alkalis are the hydroxide salts of sodium, potassium, ammonium, lithium, barium, and calcium. White phosphorus used in munitions was the most common cause of chemical burns to military personnel during times of armed conflict in the 1960s. White phosphorus also may be found in rodenticides, pesticides, and fireworks.

The body sites most often burned by chemicals are the face, eyes, and extremities. In general, chemical burns are smaller than thermal burns and the mortality rate is lower. However, wound healing and duration of hospital stay are longer. Disability and time away from work tend to be greater than that of other occupational injuries.

PATHOPHYSIOLOGY

The skin constitutes a barrier and transition zone between the internal and external environments. The outer stratum corneum layer of the skin functions as an excellent barrier against many chemicals, although some may penetrate it readily.

Chemicals can produce burns, dermatitis, allergic reaction, thermal injury, or systemic toxicity. Pathophysiologically, burns produced by all chemicals are similar because the skin has a limited variety of toxic responses.[2] Toxic reactions are described mainly on the basis of morpho-logic rather than functional responses.[3] Skin has protective mechanisms and elements, including the epidermal barrier, eccrine sweating, phagocytic cells, metabolic detoxification, immunologic processes, and melanin pigmentation. However, these protective mechanisms vary according to phenotype and may be affected by systemic or local disease.

Skin damage by chemicals may demonstrate the classic manifestations of thermal injury (erythema, blistering, or full-thickness loss). However, an acute injury may be deceptively mild, only to be followed by extensive skin damage and systemic toxicity. A superficial (first-degree) burn causes capillary and arterial dilatation. Initially, this involves only the superficial vessels, but then extends to the deeper subcutaneous vessels by both direct and reflex action. Tissue hyperemia and congestion result in symptoms of itching, burning, or pain. More extensive inflammatory reactions result in an outpouring of fluid into the extracellular space, causing edema and vesicle or bulla formation characteristic of partial-thickness (second-degree) burns. Continued chemical damage through the dermis or into the hypodermis results in a full-thickness (third-degree) burn.

Tissue damage is determined by: 1) strength/concentration of the agent, 2) manner of contact, 3) quantity of agent, 4) phase of agent (i.e., liquid vs. solid), 5) duration of contact, 6) mechanism of action, and 7) extent of penetration. Factors enhancing percutaneous absorption of chemical are body site (areas of thin skin, i.e., genitalia, face; chemical contact between skinfolds; amount of surface area exposed); integrity of skin (traumatized skin, elderly skin, dehydration, inflammation); nature of the chemical (lipid solubility, pH, concentration); and occlusion (garments, occlusive dressings).

The majority of chemical burns are caused by acids or alkalis. At similar volumes and manner of contact, alkalis usually produce far more tissue damage than acids. Acids in general cause coagulation necrosis with protein precipitation, tending to form a tough leathery eschar. The eschar typically limits deeper penetration of the agent. Alkalis produce liquefaction necrosis and saponification of lipids. The result is a poor barrier to chemical penetration and deeper, ongoing burns. Not all chemicals causing burns can be considered acid or alkali. A useful classification by Jelenko groups chemicals by the manner in which they damage protein:[4]

1. Oxidizing agents: Damage is produced when a chemical becomes oxidized in contact with tissue. Often a toxic moiety is released during this reaction.
2. Corrosives: Extensive protein denaturation is produced, resulting in soft eschar and shallow, indolent ulcers.
3. Reducing agents: Protein denaturation is produced by binding of free electrons in tissue protein.
4. Desiccants: Severe cellular dehydration is produced, and thermal injury occurs due to exothermic reaction.
5. Vesicant: Blisters are produced, tissue cytokines are liberated, local ischemia and anoxic tissue damage and pandermic inflammation occur.
6. Protoplasmic poisons: Protein is denatured by salt formation or by metabolic competition/inhibition (i.e., binding calcium or other inorganic ions is necessary for tissue viability and function).

GENERAL APPROACH

The goal of treatment is to minimize any area of irreversible injury and maximize salvage in the zone of reversible damage. With few exceptions, aggressive hydrotherapy is the cornerstone of initial treatment for chemical burns. Chemical agents may continue to damage tissue until they are removed or inactivated. Immediate removal from the offending chemical, removal of garments, and counteraction of the chemical remaining on the body by dilution, debridement, or neutralization are important measures. Dry chemical particles such as lime should be brushed away before irrigation. Sodium metal and related compounds should be initially covered with mineral oil or excised, since water can cause a severe exothermic reaction. Dilution of phenol (carbolic acid) with water may enhance penetration. For the most part, however, use of water or saline to irrigate a chemical burn should not be delayed while searching for other treatment agents and should begin at the scene of the accident. Almost universally, earlier irrigation means a better prognosis.

The amount of elapsed time to initiate dilution or removal of chemical agents relates to the depth and degree of injury. Wounds irrigated 3 min after contact with some chemicals have a twofold greater chance of becoming full-thickness burns than wounds irrigated within 1 min of chemical contact. When using agents to neutralize a chemical burn, additional tissue injury may occur through heat production. In some cases, heat may be produced by using water irrigation, but copious amounts will decrease the rate and amount of chemical reaction and dissipate the heat. Irrigation should be maintained at a gentle flow to avoid driving the chemical deeper into tissue or splashing chemical into the victim or rescuer's eyes. The time required for irrigation varies; irrigation may need to be continued for hours in the case of severe alkali burns. Use of pH indicator paper may help determine continued presence of alkali or acid in burn wounds and possible need for further irrigation. A more accurate pH result will be obtained if the test is performed 10 to 15 min after completion of irrigation. This will allow residual chemical in the deeper areas to diffuse to the surface.

After irrigation and debridement of remaining particles and devitalized tissue, topical antimicrobial agents should be used and tetanus immunization should be updated. Other than measures specific for a particular chemical burn, treatment following initial therapy is basically the same as for thermal burns. Patients sustaining extensive chemical burns require the same aggressive fluid replacement as those with thermal burns. Analgesics may be needed, and in the case of allergic responses to chemicals, antihistamines, steroids, and epinephrine may be required. Early tangential excision and surgical management of severe burns, especially from alkalis or those with ongoing tissue destruction, have been shown to reduce burn size. This method, in conjunction with persistent hydrotherapy, also reduces operative blood loss.[5] Autografts, heterografts, homografts, or synthetic material may be necessary for full-thickness burns. Hyperbaric oxygen may be utilized to assist healing of resistant burn wounds.

SPECIFIC CHEMICALS

Acids

With the exception of hydrofluoric acid, strong acids produce coagulation necrosis from the desiccating action of the acid on proteins in the superficial tissue. Injury severity is related to the physical characteristics of the acid. Most substances with a pH less than 2 are strong corrosives. Other important tissue-damaging properties of acids include concentration, molarity, and complexing affinity for hydroxyl ions. The higher each of these factors is, the greater is the tissue damage. Contact time with the skin is the most important chemical burn feature that health care professionals may alter. Instantaneous skin decontamination of 18 *M* sulfuric acid will cause no burn; however, a 1-min exposure can cause full-thickness skin damage. Examination of a patient with a significant chemical burn from these acids should not be limited to observation of the skin, because several of these acids are respiratory and mucous membrane irritants as well. Furthermore, skin absorption of some compounds may occur and result in systemic signs and symptoms.

ACETIC ACID   The dilute (<40%) acetic acid solution found in hair-wave neutralizer solutions is perhaps the most common cause of chemical burns to the scalp in women. Prolonged contact, especially with an already damaged scalp, may cause a partial-thickness burn that heals slowly because of the constant bacterial flora on the scalp.

Initial treatment is copious water irrigation. As trimming the hair is not a viable option in these patients, oral antibiotics are often given if the entire scalp is involved.

CARBOLIC ACID (PHENOL)   Phenol (carbolic acid), a corrosive organic acid used widely in industry and medicine, denatures proteins and causes chemical burns characterized by a white or brown coagulum that is relatively painless. Systemic absorption may result in life-threatening complications. Its unpleasant, acrid odor, detectable in air at 0.047 parts per million, and its low volatility, help prevent airborne exposure. Though commercially available in concentrations up to 90% even dilute solutions of 1 to 2% phenol may cause a burn if contact is prolonged. Hexylresorcinol is a bactericidal phenol derivative. Chemically related phenolic compounds that induce skin damage include cresol, creosote, and cresylic acid.

Coagulation necrosis of the involved area is common. Necrotic tissue may delay absorption temporarily, but phenol may become entrapped under the eschar. Contaminated clothing should be removed and water lavage begun immediately. Water lavage alone may be ineffective, presumably because the necrotic coagulum inhibits water penetration to the deeper layers. Paradoxically, dilute phenol penetrates tissue more readily than when concentrated.

More effective decontamination has been demonstrated with a 5- to 10-min swab with a combination of polyethylene glycol 300 (PEG 300) and industrial methylated spirits (IMS) in a 2:1 mixture. This should not only reduce the extent of cutaneous corrosion but also decrease systemic toxicity. The PEG 300 is mixed with the IMS for a more liquid (and therefore easier to use) formulation. However, the viscous PEG 300 or PEG 400 may be used alone, and, indeed, glycerol is an acceptable substitute if the PEG-IMS mixture is not available. The use of an isopropyl alcohol rinse appears to be equal to PEG-IMS in removing phenol.[6] The advantage of isopropyl alcohol is its ready availability.

CHROMIC ACID   The toxicity of chromium compounds is related to the powerful oxidizing action of the hexavalent compounds (Cr^{6+}). The chromate ion in chromic acid will produce a chronic penetrating ulcerating lesion of the skin. Associated signs and symptoms are conjunctivitis, lacrimation, ulceration of the nasal septum, and systemic chromium toxicity with liver or renal failure, GI bleeding, coagulopathy, and CNS disturbances. A 10 percent total body surface area (BSA) cutaneous burn caused by chromic acid can be fatal due to systemic toxicity. Significant symptoms may occur after only 1 to 2 percent BSA burns. Any acute skin exposure to chromic acid should be treated with copious water irrigation and observation for systemic effects. Aggressive excision has been shown to be the best method for prevention of systemic effects because depth of the burn is difficult to determine and absorption of chromium may continue.[7] Topical agents such as 5% thiosulfate and ascorbic acid are useful in preventing toxicity while preparing for surgical excision.

FORMIC ACID   Formic acid in 60% solution is used by acrylate-glue makers, cellulose formate workers, and tanning workers. Formic acid produces coagulation necrosis of the skin. Systemic effects including decreased respiration and an anion-gap metabolic acidosis have been reported.[8] Treatment includes immediate decontamination and irrigation with water. Open lesions should be treated like any damaged skin: with debridement of devitalized tissue, prevention of further damage and infection, and skin grafting if the defect is full-thickness and of a size requiring coverage.

HYDROCHLORIC AND SULFURIC ACIDS   The dermal toxicity of hydrochloric acid and sulfuric acid is so well recognized that early decontamination and water irrigation usually prevent severe burns to the skin. These acids can burn the skin dark brown or black. Toilet bowl cleaners may contain 80% solutions of sulfuric acid, and some drain cleaners may be 95 to 99% sulfuric acid solutions. Munitions, chemical, and fertilizer manufacturers commonly use 95 to 98% sulfuric acid solutions in their industrial processes. Automobile battery fluid is 25% sulfuric acid. Most household bleaches are only 3 to 6% hypochlorite solutions, which, though acidic, cause little damage unless they are in contact with skin for a prolonged time. Treatment is the same as for formic acid burns.

HYDROFLUORIC ACID Hydrofluoric acid (HF) is unique among the corrosives in its mechanism of action and degree of toxicity. HF applications include use in production of high-octane fuel, etching and frosting glass, semiconductors, microelectronics/microinstruments, germicides, dyes, plastics, tanning, and fireproofing material, and use in cleaning stone and brick buildings. It is also a very effective rust remover.

HF acts like alkalis and will cause progressive tissue loss, including bony destruction. HF produces burns in two ways. First, hydrogen ions cause direct cellular damage, often producing deep burns. Second, free fluoride ions are released, causing deeper burns and toxicity by immobilization of intracellular calcium and magnesium and poisoning of cellular enzymatic reactions. Potassium permeability is increased and results in spontaneous depolarization of nerve tissue and pain. Pain will persist until all free fluoride ions have been neutralized.

HF rapidly penetrates the skin and causes both local and potentially lethal systemic toxicity. Its systemic effects include hypocalcemia, hypomagnesemia, and hyperkalemia. The dermal effects may not be immediately noted and appear to be more related to the concentration of HF than to the duration of exposure. Solutions greater than 50% produce immediate pain and tissue destruction; solutions less than 20% may not produce signs and symptoms until 12 to 24 h after exposure. The skin may develop a blue-gray appearance with a surrounding region of erythema.

Unlike the treatment of dermal injury caused by other acids, the treatment of HF burns consists of two phases. The first, which should be immediate, is copious water irrigation of the affected skin for 15 to 30 min. This may be the only treatment that is needed if the HF solution is less than 20% concentration, the duration of exposure was very brief, and decontamination is begun immediately. Unfortunately, this is rarely the case. Severe, persistent pain denotes a more serious injury requiring the second phase of treatment.

The second phase of treatment is aimed at detoxifying the enzyme-poisoning fluoride ion. Two ions—calcium (Ca^{2+}) and magnesium (Mg^{2+})—have been shown to be beneficial in binding the fluoride and curtailing its toxic effects. However, the overwhelming clinical experience to date has been with the use of calcium gluconate, and it should be considered the agent of choice. Several therapeutic modalities are available for using calcium gluconate: topical, subcutaneous/intradermal injection, or intraarterial infusion. An intravenous regional perfusion technique based on Bier's method has been described and reported effective.[9] High-dose intravenous magnesium sulfate appears to be effective in animal models, but human data are lacking.[10]

A calcium gluconate gel made with either Surgilube (E. Fougera & Co.) or dimethyl sulfoxide (DMSO) in a 2.5 to 10% concentration may be applied directly to the affected area.[11] The main limitation of topical therapy is the impermeability of the skin to calcium. Penetration into the dermis and subcutaneous tissues may be enhanced if the formulation with DMSO is used, but DMSO can cause toxicity. The topical therapy can be used in the outpatient setting, and industries utilizing HF should keep this topical formulation on hand for emergency use.

Subcutaneous and intradermal injection of a 5% calcium gluconate solution through a 30-gauge needle into the HF-burned skin is the most widely used treatment. A maximum dose of 1.0 mL of 5% calcium gluconate per square centimeter of burned skin is recommended. Pain relief is nearly immediate, and indeed, the elimination of pain may be used as a guide for further therapy. Recurrence of pain indicates the need for further therapy. Unfortunately, injection therapy has several disadvantages: 1) only limited amounts of calcium are deliv-

ered to the tissue; 2) hyperosmolarity and inherent toxicity of free calcium ions cause more pain initially, and more tissue damage is possible if calcium is not bound to fluoride; 3) vascular compromise can result if too much fluid is injected, especially into digits; and 4) rapid penetration of HF beneath the nail requires nail removal to administer the calcium gluconate into the nailbed adequately.

Intraarterial infusion of calcium gluconate may be used to prevent tissue necrosis and stop the pain associated with HF burns. This should be performed as soon as possible after the initial burn, preferably within 6 h of insult. An intraarterial catheter should be placed in the appropriate vascular supply (the brachial artery if the entire hand is affected) and connected to a three-way stopcock to which is attached an arterial pressure-monitoring device and the infusion syringe of calcium gluconate. A 50-mL syringe may be filled with 10 mL of a 10% calcium gluconate solution and 40 mL of D5. This should be infused over 2 to 4 h. The arterial pressure-monitoring device ensures that the catheter has not dislodged from the lumen of the cannulated artery. Infusion of the calcium solution into the deep tissues may cause further tissue damage. Repeat infusion may be needed if pain recurs within 4 h. This intraarterial infusion avoids the disadvantages of local infiltration therapy; however, it has its own disadvantages: an invasive vascular procedure that 1) may result in arterial spasm or thrombosis and 2) requires more time and resources, including hospital admission.

Nebulized calcium gluconate is a recognized treatment for inhalational exposures to HF. Ocular exposure to HF requires water irrigation for at least 30 min. Treatment with calcium chloride or magnesium chloride by subconjunctival injection or irrigation may increase corneal damage. Complete and quick recovery by utilizing 1% calcium carbonate eyedrops in a patient who had sustained a large corneal erosion due to a 49% HF burn has been reported.

Iontophoresis has recently been explored as a means to enhance penetration of calcium through the dermis and tissues more effectively by using an electric field across the skin. Patches are placed on the skin and an electrical field is established, creating a gradient by which ions are transported across the skin, enhancing delivery. This technique shows promise, but limitations include time to set up the apparatus and ability to treat only small burns.[12]

Systemic toxicity related to dermal HF exposure has resulted in death. This appears to be related to myocardial irritability and subsequent ventricular fibrillation as a result of systemic acidosis, hyperkalemia, hypomagnesemia, and hypocalcemia. Cardiac monitoring, intravenous access, and electrolyte monitoring should be performed in cases of all significant HF dermal burns.

METHACRYLIC ACID Methacrylic acid found in many artificial nail cosmetic products can produce severe dermal burns, usually in preschoolers.[13]

NITRIC ACID Nitric acid is used in industry for casting iron and steel, electroplating, engraving, and fertilizer manufacturing. Upon contact with skin, nitric acid can produce tissue damage by oxidation and may turn the skin yellowish as it is burned.

OXALIC ACID Oxalic acid is used for leather tanning and blueprint paper. Like hydrofluoric acid, it poisons enzymatic processes. Oxalic acid binds calcium and prevents muscle contraction. The wounds should be irrigated with water, and intravenous calcium may be required. Serum electrolytes and renal function should be evaluated, and cardiac monitoring should be instituted after serious dermal exposure.

Alkalis

Alkalis penetrate skin much more deeply and longer than acids, with a greater danger of toxicity from systemic absorption. Wounds may initially look superficial and in 2 to 3 days become full-thickness burns. Alkalis combine with protein and lipids in tissue to form soluble protein complexes and soaps that permit passage of hydroxyl ions deep into tissue. Soft, gelatinous, friable, brownish eschars are often produced. Strong alkalis have a pH ≥12.

LYES Strong, corrosive alkalis ("lyes") include ammonium, barium, calcium, lithium, potassium (caustic potash), and sodium (caustic soda) hydroxides. Lyes are widely used in industry and are found in home products (drain and toilet cleaners, detergents, and paint removers). The urine sugar reagent tablet Clinitest (Bayer) contains anhydrous sodium hydroxide. As a mode of assault, lyes have a lower mortality rate than gunshot wounds or stabbings, but victims often suffer long-term pain, scarring, and blindness.[14] Lyes are extremely corrosive and penetrating, and burns require copious irrigation for long periods. Suicidal ingestion of lye may result in rapid death from upper airway occlusion. Late morbidity related to esophageal and gastric necrosis may be minimized by early surgical intervention with esophagogastrectomy.

Ammonium hydroxide is used in the production of synthetic fibers and extensively in agriculture. Toxicity can be severe and include mucous membrane, ocular, dermal, gastrointestinal, and inhalational/pulmonary injury. Treatment is as with other lyes, with immediate, voluminous, and persistent irrigation.[15]

LIME Lime (calcium oxide) is found in agricultural products and cements. There is considerable variability of lime content in different grades of cement, with fine to textured masonry cement having more lime than concrete. Lime is converted by water to the alkali calcium hydroxide. Upon skin contact, lime draws water out of the skin. All dry lime particles should be brushed away prior to irrigation. Paradoxically, a small amount of water may generate an exothermic reaction with tissue injury secondary to calcium hydroxide formation, so a large amount and strong stream of water (taking care to avoid splashing in eyes) should be used and will permit dissipation of heat.

PORTLAND CEMENT Portland cement, which accounts for a major proportion of the cement used in the United States, is a mixture of sand, lime, and other metal oxides. In the presence of water, calcium hydroxide, sodium hydroxide, and potassium hydroxide may all be formed. Workers who kneel in wet cement or get cement in their boots may discover burns hours after initial contact. In addition, skin may become irritated from gritty material, and a contact dermatitis may develop in individuals sensitive to the chromate contained in the material.

Metals

Foundry workers are sometimes burned by molten metal, which may spill or splash on body parts and run down into the boots. Elemental metals, sodium, lithium, potassium, magnesium, aluminum, and calcium may all cause burns. When exposed to air, some elemental metals spontaneously ignite. Water is generally contraindicated in extinguishing burning metal fragments embedded in the skin, because the explosive exothermic reaction that may result can lead to significant tissue injury. Burning metal may be extinguished with a class D fire extinguisher or smothered with sand. Covering metal fragments with mineral oil, however, appears to be the favored treatment method. Wound debridement should include excision of metal fragments that cannot be wiped away. Metal fragments should be placed in mineral oil to prevent further ignition.

Others

HYDROCARBONS Hydrocarbons will cause a fat-dissolving corrosive injury to the skin. In our present petroleum-dependent society, gasoline is a common agent of chemical burns. Patients sustaining gasoline immersion burns usually have undergone some other traumatic insult (e.g., a motor vehicle accident). Gasoline is a complex mixture of alkanes, cycloalkanes, and aromatic hydrocarbons. A hydrocarbon chemical burn resembles either a thermal scald or a partial-thickness burn.[16] Full-thickness burns secondary to prolonged contact with gasoline have been reported. Topical gasoline exposure in cold weather can result in frostbite of the digits due to rapid evaporation of gasoline resulting in heat loss from the skin. Systemic effects of the involved hydrocarbon (or what it was a solvent for) may expose the patient to greater morbidity than the skin damage. Dehydration of the skin associated with solvent contact contributes to injury. Patients should be advised not to use harsh soaps over the areas of defatting dermatitis caused by hydrocarbons, as these will cause further skin damage. Treatment involves decontamination; otherwise, management is as for a thermal burn.

Hot tar is derived from long-chain petroleum and coal hydrocarbons. Roofing tars and asphalt are heated to temperatures in excess of 500°F (260°C), and the burns sustained are usually thought of more as thermal than chemical. Cold tar can produce a liquefaction injury to tissue. Though the surface area size of the burn is usually small, solidified material stuck to skin and hair is hard to remove. If hot, the tar should be cooled to prevent continued thermal injury. Manual mechanical debridement can be painful and destructive to skin structures. Polyoxylene sorbitan (polysorbate) contained in many antibiotic ointments is an emulsifying agent that can be used to remove tar. Industrial removal agents such as De-solv-it, a citrus and petroleum distillate, are also effective in tar removal. Mayonnaise has been reported as a home remedy used topically in a similar fashion.

VESICANTS (DMSO, CANTHARIDES, AND MUSTARD GAS) DMSO, cantharides, and mustard gas are considered to be vesicant agents. Skin burns with edema and blister formation can occur due to production of ischemia and anoxic necrosis at the site of contact. DMSO is a water-soluble organic solvent that has been used industrially since the 1940s. General therapeutic interest in DMSO began in the 1960s, when it was used topically by thousands of patients for sprains, bruises, minor burns, and arthritis. Its use has declined substantially because of eye toxicity, although it is still used for research and some clinical problems. Cantharides ("Spanish Fly") is used as a veterinary aphrodisiac and occasionally by human beings as well for its supposed aphrodisiac effects. Mustard gas is a vesicant in which public interest has resurfaced because of the threat of biochemical warfare and terrorist attack. Sulfur mustard is the most widely used of these agents. The development of British anti-lewisite was initiated by the threat of the arsenical war-gas, lewisite. It was found to effectively chelate arsenic as well as donate sulfur to minimize skin damage.

Skin damage following vesicant exposure can be severe and result in deep skin penetration, edema, blisters, ulcers, and serious morbidity. Burns resulting from vesicants should be irrigated copiously with water or saline. Skin can be decontaminated by using adsorbent powders (flour, talcum powder, Fuller's earth) if the supply of water is limited. The powder adsorbs the mustard from the skin and should be wiped away with a moist towel. The military uses M258A1 kits for skin decontamination. These kits contain three sets of towelettes, one of each containing phenol, sodium hydroxide, and sodium benzenesulphonochloramine (chloramine). Chloramine produces "free" chlorine, which inactivates sulfur mustard. Povidone iodine shows great promise in the prevention and early treatment of skin damage caused by sulfur mustard. Human data are currently lacking, but in animal models both prevention of burns and immediate (<10 min) treatment of exposure yielded impressive skin protection.[17]

POTASSIUM PERMANGANATE Potassium permanganate is an oxidizing agent that is mildly irritating in dilute solution, but in concentrated solution can produce dermal burns with a thick, brownish purple eschar of coagulated protein. Burns should be copiously irrigated.

ALKYL MERCURY COMPOUNDS   Alkyl mercury compounds, which are reducing agents used in disinfectants, fungicides, and wood preservatives, can produce dermatitis or burn lesions. Lesions typically are erythematous with blister formation. The blister fluid is high in metallic mercury content. The burning process continues as long as the agent remains in contact with skin. Partial-thickness burns deepen if the blister fluid is allowed to remain, so the blisters should be debrided, drained, and copiously irrigated.

DIQUAT DIBROMIDE   Full-thickness skin burns have been reported to occur after prolonged exposure to the herbicide diquat dibromide. These burns were treated with skin grafting. It is unknown whether earlier therapy would have prevented the chain of events.

LACRIMATORS (CHLOROACETOPHENONE, CHLOROBENZYLI-DENEMALONITRILE, AND DIBENZOXAZEPINE)   Lacrimators (tear gas) such as chloroacetophenone (CN), chlorobenzylidene-malonitrile (CS), and dibenzoxazepine (CR) cause skin and mucosal irritation and contact dermatitis. The epidermal injury is limited, in contrast to the possible pulmonary parenchymal damage. Burns to the skin are treated with standard water irrigation. Ocular irritation is treated with copious water irrigation, followed by slit-lamp exam for corneal damage. Structural damage to the cornea occurs at high concentrations of these lacrimators. Pepper gas (trichloronitromethane), so named because of its pepper-like odor and propensity to induce sneezing, is used in some areas by law enforcement agencies. As with the other lacrimators, it will cause mucous membrane, ocular, and upper airway irritation (as well as bronchospasm in susceptible patients). Treatment is copious irrigation with saline and removal of the patient from the offending agent.

WHITE PHOSPHORUS   White phosphorus is a chemical used as an incendiary and in insecticides, rodenticides, and fertilizers. It can ignite spontaneously when exposed to air and is rapidly oxidized to phosphorus pentoxide. White phosphorus is commonly found in hand grenades and other warfare munitions and thus is implicated in wartime and accidental burns to military personnel. In munitions, white phosphorus is solid, but some of it may liquefy with detonation. Burns may be caused by liquid or solid forms. White phosphorus burns may be complicated by multiple traumatic injuries as a result of shell fragments and the force of weapon explosions. Because of its many uses, white phosphorus burns also occur in civilians.

Flaming droplets of inorganic phosphorus may embed beneath the skin. The heat of reaction can be directly destructive to tissue. Particles continue to oxidize slowly until either debrided, neutralized, or completely oxidized. Contaminated clothing should be removed, visible particles debrided, and burns copiously irrigated with normal saline or water. A brief rinse with 1% copper sulfate solution may be helpful. Copper sulfate combines with phosphorus to form a dark-copper phosphide coating on the particles that makes them easier to see and debride, and also impedes further oxidation. However, copper sulfate can cause hemolysis and hemoglobinuria, and should be used with caution. Inorganic phosphorus particles may reignite if allowed to dry out, so wounds should be submerged or packed with soaked dressings.

White phosphorus burns are characterized by slow healing and ongoing burning, necessitating early and aggressive treatment. Systemic toxicity is a major risk, with hypocalcemia, hyperkalemia, and hepatic and renal injury all reported. Even patients with small burns should be considered for admission or transfer to a burn center for hydration, monitoring, and further treatment.[18]

Airbag Burns

Approximately 8 percent of individuals suffering injuries related to airbag deployment are burned. Airbags deploy by ignition of a solid propellant—sodium azide—that creates an exothermic reaction leading to quick inflation of the airbag. Many other gases are created during activation, including corrosives such as sodium hydroxide, nitric oxide, ammonia, and multiple hydrocarbons. An airbag is deflated within 2 s of inflation through exhaust side ports on the bag. Burns associated with airbags include friction, thermal, and chemical burns.[19] Sodium hydroxide has been implicated in the chemical keratitis reported after airbag deployment. Sodium azide may cause cutaneous burns in addition to severe systemic effects, but its contribution to airbag chemical burns is limited. Treatment of airbag chemical burns is similar to any alkali burn: immediate and copious water irrigation.

OCULAR BURNS

Chemical burns to the eyes are common and considered true ocular emergencies requiring immediate treatment.[20] Typically, chemical burns to the eye occur in the industrial setting, in laboratories, or as a result of accidents such as battery explosion and intentional assaults. Rupture of automobile airbags with spillage of chemicals onto the face represents a new potential source of ocular as well as skin burns. Early signs and symptoms of eye burns include tearing, rubbing, redness, pain, and blepharospasm. The conjunctiva, if severely injured, may appear pale due to ischemia and destruction of vascular supply. Swelling of the corneal epithelium, clouding of the anterior chamber, pupillary dilatation, and corneal ulceration may all occur.

If the nature of the chemical is not known, pH paper should be used to determine the presence of acid or alkali. Acid quickly precipitates the superficial tissue proteins of the eye, producing the typical "ground glass" appearance of the cornea. Penetration is limited by local buffering and barrier effects of the precipitated proteins. Damage sustained secondary to acid burns in most cases is immediate and limited to the area of contact. The posterior segment of the eye rarely suffers injury, and there are usually no late effects such as cell disruption or tissue softening.

Alkali burns are more severe, and results are frequently unsightly and disastrous. In general, the higher the pH of the alkali, the more damage. In a short period, strong alkali can penetrate the cornea, anterior chamber, and the retina, with destruction of all sensory elements, thus causing complete blindness. Severe chemosis, blanched conjunctiva, and an opacified cornea obscuring view of the iris or lens may occur. The penetration of alkali can continue for hours to days, resulting in globe perforation. The conjunctiva, and scleral blood vessels and collecting veins of the anterior chamber may be destroyed, leading to secondary glaucoma. Second- and third-degree burns of surrounding tissue can complicate the burn.

Chronic inflammation of the iris and ciliary body (iridocyclitis) and adhesions between lens and iris (posterior synechiae) are possible complications of ocular burns. Other complications of eye burns include ectropion (lid deformity), cataract formation, scarring and marked revascularization of the cornea, and scarring of both palpebral and bulbar conjunctiva with resulting adhesions between the lids and globe (symblepharon).

Treatment of eye burns should begin immediately, utilizing nonsterile or tap water if needed. Immediate treatment is copious and continuous irrigation at the scene, in transport, and at the hospital. Special eye-irrigating kits may be used. In general, 1 to 2 L of NS for each eye for 30-min continuous irrigation is the minimum treatment. Neutralizing substances should not be used.

Acid burns may not require as much volume or treatment time as alkali burns. For treatment of severe alkali burns, 24 h or more of continuous irrigation has been recommended by some. Checking the pH in the conjunctival sac to see whether it has returned to normal may be helpful in determining need for further irrigation (the goal is a neutral pH of 7.4). The eyelid may have to be held open manually or with retractors, due to severe orbicularis spasm. The eyelids should be everted if they are not too edematous. It is useful to routinely sweep the fornices with a wet cotton applicator to remove any particulate matter, especially if the pH is not responding well to irrigation.

Pain control with topical anesthetics and systemic analgesics may be necessary. Cycloplegics, mydriatics, and antibiotics should be used, though the efficacy of an eye patch to encourage corneal reepithelialization is uncertain. Phenylephrine should be avoided because of its vasoconstrictive properties. The patient should be hospitalized and ophthalmology consultation obtained for severe corneal burns.

For severe corneal damage, a collagenase inhibitor such as cysteine or acetylcysteine is used to prevent loss of corneal stroma, which occurs with liberation of collagenase from injured corneal and conjunctival epithelium. Topical steroids may reduce iridocyclitis, but may also exacerbate collagenase-induced corneal ulceration. A scleral contact lens may reduce adhesions and scarring. Intraocular pressure should be checked, and agents to reduce intraocular pressure should be used if glaucoma develops. Paracentesis may be required in severe alkali burns to introduce sterile phosphate buffer solution into the anterior chamber in an attempt to reduce the pH of the inner eye. Surgery to the eye is usually not indicated during the early phase of burn management unless for corneal grafting following corneal perforation. Blepharoplasty, keratoplasty, or keratoprosthesis may be eventually required.

IATROGENIC CHEMICAL BURNS

Iatrogenic chemical burns have been caused by the use of potassium permanganate at an inappropriately high concentration to treat dermatologic problems. DMSO used as a transcutaneous vehicle for minor sprains has caused burns. Patients in the operating room may develop burns from skin-prep solutions; thimerosal, which has high mercury content, is the most common agent implicated. Mechanical abrasion of the skin from scrubbing and from pooling of the skin-prep agent under the torso or tourniquet predisposes patients to burns. Blister formation, skin sloughing, and eschar development have been reported in neonates when isopropyl alcohol pledgets were substituted for conducting paste beneath limb electrocardiograph electrodes. Silver nitrate utilized to cauterize umbilical granulomas in infants reportedly has caused periumbilical burns.

SYSTEMIC TOXICITY

Death early after severe chemical burns is usually related to hypotension, acute renal failure, and shock as a result of fluid loss. However, systemic toxicity and subsequent morbidity and mortality may also occur with some chemicals that are absorbed through denuded dermis. Acidosis, hypotension, and shock can occur with significant absorption of acids. Hypocalcemia has been reported with both oxalic acid and hydrofluoric acid burns. Profound hypocalcemia and hypomagnesemia may be accompanied by hyperkalemia, cardiac arrhythmias, and sudden death. Tannic acid, chromic acid, formic acid, picric acid, and phosphorus may cause hepatic necrosis and nephrotoxicity.

Cresol can cause methemoglobinemia, massive hemolysis, and multiple organ failure. Gasoline immersion with large surface area exposure and absorption of hydrocarbon aromatic components may result in severe pulmonary, cardiovascular, neurologic, renal, and hepatic complications. Gasoline lead additives such as tetraethyl and tetramethyl can cause lead encephalopathy. Carburetor-cleaning solvent containing phenol and methylene chloride may cause renal and hepatic failure. When absorbed, phenol (carbolic acid) can lead to intravascular hemolysis and cardiovascular, pulmonary, and central nervous system toxicity.

Sodium nitrate and potassium nitrate can cause a severe toxic methemoglobinemia from absorption with refractory cyanosis. Significant absorption of dichromate solution can result in liver failure and acute renal failure and death despite hemodialysis.

REFERENCES

1. U.S. Department of Labor and Bureau of Labor Statistics. Available at: http://stats.bls.gov. Accessed 5/30/03.
2. Luterman A, Curreri PW: Chemical burn injury, in Boswick JA (ed): *The Art and Science of Burn Care.* Rockville, MD, Aspen, 1987, pp. 233–239.
3. Rice RH, Cohen DE: Toxic responses of the skin, in Klaassen CD, Amdur MO, Doull J (eds): *Cassaret and Doull's Toxicology: The Basic Science of Poisons.* New York, McGraw-Hill, 1996, pp. 529–546.
4. Jelenko C: Chemicals that "burn." *J Trauma* 14:65, 1974.
5. Acikel C, Ulkur E, Guler MM: Prolonged intermittent hydrotherapy and early tangential excision in the treatment of an extensive strong alkali burn. *Burns* 27:293, 2001.
6. Hunter DM, Timerding BL, Leonard RB, et al: Effects of isopropyl alcohol, ethanol, and polyethylene glycol/industrial methylated spirits in treatment of acute phenol burns. *Ann Emerg Med* 21:1303, 1992.
7. Matey P, Allison KP, Sheehan MT, et al: Chromic acid burns: Early aggressive excision is the best method to prevent systemic toxicity. *J Burn Care Rehabil* 21:241, 2000.
8. Chan TC, Williams SR, Clark RF: Formic acid skin burns resulting in systemic toxicity. *Ann Emerg Med* 26:383, 1995.
9. Graudins A, Burns MJ, Aaron CK: Regional intravenous infusion of calcium gluconate for hydrofluoric acid burns of the upper extremity. *Ann Emerg Med* 30:604, 1997.
10. Williams JM, Hammad A, Cottington EC, et al: Intravenous magnesium in the treatment of hydrofluoric acid burns in rats. *Ann Emerg Med* 23:464, 1994.
11. Burkhart KK, Brent J, Kirk MA, et al: Comparison of topical magnesium and calcium treatment for dermal hydrofluoric acid burns. *Ann Emerg Med* 24:9, 1994.
12. Yamashita M, Yamashita M, Suzuki M, et al: Iontophoretic delivery of calcium for experimental hydrofluoric acid burns. *Crit Care Med* 29:1575, 2001.
13. Woolf A, Shaw J: Childhood injuries from artificial nail primer cosmetic products. *Arch Pediatr Adolesc Med* 152:41, 1998.
14. Yeong EK, Chen MT, Mann R, et al: Facial mutilation after an assault with chemicals: 15 cases and literature review. *J Burn Care Rehabil* 18:234, 1997.
15. Amshel CE, Fealk MH, Phillips BJ, et al: Anhydrous ammonia burns. Case report and review of the literature. *Burns* 26:493, 2000.
16. Hansbrough JF, Zapata-Sirvent R, Dominic W, et al: Hydrocarbon contact injuries. *J Trauma* 25:250, 1985.
17. Wormser U, Brodsky B, Green B, et al: Protective effect of povidone iodine ointment against skin lesions induced by chemical and thermal stimuli. *J Appl Toxicol* 20:S183, 2000.
18. Chou TD, Lee TW, Chen SL, et al: The management of white phosphorus burns. *Burns* 27:492, 2001.
19. Ulrich D, Noah EM, Fuchs P, et al: Burn injuries caused by airbag deployment. *Burns* 27:196, 2001.
20. Wagoner MD: Chemical injuries of the eye: Current concepts in pathophysiology and therapy. *Surv Ophthalmol* 41:275, 1997.

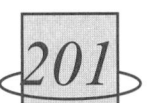

ELECTRICAL INJURIES
Raymond M. Fish

Electric shock may be defined as a sudden violent response caused by electric current flow through any part of the body or head. Electrocution is death caused by electricity. Electrical injury is tissue damage produced by the flow of electrical current through tissue. Electrical burns are cutaneous injury and necrosis resulting from electrical current flow through the skin.

EPIDEMIOLOGY

The true incidence of electrical accidents is unknown. Many persons receiving an electric shock fall from a height, have a fatal dysrhythmia, or otherwise are found dead, and in many of these cases, the occurrence or significance of the electric shock is not recognized. A fall may be attributed to the victim tripping or a sudden death may be attributed to myocardial infarction from natural causes. Medical personnel should obtain careful histories from witnesses and survivors that may help in diagnosing and treating the victim. This information may also help to prevent others from being injured from contact with the same voltage source.

The total number of electrocutions in the United States was reported to be 550 in 1998.[1] A study in Dade County, Florida, where the Dade County Medical Examiner's Office aggressively investigated possible electrical deaths, found the incidence of electrocution in that county to be 50 percent higher than that reported in the rest of the United States.[2] This apparent difference was attributed to underreporting in most of the country. Investigation of possible electrocutions included an "autopsy" of the circumstances and equipment. This study also found and explained that in nearly half of low-voltage deaths (<1000 volts AC), there will be no visible burns or electrical marks on the victims.[2]

Severe nonlethal electrical injuries account for 3 to 5 percent of admissions to burn centers, usually a result of contact with high-voltage power lines. These injuries are frequently disabling, sometimes involving amputations of one or more extremities. The incidence of minor and nonsevere electrical injuries is unknown, but up to 17,000 victims of electrical injury are estimated to be treated each year in U.S. emergency departments.

Three distinct populations are at risk for electrical injury, each accounting for approximately 20 to 25 percent of electrical injuries. The first trimodal peak occurs in toddlers who sustain electrical injuries from household electrical sockets and cords. The second peak occurs in adolescents who engage in risky behavior around electrical power lines. The third population at risk is those that work with electricity for a living. Electrical utility workers in the United States have an annual death from electrical incidence of approximately 1 per 10,000.[3]

PATHOPHYSIOLOGY

Electrical current is the movement of electrical charges; this flow is measured as amperes. Current flow is driven by an electrical potential difference; this difference is measured as volts. The intervening material resists electrical current flow; this resistance is measured as ohms. Ohms law describes the relation between current (I), voltage (V), and resistance (R): $I = V/R$. For example, in a person who grasps a grounded pipe in one hand and a wire connected to a 120-volt source in the other hand, with the total resistance from power source through person to ground of 1000 ohms, the peak current would be: $I = (120 \text{ volts})/(1000 \text{ ohms}) = 0.120$ amperes = 120 milliamperes.

Materials that allow electrical current to flow easily are called conductors. Materials that do not allow electrical current flow are called insulators. Most biologic materials conduct electricity to some extent. Tissues with high fluid and electrolyte content conduct electricity better than tissues with less fluid and electrolyte content. Bone is the biologic tissue with the greatest resistance to electrical current. Dry skin has high resistance, but sweaty or wet skin has much less resistance by a factor of 100 or more.

Electrical current can be either continuous in one direction (direct current or DC) or with periodic reversal in the direction of current flow (alternating current or AC). Alternating current is found in the electricity supplied to homes and businesses. The frequency of AC electricity is the number of complete cycles (from positive through negative back to positive) made in one second. In the United States, most AC, including household electricity, is 60 Hz (cycles per second), while in Europe and Australia, 50 Hz AC is used. Most electronic and many medical devices use DC that is supplied by batteries or power supplies that convert AC supplied from an electric socket to DC for use in the device.

Many of the physiologic effects of electric shock are related to the amount, duration, type (AC or DC), and path of current flow (Table 201-1). For current to flow through an individual, a complete circuit must be created from one terminal of a voltage source to a contact area on the body, through the subject, and then from another contact area back to the other terminal of the voltage source. Current flows through the body (and head, if the circuit includes it) from one contact area to another, along multiple, somewhat parallel paths. Unless there is just one type of tissue present, the current does not flow through a single "path of least resistance," as is sometimes claimed in medical articles. Electrical contacts on the left hand and left leg would give current flow through those limbs and the trunk, but not through the other limbs or head.

Electric current flows through multiple paths in various proportions depending on tissue type, cross-sectional area, anatomic location, and resistance. In a typical limb, nerves and blood vessels have the lowest tissue resistance per unit of cross-sectional area, followed by that of muscle (about twice the resistance of blood vessels and nerves) and then bone, with resistance roughly 3 to 12 times as high, depending on the type of bone. In a typical limb, the cross-sectional area of muscle is approximately 100 times that of blood vessels or nerves, so that the total current flow through muscle is approximately 50 times that in blood vessels or nerves. However, while only a few percent of the total current flows through nervous tissue, nerves have a higher current density (current flow per unit cross-sectional area).[4] This is one reason that nerves can be significantly injured, even though most of the current flow was through other nearby tissues with little effect.

As current flows though a resistor, energy is deposited in the form of heat. If resistance and other factors remain constant, heating from current flow through tissue is proportional to duration of current flow and the square of the current intensity according to Joule's law: energy = $I^2 \times R \times time = (V^2 \times time)/R$. Therefore, as long as the resistance remains constant (i.e., until the tissue burns and changes resistivity), heating of tissues increases according to the square of applied voltage. Direct tissue heating predictions by applying Joule's law are generally implicated as the etiology of most tissue damage from electricity.

High voltage is usually defined as greater than 1000 V, although there is evidence that the risk for serious and fatal electrical injury increases significantly with voltages above 600 V. Power lines in U.S.

TABLE 201-1   Effects of Current

Effect	Current Path	Minimum Current 60 Hz AC Milliamperes*
Tingling sensation, minimal perception	Through intact skin	0.5 to 2
Pain threshold	Through intact skin	1 to 4
Inability to let go: tetanic contractions of hand and forearm tighten grasp, decreasing skin resistance	From hand, through forearm muscles, into trunk	6 to 22
Respiratory arrest: can be fatal if prolonged	Through chest	18 to 30
Ventricular fibrillation	Through chest	70 to 4000
Ventricular standstill (asystole): in effect, cardioversion; if current stops, sinus rhythm may resume	Through chest	>2000

*Ranges are approximate and depend on various factors.
Source: Reprinted (with slight modification) with permission from Fish RM, Geddes LA: *Medical and Bioengineering Aspects of Electrical Injuries.* Lawyers and Judges Publishing Company, Inc, Tucson, AZ, p 404, 2003.

residential areas are typically 7620 V, which is stepped down by transformers to 220 V before entering the house. Urban subway electrical third rails are typically 600 V. Although high voltage is more dangerous, the general population has much greater access to low-voltage sources and these low-voltage sources account for about half of all electrical injuries and deaths.

Electrical skin burns tend to be severe with high voltages, where only a fraction of a second of contact time is necessary for severe damage.[5] Conversely, cutaneous burns tend to be minimal with household voltages (110 V) unless there is several seconds of contact time; even then the burns tend to be minor. Moreover, in low-voltage electrocution deaths, electrical burns are absent in more than 40 percent of cases because 110 V AC is capable of producing ventricular fibrillation, but deposits relatively little heat energy into the skin.[2]

Electrical current can induce sustained muscular contraction or tetany, the overall effect varies according to type (AC or DC), frequency, voltage, and extent of contact.[5,6] For example, when AC current flows though the arm, flexor tetany of the fingers and forearm overpowers that of the extensors, and if the hand and fingers are properly positioned, the hand will grasp the conductor tighter, leading to extended contact to the power source. Alternatively, if the person has not grasped the contact tightly, tetanic flexor contraction of the hand and forearm may not occur, but current flow through the trunk and legs may cause opisthotonic (arching) postures and leg movements. Such involuntary muscle contractions may be very strong, leading to the person appearing to "be thrown" from a voltage source, and produce mechanical trauma. High-voltage AC and DC contacts are also more likely to produce a single violent skeletal muscle contraction that tends to throw the victim away from the source. Forceful muscle contractions can cause fractures and joint dislocations, especially around the shoulders.[7]

Electrical current can induce immediate cardiac (arrhythmias) and neurologic (respiratory arrest and seizures) effects. Current that traverses the body vertically ("hand to foot" or "head to toe") can produce arrhythmias and respiratory arrest as can current that traverses horizontally ("hand to hand").

An electrical arc is a spark of current through the air between objects of differing electrical potential. A typical arc burn is from the electrical source to the patient. The voltages required to create an electrical arc are extreme and the temperatures created can be as high as 2500°C (4532°F), so thermal tissue destruction from an electrical arc can be excessive.

Electric control devices, such as the stun gun or Taser, produce a series of damped sinusoidal electrical impulses, typically 10 to 15 Hz, designed to induce involuntary muscle contraction and incapacitation in the victim. These electromuscular disruptive devices deliver electricity at high voltage (50,000 V for a Taser) but low amperage and low average energy.

PATIENT CARE AND RESCUER SAFETY AT THE ACCIDENT SCENE

The scene of a high-voltage electrical incident contains many hazards for rescue personnel. Power lines are almost never insulated, although a line may appear to be insulated because of atmospheric contaminants deposited on the line over time. Electrocution is possible when walking on ground near a downed power line. It is recommended that persons stay at least 9 m (30 ft) from downed power lines, though 3 m (10 ft) is sometimes suggested as a safe distance. Additionally, reapplication of voltage to downed lines sometimes occurs as circuit breakers reset, making the lines physically jump many feet with great force. It is possible to place a heavy object over downed lines to prevent "jumping," though this can be difficult and very dangerous. Metal cables that support telephone and power poles are normally grounded, but may be energized if broken or disconnected from an attachment and make contact with a nearby power line.

Victims still in contact with a source of voltage may transmit an electric current to would-be rescuers. If it can be done quickly, it is best to first turn off the source of electricity. If this cannot be done quickly, precautions must be taken to prevent electric injury to the rescuer. With voltages above about 600 volts, dry wood and other materials may conduct significant amounts of electric current and therefore cannot be used to remove the person from a voltage source. A rescuer standing on the ground touching any part of a vehicle that is in contact with a power line is likely to be killed or seriously injured. Electrical shock is not prevented in this situation by the rescuer wearing rubber gloves and boots (unless these are designed for the voltage present and have been recently tested for insulation integrity). Persons inside a vehicle in contact with a power line are likely to be killed as they step out of the vehicle, and may also receive a shock if they touch objects at different potentials inside the vehicle.

It is recommended that mouth-to-mouth breathing for lineworkers in respiratory arrest on utility power poles be initiated by rescuers while still on the pole. As soon as the patient is lowered to the ground, chest compressions can be added if there is cardiac as well as respiratory arrest.

Spinal fractures can be caused by tetanic muscle contractions, as well as by falls and other secondary trauma. Therefore, spinal immobilization during resuscitation, to the extent possible under the circumstances, should be done.

EMERGENCY DEPARTMENT EVALUATION AND TREATMENT

The usual evaluation (airway, breathing, circulation) and resuscitation for major trauma victims should be provided as appropriate. Cardiac arrhythmias can be treated according to accepted advanced life support guidelines. Cardiac monitoring should be instituted for all high-voltage patients, patients with neuromuscular or cardiac symptoms (loss of consciousness, amnesia, altered mental status, episode of tetany, chest pain, palpitations), and those with transthoracic current paths. Spinal fractures can be caused by tetanic muscle contractions, as well as by falls and other secondary trauma. Therefore, spinal immobilization should be maintained during resuscitation until adequate radiographs and examination are possible.

The physical examination should assess tissue damage and identify associated complications. A careful vascular and neurologic examination of involved extremities is important. Occult and delayed injuries occur and a normal initial assessment does not exclude serious injury.

Patients with high-voltage injury, extensive cutaneous burns, or evidence of systemic injury should have laboratory tests done: serum electrolytes, creatinine, blood urea nitrogen, creatine kinase, serum and urine myoglobin, and complete blood cell count. An electrocardiogram is recommended for the same indications as cardiac monitoring. Imaging studies (plain radiography, computed tomography, angiography) are indicated for suggested injuries.

Fluid resuscitation is commenced using isotonic crystalloid (normal saline or Ringer's lactate solution). Fluid requirements for serious electrical injuries are higher than estimates provided by thermal burn injury formula (e.g., Parklands formula) because the visible cutaneous damage underestimates the internal damage. An initial fluid volume of 20 to 40 mL/kg over the first hour is appropriate for most patients and further fluid administration is guided by clinical and hemodynamic assessment.

If there is rhabdomyolysis, fluid loading is desirable to prevent myoglobinuric renal failure. Myoglobinuria should be considered present if a urine dipstick test registers positive for hemoglobin, but the freshly spun urine sediment shows no red blood cells. In rhabdomyolysis, a serum sample has normal color, whereas in hemolysis, the serum sample has a red or brown color indicating free hemoglobin. In ambiguous cases, myoglobin can be tested for in the serum or urine.

Specific Injuries

CARDIAC ARREST Cardiac arrest is the primary cause of death from electrocution. The specific fatal arrhythmia varies; low-voltage AC is likely to produce ventricular fibrillation, whereas high-voltage AC and DC are more likely to produce transient ventricular asystole. Cardiac arrhythmias can be seen in up to 30 percent of high-voltage victims and include sinus tachycardia, premature atrial contractions, premature ventricular contractions, supraventricular tachycardia, atrial fibrillation, and first- or second-degree atrioventricular block. Arrhythmias other than ventricular fibrillation are rare if voltage is less than 220 V and water contact was not involved.

Vigorous resuscitation efforts should be initiated for cardiac arrest from electric shock because 1) many victims are young and without prior cardiovascular disease, so the chance of recovery and survival is good, and 2) it is often not possible to predict the outcome of attempted resuscitation based on age and initial rhythm in electric shock–induced cardiac arrest.[8] Usual basic or advanced resuscitation protocols should be used, with modifications for rescuer safety, patient access, and injuries that interfere with airway access.

CENTRAL NERVOUS SYSTEM INJURIES Neurologic impairment occurs in approximately 50 percent of patients with high-voltage injuries.[5,7] Transient loss of conscious is common, followed by other changes such as agitation, confusion, coma, seizures, quadriplegia, hemiplegia, asphasia, and visual disturbances.

SPINAL CORD INJURIES Spinal cord injuries can be the result of vertebral fractures, usually present on initial evaluation, and sometimes occurring at multiple levels in the same patient.[7] Delayed spinal cord injury can occur from the electrical current itself and presents as ascending paralysis, complete or incomplete spinal cord syndromes, or transverse myelitis.

With purely electrical trauma, spinal cord magnetic resonance imaging (MRI) results are not closely correlated with prognosis. With high-voltage electrical trauma, diagnosis of spinal cord injury can be hindered by altered mental status or associated severe injuries. Even in patients who are alert, a delayed onset of spinal cord dysfunction is sometimes noted. In rare cases, the initial MRI may be normal in electrical trauma patients with permanent spinal cord injury.[9] Conversely, the great majority of patients with spinal cord impairment following mechanical trauma who have a normal initial spinal MRI will have complete resolution of neurologic dysfunction.[10]

PERIPHERAL NERVE INJURIES Peripheral nerve injuries often involve the hands after touching a power source. Paresthesias may be immediate and transient or delayed in onset, appearing up to 2 years after injury.[7] Most delayed neurologic deficits after high-voltage trauma involve the spinal cord. Electrical contact with the palm produces median or ulnar neuropathy more than radial nerve injury. Brachial plexus lesions have been reported.

CUTANEOUS WOUNDS Cutaneous burns are often seen at the electrical contact areas ("entry and exit" points). The majority of serious cases have burns on either the arm or skull, paired with burns on the feet. These burns are typically painless, gray to yellow depressed areas.

After cleansing, burns of the skin can be dressed with silver sulfadiazine or mafenide acetate. Mafenide is preferred by some for full-thickness burns because of its better eschar penetration. However, if used on more than 15 to 20 percent of the body, inhibition of carbonic anhydrase by mafenide acetate can cause electrolyte and pH abnormalities. Another disadvantage of mafenide is that it is painful. Extremities with burns need careful examination for neurovascular compromise, compartment syndromes, and the need for escharotomy or fasciotomy. Extremities with burns should be splinted. The hand should be splinted in 35 to 45 degrees of extension at the wrist, 80 to 90 degrees of flexion at the metacarpophalangeal joints, and almost full extension of the proximal interphalangeal and distal interphalangeal joints. Surgical debridement of necrotic tissue should be done early, with vascular and other reconstruction as needed. Early excision and skin grafting is recommended, and a variety of commercial skin substitutes are available for use.[11]

ORTHOPEDIC INJURIES Fractures may be caused by tetanic muscle contractions or associated falls. Fractures may be missed on initial assessment because there is often pain associated with burns and other injuries, and patients are not always alert because of their injury or pain medications. All joints should be put through a full, active range of motion if possible; otherwise, passive range of motion should be tested. If such movements are not possible, radiographic study is indicated. Limited motion, fixed internal rotation, and deformities are suggestive of shoulder dislocation and fracture. Fractures and dislocations of the shoulders have been reported from sources of 110 to 440 volts AC.[7]

BLAST INJURIES Electric arcs in the industrial environment or near a power line can produce a strong blast pressure, similar to those of other explosions.[12] Cognitive complaints following blast injury sometimes resemble those that result from mild to moderate mechanical head trauma. Mechanisms of brain injury include mechanical trauma related to the blast, as well as arterial air emboli associated with blast-related alveolar disruption.

INHALATION INJURIES Chemical toxins such as ozone can be produced by coronas and arcs.[13] Acute effects of ozone include mucous membrane irritation, temporarily reduced pulmonary function, and pulmonary hemorrhage and edema. Fires and explosions associated with electric incidents may lead to inhalation of carbon monoxide and other toxic substances.

EYE INJURIES Cataract formation has been described weeks to years after electrical injury to head, neck, or upper chest.[7] Cataracts have also occurred after electric arc or flash burns. Therefore, it is important to document the absence of cataracts following such an injury. Retinal detachment, corneal burns, intraocular hemorrhage, and intraocular thrombosis may be seen after high-voltage injury.

AUDITORY SYSTEM INJURY The auditory system may be damaged by current or by hemorrhage in the tympanic membrane, middle ear, cochlea, cochlear duct, and vestibular apparatus. Delayed complications include mastoiditis, sinus thrombosis, meningitis, and brain abscess. Hearing loss may be immediate or develop later as a result of complications. Hearing should be checked in the emergency department as well as formal testing in any patient who appears to have a deficit.

ORAL BURNS An oral injury can occur in children who chew through the insulation of a power cord. The electrical arc created between the two wires can produce high temperatures and significant tissue damage. Most injuries are unilateral and involve the lateral commissure, tongue, or alveolar ridge.[5,7] Systemic complications of oral burns are uncommon. Vascular injury to the labial artery is not immediately apparent because of vascular spasm, thrombosis, and the overlying eschar. Severe bleeding from the labial artery occurs in up to 10 percent of cases when the eschar separates, usually after 5 days. For this reason, children with this injury are often admitted to the hospital.

However, some authors believe that outpatient management is adequate.[14] If parents are reliable, can monitor the child, and can be shown how to control bleeding, outpatient management may be considered. The parents need to be told that bleeding may occur up to 2 weeks later. Home care may include saline or hydrogen peroxide rinses and swabs that will debride necrotic tissue and promote formation of healthy granulation tissue. Topical petrolatum-based antibiotics may have a soothing effect. Specialty consultation should be obtained, as splinting and other measures are often needed to prevent residual deformity and dysfunction.

GASTROINTESTINAL INJURIES   There are reports in the literature of lethal intraabdominal injuries from electric current being found only at autopsy. Intraabdominal injury should be suspected in patients having burns of the abdominal wall or a report of trauma, such as in a fall or explosion. Similar to other critically ill patients, major electrical trauma patients can develop stress injury and bleeding from the gastrointestinal tract.

VASCULAR AND MUSCLE INJURY   Vascular and muscle injury occur most commonly in the setting of high-voltage injury, such as from power lines. Electrical current passing along peripheral arteries may cause early spasm and delayed thrombosis or aneurysm formation. Extensive vascular injury may produce a muscle compartment syndrome.

DISSEMINATED INTRAVASCULAR COAGULATION   Thermal injury or tissue necrosis from electrical current can cause disseminated intravascular coagulation (DIC). Low-grade DIC may be a result of hypoxia, vascular stasis, rhabdomyolysis, and release of procoagulants from damaged tissue. Treatment consists of elimination of the precipitating factor by early surgical debridement. If bleeding is present, coagulation factors should be replaced with fresh-frozen plasma or cryoprecipitate (see Chap. 219).

ELECTRONIC RESTRAINT DEVICES   Stun guns, stun belts, shock batons, Taser, and electric cattle prods (goads) generate high voltages that can be used for self-defense, as weapons, and to control violent persons. The likelihood of electrical injury is minimal with the rare potential for application of electricity to the eye that might result in ocular injury. However, falls or other forceful movements made as a result of the electric current can lead to injury. Some devices shoot wires with fishhook-like barbs on the ends that may need removal from the skin.

Although most victims do not sustain demonstrable injury from electromuscular disruptive devices, several case reports have documented death within minutes of their use, presumably from cardiac arrhythmias. Most reported deaths were associated with concomitant drug use (usually phencyclidine or cocaine), trauma as a result of struggling, or preexisting cardiac disease. Usually the main concern of the physician treating a person who has been shocked with such a nonlethal restraint device will be the issue of why the person was in need of restraint.

TREATMENT OF ELECTRIC INJURY IN PREGNANCY

A number of pregnant women who have received apparently harmless contacts with electric current have later suffered fetal damage or loss.[15] In most cases, the mechanism of fetal injury is uncertain. General recommendations for maternal and fetal monitoring after electrical shock in pregnancy include 1) fetal heart rate and uterine activity monitoring for 4 h in women beyond 20 to 24 weeks' gestation and 2) maternal cardiac and fetal heart rate and uterine monitoring for 24 h if there was loss of consciousness, if there are electrocardiogram (ECG) abnormalities, or if the woman has cardiovascular disease.[15] Fetal ultrasonography is also recommended. That said, there is no proof that monitoring or treatment can influence the fetal outcome in pregnant women following electric injury without mechanical trauma. In addition to these indications for immediate monitoring, it is recommended that ultrasonography or fetal heart Doppler be done 2 weeks after the accident.

Disposition

All patients having contact with over 600 V should be admitted for observation, even if there is no apparent injury. Routine cardiac monitoring is not required unless the initial ECG is abnormal. Patients with

symptoms (chest pain, palpations, loss of consciousness, confusion, weakness, dyspnea, abdominal pain), signs (weakness, burn with subcutaneous damage, vascular compromise), or ancillary changes (abnormal ECG, elevated creatine kinase or urine myoglobin) suggestive of systemic injury also require admission.

Adults with electrical injury caused by household voltage (110 to 220 V) have negligible risk for delayed arrhythmias.[15] Asymptomatic patients who sustain a household electrical shock can be discharged home if they have a normal ECG on presentation and normal examination findings.

Children with only hand wounds from electrical outlet injuries and no evidence of cardiac or neurologic involvement can be discharged with local wound care. A child with a home situation of equivocal safety or reliability should be considered for admission, although cardiac monitoring is not required for these "social" admissions.

ACKNOWLEDGMENTS

The author would like to thank Neil Abarbanelle, MD; Leslie A. Geddes, PhD; Barb Meyer, RN; and Uretz Oliphant, PhD, who reviewed various parts this paper and gave many helpful suggestions.

REFERENCES

1. Hiser S: *1998 Electrocutions Associated with Consumer Products.* Washington, DC, U.S. Consumer Product Safety Commission, 2001. http://www.cpsc.gov/library/shock98.pdf.
2. Wright RK, Davis JH: The investigation of electrical deaths: A report of 220 fatalities. *J Forensic Sci* 25:514, 1980.
3. Ore T, Casini V: Electrical fatalities among US construction workers. *J Occup Environ Med* 38:587, 1996.
4. Chilbert MA: Evaluation of electrical burn injury using an electrical impedance technique, in Lee RC, Cravalho EG, Burke JF (eds): *Electrical Trauma.* Cambridge, UK, Cambridge University Press, 1992, pp. 216–238.
5. Koumbourlis AC: Electrical injuries. *Crit Care Med* 30(Suppl):S424, 2002.
6. Fish RM: Electrical injury: Part I. Treatment priorities, subtle diagnostic factors, and burns. *J Emerg Med* 17:977, 1999.
7. Fish RM: Electric injury: Part II. Specific injuries. *J Emerg Med* 18:27, 2000.
8. European Resuscitation Council: Part 8: Advanced challenges in resuscitation. Section 3: Special challenges in ECC. 3G: Electric shock and lightning strikes. *Resuscitation* 46:297, 2000.
9. Arevalo JM, Lorente JA, Balseiro-Gomez J: Spinal cord injury after electrical trauma treated in a burn unit. *Burns* 25:449, 1999.
10. Ramon S, Dominguez R, Ramirez L, et al: Clinical and magnetic resonance imaging correlation in acute spinal cord injury. *Spinal Cord* 35:664, 1997.
11. Guo Z, Sheng Z, Li F: Wound management in electrical injuries. *Ann N Y Acad Sci* 888:105, 1999.
12. Capelli-Schellpfeffer M, Lee RC, Toner M, et al: Correlation between electrical accident parameters and injury. *IEEE Indus Appl Mag* 4:25, 1998.
13. Gordon LB: Electrical hazards in the high-energy laboratory. *IEEE Trans Educ* 34:231, 1991.
14. Garcia CT, Smith GA, Cohen DM, et al: Electrical injuries in a pediatric emergency department. *Ann Emerg Med* 26:604, 1995.
15. Fish RM: Electric injury: Part III. Monitoring indications, the pregnant patient, and lightning. *J Emerg Med* 18:181, 2000.

LIGHTNING INJURIES
Raymond M. Fish

EPIDEMIOLOGY

Lightning causes approximately 300 injuries each year in the United States and is the second leading cause of weather-related death, with approximately 100 reported deaths each year.[1] Reported mortality rates vary, from approximately 0.5 per million in the general U.S. population, to as high as 8.8 per million in the rural South African population.[2]

Lightning injury reporting is biased to the more severe and fatal events, and it is estimated that more unreported lightning injuries occur each year, perhaps up to several thousand cases per year. Approximately 70 to 90 percent of persons struck by lightning survive, but as many as three-quarters of these survivors will have permanent sequelae.[3,4] Livestock and other animals also suffer deaths and injuries from lightning.

Lightning most often occurs during thunderstorms in association with large cumulonimbus clouds. However, approximately 10 percent of lightning occurs without rain and when the sky is blue.[5] In addition, lightning can occur during dust storms, sandstorms, snowstorms, nuclear explosions, and in the clouds over volcanic eruptions. The U.S. locations with the highest lightning-strike mortality rates are Arizona, Arkansas, Florida, Mississippi, New Mexico, and Wyoming.[1]

A number of lightning injuries are associated with transportation; most commonly when the victim is standing outside near a vehicle. Lightning injuries are also associated with airplanes (both private and commercial) and water sports. Lightning injury from indoor telephone use has been reported. A report from Australia indicated up to 80 such injuries yearly without any reported fatalities.[6]

Even though lightning is electrical energy, lightning injuries differ substantially from high-voltage electrical injuries seen from human-generated sources; different injury patterns, different injury severity, and different emergency treatment (Table 202-1).[2,7,8]

PATHOPHYSIOLOGY

Lightning is an extremely high-voltage direct current (DC) electrical discharge. Unlike alternating current (AC) injury from human-generated sources, lightning often travels over the surface of the body in a phenomenon called *flashover,* and is less likely to cause internal cardiac injury or muscle necrosis. Wet skin may actually decrease the risk of internal injury, helping the current travel along the outside of the body. Flashover explains how victims may survive exposure to tremendous amounts of electrical current. Lightning occasionally does cause internal injury through blunt force mechanisms.

Lightning emits brief but intense thermal radiation that produces rapid heating and expansion of the surrounding air. This energy is transmitted as a blast or shock wave that can cause tympanic membrane perforation and internal organ contusion (see Chap. 9). The blast associated with lightning can tear clothing, giving the appearance of an assault.[9] Lightning may inflict thermal injury as moisture on the victim's skin is transformed into steam or through resistance heating of

metal objects on the body or in clothing pockets. Lightning is attracted to metallic objects on the victim and these are sometimes melted. Intense photic injury may damage the retina or produce cataracts.

The nature and severity varies according to the type of lightning strike. A *direct strike* occurs when the victim is struck directly by the lightning discharge, producing the most serious injuries associated with lightning strike. A *side flash* occurs when a nearby object is struck and current then traverses through the air to strike the victim. A side flash may injure multiple victims at once, as when a group huddles close to a structure that is struck. A *contact strike* occurs when lightning strikes an object the victim is holding and current is transferred from the object through the person to the ground. Lightning injuries from indoor telephone use during a lightning storm is an example of contact strike. A *ground current* occurs when lightning hits the ground and current is transferred through the ground to a nearby victim. The electrical voltage and amount of current decreases as the distance between the victim and strike point increases. This ground current can create a stride potential or step voltage between the victim's separated feet. The foot closer to the strike point will experience a higher electrical potential than the foot further away. Therefore, electrical current can enter one foot, travel up that leg, through the torso, and down the other leg and exit the other foot. This can result in isolated neurovascular injury to the legs. Recently, a fifth mechanism, where a weak *upward streamer* does not become connected to the completed lightning channel, was implicated in a fatal lightning injury.[10]

Immediate cardiac arrest from lightning strike results from direct current depolarization of the myocardium and sustained asystole. Immediate respiratory arrest after lightning strike is a result of depolarization and paralysis of the medullary respiratory center. Both cardiac and respiratory arrest may be present without evidence of external injury. Although cardiac automaticity may spontaneously return, concomitant respiratory arrest may persist and lead to a secondary hypoxic cardiac stoppage. The duration of apnea, rather than the duration of cardiac arrest, appears to be the critical prognostic factor.

DIAGNOSIS AND MANAGEMENT

Care at the Injury Scene

TRIAGE CONSIDERATIONS   Lightning can produce multiple victims because of multiple lightning strikes, stride potentials, and side

TABLE 202-1   Comparison of Lightning and Electrical Injuries

Factor	Lightning	High-Voltage AC	Low-Voltage AC
Current duration	1–3 ms	Generally brief (1–2 s), but may be prolonged	Prolonged
Typical voltage and current range	10 million to 2 billion V; 20,000–200,000 A	600–70,000 V; <1000 A	<600 V; usually <20–30 A
Current characteristics	Unidirectional (DC)	Alternating (AC)	Alternating (AC)
Current pathway	Skin flashover	Horizontal (hand to hand), vertical (hand to foot)	Horizontal (hand to hand), vertical (hand to foot)
Tissue damage	Superficial, minor	Deep tissue destruction	Sometimes deep tissue destruction
Initial rhythm in cardiac arrest	Asystole	Asystole greater than ventricular fibrillation	Ventricular fibrillation
Renal involvement	Myoglobinuria is uncommon and renal failure is rare	Myoglobinuria and renal failure are common	Myoglobinuria and renal failure occasionally
Fasciotomy and amputation	Rarely necessary	Relatively common	Sometimes necessary
Blunt injury	Explosive effect with shock wave	Being thrown from current source or falls	Tetanic contraction or falls
Immediate cause of death	Prolonged apnea	Apnea	Ventricular fibrillation

Abbreviations: AC = alternating current; DC = direct current.

flashes.[2] In contrast to multiple-victim events caused by mechanical trauma, persons with lightning injury who appear to be dead (in respiratory arrest, with or without cardiac arrest) should be treated first. Such victims often have little physical damage, and they have a reasonable chance of resuscitation.

EXAMINATION OF THE SCENE AND RESCUER SAFETY   Power lines may fall to the ground as a result of high winds or lightning-related damage to power poles or to the lines. Therefore, a person thought to have been hit by lightning may actually have been shocked by the stride potential related to a nearby power line lying on the ground. It is important that rescuers visually survey the area, especially if there is plant growth or darkness that may hide lines on the ground. While patient care should not be delayed unduly, everyone's safety may be improved by a brief survey looking for burns on the ground or nearby objects, melting of metal objects on or near the person, and unusual sounds, smells, or smoke. If a downed power line is found, safety precautions are important (see Chap. 201).

Patient physical findings suggestive of lightning injury may be subtle or nonexistent. Therefore, information about the scene of the accident may be more informative than examination of the patient, similar to other types of electrical injury. Important information about the accident scene includes: history of an electric storm in the area at the time, blast effects on nearby objects, areas of burned vegetation, melted or magnetized metal objects, and melted nylon underclothing.

Emergency Department Diagnosis and Treatment

The usual advanced cardiac and trauma treatment principles apply: assessment and stabilization of airway, breathing, and circulation. Intravenous access, supplemental oxygen, and continuous cardiac monitoring should be instituted. Lightning victims in cardiac arrest have a better prognosis than those in cardiac arrest from coronary artery disease, so aggressive resuscitative efforts are indicated.[11,12] Hypotension is not an expected finding from lightning injury and warrants an investigation for hemorrhagic blood loss.

A careful secondary examination should be done to detect occult injuries.[11] Cutaneous burns may help determine the current path and suggest potential organ injury. Initial ancillary studies include complete blood count, serum electrolytes, creatinine, blood urea nitrogen, glucose, creatine kinase, urinalysis, and electrocardiogram. Imaging studies (plain radiography, ultrasound, or computed tomography) should be obtained for suspected injuries. Other ancillary studies may be indicated according to clinical circumstances.

CARDIAC   In the victim with spontaneous circulation, hypertension and tachycardia are common findings, presumably because of sympathetic nervous system activation; specific treatment is not necessary as blood pressure and pulse rate will spontaneously decrease. Cardiac effects reported after lightning injury include global myocardial contractility depression, coronary artery spasm, pericardial effusion, and atrial and ventricular arrhythmias. The electrocardiogram (ECG) may show acute injury with ST-segment elevation and QT-interval prolongation. T-wave inversions may be seen, especially in the presence of neurologic injury. Myocardial infarction after lightning injury is unusual.

NEUROLOGIC   Many lightning strike victims are rendered unconscious or have temporary lower extremity paralysis. Seizures may result from the passage of electric current through the brain with no permanent effects, as with electroconvulsive therapy. Or, seizures may be the result of mechanical brain injury or hypoxia. The most lethal neurologic injuries involve heat-induced coagulation of the cerebral cortex, development of epidural or subdural hematoma, or intracerebral hemorrhage. Autonomic dysfunction caused by lightning may produce pupillary dilation or anisocoria not related to brain injury but has no prognostic significance in comatose lightning-strike victims.

Neurologic injury after lightning strike is usually classified as immediate and transient or delayed and permanent. However, some effects may be immediate and permanent. Transient effects that typically resolve in 24 h include loss of consciousness, confusion, amnesia, and extremity paralysis. Delayed and usually progressive disorders include seizures, spinal muscular atrophy, amyotrophic lateral sclerosis, parkinsonian syndromes, progressive cerebellar ataxia, myelopathy with paraplegia or quadriplegia, and chronic pain syndromes.

Lightning can cause intracranial injury directly when passing through the head, as well as by secondary trauma. Therefore, computed tomography (CT) scan is indicated in cases of coma, altered mental status, or persistent headache or confusion.

VASCULAR   Vasomotor spasm in an extremity is sometimes seen as a local response. Possible mechanisms include sympathetic nervous stimulation, local arterial spasm, and ischemia of peripheral nerves. Color changes, from white to blue to red, have been reported in extremities after lightning strike; presumably from cycles of vasoconstriction and vasodilatation, with pallor and cyanosis followed by hyperemia. Severe vasoconstriction is thought to be responsible for loss of pulses, mottling of skin, coolness of extremities, loss of sensation, and paralysis due to ischemia of peripheral nerves. As vasoconstriction resolves spontaneously, these signs and symptoms often resolve. Because skeletal muscle injury is rare in lightning strike, compartment syndromes are not usually a consideration and fasciotomy is not indicated. If in doubt, the presence of compartment syndrome and the need for fasciotomy may be confirmed by measuring intracompartmental pressures.

OCULAR   Ophthalmic injuries are common in lightning-strike victims, and lightning-induced cataracts are the most frequently observed ocular sequela.[13] Cataracts caused by thermal injury are generally unilateral, while cataracts induced by lightning are usually bilateral. Cataract formation has been described without evidence of current flow through the head or eyes, as after brief exposure to an electric arc. Perhaps this is a result of damage of the lens by radiant energy. Cataracts may form weeks to years after the lightning injury. Therefore, it is important to document lack of cataracts when a person has been exposed to lightning. Lightning can affect any part of the eye, producing hyphema, vitreous hemorrhage, corneal abrasion, uveitis, retinal detachment or hemorrhage, and optic nerve damage. Discomfort or visual changes suggest a careful examination with follow-up should be done.

AUDITORY   Blast effect producing tympanic membrane rupture is relatively common. Victims sustaining lightning strike along a conventional corded telephone are at higher risk for otologic injury, including persistent tinnitus, sensorineural deafness, ataxia, vertigo, and nystagmus.[6] In patients who are sleeping with an ear or eye on the ground near a lightning strike, temporary deafness or blindness can result.

MUSCULOSKELETAL   A variety of skeletal fractures can be seen from the blunt force injury associated with lightning strike. Intense myotonic contractions can produce posterior shoulder dislocations and cervical spine fractures. Rhabdomyolysis after lightning strike is unusual.

SPINAL CORD   Spinal fractures can be caused by tetanic muscle contractions, as well as by falls and other secondary trauma. Therefore, spinal immobilization should be maintained during resuscitation, to the extent possible under the circumstances, until spinal stability can be assessed. Plain-film radiography and clinical examination are usually adequate to evaluate these patients. Because spinal fractures often occur at multiple levels in the same patient, the entire vertebral column should be imaged when a fracture is found at one level. For patients with spinal cord motor or sensory findings, but without radiographic fracture, magnetic resonance imaging (MRI) may show spinal cord and ligamentous injuries not seen by plain film and CT studies.

CUTANEOUS There are six main dermatologic manifestations of lightning injury. *Lichtenberg figures* are considered pathognomonic for lightning strike and consist of a superficial feathering or ferning pattern (Figure 202-1). These figures are the result of electron showering over the skin and are not true thermal burns; they disappear in 24 h. *Flash burns* are similar to those found in arc welders, appearing as mild erythema, and may involve the cornea. *Punctate burns* look similar to cigarette burns in that they are usually smaller than 1 cm and are full-thickness burns. *Contact burns* occur when metal close to the skin is heated from the lightning current. *Superficial erythema* and *blistering burns* have been described. *Linear burns,* less than 5 cm wide, occur in areas of skin folds such as the axilla or groin. Contact, so-called entrance and exit, wounds characteristic of electrical injury from human sources are not commonly seen in lightning injuries. Cutaneous wounds are treated with standard wound or burn care; tetanus prophylaxis, cleaning, debridement, and dressing.

PREGNANCY Fetal injury and death have been noted to follow lightning strike with little or no maternal injury, presumably because amniotic fluid serves as a preferential path for current flow. In a review of 11 pregnant women who survived being struck by lightning, there were 5 cases of fetal death in utero, abortion, stillbirth, or neonatal death.[14] Placental abruption has been reported, and uterine/fetal ultrasonography is recommended for pregnant lightning-strike victims.

DISPOSITION

The majority of lightning-strike victims will have moderate to severe injuries that require admission for specialized care. For patients with minor injuries, admission for observation is recommended because of the potential delayed sequelae. For the rare patient with no neurologic injuries and normal cardiovascular evaluation, a period of monitoring in the emergency department is recommended, and discharge can be considered if no new abnormal symptoms or signs develop. Neurologic and ophthalmologic referral is recommended.

Maternal uterine activity and fetal heart rate monitoring is recommended for 4 h after a lightning strike to a pregnant woman.[7] That said, there is no evidence that fetal monitoring after lightning strike prevents fetal demise, aside from the associated physical trauma leading to abruptio placentae.

PREVENTION

Prevention of lightning injury through the development of safety guidelines was the subject of a meeting of the Lightning Safety Group in 1998.[5] The basic principles are to anticipate potential lightning storms (hot humid days), seek safer shelter when lightning is first seen or thunder heard, to use safer shelters (large structures with plumbing or electrical wiring, or fully enclosed metal vehicles), and to avoid dangerous locations (tall structures, open fields, open structures or vehicles, near or in water, contact with conductive materials).

ACKNOWLEDGMENT

The author would like to thank Neil Abarbanelle, MD, who reviewed this paper and gave many helpful suggestions.

REFERENCES

1. Centers for Disease Control: Lightning-associated injuries and deaths among military personnel—United States 1998–2001. *MMWR* 51:859, 2002.
2. Carte AE, Anderson RBV, Cooper MA: A large group of children struck by lightning. *Ann Emerg Med* 39:665, 2002.
3. Cherington M: Central nervous system complications of lightning and electrical injuries. *Semin Neurol* 15:233, 1995.
4. Muehlberger T, Vogt PM, Munster AM: The long-term consequences of lightning injuries. *Burns* 27:829, 2001.
5. Zimmerman C, Cooper MA, Holle RL: Lightning safety guidelines. *Ann Emerg Med* 39:660, 2002.
6. Andrews CJ: Telephone-related lightning injury. *Med J Aust* 157:823, 1992.
7. Fish RM: Electric injury: part III. Monitoring indications, the pregnant patient, and lightning. *J Emerg Med* 18:27, 2000.
8. Whitcomb D, Martinez JA, Daberkow D: Lightning injuries. *South Med J* 95:1331, 2002.
9. Lifschultz BD, Donoghue ER: Deaths caused by lightning. *J Forensic Sci* 38:353, 1993.
10. Cooper MA: A fifth mechanism of lightning injury. *Acad Emerg Med* 9:172, 2002.
11. Cooper MA: Emergent care of lightning and electrical injuries. *Semin Neurol* 15:268, 1995.
12. European Resuscitation Council: Part 8: Advanced challenges in resuscitation. Section 3: Special challenges in ECC. 3G: Electric shock and lightning strikes. *Resuscitation* 46:297, 2000.
13. Norman ME, Albertson D, Younger BR: Ophthalmic manifestations of lightning strike. *Surv Ophthalmol* 46:19, 2001.
14. Fatovich DM: Electric injury in pregnancy. *J Emerg Med* 11:175, 1993.

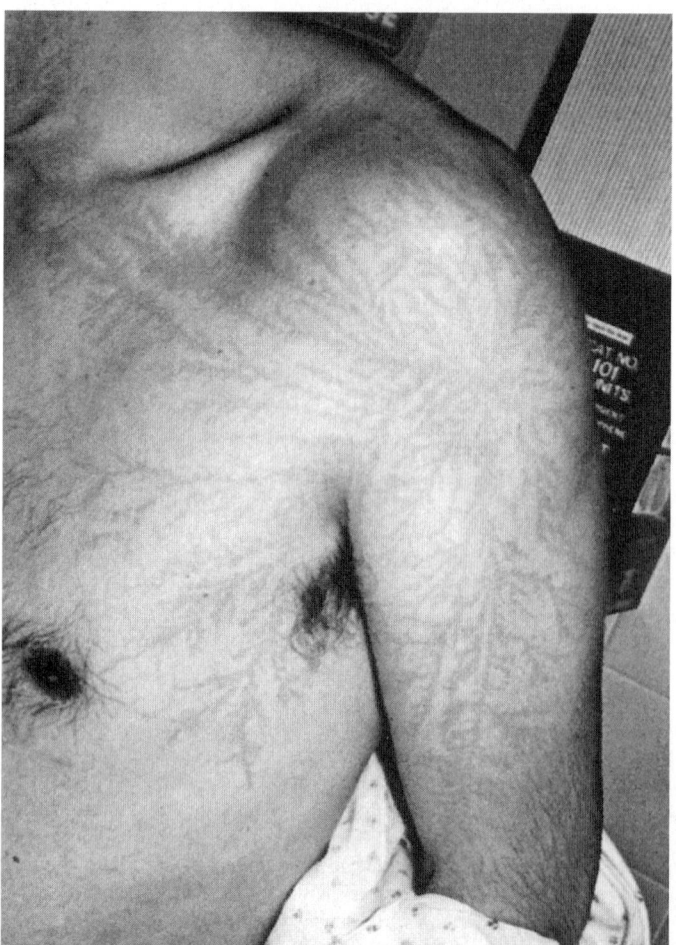

FIG. 202-1. Lichtenberg figures demonstrating the superficial ferning pattern.

203 CARBON MONOXIDE POISONING
Keith W. Van Meter

Carbon monoxide (CO) exposure and toxicity is a potentially lethal disorder with immediate and delayed side effects. Carbon monoxide is produced by incomplete combustion of carbon-containing material. Treatment of CO poisoning remains controversial because of conflicting clinical studies.

EPIDEMIOLOGY

Estimates of CO toxicity and fatality in the United States vary according to the data source and methodology. Analysis of data from the National Center for Health Statistics for calendar years 1994 to 1998 identified an average of 516 deaths each year from unintentional non-fire CO poisoning.[1] These fatality figures do not include intentional poisoning and deaths from fire and smoke inhalation, some of whom undoubtedly died from carbon monoxide toxicity. During roughly the same period, an estimated 11,000 individuals were seen in U.S. emergency departments for nonfatal nonfire CO poisoning. Unintentional CO toxicity and deaths are more common in northern climates and during the winter months.[2]

Industrial sources of CO from combustion include fossil fuel engine exhaust, gas- or coal-heater emissions, smoke from accidental fires, and fumes from cupolas of steel foundries, pulp paper mills, or formaldehyde-producing plants. Indoor burning of charcoal—particularly in some countries such as Korea, with a tradition of charcoal subfloor home heating—produces a disproportionate level of accidental CO intoxication. Interestingly, industrial sources produce slightly less environmental CO per land area than does the burning of tropical forests.[3] Little is known about the impact of low CO atmospheric levels on health. Regular cigarette smoking can produce carboxyhemoglobin (COHb) levels of 5 to 10 percent, and this chronic CO exposure is implicated in the acceleration of atherosclerosis seen in smokers. Truck drivers sitting in the cabs of their vehicles in heavy traffic can attain COHb levels similar to tobacco smokers.

CO toxicity has also been reported as a result of inhaling methyl chloride vapor, which is a component of paint stripping solutions, or from leaking "bubble" electric Christmas tree lights.[4]

PATHOPHYSIOLOGY

CO is an odorless, clear gas (in extremely high concentrations, it has a lavender odor), with a density of 0.97 that of air. In most instances, CO mixes evenly in turbulent air. A small amount of CO is endogenously produced from the metabolism of hemoglobin to bilirubin, and COHb levels rise slightly in hemolytic anemia. CO may function as an endogenous central nervous system (CNS) neurotransmitter.[5]

CO forms a ligand with respiratory pigments and enzymes such as hemoglobin, myoglobin, cytochrome P450, and cytochrome aa_3. In fact, cytochrome P450 was named after the *peak* (P) absorption of light at 450 μm when the enzyme is 50 percent saturated with CO. Respiratory enzymes have varying binding affinities for CO compared to oxygen. For example, hemoglobin binds CO 230 to 270 times as tenaciously as oxygen, myoglobin binds CO with 20 to 25 times the affinity for oxygen, and most respiratory enzymes have equal or less affinity for CO than for oxygen. In fact, cytochrome aa_3 has only one-ninth the affinity for CO as it does for oxygen.[6] When CO competes with oxygen for binding sites, it prevents utilization of oxygen by that enzyme or pigment. Thus, COHb will carry less oxygen according to the number of binding sites occupied by CO.

In addition, the binding of CO to hemoglobin also transforms the oxyhemoglobin dissociation curve from a sigmoid shape to an asymptotic shape, increasing the ability of COHb to hold on to oxygen at the remaining available heme moiety sites and reducing the availability of oxygen to metabolically active tissues (Figure 203-1). In CO toxicity, both the reduced oxygen carriage and the transformation of oxyhemoglobin dissociation curve impair tissue oxygen delivery. In effect, high COHb imposes the equivalent of a sudden "chemical" anemia in the patient.

The tolerance of the patient to this sudden chemical anemia may be worse than its hemorrhagic equivalent because of the toxic effects of CO on other respiratory pigments and enzymes. While tissue oxygen delivery is decreased, CO delivery still occurs by the dissolved CO in the circulating plasma. Experimental exchange transfusion in dogs of autologous red blood cells (RBC) exposed extracorporeally to CO be-

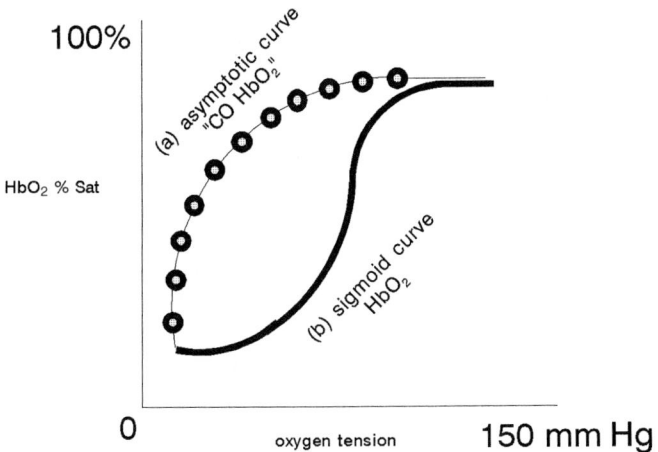

FIG. 203-1. COHb "shift to the left" reshaping of the oxyhemoglobin (HbO$_2$) dissociation curve. **(a)** Carbon monoxide–affected HbO$_2$ dissociation curve (asymptotic) and **(b)** normal HbO$_2$ dissociation curve (sigmoid).

fore transfusion, resulting in 60 percent COHb, demonstrated no signs of CO toxicity. Thus, while impairment of O$_2$ delivery by reduction of O$_2$ carriage is a part of CO toxicity, it may be that delivery of CO contributes more to the toxic effects of CO. In fact, hemoglobin may provide a protective buffer, preferentially binding CO and preventing binding to other respiratory pigments and mitochondrial cytochromes.

CO binding to mitochondrial cytochromes stops electrons—derived from aerobic metabolism of lipids, protein, and carbohydrates—from flowing through the cytochrome chain and halting the generation of adenosine triphosphate (ATP) in oxidative phosphorylation. CO binding to cytochrome aa_3 prevents the attachment of O$_2$, preventing the reduction of O$_2$ to H$_2$O. The cessation of cytochrome oxidative phosphorylation causes CO to "wreck the machine," as Haldane so aptly described the role of CO toxicity in aerobic metabolism.

CO binds strongly to intracellular pigments, such as myoglobin. In muscle with high oxygen use, such as the heart, the binding of CO to myoglobin markedly reduces the availability of oxygen for aerobic metabolism. CO poisoning of myocardial myoglobin reduces myocardial contractility, diminishes cardiac output, and further decreases tissue oxygen delivery. CO may likewise bind to neuroglobin in the human central nervous system, impairing neuronal function.[7]

CO toxicity, by imposing ischemic damage, causes white blood cells to become adherent to endothelial surfaces of tissue microvasculature upon reperfusion of ischemic tissue.[8] Immediately after reperfusion of ischemic CO-poisoned tissue, oxidative free radical products from these adherent white cells accelerate cell membrane lipid peroxidation, a process in part responsible for reperfusion injury.[9]

CLINICAL FEATURES

High-oxygen-extracting organs, such as the brain and the heart, easily become dysfunctional from CO intoxication. Neurologic symptoms and signs include fatigue, malaise, or flulike symptoms; nausea; difficulty in thinking, concentration, and memory; emotional lability; dizziness; paresthesias; weakness; vomiting; lethargy; somnolence; stroke; coma; seizure; and respiratory arrest. Cardiovascular symptoms and signs include chest pain from myocardial ischemia, palpitations from dysrhythmias, mildly to severely mottled skin from diminished circulation, poor capillary refill, hypotension, and cardiac arrest.

In a pattern of secondary injury from ischemia imposed by severe CO poisoning, the following clinical injury syndromes may occur: 1) rhabdomyolysis; 2) noncardiogenic pulmonary edema (NCPE); 3) multiorgan failure (MOF); 4) disseminated intravascular coagulation (DIC); 5) dermal blistering or increased dermal susceptibility to dermal pressure wounding; 6) circulatory shock from direct

CO-induced vasodilatation of vasculature and direct CO-induced impairment of myocardial function; 7) acute renal failure; and 8) "interval CO syndrome" of leukoencephalopathy of the centrum ovale (cerebral subcortical white matter) along with ischemic damage to basal ganglia and hippocampus.[10]

The symptoms and signs of CO toxicity are exacerbated by circumstances that increase neurologic and myocardial oxygen demand. Patients describe the onset of symptoms while at rest, with a marked increase after physical exertion. One example would be a patient who develops toxicity from using an internal combustion engine in a closed space. Starting to feel ill, the patient may walk or run outside to fresh air, only to collapse as the heart and brain are not able to deliver or utilize oxygen to meet the increased metabolic demands. CO intoxication is more severe in patients who have increased oxygen demands from the comorbidities of trauma, concurrent drug ingestion, burns, myocardial ischemia, cerebrovascular disease, or smoke inhalation.[11]

DIAGNOSIS

Signs and symptoms of CO injury correlate reasonably well with on-the-scene co-oximetry determination of COHb levels. However, by the time the patient gets to the ED after breathing air and with prehospital oxygen administration, the predictive value of COHb levels falls considerably. A very careful history, coupled with a screening neurologic examination that includes a CO neuropsychometric screening battery (CONSB), is a sensitive but not specific assay for CO intoxication. The CONSB has a good positive predictive value for discerning neurologic dysfunction or injury from CO intoxication.[12] The CONSB should be done with the patient breathing room air to be most sensitive.

Patients with CO exposure and only mild symptoms (no loss of consciousness, no cardiopulmonary symptoms, awake and cooperative) require minimal ancillary testing: a measure of COHb and possibly an electrocardiogram (ECG) to detect silent myocardial ischemia. Patients with moderate to severe exposures should have additional studies done to assess the extent of ischemic injury, including 1) COHb determination; 2) arterial blood gases (ABG), serum electrolytes, and serum lactate to detect metabolic acidosis; 3) complete blood count (CBC) and arterial oxygen content [CaO_2]; 4) an ECG if the patient has chest pain, palpitations, or dysrhythmia on the monitoring lead; 5) serum creatine phosphokinase MB isoenzyme (CK-MB) and troponin levels to detect potential myocardial ischemia; 6) serum CK, serum myoglobin, and urine myoglobin to detect skeletal muscle injury; 7) chest radiograph for patients with dyspnea, with abnormal auscultatory findings, or with multiple trauma; and 8) urine toxicologic screens when concurrent drug ingestion is suspected.

Imaging studies, such as computed tomography (CT) and magnetic resonance imaging (MRI) of the brain are modestly sensitive but nonspecific in documenting CNS ischemic injury 6 h after CO exposure.[13] Diffusion-weighted MRI brain scanning is being investigated for its utility in defining brain injury from CO intoxication. Single-photon emission computed tomography (SPECT) with radiolabeled hexamethylpropyleneamine oxime (HMPAO)–technetium 99m is immediately sensitive but not specific for acute ischemic CNS injury in CO poisoning.[14] Brain HMPAO/SPECT scan has the advantage that the radionuclide may be initially injected as the patient arrives in the ED without interrupting the resuscitation effort. The patient can be scanned later after stabilization, with a lasting "snapshot" of preresuscitation brain metabolism and perfusion. The bulk of HMPAO is taken up by the brain on first pass as it crosses the blood–brain barrier. Accordingly, the HMPAO "locks" into CNS tissue without much redistribution during the successive half-lives of the HMPAO radionuclide. The positron emission tomography (PET) brain scan may be helpful in illustrating CNS ischemic injury, but the scanner is rarely available and hard to obtain for critically ill patients.

SPECIFIC ISSUES

CO intoxication is especially harsh on the very old and very young. Pregnant patients with CO intoxication have no greater risk, but the fetus is at greater risk than the mother for ischemic injury because fetal hemoglobin has greater affinity than adult hemoglobin for CO.[15]

CO intoxication is more severe in patients with the comorbidity of multiple trauma, thermal or chemical burns, smoke inhalation, cerebral ischemia, or myocardial ischemia. CO intoxication coupled with drug intoxicants increases the risk of failure at self-evacuation from a toxic atmosphere. Further, concurrent inhalation of inert gas (natural gas), carbon dioxide, or chemical asphyxiants [nitrous oxide (NO), hydrogen sulfide (H_2S), hydrogen cyanide (HCN)] can augment ischemic insult in a CO patient. Also performing the CONSB assessment of the patient while the patient is breathing supplemental O_2 has led to false-negative normal exam results. If the CONSB is normal, the patient should have repeat evaluation on room air.

TREATMENT

The ABCs (airway, breathing, and circulation) of resuscitation apply to the seriously ill or injured victim with presumed CO intoxication. Normobaric oxygen (NBO) therapy should be administered as soon as possible with 100 percent fraction of inspired oxygen (FIO_2) by mask (nonrebreathing mask with reservoir). Patients who require ventilatory assistance should have bag-valve-mask ventilation with 100 percent oxygen until spontaneous ventilation recovery or endotracheal intubation can be performed in the field or the ED. **Pulse oximetry cannot be used to access adequacy of arterial oxygenation because the device confuses COHb for oxyhemoglobin and gives spuriously high values for percent of oxygen saturation.**[16]

Once the patient reaches the ED, decisions about further treatment are guided by the clinical evaluation (Table 203-1). Patients with only mild symptoms (nausea, headache, weakness, or flulike malaise) should receive 100 percent NBO for a period of about 4 h, with periodic reassessment. The ability of oxygen treatment to eliminate CO from the body has often been estimated using the half-life of COHb with different treatment regimens. The half-life of COHb is approximately 3 to 4 h while breathing room air, approximately 60 min by breathing 100 percent NBO, and 15 to 23 min with 100 percent hyperbaric oxygen (HBO) at 2.5 to 2.8 atmospheres of pressure [2.5 to 2.8 atmosphere absolute (ATA)]. Failure of mild symptoms to resolve after 4 h of NBO administration, if no other likely cause for the symptoms can be found, should lower the emergency clinician's threshold for the use of HBO therapy.

Major symptoms (any history of loss of consciousness, profound dip in blood pressure, amnesia, or myocardial ischemia) have tradi-

TABLE 203-1   Indications for Hyberbaric Oxygen Treatment in Acute Carbon Monoxide Poisoning

Definite Indication	Relative Indication
Altered mental status and/or abnormal neurologic examination (if patient has normal evaluation while on supplemental oxygen, temporarily take patient off oxygen and repeat evaluation)	Persisting neurologic symptoms including headache and dizziness after 4 h of 100% normobaric oxygen
History of loss of consciousness or near-syncope	Persisting acidosis
History of seizure	Concurrent thermal or chemical burns
Coma	Pregnancy with history of carbon monoxide exposure regardless of COHb level
History of hypotension during or shortly after exposure	
Myocardial ischemia	
History of prolonged exposure	
Pregnancy with COHb >15%	

tionally been an indication for initial HBO treatment. While dramatic improvement in symptoms and signs is generally seen, there is continued debate as to whether HBO is better than NBO with regard to short- and long-term outcomes.[17] Prospective, randomized studies comparing HBO and NBO have yielded conflicting results, possibly because of different entry criteria, treatment regimen, the intensity of the outcome measure, and the duration of follow-up.[17,18] There appears to be some benefit to HBO in reducing neurophysiologic sequelae, but that difference may be detectable only with specific testing and the benefit may be less apparent after 12 months of follow-up.[18]

Two recent controlled, prospective, randomized human trials yielded different results. Scheinkestel and colleagues found little difference between HBO and NBO in most neuropsychological tests at the completion of treatment, but noted that no patients in the NBO group developed **delayed neurologic sequelae, versus 4.8 percent in the HBO group. But the statistical significance of this result is questionable. Scheinkestel** used a hyperbaric regimen of 3 to 6 treatments at 2.8 ATA for 60 min (total chamber time of 100 min) over 3 to 6 days and the unconventional approach of placing all patients on continuous supplemental oxygen at 14 L/min by nonocclusive facemask for the duration of treatment (mean of 3 days).[19] Weaver and colleagues demonstrated marked reduction in neurologic sequelae at 6 weeks with hyperbaric treatment (46 percent in the NBO group versus 25 percent in the HBO group; absolute reduction 21 percent, 95% CI 6.2 to 35.9%).[20] This difference was sustained to a lesser degree at a 12-month follow-up. Weaver and colleagues used a protocol of three hyperbaric treatments 6 to 12 h apart, initiated within 24 h after the end of CO exposure, and without supplemental oxygen after the first treatment. Hyperbaric treatment duration and pressures were 1) first treatment at 3.0 ATA for 60 min followed by 2.0 ATA for 60 min, with total chamber time of 150 min, and 2) second and third treatments at 2.0 ATA for 100 min, with total chamber time of 120 min.

While the patient is being prepared for referral to a hyperbaric chamber, the patient should be maintained on 100 percent NBO. Traditional recommendations for HBO treatment for CO poisoning have sometimes stressed the use of COHb levels. **This approach is no longer advocated because of the poor correlation between clinical symptoms, morbidity, mortality, and ED COHb levels.** In addition, there is no evidence that HBO treatment based on COHb level alone is beneficial. Patients with mild to moderate symptoms improve dramatically after one HBO treatment, often becoming asymptomatic, and a common practice is to provide only one treatment. The benefit of a single treatment is unproven, retrospective analysis suggests that more than two treatments provided better outcomes than a single treatment, and the only prospective study finding benefit to HBO used three treatments. Thus, a single HBO treatment cannot be recommended.

In addition to enhancing the elimination of CO from the body, HBO treatment has several theoretical advantages over NBO treatment. HBO improves oxygen delivery to ischemic tissue and CO elimination from hemoglobin. HBO, not NBO, lessens CO-induced reperfusion injury by truncating lipid peroxidation and lessening leukocyte endothelial adherence in microvasculature.[8,9]

Complications of HBO treatment include a very low incidence of oxygen-induced seizures (approximately 1 per 1000 patients) and ear and sinus barotrauma. While possible, pulmonary barotrauma and vascular gas embolism are extraordinarily rare with clinical HBO treatment. Pregnancy is not a contraindication to HBO treatment; the only absolute contraindication to HBO treatment is an untreated pneumothorax.

The added mortality or morbidity incurred by transport to an HBO treatment facility has been established to occur in less than 5 percent of cases so handled. Both monoplace and multiplace hyperbaric chambers have critical care capability for ventilator support of endotracheally intubated patients, blood pressure monitoring, central venous manometry, and cardiac monitoring. U.S. emergency physicians can find the location of the nearest hyperbaric chamber by calling the Divers Alert Network (DAN), Duke University, Durham, NC, at 1-919-684-8111.

DISPOSITION

CO-intoxicated patients with mild symptoms (headache, nausea, flu-like symptoms, weakness, and dizziness) that remit after 4 h of 100 percent NBO may be discharged with the proviso that they return for evaluation if symptoms return. Patients should be reevaluated in 24 to 48 h. If patients with minor symptoms do not improve after 4 h of NBO therapy, they should be referred for HBO treatment. CO-intoxicated patients with the history of loss of consciousness, amnesia, myocardial ischemia, or seizure should be admitted even if symptoms improve with initial HBO treatment. CO-intoxicated pregnant patients at greater than 20 weeks' gestation should be admitted for fetal monitoring.

A subset of CO patients has "interval CO injury" or delayed development of neurologic symptomatology from 2 days to 1 month after initial improvement. Discharge instructions should include this information. Amelioration of neurologic residual injury with delayed treatment has occurred up to at least 20 days postinjury with HBO treatment. A short series of daily "tailing" low-dose HBO treatments has been anecdotally used to resolve or ameliorate lingering residual neurologic injury.

REFERENCES

1. Mah JC: Non-fire carbon monoxide deaths associated with the use of consumer products. 1998 Annual estimates. Bethesda, MD, Consumer Products Safety Commission, 1998.
2. Centers for Disease Control and Prevention: Deaths from motor vehicle–related unintentional carbon monoxide poisoning. *MMWR* 45:1029, 1996.
3. Newell RE, Rachle HG, Seiler W: Carbon monoxide and the burning earth. *Sci Am* 261(4):82, 1989.
4. Raphael M, Nadiras P, Flacke-Vordoa N: Acute methylene chloride intoxication—A case report on domestic poisoning. *Eur J Emerg Med* 9:57, 2002.
5. Dawson TM, Snyder SH: Gases as biological messengers: Nitric oxide and carbon monoxide in the brain. *J Neurosci* 14:5147, 1994.
6. Piantadosi CA: Carbon monoxide, oxygen transport and oxygen metabolism. *J Hyperbar Med* 2:27, 1987.
7. Trent JT, Watts RA, Hargrove MS: Human neuroglobin, a hemacodidanate hemoglobin that reversibly binds oxygen. *J Biol Chem* 276:30106, 2001.
8. Thom SR: Functional inhibition of leukocyte B2 integrins by hyperbaric oxygen in carbon monoxide–mediated brain injury in rats. *Toxicol Appl Pharmacol* 123:248, 1993.
9. Thom SR, Elbuken ME: Oxygen-dependent antagonism of lipid peroxidation. *Free Radic Biol Med* 10:413, 1991.
10. Gorman DF, Clayton D, Gilligan JE, Webb RK: A longitudinal study of 100 consecutive admissions for carbon monoxide poisoning to the Royal Adelaide Hospital. *Anaesth Intens Care* 20:311, 1992.
11. Goulon M, Barois A, Rapin M, et al: Carbon monoxide poisoning and acute anoxia due to breathing coal gas and hydrocarbons. *J Hyperbar Med* 1:23, 1992.
12. Messier LD, Myers RA: A neuropsychological screening battery for emergency assessment of carbon monoxide–poisoned patients. *J Clin Psychol* 47:675, 1991.
13. Pracyk JB, Stolp BW, Fife CE, et al: Brain computerized tomography after hyperbaric oxygen therapy for carbon monoxide poisoning. *Undersea Hyperbar Med* 22:1, 1995.
14. Choi IS, Kim SK, Lee SS, Choi YC: Evaluation of outcome of delayed neurologic sequelae after carbon monoxide poisoning by technetium-99m hexamethylpropylene amine oxime brain single photon emission computed tomography. *Eur Neurol* 35:137, 1995.
15. Koren G, Sharav T, Pastuszak A, et al: A multicenter, prospective study of fetal outcome following accidental carbon monoxide poisoning in pregnancy. *Reprod Toxicol* 5:397, 1991.
16. Bozeman WP, Myers RA, Barish RA: Confirmation of the pulse oximetry gap in carbon monoxide poisoning. *Ann Emerg Med* 30:608, 1997.

17. Juurlink DN, Standbrook MB, McGuigan MA: Hyperbaric oxygen for carbon monoxide poisoning. *Cochrane Database Syst Rev* 2:CD002041, 2000.

18. Thom SR, Taber RL, Mendiguren II, et al: Delayed neuropsychologic sequelae after carbon monoxide poisoning: Prevention by treatment with hyperbaric oxygen. *Ann Emerg Med* 25:474, 1995.

19. Scheinkestel CD, Bailey M, Myles PS, et al: Hyperbaric or normobaric oxygen for acute carbon monoxide poisoning: A randomized, controlled clinical trial. *Med J Aust* 170:203, 1999.

20. Weaver LK, Hopkins RO, Chan KJ, et al: Hyperbaric oxygen for acute carbon monoxide poisoning. *New Engl J Med* 347:1057, 2002.

MUSHROOM POISONING

Anne F. Brayer
Sandra M. Schneider

Mushrooms are a common toxic exposure, with more than 8400 mushroom exposures reported to poison centers in 2001.[1] More than 85 percent of these ingestions were unintentional, with nearly 70 percent occurring in children younger than age 6 years. Most reported ingestions result in little or no toxicity.[2,3]

Depending on the type of mushroom, adverse effects from ingestion range from mild gastrointestinal (GI) symptoms to major cytotoxic effects resulting in organ failure and death. Toxicity may also vary based on the amount ingested, the age of the mushroom, the season, the geographic location, and the way in which the mushroom has been prepared prior to ingestion. Individuals vary in their response to any given mushroom ingestion, so that one person may show significant effects while others may be asymptomatic ingesting the same mushroom (Table 204-1).

Mushroom toxicity is divided into early toxicity (within 2 h after ingestion) and delayed toxicity (6 h to 20 days). In general, if toxicity begins within 2 h of ingestion of a mushroom, the clinical course will most likely be benign. If symptoms begin 6 h or later after ingestion, the clinical course will likely be more serious and potentially fatal. Nearly all fatalities in the United States occur from the ingestion of the *Amanita* species *(Amanita phalloides, Amanita virosa,* and *Amanita verna)*.

Mushroom poisoning occurs among four main groups of individuals: young children who ingest mushrooms inadvertently, wild-mushroom foragers, individuals attempting suicide or homicide, and individuals looking for a hallucinatory "high." Identification of the mushroom ingested may be difficult and time-consuming. Very often, foragers will mix different species of mushrooms together, so it is not always clear that the species being identified is the same one that was ingested. In all cases, treatment should be directed by a patient's symptoms rather than by attempts at mushroom identification.

However, identification of the *Amanita* species may be helpful, but difficult, as there are many *Amanita* mushrooms that are nontoxic. *Amanita* species generally have warts on the cap (remnants of the membrane covering the emerging mushroom), which often give it a spotted appearance. The gills are "free," ending before the stem begins. The stem characteristically has a membrane ring around it and widens as it enters the soil. In most cases, the stem of the mushroom is contained in a cup or volva, which may be underground.

EARLY ONSET GASTROINTESTINAL SYMPTOMS

Pathophysiology

The most commonly ingested toxic mushrooms are those that cause GI irritation. These mushrooms can be of many types. In North America, *Chlorophyllum molybdites* is particularly common and is sometimes mistaken for an *Amanita*. Many of the so-called little brown mushrooms found commonly in lawns, and often accidentally ingested by children, are in this category. The actual toxin varies with the species of mushroom, but most toxins are poorly described.

TABLE 204-1   Mushrooms: Symptoms, Toxicity, and Treatment

Symptoms	Mushrooms	Toxicity	Treatment
Gastrointestinal symptoms			
Onset <2 h	*Chlorophyllum molybdites* *Omphalotus illudens* *Cantharellus cibarius* *Amanita caesarea*	Nausea, vomiting, diarrhea (occasionaly bloody)	IV hydration Antiemetics
Onset 6–24 h	*Gyromitra esculenta:* fall season *Amanita phalloides, Amanita verna,* and *Amanita virosa:* spring season	Initial: nausea, vomiting, diarrhea Day 2: rise in AST, ALT Day 3: hepatic failure	IV hydration, glucose, monitor AST, ALT, PT, PTT, bilirubin, BUN, creatinine For *Amanita:* activated charcoal Penicillin G 300,000–1,000,000 units/kg per d Silymarin 20–40 mg/kg per d Consider cimetidine 4–10 g/d Hyperbaric oxygen
Muscarinic syndrome Onset <30 min	*Inocybe* *Clitocybe*	SLUDGE	Supportive atropine 0.01 mg/kg repeated as needed for severe secretions
CNS excitement Onset <30 min	*Amanita muscaria* *Amanita pantherina*	Intoxication, dizziness, ataxia, visual disturbances, seizures, tachycardia, hypertension, warm dry skin, dry mouth, mydriasis (anticholinergic effects)	Supportive sedation with phenobarbital 30 mg IV or diazepam 2–5 mg IV as needed for adults
Hallucinations Onset <30 min	*Psilocybe* *Gymnopilus*	Visual hallucinations, ataxia	Supportive sedation with phenobarbital 0.5 mg/kg or, for adults 30–60 mg IV, or diazepam 0.1 mg/kg or 5 mg IV for adults
Disulfiram 2–72 h after mushroom, and <30 min after alcohol	*Coprinus*	Headache, flushing, tachycardia, hyperventilation, shortness of breath, palpitations	Supportive IV hydration β-blockers for supraventricular tachycardia Norepinephrine for refractory hypotension

Abbreviations: ALT = alanine aminotransferase; AST = aspartate aminotransferase; BUN = blood urea nitrogen; CNS = central nervous system; PT = prothrombin time; PTT = partial thromboplastin time; SLUDGE syndrome = salivation, lacrimation, urination, defecation, gastrointestinal hypermotility, and emesis.

Clinical Features

Typically, patients will present with acute onset of vomiting and diarrhea less than 2 h after ingesting the mushroom. There may be intestinal cramping, chills, headaches, and myalgias. The diarrhea is usually watery, but occasionally may be bloody, with fecal leukocytes. Most commonly, symptoms are mild and self-limited. Infrequently, the vomiting and diarrhea may lead to significant dehydration and electrolyte imbalance. The patient frequently offers the history of ingestion, but in cases where it is not, the presentation may be confused with acute gastroenteritis or acute food poisoning.

Treatment

General treatment for toxic mushroom ingestion includes GI decontamination. Activated charcoal 0.5 to 1.0 g/kg PO or via nasogastric tube is indicated for all ingestions unless toxic species can be excluded. Syrup of ipecac use may confuse the clinical picture, and is of little benefit. Treatment for ingestion of GI irritants is largely supportive, including IV fluid and electrolyte replacement when necessary. Judicious use of antiemetics is probably justified, but antidiarrheal agents are best withheld, because they may prolong the exposure to the toxin.

In most cases, the illness is self-limited, with symptoms resolving within 12 to 24 h. Rarely, symptoms may persist and hospitalization may be indicated for fluid and electrolyte replacement.

EARLY ONSET NEUROLOGIC SYMPTOMS

Pathophysiology

There are several classes of mushrooms that can cause neurologic symptoms. These include the hallucinogenic mushrooms ("magic" mushrooms) that are intentionally ingested for their mind-altering qualities. These mushrooms contain psilocybin or psilocin toxins, which are neuroactive chemicals similar to lysergic acid diethylamide (LSD). They act on serotonin-dependent neurons in the central nervous system (CNS), causing effects similar to those of LSD. Mushrooms from the *Psilocybe* genus, which are the most commonly ingested in this class, are small brown or gold mushrooms that commonly grow on dung in warmer climates and often turn a greenish blue when bruised or cut. They may also be cultivated at home from purchased spores. Nontoxic mushrooms may also be laced with phencyclidine (PCP) or LSD and sold as hallucinogenic mushrooms.

Mushrooms containing the isoxazole derivatives, ibotenic acid and muscimol, also possess neurologic effects, which are thought to be mediated by γ-aminobutyric acid (GABA) and anticholinergic activity. *Amanita muscaria* is an easily identified member of this group. It has an orange or red cap with white warts (remnants of the universal veil present in young specimens), as well as a ring (annulus) and cup (volva) on the stem. *Amanita pantherina,* another member of the group, is 5 to 14 cm in length and diameter, with a white to brown cap, and with the ring and cup on the stem. Both specimens grow under trees in woodlands throughout North America.

Clinical Features

Ingestion of hallucinogenic mushrooms usually leads to development of symptoms within 2 h. Euphoric sensation, a heightened imagination, a loss of time sensation, and visual distortions or hallucinations are common. There may be tachycardia and hypertension. Fever and seizures have rarely been reported. Symptoms typically last 4 to 6 h. There are infrequent reports of patients suffering from flashbacks for up to 4 months after ingestion.

Patients ingesting isoxazole mushrooms usually present with symptoms within 30 min of ingestion. Dizziness, mild intoxication, ataxia, muscular jerking, and difficulty with size, time, and place perceptions are common. Uncommonly, there may be anticholinergic symptoms, including tachycardia, hypertension, warm, dry skin and mucous membranes, and mydriasis. Seizures have been reported in children. Symptoms are typically self-limited, resolving within 3 to 4 h after ingestion.

Treatment

Treatment for ingestion of hallucinogenic mushrooms is largely supportive. Placing the patient in a darkened quiet room, devoid of visual stimuli, and providing reassurance are often sufficient. If sedation is required, benzodiazepines such as diazepam 0.1 mg/kg for children and 5 mg for adults, administered intravenously are preferred to phenothiazine derivatives because the latter can lower seizure threshold. The use of anticholinergic agents should be avoided, as they may aggravate the delirium.

Treatment of symptomatic ingestion of isoxazole containing mushrooms begins with GI decontamination. Syrup of ipecac may be appropriate if it can be administered within 30 to 60 min of ingestion, but caution is advised because of the potential for CNS depression and seizures. Activated charcoal administration is advised in most cases. In patients with significant vomiting and diarrhea, fluid and electrolyte replacement may be necessary. Patients who are agitated should be appropriately restrained. Sedation may be provided as necessary with benzodiazepines (diazepam or lorazepam) or phenobarbital. Seizures have been successfully treated with benzodiazepines.

For patients with severe anticholinergic symptoms, treatment with physostigmine may be considered. Physostigmine has been known to produce bradycardia, hypotension, and seizures, so administration should be reserved for severely symptomatic patients. The dosage is 1 to 2 mg intravenous slowly in adults, and 0.5 mg in children. Patients should have continuous cardiorespiratory and blood pressure monitoring during administration.

EARLY ONSET MUSCARINIC SYMPTOMS

Pathophysiology

Mushrooms containing muscarine cause neurologic symptoms and muscarinic or cholinergic effects. The symptoms are characterized by the SLUDGE syndrome (salivation, lacrimation, urination, defecation, GI hypermotility, and emesis). Mushrooms of the *Inocybe* and *Clitocybe* genus are common causes of muscarinic poisoning. The *Inocybe* mushrooms are small brown mushrooms with conical caps, typically found under hardwoods and conifers. The *Clitocybe* mushrooms are usually found individually on lawns and in parks, and are white to gray, with a cup-shaped cap. *Amanita muscaria,* despite its name, contains far less muscarine than these other families, and only rarely causes cholinergic poisoning symptoms.

Clinical Features

In addition to the SLUDGE syndrome, patients with muscarine ingestions can present with diaphoresis, muscle fasciculations, miosis, bradycardia, and bronchorrhea. Symptoms typically present within 30 min of ingestion and spontaneously resolve in 4 to 12 h.

Treatment

In most cases, symptoms are mild and self-limited. Supportive care is often sufficient. Because emesis is a common presenting symptom, activated charcoal administration is often difficult. Patients with severe vomiting may require intravenous fluid and electrolyte replacement.

Atropine is an antidote for muscarinic symptoms and can be administered in severe cases. It can be effective in treating bradycardia and hypotension unresponsive to intravenous fluids. Atropine is helpful in the treatment of diaphoresis, increased oral secretions, and bronchorrhea. It may also help reduce GI cramping, emesis, and diarrhea. The dose is 0.5 to 1.0 mg for adults and 0.01 mg/kg for children, administered intravenously. The dose can be repeated as necessary to control bronchorrhea, bradycardia, or hypotension. Large doses may be necessary to treat severe toxicity. Patients should be carefully monitored during administration. Oxygen and inhaled β-agonists (e.g., albuterol) are recommended for the treatment of patients with increased pulmonary secretions and bronchospasm.

DELAYED GASTROINTESTINAL SYMPTOMS

Pathophysiology

Two different mushrooms, *Gyromitra* and *Amanita,* cause significant toxicity, which characteristically present several hours after ingestion. *Gyromitra esculenta* (the false morel) grows primarily in the spring in North America and is also found in several European countries. It has a brown convoluted top resembling a brain and is often mistaken for the tasty morel mushroom. Gyromitrin (*N*-methyl-*N*-formylhydrazone) is a volatile heat-labile toxin and primarily responsible for symptoms. Parboiling the mushroom can partially eliminate the toxin. Gyromitrin is hydrolyzed in the stomach to form *N*-methyl-*N*-formylhydrazine (MFH) and *N*-methylhydrazine (MH). MH is chemically identical to rocket fuel, and workers exposed to MH develop CNS toxicity. MH binds to pyridoxine and interferes with enzymes that require pyridoxine as a cofactor. GABA is lowered in the CNS, which may be a possible etiology for the seizures. MFH is converted into a free radical in the liver and causes local hepatic necrosis by blocking the activity of the P450 system, glutathione, and other hepatic enzyme systems.[4] These two chemicals explain the CNS and hepatic dysfunction characteristic of gyromitrin toxicity. The etiology of the initial GI symptoms remains obscure.

Amanita phalloides, Amanita virosa, and *Amanita verna* commonly occur in the Northern Hemisphere and are particularly common in North Central Europe. Mushrooms of this species are found throughout the West Coast, Midwest, and in parts of the Northeast of the United States. Immigrants may mistake these mushrooms for edible varieties common in Eastern Asia. Mushrooms of the *Amanita* species are responsible for 95 percent of deaths associated with mushrooms. Toxic ingestions in North America occur most commonly in the autumn.

Amanita phalloides contains several amatoxins and phallotoxins. Phallotoxins are bicyclic peptides that inactivate F-actin. Although this action has been of interest to basic scientists, phallotoxins do not appear to be active in human toxicity. Amatoxins are bicyclic octapeptides that are rapidly absorbed through the intestinal mucosa. They are carried to the liver, and undergo enterohepatic circulation, which leads to prolonged toxin exposure after ingestion. Kinetic studies in humans show that α-amanitin is cleared from the plasma within 48 h.[5] Concentrations in the plasma are quite small; amatoxins are not protein bound, but actively transported into hepatocytes, where they bind to RNA polymerase II and inhibit the formation of messenger RNA. Some literature regarding studies with animals suggests that free radical formation may also be involved in toxicity.[6] Pathologic evidence of nuclear fragmentation and condensation of chromatin occur within 24 h after ingestion. Amanitin has the greatest effect on cells that undergo rapid protein synthesis and turnover, including cells of the GI mucosa, hepatocytes, and renal tubular epithelium.[7]

The diagnosis of gyromitrin toxicity is generally assumed from the clinical features and the identification of the mushroom, either by the patient or from samples. Identification of *Amanita* species generally requires a trained mycologist. The Meixner colorimetric test is used to look for the presence of amatoxin. Although it is sensitive, it is not

very specific, as other nontoxic mushrooms may test positive. Thin-layer chromatography, high-performance liquid chromatography, and radioimmunoassay have been developed to detect amatoxin. Amatoxin can be detected in plasma, urine, GI contents, and feces. However, its presence merely confirms amatoxin poisoning. Levels do not appear to correlate with clinical severity, and many patients do not have amatoxin detected, presumably because of rapid clearance.

Clinical Features

The distinct characteristic of these mushrooms is the onset of intense GI symptoms (nausea, vomiting, and diarrhea) 6 to 24 h after ingestion. In cases of *Amanita* species ingestion, the later the onset of the GI symptoms, the milder is the disease. After resolution of the initial GI symptoms, patients may develop hepatic injury.

Patients who ingest a gyromitrin-containing mushroom typically have a delayed onset of GI symptoms, which appear 6 to 8 h after ingestion. Initial GI symptoms are accompanied by neurologic symptoms, including dizziness and headache. In a mild ingestion, patients will have neurologic symptoms for several days and recover without difficulty. In severe cases, however, hepatic failure becomes symptomatic on day 3 and may result in death by as soon as day 7. Hypovolemia is common in the first phase of toxicity. Hypoglycemia occurs during the GI phase and again in the acute hepatic failure phase. Seizures, lack of coordination, and muscle cramps may occur.

Patients who ingest amatoxin-containing mushrooms also have delayed onset of GI symptoms (6 to 24 h). The gastroenteritis is intense, often requiring fluid and electrolyte replacement. Hypovolemia and hypoglycemia are quite common during the early GI phase. The gastroenteritis generally subsides after 12 h, and patients enter a second phase, where they often are asymptomatic despite ongoing liver damage. Hepatic failure becomes symptomatic on day 3 or 4, and death may follow as soon as day 7. Patients rapidly develop jaundice and right-upper-quadrant pain, and may develop a decreased level of consciousness, an elevated ammonia level, and cerebral edema. Liver enzymes, bilirubin, and prothrombin time rapidly become abnormal. Renal failure occurs either as a direct result of the toxin or as part of the hepatorenal syndrome.

In both toxicities, serum transaminases begin to increase 36 to 72 h after ingestion. Levels may be quite elevated. Prothrombin time may be elevated and unresponsive to vitamin K or fresh frozen plasma replacement. Amylase and lipase elevation suggests pancreatic damage, although symptomatic pancreatitis is rare. Abnormal laboratory findings in amatoxin poisoning include a decrease in neutrophils, lymphocytes, and platelets, and abnormal thyroid function. Hypophosphatemia (primarily noted in children), hypocalcemia, and elevated insulin levels occur. None of these laboratory abnormalities correlate with clinical disease, and their cause is unknown.

Pathologic changes are noted in both gyromitrin and amatoxin toxicity. Patients who ingest gyromitrin show diffuse hepatocellular damage and interstitial nephritis. Patients who ingest amatoxins show fatty degeneration of the liver, with intranuclear collection of lipids and extensive hepatic necrosis. Electron microscopy shows vacuolization of the mitochondria and clumping of the chromatin in the nucleoli. There are extensive lipid peroxidation changes in both the nucleus and the cytoplasm.

Toxic mushroom exposure during pregnancy has been reported.[8] In one series, a slightly lower birth weight was noted, as compared with normal controls. Most infants appeared to be healthy and developmentally normal, in keeping with the findings that amatoxins do not cross the placental barrier.[9]

The mortality rate from *Gyromitra* ingestion is estimated at 15 to 35 percent. Although historically amatoxin hepatic failure had a mortality rate as high as 50 percent, more recently mortality has been reduced to 10 to 15 percent, based on improved care for hepatic failure.

Patients who survive severe hepatic failure from amatoxin may develop signs of chronic active hepatitis with persistent elevation in liver transaminases, development of antismooth muscle antibodies, and cryoglobulins; the long-term consequences are unclear. No prolonged effects from gyromitrin toxicity have been reported.

Treatment

Most patients present with initial GI symptoms—severe vomiting and diarrhea. If a patient presents within a few hours of ingestion, gastric decontamination is indicated. Repeated doses of charcoal may be effective, particularly in the presence of amatoxin (as it undergoes enterohepatic circulation), at least for the first 24 h, but no clinical studies show the efficacy of charcoal for gyromitrin or amatoxin. Fluid and electrolyte replacement is mandatory. Glucose should be monitored and replaced, if necessary. **Hypoglycemia is one of the most common causes of death in early mushroom toxicity.**

All patients who have ingested amatoxin- or gyromitrin-containing mushrooms should be closely monitored for 48 h for the development of hepatic failure. Liver enzymes and prothrombin time should be monitored several times a day. Patients should be treated with a low-protein diet and receive standard supportive therapy for hepatic failure. Fresh-frozen plasma and vitamin K can be used for the treatment of prolonged prothrombin time; in many cases, however, coagulopathy does not respond to treatment.

Patients who develop hepatic failure should be monitored closely and, in severe cases, preparations made for liver transplantation. Although no firm criteria exist, progressive coagulopathy and encephalopathy, in spite of maximal medical therapy, are frequently listed indications for emergency liver transplantation.[10] Many patients have met this criteria and survived without transplantation, and many patients have died without achieving these "target" values. Liver transplantation, however, does provide the only option for patients in fulminant hepatic failure and has been quite successful. Auxiliary liver transplantation has also been used. In this case, a portion of the damaged liver is removed, and a temporary transplant provided, allowing time for the native liver to regenerate.[11]

Gyromitrin-Specific Treatment

The neurologic symptoms associated with gyromitrin are successfully treated with high-dose pyridoxine. *Pyridoxine* provides the cofactor required for the regeneration of GABA. High doses of pyridoxine, 25 mg/kg up to a maximum of 25 g/d, are recommended, but doses of pyridoxine in excess of 40 g are associated with severe peripheral neuropathy.[12] Pyridoxine does not affect the development or course of hepatic failure, and there is no specific therapy for gyromitrin-induced hepatic failure.

Amatoxin-Specific Treatment

Historically, there have been many anecdotal and largely ineffective treatments used to counteract this deadly toxin. Because 80 percent of the toxin is eliminated in the urine, forced diuresis may have some theoretical basis, but no clinical trials have shown efficacy. Charcoal hemoperfusion or hemodialysis may remove amatoxin, but studies have questioned their benefit.[13] Attempts to interrupt enterohepatic circulation have also been tried but are of limited usefulness. Plasmapheresis has been reported to be useful, in combination with other detoxification techniques.[14]

Thioctic acid, which has been used for many years in Europe, is a known free radical scavenger and may be effective in the treatment of acute hepatic failure of undifferentiated cause. Thioctic acid and glutathione appear to protect against microsomal lipid peroxidation and therefore may be of theoretical use in amatoxin poisoning. Animal and human studies, however, have not shown thioctic acid to be effective.

High doses of penicillin have been advocated for amatoxin poisoning because penicillin blocks the uptake of amatoxin into the liver by its shared active transport system. In addition, penicillin increases renal excretion of the toxin. Other antibiotics, such as rifampin and cephalosporins, have a similar effect in animal studies. Huge doses of penicillin G 300,000 to 1,000,000 units/kg per day, are required to decrease toxicity in animal studies. Such doses are associated with seizures, and if used, patients should be appropriately monitored. If amatoxin is suspected, penicillin should be started very soon after ingestion. Penicillin-allergic patients either should not be treated with penicillin or should undergo desensitization. Unfortunately, a retrospective review of amatoxin poisoning found little efficacy to penicillin therapy.[15]

Silymarin (silybinin), which has been used successfully in Europe to treat amatoxin ingestion, acts as a free radical scavenger and may interrupt the enterohepatic circulation of amatoxin when given orally. It is not available in the United States, but a recent study in Europe showed success in patients with amatoxin poisoning.[16]

There have been animal studies and isolated human case reports of other therapies for amatoxin poisoning. High-dose *cimetidine* 10 g/d, is effective in animals and recently was used successfully in humans.[6] Vitamin C, zinc, and thiol compounds have also been useful in animal models.

DELAYED-ONSET RENAL FAILURE

Pathophysiology

Orellanine and ortinarin A and B are nephrotoxic compounds found in species of *Cortinarius* (*C. orellanus, C. speciosissimus,* and *C. gentilis*). These toxins are heat stable, and their mechanisms of action are unknown. Mushrooms of this species are found primarily in Europe and do not represent a significant problem in the United States. A similar delayed onset of renal toxicity has been reported following the ingestion of *Amanita smithiana.*[17] This mushroom is commonly mistaken for pine mushrooms and grows commonly in the Pacific Northwest. Nephrotoxins in this mushroom are norleucine (aminohexadrenoic acid) and chlorocrotylglycine.

Clinical Features

Patients who ingest mushrooms containing nephrotoxins often initially present with gastrointestinal symptoms including nausea, vomiting and nonbloody diarrhea. Symptoms begin several hours after ingestion, and may persist for 3 days. Occasionally, paresthesias, abnormal taste, and cognitive dysfunction are reported. Symptoms of renal failure, including lumbar and flank pain, oliguria, or more rarely polyuria begin between 3 and 20 days following ingestion. There is some evidence to suggest that patients who ingest *Amanita smithiana* may develop renal failure earlier. Many patients who ingest these mushrooms never go on to develop renal dysfunction, suggesting host variability. Supportive hemodialysis may be required in as many as 30 to 50 percent of patients, but 50 percent of patients will have spontaneous return of normal renal function.

Treatment

There is no specific treatment for patients who develop renal failure from *Cortinarius* or *Amanita smithiana*. Urine output and electrolyte, calcium, magnesium, blood urea nitrogen, and creatinine levels should be monitored. Hemodialysis support is indicated for refractory hyperkalemia, refractory acidosis, uremic symptoms, or severe renal dysfunction. As spontaneous improvement is reported, renal transplant should be withheld for several months to monitor patient response. Renal transplant has been used in several patients with good success.[18]

DELAYED-ONSET DISULFIRAM REACTION

Pathophysiology

Perhaps the most interesting, but clinically least important, is a mushroom toxin contained in the *Coprinus* genus. This mushroom, which is very common in North America, is known as the "inky-cap" or "shaggy mane." It is a tall, white, thin mushroom with a shaggy cap. As the mushroom ages, the cap liquefies and blackens, and black liquid drips from the necrosing cap. The mushroom contains coprine, which is chemically related to disulfiram. Coprine causes inhibition of alcohol dehydrogenase within 2 h of ingestion, and activity may last up to 72 h. If alcohol is consumed during this "sensitive" period, patients will develop a typical disulfiram reaction. Mushrooms ingested at the same time as alcohol produce no toxicity.

Clinical Features

Because of the delay between mushroom consumption and alcohol consumption, few patients will link their symptoms to the ingestion of a mushroom. Patients present with facial flushing, diaphoresis, headache, tachycardia, nausea, and vomiting. Most symptoms are mild.

Treatment

Because alcohol is readily absorbed from the GI tract, GI decontamination has no role. Likewise, charcoal would not be expected to have great benefit. Patients occasionally become hypotensive and respond to intravenous fluids or, in refractory cases, norepinephrine. Patients should be educated about the link between the alcohol and mushroom ingestion.

REFERENCES

1. Litovitz TL, Klein-Schwart W, Rodgers GC, et al: 2001 Annual report of the American Association of Poison Control Centers Toxic Exposure Surveillance System. *Am J Emerg Med* 20:391, 2002.
2. Nordt SP, Manoguerra A, Clark RF: Five-year analysis of mushroom exposures in California. *West J Med* 173:317, 2000.
3. Hender E, May T, Beulke S: Poisoning due to eating fungi in Victoria. *Aust Fam Physician* 29:1000, 2000.
4. Michelot S, Toth B: Poisoning by *Gyromitra esculenta*: A review. *J Appl Toxicol* 11:235, 1991.
5. Jaeger A, Jehl F, Flesch F, et al: Kinetics of amatoxins in human poisonings: Therapeutic implications. *J Toxicol Clin Toxicol* 31:63, 1993.
6. Schneider SM, Borochovitz D, Krenzelok EP: Cimetidine protection against α amanitin hepatotoxicity in mice: A potential model for the treatment of *Amanita phalloides* poisoning. *Ann Emerg Med* 16:1136, 1987.
7. Vetter J: Toxins of *Amanita phalloides*. *Toxicon* 36:13, 1998.
8. Boyer JC, Hernandez F, Estorc J, et al: Management of maternal *Amanita phalloides* poisoning during the first trimester of pregnancy: A case report and review of the literature. *Clin Chem* 47:971, 2001.
9. Timar L, Czeizel AE: Birth weight and congenital anomalies following poisonous mushroom intoxication during pregnancy. *Reprod Toxicol* 11:861, 1997.
10. Beckurts KT, Holscher AH, Heidecke, et al: The role of liver transplantation in the treatment of acute liver failure following *Amanita phalloides* poisoning. *Dtsch Med Wochenschr* 122:351, 1997.
11. Rosenthal P, Roberts JP, Ascher NL, et al: Auxiliary liver transplant in fulminant failure. *Pediatrics* 100:e10, 1997.
12. Albin RL, Albers JW, Greenberg HS, et al: Acute sensory neuropathy-neuronopathy from pyridoxine overdose. *Neurology* 37:1729, 1987.
13. Mullins ME, Horowitz BZ: The futility of hemoperfusion and hemodialysis in *Amanita phalloides* poisoning. *Vet Hum Toxicol* 42:90, 2000.
14. Jander S, Bischoff J: Treatment of *Amanita phalloides* poisoning: I. Retrospective evaluation of plasmapheresis in 21 patients. *Ther Apher* 4:303, 2000.
15. Enjalbert F, Rapior S, Nouguier-Soule J, et al: Treatment of amatoxin poisoning: A 20-year retrospective analysis. *J Toxicol Clin Toxicol* 40:715, 2002.
16. Saller R, Meier R, Brignoli R: The use of silymarin in the treatment of liver diseases. *Drugs* 61:2035, 2001.
17. Warden CR, Benjamin DR: Acute renal failure associated with suspected *Amanita smithiana* mushroom ingestion: A case series. *Acad Emerg Med* 5:808, 1998.
18. Danel VC, Saviuc PF, Garon D: Main features of *Cortinarius* spp. poisoning: A literature review. *Toxicon* 39:1053, 2001.

205 POISONOUS PLANTS
Mark A. Hostetler
Sandra M. Schneider

Poisonous and injurious plants number in the hundreds and have a wide variety of toxicities. Rather than attempting a comprehensive listing, this chapter focuses on the most important plant-related encounters clinically relevant to emergency medicine, with descriptions of the most severely poisonous and commonly encountered plants (Tables 205-1 and 205-2), and those most frequently encountered during the holiday season.[1,2] Individual plants are discussed in terms of their pathophysiology, clinical features (toxidromes), and treatment.[3]

EPIDEMIOLOGY

According to statistics gathered by the American Association of Poison Control Centers (AAPCC), plants are the fourth most common reason for poison center notification and account for 5 to 10 percent of all calls received.[1-3] This high rank is a reflection of their wide availability rather than any unusually high level of innate toxicity. Children younger than 6 years of age account for 70 to 80 percent of all plant-related exposures, the vast majority of which (96 percent) are unintentional.[4] The most common plant-related call received by a poison control center is for completely nontoxic plants (21 percent) and, on average, fewer than 10 percent of patients require treatment in a health care facility. Dermatitis and gastrointestinal irritation are most common reported sequelae of plant toxicity and occur in approximately 20 percent of patients, but contrary to its emphasis in the literature, vomiting is not a common manifestation of plant ingestions.[5] Moderate effects of a more systemic nature occur in 1 percent of patients. Severe effects associated with life-threatening or disabling injuries are extremely uncommon and occur in only 0.04 percent of patients. Death as a consequence of plant-related exposures is rare, and occurs at a rate of less than 0.001 percent of patients.

Toddlers experience the world by first putting it into their mouth. Because 80 percent of the exposures occur among toddlers younger than age 6 years, and most within the home, prevention is paramount. All poisonous and injurious plants should be kept out the reach of toddlers and preschoolers. Homes should be purged of all potentially toxic plants, just as they are for medications and cleaning supplies, and children should be specifically instructed never to eat plants or wild berries.[4,6]

TREATMENT

Most plant-related exposures require no treatment, and those that do often can be managed by simple decontamination procedures. Those

TABLE 205-1   Most Highly Poisonous Plants

Castor bean *(Ricinus communis)*
Foxglove *(Digitalis purpurea)*
Jequirity bean *(Abrus precatorius)*
Oleander *(Nerium oleander)*
Poison hemlock *(Conium maculatum)*
Water hemlock *(Cicuta maculata)*
Yew *(Taxus spp)*

TABLE 205-2 Most Commonly Encountered Poisonous and Nonpoisonous Plants

Poisonous/Injurious	Nonpoisonous
Aloe spp	African violet (*Episcia reptans*)
Azalea (*Rhododendron* spp)	*Coleus* spp
Cactus spp	*Dracaena* spp
Caladium spp	Ficus plant (*Ficus* spp)
Colchicine (autumn crocus, meadow saffron)	Honeysuckle (*Lonicera* spp)
Dumbcane (*Dieffenbachia amoena*)	Jade plant (*Crassula* spp)
	Pyracantha spp
Fava beans	Rubber tree plant (*Ficus elasticus*)
Holly (*Ilex* spp)	Spider plant (*Chlorophytum* spp)
Jimsonweed (*Datura* spp)	Umbrella plant (*Schefflera* spp)
Lily of the valley (*Convallaria majalis*)	Wandering jew (*Tradescantia albiflora*)
Mistletoe (*Phoradendron flavescens*)	
Nightshade (*Solanum* spp)	
Peppers (*Capsicum* spp)	
Philodendron spp	
Poinsettia (*Euphorbia* spp)	
Poison ivy (*Toxicodendron* spp)	
Pokeweed (*Phytolacca* spp)	
Pothos (*Epipremnum* spp)	

patients with a potentially serious exposure who are asymptomatic should be observed in the ED for at least 4 to 6 h. If they remain asymptomatic, they may be discharged with appropriate instructions and follow-up. Symptomatic patients require ongoing monitoring and care and should be admitted to the hospital, because toxicity may continue to evolve. Few plants have specific antidotes.

It is recommended that all exposures be reported to the regional poison control center, so that accurate data can be collected on poisonous and injurious plant exposures, for help with plant identification, and for valuable input regarding patient management.

SEVERELY POISONOUS PLANTS

Castor Bean (*Ricinus communis*)

Ricin is a potent toxalbumin that inhibits protein synthesis and causes severe cytotoxic effects on multiple organ systems. It may be one of the most poisonous naturally occurring substances known.[7] Although present in all parts of the plant, ricin is concentrated most in the bean. Castor beans are covered by a hard, relatively impervious outer shell that must be chewed or in some way broken in order for the ricin to result in toxicity.

Symptoms include delayed gastroenteritis, which may be severe and hemorrhagic, followed by delirium, seizures, coma, and death. Beans are particularly antigenic and may cause severe hypersensitivity and cutaneous and systemic allergic reactions.

Whole-bowel irrigation (WBI) has been advocated to ensure rapid and complete decontamination of the gastrointestinal (GI) tract. Rapid elimination of the bean before erosion of the outer shell occurs may decrease or prevent the release of potent toxins. Beans should be counted to assure complete recovery. Patients should be observed for at least 8 to 12 h. Once symptomatic, supportive care involves attention to fluid, glucose, and electrolyte replacement.

Foxglove (*Digitalis purpurea*)

Foxglove contains cardiac glycosides similar in structure and action to digitalis. Its toxicity lies somewhere between lily of the valley and oleander (see "Oleander" below).

Jequirity Bean (*Abrus precatorius*)

Jequirity beans contain the toxalbumin abrin, one of the most lethal naturally occurring toxins known.[8] Children have died as a result of chewing alone (without swallowing) the beans. Chewing and swallowing just one bean may also be lethal to an adult. Symptoms include a delayed gastroenteritis, which may be severe and hemorrhagic, followed by delirium, seizures, coma, and death. Like castor bean, recovery of the intact bean by WBI is recommended. Patients should be observed for at least 8 to 12 h. Treatment is otherwise supportive, with attention to fluid replacement and monitoring of electrolytes.

Oleander (*Nerium oleander*)

Similar in structure and effect to digitalis, all parts of the plant contain the cardiac glycosides oleandrin, oleandroside, nerioside, and digitoxigenin. Cardiac glycosides act by inhibiting the sodium- and potassium-activated adenosine triphosphatase ($Na^+K^+ATPase$) pump and lead to hyperkalemia and a variety of dysrhythmias (see Chap. 174). Of all plants containing cardiac glycosides (lily of the valley, foxglove, and oleander), oleander is the most toxic.[9]

These glycosides cross-react sufficiently so that a positive serum digoxin level will qualitatively confirm ingestion. However, quantitative levels are not and should not be used to quantify the amount of ingestion or potential toxicity. Effects include nausea, vomiting, diarrhea, abdominal pain, confusion, and cardiac dysrhythmias.

Potassium levels should be closely monitored. Hyperkalemia may be severe, refractory to the usual treatments (insulin, glucose, bicarbonate), and may require hemodialysis.[10] Calcium is generally not recommended, as it may theoretically exacerbate the digitalis toxicity, although there is no published human experience. In addition to GI decontamination and routine antidysrhythmic therapy, digoxin-specific Fab antibody fragments are recommended for patients with ventricular dysrhythmias.[11]

Poison Hemlock (*Conium maculatum*)

All parts contain coniine alkaloids similar in structure and effect to nicotine, and with the ability to induce neuromuscular blockade. Symptoms occur rapidly in 15 min to 1 h after ingestion and begin with complaints of burning and dryness of the mouth. Tachycardia, tremors, diaphoresis, mydriasis, profound muscle weakness, and seizures may develop. In severe cases, ascending paralysis, rhabdomyolysis, acute renal failure, bradycardia, coma, and death occur. Although most cases are unintentional, there are some case reports of toxicity resulting from the intentional use by patients for a presumed narcotic-like effect.[12] Treatment consists of GI decontamination, activated charcoal, and supportive care which may include intravenous fluids, antidysrhythmics, and anticonvulsants.

Water Hemlock (*Cicuta maculata*)

Cicutoxin, a C_{17}-polyacetylene, is found in highest concentrations in the root, but all parts contain the poison. Its mechanism of action appears to involve inhibition of noncompetitive γ-aminobutyric acid (GABA) antagonists to GABA receptors. One mouthful may be fatal in as soon as 15 min. Initial symptoms include nausea, vomiting, and abdominal pain, followed by delirium, seizures, and death. Seizures may be severe and refractory to conventional anticonvulsant therapy. The mortality rate may be as high as 30 percent.[13] GI decontamination is important, otherwise, treatment is supportive with intravenous fluids and anticonvulsants.

Yew (*Taxus* spp)

Yew contains taxine alkaloids in the leaves and seeds, a potent toxin with effects on cardiac myocytes.[14] Case reports of near-fatal human ingestions and fatal livestock ingestions have created the reputation that yew berry ingestions are highly toxic. However, a retrospective review of *Taxus* species ingestions found that while symptoms, predominantly gastrointestinal, were common, moderate to life-threatening complications were rare (<1 percent) and there were no human fatalities.[15] Symptoms after ingestion include nausea, vomiting, and abdominal pain. Rarely, seizures, cardiac dysrhythmias, and coma occur. Treatment consists of GI decontamination, activated charcoal, fluids, anticonvulsants, and antidysrhythmics as necessary.

COMMON POISONOUS AND INJURIOUS PLANTS

Aloe (*Aloe barbadensis*)

Sap from this common succulent houseplant contains an anthraquinone that acts as a cathartic. Symptoms include abdominal pain and diarrhea within 6 to 12 h of ingestion. It may occasionally turn the urine red, and large doses may cause nephritis. There is no specific antidote. Intravenous fluids may be necessary to support GI fluid losses.

Azalea (*Rhododendron* spp)

Andromedotoxins are found in the leaves, flowers, and nectar. Potential symptoms after ingestion include salivation, lacrimation, bradycardia, hypotension, progressive paralysis, and potentially (but rarely) death. Most cases of ingestion result in minimal toxicity. In addition to GI decontamination, treatment consists of atropine for symptomatic bradycardia and fluids or vasopressors for hypotension.

Cactus

Needles or spines may embed in the skin and cause direct mechanical injury. Patients typically complain of pain and irritation at the site. Unlike other foreign bodies, such as glass, that are inert, spines contain proteinaceous material and should be removed if possible. Multiple small cactus spines may be removed by applying a thin layer of rubber cement or other similar type substance over area, allowing the material to dry, and then gently peeling it off, removing the spines that have become embedded in the adhesive. Complications such as infection and granuloma formation occur, but are uncommon.

Caladium spp

Toxicity is similar to dumbcane (calcium oxalate raphides), but less severe.

Colchicine (Autumn Crocus, Meadow Saffron, Glory Lily)

Colchicine is contained in all parts of the autumn crocus, meadow saffron, and glory lily. Colchicine causes a delayed and severe gastroenteritis, followed by severe multisystem organ failure.[16] Common effects include coagulopathy, bone marrow suppression with granulocytopenia and thrombocytopenia, cardiac dysrhythmias, cardiogenic shock, adult respiratory distress syndrome, hepatic failure, delirium, seizures, coma, and death. In addition to GI decontamination, treatment usually requires aggressive fluid resuscitation. Colchicine-specific Fab fragments are commercially available for severe poisonings.

Dumbcane (*Dieffenbachia amoena*)

These plants contain calcium oxalate crystals packaged into bundles known as raphides. In addition, these plants also contain proteolytic enzymes with antitrypsin-like activity, which stimulates the release of histamine and bradykinin. It remains unclear why some plants such as schefflera, which also contain calcium oxalate crystals, are completely nontoxic. Children who chew the leaves develop immediate burning and irritation of the oral mucosa. Cases of severe swelling, drooling, dysphagia, and respiratory compromise have been reported, but are not common.[17] Most cases of human ingestion report minor symptoms that resolve with little or no treatment. Demulsifying agents, such as cold milk or ice cream, may help and analgesics may be necessary. Steroids are considered beneficial for severe cases, although there have been no controlled trials.

Fava Beans

A portion of persons affected by glucose-6-phosphate dehydrogenase (G6PD) deficiency provide one of the few examples where genetic predisposition is associated with increased potential for toxicity after plant exposure; an estimated 10 to 20 percent of G6PD deficiency patients will develop favism after consuming fava beans. Symptoms include GI upset, fever, and headache and patients may develop hemolytic anemia with hemoglobinuria and jaundice (see Chap. 221).

Jimsonweed (*Datura* spp)

Jimsonweed (also known as thorn apple, devil's trumpet, or locoweed) is a wildly occurring weed infamous for its hallucinatory properties. Exposures most commonly are intentional and occur through experimentation.[18] All parts of the plant are toxic and contain atropine-like alkaloids (hyoscyamine, atropine, and scopolamine) capable of precipitating acute anticholinergic crises by competitive inhibition of cholinergic muscarinic receptors.

Symptoms occur within 30 to 60 min and may last for up to 48 h because of delayed gastric motility. Symptoms include hyperthermia ("hot as a hare"), flushed skin ("red as a beet"), dry skin and mucous membranes ("dry as a bone"), mydriasis ("blind as a bat"), and hallucinations or delirium ("mad as a hatter"). Tachycardia and urinary retention are also common.

Treatment includes GI decontamination with emesis or lavage, activated charcoal, and supportive care (intravenous fluids, external cooling, and restraints for patient protection). GI decontamination may be useful for up to 48 h after ingestion if the patient remains symptomatic. Physostigmine, a cholinesterase inhibitor, antagonizes both the central and peripheral effects and may be required in 30 to 40 percent of cases.[18] It should be considered for severe cases exhibiting hyperthermia, seizures, or frank psychosis. An initial dose of 0.5 mg for children or 1.0 to 2.0 mg for adults is given slowly IV over 5 min. Repeat doses may be required (see Chap. 183).

Lily of the Valley (*Convallaria majalis*)

In addition to ingestion of the plant itself, toxicity has been reported from drinking of water in which the freshly cut flowers were kept (see "Oleander" above).

Nettle (Stinging Nettle, Bull Nettle)

Nettles contain a specialized system for injecting their toxins. Stinging hairs are connected to a bladder filled with various irritants (histamine, acetylcholine, 5-hydroxytryptamine). Handling of the plant stimulates the injection of these substances via the hair tube. An immediate burning response may last for hours. Treatment is symptomatic.

Nightshade, Common or Woody (*Solanum* spp)

The glycoalkaloid solanine is present in all parts of the plant. Ingestion results in nausea, vomiting, diarrhea, and abdominal pain. Delirium, hallucinations and coma may also occur with larger doses. There is no specific treatment.

Nightshade, Deadly (*Atropa belladonna*)

This plant contains atropine-like substances with anticholinergic properties (see "Jimsonweed" above).

Peach, Apricot, Pear, Crab Apple, and Hydrangea

Amygdalin, a cyanogenic glycoside, is metabolized by the enzyme emulsin to hydrocyanic acid. In sufficient quantities, hydrocyanic acid may lead to acute cyanide toxicity. The requisite enzyme (emulsin) is present in the pits or seeds of these plants noted above and may be present to some degree in intestinal bacteria. Ingestion of large amounts of seeds or pits results in diaphoresis, nausea, vomiting, abdominal pain, and lethargy. Symptoms develop over hours. GI decontamination is needed. If symptomatic, antidotal therapy may be needed for cyanide toxicity (see Chap. 188).

Pepper (*Capsicum* spp)

Capsicum causes irritation, burning, and pain upon contact with mucous membranes as a result of depletion of substance P from terminal nerve endings. There is intense burning of the mucous membranes with contact. Patients typically self-inoculate their eye while preparing peppers. Police use pepper sprays to subdue combative individuals. In addition to cutaneous decontamination with copious amounts of water and gentle hand soap, demulsifying agents, such as cold milk or ice cream, may help. Analgesics may be necessary.

Philodendron spp

All parts contain oxalate raphides and may produce symptoms similar to dumbcane, although less severe.

Pokeweed (*Phytolacca americana*)

All parts of the plant are toxic, but especially the roots, unripe berries, and seeds. Phytotoxins (phytolaccotoxin and phytolaccine) cause direct mucosal irritation and GI symptoms. Patients complain of burning in the mouth and throat, with abdominal pain, nausea, vomiting, and profuse diarrhea that may be foamy.[19] Severe intoxications may result in coma and death. Although their safety remains somewhat controversial, ripe berries are occasionally used in pies and the leaves boiled for greens. Treatment is GI decontamination with emesis or lavage, charcoal, and supportive care consisting of fluid-electrolyte replacement.

Potato, Eggplant (*Solanum* spp)

Solanine is contained in green potatoes and in the sprouts, and is destroyed by cooking. Delayed gastroenteritis may be seen (see common nightshade above).

Pothos (Devil's Ivy, *Epipremnum* spp)

This plant has toxicity similar to dumbcane, but less severe.

Yellow Sage (*Lantana camara*)

Leaves and unripe fruit contain the toxin lantadene, which may produce dilated pupils, vomiting, diarrhea, weakness, and coma. Symptoms may be delayed for 2 to 6 h. Treatment is GI contamination and fluids for dehydration.

Toxicodendron Species (Poison Ivy, Oak, and Sumac)

These plants contain the antigenic resin urushiol. Once exposed, most, but not all, individuals develop sensitization as the antigenic resin binds with skin proteins and forms a complete antigen. Reexposure then stimulates a T-cell-mediated immune response. Reactions begin with itching, burning and redness developing over 12 to 48 h, and may progress to include varying degrees of vesiculobullous formation. Resin may remain after the plant has dried and may be aerosolized during burning. Antipruritic and topical therapies (oatmeal baths and topical steroids) are commonly used. Facial, genital, or widespread involvement requires systemic steroids for 10 to 14 days. Patients should be advised to clean under their fingernails and wash all contaminated clothing. IvyBlock, a new product recently approved by the Food and Drug Administration, contains bentoquatam and binds urushiol to prevent absorption. Skin cleansers (such as Tecnu) may be used up to 8 h after exposure to decontaminate the skin.

COMMON HOLIDAY OR SEASONAL PLANTS (POISONOUS AND NONPOISONOUS)

Holly (*Ilex* spp)

The leaves are nontoxic, whereas the berries contain a variety of toxins known as saponins. Gastroenteritis is most common effect after ingestion and may occur with as few as 2 or 3 berries, whereas 20 to 30 berries may be fatal. Treatment is GI decontamination followed by intravenous fluids to prevent dehydration.

Poinsettia (*Euphorbia pulcherrima*)

Poinsettia is a much-maligned plant ubiquitous during the Christmas holidays. Originally implicated as being toxic, recent evidence suggests that, at most, it may occasionally cause some local irritation to skin, mouth, or conjunctiva.[20]

American Mistletoe (*Phoradendron flavescens*)

All parts are poisonous and contain phoratoxin, a toxalbumin. Gastroenteritis may occur following ingestion of a large number of berries, but significant morbidity is rare.[21] Treatment is GI decontamination with fluid and electrolyte monitoring.

Easter Lily (*Lilium longiflorum*)

Toxicity has not been reported in humans.

REFERENCES

1. Krenzelok EP, Jacobsen TD: Plant exposures: A national profile of the most common plant genera. *Vet Hum Toxicol* 39:248, 1997.
2. Litovitz TL, Klein-Schwartz W, Rogers GC, et al: 2001 Annual report of the American Association of Poison Control Centers Toxic Exposure Surveillance System. *Am J Emerg Med* 20:391, 2002.
3. Mrvos R, Krenzelok EP, Jacobsen TD: Toxidromes associated with the most common plant ingestions. *Vet Hum Toxicol* 43:366, 2001.
4. Lawrence RA: Poisonous plants: When they are a threat to children. *Pediatr Rev* 18:162, 1997.
5. Krenzelok EP, Mrvos R, Jacobsen TD: Contrary to the literature, vomiting is not a common manifestation associated with plant exposures. *Vet Hum Toxicol* 44:298, 2002.
6. Krenzelok EP, Jacobsen TD, Aronis J: Those pesky berries: Are they a source of concern? *Vet Hum Toxicol* 40:101, 1998.
7. Challoner KR, McCarron MM: Castor bean intoxication. *Ann Emerg Med* 19:1177, 1990.
8. Kinamore PA, Jaeger RW, Castro FJ: Abrus and ricinus ingestion. *Clin Toxicol* 17:401, 1980.
9. Bose TK, Basu RK, Biswas B, et al: Cardiovascular effects of yellow oleander ingestion. *J Indian Med Assoc* 97:407, 1999.
10. Haynes BE, Bessen HA, Wightman WD: Oleander tea: Herbal draught of death. *Ann Emerg Med* 14:350, 1985.
11. Shumaik GM, Wu AW, Ping AC: Oleander poisoning: Treatment with digoxin-specific Fab antibody fragments. *Ann Emerg Med* 17:732, 1988.

12. Drummer OH, Roberts AN, Bedford PJ, et al: Three deaths from hemlock poisoning. *Med J Aust* 162:592, 1995.

13. Centers for Disease Control: Water hemlock poisoning—Maine, 1992. *MMWR* 43:229, 1994.

14. Wilson CR, Sauer J, Hooser SB: Taxanes: A review of the mechanism and toxicity of yew (*Taxus* spp.). *Toxicon* 39:175, 2001.

15. Krenzelok EP, Jacobsen TD, Aronis J: Is the yew really poisonous to you? *J Toxicol Clin Toxicol* 36:219, 1998.

16. Klintschar M, Beham-Schmidt C, Radner H, et al: Colchicine poisoning by accidental ingestion of meadow saffron (*Colchicum autumnale*): Pathological and medicolegal aspects. *Forensic Sci Int* 106:191, 1999.

17. Pedaci L, Krenzelok EP, Jacobsen TD, Aronis J: *Dieffenbachia* species exposures: An evidence-based assessment of symptom presentation. *Vet Hum Toxicol* 41:335, 1999.

18. Thabet H, Brahmi N, Amamou M, et al: *Datura stramonium* poisonings in humans. *Vet Hum Toxicol* 41:320, 1999.

19. Roberge R, Brader E, Martin ML, et al: The root of evil: Pokeweed intoxication. *Ann Emerg Med* 15:470, 1986.

20. Krenzelok EP, Jacobsen TD, Aronis JM: Poinsettia exposures have good outcomes: Just as we thought. *Am J Emerg Med* 14:671, 1996.

21. Krenzelok EP, Jacobsen TD, Aronis J: American mistletoe exposures. *Am J Emerg Med* 15:516, 1997.

EMERGENCY MEDICINE IN UNIQUE ENVIRONMENTS

206 WORLD TRAVELERS
Michael J. VanRooyen

Chayan C. Dey

Raghu Venugopal

"The art of being wise is the art of knowing what to overlook."
William James

The evaluation of the world traveler is a growing concern as a consequence of the increase in the popularity of transcontinental travel that allows even exotic destinations to be reached within 36 h. Greater numbers of immunologically naive travelers venture abroad each year, and more than half of these travelers travel to tropical nations whose illness burden is largely due to poverty, civil unrest, poor environmental hygiene, malnutrition, and tropical illnesses.[1] One needs a logical and organized approach to patients who have been exposed to uncommon tropical infections, since most returning travelers have neither serious nor exotic illnesses. The likely causes of acute symptoms are common problems such as upper respiratory infections, diarrheal illnesses, or reactions to stress, fatigue or new medications. The ED physician often does not routinely confirm the final diagnosis, but rather begins diagnostics and provides appropriate referral. It is important to identify local or regional travel health facilities for referral of patients who need more advanced evaluation, serologic testing, and long-term follow-up.

POPULATIONS AT RISK

Each year, some 8 million Americans travel to lesser-developed nations and up to 1 in 10 seek posttravel medical care. Most such travelers are in their early forties, although there is a rise in the number of travelers at extremes of age. Among travelers, 64 percent report one or more illnesses during travel, 26 percent are ill upon return, and 56 percent of those ill upon return develop symptoms after arrival in the United States.[2] Many disease incubation times are longer than the transit times of most modern travelers.

Travelers are at risk for certain infectious diseases based on the duration of travel, the endemic exposure, and preexisting immunity. Most travelers on vacation or business are abroad for fewer than 20 days, and less than 5 percent spend extended time overseas. A variety of travelers originate from disease-endemic nations, including tourists or newly arrived immigrants seeking U.S. domicile. Such visitors and foreign nationals are at risk for typical infectious diseases and newly emerging infections. Others at risk include nonvoluntary travelers, such as refugees and displaced persons, as well as landed immigrants with permanent U.S. residence who are returning from visiting their homeland. A high degree of clinical suspicion is warranted for this latter group because many presume they still have acquired immunity for diseases such as malaria, but remain susceptible to endemic illnesses. Western travelers also have an increasing risk of tropical illness as a result of increasing exotic adventure-type travel to remote locales that were previously inaccessible (Table 206-1).

Many travelers are exposed to diseases such as *Plasmodium falciparum* (malaria) that are uncommon in the United States, but which are leading causes of mortality overseas. Other parasitic agents, such as helminths and rickettsia, also occur with increased frequency and severity in the tropics. Helminths are discussed in Chap. 149 and rickettsia in Chap. 151. It is important to suspect when patients may be infected by a tropical infection because diagnosis often requires a unique set of tests and therapy is organism specific. Also, in all cases of suspected tropical illnesses, the potential for a bioterrorist agent should be suspected when plausible. Factors suggesting intentional releases include divergence of the disease presentation from the typical epidemiology of the community and an atypical number of patients presenting with similar clinical syndromes. Examples of diseases which could be weaponized include anthrax, plague, viral hemorrhagic fevers, and tularemia. These are discussed in detail in Chap. 7.

HISTORY

Imported disease should be suspected among recent world travelers. This is particularly important in those arriving from an endemic nation presenting with otherwise typical chief complaints. These include shortness of breath, fever, abdominal pain, diarrhea, hematuria, headache, and skin rash (Table 206-2). Noting previous medical conditions is paramount because those with risk factors such as immunosuppression, early childhood, advanced age, pregnancy, or diabetes are often less tolerant of tropical infections.

The risk of infection depends on historical aspects such as the duration of travel (suggesting specific disease incubation periods) and destination or origin (suggesting possible etiology). Knowing the region of travel can reduce the differential diagnosis of possible causative agents (Table 206-3). Other important considerations are the living conditions and locale of the traveler (rural areas have greater infectious risks), type of accommodation, and travel-related activities (suggesting possible exposure) (Table 206-4). A review of systems, pretravel immunizations and medications, high-risk behaviors, and prior medical conditions should be queried. This is relevant because proper vaccination against hepatitis A, hepatitis B, and yellow fever can effectively rule these out as causes of illness. In addition, adherence to appropriate chemoprophylaxis can significantly reduce the risk of acquiring malaria—which is the most important tropical emergency—yet the possibility of malaria should never be discounted, regardless of compliance with prophylaxis. Because of increasing malaria resistance, febrile returning travelers must be assumed to have malaria even if chemoprophylaxis was correctly used for 4 weeks after return. A history of medications, herbs, and traditional medicines consumed is also useful. The use of mefloquine prophylaxis and antipyretics can still result in late-appearing fever caused by malaria breakthrough. For tropical emergencies such as cerebral malaria, the clinician may need to depend on only what is uncovered during the patient interview, physical examination, and available diagnostic tests. When patients cannot give a full history because of altered mental status, suspect cerebral malaria or meningitis and consider early treatment for both until the diagnosis is confirmed.

PHYSICAL EXAMINATION

The physical examination should be as detailed as practically possible, even though positive physical findings may be nonspecific. Focus should be paid to evaluating the abdomen for hepatosplenomegaly or focal abdominal discomfort. Examine the patient for lymph node involvement and inspect the skin and mucosal surfaces. Ophthalmologic examination should note scleral icterus, conjunctival injection or petechiae. Imported diseases should be suspected in the presence of high fever, signs of hemorrhage, profuse diarrhea, shortness of breath, skin lesions, and neurologic disturbances. Table 206-5 lists other signs of tropical illness.[3]

TABLE 206-1   Overall Risk of Exposure to Infectious Agents

High risk (1 in 10 travelers): Diarrhea, URIs, and noninfectious illnesses such as injuries and cardiac problems
Moderate risk (1 in 200): Dengue, enteroviral infection, gastroenteritis, giardiasis, hepatitis A, malaria, salmonella, STDs, shigella
Low risk (1 in 1000): Amebiasis, ascariasis, measles, mumps, enterobiasis, scabies, TB, typhoid, hepatitis B
Very low risk (1 in >1000): HIV, anthrax, Chagas, hemorrhagic fevers, pertussis, plague, typhus, hookworm

Abbreviations: HIV = human immunodeficiency virus; STD = sexually transmitted disease; TB = tuberculosis; URI = upper respiratory illness.

TABLE 206-3   Regional Tropical Illnesses

Africa: Hookworm, malaria, HIV, dengue, brucellosis, yellow fever (and other hemorrhagic fevers), dracunculiasis, relapsing fever, tapeworm, roundworm, schistosomiasis
Central and South America: Malaria, relapsing fever, dengue, filariasis, TB, schistosomiasis, Chagas, typhus
Mexico and the Caribbean: Dengue, hookworm, malaria, cystercercosis
Australia, New Zealand: Dengue, Lyme disease, Q fever
Middle East: Hookworm, malaria, anthrax, brucellosis
Europe: Giardiasis, Lyme disease, tick-borne encephalitis, babesiosis
China and East Asia: Dengue, hookworm, malaria, strongyloidiasis, hemorrhagic fever, Japanese encephalitis

Abbreviations: HIV = human immunodeficiency virus; TB = tuberculosis.

LABORATORY TESTING

Initial investigations may include standard tests like complete blood count (CBC) with differential and platelet count, absolute eosinophil count, liver enzymes and hepatic function tests, and urinalysis; thick and thin blood smears for malaria, blood cultures, urine cultures and stool analysis for white blood cells (WBCs), ova, and parasites. Specific serologic tests may be indicated, such as erythrocyte sedimentation rate (ESR), purified protein derivative (PPD), Venereal Disease Research Laboratory (VDRL), HIV, and serology for arboviruses. The absolute eosinophil count should be elevated to greater than 500/μL in parasitic diseases such as helminths (worms). It is helpful to consult an

infectious disease specialist early in evaluation to be certain that the proper laboratory tests have been ordered.

CLINICAL DIAGNOSIS BASED ON SYNDROMIC PRESENTATION

The presentation of tropical disease is often subtle and necessitates a high degree of clinical suspicion. However, there are usually one or more hallmark symptoms or signs that most infections elicit. Hereafter, tropical conditions are categorized by their classical symptoms. These include fever, central nervous system (CNS) complaints, abdominal pain, diarrhea, skin and eye complaints, and respiratory symptoms.

TABLE 206-2   Travel-Specific Aspects of the Medical History

Pretravel information
  Previous medical condition
    Pediatric patient, diabetes, pregnancy, immunosuppression (especially HIV/AIDS)
  Pretravel consultation and preparation (self-treatment medications, vaccination history, prophylaxis, etc.)
    Type and compliance with chemoprophylaxis—particularly malaria
    History of routine childhood immunization
  Nation of birth and citizenship
Exact itinerary of departure and arrival (within the last 3–5 years may be relevant)
  Season of travel (monsoon, dry season)
Destinations visited (including locations of transit or stopovers)
  Urban or rural, altitude
Purpose of travel and activities in-country
  General purpose of visit or travel (e.g., "adventure travel" with high exposure to remote, natural elements)
  Contacts and their health
  Habitat and location of lodging (bednets, window screens)
    Crowded living or sleeping conditions
  High risk activities (e.g., medical care of refugees, spelunking in caves, cohabitation with indigenous, poor populations)
  Opiate use or intravenous drug use
  Sexual intercourse with any foreign national and very high-risk populations such as commercial sex-trade workers (dates and nature of sexual contact)
  Exposure to environment (swimming, hiking, trekking, digging, or soil contact)
  Consumption of high-risk foods (wild game or bush meat, raw or undercooked meats or fish, unpasteurized milk products, food from street vendors, natural sources of water, salads)
  Exposure to dogs, birds, or rodents
Adverse incidents
  Insect or animal bites
  Saliva from animals to open wounds
  Assault or trauma
Status and health of fellow travelers
  Possible ill contacts
In-country medical consultations sought, remedies used, and procedures (injections, acupuncture, transfusions, dental procedures, body piercing, or tattooing)

TABLE 206-4   Specific Exposures and Associated Tropical Infections

Contact/Exposure	Possible Infections
Untreated water, unpasteurized dairy products	Salmonellosis, shigellosis, hepatitis, amebiasis, brucellosis, tuberculosis
Raw or undercooked shellfish	Clonorchiasis, paragonimiasis, vibrios, hepatitis A
Raw or undercooked animal flesh	Trichinosis (e.g., pig, horse, bear), salmonella, enterohemorrhagic *E. coli*
Raw vegetables, water plants (e.g., watercress)	Fascioliasis
Animal contact (and animal products)	Rabies, Q fever, tularemia, brucellosis, echinococcosis, anthrax, plague, Nipah virus, toxoplasmosis
Rodent contact	Hantavirus, viral hemorrhagic fevers, murine (endemic) typhus, Lassa fever, plague
Arthropod vectors	
Mosquitoes	Malaria, dengue, filariasis, yellow fever, and other arboviral infections
Ticks or mites	Rickettsioses, tularemia, scrub typhus, Crimean-Congo hemorrhagic fever
Reduviid (kissing) bugs	American trypanosomiasis (Chagas disease)
Tsetse flies	African trypanososmiasis (African sleeping sickness)
Fleas	Typhus, plague
Sandflies	Leishmaniasis
Freshwater exposure	Schistosomiasis, leptospirosis
Barefoot exposure	Strongyloidiasis, cutaneous larva migrans
Sexual contacts	HIV, hepatitis B, syphilis, gonorrhea, herpes simplex
Infected persons contact	Viral hemorrhagic fever, enteric fever, meningococcal infection, tuberculosis

TABLE 206-5 Physical Findings in Selected Tropical Infections

Physical Finding	Likely Infection or Disease
Rash	Dengue fever, typhoid, typhus, syphilis, gonorrhea, Ebola, brucellosis
Jaundice	Hepatitis, malaria, yellow fever, leptospirosis, relapsing fever
Lymphadenopathy	Rickettsial infections, brucellosis, dengue, HIV, Lassa fever, leishmaniasis
Hepatomegaly	Amoebiasis, malaria, typhoid, hepatitis, leptospriosis
Splenomegaly	Malaria, relapsing fever, trypanosomiasis, typhoid, brucellosis, kala-azar, typhus, dengue fever
Eschar	Typhus, borrelia, Crimean-Congo hemorrhagic fever
Hemorrhage	Lassa, Marburg, or Ebola viruses; Crimean-Congo hemorrhagic fever; meningococcemia, epidemic louse-borne typhus

Source: Adapted from Hill DR: Health problems in a large cohort of Americans traveling to developing countries. *J Travel Med* 7:259, 2000.

Diseases Commonly Associated with Fever

Although fever is often a nonspecific symptom, it should arouse suspicion of a potentially life-threatening infection (Table 206-6).[4] It is important to differentiate diseases that may be rapidly fatal, easily treatable, and/or potentially contagious. In all cases, fever associated with confusion, hypotension, or hypoxemia necessitates emergent care. Although exotic diseases should be considered, it is more important to determine the existence of common and easily treatable infections. Even in the international tropical traveler, the most common life-threatening infectious diseases are caused by organisms causing pneumonia, meningitis, and acute gastrointestinal illness (Table 206-7).[5,6]

The fever pattern is sometimes helpful because onset, pattern, and duration can suggest a particular illness. Determining an approximate incubation period (the time between exposure and signs and symptoms) can be helpful in ruling in or out certain etiologies. For example, if fever begins more than 21 days after return, dengue, yellow fever, and other arboviruses are unlikely, irrespective of the exposure history (Table 206-8). In comparison, those acutely infected by schistosomiasis may only exhibit symptoms 5 weeks postexposure. Incubation periods should be used cautiously because some diseases have variable incubation depending on factors such as host immunity and the use of chemoprophylaxis and other medications.

Malaria

Malaria is the most important tropical disease. The classic clinical triad for all species of malaria is fever, splenomegaly, and anemia.[7,8] Fever is typically irregular for the first week and later demonstrates periodicity. Illnesses with similar presentation include viral influenza, dengue fever, meningococcal meningitis, typhoid fever, pneumococcal pneumonia, and viral hepatitis.

Patients usually have continuous symptoms initially, followed by episodic pyrexia every 2 to 3 days, depending on the infecting species. Serious infections occur primarily in young children, gravid women, individuals never previously infected (such as Western nationals), and debilitated patients with comorbid medical problems. Because associated symptoms such as headache, cough, and gastrointestinal (GI) problems mimic other conditions, malaria should be seriously considered in all febrile travelers.

Diagnosis is based on clinical presentation and confirmed with lab evidence of blood-borne protozoa. Patients with fever >38.5°C (101.4°F) of unclear origin and with recent or past travel to an endemic area should be screened by obtaining blood smears. Refer to Chap. 142 for a detailed discussion of malaria diagnosis and treatment.

Dengue Fever

Dengue is the most significant arbovirus affecting humans, and most serious febrile tropical disease after malaria. It should be suspected among febrile travelers within 2 weeks of tropical travel. Dengue may occur more than once because each of the four strains offers no cross-protective immunity. Worldwide, it annually causes an estimated 100 million cases, including 25,000 deaths. With increasing global population, transcontinental travel, and tropical urbanization, the frequency of imported dengue is predicted to rise. More than 500 laboratory-confirmed cases occurred in the last 20 years in the United States, although this is an underestimation, because many cases are self-limiting and the illness is nonreportable.[9] Also, the long serology processing time also means it usually does not aid acute diagnosis or treatment, so many physicians do not order it.

Dengue fever occurs in most urban environments in most tropical nations and is borne by the peridomestic day-biting *Aedes aegypti* mosquito. Urban dengue in the Americas, Africa, and the Indian subcontinent is usually classical dengue fever, whereas in Southeast Asia it manifests as hemorrhagic fever and shock. Classic dengue fever presents after a typically short incubation period of 4 to 7 days with sudden high fever, headache, nausea, vomiting, myalgias, and rash usually lasting a week. Facial flushing, conjunctival injection, retro-orbital pain, and facial edema (termed dengue facies) also occur. Following defervescence a fine pale morbilliform rash develops on the trunk and spreads to extremities and face. Small children may only present with a mild upper respiratory infection and classic dengue may be confused with influenza, measles, or rubella. While other causes of fever can present with a similar clinical picture, such as West Nile fever (transmitted by the *Culex* mosquito), West Nile fever causes lymphadenopathy, which is usually absent in dengue. Dengue can also cause petechial hemorrhages indistinguishable from meningococcemia.

Dengue hemorrhagic fever (DHF) preferentially occurs among infants of immune mothers, children older than age 1 year and those with second and subsequent infections. It begins as classical dengue with fever and myalgias. After 2 to 7 days as pyrexia improves, lassitude, fatigue, and shock develop with an ensuing mortality that is greater than 10 percent. Patients demonstrate hemorrhagic pleural effusions, bleeding diathesis, epistaxis, purpura, petechia, and thrombocytopenia with elevated hematocrit because of vascular permeability. DHF, if untreated, rapidly evolves into dengue septic shock (DSS) which is often fatal. DSS is heralded by abdominal pain, severe emesis, mental status changes, and alternating severe pyrexia and hypothermia. Diagnosis of dengue and DHS-DSS is based on clinical findings, and while serology is confirmatory, cross-reactivity often occurs with other flaviviruses. Enzyme-linked immunosorbent assay (ELISA) for IgM can provide a more accurate and rapid confirmation of infection by day 6 of the illness. Laboratory abnormalities include leukopenia, thrombocytopenia, and hepatic dysfunction. In uncom-plicated dengue fever, treatment is supportive and consists of oral fluids and analgesics. Only acetaminophen is recommended for managing pain and fever because aspirin and other nonsteroidal anti-inflammatory drugs (NSAIDs) are contraindicated due to anticoagulant properties. Dengue often requires intravenous hydration with LR solution or NS. Supplemental oxygen and sedation may be required.

Typhoid Fever

Enteric fever or typhoid is a serious infection diagnosed in 2 percent of febrile travelers and caused by *Salmonella typhi* and *S. paratyphi*. Once malaria has been ruled out, this is typically the cause of a febrile illness lasting greater than 10 days. Imported cases are typically among children or adolescents; recently, travelers in Mexico, Indonesia, Peru, and India accounted for more than half of imported cases. Vaccination is recommended before travel (especially to India) yet is only 75 percent effective. The disease is transmitted in a dose-related

TABLE 206-6   Tropical Infectious Diseases Causing Fever Among International Travelers

Disease	Distribution	Mode of Transmission
Incubation <14 days		
Undifferentiated fever		
Malaria	Most tropical and subtropical areas	Infected mosquito bite
Dengue	Tropics and subtropics, including urban area	Infected mosquito bite
Spotted fever	Worldwide	Infected tick or mite bite
Scrub typhus	Asia, Australia	Infected mite bite
Leptospirosis	Widespread, mostly tropics	Percutaneous contact with animal urine or contaminated soil; ingestion
Typhoid fever	Developing countries, especially Indian subcontinent	Contaminated food/water ingestion
Acute HIV infection	Worldwide	Permucosal or percutaneous exposure to infective blood or fluids
East African trypanosomiasis	Sub-Saharan East Africa	Infective tsetse fly bite
Shigella	Widespread, most common developing countries	Contaminated food/water ingestion
Salmonella	Widespread, most common developing countries	Contaminated food/water ingestion
Campylobacteria	Widespread, most common developing countries	Contaminated food/water ingestion
Fever with hemorrhage		
Meningococcemia		
Leptospirosis		
Malaria		
Viral hemorrhagic fever	Worldwide	Infected mosquito or tick bite
Other bacterial infection		
Fever with CNS involvement		
Meningococcemia		
Rabies	Common in Africa, Asia, and Latin America	Infected animal saliva exposure
Malaria		
Many viral and bacteria forms		
Arboviral encephaltitis	World wide	Infected mosquito or tick bite
Angiostrongyliasis	Widely scattered, most common in East Asia and Southeast Asia	Ingestion of contaminated food/water with snail or slug slime
Polio	Primarily Africa and parts of Asia	Ingestion of feces contaminated food/water
Fever with respiratory findings		
Influenza	Widespread; outbreaks on cruise ships	Direct or airborne transmission
SARS	China, Hong Kong, other regions in East Asia	Airborne droplet transmission
Legionellosis	Widespread; outbreaks hotels and cruise ships	Inhalation or aspiration
Q fever	Worldwide; inhalation of infective aerosol from animal source	
Incubation 14 days to 6 weeks		
Malaria		
Typhoid fever		
Hepatitis A and E	Widespread; most common in developing countries	Contaminated food/water ingestion
Acute schistosomiasis	Africa, Asia, and Latin America	Penetration of skin by cercariae
Amebic liver disease	Widespread; developing countries	Ingestion of cysts usually in feces contaminated food/water
Leptospirosis		
East African trypanosomiasis		
Q fever		
Acute HIV infection		
Incubation >6 weeks		
Malaria		
Tuberculosis	Worldwide	Inhalation
Hepatitis B	Widespread	Permucosal or percutaneous exposure to infective blood or fluids
Visceral leishmaniasis	Many parts of Africa, Asia, South America, and Mediterranean basin	Infective sand fly bite
Lymphaitic filariasis	Widespread in tropical areas	Infected mosquito bite
Schistosomiasis		
Amebic liver abscess		
Rabies		
African trypanososmiasis	Sub-Saharan Africa	Infected tsetse fly bite

Sources: Adapted from Keyston J, Humar A: Fortnightly review: Evaluating fever in travelers returning from tropical countries. *BMJ* 312:953, 1966, and from Ryan ET, Wilson ME, Kain KC: Illness after international travel. *New Engl J Med* 347:505, 2002.

fashion after food contamination by feces or urine from actively infected cases or healthy disease carriers. Incubation times and disease severity depend on bacteria dose exposure and are thus variable from 1 to 3 weeks. After ingestion, bacteria adhere to the small-bowel mucosa, invade lymphoid tissues, and disseminate via lymphatics to the bone marrow, gall bladder, and spleen to reproduce in macrophages.

Most pathology occurs in the gut as a consequence of inflammation, necrosis, and ulceration.

Typhoid fever classically begins with vague symptoms, progressive high fever with chills, headache, abdominal distention, myalgias, constipation, and prostration. Fever and headache are the most common early symptoms. The differential diagnosis includes malaria, typhus,

TABLE 206-7 Commonest Causes of Fever Following Travel to Tropical Regions

Malaria
Respiratory tract infections (pneumonia, Legionnaire disease and influenza)
Diarrheal disease
Urinary tract infection
Dengue fever
Enteric fever
Rickettsial infection
Infectious mononucleosis
Pharyngitis

Source: Ryan ET, Wilson ME, Kain KC: Illness after international travel. *New Engl J Med* 347:505–516, 2002.

viral hepatitis, amebic liver abscess, and other infective causes of enteritis. In epidemics, patients can present with acute diarrhea and vomiting, headache, and meningeal signs. Most patients, however, present with constipation rather than diarrhea. Bradycardia relative to fever is classic (but may be absent) and after several days of fever a pale red macular rash may appear on the trunk ("rose spots") among the fair-skinned. As disease progresses, splenomegaly is appreciable and complications may arise after even mild disease. Complications include small bowel ulceration, anemia, disseminated intravascular coagulopathy (DIC), pneumonia, meningitis, myocarditis, cholecystitis, and renal failure. Sequelae include epistaxis, deafness, and in 10 percent there is neurologic involvement including psychosis, ataxia, and seizures.

TABLE 206-8 Typical Incubation Periods for Selected Tropical Infections

Incubation Period	Infections Likely
<10 Days (short incubation)	Traveler's diarrhea Dengue fever and arboviral infections Yellow fever Spotted fevers Anthrax Diptheria Malaria Rabies Typhoid fever Meningococcal infections Plague Tularemia Typhus (louse and flea borne)
<21 Days (intermediate incubation)	Leptospirosis Viral hemorrhagic fevers Malaria Enteric fevers (typhoid, paratyphoid) Typhus Africa trypanosomiasis
>21 Days	Viral hepatitis (A, B, C, D, E) Malaria Acute HIV infection Amebic liver abscess Shistosomiasis (Katayama fever) Visceral leishmaniasis Filariasis
>Months	Tuberculosis Malaria caused by *Plasmodium vivax* Filariasis Viral hepatitis B, C HIV Visceral leishmaniasis Rabies Syphillis African and American (Chagas disease) trypanosomiasis

Diagnosis is clinical and confirmed by culturing blood, urine, or stool (during the second week), or by "rose spot" aspiration biopsy. Although most cultures have a low yield, bone marrow culture is most sensitive and is even possible following empirical treatment. Patients may develop leukopenia and elevated liver enzymes, though most cases have nonspecific lab values. Typhoid is treated with several antimicrobials, and chloramphenicol is the traditional drug of choice yielding a rapid and reliable cure. However, antibiotic resistance has caused ampicillin, trimethoprim-sulfamethoxazole (TMP-SMX), and chloramphenicol to be unreliable first line treatments. Current recommendations are either ceftriaxone 2 g IV every 24 h for 14 days, ciprofloxacin 400 mg IV every 12 h for 10 days, or ciprofloxacin 500 mg PO bid for 10 days. Alternatives include azithromycin 1 g PO on the first day followed by 500 mg PO per day for 6 days, azithromycin 1 g PO per day for 5 days, or cefixime 10 to 15 mg/kg IV every 12 h for 8 days. For patients with severe typhoid fever with delirium, coma, shock, or DIC, dexamethasone 3 mg/kg IV loading dose over 30 min followed by 1 mg/kg IV every 6 h for 8 doses should be administered. Supportive treatment includes intravenous rehydration, and in the event of serious GI bleeding, blood transfusion. If untreated, mortality is 10 to 15 percent, mostly occurring in young children.

Spotted Fever (Rickettsial Infections)

Spotted fevers are an underappreciated source of fever among returned travelers. They are transmitted by the bite, body fluid, or feces of ixodid arthropod ticks and are widely distributed around the world. Among the eight major rickettsial infections there is great variation in severity, and mortality without treatment approaches 25 percent and with treatment 5 percent. In particular, scrub typhus (*Rickettsia orientalis*) and African tick typhus (*R. conorii* var. *pijperi*) should be suspected after African safaris, adventure travels, and military activity. After 3 to 14 days incubation, when the tick bite may go unnoticed, patients demonstrate sudden fever, malaise, myalgias, severe headache, and nausea/vomiting. Whereas fever and centripetal rash are classic, the rash may be absent. Scrub typhus presents with a papule at the bite site later becoming necrotic and forming a crusted black "tache noire" eschar. As organisms metastasize, patients develop fever, malaise, headache, lymphadenopathy, and splenomegaly. African tick typhus presents like scrub typhus, but with less-severe symptoms. Diagnosis is clinical and serologic tests are confirmatory. Doxycycline 100 mg PO twice per d for 7 to 10 d is the empirical treatment of choice and chloramphenicol is an alternative. In severe cases, death occurs from a multiorgan toxemia within 1 to 2 weeks of illness onset if untreated. Therapy should be continued for at least 5 days and for 48 h after defervescence. Despite treatment, long-term complications are common.

Leptospirosis (Weil Disease)

This is the world's most widespread zoonotic infection and is commonly found in tropical climates. It follows mucous membrane or percutaneous exposure to fresh water contaminated by *Leptospira interrogans* from infected animals that excrete the spirochete in their urine. Infected patients typically have had contact with dogs; swam, rafted, or waded in contaminated surface water; or farmed or gardened. Outbreaks have been known to occur following flooding. While the risk to most routine travelers is low, recent ecotourists and adventure travelers have been infected following intense water exposure. During Eco-Challenge-Sabah 2000, in Malaysia, many participants were infected while swimming, kayaking, or swallowing water from the Segama River. The clinical course can be asymptomatic but often symptoms illustrate a biphasic pattern. After an incubation of 2 to 20 days, high fever, severe headache, chills, myalgias, jaundice, and nonspecific influenza-like symptoms develop along with conjunctival injection without purulent discharge. Symptoms resolve in 4 to 7 days, followed several days later by the severe, icteric "Weil disease" or aseptic meningitis lasting up to 4 weeks duration, renal failure, uveitis, rash, and, rarely, circulatory collapse caused by circulating antibodies. Isolation of leptospires from blood or cerebrospinal fluid (CSF) is diagnostic, but requires a prolonged incubation period. The illness is self-limited, but treatment reduces the severity and duration of symptoms and may prevent the second disease phase. Mild disease can be treated within the first 3 days of illness with oral amoxicillin or doxycycline, whereas more severe cases require intravenous penicillin or ampicillin. Empiric therapy with oral doxycycline or intravenous penicillin (or ampicillin) should be considered if leptospirosis is suspected.

Relapsing Fever

Relapsing fever is a bacterial infection caused by the spiral-shaped *Borrelia* species transmitted by lice or ticks. It is rare among travelers, yet should be suspected among contacts with refugee and disrupted populations in whom epidemics are common. Tick-borne disease results from a bite or tick body fluid exposure. Subsequently, *Borrelia* reproduce in body fluids and produce endotoxins affecting the liver, spleen, and capillaries. After incubation of 3 to 10 days, patients present with sudden fever, chills, headache, myalgias, and prostration, along with abdominal pain and jaundice. In severe cases, mental status changes, meningoencephalitis, myocarditis, hepatic failure, and DIC occur. After 5 to 7 days, fever may spontaneously abate, accompanied by hypotension, and near day 14, fever may recur. Such relapses number 1 to 2 among louse-borne fever, 3 to 6 among tick-borne fever, and up to 11 among African varieties. Diagnosis is made by clinical suspicion and confirmed by performing a Romanowsky-stained thick smear (similar to malaria) taken during the febrile period to identify spirochetes. Both louse-borne and tick-borne relapsing fever can be treated with a single oral dose of 500 mg tetracycline, 200 mg doxycycline, or 1 g of erythromycin.

Typhus (Epidemic Louse-Borne)

This bacteria is transmitted by the arthropod body louse and is common in Ethiopia, Mexico, Guatemala, and the Himalayas. It is also common in cold mountainous regions affected by famine, war, or mass population movement, but where adequate clothing exists to harbor the louse or lice. Louse-borne disease occurs after louse body fluids and feces are rubbed into abrasions after it is crushed or after it bites humans. Infection by the etiologic agent, *Rickettsia prowazekii,* causes high fevers and other nonspecific symptoms after an 8 to 12 day incubation period. Severe headache is common and a maculopapular rash appears between days 4 and 7, generally sparing palms and soles, and if severe, may be hemorrhagic. Diagnosis depends on serologic testing and treatment is doxycycline (100 mg PO bid) or chloramphenicol (60 to 75 mg/kg per d PO in four divided doses) to be administered for 7 days and for 48 h after defervescence. Untreated, mortality is as high as 60 percent.

Diseases Commonly Associated with Fever and Hemorrhage

Among the most feared tropical diseases are viral hemorrhagic fevers (VHFs). However, they are rare when compared to other febrile hemorrhagic infections such as leptospirosis, plague, rickettsia, and vibrio. While travel-related VHFs are public health and medical emergencies, non-travel-associated causes of fever and hemorrhage should not be discounted because *Neisseria meningitidis* is the most common temperate infection causing acute hemorrhagic fever. Among travelers, several treatable infections, including Lassa fever, malaria, meningococcemia, leptospirosis, and rickettsial infection can cause fever associated with hemorrhage. Most people with VHFs, such as dengue, hantavirus, Lassa, Ebola, Marburg, and Rift Valley, develop fever within 3 weeks after exposure. It is therefore important to establish a precise travel itinerary to estimate the incubation time. VHF usually follows the bite of infected mosquitoes, ticks, or close contact with rodent excreta.

In the event of a suspected VHF of tropical origin, control measures such as isolation in a negative-pressure room and the use of high-efficiency particulate-arresting (HEPA) respirators, gloves, and gowns is warranted. For contagious VHFs such as Marburg, Lassa, Ebola, or Crimean-Congo hemorrhagic fever, public health officials and the Centers for Disease Control and Prevention (CDC) should be immediately notified. If an intentional bioterrorism is suspected, local law-enforcement officials, the Federal Bureau of Investigation (FBI), and the CDC should be notified. The CDC Emergency Response Hotline is 1-770-488-7100.

Yellow Fever

This acute zoonotic flavivirus has a jungle monkey reservoir and its equatorial belt lies in South/Central America and Africa, yet it is notably absent in Asia throughout recorded history. Recent outbreaks in Bolivia, Kenya, and Nigeria indicate that it could reappear in the southern United States, where the mosquito vector *Aedes aegypti* (also transmitting dengue) is endemic. It is rare among travelers, because the yellow fever vaccination is mandatory in endemic areas. Outbreaks are common near tourist areas and may occur among nonimmunized adventure travelers who travel to endemic areas. Yellow fever ranges in severity from an undifferentiated self-limited flulike illness to a hemorrhagic fever fatal in 50 percent of cases. After an incubation of 3 to 6 days, patients develop fever, headache, myalgias, conjunctival injection, abdominal pain, prostration, facial flushing, and relative bradycardia. In most cases patients recover, but among others fever remission lasts a few hours to several days, followed by renewed high fever, vomiting, headache, back pain, shock, multiorgan failure, and bleeding diathesis. The classic presentation is a triad of jaundice, black emesis and albuminuria. In severe cases, hypotension, shock, and metabolic acidosis may develop, complicated by myocardial dysfunction and arrhythmias. Confusion, seizures, and coma are common in the late stages of the illness and death can occur within 7 to 10 days after onset. The diagnosis is primarily clinical, although confirmation is possible through virus identification or rising antibody titers in recovering patients. Leukopenia and albuminuria are typical, direct bilirubin levels rise, and liver enzymes are elevated for several days during when azotemia and oliguria ensue. Treatment is generally supportive, with fluid replacement and management of hematologic complications.

Lassa Fever

This arenavirus was first detected in Lassa, Nigeria, and is spread by contact with bush rat excreta. Epidemics have been associated with civil unrest and forced migration of populations. Although mostly found in rural West Africa, it has been exported to Europe and North America by infected patients and is a concern because it is highly contagious via close contact with blood and body fluids. The likelihood of travelers becoming infected is low because it is primarily a disease of rural communities where bush rats thrive.

After an incubation period of 3 to 16 days, the disease presents as a viral syndrome with insidious onset of fever, malaise, headache, sore throat, retrosternal chest pain, back pain, abdominal pain, and myalgias. Varied and nonspecific symptoms persist for 4 to 6 days, when the patient suddenly deteriorates and becomes gravely ill. Among those infected, 80 percent have few or no symptoms and 20 percent have severe multiorgan disease. The main features are high fever, severe prostration out of proportion to the fever, severe sore throat with dysphagia and yellow-white exudates, abdominal pain, diarrhea, and vomiting. Diagnosis is made by ELISA serology, culture, or immunohistochemistry, and should be carried out in a secure laboratory. Similar to Ebola, strict isolation and personal protection must be taken.

Treatment is largely supportive, but patients with severe disease may benefit from early treatment with ribavirin IV or PO, 30 mg/kg (max 2 g) initially, then 16 mg/kg (max 1 g) q6h for 4 days, followed by 8 mg/kg (max 500 mg) q6h for 6 days. Death, primarily from septic shock and multiorgan failure, can occur after 7 to 14 days. Survivors will defervesce within 10 days of disease onset and, except for sensorineural deafness, can make a complete recovery.

Diseases Commonly Associated with Fever and CNS Involvement

Febrile patients with acute mental status changes, headache (Table 206-9), nuchal rigidity and focal neurologic signs may have a number of serious infections. CNS involvement with fever in travelers returning from malaria-endemic regions requires emergent diagnosis and presumptive treatment for both malaria and meningitis. The differential diagnosis for fever with CNS involvement includes malaria, bacterial meningitis, TB, typhoid fever, rickettsial infections, and rabies. Other causes are viral encephalitides, including Japanese and West Nile encephalitis, which often present similarly.

Patients with altered mental status suspected of tropical illness may demonstrate coma, decreased level of consciousness, meningeal signs, or seizures. While seizures should arouse suspicion of cerebral malaria, cysticercosis should be suspected among those with long-term residence in Latin America with a first-time seizure. Meningococcal meningitis occurs with regularity in sub-Saharan Africa along the "meningitis belt." Aseptic meningitis may be caused by enteroviruses or, less commonly, by typhoid fever, leptospirosis, or rickettsiae. Encephalitis may be caused by an arboviral infection, such as Japanese B encephalitis.

JAPANESE ENCEPHALITIS This *Culex* mosquito-borne flavivirus occurs in an epidemic or sporadic pattern over large areas of Asia and the western Pacific. It is rarely transmitted to U.S.-bound travelers, because the vector breeds primarily in rural rice-paddy fields. Infected patients present with a sudden high fever, headache, nuchal rigidity, vomiting, and seizures (especially infants) after the incubation time of 5 to 15 days. A variety of pyramidal and extrapyramidal signs may develop soon after fever. If the outcome is fatal, it usually occurs in the first 10 days. Diagnosis is based on clinical suspicion, although virus can be isolated from CSF and antibody titers can rise. Treatment is supportive with intravenous fluid and electrolyte management, assisted respiration if necessary, anticonvulsants, and neuropsychiatric consultation during convalescence. Recovery may take months and varying degrees of residual neurologic damage may persist indefinitely. Immunization is recommended for travelers to rural, endemic regions in Asia.

CYSTICERCOSIS Cysticercosis is a systemic illness caused by dissemination of the larval form of the pork tapeworm, *Taenia solium.* The disease affects an estimated 50 million people worldwide. Endemic areas include Mexico, Latin America, sub-Saharan Africa, India, and East Asia. The incidence in the U.S. is increasing due to increased immigration from endemic areas and increased travel to endemic areas. Humans are definitive *T. solium* hosts and carry an in-

testinal adult tapeworm. Intermittent fecal shedding of egg-containing proglottids or *T. solium* eggs are ingested by the intermediate host (typically pigs). When undercooked pork is consumed, an intestinal tapeworm will again be formed, completing the life cycle of the worm.

Infestation can occur in almost any tissue. Involvement of the central nervous system, known as neurocysticercosis (NCC), is the most clinically important manifestation of the disease and may present with dramatic CNS findings. NCC is a leading cause of adult-onset seizures worldwide and an estimated 1000 new cases are diagnosed per year in the U.S. NCC is frequently asymptomatic. Symptoms are generally similar to those found with other intracranial mass lesions, and may include seizures, obstructive hydrocephalus, meningoencephalitis, and vascular accidents. Patients may also present with seizures, chronic headache, nausea and vomiting, and visual or mental status changes.

Brain CT scan is the first-line imaging study, followed by MRI as an adjunctive study. Noncontrast CT scan commonly shows calcifications of inactive disease, and can reveal mass effect or hydrocephalus. Antihelminthic agents are the mainstay of treatment, although steroids should be used in those with significant pretreatment encephalitis, hydrocephalus, or vasculitis to avoid inflammation as cysts involute, leading to worsening clinical status.

Diseases Commonly Associated with Chronic Fever

Chronic or relapsing fever lasting beyond 3 weeks following travel should first be evaluated for non-travel-related infections such as pneumonia, endocarditis, cholangitis, as well as noninfectious causes such as occult neoplasms, collagen vascular disorders (e.g., systemic lupus erythematosus and rheumatic fever), and inflammatory diseases (e.g., gout, sarcoidosis, inflammatory bowel disease). Tropical illnesses that cause chronic fever can include protozoal infections (such as trypanosomiasis, leishmaniasis, malaria), typhoid or paratyphoid and TB of the bone, CNS, gut, joints, lungs, peritoneum, and urinary tract (Table 206-10).

TABLE 206-9   Tropical Infectious Diseases Causing Severe Headache

Malaria
Rickettsial disease
Dengue fever
Typhoid fever
Human African trypanosomiasis

Source: Adapted from Guerrant RL, Walker DH, Weller PF (eds): *Essentials of Tropical Medicine.* Philadelphia: Churchill Livingstone, 2001.

TABLE 206-10   Selected Causes of Chronic and Relapsing Fevers

Etiological Organism	Organism Species
Bacterial	Bartonellosis
	Brucellosis
	Leptospirosis
	Q fever
	Relapsing fever
	Syphillis
	Tuberculosis
	Tularemia
	Typhoid fever
Fungal	Blastomycosis
	Coccidioidomycosis
	Cryptococcosis
	Histoplasmosis
Protazoan	Amebic liver disease
	Visceral leishmaniasis
	Malaria
	Human African and human American trypanosomiasis
Viral	HIV
Helminthic	Angiostrongyliasis
	Fascioliasis
	Loiasis
	Schistosomiasis
	Toxocariasis
	Trichinosis

HUMAN AFRICAN TRYPANOSOMIASIS (AFRICAN SLEEPING SICKNESS) Two kinds of trypanosomiasis exist in sub-Saharan Africa and South/Central America with different vectors, clinical manifestations and therapies. Sleeping sickness is caused by the two identical endemic protozoan subspecies, *Trypanosoma brucei gambiense* and *T. brucei rhodesiense,* transmitted by the aggressive tsetse fly, which is indigenous only to vegetation near rivers, lakes, forests, and wooded savannah. Approximately 30 cases were imported to the United States in the last century, primarily from East Africa, and is a low risk to U.S. travelers, with 1 to 2 cases imported each year, usually following intensive fly exposure during game-park exposure. After a bite, a localized inflammatory reaction occurs followed in 2 to 3 days by a painless chancre that increases in size for 2 to 3 weeks, and then gradually regresses. Trypomastigotes mature and divide in the blood and lymph after the development of the chancre and cause intermittent fever unresponsive to antimalarials. Malaise, rash, wasting, and eventual CNS involvement occurs, causing behavioral and neurologic changes, encephalitis, coma, and death. Other complications include hemolysis, anemia, pancarditis, and meningoencephalitis.

Lab findings include anemia, hypergammaglobulinemia, elevated ESR, thrombocytopenia, and hypoalbuminemia. Diagnosis is made by rapid evaluation of blood smears for the mobile parasite. Organisms can also be identified by aspiration of lymph nodes, chancres, bone marrow or by CSF examination. Treatment for *T. brucei rhodesiense* when CSF is normal (stage 1) is suramin and for *T. gambiense* is eflornithine. Treatment with CNS involvement (stage 2) first involves treating underlying health concerns, eliminating parasites outside the CNS with suramin, and then eradicating parasites in the brain with melarsoprol, which is the only available agent to treat the advanced stage (however, for *T. gambiense* eflornithine can be used). Melatsoprol is given as 3.6 mg/kg IV qd for 3 days. The three dose treatment is repeated after 7 days and again after 10 to 21 days.

AMERICAN TRYPANOSOMIASIS (CHAGAS DISEASE) The protozoan *T. cruzi* is found in up to 5 percent of emigrants from endemic parts of Latin America and is reported as far north as Texas. It is spread by the reduviid, "kissing" or "assassin" bug, typically biting nocturnally after emerging from rural adobe walls or thatched roofs. Among travelers, it is rare. It causes an acute illness and, commonly, an asymptomatic infection with complications arising years later in the heart and GI tract. It is transmitted during a blood meal when the bug defecates trypanosome-infected feces around the meal site, causing a local inflammatory reaction and trypanosome inoculation after the host rubs the organism into the bite wound, or into adjacent mucus membranes or conjunctiva. Infection can also be acquired by blood transfusion, lab accidents, and congenitally.

Unilateral periorbital edema (Romaña sign) or painful cutaneous edema at the site of skin penetration (chagoma) is followed by a toxemic phase with parasitemia causing lymphadenopathy and hepatosplenomegaly. Death can occur in this acute phase, which is generally 2 to 4 weeks but may last up to 3 months, and is often a result of cardiac damage or meningoencephalitis among infants and the immunosuppressed. Patients commonly progress into a long, asymptomatic, latent phase when ganglion cells are gradually destroyed leading to depressed cardiac and GI function. These result in asymptomatic infections or complications years later such as myocarditis, dysrhythmias, and sudden death. Chronic cardiomyopathy, megaesophagus, or megacolon occur. Chagas induced heart disease is the leading form of congestive heart failure (CHF) in much of Latin America. The acute diagnosis is from peripheral smears demonstrating motile parasites, blood culture, or muscle biopsy. In the chronic phase, serologic tests or tissue biopsy are useful. Several drugs eliminate the parasite in the acute phase, including nifurtimox (Lampit), 8 to 10 mg/kg per d PO divided qid × 120 days, other nitrofurazones, or primaquine.

LEISHMANIASIS (VISCERAL) *Leishmania* is an intracellular protozoan transmitted by *Lutzomyia* or *Phlebotomus* sandflies. It is scat-

tered throughout rural Africa, Asia, the Mediterranean basin, and Central/South America, and occasionally leads to outbreaks, such as in Brazil, India, and the Sudan, which place resident expatriates and travelers at risk. There have been several hundred cases among U.S. military personnel and their dependents in the last four decades. It is a low risk to most travelers, although European travelers to nonendemic Mediterranean nations occasionally export cases, as do 30 to 40 U.S. travelers each year, who mostly export the cutaneous form and rarely the visceral form. HIV-infected persons are at risk to both forms. Physicians should suspect leishmania among military and their families living proximal to jungles, adventure travelers, field biologists, and emigrants from endemic zones.

The infecting species determines the pathology ranging from a localized self-healing lesion to widespread, persistent and potentially destructive disease. Four major clinical syndromes are recognized (Table 206-11).

The most important diagnostic information is patient's origin and travel itinerary because endemic areas suggest the infection type. Definitive diagnosis requires isolating motile extracellular parasites aspirated from bone marrow, spleen or lymph nodes, or on smears or sections taken from the ulcer edge by punch biopsy. Stained smears can show nonmotile intracellular amastigotes (Leishman-Donovan bodies) from bone marrow, spleen, liver, lymph nodes, or blood.

Visceral disease should be treated with the effective pentavalent antimonials, either sodium stibogluconate, single daily dose of 20 mg/kg per d IM or IV for 20 to 30 days [available from the CDC (http://www.cdc.gov/ncidod/srp/drugservice/immuodrugs.htm, or 1-404-639-3670 or after hours, 1-404-639-2888)], or meglumine antimonate same dose and duration of treatment. Oral miltefosine (hexadecylphosphocholine) is also effective. Relapses with drug-resistant disease are treated with amphotericin B or pentamidine, which are not used routinely because of toxicity. Amphotericin is useful against pentavalent antimony-resistant mucocutaneous and visceral leishmania.

Diseases Commonly Associated with Abdominal and Urinary Complaints

Illnesses causing abdominal pain and diarrhea are common among world travelers, because of infecting bacteria, viruses, soil-transmitted helminths, and other parasites. Most of these infections are caused by the consumption of undercooked or fecal-contaminated foods, and are preventable by adequate hygiene, potable water, and careful food preparation.

SCHISTOSOMIASIS (BILHARZIASIS OR SNAIL FEVER) This blood fluke, found in Africa, the Middle East, South America, and Asia, infects more than 200 million people worldwide, with 20 million people suffering severe consequences. It should be suspected among travelers following long exposure to endemic zones. For most short-term trav-

TABLE 206-11   Clinical Syndromes of Leishmaniasis

Visceral leishmaniasis (Kala-azar or Black fever): the most devastating and fatal form caused by *L. donovani.* A progressive, chronic and systemic disease with high mortality if untreated but with a good prognosis if provided adequate care. Fatality is a result of secondary infections such as TB, pneumonia, and dysentery. It is typified by the pentad of fever, weight loss, hepatosplenomegaly, pancytopenia, and hypergammaglobulinemia.

Cutaneous leishmaniasis: old world disease is the most common form, and found in most of the world, whereas new world disease is only found in the Americas.

Mucocutaneous leishmaniasis (espundia): chronic and relentless disease complicated by secondary infections and pneumonia.

Diffuse cutaneous leishmaniasis: typically chronic, difficult to treat, and with few resulting deaths.

elers, the risk is generally low, although significant outbreaks now occur among adventure tourists, Peace Corps workers, and patients who swim in infested streams and lakes. The larvae are released into freshwater by snails which are intermediate hosts. Infection occurs by tiny, free-swimming cercariae that penetrate wet, unbroken skin or are ingested from slow-moving fresh water. Brief or even single exposures like washing or wading can cause infection in previously unexposed asymptomatic expatriates. Following inoculation an immediate cercarial allergic and pruritic dermatitis occurs which can last days. In the following 4 to 8 weeks, fever occurs, accompanied by headache, cough, urticaria, diarrhea, hepatosplenomegaly and hypereosinophilia (Katayama fever). Worms mature into adults in the venous blood and for the next 30 to 40 years deposit eggs into selective body tissues (*Schistosoma haematobium* in the bladder and *S. mansoni* and *S. japonicum* in the GI tract).

Symptoms follow granulomatous scarring from eggs deposited throughout the brain, skin, liver, and GI tract, and depend on the infecting species. CNS symptoms such as seizures, paralysis and acute transverse myelitis can occur if eggs ectopically migrate. *S. haematobium* leads to dysuria, frequency, and terminal hematuria, and can cause bladder scarring, calcification, and squamous cell carcinoma. *S. japonicum* and *S. mansoni* lead to hepatosplenomegaly, periportal fibrosis, hepatic granulomas, and jaundice. These two species also can cause diarrhea, abdominal cramps, acute abdominal pain, and late in the disease course, portal hypertension. *S. dermatidis*, a non-human-infecting schistosome, has cercariae that only penetrate the superficial skin, causing an irritation known as swimmer's itch.

Diagnosis is by detecting eosinophilia, and microscopic identification of eggs in the first-morning urine or stool, or in a biopsy specimen. Serologic methods such as ELISA plus Western blot may be also used. Treatment should be offered to symptomatic patients and seropositive travelers. Praziquantel 20 mg/kg PO bid for 1 day is effective for all *Schistosoma* parasites with a 70 to 85 percent cure rate. Oxamniquine 15 mg/kg in a single dose is effective against *S. mansoni* and for *S. haematobium* metriphonate 10 mg/kg PO on three occasions with intervals of 2 to 4 weeks is effective. For swimmer's itch, no treatment is required.

CLONORCHIASIS (CHINESE OR ORIENTAL LIVER FLUKE) This trematoidal disease of the bile ducts is caused by *Clonorchis sinensis* and follows ingestion of poorly cooked freshwater fish containing encysted larvae. Travelers are at low risk despite the tremendous prevalence among those living in endemic zones such as Southeast Asia. Once ingested, larvae mature into adults, migrate to bile ducts, survive for 30 or more years, and cause fibrosis. The extent of pathology is related to parasite burden, and among the millions infected, only few are symptomatic. Acute symptoms include anorexia and diarrhea, and may progress to chronic bile duct obstruction, liver tenderness and/or jaundice, and in advanced cases, biliary cirrhosis and cholangiocarcinoma. Diagnosis is made by detecting the characteristic embryonated eggs in stool or duodenal aspirate and eosinophilia is common. Serologic tests using ELISA have 70 percent sensitivity and computed tomography (CT) or abdominal ultrasonography exams are useful. Treatment of choice is praziquantel in 25 mg/kg PO tid for three doses.

Diseases Commonly Associated with Abdominal Pain and Diarrhea

Diarrhea and gastroenteritis are the most common travel ailments, affecting up to one-half of travelers (Table 206-12). Gastroenteritis can be accompanied by fever, flatulence, nausea, emesis and abdominal pain which is usually spasmodic and colicky with the exception of *Campylobacter jejuni,* which causes severe and constant pain, and cholera causing somatic muscle cramps. Nonbloody gastroenteritis is usually caused by bacteria or bacterial toxins, whereas dysentery usu-

TABLE 206-12 Common Infectious Diseases Causing Diarrhea Among Travelers

Cause	Organism	Comments
Acute (duration <2 weeks)		
Viral	Norwalk-like virus	Often not diagnosed; may
	Rotaviruses	account for 5–10% of
	Enteroviruses	acute traveler's diarrhea
Bacterial	*Escherichia coli* (enterotoxigenic or enteroaggregative)	Most common identified cause of acute traveler's diarrhea; 50–70%
	Campylobacter jejuni	
	Salmonella	
	Shigella	
	Vibrio	
	Clostriduium difficle	
Parasitic	*Giardia lamblia*	Accounts of <1–5% of
	Cryptosporidium parvum	acute traveler's diarrhea
	Entamoeba histolytica	
	Cyclospora cayetanensis	
	Isopora belli	
	Balantidium coli	
	Trichinella spiralis	
Chronic or persistent (duration >2 to 4 weeks)		
Bacterial	See above	Rare cause of chronic diarrhea
Parasitic		
Microsporidial	*Enterocytozoon bieneusi*	Almost exclusively in immunocompromised
	Encephalitozoon intestinalis	
Protozoal	*Giardia lamblia*	Most commonly identified cause
	Entamoeba histolytica	Bloody diarrhea with fever; fecal white blood cell count may be present
Helminthic	*Trichuris trichiura*	Rarely associated with chronic diarrhea;
	Strongyloides stercoralis	usually in persons with
	Fasciolopsis buski	heavy parasite burdens
	Schistosoma	

Source: Adapted from Ryan ET, Wilson ME, Kain KC: Illness after international travel. *New Engl J Med* 347:505, 2002.

ally results from toxigenic and invasive bacteria such as *Shigella, Salmonella, Campylobacter, Aeromonas, Escherichia coli,* or *E. histolytica* (Table 206-13). Acute abdominal pain among travelers should first be considered to be caused by nontravel causes with an expanded travel-based differential diagnosis. For example, intestinal obstruction that causes colicky pain as a consequence of heavy infestation by *Ascaris lumbricoides* can cause pain similar to acute appendicitis, and attempts should be made to distinguish between diagnoses. Chap. 83 more specifically addresses the etiology and workup of routine diarrheal illnesses.

AMEBIASIS Amebiasis is a fecal-oral parasite found worldwide. Pathogenic species such as *Entamoeba histolytica* are endemic to Asia, Africa, and Latin America. Amebiasis is typically spread by asymptomatic carriers whose excrement contains the encysted organism. Short-term travelers are at low risk, but longer-term travelers such as Peace Corps volunteers are at significant risk. The disease is most severe among young children, the elderly, and pregnant women.

TABLE 206-13   Causes of Diarrhea With and Without Fever or Blood

	With Fever	Without Fever
With blood	Bacillary dysentery	*Amebiasis*
	Campylobacter enterocolitis	*Balantidium coli*
	Salmonella enterocolitis	*Schistosoma*
	Escherichia coli	*Trichuris*
Without blood	*Salmonella* enteritis	*Staphylococcus aureus*
	Malaria (especially	*Escherichia coli*
	Plasmodium falciparum)	(enterotoxigenic)
	Mild shigellosis	*Clostridium perfringens*
	Campylobacter infections	Viral infections of the
	Almost any infections in	gut
	a child	Food toxins

Incubation times are typically 1 to 3 weeks for colitis and 2 weeks to several months for liver abscesses. Once cysts are ingested, amebic trophozoites invade the colon wall, lyse tissues, and cause necrotic abscesses. Symptoms range from alternating constipation and diarrhea over 1 to 3 weeks, abdominal pain, fever, dehydration, and weight loss. Extraintestinal metastases can infect the liver, skin, pericardium, lung, and the brain. Complications such as liver abscesses may present acutely with fever, right upper quadrant pain, or chronic, vague abdominal pain accompanied by weight loss. Hepatic abscesses can be fatal if rupture occurs.

Stool ova and parasites examination (O + P) is diagnostic, and organisms are found either as motile trophozoites or cysts. Stool wet mount should be performed within 30 min of specimen collection to detect trophozoites, and fixative (polyvinyl alcohol) should be used to identify cysts. It can be difficult to differentiate pathogenic organisms (*E. histolytica*) from those benign (*E. coli*) without use of stool antigen-detection tests. Serology for elevated antibody titers is 90 percent sensitive for extraintestinal disease and 80 percent sensitive for invasive colon disease. Ultrasonography or CT scans may be useful to identify hepatic abscesses. Treatment of asymptomatic cyst passers includes either iodoquinol 650 mg PO tid for 20 days, paromomycin 500 mg PO tid for 7 days, or diloxanide furoate 500 mg PO tid for 10 days. For symptomatic disease, choices include metronidazole 500 to 750 mg PO tid for 10 days or tinidazole 1 g PO bid for 3 days, followed by either iodoquinol or paromomycin in the doses and duration noted before. For liver abscess, metronidazole 750 mg PO or IV tid for 10 days followed by paromomycin 500 mg PO tid for 7 days is given.

GIARDIASIS   *Giardia lamblia* is a flagellated protozoan infecting the small intestine and biliary tree. It is distributed worldwide and is food- or waterborne by fecal contamination with encysted parasites. It is common to rural areas with poor sanitation and impure surface water, but has also occurred in day-care settings in the United States. In Eastern Europe, it is a common cause of traveler's diarrhea and is found at camping sites and rural swimming areas. Long-term residents of tropical nations are at high risk; short-term travelers are also at risk. Ingested parasites reside in the duodenum, and may lead to malabsorption because of duodenal microvilli obstruction. Symptoms include abdominal cramping, flatulence, and foul-smelling, watery diarrhea without blood or mucus. Chronic infections cause weight loss and anemia, and a common complication is lactose intolerance. Diagnosis is by stool ova and parasites showing either motile (trophozoites) or cysts. A "string test" (Entero-Test) can obtain duodenal samples but is cumbersome. Serology can demonstrate *Giardia* antigen in stool with good sensitivity and specificity. Treatment is with metronidazole (250 mg PO tid for 3 to 5 days), tinidazole (2 g PO for 1 dose), quinacrine (100 mg PO tid for 5 days), or furazolidone (100 mg PO

qid for 7 days) for children. It should be noted that treatment is not always successful regardless of drug used.

CHOLERA   Cholera is an acute diarrheal disease caused by the bacterium *Vibrio cholerae*. It is endemic and epidemic to many tropical nations. Most recently, South America, which was relatively free of epidemic disease, has seen a marked increase among travelers and its nationals. Epidemics occur after flooding or acute population displacement with disruption of the water-sanitation system. Transmission is by fecal contamination of water or food (including raw or poorly cooked seafood and shellfish). Significant bacterial ingestion is required to cause symptoms. The incubation time is 2 to 3 days and symptoms follow sodium pump inhibition by the cholera toxin. Infection is usually mild, but can be life-threatening, particularly among vulnerable populations, such as malnourished children, refugees, and those with chronic illness. Another group at risk are patients with achlorhydria or those using medications decreasing gastric acidity. Approximately 80 clinical cases of cholera are imported into the United States each year, although there are many more suspected asymptomatic carriers.[10]

Severe disease is characterized by profuse, usually painless, watery diarrhea ("rice water stools"), severe dehydration causing "dishwater hands," vomiting, leg cramps, and occasionally fever. Rapid fluid loss (up to 15 L per d) leads to extreme dehydration and shock. Without aggressive rehydration, death can occur within hours. With proper fluid resuscitation, most patients can recover uneventfully. Diagnosis is clinical and, when suspected, a rectal swab or stool specimen should be sent to a reference lab for culture confirmation. Aggressive fluid resuscitation with oral rehydration solution or intravenous fluids is imperative, accompanied by correction of metabolic acidosis and hypokalemia. Tetracycline 500 mg PO qid (drug of choice, although resistance exists) or in children, TMP-SMX 5 mg/25 mg/kg PO bid for 3 days can shorten the illness course, diminish vomiting, lessen volume resuscitation needs, and ensure that bacteria are eradicated from stool. Other antimicrobial choices include erythromycin, ciprofloxacin, and norfloxacin. Though secondary transmission is rare, close contacts should be given a tetracycline as a prophylaxis.

ASCARIS (ROUNDWORM)   *Ascaris lumbricoides* is the most common geohelminthic infection. The risk to short-term travelers is low, yet it should be suspected following ingestion of street vendor foods or vegetables fertilized by "night soil" (human feces) or animal feces. Eggs survive for years in moist soil and transmission is typically fecal-oral or via poorly cooked food. Symptoms are usually minimal; however, a dry cough or pneumonia may occur as young worms are expectorated and migrate from the lungs to the esophagus and gut. A large worm burden can lead to malnutrition, weakness, and a mass of worms may lead to bowel obstruction. Wandering ascaris also traverse internal organs leading to biliary obstruction, hepatic abscess, acute pancreatitis, acute appendicitis, or hypersensitivity pneumonitis. For details of diagnosis and treatment, see Chap. 149.

ENTEROBIASIS (PINWORM, SEATWORM)   *Enterobiasis vermicularis* is common tropical disease caused by a small intestinal parasite transmitted fecal-orally, and often acquired from contaminated objects such as toys, utensils, and bedding. It is a common disease among U.S. children, and is more likely to be peridomestic rather than following tropical travel. For more discussion of diagnosis and treatment, see Chap. 149.

TRICHURIS (WHIPWORM DISEASE)   Whipworm (*Trichuris trichiura*) is a nematode parasite of the large intestine distributed globally but most heavily in the tropics. It is a low risk among short-term travelers, but long-term travelers, former tropical residents, and visitors from the tropics are at high risk. It is obtained by ingesting contaminated soil or vegetables and is not transmissible from person to person. See Chap. 149 for diagnosis and treatment.

HOOKWORM Hookworm is a common chronic nematoidal infection caused by *Ancylostoma duodenale* and *Necator americanus*, which are globally distributed but most heavily in the tropics and subtropics. Because symptoms require large worm burdens, it is a low risk among short-term travelers. Hookworm is a significant global health problem, causing chronic, severe anemia among children. Transmission is by direct skin contact with soil contaminated by human feces, often in children with poor footwear exposed to raw sewage, allowing filariform larvae to penetrate the skin. See Chap. 149 for further diagnosis and treatment.

CESTODES (TAPEWORMS) Among the cestodes, taeniasis and cysticercosis are the most pathologic. Infections occur worldwide, but especially in the tropics, and suspicion should be raised among children, the mentally disabled, and immigrants or visitors from endemic nations. Risk to travelers is low but is increased with consumption of undercooked pork, fish, or beef. For further discussion of diagnosis and treatment, see Chap. 149.

Pork tapeworm (*Taenia solium*) infection can also cause cysticercosis when cysts (small sacs with developing worms) form throughout the body, including the brain, causing pathology depending on their location. For further discussion of cysticercosis, see Chap. 149.

STRONGYLOIDES *Strongyloides stercoralis* is a helminthic infection of the small intestine with worldwide distribution, but is most commonly found in the humid tropics. It is common in overseas military personnel, refugees, or immigrants. Among short-term travelers, the risk is low. Almost all infections cause minimal or no symptoms, yet it can be serious among those immunosuppressed or malnourished. For further discussion, see Chap. 149.

Diseases Commonly Associated with Skin or Eye Complaints

These complaints among travelers are common, nonspecific, and have many etiologies. In the evaluation of skin complaints in the international traveler, applying a few basic principles may simplify the diagnosis and management. For example, travel-related skin disease is generally caused by one of three etiologies: 1) exacerbations of previous conditions (e.g., atopic dermatitis, psoriasis); 2) environmental conditions (e.g., photosensitivity, contact allergies); or 3) infective organisms causing infestations or infections.[10] The distribution and timing of the dermatosis may aid diagnosis of rashes associated with system illness (Table 206-14).[11] Among rashes reported by travelers, most are minor problems such as sunburn, phototoxic/sensitivity reactions, insect bites, prickly heat, and are often self-limiting and necessitate symptomatic care. It has been suggested the top ten tropical travel dermatoses requiring specific therapy include: cutaneous larva migrans, pyodermas due to staphylococcal or streptococcal ecthyma, arthropod reactive dermatoses, myiasis, tungiasis, urticaria, febrile syndromes with rash, cutaneous leishmaniasis, scabies, and fungal infections.[12] The risk of serious conditions tends to increase with the amount of time spent overseas and thus, short-term travelers rarely contract dermatoses such as filariasis, Buruli ulcer, yaws, and Hansen disease. To further aid diagnosis, travelers with dermatoses can fit into 5 syndromic and morphological categories (Table 206-15).

Management includes arranging biopsy for patients with chronic ulcerative lesions. Beware of the rare patient presenting with anxiety or delusions of parasitosis regardless of travel history. Hereafter are presented dermatoses associated with tropical exposures that frequently prompt patients to seek ED attention.

ONCHOCERCIASIS (RIVER BLINDNESS) River blindness is a chronic, nonfatal filarial disease leading to subcutaneous skin changes and blindness. It is caused by a *Onchocerca volvulus*, a nematode

TABLE 206-14 Cutaneous Manifestations of Selected Infections

Appearance of Lesion	Possible Diagnosis
Maculopapular rash	Dengue fever Viral hemorrhagic fevers Leptospirosis Acute HIV infection
Erythema chronicum migrans	Lyme disease
Rose spots	Typhoid fever
Pustules	Disseminated gonococcal infection
Petechiae, ecchymoses, hemorrhage	Meningococcemia Dengue fever Viral hemorrhagic fevers Yellow fever Rocky Mountain spotted fever Epidemic louse-borne typhus Leptospirosis
Eschar	Tick or scrub typhus Anthrax
Ulcer	Tularemia Cutaneous diphtheria
Urticaria	Helminthic infections

Source: MacLean JD, Lalande RG, Ward B: Fever from the tropics, section 5, in *Travel Medicine Advisor*. Atlanta, GA: American Health Consultants, 1994, p. 271.

transmitted by the female black fly, *Simulium* sp., found near fast-moving rivers in parts of Central/South America and mostly equatorial Africa. Despite global eradication campaigns, the disease burden is increasing. It should be suspected among long-term travelers, immigrants from endemic zones, and, rarely, among short-term adventure travelers. Early treatment can prevent blindness and reduce systemic spread, because the incubation period from fly bite to microfilariae appearing in skin is often more than a year. Symptoms include intractable pruritus, altered skin pigmentation, skin nodules (typically found on the head and shoulders in South America, and pelvic girdle and lower extremities in Africa), lymphadenitis, and gradual visual impairment leading to blindness. Adult female worms reside in 2–3 cm painless nodules in skin and bones near joints, and release microfilariae that migrate through the skin, causing intense pruritus when they die, causing chronic dermatitis, edema, and skin atrophy. Skin pigment changes result in "leopard skin," while loose pelvic skin is called "hanging groin." Blindness is a result of microfilariae migrating to the eye, invading it and causing permanent damage when they die. Diagnosis is made by identification of microfilariae from a fresh skin

TABLE 206-15 Syndromic Categories of Travel-Related Dermatoses with Select Examples

Fever and rash (petechial or hemorrhagic): dengue, arboviruses, rickettsial infections (e.g., scrub typhus), meningococcemia, leptospirosis, malaria, and erythema multiforme cause by drug reaction or common infection

Papular eruptions: insect bites, persistent lesions (chiggers), scabies, allergic drug reactions, cercarial dermatitis (swimmers), *Pseudomonas* follicultis (hot-tubbing), onchocerciasis (long-term travel)

Persistent nodules: furunculosis, myiaisis (moving lesions), chancroid, syphilis, systemic parasites/fungi

Migratory swellings or skin lesions: cutaneous larva migrans, strongyloidiasis (fast-moving and often on the buttocks), urticaria from various causes, and *Loa loa* (rarely)

Ulcerative lesions: pyodermas, spider bites, chancroid and syphilis, cutaneous leishmaniasis

biopsy, nodule biopsies, or in the urine. Slit-lamp examination may reveal microfilariae in the cornea, anterior chamber, or the vitreous. Treatment is one dose of ivermectin 150 μg/kg PO, which does not kill the adult worm, but when repeatedly dosed every 6 to 12 months, reduces morbidity by killing microfilariae, suppressing microfilariae release from adults, and preventing spread to eyes and skin. Diethylcarbamazine citrate and suramin (which can kill adult worms and microfilariae) have been used but because of their potentially serious side effects, they should be avoided. Surgical removal of nodules can reduce symptoms, the incidence of worms, and if removed from the frontal scalp can help prevent progression of visual impairment and blindness.

DRACUNCZULIASIS (GUINEA WORM) Guinea worm is the largest tissue parasite and is a painful, debilitating nematoidal infection of the subcutaneous tissues. It is found in sub-Saharan Africa and Asia, and especially in dry climates. While risk among short-term travelers is low, it can occur among long-term residents in rural communities or among nonvoluntary migrants such as refugees. Guinea worm remains endemic in isolated regions in Africa such as southern Sudan, although international efforts are underway and are expected to successfully eradicate the parasite. The infection is acquired from ingestion of water contaminated by the larvae within its intermediate host, a minute crustacean copepod (*Cyclops* spp.). A year after infection, a painful swelling starts on a lower extremity (typically the foot). After 1 week, a blister appears and upon rupture, a 60–100 cm gravid female worm discharges larvae upon water contact. Fever, itching, nausea, vomiting, and diarrhea may accompany sore formation. Diagnosis is made by identifying the adult worm in the sore or finding microscopic larvae in which the sore is bathed. Although no drug exists to definitively kill the parasite, ivermectin and metronidazole with corticosteroids may be of value. Tetanus toxoid should be administered, antibiotics used for secondary wound infection, and a local antibacterial ointment and occlusive bandage should be used over the lesion. The worm can be removed slowly over a week or longer by attaching it to a thread, pulling gently a little more each day and rolling the worm around a small appliance or stick. Because the worm may measure more than a meter, care must be taken not to break it as it is removed. Aseptic surgical excision can be used to remove the adult worm if done before emergence. Prognosis is usually good unless the ulcer made by the worm becomes infected.

LOA LOA (EYE WORM) Loiasis is a filarial nematode confined to the rain forests of western and central Africa. It is a low risk to short-term travelers but should be suspected among immigrants, refugees, visiting nationals, and expatriates living several months or more in endemic zones. Among such travelers, worm burden is usually low and symptoms are related to hypersensitivity syndromes and not serious disease. The adult worms inhabit subcutaneous tissues, move about freely and can live for up to 18 years after the patient's last possible exposure. They are spread from the bite of the *Chrysops* fly and take 1 year to mature. Infections are usually asymptomatic; however, at times, infections cause painful or itchy subcutaneous swellings near the face and extremities known as Calabar swellings. The most dramatic presentation is when a worm passes across the eye under the conjunctiva, thus coining the disease "eye worm."

Patients will complain of "something in their eye," intense irritation, pain, and swelling of the periorbital tissues. The worm usually moves out of the conjunctiva in 30 min, but it takes usually several days for symptoms to subside.

Diagnosis is made by clinical presentation and by evaluating daytime-drawn blood drawn for distinctively sheathed microfilariae and high-grade eosinophilia. Treatment for microfilariae and adult worms is diethylcarbamazine citrate (DEC) 2 mg/kg PO tid for 3 weeks. In patients with very high microfilariae counts, DEC may induce sudden severe hypersensitivity and encephalitic syndrome, therefore treatment should start with a very small dose in this patient population. Surgical excision is not recommended because multiple worms may not be visible. Subconjunctival worms, however, can be removed from the eye with analgesia and fine tweezers.

CREEPING ERUPTION (CUTANEOUS LARVA MIGRANS) This erythematous "creeping eruption" commonly occurs among tropical travelers and beach resort vacationers who walk barefoot or sit in beach sand contaminated by dog feces harboring the parasite *Ancylostoma braziliense*.[13] The lesions are typically slow moving, tracking and serpiginous, and are a result of an inflammatory reaction from the worm, which is unable to complete its growth cycle in humans (it is only an effective parasite of dogs or cats). Pruritus causes sleeplessness and restlessness, and diagnosis is based on clinical presentation and eosinophilia. Treatment consists of thiabendazole 10 percent suspension topically qid for 2 to 7 days, and liquid nitrogen freezing or surgical excision is not recommended because of scarring. If a patient has multiple lesions, systemic treatment with albendazole 400 mg PO bid for 5 days is effective.

CUTANEOUS LEISHMANIASIS This is the most important cause of chronic skin ulceration in the world and is spread by sandflies in tropical and subtropical regions of Latin America, the Middle East, and Asia. This should be suspected among travelers such as military personnel, biologists, ecotourists, and adventure travelers, and should be part of the differential diagnosis of cutaneous ulcers among travelers, foreign visitors, and immigrants from endemic areas. Although there are a variety of subtypes causing varying infections, the common presentation is of a small papule slowly enlarging and forming a painless shallow skin ulcer with a noticeable rolled edge like a volcano, with a raised edge and central crater, often with a scab. Diagnosis is made by tissue biopsy of the indurated ulcer margin. Many forms are self-limiting, and treatment should be guided by clinical presentation and in concert with infectious disease consultants or CDC's Parasitic Diseases Branch.

BANCROFTIAN FILARIASIS (*WUCHERERIA BANCROFTI*) This filarial disease is caused by nematodes residing in the subcutaneous tissues and lymphatics for up to 10 years. It is common to the tropics and subtropics (especially Asia), and the risk to short-term travelers is low, although cases are imported by long-term travelers. It is transmitted by flies or mosquitoes permitting larvae to enter the puncture wound during their blood meal. Adult filariae then reside in lymphatics and produce microfilariae that migrate to the bloodstream at night. Because the incubation period is long, first symptoms usually develop after 6 months or later (up to 5 years). The most common symptom is recurrent bouts of "filarial fevers" lasting 2 to 3 weeks, associated with warmth and tenderness overlying a lymphatic vessel, followed by retrograde lymphangitis. The most frequently affected sites are extremities, breasts, and spermatic cord. As more attacks occur, lymphatics are chronically damaged and the most important consequence is the disfiguring and ostracizing condition, elephantiasis. Diagnosis depends on finding the sheathed microfilariae in a nocturnal peripheral blood smear and eosinophilia, as well as hematuria and proteinuria. Treatment is ivermectin 120 μg/kg PO for one dose which is equivalent to DEC at full dose of 2 mg/kg tid for 3 weeks. This drug is well tolerated but can cause hypersensitivity reactions because of early antigen liberation with fever, headache, nausea, and urticaria. Symptoms can be reduced by starting with a small dose and checking for reactions. Established elephantiasis may be treated surgically.

Diseases Commonly Associated with Pulmonary Complaints

Returning travelers frequently present for persistent cough, sinus congestion, and fever, and such nonspecific symptoms may be caused by travel-related causes such as malaria, typhoid fever, typhus, and dengue. Yet a search should also occur for common respiratory pathogens such as viral causes, *Streptococcus pneumoniae,* and mycoplasma. Risk factors for pulmonary disease include prolonged air travel with recirculation of dry cabin air and exposure to fellow travelers with infectious agents. Long-term travelers are at increased risk for TB which may manifest many years posttravel. The approach to respiratory problems in the returned traveler is no different than nontravel patients with regards to examination, identifying risk factors (e.g., smoking, occupational exposures, and immunization history) and workup. Additionally, travel-related risk factors should be assessed for a variety of pathogens such as viruses (viral hemorrhagic fevers), helminths (*Strongyloides, Schistosoma, Paragonimus, Ascaris*), and protozoa (*Entamoeba histolytica, Trypanosoma, Leishmania*), which may produce pulmonary symptoms or radiographic infiltrates.

SEVERE ACUTE RESPIRATORY SYNDROME (SARS) **SARS** has emerged as a serious international health threat since March 2003. Although initial cases were seen in late November 2002 in Guangdong Province in China, they were not reported. The first confirmed cases were in Hong Kong. The disease has since spread to Vietnam, Singapore, Canada, and more recently Taiwan. As of May 28, 2003, a total of 8240 cases with 745 deaths in 28 countries have been reported by WHO.

SARS is caused by a coronavirus. Although the means of transmission has not been fully understood, it is likely to be spread by "droplet infection," that is, through exposure to respiratory droplets spread by a cough or sneeze from an infected person. Laboratory tests can be used to detect the SARS-associated coronavirus (SARS-CoV), including PCR testing, serologic testing, or viral cultures.

Preventative measures are aimed at reducing close contact with infected persons and nosocomial transmission. For those in high risk areas (countries where community spread has been identified), this includes proper travel precautions and enhanced personal hygiene measures, such as hand washing and droplet precautions. Persons who have traveled from high risk areas should monitor their health for at least 10 days following their departure. Should a fever **and** respiratory symptoms occur—such as cough, shortness of breath, or difficulty breathing—medical assistance should be sought as soon as possible.

TUBERCULOSIS *Mycobacterium tuberculosis* should be considered among patients with appropriate risk factors presenting with cough, fever, diaphoresis, weight loss, and malaise. Risk factors include populations like refugees and immigrants or expatriate workers (especially health care workers) with prolonged exposure to TB-prone populations (e.g., Eastern Europe, Africa, North Korea). Exposure to multidrug-resistant mycobacteria is increased in Russia, Asia, the Dominican Republic, and Argentina. The initial management of suspected TB includes a PPD tuberculin skin test, sputum culture, and chest radiograph. See Chap. 65 for more details.

PARAGONIMUS (LUNG FLUKE DISEASE) *P. westermani* is a trematoidal infection primarily affecting the lungs. It is widely distributed, but is mostly found in Far East and Southeast Asia (China is the major endemic site). It is uncommon in short-term travelers, but should be considered among immigrants or long-term residents of Asia suspected for TB, and among travelers indulging in local exotic foods. Humans are infected by swallowing larvae contaminating raw or pickled crustaceans. Incubation lasts 6 to 12 weeks, as larvae migrate from the duodenum to the lungs where they cause cough (sometimes with rusty sputum), pleuritic chest pain, and hemoptysis. Chest pain is often present, and fever with night sweats may occur during early infections causing TB to be incorrectly diagnosed. Chest radiographs will be similar to TB (diffuse segmental infiltrates, nodules, ring cysts, or pleural effusions). Paragonimiasis should be suspected when no sputum smear acid-fast bacilli are found. If parasites do not reach the lung, patients may present with symptoms, depending on fluke location, such as abdominal pain, diarrhea, migrating subcutaneous swelling, blindness, epididymis, testicular inflammation, and a variety of cerebral symptoms. Seizures can occur in response to encysted adults residing intracranially. Diagnosis is made by finding the characteristic eggs in sputum, urine, or stool, or by serological tests such as CF, ELISA, or antigen detection. The treatment of choice is praziquantel 25 mg/kg PO tid for 3 days.

PARASITE-INDUCED BRONCHOSPASM The most common helminths causing pulmonary symptoms are *Ascaris* and *Strongyloides.* A suggestive clinical history includes recent travel and ingestion of local food of uncertain quality. Suspicion should be raised by any new pulmonary symptoms such as cough or wheezing associated with patchy infiltrates on chest radiograph and hypereosinophilia, which indicates a hypersensitivity reaction to migrating parasites. For diagnosis and treatment for each helminth, see previous respective sections.

REFERENCES

1. VanRooyen MV, Kirsch T, Clem K, et al. (eds): *Emergent Field Medicine.* New York: McGraw-Hill, 2002.
2. Hill DR: Health problems in a large cohort of americans traveling to developing countries. *J Travel Med* 7:259, 2000.
3. Keystone J, Humar A: Fortnightly review: Evaluating fever in travelers returning from tropical countries *BMJ* 312:953, 1996.
4. Ryan ET, Wilson ME, Kain KC: Illness after international travel. *New Engl J Med* 347:505, 2002.
5. Magill AJ: Fever in the returned traveler. *Infect Dis Clin North Am* 12:445, 1998.
6. MacLean JD, Lalonde RG, Ward B: Fever from the tropics, section 5, in *Travel Medicine Advisor.* Atlanta, GA: American Health Consultants, 1994, p. 27.1.
7. Centers for Disease Control and Prevention: CDC surveillance summaries: Malaria surveillance-United States, 2002. *MMWR* 51(SS-5):9, 2002.
8. Kyriacou DN, Spira AM, Talan DA, et al: Emergency department presentation and misdiagnosis of imported *Falciparum* malaria. *Ann Emerg Med* 27:696, 1996.
9. Clark GG, et al: Imported dengue—United States, 1997 and 1998. *MMWR* 49:248, 2000.
10. Tornieporth NG, Johnson WD: Infectious considerations in the world traveler. *Dermatol Clin* 15:285, 1997.
11. Suh KN, Kozarsky PE, Keystone JS: Evaluation of fever in the returned traveler. *Med Clin North Am* 83:997, 1999.
12. Caumes E, Carriere J, Guermonprez G, et al: Dermatoses associated with travel to tropical countries: A prospective study of the diagnosis and management of 269 patients presenting to a tropical disease unit. *Clin Infect Dis* 20:542, 1995.
13. Jong EC, McMullen R: Travel medicine problems encountered in emergency departments. *Emerg Med Clin North Am* 15:261, 1997.

HIGH-ALTITUDE MEDICAL PROBLEMS
Peter H. Hackett

Millions of people annually visit the mountainous areas of the western United States at altitudes over 2440 m (8000 ft). In addition, tens of thousands travel to high-altitude regions in other parts of the world.[1]

Physicians working or traveling in or near these locations are likely to encounter high-altitude illness or preexisting conditions that are exacerbated by altitude. Although the focus of this chapter is hypoxia-related problems, patients in the mountain environment also may require care for associated illnesses such as hypothermia, frostbite, trauma, ultraviolet keratitis, dehydration, and lightning injury.

High altitude is a hypoxic environment. Because the concentration of oxygen in the troposphere remains constant at 21 percent, the partial pressure of oxygen decreases as a function of the barometric pressure. In Denver (1610 m), air pressure is 17 percent less than at sea level, and therefore the air contains 17 percent less oxygen. The air of Aspen, Colorado (2438 m), has 26 percent less oxygen, and the barometric pressure on top of Mt. Everest is merely one-third that of sea level. Supplemental oxygen prevents symptoms of altitude illness during hypobaric exposure, and hypoxia, not hypobaria, is responsible for illness.

For the purposes of discussion, altitude may be divided into stages according to physiologic effects. *Intermediate altitude,* 1500 to 2440 m (5000–8000 ft), produces decreased exercise performance and increased alveolar ventilation, without major impairment in arterial oxygen transport. Acute mountain sickness starts to occur at 7000 to 8000 ft and sometimes lower in particularly susceptible individuals. Patients with cardiovascular and pulmonary diseases may become more symptomatic in this range of altitude. *High altitude,* 2440 to 4270 m (8000–14,000 ft), is associated with a decrease in arterial oxygen satu-ration, and marked hypoxemia may occur during exercise and sleep. Most cases of medical problems associated with altitude occur in this range because of the availability of overnight tourist facilities located at these heights. *Very high altitude,* 4260 to 5490 m (14,000–18,000 ft), is uncommon in the United States but is encountered by visitors to the mountainous regions of South America and the Himalayas. Abrupt ascent can be dangerous, and a period of acclimatization is required to prevent illness. *Extreme altitude,* over 5490 m (18,000 ft) is available only to mountain climbers and is accompanied by severe hypoxemia and hypocapnia. At this height, progressive physiologic deterioration eventually outstrips acclimatization, and sustained human habitation is impossible. Since hypoxemia is maximal during sleep, the sleeping altitude is the critical altitude to consider.

ACCLIMATIZATION TO HIGH ALTITUDE

Persons rendered acutely hypoxic become dizzy, faint, and rapidly unconscious if hypoxic stress is sufficient ($SaO_2 < 65\%$). These same individuals, given days to weeks to develop the exact same degree of hypoxia, are able to function quite well. While the fundamental process of this acclimatization takes place in the metabolic machinery of cells and mitochondria, acute "struggle" responses are critical while allowing the cells time to adjust.

Ventilation

Defense of alveolar PO_2 through increased ventilation is the primary initial adaptation. The hypoxic ventilatory response (HVR) is effected by the carotid body, which senses a decrease in arterial oxygenation and inputs to the central respiratory center in the medulla to increase ventilation. The vigor of this inborn response is related to successful acclimatization and increased performance. Respiratory depressants or stimulants may affect HVR, as does chronic hypoxia, which eventually blunts the response. A low hypoxic drive may allow extreme hypoxemia to develop during sleep. The initial hyperventilation is attenuated quickly by respiratory alkalosis, which acts as a brake on the respiratory center. As renal excretion of bicarbonate compensates for the respiratory alkalosis, pH returns toward normal, and ventilation continues to increase. This process of maximizing ventilation, termed *ventilatory acclimatization,* culminates after 4 to 7 days at a given altitude. With continuing ascent to higher altitudes, the central chemoreceptors reset to progressively lower PCO_2 values, and the completeness

of acclimatization can be gauged by the arterial PCO_2. Acetazolamide, which forces a bicarbonate diuresis, greatly facilitates this process. An appreciation of the normal values for blood gases and acid-base status with acclimatization at various altitudes is necessary to distinguish abnormalities (Table 207-1).

Blood

We know that within 2 h of ascent to altitude, erythropoietin is increased in plasma and, over days to weeks, results in increased red cell mass. This adaptation has no importance during initial acclimatization when altitude illness develops and, when excessive, results in chronic mountain polycythemia. Shifts in the oxyhemoglobin dissociation curve are thought to be minimal in vivo at altitude because the increase in 2,3-diphosphoglyceric acid, which is proportional to the severity of hypoxia and shifts the curve to the right, is offset by the respiratory alkalosis, which shifts the curve to the left. Naturally occurring left-shifted hemoglobin is an advantage at high altitude.

Fluid Balance

Peripheral venous constriction on ascent to altitude causes an increase in central blood volume that triggers baroreceptors to suppress antidiuretic hormone (ADH) and aldosterone and induce a diuresis. Combined with the bicarbonate diuresis from the respiratory alkalosis, this can result in decreased plasma volume and hyperosmolality (serum osmolality of 290–300 mosmol/kg) that the body appears to permit by a reset of the osmolar center of the brain. Clinically, diuresis and hemoconcentration are considered a healthy response. Antidiuresis is a hallmark of acute mountain sickness.

Cardiovascular

Stroke volume is decreased initially, and an increased heart rate maintains cardiac output. Maximum exercising heart rate declines at altitude proportional to the decrease in maximum oxygen consumption (VO_{2max}). Cardiac muscle in healthy persons is able to withstand extreme levels of hypoxemia ($PaO_2 < 30$ mm Hg) without evidence of ST-segment changes or ischemic events. Blood pressure is mildly elevated on ascent secondary to increased sympathetic tone.

The pulmonary circulation constricts with exposure to hypoxia. This is an advantage during regional alveolar hypoxia, such as pneumonia, but is a disadvantage during the global hypoxia of altitude exposure. As a result, pulmonary pressure increases. This degree of hypertension is quite variable, with those having a hyperreactive response much more susceptible to high-altitude pulmonary edema.

Cerebral blood flow transiently increases on ascent to altitude (despite the hypocapnic alkalosis), which increases oxygen delivery to the brain. This response, however, is limited by the increase in cerebral blood volume, which may increase intracranial pressure and aggravate symptoms of altitude illness.

TABLE 207-1 Blood Gases and Altitude

Altitude (meters)	PaO$_2$ (mm Hg)	SaO$_2$%	PaCO$_2$ (mm Hg)
Sea level	90–95	96	40
1524 (5000 ft)	75–81	95	35.6
2286 (7500 ft)	69–74	92–93	31–33
4572 (15,000 ft)	48–53	86	25
6096 (20,000 ft)	37–45	76	20
7620 (25,000 ft)	32–39	68	13
8848 (29,029 ft)	26–33	58	9.5–13.8

Effects on Exercise

Exercise capacity, as measured by $V_{O_{2max}}$, drops dramatically on ascent to altitude, approximately 10 percent for each 1000-m altitude gain above 1500 m. During acclimatization, submaximal endurance increases appreciably after 10 days, but $V_{O_{2max}}$ does not. The mechanism of this decrement might be lack of adequate oxygen supply to the muscle cells due to the low driving pressure for diffusion of oxygen from the capillary. Another theory suggests that the central nervous system (CNS) limits muscle activity to preserve its own oxygenation.

Limitations to Acclimatization

There are limits to acclimatization. Even those who are by nature good acclimatizers cannot tolerate the hypoxia of extreme altitude for long. Miners in South America report that they cannot live at altitudes above 5800 m because of weight loss, increasing lethargy, poor-quality sleep, weakness, and headache. High-altitude mountaineers cannot survive for more than a few days above 8000 m without supplemental oxygen because of acute deterioration in physiologic functioning. Considerable weight loss, due to loss of fat and lean body mass, is unavoidable. Other factors limiting ability to acclimatize to extreme altitude include right ventricular strain from excessive pulmonary hypertension, intestinal malabsorption, impaired renal function, polycythemia and microcirculatory sludging, and prolonged cerebral hypoxia. Even at more modest altitudes, some individuals are very slow or poor acclimatizers for reasons not entirely known but, at least in part, due to poor carotid body function and inadequate ventilation.

Sleep at High Altitude

Sleep stages III and IV are reduced at altitude, whereas sleep stage I is increased. More time is spent awake, with a significant increase in arousals, but with only slightly less rapid eye movement (REM) time. The frequent arousals are a common source of bitter complaints from skiers and others, but they are innocuous and improve with time at altitude. The typical periodic breathing (Cheyne-Stokes) in those sleeping above 2700 m (9000 ft) consists of 6- to 12-s apneic pauses interspersed with cycles of vigorous ventilation. Interestingly, the frequent awakenings are not necessarily related to the sleep periodic breathing, and neither are they related to acute mountain sickness. Presumably, the mechanism of the lighter sleep is related to cerebral hypoxia. Quality of sleep and arterial oxygenation during sleep improves with acclimatization and with acetazolamide.

HIGH-ALTITUDE SYNDROMES

High-altitude syndromes are those attributed directly to the hypoxia: acute hypoxia, acute mountain sickness, pulmonary edema, cerebral edema, retinopathy, peripheral edema, sleeping problems, and a group of neurologic syndromes. The other syndromes, not necessarily related to hypoxia, include thromboembolic events (which may be attributable to dehydration, prolonged incapacitation, polycythemia, and cold), high-altitude pharyngitis and bronchitis, and ultraviolet keratitis. Although the different hypoxic clinical syndromes overlap, all share a fundamental mechanism, all are seen in the same setting of rapid ascent in unacclimatized persons, and all respond to the same essential therapy: descent and oxygen.

Acute Hypoxia

The syndrome of acute hypoxia occurs in the setting of sudden and severe hypoxic insult, such as accidental decompression of a pressurized aircraft cabin or a failed oxygen system in a pilot or high-altitude mountaineer. Sudden overexertion precipitating arterial desaturation, acute onset of pulmonary edema, carbon monoxide poisoning, and sleep apnea may result in relatively acute hypoxia as well. Unacclimatized persons become unconscious at an arterial oxygen saturation of 50 to 60 percent, a Pa_{O_2} of less than about 30 mm Hg, or a jugular venous P_{O_2} of less than 15 mm Hg. Acute hypoxia is reversed by immediate administration of oxygen, rapid descent, and correction of the underlying cause, such as removal of the carbon monoxide source or repair of the oxygen delivery system. Symptoms of acute hypoxia reflect the sensitivity of the CNS to this insult: dizziness, lightheadedness, and dimmed vision progressing to loss of consciousness. Hyperventilation has been shown to increase the time of useful consciousness during acute alveolar hypoxia.

Acute Mountain Sickness (AMS)

INCIDENCE   AMS occurs in the setting of more gradual and less severe hypoxic insult than with acute hypoxic syndrome. Its incidence varies by location, depending on ease of access, rate of ascent, and sleeping altitude reached. One study found a 25 percent incidence of AMS in physicians attending a continuing-education meeting held at 2100 m (6900 ft) in Colorado. Other studies at resorts between 2220 and 2700 m (7200 and 9000 ft, respectively) claim an incidence between 17 and 40 percent, and a sleeping altitude of 2750 m (9000 ft) seems to be a threshold for increased attack rate.[2] Approximately 40 percent of trekkers in Nepal on the path to Mt. Everest suffer AMS, whereas climbers on Mt. Rainier have a very high incidence of 70 percent because of the rapidity of ascent.

In addition to rate of ascent and sleeping altitude, inherent factors determine individual susceptibility to AMS. Factors identified so far are low hypoxic ventilatory response and low vital capacity. Age has little influence on incidence, with children being as susceptible as adults. Women are just as likely, if not more so, to develop mountain sickness but appear to have less pulmonary edema. Susceptibility to AMS generally is reproducible in an individual on repeated exposures. Persons living at intermediate altitudes of 1000 to 2000 m already are acclimatized partially and do much better than lowlanders on ascent to higher altitudes. There is no relationship of susceptibility to AMS and physical fitness.

CLINICAL FEATURES   The diagnosis of AMS is based on the setting, symptoms, and physical findings. The setting is rapid ascent of an unacclimatized person to 2000 m (6600 ft) or higher. Typically, the person on arrival feels light-headed and slightly breathless, especially with exercise. Between 1 and 6 h later, but sometimes delayed for 1 day or more (and especially after a night's sleep), the typical symptoms of mild AMS develop; they are similar to an alcohol hangover. The headache usually is described as bifrontal and worsened with bending over and the Valsalva maneuver. Gastrointestinal symptoms include anorexia, nausea, and sometimes vomiting, and the chief constitutional symptoms are lassitude and weakness. The person with AMS is often irritable and wants to be left alone. Sleepiness and a deep inner chill also are common. If the illness progresses, headache and dyspnea become more severe, and vomiting and oliguria develop. Lassitude may progress so that the victim requires assistance for eating and dressing. The most severe form of AMS, high-altitude cerebral edema (HACE), is heralded by onset of ataxia and altered level of consciousness. Coma may ensue within 12 h if treatment is delayed. The diagnosis of AMS can be difficult in preverbal children.[3]

Physical findings in mild AMS are nonspecific. Heart rate and blood pressure are variable and usually in the normal range, although postural hypotension may be present. Localized rales are detectable in up to 20 percent of persons with AMS. Funduscopy reveals venous tortuosity and dilatation, and retinal hemorrhages are common over 5000 m or in those with pulmonary and cerebral edema. Fluid retention is a hallmark of AMS, in contrast to the usual diuresis of acclimatization, and may result in peripheral and facial edema. Differential diagnosis in this setting includes hypothermia, carbon monoxide poisoning, pulmonary or CNS infection, dehydration, and exhaustion.

The natural history of AMS at a Colorado resort (3000 m or 10,000 ft) was 15 h for mean duration of symptoms, with a range to 94 h, despite the fact that one-half of those with symptoms self-medicated. At higher sleeping altitudes, the illness may last much longer, even weeks if untreated, and is more likely to progress to pulmonary or cerebral edema. Eight percent of those with AMS at 4243 m (14,000 ft) in Nepal developed cerebral or pulmonary edema or both.

PATHOPHYSIOLOGY AMS is due to hypobaric hypoxia, but the exact sequence of events leading to illness is unclear. Figure 207-1 (left side) offers a schema for the pathophysiology. The brain enlarges in all persons ascending to high altitude because of increased cerebral blood flow and accompanying increased blood volume. Whether this is sufficient to cause the symptoms of mild AMS is unclear; in fact, the cause of mild AMS remains a mystery. However, in persons who go on to become ill with high-altitude cerebral edema, vasogenic edema is evident as increased T_2 signal on magnetic resonance imaging.[4] The leaky blood-brain barrier is due either to loss of autoregulation and overperfusion or to hypoxia-induced increased permeability via mediators such as vascular endothelial growth factor (VEGF) or bradykinin, or to a combination of the two processes. The fact that dexamethasone so effectively treats AMS also supports the notion of vasogenic edema because this is the only type of cerebral edema responsive to steroids.

The cerebral edema, interstitial pulmonary edema, peripheral edema, and antidiuresis observed in AMS all point to an abnormality of water handling by the body. The mechanism is thought to be increased renin-angiotensin, aldosterone, and ADH in contrast to the normal ADH and aldosterone suppression at high altitude and usual diuresis. A decrease in glomerular filtration also has been observed. Increased sympathetic activation is thought to play a role in the pulmonary and renal circulations, contributing to the pathophysiology (see Figure 207-1).

TREATMENT

Descent and Oxygen The goals of treatment (Table 207-2) are to prevent progression, abort the illness, and improve acclimatization; early diagnosis is essential. Initial clinical presentation does not predict eventual severity, and all persons with AMS must be observed carefully for progression. The three principles of treatment are 1) to not proceed to a higher sleeping altitude in the presence of symptoms, 2) to descend if symptoms do not abate or become worse despite treatment, and 3) to descend and treat immediately in the presence of a change in consciousness, ataxia, or pulmonary edema. Mild AMS is self-limited and generally improves with an extra 12 to 36 h of acclimatization if ascent is halted. Descent is the definitive treatment for all forms of altitude illness, although it is not always an option, nor always necessary. Remarkably, a drop in altitude of only 500 to 1000 m usually is effective promptly. Evacuation to a hospital or to sea level is unnecessary except in the most severe cases. To simulate descent, portable hyperbaric bags are being used in various locations to treat AMS. The patient is inserted into the fabric chamber, and a pressure of 2 lb/in² is achieved by means of a manual or automated pump; the pressure is equivalent to a drop in altitude of 1500 m (5000 ft). A valve system creates sufficient ventilation to avoid CO_2 accumulation or O_2 depletion.

Oxygen effectively relieves symptoms, but it often is unavailable in the field and generally is reserved for moderate to severe AMS in order to conserve supplies. Oxygen promptly relieves headache, dizziness, and most other symptoms, although ataxia may resolve more slowly. Nocturnal low-flow oxygen (0.5–1 L per min) is particularly helpful and efficient. The combination of oxygen and descent provides optimal therapy, especially in more severe cases.

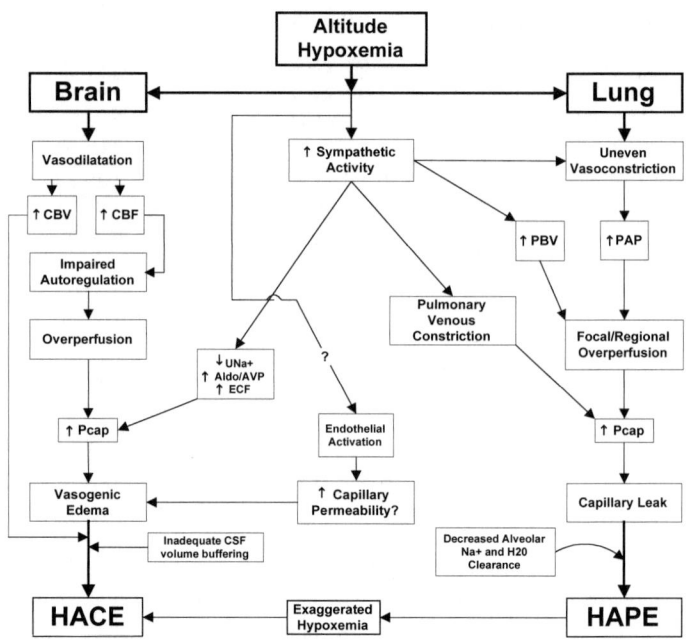

FIG. 207-1. Proposed pathophysiology of high-altitude illness. At high altitudes, hypoxemia can lead to overperfusion, elevated capillary pressure, and leakage from the cerebral and pulmonary microcirculation. Increased sympathetic activity has a central role in this process, and increased permeability of capillaries as a result of endothelial activation (inflammation) also may have a role, especially in the brain. Aldo/AVP = aldosterone/arginine vasopressin; CBF = cerebral blood flow; CBV = cerebral blood volume; CSF = cerebrospinal fluid; ECF = extracellular fluid compartment; PAP = pulmonary artery pressure; PBV = pulmonary blood volume; Pcap = capillary pressure; UNa = urinary sodium excretion. (From Hackett and Roach,[5] with permission.)

Medical Therapy Pharmacologic treatment offers an alternative to descent or oxygen in mild to moderately severe AMS. Acetazolamide is very helpful in speeding acclimatization and aborting illness, especially when used early. The drug acts by inhibiting the enzyme carbonic anhydrase, slowing the hydration of carbon dioxide to hydrogen and bicarbonate ions. In the kidney, acetazolamide reduces reabsorption of bicarbonate, causing a bicarbonate diuresis and metabolic acidosis that stimulates ventilation. The drug essentially mimics the process of ventilatory acclimatization. As a result, PaO_2 is higher, and sleep oxygenation remains high and stable, without periods of apnea. The drug also maintains cerebral blood flow despite greater hypocapnia, and because of its diuretic action, it counteracts the fluid retention of AMS. Many trials have shown its value for prevention, whereas one documented its effectiveness for treatment. **Indications for acetazolamide are 1) a history of altitude illness, 2) abrupt ascent to over 3000 m (10,000 ft), 3) for treatment of AMS, and 4) bothersome sleep periodic breathing. The dosage regimen varies; 5 mg/kg PO per d in two or three divided doses is sufficient, whether for prevention or treatment, or 125 mg PO twice daily, which is empirically effective.**[5] Treatment should be continued until symptoms of AMS resolve, and then the drug can be restarted if symptoms return. Because the drug acts by improving acclimatization, fear of masking serious illness is unwarranted. Common side effects of acetazolamide include peripheral paresthesias and sometimes nausea or drowsiness. It contains a sulfhydryl moiety, so it should not be given in patients with allergy to sulfa. Because the drug inhibits the instant hydration of CO_2 on the tongue, the carbon dioxide in carbonated beverages can be tasted, ruining the flavor of beer and other drinks.

TABLE 207-2   Suggested Treatment of High Altitude Illness

Mild AMS	Stop ascent
	Descend to lower altitude or acclimatize at same altitude
	Acetazolamide 125–250 mg PO bid to speed acclimatization
	Symptomatic treatment as necessary with analgesics and antiemetics
Moderate AMS	Immediate descent for worsening symptoms
	Low flow oxygen if available
	Acetazolamide 250 mg PO bid and/or dexamethasone 4 mg PO q6h
	Hyperbaric therapy
HACE	Immediate descent or evacuation
	Oxygen 2–4 L/min or titrated to Sao_2 >90%
	Dexamethasone 8 mg PO, IM, or IV, then 4 mg q6h
	Hyperbaric therapy if cannot descend
HAPE	Immediate descent or evacuation to medical facility
	Oxygen 4 L per min or titrated to Sao_2 >90%
	Nifedipine 10 mg PO q4–6h or 30 mg extended release q12h if no oxygen or descent
	Hyperbaric therapy if cannot descend
	Continuous positive airway pressure
	Minimize exertion and keep warm
	Dexamethasone if cerebral signs 4 mg PO q6h. Consider albuterol, 2–4 inhalations q4h
Periodic breathing	Acetazolamide 125 mg PO at bedtime as needed

Symptomatic treatment of AMS is sometimes sufficient. Aspirin 650 mg, acetaminophen 650 to 1000 mg (with or without codeine), or ibuprofen 600 to 800 mg can be effective for headache. Aspirin is also effective for prophylaxis of headache in persons not exercising.[6] Prochlorperazine 5 to 10 mg IM is useful for nausea and vomiting. A short-acting benzodiazepine such as triazolam 0.25 mg or temazepam 15 mg or the nonbenzodiazepine zolpidem 10 mg can be used to treat the complaint of frequent wakening, but these agents are potentially dangerous in ill persons because of possible respiratory depression. Combining acetazolamide with one of these agents works well for insomnia and is safe.

Dexamethasone 4 mg PO, IM, or IV every 6 h is quite effective therapy for mountain sickness, but it is best reserved for moderate to severe AMS because of potential side effects and because it does not aid acclimatization, sometimes resulting in rebound symptoms when discontinued. A short taper period may prevent this rebound phenomenon. The use of acetazolamide to speed acclimatization and a brief course of dexamethasone to treat illness can be a useful combination.

PREVENTION   Graded ascent with adequate time for acclimatization is the best prevention. A recommendation for those visiting medium-altitude resorts in the western United States is to spend a night at an intermediate altitude of 1500 to 2000 m (Denver or Salt Lake City) before sleeping at altitudes above 2500 m (8200 ft). Mountaineers and trekkers should avoid abrupt ascent to sleeping altitudes over 3000 m and then allow two nights for each 1000-m gain in camp altitude starting at 3000 m. Other preventative measures include avoiding overexertion, alcohol, and respiratory depressants and eating a high-carbohydrate diet.

Acetazolamide is a useful prophylactic agent for those with a history of AMS or for forced abrupt ascent without acclimatization stages. The drug should be started 24 h before the ascent and continued for the first 2 days at altitude. The medication then can be discontinued and started again if illness develops. Acetazolamide reduces the symptoms of AMS by approximately 75 percent in persons ascending rapidly to sleeping altitudes of over 2500 m. An alternative for those allergic to sulfa is dexamethasone 4 mg PO every 12 h starting the day of ascent and continuing for the first 2 days at altitude.

Neurologic Syndromes of High Altitude

Until recently, most neurologic events at high altitude were attributed to HACE or AMS. Clearly, this has been a diagnostic oversimplifica-

tion. Other syndromes now recognized as related to high altitude include altitude syncope, cerebrovascular spasm (migraine equivalent), cerebral arterial or venous thrombosis (infarct), transient ischemic attack, and cerebral hemorrhage. These syndromes are characterized by more focal neurologic findings than in cerebral edema, although differentiation in the field may be impossible.

Other symptoms may be due to exacerbation or unmasking of underlying disease, such as previously asymptomatic brain tumors and epilepsy. Presumably, space-occupying lesions become symptomatic because of increased brain volume at altitude. Hyperventilation (hypocapnic alkalosis), which is commonly used to induce seizure activity on electroencephalography, may explain unmasking of a seizure disorder at altitude, whereas changes in cerebral blood flow may exacerbate vascular lesions.

High-Altitude Cerebral Edema (HACE)

HACE is defined clinically as the presence of progressive neurologic deterioration in someone with AMS or high-altitude pulmonary edema (HAPE). It is characterized by altered mental status, ataxia, stupor, and progression to coma if untreated. Headache, nausea, and vomiting are not always present. Because of raised intracranial pressure, focal neurologic signs such as third and sixth cranial nerve palsies may result from distortion of brain structures and compression.

HACE usually is associated with pulmonary edema. Pathologically, necropsies have described severe, diffuse cerebral edema with multiple small hemorrhages and sometimes thrombosis.

The treatment of HACE is the same as for severe AMS: oxygen, descent, and steroids (Tables 207-2 and 207-3). Descent is the highest priority. Acetazolamide may be an adjunct, but immediate reversal of the illness is the goal; improving acclimatization comes later. In acutely ill patients who cannot descend, the combination of steroids, supplemental oxygen, and a hyperbaric bag is optimal therapy but rarely available. Persons remaining ataxic or confused after descent should be admitted to the hospital. Comatose patients require additional airway management, bladder drainage, and other coma care. For coma, the use of hyperventilation to decrease intracranial pressure is a reasonable approach, keeping in mind that the $Paco_2$ is already low and the pH high in these individuals. Additional acute hyperventilation could produce cerebral ischemia; monitoring of arterial blood gases and, if available, cerebral blood velocities by transcranial Doppler ultrasonography may be advisable. Loop diuretics such as furosemide 40 to 80 mg or bumetanide 1 to 2 mg IV may help reduce brain overhydration, but hypoperfusion and ischemia must be avoided. Hypertonic solutions of saline, mannitol, or urea have been used too infrequently to establish clinical guidelines. In the hospital setting, mannitol is worth considering in a patient who does not respond immediately. Coma may persist for days, even for weeks, after evacuation to lower altitude, and the patient may still recover, only rarely with permanent sequelae. Persistent coma is unusual, however, and mandates exclusion of other possible etiologies.

Cerebrovascular Syndromes of Altitude

Strokes, due both to infarct and hemorrhage in the arterial circulation, as well as venous thrombosis, have been reported in young, healthy persons at altitude who otherwise would not be considered at risk for such conditions. Transient ischemic attack, cortical blindness, and various focal neurologic signs, such as hemiparesis or hemiplegia of a transient nature, also occur. Because these latter events are reversible, they suggest etiologies such as vasospasm, migraine, watershed hypoxia between arterial zones, and transient ischemic attack.

Differentiation of the various neurologic syndromes may be impossible in the field, and treating as if cerebral edema were present may be reasonable, with a rapid descent to lower altitude, oxygen, steroids, and evacuation to a hospital if symptoms persist despite treatment.

TABLE 207-3   Medications for High-Altitude Illnesses

Agent	Indication	Dose	Adverse Effects	Comments
Acetazolamide	Prevention of AMS	125–250 mg PO bid beginning 24 h before ascent and continuing during ascent and to at least 48 h after arrival at highest altitude	Common: Paresthesias, polyuria, alters taste of carbonated beverages Precautions: Sulfonamide reactions possible, avoided in breast-feeding, can decrease therapeutic levels of lithium	Can be taken episodically for symptoms, no rebound effect, pregnancy category C
	Treatment of AMS	250 mg PO q8–12h		
	Pediatric AMS	5 mg/kg per day PO in divided doses q8–12h		
	Periodic breathing	125 mg PO 1 h before bed		
Dexamethasone	Treatment of AMS	4 mg every 6 hr PO, IM, or IV	Mood changes, hyperglycemia, dyspepsia	Rapidly improves AMS symptoms, can be lifesaving in HACE, may improve HACE enough to facilitate descent, no value in HAPE, pregnancy category C but preferably avoided by women who are pregnant or breast-feeding
	HACE	8 mg initially, then 4 mg q6h PO, IM, or IV		
	Pediatric HACE	1–2 mg/kg initially, then 0.25–0.5 mg/kg q6h PO, IM, or IV, not to exceed 16 mg/d		
Ginkgo biloba	Prevention of AMS	80–120 mg PO bid starting 5 days before ascent and continuing to highest altitude	Occasional headache, rare reports of bleeding	Requires further study, preparations vary, may be used by women who are pregnant or breast-feeding
Nifedipine	Prevention of HAPE	20–30 mg of extended-release formulation PO q12h	Reflex tachycardia, hypotension (uncommon)	No value in AMS or HACE, not necessary if supplemental oxygen available, pregnancy category C
	Treatment of HAPE	10 mg PO initially, then 20–30 mg of extended-release formulation PO q12h		

Abbreviations: AMS = acute mountain sickness; HACE = high-altitude cerebral edema; HAPE = high-altitude pulmonary edema.
Source: From Hackett 2001,[5] with permission.

Fortunately, focal neurologic signs usually resolve spontaneously and do not recur on reascent. However, a thorough cerebrovascular evaluation before advising reascent may be prudent.

High-Altitude Pulmonary Edema (HAPE)

HAPE is the most lethal of the altitude illnesses. Because the condition is easily reversible with descent and oxygen, the cause of death is usually lack of early recognition, misdiagnosis, or inability to descend to a lower altitude.

EPIDEMIOLOGY   The incidence of HAPE varies from less than 1 in 10,000 skiers in Colorado to 2 to 3 percent of climbers on Mt. McKinley and was reported to be as high as 15 percent in some regiments in the Indian army that were airlifted to high altitude during the Indian-Chinese war. Women appear less susceptible than men. Risk factors include heavy exertion, rapid ascent, cold, excessive salt ingestion, use of sleeping medication, and a previous history indicating inherent individual susceptibility. Genetic factors include diminished lung epithelial sodium channel activity,[7] excessive hypoxic pulmonary hypertension, and immunogenetic factors.[8] Pulmonary hypertension of any cause greatly predisposes to HAPE. As a result, HAPE has been reported in patients with intracardiac shunts (atrial septal defect, patent ductus arteriosus [PDA], patent foramen ovale), drug-induced pulmonary hypertension (phentermine), and chronic venous thrombotic disease.[9,10] Preexisting respiratory infection may predispose children to HAPE.[11]

CLINICAL FEATURES   Early in the course of illness, when the edema is still interstitial or localized, the victim develops a dry cough, decreased exercise performance, dyspnea on exertion, increased recovery time from exercise, and localized rales, usually in the right mid-lung field. Late in the course of the illness, there develops tachycardia, tachypnea, and dyspnea at rest, marked weakness, productive cough, cyanosis, and more generalized rales. As hypoxemia worsens, consciousness becomes impaired. Victims usually become comatose and then die. Early diagnosis is critical, and decreased exercise performance and dry cough are enough to raise the suspicion of early HAPE. The typical victim is strong and fit and may or may not have symptoms of AMS before the onset of HAPE. The condition typically worsens at night and is noticed most commonly on the second night at a new altitude. Unfortunately, rales may not be audible in 30 percent of persons with HAPE at rest but can be elicited immediately after a short bout of exercise. Low-grade fever is common, and tachycardia and tachypnea generally correlate with the severity of illness. On cardiac auscultation, a prominent P_2 and right ventricular heave may be appreciated. Electrocardiogram generally reveals right-axis deviation and a right ventricular strain pattern consistent with acute pulmonary hypertension. Chest x-ray findings progress from interstitial to localized alveolar to generalized alveolar infiltrates as the illness progresses from mild to severe.

PATHOPHYSIOLOGY   HAPE is a noncardiogenic, hydrostatic edema; left ventricular function is normal. Left ventricular end-diastolic pressure, wedge pressures, and left atrial pressures are low to normal, cardiac output is low, and pulmonary vascular resistance and pulmonary artery pressure are markedly elevated. The culprit in HAPE is high microvascular pressure (see Figure 207-1). Pulmonary hypertension is an essential component, but not all persons with pulmonary hypertension develop HAPE. Other factors that play a role include pulmonary venous constriction and uneven arterial vasoconstriction, leading to overperfusion of some areas of the lung vasculature. Inflammation was not present early in the course of HAPE, as measured by chemical composition of bronchoalveolar lavage fluid, but appears to be a secondary finding later in the illness.[12] Predisposed individuals have a low hypoxic ventilatory response, an abnormal pulmonary circulation response to hypoxia, and tend to suffer HAPE on repeated exposures.

TREATMENT The key to successful treatment of HAPE (see Tables 207-2 and 207-3) is early recognition, because the condition in its early stage is easily reversible. The optimal therapy depends on the environmental setting, evacuation options, availability of oxygen or hyperbaric units, and ease of descent. **Immediate descent is the treatment of choice, but this is not always possible.** During descent, exertion by the victim must be minimized. Reports of victims dying during descent probably are related to overexertion offsetting the benefit of lower altitude. Oxygen provides excellent results and can completely resolve the pulmonary edema without descent to a lower altitude, but it may require 36 to 72 h to do so. Such quantities of oxygen are rarely available to trekking, mountaineering, and skiing groups, but they may be available at ski resorts or medical facilities. Oxygen immediately lowers pulmonary artery pressure and improves arterial oxygenation. Its use is lifesaving when descent is not an option; in such cases, rescue groups should make delivery of oxygen to the victim the highest priority. As in the treatment of AMS and HACE, the portable hyperbaric bag is a very useful adjunct to therapy when immediate descent is not possible.

Bed rest may be adequate for very mild cases, and bed rest with supplemental oxygen may suffice for moderate illness, as long as the safety of the patient can be ensured by the presence of a medical facility, adequate oxygen, or immediate descent capability should the patient's condition deteriorate.[13] Because cold stress elevates pulmonary artery pressure, the patient should be kept warm. The use of an expiratory positive airway pressure (EPAP) mask has been shown to increase arterial oxygen saturation by 10 to 20 percent in HAPE patients by enhancing alveolar recruitment. The mask is lightweight, well tolerated, and may be a useful adjunct to descent.

Because oxygen and descent are so effective, experience with drugs has been limited. Several studies have demonstrated that nifedipine, either a 10-mg capsule or the 30-mg extended-release formulation, PO was of clinical benefit in reducing pulmonary artery pressure by 30 to 50 percent but increased arterial oxygen saturation only slightly. Nifedipine, at a dose of 20 mg (slow-release preparation) every 8 h while ascending, also was an effective prophylactic agent in those who have had previous episodes of HAPE.[14] Nitric oxide also lowers pulmonary artery pressure and redistributes blood away from edematous areas.[15] Nitric oxide, however, is difficult to administer. Sildenafil nearly completely blocks hypoxic pulmonary hypertension and therefore should prevent HAPE, although the study documenting this has yet to be done. Theoretically, it also should be useful for the treatment of HAPE.

None of these agents is as effective as oxygen or descent, which still remain the treatments of choice.[16] An interesting recent study showed that inhaled salmeterol twice a day reduced the incidence of HAPE by 50 percent in persons with previous repeat episodes of HAPE.[17] The mechanism is presumed to be upregulation of the epithelial sodium channel and increased clearance of alveolar fluid, a known effect of β-agonists. Although these agents have not yet been studied for the treatment of HAPE, given their likely benefit and safety and ease of use, treatment of HAPE with β-agonists is reasonable.

Hospitalization may be warranted for severe cases that do not respond immediately to descent, especially if cerebral edema is present. Intubation, high Fio₂, and positive end-expiratory pressure ventilation are rarely required. Antibiotics are indicated for coexisting infection when present. Occasionally, pulmonary artery catheterization is useful to exclude a cardiac component to the edema in persons with heart disease. The patient with HAPE who does not make the usual rapid improvement [or develops HAPE at altitudes of less than 2500 m (8200 ft)] should be evaluated for pulmonary emboli or other pulmonary circulatory abnormalities, such as congenital absence of a pulmonary artery or intracardiac shunt. Echocardiography with bubble contrast material can assess presence or absence of shunting from a patent foramen ovale or other cardiac abnormality.

Adequate discharge criteria are progressive clinical and radiographic improvement and a Pao₂ of 60 mm Hg or an Sao₂ of greater than 90 percent. Residua such as fibrosis and impaired pulmonary function tests have not been reported. An episode of HAPE is not a contraindication to subsequent ascent, but patients should be advised on staged ascent, acetazolamide and/or nifedipine prophylaxis, and recognition of early signs and symptoms.

Peripheral Edema

Swelling of the face and distal extremities is common at high altitude. Peripheral edema was reported in 18 percent of trekkers at 4200 m in Nepal and was twice as likely in women. It often was associated with AMS but not necessarily. The presence of peripheral edema should raise suspicion of altitude illness and prompt a thorough examination for pulmonary and cerebral edema. The problem can be treated with diuretics, but if left untreated, it will resolve spontaneously with descent. The mechanism is presumably similar to that of the fluid retention of AMS but with edema formation peripherally rather than in the brain and lung.

High-Altitude Retinopathy

Retinal abnormalities described at high altitude include retinal edema, tortuosity and dilatation of retinal veins, disc hyperemia, retinal hemorrhages, and rarely, cotton-wool exudates. Retinal hemorrhages are asymptomatic, except for rarely occurring macular hemorrhages, and are not considered an indication for descent unless visual changes are present. They resolve spontaneously in 10 to 14 days. Hemorrhages are common above a sleeping altitude of 5000 m and occur at lower altitudes in persons with altitude illness.

High-Altitude Pharyngitis and Bronchitis

Most unacclimatized persons exercising at altitudes over 2500 m develop a dry, hacking cough. With exposure to extreme altitudes for prolonged periods of time, a purulent bronchitis and a painful pharyngitis become nearly universal. These problems may not be of an infectious nature; high volumes of dry, cold air through the lungs may induce respiratory heat loss and cause purulent secretions on that basis alone. Bronchospasm also may be triggered by respiratory heat loss. Severe coughing spasms can result in cough fracture of the ribs.

Pharyngeal membranes become dry, painful, and cracked because of the dehydration and high ventilation. Mucosal cracks may be an entry for pathogens, or the erythema and dryness may cause discomfort strictly on a mechanical basis. Antibiotics generally are not helpful, supporting the concept of a noninfectious etiology. Breathing of steam, hard candies or lozenges to increase salivation, and forcing hydration may provide some benefit, with systemic analgesics being used as necessary. A silk balaclava or a scarf of similar material across the nose and mouth that is sufficiently porous to allow large-volume ventilation but trap some moisture and heat helps ameliorate these bothersome high-altitude conditions.

Chronic Mountain Polycythemia (CMP)

Monge disease, also called *chronic mountain sickness* (CMS), has been recognized in all high-altitude locations of the world. Both long-term high-altitude residents and lowlanders who relocate to high altitude may develop this condition after variable lengths of residence. The incidence is much higher in males and increases with age. The disease is characterized by excessive polycythemia for a given altitude, which causes symptoms such as headache, muddled thinking, difficulty sleeping, impaired peripheral circulation, drowsiness, and chest congestion. The diagnosis is made by the characteristic symptoms and a hemoglobin value greater than expected for the altitude, generally over 20 to 22 g/dL. Any problem causing hypoxemia at sea level causes greater hypoxemia at altitude, and the etiology of CMP can be traced to problems such as chronic obstructive pulmonary disease (COPD) and sleep apnea in 50 percent of patients. The etiology of pure CMP is attributed to idiopathic hypoventilation on the basis of diminished respiratory drive.

Therapy includes phlebotomy, relocation to a lower altitude, or home oxygen use. Respiratory stimulants such as acetazolamide (250 mg PO bid) and medroxyprogesterone acetate (20–60 mg PO per d) also have been employed successfully. The response to respiratory stimulants supports the role of hypoventilation in this disorder.

Ultraviolet Keratitis (Snow Blindness)

Ultraviolet light (UVA and UVB) penetrates the atmosphere to a greater degree at high altitude because of less cloud cover, less water vapor, and less particulate matter in the air. Radiation increases roughly 5 percent for every 300 m (1000 ft) gained, and it is exacerbated by reflection back from snow. UV radiation below 300 nm (UVB) is absorbed by the cornea, and high exposure levels can cause corneal burns in 1 h, although symptoms do not become apparent for 6 to 12 h. The typical symptoms of photokeratitis are severe pain, a foreign body or gritty sensation, photophobia, tearing, marked conjunctival erythema, chemosis, and eyelid swelling. UV keratitis generally is self-limited and heals within 24 h, but the condition is sufficiently painful to warrant systemic analgesics. Cold compresses also may provide some relief, and eye patches may be necessary for comfort. Prevention is obviously of great importance because this condition can be disabling, especially in hazardous terrain. Adequate sunglasses should transmit less than 10 percent of UVB light. Side shields are necessary if traveling on snow, and polarizing lenses help by absorbing glare. Makeshift protection can be fashioned by cutting narrow horizontal slits in cardboard, foam, or any available material ("Eskimo sunglasses").

ILLNESSES AGGRAVATED BY HIGH ALTITUDE

Chronic Lung Disease

COPD patients ascending to altitude often report increased dyspnea and reduced exercise ability. Those with hypoxemia, pulmonary hypertension, disordered control of ventilation, and sleep-disordered breathing at sea level may have greater problems at altitude because of the greater alveolar hypoxia. Such patients may require supplemental oxygen at altitude when they do not at sea level (and avoid having to descend), and oxygen-dependent patients at sea level may need to increase the FIO_2. The required FIO_2 can be calculated by multiplying low-altitude FIO_2 by the ratio of low-altitude barometric pressure divided by high-altitude barometric pressure. This will ensure the delivery of the same partial pressure of oxygen as at low altitude. There are no data to suggest that persons with COPD are more likely to develop AMS or HAPE, although such persons may be self-selected to avoid travel to high-altitude locations. In fact, persons with mild to moderate COPD already are partially acclimatized and may do well at modest altitude. High altitude per se does not exacerbate asthma, and persons with chronic bronchospasm often report easier breathing at high altitude due to lower air density and/or cleaner air. Patients with allergic asthma do better at high altitude because of reduced allergens.

Arteriosclerotic Heart Disease (ASHD)

The healthy heart and cardiovascular system tolerate even extreme hypoxia very well. Numerous electrocardiographic (ECG) studies,

echocardiograms, heart catheterizations, and exercise tests do not demonstrate cardiac ischemia or cardiac dysfunction in healthy persons at high altitude, even when PaO_2 was less than 30 mm Hg. Those with arteriosclerotic disease may not have the same adaptive capabilities and intuitively seem more likely to suffer from acute cardiac events. Epidemiologic data, however, do not support this supposition. Morbidity and mortality from arteriosclerotic heart disease are reduced in persons with long-term residence at high altitude, and visitors apparently do not have increased risk of acute myocardial infarction. Recent work, however, suggested earlier onset of angina at high altitude compared with sea level during the first few days at 2500 m. After 5 days, an elderly group with coronary artery disease (CAD) acclimatized well and performed at sea-level exercise capacity without increased or early-onset angina.[18] Even men with CAD and low left ventricular ejection fraction (mean 39 percent) but without overt heart failure tolerated exercise at 2500 m as well as at low altitude.[19] Congestive heart failure (CHF) may worsen in tourists arriving at the medium altitude of ski resorts, and it is related apparently to fluid retention rather than depressed ventricular function from hypoxia. Patients with CHF therefore should maintain or increase their diuretic regimen during travel to high altitude, and clinicians may want to consider administering low-flow oxygen during sleep for CHF patients, at least for the first few nights. Individuals after coronary-artery bypass graft have trekked to altitudes over 5000 m without problems.

Ascent to altitude produces a mild increase in blood pressure in normotensive and hypertensive persons secondary to increased sympathetic tone. However, the magnitude of blood pressure response is quite variable and not predictable. Patients should continue hypertensive medications at altitude, and blood pressure monitoring might be prudent. No data suggest that hypertensives have a higher risk for any of the altitude illnesses, and in general, hypertension is not a contraindication to altitude exposure.[10]

Sickle Cell Disease

Even the modest simulated altitude of a pressurized aircraft (1500–2000 m) may cause persons with hemoglobin SC and sickle-thalassemia to have a vaso-occlusive crisis. Exposure to high altitude thus requires supplemental oxygen. Sickle cell trait is not considered an increased risk, although splenic infarction syndrome during heavy exercise at altitude has been reported in those with trait.

Pregnancy

Pregnant residents of high altitude have an increased prevalence of hypertension, low-birth-weight infants, and neonatal hyperbilirubinemia. However, an increased incidence of pregnancy complications in lowlanders who visit high altitude has not been reported. The normal PaO_2 of the fetus is 29 to 33 mm Hg, and the mild maternal hypoxia induced by traveling to resort-type altitudes does not generate significantly more hypoxic stress. The few studies available suggest that exercise in pregnant women at altitudes of 2500 m is safe for mother and fetus. Based on the available data, pregnant women should be advised to avoid altitudes at which arterial oxygen saturation falls below 85 percent, which would be a sleeping altitude of about 10,000 ft. Perhaps of more concern than mild hypoxia is the fact that high-altitude locations are often remote from medical facilities, and patients need to be aware that without access to sophisticated medical care, complications could have more serious consequences.

REFERENCES

1. Hackett PH, Roach RC: High-altitude medicine, in PA Auerbach (ed): *Wilderness Medicine.* St Louis, Mosby, 2001, p 2.
2. Honigman B, Theis MK, Koziol-McLain J, et al: Acute mountain sickness in a general tourist population at moderate altitudes. *Ann Intern Med* 118:587, 1993.

3. Yaron M, Waldman N, Niermeyer S, et al: The diagnosis of acute mountain sickness in preverbal children. *Arch Pediatr Adolesc Med* 152:683, 1998.
4. Hackett PH, Yarnell PR, Hill R, et al: High-altitude cerebral edema evaluated with magnetic resonance imaging: Clinical correlation and pathophysiology. *JAMA* 280:1920, 1998.
5. Hackett P, Roach RC: High-altitude illness. *New Engl J Med* 345:107, 2001.
6. Burtscher M, Likar R, Nachbauer W, et al: Aspirin for prophylaxis against headache at high altitudes: Randomised, double blind, placebo controlled trial. *Br Med J* 316:1057, 1998.
7. Sartori C, Matthay MA, Scherrer U: Transepithelial sodium and water transport in the lung, in RC Roach, PD Wagner, PH Hackett (eds): *Hypoxia: From Genes to the Bedside.* New York, Kluwer/Plenum Academic, 2001, p 315.
8. Hanaoka M, Kubo K, Yamazaki Y, et al: Association of high-altitude pulmonary edema with the major histocompatibility complex. *Circulation* 97:1124, 1998.
9. Durmowicz A: Pulmonary edema in 6 children with Down syndrome during travel to moderate altitude. *Pediatrics* 108:443, 2001.
10. Hackett P: High altitude and common medical conditions, in T Hornbein, R Schoene (eds): *High Altitude: An Exploration of Human Adaptation.* New York, Dekker, 2001, p 839.
11. Durmowicz AG, Noordeweir E, Nicholas R, et al: Inflammatory processes may predispose children to high-altitude pulmonary edema. *J Pediatr* 130:838, 1997.
12. Swenson ER, Maggiorini M, Mongovin S, et al: Pathogenesis of high-altitude pulmonary edema: Inflammation is not an etiologic factor. *JAMA* 287:2228, 2002.
13. Hultgren HN, Honigman B, Theis K, et al: High-altitude pulmonary edema at a ski resort. *West J Med* 164:222, 1996.
14. Bärtsch P, Maggiorini M, Ritter M, et al: Prevention of high-altitude pulmonary edema by nifedipine. *New Engl J Med* 325:1284, 1991.
15. Scherrer U, Vollenweider L, Delabays A, et al: Inhaled nitric oxide for high-altitude pulmonary edema. *New Engl J Med* 334:624, 1996.
16. Hackett P, Rennie D: High-altitude pulmonary edema. *JAMA* 287:2275, 2002.
17. Sartori C, Allemann Y, Duplain H, et al: Salmeterol for the prevention of high-altitude pulmonary edema. *New Engl J Med* 346:1631, 2002.
18. Levine BD, Zuckerman JH, deFilippi CR: Effect of high-altitude exposure in the elderly: The Tenth Mountain Division study. *Circulation* 96:1224, 1997.
19. Erdmann J, Sun K, Masar P: Effects of exposure to altitude on men with coronary artery disease and impaired left ventricular function. *Am J Cardiol* 81:266, 1998.

ANTARCTIC MEDICINE
Desmond J. Lugg

Antarctica, the lands and ice sheets below the Antarctic Convergence (Antarctic Polar Front), where the cold waters from the Antarctic region meet and sink beneath the warm waters from the middle latitudes, has no indigenous population. Humans are transient visitors, spending from days to several years at a time. The first group wintered on the Antarctic Continent just over 100 years ago. Captain James Cook was most likely the first of the explorers to travel beyond the Polar Front and over the Antarctic Circle in 1773. Discoveries of seals and whales by Cook and others drew those keen to exploit the riches of the region. Scientific studies were performed in this heroic era, but it was not until the International Geophysical Year (IGY) 1957–1959 that multinational, multidisciplinary research programs burgeoned and have been maintained to the present. The advent of the Antarctic Treaty, signed in 1959 and entering into force in 1961, made Antarctica an international region; the later convention on living resources conservation and protocol on environmental protection curtailed exploitation and ensured the desirability of Antarctica as a tourist destination. The first shipboard tourist voyages came in the late 1950s.

Antarctica, with its cold, dry, windy climate, photoperiodicity, and isolation, is one of the harshest environments on earth. Despite the improved technological changes in clothing, equipment, food, and shelter, the environment is no less challenging than it was to the early explorers and exploiters. Apart from water, which needs significant energy to be "mined" from the polar ice cap, all survival needs must be taken to Antarctica, including health care. The history of medicine in Antarctica is a most interesting one.[1] No Antarctic-specific disease or ailment has been found. Since many of the persons going south are highly mobile, exotic diseases contracted in tropical or temperate areas may occur in Antarctica, consistent with the age and sex of the individual. Antarctic medicine is therefore the practice of medicine in the Antarctic region, as varied as that practice is, and not a specialty of Antarctic-specific disease states.

This chapter discusses Antarctic medicine as currently practiced by the varied groups, with particular emphasis on emergencies that may occur, whether shipboard, station, or remote field location.

POPULATION

In 2001, 18 nations operated 36 winter stations south of 60 degrees S,[2] with around a thousand scientists and support personnel spending the austral winter there; the number increases three- or fourfold in summer. In summer, over 14,000 tourists and adventure seekers travel by ship, yacht, and aircraft to indulge in observing and photographing this largely pristine wilderness and its wildlife, mountain climbing, skiing, camping, trekking, diving, skydiving, parasailing, kayaking, and running marathons. Over 60 Antarctic tour companies operate. Tourist overflights, of some 12 h duration, operate from Australia and are very popular.

EPIDEMIOLOGY

Trauma and accidents are the most common conditions, although most of these are of a minor nature. Injuries can range from abrasions, lacerations, sprains, and other musculoskeletal injuries and burns to fractures and multiple injuries causing death. Not all emergencies are simple, as illustrated by serious cases of a polio-like illness,[3] ruptured intracranial aneurysm,[4] breast cancer,[5] chest injuries, myocardial infarction,[6,6a] abdominal pain, fractured cervical vertebrae, and cold injuries.[6] After trauma and accidents, symptoms and ill-defined diseases, such as insomnia (endemic in Antarctica in the period of 24 h of sunshine in summer), dyspepsia, and headaches rate high, along with dental problems and skin diseases.

Cold-related injuries are uncommon, with most being recreational, such as snowmobiling and skiing.[7] Other conditions related to the environment, such as snow blindness and sunburn, are of low incidence.[8] Ozone depletion, known as the annual "ozone hole," is not thought to be a problem because of changed attitudes to exposing skin to sunlight, the use of goggles and sunscreen, and the presence of polar clothing covering most of the body.[9]

Diagnoses in Antarctica have included nutritional disorders (scurvy and hypervitaminosis A),[1] hepatitis, malaria, amoebic dysentery, pneumonia, anorexia nervosa, appendicitis, peptic ulcer, myocardial infarction, acute terminal ileitis, pyrexia of unknown origin, kidney stones, and gout. Mental disorders have low rates of occurrence in documented studies.[8,10] Although suggestions are made that behavioral problems are underreported,[11] many consider that much of this behavioral category consists of nonpathologic, adaptive mechanisms to the isolation and confinement. The role of alcohol in Antarctic communities reveals both positive and negative aspects.[11] Alcohol abuse does occur, and alcohol has been implicated in accidents.

Deaths in Antarctica have always been highly publicized. In the heroic era, deaths such as those of Scott and his four colleagues on the return from the South Pole, Mawson's two sledging companions on the Australasian Antarctic Expedition in 1911–1914, and three members of the Ross Sea Party of Shackleton's Trans-Antarctic Expedition in 1914–1917 took from months to years to reach the public press but are now classic descriptions of human endurance. In marked contrast are the recent real-time press releases of the crash of the Air New Zealand tourist flight on Mount Erebus in November 1979 with the loss of 257 lives, the deaths of 3 sky divers, and the death of a young woman from diabetes while traveling on a yacht in Antarctic waters. Deaths on national expeditions have resulted from myocardial infarction, appendicitis, perforated gastric ulcer, cerebral hemorrhage, alcohol poisoning, head injuries, hypothermia, drowning, crush injuries, falls into crevasses, burns, pulmonary embolism, and carbon monoxide poisoning. Most national programs have had deaths. Examples are 17 fatalities on the Australian National Antarctic Research Expeditions (ANARE) between 1947 and 2002 and 57 on the U.S. Antarctic program since 1946,[11] 3 in the last 10 years.[27] The case report of a recent tourist death probably from septic shock secondary to respiratory tract infection and suspected vertebral fracture illustrates that health risks are present even for those on cruise ships in Antarctica[12] (Table 208-1).

HEALTH CARE SERVICES

Each nation and group traveling to Antarctica has assessed the risks to their particular group and has developed health care services in response to the perceived needs. They range from multidisciplinary medical teams and elaborate medical suites and equipment at some stations to no medical or paramedical staff and very basic equipment and supplies at others. Each should be self-sufficient because of the cost in terms of both financial and the diversion of scientific and support personnel from their work. Countries involved in Antarctica have chosen different models of health care: civilian, military, contract, within the national polar organization, or combination of these. Determining factors include the number and skills of the medically trained staff, the degree of physical isolation, and medical logistics capabilities, especially the ability to provide medical evacuation by ship or aircraft.[27] Medical services for the younger, more adventurous tourists cater to traumatic injuries, whereas on traditional tourist ships, older passengers need support for age-related medical problems.[12,13] The International Association of Antarctic Tour Operators (IAATO), the voluntary self-regulating body for Antarctic tourism founded in 1991, is currently developing standards for its members' medical services.[14]

Some Antarctic medical practices have an evidence base of over 50 years, with a resulting emphasis on preventive medicine.[8] This is arguably the most important factor and has been the cornerstone of "best practice" services in Antarctica, where logistic constraints prevent timely evacuation and resupply. Physicians who have wintered over and been the sole medical providers consider that two-doctor teams

would be preferable. As well as having an "on the spot" second opinion, this also brings a wider range of skills and experience to medical management in isolation. Although a number of nations used two-doctor teams in the past, few continue this practice today. All doctors would prefer medical evacuation capability, but limited numbers of groups have this luxury, even in summer. Without such capability, the Antarctic physician must rely on his own skills, the supplies and equipment at hand, and the assistance of telemedicine. Specialist advisors in the home country must know the doctor's skills and capabilities, as well as the limitations of the pharmaceuticals and equipment, preferably having seen the medical facilities in Antarctica at first hand. Planning is very important, and the risk-benefit ratio of every potential procedure must have been assessed.

Predeparture Medical Screening

Predeparture screening was advocated in the heroic era.[15] Nations practicing preventive medicine have a rigorous predeparture medical screening, some having psychological or psychiatric assessment. This contrasts with many tourist operations.[12,13]

Guidelines for screening vary between groups, with the most rigorous rejecting persons with specific conditions such as asthma, coronary artery disease, diabetes, and epilepsy and those whose continuing good health depends on medications. Waivers are granted for some groups. Most standards or guidelines are under constant or annual review to guarantee that the latest medical knowledge is taken into account. Investigations vary between groups and may include blood donor screening, electrocardiogram (stress electrocardiogram for some above a certain age), chest x-ray, and laboratory tests.

Selection and Training of Medical Staff

In selecting a doctor for the austral winter-over, account must be taken of the likelihood and consequences of medical events and the needed medical skills. In addition, one must assess the physician's personality and ability to deal with the demands of the practice with its isolation, confinement, and separation from family, friends, and colleagues. No one medical specialty is considered best for the Antarctic because it is the combination of personal attributes for the environment as well as medical expertise and experience of the individual that is important— a true "supergeneralist."

Experience in a number of fields is desirable. With the possibility of cold injury and the presence of scientific chemicals and allied materials, many deemed hazardous, occupational and environmental skills are useful. Knowledge of nutrition is often needed and certainly public health principles if food poisoning or water pollution occurs. Emergency medicine skills prepare for the accidents and acute conditions, while diving and aviation medicine are an advantage for such programs. For stations and groups that are completely isolated, predeparture training of physicians in surgery, anesthesiology, radiology, dentistry, and laboratory techniques is desirable. Medical training of lay staff is also important. In locations that are accessible by sea or air, a lower level of skill may be acceptable. Medical handbooks and first aid manuals are particularly useful to assist in orientation processes.[16,17] With many hazards confronting all groups, preventive aspects are important for all individuals. Predeparture training in both general medical and work-related areas is also important for all; for those spending larger periods of time in Antarctic isolation, reentry into society also should be covered.

One topic rarely discussed is what happens if the doctor becomes ill. This is important not only for the patient but also for the group, especially if evacuation cannot be accomplished. Such scenarios are vividly illustrated by the description by Rogozov of his self-operation for appendicitis in 1961[18] and the difficulties and management of the highly publicized medical evaluation of doctors from the South Pole.[5,6a] Evacuation of patients has been achieved in all months of the

TABLE 208-1 ANARE Health Register, 1988–1997

Disorder	Number	Percent
Injury and poisoning	3910	42.0
Respiratory	910	9.7
Skin, subcutaneous	899	9.6
Nervous system/sensory	702	7.5
Digestive	691	7.4
Infection/parasitic	682	7.3
Musculoskeletal	667	7.1
Ill-defined symptoms	335	3.6
Mental	217	2.3

Source: Adapted from Lugg, DJ. Antarctic Medicine. *JAMA* 283(16); 2082, 2000.

year from the U.S. McMurdo Station and recently during winter-over from Pole Station.[6a] Preventive principles have even been extended to predeparture prophylactic appendectomy for physicians.[10]

Telemedicine and Medical Informatics

Medical communications have always been of utmost importance both within Antarctica and to the outside world, allowing solo practitioners to advise patients remote from them, as well as giving them access to a range of skills, ideas, and experience of medical specialists. Despite communications being subject to radio blackouts of polar cap absorption (PCA), they were the cornerstone of many medical systems.[19] Simple, cheap, and effective solutions allowed data, clinical and microscopic photos, x-rays, and electrocardiograms to be transmitted from Antarctica to the countries of origin of expeditions for over 50 years.[4,6,19] Today, with satellite systems, medical imaging and the transmission of medical and biomedical data are daily occurrences, unaffected by PCA blackouts. Many groups have access to phone, fax, e-mail, data circuits, and the World Wide Web. The system, in addition to providing clinical and peer support, has been innovative in education and continuing training of doctors with access to databases, electronic journals, and universities.

Hand-written medical logs from the 1940s onward were surveyed in the 1970s for epidemiology. For the last 15 years, medical informatics has come to the fore, with health registers containing data on all health events; coded information relating to each consultation with diagnosis, treatment, procedure performed, and pharmaceutical prescribed is transmitted in real time from Antarctica.[20] This has enabled researchers to quantify the occurrence of injuries in Antarctica; to compare incidence rates; to assess temporal, seasonal, and occupational trends; and to identify high-risk groups.[7,21] Accurate usage records also assist in inventory control and planning.

Laboratory and Diagnostic Equipment

Routine diagnosis and treatment present a challenge to physicians, and it is important that they have access to facilities that can assist. Diagnostic facilities range from the basic to more sophisticated laboratory tests. It is important that every piece of equipment is assessed for its usefulness and not for the fact that it is nice to have. A solo practitioner with a very ill patient does not have a lot of time to operate laboratory equipment that takes considerable time to arrive at a result. Considerable planning must go into the "ideal" diagnostic armamentarium, with emphasis on what will assist. Equipment that works in a major teaching hospital may not work in a small boat or ship in Antarctica. Dry-chemistry analyzers have increased laboratory services in Antarctica, but difficulties still exist for their operation in simple ways such as shelf life of components and storage temperatures.[22]

UNIQUENESS OF PRACTICE

In most Antarctic groups, the doctor lives and works with the group. The potential patients therefore see their physician at close quarters and also the medical system and what it could provide should they become ill or injured. This often puts stress on both the doctor and the patient. Patients are aware of the difficulties of supply, the problems of storage of pharmaceuticals (some do not survive freezing or dramatic temperature changes), the short shelf life of some pharmaceuticals, and the lack of equipment and skills. In most cases this can be overcome by clear advice at the outset of what can be done and whether evacuation can be accomplished. Doctors, too, are well aware of perceptions of danger, risk taking, and outcomes in remote Antarctica.[23] In addition, most staff are very perspicacious patients.[24]

Doctors in Antarctica must be past masters of improvisation in managing health and related issues. The successful use of cyanoacrylate tissue adhesive for the painful spontaneous skin disorder "polar hands,"[25] the manufacture of glasses from perspex, the manufacture of toothpaste, the unconventional repair of dentures and equipment, and the disassembly of an x-ray machine so that it could be flown by helicopter to a tourist ship to confirm a suspected diagnosis[13] are a few of the documented cases.

RESEARCH

In Antarctic medicine there has always been a close association between clinical practice and research. The prime responsibility of doctors is health care, and they are in a unique position to integrate clinical and evidence-based observation of their colleagues, especially during winter. The multidisciplinary research has centered on human interaction with the Antarctic environment.[10] Despite the inability to replicate space-specific effects of radiation, altered atmosphere, and weightlessness in Antarctica, the isolation, confinement, and total reliance on technology make Antarctica an excellent analogue for studies on long-duration space missions. The finding of an altered immune status in Antarctic wintering personnel, although not associated with any specific disease, has important health implications should viral disease occur. Further studies, however, have given evidence that such subjects have normal antibody production.[26] These studies illustrate the close nexus between Antarctic medicine and research.

INTERNATIONAL COLLABORATION

There has always been excellent collaboration in Antarctica, especially with medical evacuations.[8] The Scientific Committee on Antarctic Research (SCAR) has had an active Working Group on Human Biology and Medicine for nearly 30 years. The continuing process of physicians of different national Antarctic programs sharing data, diagnostic dilemmas, management of difficult cases, experiences of pharmaceuticals, and equipment has led to improved standards of care. The decades of collective experience of the working group has greatly assisted nations establishing health care for the first time. The SCAR working group has been particularly active since 1974 in guidelines for Antarctic predeparture screening for national groups.

GUIDELINES FOR HEALTH CARE SERVICES IN ANTARCTICA

The following guidelines on staffing, training, facilities, medical equipment, and pharmaceuticals are not definitive. Organizers of health care must take into account the following:

1. Area of Antarctica—isolation factor
2. Numbers of people, their ages, sex, and medical status
3. Length of stay (winter, summer, ship visit, overflight)
4. Presence of medical practitioner(s), paramedical staff
5. Facilities available
6. Communications
7. Risk factors
8. Medivac capability and plan efficiently and effectively to cover all contingencies

Staffing and Training

Ideally, a medical practitioner should accompany all groups and should have the skills and adequate predeparture training to manage all medical, surgical, and dental emergencies to the level of care decided on. A doctor is a must for a wintering group. Additional personnel should receive training in assisting in emergency care and, if surgery is contemplated, maintenance of anesthesia and sterile operating theater techniques to assist the doctor. If paramedics are used instead of doctors, they should be adequately briefed and trained. In the case of small, isolated summering or wintering groups, predeparture training for all should include first aid and occupational health and safety.

Facilities

An adequate medical area should be provided to cope with the needs of each group. If a doctor is present, serious consideration should be given to operating facilities. Such facilities are vital for initial management of burns and much of the trauma sustained, even if the patient is ultimately evacuated. All vessels, both national expedition and tourist, require adequate facilities.

Equipment

The following list is an *aide memoire* for equipment selection. The amount and sophistication depend on factors mentioned earlier, as well as on the skills of the staff.

1. Medical library
2. Examination equipment
3. Ward equipment (suction, nasogastric tubes, Foley catheters, etc)
4. Emergency and resuscitation equipment including stretcher, defibrillator/electrocardiograph, and transfusion supplies
5. Instruments for surgical, orthopedic, obstetrics/gynecology, and dental procedures
6. Suture material
7. Sterilizing equipment (autoclave)
8. Laboratory and diagnostic equipment
9. Anesthetic equipment (including a pulse oximeter)
10. X-ray equipment and supplies, ultrasound
11. Operating theater equipment, including soft goods
12. Dressing, bandages, etc.
13. Splints and traction equipment
14. Physiotherapy and rehabilitation (ultrasound)
15. Medical gases
16. Training equipment
17. Telemedicine equipment

Pharmaceuticals

A complete range of pharmaceuticals should be selected to cover the following:

1. Cardiovascular system
2. Respiratory system
3. Alimentary system
4. Analgesics, anti-inflammatory (nonsteroid), etc.
5. Narcotics, hypnotics, psychotropics, anticonvulsants
6. Antidotes
7. Antiallergics
8. Endocrine drugs
9. Vitamins and minerals
10. Hematopoietic system
11. Urinary system
12. Gynecologic drugs
13. Sera, vaccines
14. Dermatologic preparations
15. Ophthalmic preparations
16. ENT preparations
17. Intravenous fluids
18. Anesthetics and allied drugs
19. Diagnostic and laboratory agents
20. Antibiotics and allied drugs

MEDICOLEGAL

This is a complex issue and far beyond the Good Samaritan principle and the extent of national expeditions providing medical care for nongovernment activities.[11] This starts in the country of origin of the groups and extends to disability legislation and whether medical selection legally can disqualify those with preexisting conditions. Many groups face the dilemma by giving waivers instead of arguing a case that Antarctica is different. A number of countries have legislation covering areas of Antarctica (the so-called Frozen Claims of the Antarctic Treaty), but whether this pertains only to citizens of the claimant nation or beyond probably will require legal testing in the courts.

Despite increasing standards of health care in Antarctica, which are in part a reflection of community attitudes and the expectations of groups in Antarctica and their families at home, it is unrealistic to expect the standard to be that of best practice in teaching hospitals. Availability of and short shelf life of pharmaceuticals; levels of skills, equipment, and diagnostic and laboratory tests; correct servicing of equipment; and status of medical assistants, especially if dispensing drugs in the absence of a doctor, are but some of the areas that prevent Antarctic medicine from reaching the standard of teaching hospitals. When one adds international patients, issues of medical confidentiality in isolated small groups, the status of walking blood banks, the ability to screen adequately for all viruses, the potential sexual misconduct of a sole doctor who enters a relationship with a fellow member of the group (all of whom are potential patients), issues of pregnancy and management, and who doctors the doctor, then there is a medicolegal situation beyond belief. It is considered that common sense will prevail and that many of these will become nonissues in the situation of Antarctic medicine and its rather basic nature. However, in this litigious society, one cannot be certain, and the next decade therefore will be interesting because already government agencies and doctors have been sued.

REFERENCES

1. Lugg DJ: Antarctic medicine, 1775–1975. Part I. *Med J Aust* 2:295, 1975. Part II. *Med J Aust* 2:335, 1975.
2. Stations of SCAR nations operating in Antarctic, Winter 2001. *SCAR Bull* 145:7, 2002.
3. Budd GM: A polio-like illness in Antarctica. *Med J Aust* 1:483, 1962.
4. Pardoe R: A ruptured intracranial aneurysm in Antarctica. *Med J Aust* 1:344, 1965.
5. Nielsen J, Vollers M: *Icebound.* New York, Hyperion, 2001.
6. Taylor D, Gormly P: Emergency medicine in Antarctica. *Emerg Med* 9(3):237, 1997.
6a. Ogle JW, Dunckel GN: Clinical medicine: Defibrillation, thrombolysis following a myocardial infarct in Antarctica. *Aviat Space Environ Med* 73:694, 2002.
7. Cattermole TJ: The epidemiology of cold injury in Antarctica. *Aviat Space Environ Med* 70:135, 1999.
8. Lugg DJ: *Antarctica: Australia's Remote Medical Practice.* Kingston, Australian Antarctic Division, 1993.
9. Lugg DJ, Roy CR: UBV and health effects in Antarctica. *Polar Res* 18(2):353, 1999.
10. Lugg DJ: Antarctic medicine. *JAMA* 283(16):2082, 2000.
11. Carlisle B, Shen B: Polar medicine, in Auerbach PS (ed): *Wilderness Medicine,* 4th ed. St. Louis, Mosby, 2001, p. 226.
12. Lamberth PG: Death in Antarctica. *Med J Aust* 175:583, 2001.
13. Levinson JM, Ger E (eds): *Safe Passage Questioned: Medical Care and Safety for the Polar Tourist.* Centreville, MD, Cornell Maritime Press, 1998.
14. Curry CM: Death in Antarctica. *Med J Aust* 176:451, 2002.
15. Macklin AH: Appendix V, Medical, in Wild F: *Shackleton's Last Voyage: The Story of the Quest.* London, Cassell, 1923, p. 352.
16. Grant IC (ed): *Kurafid: The British Antarctic Survey Medical Handbook.* Cambridge, England, BAS/Boeing Publishers, 2001.
17. Gormly PJ: *ANARE First Aid Manual,* 6th ed. Kingston, Australia, Australian Antarctic Dvision, 1998.
18. Rogozov KI: Self operation. *Soviet Antarctic Exp Inform Bull* 4:233, 1964.
19. Sullivan P, Lugg DJ: Telemedicine between Australia and Antarctica: 1911–1995. SAE Technical Paper 951616. Presented at the 25th International Conference on Environmental Systems, San Diego, CA, July 12, 1995.

20. Sullivan P, Gormly P: The Australian National Antarctic Research Expedition's (ANARE) health register, in Peasley K (ed): *Proceedings of the National Centre for Classification in Health (NCCH)*, 6th Annual Conference, Hobart, September 1999. Lidcombe, Australia, NCCH, 1999, p. 36.
21. Cattermole TJ: The incidence of injury with the British Antarctic Survey, 1986–1995. *Int J Circumpolar Health* 60(1):72, 2001.
22. Kibby J, Sullivan P: Evaluation and use of a dry chemistry analyzer in Antarctica. *Int J Circumpolar Health* 56(4):142, 1997.
23. Plowright RK: Crevasse fall in the Antarctic: A patient's perspective? *Med J Aust* 173:576, 2000.
24. Burns R, Sullivan P: Perceptions of danger, risk taking and outcomes in a remote community. *Environ Behav* 32(1):32, 2000.
25. Ayton JM: Polar hands: Spontaneous skin tissues closed with cyanoacrylate (Histoacryl Blue) tissue adhesive in Antarctica. *Arctic Med Res* 52:127, 1993.
26. Shearer WT, Lugg DJ, Rosenblatt HM, et al: Antibody responses to bacteriophage φχ-174 in humans exposed to the Antarctic winter-over model of space flight. *J Allergy Clin Immunol* 107:160, 2001.

SPACE MEDICINE
David Williams

When once you have tasted flight, you will forever walk the earth with your eyes turned skyward, for there you have been, and there you will always long to return.

Leonardo da Vinci

INTRODUCTION

Space flight confronts some of the most challenging clinical, engineering, and technological problems of our time. Space medicine has grown significantly since the Mercury program, when the primary focus was on medical selection of astronauts, into an area of clinical practice requiring a unique set of knowledge, judgment, and clinical skills. Currently the delivery of health care in space is a combination of preflight medical selection of astronauts, wellness programs to optimize crew readiness for flight, health stabilization programs prior to launch, on-orbit countermeasures and conditioning programs, a system of clinical care provided by crew medical officers (CMOs) supported by flight surgeons (FS) in mission control, and postflight rehabilitation programs.

For the purposes of human space travel, the border to space has been set at 80 km (50 miles). In the United States, the term *astronaut* is used for individuals who have traveled above this altitude. Aerodynamic aircraft control is no longer effective beyond approximately 80 km above the earth's surface, and the vacuum and temperature extremes of space require complex environmental control and life support systems (ECLSS) for crew survival. Microgravity affects virtually every organ system. There are three primary sources of ionizing radiation that exist in the space environment: galactic cosmic rays (GCR), trapped belt radiation, and solar particle events (SPE). As mission duration and altitude increase, radiation shielding and specific radiation countermeasures become necessary.

Early in the history of human space exploration, a life science research program was implemented to study the physical challenges of space flight and physiologic adaptations that would occur in microgravity. The term *bioastronautics* was initially used to describe the study of the biological and medical effects of space flight on living organisms, with a particular focus on human adaptation to space. Prior to the first human space flights, the primary clinical question dealt with the survivability of space flight. Concerns were expressed about a number of issues ranging from cardiovascular, neurovestibular, and musculoskeletal changes to fears that astronauts would aspirate saliva and be unable to swallow in microgravity. The first human flights in 1961 demonstrated that humans could survive short-duration space travel with minimal adverse effects. This information was critical to the later declaration that the National Aeronautics and Space Administration (NASA) would land humans on the moon and safely return them to earth.

SPACE PROGRAMS

Early spacecraft from Mercury through Apollo-Soyuz were based on a ballistic capsule design with thermal barriers to protect the vehicle during reentry, and a series of parachutes to slow the vehicle for landing in the ocean. During the Mercury and Gemini programs, an environmental control system (ECS) was designed to maintain pressurization and thermal control of the capsule with crew members wearing space suits. Later in the Apollo, Skylab, and Apollo-Soyuz programs, crew wore space suits only for the launch and re-entry phases of space flight.

Mercury

The Mercury spacecraft provided a 28-h flight capability based on an oxygen consumption of 500 mL per min at standard temperature and pressure. Cabin pressurization was maintained at 5.1 psi. This pressure was chosen as the best compromise to provide necessary oxygen partial pressure, efficient use of the oxygen supply for emergency modes of operation, a pressure offering small differential change during sudden decompression emergencies, and a level at which decompression sickness would be minimal. The astronauts breathed 100 percent oxygen for 2 h prior to launch to reduce the risk of decompression sickness while transitioning from an ambient pressure of 14.7 psi at the launch site to 5 psi in the spacecraft in orbit.

A heat exchanger was designed as part of the suit pressure control system to accommodate astronaut metabolic heat production of 500 BTU per h. Potable water consisted of a flexible water pouch containing 2.7 kg of water with a flexible hose and drinking tube.

The primary medical conclusions from Project Mercury revealed few areas of significant clinical concern.[1] There was no evidence of deterioration in pilot performance and all measured physiologic functions remained within normal limits during the mission. An orthostatic rise in heart rate and fall in blood pressure were noted postflight and it persisted for 7 to 19 h after landing. There was no evidence of abnormal sensory or psychological response in any phase of flight and the radiation dose received was considered medically insignificant.

Still, many questions needed to be answered about the ability of astronauts to perform complex tasks on longer-duration missions, to pilot and dock spacecraft on orbit and perform spacewalks or extravehicular activities (EVAs).

Gemini

A new spacecraft that accommodated two astronauts was developed for the Gemini program with enhanced ECS capabilities to support longer missions.[2] The longest Gemini mission lasted close to 14 d, compared to the single-crewman Mercury missions that lasted a maximum of a day and a half.

The Gemini spacecraft ECS maintained a 100 percent oxygen atmosphere, controlled the temperature of the crew and spacecraft equipment, and provided a drinking water supply and means of disposing of waste fluids. Clinical studies showed no oxygen toxicity with exposure of humans for 14 d to the 100 percent oxygen at 5 psi. Gemini introduced a flight crew equipment system to support the longer missions. A food system consisting of vacuum packed freeze-dried rehydratable foods and beverages were provided to maintain between 2000 and 2500 calories per day. A urine collection system consisting of a portable receiver with a latex condom catheter and a defecation system consisting of individual plastic bags with adhesive-lined circular tops and a disinfectant packet to eliminate bacterial growth were flown. In-flight use required considerable care and effort. The personal hygiene system included tissues in fabric dispenser packs, fabric towels, wet cleaning pads, and toothbrushes and chewing gum for oral hygiene.

The first NASA EVAs were performed in the G4C suit during the Gemini 4 mission.[3] EVAs were accomplished on five of the ten Gemini missions, with important findings that facilitated the development of the more complex Apollo EVAs that would later be done in space and on the lunar surface. A small chest pack called the *ventilation control module* was developed for control of the space suit pressurization and ventilation, and suit pressure was maintained at 4.2 psi. The 100 percent oxygen environment of the spacecraft and the small change in cabin pressure from 5.1 to 4.2 psi minimized the risk of decompression sickness. During the initial egress activities and during ingress, the oxygen flow in the space suit did not keep the EVA pilot cool and overheating and visor fogging occurred.

Preflight quarantine was rejected as impractical in the Gemini program and a number of the astronauts developed short-lived flu-like syndromes; one was exposed to mumps and there was one incident of streptococcal pharyngitis that developed in the immediate preflight period. A drug kit was made available for in-flight prescription and aspirin was used in-flight for occasional mild headaches and for relief of muscular discomfort. Decongestants were used to relieve nasal congestion and alleviate the necessity for frequent clearing of the ears prior to reentry. Motion sickness medication was taken in one instance prior to reentry to reduce motion sickness resulting from motion of the spacecraft in the water. An inhibitor of gastrointestinal motility was prescribed when necessary to assist in avoiding in-flight defecation.

The medical findings from the Gemini Program extended the Project Mercury findings that humans can tolerate exposure to the space environment quite well.[4] No significant performance detriment was noted. Once again, postflight orthostatic hypotension persisting for some 50 h was observed during tilt table tests. A decrease in red cell mass of the order of 5 to 20 percent was noted, and bone demineralization was observed as a percentage change in the density of the calcaneus. No adverse psychological reactions were observed even during 14 days' confinement in a restrictive cabin environment, and no vestibular disturbances were reported.

Apollo

The Apollo Program accomplished the goal of landing humans on the moon and safely returning them to earth less than a year after the first manned flight test of the Apollo vehicle.[5] The three-person Apollo spacecraft consisted of a command module (CM), service module (SM), and lunar excursion module (LEM). The SM was mounted below the CM and contained the main propulsion system and stowage for most of the consumables. The SM was jettisoned prior to reentry into the earth's atmosphere at the end of the mission. The LEM was a two-staged vehicle with the ascent stage made up of three sections: the crew compartment, midsection, and aft equipment bay.

The Apollo CM ECS was composed of the oxygen subsystem, pressure suit circuit subsystem, water subsystem, coolant subsystem, and waste management subsystem. As in Mercury and Gemini, a 100 percent oxygen atmosphere was used with a cabin pressure of 5 psi and normal shirtsleeve environment except for launch and entry. Tragically, this environment led to the catastrophic loss of the Apollo 1 vehicle and crew in a fire on the launch pad during vehicle testing. This led to a redesign of the ECS such that the CM was launched with 60 percent oxygen/40 percent nitrogen gas composition that was eventually raised to 100 percent oxygen during the mission. The atmospheric pressure and composition after launch remained between 4.71 and 5.1 psi, including the time in the lunar module.

Carbon dioxide levels in the spacecraft were regulated to 3.8 mm Hg with a maximum limit of 7.6 mm Hg and an emergency limit of 15.0 mm Hg. Carbon dioxide levels recorded by sensors in the CM and LEM remained well below these limits except for the return flight of the Apollo 13 spacecraft, when they rose to a maximum of 14.9 mm Hg in the LEM. Temperature and humidity in the Apollo CM was regulated to between 70° and 80°F with a relative humidity of 40 to 70 percent. During the Apollo 13 mission the LEM ECS provided a habitable environment for approximately 83 h, after which cabin temperatures ranged between 49° and 55°F.

The primary medical objectives of Apollo were to ensure crew safety and health by identifying, minimizing, or eliminating potential crew health hazards. An important additional objective was to prevent terrestrial contamination from material brought back from the lunar surface. Supplemental objectives included continuing research to understand the biomedical changes affecting the body during space flight. A preflight medical program was implemented during the Apollo missions with the implementation of a health stabilization program and other preventive measures after Apollo 13. Determination of individual drug sensitivities to the contents of the Apollo medical kits was performed on all astronauts and a baseline data collection program was implemented to compare with postflight data for determination of the effects of space flight.

Significant in-flight medical observations[6] from the Apollo program included upper respiratory tract infections (prior to preflight quarantine), space motion sickness, skin and eye irritation from fiberglass insulation, contact dermatitis, facial and inguinal rashes, cardiac dysrhythmias, fatigue, dehydration, anorexia, urinary tract infection, shoulder strain from drilling for lunar specimens, and possible mild decompression sickness. A number of factors predisposed to sleep disruption, including noise from thruster firings or communication with the ground, staggered sleep periods, excitement, the unfamiliar sleep environment, and the command pilot syndrome reported by some of the command pilots when alone in lunar orbit awaiting the return of the LM.

Crew nutrition was a concern due to inadequate food consumption to maintain metabolic balance during some of the missions (caloric intake was less than calories expended, with loss of tissue fluid and electrolytes). Meal preparation and consumption required too much time and effort relative to other mission tasks. Reconstitution of dehydrated foods affected its taste, and in some cases it contained large quantities of undissolved hydrogen and oxygen gas. Weight losses of 2 to 3 kg were observed. Dehydration was an issue after the explosion of the SM oxygen tank during the flight of Apollo 13 that required the crew to use the LEM as a lifeboat to return from the aborted lunar mission.

Despite the complexity of the CM EVAs and the 14 lunar surface EVAs, no problems were experienced by any of the astronauts.

Skylab

The successful conclusion of the Apollo program represented a tremendous technological and human achievement. Space medicine had evolved significantly over a period of 10 years, yet the discipline was still in its infancy. The major focus of space biomedical research following Apollo was on the physiologic adaptation of humans to space in both short- and long-duration missions. Long-duration missions are defined as those lasting longer than 30 days. By the end of the Apollo program, the longest NASA missions were 2 weeks.

Skylab was developed as an orbiting space station to provide a research platform to extend human capability during long-duration space flight. Launched to an altitude of 270 miles, it provided a shirtsleeved environment pressurized to 5 psi: 3.7 psi oxygen and 1.3 psi nitrogen. It was equipped to house three astronauts for up to 3 months in a volume of 294 cubic meters.[7] This was huge in comparison to the Mercury, Gemini, and Apollo spacecraft, whose volume ranged between 1 and 8 cubic meters. The mission duration for Skylab-2 was 28 days, Skylab-3 59 days, and Skylab-4 84 days.

The biomedical objectives of Skylab included determining human physiologic responses and behavioral performance in space and during the postflight readaptation to the terrestrial environment, after a series of progressively longer missions. Enhanced clinical capability was provided during the mission with the in-flight medical support system (IMSS). The IMSS consisted of diagnostic and therapeutic equipment to optimize the capability for mission completion in the event of an illness or injury by diagnosing and treating the affected astronaut in space. For diagnostic purposes, the standard clinical tools (stethoscopes, sphygmomanometers, thermometers) were provided, in addition to lab equipment for blood analysis, urinalysis, and microbiological work. For therapeutic purposes the IMSS was supplied with an assortment of drugs, both oral and injectable, for the treatment and prevention of infection, disease, and allergies. The IMSS was also outfitted with a surgery kit for the care of minor injuries.

Space motion sickness was reported by some of the astronauts and was treated with prophylactic medication early in the flight. Symptoms were reported to last up to 4 days, but typically resolved within 48 h of being in space. Anecdotal reports from the Skylab crews suggested that space motion sickness could not be predicted with the usual ground-based tests, but could be alleviated somewhat by prophylactic administration of medications early in the mission.

The cardiovascular response of the astronauts to provocative orthostatic stress was examined for the first time on orbit. The crews were tested using a lower-body negative pressure (LBNP) device before, during, and after all Skylab missions. LBNP during the mission imposed a negative 50 mm Hg orthostatic stress for 25 min. This provided an orthostatic challenge similar to standing in a 1 G environment and showed the familiar indices of reduced cardiovascular efficiency. This was found to stabilize after 4 to 6 weeks with no apparent impairment of crew health or performance. Bone density studies did not show mineral losses in the upper extremities, but bone loss occurred in the lower extremities at a rate of approximately 1.5 percent per month, comparable to rates observed in bed rest studies. Evidence of muscle loss was obtained from anthropometric studies, revealing a marked loss in leg volume, most of which was restored within 21 days of landing. One-third of the loss was attributed to partial atrophy of the leg muscles, while the remainder was attributed to fluid loss.

As in the case of Apollo, fatigue was an issue for some of the Skylab crews. Sleeping compartments were not sufficiently isolated from each other and from the waste management compartment for optimum noise control. Mobility and restraint systems were also found to be major factors in the perceived habitability of the station and suggested that further research on human factors would help improve performance in microgravity. The Skylab program conclusions suggested that with sufficient attention to such issues as food service, waste management, and sleep arrangements, a spacecraft can provide satisfactory living and working quarters for long periods of time.

Space Shuttle

Following completion of Skylab, attention shifted to developing a new launch vehicle. The space shuttle, or space transportation system (STS), was developed as a multipurpose vehicle to deliver crew and payloads to low earth orbit, to rendezvous and dock with orbiting space stations, and to function as an autonomous microgravity research platform. The maximum G forces during the launch are limited to 3 G's and occur in the last minute of powered flight.

The shuttle atmosphere is maintained at 14.7 psi, with a P_{O_2} of 3.2 ± 0.25 psi (165 mm Hg) and a P_{CO_2} below 7.6 mm Hg (0.15 psi). Mission rules require that oxygen masks be donned if oxygen pressure falls below 2.34 psi (121 mm Hg) or if carbon dioxide levels exceed 15 mm Hg. Water vapor pressure of 10 mm Hg is optimal for habitability and is controlled between 6 and 14 mm Hg. Ambient temperatures within the shuttle range from 18° to 27°C. The crew members wear launch and entry suits during the dynamic flight phases of the mission to support crew escape in the event of emergency.

The shuttle has sophisticated systems including onboard computers, communications capability, electrical systems, guidance, navigation and control systems, mechanical systems, orbital and aerodynamic maneuvering systems, and robotic and rendezvous/docking systems. The aviation skills required of the shuttle commander and pilot during all phases of flight are significant, but entry and landing are most critical, in part due to the physiologic deconditioning that occurs even on short-duration missions.

Biomedical research on the shuttle was organized to develop a series of countermeasures to prevent the deleterious effects of space flight. The research capability of the shuttle was augmented by the Spacelab and SpaceHab modules that could be installed in the payload bay of the orbiter. The additional workspace provided by these modules turns the shuttle into an orbiting laboratory for short-duration microgravity research. A number of shuttle missions have focused on space life science research, including SLS1 and SLS2, the International Microgravity Laboratory missions, the Life and Microgravity Science mission, and more recently Neurolab.

From 1990 to 1995 a robust research program[7] to evaluate extending the duration of shuttle flights was implemented. Forty-six different experiments were flown on 42 different shuttle flights with 133 astronauts participating in the research protocols. The results of these studies, when combined with previous physiologic research, helped develop and evaluate a series of new countermeasures.

Mir

Eight flights between 1995 and 1998 were conducted to send and return seven NASA astronauts to the Russian Mir space station. The average mission duration was 131 days and 25 experiments were conducted in phase 1A and 26 experiments in phase 1B. Data were collected from both astronaut and cosmonaut participants. Many benefits arose from the program in addition to the life science research objectives. NASA gained further rendezvous, docking, and long-duration operational experience that would help reduce the risks associated with developing and assembling the International Space Station (ISS).

PHYSIOLOGIC ADAPTATIONS TO MICROGRAVITY

Cardiovascular Responses

Cardiovascular studies documented the prevalence of a number of benign atrial and ventricular dysrhythmias and helped establish normative values for heart rate and blood pressure on missions lasting 10 days or less. Extensive postflight studies of orthostatic intolerance were conducted, and the results suggested that decreased plasma volume plays a role, but decreased total peripheral resistance is an important determinant of pre-syncope.[8] Use of a liquid-cooled garment as part of the launch and entry suit was found to be critical in preventing peripheral vasodilatation, and fluid-loading protocols were developed and utilized prior to reentry to maintain preload. Early inflation of G suits during entry was also found to be very helpful as the gravitational vector (+Gz) runs from head to toe when the crew are seated for entry and landing.

Aerobic and Muscular Capacity

Functional performance assessments revealed decreased (10 to 20 percent) aerobic capacity for all subjects, with a protective benefit documented for subjects who exercise for 20 min or more at 60 to 80 percent preflight maximum work levels at least three times per week. Decreases in muscle strength ranging from 10 to 20 percent were noted in the legs and postural muscles of the trunk. Muscle morphology changed rapidly in response to microgravity, with decreases noted in both type 1 and type 2 fibers.

Neurovestibular Adaptations

Neurovestibular and neuromuscular assessments revealed that experienced astronauts with multiple space flights had better adaptation to space and better postflight performance, suggesting retained learning.[9]

Metabolic Adaptations

Total energy requirements were documented to be similar for short-duration flight and a normal terrestrial activity level. Energy intake decreased in flight, partly due to space motion sickness, and most subjects lose body mass to some degree. All subjects were noted to lose 1 to 2 L of total body water, and it was felt that the renal stone risk increased immediately in flight and postflight due to decreased fluid intake.

Infections and Environmental Hazards

Changes in the shuttle environment were documented, revealing a moderate increase in bacterial levels during the mission. Fungal levels generally decreased due to the relatively low humidity of the shuttle. Although volatile organic hydrocarbons were generally below required levels, the necessity for monitoring real-time levels of combustion products led to the development of a combustion product analyzer.

Countermeasures

The Extended Duration Orbiter Medical Project (EDOMP) program demonstrated the need for a comprehensive countermeasures program that would include at least the following protocols: fluid/salt loading; pharmacologic, aerobic and resistive exercise; and nutritional, environmental, mechanical, and special countermeasure training for crews. Important lessons were learned about the need to monitor and maintain an appropriate cabin atmosphere, levels of potentially toxic environmental contaminants, the acoustic environment, the radiation environment, water quality, flight crew equipment, clothing, sleep quarters, exercise equipment, food, family support, and behavioral support. These lessons were not only important in extending the duration of shuttle missions; they helped prepare for the NASA/Mir long-duration missions. Current countermeasures are often specifically developed for each crew member to optimize their efficacy for astronauts of both genders and different ages. Although preliminary data suggests that the efficacy of these countermeasures is considerably improved over those in previous use, further research to improve efficacy will be critical to minimize the risk of long-duration space travel beyond low earth orbit.[10]

ILLNESS AND INJURY IN SPACE

Many of the deleterious physiologic changes associated with the transition to microgravity cause clinical conditions that are similar to terrestrial diseases. The bone loss and muscle wasting induced in long-duration space travel are similar to those noted in patients during prolonged bed rest, immobilization, or those with spinal cord injuries. The combination of increased calcium turnover and dehydration seen in astronauts increases the risk of kidney stones.

Once the physiologic adaptations to space have stabilized, it is not known if these adaptations alter the pathophysiology and clinical course of a particular illness. For instance, it has been suggested that a transient increase in intracranial pressure associated with the cephalad fluid shift early in flight results in the characteristic headache, nausea, and vomiting associated with space motion sickness. The combination of such physiologic changes with those associated with a significant closed head injury could be significant. Similarly, the hemodynamic response to blood loss may be altered by the cardiovascular and hematologic changes that have been described in both short- and long-duration crews.

Decompression illness (DCI) in a terrestrial environment is caused by rapid changes in ambient pressure, resulting in the formation of bubbles from gases saturated in the tissue. Preparation for EVA involves transitioning from the ambient pressure of the shuttle or ISS to the final 4.3 psi suit pressure. To prevent DCI, astronauts prebreathe 100 percent oxygen for up to 4 h, depending on the protocol used. It is of interest that the protocols evaluated for use in space have been associated with up to a 20 percent incidence of DCI in terrestrial studies, yet no DCI has been reported in space. The relative absence of tissue bubble micronuclei in microgravity has been proposed as a possible explanation. In a terrestrial gravitational environment, moving the extremities against the resistance of gravity will cause small tissue gas micronuclei that can produce evolved tissue gas when subjected to sufficient decompression stress. In the absence of gravity, these micronuclei are either less frequent or do not exist, a phenomenon that would protect against developing DCI. This has been referred to as the *adynamia model*[11] and is currently an area of great research interest due to the large number of EVAs required to build the ISS.

The biomechanics of blunt trauma may also be affected in space, depending on whether the astronaut is inside the spacecraft or performing an EVA. Typically, blunt trauma results from the dissipation of force and transfer of energy to tissue following impact with a fixed or moving object. Objects in space have no weight, yet they still possess mass, an important point when moving a 400-kg object in space with one hand. Significant crushing injuries are a major concern as astronauts move large objects with significant mass within the space station. During an EVA, whether in microgravity or on the surface of another planetary body, crew members wear protective space suits. It is unknown to what degree the space suit would help dissipate force, although their resemblance to an exoskeleton suggests there may be some protective effect.

HEALTH CARE SYSTEM IN SPACE

The delivery of health care in space[12,13] is a team effort. All crew members have sufficient first aid training to act as first responders, and extended medical training is provided to the crew medical officers (CMOs). The majority of CMOs are not health care professionals, although when a career astronaut that is also a physician is assigned to a crew, they are automatically designated the CMO for the flight. CMOs are supported by flight surgeons (FS) sitting on console in mission control and are an important link in the chain of clinical care from space to terrestrial definitive medical care facilities. In the event of significant illness or injury in one of the astronauts on a space station or spacecraft in low earth orbit, the CMO would perform a focused history and physical examination, arrive at a primary diagnosis, and begin treatment as required. The CMO communicates his or her findings to the FS as soon as possible, and may initiate further diagnostic or therapeutic procedures at the request of the FS. Consultative support is available to the FS if necessary.

Some clinical conditions may require mission termination to return the crew member if consumables are depleted in treating the patient, if the treatment is not possible in space, or if the clinical condition of the patient warrants evacuation. Preparation of the shuttle and patient for reentry and landing results in a transport time of between 6 and 24 h to landing at the Kennedy Space Center. Upon landing the patient would be reassessed, treated, and stabilized by the medical support team, and transferred to a definitive medical care facility.

Shuttle On-Board Medical System

The shuttle on-board medical system (SOMS) includes two kits designed to support the delivery of basic life support, first aid, and ambulatory medical care. The emergency medical kit and the medications and bandages kit are stowed on the mid-deck for each orbiter flight. The two soft stowage kits are similar to the jump packs used by many prehospital personnel and include a number of pallets that may be attached with Velcro to the medical worksite. Six pallets are included in the two kits, including injectable drugs, emergency items, diagnostic and therapeutic items, oral drugs, bandage items, and topical medications. The kits can be taken to the location of the ill crew member in the event of a serious injury or illness requiring immediate resuscitation. As in a terrestrial environment, ambulatory patients would be brought to a medical facility, in this case the mid-deck area, for definitive diagnosis and treatment.

One of the unique challenges in providing medical care in a microgravity environment is the need to restrain the patient, CMO, and medical supplies. The configuration of each of the pallets is designed to facilitate their use in microgravity, with extensive use of Velcro and individual pouches for restraint of instruments. Injectable medications are provided in preloaded syringes, and oral medications are stowed in single-dose dispensers.

Advanced cardiac life support (ACLS) capability was developed for the phase 1 NASA-Mir program and has also been flown on dedicated life sciences shuttle flights.[14] The additional equipment includes an advanced airway management kit, defibrillator, and crew medical restraint system. Numerous flights on the KC-135 training aircraft were used to develop and validate procedures to implement resuscitation protocols in microgravity.

ISS Crew Health Care System

The medical capability of the ISS was designed to support the health care needs of long-duration missions. The three main subsystems of the crew health care system (CHeCs) provide physiologic countermeasures, environmental monitoring capability, and a clinical capability to prevent, diagnose, and treat illnesses and injuries during a mission. The countermeasures system (CMS) provides a capability to evaluate crew fitness, implement exercise countermeasures, and monitor crew response to the countermeasures during the mission. The environmental health system (EHS) monitors air and water quality for chemical and microbial contaminants, and monitors radiation levels as well as surface microbial contamination. The health maintenance system (HMS) enables the FS to periodically assess crew health, provides resuscitative and ambulatory care in the event of illness or injury, and is the first link in the chain of clinical care to stabilize and medically evacuate crew to a terrestrial definitive medical care facility.

The primary purpose of the CMS is to prevent the cardiovascular deconditioning, disuse bone loss, and muscle atrophy associated with long-duration space flight. Prescribed exercise protocols are individually developed and performed daily by all ISS crew members except on the day of an EVA or within 24 h of a periodic fitness assessment. The CMS exercise equipment includes a vibration-isolated treadmill and cycle ergometer as well as a resistive exercise device. Heart rate, blood pressure, and electrocardiographic monitoring are provided to evaluate the efficacy of the exercise protocols. Treadmill exercise seems to provide additional benefit in promoting gaze stability and lower extremity proprioceptive training, facilitating neurovestibular readaptation that helps astronauts ambulate after landing.

The closed loop life support systems used in spacecraft are very reliable and provide a shirt-sleeved environment for crew members to live and work in. However, qualitative and quantitative monitoring are crucial to monitor potential toxicologic and microbial contamination of the environment. Periodic water sampling for onboard microbial and toxic contaminants is performed. Samples are obtained for return on the shuttle for terrestrial analysis to validate the data obtained in flight. Kits have been designed for collection of surface samples from different locations throughout the ISS for determination of microbial and fungal contamination. A microbial air sampler is used to record airborne microbial contaminants in the different modules of the ISS.

Radiation monitoring consists of area and personal dosimeters to document dose variation in different areas of the ISS, as well as individual mission doses. Postflight biodosimetry is performed on long-duration astronauts to determine the biological consequences of the prolonged low-dose radiation exposure characteristic of space flight.

The HMS provides a clinical capability similar to that found in many primary care clinics. It is routinely used to prevent, diagnose, and treat minor medical problems, and could be instrumental in saving the life of an acutely ill or injured astronaut. There are five components to the HMS: the ambulatory medical pack (AMP), crew contamination protection kit (CCPK), the advanced life support (ALS) pack, crew medical restraint system (CMRS), and respiratory support pack. The AMP contains individual diagnostic and therapeutic pallets, including a stethoscope, sphygmomanometer, and portable clinical blood analyzer, in addition to medications, bandages, minor surgical instruments, and suture materials. Crew protection from toxic and nontoxic particulates and liquids is provided in the CCPK. The most frequently used item is the space station eyewash system for removal of ocular foreign bodies. In the absence of gravity, small airborne particles are present that can injure the eye. The CCPK also includes goggles, masks, gloves, and multiple waste bags for containment of contaminated material.

The ALS pack, defibrillator, and respiratory support pack provide limited resuscitative capability to manage life-threatening medical and surgical problems. The crew medical restraint system is an integral component of the suite of critical care hardware on the ISS, as it is required to isolate the spacecraft from electrical shocks during defibrillation. It can be deployed within 2 min and provides additional restraints for the CMO. The combined defibrillator and transcutaneous pacer is interfaced through a data interface module to downlink ECG and heart rate data to the FS in mission control.

In addition to the diagnostic capability provided in the HMS, the CMO may use equipment from the human research facility (HRF) for diagnostic purposes. An ultrasound with color Doppler capability is one of many biomedical research devices on the ISS and provides an important noninvasive diagnostic capability to the CMO. Due to the limited imaging capability on the ISS, terrestrial evaluations of nonstandard uses of ultrasound to augment on-orbit diagnostic capabilities have revealed potential value in diagnosing extremity trauma,[15] pneuomothoraces,[16] and dental abscesses.

Medical Events in Space Flight

The combined space flight experience of Russian cosmonauts and NASA and international astronauts has been 25,265 person-days in space by 418 people over 40 years. Up to STS-108, there were 5496 person-days on the shuttle (1981 to 2001) in comparison to the long-duration Skylab experience (504 person-days) and the NASA Mir program (849 person-days). Considering the risks associated with training astronauts and the potential for illness and injury during short- and long-duration missions, it is not surprising that a number of medical events have been reported.

Training for space flight occurs in a wide range of environments, including high-performance jets, simulators, and underwater. It includes extensive physical training and survival training in extreme terrestrial environments. Fatalities have occurred in high-performance jets and during development testing of spacecraft. Successful ejections from the lunar landing research/training vehicle occurred during the Apollo program, and other aviation incidents have included ejections from high-performance jet aircraft, and in one case minor injuries associated with a helicopter crash in flight training. Cases of soft tissue injury, minor extremity trauma, overuse syndromes, and barotrauma have occurred during shuttle and ISS training. The rigorous attention given to safety and training as well as the excellence of facilities, aircraft, and hardware have all been critical in preventing further significant training-related injuries.

Medical events related to space flight may be categorized based upon their occurrence during a particular phase of flight. Events during ascent and re-entry, the dynamic phases of flight, range from relatively insignificant to catastrophic. Fatalities have occurred in both the Russian and U.S. space programs during the launch, ascent, or entry phases of flight. These fatalities have resulted from the failure of specific spacecraft systems that led to either destruction of the vehicle or loss of environmental control. The probability of such events is as low as reasonably achievable due to the appropriate attention given to safety and risk reduction. Improvements in spacecraft design, redundancy, mission support, and flight rules have played key roles in continuing to optimize the safety of human space travel.

Medical events in space are frequent, usually minor, self-limited medical problems. In a review of shuttle missions from 1981 to 1998,[17] 439 male and 69 female astronauts participated in 89 missions, accumulating 4443 days of space flight experience. Overall, 98 percent reported some type of medical problem during the mission, with space motion sickness (79 percent) and headache (67 percent) being the most frequent. The remaining symptoms reported involved respiratory complaints (64 percent), facial fullness (59 percent), gastrointestinal problems (32 percent), and musculoskeletal problems (26 percent). Ocular foreign bodies have been a problem during short-duration missions and were readily treated with the emergency eye-wash kit.

Clinical experience from the NASA Phase 1 Mir program documented skin rashes and infections, crew fatigue, sleep disorders, urinary retention, dental problems, back pain, temporary hearing threshold shifts due to the acoustic environment, minor musculoskeletal injury, and benign dysrhythmias.[18] A fire on the Mir station led to thermal injuries in some of the crew and the collision with the Progress spacecraft resulted in sudden decompression of a module.[19] These environmental hazards and the associated risk of trauma are of significant clinical concern and re-emphasize the need ensure optimum crew safety at all times.

Resuscitation in Microgravity

Electric shock, anaphylaxis, cardiac dysrhythmia, DCI, toxic exposures, trauma, and clinical deterioration of medical or surgical events could all result in situations requiring some degree of resuscitative support. Procedure validation on the KC-135 has documented successful animal resuscitation using a porcine model in microgravity. End-tidal CO_2 measurements during CPR documented the efficacy of chest compressions in producing blood circulation in these trials. Limitations exist in extrapolating this data to space due to the potential impact of the physiologic changes associated with short- and long-duration missions on the efficacy of resuscitation.

In most circumstances the patient would be brought to the HMS where the CMRS, ALS pack, and defibrillator could be readily deployed. It is possible to establish unresponsiveness, open the airway, and verify respiratory and circulatory activity quite readily in any location on the space station. Moving the patient in microgravity to the medical work site is analogous to performing an aquatic rescue on a drowning victim, without the need to move against the resistance of the water. To perform CPR and defibrillate the patient, the CMRS must be deployed with the patient and CMO restrained. The CMO gets into position to perform cardiac compression with the feet pushing against the opposite surface of the module to provide the appropriate body positioning for performing chest compressions.

Rapid sequence defibrillation, intubation, and intravenous access are performed in the CMRS if required. It is anticipated that performing these medical procedures in microgravity will be associated with additional delays due to the difficulty manipulating the patient and equipment. Depending upon the ACLS protocol and the time to establish intravenous access, initial endotracheal drug administration will be followed by subsequent intravenous doses. A constant infusion pump is used to administer the intravenous fluids and volume replacement if required. Limited consumables can be a significant constraint

to resuscitation in space. This limitation may be mitigated by the ready availability of a crew return vehicle with medical evacuation capability.

Blood loss on orbit presents a unique clinical challenge[20] in the absence of blood replacement products, relatively prolonged transport times in comparison to terrestrial prehospital care, and limited capability for volume replacement. Hemorrhagic shock would most likely occur following blunt trauma, although gastrointestinal bleeding and uncontrolled epistaxis could present significant clinical challenges to the CMO and FS.

Surgery in Microgravity

Experience performing surgical procedures in microgravity is limited. The KC-135 has been used to demonstrate the efficacy of a wide range of surgical procedures, including laparoscopic surgery,[21,22] yet caution must be used in applying the results to the space environment. Animal dissections have been performed on a number of life science missions, including the successful reversible administration of a general anesthetic to perform research protocols.[23] The lessons learned reaffirm KC-135 findings documenting the need for patient, operator, and instrument restraint. A number of techniques have been proposed to restrain instruments in microgravity, including Velcro, magnets, and customized minor surgical trays. Customized kits with individual pockets for each surgical instrument were used successfully on the Neurolab mission.

Hemostasis in space does not present any different challenges than those confronting terrestrial surgeons.[24] Direct pressure, cauterization, and wound repair are all equally effective in space. Small or moderate amounts of blood form a dome on adjacent tissues in the absence of gravity. Profound venous and arterial bleeding rapidly produces large domes of blood that temporarily obscure the operative field until hemostasis is achieved and the blood is removed with gauze squares or suction. Uncontrolled arterial bleeding travels in a straight line until hitting a surface. Personal experience performing complex animal dissections, both on the KC-135 and in space, has confirmed that hemostasis does not pose any unique problems in microgravity. Anecdotal data suggest that clotting and wound healing appear normal in space, although confirmatory studies are required.

EVA Medical Support

The medical issues associated with astronauts performing spacewalks fall into several categories: pressure related, suit related, or task related. The transition from 14.7 psi to 4.3 psi in the NASA space suit or 5.7 psi in the Russian space suit is associated with a risk of DCI. A number of different prebreathing protocols exist for the NASA space-suit, and are chosen for operational reasons, while a 30-min 100 percent oxygen prebreathing protocol is used for the Russian Orlan space-suit. Barotrauma and DCI are the two pressure-related clinical concerns during spacewalks. Difficulty equalizing pressure in the ears or sinuses may be encountered and is often prevented by the prophylactic use of oral and nasal decongestants. There have not been any cases of DCI formally reported in either the NASA or Russian space program, although there is one anecdotal mention of isolated joint pain unrelated to an EVA in an Apollo astronaut that was described in a lay publication. To date it has not been possible to objectively validate the efficacy of prebreathing protocols in space. New noninvasive Doppler bubble detection devices may prove useful in this area, but must be certified for use in the 100 percent oxygen environment found in the spacesuit.

Some astronauts have reported minor symptoms related to pressure points in the spacesuit. Considerable effort is spent preflight to optimize suit fit and provide padding in potential areas of irritation. Eye irritation from the anti-fog compound used on the suit helmet visor has also been reported. This typically arises if the mouth seal of the in-suit drink bag leaks and water droplets contact the visor and then enter the astronaut's eyes. Nonirritating anti-fog compounds eliminate this problem.

Astronauts perform a wide range of servicing and construction tasks during a spacewalk. It is not unusual to move large objects that weigh hundreds of kilograms manually while performing EVA tasks. In fact, three astronauts on an early shuttle mission were positioned in the payload bay of the shuttle to manually retrieve a satellite after rendezvous with the shuttle. Despite the evident skill of the astronauts, working with massive payloads introduces the risk of musculoskeletal injury, crushing injuries, and overuse syndromes. Extensive training and crew experience in managing massive payloads has played a critical role in preventing these injuries to date.

Spacewalks during the Apollo program were performed both in space and on the lunar surface. The potential for trauma related to working in a space suit while in the partial gravitational environment of another planet is another area of concern. Minor shoulder strain was reported by one of the Apollo astronauts on the lunar surface while drilling for lunar specimens. Astronauts successfully explored the lunar surface both on foot and in the lunar rover without difficulty.

FUTURE OF SPACE MEDICINE

Space medicine has undergone a gradual evolution from developing and implementing selection and retention standards to minimize the probability of disease in astronauts in space, to providing clinical support for short-duration missions in and beyond low earth orbit, and most recently to supporting a permanent human presence in space on the ISS.[25] The space station not only serves as an orbiting laboratory and technology development platform, it provides clinicians with a unique opportunity to conduct research to optimize crew safety, health, and performance that will be critical in reducing the biomedical risk of extended missions of human space exploration. Spacefaring nations worldwide have sought to extend the accessibility to space for the purposes of research and technological development, commercial utilization, educational outreach, transportation, and exploration. While medical certification standards for professional astronauts and cosmonauts are extremely rigorous, less stringent standards have been developed for space flight participants to enable greater accessibility to space for lay people. Space medicine practitioners will play a critical role in helping engineers optimize the design of space planes to minimize the physiologic challenges experienced by travelers during short episodes of microgravity.

Dr. Williams flew on the STS-90 in April–May 1998. He was also on the first NASA Aquarius mission. He is currently training for his next shuttle flight.

REFERENCES

1. Mills Link M: Mercury medical operations, in *Space Medicine in Project Mercury.* Washington, NASA Scientific and Technical Information Division, 1965.
2. Collins DR, Dotts HW, Hoyler WF, Hecht KF: Spacecraft development, in Gilruth RR, Low GM (eds): *Gemini Midprogram Conference Including Experiment Results.* Houston, TX, Johnson Space Center, NASA, 1966.
3. Machell RM, Shows JC, Corrreale JV, et al: Crew station and extravehicular equipment, in Gilruth RR, Low GM (eds): *Gemini Midprogram Conference Including Experiment Results.* Houston, TX, Johnson Space Center, NASA, 1966.
4. Berry CA, Coons DO, Catterson AD, Kelly GF: Man's response to long-duration flight in Gemini spacecraft, in Gilruth RR, Low GM (eds): *Gemini Midprogram Conference Including Experiment Results.* Houston, TX, Johnson Space Center, NASA, 1966.
5. Johnston RS, Hull WE: Apollo missions, in Johnston RS, Dietlein LF, Berry CA (eds): *Biomedical Results of Apollo.* Washington, NASA Scientific and Technical Information Office, 1973.
6. Hawkins WR, Zieglschmid JF: Clinical aspects of crew health, in Johnston RS, Dietlein LF, Berry CA (eds): *Biomedical Results of Apollo.* Washington, NASA Scientific and Technical Information Office, 1973.
7. Sawin CF, Taylor GR, Smith WL (eds): *Extended Duration Orbiter Medical Project Final Report.* Houston, TX, NASA, 1999.
8. Buckey JC, Lane LD, Levine BD, et al: Orthostatic intolerance after spaceflight. *J Appl Physiol* 81:7, 1996.
9. Lathan CE, Clement G: Response of the neurovestibular system to spaceflight, in Churchill SE (ed): *Fundamentals of Space Life Sciences.* Krieger Publishing, 1997.
10. Williams DR: Optimizing human performance through research and medical innovations. *Nutrition* 18:794, 2002.
11. Conkin J, Powell MR: Lower body adynamia as a factor to reduce the risk of hypobaric DCS. *Aviat Space Environ Med* 72(3):202, 2001.
12. Logan JS: Operational medicine and health care delivery, in Churchill SE (ed): *Fundamentals of Space Life Sciences.* Krieger Publishing, 1997.
13. Williams DR: The biomedical challenges of space flight. *Ann Rev Med* 54:245, 2003.
14. Marshburn T: Resuscitation and Stabilization in Microgravity-Cardiac Resuscitation. Presented at the Institute of Medicine Review of Space Medicine, Johnson Space Center, February 22–24, 2000.
15. Dulchavsky SA, Henry SE, Moed BR, et al: Advanced ultrasonic diagnosis of extremity trauma: the FASTER examination. *J Trauma* 53:28, 2002.
16. Dulchavsky SA, Schwarz KL, Kirkpatrick AW, et al: Prospective evaluation of thoracic ultrasound in the detection of pneumothorax. *J Trauma* 50:201, 2001.
17. Billica R, Marshburn T, Wear M: In-flight Medical Events for Astronauts during the Space Shuttle Program: STS-1 through STS-89. Presented at the Institute of Medicine Review of Space Medicine, Johnson Space Center, February 22, 2000.
18. Marshburn T: Phase 1 Mir Clinical Experience. Presented at the Institute of Medicine Review of Space Medicine, Johnson Space Center, February 22–24, 2000.
19. Shayler DJ: *Disasters and Accidents in Manned Spaceflight.* Chichester, UK, Springer Praxis Publishing, 2000.
20. Kirkpatrick AW, Dulchavsky SA, Boulanger BR, et al: Extraterrestrial resuscitation of hemorrhagic shock: Fluids. *J Trauma* 50:162, 2001.
21. Campbell MR, Billica RD, Jennings R, Johnson SL: Laparoscopic surgery in weightlessness. *Surg Endosc* 10:111, 1996.
22. Campbell MR, Kirkpatrick AW, Billica RD, et al: Endoscopic surgery in weightlessness: The investigation of basic principles for surgery in space. *Surg Endosc* 15:1413, 2001.
23. Buckey JC, Williams D, Riley D: Surgery and recovery in space, in Buckey JC, Homick JL (eds): *The Neurolab Spacelab Mission: Neuroscience Research in Space.* NASA Publications, Houston, TX, 2003.
24. Williams DR: Resuscitation and Stabilization in Microgravity-Surgical Technique. Presented at the Institute of Medicine Review of Space Medicine, Johnson Space Center, February 22–24, 2000.
25. Nicogossian A, Pober D: The future of space medicine. *Acta Astronaut* 49(340):529, 2001.

HYPOGLYCEMIA
William J. Brady
Richard A. Harrigan

Although there is no universally accepted definition of hypoglycemia, it is generally defined as: 1) symptoms consistent with the diagnosis, that 2) usually occur with a serum glucose level of less than 50 to 60 mg/dL, and (3) resolve following glucose administration. Up to 20 percent of patients with diabetes mellitus using insulin or oral hypoglycemic agents (OHAs) will experience symptoms of hypoglycemia in their lifetime, requiring ED evaluation and therapy.[1–3] If one considers all patients with altered mentation arriving at the ED, hypoglycemia is the underlying process in approximately 7 percent. From the perspective of the diabetic patient, hypoglycemia occurs frequently within this population; approximately 25 percent of diabetes patients will experience hypoglycemia on a regular basis.[4] In addition to diabetes, other clinical settings associated with hypoglycemia include sepsis, liver disease, alcohol intoxication, starvation, and certain toxic ingestions. Hypoglycemia should be considered in the differential diagnosis in any patient with altered mental status or focal neurologic signs.

PATHOPHYSIOLOGY

Blood glucose homeostasis involves complex neural, metabolic, and hormonal interactions. The central nervous system (CNS) requires a continuous supply of carbohydrate fuel for normal function and uses approximately 150 g/d of glucose. The CNS has a small reservoir of glucose that is sufficient for only a few minutes of normal brain function. Despite these stringent demands, the body normally functions quite well in maintaining plasma glucose levels within a narrow range despite constant changes in glucose intake and/or utilization.

The primary glucoregulatory organs are the liver, the pancreas, adrenals, and pituitary gland. These organs maintain glucose control by the release and interaction of various hormonal agents, including insulin, glucagon, the catecholamines epinephrine and norepinephrine, cortisol and other glucocorticoids, and growth hormone. Insulin is the major metabolic regulatory factor, acting predominantly on the liver, skeletal muscle, and adipose tissue. Insulin suppresses endogenous glucose production, stimulates glucose use, and increases glucose storage in the form of glycogen, thus lowering the plasma glucose concentration.

The first defense against the development of hypoglycemia is a decrease in insulin secretion. Glucagon and epinephrine are also important for the acute protection against hypoglycemia. Both of these counterregulatory hormones are the only agents capable of stimulating hepatic glucose production within minutes of their release into circulation, primarily by glycogenolysis—the release of glucose from its intracellular storage, depot glycogen. The effect of these two hormones beyond the immediate period after their release—ranging from several hours to several days—is felt predominantly through their effect on gluconeogenesis—the production of glucose from other metabolic substrates. Glucagon is thought to be the major counterregulatory hormone while epinephrine is important under certain conditions, especially during glucagon deficiency and in the generation of warning symptoms of hypoglycemia. Epinephrine also stimulates hepatic glucose production, and also limits glucose use. In contrast to glucagon and epinephrine, glucocorticoid and growth hormone responses are largely involved in the protection against prolonged hypoglycemia over days to weeks.

Hormonal responses are largely determined by glucose intake and vary between the fed and the fasting states. The fed state extends for up to 3 h after the ingestion of food. In the fed state, glucose absorption from the gut stimulates the release of insulin from the pancreas, causing a shift of carbohydrate from the circulation into the various tissues for either consumption or storage. In certain cases, after entry into the cell, glucose is immediately used for energy production by glycolysis, with the glycolytic products proceeding on to the tricarboxylic acid cycle and down the electron transport chain, generating additional ATP. If the glucose is destined for fuel storage, it may take various forms, depending on the host tissue location: glycogen in the liver, triglycerides in adipose tissue, and protein in muscle. Insulin also acts on the liver to decrease glucose output by inhibiting glycogenolysis and gluconeogenesis. It inhibits lipolysis and promotes lipogenesis in adipose cells, and encourages the uptake of amino acids and inhibits proteolysis.

The fasting period is the interval between feedings, beginning approximately 4 h after eating and extending up to the next meal. In fasted individuals, the maintenance of normal blood glucose levels depends on an adequate supply of endogenous gluconeogenic substrates (amino acids, glycerol, and lactate), functionally intact hepatic glycogenolytic and gluconeogenic enzymatic systems, and normal endocrinologic function for integrating and modulating these processes. Hypoglycemia may result if any part of this system is disrupted. During fasting, relatively low insulin levels initiate the mobilization of these various stored fuels from host tissue sources. The most readily and rapidly available source of glucose is hepatic glycogen. Glucose is formed by glycogenolysis, which is potentiated in the liver by glucagon and epinephrine. The glycogen reserve is limited and will be depleted after 24 to 48 h of fasting in healthy patients, and possibly earlier in malnourished individuals. With continuation of fasting (approximately 4 to 6 h), gluconeogenesis becomes the primary source of blood glucose required for CNS metabolism and other bodily processes. Gluconeogenesis, occurring primarily in the liver, uses various metabolic substrates to generate an additional glucose supply. Amino acids are mobilized from muscle tissue by proteolysis, which is facilitated by low insulin levels and mediated by cortisol and glucagon. Lactate, from recycled glucose, and glycerol, from lipolysis, are minor yet important substrates for gluconeogenesis. During nonprolonged overnight fasting, 90 percent of gluconeogenesis occurs via proteolysis with conversion of amino acids to glucose.

If fasting is prolonged beyond the functional capabilities of both gluconeogenesis and glycogenolysis, the mobilization of other fuel stores is initiated with a decline in plasma insulin levels, thus removing the insulin-mediated inhibitory action on lipolysis and proteolysis; alternative fuel stores are then mobilized. Fat stores in the form of triglycerides are a major source of energy. Lipolysis, potentiated by a relative decline in serum insulin levels and the presence of both epinephrine and growth hormone, produces free fatty acids and glycerol. Most tissues, except the CNS and cellular blood elements, use free fatty acids as a source of energy, simultaneously allowing the body to conserve glucose for brain metabolism and sparing protein from catabolism for gluconeogenesis. The released glycerol may also be converted to glucose in the liver.

Hypoglycemia unawareness—the development of low serum sugar values without the physiologic ability to react—places individuals at greater risk for coma and other neurologic sequelae. Extremes of age, comorbidity, medications, autonomic neuropathy, and the degree of serum sugar control are some factors affecting awareness of hypoglycemia. It has been suggested that elderly patients are more likely to experience hypoglycemia without an awareness of the event. As an example, the presence of previous stroke in older patients could increase the chance of unrecognized hypoglycemia. β-Adrenergic receptor antagonists block the effects of epinephrine, therefore contributing to patient unawareness of hypoglycemia. Furthermore, patients with diabetes mellitus and autonomic neuropathy demonstrate blunted counterregulatory responses to hypoglycemia.[5,6] Although somewhat counterintuitive, increasingly rigid control of the serum glucose in patients with diabetes mellitus without neuropathy may also have reduced responsiveness of the counterregulatory hormones, potentiating an unawareness of hypoglycemia.[7] Such a clinical unawareness may result from either a lack of CNS recognition of hypoglycemia or impaired autonomic response to low serum sugar.

CLINICAL FEATURES

Common underlying etiologies among adults likely to be encountered in an ED are diabetic medical therapy, ethanol use, and sepsis.

Common scenarios in diabetic patients include inadequate food intake, increased physical exertion, incorrect medication dosing, or drug interactions. The characteristics of diabetic patients who are more likely to experience hypoglycemia include male gender, adolescent and very elderly age groups, African American heritage, a past history of hypoglycemia, "intensive" diabetic medical therapy, insulin use [compared with oral hypoglycemic agent (OHA) therapy], polypharmacy (more than five agents), and recent hospitalization.[1–3] A recent report notes that insulin therapy, lower hemoglobin A_{1c} levels, younger patient age, and report of past hypoglycemia are also associated with increased prevalence of hypoglycemia.[4]

Table 210-1 compares diabetic medical therapies and their propensity for hypoglycemia. Metformin, a biguanide, improves the end-organ sensitivity to insulin and acts by a number of mechanisms in diabetic patients, including a reduction in hepatic glucose output and enhanced peripheral glucose uptake. Metformin is considered an antihyperglycemic drug rather than a hypoglycemic agent such as the sulfonylureas (OHA) and insulin. Hypoglycemia is rarely, if ever, encountered in patients using only metformin. Three other new classes of medications, which are uncommonly associated with hypoglycemia, include the nonsulfonylurea secretagogues (repaglinide, nateglinide), the α-glucosidase inhibitors (acarbose, miglitol), and the thiazolidinediones (troglitazone, rosiglitazone, pioglitazone). The nonsulfonylurea secretagogues repaglinide and nateglinide increase pancreatic insulin secretion and target postprandial hyperglycemia; they are frequently used either as monotherapy or in combination with metformin. These agents are associated with hypoglycemia—though less often as compared to the OHAs. The α-glucosidase inhibitors acarbose and miglitol decrease gut absorption of carbohydrate; hypoglycemia has not been reported in association with either agent. The thiazolidinediones rosiglitazone and pioglitazone increase use of peripheral glucose; they are not associated with the development of hypoglycemia.

The nonselective β-blocker agents impair glycogenolysis and the hyperepinephrinemic response to lowered serum sugar levels, thus predisposing individuals to hypoglycemia. Hypoglycemia resulting from the sole ingestion of such adrenergic-blocking agents is rare.

At least one study in the past showed that approximately 50 percent of patients treated for hypoglycemia in an urban ED were acutely intoxicated with ethanol or were chronic alcohol abusers. Alcohol inhibits hepatic gluconeogenesis, which becomes problematic when a patient has not eaten for a prolonged period and the glycogen stores have been depleted by glycogenolysis. A 12-h fast is often sufficient for severely malnourished alcoholics to become hypoglycemic. Hypoglycemia has also been produced in healthy adults by infusing 75 g of alcohol after a 36-h fast. Rapid bedside serum glucose determinations should be performed on all patients with any mental status abnormality or evidence of alcohol use.

Sepsis may cause hypoglycemia by inhibition of gluconeogenesis and by increased responsiveness to insulin. Systemic hypoperfusion, often associated with sepsis, increases peripheral glucose use while metabolic acidosis decreases gluconeogenesis. The multiorgan failure associated with the sepsis syndrome not infrequently includes hepatic dysfunction and an increased potential for hypoglycemia.

Patients with hypoglycemia may have a wide array of symptoms and signs. The clinical manifestations of hypoglycemia are divided into two broad categories: *neuroglycopenic and hyperepinephrinemic* (also known as the autonomic or sympathomimetic findings). As glucose is the main energy source for CNS function, it is not surprising that most episodes of symptomatic hypoglycemia include neurologic dysfunction. With a decline in serum sugar, the brain quickly exhausts its reserve supply of carbohydrate fuel, resulting in CNS dysfunction. This manifests most commonly by alterations in consciousness, lethargy, confusion, combativeness, agitation, and unresponsiveness. Other neuroglycopenic manifestations include seizures and focal neurologic deficits.

A rapid fall in blood glucose levels or the hypothalamic sensing of neuroglycopenia causes the release of the counterregulatory hormones, primarily the catecholamines epinephrine and norepinephrine. Their release is responsible for the hyperepinephrinemic findings, including anxiety, nervousness, irritability, nausea, vomiting, palpitations, and tremor.

TABLE 210-1 Diabetic Medical Therapy, Mechanism of Action, and Expected Glycemic Response

Agent (Examples)	Mechanism of Action	Expected Glycemic Response
Insulin (Regular, NPH, Lente, Ultra-lente)	Direct tissue effect	Hypoglycemia

Sulfonylurea (OHA)
  First generation: chlorpropamide, tolbutamide, tolazamide
  Second generation: glyburide, glipizide, glimepiride
	Increased pancreatic insulin secretion	Hypoglycemia

Nonsulfonylurea secretagogues (repaglinide, nateglinide)	Increased pancreatic insulin secretion	Hypoglycemia *(less than OHAs)*
Biguanides (metformin)	Decreased hepatic glucose production	No hypoglycemia
α-Glucosidase inhibitors (acarbose, miglitol)	Decreased gastrointestinal tract glucose absorption	No hypoglycemia
Thiazolidinediones (troglitazone,* rosiglitazone, pioglitazone)	Increased peripheral tissue glucose use	No hypoglycemia

*Removed from the market because of idiosyncratic hepatocellular injury.
Abbreviation: OHA = oral hypoglycemic agent.

The term "hyperepinephrinemic" is a misnomer in that cholinergic factors resulting from autonomic nervous system stimulation are also noted in certain patients. Stimulation of the cholinergic nervous system also occurs and may result in manifestations such as sweating, changes in pupillary size, bradycardia, and salivation.

The rapidity of onset of the hypoglycemic event determines in part the presentation. A gradual onset of hypoglycemia results from a relatively slow decrease in the serum glucose and the development of the neuroglycopenic signs and symptoms. Conversely, a sudden drop in the blood sugar level will produce anxiety, diaphoresis, tremor, and the other hyperepinephrinemic findings. In most cases of hypoglycemia, however, CNS dysfunction predominates with some degree of alteration in the level of awareness, accompanied by diaphoresis and tachycardia.

DIAGNOSIS

Hypoglycemia should always be considered early (including the prehospital setting) as a potential cause of altered mentation. Failure to determine the blood glucose level early in the evaluation can result in a delayed or missed diagnosis with associated morbidity because of CNS injury or unnecessary invasive procedures and therapies. A recent investigation of children requiring advanced resuscitation on ED arrival reported that 18 percent of these patients had hypoglycemia.[8] Hypoglycemia has been misdiagnosed as stroke, transient ischemic attack, seizure disorder, traumatic head injury, brain tumor, narcolepsy, multiple sclerosis, psychosis, sympathomimetic drug ingestion, hysteria, altered sleep patterns and nightmares, and depression.[5,7] Although uncommon, bradycardia has also been reported.

The use of bedside testing is preferred in that the result is immediately available to the clinician and as such may alter therapeutic and diagnostic plans. The accuracy of bedside reflectance tests is acceptable though less reliable at extremely low and high glucose levels. If possible, immediately prior to intravenous dextrose therapy, a serum sample should be obtained and sent to the lab for confirmation. Glucose values of whole blood are approximately 15 percent less than that of serum or plasma. This discrepancy is a result of the relatively low glucose concentration in red blood cells—with storage, equilibration occurs. Venous blood has a 10 percent lower glucose concentration when compared with either capillary or arterial blood. Finally, the collecting tube should contain fluoride to inhibit in vitro glycolysis before the sample is assayed.

TREATMENT

Initial management is the administration of 1 g/kg body weight dextrose, as D50W in adults. This can be followed by the infusion of D10W at a rate to maintain the serum glucose above 100 mg/dL. Repeat bedside glucose determination should be done every 30 min for the first 2 h, to detect rebound hypoglycemia. Oral replacement is best, however. A total of 300 g (1200 cal) of carbohydrate should be given PO, as sodas, juices, sandwiches, or snacks. A total of 50 mL of D50W contains only 100 cal. Whereas some suggest that each ampule of glucose (50 g of a D50W solution) will raise the serum glucose by 60 mg/dL,[9] others feel that prediction of pre- and posttreatment levels is impossible.[10]

Glucagon, 1 mg IM or IV, can be used in diabetics or in those in whom intravenous access is not readily obtainable. Response to glucagon therapy is generally slower when compared with intravenous dextrose, requiring 7 to 10 min prior to normalization of mental status; additionally, the response to glucagon administration may be short-lived. **The condition of alcoholics, the elderly, and others with depleted glycogen stores will generally not improve with glucagon.** Fructose and lactose should not be used to correct hypoglycemia in that these sugars do not cross the blood-brain barrier effectively and require extensive metabolic conversion.

If hyperglycemia is maintained by slow administration of dextrose, the infusion may be reduced and eventually withdrawn. Failure to re-

spond to parenteral glucose administration should prompt consideration of other causes of hypoglycemia, such as sepsis, toxin, insulinoma, hepatic failure, or adrenal insufficiency.

Octreotide, a synthetic analogue of somatostatin, inhibits the release of insulin and has been used in the treatment of sulfonylurea-induced hypoglycemia. One recent report describes the use of octreotide in patients who ingested excessive amounts of sulfonylurea OHA.[11] These patients, prior to octreotide administration, had experienced recurrent hypoglycemia. Soon after the initiation of octreotide therapy, serum sugar levels stabilized with a significant reduction in recurrent hypoglycemia. It is administered subcutaneously at an initial dose of 50 to 125 μg. Constant infusions (125 μg/h) and repeat dosing (50 to 100 μg at 6- to 12-h intervals) have been employed successfully. The optimal dose, frequency of administration, and duration of therapy have not been defined. Intravenous glucose is still the most appropriate therapy for hypoglycemia. **Octreotide is only recommended after initial glucose therapy has been initiated in the sulfonylurea ingestion.** It should be considered when OHA induced hypoglycemia is not responding to dextrose therapy. It is primarily designed to reduce the chance of recurrent hypoglycemia.

A total of 100 mg parenteral thiamine should be given in conjunction with glucose, because, historically, the administration of glucose without thiamine in severe nutritional deficiency states could precipitate Wernicke encephalopathy. Today, this is rare. Thiamine acts as a coenzyme in several reactions in intermediary metabolism, specifically in the conversions of pyruvate to acetyl coenzyme A (linking glycolysis to the tricarboxylic acid cycle) and α-ketoglutarate to succinate (a reaction in the tricarboxylic acid cycle). As thiamine reserves disappear, the reactions halt, removing the CNS's main source of ATP and causing the acute development of Wernicke syndrome. Steroid administration should be considered for hypoglycemia that is either resistant to aggressive glucose replacement therapy or associated with the signs of adrenal insufficiency (see Chap. 217). The dose is 100 to 200 mg hydrocortisone intravenously in adults.

Studies in the early 1980s suggested that hyperglycemia at the time of hospital admission is associated with poor neurologic recovery in stroke patients[12] and survivors of out-of-hospital cardiopulmonary arrest.[13] Similar concern has been voiced regarding the association of worsened neurologic outcome and hyperglycemia in patients with acute head injury.[14,15] It is theorized that hyperglycemia accentuates local tissue damage by continued or increased anaerobic metabolism, lactate production, and intracellular acidosis. Acidosis may trigger a cascade that includes calcium entry into cells, lipolysis, and cytotoxic fatty acid release, culminating in neuronal death. The clinical significance of this issue has not yet been demonstrated; it is a known fact, however, that **untreated hypoglycemia is deleterious to the medically or traumatically injured brain.** Information from these retrospective studies should not alter the management of hypoglycemia at this time.

DISPOSITION

Factors affecting disposition (Table 210-2) include:

1. The patient's current mental status as well as the level of consciousness during observation in the ED;
2. Serial determinations of the serum glucose;
3. Both the timing and extent of the response to resuscitative therapy;
4. The need for additional replacement therapy;
5. Comorbidities;
6. The patient's social situation;
7. Any psychiatric issues;
8. The agent ingested; and
9. Cause of hypoglycemia.

Either continued or recurrent mental status alteration, recurrent hypoglycemia, or a downward trend in serial glucose values during ED

TABLE 210-2   Admission Guidelines in the ED Hypoglycemic Patient

Issue Under Consideration	Indication (Relative/Absolute)	In-patient Location (Noncritical Care Setting vs Critical Care Setting)
Medication etiology: non–short-acting insulins and all OHA	Absolute	Variable
Continued/recurrent mental status change	Absolute	Critical care setting
Continued/recurrent hypoglycemia	Absolute	Likely critical care setting
Requirement for frequent/continuous glucose administrations	Absolute	Critical care setting
Etiology of event: sepsis, severe malnutrition, toxicologic response to ingestion with other body system failures	Absolute	Critical care setting
Psychiatric (i.e., intentional ingestion) etiology	Absolute	Variable
Lack of 1) responsible adult supervision, 2) motivated patient or caretaker, and 3) identified physician care as outpatient	Absolute	Likely noncritical care setting
Patient age: neonate/infant and very elderly	Relative	Variable
Lack of "reactive" hyperglycemia despite adequate glucose replacement therapy	Relative	Variable
Significant comorbidities (renal, hepatic failure)	Relative	Variable
History of hypoglycemia	Relative	Variable

observation despite adequate replacement therapy demands admission to the hospital. Also, any patient requiring large doses of dextrose as both bolus and infusion should be admitted. An inpatient disposition in a critical care setting is likely warranted in cases involving the following etiologies: massive insulin or OHA ingestion, marked malnutrition, sepsis, acute liver failure, or any other event associated with the tendency toward profound hypoglycemia. Furthermore, patients without proper outpatient supervision should be admitted for observation.

The case suitable for outpatient observation is characterized by a responsible adult who will monitor the patient's mental status frequently on a regular basis, coupled with a motivated patient who will perform serum glucose determinations frequently and who can maintain oral feeding. Patients managed in a chronic care facility with adequate nursing supervision may also be managed out-of-hospital in such a setting, assuming that they have remained stable during ED observation. The use of this option is at the discretion of the treating physician's review who has reviewed all facets of the clinical presentation. The suspected or known *intentional* ingestion of either insulin or OHA must be admitted for ongoing medical and psychiatric care.

The particular medication agent ingested must be considered in disposition decisions as well. Short-acting insulin preparations do not always demand hospitalization, whereas intermediate- and long-acting preparations likely will require admission for ongoing observation and, at times, continued supportive care. Care must be exercised in large short-acting insulin exposures in that the pharmacodynamics of such insulin preparations are altered with massive doses. The expected short half-life may not be encountered. OHAs also represent a possible indication for hospitalization due to relatively long serum half-life with a prolonged tendency toward the development of hypoglycemia. Patients with OHA excess and end-stage renal disease may experience prolonged periods of hypoglycemia and therefore warrant inpatient management.[16] Low serum glucose may develop as long as 16 h after ingestion, although the majority of patients will become symptomatic within 8 h of exposure. A single tablet ingestion by a child can produce significant hypoglycemia. Finally, if any doubt exists as to the need for inpatient observation, admission for short-term observation is justified. If a patient is discharged, follow-up should be provided within a reasonably short period of time with the primary care physician.

The above recommendations are largely based on retrospective data, practice patterns, anecdote, and medical "common sense"; they lack significant support in the medical literature. One recent investigation, which compared the outcome of diabetic hypoglycemic patients who refused emergency medical services (EMS) transport with those individuals transported to the ED, does support the contention that many patients with hypoglycemia experience prompt, rapid return to the nonhypoglycemic state. Of 517 instances, 374 patients, the vast majority (72 percent), refused EMS transport. The rates of relapse did not differ between those patients refusing and accepting EMS transportation to the ED, and the nontransported patients did not suffer significant morbidity or mortality after termination of prehospital medical care. While the out-of-hospital treatment of hypoglycemic patients may be safe and effective,[17] it should be noted that patients refusing transport may self-select for lower likelihood of adverse outcome. The treating clinician must weigh numerous factors and exercise medical judgment in arriving at the appropriate, safe disposition for the patient.

REFERENCES

1. Hayward RA, Manning WG, Kaplan SH, et al: Starting insulin therapy in patients with type 2 diabetes: Effectiveness, complications, and resource utilization. *JAMA* 278:1663, 1997.
2. Anonymous: Hypoglycemia in the Diabetes Control and Complications Trial: The Diabetes Control and Complications Trial Research Group. *Diabetes* 46:271, 1997.
3. Shorr RI, Ray WA, Daugherty JR, Griffin MR: Incidence and risk factors for serious hypoglycemia in older persons using insulin or sulfonylureas. *Arch Intern Med* 157:1681, 1997.
4. Miller CD, Phillips LS, Ziemer DC, et al: Hypoglycemia in patients with type 2 diabetes mellitus. *Arch Intern Med* 161:1653, 2001.
5. Fanelli C, Pampanelli S, Lalli C, et al: Long-term intensive therapy of IDDM patients with clinically overt autonomic neuropathy: Effects on hypoglycemia awareness and counterregulation. *Diabetes* 46:1172, 1997.
6. Segel SA, Paramore DS, Cryer PE: Hypoglycemia-associated autonomic failure in advanced type 2 diabetes. *Diabetes* 51:724, 2002.
7. Boyle PJ, Kempers SF, O'Connor AM, Nagy RJ: Brain glucose uptake and unawareness of hypoglycemia in patients with insulin-dependent diabetes mellitus. *New Engl J Med* 333:1726, 1995.
8. Losek JD: Hypoglycemia and the ABC'S (sugar) of pediatric resuscitation. *Ann Emerg Med* 35:43, 2000.
9. Hoffman RS, Goldfrank LR: The poisoned patient with altered consciousness: Controversies in the use of a "coma cocktail." *JAMA* 274:562, 1995.

10. Balentine JR, Gaeta TJ, Kessler D, et al: Effect of 50 milliliters of 50 percent dextrose in water administration on the blood sugar of euglycemic volunteers. *Acad Emerg Med* 5:691, 1998.
11. MacLaughlin SA, Crandell CS, McKinney PE: Octreotide: An antidote for sulfonylurea-induced hypoglycemia. *Ann Emerg Med* 36:133, 2000.
12. Pulsinelli WA, Levy DE, Sigsbee B, et al: Increased damage after ischemic stroke in patients with hyperglycemia with or without established diabetes mellitus. *Am J Med* 74:540, 1983.
13. Longstreth WT, Inui TS: High blood glucose level on hospital admission and poor neurological recovery after cardiac arrest. *Ann Neurol* 15:59, 1984.
14. Lam AM, Winn HR, Cullen BF, et al: Hyperglycemia and neurologic outcome in patients with head injury. *J Neurosurg* 75:545, 1991.
15. Young B, Ott L, Dempsey R, et al: Relationship between admission hyperglycemia and neurologic outcome of severely brain-injured patients. *Ann Surg* 210:466, 1989.
16. Krepinsky J, Ingram AJ, Clase CM: Prolonged sulfonylurea-induced hypoglycemia in diabetic patients with end-stage renal disease. *Am J Kidney Dis* 35:500, 2000.
17. Socransky SJ, Pirrallo RG, Rubin JM: Out-of-hospital treatment of hypoglycemia: Refusal of transport and patient outcome. *Acad Emerg Med* 5:1080, 1998.

DIABETIC KETOACIDOSIS
Michael E. Chansky
Cary L. Lubkin

Diabetic ketoacidosis (DKA) is an acute, life-threatening complication of diabetes mellitus. DKA occurs predominantly in patients with type I (insulin-dependent) diabetes mellitus but is also well described in type II (non-insulin-dependent) diabetes mellitus.[1] DKA accounts for 24 percent of all diabetic admissions and has an incidence among diabetics in the United States of 15 episodes per 1000 patients.[2] Europe has a comparable incidence. Between 20 and 30 percent of cases oc-

cur in patients with new-onset diabetes. Better understanding of pathophysiology and an aggressive, uniform approach to diagnosis and management have reduced mortality to less than 5 percent of reported episodes.[3] However, mortality is higher in the elderly due to underlying renal disease or coexisting infection.

PATHOPHYSIOLOGY

In simplest terms, DKA represents the body's response to cellular starvation brought on by relative insulin deficiency and counterregulatory or catabolic hormone excess (Figure 211-1). Insulin is the only anabolic hormone produced by the endocrine pancreas and is responsible for the metabolism and storage of carbohydrates, fat, and protein. Counterregulatory hormones include glucagon, catecholamines, cortisol, and growth hormone. The lack of insulin and the exces counterregulatory hormones result in hyperglycemia (due to excess production and underutilization of glucose), osmotic diuresis, prerenal azotemia, ketone formation, and a wide-anion gap metabolic acidosis.[3,4]

Insulin

Ingested glucose is the primary stimulant of insulin release from the β-cells of the pancreas. Insulin's main action occurs at the three principal tissues of energy storage and metabolism (i.e., liver, adipose tissue, and skeletal muscle). Insulin acts on the liver to facilitate the uptake of glucose and its conversion to glycogen while inhibiting glycogen breakdown (glycogenolysis) and suppressing gluconeogenesis. The net effect of these actions is to promote the storage of glucose in the form of glycogen. Insulin's effect on lipid metabolism is to increase lipogenesis in the liver and adipose cells by the production of triglycerides from free fatty acids and glycerol while inhibiting the breakdown of triglycerides. Insulin stimulates the uptake of amino acids into muscle cells with subsequent incorporation into muscle protein while preventing the release of amino acids from muscle and hepatic protein sources.

FIG. 211-1. Pathogenesis of DKA secondary to relative insulin deficiency and counterregulatory hormone excess.

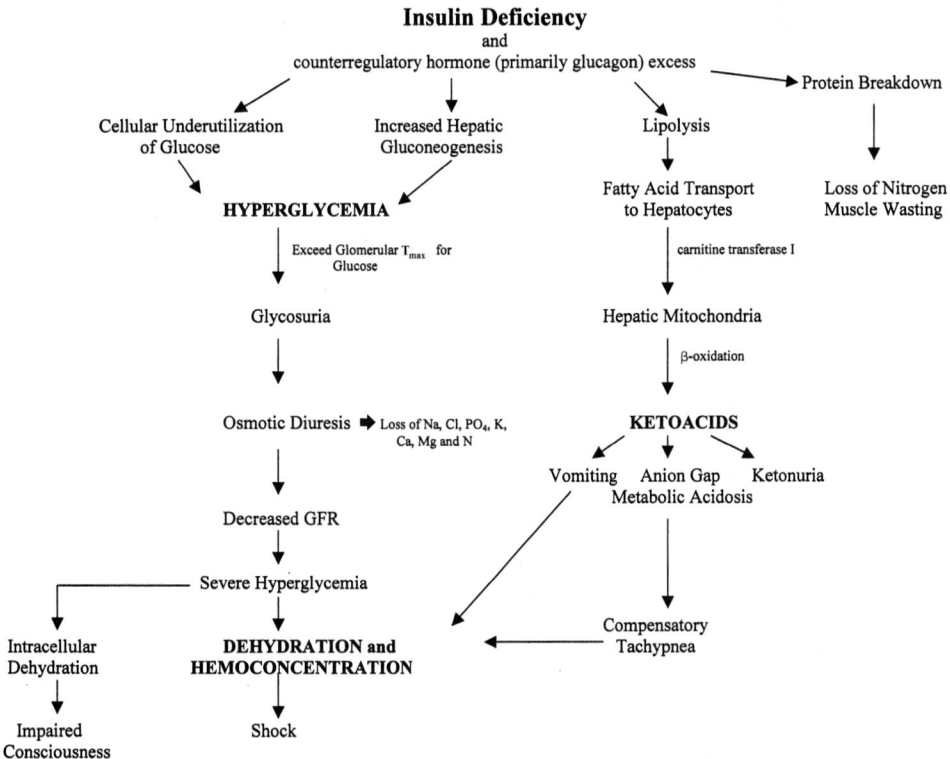

Deficiency in insulin secretion due to loss of islet cell mass is the predominant lesion in diabetes mellitus, and it may be partial or total. In the initial stages of diabetes mellitus, the secretory failure of β cells impairs fuel storage and may be evident only during a glucose-tolerance test. As the disease progresses and levels of insulin decrease, fuel stores are mobilized during fasting, resulting in hyperglycemia. When pancreatic β-cell reserve is present, hyperglycemia may trigger an increase in insulin and a return to normal glucose concentration. With further disease progression, hyperglycemia can no longer trigger an increase in insulin activity. Despite the presence of elevated intravascular glucose, in the absence of insulin, the cells are unable to use glucose as a fuel source. The body responds by breakdown of protein and adipose stores to try to produce a usable intracellular fuel. Loss of the normal physiologic effects of insulin leads to secretion of catabolic hormones and resulting hyperglycemia and ketonemia.

Counterregulatory Hormones

The response to cellular starvation seen with insulin insufficiency is increased levels of glucagon, catecholamines, cortisone, and growth hormone. Glucagon is the primary counterregulatory hormone. The catabolic effects of these hormones include increased gluconeogenesis and glycogenolysis, breakdown of fats into free fatty acids and glycerol, and proteolysis with increased levels of amino acids. Increased levels of glucogenic precursors, such as glycerol and amino acids, facilitate gluconeogenesis, worsening hyperglycemia.

Free fatty acids released in the periphery are bound to albumin and transported to the liver, where they undergo conversion to ketone bodies. The primary ketone bodies β-hydroxybutyric acid (βHB) and acetoacetic acid (AcAc) account for the metabolic acidosis seen in DKA. The two are in equilibrium: $AcAc + NADH = \beta HB + NAD$. AcAc is metabolized to acetone, another major ketone body. Depletion of baseline hepatic glycogen stores tends to favor ketogenesis. Low insulin levels decrease the ability of the brain and cardiac and skeletal muscle to use ketones as an energy source, also increasing ketonemia. The persistently elevated serum glucose level eventually causes an osmotic diuresis. The resulting volume depletion worsens hyperglycemia and ketonemia.

The renin-angiotensin-aldosterone system, activated by volume depletion, exacerbates renal potassium losses already occurring from osmotic diuresis. In the kidney, chloride is retained in exchange for the ketoanions being excreted. This loss of ketoanions represents a loss of potential bicarbonate. In the face of marked ketonuria, a superimposed hyperchloremic acidosis is also present. The presence of a concurrent hyperchloremic metabolic acidosis can be detected by noting a $[HCO_3^-]$ lower than explainable by the amount the anion gap has increased (see Chap. 25). As adipose tissue is broken down, prostaglandins PGI_2 and PGE_2 are produced. Both account for the paradoxical vasodilation that occurs despite profound levels of volume depletion. They may be responsible for the fact that acute renal failure and extremity gangrene rarely develop in DKA despite volume depletion.

DKA in Pregnancy

Several physiologic changes in pregnant patients make them more prone to DKA. Maternal fasting serum glucose levels are normally lower, which leads to relative insulin deficiency and an increase in baseline free fatty acid levels in the blood. Pregnant patients normally have increased levels of counterregulatory hormones. In addition, the chronic respiratory alkalosis seen in pregnancy leads to decreased bicarbonate levels due to a compensatory renal response, resulting in a decrease in buffering capacity. Pregnant patients also have an increased incidence of vomiting and infections (e.g., urinary tract infections, sinusitis, and otitis media), which are frequent precipitants of DKA. In addition, DKA is triggered at lower sugar levels in the pregnant population.[5] Maternal acidosis causes fetal acidosis, decreases

uterine blood flow and fetal oxygenation, and shifts the oxygen-hemoglobin dissociation curve to the right. Maternal hypokalemia also can lead to fetal dysrhythmias and death.

Causes of Diabetic Ketoacidosis

Factors known to precipitate DKA include omission of daily insulin injections and a variety of stressful events, such as infection, stroke, myocardial infarction, trauma, pregnancy, hyperthyroidism, pancreatitis, pulmonary embolism, surgery, and steroid use. Studies have shown that errors in insulin usage are a much more common precipitant than previously thought, especially in the younger population.[6] In approximately 25 percent of patients, no clear precipitating cause is found.[7]

CLINICAL FEATURES

The clinical manifestations of DKA are related directly to the three primary metabolic derangements-hyperglycemia, volume depletion, and acidosis. Hyperglycemia causes an increased osmotic load with movement of intracellular water into the vascular compartment. The ensuing osmotic diuresis gradually leads to volume loss in addition to renal losses of sodium, chloride, potassium, phosphorous, calcium, and magnesium. Initially, patients may compensate by increasing their fluid intake. In this initial period, polyuria and polydipsia are usually the only symptoms until ketonemia and acidosis develop. As acidosis progresses, the patient develops a compensatory augmented ventilatory response. Increased ventilation is stimulated physiologically by acidemia to diminish the P_{CO_2} and thus counters the metabolic acidosis. The acidosis combined with the effects of PGI_2 and PGE_2 lead to peripheral vasodilation despite profound levels of volume depletion. Prostaglandin release is also felt to play a role in the often unexplained nausea, vomiting, and abdominal pain that are seen frequently at presentation, especially in children. Vomiting, which may be a maladaptive physiologic response to diminish the acid load, unfortunately exacerbates the potassium losses and contributes to rapidly progressive volume loss, weakness, and weight loss. As volume depletion progresses, poor absorption of subcutaneous insulin renders its administration ineffective. Mental confusion or coma may be apparent at the time of presentation; these symptoms are much more likely with a serum osmolarity of greater than 340 mosm/L. If the serum osmolarity is less than 340 mosm/L in a comatose patient, another cause of the coma should be sought.

Abnormal vital signs may be the only significant physical findings at the time of presentation. Tachycardia and either significant orthostasis or hypotension are usually present. Poor skin turgor denotes significant volume depletion. With severe acidemia, Kussmaul respirations may be observed. Acetone produces the characteristic fruity odor on the breath found in some patients. The absence of fever does not exclude infection as a source of the patient's ketoacidosis. Hypothermia is present occasionally because of the aforementioned peripheral vasodilation.

Abdominal pain and tenderness can be due to gastric dilatation, ileus, or pancreatitis. Due to the frequency of abdominal pain and the presence of an elevated serum amylase level in both DKA and pancreatitis, distinguishing the diagnoses may be difficult. An elevated serum lipase level is more specific to pancreatitis and should be used to differentiate the two conditions.

ANCILLARY TESTS

When DKA is suspected, initial steps should include a test-strip glucose determination, a urine test strip, an electrocardiogram (ECG), venous blood gas determinations, and a normal saline intravenous drip. Almost all patients with DKA present with a blood glucose level greater than 300 mg/dL. Patients who present just after receiving insulin or who have impaired gluconeogenesis (e.g., in alcohol abuse or liver failure) may have lower initial serum glucose levels.[4] Elevated serum levels of βHB and AcAc cause acidosis and ketonuria. The **nitroprusside** reagent normally used to detect urine and serum ketones **only detects AcAc.** Acetone is only weakly reactive and βHB not at all. NADH accumulation in mitochondria, as may occur with lactic acidosis or alcohol metabolism, favors the βHB side of the equation noted earlier. The enzymatic test for βHB is reliable but not widely available. Paradoxically, as the patient is being treated and clinically improves, measured ketone levels will increase as the body converts the more acidic βHB to AcAc. Therefore, ketones need only be checked initially in the urine. Serum electrolytes should be examined carefully for multiple metabolic abnormalities. Elevated serum ketone levels lead to a wide-anion-gap metabolic acidosis. Hyperchloremic acidosis also occurs on the basis of ketoanion exchange for chloride in the urine; this is especially true in patients who maintain good hydration status and glomerular filtration rate despite ketoacidosis. Metabolic alkalosis also can occur secondary to vomiting, osmotic diuresis, and concomitant diuretic use. Some patients with DKA may present with normal-appearing [HCO$_3^-$] or even alkalemia if these other alkalotic processes are severe enough to mask the acidosis. In such situations, **an elevated anion gap may be the only clue to the presence of an underlying metabolic acidosis** otherwise masked by the concomitant volume contraction-related metabolic alkalosis.

Arterial blood gases (ABGs) have been used traditionally to help determine precise acid-base status in order to direct treatment, but venous pH is just as helpful. A decreased Pco$_2$ determination usually reflects respiratory compensation for metabolic acidosis. If it is lower than explained by the degree of acidosis, as indicated by the [HCO$_3^-$], a primary respiratory alkalosis exists, which may be an early indication of pulmonary disease (e.g., pneumonia, pulmonary embolus) as a possible trigger of the DKA or associated sepsis. (Chap. 25 details how compensatory changes in Pco$_2$ can be distinguished from a primary respiratory alkalosis.) Recent studies have shown a strong correlation between venous and arterial pH in patients with DKA.[8] Venous pH obtained during routine phlebotomy potentially can be used to avoid ABGs, which are painful and may cause arterial vascular complications. Also, serial venous blood draws, should they be necessary to follow acid-base status, are more easily tolerated.

Total body potassium is depleted by renal losses. However, the measured serum potassium level is normal or elevated in most patients[3] because of two important factors: extracellular shift of potassium secondary to acidemia and increased intravascular osmolarity caused by hyperglycemia.[9] Prerenal azotemia also contributes by interfering with kaliuresis. Osmotic diuresis leads to excessive renal losses of sodium chloride in the urine. However, the presence of hyperglycemia tends to artificially lower the serum sodium levels. The standard teaching is that 1.6 mEq should be added to the reported sodium value for every 100 mg of glucose over 100 mg/dL. However, the correction factor is probably 2.4, especially for blood glucose levels over 400 mg/dL.[10] Osmotic diuresis also causes urinary losses and total-body depletion of phosphorous, calcium, and magnesium. Be aware that hemoconcentration frequently leads to initially elevated levels of these electrolytes in serum. As therapy progresses, lower serum levels of each will be evident.

Serum creatinine frequently may be elevated factitiously if the laboratory assays for creatinine and AcAc interfere. Some elevation in creatinine is expected due to prerenal azotemia. Liver function studies may be elevated because of fatty infiltration of the liver, which gradually corrects as the acidosis is treated. Creatine phosphokinase (CPK) and amylase are also frequently elevated at the time of presentation. Leukocytosis is often present because of hemoconcentration and stress. However, an absolute band count of 10,000 μL or more has been shown to reliably predict infection in this population.[11]

ECG changes of hyperkalemia or hypokalemia may be seen. These changes are often transient because of the rapidly changing metabolic status. The ECG also should be evaluated for ischemia because myocardial infarction may precipitate DKA. The underlying rhythm is usually sinus tachycardia.

DIFFERENTIAL DIAGNOSIS

Although the exact definition of DKA is variable, most experts agree that a blood glucose level greater than 250 mg/dL, a bicarbonate level of less than 15 mEq/L, and an arterial pH of less than 7.3 with moderate ketonemia constitute the diagnosis.[3,4]

The differential diagnosis of metabolic coma in a diabetic patient includes hypoglycemia, nonketotic hyperosmotic coma, alcoholic ketoacidosis, lactic acidosis, and other causes of wide-anion gap acidosis. A rapid differentiation can be made in the ED using a glucose reagent strip, a urine test strip for ketones, and blood gas analysis. As an initial rapid diagnostic step, the finding of an elevated glucose level with the concomitant detection of ketones (by point-of-care testing methods) and the presence of metabolic acidosis on venous or arterial blood gas analysis have few rival diagnoses other than DKA. Evaluation of the anion gap is usually superior to pH or [HCO$_3^-$] determination alone because "widening" of the anion gap is independent of potentially masking effects of concurrent acid-base disturbances. The clinician who is not well acquainted with the nuances of blood gas interpretation (see Chap. 25) will be confused when the pH and [HCO$_3^-$] are close to normal. Although the pH and [HCO$_3^-$] are usually examined in addition to the anion gap, both of the former can be affected by concurrent acid-base disturbances such as a metabolic alkalosis or respiratory alkalosis. Patients with hyperosmolar, nonketotic coma tend to be older, have a more prolonged course, and have prominent mental status changes. Their serum glucose levels generally are much higher (>600 mg/dL), and they have little to no anion-gap metabolic acidosis.[3]

The differential diagnosis of DKA (see Table 211-1) includes any entity that causes a high-anion-gap metabolic acidosis. These include alcoholic or starvation ketoacidosis, uremia, lactic acidosis, and various ingestions (e.g., methanol, ethylene glycol, and aspirin). The ketosis in alcoholic ketoacidosis and starvation ketosis tends to be milder, and the serum glucose level is usually low or normal. βHB predominates in alcoholic ketoacidosis, so the urinary ketone test may be negative. If an ingestion cannot be excluded, serum osmolarity or drug-level testing is required. Depending on the hemodynamic status, lactic acidosis (poor perfusion) may occur simultaneously with DKA; in these cases, determination of the serum lactate level is indicated. Patients on metformin with new-onset renal insufficiency are at risk for developing type B (aerobic) lactic acidosis. The absence or presence of only moderate ketonemia should elicit a search for lactic acidosis because its presence favors the undetected βHB as the predominant ketone.

TREATMENT

The diagnosis of DKA should be suspected at triage, and aggressive fluid therapy should be initiated prior to receiving the laboratory results[3] (Figure 211-2). Patients should be placed on a monitor in an acute care setting immediately and have at least one large-bore (16- to 18-gauge) intravenous line of NS running, a second intravenous line of ½NS at minimal rate to keep the intravenous line open. Obtain a rapid bedside glucose determination, a urine test strip, and an ECG. A complete blood count (CBC); determination of electrolyte, phosphate, magnesium, and calcium levels; blood cultures; and other

TABLE 211-1 Differential Diagnosis for DKA

Alcoholic ketoacidosis
Starvation ketoacidosis
Uremia
Lactic acidosis
Ingestions
  Salicylates
  Ethylene glycol
  Methanol

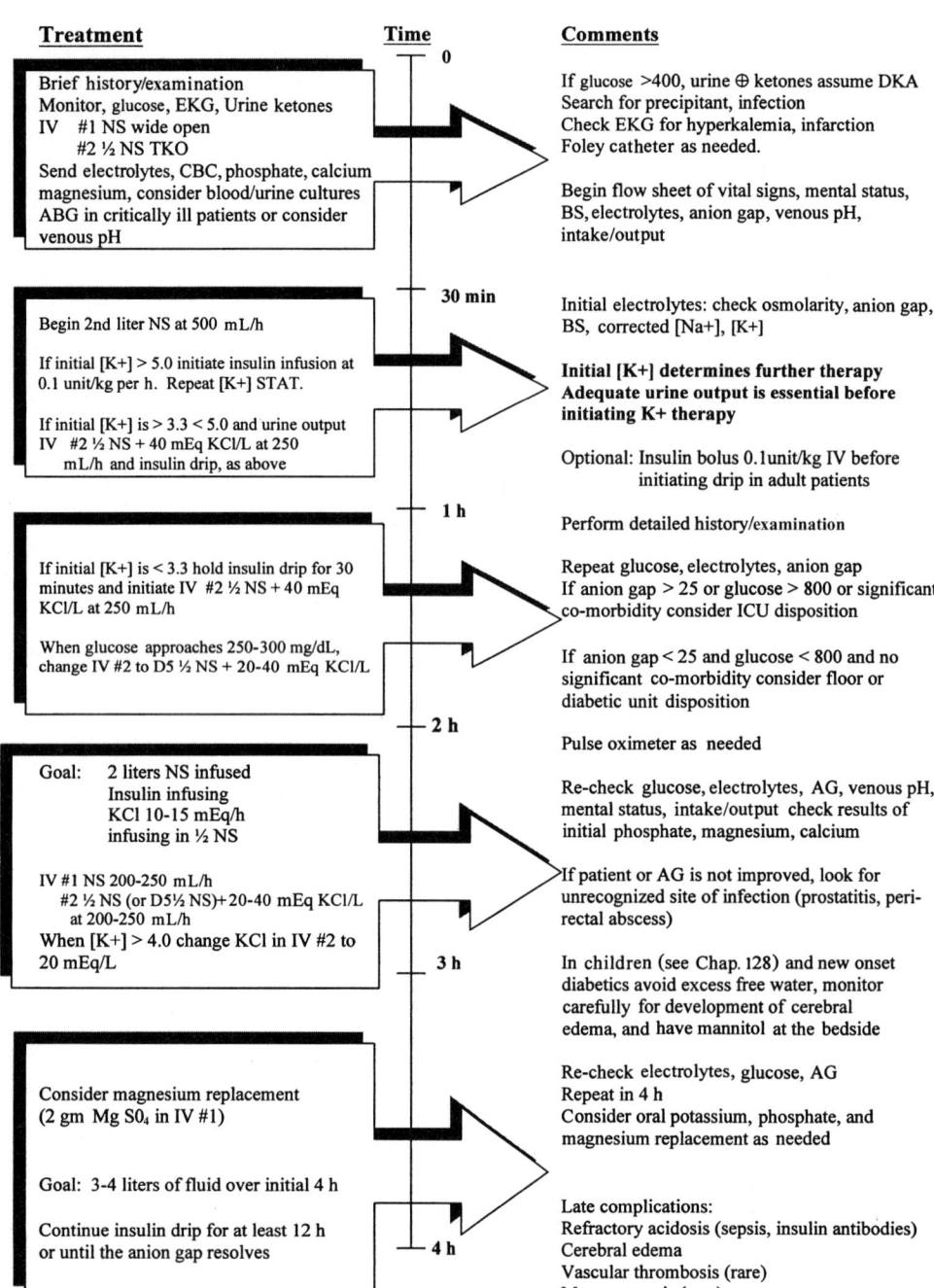

FIG. 211-2. Time line for the typical adult patient with suspected DKA.

laboratory tests should be done as indicated. Arterial blood gas determinations are optional and are only required for the diagnosis and monitoring of critically ill patients. Consider using venous pH determinations (approximately 0.03 lower than arterial pH)[8] for monitoring critically ill patients. The goals of therapy include volume repletion, reversal of the metabolic consequences of insulin insufficiency, correction of electrolyte and acid-base imbalances, recognition and treatment of precipitating causes, and avoidance of complications. Metabolic disturbances should be corrected at the rate of occurrence or over 24 to 36 h.

Meeting the goals of safely replacing deficits and supplying missing insulin requires frequent (every 1–2 h) monitoring of electrolytes (glucose, potassium, and anion gap), vital signs, level of consciousness, and volume input/output until recovery is well established. Resolving hyperglycemia alone is not the end point of therapy. Con-

comitant resolution of the metabolic acidosis (or inhibition of ketoacid production) signifies resolution of DKA. Normalization of the anion gap usually requires 8 to 16 h and reflects clearance of ketoacids. **The order of therapeutic priorities is volume first and foremost** and then insulin and/or potassium, phosphate, magnesium, and bicarbonate.

Fluid Administration

Rapid fluid administration is the single most important initial step in the treatment of DKA.[3] Fluid helps restore intravascular volume and normal tonicity, perfuse vital organs, improve glomerular filtration rate (GFR), and lower serum glucose and ketone levels. The average adult patient has a water deficit of 100 mL/kg (5–10 L) and a sodium deficit of 7 to 10 mEq/kg.[3] NS is the most frequently recommended fluid for initial volume repletion, even though the extracellular fluid of the patient is hypertonic initially. NS does not provide "free water" to correct intracellular fluid loss, but it does prevent an excessively rapid fall in extracellular osmolarity and the resulting devastating transfer of excessive water into the central nervous system (CNS). After initial resuscitation with NS, most authors favor alternating the administration of NS with $\frac{1}{2}$NS[3] or using two intravenous lines—one with NS and the other with $\frac{1}{2}$NS.

Based on clinical suspicion alone and prior to initial electrolyte results, the first liter of NS should be administered well within the first 30 min unless there are mitigating circumstances. In general, the first 2 L are administered rapidly over 0 to 2 h, the next 2 L over 2 to 6 h, and then 2 L more over 6 to 12 h. This replaces approximately 50 percent of the total water deficit over the first 12 h, with the remaining 50 percent water deficit to be replaced over the subsequent 12 h. The blood glucose and ketone body concentrations begin to fall after fluid administration and before implementation of any other therapeutic modality. Hydration alone will reduce the glucose concentration somewhat over 12 to 14 h.[4] Tissue perfusion is restored with volume repletion, improving the effectiveness of insulin. The subsequent rise in GFR allows for glucose and ketone body clearance, lowering serum glucose concentration and osmolarity. The patient's blood glucose level needs to be monitored carefully, and D5 is added to the rehydration solution when the glucose level is 250 to 300 mg/dL.

The fluid should be changed to a hypotonic solution ($\frac{1}{2}$NS or D5$\frac{1}{2}$NS if blood glucose level is less than 300 mg/dL) after initial replacement of intravascular volume with NS. Patients presenting without extreme volume depletion can be managed safely with a modest fluid replacement regimen (500 mL/h for 4 h).[12] Monitoring central venous pressure or pulmonary artery wedge pressure should be considered during fluid replacement in elderly patients or in those with heart disease. Although a common pitfall is failure to give adequate volume replacement, excess fluid may contribute to the development of adult respiratory distress syndrome and cerebral edema.[13]

Insulin

Initial volume repletion reduces the level of counterregulatory hormones, replaces vital fluid and electrolytes, and more important, makes cells more responsive to insulin. It is generally accepted that the "ideal way" to administer insulin is by continuous intravenous infusion of small doses of regular insulin through an infusion pump.[3,14] This approach appears to be more physiologic, helps produce a more linear fall in serum glucose and ketone body levels, and is associated with less severe metabolic complications (hypoglycemia, hypokalemia, and hypophosphatemia).

Low-dose regular insulin administration by an infusion pump is simple and safe, ensures a steady blood concentration, and allows flexibility in adjusting the insulin dose. Insulin inhibits gluconeogenesis, lipolysis, catabolic hormone secretion, and the production of ketoacids, in addition to promoting potassium, glucose, and phosphate uptake in tissues. After the initial fluid bolus, insulin is administered at 0.1 unit/kg per h. The effect of insulin begins almost immediately after initiation of the infusion. A loading dose has not been proven necessary. The desired gradual decrease in serum glucose level is secondary to improved renal perfusion as fluids are administered and insulin receptors become saturated. Recent reviews have different recommendations regarding the use of an insulin loading or priming dose.[3,4,7] An intravenous loading dose is not recommended in children and is optional in adults. The half-life of insulin given IV is 4 to 5 min, with an effective biologic half-life at the tissue level of approximately 20 to 30 min. Because insulin binds to plastic tubing, the first 25 mL of a prepared insulin solution (100 units of regular insulin in 100 mL of NS) should be discarded, and the drip should be placed into an established intravenous line on an infusion pump at the port closest to the skin. Serious complications with continuous intravenous

low-dose insulin infusions are minimal. Frequent monitoring is required to ensure that insulin is being administered in the desired amount.

Intramuscular or subcutaneous administration of regular insulin in DKA is to be avoided.[15] Insulin absorption may be erratic in the volume-depleted, vasoconstricted patient, delaying the achievement of adequate insulin levels. Furthermore, delayed absorption can produce deposits of insulin that may be absorbed later, causing hypoglycemia.

The incidence of nonresponse to low-dose continuous intravenous insulin administration is 1 to 2 percent. Infection is the primary reason for failure to respond. If the patient fails to respond to low-dose insulin therapy, i.e., a decrease of the serum glucose level by 50 to 70 mg/dL in the first hour (assuming adequate hydration), the infusion rate should be doubled or an intravenous bolus (0.2–0.4 units/kg) administered.[3]

The insulin infusion should continue until ketonemia has cleared and the anion gap has normalized. As noted previously, there is conversion from βHB to AcAc, with "increasing ketones" measurable in the serum and urine. Therefore, the anion gap is the most accurate determinant of ongoing recovery. Resolution of hyperglycemia usually occurs earlier than the anion gap, and it may be necessary to administer glucose from the beginning of insulin therapy or shortly after its institution. In most patients, continuous intravenous insulin therapy should continue for at least 12 h (or until resolution of the anion gap), and an overlap period in which subcutaneous insulin is initiated should precede discontinuation of the insulin.

In the rare patient with initial hypokalemia (<3.3 mEq), insulin can precipitate life-threatening hypokalemic effects.[3] While there are no studies supporting the administration of potassium prior to insulin therapy, the American Diabetes Association (ADA) suggests that parenteral potassium should be administered (10–15 mEq/h) 30 min prior to insulin.[3]

Potassium

Patients in DKA usually present with profound total-body potassium deficits in the range of 3 to 5 mEq/kg.[3] This deficiency is created by insulin deficiency, metabolic acidosis, osmotic diuresis, and frequent vomiting. Only 2 percent of total-body potassium is intravascular. The initial serum concentration is usually normal or high because of the intracellular exchange of potassium for hydrogen ions during acidosis, the total-body fluid deficit, and the diminished renal function. Initial hypokalemia indicates severe total-body potassium depletion, and large amounts of potassium are necessary for replacement in the first 24 to 36 h.

The goals of potassium replacement are to maintain a normal extracellular potassium concentration during the acute phases of therapy and to replace the intracellular deficit over a period of days. During initial therapy for DKA, the serum potassium concentration may fall rapidly, primarily due to the action of insulin promoting reentry of potassium into cells and, to a lesser degree, the dilution of extracellular fluid, correction of acidosis, and increased urinary loss of potassium. If these changes occur too rapidly, precipitous hypokalemia may result in fatal cardiac arrhythmias, respiratory paralysis, paralytic ileus, and rhabdomyolysis. The development of severe hypokalemia is potentially the most life-threatening electrolyte derangement during the treatment of DKA.[3]

Early potassium replacement is now a standard modality of care. Potassium is not added blindly to the first liter of NS administered to restore circulation because giving potassium rapidly to a patient in a hyperkalemic potentiating state (i.e., acidemia, insulin deficiency, renal insufficiency), may dangerously increase the extracellular potassium level and precipitate fatal ventricular tachycardia or fibrillation. The patient's initial ECG often provides early evidence of hyperkalemia: progressively manifested by peaked T waves, a prolonged PR interval, an absent P wave, an increasing QRS interval, and lastly, a sine-wave pattern. The initial measurement of serum electrolytes and the presence of urine output determine initial potassium therapy. As a general guideline, an initial serum potassium level greater than 3.3 mEq/L and less than 5.0 mEq/L (prior to fluid resuscitation and insulin) coupled with urine output calls for 10 mEq KCl per hour replacement in intravenous fluid for at least 4 h. Because the most rapid changes occur during the first few hours of therapy, the plasma potassium level initially is measured every 1 to 2 h. If oliguria is present (fortunately, this is rare secondary to the protective osmotic diuresis), renal function must be evaluated and potassium replacement must be decreased. An initial serum potassium level greater than 5.0 mEq/L usually reflects a more profound acidemia. Intravenous potassium replacement is withheld until the serum potassium level is documented to be below 5.0 mEq/L and urine output is established. Fluid and insulin therapy alone usually will lower the serum potassium level rapidly. Correction of the acidosis predicts a change in serum potassium concentration. For each 0.1 change in pH, serum the potassium concentration changes approximately 0.5 mEq/L inversely. This can be used as a guide for estimating the serum potassium concentration when pH balance is restored.

Initial hypokalemia (<3.3 mEq/L) necessitates more aggressive replacement prior to insulin therapy.[3] In this setting, potassium should be given IV at 15 to 20 mEq/h, with insulin initiated 30 min later. There is no documented advantage to using potassium phosphate over potassium chloride; excessive use of potassium phosphate may result in metastatic precipitation of calcium phosphate in tissues.

The goal is to maintain serum potassium levels within the normal range of 4 to 5 mEq/L and avoid life-threatening hyper- or hypokalemia. Oral potassium replacement is safe and effective and should be used as soon as the patient can tolerate oral fluids. During the first 24 h, potassium chloride 100 to 200 mEq is usually required. Occasionally, as much as 500 mEq is necessary.

Phosphate

Phosphate plays an integral role in the conversion of energy from adenosine triphosphate (ATP) and in the delivery of oxygen at the tissue level through 2,3-diphosphoglyceric acid (2,3-DPG). In addition, many important enzymes, cofactors, and biochemical intermediates depend on phosphate. Phosphate is primarily intracellular, and it shifts to the extracellular compartment during DKA. Serum levels often are normal or increased on presentation and do not reflect the total-body phosphate deficits secondary to enhanced urinary losses.[7] Phosphate (similar to glucose and potassium) reenters the intracellular space during insulin therapy, resulting in low phosphate concentrations. Hypophosphatemia is usually most severe 24 to 48 h after the start of insulin therapy. Acute phosphate deficiency (<1.0 mg/dL) has been associated with a variety of clinical disorders, including hypoxia, rhabdomyolysis, hemolysis, respiratory failure, and cardiac dysfunction. Fortunately, all are extremely rare during therapy of DKA.[15]

The role of phosphate replacement during the treatment of DKA remains controversial. No clinical trial has demonstrated significant benefits from routine intravenous phosphate therapy.[3,7] In general, intravenous therapy should be withheld unless the serum phosphate concentration is less than 1 mg/dL. Hypophosphatemia can be corrected safely and effectively with oral replenishment, which may cause diarrhea.

There is no established role for initiating intravenous potassium phosphate in the ED. Significant hypo-phosphatemia tends to develop many hours into therapy, after the patient is already admitted. Several undesirable side effects from intravenous phosphate administration have been reported. These include hyperphosphatemia, hypocalcemia, hypomagnesemia, metastatic soft tissue calcifications, and hypernatremia and volume loss from osmotic diuresis. If deemed necessary (a phosphate level of less than 1.0 mg/dL early in therapy and/or patient vomiting), intravenous phosphate replacement should be done by or in consult with experienced physicians in an intensive care

unit (ICU) setting. Serum phosphate, calcium, and magnesium levels should be monitored during therapy of DKA, but again, the case for routine early parenteral phosphate replacement in the ED has not been made.

Magnesium

Ongoing osmotic diuresis may cause significant depletion of magnesium stores (from bone) and hypomagnesemia. Hypomagnesemia may inhibit parathyroid hormone secretion, causing hypocalcemia and hyperphosphatemia. Symptomatic hypomagnesemia in DKA (hyperreflexia, positive Chvostek or Trousseau signs) is rare, as is the need for intravenous therapy. If the serum magnesium concentration is less than 1.2 mg/dL or symptoms are suggestive of hypomagnesemia, magnesium can be given orally in the form of magnesium oxide or parenterally as magnesium sulfate. Serum magnesium and calcium concentrations should be monitored on presentation and 24 h into therapy unless symptoms suggestive of hypomagnesemia or hypocalcemia occur.

Bicarbonate

The role of bicarbonate in DKA has been debated for decades. Arbitrary initial pH levels to use bicarbonate are still currently recommended in many texts. To date, not a single study clearly demonstrates improved clinical outcome using bicarbonate in the treatment of DKA. Acidotic patients routinely recover from DKA without alkali therapy. **Routine use of supplemental bicarbonate in the treatment of DKA is not recommended.**[7,16–18]

Severe metabolic acidosis is associated with numerous cardiovascular (impaired contractility, vasodilation, hypotension) and neurologic (cerebral vasodilation and coma) complications.[12] Theoretical advantages of bicarbonate include improved myocardial contractility, elevated ventricular fibrillation threshold, improved catecholamine tissue response, and decreased work of breathing.[16] These theoretical advantages are outweighed by the possible disadvantages of bicarbonate administration in DKA: severe and worsening hypokalemia, paradoxical CNS acidosis, worsening intracellular acidosis, impaired (shift to left) oxyhemoglobin dissociation, hypertonicity and sodium overload, delayed recovery from ketosis,[17] elevation of lactate levels,[16] and possible precipitation of cerebral edema.[13] During routine therapy of DKA, hydrogen ion production ceases when ketogenesis stops; excessive hydrogen ions are eliminated through the urine and respiratory tract. Ketone body metabolism results in the endogenous production of alkali. Children with initial pH values as low as 6.73 have been shown to recover promptly from DKA without bicarbonate.[16]

Severe acidosis (pH <7.0) and worsening pH despite aggressive therapy for DKA should prompt the clinician to rule out other causes of metabolic acidosis (i.e., lactate from sepsis, bowel infarction, metformin or methanol ingestion, etc.). The potential benefits of bicarbonate in the elderly with cardiovascular instability and DKA must be balanced against the potential disadvantages.[3,7]

OUTCOMES, COMPLICATIONS, AND MORTALITY

Complications Related to Acute Disease

A critically ill, lethargic patient is at risk for aspiration, and airway protection should be instituted. In general, the greater the presenting serum osmolality, blood urea nitrogen, and blood glucose concentrations, the greater is the mortality. There is also increased mortality for patients presenting with a serum bicarbonate level of less than 10 mEq/L.

Of the factors responsible for precipitating DKA, infection and myocardial infarction are the main contributors to high mortality. The mortality rate of DKA is high when myocardial infarction is the precipitating event. Additional factors that reduce the chances of survival include old age, severe hypotension, prolonged and severe coma, and underlying renal and cardiovascular disease. Severe volume depletion leaves the elderly at risk for vascular stasis and deep venous thrombosis. Prophylactic heparin should be instituted in high-risk patients.

Complications Related to Therapy

Major complications related to therapy of DKA include hypoglycemia, hypokalemia, hypophosphatemia, adult respiratory distress syndrome (ARDS), and cerebral edema. The goal of therapy, i.e., a gradual return to normal metabolic balance, will mitigate these possible outcomes to some extent.

ARDS is a rare complication of therapy. Aggressive fluid therapy decreases plasma oncotic pressure and raises left atrial end-diastolic pressure, favoring a shift of fluid across the pulmonary capillary membrane. Elderly patients with rales on chest examination may be at increased risk and should be monitored closely for this complication with continuous pulse oximetry and serial examinations; they also should receive lower rates of fluid administration.

Cerebral edema tends to occur between 4 and 12 h after the start of therapy but may develop as late as 48 h after.[19] It is often seen when the patient appears to be improving clinically and biochemically.[7,19] The true incidence of clinically apparent cerebral edema is unknown but estimated to be 0.7 to 1.0 per 100 episodes of DKA in children.[7] Cerebral edema complicating DKA has a reported mortality of 70 percent. One hypothesis is that the osmotic diuresis promotes loss of water and sodium from both intra- and extracellular spaces. Hyperglycemia leads to a hyperosmolar extracellular state. Brain cells enzymatically produce osmotically active particles or idiogenic osmoles that protect cells from further loss of water and shrinkage. During therapy with intravenous fluid and insulin, water moves into brain cells faster then idiogenic osmoles can dissipate, promoting cellular swelling.[7,13,19] Subclinical brain swelling has been reported in asymptomatic children during treatment of DKA.[13]

Multiple studies and reviews have found no specific presentation or treatment variables that predict or contribute to the development of cerebral edema.[13,19] Young age and new-onset diabetes are the only identified potential risk factors. Excessive initial fluid administration of greater than 4 L/m^2 of body surface area per day has been associated with cerebral edema.[13,19] Initial "corrected" hypernatremia may be a risk factor in children as well. Recent data suggest that children who develop cerebral edema initially may have a relatively normal serum osmolarity and subsequently develop progressive hyponatremia and/or a trend toward a declining serum sodium level before developing cerebral edema.[20] Approximately one-half of the patients who developed cerebral edema had premonitory symptoms of severe headache, incontinence, change in arousal or behavior, pupillary changes, blood pressure changes, seizures, bradycardia, or disturbed temperature regulation. Any change in neurologic function early in therapy should prompt the clinician to immediately administer mannitol (1–2 g/kg), which should be at the bedside of high-risk patients. Mannitol should be given prior to obtaining confirmatory computed tomographic (CT) scans[7,19] because serious morbidity and mortality may be prevented. Other aggressive measures such as intubation, hyperventilation, and fluid restriction may be necessary. Gradual replacement of water and sodium deficits and slow correction of hyperglycemia may lessen the risk.

Late Complications

Metabolic acidosis refractory to routine therapy may be secondary to unrecognized infection (lactic acidosis), insulin antibodies, or improper preparation or administration of the insulin drip. Shock that is unresponsive to aggressive fluid therapy suggests gram-negative bacteremia or silent myocardial infarction. Hyperchloremic non-anion-

gap metabolic acidosis develops in virtually every patient during therapy due to rapid volume expansion in the face of reduced bicarbonate. In addition, bicarbonate equivalents are excreted in the urine as ketones and replaced with chloride provided by the NS. This emphasizes the importance of monitoring the anion gap during therapy, not the bicarbonate concentration. The non-anion-gap metabolic acidosis (should it be present) resolves during recovery as bicarbonate is regenerated and excess chloride excreted in the urine.

Late vascular thrombosis may occur in any muscular artery, although the cerebral vessels appear to be most susceptible.[15] Volume depletion, low cardiac output, increased blood viscosity, and underlying atherosclerosis may predispose the elderly to this rare complication. Thrombosis may occur several hours or days after institution of therapy and after resolution of ketoacidosis.

Mortality in DKA results mainly from sepsis or pulmonary and cardiovascular complications in the elderly and fatal cerebral edema in children and young adults (<28 years old).[7] Age-adjusted death rates per 100,000 diabetic population for DKA and DKA-related deaths declined between 1980 and 1996. Overall, both the age-adjusted DKA death rate and the DKA-related death rate were 34 percent lower in 1996 than in 1980. This trend was seen in all age groups except in those aged less than 45 years. The highest death rates were among persons aged 75 years and older, followed by persons aged less than 45 years. Among race-sex groups, DKA death rates were highest among black males, followed by black females and then by whites. In 1996, the age-adjusted DKA death rate for black males was almost twice that for white males.[2]

DISPOSITION

The great majority of patients require hospitalization in a monitored setting where there is nursing experience with insulin drips. In many institutions, patients are cared for initially in an ICU or intermediate care unit. A select group of patients with an anion gap of less than 25, a glucose level of less than 600 mg/dL, and no comorbidity at the time of disposition decision may be managed safely on an inpatient unit with nursing expertise using insulin drips and managing diabetic patients. Patients presenting early in the course of their illness who can tolerate oral liquids may be managed safely in the ED or observation unit and discharged after 4 to 6 h of therapy. The anion gap on discharge should be less than 20.

REFERENCES

1. Westphal SA: The occurrence of diabetic ketoacidosis in non-insulin-dependent diabetes and newly diagnosed diabetes and newly diagnosed diabetic adults. *Am J Med* 101:19, 1996.
2. Centers for Disease Control and Prevention: *Diabetes Surveillance, 1999: Diabetic Ketoacidosis.* Atlanta, GA, US Department of Health and Human Services, 1999, pp 1-2.
3. American Diabetes Association: Clinical practice recommendations 2002. *Diabetes Care* 25(suppl 1):S1, 2002.
4. Umpierrez GE, Khajavi M, Kitabchi AE: Review: Diabetic ketoacidosis and hyperglycemic hyperosmolar nonketotic syndrome. *Am J Med Sci* 311(5):225, 1996.
5. Chauhan SP, Perry KG Jr: Management of diabetic ketoacidosis in the obstetric patient. *Obstet Gynecol Clin North Am* 22(1):143, 1995.
6. Thompson CJ, Cummings F, Chalmers J, et al: Abnormal insulin treatment behavior: A major cause of ketoacidosis in the young adult. *Diabet Med* 12:429, 1995.
7. Lebovitz HE: Diabetic ketoacidosis. *Lancet* 345:767, 1995.
8. Brandenburg MA, Dire DJ: Comparison of arterial and venous blood gas values in the initial emergency department evaluation of patients with diabetic ketoacidosis. *Ann Emerg Med* 31(4):459, 1998.
9. Adrogue HJ, Lederer ED, Suki WN, et al: Determinants of plasma potassium levels in diabetic ketoacidosis. *Medicine* 65(3):163, 1986.
10. Hillier TA, Abbott RD, Barrett EJ: Hyponatremia: Evaluating the correction factor for hyperglycemia. *Am J Med* 106:399, 1999.

11. Slovis CM, Mork BGC, Slovis RJ, et al: Diabetic ketoacidosis and infection: Leukocyte count and differential as early predictors of serious infection. *Am J Emerg Med* 5(1):1, 1987.

12. Adrogue HJ, Barrero J, Eknoyan G: Salutary effects of modest fluid replacement in the treatment of adults with diabetic ketoacidosis. *JAMA* 262(15):2108, 1989.

13. Krane EJ, Rockoff MA, Wallman JK, et al: Subclinical brain swelling in children during treatment of diabetic ketoacidosis. *New Engl J Med* 312: 1147, 1985.

14. Butkiewicz EK, Leibson CL, O'Brien PC, et al: Insulin therapy for diabetic ketoacidosis. *Diabetes Care* 18(8):1187, 1995.

15. Foster DW, McGarry JD: The metabolic derangements and treatment of diabetic ketoacidosis. *New Engl J Med* 309:159, 1989.

16. Green SM, Rothrock SG, Ho JD, et al: Failure of adjunctive bicarbonate to improve outcome in severe pediatric diabetic ketoacidosis. *Emerg Med* 31:41, 1998.

17. Okuda Y, Adrogue HJ, Field JB, et al: Counterproductive effects of sodium bicarbonate in diabetic ketoacidosis. *J Clin Endocrinol Metab* 81:314, 1996.

18. Viallon A, Zeni F, Lafond P, et al: Does bicarbonate therapy improve the management of severe diabetic ketoacidosis? *Crit Care Med* 27(12):2690, 1999.

19. Edge J: Cerebral oedema during treatment of diabetic ketoacidosis: Are we any nearer finding a cause? *Diabetes Metab Res Rev* 16:316, 2000.

20. Hale PM, Rezvani I, Braunstein AW, et al: Factors predicting cerebral edema in young children with diabetic ketoacidosis and new onset type I diabetes. *Acta Paediatr* 86:626, 1997.

DIABETES MELLITUS

Micheal D. Rush
Sonia Winslett
Kimberley Dawn Wisdom

Diabetes mellitus is a group of metabolic diseases characterized by deficiency of insulin production, deficiency of insulin action, or a combination of the two deficiencies resulting in hyperglycemia. Chronic hyperglycemia resulting from all forms of diabetes is a final common precipitant of long-term complications involving the eye, the nervous system, the kidneys, and the immune system that collectively can be grouped as microvascular sequelae. These microvascular sequelae are leading causes of blindness, chronic renal failure, and lower extremity amputation. Hyperglycemia and diabetes, along with obesity, hypertension, and dyslipidemia, collectively known as the *dysmetabolic syndrome* or *metabolic syndrome X,* also predispose individuals to accelerated atherogenesis and endothelial damage. These effects are integral to the macrovascular complications of diabetes: cardiovascular, cerebrovascular, and peripheral vascular disease. Emergency physicians are called on frequently to evaluate and treat the complications of diabetes and may in some cases make the initial diagnosis. Early diagnosis and treatment are essential in preventing long-term complications of the disease.

CLASSIFICATION/DEFINITIONS

Diabetes can be grouped into four major categories.[1] *Type 1 diabetes* [older terminology: *insulin-dependent diabetes mellitus* (IDDM) or *juvenile-onset diabetes mellitus* (JODM)] is defined by a deficiency of insulin secretion. The disease is believed to be caused by autoimmune-mediated destruction of pancreatic β-cells in the islets of Langerhans, or it may be idiopathic. There is a genetic predisposition to autoimmune type 1 diabetes and possible links with viral infections or other environmental factors (such as absence of breast-feeding, diet, and factors related to low socioeconomic status). Rates of β-cell destruction vary, and some patients may retain some residual β-cell function throughout their lives. Individuals with type 1 diabetes frequently require insulin therapy to sustain life and are prone to diabetic ketoacidosis (DKA).

Type 2 diabetes [older terminology: *non-insulin-dependent diabetes mellitus* (NIDDM) or *adult-onset diabetes mellitus* (AODM)] is defined as a combination of resistance to the action of insulin by the target organs and tissues with a relative inadequacy of compensatory insulin secretion and, in many cases, eventual β-cell failure. Type 2 diabetes is also believed to have a strong genetic predisposition. However, lifestyle issues such as a diet low in fiber and high in fat and simple carbohydrates (sugars, processed starches) combined with lack of exercise and obesity, also can have an impact on the development and severity of the disease and likely account for the alarming increase in both developed and developing countries. Patients with type 2 diabetes can have a variety of initial presentations such as life-threatening hyperglycemic, hyperosmolar, nonketotic syndrome (HHNS) or microvascular (retinopathy, nephropathy, neuropathy) or macrovascular complications (heart disease, cerebrovascular disease). Patients may have type 2 diabetes for years prior to having clinical symptoms. Type 2 patients often require insulin at some point in their course for adequate glycemic control. Therapy of type 2 diabetes typically is initiated stepwise from diet/exercise to oral agents to insulin or combination oral agent—insulin therapies. Data from the United Kingdom Prospective Diabetes Study (UKPDS) suggests that up to 75 percent of patients will need multiple steps of therapy by 9 years' disease duration to maintain glycemic control (i.e., glycosylated hemoglobin A_{1C}) ≤ 7 percent.[2]

Unlike type 1 diabetes, type 2 diabetes can be prevented or delayed. A lifestyle intervention involving a low-fat, low-calorie diet high in fiber and low in simple carbohydrates, regular exercise up to 2.5 h weekly, and as little as a 7 percent weight reduction reduced the incidence of new cases of type 2 diabetes in prediabetes patients at high risk [impaired fasting glucose (IFG) or impaired glucose tolerance (IGT)] by 58 percent over a mean follow-up period of approximately 3 years.[3]

The third category represents *secondary* causes for diabetes, which are listed in Table 212-1. Collectively, patients with secondary diabetes represent only about 1 percent of all diabetes cases.

The fourth group, *gestational diabetes mellitus* (GDM), is present only during pregnancy and complicates about 4 percent (about

TABLE 212-1 Causes/Diseases Associated with Hyperglycemia or Secondary Diabetes (Most Common Entities Listed)

Genetic defects in β islet cell function or insulin action
Diseases of the exocrine pancreas
    Pancreatitis
    Cystic fibrosis
    Hemochromatosis
Endocrinopathies
    Acromegaly
    Cushing syndrome
    Hormone secreting tumors of thyroid, pancreas, adrenal glands
Drugs/chemicals
    Glucocorticoids
    Thiazide diuretics
    β-Adrenergic receptor agonists
    Thyroid hormone
    Dilantin
    Interferon-α
    Nicotinic acid
Infections
    CMV
    Congenital rubella
Genetic syndromes
    Down syndrome
    Kleinfelter syndrome
    Turner syndrome
    Porphyria

135,000) of pregnancies in the United States annually. Excellent glycemic control is essential in preventing fetal cardiac and central nervous system (CNS) abnormalities, as well as fetal macrosomia.[1]

EPIDEMIOLOGY

It is estimated that 100 million people worldwide have diabetes, with 85 to 90 percent of cases being type 2. It is projected that by the year 2010, this number will increase to 215 million. In most developed countries, diabetes is one of the five leading causes of death.[4]

According to data collected from 1997 to 1999 by the National Health Information Survey (NHIS), approximately 17 million Americans, or 6.2 percent of the total U.S. population in year 2000, have diabetes mellitus, with 90 to 95 percent of cases classified as type 2 (NIDDM). Of these, 11.1 million have had their diabetes diagnosed by a physician, whereas 5.9 million are undiagnosed and do not know they have the disease. Approximately 1 million new cases of diabetes of all types were diagnosed each year in the United States from 1997 to 1999, with 90 to 95 percent diagnosed as type 2 diabetes.[4] Prevalence of diabetes rose approximately 33 percent from 1990 to 1998 in the United States. In part, this was due to an increase in the population older than age 65, the group with highest diabetes prevalence, but was related most strongly to the epidemic levels of obesity.[5] An additional 6.9 percent, or 13.4 million people in the U.S. population, has IFG (newer terminology: *prediabetes*) and is at high risk to develop the disease.[6]

Incidence rates for type 1 diabetes worldwide range from less than 0.1 per 100,000 per year in China to a high of 36.5 per 100,000 per year in Finland. Scandinavian/European countries tend to have much higher incidence rates for type 1 diabetes versus Asian and South American countries, with the rest of the world in the intermediate range. North Americans with ancestry in these ethnic groups likely would exhibit similar trends.[7]

In the United States, the prevalence of type 1 diabetes is slightly higher among men than among women. For type 2 diabetes, prevalence is roughly equal between sexes. For type 1 diabetes, non-Hispanic whites are affected most commonly, followed by African-Americans and Hispanic Americans. For type 2 diabetes, Americans of African, Mexican, Japanese, and Native American ethnicity are at higher risk than non-Hispanic whites.

In 1999, diabetes was estimated to account for 19 percent of all deaths in the United States in people aged 25 or older. The overall risk of death from diabetes is about twice that of people without diabetes, with a much higher risk ratio of 3.6 in people aged 25 to 44 years versus 1.5 in those aged 65 to 74 years. Ischemic cardiovascular disease is the most common cause of death in type 2 diabetes, and a person with diabetes has a two- to fourfold greater chance of death from cardiovascular disease than adults without diabetes.[4,8] Generally, a middle-aged person with type 2 diabetes can expect 5 to 10 years of decreased life expectancy because of the disease. African, Hispanic, and Native American ethnicity increase the risk of death from diabetes versus non-Hispanic whites. DKA and coma are the most common causes of death in the early years of type 1 diabetes, with renal disease becoming more common up to age 30 and cardiovascular disease more common after age 30. Diabetes ranks sixth in the leading underlying causes of death listed on death certificates in the United States.[4,8]

RISK FACTORS

Type 1 Diabetes

There is a genetic predisposition for type 1 diabetes, particularly if the father (three times more likely than if the mother) has type 1. Certain HLA antigens (HLA-DR3 and HLA-DR4) located on chromosome 6 are present in 95 percent of type 1 diabetics. Type 1 diabetes patients also have a higher prevalence of islet cell cytoplasmic antibodies

(ICAs), antibodies to insulin, and antibodies to the enzyme glutamic acid decarboxylase. Since concordance of type 1 diabetes occurs in only about 36 percent of monozygous twins, environmental factors also must play a role in the development of type 1 disease.

Dietary factors—such as breast-feeding for less than 3 months or not breast-feeding at all; exposure to cow's milk proteins, casein, and bovine serum albumin at age younger than 3 months; and exposure to food additives such as nitrates and nitrosamines—also have been associated with increased risk for development of type 1 diabetes.

Viral infections, especially coxsackie B group, are strongly associated with type 1 diabetes. Coxsackie B virus is isolated routinely from the sera of patients newly diagnosed with type 1 disease. Other viral infections with possible epidemiologic associations with type 1 diabetes include congenital rubella, cytomegalovirus (CMV), and mumps.

Older maternal age, birth order, and lower socioeconomic status also may contribute to development of type 1 diabetes, but results of studies are conflicting.

Type 2 Diabetes

Twin studies in type 2 diabetes establish a strong genetic link, with concordance rates of 34 to 100 percent for monozygous twins. Risk factors for type 2 diabetes are presented in Table 212-2.

PATHOPHYSIOLOGY

Type 1 diabetes results from destruction of insulin-producing pancreatic beta cells and absolute insulin deficiency. Type 2 diabetes begins with the development of insulin resistance and increased insulin production.

The organs and tissues that are most affected by diabetes—the retina, the kidney, and the nerves—all readily take up glucose, leading to its intracellular accumulation and subsequent metabolic end products. Two major mechanisms leading to microvascular complications from hyperglycemia are the increased formation and accumulation of sorbitol and other polyols by the aldose reductase pathway, and the formation of advanced glycosylation end products (AGEs) due to reactions of excess glucose with various cellular proteins.

Sorbitol formed from glucose through the aldose reductase pathway competitively inhibits *myo*-inositol formation, which causes a decrease in uptake of phosphoinositides into cell membranes, which in turn decreases $Na^+K^+ATPase$ activity. The ultimate clinical effect is slowed nerve conduction. This decrease in the synthesis of *myo*-inositol may be the common metabolic link to membrane damage in neuropathy, retinopathy, and nephropathy.

Glycosylation and the subsequent formation of AGEs is another major explanation for diabetic microvascular pathology. Chemical cross-links form between excess glucose and various cellular proteins, altering their structure and function; most notable of these is glycosy-

TABLE 212-2 Risk Factors for Type 2 Diabetes

Pre-diabetes: IFG (FPG ≥ 110 mg/dL <126 mg/dL) or IGT (plasma glucose 2 h following 75-g glucose load of ≥140 mg/dL but <200 mg/dL)
Prior gestational diabetes or giving birth to infant >9 lb
Hypertension ≥140/90 mm Hg
Dyslipidemia: HDL ≤35 mg/dL and/or triglycerides ≥250 mg/dL
Sedentary lifestyle, lack of regular physical activity
Diet: High fat, high calorie, high simple carbohydrates (sugars, simple starches), low fiber
Overweight/obesity: BMI ≥25 kg/m²
Centripetal obesity
Low birth weight
Low socioeconomic status

Abbreviations: BMI = body mass index; FPG = fasting plasma glucose; IFG = impaired fasting glucose; IGT = impaired glucose tolerance.

lated hemoglobin (HbA$_{1c}$), which forms proportional to glucose concentrations in the blood over time and is now used as a measure of glucose control in diabetes therapy. AGEs are thought to play a role in diabetic microvascular complications by effects on the structure and function of extracellular matrix and its interaction with the cell. An example of this is AGE formation on collagen, which, by trapping low-density lipoproteins, may be a contributor to accelerated atherogenesis seen in diabetes clinically.[9] A second potential mechanism for the pathogenesis of AGE formation from hyperglycemia is by action on AGE-specific receptors, which alters levels of various hormones and cytokines, such as nitric oxide, ultimately leading to vascular proliferation and decreased elasticity in existing vessels. Intracellularly, AGE formation on DNA molecules leads to subsequent mutations and other harmful effects on gene expression in mammalian cell cultures in vitro. Ongoing clinical trials using aminoguanidine, an inhibitor of AGE formation, show promise in the prevention and treatment of microvascular complications of diabetes.

Accelerated atherogenesis in diabetes is multifactorial and is related to hyperglycemia, hyperlipidemia, insulin resistance, formation/activation of AGE, modification/oxidation of lipoproteins, platelet/coagulation factor activation, and endothelial injury (Figure 212-1).

CLINICAL FEATURES

Type 1 diabetes frequently presents as DKA, often associated with an acute infection or other significant physiologic stress, in children, adolescents, or young adults. Type 2 diabetes can be present for years prior to the onset of clinical symptoms. It also may present suddenly with HHNS or DKA. Frequently, type 2 diabetes is only diagnosed concurrently with the initial presentation of a macrovascular, microvascular, or infectious complication of the disease.

Classic diabetes signs and symptoms may include polyuria, polydipsia, fatigue, polyphagia, unexplained weight loss, poor wound healing, blurred vision, and a higher prevalence of certain infections, especially candidal vaginitis and balanitis, recurrent/severe urinary tract infections, recurrent skin and skin structure infections, and malignant otitis externa. The presence of any of these symptoms or infections should lead an emergency clinician to check the patient's blood glucose level.

Documentation of the medical history of patients with diabetes in the emergency department should be complaint-directed but generally also should include questions on access to and frequency of home blood glucose monitoring, frequency and causes, if known, of recent hyperglycemia or hypoglycemia, recent glycosylated hemoglobin A$_{1C}$ values, presence of and therapy for microvascular and macrovascular complications of diabetes, recent adjustments by the patient or the patient's physician in their glycemic control regimen, any problems with adherence to therapy, and symptomatology suggestive of complications.

Symptoms suggestive of potential complications or poor glucose control include visual changes, neurologic symptoms (especially numbness, dizziness, and weakness), chest pain, gastrointestinal symptoms, and genitourinary symptoms (especially overflow incontinence, changes in amount of urine, and sexual dysfunction). A thorough history of any recent or concurrent chronic medical illness, injury, or infection should be obtained. Current medications, diet and exercise history, and social history are also important components of the evaluation of diabetes patients. Medications such as diuretics or β-adrenergic agonists may adversely affect glycemic control, and β-adrenergic blockers may adversely affect awareness of hypoglycemia. Poor living conditions or the inability to afford home blood glucose monitoring or medications affect treatment compliance. Psychiatric disorders and substance abuse should be considered. Finally, diabetic patients should be fed according to schedule, and they should receive their diabetic medication while being evaluated in the emergency department if they are not metabolically decompensated.

Key elements of the physical examination of patients with diabetes are presented in Table 212-3. Physical examination should be tailored to the patient's chief complaint. However, it generally should include blood pressure measurement, funduscopy (to look for hemorrhage or proliferative retinopathy), cardiovascular examination (including auscultation of the carotids and abdomen for bruits and assessment of peripheral pulses), extremity examination (especially the feet for signs of skin breakdown, acute vascular disease, or infection), skin examination (including intertriginous areas to assess for irritations and infections, especially around peripheral insulin injection sites, and in the hands to assess lancet puncture sites), and a neurologic examination (to screen for neuropathy). In children, measurements of height,

TABLE 212-3 Key Elements of Physical Examination in Patients with Diabetes

Vital Signs
   Temperature—fever, hypothermia (sepsis, hypoglycemia)
   Pulse—tachycardia or bradycardia
   Respirations—Kussmaul, tachypnea
   Blood pressure—hypertension or hypotension
HEENT
   Visual acuity—decreased acuity may be early retinopathy or detachment, may affect ability to dose insulin and other medications, have low threshold to measure intraocular pressures as incidence/prevalence of glaucoma is increased in diabetes
   Funduscopy—vessel proliferation/hemorrhage, cotton wool exudates
Cardiovascular
   Auscultation for bruits over carotids and abdomen
   Assessment of peripheral pulses and adequacy of circulation
Extremities
   Thorough extremity exam—especially the feet focusing on signs of abnormal wear/skin breakdown, abnormal sensation (proprioception and light touch), acute vascular disease, and infection (tinea, cellulitis, ulcers)
   Examine hands at sites of lancet punctures for glucose checks
Skin
   Insulin injection sites—lipodystrophy, scars, infection
   Skin structures—folliculitis, cellulitis, intertrigo, tinea, nonhealing wounds
Pediatric considerations:
   Height, weight, and measures of sexual maturity should be obtained and compared with normal individuals for age

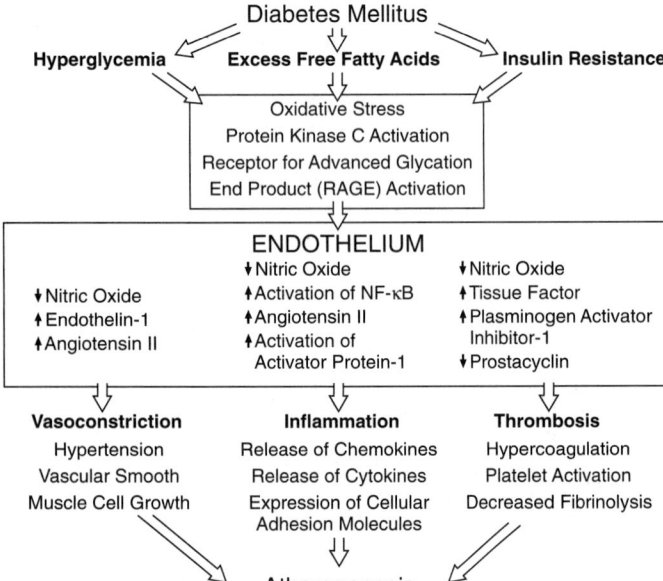

FIG. 212-1. Endothelial dysfunction in diabetes.

weight, and sexual maturity should be obtained and compared with normal children for age.[10] **Testing of visual acuity may reveal the patient's inability to measure a self-administered insulin dose.**

DIAGNOSIS

The diagnostic criteria for diabetes have been revised recently, lowering the serum glucose values at which the diagnosis can be made, and include an intermediate category for patients whose glucose levels do not meet criteria for diagnosis of diabetes but which are significantly abnormal. These changes reflect advances in knowledge of what levels constitute abnormality significant enough to produce the complications of diabetes. Replacing the old term of *borderline* diabetes are IFG (newer terminology: *prediabetes;* fasting plasma glucose level ≥ 110 but <126 mg/dL) and IGT, which constitute a group of patients who are generally euglycemic in everyday life but manifest hyperglycemia on oral glucose tolerance tests (fasting plasma glucose level ≥ 140 but <200 mg/dL) 2 h after an oral 75-g glucose load. In nonpregnant patients, these categories are not diagnostic entities in themselves but represent a group of patients at high risk of developing diabetes.

The diagnosis of diabetes can be established in three ways. Two of these may be feasible in the ED, and the methods are summarized in Table 212-4.[1] It is not unreasonable to test blood glucose in the emergency department in patients with certain presentations such as unexplained cellulitis, foot ulcers, frequent candidal infections, and unexplained neuropathy.

THERAPY

Therapy for diabetes can best be divided into acute therapy of severe hyperglycemia and life-threatening metabolic decompensation, and the day-to-day prevention of hyperglycemia through insulin, oral agents, or combination therapy.

DKA and hyperosmolar hyperglycemic nonketotic syndrome (HHNS) are the acute life-threatening entities involving metabolic decompensation, with primarily type 1 diabetes in the case of DKA and type 2 diabetes with HHNS. DKA and HHNS, however, can be seen in either type of diabetes. Acute hyperglycemia and chronic hyperglycemia represent intermediates between good glycemic control and the development of life-threatening metabolic decompensation, as well as macrovascular and microvascular complications of diabetes. DKA and HHNS are discussed elsewhere in this book (Chaps. 211 and 214, respectively).

TABLE 212-4   Criteria for the Diagnosis of Diabetes Mellitus

Symptoms of diabetes plus casual plasma glucose concentration ≥200 mg/dL (11.1 mmol/L). *Casual* is defined as any time of day without regard to time since last meal. The classic symptoms of diabetes include polyuria, polydipsia, and unexplained weight loss.

or

FPG ≥126 mg/dL (7.0 mmol/L). *Fasting* is defined as no caloric intake for at least 8 h.

or

2-h PG ≥200 mg/dL (11.1 mmol/L) during an OGTT. The test should be performed using a glucose load containing the equivalent of 75 g anhydrous glucose dissolved in water.

Note: In the absence of unequivocal hyperglycemia with acute metabolic decompensation, these criteria should be confirmed by repeat testing on a different day. OGTT is not recommended for routine clinical use.

Abbreviations: FPG = fasting plasma glucose; PG = plasma glucose; OGTT = oral glucose tolerance test.

Source: Copyright © 2002 by the American Diabetes Association. From *Diabetes Care* 25(1):S5–S20, 2002. Reprinted with permission from the American Diabetes Association.

ACUTE HYPERGLYCEMIA

Acute hyperglycemia, defined as a blood glucose level of greater than 300 mg/dL, can represent impending metabolic decompensation. High glucose levels, if present chronically, represent high risk for development of both macrovascular and microvascular complications of diabetes. Acute hyperglycemia and associated electrolyte abnormalities should be treated, and precipitating causes identified.

Clinical Features

The history and physical examination should focus on finding an underlying cause for the hyperglycemia and include a thorough medication history to ascertain the potential contributions of glucose-altering medications, most commonly corticosteroids, sympathomimetics, diuretics, anticonvulsants, salicylates, and β-adrenergic receptor agonists. A thorough evaluation for infections is indicated, with pneumonia, urinary tract, and foot/skin structure infections being the most common. Acute coronary or CNS ischemia is also a common cause of acute hyperglycemia. In sexually active females, a pelvic examination should be performed to rule out cervicitis or pelvic inflammatory disease as an occult precipitating factor. Finally, and only after the above precipitants have been excluded, changes in or noncompliance with insulin or oral hypoglycemic therapy may be the etiology for the hyperglycemia.

Younger adults may complain only of polyuria and/or polydipsia as symptoms, whereas elderly diabetics may present severely volume depleted, with acute mental status changes, hypovolemic shock, and acute renal insufficiency or failure.

Determination of serum electrolyte, blood urea nitrogen, and serum creatinine levels is indicated in the clinical assessment of acute hyperglycemia. Clinicians experienced in acid-base interpretation should be able to diagnose abnormalities based on venous electrolyte and bicarbonate levels and anion gap, only using respiratory rate and pulse oximetry to guide the rare need for arterial blood gas determination. Capillary blood glucose measurement is indicated every 1 to 2 h during therapy, with the caveat that capillary blood glucose (glucometer) determination may be inaccurate at low (<30 mg/dL) or high (>400 mg/dL) levels. Coefficients of analytic variation within glucometer systems have been found to range from 4 to 33 percent. Ideally, analytic and user errors should be no more than 10 percent.[11]

Therapy

Therapy for simple acute hyperglycemia is similar to that for DKA and HHNS and includes volume repletion, intravenous regular insulin therapy, correction of electrolyte imbalance, and specific therapies directed toward any identified underlying cause of hyperglycemia.

The cornerstone of therapy for acute hyperglycemia is restoration of intravascular volume and reperfusion of vital organs, especially the kidneys. Infusion of NS at a rate of 500 to 1000 mL/h should be initiated as soon as possible unless specific entities such as myocardial infarction with cardiogenic shock, acute renal failure, or stroke with cerebral edema contraindicate aggressive volume resuscitation. More moderate intravenous fluid infusion rates actually have been shown to improve hyperglycemia and metabolic acidosis faster and with fewer complications in the setting of DKA.[12] If the patient is hypotensive, 1 to 2 L of NS may be infused wide open to restore blood pressure. The use of two intravenous lines, 18 gauge or larger, is advisable to facilitate fluid resuscitation and correction of electrolyte imbalance. Volume resuscitation should be geared to the end point of lowering the serum glucose level, restoring organ perfusion, and replacing extracellular volume depletion. In patients with a history of congestive heart failure or chronic renal insufficiency, reassessment of status and need for further therapy should occur more frequently (approximately every hour or every 500 mL of intravenous fluid). Once improvement is noted in vital signs and hyperglycemia (~250 mg/dL or less) and adequate urine output of at least 30 to 50 mL/h is ensured, intravenous fluids may be reduced to maintenance levels with D5$\frac{1}{2}$NS or discontinued if the patient is taking oral fluids well.

Regular human insulin is administered IV because absorption of subcutaneous insulin in a volume-depleted patient can be erratic and unpredictable. Subcutaneous administration of insulin in non-volume-depleted patients is acceptable. Pharmacology of regular human insulin and insulin lispro is nearly identical except that insulin lispro has a significantly shorter onset of action and duration of action when compared with regular insulin and may lower glucose levels more rapidly.[13] Insulin lispro would appear to be an excellent alternative to regular human insulin; however, insulin lispro does not currently have Food and Drug Administration (FDA) approval for intravenous administration, although many clinicians do use it.

It should be noted that there are currently no randomized clinical trials comparing route, type of insulin, or type and rate of intravenous fluids used in the treatment of acute hyperglycemia in the emergency department setting. Thus recommendations are based on available laboratory studies, clinical studies of related entities (DKA, HHNS), and clinical experience. Typically, an initial bolus dose of 0.1 to 0.15 units/kg IV or SC of regular human insulin or insulin lispro is given, which may be repeated in 1 to 2 h if glucose levels have not fallen at least 50 to 75 mg/dL in the first hour. While an intravenous bolus priming dose of insulin may speed the onset of ketone body metabolism and may be advantageous in overcoming the lag time for the low volumes delivered in insulin infusions reaching the patient, no advantage in the outcome of patients with DKA or HHNS has been demonstrated. Thus a patient simply may be started on a regular human insulin infusion of 0.1 to 0.15 units/kg of ideal body weight per hour, with hourly capillary blood glucose monitoring to assess therapy. The blood glucose level generally will decrease much more rapidly in patients with type 2 diabetes than in those with type 1. Once the capillary blood glucose level reaches 250 mg/dL or less and there is significant improvement of symptoms, patients are at low risk for acute metabolic decompensation, assuming treatment of any underlying cause for hyperglycemia has been initiated.

The most significant electrolyte disorder in acute hyperglycemia is hypokalemia. There is frequently a total-body deficit of potassium secondary to severe extracellular volume loss. Appropriate volume therapy further promotes urinary losses. The presence of metabolic acidosis, which elevates the serum potassium level, may mask true potassium deficits, leading to nearly normal serum potassium levels initially. While fluid administration should be aggressive, rapid correction of metabolic acidosis with large volumes of intravenous fluids and sodium bicarbonate may drop serum potassium levels precipitously, and in particular bicarbonate should be avoided. However, potassium replacement should remain a priority as soon as the potassium level is at or below 5.5 mEq/L if renal function is ensured. Potassium levels of less than 3.3 mEq/L represent severe deficit and need emergent supplementation even in the face of compromised renal function to prevent lethal dysrhythmias. Total-body potassium deficits in the range of 3 to 5 mEq/kg are typical for DKA. Potassium repletion should be geared to serum potassium levels and usually can be accomplished by adding 20 to 30 mEq potassium chloride (KCl) per liter to the intravenous infusion if the [K$^+$] level is 3.3 to 5.0 mEq/L. Potassium also can be replaced orally with multiple doses of 20 to 40 mEq KCl if the patient is not vomiting. In the presence of severe hypokalemia, 10 mEq of KCl per 50 mL of NS may be administered IV every 15 min. Plan for approximately 100 mEq of KCl supplementation for each 1 mEq/L deficit. Measure serum potassium every 2 h during the initial 8 h of therapy. An electrocardiogram also may be useful in assessing for severe hypo- or hyperkalemia if the serum potassium level is not immediately available.

Phosphate therapy is not without complications, and **there is no routine indication for phosphate supplementation** in the treatment

of acute hyperglycemia, DKA, or HHNS. Patients with hyperglycemia refractory to therapy, severe electrolyte disturbance, significant prerenal azotemia or increase in baseline blood urea nitrogen and creatinine, or a serious underlying cause should be admitted to the hospital for further workup and therapy.

PRINCIPLES OF LONG-TERM THERAPY FOR HYPERGLYCEMIA

The general guiding principle of diabetes therapy is to lower glucose levels on a consistent basis to normal or near normal. Keeping glucose levels at or near normal in patients with type 1 diabetes (HbA$_{1C}$ ≤ 7.0 percent; normal: 4.0–6.0 percent) dramatically reduces the risk of developing both the microvascular and macrovascular complications of diabetes.[14] Intensified hypertension control, glycemic control, and serum cholesterol control in type 2 diabetes are cost-effective in reducing morbidity and mortality from cardiovascular disease. Intensified blood pressure control actually reduces health care costs in patients with type 2 diabetes.[15]

Intensive insulin therapy is indicated for well-motivated patients who administer multiple daily injections, usually as a single injection of a basal long-acting insulin such as ultralente or insulin glargine at bedtime coupled with short-acting lispro, aspart, or regular insulin injections before meals. Insulin also can be administered as a continuous subcutaneous insulin infusion (CSII) by means of a small pump that delivers insulin subcutaneously into the abdominal wall through a butterfly needle. Insulin usually is infused at a continuous basal rate, with preprogrammed or patient-initiated boluses given just before meals. Both hypoglycemia and ketoacidosis are more frequent in patients with CSII. For emergency department patients with CSII who develop hypoglycemia, marked hyperglycemia, or DKA, it is best to shut off the pump in the ED while standard glucose or insulin therapy is administered.

Intensive therapy generally is not indicated for patients with autonomic insufficiency, adrenal or pituitary insufficiency, and atherosclerotic coronary or cerebrovascular disease; for patients taking β-blocker medication; for patients with counterregulatory hormone deficiency; for the elderly or small children; for patients with psychiatric disorders; and for unreliable, chronically noncompliant patients.[14]

Glycemic control in type 2 patients is staged. Stage 1 is diet modification and weight reduction. Stage 2 includes various oral antidiabetic medications. Figure 212-2 represents the various pharmacologic approaches to therapy of type 2 diabetes.[16] Stage 3 represents insulin requirement resulting from β-cell failure, alone or in combination with oral agents. The indications for insulin therapy in type 2 diabetes are presented in Table 212-5.[17] Initiating this therapy in patients who are failing oral agent therapy involves continuing the oral agent at the usual dose and adding an evening subcutaneous injection of 5 to 10 units of NPH insulin in lean patients [≤25 kg/m^2 body mass index (BMI)] and 10 to 15 units in obese patients.[17] Caution should be used in prescribing oral agents to the elderly or to patients with impaired renal or hepatic function. Once the symptoms of acute hyperglycemia are controlled and underlying causes or exacerbating factors are sought out and treated, initiation of oral hypoglycemic and/or insulin therapy in patients with new-onset type 2 diabetes usually can be left to the primary care provider at 24 to 48-h follow-up if admission was not warranted. If the patient is overweight/obese (BMI ≥ 25 kg/m^2) and renal function is adequate (serum creatinine level ≤ 1.4 mg/dL), metformin, which inhibits hepatic gluconeogenesis and confers little risk of hypoglycemia, may be initiated safely at a dosage of 500 mg PO once a day, increasing by 500 mg each week until the maximum of 500 mg four times a day has been reached. This is until the patient can receive a diabetes education session, learn to test their his or her glucose, and recognize symptoms of hypoglycemia prior to starting an oral hypoglycemic agent, insulin, or a combination regimen.

A working knowledge of the pharmacology, including time to peak effect and duration of action of the various insulin and oral hypo-

FIG. 212-2. Pharmacologic approaches to the major metabolic defects of type 2 diabetes mellitus.

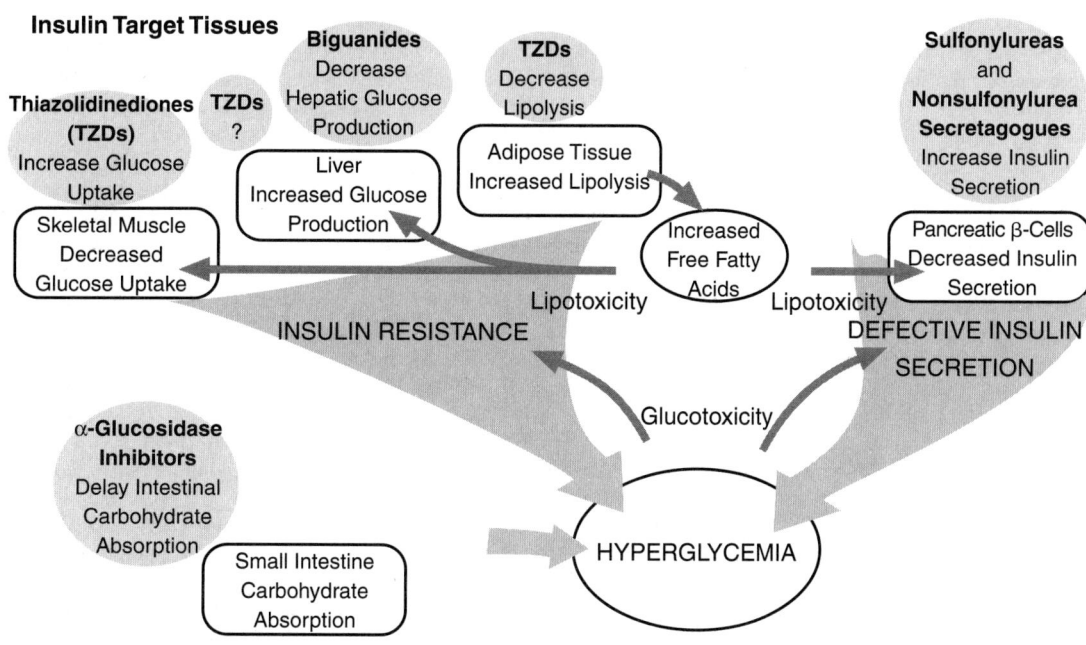

glycemic preparations, should enable the emergency physician to make adjustments in a patient's usual insulin or oral hypoglycemic regimen, especially if the patient arrives with a home blood glucose diary. Table 212-6 presents the various forms of insulin commonly prescribed, time to onset of action, time to peak effect, and their durations of action when given SC. **It is a good general rule not to change the total number of units of insulin by more than a 10 percent increase or decrease in a single day.** Adjustment of oral agent dosage generally can be left to the primary care provider because it requires careful and close monitoring. If this option is not readily available, oral hypoglycemic agent dosing generally should not exceed a 20 percent increase or decrease. If the patient is not doing regular home glucose monitoring, be sure that he or she has the equipment and the knowledge to test regularly during the adjustment period to avoid severe hypoglycemia or hyperglycemia. When the availability of a primary physician is in question, some EDs are able to provide a home health nurse for teaching and assessment.

Self-monitoring of blood glucose is recommended for all patients whose diabetes is managed with insulin and may be indicated for patients with type 2 diabetes who are initiating or changing their oral therapeutic regimens. Glucose measurements are indicated prior to meals and at bedtime at a minimum to guide intensive management regimens.

If a patient is unwilling or unable to test his or her blood glucose regularly during an adjustment and is not at high risk for metabolic decompensation, any adjustment of regimen and further education should be left to a primary care provider or endocrinologist.

TABLE 212-5 Indications for Insulin Therapy in Type 2 Diabetes

FPG consistently ≥300 mg/dL with ketonuria or ketonemia.
Temporary 6–8 week therapy for FPG ≥300 mg/dL and symptoms such as polyuria, polydipsia, weight loss at onset of type 2. Many patients can then be converted to oral therapy or continue insulin if comfortable and compliant.
Patient desires insulin as initial therapy after reviewing available options with PCP.
In women whose gestational diabetes is not controlled with diet or in women with type 2 diabetes who become pregnant. *All oral antidiabetic medications are contraindicated in pregnancy.*

Abbreviations: FPG = fasting plasma glucose; PCP = primary care physician.
Source: From Medaliar S, Edelman SV: Insulin therapy in type 2 diabetes. *Endocrinol Metab Clin North Am* 30:935, 2001, with permission.

COMPLICATIONS OF DIABETES MELLITUS

Cardiovascular Complications

Heart disease is the leading cause of diabetes-related deaths, accounting for approximately 40 percent of deaths in men with diabetes and nearly 32 percent in women.[18] A diabetic is two to four times more likely to have ischemic heart disease or stroke than a nondiabetic, and the risk of a first myocardial infarction in a study that compared incidence rates of myocardial infarction in control versus patients with diabetes over 7 years was six times that of patients without diabetes.[19] Odds ratios for stroke in patients with diabetes are increased 3.3 to 23.1 times, with the worst odds ratios noted in younger patients.[20]

Factors contributing to cardiac dysfunction in diabetes are increased incidence of atherosclerosis of the coronary arteries, autonomic neuropathy, and microvascular disease (associated with hypertension and renal disease). Diabetics are prone to "silent"(pain-free) myocardial infarction or infarction associated with atypical symptoms, such as weakness. Even in the absence of vascular disease and hypertension, some diabetic patients develop cardiomegaly, with systolic and diastolic ventricular dysfunction that may evolve into congestive heart failure. Diabetic cardiomyopathy may be a direct effect of insulin deficiency or resistance on myocardial cell function. The detrimental effects of diabetes mellitus on the heart are more prominent in young diabetics and women. Women usually have a lower risk of coronary artery disease, but diabetes renders them more vulnerable to reinfarction and death after myocardial infarction and congestive heart failure. Vascular disease in patients with diabetes may be either nonspecific (atherosclerosis of large vessels) or specific (microangiopathic disease in

TABLE 212-6 Common Insulin Preparations: Onset, Peak, and Duration

Preparation	Onset of Action	Peak	Duration
Lispro/Aspart	5–15 min	1–2 h	4–6 h
Regular human	30–60 min	2–4 h	6–10 h
NPH/Lente	1–2 h	4–8 h	10–20 h
Ultralente	2–4 h	Variable	16–20 h
Glargine	1–2 h	No peak/flat	Approx. 24 h

small vessels) for diabetes.[14] Therapy to reduce cardiovascular risk in type 1 and especially type 2 diabetic patients also must involve aggressive blood pressure control to 130/80 mm Hg or less, reduction of serum cholesterol to less than 200 mg/dL, and antiplatelet therapy with aspirin or clopidogrel (if the patient is aspirin-allergic or aspirin-sensitive), in addition to excellent glycemic control (HbA$_{1C}$ < 7 percent if possible). Angiotensin-converting enzyme inhibitors (ACEIs) have been shown to slow the progression of diabetes-related nephropathy and reduce cardiovascular events and mortality in patients with diabetes at high risk for heart disease.[21] Aspirin therapy is indicated in type 1 or 2 diabetic patients over 30 years of age as a primary prevention therapy for ischemic heart disease and as secondary prevention for patients with a history of macrovascular complications. It should not be used in anyone younger than 21 years of age because of the risk of Reye syndrome.[22]

There is a risk for intraocular bleed from thrombolytic administration (for cardiac events) to a diabetic with proliferative retinopathy. Even though the risk of intraocular bleed is low, **proliferative retinopathy is an absolute contraindication to thrombolytic therapy.** The challenge to the emergency physician is expedient evaluation for proliferative retinopathy while simultaneously evaluating the need for thrombolytics.

Retinopathy

Diabetic retinopathy is the leading cause of new cases of blindness in patients aged 25 to 74 in the United States. Patients with this complication are 29 times more likely to become blind than those without retinopathy. Glaucoma and cataracts, also more common in diabetes, can contribute to new cases of blindness. An estimated 97 percent of diabetics taking insulin (types 1 and 2) and 80 percent of diabetics who do not take insulin (type 2 only) who have had their diabetes for 15 years or longer have some diabetic retinopathy. Among those with this complication, 40 percent of insulin-using and 5 percent of non-insulin-using diabetics have the most severe form—proliferative retinopathy—that frequently leads to blindness. In diabetes patients without eye disease, intensive glucose control lowers the risk of developing proliferative retinopathy by more than 75 percent compared with patients who do not practice intensive glucose control. Among patients with mild retinopathy, the risk for sustained retinopathy, progression to proliferative retinopathy, or need for laser photocoagulation can be reduced by more than 50 percent.

In the ED, history of any visual changes, low visual acuity, and the presence of visual field defects should arouse suspicion for retinopathy. A nondilated retinal examination frequently can reveal "cotton wool" exudates, microaneurysms, and vascular proliferation consistent with diabetic retinopathy (Table 212-7). A red and/or painful eye in association with headache or simply unexplained headache in patients with diabetes should prompt measurement of intraocular pressure to rule out acute glaucoma. The presence of these findings should prompt an immediate referral to an ophthalmologist for further examination and therapy. A baseline dilated funduscopic examination is in-

dicated 5 years after onset if age of onset is below 30 years and yearly thereafter. Those over age 30 at diagnosis should be examined at the time of diagnosis and yearly thereafter.

Laser photocoagulation of proliferative retinopathy has been proven to be efficacious in preventing blindness from proliferative retinopathy, particularly in patients with macular edema. Vitrectomy may be necessary to preserve vision in patients with severe proliferative retinopathy with vision loss secondary to retinal hemorrhage and detachment or vitreous hemorrhage.

Nephropathy

Diabetic nephropathy is one of the leading causes of end-stage renal disease. Approximately 43 percent of new cases of renal failure each year are due to diabetic nephropathy.[4] Incidence approaches 40 percent lifetime in type 1 diabetes and 4 to 20 percent in type 2 diabetes. Since the overwhelming majority of diabetics are type 2, most patients with nephropathy will have this form of the disease. Hyperglycemia leads to glomerular hypertension and hyperfiltration, which in turn lead to deposition of protein in the mesangium. These protein deposits ultimately lead to sclerosis of the glomerulus and renal failure. The most useful clinical marker for nephropathy is the presence and degree of microalbuminuria. Patients with albumin excretion rates of as little as 30 mg/d are at high risk for developing diabetic nephropathy and subsequent renal failure. (Unfortunately, standard urine test strips do not give positive results until the urinary excretion of albumin has reached extremely high levels.) A special, more costly test strip and/or radioimmunoassay must be used to test for microalbuminuria. All diabetes patients should be screened for microalbuminuria at diagnosis and at least yearly thereafter. In addition to being a marker for nephropathy, microalbuminuria also has been shown to be associated with high risk for coronary ischemic events. Intensive insulin therapy reduces the likelihood of developing microalbuminuria, the clinical herald of diabetic nephropathy, by 60 percent. This benefit is maintained for at least 4 years.[23] Each point of reduction in HbA$_{1C}$ when above normal represents a decrease in the risk of microvascular complications by 35 percent.[14] ACEIs have been shown to delay both the onset and the progression of diabetic nephropathy independent of their effect on controlling blood pressure. Overall prevention of nephropathy involves a combination of glycemic control, effective treatment of hypertension to 130/80 mm Hg or less, restriction of dietary protein, and avoidance of nephrotoxic drugs or dyes.

Blood pressure control, ideally to 130/80 mm Hg or less, is crucial to slowing the progression of nephropathy. Nondihydropyridine calcium channel blockers (e.g., diltiazem, verapamil) and ACEIs are the best agents to begin therapy in patients with diabetes. β-Blockers also may be a good choice if balancing the tendency toward hyperglycemia with cardioprotective and renal protective effects or if CHF with an ejection fraction of greater than 25 percent is present. Thiazide diuretics have side effects such as hyperglycemia, hypokalemia, and hyperlipidemia that make them unattractive. Dihydropyridine calcium channel blockers such as nifedipine and amlodipine actually may increase proteinuria and are best avoided in patients with diabetes. Patients with nephropathy are encouraged to eat a lower-protein diet (0.6–0.8 g/kg ideal body weight per day). Drugs with nephrotoxic potential, such as the nonsteroidal anti-inflammatory drugs (NSAIDs), should be avoided. NSAIDs should be used sparingly and in short courses in diabetic patients without evidence of nephropathy.

Neuropathy

Neuropathy can be divided into peripheral neuropathy and autonomic neuropathy. The degree of functional and structural neural damage is related directly to the degree and duration of hyperglycemia. Approximately 42 percent of patients with type 2 diabetes will develop symptomatic polyneuropathy in the 10 years after diagnosis.[24] Symptomatic peripheral neuropathy results from loss of both myelinated and un-

TABLE 212-7   Changes in the Diabetic Retina

Background (Simple)	Proliferative
Increased capillary permeability	New vessels
Capillary closure and dilation	Scars (retinitis proliferans)
Microaneurysms	Vitreal hemorrhage
Arteriovenous shunts	Retinal detachment
Dilated veins	
Hemorrhages	
Cotton-wool spots	
Hard exudates	

myelinated nerve fibers and blunted nerve fiber reproduction, resulting in abnormal firing of sensory neurons. Usually bilateral, it often consists of symmetrical stocking/glove loss in the distal extremities. Symptoms run a spectrum from numbness to dysesthesias/paresthesias to constant burning pain. Physical examination also may demonstrate loss of vibratory sense and deep tendon reflexes.

Intensive glycemic control reduced the incidence of clinical neuropathy by 60 percent in the Diabetes Control and Complications Trial (DCCT) and approximately 35 percent with each 1 percent reduction in HbA$_{1C}$ in the UKPDS.[14] Drugs that have been proven effective in treating the pain associated with diabetic neuropathy include tricyclic antidepressants, especially amitriptyline, topical capsaicin, phenytoin, neurontin, and carbamazepine. Narcotic analgesics have a high abuse potential in this setting, so their use should be avoided. NSAIDs also should be avoided secondary to potential nephrotoxicity. Sensory nylon monofilament testing (Semmes-Weinstein) is a useful screening tool for early neuropathy.[25] Diabetic patients with depressed or absent Achilles' reflex or loss of vibratory sensation in the foot are at high risk for developing foot ulcers. Pain often subsides with time as neurons become destroyed.[24]

Diabetic mononeuropathy usually affects a large peripheral nerve (femoral, obturator, sciatic, median, or ulnar) or an isolated cranial nerve (usually the third, fourth, or sixth). Patients present with sudden onset of symptoms related to the involved nerve. It may be difficult in the emergency department to differentiate the signs and symptoms of diabetic mononeuropathy from a transient ischemic attack or cerebrovascular accident.

Autonomic neuropathy represents the clinical entities of gastroesophageal reflux disease (GERD), gastroparesis, neurogenic bladder, impotence and sexual dysfunction, autonomic diarrhea (nocturnal, often with incontinence), and orthostatic hypotension. Symptoms of GERD include dysphagia, chest pain, and heartburn. GERD may be difficult to differentiate from acute coronary syndrome in the emergency department and usually will respond to antacids, H$_2$-receptor blockers, or proton pump inhibitors. Gastroparesis, which is associated clinically with nausea, vomiting, bloating, and easy satiety, has been shown to respond to erythromycin or metoclopramide, which decrease gastric emptying time. Severe cases may not respond to medication. Autonomic diarrhea, defined as at least 3 weeks of increased stool frequency and/or liquidity, usually will respond to traditional antidiarrheal medicines.

Constipation is probably the most common gastrointestinal symptom in diabetes patients. Treatment includes dietary fiber supplementation and stool softener. Neurogenic bladder, inadequate or spastic emptying of the bladder, may respond to bethanechol therapy. Erectile dysfunction may be treated successfully with the new oral agent, sildenafil, but this drug is contraindicated in patients using any form of organic nitrate therapy and should be used with caution in patients with known coronary artery disease. Symptomatic orthostasis can be treated by increasing salt intake (in the absence of hypertension) or by using elastic stockings (which should be fitted by a specialist), or the symptoms may respond to fludrocortisone, which increases arterial tone and expands intravascular volume.

Infections

Diabetic patients who achieve and maintain excellent glycemic control (HbA$_{1C}$ < 7 percent) are probably not significantly more susceptible to infection than the general population. A number of factors related to both the associated defects in immunity and disease-specific effects may account for the increased prevalence of certain infections and poor wound healing in patients with diabetes.

There are possible epidemiologic associations between diabetes and urinary tract infections (UTIs), candidal vulvovaginitis, cystitis, and balanitis, pneumonia, influenza, chronic bronchitis, pneumococcal bacteremia, primary and reactivation tuberculosis, rhinocerebral mucormycosis, malignant otitis externa, lower extremity skin and soft tissue structure infections, surgical wound infections, and Fournier

gangrene.[26] However, only a few of these conditions (UTI and other urogenital infections; staphylococcal, streptococcal and candida skin infections) have been shown to be more frequent in diabetic patients than control groups in retrospective or prospective studies.

There are several impairments seen in polymorphonuclear leukocytes in diabetic patients, including impaired migration, phagocytosis, intracellular killing, and chemotaxis, that lead to an intrinsic decrease in immunity and in the ability to heal wounds properly. Disease-specific factors such as neuropathy, impairments in bladder emptying, and poor local circulation may further hinder the immune response. Although there are few controlled outcome studies, it is probably prudent to have a low threshold for initiating intravenous antibiotics and hospitalization of diabetic patients with upper urinary tract, lower respiratory tract, or skin (cellulitis/erysipelas) and skin structure (abscesses, furuncles, ulcers, and boils) infections. However, the availability of home intravenous infusion therapy and the development of oral antibiotics with excellent antimicrobial coverage provide outpatient alternatives for the management of uncomplicated infections.

Immunizations are recommended according the Centers for Disease Control and Prevention (CDC) Advisory Committee on Immunization Practices (ACIP; http://www.cdc.gov/nip/recs/adult-schedule.pdf) for patients with diabetes, especially those with evidence of complications, against influenza annually in the fall and once with the pneumococcal polyvalent vaccine. Repeat pneumococcal vaccination is indicated only for patients older than 64 years of age if their initial vaccination was more than 5 years ago.

There is little in the literature to guide the emergency physician when confronted with a febrile patient with diabetes and no obvious source of infection. Given the potential for problems with host defects in immunity in patients with poor glycemic control, and given that many infections associated with diabetes can be catastrophic, **fever without a clear source is a good reason to admit the patient.** Some serious diabetic infectious complications are discussed below.

RHINOCEREBRAL MUCORMYCOSIS Rhinocerebral mucormycosis is an invasive fungal infection of the nasal and paranasal sinuses; sometimes involving the palate and adjacent tissues. An estimated 70 percent of these infections occur in patients with DKA; the other 30 percent in immunocompromised patients without diabetes. The onset is sudden and rapidly progressive; patients present with periorbital or perinasal pain; blood-tinged nasal discharge; unilateral headache; increased tearing; swelling of eyelids and conjunctiva, and decreased vision. Physical signs can include black eschar on the nasal mucosa or hard palate due to ischemia, proptosis, and if the infection progresses, cranial nerve involvement or seizures. The organism has a propensity for vascular occlusion; therefore, cavernous sinus thrombosis, as well as brain abscesses, can occur.[26]

Mortality is high (up to 50 percent); therefore, prompt diagnosis and immediate, aggressive therapy must be initiated. Acidosis must be corrected and an otolaryngologist consulted for extensive debridement of necrotic tissue and drainage of sinuses or abscesses. Computed tomography (CT) or magnetic resonance imaging (MRI) should be obtained to both determine the extent of the infection and rule out an intracranial process. Amphotericin B is the drug of choice. Even with aggressive therapy, only 50 to 85 percent of patients are cured.

MALIGNANT OTITIS EXTERNA Unlike other serious infections in patients with diabetes mellitus, well-controlled glucose levels are present in up to half, and systemic toxicity is often absent. Microangiopathy in the external auditory canal of diabetic patients is thought to be a predisposing factor. Patients present with unilateral otalgia, decreased hearing, purulent discharge, and sometimes fever (see Chap. 239). Examination finds a tender, inflamed external auditory canal, and almost all patients have a mass of granular-appearing tissue. The infection can progress to osteomyelitis of the mastoid, temporal bone, or base of skull and meningitis, venous sinus thrombosis, or subdural emphysema. MRI or CT can define the extent of anatomic involvement.[26]

Infection is frequently due to *Pseudomonas aeruginosa,* but staphylococci, fungi, and other gram-negative organisms have been isolated. Parenteral antibiotics, imipenem, meropenem, ciprofloxacin, or the combination of a third-generation cephalosporin (ceftazidime) and an antipseudomonal penicillin (ticarcillin) is indicated for 4 to 6 weeks. Early surgical debridement and frequent cleansing are critically important.[26]

CHOLECYSTITIS Patients with diabetes have a predisposition to cholelithiasis. When acute cholecystitis develops in patients with diabetes, it is associated with higher morbidity and mortality rates. In addition, the greater chance (up to 25 percent) of developing emphysematous cholecystitis is associated with a higher incidence of gangrenous gallbladder that is more likely to perforate. Abdominal radiographs may reveal gas in the gallbladder and biliary tree. Unexplained fever, with or without abdominal pain, should be evaluated with ultrasound for cholecystitis. The causative agents are most frequently a *Clostridium* species in addition to streptococci, *Escherichia coli,* and *Pseudomonas.* Despite prompt treatment and surgery, the mortality rate (15 percent) is 3 to 10 times higher than that for ordinary cholecystitis.[26]

PYELONEPHRITIS, PERINEPHRIC ABSCESS, AND PAPILLARY NECROSIS Diabetics are at increased risk for two serious renal infections: emphysematous pyelonephritis and perinephric abscess. Emphysematous pyelonephritis is a rare, life-threatening infection with gas production in and around the kidney. Over 70 percent of these patients will have diabetes. Patients with emphysematous pyelonephritis are ill with fever, flank pain, and sometimes a palpable mass. Bacteremia is often present. Aggressive treatment with parenteral antibiotics and nephrectomy is required. Even then, the mortality rate is still about 40 percent. Patients presumed to have pyelonephritis but who fail to respond to parenteral antibiotics should be evaluated for renal papillary necrosis and perinephric abscess. Symptoms of flank pain suggesting renal colic always should be evaluated fully to exclude infection or papillary necrosis. Thirty-five percent of patients with perinephric abscess will have diabetes. Patients usually do not respond completely to parenteral antibiotics, and surgical drainage often is required. Even with surgical drainage, mortality is about 20 percent.

About 50 percent of patients who develop renal papillary necrosis have diabetes. Patients may be asymptomatic and not notice the sloughed papillary tissue excreted in their urine, or they may present with symptoms similar to acute pyelonephritis. Renal infection with ureteral obstruction may develop into sepsis and septic shock in these diabetic patients. Necrotic tissue fragments, when seen in the urine along with red and white blood cells and bacteria, are suggestive of the diagnosis. Ureteral obstruction can be detected with ultrasound and helical CT. An intravenous pyelogram should be avoided, especially in cases of preexisting renal disease. Treatment consists of aggressive intravenous antibiotics, urinary drainage, and if the condition is severe, surgery to remove necrotic tissue.[26]

Diabetes-Related Foot and Lower Extremity Ulcers

Foot and lower extremity ulcers and associated infections are a major source of morbidity in the diabetic population, affecting some 15 percent of diabetic patients during their lifetime. The complications account for 20 percent of diabetes-related admissions and nearly 60 percent of all lower extremity amputations in the United States. A pathologic triad of neuropathy, premature atherosclerotic vascular disease, and impaired immunity combines to make diabetic foot ulcers a multidisciplinary treatment challenge.

Peripheral neuropathy predisposes the foot to ulceration, infection, and joint degeneration (Charcot joints) through the mechanisms of lack of sensation, diminished or absent proprioception, anhidrosis, and poor circulatory and thermal regulation. Risk factors for foot and lower extremity ulcers include high HbA_{1C} levels, older age, longer

duration of diabetes, foot deformities, smoking, retinopathy, peripheral neuropathy, albuminuria, and low diastolic blood pressure. Preventing foot ulcers involves education on foot care and proper fitting of footwear, combined with good glycemic control to limit development of neuropathy and premature vascular disease.

A thorough clinical examination of the diabetic patient's feet should be performed during all emergency department visits even for unrelated complaints. Hair and nail growth, calluses, corns, deformities, erythema, swelling, sensation, and vascular function should be assessed. Any ulcerations found should be unroofed surgically and probed using a blunt-ended rigid probe to determine the depth and possible bone, joint, or tendon involvement and rule out deep abscess. The ability to probe to bone through the ulcer suggests the strong possibility of osteomyelitis and deep-space soft tissue infection.

Foot ulcers can be classified into non-limb-threatening, limb-threatening, and life-threatening infections. *Non-limb-threatening infection* is defined as small (under 2 cm of cellulitis or inflammation), does not involve deep structures or bone, and is the result of recent injury to a well-perfused limb. *Limb-threatening infection* (more than 2 cm of cellulitis or inflammation) with associated ascending lymphangitis, deep ulceration or abscess, large area of necrotic tissue, involvement of deep structures or bone, gangrene, or critical lower extremity ischemia is defined by the absence of palpable pulses. *Life-threatening infection* has clinical signs of sepsis, including fever, leukocytosis, hypotension, tachycardia, tachypnea, altered mental status, and metabolic abnormalities ranging from hypoglycemia to DKA and HHNS.

Management of foot ulcers that do not appear infected and do not expand to the deep structures or bone on exploration should include avoidance of weight bearing and nonadherent padded dressings. Follow-up referral with a specialist in diabetes-related foot care should occur within a few days to consider the need for debridement, full contact casting, further evaluation of any bony deformity or neuropathy, and evaluation for peripheral vascular disease. Constrictive dressings, such as an Unna paste boot (alkaline methylene blue), and tight-fitting

TABLE 212-8 Antimicrobial Therapy in Infected Diabetes-Related Lower Extremity Ulcers

Non-limb-threatening*
  (May give initial dose as IV equivalent)
  Cephalexin 500 mg PO qid, 10-day course (cefazolin 1 g IV) *or*
  Clindamycin 300 mg PO qid, 10-day course (clindamycin 900 mg IV) *or*
  Dicloxacillin 500 mg PO qid, 10-day course *or*
  Amoxicillin-clavulanate 875 mg PO bid, 10-day course
Limb-threatening*
  More than 2 cm of cellulitis/inflammation
  Ascending lymphangitis
  Deep structure involvement
  Large areas of necrosis
  Gangrene
  Lower extremity ischemia with decreased or absent pulses
  Oral regimen: Fluoroquinolone and clindamycin *Close follow-up!*
  IV regimens:
    Ampicillin-sulbactam 3 g IV q6h *or*
    Ticarcillin-clavulanate 3.1 g IV q8h *or*
    Second-generation cephalosporin (cefoxitin, cefotetan) 1–2 g IV q12h *or*
    Ciprofloxacin 400 mg IV q12h and clindamycin 900 mg IV q6h
Life-threatening*
  IV regimens:
    Imipenem-cilastatin 1 g q6h *or*
    Ampicillin-sulbactam 3 g q8h + antipseudomonal aminoglycoside
      tobramycin 5–7 mg/kg qd *or*
    Vancomycin 1 g q12h + metronidazole 500 mg q6h + aztreonam 2 g q8h

*See text for definitions.
Note: Adjust all dosages for renal/hepatic function and monitor blood levels where appropriate.
Abbreviations: DKA = diabetic ketoacidosis; HHNS = hyperglycemic, hyperosmolar nonketotic syndrome.

TABLE 212-9   Disposition/Guidelines for Hospital Admission

Inpatient care for the diabetic patient is generally appropriate for the following clinical situation:

Life-threatening metabolic decompensation such as diabetic ketoacidosis or hyperglycemic, hyperosmolar, nonketotic syndrome.

Newly diagnosed diabetes in children or adolecents.

Chronic, poor metabolic control that necessitates close monitoring to determine the cause of the poor control, with subsequent modification of the therapeutic plan.

Severe chronic complications of diabetes, such as chronic renal insufficiency or failure, atherosclerotic cardiovascular disease, infected lower extremity ulcers, retinopathy with acute loss of vision, neuropathy with intractable pain or affecting ability to ambulate, and autonomic neuropathy, i.e., gastroparesis with intractable nausea and vomiting that require admission for intensive therapy or to prevent metabolic decompensation.

Conditions that impact adversely on diabetes control or are complicated by the presence of diabetes, such as acute asthma or chronic obstructive pulmonary disease exacerbations requiring high does of corticosteroids as therapy.

Uncontrolled or newly discovered diabetes during pregnancy.

Institution of insulin pump or other intensive insulin regimens for glycemic control.

Hyperglycemia (>400 mg/dL) associated with severe volume depletion.

Hyperglycemia that does not respond to appropriate interventions or with associated metabolic deterioration.

Hypoglycemia with neuroglycopenia (altered level of consciousness, altered behavior, coma, seizure) that does not rapidly resolve with correction of hypoglycemia.

Hypoglycemia resulting from long-acting oral hypoglycemic agents.

Hypoglycemia with adequate resolution of symptoms but no responsible adult to be with the patient for the next 12 h.

Recurrence of hypoglycemia despite interventions.

Admissions for complications of diabetes should be driven by the appropriate care for the particular diagnostic entity, such as infected lower extremity ulcer, renal failure, congestive heart failure, or unstable angina.

Admissions for other medical conditions should be considered if rapid initiation of glucose control can improve outcome, such as in pregnancy, infections, or surgery. Also, consider admission if the medical illness can lead to acute onset of retinal, renal, neurologic, or cardiovascular complications of diabetes, for example, hypertensive urgency/emergency. These guidelines may result in admissions for diabetic patients for conditions that may be treated on an outpatient basis in the nondiabetic population.

Fever without an obvious source in patients with poorly controlled diabetes.

Source: Adapted from the American Diabetes Association,[28] with permission.

shoes should be avoided. Avoidance of weight bearing on the affected limb is critical to avoid progression to infection and for proper healing.

Radiographs of the foot are indicated for all ulcers to exclude subcutaneous gas, foreign bodies, osteomyelitis, and Charcot joints. Swab cultures of foot ulcers may provide misleading results. Culture of tissue excised from the base of the ulcer provides the most accurate identification of the bacteria involved. Commonly isolated organisms include *Bacteroides* species, *Staphylococcus aureus, Staphylococcus epidermidis, Enterococcus, E. coli, Proteus mirabilis,* and *Pseudomonas aeruginosa.* Empirical antibiotic therapy should be directed against these organisms.

In choosing antibiotic therapy for these infections, severity should be taken into account[27] (Table 212-8). The use of aminoglycosides generally should be avoided whenever possible because of their associated nephrotoxicity. For limb-threatening and life-threatening infections, immediate surgical consultation is indicated for incision and debridement, possible revascularization, or amputation.[27]

Skin and Soft Tissue Complications

Skin infections such as cellulitis, furuncles, and carbuncles and candidiasis occur more commonly in patients with diabetes. Serious infections usually develop due to the combination of poorly controlled serum glucose, vascular insufficiency, and tissue hypoxia. These infections may spread rapidly with dramatic skin changes. The worst of these infections is necrotizing fasciitis.

NECROTIZING FASCIITIS   Necrotizing fasciitis is a rapidly progressive infection of the skin and soft tissues that is more common in diabetic patients (see Chap. 152). It can occur anywhere on the body but is associated most commonly with the extremities and the abdominal wall. Fournier gangrene is a form of necrotizing fasciitis involving the male genitalia and perineum. On clinical evaluation, pain is usually severe and out of proportion to the visible degree of erythema, swelling, and palpable tenderness. Later skin changes include the formation of bullae and eschar. Crepitus is noted in up to half of patients. Radiographs may reveal gas in the tissues in up to 75 percent of patients. Necrotizing fasciitis has been classified as type 1, typically caused by a combination of anerobe (usually *Bacteroides fragilis* or *Clostridium* sp.) and facultative aerobe (usually *E. coli*), or type 2, typically caused by group A streptococci with or without concurrent *S. aureus* infection. Treatment involves immediate surgical consultation for aggressive debridement of necrotic tissue and IV antibiotics: penicillin G 6 million units IV every 6 h plus clindamycin 900 mg IV every 8 h plus gentamicin 5 mg/kg IV every day. Synthetic penicillins plus β-lactamase inhibitors (ampicillin-sulbactam, ticarcillin-clavulanic acid) and third-generation cephalosporins also may be effective in combination with clindamycin. Vancomycin and/or fluoroquinolones may be reasonable alternatives in the penicillin-allergic patient.

Hemodynamic support and correction of ketoacidosis and/or hyperglycemia are required to create optimal conditions for healing postoperatively.[26]

DISPOSITION AND INDICATIONS FOR HOSPITAL ADMISSION

Guidelines for admission considerations are listed in Table 212-9. These guidelines may result in admissions for diabetic patients for conditions that may be treated on an outpatient basis in the nondiabetic population.[28]

Patients who present with new-onset type 2 diabetes or type 1 diabetes without evidence of metabolic decompensation, acute hypoglycemia, or hyperglycemia and do not meet the aforementioned criteria for admission should see their primary care provider within 24 to 48 h as a general rule to arrange for general education and dietary evaluation and to initiate appropriate therapy for glycemic control. General discharge instructions for all diabetic patients, new or established, are detailed in Table 212-10.

TABLE 212-10   Discharge Instructions and Follow-Up Care

Follow a healthy diet.

Self-monitor blood glucose regularly.

Take insulin or oral hypoglycemics as directed.

Reduce weight where appropriate.

Cease smoking where appropriate.

Exercise regularly in the absence of contraindications, such as foot ulcers.

Practice good general foot care (check regularly for minor trauma and hot spots, keep nails trimmed properly, and wear well-fitted shoes).

Wearing a Medic-alert bracelet or necklace.

Be able to recognize symptoms of high blood sugar, such as frequent urination, thirst, dizziness, headache, nausea or vomiting, abdominal pain, lethargy, or blurry vision.

Be able to recognize symptoms of low blood sugar, including fatigue, headache, drowsiness, agitation, pale or moist, visual changes, or loss of consciousness.

Know how to help yourself or others with low blood sugar by self-administering or giving an awake person (who can swallow without gagging or choking) candy, fruit juice, or sugar or by calling an emergency phone number (e.g., 911) if the affected person is not able to respond.

REFERENCES

1. Expert Committee on the Diagnosis and Classification of Diabetes Mellitus: Report of the Expert Committee on the Diagnosis and Classification of Diabetes Mellitus. *Diabetes Care* 25(suppl 1):S5, 2002.
2. Turner RC, Cull CA, Frighi V, et al: Glycemic control with diet, sulfonylurea, metformin, or insulin in patients with type 2 diabetes mellitus: Progressive requirement for multiple therapies. *JAMA* 28:2005, 1999.
3. Diabetes Prevention Program Research Group. Reduction in the incidence of type 2 diabetes with lifestyle intervention or metformin. *New Engl J Med* 346:393, 2002.
4. National Diabetes Statistics: General Information and National Statistics on Diabetes in the United States, 2000. NIH Publication No. 02-3892. March 2002; accessed online April 3, 2002 at http://www.niddk.nih.gov/health/diabetes/pubs/dmstats/htm.
5. Mokdad AH, Ford ES, Bowman BA, et al: Diabetes trends in the United States: 1990–1998. *Diabetes Care* 23:1278, 2000.
6. Harris MI, Flegal KM, Cowie CC, et al: Prevalence of diabetes, impaired fasting glucose, and impaired glucose tolerance in U.S. adults. *Diabetes Care* 21:518, 1998.
7. Karvonen M, Viik-Kajander M, Moltchanova E, et al: Incidence of childhood type 1 diabetes worldwide. *Diabetes Care* 23:1516, 2000.
8. Gu K, Cowie CC, Harris MI: Mortality in adults with and without diabetes in a national cohort of the U.S. population, 1971–1993 *Diabetes Care* 21:1138, 1998.
9. Brownlee M, Vlassara H, Cerami A: Non-enzymatic glycolysation products on collagen covalently trap low-density lipoproteins. *Diabetes* 34:938, 1985.
10. American Diabetes Association: Standards of medical care for patients with diabetes mellitus (position statement). *Diabetes Care* 25(suppl 1):S33, 2002.
11. Johnson RN, Baker JR: Analytical error of home glucose monitors: A comparison of 18 systems. *Ann Clin Biochem* 36:72, 1999.
12. Adrogue HJ, Barrero J, Eknoyan G: Salutary effects of modest fluid replacement in the treatment of adults with DKA. *JAMA* 262:2108, 1989.
13. Holleman F, van den Brand JJ, Hoven RA, et al: Comparison of LysB28, ProB29-human insulin analogue and regular human insulin in the correction of incidental hyperglycemia. *Diabetes Care* 19:1426, 1996.
14. UK Prospective Diabetes Study Group: Intensive blood-glucose control with sulphonylureas or insulin compared with conventional treatment and risk of complications in patients with type 2 diabetes. *Lancet* 352:837, 1998.
15. Cost-effectiveness of intensive glycemic control, intensified hypertension control, and serum cholesterol level reduction for type 2 diabetes. *JAMA* 287:2542, 2002.
16. Inzucchi SE: Oral antihyperglycemic therapy for type 2 diabetes. *JAMA* 287:360, 2002.
17. Medaliar S, Edelman SV: Insulin therapy in type 2 diabetes. *Endocrinol Metab Clin North Am* 30:935, 2001.
18. Gu K, Cowie CC, Harris MI: Mortality in adults with and without diabetes in a national cohort of the U.S. population, 1971–1993. *Diabetes Care* 21:1138, 1998.
19. Haffner SM, Lehto S, Ronnemaa T, et al: Mortality from coronary heart disease in subjects with type 2 diabetes and in nondiabetic subjects with and without prior myocardial infarction. *New Engl J Med* 339:229, 1998.
20. Rohr J, Kittner S, Feeser B, et al: Traditional risk factors and ischemic stroke in young adults. *Arch Neurol* 53:603, 1996.
21. Heart Outcomes Prevention Evaluation Study Investigators: Effects of an angiotensin-converting-enzyme inhibitor, ramipril, on cardiovascular events in high-risk patients. *New Engl J Med* 342:145, 2000.
22. American Diabetes Association: Aspirin therapy in diabetes (position statement). *Diabetes Care* 25:S78, 2002.
23. The Diabetes Control and Complications Trial/Epidemiology of Diabetes Interventions and Complications Research Group: Retinopathy and nephropathy in patients with type 1 diabetes four years after a trial of intensive therapy. *New Engl J Med* 342:381, 2000.
24. Partanen J, Niskanen L, Lehtinen J, et al: Natural history of peripheral neuropathy in patients with non-insulin dependent diabetes mellitus. *New Engl J Med* 333:89, 1995.
25. Armstrong DG, Lavery LA, Vela SA, et al: Choosing a practical screening instrument to identify patients at risk for diabetic foot ulceration. *Arch Intern Med* 158:289, 1998.
26. Joshi N, Caputo GM, Weitekamp MR, et al: Infections in patients with diabetes mellitus. *New Engl J Med* 341:1906, 1999.
27. Caputo GM, Cavanagh PR, Ulbrecht JS, et al: Assessment and management of foot disease in patients with diabetes. *New Engl J Med* 33:854, 1994.
28. American Diabetes Association: Hospital admission guidelines for diabetes mellitus (position statement). *Diabetes Care* 25(suppl 1):S109, 2002.

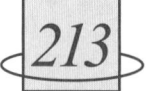

ALCOHOLIC KETOACIDOSIS

William A. Woods
Debra G. Perina

Alcoholic ketoacidosis (AKA) is a wide-anion-gap acidosis most often associated with acute cessation of alcohol consumption after chronic alcohol abuse. The metabolism of alcohol with little or no glucose sources results in the elevated levels of ketoacids that typically produce the metabolic acidosis present in this illness. Although usually seen in chronic alcoholics, ketoacidosis has been described in first-time drinkers who binge drink, particularly in association with volume depletion from poor oral intake and vomiting.

EPIDEMIOLOGY

There are no gender differences. The age of presentation is variable but usually between 20 and 60 years. Patients often experience repeated episodes of ketoacidosis, with 23 percent of patients having more than one episode of AKA in one series.[1] The true incidence of this illness is unknown but most likely mirrors the incidence of alcoholism in the population.[1] This illness may be more prevalent than previously suspected. One study indicated that analysis of serum chemistries of alcoholics arriving at emergency departments with complaints related to excessive alcohol intake incidentally found ketoacidosis in 25 percent of patients.[2] Although with proper treatment this illness is self-limited, poor outcomes can occur. Medical examiner literature notes that 7 to 25 percent of deaths in known alcoholics are from AKA.[2–4]

PATHOPHYSIOLOGY

The pathophysiology of AKA is complex and not entirely understood. The key features of AKA are an ingestion of a large quantity of alcohol, relative starvation, and volume depletion. To begin to understand this disorder, it is necessary to understand ethanol metabolism (Figure 213-1). Ethanol metabolism requires nicotinamide adenosine dinucleotide (NAD) and the enzymes alcohol dehydrogenase and aldehyde dehydrogenase to convert ethanol to acetyl coenzyme A. Acetyl coenzyme A can be metabolized directly (resulting in ketone production), used as substrate for the Krebs cycle, or used for free fatty acid synthesis.

The pathologic state of AKA can occur when NAD is depleted, aerobic metabolism in the Krebs cycle is inhibited, glycogen stores are depleted, and lipolysis is stimulated. The lactate-pyruvate ratio is in the range of 20:1.[5] All these conditions are met in the recently intoxicated, volume-contracted patient with underlying poor nutrition and liver disease. Ethanol metabolism results in a higher ratio of NAD to NADH. When glycogen stores are depleted in a patient stressed by concurrent illness or volume depletion, insulin secretion is suppressed. On the other hand, under these same conditions, glucagon, catecholamine, and growth hormone secretion are all stimulated. This hormonal milieu inhibits aerobic metabolism in favor of anaerobic metabolism and promotes lipolysis. Hence the acetyl coenzyme A is metabolized to ketones.

The relative deficiency of NAD has another effect. NAD is used in the conversion of β-hydroxybutyrate (βHB) to acetoacetate. Acetoacetate is rapidly converted to acetone, which is excreted in the urine. Due to the imbalance of NAD and NADH, βHB is the predominant ketone product formed. Normally, the ratio of acetoacetate to βHB is 1:1, however, in AKA it is 1:7, although it can be higher.[5]

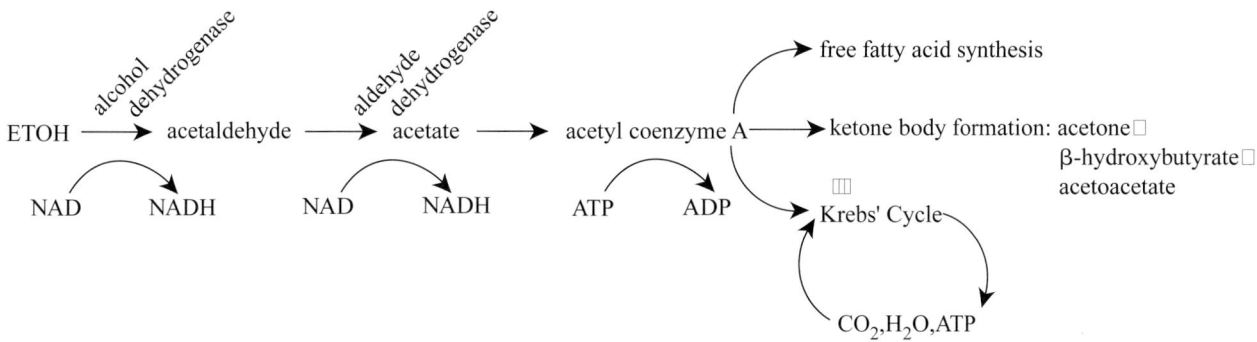

FIG. 213-1. Ethanol metabolism.

Ketone production can be further stimulated in malnourished, vomiting patients or in those who are hypophosphatemic. Both these conditions are seen commonly in alcoholic patients with AKA.

CLINICAL FEATURES

AKA typically occurs after an episode of heavy drinking followed by an acute decrease in alcohol and food intake and vomiting. The nausea, vomiting, and abdominal pain that may be associated with gastritis or pancreatitis may exacerbate the progression of this illness. As anorexia continues, the symptoms worsen, leading the patient to seek health care. Symptoms are nonspecific, making diagnosis difficult without laboratory studies as confirmation (Table 213-1).

There are no specific physical findings associated solely with AKA. The most common findings are tachycardia, tachypnea, and diffuse, mild to moderate abdominal tenderness. Volume depletion resulting from anorexia, diaphoresis, and vomiting may explain the frequently seen tachycardia and hypotension. Most patients are alert at presentation. Mental status changes in patients with ketoacidosis should alert clinicians to other potential causes, such as toxic ingestion, hypoglycemia, alcohol-withdrawal seizures, postictal state, or unrecognized head injury.

LABORATORY

Alcohol levels are usually low or undetectable at the time of presentation, but some patients may present with an elevated blood alcohol level, making diagnosis more challenging. An elevated anion gap caused by ketones is essential for diagnosing AKA. Since βHB predominates, the degree of ketonemia may not be appreciated, depending on the method of ketone detection (see Chap. 211 for a complete discussion). The initial anion gap is usually 16 to 33, with a mean of 21.[2] Patients frequently have mild hypophosphatemia, hyponatremia, and/or hypokalemia. Severe derangements are rare but have been reported. Most patients also will have elevated bilirubin and liver en-zyme levels due to liver disease from a long history of chronic ethanol use. Blood urea nitrogen and creatine kinase levels frequently are elevated due to relative volume depletion. Serum lactate levels can be mildly elevated. Glucose levels most often are only mildly elevated, but a subset of patients will have hypoglycemia. On rare occasions, the glucose level may be greater than 200 mg/dL.

Acid-Base Balance

Serum pH is typically acidemic, but the pH may be normal or even alkalemic early in the course of the illness.[6] In one study, 15 percent of patients were alkalemic, 30 percent had normal pH, and 55 percent had acidemia.[1] The degree of acidosis is typically less than that seen in patients with diabetic ketoacidosis. If the acidosis is mild and the patient also has a primary respiratory alkalosis (i.e., due to fever, sepsis, or alcohol withdrawal), then the pH may be normal or even alkalemic. Similarly, contraction metabolic alkalosis may mask the presence of a concurrent wide-anion-gap acidosis and result in a "normal" or even elevated serum bicarbonate level, rendering the pH normal or alkalemic. Since volume loss, whether due to poor volume intake or vomiting, is virtually always present in AKA, some degree of metabolic alkalosis is present.

Without routine evaluation of the anion gap in every patient at risk for AKA, the diagnosis can be easily missed. An anion gap greater than the patient's baseline (or greater than 15 in any case) signifies the presence of a wide-anion-gap acidosis regardless of the actual [HCO_3^-] or the pH, even if the patient is alkalemic. For example, a common serum chemistry result in a patient with AKA may be along the following lines: [Na^+], 145; [Cl^-; 95; [K^+], 4.1; and [HCO_3^-], 25 all in mEq/L. In this example, the anion gap (25, excluding K^+) is elevated by at least 10, yet the [HCO_3^-] and electrolyte levels are normal. The only explanation is that a mixed acid-base abnormality of approximately equal but opposing magnitudes exists. Arterial blood gas determination is not needed to arrive at the correct diagnosis for this relatively complicated acid-base disturbance. (For a more detailed discussion, the reader is referred to Chap. 25.)

Ketones

The standard test for ketone detection is the serum or urine nitroprusside test. While βHB is the predominant ketone present in AKA, acetoacetate is the only ketone normally detected by the nitroprusside test. Since patients with AKA may have only mildly elevated acetoacetate levels, it is important not to exclude the diagnosis of AKA with a negative or only weakly positive test. As treatment progresses and NAD is replenished, the acetoacetate levels actually may increase, and the nitroprusside test will reflect an increasingly positive reaction. This natural progression should be expected and does not indicate a worsening of the patient's condition. The clinical application of this test is thus quite variable. Most authors suggest measuring βHB and acetoacetate levels only if the diagnosis is unclear or other ways are not available to follow the patient's response to therapy.[6]

TABLE 213-1   Common Symptoms and Signs in Alcoholic Ketoacidosis

Symptoms	%	Signs/Anion Gap	%
Nausea	76	Tachycardia	56
Vomiting	73	Tachypnea	49
Abdominal pain	62	Abdominal tenderness	43
Shortness of breath	20	Heme-positive stool	18
Tremulousness	20	Hepatomegaly	18
Hematemesis	19	Altered mental status	15
Dizziness	19	Hypotension	12

Source: From Wrenn et al[1] and Soffer and Hamburger,[2] with permission.

DIAGNOSIS

The diagnosis is easily established in the classic presentation of the chronic alcoholic with recent anorexia, vomiting, abdominal pain, unexplained metabolic acidosis with a positive nitroprusside test, elevated anion gap, and a low or mildly elevated serum glucose level. However, classic presentations are uncommon. Establishing this diagnosis can be difficult for several reasons. First, the blood alcohol level may be zero, and the patient may not voluntarily provide the history of alcohol consumption. Second, urine nitroprusside testing may be negative or weakly positive despite significant ketoacidosis. Finally, the pH may vary from significant acidemia to mild alkalemia. However, a widened anion gap is invariable.

Initial laboratory studies include determination of electrolyte, blood urea nitrogen (BUN), and creatinine levels; hepatic and pancreatic enzyme levels; white blood cell count; hematocrit; and urinalysis. The anion gap should be calculated. Determination of serum lactic acid level and serum osmolarity also may be helpful if the diagnosis is in doubt. Further laboratory studies may be needed to delineate the cause of the increased anion-gap acidosis if other ingestions besides ethanol are suspected (see "Differential Diagnosis" below). An arterial blood gas determination is unnecessary unless a primary respiratory acid-base disturbance is suspected (Table 213-2).

Differential Diagnosis

The differential diagnosis for AKA is very broad. It is essentially the differential diagnosis of wide-anion-gap metabolic acidosis. Lactic acidosis, uremia, and other ingestions (particularly methanol and ethylene glycol) should be considered. A mild lactic acidosis is occasionally present in AKA related to ethanol metabolism, but it is comparatively inconsequential. Lactic acidosis related to anaerobic metabolism (e.g., hypotension, sepsis, or tissue ischemia or associated with methanol, ethylene glycol, and salicylic acid) is usually markedly more severe and less readily masked by concurrent metabolic alkalosis. Both salicylic acid poisoning and sepsis often present with triple acid-base disturbances (metabolic acidosis, metabolic alkalosis, and respiratory alkalosis). Other potential etiologies, such as renal failure or diabetic ketoacidosis, can be ascertained from the serum chemistries, with an elevated creatinine, BUN, or blood sugar level greater than 300 mg/dL, respectively. Differentiation of AKA from starvation ketosis is an academic exercise and unimportant because underlying pathophysiology, treatment, and implications are similar.

Differentiating AKA from other alcohol ingestions should not be difficult. Methanol and ethylene glycol ingestions do not produce ketosis, but acidosis tends to be severe. Since patients with AKA have a negative urine nitroprusside test in approximately 15 percent of cases,[1] **the absence of urinary ketones cannot be used to exclude a diagnosis of AKA** if concurrent methanol or ethylene glycol ingestion is suspected. Isopropyl alcohol ingestion results in production of ketones and is on occasion associated with a mild lactic acidosis. However, the presence of an osmolal gap (which is a feature of isopropyl, methanol, and ethylene glycol poisonings) may help in differentiating pure AKA from other concurrent mixed ingestions. Remember, ethanol is osmotically active and, if present, also will contribute to production of an os-

molal gap. If the blood alcohol level is known, then its contribution to any osmolal gap can be calculated. If the entire osmolal gap cannot be attributed to the ethanol level, then isopropyl alcohol (mild or no acidosis), methanol, or ethylene glycol (severe acidosis) may well be the explanation. Each 100 mg/dL of ethanol raises the osmolal gap by 22. (Details of osmolal gap are discussed in Chap. 27.)

Patients with AKA often have concurrent illnesses that may have promoted the alcohol cessation and anorexia. Thus a thorough investigation for underlying illnesses should be performed. Common concurrent illnesses are pancreatitis, gastritis or upper gastrointestinal bleeding, seizures, alcohol withdrawal, pneumonia, sepsis, and hepatitis.

TREATMENT

Therapy is aimed at both glucose administration and volume repletion. The fluid of choice is D5NS. Glucose stimulates insulin production, which stops lipolysis and halts the further formation of ketones. Glucose also increases the oxidation of NADH to NAD, thereby further stopping ketone production. Patients with AKA are not hyperosmolar, and unlike treatment of diabetic ketoacidosis, cerebral edema is of little concern with large volumes of fluid administration. Even with vigorous fluid resuscitation, no cases of cerebral edema have been reported among those being treated for AKA.

Insulin is of no proven benefit and can be dangerous because patients often have depleted glycogen stores and normal or low glucose levels. Sodium bicarbonate is not indicated unless patients are severely acidemic, with a pH of 7.1 or lower. As noted, this level of acidemia is unlikely to be explained by AKA alone. A vigorous search for an alternate explanation must be undertaken. Hypophosphatemia is seen frequently in chronic alcoholic patients and can retard the resolution of acidosis because phosphorus is necessary for mitochondrial utilization of glucose to produce NADH oxidation. However, phosphate replacement generally is unwarranted as part of this treatment in the emergency department unless very low levels are encountered (<1.0 mg/dL). Oral replenishment is safe and effective. Nitroprusside tests correlated with clinical status may be used to help guide therapy because an increasingly positive reaction signifies improvement. To prevent the theoretical precipitation of Wernicke disease, all patients should receive 50 to 100 mg of thiamine prior to the administration of glucose. Concomitant administration of magnesium sulfate and multivitamins should be considered and guided by laboratory results. Acidosis may clear within 12 to 24 h. Patients with an uncomplicated emergency department course may be safely discharged home if there is resolution of acidosis over time and the patient is able to tolerate oral fluids. Patients with a complicated course, underlying illnesses, or persistent acidosis should be admitted for further evaluation and treatment.

REFERENCES

1. Wrenn KD, Slovis CM, Minion GE, Rutkowski R: The syndrome of alcoholic ketoacidosis. *Am J Med* 91:119, 1991.
2. Soffer A, Hamburger S: Alcoholic ketoacidosis: A review of 30 cases. *J Am Med Women's Assoc* 37:106, 1982.
3. Thomsen JL, Simonsen KW, Felby S, Frohlich B: A prospective toxicology analysis in alcoholics. *Forensic Sci Int* 90:33, 1997.
4. Iten PX, Meier M: β-Hydroxybutyric acid: An indicator for an alcoholic ketoacidosis as cause of death in deceased alcohol abusers. *J Forens Sci* 45(3):624, 2000.
5. Umpierrez GE, DiGirolamo M, Tuvlin JA, et al: Differences in metabolic and hormonal milieu in diabetic- and alcohol-induced ketoacidosis. *J Crit Care* 15(2):52, 2000.
6. Elisaf M, Merkouropoulos M, Tsianos EV, Siamopoulos KC: Acid-base and electrolyte abnormalities in alcoholic patients. *Miner Electrolyte Metab* 20:274, 1994.

TABLE 213-2   Diagnostic Criteria for Alcoholic Ketoacidosis*

Glucose level less than 300 mg/dL
Vomiting
Recent ethanol intake, with decline over 1 to 3 days
Wide-anion-gap metabolic acidosis without alternate explanation

---

*The absence of ketones in the urine based on the nitroprusside test does not exclude the diagnosis (see text).
Source: From Soffer and Hamburger,[2] with permission.

214 HYPEROSMOLAR HYPERGLYCEMIC STATE
Charles S. Graffeo

The disease process discussed in this chapter is frequently referred to as *nonketotic hyperosmolar coma* to characterize the syndrome of severe hyperglycemia, hyperosmolality, and a relative lack of ketonemia in patients with poorly controlled or undiagnosed type 2 diabetes mellitus. The literature is replete with a score of other acronyms for this syndrome. The nomenclature used by the American Diabetes Association, *hyperosmolar hyperglycemic state* (HHS) and *hyperosmolar hyperglycemic nonketotic syndrome* (HHNS) are both commonly used and more appropriate. This chapter uses the HHNS designation. Placing emphasis on the presence or lack of coma is likely to underestimate the severity of disease, and thus "coma" should be excluded from the nomenclature. In fact, less than 10 percent actually present with coma.[1]

In general, HHNS is "defined" by severe hyperglycemia with serum glucose usually greater than 600 mg/dL, an elevated calculated plasma osmolality of greater than 315 mOsm/kg, serum bicarbonate greater than 15, an arterial pH greater than 7.3, and serum ketones that are negative to mildly positive in a 1:2 dilution.[2] These values, however, are fairly arbitrary. A profound metabolic acidosis and even moderate degrees of ketonemia may be found in HHNS. The importance of recognizing the potential for a variety of mixed acid-base patterns in patients presenting with HHNS cannot be overemphasized.

Many authors propose that HHNS and diabetic ketoacidosis (DKA) should be viewed as similar disease processes with the fundamental difference being in the metabolism of lipids during a period of relative insulin deficiency. Shared features of both include hyperglycemia, hyperosmolality, severe volume depletion, electrolyte disturbances, and sometimes acidosis. The acidosis associated with HHNS is more likely to be due to tissue hypoperfusion (lactic acidosis), starvation ketosis, and azotemia, in various combinations. In contrast, patients with DKA at similar levels of tissue perfusion have much higher levels of lipolysis with the release and subsequent oxidation of free fatty acids (FFA) to ketone bodies, β-hydroxybutyrate and acetoacetate, which contribute additional anions, resulting in a more profound acidosis. The inhibition of lipolysis and FFA metabolism characteristic of HHNS is poorly understood. A comparison of the laboratory features of DKA and HHNS is shown in Table 214-1.

Knowledge of the diagnostic criteria for diabetes can be an aid for identification of undiagnosed diabetes (Table 212-4).[3] Early identification of those at risk for HHNS is the most effective means of preventing serious complications. Patients with any evidence of unexplained hyperglycemia should be made aware of this potentially significant finding and referred for further evaluation. Caretakers of those without easy access to water such as nonambulatory nursing home patients must be particularly vigilant of the hydration status of such individuals. It is impaired access to water that is the fundamental risk factor for developing HHNS.

EPIDEMIOLOGY

The basic epidemiology of diabetes is discussed in Chap. 212. Although HHNS occurs much less frequently than DKA, mortality rates are much higher. The reported range of mortality in HHNS is approximately 15 to 30 percent versus approximately 5 percent in DKA.[4] However, mortality for HHNS increases substantially with advanced age and concomitant illness.

PATHOPHYSIOLOGY

The basic pathophysiology of diabetes is discussed in Chap. 212. The development of HHNS is attributed to three main factors: 1) decreased insulin utilization, 2) increased hepatic gluconeogenesis and glycogenolysis, and 3) impaired renal excretion of glucose.

During a state of poorly controlled type 2 diabetes mellitus, inadequate tissue utilization of glucose caused by insulin resistance results in hyperglycemia. In the absence of an adequate peripheral response to insulin, hepatic glycogenolysis and gluconeogenesis occurs, further elevating serum glucose. As serum glucose concentration increases, it creates an osmotic gradient, attracting water from the intracellular space and into the intravascular compartment. This initial increase in intravascular volume is accompanied by a temporary increase in the glomerular filtration rate (GFR). As serum glucose concentration exceeds approximately 180 mg/dL, the capacity of the kidneys to reabsorb glucose is exceeded, and glucosuria and a profound osmotic diuresis occur.

Patients with free access to water are often able to prevent profound volume depletion by replacing lost water with large free water intake. If this water requirement is not met (as may occur in a nonambulatory nursing home patient), volume depletion occurs. During osmotic diuresis, urine produced is markedly hypertonic. Still, significant urinary loss of sodium and potassium, as well as more modest losses of calcium, phosphate, magnesium, and urea, also occur. As volume depletion progresses, renal perfusion decreases and the GFR is reduced.

TABLE 214-1 Diagnostic Criteria for DKA and HHNS

	DKA			HHNS
	Mild	Moderate	Severe	
Plasma glucose (mg/dL)	>250	>250	>250	>600
Arterial pH	7.25–7.30	7.00–7.24	<7.00	>7.30
Serum bicarbonate (mEq/L)	15–18	10 to <15	<10	>15
Urine ketone*	Positive	Positive	Positive	Small
Serum ketones*	Positive	Positive	Positive	Small
Effective serum osmolarity (mOsm/L)†	Variable	Variable	Variable	>320
Anion gap‡	>10	>12	>12	<12
Alteration in sensoria or mental obtundation	Alert	Alert/drowsy	Stupor/coma	Stupor/coma

*Nitroprusside reaction method.
†Calculation: 2(measured [Na$^+$] (mEq/L)) + glucose (mg/dL)/18.
‡Calculation: [Na$^+$](mEq/L) − [Cl$^-$] + [HCO$_3^-$]) (mEq/L). See text for details.
Source: ADA,[2] with permission.

Renal tubular excretion of glucose is consequently impaired, which further worsens the hyperglycemia. A sustained osmotic diuresis may result in total body water losses that often exceed 20 to 25 percent of total body weight, or approximately 8 to 12 L in a 70-kg patient.

The reason for the absence of ketoacidosis in HHNS is not clearly understood. Though some degree of a starvation ketosis does occur, clinically significant ketoacidosis does not. This lack of ketoacidosis in HHNS has been attributed to three possible mechanisms: 1) lower levels of counterregulatory hormones, 2) higher levels of endogenous insulin, which strongly inhibits lipolysis, and 3) inhibition of lipolysis by the hyperosmolar state.

There is controversy about the role that counterregulatory hormones glucagon, cortisol, growth hormone, and epinephrine play in HHNS. When compared with DKA, glucagon and growth hormone levels have been shown to be lower, which may help prevent lipolysis. When compared with DKA, significantly higher levels of insulin are found in the peripheral and portal circulation in HHNS. Though these levels of insulin are insufficient to overcome hyperglycemia, they appear to be sufficient to inhibit lipolysis.[5] Finally, there have also been limited experimental animal studies that have shown that both the hyperosmolar state and severe hyperglycemia inhibit lipolysis in adipose tissue.

CLINICAL FEATURES

The typical patient with HHNS is usually elderly, and is often referred by a caretaker for abnormalities in vital signs and or mental status. Patient complaints may include weakness, anorexia, fatigue, cough, dyspnea, or abdominal pain. Many will have either undiagnosed or poorly controlled type 2 diabetes that has been precipitated by an acute illness. Pneumonia and urinary tract infection account for 30 to 50 percent of cases. Noncompliance with or under-dosing of insulin has been identified as a common precipitant as well, at least in some populations.[6] Those predisposed to HHNS often have some level of baseline cognitive impairment, such as senile dementia, and self-referral for medical treatment during early stages of illness is rare. In general, any patient with hyperglycemia, an impaired means of communication, and limited access to free water intake is at major risk for HHNS. The presence of hypertension, renal insufficiency, or cardiovascular disease is common in this patient population, and medications commonly used to treat these diseases, such as diuretics and β-blockers, predisposes to the development of HHNS.

Typically, an insidious state of progressive hyperglycemia, or hyperosmolarity and osmotic diuresis develops, which usually goes unchecked. Alterations in vital signs and cognition follow and signal a severity of illness that is often advanced. A host of metabolic and iatrogenic causes have been identified (Table 214-2), including many commonly prescribed drugs that may predispose to hyperglycemia, volume depletion, or other effects leading to HHNS (Table 214-3).

Physical Findings

The physical manifestations associated with HHNS are nonspecific. Generally, clinical signs of volume depletion such as poor skin turgor, dry mucous membranes, sunken eyeballs, and hypotension will corre-

TABLE 214-2   Conditions That May Precipitate Hyperosmolar Hyperglycemic State

Diabetes	Infection
Parental or enteral alimentation	Myocardial infarction
Gastrointestinal hemorrhage	Severe burns
Pulmonary emboli	Renal insufficiency
Pancreatitis	Peritoneal or hemodialysis
Heat-related illness	Cerebrovascular events
Mesenteric ischemia	Rhabdomyolysis

TABLE 214-3   Drugs That May Predispose Individuals to the Development of Hyperosmolar Hyperglycemic State

Diuretics	Glucocorticoids
Lithium	Neuroleptics
β-Blockers	Phenytoin
Mannitol	Didanosine
Chlorpromazine	Calcium-channel blockers
Cimetidine	Pentamidine

late with degree of hyperglycemia and hyperosmolality and duration of physiologic imbalance.

A wide range of findings from subtle changes in vital signs and cognition to clear evidence of profound shock and coma may occur. Normothermia or hypothermia is common due to vasodilation. HHNS may unexpectedly be found in non-diabetics who present with an acute medical insult such as a cerebrovascular accident (CVA), severe burns, myocardial infarction, infection, pancreatitis, or other acute illness. Up to 15 percent may present with seizures. These are typically focal, though generalized seizures, which are often resistant to anticonvulsants, may occur.[7]

Other central nervous system (CNS) symptoms may include tremor, clonus, hyperreflexia or hyporeflexia, a positive plantar response, reversible hemiplegia, or hemisensory defects (without CVA or structural intracerebral lesion). The degree of lethargy and coma is proportional to the level of osmolality. Those with coma tend to have higher osmolality, hyperglycemia, and greater volume contraction.[8] In view of the age of the patient population, it is not surprising that the misdiagnosis of stroke or organic brain disease is common.

Laboratory Tests

Essential laboratory tests should include serum glucose, electrolytes, calculated and measured serum osmolality, blood urea nitrogen (BUN), ketones, and creatinine, as well as complete blood count. In view of the frequency of precipitating causes and underlying medical conditions associated with HHNS, a broad range of ancillary studies should be considered. These should include blood cultures, sputum collection, urinalysis and culture, liver and pancreatic enzyme determinations, cardiac enzymes, thyroid function, coagulation profiles, chest x-ray, and electrocardiogram. Other ancillary studies such as computed tomography of the head, lumbar puncture, and toxicologic studies should also be considered. Arterial blood-gas determination is of added value only if there is suspicion of a respiratory component to the acid-base abnormality, as both P_{CO_2} and pH can be predicted from $[HCO_3^-]$ concentration obtained in venous electrolytes (see Chap. 25, "Acid-Base Disorders").

In general, electrolyte abnormalities initially reflect a contraction alkalosis due to profound water deficit. As many as 50 percent of patients with HHNS will have an increased anion gap metabolic acidosis (lactic acidosis, azotemia, starvation ketosis, severe volume contraction). Acute or concurrent illnesses, however, such as ischemic bowel, will contribute anions such as lactic acid, causing varying degrees of an anion-gap metabolic acidosis. Initial serum electrolyte determinations can be reported as seemingly normal because the concurrent presence of both metabolic alkalosis and acidosis may result in each cancelling out the other's effect. A lack of careful analysis of serum chemistries may lead to a delayed appreciation of the severity of the underlying abnormalities, including volume loss. Serum sodium is suggestive but not a reliable indicator of degree of volume contraction. Although the patient is certainly total body sodium depleted, the serum sodium (even corrected for the glucose elevation) may be low, normal, or elevated. Measured serum sodium, however, is often reported as factitiously low due to the dilutional effect of hyperglycemia. It is important to correct for this effect. Serum sodium decreases by approximately 1.6 mEq for every 100 mg/dL increase in serum glucose above 100 mg/dL or:

$$\text{corrected } [Na^+] = \text{measured } [Na^+] + \frac{1.6 \times [\text{glucose} - 100]}{100}$$

Elevated corrected serum sodium during severe hyperglycemia is usually explainable only by profound volume contraction. Normal sodium level or mild hyponatremia usually (but not invariably) suggests modest dehydration.

Serum osmolarity has also been shown to correlate with severity of disease as well as neurologic impairment and coma.[2] A calculated effective serum osmolarity excludes osmotically inactive urea, which is usually included in laboratory measures of osmolarity. The formula for calculated effective osmolarity (mOsm/L) is:

$$2[Na^+] + \frac{\text{glucose}}{18}$$

Normal serum osmolarity range is approximately 275 to 295 mOsm/kg. Values above 300 mOsm/kg are usually indicative of significant hyperosmolarity and those above 320 mOsm are commonly associated with alterations in cognitive function. Osmolarity (mOsm/L) and osmolality (mOsm/kg) are discussed in detail in Chap. 27.

Hypokalemia probably poses the most immediate electrolyte-based risk and should be anticipated. Total body deficits of 500 to 700 mEq/L are not uncommon. Initial values may be reported as normal during a period of severe volume contraction and with metabolic acidosis when intravascular $[H^+]$ ions are exchanged for intracellular $[K^+]$ ions. The presence of acidemia may mask a potentially life-threatening $[K^+]$ deficit. As intravascular volume is replaced and acidemia reversed, $[K^+]$ losses become more apparent. Patients who have low serum $[K^+]$ during the period of severe volume contraction are at greatest risk for dysrhythmia. The importance of $[K^+]$ replacement during periods of volume repletion and insulin therapy cannot be overemphasized.

Both prerenal azotemia and renal azotemia are common, with plasma BUN:creatinine ratios often exceeding 30:1. Leukocytosis is variable and a weak clinical indicator. When present, it is usually due to infection or hemoconcentration. Hypophosphatemia may occur during periods of prolonged hyperglycemia. Acute consequences such as CNS abnormalities, cardiac dysfunction, and rhabdomyolysis are rare and usually associated with serum phosphate levels below 1.0 mg/dL. Routine replacement of phosphate or magnesium, unless severe, is usually unnecessary. Both electrolytes tend to normalize as metabolic derangements are addressed. When necessary, gradual replacement minimizes the risks of complications such as renal failure or hypocalcemia. Metabolic acidosis is of a wide-anion-gap type, often due to lactic acidosis from poor tissue perfusion, resulting in uremia, mild starvation ketosis, or all three.

TREATMENT

Improvement of tissue perfusion is the key to effective recovery in HHNS. Treatment includes correction of hypovolemia, identifying and treating precipitating causes, correcting electrolyte abnormalities, and gradual correction of hyperglycemia and osmolarity. What cannot be overstated is the importance of a judicious therapeutic plan that adjusts for concurrent medical illnesses such as left ventricular dysfunction or renal insufficiency commonly found in this patient population. Due to the potential for complications (noted below), rapid therapy should be reserved for potentially life-threatening electrolyte abnormalities only. A protocol for treating severely ill patients likely requiring ICU-level care is shown in Figure 214-1.

Fluid Resuscitation

Initial fluid resuscitation should be aimed at reestablishing adequate tissue perfusion and decreasing serum glucose. Replacement of in-

travascular fluid losses alone can account for reductions in serum glucose of 35 to 70 mg/h on average, or up to 80 percent of the necessary reduction.

The average fluid deficit in HHNS is in the range of 20 to 25 percent of total body water (TBW) or 8 to 12 L. In the elderly, about 50 percent of body weight is due to TBW. By using the patient's usual current weight in kilograms, normal TBW and water deficit can be calculated. One-half of the fluid deficits should be replaced over the initial 12 h and the balance over the next 24 h when possible. The actual rate of fluid administration should be individualized for each patient based on the presence of renal and cardiac impairment. Initial rates of 500 to 1500 mL per h during the first 2 h, followed by rates of 250 to 500 mL per h are usually well tolerated. Patients with cardiac disease may require a more conservative rate of volume repletion. Renal and cardiovascular function should be carefully monitored. Central venous and urinary tract catheterization should be considered in patients with preexisting renal or cardiac disease.

However, rate of fluid administration may need to be limited in children. Historically, a limited number of reports of cerebral edema occurring during or soon after the resuscitation phase of patients with both DKA and HHNS have been described.[9] Most cases have occurred in children with DKA, and the mechanism is unclear. In one review, cerebral edema was found with similar frequency before treatment with replacement fluids.[10] In a more recent study of cerebral edema in children with DKA, rehydration during the first 4 h at a rate greater than 50 mL/kg was associated with an increased risk of brain herniation.[11] There is little credible data on incidence or clinical indicators that may predispose to cerebral edema in HHS patients. However, current recommendations based on available data include limiting the rate of volume repletion during the first 4 h to <50 mL/kg of NS. Mental status should be closely monitored during treatment and computed tomographic brain imaging should be obtained with any evidence of cognitive impairment.

Most authors agree that the use of isotonic saline (NS) is the most appropriate initial crystalloid for the replacement of intravascular volume.[2] It is hypotonic to the patient's serum osmolality and will more rapidly restore plasma volume. Once hypotension, tachycardia, and urinary output improve, $\frac{1}{2}$NS can be used to replace the remaining free water deficit.

Electrolytes

Potassium deficits pose the most immediate electrolyte-based risk for a bad outcome. On average, potassium losses range from 4 to 6 mEq/kg, though deficits as high as 10 mEq/kg body weight have been reported. Despite these total body deficits, initial serum laboratory measurements may be normal or even high in the presence of acidemia. Patients whose initial serum potassium measurements are low (<3.3 mEq/L) are at highest risk for cardiac dysrhythmia and respiratory arrest and should be treated with urgency. Insulin therapy can precipitously lower intravascular potassium further and $[K^+]$ must be vigorously replaced.

When adequate urinary output is assured, potassium replacement should begin. In general, potassium should be replaced at a rate of 10 to 20 mEq per h, though life-threatening hypokalemia may warrant utilizing infusion rates of up to 40 mEq per h. (Rates over 20 mEq per h require central line administration.) Some authors feel that potassium infusion through a central venous catheter poses a risk for conduction defects and should be avoided although evidence for safe administration by this route exists.[12] If properly diluted, peripheral infusions of potassium through two peripheral intravenous lines are well tolerated. Monitoring of serum potassium should occur every hour until a steady state has been achieved.

Sodium deficits are replenished fairly rapidly, considering the amount of NS and $\frac{1}{2}$NS given during fluid replacement. Phosphate and magnesium levels should be measured. Current guidelines suggest

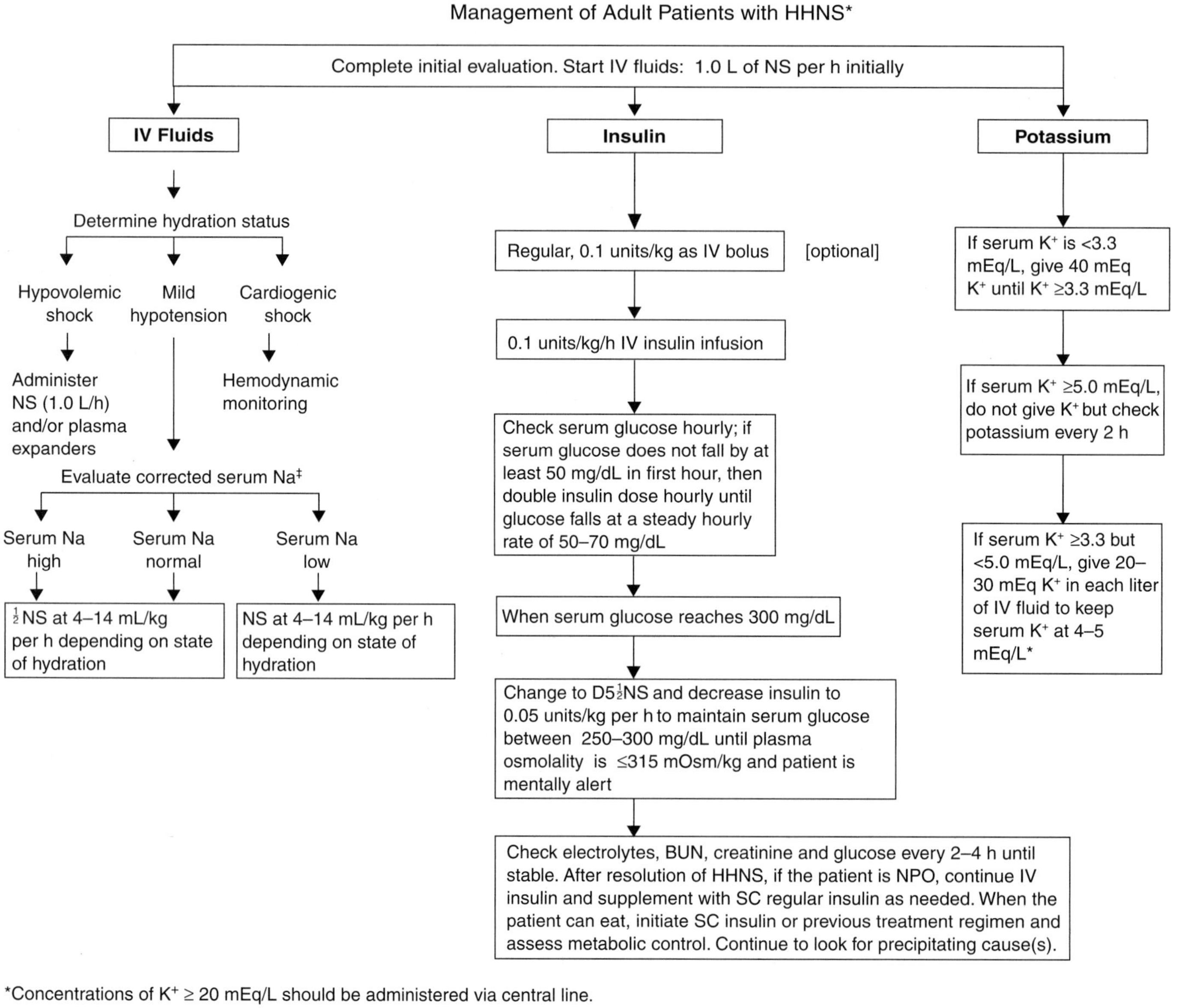

Management of Adult Patients with HHNS*

Complete initial evaluation. Start IV fluids: 1.0 L of NS per h initially

IV Fluids

Determine hydration status

Hypovolemic shock | Mild hypotension | Cardiogenic shock

Administer NS (1.0 L/h) and/or plasma expanders

Hemodynamic monitoring

Evaluate corrected serum Na‡

Serum Na high | Serum Na normal | Serum Na low

½NS at 4–14 mL/kg per h depending on state of hydration

NS at 4–14 mL/kg per h depending on state of hydration

Insulin

Regular, 0.1 units/kg as IV bolus [optional]

0.1 units/kg/h IV insulin infusion

Check serum glucose hourly; if serum glucose does not fall by at least 50 mg/dL in first hour, then double insulin dose hourly until glucose falls at a steady hourly rate of 50–70 mg/dL

When serum glucose reaches 300 mg/dL

Change to D5½NS and decrease insulin to 0.05 units/kg per h to maintain serum glucose between 250–300 mg/dL until plasma osmolality is ≤315 mOsm/kg and patient is mentally alert

Check electrolytes, BUN, creatinine and glucose every 2–4 h until stable. After resolution of HHNS, if the patient is NPO, continue IV insulin and supplement with SC regular insulin as needed. When the patient can eat, initiate SC insulin or previous treatment regimen and assess metabolic control. Continue to look for precipitating cause(s).

Potassium

If serum K⁺ is <3.3 mEq/L, give 40 mEq K⁺ until K⁺ ≥3.3 mEq/L

If serum K⁺ ≥5.0 mEq/L, do not give K⁺ but check potassium every 2 h

If serum K⁺ ≥3.3 but <5.0 mEq/L, give 20–30 mEq K⁺ in each liter of IV fluid to keep serum K⁺ at 4–5 mEq/L*

*Concentrations of K⁺ ≥ 20 mEq/L should be administered via central line.

FIG. 214-1. Protocol for the management of severely ill adult patients with HHNS. Diagnostic criteria for HHS: blood glucose >600 mg/dL, arterial pH >7.3, bicarbonate >15 mEq/L, mild ketonuria or ketonemia, and effective serum osmolality >320 mOsm/kg H_2O.
*History and physical examination, appropriate ancillary studies.
[Adapted with permission from the American Diabetes Association. *Diabetes Care* 24:131, 2001.]

administering one-third of the [K⁺] replacement as potassium phosphate to avoid excessive chloride administration and to prevent hypophosphatemia. However, unless severe, alleviation of hypophosphatemia or hypomagnesemia should occur after the patient is admitted and usually in an ICU setting.

Insulin

Volume repletion should precede insulin therapy. If insulin is administered prior to fluids, intravascular volume may be further depleted. Insulin causes a shift of osmotically active glucose into the intracellular space, bringing free water with it. This fluid shift may further deplete the intravascular compartment and precipitate vascular collapse.

The absorption of insulin by the intramuscular or subcutaneous route is unreliable in patients with HHNS, and a continuous infusion of regular insulin should be given. While initiation of insulin therapy with a bolus (0.1 units/kg) is common, there is no proven benefit over a simple continuous infusion (0.1 units/kg). Insulin for infusion ideally should be mixed in a 1:1 ratio (e.g., 250 units or regular insulin in

250 mL of NS). Pump infusion rates will thus correlate exactly to the hourly rate of units of insulin required. Steady states utilizing infusion pumps occur within 30 min of infusion. This usually results in a decrease in the plasma concentration of glucose of 50 to 75 mg/dL per h, provided adequate hydration is being provided. With adequate hydration, the insulin infusion may be doubled every hour until a steady glucose decline between 50 and 75 mg per h is achieved. Some patients will demonstrate insulin resistance and require higher doses. Once serum glucose decreases to less than 300 mg/dL, the intravenous solution should be changed to D5½NS, and the insulin infusion should be reduced to half or 0.05 units/kg per h.

DISPOSITION

When considering the patient population likely to develop HHNS, most will require ICU monitoring for the initial 24 h of care. Patients without significant comorbid conditions, who demonstrate a good response to initial therapy as evidenced by documented improvement in vital signs, urine output, electrolyte balance, and mentation, may be considered for step-down admission. Utilizing data flow sheets to track pH, vital signs, and key lab values is very useful for ED management and determining appropriate disposition.

REFERENCES

1. Lorber DL: Nonketotic hypertonicity in diabetes. *Endocrinologist* 3:29, 1993.
2. American Diabetes Association: Hyperglycemic crises in patients with diabetes mellitus. *Diabetes Care* 25(Suppl. 1):S100, 2002.
3. Report of the Expert Committee on the Diagnosis and Classification of Diabetes Mellitus: *Diabetes Care* 25:5, 2002.
4. Centers for Disease Control and Prevention: National Diabetes Fact Sheet: National Estimates and General Information on Diabetes in the United States. Atlanta, U.S. Department of Health and Human Services, Centers for Disease Control and Prevention, 1997.
5. Chaupin M, Charbonnel B, Chaupin F: C-peptide blood levels in ketoacidosis and in hyperosmolar non-ketotic diabetic coma. *Acta Diabet Lat* 18:123, 1981.
6. Umpierrez GE, Kelly JP, Navarrete JE, et al: Hyperglycemic crises in urban blacks. *Arch Intern Med* 157:669, 1997.
7. Wachtel TJ, Tetu-Mouradjian LM, Goldman DL, et al: Hyperosmolality and acidosis in diabetes mellitus: A three year experience in Rhode Island. *J Gen Intern Med* 6:495, 1991.
8. Guisado R, Arieff AI: Neurologic manifestations of diabetic comas: Correlation with biochemical alterations in the brain. *Metabolism* 24:665, 1975.
9. Silver SM, Clark EL, Schroeder BM, et al: Pathogenesis of cerebral edema after treatment of diabetic ketoacidosis. *Kidney Int* 51:1237, 1997.
10. Hoffman WH, Steinhart CM, Gammal TE, et al: Cranial CT in children and adolescents with diabetic ketoacidosis. *AJNR* 9:733, 1988.
11. Mahoney CP, Vlcek BW, DelAguila M: Risk factors for developing brain herniation during diabetic ketoacidosis. *Pediatr Neurol* 21:721, 1999.
12. Hamill RJ, Robinson LM, Wexler HR, Moote C: Efficacy and safety of potassium infusion therapy in hypokalemic critically ill patients. *Crit Care Med* 19:694, 1991.

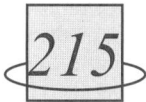

HYPERTHYROIDISM AND THYROID STORM
Horace K. Liang

Hyperthyroid states may result from various disorders. Manifestation of disease may range from patients with subtle, nonspecific complaints to individuals presenting with life-threatening emergencies. Recognition and subsequent empirical treatment of thyroid storm are clinical decisions.

NORMAL THYROID STATE

Regulation of synthesis and release of thyroid hormone is under the control of the anterior pituitary gland via thyroid-stimulating hormone (TSH, thyrotropin). Regulation of TSH, in turn, is by hypothalamic thyrotropin-releasing hormone (TRH) and also by means of a feedback loop to the pituitary by circulating T_4 (thyroxine) and T_3 (triiodothyronine) levels. Thyroid hormone production depends on an adequate iodine intake and synthesis of thyroglobulin. Thyroid hormones, following release from the thyroid, are reversibly bound to various circulating plasma proteins, of which thyronine-binding globulin (TBG) is the major constituent. The free, unbound portions of the hormone are biologically active. Normally, T_4 is the predominant circulating hormone. T_4 is peripherally deiodinated to T_3 and is responsible for producing 80 percent of the circulating T_3 hormone. Free T_3 is biologically more active than T_4 but has a shorter half-life (1 day versus 1 week).

Thyroid hormone exerts its action on a wide host of metabolic processes. It appears that most actions of thyroid hormone are at the cellular level and mediated by nuclear receptors for T_3. Binding of these receptors modulates expression of specific target genes and subsequent protein synthesis. Thyroid hormone also may mediate cellular metabolism.

HYPERTHYROIDISM

Hyperthyroidism occurs at all ages but is less common under the age of 15. It is 10 times more common in women than in men, with an annual incidence of about 1 per 1000 women.[1] Causes of hyperthyroidism are shown in Table 215-1. Graves disease is by far the most common etiology, accounting for more than 80 percent of cases of hyperthyroidism in the United States. Toxic multinodular and toxic (adenoma) nodular goiters are the next most frequent etiologies. Graves disease is common in the third and fourth decades of age. It is characterized by hyperthyroidism due to an autoimmune thyroid-stimulating antibody that activates the thyrotropin receptor on thyroid cells. Graves disease also is associated with diffuse goiter, ophthalmopathy, and local dermopathy. In contrast, toxic multinodular goiter usually occurs in a somewhat older population, commonly with a previous history of simple goiter. Often these patients have milder symptoms of thyrotoxicosis. Less common etiologies of hyperthyroidism are thyroiditis, pituitary tumors, metastatic thyroid cancer, and dermoid tumors or teratomas of the ovary. Medication-induced hyperthyroidism may be due to iodine ingestion, lithium therapy, or thyroid medication (thyrotoxicosis factitia).

Amiodarone, an effective iodine-rich antiarrhythmic drug, may cause both hyper- and hypothyroidism.[2] Amiodarone-induced thyrotoxicosis (AIT) has proved to be difficult to treat until recently because of incompletely understood mechanism of AIT pathogenesis.[3] There are two major forms of AIT. Type I occurs in an abnormal thyroid, while type II develops in an apparently normal thyroid. The treatment approach is different based on type (see below).

Classically, patients with hyperthyroidism may complain of heat intolerance, palpitations, weight loss, sweating, tremor, nervousness, weakness, and fatigue (Table 215-2).[4] Sinus tachycardia (the most common rhythm disturbance), widened pulse pressure, and increased cardiac output resemble a state of increased adrenergic activity despite a normal or low serum concentration of catecholamines.[5] An individual with hyperthyroidism exhibiting only mild symptoms may be safely referred for further evaluation as an outpatient. Clinical suspicion of hyperthyroidism is confirmed by thyroid function tests. An elevated free T_4 level and a low or undetectable TSH level are consistent with a diagnosis of hyperthyroidism. In some cases of Graves disease,

TABLE 215-1   Causes of Thyrotoxicosis

Primary hyperthyroidism
   Graves disease (toxic diffuse goiter)
   Toxic multinodular goiter
   Toxic nodular (adenoma) goiter
   Iodine intake (Jod-Basedow disease)
Central hyperthyroidism
   Pituitary adenoma
Thyroiditis
   Subacute painful (de Quervain)
   Silent subacute
   Postpartum
   Radiation thyroiditis
Nonthyroidal disease
   Ectopic thyroid tissue (struma ovarii)
   Metastatic thyroid cancer
Drug-induced
   Lithium
   Iodine (including radiographic contrast agents)
   Amiodarone
   Excessive thyroid hormone ingestion (thyrotoxicosis factitia)

TABLE 215-2 Signs and Symptoms of Symptoms of Hyperthyroidism

Symptoms	Signs
Weakness	Goiter/thyroid bruit
Fatigue	Hyperkinesis
Heat intolerance	Ophthalmopathy
Nervousness	Lid retraction/stare
Increased sweating	Lid lag
Tremor	Tremor
Palpitation	Warm, moist skin
Increased appetite	Muscle weakness
Weight loss	Hyperreflexia
Hyperdefecation	Tachycardia/arrhythmia
Dyspnea	Systolic hypertension
Menstrual abnormalities	Widened pulse pressure

Source: From Tietgens and Leinung.[4]

T_4 may be normal and TSH decreased, but the patient appears to be thyrotoxic. A T_3 level should be determined to rule out T_3 toxicosis. Patients with hyperthyroidism secondary to pituitary adenomas will have elevated TSH level.

Palliative treatment for mild hyperthyroidism can be accomplished by using various β-blocker medications, the most common of which is propranolol. The goal of therapy includes decreased heart rate, decreased tremor, increased muscle strength, and an overall improvement in the patient's sense of well-being. Treatment of Graves disease may include long-term antithyroid medication (e.g., propylthiouracil, methimazole, or carbimazole), radioactive iodine (^{131}I), or subtotal thyroidectomy.[6] A successful regiment for type I AIT is methimazole (30 mg per d) and potassium perchlorate (1 g per d). Type II is treated with glucocorticoids.[7] Thyrotoxicosis exacerbation is treated with (increasing) glucocorticoids for either type.[2] Toxic multinodular goiter and solitary adenomas also may be treated with radioiodine. Hyperthyroidism due to thyroiditis is usually self-limited, and therapy is rarely needed. Common etiologies of thyroiditis are subacute (painful) thyroiditis (due to viral etiologies), silent thyroiditis (due to lymphocytic infiltrates), and postpartum thyroiditis (due to transient immune destruction). Thyrotoxicosis factitia may be suspected with the absence of thyromegaly, a low serum thyroglobulin level, and decreased or absent radioactive uptake with thyroid scanning. Hyperthyroidism during pregnancy is almost always due to Graves disease. Often Graves disease will improve with progression of gestation. The lowest amounts of medication should be used in order to maintain the euthyroid state. Treatment options include propylthiouracil (fewer fetal anomalies than methimazole), although neonatal goiter has been reported with its use. Administration of radioiodine is contraindicated in pregnant women or those who are breast-feeding.[8]

THYROID STORM

The life-threatening hypermetabolic state due to hyperthyroidism is termed *thyroid storm*. This is a rare occurrence but constitutes a medical emergency. The diagnosis is based on clinical suspicion, treatment is initiated empirically, and the patient is admitted to an appropriately monitored setting. The differential diagnoses are listed in Table 215-3. Classically, thyroid storm occurs as a result of either previously unrecognized or poorly treated hyperthyroidism. Etiologies that precipitate thyroid storm are often recognized (Table 215-4), but the pathophysiology is not clearly understood. Most studies have not

TABLE 215-3 Differential Diagnosis for Thyroid Storm

Sepsis
Sympathomimetic ingestion (cocaine, amphetamine)
Heat stroke
Delirium tremens
Malignant hyperthermia
Malignant neuroleptic syndrome
Hypothalamic stroke
Pheochromocytosis
Medication withdrawal*

*Including illicit drugs (e.g., cocaine, opioids).

demonstrated differences in thyroid hormone levels in patients with symptomatic, uncomplicated hyperthyroidism and thyroid storm. Some studies have noted higher levels of free T_4 in individuals who have presented with thyroid storm. Enhanced sympathetic nervous system activity explains many of the presenting clinical findings of thyroid storm. Mortality rates despite treatment are high (10-75 percent). The signs and symptoms of thyroid storm are listed in Table 215-5. The classic mark of this disease is fever, sinus or supraventricular tachycardia out of proportion to the fever, changes in normal mental status (e.g., confusion, delirium, or coma), and gastrointestinal symptoms.[9]

Laboratory analysis is usually not helpful. Thyroid function tests are not routinely available to the emergency physician. Nonspecific laboratory findings may include leukocytosis, hyperglycemia, and increased transaminases and bilirubin. Further laboratory studies are aimed at potential underlying precipitants.

Treatment

Initial treatment of thyroid storm is stabilization, airway protection, oxygenation, intravenous fluids, and monitoring. Specific therapy is outlined in Table 215-6. β-Blockers are used to treat the severe adrenergic symptoms. Administration of propranolol has the additional benefit of inhibiting peripheral conversion of T_4 to T_3. If there is a contraindication to propranolol administration (e.g., asthma, congestive heart failure, chronic obstructive pulmonary disease), a selective $β_1$ medication (esmolol) may be substituted. Guanethidine (which inhibits norepinephrine release at the sympathetic junction) or reserpine (which depletes stored catecholamines both centrally and peripherally, including the adrenal medulla) may be considered as alternative therapy. Additional treatment goals are directed toward decreasing synthesis of additional hormone by the administration of propylthiouricil (PTU) or methimazole (MMI). PTU also decreases T_4-to-T_3 conversion.

After PTU administration has been initiated, treatment is then directed toward decreasing the release of preformed thyroid hormone by the administration of iodine. **It is important to not administer iodine until the synthetic pathway has been blocked.** Otherwise, the addition

TABLE 215-4 Precipitants of Thyroid Storm

Infection
Trauma
Diabetic ketoacidosis
Myocardial infarction
Cerebrovascular accidents
Pulmonary thromboembolic disease
General surgery
Withdrawal of thyroid medication
Iodine administration
Palpation of the thyroid gland
Ingestion of thyroid hormone
Unknown etiology in 20–25% of cases

TABLE 215-5   Presenting Signs and Symptoms of Thyroid Storm

Fever
Tachycardia
Arrhythmia
Congestive heart failure
Central nervous system dysfunction
    Agitation
    Confusion
    Delirium
    Stupor
    Coma
    Seizure

of iodine will promote further hormone production. Various iodine-containing preparations, including iodine-containing radiographic contrast material [iopanoate (Telepaque) and iopodate (Oragrafin)] have been used for this purpose. Administration of lithium should be considered in patients with a prior history of iodine allergies. Note that many of the drugs used to treat thyroid storm are oral preparations and subsequently may need to be administered by naso- or orogastric tube. In cases where clinical deterioration occurs despite appropriate therapy, direct removal of circulating thyroid hormone has been accomplished by exchange transfusion, plasma transfusion, plasmapheresis, and charcoal plasmaperfusion. Cholestyramine also has been reported to modestly decrease circulating thyroid hormone levels. Other therapeutic goals include treatment of hyperthermia with cooling blankets, ice packs, and antipyretics (acetaminophen). Avoidance of salicylates has been recommended because of displacement of T_4 from TBG, thereby increasing free T_4. The empirical use of corticosteroids has been suggested to treat potential adrenal insufficiency that may occur with such a hypermetabolic state.

Comorbid factors that may have been a precipitant to thyroid storm also must be addressed. Electrocardiograms, chest radiographs, urinalysis, blood cultures, and administration of empirical antibiotics always should be considered in patients presenting in thyroid storm. Standard therapy for heart failure due to ischemic or hypertensive heart disease may be used. All patients should be admitted to an appropriately monitored setting for further evaluation and care. Definitive therapy is usually radioiodine administration once the patient is stable and euthyroid.

TABLE 215-6   Drug Treatment of Thyroid Storm

Decrease de novo synthesis:	
Propylthiouracil	600–1000 mg PO initially, followed by 200–250 mg q4h
Methimazole	40 mg PO initial dose, then 25 mg PO q6h
Prevent release of hormone (after synthesis blockade initiated):	
Iodine	Iapanoic acid (Telepaque) 1 g IV q8h for the first 24 h, then 500 mg IV bid *or*
	Potassium iodide (SSKI) 5 drops PO q6h *or*
	Lugol solution 8–10 drops PO q6h
Lithium carbonate	800–1200 mg PO per d
Prevent peripheral effects:	
β-blockade	Propranolol (IV) titrate 1 to 2 mg q5min prn (may need 240–480 mg PO per d) *or*
	Esmolol (IV) 500 μg/kg IV bolus, then 50–200 μg/kg per min maintenance
Guanethidine	30–40 mg PO q6h
Reserpine	2.5–5 mg IM q4–6h
Other considerations:	
Corticosteroids	Hydrocortisone 100 mg IV q8h *or* Dexamethasone 2 mg IV q6h
Antipyretics	Cooling blanket Acetaminophen 650 mg PO q4h

REFERENCES

1. Lazarus JH: Hyperthyroidism. *Lancet* 349:339, 1997.
2. Martino E, Safran M, Aghini-Lombardi F, et al: Environmental iodine intake and thyroid dysfunction during chronic amiodarone therapy. *Ann Intern Med* 101:28, 1984.
3. Bartalena L, Brogioni S, Grasso L, et al: Treatment of amiodarone-induced thyrotoxicosis, a difficult challenge: Results from a prospective study. *J Clin Endocrinol Metab* 81:2930, 1996.
4. Tietgens ST, Leinung MC: Thyroid storm. *Med Clin North Am* 79:169, 1995.
5. Klein I, Ojamaa K: Thyroid hormone and the cardiovascular system. *New Engl J Med* 344:501, 2001.
6. Weetman A: Graves disease. *New Engl J Med* 343:1236, 2000.
7. Bogazzi F, Bartalena L, Cosci C, et al: Treatment of type II amiodarone-induced thyrotoxicosis by either iopanoic acid or glucocorticoids: A prospective, randomized study. *J Clin Endocrinol Metab* 88:1999, 2003.
8. Roti E, Minelli R, Salvi M: The management of hyperthyroid and hypothyroidism in the pregnant woman. *J Clin Endocrinol Metab* 81:1679, 1996.
9. Ringel M: Management of hypothyroidism and hyperthyroidism in the intensive care unit. *Crit Care Clin* 17:115, 2001.

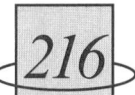

216 HYPOTHYROIDISM AND MYXEDEMA COMA
Horace K. Liang

Hypothyroidism arises from many etiologies. The severe manifestation of extreme hypothyroidism, myxedema coma, is a rare, potentially life-threatening illness. Correct diagnosis requires a high degree of clinical suspicion, and initiation of treatment is an empirical decision.

HYPOTHYROIDISM

Normal thyroid physiology was discussed in Chap. 215. Hypothyroidism occurs when there is insufficient hormone production or secretion. A general hypometabolic state is the principal feature of this disease. Hypothyroidism occurs more frequently in women than in men. The prevalence of hypothyroidism in women ranges from 0.6 to 5.9 percent.[1] The most common etiologies of hypothyroidism are primary thyroid failure due to autoimmune diseases (of which Hashimoto thyroiditis is most common), idiopathic causes, after ablative therapy, and iodine deficiency.[2] Hypothyroidism may be transient as in some cases of thyroiditis such as subacute or silent thyroiditis. The pathophysiology of this entity is unclear but may be viral in origin. Postpartum thyroiditis occurs within 3 to 6 months postpartum and reportedly occurs in 2 to 16 percent of women.[1] Secondary (due to pituitary tumors, infiltrative disease, or hemorrhage) or tertiary (hypothalamic disease) etiologies of hypothyroidism are less common (Table 216-1). Several medications have been reported to induce hypothyroidism. Amiodarone-associated hypothyroidism has been reported to occur from 1 percent to as high as 32 percent of patients.[3] The mechanism is probably the large amount of iodine that is released by metabolism of the drug, which then inhibits thyroid hormone synthesis, release, and inhibition of triiodothyroxine (T_4) to triiodothyronine (T_3) conversion. Lithium acts similarly to iodine and decreases thyroid hormone release. When initiating lithium therapy, especially in patients with prior hypothyroidism, careful monitoring of thyroid function is required.

Primary hypothyroidism usually has an insidious onset (findings are shown in Table 216-2). Hemodynamic changes are opposite those of hyperthyroidism but are accompanied by fewer signs and symptoms.[4] Patients with suspected uncomplicated hypothyroidism may be evaluated as outpatients. Typical laboratory findings in primary hypothyroidism include low T_4 and high thyrotropin [thyroid-stimulating

TABLE 216-1   Etiologies of Hypothyroidism

Primary
   Autoimmune etiologies (Hashimoto)
   Idiopathic
   After ablation (surgical, radioiodine)
   After external radiation
   Iodine deficiency
   Thyroiditis (subacute, silent, postpartum)*
   Infiltrative disease (lymphoma, sarcoid, amyloidosis, tuberculosis)
   Congenital
Secondary (pituitary)
   Panhypopituitarism
Tertiary (hypothalamic)
   Neoplasms
   Infiltrative
Drugs
   Amiodarone
   Lithium
   Iodine (in patients with pre-existing autoimmune disease)
   Antithyroid medication

*Self-limited etiologies, often preceded by hyperthyroid phase.

hormone (TSH)] levels. T_3 is un unreliable indicator of hypothyroidism and is not measured routinely. There is little urgent need for obtaining thyroid function tests, and typically they are not available during the emergency department visit. However, obtaining blood for testing in the emergency department may be helpful to the patient's health provider in follow-up care. In many cases, elderly patients with hypothyroidism may exhibit a paucity of symptoms. Because of the high prevalence of hypothyroidism in women over the age of 60 years of age, it is recommended that they be screened routinely with a serum TSH measurement.

Treatment

Treatment of primary uncomplicated hypothyroidism is with thyroxine administration. Initiation of oral therapy begins at a dose of 50 to 100 μg/d and is increased gradually. The average daily adult dose is 75 to 150 μg. Elderly patients with underlying heart disease are treated with lower initial dosages. Monitoring of therapy is by achieving appropriate serum thyrotropin levels after 6 to 8 weeks of therapy. If hypothyroidism is due to less common secondary etiologies, initiation of thyroid hormone replacement may exacerbate preexisting adrenal insufficiency. Therefore, the etiology of hypothyroidism (primary versus secondary failure) should be determined prior to initiating thyroxine replacement. Initiation of therapy in the emergency department is rarely warranted. Clinical clues that may differentiate primary and secondary hypothyroidism are listed in Table 216-3.[5]

MYXEDEMA COMA

Myxedema coma is a rare clinical state in which an individual with long-standing preexisting hypothyroidism presents with life-threaten-

TABLE 216-2   Symptoms and Signs of Hypothyroidism

Symptoms	Signs
Fatigue	Hoarseness
Weight gain	Hypothermia
Cold intolerance	Periorbital puffiness
Depression	Delayed relaxation of ankle jerks
Menstrual irregularities	Loss of outer third of eyebrow
Constipation	Cool, rough, dry skin
Joint pain	Nonpitting edema
Muscle cramps	Bradycardia
Infertility	Peripheral neuropathy

TABLE 216-3   Differentiation of Primary and Secondary Hypothyroidism

Primary	Secondary
Previous thyroid operation	No prior thyroid operation
Obese	Less obese
Hypothermia more common	Hypothermia less common
Voice course	Voice less course
Pubic hair present	Pubic hair absent
Skin dry and course	Skin fine and soft
Heart increased in size	Heart usually normal
Normal menses and lactation	Traumatic delivery, no lactation, amenorrhea
Sella turcica normal	Sella turcica may be increased in size
Serum TSH increased	Serum TSH decreased
Plasma cortisol normal	Plasma cortisol decreased
No response to TSH	Good response to TSH
Good response to levothyroxine without steroids	Poor response to levothyroxine without steroids

Source: From Senior et al.[5]

ing decompensation. In reality, few patients present comatose with severe myxedema. Affected patients are commonly in the geriatric population. Various etiologies that may precipitate this syndrome include infection, cold exposure, drugs (sedatives, lithium, amiodarone), trauma, stroke, congestive heart failure (CHF), inadequate thyroid hormone replacement, and previously undiagnosed hypothyroidism. The clinical presentation is one of a severe decompensated metabolic state that may include an alteration in mental status, hypothermia, bradycardia, hypoventilation, and even cardiovascular collapse (Table 216-4). These findings are not only secondary to a decline in metabolic function but also due to neurovascular and cardiovascular adaptations. Some of these adaptations are similar to those which occur in euthyroid patients exposed to a cold environment (decline in oxygen consumption and heat generation and redistribution of blood flow centrally). In addition, there is a change in end-organ responsiveness to catecholamines and a decline in cardiac performance. This is due to an absolute diminution in β-adrenergic receptors (decreased inotrope and chronotrope activity). There is also relatively increased α-adrenergic responsiveness resulting in mild diastolic hypertension. Increased CO_2 retention occurs because of decreased respiratory muscle strength and diminished ventilatory drive in response to hypercapnia. There is also decreased free-water clearance, resulting in a dilutional hyponatremia, impaired gluconeogenesis, and decreased drug clearance that predisposes patients to drug toxicity from medication.

Diagnosis of myxedema coma requires high clinical suspicion. A patient suspected of presenting with myxedema coma commonly has a prior history of primary hypothyroidism or previous thyroid surgery.

TABLE 216-4   Clinical Presentation of Myxedema Coma

Decreased mental status
Hypothermia
Bradycardia
Hypoventilation
Periorbital edema
Nonpitting edema
Delayed deep tendon reflexes
Hypoglycemia
Hyponatremia

Medication noncompliance or coexisting stressors such as cold exposure, severe infection, or the addition of new medications may precipitate the onset of myxedema coma. The decline in function is usually gradual and insidious in onset. The physical examination may confirm a history of long-standing hypothyroidism. In addition, there also may be clinical findings of hypothermia, hypoventilation, hypotension, bradycardia, and alteration or deterioration of the patient's mental status.

Laboratory evaluation of the patient with suspected myxedema coma may reveal anemia; hyponatremia; hypoglycemia; elevated transaminases, creatine phosphokinase (CPK), and lactate dehydrogenase (LDH); hypercholesterolemia; and arterial blood gas abnormalities (decreased PO_2 and increased PCO_2). The electrocardiogram may demonstrate sinus bradycardia, prolongation of the QT interval, and low voltage with flattening or inversion of T waves. A chest radiograph may demonstrate an increased cardiac contour due to the presence of a pericardial effusion.

Treatment of Myxedema Coma

There are no prospective studies on the optimal therapy for patients in myxedema coma. Therefore, treatment recommendations are not uniform.[6] However, initial therapy is directed toward stabilization. The patient may require endotracheal intubation and mechanical ventilation for airway protection and correction of hypoventilation, hypercapnia, and hypoxia. Correction of hypothermia is directed toward decreasing further heat loss. Cautious use of gentle passive external rewarming should be initiated. Hypotension due to reversal of the patient's hypothermic vasoconstriction should be avoided.

Specific therapy includes intravenous levothyroxine, which is recommended by most authors. An initial intravenous bolus of levothyroxine (Table 216-5) is administered and followed by a reduced daily dose until the patient can take oral medication. This has the advantage of repleting the thyroxine pool and allowing the hormone to slowly enter tissues. Other authors suggest that in ill patients there may be decreased T_4-to-T_3 conversion, and thus they recommend T_3 as the initial replacement hormone.

Routine administration of glucocorticoid is recommended to avoid the potential of precipitating adrenal crisis in patients with unrecognized adrenal insufficiency or hypothyroidism secondary to hypopituitarism. If possible, a baseline cortisol level should be sent to the laboratory prior to initiating therapy. Correction of hyponatremia is by means of fluid restriction. Severe hyponatremia has been treated successfully with hypertonic saline administration.

A search for a precipitating etiology must be initiated, and any such disorder should be treated aggressively. Infection is a common precip-

itant of myxedema coma. If possible, appropriate cultures should be obtained prior to initiating empirical antibiotic therapy.

All patients presenting with a suspected diagnosis of myxedema coma should be admitted to an appropriately monitored inpatient bed for further evaluation and treatment.

REFERENCES

1. Mulder JE: Thyroid disease in women. *Med Clin North Am* 82(1):103, 1998.
2. Lindsay RS, Toft AD: Hypothyroidism. *Lancet* 349:413, 1997.
3. Harja KJ, Licata AA: Effects of amiodarone on thyroid function. *Ann Intern Med* 126:63, 1997.
4. Klein I, Ojamaa K: Thyroid hormone and the cardiovascular system. *New Engl J Med* 344:50, 2001.
5. Senior RM, Birge SJ, Wessler S, et al: The recognition and management of myxedema coma. *JAMA* 217:61, 1971.
6. Ringel M: Management of hypothyroidism and hyperthyroidism in the intensive care unit. *Crit Care Clin* 17(1):115, 2001.

217 ADRENAL INSUFFICIENCY AND ADRENAL CRISIS
Charles N. Schoenfeld

The adrenal glands are divided into the medulla and cortex. The medullary portion is controlled by the nervous system and, when stimulated, secretes epinephrine and norepinephrine into the adrenal veins.

The adrenal cortex secretes steroids that contribute to the control of glucose, protein, and fat metabolism; act to maintain vascular tone and cardiac contractility; aid in the maintenance of total-body water and sodium-potassium balance; and provide androgenic effects. In steady-state conditions, this secretion is cyclic and controlled by a complex series of interactions involving the time of day, the hypothalamic-pituitary-adrenal (HPA) axis, the renin-angiotensin system, and serum potassium levels. During times of stress (e.g., sepsis, trauma, major surgery, hypoxia, hypoglycemia, and burns), the basal secretion of glucocorticoids and, to a lesser extent, mineralocorticoids is increased by as much as 5 to 10 times. While the exact mechanisms by which stressful events stimulate the HPA axis are unknown, the effect is nearly immediate, occurring in minutes.

Failure of the adrenal glands to produce the essential basal secretion of these steroids results in *adrenal insufficiency* (AI), an insidious wasting disease. Failure to respond to the increased demands created by stress or the sudden inability to secrete these essential steroids results in the life-threatening condition of *adrenal crisis* (AC). Of the three types of steroids normally secreted, the absence of glucocorticoids is the most critical in adrenal crisis—making their repletion the mainstay of therapy.

CORTICOSTEROIDS

The adrenal gland produces more than 50 different steroids, grouped into three classes according to their effects. These are glucocorticoids, mineralocorticoids, and androgenic steroids.

Glucocorticoids

Cortisol, the most abundant steroid produced by the adrenals, is representative of this class. The glucocorticoids are involved in the regulation of glucose, protein, and fat metabolism. They are active in the synthesis of medullary catecholamines as well as β-adrenergic receptors and thus play an important role in the maintenance of vascular tone and cardiac contractility. Other hemodynamic effects include maintaining endothelial integrity and controlling vascular permeability.

TABLE 216-5   Treatment of Myxedema Coma

Recognition
Supportive measures including ventilatory support
Thyroid replacement
    Levothyroxine: 300–500 μg slow IV initial dose; then
        50–100 μg IV per day *or*
    T_3: 25 μg IV or PO q8h *or*
    Combination of thyroxine plus T_3
Glucocorticoid
    Hydrocortisone: 100 mg IV q8h
Hypothermia
    Prevent additional loss
    Passive external rewarming
Electrolyte correction
    Gentle fluid restriction for dilutional hyponatremia
    Hypertonic saline for severe hyponatremia
Hypoglycemia
    Dextrose-containing IV solution
    Monitoring
Aggressive treatment of precipitating cause
Admit the patent to a monitored setting

Cortisol secretion by the adrenal cortex is controlled by the HPA axis. In the nonstressed state, the hypothalamus secretes corticotropin-releasing (CR) hormone and arginine vasopressin (AV) in a circadian rhythm, with maximal secretion occurring between 2 and 4 A.M. This stimulates the anterior pituitary to release adrenocorticotropic hormone (ACTH), which causes the adrenal cortex to produce and release cortisol, with peak cortisol levels occurring around 8 A.M. and declining throughout the day. Total daily production of cortisol is approximately 25 mg in the nonstressed state, of which only 5 to 10 percent is free and physiologically active. The remainder is bound to plasma proteins, principally (80 percent) cortisol-binding globulin. There is evidence that this bound cortisol is uncoupled from these proteins during times of serious illness, increasing the availability of the active form of cortisol.[1]

Cortisol, as well as exogenous corticosteroids, is involved in a negative feedback loop with the hypothalamus. Rising levels of cortisol inhibit the release of CR and AV, thus reducing the release of ACTH from the pituitary. This mechanism plays a crucial role in the development of secondary adrenal insufficiency (see below).

Mineralocorticoids

Aldosterone is the principal mineralocorticoid produced by the adrenals. While ACTH has a minor influence on its secretion, the primary regulators are the renin-angiotensin system and serum potassium levels. The juxtaglomerular apparatus, stimulated by the diminished glomerular filtration seen in volume depletion, releases prorenin. This ultimately causes the release of aldosterone from the adrenals, which results in the resorption of sodium and water in the distal tubules at the expense of potassium loss. Minor degrees of hyperkalemia directly stimulate the adrenals to secrete aldosterone. The net result is to increase serum volume while depleting potassium.

Adrenal Androgens

Adrenal androgens are under the control of ACTH and exhibit the same diurnal rhythm as cortisol. While they are a minor contributor to total androgen levels in the male, they are a significant source in the female—leading to some of the signs of adrenal insufficiency in these patients (see below).

ADRENAL INSUFFICIENCY

The signs and symptoms of adrenal insufficiency may occur because of failure of the adrenal glands (primary AI) or failure of the HPA axis (secondary AI), the latter most commonly due to suppression of the HPA axis by the chronic administration of exogenous glucocorticoids. Some authors divide secondary AI into that caused by pituitary failure (secondary AI) and that caused by hypothalamic dysfunction (tertiary AI). For the purposes of this chapter, any failure of the HPA axis will be considered secondary AI.

Primary Adrenal Insufficiency

Because of the functional reserve of the adrenals, 90 percent of the glands must be destroyed in order for AI to become manifest clinically. It is characterized by the loss of all three types of adrenal steroids. Table 217-1 lists the principal causes of primary AI.

The spectrum of causes of primary AI is changing. Addison disease, once considered idiopathic, is now recognized as being most commonly the result of autoimmune disorders.[2] This may occur as an isolated process or as a component of autoimmune polyglandular syndrome types I and II.

Worldwide, tuberculosis is the most common infectious cause of primary AI. In the United States, however, infection with the human immunodeficiency virus (HIV) is the most common cause.[1] While 50

TABLE 217-1 Causes of Primary Adrenal Insufficiency

Autoimmune
Infectious
   HIV
   Tuberculosis
   Systemic fungal infections
Infiltrative diseases
   Amyloidosis
   Sarcoidosis
   Hemosiderosis
Hemorrhage/thrombosis
   Anticoagulant therapy
   Overwhelming sepsis (including Waterhouse-Friderichsen syndrome)
   DIC
Metastasis
Adrenoleukodystrophy

percent of HIV-infected patients show some degree of destruction of the adrenals, less than 5 percent will have clinical AI.[3] HIV may cause AI via opportunistic infections (principally cytomegalovirus), the use of medications such as ketoconazole, or by inhibition of the HPA axis by cytokines released by macrophages.

Thrombosis and/or hemorrhage of the adrenals may occur as a complication of anticoagulation therapy, sepsis, or disseminated intravascular coagulation or in antiphospholipid syndrome. Infiltrative diseases such as amyloidosis and hemosiderosis are uncommon causes of primary AI, as is bilateral metastasis from cancer. Adrenoleukodystrophy is an inherited disorder of very-long-chain fatty acid metabolism. It is an X-linked disorder and is characterized by AI and progressive neurologic symptoms caused by demyelination.

Secondary Adrenal Insufficiency

Secondary AI occurs when the HPA axis fails to secrete corticotropin and/or ACTH. This causes a deficiency of glucocorticoids and adrenal androgens. The secretion of mineralocorticoids is unaffected, however. Table 217-2 lists the principal causes of secondary AI.

By far the most common cause of secondary AI is the chronic administration of exogenous glucocorticoids.[2,4] This suppresses the diurnal hypothalamic release of CR and AV, leading to failure of the anterior pituitary to secrete ACTH, which in turn results in adrenal atrophy. As a result, the adrenals cannot respond to acute stressful events. This HPA axis suppression appears to be both time- and dose-related and usually is reversible, although recovery may take up to a year. It is generally believed that a short course (<2 to 3 weeks) of supraphysiologic doses of glucocorticoids is unlikely to suppress the HPA axis. Doses of less than 5 mg of prednisone (or its equivalent) daily are also unlikely to cause secondary AI.[4]

Less commonly, secondary AI is caused by infiltrative diseases or tumors that involve the hypothalamus or pituitary. Postpartum necrosis (Sheehan syndrome), hemorrhage into an adenoma, or head

TABLE 217-2 Causes of Secondary Adrenal Insufficiency

Exogenous glucocorticoid therapy
Infiltrative
   Sarcoidosis
   Histiocytosis X
   Hemosiderosis
Tumors
   Primary pituitary or hypothalamic
   Local invasion (craniopharyngioma)
   Metastatic
Postpartum pituitary necrosis (Sheehan syndrome)
Head trauma
Pituitary surgery or irradiation

trauma may abruptly destroy the pituitary. These forms of secondary AI generally are associated with focal neurologic findings, visual field cuts, diabetes insipidus, or findings of panhypopituitarism.

CLINICAL PRESENTATION

Adrenal insufficiency may present as a slowly progressive wasting disease (chronic AI) or as an acute life-threatening illness (adrenal crisis). The clinical manifestations of each are remarkably different.

Chronic Adrenal Insufficiency

The signs and symptoms of chronic AI are nonspecific and may mislead the clinician into an incorrect diagnosis. Fatigue, anorexia, weight loss, and loss of libido are common and may lead to a diagnosis of depression. Abdominal pain, nausea, vomiting, and diarrhea are also seen frequently, suggesting a primary gastrointestinal disorder. Fortunately, there are other findings that should raise the suspicion of chronic AI. Indeed, for the observant physician there are clues that suggest whether the AI is primary or secondary.

Hyperpigmentation is seen in primary AI due to elevated levels of ACTH and its effect on melanocytes. It may be particularly noticeable over pressure points and in the axillae, palmar creases, perineum, and oral mucosa. It characteristically develops early in the course of AI. In contrast, patients with secondary AI commonly exhibit a pallor out of proportion to their degree of anemia.

Low blood pressure and orthostasis are common findings. The habitus of patients with chronic AI generally is cachectic. In women, the loss of adrenal androgens results in thinning of axillary and pubic hair.

Hyponatremia, usually mild but occasionally marked (serum Na^+ <120 mEq/L), may be seen in both primary and secondary AI. In primary AI it is due to the lack of aldosterone and sodium wasting. In secondary AI it is due to increased vasopressin secretion and water retention.

Hyperkalemia, due to a loss of aldosterone, is seen in primary AI and generally is mild. This also may be associated with a mild azotemia and metabolic acidosis. Since aldosterone secretion is maintained in secondary AI, hyperkalemia does not occur.

Normocytic anemia, lymphocytosis, and eosinophilia are seen in both primary and secondary AI. Similarly, hypoglycemia is seen in both types of AI.

Secondary AI is commonly associated with other neurologic signs and symptoms. Headaches, visual field cuts, diabetes insipidus, or other signs of hypopituitarism may occur.

Adrenal Crisis

In contrast to the indolent and progressive course of chronic AI, AC presents as a life-threatening emergency in which the primary manifestation is hypotension. It can occur in either primary or secondary AI. The hypotension in AC typically is resistant to catecholamine and IV fluid administration and, if the missing cortisol is not replaced, will lead to death.

Adrenal crisis occurs when the body undergoes a significant stress and the adrenals are unable to respond by increasing cortisol secretion. It may be seen in a patient with known chronic AI or unrecognized chronic AI or in whom the adrenals or HPA axis fails abruptly.

Abrupt failure of the adrenals usually occurs as a consequence of hemorrhage or thrombosis of the glands. This may occur as a complication of anticoagulant therapy, disseminated intravascular coagulation, sepsis (Waterhouse-Friderichsen syndrome), or other overwhelming stress. Patients generally have abdominal and flank pain in addition to resistant hypotension, mimicking the presentation of ruptured abdominal aortic aneurysm.

Catastrophic failure of the HPA axis may occur as a result of head trauma, hemorrhage of a pituitary adenoma, or in the postpartum period (Sheehan syndrome). Patient's generally will have other neurologic deficits, headache, visual field cuts, and diabetes insipidus.

DIAGNOSIS

Adrenal crisis is relatively rare, and few emergency physicians have recognized experience with such patients. A multitude of diagnostic studies are used to confirm the presence of AI, but the results are rarely available to the emergency physician and thus of little utility in the management of these patients.

Measurement of plasma cortisol levels between 8 and 9 A.M. can rule in (level <83 nmol/L) or rule out (level >525 nmol/L) AI.[2] The short corticotropin stimulation test is the most commonly used test to assess for AI. After measuring plasma cortisol levels, 250 g of cosyntropin is injected (IM or IV), and plasma cortisol levels are measured at 60 min. AI is excluded if the basal or poststimulation level exceeds 550 nmol/L. Other studies include the insulin-induced hypoglycemia test, the short metyrapone stimulation test, and the CR hormone test.

TREATMENT

Stable Patient

Emergency department management of patients with known or suspected AI varies according to the clinical situation. Hemodynamically stable patients in whom the diagnosis of AI is to be excluded are best

TABLE 217-3 Guidelines for Adrenal Supplementation Therapy

Medical or Surgical Stress	Corticosteroid Dosage
Minor	
Inguinal hernia repair	25 mg hydrocortisone or 5 mg
Colonoscopy	methylprednisolone IV on
Mild febrile illness	day of procedure only
Mild–moderate nausea/vomiting	
Gastroenteritis	
Moderate	
Open cholecystectomy	50–75 mg hydrocortisone or
Hemicolectomy	10–15 mg methylprednisolone IV
Significant febrile illness	on day of procedure
Pneumonia	Taper quickly over 1–2 days to usual
Severe gastroenteritis	dose
Severe	
Major cardiothoracic surgery	100–150 mg hydrocortisone or
Whipple procedure	20–30 mg of methylprednisolone
Liver resection	IV on day of procedure
Pancreatitis	Rapid taper to usual dose over next
	1–2 days
Critically ill	
Sepsis-induced hypotension or shock	50–100 mg hydrocortisone IV q6–8 h or 0.18 mg/kg per h as a continuous infusion and 50 μg/d fludrocortisone until shock resolves May take several days to a week or more Then gradually taper, following vital signs and serum sodium

Source: Coursin DB, Wood KE: Corticosteroid supplementation for adrenal insufficiency. *JAMA* 287(2):236, 2002, with permission.

managed by an internist. A short corticotropin stimulation test could be performed, but it is most reliable if done before 10 A.M., and the results will not be available to the emergency physician. Other tests of adrenal function are much too time-consuming and cumbersome to warrant their use in the ED.

Stress or Rescue Management

Consideration of stress or rescue doses of corticosteroids is mandatory in patients with known or strongly suspected (e.g., chronic high-dose steroid use) AI when they are acutely stressed or about to undergo various procedures. Traditionally, these patients received corticosteroids in dosages similar to those used in the treatment of AC. However, there is evidence that this is both unnecessary and potentially harmful.[4] A more physiologic approach (Table 217-3) is to base the dose of supplemental therapy on the severity of the stressful event. Patients receiving 5 mg/d of prednisone (or its equivalent) do not require additional corticosteroids regardless of the degree of stress because the HPA axis is not suppressed at this dose.

The treatment of AC, whether primary or secondary, requires only the use of glucocorticoids. Mineralocorticoids are not needed. Intravenous hydrocortisone is given as a 100-mg bolus, and then an infusion of 200 mg is given over the next 24 h. Several liters of D5NS may be required to correct hypovolemia and hypoglycemia.

Any patient in whom AC is suspected should receive 100 mg hydrocortisone intravenously. The presence of unexplained hyponatremia and hyperkalemia in the setting of hypotension unresponsive to catecholamine and fluid administration is strong evidence of AC. Two decades ago, dexamethasone was proposed for all patients in cardiac arrest, but it was not shown to be of clear benefit.

ACKNOWLEDGMENT

Parts of this chapter are based on the previous contribution of Gene Ragland, M.D.

REFERENCES

1. Zaloga GP, Marik P: Hypothalamic-pituitary-adrenal insufficiency. *Crit Care Clin* 17:25, 2001.
2. Oelkers W: Adrenal insufficiency. *New Engl J Med* 335:1206, 1996.
3. Carey RM: The changing clinical spectrum of adrenal insufficiency. *Ann Intern Med* 127:1103, 1997.
4. Coursin DB, Wood KE: Corticosteroid supplementation for adrenal insufficiency. *JAMA* 287:236, 2002.

HEMATOLOGIC AND ONCOLOGIC EMERGENCIES

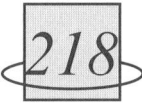

218 EVALUATION OF ANEMIA AND THE BLEEDING PATIENT
Robin R. Hemphill

EVALUATION OF THE PATIENT WITH ANEMIA

Anemia is a common problem, affecting an estimated one-third of the world's population. By itself, anemia is not so much a disease as a symptom of an underlying process. Worldwide, the most common causes of anemia include iron deficiency, thalassemia, hemoglobinopathies, and folate deficiencies. Within the United States, the most common causes are iron deficiency, thalassemia, and anemia of chronic disease. Not only is anemia common in the general population, the prevalence of anemia increases with age. Given the ubiquity of this entity, patients with anemia will present to the ED, some of whom will be symptomatic from their anemia, while in others this will be a spurious finding.

Pathophysiology

Anemia is defined as a reduced concentration of red blood cells (RBCs).[1] In healthy persons, normal erythropoiesis ensures that the number of RBCs present is adequate to meet the body's demand for oxygen and that RBC destruction equals production. The average life span of the circulating erythrocyte is approximately 120 days. Any process or condition that impairs the production, increases the rate of destruction, or increases the loss of erythrocytes will result in anemia if the body cannot produce enough new RBCs to keep up with the loss. More than one mechanism may be present in a single patient.

Quantification of the RBC concentration is reflected in the RBC count per µL, hemoglobin concentration, or hematocrit (percentage of RBC mass to blood volume). Normal RBC values for adults vary slightly between males and females (Table 218-1). Based on pathophysiologic mechanisms, there are three categories of anemia (Table 218-2).

Compensatory Mechanisms in Anemia

The body may respond to the development of anemia in several ways. These compensatory mechanisms vary dependent upon the rapidity of onset, the degree of anemia, and the underlying condition of the patient. In acute onset anemia, if there is loss of intravascular volume, then peripheral vasoconstriction and central vasodilatation will help preserve blood flow to vital organs. As the anemia worsens, systemic small-vessel vasodilatation allows increased blood flow to tissues. Both of these compensatory actions result in decreasing systemic vascular resistance, increasing cardiac output, and tachycardia. Along with these changes, the RBCs enhance their ability to release oxygen to the tissues. If the anemia is more chronic in nature, there should be an increase in plasma volume that will maintain the total blood volume at a constant level. Finally, anemia will result in the stimulation of erythropoietin that should stimulate new erythrocyte production. New reticulocytes should begin to appear in the blood within 3 to 7 days.

Clinical Features

Regardless of the cause of anemia, many of the clinical manifestations are the same. The severity of symptoms and signs related to anemia depend on several factors: the rate of development of anemia, the extent of anemia that is present, the age of the patient, the general physical condition of the patient, and other existing comorbid illnesses that may be present.

Patients with chronic and slowly developing anemia may have almost no complaints even with hemoglobin levels as low as 5 to 6 g/dL. More typically, people will begin to be symptomatic at about 7 g/dL. Patients with chronic anemia may complain of weakness, fatigue, lethargy, dyspnea with minimal exertion, palpitations, and orthostatic symptoms. Physical examination findings that may be present in patients with significant chronic anemia include orthostatic hypotension; tachycardia; skin, nail bed, and mucosal pallor; systolic ejection murmur; bounding pulse; and widened pulse pressure. Evidence of jaundice and hepatosplenomegaly should lead one to consider a hemolytic anemia as the cause of symptoms. Unusual skin ulcerations or evidence of peripheral neuropathy may be evidence of nutritional abnormality. Additional manifestations may depend upon comorbid illnesses. Thus, a patient with preexisting angina may find that these symptoms are markedly worsened when anemia is present.

Patients who develop anemia in a rapid fashion may have all of the symptoms mentioned above, but frequently these symptoms will be more pronounced. Additionally, these patients may have hypotension; resting and exertional dyspnea; palpitations; diaphoresis; anxiety; severe weakness that may progress to lethargy; and altered mental status. They may also complain of thirst and will usually have decreased urine output. Again, comorbid illnesses may be worsened. Loss of more than 40 percent of blood volume leads to severe symptoms that are due more to intravascular volume depletion than to anemia.[2] In healthy patients, coronary artery blood flow usually is not limited until

TABLE 218-1 Normal Red Blood Cell (RBC) Values for Adults

	Male	Female
RBC count (million/µL)	4.5–6.0	4.0–5.5
Hemoglobin; Hgb (g/dL)	14–17	12–15
Hematocrit; Hct (%)	42–52	36–48
Mean corpuscular volume; MCV (fL)	78–100	78–102
Mean cellular hemoglobin; MCH (pg/cell)	25–35	25–35
Mean corpuscular hemoglobin concentration; MCHC (g/dL)	32–36	32–36
Red cell distribution width; RDW (%)	11.5–14.5	11.5–14.5
Reticulocytes (%)	0.5–2.5	0.5–2.5

Note: Normal values may vary depending upon the equipment used, patient's age, and the altitude of the equipment location.

TABLE 218-2 Classification of Anemias

Loss of red blood cells by hemorrhage
  Blood loss, acute or chronic
Increased destruction
  Hereditary hemolytic anemias
  Acquired hemolytic anemias
Impaired production
  Hypochromic anemia
  Aplastic or myelodysplastic anemias
  Megaloblastic anemia
Dilutional

the hemoglobin is 50 percent or less of normal. Keep in mind that the hemodynamic response to anemia may be altered by the use of ethanol, prescription drugs, or recreational drugs.

Diagnosis

The diagnosis of anemia is established by the finding of a decreased RBC count, hemoglobin, and hematocrit on the routine complete blood count (CBC).[3,4] Other than in patients who are acutely hemorrhaging, it is rarely essential that a specific cause of anemia be established in the ED. However, appropriate workup can be initiated in the ED to help expedite a diagnosis and should be started before the transfusion of packed red blood cells (PRBCs).

The basic evaluation of a patient newly diagnosed with anemia includes the following: review of the RBC indices provided with the CBC, reticulocyte count, and review of the peripheral blood smear (Table 218-3). The mean cellular volume (MCV) is the most useful guide to the possible etiology of an anemia. The reticulocyte count reflects activity in the bone marrow and, along with the MCV, can help classify an anemia quickly and helps provides an initial approach to the differential diagnosis (Figure 218-1). The red cell distribution width (RDW) measures the size variability of the RBC population and in early deficiency anemias (iron, vitamin B_{12}, or folate), may be increased before the MCV becomes abnormal. If not already done as part of the general evaluation, questions should be asked and findings sought for the two most common sources of blood loss: gastrointestinal (e.g., checking the stool for occult blood) and uterine bleeding.

Treatment

The treatment of anemia depends on the etiology, the symptoms, and the clinical status of the patient. In the ED, anemia that requires the most urgent attention results from acute blood loss. All patients who have ongoing blood loss and anemia should have blood typed and cross-matched so that it is available for transfusion if needed. The decision to transfuse PRBCs has to be individualized for each patient with consideration of clinical symptoms, objective signs, age of the patient, presence of comorbid disease, and the likelihood of further blood loss[5,6] (see Chap. 223). In general, patients who are symptomatic and hemodynamically unstable and have evidence of tissue hypoxia and/or limited cardiopulmonary reserve should have PRBCs transfused. In most settings, patients with anemia resulting from acute blood loss are transfused at hemoglobin levels of 7 g/dL, if not at higher levels, as dictated by patient considerations discussed earlier.

ED patients with chronic anemia or a newly diagnosed anemia of uncertain etiology not caused by acute blood loss may not require immediate transfusion unless they are hemodynamically unstable, hypoxic, or have acidosis or ongoing cardiac ischemia. In a patient with newly diagnosed anemia of uncertain etiology, it is important that laboratory studies required for hematologic evaluation are obtained prior to transfusion. Consultation with a hematologist may be beneficial to guide this evaluation. The evaluation of some patients with chronic anemias or anemias of uncertain etiology can be made more difficult by transfusion, so transfusion should not be undertaken unless specifically indicated.

Disposition

Any patient with anemia from ongoing blood loss should be admitted to the hospital for further evaluation and treatment. Patients with isolated anemia that is chronic or newly diagnosed and not related to blood loss do not necessarily require admission if they are asymptomatic, hemodynamically stable, have minimal comorbid disease, and close follow-up can be arranged. Patients newly diagnosed with anemia who also have abnormalities in the white blood cell or platelet count should have immediate hematologic consultation and probable admission.

THE BLEEDING PATIENT

Most bleeding that is seen in the ED is a result of trauma—local wounds, lacerations, or other structural lesions. The majority of traumatic bleeding occurs in patients with normal hemostasis. With careful attention to the history and physical findings, patients with pathologic bleeding often can be readily identified.[7] Generally speaking, patients who manifest spontaneous bleeding from multiple sites, bleeding from untraumatized sites, delayed bleeding several hours after trauma, and bleeding into deep tissues or joints should have the possibility of a bleeding disorder considered.

Important historical data for the presence of a congenital bleeding disorder include the presence or absence of unusual or abnormal bleeding in the patient and other family members and the possible occur-

TABLE 218-3   Tests in the Evaluation of Anemia

Test	Interpretation	Clinical Correlation
MCV (mean corpuscular volume)	Measure of the average red blood cell size	Decreased MCV (microcytosis) is seen in chronic iron deficiency, thalassemia, anemia of chronic disease Increased MCV (macrocytosis) is seen in B_{12} or folate deficiency, alcohol abuse, liver disease, phenytoin, some HIV drugs
MCH (mean corpuscular hemoglobin)	Measure of the amount of hemoglobin in average red blood cell	
MCHC (mean corpuscular hemoglobin concentration)	Measure of hemoglobin concentration in average red blood cell	
Reticulocyte count	These red blood cells of intermediate maturity are a marker of production by the bone marrow	Decreased reticulocyte count reflects impaired red blood cell production Increased counts are a marker of accelerated red cell production
Peripheral blood smear	Allows visualization of the red blood cell morphology Allows evaluation for abnormal cell shapes Allows examination of the white blood cells and platelets	
Direct and indirect Coombs test	Direct Coombs test is used to detect antibodies on red blood cells Indirect Coombs test is used to detect antibodies in the sera	Direct Coombs test is positive in autoimmune hemolytic anemias, transfusion reactions, and some drug-induced hemolytic anemias Indirect Coombs test is routinely used in compatibility testing prior to transfusion

FIG. 218-1. Flow chart for the evaluation of anemia.

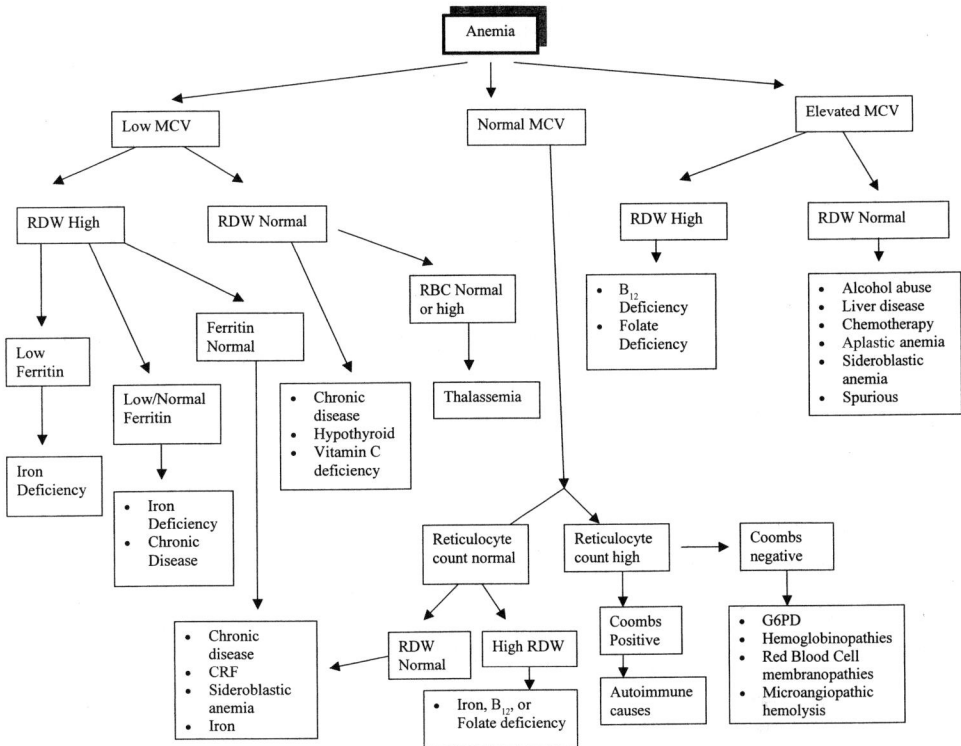

rence of excessive bleeding after dental extractions, surgical procedures, or trauma. Many patients with abnormal bleeding have an acquired disorder. Questioning about liver disease and drug use (particularly ethanol, aspirin, nonsteroidal anti-inflammatory drugs, warfarin, antibiotics, and other aspirin-containing products) may be helpful.

The site of bleeding may provide an indication of the hemostatic abnormality. Mucocutaneous bleeding, including petechiae, ecchymoses, epistaxis, gastrointestinal, genitourinary, or heavy menstrual bleeding is characteristic of qualitative or quantitative platelet disorders. Purpura is often associated with thrombocytopenia and commonly indicates a systemic illness. Bleeding into joints and potential spaces, such as between fascial planes and into the retroperitoneum, as well as delayed bleeding, is most commonly associated with coagulation factor deficiencies. Patients who demonstrate both mucocutaneous bleeding and bleeding in deep spaces may have disorders such as disseminated intravascular coagulation, where both platelet abnormalities and coagulation factor abnormalities are present.

Review of Normal Coagulation

The normal hemostatic system consists of a complex process that limits blood loss by the formation of a platelet plug (primary hemostasis) and the production of cross-linked fibrin (secondary hemostasis), which strengthens the platelet plug. These reactions are counterregulated by the fibrinolytic system, which limits the size of fibrin clot that is formed, thereby preventing excessive clot formation. Congenital and acquired abnormalities occur in all these systems. The affected patients may have excessive hemorrhage, excessive thrombus formation, or both.

PRIMARY HEMOSTASIS   Primary hemostasis is the platelet interaction with the vascular subendothelium that results in the formation of a platelet plug at the site of injury. Required components for this to occur are normal vascular subendothelium (collagen), functional platelets, normal von Willebrand factor (connects the platelet to the endothelium via glycoprotein I_B), and normal fibrinogen (connects the platelets to each other via glycoprotein II_B-III_A) (Figure 218-2).

SECONDARY HEMOSTASIS   Secondary hemostasis describes the reactions of the plasma coagulation proteins by a tightly regulated mecha-

nism. The final product is cross-linked fibrin, which is insoluble and strengthens the platelet plug formed in primary hemostasis (Figure 218-3).

THE FIBRINOLYTIC SYSTEM   This complex system regulates the hemostatic mechanism by limiting the size of fibrin clots that are formed (Figure 218-4). The principal physiologic activator is tissue plasminogen activator (tPA), which is released from endothelial cells. Tissue

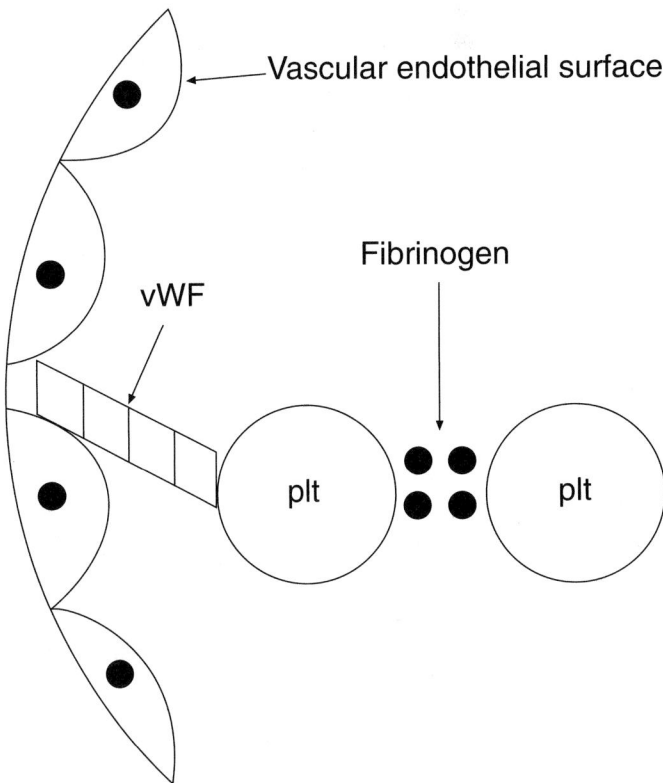

FIG. 218-2. Primary hemostasis. See text for details. plt = platelet; vWF = von Willebrand factor.

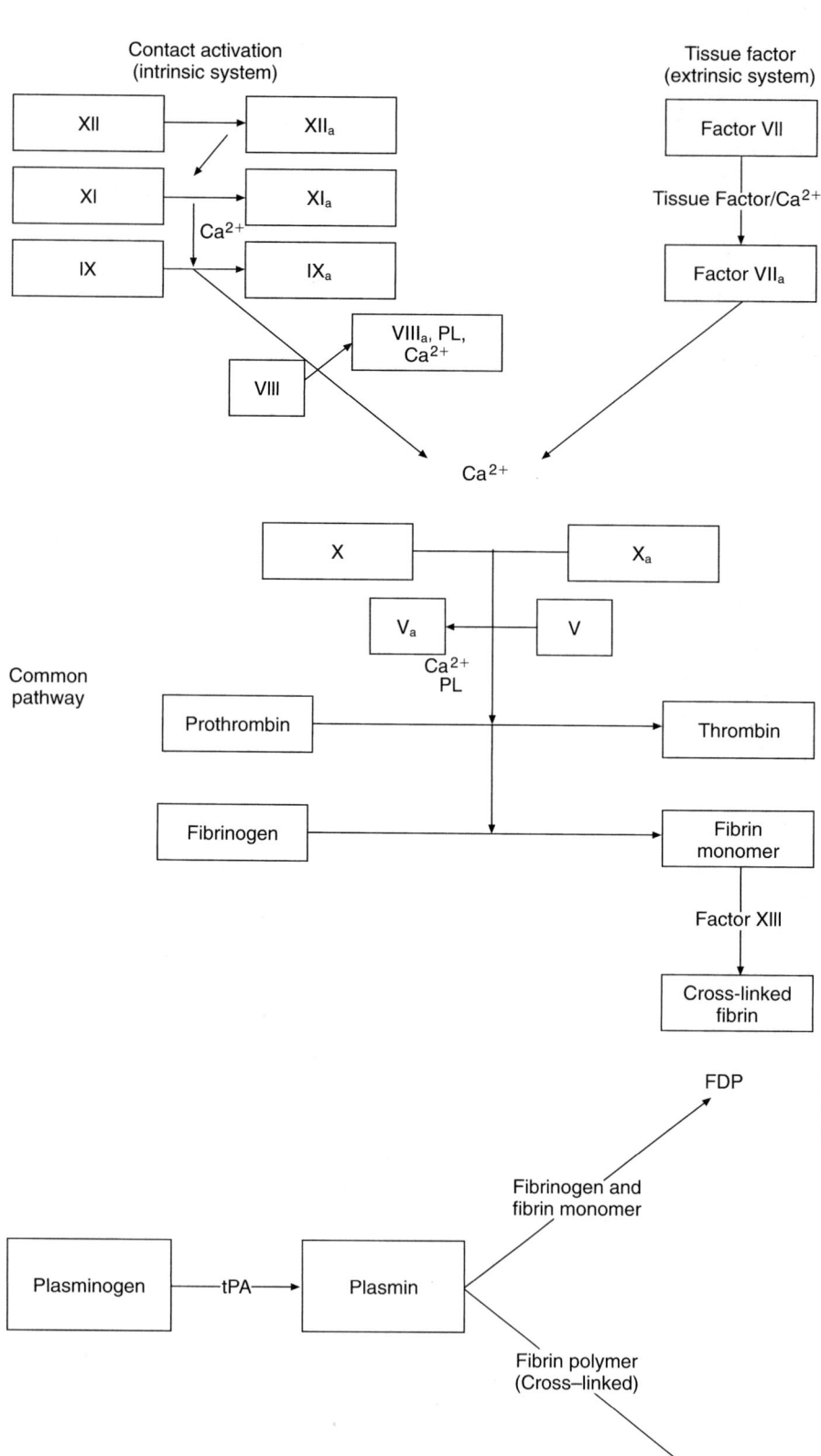

FIG. 218-3. Secondary hemostasis, also known as the coagulation cascade. The inactivated coagulation proteins (factors) are indicated by roman numerals; after the reaction occurs, the factor is activated and designated by subscript a. There are two independent activation pathways. The contact system is known as the *intrinsic pathway*, and the tissue factor system is known as the *extrinsic pathway*. The pathways merge at the point of activation of factor X. This begins the common pathway that generates the final product, cross-linked fibrin. Ca^{2+} = calcium; fibrinogen is factor I; PL = phospholipid surface (often platelets); prothrombin is factor II.

FIG. 218-4. The fibrinolytic pathway. See text for details. FDP = fibrin degradation product; tPA = tissue plasminogen activator.

plasminogen activator converts plasminogen, which is synthesized in the liver and adsorbed in the fibrin clot, to plasmin. Plasmin degrades fibrinogen and fibrin monomer into low-molecular-weight fragments known as fibrin degradation products (FDPs) and cross-linked fibrin into D-dimers.

Other physiologic inhibitors of hemostasis with clinical relevance include antithrombin III and the protein C–protein S system. Antithrombin III is a protein that forms complexes with all the serine protease coagulation factors (factors XII_a, XI_a, IX_a, and thrombin), thereby inhibiting their function. Heparin potentiates this interaction, and this is the basis for its use as an anticoagulant. Proteins C and S are vitamin K–dependent factors

that are produced in the liver. Activated protein C binds to the cell-surface-bound protein S and this complex is capable of inactivating the two plasma cofactors factors V_a and VIII_a, and inhibiting their participation in the coagulation cascade. Deficiency or defects in antithrombin III, protein C, and protein S produce a potentially hypercoagulable condition and predispose the patient to arterial and venous thromboses.

Diagnosis

The basic laboratory parameters that should be obtained in a patient with a suspected bleeding disorder are a complete blood count and

TABLE 218-4 Tests of Hemostasis

Screening Tests	Normal Value	Measures	Clinical Correlations
PRIMARY HEMOSTASIS			
Platelet count	150,000–300,000/μL	Number of platelets per μL	Decreased platelet count (thrombocytopenia)—bleeding usually not a problem until platelet count <50,000/mL; high risk of spontaneous bleeding including CNS with count <10,000/μL; usually due to decreased production or increased destruction Elevated platelet count (thrombocytosis)—commonly reactive to inflammation or malignancy, or in polycythemia vera; can be associated with hemorrhage or thrombosis
Bleeding time (BT)	2.5–10 min (template BT)	Interaction between platelets and the subendothelium	Prolonged BT caused by: Thrombocytopenia (platelet count <50,000/μL) Abnormal platelet function (vWD, ASA, NSAIDs, uremia, liver disease)
SECONDARY HEMOSTASIS			
Prothrombin time (PT) and International Normalized Ratio (INR)	11–13 s, depending on reagent; INR 1.0	Extrinsic system and common pathway—factors VII, X, V, prothrombin, and fibrinogen	*Prolonged PT*—most commonly caused by: Use of warfarin (inhibits vitamin K–dependent factors II, VII, IX, and X) Liver disease with decreased factor synthesis Antibiotics, some cephalosporins, (moxalactam, cefamandole, cefotaxime, cefoperazone) that inhibit vitamin K–dependent factors
Activated partial thromboplastin time (aPTT)	22–34 s Depends on type of thromboplastin used; "activated" with Kaolin	Intrinsic system and common pathway including factors XII, XI, IX, VIII, X, V, prothrombin, and fibrinogen	*Prolongation of aPTT* most commonly caused by: Heparin therapy Factor deficiencies; factor levels have to be >30% of normal to cause prolongation
Thrombin clotting time (TCT)	10–12 s	Conversion of fibrinogen to fibrin monomer	*Prolonged TCT* caused by: Low fibrinogen level (DIC) Abnormal fibrinogen molecule (liver disease) Presence of heparin, FDPs or a paraprotein (multiple myeloma); these interfere with the conversion Very high fibrinogen level (acute phase reactant)
"Mixes"	Variable	Performed when one or more of the above screening tests is prolonged; the patient's plasma ("abnormal") is mixed with "normal" plasma and the screening test is repeated	*If the "mix" corrects* the screening test, one or more factor deficiencies are present. *If the "mix" does not correct the screening test*, an inhibitor is present
OTHER HEMOSTATIC TESTS			
Fibrin degradation products and D-dimer (evaluate fibrinolysis)	Variable	*FDPs* measure breakdown products from fibrinogen and fibrin monomer; normal <2.5 μg/L *D-Dimer* measures breakdown products of cross-linked fibrin; normal <500 μg/L	Levels of these are elevated in DIC, thrombosis, pulmonary embolus, liver disease
Factor level assays	60–130% (0.60–1.30 units/mL)	Measures the percent activity of a specified factor compared to normal	Used to identify specific factor deficiencies and in therapeutic management of patients with deficiencies
Inhibitor screens	Variable	Verifies the presence or absence of antibodies directed against one or more of the coagulation factors	*Specific inhibitors*—directed against one coagulation factor, most commonly against factor VIII; can be in patients with congenital or acquired deficiency *Nonspecific inhibitors*—directed against more than one of the coagulation factors; example is lupus-type anticoagulant

Abbreviations: ASA = aspirin; CNS = central nervous system; DIC = disseminated intravascular coagulation; FDPs = fibrin degradation products; NSAIDs = nonsteroidal anti-inflammatory drugs; vWD = von Willebrand disease.

platelet count, prothrombin time, and activated partial thromboplastin time (Table 218-4).[7,8] The results of these tests coupled with clinical evaluation should enable one to formulate a differential diagnosis. Additional coagulation studies are ordered as indicated (see Table 218-4). Hematologic consultation should be sought if the differential diagnosis or the laboratory approach is unclear.

ACKNOWLEDGMENT

Thank you to the previous author, Mary Eberst, for her work.

REFERENCES

1. Beutler E: The common anemias. *JAMA* 259:2433, 1988.
2. Baron BJ, Scalea TM: Acute blood loss. *Emerg Med Clin North Am* 14:35, 1996.
3. Hermiston ML, Mentzer WC: A practical approach to the evaluation of the anemic child. *Pediatr Clin North Am* 49:877, 2002.
4. Hord JD: Anemia and coagulation disorders in adolescents. *Adolesc Med* 10:359, 1999.
5. Goldhill D, Boralessa H: Anemia and red cell transfusion in the critically ill. *Anaesthesia* 57:527, 2002.
6. Crosby E: Re-evaluating transfusion trigger: How low is safe? *Am J Ther* 9:411, 2002.
7. Sallah S, Kato G: Evaluation of bleeding disorders. A detailed history and laboratory tests provide clues. *Postgrad Med* 103:209, 1998.
8. Hemphill RR: Hematologic emergencies and life-threatening bleeding disorders: Differential diagnosis, evaluation and management. *Emerg Med Report* 22:183, 2001.

219 ACQUIRED BLEEDING DISORDERS
Mary A. Wittler
Robin R. Hemphill

ACQUIRED PLATELET DEFECTS

Acquired platelet defects can be either quantitative or qualitative. Quantitative defects, resulting in thrombocytopenia, are caused by decreased production, increased destruction, splenic sequestration or a combination of the three (Table 219-1).[1] A decreased platelet count is commonly manifested by the presence of nonpalpable petechiae. These are most prominent in the lower extremities and in areas where blood flow is restricted. Other findings typical of thrombocytopenia include purpura, mucosal bleeding, hemoptysis, hematuria and hematochezia, whereas deep tissue bleeding is less common.

When platelet levels decrease to below 10 to 20,000/μL, the risk of spontaneous bleeding becomes concerning, particularly for intracranial bleeding. Additional risk factors for bleeding include age, comorbid illnesses (i.e., renal disease, liver disease, connective tissue disease, peptic ulcer disease, hypertension), fall risk, and lifestyle activity. With the exception of a few disease processes, platelet transfusion should be considered when counts fall below 10,000/μL (higher if other comorbid illness are present).[2] The cause of the platelet deficiency may also influence the risk of bleeding. At a given platelet level, patients with idiopathic thrombocytopenic purpura bleed less than patients with aplastic anemia. Research suggests that the younger platelets present in idiopathic thrombocytopenic purpura are more effective in hemostasis due to increased metabolic activity.

During the initial evaluation of a patient who exhibits signs of bleeding the circulatory stability should be assessed and secured. Once this is done, the history and physical examination, along with directed laboratory testing, may help limit the differential. Family history is important, but recent illness, current complaints and recent medications are likely of greater relevance in the patient who appears to have a platelet disorder. Physical examination should evaluate for additional bleeding sites, the type of bleeding, and assess the size of the spleen.

TABLE 219-1 Pathophysiology of Acquired Thrombocytopenia

Mechanism	Associated Clinical Conditions
Decreased platelet production	Marrow infiltration (tumor or infection)
	Aplastic anemia
	Viral infections (measles)
	Drug (thiazides, estrogens, ethanol, interferon-α, chemotherapeutic agents)
	Radiation
	Vitamin B_{12} and/or folate deficiency
Increased platelet destruction	Idiopathic thrombocytopenic purpura
	Thrombotic thrombocytopenic purpura
	Hemolytic uremic syndrome
	Disseminated intravascular coagulation
	Viral infections (HIV, mumps, varicella, EBV)
	Drugs (heparin, protamine)
Splenic sequestration	Hypersplenism
	Hypothermia
Platelet loss	Excessive hemorrhage
	Hemodialysis
	Extracorporeal circulation

Abbreviations: EBV = Epstein–Barr virus; HIV = human immunodeficiency virus.

A complete blood cell count (CBC) will establish whether a low platelet count is present. The CBC will also determine whether other hematologic cell lines are affected. Platelet clumping can occur in some individuals, yielding a falsely low platelet count. In vitro platelet clumping results from cold-dependent or ethylenediaminetetraacetic acid (EDTA)-dependent agglutinins. This can be detected by examining the peripheral smear, which will show clumps of platelets. A correct platelet count can be obtained by collecting the blood in a citrated or heparin-anticoagulated sample tube. A peripheral smear should be done to evaluate the morphology of the platelets as well as the other cell lines.

Thrombocytopenia from Decreased Platelet Production

Neonatal infections, such as cytomegalovirus (CMV) or rubella, may include thrombocytopenia, but generally infants with these disorders have other problems as well. In the older child or adult, if multiple cell lines are affected, the differential diagnosis includes aplastic anemia, marrow infiltration from lymphoma or leukemia, or myelofibrosis. A drug history is important as many medications have been implicated as impairing platelet production (Table 219-2).[3] Chronic alcohol use is a common cause of thrombocytopenia and will generally resolve if the patient abstains from drinking for 7 days. Usually the history and physical examination will determine the most likely source of thrombocytopenia; however, a bone marrow biopsy may be needed if no immediate cause is identified.

Thrombocytopenia from Increased Platelet Destruction

IMMUNE CAUSES OF PLATELET DESTRUCTION Antibody-mediated platelet destruction can be related to medications, infections, or autoimmune diseases. A review of the patient's age, prior medical history, medications, and concurrent symptoms may suggest an immune-mediated cause. Two of the more common antibody-mediated thrombocytopenic disorders are idiopathic thrombocytopenic purpura (ITP) and drug-induced immune thrombocytopenia.[3,4]

Idiopathic Thrombocytopenic Purpura ITP is an acquired autoimmune disease that results in the rapid destruction of platelets. It is characterized by thrombocytopenia, the presence of purpura or petechiae, a normal bone marrow, and no other identifiable cause for the

TABLE 219-2   Drugs Which Produce Thrombocytopenia or Impair Platelet Function

Produce Thrombocytopenia	Impair Function (Prolong Bleeding Time)
Heparin 4+	Aspirin
Gold salts 4+	Nonsteroidal anti-inflammatory drugs
Sulfa-containing antibiotics 4+	Antiplatelet agents: ticlopidine and
Quinine and quinidine 4+	clopidogrel
Ethanol (chronic use) 4+	Penicillins and cephalosporins
Aspirin 3+	Calcium channel blockers
Indomethacin 3+	Propranolol
Valproic acid 3+	Nitroglycerin
Heroin 3+	Antihistamines
Thiazides 2+	Phenothiazines
Furosemide 2+	Tricyclic antidepressants
Procainamide 2+	
Digoxin 2+	
Cimetidine and ranitidine 2+	
Phenytoin 1+	
Penicillins/cephalosporins 1+	

Note: 4+ to 1+ indicates relative incidence, from more frequent to less frequent, based on case reports.

thrombocytopenia.[4,5] Platelet destruction is mediated by the production of autoantibodies that attach to circulating platelets and the antibody-coated platelets are removed by the reticuloendothelial system. The bone marrow will usually respond by increasing platelet production. However, in some cases, the same antibodies that bind to the platelets will also bind to the megakaryocytes, limiting the bone marrow response. Despite the presence of antibodies, the circulating platelets function properly and many people with ITP may not have significant bleeding despite very low platelet counts.

ITP presents in all age groups and may have an acute or chronic course. Acute ITP is more common among younger children, affects males and females equally, and typically resolves in 1 to 2 months. Chronic ITP lasts more than 3 months, is more common in adults, has a female predilection, and rarely remits spontaneously or with treatment. Additionally, patients with chronic ITP are more likely to exhibit an underlying disease or autoimmune disorder, such as HIV, systemic lupus erythematosus (SLE), Graves' disease, Hashimoto thyroiditis, or antiphospholipid antibody syndrome.

The most common sign of ITP is the development of petechiae. Mild epistaxis, gingival bleeding, and menorrhagia in women of childbearing age may also be seen. Except for the petechiae and bruising, the patient should have a normal physical examination. The presence of lymphadenopathy, hepatosplenomegaly, pallor, or hyperbilirubinemia should suggest an alternative diagnosis such as leukemia, lymphoma, systemic lupus erythematosus, infectious mononucleosis, or hemolytic anemia.

Laboratory testing includes a CBC with platelets and a peripheral blood smear. The CBC should demonstrate normal cell lines except for the platelets. In some patients with bleeding, a mild anemia may be present, but the red cell indices should be normal. The peripheral blood smear should show large, well-granulated platelets, although few in number. The diagnosis of ITP is based primarily on the history, physical examination, CBC, and peripheral smear. If the evaluation supports the diagnosis of ITP and there are no atypical findings suggesting a different disease, then additional testing in the ED is not required.

For all patients with ITP, bleeding risks should be minimized, including: avoiding the use of antiplatelet medications [i.e., aspirin and nonsteroidal anti-inflammatory drugs (NSAIDs)]; avoiding unnecessary invasive procedures; maintenance of good blood pressure control; treatment of exacerbating comorbid conditions (i.e., liver disease, renal disease); and addressing fall risks. Treatment of ITP depends upon severity, age, and presence of bleeding.[5,6] **Asymptomatic patients**

who are otherwise healthy with platelet counts >50,000/µL require no treatment. Patients with platelet counts <20,000 to 30,000/µL and patients with platelet counts <50,000/µL with bleeding or significant risk factors for bleeding require treatment. Initial therapy in adults with ITP is prednisone started at 60 to 100 mg/d and tapered after the platelet count reaches normal.[6] Steroid treatment failure is defined by 1) treatment with steroids for a period of 4 to 6 weeks without the return of platelets to >30,000 to 50,000/µL; 2) platelet counts that have not normalized after 6 to 8 weeks of treatment; or 3) falling platelet counts after tapering the steroid dose. For these patients, the main alternative therapy is splenectomy, which produces long-standing remission in approximately 65 percent of patients.

For life-threatening bleeding, stabilization and control of local bleeding should be implemented. In addition, the current recommendation is to initiate high-dose steroid therapy (methylprednisolone 1 to 2 g/d IV for 2 or 3 days). Intravenous immunoglobulin may be given alone or in combination with steroids. Platelets should be transfused as needed following the first dose of methylprednisolone or immunoglobulin; holding the platelet transfusion until the first dose of either is completed generally results in a greater rise in the platelet count. Red cells should be transfused as needed. Conjugated estrogen, 25 mg intravenously once, can be given for severe uterine bleeding.

Hospitalization is required for ITP-related bleeding. However, outside of this obvious indication, the necessity for hospitalization is less clear. Hospitalization is generally not required for asymptomatic patients with platelet counts >20,000 to 30,000/µL. Hospitalization is prudent when arranging patient follow-up is difficult, when compliance is in doubt, or when significant additional bleeding risk factors are present.

Drug-Related Causes of Thrombocytopenia   Multiple medications have been implicated in causing immune mediated destruction of platelets.[3] While the exact mechanisms have not always been determined, certain medications appear to bind to the platelet membrane causing a structural change that then stimulates an immune response (see Table 219-2). Presentation is identical to ITP.

NONIMMUNE CAUSES OF PLATELET DESTRUCTION   Increased platelet destruction can occur from nonimmune mediated causes (see Table 219-1). In thrombotic thrombocytopenic purpura (TTP) and hemolytic uremic syndrome (HUS), thrombotic microangiopathy occurs when vessel injury results in the deposition of platelet-fibrin thrombi.[7] Disseminated intravascular coagulation (DIC) is a well-described cause of platelet destruction. Additionally, certain bacterial, rickettsial, and viral infections can cause direct toxic effects on platelets. Thrombocytopenia specific to pregnancy may be a result of the HELLP (hemolysis, elevated liver enzymes, and low platelets) syndrome, preeclampsia, or gestational thrombocytopenia.[8] Gestational thrombocytopenia occurs in 5 to 8 percent of pregnancies and is generally benign.

Platelet Sequestration

The last major cause of thrombocytopenia is platelet sequestration. In patients with marked splenomegaly, platelet counts as low as 40,000/µL are common. However, isolated splenomegaly rarely results in clinically significant hemorrhage without the presence of another concomitant hemorrhagic disorder, and splenectomy is rarely indicated.

Qualitative Platelet Abnormalities

Several disease processes can cause acquired qualitative or functional abnormalities of platelets (Table 219-3). In the myeloproliferative diseases, platelets are often dysfunctional, even if the platelet count is elevated. Patients can develop prolonged bleeding times or clinically significant bleeding. To control acute bleeding, transfusion should be

TABLE 219-3 Clinical Conditions Associated with Qualitative Platelet Abnormalities

Uremia
Liver disease
Disseminated intravascular coagulation
Antiplatelet antibodies (ITP, SLE)
Cardiopulmonary bypass
Myeloproliferative disorders (PCV, CML)
Dysproteinemias (multiple myeloma, Waldenström macroglobulinemia)
Preleukemias, AML, ALL
von Willebrand disease (congenital or acquired)

Abbreviations: ALL = acute lymphocytic leukemia; AML = acute myelogenous leukemia; CML = chronic myelogenous leukemia; ITP = idiopathic thrombocytopenic purpura; PCV = polycythemia vera; SLE = systemic lupus erythematosus.

considered to raise the level of normal platelets to 50,000 /μL. In macroglobulinemia and related disorders, the elevated level of viscous proteins interferes with platelet function. Patients with clinically significant bleeding may require plasmapheresis to reduce the protein level and correct hemostatic function.

Many commonly used drugs can influence platelet function and should be avoided in clinical conditions characterized by altered platelet function (see Tables 219-2, and 219-4). Of these, the most commonly used are aspirin—which produces an irreversible impairment in platelet aggregation—and the NSAIDs, clopidogrel, and ticlopidine—which produce temporary impairment in platelet adhesion and aggregation (see Chap. 224).

Thrombocytosis, a platelet count above 500,000 /μL, can be seen in many disorders, including inflammatory reactions, malignancy, polycythemia, and postsplenectomy. Platelet function can be normal or abnormal depending upon the underlying condition. With abnormal platelet function, thrombocytosis can be associated with bleeding (mucosal, ecchymoses, gastrointestinal) or thromboembolic (deep vein thrombosis, portal or mesenteric thrombosis, splenic vein thrombosis) manifestations. However, these events are unusual, even with platelet counts in excess of 1 million/μL.

ANTICOAGULANTS AND FIBRINOLYTICS

These agents are discussed in detail in Chap. 224. Patients with acquired bleeding disorders should be carefully assessed before administration of anticoagulants or fibrinolytics.

LIVER DISEASE

Acute and chronic diseases of the liver can be associated with many hemostatic abnormalities.[9] Hepatocytes synthesize all of the coagulation factors and related regulatory proteins, with the exception of factor VIII. Diseases affecting the hepatic parenchyma may result in a decreased synthesis of these factors, including the vitamin K–dependent carboxylation of factors II (prothrombin), VII, IX, and X. Because vitamin K is a fat-soluble vitamin, malabsorption can occur with processes that interfere with the absorption of fat-soluble vitamins, including impaired bile acid metabolism (i.e., primary biliary cirrhosis), intrahepatic or extrahepatic cholestasis, and treatment with bile acid binders.

TABLE 219-4 Duration of Antiplatelet Activity

Drug	Onset	Duration of Effect
Aspirin	1 h	Platelet life span (8 d)
Most NSAIDs	1 h	1 d
Piroxicam	1 h	2 d
Ticlopidine or clopidogrel	1–2 d	4–10 d

Thrombocytopenia in severe liver disease is most often caused by portal hypertension, which leads to congestive hypersplenism and splenic sequestration. Splenic sequestration decreases the effective circulating platelet number. Alone, this thrombocytopenia is not usually clinically significant, but can have additive effects to other hemostatic abnormalities present in liver disease. Patients with significant liver disease have increased fibrinolysis as a result of decreased synthesis of α_2-plasmin inhibitor, which is produced by the liver. As α_2-plasmin inhibitor is the major inhibitor of plasmin, a deficiency results in unregulated plasmin activity and increased fibrinolysis. Characteristics of increased fibrinolysis include low fibrinogen levels and a mild elevation of fibrin degradation products (FDPs) and D-dimers. In some patients with liver disease, abnormal fibrinogen molecules are synthesized. These abnormal fibrinogen molecules are converted to abnormal fibrin molecules that do not polymerize correctly.

Distinguishing DIC from the coagulopathy of severe liver disease is difficult. Abnormal laboratory values, including decreased platelets, decreased coagulation factors, and hypofibrinogenemia can be present in both conditions. The D-dimer assay should be normal in liver disease (see DIC discussion below). Patients with mild to moderate hepatic dysfunction frequently have subclinical hemostatic abnormalities. Those with severe liver disease may have life-threatening bleeding. Laboratory studies that should be obtained include a hematocrit, prothrombin time (PT), aPTT, and platelet count. Fibrinogen levels and measurement of FDP and/or D-dimers may also be considered. In general, prolongation of the PT and hypofibrinogenemia with a plasma fibrinogen level <100 mg/dL are poor prognostic signs in patients with liver disease.

Patients who have liver disease and laboratory abnormalities without clinically significant bleeding usually require only close observation. If there is clinically significant bleeding or a pending invasive procedure or surgery, the coagulopathic state will need to be treated. Packed red blood cells should be transfused to maintain an adequate hemoglobin level and to maintain hemodynamic stability. Oral or intravenous vitamin K should be given to all patients with liver disease and active bleeding. For patients with prolonged PT and aPTT and active bleeding or pending procedure, FFP can be used to temporarily replace coagulation factors. The volume needed to completely replenish the coagulation factors may limit the use of FFP. Each FFP unit is 200 to 250 mL and contains approximately 200 to 250 units of each coagulation factor. Because the half-life of several of the clotting factors is 12 h or less, additional doses of FFP may be required. Cryoprecipitate may be used to replace fibrinogen in patients with active bleeding and fibrinogen levels <100 mg/dL. Platelet transfusions may be appropriate if bleeding is present with low counts. Desmopressin (DDAVP), a synthetic analogue of vasopressin, shortens the prolonged bleeding time in some patients with liver disease. Although controlled trials are lacking, there appear to be few side effects. The dose is 0.3 μg/kg (maximum 20 μg) SC or IV every 12 h up to three doses. Intranasal desmopressin may also be effective in this setting at a dose of 3 μg/kg (maximum 300 μg).

RENAL DISEASE

Hemostatic abnormalities are commonly present in patients with renal disease related to multiple abnormalities in hemostasis, including quantitative and qualitative platelet abnormalities and clotting factor abnormalities.[10] Platelet counts are usually normal, although mild thrombocytopenia may occur. Clinically significant bleeding may occasionally occur with dialysis-induced thrombocytopenia. Retention of uremic toxins causes inhibition of platelet aggregation.

Management of these hemostatic defects is aimed at both prevention and directed at treatment of acute bleeding. Preventative measures include optimizing nutrition; folate, vitamin B_{12} and iron repletion; optimizing dialysis; and correction of anemia with recombinant human erythropoietin (rHuEPO). Acute bleeding can be treated with dialysis, transfusion of red blood cells, DDAVP, conjugated estrogens, cryoprecipitate transfusion, and (rarely) platelet transfusion. Dialysis improves platelet function transiently for 1 to 2 days. Optimally, patients are well dialyzed three times per week. In uremic patients with prolonged bleeding times, most will have shortening or normalization of the bleeding time when treated with desmopressin. Side effects associated with desmopressin are generally mild and include headache, flushing, minor hypotension, tachycardia, nausea, abdominal cramps, and local site reaction. Conjugated estrogens also improve both the bleeding time and clinical bleeding in more than 80 percent of uremic patients treated. Platelet transfusions are not routinely used in this setting because the infused platelets quickly acquire the uremic defect. Cryoprecipitate and platelet infusions are only indicated for life-threatening bleeding used in combination with packed red blood cells, desmopressin and conjugated estrogens.

DISSEMINATED INTRAVASCULAR COAGULATION

DIC is an acquired syndrome characterized by activation of the coagulation system resulting in fibrin formation.[11] Activation of the fibrinolytic system also occurs, resulting in the breakdown of fibrin clots, consumption of coagulation factors, and bleeding. DIC is associated with a wide variety of disorders and may be acute and life-threatening, or chronic and compensated (Table 219-5).

Pathogenesis

Although the diseases triggering DIC are diverse, the commonality of these illnesses is the activation of tissue factor, a substrate in the extrinsic pathway of the coagulation cascade. The deregulated formation of thrombin is central to the pathogenesis of DIC (Figure 219-1). Thrombin generation results in small fibrin clots formed and deposited in the microcirculation, thereby leading to the thrombotic occlusion of vessels and eventually end-organ dysfunction. Widespread activation of the coagulation system leads to consumption of circulating platelets and coagulation factors. Production of thrombin and fibrin indirectly activates tissue plasminogen activator (tPA) and the counterregulatory fibrinolytic system. Plasmin is produced from plasminogen, which then degrades fibrin and results in the generation of FDP. Normally, the fibrinolytic system plays a homeostatic role and is balanced with the coagulation system, but in DIC, the degree of fibrinolytic activation is excessive and can result in pathologic bleeding.

Clinical Features

Clinical features of DIC vary with the underlying precipitating medical illness. The clinical complications of DIC are bleeding, thrombosis, purpura fulminans, and multiple organ failure. Although hemorrhage and thrombosis may occur simultaneously, in an individual patient, one usually predominates and the most common manifestation is bleeding. Bleeding can range from petechiae and ecchymoses to widespread bleeding from the gastrointestinal tract, genitourinary tract, surgical wounds, mucocutaneous sites and venipuncture sites. Intravascular coagulation and fibrin deposition can cause multiple organ failure. Clinical signs of this include mental status changes, focal ischemia or gangrene, oliguria, renal cortical necrosis and adult respiratory distress syndrome (ARDS). Purpura fulminans occurs when there are widespread arterial and venous thromboses and is most commonly seen with significant bacteremia. In chronic DIC, the pathophysiology of disease is essentially the same, but the consumption of coagulation factors and platelets is balanced by hepatic production.

Laboratory

The typical laboratory results in acute DIC include prolonged PT, low platelet count, and/or low fibrinogen level (Table 219-6). The most commonly observed abnormality is thrombocytopenia; a progressive drop in the platelet count is sensitive, although not specific, for DIC. Depletion of coagulation factors is reflected by prolonged clotting times. Fibrinogen levels may remain normal because fibrinogen is an acute-phase reactant. A fibrinogen level <100 mg/dL is associated

TABLE 219-5   Common Conditions Associated with Disseminated Intravascular Coagulation

Clinical Setting	Comments
Infection Bacterial Viral Fungal	Probably the most common cause of DIC; 10–20% of patients with gram-negative sepsis have DIC; endotoxins stimulate monocytes and endothelial cells to express tissue factor; Rocky Mountain spotted fever causes direct endothelial damage; DIC more likely to develop in asplenic patients or those with cirrhosis; septic patients are more likely to have thrombosis than bleeding.
Carcinoma Adenocarcinoma Lymphoma	Malignant cells may cause endothelial damage and allow the expression of tissue factor as well as other procoagulant materials; most adenocarcinomas tend to have thrombosis (Trousseau syndrome), except prostate cancer tends to have more bleeding; DIC is often chronic and compensated.
Acute leukemia	DIC most common with promyelocytic leukemia; blast cells release procoagulant enzymes, there is excessive release at time of cell lysis (chemotherapy); more likely to have bleeding than thrombosis.
Trauma	DIC especially with brain injury, crush injury, burns, hypothermia, hyperthermia, rhabdomyolysis, fat embolism, hypoxia.
Liver disease	May have chronic compensated DIC; acute DIC may occur in the setting of acute hepatic failure, tissue factor is released from the injured hepatocytes.
Pregnancy	Placental abruption, amniotic fluid embolus, septic abortion, intrauterine fetal death (can be chronic DIC); can get DIC in HELLP (hemolysis, elevated liver enzymes, low platelets) syndrome.
Vascular disease	Large aortic aneurysms (chronic DIC can become acute at time of surgery), giant hemangiomas, vasculitis, multiple telangiectasias.
Envenomation	DIC can develop with bites of rattlesnakes and other vipers; the venom damages the endothelial cells; bleeding is not as bad as expected from laboratory values.
Adult respiratory distress syndrome (ARDS)	Microthrombi are deposited in the small pulmonary vessels, the pulmonary capillary endothelium is damaged; 20% of patients with ARDS develop DIC and 20% of patients with DIC develop ARDS.
Transfusion reactions Acute hemolytic reaction Massive transfusion	DIC with severe bleeding, shock, and acute renal failure.

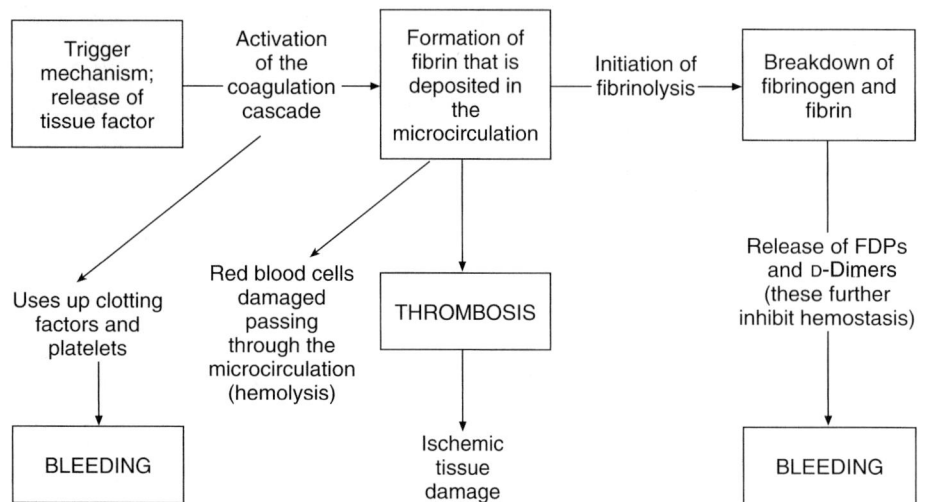

FIG. 219-1. Pathophysiology of disseminated intravascular coagulation. Refer to text for details. FDPs = fibrin/fibrinogen degradation products.

with increased bleeding manifestations. FDP and D-Dimer may help differentiate DIC from other causes of prolonged coagulation times and low platelets. D-Dimer is a test that indicates excessive cross-linked fibrin breakdown and may be more specific in diagnosing DIC than FDP. Additional laboratory findings include increased lactic acid dehydrogenase, decreased haptoglobin levels, and a peripheral smear with schistocytes. Chronic DIC will have minor abnormalities of the screening assays, reflecting the limited consumption of coagulation factors that are being replaced by hepatic synthesis.

TABLE 219-6 Laboratory Abnormalities Characteristic of Disseminated Intravascular Coagulation

Studies	Result
MOST USEFUL	
Prothrombin time	Prolonged
Platelet count*	Usually low
Fibrinogen level†	Low
HELPFUL	
Activated partial thromboplastin time	Usually prolonged
Thrombin clot time‡	Prolonged
Fragmented red blood cells§	Should be present
FDPs and D-dimers¶	Elevated
*Specific factor assays***	
Factor II	Low
Factor V	Low
Factor VII††	Low
Factor VIII‡‡	Low, normal, high
Factor IX	Low (decreases later than other factors)
Factor X	Low

*Platelet count usually low, most important that it is falling if it started at an elevated level.

†Fibrinogen level correlates best with bleeding complications; it is an acute phase reactant so it may actually start out at an elevated level; fibrinogen level <100 mg/dL correlates with severe DIC.

‡Not a sensitive test, prolonged by many abnormalities.

§Fragmented red blood cells and schistocytes are not specific for DIC.

¶Levels may be chronically elevated in patients with liver or renal disease.

**The factors in the extrinsic pathway are most affected (VII, X, V, and II).

††Factor VII is usually low early because it has the shortest half-life.

‡‡Factor VIII is an acute phase reactant so its level may be normal, low, or elevated in DIC.

Abbreviations: DIC = disseminated intravascular coagulation; FDP = fibrin degradation products.

Differential Diagnosis

Primary fibrinolysis is a rare syndrome whereby plasmin and fibrinolysis are independently generated without the production of thrombin. Severe liver disease will also manifest with coagulation abnormalities and low platelets. These two entities can be differentiated from DIC on the basis of clinical history and laboratory tests. The hematologic abnormalities in liver disease should be relatively stable in contrast to the worsening abnormalities associated with acute DIC. Additionally, the D-dimer assay will usually be normal or minimally elevated in both primary fibrinolysis and liver disease, but elevated in DIC.

Treatment

Treatment of DIC rests on supportive measures and management of the underlying illness.[11] Circulatory stabilization requires fluid, red cells, and, sometimes, inotropic agents. If possible, the underlying cause of the DIC needs to be treated. Secondary treatment involves replacement therapy with platelets, fibrinogen, and coagulation factors. Many patients with DIC require no specific therapy if evidence of bleeding or thrombosis is lacking and laboratory studies are not deteriorating. Replacement therapy should only occur in patients with documented DIC with bleeding or an impending invasive procedure. Fibrinogen repletion should be considered in the patient who has hypofibrinogenemia and significant bleeding. The goal of treatment is to raise the plasma fibrinogen level to 100 to 150 mg/dL with cryoprecipitate. Each unit of cryoprecipitate contains approximately 200 to 250 mg of fibrinogen and is usually transfused in 10-unit increments. Platelet repletion should be considered in the patient with a platelet count less then 50,000/μL with bleeding, or with a platelet count less than 20,000/μL without bleeding. Typically, 6 units of random donor platelets (or one apheresis unit) are given at a time. FFP is used to replace clotting factors for DIC-associated bleeding with prolonged PT and aPTT. Each unit of FFP contains 200 to 250 units of each factor. A patient is usually transfused with 10 to 15 mL/kg, or in increments of 2 to 4 units of FFP. Patients with DIC also should be given vitamin K and folate.

Heparin administration usually has a limited role in the treatment of acute DIC, and it is usually considered in patients with documented DIC in whom thromboembolic complications predominate the clinical picture (i.e., purpura fulminans). The role of heparin in treatment of acute promyelocytic leukemia and advanced liver disease remains controversial. Heparin should also be considered in patients with chronic DIC and thrombosis (i.e., solid tumors). Low-molecular-weight heparin may be just as efficacious as unfractionated heparin. Antifibrinolytic agents, including ε-aminocaproic acid (EACA), are used with great caution in DIC. Although these drugs may reduce bleeding, their use is associated with serious and/or fatal thromboembolic complications. Antifibrinolytic agents should be restricted to patients who have documented hypofibrinogenemia and fibrinolysis. When used, antifibrinolytic agents are given together with heparin or after heparin infusion to minimize the potential for thrombosis. Because several of the regulatory pathways of anticoagulation are dysfunctional and/or ineffective in DIC, current research is focusing on the use of antithrombin III concentrate replacement, protein C concentrate replacement, and tumor factor inhibitors.

INFECTION WITH HUMAN IMMUNODEFICIENCY VIRUS

The more common hemostatic abnormalities observed in patients infected with HIV-1 are thrombocytopenia and acquired circulating anticoagulants.[12,13]

Thrombocytopenia is one of the earliest findings in asymptomatic HIV-1–infected individuals.[12] For patients with fully developed AIDS, 30 to 45 percent will have mild to moderate thrombocytopenia at some time during the course of their illness. Clinically significant bleeding is unusual, with the common manifestations being easy bruising, petechiae, and mucosal bleeding. The thrombocytopenia is secondary to increased peripheral platelet destruction and decreased platelet production. The increased platelet destruction is likely immune mediated. HIV-1 also directly infects bone marrow megakaryocytes, resulting in decreased thrombopoiesis. Additionally, drugs used to treat HIV-related illnesses can contribute to thrombocytopenia, including trimethoprim-sulfamethoxazole, ganciclovir, and fluconazole. TTP is an uncommon but well-described complication of HIV-1 infection and may be the initial manifestation of infection. It is characterized by the pentad of fever, thrombocytopenia, neurologic symptoms, renal insufficiency, and microangiopathic hemolytic anemia (see Chap. 222).

Antiphospholipid antibodies, including lupus anticoagulant and anticardiolipin antibodies, are a common hemostatic abnormality in HIV-1–infected patients.[13] Patients with lupus anticoagulant will have a prolongation of the aPTT that does not correct after mixing with normal plasma. Often a transient defect, the lupus-type anticoagulant may appear with an acute opportunistic infection and disappear when the infection is treated. Anticardiolipin antibodies are detected by enzyme-linked immunosorbent assay (ELISA) and do not affect the basic hemostatic screening tests. One or both of these antibodies occur in 22 to 82 percent of patients with HIV-1 infection. While these antibodies do not predispose a patient to clinical bleeding, concomitant hemostatic abnormalities such as platelet dysfunction or hypoprothrombinemia (associated with the lupus-type anticoagulant) may lead to bleeding manifestations. Whereas HIV-negative patients who have antiphospholipid antibodies are predisposed to thrombosis, HIV-positive patients with antiphospholipid antibodies rarely manifest thrombosis.

CIRCULATING ANTICOAGULANTS

Acquired inhibitors of blood coagulation, also known as circulating anticoagulants, are antibodies directed against one or more of the coagulation factors.[14] While inhibitors may develop spontaneously in previously healthy patients with normal hemostasis, most inhibitors develop in patients with hereditary bleeding disorders who receive transfusion of plasma products. Inhibitors have been described for most of the coagulation factors; the two most common inhibitors are factor VIII inhibitors and antiphospholipid antibodies. Factor VIII inhibitors are "specific" inhibitors, directed only against factor VIII as opposed to antiphospholipid antibodies, including lupus anticoagulant and anticardiolipin antibodies, which are "nonspecific" inhibitors directed against several of the coagulation factors.

Factor VIII Inhibitors

Factor VIII inhibitors most commonly develop in patients with hemophilia A (Chap. 220), but can also develop spontaneously in patients with previously normal hemostasis. This latter group includes the development of inhibitors in the elderly having no underlying disease, postpartum patients, and patients with autoimmune disorders or underlying disease processes. The incidence of spontaneously arising inhibitors is estimated at 0.2 to 1.0 per 1 million persons per year. Although uncommon, it is important to recognize this clinical entity because the mortality rate approaches 22 percent. Inhibitors can develop in association with autoimmune disorders [systemic lupus erythematosus (SLE), rheumatoid arthritis, ulcerative colitis], lymphoproliferative disorders (multiple myeloma, Waldenström macroglobulinemia, benign monoclonal gammopathy of uncertain significance), and in patients with allergic drug reactions (penicillins, sulfonamides, phenytoin).

Patients without a prior bleeding history who develop factor VIII inhibitors can present with massive spontaneous bruises, ecchymoses and hematomas. Laboratory studies classically show a normal PT, normal thrombin clotting time (TCT), and a greatly prolonged aPTT that does not correct with "mixing." A factor VIII-specific assay will show very low or absent factor VIII activity. Other factor specific assays should be normal or only slightly decreased. Quantitative measurement of the inhibitor by the Bethesda Inhibitor Assay is important for the emergency management of bleeding episodes. Treatment of factor VIII inhibitors focuses on using long-term management to suppress antibody production and treatment of acute bleeding episodes. Long-term management is directed at the suppression of antibody production via steroids, intravenous immunoglobulin, or cytotoxic agents. A hematologist should direct the management of an acute, clinically significant bleeding episode. Conservative therapies should be considered, including compression and immobilization of the bleeding site and possible administration of ε-aminocaproic acid. Additionally, the use of aspirin, NSAIDs, and intramuscular injections should be avoided. Other treatment options include factor VIII concentrates (porcine factor VIII, human purified factor VIII, recombinant factor VIII), factor IX complex concentrates, purified prothrombin complex concentrates, recombinant factor VIIa concentrates, and plasmapheresis.

Antiphospholipid Antibody Syndrome

The antiphospholipid antibody syndrome is defined by the presence of the lupus anticoagulant or anticardiolipin antibodies plus one or both of the following clinical criteria: thrombosis (arterial or venous) and/or complications with pregnancy (recurrent fetal loss or recurrent premature births at <34 weeks estimated gestational age).[15] The lupus anticoagulant is an antiphospholipid antibody that, in vitro, prolongs many of the coagulation reactions. In vivo, the lupus anticoagulant inhibits anticoagulant pathways, resulting in thrombosis. **Lupus anticoagulant is a misnomer because the majority of affected patients do not have lupus (it is present in only 5 to 15 percent of patients with SLE) and the majority of patients develop thrombosis rather than bleeding.** Aside from SLE, other conditions associated with the development of lupus anticoagulants include other autoimmune disorders, drug reactions (especially procainamide and phenothiazine), malignancies, and patients with HIV-1 infection.

Primary antiphospholipid syndrome includes affected patients who have no underlying disease state. Secondary antiphospholipid syndrome includes affected patients with an underlying autoimmune process or other disease state. Frequently, patients who have lupus anticoagulant also have anticardiolipin antibodies, which, like lupus anticoagulant, is an antiphospholipid antibody that, in vitro, prolongs many of the coagulation reactions. Although frequently present simultaneously, lupus anticoagulant and anticardiolipin antibodies may occur independently of each other. Therefore, both should be tested when evaluating for an antiphospholipid syndrome.

Laboratory studies of patients with the lupus anticoagulant typically show a normal or slightly prolonged PT (0.5 to 3.0 s), prolongation of the aPTT (not usually more than 10 to 15 s prolonged), and a normal TCT. The prolonged aPTT will not correct with mixing equal parts of the patient's plasma with normal plasma. Some patients with lupus anticoagulant develop antibodies that bind to prothrombin, resulting in a hypoprothrombinemia (factor II deficiency). Excessive prolongation of the PT (i.e., 18 to 20 s) is suggestive of a concomitant hypoprothrombinemia. Factor-specific assays will show a decrease in all the factor levels, although none are extremely low. There are multiple tests available to detect the presence of the lupus anticoagulant, including the dilute Russell viper venom time (dRVVT), the kaolin clotting time, the dilute phospholipid time, and the tissue thromboplastin inhibition test. Multiple tests should be employed to increase the number of patients identified. Patients suspected of having lupus anticoagulant should also be tested for anticardiolipin antibodies as measured by an ELISA.

Many patients with lupus anticoagulant and anticardiolipin antibodies are asymptomatic, with abnormalities discovered only on routine coagulation screening tests. If symptomatic, the major clinical manifestations are thromboembolism, pregnancy complications, and thrombocytopenia. Patients are more likely to develop venous as opposed to arterial thrombosis. Additionally, patients may develop nonbacterial aortic or mitral valvular lesions with resulting systemic embolization. Patients who remain positive for lupus anticoagulant have a 50 percent recurrence of arterial or venous thrombosis within 2 years. Complications during pregnancy include recurrent fetal loss and premature labor. Recurrent fetal loss usually occurs at an estimated gestational age >10 weeks, but can occur earlier. The likely mechanism for recurrent fetal loss is thrombosis of placental vessels and placental infarction. Additionally, premature delivery at <34 weeks is thought to be secondary to uteroplacental insufficiency. Approximately 40 to 50 percent of patients develop thrombocytopenia. Bleeding is rare, and if present, it is usually secondary to another process, such as hypoprothrombinemia (usually patients with SLE), significant thrombocytopenia, or uremia.

Asymptomatic patients diagnosed with the lupus anticoagulant or anticardiolipin antibodies require no treatment. However, risk factors for the development of thromboembolism, including vascular stasis, vessel injury, and hypercoagulable states should be minimized. Additionally, treatment of concurrent underlying disorders or autoimmune diseases may result in the reduction or disappearance of the antiphospholipid antibody. Corticosteroids are not recommended unless there is an associated autoimmune disorder. Patients who sustain a thrombotic event, whether arterial or venous, are managed with long-term anticoagulation by using oral anticoagulants. Aspirin alone fails to prevent recurrent thrombosis. Pregnant patients with the lupus anticoagulant or anticardiolipin antibody can be treated with low- or intermediate-dose heparin with or without daily aspirin. LMWHs are likely to be as efficacious as unfractionated heparin and a safe, convenient alternative.

ACKNOWLEDGMENT

We wish to recognize the contributions of Mary Eberst, MD, for chapter content in previous editions.

REFERENCES

1. McCrae KR, Bussel JB, Mannucci PM, et al: Platelets: An update on diagnosis and management of thrombocytopenic disorders. *Hematology* (Am Soc Hematol Educ Program) 282, 2001.
2. Rebulla P: Platelet transfusion trigger in difficult patients [erratum appears in *Transfus Clin Biol* 9:109, 2002]. *Transfus Clin Biol* 8:249, 2001.
3. Greinacher A, Eicheler P, Lubenow N, Kiefel V: Drug-induced and drug-dependent immune thrombocytopenias. *Rev Clin Exp Hematol* 5:166, 2001.
4. Cines DB, Blanchette VS: Immune thrombocytopenic purpura. *New Engl J Med* 346:995, 2002.
5. Bolton-Maggs PH: Idiopathic thrombocytopenic purpura. *Arch Dis Child* 83:220, 2000.
6. George JN: Initial management of adults with idiopathic (immune) thrombocytopenic purpura. *Blood Rev* 16:37, 2002.
7. Moake JL: Thrombotic microangiopathies. *N Engl J Med* 347:589, 2002.
8. McCrae KR: Thrombocytopenia in pregnancy: Differential diagnosis, pathogenesis, and management. *Blood Rev* 17:7, 2003.
9. Amitrano L, Guardascione MA, Brancaccio V, Balzano A: Coagulation disorders in liver disease. *Semin Liver Dis* 22:83, 2002.
10. Opatrny K: Hemostasis disorders in chronic renal failure. *Kidney Int Suppl* 62:S87, 1997.
11. Levi M, ten Cate H: Disseminated intravascular coagulation. *New Engl J Med* 341:586, 1999.
12. Scaradavou A: HIV-related thrombocytopenia. *Blood Rev* 16:73, 2002.
13. Saif MW, Greenberg B: HIV and thrombosis: A review. *AIDS Patient Care STDS* 15:15, 2001.
14. Sallah S: Inhibitors to clotting factors. *Ann Hematol* 75:1, 1997.
15. Levine JS, Branch DW, Rauch J: The antiphospholipid syndrome. *New Engl J Med* 346:752, 2002.

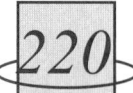

220 HEMOPHILIAS AND VON WILLEBRAND DISEASE
Robin R. Hemphill

Hemophilias are bleeding disorders due to deficiency or defect in one of the factors present in the clotting cascade.[1] The most common factor abnormalities are of factor VIII (hemophilia A or classic hemophilia) or factor IX (hemophilia B or Christmas disease). von Willebrand disease is a related hereditary deficiency, a defect in a portion of the factor VIII complex.[2]

The hereditary disorders typically appear early in life and adult patients will usually be able to relate a history of a bleeding disorder in themselves or their family. However, patients with mild forms of inherited disease may be unaware of a bleeding disorder until stressed by significant trauma or development of another hemostatic problem. Because of new mutations, patients with congenital coagulopathies may not have a family history of bleeding.

Systemic bleeding disorders should be suspected in patients with severe bleeding related to trivial trauma or minor surgery, or spontaneous bleeding, particularly when the bleeding occurs in joints or muscle. Unusual bleeding or bruising at multiple areas should also raise concern about a coagulopathy. Medications can be responsible for unmasking a mild bleeding diathesis and a complete inquiry of current and recent medication use is warranted.

The pattern of bleeding can suggest a likely etiology. For example, patients with easy bruising, gingival bleeding, epistaxis, hematuria, gastrointestinal bleeding, or heavy menses are more likely to have a deficiency or dysfunction of the platelets. Conversely, patients with spontaneous deep bruises, hemarthrosis, retroperitoneal bleeding, or intracranial bleeding are more likely to have a coagulation factor deficiency. In factor-deficient patients, bleeding associated with trauma may be delayed. This is presumed to be due to the instability of the initial platelet thrombus that is inadequately stabilized by fibrin clot formation. Patients with von Willebrand disease may present with features of both platelet and clotting factor problems.

HEMOPHILIA

Hemophilia is a disorder of coagulation caused primarily by a deficiency or defect in one of two circulating plasma proteins.[1,2] Hemophilia A or "classic" hemophilia is caused by a deficiency of factor VIII and is the most common cause of hemophilia in the United States, affecting 1 in 10,000 males. Hemophilia B or Christmas disease is caused by a deficiency of factor IX and is less common, affecting approximately 1 in 25,000 to 35,000 males. Together these forms of hemophilia make up about 99 percent of patients with inherited coagulation factor deficiencies. Hemophilia A and B are clinically indistinguishable from each other, and specific factor testing must be done to identify the specific type of hemophilia.

Both hemophilia A and B are X-linked recessive disorders, therefore this is overwhelmingly a disease of men with women being asymptomatic carriers. However, approximately one-third of new cases of hemophilia A and one-fifth of new cases of hemophilia B arise from a spontaneous gene mutation.

Bleeding manifestations in patients with all forms of hemophilia are directly attributable to the decreased plasma levels of either factor VIII or IX. Individuals with factor levels below 1 percent of normal are classified as having severe disease, and these people will experience severe spontaneous bleeding episodes and difficult-to-control bleeding related to traumatic events. Patients with levels of 1 to 5 percent of normal are classified as having moderate disease. They may bleed spontaneously, but most commonly their bleeding is related to a traumatic event. Patients with factor levels of 5 to 25 percent of normal are classified as having mild disease. They will usually bleed only after trauma. Those with factor levels of 25 to 50 percent may never be aware that they have hemophilia, or they might manifest unusual bleeding only after major surgery or severe trauma. Unless there is another underlying disease, patients with hemophilia do not have problems with minor cuts and abrasions. Treatment of patients with hemophilia relies on either the replacement of missing factors, or for those who have mild factor VIII deficiency, stimulating the body to secrete additional clotting factor from intracellular stores.

Bleeding is the major complication of hemophilia, but as a result of exposure to blood products, many hemophiliacs have chronic viral hepatitis or are infected with the human immunodeficiency virus (HIV). Fortunately, as a result of newer viral inactivation procedures, there have been few seroconversions resulting from the use of currently available factor replacement products.

Clinical Manifestations

Depending on the severity of the disease, both types of hemophilia are characterized by easy bruising and recurrent bleeding into the joints and muscles. While the joints and muscles are the most common areas into which bleeding occurs, hemorrhage may also occur in the abdomen, retroperitoneum, or the central nervous system (Table 220-1). Any trauma or surgical procedure can result in prolonged and difficult-to-control bleeding.

TABLE 220-1   Common Bleeding Manifestations in Patients with Hemophilia

Site	Comments
Hemarthroses	Leads to joint destruction and chronic arthropathy if not treated aggressively
Hematomas	Bleeding into soft tissues or muscle; this bleeding can dissect along fascial planes; most dangerous near in the neck (airway compromise), limbs (compartment syndromes), and retroperitoneum (massive blood loss)
Mucocutaneous bleeding	Spontaneous bleeding uncommon from the oropharynx, gastrointestinal tract, epistaxis, or hemoptysis; delayed bleeding after dental extractions is common
Central nervous system	Intracranial bleeding is the most common cause of hemorrhagic death in hemophiliacs with a reported 34% mortality, subdural hematomas occur spontaneously or with minimal trauma
Hematuria	Common, usually not serious, and the source is rarely found
Pseudotumor	Bone cysts that result from unresolved hematomas; usually have to be removed surgically

While adults often know that they have hemophilia, young children may not have been diagnosed at the time that they present to the ED. A family history may reveal bleeding disorders. Hemophilia should be suspected in any infant or child that presents with excessive bruising or with significant bleeding into the joints, muscles, or central nervous system that is spontaneous or out of proportion to the history of trauma. Because factor level determines the severity of disease, those with mild hemophilia may come to medical attention only when they have a significant surgical procedure or trauma or have started a medication with antihemostatic effects. In addition, excessive bruising and bleeding out of proportion to the described trauma should raise consideration of child abuse, a condition much more common than hemophilia.

Laboratory Testing

In patients with hemophilia, the prothrombin time (PT), which measures the extrinsic coagulation cascade, will be normal, while the activated partial thromboplastin time (aPTT), which measures the intrinsic coagulation cascade, will be abnormal. However, if the factor VIII level in hemophilia A or factor IX level in hemophilia B is greater than 30 percent of normal activity (mild hemophilia), the aPTT may be normal. **Bleeding time in both forms of hemophilia will be normal.** Specific factor assays can be done to help determine the exact nature of the clotting deficiency if the diagnosis is new. Coagulation studies are unlikely to yield new information in the known hemophiliac and are not routinely indicated when the patient presents with mild to moderate bleeding episodes.

Initial Assessment

A general principle in managing major or life-threatening bleeding in a hemophilic patient is early and complete factor replacement, before or at the same time as other resuscitative and diagnostic maneuvers. Spontaneous or traumatic bleeding into the neck, tongue, retropharynx, or pharynx has a high potential for airway compromise. Airway management, including oral intubation, is appropriate if there is the potential for airway compromise. Bleeding into the central nervous system (CNS) can occur spontaneously as well as after trauma. Any patient with hemophilia who complains of a new headache, localizing neurologic symptoms, or a blunt head injury requires immediate factor replacement therapy followed by urgent computed tomographic (CT) scanning of the head. If the neurologic deficit localizes to a region within the spinal cord, magnetic resonance imaging (MRI) is appropriate. Hemophilic patients with complaints of back, thigh, groin, or abdominal pain may have bleeding into the retroperitoneum. Again, immediate factor replacement and CT scanning are indicated. If a hemophiliac patient requires transfer, factor replacement should be initiated before transfer and not be delayed by attempts to obtain imaging. Even in the patient who initially appears well, transport to specialized centers should be considered for intracranial, intrathoracic, retroperitoneal, or intraabdominal bleeding.

At times the initial manifestations of bleeding can be subtle. Simple injuries such as ankle and wrist sprains may at first appear benign but can be complicated by bleeding. Compartment syndromes can result from muscle bleeds within the fascial compartments of the extremities, both spontaneously and after minimal trauma to an extremity. If compartment syndrome is a concern, the compartment pressures can be safely measured after the patient has received factor replacement.

One of the most common manifestations of hemophilia is hemarthrosis. There may or may not be clinical evidence of an acute hemarthrosis, but patients can reliably report when bleeding is occurring. Prompt treatment of hemarthroses can prevent or reduce the long-term sequelae of hemophilic arthropathy. If a large hemarthrosis is already present, consultation with an orthopedist for appropriate splinting and rehabilitation may improve the outcome once the bleeding has been controlled. Infants with hemophilia are difficult to evaluate. If an infant is irritable and no other source is found, there should be a presumption of occult bleeding.

Many patients and their families have a very sophisticated understanding of their disease. Patients will know to seek treatment at the first symptom when there may initially be little outward evidence of pathology. Despite minimal findings, patient concerns should be taken seriously. Many will have a detailed management plan for acute bleeding episodes in the medical record that should be consulted. A specific point needs to be made about pain management. Many of the above conditions are terribly painful. Pain control needs to be aggressively addressed. Even with a history of opiate abuse, if there is an obvious site of contained bleeding, the patient should receive analgesics.

When treating patients with hemophilia for other reasons, certain principles need to be kept in mind. Central lines, including femoral lines and external jugular lines, should not be placed in patients with hemophilia without factor replacement therapy. Similar rules apply to arterial blood gases or lumbar puncture. Patients with hemophilia should never receive intramuscular injections unless factor replacement is given and maintained for several days. Patients undergoing invasive procedures will also require factor replacement. Do not give compounds that contain aspirin or nonsteroidal anti-inflammatory agents for pain relief. If there is ever doubt or concern about the need for factor replacement in a hemophiliac, a hematologist should be consulted.

Treatment

Factor replacement therapy is effective in controlling hemorrhage in hemophilia.[3] There are now two different treatment options: recombi-

nant factor replacement or plasma-derived and purified factor replacement (Table 220-2). The highest level of purity comes from the recombinantly produced factors. However, the cost of these products is high and they are not available everywhere. While the purity of the plasma-derived factors has improved, it does remain possible for even the treated plasma-derived products to potentially transmit viruses such as hepatitis A and the highly heat resistant parvovirus. Another concern with the plasma-derived factors is that some of the preparations may contain other coagulation factors. Prolonged use of the less pure concentrates may increase the risk of DIC, or in some cases cause paradoxical clotting.

The choice of which product to use in replacement therapy is dependent on considerations of safety, the cost, and the availability.[4] The recombinant forms cost two to three times as much as the plasma-derived factors and occasionally there are shortages of these factors. However, because the recombinant forms are perceived to be safer, approximately 60 percent of patients with severe hemophilia in the U.S. receive these preparations.

The dosing regimen used in the hemophilic patient is based on the clotting factor volume of distribution, the half-life of the factor, and the hemostatic level of factor required to control the bleeding (Table 220-3).[5] Clotting factor is dosed in units of activity. One unit of factor represents the amount of factor present in 1 mL of normal plasma. In the case of hemophilia A, one unit of factor VIII per kg of body weight raises the plasma level by approximately 0.02 U/mL (2 percent). The half-life of factor VIII is approximately 8 to 12 h. For hemophilia B, one unit of factor IX per kilogram of body weight will raise the plasma level by approximately 0.01 U/mL (1 percent). The half-life of factor IX

TABLE 220-2 Available Products for Hemophilia Treatment

Hemophilia Type	Available Products	Comments
Hemophilia A	*Human plasma-derived factor VIII products* Koate-HP (gel chromatography, solvent and detergent purified) Humate-P (heat treated) Alphanate (solvent and detergent purified)	All have a low risk of HIV and hepatitis transmission
	Human plasma-derived factor VII with immunoaffinity purification Hemofil M (monoclonal, solvent and detergent purified) Monoclate-P (monoclonal and heat treated)	Both have reduced amounts of vWF; Monoclate-P is highly purified source of factor VIII
	Recombinant factor VIII products Recombinate (recombinant DNA product) Gelixate (recombinant DNA product) Bioclate (recombinant DNA product) Kogenate (recombinant DNA product)	Low to no risk of HIV and hepatitis transmission
	Porcine factor VIII products Antihemophilic factor (cryoprecipitate fractionation, screened for porcine viruses) Hyate C (cryoprecipitate fractionation, screened for porcine viruses)	No evidence that human viral infection occurs
Hemophilia B	*Factor IX complex products* Koyne-80 factor IX complex (heat treated) Proplex T factor IX complex (heat treated) Profilnine SD (solvent and detergent purified) Bebulin VH (two-step vapor heat treatment)	Propex T: HIV seroconversion has occurred Other products have low risk of HIV and hepatitis transmission
	Activated factor IX complex products Autoplex T (heat treated) Feiba VH (two-step vapor heat treatment)	Low risk of HIV and hepatitis transmission
	Purified factor IX products Alpha Nine SD (solvent and detergent purified, polysorbate) Mononine (monoclonal antibody purification, ultrafiltration)	Low risk of HIV and hepatitis transmission
	Recombinant factor IX products BeneFIX (recombinant DNA product)	No known risk of transmission

Abbreviation: vWF = von Willebrand factor.

TABLE 220-3   Initial Factor Replacement Guidelines in Severe Hemophilia

Site	Minimum Initial Factor Level	Hemophilia A Initial Dose	Hemophilia B Initial Dose	Details
Deep muscle	40–50%	20–40 U/kg	40–60 U/kg	Admit, monitor total blood loss, watch for compartment syndrome Duration of replacement: 1–3 days
Joint	30–50%	20–40 U/kg	30–40 U/kg	Orthopedic consult for splinting, physical therapy, and follow-up Duration of replacement: 1–3 days
Epistaxis	80–100%	40–50 U/kg	80–100 U/kg	Local measures should be used Replacement is given until bleeding resolves
Oral mucosa	50%	25 U/kg	50 U/kg	Local measures and antifibrinolytic therapy will decrease need for additional factor replacement Duration of replacement: 1–2 days
Gastrointestinal bleeding	100%	40–50 U/kg	80–100 U/kg	Consultation with a gastroenterologist for endoscopy to locate potential lesion is appropriate Duration of replacement: 7–10 days
Central nervous system	100%	50 U/kg	100 U/kg	Neurosurgical consultation should be done early Lumbar puncture requires factor replacement

is approximately 16 h. Calculation of the amount of factor needed can be done using the patient's weight and the desired increase in factor:

Factor VIII required = weight in kg × 0.5 × (% change in factor activity needed)

Factor IX required = weight in kg × 1.0 × (% change in factor activity needed)

To avoid wasting factor, round off all doses to the closest vial.

When major bleeding occurs in the central nervous system, gastrointestinal tract, neck, throat, in a large muscle, or when a severe injury is present, factor replacement levels between 80 and 100 percent are necessary. In these cases therapy will need to continue for days or weeks. Factor replacement can be given as bolus therapy or as a continuous therapy. Continuous therapy may help decrease the total amount of factor required, but is best administered by those familiar with this method.[6]

When less severe bleeding occurs in soft tissue, muscle, or joints, the appropriate factor replacement level is from 30 to 50 percent. Usually three doses over 1 to 2 days are sufficient to control bleeding and prevent additional bleeding, although the clinical picture should be reassessed to ensure that the expected improvement is seen. In addition to factor replacement, extremity and joint bleeding may benefit from splinting followed by physical therapy.

There may be rare instances in which a patient presents with what appears to be a previously undiagnosed bleeding disorder. In these cases the use of a specific factor may not be possible, and the emergency physician may need to use fresh-frozen plasma (FFP) or cryoprecipitate (contains factor VIII and vWF; use is only appropriate if there is strong suspicion that the bleeding presentation is due to hemophilia A or von Willebrand disease) to control bleeding until definitive studies can be done. As is true of the other replacement factors, the measures used to purify FFP and cryoprecipitate have improved, and the risk of transmitting diseases such as HIV and hepatitis is far less than in the past. Each bag of cryoprecipitate contains about 100 units of factor VIII and variable amounts of von Willebrand factor (vWF). FFP contains all of the plasma clotting factors with an average concentration of 1 U/mL. However, one unit of FFP will only raise the factor levels by 3 to 5 percent, so volume overload can complicate extensive factor replacement using FFP. FFP is the most appropriate choice if there is no family history to suggest the type of bleeding disorder.

Specific Problems

ORAL AND MUCOSAL BLEEDING   Bleeding from the mouth is common in hemophiliacs, particularly children. This bleeding is worsened by the fact that saliva contains fibrinolysins. For an oral bleed, the area should be identified and then cleaned of inadequate clot, and a dry topical thrombin placed on the bleeding site. Initial factor replacement should be 80 to 100 percent. However, additional therapy may still be needed to prevent bleeding when the clot falls off. For oral or mucosal bleeding, antifibrinolytic agents such as epsilon-aminocaproic acid (EACA) and tranexamic acid are useful adjunctive therapy to factor replacement. For very superficial mucosal injuries, it may be possible to manage the bleeding with antifibrinolytic therapy alone. Patients should be closely monitored to ensure response. The dose of EACA is 75 to 100 mg/kg q6h for children, and 6 g q6h for adults, given PO or IV. Topical hemostatic agents used to help control oral or nasal bleeding include microfibrillar collagen hemostats, thrombin, and absorbable gelatin sponges.

MILD HEMOPHILIA A   Patients with mild hemophilia A (factor levels of 5 percent of normal or greater) who have mild bleeding may not always require factor replacement. Rather, they may be given desmopressin (DDAVP).[7] Desmopressin is believed to cause release of von Willebrand factor from endothelial storage sites. The increased amount of vWF is capable of carrying additional amounts of factor VIII in the plasma. This medication is well tolerated and patients can administer it at home by the subcutaneous route. When giving intravenous desmopressin, the dose is 0.3 μg/kg (maximum dose 20 μg) over 30 min. A concentrated intranasal form of desmopressin is also an option for use in hemophilia. For children older than age 5, a single spray in a single nostril (150 μg total dose) is adequate. For adolescents and adults, a single spray in each nostril is used (300 μg total dose). This dose of intranasal DDAVP will increase the factor VIII level by 2 to 3 times. This treatment can be repeated in 8 to 12 h, but the patient's stores of factor VIII will become depleted, and subsequently the effect will be less. DDAVP is an antidiuretic agent, and fluid restriction may be needed during use.

INHIBITORS   Inhibitors, antibodies against replacement factors, tend to occur most commonly in severe hemophiliacs because of frequent factor replacement. Inhibitors not only interfere with the effectiveness of factor replacement therapy but can cause anaphylaxis during factor administration in patients with hemophilia B.[8] Inhibitors occur in 10 to 25 percent of those with hemophilia A and 1 to 2 percent of those with hemophilia B. The use of factor replacement in hemophilic patients with inhibitors is guided by the concentration of inhibitor [measured in Bethesda inhibition assay (BIA) units] and the type of response the patient has to factor concentrates.

Patients with inhibitors are more difficult to treat during bleeding episodes, but options do exist (Table 220-4).[9] In patients with an inhibitor titer less than 5 BIA and who are not vigorous antibody responders, an increased dose of factor can be given in an attempt to overwhelm the existing antibody. Alternative therapies include porcine factor VIII, prothrombin complex concentrates that circumvent the factor deficiency, activated prothrombin complex concentrates, and recombinant activated factor VII (rfVIIa). The rfVIIa is thought to act by competing against normal plasma-nonactivated factor VII for tissue binding, thus enhancing thrombin generation, and by binding to activated platelets, thereby activating factors IX and X on the platelet surface in the absence of tissue factor. Given the complexity of treating these patients, consultation or transfer to a hemophiliac center is recommended.

Indications for Hospital Admission

Hemophilic patients with bleeding episodes will require hospital admission in these situations:

Bleeding involving the CNS, neck, pharynx, retropharynx, or retroperitoneum
Potential compartment syndrome
Treatment requiring more than three doses (relative indication)
Inability to use or lack of access to factor replacement
Inability to control pain with oral analgesics

VON WILLEBRAND DISEASE

von Willebrand disease (vWD) is the most common congenital bleeding disorder, present in 1 percent of the population.[10] This disease is a group of disorders caused by abnormalities of vWF.[11] The disease is heterogeneously inherited and expressed and, although there are multiple subtypes, can be classified into three major groups (Table 220-5). Type I is the most common and is a partial quantitative disease, type II is qualitative (abnormal function), and type III is a severe and almost complete deficiency of vWF (this type is a rare autosomal recessive form). vWF is a glycoprotein that unlike most other coagulation factors, is synthesized, stored, and then secreted by the vascular endothelial cells.

von Willebrand factor serves two key roles in normal hemostasis.[11] It is a cofactor for platelet adhesion as well as the carrier protein for factor VIII. Circulating vWF does not bind directly to platelets, but when exposed to the subendothelial matrix, vWF undergoes a structural change, allowing it to bind to platelet glycoprotein Ib. This inter-action between vWF and platelet glycoprotein Ib leads to platelet activation and adhesion to other platelets, as well as to the damaged endothelium. The vWF is also a carrier protein for factor VIII. When vWF is absent, the half-life of factor VIII will decrease because vWF protects the factor VIII from proteolytic degradation within the plasma. If vWF fails to bind factor VIII due to defect or severe deficiency, the clinical presentation is similar to hemophilia A.

Clinical Manifestations

Skin and mucosal bleeding symptoms are common in people with vWD, particularly in children and adolescents. This includes recurrent epistaxis, gingival bleeding, unusual bruising, gastrointestinal bleeding, and menorrhagia in young women. Hemarthrosis is not typical unless severe disease is present. In mild cases of vWD the patient may be unaware of the disease until they have a surgical procedure or traumatic event and unexpected bleeding occurs.

Laboratory Tests

Diagnostic tests used to diagnose von Willebrand disease include bleeding time, aPTT, factor VIII coagulant activity, vWF antigen, and vWF activity. It is possible for some laboratory tests to be normal even in those with disease. However, the common abnormalities include prolonged bleeding time, low or normal vWF antigen, and low vWF activity. The PT should be normal and about half of patients have a mildly prolonged aPTT. Variability in vWF levels can sometimes make vWD difficult to differentiate from mild hemophilia A. The patient's blood type also affects the vWF, with blood type O having as much as a 30 percent reduction in vWF levels compared to the other blood types.

Treatment

von Willebrand disease is relatively common, and in addition to bleeding episodes, the presence of vWD has influence on treatment for other medical problems.[12] Medications with known antiplatelet effects should be avoided, including aspirin, nonsteroidal anti-inflammatory drugs (NSAIDs), antiplatelet agents, heparin, and some antibiotics.

NONTRANSFUSIONAL THERAPIES Desmopressin (DDAVP) has become a mainstay of therapy for many patients with type I vWD.[7,12] For the other types of vWD, DDAVP may still work in conjunction

---

TABLE 220-4   Replacement Therapy for Hemophilia A and B in Patients with Inhibitors

Type of Product	Hemophilia A Dose	Hemophilia B Dose	Comments
Factor VII concentrates	5000–10,000 unit bolus followed by a continuous infusion	Not applicable	
Prothrombin complex concentrates (PCCs), contain factors II, VII, IX, X	75–100 U/kg	75–100 U/kg	Risk of DIC, thromboembolic disease, and low risk of hepatitis transmission
Activated prothrombin complex concentrates (aPPCs), contain factors II, VII, IX, X, with variable amounts of activated factors VIIa, IXa, and Xa	75–100 U/kg	Approximately 75 U/kg	Similar risks as with the PCCs
Recombinant factor VIIa (NovoSeven)	Variable	Variable	No risk of viral transmission
Porcine factor VIII (Hyate C)	Variable	Not applicable	Patients may develop inhibitors
Highly purified factor IX concentrates	Not applicable	Variable	

Abbreviation: DIC = disseminated intravascular coagulation.

TABLE 220-5   Simple Classification and Treatment of von Willebrand Disease

Type	Frequency	Defect	Treatment
I	70–80% of cases	All the multimeric forms are present, but in decreased quantity (about 20–50% normal levels)	Desmopressin (DDAVP) and if no response, consider the measures below
II	10–15% of cases	The von Willebrand molecule is abnormal and dysfunctional	Factor VIII concentrates or cryoprecipitate
III	Less than 10% of cases	Almost no von Willebrand factor present	Factor VIII concentrates or cryoprecipitate

with plasma products that contain vWF. Desmopressin induces the release of vWF from storage sites within the endothelium. In responsive individuals it causes a transient two- to fourfold increase in vWF. Desmopressin also seems to have an effect on the endothelium that promotes hemostasis. The dose is 0.3 μg/kg (maximum 20 μg) of body weight, administered SC or IV every 12 h to a total of three or four doses; after four doses, tachyphylaxis develops. A concentrated form of desmopressin is also available as an intranasal spray. For children older than age 5, a single spray in a single nostril is adequate (150 μg total dose). For adolescents and adults, administer a single spray in each nostril (300 μg total dose). Again, the number of times this can be used is limited.

TRANSFUSIONAL THERAPIES   Plasma derivatives that contain vWF are used for those type I patients that do not (or no longer) respond to DDAVP or have type II or III vWD.[12] The chosen product needs to have vWF in the high-molecular-weight form to be effective. Cryoprecipitate meets this objective (contains factor VIII and vWF), but there is concern about the potential for viral transmission. The administration of 10 bags of cryoprecipitate every 12 to 24 h will usually control bleeding. Because of the risk of viral contamination, factor VIII products that contain multimeric vWF and have undergone viral inactivation processes are preferred. Humate-P is an intermediate-purity factor VIII concentrate that has significant amounts of vWF, and can be used to treat bleeding episodes. Cryoprecipitate from a limited number of donors is another possibility. Platelet transfusions may benefit patients with certain types of vWD (type III) who do not respond to vWF-containing plasma products.

ADDITIONAL THERAPY   Patients with a history of vWD and have significant epistaxis should receive the normal measures taken to control bleeding. If these are not successful, intranasal application of porcine strips (Surgicel) or porcine strips sprinkled with microfibrillar collagen (Avitene) may help control bleeding. Cauterization is necessary in some cases.

Menorrhagia is a common complaint in young women with vWD. Birth control pills can help raise vWF levels and limit the degree of menstrual bleeding. DDAVP may also be used in responsive individuals.

For dental injury or planned procedures in the oral cavity, an antifibrinolytic agent should be used. EACA can be taken orally and tranexamic acid can be made into a mouthwash. These may be used for 5 to 10 days after the injury or surgical procedure.

ACKNOWLEDGMENT

Thank you to the previous author, Mary Eberst, for her work.

REFERENCES

1. Mannucci PM, Tuddenham EG: The hemophilias—from royal genes to gene therapy. *New Engl J Med* 344:1773, 2001 [erratum in *New Engl J Med* 345: 384, 2001].
2. Hemphill RR: Hematologic emergencies and life-threatening bleeding disorders: Differential diagnosis, evaluation, and management. *Emerg Med Report* 22:191, 2001.
3. Petrini P: Treatment strategies in children with hemophilia. *Paediatr Drugs* 4:427, 2002.
4. Mannucci PM, Giangrande PL: Choice of replacement therapy for hemophilia: Recombinant products only? *Hematol J* 1:72, 2000.
5. Bjorkman S, Berntrop E: Pharmacokinetics of coagulation factors: Clinical relevance for patients with hemophilia. *Clin Pharmacokinet* 40:815, 2001.
6. Stachnik JS, Gabay MP: Continuous infusion of coagulation factor products. *Ann Pharmacother* 36:882, 2002.
7. Seremetis SV, Aledort LM: Desmopressin nasal spray for hemophilia A and type I von Willebrand disease. *Ann Intern Med* 126:744, 1997.
8. Warrier I, Ewenstein BM, Koerper MA, et al: Factor IX inhibitors and anaphylaxis in hemophilia B. *J Pediatr Hematol Oncol* 19:23, 1997.
9. Shapiro A: Inhibitor treatment: State of the art. *Semin Hematol* 38(Suppl 12):26, 2001.
10. Federici AB, Mannucci PM: Advances in the genetics and treatment of von Willebrand disease. *Curr Opin Pediatr* 14:23, 2002.
11. Budde U, Schneppenheim R: Von Willebrand factors and von Willebrand disease. *Rev Clin Exp Hematol* 5:335, 2001.
12. Mannucci PM, Federici AB: Management of inherited von Willebrand disease. *Best Pract Res Clin Haematol* 14:455, 2001.

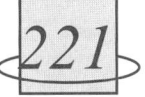

HEREDITARY HEMOLYTIC ANEMIAS
Robin R. Hemphill

The hereditary hemolytic anemias are characterized by defects of hemoglobin or the red cell membrane that result in premature destruction of red cells. These disorders include hemoglobins that tend to gel or crystallize, unstable hemoglobin with abnormal oxygen-binding properties, hemoglobin that is readily oxidized to methemoglobin, and hemoglobin chains that are synthesized at unequal rates. This chapter discusses the common inherited hemolytic anemias: sickle cell anemia and its variants, thalassemia, glucose-6-phosphate dehydrogenase deficiency, and hereditary spherocytosis.

SICKLE CELL ANEMIA (SCA)

Pathophysiology

The normal adult red blood cell (RBC) contains three forms of hemoglobin (Hb): HbA, HbA$_2$, and HbF (fetal hemoglobin) (Table 221-1). Normal hemoglobin consists of a tetramer of four polypeptide chains: two α-globin chains and two non-α-globin chains. Hemoglobin A accounts for about 96 to 98 percent of adult hemoglobin and consists of two α- and two β-globin chains ($\alpha_2\beta_2$). HbA$_2$ accounts for about 2 to 3.5 percent of adult hemoglobin and is composed of two α- and two δ-globin chains ($\alpha_2\delta_2$). Fetal hemoglobin is composed of two α- and two γ-globin chains ($\alpha_2\gamma_2$). HbF production peaks in utero and starts declining just before birth and continues to decline, reaching a baseline at about 48 weeks of age. Because of the 120-day life span of the normal RBC, HbF is the predominant hemoglobin in the circulation for about the first 4 months of life. The α-globin chains are coded by four genes on chromosome 16, whereas the β-, γ-, and δ-globin chains are coded by two genes each on chromosome 11. A *hemoglobinopathy* is an inherited disease resulting from the presence of one or more abnormal hemoglobins.

TABLE 221-1 Composition of Normal Human Hemoglobin and Hemoglobin Variants

Syndrome	Types of Hemoglobin Present	Percent	Hemoglobin Tetramer Composition (Globin Chains)
Normal adults	HbA	96–98%	$\alpha\alpha/\beta\beta$
	HbA$_2$	3–3.5%	$\alpha\alpha/\delta\delta$
	HbF	0.5–0.8%	$\alpha\alpha/\gamma\gamma$
Sickle cell trait (heterozygous)	HbA	60–65%	$\alpha\alpha/\beta\beta$
	HbAS	35–40%	$\alpha\alpha/\beta\beta$-sickle
	HbF	0.5–0.8%	$\alpha\alpha/\gamma\gamma$
Sickle cell disease (homozygous)	HbSS	80–90%	$\alpha\alpha/\beta$-sickle β-sickle
	HbA$_2$	2–4%	$\alpha\alpha/\delta\delta$
	HbF	2–20%	$\alpha\alpha/\gamma\gamma$

SCA is caused by the substitution of the amino acid valine for glutamine at position 6 in the β-globin chain.[1] This is the most common variant of hemoglobin and is known as *hemoglobin S* (HbS). As a result of this mutation, deoxygenated HbS polymerizes, deforming the RBC and producing the characteristic sickled appearance. The distorted cell results in premature RBC destruction and also increases the viscosity of blood, leading to obstruction within the microvasculature.[2] The overall effect is chronic ongoing hemolysis and episodic periods of vascular occlusion, resulting in tissue ischemia affecting most organ systems.

This defect is inherited as an autosomal recessive trait, and disease is seen in patients who are homozygous for the sickle gene (*HbSS*). **People with sickle cell trait** (*HbAS,* heterozygous with one gene for normal β-globin chain and one gene for a β-globin chain with the sickle mutation) **have a normal life span and usually are asymptomatic,** except in rare cases of severe physiologic stress, when they may suffer an acute pain crisis, splenic infarction, or cerebrovascular complications. Approximately 8 percent of the African-American population caries sickle cell trait (heterozygous for the sickle cell gene), and approximately 0.15 to 0.2 percent of African-American newborns have sickle cell disease (SCD) (homozygous for the sickle gene). A lesser percentage of individuals of Middle Eastern, eastern Mediterranean, and Indian descent may have the HbS gene. While sickle cell anemia accounts for the majority of disease, other sickle cell disorders can result from the coinheritance of a sickle cell gene and β-thalassemia or other hemoglobin abnormality.

The pathophysiologic effects of SCD are due to the polymerization of deoxygenated HbS that deforms the red cell into a sickled shape that causes microvascular sludging and obstruction (vasoocclusion). This obstruction worsens hypoxia and causes acidosis in the microcirculation that contributes to further sickling. The sickling process is reversible initially when the HbS is reoxygenated, but with repeated episodes of sickling, the red cell membrane is permanently damaged, and the cell remains irreversibly sickled. Anywhere from 5 to 50 percent of the circulating erythrocytes in a patient with SCD can be irreversibly sickled cells (ISCs). The sickling process is inhibited by the presence of fetal hemoglobin (HbF) and other hemoglobin variants. Structural and antigenic changes on the RBC membrane cause an increased abnormal tendency for the RBC to catalyze plasma coagulation factors and adhere to vascular endothelium in sickle cell disease. Paradoxically, ICSs loose this heightened ability for vascular endothelial adherence, and patients with high levels of circulating ISCs have fewer vasoocclusive crises. As stated earlier, the abnormal shape of the RBCs causes a decreased life span and yields a chronic hemolytic anemia. The combination of hemolytic anemia and recurrent vasoocclusive events provides the basis for this chronic disease.

Patients with SCD have a significantly decreased life span that in the past was predominantly due to early death from infection. Prevention and treatment of infections have improved the life span of SCD patients, but complications related to the disease continue to reduce life span.

Clinical Presentations

Because newborn screening takes place in the United States and most developed countries, most patients that present to the ED will already know that they have sickle cell trait or disease. Infants are protected from sickle cell complications during their initial six months of life largely due to the continuing presence of significant amounts of HbF. The continued presence of HbF in adults with SCD is protective, and the level of HbF inversely correlates with the frequency and severity of SCD complications. SCD should be considered in any child of African, Middle Eastern, or Indian descent with a presentation of unexplained pain or swelling in the extremities, anemia, or splenomegaly. The peripheral smear can be normal, and absence of anemia does not exclude the diagnosis in children younger than 4 years of age. Screening tests (such as hemoglobin solubility or sickle cell preparation) are not reliable before 6 months of age, may be falsely negative with severe anemia, and will not distinguish sickle cell trait from SCD. Accurate diagnosis requires hemoglobin electrophoresis. SCD patients typically present to the emergency department because of complications, most commonly vasoocclusive painful crisis (Table 221-2).

VASOOCCLUSIVE PAIN CRISIS Acute painful sickle crisis is a common problem, and the average patient with SCD will have one to four severe attacks per year. The initiating event may not be identifiable, but stressors such as infection, cold, dehydration, and altitude have been implicated. As a result of intravascular sickling and small vessel occlusion, infarction of bone, viscera, and soft tissue occurs. This is manifested as diffuse bone, muscle, and joint pain and, in some cases, symptoms related to a specific affected organ. Initial management of these patients includes aggressive pain management and hydration and an assessment of the cause of the current crisis as well as a search for additional complications.[1]

Supplemental oxygen is used commonly for painful crises, but unless the patient is systemically hypoxemic, it has not been proven to be of routine benefit. Treatment of acute pain requires opioids, and severe pain should be treated with parenteral agents, commonly intravenously in the United States and subcutaneous in the United Kingdom.[3,4] A potent opioid, such a morphine or diamorphine, is recommended, and meperidine, with the potential for neurotoxicity from the metabolite normeperidine, is not recommended. Some patients, because of prior opioid treatment, may be very tolerant, and large doses may be required. Regular doses of analgesics for a few hours to several days typically are required. Patient-controlled analgesia can be used in selected patients. Nonsteroidal anti-inflammatory drugs can be used for their additive effect in pain management of sickle cell crisis.[4] SCD patients with a painful crisis have an absolute or relative hypovolemia due to

TABLE 221-2 Emergencies in Sickle Cell Disease

Vasoocclusive crises	Musculoskeletal pain (typical painful crisis)
	Dactylitis (hand-foot syndrome)
	Acute chest pain syndrome
	Stroke
	Priapism
Hematologic crises	Splenic sequestration
	Aplastic crisis
	Hemolytic crisis
Infections	Pneumonia
	Meningitis
	Sepsis
	Osteomyelitis
	Urinary tract infections

their disease (deficient renal concentrating ability) or crisis (anorexia, vomiting, fever), so aggressive oral or intravenous rehydration is done commonly. Research into therapies to shorten the duration or severity of painful crises has found small but statistically significant benefit with induced hyponatremia and purified poloxamer 188.[5,6] However, no current approach to shortening the duration and severity of a painful sickle cell crisis has proven reliable, safe, and appropriate for routine use. A common and recommended practice is to develop an individualized assessment and treatment protocol for specific patients who frequently present to the emergency department with painful crises.[7]

Simple or exchange transfusion to reduce the concentration of HbS-containing RBCs to below 30 percent can prevent or reverse the vasoocclusive process.[8] Transfusion should avoid raising the hematocrit above 36 percent in sickle cell patients. However, transfusion carries significant expense, the risk of blood-borne disease transmission, and the potential for iron overload and exposes the patient to the minor RBC antigens with the potential to induce antibodies that prevent or complicate future transfusions. Transfusion for sickle cell crisis or complications is reserved for specific indications, such as aplastic crisis, pregnancy, stroke, respiratory failure, general surgery, and priapism.[8–10]

Hydroxyurea has been used to reduce the frequency and severity of painful crises.[11] The major side effect is bone marrow, hepatic, and renal toxicity. Hydroxyurea has not been approved for use in children. Daily prophylactic penicillin V reduces the incidence of infections and reduces mortality from sepsis in children.[12] A number of emerging therapies are being studied for prevention and treatment of SCD crises and complications.[13]

Generally, a complete blood count and reticulocyte count help to assess the degree of anemia and ensure that the marrow is still producing red cells. If the reticulocyte count is not available, the presence of polychromasia in the peripheral blood smear can be used to provide evidence of continued RBC production. It is not uncommon for the sickle cell patient to have a low-grade temperature as well as an elevated white blood cell (WBC) count. This combination can make it difficult to differentiate whether an infection is present during a crisis. If the WBC count has a left shift and is elevated above 20,000/μL, a potential infection should be considered. Because of the chronic hemolysis, mild elevations in bilirubin and serum lactate dehydrogenase (LDH) levels are common.

Specific issues with an acute vasoocclusive crisis include the following:

Bone Pain   Bone pain is common during a sickle cell crisis and may include the back and the extremities.[14] Usually the pain will be diffuse, and there will be no physical findings. However, redness, warmth, or swelling suggests infection (cellulitis or osteomyelitis). The complaint of localized pain to the hip with difficulty ambulating raises the possibility of aseptic necrosis of the femoral head, and approximately 30 percent of SCA patients develop hip pathology by age 30. Bone infarctions may cause symptoms similar to osteomyelitis.[15] Joint effusions are seen occasionally as a complication of sickle cell crisis, but arthrocentesis is often necessary to determine if the joint is infected. Plain radiographs may show evidence of aseptic necrosis or osteomyelitis, whereas bone infarcts usually are not visible on radiographs. A bone scan or magnetic resonance imaging (MRI) may be necessary to differentiate infection from infarction.

In young children, an early manifestation of SCD is dactylitis (hand-foot syndrome). The syndrome is thought to be due to infarction of the red marrow with associated periosteal inflammation. The syndrome manifests as fever and painful swelling of the hands, feet, or both, and some redness and warmth may be present. As the child grows, the hematopoietic tissue in the metacarpal and phalangeal marrow is replaced by fatty tissue, making this entity less likely.

Chest Syndrome   The acute chest syndrome is used to describe a sickle cell crisis with pulmonary symptoms and a new pulmonary infiltrate found on radiograph.[16] The patient may have pleuritic chest pain, shortness of breath, fever, nonproductive cough, and tachypnea. The exact etiology of the chest syndrome is unclear, but infection, infarction (ribs and/or lung), and pulmonary fat embolism (from ischemic marrow fat necrosis) all have been implicated. It can be difficult to distinguish pneumonia from pulmonary infarction. A chest radiograph is not required routinely in all patients with painful sickle cell crisis but is indicated in those with pulmonary symptoms, decreased Sao$_2$, or signs of fever.[17] The onset of acute chest syndrome may be associated with a fall in hemoglobin level from the normal baseline. Pulmonary infiltrates may be present in one lobe or be diffuse and bilateral, and pleural effusions also may be present. Severe cases may progress rapidly to respiratory failure. The initial chest radiograph may be normal, so the patient with pulmonary symptoms may require serial radiographs.

Treatment involves close monitoring of fluid status, oxygen, and pain control. Therapy should assume the cause to be both pulmonary infarction from microvascular occlusion and infection.[18] Broad-spectrum antibiotics to cover *Streptococcus pneumoniae* and *Mycoplasma pneumoniae* are recommended. In severe cases, simple transfusion or exchange transfusion can be done. The acute chest syndrome is currently the leading cause of death from SCD in the United States.

Abdominal Crisis   Generalized and constant abdominal pain is a common complaint during an acute sickle cell crisis, and it may be difficult to distinguish between infarction of the abdominal and retroperitoneal organs associated with a sickle cell crisis versus a focal abdominal problem such as cholecystitis or appendicitis. Frequently the patient can determine that the pain is similar to prior episodes. If there is doubt, repeated abdominal examinations should be done to assess for progression of tenderness and peritoneal signs (e.g., rebound). Patients with a typical vasoocclusive episode should not have evidence of peritonitis.

Hepatic infarction may cause the acute onset of jaundice and abdominal pain and can be difficult to distinguish from hepatitis or cholecystitis. Biliary disease is common because pigment-related cholelithiasis is seen in 30 to 70 percent of sickle cell patients. Both hepatic infarction and biliary obstruction should show elevations of liver enzymes and bilirubin. Severe right upper quadrant pain and marked elevations of bilirubin may be due to intrahepatic cholestasis, which rarely may progress to hepatic failure. When there is a concern for biliary disease or other intra-abdominal pathology, ultrasound or computed tomographic (CT) scanning of the abdomen and pelvis is useful.

Genitourinary System   Vasoocclusive events involving the kidneys are common but often asymptomatic.[19] Infarction in the renal medulla may cause flank pain, renal colic-type pain, and costovertebral angle tenderness, mimicking pyelonephritis. Papillary necrosis may result in either gross or microscopic hematuria, but RBC casts are uncommon. Renal imaging studies generally are necessary for correct diagnosis. Both renal medulla infarction and papillary necrosis are treated with intravenous fluids and close monitoring of hemoglobin levels to ensure that anemia does not worsen. Priapism occurs in up to 30 percent of males with SCD. Initial treatment is fluid hydration, pain control, and transfusion (see Chap. 95). Early involvement of the urologist is important. Urinary tract infections are more common in SCD patients, and urinalysis is recommended when these patients present to the emergency department.

Additional Systemic Manifestations of SCD

SPLENIC INFARCTION   The spleen is particularly susceptible to the effects of sickled cells. Over time, microinfarctions result in a spleen that is essentially nonfunctional. The Cooperative Study for Sickle Cell Disease demonstrated that the proportion of children with sickle cell disease who are functionally asplenic is 14 percent at 6 months and 94 percent by the age of 5 years. This renders these patients at risk for serious infections and sepsis from encapsulated organisms. Therefore, immunizations, prophylactic penicillin therapy, and parental education are critical to minimize the risk of infection and prompt early evaluation of fever in these patients.[12,20] As sickle cell patients age, their risk of overwhelming sepsis decreases, but they remain predisposed to infection.

SPLENIC SEQUESTRATION   Splenic sequestration is more common in children than in adults and remains an important cause of morbidity and mortality. This syndrome manifests by the sudden enlargement of the spleen with an acute fall in the hemoglobin level due to sequestration of the blood volume within the spleen. Symptoms include tachycardia, hypotension, pallor, lethargy, and abdominal fullness. Left upper quadrant pain may or may not be present. The spleen is usually enlarged and firm. Platelets also may be sequestered, resulting in moderate thrombocytopenia. Reticulocyte count should remain elevated.

Therapy includes volume resuscitation, which may mobilize some of the RBCs trapped within the spleen. Transfusion or exchange transfusion may be necessary. Rarely, splenectomy is necessary. Search for a precipitating infection should be done. Unfortunately, recurrence of this syndrome is common.

HEMOLYTIC ANEMIA   Patients with SCD have a chronic hemolytic process due to the shape of the red cells. The baseline hemoglobin level is often between 6 and 9 g/dL, and the reticulocyte count is between 5 and 15 percent. With infections, the hemolytic process may worsen, and hemoglobin may drop from the previous baseline. Typically, reticulocytosis will increase in response to the increased RBC destruction, but it may not be enough to compensate for the increased hemolysis. Acutely, the patient may notice symptoms of worsening fatigue, shortness of breath, dyspnea on exertion, and scleral icterus. These symptoms may be worsened if other comorbid diseases are present. It is uncommon for the hemolysis to be so severe as to require transfusion.

APLASTIC CRISIS   Generally, the increased production of RBCs by the bone marrow is able to compensate for the increased rate of destruction. Aplastic crisis results when the production of RBCs declines significantly, producing a rapid decrease in the hemoglobin level with reticulocytopenia. The most common cause of aplastic crisis appears to be infection, specifically parvovirus. Folate deficiency and bone marrow necrosis also may play a role. Aplastic crisis is more common in pediatric patients than in adults. Patients generally will present with increasing fatigue and pallor and no evidence of increased hemolysis. The hemoglobin level will be unusually low, and few or no reticulocytes will be present (reticulocyte count typically <0.5 percent). The WBC and platelet levels are usually normal. Generally, this syndrome is self-limiting, and the marrow will begin producing RBCs spontaneously within a week. Transfusion may be required in the interim.

NEUROLOGIC DISORDERS   Complications of SCA include stroke, subarachnoid hemorrhage, and isolated functional loss.[21] Strokes usually develop abruptly with little warning but may occur during episodes of vasoocclusive pain. In some cases, vague symptoms consistent with a transient ischemic attack may be present and should be assumed to be potential warnings of impending stroke. The cause of stroke in most patients is cerebral infarction due to occlusion or narrowing of large cerebral vessels. The exact mechanism by which SCD causes endothelial damage in these large vessels is not clear. Approximate 10 percent of patients with SCA experience a stoke before age 20. Acute treatment is emergent simple or partial exchange transfusion. Cerebral aneurysms are also more common in sickle cell patients, perhaps due to local vessel occlusion or ischemia. Therefore, if symptoms of stroke due not improve with transfusion or the history

suggests that subarachnoid hemorrhage may be present, head CT scanning followed by lumbar puncture (if the head CT scan is normal) is indicated. Unfortunately, children who suffer a stroke are at 70 to 90 percent risk for recurrence. Chronic transfusion therapy is indicated to prevent recurrent stoke after the initial event.[10]

INFECTIONS   Patients with SCA are functionally asplenic after early childhood, making them susceptible to infections from encapsulated organisms, such as *Haemophilus influenzae* and *Streptococcus pneumoniae*. Other common infections associated with SCA include pneumonia caused by these organisms as well as *Mycoplasma pneumoniae*, meningitis, and osteomyelitis due to *Salmonella typhimurium*, *Staphylococcus aureus*, and *Escherichia coli*. While low-grade fever is not uncommon during an acute crisis, unexplained fevers of 38°C (101°F) or higher require evaluation for bacterial infection and consideration for early treatment with broad-spectrum antibiotics. In addition to *H. influenzae* immunization, patients with SCD should be encouraged to receive yearly influenza vaccinations and remain up to date with the pneumococcal immunization, and children should be on prophylactic penicillin.[12,20]

CARDIAC   Cardiomegaly is common and correlates with the degree of chronic anemia. Additionally, cardiac dysfunction may occur from microinfarcts and hemosiderin deposition from hemolysis and blood transfusion. Because of the chronic anemia, enhanced cardiac contractility is present to maintain adequate systemic oxygen delivery, producing a widely radiating systolic ejection murmur.

DERMATOLOGIC   Chronic, poorly healing leg ulcers around the malleoli are common in older sickle cell patients. Minor injury, impaired microcirculation due to repeated sickling episodes and microinfarcts, and infections all contribute to the development and persistence of these ulcers.

Disposition

Most painful crises last 2 to 3 days. Patients with an adequate clinical response and no indications for hospital admission can be discharged with oral pain medications and referred for follow-up with their primary care physician in the next 24 to 48 h. Patients also should receive instructions to return for the recurrence of severe pain, inability to take in fluids, fever, or other new and concerning symptoms. The following are some guidelines for hospital admission for sickle cell patients:

Patients with pulmonary or neurologic manifestations of their disease
Patients with evidence of significant bacterial infection
Patients with splenic sequestration or aplastic crisis
Patients in whom pain remains poorly controlled
Patients who are unable to maintain adequate hydration

VARIANTS OF SICKLE CELL DISEASE

Sickle Cell–Hemoglobin C (HbSC) Disease

Hemoglobin C results from a single point mutation in the β-chain gene; lysine is substituted for glutamic acid at the sixth position. The prevalence of the HbC gene is approximately 0.02 percent in African-Americans and 0.03 percent in northern Africans. Deoxygenated HbC has the tendency to precipitate inside the RBC, forming crystals that decrease cell deformability and increase blood viscosity. Patients with HbC trait (heterozygous for the HbC gene, or *HbAC*) are asymptomatic, and those with HbC disease (homozygous for the HbC gene, or *HbCC*) typically have a mild hemolytic anemia, abundant target cells, sporadic episodes of musculoskeletal pain, splenomegaly, dental infarctions, and angioid retinopathy. The heterozygous sickle cell variant, HbSC, results when the gene for HbS is inherited from one parent and the gene for HbC is inherited from the other parent. These individuals have almost equal amounts of HbS and HbC but no HbA. Because HbC does not polymerize as readily as HbS, HbSC disease generally has less severe clinical consequences, and patients with HbSC disease live, on average, 20 years longer than those with SCD. These patients have less severe hemolytic anemia and, as a consequence, milder reticulocytosis. The peripheral smear shows abundant target cells and a few sickle cells, and HbC may be seen precipitated as a rhomboid crystal in the RBCs. The complications of HbSC disease are similar to SCD, although usually less severe. As opposed to SCD, adult patients with HbSC disease often have splenomegaly. HbSC disease patients are susceptible to a proliferative retinitis that may lead to loss of vision.

Sickle Cell–Hemoglobin D (HbSD) Disease

There are a number of hemoglobins termed HbD based on their migration location on hemoglobin electrophoresis. The most common form, HbD-Los Angeles (also called D-Punjab) has substitution of glycine for glutamic acid at position 121 in the β-chain. By itself, HbD is of no clinical consequence; patients with HbD trait (heterozygotes, *HbAD*) are normal, and homozygotes (*HbDD*) have some decreased RBC osmotic fragility and target cells on peripheral blood smear but normal hemoglobin levels and no clinical symptoms. Patients with the heterozygous sickle variant, HbSD disease, are usually clinically similar to patients with SCD, having chronic hemolytic anemia, recurrent painful crises, and susceptibility to splenic sequestration and infections.

Sickle Cell–Hemoglobin O-Arab (HbSO-Arab) Disease

Hemoglobin O-Arab is a hemoglobin variant found in the Balkans and the Middle East and occasionally in African-Americans with a substitution of lysine for glutamic acid at position 121 of the β-chain. Patients heterozygous for hemoglobin O-Arab (HbAO-Arab) have no clinical problems. Patients homozygous for hemoglobin O-Arab (*HbOO-Arab*) or heterozygous for sickle cell-hemoglobin O-Arab (*HbSO-Arab*) are clinically similar to patients with SCD, having severe hemolytic anemia and recurrent vasoocclusive crises, and children have the potential to develop sickle cell dactylitis and splenic sequestration crises.

THALASSEMIAS

The thalassemias are a diverse group of disorders characterized by defective synthesis of globin chains that results in the inability to produce normal adult hemoglobin.[22] The hallmark of these disorders is a microcytic, hypochromic, hemolytic anemia. These disorders are most common in those of Mediterranean, Middle Eastern, African, and Southeast Asian descent. Like sickle cell trait, the abnormalities found in thalassemia trait are thought to be protective against malaria.

The β-thalassemias have diminished production of the β-globin chain, which allows unmatched α-globin chains to accumulate as $α_4$ tetramers in the immature RBC. These tetramers are very insoluble, and their precipitation damages the developing erythroid precursor cells, resulting in early death. The cells that are produced have decreased hemoglobin, which accounts for the hypochromia and target cell formation. Patients with α thalassemia develop an excess of β-globin chains that accumulate as $β_4$ tetramers called *hemoglobin H* (HbH). HbH is more soluble and stable so that in severe α thalassemia, ineffective erythropoiesis is less of a problem, and increased destruction of the cells due to the structural abnormality is more prominent.

Both forms of thalassemia are characterized by differing extremes of anemia depending on the amount of ineffective erythropoiesis and premature destruction of the circulating RBCs. The hypoxia associated with severe anemia triggers compensatory mechanisms in an attempt to increase RBC production. This causes enlargement of the reticuloendothelial organs and expansion of the bone marrow cavity, leading to osteopenia. The complications of increased RBC production are

compounded by the complications that result from the chronic destruction of peripheral RBCs.

The β-thalassemias have two clinical syndromes representing mutations in one or both β-globin genes: β-thalassemia major (Cooley anemia) and β-thalassemia minor. Because there are four α-globin genes, two each inherited from the parents, the genetics and clinical consequences of the α-thalassemias are determined by five genotypic possibilities: Normal is αα/αα, the silent carrier is α-/αα, the homozygous α-thalassemia trait is α-/α-, and the heterozygous α-thalassemia trait is --/αα. Hemoglobin H disease is α-/-- and homozygous α-thalassemia is --/--. The most severe form of α-thalassemia occurs when there is a defect in all the α-globin chain genes, called *hemoglobin Bart's,* that is incompatible with life, producing stillborn or severely distressed infants. Outside of this most severe form, individuals with either α or β-thalassemia can be minimally to severely affected due to the specific genotype and whether the mutation produces complete or partial reduction in globin chain production.

α-Thalassemia Carrier and Trait

These patients have no clinical symptoms or physical findings. Patients with α-thalassemia trait are detected by the finding of microcytic RBCs and a normal hemoglobin level.

Hemoglobin H Disease

This is a disorder in which one α-globin chain gene is still functional. Hemoglobin H disease usually presents in the neonatal period with a severe hypochromic anemia. Later in life the clinical picture includes a hypochromic, microcytic anemia with jaundice and hepatosplenomegaly. These patients may not require regular transfusions, but in conditions of increased oxidative stress (that may cause precipitation of the unstable hemoglobin H, resulting in hemolysis) or infection, a transfusion may be necessary. Most of these people will know their diagnosis, and the emergency physician need only provide supportive care and blood transfusion when necessary. Medications that may precipitate hemolysis should be avoided in this population (Table 221-3).

TABLE 221-3   Drugs That Produce Oxidative Stress on Red Blood Cells

Sulfonamides	Sulfacetamide
	Sulfamethoxazole
	Sulfanilamide
	Sulfapyridine
Antimalarials	Primaquine
	Chloroquine
	Pamaquine
	Pentaquine
Urinary agents	Nitrofurantoin
	Nalidixic acid
	Phenazopyridine
Miscellaneous antibiotics	Ciprofloxacin niridazole
	Norfloxacin
	Chloramphenicol
Mothballs	Naphthalene
Miscellaneous	Vitamin K analogues
	Methylene blue
	Acetanilid
	Doxorubicin
	Isobutyl nitrite
	Phenylhydrazine

β-Thalassemia Minor (β-Thalassemia Trait)

Patients with this form of thalassemia are heterozygous for the β-globin mutation and have only mild microcytic anemia. Splenomegaly may be present but is not common. On blood smear, these patients may have microcytosis and hypochromia as well as basophilic stippling. An elevated HbA₂ level, typically 4 to 6 percent, confirms the diagnosis. These patients generally will not have clinical manifestations and may only come to attention during an evaluation for a mild anemia.

β-Thalassemia Major (Cooley Anemia)

In this disorder, both β-globin genes are defective, and production of β-globin chains is severely impaired.[23] β-Thalassemia major is characterized by a severe anemia that begins within the first year of life. These children develop hepatosplenomegaly, jaundice, expansion of the erythroid marrow (causing bone changes and osteoporosis), and increased susceptibility to infection. The anemia is severe and requires regular and lifelong blood transfusions. These transfusions and enhanced iron absorption eventually cause iron overload, which, if untreated, results in hemochromatosis with cardiac, hepatic, and endocrine dysfunction.

The RBCs of these children show a low mean corpuscular volume with microcytic and hypochromic cells. Variation in size and shape of the RBCs will be notable (increased red blood cell distribution width), as will be the presence of nucleated cells. This diagnosis should be considered in any child with a severe microcytic anemia and the appropriate ethnic background. For those with a known diagnosis who present to the emergency department with significant symptoms related to anemia or hemolysis, transfusion should be considered along with a search for precipitating events.

Sickle Cell–β-Thalassemia Disease

This heterozygous sickle cell variant occurs when the gene for sickle hemoglobin is inherited from one parent and the gene for β-thalassemia is inherited from the other parent. The frequency of sickle cell–β-thalassemia disease is 2 per 3200 African-American births. The severity of the disease depends on the type of β-thalassemia gene that is inherited. Between 80 and 90 percent of affected individuals have a β-thalassemia gene that results in the production of some normal beta chains; thus some normal HbA is made. These patients have a mild hemolytic anemia with near-normal hemoglobin levels, few crises, and minimal organ damage. Those 10 to 20 percent of patients who inherit a β-thalassemia gene that produces no beta chains and therefore no normal hemoglobin have severe hemolytic anemia and vasoocclusive symptoms comparable with patients with SCD.

GLUCOSE-6-PHOSPHATE DEHYDROGENASE DEFICIENCY

Glucose-6-phosphate dehydrogenase (G6PD) is an enzyme responsible for the production of nicotinamide adenine dinucleotide phosphate (NADPH), a required cofactor for maintaining glutathione in its reduced state.[24] RBCs rely on G6PD activity because it is the only source of NPDPH that prevents oxidative damage to intraerythrocytic hemoglobin. There are over 300 variant mutations described for G6PD, with the highest prevalence in individuals of African, Asian, or Mediterranean descent. The gene for G6PD is carried on the X chromosome, so males are affected when they are hemizygous. Females must carry two defective genes to be severely affected, but because expression of this gene is variable, women with even one gene may still show some symptoms. The severity of G6PD disease is related to the magnitude of enzyme deficiency; severe cases have less than 10 percent of normal enzyme activity, and moderate cases have 10 to 60 percent of normal activity. G6PD deficiency is seen in approximately 10 to 15 percent of black males in the United States and a lesser percentage of those of Mediterranean descent.

G6PD-deficient RBCs are susceptible to oxidative stress; oxidization of the hemoglobin sulfhydryl groups causes hemoglobin to precipitate within the cell. The precipitated hemoglobin is recognized by the presence of Heinz bodies on the peripheral blood smear. The affected RBC is removed from the circulation by the spleen. Oxidant damage also occurs at the RBC membrane, producing both extravascular and intravascular hemolysis.

A history of neonatal jaundice 1 to 4 days after birth is common. In severe variants, the patient may have a severe chronic hemolytic anemia. In the more common variants of G6PD deficiency, the patient is usually asymptomatic, except for acute hemolytic crises that occur due to bacterial and viral infections, exposure to oxidant drugs, metabolic acidosis (such as diabetic ketoacidosis), renal failure, and in some patients, ingestion of fava beans[23] (see Table 221-3). These episodes are usually self-limited and well tolerated because only the older RBCs will hemolyze. There is an increased incidence of pigmented gallstones and splenomegaly in patients with G6PD deficiency.

The diagnosis of G6PD deficiency can be established by the demonstration of decreased enzyme activity through quantitative assay. Treatment for this disease is supportive and preventative. In patients with known G6PD deficiency, infections should be treated aggressively and oxidant drugs avoided. The drugs most commonly associated with oxidant stress are sulfonamides, antimalarials, and nitrofurantoin. HIV-positive patients should be screened for this defect because of the common use of sulfamethoxazole for the treatment and prophylaxis of *Pneumocystis carinii* pneumonia.

HEREDITARY SPHEROCYTOSIS

Hereditary spherocytosis (HS) is the result of an erythrocyte membrane defect and is the most prevalent hereditary hemolytic anemia among people of northern European descent.[25] The disease typically is inherited in an autosomal dominant pattern, although a less common autosomal recessive variant exists, and up to 20 percent of HS patients are the result of an apparent spontaneous mutation. The abnormal shape of the RBC results from molecular abnormalities in the cytoskeleton of the cell membrane, most commonly from mutations in the genes for the proteins spectrin and ankyrin. These abnormalities result in RBCs with a microspherocytic shape, which is not pliable enough to pass through the spleen. This results in an increased rate of destruction and a compensatory increase in RBC production. The clinical spectrum of HS is divided into those with 1) mild disease, occurring in 20 to 30 percent with an autosomal dominant inheritance, 2) moderate disease, occurring in 60 to 75 percent with primarily autosomal dominant inheritance, and 3) severe, occurring in about 5 percent with an autosomal recessive inheritance.

Neonatal jaundice during the first week of life occurs in 30 to 50 percent of HS patients. After the neonatal period, the symptoms and signs depend on the severity of ongoing hemolysis. Patients with mild disease usually have a normal hemoglobin level and little or no splenomegaly but are susceptible to hemolytic or aplastic episodes triggered by infection. Patients with moderate disease have mild to moderate anemia, modest splenomegaly, periodic episodes of hemolysis with jaundice, and an increased incidence of pigmented gallstones. The rare patient with severe HS has significant hemolytic anemia requiring episodic blood transfusions, chronic jaundice, and an enlarged spleen.

The peripheral blood smear shows spherocytes with a normal to low mean corpuscular volume and increased mean corpuscular hemoglobin concentration (>36 percent). The diagnosis of HS is established by the osmotic fragility test. In severe cases, splenectomy generally will reverse the anemia, except in the unusual cases of autosomal recessive variants. After splenectomy, spherocytes are still present.

ACKNOWLEDGMENT

We would like to acknowledge Mary Eberst for her contribution to these chapters in previous editions.

REFERENCES

1. Ballas SK: Sickle anaemia: Progress in pathogenesis and treatment. *Drugs* 62:1143, 2002.
2. Frenette PS: Sickle cell vasoocclusion: A multistep and multicellular paradigm. *Curr Opin Hematol* 9:101, 2002.
3. Marlowe KF, Chicella MF: Treatment of sickle cell pain. *Pharmacotherapy* 22:484, 2002.
4. Okpala I, Tawil A: Management of pain in sickle-cell disease. *J R Soc Med* 95:456, 2002.
5. Rosa RM, Bierer BE, Thomas R, et al: A study of induced hyponatremia in the prevention and treatment of sickle-cell crisis. *New Engl J Med* 303:1138, 1980.
6. Orringer EP, Casella JF, Ataga KI, et al: Purified poloxamer 188 for treatment of acute vasoocclusive crisis of sickle cell disease: A randomized controlled trial. *JAMA* 286:2099, 2001.
7. Okpala I, Thomas V, Westerdale N, et al: The comprehensiveness care of sickle cell disease. *Eur J Haematol* 68:157, 2002.
8. Telen MJ: Principles and problems of transfusion in sickle cell disease. *Semin Hematol* 38:315, 2001.
9. Riddington C, Williamson L: Preoperative blood transfusions for sickle cell disease. *Cochrane Database Syst Rev* 3:CD003149, 2001.
10. Riddington C, Wang W: Blood transfusion for preventing stoke in people with sickle cell disease. *Cochrane Database Syst Rev* 1:CD003146, 2002.
11. Davies S, Olujohungbe A: Hydroxyurea for sickle cell disease. *Cochrane Database Syst Rev* 2:CD002202, 2001.
12. Riddington C, Owusu-Ofori S: Prophylactic antibiotics for preventing pneumococcal infection in children with sickle cell disease. *Cochrane Database Syst Rev* 3:CD003427, 2002.
13. Vichinsky E: New therapies in sickle cell disease. *Lancet* 360:629, 2002.
14. Smith JA: Bone disorders in sickle cell disease. *Hematol Oncol Clin North Am* 10:1345, 1996.
15. Wong AL, Sakamoto KM, Johnson EE: Differentiating osteomyelitis from bone infarction in sickle cell disease. *Pediatr Emerg Care* 17:60, 2001.
16. Vichinsky EP, Neumayr LD, Earles AN, et al: Causes and outcomes of the acute chest syndrome in sickle cell disease. *New Engl J Med* 342:1855, 2000; erratum in *New Engl J Med* 343:824, 2000.
17. Morris C, Vichinsky E, Styles L: Clinical assessment of acute chest syndrome in febrile patients with sickle cell disease: Is it accurate enough? *Ann Emerg Med* 34:64, 1999.
18. Minter KR, Gladwin MT: Pulmonary complications of sickle cell anemia: A need for increased recognition, treatment, and research. *Am J Respir Crit Care Med* 164:2016, 2001.
19. Bruno D, Wigfall DR, Zimmerman SA, et al: Genitourinary complications of sickle cell disease. *J Urol* 166:803, 2001.
20. Wong WY: Prevention and management of infection in children with sickle cell anaemia. *Paediatr Drugs* 3:793, 2001.
21. Prengler M, Pavlakis SG, Prohovnik I, Adams RJ: Sickle cell disease: The neurologic complications. *Ann Neurol* 51:543, 2002.
22. Scjroer SL: Pathophysiology of thalassemia. *Curr Opin Hematol* 9:123, 2002.
23. Wonke B: Clinical management of beta-thalassemia major. *Semin Hematol* 38:350, 2001.
24. Mehta A, Mason PJ, Vulliamy TJ: Glucose-6-phosphatase dehydrogenase deficiency. *Baillieres Best Pract Clin Haemtol* 13:21, 2000.
25. Bolton-Maggs PH: The diagnosis and management of hereditary spherocytosis. *Baillieres Best Pract Clin Haemtol* 13:327, 2000.

ACQUIRED HEMOLYTIC ANEMIA
Patty Chu
Robin R. Hemphill

Acquired hemolytic anemia is characterized by the destruction of red blood cells (RBCs) not due to a genetic or congenital disorder of hemoglobin synthesis or RBC membrane. The acquired hemolytic anemia disorders can produce disease of varying severity from asymptomatic, mild illness to fulminant, potentially fatal hemolysis. Hemolytic anemia can exist in isolation or as part of a larger clinical syndrome. The hemolytic process can be idiopathic, triggered by sundry precipitants, present as a complication of known systemic illness, or herald systemic illness that has yet to be diagnosed. The patient with hemolytic anemia requires timely clinical and laboratory diagnosis, rapid determination of related pathology as part of a known clinical syndrome, initiation of cause-specific treatment made with specialty consultation, and likely hospital admission to carry out treatment and pursue the possibility of underlying illness. Acquired causes of hemolysis can be categorized according to mechanism (Table 222-1).

Presenting symptoms and signs of hemolytic anemia can include weakness or fatigue, dizziness, dyspnea on exertion, tachycardia, new or accentuated cardiac murmur, abdominal pain, pallor, and jaundice. When fever and lymphadenopathy are prominent, an underlying systemic disease should be suspected. Splenomegaly in the setting of hemolysis suggests that RBC destruction has been ongoing for weeks to months. Hepatomegaly may occur with significant hemolysis. Darkening of the urine is caused by intravascular hemolysis and hemoglobinuria.

The diagnosis of hemolytic anemia requires interpretation of laboratory data (Table 222-2). In general, hemolysis is corroborated by spherocytes or schistocytes on peripheral smear, a decreased hematocrit indicating anemia, an increased reticulocyte count indicating enhanced RBC production, increased unconjugated (indirect) bilirubin secondary to excessive hemoglobin breakdown, increased serum lactate dehydrogenase (LDH) as a nonspecific marker of RBC destruction, and decreased haptoglobin, a serum protein that binds free hemoglobin and serves as a sensitive marker of intravascular hemolysis.

TABLE 222-1   Etiologies of Acquired Hemolytic Anemia

Immune-mediated
  Autoimmune
    Warm-type antibody
    Cold-type antibody
      Cold agglutinin syndrome (CAS)
      Paroxysmal cold hemoglobinuria (PCH)
    Mixed-type (warm and cold antibody)
  Alloimmune
    Hemolytic disease of the newborn
    Hemolytic transfusion reaction
  Drug-related
    Autoimmune type
    Drug adsorption type
    Neoantigen type
Microangiopathic
  Thrombotic thrombocytopenic purpura (TTP)
  Hemolytic-uremic syndrome (HUS)
  Pregnancy-associated
    Preeclampsia/eclampsia
    HELLP syndrome
    TTP/HUS
  Disseminated intravascular coagulation
  Malignant hypertension
  Malignancy
  Immune complex vasculitis
Macrovascular
  Prosthetic heart valve
  Intracardiac patch
  Coarctation of the aorta
  Extracorporeal circulation (cardiovascular bypass or hemodialysis)
Toxin-mediated
  Infectious etiology
  Envenomation
  Copper toxicity (Wilson disease)
Drug-induced (without immune-related mechanism)
  Methemoglobin-mediated
Mechanical damage
  Heat denaturation
  March hemoglobinuria (exertion-related)

TABLE 222-2   Ancillary Tests Used in the Evaluation of Hemolytic Anemia

Test	Finding	Interpretation
WBC	Leukocytosis	Common finding in hemolysis
	Leukocytosis *and* thrombocytopenia	Consider Evans syndrome (idiopathic thrombocytopenic purpura and AIHA)
Platelet count	Thrombocytopenia	TTP and HUS <20,000 /μL
		HELLP <100,000 /μL
	Thrombocytopenia *and* leukopenia	Consider Evans syndrome
Hematocrit	Anemia	Expected with significant hemolysis
Reticulocyte count	Elevated	Expected bone marrow response to hemolysis
	Decreased	Bone marrow suppression (hyperhemolytic transfusion reaction, early hemolysis, HIV-associated hemolysis)
Mean corpuscular volume	Elevated	Juvenile RBC population (reticulocytosis)
		Vitamin B_{12} or folate deficiency
WBC differential	Lymphocytosis	Lymphoproliferative disorder (secondary HA)
	Eosinophilia	Inflammatory or infectious condition (secondary HA)
	Neutrophilia or bandemia	Infectious disorder (secondary HA)
	Atypical lymphocytosis	CMV or EBV infection (secondary HA)
Peripheral smear	Spherocytes	RBC membrane destruction (probable immune HA)
	Schistocytes	RBC fragmentation
		MAHA or macrovascular HA
	Agglutination	IgM Ab present (CAS)
Direct antigen (direct Coombs) test	Positive	IgG or compliment present on RBC surface, consistent with AIHA, does not test for IgM on RBC surface
Indirect antibody (indirect Coombs) test	Positive	Anti-RBC IgG antibodies found in serum or eluted off red cells
Haptoglobin	Decreased	Binds to free hemoglobin, indicates intravascular hemolysis
	Increased	Acute phase reactant
Lactate dehydrogenase (LDH)	Increased	Elevated in hemolysis
		Isoenzyme LDH-1 found in RBCs
Unconjugated (indirect) bilirubin	Increased	Indicates enhanced hemoglobin catabolism
Coagulation studies: PTT, PT/INR, fibrinogen, fibrin split products, D-dimer	Elevated	Coagulopathy
		DIC
	Normal	TTP/HUS
Free serum hemoglobin	Increased	Intravascular hemolysis
Urine hemoglobin	Present	Intravascular hemolysis
ESR	Elevated	Systemic inflammatory or infections condition (secondary HA)
		Elevated in severe anemia
C-reactive protein	Elevated	Acute phase reactant
		Systemic inflammatory or infectious condition (secondary HA)

Abbreviations: CAS = cold agglutinin syndrome; CMV = cytomegalovirus; DIC = disseminated intravascular coagulation; EBV = Epstein-Barr virus; ESR = erythrocyte sedimentation rate; HA = hemolytic anemia; HUS = hemolytic-uremic syndrome; MAHA = microangiopathic hemolytic anemia; TTP = thrombotic thrombocytopenic purpura.

IMMUNE-MEDIATED

The immune-mediated hemolytic anemias traditionally have been divided into three categories: autoimmune, alloimmune, and drug-related (see Table 222-1).

Autoimmune Hemolytic Anemia

Individuals with autoimmune hemolytic anemia (AIHA) make antibodies against their own RBCs or against the body's higher-incidence antigens.[1,2] AIHA is thought to occur because of generalized immune system dysfunction. The overall incidence of AIHA is approximately 1 to 3 cases per 100,000 people per year. The incidence of AIHA in infants and children is less, approximately 0.2 cases per 100,000 per year in those under age 20 years. AIHA in children is commonly associated with viral or respiratory infections, is mediated by IgG, and causes acute, fulminant hemolysis. Pregnancy carries a five times

greater risk of developing autoantibodies, but significant RBC destruction is not common.[3]

Diagnosis of AIHA requires evidence of an autoantibody on the patient's RBCs in the form of a positive direct antigen test (DAT or direct Coombs test) *and* identification of an autoantibody, either after elution (washing off) of the antibodies from a patient's RBCs or detecting the autoantibodies in the patient's serum (indirect Coombs test). The DAT is performed by combining the patient's anticoagulated RBCs with anti-IgG and anti-C3d (complement) antibodies to detect the presence of IgG and/or complement on the RBC surface. The DAT itself is not specific for AIHA (Table 222-3). The indirect Coombs test looks for the presence of antibodies in the patient's serum, testing against normal RBCs bearing specific surface antigens. Serologic evidence of autoantibodies should be correlated with clinical and other routine laboratory evidence of hemolytic anemia, including decreased hematocrit, decreased haptoglobin in the setting of intravascular hemolysis, elevated reticulocyte count, elevated unconjugated (indirect)

TABLE 222-3 Differential Diagnosis of Positive Direct Antigen (Direct Coombs) Test

Autoimmune hemolytic anemia
Hemolytic transfusion reaction, acute or delayed
Hemolytic disease of newborn
Transplantation
Drug-related hemolytic anemia
Intravenous immunoglobulin therapy
Rh immunoglobulin therapy (RhoGAM)
Antilymphocyte globulin therapy
Antithymocyte globulin therapy
Sickle cell disease
β-Thalassemia
Renal disease
Multiple myeloma
Hodgkin disease
Autoimmune disease(s)
HIV/AIDS

TABLE 222-4 Causes of Warm Antibody Hemolytic Anemia

Lymphoproliferative disease
  Chronic lymphocytic leukemia
  Lymphoma/Hodgkin disease
  Waldenström macroglobulinemia
  Multiple myeloma
Autoimmune disease/collagen-vascular disease
  Systemic lupus erythematosus
  Rheumatoid arthritis
  Polyarteritis nodosa
  Pernicious anemia
  Scleroderma
  Ulcerative colitis/Crohn disease
Infection (can be associated with warm or cold or often both)
  Infectious mononucleosis
  CMV
  Viral hepatitis
  Malaria
  Pediatric viral respiratory illness
Immunodeficiency syndrome
  HIV
  Congenital syndromes
    X-linked agammaglobulinemia
    Common variable immunodeficiency
    IgA deficiency
    Wiskott-Aldrich syndrome
    Dysglobulinemia
Nonlymphoid tumors
  Ovarian carcinoma and dermoid cysts
  Teratomas
  Kaposi sarcoma
  Thymoma

bilirubin, elevated LDH, and/or hemoglobinuria, to make the diagnosis of AIHA.

AIHA can be divided into primary and secondary varieties. Primary refers to cases without an underlying etiology (idiopathic), and secondary refers to cases of AIHA seen with an underlying disorder. Primary AIHA is more common in women, with peak incidence during the fourth and fifth decades. Many cases initially labeled idiopathic are found later to be associated with significant underlying pathology, such as a lymphoproliferative or autoimmune disorder. Thus all patients with AIHA, especially of the chronic variety, need regular follow-up. The hemolytic process in AIHA can take place within the vascular space or in the liver or spleen. AIHA is also divided into autoantibody type: warm-type, cold-type, and mixed-type.

WARM ANTIBODY AIHA Warm-type AIHA comprises 70 percent of AIHA cases and is usually mediated by an IgG antibody directed against surface antigens of the Rh-erythrocyte system. Autoantibodies of the warm type react most strongly near 37°C, with less affinity for RBC antigens at lower temperatures. These autoantibodies, when eluted or washed off the patient's RBCs, usually are panreactive with RBC panels. Thus these autoantibodies hemolyze not only the patient's own RBCs but also transfused RBCs from another individual (allogenic). Alloimmune-mediated hemolytic anemia, as described below, is characterized by specific autoantibodies triggered by and only reactive against allogeneic RBCs and their antigens; the patient's own RBCs are not damaged. In distinction, warm-type autoantibodies produce hemolysis in both the patient's RBCs and the transfused RBCs. Warm-type autoantibody-mediated hemolysis is predominantly extravascular, occurring in the spleen.

Warm-type AIHA carries a 2:1 female preference but has no racial predilection. About half of warm-type AIHA cases can be labeled as primary or idiopathic, but as mentioned earlier, an initial designation as primary may later be revised on discovery of an associated disease process. Secondary cases most often are associated with lymphoproliferative disorders (in about half) or a systemic autoimmune disease (Table 222-4).

Chronic lymphocytic leukemia is the most common lymphoproliferative disorder associated with warm-type AIHA, accounting for up to 25 percent of patients affected. Hemolytic anemia can precede the development of other systemic effects and diagnosis of lymphoma, Hodgkin disease, and systemic lupus erythematosus (SLE) by up to 3 years. Up to 4 percent of Hodgkin patients will have DAT-positive hemolytic anemia. Warm-type AIHA is seen uncommonly in patients with ulcerative colitis, most often occurring during or after a flare of colitis. Viral-induced warm-type AIHA is often mild and self-limited. Infection may produce warm- or cold-type AIHA as well as mixed-type. Warm-type AIHA associated with human immunodeficiency virus (HIV) infection is uncommon but likewise mild.

High-dose corticosteroids constitute first-line therapy for patients with warm-type AIHA. The initial dose typically is oral prednisone 1 to 1.5 mg/kg per d for 1 to 3 weeks.[4] Improvement usually is noted within 1 week of initiating treatment, and 70 to 80 percent of patients are better within 3 weeks. Once the hemoglobin level stabilizes, the steroids can be tapered. Complete remission is achieved in 15 to 20 percent of new-onset cases of warm-type AIHA, and about half of patients will need low-dose prednisone for several months. If no improvement is noted within 3 weeks of initiating steroid therapy or if a chronic prednisone dose of more than 15 mg/d is needed to maintain a hematocrit of greater than 30 percent, the case should be deemed a steroid failure and alternative therapies considered. Between 10 and 20 percent of steroid-treated patients either will fail to respond adequately or will require unacceptably high doses to maintain the desired response. Such patients are treated with either splenectomy or cytotoxic drugs.

Splenectomy removes both the main site of extravascular hemolysis in IgG-mediated AIHA and a major site of general autoantibody production. Splenectomy produces a 65 to 70 percent response rate and has the potential for long-term remission or a complete cure. At the very least, if incomplete remission is achieved or if relapse occurs, patients after splenectomy may require lower doses of corticosteroids. The most feared complication of splenectomy is overwhelming postsplenectomy infection (OPSI) with encapsulated bacteria. **Splenectomized patients should receive pneumococcal and meningococcal vaccinations** and should be considered for daily penicillin prophylaxis.

Cytotoxic drugs produce a 40 to 60 percent response rate and have been used both for patients who have failed steroids and for those who have failed splenectomy. Some sources suggest saving cytotoxic agents for those who have failed a second trial of lower-dose steroids after splenectomy. The cytotoxic drugs may be used with or without steroids. Once the desired response is achieved, the steroids once again can be tapered slowly, followed by tapering the cytotoxic agent as tolerated. Cytotoxic drugs have significant side effects, including bone marrow suppression, gastrointestinal intolerance, secondary malignancy development, hemorrhagic cystitis, alopecia, and sterility. Conflicting reports exist as to the efficacy of using cyclosporine, and its use requires careful monitoring for the development of nephrotoxicity. Rituximab, a genetically engineered chimeric murine-human anti-CD20 monoclonal antibody, is useful in severe, refractory cases of both warm- and cold-type AIHA, but the associated side effects can be serious or even fatal.

Severe hemolysis in cases of warm-type AIHA may be treated with plasma exchange as a transient stabilizing measure while waiting for steroids or cytotoxic agents to take effect. Intravenous immunoglobulin may be used as adjunctive treatment in children who cannot tolerate the side effects of chronic high-dose steroids or cytotoxic agents. Danazol, an attenuated androgen with fewer side effects than glucocorticoids, can produce remission in occasional patients. Vincristine-loaded platelets may bring about selective splenic macrophage injury, preventing the extravascular hemolysis that defines warm-type AIHA.

For patients with life-threatening anemia or for those at high-risk for cardiac or cerebrovascular ischemic complications, RBC transfusion of the *least incompatible* units may be transfused slowly with close monitoring. Transfusion may precipitate further production of autoantibodies as well as introduce a source for the production of allogeneic antibodies. In both warm- and cold-type AIHA, secondary cases may not respond to aggressive therapy unless the underlying illness is treated appropriately.

COLD ANTIBODY AIHA   In cold-type AIHA, the autoantibodies produced are usually IgM and most strongly hemolytic at 0 to 4°C. The presence of cold-type autoantibodies leads to clumping or agglutination of RBCs on peripheral smear at cooler temperatures. This IgM-mediated disease is associated with the complement fixation on the RBC surface and the subsequent triggering of the complement cascade. Hemolysis occurs in both the extravascular and intravascular spaces after massive autoantibody production and complement activation. Instead of splenic macrophages, Kupffer cells in the liver are responsible for most of the extravascular RBC destruction. The two common cold-type AIHA disorders are cold agglutinin syndrome and paroxysmal cold hemoglobinuria. Fifty percent of secondary cold-type AIHA cases are associated with lymphoproliferative disorders, with infection the next leading secondary cause.

Cold Agglutinin Syndrome (CAS), accounting for up to one-third of all AIHA cases, is typically IgM-mediated but rarely has been found to be IgG- or IgA-mediated. Autoantibodies in the CAS are directed against the I/i blood group antigens, which are related to ABO antigens. CAS autoantibodies bind to RBC surface antigens in the cooler peripheral circulation and initiate the steps of the complement cascade. During the early phases of complement cascade activation, extravascular hemolysis takes place in the Kupffer cells, and during terminal stages of complement cascade activation, intravascular hemolysis occurs.

Primary CAS is seen in older adults, particularly females, with a peak incidence at age 70. The hemolysis associated with the primary and chronic secondary forms of CAS tends to be mild and stable with hemoglobin levels of 9 to 12 g/dL, and symptoms typically are mild. Secondary CAS also can present as an acute attack, such as that seen in patients who have preceding infectious illnesses, including *Mycoplasma pneumoniae,* Epstein-Barr virus (EBV), adenovirus, cytomegalovirus (CMV), influenza, varicella-zoster virus (VZV), HIV, *Escherichia coli, Listeria monocytogenes,* and *Treponema pallidum.* Symptom onset corresponds with the peak antibody response to infection, usually 2 to 3 weeks after the onset of illness. As the original illness itself resolves, the triggered cold-type AIHA resolves approximately 2 to 3 weeks later. In cases of severe hemolysis, pallor, jaundice, hemoglobinuria, and/or renal failure can occur. Chronic cold-type AIHA associated with lymphoproliferative diseases, such as chronic lymphocytic leukemia (CLL), lymphomas, and Waldenström macroglobulinemia, produces high autoantibody levels with the potential for significant hemolysis.

Cold weather exacerbates CAS; more episodes of acute hemolysis are seen during winter. Patients are apt to develop acrocyanosis because the peripheral circulation typically is cooler than the central circulation. Raynaud phenomenon, vascular occlusion, and tissue necrosis may complicate CAS. Clumping of cold agglutinins will elevate the mean corpuscular volume (MCV) and decrease the RBC count. Peripheral smear findings include the spherocytosis caused by RBC membrane destruction, as well as anisocytosis, poikilocytosis, polychromasia, and agglutination. As with other forms of hemolytic anemia, patients will have elevated LDH and unconjugated bilirubin levels with moderate disease and decreased haptoglobin, hemoglobinemia, and hemoglobinuria with severe, intravascular hemolysis.

In primary and chronic CAS with mild anemia, treatment is symptomatic and involves simply keeping the extremities as well as the nose and ears warm in cold weather. Patients with CAS should take a daily folate supplement. Treatment for severe hemolysis has been successful with immunosuppressive or cytotoxic agents, such as chlorambucil, cyclophosphamide, interferon-α, and fludarabine. The major side effect with such treatment is bone marrow suppression. Plasmapheresis, as in warm-type AIHA, may prove helpful as a temporizing measure by removing autoantibodies, particularly because auto-IgM has an intravascular distribution, but such therapy should be combined with immunosuppressive agents. Unlike warm-type AIHA, CAS rarely responds to steroids, although such treatment may be considered in atypical cases. Because splenic macrophages play a lesser role in IgM-mediated cold antibody disease, splenectomy is not particularly helpful for cold antibody-mediated extravascular hemolysis.

Treatment of secondary CAS depends on the underlying illness, whether it is chemotherapy for lymphoproliferative disease or antibiotics for a nonviral infection. Infection-related cold antibody disease does not require immunosuppressive therapy because the hemolytic anemia is usually self-limited. As with warm-type AIHA, rituximab may prove helpful.

RBC transfusion can be performed for patients at risk for significant cardiac or cerebrovascular ischemia, but transfused blood should be kept at 37°C using a blood warmer. Transfusions should be limited because they may worsen ongoing hemolysis; in addition to the risk of producing alloantibodies to transfused RBCs, most cold antibodies act against the I group antigens, which are found on most donor RBCs. Donor complement in the transfused product also may exacerbate ongoing hemolysis. There is limited experience using intravenous immunoglobulin in the treatment of CAS.

Paroxysmal Cold Hemoglobinuria (PCH) is caused by a biphasic IgG autoantibody called the *Donath-Landsteiner antibody.*[5] The PCH autoantibody is directed against the P antigen system found on most RBCs. On binding, this potent autoantibody fixes complement not only at low temperatures, but it also can bind certain complement components at normal physiologic temperatures, causing clinically significant hemolysis at low autoantibody titers. Thus hemolysis may occur at both cold and normal temperatures. Symptoms include high fever, chills, headache, abdominal cramps, nausea and vomiting, diarrhea, and leg and back pain that develops with cold exposure. Cold urticaria also may develop, as well as extremity paresthesias and Raynaud phenomenon.

Primary PCH and PCH secondary to congenital or late-stage syphilis are characterized by chronic disease with cold-induced relapses; patients with chronic, relapsing disease should be tested for syphilis. Secondary PCH caused by other infectious agents is most common in children and is one of the more common causes of childhood hemolytic anemia. Postinfection PCH is usually seen after a preceding upper respiratory infection (URI) and has been associated with measles, mumps, EBV, CMV, VZV, adenovirus, influenza A, *M. pneumoniae, Haemophilus influenzae,* and *E. coli.* Most cases of postinfectious PCH are self-limited, but severe cases may take weeks to resolve. With severe hemolysis, hemoglobinuria is common, and methemoglobinuria may be seen. Acute renal failure may develop as a complication of PCH.

Patients with PCH should be kept warm. Steroids can be considered in children with severe hemolytic anemia, but since infection-related PCH tends to be self-limited, benefit is uncertain. PCH secondary to syphilis responds to effective antibiotic treatment. Splenectomy is not helpful, and plasmapheresis should be used only as a temporizing measure in life-threatening cases. RBC transfusion should be limited to cases of severe hemolysis because most donor units are P antigen-positive and may stimulate further production of PCH autoantibodies. Transfusion in cases of cold-type AIHA, whether CAS or PCH, always should be performed using a blood warmer.

MIXED-TYPE AIHA Mixed-type AIHA presents as primary or secondary disease—most commonly lymphoproliferative and autoimmune diseases. The course of illness is usually chronic with severe exacerbations. Like warm-type AIHA, mixed-type AIHA is steroid-responsive, can be treated with splenectomy, and responds to cytotoxic therapy. Relapses are not triggered by cold exposure, so acrocyanosis and Raynaud are not seen characteristically. As with any secondary AIHA, treatment of the underlying disorder will reduce hemolytic activity.

Alloimmune Hemolytic Anemia

Alloimmune hemolytic anemia requires exposure to allogeneic RBCs with subsequent alloantibody formation. In the laboratory, alloantibodies react specifically with the allogenic RBCs that triggered their production; these antibodies do not react against a patient's own RBCs.

A well-known example of this is when the RhD-negative maternal immune system develops IgG alloantibodies on exposure to RhD-positive fetal RBCs.[6] The maternal alloantibodies can then cross the placenta to inflict fetal RBC destruction in a condition termed *hemolytic disease of the newborn* (HDN). Anemia can range from mild to potentially fatal, producing intrauterine fetal death. The term *hydrops fetalis* has been used to describe the anatomic changes seen in severe HDN. Transplacental or fetomaternal hemorrhage, the inciting stimulus for maternal alloantibody formation, may occur during amniocentesis, chorionic villus sampling, delivery, or abortion (threatened or otherwise) or even during external cephalic version. By still uncertain mechanisms, administration of anti-D IgG (RhoGAM) with any fetomaternal hemorrhage event and soon after delivery will suppress maternal alloantibody formation and prevent HDN. Treatment of established HDN employs intrauterine and intravascular fetal transfusion and may include plasma exchange and/or intravenous immunoglobulin therapy.

Most adults who develop alloimmune hemolytic anemia have a history of RBC transfusion, which sensitizes patients to allogeneic RBC antigens. A subsequent transfusion can result in immediate alloantibody production, resulting in the fever, chest and flank pain, tachypnea, tachycardia, hypotension, hemoglobinuria, and oliguria seen in the hemolytic transfusion reaction. In patients with high alloantibody titers, the hemolytic reaction can be immediate. Delayed alloantibody-mediated hemolysis is possible, with hemolytic transfusion reaction (HTR) symptoms presenting 3 to 7 days after transfusion (see Chap. 223).

DRUG-RELATED

Drug-related hemolytic anemia can be divided into three types: autoimmune, drug adsorption, and neoantigen. Steroids can be used in cases of drug-related severe hemolysis. RBC transfusion will aggravate hemolysis if the recipient's serum contains antibodies against antigens found on the transfused RBCs.

Autoimmune Drug-Related Hemolytic Anemia

In autoimmune drug-related hemolytic anemia, the offending drug triggers formation of autoantibodies that bind with self RBC antigens,

leading to a hemolytic process serologically indistinct from that seen in warm-type AIHA.[7] The diagnosis is proven when the hemolytic process abates on withdrawal of the offending drug. The classic and first example of autoimmune-type drug-related hemolytic anemia was discovered in the mid-1960s, when alpha-methyldopa was found to stimulate production of autoantibodies. Other drugs implicated in the formation of autoantibodies against RBCs include levodopa, mefenamic acid, procainamide, diclofenac, quinidine, phenacetin, and the second- and third-generation cephalosporins (particularly cefotetan and ceftriaxone). Up to 71 drugs have been associated with development of a positive DAT (direct Coombs test); however, significant hemolysis is seen only occasionally. An extended drug exposure usually is required for autoantibodies to form. Importantly, a positive DAT (direct Coombs test) does not indicate that hemolysis will occur or that a drug must be discontinued. Within days of stopping the offending drug, hemolysis usually stops, although it may take months to see full resolution of the process.

Drug Adsorption–Type Hemolytic Anemia

Drug adsorption–type hemolytic anemia requires that the drug incite the formation of antidrug antibodies and that the drug bind to the RBC with significant affinity. Antibodies formed against the drug will in turn react against the drug-bound RBCs, producing hemolysis. This type of hemolysis also has been called *drug-requiring* because the absence of the offending drug eliminates the hemolytic reaction completely.

Neoantigen-Type Drug-Related Hemolytic Anemia

Neoantigen-type drug-related hemolytic anemia involves weak binding of the offending drug to normal RBCs. The body's immune system, seeing the formed immune complexes as foreign, will generate an immune response, which then produces hemolytic disease. The classic causative agent is penicillin. Isolated cases of diphtheria-tetanus-pertussis (DTP) vaccination in children have been associated with hemolysis, possibly via this neoantigen mechanism.[8]

MICROANGIOPATHIC SYNDROMES: THROMBOTIC THROMBOCYTOPENIC PURPURA (TTP) AND HEMOLYTIC UREMIC SYNDROME (HUS)

Both TTP and HUS involve platelet aggregation in the microvascular circulation via the mediation of von Willebrand factor (vWF), leading to thrombocytopenia, often with platelet counts of less than 20,000/μL. Microangiopathic hemolytic anemia (MAHA) or schistocyte-forming hemolysis develops as RBCs are fragmented during travel through these occluded arterioles and capillaries.[9] TTP and HUS are clinical syndromes with characteristic features, but overlap does occur, making differentiation sometimes difficult. TTP is traditionally more common in adults, whereas HUS is more common in children. TTP typically induces more prominent neurologic deficits with deposition of platelet aggregates in a broader, systemic distribution, whereas HUS more specifically impairs the renal system. However, TTP may present with significant renal compromise, whereas HUS can cause important extrarenal complications, obscuring the line between the two. In general, adults presenting with clinical and laboratory evidence of MAHA accompanied by thrombocytopenia should be treated as though they have TTP once other diagnoses have been excluded (Table 222-5) because untreated TTP has a 80 to 90 percent mortality.

Because of the significant hemolytic anemia, pallor, jaundice or scleral icterus, fatigue, and dyspnea on exertion are common. With significant thrombocytopenia, purpura or mucosal bleeding may be evident. Focal neurologic deficits (often vacillating), aphasia, seizure, coma, visual disturbance, chest pain, cardiac conduction disorders, abdominal pain, oliguria, and hypertension indicate end-organ involvement.

TABLE 222-5   Differential Diagnosis for TTP/HUS

Sepsis
Metastatic cancer
Systemic vasculitis
Preeclampsia/eclampsia
Evans syndrome
Heparin-induced thrombocytopenia with thrombosis
Malignant hypertension

Thrombotic Thrombocytopenic Purpura

TTP is classically comprised of the following pentad: 1) thrombocytopenia, 2) MAHA, 3) fever, 4) renal impairment, and 5) neurologic impairment.[10] It is uncommon to see all five features in any one patient, but if present, severe end-organ ischemia or damage likely has taken place. Thrombocytopenia and MAHA are the most common features, and fever is the least frequent finding.

A key pathophysiologic role in TTP is played by the vWF-cleaving metalloprotease ADAMTS-13.[11] Endothelial cells and megakaryocytes normally make monomers of vWF that are joined to form larger vWF multimers. Under usual conditions, ADAMTS-13 cleaves these multimers before being allowed to enter the circulation or rest on the surface of endothelial cells. In cases of familial TTP or Upshaw-Schulman syndrome, a severe deficiency in ADAMTS-13 activity has been found to promote the adherence of unusually large vWF multimers to the surfaces of endothelial cells. These large vWF multimer strings attract circulating platelets, resulting in the formation of platelet thrombi; the larger the multimers, the greater is the affinity for platelets. The normal process of cleaving multimers is key to maintaining laminar microvascular blood flow. Microvascular platelet thrombi generate turbulent RBC flow through occluded vessels with subsequent RBC shear or hemolysis (MAHA). Tissue ischemia and necrosis follow, causing end-organ damage.

About 50 to 80 percent of patients with acquired TTP have presumed autoantibodies against ADAMTS-13. In those without autoantibodies, altered enzyme production, survival, or activity is presumed to produce TTP. Patients with many disorders associated with TTP or MAHA have been identified as having lower levels of ADAMTS-13 activity: liver disease, metastatic cancer, chronic metabolic disease, chronic inflammatory disease, pregnancy, and the neonatal period. Overall, ADAMTS-13 deficiency has been shown to play a definitive role in the pathogenesis of familial-type TTP and is suspected to play a central role in cases of acquired TTP.

Pregnancy is the most common precipitating event for TTP. Preeclampsia has some features similar to TTP, but because delivery is the treatment for preeclampsia but fails to alter the course of TTP, it is important to distinguish between the two entities. TTP usually presents earlier during pregnancy, around 23 to 24 weeks, whereas preeclampsia more commonly presents in the third trimester. Second-trimester preeclampsia is associated with molar pregnancies. The maternal mortality rate in cases of TTP has been reduced significantly with the use of plasma-exchange therapy, but fetal mortality has remained high secondary to placental microvascular occlusion and resulting infarction. TTP may relapse with a subsequent pregnancy, so affected women should be counseled accordingly.

Other triggers of TTP include infection (particularly HIV), vaccination, and autoimmune disorders such as SLE. Several drugs have been associated with TTP, including quinidine, cyclosporine, and tacrolimus.[12] Ticlopidine and clopidogrel, two thienopyridine antiplatelet agents commonly used in patients with cardiac and cerebrovascular disease, have received attention for their TTP-inciting potential, presumably due to the ability of either drug to incite the development of autoantibodies against ADAMTS-13 within 2 weeks of starting treatment. Most patients with thienopyridine-associated TTP have developed the illness within 1 month of drug initiation. TTP has been seen more commonly with ticlopidine than with clopidogrel, with an incidence between 1 in 1600 and 1 in 5000. Thus clopidogrel has become the thienopyridine of choice.

A particularly refractory form of TTP has been linked with the post-bone marrow transplant (BMT) and postchemotherapy settings. As opposed to most other patients with TTP, post-BMT or postchemotherapy TTP patients have not been shown to have ADAMTS-13 deficiency, so the mechanism of disease may be immune-mediated or cytotoxic endothelial damage. Patients undergoing BMT are exposed to many known triggers of TTP, including infection and drugs, as well as endothelial damage from both chemotherapy and graft-versus-host disease. The chemotherapeutic agents mitomycin, cisplatin, gemcitabine, and bleomycin also have been associated with TTP.

TTP is still a clinical diagnosis, but characteristic laboratory findings include severe anemia, thrombocytopenia of less than $20,000/\mu L$, schistocytes or helmet cells on peripheral smear, decreased haptoglobin, elevated reticulocyte count, and elevated unconjugated (indirect) bilirubin seen with intravascular hemolysis. The DAT (direct Coombs test) is characteristically negative because the hemolysis seen in TTP does not involve anti-RBC autoantibodies. TTP thrombi do not involve fibrin, so TTP is distinguished from DIC based on normal coagulation studies.[13] Preeclampsia is associated with a reduced plasma AT III level as opposed to TTP. Renal function should be assessed, and cultures should be obtained as appropriate. ADAMTS-13 activity measurement is still too time- and labor-intensive for general use and is only available in specialty laboratories.

Familial-type TTP can be prevented with a periodic infusion of platelet-poor fresh frozen plasma (FFP), cryoprecipitate-poor plasma (from which vWF has been removed; also known as *cryosupernatant*), or plasma pretreated with detergent and solvent. All these products contain the ADAMTS-13 metalloprotease. An acute attack also can be treated with an infusion of one of these products; an ADAMTS-13 level of 5 percent of normal is sufficient to thwart an attack of TTP.

Acquired TTP is treated with daily plasma exchange consisting of 1) plasmapheresis to remove large vWF multimers and autoantibodies and 2) plasma infusion to give the patient back one calculated daily volume of FFP or cryosupernatant. Cryosupernatant may prove more advantageous to use due to its lack of vWF. Infusion can be initiated with FFP and then converted to cryosupernatant in refractory cases, or treatment can employ cryosupernatant initially. The use of plasma exchange has decreased TTP mortality rates from 90 percent down to 10 to 20 percent. Plasma exchange, presumably by removing vWF multimers and autoantibodies, is superior to plasma infusion alone, with improved response and lower mortality rates. If plasmapheresis cannot be performed immediately, initial FFP infusion should be started, but infusion should never replace exchange. Plasma exchange is performed daily until several days after remission is achieved, usually seen within 1 week, but it may require up to 4 weeks. Remission is defined by normalization of the platelet count and LDH combined with clinical resolution of tissue ischemia and thrombosis. Plasma exchange requires the placement of a central venous catheter and thus carries the same risks: hemorrhage, line-site thrombosis, line sepsis, and pneumothorax. Infusion of plasma carries a small risk of blood-borne pathogen transmission.

Corticosteroids, usually prednisone 1 to 2 mg/kg per d, may be helpful in the presence of a high autoantibody titer and if plasma exchange does not provide the desired response. Splenectomy can induce long-term remission or cure in cases of plasma-exchange failure by removing a site of autoantibody production and removing a site of microvascular occlusion mitigating MAHA. In post-BMT and postchemotherapy patients, running the patient's plasma through a staphylococcal protein A column, known as *immunoadsorption,* can remove immune complexes from patients with immune-mediated TTP. Post-BMT patients often change immunosuppressive drugs when TTP is considered drug-related. Vincristine, intravenous immunoglobin, azathioprine, cyclosporine, and rituximab have been investigated as possible therapies.

Supportive measures may be needed to address systemic complications associated with TTP, including RBC transfusion in the setting of significant MAHA, anticonvulsants for seizures, antihypertensives for hypertension, and hemodialysis in cases of severe renal insufficiency. Platelet transfusions should be avoided, except for life-threatening bleeding or intracranial hemorrhage, because thrombosis may worsen acutely, leading to rapid renal failure and potentially death. Aspirin can worsen hemorrhagic complications in the setting of severe thrombocytopenia and also should be avoided. Heparin has not been shown beneficial in TTP or HUS. Relapse after appropriate treatment may be as high as 30 percent, and maintenance therapies have not been shown to prevent relapse.

Hemolytic Uremic Syndrome

HUS is a disease primarily of early childhood, with a peak incidence between 6 months and 4 years of age.[14] The adult form of HUS may be very difficult to distinguish from TTP. Overall mortality rate is 5 to 15 percent, with a worse prognosis in older children and adults. HUS is one of the most common causes of acute renal failure in childhood and is characterized by acute renal failure, microangiopathic hemolytic anemia, fever, and thrombocytopenia.

In children, HUS often follows a viral or bacterial illness. Although several infectious agents have been implicated, infection with *Escherichia coli* serotype O157:H7 is a well- recognized agent associated with HUS. On ingestion, *E. coli* O157:H7 produces a toxin that is absorbed into the systemic circulation. The toxin then binds with greatest affinity to receptors found on the surfaces of glomerular and renal tubular epithelial and endothelial cells and to a lesser extent to receptors lining cerebral and colonic epithelial and endothelial cells. The result is targeted renal microvasculature damage leading to the formation of platelet thrombi, mediated by vWF multimers (as in TTP), with subsequent MAHA via shear mechanism and renal tissue ischemia and necrosis. The toxin also potentiates release of the large vWF multimers and upregulates high-affinity receptors to continue the cycle of thrombosis and hemolysis. Onset of HUS is typically 2 to 14 days after diarrhea develops. Bewteen 20 and 40 percent of *E. coli* O157:H7-infected patients will have bloody diarrhea, whereas 15 percent of children and 5 percent of adults will go on to develop HUS. Other organisms implicated in HUS include *Shigella, Yersinia, Campylobacter, Salmonella, Streptococcus pneumoniae,* varicella, echovirus, and coxsackieviruses A and B.

Like TTP, HUS is pathologically identified by microthrombi consisting of platelet aggregates that occlude the arterioles and capillaries. In HUS, the microthrombi are confined mostly to the kidneys; in TTP, they occur throughout the microcirculation. Like TTP, HUS is a clinical diagnosis. Laboratory studies reflect the presence of MAHA. Thrombocytopenia may be present but generally not to the degree seen in TTP. The serum creatinine level may be markedly elevated, and urine, if present, will contain protein and red blood cells (although the urine can be normal). Coagulation studies usually are normal.

Mild HUS with less than 24 h of urinary symptoms requires only fluid and electrolyte correction and supportive care. Steroid therapy may be beneficial. In the setting of more severe disease, plasma exchange or infusion has been performed with equivocal results. Patients whose disease resembles TTP may respond to plasma therapy. The overall low mortality of HUS makes use of plasma exchange questionable. Hemodialysis may be required in the setting of acute renal failure, especially in adults, in whom acute renal failure tends to be more severe. A shorter duration of dialysis therapy is associated with increased likelihood of recovery from HUS. Infection with *E. coli* O157:H7 should not be treated with antimotility drugs because these agents appear to increase the risk of developing HUS. The use of antibiotics for treatment of *E. coli* O157:H7 is controversial. A recent meta-analysis found no evidence that antibiotic treatment increased or decreased the risk of developing HUS.[15]

PREGNANCY-ASSOCIATED HEMOLYSIS

HELLP Syndrome

A complication of preeclampsia known as the HELLP syndrome is comprised of hemolysis, elevated liver tests, and low platelets.[16] The incidence of HELLP is about 1 in 1000 pregnancies.[17] Endothelial cell dysfunction resulting from the release of vasoactive agents leads to the formation of microvascular platelet-fibrin thrombi in the preeclamptic patient and subsequent MAHA as RBCs pass through occluded vessels. Initially, pathologic changes occur predominately in the liver, as opposed to pathologic changes predominately seen in the CNS and kidneys from TTP and HUS, respectively. In the HELLP syndrome, widespread vascular occlusion may produce systemic end-organ damage, and excess coagulation cascade stimulation may progress to DIC. Right upper quadrant or epigastric pain may be seen in up to 90 percent of patients with HELLP syndrome and indicates the potential for hepatic rupture, the most ominous complication of HELLP.

Diagnosis of HELLP is made based on laboratory data. A decreased serum haptoglobin level (see Table 222-2) is the most sensitive marker for MAHA in the setting of HELLP.[18] A decreased serum haptoglobin level may precede the onset of thrombocytopenia by 1 to 2 days, making it that much more valuable a marker to monitor in the HELLP syndrome.[19] Unfortunately, classic markers of hemolysis such as schistocytes on the peripheral smear, elevated indirect bilirubin and LDH levels, hemoglobinemia, and hemoglobinuria are less reliable in the setting of the HELLP syndrome and may be seen only in late-stage or severe cases; their absence does not rule out hemolysis.

Timely delivery is the definitive treatment for the HELLP syndrome.[17] Medical treatment of the HELLP syndrome includes supportive measures for complications such as seizures and hypertensive crisis. Steroids may be of use beyond inducing fetal lung maturity, but their use in the HELLP syndrome is still investigational and the mechanism is uncertain. The clinical and laboratory findings of the HELLP syndrome may extend up to 6 days postpartum.[17]

Pregnancy-Associated TTP

Pregnancy-associated TTP usually occurs in the antenatal period. As mentioned earlier, it is important to distinguish between preeclampsia/HELLP and TTP because the course of TTP is not altered by delivery but can be improved dramatically by initiation of plasma exchange therapy. Onset of TTP in the postpartum period requires a search for retained products of conception.

Pregnancy-Associated HUS

Pregnancy-associated HUS usually occurs during the postpartum period and is characterized by abrupt onset of acute renal failure, MAHA, and hypertension after a usually normal, complication-free delivery. Coagulation studies in both TTP and HUS should be normal, distinguishing these disorders from DIC.

MALIGNANCY-ASSOCIATED HEMOLYSIS

Patients with widely disseminated cancer may develop MAHA. Those at particular risk include patients with gastric cancer, followed by, in no particular order, patients with lung, breast, colon, prostate, and hepatic neoplasms. Malignancy-associated MAHA is attributed to microvascular fibrin deposition and resulting RBC shear-injury as blood passes through occluded arterioles and capillaries. In contrast to other forms of MAHA, malignancy-associated hemolysis may target the pulmonary circulation, with intimal proliferation in the pulmonary microvasculature leading to elevation in pulmonary artery pressures. Up to half of malignancy-associated MAHA cases may be associated with DIC. MAHA itself portends a poor prognosis for the cancer patient, and the only known treatment for such cases is chemotherapy to treat the underlying malignancy.

HEMOLYSIS AND IMMUNE-COMPLEX DISEASE

Immune-complex deposition in the setting of collagen-vascular disease triggers the coagulation cascade, creating fibrin in the systemic microvasculature. The result is endothelial damage and RBC shear producing MAHA. SLE, polyarteritis nodosa, Wegener granulomatosus, and scleroderma may be complicated by MAHA.

HEMOLYSIS IN MALIGNANT HYPERTENSION

MAHA in the setting of malignant hypertension occurs via poorly understood mechanisms. The process has been attributed largely to fibrinoid necrosis occurring in systemic arterioles as a result of severely elevated blood pressure. MAHA abates with normalization of blood pressure.

MACROVASCULAR HEMOLYSIS

The presence of a prosthetic heart valve sets the stage for turbulent blood flow with high shear-stress across the prosthetic valve.[20] Intravascular hemolysis occurs in up to 85 percent of people with normally functioning mechanical prosthetic valves, although it is less frequent in patients with bioprosthetic compared with mechanical heart valves. Stentless aortic prosthetic valves produce less hemolysis, encouraging researchers that prosthetic valves can be modified even further to reduce the incidence of hemolysis and its resulting complications. Severe hemolysis may require replacement of an implicated prosthetic valve. Macrovascular hemolysis also may be seen after intracardiac patch repair, aortofemoral bypass, in patients with coarctation of the aorta, in patients with severe aortic valve disease, and with extracorporeal circulation, as in cardiopulmonary bypass or hemodialysis.[21] Patients with ongoing mild hemolysis should receive supplemental iron and folate.

DIRECT TOXIC EFFECTS CAUSING HEMOLYSIS

Infections

Destruction of RBCs commonly occurs in the course of many infectious diseases. Malaria is the world's most common cause of hemolytic anemia, with RBC hemolysis resulting from direct parasitization of the RBCs. Hemolysis also results from direct parasitization of RBCs in babesiosis and infection with *Bartonella henselae*. *H. influenzae* type b infection can produce hemolysis by altering the RBC surface; the capsular polysaccharide of the bacterium binds to the RBC surface, and then antibodies destroy the bacterium as well as the RBC. *Clostridium perfringens (welchii)* infection can result in severe hemolysis by direct lysis of red blood cells. The organism releases enzymes that acutely degrade the phospholipids of the RBC membrane bilayer and the proteins in the structural membrane. Many viral infections can be accompanied by hemolytic anemia, including measles, CMV, herpes simplex virus, VZV, coxsackievirus, and HIV.

Toxin-Induced Hemolysis

Acute intravascular hemolysis can occur following bites/stings of bees, wasps, the southern black widow spider, and the brown recluse spider. American pit vipers and coral snake bites are known to cause coagulation abnormalities but rarely cause hemolysis. Conversely, the bite of the cobra snake does cause intravascular hemolysis.

MECHANICAL DAMAGE CAUSING HEMOLYSIS

Uncommonly, march hemoglobinuria occurs predominantly in young males after significant exertion against a hard surface, such as concrete. Damage to RBCs from direct impact causes transient red or dark urine lasting up to a few hours after exercise. Runners, particularly beginners and those with a heavy stride, as well as soldiers, karate participants, and conga drummers, may develop march hemoglobinuria. Anemia is not usually seen because less than 1 percent of the body's RBCs are damaged. Patients are advised to wear thick-soled shoes and change exercise style to prevent further episodes.

ACKNOWLEDGMENT

Thank you to the previous author, Mary Eberst, for her work.

REFERENCES

1. Gehrs BC, Friedberg RC: Autoimmune hemolytic anemia. *Am J Hematol* 69:258, 2002.
2. Dacie SJ: The immune haemolytic anaemias: A century of exciting progress in understanding. *Br J Haematol* 114:770, 2001.
3. Hoppe B, Stibbe W, Bielefeld A, et al: Increased RBC autoantibody production in pregnancy. *Transfusion* 41:1559, 2001.
4. Petz LD: Treatment of autoimmune hemolytic anemias. *Curr Opin Hematol* 8:411, 2001.
5. Bessler M, Schaefer A, Keller P: Paroxysmal nocturnal hemoglobinuria: Insights from recent advances in molecular biology. *Transfus Med Rev* 15:255, 2001.
6. Urbaniak SJ, Greiss MA: RhD hemolytic disease of the fetus and the newborn. *Blood Rev* 14:44, 2000.
7. Wright MS: Drug-induced hemolytic anemias: Increasing complications to therapeutic interventions. *Clin Lab Sci* 12:115, 1999.
8. Downes KA, Domen RE, McCarron KF, Bringelsen KA: Acute autoimmune hemolytic anemia following DTP vaccination: Report of a fatal case and review of the literature. *Clin Pediatr* 40:355, 2001.
9. Moake JL: Thrombotic microangiopathies. *New Engl J Med* 347:589, 2002.
10. Elliott MA, Nichols WL: Thrombotic thrombocytopenic purpura and hemolytic uremic syndrome. *Mayo Clin Proc* 76:1154, 2001.
11. Levy GG, Nichols WC, Lian EC, et al: Mutations in a member of the ADAMTS gene family cause thrombotic thrombocytopenic purpura. *Nature* 413:488, 2001.
12. Medina PJ, Sipols JM, George JN: Drug-associated thrombotic thrombocytopenic purpura-hemolytic uremic syndrome. *Curr Opin Hematol* 8:286, 2001.
13. Levi M, Ten Cate H: Disseminated intravascular coagulation. *New Engl J Med* 341:586, 1999.
14. Corrigan JJ, Boineau FG: Hemolytic-uremic syndrome. *Pediatr Rev* 22:365, 2001; erratum in *Pediatr Rev* 23:0, 2002 (online journal).
15. Safdar N, Said A, Gangnon RE, Maki DG: Risk of hemolytic uremic syndrome after antibiotic treatment of *Escherichia coli* O157:H7 enteritis: A meta-analysis. *JAMA* 228:996, 2002.
16. Rath W, Faridi A, Dudenhausen JW: HELLP syndrome. *J Perinat Med* 28:249, 2000.
17. Abraham KA, Connolly G, Farrell J, Walshe JJ: The HELLP syndrome, a prospective study. *Renal Fail* 23:705, 2001.
18. Wilke G, Rath W, Schutz E, et al: Haptoglobin as a sensitive marker of hemolysis in HELLP-syndrome. *Int J Gynaecol Obstet* 39:29, 1992.
19. Schrocksnadel H, Sitte B, Steckel-Berger G, Dapunt O: Hemolysis in hypertensive disorders of pregnancy. *Gynecol Obstet Invest* 34:211, 1992.
20. Mecozzi G, Milano AD, De Carlo M, et al: Intravascular hemolysis in patients with new-generation prosthetic heart valves: A prospective study. *J Thorac Cardiovasc Surg* 123:550, 2002.
21. Wright G: Haemolysis during cardiopulmonary bypass: Update. *Perfusion* 16:345, 2001.

TRANSFUSION THERAPY
Sally A. Santen

Effective and safe blood transfusion began in the early to middle twentieth century when preservative solutions were developed and blood group types were identified. Continued advances in transfusion medicine have improved our understanding of the benefits and risks of blood component replacement.[1] Currently available products are purified so that precise factor or component replacement is common practice. While there have been significant advances in individual factor and component replacement, development of hemoglobin substitutes has been less successful.

Transfusion in the emergency department typically is done for acute blood loss and circulatory shock. As medical care is moved to outpatient settings and emergency departments become more crowded, emergency physicians may be responsible for transfusion therapy that was once relegated to inpatient settings. An understanding of the available blood products, their indications, and potential complications of transfusions is important for safe and effective transfusion practice (Table 223-1).

TRANSFUSION OF AVAILABLE BLOOD PRODUCTS

Packed Red Blood Cells (PRBCs)

An adult's total blood volume is estimated to be 2.5 L/m^2, 75 mL/kg, or approximately 5 L in a 70-kg person. Fresh whole blood transfusion would be ideal to replace acute blood loss; however, during the storage of whole blood, platelets and other factors become inactive. In addition, the storage life of whole blood is less than that individual components. Therefore, by necessity and convenience, whole blood is fractionated to its components for storage and transfusion.

PRBCs are prepared by the centrifugation of whole blood to remove about 80 percent of the plasma; then a preservative solution is added, most commonly citrate-phosphate-dextrose (CPD) with additional nutrients adenosine, glucose, and mannitol. Each unit of PRBCs has a hematocrit of 55 to 80 percent and a volume of approximately 250 mL (see Table 223-1). Transfusion of 1 unit of PRBCs into a typical adult will increase the hematocrit by 3 percent or the hemoglobin by 1 g/dL.

The primary reason for transfusion of PRBCs is to increase oxygen-carrying capacity.[2] The two indications for emergency PRBC transfusion are acute blood loss and profound anemia with impaired oxygen delivery. It is difficult to set a transfusion threshold that holds true for all patients.[3–7] Based on animal and human studies, lactic acid production increases, oxygen extraction ratio exceeds 50 percent, and the mortality rate starts to increase in otherwise stable patients with hemoglobin levels of 3.5 to 4.0 g/dL. In an animal model of coronary stenosis, adverse cardiac effects are seen with hemoglobin levels of 6.0 g/dL. Therefore, practice guidelines often use this level as a threshold for PRBC transfusion. However, there are reports of Jehovah's Witnesses who tolerate surgery with hemoglobin levels below 6.0 g/dL provided that intravascular volume is maintained.

The American College of Surgeons classifies hemorrhage according to estimated blood volume loss correlated with clinical findings. *Class II hemorrhage* corresponds to an estimated 15 to 30 percent blood volume loss with clinical manifestations of tachycardia, decreased pulse pressure, restlessness, and anxiety. While young, healthy patients can tolerate blood loss of up to 25 to 30 percent or 1500 mL when treated with crystalloid, older patients and patients with chronic illness such as cardiac diseases may not tolerate similar blood loss without cardiac or neurologic decompensation. Additionally, patients at most risk for end-organ damage are likely to have complicating factors such as medications (β-blockers), pacemakers that may alter the body's usual response to hypovolemia, and decreased oxygen-carrying capacity related to other comorbid conditions. *Class III hemorrhage* is an estimated 30 to 40 percent blood volume loss with clinical manifestations of tachycardia, tachypnea, systolic hypotension, and mental status changes. During hemorrhage, hematocrit values or hemoglobin levels lag behind the clinical signs or physiologic parameters in assessing the adequacy of oxygen-carrying capacity and delivery. Therefore, patient status is more useful than hemoglobin level to determine if crystalloid resuscitation alone is effective or if PRBC replacement is needed.

The second indication for transfusion is anemia.[2] The use of PRBCs to treat anemia depends on the severity, duration, and rate of change of the anemia, as well as the patient's ability to compensate for the diminished oxygen-carrying capacity. Patients with chronic anemia have developed compensation mechanisms so that chronic anemia is better tolerated than acute anemia. The threshold for transfusion in anemia is inexact, although various consensus panels have recommended transfusion for hemoglobin levels of less than 7 g/dL, whereas patients with hemoglobin levels greater than 10 g/dL rarely will benefit from transfusion.[4–6] In intermediate ranges, patients with cardiac or vascular diseases may benefit from transfusion at a higher threshold. Transfusion thresholds for children may be higher and depend on the etiology of their anemia.

Red blood cell replacement usually is done with PRBCs. Depending on the urgency of transfusion, most patients can be typed (ABO and RhD blood group type) and cross-matched against the blood intended for transfusion. The blood type can be determined in about 15 min, whereas to perform a type and cross-match, it takes approximately 1 h. In critical patients, type O RhD$^-$ (universal donor) may be transfused because the red cells do not contain blood group antigens. Type O RhD$^+$ blood also may be used if type O RhD$^-$ is not available but is not the blood of choice for women of child-bearing potential. If an RhD$^-$ patient is transfused with 1 unit of RhD$^+$ PRBCs, approximately 80 percent will develop anti-D antibodies. Because **the effect**

TABLE 223-1 Characteristics of Blood Products and Doses

Component	Shelf Life	Volume/Unit	Approximate Content/Unit*	Typical Dose	Dosage Effect
PRBC	21–42 days	250–350 mL	Red cells 65–80% Plasma 20–35%	2 units or 15 mL/kg	Raises hemoglobin concentration about 2 g/dL
Platelets (random donor platelet concentrate)	5 days	50–60 mL	Platelets 7.5 × 10^{10}	6 units or 5 mL/kg	Raises platelet count about 50,000/μL
Platelets (apheresis collected single donor platelet concentrate)	5 days	250–300 mL	Platelets 3 to 6 × 10^{11}	One unit	Raises platelet count about 50,000/μL
FFP	1 year frozen and 24 h thawed	200–250 mL	Each coagulation factor 200–250 units and fibrinogen 400–500 mg	4 units or 15 mL/kg	Raises most coagulation factors levels about 20%
Cryoprecipitate	1 year frozen	20–50 mL	Factor VIII 80 units, fibrinogen 225 mg, and von Willebrand factor variable amounts	10 units or 1 unit/5 kg	Raises fibrinogen 75 mg/dL

*Blood-derived components often contain WBCs, RBCs, platelets, and plasma unless they have been specially prepared.

of 1 unit of PRBCs is small (increase in hematocrit of 3 percent and hemoglobin of 1 g/dL) and clinically inconsequential, it is standard practice to transfuse a minimum of 2 units and raise the hematocrit by 6 percent and hemoglobin level by 2 g/dL. In children, 15 mL/kg of PRBCs will raise the hematocrit 6 percent and hemoglobin level by about 2 g/dL.[8]

PRBCs may be further treated to meet specific uses: leukocyte-reduced PRBCs, irradiated PRBCs, washed PRBCs, and frozen PRBCs. Leukocyte-reduced PRBCs have had 70 to 85 percent of the leukocytes removed. The advantages of leukocyte-reduced PRBCs is 1) to prevent or avoid nonhemolytic febrile reactions due to antibodies to white blood cells (WBCs) and platelets if the patient has been exposed to previous transfusions or pregnancies, 2) to prevent sensitization in patients who may be eligible for bone marrow transplantation, and 3) to minimize the risk of virus transmission such as human immunodeficiency virus (HIV) and cytomegalovirus (CMV). The leukocytes can be reduced by filtration or other methods before storage of the PRBCs or during transfusion. Irradiation of PRBCs eliminates the capacity of T cells to proliferate, thereby preventing the donor's T cells from reacting to the recipient's cells and causing graft-versus-host disease. Irradiated cells should be considered in transplant patients, neonates, and immunocompromised patients. Washed PRBCs are indicated in patients who have a hypersensitivity to plasma, such as IgA deficiency. For rare blood types, PRBCs may be frozen and saved for up to 10 years for later use.[1] This is more expensive than normal storage, and once thawed, the blood must be washed and transfused within 24 h.

One unit of PRBCs, about 250 mL in volume, generally is transfused over 1 to 2 h. However, blood may be transfused more rapidly in patients with hemodynamic instability. During standard transfusions, the initial rate is slower over the first 30 min so that if there is incompatibility, the transfusion may be stopped.

Platelet Transfusion

Platelet transfusions may be used either prophylactically to prevent bleeding or therapeutically when patients with thrombocytopenia are actively bleeding.[9,10] Platelets are collected from whole blood donations or from single donors using apheresis techniques. One random-donor platelet concentrate prepared from 500 mL of donated whole blood contains an average of 7.5×10^{10} platelets (see Table 223-1). One apheresis-collected single-donor platelet concentrate generally contains 3 to 6×10^{11} platelets depending on local collection practice. Platelets should be given according to ABO compatibility, if available. A dose of one random-donor platelet concentrate per 10 kg (approximately six to eight random-donor platelet concentrates for an adult) or one apheresis—collected single—donor platelet concentrate in an adult will increase the platelet count by about 50,000/μL. Response to platelet transfusions is variable; therefore, platelet levels should be checked at 1 and 24 h. Failure of platelets to rise appropriately may be due to increased consumption of platelets from an underlying process, destruction due to platelet antibodies, or sequestration due to hypersplenism. Transfused platelets should survive 3 to 5 days unless there is a consumptive process.

The etiology of thrombocytopenia is important in the decision to transfuse platelets.[9,10] With idiopathic thrombocytopenic purpura, an antiplatelet antibody-mediated consumptive process, the platelets are larger, younger, and more functional, so prophylactic transfusion is rarely indicated despite very low platelet counts. However, with platelet hypoplasia, platelet function is impaired, making the risk of bleeding greater. Patients with comorbid diseases such as infection, fever, medications, and central nervous system (CNS) involvement may be more likely to bleed or be at higher risk if they bleed; therefore, the threshold for platelet transfusion is higher. The dose of platelets should reflect the indication. In general, spontaneous bleeding is possible, and prophylactic transfusion is indicated with platelet counts of less than 10,000/μL. Platelet counts of greater 50,000/μL rarely cause significant bleeding.

Indications for platelet transfusions include:

Platelet count <10,000/μL in asymptomatic patients
Platelet count <15,000/μL with a coagulation disorder or minor bleeding
Platelet count <20,000/μL with major bleeding
Platelet count <50,000/μL with an invasive procedure (thoracentesis, paracentesis) or general surgery required or during massive transfusion (1 to 2 blood volumes)
Platelet count <100,000/μL with neurologic or cardiac surgery

It is not possible to provide clear recommendations for patients with nonfunctioning platelets (antiplatelet medications, uremia, von Willebrand disorder, or hyperglobulinemia) and active bleeding. In von Willebrand disorder, normal platelets can deliver von Willebrand factor to the bleeding site. Conversely, in uremic patients, the transfused platelets may not function better than native platelets. In these complex cases, it is helpful to consult with a hematologist for the best recommendations.

Like PRBCs, platelets can be leukocyte-reduced or washed. Patients who have had repeated transfusions may become alloimmunized and refractory to platelet transfusion, noted by the lack of expected rise of platelet count after transfusion. Such patients need HLA- or cross-matched platelets. Other disorders may affect the efficacy of platelet transfusion, including duration of platelet storage, bacterial sepsis, antibiotics, graft-versus-host disease, disseminated intravascular coagulation (DIC), and splenomegaly.

Relative contraindications to the transfusion of platelets are disorders associated with platelet activation, such as thrombotic thrombocytopenic purpura (TTP) or heparin-induced thrombocytopenia, where transfusion may worsen thrombosis. In these diseases, procedures may necessitate platelet transfusion but should be performed in consultation with hematology.

Fresh Frozen Plasma Transfusion

Fresh frozen plasma (FFP) is plasma obtained after the separation of whole blood from RBCs and platelets and then frozen within 6 h.[11] Each unit of FFP is 200 to 250 mL and contains about 1 unit of each coagulation factor and 2 mg of fibrinogen per milliliter (see Table 223-1). FFP is appropriate for rapid replacement of multiple coagulation deficiencies such as in liver failure, warfarin overdose, DIC, and massive transfusion in bleeding patients. It should be considered when there is bleeding and the standard coagulation tests [prothrombin time/International Normalized Ratio (PT/INR) or activated partial thromboplastin time (aPTT)] are elevated 1.5 times control. Administration of FFP prophylactically to nonbleeding patients is not indicated, and prophylaxis is not always needed for some procedures in patients with a coagulopathy. For example, patients undergoing paracentesis and thoracentesis are not at increased risk of bleeding until the PT, INR, or aPTT are greater than 2 times control. During massive transfusions, replacement of an entire blood volume leaves only about one-third of normal factors, and although PT and aPTT may be abnormal, clinical coagulopathy does not always occur.

Indications for FFP transfusion include:

Rapid reversal of warfarin over-anticoagulation
Bleeding and multiple coagulation defects as evidenced by prolonged PT/INR/aPTT greater than 1.5 control (liver disease, DIC)
Correction of coagulation defects for which no specific factor is available (Table 223-2) (Specific factor replacement is safer and better but may not always be available.)
Transfusion of more than a total of one blood volume with evidence of active bleeding and prolonged PT/aPTT

Other possible indications for FFP in consultation with a hematologist include TTP, antithrombin III deficiency, and hereditary angioedema (FFP contains C1 esterase).[12]

TABLE 223-2 Replacement Therapy for Congenital Factor Deficiencies

Coagulation Factor	Incidence*	Replacement Therapy
Factor I (fibrinogen)	150 cases	Cryoprecipitate
Factor II (prothrombin)	>30 cases	FFP for minor bleeding episodes Prothrombin complex concentrate† for major bleeding
Factor V	150 cases	FFP
Factor VII	150 cases	FFP for minor bleeding episodes Prothrombin complex concentrates for major bleeding Recombinant factor VII$_A$ (experimental)
Factor VIII‡	1 in 10,000 males	Factor VIII concentrates (cryoprecipitate or FFP if not available) Desmopressin for those with mild hemophilia
von Willebrand disease	up to 1 in 100 persons	Desmopressin (or some factor VIII concentrates or cryoprecipitate)
Factor IX‡	1 in 30,000 males	Factor IX concentrates
Factor X	1 in 500,000	FFP for minor bleeding episodes Prothrombin complex concentrates for major bleeding
Factor XI§	3 in 10,000 Ashkenazi Jews 1 in 1,000,000 in general	FFP
Factor XII	Several hundred cases	Replacement not required
Factor XIII	>100 cases	FFP or cryoprecipitate

*Incidence as of 1998.
†See Chap. 220 for details concerning prothrombin complex concentrates.
‡See Chap. 220 for detailed management recommendations for patients with hemophilia A and hemophilia B.
§Factor XI levels correlate poorly with bleeding complications; many patients have low levels, but no bleeding complications.
Abbreviation: FFP = fresh frozen plasma.

The efficacy of transfused coagulation factors varies, so the increase in specific coagulation factors seen after FFP infusion also varies. In general, 1 unit of FFP will increase most coagulation factors by 3 to 5 percent in a 70-kg adult. The common adult dose of 7 to 8 mL/kg (or 2 units of FFP in a 70-kg individual) will only increase coagulation factors by 10 percent, a clinically inconsequential benefit in most circumstances. For clinically relevant correction of coagulation factor deficiencies, a dose of 15 mL/kg (or 4 units in a 70-kg adult) is required (see Table 223-1). As indicated by the name, FFP is stored frozen, and there may be a delay while it is thawed. FFP should be ABO-compatible. After transfusion, bleeding and coagulation studies should be reevaluated. If coagulation factor consumption is present, repeated FFP transfusion should be guided by the PT/INR/aPTT response.

Cryoprecipitate Transfusion

Cryoprecipitate is the cold insoluble protein fraction of FFP. Each unit of cryoprecipitate is about 20 to 50 mL and contains about 225 mg of fibrinogen and 80 units of factor VIII and von Willebrand factor (vWF). It also contains some factor XIII and fibronectin. With the de-

velopment of recombinant factor VIII products for use in hemophilia, the primary role of cryoprecipitate is now replacement of fibrinogen or vWF. Bleeding patients with fibrinogen levels below 100 mg/dL due to severe liver disease, DIC, and dilutional coagulopathy may benefit from cryoprecipitate, although there is little evidence of improved clinical outcomes. The dose of cryoprecipitate is 1 unit of cryoprecipitate per 5 kg, which will raise the fibrinogen level by about 75 mg/dL. Usually 10 units are given at a time.

Indications for cryoprecipitate transfusion include:

Bleeding with a fibrinogen level of less than 100 mg/dL
Bleeding in some subtypes of von Willebrand disease that are unresponsive to desmopressin (DDAVP)

Other Plasma-Derived Products

Immunoglobulin for intravenous administration (IVIG) is a pooled IgG product that has been virally attenuated. Labeled indications for IVIG are idiopathic thrombocytopenic purpura, pediatric HIV infection, primary humoral immunodeficiency, and several new and off-label treatments such as Kawasaki disease and autoimmune disorders. Dose and administration vary by indication. Adverse reactions include anaphylaxis, especially in IgA deficiency (rare); febrile reactions; headache; and renal failure. Some patients develop transient positive serology to hepatitis C and cytomegalovirus.

Albumin is a virally inactivated purified plasma protein that normally accounts for 50 percent of circulating protein and 75 percent of plasma oncotic pressure. Albumin transfusion in patients with decreased oncotic pressures may transiently increase oncotic pressure, but the albumin rapidly distributes to extravascular spaces. Therefore, due to the cost and the lack of proven efficacy over crystalloid, there is no advantage to using albumin for volume resuscitation.[13,14]

Antithrombin III (AT III) is a coagulation inhibitory protein. Deficiency can be acquired or congenital and usually is associated with difficult-to-treat thrombosis. AT III replacement is indicated in AT III deficiency-related thrombosis and for thrombosis prophylaxis. This product should be considered in AT III-deficient patients when difficulty is encountered in achieving adequate heparinization or recurrent thrombosis is observed despite adequate anticoagulation. It is also reasonable to treat AT III-deficient subjects with concentrate before major surgeries or in obstetric situations where the risks of bleeding from anticoagulation are unacceptable. Currently, AT III therapy is under investigation in sepsis, DIC, and other thrombotic diseases. The dose depends on the indication. An infusion of 50 units (1 unit is the amount of AT III in 1 mL of pooled plasma) of AT III concentrate per kilogram usually will raise the plasma antithrombin III level to about 120 percent of normal in a congenitally deficient individual. Plasma AT III levels should be monitored to ensure that they remain above 80 percent. Subsequent administration of AT III at 60 percent of the initial dose at 24-h intervals is recommended to maintain AT III levels in the normal range.

Massive Transfusion

Massive transfusion is defined as the replacement of one blood volume or about 10 units of PRBCs within a 24-h period. Patients receiving less than one blood volume rarely need hemostatic factor (FFP, platelets) replacement. In patients receiving two blood volumes or more than 20 units of PRBCs, transfusing coagulation factors and platelet may be empirically helpful. For patients who receive one to two times total blood volume, hemostatic factor replacement should be guided by the considerations noted above: 1) if the platelet count is below 50,000/μL, platelet transfusion is warranted; 2) if the INR is greater than 1.5, FFP may be given; and 3) if the fibrinogen level is below 100 mg/dL, it may be replaced with cryoprecipitate.

In massive transfusion, hypothermia is a risk, and blood and crystalloid as well as the patient should be warmed. Hypocalcemia from the preservative citrate chelating calcium is rare but should be considered in massive transfusion and symptoms or signs of hypocalcemia.

COMPLICATIONS OF BLOOD TRANSFUSIONS

The need for blood transfusions in the emergency department is common. Many are emergent due to hemorrhage, whereas others are less urgent and occur in the setting of an observation unit or prolonged emergency department stays. Up to 20 percent of all transfusions may lead to some type of adverse reaction.[1] Although most of these reactions are minor, some are life-threatening (Table 223-3). In critically ill patients, transfusion reactions may be difficult to identify; therefore, attention should be paid to unexpected changes in patient status during a transfusion.

Infectious Complications of Blood Transfusion

Improved blood donor screening, serologic testing, safer handling of blood products, and viral inactivation of many blood products have reduced the risk of infection from blood transfusion.[1,15] However, risks remain, and patients need to be informed of the hazards associated with transfusions.

Donor blood is screened for the most concerning viral agents (Table 223-4). However, there is still a small risk of viral transmission[1,15] (Table 223-5). Most cases of transmission are thought to occur during the window period between infection and antibody production in the donor. This window is reduced by the use of antigen testing but is still not eliminated completely.

The prevalence for CMV antibodies in the general population is between 50 to 80 percent. Therefore, blood is not tested routinely for CMV unless the recipient is seronegative and either pregnant, a potential or present transplant candidate, immunocompromised, or a premature infant. Use of leukocyte-reduced blood components further decreases the risk of CMV transmission to susceptible populations because most of the virus resides in the leukocytes.

Many other infections also can be transmitted by blood transfusion, including the hepatitis viruses, West Nile virus, and other bacteria (occurs if the donor was bacteremic during donation). Additionally, blood can become contaminated during storage or processing. Bacterial sepsis that results from RBC transfusion is most commonly due to *Yersinia enterocolitica*, which is able to grow easily in refrigerated blood.[16] The risk of bacterial sepsis is estimated to be 1 in 500,000 units of PRBCs transfused and 1 in 40,000 units for random-donor platelet concentrates.[1]

Hemolytic Transfusion Reactions

Hemolytic transfusion reactions occur when the recipient's antibodies recognize and induce hemolysis in the donor's RBCs. The reaction is usually acute when antibodies already exist but can be delayed when there is an amnestic response to a transfused RBC-antigen to which the recipient is already sensitized. Immediate transfusion reactions are caused most commonly by ABO incompatibility and usually are the result of technical errors made during the collection of blood, in pretransfusion testing, or in patient identification. The majority of transfusion fatalities are acute hemolytic reactions due to human error of incorrect cross-matching or inadvertent administration of the wrong blood. The risk of acute hemolytic transfusion reaction due to incompatible blood is 1 to 4 per 1 million units transfused and has a high fatality rate.[1]

With acute hemolytic reaction, most of the transfused cells are destroyed, which may result in activation of the coagulation system with DIC and release of anaphylotoxins and other vasoactive amines. Evidence of this type of reaction includes back pain, pain at the site of the transfusion, headache, alteration of vital signs (fever, hypotension, dyspnea, tachycardia), chills, bronchospasm, pulmonary edema, bleeding due to developing coagulopathy, and evidence of new or worsening renal failure. Recognition of transfusion reactions in critically ill patients who already may be hypotensive and tachycardiac is difficult and requires a high degree of suspicion.

TABLE 223-3 Acute Transfusion Reactions: Recognition, Management, Evaluation

Reaction Type	Signs and Symptoms	Management	Evaluation
Acute intravascular hemolytic reaction	Fever, chills, low back pain, flushing, dyspnea, tachycardia, shock, hemoglobinuria	Immediately stop transfusion IV hydration to maintain diuresis; diuretics may be necessary Cardiorespiratory support as indicated Can be life threatening	Retype and crossmatch Direct and indirect Coombs tests CBC, creatinine, PT, aPTT Haptoglobin, indirect bilirubin, LDH, plasma free hemoglobin Urine for hemoglobin
Acute extravascular hemolytic reaction	Often have low-grade fever but may be entirely asymptomatic	Stop transfusion Rarely causes clinical instability	Hemolytic workup as above to rule out the possibility of intravascular hemolysis
Febrile nonhemolytic transfusion reaction	Fever, chills	Stop transfusion Manage as in intravascular hemolytic reaction (above) because cannot initially distinguish between the two Can treat fever and chills with acetaminophen and meperidine Usually mild but can be life threatening in patients with tenuous cardiopulmonary status Consider infectious work-up	Hemolytic workup as above because initially cannot distinguish the etiology
Allergic reaction	If mild, urticaria, pruritus If severe, dyspnea, bronchospasm, hypotension, tachycardia, shock	Stop transfusion If mild, reaction can be treated with diphenhydramine; if symptoms resolve, can restart transfusion If severe, may require cardiopulmonary support; do not restart transfusion	For mild symptoms that resolve with diphenhydramine, no further workup is necessary, although blood bank should be notified For severe reaction, do hemolytic workup as above because initially will be indistinguishable from a hemolytic reaction

Abbreviations: aPTT = activated partial thromboplastin time; CBC = complete blood count; LDH = lactate dehydrogenase; PT = prothrombin time.

TABLE 223-4   Required and Optional Laboratory Testing of Donated Blood Required

ABO antigens
RhD antigens
RBC antibody screen
Serologic tests for syphilis (RPR), not that syphilis is thought to be transmitted by blood transfusion, but that it is a marker for other sexually transmitted bloodborne infections. If RPR is positive, then FTA-ABS is run. RPR positive, blood not used; FTA positive, then donor notified.
Hepatitis B surface antigen (RIA or ELISA, RPHA)
Anti-hepatitis B core antibody
Hepatitis C antibody
HIV-1,2 antibody
HIV-1 p24 antigen
HTLV (human T-cell lymphotrophic virus) type I and II antibody
Optional
    CMV antibody
    HLA antibody
    Other RBC antigens

Ongoing transfusion should be stopped immediately on first indication of potential problems. While laboratory confirmation is being performed, the sequelae of hemolysis are treated supportively. Renal function (serum creatinine, urinalysis), electrolytes, and coagulation status (PT/INR/aPTT) should be checked. It is critical to maintain renal blood flow with fluids, mannitol, and furosemide as needed. Shock should be treated with volume and vasopressors to support blood pressure. Coagulopathy should be treated with FFP. Heparin or steroids may be helpful.

The remaining donor blood should be sent, along with a posttransfusion blood specimen from the recipient, to the blood bank. Diagnosis is made by evidence of hemolysis (hemoglobinuria or hemoglobinemia) and by blood incompatibility. In rechecking the blood type and cross-match, the patient's serum is tested for blood group alloantibodies, and the donor's plasma is tested for the presence of antibodies that react with the patient's blood. In transfusion reactions, serum haptoglobin will be decreased, serum lactate dehydrogenase will be elevated, and a direct antigen (Coombs) test usually will be positive. The blood bank will be able to test the blood, review records, confirm blood types, and determine if the patient's syndrome is from a transfusion reaction.

Risk of morbidity and mortality is proportional to amount of blood received prior to recognition of the transfusion reaction. Therefore, **in nonemergent blood transfusions, the initial rate of blood transfusion is low for the first 30 min to allow for identification of a transfusion reaction** while minimizing the volume of blood transfused. The best medicine is prevention by strict adherence to detail in obtaining blood for cross-match and initiating transfusion.

Extravascular delayed hemolytic reactions occur in about 1 per 1000 PRBC units transfused.[1] Hemolysis most commonly occurs in

TABLE 223-5   Risk of Infections from Transfusion of Blood Products

Etiology	Estimated Frequency: One Infection per Number of Units Transfused (95% CI)
HIV-1	1:1,000,000 (200,000–2,000,000)
HIV-2	Unknown
HTLV-I/II	1:500,000 (250,000–2,000,000)
Hepatitis B	1:40,000 (30,000–250,000)
Hepatitis C	1:40,000 (30,000–150,000)
Parvovirus B19	1:10,000
Bacterial contamination	1:12,000 random-donor platelet concentrates 1:500,000 PRBCs

the spleen and occasionally in liver and bone marrow. This type of reaction is less serious and rarely fatal. It may be determined by a positive Coombs test, elevated unconjugated (indirect) bilirubin level, and poor response to transfusion. Treatment is supportive.

Febrile Transfusion Reactions

Febrile transfusion reactions are characterized by onset of fever during or within a few hours of a blood transfusion.[17] This type of reaction is one of the more common transfusion-related complications and is more common in multiparous women or multiply transfused patients. The clinical presentation can range from a mild elevation in temperature to fever along with rigors, headache, myalgias, tachycardia, dyspnea, and chest pain. Initially, it may be difficult to differentiate a febrile reaction from the more serious hemolytic transfusion reaction or sepsis.

Febrile transfusions result from a combination of recipient antibody against donor leukocytes and the release of cytokines that are produced during storage. For non-leukocyte-reduced platelets, the risk of fever during transfusion is about 20 percent, and with leukocyte reduction, the incidence of febrile reactions is about 2 percent. For the first-time febrile reaction or in any severe reaction, the transfusion should be stopped and the product returned to the blood bank. Laboratory investigation similar to that done for possible hemolytic transfusion should be done, and blood cultures should be obtained.

The febrile transfusion reaction is usually self-limited and will respond to antipyretics. Premedication with diphenhydramine and acetaminophen may help prevent these reactions. For patients with recurrent febrile reactions, the use of leukocyte-reduced blood products may be helpful, as well as pretreatment with antipyretics.

Allergic Transfusion Reactions

Allergic transfusion reactions are associated with the onset of urticaria and pruritus during the transfusion and occur in approximately 1 percent of transfusions. Fortunately, only a small percentage of patients will have more severe reactions, such as bronchospasm, wheezing, and anaphylaxis. These reactions are caused by an immune response to plasma proteins.

Conservative therapy with an antihistamine usually will control the symptoms. The transfusion usually does not have to be stopped. For more severe symptoms, the transfusion may need to be stopped and more aggressive management initiated. In patients with IgA deficiency, more severe anaphylactoid reactions can occur in response to exposure to the IgA in donor products. Washing the plasma from the cells minimizes this type of reaction.

Transfusion-Related Acute Lung Injury

Transfusion-related acute lung injury is an uncommon but complex process that is thought to be due to granulocyte and antibody deposition within the lung.[18] This injury results in the appearance of bilateral pulmonary infiltrates due to noncardiogenic pulmonary edema, usually within 4 h of transfusion. The presentation will be similar to a patient with adult respiratory distress syndrome and diagnosed by diffuse patchy infiltrates on chest radiograph and then excluding other etiologies. By itself, this lung injury is self-limiting and generally resolves spontaneously with only supportive care.

Hypervolemia

Transfusion of blood products can cause rapid volume expansion that patients with limited cardiovascular reserve such as infants, severe chronic compensated anemia, and the elderly may have difficulty managing. Patients may develop dyspnea, hypoxia, and pulmonary edema. Recognition of the potential for volume overload is the best prevention so that blood can be transfused slowly, the patient monitored carefully, and treatment with diuretics may be initiated when necessary. The usual rate of transfusion is 2 to 4 mL/kg per h, but it can be slowed to 1 mL/kg per h in more delicate patients.

Electrolyte Imbalance

Electrolyte imbalances of hypocalcemia, hyperkalemia, or hypokalemia due to large-volume transfusions or altered excretion are uncommon. The anticoagulant citrate chelates calcium and is a component of many blood preservatives. Rarely with massive transfusions, hypocalcemia will develop. In patients with normal hepatic function, the infused citrate is metabolized to bicarbonate. Rarely, the excess bicarbonate causes alkalemia, driving potassium into the cells and causing hypokalemia. The potassium content in stored blood products increases during storage, and uncommonly, patients with renal insufficiency or neonates can develop hyperkalemia.

Delayed Complications

Many of the preceding complications can have delayed presentations. Furthermore, in patients with impaired immune systems, alloimmunization to class I HLA antigens can occur, having an impact on treatment and later transfusions. Immunocompetent T lymphocytes of donor blood can identify recipient cells as foreign and cause GVH disease, but this can be prevented by irradiation of blood products prior to transfusion.

ACKNOWLEDGMENT

We would like to acknowledge Mary Eberst for her contribution to these chapters in previous editions.

REFERENCES

1. Goodnough LT, Brecher ME, Kanter MH, AuBuchon JP: Transfusion medicine: I. Blood transfusion. II. Blood conservation. *New Engl J Med* 340:438, 525, 1999.
2. Blajchman MA, Hebert PC: Red blood cell transfusion strategies. *Transfus Clin Biol* 8:207, 2001.
3. Crosby E: Reevaluating the transfusion trigger: How low is safe? *Am J Ther* 9:411, 2002.
4. Hill SR, Carless PA, Henry DA, et al: Transfusion thresholds and other strategies for guiding allogeneic red blood cell transfusion. *Cochrane Database Syst Rev* 2:CD002042, 2002.
5. Carson JL, Hill S, Carless P, et al: Transfusion triggers: A systematic review of the literature. *Transfus Med Rev* 16:187, 2002.
6. Myhre BA: Clinical commentary: The transfusion trigger: The search for a quantitative holy grail. *Ann Clin Lab Sci* 31:359, 2001.
7. Tan IK, Lim JM: Anaemia in the critically ill: The optimal haematocrit. *Ann Acad Med Singapore* 30:293, 2001.
8. Roseff SD, Luban NLC, Manno CS: Guidelines for assessing the appropriateness of pediatric transfusion. *Transfusion* 42:1398, 2002.
9. Rebulla P: Revisitation of the clinical indications for the transfusion of platelet concentrates. *Rev Clin Exp Hematol* 5:228, 2001.
10. Rebulla P: Platelet transfusion trigger in difficult patients. *Transfus Clin Biol* 8:249, 2001; erratum in *Transfus Clin Biol* 9:109, 2002.
11. Bianco C: Choice of human plasma preparations for transfusion. *Transfus Med Rev* 13:84, 1999.
12. Fay A, Abinun M: Current management of hereditary angio-oedema (C'1 esterase inhibitor deficiency). *J Clin Pathol* 55:266, 2002.
13. Wilkes MM, Navickis RJ: Patient survival after human albumin administration. A meta-analysis of randomized, controlled trials. *Ann Intern Med* 135:149, 2001.
14. Alderson P, Bunn F, Lefebvre C, et al: Human albumin solution for resuscitation and volume expansion in critically ill patients. *Cochrane Database Syst Rev* 1:CD001208, 2002.
15. Dodd RY: Current viral risks of blood and blood products. *Ann Med* 32:469, 2000.
16. Kopko PM, Holland PV: Mechanisms for severe transfusion reactions. *Transfus Clin Biol* 8:278, 2001.
17. Heddle NM: Pathophysiology of febrile nonhemolytic transfusion reactions. *Curr Opin Hematol* 6:420, 1999.
18. Popovsky MA: Transfusion and lung injury. *Transfus Clin Biol* 8:272, 2001.

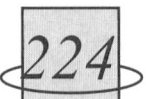

224 ANTICOAGULANTS, ANTIPLATELET AGENTS, AND FIBRINOLYTICS

Jim Edward Weber
F. Michael Jaggi
Charles V. Pollack, Jr.

Antithrombotic therapy is standard for numerous arterial and venous thromboembolic conditions, including acute myocardial infarction (AMI)—both ST-segment elevation MI (STEMI) and non-ST-segment elevation MI (NSTEMI)—unstable angina pectoris, deep venous thrombosis (DVT), pulmonary embolism (PE), and transient ischemic attack (TIA) or cardiovascular accident (CVA). Moreover, antithrombotic agents help prevent occlusive vascular disease in patients at risk for thrombosis. These agents, however, also have the potential to cause life-threatening complications, primarily uncontrolled hemorrhage. This chapter provides an overview of antithrombotic agents, including mechanisms of action, indications, and contraindications, as well as evaluation and management of acute bleeding complications. Detailed management of thromboembolic disorders is discussed in their respective chapters.

Hemostasis is initiated by platelet interaction with the vascular subendothelium and continues with a series of plasma coagulation proteins reactions that generate the final product of cross-linked fibrin, an insoluble protein, meshed with the initial platelet plug (see Chap. 218). Arterial thrombi, composed primarily of platelets bound by thin fibrin strands, develop under high-flow conditions, especially at sites of ruptured atherosclerotic plaques. Both anticoagulants and platelet-inhibiting drugs may effectively prevent and treat arterial thrombosis. In contrast, venous thrombi form in areas of sluggish blood flow, and are composed mainly of red blood cells and large fibrin strands. Anticoagulant drugs are effective in preventing and treating venous thromboembolism, while platelet-suppressing agents are less useful.

Both arterial and venous thrombi may result in local vascular obstruction or distant embolization. Antithrombotic agents interfere with these processes either by preventing formation of the platelet-fibrin net (blocking thrombin activation or platelet function) or by accelerating clot breakdown (fibrinolysis). Antithrombotic agents are classified by mechanism of action. Anticoagulants block the synthesis and activation of clotting factors, interfering with the coagulation cascade at one or more steps. Antiplatelet agents interfere with platelet activation or aggregation. Fibrinolytics (often but inaccurately referred to as thrombolytic agents) enzymatically dissolve the fibrin component of thrombi.

ANTICOAGULANTS

Warfarin

PHARMACOLOGY OF WARFARIN   Oral anticoagulants are used to 1) stop further thrombosis when the condition already exists (e.g., DVT), 2) reduce the risk of embolism in patients with thrombotic disease (e.g., DVT or left ventricular mural thrombus), and 3) prevent thrombi from forming in patients with risk factors for their development (e.g., prolonged immobilization or venous disease) (Table 224-1). Sodium warfarin, a hydroxycoumarin compound, is the most

TABLE 224-1 Antithrombotic Therapy Guidelines

Clinical Indication	Comments
Treatment of DVT and PE	In most cases, heparin and warfarin can be started simultaneously, with an overlap of 3–5 days.
Unfractionated heparin: 80 U/kg IV bolus, then 18 U/kg per h continuous infusion, with the aPTT checked after 6 h and the infusion adjusted to maintain the aPTT 1.5–2.5 times control *with* concurrent institution of warfarin.	Warfarin should be continued for at least 3 months.
Enoxaparin: 1 mg/kg SC bid or 1.5 g/kg SC per d	
SK: 250,000 units IV bolus, then 100,000 U/h continuous infusion for 1–3 d	
Alteplase: 15 mg bolus, then 0.75 mg/kg over 30 min (maximum 50 mg), then 0.50 mg/kg over 60 min (maximum 35 mg)	
Urokinase: 4400 U/kg IV bolus then 4400 U/kg per h continuous infusion for 1–3 d	
Prophylaxis of DVT and PE	
Unfractionated heparin: 5000 units SC bid or tid	
Ardeparin: 50 U/kg SC bid	
Dalteparin: 2500 to 5000 units SC per d	
Enoxaparin 30 mg SC bid or 40 mg SC per d	
STEMI	All postmyocardial infarction patients should receive aspirin 160–325 mg/d for an indefinite period (unless contraindicated or if on warfarin).
Aspirin (nonenteric coated): 160–325 mg PO per d	Optimal strategies are unclear. Research is evolving rapidly.
Unfractionated heparin: 60 U/kg IV bolus, then 12 U/kg per h continuous infusion adjusted to keep aPTT 1.5–2.5 times control *or* 17,500 units SC bid	
Enoxaparin: 1 mg/kg SC bid	
Patients at high risk for mural thrombosis or systemic embolism: heparin, then warfarin for 1–3 months (INR 2.0–3.0)	
Streptokinase: 1–1.5 million units IV over 60 min	
Alteplase: 15 mg bolus, then 0.75 mg/kg over 30 min (maximum 50 mg), then 0.50 mg/kg over 60 min (maximum 35 mg)	
Reteplase: 10 units IV bolus, then a second dose at 30 min	
Tenecteplase: weight-tiered single bolus (approximately 0.5 mg/kg with maximum of 50 mg) over 5 s	
Unstable angina or NSTEMI	
Aspirin: 162 mg PO per d	
Clopidogrel: 75 mg PO per d	
Heparin: 60 U/kg IV bolus, then 12 U/kg per h continuous infusion to keep aPTT 1.5–2.5 times control	
Enoxaparin 1 mg/kg SC bid	
Glycoprotein IIb-IIIa inhibitor depending upon risk and whether PCI is planned	
Peripheral vascular disease	
Aspirin: 160–325 mg/d for all patients with peripheral vascular disease	
Acute stroke	Use of fibrinolytics in acute CVA requires *strict* adherence to national guidelines and should be done with informed consent.
Alteplase: 90 mg over 1 h, with 0.9 mg/kg as initial bolus, if within 3 h of symptom onset and no intracranial hemorrhage on brain CT	Adjunctive use of anticoagulants must be avoided for 48 h.
Heparin: for acute cardioembolic stroke, small to moderate size, no hemorrhage on CT or MRI	Some evidence suggests that clopidogrel may be the preferred agent in patients with completed stroke.
Delay anticoagulation: for large-size stroke or poorly controlled hypertension	
Aspirin: 81 mg PO per d for completed stroke	
Clopidogrel: 75 mg PO per d	
Ticlopidine: 250 mg PO per bid	
TIA	Use clopidogrel or ticlopidine if "aspirin-failure" or aspirin allergic.
Aspirin: 81 mg PO per d	
Clopidogrel: 75 mg PO per d	
Ticlopidine: 250 mg PO bid	

Abbreviations: aPTT = activated partial thromboplastin time; AMI = acute myocardial infarction; CT = computed tomography; CVA = cerebrovascular accident; DVT = deep venous thrombosis; INR = International Normalized Ratio; MRI = magnetic resonance imaging; NSTEMI = non-ST-segment elevation myocardial infarction; PCI = percutaneous coronary intervention; PE = pulmonary embolism; SK = streptokinase; STEMI = ST-segment elevation myocardial infarction; TIA = transient ischemic attack.

widely used oral anticoagulant in North America. Readily absorbed from the gut, it reaches peak blood concentrations in 90 min and has a circulating half-life of 36 to 42 h. Warfarin is bound to albumin, metabolized by the liver, and excreted in the urine. Warfarin blocks activation of vitamin K and thereby interferes with hepatic carboxylation of coagulation factors II, VII, IX, and X. Without these vitamin K-dependent cofactors, the extrinsic coagulation pathway is blocked. Warfarin also blocks the synthesis of the antithrombotic proteins C

and S; proteins that inhibit the function of factors V and VII in the co-agulation cascade.

Warfarin dosing is guided by measurement of the International Normalized Ratio (INR), a standardized measurement of prothrombin time (PT), with a desired therapeutic range of 2 to 3 in most cases.[1] Drugs and food that interfere with warfarin absorption, binding to albumin, or hepatic metabolism can have a profound effect on warfarin activity (Table 224-2). Warfarin is contraindicated in pregnancy

TABLE 224-2 Warfarin Interactions

Consideration	Prothrombin Time (PT) or INR*
Major	
Vitamin K malabsorption or dietary deficiency	↑
Excess vitamin K	↓
Reduced gut bacteria (antibiotics)	↑
Decreased warfarin absorption	↓
Altered warfarin metabolism (cytochrome P450)	↑ or ↓
Drug effects	↑ or ↓
Other	
Decreased clotting factor production (liver disease)	↑
Increased metabolism of clotting factors (fever)	↑
Confounding technical or laboratory factors (e.g., phlebotomy, handling in transport, thromboplastin reagents)	↑ or ↓

*↑ = Prothrombin time (PT) or International Normalized Ratio (INR) prolonged; ↓ = PT or INR decreased.

because it is teratogenic (especially during the sixth to twelfth week of gestation) and causes fetal hemorrhage.

Protein C has a short half-life (8 h), and its plasma level falls quickly after starting warfarin. The coagulation factors have variable half-lives; from about 7 h for factor VII to about 60 h for prothrombin (factor II). The phase delay between the fall in protein C (an antithrombotic protein) and the fall in the affected four coagulation factors (prothrombotic proteins) results in a transient state of increased thrombogenesis at the start of warfarin therapy that lasts for about 24 to 36 h. This potential hypercoagulable state is reduced but not eliminated by initiating warfarin therapy with 5 mg/d doses.[2] For patients in whom sudden intravascular thrombosis can be fatal (e.g., those with a prosthetic heart valve), anticoagulation should be ensured with a heparin product (unfractionated or low molecular weight) before starting oral warfarin. Thus, a noncompliant patient with a prosthetic heart valve who has stopped oral anticoagulants should not simply be discharged with instructions to restart warfarin.

There is also a prothrombotic rebound during warfarin withdrawal. During the first 4 days after cessation of therapy, factors VII and IX increase more rapidly than proteins C and S, resulting in an imbalance between provokers and inhibitors of coagulation.[3] This potential hypercoagulable condition appears to exist biochemically, although prospective studies have shown no increased incidence of clinical episodes of thrombosis with sudden termination of warfarin therapy compared to gradual tapering during this interval. Thromboembolic events that occur in patients after warfarin discontinuation are related more to the underlying condition than to the method of termination.

COMPLICATIONS AND MANAGEMENT The two major complications of warfarin therapy are major bleeding episodes and skin necrosis. The most important factor influencing the risk of bleeding is the intensity of anticoagulant therapy. For most purposes, the target INR is 2.0 to 3.0, except for patients with mechanical heart valves and antiphospholipid antibody syndrome, who require more intense anticoagulation with an INR of 2.5 to 3.5. The risk of clinically significant bleeding is increased when the INR is in the 3.0 to 4.5 range, and an exponential increase in bleeding events occurs when the INR is >5.0. Reversal with vitamin K₁ or factor replacement may be necessary for major hemorrhage. Skin necrosis occurs primarily in patients with protein C deficiency. This complication usually develops 3 to 8 days after starting treatment and is caused by thrombosis of small cutaneous vessels. Treatment includes discontinuation of warfarin, administration of UFH or LMWH, vitamin K₁ administration, and screening for protein C and S deficiencies.

Bleeding is the most common complication of warfarin treatment. Risk factors for bleeding include hypertension, anemia, prior cerebrovascular disease, gastrointestinal lesions, and renal disease. Medications that increase warfarin activity and antiplatelet medications can also increase bleeding risks (see Table 224-2). The relationship between advanced age and warfarin-associated bleeding is controversial. Elderly individuals who are otherwise good candidates for anticoagulant therapy should not have it withheld because of their age. However, elderly patients require more frequent and careful monitoring.

Two general principles are important when warfarin-treated patients bleed with a prolonged INR: 1) attempt to identify and attenuate the cause of bleeding, and 2) lower the intensity of the anticoagulant effect. In patients with a high INR *without* clinically evident bleeding, cessation of warfarin, careful observation, and periodic monitoring is the safest course.[4] With clinically significant bleeding, however, reversal may be required, but the speed and extent of reversal must be balanced against the risk of recurrent thromboembolism in patients who require therapeutic anticoagulation. For example, an over-anticoagulated patient with a prosthetic mitral valve may develop fatal thrombosis if rapidly and fully reversed.

Three approaches can be taken to reverse warfarin-induced coagulopathy. The first is to stop warfarin therapy; the second is to administer vitamin K₁ (PO, SC, or IV); the third is to administer fresh-frozen plasma (FFP) or prothrombin concentrate (see Table 224-3). One mg of oral vitamin K₁ decreases the INR faster than 1 mg of subcutaneous vitamin K₁ in asymptomatic patients with elevated INR values while receiving warfarin. To reduce the risk of hemorrhage, 1 mg of oral vitamin K₁ should be considered for asymptomatic patients who are receiving warfarin and who present with an INR of 4.5 to 9.[5] Reversal is significant by 16 h, and the INR is within the therapeutic range by the second day. While subcutaneous vitamin K₁ (1 to 2 mg) reverses warfarin, with a measurable effect on the INR usually by 8 to 12 h, the response may be less predictable and delayed when compared to oral administration. At least some normal liver function is required for vitamin K₁ to be effective and to reverse the coagulopathy associated with warfarin. Low-dose oral and subcutaneous vitamin K₁ carry a small risk for patients who require therapeutic anticoagulation, and it is recommended that the emergency physician consult an appropriate specialist before using either approach.

Intravenous vitamin K₁ carries a rare but serious, non-dose-dependent risk of anaphylaxis, and should not be used for routine reversal of therapeutic over-anticoagulation. For patients who require continued anticoagulation, intravenous administration carries the risk of overcorrection not associated with oral or subcutaneous use. Intravenous vitamin K₁ should be restricted to those patients with life-threatening bleeding or with an INR >20, and for symptomatic patients poisoned by an ingestion of warfarin (suicidal overdose) or a rodenticide (brodifacoum). Generally, such patients do not require therapeutic anticoagulation, and reversal does not carry the risk of recurrent thrombosis. Because of the long half-life of these superwarfarin rodenticides, significantly poisoned patients may require treatment with high doses of vitamin K₁, up to 125 mg/d, for several weeks.

From the standpoint of the risk of recurrent thrombosis, the safest method of reversing therapeutic over-anticoagulation is with coagula-

TABLE 224-3 Emergency Treatment of Bleeding Complications of Antithrombotic Therapy

Agent	Management
Warfarin	
INR <5.0 without clinically evident bleeding	Cessation of warfarin administration and observation with serial PT/INR
INR 5–9 and no significant bleeding	Hold warfarin, may resume at lower dose once INR therapeutic Oral vitamin K_1 1–2 mg if patient at increased bleeding risk
INR >9 and no significant bleeding	Hold warfarin and monitor INR frequently Oral vitamin K_1 2–4 mg
INR >20 *or* clinically significant bleeding (major or life-threatening)	FFP: 10–15 mL/kg to acutely restore coagulation factors to ≥30% of normal Vitamin K_1: 5–10 mg slow IV infusion Vitamin K_1 therapy requires 12–24 h for full effect and may require >1 treatment Vitamin K_1 may induce unwanted thrombosis and/or overcorrection
Heparin	
Clinically significant/bleeding	Immediate cessation of heparin administration Supratherapeutic aPTT not always present Anticoagulation effect lasts up to 3 h from last dose
Minor bleeding	Observation with serial aPTT may be sufficient
Major bleeding	Protamine: 1 mg per 100 units of heparin, given slowly IV over 1–3 min to a maximum of 50 mg over any 10-min period Protamine may need to be repeated Protamine has anaphylaxis risk Protamine does not reverse LMWH (e.g., enoxaparin)
Aspirin and NSAID	
Clinically significant bleeding: correlates poorly with BT **Other Antiplatelet Agents**	Cessation of aspirin or NSAID administration Platelet transfusion to increase count by 50,000 (typically requires at least 6 units of random donor platelets) Aspirin inhibition lasts for life of affected platelets so repeat platelet transfusions sometimes required NSAID platelet inhibition typically lasts less than 1 day
Fibrinolytics	
Minor external bleeding	Manual pressure
Significant internal bleeding	Immediate cessation of fibrinolytic agent, antiplatelet agent, and/or heparin Reversal of heparin with protamine as above Typed and cross-matched blood ordered with verification of aPTT, CBC, TCT, and fibrinogen level Volume replacement with crystalloid and PRBC as needed
Massive bleeding with hemodynamic compromise	All measures listed for significant internal bleeding, above Cryoprecipitate: 10 units and recheck fibrinogen level If fibrinogen level <100 mg/dL, repeat cryoprecipitate If bleeding remains after cryoprecipitate or despite fibrinogen level >100 mg/dL: administer 2 units of FFP If bleeding continues after FFP: check BT If BT <9 min: give ϵ-aminocaproic acid 5 g IV over 60 min, then 1 g/h infusion for 8 h or until bleeding stops or tranexamic acid 10 mg/kg q6–8h If BT >9 min: give ϵ-aminocaproic acid or tranexamic acid as above with 10 units of random donor platelets
Intracranial hemorrhage	All measures listed for significant internal and massive bleeding Immediate neurosurgery consultation.

Abbreviations: aPPT = activated partial thromboplastin time; BT = bleeding time; CBC = complete blood count; INR = international normalized ratio; LMWH = low-molecular-weight heparin; FFP = fresh-frozen plasma; NSAID = nonsteroidal anti-inflammatory drug; PRBC = packed red cells; PT = prothrombin time; TCT = thrombin clotting time.

tion factor infusion using either FFP or factor concentrates. A dose of FFP 10 to 15 mL/kg (typically 3 to 4 units) will acutely restore coagulation factor levels to at least 30 percent of normal in most adults, and will control most bleeding without undue risk. Reversal of anticoagulation with FFP is usually safe for short periods, regardless of indication for anticoagulant therapy.[6] For patients with life-threatening hemorrhage and who require rapid, complete reversal, coagulation factor concentrates are more reliable and preferred.[7]

Heparin

PHARMACOLOGY OF UNFRACTIONATED HEPARIN Unfractionated heparin (UFH) is a heterogeneous mixture of polysaccharides ranging in molecular weight from 2000 to 40,000 Da. The anticoagulant effect of UFH requires binding to antithrombin III (ATIII). The heparin-ATIII complex is capable of inhibiting multiple steps in the extrinsic and common coagulation pathways, including factors Xa,

IXa, XIa, and XIIa, and thrombin (factor IIa). UFH inhibition of thrombin is dependent upon saccharide chain length, with shorter chain lengths (<18 saccharide units) possessing greater anti-Xa activity and longer chain lengths having greater antithrombin activity. These wide variations in chain lengths in UFH likely contribute to the unpredictable nature of its dose-response relationship.

UFH must be given parenterally (IV or SC). Its half-life (30 to 150 min) depends on the dose and route. Weight-based intravenous heparin-dosing protocols are the most reliable approach for achieving a therapeutic effect and preventing further thrombosis during acute thromboembolic events. The subcutaneous method is not recommended for the treatment of acute thromboembolic disease because the bioavailability of subcutaneous UFH ranges from 10 to 90 percent, depending on the dose. However, subcutaneous UFH can be used to prevent thromboembolism with a 60 to 70 percent risk reduction for DVT and fatal PE (see Table 224-1). Because UFH interferes with most laboratory investigations for hypercoagulable states, these tests should ideally be ordered before the patient is anticoagulated. Neither UFH nor low-molecular-weight heparin (LMWH) crosses the placenta; consequently, both are safe to use in pregnancy.

Despite extensive use in clinical practice over several decades, UFH continues to possess several important limitations. UFH has an unpredictable anticoagulation effect, requires frequent monitoring, and is inactivated by plasma proteins and platelet factor-4 (PF₄). The unpredictable inhibition of thrombin by UFH is attributable to a low bioavailability from extensive nonspecific binding to serum proteins, macrophages, and endothelial cells. The anticoagulant effect of heparin can be monitored with the activated partial thromboplastin time (aPTT), which is widely available from clinical laboratories (see Table 224-1).[8] There is not a linear relationship between heparin concentration, the anticoagulant activity of heparin (as measured by its antifactor Xa activity), and the aPTT. For most purposes, a therapeutic range for heparin can be either an aPTT of 1.5 to 2.5 the "normal" value, a heparin level of 0.2 to 0.4 U/mL when assayed by protamine titration, or 0.3 to 0.7 U/mL when assayed for anti-Xa activity.[8] UFH can increase the PT and INR by a variable amount, depending on the heparin concentration and the thromboplastin reagent used in the assay. Typically, therapeutic concentrations of heparin increase the PT by approximately 1 to 5 s.

PHARMACOLOGY OF LOW-MOLECULAR-WEIGHT HEPARIN FRACTION
The LMWH has made a significant contribution to the advancement of anticoagulation therapy. Both UFH and LMWH exert their anticoagulant effect by activating ATIII.[9] Their interaction with ATIII is mediated by a unique pentasaccharide sequence that is randomly distributed along the heparin chains. When ATIII interacts with the pentasaccharide sequence on the heparin molecule, it undergoes a conformational change that allows it to bind thrombin 1000 times faster. This coupling with thrombin requires an additional 13-saccharide group that brings the key binding regions of ATIII and thrombin into contact. However, only the specific pentasaccharide sequence is necessary to bind to ATIII for effective inhibition of factor Xa. UFH binds factor Xa and thrombin in roughly equal proportions (anti-Xa: anti-IIa ratio = 1.0) because chains of at least 18 residues predominate. In contrast, LMWH are manufactured from UFH through depolymerization using either a chemical or an enzymatic process. This results in a smaller molecule (4000 to 5000 Da) with less than half containing the required 13-saccharide residues to bind ATIII and thrombin. The shorter chains results in a reduced ability to inactivate thrombin and enhanced affinity for inactivating factor Xa.

There are many clinical advantages associated with the use of LMWH (Table 224-4). The plasma half-life of LMWH is two to four times as long as UFH, allowing for once- or twice-daily dosing. LMWH has a decreased binding to plasma proteins, endothelial cells, and macrophages, thus yielding a more predictable anticoagulant and dose-response relationship. This allows for subcutaneous administra-

TABLE 224-4 Advantages of LMWH Over Unfractionated Heparin

Pharmacologic Effects	Clinical Benefit
Quick and predictable SC absorption	More reliable level of anticoagulation
More stable dose response	
Resistance to inhibition by PF₄	Eliminates need for monitoring
Decreased antiheparin antibody production by 70%	Decreased incidence of thrombocytopenia
Greater anti-Xa activity	Greater antithrombotic effects
Less antithrombin activity	Potential to reduce bleeding
Ease of administration	Absence of "rebound"
	Outpatient therapy

Abbreviations: LMWH = low-molecular-weight heparin; PF₄ = platelet factor-4.

tion of fixed dosages. Laboratory monitoring of these agents is generally unnecessary except in patients with renal insufficiency and obesity. LMWH is cleared by the kidneys, and toxicity can occur in patients with significant renal impairment. LMWH therapy may be monitored by anti-Xa activity.[10] Anti-Xa activity and half-life is prolonged with decreasing renal function, resulting in a higher tendency for hemorrhagic complications. Because of the lack of clear dosing guidelines, these agents should be dosed with caution in patients with renal impairment. LMWH dosing in obese patients has not been specifically addressed in large clinical trials. Safety data in the obese population are thus derived from studies in the ACS population.[11] In these trials, LMWH dosing was based on total body weight up to a maximum of 160 kg. In patients over 160 kg, the use of anti-Xa activity should be considered.

Enoxaparin, dalteparin, and ardeparin are the most widely available of the LMWH products. Current indications for LMWH use are treatment of DVT, PE, unstable angina, and AMI. Only enoxaparin is approved for outpatient management of DVT. Although acquisition costs of LMWH are higher than for UFH, formal studies of cost-effectiveness suggest that LMWH use pays for itself, and may ultimately be cost-saving. This cost benefit can be magnified if patients with DVT are treated primarily in the outpatient setting.

COMPLICATIONS AND MANAGEMENT

Unfractionated heparin The two major complications of UFH are major bleeding episodes and HIT. Up to one-third of patients receiving heparin develop some form of bleeding complication, with a 2 to 6 percent risk for major bleeding. An increased risk (up to 20 percent) for major bleeding is associated with a number of comorbid conditions, including recent surgery or trauma, renal failure, alcoholism, malignancy, liver failure, and gastrointestinal bleeding, as well as the concurrent use of warfarin, fibrinolytics, steroids, or antiplatelet drugs.

Bleeding in patients being treated with UFH is treated according to the clinical severity and aPTT level.[12] Unfortunately, heparin-associated bleeding is not always reflected by a supratherapeutic aPTT. If bleeding develops during UFH therapy, UFH administration should be stopped immediately. While UFH half-life is dose dependent (30 to 150 min), its anticoagulation effect can last up to 3 h. Thus, observation may be appropriate in less-severe cases, with serial aPTT used to determine when therapy may be resumed. While protamine can reverse the anticoagulant effect of UFH (a ratio of 1 mg intravenous protamine neutralizes 100 units of UFH administered in the prior 4 h), the adverse effects of protamine are significant. **Protamine should be given slowly intravenously over 1 to 3 min and should not exceed 50 mg in any 10-min period.** However, because the half-life of protamine is short, a heparin rebound may occur, requiring a second treatment. Allergic reactions are possible, and **approximately 0.2 percent of patients receiving protamine develop anaphylaxis, which has a**

30 percent mortality rate. Thus, protamine should be reserved for major bleeding complications.

There are two types of HIT: type I and type II. HIT type I is the more common type, and is caused by UFH-induced direct platelet aggregation. It occurs early (1 to 5 days) and is usually transient and benign. HIT type II is caused by IgG or IgM autoantibody formation directed against both heparin and PF_4. Thus platelet activation occurs, producing both thrombocytopenia and a tendency for thrombosis. Thrombosis may involve the skin (similar to warfarin-induced cutaneous necrosis), major arteries (e.g., ischemic limbs), or the veins (e.g., recurrent DVT or PE). The onset of HIT type II is usually 5 to 12 days after UFH treatment is started, but may be sooner for patients who developed the antibody from a previous exposure. Overall, the incidence of HIT type II is between 1 and 3 percent in patients treated with UFH, but is significantly less in patients treated with LMWH products. The platelet count nadir is often modest, typically 20,000 to 150,000/μL. However, a drop of 50 percent from baseline is concerning, even if the platelet count is normal. It is important to assess for recent use of UFH or LMWH before instituting therapy for a new DVT that may in fact be a thrombotic complication of HIT.

In HIT type II, UFH therapy must be stopped as soon as the condition is recognized. Protamine is not effective against the immune-mediated response. The platelet count generally returns to normal in 4 to 6 days. During the recovery phase, however, the risk of arterial or venous thrombosis is substantially elevated, and the potential complications include gangrene, stroke, and death. It is unclear whether such patients should ever be exposed to UFH again. Thrombocytopenia appears to be less common with porcine UFH than with bovine UFH. LMWH are not recommended for use in treating HIT because of cross-reactivity between LMWH and the antiplatelet antibody. Additionally, warfarin should not be started until the patient is sufficiently anticoagulated by an alternative measure to avoid precipitating arterial or venous thrombosis or producing skin necrosis. Prophylactic transfusion of platelets is not indicated because bleeding is not usually a manifestation of HIT type II, and platelet transfusion may precipitate thrombosis. Anticoagulation with a DTI should be considered in patients with clinically suspected HIT type II, even in the absence of symptomatic thrombosis.

Low-molecular-weight heparins   In general, LMWH preparations cause less bleeding than does UFH. Reported side effects of LMWH include bleeding, HIT, local skin reaction, pruritus, and rare skin necrosis. Protamine will neutralize the antithrombin effect of LMWH, but incompletely reverses factor Xa inhibition. In the event of bleeding, 1 mg of protamine can neutralize 1 mg of enoxaparin and 100 units of dalteparin. The use of FFP and packed red blood cells should be considered in patients with ongoing or life-threatening bleeding.

Hirudin and Analogues

PHARMACOLOGY OF HIRUDIN AND HIRUDIN ANALOGUES Direct thrombin inhibitors (DTIs), hirudin and hirudin analogues, have several potential advantages over heparin. Unlike heparin, DTIs are capable of inhibiting both circulating and clot bound thrombin, do not inhibit other coagulation pathway or fibrinolytic enzymes, do not require ATIII as a cofactor, and are not inactivated by PF_4 or plasma proteins. Therefore, DTIs have a more predictable anticoagulant effect than UFH. Hirudin is a 65-amino-acid polypeptide, originally derived from the salivary gland of the medicinal leech *Hirudo medicinalis*. It is now prepared by recombinant technology. Recombinant hirudin has been modified into a number of available analogues. Currently, hirudin, lepirudin, and argatroban are currently FDA-approved for anticoagulation in patients with HIT. In the setting of AMI, unstable angina, or primary coronary intervention (PCI), hirudin reduced the incidence of death and reinfarction at 24 h, but not at 30 days postadmission. Although there were no significant differences in the inci-

dence of serious or life-threatening hemorrhagic complications, hirudin was associated with a higher incidence of moderate bleeding.[13] Currently, hirudin is approved only for patients with history of or at risk for HIT.

Synthetic analogues of hirudin are currently being studied as alternatives to heparin for the treatment of unstable angina, post-PCI use, postsurgical DVT prevention, and as an adjunct to fibrinolytic therapy. Currently, bivalirudin and argatroban are approved for use in the catheterization laboratory as an anticoagulant during PCI. In addition to hirudin, lepirudin and argatroban are used for antithrombotic treatment in patients with HIT.

COMPLICATIONS AND MANAGEMENT   The primary adverse effect of DTIs is bleeding and the majority of bleeding events occur at invasive sites. Because the half-life of hirudin and its analogues is relatively short (<2 h), and an antidote is not currently available, management of DTI-related hemorrhage may require only stopping the intravenous infusion and waiting, with coagulation factor replacement using FFP or prothrombin concentrates if bleeding persists.

ANTIPLATELET AGENTS

Aspirin and NSAIDs

PHARMACOLOGY   Aspirin irreversibly blocks cyclooxygenase, an enzyme that in the platelet catalyzes the conversion of arachidonic acid to thromboxane A_2, and in the blood vessel wall promotes prostacyclin synthesis. The net effect of aspirin in ischemic arterial beds depends on the balance between thromboxane A_2, a potent vasoconstrictor and platelet-aggregation agent, and prostacyclin, a vasodilator and platelet-aggregation inhibitor. An antithrombotic effect can be seen with doses as low as 30 mg. Because prostacyclin synthesis is stimulated at lower aspirin levels than is thromboxane A_2 conversion, treatment plans often use low-dose strategies (e.g., 81 to 162 mg/d). For more rapid antiplatelet effect, a medium or higher initial dose (e.g., 162 to 325 mg) is indicated (see Table 224-1).

Aspirin is quickly absorbed in the upper gastrointestinal tract, reaches peak blood concentrations in 15 to 20 min, and circulates with a half-life of 30 to 60 min. However, its antiplatelet effect is irreversible and lasts for the life span of the platelet (about 10 days).

Side effects of aspirin use are mainly gastrointestinal and dose related, and may be reduced with concomitant use of antacids, enteric coating, and buffering agents. Aspirin should be avoided in patients with known hypersensitivity and used cautiously in those with bleeding disorders or severe hepatic disease. Active gastrointestinal hemorrhage (e.g., bleeding peptic ulcer) is a contraindication to aspirin use. However, in AMI and unstable angina with occult gastrointestinal bleeding (e.g., guaiac-positive stool), most experts favor aspirin use with careful monitoring. Non–enteric-coated aspirn should be considered when prompt onset of action is necessary, as in patients with ongoing chest pain. Aspirin therapy is also associated with a slightly increased risk of hemorrhagic stroke (12 per 10,000 over 3 years), but this risk is balanced by a tenfold reduction in the risk of myocardial infarction and a threefold reduction in the risk of ischemic stroke.[14]

Nonsteroidal anti-inflammatory agents reversibly inhibit platelet cyclooxygenase and inhibition of platelet aggregation usually lasts less than 24 h. The exception is piroxicam, which has a 2-day half-life.

COMPLICATIONS AND MANAGEMENT   Upper gastrointestinal irritation is the most common side effect of aspirin therapy, while life-threatening gastrointestinal bleeding is uncommon.[15] As noted earlier, intracranial hemorrhage, the most feared complication of anticoagulation and antithrombotic therapy, appears to occur rarely with aspirin alone.[14] Some patients are markedly sensitive to aspirin, such that even low doses lead to markedly prolonged bleeding times and risk of severe clinical hemorrhage, particularly related to surgery or trauma. Uremic patients are especially sensitive to bleeding induced by aspirin. The combination of alcohol and aspirin can also prolong a patient's bleeding time (BT).

Unfortunately, the BT is a poor test to confirm bleeding complications of aspirin. If aspirin-associated bleeding is suspected [e.g., persistent oozing after tooth extraction despite normal platelet count (>100,000/μL) and coagulation studies], further workup should include obtaining a careful history for ingestion (significant unintentional ingestion may occur because some 300 over-the-counter medications contain aspirin), and confirmed with a salicylate level if needed. Management of acute aspirin-induced or NSAID-induced hemorrhage involves the transfusion of enough normal platelets to increase the platelet count by 50,000/μL. Because of the irreversible effect of aspirin on platelets, the hemostatic compromise might last for 4 to 5 days after aspirin has been discontinued, and platelet transfusions may have to be repeated daily, whereas NSAID-induced platelet dysfunction typically resolves within 1 day after halting use.

Clopidogrel and Ticlopidine

PHARMACOLOGY OF PLATELET MEMBRANE ALTERING AGENTS
During platelet aggregation, fibrinogen forms a bridge between adjacent platelets by binding to the glycoprotein platelet-surface receptor, labeled IIb-IIIa. A variety of agents that interfere with the platelet membrane and the glycoprotein (GP) IIb-IIIa receptor have been introduced into clinical practice during the past few years.

Clopidogrel and ticlopidine selectively inhibit platelet aggregation induced by adenosine diphosphate (ADP). Specifically, they appear to irreversibly inhibit the binding of ADP to the receptor mediating inhibition of platelet adenylate cyclase, thereby deforming the region of the platelet membrane next to its fibrinogen receptor and rendering it ineffective. Clopidogrel has been approved for the treatment of unstable angina, NSTEMI, secondary prevention of AMI and CVA, and in established peripheral artery disease.[16] Although clopidogrel is generally well tolerated, side effects include dyspepsia, rash, and diarrhea. Ticlopidine is associated with hematologic problems, such as neutropenia, idiopathic thrombocytopenic purpura, and, rarely, thrombotic thrombocytopenic purpura (TTP). Ticlopidine-related TTP occurs most often during the first 2 weeks of therapy. Clopidogrel should be considered for administration in hospitalized patients with NSTEMI or unstable angina who have a history of ASA hypersensitivity or major gastrointestinal intolerance.

COMPLICATIONS AND MANAGEMENT
TTP has rarely been reported, even after as little as 2 weeks of exposure. If quick reversal of pharmacologic effects is needed, platelet transfusion should be considered.

Abciximab, Eptifibatide, and Tirofiban

PHARMACOLOGY OF GLYCOPROTEIN IIB-IIIA RECEPTOR INHIBITORS
Damaged platelets activate several receptor sites, most notably the GP IIb-IIIa receptors. Once activated, a single fibrinogen molecule is capable of binding two GP IIb-IIIa receptor sites on adjacent platelets. Thus, GP IIb-IIIa receptors represent the final common pathway for platelet activation and aggregation.

Three parenteral GP IIb-IIIa receptor inhibitors are currently available for the treatment of unstable angina, NSTEMI, and high-risk patients undergoing PCI. Abciximab (a monoclonal antibody), eptifibatide (a synthetic peptide), and tirofiban (a nonsynthetic peptide) inhibit platelet aggregation, prevent thrombosis, and may augment thrombolysis. These agents are administered as an initial loading-dose bolus for abciximab and eptifibatide, and as a 30-min infusion for tirofiban, followed by a constant intravenous infusion. Abciximab is a noncompetitive GP IIb-IIIa inhibitor with a much longer platelet effect than its plasma half-life of 10 min; platelet function will return to normal within 48 h after discontinuing the infusion. Eptifibatide is a competitive GP IIb-IIIa inhibitor with a plasma half-life of approximately 2.5 h. Tirofiban is also a competitive GP IIa-IIIb inhibitor with a plasma half-life of approximately 2 h. Platelet functional recovery after stopping either eptifibatide or tirofiban infusion is seen in 3 to 5 h.

Improved outcome has been demonstrated in high risk unstable angina and NSTEMI patients with GP IIb-IIIa blockade who undergo PCI.[17] Glycoprotein IIb-IIIa antagonists are recommended for such patients when catheterization and PCI are planned.[18] Although a "time-dependent benefit window" for GP IIb-IIIa therapy has not been clearly established for unstable angina or NSTEMI, in patients undergoing PCI, a time-to-treatment benefit has been demonstrated with prompt initiation of eptifibatide and in the ED setting. The 2002 American College of Cardiologists (ACC)/American Heart Association (AHA) Guidelines state that the GP IIb-IIIa agent may "also be administered just prior to PCI."[18] In institutions with ready access to a catheterization laboratory, emergency physicians can expedite definitive management by initiating aggressive medical therapy in consultation with interventional cardiologists. In institutions without an on-site catheterization laboratory, emergency physicians should initiate medical therapy and transfer arrangements in collaboration with the accepting interventional cardiologist. In patients not undergoing PCI, GP IIb-IIIa antagonists are appropriate for high-risk patients, but are not recommended for low-risk patient groups.[18]

COMPLICATIONS AND MANAGEMENT
Patients receiving GP IIb-IIIa inhibitors have increased risk for bleeding complications (particularly if heparin is also used and usually related to catheterization or coronary artery bypass surgery) but have no increased risk of intracranial hemorrhage. Treatment of major hemorrhage in patients on GP IIb-IIIa inhibitors requires red cell and platelet transfusions, and replacement of coagulation factors as needed.

FIBRINOLYTICS

Although mechanisms vary, each fibrinolytic agent eventually converts plasminogen to plasmin, which then enzymatically breaks apart the fibrin component of thrombi. Currently approved fibrinolytic agents include streptokinase, anistreplase, alteplase, reteplase, and tenecteplase.

Streptokinase and Antistreplase (First Generation)

Streptokinase (SK), derived from β-hemolytic streptococci, binds to and activates circulating plasminogen, converting it to plasmin, which in turn attacks fibrin, leading to thrombus dissolution. Circulating fibrinogen also undergoes plasmin-induced lysis, producing a state of "systemic fibrinolysis." SK is administered as a slow infusion (usually 1.0 to 1.5 million U IV over 60 min) and has a serum half-life of approximately 23 min, but in most patients systemic effects persist for up to 24 h. Because of the prolonged fibrinolytic state and increased risk of hemorrhage, anticoagulation with heparin is usually delayed following treatment with SK. Anistreplase, a modified active plasminogen-streptokinase complex, has an effect similar to that of SK, but its chief advantage is that it can be administered as a slow bolus (usually 30 mg IV over 5 min) and has a serum half-life of approximately 90 min. Anistreplase has similar benefits and adverse effects compared to SK. Both SK and anistreplase are antigenic, and allergic reactions occur in approximately 6 percent of patients treated with SK and subcutaneous heparin. Antibodies to SK develop approximately 5 days after treatment and persist for 6 months; retreatment with SK or anistreplase is not advised during this interval. In addition, SK or anistreplase should not be administered within 12 months of a streptococcal infection.

Alteplase or Tissue Plasminogen Activator (Second Generation)

Alteplase or tissue plasminogen activator (tPA) is a naturally occurring enzyme in vascular endothelial cells that directly cleaves a specific peptide bond in plasminogen, converting it to active plasmin, with subsequent fibrinolysis. Alteplase has binding sites for fibrin, which would suggest specificity for activity in the thrombus and less systemic fibrinolysis. Despite the in vitro clot specificity of alteplase, its clinical side-effect profile is comparable to that of other fibrinolytics. The serum half-life of alteplase is less than 5 min, and it produces a shorter fibrinolytic state than does SK. Heparin is commonly administered shortly after the completion of alteplase infusion. Unlike SK and anistreplase, alteplase is not antigenic; allergic reactions occur in fewer than 2 percent of patients treated with alteplase and intravenous heparin. Depending on the indication, alteplase is given as a weight-based dose via an intravenous infusion over 60 to 90 min.

Reteplase and Tenecteplase (Third Generation)

Both reteplase and tenecteplase (TNK) were created from modifications of the parent alteplase molecule, with the intent of improving both efficacy and safety. Reteplase is a deletion mutant of tPA in which the fibronectin finger (high-affinity fibrin binding), epidermal growth factor (EGF), and kringle-1 (receptor binding) regions of the wild-type tPA molecule have been deleted. These modifications prolong the half-life of reteplase to 18 min, nearly fourfold longer than alteplase, allowing for bolus administration of reteplase as opposed to infusion administration of alteplase. The double-bolus reteplase regimen results in superior coronary blood flow compared to the accelerated alteplase regimen, although mortality rates are similar.

TNK resulted from creating amino acid substitutions in four different regions of the tPA molecule, with the intention of producing a molecule with an extended half-life, higher level of fibrin specificity, and superior potency. The long half-life of TNK (approximately 20 min) allows for single-weight tiered bolus dosing over 5 to 10 s. The specific amino acid substitutions also resulted in a molecule with 14-fold greater fibrin specificity than alteplase in an effort to reduce systemic plasmin generation. Point mutations in the TNK molecule have resulted in plasminogen activator inhibitor-1 resistance 80 times greater than alteplase, thus allowing for longer association of TNK with the fibrin-rich clot. In addition, no increase in thrombin–antithrombin complex was seen following administration of TNK, in contrast to a fourfold increase following administration of streptokinase and a twofold increase after administration of alteplase.[17]

Despite theoretical advantages associated with genetic modification, neither reteplase nor tenecteplase demonstrate an absolute mortality benefit in AMI. However, bolus-dose fibrinolytics result in significantly fewer medication errors, when compared to more complicated regimens.[19]

Indications for Fibrinolytic Therapy

ACUTE MYOCARDIAL INFARCTION   The National Heart, Lung, and Blood Institute has established the principle that routine STEMI patients should receive emergency reperfusion therapy, either fibrinolytic therapy initiated within 30 min or PCI within 90 min after arrival in the emergency department. There are four general criteria for emergent fibrinolytic therapy in AMI: 1) clinical presentation consistent with AMI within 12 h of symptom onset; 2) an electrocardiogram showing ST-segment elevation in two or more contiguous leads or new-onset left bundle-branch block; 3) absence of contraindications (Table 224-5); and 4) absence of cardiogenic shock. PCI, if available within 60 to 90 min of presentation, is preferred over peripheral fibrinolytic therapy for AMI with cardiogenic shock. Important additional considerations, however, include patient age, location of the infarct, relative contraindications to fibrinolysis, and duration of symptoms within the 12-h criterion.

TABLE 224-5   Contraindications to Fibrinolytic Therapy

Absolute
Active or recent internal bleeding ($\leq$14 d)
CVA <2–6 months or hemorrhagic CVA
Intracranial or intraspinal surgery or trauma <2 months
Intracranial or intraspinal neoplasm, aneurysm, or arteriovenous malformation
Known severe bleeding diathesis
On anticoagulants (warfarin with PT >15 s, heparin with increased aPTT)
Uncontrolled hypertension (i.e., blood pressure >185/100 mm Hg)
Suspected aortic dissection or pericarditis
Pregnancy
Relative*
Active peptic ulcer disease
Cardiopulmonary resuscitation >10 min
Hemorrhagic ophthalmic conditions
Puncture of noncompressible vessel <10 d
Advanced age >75 years
Significant trauma or major surgery >2 weeks and <2 months
Advanced kidney or liver disease

*Concurrent menses is *not* a contraindication.
Abbreviations: aPTT = activated partial thromboplastin time; CVA = cerebrovascular accident; PT = prothrombin time.

Patients who do *not* meet all four eligibility criteria (e.g., because symptoms have been present for >12 h or relative contraindications to fibrinolytic therapy are present) may still derive benefit from fibrinolytic therapy provided that no absolute contraindications are present and the differential diagnosis does not include disorders in which fibrinolytic therapy is harmful (e.g., aortic dissection). Under such circumstances, consultation with the physician who will assume continued definitive care of the patient (e.g., a cardiologist or internist) is reasonable and appropriate before initiating fibrinolysis.

The rapid administration of fibrinolytic therapy is of greater importance than the specific agent used. Bolus-dose fibrinolytics have the added benefit of reducing medical errors. However, despite early studies that demonstrated improvement in patient survival, recent trials investigating newer fibrinolytic agents have not achieved significant improvement in 30-day mortality and stroke rates. Defining additional mortality benefit is the subject of much debate. Most clinicians in the United States accept a 1 percent absolute difference as clinically relevant; the level of benefit found favoring alteplase versus SK. Fibrinolytic studies underscore the important relationship between restoration of normal coronary flow and survival benefit. However, an additional 1 percent mortality benefit would require near-normal coronary blood flow [Thrombolysis in Myocardial Infarction (TIMI)-3 grade] rates after fibrinolytic therapy to approach 80 percent. Most new fibrinolytic agents are only capable of generating TIMI-3 flow rates of approximately 60 to 70 percent, suggesting that additional mortality reduction is unlikely with fibrinolytics alone.

Prehospital fibrinolytic administration has a sound theoretical basis, given the critical relation between time to successful reperfusion and outcomes. Nonrandomized trials comparing prehospital administration of reteplase to hospital administration for STEMI have found the prehospital group is more likely to receive their first bolus within 30 min and achieve complete ST-segment resolution sooner.[20] Although such studies have been underpowered to determine a mortality benefit, there is a trend for lower mortality at 7 days or hospital discharge favoring prehospital fibrinolytic therapy. A prehospital strategy of electrocardiography, confirmation of fibrinolytic eligibility and administration of bolus-dose lytic appears feasible in accelerating the time to reperfusion in patients with STEMI. Although prehospital fibrinolytic therapy for AMI remains investigational, in rural and remote communities, such therapy seems medically reasonable when excessive delays (>30 min) until arrival at the hospital may occur.

DEEP VENOUS THROMBOSIS OR PULMONARY EMBOLISM
Although DVT and PE are a continuum of one disease, venous thromboembolism (VTE), management options are discussed separately. Therapy for VTE should start with an agent that has immediate anticoagulant effect (either UFH or LMWH) and it should be given at adequate dosage. Failure to reach the prescribed intensity of anticoagulation in the first 24 h of treatment is correlated with an increased risk of VTE recurrence during the next 3 months.

DVT In a patient with DVT, the goals of therapy are the prevention of pulmonary embolism and the restoration of venous patency and valvular function in order to prevent the postphlebitic syndrome. Anticoagulation, with the dose adjusted for body weight, using intravenous UFH with aPTT monitoring or subcutaneous LMWH, are both suitable options. LMWH preparations are as safe and as effective as standard heparin for the treatment of acute DVT, with a lower incidence of bleeding complications. Alternatively, recent well-controlled studies demonstrated that selected patients with DVT may safely and effectively be treated entirely at home or after a brief hospitalization. Therapeutic anticoagulation with either agent along with initiation of a vitamin K antagonist (e.g., warfarin) on the first day of treatment is standard practice. The INR should be therapeutic (target INR 2.0 to 3.0) for 2 consecutive days before the discontinuation of the UFH or LMWH. The duration of warfarin therapy following an acute DVT is typically 3 months.

The risks and benefits of fibrinolytic therapy in DVT remain uncertain. Systemic fibrinolytic therapy for DVT has shown some promise in reducing the incidence and morbidity of postphlebitic syndrome. Catheter-directed fibrinolysis has also shown some promise in the hands of highly skilled interventional radiologists. Controlled trials are lacking, and thus no formal guidelines exist regarding the use of fibrinolytic agents when treating patients with DVT.

PE Antithrombotic drugs, mechanical devices, and fibrinolytics are all used to some extent in treating this life-threatening condition. The goals of treatment are to prevent death from the embolus and to prevent any further recurrence. Occasionally, empiric therapy may be initiated based on clinical suspicion alone before diagnostic testing.

Both UFH as well as LMWH are indicated for the treatment of pulmonary embolism. A number of studies have found that LMWH is at least as effective and as safe as UFH in the treatment of PE. As with DVT, recent studies suggest that outpatient treatment of PE in a highly selective patient population is possible. Regardless of which heparin product is used, timely administration and adequate dosing are essential to good patient outcomes. Provided the patient is hemodynamically stable, adequate anticoagulation with UFH or LMWH, along with a vitamin K antagonist (e.g., warfarin), initiated during the first 24 h is standard practice. Warfarin is continued for a minimum of 3 months. The total duration of therapy is dependent upon the etiology of the thrombus.

Thrombolytic agents provide a more rapid lysis of pulmonary emboli and reduction of pulmonary hypertension than heparin.[21] Whether or not these advantages result in improved clinical outcomes and outweigh the increased risk of bleeding complications is controversial. No conclusive clinical outcome studies aimed at comparing thrombolysis with standard treatment in patients with pulmonary embolism are available. A recent meta-analysis concluded that in patients with pulmonary embolism, thrombolysis had a lower composite end point of death/reoccurrence than did heparin treatment.[21] However, the risk of intracerebral hemorrhage and other serious bleeding complications were significantly higher in patients treated with thrombolytic therapy. Other opinions suggest that there was no evidence that thrombolytic therapy decreases the mortality or the rate of reoccurrence of PE.[22] Advocates for the more liberal use of thrombolytic therapy suggest that in the presence of right ventricular strain as evidenced by echocardiography, patients may achieve better outcomes. As published in the American College of Chest Physicians (ACCP) guidelines, the use of thrombolytic agents in treating VTE is highly individualized.[23] However, most authorities agree that thrombolytic therapy may play a role in patients with massive PE complicated by hemodynamic collapse.

Currently approved fibrinolytic agents for PE include alteplase, streptokinase, and urokinase. The antigenicity and high incidence of bleeding complications associated with the 24-h infusion of SK make it a less-attractive alternative. Full anticoagulation with UFH or LMWH is not a contraindication to fibrinolysis for PE.

Vena cava filter devices are indicated for patients with contraindications to anticoagulation therapy, patients who have failed anticoagulation therapy, and patients who are at high risk of mortality from recurrent pulmonary embolism. There are a number of different devices available and most are placed percutaneously. Complications include filter migration, thrombosis, and perforation of the inferior vena cava. Anticoagulation therapy is recommended whenever possible as an adjunctive therapy with filters to help prevent thrombosis of the filter and further DVT.

ISCHEMIC STROKE The use of fibrinolytics for acute ischemic stroke to restore cerebral blood flow and to improve neurologic outcome is controversial. Only alteplase has been shown to benefit carefully selected patients with acute ischemic stroke if given within 3 h of the onset of stroke symptoms. The benefit was greater if alteplase was given within 90 min from stroke onset as measured by 24-h and 3-month outcomes.[24] Benefits are sustained up to 1 year in treated patients.[25] Conversely, there is no reduction in mortality.[25] One reason for this lack of mortality reduction is that alteplase increases the absolute risk of conversion to intracerebral hemorrhage by 6 percent, and the majority of these patients died.[26] Currently, alteplase can be recommended only if the protocol used in the National Institutes of Neurological Disorders and Stroke Tissue Plasminogen Activator Stroke Trial is strictly followed. Physicians are advised to obtain informed consent from patients or their proxies in all cases. It is best to have an emergency department policy developed in cooperation with neurologists concerning the administration of alteplase for acute CVA.

Contraindications to the use of alteplase for acute stroke include patients with rapidly improving neurologic signs or minor symptoms, significant pretreatment hypertension (blood pressure >185/110 mm Hg or requiring aggressive therapy to control), seizure at onset, or symptoms suggestive of subarachnoid hemorrhage.

Complications and Management

Compared with fibrinolytic therapy, PCI (angioplasty and/or stent placement) are the favored reperfusion strategies for high-risk patients presenting with STEMI. Unfortunately, not all patients have expeditious access to PCI. In such cases, thrombolytic therapy remains a good alternative for most patients. The most significant complications of fibrinolytic therapy are hemorrhagic, and the most catastrophic complication is intracranial hemorrhage, seen in at least 1 to 3 percent of patients.[27] Fibrinolytics should not be given to any patient with an absolute contraindication (see Table 224-5). In patients with a relative contraindication, careful weighing of potential risks and benefits of fibrinolysis in consultation with the physician who will assume in-hospital care of the patient is indicated.

Allergic reactions and anaphylaxis from SK and anistreplase should be treated with diphenhydramine 50 mg and methylprednisolone 125 mg IV. Hypotension occurs in up to 10 percent of patients treated with either SK or tPA, and is treated by slowing the fibrinolytic infusion rate and administering intravenous crystalloid, paying close attention to the patient's volume status.

To minimize the bleeding risks associated with fibrinolytic therapy, the following precautions should be observed: 1) avoid all unnecessary needle sticks; 2) avoid any arterial punctures; 3) limit venous access to easily compressible sites (e.g., avoid central lines, especially the jugular or subclavian veins); and 4) avoid both nasogastric tubes and nasotracheal intubation.

Careful monitoring of the patient is crucial. The hematocrit should be checked every 4 to 6 h after fibrinolytic therapy is initiated. A fall in hematocrit of greater than 2 percent should prompt a search for the source of blood loss. Most bleeding episodes (more than 70 percent) occur at vascular puncture sites, but intracranial, intrathoracic, retroperitoneal, gastrointestinal, genitourinary, or soft tissue extremity hemorrhage may occur.

External bleeding at any site should be controlled with prolonged manual pressure. Significant bleeding, especially from an internal site, mandates discontinuation of the fibrinolytic agent, antiplatelet agent, and heparin. Volume replacement using NS or LR solution should be provided as necessary and supplemented with red blood cell transfusions if clinically indicated. The thrombin time, aPTT, platelet count, and fibrinogen level should be checked. Heparin administered within 4 h of the onset of bleeding can be reversed with protamine.

Massive bleeding with hemodynamic compromise necessitates coagulation factor replacement in addition to the interventions recommended above. Ten units of cryoprecipitate (rich in fibrinogen) should be administered and the fibrinogen level rechecked. If the fibrinogen level is less than 100 mg/dL, the dose of cryoprecipitate should be repeated. If bleeding continues after cryoprecipitate or if bleeding persists despite a fibrinogen level above 100 mg/dL, 2 units of FFP should be given. If bleeding persists after appropriate cryoprecipitate and FFP treatments, a BT should be checked. If it is more than 9 min, 10 units of random donor platelets should be administered, followed by an antifibrinolytic agent (e.g., ε-aminocaproic acid or tranexamic acid); if the BT time is less than 9 min, platelets are unnecessary, but an antifibrinolytic agent should still be administered for continuing hemorrhage.

Fibrinolytic-associated intracranial hemorrhage requires an aggressive response. Immediately discontinue the fibrinolytic agent, antiplatelet agent, and heparin. Administer protamine in the dose outlined above if the patient received heparin. The patient should also receive cryoprecipitate, FFP, platelet transfusion, and an antifibrinolytic agent (e.g., ε-aminocaproic acid or tranexamic acid).

REFERENCES

1. Ansell J, Hirsh J, Dalen J, et al: Managing oral anticoagulant therapy. *Chest* 119(Suppl 1):22S, 2001.
2. Crowther MA, Ginsberg JB, Kearon C, et al: A randomized trial comparing 5-mg and 10-mg warfarin loading doses. *Arch Intern Med* 159:46, 1999.
3. Hirsh J, Dalen J, Anderson DR, et al: Oral anticoagulants: Mechanism of action, clinical effectiveness, and optimal therapeutic range. *Chest* 119(Suppl 1):8S, 2001.
4. Glover JJ, Morrill GB: Conservative management of over anticoagulated patients. *Chest* 108:987, 1995.
5. Crowther MA, Douketis JD, Schnurr T, et al: Oral vitamin K lowers the international normalized ratio more rapidly than subcutaneous vitamin K in the treatment of warfarin-associated coagulopathy: A randomized controlled trial. *Ann Intern Med* 137:251, 2002.
6. Makris M, Greaves M, Phillips WS, et al: Emergency oral anticoagulant reversal: The relative efficacy of infusions of fresh frozen plasma and clotting factor concentrate on correction of the coagulopathy. *Thromb Haemostat* 77:477, 1997.
7. Levine MN, Raskob G, Landefeld S, Hirsh J: Hemorrhagic complications of anticoagulant treatment. *Chest* 119(Suppl 1):108S, 2001.
8. Olson JD, Arkin CF, Brandt JT, et al: College of American Pathologists Conference XXXI on Laboratory Monitoring of Anticoagulant Therapy: Laboratory monitoring of unfractionated heparin therapy. *Arch Pathol Lab Med* 122:782, 1998.
9. Pineo GF, Hull RD: Unfractionated and low-molecular-weight heparin: Comparisons and current recommendations. *Med Clin North Am* 82:587, 1998.
10. Laposata M, Green D, Van Cott EM, et al: College of American Pathologists Conference XXXI on Laboratory Monitoring of Anticoagulant Ther-

apy: The clinical use and laboratory monitoring of low-molecular-weight heparin, danaparoid, hirudin and related compounds, and argatroban. *Arch Pathol Lab Med* 122:799, 1998.
11. Cohen M, Antman EM, Gurfinkel EP, et al: The ESSENCE (Efficacy and Safety of Subcutaneous Enoxaparin in Non-Q-wave Coronary Events) and TIMI 11B Investigators: Enoxaparin in unstable angina/non-ST-segment elevation myocardial infarction: Treatment benefits in prespecified subgroups. *J Thrombosis Thrombolysis* 12:199, 2001.
12. Hirsh J, Warkentin TE, Shaughnessy SG, et al: Heparin: Mechanism of action, pharmacokinetics, dosing considerations, monitoring, efficacy, and safety. *Chest* 119(1 Suppl):64S, 2001.
13. The Global Use of Strategies to Open Occluded Coronary Arteries (GUSTO) IIb investigators: A comparison of recombinant hirudin with heparin for the treatment of acute coronary syndromes. *New Engl J Med* 335:775, 1996.
14. He J, Whelton PK, Vu B, Klag MJ: Aspirin and risk of hemorrhagic stroke: A meta-analysis of randomized controlled trials. *JAMA* 280:1930, 1998.
15. Hirsh J, Dalen JE, Fuster V, et al: Platelet-active drugs: The relationship among dose, effectiveness, and side effects. *Chest* 119(Suppl 1):39S, 2001.
16. The Clopidogrel in Unstable Angina to Prevent Recurrent Events (CURE) trial investigators: Effects of clopidogrel in addition to aspirin in patients with acute coronary syndromes without ST-segment elevation. *New Engl J Med* 345:494, 2001.
17. Cannon CP, Weintraub WS, Demopoulos LA, et al: Comparison of early invasive and conservative strategies in patients with unstable coronary syndromes treated with the glycoprotein IIb-IIIa inhibitor tirofiban. *New Engl J Med* 344:1879, 2001.
18. Braunwald E, Antman EM, Beasley JW, et al: ACC/AHA guidelines for the management of patients with unstable angina and non-ST-segment elevation myocardial infarction: A report of the American College of Cardiology/American Heart Association Task Force on Practice Guidelines (Committee on the Management of Patients with Unstable Angina). *J Am Coll Cardiol* 26:970, 2000. Updated March 2002, at www.acc.org and www.americanheart.org.
19. Cannon CP: Thrombolysis medication errors: Benefits of bolus thrombolytic agents. *Am J Cardiol* 85:17C, 2000.
20. Morrow DA, Antman EM, Sayah A, et al: Evaluation of the time saved by pre-hospital initiation of reteplase for ST-elevation MI: Results of the Early Retavase (ER-TIMI 19) Trial. *J Am Coll Cardiol* 40:71, 2002.
21. Agnelli G, Becattini C, Kirschstein T: Thrombolysis vs heparin in the treatment of pulmonary embolism: A clinical outcome-based meta-analysis. *Arch Intern Med* 162:2537, 2002.
22. Dalen JE: The uncertain role of thrombolytic therapy in the treatment of pulmonary embolism. *Arch Intern Med* 162:2521, 2002.
23. Hyers TM, Angelli G, Hull RD, et al: Antithrombotic therapy for venous thromboembolic disease. *Chest* 119(Suppl 1):176S, 2001.
24. Marler JR, Tilley BC, Lu M, et al: Earlier treatment associated with better outcome: The NINDS-TPA Stroke Study. *Neurology* 55:1649, 2002.
25. Kwiatkowski TG, Libman RB, Frankel M, et al: Effects of tissue plasminogen activator for acute ischemic stroke at one year. *New Engl J Med* 340:1781, 1999.
26. The NINDS-TPA Stroke Study group: Intracerebral hemorrhage after intravenous tPA therapy for ischemic stroke. *Stroke* 28:2109, 1997.
27. Levine MN, Goldhaber SZ, Gore JM, et al: Hemorrhagic complications of thrombolytic therapy in the treatment of myocardial infarction and venous thromboembolism. *Chest* 108(Suppl 4):291S, 1995.

EMERGENCY COMPLICATIONS OF MALIGNANCY
Paul Blackburn

Most cancer patients experience at least one emergency during the course of the disease, and emergency physicians are increasingly being confronted with complications related to cancer or its treatment. The approach to the patient with potential complications may be confounded by many variables. Patients may be uncomfortable discussing their disease or its extent or may not be knowledgeable concerning the condition or its therapy. The emergency physician may be unfamiliar with the large number or combinations of chemotherapeutic agents or with the complex classification and staging of malignancies. The biologic variation in cancer progression and response to treatment makes for imprecise prognostic predictions in individual patients.

Trends in cancer management include an aging population with a concomitant increased prevalence of malignant disease, aggressive chemotherapeutic regimens with broader applications, and longer patient survival. All place demands on the ability of the emergency physician to recognize and treat a broad spectrum of oncologic emergencies.

Emergencies related to cancer or its therapy can be broadly categorized into those created by local tumor effects, due to biochemical derangement, from hematologic derangement, or related to therapy (Table 225-1).

RELATED TO LOCAL TUMOR EFFECTS

Pathologic Fractures

Anatomic disruption of diseased bone resulting from normal but stressful activity is termed a *pathologic fracture*. The skeleton is most commonly affected by metastases, mostly in the axial skeleton and proximal aspect of the limbs, where the red marrow is located.[1] Patients present with bone pain and history of a primary cancer. Only rarely will the fracture represent the first evidence of malignancy. Plain radiographs are usually sufficient for initial imaging. Computed tomography evaluates the three-dimensional bone integrity and soft tissue extension, whereas magnetic resonance imaging delineates soft tissue and bone marrow involvement.[2]

The goals of treatment are pain relief and restoration of ambulation or function, through IV narcotics and fracture immobilization. Nondisplaced fractures in non-weight-bearing bones are occasionally managed conservatively, but most are treated surgically. Criteria for hospitalization include those with neurologic deficits, fractures through lesions of unknown origin involving the hip or femur (the most disabling fractures), comminuted or irreducible fractures, and those with hemodynamic compromise.[2]

Acute Spinal Cord Compression

Up to 20 percent of patients with neoplastic involvement of the vertebral column and 5 to 10 percent of all patients with cancer will develop spinal cord compression. Patients present with unrelenting, progressive back pain that usually worsens when supine, unlike most other musculoskeletal cases of back pain. The thoracic vertebrae are most often involved. Weakness is most apparent in the proximal extremity musculature and may progress to complete paralysis. Sensory changes initially may be confined to a band of hyperesthesia around the trunk at the involved spinal level or eventually become anesthetic distal to the level. Urinary retention (with overflow incontinence), fecal incontinence, and impotence are late manifestations.[2]

Plain films may identify the level of vertebral collapse and deformity. Magnetic resonance imaging is the imaging tool of choice to define the site and degree of cord compression and to identify the presence of additional vertebral lesions. Computed tomography with or without myelography is used when magnetic resonance imaging is contraindicated or inaccessible.[2]

Initial pain control is done with narcotic analgesics. Definitive pain control is achieved through the use of corticosteroids, radiation therapy, surgery, or a combination of modalities and will depend on the life expectancy of the patient, extent of disease, and degree of motor impairment (ambulatory vs. nonambulatory vs. paraplegic status). The usual steroid dose is dexamethasone 10 mg IV bolus, followed by 4 mg PO or IV every 6 h.[2]

Upper Airway Obstruction

Malignancy-related airway obstruction is insidious, rarely an emergent problem, and due to tumors arising in the oropharynx, neck, and superior mediastinum. Acute compromise may occur due to supervening infection, hemorrhage, or inspissated secretions. Soft tissue plain films may assist in defining the soft tissue architecture. Due to the distortion of local anatomy, fiberoptic laryngoscopy is often necessary to evaluate the airway lumen size. If immediate airway control is required, options include cricothyrotomy, jet insufflation, or emergency tracheostomy.

Malignant Pericardial Effusion with Tamponade

The most common sources of malignant pericardial effusions are breast and lung cancer, although other malignancy-related etiologies include mediastinal radiation, infection, and certain chemotherapeutic agents. Symptoms of pericardial effusion are a function of accumulation rate and total volume. Collections greater than 500 mL may be well tolerated with gradual development. Sudden accumulation or hemorrhage may cause dyspnea, chest pain, or hypotension.

Classic features of cardiac tamponade are 1) hypotension and narrowed pulse pressure, 2) jugular venous distention, 3) diminished heart sounds, 4) pulsus paradoxus greater than 10 mm Hg, 5) low QRS voltage on the electrocardiogram, and 6) cardiomegaly without radiographic evidence of congestive heart failure. Diagnosis of the pericardial effusion can be confirmed with echocardiography or bedside transthoracic ultrasound. Although sonographic features of pericardial tamponade may be seen, the absence of these features does not exclude tamponade, and the decision to emergently intervene is made by evidence of inadequate cardiac output.

Emergency pericardiocentesis can be lifesaving, although classic blind pericardiocentesis has been associated with mortality rates of up to 6 percent. Echo-guided pericardiocentesis is safe, effective, and well tolerated, and Doppler mode allows evaluation of the hemodynamic effects of the effusion and treatment.[3] Care of the stable patient should include discussion with an oncologist. The tumor type, symptom severity, and prognosis are considered in determining a treatment plan that might include systemic chemotherapy, intrapericardial chemotherapy or sclerotherapy, or creation of a pleuropericardial window.

Superior Vena Cava Syndrome

Superior vena cava (SVC) syndrome occurs by compression of the thin-walled SVC carrying blood at low pressure through the nondis-

TABLE 225-1 Emergency Complications of Malignancy

Related to local tumor effects
  Pathologic fractures
  Acute spinal cord compression
  Upper airway obstruction
  Malignant pericardial effusion with tamponade
  Superior vena cava syndrome
Related to biochemical derangement
  Hypercalcemia
  SIADH, hyponatremia
  Adrenocortical insufficiency
  Tumor lysis syndrome
Related to hematologic derangement
  Granulocytopenia and infection
  Hyperviscosity syndrome
  Thromboembolism
Related to therapy
  Chemotherapy-induced nausea and vomiting
  Pain control
  Systemic therapy emergencies
  Renal and urologic syndromes

Abbreviation: SIADH = syndrome of inappropriate antidiuretic hormone.

tensible mediastinum by primary tumor or superior mediastinal nodes. Up to 97 percent of patients with SVC syndrome have a malignant cause, with lung cancer accounting for 65 to 80 percent of cases. Those diagnosed with SVC syndrome usually do not die of the syndrome itself but of the underlying disease.[4]

Symptoms are usually easy to recognize, the most common being facial swelling, with venous engorgement of the trunk, upper extremities, and neck. The skin may have a slightly violet hue, mimicking cyanosis. Dyspnea, orthopnea, and cough are common complaints, as are headache, nausea, dizziness, and visual disturbances. Neurologic involvement with obtundation, seizures, or coma may be secondary to metastatic disease and cerebral edema from venous occlusion. The more rapid the compression onset, the more severe the symptoms due to lack of time for collateral vessel development. Histologic diagnosis is desirable before definitive treatment is initiated, if possible. Sputum cytology is the simplest method and can yield a diagnosis in two-thirds of patients.

Initial management is head elevation, rest, cautious administration of fluids, and supplemental oxygen. Diuretics (furosemide 40 mg IV) for temporary relief of symptoms and glucocorticoids (methylprednisolone 125 mg IV, or dexamethasone 16 to 20 mg IV) are often recommended, but their roles are unclear. Most patients with SVC syndrome are treated nonoperatively with radiotherapy, chemotherapy, or both. In addition, vena caval stents, adjuvant therapy with anticoagulants, and surgical procedures may be considered after stabilization.

RELATED TO BIOCHEMICAL DERANGEMENT

Hypercalcemia

Hypercalcemia is one of the most common metabolic complications of malignancy, occurring in 20 to 30 percent of patients at some time during the course of their disease and more commonly in patients with advanced disease.[5–6]

Symptoms are referable to almost any organ system and depend on the level of plasma calcium, the rate of rise, and the general medical condition of the patient. Gastrointestinal symptoms such as anorexia, nausea, vomiting, and constipation are early, frequent features that may be mistakenly attributed to underlying disease or therapy. Neurologic manifestations occur in more than 50 percent of patients, including cognitive and behavioral changes, altered mental status, and neuromuscular disturbance. Psychiatric symptoms may resemble schizophrenia or mania. Renal involvement includes polydipsia and polyuria due to interference with antidiuretic hormone (ADH) action at the distal nephron, causing a diabetes insipidus-like syndrome. The resulting dehydration further exacerbates the existing dehydration.[5]

Normal calcium regulation is through the interaction of parathyroid hormone (PTH), calcitonin, and $1,25(OH)_2$ vitamin D. In malignancy, the breakdown of normal regulation leads to increased bone resorption in all cases and occasionally to decreased renal excretion of calcium. The most common cause of hypercalcemia of malignancy is by production of a PTH-related peptide that is structurally similar to PTH. The PTH-related peptide binds to PTH receptors, thereby mobilizing calcium from bones and increasing renal reabsorption of calcium.[5,6] Some malignancies, such as multiple myeloma, secrete a factor or factors that stimulate osteoclasts to resorb bone.[5]

Significant hypercalcemia is a true metabolic emergency. Due to the invariable dehydration present, continuous administration of intravenous isotonic saline at a rate based on severity of hypercalcemia, degree of dehydration, and ability to tolerate volume expansion is initiated and will result in a modest decrease in the plasma calcium. Clinical improvement will improve over 24 to 48 h but rarely normalizes the level. Forced saline diuresis with large doses of furosemide 80 to 100 mg IV every 2 h, increases renal excretion of calcium, but only after adequate hydration. Calcitonin 4 to 8 U/kg SC or IM every 6 to 12 h, lowers plasma calcium within 2 to 4 h. It may cause a hypersensitivity response, and tachyphylaxis develops within 3 days.[5,6] Glucocorticoids may

blunt the tachyphylaxis and may be helpful in the short term in and of themselves, especially with sensitive tumors such as lymphoma and myeloma.[5–7] Bisphosphonates are potent inhibitors of bone resorption and produce a sustained decrease in calcium for approximately 2 to 4 weeks beginning 12 to 48 h after administration. Bisphosphonate is given slowly to prevent precipitation of bisphosphonate-calcium complexes in the kidney and subsequent renal failure. Gallium nitrate, mithramycin, and plicamycin are used infrequently due to their toxicity.[5,6] Dialysis is indicated for those with profound mental status changes, renal failure, or unable to tolerate a saline load.[6–8]

Syndrome of Inappropriate ADH, Hyponatremia

Ectopic secretion of ADH may be present with a variety of malignancies or from stimulation of ADH release from chemotherapy, narcotics, carbamazepine, and selective serotonin reuptake inhibitors.[8] Regardless of the etiology, the syndrome of inappropriate ADH consists of hyponatremia, less than maximally dilute urine, excessive urine sodium excretion ($U_{Na} > 30$ mEq/L), and decreased serum osmolality, all in the presence of euvolemia, absence of diuretic therapy, and normal renal, adrenal, and thyroid function (see Chap. 27).

Hyponatremia is the most common electrolyte abnormality in cancer patients. Signs and symptoms are primarily neurologic and correlate with severity and with rapidity of development. Anorexia, nausea, and malaise are the earliest findings, followed by headache, confusion, obtundation, seizures, and coma. Seizures are tonic clonic and, if recurrent, require treatment with hypertonic saline. Focal seizures require more in-depth evaluation. Life-threatening symptoms are nearly invariably present with sodium concentrations below 105 mEq/L.[8]

Water restriction is the mainstay of treatment. Patients with sodium levels above 125 mEq/L are generally asymptomatic and can be managed with water restriction of 500 mL per d and close follow-up. More severe symptoms may require furosemide (0.5 to 1.0 mg/kg) administration, with concomitant administration of NS to maintain euvolemia and effect a net free water clearance. Demeclocycline (300 to 600 mg bid) is a tetracycline derivative that will induce a drug-induced diabetes insipidus, allowing continued water intake and improvement in sodium level. Three percent hypertonic saline (51 mEq sodium/dL) can be given, with or without furosemide, for rapid correction. The hypertonic saline amount must be carefully calculated to avoid volume overload or too rapid correction, with subsequent osmotic demyelination syndrome (central pontine myelinolysis). The rate of correction of hyponatremia is controversial, but a rate of 0.5 mEq/L per h, with not more than a 12- to 15-mEq increase in the first 24 h, is recommended (see Chap. 27). Coincident hypokalemia requires repletion, because plasma potassium elevation can raise the serum sodium concentration.[8]

Adrenal Insufficiency

Adrenal insufficiency may be related to adrenal gland replacement by metastases or suppression from glucocorticoid administration, with adrenal function insufficient to support the patient stressed by infection, metabolic disruption, or surgery. Adrenal crisis with vasomotor collapse may be sudden and fatal. Clues to possible adrenal insufficiency may include mild hypoglycemia, hyponatremia, hyperkalemia, and eosinophilia. The stressed and steroid dependent patient empirically should be given intravenous steroids with glucocorticoid and mineralocorticoid effects. Appropriate emergency stress doses of hydrocortisone hemisuccinate are 200 to 500 mg IV (see Chap. 217). In suspected cases of adrenal insufficiency, a serum cortisol should be drawn before steroid treatment.

Tumor Lysis Syndrome

Tumor lysis syndrome is a set of metabolic abnormalities resulting from acute destruction of neoplastic cells, with release of intracellular contents into the circulation overwhelming the body's homeostatic mechanisms for handling potassium, calcium, phosphorus, and uric acid. Abnormalities may occur individually or in combination. It is more common with hematologic malignancies and may occur spontaneously or after cytotoxic therapy. Morbidity (primarily renal failure) depends on the type and extent of tumor, treatment type, and pre-existing renal function. Prophylaxis with intravenous fluids and allopurinol has greatly reduced the incidence of tumor lysis syndrome.

Catabolism of DNA and RNA produces uric acid, which may precipitate in the renal tubules. Malignant cells may contain up to four times the amount of phosphorus as normal cells. As phosphate increases, it combines with calcium and precipitates in soft tissue and renal tubules, leading to hypocalcemia and renal failure. Hyperkalemia is the most life-threatening derangement of tumor lysis syndrome. The sudden increase in potassium results in the well-described presentation of cardiac arrhythmias and death.[6–8]

Treatment of hyperuricemia includes urine alkalinization through addition of sodium bicarbonate to intravenous fluids or administration of acetazolamide, with a goal of urine pH at or above 7.0. Excessively alkaline urine increases the likelihood of calcium phosphate precipitation in the renal tubules. Hyperkalemia is treated with the usual regimen of β-adrenergic agonists, glucose, insulin, and sodium-potassium exchange resin (see Chap. 27). Calcium administration is to be avoided unless there is evidence of cardiovascular instability (electrocardiographic changes) or neuromuscular irritability (Chvostek or Trousseau sign), because supplemental calcium may cause metastatic precipitation of calcium phosphate. Hyperphosphatemia is managed with phosphate binders (limited effect) or by the administration of glucose and insulin. Hemodialysis is effective in correcting all abnormalities of tumor lysis syndrome, although the large phosphate burden may require repeat dialysis at 12- to 24-h intervals.[8]

RELATED TO HEMATOLOGIC DERANGEMENT

Granulocytopenia and Infection

A febrile, neutropenic patient is an absolute medical emergency. Neutropenia, or an absolute neutrophil count of fewer than 500/μL, is the most frequent factor predisposing patients with cancer to infection, especially bacteremia. If untreated, the mortality rate of a neutropenic patient with a bacteremic infection is about 50 percent.[6] The most common presenting symptom is fever, defined as a temperature of 38.3° C on one occasion or 38.0° C for longer than 1 h.

Due to an impaired inflammatory response and granulocytopenia, the usual findings of infection may be muted or masked. Signs of infection, such as purulence, may not develop, and erythema or pain may be the only findings. During the physical examination, all portals of entry, including mucosal surfaces, must be inspected. Funduscopic examination may show evidence of disseminated infection or papilledema. Manifestations of pneumonia may be auscultatory only, because granulocytopenia may preclude development of a visible infiltrate on chest radiograph. A detailed skin examination, in particular the perirectal area of acute leukemia patients, is important. **Digital rectal examination is relatively contraindicated in neutropenic patients and should be withheld until after initial antibiotic administration.** Clotted catheters represent a high risk of infection due to bacterial colonization, and central venous catheters may be associated with the development of endocarditis.[9]

To evaluate for occult infection, ancillary tests include blood and urine cultures and chest radiograph. Sputum, stool, and wound drainage Gram's stain and culture should be obtained if productive cough, diarrhea, or wound drainage is present. Lumbar puncture is not routine, because the incidence of meningitis is not increased with neutropenia.

The choice of initial empiric antimicrobial therapy should be broad spectrum to cover the range of potential bacterial pathogens. There are several combination regimens in use. Bacteremia is most frequently due to aerobic gram-positive cocci (coagulase-negative staphylococci, viridans streptococci, or *Staphylococcus aureus*) or aerobic gram-negative bacilli (*Escherichia coli, Klebsiella pneumoniae,* or *Pseudomonas aeruginosa*). An aminoglycoside combined with an antipseudomonal β-lactam has become standard for empiric treatment. Vancomycin should be added if the following are present: severe mucositis, catheter infection, quinolone prophylaxis, hypotension, institutions with methicillin-resistant *S. aureus,* or known colonization with resistant gram-positive organisms.[6–9] Fungi are common secondary infections in those who have received courses of broad-spectrum antibiotics.[9]

Hyperviscosity Syndrome

Hyperviscosity syndrome describes a group of pathologic conditions in which blood flow is impaired due to abnormal blood characteristics. The flow properties of blood are dependent on its fluid and cellular contents. Abnormal plasma contents are most commonly Waldenström macroglobulinemia, followed by immunoglobulin A myeloma. Hyperproduction of any cell line can lead to hyperviscosity.[10] Polycythemia (with a hematocrit >60 percent) and leukemias (with a white blood cell count >100,000/μL or a leukocrit >10 percent) often are associated with clinically significant hyperviscosity. Dehydration will exacerbate the effects of all hyperviscosity syndromes.

Initial symptoms are vague and may include fatigue, abdominal pain, headache, or, most commonly, altered mental status. Thrombosis may occur, with the creation of focal or unusual findings. Specific physical findings other than retinal hemorrhages, exudates, and "sausage-linked" vessels are rare. The diagnosis depends on a high index of suspicion coupled with laboratory findings. The peripheral blood smear may reveal *rouleaux* formation (red cells stacked like coins). The laboratory may be unable to perform serological testing due to serum stasis in the analyzers. Serum viscosity and protein electrophoresis can be diagnostic.

Initial therapy consists of intravascular volume repletion, early involvement of a hematologist, and emergency plasmapheresis. When coma is present and the diagnosis established, a temporizing measure can be a two-unit (1000 mL) phlebotomy with concomitant volume replacement with 2 to 3 L of NS.

Thromboembolism

Thromboembolism occurs with all tumor types and is the second leading cause of death in cancer patients. Symptomatic deep venous thrombosis (DVT) occurs in approximately 15 percent of all patients with cancer and up to 50 percent of those with advanced malignancies.[11] A hypercoagulable state, decreased proteins C, S, and antithrombin III, the effect of metastases on activation of the coagulation pathway, chemotherapy, invasive procedures, and long-term venous catheterization increase thromboembolism risk.[12]

Coagulation activation may contribute to the tumor progression; as such, anticoagulants may have anticancer activity. Treatment with low molecular weight heparin (LMWH) or unfractionated heparin as a bridge to chronic warfarin therapy is appropriate for most newly diagnosed cases of DVT, although some recommend the use of LMWH in view of data suggesting a survival advantage for cancer patients receiving LMWH. **Cancer patients do not appear at increased risk for anticoagulant-related bleeding complications, including those with brain metastases.** More frequent monitoring of the International Normalized Ratio is required, because warfarin is more difficult to control than in other patients.[11] Thrombolytic therapy for treatment of DVT is not indicated, because anticoagulant therapy alone is generally successful.

A pulmonary embolus with hemodynamic stability is treated with unfractionated heparin or LMWH. Because of the high mortality rate for pulmonary embolus and hemodynamic instability, right ventricular fail-

TABLE 225-2   Antiemetic Agents (Adult Dosages)

Class and Agent	Dose	Comments
Dopamine receptor antagonists		
Metoclopramide	10 mg IV or IM	Dose-related extrapyramidal side effects
Promethazine	25 mg IV	IV use common but not approved
Serotonin (5-HT$_3$) antagonists		
Dolasetron	1.8 mg/kg up to 100 mg IV	Constipation, headaches (all)
Granisetron	10 μg/kg IV over 5 min	
Ondansetron	32 mg IV over 15 min	
Corticosteroids		
Dexamethasone	20 mg IV	Mechanism unknown, no immunosuppression
Benzodiazepines		
Lorazepam	1–2 mg IV	Sedation, anxiolysis
Histamine receptor antagonists		
Diphenhydramine	50 mg IV or IM	Minor therapeutic effect

ure, or thrombus in the right atrium or ventricle, thrombolytic therapy is recommended. Of the available agents, no agent or dosing range has currently been shown to be superior to another. Less ill patients should not receive thrombolytic therapy, because major bleeding can occur in 20 percent of patients, and there is no improvement in mortality. However, a blocked indwelling catheter due to catheter tip thrombosis can be treated with a local infusion of low-dose thrombolytic therapy.[12] This is best done with the approval of the local specialist.

RELATED TO THERAPY

Chemotherapy-Induced Nausea and Vomiting

Nausea and vomiting can be debilitating to an already compromised patient. Commonly used antiemetics include benzodiazepines, corticosteroids, dopamine antagonists, neuroleptics, and serotonin (5-HT$_3$) receptor antagonists (Table 225-2). Although there is no definite superiority for any group or combination of agents, the most common regimens are a combination of metoclopramide or a 5-HT$_3$ receptor antagonist plus dexamethasone. Although lorazepam has no direct antiemetic efficacy, its addition will provide sedation and anxiolysis and a measurable decrease in emesis.[13]

Pain Control

The pain associated with cancer requires aggressive treatment and avoidance of "oligoanalgesia," a term describing the underuse of analgesics. Physicians are generally poor at adequately treating pain, with the usual reasons given as fear of adverse effects, such as respiratory depression or addiction with prolonged courses of treatment. The concern of causing addiction in the patient with significant cancer-related pain should be disregarded. First-line therapy should be parenteral opioids, which allows for a more rapid onset of action and titratability. Nonopioid analgesics (aspirin, acetaminophen, other nonsteroidal agents) may act as adjuvants, allowing lower narcotic dosages, and should be concomitantly administered if there are no contraindications.[14] Corticosteroids also can be used as opioid adjuvants, usually in patients in the terminal phases of cancer, although drug, dose, route, and schedule are not standardized.[7]

Systemic Therapy Emergencies

The two emergencies related to systemic therapy are drug extravasation and hypersensitivity reactions. Most chemotherapeutic agents cause different degrees of local tissue injury when extravasated. If extravasation occurs through a peripheral line, the infusion is stopped and aspiration through the line is attempted. If an antidote exists, it is administered

through the original line while avoiding pressure to the area to prevent further dispersion of material (Table 225-3). Conservative measures include rest and elevation. There are no indications for corticosteroids or the use of bicarbonate to alter local pH. Hyaluronidase injected locally has been shown to enhance absorption of some drugs. Topical dimethyl sulfoxide has been proposed as an antidote, because of its potent free radical-scavenging properties, plus its possible capacity to hasten the removal of drug from tissue. Hypersensitivity reactions are treated in the usual manner with epinephrine, H$_1$ and H$_2$ blockers, intravenous fluids, nebulized albuterol, and steroids as needed.[15]

Renal and Urologic Syndromes

Urologic emergencies in cancer patients are common and consist of bladder hemorrhage, obstruction, and infection.

Bladder hemorrhage may be a presenting sign of malignancy or secondary to tumor invasion, chemotherapy, radiation therapy, or infection. It can evolve into a life-threatening emergency, with clot retention, obstruction, or hemodynamic instability. Initial treatment is a multiple-hole bladder catheter with continuous saline lavage and, occasionally, endoscopic clot evacuation in the operating room, if required. Methods of controlling bleeding have included intravesicular agents (alum, prostaglandins, phenol, and silver nitrate), iced saline lavage, and oral or parenteral aminocaproic acid, all with different degrees of success.

TABLE 225-3   Antidotes for Extravasated Cytotoxic Drugs

Drug	Antidotes	Comments
Anthracyclines	Dimethyl sulfoxide	Apply topically, allow to dry, repeat
	Ice packs	Repeat every 6–8 h
Mitomycin	Dimethyl sulfoxide	Apply topically, allow to dry, repeat
Cisplatin, mechlorethamine	Sodium thiosulfate	Prepare 0.17 mol/L solution: mix 4 mL 10% wt/vol sodium thiosulfate with 5 mL sterile water, inject into extravasation site
Vinca alkaloids	Hyaluronidase	Reconstitute with normal saline, inject 150–900 U into extravasation site
	Warm packs	
Paclitaxel	Hyaluronidase	Reconstitute with normal saline, inject 150–900 U into extravasation site
	Ice packs	

Obstruction of the ureters may be due to direct tumor invasion or compression, retroperitoneal lymph node encasement, or, rarely, by direct metastases. Surgery, chemotherapy, or radiation therapy may cause retroperitoneal fibrosis with compression. Clinically, acute unilateral obstruction will appear identical to ureterolithiasis, whereas chronic unilateral obstruction is a silent event incidentally discovered as hydronephrosis on computed tomography. Bilateral chronic ureteral obstruction will present with decreased urine output and uremia. Urologic consultation for relief of obstruction is required.

Lower tract obstruction can be caused by mechanical or neurophysiologic factors. The combination of antiemetic and pain medications with hydration may precipitate urinary retention in those with preexisting prostatism. Relief is obtained with bladder catheters, with a coudé tip if passage of standard catheters cannot be accomplished.

REFERENCES

1. Coleman RE: Skeletal complications of malignancy. *Cancer* 80(suppl):1588, 1997.
2. Manglani HH, Rex AWM, Picciolo A, et al: Orthopedic emergencies in cancer patients. *Semin Oncol* 27:299, 2000.
3. Tsang TS, Seward JB, Barnes ME, et al: Outcomes of primary and secondary treatment of pericardial effusion in patients with malignancy. *Mayo Clin Proc* 75:248, 2000.
4. Wudel LJ, Nesbitt JC: Superior vena cava syndrome. *Curr Treat Options Oncol* 2:77, 2001.
5. Grill V, Martin TJ: Hypercalcemia of malignancy. *Rev Endocr Metab Disord* 1:253, 2000.
6. Krimsky WS, Behrens RJ, Kerkvliet GI: Oncologic emergencies for the internist. *Cleve Clin J Med* 69:209, 2002.
7. Woolridge JE, Anderson CM, Perry MC, et al: Corticosteroids in advanced cancer. *Oncology* 15:225, 2001.
8. Flombaum CD: Metabolic emergencies in the cancer patient. *Semin Oncol* 27:322, 2000.
9. Quadri TL, Brown AE: Infectious complications in the critically ill patient with cancer. *Semin Oncol* 27:335, 2000.
10. Kwann HC, Bongu A: The hyperviscosity syndromes. *Semin Thromb Hemost* 25:199, 1999.
11. Ornstein DL, Zacharski LR: Cancer, thrombosis, and anticoagulants. *Curr Opin Pulmon Med* 6:301, 2000.
12. Lee AY: Treatment of venous thromboembolism in cancer patients. *Thromb Res* 102:V195, 2001.
13. Oettle H, Riess H: Treatment of chemotherapy-induced nausea and vomiting. *J Cancer Res Clin Oncol* 127:340, 2001.
14. Blackburn PA, Vissers R: Pharmacology of emergency department pain management and conscious sedation, in Pollack C (ed): *Emergency Medicine Clinics of North America*. Philadelphia, WB Saunders, 2000, p. 803.
15. Albanell J, Baselga J: Systemic therapy emergencies. *Semin Oncol* 27:347, 2000.
16. Russo P: Urologic emergencies in the cancer patient. *Semin Oncol* 27:284, 2000.

THE NEUROLOGIC EXAMINATION IN THE EMERGENCY SETTING

J. Stephen Huff

Andrew D. Perron

The key to evaluation of patients with neurologic problems is the medical history; in most patients, the physical examination confirms thoughts formulated during history taking. Time of onset, symptom progression, associated symptoms, and exacerbating factors are key historical points. Another axiomatic point is that the neurologic examination does not exist in isolation from the general physical examination or imaging procedures. Rarely does the neurologic examination delineate a problem not suggested by the patient's history or general physical examination. Few findings of the neurologic examination are pathognomonic of clinical conditions or sufficiently specific that examination alone secures the diagnosis. Further complicating the value of the neurologic examination are that the sensitivity and specificity of different examination techniques have not been rigorously investigated and the degree of interobserver variability is not known.

The idea of performing a "complete" examination in the emergency department is misleading, because most frequently a "complete" examination is neither required nor appropriate. An adequate examination is one that is sufficient for the task at hand. The examination detailed in this chapter is arbitrarily divided into eight sections, and basic and advanced levels are described for each section. Much of this information should be a review for the reader, but it is hoped that this simple framework will help with organization and in the approach to the patient.

Examination of children follows the same framework as that for adults, but even more information is gathered indirectly by observation. For example, interacting with a child playing with a toy or other object allows the examiner to assess vision, extraocular motion, coordination, and strength as the child reaches for and grasps the toy.

Traditional neurologic formulation follows a three-tiered approach: 1) Is there a lesion of the nervous system? 2) Where is the lesion? 3) What is the lesion? History is the key to answering these questions, with the physical examination useful for confirmation. Findings should be clearly documented without the use of ambiguous terms or abbreviations. After data gathering by history and physical examination, the clinician might formulate possible answers to these questions by integrating historical information and physical examination findings. There may very well be only tentative answers, but formulation will guide the tempo of workup and follow-up. The brevity of this chapter allows only an introduction to problem formulation, but more information is available in chapters on specific disease processes in this book and in other references listed at the end of this chapter.

ORGANIZATIONAL FRAMEWORK

Organization of the neurologic examination along a framework of subsections is a convenient technique. At the bedside, the clinician can mentally review the framework as he or she examines the patient and selects additional tests to explore possibilities suggested by the history. Some of the tests grouped in a section test several aspects of the nervous system function, and listing of tests in a particular section is for organizational convenience. The clinician should keep this organization in mind while at the bedside. For example, visual field testing, although technically a test of higher cortical function, is listed with cranial nerve testing, because the examining physician may find it easier

to evaluate visual fields during that portion of the examination dealing with cranial nerve function. One organizational scheme divides the examination into eight elements:

1. Mental status testing
2. Higher cerebral functions
3. Cranial nerves
4. Sensory examination
5. Motor system
6. Reflexes
7. Cerebellar testing
8. Gait and station

Mental Status Testing

BASIC   A mental status examination, however informal, is part of every patient encounter. The observation may be brief and descriptive, such as, "The patient is awake, alert, and conversant," or it may be quite detailed. Mental status assesses the emotional and intellectual functioning of the patient. It is quite important to make some assessment of mental status, because the patient with an abnormal mental status cannot be relied on for an accurate history of the medical problem.

Major elements of mental status testing are assessment of appearance and assessment for thought disorders or abnormal thought content, such as hallucinations, mood, insight, and testing of the sensorium. *Sensorium* is a term for the appropriate awareness and perception of consciousness. Mental status testing is covered more fully in Chap. 229.

One key element in mental status testing is attention and memory assessment. Attention testing is best performed with digit repetition. The average adult of normal intelligence should be able to repeat six or seven digits forward and four or five digits backward. Failure to do so may suggest confusion, delirium, or a problem with language perception. Often this represents a problem with attention rather than with memory. Memory is a complex process but is often simply broken into long-term and short-term activities. *Long-term memory* is recall of events of some months or years ago. *Short-term memory* is assessed by asking about events of the day or by three-object recall at 5 min. The patient is verbally presented with three items in a neutral tone and asked to repeat; reassessment at 5 min gives a gross assessment of short-term memory function. Failure to repeat the items immediately after presentation is likely an indication of an attention problem rather than of a memory problem.

ADVANCED   Evaluation by screening tools, such as the Mini-Mental State Examination and the Quick Confusion Scale, are described in Chap. 229. Other screening tests for depression, substance abuse, and other problems are outside the scope of this chapter.

SPECIAL CIRCUMSTANCES   In general, patients with abnormal mental status, in particular attention problems or disorientation, are more likely to have "organic," i.e., medical, problems than "functional," i.e., psychiatric, etiologies.

Higher Cerebral Functions

Higher cerebral functions concern maneuvers that test neurologic functions that are thought to reside in the cerebral cortex. Language defines dominant hemisphere function. The majority of the population is right-handed; for 90 percent of these patients, the left hemisphere is where language functions reside; hence, they are referred to as left-hemisphere dominant. Even in left-handed patients, most have the left hemisphere dominant for speech. Thus, a large cortical stroke affecting the cortex of the dominant hemisphere (the left hemisphere in most patients, whether they are left- or right-hand dominant) likely will affect language functions.

The nondominant hemisphere is concerned with spatial relationships. Often a nondominant hemispheric problem is suspected in the ED when the patient has consistent visual inattention to a care provider approaching from one side (usually the left, because most patients are left-hemisphere dominant).

Higher cerebral function pragmatically involves the assessment of language. For a patient with speech that is difficult to understand, a fundamental distinction must be made between the presence of *dysarthria* and a *dysphasia* (aphasia and dysphasia are often used interchangeably in clinical practice). A dysarthria is a mechanical disorder of speech resulting from difficulty in the production of sound from weakness or incoordination of facial or oral musculature; this may result from a motor system problem (cortical, subcortical, brainstem, cranial nerve, or cerebellar), but it does not represent a disorder of higher cerebral function. Dysphasia is a problem of language resulting from cortical or subcortical damage; the portion of the brain concerned with comprehension, processing, or producing language is impaired.

There are many different types of aphasias, but a simplified scheme is sufficient for assessment. A descriptive scheme that discriminates aphasias into fluent, nonfluent, and mixed patterns is adequate for testing in the ED and for communicating with other physicians.

BASIC   Normal conversation monitoring for correct responses is the common screening examination for a language disorder. If suspicion of a language disorder exists, a series of assessments allows confirmation and categorization of the aphasia.

Comprehension is tested initially by the ability to follow simple commands. Asking the patient to identify common objects may be part of the assessment. Objects commonly available, such as a watch, a pen, or a glass, may be used as a stimulus. The patient may be queried regarding the names of different parts of the objects. The inability to name objects is of little localizing value other than to note a dominant hemisphere problem. The patient also may be asked to demonstrate how an object is used in the case of a pen or watch. The inability to show how an object is used, assuming hearing and motor functions are intact, may represent an apraxia, defined as the inability to perform a willed act.

In a nonfluent aphasia (a rough synonym is motor or expressive aphasia), the speed of language and the ability to find the correct words may be impaired. A common type of nonfluent motor aphasia is known as *Broca aphasia,* from localization to the eponymous portion of the dominant cortex. Speech is halting and slow, with stops between words or word fragments.

In a fluent aphasia (a rough synonym is auditory or receptive aphasia), the quantity of word production is normal or even increased. Sentences may have normal grammatical structure with normal rhythm, and intonation may be clearly articulated. However, language is impaired and the listener is struck by peculiarities of conversation that may lack content. Incorrect words may be substituted within sentences that may be sound-alike words or words with similar yet incorrect meanings. A global or mixed aphasia involves elements of fluent and nonfluent aphasias and is the most common type encountered in clinical practice.

Nondominant hemisphere problems may show problems of higher function, such as sensory discrimination, or auditory or visual inattention.

ADVANCED   Testing of mental status and cognitive function may require appreciation of cultural context and language barriers. Further assessment of comprehension may involve showing the patient a picture (there are some standard stimuli, but almost any magazine photo will suffice for testing) and asking for the patient's interpretation of the picture while noting if the content is correctly described and if the sentence structure and word selection of the descriptions are correct.

Assessing the ability of the patient to repeat a phrase may be a key point in delineating some types of fluent aphasias. Typically, the ability to repeat short words is more impaired than the ability to repeat longer words. A classic test involves the patient repeating the phrase, "No ifs, ands, or buts." In one type of fluent aphasia, Wernicke aphasia, comprehension is impaired, as is repetition.

Paraphasic errors may be further characterized in patients with fluent aphasia. A literal paraphasic error is one in which part of a word is replaced by an incorrect sound. The use of *spool* when *spoon* is meant is an example of this type of literal paraphasic error. At times the errors may reach the point when the substitutions are not understandable and a neologism is produced, i.e., a meaningless collection of syllables that takes the place of a word in conversation. Verbal paraphasic errors involve substitution of one correct word for another; for example, a patient may wish to use *spoon* in a sentence and substitute *fork* or even *bike;* the word is a correct word, but the meaning of the sentence is transformed erroneously.[1]

A patient who is aphasic in speaking also will be aphasic in written communication. Writing and drawing simple constructions may be revealing in selected patients. A sequence of simple commands such as requesting the patient to draw a circle and then placing numbers correctly on it as if placing numbers on a clock may reveal constructional errors. A response consistent with a problem in the nondominant hemisphere might be to number half the clock face and stop or to place all the numbers around one-half of the circle.

Impairment of sensory perception on a cortical level may involve the inability to distinguish objects by feeling alone. Implied in this testing is that the primary sensory modalities (sharp, light touch, etc.) are intact. In cases of nondominant hemisphere lesions, the ability to identify objects placed in a hand, such as a coin, may be impaired.

SPECIAL CIRCUMSTANCES   Fluent aphasias at times so impair communication that the patient is thought to be intoxicated or psychotic from severe psychiatric illness. Attention to the speech may give a first clue and then further constructional or language testing may reveal the aphasia.

Cranial Nerves

BASIC   A survey of the cranial nerves is part of the neurologic examination. Much information may be gathered informally. Facial asymmetry (cranial nerve VII) at rest or with movement may be observed. Lingual movement (XII) and other facial movements may be inferred during conversation if articulation is good. However, a more formal approach often is used in assessment. Most examiners start sequentially with cranial nerve II in testing; cranial nerve I (olfactory) testing has infrequent application in emergency medicine.

Cranial nerve II is the optic nerve with afferent function of light and visual perception. The optic nerve head is visible with direct ophthalmoscopy and may be inspected for any abnormalities. Common tests for optic nerve function include visual acuity and stimulation for pupillary reactivity. The response to bright light stimulation involves direct and indirect (consensual) pupillary responses. This is a reflex arc, with the afferent limb being cranial nerve II and brainstem interneurons and the efferent limb of the arc being cranial nerve III, which carries the pupilloconstrictors. A bright light shone into one eye should cause a brisk constriction of equal magnitude in both pupils. In the swinging flashlight test, the pupils are observed as the light is slowly moved from one pupil to the other. A seemingly paradoxical dilation of one pupil as the light is moved onto that pupil may indicate optic nerve dysfunction of that eye; this is referred to as an *afferent pupillary defect.*

Cranial nerves III, IV, and VI are concerned with extraocular eye movements. Tracing an object through a full-H pattern allows assessment of the different cranial nerves. Cranial nerve VI innervates the lateral rectus muscle, which abducts the globe moving it laterally away from the midline; this lateral movement will be impaired or lost in the case of a cranial nerve VI palsy. In fact, the unopposed adduction movement of medial rectus muscle innervated by cranial nerve III may result in the globe being adducted. Cranial nerve III innervates the extraocular muscles that adduct each eye and those that elevate and depress the globe. Impairment of cranial nerve III will reveal several abnormalities of extraocular movement, reflecting weakness in the innervated muscles. A complete paresis of cranial nerve III will show a dilated pupil in a globe deviated downward and outward. An isolated cranial nerve IV weakness may be hard to detect; cranial nerve IV supplies the superior oblique muscle that elevates and intorts the globe. Often, only subtle abnormalities of elevation are present.

Cranial nerve III also carries the parasympathetic pupilloconstrictors to the eye; a lesion of cranial nerve III may impair those fibers, resulting in unopposed dilatation (by functioning sympathetic fibers reaching the eye by a circuitous path) and a pupil larger than in the unaffected eye. Ptosis from levator paralysis is another finding of cranial nerve III paresis.

Cranial nerve V has motor and sensory functions. It supplies the muscles of mastication and is assessed by appreciating the masseter bulk. The sensory component of cranial nerve V supplies the cornea; the corneal reflex is a reflex arc of cranial nerves V to VII. Cranial nerve VII supplies the muscles for facial movement.

Cranial nerve VIII has auditory and vestibular afferent components. Cranial nerves IX and X are tested by observing pharyngeal musculature and gag reflexes. Cranial nerve XII controls lingual movement and can be assessed by asking the patient to stick out the tongue and observing for any asymmetry of motion. Cranial nerve XI is assessed by a shoulder shrug.

ADVANCED   In about 20 percent of the population, some degree of physiologic anisocoria is present. Small differences in pupillary size in otherwise asymptomatic patients likely represent this normal variant. A peripheral lesion of cranial nerve VII will cause complete facial paralysis on the same side as the lesion. A cortical lesion (often stroke) results in weakness of the lower and mid-face, with preservation of motor function in the upper face ("central seventh pattern"), because of the bilateral cortical upper motor neuron innervation of the forehead musculature present in most patients.

SPECIAL CIRCUMSTANCES   In the comatose patient, a unilaterally dilated pupil that is unreactive or reacts sluggishly to light may represent third nerve dysfunction or paresis from impingement of the oculomotor (III) nerve at the tentorium; this finding is consistent with the uncal herniation syndrome.

Sensory Examination

BASIC   The sensory examination may be the most time-consuming portion of the overall examination, but it is key in some patients with sensory complaints. The primary sensory modalities are light touch, pinprick, position, vibration, and temperature sense. Because of variability in neuroanatomy, at times dissociation of these modalities occur and allow localization of problems to anatomic areas within the central nervous system.

Practically, in the screening examination, establishing that touch or pinprick is perceived in all extremities is often the only sensory examination assessment needed. However, if this is not intact or if peripheral nerve or spinal cord injury is suspected, additional examination is necessary.

Position testing is best used for the detection of peripheral neuropathy or if posterior column spinal cord disease is suspected. Position and vibration sensations are conveyed in the posterior columns of the spinal cord, so that there is little utility in testing both modalities.

ADVANCED   Spinal cord dermatome levels are illustrated in Figure 226-1. If sensory alteration conforms to a level or selectively involves specific dermatomes, further localization to the peripheral nerve or nerve root may be possible.

If primary sensory modalities have been demonstrated to be intact, then testing of higher sensory functions may be pursued; these are covered in the section on higher cerebral functions.

SPECIAL CIRCUMSTANCES   A few patterns of sensory loss are worthy of special mention. In cervical spinal cord injury or compression, an area of apparent sensory demarcation often appears to be just above the nipples. This transverse sensory level suggests a spinal cord lesion in the low cervical to high thoracic area. Most cervical dermatomes are represented in the upper extremity and not in the trunk (see Figure 226-1), and further testing is necessary to delineate the sensory level.

With suspected spinal cord injury, it is important to test the area of the perineum for sensation. The sacral dermatomes are distributed in an onion skin pattern around the perineum and represented only in that region. **The demonstration of a preserved island of sensation around the perineum may be the only sign of an incomplete spinal cord injury, which has a different prognosis than a complete spinal cord injury.**

Some general comments may be made about patterns of sensory alterations. In general, a hemi-body sensory loss or alteration suggests that cortical or subcortical lesions may be present. A localized problem in one limb suggests a peripheral nerve or nerve root problem, although there are other possible locations of abnormalities in the central nervous system. More information may be found in a recent monograph on new-onset sensory alteration.[2]

Motor System

There is more to evaluation of the motor system than simple assessment of strength. Muscle bulk and muscle tone are basic areas of assessment. The presence of any tremor should be noted and described. Is the tremor fine or coarse? Is it worse with activity?

BASIC   Muscle tone may be characterized as normal, decreased, or increased. Movement of muscle groups and appreciating any resistance to movement comprise the process of assessing tone. The patient is requested to relax and not resist. Increased tone may be appreciated by greater than normal resistance to passive motion. At times the resistance will be increased, seemingly with the muscle transiently catching and then releasing to the movement (cogwheeling). Axial or truncal tone may be assessed by standing behind the patient, grasping the shoulders, and gently moving the shoulders forward and then backward. A patient with normal tone will offer little resistance to repeated motions, and some spontaneous swing of the arms will be noted. A patient with increased axial tone (e.g., Parkinson disease) may turn en bloc without the arm swing.

Simply having the patient hold the arms outstretched with palms upward and observing for any inward rotation or downward drift is a very sensitive sign for weakness (pronator drift); this also may be assessed in unresponsive patients (Figure 226-2). If both arms are held outright at the same time, comparison is easy, with observation of the upper extremity of one side as opposed to the other. A similar maneuver may be performed in the lower extremities. Another sensitive test for a subtle hemiparesis is the forearm rolling technique; the patient is asked to move the arms around each other in a tight circle in front of the trunk; the movements should be small and rapid. Asymmetry or slowness with one arm suggests a weak limb.[3]

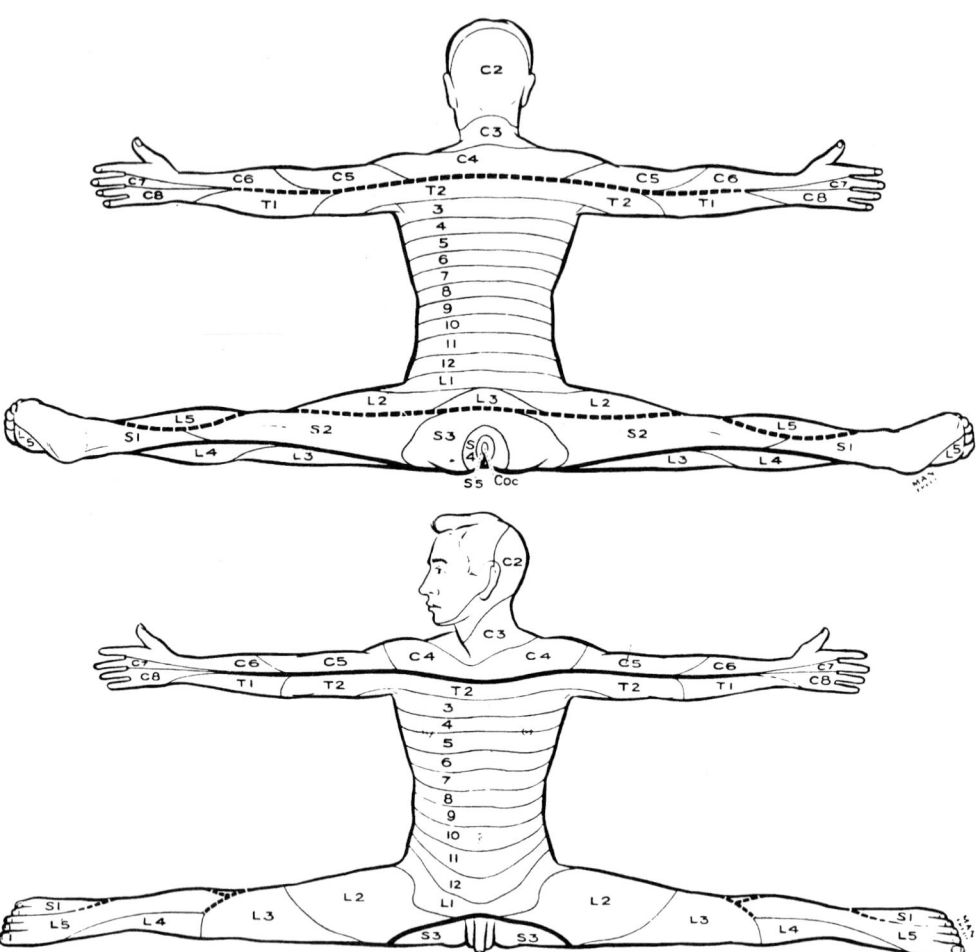

FIG. 226-1. Sensory dermatomes. (Reproduced with permission from DeMyer W: *Technique of the Neurologic Examination: A Programmed Text.* New York, McGraw-Hill, 1994.)

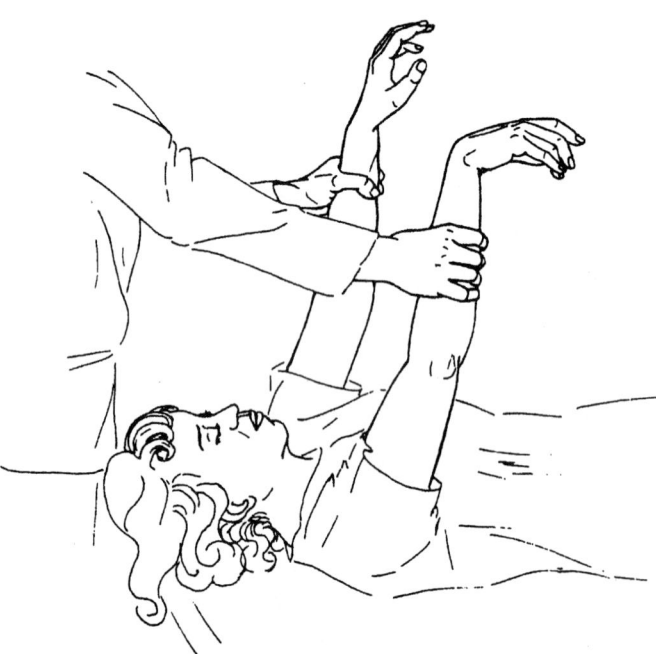

FIG. 226-2. Testing for weakness in the comatose patient; diagram illustrates assessment of muscular tone in a patient with a right hemiplegia. A similar maneuver may be used in the conscious patient. (Reproduced with permission from DeMyer W: *Technique of the Neurologic Examination: A Programmed Text.* New York, McGraw-Hill, 1994.)

Assessment and recording of other motor strength is best done by description of the stimulus and response. For example, the fact that the patient is able to strongly resist elbow extension or elbow flexion against the examiner is an appropriate notation.

ADVANCED   Observation of the muscles at times may be very informative. Muscle mass or bulk should be comparable with muscle groups of the extremities. If weakness or paralysis has been present for some time, muscle wasting or atrophy may be present. Brief, rapid twitches of small parts of a muscle may represent fasciculations; fasciculations may indicate a process involving the lower motor neurons.

A formal rating scale for muscle strength exists but is not straightforward to apply. A rating of five is assigned for normal strength, and a rating of four indicates weakness and the ability to contract the muscle against some resistance. Thus, a tremendous range of strength is covered within the range of the four rating; rating is often further roughly quantified by adding 4+ and 4− to that rating range. A rating of zero represents complete paresis, and a rating of one indicates a minimal flicker of contraction. A rating of two is assigned for active movement of a muscle with gravity eliminated by limb repositioning, e.g., so that elbow flexion and contraction are demonstrated by a horizontal rather than by a vertical movement. A value of three is assigned to a muscle able to voluntarily demonstrate full motion against gravity only. It is better for the examiner to describe the strength of a muscle by noting the amount of resistance than by invoking what may be a little-used scale and erroneously applying a rating.

Listings of some muscle innervations, actions to test, and dermatomal representations may be found in Tables 226-1 and 226-2.

TABLE 226-1   Muscle Innervation: Shoulder and Upper Extremity

Nerve	Action to Test	Muscle*
Long thoracic	Forward shoulder thrust	Serratus anterior
Dorsal scapular	Elevate scapula	Levator scapulae
Suprascapular	Arm external rotation	Infraspinatus; C5, C6
Axillary	Abduct arm (>90 degrees)	Deltoid; C5
Musculocutaneous	Flex and supinate arm	Biceps brachii
Ulnar	Ulnar flexion of hand Flex DIP of fingers 4 and 5 Thumb adduction Abduction of finger 5 Opposition of finger 5 Flexion of finger 5 Finger abduction and adduction Flex PIP and extend DIP of fingers 4 and 5	Flexor carpi ulnaris; C7, C8,† T1 Flexor digitorum profundus Adductor pollicis; C7, C8† Abductor digitorum minimi Opponens digitorum minimi Flexor digitorum minimi brevis Interossei; C8, T1† Lumbricals 3 and 4
Median	Forearm pronation Radial hand flexion Hand flexion PIP flexion of fingers 2–5 Abduct thumb at the MCP Flex proximal phalanx thumb	Pronator teres Flexor carpi radialis; C7, C8, T1 Palmaris longus Flexor digitorum superficialis Abductor pollicis brevis Flexor pollicis brevis; C7, C8†
Anterior interosseous	Flex DIP fingers 2–5 Flex thumb IP Oppose thumb Flex PIP and extend DIP of fingers 2 and 3	Flexor digitorum profundus (radial) Flexor pollicis longus Opponens pollicis; C8, T1† Lumbricals 1 and 2
Posterior interosseous	Extension of digits 2–5 Ulnar hand extension Thumb abduction Thumb extension Index finger extension	Extensor digitorum Extensor carpi ulnaris Abductor pollicis longus Extensor pollicis longus and brevis Extensor indicis proprius
Radial	Forearm extension Forearm flexion Radial hand extension Forearm supination	Triceps brachii; C6, C7,† C8 Brachioradialis; C5, C6 Extensor carpi radialis Supinator

*Dermatomal representations are listed after some muscles.
†Predominant dermatome.
Abbreviations: DIP = distal interphalangeal joint; IP = interphalangeal joint; PIP = proximal interphalangeal joint.

SPECIAL CIRCUMSTANCES   Although not classically described as part of the motor system examination, information regarding bladder tone and function is at times vital to the examiner. In patients with complaints of incontinence and low back pain, for example, discovery of a probable neurogenic bladder by demonstrating large postcatheterization residual urine volume might be a key to diagnosis of spinal cord compression. A normal value is less than 75 mL.

Reflexes

Elicitation of muscle stretch reflexes is arguably the least important part of the neurologic examination and offers little value when used in isolation. Correctly termed *muscle stretch reflexes,* the jerk or involuntary motor movement follows the stretching of intrafusal muscle spindle fibers by the strike of the reflex hammer and the involuntary muscle contraction that follows. Muscle stretch reflexes serve mainly to weight evidence collected in other parts of the history or physical examination.

Depending on the force of the reflex hammer strike and local impact factors, an elicited reflex may seemingly change from moment to moment. The patient should be relaxed, and the muscle tested should be relaxed. Often several reflex strikes are performed. The best response is the value recorded.

BASIC   Muscle stretch reflexes are graded on a scale from one to four that is not rigorously defined, with zero representing the absence of reflex, two or three being normal, and four representing hyperactive reflexes. Patterns of reflex abnormalities, e.g., upper versus lower extremity, left versus right, may suggest a location of a problem within the central or peripheral nervous system.

A toe that moves upward in response to a mildly noxious stimulation applied to the lateral plantar or lateral aspect of the foot defines Babinski response. The application of stimuli should not be hard or forceful. In adults, the normal response of the toe is to move downward to plantar stimulation.

ADVANCED   Clonus is the rhythmic oscillation of a body part, typically the ankle, elicited by a brisk stretch (Figure 226-3). It may be thought of as one sign of a spasticity in addition to Babinski response, increased muscle tone, and hyperactive muscle stretch reflexes. It may be seen in conditions of metabolic disturbance and primary neurologic dysfunction.

SPECIAL CIRCUMSTANCES   Principles of interpretation are that disease processes involving upper motor neurons or their processes (cortical or spinal cord injuries) result in hyperactive reflexes, Babinski response, and clonus. Processes injuring lower motor neurons,

TABLE 226-2 Muscle Innervation: Hip and Lower Extremity

Nerve	Action to Test	Muscle*
Femoral	Hip flexion Leg extension	Iliopsoas; T12, L1,† L2, L3 Quadriceps femoris; L2, L3,† L4
Obturator	Thigh adduction	Pectineus Adductor longus, brevis, magnus; L2, L3, L4 Gracilis
Superior gluteal	Thigh abduction Thigh flexion Lateral thigh rotation	Gluteus medius and minimus Tensor fascia lata Piriformis
Inferior gluteal	Thigh abduction	Gluteus maximus
Sciatic (trunk)	Leg flexion	Biceps femoris; L5,† S1, S2 Semitendinosus Semimembranosus
Deep peroneal	Foot dorsiflexion and supination Toes 2–5 and foot extension Great toe and foot dorsiflexion	Tibialis anterior; L4, L5 Extensor digitorum longus/brevis Extensor hallucis longus
Superficial peroneal	Plantar flexion foot and eversion	Peroneus longus/brevis; L5, S1
Tibial	Plantar flexion and inversion Flex distal phalanx toes 2–5 Flex distal phalanx great toe Flex middle phalanx toes 2–5 Flex proximal phalanx great toe Knee flexion and ankle plantar flexion Ankle plantar flexion	Posterior tibialis Flexor digitorum longus Flexor hallucis longus Flexor digitorum brevis Gastrocnemius; L5, S1,† S2 Flexor hallucis brevis Plantaris, soleus
Pudendal	Voluntary pelvic floor contraction	Perineal and sphincters; S3, S4

*Dermatomal representations are listed after some muscles.
†Predominant dermatome.

their axons, peripheral nerve roots, peripheral nerves, or the muscles themselves may result in hypoactive reflexes. However, in spinal cord injury or stroke, reflexes may take several hours or even days to become hyperactive, so the absence of these signs is not valuable in excluding acute spinal cord injury.

Spinal cord emergencies are high-risk clinical scenarios. A recent report noted that emergency physicians erroneously derive false reassurance from the absence of pathologic reflexes.[4] Although the presence of Babinski signs and hyperreflexia are understood to be cardinal signs of upper motor neuron syndrome, the absence of these signs does not reliably exclude a diagnosis of spinal cord compression, and the diagnosis should be pursued if historical or other physical examination findings suggest the possibility of this critical diagnosis.

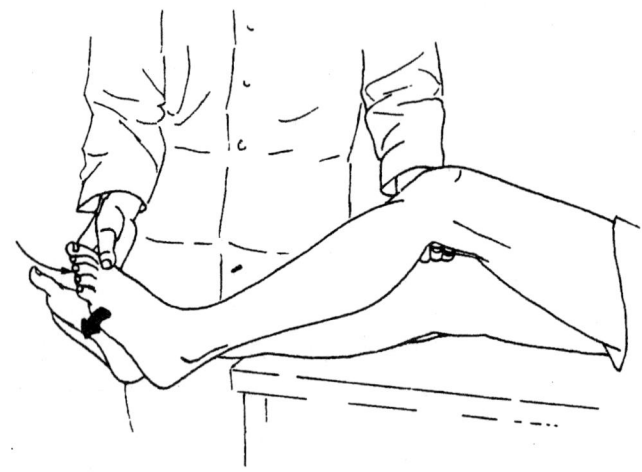

FIG. 226-3. Method for eliciting ankle clonus. (Reproduced with permission from DeMyer W: *Technique of the Neurologic Examination: A Programmed Text*. New York, McGraw-Hill, 1994.)

Cerebellar Testing

The cerebellum is concerned with involuntary activities of the central nervous system and may be simply thought of as a structure that helps with smoothing muscle movements and aiding with movement coordination. Very simply, the central cerebellar structures may be thought of as controlling coordination of posture and truncal movements, i.e., *axial coordination*. The lateral cerebellar structures are more coordinated with movements of the extremities, i.e., *appendicular coordination*.

BASIC   Rapidly alternating movements may be assessed by a variety of maneuvers. Hand-slapping tests, asking the patient to rapidly pronate and then supinate the forearm, and slapping the thigh with each movement is a commonly used test. The movements are normally small, and the hand slapping should be symmetric. Rapid pronation and supination of the hands is another test for dystaxia and dysmetria; the movements should be equal with both hands (Figure 226-4).

ADVANCED   Although usually included in cranial nerve testing, eye movements are useful in assessing cerebellar function, and abnormalities in their movements may suggest cerebellar dysfunction. Tracking an object slowly should show smooth, slow eye movements; breakup of the smooth movement may be evident and is analogous to the decompensation of movements that may occur in isolated cerebellar impairment. Similarly, if a patient is asked to look back and forth between two objects (finger-to-nose testing involves the patient looking back and forth quickly between the examiner's outstretched finger and nose), the eyes should quickly and conjugately look at the target without overshoot. These faster, or saccadic, movements are, at least in part, reflective of cerebellar function. *Nystagmus* refers to rapid involuntary movements of the eyes that may be present with primary (straight-ahead) gaze or provoked by looking at extremes of gaze. Course nystagmus or other abnormalities of eye movements are at times present with cerebellar problems (see Chap. 238 for a discussion of nystagmus).

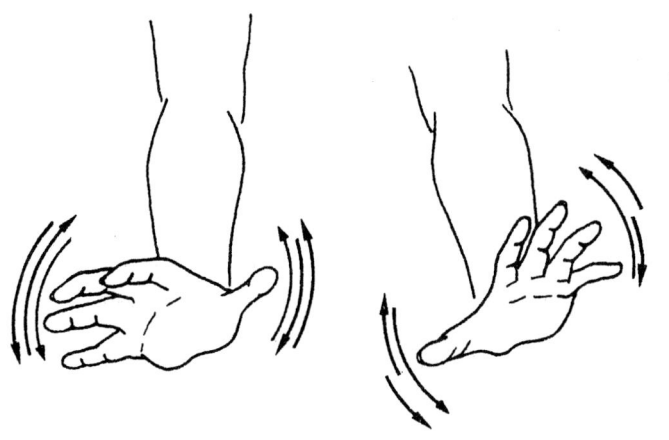

FIG. 226-4. Pronation and supination test: cerebellar testing. (Reproduced with permission from DeMyer W: *Technique of the Neurologic Examination: A Programmed Text.* New York, McGraw-Hill, 1994.)

Gait and Station

BASIC   It has been said that, if only one neurologic test could be performed, observation of the patient walking would be the most informative. The posture that the patient assumes when stationary defines the station of the patient. A variety of abnormal gaits and postures are discussed further in Chap. 230, "Ataxia and Gait Disturbances," as are different techniques of physical examination.

SPECIAL CIRCUMSTANCES   Cerebellar infarction or hemorrhage is a true emergency, because expanding lesions in the posterior fossa may rapidly compress the brainstem, causing apnea and death. However, rapid recognition and surgical intervention have been shown to have good outcomes, unlike most other intraparenchymal brain hemorrhages. Patients with cerebellar hemorrhage may have severe nausea and vomiting and be massively diaphoretic. Their clinical condition is such that fine neurologic examination is simply not possible. One feature common in many patients with cerebellar hemorrhage is the sudden inability to walk. The examiner should keep the possibility of cerebellar injury in mind when evaluating a patient with sudden onset of symptoms that include the inability to walk.

ACKNOWLEDGMENTS

The authors acknowledge the work of Dr. Greg Henry and Dr. Hugh S. Mickel, authors of chapters on this topic in previous editions of the study guide. Their chapters served as a check for completeness and provided some tabular information. J. Stephen Huff also thanks Dr. William DeMyer of Indiana University whose instruction in the neurologic examination years ago stimulated an interest in this area.

REFERENCES

1. Geswind N: Current concepts: Aphasia. *New Engl J Med* 25:654, 1971.
2. Huff JS: New-onset sensory loss or alteration. *Emerg Med Clin North Am* 16:811, 1998.
3. Sawyer RN, Hanna JP, Leigh RJ: Asymmetry of forearm rolling as a sign of unilateral cerebral dysfunction. *Neurology* 43:1596, 1993.
4. Glick TH: Spinal cord emergencies: False reassurance from reflexes. *Acad Emerg Med* 5:1041, 1998.

A variety of comprehensive references of different complexity are available for the neurologic examination and are listed below.
Brazis PW, Masdeu JC, Biller J: *Localization in Clinical Neurology.* Philadelphia, Lippincott, Williams & Wilkins, 2001.
DeMyer W: *Technique of the Neurologic Examination: A Programmed Text.* New York, McGraw-Hill, 1994.
Patten J: *Neurological Differential Diagnosis.* New York, Springer, 1995.

HEADACHE AND FACIAL PAIN
Christopher J. Denny
Michael J. Schull

HEADACHE

Headache represents up to 4 percent of all emergency department visits.[1] Emergency physicians generally are concerned with identifying those patients whose headaches are caused by life-threatening conditions. Most patients, however, have benign primary headache syndromes and are concerned with receiving rapid and effective treatment for their headaches.

Epidemiology

Migraine headaches have prevalence rates of approximately 17 percent in women and 5 percent in men. Most emergency department patients have benign primary headache syndromes, but approximately 3.8 percent have serious or secondary pathology.[1]

Classification

For practical purposes, headaches generally are divided into primary headache syndromes, including migraine, tension-type, and cluster headaches, and secondary causes. The most common causes are listed in Table 227-1.

Pathophysiology

The brain parenchyma is largely insensate to pain. Pain may originate from large cranial vessels, proximal intracranial vessels, and the dura mater. Anterior vessels are innervated by branches of the ophthalmic division of the trigeminal nerve, whereas contents of the posterior fossa are innervated by branches of the C2 nerve roots.[2]

Approach to Patients with Headache in the Emergency Department

The 1996 American College of Emergency Physicians' (ACEP's) Clinical Policy for Adults with Headache groups all causes of headache into four broad categories[3] (Table 227-2). Evaluation of the headache patient has four essential objectives:

1. To appropriately select patients for emergency investigation and treatment of suspected critical secondary headache causes
2. To diagnose and effectively treat patients with generally benign and reversible secondary headache causes
3. To provide effective treatment for primary headache syndromes
4. To provide appropriate disposition and follow-up (including outpatient investigations and referral as necessary) for all discharged patients

The central role played by the history in the evaluation of the headache patient is emphasized in the guidelines published by ACEP and those of other groups. Patients with an atypical history, a substantial change from a previous headache pattern, or certain high-risk features, as summarized below, require emergency department evaluation.[3,4]

HISTORY

Headache Pattern   Important features include: first severe headache, worst headache ever, steady worsening over several days, or significant differences from prior headaches in terms of duration, severity, or associated symptoms.[3]

Onset   Sudden-onset headache, especially if it begins during exertion (including coughing, defecation, etc.), is an independent predictor of

TABLE 227-1 Etiology of Headache

CRITICAL SECONDARY CAUSES

Vascular
    Subarachnoid hemorrhage
    Intraparenchymal hemorrhage
    Epidural hematoma
    Subdural hematoma
    Stroke
    Cavernous sinus thrombosis
    Arteriovenous malformation
    Temporal arteritis
    Carotid or vertebral artery dissection
CNS infection
    Meningitis
    Encephalitis
    Cerebral abscess
Tumor
Pseudotumor cerebri
Ophthalmic
    Glaucoma
    Iritis
    Optic neuritis
Drug-related
    Nitrates and nitrites
    Monoamine oxidase inhibitors
    Alcohol withdrawal
Toxic
    Carbon monoxide poisoning
Endocrine
    Pheochromocytoma
Metabolic
    Hypoxia
    Hypoglycemia
    Hypercapnia
    High-altitude cerebral edema
    Preeclampsia

REVERSIBLE SECONDARY CAUSES

Non-CNS infections
    Focal
    Systemic
    Sinusitis
    Odontogenic
    Otic
Drug-related
    Chronic analgesic use
    Monosodium glutamate
Miscellaneous
    Post–lumbar puncture

PRIMARY HEADACHE SYNDROMES

Migraine
Tension
Cluster

TABLE 227-2 ACEP Headache Categories

Headache Category	Examples
I. Critical secondary causes requiring emergent identification and treatment	Subarachnoid hemorrhage, meningitis, brain tumor with raised ICP
II. Critical secondary causes not necessarily requiring emergent identification or treatment	Brain tumor without raised ICP
III. Generally benign and reversible secondary causes	Sinusitis, hypertension, post–lumbar puncture headache
IV. Primary headache syndromes	Migraine, tension type, or cluster

Abbreviations: ACEP = American College of Emergency Physicians; ICP = intracranial pressure.

ness, persistent visual disturbance, fever, or seizure(s).[3] The history also should include a search for symptoms of nonneurologic conditions causing headache, such as visual change and eye pain, suggestive of glaucoma or iritis; jaw claudication, suggestive of temporal arteritis; or congestion and facial pain, suggestive of sinusitis.[3]

Other History Medications [e.g., nitroglycerin, chronic analgesic use, monoamine oxidase inhibitors (MAOIs), or anticoagulants], a remote history of trauma, or toxic exposures (e.g., carbon monoxide) may be important causes. Prior headache history, results of any previous neuroimaging, and comorbid conditions such as malignancies, AIDS or HIV seroconversion, coagulopathy, and hypertension should be sought.[3]

Family History Migraine headaches occur more commonly in patients with a family history of migraines or motion sickness.[2] Headache patients should be asked about relatives with SAH because the risk of ruptured intracranial aneurysm in first- and second-degree relatives is up to four times higher than in the general population.[6]

PHYSICAL EXAMINATION Aspects of the general appearance and vital-sign abnormalities are warning signs of a possible serious cause. Fever suggests infection, such as meningitis or sinusitis, but also can occur in SAH. Marked hypertension should raise suspicion of a hypertensive urgency or emergency.

A focused examination looking for important nonneurologic causes of headache should be undertaken. In the head and neck, the sinuses should be examined for evidence of sinusitis; the temporal arteries palpated for tenderness or reduced pulsation, suggestive of temporal arteritis; and the dentition and temporomandibular joints examined for tenderness.[3] An eye examination should be carried out to exclude acute glaucoma, visual field defects, or iritis. Funduscopy may reveal papilledema or the absence of venous pulsations, both signs of raised intracranial pressure (ICP) or subhyaloid hemorrhage (gravity-dependent venous hemorrhage between the retina and vitreous membrane, convex at the bottom and flat at the top when the patient is examined sitting), which is highly suggestive of SAH.

Finally, a careful neurologic examination is mandatory, focusing on the mental status, cranial nerves, motor and sensory examinations, reflexes, gait, and cerebellar testing. Evidence of meningeal irritation should be assiduously ruled out. Papilledema, altered mental status, or focal neurologic deficits are predictive of raised ICP. An abnormal neurologic examination in the setting of a headache requires emergent neuroimaging.[1,3,4]

SPECIAL CONSIDERATIONS

intracranial pathology, and up to 25 percent of such headaches are caused by subarachnoid hemorrhages (SAHs).[1]

Headache Location The location of the headache is nonspecific and should not be relied on for diagnosis. Migraines are most commonly unilateral and tension-type headaches bilateral, but the reverse also may be true.[5] Occipitonuchal location of headache among emergency department patients is an independent predictor of intracranial pathology, although its positive predictive value is only 16 percent.[1] It is, however, the most common location for the headache of an acute SAH.

Associated Symptoms Other important features include a history of syncope, altered level of consciousness, confusion, neck pain or stiff-

Women Migraine headaches are more common in women and are influenced by hormonal factors. Menarche, menstruation, oral contraceptive use, pregnancy, and menopause all may affect migraine. Higher estrogen levels generally are associated with improved symptoms.

Pregnancy Preeclampsia should be considered in pregnant women. Pregnancy improves migraine symptoms in 60 to 70 percent of patients.

Older Age New onset of headaches in patients over 50 years of age is worrisome and may herald the presence of a secondary cause.[1] However, one study of new-onset headache in older patients still found primary headache syndromes to be the most common diagnosis.

Children (See Chap. 130)

HIV and Other Causes of Immunosuppression Specific consideration of space-occupying lesions such as toxoplasmosis and central nervous system (CNS) lymphoma is prudent in the immunosuppressed patient. Altered mental status, new seizure activity, and greater than 3 days of headache are high-risk criteria.[7]

USING CLINICAL DATA TO GUIDE DECISION MAKING (SEE ALSO CHAP. 237)

Data obtained from the history and physical examination allow patients to be classified according to the ACEP groupings (see Table 227-2). Patients suspected of having critical secondary causes of headache (see Table 227-1) should undergo emergent investigations, as outlined below, and have appropriate consultation and treatment initiated. Those with a benign and reversible secondary cause or an urgent but not emergent secondary etiology can have diagnostic tests and specific treatments initiated in the ED or as outpatients, as appropriate.

The 2002 ACEP Clinical Policy on Acute Headache differentiates between the use of neuroimaging for the identification of life-threatening etiologies versus its use in diagnosis for disposition.[8] The policy grades these recommendations based on the quality of evidence for or against an intervention. There were no level A recommendations (i.e., those which reflect a high degree of certainty). Level B recommendations are for emergent neuroimaging of new focal deficits, acute sudden onset of headache, and in HIV-positive patients presenting with a new headache. In patients older than 50 years of age with new headache and a normal neurologic examination, there are level C recommendations for consideration of urgent neuroimaging. The largest group of emergency department headache patients has assessments that suggest a benign primary headache syndrome, and the objective for these patients is to provide effective therapeutic relief.

Appropriate follow-up should be ensured for all discharged patients. Outpatient investigation and referral may be required, especially in cases such as poorly controlled primary headache syndromes or occasionally a patient with a suspected critical secondary cause not needing emergent investigation (e.g., suspected brain tumor without raised ICP). In cases such as the latter, outpatient workup is appropriate only if the physician is confident that the patient will not be lost to follow-up.

Diagnostic Adjuncts

COMPUTED TOMOGRAPHY

The emergency department patient whose headache requires emergent investigation usually begins with a non-contrast-enhanced computed tomographic (CT) scan.[3] The use of contrast material increases the time, expense, and risk of adverse effects (minor 10 percent, severe 0.1 percent),[4] and the non-contrast-enhanced CT scan usually adequately excludes critical lesions or mass effects requiring emergent interventions. In particular, the non-contrast-enhanced CT scan is the best neuroimaging test for diagnosing an acute SAH, although a negative CT scan alone cannot exclude SAH. When there is strong suspicion of small lesions likely to be missed without contrast (e.g., in an AIDS patient suspected of cerebral toxoplasmosis or suspected small brain mass), then a CT with intravenous contrast material or magnetic resonance imaging (MRI) may be needed.[4] Chap. 237 provides a detailed review of the various neuroimaging techniques and their indications.

LUMBAR PUNCTURE (LP)

See Chap. 235 for a description of this procedure. LP is required in cases such as suspected meningitis or suspected SAH with a normal CT scan.[9] Contraindications to LP include the suspicion of raised ICP, which can be excluded by a combination of the absence of papilledema, normal level of consciousness, and normal findings on neurologic examination. **Absence of papilledema by itself is unreliable** because papilledema may not be apparent in rapidly developing ICP. Venous pulsations seen at the disc margins on funduscopic examination with the patient upright reliably insures a normal ICP. If these conditions are met, then a CT scan is not required prior to LP, especially if the CT scan is likely to be delayed.

MAGNETIC RESONANCE IMAGING (MRI)

The cost and restricted availability of MRI limit its utility in the emergency investigation of headache. MRI is more sensitive than CT scanning in evaluating brain injuries, such as diffuse axonal injuries, small parenchymal contusions, isodense subdural hemorrhages, and most tumors.[4] In acute SAH, however, MRI is no more sensitive than CT scanning in the first few days following a bleed. CT scanning and LP are adequate for the large majority of emergency department headache patients requiring emergent investigation.

Life-Threatening Causes of Headache

SUBARACHNOID HEMORRHAGE

Epidemiology SAH (see Chap. 228) has an annual incidence of approximately 1 per 10,000 in the United States.[6] Of all sudden, severe headaches presenting to the ED with a normal neurologic examination, 12 percent have SAH.[10] SAH occurs in young people, with a median age of 50 years. Mortality rates from SAH are high; 50 percent of patients die within 6 months.

Clinical Features At the time of presentation, almost half of patients with SAH have normal findings on neurologic examination, including normal vital signs, normal level of consciousness, and no neck stiffness. The headache of SAH is most commonly severe and of sudden onset, but it also may be more subtle. The most common location for the headache is occipitonuchal. Many presentations are atypical and may mislead the clinician. For example, sudden-onset intense neck pain may be mistakenly attributed to radiculopathy. Also, resolution of the pain even without treatment does not exclude the diagnosis. Beware of radiation of pain down along the cervial spine because this suggests tracking of subarachnoid blood down the spinal canal.

Diagnosis Investigation of suspected SAH usually begins with a plain CT scan of the head. Retrospective studies suggest that the sensitivity of newer-generation CT scans may be in excess of 93 percent for the detection of SAH when symptom presentation is within 24 h and may be even higher if performed within 12 h of symptom onset.[11] However, no study has convincingly shown that CT scanning alone can exclude SAH, even within 12 h.[12] The sensitivity of CT scanning falls to slightly over 80 percent after 24 h and decays rapidly thereafter. Older-generation CT scanners were less sensitive among patients who were alert compared with those with an altered sensorium. It remains unclear whether this finding holds with new-generation scanners.[13]

Most authorities consider an LP to be mandatory following a negative CT scan. An alternate view suggests that LP may be unnecessary when the pretest probability is very low. However, this view has itself been challenged on the basis that so-called low-probability patients (isolated severe headache and absence of neurologic findings) may still have up to a 12 percent chance of SAH and that CT scanning may be less sensitive in these patients.[14] Thus, given the potential for catastrophic outcome, it remains prudent to perform an LP on all patients suspected of SAH in whom the CT scan was negative.

The "gold standard" for the diagnosis of SAH is the presence of xanthochromia in the cerebrospinal fluid (CSF) supernatant. If LP is performed 12 h or longer after onset of headache (allowing sufficient time for xanthochromia to develop) and spectrophotometry is used for CSF analysis, then xanthochromia is nearly 100 percent sensitive for up to 2 weeks following a bleed. Naked-eye detection of xanthochromia may yield a false-negative result in 50 percent of cases, yet this remains the laboratory standard in many hospitals across North America. If a patient presents to the emergency department less than 12 h after the onset of headache, some authors argue that LP should not be delayed.[10] Others suggest that delaying LP optimizes the detection of xanthochromia, which simplifies interpretation of CSF results. Traumatic taps occur in up to 20 percent of LPs. In LPs with questionable red blood cell counts, the presence of xanthochromia suggests a SAH, whereas its absence in a delayed LP suggests the blood may be due to the procedure itself. Regardless of LP timing, persistently bloody CSF or the presence of xanthochromia mandates CNS vascular imaging.

Treatment Treatment for SAH diagnosed as a "stroke syndrome" is discussed in Chap. 228. Neurosurgical consultation is appropriate. The Hunt and Hess classification (Table 227-3) is one of several scales that can be used to assess prognosis and determine eligibility for surgery. Patients presenting with headache and without major neurologic complaints or findings are likely to be of grade I or II severity and thus are appropriate candidates for angiography and surgical intervention. However, the Glasgow Coma Scale (see Figure 255-2) and the World Federation of Neurological Surgeons (WFNS) scale can also be used to predict mortality.[15,16]

Nimodipine (60 mg PO q6h) appears to decrease incidence and severity of vasospasms that may cause cerebral ischemia. If the patient cannot take oral medications, initiation of this medication is delayed.

Prophylactic phenytoin loading is recommended to avoid seizures, which can cause increased intracranial pressure. For similar reasons, nausea and vomiting should be treated with standard antiemetics.

MENINGITIS (SEE ALSO CHAP. 235) All forms of meningitis can cause headache. In viral or bacterial meningitis, the headache may be severe and of rapid onset, and it is usually accompanied by fever and meningismus. Opportunistic infections in immunocompromised patients, such as cryptococcal meningitis, may present with a more insidious onset of headache, and fever and neck stiffness may be absent. An LP is required if there is any suspicion of meningitis, and it need not be preceded by a CT scan in patients with normal findings on neurologic examination, a normal level of consciousness, and no papilledema. If the LP must be delayed for any reason and bacterial meningitis is suspected, antibiotics should be started immediately.

TABLE 227-3 Hunt and Hess Classification of Subarachnoid Hemorrhage

Classification	Symptoms
Grade I	Asymptomatic or minimal headache and mild nuchal rigidity
Grade II	Moderate to severe headache, nuchal rigidity, no neurologic deficit other than cranial-nerve palsy
Grade III	Drowsiness, confusion, or mild focal deficit
Grade IV	Stupor, moderate to severe hemiparesis, possible early decerebrate rigidity, vegetative disturbance
Grade V	Deep coma, decerebrate rigidity, moribund appearance

Source: Hunt WE, Hess RM: Surgical risk as related to time of intervention in the repair of intracranial aneurysms. *J Neurosurg* 28:14, 1968.

INTRAPARENCHYMAL HEMORRHAGE AND CEREBRAL IS-CHEMIA About 55 percent of patients with intraparenchymal hemorrhage report headache at the onset of their symptoms. Only 17 percent of ischemic stroke patients and 6 percent of patients with transient ischemic attacks (TIAs) complain of headache. Other neurologic signs and symptoms are present in most patients.

SUBDURAL HEMATOMA (SDH) A history of remote trauma in a patient with a headache should raise suspicion of a subacute or chronic subdural hematoma. A low threshold for initiating investigations is appropriate for high-risk patients, including patients on anticoagulants, chronic alcoholics, and the elderly, in whom there may be no clear history of trauma.[3] If a plain CT scan of the head appears normal yet the clinician has grounds to suspect a subacute or chronic SDH (which may appear isodense to brain parenchyma), then a contrast-enhanced CT scan or MRI of the head should be considered.

BRAIN TUMOR Up to 70 percent of patients with brain tumors complain of headache at the time of diagnosis, and only about 8 percent have abnormal findings on neurologic examination. The headache may be unilateral or bilateral, intermittent or continuous. The classic headache of brain tumors (worse in the morning, associated with position and nausea and vomiting) occurs in only a few. If headache is suspected of being due to a tumor and 24-h follow-up can be ensured, a reliable patient with normal findings on neurologic examination, including absence of papilledema, can be investigated as an outpatient.[3]

Secondary Causes of Headache

TEMPORAL ARTERITIS

Epidemiology Temporal arteritis (TA) occurs almost exclusively in patients over 50 years of age. In this age group, there is an annual incidence rate of 15 to 30 cases per 100,000 persons, and it occurs more commonly in women.[17]

Pathophysiology TA is a systemic panarteritis that selectively involves arterial walls with significant amounts of elastin.

Clinical Features Headache is the most common symptom of TA, reported in 60 to 90 percent of patients. The headache is most often severe and throbbing and usually located over the frontotemporal region. Other strongly suggestive features include jaw claudication or evidence of polymyalgia rheumatica, with which TA is strongly associated. The involved temporal artery may be nonpulsatile or tender or have a diminished pulse. The most serious complication is loss of vision, usually due to ischemic optic neuritis.[17]

Diagnosis The diagnosis is established by fulfilling three of the five following criteria: age over 50 years, new-onset localized headache, temporal artery tenderness or decreased pulse, erythrocyte sedimentation rate over 50 mm per h, and abnormal arterial biopsy findings.[17]

Treatment In order to prevent loss of vision, treatment should begin immediately with 40 to 60 mg PO per d of prednisone when TA is suspected clinically. Patients should be referred urgently for definitive diagnosis and follow-up.[17]

OPHTHALMIC DISORDERS (SEE ALSO CHAP. 238) Acute glaucoma may present with headache, and in other eye disorders, such as iritis or optic neuritis, some patients may describe eye or supraciliary pain as headache. These conditions usually can be distinguished by a careful history and eye examination, including measurement of intraocular pressure when necessary.[3]

HYPERTENSION (SEE ALSO CHAP. 57) Hypertension may cause headaches, with higher diastolic pressures generally associated with more severe headaches. Physicians should be cautious prior to making this diagnosis, however, because hypertension also may occur as a sign of other secondary headache conditions (e.g., stroke, pheochromocytoma, or preeclampsia) or simply may be secondary to the pain and anxiety associated with a primary headache syndrome.[3] When other secondary causes of headache, including hypertensive emergency, have been excluded, reduction of the blood pressure should result in improvement or resolution of the headache. While some consider isolated headache associated with hypertension as evidence of possible end-organ involvement, most such patients can be discharged following complete resolution of symptoms and blood pressure reduction if follow-up in the next 24 to 48 h can be arranged.

SINUSITIS (SEE ALSO CHAP. 241) Infection of the sinuses may result in facial pain or headache. Maxillary sinusitis, by far the most common type, causes pain over the anterior aspect of the face rather than headache. Involvement of other sinuses can cause headache: frontal sinusitis over the forehead, ethmoid sinusitis behind and between the eyes, and sphenoid sinusitis cause a diffuse headache. The headache frequently varies with head position. Symptoms predictive of sinusitis include colored nasal discharge, maxillary toothache, and poor response to decongestants, while reliable signs include purulent nasal discharge and abnormal transillumination (not easy to do properly in the ED). Regardless of plain sinus x-ray findings, patients with four or more of the above-mentioned features have a very high likelihood of sinusitis, while those with fewer than two features are very unlikely to have sinusitis.

DRUG-RELATED AND TOXIC OR METABOLIC HEADACHES Various drugs, such as nitrates, MAOIs, or chronically used analgesics, may cause headache. Metabolic conditions such as hypoxia, hypercapnia, and hypoglycemia and toxins such as monosodium glutamate and carbon monoxide may cause headache as well. Withdrawal from alcohol also may result in headache. Such headaches can be identified either in the history or through appropriate laboratory testing (glucometer, arterial blood gases, and carboxyhemoglobin levels).[3]

BENIGN INTRACRANIAL HYPERTENSION (PSEUDOTUMOR CEREBRI) A rare entity, benign intracranial hypertension (BIH), should be considered in a young, obese patient presenting with long-standing headaches. Nausea, vomiting, and visual disturbance also may be present. While its cause is unknown, BIH has been linked to the use of oral contraceptives, vitamin A, and tetracycline and to thyroid disorders. BIH is characterized by papilledema, a normal level of consciousness, normal CT scan findings, and markedly elevated CSF pressure on LP. The only serious adverse outcome is the potential for visual loss. Initial treatment is usually with acetazolamide or steroids. When these fail, repeated LPs to drain CSF or surgery (CSF shunts or optic nerve sheath fenestration) may be tried.

INTERNAL CAROTID AND VERTEBRAL ARTERY DISSECTION While rare, dissection of the internal carotid or vertebral artery is frequently associated with headache. Dissection may be spontaneous or the result of trauma and generally occurs in younger patients (median age 40 years). Internal carotid artery dissection may be suspected in a patient with unilateral anterior neck pain or headache, usually around the eye or frontal area. Most patients present with or eventually develop neurologic signs, such as TIA, stroke, Horner syndrome, transient monocular blindness, or cranial nerve palsies. Vertebral artery dissection typically presents with marked occipital or posterior neck pain associated with signs of a brainstem TIA or stroke. Diagnosis is usually made by angiography. Duplex scanning and MRI also may identify vessel abnormalities. SAH may be caused by dissection through the adventitia of the vessel, and this must be excluded prior to initiating anticoagulant therapy.

POST–LUMBAR PUNCTURE HEADACHE Between 10 and 36 percent of patients who undergo LP develop a headache within 24 to 48 h due to a persistent CSF leak from the dura. The incidence of post-LP headaches can be minimized through the use of smaller-bore needles with noncutting tips in order to spread, rather than cut, dural fibers. Post-LP headache can be treated with simple analgesics, intravenous fluids, and intravenous caffeine. If this treatment fails, a blood patch may be required. This procedure involves an epidural injection of autologous blood at the level of the LP to "patch" the CSF leak.

Primary Headache Syndromes

The term *primary headache* includes all forms of migraine, tension-type, and cluster headaches. There is considerable clinical overlap in primary headache syndromes, and it has been suggested that they share a pathophysiology and represent different ends of a clinical spectrum.[5]

MIGRAINE

Epidemiology Migraine headaches are common, with onset usually in the early teens or even younger. Prevalence is estimated at approximately 5 percent for males and 15 to 17 percent for females. Prevalence peaks in both sexes at around 40 years of age and then declines gradually.[18]

Pathophysiology Early theories postulated abnormal vasculature as the root cause of migraine headaches, with vasoconstriction being responsible for the aura and rebound vasodilatation the cause of the pounding headache. It now seems clear that migraines are a primary response of brain tissue to some trigger, resulting in dysfunction of brainstem pathways that normally modulate sensory input, whereas the disordered activity of blood vessels is secondary.[2]

Auras are thought to be due to primary neuronal dysfunction, with the neurologic symptoms resulting from a slowly spreading wave of neuronal hypoactivity traveling across brain tissue. There is a corresponding decrease in local blood flow where neuronal activity is reduced. This reduction in blood flow does not follow vascular territories, which makes it unlikely to be vasospastic in origin.[2]

Animal models suggest that the headache of migraine is related to activation of sensory axons, leading to the release of various peptides. This causes sterile neurogenic inflammation in pain-sensitive arteries, the dura, and meningial tissues and promotes local vasodilatation. The release of these peptides and the resulting inflammation and plasma extravasation can be blocked by sumatriptan, a selective agonist of 5-HT$_{1D}$ (serotonin) receptors, as well as by ergots, indomethacin, and others. Sumatriptan also has direct vasoconstricting effects. Both mechanisms may explain its efficacy at revealing migraine headache. The neurophysiologic pathways linking auras and headaches are still poorly understood.

The actual triggers for these complex mechanisms are unknown, although enhanced excitability of occipital cortex neurons in migraine patients has been proposed.[2]

Clinical Features Migraine without aura accounts for most migraines. The headache generally is slow in onset and lasts from 4 to 72 h. It is typically unilateral and pulsating and worsened by physical activity. Nausea, vomiting, and photo- or phonophobia frequently accompany the headache. The scalp may or may not be tender. These features, however, are not entirely sensitive (migraines need not be unilateral or pulsating) or specific (the same features can be present in tension-type headaches).[5] Suspicion that a different etiology may be underlying should be raised when a patient presents with a "migraine" that is significantly different from prior headaches. The headache in migraine with aura is similar but is preceded or accompanied by an aura that develops gradually over minutes, usually lasts 60 min, and is fully reversible.

Visual auras are the most common, usually consisting of scintillating scotomata (i.e., dark spots) or flashing lights, but virtually any neurologic symptom or sign can occur. Other "typical" auras include hemiparesthesia, hemiparesis, aphasia, or other speech difficulties. Rarer types of auras include those with brainstem symptoms (basilar migraine), those lasting longer than 60 min (migraine with prolonged aura), and aura without accompanying headache (migraine aura without headache). Auras should be distinguished from migraine prodromes, which occur many hours prior to the headache and can consist of lethargy, hyperactivity, yawning, depression, food craving, polyuria, or rarely fluid retention.

Other, less common forms of migraine include *ophthalmoplegic migraine,* in which headache overlaps with paresis of one or more of cranial nerves III, IV, and VI, or retinal migraine, with sudden monocular scotoma or blindness associated with headache. Rarely, migrainous infarction may occur (previously called *complicated migraine*), characterized by an aura lasting more than 7 days or neuroimaging evidence of cerebral infarction.

Clearly, in a patient who presents with a focal neurologic deficit and headache, migraine of any sort must be a diagnosis of exclusion unless the patient has a clear history of previous similar migraines, including the neurologic deficit, and normal results of prior investigations. Given that they rarely last more than 60 min, the aura and deficits would be expected to resolve in migraine patients prior to discharge from the emergency department.

Treatment There is a wide spectrum of clinical practice and no clear consensus on the best therapy for migraine. This reflects the fact that, to date, no migraine treatment has been shown to be superior in all respects. Although there is ongoing use of opiate medications as abortive migraine therapy in the emergency department, several guidelines suggest instead using more migraine-specific therapy.[2]

At present, several nonopioid abortive therapeutic options are available (Table 227-4) based on a review of emergency department randomized, controlled trials (RCTs) and consensus guidelines. Dihydroergotamine (DHE), a 5-HT$_{1B/1D}$ (serotonin) receptor agonist, is highly effective in relieving headaches and is an appropriate first-line therapy for migraine. However, DHE causes vomiting in a significant proportion of patients, probably due to its affinity for other serotonin and dopamine receptors. Patients therefore should be pretreated with an antiemetic, such as metoclopramide or prochlorperazine.

The triptans (e.g., sumatriptan) are more selective 5-HT$_{1D}$ agonists than DHE and cause less nausea and vomiting.[19] These agents have three potential mechanisms of action: cranial vasoconstriction, peripheral neuronal inhibition, and inhibition of transmission through second-order neurons of the trigeminocervical complex.[2] However, emergency department–based studies have shown that subcutaneous sumatriptan results in frequent but short-lived minor adverse effects (e.g., sensations of heat, tingling, chest discomfort, and injection-site reactions), is more costly, and has a higher 24-h recurrence/relapse rate than treatment with DHE.[19] While sumatriptan still may be useful for migraines unresponsive to other medications, it should not be given within 24 h of the administration of DHE or other ergots because both cause vasoconstriction.

Other migraine drugs studied in emergency department–based RCTs and shown to be effective include several dopamine-antagonist antiemetics: metoclopramide, chlorpromazine, prochlorperazine, ketorolac, and droperidol[20] (see Table 227-4). Regardless of the medication chosen, patients should be placed in a darkened, quiet area in order to lessen the associated phono- and photophobic symptoms. Given that patients may have been vomiting and had poor oral intake for hours or days prior to their arrival in the emergency department, intravenous rehydration is also frequently of benefit.

Dexamethasone has been touted as effective in reducing the rate of recurrent migraine following standard treatment. In one emergency department–based RCT, patients received either 20 mg intravenous dexamethasone or placebo after standard migraine therapy. A significant reduction in the rate of 48- to 72-h recurrent migraine was found in the dexamethasone group as compared with the placebo group.[21]

Special mention is reserved for the use of opioid analgesics in migraine. Meperidine is still used as an acute migraine treatment despite several studies that have shown it to be less effective than other agents.[22] The frequent use of opioids in chronic and recurrent headache conditions may lead to adverse effects and may even exacerbate headaches. Today the indications for opioid use in the treatment of migraine are declining.

Special Considerations

PREGNANT WOMEN Migraines generally improve during pregnancy, especially after the first trimester. Nonpharmacologic therapy,

TABLE 227-4   Treatment Options for Migraine Headache

Drug	Dosing and Adjuncts	Contraindications (CI), Precautions (PC), and Notes
Dihydroergotamine (DHE)	1 mg IV over 3 min; pretreat with metoclopramide or chlorpromazine or prochlorperazine to reduce nausea and vomiting	CI: Pregnancy, hypertension (uncontrolled), coronary artery disease, recent sumatriptan use, hemiplegic or basilar migraine PC: May cause nausea, vomiting, diarrhea, abdominal pain
Sumatriptan (Imitrex)	6 mg SC	CI: Pregnancy, hypertension (uncontrolled), coronary artery disease, ergot use in past 24 h, MAOI use, hemiplegic or basilar migraine PC: Minor adverse effects; rarely, coronary artery spasm, myocardial infarction, dysrhythmias
Ketorolac	30 mg IV or 60 mg IM	CI: History of peptic ulcer disease (especially in the elderly) PC: Class B in pregnancy, avoid in third trimester
Chlorpromazine	Pretreat with NS bolus to minimize hypotension; 7.5 mg IV	PC: Class C in pregnancy, may cause hypotension, drowsiness, dystonic reactions. Note: effective antiemetic
Prochlorperazine	5–10 mg IV or PR	PC: Class C in pregnancy, may cause drowsiness, dystonic reactions Note: effective antiemetic
Metoclopramide	10 mg IV	PC: Class B in pregnancy, may cause drowsiness, dystonic reactions Note: effective antiemetic
Droperidol	2.5 mg IV slow, or 2.5 mg IM	PC: Cases of QT-interval prolongation and/or torsades de pointes have been reported
Magnesium sulfate	2 g IV over 30 min	Note: nonvalidated but occasionally useful therapy
Methylprednisolone	125 mg IV or IM	Note: nonvalidated but occasionally useful rescue therapy

Abbreviation: MAOI = monoamine oxidase inhibitor.

such as rest and ice, should be tried first, but in patients with intractable headache or nausea and vomiting, medications may be used. Acetaminophen and nonsteroidal anti-inflammatory drugs (NSAIDs) are considered class B by the U.S. Food and Drug Administration (i.e., no evidence of risk in pregnant women, but there are no controlled trials) and can be used. However, NSAIDs should not be used in the third trimester because they inhibit labor and decrease amniotic fluid volume. Metoclopramide, another class B drug, can be very useful, especially if there is significant nausea and vomiting. Akathisia is a potential side effect of metoclopramide.

PREVENTIVE THERAPY Nonpharmacologic therapies include education of the patient about the disorder, its mechanisms, approaches to treatment, and changes in lifestyles involved in the avoidance of triggers of migraine.[2] Initiating pharmacologic preventive therapy is best done in collaboration with the family physician and/or the patient's neurologist.

TENSION-TYPE HEADACHES Previously, extracranial muscle tension was thought to be a causative factor in tension-type headaches. However, this relationship has been questioned, given the problem of demonstrating muscle tension and the difficulty of determining whether it is a cause or merely an epiphenomenon. More recent theories suggest that tension-type headaches and migraines may share a common pathophysiology and that they represent different ends of a clinical spectrum.[5]

Tension-type headaches are defined in such a way as to distinguish them from migraines. Therefore, they are described as bilateral, nonpulsating, not worsened by exertion, and not associated with nausea or vomiting. However, patients with severe tension-type headaches may indeed have nausea and vomiting, and mild migraine easily may fit the description of a tension-type headache.[5]

Treatment for mild headaches consists of simple analgesics or NSAIDs. For severe tension-type headaches, treatment is the same as for migraines, given the difficulty of distinguishing between the two entities.

CLUSTER HEADACHES Cluster headaches are generally rare (prevalence rates of 0.4 percent of the general population), and they are very short-lived, even without treatment. Unlike other primary headaches, they are more common in men, and onset is usually after 20 years of age.

Dysfunction of the trigeminal nerve is believed to cause cluster headaches, and the fact that they respond to 5-HT$_{1D}$ agonists suggests a common mechanism with migraines.

Cluster headaches are characterized by very severe unilateral orbital, supraorbital, or temporal pain lasting 15 to 180 min. The pain is such that patients rarely can lie still, and most are pacing and restless. The headaches are associated with at least one of the following signs on the ipsilateral side: conjunctival injection, lacrimation, nasal congestion, rhinorrhea, facial swelling, miosis, or ptosis. They tend to occur in clusters, i.e., daily on the same side of the face for several weeks, before remitting for anywhere from weeks to years.

Given the short duration of cluster headaches, any medication used in their treatment must act very rapidly. High-flow oxygen is effective in up to 70 percent of patients, and DHE and sumatriptan also have been shown to be rapidly effective. Oral agents are unlikely to be effective for acute attacks, given the long time for absorption and the short duration of cluster headaches, but NSAIDs may be useful in reducing the frequency and severity of future attacks.

Disposition of Patients with Primary Headache Syndromes

Regardless of the type of primary headache, poor response to treatment should heighten suspicion of a secondary cause and prompt emergent investigations. However, improvement of a presumed primary headache as a result of treatment does not exclude secondary causes.[3] Patients who respond well to emergency department management usually can be discharged with appropriate follow-up. Occasionally, a patient with intractable migraine may require admission for more aggressive pain control.

CRANIAL AND FACIAL PAIN DISORDERS

Temporomandibular Disorder

Temporomandibular disorder (TMD) refers to persistent discomfort due to dysfunction of the temporomandibular joint (TMJ), surrounding muscles, and ligaments. Symptoms include TMJ noise and pain on movement, limited jaw movements, locking of the jaw on opening, bruxism, and tongue, lip, or cheek biting. Headache may be associated with TMD as well, but in patients with headache and bruxism, it is often not clear which is cause and which is effect. Patients with TMD usually can locate their pain in the TMJ area. It is usually acute and associated with jaw movement. More diffuse symptoms may be the result of dysfunction of the muscles and ligaments used for mastication. Effective management of TMD often requires a multidisciplinary team, and improvement usually occurs with conservative measures. Simple radiographs of the TMJs are of little use in the emergency department because the diagnosis of TMD frequently requires more sophisticated imaging techniques. Simple analgesics or NSAIDs can be tried as an initial treatment.

Trigeminal Neuralgia (Tic Douloureux)

Trigeminal neuralgia is characterized by paroxysms of severe unilateral pain in the trigeminal nerve distribution lasting only seconds, with normal findings on neurologic examination. There is no pain between paroxysms. Treatment can be medical or surgical. Carbamazepine is a very effective treatment. If it fails, the patient is unlikely to have trigeminal neuralgia. Patients with trigeminal neuralgia may present to the emergency department because symptoms are of recent onset or recurrent, and they should be started or restarted on carbamazepine. Pain control is rarely an issue because the paroxysms are so brief. Patients with intractable symptoms despite medical therapy should be referred to a neurologist or neurosurgeon.

REFERENCES

1. Ramirez-Lassepas M, Espinosa CE, Cicero JJ, et al: Predictors of intracranial pathologic findings in patients who seek emergency care because of headache. *Arch Neurol* 54:1506, 1997.
2. Goadsby PJ, Lipton RB, Ferrari MD: Migraine: Current understanding and treatment. *New Engl J Med* 346:257, 2002.
3. American College of Emergency Physicians: Clinical policy for the initial approach to adolescents and adults presenting to the emergency department with a chief complaint of headache. *Ann Emerg Med* 27:821, 1996.
4. Frishberg BM: The utility of neuroimaging in the evaluation of headache in patients with normal neurological examinations. *Neurology* 44:1191, 1994.
5. Solomon S: Diagnosis of primary headache disorders: Validity of the International Headache Society criteria in clinical practice. *Neurol Clin* 15:15, 1997.
6. Schievink WI: Intracranial aneurysms. *New Engl J Med* 336:28, 1997.
7. Rothman RE, Keyl PM, McArthur JC, et al: A decision guideline for emergency department utilization of noncontrast head computed tomography in HIV-infected patients. *Acad Emerg Med* 6:1010, 1999.
8. American College of Emergency Physicians: Clinical policy: Critical issues in the evaluation and management of patients presenting to the emergency department with acute headache. *Ann Emerg Med* 39:108, 2002.
9. Gopol AK, Whitehouse JD, Dimel DL, et al: Cranial computed tomography before lumbar puncture: A prospective clinical evaluation. *Arch Intern Med* 159:2681, 1999.
10. Edlow JA, Caplan LR: Avoiding pitfalls in the diagnosis of subarachnoid hemorrhage. *New Engl J Med* 342:29, 2000.

11. Sidman R, Connolly E, Lemke T: Subarachnoid hemorrhage diagnosis: Lumbar puncture is still needed when the computed tomography scan is normal. *Acad Emerg Med* 3:827, 1996.

12. Morgenstern LB, Luna-Gonzales H, Huber JC: Worst headache and subarachnoid hemorrhage: Prospective, modern computed tomography and spinal fluid analysis. *Ann Emerg Med* 32:297, 1998.

13. Sames TA, Storrow AB, Finkelstein JA, Magoon MR: Sensitivity of new generation computed tomography in subarachnoid hemorrhage. *Acad Emerg Med* 3:16, 1996.

14. Schull MJ: Lumbar puncture first: An alternative model for the investigation of lone acute sudden headache. *Acad Emerg Med* 6:131, 1999.

15. Oshiro EM, Walter KA, Piantadosi S, et al: A new subarachnoid hemorrhage grading system based on the Glasgow Coma Scale: A comparison with the Hunt and Hess and World Federation of Neurological Surgeons Scales in a Clinical Series. *Neurosurgery* 41(1):140, 1997.

16. Chiang VL, Claus FB, Awad IA: Toward more rational prediction of outcome in patients with high-grade subarachnoid hemorrhage. *Neurosurgery* 46(1):28, 2000.

17. Hellmann DB: Temporal arteritis: A cough, toothache, and tongue infarction. *JAMA* 287:2996, 2002.

18. Vinson DR: Treatment patterns of isolated benign headache in US emergency departments. *Ann Emerg Med* 39:215, 2002.

19. Akpunonu BE, Mutgi AB, Federman DJ, et al: Subcutaneous sumatriptan for the treatment of acute migraine in patients admitted to the emergency department: A multicenter study. *Ann Emerg Med* 25:464, 1995.

20. Miner JR, Fish SJ, Smith SW, et al: Droperidol vs prochlorperazine for benign headaches in the emergency department. *Acad Emerg Med* 8:873, 2001.

21. Innes GD, MacPhail I, Dillon EC, et al: Dexamethasone prevents relapse after emergency department treatment of acute migraine: A randomized clinical trial. *Can J Emerg Med* 1:26, 1999.

22. Carleton SC, Shesser RF, Pietrzak MP, et al: Double blind multicenter trial to compare the efficacy of intramuscular dihydroergotamine plus hydroxyzine versus intramuscular meperidine plus hydroxyzine for the emergency treatment of acute migraine headache. *Ann Emerg Med* 32:129, 1998.

228 STROKE, TRANSIENT ISCHEMIC ATTACK, AND OTHER CENTRAL FOCAL CONDITIONS

Phillip A. Scott

Caroline A. Timmerman

Stroke is the third leading cause of death and the leading cause of disability in the United States. More than 700,000 Americans are afflicted yearly; of these, almost 20 percent will die within the first year. Although stroke is considered to be a disease of the elderly, one third of patients are younger than 65 years of age.[1] Research suggests early diagnosis and management of patients arriving with stroke at the emergency department may lessen the impact of this disease.

STROKE TYPE

The term "stroke" refers to any disease process that disrupts blood flow to a focal region of brain and that may be ischemic or hemorrhagic in nature. Approximately 80 percent are ischemic in nature with the remainder caused by hemorrhage within the cranial vault. Injury is dependent on the mechanism and is related to the loss of oxygen and glucose substrates necessary for high-energy phosphate production and the presence of mediators of secondary cellular injury. Subsequent factors, such as edema and mass effect, may exacerbate the initial insult.

Ischemic Stroke

Ischemic stroke can be subdivided into three major etiologies: thrombosis, embolism, and hypoperfusion. *Thrombosis* is the most common and occurs as a result of narrowing of the vascular lumen, with subse-

quent platelet adhesion and clot formation. Narrowing because of atherosclerotic disease is the most common cause of thrombotic stroke in the United States, and results from plaque development following vascular injury, with resultant arterial hyperplasia and fibrous deposition in the subintimal region. Other causes of thrombotic stroke include vasculitis, dissection, polycythemia, and hypercoagulable states. Less common effectors of vessel injury and narrowing are infectious diseases, such as HIV, syphilis, tuberculosis, aspergillosis, and trichinosis.

The signs and symptoms of thrombotic stroke usually develop gradually over minutes to hours and may wax and wane in severity. Often there is a history of similar but transient symptoms that have occurred in the past, suggesting a transient ischemic attack (TIA) in the same vascular distribution.

One-fifth of ischemic strokes are due to *embolism*. Intravascular material from a proximal source is released, subsequently occluding a distal vessel. In contrast to thrombotic stroke, there is no intrinsic vascular disease in the occluded vessel. Thus, emboli are less adherent and more likely to fragment or move distally than thrombotic occlusions. Cardiac sources of emboli include valvular vegetations, mural thrombi (caused by atrial fibrillation, myocardial infarction, or dysrhythmias), paradoxical emboli (caused by an atrial or ventricular septal defect), or cardiac tumors (myxomas). Artery-to-artery emboli occur when a platelet-fibrin clump is dislodged from a tight stenotic lesion or from a large-vessel atherosclerotic plaque. Rarer causes of embolic stroke include fat emboli, particulate emboli from intravenous drug injection, and septic emboli.

Systemic *hypoperfusion* is a less common mechanism of ischemic stroke and is typically caused by cardiac failure. Hypoperfusion leads to a more diffuse injury pattern compared to thrombosis or embolism and is typically located in watershed regions at the periphery of the cerebral vascular supply territories. Clinical findings often wax and wane with hemodynamic parameters.

Hemorrhagic Stroke

Hemorrhagic strokes are typically divided into two subtypes: intracerebral (ICH) and nontraumatic subarachnoid (SAH) hemorrhage. In ICH, which is the more common form, bleeding occurs directly into brain parenchyma from small arterioles previously weakened by elevated blood pressure. Increasing age and a history of prior stroke are leading risk factors for developing ICH. Race also plays a prominent role, with Asians and blacks having a higher incidence relative to whites. Tobacco and alcohol abuse are additional risk factors. Amyloidosis is another major cause of ICH, especially among elderly patients with lobar or multiple hemorrhages. Other causes of ICH include bleeding diathesis because of anticoagulant or thrombolytic use, vascular malformations, and cocaine use.

In SAH, blood leaks from a cerebral vessel into the subarachnoid space. SAHs result from berry aneurysm rupture, most commonly occurring at arterial bifurcations, or rupture of an arteriovenous malformation.

PATHOPHYSIOLOGY

Anatomy

The vascular supply to the brain is divided into anterior and posterior circulations. The anterior circulation, supplying blood to four-fifths of the brain, originates from the carotid system. The common carotid arteries divide into the right and left internal and external carotid arteries at the level of the angle of the mandible. The internal carotid arteries then course intracranially along the sella turcica within the cavernous sinus. The first branch off the internal carotid artery is the ophthalmic artery, supplying the optic nerve and retina. Sudden onset of painless monocular blindness (amaurosis fugax) identifies the stroke as involving the anterior circulation (specifically, the carotid artery) at or below the level of the ophthalmic artery. The internal carotid arteries terminate by branching into the anterior and middle cerebral arteries at the circle of Willis. The anterior circulation supplies blood to the optic nerve, retina, and frontoparietal and anterotemporal lobes of the brain.

The posterior circulation is derived from the two vertebral arteries that ascend through the transverse processes of the cervical vertebrae. The vertebral arteries enter the cranium through the foramen magnum, supplying the cerebellum via the posteroinferior cerebellar arteries. They join to form the basilar artery, which branches to form the posterior cerebral arteries. The posterior circulation supplies the brainstem, cerebellum, thalamus, auditory and vestibular functions of the ear, medial temporal lobe, and the visual occipital cortex.

The anterior and posterior circulations join at the circle of Willis, potentially allowing collateral flow around an area of occlusion. A patient with excellent collateral blood flow from the contralateral hemisphere may have minimal clinical deficits despite a complete carotid occlusion. In contrast, a patient with poor collateral flow may be hemiplegic with the same lesion.

Ischemic Stroke

Neurons are exquisitely sensitive to changes in cerebral blood flow and die within minutes of complete cessation. Despite complete occlusion of a cerebral vessel during an ischemic stroke, some perfusion may remain due to collateral flow and variations in local tissue pressure gradients. Cells vary from irreversibly injured neurons in the center of the ischemic region to reversibly injured neurons in the periphery (the penumbra). The degree and duration of occlusion determine the viability of the cells in the penumbra. Theoretically, the earlier reperfusion occurs, the greater the chance of survival. The use of intravenous and intraarterial thrombolytic therapy and the use of neuroprotective agents, are based on this rationale.

Hemorrhagic Stroke

In ICH and SAH, intracranial pressure (ICP) rises following vascular rupture with a corresponding short-term decrease in global perfusion. After these immediate changes, ICP and perfusion gradually improve, although they do not return to baseline. A marked reduction in perfusion occurs near the hematoma in ICH and is probably a result of local compression. Areas of the brain remote from the hemorrhage also have alterations in perfusion, thought to be secondary to vasoconstriction mediated by blood breakdown products or neuronal mechanisms (diaschisis).

CLINICAL FEATURES

The clinical presentation of stroke is often subtle and varied. Armed with an understanding of the various stroke types and anatomy, the history taking and physical examination should be aimed at diagnosing stroke, and determining the underlying cause and the location of the lesion. For example, strokes within the middle cerebral artery (MCA) distribution have the potential for benefit from early treatment with intraarterial thrombolysis (discussed later). Also newer approaches that use mechanical clot disruption catheters (e.g., jet-pulse venturi effect, ultrasound, vacuum, rotation) are in clinical trial, and are directed at larger MCA territory infarcts. Proximal MCA strokes have a higher likelihood of developing cerebral edema.

History

A history of hypertension, coronary artery disease, and diabetes mellitus are all suggestive of underlying atherosclerotic disease and vessel thrombosis. In contrast, atrial fibrillation, valvular replacement, or recent myocardial infarction suggest embolism.

Patients should be thoroughly questioned regarding recent history of TIAs, because this can help differentiate stroke types. A transient neurologic deficit in the same vascular distribution is suggestive of underlying vascular disease consistent with a thrombotic stroke, in contrast to multiple TIAs involving different vascular distributions, which suggest embolism.

Sudden onset of symptoms suggest an embolic or hemorrhagic stroke, whereas a stuttering or waxing and waning deficit suggests a thrombotic or hypoperfusion related stroke. Concomitant complaints such as headache, vomiting, or recent trauma should be recorded. Headache occurs in the majority of patients with hemorrhage but in a minority of those with ischemic stroke. A recent history of neck injury, such as in a motor vehicle accident, chiropractic manipulation or a sports-related injury, suggests a carotid dissection. A history of straining or coughing immediately preceding symptoms suggests ruptured aneurysm.

Physical Examination

If a patient is febrile, a potential infection should be investigated. An infection may be the cause of a patient's deterioration or may be a complication of the stroke (e.g., aspiration pneumonia). The skin should be examined for signs of emboli (Janeway lesions and Osler nodes) or bleeding dyscrasia (ecchymosis or petechiae). A funduscopic examination should be completed to identify signs of papilledema (suggesting a mass lesion, cerebral vein thrombosis or hypertensive crisis), pre-retinal hemorrhage (consistent with SAH), or evidence of hypertensive retinopathy. Findings suggestive of possible cardiac or vascular disease such as rales, an S3 gallop, or carotid bruit should be identified.

Neurologic Examination

The goal of the neurologic examination is to localize the central nervous system (CNS) lesion and exclude other neurologic disease processes. The National Institutes of Health (NIH) stroke scale is a 15-item neurologic evaluation (range 0–42) that is reproducible and correlates to infarct volume (Table 228-1).[2,3] It allows a serial, standardized neurologic evaluation of a patient by either a nurse or a physician. The basic neurologic assessment can be broken down into six major areas: 1) level of consciousness; 2) visual assessment; 3) motor function; 4) sensation and neglect; 5) cerebellar function; and 6) cranial nerves. Many of these elements are contained in the NIH stroke scale.

LEVEL OF CONSCIOUSNESS A patient's level of alertness should be evaluated by asking simple questions (birth date or month of the year) and by having the patient follow simple commands (close their eyes, make a fist, show me two fingers).

VISUAL ASSESSMENT Evaluation of visual fields and extraocular movements can provide information regarding occipital lobe or brainstem lesions. Visual fields can be tested by confrontation, using finger counting or visual threat as appropriate. Gaze palsy can be assessed by evaluating both voluntary and reflex eye movements (oculocephalic maneuver).

MOTOR FUNCTION Upper extremity motor weakness is best determined by testing for pronator drift. The test is considered positive if one arm pronates or drifts lower than the other within 10 s. Lower extremity strength can be similarly evaluated by a patient's ability to elevate each leg 45 degrees individually for 5 s while lying in bed. For subtle signs of lower extremity weakness, observe the patient's gait or have patients walk on their toes and then on their heels.

CEREBELLAR FUNCTION Cerebellar function is tested by observing a patient's gait, finger-to-nose and/or heel-to-shin testing. These

TABLE 228-1 **National Institute of Health Stroke Scale (NIHSS)**

Category	Patient Response	Score
LOC questions	Answers both correctly	0
	Answers one correctly	1
	Answers none correctly	2
LOC commands	Obeys both correctly	0
	Obeys one correctly	1
	Obeys none correctly	2
Best gaze	Normal	0
	Partial gaze palsy	1
	Forced deviation	2
Best visual	No visual loss	0
	Partial hemianopsia	1
	Complete hemianopsia	2
	Bilateral hemianopsia	3
Facial palsy*	Normal	0
	Minor facial weakness	1
	Partial facial weakness	2
	No facial movement	3
Best motor arm	No drift	0
Right _____	Drift <10 secs	1
Left _____	Falls <10 secs	2
	No effort against gravity	3
	No movement	4
Best motor leg	No drift	0
Right _____	Drift <5 secs	1
Left _____	Falls <5 secs	2
	No effort against gravity	3
	No movement	4
Limb ataxia*	Absent	0
	Ataxia in 1 limb	1
	Ataxia in 2 limbs	2
Sensory	No sensory loss	0
	Mild sensory loss	1
	Severe sensory loss	2
Neglect	Absent	0
	Mild	1
	Severe	2
Articulation	Normal	0
	Mild	1
	Severe	2
Language	Normal	0
	Mild aphasia	1
	Severe aphasia	2
	Mute or global aphasia	3

*Items deleted from the modified NIHSS.[3]

tests are all performed with the patient's eyes open and then closed to differentiate from posterior column disease (see Chap. 226).

SENSATION AND NEGLECT Sensory deficits and neglect should be evaluated by pinprick testing, having the patient identify numbers gently written on the palm (graphesthesia), and by double-simultaneous extinction (the physician touches the patient's right and left limbs individually and then simultaneously). The double-simultaneous extinction test is positive if the patient feels the sensation in either limb individually but only on one side when touched simultaneously. Neglect can be further confirmed by having the patient draw a box or house. Patients with neglect will often omit figures on one side of the drawing.

LANGUAGE *Dysarthria* is a disturbance in articulation and is caused by paralysis or incoordination of muscles used for speech. Dysarthric speech is often slurred. Repetition of simple phrases may identify subtle cases. In contrast, *aphasia* is caused by a disturbance in processing language (either written or spoken) and can be receptive (difficulty in comprehension), expressive (difficulty in communicating thoughts), or both. Receptive aphasia can be tested by having patients follow simple commands (either vocal or written). Having patients identify simple objects or describe what is happening in a magazine picture assists in evaluating an expressive aphasia. Patients with expressive aphasia will use inappropriate words or use nonfluent sentences, whereas the words of patients with dysarthria will be slurred.

CRANIAL NERVES Cranial nerves should be individually tested in all patients to identify possible brainstem involvement. Anterior circulation strokes, which cause contralateral motor deficits, while brainstem involvement causes ipsilateral cranial nerve deficits with contralateral motor weakness. In facial nerve weakness caused by a CNS lesion, the patient retains the ability to wrinkle the forehead. Inability to move the upper and lower face can be a result of Bell's palsy or Genu VII palsy (see Chap. 238). Genu VII palsy is a stroke involving Cranial Nerve VI and VII as it "genuflects" around the sixth nerve nucleus. The upper and lower face are paralyzed but there is also inability to abduct the ipsilateral eye.

STROKE SYNDROMES

Physical findings often follow classic patterns that can assist in localizing the lesion.

Transient Ischemic Attack

A TIA is a neurologic deficit that resolves within 24 h (although most resolve within 30 min) and is most commonly associated with thrombotic strokes. The incidence of prior TIAs ranges from 50 to 75 percent in patients with subsequent thrombotic, extracranial carotid artery strokes, but only 10 percent in all other stroke types. Many clinical TIAs may in fact be associated with computed tomography (CT) findings of infarction. Recent data suggest that more than 10 percent of patients with TIA may return to the ED with a stroke within 90 days, with half of these in just 2 days.[4]

Ischemic Stroke Syndromes

ANTERIOR CEREBRAL ARTERY INFARCTION Lesions of the anterior cerebral artery cause contralateral leg weakness greater than arm weakness with mild cortical sensory deficits. Patients may perseverate with speech or motor actions and respond slowly. Anarthria (speechlessness) with paraplegia may occur in a bilateral parasagittal infarct if the anterior cerebral arteries originate from an occluded common trunk.

MIDDLE CEREBRAL ARTERY INFARCTION A stroke involving the MCA territory presents with contralateral weakness and numbness variably affecting the face and arm greater than the leg. If the dominant hemisphere is involved, aphasia (receptive, expressive, or both) is often present. In right-handed patients, and in up to 80 percent of left-handed patients, the left hemisphere is dominant. Inattention, neglect, or extinction on double-simultaneous stimulation localize the lesion to the nondominant hemisphere. Constructional apraxia in these patients can be demonstrated by the inability to draw a clock and fill in the appropriate numbers. Patients may be dysarthric but typically are not aphasic. A homonymous hemianopsia and gaze preference toward the side of the infarct may also be found.

POSTERIOR CEREBRAL ARTERY INFARCTION   Patients with posterior cerebral artery (PCA) infarcts may be unaware of their deficits until formally tested. Motor involvement is minimal, and visual cortex abnormalities may go unrecognized. Light-touch and pinprick sensory modalities, however, may be significantly reduced. The anastomoses of branches of the PCA with arteries from the anterior cerebral artery and MCA territories are common locations of watershed infarcts in hypotensive states.

VERTEBROBASILAR SYNDROME   The posterior circulation supplies blood to the brainstem, cerebellum, and visual cortex. Signs and symptoms attributable to a stroke in this distribution may be subtle. They include findings such as dizziness, vertigo, diplopia, dysphagia, ataxia, cranial nerve palsies, and bilateral limb weakness, singly or in combination. **The hallmark of posterior circulation stroke is crossed neurologic deficits (i.e., ipsilateral cranial nerve deficits with contralateral motor weakness).**

The lateral medullary (Wallenberg) syndrome is a specific posterior circulation infarct involving the vertebrobasilar arteries and/or the posterior inferior cerebellar artery. In its pure form, it has a good prognosis. Presenting signs include ipsilateral loss of facial pain and temperature sensation with contralateral loss of these senses over the body, and gait and limb ataxia. Partial ipsilateral loss of cranial nerves V, IX, X, and XI in varying combinations are also present. Ipsilateral Horner syndrome (ptosis, miosis, and anhidrosis) may be present from disruption of the reticulospinal tracts to the sympathetic outflow.

BASILAR ARTERY OCCLUSION   Occlusion of the basilar artery causes severe quadriplegia, coma, and the *locked-in syndrome.* The locked-in syndrome occurs with lesions in the pontine tectum with complete muscle paralysis except for upward gaze.

CEREBELLAR INFARCTION   An important subset of posterior circulation strokes involve the cerebellum. Patients commonly present following a "drop attack" with the sudden onset of inability to walk or stand. This is often accompanied by vertigo, headache, nausea, vomiting, and neck pain. Cranial nerve abnormalities are often present. Bone artifact on CT imaging of the posterior fossa can obscure imaging, and an MRI or MRA should be obtained for diagnosis. Typically, after a delay of 6 to 12 h, cerebral edema will develop with subsequent increased brainstem pressure and decreased level of consciousness. Treatment of elevated ICP and emergent surgical decompression may be lifesaving.

LACUNAR INFARCTION   Lacunar infarcts are pure motor or sensory deficits caused by infarction of small penetrating arteries and are commonly associated with chronic hypertension. Lesions are primarily located in the pons and the basal ganglia.

ARTERIAL DISSECTION   Dissections are often associated with severe trauma but can occur from such mild events as turning the head sharply. Hypertension is a risk factor in spontaneous dissection. Patients may complain of severe neck pain or headache hours to days prior to onset of neurologic deficits. Dissections may occur in the carotid or vertebral circulation. Diagnosis is difficult as the extracranial vessels may not be well visualized on CT scans.

Hemorrhagic Stroke Syndromes

INTRACEREBRAL HEMORRHAGE   ICH may be clinically indistinguishable from cerebral infarction. Headache, nausea, and vomiting often precede the neurologic deficit and the patient's condition may quickly deteriorate necessitating emergent intubation. Bleeding is usually localized to the putamen, thalamus, pons, or cerebellum (in order of decreasing frequency) in patients with hypertensive ICH. Lobar hemorrhages are suggestive of amyloid angiopathy and are associated with a better prognosis.

CEREBELLAR HEMORRHAGE   A patient presenting with sudden onset of dizziness, vomiting, marked truncal ataxia, and inability to walk must be immediately suspected of having a cerebellar infarction or hemorrhage. These findings may be associated with gaze palsies and increasing stupor. Patients may rapidly progress to coma and herniation unless surgical decompression and/or hematoma evacuation are quickly initiated. However, with appropriate surgical treatment, the prognosis is good.

SUBARACHNOID HEMORRHAGE   SAHs frequently develop focal findings, possibly related to location of an aneurysm, but often there is no adequate explanation. Overall, SAH occurs more commonly in women, however men have a higher incidence in the under-forty population. Patients typically present with a severe, constant headache often occipital or nuchal in location. A recent history suggestive of a "sentinel hemorrhage" can be obtained in many cases. Vomiting often presents with the onset of headache, and patients may have a decreased level of consciousness. Presentation is usually sudden, and a careful history may reveal activities associated with elevated blood pressures such as defecation, intercourse, or coughing at stroke onset. Occasionally, the pain is only nuchal, misleading clinicians to consider only musculoskeletal etiologies. See Chap. 227 for detailed discussion regarding diagnostic approach.

DIAGNOSIS

Critical Pathway

Specific critical pathways similar to those used for AMI (door, data, decision, drug) should be used to speed the evaluation of patients with suspected acute stroke. Triage personnel should be educated to identify patients with symptoms of acute stroke and initiate standing orders. These include electrocardiogram; CBC; coagulation profile; type and screen; serum electrolytes, glucose, and renal function studies. An emergency noncontrast CT of the head should be ordered. The emergency physician should be notified of a potential acute stroke, and the acute stroke team notified if available.

There must be careful identification of the time of symptom onset, defined as *the last moment the patient was known to be normal.* Taking the patient and family chronologically through the events immediately prior to the stroke is a particular help in unclear cases. Thrombolytic use in stroke is not recommended when the time of onset cannot be reliably ascertained. Strokes recognized upon awakening should be timed from when the patient was last known to be without symptoms. A review of alteplase (rtPA) inclusion and exclusion criteria (Table 228-2) should be completed. Relative exclusion and inclusion criteria for rtPA administration based upon CT findings are shown in Table 237-2.

Diagnostic Tests

An emergent noncontrast CT of the head is essential to quickly differentiate hemorrhage from ischemia. **Most acute ischemic strokes will not be visualized by routine CT for at least 6 h**, depending on the size of the infarct. However, hypodensity indicating infarct should appear within 24 to 48 h. CT identifies almost all parenchymal hemorrhages greater than 1 cm in diameter and up to 95 percent of subarachnoid hemorrhages (if obtained within 12 h of symptom onset). This information is crucial for subsequent therapeutic decisions. If subarachnoid hemorrhage is still strongly suspected after a nondiagnostic CT scan, lumbar puncture is indicated. CT can also identify other life-threatening intracranial processes, such as abscess, tumor, and subdural or epidural hematoma.

TABLE 228-2   Criteria for Intravenous Thrombolysis in Ischemic Stroke

Inclusion	Exclusion*
Age 18 years or older	Minor stroke symptoms
Clinical diagnosis of ischemic stroke	Rapidly improving neurologic signs
Time since onset *well established* to be less than 3 h	Prior intracranial hemorrhage
	Blood glucose <50 mg/dL or >400 mg/dL
	Seizure at onset of stroke
	GI or GU bleeding within preceding 21 days
	Recent myocardial infarction
	Major surgery within preceding 14 days
	Sustained pretreatment SBP >185 mm Hg or DBP >110 mm Hg
	Previous stroke within preceding 90 days
	Previous head injury within preceding 90 days
	Current use of oral anticoagulants or PT >15 s or INR >1.7
	Use of heparin within preceding 48 h and a prolonged PTT
	Platelet count <100,000/μL

*Caution is advised before giving rtPA to persons with severe stroke (NIH Stroke Scale Score greater than 22).
Abbreviations: DBP = diastolic blood pressure; GI = gastrointestinal; GU = genitourinary; INR = international normalized ratio; PT = prothombin time; PTT = partial prothrombin time; SBP = systolic blood pressure.
Source: Adams HP, Brott TG, Furlan AJ, et al: Guidelines for thrombolytic therapy for acute stroke: A supplement to the guidelines for the management of patients with acute ischemic stroke. *Circulation* 94:1167, 1996.

An electrocardiogram should be obtained in all patients with suspected stroke to identify atrial fibrillation or acute myocardial infarction. Patients with untreated chronic atrial fibrillation have an associated 6 percent risk of stroke per year. In the first month following a myocardial infarction, the risk of stroke is 2.5 percent.

Blood tests that may be helpful include a complete blood count with platelet count, coagulation studies, toxicologic screen, and cardiac enzymes. A hematocrit can identify polycythemia, which can affect blood flow by increasing viscosity. A platelet count can identify thrombocytosis or thrombocytopenia that may precipitate thrombosis or hemorrhage, respectively. Coagulation studies are especially helpful in patients with hemorrhagic stroke to exclude coagulopathy or excessive anticoagulation with warfarin. A toxicologic screen for cocaine or amphetamine use should be obtained in patients with either ischemic or hemorrhagic stroke in which substance abuse is suspected, particularly young adults with stroke. Serum electrolytes are necessary to detect hyponatremia. Determination of cardiac enzymes will assist evaluation for a possible myocardial infarction.

Other diagnostic tests that may be of assistance, depending on the circumstances, include an echocardiogram, carotid duplex scanning, angiogram, and magnetic resonance imaging (MRI) or magnetic resonance imaging angiography (MRA). Few of these help with ED evaluation or treatment. An echocardiogram can identify a mural thrombus, tumor, or valvular vegetation in patients with a suspected cardioembolic stroke. Carotid duplex scanning may be helpful in patients with worsening neurologic deficit or crescendo TIAs with known or suspected high-grade carotid stenosis. Such patients may be candidates for emergent carotid endarterectomy or consideration of anticoagulation. Angiography is the definitive test to demonstrate stenosis or occlusion of both large and small blood vessels of the head and neck. It can detect subtle arterial abnormalities, such as dissection, which may be missed with other imaging techniques. Angiography remains the "gold standard" for demonstrating the cause of SAH and for defining the anatomic relationships of aneurysms.

MRI currently has a limited role in the emergency department evaluation of stroke because of access issues, delays for patient screening, and patient ability to cooperate. MRI will visualize ischemic infarcts earlier than CT and is more effective than CT at identifying acute posterior circulation strokes. Previously, MRI was considered less accurate at differentiating ischemia from hemorrhage, but new data suggests T2-weighted MRI sequences may be superior in detecting microbleeds, although this remains to be confirmed.[5] Emergent MRI should be considered when a dural sinus thrombosis is suspected or confirmation of a brainstem lesion is required. MRA enables demonstration of large vessel occlusions at the base of the skull, but small intracranial vascular occlusion may not be readily apparent. Improvement in MRA speed and resolution may allow greater use of this technology, and MRAs may replace the need for angiograms in the future.

Differential Diagnosis

Although strokes are the most common cause of focal neurologic deficits, other causes must be considered (Table 228-3). All patients with neurologic deficits should have their blood glucose checked for hypoglycemia. Bell palsy usually occurs in younger patients, is associated with upper and lower facial paralysis has no associated extraocular muscle involvement, and does not involve the extremities. Epidural or subdural hematoma can mimic an acute stroke and are usually associated with trauma. However, minor traumatic events may be overlooked, especially in those at risk (e.g., alcoholics). Although stroke can present with marked hypertension, one can usually differentiate stroke from hypertensive encephalopathy by history and physical examination. Unlike stroke, the onset of hypertensive encephalopathy is more gradual, and focal neurologic deficits, if present, are superimposed upon global cerebral dysfunction. Other diseases mimicking stroke include meningoencephalitis and hyperosmotic coma. Diabetic ketoacidosis (DKA), may be associated with infarction and arterial thrombosis, but also may rarely mimic stroke. Another stroke mimic is Wernicke encephalopathy, with its triad of ataxia, ophthalmoplegia, and confusion, typically found in chronic alcoholics. Multiple sclerosis, presenting commonly in the third and fourth decades of life, with a female predominance, may present with focal deficits, depending on the area of demyelination. The onset of symp-

TABLE 228-3   Differential Diagnosis of Acute Stroke

Epidural/subdural hematoma*
Hyponatremia*
Postictal paralysis (Todd paralysis)
Hypertensive encephalopathy*
Brain tumor/abscess*
Meningitis/encephalitis*
Hyperosmotic coma*
Wernicke encephalopathy*
Labyrinthitis*
Drug toxicity (lithium, phenytoin, carbamazepine)*
Bell palsy
Complicated migraine
Ménière disease
Demyelinating disease (multiple sclerosis)

*Critical diagnoses that must be considered.

toms, however, is more gradual than those in acute stroke. Ménière disease may be distinguished by its paroxysmal course of vertigo, tinnitus, and deafness. Drug toxicity may also masquerade as acute stroke, with lithium toxicity inducing dysarthria, cranial nerve deficits, and confusion. Phenytoin and carbamazepine toxicity may present with ataxia, vertigo, nausea, and abnormal reflexes.

SPECIFIC ISSUES THAT IMPACT EVALUATION AND TREATMENT

Sickle Cell Disease

Stroke occurs by age 20 years in more than 10 percent of patients with sickle cell anemia, and is the most common cause of ischemic stroke in children. The risk is inversely proportional to age, with the highest incidence noted between ages 2 and 5 years. Symptoms are similar to those in patients without sickle cell disease and range from brief TIAs to hemiparesis, depending on the vascular territory involved and duration of ischemia. Cerebral aneurysms also occur with increased frequency in patients with sickle cell anemia, and careful evaluation for SAH is mandated for patients presenting with headache and neurologic findings.

Emergent management of stroke in patients with sickle cell anemia includes supportive care with oxygen, intravenous fluids, and immediate CT scanning to evaluate for ruptured cerebral aneurysm or ICH. Initial laboratory studies should include a type and cross-match. Lumbar puncture is indicated in patients with suspected SAH and a nondiagnostic CT. If SAH is established, it is recommended delaying arteriography until hemoglobin S levels are below 30 percent of the total hemoglobin concentration and generous hydration is established. This may avoid increased sickling as a result of vasospasm from hyperosmolar contrast media.

In sickle cell patients with ischemic stroke, emergent simple or exchange transfusion should begin as soon as blood is available to reduce hemoglobin S to less than 30 percent. This is targeted toward improving blood flow and oxygen delivery to the infarct zone. The same therapy is indicated in hemorrhagic stroke in order to reduce vasospasm and secondary ischemic infarction. The efficacy of aspirin or warfarin therapy following ischemic stroke in this population has not been established. Early consultation with a hematologist and a neurologists are in order, and admission to an intensive care unit (ICU) setting indicated for close neurologic monitoring. Patients with TIA should also undergo similar exchange transfusion to the same target hemoglobin S levels.[6]

Young Adults with Stroke

Particular care should be exercised when evaluating the young adult (ages 15 to 50 years) with acute stroke. In this group, arterial dissection accounts for 20 percent of all ischemic strokes and may often be preceded by only minor trauma. The young adult with a cardioembolic event may have mitral valve prolapse, rheumatic heart disease, or paradoxical embolism as the originating cause. Migrainous stroke (infarction associated with typical migraine attack, among those with established recurrent migraines) in this age group is also a possibility. Air embolism should be considered in patients with a history of recent scuba diving or an invasive medical procedure. Such patients should be placed in a supine position and also placed on 100 percent oxygen. Emergent recompression in a hyperbaric chamber is indicated. Finally, some members of this population are at risk for ischemic stroke from substance abuse, with heroin, cocaine, amphetamines or other sympathomimetic drugs often implicated.

Pregnancy

While early pregnancy itself has not been associated with an increased risk of stroke, the peripartum and postpartum periods (up to 6 weeks after birth) have been identified as having an increased incidence of both ischemic and hemorrhagic stroke. Potential contributors to this increased risk include the presence of preeclampsia/eclampsia and the decrease in blood volume and alterations in hormonal status following birth.[7] Treatment should be targeted toward the underlying etiology.

The Elderly

The fastest growing population in the United States are those aged 85 years and older. The Census Bureau estimates a fivefold increase in this group to 18.2 million by 2050. There are no age-related limitations on the use of thrombolytic therapy.[8] In elderly patients with ICH, particular consideration should be given to amyloid angiopathy as a pathologic cause because of its increased incidence in the elderly.

Medicolegal Issues

At the time of this writing, initiation of anticoagulation in ischemic stroke or TIA is without a uniform consensus and is a matter of individual physician preference. With FDA approval of alteplase for the treatment of acute (0 to 3 h from symptom onset) ischemic stroke, the need for early identification of stroke in the emergency department has assumed increased importance. Delays in patient evaluation may prevent use of thrombolytic therapy when appropriate and place the physician at potential medicolegal risk. The development of ED systems to coordinate care of these patients is strongly recommended.

TREATMENT OF ISCHEMIC STROKE

General Management

Upon entry of patients with ischemic stroke into the emergency medical services (EMS) or emergency department setting, priority should be given to airway management and oxygenation. Generally, all patients should be placed on oxygen. The head of the bed should be slightly elevated, and a cardiac monitor and intravenous access established. Unless there is hypotension, fluids should be administered judiciously to prevent cerebral edema. Volume depletion in patients with ischemic stroke deserves prompt treatment, as it may contribute to decreased cerebral blood flow in the ischemic region. Careful examination of the scientific evidence for avoidance of glucose containing fluids is weak, and no causation of effect has been shown. Still, general practice is to avoid glucose-containing solutions except in those with proven hypoglycemia. Patients with fever should have antipyretics promptly administered. Experimental studies suggest hyperthermia increases CNS metabolic demands, whereas hypothermia has demonstrated neuroprotective effects.

The use of anticonvulsants is not recommended for seizure prophylaxis in ischemic stroke. If seizures occur, the patient should be treated acutely with benzodiazepines (e.g., lorazepam 2 to 4 mg IV, or diazepam 5 to 10 mg IV) and then given a loading dose of fosphenytoin (18 mg/kg IV at 25 mg/min).

Hypertension

A cautious approach to the management of elevated blood pressure is recommended in acute ischemic stroke. In general, frequent monitoring of blood pressure in hypertensive stroke patients is indicated and only persistent, severe hypertension (greater than 220 mm Hg systolic or more than 130 mm Hg mean arterial pressure) should be considered for treatment. Pharmacologic lowering of systemic blood pressure may reduce perfusion to the penumbra, converting an area with reversible injury to an area of infarction. Recommended agents include parenteral drugs that are easily titrated and that have minimal effects on cerebral blood vessels, such as labetalol or enalaprilat. Sublingual use of calcium-channel antagonists should be avoided.[9]

In hypertensive patients being considered for thrombolytic stroke therapy, the use of nitroglycerin paste or labetalol is acceptable to reduce blood pressure below 185/115 mm Hg to allow treatment. **Requirements for more aggressive treatment exclude the use of tissue plasminogen activator** in stroke patients. Following the use of recombinant tissue-type plasminogen activator (rtPA) in acute stroke, however, aggressive treatment with the aforementioned agents or, if control is inadequate, nitroprusside is warranted to maintain the blood pressure below 185/115 mm Hg. Hypertension is a significant cofactor in the risk of ICH in patients treated with thrombolytics.[10]

Thrombolysis

BACKGROUND The NIH/National Institutes of Neurological Disorders and Stroke (NINDS) study was a randomized, double-blind, placebo-controlled trial conducted at 40 geographically diverse hospitals (30 community and 10 university settings) comparing intravenous rtPA against placebo in 624 patients meeting specific enrollment criteria, including treatment within 3 h of symptom onset. Neurologists in private practice treated many patients in the trial, and some were evaluated and treated by emergency physicians. At 3 months, patients treated with rtPA were at least 30 percent more likely to have minimal or no disability as measured by four different neurologic outcome scales, with an absolute increase in favorable outcome of 11 to 13 percent. Benefit was found regardless of ischemic stroke subtype and has been demonstrated to continue for up to 1 year following therapy. Symptomatic ICH attributable to drug occurred in 6.4 percent of treated patients compared with 0.6 percent in the placebo group. The mortality rate at 3 months was not significantly different between treatment and placebo groups (17 percent, rtPA patients; 21 percent, placebo; $p = 0.3$), but the percentage of patients left severely disabled was lower in those receiving rtPA.[11]

Four other trials of intravenous thrombolysis have been published, and their conflicting results have generated debate over the role of thrombolysis in stroke. One of these, the European Cooperative Acute Stroke Study (ECASS), also evaluated the use of rtPA, although at a higher dosage (1.1 mg/kg; maximum dose, 100 mg) and longer time window (0 to 6 h). Although this study failed to demonstrate a difference in its primary end points between treatment and placebo groups, it must be considered that 109 of the 620 enrolled patients had major protocol violations. After excluding protocol violators, neurologic recovery at 3 months was significantly better for patients treated with rtPA.[12] The three trials of intravenous streptokinase in ischemic stroke were all halted prematurely for safety considerations. Potential explanations of the increased risk include the use of streptokinase itself, the high dosage used (1.5 million units), the allowance of concurrent heparin and aspirin use, and the time to treatment (the majority of patients were treated within 3 to 6 h).[13–15]

The FDA approved the use of intravenous rtPA in acute ischemic stroke in 1996 and approval was granted in Canada in 1999. The American Heart Association and the American Academy of Neurology support its use under appropriate conditions. The American College of Emergency Physicians has endorsed the principle that "intravenous tPA may be an efficacious therapy for the management of acute ischemic stroke if properly used incorporating the guidelines established by the NINDS," but did not endorse its use where systems are not in place to meet those guidelines.[16] The time-critical nature of thrombolytic therapy highlights the need for the involvement of emergency medicine in a coordinated, multidisciplinary approach to the treatment of stroke patients.

The use of intraarterial delivery of thrombolytics remains investigational. Advantages include specific evaluation of the occluded vascular territory, use of lower total doses of thrombolytic drugs, and the possibility of mechanical clot disruption. Studies evaluating prouroki-

nase given within 6 h of symptom onset found superior recanalization compared with placebo but with high rates of hemorrhagic complications.[17] Intraarterial thrombolysis may have a unique role in the treatment of patients with acute or subacute brainstem infarcts. Numerous cases have been reported where late intraarterial thrombolysis in the posterior circulation successfully restored function, suggesting this region may tolerate longer periods of ischemia.

DOSE AND COMPLICATIONS **The total dose of rtPA is 0.9 mg/kg, with a maximum dose of 90 mg; 10 percent of the dose is administered as a bolus, with the remaining amount infused over 60 min.** Blood pressure and neurologic checks should be assessed every 15 min for 2 h after starting the infusion. Table 228-4 outlines the emergent management of hypertension following thrombolytic administration. **No aspirin or heparin is given in the initial 24 h following treatment.** Patients should be admitted to an ICU setting familiar with the use of thrombolytic drugs and neurologic monitoring. Intracerebral bleeding should be suspected as the cause of any neurologic worsening until repeat CT imaging is obtained.

If bleeding is suspected, a CBC with platelet count, coagulation studies, fibrinogen and type- and cross-match for packed red blood cells, cryoprecipitate or fresh-frozen plasma, and platelets should be obtained. An emergent hematology and neurosurgical consultation, as necessary, is appropriate. Patients may be cared for at hospitals without in-house neurosurgical availability as long as access, or transport, to neurosurgical care can be arranged while a patient is stabilized. Chap. 224 discusses treatment of bleeding complications in detail.

Antiplatelet Agents

For the majority of stroke patients thrombolytic treatment will not be a consideration. In these patients, and those with TIAs, *antiplatelet strategies form the cornerstone for secondary stroke prevention.* Aspirin is the prototypical agent, decreasing the synthesis of thromboxane A_2 by irreversibly inhibiting cyclooxygenase for the life of the platelet, causing decreased platelet aggregation. Both the International Stroke Trial (IST) and Chinese Acute Stroke Trial (CAST) studies

TABLE 228-4 Emergent Management of Hypertension Following the Use of rtPA in Acute Stroke

Monitor arterial blood pressure during the first 24 h after starting treatment.
    Every 15 min for 2 h after starting the infusion, then every 30 min for
      6 h, then every 60 min for 24-h total
If SBP is 180–230 mm Hg or DBP is 105–120 mm Hg for two or more
readings 5–10 min apart:
    Give IV labetalol 10 mg over 1–2 min; the dose may be repeated or
      doubled every 10–20 min up to a total dose of 150 mg
    Monitor blood pressure every 15 min during labetalol treatment and
      observe for hypotension
If SBP is >230 mm Hg or if DBP is 121–140 mm Hg for two or more
readings 5–10 min apart:
    Give IV labetalol 10 mg over 1–2 min; the dose may be repeated or
      doubled every 10–20 min up to a total dose of 150 mg
    Monitor blood pressure every 15 min during labetalol treatment and
      observe for hypotension
    If no satisfactory response, infuse sodium nitroprusside (0.5–1.0 μg/kg per
      min); continuous arterial monitor advised
If DBP is >140 mm Hg for two or more readings 5–10 min apart:
    Infuse sodium nitroprusside (0.5–1.0 μg/kg per min); continuous arterial
      monitor advised

Abbreviations: DBP = diastolic blood pressure; SBP = systolic blood pressure.
Source: Adams HP, Brott TG, Furlan AJ, et al: Guidelines for thrombolytic therapy for acute stroke: A supplement to the guidelines for the management of patients with acute ischemic stroke. *Circulation* 94(5):1167, 1996. Copyright © American Heart Association.

demonstrated significant reduction in mortality rates and stroke recurrence in aspirin treated patients. Aspirin reduces stroke risk 20 to 25 percent compared to placebo.[18,19] No dose-effect response has been identified,[20] suggesting lower doses may be equally effective and better tolerated. Thus, initiation of aspirin therapy with doses of 50 to 300 mg in the ED is reasonable and offers a substantial cost advantage compared to other antiplatelet agents, and will not interfere with subsequent thrombolytic consideration.

Dipyridamole acts by phosphodiesterase inhibition thereby increasing cyclic adenosine monophosphate and inhibiting platelet function. Dipyridamole alone (200 mg PO bid) reduces the risk of stroke or death by 15 percent, as compared to placebo in patients with prior stroke or TIA. When combined with aspirin (50 mg PO per d), a 37 percent relative risk reduction compared to placebo can be expected.[21]

Clopidogrel acts via inhibition of adenosine diphosphate-dependent platelet activation and is, at best, marginally superior to aspirin with fewer side effects than its pharmacologic predecessor, ticlopidine. The use of clopidogrel (75 mg PO per d) in patients with atherosclerotic vascular disease resulted in a statistically significant but minimal (0.5 percent absolute) reduction in the annual risk of ischemic stroke, myocardial infarction, or vascular death when compared with aspirin (325 mg PO per d).[22] No combination studies have been reported. The use of clopidogrel is ideal for those patients who cannot tolerate, or fail, aspirin therapy. The selection of a particular antiplatelet regimen is a multifactorial decision based on comorbid conditions, prior drug use and cost. Aspirin remains a reasonable initial choice in the patient with a first-ever stroke or TIA.

Anticoagulants

Often, in the emergent setting, the etiology of a presenting stroke is unknown and the clinician must treat based on their best presumption as to etiology. The goal in treating these patients is to limit stroke progression and/or recurrent thromboembolism. Although used in this role, benefits of unfractionated heparin (UFH) in any stroke patient population remains unproven. Indeed, recently published studies have called into doubt its effectiveness. Although patients receiving heparin can expect significantly fewer recurrent ischemic strokes, this benefit is offset by an increased intracranial hemorrhage.[4] Thus, a decrease in death or nonfatal recurrent stroke is inapparent.

Multiple studies of low-molecular-weight heparin (LMWH) and heparinoids have found similarly disappointing results as with UFH. As of this writing, **the use of UFH, LMWH, or heparinoids to treat a specific stroke subtype or TIA cannot be recommended based on available evidence** and its use is at the discretion of the treating physician, preferably within the context of a clinical trial. In patients with atrial fibrillation and TIA, adjusted-dose oral anticoagulation with warfarin is the therapy of choice for stroke prevention.

Cerebellar Infarction

Early neurosurgical consultation is needed in the treatment of all patients with cerebellar infarction. Cerebellar swelling can lead to rapid deterioration with herniation, and consultation is required to determine the need for emergency posterior fossa decompression in these patients.

Transient Ischemic Attack

Patients with new onset TIAs should be admitted for evaluation of cardiac sources of emboli or high grade stenosis of the carotid arteries. Heparin is not recommended as routine therapy, either acutely or long term, for patients with TIAs. Some suggest UFH use may be considered in patients with recent TIAs who are at high risk for recurrence. These include patients with 1) known high-grade stenosis in the ap-

propriate vascular distribution for the symptoms, 2) a cardioembolic source (except infective endocarditis), 3) TIAs of increasing frequency (crescendo TIAs), and 4) TIAs despite antiplatelet therapy. No conclusive data exist to support or refute this practice and its use is at discretion of the admitting physician. Urgent carotid endarterectomy should be considered for TIAs that resolve within the first 6 h and are associated with greater than 70 percent stenosis of the carotid artery. Endarterectomy has been shown to significantly reduce the risk of future strokes in these patients.[23] The role of angioplasty and cerebral artery stenting are unclear at this time.

TREATMENT OF INTRACEREBRAL HEMORRHAGE

To date, there are no large randomized studies evaluating the appropriate management of blood pressure in ICH. Current recommendations are that only severe hypertension (i.e., greater than 220 mm Hg systolic or more than 120 mm Hg diastolic) be treated. When treated, blood pressure should be lowered gradually to prehemorrhage levels using either labetalol or nitroprusside. The exceptions to this rule are cases of ICH associated with cardiac failure or arterial dissection, in which more rapid reduction is required. If a patient is known to have chronic hypertension, the blood pressure should not be lowered to normotensive levels but rather to an approximation of the patient's usual hypertensive blood pressure.

The patient's head should be elevated 30 degrees to the horizontal. The use of hyperventilation and osmotherapy with mannitol (0.25 to 1.0 g/kg IV), and furosemide (10 mg IV) is recommended in patients with evidence of increased intracranial pressure with features such as mass effect, midline shift, or herniation. The target Pa_{CO_2} is 30 to 35 mm Hg, while the target serum osmolality is $\leq$310 mOsm/kg. Steroids are not indicated. ICP monitors should be considered in (but not limited to) patients with a Glasgow Coma Scale score of <9, and in all patients whose condition is thought to be deteriorating because of elevated ICP. Intraventricular devices allow direct reduction of ICP by cerebrospinal fluid drainage. Seizure prophylaxis with phenytoin should also be considered.

The role of acute surgical intervention remains controversial and depends on the neurologic status of the patient as well as the size and location of the hemorrhage. Surgical decompression and hematoma evacuation may be lifesaving in patients with cerebellar hematomas greater than 3 cm in diameter or those near the brainstem.

TREATMENT OF SUBARACHNOID HEMORRHAGE

Rebleeding and vasospasm are the major complications in SAH. Risk of rebleeding is greatest in the first 24 h. In patients with elevated blood pressures, lowering systolic blood pressure to 160 mm Hg and/or maintaining a mean arterial pressure of 110 mm Hg is associated with lower risk of rebleeding and a decreased mortality rate. Current recommendations are that blood pressure should be maintained at prehemorrhage levels.

Cerebral ischemia caused by vasospasm occurs from 2 days to 3 weeks after aneurysm rupture. Nimodipine, given PO 60 mg every 6 h, reduces the incidence and severity of vasospasm and should be given to all patients with SAH. In patients who have difficulty swallowing, it may be advisable to delay initiation of this medication, although if there are no contraindications it may be started in the ED.

Seizures and persistent vomiting can cause elevations in systemic and intracranial pressure. Prophylactic phenytoin loading is recommended. Nausea and vomiting should be promptly treated with antiemetics. Pain should be appropriately managed.

Usually, candidates for early angiography and surgical intervention are stable patients with good neurologic condition (Hunt and Hess grades 1 to 3). However, there is little published evidence that this regimen reduces the long-term morbidity or mortality rates. Alternative approaches for patients with appropriate aneurysms include endovascular obliteration through the use of intraluminal platinum coils or detachable balloon embolization.

REFERENCES

1. American Heart Association: *2002 Heart and Stroke Facts Statistical Update.* Dallas, American Heart Association, 2001.
2. Brott T, Adams HP, Olinger CP, et al: Measurements of acute cerebral infarction: A clinical examination scale. *Stroke* 20:864, 1989.
3. Meyer BC, Hemmen TM, Jackson CM, et al: Modified National Institute of Health Stroke Scale for use in Stroke Clinical Trials. *Stroke* 33:1261, 2002.
4. Johnston SC, Gress DR, Browner WS, et al: Short-term prognosis after emergency department diagnosis of TIA. *JAMA* 284:2901, 2000.
5. Kidwell C, Saver J, Villablance J, et al: Magnetic resonance imaging detection of microbleeds before thrombolysis: An emerging application. *Stroke* 33:95, 2002.
6. Reid CD, Charache S, Lubov B, et al (eds): *Management and Therapy of Sickle Cell Disease,* 3rd ed. Bethesda, MD, National Heart, Lung and Blood Institute, NIH Publication 96-2117, revised December 1995.
7. Kittner SJ, Stern BJ, Feeser BR, et al: Pregnancy and the risk of stroke. *New Engl J Med* 335:768, 1996.
8. Tanne D, Gorman MJ, Bates VE, et al: Intravenous tissue plasminogen activator for acute ischemic stroke in patients aged 80 years and older: The TPA stroke survey experience. *Stroke* 31:370, 2000.
9. Adams HP Jr, Brott TG, Furlan AJ, et al: *Guidelines for the Management of Patients with Acute Ischemic Stroke: American Heart Association Medical/Scientific Statement 1994.* Dallas, TX, American Heart Association, 1994.
10. Gebel JM, Sila CA, Sloan MA, et al: Thrombolysis-related intracerebral hemorrhage: A radiographic analysis of 244 cases from the GUSTO-1 trial with clinical correlation. *Stroke* 29:563, 1998.
11. National Institute of Neurological Disorders and Stroke rt-PA Stroke Study Group: Tissue plasminogen activator for acute ischemic stroke. *New Engl J Med* 333:1581, 1995.
12. Hacke W, Kaste M, Fieschi C, et al: Intravenous thrombolysis with recombinant tissue plasminogen activator for acute hemispheric stroke: The European Cooperative Acute Stroke Study (ECASS). *JAMA* 274:1017, 1995.
13. Multicenter Acute Stroke Trial-Europe Study Group: Thrombolytic therapy with streptokinase in acute ischemic stroke. *New Engl J Med* 335:145, 1996.
14. Multicentre Acute Stroke Trial-Italy (MAST-I) Group: Randomised controlled trial of streptokinase, aspirin, and combination of both in treatment of acute ischaemic stroke. *Lancet* 346:1509, 1995.
15. Donnan GA, Davis SM, Chambers BR, et al: Streptokinase for acute ischemic stroke with relationship to time of administration. *JAMA* 276:961, 1996.
16. Anonymous. ACEP Policy Statement: *Use of Intravenous tPA for the Management of Acute Stroke in the Emergency Department.* American College of Emergency Physicians [Internet]. Available at: http//www.acep.org/1,5006,0.html. Accessed 5/15/03.
17. del Zoppo GJ, Higashida RT, Furlan AJ, et al: PROACT: A phase II randomized trial of recombinant pro-urokinase by direct arterial delivery in acute middle cerebral artery stroke. *Stroke* 29:4, 1998.
18. International Stroke Trial Collaborative Group: The International Stroke Trial (IST): A randomised trial of aspirin, subcutaneous heparin, both, or neither among 19,435 patients with acute ischaemic stroke. *Lancet* 349:1569, 1997.
19. Anonymous. CAST: Randomised placebo-controlled trial of early aspirin use in 20,000 patients with acute ischaemic stroke. CAST (Chinese Acute Stroke Trial) Collaborative Group. *Lancet.* 349(9066):1641, 1997.
20. Tijssen JGP: Low-dose and high-dose acetylsalicylic acid, with and without dipyridamole: A review of clinical trial results. *Neurology* 51(Suppl 3):S15, 1998.
21. Diener HC, Cunha L, Forbes C, et al: European Stroke Prevention Study: 2. Dipyridamole and acetylsalicylic acid in the secondary prevention of stroke. *J Neurol Sci* 143:1, 1996.
22. CAPRIE Steering Committee: A randomised, blinded trial of clopidogrel versus aspirin in patients at risk of ischaemic events (CAPRIE). *Lancet* 348:1329, 1996.
23. Feinberg WM, Albers GW, Barnett HJM, et al: *Guidelines for the Management of Transient Ischemic Attacks. American Heart Association Medical/Scientific Statement, 1994.* Dallas, American Heart Association, 1994.

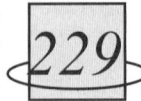

ALTERED MENTAL STATUS AND COMA
J. Stephen Huff

Disorders of consciousness may be divided into processes that affect either arousal functions, content of consciousness functions, or combinations of both functions. Arousal behaviors include wakefulness and basic eyes-open, alerting functions. Anatomically, neurons responsible for these arousal functions reside in the reticular activating system, a collection of neurons scattered through the midbrain, pons, and medulla. Content of consciousness includes self-awareness, language, reasoning, spatial relationship integration, emotions, and the myriad complex integration functions that we regard basic to being human. The neuronal structures responsible for the content of consciousness reside in the cerebral cortex. Dementia is failure of the content portions of consciousness with relatively preserved alerting functions. Delirium is an arousal system dysfunction, and content of consciousness is affected as well. Coma is failure of both arousal and content functions. Psychiatric disorders and altered mental states may share features such as hallucinations or delusion; some distinctions between the different states are summarized in Table 229-1.[1]

Mental status is the clinical state of emotional and intellectual functioning of the individual. The mental status evaluation may be divided into six categories (Table 229-2). Testing the mental status is done both formally and informally during patient evaluation.[2] The higher mental or cognitive functions need specific tests for assessment; screening tests are described in the following section.

DELIRIUM

Delirium, acute confusional state, acute cognitive impairment, acute encephalopathy, and other synonyms refer to a transient disorder with impairment of attention and cognition. Delirium represents a form of brain failure, but the patient is more alert than in coma. Alerting functions are working, perhaps overworking. The patient may have difficulty in focusing, shifting, or sustaining attention. The formal definition also includes disturbed wake-sleep cycles and a fluctuating course of confusion (see Table 229-1).

The incidence of delirium in emergency department populations is not clear. It is estimated that 10 to 25 percent of elderly hospitalized patients have delirium at the time of admission.[3] Recent literature suggests that up to one-quarter of all emergency department patients aged 70 or older have impaired mental status or delirium, and notes that routine evaluation is not satisfactory to identify many of these patients.[4,5]

Pathophysiology

Delirium always has an organic cause. Pathologic mechanisms are complex and are thought to involve widespread neuronal or neurotransmitter dysfunction. There are four general causes:

1. Primary intracranial disease
2. Systemic diseases secondarily affecting the central nervous system (CNS)
3. Exogenous toxins
4. Drug withdrawal[1]

Clinical Features

Delirium or acute confusional state develops quickly, generally over days. Attention, perception, thinking, and memory are all distorted to varying degrees. Alertness is reduced as manifested by difficulty maintaining attention and focusing concentration. The patient may appear quite awake, but attention is impaired. Activity levels may be either increased or decreased. Three variants are described: hypoalert-hypoactive, hyperalert-hyperactive, and mixed. The patient with the mixed variety may fluctuate rapidly between hypoactive and hyperac-

TABLE 229-1   Features of Delirium, Dementia, and Psychiatric Psychosis

Characteristic	Delirium	Dementia	Psychiatric
Onset	Over days	Insidious	Sudden
Course over 24 h	Fluctuating	Stable	Stable
Consciousness	Reduced	Alert	Alert
Attention	Disordered	Normal	May be disordered
Cognition	Disordered	Impaired	May be impaired
Orientation	Impaired	Often impaired	May be impaired
Hallucinations	Visual and/or auditory	Often absent	Usually auditory
Delusions	Transient, poorly organized	Usually absent	Sustained
Movements	Asterixis, tremor may be present	Often absent	Absent

Source: Modified from Lipowski.[1]

tive states. Symptoms may be intermittent and it is not unusual for different caregivers to witness completely different behaviors within a brief time span.[3] The sleep-wake cycles are often disrupted with increased somnolence during the day and agitation at night. The increased nocturnal agitation is commonly referred to as "sundowning." Evidence of organic disease such as tremor, asterixis, tachycardia, sweating, hypertension, or emotional outbursts may be present. Hallucination, delusions, and illusions may be present. Hallucinations tend to be visual, though auditory hallucinations can also occur.

Diagnosis

Both historical and physical findings are necessary to confirm the diagnosis of delirium. The history is needed to confirm the acuity of the change in behavior and reveal the fluctuating confusion consistent with the delirium. The history from caregivers, spouse, or other family members is the primary method for diagnosing delirium.[3] The acute onset of attention deficits and cognitive abnormalities with fluctuating severity through the day and worsening at night is virtually diagnostic of delirium. Medication history, including over-the-counter medications, should be examined in detail. In the elderly, medication side effects or toxicity may be observed in what are ordinarily regarded as therapeutic and safe doses. General physical examination is directed at discovering the underlying process, such as pneumonia. Ancillary testing, should include serum electrolytes hepatic and renal studies; urinalysis; blood count; and a chest radiograph. Cranial CT should be done followed by lumbar puncture if meningitis or subarachnoid hemorrhage is in consideration.

TABLE 229-2   Six Elements of Mental Status Evaluation

Appearance, behavior, and attitude
  Is dress appropriate?
  Is motor behavior at rest appropriate?
  Is the speech pattern normal?
Disorders of thought
  Are the thoughts logical and realistic?
  Are false beliefs or delusions present?
  Are suicidal or homicidal thoughts present?
Disorders of perception
  Are hallucinations present?
Mood and affect
  What is the prevailing mood?
  Is the emotional content appropriate for the setting?
Insight and judgement
  Does the patient understand the circumstances surrounding the visit?
Sensorium and intelligence
  Is the level of consciousness normal?
  Is cognition or intellectual functioning impaired?

Source: Modified from Zun and Howes.[2]

One key tool for detecting delirium is the mental status examination. The Mini-Mental State Examination (MMSE) is probably the most widely used test, though frequently only parts are administered in ED (Table 229-3).[6] This test is valuable in directing the physician to study aspects of attention and memory that might not otherwise be formally tested. Age, education, chronic cognitive impairment, and verbal abilities may all affect scores. Several other shorter evaluation systems have been proposed. The Quick Confusion Scale (QCS) has been tested in ED patients, correlates well with the MMSE, and takes less time to administer (Table 229-4).[7]

Depression may resemble a hypoactive delirium, with withdrawal, slowed speech, and poor results in cognitive testing present in both conditions. However, rapid fluctuation of symptoms is common in delirium but absent in depression. Additionally, clouding of consciousness is absent in patients with depression; usually testing will find patients oriented and able to perform commands.[3]

Treatment

Treatment is directed at the underlying cause. Common medical causes of delirium are listed in Table 229-5, and multiple causes may be present in a patient.

Environmental manipulations such as adequate lighting and psychosocial support may be helpful in enhancing the patient's ability to interpret the surroundings correctly.[3] Sedation may be needed at times to relieve severe agitation. Haloperidol is a frequent initial choice at a dose of 5 to 10 mg PO, IM, or IV; 1 to 2 mg in the elderly. This may be repeated at 20- to 30-min intervals as the clinical situation indicates. Benzodiazepines such as lorazepam 0.5 to 2 mg PO, IM, or IV may be used in combination with haloperidol in doses of 1 to 2 mg, the dose varying widely because of the age and size of the patient and the degree of agitation. Any institutional confinement or restraint policies should be appropriately addressed. Sedation or restraint is no substitute for diagnostic activities and specific illness-targeted therapy.

Disposition

Unless a readily reversible cause for the acute mental status change is discovered, treatment initiated, and improvement is seen, the majority of patients will be hospitalized for further treatment and possibly additional diagnostic testing. This decision will be individualized to the patient, the resources in the home or health care facility, and the safety of the patient.

DEMENTIA

Dementia implies a loss of mental capacity. The individual who once functioned at a certain psychosocial level with certain cognitive abilities

TABLE 229-3   The Mini-Mental State Examination

Maximum Score	Score	
		ORIENTATION
5	( )	What is the: (year) (season) (date) (day) (month)?
5	( )	Where are we: (state) (county) (town) (hospital) (floor)?
		REGISTRATION
3	( )	Name 3 objects; ask patient to repeat.
		ATTENTION AND CALCULATION
5	( )	The serial 7 test; 1 point for each correct. Stop after 5 answers. Option: spell "world" backwards.
		RECALL
3	( )	Ask for the 3 objects repeated above. 1 point scored for each correct object recalled.
		LANGUAGE
9	( )	Name a pencil and watch (2 points)
		Repeat the following, "No if's, ands, or buts." (1 point)
		Follow 3 stage command: "Take a paper in your right hand, fold it in half, and put it on the floor." (3 points)
		Read and follow the following printed command:
		"Close your eyes" (1 point)
		Write a sentence (1 point)
		Copy design (1 point)

SCORING: A score of 23 or less may indicate the presence of dementia or another cognitive disorder and suggests the need for further testing and evaluation.

Instructions for Administering the Mini-Mental State Examination

Orientation: Ask for the date. Specifically ask for any omitted information. One point for each correct answer.

Registration: Ask permission to test memory. Name 3 unrelated objects clearly and slowly about 1 s apart. After you have said all 3, ask the patient to repeat. The first repetition determines the score. In order to test recall (discussed below) the examiner should repeat the items in order up to 6 times, until the patient can repeat all 3. If the patient is unable to do this, recall can't be tested.

Attention and calculation: Ask the patient to begin with 100 and count backwards by 7. Stop after 5 subtractions and score correct answers. If the patient cannot calculate, ask him or her to spell "world" backwards. The score is the number of letters in correct order.

Recall: Ask the patient if he or she can recall the 3 words previously asked to remember. Score 0–3.

Language: Naming: Show the patient a wristwatch and pencil and ask name. Score 0–2.
  Repetition: Ask the patient to repeat a sentence. Allow one trial. Score 0 or 1.
  3-Stage command: Give the patient a piece of paper and repeat the command. Score 1 point for each portion of the command correctly performed.
  Reading: Print clearly on a piece of paper in large letters the command, "Close your eyes." Ask the patient to read and perform the command. Score 1 point if the eyes are closed.
  Writing: Give the patient a blank piece of paper and ask him or her to write a sentence of his or her own choosing. It must contain a subject and a verb to be scored 1 point. Punctuation does not matter for scoring purposes.
  Copying: On a clean piece of paper, draw intersecting pentagons, each side 1 inch, and ask the patient to copy exactly. All 10 angles must be present and the 2 figures must intersect to score 1 point. Any rotation of the figures or tremor is ignored.

Source: Modified from Folstein and Folstein.[6]

is now failing and behavioral problems have developed. Most dementias are idiopathic and are termed *dementia of the Alzheimer disease* (DAT). The other large category is vascular dementia. However, many other disorders more treatable than Alzheimer disease (AD) or vascular dementia may also cause dementia or simulate dementia. The largely untreatable dementias are thus diagnoses of exclusion.

The typical course of dementia is slow with insidious symptom onset; the abrupt onset of symptoms or rapidly-progressing symptoms should prompt a search for another organic process. Presentation to the ED is usually precipitated by some sentinel occurrence or event. Patients may be brought to the ED as a consequence of caregiver burnout. The behavioral symptoms of patients with Alzheimer may be disruptive to the home environment and distressing to the patient and caregivers. Hallucinations, delusions, repetitive behaviors, and depression are all common. Patients may misidentify other people and family members may be regarded as strangers, sometimes with apparent great fear.

Pathophysiology

The majority of cases of dementia in the United States are due to AD. Alzheimer is a neurodegenerative disorder of unknown etiology. The pathophysiology is complex, with a reduction in neurons in the cerebral cortex as well as increased amyloid deposition and the production of neurofibrillary tangles and plaques. Other neurodegenerative diseases have their own unique pathologies.

Vascular dementia accounts for the next largest number of individuals with dementia. The pathology is that of cerebrovascular disease with multiple infarctions. A listing of different dementias is provided in Table 229-6.

Clinical Features

Impairment of memory, particularly recent memory, is gradual and progressive. Remote memories are often preserved. Impairment of memory and orientation with preservation of motor and speech abilities is said to be characteristic of the onset of AD. Degenerative dementias such as AD may be divided into early, middle, and late stages. Early in the disease, complaints of memory loss, naming problems, or forgetting items are common. The middle stage shows progression of these problems plus loss of reading, decreased performance in social situations, and losing directions. The late stage of the illness may include extreme disorientation, inability to dress and perform self-care, and personality change. Typically, the onset of symptoms is slow and gradual; if the onset of symptoms is acute, the possibility of a reversible process is increased. Clinical features of AD or other demen-

TABLE 229-4   The Quick Confusion Scale

Item	Score (Number Correct)	× (Weight)	=	(Total)
What year is it now?	0 or 1 (Score 1 if correct, 0 if incorrect)	× 2	=	_____
What month is it?	0 or 1	× 2	=	_____
Present memory phrase: "Repeat this phrase after me and remember it: John Brown, 42 Market Street, New York."				
About what time is it? (Answer correct if within 1 hour)	0 or 1	× 2	=	_____
Count backwards from 20 to 1	0, 1, or 2	× 1	=	_____
Say the months in reverse	0, 1, or 2	× 1	=	_____
Repeat memory phrase (each underlined portion correct is worth 1 point)	0, 1, 2, 3, 4, or 5	× 1	=	
Final Score is the Sum of the Totals			=	_____

15 is the top score; a score less than 15 may indicate the need for additional assessment.
Scores highest number in category indicates correct response; lower scoring indicates increased number of errors.
Item 1. "What year is it now?"
Score 1 if answered correctly, 0 if incorrect.
Item 2. "What month is it?"
Score 1 if answered correctly, 0 if incorrect.
Item 3. "About what time is it?"
Answer considered correct if within 1 hour; score 1 if correct, 0 if incorrect.
Item 4. "Count backwards from 20 to 1"
Score 2 if correctly performed; score 1 if one error, score 0 if 2 or more errors.
Item 5. "Say the months in reverse"
Score 2 if correctly performed; score 1 if one error, score 0 if 2 or more errors.
Item 6. Repeat memory phrase
"John Brown, 42 Market Street, New York"
Each underlined portion correctly recalled is worth 1 point in scoring; score 5 if correctly performed; each error drops score by one.
Final score is sum of the weighted totals; items one, two, and three are multiplied by 2 and summed with the other item scores to yield the final score.
Source: From Huff et al.[7]

tias may include affective symptoms such as depression and anxiety, behavioral disorders, and speech difficulties.

Vascular or multi-infarct dementia has symptoms similar to AD, but may have findings on physical examination of exaggerated or asymmetric deep tendon reflexes, gait abnormalities, or weakness of an extremity.

Diagnosis

The history of memory problems is usually one of slow progression without landmark occurrences. If specific dates of worsening are noted, the possibility of a vascular dementia increases. Family history may be significant. One inherited dementia, Huntington disease, has a clear autosomal dominant pattern of inheritance.

General physical examination does not determine the diagnosis of dementia, but may be helpful in identifying associated causes.[8] The presence of focal neurologic signs may suggest vascular dementia or a mass lesion. Increased motor tone and other extrapyramidal signs such as rigidity or a movement disorder may suggest Parkinson disease. Mental status testing should be performed as outlined above and summarized in Tables 229-2, 229-3, and 229-4.

For diagnosis, the American Academy of Neurology practice parameter[9] in 1994 recommends complete blood count, serum electrolytes, calcium, glucose, BUN, creatinine, and liver function tests. However, no studies have been done to evaluate these recommendations. In 2001, an evidence-based review suggested the use of thyroid function tests, serum vitamin B_{12}, and serology for syphilis (only if at risk).[10] Other laboratory tests that are optional and may be helpful in certain circumstances include erythrocyte sedimentation rate, serum folate level, HIV testing, chest x-ray, urinalysis. Neuroimaging such as

CT or MRI should be considered in every patient at some point in the diagnostic evaluation. Lumbar puncture should be performed if the diagnosis is not readily apparent.

Diagnosis of probable vascular dementia again requires signs of cerebrovascular disease. The relationship between stroke and cognitive decline must be temporally related, with dementia within 3 months of the stroke or abrupt deterioration in memory and other cognitive abilities. A fluctuating, stepped course suggests vascular dementia.[11]

The possibility of a comorbid condition suddenly worsening cognitive functioning should be strongly considered and often is the thrust of investigation in the ED. Urinary tract infection, congestive heart failure, or hypothyroidism are just a few of the conditions that may cause a mildly demented but functioning individual to rapidly deteriorate. The symptoms overlap with those of delirium as discussed above. The differential diagnosis is particularly important for consideration of depression imitators, the so-called treatable causes of dementia (see Table 229-6).

Depression may coexist with dementia; however, depression imitating dementia (pseudodementia) should also be considered. Appropriate inpatient or outpatient follow-up may be arranged for further psychiatric evaluation. If the patient is thought to be seriously depressed, consideration should be given to hospital admission.

Treatment

All types of dementia are treatable at least to some degree by environmental or psychosocial interventions. Antipsychotic drugs have been used for management of the psychotic and nonpsychotic behaviors, but treatment remains problematic because of adverse drug effects. Use of these drugs should be selective and reserved for patients with

TABLE 229-5   Important Medical Causes of Delirium in Elderly Patients

Infection	Pneumonia
	Urinary tract infection
	Meningitis or encephalitis
	Sepsis
Metabolic/toxic	Hypoglycemia
	Alcohol ingestion
	Electrolyte abnormalities
	Hepatic encephalopathy
	Thyroid disorders
	Alcohol or drug withdrawal
Neurologic	Stroke or TIA
	Seizure or postictal state
	Subarachnoid hemorrhage
	Intracranial hemorrhage
	Mass CNS lesion
	Subdural hematoma
Cardiopulmonary	Congestive heart failure
	Myocardial infarction
	Pulmonary embolism
	Hypoxia or CO_2 narcosis
Drug-related	Antiemetics
	Antihistamines
	Antiparkinsonian agents
	Antipsychotics
	Antispasmodics
	Muscle relaxants
	Tricyclic antidepressants
	Digoxin
	Sedative-hypnotics
	Narcotic analgesics

TABLE 229-6   Classification of Dementia by Cause

Degenerative
  Alzheimer disease
  Huntington disease
  Parkinson disease, others
Vascular
  Multiple infarcts
  Hypoperfusion (cardiac arrest, profound hypotension, others)
  Subdural hematoma
  Subarachnoid hemorrhage
Infectious
  Meningitis (sequelae of bacterial, fungal, or tubercular)
  Neurosyphilis
  Viral encephalitis (herpes, HIV), Creutzfeldt-Jakob disease
Inflammatory
  Systemic lupus erythematosus
  Demyelinating disease, others
Neoplastic
  Primary tumors and metastatic disease
  Carcinomatous meningitis
  Paraneoplastic syndromes
Traumatic
  Traumatic brain injury
  Subdural hematoma
Toxic
  Alcohol
  Medications (anticholinergics, polypharmacy)
Metabolic
  Vitamin B_{12} or folate deficiency
  Thyroid disease
  Uremia, others
Psychiatric
  Depression
Hydrocephalus
  Normal-pressure hydrocephalus (communicating hydrocephalus)
  Noncommunicating hydrocephalus

Source: Modified from Fleming et al.[8]

persistent psychotic features or those with extreme disruptive or dangerous behaviors.[12] Treatment is best coordinated with caregivers that are in a position to monitor the patient's behavior patterns over time.

Treatment of vascular dementia is limited to treatment of risk factors including hypertension.

Normal-pressure hydrocephalus (NPH) is suggested by the presence of excessively large ventricles on head CT and can prompt consideration of a trial of ventricular shunting. The clinical suspicion of NPH should be increased with the presence of urinary incontinence and gait disturbance at a relatively early point in the disease. Improvement in some individuals may be striking, but controversies remain on patient selection and the duration of improvement.

Disposition

A new diagnosis of dementia may be entertained in the ED, but the decision making and depth of the diagnostic evaluation will usually exceed the time available during the ED stay. A decision to admit or arrange an outpatient diagnostic plan is the usual course in the ED after the major differential diagnostic possibilities have been eliminated. Attention should be directed toward the presence of delirium or a treatable cause of dementia. The existence of comorbid medical problems, a rapidly progressive or atypical clinical course, or an unsafe or uncertain home situation should prompt consideration for admission.

COMA

Introduction

Coma is a state of reduced alertness and responsiveness from which the patient cannot be aroused.[13] The Glasgow Coma Scale (see Table 255-2) is a widely used clinical scoring system for alterations in consciousness. Advantages are a simple scoring system and assessment of separate verbal, motor, and eye-opening functions. Disadvantages include lack of acknowledgement of hemiparesis or other focal motor signs and lack of testing of higher cognitive functions. Causes of coma likely to be encountered in the ED are noted in Table 229-7.

Pathophysiology

The pathophysiology of coma is complex for clinical purposes. Coma can result from deficiency of substrates needed for neuronal function (as with hypoglycemia or hypoxia). With systemic causes, the brain is globally affected and signs that localize dysfunction to a specific area of the brainstem or cortex will usually be lacking. In primary CNS causes, coma may result from brainstem disease such as hemorrhage or from bilateral cortical dysfunction. Signs localizing to specific areas of CNS dysfunction such as hemiparesis or cranial nerve abnormalities may be present. Unilateral hemispheric disease, such as stroke, should not by itself result in coma. The function of either the brainstem and/or both hemispheres must be impaired for unresponsiveness.

A traditional view of reduced consciousness from mass lesions invokes secondary compression of the brainstem by physical shifting of brain tissue. In the uncal herniation syndrome, the medial temporal lobe shifts to compress the upper brainstem, resulting in progressive drowsiness followed by unresponsiveness. The ipsilateral pupil will be sluggish, eventually becoming dilated and nonreactive on the postulated basis of third cranial nerve compression by the medial temporal lobe. Other signs of progressive third nerve dysfunction include loss of extraocular movements. Hemiparesis may develop ipsilateral to the mass from compression of the descending motor tracts in the opposite cerebral peduncle. A central herniation syndrome is also described

TABLE 229-7   Differential Diagnosis of Coma

Coma from Causes Affecting the Brain Diffusely
  Encephalopathies
    Hypoxic encephalopathy
    Metabolic encephalopathy
      Hypoglycemia
      Hyperosmolar state (e.g., hyperglycemia)
      Electrolyte abnormalities (e.g., hyper- or hyponatremia, hypercalcemia)
      Organ system failure
        Hepatic encephalopathy
        Uremia/renal failure
        Endocrine (e.g., Addison, hypothyroid, etc)
        Hypoxia
        CO_2 narcosis
    Hypertensive encephalopathy
  Toxins
  Drug reactions (e.g., neuroleptic malignant syndrome)
  Environmental causes—hypothermia, hyperthermia
  Deficiency state—Wernicke encephalopathy
  Sepsis
Coma from Primary CNS Disease or Trauma
  Direct CNS trauma
  Vascular disease
    Intraparenchymal hemorrhage (hemispheric, basal ganglia, brainstem, cerebellar)
  Subarachnoid hemorrhage
  Infarction
    Hemispheric, brainstem
  CNS infections
  Neoplasms
  Seizures
    Nonconvulsive status epilepticus
    Postictal state

characterized by progressive loss of consciousness, loss of brainstem reflexes, decorticate posturing, and irregular respirations.

The herniation syndromes serve as models, but their exact mechanism has been questioned. The amount of midline shift of structures as evaluated by neuroimaging seemingly correlates with the level of consciousness without invoking physical herniation. For example, given an acute lesion, the patient may be awake with up to 3 to 4 mm of pineal shift with unresponsiveness deepening as the pineal shift increases to 10 mm.

Ischemia from vascular compression is undoubtedly a factor in cerebral edema and increased intracranial pressure (ICP). Increased ICP may be localized to specific regions of the brain, perhaps initiating a herniation syndrome or midline shift as described above. Increased ICP may also occur diffusely, resulting in diffuse CNS dysfunction. Cerebral blood flow (CBF) is constant at mean arterial pressures (MAPs) of 50 to 100 mm Hg through the process of cerebral autoregulation. At MAPs outside this range, CBF will be reduced and ischemia may develop. Cerebral perfusion pressure (CPP) is equal to the MAP minus the intracranial pressure (CPP = MAP − ICP). It follows that in extreme uncontrolled elevation of the ICP, cerebral perfusion pressure is lost as the ICP approaches the MAP, and ischemia will develop.

Clinical Features

The clinical features of coma vary both with the depth of coma and the etiology. For example, a patient in coma with a hemispheric hemorrhage may still have some muscle tone; careful examination may allow detection of decreased muscle tone on the side of the hemiparesis. The eyes may conjugately deviate toward the side of the hemorrhage. With expansion of the hemorrhage and surrounding edema, increase in ICP, or brainstem compression, unresponsiveness may progress to a complete loss of motor tone and loss of the ocular findings as well.

A variety of abnormal breathing patterns may be seen in the comatose patient. They are of interest, but offer little information in the acute setting. Pupillary findings, the results of other cranial nerve evaluation, hemiparesis, and response to stimulation are all part of the clinical picture that need to be assessed. These findings help the clinician sort the cause of the coma into a likely large general category—diffuse CNS dysfunction (toxic-metabolic coma) or focal CNS dysfunction (structural coma). A further division of structural coma is into hemispheric (supratentorial) and posterior fossa coma, and is often possible at the bedside.

Toxic and metabolic causes of coma result from a wide range of clinical conditions. In general, the diffuse CNS dysfunction is reflected by the lack of physical examination findings that might point to a specific region of dysfunction within the brain. For example, in toxic-metabolic coma, if the patient is having either spontaneous movements or reflex posturing, the movements are symmetric without evidence of hemiparesis. Muscle stretch reflexes, if present, are symmetric. Pupillary response is generally preserved in toxic-metabolic coma; typically the pupils are small but reactive. If extraocular movements are present, again they are symmetric. However, if extraocular movements are absent, this sign is of no value in differentiating toxic-metabolic from structural coma. A notable exception is severe sedative poisoning as with barbiturates; the pupils may be large, extraocular movements absent, muscle tone flaccid, and the patient apneic simulating the appearance of brain death.

Coma from lesions of the hemispheres, or supratentorial masses, may present with progressive hemiparesis or asymmetric muscle tone and reflexes. The hemiparesis may be suspected with asymmetric responses to stimuli or asymmetric extensor or flexor postures. The uncal herniation syndrome, as described above, is an example of a supratentorial syndrome. Frequently, however, large acute supratentorial lesions are seen without the features consistent with temporal lobe herniation. Coma without lateralizing signs may result from decreased cerebral perfusion secondary to increased intracranial pressure. Reflex changes in blood pressure and heart rate may be observed with increased ICP or brainstem compression. Hypertension and bradycardia in a comatose patient may represent the Cushing reflex from increased ICP.

Posterior fossa or infratentorial lesions comprise another structural coma syndrome. An expanding mass, such as cerebellar hemorrhage or infarction, may cause abrupt coma, abnormal extensor posturing, loss of pupillary reflexes, and loss of extraocular movements. The anatomy of the posterior fossa leaves little room for accommodating an expanding mass. Early brainstem compression with loss of brainstem reflexes may develop rapidly. Another infratentorial cause of coma is pontine hemorrhage, which may present with the unique signs of pinpoint-sized pupils.

Pseudocoma or psychogenic coma is occasionally encountered and may present a perplexing clinical problem. Adequate history and observation of responses to stimulation will reveal findings that differ from the syndromes described above. Pupillary responses, extraocular movements, muscle tone, and reflexes will be shown to be intact on careful examination. Tests of particular value are observing the response of the patient to manual eye-opening (there should be little or no resistance in the truly unresponsive patient) and extraocular movements. Specifically, if avoidance of gaze is consistently seen with the patient always looking away from the examiner, or if nystagmus is demonstrated with caloric vestibular testing, this is strong evidence for nonphysiologic or feigned unresponsiveness.

Diagnosis

In the approach to the comatose patient, stabilization, diagnosis, and treatment actions overlap and are often performed simultaneously. Examination, laboratory procedures, and neuroimaging allow determination of the cause of coma in almost all patients in the ED. As with any patient, airway, breathing, and circulation need to be immediately addressed. Reversible causes of coma, such as hypoglycemia or opiate overdose, should always be considered. Exploit all possible historical sources (EMS personnel, caregivers, family, witnesses, medical records, etc.) to aid in diagnosis.

The tempo of onset of the coma is of great diagnostic value. Abrupt coma suggests abrupt CNS failure with possible causes such as catastrophic stroke or seizures. A slowly progressive onset of coma may suggest a progressive CNS lesion such as tumor or subdural hematoma. Metabolic causes such as hyperglycemia may also develop over several days.

General examination and vital signs (including oxygen saturation and temperature) should receive special attention following stabilization and resuscitation. General examination may reveal signs of trauma or suggest other diagnostic possibilities for the unresponsiveness. For example, a toxidrome may be present that suggests diagnosis and therapy, such as the hypoventilation and small pupils found with opioid overdose.

Neurologic testing deviates from the standard examination. Fine tests of weakness in the alert patient, such as testing for pronator drift of the outstretched upper extremities, are not possible in the unresponsive patient. However, assessment of cranial nerves through pupillary examination, corneal reflexes, and oculovestibular reflexes may suggest focal CNS lesions. Observation for abnormal extensor or flexor postures are nonspecific for localization or etiology of coma, but suggest profound CNS dysfunction. Again, asymmetric muscle tone or reflexes raise the suspicion of a focal lesion. The goal of the physician is to rapidly determine if the CNS dysfunction is from diffuse impairment of the brain or if signs point to a focal (and perhaps surgically treatable) region of CNS dysfunction.

CT scanning is the neuroimaging procedure of choice. Acute hemorrhage is readily identified as are midline shifts and mass lesions. Lumbar puncture should be done if CT scan is negative, to identify CNS bleeding or infection. Basilar artery thrombosis should be suspected in the comatose patient with a "normal" head CT, where the only finding may be a hyperdense basilar artery. MRI or angiography are needed to make the diagnosis.

Specific Issues

Airway issues of importance in the comatose patient include concerns for cervical spine injury and increased intracranial pressure. If trauma is suspected, stabilization of the cervical spine during the diagnostic process must be maintained. Issues of intubation in the head-inured patient or other comatose patient with suspected increased intracranial pressure need modification of rapid sequence intubation techniques that are discussed at length in Chap. 19. If protection of the airway is at all in doubt, seizure is a possibility, or the coma state is likely prolonged, it may be prudent to intubate the patient.

In the pediatric patient, causes of coma differ from the adult. Toxic ingestions, infections, and child abuse all assume a greater frequency and importance.

Nonconvulsive status epilepticus or subtle status epilepticus is an area of increasing interest. Patients who have had generalized seizures and remain unresponsive may be in a continuing state of electrical seizures without corresponding motor movements. This has been termed *electromechanical dissociation of the brain and body.* If the motor activity of the seizure has been stopped and the patient is not awakening within 30 min, the existence of this subtle status epilepticus should be considered and urgent EEG or neurologic consultation sought.

Treatment

Treatment of coma involves identification of the etiology of the brain failure and initiation of specific therapy directed at the underlying cause. Brain-saving procedures should be performed while diagnostic steps are taking place. Again, stabilization with attention to airway, ventilation, and circulation assume priority. Attention to readily reversible causes of coma such as hypoglycemia and opioid toxicity demand priority.

The "coma cocktail" that was routinely given to all comatose patients has come under scrutiny. While hypoglycemia is common, with rapid glucose determinations, empiric administration of dextrose is not always necessary. It has been axiomatic that thiamine should be administered before glucose infusions, and this certainly is true of the patient with a suspected history of alcohol abuse or malnutrition, but this may not be necessary in all patients. Some suggest that naloxone, an opiate antagonist, need not be administered if clinical signs of the opioid are not present. Routine use of flumazenil in unknown coma is not recommended.[14]

Several rapid decisions face the emergency physician. An early decision involves assigning the patient into probable structural coma etiology versus toxic-metabolic etiology. History and physical examination will allow that initial categorization with many patients, but liberal use of CT scanning is encouraged since exceptions to the tentative clinical diagnosis are frequent.

If history, physical examination, or neuroimaging suggests increased intracranial pressure, specific steps may be indicated to reduce or ameliorate any further rise in ICP. Any noxious stimulus including "bucking" the ventilator will increase ICP; paralysis and sedation should be liberally used. A general recommendation is to keep the head elevated about 30° and midline to aid in venous drainage. Osmotic diuretics such as mannitol (0.5 to 1 g/kg) will decrease intravascular volume and brain water and may transiently reduce ICP. In cases of brain edema associated with tumor, steroids such as dexamethasone will reduce edema over several hours. Hyperventilation with reduction of $Paco_2$ will reduce cerebral blood volume and transiently lower ICP. Current recommendations are to avoid prophylactic hyperventilation ($Paco_2 \leq 35$ mm Hg) during the first 24 h after brain injury. Brief hyperventilation may be necessary for refractory intracranial hypertension. Data to recommend specific therapy is lacking and preferences among individuals and institutions vary greatly; early communication is encouraged with consultants and admitting physicians.

Disposition

Patients with readily reversible causes of coma, such as insulin-induced hypoglycemia, may be discharged if home care and follow-up care are adequate and a clear cause for the episode is suspected. For patients with enduring altered consciousness, admission will be necessary. Most systems depend on emergency physicians to stabilize the patient and correctly assign a tentative diagnosis so the patient may be admitted to the proper specialty service. If the appropriate service is not available, transfer should be considered after stabilization.

REFERENCES

1. Lipowski Z: Delirium in the elderly patient. *New Engl J Med* 320:578, 1989.
2. Zun L, Howes DS: The mental status evaluation: Application in the emergency department. *Am J Emerg Med* 6:165, 1988.
3. Rummans TA, Evans JM, Krahn LE, et al: Delirium in elderly patients: Evaluation and management. *Mayo Clin Proc* 70:989, 1995.
4. Hustey FM, Meldon SW: The prevalence and documentation of impaired mental status in elderly emergency department patients. *Ann Emerg Med* 39:248, 2002.
5. Sanders AB: Missed delirium in older emergency department patients: A quality-of-care problem. *Ann Emerg Med* 39:338, 2002.
6. Folstein MF, Folstein SE: "Mini-mental state:" A practical method for grading the cognitive state of patients for the clinician. *J Psychiatr Res* 12:189, 1975.
7. Huff JS, Farace E, Brady WJ, et al: The quick confusion scale in the ED: Comparison with the mini-mental state examination. *Acad Emerg Med* 19:461, 2001.

8. Fleming KC, Adams AC, Petersen RC: Dementia: Diagnosis and evaluation. *Mayo Clin Proc* 70:1093, 1995.
9. Practice parameter for diagnosis and evaluation of dementia (summary statement). Report of the Quality Standards Subcommittee of the American Academy of Neurology. *Neurology* 44:2203, 1994.
10. Knopman DS, DeKosky ST, Cummings JL, et al: Practice parameter: Diagnosis of dementia (an evidence-based review): Report of the Quality Standards Subcommittee of the American Academy of Neurology. *Neurology* 56:1143, 2001.
11. Gold G, Giannakopoulos P, Montes-Paixao C, et al: Sensitivity and specificity of newly proposed clinical criteria for possible vascular dementia. *Neurology* 49:690, 1997.
12. Borson S, Raskind MA: Clinical features and pharmacologic treatment of behavioral symptoms of Alzheimer's disease. *Neurology* 48(Suppl 6):S17, 1997.
13. Giacino JT, Ashwal S, Childs N, et al: The minimally conscious state: definition and diagnostic criteria. *Neurology* 58:349, 2002.
14. Hoffman RS, Goldfrank LR: The poisoned patient with altered consciousness: Controversies in the use of a "coma cocktail." *JAMA* 274:562, 1994.
15. Richardson PG: Basilar artery thrombosis. *Emerg Med* (Fremantle) 13:367, 2001.

230 ATAXIA AND GAIT DISTURBANCES
J. Stephen Huff

Ataxia and gait disturbances may be symptoms of a variety of disease processes and generally are not diagnoses themselves. Ataxia is the failure to produce smooth intentional movements. Gait disorders include ataxic gait, as well as a variety of other conditions. The presenting complaint may be articulated by the patient or family as weakness, dizziness, stroke, falling, or another nonspecific or even inaccurate chief complaint. These symptoms must always be viewed in the context of the patient's overall clinical picture. For example, in a patient with the inability to walk, hemiplegia would not be considered primarily a gait disturbance. However, if the intraparenchymal hemorrhage were in the cerebellum, the inability to walk may be one of the dominating signs and symptoms. In this chapter, acute ataxia and disorders of gait are emphasized; chronic or progressive forms are covered only in a list.

PATHOPHYSIOLOGY

Ataxia or gait disturbances may result from many conditions that affect different elements of the central and peripheral nervous systems as well as systemic conditions (Table 230-1). Clinicians tend to think that these disorders result primarily from cerebellar lesions. Cerebellar lesions may indeed cause ataxia, but isolated lesions of the cerebellum are not the most common cause of these complaints.

Ataxia may be roughly categorized into two types. *Motor ataxias* (also referred to as cerebellar ataxia) are usually caused by disorders of the cerebellum; the sensory receptors and afferent pathways are intact, but integration of the proprioceptive information is faulty. Involvement of the lateral cerebellum (one of the cerebellar hemispheres) may lead to a motor ataxia of the ipsilateral limb. Lesions affecting primarily the midline portion of the cerebellum often cause problems with axial muscle coordination reflected in difficulty maintaining a steady upright standing or sitting posture.

There are many reports of lesions in what would seem to be unlikely locations producing motor ataxia. Supratentorial infarctions, particularly small deep infarctions or lacunae of the posterior limb of the internal capsule, have been reported to cause isolated hemiataxia. It is postulated that interruption of either ascending or descending cerebellar to cortical pathways are the cause of this motor-type ataxia.[1] Small infarctions or hemorrhages in thalamic nuclei may produce a

TABLE 230-1   Common Etiologies of Acute Ataxia and Gait Disturbances

Systemic conditions
  Intoxications with diminished alertness
    Ethanol
    Sedative-hypnotics
  Intoxications with relatively preserved alertness (diminished alertness at higher levels)
    Phenytoin
    Carbamazepine
    Valproic acid
    Heavy metals—lead, organic mercurials
  Other metabolic disorders
    Hyponatremia
    Inborn errors of metabolism
Disorders predominantly of the nervous system
  Conditions affecting predominantly one region of the central nervous system
    Cerebellum
      Hemorrhage
      Infarction
      Degenerative changes
      Abscess
    Cortex
      Frontal tumor, hemorrhage, or trauma
      Hydrocephalus
    Subcortical
      Thalamic infarction or hemorrhage
      Parkinson's disease
    Spinal cord
      Cervical spondylosis
      Posterior column disorders
  Conditions affecting predominantly the peripheral nervous system
    Peripheral neuropathy
    Vestibulopathy

clinical picture of motor- or cerebellar-like ataxia with hemisensory loss. These effects are seen contralateral to the lesion.[2] Lesions affecting the frontal lobe, such as tumor or hydrocephalus, may cause a motor ataxia of the contralateral extremities through poorly understood mechanisms.[3]

Sensory ataxia occurs with a failure in transmission of proprioception or position sense information to the central nervous system (CNS). This may arise from disorders affecting the peripheral nerves, spinal cord, or cerebellar input tracts. Coordinated motor performance is faulty even though motor systems and the cerebellum are intact. Sensory ataxia may be compensated to a degree, consciously with visual sensory information. Loss of this visual information leads to the observation that symptoms of sensory ataxia often worsen in poor lighting conditions and may by brought out during examination (see below).

CLINICAL FEATURES

Historical information should be collected about the entire symptom constellation in addition to any complaints of headache, nausea, fever, weakness, or numbness. A history of febrile illness, medication history, or family history may be a key element leading to a correct diagnosis in individual cases. The nature of onset of symptoms and the time course of the process guide the pace of investigations. For example, abrupt onset of gait difficulty in a patient with severe headache, drowsiness, nausea, and vomiting should suggest an acute process within the CNS, possibly a hemorrhage into the cerebellum. The possible consequences of that diagnosis are severe and may require immediate attention. At the other extreme, a patient without significant medical history who is brought to the emergency department with a stumbling gait after an episode of binge drinking requires examination but may need nothing other than observation unless history or physical examination suggest trauma or some alternative cause for the symptoms.

The following discussion of the neurologic examination assumes that the gait disorder is the dominating abnormality, but examination including testing of cranial nerves, mental status, sensation, or the motor system is necessary and may yield findings that lead to an unanticipated diagnosis.

General physical examination of a patient with ataxia or gait disturbance should include determination of orthostatic vital signs; besides hypovolemia, orthostatic hypotension may be present in patients with diabetic neuropathy and other neurologic syndromes. Especially in the elderly, volume replacement for simple hypovolemia may correct many symptoms of unsteadiness.

Gait testing is one of the most important parts of the directed neurologic examination. Observing the patient sit upright in the stretcher, rise, stand, walk, and turn gives information about many parts of the nervous system. The patient should be asked to walk at a normal speed, then walk on the heels, and then toes. Tandem gait is toe-to-toe walking and also tests many elements of the nervous system. Do not assume a normal examination without observing ambulation.

Cerebellar functions are tested by asking the patient to perform smooth voluntary movements and rapidly alternating movements; dyssynergia (breakdown of movements into parts), dysmetria (inaccurate fine movements), or dysdiadochokinesia (clumsy rapid movements) may be indicative of a problem in the lateral cerebellum. The rapid thigh-patting test particularly examines rapidly alternating movements. This is correctly performed by asking the patient to pat the thigh with the palm then the back of the same hand in alternating fashion, making a sound with each rapid slap. The maneuver is performed with each hand in turn. The familiar finger-to-nose test (*dyssynergia*) may be helpful in distinguishing between cerebellar and posterior column lesions. Performing this test with the eyes closed tests proprioception in the upper extremity. A test for cerebellar function that emphasizes the lower extremities (and another part of the cerebellum) is the familiar heel-to-shin test (also dyssynergia). In cerebellar disease, the knee may initially overshoot. In posterior column disease, there may be difficulty locating the knee, but the movement down the shin typically weaves from side to side or falls off. Another test commonly used for cerebellar function is the *Stewart–Holmes rebound sign* (sudden release of the flexed forearm may rebound back and forth in several cycles).

The *Romberg test* is primarily a test of sensation and, if positive, may distinguish sensory from motor ataxia. With the patient standing with arms outstretched and the eyes open, the patient is observed for signs of unsteadiness. The feet should be narrowly spaced, and the posture should be easily maintained. The inability to maintain a steady standing posture (or, in extreme cases, a seated position) confirms that an ataxia is present but does not yet give any information about the type of ataxia. The patient is then asked to close the eyes with the resulting loss of visual orienting information. If the ataxia worsens with this loss of visual input, then the Romberg sign is present or positive, suggesting sensory ataxia with a problem of proprioceptive (posterior column, vestibular dysfunction), or a peripheral neuropathy. In patients who show little or no change in their unsteadiness with eye closure (Romberg test–negative), a motor ataxia is suggested with possible localization of that problem to the cerebellum. Note that many normal individuals will have some small increase in unsteadiness with eye closure. Further neurologic examination is indicated to confirm the suspicion of sensory etiology of the ataxia.

In the last century, tabes dorsalis (neurosyphilis) was a common cause of sensory ataxia. In tabes dorsalis, the posterior columns and posterior spinal roots degenerate, primarily in the lumbosacral region. The loss of proprioceptive information from the lower extremities renders the patient dependent on visual cues for correct gait. The classic description paints the picture of a patient who walks slowly with wide gait while staring at the ground. In darkness or with interruption of vi-

sion, the patient is unable to walk. The gait in this condition is peculiar with the foot first raised and then slapped to the ground with each step. These abnormalities reflect the loss of proprioceptive information from the posterior roots and posterior columns. The possibility of vitamin B_{12} deficiency should be a consideration in patients with evidence of posterior column disease. If left untreated, an initial unsteady gait may progress to weakness, spasticity, and ataxia. The finding of a megaloblastic anemia may be a clue, but the neuropathy may precede the anemia.

Sensory examination in a patient with unsteady movements should include position or vibration testing (posterior columns), as well as testing sensation to pinprick. Testing of the deep tendon reflexes will serve largely to discover asymmetry or spasticity that might suggest an alternative diagnosis. Acute cerebellar injury may result in muscle hypotonia for a few days or weeks.[4]

Nystagmus is seen in many different disorders due to lesions in a variety of different locations of the CNS, but the presence of nystagmus does suggest that the pathologic process is intracranial and not in the spinal cord or peripheral nervous system (see Chap. 231).

No organized classification scheme exists for gait disorders, and different authors categorize abnormal gaits in descriptive terms. A brief summary of some of the more commonly used terms follows. A *cerebellar* or *motor ataxic* gait is wide-based with unsteady and irregular steps; compensation to barriers in the environment may be lacking. The gait of sensory ataxia resulting from loss of proprioception is notable for abrupt movement of the legs and slapping impact of the feet with each step.

An *apraxic* gait is one in which the patient seemingly has lost the ability to initiate the process of walking, a sort of "ignition failure." Apraxia describes the inability of a patient to perform a voluntary act even though the motor system and understanding are intact. This may occur with right or nondominant hemispheric lesions. Frontal lobe dysfunction may result in a similar gait. This may be seen in normal pressure hydrocephalus.

Footdrop from peroneal muscle weakness is reflected in an *equine* (high-stepping) gait. The high stepping from hip flexion is necessary for the foot to clear the ground.

The term *festinating* gait is used to describe narrow-based miniature shuffling steps. Once the walk begins, the steps may become more rapid. This is common in Parkinson disease and may be accompanied by other elements of Parkinson disease, such as increased muscle tone, lack of facial expression, slow movements (bradykinesia), and tremor.

An abnormal gait with outward swinging or circumabduction of the leg suggests a mild hemiparesis reflecting the asymmetric weakness of the proximal lower extremity muscles. The examination should then be directed to find other signs of hemiparesis. Bilateral weakness of the trunk and pelvic girdle muscles may result in a waddling gait from failure to maintain the normal position of the pelvis relative to the lower extremities.

A *functional* gait disorder is one in which the patient is unable to walk normally, though all motor pathways, sensory pathways, and cerebellar functions may be demonstrated to be functioning normally. The underlying problem is often a conversion disorder. These gaits may be bizarre, at times resembling a person balancing on a tightrope and seemingly threatening to fall but not falling. The wildness of flailing movements without falling actually demonstrates that the strength, balance, and coordination are intact. This dramatic functional gait is termed *astasia-abasia*.

A unifying concept defines gait disorders according to the level of processing of neurologic information (Table 230-2).[5] Low-level gait disturbance refers to disorders of proprioception or dysfunction of the musculoskeletal system. Middle-level gait disturbance causes distortion of appropriate interaction of postural and motor processes or synergies. This might include stroke with paralysis, cerebellar dysfunction, or diseases of the basal ganglia such as Parkinson disease. On

TABLE 230-2 Classification of Gait Disorders

Low-level gait disorders
  Musculoskeletal problems
    Arthritic gait or other joint or skeletal problems
    Muscle weakness
  Peripheral sensory problems
    Sensory ataxic gait
    Vestibular problems
Middle-level gait disorders
  Hemiplegia
  Paraplegia
  Motor or cerebellar ataxia
  Parkinson disease
  Dystonia, chorea, other movement disorders
High-level gait disorders
  Senile gait (cautious gait)
  Frontal ataxic gait
  Apraxic gait (gait ignition failure)
  Frontal disequilibrium

Note: "Level" refers to the level of processing of sensorimotor information.
Source: Modified from Nutt JG, Marsden CD, Thompson PD: Human walking and higher-level gait disorders, particularly in the elderly. *Neurology* 43:268, 1993, with permission.

examination, patients might have findings of spasticity, muscular tone, paralysis, or abnormal movements. High-level gait disturbances seemingly involve structures or processes that choose the appropriate responses for the support surface, body position in space, and intention of the patient. Cautious gait, apraxic gait, and the frontal gait disorder conceptually fall into this group with pathology that correlates with lesions in the frontal cortex or thalamus. This latter group is the least understood and the source of clinical confusion. This classification scheme is not ideal but does allow a thoughtful approach to patient diagnosis.

DIAGNOSIS

Assuming a primary complaint of ataxia, the first task is to determine whether the ataxia is sensory or motor and whether the primary process is systemic or within the nervous system. If within the nervous system, the next question is one of localization to the peripheral nervous system versus the CNS and perhaps to a more specific anatomic location. Finally, the tempo of the illness, comorbid diseases, and other clinical findings guide investigations and may allow a disease-specific diagnosis.

A patient with acute gait failure over hours to days needs thorough evaluation in the emergency department, consultation if available, and possible admission, in contrast to a patient with gradual loss of abilities over weeks or months where outpatient referral and evaluation may be appropriate.

SPECIFIC ISSUES THAT IMPACT EVALUATION AND TREATMENT

The Geriatric Patient

The gait changes with advancing age. A typical constellation includes gait slowing, shortening of the stride, and widening of the base. This results in the appearance of a guarded gait, that is, the gait of someone about to slip and fall. Many patients are aware of the loss of speed and adaptive balance and acknowledge the need to be careful. The nature of this *senile* gait is not fully understood but may represent a mild degree of neuronal loss, failing proprioception, slowing of corrective responses, or weakness of the lower extremities. Senile gait disorder is thought to exist in up to one-quarter of the elderly population. Some authorities divide this disorder into components of gait ataxia with

mild truncal instability and widened gait, and gait slowing with diminished spontaneous arm swing and bradykinesia.[6] However, elements of the senile gait are also found in neurodegenerative diseases, and caution is urged to consider the possible presence of a neurodegenerative disorder such as Parkinson disease in elderly patients with gait impairment.[6] Patients unable to walk or care for themselves need admission for supportive care.

The Alcoholic Patient

A history of alcoholism or malabsorption problem in the patient with ataxia or gait disorder should raise the possibility of a potentially remedial nutritional problem. If acute motor ataxia is present with confusion or eye movement abnormalities, the possibility of *Wernicke disease* should be considered and intravenous thiamine administration should be initiated promptly. The entity of alcoholic cerebellar degeneration (sometimes referred to as *rostral vermis syndrome,* since a portion of the cerebellar vermis is preferentially affected) may represent the same nutritional deficiency and not direct toxic effects of alcohol.

Children

In evaluating children with acute ataxia or gait disorder, examination must exclude weakness and musculoskeletal disorders. The child may be awake, alert, and playful but is visibly unsteady or wobbly sitting on a stretcher. The differential diagnosis is extensive (Table 230-3). Acute or deteriorating presentation generally mandates aggressive search for underlying etiology and likely inpatient management.

Intoxications are a cause of ataxia in children, and the ingestion may be surreptitious. Though ethanol may be suspected by odor, other drugs such as phenytoin or carbamazepine will not be detected in that

TABLE 230-3 Causes of Acute Ataxia in Children, Roughly in Order of Frequency

Cause	Example
Drug intoxication	Ethanol Isopropyl alcohol Phenytoin Carbamazepine Sedatives Lead, mercury
Infection and inflammation	Varicella Coxsackievirus A and B Mycoplasma Echovirus Postinfectious inflammation Postimmunization
Neoplasm	Neuroblastoma Other central nervous system tumors
Trauma	Subdural or epidural posterior fossa hematoma
Congenital or hereditary	Pyruvate decarboxylase deficiency Friedreich ataxia Hartnup disease
Hydrocephalus	
Cerebellar abscess	
Labyrinthitis/vestibular neuronitis	
Meningoencephalitis	
Idiopathic	

Source: Modified from Belcher RS: Preeruptive cerebellar ataxia in varicella. *Ann Emerg Med* 27:511, 1996, and Chutorian AM, Pavlakis SG: Acute ataxia, in Pellock JM, Myer EL (eds): *Neurologic Emergencies in Infancy and Childhood.* Boston: Butterworth-Heinemann, 1993, p. 208, with permission.

manner. History should include queries about any medications in the household.

Unusual metabolic disorders such as pyruvate decarboxylase complex deficiency may present with ataxia. Family history may or may not suggest a metabolic disorder. Typically, the onset is gradual, but abrupt decompensations may occur. Other systemic or CNS abnormalities will be present.

Posterior fossa mass lesions and other CNS masses may present with ataxia, though usually some abnormality of cranial nerves or strength will be discovered with careful examination. Attention is needed to exclude abnormalities on physical examination that might suggest problems not localized to the cerebellum. Abnormal ocular movements should increase the suspicion of a mass lesion.

Rarely, acute ataxia may follow immunizations, viral illnesses, or varicella but also has been rarely reported in the preeruptive phase of varicella.[7] Most children are in the 2- to 4-year-old range. The onset of gait ataxia is abrupt, and only occasionally is fever present at the time ataxia begins. The latency from the prodromal illness to the onset of ataxia is from 2 days to 2 weeks. Other neurologic findings encountered included truncal ataxia, dysmetria, and, uncommonly, cranial nerve abnormalities. Varicella patients appear to have uniform excellent recovery compared with patients with acute cerebellar ataxia from other causes that may have some residual problems.[8] Little workup is needed if the ataxia occurs in the convalescent phase of varicella, and antiviral medications are not indicated. Otherwise, neuroimaging, lumbar puncture, and consultation are advisable. One study showed that while roughly half of the patients had cerebrospinal fluid inflammatory changes with pleocytosis or elevated immunoglobulin G index, magnetic resonance imaging (MRI) identified inflammatory changes in the cerebellum in only a minority of cases.[8] Another small report noted MRI abnormalities not only in the cerebellum, but also in other areas of the CNS. This "syndrome" may in fact consist of several subgroups, some of which involve transient demyelination.[9]

REFERENCES

1. Luijckx GJ, Baiten J, Lodder J, et al: Isolated hemiataxia after supratentorial brain infarction. *J Neurol Neurosurg Psychiatry* 57:742, 1994.
2. Solomon DH, Barohn RJ, Bazan C, Grissom J: The thalamic ataxia syndrome. *Neurology* 44:810, 1994.
3. Terry JB, Rosenberg RN: Frontal lobe ataxia. *Surg Neurol* 44:583, 1995.
4. Diener H-C, Dichgans J: Pathophysiology of cerebellar ataxia. *Move Disord* 7:95, 1992.
5. Nutt JG, Marsden CD, Thompson PD: Human walking and higher-level gait disorders, particularly in the elderly. *Neurology* 43:268, 1993.
6. Waite LM, Broe GA, Creasy H, et al: Neurologic signs, aging, and the neurodegenerative syndromes. *Arch Neurol* 53:498, 1996.
7. Belcher RS: Preeruptive cerebellar ataxia in varicella. *Ann Emerg Med* 27:511, 1996.
8. Connolly AM, Dodson WE, Prensky AL, Rust RS: Course and outcome of acute cerebellar ataxia. *Ann Neurol* 35:673, 1994.
9. Maggi G, Varone A, Aliverti F: Acute cerebellar ataxia in children. *Child Nerv Syst* 13:542, 1997.

231 VERTIGO AND DIZZINESS
Brian Goldman

Recent evidence suggests that as many as one in five adults aged 18 to 64 years reported dizziness during the past month.[1] To patients, dizziness may mean vertigo, syncope, presyncope, weakness, giddiness, anxiety, or a disturbance in mentation.

Vertigo is the perception of movement (rotational or otherwise) where no movement exists. *Syncope* is a transient loss of consciousness that is accompanied by loss of postural tone with spontaneous re-

covery. *Near-syncope* is defined as light-headedness signifying an impending loss of consciousness. *Psychiatric dizziness* is defined as a sensation of dizziness not related to vestibular dysfunction that occurs exclusively in combination with other symptoms as part of a recognized psychiatric symptom cluster.[2] *Disequilibrium* refers to a feeling of unsteadiness, imbalance, or a sensation of "floating" while walking.

PATHOPHYSIOLOGY

The central nervous system (CNS) coordinates and integrates sensory input from the visual, vestibular, and proprioceptive systems. The three streams of information help form an impression of the orientation of the head and body as well as the perception of motion. Vertigo arises from a mismatch of information from two or more of the involved senses, which, in turn, can be caused by dysfunction in the sensory organ or its corresponding pathway.

Visual inputs provide spatial orientation. Proprioceptors help relate body movements and indicate the position of the head relative to that of the body. The vestibular system (via the otoliths) establishes the body's orientation with respect to gravity. The cupulae contain sensors that track rotary motion. The presence of embedded otoconia or particles on the cupulae may transform them into linear motion sensors capable of sensing gravity. The three semicircular canals sense orientation to movement and head tilts and are filled with a fluid called *endolymph*. The endolymphatic sac produces glycoproteins that create an osmotic sink necessary to maintain flow. The movement of fluid in the semicircular canals causes specialized hair cells inside the canals to move, causing afferent vestibular impulses to fire. Sensory input from the vestibular apparatus travels to the nucleus of the eighth cranial nerve (Figure 231-1).

The CNS structures involved in integrating sensory input from all three sensory modalities include the medial longitudinal fasciculus, the red nuclei, the cerebellum, and the parietal lobes and superior temporal gyrus of the cerebral cortex. Connections between these structures and the oculomotor nuclei that drive the vestibuloocular reflex (VOR) complete the system. The VOR prevents retinal slip and thus visual blurring that otherwise would result from head movements and body sway.

Ordinarily, there is balanced input from the vestibular apparatus on both sides of the body. Asymmetrical activity may result in vertigo. Causes of assymetical activity include unilateral lesions of the vestibular apparatus as well as excessive unilateral firing due (for instance) to abnormal motion of the endolymph. Rapid head movements induce vertigo by accentuating the imbalance. Symmetrical bilateral damage does not usually produce vertigo but may lead to truncal or gait instability.

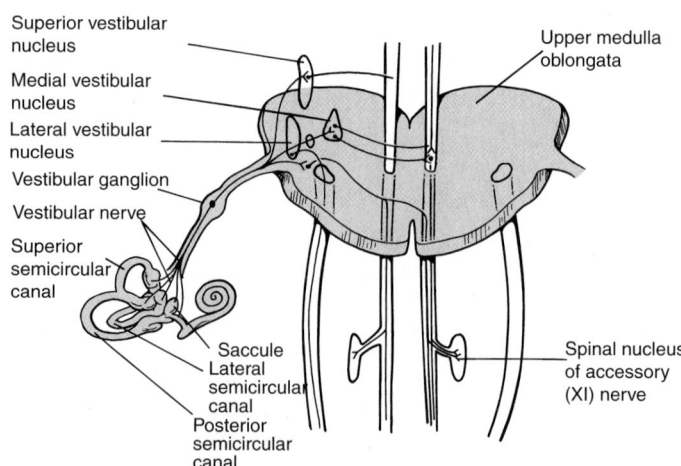

FIG. 231-1. Vestibular innervation.

The most striking clinical sign associated with vertigo is nystagmus. *Nystagmus* is a rhythmic movement of the eyes that has both a fast and a slow component, with direction named by its fast component. The slow component is due to the vestibuloocular reflex and is generated by excitation of the semicircular canal, producing eye movement away from that canal. The fast component of nystagmus is caused by the cortex, which exerts a quick corrective movement in the opposite direction. With disorders of the vestibular apparatus, the sensation of vertigo is usually associated with nystagmus. The nystagmus of vestibular injury or dysfunction is provoked when the affected side is in the dependent position, and the characteristic pattern is vertical and rotational or horizontal. When horizontal nystagmus is present, its slow-beating component points to the injured labyrinth. Vertical nystagmus by itself (and not associated with a rotational component) usually indicates a brainstem abnormality. However, an atypical pattern of nystagmus in the absence of other signs of CNS disease does not necessarily indicate central pathology.[3]

The prevalence of vertigo and dizziness is greatest in the elderly. Decreases in visual acuity, proprioception, and vestibular input often occur with aging. The risk of near-syncope also increases with age due to causes such as dysrhythmias, orthostatic hypotension, and autonomic dysfunction. In addition, as people age, they are more likely to have free-floating otoconia within the semicircular canals, a condition that is believed to increase the risk of benign paroxysmal positional vertigo (BPPV).[4] The elderly are also more likely to be taking medications, many of which, alone or in combination, can cause "dizziness."

Physiologic Vertigo

Physiologic vertigo is vertigo not caused by disease of the cochleovestibular system. It results from a mismatch among visual, proprioceptive, and vestibular input. This may be the pathogenesis of motion sickness as well as the transient vertigo associated with watching a film that captures the visual sensation of motion without the corresponding vestibular or proprioceptive input *(visual vertigo)*. Visual vertigo can be triggered by complex visual environments such as shopping malls (due in part to the ceiling height of shopping malls as well as the large number of objects in motion) and by viewing complex floor or wallpaper patterns.

CLINICAL FEATURES

The conditions that cause vertigo are summarized in Table 231-1. Vertigo is usually categorized into peripheral and central causes. There is no valid measurement of the severity of vertigo. Peripheral vertigo is caused by disorders affecting the vestibular apparatus and the eighth cranial nerve, whereas central vertigo is caused by disorders affecting central structures, such as the brainstem and the cerebellum. The classic characteristics distinguishing peripheral and central vertigo are found in Table 231-2 and in reality are not so distinct. For example, vertigo due to stroke or cerebellar hemorrhage certainly would have an acute (rather than insidious) presentation yet be of central origin. Similarly, severity and even accentuation with certain head positions, while suggestive, does not uniformly distinguish underlying pathology. Figure 231-2 shows how the nystagmus pattern itself may help to differentiate peripheral and central vertigo. Peripheral nystagmus is increased by removal of fixation, but central nystagmus generally (though not always) decreases with fixation.

Although disorders causing peripheral vertigo tend to produce more distressing symptoms, they are seldom life-threatening. Disorders causing central vertigo may produce less distressing symptoms and have a slower onset than those due to peripheral vertigo, but they are generally of a more serious nature, requiring urgent or semiurgent diagnostic imaging or consultation with a neurologist or neurosurgeon.

TABLE 231-1 An Etiologic Classification of Vertigo

Vestibular/otologic	Benign paroxysmal positional vertigo
	Traumatic: after head injury
	Infection: labyrinthitis, vestibular neuronitis, Ramsay Hunt syndrome
Syndrome	Ménière syndrome
	Neoplastic
	Vascular
	Otosclerosis
	Paget disease
	Toxic or drug-induced: aminoglycosides
Neurologic	Vertebrobasillar insufficiency
	Lateral Wallenburg syndrome
	Anterior inferior cerebellar artery syndrome
	Neoplastic: cerebellopontine angle tumors
	Cerebellar disorders: hemorrhage, degeneration
	Basal ganglion diseases
	Multiple sclerosis
	Infections: neurosyphilis, tuberculosis
	Epilepsy
	Migraine headaches
	Cerebrovascular disease
General	Hematologic: anemia, polycythemia, hyperviscosity syndrome
	Toxic: alcohol
	Chronic renal failure
	Metabolic: thyroid disease, hypoglycemia

DIAGNOSIS

History

An approach to vertigo is shown in Figure 231-3. A key portion of the history is the unprompted description of what the patient means by "dizziness." It is important to avoid leading questions because they may bias the patient's responses. If patients have difficulty describing the dizziness, it is useful to ask them to describe the initial episode in detail. Often this is the most vivid episode, and the patient is more likely to recall key precipitants. Further history taking depends on how the dizziness is categorized.

If the patient has experienced true vertigo, the next step is to determine whether the vertigo is of peripheral or central origin. Although the symptoms of central vertigo may not be severe, they are more likely to indicate potentially life-threatening disorders. The temporal pattern and precipitating causes can help to distinguish the different etiologies of vertigo (Table 231-3). Peripheral vertigo is more likely

TABLE 231-2 Differentiating Peripheral from Central Vertigo

	Peripheral	Central
Onset	Sudden	Sudden or slow
Severity of vertigo	Intense spinning	Ill defined, less intense
Pattern	Paroxysmal, intermittent	Constant
Aggravated by position/movement	Yes	Variable
Associated nausea/diaphoresis	Frequent	Variable
Nystagmus	Rotatory-vertical, horizontal	Vertical
Fatigue of symptoms/signs	Yes	No
Hearing loss/tinnitus	May occur	Does not occur
Abnormal tympanic membrane	May occur	Does not occur
CNS symptoms/signs	Absent	Usually present

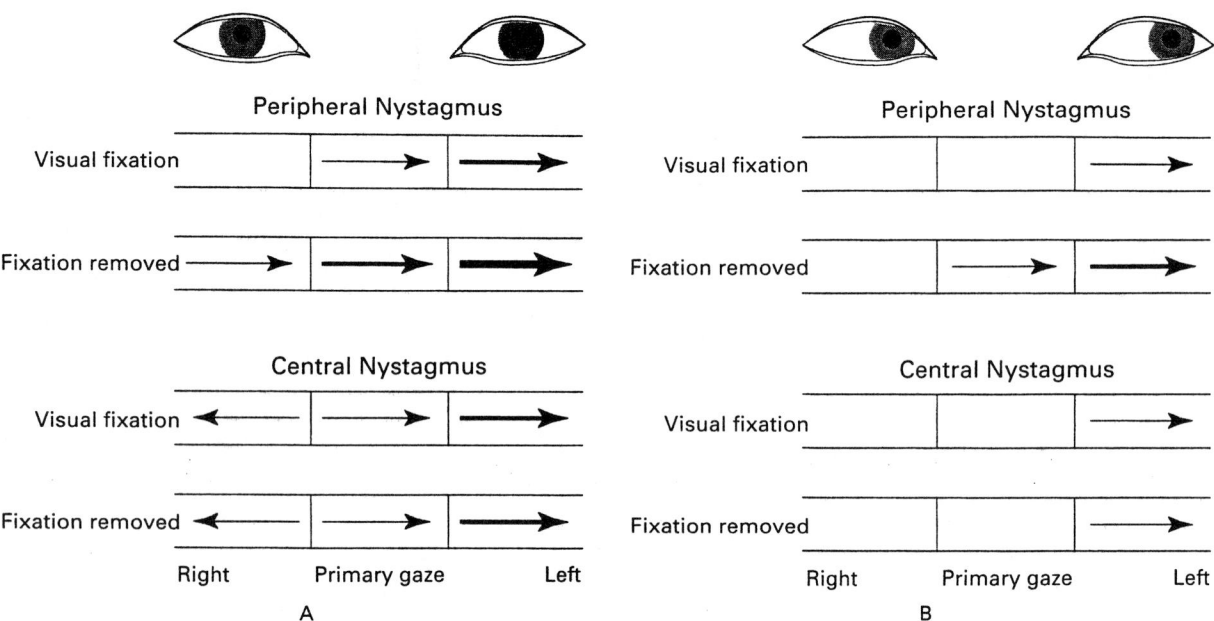

FIG. 231-2. Schematic drawing of peripheral and central vestibular nystagmus with and without visual fixation. The direction of the arrows indicates the horizontal direction of the fast phase of the nystagmus (a torsional component is not shown). The thickness of the arrows represents the relative intensity of the nystagmus. **A.** Findings typical of peripheral nystagmus, which remains in the same direction when the direction of gaze changes, and central nystagmus, which changes direction when the direction of gaze changes. Removal of visual fixation increases the intensity of peripheral nystagmus but not of central nystagmus. **B.** Removal of fixation helps to differentiate peripheral from central nystagmus when the nystagmus is predominantly in one direction of gaze during fixation. With removal of fixation, peripheral nystagmus may increase in intensity and become apparent in more than one direction of gaze. (Reprinted with permission from Hotson JR, Baloh AW: Acute vestibular syndrome. *New Engl J Med* 339:680, 1998. © 1998 Massachusetts Medical Society. All rights reserved.)

than central vertigo to be intense and to be associated with nausea, vomiting, diaphoresis, tinnitus, hearing loss, and photophobia. Central vertigo is more likely to be associated with neurologic symptoms and signs such as diplopia, dysarthria, and bilateral visual abnormalities. An associated headache or history of headache suggests migraine or a space-occupying lesion. Inquiry into history of head trauma and medications is required because these can precipitate episodes of dizziness or interfere with central adaptation. **Again, while these classic differentiations are useful, they are not invariable, and thus the clinician should not be reassured that a central cause is not present when symptoms appear more consistent with benign peripheral etiology.**

Physical Examination

Patients with vertigo should have ear, neurologic, and vestibular examinations. The external auditory canal and tympanic membrane should be examined for evidence of otitis media, cholesteatoma, and other pathology. Insufflation of air by use of a pneumatic otoscope that precipitates a burst of vertigo with nystagmus is diagnostic of an inner ear fistula. Hearing should be screened by whispering questions to the patient in one ear while lightly covering or rubbing one's fingers in front of the contralateral ear. Webber and Rinne testing also should be done if indicated. Other cranial nerves should be examined in detail as appropriate. Where central vertigo is considered, note abnormalities such as absent corneal reflex, facial paresis, difficulty swallowing, dysphonia, and depressed gag reflex. Test for limb as well as truncal ataxia. The vestibulospinal system and cerebellum are tested by tandem gait and Romberg testing. Proprioception and vibration also should be tested.

Nystagmus is the principal objective sign of vertigo. The eyes should be examined for spontaneous nystagmus, and the direction of such nystagmus should be noted. Because visual fixation can suppress nystagmus, the patient ideally should be wearing a pair of Frenzel

glasses, which are high-diopter lenses in a frame equipped with a light source. Examine for nystagmus while testing extraocular movements to 40 degrees from the midline. Note that several beats of nystagmus at the extremes of lateral gaze are a normal finding. Nystagmus on gaze testing suggests peripheral or central vertigo. The nystagmus pattern and behavior can assist in determining whether the lesion is central or peripheral (Figure 231-2).

The diagnosis of BPPV is aided by the Dix-Hallpike position test. This test should not be performed on patients with carotid bruits. It may be performed on patients with cervical spondylosis, provided that the neck is not hyperextended. The patient should be cautioned that the test might provoke vertigo. Pretreatment with 50 mg dimenhydrinate IM or IV may make the test more tolerable but will not obliterate nystagmus. Patients should keep their eyes open at all times and stare at the examiner's nose or forehead. The initial position of the patient on the examining table is upright and seated, close enough to the head of the table so that when the patient lies down, the head will be able to extend backward an additional 30 to 45 degrees. To test the right posterior semicircular canal, the head is initially rotated 30 to 45 degrees to the right. Keeping the head in this position, the patient is rapidly brought to the recumbent position until the head is 30 to 45 degrees below the level of the stretcher or examining table. A positive test is indicated by rotatory nystagmus following a latency of 1 to 5 s; the nystagmus exhibits rapid eye torsions toward the affected ear and lasts for 10 to 40 s. The patient is then returned to the upright sitting position, and the test is repeated on the left side. The side exhibiting the positive test is the side of the lesion.

Patients with suspected near-syncope should be tested for orthostatic hypotension. This maneuver is not definitive because orthostatic blood pressure measurements are notoriously unreliable, especially in elderly patients and even in patients with documented blood pressure changes. On cardiac examination, note the heart rate and rhythm, and evaluate the patient for evidence of valvular disease.

FIG. 231-3. Guideline approach to vertigo. MS = Multiple sclerosis; URI = Upper respiratory infection.

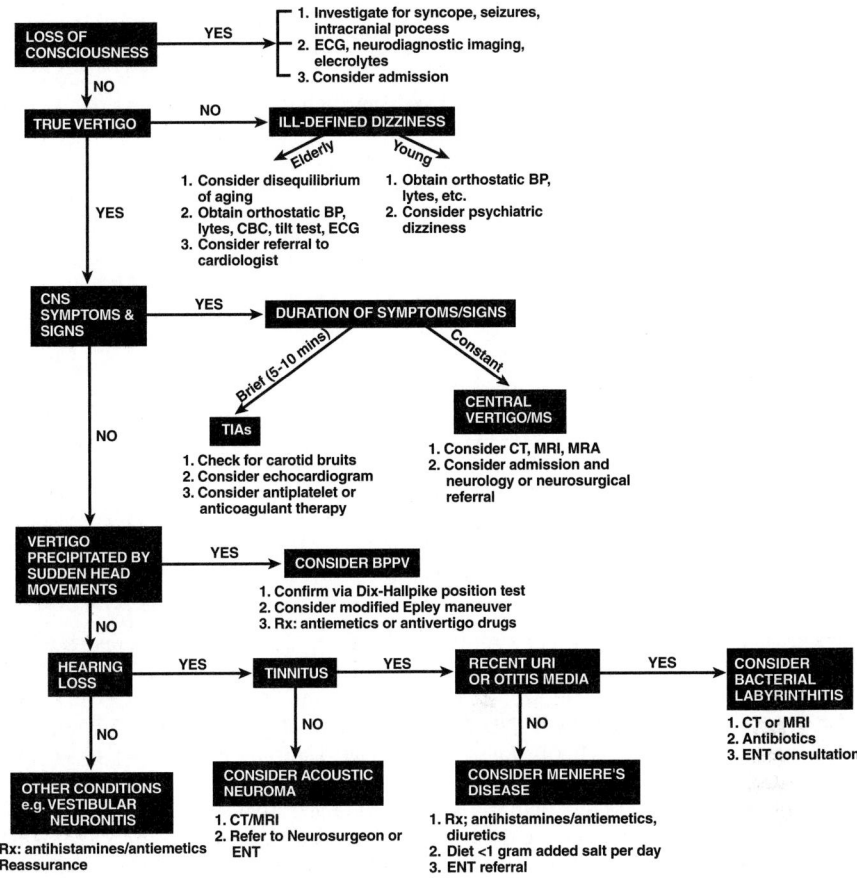

Ancillary Tests

Most patients with peripheral vertigo do not require emergent laboratory investigations. For suspected bacterial labyrinthitis, obtain a complete blood count (CBC) and blood cultures. Vertigo associated with a closed head injury warrants a computed tomographic (CT) scan or magnetic resonance imaging (MRI) to exclude intracranial bleeding. Patients with near-syncope should have an electrocardiogram (ECG) and cardiac monitoring as well as a CBC if anemia is suspected. Ambulatory Holter monitoring is indicated for suspected cardiac dysrhythmias. Emergent echocardiography generally is not indicated unless symptomatic valvular heart disease (such as aortic stenosis) or conditions causing compromised cardiac output are suspected. Electrolytes, glucose, and renal function tests are occasionally of value in patients with nonvertiginous dizziness, such as disequilibrium of aging. Outpatient thyroid testing may be of use if anxiety due to thyrotoxicosis is suspected.

Patients with suspected central vertigo may require more urgent investigations. If a cerebellar hemorrhage, infarction, or tumor is suspected, a CT scan or MRI should be obtained immediately. In the case of suspected vertebral artery dissection, magnetic resonance angiography (MRA) may be superior to conventional angiography. Patients with suspected vertebrobasilar insufficiency (VBI) require an ECG, cardiac monitoring. Echocardiography is appropriate if cardiac emboli are suspected although this need not be performed in the ED. With VBI, it is sufficient to leave investigations such as duplex ultrasound of the cartotids and MRI with MRA to the consulting neurologist. A psychiatric assessment for consideration of panic and/or mood disorders may be warranted in patients with persistent unexplained dizziness. In addition, patients with agoraphobia suggestive of space and motion discomfort (SMD) might warrant a full neurologic assessment. Detailed testing of cochleovestibular function can be left to the otologist or ear, nose, and throat (ENT) specialist.

SYMPTOMATIC TREATMENT

In general, short-term treatment with pharmacotherapy is the mainstay for patients with peripheral vertigo (Table 231-4). However, prolonged treatment with such medications may exacerbate symptoms in patients with nonvertiginous dizziness. Specific treatment varies somewhat with the etiology of peripheral vertigo.

Drug Therapy

The goals of pharmacotherapy are the reduction or elimination of vertigo, the enhancement or noncompromise of vestibular compensation, and the reduction of accompanying symptoms such as nausea, vomiting, and anxiety. Many of the agents used in the treatment of vertigo may suppress both vertigo and vestibular compensatory mechanisms.

Drugs with anticholinergic effects can be quite effective in the treatment of vertigo. The current agent of choice is transdermal scopolamine.

TABLE 231-3   Temporal Patterns Seen in Vertigo

Pattern	Conditions
Seconds	BPPV,* postural hypotension
Minutes	TIAs†
Hours	Ménière disease
Days	Viral labyrinthitis
Constant	Nonspecific dizziness

*Benign paroxysmal positional vertigo.
†Transient ischemic attacks.

TABLE 231-4 Pharmacotherapy of Vertigo and Dizziness

Category	Drug	Dosage	Indications	Advantages	Disadvantages
Anticholinergics	Scopolamine	0.5 mg transdermal patch (behind ear) q3–4d	Vertigo, nausea	Useful if patient is vomiting	Sometimes difficult to obtain
Antihistamines	Dimenhydrinate	50–100 mg IM, IV, or PO q4h	Vertigo, nausea	Inexpensive	Drowsiness/anticholinergic effect
	Diphenhydramine	25–50 mg IM, IV, or PO q4h	Vertigo, nausea	Inexpensive	Drowsiness/anticholinergic effect
	Meclizine	25 mg PO q6–12h	Vertigo, nausea		Drowsiness/anticholinergic effect
Antiemetics	Hydroxyzine	25–50 mg PO q6h	Vertigo, nausea	Inexpensive	Drowsiness/anticholinergic effect
	Metoclopramide	10–20 mg IV, PO q8h	Vertigo, nausea	Effective, versatile	Occasional extrapyramidal effect
	Promethazine	25 mg IM, PO, or PR q6–8h	Vertigo, nausea	Useful if vomiting	Occasional extrapyramidal effect
Benzodiazepines	Diazepam	2–5 mg PO q6–12h	Central vertigo, anxiety related to peripheral vertigo	Inexpensive	Dependency, may impair vestibular compensation
	Clonazepam	0.5 mg PO q12h	Central vertigo, anxiety related to peripheral vertigo	Inexpensive	Dependency, may impair vestibular compensation
Calcium antagonists	Cinnarizine	150 mg PO od	Peripheral vertigo, migraine	Nonsedating	Lesser clinical experience
	Nimodipine	30 mg PO tid	Peripheral vertigo	Nonsedating	Lesser clinical experience
	Flurarazine	20 mg PO tid	Ménière	Well tolerated	Not available in United States
Vasodilators	Betahistine	8–16 mg PO tid	Peripheral vertigo	Well tolerated	Little evidence of efficacy

Antihistamines are the most commonly prescribed drugs for the treatment of vertigo. Such agents possess anticholinergic effects. Some antihistamines such as astemizole (see Table 231-5) have antivertigo properties without appreciable anticholinergic effects, suggesting a unique central action. H_1 antihistamines are considered effective against vertigo, but H_2 antihistamines are not. Calcium channel blockers such as cinnarizine and nimodipine (see Table 231-5) have been shown to be useful in the treatment of peripheral vertigo. Calcium channel blockers are known to possess antihistaminic and antidopaminergic activity. They also may act by suppressing sensory input from the vestibular apparatus. Calcium channel blockers are indicated for the symptomatic relief of vertigo in patients not responding to scopolamine or antihistamines or for whom such drugs are contraindicated. Calcium channel blockers are also useful in managing vertigo in association with migraine headaches. Antidopaminergic (neuroleptic) agents such as promethazine and metoclopramide are indicated as second-line treatment for patients who fail to respond to transdermal scopolamine and antihistamines. They also have been shown to be effective in the treatment of vertigo. Such agents reduce neurovegetative symptoms such as nausea and vomiting by blocking dopaminergic receptors in the area postrema of the brainstem. They also possess antihistamine and anticholinergic effects. Prochlorperazine and chlorpromazine should not be used in the management of vertigo because they tend to cause excessive orthostatic hypotension, which can exacerbate symptoms. Ondansetron, a serotonin 5-HT_3 receptor antagonist, has not been shown to be effective in the management of nausea related to motion.[5,6] Small doses of benzodiazepines such as diazepam and clonazepam may be used sparingly in the management of severe anxiety accompanying vertigo. Benzodiazepines bind to γ-aminobutyric acid (GABA) receptors in the brainstem, and thus may act centrally to suppress vestibular responses and to impair vestibular compensation.

There are several recognized complications of symptomatic therapy. Antihistamines can cause sedation and anticholinergic adverse effects. Antidopaminergic neuroleptic agents can induce or exacerbate orthostatic hypotension. These drugs also can cause somnolence and acute dystonia and can exacerbate anticholinergic adverse effects. Because of overlapping anticholinergic and antidopaminergic effects, anticholinergic, antihistaminic, and neuroleptic drugs should never be used in combination.

Patients with nonvertiginous dizziness and disequilibrium of aging should not be treated with antivertigo medication.

Vestibular Rehabilitation Exercises

Vestibular exercises are indicated for patients with BPPV, chronic vertigo, and psychiatric dizziness.[7] They are relatively simple to teach and can be quite helpful in giving patients a measure of control over their own symptoms. The principle behind vestibular exercises is the fatiguing response observed with Dix-Hallpike testing. Exercises developed by Brandt and Daroff have been shown to be efficacious.[8] Such exercises can be repeated by the patient at 3-hourly intervals at home.

DISORDERS CAUSING PERIPHERAL VERTIGO

Peripheral vertigo is noted for its abrupt (often explosive) onset. It is an intense sensation of spinning or hurtling toward the ground or surrounding walls. It is typically worsened by rapid movement and by changes in head position. It is frequently associated with nausea, often severe vomiting, diaphoresis, and bradycardia and hypotension.

Benign Paroxysmal Positional Vertigo

BPPV is a frequent diagnosis for patients presenting to dizziness clinics. The incidence of BPPV is conservatively estimated at 64 patients per 100,000 per year.[9] BPPV is defined as a mechanical disorder of the inner ear causing transient vertigo (with autonomic symptoms) and associated nystagmus that is precipitated by certain head movements. The condition was described first by Barany in 1921; most of the essential clinical features were described by Dix and Hallpike in 1952.[10]

TABLE 231-5 Supportive Findings in Benign Paroxysmal Positional Vertigo

Latency period of 1–5 s between the provocative head position and onset of nystagmus.

The intensity of nystagmus increases to a peak before slowly resolving.

Duration of vertigo and nystagmus ranges from 5–40 s.

If nystagmus is produced in one direction by placing the head down, then the nystagmus reverses direction when the head is returned to the sitting position.

Repeated head positioning causes both the vertigo and accompanying nystagmus to fatigue and subside.

The most widely accepted hypothesis to explain BPPV is known as *canalolithiasis*. According to this hypothesis, BPPV is caused by inappropriate activation of the posterior semicircular canal (typically unilateral) by the presence of free-floating particles or otoconia. The otoconia become displaced from the utricular macula by aging, head trauma, or labyrinthine disease. Because the particles are heavier than the surrounding endolymph, they tend to collect in the long arm of the posterior semicircular canal, the most dependent part of the endolymph system. Once the particles clump in sufficient mass, changes in head position cause gravitation of the particles, which creates a hydrodynamic drag (or plunger effect) on the endolymph, causing the cupula to be displaced. This results in inadvertent neural firing, causing both vertigo and nystagmus.

BPPV can occur at any age, but the average age of onset is in the midfifties. Women are twice as likely to be affected as men. The onset is sudden, and an attack typically is precipitated by rolling over in bed, assuming a supine position, leaning forward, looking up at the sky or ceiling, or turning the head. Nausea is often present. Because the symptoms fatigue, they tend to be worse in the morning and become less pronounced as the day progresses. Patients may eliminate the offending activities. There is no associated hearing loss or tinnitus and no physical findings on examination of the external auditory canal.

Several findings support a diagnosis of BPPV (Table 231-5). There is a latency period of 1 to 5 s between assuming the offending head position and onset of vertigo and nystagmus. Both the vertigo and nystagmus crescendo to a peak of intensity and then subside within 5 to 40 s. BPPV is diagnosed using the Dix-Hallpike position test described earlier.[10] The response to repeated provocative testing fatigues, causing the vertigo and nystagmus to disappear.[11]

Some patients with BPPV have a negative Dix-Hallpike test. Instead, they have anterior semicircular canalithiasis and may exhibit positional down-beating nystagmus when the head is lowered as described earlier but not turned to one side or the other (the so-called straight head-hanging maneuver).[12]

The treatment of BPPV includes the use of transdermal scopolamine as well as antihistamines. In addition, the particle-repositioning maneuver (or Epley maneuver) may be attempted by emergency physicians, but few have any experience with this, and the diagnosis is rarely established conclusively in the emergency department. The principle behind the particle-repositioning maneuver is to use gravity to induce the particles to move along the semicircular canals until they end up inside the utricle, where they are unlikely to cause vertigo. The maneuver is indicated in patients who have a history suggestive of BPPV plus a positive Dix-Hallpike position test. The affected ear is determined by the side on which the Dix-Hallpike position test is positive. An antihistamine or antiemetic should be administered prior to the maneuver for the patient's comfort. The patient is seated as in the Dix-Hallpike position test, and the head is turned 45 degrees toward the affected ear. The patient is gently brought to the recumbent position with the head hanging 30 to 45 degrees below the examining table. The head is gently rotated 45 degrees to the midline. The head is then rotated a further 45 degrees to the unaffected side. The patient rolls onto the shoulder of the unaffected side, at the same time rotating the head a further 45 degrees. The patient is returned to the sitting position, and the head is returned to the midline.

Each portion of the maneuver should be done slowly (about 5 min) and evenly to permit the particles to traverse their intended course. If the maneuver is done correctly, nystagmus in the same direction as that observed during Dix-Hallpike position testing may be observed. If nystagmus in the opposite direction is observed, then the particles have moved back toward the cupula; this portends an unsuccessful maneuver. The maneuver is repeated several times until both the vertigo and the accompanying nystagmus have disappeared. A Cochrane Review concluded that the Epley maneuver is a safe and effective treatment for posterior canal BPPV. However, there is no good evidence to conclude that the maneuver provides long-term resolution of symptoms.[13]

Adverse effects include light-headedness and exacerbation of vertigo (caused by backsliding of the particles). The Epley maneuver should not be performed on patients with cervical spondylosis or back pain that might be exacerbated.

Most episodes of BPPV resolve spontaneously after a few days. Patients with persistent symptoms should be referred to an otolaryngologist.

Ménière Disease

Ménière disease is a disorder associated with an increased endolymph within the cochlea and labyrinth. It occurs equally in men and women. The first attack of Ménière disease usually occurs in patients aged 65 years and older. Rarely, the disease may begin in childhood. The disease is usually unilateral initially but often becomes bilateral over time. The precise pathogenesis is unknown, but evidence suggests that patients have difficulty regulating the volume, flow, and composition of endolymph. Histologic studies have demonstrated that the endolymphatic sac contains immunologically active tissue, raising the possibility of an autoimmune mechanism. As with BPPV, the onset of vertigo is usually sudden. However, the duration of vertigo ranges from 20 min to 12 h (typically 2 to 8 h). It is associated with nausea, vomiting, and diaphoresis. The frequency of attacks can vary from several times per week to several times per month. Other associated symptoms include roaring tinnitus, diminished hearing, and fullness in one ear. Between attacks, the patient is usually well, although deafness may persist. Increasingly, the diagnosis of Ménière disease is confirmed by the introduction of glycerol, an osmotic agent, into the inner ear. A positive glycerol tested is heralded by temporary improvement in postural control as well as a decrease in vertigo.[14]

Patients with Ménière disease usually are managed by an otolaryngologist. Ménière disease is managed symptomatically with antihistamines as well as with a combination of the diuretics triamterene and hydrochlorthiazide (the latter two drugs are used in confirmed cases only). Flunarizine, a calcium channel blocker (not available in the United States at the time of this writing) is second-line treatment in the management of vertigo associated with Ménière disease (see Table 231-4). Betahistine, a structural analogue of histamine, has been used widely in Europe for the treatment of vertigo due to Ménière disease. Betahistine is believed to act by reducing the asymmetrical functioning of sensory vestibular organs as well as by increasing vestibulocochlear blood flow. The dosage of betahistine is 8 to 16 mg PO three times daily. None of these drug treatments improves hearing. A salt-restricted diet (<1 g/d of added salt) is recommended for patients with a confirmed diagnosis. Intratympanic steroid injections, as well as transtympanic gentamicin administered via round-window microcatheter, also can offer significant relief to symptomatic patients.

Perilymph Fistula

A perilymph fistula is an opening in the round or oval window that permits pneumatic changes in the middle ear to be transmitted to the vestibular apparatus. Trauma, infection, or a sudden change in the pressure inside the ventricular system may cause the tear. The diagnosis is suggested by the sudden onset of vertigo associated with flying, scuba diving, severe straining, heavy lifting, coughing, or sneezing. Associated symptoms may include hearing loss. The diagnosis is confirmed by nystagmus elicited by pneumatic otoscopy (Hennebert sign). Hearing loss is confirmed by audiology testing.

Perilymph fistula is managed with symptomatic treatment and bed rest, with referral to an ENT specialist for surgical repair. Fistulas associated with hearing loss of less than 14 days' duration may benefit from rapid surgical intervention.

Vestibular Neuronitis

Vestibular neuronitis is a disorder of suspected viral etiology. Unlike BPPV and Ménière disease, vestibular neuronitis typically lasts several days and does not recur. The onset is usually sudden, and the patient is otherwise well except for possible symptoms of a viral illness. The vertigo is often so intense that the patient requires several days of bed rest; symptoms usually decrease dramatically, with complete resolution over several weeks. Elderly patients may have persistent unsteadiness of gait. Unilateral loss of hearing and tinnitus may occur. Up to one-third of patients have positional nystagmus.

Vestibular neuronitis is treated symptomatically. Antihistamines and antinausea drugs should be used at the outset and withdrawn after several days, if possible.

Vestibular Ganglionitis

This disorder is believed to be caused by a neurotrophic virus such as varicella zoster that can be reactivated years following an initial infection. Typical histopathologic changes associated with a viral inflammatory process have been identified in the vestibular ganglion. This disorder may be mistaken for more commonly diagnosed conditions such as BPPV and Ménière disease. Multiple ganglia may be involved. Herpes zoster oticus, also known as the Ramsay Hunt syndrome, is a neuropathic disorder thought to be associated with vestibular ganglionitis. It is characterized by deafness, vertigo, and facial nerve palsy. The diagnosis is confirmed by the presence of grouped vesicles on an erythematous base inside the external auditory canal. Patients with this disorder are managed with a combination of symptomatic treatment and antiviral therapy (if diagnosed within 72 h of the appearance of vesicles).

Labyrinthitis

Labyrinthitis is an infection of the labyrinth that produces peripheral vertigo associated with hearing loss. The infection may be viral, in which case the clinical course is similar to that of vestibular neuronitis. Cases reportedly have been associated with measles and mumps. Bacteria also may cause labyrinthitis. Although unusual, an infection within the labyrinth can develop from otitis media, in which bacteria and toxins diffuse across the membrane of the round window. A cholesteatoma can erode into the inner ear, creating a portal of entry for bacteria. Other possible antecedents for bacterial labyrinthitis include otitis media with fistula, meningitis, mastoiditis, and dermoid tumor. The hallmarks of this disease include sudden onset of vertigo with associated hearing loss and middle ear findings. Serous labyrinthitis occasionally may produce vertigo.

Patients with bacterial labyrinthitis may benefit from symptomatic treatment but also require antibiotics (see Chap. 235) and referral to an otologist or ENT specialist for likely admission and possible surgical drainage.

Ototoxicity

Aminoglycoside antibiotics produce hearing loss and peripheral vestibular dysfunction by accumulating inside the endolymph, where they cause the death of cochlear and vestibular hair cells. However, since both inner ears are affected, vertigo is uncommon. Typical clinical manifestations include ataxia and oscillopsia, which is defined as an inability to maintain visual fixation while moving. The damage is irreversible but is dose- and duration-dependent. Loop diuretics (furosemide and ethacrynic acid) also cause irreversible vestibular and ototoxicity. Cytotoxic agents associated with vestibular damage include vinblastine and cisplatin. Recent evidence suggests that the topical administration of D-methionine to the round window membrane may protect against the ototoxic effects of cisplatin. Newer platins such as carboplatin have been shown to induce less ototoxicity than cisplatin. The antiarrhythmic drug quinidine and antimalarial drugs derived from quinine, such as chloroquine and mefloquine, also can cause vestibular symptoms that may be irreversible (Table 231-6). In

TABLE 231-6   Ototoxic and Vestibulotoxic Agents

Agent	Dose Dependent	Reversible
Aminoglycosides	Yes	No
Erythromycin	No	Yes
Minocycline	No	Yes
Fluoroquinolones	No	Yes
NSAIDs, salicylates	Yes	Yes
Loop diuretics	No	Can be irreversible
Cytostatic drugs	Yes	No
Antimalarials	No	Yes

one study, 96 percent of healthy adults had vertigo while taking mefloquine. However, the symptoms resolved within 3 weeks of cessation of therapy in 77.3 percent of patients.[15]

Reversible causes of vestibular damage and ototoxicity include NSAIDs, salicylates, minocycline, erythromycin, and some fluoroquinolones. Tinnitus as well as alterations in the perception of sounds have long been known to be associated with salicylate ingestion. There have also been rare case reports of sudden hearing loss associated with the use of NSAIDs including ketorolac, naproxen, and piroxicam. In the cases of naproxen as well as piroxicam, tinnitus has been associated with hearing loss.[16–18] Isolated cases of unsteady gait have been observed with antiviral drugs such as abacavir, as well as antiparasitic agents.

Numerous solvents and other chemicals can cause both peripheral and central vestibular symptoms. These include propylene glycol, mercury, and hydrocarbons. Drugs that sometimes induce a central vestibular syndrome include anticonvulsants, tricyclic antidepressants, neuroleptics, opiates, and alcohol.[19] Phencyclidine is a recreational drug that causes central vestibular symptoms, including nystagmus and ataxia. Drugs causing irreversible cerebellar toxicity include phenytoin and toluene, as well as cancer chemotherapeutic agents. In general, most patients adapt to vertigo that is chronic by relying on increased sensory input from unaffected modalities such as proprioception and vision. However, certain drugs that are used as antivertigo therapy may exacerbate preexisting chronic vertigo by delaying or inhibiting such compensation. These drugs include alcohol, benzodiazepines, barbiturates, and neuroleptics. Thus, with chronic vertigo, antivertigo therapy should not be used on a long-term basis. Patients with suspected ototoxicity should be referred to an otolaryngologist.

Eighth-Nerve Lesions

Lesions of the eighth cranial nerve may produce mild vertigo. Meningiomas and acoustic schwannomas are typical causes. The onset of vertigo is usually gradual, remaining constant until central compensation can take place. The vertigo is usually preceded by hearing loss. Such patients require urgent diagnostic imaging as well as referral to a neurosurgeon.

Cerebellopontine Angle Tumors

Vertigo is sometimes associated with tumors of the cerebellopontine angle. Such tumors include acoustic neuromas, meningiomas, and dermoids. They usually present with a cluster of findings including deafness and ataxia as well as ipsilateral facial weakness, loss of the corneal reflex, and cerebellar signs. Such patients require urgent diagnostic imaging as well as referral to a neurosurgeon.

Posttraumatic Vertigo

Vertigo and gait unsteadiness are common complaints following a head injury. Acute posttraumatic vertigo is caused by a direct injury to the labyrinthine membranes. The onset of vertigo is immediate and is accompanied by nausea and vomiting. Such patients may have sustained a concomitant fracture of the temporal bone. Vertigo associated with a closed head injury warrants a CT scan or MRI to exclude an extradural or intradural hematoma. Vertigo due to direct labyrinthine trauma tends to resolve within several weeks. Closed head trauma also can displace otoconia from the utricular maculae, precipitating an attack of BPPV. Some patients with a history of a closed head injury develop a postconcussive syndrome that can be associated with unsteadiness of gait and a vague sense of dizziness. Patients with this condition usually are treated symptomatically. Those who fail to improve usually are referred to a neurologist or neurosurgeon.

Vertigo Following Cochlear Implantation

As many as three-quarters of adults who undergo cochlear implantation experience vertigo postoperatively. Such patients generally respond to symptomatic therapy as well as vestibular rehabilitation exercises.[20]

DISORDERS CAUSING CENTRAL VERTIGO

Central vertigo is caused by disorders affecting the cerebellum and the brainstem. Central vertigo is gradual in onset and mild in intensity; the symptoms are not provoked by changes in position. Central vertigo is unlikely to be associated with nausea, vomiting, or diaphoresis. Unlike conditions causing peripheral vertigo, both tinnitus and hearing impairment are unlikely. Nystagmus is more likely to be vertical than horizontal or rotatory and may be present in the absence of vertigo. However, a finding of vertical nystagmus does not necessarily imply a central etiology unless accompanied by signs of brainstem disease, such as ataxia, blurred vision, long tract signs, dysphagia, dysarthria, and diplopia.

Cerebellar Hemorrhage and Infarction

Cerebellar hemorrhage typically causes symptoms such as acute vertigo and ataxia. Headache, nausea, and vomiting may or may not be present. Instead of intense vertigo, patients tend to complain of a sense of side-to-side or front-to-back motion. Patients may have truncal ataxia and may not be able to sit without support. Romberg testing and tandem gait will be abnormal. Occasionally, there may be a sixth cranial nerve palsy or conjugate eye deviation away from the side with the hemorrhage. Cerebellar infarction has a similar clinical presentation. When suspected, both conditions require urgent diagnostic imaging as well as referral to a neurosurgeon or neurologist as appropriate.

Wallenberg Syndrome

A lateral medullary infarction (Wallenberg syndrome) of the brainstem can cause vertigo as part of its clinical presentation. Classic ipsilateral findings include facial numbness, loss of corneal reflex, Horner syndrome, and paralysis or paresis of the soft palate, pharynx, and larynx (causing dysphagia and dysphonia). Contralateral findings include loss of pain and temperature sensation in the trunk and limbs. Occasionally, lesions of the sixth, seventh, and eighth cranial nerves can occur, causing vertigo, nausea, vomiting, and nystagmus. Such patients usually require urgent diagnostic imaging and referral to a neurologist.

Vertebrobasilar Insufficiency

Transient ischemic attacks (TIAs) of the brainstem due to vertebrobasilar insufficiency (VBI) can produce vertigo. Such patients have typical risk factors for cerebrovascular disease. Orthostatic signs should be determined, as orthostasis can worsen symptoms of VBI. As

with TIAs in general, the vertigo may be of sudden onset and typically lasts from minutes to hours. By definition, the episode should resolve completely within 24 h. VBI-induced vertigo can present by itself or be accompanied by diplopia, dysphagia, dysarthria, bilateral long-tract signs, and bilateral loss of vision. **Unlike other causes of central vertigo, VBI may be provoked by position.** Turning the head partially occludes the ipsilateral vertebral artery. If the contralateral artery is stenotic, head turning could cause transient ischemia to the brainstem, resulting in VBI. A sufficient loss of brainstem circulation caused by a head turn could affect the reticular activating system, causing near-syncope or syncope. Patients with VBI should have diagnostic imaging in the emergency department, as well as referral to a neurologist for investigation and treatment of TIAs.

Vertebral Artery Dissection

Vertebral artery dissection can lead to strokes involving the posterior circulation. Symptoms of vertebral artery dissection include headache, vertigo, and a unilateral Horner syndrome. Sudden (and often violent) rotation or extension of the neck may precipitate a dissection of the vertebral artery in susceptible patients. Such injuries reportedly have occurred following high-velocity motor vehicle accidents, diving injuries, coughing, sneezing, and chiropractic neck adjustments.[21] Such patients require urgent diagnostic imaging plus referral to a neurosurgeon.

Multiple Sclerosis

Demyelinating disease can present with vertigo that tends to last several hours to several days or weeks and is usually nonrecurrent. The vertigo is not usually intense; the nystagmus is often more prominent than the vertigo reported by the patient. Ataxia or optic neuritis may be present or may have occurred previously. The diagnosis usually is made using MRI as well as vestibular evoked myogenic potentials. Patients with vertigo due to demyelination require urgent referral to a neurologist.

Neoplasms

Neoplasms of the fourth ventricle can cause brainstem signs and symptoms, including vertigo. Such tumors include ependymomas in younger patients and metastases in older patients. Obviously, these patients require diagnostic imaging while in the emergency department and should be referred to a neurosurgeon.

Migraine-Related Dizziness and Vertigo

Vertigo can be a symptom of an aura, an analogue or equivalent of the headache phase itself, or as an associated symptom with the migraine prodrome. Basilar migraine is a migraine headache in which the aura is associated with clinical manifestations similar to those of VBI. The etiology of migraine-related vertigo remains somewhat unclear. The International Headache Society's diagnostic criteria for basilar migraine[22] are shown in Table 231-7. Vertigo as an aura should develop over 5 to 20 min and should subside within 60 min. Vertigo as a symptom of a migraine aura may precede the headache or may occur in the absence of a headache.

A strong association has been found between migraine and cochleovestibular disturbances. Such patients may complain of episodes of constant vertigo, positional vertigo, or nonvertiginous dizziness. In cases of true vertigo, the vertigo may accompany the headache or may occur independently. Some patients complain of vertigo lasting from several minutes to 2 h, whereas others experience vertigo lasting longer than 24 h. The diagnostic criteria for migraine-related vertigo include a history of vertigo not attributable to other known conditions and a present or past history of migraine or a strong

TABLE 231-7   Diagnostic Criteria for Basilar Migraine*

Bilateral visual symptoms in both the nasal and temporal fields
Vertigo
Tinnitus
Decreased hearing
Diplopia
Dysarthria
Ataxia
Bilateral paresis
Bilateral paresthesias
Decreased level of consciousness

*Fulfills criteria for migraine with aura (two or more of the above aura symptoms).
Source: From Ref. 22, with permission.

family history. Often it is difficult to distinguish vertigo associated with migraine and vertigo associated with Ménière disease. Frequently, patients who fail to respond to therapy specific for Ménière disease may benefit from therapy for vertigo associated with migraine headaches.

Patients with vertiginous migraine headaches are managed symptomatically with antivertigo therapy; migraine prophylactic agents such as β-blockers and calcium channel antagonists may be instituted as well (see Chap. 227). Patients with migraine-related vertigo and dizziness can be managed symptomatically. However, ergotamine preparations or sumatriptan should not be used in basilar migraine. They should be referred to a neurologist for definitive management.

OTHER CONDITIONS

Disequilibrium of Aging

Disequilibrium of aging is a condition manifesting as ill-defined dizziness and gait unsteadiness. It is associated with age-related loss of hearing, balance, proprioceptive input, and vision. Other factors include a decline in central integration and processing, as well as a decrease in motor responses. Approximately 50 percent of individuals over the age of 70 experience imbalance and frequent falls. Symptoms may be precipitated or exacerbated by diminished ambient light (with worsening of symptoms at night), unfamiliar surroundings, and the use of benzodiazepines and drugs with anticholinergic effects such as tricyclic antidepressants and neuroleptic agents. Such patients should be referred to an internist or gerontologist.

Near-Syncope

Near-syncope is a feeling of light-headedness that, in its most severe form, leads to loss of consciousness (syncope). The most common categories of near-syncope include vasovagal, situational, and orthostatic hypotension; drug-induced syncope; and cardiac causes (cardiac dysrhythmias and valvular heart disease). The cause of near-syncope is not determined in a significant percentage of patients. Recent evidence suggests that most patients with unexplained presyncope may have subclinical vasovagal presyncope. Positive upright tilt testing, in which the patient is placed in the passive upright position at 60 degrees for 45 min, generally is recommended. The end points of a positive tilt test include the development of syncope or presyncope associated with hypotension, bradycardia, or both. In normal subjects, tachycardia usually results from a passive tilt test.[23]

Syncope and near-syncope in the elderly may be associated with micturition, defecation, postural changes, meals, laughing, coughing, and swallowing. Orthostatic hypotension is extremely common in the elderly and is associated with volume depletion, venous insufficiency, poor conditioning, polyneuropathy, preganglionic autonomic dysfunction (Shy-Drager syndrome), and the use of such medications as vasodilating drugs, diuretics, other antihypertensive agents, and antiparkinsonian and anticholinergic medications; polypharmacy is a relatively common factor.

Orthostatic tachycardia syndrome is a relatively mild disorder associated with a fall in blood pressure in which patients experience near-syncope, nonvertiginous dizziness, and symptoms suggestive of a TIA. The pathogenesis is thought to be mild autonomic dysfunction. Findings on tilt testing include an increase in heart rate of 30 beats/min over baseline within the first 10 min of testing (unassociated with profound hypotension) along with recurrence of the symptom complex.[24] Unless debilitated, such patients should be referred to a cardiologist, internist, or gerontologist for outpatient management.

Convulsive Disorders

Nonconvulsive status epilepticus (NCSE) is characterized by altered mental status without loss of consciousness or tonic-clonic phenomena yet associated with electroencephalographic (EEG) evidence of seizure activity. Some patients with NCSE may complain of nonvertiginous dizziness. Symptoms may last for hours to days. The diagnosis is made by electroencephalography as well as by determining the underlying mechanism for the seizure. Patients with suspected convulsive disorders should be treated symptomatically while in the emergency department and referred to a neurologist for further assessment.

Hyperventilation Syndrome

Patients with primary hyperventilation may experience nonvertiginous dizziness or near-syncope during an episode. Such symptoms usually can be reproduced by asking the patient to hyperventilate. Such patients are managed by the emergency physician.

Psychiatric Dizziness

Psychiatric dizziness is dizziness that presents as part of a recognized psychiatric disorder or symptom complex that is not related to known vestibular disorders. Dizziness is the second most common symptom reported by patients with panic disorder.[25] In the emergency setting, a diagnosis of psychiatric dizziness should only be made when the evidence is overwhelming and when other more serious causes of dizziness have been ruled out.

DISPOSITION

In general, patients with peripheral vertigo may be discharged from the emergency department, once symptoms are controlled. All patients with a first episode of peripheral vertigo should be referred to their primary care physician or an otolaryngologist for further testing. Patients with BPPV who have had a particle-repositioning maneuver should be referred to an otologist or ENT specialist for follow-up.

Patients with suspected central causes of their vertigo almost always require urgent diagnostic imaging and neurologic or neurosurgical consultation while in the emergency department. Patients in whom less urgent causes of central vertigo remain within the differential diagnosis (such as multiple sclerosis and migraine headache) may be referred for neurologic consultation on an outpatient basis. Patients with near-syncope should be referred on an outpatient basis to a cardiologist for tilt testing, an echocardiogram, and Holter monitoring. Elderly patients should be referred for admission to a cardiologist if they have symptomatic coronary artery or valvular disease, exhibit a potentially life-threatening dysrhythmia, or have a past history of syncopal episodes.

Outpatient psychiatric consultation may be considered for patients with dizziness not related to vestibular dysfunction that occurs exclusively in combination with other symptoms as part of a recognized psychiatric symptom cluster or for patients in whom dizziness appears to be amplified by psychogenic overlay.

REFERENCES

1. Yardley L, Owen N, Nazareth I, Luxon L: Prevalence and presentation of dizziness in a general practice community sample of working age people. *Br J Gen Pract* 48:1131, 1998.
2. Furman JM, Jacob RG: Psychiatric dizziness. *Neurology* 48:1161, 1997.
3. Chang MB, Bath AP, Rutka JA: Are all atypical positional nystagmus patterns reflective of central pathology? *J Otolaryngol* 30:280, 2001.
4. Parnes LS, McClure J: Free-floating endolymph particles: A new operative finding during posterior semicircular canal occlusion. *Laryngoscope* 102:988, 1992.
5. Levine ME, Chillas JC, et al: The effects of serotonin (5-HT$_3$) receptor antagonists on gastric tachyarrhythmia and symptoms of motion sickness. *Aviat Space Environ Med* 71(11Pt1):1111, 2000.
6. *CPS 2000 Compendium of Pharmaceuticals and Specialties.* Canadian Pharmacists Association, Ottawa, Canada, p 1926.
7. Beynon GJ: A review of management of benign paroxysmal positional vertigo by exercise therapy and by repositioning maneuvers. *Br J Audiol* 31:11, 1997.
8. Yardley L, Luxon LM: Treating dizziness with vestibular rehabilitation. *Br Med J* 308:1252, 1994.
9. Froehling DA, Silverstein MD, Mohr DN, et al: Benign positional vertigo: Incidence and prognosis in a population-based study in Olmsted County, Minnesota. *Mayo Clin Proc* 66:596, 1991.
10. Dix MR, Hallpike CS: The pathology, symptomatology and diagnosis of certain common disorders of the vestibular system. *Proc R Soc Med* 45:341, 1952.
11. Hughes CA, Proctor L: Benign paroxysmal peripheral vertigo. *Laryngoscope* 107:607, 1997.
12. Bertholon P, Bronstein AM, Davies RA, et al: Positional down beating nystagmus in 50 patients: Cerebellar disorders and possible anterior semicircular canalithiasis. *J Neurol Neurosurg Psychiatry* 72:366, 2002.
13. Hilton M, Pinder D: The Epley (canalith repositioning) maneuver for benign paroxysmal positional vertigo (Cochrane Review). *Cochrane Database Syst Rev* (1):CD003162, 2002.
14. Di Girolamo S, Picciotti P, Sergi B, et al: Postural control and glycerol test in Meniere's disease. *Acta Otolaryngol* 121:813, 2001.
15. Rendi-Wagner P, Noedl H, Wernsdorfer WH, et al: Unexpected frequency, duration and spectrum of adverse effects after therapeutic dose of mefloquine in healthy adults. *Acta Trop (Basel)* 81:167, 2002.
16. McKinnon BJ, Lassen LF: Naproxen-associated sudden sensorineural hearing loss. *Mil Med* 163(11):792, 1998.
17. Vernick DM, Kelly JH: Sudden hearing loss associated with piroxicam. *Am J Otol* 7:97, 1986.
18. Schaab KC, Dickinson ET, Setzen G: Acute sensorineural hearing loss following ketorolac administration. *J Emerg Med* 13:509, 1995.
19. Rascol O, Hain TC, Brefel C, et al: Antivertigo medications and drug-induced vertigo: A pharmacological review. *Drugs* 50:777, 1995.
20. Steenerson RL, Cronin GW, Gary LB: Vertigo after cochlear implantation. *Otol Neurotol* 22:842, 2001.
21. Rothwell DM, Bondy SJ, Williams I: Chiropractic manipulation and stroke: A population-based case-control study. *Stroke* 32:1054, 2001.
22. Headache Classification Committee of the International Headache Society: Classification and diagnostic criteria for headache disorders, cranial neuralgias and facial pain. *Cephalagia* 8:19, 1988.
23. Sheldon R, Koshman ML: A randomized study of tilt test angle in patients with undiagnosed syncope. *Can J Cardiol* 17:1051, 2001.
24. Grubb BP, Kosinski DJ, Boehm K, Kip K: The postural orthostatic tachycardia syndrome: A neurocardiogenic variant identified during head-up tilt table testing. *Pacing Clin Electrophysiol* 20:2205, 1997.
25. Asmundson GJG, Larsen DK, Stein MB: Panic disorder and vestibular disturbance: An overview of empirical findings and clinical implications. *J Psychosom Res* 44:107, 1998.

SEIZURES AND STATUS EPILEPTICUS IN ADULTS
Christina L. Catlett

INTRODUCTION

A seizure is an episode of abnormal neurologic function caused by an inappropriate electrical discharge of brain neurons. The seizure is the clinical attack experienced by the patient; some patients with "epileptic" electroencephalographic (EEG) discharges may not experience any overt clinical symptoms. Conversely, some seizure-like clinical episodes may be due to causes other than abnormal brain electrical activity; such attacks, however impressive, are not true seizures (see below).

Epilepsy is a clinical condition in which an individual is subject to recurrent seizures; it implies a more or less fixed condition of the brain responsible for the seizures. Ordinarily, the term *epileptic* is not used to refer to an individual with recurrent seizures caused by reversible conditions such as alcohol withdrawal, hypoglycemia, or other metabolic derangements.

Seizures referred to as *primary* or *idiopathic* occur in patients who are otherwise normal and in whom no evident cause for the attacks can be discerned. Seizures that occur as a consequence of some other identifiable neurologic condition, such as a mass lesion, are referred to as *secondary* or *symptomatic.* Any individual can have a seizure under appropriate conditions. Electrical stimulation of the brain, convulsant potentiating drugs, profound metabolic disturbances, or a sharp blow to the head may induce seizures (termed *reactive seizures*) in otherwise normal individuals. Such attacks are generally self-limited, and such persons are not considered to have a seizure disorder or epilepsy.

There are approximately 100,000 new cases diagnosed in the United States each year. An estimated 6 to 10 percent of individuals will experience at least one seizure during their lives, and 1 to 2 percent of persons are subject to recurrent seizures. Hauser and Hesdorffer[1] from the Epilepsy Foundation of America analyzed reports of incidence and prevalence of seizures and epilepsy worldwide and deduced an overall age-adjusted incidence of 30.9 to 56.8 per 100,000. Incidence rates are highest among people less than 20 years old, with a second peak in incidence in those older than 60 years, reflecting a difference in seizure etiology between these two groups. There is a slightly higher male predominance (estimated 1.1 to 1.7 greater incidence).

The mechanisms involved in generating clinical seizures appear to be multifactorial, requiring intense and prolonged neuronal electrical discharges, and failure or inhibition of normal protective mechanisms. Scars from previous insults, such as penetrating head trauma or stroke, can act as epileptogenic foci. Factors such as medical noncompliance, fever, sleep deprivation, convulsant drugs, alcohol withdrawal, and infection can lower the seizure threshold.

SEIZURE CLASSIFICATION

Many attempts have been made to provide a clinically useful classification of seizure types, both to facilitate communication among physicians and to provide a basis for treatment decisions. Formerly, seizures were identified using the terms grand mal, petit mal, and psychomotor. The International League Against Epilepsy[2] recommends dividing seizures into two major groups: *generalized seizures* and *partial seizures* (Table 232-1). When there is inadequate data to categorize the seizure, the seizure is considered *unclassified.*

TABLE 232-1   Classification of Seizures

Generalized seizures (consciousness always lost)
Tonic-clonic seizures (grand mal)
Absence seizures (petit mal)
Myoclonic seizures
Tonic seizures
Clonic seizures
Atonic seizures
Partial (focal) seizures
Simple partial (no alteration of consciousness)
Complex partial (consciousness impaired)
Partial seizures (simple or complex) with secondary generalization
Unclassified (due to inadequate information)

Generalized Seizures

Generalized seizures are thought to be caused by a nearly simultaneous activation of the entire cerebral cortex, perhaps caused by an electrical discharge originating deep in the brain and spreading outward. The attacks begin with abrupt loss of consciousness. This may be the only clinical manifestation (as in absence attacks), or there may be a variety of motor manifestations (myoclonic jerks, tonic posturing, clonic jerking of the body and extremities, etc.).

Generalized tonic-clonic seizures (grand mal) are the most familiar and dramatic of the generalized seizures. They begin with abrupt loss of consciousness; there is usually no warning or aura. In a typical attack, the patient suddenly becomes rigid, trunk and extremities are extended, and the patient falls to the ground. Patients are often apneic during this period and may be deeply cyanotic. They often urinate and may vomit. As the rigid (tonic) phase subsides, there is increasing coarse trembling that evolves into a symmetrical rhythmic (clonic) jerking of the trunk and extremities. As the attack ends, the patient is left flaccid and unconscious, often with deep, rapid breathing. Typical attacks last from 60 to 90 s (occasionally longer). Bystanders generally overestimate the duration of the seizure. Consciousness returns gradually, and postictal confusion and fatigue may persist for several hours or longer.

Absence seizures (petit mal) are very brief, generally lasting only a few seconds. The patients suddenly lose consciousness without losing postural tone. They appear confused, detached, or withdrawn, and current activity ceases. They may stare and have twitching of their eyelids. They do not respond to voice or to other stimulation, exhibit voluntary movements, or lose continence. The attack ceases abruptly, and the patients are able to resume their previous activity with no postictal symptoms. Both the patients and witnesses may be unaware that anything has happened. Classic absence seizures are limited to school-aged children and are often attributed by parents and teachers to daydreaming or not paying attention. The attacks may be very frequent, sometimes occurring 100 or more times daily, and may result in poor school performance. Petit mal attacks may occur alone or in association with other kinds of seizures. They usually resolve as the child matures. Similar attacks in adults are more likely to be minor complex partial seizures and should not be called absence. The distinction is important, because the causes and treatment of the two seizures are quite different.

There are four less-common seizure classifications with which the clinician should be familiar. *Myoclonic seizures* are characterized by brief, shock-like muscular contractions that may be generalized or limited to one or more extremities. *Clonic seizures* involve repetitive clonic jerks without the tonic element. *Tonic seizures* have a prolonged, strained contraction of the body with deviation of the head and eyes. The patient becomes pale, flushed, then cyanotic, and the body may rotate around in position. *Atonic seizures* are characterized by a sudden loss of postural tone in the head, trunk, and/or limbs, which may be associated with a brief loss of consciousness.

Partial (Focal) Seizures

Partial seizures are due to electrical discharges, which begin in a localized region of the cerebral cortex; the discharge may remain localized or may spread to involve nearby cortical regions or the entire cortex. Focal seizures are generally thought to be *secondary* seizures, their occurrence implying a localized structural lesion of the brain.

In *simple partial focal seizures,* the seizure remains localized, and consciousness and mentation are not affected. It is possible to deduce the likely location of the initial cortical discharge from the clinical features at the onset of the attack. Unilateral tonic or clonic movements, often limited to one extremity, suggest a focus in the motor cortex, while tonic deviation of the head and eyes suggests a frontal lobe focus. Sensory hallucinations (e.g., paresthesias or numbness) suggest a discharge in the sensory cortex. Visual symptoms, especially flashing lights or distortions of vision, suggest an occipital focus. Bizarre olfactory or gustatory hallucinations suggest a focus in the medial temporal lobe. Such sensory phenomena, known as *auras,* are often the initial symptoms of attacks that then become more widespread, and that are termed *secondary generalization.*

Complex partial seizures are focal seizures in which consciousness and/or mentation *are* affected. They are often caused by a focal discharge originating in the temporal lobe and are sometimes referred to as *temporal lobe seizures.* Because of their alterations of thinking and behavior, they are occasionally called *psychomotor seizures.* As such seizures may originate from brain regions other than the temporal lobes, and to avoid any confusion with psychiatric illness, the term complex partial seizures is preferred. Often thought to be rare, they are in fact quite common.

Because of their frequently bizarre symptoms, complex partial seizures are commonly misdiagnosed as psychiatric problems. Their symptoms may include automatisms, visceral symptoms, hallucinations, memory disturbances, distorted perception, and affective disorders. Automatisms are typically simple, repetitive, purposeless movements such as lip smacking, fiddling with clothing or buttons, or repeating short phrases. More complex behaviors may occur, but well-organized, purposeful activity is unlikely. Visceral symptoms often consist of a sensation of "butterflies" rising up from the epigastrium. Hallucinations may be olfactory, gustatory, visual, or auditory. There may be complex distortions of visual perception, time, and memory. Affective symptoms may include intense sensations of fear, paranoia, depression, or rarely, elation or ecstasy.

As noted, a focal seizure discharge may spread to involve both hemispheres, mimicking a typical generalized seizure. This is termed *secondary generalization.* For the purpose of classification, diagnosis, and treatment, such attacks are regarded as focal seizures. In some patients, the discharge may spread so rapidly that no focal symptoms are evident, and the correct diagnosis may depend on demonstration of the focal discharge on an EEG recording.

CLINICAL EVALUATION OF SEIZURE PATIENTS

History

When a patient presents after an event, the first step is to determine whether the attack was truly a seizure. A careful history of the details of the attack should be obtained from the patient, if possible, and from any bystanders who actually witnessed the attack. Only a physical description of the attack should be sought as witnesses, even physicians, may mislabel the activity and mistake nonseizure activity as a seizure.

Important avenues of inquiry include preceding aura, abrupt or gradual onset, progression of motor activity, loss of bowel or bladder control, and whether the activity was local or generalized, symmetrical or not. Finally, the duration of the attack and any postictal confusion or lethargy should be sought. The patient should be asked whether he or she has any recollection of the attack.

Next, the clinical context in which the attack occurred should be determined. If the patient is a known epileptic, the baseline seizure pattern should be established. In patients presenting with an attack consistent with their previously documented seizures, the history should be directed toward factors that may have precipitated epileptic activity. Missed doses of antiepileptics or recent alterations in medication, including dosage change or conversion from brand name to generic formulation, may be the inciting element. Other possible factors that might provoke a seizure include sleep deprivation, alcohol withdrawal, infection, electrolyte disturbances, and use or cessation of other drugs.

If there is no previous history of seizures, a more detailed inquiry is needed. Symptoms that might suggest previous unwitnessed or unrecognized seizures, such as blank or staring spells in school, involuntary movements, unexplained injuries, nocturnal tongue biting, and enuresis may be clues to a more longstanding problem. A history of recent or remote head injury should be sought. Persistent, severe, or sudden headache should prompt a search for intracranial pathology. Concurrent pregnancy or recent delivery suggests the possibility of eclampsia. A history of metabolic derangements or electrolyte abnormalities, hypoxia, systemic illness (especially cancer), coagulopathy or anticoagulation, drug ingestion or withdrawal (licit and illicit), and alcohol use may help identify factors that predispose patients to seizures (Table 232-2).

Physical Examination

The general physical examination should be directed toward discovering any injuries, especially to the head or spine, that might have resulted from the seizure. Seizures may cause injuries such as fractures, sprains, and bruises; posterior dislocations of the shoulder can occur and may be overlooked. Tongue lacerations and pulmonary aspiration are frequent sequelae. A search for any systemic illness or derangements (see Table 232-2) that may have caused the attack should be undertaken. Temperature should be noted, and a bedside glucose determination should be obtained.

A directed neurologic examination should be performed with subsequent serial examinations as appropriate. Level of consciousness and mentation should be followed closely. Profound obtundation that improves steadily is likely benign. Progressive deterioration is not an expected sequela of any benign process and requires prompt intervention. Signs of increased intracranial pressure should be sought. Any focal neurologic deficit should be noted. A transient focal deficit (usually unilateral) following a simple or complex focal seizure is referred to as *Todd paralysis,* and should resolve within 48 h. If the patient's symptoms cannot be readily attributed to a benign cause, further urgent evaluation (see below) is warranted.

Differential Diagnosis

Many episodic disturbances of neurologic function may be mistaken for seizures (Table 232-3). A complete review of these conditions is too lengthy for inclusion here, but several of the more important entities should be mentioned. Of these, syncope is clearly of the highest order for consideration.

TABLE 232-2 Causes of Secondary Seizures

Trauma (recent or remote)
Intracranial hemorrhage (subdural, epidural, subarachnoid, intraparenchymal)
Structural abnormalities
    Vascular lesion (aneurysm, arteriovenous malformation)
    Mass lesions (primary or metastatic neoplasms)
    Degenerative diseases
    Congenital abnormalities
Infection (meningitis, encephalitis, abscess)
Metabolic disturbances
    Hypo- or hyperglycemia
    Hypo- or hypernatremia
    Hyperosmolar states
    Uremia
    Hepatic failure
    Hypocalcemia, hypomagnesemia (rare)
Toxins and drugs (many)
    Cocaine, lidocaine
    Antidepressants
    Theophylline
    Alcohol withdrawal
    Drug withdrawal
Eclampsia of pregnancy (may occur up to 8 weeks postpartum)
Hypertensive encephalopathy
Anoxic-ischemic injury (cardiac arrest, severe hypoxemia)

TABLE 232-3 Paroxysmal Disorders: Differential Diagnosis

Seizures
Syncope
Pseudoseizures
Hyperventilation syndrome
Migraines
Movement disorders
Narcolepsy/cataplexy

Syncope usually is attended by premonitory symptoms such as dizziness, diaphoresis, nausea, and "tunnel vision." Patients often are aware that they are going to faint and can clearly describe the onset of the attacks. Cardiac syncope, however, may occur suddenly without any warning. Injury or incontinence may attend syncope; in addition, some patients may experience brief tonic-clonic activity. Recovery is usually rapid, with few or no postictal-like symptoms.

Pseudoseizures, or nonepileptic seizures, are common and may be extremely difficult to distinguish from true seizures in the emergency department. They may occur as well in a patient who has a documented seizure disorder. They are psychogenic, rather than neurogenic, in origin, and are not accompanied by an alteration in brain activity. They are often associated with a conversion disorder, panic disorder, psychosis, impulse control disorder, Munchausen syndrome, or malingering. The patients are usually female, and there may be a history of physical or sexual abuse. The diagnosis of pseudoseizures should be suspected when seizures occur regularly in response to emotional upset or when seizures only occur with witnesses present. The attacks are often very bizarre and highly variable. Patients often are able to protect themselves from noxious stimuli during the attack. Characteristic movements include side-to-side head thrashing, rhythmic pelvic thrusting, and clonic extremity motions that are alternating rather than symmetric. Incontinence and injury are uncommon, and there is usually no postictal confusion. The examiner may be able to provoke or arrest the seizure by suggestion (through injection of saline, for example). Accurate diagnosis of pseudoseizures may require prolonged EEG or video monitoring to demonstrate the presence of normal EEG activity during an attack. The lack of lactic acidosis, as evidenced by the presence of an anion gap acidosis on serum electrolytes drawn within 10 to 15 min of the cessation of seizure-like activity, makes generalized seizures unlikely.

Hyperventilation syndrome is common and is often misdiagnosed as a seizure disorder. A careful history will reveal the gradual onset of the attacks with shortness of breath, anxiety, and perioral numbness. Such attacks may progress to involuntary spasm (especially carpopedal) of the extremities and even loss of consciousness. The episodes often are reproduced easily by asking the patient to hyperventilate.

Movement disorders, such as dystonia, chorea, myoclonic jerks, tremors, or tics, may occur in a variety of neurologic conditions. Consciousness is always preserved during these movements. Though involuntary, the movements can often be temporarily suppressed by the patient.

Migraines may be preceded by an aura similar to that seen in some partial seizures. The most common migraine aura is the scintillating scotoma. Migraines may also be accompanied by focal neurologic symptoms such as homonymous hemianopsia and hemiparesis. However, there is no active movement disorder seen.

Narcolepsy is characterized by brief attacks of uncontrollable daytime sleepiness. Patients are able to feel their attacks coming on and can sometimes control them with judiciously timed naps. Other symptoms of narcolepsy include vivid dreams, often at the onset of sleep or immediately upon awakening, and attacks of sleep paralysis. An associated symptom is *cataplexy,* characterized by a sudden brief loss of postural muscle tone that is often triggered by emotional upset, laughter, or crying. The patient collapses but remains fully conscious; there are no involuntary movements.

Clinical features that help to distinguish seizures from other kinds of mimicking attacks include:

1. Abrupt onset and termination. Although some focal seizures are preceded by auras that last 20 to 30 s (or more), most attacks begin abruptly. Attacks reported to develop over several minutes or longer should be regarded with suspicion. Most seizures last only 1 or 2 min, unless the patient is in status epilepticus.
2. Lack of recall. Except for simple partial seizures, patients usually cannot recall the details of an attack.
3. Movements or behavior during the attack generally are purposeless or inappropriate. Rare exceptions have been described.
4. Most seizures, except for simple absence attacks (petit mal) or simple partial seizures, are followed by a period of postictal confusion and lethargy.

Although a clinical diagnosis of seizures often can be made with a high degree of certainty, there are occasions when the presentation is not convincing. In such cases it is better to admit uncertainty and provide follow-up to determine the exact diagnosis, and not to use the term seizure or begin inappropriate and potentially hazardous treatment. Multiple EEG recordings, prolonged EEG monitoring, and neurologic evaluation may be necessary.

Laboratory Examination

The need for laboratory studies must be assessed on an individual basis. In a patient with a well-documented seizure disorder who has had a single unprovoked seizure, the only test that may be needed is an anticonvulsant level.

In the case of a patient with a first seizure or when the history is unclear, more extensive studies may be helpful. A serum glucose should be obtained, and serum electrolytes, blood urea nitrogen (BUN), creatinine, calcium, magnesium, a pregnancy test, and a toxicology screen may be indicated depending on the clinical context. If the patient's urine is positive for hemoglobin, but there are no red cells in the urine, a CPK should be done to rule out rhabdomyolysis.

If blood is drawn soon after the event, the patient should demonstrate a wide anion gap metabolic (lactic) acidosis following a major seizure, which should correct spontaneously within 1 h.[3] The majority will clear within 30 min and some will clear in as little as 15 min. If the diagnosis is in doubt, serum lactate can be drawn within 15 min of the episode. The blood prolactin level may also be elevated for a brief period (15 to 60 min) immediately following a seizure and may be helpful in distinguishing a true seizure from a pseudoseizure;[4] a normal prolactin level, however, is not helpful.

The presence of anticonvulsant drugs in the blood of a patient from whom no history is available suggests (but does not prove) the presence of a seizure disorder. Anticonvulsant drug levels must be interpreted with caution, as the time the last dose was taken needs to be known to properly interpret levels. The usual therapeutic and toxic levels indicated in laboratory reports are helpful only as rough guides. **The therapeutic level of a drug is that level that provides adequate seizure control without unacceptable side effects.** A phenytoin level of 15 μg/mL may be toxic in a given patient; conversely, a phenytoin level of 24 μg/mL in another may result in excellent seizure control and be well tolerated. A marked change in previously stable drug levels may indicate noncompliance, a change in medication (e.g., from one brand name or generic to another), malabsorption of a drug (as in severe diarrhea or vomiting), or ingestion of a potentiating or competing drug. Minimal amounts of a standard seizure medication most likely indicates a compliance problem.

Radiographic Studies

The issue of neuroimaging following seizures remains controversial. In 1996, the American College of Emergency Physicians (ACEP)[5] in conjunction with a panel of neurologists, neurosurgeons, and neuroradiologists, developed a practice parameter outlining the role and timing of neuroimaging following seizures. In patients with a febrile seizure or seizure typical of their documented epilepsy, radiographic studies usually are not indicated. However, for patients with a first seizure or a change in their established seizure pattern, CT scanning of the head is appropriate to identify a structural lesion. Table 232-4 lists guidelines for emergent CT scanning following a seizure. Noncontrast CT is an appropriate screening tool.[6]

If the patient does not meet the criteria in Table 232-4, has recovered from the seizure, and no metabolic cause for the seizure has been identified, a head CT may be obtained in the outpatient setting in conjunction with close follow-up with a neurologist.

Because many important processes, such as metastatic or primary tumors or vascular anomalies, may not be evident on noncontrast studies, a follow-up enhanced CT or MRI may be arranged. MRI is more sensitive than CT in detecting subtle alterations of brain structure and is often the study of choice in the evaluation of patients with seizures. In patients with an uncomplicated first seizure, it is reasonable to omit the CT scan and obtain an MRI instead. Consultation with a neurologist or radiologist may be helpful in choosing the best approach and avoiding unnecessary examinations.

Other radiographic studies may be indicated in some cases. Radiographs of the cervical spine or neck should be obtained if there is suspicion for head or neck trauma. Chest radiographs may reveal primary or metastatic tumors. There may be evidence of aspiration, although related radiographic findings are usually delayed. Skull x-rays are generally not indicated. Special examinations, such as cerebral angiography, are rarely part of the emergency department evaluation.

ELECTROENCEPHALOGRAPHY

While EEG may be very helpful, it is not readily available in most emergency departments. Emergency EEG can be considered in the evaluation of a patient with persistent, unexplained, altered mental status to rule out nonconvulsive status epilepticus; to evaluate a paroxysmal attack when a seizure is suspected; or in status epilepticus to detect ongoing seizures after paralysis for intubation or induction of general anesthesia. Patients in whom an EEG is warranted emergently should be admitted to the appropriate service and setting, and the EEG should be performed there if possible.

In the outpatient setting, the EEG may be used to distinguish specific epileptic syndromes. The diagnostic yield of EEG recordings can be increased by appropriate patient preparation (especially sleep deprivation) or by activation techniques such as hyperventilation, photic stimulation, and sleep recordings. More elaborate examinations, such as 24-h recordings or video-EEG recordings, may also be used. Consultation with a neurologist ensures that the appropriate studies are chosen.

TREATMENT

Certain general measures should be taken for any seizure patient. A patent airway must be assured and vital signs should be stabilized. Initial

TABLE 232-4   ACEP Recommendations for Obtaining Emergent Neuroimaging Following a Seizure[5]

New focal deficits
Persistent altered mental status
Recent head trauma
First seizure
Coagulopathy/platelet disorder/anticoagulation therapy
HIV-positive/immunosuppression
Meningismus
Alcoholism
Change in seizure pattern

interventions should include an intravenous line, oxygen, pulse oximetry, bedside glucose determination, and a cardiac monitor if warranted. Intubation should be considered for prolonged seizures, persons that require GI decontamination, and patients who may need to be transferred off site. In and of themselves simple seizures do not usually warrant intubation. Standard measures for management of any unconscious patient should be employed (see Chap. 229). The likelihood of trauma should be assessed. Care should be taken to identify and treat any underlying metabolic disorder.

The first objective is to make an accurate diagnosis; only in patients with status epilepticus is it necessary to initiate specific treatment (for seizures) before diagnostic evaluation has been completed.

Specific management is reviewed below for four clinical situations: the patient who is actively seizing; the patient with previous epilepsy who has a seizure; the patient with a first seizure; and status epilepticus.

The Active Seizure

Usually, little is required during the course of an actual seizure other than to protect the patient from injury. Gentle but firm restraint should be used to prevent falls. If possible, the patient should be turned to one side to reduce the risk of aspiration. It is usually not possible to insert a bite block between the teeth without using considerable force and risking damage to teeth. It is usually not necessary or even possible to ventilate a patient effectively during a seizure, but once the attack subsides, ensure a clear airway. Suction and airway adjuncts should be readily available. Seizure activity should be observed to determine if it is focal. **There is no indication for intravenous anticonvulsant medications during the course of an uncomplicated seizure.** Expectant treatment is best. Unnecessary sedation at this point will complicate evaluation and result in a prolonged decrease in level of consciousness. Seizures that fail to abate are considered status epilepticus (see below).

Patients with Previous Seizures

Proper management of a patient with a well-documented seizure disorder who presents after one or more seizures depends on the particular circumstances of the case. Potential precipitants that may lower seizure threshold should be sought. Many such seizures occur because of failure to take anticonvulsant medication as prescribed. Some anticonvulsants have short serum half-lives (Table 232-5), and missing even a single dose may result in a sharp drop in serum levels.

If anticonvulsant levels are very low, supplemental doses may be appropriate, and the patient may be restarted on their regular regimen or require adjustment. Without a loading dose, the patient may not achieve anticonvulsant effects for 2 d to 3 weeks (see Table 232-5). An oral loading dose of phenytoin (usually 18 mg/kg PO, divided into three doses given q2h) will achieve therapeutic serum concentrations

in 2 to 24 h. Alternatively, 10 to 20 mg/kg of intravenous phenytoin (no faster than 25 mg/min) achieves anticonvulsant effects in 1 to 2 h. The dose of fosphenytoin is 10 to 20 mg phenytoin equivalent (PE) at a maximum IV rate of 150 mg per min. Loading doses of carbamazepine are not generally given.

In the known or suspected noncompliant patient, it is common practice for some clinicians to initiate antiepileptic loading (in full or half dosing) prior to, or in lieu of, a serum anticonvulsant level. This has the advantage of potentially shortening the length of stay of the patient in the ED, but could result in toxic levels of anticonvulsant if indeed the patient has some medication in their system. **If anticonvulsant levels are adequate and the patient has had a single attack, specific treatment may not be needed if the pattern and frequency of occurrence falls within the expected range for the patient.** Even well-controlled patients may have occasional breakthrough seizures. Any precipitants that have lowered the seizure threshold should be identified. If there has been a recent change in the frequency or pattern of breakthrough seizures, conditions affecting the seizure threshold should be sought. If none is found, a change in or adjustment of medication may be needed. The patient's primary care physician or neurologist should be made aware of the situation and participate in decision making.

If a medication's maintenance dose is increased, only very small increments should be made, and follow-up within 1 to 3 d should be provided, because even small dose changes may result in dramatic increases in serum levels.

The Patient with a First Seizure

There has been considerable controversy about the appropriate management of a patient who has experienced an apparent first seizure. The decision to begin outpatient treatment with antiepileptics depends on the risk of recurrent seizures weighed against the risk/benefit ratio of anticonvulsant therapy. Previous studies have suggested a risk of recurrence ranging from 23 to 71 percent. The most important predictors of the risk of recurrence were the etiology of the seizure and the results of the EEG.[7] In patients with idiopathic seizures and a normal neurologic examination, the risk of a recurrent seizure within 2 years is 24 percent if the EEG was normal and 48 percent if the EEG is abnormal. In patients with previous neurologic injury or illness, the risk is 48 percent if the EEG was normal, and 65 percent if the EEG is abnormal. Neither family history, age, sex, nor the presence of status epilepticus at the time of the first seizure was a strong predictor of the risk of recurrence. Unfortunately, EEG results are often not available to the emergency physician who must make a treatment decision.

A randomized multicenter clinical trial of 397 patients demonstrated that treatment of first unprovoked seizures appears to reduce the risk of recurrent seizures from 51 to 25 percent during 2 years of follow-up.[8] Some general recommendations can be made based on these studies.[7,8] Patients with secondary seizures due to an identifiable

TABLE 232-5   Properties of Commonly Used Anticonvulsant Drugs

Drug	Oral Dose, mg per d*	Therapeutic Level, µg/mL†	Days to Reach Steady State‡	Serum Half-Life, h
Phenytoin	300–600 divided tid	10–20	5–10	7–42
Carbamazepine	400–1200 divided tid or qid	6–12	2–4	12–17
Phenobarbital	60–200 qd	10–40	14–21	48–144
Primidone	750–2000 divided tid or qid	5–12	4–7	10–21
Valproic acid	15–60 mg/kg per d divided bid or tid	50–150	2–4	12–18

*Average therapeutic dose. Initiation dosing may be different. Daily dose is individualized. Drug-drug interactions may dramatically change daily doses in patients receiving multiple drugs.

†See text for definition of therapeutic and toxic levels.

‡Indicates time required to establish stable serum levels after any change in dose.

neurologic condition should generally be treated, as their risk of recurrence is quite high (48 to 65 percent). In patients with idiopathic seizures, the decision is less clear. Their risk of recurrence may be as low as 24 percent if the EEG is normal. Given the expense, inconvenience, and potential side effects, initiation of treatment in the ED should be made on consultation with a neurologist.

The ideal initial antiepileptic regimen is a single-drug therapy that controls seizures with minimum toxicity. If treatment is initiated, drug selection is based on the type of seizure. For generalized or partial seizures, either phenytoin or carbamazepine would be an appropriate choice for most adults (see above for dosing information). Both drugs are equally efficacious and have similar side effect profiles. Valproic acid, phenobarbital, and primidone may also be used.

Determining Need for Consultation and Admission

ACEP guidelines[6] recommend *neurologic consultation* in the emergency department (or urgently on the floor if the patient is admitted) in certain situations (Table 232-6). Hospital admission recommendations are shown in Table 232-7. Alcohol- or drug-related seizures do not necessarily require admission, although detoxification or withdrawal should be addressed.

Disposition

There are no evidence-based rules for how long a patient must be observed prior to discharge. Some clinicians discharge patients with nontherapeutic anticonvulsant levels after administration of a loading dose of an anticonvulsant if vital signs are normal and the mental status is at baseline. Peak effect can be expected soon after intravenous loading of phenytoin and thus it is preferred. While there is no proscription regarding oral loading of medication, time to peak effect compared to intravenous loading is considerably delayed. If the patient has a subsequent seizure in the next few hours, it will be unclear if an inadequate level remains an issue, or whether the patient is seizing despite adequate levels. Those given oral loading doses should be warned of continued risk for seizures until anticonvulsant effect has been achieved. Such patients should be discharged with a reliable family member or friend, with imperative medical follow-up arranged within a week.

Patients should be instructed to take precautions to minimize the risks for injury from further seizures. Swimming should be avoided. Working with hazardous tools or machines and working at heights should be avoided. The emergency physician should be familiar with driving regulations and reporting requirements, which vary from state to state. Regardless of local laws, it is prudent to advise patients against driving and other hazardous activity until they have stabilized and have been seen in follow-up. The emergency department record should reflect the precise instructions given to the patient.

SPECIAL CONSIDERATIONS

Seizures in the HIV-Positive Patient

Seizures are a common manifestation of CNS disease in patients infected with HIV, although the etiology of seizures in this population dif-

TABLE 232-6   ACEP Guidelines for Obtaining Neurology Consultation[6]

New onset seizures
Focal neurologic examination
Persistent altered mental status
New intracranial lesion
Marked change in seizure pattern
Poorly controlled seizures
Pregnant patient

TABLE 232-7   ACEP Guidelines for Hospital Admission of Patients with New-Onset Seizure[6]

Persistent altered mental status
CNS infection
New focal abnormality
New intracranial lesion
Underlying correctable medical problem
   Significant hypoxia
   Hypoglycemia
   Hyponatremia
   Dysrhythmia
   Significant alcohol withdrawal
Acute head trauma
Status epilepticus
Eclampsia

fers somewhat from immunocompetent patients (Table 232-8). Mass lesions, HIV encephalopathy, and meningitis are seen more frequently.[9] The most common mass lesion is caused by toxoplasmosis, followed by lymphoma. Cryptococcal, bacterial, or aseptic meningitis, or encephalitis due to herpes simplex, varicella zoster, or cytomegalovirus may cause seizures. HIV encephalopathy or AIDS dementia complex is an underrecognized etiology of seizures for HIV-infected patients. Other etiologies to consider are progressive multifocal leukoencephalopathy, CNS tuberculosis, cysticercosis, and neurosyphilis.

While the evaluation of seizures in HIV-positive patients should include a search for metabolic or toxicologic causes, there is also a high incidence of space-occupying lesions. If no space-occupying lesion is identified on noncontrast head CT scan, and there is no evidence of increased intracranial pressure, a lumbar puncture should be performed to exclude meningitis. Finally, if the initial head CT scan is negative or no other explanation for seizures is found, a contrast-enhanced head CT or an MRI should be obtained on an urgent basis, either on the floor if the patient is admitted, or arranged by the primary physician as part of the disposition. Some HIV patients will have no discernible cause for seizures after a thorough evaluation, particularly if the neurologic examination in the interictal period is normal.

Treatment of the first-time seizure in the HIV patient is controversial. Most authorities recommend treatment with phenytoin or phenobarbital because the seizure recurrence rate in this population is high, but there is a 10 percent incidence of hypersensitivity reactions to phenytoin in patients with HIV.

Seizures and Neurocysticercosis

Neurocysticercosis is caused by CNS infection with the larval stage of the tapeworm *Taenia solium*. It is the most common cause of secondary epilepsy in the developing world. Cases in the United States are increasing, with over 1000 cases diagnosed each year, due to immigration from endemic areas, particularly Latin America.[10]

TABLE 232-8   Causes of Seizures in the HIV Patient

Mass lesion
   Toxoplasmosis
   Lymphoma
Meningitis/encephalitis
   Cryptococcal
   Bacterial/aseptic
   Herpes zoster
   Cytomegalovirus
HIV encephalopathy/AIDS dementia complex
Progressive multifocal leukoencephalopathy
CNS tuberculosis
Cysticercosis
Neurosyphilis

Neurocysticercosis exists in several different forms, which vary in their presentation, pathology, and treatment. Ten to twenty percent of patients develop cysticerci in the ventricles and present with obstructive hydrocephalus. These patients are commonly managed by ventriculoperitoneal shunting. Cysticerci in the basilar cisterns may cause arachnoiditis; patients will present with meningeal signs or communicating hydrocephalus. These patients are managed with anti-inflammatory drugs, particularly steroids, and shunting if needed. The use of antiparasitics (praziquantel and albendazole) in neurocysticercosis is controversial, and is dependent upon the number, location, and viability of the parasites within the CNS.[11,12]

The most common form of disease involves parasitic invasion of brain parenchymal tissue. The natural history of parenchymal neurocysticercosis begins with the establishment of cysts by the parasite, which may remain asymptomatic for several years. Host response eventually causes localized edema and inflammation. Over 1 to 2 years, the cyst degenerates and becomes fibrotic, leaving a focal area of scarring and calcification.

Patients with neurocysticercosis may present with headaches or signs of increased intracranial pressure such as nausea or vomiting, altered mental status, or visual changes. Seizures are the most common clinical manifestation of neurocysticercosis and may be focal, focal with secondary generalization, or generalized. They usually develop as a result of the host response. Most patients present with seizures during the inflammatory phase. These seizures are easily controlled with antiepileptics and management is as previously discussed for secondary seizures. Patients who develop scarring and calcifications are more likely to have recurrent seizures and may need to be maintained on antiepileptics such as phenytoin, phenobarbital, and carbamazepine.

In most cases, neuroimaging in neurocysticercosis is not diagnostic. CT scan or MRI may reveal a 1- to 2-cm cystic lesion with thin walls and a 1- to 3-mm mural nodule (the parasite), a localized area of ringlike enhancement with edema, a calcified lesion, or hydrocephalus. Definitive diagnosis relies on a combination of the patient's clinical picture, exposure history, serologic testing, and neuroimaging.

Seizures in Pregnancy

The management of seizures (or control of epilepsy) during pregnancy requires a multidisciplinary approach. Antiepileptic drugs have been associated with neural tube defects, fetal facial dysmorphism, cleft lip and palate, heart defects, and digital defects. Despite the potentially teratogenic effects of anticonvulsants, the risks of uncontrolled seizures to the mother and fetus warrant continuation of seizure medications in the known epileptic during pregnancy.

Reduction of risk to the fetus can be accomplished by single-drug regimens, splitting dosing to avoid high peak levels of drugs, and supplementation of folic acid and vitamin K to reduce the risk of neural tube defects and neonatal hemorrhage. Lack of compliance due to the mother's concern for drug toxicity or nausea and vomiting associated with pregnancy can be a problem.

Initial evaluation of a pregnant woman with a seizure is generally as discussed above, with some important distinctions. An obstetric evaluation is needed to determine gestational age and fetal well-being. Since pregnancy is a hypercoagulable state, stroke as an etiology for the seizure should be considered. Head CT scan may be performed with lead shielding of the abdomen. MRI is also considered safe in pregnancy at this time.

When a woman beyond 20 weeks of gestation develops seizures in the setting of hypertension, edema, and proteinuria, her condition is referred to as *eclampsia*. Attention should be paid to signs and symptoms associated with eclampsia such as headache, blurry vision, confusion, hyperreflexia, and epigastric pain. Eclampsia can occur during the post-partum period, usually over the first few days. Rarely, eclampsia may occur up to 3 weeks post-partum.[13]

The decision to initiate treatment for a first-time seizure in a pregnant female is complex and should involve the obstetrician and neurologist. The emergency physician should not make definitive treatment decisions alone.

Although a healthy fetus should tolerate a single generalized seizure, there are two situations, eclampsia and status epilepticus, which can be life-threatening to both the mother and the fetus. Although not an anticonvulsant per se, magnesium sulfate (4 to 6 g IV followed by 1 to 2 g per h IV drip) has long been used to treat eclampsia with good results. Studies indicate that in eclamptic women, magnesium sulfate compared to diazepam and phenytoin resulted in more than a 50 percent reduction in recurrence of seizures, and a lower incidence of pneumonia, ICU admission, and assisted ventilation.[14,15] The definitive treatment of eclampsia is delivery of the fetus. This topic is discussed in greater detail in Chap. 106.

Status epilepticus treatment should proceed as for any nonpregnant patient, but should include fetal monitoring as well as assistance from an obstetrician, and neonatologist if delivery is a possibility. Lorazepam and diazepam are the two benzodiazepines of choice; phenytoin, fosphenytoin, or phenobarbital may be used as second-line choices (see Figure 232-1 for doses). EEG should be used to confirm seizure cessation. Because both the seizure and the treatments can cause respiratory depression or hypotension, close monitoring is necessary.

Seizures in the Alcohol Abuser

Seizures and alcohol are associated through missed doses of medication; sleep deprivation as an epileptogenic trigger; propensity for head injury; toxic coingestions; electrolyte abnormalities; and alcohol withdrawal seizures.

The *alcohol withdrawal syndrome* involves a spectrum of symptoms that follow reduction or cessation of alcohol. Minor symptoms of alcohol withdrawal, which usually begin 6 to 8 h after cessation of drinking, include tremulousness, nausea, anxiety, tachycardia, hypertension, and insomnia. When autonomic hyperactivity becomes more pronounced, disorientation, visual or tactile hallucinations, paranoid

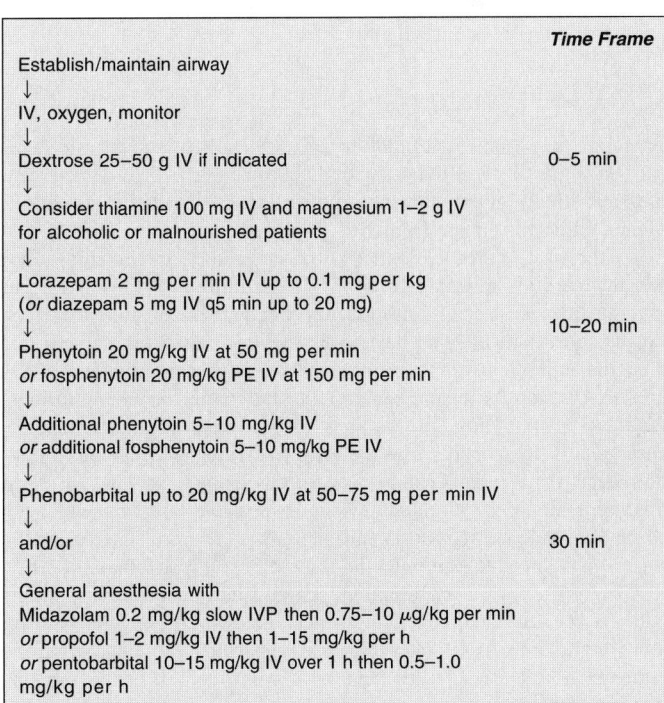

FIG. 232-1. Guidelines for management of status epilepticus. (Adapted from Lowenstein DH, Alldredge BK: Status epilepticus. *New Engl J Med* 338:970, 1998.)

ideation, or delirium may occur, in the symptom complex of *delirium tremens* (DTs). If left untreated, approximately 5 percent of patients who withdraw from alcohol will proceed to DTs, which usually begin 3 to 5 days after cessation of alcohol (see Chap. 295). Prior to the advent of intensive care settings and benzodiazepines, mortality from DTs was as high as 35 percent; currently, with advanced treatment modalities, mortality estimates are from 5 to 15 percent.

Classic *alcohol withdrawal seizures* usually occur within 6 to 48 h after reduction or cessation of alcohol, but may occur up to 1 week later. The seizures are generalized, and the interval EEG is usually normal. There may be several seizures occurring over several hours.

The alcohol-abusing patient with a first seizure should be evaluated and treated as any patient with a first-time seizure (see previous discussion), with additional evaluation for toxic-metabolic abnormalities and intracranial bleeding. Cervical spine precautions may be appropriate. Head CT should be considered when the diagnosis is in doubt, or there are concurrent considerations such as trauma, focality, or persistent depressed sensorium.

Most authorities agree that patients with alcohol withdrawal seizures usually do not require chronic anticonvulsant therapy. Acute or chronic treatment with phenytoin is neither necessary nor effective.[16] Use of benzodiazepines such as valium (5 to 10 mg IV then q5 to 15 min as needed) or lorazepam (2 to 4 mg IV then q5 to 15 min as needed), in doses sufficient to manage withdrawal symptoms will usually afford adequate protection from acute seizures. The exception is withdrawal that is complicated by status epilepticus, which requires prompt treatment. Patients with epilepsy exacerbated by alcohol withdrawal should be managed as any other seizure patient with recurrent seizures.

If the clinical presentation and evaluation are consistent with alcohol withdrawal seizures, and the patient remains stable and seizure-free for several hours, the patient may be discharged and referred for detoxification. Outpatient detoxification with a benzodiazepine regimen is most appropriate for patients with mild to moderate withdrawal symptoms, no significant medical or psychiatric problems, no concurrent drug use, and no history of DTs. Since 90 percent of patients with alcohol withdrawal seizures have one or two seizures within a 6-h window, patients with more than two seizures should be admitted for observation and further investigation.

STATUS EPILEPTICUS

There are an estimated 120,000 to 200,000 cases of status epilepticus per year in the United States, with 55,000 deaths. In 12 to 30 percent of these, status epilepticus is the first epileptic event.[17,18] Estimations of acute mortality range from 1 to 10 percent.

In the past, status epilepticus was defined as either continuous seizure activity for 30 min or more, or two or more seizures that occur without full recovery of consciousness between the attacks. Recently, Lowenstein and colleagues have recommended revising the time frame of status epilepticus to 5 or more mins of seizure activity.[19] It remains unclear how long a seizure can continue before permanent neurologic sequelae ensue. Although this question has never been satisfactorily answered, it does appear that the longer seizures are allowed to continue, the more likely that permanent CNS injury will result. Thus treatment should be initiated as soon as possible in all patients with continuous seizure activity lasting more than 10 min. The longer the seizure is allowed to continue, the more difficult it will be to control.

The diagnosis of status epilepticus is usually obvious in patients with continuous tonic-clonic movements. However, convulsive activity may gradually lessen over time or with partial treatment, giving the impression that the seizures have been controlled. This is known as *nonconvulsive status epilepticus*. The incidence of nonconvulsive status epilepticus is unknown, as the condition is probably underrecognized. Nonconvulsive status epilepticus should be suspected in a critically ill patient with altered mental status of unknown etiology,

especially if the patient has subtle motor activity (nystagmus, or twitching of the face, hands, or feet). An EEG is confirmatory.

Any type of seizure may occur continuously or in rapid succession, fulfilling the criteria for status epilepticus. *Epilepsia partialis continua* is repeated partial seizures without loss of consciousness and often with one's ability to follow simple commands retained. Altered mentation, diminished responsiveness, confusion, amnesia, or dream-like states without motor symptoms suggest continuous absence seizures.

Treatment

The goal of treatment of convulsive status epilepticus and epilepsia partialis continua is seizure control within 30 min of presentation (see Figure 232-1). Morbidity is due to hypoxemia, hyperthermia, circulatory collapse, and eventual neuronal injury.

A brief history and physical examination should be directed toward discovery of the cause of the seizures and to any injury that may have resulted. Any of the causes of seizures (see Table 232-2) may result in status epilepticus; in many patients, no specific etiology is found.

A large-bore IV line should be established and a bedside glucose determination made. Use of an IV fluid without glucose will facilitate administration of anticonvulsant drugs (glucose is not compatible with phenytoin). The patient should be placed on oxygen, a cardiac monitor, and a pulse oximeter.

Endotracheal intubation is recommended when status epilepticus is diagnosed. If a paralytic agent is used to assist with intubation, a short-acting agent such as vecuronium should be used so the physician can monitor ongoing seizure activity.

Initial laboratory evaluation should include blood glucose, a metabolic panel including calcium and magnesium, and if appropriate, a pregnancy test, a toxicology screen, and anticonvulsant levels.

Thiamine (100 mg) and glucose (25 to 50 g) should be given IV if hypoglycemia is suspected or confirmed. There is no benefit to giving additional glucose to normoglycemic patients. Rectal temperature should be monitored, and hyperthermia should be treated with passive cooling. A urinary drainage catheter should be placed to monitor urine output and a nasogastric tube to minimize aspiration.

If ingestion is suspected as the cause of seizures, GI decontamination (as appropriate) should ensue. Emergency lumbar puncture should not be attempted during status epilepticus. If bacterial meningitis is suspected, empiric antibiotic therapy should be started. It should be noted that status epilepticus can induce a brief peripheral leukocytosis as well as a mild CSF pleocytosis. Radiographic studies (such as a CT scan) will usually need to be delayed until the seizures are controlled.

Anticonvulsant Drugs in Status Epilepticus

The drugs most often used in the therapy of status epilepticus are the benzodiazepines (diazepam or lorazepam), phenytoin or fosphenytoin, and phenobarbital (see Figure 232-1).

Benzodiazepines are used in patients with continuous or very frequent seizures to temporarily control the seizures until more specific agents can be given. **Intravenous lorazepam** (4 to 8 mg) and IV diazepam (10 to 20 mg) have equal efficacy in controlling status epilepticus.[20] Although diazepam has a slightly faster onset, (2 min vs. 3 min), lorazepam has a significantly longer duration of action (12 to 24 h vs. 15 to 30 min), is associated with fewer seizure recurrences, and **is thus considered the initial agent of choice.** Lorazepam is also more effective than phenytoin or phenobarbital as the initial drug.[21] Respiratory depression and hypotension may occur when benzodiazepines are used, especially in young children and in patients who have taken alcohol, barbiturates, narcotics, or other sedatives. Although diazepam enters the brain readily, it is redistributed quickly to fatty tissues, so serum concentrations fall rapidly. Therefore a longer-acting agent such as phenytoin should follow diazepam.

Phenytoin is the most important drug used in the management of status epilepticus. It may be given immediately after a benzodiazepine or may be used as primary therapy in patients whose seizures are less frequent. The recommended loading dose is 18 to 20 mg/kg IV; note that doses well in excess of the usual 1000 mg are required for many adults. A smaller loading dose (15 mg/kg) may be used in the elderly, but the loading dose is not reduced in patients with renal or hepatic disease. Due to myocardial depression effects, phenytoin should be infused at a rate of 25 mg per min. Phenytoin should not be mixed with any glucose-containing intravenous fluid and should not be given intramuscularly due to erratic absorption. The drug is contraindicated in the presence of second- or third-degree AV block. Adverse effects include significant infusion-site reactions, hypotension, and cardiac dysrhythmias, so continuous cardiac monitoring is needed. If side effects develop, the infusion should be stopped and may be restarted at a lower rate when the side effects have resolved; in some cases, patients are unable to tolerate the drug.

Fosphenytoin is a water-soluble prodrug of phenytoin that is rapidly converted to phenytoin in the plasma. In status epilepticus, fosphenytoin has similar time of onset, effectiveness, and cardiac effects as phenytoin. Its advantages include fewer infusion-site reactions due to the lack of propylene glycol and ethanol as the diluents. Secondly, fosphenytoin may be infused at a faster rate. Fosphenytoin dosing is expressed as "phenytoin equivalents (PE)" to prevent confusion. The loading dose is 15 to 20 PE per kg, which can be infused at 100 to 150 mg PE per min. Unlike phenytoin, fosphenytoin can be given intramuscularly, which is useful if the patient is not in status epilepticus. The only apparent drawback is the cost. Fosphenytoin can cost 10 to 60 times more than phenytoin.

Phenobarbital (up to 20 mg/kg IV) can be used as a third-line drug in patients who are unable to tolerate phenytoin or in patients whose seizures are not controlled despite full loading doses of benzodiazepines and phenytoin. However, patients who do not respond to lorazepam and phenytoin are unlikely to respond to phenobarbital.[22] Because of very slow elimination, large doses of phenobarbital may result in prolonged obtundation. Respiratory depression and hypotension are common, especially at higher doses or when diazepam or lorazepam is also given.

In some patients, seizure control is not obtained with these regimens and further treatment is needed.

Refractory Status Epilepticus

The standard regimens of benzodiazepines, phenytoin, and phenobarbital suffice to control status epilepticus within 30 min of presentation in most patients. In some (generally patients with structural lesions, anoxic injuries, metabolic encephalopathy, or CNS infections), seizures continue for more than 60 min despite first- and second-line treatment. In one study, 31 percent of patients with status epilepticus developed refractory status epilepticus (RSE).[22]

Various approaches to refractory status epilepticus have been advocated, including intravenous infusions of midazolam, propofol, or barbiturates to induce anesthesia (see Figure 232-1).[23–26] These modalities are best used in an intensive care setting, as advanced respiratory and cardiovascular support, as well as continuous EEG and invasive hemodynamic monitoring, may be needed. Consultation from an anesthesiologist and neurologist should be obtained.

Anesthesia may be induced to treat RSE by administering infusions of midazolam or propofol for 12 to 24 h. General anesthesia may also be obtained with intravenous barbiturates such as thiopental and pentobarbital. Midazolam and propofol have the advantage over barbiturates of having a short half-life and rapid clearance, allowing for earlier extubation and earlier clinical assessment; midazolam also causes less hypotension.[22–24] Intravenous valproate has also been advocated as a treatment modality.[26]

Neuromuscular blocking agents (usually pancuronium or vecuronium) are sometimes helpful. These drugs will abolish tonic-clonic movements and may facilitate ventilation and other measures, but they have no effect on abnormal neuronal activity. EEG monitoring is necessary to assess the effectiveness of anticonvulsant therapy when neuromuscular blockers are utilized.

REFERENCES

1. Hauser WA, Hesdorffer DC: *Epilepsy Frequency, Causes and Consequences.* New York, Demos, 1990.
2. Commission on Classification and Terminology of the International League against Epilepsy: Proposal for revised clinical and electroencephalographic classification of epileptic seizures. *Epilepsia* 22:489, 1981.
3. Orringer LE, Eustace JC, Wunsch CD, et al: Natural history of lactic acidosis after grand mal seizures; A model for the study of an anion gap acidosis not associated with hyperkalemia. *New Engl J Med* 297:796, 1977.
4. Rao ML, Stefan H, Bauer BJ: Epileptic but not psychogenic seizures are accompanied by simultaneous elevation of serum pituitary hormones and cortisol levels. *Neuroendocrinology* 49:33, 1989.
5. American College of Emergency Physicians, American Academy of Neurology, American Association of Neurologic Surgeons, and American Society of Neurology: Practice parameter: Neuroimaging in the emergency patient presenting with seizure (summary statement). *Ann Emerg Med* 28:114, 1996.
6. American College of Emergency Physicians: Clinical policy for the initial approach to patients presenting with a chief complaint of seizure who are not in status epilepticus. *Ann Emerg Med* 29:706, 1997.
7. Berg AT, Shinnar S: The risk of seizure recurrence following a first unprovoked seizure: A quantitative review. *Neurology* 41:965, 1991.
8. First Seizure Trial Group: A randomized clinical trial on the efficacy of antiepileptic drugs in reducing the risk of relapse after a first unprovoked tonic-clonic seizure. *Neurology* 43:478, 1993.
9. Pesola GR, Westfal RE: New-onset generalized seizures in patients with AIDS presenting to an emergency department. *Acad Emerg Med* 5:905, 1998.
10. Modi G, Modi M, Martinus I, et al: New-onset seizures associated with HIV infection. *Neurology* 55:1558, 2000.
11. White AC: Neurocysticercosis: Updates on epidemiology, pathogenesis, diagnosis, and management. *Annu Rev Med* 51:187, 2000.
12. Garcia HH, Evans CA, Nash TE, et al: Current consensus guidelines for treatment of neurocysticercosis. *Clin Microb Rev* 15:747, 2002.
13. Mattar F, Sibai BM: Eclampsia VIII. Risk factors for maternal morbidity. *Am J Obstet Gynecol* 182:307, 2000.
14. The Eclampsia Trial Collaborative Group: Which anticonvulsant for women with eclampsia? Evidence from the Collaborative Eclampsia Trial. *Lancet* 345:1455, 1995.
15. Witlin AG, Sibai BM: Magnesium sulfate therapy in preeclampsia and eclampsia. *Obstet Gynecol* 92:883, 1998.
16. Rathlev NK, D'Onofrio G, Fish SS, et al: The lack of efficacy of phenytoin in the prevention of alcohol-related seizures. *Ann Emerg Med* 23:513, 1994.
17. Lowenstein DH, Alldredge BK: Status epilepticus. *New Engl J Med* 338:970, 1998.
18. Hauser WA: Status epilepticus: Epidemiologic considerations. *Neurology* 40(Suppl 2):9, 1990.
19. Lowenstein DH, Bleck T, Macdonald RL: It's time to revise the definition of status epilepticus. *Epilepsia* 40:120, 1999.
20. Leppik IE, Derivan AT, Homan RW, et al: Double-blind study of lorazepam and diazepam in status epilepticus. *JAMA* 249:1452, 1983.
21. Treiman DM, Meyers PD, Walton NY, et al: A comparison of four treatments for generalized convulsive status epilepticus. *New Engl J Med* 339:792, 1998.
22. Mayer SA, Claassen J, Lokin J, et al: Refractory status epilepticus, frequency, risk factors, and impact on outcome. *Arch Neurol* 59:205, 2002.
23. Parent JM, Lowenstein DH: Treatment of refractory generalized status epilepticus with continuous infusion of midazolam. *Neurology* 44:1837, 1994.
24. Stecker MM, Kramer TH, Raps EC, et al: Treatment of refractory status epilepticus with propofol: Clinical and pharmacokinetic findings. *Epilepsia* 39:18, 1998.
25. Prasad A, Worrall BB, Bertram EH, et al: Propofol and midazolam in the treatment of refractory status epilepticus. *Epilepsia* 42:380, 2001.
26. Sinha S, Naritoku DK: Intravenous valproate is well tolerated in unstable patients with status epilepticus. *Neurology* 55:722, 2000.

ACUTE PERIPHERAL NEUROLOGIC LESIONS
Michael M. Wang

When confronted with a patient with neurologic complaints, one should first localize the problem anatomically based on the history and physical examination. An initial distinction that should be made is whether the pathologic process involves the peripheral or central nervous system. Sometimes, the distinction is not clear.

HALLMARKS OF PERIPHERAL NERVOUS SYSTEM DISORDERS

The peripheral nervous system serves sensory, motor, and autonomic functions. The patient with a peripheral nerve problem thus may have symptoms reflecting disorder of any or a combination of these functions. Sensory symptoms may include numbness, tingling, dysesthesias, pain, or ataxia caused by proprioceptive dysfunction. Motor symptoms are predominantly weakness. Autonomic disability can include orthostatic symptoms, bowel or bladder dysfunction, gastroparesis, or sexual dysfunction.

On physical examination, the most important finding in a peripheral nerve process is reduction or absence of reflexes. The sensory examination, which includes tests of proprioception, vibratory sensation, and pain and temperature sensibility, is also often abnormal. When the motor system is involved, wasting and fasciculations may be seen in addition to weakness. Autonomic dysfunction can cause hair loss, anhidrosis, pupillary dysfunction, orthostatic hypotension, and tachy- and bradyarrhythmias.

Similar symptoms and signs may be seen in disorders of the central nervous system (CNS). Weakness and numbness can be seen in both peripheral and central disorders. Hyporeflexia sometimes occurs with acute central lesions, but hyperreflexia and spasticity invariably develop later. Peripheral nervous system disorders, like CNS diseases, can affect bulbar structures, resulting in diplopia, dysarthria, or dysphagia. Nevertheless, CNS disorders frequently have other features that are not seen in peripheral diseases. For example, aphasia, apraxia, and visual loss are hallmarks of cortical disease. Signs on examination, such as hyperreflexia and clear lateralization of weakness, should prompt evaluation for CNS disorders.

LOCALIZATION OF NEUROLOGIC DISEASE

Once a peripheral disorder has been established, it is necessary to determine which part of the peripheral nervous system is involved. A localized process, such as numbness and tingling of the fifth and half of the fourth digits of one hand, strongly suggests a focal lesion (ulnar nerve). The lesion may involve the nervous system at a number of locations: the nerve, plexus, or root. Basic knowledge or the aid of an anatomy text or neurology handbook should be sufficient to accurately localize focal lesions of these types. Figure 233-1 shows a schematized view of the peripheral nervous system and illustrates the signs associated with disease of specific parts of the neuromuscular system. Most muscle-related processes result in weakness of large proximal muscles, and patients may have a difficult time lifting their arms over their heads or arising from a seated position. Pain and tenderness of the muscles occur commonly in muscle disorders (although usually these are not predominant symptoms and if not accompanied by weakness rarely indicate myopathy), and creatine kinase (CK) is usually elevated, sometimes dramatically. Diseases that affect other components of the peripheral nervous system seldom cause muscle tenderness and elevations in CK. Neuromuscular junction processes also affect large proximal muscles and frequently affect the bulbar musculature, resulting in pupillary dysfunction, diplopia, dysarthria, or dysphagia. Unlike muscle and neuromuscular junction disorders,

neuropathies frequently affect both the motor and sensory systems; because these diseases most severely affect longer nerves, distal power is reduced most dramatically. Polyradiculopathy, which frequently follows a progressive and stepwise course, usually results in electrical pain sensations, assorted sensory abnormalities, areflexia, and weakness.

Once localization of the peripheral problem is accomplished, efforts should be made to pinpoint the etiology. Specific historical points that always should be addressed include the time course of the illness, diurnal fluctuations (if any), other systemic symptoms or conditions, a review of medications, and antecedent illnesses. A serum chemistry and metabolic profile and CK are useful blood tests in the ED. Further testing is usually deferred in the acute setting, but may include a variety of blood tests, nerve conduction studies, electromyography, lumbar puncture, and nerve/muscle biopsy.

TREATMENT: GENERAL CONSIDERATIONS

Management of peripheral nervous system disorders depends on the specific diagnosis. However, a few general remarks about care should be made. When a peripheral disorder is suspected or diagnosed in the ED, one should arrange for neurologic consultation for further specific treatments. Many neuromuscular disorders are difficult to diagnose and require complex treatments such as immunomodulation with intravenous immunoglobulin, immunosuppressive drugs, and plasmapheresis.

Careful supportive care is mandatory for severe, life-threatening neuromuscular diseases and should begin in the ED. Patients with the potential for respiratory failure, aspiration, and cardiac dysrhythmias should be monitored appropriately. Where the presentation warrants, baseline forced vital capacity or negative inspiratory pressure should be measured in the ED to assess whether there is need for imminent respiratory support or admission to an intensive care unit.

With few exceptions, admission to the hospital is generally required for acute peripheral neurologic conditions in which there is danger of respiratory or autonomic compromise, or in cases of debilitating or rapidly progressing weakness. Specific indications for hospital admission are discussed below for individual diseases.

SPECIFIC NEUROMUSCULAR DISORDERS

The number of neuromuscular disorders is extensive and cannot be discussed fully in this text; consequently, this section covers the most common and most important disorders to recognize and the diseases that have acute therapies available.

Myopathies

Polymyositis is an inflammatory myopathy that affects individuals older than age 30 years, with a slight propensity for women. Usually, patients present with chronic complaints of proximal symmetric weakness, although the disorder occasionally presents subacutely. Some patients will have dysphagia, and a few will progress to respiratory failure. There may be muscle pain and tenderness. On examination, there is reduced proximal strength, which may best be tested by asking the patient to arise from a chair with his or her arms crossed or to lift a light object over his or her head. There is no sensory loss, and unless weakness is profound, reflexes should be intact. If deep tendon reflexes are diminished, neuropathy should be considered. Laboratory testing may reveal an elevated erythrocyte sedimentation rate (ESR), leukocytosis, and CK. The differential diagnosis includes Lambert–Eaton myasthenic syndrome, inclusion body myositis, toxic myopathies, dermatomyositis, endocrinopathies, and an assortment of muscular dystrophies.

Patients with newly suspected polymyositis should be assessed for potential respiratory compromise and aspiration risk in the ED. Ad-

FIG. 233-1. Schematic of the neuromuscular system and typical findings with disease of each component of the system. DRG = dorsal root ganglion; NMJ = neuromuscular junction.

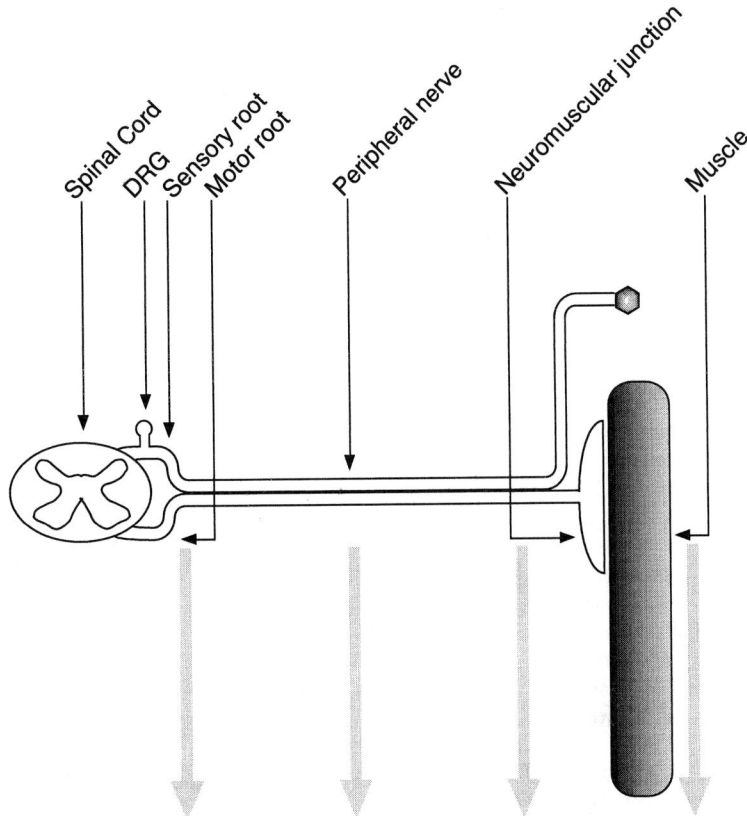

mission is usually warranted in newly suspected cases. Further diagnostic studies likely pursued under the direction or consultative advice of a neurologist typically include electromyography (EMG) and muscle biopsy. Long-term treatment consists of immunosuppressive agents such as steroids and methotrexate.

Dermatomyositis, unlike polymyositis, can affect children and, like polymyositis, affects mostly women. The clinical manifestations of dermatomyositis are similar to those of polymyositis, except for the usual appearance of a violaceous rash typically over the face and hands. The neurologic examination shows a myopathic distribution of weakness without sensory or reflex abnormalities in most cases. The laboratory findings are also similar, with an elevated ESR and CK in most instances. Despite similarities in the clinical presentation compared with polymyositis, the pathology and pathophysiology of the two disorders are quite distinct.[1] Treatment is aimed at immunosuppression.

OTHER MYOPATHIES   A large number of substances, including environmental (alcohol), occupational, and pharmacologic agents [steroids, cholesterol-lowering drugs, AZT (azidothymidine)], can cause myopathy. Table 233-1 summarizes several important medication-induced myopathies. Although usually chronic, some present subacutely and cause a predominantly proximal pattern of weakness with normal sensation and preserved tendon reflexes (except with severe weakness). CK is usually elevated. Viral myositis causes an acute myopathy, occasionally involving the heart, and is usually associated with a febrile illness, myalgia, and elevated CK levels. An important cause of both acute and chronic myositis is HIV infection (see below). Trichinosis should be suspected in patients with myalgias, bulbar and proximal muscle weakness, facial edema, and eosinophilia; symptoms occur within days of ingesting undercooked pork. Definitive diagnosis is made on visualization of parasitic cysts on muscle biopsy.

TABLE 233-1 Some Drugs That Cause Myopathy

Chloroquine	ε-Amino-caproic acid	Thiazides
Emetine	D-Penicillamine	Amphotericin
Corticosteroids	Chlorpromazine	Amphetamines
Amiodarone	Zidovudine	Toluene
Adriamycin	Colchicine	Ethanol
Procainamide	Vincristine	Phencyclidine
Perhexilene	Clofibrate	
Imipramine	Lovastatin	

Source: Kuncl RW, Wiggins WW: Toxic myopathies. *Neurol Clin* 6:593, 1988.

Disorders of the Neuromuscular Junction

Myasthenia gravis is discussed in Chap. 234.

BOTULISM   Ingestion of foods contaminated with *Clostridium botu-linum* toxin causes botulism, an acute disease marked by weakness and gastrointestinal slowing. Adults whose disease is caused not by bacterial infestation but by ingestion of botulinum toxin may report exposure to foods such as home-canned vegetables in the preceding 1 to 2 days. Unlike adults, infants, whose guts are not colonized fully, are susceptible to infection with viable bacteria that elaborate toxin. Parents of infants should be questioned for possible ingestion of *C. botulinum* spores, commonly transmitted by feeding honey. Infants may present with poor sucking. Botulism caused by infection through a wound is rare. With botulism, mentation is normal, but there may be bulbar weakness. The extraocular movements are sometimes abnormal, and an important diagnostic clue is the absence of the pupillary light reflex, which distinguishes this disorder from myasthenia gravis. There is proximal limb weakness, sensation is intact, and reflexes generally are normal except in the case of severe weakness.

Botulism is treated with antibiotics (infants only) and immune serum (adults and infants), which is obtained from the Centers for Disease Control and Prevention (Atlanta). The serum, derived from immunized horses, is first used in skin tests to exclude hypersensitivity. The antiserum is generally available at quarantine sites at major U.S. airports. Patients should be admitted to the hospital for treatment, monitoring, and testing. In cases where the diagnosis is not clear, treatment with immune serum, which has potential morbidity, should be withheld until electrodiagnostic studies are performed. Nerve conduction studies show an incremental response on repetitive nerve stimulation.

Acute Peripheral Neuropathies

Guillain-Barré syndrome (GBS) affects individuals of all ages and is the most common form of acute generalized neuropathy. Frequently, patients report an antecedent viral illness, especially gastroenteritis. There is an association between acute *Campylobacter jejuni* infection and development of GBS. Sometimes the patient first notices numbness and tingling of the lower extremities. This is followed by weakness of thighs, legs, and then arms. There are numerous variants of the syndrome, and some patients may experience facial weakness, which can mimic Bell palsy, ophthalmoparesis, severe shooting pains, or ataxia caused by proprioceptive difficulty. In most, but not all, cases, GBS is caused by an autoimmune attack on myelinated motor nerves.

In classic cases, there is symmetric extremity weakness, more pronounced in the legs. Despite subjective sensory disturbances, sensation on examination is usually normal. The hallmark finding in GBS is the lack of deep tendon reflexes. In variant cases, there may be ophthalmoplegia and pupillary disturbances. Occasionally, there may be facial weakness involving the forehead. Autonomic instability, marked by brady- and tachycardia or blood pressure fluctuation, may be apparent in a few cases. Where ophthalmoparesis is present, there may be a marked limb ataxia, and the patient may not be able to walk or stand despite reasonable strength. In all forms of the disease, there is a chance of developing respiratory failure and lethal autonomic fluctuations.

Lumbar puncture should be performed when acute disease is suspected. The classic laboratory finding in GBS is a high cerebrospinal fluid (CSF) protein with normal glucose and cell count. However, the protein will not be elevated until after the first week of symptoms and may not be elevated even after 1 week. Although many patients will have a modest CSF pleocytosis (up to 100 lymphocytes/μL), the presence of cells in the CSF should prompt consideration of other systemic diseases sometimes associated with GBS, such as HIV infection, lupus, and lymphoma.

Lyme disease can present with a clinical picture similar to GBS and would be suggested by a CSF pleocytosis in combination with a history of tick bites or the presence of CSF Lyme antibodies. Carcinomatous meningitis also can present with similar symptoms but will be evident with malignant cells in the CSF or extremely high protein or low glucose levels. *Tick paralysis* mimics GBS, and all patients with suspected GBS should be examined thoroughly for ticks. Acute intermittent porphyria (discussed below) and spinal cord compression should be considered in the differential diagnosis; the presence of upper motor neuron signs and bowel and bladder incontinence would suggest the latter.

Patients with GBS should be admitted to the hospital for monitoring and treatment. When forced vital capacity (FVC) is under 1 L, the patient should be intubated. No specific treatment is warranted in the ED; treatment is composed of plasma exchange or intravenous immunoglobulin, which both have been shown in controlled studies to shorten the duration of the illness.[2]

Acute intermittent porphyria is a rare autosomal dominant condition in which patients suddenly experience the symptom triad of weakness, psychosis, and abdominal pain. Seizures can occur. The three occasionally occur together, but in many cases occur independently. The disease activates acutely in flares that are usually precipitated by medications such as barbiturates, phenytoin, sulfonamides, and estrogen.

The major neurologic findings are weakness and diminished reflexes, particularly of the lower extremities, which are the direct consequence of an acute peripheral neuropathy. There may be sensory findings such as diminished pain and temperature sensation, although these signs are usually outweighed by motor deficits. In the acute setting, basic ancillary laboratory studies may be normal. Further testing reveals elevation in urine δ-aminolevulinic acid and porphobilinogen.

The key management issue is recognition of the disorder and identification and discontinuation of the offending drug. Care also must be taken to avoid overtreatment of symptoms such as pain and seizures with medications that may exacerbate the illness. Other treatment modalities include supportive care, glucose infusions to prevent heme biosynthesis, vitamin B_6, and hematin (4 mg/kg IV daily for 1 to 2 weeks). The differential diagnosis includes other disorders that cause pain and lower extremity weakness. Spinal cord compression causes back pain, which frequently radiates around the trunk and is followed by lower extremity weakness, but reflexes in this situation are brisk with upgoing toes (positive Babinski reflex). An aortic aneurysm or dissection also can cause abdominal pain and lower extremity weakness if spinal arteries are occluded by the expanding aneurysm.

Focal Neuropathies

The most common entrapment neuropathies are discussed below. For the most part, the nerve damage is reversible, and referral to the appropriate specialist for relief on entrapment is necessary.

Carpal tunnel syndrome (CTS) is the most commonly seen entrapment neuropathy. Patients describe intermittent pain and/or numbness in the thumb and first two fingers, prominently at night. Symptoms frequently awaken the patient from sleep, occur in both hands independently, and may be poorly localized (i.e., numbness is often described going up to the elbow). The symptoms usually can be reproduced by compression of the nerve over the carpal tunnel or by tapping on the nerve, although these signs are neither sensitive nor specific. Occasionally, these symptoms are mistaken for cerebrovascular disease until a history of bilateral, repeated, and stereotypical nocturnal occurrence is obtained. When symptoms become long-standing and severe, weakness of the thenar musculature develops. Wrist splints worn at night are useful in the conservative management of CTS. Patients should be referred to a hand surgeon as an outpatient for further diagnostics and management. A carpal tunnel release may be performed in patients who fail to respond to conservative management.

Ulnar nerve entrapment, usually occurring at the elbow, produces numbness in the fifth digit and medial half of the fourth finger, but symptoms are frequently poorly localized. Weakness and wasting of the hypothenar muscles occur very late in the course. The patient should be referred to a specialist for electrodiagnostic confirmation because occasionally, C8 radiculopathy can mimic this common condition. Severe cases are treated surgically with ulnar nerve transposition.

Entrapment of the deep peroneal nerve at the fibular head can cause footdrop and numbness of the web between the great and second toes. This condition occurs in the setting of injury to the leg, rapid weight loss, or habitual crossing of the legs. Peroneal entrapment should be confirmed by EMG to be differentiated from lumbar root disease or motor neuron disease. Almost all cases are treated conservatively and improve without specific therapy.

Meralgia paresthetica is entrapment of the lateral cutaneous nerve of the thigh. The diagnosis is often overlooked in the ED, being mistaken for a hip-related orthopedic disorder. Patients describe numbness and dysesthesias of the lateral aspect of the upper leg. This occurs after weight loss and notably following pelvic surgery or obstetric procedures where the legs are abducted and flexed for a prolonged period of time. Tricyclic antidepressants (TCA) are useful in the management of the dysesthesias associated with meralgia paresthetica. The condition resolves without sequelae and requires no specific therapy.

Mononeuritis multiplex is a syndrome of multiple nerve dysfunctions caused by a vasculitis. Patients experience multiple deficits in a stepwise fashion, usually involving both sides of the body. For example, a patient may experience wristdrop on the right, followed by footdrop on the left, and then footdrop on the opposite side a few weeks later. This condition requires urgent referral to a neurologist to determine the etiology and initiate treatment, usually in collaboration with a rheumatologist. Frequently this disorder is caused by a systemic vasculitis, and a thorough serologic examination and nerve biopsy are required to establish specific treatment plans. The condition must be differentiated from multiple compression neuropathies and from multifocal motor neuropathy.

Bell palsy should be viewed as a diagnosis of exclusion. It is the most common cause of acute facial paralysis but is similar to other processes that are important to recognize. Patients with Bell palsy complain of sudden facial weakness, difficulty with articulation, problems keeping an eye closed, or inability to keep food in the mouth on one side. Because the seventh cranial nerve also serves other functions, the patient may have variable degrees of dry eye, metallic taste of the mouth, and facial pain, commonly around the ear. The examination is notable for one-sided weakness of the face involving the forehead. There may be decreased sensation along the external acoustic meatus (Hitselberger sign). Other cranial nerves are normal. Diminished reflexes suggest a different diagnosis.

Several alternative diagnoses should be considered. Stroke can lead to sudden facial weakness that involves only the lower face but also leads to neurologic involvement below the neck or other cranial neuropathies. Lyme disease and GBS can cause facial paralysis, as discussed elsewhere in this chapter. In patients with cancer, facial weakness may herald the metastatic spread of malignancy. The ear should be inspected carefully to rule out ulcerations caused by cranial herpeszoster activation (Ramsay Hunt syndrome), which should be treated with oral acyclovir. Facial paralysis also can be seen in sarcoidosis, collagen vascular disease, and polio. All patients with facial weakness

should be screened for HIV risk factors, since seventh nerve palsy can occur at the time of seroconversion.

The treatment of Bell palsy with steroids is controversial. Most neurologists argue in favor of a short course of prednisone in individuals with low risk for complications from corticosteroids. The recommended dose is 50 mg PO per d for 7 days. More recent studies[3] suggest that steroids in combination with acyclovir (200 mg PO five times a day for 10 days) leads to better outcomes. If the patient is seen more than a week after paresis began, steroids generally are not given.

Eye care must be meticulous to avoid corneal abrasions. Patients are instructed to tape the affected eye so that the palpebral fissure is narrowed to prevent drying of the cornea. Patients should apply ocular lubricants and patch the eye before sleeping.

Lyme disease affects individuals exposed to the tick-borne pathogen *Borrelia burgdorferi.* Although its neurologic manifestations are multiple, one of the most common sites of involvement is the peripheral nervous system. A comprehensive discussion of Lyme disease can be found in Chap. 145. Neurologic complications ensue the weeks following initial manifestations such as fatigue and arthralgias. A common neurologic sign is seventh nerve palsy, which should not be confused with Bell palsy. Lyme disease affects the peripheral nerves and the nerve roots. The patient may describe the acute or subacute progression of weakness and sensory loss, sometimes associated with radicular pain. On examination, the patient will have one of several signs. Unless there is encephalitis (a rare complication of Lyme disease), mental status will be normal. Apart from seventh nerve involvement, there may be weakness in the limbs, and if there is localized radicular inflammation, there will be a patchy myotomal pattern. Similarly, depending on the regional involvement of the disease, selected deep tendon reflexes will be diminished. Laboratory features suggestive of Lyme disease include serum and CSF Lyme antibodies. A CSF pleocytosis and increased protein with a normal glucose is the most common abnormality. When the diagnosis is made with confidence and other entities such as syphilis, carcinomatous meningitis, and sarcoidosis excluded, a minimum 3-week course of intravenous antibiotics, either ceftriaxone or doxycycline, is given.

Plexopathies

Brachial neuritis is an acute condition that tends to affect younger individuals, with a slight male predominance. Patients report excruciating shoulder, back, or arm pain followed by weakness of the arm or shoulder girdle. In a third of cases, it is bilateral. The cause is idiopathic, but cases have been reported following immunizations or viral infections. On examination, the patient has weakness in various distributions of the brachial plexus. The upper trunk is the preferred site of involvement, affecting strength of proximal arm and shoulder musculature. The anterior interosseous nerve is also affected preferentially, causing inability to form a pincer with the index finger and thumb. Sensory abnormalities are found but are not as profound as the motor dysfunction. Reflexes are diminished in the affected limb.

The differential diagnosis includes multiple cervical radiculopathies, Pancoast tumors, and neoplastic or inflammatory infiltration of the plexus. The diagnosis is usually clear, because a history of pain followed by weakness that plateaus in a week or two makes other diagnoses unlikely. A chest radiograph should be performed to look for mass lesions involving the brachial plexus. CSF analysis is required if there is a suspicion of other etiologies. Spine imaging and EMG may be performed outside the ED setting.

The management of brachial plexitis is conservative, and no therapies have been shown to affect the course of the illness. The prognosis is good, with most patients experiencing full recovery in months. If careful follow-up with a neurologist can be arranged and other causes or symptoms are excluded, admission to the hospital is elective.

Lumbar plexopathy, or diabetic amyotrophy, occurs in diabetic patients and presents with back pain followed by weakness. Patients

TABLE 233-2   A Framework to Approach Chronic Neuropathies

| Etiologies | PREDOMINANT SYMPTOMS | | | |
	Sensory	Motor	Sensory and Motor	Autonomic
Infectious	HIV Leprosy	Lyme	Syphilis Lyme	Chagas disease *(American trypanosomiasis)*
Medications	Cisplatin	Dapsone	INH	Vincristine
Toxins	Arsenic Alcohol	Lead	Alcohol	
Nutritional	Beriberi		B_{12} deficiency	
Metabolic	Diabetes		Uremia	Diabetes
Neoplastic	Paraneoplastic ganglionopathy		Paraneoplastic polyneuropathy	
Hereditary	Hereditary sensory neuropathy		Charcot-Marie-Tooth	Amyloidosis Riley-Day
Inflammatory	Sjögren disease	CIDP	Mononeuritis multiplex	
Paraproteinemias, dysproteinemias	Anti-MAG sensory neuropathy	Anti-G_{M1} motor neuropathy	Waldenstrom macroglobulinemia	Amyloidosis

Note: Examples of a variety of causes of chronic neuropathy. This table is meant to illustrate the major classes of etiologies and the usefulness of classifying neuropathy by symptom complex. Syndromes of pure symptomatology (e.g., pure motor neuropathy) are rare but suggest a small number of potential causes. Note that the table is incomplete and does not necessarily list the most common neuropathies in each class. Many neuropathies present with distinct symptoms from those described above. Para- and dysproteinemias are assumed, but have not been proven, to be causative etiologies of nerve dysfunction.

report the acute onset of ipsilateral back pain, followed within days by progressive leg weakness. Sensory findings are absent. The examination reveals decreased leg power in a variety of patterns reflecting impairment of plexus function with relatively symmetric sensation. There may be muscle wasting in affected limbs in long-standing disease. Deep tendon reflexes may be diminished on the affected side. Bowel and bladder functions are not affected.

Laboratory studies are generally not helpful in the emergency setting. In the ED, routine plain films of the lumbar spine are useful to screen for spine compression from degenerative or neoplastic disease, and MRI is usually ultimately needed. The differential diagnosis also includes the cauda equina and conus medullaris syndromes and compression from arteriovenous malformations. Computed tomography (CT) scanning of the abdomen is useful to exclude aortic aneurysm and psoas muscle masses, which also lead to asymmetric lower extremity weakness. Patients with acute weakness from lumbar plexopathy should be admitted to the hospital for testing and rehabilitation to definitely determine the cause of weakness.

HIV-Associated Peripheral Neurologic Disease

HIV infection, its complications, and its pharmacologic treatments are associated with a number of peripheral neurologic disorders. Fortunately, the most common of these, HIV neuropathy and drug-induced neuropathy, are chronic processes that do not cause sudden disability or symptoms. HIV-infected patients also have a higher rate of mononeuritis multiplex and an inflammatory myopathy resembling polymyositis.

Occasionally, patients will complain of weakness that progresses over the course of days. Patients in the early stages of HIV infection have greater susceptibility to GBS. The presentation is similar to that of the non–HIV-infected patient, except that a CSF pleocytosis is seen commonly. Such patients should be treated as discussed earlier.

CYTOMEGALOVIRUS RADICULITIS   In the latter stages of AIDS, patients may suffer from an acute radiculitis caused by cytomegalovirus (CMV) infection. These patients almost always have

evidence of CMV infection elsewhere in the body and may have ongoing CMV retinitis. Patients become acutely weak, with primarily lower extremity involvement, and may have variable degrees of bowel and bladder dysfunction. The examination shows primarily lower extremity weakness and hyporeflexia, with decreased sensation in the lower extremities and groin. Rectal tone may be impaired. Lumbar puncture reveals a pleocytosis with predominantly polymorphonuclear cells and modestly increased protein; viral DNA is detected by polymerase chain reaction in most patients and is highly specific. MRI of the lumbosacral spine demonstrates swelling and clumping of the cauda equina. Imaging of these patients is mandatory to exclude mass lesions of the lower spine or nerve roots. The treatment of CMV radiculitis is intravenous ganciclovir, started at 5 mg/kg every 12 h for 3 to 6 weeks, which may be initiated prior to definitive diagnosis.

CHRONIC CONDITIONS

Neuropathies can also be chronic or subacute associated with an underlying medical disorder. A detailed discussion of neuropathies associated with underlying medical illness is worthy of an entire text. The interested reader is referred to standard neurology texts.[4] Table 233-2 shows the expected presentations for some diseases associated with peripheral neuropathies.

REFERENCES

1. Dalakas M: Polymyositis, dermatomyositis, and inclusion body myositis. *New Engl J Med* 325:1487, 1991.
2. van der Meche FGA, Schmitz PIM, and the Dutch Guillain-Barré Study Group: A randomized trial comparing intravenous immune globulin and plasma exchange in Guillain-Barré syndrome. *New Engl J Med* 326:1123, 1992.
3. Adour KK, Ruboyianes JM, Von Doersten PG, et al: Bell's palsy treatment with acyclovir and prednisone compared with prednisone alone: A double-blind, randomized, controlled trial. *Ann Otol Rhinol Laryngol* 105:371, 1996.
4. Victor M, Adams RD, Ropper AH: *Principles of Neurology*, 7th ed. New York: McGraw-Hill, 2001.

CHRONIC NEUROLOGIC DISORDERS
Edward P. Sloan

AMYOTROPHIC LATERAL SCLEROSIS

Amyotrophic lateral sclerosis (ALS), often referred to as Lou Gehrig disease, causes rapidly progressive muscle atrophy and weakness resulting from the degeneration of both upper and lower motor neurons. ALS causes varying degrees of spasticity, hyperreflexia, and muscle paralysis, eventually leading to pulmonary complications and the need for mechanical ventilatory support. Because there is no curative therapy for this disease, symptomatic management is directed at preventing pulmonary infections and forestalling terminal respiratory failure.

Epidemiology

There are two forms of ALS, the most common of which is sporadic ALS (sALS). The worldwide annual incidence rate for sALS is 0.6 to 2.0 per 100,000, and the prevalence is 4 to 6 per 100,000.[1] In the United States, 5600 new cases are diagnosed each year, causing an estimated prevalence of 30,000 U.S. ALS patients. The mean age of onset for sALS is 56 years, with a slightly higher incidence in men. Familial ALS (fALS) is genetically present in only 149 patients from 53 families worldwide (including a rare juvenile form), and there is an endemic focus of ALS in the western Pacific, especially Guam. The incidence of fALS is only 10 percent of that of sALS, with a 1.5-fold higher disease rate for men. In fALS patients, 20 percent have a change in the superoxide dismutase (SOD1) gene, which suggests the ability to test for the disease prior to symptom onset. There are no race differences with either of the forms of ALS. There is a higher prevalence of ALS in individuals older than age 60 years, and the annual worldwide ALS mortality rate is 1 per 100,000.

Pathophysiology

The most likely cause of ALS is a genetic superoxide dismutase dysfunction causing an abnormal response to a variety of environmental insults. Current theories of cell death in ALS include excitotoxins such as glutamate, free radicals, heavy metals, viral agents, and autoimmune reactions to tissues such as spinal cord collagen. Programmed cell death as a result of apoptosis is also being studied as a possible cell death etiology.

Gross central nervous system (CNS) pathology includes frontal cortical atrophy, degeneration of the corticospinal and spinocerebellar tracts, a reduction in large cervical and lumbar motor neurons, and cranial nerve nuclei degeneration. Both motor and sensory peripheral nerves are noted to undergo axonal degeneration and segmental demyelination, including motor end plate and axon terminal involvement.

Clinical Presentation

Upper motor neuron dysfunction causes limb spasticity, hyperreflexia (including Babinski sign and a brisk jaw-jerk reflex), and emotional lability. Lower-motor-neuron dysfunction causes limb muscle weakness, atrophy, cramps, fasciculations, dysarthria, dysphagia, and difficulty in mastication. At the time of initial presentation, asymmetric extremity cramping, fatigue, weakness, muscle fasciculations, and atrophy can be seen, especially in the upper extremities.[2] Patients with fALS more often present with isolated lower-extremity weakness and atrophy at the time of diagnosis. Despite these profound motor findings, sensory and cognitive function is usually spared. Regardless of the initial symptoms, widespread motor and respiratory dysfunction

progresses within weeks to months. Significant extremity atrophy occurs, as well as fasciculations, hyperreflexia, foot drop, and claw deformity of the hand. Patients also may develop monotonous speech caused by tongue atrophy, despite the relative sparing of facial and eye movements. Some patients eventually diagnosed as having ALS present initially with cervical or back pain consistent with an acute compressive radiculopathy. Despite successful operative intervention, these patients develop significant muscle wasting consistent with motor neuron dysfunction shortly after the procedure.[3]

Progressive respiratory muscle weakness initially causes exertional dyspnea and eventual dyspnea at rest. Dementia and parkinsonism also may occur in up to 15 percent of patients, especially those with fALS. Other cognitive problems such as apathy, poor attention and motivation, and altered social skills may be noted in ALS patients.

Clinical Diagnosis

The clinical diagnosis of ALS is suggested when there are signs of both upper and lower motor neuron dysfunction without other CNS dysfunction. ALS-like symptoms can be seen with other systemic illnesses such as diabetes, dysproteinemia, thyroid and parathyroid dysfunction, vitamin B_{12} deficiency, heavy metal toxicity, and vasculitis, as well as CNS and spinal cord tumors. The diagnosis of ALS also requires that other inflammatory neuropathies such as myasthenia gravis be excluded. The World Federation of Neurology developed the El Escorial criteria for the diagnosis of ALS.[4]

Electromyography (EMG) demonstrates decreased muscle action potential amplitude and decremental responses to repetitive nerve stimulation, making it the most useful diagnostic test. Nerve conduction velocity studies, magnetic resonance imaging (MRI), spinal fluid analysis, and neuromuscular biopsies are also useful diagnostic studies.

Disease Management

Therapy is designed to enhance muscle function, especially those that support breathing, swallowing, and speech, in order to avoid malnutrition, recurrent aspiration, or choking. Riluzole is a drug that delays disease progression by preventing cell toxicity through modulation of the excitotoxin glutamate.[5] It is most useful in patients with a clear diagnosis of ALS whose symptoms have been present for less than 5 years, with a forced vital capacity (FVC) >60 percent of predicted, without tracheostomy. An FVC below 25 mL/kg or a 50 percent FVC decrease increases the risk of aspiration pneumonia and respiratory failure. Optimizing pulmonary function, including the eventual use of long-term assisted ventilation, is an important part of enhancing the quality of life as diaphragm weakness progresses.[6]

Emergency Diagnosis and Management

Patients with ALS most often will not present to the ED undiagnosed unless there is extremely rapid disease progression or a long period without medical care. Emergency management usually is required for acute respiratory failure, aspiration pneumonia, choking episodes, or trauma related to extremity weakness. **Blood gas determination does not reliably predict impending respiratory failure,** because mild hypoxia and hypercarbia may exist throughout the disease course. Although no acute therapies exist for worsening ALS, therapies that optimize pulmonary function (e.g., nebulized medications, steroids, antibiotics, assisted ventilation, intubation) are indicated. Because the need for long-term ventilatory assistance rarely reverses, it is important to establish the patient's preference regarding intubation via a living will or the power of attorney for health care. Hospitalization is indicated with impending respiratory failure, pneumonia, the inability to control secretions, or a worsening overall status that requires social service intervention for long-term placement.

Long-Term Outcome

ALS causes a consistent, predictable deterioration in motor function, leading to tracheostomy in most patients within 2 to 4 years. ALS leads to complete respiratory failure in 80 percent and complete limb paralysis in 45 percent of patients. Although early diagnosis and aggressive management have increased the median survival of sALS, 50 percent of patients die within 3 years of diagnosis, and only 10 percent survive beyond 10 years. The use of riluzole in the ALS patients described above increased 12-month survival from 58 to 74 percent, with the greatest survival improvement seen in those with extensive bulbar symptoms (as opposed to those with primary limb symptoms). Patients diagnosed prior to age 40 years may survive up to four times than those diagnosed after age 60 years, especially if swallowing and airway control are spared. Survival in fALS is shorter, with a median survival of 2 years and a 23 percent 5-year survival rate. Long-term outcome is currently being followed in a longitudinal European survey termed the European ALS Health Profile Study.

MYASTHENIA GRAVIS

Myasthenia gravis (MG) is an autoimmune disease characterized by muscle weakness and fatigue, seen especially with repetitive use of voluntary muscles. Acetylcholine receptor (AChR) antibodies impair receptor function at the neuromuscular junction, causing muscle weakness, most often in proximal muscles. This weakness is generally relieved by rest, and requires long-term immunotherapy. Because the mechanism and optimal therapies for MG are well understood, much of the morbidity and mortality associated with the disease can be minimized. The diagnosis of cholinergic and myasthenic crises, and the aggressive management of respiratory complications associated with a myasthenic crisis are the most important issues for MG patients and emergency physicians.

Epidemiology

The incidence of MG is 0.4 per 100,000, and the prevalence is estimated to be 10 to 15 per 100,000.[7] There are approximately 25,000 cases in the United States and 100 million cases worldwide. The most common age of onset for females is in the second and third decades. In males, the peak onset age is in the seventh and eighth decades. Although females were believed to have up to fourfold higher disease prevalence, as the population has aged, the higher prevalence has shifted to males. There is a slightly higher prevalence in the African American population. Although family members of patients with MG are much more likely to develop MG, the disease is not transmitted by traditional Mendelian inheritance.

Pathophysiology

MG is the most well understood of the human autoimmune disorders. In the normal neuromuscular junction, acetylcholine (ACh) release by the nerve fiber causes a localized end-plate potential that leads to muscle fiber contraction. In MG there is a marked decrease in the number and function of the muscle fiber AChR, despite normal nerve anatomy and function. Failure to respond to ACh stimulation causes decreased muscle fiber potential amplitudes, causing some fibers to fail to function and leading to decreased muscle strength. The autoimmune etiology of MG is demonstrated by the consistent presence of AChR autoantibodies in nearly all MG patients. These antibodies react to the AChR, can be transferred and cause the disease, and can be induced by immunization with AChR proteins. Similarly, disease severity can be correlated with AChR autoantibody levels. These autoantibodies cause accelerated AChR degradation, as well as receptor dysfunction and blockade, through complement activation.

The etiology of the pathologic autoimmune response is believed to be caused by dysfunction of either the thymus gland or the immune response to exogenous infectious antigens. The thymus is found to be abnormal in 75 percent of MG patients, most often with hyperplasia or the presence of a thymoma. Thymectomy resolves or improves the symptoms in most MG patients, especially those with a thymoma. It is likely that the AChR autoantibodies arise following exposure to similar antigens, such as those caused by herpes simplex virus or bacteria infection, causing a pathologic attack on the AChR proteins.

Clinical Presentation

The symptoms of MG can mimic the symptoms seen in many other chronic neurologic disorders, such that some call it "the great imitator." Prior to the establishment of a definitive diagnosis, most MG patients have general weakness, especially of the proximal extremities muscle groups, neck extensors, and facial or bulbar muscles. Although ptosis and diplopia are the most common presenting symptoms, limb weakness and oropharyngeal symptoms such as dysphagia and dysarthria also can be seen initially or occur over time. These symptoms can fluctuate throughout the day, usually worsening as the day progresses or with prolonged muscle group use, such as with prolonged reading or prolonged chewing during a meal. The maximum extent of this weakness usually becomes manifest within the first year after the time of diagnosis. Despite the presence of profound muscle weakness, there usually is no deficit in sensory, reflex, or cerebellar functioning. MG in elderly patients can be misdiagnosed as ischemic stroke, especially when new-onset facial weakness is seen.[8]

Although the weakness seen in MG patients is focal and mild to moderate in severity, in rare instances undiagnosed MG patients may present with extreme weakness in the muscles of respiration, resulting in respiratory failure. This life-threatening situation, termed *myasthenic crisis,* can be seen prior to MG diagnosis or as a result of inadequate drug therapy or drug tolerance. The complications associated with the respiratory failure seen in acute myasthenic crisis are the leading cause of death in MG patients, but are fortunately rare, given the understanding of the disease and the available therapies.

Clinical Diagnosis

The diagnosis of MG should be considered in any patient who complains specifically of ocular disturbances or proximal limb muscle weakness not associated with systemic causes of generalized fatigue. Involvement of the facial muscles, muscles of mastication, and those that facilitate swallowing all may suggest MG, as well as the observations that the symptoms worsen as the day progresses and that rest alleviates the symptoms. Other causes of symptoms that suggest MG include congenital MG, Lambert-Eaton syndrome (seen with small cell lung tumors), drug-induced myasthenia (e.g., penicillamine, procainamide, quinines, aminoglycosides), botulism, thyroid disorders, and other causes of ocular disorders, such as progressive external ophthalmoplegia or intracranial mass lesions.

The diagnosis of MG is established through the administration of edrophonium chloride (an acetylcholinesterase inhibitor), EMG, and serologic testing for AChR antibodies. In the presence of abnormal neuromuscular transmission, edrophonium or neostigmine is expected to improve muscle strength in objectively weak limb, ocular, and pharyngeal muscles. Because these drugs can actually cause profound weakness in the presence of other disorders that impair neuromuscular transmission, one must be ready to provide ventilatory support or intubation as a complication of pharmacologic testing. EMG testing with repetitive nerve stimulation demonstrates a rapid reduction in the size of the muscle action potential, a finding that correlates with the clinical observation of enhanced weakness with prolonged or repetitive muscle use. AChR antibody testing is the most specific test for MG, but up to 15 percent of MG patients may have undetectable AChR antibody titers, especially those who have isolated ocular disturbances. Other useful tests in the diagnosis of MG include mediastinum thymus imaging, laboratory testing for lupus, thyroid disorders, and tuberculosis, as well as pulmonary function testing.

Disease Management

The management of MG includes the administration of acetylcholinesterase inhibitors, thymectomy, chronic immune suppression, and acute immune modulation using plasma exchange or intravenous immunoglobulin, when indicated. MG patients, especially those with a thymoma, show a favorable response to thymectomy.[9] Most show improvement with oral corticosteroids, although some patients initially become weaker prior to symptom improvement when high-dose steroids are administered. The use of azathioprine with oral prednisolone provides for fewer treatment failures and complications, longer remissions, and the need for a lower overall steroid dose.[10] Severe MG symptoms, such as those that would require hospital admission, might require the use of intravenous immunoglobulins or a combination of high-dose steroids and plasma exchange.

Muscle weakness usually does not return to normal even with the use of these immunomodulators, and there can be great temporal variability in the nature and amount of MG patient muscle weakness. Variability in the amount of muscle weakness can be seen in response to asthma exacerbations, infections, menstruation, pregnancy, emotional stress, hot weather, and other disorders that alter the response to medication, such as pulmonary, renal, and gastrointestinal disease.

Emergency Diagnosis and Management

Several drugs used in the ED are known to affect neuromuscular function, and caution must be exercised with their use in MG patients (Table 234-1). If a drug is absolutely necessary, such as steroids for status asthmaticus, equipment for emergency endotracheal intubation should be immediately available because respiratory failure can develop rapidly. MG patients being treated in the ED for other conditions should receive their usual dose of cholinergic inhibitors such as pyridostigmine. The suggested dose is often 60 to 90 mg PO every 4 h. If a dose has been missed, the next dose is usually doubled. If the patient cannot take oral medications or is intubated, one-thirtieth the oral dose of pyridostigmine is given by slow intravenous infusion. Neurology consultation generally is needed to determine the optimal intravenous dose, rate of infusion, and timing of repeat doses.

The most significant ED complication of MG is respiratory failure, which is usually precipitated by infection, surgery, or the rapid tapering of immunosuppressive drugs. Although intubation should be considered in patients with a low FVC or in the presence of abnormal blood gas analysis, this decision is made primarily on clinical grounds. Because of the increased sensitivity of MG patients to neuromuscular junction inhibitors, **if avoidable, patients preferably should not receive either depolarizing or nondepolarizing paralytic agents** in preparation for intubation. Patients with myasthenia are extremely sensitive to these agents, and the paralytic effects can be expected to persist at least two to three times longer than in normal patients. Short-acting agents such as etomidate, fentanyl, or propofol can be used instead of these agents, and can be used in smaller doses.[11] If paralytic agents are necessary, some authors recommend using one-half the dose of these agents, although there are no clinical studies supporting this recommendation.

Myasthenic crisis, which occurs because of disease exacerbation or inadequate drug therapy, must be distinguished from cholinergic crisis, which is caused by excessive cholinergic drug therapy. This differentiation can be made in the emergency department by the use of the Tensilon test. Edrophonium chloride (Tensilon) is used for this purpose because of its rapid onset (30 s) and the short effects duration (5 to 10 min). A positive result, one that suggests that the symptoms are caused by a myasthenia exacerbation, is characterized by the resolution of muscle weakness within a few minutes. To ensure that the patient does not react adversely to the edrophonium test (as a result of excessive baseline cholinergic effects), 1 to 2 mg IV should first be injected. The occurrence of muscle fasciculations, respiratory depression, or cholinergic symptoms within a few minutes of this test dose of edrophonium suggests that the baseline muscle weakness is related to a cholinergic crisis and that further edrophonium administration is contraindicated. If there is no evidence of adverse cholinergic effects, up to 10 mg of edrophonium can then be administered in order to demonstrate benefit in the face of a presumed myasthenic crisis.

If muscle weakness is improved with the edrophonium, the Tensilon test is considered positive, indicating a myasthenic crisis. Neostigmine can then be given parenterally or PO. Intramuscular or subcutaneous neostigmine is given in 0.5 to 2 mg doses, with clinical effectiveness by 30 min, lasting for up to 4 h. Alternatively, 15 mg neostigmine tablets can be given, each having a clinical effect comparable with that of a 0.5 mg parenteral neostigmine injection.

TABLE 234-1 Drugs That Should Be Used With Caution in Myasthenia Gravis

Steroids	Kanamycin*	Amitriptyline	Lidocaine	**Others**
ACTH*	Gentamicin	Droperidol	Dilantin	Amantadine
Methylprednisolone*	Tobramycin	Haloperidol	Trimethaphan	Diphenhydramine
Prednisone*	Dihydrostreptomycin*	Imipramine	**Local Anesthetic**	Emetine
Anticonvulsants	Amikacin	Paraldehyde	Lidocaine*	Diuretics
Dilantin	Polymyxin A	Trichlorethanol	Procaine*	Muscle relaxants
Ethosuximide	Polymyxin B			CNS depressants
Trimethadione	Bacitracin	**Antirheumatics**	**Analgesics**	Respiratory depressants
Paraldehyde	Sulfonamides	D-Penicillamine	Narcotics	Sedatives
Magnesium sulfate	Viomycin	Colchicine	Morphine	Procaine*
Barbiturates	Colistin	Chloroquine	Dilaudid	Tranquilizers
Antimalarials	Colistimethate*		Codeine	
Chloroquine*	Lincomycin	**Cardiovascular**	Pantopon	**Neuromuscular blocking**
Quinine*	Clindamycin	Quinidine*	Meperidine	**agents**
IV Fluids	Tetracycline	Procainamide*		Tubocurarine
Na lactate solution	Oxytetracycline	Beta blockers	**Endocrine**	Pancuronium
Antibiotics	Rolitetracycline	Propranolol	Thyroid replacement*	Gallamine
Aminoglycosides		Oxprenolol		Dimethyl tubocurarine
Neomycin*	**Psychotropics**	Practolol	**Eyedrops**	Succinylcholine
Streptomycin*	Chlorpromazine*	Pindolol	Timolol*	Decamethonium
	Lithium carbonate*	Sotalol	Ecothiopate	

*Case reports implicate drugs in exacerbations of myasthenia gravis.
Source: This table is a modified version of the table from Adams SL, Matthews J, Grammer LC: Drugs that may exacerbate myasthenia gravis. *Ann Emerg Med* 13:532, 1984, with permission.

In children, the total edrophonium intravenous dose is 0.15 mg/kg, not to exceed 10 mg. To test hypersensitivity in children, an initial intravenous edrophonium dose one-tenth that of the total dose can be given. For children weighing up to 75 lb (34 kg), a test dose of 1 mg is appropriate, and a total dose of 5 mg can be used in 1-mg increments. In infants, or when intravenous access is not available in children up to 75 lb, an intramuscular edrophonium test dose of 0.5 to 2 mg can be given.

Caution should be exercised when administering edrophonium to patients with cardiac disease, because it may cause bradycardia, atrioventricular (AV) block, atrial fibrillation, and cardiac arrest. Although atropine will counteract these muscarinic effects of edrophonium, it is ineffective in reversing the nicotinic effects, such as skeletal muscle paralysis, that can occur in the face of a cholinergic crisis.

Acute respiratory failure can result from either acute myasthenic or acute cholinergic crisis. Cholinergic crisis patients who fail the Tensilon test may require immediate intubation and management of excessive secretions and acute bronchospasm. When determining final disposition, the emergency physician also must consider other complications of muscle weakness in MG patients, such as impaired swallowing, aspiration pneumonia, dehydration, and decubitus ulcers.

MULTIPLE SCLEROSIS

Multiple sclerosis (MS) is a neurologic disorder that causes variable motor, sensory, visual, and cerebellar dysfunction as a result of multifocal areas of CNS myelin destruction. Paresthesias, gait difficulty, extremity weakness, poor coordination, and visual disturbances occur most often with a relapsing and remitting clinical course. Despite the lack of a definitive cure, immunosuppression and immunomodulation provide adequate symptomatic relief in the majority of MS patients, such that most sustain only mild to moderate lifetime morbidity without a reduction in overall life expectancy.

Epidemiology

Three clinical courses are noted in patients with MS. Up to 80 percent of MS patients have a relapsing and remitting course, with relapses lasting weeks to months. The remaining patients have either a relapsing and progressive course or a chronically progressive clinical course, the latter of which is more common with advanced age. The incidence of MS is 3.2 to 8 per 100,000, and the prevalence may be greater than 200 per 100,000.[12] In the United States, the peak age of onset for either sex is during the third decade of life. Females are two to three times more likely to contract MS, and they do so at a younger age than do men. Males, however, are more likely to have a chronically progressive disease course from the time of symptom onset. MS is two times more likely in whites than in blacks, and is rare in Asian populations. There is a geographic MS distribution, with temperate climates of economically developed countries experiencing a higher prevalence. Communities of northern Europe and the United States have prevalence rates of up to 173 per 100,000 in the white population. In the northern hemisphere there is a diminishing MS prevalence gradient that runs from north to south, while the opposite is true in the southern hemisphere. In general, 5 to 10 percent of MS patients will sustain a malignant course, and 20 to 35 percent will have a very benign disease course. Although pregnancy reduces the MS relapse rate by 50 percent, relapse risk increases up to sixfold during the postpartum period.

Pathophysiology

Although the etiology of MS is unknown, it is best described as an inflammatory disorder resulting in scattered neuron demyelination. The most frequently postulated theory for MS is a genetic predisposition triggered by a virus (such as herpes or human T-cell leukemia virus type I), heavy metals, or other environmental toxins that induce an immune-mediated neuronal inflammation and demyelinization.[13] MS causes a dysfunction in oligodendrocytes such that the axonal myelin sheaths are damaged, slowing nerve impulse conduction. These scattered cerebral and spinal plaques cause gliosis primarily in the white matter, with relative axon sparing.

These plaques occur in multiple areas, including the cerebrum, brainstem, spinal cord, and cranial nerves. The brain may have variable amounts of atrophy and ventricular dilatation. Nerves in the corticospinal tracts, posterior columns, and spinothalamic tracts will cause upper motor neuron, proprioception/vibration, and pain/temperature dysfunction, respectively. Cranial nerve dysfunction most often causes optic neuritis, as well as facial motor and sensory deficits.

Clinical Presentation

MS is suggested when a young person presents multiple times with neurologic symptoms that suggest different areas of pathology, often with resolution of the prior symptoms. Most MS patients will have more severe lower extremities symptoms as compared with the upper extremities. For example, a young person might complain of an inability to walk on a street without tripping over a curb or a sense of clumsiness with physical activity.

The physical examination may reveal decreased strength, increased tone, hyperreflexia, clonus, Babinski reflex, a decrease in both vibration sense and joint proprioception, as well as a reduction in pain and temperature sensation. Although sensory and motor deficits are present initially in only one-third of patients, all patients will experience these findings at some point during the disease course. Patients describe these deficits as a heaviness, weakness, stiffness, or extremity numbness. *Lhermitte sign* is commonly experienced during the course of MS and is described as an electric shock sensation, a vibration, or a pain radiating down the back and often into the arms or legs resulting from the flexion of the neck. Rarely, patients with established MS may present with complete or near-complete loss of motor function, termed *acute transverse myelitis*. Cerebellar lesions may cause a kinetic tremor, dysmetria, or truncal ataxia. Vertigo may be seen as a result of brainstem MS lesions.

Optic neuritis, which usually causes acute or subacute central vision loss, may be the initial sign of MS in up to 30 percent of patients. The loss, which occurs over several days and is usually unilateral, often is preceded by retrobulbar pain or extraocular muscle pain that may be reproduced with periorbital palpation. Optic neuritis may cause an afferent pupillary defect, or Marcus Gunn pupil. Although funduscopy is most often normal in the acute setting, the optic disk may be noted to have pallor due to axonal loss and gliosis. Although the ocular pain most often resolves over several days, it may take up to months for the visual disturbances to resolve. Most MS patients at some time experience blurred vision, compromised color vision, and/or eye pain due to optic neuritis. In fact, visual acuity may worsen due to increases in body temperature, known as *Uhthoff phenomenon.* Nystagmus and diplopia are often seen in MS, as is internuclear ophthalmoplegia. Internuclear ophthalmoplegia usually causes abnormal adduction bilaterally and horizontal nystagmus. When bilateral internuclear ophthalmoplegia is seen acutely in an otherwise healthy young person, it is highly suggestive of MS.

Dysautonomias can cause vesicourethral dysfunction, resulting in urinary retention, urgency, frequency, detrusor-external sphincter dyssynergia, and stress or overflow incontinence. Gastrointestinal dysfunction can cause constipation and fecal incontinence in MS patients. Sexual dysfunction, especially in males, may be the presenting MS symptom and is correlated with other types of urologic dysfunction. Cognitive and emotional changes, including dementia, decreased motivation, depression, and bipolar mood disorders occur in most MS patients. Cerebral MS, which affects only 5 percent of MS patients, can cause a severe, disabling decrease in intellect as well as focal seizures.

MS symptoms often will worsen with increases in body temperatures, as seen with exercise, fever, or even hot baths. Most initial MS attacks or exacerbations will progress over several days, peaking at about 1 week, with resolution over several weeks to months. Complete recovery from an acute attack or exacerbation occurs more commonly early in the course of the disease.

Clinical Diagnosis

The diagnosis of MS is clinically based, relying heavily on the neurologic history and physical examination. The diagnosis is suggested when a patient has either two or more prolonged or worsening episodes of neurologic dysfunction that suggest distinct white matter pathology or spinal cord dysfunction in two or more distinct locations.[14] Optic, cerebrospinal fluid (CSF), and neuroimaging findings, as well as typical features such as dysautonomias all suggest the diagnosis of MS. Symptoms that mimic MS are seen with systemic lupus erythematosus, Lyme disease, neurosyphilis, HIV disease, and Guillain-Barré syndrome, which is associated with peripheral nervous system demyelination.

Nearly all MS patients will demonstrate some CNS pathology by MRI. T2-weighted scans demonstrate either discrete lesions in the supratentorial white matter or homogeneous borders surrounding the ventricles. Although computed tomography (CT) is not as sensitive as MRI, it may show cerebral atrophy, ventricular enlargement, and low-density focal lesions in the cerebrum, brainstem, or optic nerves. CSF protein and gamma-globulin concentrations are elevated in many MS patients. A slight increase in CSF white blood cells (up to $25/\mu L$) is also seen, most of which are T lymphocytes. Evoked potentials demonstrate scattered slowing in CNS pathway conduction in the majority of MS patients.

Disease Management

The long-term management of MS is directed at slowing the progression of the disease and providing symptomatic relief during exacerbations. In order to modify the frequency and severity of MS exacerbations, immunomodulation with glucocorticoids, interferon-β, and glatiramer, as well as immunosuppression with mitoxantrone are recommended for subsets of MS patients.[15] High-dose methylprednisolone therapy shortens the duration of exacerbations, and may be most effective early in the disease course.[16] Diets high in fruits, vegetables, and grains may protect against the development of MS symptoms. Because relapses are less common during pregnancy, the use of the pregnancy hormone estriol has preliminarily been shown to be beneficial in female MS patients.[17]

Emergency Diagnosis and Management

Emergency therapy is directed at minimizing the complications of acute MS exacerbations, such as respiratory distress, optic neuritis, pulmonary infections, severe constipation, and worsening muscle weakness. Airway management with endotracheal intubation should use rapid sequence induction and the Sellick maneuver because of an increased aspiration risk as a consequence of decreased gastric motility. Also, because many MS patients have labile autonomic nervous system function, they are at greater risk of developing hypotension in the settings of rapid sequence induction, emergent intubation, and surgical anesthesia. Seizures can be treated with the standard benzodiazepine and phenytoin drugs. Fever must be reduced in order to minimize the weakness caused by elevated temperature. Urinary tract infections and pyelonephritis must be excluded during any MS exacerbation, especially in patients with residual urine volumes greater than 100 mL. A postvoid residual urine determination, a urine culture, and antibiotic therapy all should be provided whenever there is clinical evidence of an urinary tract infection or significant bacteriuria.

When feasible, discharged patients should manage elevated residual urine volumes with intermittent sterile catheterization as opposed to placement of a urinary drainage catheter.

Hospitalization is indicated for any exacerbation that puts the MS patient at risk of further complications or when intravenous antibiotic or steroid therapy needs to be initiated. Admission is also indicated when depression and a significant risk of suicide require inpatient management.

LAMBERT-EATON MYASTHENIC SYNDROME

Lambert-Eaton myasthenic syndrome (LES), like myasthenia gravis, is an autoimmune disorder that causes fluctuating weakness and fatigue, especially of the proximal limb muscles. It is 100 times less common than MG, and unlike patients with MG, LES patients may show some improvement in strength with sustained or repeated exercise. For example, when an LES patient is asked to grasp the examiner's hand, the squeeze becomes more forceful over several seconds, termed *Lambert sign*. Patients often complain of myalgias, muscle stiffness, paresthesias, metallic tastes, and autonomic symptoms (e.g., dry mouth and impotence) caused by muscarinic cholinergic insufficiency. Although eye movements are unaffected, the pupillary reaction can be abnormal, and the reflexes can be diminished. The sensory examination can be normal, but because LES is associated with malignancy, paraneoplastic or chemotherapy-induced neuropathy can lead to a superimposed sensory deficit. LES is predominantly a disease associated with older men with a history of cigarette smoking and lung cancer, although it can occur in younger women without an associated neoplasm. When seen with a neoplasm, it can precede detection of the malignancy by several years. EMG and single-fiber EMG examinations are abnormal in LES patients as a result of diseased calcium channels at the cholinergic nerve terminals. Serum tests are highly specific for antibodies top the voltage-gated calcium channels.

Only in rare cases does LES progress to respiratory or bulbar failure, such that the acute treatment of LES patients, as with the other chronic neurologic disorders, is mainly supportive. Treatment of the neoplasm can markedly improve LES symptoms, as can treatment with cholinesterase inhibitors such as pyridostigmine. Neuromuscular transmission can also be enhanced with 3,4-diaminopyridine (DAP). Immunosuppression with corticosteroids and azathioprine also can be used to reduce symptom severity.[18] Hospital admission is required when infectious complications occur or when severely disability requires inpatient immunotherapy with IV immunoglobulin or plasma exchange.

PARKINSON DISEASE

Parkinson disease (PD) is the most common of the chronic neurodegenerative diseases. It is an extrapyramidal movement disorder characterized by the presence of a resting tremor, cogwheel rigidity, bradykinesias or akinesias, and impaired postural reflexes. Although the exact disease etiology is unknown, PD patients consistently have a reduced number of functional dopaminergic receptors in the substantia nigra. Drug therapy is designed to enhance central dopaminergic activity, thus decreasing the relative excess in central cholinergic activity. Even though multiple drug and surgical therapies can be used to minimize PD symptoms, the disease still progresses without symptom remission in most patients.

Epidemiology

Epidemiologic studies suggest that PD is caused primarily by environmental factors in patients who possibly may have a genetic predisposition to the disease. The overall U.S. incidence is 16 cases per 100,000 persons and is as high as 200 per 100,000 in patients in their seventh and eighth decades of life, affecting up to 1.5 million Americans.[19]

The average onset age is between 55 and 60 years, with the peak age of onset between 70 and 79 years.

Pathophysiology

PD is characterized by consistent CNS changes, including the presence of cellular cytoplasmic inclusions termed *Lewy bodies,* and extracellular pigment granules that stimulate macrophage activity. An oxidative phosphorylation disturbance and free radical formation is thought to be one possible mechanism for these changes. In the pigmented areas of the midbrain, especially the substantia nigra, there is depigmentation, dopaminergic neuron loss, and gliosis. These cellular changes result in the loss of functional dopaminergic receptors, causing a decrease in the overall level of striatal dopamine.

Clinical Presentation

The clinical diagnosis of PD is based on the presence of one or more of four hallmark neurologic signs identified in the mnemonic *TRAP:* resting *tremor,* cogwheel *rigidity,* bradykinesia or *akinesia,* and impairment in *posture* and equilibrium. Besides these signs, there also may be facial and postural changes, voice and speech abnormalities, depression, and muscle fatigue. Prior to the diagnosis of PD, most patients will have symptoms for months to years, including a general feeling of slowness or stiffness and/or difficulties with handwriting and other skills that require manual dexterity.

Most often patients will complain initially of a unilateral resting tremor of the upper extremity. The tremor is a repetitive low amplitude movement of the fingers and thumb that occurs five or more times per minute, described as "pill rolling." These tremors, which also can be seen in the legs or face, most often dissipate when intentional movement is performed, which differentiates it from the kinetic tremor of other neurologic disorders. The resting tremor of PD will become less prominent as the patient performs the finger-to-nose test and resumes once this purposeful movement is ended and the limb is supported and at rest. Cogwheel rigidity is elicited by causing passive movement of the limb through a full range of motion. As the limb is moved, the muscles will develop an increased tone, and a ratchet-like movement is noted. Bradykinesia, the general sense of slowness of voluntary movement, is often felt to be the most debilitating symptom of PD. The most severely affected PD patients can develop akinesia, the inability to perform the movements necessary for daily living, such as turning over in bed, rising from a seated position, or walking. When PD impairs postural reflexes, patients may have an impaired ability to turn or change direction while walking or may lose their balance and fall.

Clinical Diagnosis

The clinical diagnosis of PD is easy to recognize, given the presence of the TRAP symptoms. Once noted, the patient should be questioned about any family history of neurologic disorders, a prior history of encephalitis or other CNS infections, concurrent drug use, and any exposure to toxins or street drugs. The symptoms of PD also can be seen in postencephalitis patients and those with other infections such as neurosyphilis, subacute spongiform encephalopathy, and AIDS. Parkinsonism also can occur as a result of street drugs, toxins, neuroleptic drugs, hydrocephalus, head trauma, and with more rare and complex neurologic disorders.

Although once thought to be a common cause of parkinsonism, cerebral infarction is now considered an unusual cause of these symptoms.

In drug-induced PD, akinesia is the most common sign, with resting tremor less commonly observed. Other characteristics of drug-induced parkinsonism include a history of drug ingestion known to interfere with central dopamine activity, short interval between symptom onset and maximal disability, bilateral presentation of motor dysfunction, and the presence of other drug-related motor abnormalities.

There is no definitive laboratory or neuroimaging study that is pathognomonic for PD. Although positron emission tomographic (PET) scans may be useful in demonstrating this CNS pathology, CT and MRI most often only show CNS atrophy.

Disease Management

Although currently available therapies do not change the underlying pathology of PD, their use can significantly reduce symptoms. These drugs include anticholinergics such as trihexyphenidyl and benztropine; drugs that increase central dopamine levels such as amantadine, levodopa, and carbidopa; and dopamine receptor agonists such as bromocriptine and pergolide. When PD symptoms cause severe motor dysfunction, the monoamine oxidase inhibitor selegiline and the catechol methyltransferase inhibitors entacapone and tolcapone may be effective through beneficial dopamine metabolism.

Levodopa, which is converted into dopamine by decarboxylases that are present peripherally, can cause symptoms such as anorexia, nausea, and vomiting due to increases in peripheral dopamine levels. When levodopa is combined with carbidopa, a peripheral decarboxylase inhibitor, smaller doses of levodopa are required for effectiveness, reducing side effects. Over time, the effectiveness of levodopa will diminish, requiring the additional use of dopamine receptor agonist therapy. PD patients who are fully mobile, in the "on" state, can suddenly convert to the "off" state and become akinetic, especially in the morning shortly after rising and prior to taking the initial daily dose. This "on-off" phenomenon is treated by the use of controlled-release preparations of the combined carbidopa-levodopa therapy.

When drug therapy effectiveness diminishes over time, or when significant motor or psychiatric complications occur, a "drug holiday" lasting about 1 week is often attempted. Despite the fact that withdrawal of dopaminergic therapy can worsen PD symptoms, functioning actually can improve once therapy is resumed, lasting weeks to months.

The treatment for drug-induced parkinsonism, which most often causes akinesia, is termination of the causative agents, which presumably either acts to block central dopamine receptors (neuroleptics, metoclopramide) or reduce central dopamine levels (reserpine). Patients who are refractory to optimal drug therapy for all types of PD may benefit from pallidotomy, a stereotactic neurosurgical procedure that enhances medical therapy effectiveness and reduces dyskinesia severity.[20,21] Thalamic stimulation or thalamotomy are useful for PD patients with severe tremor.

Emergency Diagnosis and Management

Although most PD patients present to the ED already diagnosed, some might present undiagnosed with motor or sensory symptoms that may not be related immediately to the diagnosis of PD. Patients may experience motor symptoms such as freezing episodes, dysphagia, or abnormalities of whole-body movement. Sensory complaints may include akathisias, paresthesias, muscles aches, or extremity pain. Although severe pain is usually related to the loss of medication efficacy, it can be the prominent symptom of undiagnosed PD.

Complications related to the motor, gait, and truncal disabilities of PD include deep venous thrombosis, pulmonary embolism, aspiration pneumonia, compressive neuropathies, and trauma related to falls. Autonomic disturbances such as orthostatic hypotension, intestinal motility disorders, and bladder dysfunction can occur, as well as facial seborrhea. Behavior abnormalities caused by frontal lobe dysfunction and dementia also are seen.

Dyspnea, respiratory distress, and pneumonia are more likely during the "off" periods, when drug efficacy is reduced. The most common cause of death in severe PD is respiratory failure.

Dopaminergic therapy toxicities can include cardiac dysrhythmias, orthostatic hypotension, dyskinesias, and dystonias. Psychiatric and sleep disturbances, including nightmares, auditory and visual hallucinations, paranoia, and frank psychosis, is related to the treatment dose and duration, and can be improved by a reduction in dosage or a drug holiday. Depression and panic attacks are common, and can occur in PD patients independent of dopaminergic therapy.

Psychotropics that are known to cause tardive dyskinesia, such as haloperidol, must be used cautiously in patients with PD because of an increased risk of this complication. Patients may manifest lingual, facial, or buccal dystonias and choreic movements similar to those seen with Huntington chorea or tardive dyskinesia. These drug effects unfortunately are relatively common but can also be alleviated with a drug holiday or a decrease in levodopa dosage. Adjustment of chronic PD therapies should be done in consultation with the patient's primary care physician, who can often help to determine which symptoms reflect dopaminergic excess and whether prior drug holidays have improved the patient's symptoms.

POLIO MYELITIS AND POSTPOLIO SYNDROME

Poliomyelitis is a neurotropic enterovirus that causes paralysis through motor neuron destruction, muscle denervation, and atrophy. Indigenously acquired wild poliovirus was eradicated from the United States in 1979, and from the Western Hemisphere in 1991. However, the disease is occasionally still seen among those originating from other populations.[22] Postpolio syndrome, termed *postpoliomyelitis progressive muscular atrophy* (PPMA), is an important sequelae of acute poliomyelitis. This disorder is characterized by the recurrence of motor symptoms following a latent period of several decades after the resolution of the motor symptoms caused by the initial infection.

Epidemiology

Poliomyelitis, an infection caused by a group of enteroviruses, leads to significant striated muscle paralysis in less than 5 percent of infected patients.[23] Prior to mass immunization, virtually all children were exposed to and developed antibodies to this enterovirus infection by age 4 years. A 1952 polio epidemic caused 14 new cases of paralytic polio per 100,000 persons, a rate similar to that seen in developing countries that are unable to provide mass immunization. Polio rates as high as 600 cases per 100,000 were seen as recently as the early 1980s in India. Mass immunization with the inactivated poliovirus vaccine or attenuated oral poliovirus (OPV) has dramatically reduced the incidence of polio, which was 0.003 cases per 100,000 persons in the United States in 1981. Polio outbreaks still occur in populations that are not consistently immunized, such as were seen in the 1979 U.S. Amish epidemic, which was caused by the wild poliovirus type 1. Outbreaks also have been seen in association with inadequate immunization with modified poliovirus type 3, as was seen in the Finland outbreak in 1984–1985. With the use of OPV, some immunized children will develop polio, as will some young adults who are exposed to children who have been vaccinated with the OPV vaccine. Immunocompromised patients are at greater risk for contracting polio after exposure to children who were vaccinated with the OPV vaccine. In developing countries, recent intramuscular injections, tonsillectomy, and strenuous exercise all are associated with increased polio infection severity.

The prognosis for most enteroviral CNS infections is favorable with the exception of paralytic poliomyelitis and those enteroviral infections which occur during the first year of life.

PPMA is expected to afflict up to 100,000 of the 250,000 U.S. adults with a prior history of polio. Because the majority of these polio cases occurred prior to mass immunization, these patients most likely will be older than age 50 years. There is no gender predisposition for PPMA. Although PPMA most often occurs after a stable, disease-free period of 20 to 30 years, there are risk factors that predict an earlier onset of postpolio syndrome. These include greater age at the time of initial polio infection, greater residual motor disability, residual bulbar or respiratory signs, and the occurrence of recent injuries that require limb immobilization.

Pathophysiology

In developed countries the viral transmission is oral to oral, whereas in developing countries where the sanitation is poor the transmission is fecal to oral. Acutely, the polio enterovirus enters the body via the gastrointestinal tract and reproduces in the gastrointestinal lymphoid tissue, termed *gut-associated lymphoid tissue.* Oral secretion of the virus takes place for several days and stool excretion for several weeks.

At a critical concentration, the virus spreads to the large motor nuclei of the spinal cord, the brainstem, and the reticular formation. The vestibular and brainstem motor nuclei, hypothalamus, thalamus, cerebellum, and the precentral motor cerebral cortex also can be infected by the poliovirus. The infected neurons sustain Nissl granule dissolution and disruption, causing neuronal loss and gliosis. Most affected neurons have an altered morphology, and half are destroyed during the first week of acute paralysis. Neuron loss then causes a cycle of muscle denervation and reinnervation, resulting in lost muscle function.

The pathology of the postpolio syndrome remains unclear. The motor neuron degeneration seen in PPMA is thought not to be a result of the loss in whole motor neurons, as is seen in ALS, but rather a result of a dysfunction in the individual nerve axons in surviving motor neurons. It is suggested that postpolio fatigue is similar to that seen in chronic fatigue syndrome, both of which may cause fatigue by causing a relative depletion of central dopamine.[24] Although bromocriptine, amantadine, and pyridostigmine all have been studied in PPMA, none have been shown to be effective in minimizing patient symptoms.[25,26]

Clinical Presentation

Polio infection remains asymptomatic in more than 90 percent of cases. The majority of symptomatic polio infections involve only a minor viral illness that causes no paralysis, termed *abortive polio.* After an incubation period of a few days, symptoms may include fever, malaise, headache, sore throat, and gastrointestinal symptoms. Some of the patients who experience the minor viral illness, especially young children, may develop aseptic meningitis as the infection resolves. Only 1 to 2 percent of all poliovirus infections result in the major illness associated with neurologic involvement. Often there is resolution of the minor viral illness symptoms prior to development of neurologic symptoms, such that it is difficult to identify the preceding minor viral illness. Muscle pain, stiffness, and weakness during the early viral syndrome may suggest the later occurrence of paralysis. Because exercise can exacerbate the severity of the subsequent paralysis, patients with these symptoms suspected of having polio should be advised to avoid exercise.

When the major illness occurs, most commonly the spinal cord anterior horn cells are affected, causing asymmetric proximal limb weakness, especially in the lower extremities. Flaccid and weak muscles, absent tendon reflexes, and fasciculations, characterize spinal polio. Although polio patients note pain, paresthesias, and transient sensory abnormalities, sensory deficits are usually not found on clinical examination. Maximal paralysis usually occurs within five days, and muscle wasting then occurs over several weeks. Autonomic dysfunction, including sweating disturbances, urine retention, delayed gastric emptying, and constipation, is commonly found. Most spinal polio patients will demonstrate improved motor function, with resolution of the paralysis occurring within the first year after the acute infection.

Up to 20 percent of polio patients with paralysis will develop bulbar polio, which can cause speech, swallowing, facial muscle, and extraocular muscle dysfunction. Acute polio infection also can cause encephalitis and can disturb the reticular formation, resulting in cardiac dysrhythmias, blood pressure alterations, hypoxia, and hypercarbia. Patients who survive the acute episode of encephalitis normally will recover without residual affects.

Patients who present with postpolio syndrome complain of muscle fatigue, joint pain, worsening of skeletal deformities, or weakness in muscles that were spared during the initial viral infection.[27] These complaints occur on average 30 years after maximal resolution of the neurologic symptoms caused by the initial polio infection. When muscle weakness is observed, atrophy, pain, and fasciculations may be noted both in previously unaffected muscle groups and in those previously involved. Patients with PPMA also may present with new bulbar, respiratory, or sleep difficulties. For example, laryngeal muscle weakness can cause progressive dyspnea, dysphagia, and/or hoarseness. Some patients complain of abnormal movements in sleep that disturb normal sleep, requiring therapy with benzodiazepines or dopaminergic drugs.[28] These symptoms occur independent of any concurrent neurologic, orthopedic, psychiatric, or systemic medical illness.

Clinical Diagnosis

Acute paralytic poliomyelitis should be considered whenever an at-risk patient (see above) presents with an acute febrile illness, aseptic meningitis, and asymmetric flaccid paralysis associated with the loss of deep tendon reflexes and normal sensation. As with other causes of aseptic meningitis, the CSF reveals pleocytosis during the first week after paralysis onset. The CSF white cell count can elevate into the hundreds, with a predominance of neutrophils early in the disease course. These cells allow noninflammatory causes of paralysis to be excluded from the differential diagnosis. Although the poliovirus can be cultured from the CSF early in the disease course, throat and rectal swabs will provide a greater yield. When a particular viral serotype is identified, serial serum antibody titers can be used to verify the cultures.

The most important cause of paralysis that must be excluded is Guillain-Barré syndrome, which, unlike the acute polio infection, causes more symmetric muscle weakness. Acute paralysis can result from peripheral neuropathies caused by infectious mononucleosis, Lyme disease, or porphyria. Paralysis also can result from inflammatory myopathies, electrolyte abnormalities, toxins, or other viruses, such as coxsackieviruses, mumps, echoviruses, and nonpolio enteroviruses. Paralysis also can result from acute spinal cord compression, vascular lesions, and transverse myelitis, all of which should produce a sensory level and sphincter disturbances. In children, it is necessary to exclude spinal muscular atrophy, which can be undiagnosed until it is manifested by dramatic limb weakness caused by an acute febrile illness.

To diagnose postpolio syndrome, the patient should have a history of acute paralytic poliomyelitis with stable recovery of motor function associated with residual muscle atrophy, weakness, and areflexia with normal sensation in at least one limb. Additionally, there should be new muscle symptoms or weakness not attributable to an acute injury, neuropathy, radiculopathy, or systemic, neurologic, or psychiatric illness.

Disease Management

Treatment of the new muscle weakness seen with postpolio patients is primarily symptomatic, with the use of analgesic and anti-inflammatory medications. The onset of new weakness that is severe enough to cause the complications seen with the other chronic neurologic disorders such as ALS, MG, or MS is not to be expected. However, dyspnea, respiratory dysfunction, sleep disorders, and psychiatric disorders all must be addressed in patients with worsening PPMA.[29]

ACKNOWLEDGMENT

The author would like to thank James M. Edwards for his assistance in collecting information for this chapter.

REFERENCES

1. Chancellor AM, Warlow CP: Adult onset motor neuron disease: Worldwide mortality, incidence and distribution since 1950. *J Neurol Neurosurg Psychiatry* 55:1106, 1992.
2. Swash M: Early diagnosis of ALS/MND. *J Neurol Sci* 160(Suppl 1):S33, 1998.
3. Sostarko M, Vranjes D, Brinar V, Brzovic Z: Severe progression of ALS/MND after intervertebral discectomy. *J Neurol Sci* 160(Suppl 1):S42, 1998.
4. Wilbourn AJ: Clinical neurophysiology in the diagnosis of amyotrophic lateral sclerosis: the Lambert and the El Escorial criteria. *J Neurol Sci* 160(Suppl 1):S25, 1998.
5. Practice advisory on the treatment of amyotrophic lateral sclerosis with riluzole: Report of the Quality Standards Subcommittee of the American Academy of Neurology. *Neurology* 49:657, 1997.
6. Miller RG, Rosenberg JA, Gelinas DF, et al: Practice parameter: The care of the patient with amyotrophic lateral sclerosis (an evidence-based review): Report of the Quality Standards Subcommittee of the American Academy of Neurology: ALS Practice Parameters Task Force. 52:1311, 1999.
7. Jacobson DL, Gange SJ, Rose NR, Graham NM: Epidemiology and estimated population burden of selected autoimmune diseases in the United States. *Clin Immunol Immunopathol* 84:223, 1997.
8. Kleiner-Fisman G, Kott HS: Myasthenia gravis mimicking stroke in elderly patients. *Mayo Clin Proc* 73:1077, 1998.
9. Gronseth GS, Barohn RJ: Practice parameter: Thymectomy for autoimmune myasthenia gravis (an evidence-based review): Report of the Quality Standards Subcommittee of the American Academy of Neurology. *Neurology* 55:7, 2000.
10. Palace J, Newsom-Davis J, Lecky B: A randomized double-blind trial of prednisolone alone or with azathioprine in myasthenia gravis. Myasthenia Gravis Study Group. *Neurology* 50:1778, 1998.
11. Barrons RW: Drug-induced neuromuscular blockade and myasthenia gravis. *Pharmacotherapy* 17:1220, 1997.
12. Weinshenker BG: Epidemiology of multiple sclerosis. *Neurol Clin* 14:291, 1996.
13. Sobel RA: The pathology of multiple sclerosis. *Neurol Clin* 13:1, 1995.
14. Poser CM, Brinar VV: Diagnostic criteria for multiple sclerosis. *Clin Neurol Neurosurg* 103:1, 2001.
15. Goodin DS, Frohman EM, Garmany GPJ, et al: Disease modifying therapies in multiple sclerosis: Report of the Therapeutics and Technology Assessment Subcommittee of the American Academy of Neurology and the MS Council for Clinical Practice Guidelines. *Neurology* 58:169, 2002.
16. Sellebjerg F, Frederiksen JL, Nielsen PM, Olesen J: Double-blind, randomized, placebo-controlled study of oral, high-dose methylprednisolone in attacks of MS. *Neurology* 51:529, 1998.
17. Sicotte NL, Liva SM, Klutch R, et al: Treatment of multiple sclerosis with the pregnancy hormone estriol. *Ann Neurol* 52:421, 2002.
18. Pascuzzi RM: Myasthenia gravis and Lambert-Eaton syndrome. *Ther Apher* 6:57, 2002.
19. Tanner CM, Goldman SM: Epidemiology of Parkinson's disease. *Neurol Clin* 14:317, 1996.
20. Hallett M, Litvan I: Evaluation of surgery for Parkinson's disease: A report of the Therapeutics and Technology Assessment Subcommittee of the American Academy of Neurology. The Task Force on Surgery for Parkinson's Disease. *Neurology* 53:1910, 1999.
21. Uitti RJ, Wharen REJ, Turk MF: Efficacy of levodopa therapy on motor function after posteroventral pallidotomy for Parkinson's disease. *Neurology* 51:1755, 1998.
22. MMWR Poliomyelitis Prevention in the United States: Introduction of a sequential vaccination schedule of inactivated poliovirus vaccine followed by oral poliovirus vaccine recommendations of the Advisory Committee on Immunization Practices (ACIP). 46(RR-3):1, 1997.
23. Jubelt B: Enterovirus and mumps virus infections of the nervous system. *Neurol Clin* 2:187, 1984.
24. Bruno RL, Creange SJ, Frick NM: Parallels between post-polio fatigue and chronic fatigue syndrome: A common pathophysiology? *Am J Med* 105:66S, 1998.
25. Bruno RL, Zimmerman JR, Creange SJ, et al: Bromocriptine in the treatment of post-polio fatigue: A pilot study with implications for the pathophysiology of fatigue. *Am J Phys Med Rehabil* 75:340, 1996.
26. Trojan DA, Collet JP, Shapiro S, et al: A multicenter, randomized, double-blinded trial of pyridostigmine in postpolio syndrome. *Neurology* 53:1225, 1999.

27. Wekre LL, Stanghelle JK, Lobben B, Oyhaugen S: The Norwegian Polio Study 1994: A nationwide survey of problems in long-standing poliomyelitis. *Spinal Cord* 36:280, 1998.
28. Bruno RL: Abnormal movements in sleep as a post-polio sequelae. *Am J Phys Med Rehabil* 77:339, 1998.
29. Stanghelle JK, Festvag LV: Postpolio syndrome: A 5-year follow-up. *Spinal Cord* 35:503, 1997.

235 CNS INFECTIONS
Keith E. Loring

BACTERIAL MENINGITIS

In cases of bacterial meningitis, the two most critical actions in the emergency department are to suspect it and to begin empirical treatment promptly. In the emergency department it is often impossible to distinguish with certainty bacterial meningitis from meningitis due to viruses, fungi, and other organisms or those due to neoplastic, toxic, and autoimmune processes from bacterial meningitis on the basis of clinical findings and sometimes even lumbar puncture (LP) results. If the clinical situation and the emergency physician's practice environment permit, the diagnostic groundwork can be laid for establishing alternative diagnoses. Prompt initiation of therapy must take priority over all diagnostic maneuvers when bacterial meningitis is part of the differential diagnosis.

Epidemiology

Attack rates of meningitis are age-specific, ranging from almost 400 per 100,000 in neonates to 1 to 2 per 100,000 in adults. Two-thirds of cases are in children.[1] Long-term complications, such as cognitive deficits, epilepsy, hydrocephalus, and hearing loss, affect about a quarter of survivors. Prior to 1985, three species accounted for the majority of bacterial meningitis: *Haemophilus influenzae* (45 percent), *Streptococcus pneumoniae* (18 percent), and *Neisseria meningitidis* (14 percent). However, the specific cause of bacterial meningitis has changed dramatically in the era of vaccination against *H. influenzae* type b. From 1991 to 1996 alone, the incidence of *H. influenzae* meningitis in children younger than 5 years of age dropped from a rate of 100 per 100,000 to less than 0.3 and has remained at that level through 2000. Hence *S. pneumoniae* and *N. meningitidis* have become the predominant causes of meningitis in children 1 month of age or older.[2] Antibiotic resistance of *S. pneumoniae* to penicillins and ceftriaxone is becoming more prevalent in the United States. While such resistance has been encountered to date mostly in children, the clinician should consider modifying antibiotic selection for both children and adults with suspected pneumococcal meningitis (Table 235-1). The following discussion focuses on bacterial meningitis in adults.

Pathophysiology

Bacterial meningitis begins with the entry of organisms into the well-defended subarachnoid space. The ability to infect the subarachnoid space is not shared equally by all bacteria. The dominance of three organisms—*S. pneumoniae, H. influenzae* type b, and *N. meningitidis*—that cause over two-thirds of bacterial meningitis is not accidental. These encapsulated organisms share the ability to invade the host through the upper airway, survive dissemination through the bloodstream, and then gain access to the subarachnoid space. The subcapsular constituents of these organisms are a strong trigger of inflammatory cascades in the host. Inflammation produces the clinical picture of fever, meningismus, and eventually altered mental status that are the hallmarks of the disease. Stimulation of pain-sensitive structures in meninges and posterior spinal roots leads to headache and meningeal signs. The brain and meninges, encased in the fixed-volume skull, become edematous. Cerebrospinal fluid (CSF) drainage is reduced by interference with its flow in the subarachnoid pathways as well as its absorption by the arachnoid granulations. Hence the quantity of CSF increases, causing communicating or noncommunicating hydrocephalus. Intracranial blood vessels expand initially, increasing the volume occupied by that compartment. The brain itself swells by several mechanisms. Disruption of the blood-brain barrier allows entry of protein and ultimately water (vasogenic edema), simultaneously hydrocephalus forces CSF into the periventricular parenchyma (interstitial edema). Eventually, cell membrane homeostasis may be compromised, leading to increased intracellular water (cytotoxic edema).

The sum of these expanded volumes overwhelms the compensatory displacement of CSF into the more compliant spinal compartment, and intracranial pressure rises as a result. Since brain perfusion depends on arterial pressure exceeding tissue pressure (in this case, intracranial pressure), ischemia may develop. Diminished perfusion is all the more likely because the vascular supply is burdened with an inflammatory infiltrate whose functional and structural consequences include faulty autoregulation, inflammatory narrowing, and a prothrombotic milieu. There are some variations on the pathophysiologic

TABLE 235-1   Guidelines for Empirical Treatment of Bacterial Meningitis* with No Organisms on Gram Stain

Patient Category	Potential Pathogens	Empirical Therapy
AGE		
18–50 years	*S. pneumoniae, N. meningitidis*	Ceftriaxone 2 g IV q12h plus vancomycin or rifampin if *S. pneumoniae* resistance possible
Older than 50 years	*S. pneumoniae, N. meningitidis, L. monocytogenes,* aerobic gram-negative bacilli	Ceftriaxone 2 g IV q12h plus ampicillin 2 g IV q4h plus vancomycin or rifampin if *S. pneumoniae* resistance possible
SPECIAL CIRCUMSTANCES		
CSF leak with history of closed head trauma	*S. pneumoniae, H. influenzae,* group B streptococcus	Ceftriaxone 2 g IV q12h
History of recent penetrating head injury, neurosurgery, CSF shunt	*S. aureus, S. epidermidis,* diphtheroids, aerobic gram-negative bacilli	Vancomycin 25 mg/kg IV load (max infusion rate 500 mg per h), then 19 mg/kg at intervals dictated by Matzke nomogram plus ceftazidime 2 g IV q8h†
Immunocompromised host	*S. pneumoniae, N. meningitidis, L. monocytogenes,* aerobic gram-negative bacilli	Vancomycin 25 mg/kg IV load (max infusion rate 500 mg per h), then 19 mg/kg at intervals dictated by Matzke nomogram plus ampicillin 2 g IV q4h plus ceftazidime 2 g IV q8h†

*For pediatric meningitis treatment, see Chap. 116.
†Matzke GR, Kovarik JM: Evaluation of the vancomycin-clearance: Creatinine-clearance relationship for predicting vancomycin dosage. *Clin Pharm* 4:311, 1985.
Source: From Quagliarello and Scheld,[1] with permission.

themes just described. For example, organisms sometimes gain entry to the CSF not by hematogenous seeding but through direct contiguity. Such direct spread may be from infected parameningeal structures (e.g., brain abscess, otitis media, and sinusitis), traumatic or congenital communications with the exterior, or neurosurgery. The bacteriologic characteristics of these infections may vary. Immunologic deficiency states are increasingly common and predispose to yet other organisms. The clinical and pathophysiologic effects of organisms other than *S. pneumoniae, H. influenzae* type b, and *N. meningitidis* depend on their capacity to stimulate the host's immune processes and the host's response.

Clinical Features

SIGNS AND SYMPTOMS   About 25 percent of adult cases are classic and fulminant, and there is little diagnostic challenge. The patient presents with rapidly developing fever, headache, stiff neck, photophobia, and altered mental status. Seizures occur in 25 percent of adults and in at least that proportion of children. In some patients, typically the very young and the elderly, the clinical features may be nonspecific.

Certain historic data should increase the suspicion of meningitis and suggest specific pathogens. Several areas deserve special attention: living conditions, trauma, immunocompetence, immunization history, and antibiotic use. Army barracks and college dormitories are typical environments in which clusters of cases due to *N. meningitidis* occur. Day-care centers may become a source for multiple cases due to *H. influenzae* type b. A history of head trauma *(S. pneumoniae)* or neurosurgery (staphylococcal species or gram-negative rods) may be significant. Conditions that affect immunocompetence (e.g., history of surgical or functional splenectomy, glucocorticoid therapy, and HIV infection) should be sought. On the other hand, a history of immunization to *H. influenzae* type b in the past will make meningitis due to this organism unlikely. It is important to inquire about recent exposure to antibiotics, which may influence the clinical course and CSF findings.

Examination must include assessment for meningeal irritation with resistance to passive neck flexion, Brudzinski sign (flexion of the hips and knees in response to passive neck flexion), and Kernig sign (contraction of the hamstrings in response to knee extension while the hip is flexed). Examination of the skin is also crucial for seeking the purpuric rash characteristic of meningococcemia and, less commonly, other pathogens. Cutaneous stigmata suggesting microembolization (e.g., petechiae, splinter hemorrhages, and pustular lesions) should be aspirated when possible for Gram stain and culture. Paranasal sinuses should be percussed, and the ears should be examined for evidence of primary infection. Fundi must be assessed for papilledema or absence of venous pulsation (patient should be sitting upright), indicating increased intracranial pressure. Neurologic examination should seek evidence of focal neurologic dysfunction, such as disordered eye movements, homonymous visual field deficits, facial asymmetry, and hemiparesis.[3,4]

Diagnosis

The differential diagnoses may be categorized into parenchymal or meningeal disorders. When fever and focal neurologic symptoms and signs predominate, parenchymal central nervous system (CNS) infections are concerns (e.g., brain abscess, viral encephalitis, cerebral toxoplasmosis, and other parenchymal processes). When meningeal signs predominate, other infectious meningitides, meningeal neoplasm, CNS vascularity, and subarachnoid hemorrhage are possible.

For evaluation of parenchymal brain infections, LP is unhelpful and potentially dangerous because it can lead to transtentorial or tonsillar herniation. A cranial computed tomographic (CT) scan should be done first if the patient exhibits papilledema or focal neurologic signs. A cranial CT scan is also the preferred initial mode in diagnosing subarachnoid hemorrhage.

For meningeal disorders other than subarachnoid hemorrhage, CSF examination is most helpful. LP should be carried out as soon as it is deemed safely possible; however, its timing should not impede the early administration of empirical antibiotic therapy. Appropriate sequencing of LP, cranial imaging studies, and initiation of empirical antibiotics are discussed further below. Blood cultures (two specimens drawn 15 min apart) yield the responsible organism in only around 50 percent of cases of bacterial meningitis. Thus, for bacteriologic diagnosis, CSF analysis is paramount.

Typical CSF findings for bacterial, viral, neoplastic, and fungal meningitides are displayed in Table 235-2, but there is considerable overlap in findings. Some infectious agents (e.g., *Mycoplasma, Listeria,* spirochetes, syphilis, *Leptospira,* and *Borrelia*) produce CSF alterations that are less pronounced than those outlined for bacteria in Table 235-2. An aseptic profile, suggesting viral infection, is typical of partially treated bacterial infections (one-third or more of pediatric cases have received antimicrobial treatment before presenting with meningitis). The same is true of untreated bacterial infections adjacent to but not communicating with the subarachnoid space, such as abscesses of the brain and subdural or epidural spaces. The percentage of polymorphonuclear cells may be higher in early viral meningitis, and glucose levels may be reduced in some viral cases.

Additional testing can include viral cultures in suspected viral meningitis, tests for *Borrelia* antibodies in patients with possible Lyme disease, india ink or serum cryptococcal antigen in immunocompromised patients, acid-fast stain and culture for mycobacteria in tuberculous meningitis, and latex agglutination or counterimmune electrophoresis for bacterial antigens in potentially partially treated bacterial cases. Assays are most widely available for *S. pneumoniae,* other group B streptococci, *H. influenzae* type b, and *N. meningitidis.* Rarely, CSF may be normal or nearly so in very early bacterial meningitis, especially during meningococcemia. Empirical antibiotic treatment, admission, and repeated LP are appropriate if clinical suspicion is great despite negative initial CSF results.

LUMBAR PUNCTURE   LP can be performed safely if intracranial mass lesions and coagulopathy are unlikely on historical or clinical grounds (Table 235-3). Coagulopathy is considered a relative contraindication to LP. At least one major authority asserts that LP may be performed even in the presence of known coagulopathy when the results are felt to provide essential information, as may be the case in suspected meningitis.[5] Infusion of clotting factors in the hemophiliac patient is desirable if conditions permit and appears to mitigate related complications.[6] There is no standard agreement regarding safe performance of lumbar puncture based on a given platelet level. Again, if the clinical situation allows, infusion of platelets may be desirable in cases of severe thrombocytopenia.[5] Lumbar puncture is contraindicated if there is infection in the overlying skin.

If a delay is anticipated for any reason, then blood cultures should be obtained, and empirical antibiotic therapy should be instituted promptly. LP can then proceed if no intracranial mass lesion and no mass effect are found on CT scan. Antibiotic therapy given up to 2 h prior to LP will not decrease the diagnostic sensitivity if CSF bacterial antigen assays are obtained along with CSF culture. However, at 2 h after antibiotic administration, the CSF likely will be sterilized in meningococcal disease but not until 4 h after antibiotic administration in pneumococcal disease.[7,8]

Local anesthetic should be used to improve patient comfort, relaxation, and cooperation. Anxiolitics such as benzodiazepines, which are helpful adjuncts in the performance of painful procedures, can cloud the patient's sensorium and confuse subsequent clinical assessment. The L3–L4 interspace should be punctured (L4–L5 in newborn infants) while the patient is curled as tightly as possible in a fetal position. In

TABLE 235-2   Typical Spinal Fluid Results for Meningeal Processes

Parameter (Normal)	Bacterial	Viral	Neoplastic	Fungal
OP (<170 mm CSF)	>300 mm	200 mm	200 mm	300 mm
WBC (<5 mononuclear)	>1000/μL	<1000/μL	<500/μL	<500/μL
% PMNs (0)	>80%	1–50%	1–50%	1–50%
Glucose (>40 mg/dL)	<40 mg/dL	>40 mg/dL	<40 mg/dL	<40 mg/dL
Protein (<50 mg/dL)	>200 mg/dL	<200 mg/dL	>200 mg/dL	>200 mg/dL
Gram stain (−)	+	−	−	−
Cytology (−)	−	−	+	+

Abbreviations: OP = opening pressure; PMNs = polymorphonuclear cells; WBC = white blood cells.
Source: From Greenlee JE: Approach to diagnosis of meningitis: Cerebrospinal fluid evaluation. *Infect Dis Clin North Am* 4:583, 1990.

adults, a line drawn between the iliac crests crosses the spine at the L3–L4 interspace. Alternatively, the patient may be seated on the edge of a bed or cart leaning over a tray stand. The latter technique is particularly useful when landmarks are uncertain, as they may be in an obese patient. The site should be prepared with povidone-iodine and allowed to dry thoroughly to avoid introduction of bacteria by puncture and the production of chemical arachnoiditis. A 2½-in. 22-gauge needle should be used in children and a 3½-in. 20-gauge needle in adults. The use of larger-gauge needles will greatly increase the risk of post-LP CSF leak and resulting headache. Although useful, the opening pressure is not critical for interpretation of the procedure. To obtain meaningful results, the pressure must be measured with the patient lying extended on his or her side. Pressures measured with the patient still curled in extreme flexion or while sitting will be artificially elevated. Normal pressure is less than 170 mm CSF. Careful repositioning (straightening the curled patient or helping the seated patient to a lying position on his or her side) is performed safely with the needle in situ.

Four tubes, each containing at least 1 mL of CSF, typically are obtained. More volume—up to 5 mL—may be preferable in patients who are immunocompromised. Red and white blood cell counts with differential counts are requested for tubes 1 and 4. The two-tube assessment helps detect a traumatic tap because the rate of bleeding changes rapidly, causing a difference in red blood cell count between the two tubes. Tube 4 also may be used for culture and Gram stain. Tube 2 is sent for determination of protein and glucose levels. Tube 3 should be saved for other studies, discussed below, if necessary. Closing pressure determination is not routinely necessary.[9]

Treatment

Ideal management has several goals. The first priority is the rapid administration of a bactericidal antibiotic that gains rapid entry to the subarachnoid space. A secondary priority in some cases is use of an anti-inflammatory agent to suppress the normal inflammatory processes, which are amplified by antibiotic-induced bacteriolysis. A

TABLE 235-3   Considerations for Lumbar Puncture without Neuroimaging*

Age <60
Immunocompetent
No history of CNS disease
No recent seizure (<1 wk)
Normal sensorium and cognition
No papilledema
No focal neurologic deficits

*Coagulopathy is a separate consideration for lumbar puncture.
Source: From Hasbun R, Abrahams J, Jeleel J, et al: Computed tomography of the head before lumbar puncture in adults with suspected meningitis. *New Engl J Med* 345:1727, 2001.

final concern is to counter the adverse effects of increased intracranial pressure and vasculopathy, which may lead to brain ischemia. Agents to which local bacterial resistance has developed should be avoided. Currently, for example, about 30 percent of *H. influenzae* type b isolates are resistant to ampicillin. **Bacteriostatic agents should not be used alone or in combination with a bactericidal agent because they are antagonistic.** Agents of current choice for given bacterial meningitides are indicated in Table 235-1.

Empirical treatment for bacterial meningitis *is based on the likelihood of certain pathogens* (see Table 235-1) and results of CSF Gram stain, the patient's age, and certain risk factors, if available.[10–12] For patients aged 18 to 50 years with no organisms evident on Gram stain, ceftriaxone 2 g IV every 12 h is the current recommendation.

For patients with Gram stain suggestive of *S. pneumoniae* (gram-positive cocci in clusters), a broad-spectrum cephalosporin and vancomycin should be given to ensure coverage of resistant organisms. For patients >50 years or the immunosuppressed, ampicillin should be given to treat against *Listeria monocytogenes*. For gram-negative cocci, presumed *N. meningitidis*, penicillin G is still effective. For gram-positive rods, *Listeria monocytogenes* is the presumed agent, and the recommended regimen is ampicillin and gentamicin. For gram-negative rods, the recommendation is ceftazidime and an aminoglycoside. If herpes simplex is suspected, acyclovir 10 mg/kg ideal body weight (IBW) is given every 8 h. Dosage should be decreased in renal insufficiency.

A number of inflammation suppressants have been shown to improve outcome in experimental bacterial meningitis, but only glucocorticoids, and specifically dexamethasone, have been tested in clinical trials. The use of steroids in pediatric meningitis is discussed in Chap. 116.

The question of steroid use for adults in the emergency department is inadequately answered.[13,14] Dexamethasone given to adults with bacterial meningitis (10 mg IV 15 min prior to antibiotic administration) appears to decrease the morbidity and mortality of meningitis due to *S. pneumoniae*, but not for *N. meningitides*. The problem in the emergency department, however, is that because administration of antibiotics usually appropriately precedes diagnosis, we rarely deal with *known* bacterial meningitis. As noted antibiotic administration should never be delayed in *suspected* bacterial meningitis, especially in cases where neurologic decompensation or clear toxicity is present. Additionally, many patients ultimately prove to have a viral etiology and potentially may be harmed by the administration of steroids.

Also important in management is surveillance for and correction of complications, including seizures, hyponatremia, hydrocephalus, and cerebrovascular accidents. General treatment measures include maintenance of normal blood volume. Hypotonic fluids should be avoided. The serum sodium level should be monitored serially to detect the syndrome of inappropriate antidiuretic hormone or cerebral salt wasting. Hyperpyrexia should be treated. Coagulopathies should be corrected using specific replacement therapies. Phenytoin loading is indicated in patients who develop seizures. For marked cerebral edema, as evidenced by clinical or CT findings, the following are indicated: head elevation, hyperventilation to a $Paco_2$ of 25 to 30 mm Hg, and use of mannitol. Measurements of intracranial and systemic arterial pressure are useful in severe cases to enable monitoring of cerebral perfusion pressure.

Chemoprophylaxis is indicated for high-risk contacts of patients with documented *N. meningitidis* or *H. influenzae* type b infection, including household contacts; school or day-care contacts in the previous 7 days; those who have had direct exposure to the patient's secretions through kissing, shared utensils, or shared toothbrushes; and those who have performed mouth-to-mouth resuscitation or have intubated the patient while unprotected with a face mask. Other health care providers do not require prophylaxis. First-line treatment is with rifampin 10 mg/kg (to a maximum of 600 mg per dose) every 12 h for four doses. Alternatives are ceftriaxone, ciprofloxacin, and sulfisoxazole. High-risk contacts should be instructed to return at once if they develop symptoms. For moderate- to low-risk contacts, single-dose ciprofloxacin 500 mg is recommended.[11]

VIRAL MENINGITIS

A number of viruses can cause aseptic meningitis, including nonpolio enteroviruses, mumps, cytomegalovirus, herpes simplex virus (HSV), lymphocytic choriomeningitis, adenovirus, and HIV. Specific diagnosis depends on isolation of the virus or positive results on immunoassay of the CSF. Nonpolio enteroviruses (echovirus, coxsackievirus, and enterovirus) account for about 85 percent of all cases of viral meningitis in the United States.

While the diagnosis of viral meningitis is often straightforward (see Table 235-2), there can be overlap of CSF findings with early bacterial meningitis and partially treated bacterial meningitis, making specific diagnosis for some cases difficult in the emergency department. Neutrophils may predominate in the CSF for the first 24 h in viral meningitis. Standard references report up to a 10 percent incidence of lymphocytic predominance in CSF with bacterial meningitis, more common with *L. monocytogenes* and in neonatal meningitis. Depending on clinical diagnostic certainty, a range of approaches can be employed in the management of presumed viral meningitis, from admission with empirical antibiotic therapy until culture results return to discharge from the emergency department with follow-up in 24 h.

VIRAL ENCEPHALITIS

Viral encephalitis is a viral infection of brain parenchyma that produces an inflammatory response. It is distinct from, although often coexists with, viral meningitis, in which the infectious agent and inflammatory response are in the subarachnoid space. Clinically, the distinction is made by the presence of neurologic abnormality in encephalitis, whereas only meningeal symptoms and signs (e.g., photophobia, headache, and stiff neck) occur in meningitis. The true incidence of viral encephalitis is difficult to estimate because of the variability of clinical expression, ranging from profound neurologic involvement to clinically silent cases, as well as variability in reporting policies. Several thousand cases are reported yearly in the United States.

Epidemiology

The incidence of the various types of viral encephalitis varies from year to year, depending on whether sporadic or epidemic outbreaks occur. In relative terms, the incidence is about one-tenth that of bacterial meningitis. In North America, viruses that cause encephalitis include the arboviruses, HSV-1, herpes zoster, Epstein-Barr virus (EBV), cytomegalovirus (CMV), and rabies. Arboviruses account for 10 percent of cases during times of sporadic, isolated cases but can ac-

count for up to 50 percent of cases during epidemic outbreaks. Historically, the four most common arboviral encephalitides in the United States have been La Crosse encephalitis (LAC), St. Louis equine encephalitis (SEE), western equine encephalitis (WEE), and eastern equine encephalitis (EEE). However, after the 1999 outbreak of the West Nile virus (WNV) in New York State—its first appearance in the western hemisphere—this pathogen has become widely recognized as part of the differential diagnosis. Of these viruses, LAC is diagnosed most frequently, with a reported average annual incidence of 75. It is seen in the midwestern and eastern United States exclusively. Ninety percent of reported cases occur in children. SEE is seen throughout the United States in periodic outbreaks, with the yearly incidence ranging from 20 reported cases to 2000. It is seen primarily in young children and the elderly and has a 20 percent mortality rate in the latter. WEE prevails in the western United States and Canada. Disease is most severe in the very young, causing seizures in 90 percent of affected infants and permanent neurologic deficits in 50 percent. EEE, the most devastating of these arboviral infections, is prevalent in the Atlantic and Gulf Coast regions. It tends to occur in sporadic epidemics and has a mortality rate of nearly 70 percent. WNV, only under surveillance since 1999 and then initially found only in New York, spread to 27 states in 2002. It leads to clinical disease in roughly 20 percent of those infected, the majority of these suffering a mild febrile illness. Neurologic sequelae are relatively uncommon, but it can lead to significant morbidity in the extremes of age.[15]

HSV-1 and HSV-2 encephalitides occur in 1 in 250,000 to 1 in 500,000 cases annually in the United States, respectively. HSV-1 disease typically is seen in older children and adults as reactivation disease, whereas HSV-2 disease is seen in neonates as a result of perinatal transmission and generally leads to devastating neurologic outcomes.

Pathophysiology

Entry portals are highly specific for the encephalitis-producing viruses. The arboviruses (*arbo* meaning "arthropod-borne") are transmitted by mosquitoes and ticks, and rabies is transferred by the bite of an infected animal. Impaired immune status may play a role in herpes zoster and CMV encephalitis. Common to all is preliminary viral invasion of the host at a site where replication takes place that is outside the CNS. Most viruses then reach the nervous system hematogenously during viremia. However, at least three important viruses—rabies, HSV, and herpes zoster virus (HZV)—reach the spinal cord and eventually the brain by traveling backward within axons from a distal site where they have gained access to nerve endings.

Once in the brain, the virus enters neural cells. Neurologic dysfunction and damage are caused by the disruption of neural cell functions by the virus and by the effects of the host's inflammatory responses. Gray matter is predominantly affected, resulting in cognitive and psychiatric signs, lethargy, and seizures. Multifocal white matter damage occurs predominantly in postinfectious encephalomyelitis and rarely during acute encephalitis. Sensorimotor deficits referable to one hemisphere or to the spinal cord are more typical of this immune-mediated pathologic process, which may follow viral encephalitis and meningitis of any type.

Clinical Features

Encephalitis should be considered in patients presenting with the following clinical features singly or in combination: new psychiatric symptoms, cognitive deficits (e.g., aphasia, amnestic syndrome, or acute confusional state), seizures, and movement disorders. Features of meningeal involvement, such as headache and photophobia, are usually but not invariably present. The same is true for fever.

Patients with HZV, EBV, or CMV encephalitis (lymphadenopathy and hepatosplenomegaly) often will have a history of and/or show signs typical of clinical syndromes caused outside the CNS by these viruses. Other circumstances of the case may suggest both the broad diagnosis of encephalitis and a specific viral cause (Table 235-4). For example, a late-summer encephalopathy suggests the possibility of an arbovirus encephalitis, and an animal bite for which no antirabies treatment was obtained has obvious relevance.

Signs of meningeal irritation and increased intracranial pressure should be sought. Neurologic findings reflect the areas of involvement. A careful assessment of cognition is crucial. Sensorimotor deficits are not typical. Encephalitides may show special regional tropism. HSV involves limbic structures of the temporal and frontal lobes, with prominent psychiatric features, memory disturbance, and aphasia. Some arboviruses predominantly affect the basal ganglia, causing choreoathetosis and parkinsonism. Involvement of the brainstem nuclei that control swallowing leads to the hydrophobic choking response characteristic of rabies encephalitis.

Diagnosis

Diagnosis rests on imaging studies using magnetic resonance imaging (MRI) or CT scan if MRI is not reasonably available, electroencephalography (EEG), and LP. Imaging not only excludes other potential lesions, such as brain abscess, but also may display findings that are highly suggestive of HSV encephalitis, a treatable infection, with involvement of medial temporal and inferior frontal gray matter. MRI is more sensitive than CT scan in this regard. EEG is quite useful in establishing the broad diagnosis as well. Almost by definition, the EEG findings are abnormal in encephalitis, in contrast to isolated viral meningitis or to a primary psychiatric disorder. Furthermore, HSV produces an almost pathognomonic picture, with the EEG showing periodic, usually asymmetric, sharp waves in the setting of acute febrile encephalopathy. These findings can be present before any abnormality is visible on MRI. Realistically, LP is the most useful diagnostic procedure in the emergency department once imaging studies, if clinically indicated and available, rule out the risk of uncal herniation. Findings of aseptic meningitis are typical on CSF examination. It is at least theoretically possible to have encephalitis without meningitis, but it is quite rare.

The differential diagnosis depends on the nature of the presentation. When fever and meningeal symptoms predominate, bacterial meningitis is suspected. In less fulminant meningeal cases, Lyme disease; tuberculous, fungal, and neoplastic meningitis; and subacute subarachnoid hemorrhage are part of the differential diagnosis. When parenchymal features are prominent, brain abscess, bacterial endocarditis, postinfectious encephalomyelitis, and toxic or metabolic encephalopathies should be considered.

The clear diagnostic imperative in the emergency department is to exclude the most immediately life-threatening alternative processes requiring immediate treatment. The two most important are bacterial meningitis and acute subarachnoid hemorrhage. Once this is accomplished satisfactorily, the mandate is less definite. Of the viruses causing encephalitis, only HSV has been shown by clinical trial to be responsive to antiviral therapy at this time. HSV can be isolated in as many as 50 percent of neonatal infections but is found rarely in older children and adults. The polymerase chain reaction (PCR) analysis of CSF has 95 percent sensitivity and 100 percent specificity in the diagnosis of HSV infection with respect to brain biopsy. Regardless of diagnostic approach, because current antiviral treatment is relatively free of risk and side effects, empirical therapy is recommended in cases of clinical encephalitis.[16] Of the other viral encephalitides, CSF culture results are positive for 50 to 70 percent of patients with enteroviral meningitis but for a much smaller percentage of those with isolated enteroviral encephalitis. The use of PCR techniques for the enteroviruses is also showing promise for CNS diagnosis in the future.

Treatment

The agent of choice for HSV disease is acyclovir 10 mg/kg every 8 h for 14 to 21 days. Based on anecdotal data, patients with HZV and CMV encephalitis also may benefit from antiviral therapy: acyclovir for HZV and ganciclovir for CMV encephalitis.

Prognosis depends on the virus and host. Rabies encephalitis, while rare, continues to be neurologically devastating and usually fatal. EEE and HSV encephalitis also have high mortality rates and frequently produce residual deficits. For the others, adverse outcome is seen mainly in elderly patients or in those with compromising preexisting systemic or neurologic conditions.

Disposition

Patients with encephalitis in general should be admitted. The outcome in cases of HSV encephalitis is related to the neurologic condition at the time that antiviral therapy is initiated. Patients who are already in coma do very poorly, making timely diagnosis and therapy priorities for this form of encephalitis. Empirical initiation of acyclovir 10 mg/kg in the emergency department in encephalitis suspects should be highly considered.

BRAIN ABSCESS

A brain abscess is a focal pyogenic infection. When fully developed, it is composed of a central pus-filled cavity ringed by a layer of granulation tissue and an outer fibrous capsule. Surrounding this is edematous brain tissue infiltrated with inflammatory cells. It is a pathologic

TABLE 235-4   Viral Pathogens Causing Encephalitis in North America

Virus	Clinical Clues	Diagnosis	Prognosis
HSV-1	"Psychiatric" presentation	MRI, EEG, PCR of CSF, biopsy	30% die, 30% have deficits
Herpes zoster	Shingles, chickenpox, immunosuppressed state	Skin vesicle or CSF culture, serology	10–20% die
EBV	Mononucleosis	Serology	5–10% die
Rabies	Animal bite	Saliva or CSF culture, biopsy, serology	90% die
Arboviruses	Seasonal		
La Crosse	Midwest, children	CSF or blood culture, serology	Good
St. Louis	Midwest, older urban dwellers	As above	5–10% die
Western equine	West, outside workers	As above	5–10% die
Eastern equine	Southeast, outside workers	As above	50% die
WNV	East, urban dwellers	CSF or IgM serology	15% mortality among hospitalized patients

Abbreviations: CSF = cerebrospinal fluid; EBV = Epstein-Barr virus; EEF = electroencephalogram; HSV-1 = herpes simplex virus 1; MRI = magnetic resonance imaging; PCR = polymerase chain reaction; WNV = West Nile virus.
Source: From Bale JR Jr: Viral encephalitis. *Med Clin North Am* 77:25, 1993, with permission.

response typical of a relatively competent immune system against a bacterial invader. Focal brain infections due to other organisms, such as granulomas due to tuberculosis, necrotic lesions of toxoplasmosis in immunocompromised patients, or cystic lesions of cysticercosis, are not abscesses in the pathologic sense. These nonpurulent focal lesions are not considered here.

Epidemiology

Brain abscess is rather uncommon. The rate has fallen gradually over the past century, probably reflecting the effect of antibiotics on predisposing conditions such as otitis media. Mortality rates for diagnosed cases also have fallen.

Age distribution corresponds to the various predisposing conditions. Most patients with brain abscess related to a paranasal sinus focus are in the 10- to 30-year-old range. When the source is otic, a bimodal incidence occurs in ages younger than 20 and older than 40 years. Twenty-five percent of cases occur in children under 15 years of age, with the majority occuring in the 4- to 7-year-old range. Pockets of higher incidence occur along the lines of age, origin of initial infection, and in some cases, gender.

Pathophysiology

Organisms reach the brain by one of three known routes: hematogenously (one-third of cases); from contiguous infections of middle ear, sinus, or teeth (one-third of cases); or by direct implantation by neurosurgery or penetrating trauma (about 10 percent of cases). The route is unknown in about 20 percent. Circumstances that reduce oxygenation of brain parenchyma are important predisposing factors for bacterial invasion. For example, spread from a contiguous infection usually involves intervening cerebral thrombophlebitis, with congestive ischemic hypoxemia of tissue destined to become infected. Hematogenous seeding is facilitated by systemic hypoxemia, as in congenital heart diseases with right-to-left shunt and chronic pulmonary suppuration. This is demonstrated by the prominent role of anaerobic bacteria in brain abscesses. The source of brain abscess should be identified for the dual purpose of eliminating the source itself and gaining insight into the probable bacteriologic characteristics of the abscess. For example, gram-negative rods, especially *Bacteroides,* are the usual pathogens in otogenic brain abscesses, which are typically single and located in the adjacent temporal lobe or cerebellum. Anaerobic and microaerophilic streptococci are the most common pathogens in sinogenic and odontogenic abscesses and are located more typically in the frontal lobes. Abscesses formed from hematogenous spread are often multiple and polymicrobial, with anaerobic and microaerophilic streptococci commonly represented. Staphylococci are typical pathogens in abscesses due to direct implantation. Gram-negative rods are also suspected in cases related to a neurosurgical procedure.

Clinical Features

Presenting features of brain abscess are notoriously nonspecific. Patients rarely appear acutely ill, and the classic triad of headache, fever, and focal neurologic deficit is present in less than one-third of all patients. As a result, the diagnosis is often delayed. Symptoms reflect the infectious and neurologic (focal and mass effect–producing) aspects of the disease. The most common symptom is headache, which is a complaint in almost all cases. Fever is present in about half of all cases, and neck stiffness occurs in fewer than half. Toxic appearance is rare until late in the disease process. Focal neurologic symptoms, such as hemiparesis or seizures, are present in about a third. Other symptoms of increased intracranial pressure, such as vomiting, confusion, or obtundation, are present in about half of cases. The presentation may be dominated by the origin of the infection (e.g., ear or sinus pain).

Meningeal signs and papilledema are uncommon. Focal neurologic signs reflecting the site of the lesion (e.g., frontal lobes, hemiparesis; temporal lobes, homonymous superior quadrant visual field deficits or aphasia; or cerebellum, limb incoordination or nystagmus) are present in about 60 percent of patients on careful examination. Discovery of potential sites of origin may raise suspicion of brain abscess when the presentation is otherwise nonspecific (e.g., otitis media, sinus tenderness, evidence of pulmonary suppuration, or right-to-left shunting) in a patient with subacute headache and lethargy.

Diagnosis

Brain abscess is diagnosed by imaging studies. CT scan with contrast infusion classically demonstrates one or several thin, smoothly contoured rings of enhancement surrounding a low-density center and surrounded by white matter edema. Early in the course, a ring may be thicker and less well defined, with the only CT finding being an area of focal hypodensity. Suspected brain abscess is one of the rare instances in the emergency department when a contrast-enhanced study is preferred over a non-contrast-enhanced study. MRI usually demonstrates a ring even without gadolinium enhancement. Both types of studies are highly sensitive, and one imaging modality has no real advantage over the other except that CT scans usually are more readily available in the emergency department. Other studies, such as blood analysis, EEG, and CSF examination, are too nonspecific for definitive diagnosis, and LP is contraindicated when suspicion is high and when focal neurologic signs are present. Cultures of blood or other sites of infection may guide future management and always should be obtained.

Differential diagnosis of the clinical presentation is broad because of its nonspecific and variable nature. A sudden onset with focal features may suggest cerebrovascular disease. Prominent fever, stiff neck, and confusion may suggest meningitis. A protracted course with features of increased intracranial pressure may suggest neoplasm. Brain neoplasm, subacute brain hemorrhage, other focal lesions, and other focal brain infections, such as toxoplasmosis, may mimic the imaging findings of brain abscess. Biopsy or aspiration for confirmation of diagnosis as well as for bacteriologic studies is necessary in most cases.

Treatment

The cornerstone of early emergency department treatment of brain abscess is administration of antibiotics (Table 235-5). The susceptibility of the likely pathogen and the penetration of the agent into the lesion should be considered when choosing an antibiotic. The bacteriologic characteristics of the lesion may be inferred if the origin is obvious. Initial empirical antibiotic choice should take advantage of such information. Initial treatment in a suspected otogenic case is with a third-generation cephalosporin such as cefotaxime (2 g IV every 6 h) or trimethoprim-sulfamethoxazole with metronidazole or chloramphenicol. For presumed abscess of sinogenic or odontogenic origin, high-dose penicillin and metronidazole is a good choice (see Table 235-5). Penicillin is also appropriate for an abscess of hematogenous origin. Chloramphenicol or metronidazole, which by virtue of their lipophilic nature penetrate abscesses very well, can be added to penicillin. When communication with the exterior is suspected, as in penetrating trauma or after neurosurgery, nafcillin or vancomycin are indicated. Addition of ceftazidime may be required if gram-negative aerobes are suspected. For patients in whom no mechanism is apparent or suspected, the combination of a third-generation cephalosporin such as cefotaxime and metronidazole provides good coverage.

Most patients require a neurosurgical procedure for diagnosis and bacteriologic analysis, if not for definitive treatment. Total excision has become necessary less often with the availability of imaging techniques for following the course of abscesses treated medically after surgical aspiration. In patients in whom intracranial pressure is high,

TABLE 235-5 Guidelines for Empirical Treatment of Brain Abscess Based on Presumed Source

Presumed Source	Primary Empirical Therapy	Alternative Therapy
Otogenic	Cefotaxime 2 g IV q8h	TMP-SMX* 5 mg/kg IV q6h based on TMP and metronidazole 1 g IV load then 500 mg IV q6h or chloramphenicol
Sinogenic or odontogenic	Penicillin 24 million units/day IV divided q4h and metronidazole 1 g IV load then 500 mg IV q6h	Penicillin (same dose) and chloramphenicol 100 mg/kg per d divided q6h
Penetrating trauma or neurosurgical procedures	Nafcillin 2 g IV q4h and ceftazidime 2 g IV q8h if gram-negative aerobes suspected	Vancomycin 15 mg/kg IV q6h (max 1 g/dose; monitor serum levels) and ceftazidime 2 g IV if gram-negative aerobes suspected
Hematogenous	Penicillin 24 million units/day IV divided q4h and metronidazole 1 g IV load then 500 mg IV q6h	Penicillin (same dose) and chloramphenicol 100 mg/kg per d divided q6h
No obvious source	Cefotaxime 2 g IV q6h and metronidazole 1 g IV load then 500 mg IV q6h	No recommendation

*Trimethoprim-sulfamethoxazole.
Source: From Heilpern and Lorber,[17] with permission.

excision is still carried out. The role of glucocorticoids is controversial. Steroids may produce temporary improvement of increased intracranial pressure.[17,18]

REFERENCES

1. Quagliarello VJ, Scheld WM: Bacterial meningitis: Pathogenesis, pathophysiology, and progress. *New Engl J Med* 327:864, 1992.
2. Bath S, Bisgard K, Murphy T: Progress toward elimination of *Haemophilus influenzae* type b invasive disease among infants and children—United States 1998–2000. *MMWR* 51:235, 2002.
3. Durand ML, Calderwood SB, Weber DJ, et al: Acute bacterial meningitis in adults: A review of 493 episodes. *New Engl J Med* 328:21, 1993.
4. Ashwal S, Tomasi L, Schneider S, et al: Bacterial meningitis in children: Pathophysiology and treatment. *Neurology* 42:739, 1992.
5. Kooiker JC: Spinal puncture and cerebrospinal fluid examination, in Roberts JR, Hedges JR (eds): *Clinical Procedures in Emergency Medicine*. Philadelphia, WB Saunders, 1998, p 1054.
6. Silverman RS, Kwiatkowski T, Bernstein S, et al: Safety of lumbar puncture in patients with hemophilia. *Ann Emerg Med* 22:1793, 1993.
7. Talan DA, Zibulewsky J: Relationship of clinical presentation to time to antibiotics for the emergency department management of suspected bacterial meningitis. *Ann Emerg Med* 22:1733, 1993.
8. Kanegaye JT, Soliemanzadeh P, Bradley JS: Lumbar puncture in pediatric bacterial meningitis: Defining the time interval for recovery of cerebrospinal fluid pathogens after parenteral antibiotic pretreatment. *Pediatrics* 108:1169, 2001.
9. American Academy of Neurology Quality Standards Subcommittee, Daube JR, Frishber BM, et al: *Practice Parameters: Lumbar Puncture*. Minneapolis, American Academy of Neurology, 1992.
10. Begg N, Cartwright KAV, Cohen J, et al: Consensus statement on diagnosis, investigation, treatment and prevention of acute bacterial meningitis in immunocompetent adults. *J Infect* 39:1, 1999.
11. Quagliarello VJ, Scheld WM: Treatment of bacterial meningitis. *New Engl J Med* 336:708, 1997.
12. Choi C: Bacterial meningitis in aging adults. *Clin Infect Dis* 33:1384, 2001.
13. Wald ER, Kaplan SI, Mason EO Jr, et al: Dexamethasone therapy for children with bacterial meningitis. *Pediatrics* 95:21, 1995.
14. de Gans J, van de Beek D: Dexamethasone in adults with bacterial meningitis. *New Engl J Med* 347:1549, 2002.
15. Provisional Surveillance Summary of the West Nile Virus Epidemic—United States. *MMWR* 51:1129, 2002.
16. Rowley AH, Whitley RJ, Lakeman FD, et al: Rapid detection of herpes simplex-virus DNA in cerebrospinal fluid of patients with herpes simplex encephalitis. *Lancet* 335:440, 1990.
17. Heilpern KL, Lorber B: Focal intracranial infections. *Infect Dis Clin North Am* 10:879, 1996.
18. Seydoux C, Francioli P: Bacterial brain abscesses: Factors influencing mortality and sequelae. *Clin Infect Dis* 15:394, 1992.

236

COMPLICATIONS OF CENTRAL NERVOUS SYSTEM DEVICES
Joseph Pagane
Jay Ladde

CEREBROSPINAL FLUID SHUNTS

Hydrocephalus has an incidence of 3 cases per 1000 live births. Mechanical shunting is the primary treatment as there is usually no alternative corrective surgical or medical therapy for this disorder. The shunting of cerebrospinal fluid (CSF) was first described in 1895, but it was not until the 1950s that shunting ventricular CSF became a routine procedure.[1,2] Each year there are approximately 18,000 CSF shunts inserted, making it the most common pediatric neurosurgical procedure performed in the United States.[1] The CSF shunt is also the neurosurgical procedure with the highest incidence of postoperative complications,[1,2] with a 39 percent 1-year and a 52 percent 2-year failure rate being reported following initial shunt placement.[3] Many types of CSF shunt systems exist (Figures 236-1 and 236-2). Most systems consist of three components beginning with a silastic tube passed into the ventricle via a burr hole. This tubing is tunneled subcutaneously to a valve chamber. The valve chamber, the second component, establishes a pressure gradient that ensures drainage of fluid away from the ventricle. The valve chamber, or in some cases a separate reservoir, allows access to the shunt system for patency testing, pressure measurement, CSF sampling, medication injection (e.g., chemotherapy, antibiotics), or contrast administration. Distal tubing, which is the third component, connects the valve chamber to a drainage point. The most common drainage site is the peritoneal cavity. Other drainage sites include the right atrium, gallbladder, pleural cavity, and ureter.

Shunt Malfunction

Shunt malfunctions are the most common complications encountered with CSF shunts, occurring in up to 67 percent of patients during their lifetime. Obstruction is the most common type of shunt malfunction and most commonly occurs in the proximal tubing followed by the distal tubing, and, finally, the valve chamber. Proximal obstructions usually occur within the first 2 years after shunt insertion. Causes include tissue debris, choroid plexus, clot, infection, catheter-tip migration, or following a localized immune response to the tubing. Kinking or disconnection of the tube, pseudocyst formation, or infection can cause distal obstruction. Distal obstruction is the most frequently encountered obstruction in shunts in place for longer than 2 years.[1,2]

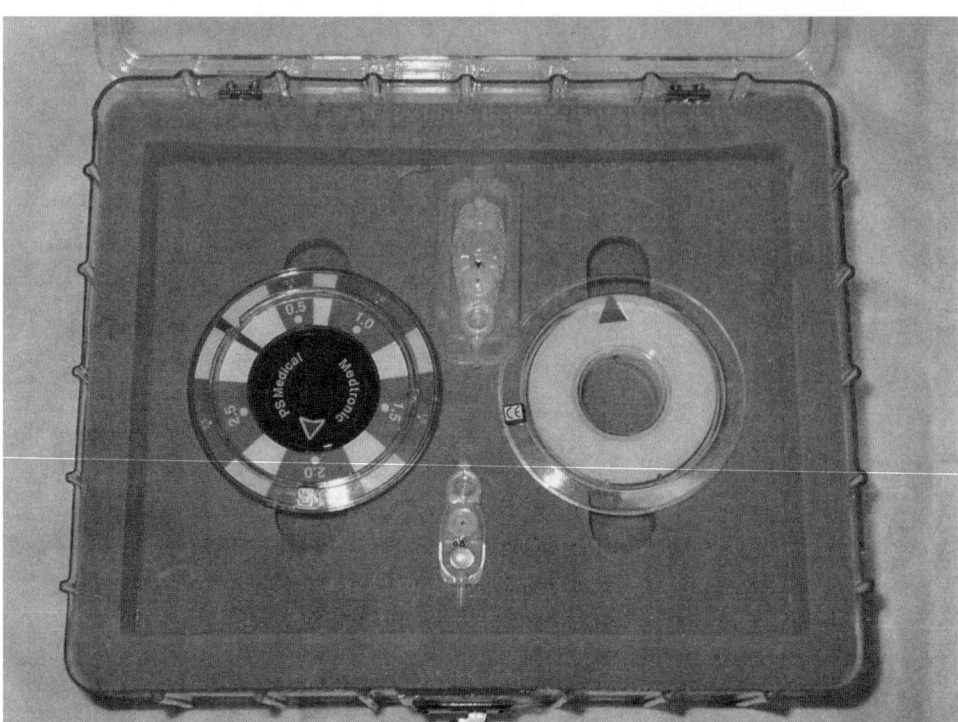

FIG. 236-1. Example of shunt kit. Circular objects on the left are a locator and a pressure/performance indicator. Circular object on right is an adjustment tool. All three are needed to adjust the settings. Two sizes of valves are shown in the middle.

SLIT VENTRICLE SYNDROME   Overdrainage and the slit ventricle syndrome are seen in approximately 5 percent of shunted patients. Because of overdrainage, the tissues actually occlude the orifices of the proximal shunt apparatus. As intracranial pressure increases, the same occluding tissue is disengaged, allowing drainage to resume. This phenomenon is cyclical and is responsible for the episode or waxing and waning aspect of the presenting complaint. Patients present with episodes of elevated intracranial pressure caused by a transient obstruction of the ventricular catheter from a collapsed ventricle. Decreased cerebral compliance may prevent the ventricles from fully expanding as intracranial pressure and volume increase, further contributing to ventricular collapse. Currently used shunt systems with antisiphon devices and improved shunt valves have a lower rate of this complication.[1,2]

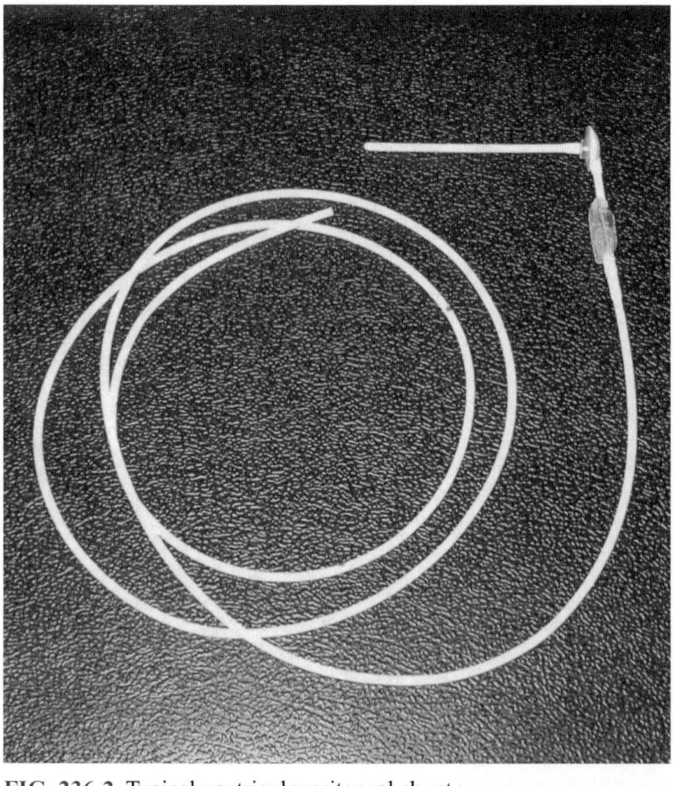

CLINICAL PRESENTATION   Symptoms of shunt malfunction usually develop over several days although rapid deterioration within 24 h has been reported. Clinical features include mental status changes; headache; nausea; vomiting; abdominal pain; lethargy; decreased intellectual performance; ataxia; coma; and autonomic instability. Often, the presenting complaint is vague. No single sign or symptom is accurate in predicting shunt malfunction. Recent analysis of signs and symptoms demonstrated that a decrease in level of consciousness and erythema at the surgical site had the highest correlation with shunt malfunction and infection.[3] As intracranial pressure increases, paralysis of upward gaze or sundowning, dilated pupils and papilledema may develop. "Sundowning" is caused by impingement of the brainstem by the third ventricle as it engorges. Symptoms of slit ventricle syndrome are exacerbated or precipitated by standing or exercise caused by excessive CSF drainage and relieved by lying down or the Trendelenburg position.

SHUNT EVALUATION   Identification of shunt type is important although frequently difficult. Many different types exist and appropriate assessment is dependent on the apparatus implanted. Shunt function is evaluated by manual testing and radiologic studies. Palpation of the shunt allows the physician to locate the valve chamber. Shunt patency is evaluated somewhat differently for each type of device depending on such features as valves, dome or cylinder-shaped reservoirs. Generally, testing follows intuitive expectations but may yet prove perplexing to inexperienced clinicians. For a simple device, once the chamber is located, it is gently compressed and observed for refill. Difficulty compressing the chamber indicates distal flow obstruction, while slow refill, defined as greater than 3 s, following compression indicates a proximal obstruction. Clinicians should realize that **compression is inaccurate in identifying shunt obstruction** as up to 40 percent of obstructed shunts have normal refill during manual palpation.[2] In any case, further evaluation is required.

FIG. 236-2. Typical ventriculoperitoneal shunt.

A shunt series of plain films includes an anteroposterior and lateral radiographs of the skull, and an anteroposterior view of the chest and abdomen (for ventriculoperitoneal shunts). While plain radiography will identify kinking, migration or disconnection of the shunt system, computed tomography (CT) is required to evaluate ventricular size. Comparison to previous CT scans is needed as many shunted patients have an abnormal baseline ventricular size. In one series, using CT, or both CT and plain films, 25 percent of patients with documented shunt malfunction had no radiologic evidence of shunt malfunction.[4] Therefore, in patients with suggestive clinical features, unimpressive CT and/or shunt series cannot be relied on to exclude shunt obstruction. In this instance, neurosurgical consultation should be obtained whenever shunt malfunction is suspected.

A shunt tap may need to be performed to make the diagnosis of shunt malfunction, exclude infection, or to alleviate life threatening increased intracranial pressure. The shunt tap should be performed by a neurosurgeon if available. Emergency physicians should be prepared to perform a shunt tap if a neurosurgeon is unavailable or if a shunt tap is needed to control life-threatening increased intracranial pressure.

To perform a shunt tap, locate and sterilely prepare the site over the valve system or reservoir. Shave the scalp. A 23-gauge needle or butterfly attached to a manometer is inserted into the reservoir. If no fluid returns or flow ceases, a proximal obstruction is likely. The opening pressure should be measured while occluding the reservoir outflow. An opening pressure of 20 cm H_2O or greater indicates a distal obstruction, while low pressures indicate a proximal obstruction. The normal basal intracranial pressure is around 12 ± 2 cm H_2O.

MANAGEMENT Surgical intervention is generally required for shunt obstruction. As a temporizing measure intracranial pressure can be lowered by standard methods-hyperventilation and osmotic diuresis (mannitol). If these measures fail and surgical intervention is not immediately available, one can lower intracranial pressure when the malfunction is distal by removing CSF via the reservoir as previously described. To prevent choroid plexus bleeding, CSF is removed slowly, and the process is discontinued when intracranial pressure reaches 10 to 20 cm H_2O. Stable patients with suspected obstruction require admission and neurosurgical consultation. Patients should be observed for any neurologic changes, abdominal complaints, or development of fever.

Shunt Infection

With improved techniques and shunts, infection rates have decreased to 5 to 8 percent per procedure.[2] The highest rates of infection are found in the very young and old, and in patients who have had multiple shunt revisions. There is no association between shunt type and infection rates.

Half of all shunt infections present within the first 2 weeks of placement, 70 percent present within 2 months, and 80 percent within 6 months of placement. CSF shunt infections can be categorized into internal and external infections. External infections involve the subcutaneous tract around the shunt, which is usually tender and there is often an associated fluid collection within the skin. An internal infection involves the shunt and the CSF contained within that shunt. Patients with CSF shunts have a higher risk of developing meningitis from typical pathogens (e.g., *Haemophilus influenzae, Streptococcus pneumoniae,* and *Neisseria meningitidis*) as compared to the general population. This increased risk may be due to disruption of the blood-brain barrier by foreign material.

If diagnosed and treated in a timely fashion, mortality from shunt infections is low. However, if ventriculitis develops, mortality is 30 to 40 percent, underscoring the need for prompt diagnosis and aggressive management.[1,2]

BACTERIOLOGY CSF shunt infections are typically caused by low-virulence organisms. The most commonly cultured agent is *Staphylo-coccus epidermidis,* which accounts for 50 percent of all shunt infections; *S. aureus,* the next most commonly cultured agent, accounts for 25 percent of all shunt infections. Gram-negative, anaerobic, and mixed infections account for approximately 5 to 10 percent of shunt infections. Gram-negative infections are associated with the highest mortality.

CLINICAL FEATURES The clinical presentation varies with the virulence of the organism and the severity of the infection. Typically, patients will present with obstructive and possibly meningeal symptoms, including mental status changes, headache, nausea, vomiting, and irritability. Fever, meningismus and abdominal pain may also be present. Unfortunately, these signs are not universally present. In fact, the finding of fever is highly variable and meningismus may only be present in only a third of patients with shunt infection.[2] Abdominal pain may be the predominant symptom in patients with ventriculoperitoneal shunts. Swelling, erythema, and tenderness along the site of the shunt tubing are highly suggestive of external shunt infection.

EVALUATION To exclude CSF shunt infection, a shunt tap is required (Figure 236-3) (see "Shunt Malfunction: Shunt Evaluation" above). This procedure should be performed by a neurosurgeon or by an emergency physician only after consultation with a neurosurgeon. **A traditional lumbar puncture often misses CSF shunt infection** and has no meaningful role in the evaluation when shunt infection is suspected.

Analysis of fluid from infected CSF shunts usually reveals an elevated leukocyte count, elevated protein, and normal glucose. Almost one-fifth of patients evaluated for shunt malfunction may have positive CSF culture despite normal CSF analysis. Other (non-CSF) lab values are rarely helpful in diagnosing CSF shunt infection. CT scan and plain radiographs of the shunt (shunt series) are required to exclude mechanical shunt malfunction, which often coexists with shunt infection.[4] Abdominal ultrasonography or CT scan are indicated if an abdominal fluid collection, pseudocyst, or abscess is suspected.

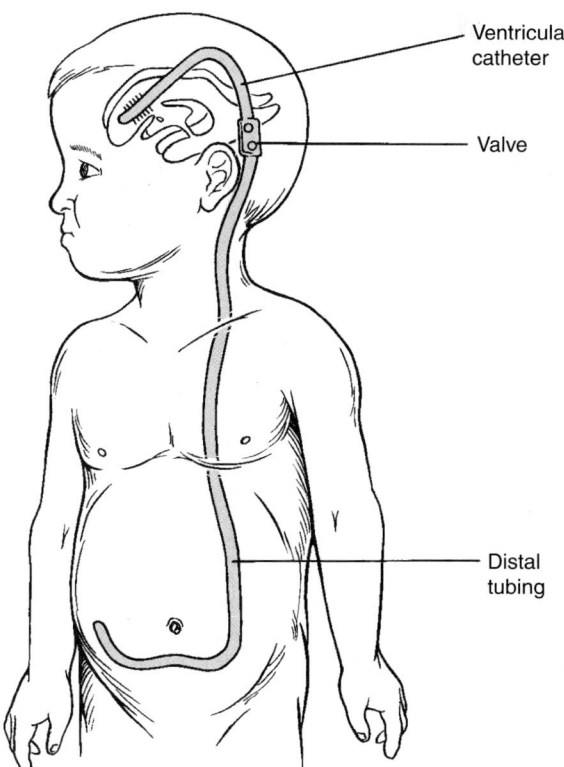

FIG. 236-3. Ventriculoperitoneal shunt system.

MANAGEMENT   All patients with CSF shunt infection or suspected shunt infection require emergent neurosurgical consultation and admission. Most neurosurgeons advocate replacement of the infected shunt, external CSF drainage, and administration of intravenous and intrathecal antibiotics. This combination of therapy has a 96 percent success rate. Until the infecting agent is identified, broad-spectrum antibiotics effective against typical pathogens are recommended (e.g., intravenous third-generation cephalosporin and aminoglycoside, plus intravenous or intrathecal vancomycin). Meningitis caused from typical pathogens has been successfully treated with antibiotics alone.

CHANGES IN AVAILABLE TECHNOLOGY

Many new types of shunts are being clinically tested and some have received FDA approval. Among these, are shunts with magnetically adjustable valves and antimicrobial impregnated shunt systems.

The adjustable valve allows for non-invasive adjustments to valve pressure/performance levels. The valve can be adjusted/tested using a locator and indicator tool to determine the pressure programmed into the valve. An adjustment tool can then be used to dial up or down the valves pressure/performance as needed. Typical nonadjustable pressure type valves are available in low, medium and high settings. These valves open at a pressure gradient of 2 to 4, 4 to 6, and 8 to 10 cm H_2O for the low, medium, and high settings, respectively. The adjustable valves will typically have five preset pressure settings that can be selected or adjusted as clinically warranted. The patient/family should be given a card that will report initial setting and any subsequent adjustments. Pressure setting can also be confirmed by radiography as the dials on the valve are radiopaque.

Exposure to strong magnetic fields and **some magnetic resonance imagings (MRIs) can change the valve pressure setting,** so all patients should have the setting verified after any exposure to strong magnetic fields.

Antimicrobial impregnated catheter systems are being produced to prevent bacterial colonization of newly implanted systems. These systems can diffuse some combination of antimicrobials (clindamycin and rifampin) to reach concentrations high enough to prevent colonization for up to a 1-month period.

Efficacy and complication rates for these new systems are not yet available.

HALO DEVICES

The halo vest provides one of the most rigid types of cervical immobilization available. The halo vest consists of a lightweight radiolucent ring attached to a lightweight adjustable vest. Current vests allow adjustment of the cervical spine in multiple planes. Titanium pins that do not interfere with MRI are stronger, lighter, and more expensive than older stainless steel pins. Pins are usually tightened to 6 to 8 lb.[5,6]

Indications

Halo devices are indicated for stabilization of an unstable cervical spine, including fractures, dislocations, subluxations, and alignment of severe kyphotic and scoliotic spines. A halo is not applied if there is a sensory deficit that extends beneath the halo vest as this leads to a higher risk of skin breakdown and infection. Pin sites are chosen to avoid nerve, vessels, and muscle while attempting to place the pins in the thickest area of calvaria possible. Four pins are usually used. The anterior pins are placed in the frontal or temporal regions. Posterior pins are placed relatively opposite to the anterior pin sites.

Complications

Pin loosening is the most common complication encountered in the emergency department. It occurs in 36 to 60 percent of patients with halo devices.[5–7] Neurosurgical consultation should be obtained, and infection of the pin site excluded. If resistance is met within the first rotations, the pin can usually be retightened to 6 to 8 lb. If no resistance is met, the pin has to be removed. This is usually done by the neurosurgeon after placement of a new pin is completed to avoid any loss of stability in the halo device.

If pin loosening has caused movement of the halo device, assume that the cervical spine is unstable, immobilize the cervical spine using an alternate technique, and obtain plain radiographs to assess for proper alignment. Tangential plain radiographs, CT, or MRI can be used to exclude penetration of a pin through the inner table of the skull.

Pin-site infection is the second most frequently encountered complication. It occurs in approximately 20 to 22 percent of patients with halo devices.[5–7] Careful examination is required to differentiate a localized pin-site infection from less common, more serious infection, such as cellulitis, osteomyelitis, and abscess formation. Patients with cellulitis often have fever, and systemic signs and symptoms of infection. Patients with osteomyelitis usually have a prolonged infection, pin-site loosening, and radiologic abnormalities. Patients who develop an abscess usually have neurologic changes and evidence of intertable penetration (CSF leak, trauma), although cases of asymptomatic brain abscess associated with pin-site infection or pin tightening after late pin loosening have been reported.[8] Local pin-site infections are commonly managed with local wound care. The skin around the pin site must be pulled away to allow thorough cleaning of the skin beneath the pin and skin-pin interface with soap and water four times a day. Culture the wound site. If antibiotics are administered, agents effective against skin pathogens (e.g., *Staphylococcus* and *Streptococcus* species) are used. If local infection does not respond to treatment, or if cellulitis, osteomyelitis, or abscess is suspected, neurosurgical consultation is required for admission, intravenous antibiotics, and possible surgical intervention.

Pin-site discomfort occurs in 18 percent of patients.[5–7] It is most commonly a result of local inflammation. However, infection (localized or systemic) must be considered in each patient. Sensory and motor deficits or paresthesias indicate nerve damage or pressure, while painful mastication indicates temporalis muscle inflammation. If infection is excluded, a short course of analgesics is recommended. Neurosurgical consultation is required if pain continues or a serious complication is suspected.

Ring migration and/or loss of immobilization occurs in 10 to 13 percent of patients.[5–7] Suspect loss of immobilization in patients complaining of neck pain and or mobility, and change in fit or position of the ring or vest. Immediately immobilize the cervical spine using an alternative technique (e.g., hard collar plus backboard). Obtain plain films to assess for changes in alignment and neurosurgical consultation for reapplication of the halo device.

Skin breakdown and pressure sores occur in 4 to 11 percent of patients.[5–7] If present, the vest should be inspected for adequate padding and strap position. Urgent referral to a neurosurgeon for refitting may be required.

Dysphagia occurs in 2 percent of patients.[5–7] Immobilization holding the head in exaggerated extension is the usual cause of the dysphagia. Halo adjustment will remedy this problem. Alternatively, dysphagia can occur following anterior displacement of a bone graft. This diagnosis can be made by plain films and/or a swallowing study and will require emergency surgical intervention.

Dural punctures occur in 1 percent of patients and are a result of halo system trauma.[5–8] Symptoms include headache, malaise, or visual changes. Physical exam may reveal a CSF leak or evidence of skull fracture. All patients require admission and neurosurgical consultation. Treatment includes elevation of head, intravenous antibiotics, and pin removal.

Cardiopulmonary resuscitation is rarely required in patients with halo devices. To perform chest compressions, remove the anterior portion of the vest. Instructions for removing the halo vest are printed on the front of most vests. Intubation is performed with the halo in place. If orotracheal intubation is unsuccessful, attempt nasotracheal intubation (if respirations are present) or cricothyrotomy.

OTHER CENTRAL NERVOUS SYSTEM DEVICES

Intrathecal Baclofen Infusions

Generalized dystonia occurs in 15 to 25 percent of patients with cerebral palsy. These patients typically respond poorly to medical and surgical treatment plans aimed at controlling their dystonia. Baclofen, a γ-aminobutyric acid agonist that acts at the level of the spinal cord by impeding the release of excitatory neurotransmitters, decreases spasticity. Oral baclofen offers patients only mild relief because of its inability to cross the blood-brain barrier and because it is poorly lipid soluble. Intrathecal administration is more effective, requires lower doses, and leads to higher CSF levels. Intrathecal baclofen reduces spasticity, improves gait, sitting ability, and upper extremity function in most patients.[9–12] Complications observed in patients receiving continuous intrathecal baclofen include hypotension; bradycardia; apnea; oversedation; respiratory depression; pump pocket effusions; mechanical failure; catheter extrusion; kinking; dislodgement; local infection; meningitis; and CSF fistula formation. Newly available intrathecal catheters cause fewer complications compared to original catheters. More experience is needed with continuous intrathecal baclofen to determine the long-term benefits. Complication occur in approximately 20 to 38 percent of cases, while infection requiring removal occurs in approximately 5 percent of cases.[9–13] Concerns about baclofen pumps should always be directed to the neurologist.

Implantable CNS Stimulators

The pathogenesis of Parkinson disease is thought to involve unregulated activity of the subthalamic nucleus and globus pallidus intermedius. Neurophysiologists have shown that high-frequency stimulation can reversibly inactivate nerve conduction in these areas.[14,15]

High-frequency stimulation with implantable CNS devices are being used for suppression of parkinsonian and essential tremors. Neurostimulation is typically used if drug therapy has failed to control tremors. Neurostimulation is as efficient at controlling tremors as classic thalamotomy, but is less invasive.

Limited studies suggest that neurostimulation has a lower risk of physical or cognitive impairment compared to thalamotomy Reported complication rates range from 7 to 65 percent, with a decline in the number of reported complications as user experience increases.[16] Patients may present to the emergency department with varied complaints including problems related to the subcutaneous pulse generator, temporary or permanent paresthesias, dysarthria, dysequilibrium, or failure of the neurostimulator to suppress tremors. Neurosurgical consultation is needed as these complaints may represent lead displacement or migration requiring surgical correction or replacement. If the diagnosis remains uncertain, observation may be required with the stimulator in the off position to help differentiate mechanical failure from an acute neurologic deficit.[14–16]

Spinal Cord Stimulation

Spinal cord stimulation is an established modality for treating chronic back pain, angina pectoris, and the pain syndromes associated with vascular disease. Multicontact electrodes are placed in the epidural space, and the distal end of the electrode is connected to an internalized pulse generator. The therapeutic response is thought to be a result of stimulation of one of several dorsal tracts. Reported complications include the need for surgical revision and infection. Surgical revisions

have been reported to be as high as 50 percent within 3 years of implantation.[17] The most common reasons for revision include electrode replacement or repositioning, generator replacement, cable failure, and implant removal. Infection at the either the generator, cable, or electrode are reported to be as high as 8.6 percent.[17]

REFERENCES

1. Blount JP, Campbell JA: Complications in ventricular cerebrospinal fluid shunting. *Neurosurg Clin N Am* 4:633, 1993.
2. Key CB, Rothrock SG: Cerebrospinal fluid shunt complications: An emergency medicine perspective. *Pediatr Emerg Care* 11:265, 1995.
3. Garton HJ: Predicting shunt failure on the basis of clinical symptoms and signs in children. *J Neurosurg* 94:202, 2001.
4. Iskandad BD, McLaughlin C: Pitfalls in the diagnosis of ventricular shunt dysfunction: Radiology reports and ventricular size. *Pediatrics* 101:1031, 1998.
5. Manthey DE: Halo traction device. *Emerg Med Clin North Am* 12:771, 1994.
6. Botte MS, Bynne TP: The halo skeletal fixator: Current concepts of application and maintenance. *Orthopedics* 18:463, 1995.
7. Glaser JN, Whitehall R: Complications associated with the halo vest. *J Neurosurg* 65:762, 1986.
8. Kameyama O: Asymptomatic brain abscess as a complication of halo orthosis: Report of a case and review of the literature. *J Orthop Sci* 4:39, 1999.
9. Albright AL, Barry MJ: Infusion of intrathecal baclofen for generalized dystonia in cerebral palsy. *J Neurosurg* 88:73, 1998.
10. Armstrong RW, Steinbok P: Intrathecally administered baclofen for treatment of children with spasticity of cerebral origin. *J Neurosurg* 87:409, 1997.
11. Albright AL: Intrathecal baclofen in cerebral palsy movement disorders. *J Child Neurol* 11:29, 1996.
12. Albright AL: Baclofen in the treatment of cerebral palsy. *J Child Neurol* 11:77, 1996.
13. Albright AL: Intrathecal baclofen in the treatment of dystonia. *Dev Med Child Neurol* 43:652, 2001.
14. Krack P, Pollack P: Opposite motor effects of pallidal stimulation in Parkinson's disease. *Ann Neurol* 43:180, 1998.
15. Benabid AL, Pollack P: Acute and long-term effects of subthalamic nucleus stimulation in Parkinson's disease. *Sterotact Funct Neurosurg* 62:76, 1994.
16. Joint C: Hardware related problems of deep brain stimulation. *Mov Disord* 17:5175, 2002.
17. Kayad: Spinal cord stimulation a long term evaluation in patients with chronic pain. *Br J Neurosurg* 15:335, 2001.

APPROACH TO NEUROIMAGING IN THE EMERGENCY DEPARTMENT
Maria G. Matheus
Norman J. Beauchamp, Jr.

GENERAL OVERVIEW OF COMMON TECHNIQUES

Although a more thorough discussion of techniques is provided in other chapters of this textbook, a brief introduction to the more common techniques will be beneficial to understanding the optimal approach to cranial neuroimaging.

Plain films remain the first-line imaging technique. X-rays generate two-dimensional images based on attenuation of a collimated beam. The attenuation is proportional to the electron density of the structures through which it passes, with the final image reflective of tissue density. This results in high spatial resolution and thus sensitivity for the detection of fractures. However, detection of abnormalities requires that there be no obscuration of the region of interest by overlying bone or other dense material. Thus whereas a skull fracture of the calvaria is often readily detected, a fracture involving the skull base is typically obscured due to overlying bone. Plain films also provide a coarse view of the extracranial soft tissues, but intracranial soft tissues are obscured. Because the primary goal of ED neuroimaging is the detection of intracranial soft tissue abnormalities, the role of plain films is largely limited to the primary assessment of spinal trauma, the assessment of some facial fractures, assessment of some subtle, linear skull fractures oriented in the axial plane of acquisition, or as part of the skeletal survey for child abuse.

Computed tomography (CT) has largely supplanted plain films for neuroimaging. CT images are generated using a rotating x-ray tube that projects a collimated beam through the brain with resultant attenuation of the beam proportional to the electron density (tissue density) of the tissue through which it passes. Thus rather than interrogating the tissue of interest from one direction (as in conventional x-rays), computerized processing of the circumferentially projected attenuated rays enables reconstruction of tissue maps largely unobscured by overlying tissues. Differentiation of adjacent tissues such as bone, gray and white matter, and cerebrospinal fluid (CSF) is possible due to perceptible differences in tissue density. Vasogenic and cytotoxic edema and hemorrhage alter the density of the tissue affected, making CT highly sensitive in the detection of disease. Further, the fine anatomic detail enables detection of morphologic alterations such as fractures and parenchymal swelling.

Magnetic resonance imaging (MRI) involves placing a patient inside an externally applied magnetic field. The nuclei of the tissues are aligned by the powerful magnetic field. Due to its odd number of nuclides and its abundance in our bodies, hydrogen is the major element responsible for the signal production in MRI. The "magnetized" hydrogen atoms are "energized" by the input of an applied radiofre-quency pulse, and the pattern of energy released provides information about the biophysical properties of the tissue being evaluated. Depending on the way that the radiofrequency pulse is applied, different sequences in an MRI are generated. The different MR sequences allow the characterization of shifts in water (hydrogen) distribution. All pathologic processes alter the biophysical properties (shift in water distribution of the affected tissue). Detectable changes in the biophysical properties occur prior to a detectable change in tissue density. Thus MRI is more sensitive than CT in detecting parenchymal pathologic processes such as cerebral ischemia, infection, or metastases. Equally important is that the presence of certain blood products (deoxy- and methemoglobin, hemosiderin) develops over time postbleeding. These cause a detectable alteration in local magnetic field. MRI and CT thus are nearly equivalent in the detection of fresh bleeding, but MRI is much more sensitive in the detection of static blood. Blood becomes CT isodense with the brain parenchyma around 7 to 10 days postbleed, but can generate an abnormal magnetic field for months to years. Lastly, MRI enables multiplanar acquisition while the patient remains supine. In the majority of the available CTs, imaging requires patient positioning specific for the plane of interest. This can be difficult for the very young, the elderly, and for trauma patients. Multidetector CT can acquire the images in an axial plane and reconstruct the images in a multiplanar isotropic fashion.

Notably, cortical bone is relatively depleted of hydrogen. Thus the cortex of bone is nearly invisible on MRI. Although this is of benefit in that parenchyma can be assessed without compromise from adjacent dense bone (e.g., infratemporal region and posterior fossa assessment is slightly limited in CT due to artifact from the adjacent skull base) (Figures 237-1A and 237-1B), MRI is inadequate for the assessment of bone integrity. Compared to CT, MRI may not be available to

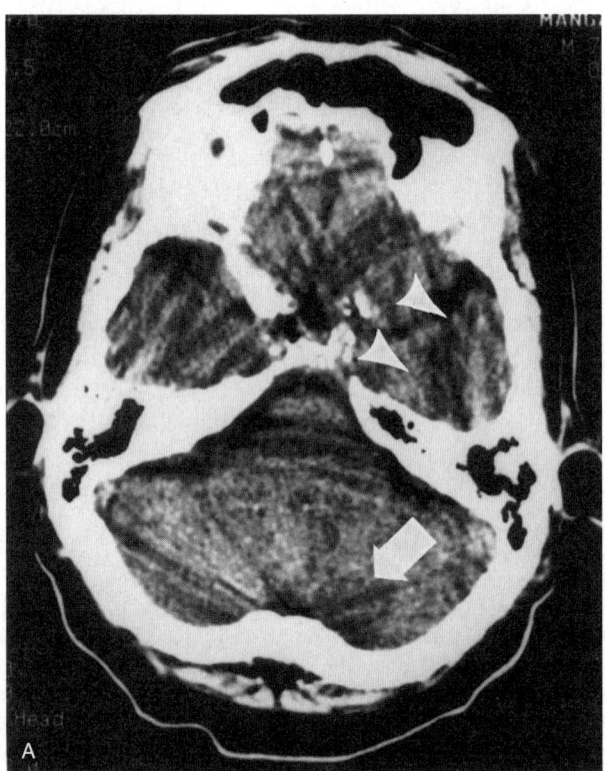
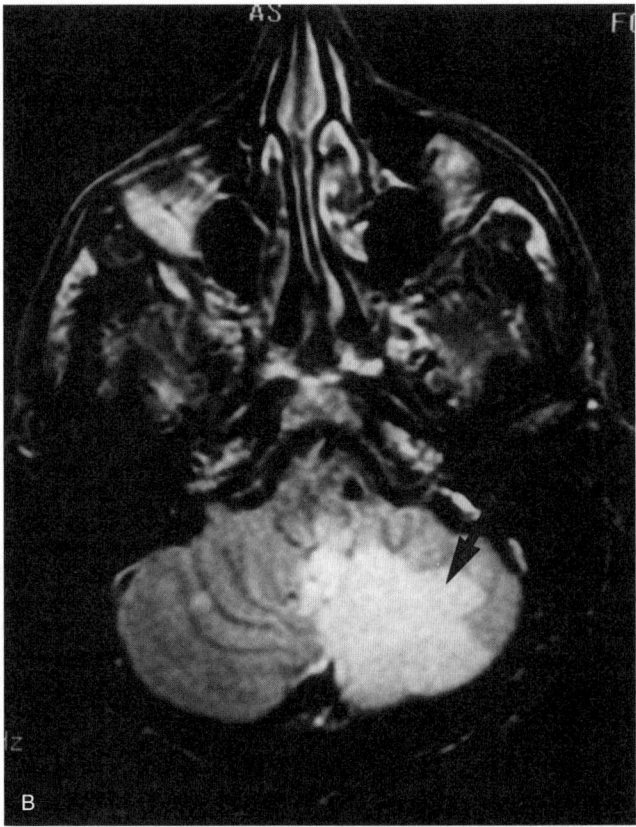

FIG. 237-1. A. Axial CT obtained in a patient presenting with a left cerebellar infarct. Initial CT demonstrates a focal area of decreased attenuation in the left cerebellar hemisphere that is difficult to detect due to artifact generated by adjacent bone *(arrow)*. Incidental note is made of similar obscuration of the inferior temporal lobe by artifact *(arrowheads)*. **B.** Axial MRI clearly demonstrates an area of infarction in the left cerebellum. Visualization is clear with no artifact generated despite proximity to bone.

many emergency departments. MRI is also contraindicated in the presence of devices such as pacemakers, cochlear implants, and metallic foreign matter near vital structures; requires greater patient cooperation; and prevents monitoring of critically ill patients. As a result, despite its superior sensitivity to most pathologic processes, MRI plays an important but more limited role when compared to CT in the ED.

Ultrasound generates images based on transmittance of sound waves. In general, sonographic imaging enables evaluation of soft tissue structures provided that air or bone does not obscure the area of interest. In neuroimaging, most of the structures of interest are obscured by the calvaria. However, in infants, patency of the fontanelle provides an adequate sonographic window, enabling high sensitivity for the detection of intracranial masses, hemorrhages, or hydrocephalus. In infants and very young children, ultrasound is the study of choice for intracranial assessment. Ultrasound can also be used to assess traumatic globe injury or masses. However, this technique is highly operator-dependent, is limited in the assessment of the orbital apex, and is typically performed by an ophthalmologist. Finally, ultrasound images can be generated in which flowing blood produces color images scaled to flow velocity. These images give information on lumen caliber and hemodynamic alterations (such as occur with a distal occlusion or proximal stenosis). Ultrasound has become the screening technique of choice in assessing common carotid bifurcation atherosclerotic disease. Transcranial Doppler and power Doppler ultrasound enable assessment of the most distal aspects of the internal carotid arteries, the proximal cerebral arteries, the circle of Willis, and the superficial parenchyma. Assessment of the posterior circulation and deeper parenchyma remains limited.

The vasculature can also be assessed noninvasively with CT angiography (CTA) or MR angiography (MRA). CTA and MRA are appealing techniques because they are noninvasive and can be incorporated into a comprehensive CT or MR examination with minimal additional time or difficulty (Figures 237-2A and 237-3B). MRA utilizes a gradient echo pulse sequence that results in increased intravascular signal intensity with normal flow. CTA is performed following the peripheral venous administration of iodinated contrast. An image similar to a conventional arteriogram can be reconstructed from the axial images. Both are sensitive to large vessel occlusion or narrowing in the internal carotid, vertebral, basilar, and first and second segments of the anterior, middle, and posterior cerebral arteries. Furthermore, both techniques can be modified to look at venous structures (i.e., CT venography or MR venography). CTA requires less patient cooperation, with an assessment of the vasculature complete in approximately 30 s. However, vascular detail is limited when vessels are in direct apposition to bone. Vascular assessment with MRA is not limited in the presence of bone. It is useful for assessing the vertebral arteries as they course through the bony transverse foramina and skull base, and in assessing the cephalad course of the internal carotid artery.

Both CTA and MRA techniques have greatly improved in the last decade, but resolution is still considered inferior to catheter angiography. Both noninvasive methods approach 90 percent accuracy for detection of aneurysms larger than 3 mm, but for small aneurysms (less than 3 mm) the sensitivity of these methods drops sharply to 61 percent and 38 percent for CTA and MRA, respectively.[1] CTA can assess the neck of the aneurysm, enabling appropriate planning for endovascular therapy. The primary use of both techniques is as a screening tool for vascular occlusion, and generally they should be supplemented with catheter angiography when clinical suspicion remains (see Figures 237-3A and 237-3B).

Catheter angiography utilizes plain x-rays in conjunction with administration of intraarterial contrast through a catheter placed in the femoral artery and positioned proximal to the vasculature to be assessed. The intraarterial contrast delineates vascular anatomy and

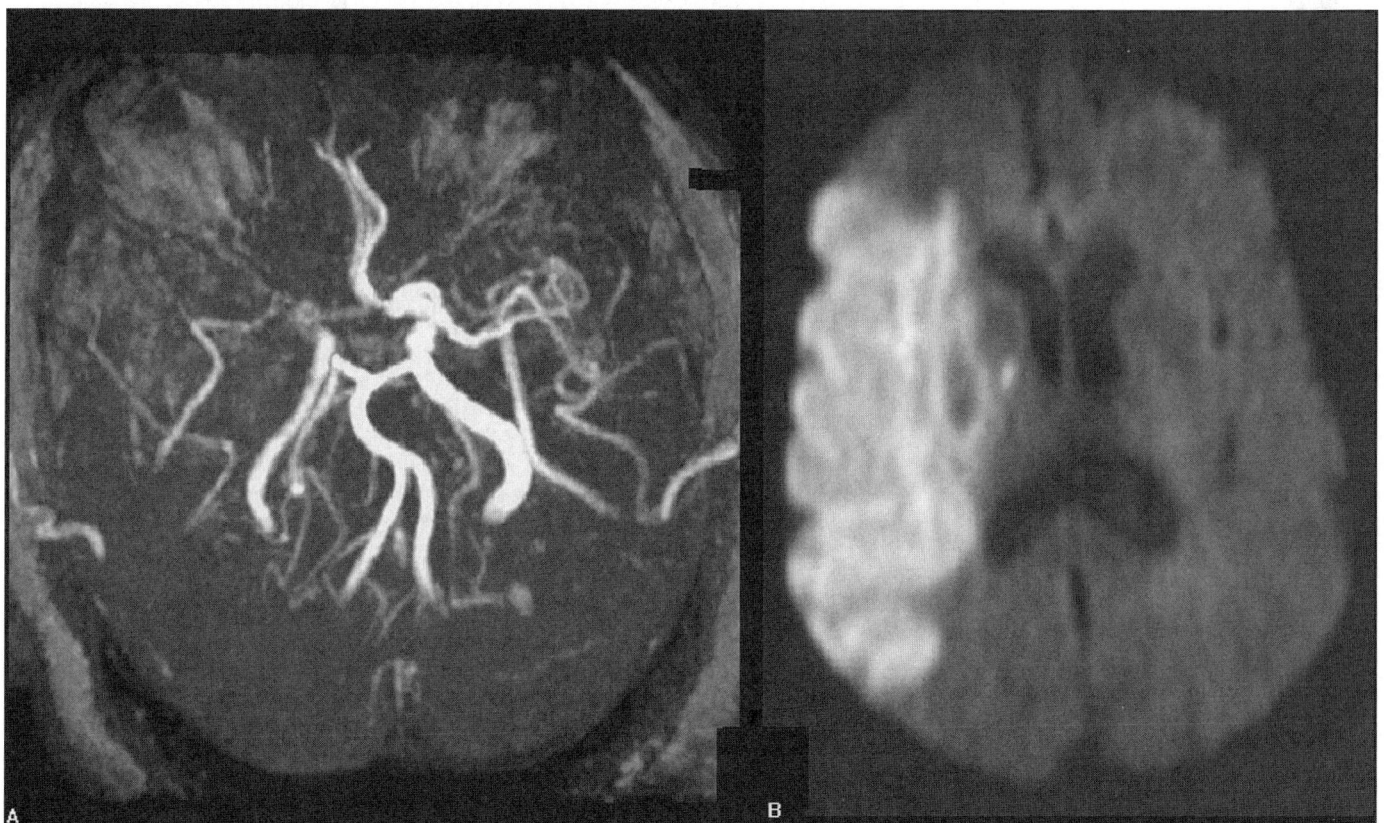

FIG. 237-2. A. MR angiogram demonstrates occlusion of the right internal carotid artery. **B.** MR diffusion-weighted image of the same patient, less than 6 h after the onset, demonstrates conspicuous high signal intensity in right frontotemporal region and basal ganglia corresponding to an infarcted area with restriction of the water's random motion. The image has low resolution but high contrast and the lesion is easily seen.

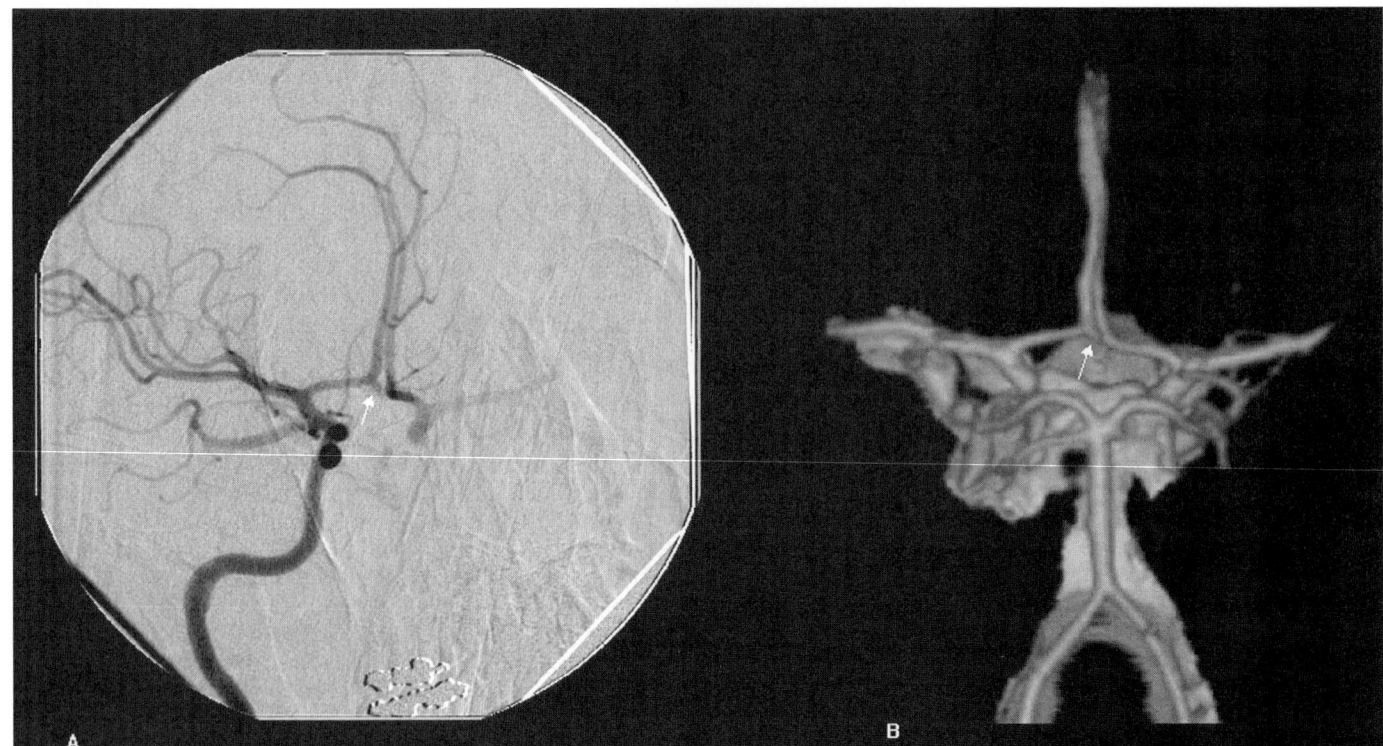

FIG. 237-3. A. Oblique view from a catheter angiogram demonstrates a small anterior communicating artery aneurysm less than 3 mm in diameter *(arrow).* **B.** In the same patient, CT angiogram shows a small irregularity in the anterior communicating artery *(arrow).* The small size of the aneurysm, the overlapping of the vessels, and its proximity with the clinoid process and sphenoid bone made the assessment of the aneurysm on the CTA image difficult.

detects pathologic changes such as narrowing and occlusion. It is the definitive procedure for assessment of the intra- and extracranial vasculature. However, there is a 1 to 2 percent risk of stroke associated with catheter angiography.

Near-infrared spectroscopy (NIRS) measures changes in absorbance of an infrared light beam projected transcranially. Specifically, near-infrared light (700 to 1000 nm) has relatively good transcranial penetration, and hemoglobin (Hb) has characteristic absorption spectra. The absorbance of light is dependent on the presence of Hb and the oxygen content of the Hb. Thus this technology can be used to assess for the presence of hemorrhage and to assess the oxygen state of the superficial microcirculation. For example, in one investigation, 24 of 27 patients with delayed traumatic intracranial hemorrhages demonstrated increases in the NIRS absorbance.[2] NIRS units are portable and relatively inexpensive, but the role for NIRS remains to be determined.

Radioisotope scans are performed following the administration of radioisotopes that emit photons. Photon imaging studies can be used to assess ventriculoperitoneal shunt patency, CSF leaks, hydrocephalus, Ommaya reservoirs, and brain death. Anatomic scans can also be performed that enable detection of space-occupying lesions. In general, nuclear medicine neuroimaging studies are infrequently utilized in the ED setting due to the superior resolution, increased availability, and expedience of CT and MR.

The remainder of this review focuses on guiding principles for the assessment of the most common emergency neurologic complaints.

HEADACHE

Subarachnoid Hemorrhage

Recommendations for which subset of patients with acute headache requires some form of neuroimaging are as varied as they are numerous. However, neuroimaging has been accepted as the standard of care in specific clinical situations (Table 237-1). In addition to atypical headache (associated with neurologic signs), severity of headache is an indicator for imaging. Specifically, acute onset of the "worst headache of my life" raises concern for subarachnoid hemorrhage. Identification is essential because rupture of an intracranial aneurysm is the most common cause of nontraumatic subarachnoid hemorrhage. Furthermore, if subarachnoid hemorrhage (SAH) remains undetected, there is a 50 percent 2-week risk of rebleeding with an associated 50 percent mortality. In this instance, nonenhanced head CT is the recommended study (Figure 237-4). Its sensitivity in the detection of SAH is within 93 to 100 percent if performed within 12 to 24 h of the event.[3] In addition to the demonstration of high-density acute blood in the subarachnoid spaces, it also demonstrates other manifestations of SAH, including intraventricular and intraparenchymal hemorrhage and hydrocephalus. With small amounts of acute hemorrhage, SAH can be overlooked and the sensitivity of CT decreases to about 80 percent after 24 h,[3] and continues to diminish significantly over time to less than 30 percent 3 days postrupture.

Conventional MRI technique (conventional gradient and spin-echo T1- and T2-weighted images) does not demonstrate SAH well. FLAIR sequence (fluid attenuation inversion recovery sequence) is an MRI technique that enables identification of SAH in subacute and even in acute periods, because the CSF signal becomes brighter in the presence

TABLE 237-1   Considerations for Nonenhanced Head CT for Headache

Unexplained mental status change or focal neurologic signs
"Worst headache of life" of sudden onset
Unexplained fever
Meningismus
Extremes of vital signs (blood pressure, bradycardia, or respiratory rate, although seldom an isolated finding)

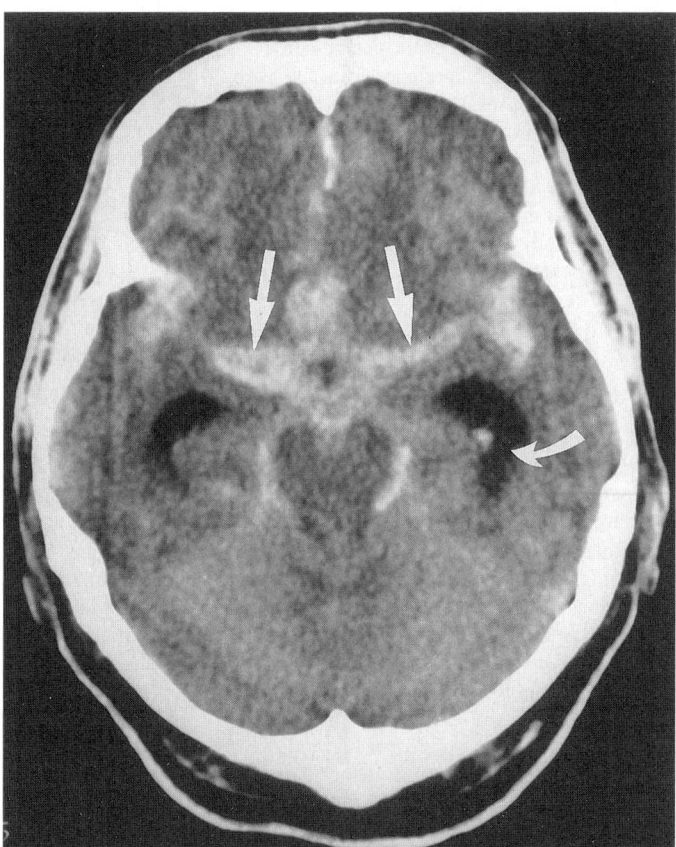

FIG. 237-4. Axial CT demonstrates areas of increased density compatible with subarachnoid hemorrhage (SAH) *(straight arrows)*. There is also early hydrocephalus with the temporal horns dilated *(curved arrow)*.

of blood. Unfortunately FLAIR imaging is somewhat limited in the posterior fossa and around the circle of Willis because of motion artifact. FLAIR is useful for SAH surrounding the hemisphere.[4] If the CT is negative and FLAIR is not available, lumbar puncture is necessary. A positive CT or lumbar puncture requires conventional angiography.

Headache and Fever

Headache associated with unexplained fever is also an indication for neuroimaging, particularly when there is associated meningismus and photophobia. Although diagnosis is made by lumbar puncture, imaging is typically recommended to exclude mass effect or hydrocephalus. Despite the absence of scientific validation, it has become the standard of care to precede lumbar puncture with nonenhanced CT (NECT) of the head. Secondary hydrocephalus tends not to obviate performing lumbar puncture, but it will lead the physician to performing a low-volume lumbar puncture. Further, it can alert to the possible need for shunt placement.

Hydrocephalus

Acute or recurrent hydrocephalus can present with headache as well as nausea, incontinence, and ataxia. There is generally an increase in the intraventricular volume. Hydrocephalus can be caused by a number of processes, including prior subarachnoid hemorrhage, prior trauma, meningitis, masses obstructing the ventricular system, or masses external to the ventricles but causing obstructing compression due to size or edema. In the evaluation of patients with suspected hydrocephalus, NECT is an adequate evaluation. It will enable detection of patients requiring emergency placement of intraventricular shunt catheters. If hydrocephalus is identified and the etiology remains undefined, a contrast-enhanced MRI examination with its superior ability to image

in multiple planes should be performed. Lastly, in examining patients with an intraventricular shunt catheter and suspected recurrent hydrocephalus, the NECT should be accompanied with a plain film shunt series. The latter will detect possible kinks or disruptions of the catheter (see Chap. 236 for detailed discussion).

Mass CNS Lesion

Generally, an intraparenchymal mass large enough to cause headache will be associated with neurologic signs prior to, or concurrent with, the development of headache. Thus in instances in which tumors are associated with headache, they are large and readily detectable on NECT; indirect effects, such as obstruction of CSF outflow, will also be evident on NECT.

MENTAL STATUS CHANGE

The issue of whether to image patients under the influence of alcohol or other substances in order to consider other etiologies as a possible explanation for mental status change frequently arises in ED practice. The approach is discussed in detail in Chap. 229. Generally, patients with a Glasgow Coma Scale (GCS) score of 13 or less, those that fail to improve with time, or those in whom alcohol or drug levels are not in keeping with the clinical findings, require imaging.

CNS Tumor

An initial NECT can be performed in patients with mental status changes who also have a known primary tumor, or who have a suspected metastasis or primary brain tumor. This will suffice to detect lesions resulting in mental status change, such as marked cerebral edema, herniation, and intracranial hemorrhage, that require emergent intervention. However, the optimal choice of imaging is based on the availability of imaging resources as well as the clinical suspicion. For example, contrast MRI is the more sensitive test and is typically required for patients in whom clinical concern persists, even if the initial CT is normal. However, if MRI resources are immediately available and the patient is stable, it could be more appropriate in some instances of high suspicion to proceed directly to MRI and avoid unnecessary time delay and additional imaging costs to the patient. Contrast-enhanced CT subjects patients to the small but unnecessary risk of iodinated contrast and is less sensitive than MRI.

Encephalitis

Proceeding directly to imaging with MRI when available is also indicated with certain cerebral infections. Encephalitis presents as acute mental status change and fever. Herpes encephalitis from HSV-1 is a particularly devastating form, but it can have a good clinical outcome if diagnosed and treated early in the course of the disease. Herpes often has a characteristic appearance in which the temporal lobes are first affected (Figure 237-5). Due to the difficulties assessing parenchyma in direct apposition to bone structures, detection of the subtle early findings of cytotoxic edema involving the temporal lobes can be difficult when utilizing NECT in the first 3 days. Sensitivity is not increased by the addition of intravenous contrast. Conversely, MR is highly sensitive to the early manifestations of encephalitis. It is often positive in the first 24 h and can be helpful in expeditious diagnosis.

HIV-Positive Patient

The approach to imaging the HIV-positive patient with mental status change is greatly debated. There is a tendency to provide an emergent screening examination with NECT followed by nonemergent performance of contrast-enhanced MRI as indicated. Using this approach, processes creating vasogenic edema and those requiring immediate intervention, such as toxoplasmosis and lymphoma, will undoubtedly be

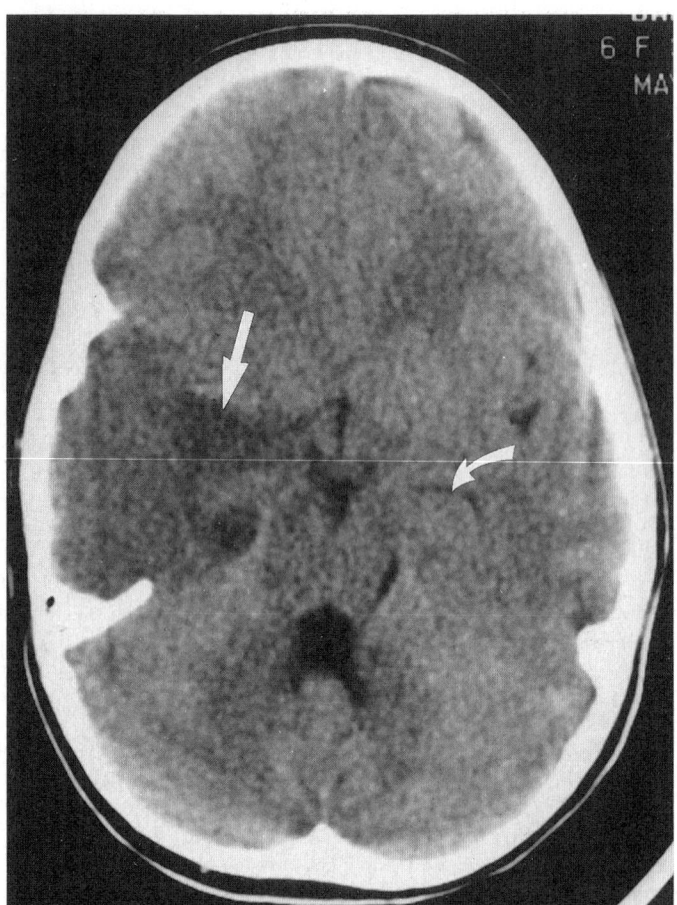

FIG. 237-5. Axial CT scan demonstrates decreased attenuation in the right temporal lobe *(straight arrow)*. In a young patient with acute-onset mental status change, this is highly suggestive of herpes encephalitis. Note the normal left temporal horn *(curved arrow)* as compared to the effaced right temporal horn.

detected. However, further investigation using contrast MRI is often requested to better characterize these lesions and for the detection of HIV encephalopathy and progressive multifocal leukoencephalopathy. A cost-effective approach of proceeding directly to MRI has also been recommended. This largely depends on the institutional availability of MRI and the management practices of clinicians.

SEIZURES

In recurrent seizures, determination of a sole cause such as noncompliance typically eliminates the need for imaging. Similarly, neuroimaging is not indicated for the evaluation of children with simple febrile seizures. However, the optimal approach for the evaluation of first-time seizures is debated.[5,6] The American College of Emergency Physicians Special Panel suggests CT scanning for first-time seizures.

CT is nearly 100 percent sensitive for etiologies of seizures that require emergent intervention, such as brain abscesses, hemorrhage, or other space-occupying lesions. However, the neurologist may additionally request multiplanar MRI emergently or electively, depending on the clinical situation, although not necessarily while the patient is in the ED.

STROKE

Determining the optimal approach to imaging cerebral infarction is becoming increasingly complex, and is thus relevant to the discussion of modality selection in neuroimaging.

U.S. Food and Drug Administration (FDA) guidelines require performance of a NECT prior to the institution of thrombolytic therapy.

Intravenous contrast administration is of limited value in the CT evaluation of acute stroke. Contrast enhancement is generally not seen during the first 3 days. Experience from the European Cooperative Acute Stroke Trial (ECASS) has demonstrated that efficacy of treatment is contingent on accurate CT interpretation.[7] Specifically, treated patients who had evidence of infarction on CT had a worsened outcome. Such patients should be excluded from treatment. However, identifying this contraindication can be challenging because the signs of infarction initially are quite subtle. For example, trained readers did not detect 12 percent of areas of advanced infarction in the ECASS study.[7] Optimal treatment is most likely to occur when all members of the treatment team are familiar with the early signs of infarction (Table 237-2). Briefly, the presence of hemorrhage or evidence of progressive infarct are contraindications to treatment (Figure 237-6). The sensitivity of CT for the detection of hemorrhage has been previously discussed. An important sign of acute stroke is the hyperdense middle cerebral artery sign (HMCAS). This may correspond to a thrombus. The early CT findings of infarction are due to cytotoxic edema—cellular injury with influx of fluid in the intracellular space. The four CT signs that can be seen in the acute period are: 1) blurring of the clarity of the internal capsule; 2) loss of distinctness of the insular ribbon cortex; 3) loss of differentiation between the cortical gray and the subjacent white matter; and 4) swelling of the cortical gray matter resulting in effacement of interposed sulci. In addition to the attenuation changes, morphologic changes occur due to the accumulation of intracellular fluid, causing swelling of the cortical gyri. This results in effacement of the spaces demarcated by the gyral infoldings (sulci) and is referred to as "sulcal effacement." The extent of these changes determines whether treatment with thrombolysis is indicated.

MR has a greater sensitivity and specificity than CT for the acute changes of stroke. In the first 24 h, over 80 percent of MR scans are positive as compared to 60 percent of CT scans. MR is particularly superior for the detection of stroke in the posterior fossa, where CT is limited due to a beam-hardening artifact from the adjacent skull base (see Figure 237-1). The earliest MR changes are morphologic swelling of the gray matter, increased signal intensity on the T2-weighted images and spin density-weighted images (referred to as T2 hyperintensity), and loss of normal intravascular flow voids (see Chap. 305 for details on the physics of MR). More importantly, MRI can be combined with MRA for the detection of large-vessel occlusion (see Figure 237-2A).

Newer MRI techniques can provide physiologic information about brain tissue. Diffusion-weighted sequences (MRD) are pulse sequences sensitive to small-scale water-molecule motion (i.e., diffusion). The principle is to apply sequential gradient pulses to a spin-echo sequence. Image construction is based on the degree of signal

TABLE 237-2   CT Appearance Exclusion and Inclusion Criteria for the Administration of Recombinant Tissue Plasminogen Activator (rtPA) in Patients Presenting within 3 Hours of Ictus

Grade 0—Normal CT
Grade 1—Possible early signs of infarction: May still give rtPA depending
  on the clinician's judgment
  Vague blurring of gray-white boundaries
  Slight attenuation of the insular ribbon
  Slight indistinctness of basal ganglia gray matter
  Suggestion of crowding of sulci
Grade 2—Subtle but definite signs of early infarction: likely will not treat
  Same as above except findings are distinct
Grade 3—Prominent signs of early infarction: contraindication to treatment
  Mass effect—i.e., ventricular effacement, subfalcine or uncal herniation
  Clearly-demonstrated hypodensity
  Intracranial hemorrhage
  Note: In the ECASS study, the major early signs of infarction included:
  diffuse swelling of the affected hemisphere and effacement of the cerebral
  sulci in more than 33% of the middle cerebral artery territory.

Note: Based on recommendations by the American Heart Association and experience from the NINDS and ECASS Trials.

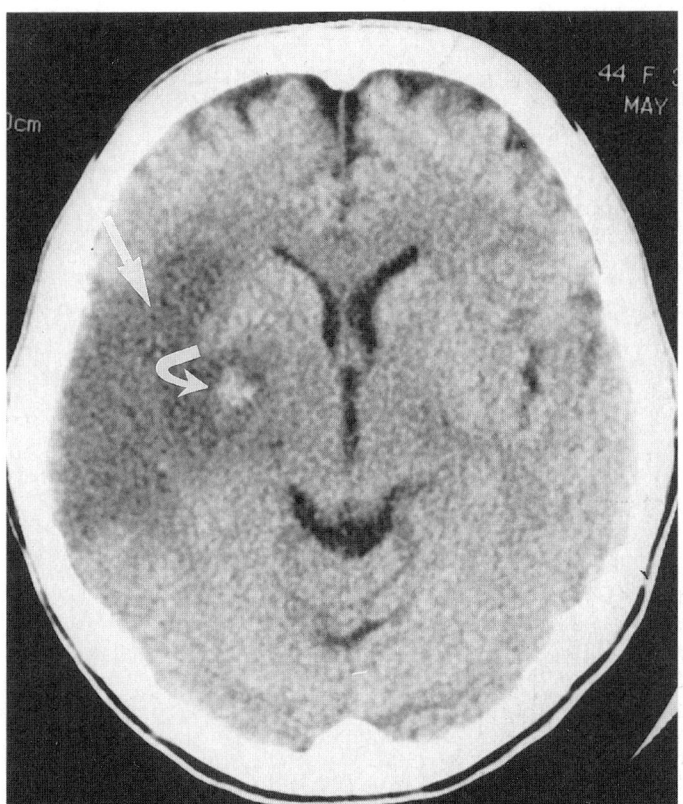

FIG. 237-6. Axial CT demonstrating clear evidence of decreased attenuation compatible with infarction *(straight arrow).* Also, there is a focal area of hemorrhage *(curved arrow),* which further obviates thrombolysis.

drop, proportional to microscopic water motion (Brownian motion). Areas with restricted motion, such as areas of acute infarction, undergo loss of signal at a slower range than does normal tissue. These changes can be detected within the first hour of infarction as conspicuous high signal intensity in diffusion-weighted sequences (see Figure 237-2B). Mathematical tools can create an ADC map (apparent diffusion coefficient map), which compares normal and affected tissue and highlights the area of infarction as dark.[8]

The mechanism of abnormal diffusion is thought to be due to: 1) alterations in the sodium/potassium pump that lead to increased intracellular water accumulation and restriction of normal random motion; or 2) a decrease in the extracellular space with increased tortuosity of the extracellular compartment.

MR perfusion is a physiologic imaging method useful to demonstrate hyperacute cerebral infarction. It is performed following the bolus administration of intravascular contrast, with changes in signal intensity that can reflect the status of the cerebral microvasculature.[9] Perfusion can be combined with echo planar spin-echo and gradient echo-techniques and can improve vessel visualization. Diffusion and perfusion MR techniques together can dramatically improve the ability to determine extent of infarction and thus should improve the safety profile of recombinant tissue-type plasminogen activator (rtPA) administration.

Neither clinical examination nor conventional CT or conventional MRI techniques provide information on the ischemic penumbra. MR perfusion, CT perfusion, and MR spectroscopic (MRS) imaging appear capable of providing this information (see Chap. 305). When ischemia is present, MR perfusion imaging shows a delay in peak signal loss in the affected area. The region with hypoperfusion does not necessarily correspond in size with the infarcted area. The mismatch in size between the area with cytotoxic edema (visualized in the diffusion-weighted images) and the hypoperfused area may correlate with the penumbra area (tissue that could be saved with early reperfusion). CT perfusion correlates the early stroke signs visualized by NECT with the perfusion maps acquired after contrast injection to assess penumbra area.[10]

MRS generates maps of hydrogen spectra containing major resonances from *N*-acetyl aspartate (NAA), choline, creatine, and lactate.[11] Signals from lactate are not normally detected, but are demonstrated in the presence of ischemia and acute infarction, possibly due to a conversion of aerobic to anaerobic glycolysis in the infarcted tissue. Clinical MRS can demonstrate low or normal levels of metabolites (NAA, choline, and creatine) and elevated lactate in the infarcted area. Peripheral areas which demonstrate low levels of metabolites without lactate buildup are felt to be the penumbra.

HEAD TRAUMA

Debate remains whether imaging is required for patients with a GCS of 15. Clear indications for neuroimaging include GCS less than 15; unexplained transient or persistent loss of consciousness; other forms of altered sensorium; focal neurologic signs; depressed skull fractures; seizure; persistent variations; progressive headache; and penetrating injuries.[12] In these instances, NECT plays an essential role for diagnosis and for detecting processes that require emergent intervention, such as epidural and subdural hematomas, increased intracranial pressure, and depressed skull fractures. Although discussed elsewhere, a number of points related to optimal imaging are worthy of emphasis.

The differential density of blood facilitates the detection of intraparenchymal and extraaxial hemorrhage. Density is displayed on a relative scale referred to in Hounsfield units (HU). For example, water or CSF is assigned a value of zero, bone or metal varies between 100 and 1000 HU (hyperdense), fat is approximately −100 HU (hypodense), and air is −1000 HU. Further, acute blood has a density of 60 to 100 HU, and normal brain parenchyma has a density of approximately 35 (white matter) to 40 HU (gray matter). This differential density enables the increased density of blood or the decreasing density with accumulating edema to be detectable. Images are filmed in a manner that accentuates differences in the parenchymal range of densities. To optimize sensitivity for detecting parenchymal injuries, a gray scale is assigned such that regions of higher density are not easily differentiated. As such, blood in proximity to bone can be difficult to detect using parenchymal windows (Figures 237-7A and 237-7B).

When evaluating for the presence of subdural and epidural collections, it is important that images are formatted in a fashion so that the high densities are also distinguishable (i.e., blood windows). At many institutions it may not be routine to print these windows due to associated added film costs, but at a minimum, images should be reviewed on the CT console to exclude small blood collections. This is particularly true in children, in whom subdural hematomas can be a marker of intentional trauma. Detection is also facilitated by attention to the subtle secondary signs of extraaxial blood, including loss of sulcal demarcation, mass effect on a ventricle, or displacement of the gray-white junction from the inner table (see Figure 237-7). These secondary signs are also important because not all acute blood is hyperdense. In anemic patients (hemoglobin level 8 to 10 g/dL) or patients with a coagulopathy, acute blood may be isodense and thus difficult to visualize.

Occasionally, MRI can be of value in assessing trauma patients. For example, in assessing for small acute subdural hematomas or for subacute/chronic hematomas, CT may be limited due to the hematoma's proximity to bone or because over time the density of blood becomes isodense to normal brain (subacute) or to normal CSF (chronic) (see Figure 237-7B). However, these blood products will remain abnormal with MRI for months to years. This can be of value in children when new and old coexistent extraaxial hematomas are essentially pathognomonic for child abuse.

MRI is also more sensitive in detecting diffuse axonal injury in which differential movement of parenchyma results in neuronal shearing. Diffuse axonal injury should be suspected when coma occurs immediately after severe injury and the degree of compromise is out of proportion to the CT findings. MRI may be beneficial in that it will show multiple punctate areas of blood products below the threshold of CT detection. Specific anatomic structures that tend to be involved

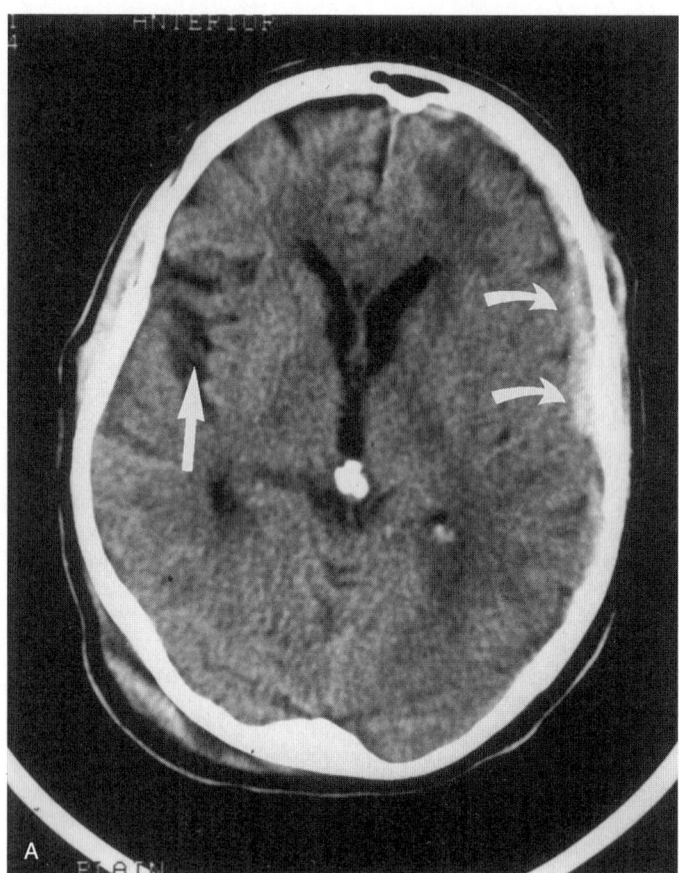
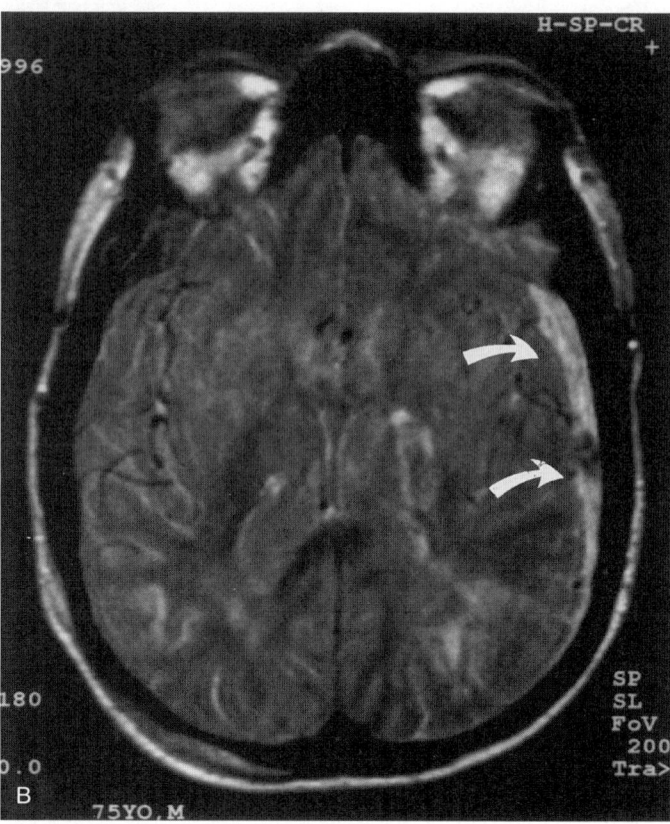

FIG. 237-7. A. Axial CT demonstrates a somewhat subtle left subdural hematoma *(curved arrows)*. Note secondary signs of mass effect with the contralateral sylvian fissure detectable but compressed on the side of the subdural hematoma *(straight arrow)*. **B.** Axial MRI demonstrating the increased conspicuity of blood due to the lack of obscuration by adjacent bone.

include the corpus callosum, adjacent to the superior cerebellar peduncle, the internal capsule, and gray-white matter junction.[13]

Intra- or extracranial arterial dissection may be the result of trivial trauma, blunt trauma, or penetrating injury. MRI can detect the presence of an acute dissection with T1 hyperintense blood seen in the vessel wall. In combination with MR angiography, it provides a fairly sensitive screening for a dissection. It enables an adequately sensitive but noninvasive method for vascular assessment and simultaneous assessment of the brain parenchyma and the extraaxial spaces. Other vascular lesions associated with trauma are pseudoaneurysms, which may occur in any dissected vessel, both intracranially and extracranially, and are prone to bleed. Catheter angiography remains the gold standard, but should be restricted to those patients with equivocal or abnormal MRA or CTA findings or a high level of clinical suspicion.

Catheter angiography is also recommended in all patients with penetrating injuries to zone 1 and zone 3 of the neck, although assessment of zone 3 injuries is slightly more equivocal.[14] Angiography is needed to evaluate vessels of the thoracic inlet and those above the mandible, because they are not accessible to visual inspection. Further, when indicated, surgical exploration will require a vascular road map. Zone 2 injuries can be observed without angiography, but angiography is recommended for expanding hematomas or where there is the development of respiratory or neurologic compromise.[15]

REFERENCES

1. White PW, Wardlaw JM, Easton V: Can noninvasive imaging accurately depict intracranial aneurysms? A systematic review. *Radiology* 217:361, 2000.
2. Gopinath SP, Robertson CS, Contant CF, et al: Early detection of delayed traumatic intracranial hematomas using near infrared spectroscopy. *J Neurosurg* 83:438, 1995.
3. Sedman R, Connolly E, Lemke T: Subarachnoid hemorrhage diagnosis: Lumbar puncture is still needed when the computed tomography scan is normal. *Acad Emerg Med* 3:827, 1996.
4. Noguchi K, Ogawa T, Seto H, et al: Subacute and chronic subarachnoid hemorrhage: Diagnosed with fluid-attenuated inversion-recovery MR imaging. *Radiology* 203:252, 1997.
5. Sujit S, Riviello JJ, Harper MB, et al: The role of emergent neuroimaging in children with new-onset afebrile seizures. *Pediatrics* 111:1, 2003.
6. Mower WR, Biros MH, Talan DA, et al: Selective tomographic imaging of patients with new onset seizure disorders. *Acad Emerg Med* 9:43, 2002.
7. Larrue V, Kummer RV, Muller A, et al: Risk factors for severe hemorrhagic transformation in ischemic stroke patients treated with recombinant tissue plasminogen activator. (ECASS II). *Stroke* 32:438, 2001.
8. Provenzale J, Sorense G: Diffusion-weighted imaging in acute stroke: Theoric considerations and clinical applications. *Am J Roentgenol* 173:1459, 1999.
9. Patel M, Siewert B, Warach S, et al: Diffusion and perfusion imaging techniques. *Magn Reson Imaging Clin N Am* 3:425, 1995.
10. Lee KH, Lee SJ, Cho SJ, et al: Usefulness of triphasic perfusion computed tomography for intravenous thrombolysis with tissue-type plasminogen activator in acute ischemic stroke. *Arch Neurol* 57:1000, 2000.
11. Baker PB, Gillard JH, van Zijl PCM, et al: Acute stroke: Evaluation with serial proton MR spectroscopic imaging. *Radiology* 192:723, 1994.
12. Stein SC, Ross SE: The value of CT scans in patients with low-risk head injuries. *Neurosurgery* 26:638, 1990.
13. Go JL, Ze CS: Clinical evaluation of patients with head trauma. *Neuroimaging Clin N Am* 12:165, 2002.
14. Jurkovich GH, Zingarelli W, Wallace J: Penetrating neck trauma: Diagnostic studies in the asymptomatic patient. *J Trauma* 25:819, 1985.
15. Golueke PJ, Goldstein AS, Sclafani SJA, et al: Routine versus selective exploration of penetrating neck injuries: A randomized prospective study. *J Trauma* 24:1010, 1984.

EYE, EAR, NOSE, THROAT, AND ORAL SURGERY

OCULAR EMERGENCIES
John D. Mitchell

A wide range of ocular emergencies, conditions, and manifestations of systemic illness are encountered regularly in the ED. The emergency physician should be comfortable with the use of a slit lamp, Tonopen or Schiøtz tonometer, and direct ophthalmoscope and be familiar with ocular anatomy (Figures 238-1 and 238-2) and basic neuro-ophthalmology. The approach to the patient should proceed in typical fashion with a good history and physical examination, with treatment of life-threatening conditions taking priority.

EYE EXAMINATION

History

A detailed history of the chief complaint and circumstances surrounding the onset should be obtained. The past ocular and medical history will provide additional information and help focus the physical examination so as to arrive at the differential diagnosis. For example, a history of sudden, painless monocular visual loss associated with a history of atrial fibrillation or carotid stenosis would suggest a central retinal artery occlusion, whereas a history of eye pain occurring while hammering metal on metal would suggest a projectile corneal or intraocular foreign body. Past visual acuity and the need for glasses or contact lenses provide information on acuity testing expectations. Use of soft contact lenses, especially the extended-wear type, is associated with a higher incidence of corneal ulceration from microbial infection. "Flashing lights" and a "curtain or veil" obstructing a portion of the visual field suggests a retinal detachment. A history of diabetes or chronic hypertension and acute isolated sixth-nerve palsy suggests an ischemic cranial neuropathy.

Physical Examination

The physical examination typically proceeds in a sequential fashion unless the circumstances require otherwise (i.e., chemical ocular injuries require intervention *prior* to assessment of visual acuity). The glossary of terms and abbreviations in Table 238-1 is useful in documenting the findings. The typical eye examination sequence is as follows: Visual acuity, external eye, visual fields, pupils, ocular motility, anterior pigment, fundus, and intraocular pressure.

VISUAL ACUITY An attempt should be made to assess visual acuity in each eye individually in all conscious and alert patients. If the patient uses glasses or contacts but the glasses are not available, pinhole testing can be performed to obtain an estimate of corrected visual acuity. The pinhole allows only parallel rays (collimated light) to fall on the macula, thereby reducing the refractive error and allowing an estimate of the person's corrected visual acuity.

Distance charts are preferable but are not practical with patients confined to a stretcher. Nearsighted patients and those under age 45 can use a near card to test their visual acuity. Patients in their midforties or older may require reading glasses or bifocals to read a near card because of presbyopia. If the bifocals are not available, again, a pinhole occluder can be used with a near card. Corneal abrasions or foreign bodies can cause severe photophobia, pain, and tearing, so a top-

ical anesthetic can reduce discomfort sufficiently to allow a more accurate assessment of visual acuity. Documentation of best acuity in each eye and whether prosthetic devices were used (glasses, pinhole) should be noted. If the patient cannot read the chart or near card, ask how many fingers you are holding up, and record the furthest distance at which the fingers can be counted correctly (e.g., at 4 ft). If the patient is unable to count fingers, assess ability to detect hand motion 1 to 2 ft in front of the eye. If the patient is unable to detect hand motion, turn off all the lights in the room, fully occlude the contralateral eye, and test for light perception. In recording the results of visual acuity testing, refer to Table 238-1.

EXTERNAL EYE Examine the periorbital skin and lids for trauma, infection, dysfunction, deformity, crepitus, or proptosis. Subcutaneous emphysema can be found with blowout fractures of the medial orbital wall (ethmoid). The orbital rims should be palpated for step-off deformities in trauma cases.

CONFRONTATION VISUAL FIELDS Test the gross confrontation visual field of each eye with all visual complaints, including "blurred" vision. Bitemporal hemianopia can occur in pituitary adenoma, homonymous hemianopia is associated with some cerebrovascular accidents (CVAs), and monocular field cuts are sometimes seen with large retinal detachments.

PUPILS Pupil assessment should be performed under slightly dim light to test for an afferent pupillary defect (Figure 238-3). A positive afferent pupillary defect indicates an optic nerve disorder. It is important to note that the pupils will be equal in size *prior* to testing because of the consensual light response. Therefore, an afferent pupillary defect does not cause a baseline anisocoria and will be discovered only if specifically tested for. Causes of unequal pupils (anisocoria) can range from an acute emergency (posterior communicating artery aneurysm) to chronic baseline conditions such as previous intraocular trauma or surgery, or can be idiopathic. A careful history is important to determine whether anisocoria is preexisting. Ocular medications such as pilocarpine can cause extreme miosis, resulting in small, nonreactive pupils. Some patients with uveitis will be using a cycloplegic agent (scopolamine, cyclopentolate, or atropine) and have a chemically dilated, unreactive pupil. **It is not worthwhile to attempt to "reverse" a chemically altered pupil in the ED** as a diagnostic test because the results are variable and unreliable.

OCULAR MOTILITY Eye movements are controlled by the six extraocular muscles attached to each eye (Figures 238-4 and 238-5). These muscles are innervated by cranial nerves III, IV, and VI. Cranial nerve IV controls the superior oblique muscle, cranial nerve VI controls the lateral rectus muscle, and all other extraocular muscles are controlled by cranial nerve III. Ocular motility can be impaired by restriction, interrupted or decreased innervation, or trauma. Examples of restriction include thyroid orbitopathy, myositis, and mechanical entrapment of a muscle secondary to an orbital blowout fracture. Cranial nerve palsies or paresis may be caused by stroke, myasthenia gravis, diabetes, hypertension, tumors, aneurysms, infections, and trauma. Penetrating or blunt traumatic injury to an extraocular muscle also can result in motility disturbance. Diplopia may develop, especially when the patient is attempting to look in the direction of the malfunctioning muscle. Ocular alignment should be evaluated in primary gaze initially (looking straight ahead), followed by testing in all fields of gaze.

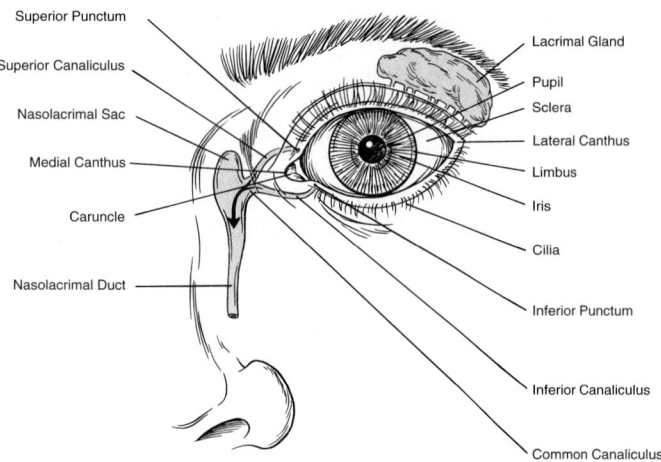

FIG. 238-1. Anatomic diagram of eye and adnexa.

ANTERIOR SEGMENT   The conjunctiva, cornea, anterior chamber, iris, lens, and ciliary body make up the anterior segment. All these structures except the ciliary body can be inspected directly by slit-lamp examination. A slit lamp is a biomicroscope that affords an excellent view of these structures and should be used whenever possible (Figure 238-6). The conjunctiva should be inspected for hemorrhages, discharge, inflammation, trauma, and foreign bodies. The upper lid always should be everted anytime a foreign-body sensation or abrasion is present. The cornea should be assessed by narrowing the light source to produce a slit beam and optically sectioning the cornea (Figure 238-7), which allows an oblique section to be seen and facilitates evaluation of the entire corneal thickness. This is a particularly important technique when one is trying to determine if a corneal foreign body has caused a full-thickness penetration.

Fluorescein dye should be instilled and the cobalt-blue filter used to identify corneal abrasions, dendrites, and perforations. The *modified Seidel test* is useful in identifying corneal perforations. The eye is anesthetized and held open, and the cobalt-blue filter is used to observe the eye while a moistened fluorescein strip is "painted" across the suspicious site. Leakage of aqueous humor through a penetrating

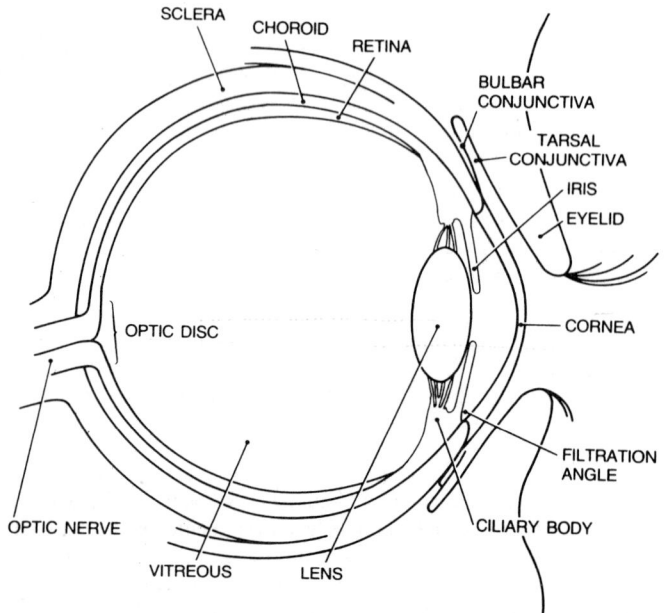

FIG. 238-2. Horizontal cross-sectional diagram of eye.

TABLE 238-1   Glossary of Terms, Abbreviations, and Notations

AC: Anterior chamber, the first portion of the anterior segment.

Anisocoria: Unequal pupil size under equal lighting conditions.

Anterior segment: Consists of the anterior chamber and posterior chamber. Aqueous humor is produced in the posterior chamber of the anterior segment and circulates through the pupil into the anterior chamber of the anterior segment.

APD: Afferent pupillary defect (see Figure 238-3).

CF: Counting fingers (visual acuity assessment).

CVF: Confrontation visual fields.

EOM: Extraocular muscle.

HM: Hand motion (visual acuity assessment).

Hyphema: Red blood cells in the anterior chamber.

Hypopyon: White blood cells in the anterior chamber.

INO: Internuclear ophthalmoplegia.

IOFB: Intraocular foreign body.

IOP: Intraocular pressure (mm Hg).

Limbus: Circumferential border where clear cornea ends and white sclera begins.

NLP: No light perception (blind).

OD: Oculus dexter (right eye).

OS: Oculus sinister (left eye).

OU: Oculus uterque (each eye).

PH: Pinhole visual acuity.

RD: Retinal detachment.

Tonopen: A handheld, pen-shaped device for measuring intraocular pressure.

T_{tono}: Tension (IOP) with subscript representing method used (tono = Tonopen, S = Schiøtz, A = applanation).

V_{Ac}: Visual acuity with correction (glasses or contact lenses).

V_{As}: Visual acuity without correction.

Note: By convention, in documenting the visual acuity (V_A) or IOP, the right eye is listed above the left, as follows:

$$V_{Ac} < \frac{20/20}{20/30}$$

This represents a visual acuity *with* glasses/contacts of 20/20 right eye and 20/30 left eye.

$$V_{As} < \frac{20/400 \to 20/30}{CF \text{ at } 8 \text{ ft} \to 20/40}$$

This represents a visual acuity *without* glasses/contacts of 20/400 in the right eye, improving to 20/30 with pinhole testing; counting fingers at 8 ft in the left eye, improving to 20/40 with pinhole testing.

$$T_{tono} < \frac{14}{15}$$

This represents an IOP of 14 mm Hg in the right eye and 15 mm Hg in the left eye measured by Tonopen.

wound will appear as a lime-green fluid oozing onto the dark violet corneal surface (Figure 238-8, **Plate 3**).

The anterior chamber should be checked for clarity and the presence of a hyphema (Figure 238-9, **Plate 4**) or hypopyon (Figure 238-10, **Plate 5**). Cell and flare may be present in acute injuries or in chronic uveitis/iritis conditions and should be checked for as follows: The slit beam should be shortened to about 1 mm, and all the room lights should be out. The high-magnification position should be selected. The incident light source should create an angle of 45 to 60 degrees with the objective (similar to optical sectioning). The light beam should be focused on the pupillary margin. Then pull back on the joy stick to focus on the cornea. Then move the focus inward halfway between the iris and cornea, with the pupillary aperture as a dark backdrop. This will place your focus in the center of the aqueous humor, and the light beam will illuminate cells slowly drifting up and down in the aqueous convection currents. Flare typically is described as the appearance of "headlights in a fog" and represents the ability to see the course of the normally transparent light beam through the aqueous hu-

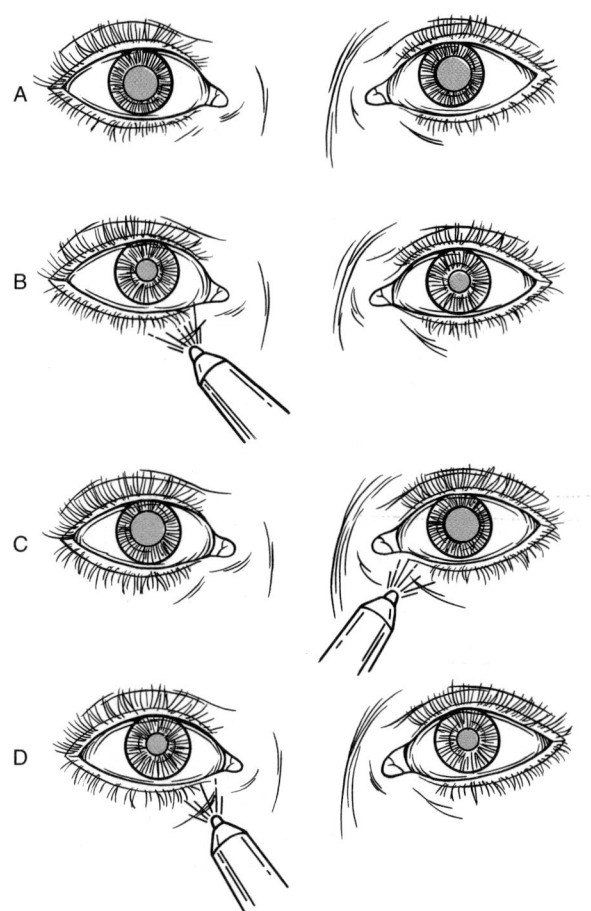

FIG. 238-3. **A.** "Swinging-flashlight test" revealing an afferent pupillary defect (Marcus-Gunn pupil) of the left eye. **C.** The test is positive when the affected pupil dilates in response to light. Conditions with an afferent pupillary defect (AFD) include optic neuritis and central retinal artery occlusion.

mor. This is caused by increased aqueous protein content, which is common with inflammatory conditions.

The iris should be inspected for tears and foreign bodies if trauma occurred. The lens likewise should be inspected for injury, subluxation, and foreign bodies.

FUNDUS   The optic nerve, macula, and retina can be viewed with a direct ophthalmoscope in the emergency department. A dilated pupil makes it easier to see these structures, and unless the patient has a rare

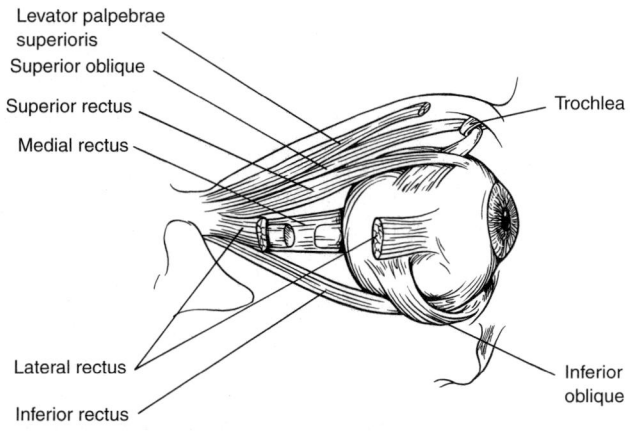

FIG. 238-4. Extraocular muscles of the eye.

contraindication (narrow angles without a previous peripheral iridectomy), dilation can be performed if a posterior segment view is needed. Dilation can be achieved by using one drop of 1% tropicamide (Mydriacyl) in Caucasians and one drop each of 1% tropicamide and 2.5% phenylephrine (Neo-Synephrine) in all others. A dilated examination is particularly important if an intraocular foreign body, central retinal artery occlusion (CRAO), or retinal detachment is suspected. A vitreous hemorrhage from diabetes or trauma can obscure or significantly reduce the view of the posterior pole. In these patients, an ophthalmologist may need to perform an ultrasound-B scan to evaluate the posterior segment. An indirect ophthalmoscope provides an excellent three-dimensional view of the optic nerve and retina but requires extensive practice to use and generally is not a tool for the non-ophthalmologist.

INTRAOCULAR PRESSURE   The eye remains consistently "inflated" because of a delicate balance between intraocular aqueous fluid production and outflow. Intraocular pressure (IOP) or tension can decrease due to reduced ciliary body production (some cases of iritis and uveitis) or loss of globe integrity (perforating injury). An increase in IOP occurs when intraocular fluid production exceeds outflow (glaucoma, hyphema). The normal IOP is 10 to 21 mm Hg, and three main methods are used to achieve a measurement. Applanation tonometry is the method preferred by ophthalmologists and physicians trained in using this slit-lamp attachment. Practice and previous experience are recommended, however. The Tonopen, a handheld instrument for measuring IOP, has gained popularity because it is easier for a non-ophthalmologist to use and has reasonable accuracy for identifying elevated IOP. The Schiøtz tonometer is another instrument that can be used readily if a Tonopen is not available. All methods require an anesthetized cornea and a cooperative patient. Avoid any pressure on the globe with your fingers when holding the lids open because this will cause a falsely high reading. The lids should be held open, with the fingers compressing the lids against the bony rims of the orbit. The method used always should be recorded. In recording the IOP, refer to Table 238-1.

INFECTIONS

Lids

STYE (EXTERNAL HORDEOLUM)   A stye is an acute staphylococcal infection of an oil gland associated with an eyelash. It is located at the lash line and has the appearance of a small pustule. Warm compresses and erythromycin ophthalmic ointment twice daily for 7 to 10 days is usually sufficient treatment.

CHALAZION (INTERNAL HORDEOLUM)   A chalazion is an acute or chronic inflammation of the eyelid secondary to blockage of one of the meibomian oil glands in the tarsal plate. A reddened, tender lump develops in the lid or at the lid margin.

Initial conservative treatment:

1. Warm, moist compresses three to four times a day
2. Erythromycin ophthalmic ointment applied to lid margins four times daily
3. Consider doxycycline 100 mg PO twice daily for 14 to 21 days if chronic and recurrent
4. Ophthalmology referral after 4 to 6 weeks, earlier if it worsens

Chronic inflammation will induce a cystic wall, and a discrete lump develops that is usually both palpable and visible in the lid. Chalazions can cycle between being quiet or acutely inflamed. The patient with a chronic, recurrent chalazion should be referred to an ophthalmologist for surgical excision and curettage, which is the definitive procedure.

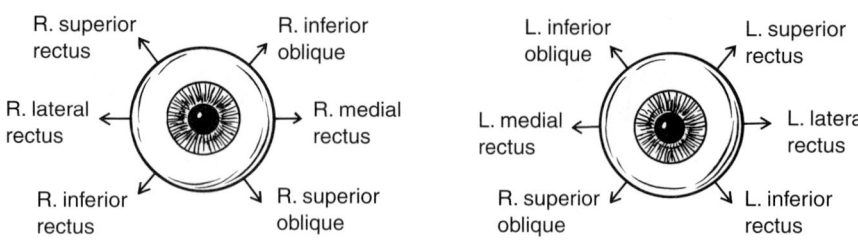

FIG. 238-5. Arrows indicate direction of ocular movement by each muscle. Cranial nerve IV, superior oblique muscle; cranial nerve VI, lateral rectus muscle; cranial nerve III, superior rectus, inferior rectus, inferior oblique, and medial rectus muscles.

Conjunctivitis

BACTERIAL CONJUNCTIVITIS Bacterial conjunctivitis generally presents with a mucopurulent discharge and inflammation of the conjunctiva. Often the eyelids are stuck together on awakening. The condition can be monocular or binocular. The cornea is clear *without* fluorescein staining. Frequently there is a history of recent exposure to someone with "pink eye." Treatment consists of a topical ocular antibiotic four times daily for 5 to 7 days. Treatment with a broad-spectrum agent is safe for patients 2 months of age and older; Polytrim (trimethoprim and polymyxin B), for example, is very effective and avoids potential allergies to sulfa and neomycin preparations. Wearers of soft contact lenses should be treated with a fluoroquinolone (Ciloxan, Ocuflox) or aminoglycoside (Tobrex) to treat *Pseudomonas*. With the expanding choices of well-tolerated topical antibiotic drops, gentamicin is now seldom used by ophthalmologists because of the high incidence of ocular irritation.

Treatment:

1. Fluorescein stain of the cornea (especially infants) to avoid missing a corneal abrasion, ulcer, or dendrite
2. *Non-contact lens wearer:* broad-spectrum topical antibiotic (Polytrim or erythromycin), one drop four times daily for 5 to 7 days
3. *Contact lens wearer:* fluoroquinolone (Ciloxan or Ocuflox) or aminoglycoside (Tobrex) for *Pseudomonas* coverage, one drop four times daily for 5 to 7 days

VIRAL CONJUNCTIVITIS Viral conjunctivitis tends to follow an antecedent upper respiratory infection and often will have a palpable preauricular node, which aids in confirming the diagnosis. Generally, one eye will be involved initially, with the other eye becoming involved within days. The discharge tends to be watery, and the conjunctiva is reddened and edematous (chemosis). The cornea is clear, with occasional punctate staining with fluorescein dye (multiple tiny dots of stain uptake seen only on slit-lamp examination). It is important to stain the cornea to avoid missing a herpes dendritic keratitis. Treatment consists of cool compresses; Naphcon-A, one drop three times daily and as needed for redness and conjunctival congestion; and artificial tears five or six times a day. Viral conjunctivitis can take 1 to 3 weeks to run its course and is highly contagious. The physician examining a patient with possible conjunctivitis should wear gloves in order to avoid self-contamination. If, after a history and physical examination, it is still uncertain if the conjunctivitis is viral or bacterial, it is not unreasonable to add an antibiotic eyedrop until the patient can be reexamined by an ophthalmologist.

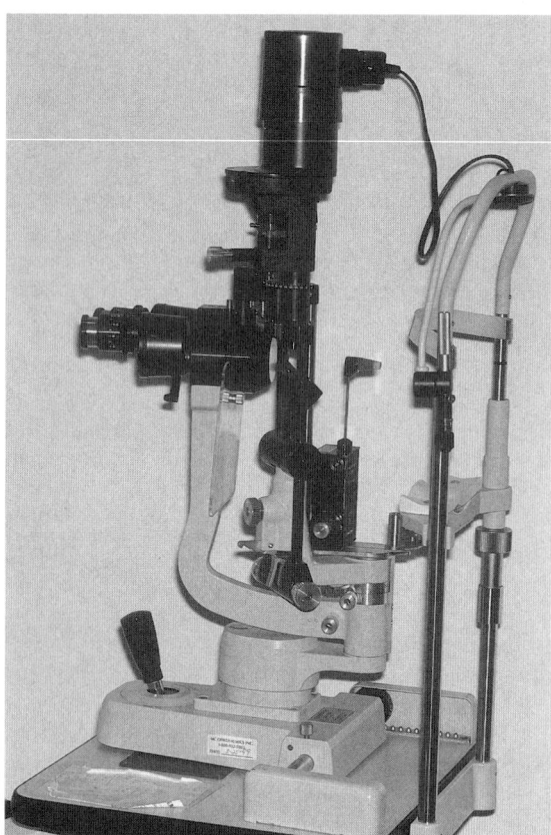

A

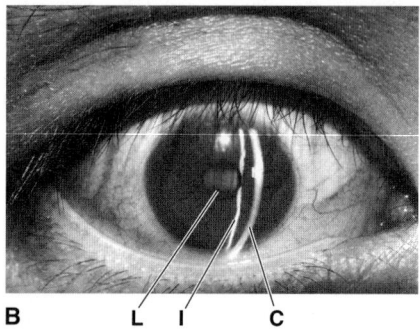

B   L   I   C

FIG. 238-6. A. The slit lamp provides a magnified view of the eye. **B.** A thin slit can demonstrate the cornea *(C)*, iris *(I)*, and lens *(L)*.

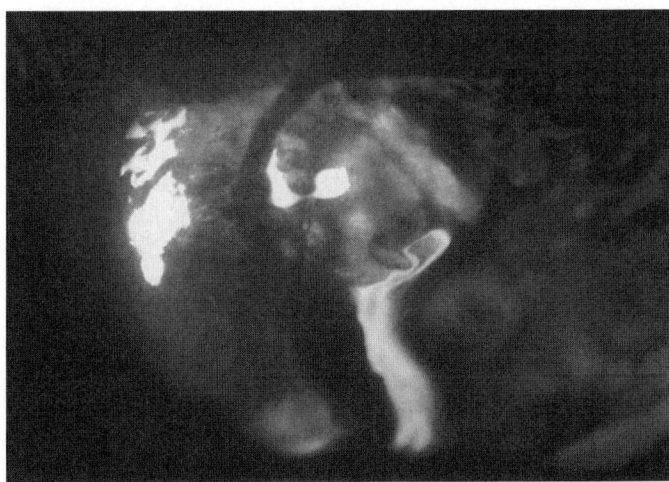

FIG. 238-8. (PLATE 3). Positive Seidel test showing aqueous leaking through a full-thickness corneal wound. Aqueous will turn fluorescein lime-green under a cobalt-blue light as it oozes through the wound while being observed at the slit lamp.

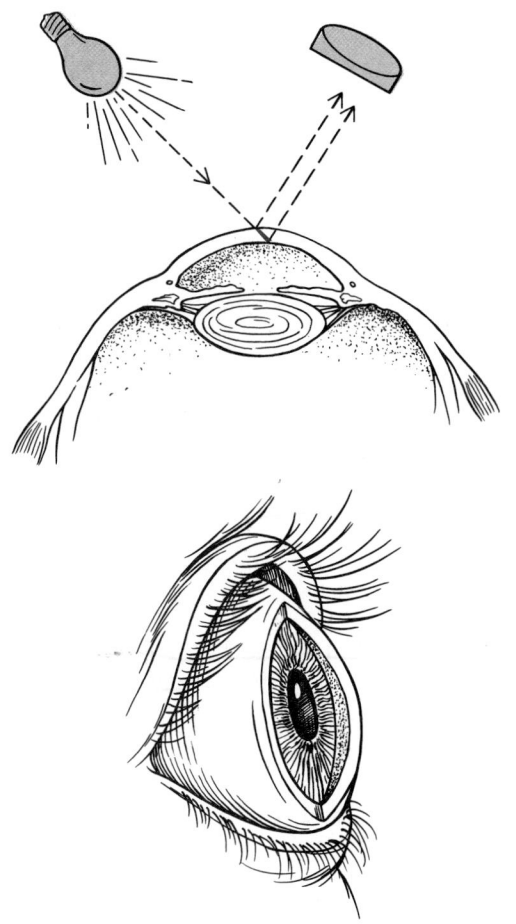

FIG. 238-7. Optical sectioning. By creating an angle of 45 to 60 degrees between the slit-beam light source and the observer's biomicroscope objective, the cornea can be optically "sectioned" obliquely. This allows a cross-sectional view of the cornea and is helpful in ascertaining depth of penetration of corneal foreign bodies and injuries.

Treatment:

1. Fluorescein stain the cornea to avoid missing a herpes dendrite
2. Cool compresses four times daily
3. Naphcon-A one drop three to four times daily or as needed for conjunctival congestion/itching
4. Consider a topical antibiotic if there is uncertainty as to whether an infection is viral or bacterial
5. Ophthalmology follow-up in 7 to 10 days if cornea is clear

ALLERGIC CONJUNCTIVITIS Allergens can cause ocular discharge, redness, and itching. Itching is a very common and consistent symptom seen with allergic conjunctivitis. Treatment consists of cool compresses four times daily, antihistamine/decongestant drops (Patanol, Zaditor, or Alocril twice daily or Naphcon-A four times daily), and artificial tears as needed.

NEONATAL CONJUNCTIVITIS (OPHTHALMIA NEONATORUM) THIS CONDITION IS DISCUSSED IN CHAP. 117.

Herpes Simplex Virus (HSV)

HSV can affect the eyelids, conjunctiva, and cornea. Skin involvement has typical vesicular eruptions, and the conjunctiva also can become inflamed. Ocular HSV alternately can present with only corneal findings on physical examination. The dendrite of herpes keratitis is an ep-

ithelial defect that can be seen with fluorescein staining and has a linear branching pattern with terminal bulbs (Figure 238-11, **Plate 6**). An initial outbreak of HSV involving the lids and conjunctiva can be treated with an oral acyclovir derivative such as Zovirax or Famvir and topical antiviral drops (Viroptic five times a day without corneal involvement, nine times a day with corneal involvement). Erythromycin ophthalmic ointment can be added to prevent secondary infection of the vesicular eruption. HSV keratitis can progress to corneal scarring and requires prompt treatment with topical antiviral agents. Viroptic—one drop nine times a day—represents standard treatment, and Vira-A ointment five times a day or Stoxil can be substituted for those who are allergic to Viroptic. Topical steroids should be strictly avoided, and all patients should be referred to an ophthalmologist for outpatient follow-up.

Treatment:

1. If the initial outbreak is less than 3 to 4 days old, consider oral acyclovir-class medications.
2. Erythromycin ophthalmic ointment four times daily to skin and conjunctival lesions to avoid secondary bacterial infection
3. HSV *without* corneal involvement: Viroptic one drop five times a day
4. HSV *with* corneal involvement: Viroptic one drop nine times a day
5. Ophthalmology follow-up in 1 to 3 days

Herpes Zoster Ophthalmicus

Herpes zoster ophthalmicus (HZO) represents shingles in the trigeminal nerve distribution with ocular involvement. When the cutaneous lesions include the tip of the nose (Hutchinson sign), the nasociliary nerve is involved, and the eye frequently becomes inflamed. An iritis can occur with photophobia and pain. Cutaneous lesions and conjunctival involvement are treated with erythromycin ointment to prevent secondary bacterial infection. The cornea can have a pseudodendrite, which is a poorly staining mucous plaque with no epithelial erosion (unlike HSV, which has a true dendrite with epithelial erosion and staining). The anterior chamber on slit-lamp examination can show manifestations of iritis (cell and flare). Iritis can be treated with topical steroids such as prednisolone acetate 1% (Pred Forte) one drop four to five times a day, and pain reduction can be achieved with topical cycloplegic agents (scopolamine 0.25% one drop three times daily or cyclopentolate 1% one drop three times daily). If HZO is diagnosed, admission and intravenous acyclovir should be considered, especially if any intracranial symptoms are present.

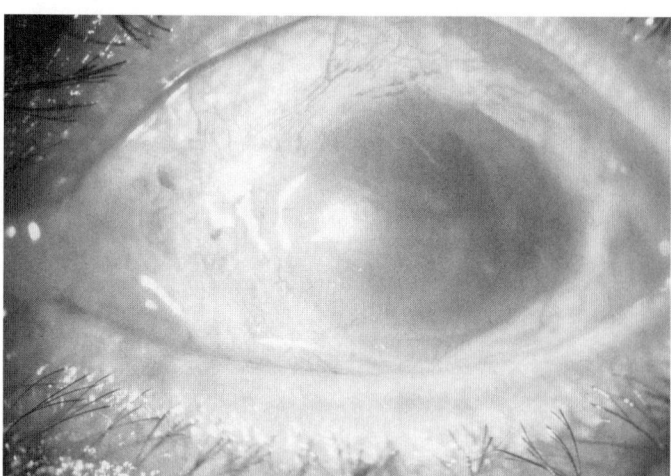

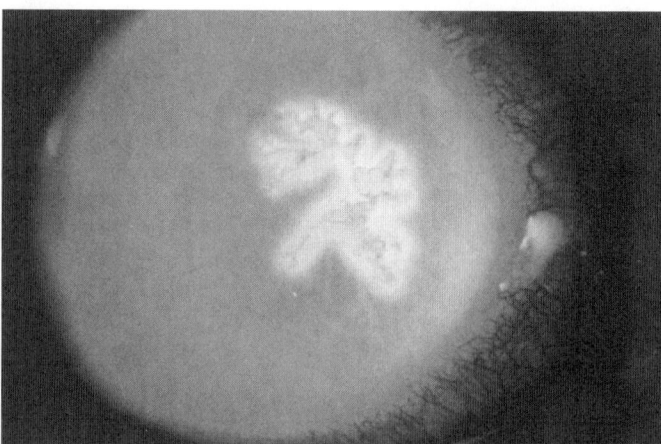

FIG. 238-9. (PLATE 4). Hyphema secondary to blunt trauma. Note the blood filling the lower half of the anterior chamber and hazy appearance of cornea suggesting increased IOP.

FIG. 238-11. (PLATE 6). Herpes simplex corneal dendrite seen with fluorescein staining and cobalt-blue light.

Treatment:

1. Erythromycin ophthalmic ointment to lesions to prevent secondary infection
2. Oral narcotic analgesia if necessary
3. Prednisolone acetate (1%) (Pred Forte) one drop five times a day if iritis is present and *no corneal epithelial defect* is seen on fluorescein staining and slit-lamp examination
4. Cycloplegic pain reduction with 0.25% scopolamine or 1% cyclopentolate one drop three times daily
5. Consideration for admission and intravenous acyclovir; dosage 30 mg/kg per d divided in three doses if creatinine is below 2 mg/dL

Preseptal Cellulitis (Periorbital Cellulitis)

Preseptal cellulitis is a periocular superficial cellulitis that has not breached the orbital septum. The eyelids become edematous, warm, and red. The eye itself is not involved, with *acuity and pupillary reaction maintained* and *full ocular motility preserved*. The majority of cases occurring in children and adults are the result of inoculation sec-

ondary to skin infection or trauma (see Chap. 122). The offending agent is usually *Staphylococcus aureus*. Oral antibiotics can be adequate if there is no orbital involvement, but if the latter is suspected, then intravenous antibiotics, computed tomographic (CT) scanning, and possible admission should be considered.

Preseptal cellulitis in children under 5 years of age is a special circumstance due to the association with bacteremia, septicemia, and meningitis and warrants a complete diagnostic evaluation, including blood cultures and intravenous antibiotics. Although *S. aureus* is still the most common organism, often the cause is bacteremic spread of *H. influenzae* from otitis media or pneumonia. The incidence of *H. influenzae* preseptal cellulitis has been decreasing with the use of *H. influenzae* type b vaccine. Consultation with a pediatrician is recommended for consideration of admission.

Treatment:

1. Ascertain no restriction of ocular motility, no proptosis, no pain with eye movement, and preserved pupillary response and acuity
2. *Children older than 5 years of age:* Amoxicillin/Clavulanate 20 to 40 mg/kg per d orally divided into three doses
3. *Adults:* Amoxicillin/Clavulanate 500 mg PO three times daily
4. Regarding those younger than 5 years of age or in severe cases, admit for IV antibiotics and systemic workup
5. *Children:* Ceftriaxone 100 mg/kg per d IV divided into two doses plus vancomycin 40 mg/kg per d IV divided three doses
6. *Adults:* Ceftriaxone 1 to 2 g IV every 12 h plus vancomycin 0.5 to 1.0 g IV every 12 h

Orbital Cellulitis (Postseptal Cellulitis)

Orbital cellulitis is an *orbital* infection; therefore, it is deep to the orbital septum. This is a serious ocular infection that has the potential to be life-threatening. *S. aureus* is the most common pathogen; however, *H. influenzae* should be considered in young children and mucormycosis in diabetics and immunocompromised patients. Polymicrobial infection is common. Orbital extension of paranasal sinus infection (especially ethmoid sinusitis) is the most frequent source. Orbital and sinus CT scans should be performed in the ED. If the CT scan is negative, an enhanced CT scan should be performed looking for a subperiosteal abscess. Diagnostic clinical findings that help distinguish this infection from preseptal cellulitis include extraocular muscle (EOM) motility impairment, pain, fever, and occasionally, proptosis. Decreased visual acuity is a late finding. Cavernous sinus

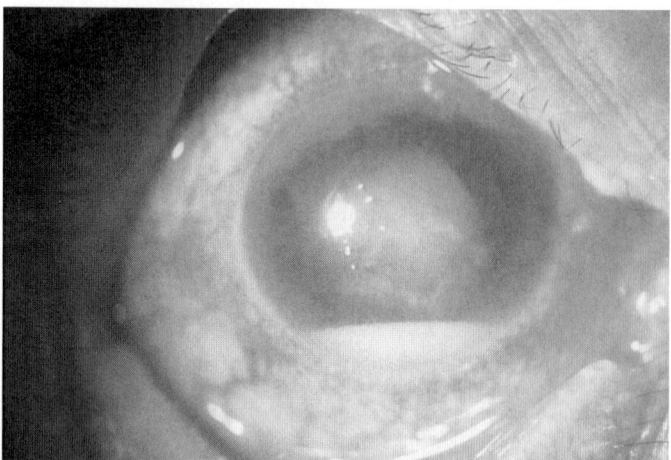

FIG. 238-10. (PLATE 5). Corneal ulcer with hypopyon. The ulcer is seen as a shaggy white corneal infiltrate surrounding the borders of the epithelial defect. The hypopyon represents the accumulation of white cells layering out in the lower one-sixth of the anterior chamber.

thrombosis also can occur. Patients require a full workup, admission, and intravenous antibiotics.

Treatment:

1. Intravenous cefuroxime alone or intravenous penicillin plus nafcillin or chloramphenicol plus nafcillin. In penicillin-allergic patients vancomycin or a cephalosporin can be substituted.
2. Contrast-enhanced CT scans of the orbits and paranasal sinuses and admission.

Corneal Ulcer

A corneal ulcer is a serious infection involving multiple layers of the cornea. Corneal ulcers develop secondary to breaks in the epithelial barrier, allowing infectious agents to gain access to the underlying corneal stroma. The initial disruption of the epithelial layer can be due to desquamation, trauma, or direct microbial invasion. Exposure keratitis from incomplete lid closure secondary to Bell palsy can cause corneal desiccation and sloughing of the epithelium, allowing bacteria to gain access to the underlying stroma and create an ulcer. Trauma can also breach the epithelium and inoculate the cornea. Wearing of soft contact lenses is a very common cause of corneal ulcers, and the incidence increases dramatically in those who use extended-wear lenses and wearers who sleep with them in place.

Typically, the patient will have a painful red eye, with tearing and occasionally photophobia. Examination reveals a staining epithelial defect and a white, hazy infiltrate underlying the defect and spreading into adjacent stroma. Occasionally, a hypopyon is also present on slit-lamp examination (see Figure 238-10), signifying an intraocular inflammatory response. Corneal ulcers need to be treated aggressively with topical antibiotics. A fluoroquinolone such as ciprofloxacin (Ciloxan) or ofloxacin (Ocuflox), one drop every hour in the affected eye, is the recommended treatment. A topical cycloplegic agent such as cyclopentolate 1% (Cyclogyl), one drop three times daily, also can help with pain control. The eye *should not be patched* because of the risk of *Pseudomonas* infection, which can cause rapid, aggressive ulceration with corneal melting and perforation. All corneal ulcers should be referred to an ophthalmologist to be seen within 12 to 24 h.

Treatment:

1. Ciloxan or Ocuflox, one drop every hour
2. No patching
3. Topical cycloplegic (1% cyclopentolate or 0.25% scopolamine) three times daily
4. Ophthalmology referral within 24 h

TRAUMA

Superficial Trauma

SUBCONJUNCTIVAL HEMORRHAGE The fragile conjunctival vessels can rupture from trauma, sudden Valsalva pressure spikes (sneezing, coughing, vomiting, straining), hypertension, or spontaneously with no discernible etiology. No treatment is necessary, and the hemorrhage usually resolves within 2 weeks. If multiple recurrent episodes occur, coagulation studies and further investigation are warranted.

CONJUNCTIVAL ABRASION Superficial conjunctival abrasions without any other associated ocular injury only require erythromycin ointment twice daily for 2 to 3 days or no treatment if very small. The lid should be everted and the fornix inspected under magnification for any residual particulate matter or organic debris.

CORNEAL ABRASION Abrasions of the cornea are associated with pain, photophobia, and tearing. They can be the result of trauma or contact lens wear. Visual acuity assessment can be difficult because of the patient's extreme discomfort. A drop of a topical anesthetic often will reduce the discomfort temporarily and facilitate visual acuity testing. A corneal epithelial defect will be present and is best seen with fluorescein staining and examination with a cobalt-blue light. The eyelid should be everted and inspected for foreign bodies. Examine the cornea for possible full-thickness injury (optical sectioning), and assess the anterior chamber with the slit lamp, looking for any associated injury. Adequate and persistent cycloplegia is essential to controlling pain. Reduction of ciliary spasm contributes significantly to pain relief and in most cases eliminates the need for narcotic pain medication. By the same token, inadequate cycloplegia almost mandates the need for oral analgesics. If an abrasion is larger than 2 mm or very painful, consider having the patient instill a cycloplegic agent (cyclopentolate 1%, homatropine 5%, or scopolamine 0.25%) one drop every 6 to 8 h at home to help control discomfort. Scopolamine dilates the pupil for several days and usually is reserved for very large, painful abrasions. Cyclopentolate 1% (Cyclogyl) one drop three times daily does an excellent job of providing cycloplegia and wears off within 24 h of discontinuation. Erythromycin ophthalmic ointment should be instilled and an eye patch may be placed, if desired, provided that the abrasion was not from an organic source or from the wearing of soft contact lenses. Abrasions will heal with or without a patch, and ophthalmologists will treat patients either way. Some patients appear to be more comfortable with an eye patch for the first 12 to 18 h, but this is not uniform, and the physician can make an individual decision with the patient. **Abrasions from organic sources have for fungal infections potential and should not be patched. Abrasions related to the wearing of soft contact lenses pose a risk of *Pseudomonas* infection and likewise should not be patched.** These patients should be treated with tobramycin ointment four times daily, followed by a fluoroquinolone (Ciloxan, Ocuflox) drop or tobramycin drop four times daily once the epithelial defect starts to close. Do not prescribe a topical anesthetic for pain relief as most anesthetics cause corneal toxicity when dosed recurrently and can lead to visual loss.

Documenting the Dimensions of a Corneal Abrasion Some slit lamps (Haag-Streit) have a measuring dial attached to the mechanism that varies the length of the slit beam. If your slit lamp is equipped with this feature, you can vary the length of the slit beam on the cornea until it corresponds to the length or width of the abrasion. The reading on the wheel equals the length of the slit beam in millimeters. This additional feature allows you to document the dimensions of the abrasion precisely, thereby enabling subsequent examiners to evaluate the wound's healing response objectively.

Treatment:

1. Identify the source of the abrasion if possible.
2. Cycloplegia (cyclopentolate 1%, or homatropine 5%) one drop now and repeat every 6 to 8 h as needed for pain. Warn the patient that the pupil will dilate and lose its ability to focus at near and that the drop will burn for 10 to 15 s when placed in the eye.
3. *Not related to contact lens wear:* Erythryomycin ophthalmic ointment and eye patch, or no patch and erythromycin ointment four times daily.
4. *Related to contact lens wear:* Tobramycin ophthalmic ointment four times daily. *No patch.*
5. *Organic source:* Erythromycin ophthalmic ointment four times daily. *No patch.*
6. Ophthalmology referral or reexamine next day.

CONJUNCTIVAL FOREIGN BODIES Conjunctival foreign bodies usually can be removed with a moistened cotton-tipped applicator after anesthetizing the eye with a topical anesthetic. The upper eyelid should be everted and inspected under the highest magnification available to avoid missing any additional foreign bodies. Frequently, small wooden particles such as sawdust will blend into the conjunctiva when moistened by the tears and be difficult to find without slit-lamp magnification. Small, fine vertical corneal abrasions seen only with fluorescein staining often will alert the physician to the presence of a foreign body embedded in the tarsal conjunctiva of the upper lid.

CORNEAL FOREIGN BODIES   Foreign bodies should be removed carefully under the best magnification available. The slit lamp provides sufficient magnification and allows both hands to be free for use. A history consistent with high-velocity ocular impact (i.e., hammering metal on metal) should alert you to the possibility of a penetrating injury. The cornea should be inspected using "optical sectioning" (see Figure 238-7) to assess depth of penetration *prior to* removal. **Full-thickness corneal foreign bodies should not be removed in the ED and require an ophthalmology consult.** Fortunately, most corneal foreign bodies are superficial and can be removed easily and safely. A "golf-club spud" is a handy tool for this task, but a small 30- to 25-gauge needle under slit-lamp magnification or a moistened cotton-tipped applicator will work most of the time. A topical anesthetic should be instilled prior to removal, and it is helpful to also instill an anesthetic drop in the unaffected eye to suppress reflex blinking during removal. Many slit lamps have an attached "fixation light" that is mobile and can be moved in front of the unaffected eye to give the patient a steady target to concentrate on. This reduces the random movements that can occur when you are trying to remove the foreign body. The eyelids can be held open with your fingers, or a wire eyelid speculum can provide excellent support during the procedure.

Metallic foreign bodies can create rust rings that are toxic to the corneal tissue. If a rust ring is present, the spud or an ophthalmic burr can be used to remove superficial rust. Even if a thorough job is done initially, the next day more rust often can be seen, requiring additional burring. It is therefore not necessary to remove all the rust aggressively in the emergency department if the patient can be seen by an ophthalmologist the next day. The rust-ring area can soften overnight and be removed in the office the next day. The deeper the stromal involvement, the higher is the risk of corneal scarring; therefore, only a superficial burring should take place in the emergency department. **No emergency department drill burring should take place if the rust ring is located in the visual axis (pupil) owing to the risk of causing visually significant scarring.** Such conditions require that an ophthalmologist remove the stromal rust in the office within 24 h. As with any foreign body of the eye, the lid should be everted and inspected under magnification to ensure that no additional foreign bodies are present. The corneal abrasion that will be present after removal of a foreign body should be treated as discussed previously with adequate cycloplegia, antibiotic ointment, and optional patching.

Treatment:

1. Instill topical anesthetic in *both eyes* to suppress the blink reflex.
2. Test visual acuity (sometimes easier after an anesthetic drop is administered).
3. Assess if this is a full-thickness or penetrating injury.
4. Remove the foreign body under slit-lamp magnification, and remove superficial rust if possible.
5. Use a burr if available, but avoid burring in visual axis, and avoid removal of deeply lying rust.
6. Evert the lid to rule out additional foreign bodies.
7. Treat resulting corneal abrasion with topical cycloplegia, erythromycin ointment, and optional patching (see "Conjunctival Abrasion" above).
8. Referral to an ophthalmologist, to be seen the next day.

Lid Lacerations

Full-thickness lid lacerations should be repaired by an ophthalmologist, if at all possible, within 24 h. Proper alignment of the lid margin during repair under magnification (loupe or microscope) is essential to preserve proper lid function and even corneal wetting with each blink. Notching of the lid can result in improper lid closure. Very small lacerations (<1 mm) at the lid edge only, do not need suturing and can heal spontaneously. Any laceration >1 mm needs repair. Notching of the lid can result in improper lid closure. If there is no opportunity for the patient to see an ophthalmologist, repair should be performed as in Figure 238-12. One 6-0 silk vertical mattress suture, using the meibomian gland orifices as a landmark, or two 6-0 silk sutures (one approximating the anterior and the other the posterior lamella) are used to repair the lid margin. The ends of the silk sutures should be left long enough to tuck under the more distal skin sutures to avoid corneal irritation. The tarsus should be repaired with 5-0 Vicryl from the external side so as to approximate the wound without the need for sutures on the conjunctival side of the lid (which would abrade the cornea with each blink). Skin closure can be performed with 6-0 or 7-0 monofilament or silk suture. Deep lacerations medial to the punctum potentially can transect the canalicular system. These injuries need to be seen by an ophthalmologist for evaluation of the nasolacrimal duct system's integrity. If a canalicular laceration is discovered, the patient will need to go to the operating room within 24 to 36 h for repair and Silastic tube stenting (Figure 238-13). Because a meticulous repair by an experienced eye surgery team is preferable, it is not unreasonable for the ophthalmologist to discharge a patient seen late in the evening or on the weekend with arrangements for surgical repair to take place within the next 36 h. Patients discharged pending repair should be placed on oral and topical antibiotics and told to use cold compresses. Oral cephalexin (Keflex) 500 mg twice or four times daily and topical erythromycin ophthalmic ointment four times daily are reasonable choices.

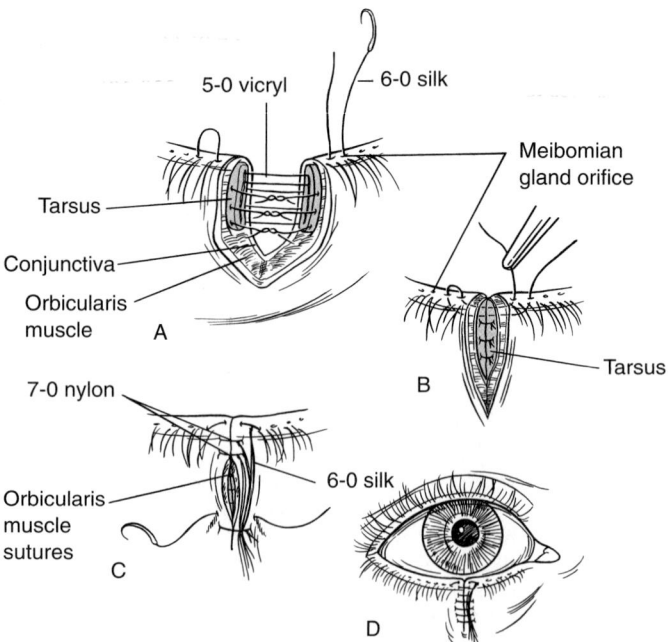

FIG. 238-12. Full-thickness lid repair. 6-0 silk is used for lid margin. 5-0 Vicryl is used to approximate the tarsal plate. The Vicryl sutures should not pass through the conjunctiva on the inside of the eyelid to avoid mechanical abrasion of the cornea during blinking. 7-0 Nylon is used for skin closure, and the lid margin silk suture tail can be incorporated into these sutures to avoid corneal irritation.

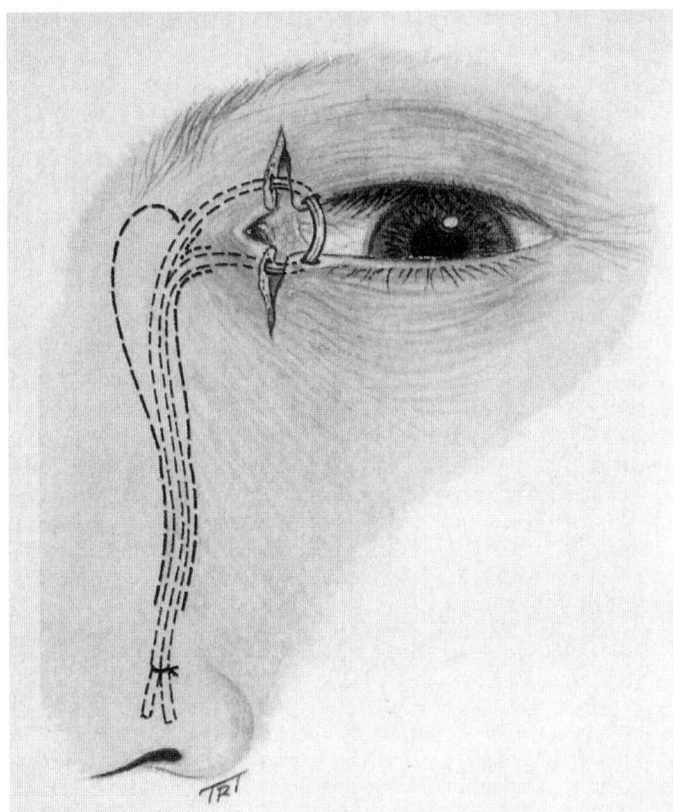

FIG. 238-13. Traumatic canalicular laceration repair requires microsurgical stenting to reestablish patency.

Partial-thickness lid lacerations can usually be repaired in the ED with referral for ophthalmologic evaluation in 2 to 3 days. It is important to have the suture ends closest to the cornea tucked under more distal sutures to avoid corneal irritation (see Figure 238-12).

Blunt Trauma

After sustaining blunt trauma, the eyelids frequently are swollen shut, and the globe is difficult to visualize. Trying to pry the eyelids open with your fingers can be frustrating; it increases the IOP and usually results in obtaining an unsatisfactory view of the globe. A wire or adjustable eyelid speculum can help tremendously. Insertion of the eyelid speculum provides a significantly improved view of the cornea and anterior chamber and allows your hands to remain free for examination of the globe at the slit lamp. If a speculum is not available, try your best to assess the patient's visual acuity and the integrity of the globe and anterior chamber. If the anterior chamber is flat, a ruptured globe is certain, and no further attempts to assess the eye should be made. A metal shield should be placed and an ophthalmologist consulted. A hyphema is also evidence of significant ocular trauma and necessitates an ophthalmology consult. If the globe appears intact and vision is preserved, next check ocular motility. Restricted upgaze or lateral gaze suggests a blowout fracture with entrapment (see "Blowout Fractures" below). Feel the orbital rim above and below for step-off deformities. Test for cutaneous sensation along the distribution of the inferior orbital nerve (below the eye and ipsilateral side of the nose). Perform a slit-lamp examination with fluorescein staining to check for abrasions, lacerations, foreign bodies, hyphema, iritis, and lens dislocation. Traumatic iritis is common, causing cell and flare to be seen on slit-lamp examination. If no corneal epithelial defect is seen, iritis can be treated with one drop of Pred Forte four to five times a day. The pupil can be constricted or dilated after sustaining trauma. It is important to look for pupillary irregularity because the pupil often will peak toward the site of a penetration or rupture. If the anterior chamber is of normal depth and not shallow, one drop of Mydriacyl 1% will dilate the pupil and allow an easier funduscopic view. Non-Caucasian brown-eyed individuals frequently will require an additional drop of phenylephrine 2.5% to achieve adequate dilation. If vision and ocular anatomy and function are preserved, outpatient follow-up by an ophthalmologist in the next 48 h should be planned. If a ruptured globe is suspected (blind eye, flat anterior chamber, obvious full-thickness laceration, intraocular foreign body), no attempts at eye manipulation or IOP measurement should take place, and an ophthalmologist should be consulted.

Treatment:

1. Assess globe integrity and vision.
2. If a ruptured globe is suspected, do not attempt to check IOP; place a protective metal eye shield, check tetanus status, administer intravenous cephalosporin, let the patient take nothing by mouth, and call ophthalmology.
3. If a ruptured globe is not suspected, proceed with the following.
4. Check eye motility and cutaneous sensation.
5. Obtain a facial/orbital CT scan if a blowout fracture or orbital/intraocular foreign body is suspected. Treat accordingly.
6. Slit-lamp examination of corneal, conjunctival, scleral, and anterior chamber structures.
7. Dilate if anterior chamber depth is normal for funduscopic view. *Caucasians:* Mydriacyl 1%, one drop. *All others:* Mydriacyl 1%, one drop, plus phenylephrine 2.5%, one drop.
8. Ophthalmology referral within 48 h if no injuries are found.

HYPHEMA   Blood in the anterior chamber is referred to as a *hyphema* (see Figure 238-9). Hyphemas generally can be classified as either traumatic or spontaneous. Traumatic hyphemas usually are the result of bleeding from a ruptured iris root vessel. Both blunt and penetrating trauma can cause hyphemas. Spontaneous hyphemas frequently are associated with sickle cell disease. All hyphemas, regardless of etiology, should be seen by an ophthalmologist. ED management consists of assessing concomitant injury (ruptured globe, intraocular foreign body) and managing rises in IOP. The patient's head should be elevated to promote settling of suspended red blood cells inferiorly so as not to clog the entire 360 degrees of trabecular meshwork. The pupil should be dilated to avoid "pupillary play" (constriction and dilation movements of the iris in response to changing lighting conditions). Because an iris vessel is usually involved, pupillary activity can put the vessel on stretch, promoting additional bleeding. Pupillary dilation *does not* compromise the angle and aqueous outflow in normal individuals, and many ophthalmologists choose to dilate hyphemas for the preceding reasons. IOP control is important and consists of topical β-blockers, intravenous mannitol, topical α-adrenergic agonists (apraclonidine), and oral, topical, or intravenous carbonic anhydrase inhibitors (CAIs) such as Diamox and Trusopt. **In patients suspected of having sickle cell disease (either by history or if the hyphema was spontaneous), carbonic anhydrase inhibitors should be strictly avoided.** CAIs will lower the aqueous pH in the anterior chamber, causing the red blood cells to sickle and become less flexible, thereby clogging outflow through the trabecular meshwork and increasing IOP.

Rebleeding can occur 3 to 5 days later in up to 30 percent of cases, sometimes causing potentially blinding elevations of IOP and necessitating surgical anterior chamber "washouts." Because of this risk, some ophthalmologists believe in admitting all patients with hyphemas, whereas others will choose to follow them closely as outpatients. Generally, those with hyphemas occupying one-third or less of the anterior chamber can be followed closely as outpatients. Because of the variance in treatment philosophy, the emergency physician should not assume responsibility for disposition. This decision should be made by the ophthalmologist on call after he or she has examined the patient.

Treatment:

1. Elevate the patient's head.
2. Administer atropine 1% one drop three times daily.
3. Administer prednisolone acetate 1% (Pred Forte) one drop four times daily.
4. If the globe is intact, measure IOP.
5. If IOP is greater than 30 mm Hg, administer topical β-blocker (Timoptic 0.5%), one drop. Give oral or intravenous acetazolamide (Diamox) 500 mg and add mannitol 1 to 2 g/kg IV if there is no response to the preceding.
6. If IOP is greater than 24 mm Hg and the patient is sickle cell trait-positive, treat as above *except avoid Diamox.*
7. Arrange for an ophthalmology consult.

BLOWOUT FRACTURES   The most frequent sites of orbital blowout fractures are the inferior wall (maxillary sinus) and medial wall (ethmoid sinus). A Waters' view x-ray frequently will show a cloudy maxillary sinus on the side of the trauma. This represents blood and fluid in the maxillary sinus from fracture of the orbital floor. Fractures of the medial wall can be associated with subcutaneous emphysema, sometimes exacerbated by sneezing or blowing the nose. Fractures of the inferior wall with entrapment of the inferior rectus muscle can cause restriction of upgaze and diplopia (Figure 230-14). Isolated blowout fractures with or without entrapment do not require immediate surgery and can be referred to ophthalmology, plastic surgery, oral maxillofacial (OMF) surgery or otolaryngology (depending on the local referral patterns) for repair within the next 3 to 10 days. CT scanning with 1.5-mm cuts of the orbit should take place, and oral antibiotics (Cephalexin 250 to 500 mg four times daily for 10 days) are often recommended because of the presence of sinus wall fractures. **All blowout fractures with normal initial eye examination in the emergency department should be referred to an ophthalmologist for an outpatient full dilated examination to rule out any unidentified retinal tears or detachments.** About one-third of blowout fractures are associated with ocular trauma (abrasion, traumatic iritis, hyphema, lens dislocation/subluxation, retinal tear or detachment); therefore, a careful eye examination in the ED and referral to an ophthalmologist are essential.

Penetrating Trauma/Ruptured Globe

Penetrating ocular trauma can occur from numerous sources (BB pellets, lawn mower projectiles, hammering, knife and gunshot wounds). Any projectile injury has the potential for penetrating the eye. Any lid laceration from a sharp object, especially if it involves the upper and lower eyelid, has the potential to have lacerated the globe and requires a slit-lamp examination. Clues to a ruptured globe or intraocular foreign body include shallow anterior chamber, hyphema, irregular pupil, significant reduction in preinjury visual acuity, and poor view of the optic nerve and posterior pole on direct ophthalmoscopy. It is not unreasonable to dilate the eye with Mydriacyl 1% and phenylephrine 2.5% to obtain a better view of the posterior segment of the eye, facilitating identification of an intraocular foreign body or retinal detachment. A modified Seidel test is helpful in identifying wound leaks (see Figure 238-8). Any penetrating injury is considered a ruptured globe and mandates an eye shield and ophthalmology consultation. Tetanus status should be determined and intravenous cephalosporin administered. Do not attempt to measure IOP if a ruptured globe is suspected. A Waters view x-ray, orbital CT scans or ultrasonography can be helpful in locating and confirming the presence of orbital and intraocular foreign bodies.

Treatment:

1. If a ruptured globe is suspected, do not attempt to check IOP; place a protective metal eye shield, check tetanus status, administer intravenous cephalosporin, caution the patient to take nothing by mouth, and call ophthalmology.
2. Obtain a Waters' view x-ray and/or orbital CT scans if foreign bodies are suspected.

Chemical Trauma

CHEMICAL OCULAR INJURY   A chemical injury to the eye is a true ocular emergency. The potential for chemical injury requires immediate recognition and treatment in the field and by the triage nurse. Immediate intervention consists of copious irrigation with at least 1 to 2 L of saline. Topical anesthesia and placement of a Morgan lens allow the irrigation to be delivered effectively and directly to the corneal surface. **This is one situation where a delay even to assess visual acuity is inappropriate.** Litmus paper or the pH portion of a urine dipstick can be used to assess the pH of the tears in the lower cul-de-sac. Irrigation should continue until pH testing improves to the range of 7.5 to 8 (see Chap. 181 for details). Both acid and alkali burns can be blinding; however, the majority of acid burns tend to coagulate proteins, thereby limiting the depth of penetration. Alkali burns (lye, ammonia) can rapidly penetrate the cornea, and aqueous pH can rise within minutes of exposure, causing damage to intraocular structures such as the iris and lens. After copious irrigation has been administered and the pH of the tears is close to normal, the eye should be inspected for any particulate matter, and visual acuity should be assessed. A topical cycloplegic agent such as 0.25% scopolamine or 1% cyclopentolate should be used three times daily for pain reduction if an epithelial defect is present. Erythromycin ophthalmic ointment should be instilled four times daily if both eyes are affected. If only one eye is affected and an epithelial defect is present, adding a pressure patch for the first 12 to 24 h sometimes will make the eye more comfortable. **Any patient with corneal clouding or an epithelial defect after irrigation should receive prompt ophthalmology referral.**

Patients with chemosis (edema of the bulbar conjunctiva overlying the white sclera) and no corneal or anterior chamber findings should be treated after irrigation with erythromycin ointment four times daily and referred for an ophthalmologic examination in the next 48 h. These patients are considered to have "chemical conjunctivitis."

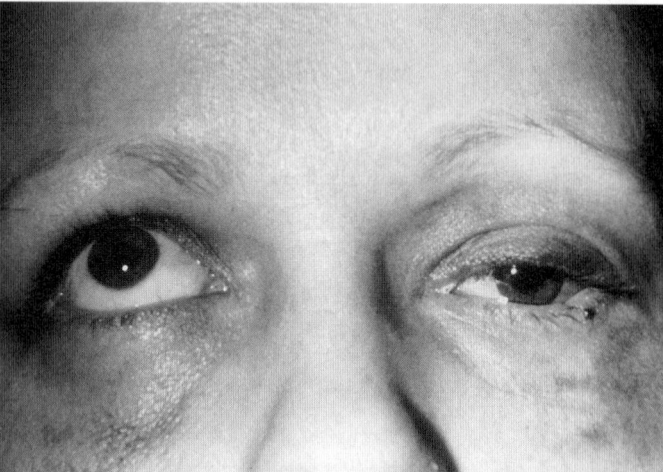

FIG. 238-14. Inferior wall blowout fracture of the left eye with entrapment of the inferior rectus muscle. The patient's left eye is unable to look upward, causing diplopia on upgaze.

Treatment:

1. Immediate copious irrigation with a minimum of 1 to 2 L of saline or until tear pH is 7.5 to 8.
2. If there is no corneal epithelial defect and the anterior segment is normal, administer erythromycin ointment four times daily.
3. If there is a corneal epithelial defect or there is clouding, administer erythromycin ointment, cycloplegia (cyclopentolate 1% or scopolamine 0.25%), and optional eye patching.
4. Provide for ophthalmology referral in the ED or within 24 h.

CYANOACRYLATE (SUPER GLUE/CRAZY GLUE)   Cyanoacrylate adhesives are commonplace and often easily accessible to children. Accidental instillation into the eye and adnexa can cause the lids to adhere and adhesive clumps to form on the cornea. Most of the time these accidental instillations are not permanently harmful to the eye. Medicinal-grade cyanoacrylates are used occasionally directly on the cornea to seal corneal perforations and are not considered toxic to the cornea. The only concern is the mechanical abrasive effect of hard, irregular glue aggregates rubbing against the cornea with eye movement and blinking. Erythromycin is instilled heavily into the eye and on the surface of the eyelids to moisten, lubricate, and provide antibiotic coverage. Initial debridement of the surface glue clump should be limited to easily removable pieces. The glue will loosen and become easier to remove in a few days. Referral to an ophthalmologist should take place within 24 to 48 h.

Treatment:

1. Moisten the glue with erythromycin ointment, and remove as much as can be removed easily without causing damage to underlying tissue.
2. Apply erythromycin ointment heavily into eye (if not glued completely shut) and eyelids five or six times a day.
3. Refer to ophthalmologist in the next 24 to 48 h.

ULTRAVIOLET KERATITIS ("WELDER'S FLASH")   Pain, tearing, photophobia, and foreign-body sensation typically occur 6 to 12 h after unprotected ocular exposure to welding or sun-tanning lights. The history is diagnostic in these cases. Slit-lamp examination with fluorescein staining shows superficial punctate keratitis; this appears as numerous small microdots of staining on the corneal surface seen under high magnification using the cobalt-blue light. Treatment consists of cycloplegia, erythromycin ointment, and pressure patching overnight. Oral narcotic analgesia sometimes is necessary.

Treatment:

1. Instill cycloplegic agent: 1% cyclopentolate or 0.25% scopolamine, one drop in each eye; this may be repeated by the patient every 6 to 8 h if needed for pain reduction.
2. Erythromycin ophthalmic ointment now, then four times daily once the patch is removed.
3. Pressure patching for comfort for the first 24 h; bilateral is preferable but seldom practical.
4. Consider oral narcotic analgesia if pain is severe.
5. Ophthalmology referral within 48 h (this condition is usually self-limited, with complete recovery).

ACUTE VISUAL REDUCTION/LOSS

Painful Visual Reduction/Loss

ACUTE ANGLE-CLOSURE GLAUCOMA   Acute angle-closure glaucoma presents with cloudy vision, eye ache and/or headache, increased IOP, and frequently, nausea and vomiting. Abdominal symptoms sometimes can be misleading and delay the diagnosis. Acute angle closure typically occurs in a patient with *no* previous history of glaucoma, but with undiagnosed narrow anterior chamber angles.

When the pupil becomes mid-dilated and the iris leaflet touches the lens, "pupillary block" suddenly develops. This prevents circulation of the aqueous humor from the posterior chamber (where it is produced by the ciliary body) through the pupil and into the anterior chamber (where it is filtered out of the eye through the trabecular meshwork located in the angle). The continuous production of aqueous humor in the posterior chamber is trapped, and the increasing hydrostatic pressure bows the iris forward, further compromising the angle and inhibiting outflow (Figure 238-15). IOP rises and eventually exceeds the capacity of the corneal pump mechanism, causing the cornea to become edematous and less transparent. This explains the foggy vision or halos patients complain of and the hazy appearance of the cornea on physical examination. The pupil is *mid-dilated and nonreactive* (Figure 238-16). Pressures as high as 50 mm Hg and greater are not uncommon. Treatment, aimed at pressure reduction, consists of using suppressants of aqueous humor production such as topical β-blockers, α-adrenergic agonists (apraclonidine), and oral or intravenous CAIs (acetazolamide). Because patients frequently are nauseated, intravenous CAIs are preferable to oral ones. Intravenous mannitol is very good at quickly lowering IOP and should be considered an adjunct to treatment if there are no contraindications. Pilocarpine frequently will not cause the iris to constrict during the acute attack until the pressure is reduced. This is due to pressure-induced ischemic paralysis of the iris. Pilocarpine 1% or 2% should be added once the pressure is reduced to make the pupil miotic, thereby pulling the peripheral iris away from the angle. This maneuver will help protect against recurrence until an ophthalmologist can perform the definitive treatment procedure of creating a peripheral laser iridectomy.

Treatment:

1. Identify mid-dilated, nonreactive pupil with increased IOP.
2. Topical β-blocker (Timoptic 0.5%), one drop.
3. Topical α-agonist (Iopidine 0.1%), one drop.
4. Topical steroid (Pred Forte 1%), one drop every 15 min for four doses, then hourly.
5. CAI (acetazolamide) 500 mg IV or PO.
6. Mannitol 1 to 2 g/kg IV.
7. Recheck IOP hourly.

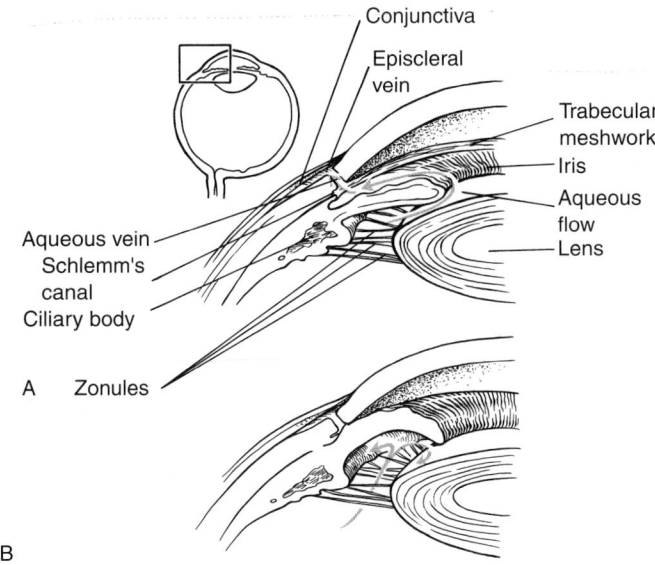

FIG. 238-15. A. Normal flow of aqueous from ciliary body, through the pupil and out through the trabecular meshwork and Schlemm's canal located in the anterior chamber angle. **B.** Angle-closure glaucoma with pupillary block. Iris leaflet bows forward, blocking the chamber angle and prohibiting aqueous outflow. Meanwhile, aqueous production continues and IOP rises.

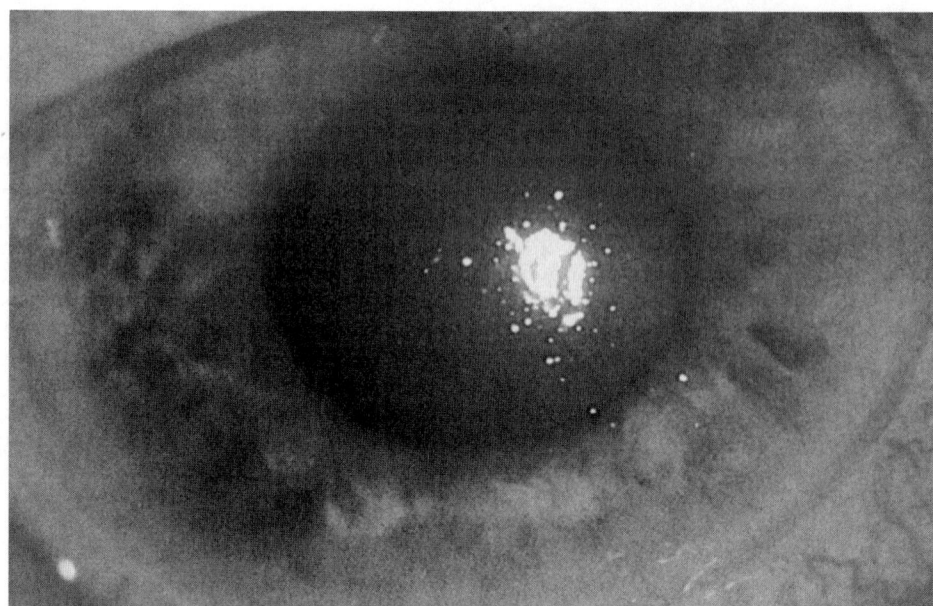

FIG. 238-16. Acute angle-closure glaucoma. Pupil is mid-dilated and nonreactive. The cornea is hazy due to stromal edema.

8. Topical pilocarpine 1% to 2%, one drop four times daily once IOP is below 40 mm Hg.
9. Consult ophthalmology.

OPTIC NEURITIS   Optic neuritis is the most common cause of acute reduction of vision due to optic nerve dysfunction in patients 20 to 40 years of age. Women are affected more frequently than men. Reduction of vision is rapid and frequently painful (especially with eye movement). Color vision is affected commonly more than visual acuity. The red desaturation test is helpful in identifying optic neuropathies. (Have the patient look with one eye at a dark red object; then test the other eye to see if the object looks the same color. The affected eye often will see the red object as pink or lighter red.) An afferent pupillary defect (APD; see Figure 238-3) is commonly present. Visual acuity can range from mildly reduced to no light perception (NLP). If the optic disc is swollen and edematous on the affected side (papillitis), the patient is said to have anterior optic neuritis. If the head of the optic nerve is normal in appearance, the patient is said to have retrobulbar neuritis. The Optic Neuritis Treatment Trial (ONTT) showed that 1 year after an attack of optic neuritis, there was no difference in visual outcome between the patients treated with intravenous steroids and those given a placebo. Treatment with intravenous steroids, however, was associated with a slightly lower 2-year risk of subsequent development of multiple sclerosis, especially in patients whose MRI showed periventricular white matter lesions. For this reason, some physicians will consider intravenous steroids for any attack of optic neuritis, although no treatment is also acceptable. *Initial treatment with oral steroids is contraindicated* and, for unexplained reasons, had the least favorable outcome in the ONTT. Children can develop optic neuritis with similar initial findings, except that the majority of them tend to have bilateral optic nerve swelling (simulating papilledema) and a viral illness is frequently associated with an attack. Subsequent development of multiple sclerosis occurs less frequently in children.

Treatment:

1. Check visual acuity, do red desaturation test, APD, eye pain with movement.
2. Check optic nerve head for papillitis (usually unilateral), may be bilateral in children or normal in retrobulbar neuritis.

3. Discuss with ophthalmologist or neurologist whether to treat with intravenous steroids or discharge without treatment. *Steroid regimen:* methylprednisolone 250 mg IV four times daily for 3 days, followed by oral prednisone 1 mg/kg per d for 11 days.

Painless Visual Reduction/Loss

CENTRAL RETINAL ARTERY OCCLUSION   Sudden, profound, painless, monocular loss of vision is characteristic of a central retinal artery occlusion (CRAO). The event is often preceded by episodes of amaurosis fugax. The first branch off the internal carotid artery is the ophthalmic artery, which supplies the central retinal artery, which, in turn, provides the blood supply to the inner retina. If the central retinal artery becomes occluded, the retina will infarct and become pale, less transparent, and edematous. The macula is the thinnest portion of the retina, and the intact underlying choroidal circulation remains visible through this section of retina, creating the illusion of a "cherry red spot." In fact, the macular area tends to maintain its normal color, whereas the surrounding ischemic retina turns pale, thus causing this classic finding on funduscopy (Figure 238-17, **Plate 7**). An APD is a common finding associated with a CRAO. Causes include embolus (carotid and cardiac), thrombosis, giant cell arteritis, vasculitis (lupus), sickle cell disease, and trauma. Often the patient will have atrial fibrillation. The retina will sustain irreversible damage within 90 min of total occlusion, so treatment should begin immediately. Unfortunately, response to therapy is rare, but because the visual loss is usually so profound, every attempt should be made to reestablish circulation to the retina. Treatment in embolic cases (the majority) is aimed at trying to convert a CRAO into a branch retinal artery occlusion (BRAO). In the attempt to dislodge the embolus from the central artery and into one of its retinal branches, the other retinal branches may become reperfused, thereby reducing the size of the infarct. Maneuvers include digital massage, IOP-lowering drugs, and vasodilation techniques (breathing into a paper bag to increase $Paco_2$). An ophthalmologist should be consulted immediately to evaluate the patient and decide whether performing an IOP-lowering anterior chamber paracentesis is indicated.

Treatment:

1. Consult ophthalmology the moment the diagnosis is made.

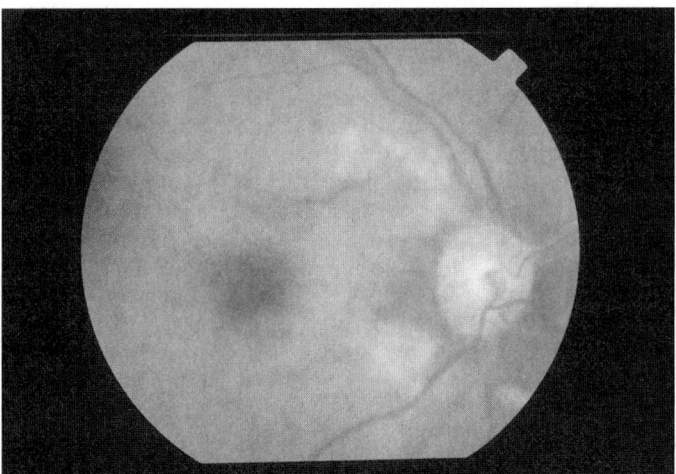

FIG. 238-17. (PLATE 7). Central retinal artery occlusion. Note macular "cherry red spot" and retinal pallor between macula and disc. The retinal veins appear normal size, but the arteries are barely visible and attenuated.

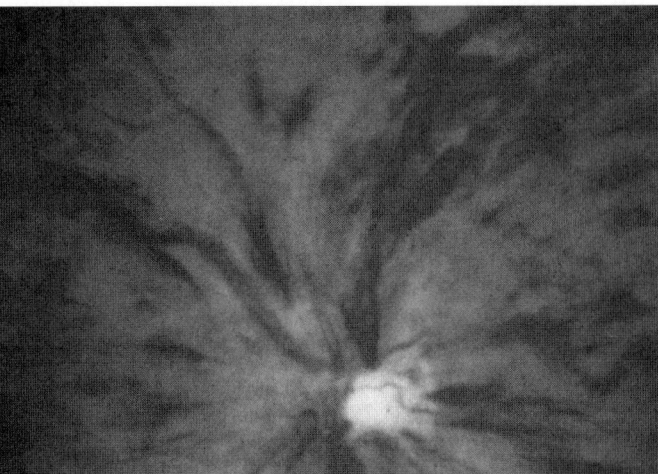

FIG. 238-18. (PLATE 8). Central retinal vein occlusion "blood and thunder fundus." Note diffuse retinal hemorrhages in all retina quadrants and blurred disc margins.

2. Administer ocular massage: firm, steady digital pressure on the globe through closed lids for about 15 s, followed by sudden release of pressure. This may be repeated several times.
3. Administer topical β-blocker (Timoptic 0.5%), one drop.
4. Give acetazolamide 500 mg IV or PO.
5. Consider having the patient breathe into a paper bag for 5 to 10 min if there are no respiratory contraindications.

CENTRAL RETINAL VEIN OCCLUSION   Thrombosis of the central retinal vein causes retinal venous stasis, edema, and hemorrhage. Loss of vision is variable, painless, monocular, and rapid. Funduscopic examination typically reveals optic disc edema and diffuse retinal hemorrhages in all quadrants ("blood-and-thunder fundus") (Figure 238-18, **Plate 8**). The contralateral optic nerve and fundus generally are normal, which helps distinguish central retinal vein occlusion (CRVO) from papilledema, and the diffuse retinal hemorrhages help distinguish it from optic neuritis (the peripheral retina is normal in optic neuritis). Typically patients have a history of hypertension, although hypercoagulable disorders, vasculitis, and glaucoma also may be associated. No specific treatment is available, although the addition of aspirin 60 to 325 mg daily is reasonable. Patients should be referred to an ophthalmologist for confirmation of the diagnosis and monitoring of ischemia-induced neovascularization.

Treatment:

1. Ophthalmology referral.
2. Consider aspirin 60 to 325 mg/d PO.

FLASHING LIGHTS (PHOTOPSIAS) AND FLOATERS   Complaints about new onset flashing lights and/or floaters commonly cause patients to seek urgent medical attention. The first distinction to make is if the symptoms are monocular or binocular. Binocular complaints are almost always intracranial (i.e., ophthalmic migraines) whereas monocular complaints are almost always related to the symptomatic eye.

The posterior segment of the eye is a large cavity filled with vitreous gel. As a person ages, this gel eventually contracts centrally and separates from the posterior wall of the eye. The vitreous is very sticky and tugs on the retina prior to separation. The mechanical traction stimulates the retina and the brain perceives this stimulation as light. This process takes place in every one eventually. The average age of onset is 55 years of age, but can occur as early as the twenties in se-

verely nearsighted people. If the vitreous gel separates successfully, then floaters occur. These may persist for years until the gel liquefies enough for the floaters to sink below the visual axis. If the gel creates enough traction on the retina prior to separation that it tears a hole in the retina, then fluid can go through the retinal hole and start to peel the retina off like wallpaper. In this case a dark veil or curtain will be perceived by the patient, blocking a segment of their visual field in the affected eye. This is an emergent condition requiring a retina specialist to evaluate and treat the patient.

Diagnosing a retinal detachment or tear requires a dilated indirect ophthalmoscopic evaluation by an ophthalmologist. It is very difficult for a non-ophthalmologist to comprehensively examine the retina. A retinal tear will be almost impossible for an emergency physician to see. A large retinal detachment will appear as a pale billowing parachute on dilated funduscopic examination. The history and symptoms are the most useful.

1. Ascertain if symptoms are monocular.
2. Assess visual acuity in the affected eye and ask about subjective changes.
3. If the visual acuity is baseline and the patient only perceives flashes and floaters and no sectoral vision loss is present, then dilate and view posterior pole to rule out hemorrhages, papilledema, or overt pathology. If it appears normal then contact ophthalmology to arrange a full evaluation with 24 h.
4. If the patient has a definite monocular visual field cut, then a retinal detachment is highly suspected and ophthalmology should be consulted. Most diagnosed retinal detachments are repaired within 24 h, unless the macula has detached. If the macula has come off and the vision is CF or HM, then the repair is less urgent.

GIANT CELL ARTERITIS (TEMPORAL ARTERITIS)   Giant cell arteritis (GCA) is a systemic vasculitis involving medium-sized arteries in the carotid circulation and can include the aorta and its primary branches. GCA can cause a painless ischemic optic neuropathy with devastating visual consequences and rapid contralateral involvement if not diagnosed and treated promptly. Patients are generally over 50 years of age and frequently have a history of polymyalgia rheumatica. Women are affected more commonly than men. Symptoms may include headache, jaw claudication, myalgias, fatigue, fever, anorexia, and temporal artery tenderness. Up to 33 percent may have associated neurologic symptoms such as transient ischemic attacks or stroke. The patient can develop rapid and profound visual loss, with the contralateral eye becoming involved within days to weeks. The physical examination frequently will reveal an APD if the optic nerve circulation is involved. An elevated Westergren sedimentation rate is usually present, with the majority of biopsy-proven cases in the range of 70 to 110 mm/h. The added presence of an elevated C-reactive protein also suggests the diagnosis. Treatment consists of several doses of intravenous steroids followed by oral steroids. Steroids should not be delayed while waiting for a temporal artery biopsy to be performed. Biopsies will still be positive a week after initiation of steroid therapy.

Treatment:

1. Order sedimentation rate and C-reactive protein.
2. Consult patient's personal physician.
3. If highly suspicious or any visual loss, admit for methylprednisolone 250 mg IV every 6 h for 3 days and temporal artery biopsy.
4. If not suspicious and no visual involvement, prednisone 80 to 100 mg/d PO and close outpatient monitoring.

NEURO-OPHTHALMOLOGY

Approximately 38 percent of all the neurons in the brain have some association with the visual system; therefore, an understanding of neuro-ophthalmology is essential.

Bell Palsy

Bell palsy is a dysfunction of peripheral cranial nerve (CN) VII commonly of viral origin. It is palsy of the ipsilateral upper and lower face. The orbicularis muscles are involved frequently, resulting in incomplete closure of the eyelids on the affected side. If the eye rolls up under the upper lid on attempted blinking *(Bell phenomenon),* the cornea will be moistened, and the risk of corneal exposure keratitis and subsequent ulceration will be less. These patients should still use viscous topical wetting agents, such as Celluvisc or Lacrilube, to keep the corneal epithelium from breaking down. Ophthalmology referral for outpatient monitoring of the cornea is warranted. Etiology and treatment of Bell palsy is discussed in Chap. 143.

Genu VII Bell palsy is a CVA masquerading as a peripheral seventh-nerve Bell palsy. It is a stroke involving CN VI and the ipsilateral CN VII as it "genuflects" around the sixth nerve nucleus. This results in a CN VII palsy identical to a typical Bell palsy (affecting the upper and lower face ipsilaterally) but with the added finding of the patient's inability to abduct the ipsilateral eye (CN VI palsy). This underscores the importance of EOM testing in all Bell palsy patients to avoid misdiagnosis of a CVA.

Treatment:

1. Test ipsilateral abduction (rule out genu VII Bell palsy).
2. Have the patient use eye lubricants every 2 h (Celluvisc or artificial tears) and ointment at bedtime.
3. Consider oral steroids and acyclovir.
4. Refer to ophthalmology for outpatient monitoring of cornea.

Diabetic/Hypertensive Cranial Nerve Palsies

Chronic diabetes and hypertension eventually can create vascular compromise to the vasa nervorum of any cranial nerve. Frequently, the patient will present with new-onset diplopia, and an isolated CN III or VI palsy will be found on physical examination. The cranial nerve palsy can be painful or painless. The *pupil is spared* in acute diabetic CN III palsy due to vascular compromise of the central nerve fibers (the efferent pupillomotor fibers run in the periphery of the nerve) (Figure 238-19). EOM testing will reveal an inhibition of ipsilateral medial gaze, upward gaze, and downward gaze as well as ptosis in an acute CN III palsy. Lateral gaze (abduction) will be preserved, and diplopia will be worse when the patient attempts to look toward the contralateral side due to the inability to adduct the eye (medial rectus dysfunction). In an acute CN VI palsy, lateral gaze will be diminished (abduction) on the ipsilateral side, and diplopia will be worse when the patient is trying to look to the affected side (lateral rectus dysfunction). If no other associated neurologic symptoms or findings are present and the blood sugar and blood pressure are under control, the patient can be discharged with ophthalmology and/or neurology follow-up. Many palsies will resolve or improve over the following 3 months. Neuroimaging is generally done in the ED to rule out an intracranial lesion.

Posterior Communicating Artery (PCA) Aneurysm

Acute CN III palsy with *ipsilateral pupillary dilatation* is a PCA aneurysm until proven otherwise. Concomitant headache is a frequent but not absolute finding. Expansion of an aneurysm of the posterior communicating artery frequently causes compression of the outer fibers of CN III. The pupillomotor fibers are located in the outer portion of CN III; therefore, the pupil becomes dilated on the affected side (see Figure 238-19). These patients require emergent blood pressure reduction, neuroimaging, and neurosurgical consultation.

Internuclear Ophthalmoplegia (INO)

A stroke or demyelinating disease involving the medial longitudinal fasciculus (MLF) will cause the patient to experience diplopia, most noticeable when he or she attempts to look to the side opposite the lesion. EOM testing reveals an ipsilateral adduction weakness (medial rectus muscle only—not a CN III palsy).

For example, if a patient has experienced a right (MLF) stroke, the right medial rectus muscle will not function when he or she attempts a leftward gaze, and the patient will not be able to adduct the right eye. The left eye will abduct but may experience some nystagmus on leftward gaze. The patient will be able to look to the right without difficulty unless there is bilateral involvement. The patient also will be able to look up and down, revealing that the superior and inferior rectus muscles are functioning and that this is not a CN III palsy.

Treatment:

1. Same as with any newly diagnosed CVA.
2. Consider demyelinating disease if the patient is young.

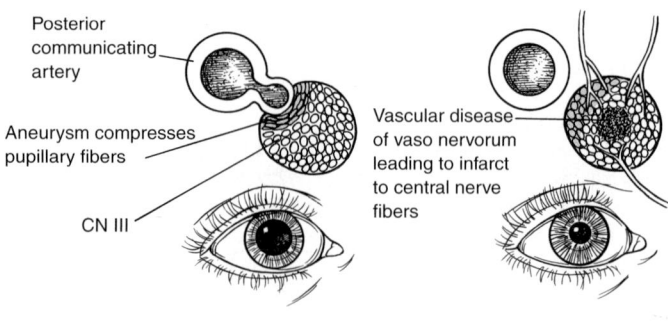

FIG. 238-19. Posterior communicating artery aneurysm compresses the peripherally located pupillomotor fibers of CN III, causing a nerve palsy and pupillary dilatation. Diabetes and hypertension can cause microvascular compromise of the central nerve fibers causing a nerve palsy with pupil sparing.

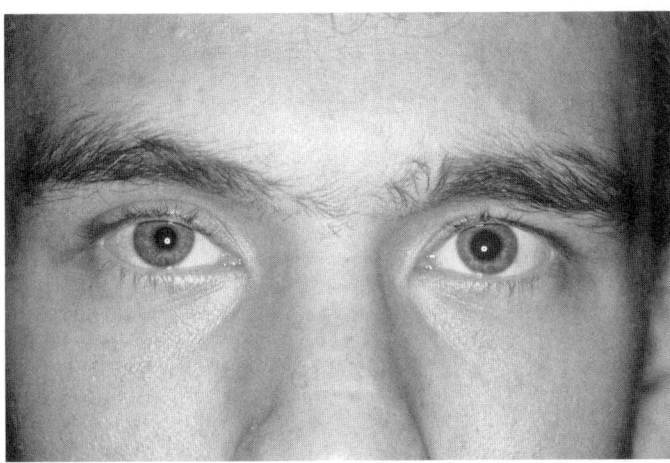

FIG. 238-20. Horner syndrome. Note ptosis and miosis of the right eye. This patient sustained an acute right carotid artery dissection after being hit in the neck with a football.

Horner Syndrome

The physical findings of ipsilateral ptosis and miosis and anhydrosis are characteristic of Horner syndrome (Figure 238-20). Interruption of the sympathetic nerve impulses controlling the Mueller muscle in the upper eyelid and the iris dilators causes these classic findings. Interruption can occur anywhere along the pathway from the brainstem to the sympathetic plexus surrounding the carotid artery (Figure 238-21). It is very important to determine whether this syndrome is acute or chronic. Patients with chronic disease can be evaluated on an outpatient basis, but all cases of acute disease require a full emergent evaluation. Workup includes a chest x-ray, CT scan of the brain and cervical region, and a carotid angiogram if a carotid dissection is suspected (acute Horner syndrome with neck pain).

Causes of Horner syndrome include, in adults, CVA, tumors, internal carotid dissection, herpes zoster, and trauma. In children, the causes include neuroblastoma, lymphoma, and metastasis. Neck pain and acute Horner syndrome suggest carotid dissection and can occur spontaneously (usually above age 30) or as a result of blunt or penetrating neck injury.

Treatment:

1. Determine whether the condition is chronic or acute.
2. *Chronic:* Outpatient workup by personal physician.
3. *Acute:* Evaluate for CVA, tumor, or carotid dissection.

Papilledema

Papilledema generally is defined as bilateral edema of the head of the optic nerve due to increased intracranial pressure (ICP). It is a common finding in malignant hypertension, pseudotumor cerebri, intracranial tumors, and hydrocephalus. Any disease process that increases the ICP and thereby inhibits vascular or axoplasmic flow in the optic nerve causes congestion and edema of the nerve head. When only one nerve head is involved, it generally is not related to increased ICP (except in the rare Foster-Kennedy syndrome). Monocular optic nerve edema or binocular involvement not associated with increased ICP is usually referred to as *optic nerve edema* or, if inflammatory in origin, *papillitis* (i.e., optic neuritis). Frequently, the term *papilledema* has been used interchangeably in the literature to refer to monocular or binocular nerve head edema; however, most neuro-ophthalmologists reserve the term *papilledema* for bilateral nerve involvement due to increased ICP. Regardless of the etiology, the clini-

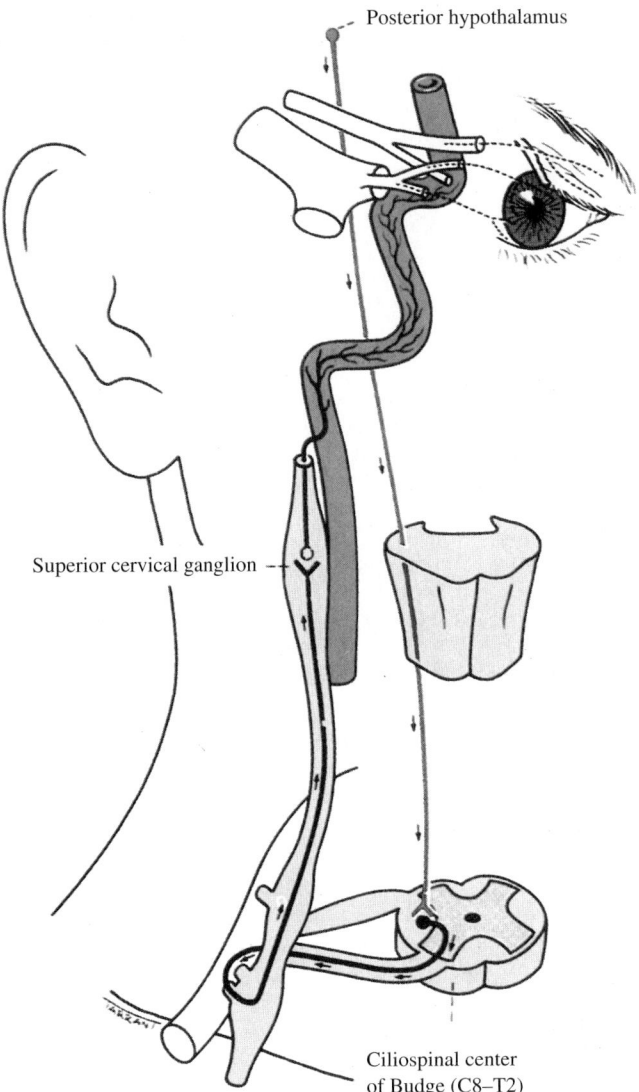

FIG. 238-21. Sympathetic nerve pathway of the eye. An interruption anywhere along this pathway can cause Horner syndrome.

cal findings on ophthalmoscopy of papilledema and papillitis are identical: The disc margins are blurred, the cup is diminished or absent, and the nerve head is elevated with vascular congestion (Figure 238-22, **Plate 9**). Frequently, flame-shaped hemorrhages are seen on or adjacent to the nerve head. A distinguishing feature of papilledema is prolonged preservation of visual acuity (frequently patients are visually asymptomatic). In this respect they differ markedly from patients with optic neuritis, who generally present with decreased visual acuity.

Pseudotumor Cerebri (Idiopathic Intracranial Hypertension)

Increased ICP, papilledema, normal CSF, and normal CT/MRI characterize pseudotumor cerebri. Most patients are 20- to 30-year-old obese women, although this condition can occur at any age. Patients complain of nausea, vomiting, headaches, and transient visual obscurations. They can develop CN VI paresis, causing horizontal diplopia (double vision on lateral gaze). A number of conditions (pregnancy) and exogenous agents (oral contraceptives, vitamin A, tetracycline,

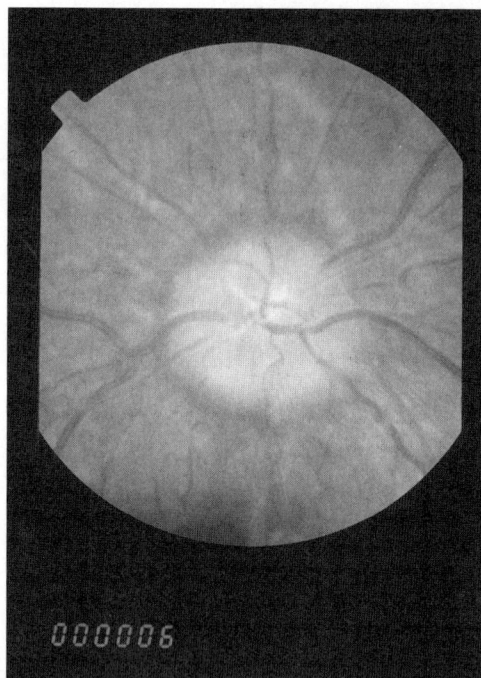

FIG. 238-22. (PLATE 9). Optic nerve head edema. Vascular congestion, elevation of the nerve head, and blurred disk margins are characteristically seen in papilledema, papillitis, and compressive lesions of the optic nerve.

nalidixic acid, and corticosteroid withdrawal or prolonged use) have been associated with this poorly understood disease. It can be self-limited, but the recurrence rate can be as high as 40 percent, and permanent loss of visual field can occur. Treatment is aimed at weight reduction and use of diuretics. Serial lumbar punctures sometimes are performed to reduce ICP.

Treatment:

1. Identify papilledema.
2. Perform neuroimaging of brain (CT/MRI).
3. If CT/MRI is normal, perform lumbar puncture and record opening pressure; send CSF for routine diagnostics.
4. If ICP is elevated and scans and CSF are normal, discuss with ophthalmologist/neurologist institution of diuretics (acetazolamide 500 mg PO twice daily) and outpatient visual field monitoring.

BIBLIOGRAPHY

Rhee D, Pyfer M: *The Wills Eye Manual: Office and Emergency Room Diagnosis and Treatment of Eye Disease,* 3d ed. Philadelphia, Lippincott, Williams & Wilkins, 1999.

Kanski J: *Clinical Ophthalmology: A Systematic Approach,* 3d ed. London, Butterworth-Heinemann, 1994.

Kline L: *Optic Nerve Disorders: Ophthalmology Monographs,* no 10. San Francisco, American Academy of Ophthalmology, 1996.

Liesegang T, Deutsch T, Grand MG: *Basic and Clinical Science Course, 2001-2002.* San Francisco, Foundation of the American Academy of Ophthalmology, 2001.

Spalton D, Hitchings R, Hunter P: *Atlas of Clinical Ophthalmology,* 2d ed. London, Mosby-Year Book Europe, 1994.

Trobe J: *The Physician's Guide to Eye Care.* San Francisco, American Academy of Ophthalmology, 1993.

Vaughan D, Asbury T, Riordan-Eva P: *General Ophthalmology,* 14th ed. Norwalk, Appleton & Lange, 1995.

Wright K: *Textbook of Ophthalmology.* Baltimore, Williams & Wilkins, 1997.

Yanoff M, Duker J: *Ophthalmology.* St Louis, Mosby, 1999.

239 COMMON DISORDERS OF THE EXTERNAL, MIDDLE, AND INNER EAR
Anne Tintinalli
Michael Lucchesi

NORMAL ANATOMY

External Ear

The auricle, or pinna, is the visible external portion of the ear, whose trumpet shape enables it to collect air vibrations. It consists of a thin plate of elastic cartilage with a tightly adherent covering of skin. The external auditory canal (EAC) is an S-shaped skin-lined tube that extends from the auricle to the tympanic membrane. The outer one-third of the EAC is composed of an incomplete cartilaginous tube. Its thick skin contains hair follicles and apocrine and sebaceous glands. The inner two-thirds of the canal is composed of bone covered by a thin layer of tightly adherent skin, which is easily torn by minimal trauma.

The blood supply to the external ear is derived from the posterior auricular, superficial temporal, and deep auricular arteries. Venous drainage of the external ear is into the superficial temporal and posterior auricular veins and then into the external jugular vein. The posterior auricular vein frequently connects to the sigmoid sinus, providing a route for extension of infection into the intracranial cavity.

Middle Ear

The middle ear is an air-containing cavity in the petrous temporal bone. It contains the auditory ossicles, which transmit vibrations of the tympanic membrane (TM) to the perilymph of the internal ear. It communicates with the nasopharynx anteriorly via the eustachian tube and with the mastoid air spaces posteriorly via the aditus ad antrum (Figure 239-1).

The TM is a thin, pearly gray, fibrous membrane, which, when illuminated, produces a cone-shaped light reflex anteroinferiorly. Superiorly, the pars flaccida is the relatively slack portion of the membrane between the malleolar folds; the remainder of the membrane is tense and is called the pars tensa. The auditory ossicles are the malleus, incus, and stapes. Both the incus and the handle and lateral processes of the malleus are typically visible through the TM (Figure 239-2). Figure 239-1 shows the relationships of the facial nerve, sigmoid sinus, and internal carotid artery to the middle ear.

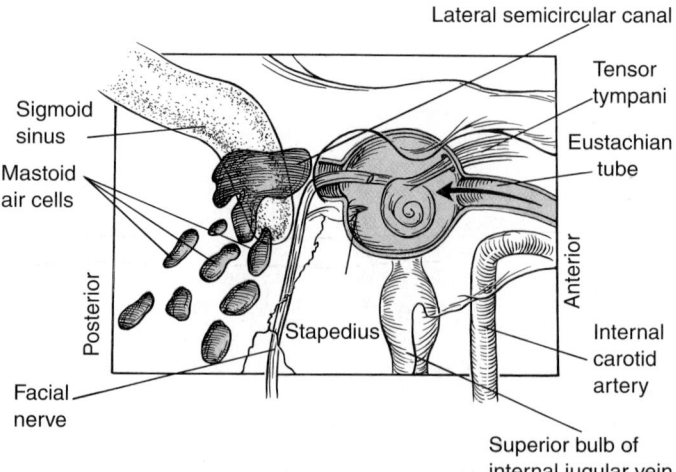

FIG. 239-1. Sagittal section of the middle ear and related structures.

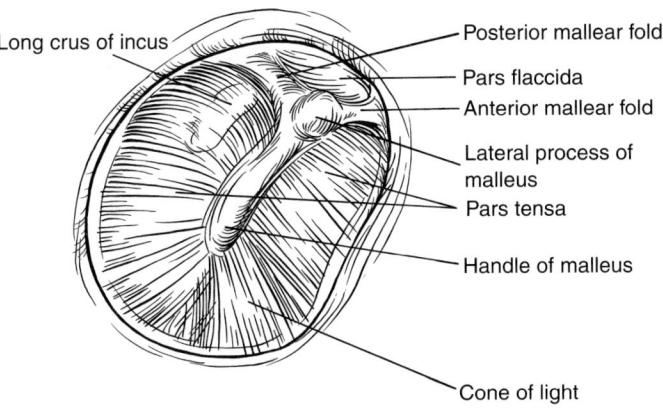

FIG. 239-2. Right tympanic membrane as seen through the otoscope.

Labels: Long crus of incus, Posterior mallear fold, Pars flaccida, Anterior mallear fold, Lateral process of malleus, Pars tensa, Handle of malleus, Cone of light

TABLE 239-1   Causes of Otalgia

Primary	Referred	Neuralgias
Trauma	Dental	Trigeminal
Infection	TMJ disease	(Tic douloureux)
Otitis externa	Abscessed teeth	Herpetic geniculate
Otitis media	Malocclusion	(Ramsay Hunt
Mastoiditis	Bruxism	syndrome)
Bullous myringitis	Trauma	
Foreign bodies	Retro- and oropharyngeal	
Cerumen impaction	Tonsillitis	
Cholesteatoma	Abscess	
Neoplasms	Neoplasm	
	Nasal cavity	
	Sinusitis	
	Deviated septum	
	Throat and neck	
	Foreign body	
	Thyroid disease	
	Cervical strain	
	Neoplasm	

Inner Ear

The inner ear consists of the cochlea, which contains the auditory sensory receptors, and the vestibular labyrinth, which contains balance receptors. Cristae in the semicircular canals detect angular acceleration and macules detect linear acceleration. Afferent nerves from the vestibular labyrinth connect to brainstem nuclei to maintain smooth movement of the eyes during head movement and to the cerebellum to control oculomotor and postural functions. Blood supply is from the vertebrobasilar system (Figure 239-3). The otolithic organs (utricle and saccule) lie in the vestibule. The internal auditory artery divides into the common cochlear artery and the anterior vestibular artery. The anterior vestibular artery provides the blood supply to the anterior and horizontal semicircular canals but not to the cochlea. Isolated occlusion of the anterior vestibular artery may therefore cause acute ves-tibular syndrome without hearing loss.

COMMON EAR COMPLAINTS

Otalgia

Primary otalgia is caused by auricular and periauricular disease, while referred otalgia is caused by disease originating from remote structures. Referred otalgia is common because of the multiple cranial nerves and branches of the cervical plexus that supply sensory innervation to both the ear and other structures of the head and neck. The sensory innervation of the ear is mediated by the fifth, seventh, ninth, and tenth cranial nerves, as well as by the cervical plexus, with much overlapping and variability. Table 239-1 lists common causes of primary and referred otalgia.

PRIMARY OTALGIA   The mandibular division of the trigeminal nerve mediates sensory innervation from the anterior outer ear: the au-

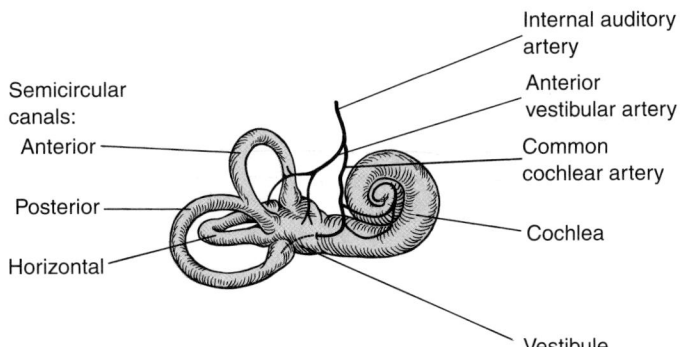

FIG. 239-3. Schematic of the bony labyrinth containing the vestibular and auditory sensory organs.

Labels: Semicircular canals: Anterior, Posterior, Horizontal; Internal auditory artery; Anterior vestibular artery; Common cochlear artery; Cochlea; Vestibule

ricle, tragus, EAC, and external surface of the TM. The facial nerve carries sensory innervation from the EAC and the skin behind the auricle. The glossopharyngeal nerve and the auricular branch of the vagus nerve (the Arnold nerve) carry sensory input from the medial ear structures. Branches of the second and third cervical nerves form the greater auricular and lesser occipital nerves, which receive input from the skin over the parotid gland and behind the ear, respectively.

Disease from any portion of the ear or its surrounding skin and structures may result in primary otalgia. A history and physical examination of the external ear, EAC, and TM will usually identify the cause of primary otalgia, with specific therapy as appropriate.

REFERRED OTALGIA   The maxillary and mandibular divisions of the trigeminal nerve receive sensory input from the nasopharynx, paranasal sinuses, teeth, parotid gland, and muscles of mastication. The facial nerve carries sensory innervation from the nasal mucosa and the ethmoid and sphenoid sinuses. The glossopharyngeal nerve carries sensory innervation from the nasopharynx, eustachian tube, soft palate, posterior pharynx, and tonsils. The vagus nerve mediates sensation from the valleculae and piriform sinuses, from the larynx via the superior laryngeal nerve, and from the cervical esophagus and trachea via the recurrent laryngeal nerve.

Abscessed and impacted teeth, usually mandibular molars, frequently cause ear pain. Malocclusion, bruxism, mandibular trauma, temporomandibular joint (TMJ) disorders, and ill-fitting dentures are frequent causes of otalgia.[1] Trigeminal neuralgia, or tic douloureux, causes severe unilateral facial pain. Herpetic geniculate neuralgia, or Ramsay Hunt syndrome, is herpes zoster of the EAC and auricle with facial palsy, which may persist long after the disappearance of the vesicles (postherpetic neuralgia).

The diagnosis of the source of referred otalgia requires a history and physical examination that encompasses the nasal and oral cavities, nasopharynx, oropharynx, throat, and neck. Again, further evaluation and treatment depend upon diagnosis.

Tinnitus

Tinnitus is the perception of sound without external stimulation. It may be constant, pulsatile, high- or low-pitched, hissing, clicking, or ringing. It is most prevalent between the ages of 40 and 70 years and has no gender predominance.[2]

Tinnitus is divided into two types: objective and subjective. Objective tinnitus may be heard by the examiner. Subjective tinnitus is more common. Its exact mechanism is unknown, although it is believed to result from damage to cochlear hair cells. Table 239-2 outlines causes of tinnitus.[2]

Pharmacologic side effects are the cause of tinnitus in at least 10 percent of cases.[2] The most commonly implicated drugs are aspirin (which may produce tinnitus in doses as low as 1.5 g per d) and aspirin-containing compounds, nonsteroidal anti-inflammatory drugs, and antibiotics, particularly aminoglycosides. (See Table 239-3 for a list of common ototoxic agents.)

Accurate diagnosis usually requires referral to an otolaryngologist. Many medications have been suggested as therapies, but antidepressants are currently the only class of drug found to be useful in alleviating tinnitus for which no correctable cause can be found.

SUDDEN HEARING LOSS

Sudden hearing loss (SHL) is hearing loss occurring over 3 days or less. The incidence increases with increasing age, and there is no gender predominance. Indicators of poor prognosis include more severe hearing loss on presentation and the presence of vertigo. Although most cases of SHL are idiopathic, other causes include infection, vascular causes, and trauma, as well as metabolic disturbances and ototoxic drugs (Table 239-4).[3]

Viral infections, most typically mumps, have long been associated with SHL. Because of the terminal branches and interosseous location of the blood supply to the inner ear, the ear is uniquely vulnerable to a variety of vascular and hematologic diseases. Cogan syndrome is an autoimmune disorder that presents with a bilateral hearing loss classically associated with tinnitus and vertigo. SHL may also be caused by rupture of the tympanic membranes.

Many common medications have been implicated in SHL (see Table 238-3).[4–10] Although a variety of mechanisms are responsible for medication-induced SHL, a general rule is that risk of hearing loss increases with increasing dosage and length of use and is further aggravated by factors that impair drug metabolism and excretion, such as renal insufficiency.

The evaluation of SHL begins with a complete history and physical examination. Sudden conductive hearing loss results from obstruction of the EAC or from disturbances of the TM or ossicles. An evaluation of all current medications for possible ototoxic agents is necessary. A history of trauma or recollection of a "popping" noise preceding the hearing loss may indicate perforation of the TM. Coexistent tinnitus or vertigo may point to Ménière disease. Systemic illness should be considered.

The differential diagnosis includes both potentially reversible and potentially ominous causes (see Table 239-4). If the physical examination does not identify the cause, emergency otolaryngologic consultation is necessary.

TABLE 239-3 Common Ototoxic Agents

Loop diuretics	Topical agents
Ethacrynic acid	Solvents
Furosemide	Propylene glycol
Bumetanide	Antiseptics
Salicylates	Ethanol
NSAIDs	Antibiotics
Quinine	Polymyxin B
Antibiotics	Neomycin
Aminoglycosides	
Erythromycin	
Vancomycin	
Chemotherapeutic agents	
Cisplatin	
Carboplatin	
Vinblastine	
Vincristine	

Abbreviation: NSAID = nonsteroidal anti-inflammatory drug.

INFECTIONS

Otitis Externa

Otitis externa includes infections and inflammation of the EAC and auricle. It is divided into acute diffuse and malignant types.

ACUTE DIFFUSE OTITIS EXTERNA

Definition and Diagnosis Also known simply as otitis externa (OE) or swimmer's ear, this infection is characterized by pruritus, pain, and tenderness of the external ear. Physical signs include erythema and edema of the EAC, which may spread to the tragus and auricle. Other signs are clear or purulent otorrhea and crusting of the EAC. As the disease progresses, the pain may become intolerable and occur with mastication or any movement of the periauricular skin. Increasing edema eventually narrows the EAC lumen and may cause hearing impairment. In severe cases, infection may spread to the periauricular soft tissues and lymph nodes, and there may be lateral protrusion of the auricle secondary to inflammation.

Pathophysiology Predisposing factors for the development of OE are trauma to the skin of the EAC and elevation of the local pH. Constant contact with water, from swimming or bathing in hot tubs, pools, or freshwater lakes is associated with the development of OE, as is living in a humid environment. Trauma is most commonly caused by scratching or by overzealous disimpaction of cerumen. Cerumen is an

TABLE 239-2 Common Causes of Tinnitus

Objective	Subjective
Vascular	Sensorineural hearing loss
AV malformations	Hypertension
Arterial bruits	Conductive hearing loss
Mechanical	Head trauma
Enlarged eustachian tube	Medication
Palatomyoclonus	TMJ disorders
Stapedial muscle spasm	Depression, stress
	Neurologic
	Acoustic neuroma
	Multiple sclerosis
	Benign intracranial hypertension
	Ménière disease
	Cogan syndrome

Abbreviations: AV = arteriovenous; TMJ = temporomandibular joint.

TABLE 239-4 Causes of Sudden Hearing Loss

Infection	Rheumatologic
Mumps	Temporal arteritis
Epstein-Barr virus	Polyarteritis nodosa
Herpes	Wegener granulomatosis
Cytomegalovirus	Other
Syphilis	Ménière disease
Labyrinthitis	Cogan syndrome
Hematologic and vascular	Acoustic neuroma
Leukemia	Pharmacologic
Sickle cell anemia	Cochlear rupture
Polycythemia	Conductive
Berger disease	Otitis externa
Cerebral aneurysm	Otitis media
Metabolic	Ruptured tympanic membrane
Diabetes mellitus	Neoplasms
Hyperlipidemia	Otosclerosis

acidic mixture of sebaceous and apocrine gland secretions and desquamated epithelial cells. It forms a physical barrier that protects the EAC skin from violation, while the acidic pH has antimicrobial properties.

Microbiology   The most common organisms implicated in OE are _Pseudomonas aeruginosa_ and _Staphylococcus aureus_,[11] although one study found a polymicrobial etiology in one-third of patients and an anaerobic bacterial etiology in one-quarter, with _Bacteroides_ species predominating. Interestingly, the microbial pathogen is often not isolated from suspect water samples.[12–14]

Otomycosis, or fungal OE, accounts for approximately 10 percent of cases, with a high percentage found in tropical climates. A history may reveal the presence of diabetes, HIV, or other immunocompromised states, or previous long-term therapy with antibiotics. Most (80 to 90 percent) of otomycosis is caused by _Aspergillus_ species, and physical examination may reveal a black, blue-green, or yellow discoloration of the EAC. The second most common fungal pathogen is _Candida_.[15]

Noninfectious causes include contact dermatitis from topical medications or resins in hearing aids, seborrhea, and psoriasis. Although not generally an occupational disease, OE resulting from mite infestation has been reported in poultry workers.[16]

Treatment   The treatment of OE involves analgesia, cleansing of the EAC, acidifying agents, topical antimicrobials, and sometimes steroids. Cleansing may be done with gentle irrigation using hydrogen peroxide, and gentle debridement by the physician with a suction aspirator such as a Frazier suction.

A variety of topical agents exist that combine an antimicrobial agent with either an acid and/or a steroid. Table 239-5 lists the components of many otic preparations. No single agent is more effective than the others, and there are many considerations to guide the choice of agent, including the risk of ototoxicity, cost, and compliance. A commonly prescribed agent, Cortisporin, is a combination of neomycin (an aminoglycoside), polymyxin B, and hydrocortisone. Although there are few established cases of ototoxicity, there is a theoretical risk of both auditory and vestibular toxicity with the use of aminoglycosides, polymyxin, and acetic acid preparations.[3,4,17] Although this risk appears to be negligible in the presence of an intact TM, there is evidence of systemic absorption of topical aminoglycosides.[18,19] A consensus panel of the American Academy of Otolaryngology-Head and Neck Surgery has concluded that nonototoxic ototopical antibiotics should be considered as first-line therapy in the treatment of OE, particularly when the integrity of the TM is unknown or in the presence of a known TM perforation or tympanostomy tubes. Both available ototopical quinolones, ofloxacin and ciprofloxacin, have both antistaphylococcal and antipseudomonal activity, and have

TABLE 239-5   Some Common Topical Otic Preparations

Preparation	Constituents	Comments
CiproHC Otic	Ciprofloxacin Hydrocortisone	Not safe with perforation
Cortisporin Otic	Neomycin Polymixin B Hydrocortisone	Use suspension* only theoretical potential for ototoxicity
Floxin Otic	Ofloxacin	Safe with perforations; 5 drops bid
Otic Domeboro	2% Acetic acid solution	pH 4.5–6.0
VoSol HC Otic	Acetic acid Hydrocortisone	pH 3.0

*Solution is thinner and more easily absorbed through the round window or a perforation.

been shown to be as effective at treating OE as Cortisporin. In addition, topical ofloxacin has been approved by the Food and Drug Administration (FDA) for use in infants and children, and is the only ototopical antibiotic approved by the FDA for use with an open middle ear.[17]

The burning associated with the acidic preparations may reduce compliance. Patients unable to tolerate the low pH of otic preparations may instead use the slightly more alkaline ophthalmic drops.

If cost is a factor and there are no known contraindications, Cortisporin drops may be used as they are less expensive than the quinolones. In this case, Cortisporin Otic _Suspension_ should be used and not the solution; theoretically, this has less chance of middle ear penetration and resultant ototoxicity.

The medication should be instilled into a cleansed ear while it is facing up, with this position held for 3 min. If edema of the EAC obstructs the lumen, a commercial wick or piece of gauze may be inserted into the EAC and kept moist with the otic drops.

Bacterial and fungal cultures may guide treatment of nonresponsive cases. Oral antibiotic therapy should be reserved for febrile patients and those with periauricular extension. All patients with OE should be taught to avoid predisposing factors in order to eliminate recurrences. Strategies include ear plugs while swimming or bathing (cotton wool impregnated with petroleum jelly or commercial ear plugs), brief use of a hair dryer to remove EAC water, and avoidance of cotton-tipped applicators or other devices to remove cerumen.

Specific treatment of otomycosis consists of antifungal agents such as clotrimazole. _Aspergillus_ is not sensitive to most oral antifungals with the exception of itraconazole.[11] With noninfectious OE, removal of the offending agent is the first step in treatment. Topical steroid drops may be used for seborrhea and psoriasis.

Finally, all patients should be instructed to follow up with their primary physician or an otolaryngologist if the condition worsens at any time or does not respond to treatment in 1 week, to be evaluated for the more serious disease of malignant otitis externa.

MALIGNANT OTITIS EXTERNA

Definitions   Malignant otitis externa (MOE) is a potentially life-threatening infection of the EAC with variable extension to the skull base. It is almost always caused by _P. aeruginosa_. The term _MOE_ actually refers to a spectrum of disease. When it is limited to the soft tissues and cartilage, it is called necrotizing otitis externa (NOE). When there is involvement of the temporal bone or skull base it is called skull-base osteomyelitis (SBO).

Pathophysiology   MOE begins as a simple otitis externa that then spreads to the deeper tissues of the EAC and infects cartilage, periosteum, and bone, with the normal anatomy of the ear serving as the conduit for the spread of infection. The cartilaginous floor of the EAC has clefts, known as the fissures of Santorini, through which the infection may spread to deeper structures. The parotid gland and TMJ are anterior, the mastoid air cells are posterior, and the skull base, carotid artery, jugular bulb, and sigmoid sinus are inferomedial. Infection may spread to any of these structures as well as to the seventh cranial nerve as it exits the stylomastoid foramen and the ninth, tenth, and eleventh cranial nerves at the jugular foramen.

The typical patient with MOE is the elderly diabetic, although it is now seen more often in the patient with HIV. The presence of an impaired immune response, which is further compromised in the elderly, may predispose to the onset of pseudomonal infection. Furthermore, the cerumen of diabetic patients has been found to have a higher pH than that of normal controls; this represents an additional breakdown in local defense mechanisms. Finally, the small blood vessel disease of diabetics may lead to cartilaginous degeneration, further promoting the spread of infection.

Microbiology   The most common causative organism of MOE is *P. aeruginosa. Aspergillus* has been reported to cause SBO, usually in patients who are immunosuppressed because of AIDS or other causes. *Aspergillus* SBO also has a different presentation than typical pseudomonal SBO in that the infection generally begins in the middle ear rather than in the EAC.

Diagnosis   Any elderly, diabetic, HIV, or otherwise immunocompromised patient presenting with OE or any person with persistent OE despite 2 to 3 weeks of topical antimicrobial therapy should be suspected of having MOE. The typical presentation is similar to that of OE: otalgia and edema of the EAC with or without otorrhea. The otalgia may be out of proportion for routine OE. Granulation tissue may be evident on the floor of the EAC near the bone-cartilage junction.

The history and physical examination should also be directed toward determining the extent of progression of the disease by identifying involvement of nearby structures. Parotitis may be present, and trismus indicates involvement of the masseter muscle or TMJ. Cranial nerve involvement is a serious sign. The history and examination should specifically rule out facial palsy and hoarseness or dysphagia. The seventh cranial nerve is usually the first affected, and the presence of dysfunction of the ninth, tenth, or eleventh cranial nerve implies even more extensive disease. Lateral or sigmoid sinus thrombosis and meningitis are also possible complications.

Certain patients may have an atypical clinical presentation and require special mention. MOE in children tends to be rapidly progressive, so children may be ill appearing upon presentation, with fever, leukocytosis, and even bacteremia. Also, the TM, middle ear, and facial nerve are more likely to be involved in children than in adults. AIDS patients with MOE tend to be younger, have etiologic organisms other than *Pseudomonas,* and tend to have a worse prognosis than patients without AIDS.

Diagnosing MOE depends first on having a high index of suspicion. Emergent otolaryngologic consultation is necessary. The next step involves radiographic confirmation and staging of the disease with computed tomography (CT) of the head, focusing on the EAC and temporal bone.

Treatment   Once the diagnosis of MOE has been made, the patient should be admitted to the hospital for parenteral antibiotics. Therapy with an aminoglycoside and antipseudomonal penicillin, or cephalosporin, or quinolone is standard, and should be initiated in the ED. Selected cases may be managed with oral quinolones, depending on the otolaryngologist's preference.

The ultimate prognosis of MOE is primarily based on the stage of disease at presentation. Earlier stages are likely to completely resolve with a single course of antibiotic therapy, while more advanced stages may require surgical debridement and may ultimately prove fatal.

Otitis Media

EPIDEMIOLOGY

Otitis media (OM) is primarily a disease of infancy and childhood (see Chap. 121). Although adults may present with OM, its incidence and prevalence peak in the preschool years and then decrease with increasing age. There is little or no literature to suggest that the diagnosis or management of OM in adults differs from that in children. The decrease in incidence of OM from childhood through adolescence is thought to be due to the changing anatomy of the eustachian tube. Between infancy and adulthood the eustachian tube angle and length both increase, promoting drainage of the middle ear and offering a greater physical barrier to the migration of bacteria from the nasopharynx to the middle ear.

MICROBIOLOGY

The most common bacterial pathogens in acute OM are *Streptococcus pneumoniae, Haemophilus influenzae,* and *Moraxella catarrhalis.* The predominant organisms involved in chronic OM are *Staphylococcus aureus, P. aeruginosa,* and anaerobic bacteria.[20] This pattern may change, however, with increasing use of pneumococcal vaccines. The heptavalent pneumococcal vaccine recently approved for use in the United States may provide protection against *S. pneumoniae* serotypes responsible for up to 86 percent of bacterial isolates causing OM, including >95 percent of drug-resistant isolates.[21] Viruses probably play a role in the pathogenesis of OM in that they may promote bacterial superinfection by impairing eustachian tube function and other host defense mechanisms. They may also interfere with host response to antimicrobial drugs.

DIAGNOSIS

The patient with OM presents with otalgia with or without fever. Otorrhea and hearing loss are variably present, while tinnitus, vertigo, and nystagmus are uncommon. The TM may be retracted or bulging. It may be red in color, indicating inflammation, or it may be yellow or white, as a result of middle ear fluid. Pneumatic otoscopy demonstrates impaired mobility. The facial nerve should always be assessed because of its proximity to the middle ear.

TREATMENT

There are no treatment guidelines specifically for adults, and recommendations for children are commonly used. Amoxicillin has been effective against all three major pathogens, but currently approximately 30 percent of *H. influenza* and up to 80 percent of *M. catarrhalis* have developed β-lactamase, conferring resistance to amoxicillin. In all, resistant strains account for approximately 10 percent of all cases of acute OM.[21–23]

The preferred initial treatment is still amoxicillin. The dose in adults (weighing >40 kg) is 500 to 875 mg PO every 12 h, or 250 to 500 mg PO every 8 h, for 7 to 10 days. Alternative agents include trimethoprim-sulfamethoxazole, azithromycin, or cefuroxime (second-generation cephalosporin). For OM unresponsive to initial therapy after 72 h, cefuroxime or amoxicillin-clavulanate may be given.

Because pain usually continues for 8 to 24 h after the initiation of antibiotics, the addition of acetaminophen or ibuprofen analgesia is appropriate. OM with effusion requires treatment with the same antimicrobials, but for 3 weeks, and prednisone may be added.[20]

Adults with simple acute OM should receive follow-up to assess treatment efficacy and to ensure that there is no anatomic obstruction to the eustachian tube, as for example, from occult neoplasm. Any patient who presents with complications of OM or who appears septic should have urgent consultation for diagnostic and therapeutic tympanocentesis and possible admission for intravenous antibiotics.

Complications

Complications of OM can be divided into intratemporal and intracranial types. Perforation of the TM is a common intratemporal complication and most often occurs in the pars tensa from the increased pressure of middle ear secretions, with resultant otorrhea. Healing usually occurs in 1 week, although a chronic perforation may result. A temporary conductive hearing loss may occur with OM secondary to fluid in the middle ear. The hearing loss resolves as the fluid is resorbed. Acute serous labyrinthitis may occur when bacterial toxins enter the inner ear via the round window. Facial nerve paralysis is an uncommon complication but requires emergent otolaryngology consultation.

ACUTE MASTOIDITIS

One of the most serious complications of acute OM is acute mastoiditis. This occurs as infection spreads from the middle ear to the mastoid air cells via the aditus ad antrum. When this opening becomes blocked, the mastoid cavity becomes a closed space, and the mastoid air cells become filled with fluid and inflamed. Spread through venous channels to the overlying periosteum is referred to as *acute mastoiditis with periostitis.* In addition to otalgia and fever, patients with mastoiditis will have postauricular erythema, swelling, and tenderness, with protrusion of the auricle and obliteration of the postauricular crease. Although the diagnosis can usually be made based on the history and physical examination, certain radiographic tests are indicated. Mastoid radiographs will demonstrate mastoid clouding because of fluid accumulation, and CT may delineate the extent of bony involvement. Mastoiditis requires admission for intravenous antibiotics, tympanocentesis, and myringotomy. Cefuroxime is frequently chosen as an initial empiric agent.[24] Incision and drainage of subperiosteal abscess or mastoidectomy may ultimately be indicated.

INTRACRANIAL COMPLICATIONS   Intracranial complications of OM are more likely with chronic than with acute OM and are, in general, decreasing with the widespread use of antibiotics in the treatment of OM. However, suppurative intracranial extension is a severe complication, and suggestive signs and symptoms should be investigated appropriately. Meningitis and brain abscess are the most common intracranial complication of OM; the most prevalent causative organisms are *S. pneumoniae* and *H. influenzae* type b. Extradural abscess and subdural empyema are also potential complications.

LATERAL SINUS THROMBOSIS   Lateral sinus thrombosis (LST) is another ominous complication of acute OM. It arises from extension of infection and inflammation in the mastoid, with eventual inflammation of the adjacent lateral or sigmoid sinus. Reactive thrombophlebitis with mural clot formation, intraluminal empyema, or perforation of the venous wall may occur. A high index of suspicion is necessary to diagnose LST because the common clinical findings are similar to those found in acute OM or mastoiditis.

Headache is the most common symptom, with papilledema, sixth-nerve palsy, and vertigo being less frequently present. Angiography with venous phase and magnetic resonance imaging (MRI) are more sensitive than CT in diagnosing LST. Although in the majority of cases of LST no bacterial isolates are recovered, antibiotic therapy is the initial treatment of choice. The agent should cover *Staphylococcus, Streptococcus,* and upper respiratory anaerobes, and have good penetration of the blood-brain barrier. A combination of intravenous penicillin or nafcillin, ceftriaxone, and metronidazole has been recommended as an initial empiric regimen.[25] Most patients will also require surgical intervention.

CHOLESTEATOMA   A serious complication associated with chronic OM is cholesteatoma. Aural cholesteatoma is composed of epidermis and exfoliated keratin within pneumatized spaces of the temporal bone. It is an erosive, expanding lesion originating within the middle ear or mastoid air cells. As the cholesteatoma expands, it may erode the ossicular chain, bony labyrinth, or facial nerve canal. Cholesteatomas are often infected and their intracranial extensions may be life-threatening.

Bullous Myringitis

DEFINITION   Bullous myringitis is a painful condition of the ear characterized by bulla formation on the TM and deep EAC. Its epidemiology, etiology, and pathology are poorly understood. It may occur at any age, frequently after an upper respiratory tract infection.

PATHOPHYSIOLOGY   The blisters are believed to occur between the highly innervated outer epithelium and the inner fibrous layer of the TM, explaining the severe otalgia. The blisters may be blood-filled, serous, or serosanguineous. Middle ear effusions may be present, either sympathetic in origin or as a result of medial rupture of bullae. Otorrhea as a result of ruptured bullae is short-lived. A reversible hearing loss is commonly associated with the condition and may be conductive, sensorineural, or mixed.

MICROBIOLOGY   Although bullous myringitis was originally associated with influenza epidemics, since then numerous pathogens have been implicated in its etiology, including *Mycoplasma pneumoniae, Chlamydia psittaci,* and numerous viral pathogens. Herpes simplex has not been implicated as a causative agent.[26]

DIAGNOSIS   Patients with bullous myringitis typically present with severe, throbbing otalgia, often with hearing loss. Otoscopy reveals multiple fluid-filled blisters, which may be yellow to red in color. There may be bloody otorrhea or hemotympanum.

TREATMENT   As the etiologic agent of bullous myringitis remains elusive, treatment of the condition consists of warm compresses and systemic analgesia with acetaminophen or nonsteroidal anti-inflammatory drugs (NSAIDs). Oral antibiotics may be added in cases with an associated middle ear effusion, because some of these may represent a concomitant otitis media.

TRAUMA TO THE EAR

Although trauma to the ear is rarely life-threatening, its associated morbidity is significant and includes hearing loss and poor cosmetic outcome.

Abrasions can cause partial loss of the covering epidermis. Abrasions that do not penetrate to the underlying perichondrium should be thoroughly irrigated with normal saline. If there are any embedded foreign bodies, they should be meticulously removed to prevent infection and "tattooing" of the wound. A topical antimicrobial ointment with a contoured nonpressure dressing should be applied. The wound should be reevaluated in 24 h. Lacerations of the auricle require delicate closure with careful realignment to maintain the natural contour (see Chap. 42). Prior to closure, a thorough examination is required to determine the magnitude of the injury, followed by cleansing and irrigation with normal saline. Further exploration can be done with a sterile cotton swab to determine the actual extent of the injury and explore for any remaining foreign bodies. In simple lacerations not involving the perichondrium or cartilage, the skin can be approximated with everting nylon sutures. In lacerations involving the cartilage, the perichondrium should be sutured using 5–0 or 6–0 absorbable sutures. If debridement is necessary, the otolaryngologist may be consulted. After skin closure, an antimicrobial ointment and a firm, contoured, nonpressure dressing should be applied. Complete or partial avulsion injuries, especially those involving tissue loss exposing large areas of cartilage, should be referred to an otolaryngologist or plastic surgeon.

Thermal Injuries

FROSTBITE   With its position of prominence and large surface area, the auricle is extremely susceptible to extremes in temperature. The thin subcutaneous tissue makes the auricle particularly susceptible to cold-induced injury. In frostbite, the ear will initially appear pale. In superficial frostbite injuries, the underlying tissue remains soft and pliable. In deep injuries, the underlying tissue is very hard. With rewarming, the ear may become painful, with edema and blister formation. If blisters do form, they should be allowed to reabsorb spontaneously. The ear should be aseptically and quickly rewarmed with saline-soaked gauze that has been warmed to 38° to 40°C (100.4° to 104°F). The rewarming process may be very painful and analgesics will be necessary.

BURNS   Burns of the upper body occur frequently, with burns of the face and neck representing approximately 30 percent of all burn injuries. In one study of patients sustaining significant facial burns, 42 percent suffered burns to the ears. Direct thermal burns may be severe enough to cause necrosis and sloughing of the entire external ear. Even with lesser injury, disruption of the auricular skin can lead to damage of the underlying cartilage, which, once damaged, is particularly susceptible to infection. Factors that affect the healing of burn injuries include the depth of the burn, development of infection, and external pressure or friction on the burned auricle.

Burns more severe than first-degree should be seen in consultation with a burn unit or an otolaryngologist. If the burn is an isolated injury and a mild second-degree type, treatment in the ED should consist of meticulous cleaning and irrigation with normal saline, application of a non–sulfa-containing antimicrobial ointment, and a nonpressure dressing. Silver sulfadiazine ointment can cause skin pigmentation changes and for cosmetic reasons should not be used above the clavicles. Referral should be made within 24 h. Substantial second-degree burns with blistering or any third-degree burns should be referred to a burn center for further management.[27]

Osteochondritis is a potentially disfiguring complication of otic burns. Chondritis may occur in up to 20 percent of significant otic burns and may appear anywhere from 2 to 5 weeks after the injury. The hallmarks of chondritis consist of helical dull pain followed by erythema, edema, exquisite tenderness to palpation, and an increase in the auriculocephalic angle (lateral protrusion of the ear from the head). Once chondritis is present, treatment must be aggressive to preserve ear architecture; it usually consists of surgical debridement. Systemic antibiotics alone are generally considered ineffective.

Hematoma

A hematoma can develop from almost any type of trauma to the ear. As a result of the lack of subcutaneous fat on the anterior surface of the auricle, blunt force applied to this area tends to shear the perichondrium from the underlying cartilage and tear the adjoining blood vessels. The cartilage depends on the perichondrial blood vessels for viability. Any separation can result in necrosis. In addition, a subperichondral collection can lead to stimulation of the overlying perichondrium, which can result in an asymmetrical formation of new cartilage and deformity of the auricle. The resultant deformed auricle has been referred to as "cauliflower ear," which is commonly associated with boxers. The auricular hematoma itself presents as a painful swelling after trauma, which obscures the normal contour of the ear. The hematoma may accumulate immediately or several hours after injury. In the past, the advised treatment was aspiration of the hematoma. More current literature suggests that aspiration alone does not completely evacuate the clot and therefore leads to deformity and increased morbidity. The goal of treatment is to remove the fluid collection and maintain pressure in the area for several days to prevent reaccumulation of fluid. After local anesthesia, and using sterile technique, a semicircular incision should be made through the skin with caution not to violate the underlying perichondrium. The incision should be the minimal necessary to drain the underlying hematoma and positioned in an area with the least exposure (the inner curvature of the helix or anthelix). The hematoma can then be removed by gentle suction or curettage.[28,29]

A dental roll or a firm sterile pledget can then be placed over the resutured site with through-and-through sutures connected to a similar bolster on the opposite side. A nonpressure dressing with antibiotic ointment should then be applied and the patient given instructions as to reevaluation within 24 h to assure there has been no reaccumulation. Prophylactic antibiotics can be reserved for immunocompromised patients and should cover *P. aeruginosa* and *S. aureus*, the two likely participants in posttraumatic chondritis.

Foreign Bodies

Foreign bodies in the external canal are commonly seen in the emergency department. Variations can include anything from cotton, pencil erasers, or pieces of toys to illicit drugs and insects. Organic materials such as beans, seeds, and vegetable matter may conform to the contour of the canal or expand if moistened, complicating the process of removal. Insects that crawl into the ear can actually survive for a long period of time, causing a local inflammation and a great deal of distress to the patient.

The evaluation of a patient with a foreign body in the ear should begin with calming the patient and placing the patient in the reclined position. Occasionally, the complaint may be sudden pain while in the recumbent position, as in the case of an embedded insect. Most of the time, the history will reveal the type of material in the ear. A thorough examination and visualization of the complete tympanic membrane is mandatory. Inability to visualize the entire canal, contact of the foreign body with the tympanic membrane, or the presence of a perforation mandates the use of an operative microscope and speculum, with obvious consultation. Foreign bodies in children medial to the bony isthmus often require conscious sedation or even general anesthesia for safe extraction. Cerumen loops, a right-angle hook, and alligator forceps are the instruments of choice for the removal. Live objects should be drowned with a 2 percent lidocaine solution or viscous lidocaine, which immediately paralyzes the bug and provides modest topical anesthesia. The liquid can then be suctioned out with butterfly tubing and the insect removed with gentle suction or forceps under direct visualization. Care must be taken to assure that no debris of the insect remains in the canal. Irrigation with room-temperature water is adequate for small particles such as hard sand or cerumen and can mobilize distally positioned objects. Irrigation should not be used unless the tympanic membrane is completely visualized and free of perforation, and it can be used only for nonorganic matter, which will not expand when moistened.

Complete inspection of the ear canal after removal of the foreign body is important to exclude more significant injury to the canal skin, tympanic membrane, and ossicles caused by the foreign body or its extraction. Small abrasions heal spontaneously. Topical antibiotics should be considered in cases where there was more serious cutaneous damage or where the foreign body consisted of organic material (see Table 239-5).

Cerumen Impaction

Occasionally, the diagnosis is made as patients present with unrelated complaints, but more often, patients complain of decreased hearing, a sensation of pressure or fullness in the ear, dizziness, tinnitus, or pain. The symptoms are often precipitated by the use of cotton-tipped applicators. Most of the time, cerumen loops can be used. In the particularly difficult cases, or where cerumen is completely occluding the canal, softening of the cerumen can be accomplished with half-strength hydrogen peroxide, sodium bicarbonate drops, mineral oil, or over-the-counter preparations such as Debrox or Cerumenex for 30 min. If irrigation is the treatment of choice, it can usually be accomplished with a metal ear syringe, a flexible 18-gauge IV catheter, or a syringe attached to the tubing of a butterfly infusion catheter. Body-temperature irrigant is the solution of choice. The catheter should be inserted into the cartilaginous canal (distal third) and a gentle, pulsatile flow should be inserted along the superior portion of the external auditory canal; in this way the pressure of the stream is directed toward the wall of the canal and not the TM. Irrigation of the canal when the middle ear is not infected often causes a temporary redness of the tympanic membrane; therefore, the subsequent diagnosis of otitis media should be made with caution.

The most common iatrogenic injury associated with syringing of the ear is traumatic TM perforation. Predisposing factors include previous ear surgery, a previous or current history of OM, and severe OE. When in doubt, it is safer to defer the procedure to an otolaryngologist. When determining if a perforation has occurred, it is important to rely on symptoms (sudden hearing loss, severe otalgia, or vertigo) rather than signs, as visualization of the TM may be impaired by the irrigating fluid and debris. In case of suspected perforation, reassurance, analgesia and otolaryngology referral in 1 to 2 weeks are indicated. Prophylactic antibiotics are not necessary.[30] If injury to ossicles is suspected, emergency consultation is needed.

Tympanic Membrane Perforation

Tympanic membrane perforations can occur as a result of blunt, penetrating, acoustic, or baro- trauma. When it is secondary to blunt or noise trauma, the perforation almost always occurs in the pars tensa, usually anteriorly or inferiorly. The pars tensa, the largest area of the tympanic membrane, is only a few cell layers thick.

The patient usually complains of an acute onset of pain and hearing loss, with or without bloody otorrhea. There may also be associated vertigo and tinnitus, but this is usually transient unless there has been injury to the inner ear or rupture of the round or oval windows. In evaluating these injuries, the canal must be cleared of blood and debris. The tympanic membrane should be completely visualized. Most tympanic membrane perforations heal spontaneously. Patients with perforations secondary to blunt or noise trauma that are isolated injuries can be safely discharged and referred to a specialist for further evaluation and a formal audiogram as soon after the injury as possible. Patients should be instructed not to allow water to enter the canal of the ear. They do not need topical or systemic antibiotics. Perforations in the posterosuperior quadrant or those secondary to penetrating trauma have a greater likelihood of damaging the ossicular chain or, in the case of the latter, a retained foreign body and should be referred to an otolaryngologist within 24 h.

Lightning fatally strikes approximately 600 persons annually in the United States and leaves thousands more survivors with permanent sequelae. Although the blast effect associated with a lightning strike plays a part in perforations, conducted electrical current from cutaneous sites via the external auditory canal and into the middle or inner ear structures is another hypothesized mechanism for lightning-induced otologic injuries.[29] Tympanic membrane perforation is the most common sequela.

Barotrauma

Barotrauma to the middle ear, also called barotitis media, is discussed in Chap. 196.

REFERENCES

1. Kreigsberg MK, Turner J: Dental causes of referred otalgia. *Ear Nose Throat J* 66:398, 1987.
2. Seidman JD, Jacobsen GP: Update on tinnitus. *Otolaryngol Clin North Am* 29:455, 1996.
3. Hughes GB, Freedman MA, Haberkamp TJ, Guay ME: Sudden sensorineural hearing loss. *Otolaryngol Clin North Am* 29:393, 1996.
4. Rohn GN, Meyerhof WL, Wright GC: Ototoxicity of topical agents. *Otolaryngol Clin North Am* 26:747, 1993.
5. Schweitzer VG: Ototoxicity of chemotherapeutic agents. *Otolaryngol Clin North Am* 26:759, 1993.
6. Jung TTK, Rhee C, Lee CS, et al: Ototoxicity of salicylate, nonsteroidal anti-inflammatory drugs, and quinine. *Otolaryngol Clin North Am* 26:791, 1993.
7. Brummett RE: Ototoxicity of vancomycin and analogues. *Otolaryngol Clin North Am* 26:821, 1993.
8. Brummett RE: Ototoxicity liability of erythromycin and analogues. *Otolaryngol Clin North Am* 26:811, 1993.
9. Matz GJ: Aminoglycoside cochlear ototoxicity. *Otolaryngol Clin North Am* 26:705, 1993.
10. Rybak LP: Ototoxicity of loop diuretics. *Otolaryngol Clin North Am* 26:829, 1993.
11. Selesnick SH: Otitis externa: Management of the recalcitrant case. *Am J Otolaryngol* 15:408, 1994.
12. Brook I, Frazier EH, Thompson DH: Aerobic and anaerobic microbiology of external otitis. *Clin Infect Dis* 16:955, 1992.
13. van Asperen IA, de Rover CM, Schijven JF, et al: Risk of otitis externa after swimming in recreational fresh water lakes containing *Pseudomonas aeruginosa. BMJ* 311:1407, 1995.
14. Agius AM, Pickles JM, Burch KL: A prospective study of otitis externa. *Clin Otolaryngol* 17:150, 1992.
15. Bojrab DI, Bruderly T, Abdurazzak Y: Otitis externa. *Otolaryngol Clin North Am* 29:761, 1996.
16. Rossiter A: Occupational otitis externa in chicken catchers. *J Laryngol Otol* 111:366, 1997.
17. Harnley MT, Denneny JC, Holzer SS: Use of ototopical antibiotics in treating 3 common ear diseases. *Otolaryngol Head Neck Surg* 122:934, 2000.
18. Lancaster JL, Mortimore S, McCormick M, et al: Systemic absorption of gentamicin in the management of active mucosal chronic otitis media. *Clin Otolaryngol* 24:435, 1999.
19. Lancaster JL, Makura ZG, Porter G et al: Topical aminoglycosides in the management of active mucosal chronic suppurative otitis media. *J Laryngol Otol* 113:10, 1999.
20. Brook I: Otitis media: Microbiology and management. *J Otolaryngol* 23:269, 1994.
21. Joloba ML, Windau A, Bajaksouzian S, et al: Pneumococcal conjugate vaccine serotypes of *Streptococcus pneumoniae* isolates and the antimicrobial susceptibility of such isolates in children with otitis media. *Clin Infect Dis* 33:1489, 2001.
22. Canafax DM, Giebink GS: Clinical and pharmacokinetic basis for the antimicrobial treatment of acute otitis media. *Otolaryngol Clin North Am* 24:859, 1991.
23. Kempthorne J, Giebink GS: Pediatric approach to the diagnosis and management of otitis media. *Otolaryngol Clin North Am* 24:905, 1991.
24. Myer CM III: The diagnosis and management of mastoiditis in children. *Pediatr Ann* 20:662, 1991.
25. Garcia RDJ, Baker AS, Cunningham MJ, Weber AL: Lateral sinus thrombosis associated with otitis media and mastoiditis in children. *Pediatr Infect Dis J* 14:617, 1995.
26. Marais J, Dale BAB: Bullous myringitis: A review. *Clin Otolaryngol* 22:497, 1997.
27. Skedros D, Goldfarb LW: Chondritis of the burned ear: A review. *Ear Nose Throat J* 71:359, 1990.
28. Starck WJ, Kaltman SI: Current concepts in the surgical management of traumatic auricular hematoma. *J Oral Maxillofac Surg* 50:800, 1992.
29. Templer J, Renner GJ: Injuries of the external ear. *Otolaryngol Clin North Am* 23:1003, 1990.
30. Blake P, Matthews R, Hornibrook J: When not to syringe an ear. *N Z Med J* 111:422, 1998.

240   FACE AND JAW EMERGENCIES
Robert Haddon
W. Franklin Peacock IV

FACIAL INFECTIONS

Facial infections can be organized from most superficial to most deep. A given infection may traverse more than one layer or space depending on its source, duration, and host. Further, infections of the upper and lower face form distinct clinical groups.[1] Sinusitis and periorbital and orbital cellulitis are covered in Chaps. 241 and 238, respectively.

Impetigo

Impetigo is a superficial epidermal infection characterized by amber crusts at the sites of minor skin trauma. *Streptococcus pyogenes* (group A β-hemolytic streptococci) predominates, often mixed with *Staphylococcus aureus. S. aureus* is the sole isolate in 10 percent of cases. Treatment should cover both pathogens and includes topical mupirocin ointment either alone or in combination with cephalexin, amoxicillin-clavulanate, dicloxacillin, cefuroxime, or clindamycin.[2,3] Lesions should be cleaned and, if practical, covered. The importance of handwashing should be emphasized to the patient and family members.

Erysipelas

Erysipelas involves both the epidermis and dermis, usually on the face. Classically, it has a red, raised, puffy appearance with a sharply defined, palpable border that advances rapidly. Erysipelas is usually caused by *S. pyogenes*. First-line treatment is either amoxicillin-clavulanate or ampicillin-sulbactam. If these cannot be used, use cefuroxime (PO or IV), vancomycin with ceftriaxone IV, or gatifloxicin, gemifloxacin, or moxifloxacin.[2,3]

Cellulitis

Cellulitis is a diffuse, spreading infection of the skin.[4] Other definitions include subcutaneous tissue as well,[2] but the general sense is of a superficial soft tissue infection that lacks either vertical or horizontal constraint. Because this infection evolves, its precise definition may hinge on the time of its diagnosis.

PATHOPHYSIOLOGY   Bacteria may enter the soft tissues from any skin violation. The patient's risk for cellulitis is increased by immunosuppression, systemic disease (e.g., diabetes), or vascular compromise such as that caused by past radiation treatment. Medical appliances and foreign bodies impair local defenses. Decorative facial piercing combines a foreign body with a renewable source of bacteria. Facial cellulitis is caused most commonly by *S. pyogenes* and *S. aureus* and in children may be caused by *Haemophilus influenzae* and *S. pneumoniae*.[2] Less commonly, cellulitis may represent extension from deep-space infections (see "Masticator Space Infections" below).

CLINICAL FEATURES   The history should address events and exposures, both recent and remote, that predispose to cellulitis. Ask about chronic illness, trauma, arthropod bites, allergen exposure, dental caries, painful mastication, surgical history, and radiation exposure. Obtain an occupational history, which may help identify unusual pathogens. Perform a thorough head and neck examination. Check for prostheses, nasal drainage, and changes in vision or phonation. Be alert for signs of systemic, occult, or invasive disease, including fever, headache, vomiting, trismus, draining sinus tracts, and airway compromise.

DIAGNOSIS   Cellulitis is diagnosed clinically, defined by pain, erythema, edema, warmth, and diminished function. The differential diagnosis includes insect envenomation, trauma, dental caries with abscess formation, occult head and neck infection, orbital or periorbital cellulitis, sinusitis with erosion of the bony cortex, otitis externa, impetigo, erysipelas, viral exanthems (e.g., erythema infectiosum or "fifth disease"), parotitis, systemic lupus erythematosus, herpes zoster, dermatitides, angioneurotic edema, contact dermatitis (e.g., cosmetics or poison ivy), allergy,[1,5] vancomycin flushing reaction, and occupational or recreational ultraviolet radiation burns.

Anthrax infections of the face and hands have been reported and are expected when the rare occupational case occurs.[6] In the 2001 bioterror attack victims, cutaneous lesions occurred on forearm, neck, chest, and fingers.[7] Cutaneous anthrax appears as a papule that becomes a vesicle in 1 to 2 days. The vesicle ulcerates and forms the classic black eschar early in the second week of illness. Especially on the face, anthrax lesions are surrounded by a surprisingly large area of edema.[8] The absence of these features and an implausible exposure history are useful in reassuring anthrax-fearing patients with minor skin infections.

TREATMENT   Administer analgesics and antipyretics as needed. Select antibiotics to cover staphylococcal and streptococcal species. When possible, remove foreign bodies and appliances from the affected area. Amoxicillin-clavulanate or ampicillin-sulbactam are the first-choice antibiotics (Table 240-1). Vancomycin and/or cephalosporins also may be used.[2] If there is not an obvious point of entry, evaluate the patient for an abscess or other deep infection. Hos-

TABLE 240-1   Antibiotic Therapy for Facial Infections

Impetigo	Topical mupirocin ointment alone or in combination with cephalexin, amoxicillin-clavulanate, dicloxicillin, cefuroxime, or clindamycin
Erysipelas	Amoxicillin-clavulanate or ampicillin-sulbactam; if these cannot be used, use cefuroxime (oral or IV), vancomycin with ceftriaxone IV, or gatifloxicin, gemifloxacin, or moxifloxacin
Cellulitis	Amoxicillin-clavulanate or ampicillin-sulbactam; vancomycin and cephalosporins are alternatives
Suppurative parotitis	Amoxicillin-clavulanate or ampicillin-sulbactam; if penicillin-allergic, clindamycin or the combination of cephalexin with metronidazole, or vancomycin with metronidazole; if hospitalized or nursing home patients, consider vancomycin
Masticator space infection	Inpatient: intravenous clindamycin is recommended; alternatives include ampicillin-sulbactam, cefoxitin, or the combination of penicillin with metronidazole; outpatient: oral clindamycin or amoxicillin-clavulanate for 10 to 14 days

pitalization should be considered for the following conditions: systemic signs of sepsis; antibiotic intolerance for any reason, including emesis; immunosuppression; extensive areas of erythema or induration; unremovable appliances or foreign bodies; or inability to comply with the outpatient regimen. Patients at the extremes of age should be hospitalized more readily.

Otherwise, outpatient therapy is appropriate. Instruct the patient to return to the emergency department for fever, difficulty swallowing or breathing, inability to take or to tolerate the antibiotic, or any worsening of the condition. If the cellulitis progresses, admission for inpatient antibiotic therapy is warranted.

SALIVARY GLANDS

There are three groups of salivary glands: the parotid, the submandibular, and the sublingual. The facial nerve passes through the superficial portion of the parotid gland, and the parotid (Stensen) duct opens into the mouth opposite the upper second molar. The submandibular and sublingual glands lie below the plane of the tongue. The submandibular ducts open into the mouth at either side of the frenulum of the tongue. The multiple sublingual ducts open into the sublingual fold or directly into the submandibular duct.

Disorders of the salivary glands may be infectious, neoplastic, immunologic, or traumatic. Only the most common disorders are discussed here. It is important initially to answer several questions:

1. Which glands are involved, and are single or multiple glands affected (multiple gland involvement suggests infection)?
2. What is the location of pain and tenderness, and is there a palpable mass (palpable mass suggests tumor or obstruction by stone)?
3. What is the acuity of symptoms and their precipitants (suppurative parotitis and obstruction have an acute onset)?
4. Are symptoms persistent or recurrent?
5. Are there associated problems such as dry mouth or eyes, joint symptoms, diabetes, or orchitis?

Viral Parotitis

Mumps is caused by the paramyxovirus and is most common in children under the age of 15 years. Vaccination has reduced its incidence substantially.[9,10] The virus is spread by airborne droplets, incubates in the upper respiratory tract for 2 to 3 weeks, and then spreads systemically. At this stage, one-third of patients experience a prodrome of fever, malaise, headache, myalgias, arthralgias, and anorexia during a 3- to 5-day period of viremia.[9] The classic salivary gland swelling then follows. Bilateral parotid involvement occurs in 75 percent. The gland is tense and painful, but erythema and warmth are notably absent.[9] Mumps is diagnosed clinically. Amylase levels will be elevated, and cell counts show leukocytopenia with lymphocytosis.[9] Viral serology can be obtained but routinely will not affect management. Treatment is supportive, and salivary gland swelling typically lasts from 1 to 5 days. The patient is contagious for 9 days after the onset of parotid swelling, and children with mumps should be excluded from school or day care for this interval. Viral parotitis may be caused less commonly by influenza, parainfluenza, coxsackieviruses, echoviruses, lymphocytic choriomenigitis virus, and even HIV.[9]

Mumps is usually benign in children but can be severe in adults. Unilateral orchitis affects 20 to 30 percent of males, whereas oophoritis affects only 5 percent of females. Other mumps complications include mastitis, pancreatitis, aseptic meningitis, sensorineural hearing loss, myocarditis, polyarthritis, hemolytic anemia, and thrombocytopenia.[9]

Suppurative Parotitis

Suppurative parotitis is a potentially fatal bacterial infection that occurs in patients with compromised salivary flow. It is caused by the retrograde migration of oral bacteria into the salivary ducts and parenchyma.[9] In contrast to mumps, the onset is rapid, and the skin over the parotid gland is red and tender. Also in contrast to mumps, pus may be expressed from Stensen duct. There is often fever and trismus.

There are many predisposing factors to suppurative parotitis. These include recent anesthesia, dehydration, prematurity or advanced age, sialolithiasis, oral neoplasms, salivary duct strictures, tracheostomy, and ductal foreign body.[9] Medications that cause either systemic dehydration or decrease salivary flow specifically can cause parotitis. These include diuretics, antihistamines, tricyclic antidepressants, phenothiazines, beta blockers, and barbiturates.[9] Several chronic illnesses also predispose patients to suppurative parotitis. These are HIV infection, hepatic failure, renal failure, diabetes mellitus, hypothyroidism, malnutrition, Sjögren syndrome, depression, anorexia, bulimia, hyperuricemia, and cystic fibrosis.[9]

The diagnosis of parotitis is clinical. Parotitis can be distinguished from cellulitis by the drainage from Stensen duct. Lymphangitis usually has a source distinct from the salivary gland. Imaging is not needed unless the patient fails to improve after 48 h of treatment.[9] If at that point computed tomographic (CT) scan or ultrasound reveals an abscess, consult an ear, nose, and throat (ENT) specialist to consider surgical drainage. The serum amylase level typically is normal, and a peripheral smear shows a neutrophilic leukocytosis.[9]

Suppurative parotitis is usually caused by *S. aureus* and less often by *S. pneumoniae, S. pyogenes,* and *H. influenzae.*[2,9] Anaerobes such as *Bacteroides* species, peptostreptococci, and fusobacteria are found in up to 43 percent of isolates. Accordingly, antibiotics effective against both staphylococci and anaerobes are needed (see Table 240-1). The first choice is amoxicillin-clavulanate or ampicillin-sulbactam.[2,9] In penicillin-allergic patients, use clindamycin or a combination of cephalexin with metronidazole or vancomycin with metronidazole. In hospitalized or nursing home patients, the possibility of methicillin-resistant *S. aureus* (MRSA), for which vancomycin is appropriate,[9] must be considered. In the compromised host, gram-negative organisms such as *Escherichia coli* and *Pseudomonas* may be seen. Cultures of Stensen duct drainage can guide therapy in the patient not responding to first-line antibiotics.[9]

Since suppurative parotitis is caused by states of decreased salivary flow, treatment should optimize salivary flow. Hydrate the volume-depleted patient. Massage and apply heat to the affected gland. Stimulate salivation using sialagogues such as lemon drops. When possible, discontinue drugs that cause dry mouth, and attempt to correct underlying medical problems.

Outpatient treatment is appropriate if the patient is hemodynamically stable, able to take oral liquids and antibiotics, and can comply with the treatment regimen.

Sialolithiasis

Salivary calculi can be seen at any age but usually are symptomatic in men between the third and sixth decades.[11] More than 80 percent of stones occur in the submandibular gland, with most of the remainder in the parotid. Submandibular sialoliths are more common in the submandibular (Wharton) duct because of both its more viscous secretions and its uphill course.[11] Sialoliths develop when an organic matrix begins to gel in a relatively stagnant duct and is then seeded with calcium carbonate and calcium phosphate.

The symptoms of pain, swelling, and tenderness may resemble those of parotitis. It may be hard to distinguish the two, and at times they may coexist. However, the pain and swelling of ductal obstruction is exacerbated by meals and may develop over the course of minutes when eating.

The diagnosis of sialolithiasis is usually clinical. Predominately unilateral, the stone may be palpated within the duct, and the gland will be firm.[11] Intraoral radiographs are more sensitive than extraoral films in identifying salivary calculi. Sialography is highly sensitive for stones but is contraindicated when infection is possible. Ultrasound and thin-cut CT scans also will identify sialoliths but are not necessary emergently. A conservative course of treatment should precede imaging studies.

The initial management of sialolithiasis consists of analgesics, antibiotics if there is concurrent infection, massage, and sialagogues such as lemon drops.[11] Outpatient management is the rule. Palpable stones in the distal duct may be digitally "milked" from the duct. They also may be removed electively either by dilation or by incision of the ductal orifice.

Complications of salivary duct obstruction include recurrent or persistent obstruction, strictures, infection, and gland atrophy.[11]

Salivary Gland Enlargement

Salivary gland enlargement can result from a large number of conditions. Beyond those already covered, additional causes include infections such as HIV, tuberculosis, actinomycosis, cat scratch disease, and branchial cleft cyst abscess.[12] Nutritional, toxic, and metabolic causes include malnutrition with vitamin deficiency, phenothiazine use, alcoholism, diabetes mellitus, hypothyroidism, pregnancy, and obesity.[12] Neoplastic lesions may present with enlarged salivary glands. Less than 3 percent of all head and neck tumors are found in the salivary glands. Most salivary neoplasms occur in the parotids, and 75 percent of these are benign.

Most cases of salivary gland enlargement do not require emergency intervention. However, the patient should be directed to appropriate follow-up for definitive diagnosis and treatment, based on the suspected underlying cause.

MASTICATOR SPACE INFECTION

Pathophysiology

The masticator space consists of four potential spaces bounded by the muscles of mastication (Figure 240-1). These spaces include the masseteric (or submasseteric), superficial temporal, deep temporal, and pterygomandibular spaces.[13] Since they are contiguous, it is rare for one to be infected alone.

The masseteric space is bounded by the masseter muscle and the ascending ramus of the mandible. Infection of the masseteric space arises most frequently from soft tissue infection around the third molar. It also may follow third molar surgery and mandibular fractures.[13]

The pterygomandibular space is bounded by the medial pterygoid muscle and the medial aspect of the ascending ramus of the mandible. It is bounded superiorly by the lateral pterygoid. Again, common sources of infection in this space are third molar disease and mandibular

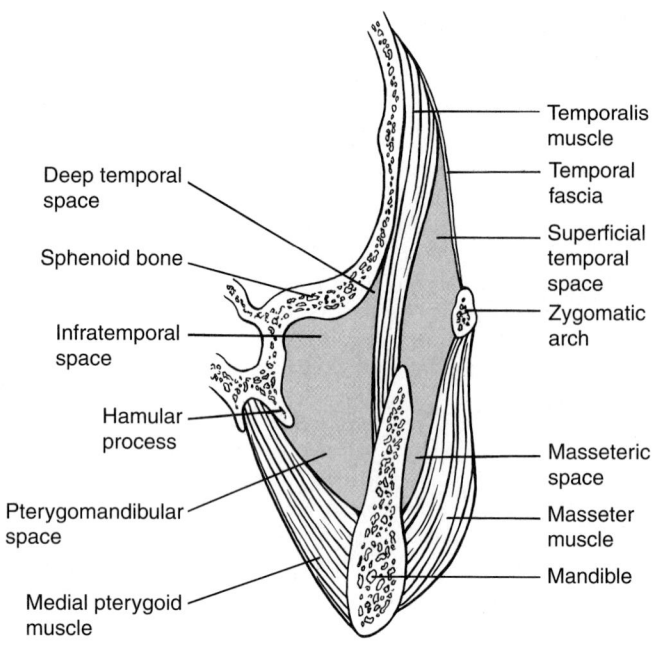

FIG. 240-1. Masticator space.

Deep temporal space

Sphenoid bone

Infratemporal space

Hamular process

Pterygomandibular space

Medial pterygoid muscle

Temporalis muscle

Temporal fascia

Superficial temporal space

Zygomatic arch

Masseteric space

Masseter muscle

Mandible

block injections.[13] Infections within this space may spread to the lateral pharyngeal space, which can then be complicated by airway compromise.

The temporal spaces lie between the temporal fascia and the temporal bone and are divided into superficial and deep by the plane of the temporalis muscle. Maxillary molar infections may spread to the deep temporal (infratemporal) space, or it may become infected by extension from elsewhere within the masticator space. The deep temporal space is one of the potential sources of cavernous sinus thrombosis. Because all the subordinate spaces of the masticator space communicate and ultimately communicate with the tissue planes that extend down the neck to the mediastinum, the extent of the infection should be defined efficiently and treatment begun promptly.

Infections of the masticator space are polymicrobial and generally anaerobic, although aerobic oral streptococcal species may predominate briefly.[2,13] Typical organisms include species of *Streptococcus, Peptostreptococcus, Bacteroides, Prevotella, Porphyromonas, Fusobacterium, Actinomyces, Veillonella,* and anaerobic spirochetes.[2,13]

Clinical Features

The most frequent acute clinical findings are facial swelling, pain, erythema, and trismus. In chronic infection, the patient can be afebrile but may complain of variable trismus.[14] Constitutional signs may include fever, malaise, dehydration, dysphagia, nausea, or vomiting. In more advanced cases, systemic signs of sepsis are present.

History and physical examination features are variable. When infection occurs in the masseteric space, there is posteroinferior facial swelling with mild to moderate trismus. If the temporal space is infected, there is soft tissue swelling over the temporalis and significant trismus. Trismus without swelling suggests pterygomandibular space abscess.

Contrast-enhanced CT scanning is the preferred imaging tool for masseteric and related deep space infections.[13,14] Not only can the extent of an abscess be seen, but CT scan can distinguish more reliably between cellulitis and abscess in all spaces except the retropharyngeal.[13] The differential diagnosis includes other sources of lateral jaw pain such as angina, masticator space neoplasm, temporomandibular joint (TMJ) dysfunction, referred dental pain, pharyngeal infection, tonsillitis or peritonsillar abscess, and otitis media or externa. History and physical examination usually will exclude these clinically.

Treatment

The patient's condition determines therapy. Airway compromise is rare in unilateral masticator space infection but should be considered. Emergent ENT consultation is required with airway compromise, severe trismus, abscess or phlegmon visible on CT scan, vomiting, palpable abscess, large or diffuse areas of cellulitis, large areas of induration, or systemic signs of sepsis.

Antibiotics should be administered in the emergency department (see Table 240-1). For patients requiring hospitalization, intravenous clindamycin is recommended. Alternatives include ampicillin-sulbactam, cefoxitin, or the combination of penicillin with metronidazole.[2,13] For outpatient management, oral clindamycin or amoxicillin-clavulanate is appropriate. Antibiotics should be continued for 10 to 14 days. Because of increased resistance, the macrolides (e.g., erythromycin) are generally no longer used for masticator space infections.[13]

Stable afebrile patients with minimal symptoms, only slight trismus, no palpable abscess or induration, and without vomiting or systemic signs of infection may be considered for discharge on oral antibiotics and analgesics. Follow-up should be arranged in 24 h.

TEMPOROMANDIBULAR JOINT DYSFUNCTION AND FRACTURE

The TMJ combines both a hinge and gliding action. The articular surfaces are separated by the articular disk, or meniscus, which assists in the hinge action between the mandibular condyle and the disk and in the gliding action between the disk and temporal bone. The masseter, temporalis, and medial pterygoid close the mandible. The jaw is opened by forward traction on the mandibular neck by the lower portion of the lateral pterygoid, with assistance from the digastric, mylohyoid, and geniohyoid muscles.[15]

Anatomic internal derangement may occur as the result of intracapsular disk displacement. This may be the result of a direct blow to the jaw or secondary to jaw hypermobility with chronic injury. The TMJ always should be assessed in patients who have direct jaw trauma or acute dental injury.

Chronic TMJ dysfunction probably results from a variety of causes, either singly or in combination, and includes neuromuscular disturbance, anatomic deviations as a result of trauma or congenital formation, dental abnormalities, or TMJ manifestations of systemic disease.[17] Most studies have found no significant correlation between occlusal parameters or bruxism and signs or symptoms of TMJ disorders.[16,18] Degenerative joint disease may result from chronic internal derangement or secondarily as the result of a systemic disease such as rheumatoid arthritis or systemic lupus erythematosus.

The patient's chief complaint is usually of pain localized to one of the muscles of mastication. The masseter is the most frequently identified painful area, followed by the temporalis, sternocleidomastoid, splenius capitus, and trapezius.[16] Physical findings may include limitation in the range of motion of the mandible. Isolated clicking without pain or other dysfunction is not diagnostically sufficient.[16] Palpate the muscles of mastication to find areas of sensitivity, induration, rigidity, and swelling. The condylar heads may be palpated just anterior to the tragus with the teeth together and then with the teeth apart. Perform a careful head and neck examination to exclude more serious causes of facial pain.

In the setting of acute trauma, the panoramic x-ray view of the mandible is usually the initial radiographic evaluation of the TMJ. This also provides information about the teeth and other parts of the jaw that may be contributing to pain.[19] The panoramic view, combined with a frontal projection, can identify medial displacement of a condylar fracture.[19] CT scanning is appropriate in the assessment of potentially complex fractures, infections, and neoplastic disease. For chronic conditions, there is no acute need for x-rays. TMJ disk condition and position are best evaluated in a nonemergency setting using magnetic resonance imaging (MRI).[19]

Acute fracture is managed by the oral maxillofacial surgeon. For chronic conditions, the patient should be advised to eat soft foods until follow-up and more definitive treatment can be provided.

DISLOCATION OF THE MANDIBLE

The mandible can be dislocated in an anterior, posterior, lateral, or superior direction. Anterior dislocation is most common and occurs when the mandibular condyle is forced in front of the articular eminence. Muscular spasm then traps the mandible in anterior dislocation. The following factors predispose patients to symptomatic anterior dislocation: a shallow glenoid fossa, increased muscle tone, and a loss of joint capsule tone from previous trauma. Spasm of the temporalis and lateral pterygoid muscles tends to prevent reduction once dislocation has occurred. Dislocations are usually bilateral, but unilateral dislocations are seen.[15]

Anterior dislocations are classified as acute, chronic recurrent, or chronic.[15] Patients usually present quickly after an anterior dislocation occurs because of pain. When presented with a chronic recurrent dislocation, look for predisposing factors such as dystonic reactions and hypermobility syndromes (e.g., Marfan's or Ehlers-Danlos syndromes). Chronic dislocations, where the condyle remains displaced from the fossa for an extended time, occur in patients who do not obtain prompt medical treatment.[15]

Posterior dislocations are rare. They follow a direct blow to the chin that does not break the condylar neck. In this dislocation, the mandibular condyle is thrust up against the mastoid, and the condylar head may prolapse into the external auditory canal.[15]

Lateral dislocations are often associated with mandibular fracture. With a lateral dislocation, the condylar head is forced laterally and then superiorly into the temporal space. Superior dislocations occur from a blow to the partially open mouth that forces the condylar head upward. Associated injuries include cerebral contusions, facial nerve palsy, and deafness.

Clinical Features

Patients with acute jaw dislocation usually present with severe pain, difficulty in speaking or swallowing, or malocclusion. There may be loose or missing teeth and areas of sensory deficit at the chin or mouth.

With anterior dislocation, pain is localized anterior to the tragus. Frequently, the symptoms are reported to have begun acutely following extreme mouth opening. Anterior dislocation has been reported to have occurred after laughing, yawning, vomiting, taking a large bite, trauma, oral sex, dental extraction, general anesthesia, and tonsillectomy.[15] In contrast to anterior dislocation, all other types of mandibular dislocation tend to require significant trauma.

All patients with possible mandibular dislocation should have a good head, neck, and dental examination. With anterior dislocations, there is a visible and palpable preauricular depression from the displacement of the mandibular condyle. There also will be difficulty with jaw movement. If the dislocation is unilateral, there is deviation of the jaw away from the dislocation.

When a posterior dislocation is considered, examine the external auditory canal. Confirm that hearing is at baseline. With lateral dislocations, the condylar head is palpable in the temporal space, and there are always signs of jaw fracture (e.g., malocclusion). When a superior dislocation is suspected, a thorough examination is needed, especially focusing on the head, neck, and nervous systems.

In the cooperative patient with a spontaneous nontraumatic anterior dislocation, the diagnosis is based on clinical grounds. In other dislocations, radiographs may be needed to confirm the clinical suspicion. With significant trauma, radiographs should be obtained to exclude fracture. The panoramic view usually demonstrates the pathology and excludes other mandibular injury. In patients with more serious trauma, where there may be a superior dislocation or intracranial injury, a CT scan will provide more information.

The differential diagnosis of jaw dislocation includes mandibular fracture, traumatic hemarthrosis, acute closed locking of the TMJ meniscus, and TMJ dysfunction.[15]

Treatment

Reduction may be attempted in closed anterior dislocations without fracture. Most attempts are made easier with analgesia. A short-acting intravenous muscle relaxant (e.g., midazolam) helps to decrease muscle spasm.[21] Appropriate airway and hemodynamic monitoring is required. Consider using narcotic analgesia. Conscious sedation also has been used successfully.[20] Alternatively, local anesthetic can be placed into the joint space. Using aseptic technique, place a 21-gauge needle into the preauricular depression just anterior to the tragus and inject 2 mL of 2% lidocaine[15] (Figure 240-2).

There are two methods for reducing an anterior mandibular dislocation.[15] The most commonly used technique requires the patient to be firmly seated with the head against the wall or chair back, positioned so that the examiner's flexed elbow is at the level of the patient's mandible. Facing the patient, the examiner places his or her gloved thumbs in the patient's mouth, over the occlusal surfaces of the mandibular molars, as far back as possible. The fingers should curve beneath the angle and body of the mandible. Using the thumbs, the examiner applies pressure downward and backward. Slightly opening the jaw may help disengage the condyle from the anterior eminence (Figure 240-3). When the dislocation is bilateral, it may be easier to relocate one side at a time. Some suggest that the examiner wear gauze over the thumbs for protection, should the mandible snap closed after reduction.[15]

The second technique requires the examiner, standing behind the recumbent patient, to place the thumbs on the molars and to apply downward and backward pressure.[15]

The patient should be able to close his or her mouth immediately after a successful reduction. Postreduction radiographs usually are not required unless the procedure was difficult or traumatic or there is significant postreduction pain. Complications from the reduction itself are unusual but can include iatrogenic fracture or avulsion of the articular cartilage.[20]

Disposition

Patients with dislocations that are open, superior, associated with fracture, have any nerve injury, or are unreducible by closed technique should be referred emergently to a head and neck or oral surgeon.

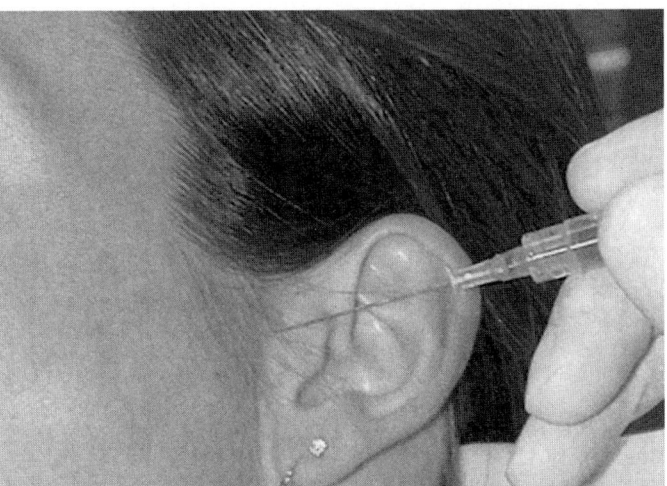

FIG. 240-2. Site for injection of local anesthesia for reduction of dislocated mandible.

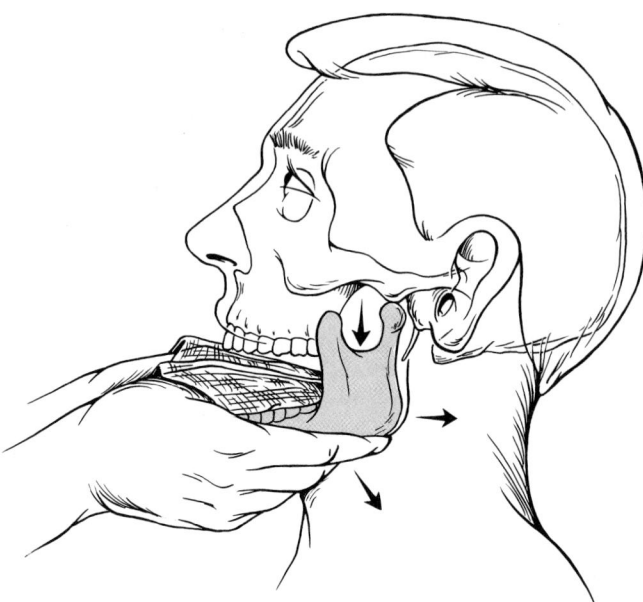

FIG. 240-3. Maneuver for mandibular relocation in a seated patient. The examiner should wear gloves for this procedure.

Following successful reduction of an acute dislocation, patients are placed on a soft diet and cautioned against opening their mouths more than 2 cm for the following 2 weeks.[21] They should be instructed to support the mandible with a hand when they yawn. Nonsteroidal analgesics may help the initial discomfort. After reduction, elective referral to an oral maxillofacial surgeon is recommended. In severe cases, intermaxillary fixation may be required to control jaw motion during healing. Chronic dislocations may require operative intervention.

REFERENCES

1. Beiderman GR, Dodson TB: Epidemiologic review of facial infections in hospitalized pediatric patients. *J Oral Maxillofac Surg* 52:1042, 1994.
2. Fairbanks DN: *Antimicrobial Therapy in Otolaryngology Head and Neck Surgery,* 10th ed. New York, American Academy of Otolaryngology Head and Neck Surgery Foundation, 2001.
3. Magnussen CR: Skin and soft tissue infections, in Reese RE, Betts RF (eds): *A Practical Approach to Infectious Disease,* 4th ed. Boston, Little, Brown, 1996, pp 96–132.
4. Berger TG: Skin, hair and nails, in Tierney LM, McPhee SJ, Papadakis MA (eds): *Current Medical Diagnosis and Treatment,* 39th ed. New York, Lange Medical Books/McGraw-Hill, 2000, p 163.
5. Middleton DB, Ferrante JA: Periorbital and facial cellulitis. *Am Fam Phys* 21:98, 1980.
6. Human anthrax associated with an epizootic among livestock—North Dakota, 2000. *MMWR* 50(32):677, 2001.
7. Update: Investigation of bioterrorism-related anthrax and interim guidelines for clinical evaluation of persons with possible anthrax. *MMWR* 50:941, 2001.
8. Pile JC, Malone JD, Eitzen EM: Anthrax as a potential biological warfare agent. *Arch Intern Med* 158:429, 1998.
9. McQuone SJ: Acute viral and bacterial infections of the salivary glands. *Otolaryngol Clin North Am* 32:793, 1999.
10. Gold E: Almost extinct diseases: Measles, mumps, rubella and pertussis. *Pediatr Rev* 17:120, 1996.
11. Williams MF: Sialolithiasis. *Otolaryngol Clin North Am* 32:819, 1999.
12. Krause GE, Meyers AD: Management of parotid swelling. *Compr Ther* 22:256, 1996.
13. Flynn TR: The swollen face. *Emerg Med Clin North Am* 18:481, 2000.
14. Mandel L: Diagnosing protracted submasseteric abscess: The role of computed tomography. *J Am Dent Assoc* 127:1646, 1996.
15. Luyk NH, Larsen PE: The diagnosis and treatment of the dislocated mandible. *Am J Emerg Med* 7:329, 1989.
16. Marbach JJ: Medically unexplained chronic orofacial pain. *Med Clin North Am* 83:691, 1999.
17. Talley RL, Murphy GJ, Smith SD, et al: Standard for the history, examination, diagnosis, and treatment of temperomandibular disorders (TMD): A position paper of the American Academy of Head Neck, and Facial Pain. *Craniology* 8:60, 1990.
18. Mitchell RJ: Etiology of temporomandibular disorders. *Curr Opin Den* 1:471, 1991.
19. Brooks SL, Brand JW, Gibbs SJ, et al: Imaging of the temporomandibular joint: A position paper of the American Academy of Oral and Maxillofacial Radiology. *Oral Surg Oral Med Oral Pathol Oral Radiol Endod* 83:609, 1997.
20. Totten VY, Zambito RF: Propofol bolus facilitates reduction of luxed temporomandibular joints. *J Emerg Med* 16:467,1998.
21. Undt G, Kermer C, Piehslinger E, Rasse M: Treatment of recurrent mandibular dislocation: I. Leclerc blocking procedure. *Int J Oral Maxillofac Surg* 26:92, 1997.

NASAL EMERGENCIES AND SINUSITIS
Thomas A. Waters
W. Franklin Peacock IV

EPISTAXIS

Introduction

Because the blood supply of the nasal mucosa ultimately originates from the carotid arteries, acute epistaxis is potentially very serious, especially when the patient is frail or elderly. Up to 60 percent of patients may experience at least one episode of epistaxis in their lifetimes.[1] Still, most cases of epistaxis are self-limited and can be managed conservatively.

Epistaxis has an increased incidence during the dry, cold winter months,[2–4] due to abrupt temperature changes and exposure to dry heat.

The origin of epistaxis can be broadly divided into anterior and posterior categories. Anterior epistaxis is more common in the young, while posterior is most common in the older patient. Determining the site of bleeding helps guide treatment.

The nose functions to warm and humidify air and therefore requires a vigorous blood supply (Figure 241-1). Its blood supply originates from both the internal and external carotid arteries. The posterior and inferior aspects of the nasal cavity are supplied by the sphenopalatine artery, which is a branch of the maxillary artery. The internal carotid artery gives rise to the ophthalmic artery, which supplies the anterior-superior nasal cavity by the anterior and posterior ethmoidal arteries. The nasal septum receives its blood supply from multiple arteries. The superior labial branch of the facial artery supplies the vestibule and inferior-anterior septum. The posterior and superior septum is supplied by branches of the sphenopalatine, anterior ethmoidal, and posterior ethmoidal arteries. These all join to form Kiesselbach plexus (Little area).

Anterior Epistaxis

Anterior epistaxis represents 90 percent of all nosebleeds, with the majority originating from Kiesselbach plexus.[5] This area has been referred to as the picking zone, and is also the area most prone to drying and cracking from the environment. Anterior nosebleeds can result from any process that causes mucosal hyperemia. Hereditary hemorrhagic telangiectasia (HHT), or Osler-Weber-Rendu disease, is an unusual but severe cause of recurrent anterior nosebleeds. HHT is an autosomal-dominant disorder, characterized by mucosal telangiectasia throughout the airway and gastrointestinal tract.

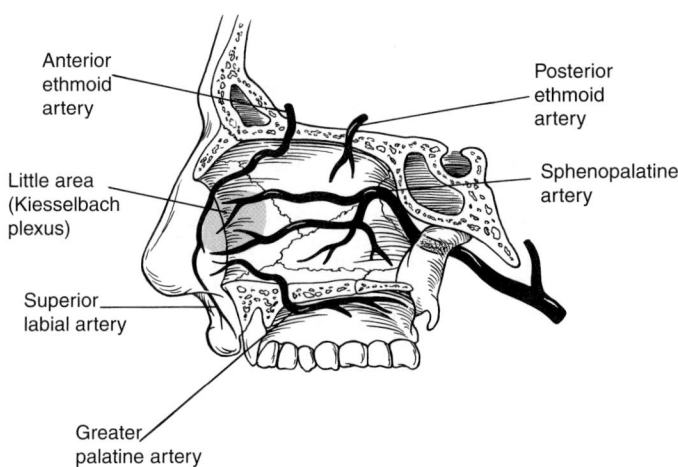

FIG. 241-1. Arterial blood supply to the nasal cavity. The most common site of nasal hemorrhage is at Little area, located on the nasal septum. The most common origin of posterior epistaxis is from the sphenopalatine artery.

Anterior epistaxis is fairly common in children. In a study of 1218 children aged 11 to 14, 6 percent had experienced epistaxis. The most common cause is idiopathic or related to upper respiratory infections. Treatment is by direct pressure. In the rare case when packing is required, conscious sedation may be needed.

Clinical Features

The history can provide valuable insight as to the location of the epistaxis. Questions that are important to ask include:

1. Is one side bleeding, or both? (anterior epistaxis is usually unilateral)
2. Do you have a sensation of blood in the back of the throat? (more often associated with posterior epistaxis)
3. Do you have a history of previous epistaxis, trauma, head/neck tumor, radiation therapy, or head/neck surgery? (suggests the need for otolaryngologic consultation)
4. Is there a family history of bleeding disorders? (clotting studies may be needed)
5. Are you using anticoagulants, nonsteroidal anti-inflammatory drugs (NSAIDs), or aspirin? (clotting studies or medication change may be needed)

In anterior epistaxis one can often directly visualize the area of bleeding. However, proper lighting and suction are essential. Adequate lighting is best achieved by the use of an ENT headlamp or by a head mirror. Universal precautions must be observed by the examiner and the patient's clothing should also be protected. The patient should be seated in a chair leaning forward with the head inclined anteriorly. This helps to visualize the nasal cavity and minimizes retropharyngeal blood flow, which decreases gagging. The assessment of the patient must include complete vital signs, as well as a thorough examination of the oropharynx and nasopharynx. Additionally, a general physical overview is necessary to evaluate for signs of systemic coagulopathy.

Laboratory investigation is not routinely required, unless there are multiple or prolonged episodes of hemorrhage, if there is clinical suspicion of anemia, or if coagulopathy is suggested by history or physical examination.

Treatment

The treatment of anterior epistaxis includes direct pressure, vasoconstrictive agents, nasal packing, and cautery. Even though the blood pressure may be elevated with acute epistaxis, stabilization should focus on direct hemorrhage control. Once bleeding has been stopped and

patient anxiety is relieved, elevated blood pressure usually spontaneously resolves. Persistent or extremely high elevations of blood pressure can then be addressed (see Chap. 57).

Most episodes of anterior epistaxis can be managed by direct pressure to the nose. This is achieved by compressing the elastic areas of the nose between the thumb and middle phalanx of the index finger. Pressure must be continuously maintained for 10 to 15 min, and confirmed with a clock, as patients frequently underestimate the amount of time that has elapsed. Premature release of pressure to see if the bleeding has stopped will not allow adequate clot formation and may result in continued bleeding. At least two adequate attempts at direct pressure should be made before moving to cautery or packing.

Vasoconstrictive agents may be used with all other treatment modalities and should be instilled into the nose before pressure is applied. Table 241-1 lists the common agents. These compounds can be instilled into the nasal cavity by a spray bottle, atomizer, or cotton swab. Have the patient completely blow out the nose to remove any clot before instillation of vasoconstrictors, to ensure that the medication reaches the nasal mucosa.[4] If the area of bleeding can be visualized, the vasoconstrictor can be topically applied with cotton swabs or pledgets using gentle direct pressure.

If the source of bleeding is easily visualized anteriorly, careful cautery using silver nitrate sticks can be attempted. After bleeding has stopped, the tip of the silver nitrate stick is gently and briefly applied to the bleeding site. Chemical cautery can lead to septal perforation if used overzealously. **Electrical and thermal cautery are best left for the otolaryngologist.** It is difficult to control or estimate the depth of cautery achieved with the battery-powered cautery devices available. Significant trauma can occur to the nasal mucosa, septal cartilage, and the skin surrounding the nares.

Anterior Nasal Packing

Anterior nasal packing is performed on any patient in whom direct pressure, vasoconstrictors, or silver nitrate application are unsuccessful in controlling epistaxis. Either nasal tampons or an anterior gauze pack can be used.

Preformed nasal tampons or sponges made of synthetic material that expands to many times its original size after hydration are generally used (Figure 241-2). They are commercially available in 5- and 10-cm lengths, for anterior and posterior packing, respectively. A drawstring at the distal end is taped to the face to secure the tampon and prevent inadvertent aspiration. Insertion of the device can be facilitated by coating the tampon with water soluble antibiotic ointment, and by mucosal pretreatment with a topical anesthetic and vasoconstrictor. The ointment decreases the number of nasal bacteria,[5] and will also help delay tampon expansion until after the tampon is in place. The nasal tampon is then inserted along the floor of the nasal cavity against the septum. If the tampon has not expanded within 30 s of placement, it should be gently irrigated (while in place) with 10 mL of normal saline in order to promote expansion. The drawstring should then be taped to the face or nose.

Placement of a traditional anterior nasal pack may be considered when the bleeding is difficult to control or other methods fail. The technique detailed in Figure 241-3 is preceded by preparing the nasal mucosa as before placement of the nasal tampon (see above).

TABLE 241-1 Vasoconstrictive and Anesthetic Agents Used in Epistaxis

Phenylephrine 0.5–1.0% concentration mixed with 4% lidocaine*
Oxymetozaline 0.05% concentration mixed with 4% lidocaine*
Epinephrine 0.25 mL of 1:1000 concentration mixed with 20 mL of 4% lidocaine*

*The maximum dose of lidocaine applied to the nasal mucosa should not exceed 4 mg/kg.

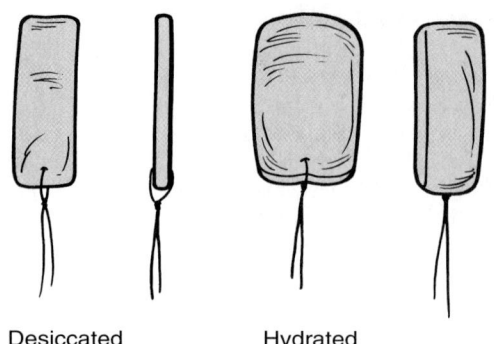

Desiccated   Hydrated

FIG. 241-2. The Merocel nasal sponge in its desiccated (*left*) and hydrated (*right*) forms.

Even a properly placed anterior nasal pack may fail to control bleeding. If bleeding continues or recurs, the pack should be replaced. If after replacement bleeding still persists, a posterior nosebleed must be considered and a posterior pack applied (see below). For refractory epistaxis, otolaryngologic consultation should be obtained.

Complications associated with anterior nasal packing include: dislodgment of the pack, persistent bleeding, sinusitis, septal necrosis, and rarely, toxic shock syndrome (see Chap. 142). Patients may also experience reflux of blood through the lacrimal puncta and need to be warned about this. No specific therapy is needed.

Disposition

Discharge instructions should include the following:

1. Do not manipulate the external nares or insert any foreign object into the nasal cavity. An exception is made for patients with no packing, in which case the patient may apply petrolatum jelly or triple antibiotic ointment to the nasal mucosa twice daily for 3 to 4 days to prevent mucosal drying.
2. **Do not use aspirin or NSAIDs for 3 to 4 days.**
3. If bleeding recurs where no packing has been inserted, home measures may be tried before returning to the ED. Patients may be advised to use an over-the-counter vasoconstrictor nasal spray (such as phenylephrine or oxymetazoline) and pinch their nose, using proper technique, for 10 to 15 min. If the bleeding continues, compression may be repeated. If after three attempts the bleeding continues, the patient should return to the ED. Patients with an anterior pack should return if bleeding occurs around it, or if there is a sensation of blood trickling down the back of the throat. They should be advised to leave the pack in place.

Any patient who has undergone nasal packing may be considered for prophylaxis against staphylococcal or streptococcal infections and for sinusitis. Coating the pack with antibiotic ointment before placement can decrease the amount of nasal bacteria and the frequency of bacteremia.[5] Cephalexin (250 or 500 mg PO qid) or amoxicillin-clavulanate (250 or 500 mg PO tid) can be given. In the penicillin-allergic patient, clindamycin (150 to 300 mg PO qid) or trimethoprim-sulfamethoxazole DS (1 tablet PO bid) can be used as a second choice.[5]

Nasal packing should be removed after 2 to 3 days. When nasal tampon removal is planned, the pack should first be rehydrated with 10 mL of NS. The drawstring is then grasped and the tampon gently removed.

POSTERIOR EPISTAXIS

Posterior epistaxis is far less common than anterior epistaxis.[6] It is more common in the elderly and is believed to be due to arteriosclerosis of the large posterior nasal cavity vessels and underlying hypertension.

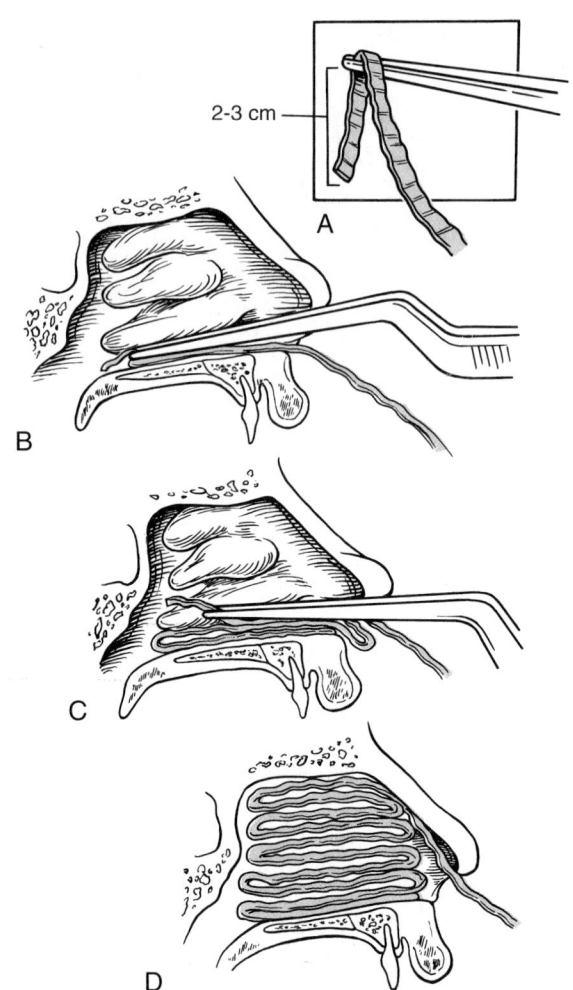

FIG. 241-3. The key to placement of an anterior nasal pack that will control epistaxis adequately and stay in place is to lay the packing into the nasal cavity in an accordion-like manner, so that part of each layer of packing lies anteriorly, preventing the gauze from falling posteriorly into the nasopharynx. **A.** The first layer of ¼-in. petrolatum-impregnated gauze strip is grasped approximately 2 to 3 cm from its end. **B.** The first layer is then placed on the floor of the nose through the nasal speculum (not pictured here). The bayonet forceps and nasal speculum are then withdrawn. **C.** The nasal speculum is reintroduced on top of the first layer of packing, and a second layer is placed in an identical manner. After several layers have been placed, it is often useful to reintroduce the bayonet forceps to push the previously placed packing down onto the floor of the nose, making it tighter and more secure. **D.** A complete anterior nasal pack can tamponade a bleeding point anywhere in the anterior nasal cavities and will stay in place until removed by the physician or patient.

The most common site of bleeding is posterior to the inferior turbinate, about 6 to 7.5 cm posterior to the vestibule, and emanates from branches of the sphenopalatine artery. The actual bleeding site can only be visualized with a nasopharyngoscope.

Bleeding is typically more profuse than with anterior epistaxis, and may be more difficult to control because the site of hemorrhage is closer to the choanae and blood is more likely to reflux to the unaffected side. Blood can often be seen flowing down the posterior oropharynx or from both nares. A complete set of vital signs, a thorough head, neck, and naso- and oropharyngeal examination, and general physical examination to search for evidence of systemic coagulopathy should be performed. An intravenous line and laboratory studies including complete blood count, blood type, and antibody screening, and coagulation studies are often warranted.

Posterior Nasal Packing

The treatment of posterior epistaxis is posterior nasal packing. Direct pressure is ineffective, and blind attempts at chemical, heat, or electrocautery can cause injury and more bleeding. The application of vasoconstrictors and anesthetic agents in the treatment of posterior epistaxis is the same as for anterior bleeding.

Posterior nasal packing is most often accomplished by the use of commercial devices, such as 10-cm nasal sponges, the Nasostat epistaxis balloon (Sparta Surgical Corp., Hayward, CA), or the Storz epistaxis catheter (Storz Instrument, St. Louis, MO). The use and insertion of the nasal tampons in posterior epistaxis is the same as discussed above for anterior epistaxis. A 10-cm sponge is utilized to obtain both anterior and posterior tamponade.

The procedure for insertion of a commercial nasal catheter for posterior epistaxis control is as follows:

1. The nasal cavity is prepared using vasoconstrictors and anesthetic agents.
2. A test is performed for leakage by filling the anterior balloon with 25 mL of water and the posterior balloon with 8 mL of water. If no leak is detected, the water is removed.
3. The device is lubricated with 4 percent lidocaine jelly and inserted into the nasopharynx. The patient opens his or her mouth, and the catheter is advanced until the distal balloon tip is visible in the posterior pharynx.
4. The posterior balloon is slowly filled with 4 to 8 mL of water, and the device is pulled anteriorly so that it wedges in the posterior nasopharynx.
5. While gentle traction is maintained, the anterior balloon is slowly inflated with 10 to 25 mL of water, providing anterior tamponade. Inflation should be stopped immediately if the patient complains of significant pain. However, some discomfort is usually present.
6. Bilateral packing may be necessary to control hemorrhage.
7. Analgesics are usually required.

If a commercial device is not available, a Foley catheter can be used to construct a posterior pack. The placement of the Foley catheter is similar to the procedure described above, but with slight differences. The tip of the Foley catheter must be trimmed off to avoid stimulation of the posterior pharynx. The Foley catheter must be pulled anteriorly and held in the forward position by a transverse clamp across the catheter, external to the nasal septum. Ensure that alar necrosis does not result by inserting padding between the nasal alae and the clamp. After placement of a Foley catheter, the anterior nasal cavity is packed to prevent accumulation of a large clot that would represent an aspiration risk.

The procedure of inserting a posterior nasal pack is very uncomfortable and stressful to the patient. After placement, the patient often continues to have significant discomfort and may require analgesia and sedation. Complications of posterior nasal packs include difficulty swallowing, eustachian tube dysfunction, otitis media, sinusitis, nasal synechiae, cardiac arrhythmias, cardiac arrest, accidental dislodgment into the airway, or aseptic necrosis of the nasal alae, columella, palate, and nasal mucosa. In patients with altered mental status, severe chronic obstructive pulmonary disease, or severe congestive heart failure, posterior nasal packing can result in hypoxia. Therefore, **admission should be considered for patients with significant comorbidities and posterior epistaxis.**

If epistaxis is refractory to the above, otolaryngologic consultation is needed. If packing by the consultant is ineffective, arterial ligation or embolization may be necessary.

Disposition

Because of the potential for serious morbidity and mortality associated with posterior packing, patients are usually admitted for observation. They may need sedation secondary to severe discomfort and require monitoring for hypoxia. Prophylactic antibiotics are generally given (see anterior packing, above).

NASAL FRACTURE

Any significant central midface trauma should be considered highly suspicious for the presence of a nasal bone fracture. A direct impact is most likely to cause a fracture because there is no soft tissue to dissipate the force of the blow. The pathomechanics of the resulting fracture vary according to the site, direction, and intensity of impact, as well as the characteristics of the bone that is struck. In younger patients, bones are denser and more elastic, whereas in older patients, bones are less dense and more brittle.

A careful history can usually ascertain the severity of trauma incurred. In cases in which the forces involved are severe, suspicion of cervical spine injury or closed-head injury takes precedence over any concurrent nasal fracture. Findings suggestive of a nasal fracture include swelling, tenderness, crepitance, ecchymosis, or nasal deformity. Indirect evidence of nasal fracture includes periorbital ecchymosis, epistaxis, and rhinorrhea. A general physical examination, specifically focused on the head, neck, and neurologic system, is necessary to exclude associated injury. After spraying the nasal mucosa with a vasoconstricting agent, search for defects in the mucosa, septal hematoma, and bony displacement. Finally, palpate the injured nose, checking for crepitance, stepoffs, and instability that suggest orbital or midface fracture.

The diagnosis of nasal fracture is clinical. Nasal radiographic studies are usually not required for either diagnosis or management. If there is associated facial bone injury, radiographic imaging selection may be driven by the requirements of collateral testing (e.g., facial bone CT scan to exclude orbital fracture).

Complications

The complications of a nasal fracture include nasal deformity, deviated nasal septum, septal hematoma, cribriform plate fracture, and associated facial, head, or spinal injuries. A septal hematoma is a rare complication. It is a collection of blood beneath the septal perichondrium. Easily visualized using an otoscope, it appears as a bluish, fluid-filled sac overlying the septum. The hematoma is easily managed by making an incision for drainage, followed by packing the nasal cavity to prevent reaccumulation (see Figure 241-3). If undiagnosed or left untreated, it may progress to an abscess or result in avascular necrosis of the cartilaginous septum within several days. Septal avascular necrosis is associated with the cosmetic complications of saddle nose deformity, retraction, and changes in phonation.

Fracture through the cribriform plate of the ethmoid bone is associated with a cerebrospinal fluid (CSF) leak via torn meninges. It represents a violation in the integrity of the subarachnoid space. Although rare, CSF rhinorrhea is suspected when there is a clear nasal discharge following facial injury. In major trauma, it is usually seen within the first week as cerebral edema resolves, but it may be delayed days to weeks. If untreated, possible sequelae include meningoencephalitis or brain abscess.

The identification of CSF rhinorrhea can be difficult in nasal injuries because it is not unusual for there to be a clear transudate from the traumatized nasal mucosa. One method of detecting CSF is to put a drop of the suspected liquid on a piece of filter paper and see if a clear area surrounds a central blood stain. **The glucose content of both CSF and nasal secretions can be similar.** All patients with suspected CSF rhinorrhea should undergo a head CT scan and urgent neurosurgical consultation. If a fracture of the cribriform plate is clinically suspected, the patient should be placed in an upright position, intranasal packing avoided, and immediate neurosurgical consultation obtained. Furthermore, the patient should be instructed to avoid coughing, sneezing, nose blowing, and straining.

Other injuries often seen with nasal trauma are fractures of the orbital wall, sinuses, and zygoma. Be suspicious of cervical spine damage or closed head injury in any patient with significant facial trauma.

Treatment and Disposition

A simple, minimally or nondisplaced nasal fracture requires no specific treatment other than analgesia, nasal decongestants, and protection from further injury. If significant epistaxis occurs, nasal packing can be placed as previously discussed, but is usually unnecessary. For extreme nasal displacement, emergency consultation is needed for realignment.

Discharge instructions include intermittent ice application for 24 to 48 h, elevation of the head (even while sleeping), and over-the-counter decongestants as needed. Patients may require head-injury instructions and advice to be alert for CSF rhinorrhea. Patients are also offered follow-up with an appropriate specialist at about 1 week, after edema has subsided. Although nondisplaced fractures rarely need further treatment, follow-up can address the cosmetic importance of the injury.

NASAL FOREIGN BODIES

Children frequently insert foreign bodies that may require removal into their nares. Items placed in the nasal cavity are limited only by the child's imagination, and are most often food, paper, and pieces of toys.[7] Dried beans and vegetable matter are particularly concerning because they tend to absorb fluid and swell, increasing discomfort and making removal difficult. Other common foreign bodies include rocks, buttons, and small batteries.

Many children are reluctant to admit to placing a foreign body in their nose for fear they will elicit displeasure from their parents or the physician. In most cases, the insertion of the foreign body is actually observed by the caregiver, or the child reports the presence of a foreign body.[8] Suspect a nasal foreign body in the following circumstances:

1. Sensation of unilateral nasal obstruction
2. Persistent, foul-smelling rhinorrhea despite proper antibiotic treatment
3. Persistent unilateral epistaxis

In addition to a nasal examination, a complete head and neck physical examination is performed. The ears are also carefully checked for foreign bodies, and the lungs auscultated for wheezing.

Treatment

If the child is cooperative and the foreign body visible, it is possible to remove the object in the ED. In small or uncooperative children, a papoose board may be used for restraint. The nasal mucosa is generally prepared with vasoconstrictors and anesthetics (1 mL of phenylephrine mixed with 3 mL of 4 percent xylocaine). In uncooperative children, aerosolized adrenaline (racemic epinephrine) can be used to decongest the nasal mucosa and loosen the foreign body.[9] When administered in the aerosolized form by the parent, it causes little or no distress to the child. Following this, visualization with an appropriate-sized nasal speculum is attempted.

If the object appears loose after vasoconstriction, an attempt to remove it can be made using a number of different techniques including:

1. Positive pressure technique
2. Removal by a suction catheter
3. Grasping the object with bayonet or alligator forceps
4. Passing a curette beyond the object, rotating the instrument, and pulling the foreign body out
5. Passing a Fogarty vascular catheter past the foreign body, inflating the balloon, and removing the catheter and foreign body

The latter four techniques are all acceptable, but require a cooperative child, physical restraint, or conscious sedation to prevent damage to the nasal mucosa. Regardless of the technique utilized, the airway must be protected and appropriate material for managing airway ob-

struction should be immediately available. The examiner should be careful not to advance the foreign body deeper into the nasopharynx.

POSITIVE PRESSURE TECHNIQUE The successful use of this method is well documented.[9–11] It can be performed in both cooperative and uncooperative patients, and is the least invasive. After vasoconstrictors, positive pressure can be applied by the patient if cooperative (i.e., blow the nose) or the caregiver. If the caregiver is performing the removal, they are instructed to give a puff of air to the mouth of the child while occluding the unobstructed nare with a finger. The foreign body is usually expressed from the nose onto the cheek of the caregiver. Repeated attempts may be necessary.

Despite anxiety generated in the mind of the parent, most patients with nasal foreign bodies can be discharged home even if removal attempts are unsuccessful. Admission need only be considered if the patient exhibits constitutional symptoms such as fever, malaise, or lethargy. If attempts to remove the foreign body are unsuccessful, the patient should follow-up with an otolaryngologist the next day. If foreign body removal was successful, no further follow-up or treatment is required.

SINUSITIS

Pathophysiology

There are six nasal sinuses: two maxillary, two frontal, one sphenoidal, and the ethmoidal air cells. Sinusitis occurs when there is an acute obstruction of the normal drainage mechanisms of the sinuses. Efficiency of sinus drainage consists of three elements: ostial patency, ciliary apparatus function, and the quality of the nasal secretions. Inflammatory edema causes obstruction or mucociliary drainage at the osteomeatal complex, followed by reabsorption of the air in the sinus, resulting in negative pressure. Negative pressure causes a collection of transudate within the sinus cavity. If bacteria are present, suppuration results.

Acute sinusitis is acute inflammation of the paranasal sinuses of less than 3 weeks duration. Viral upper respiratory tract infections and allergic rhinitis are the most common initiating factors in acute sinusitis.[12] Bacterial sinusitis is most commonly caused by *Streptococcus pneumoniae, Haemophilus influenzae,* and *Moraxella catarrhalis.*[13] Immunocompromised patients may be infected with the usual pathogens, opportunistic bacteria, or fungi.

Chronic sinusitis results from unresolved acute sinusitis of more than 3 weeks duration. In chronic sinusitis, polymicrobial anaerobic species are found in most cases.

Clinical Features

The consensus definition of acute bacterial sinusitis is as follows:[12] (1) symptoms for 7 days or more; (2) sinus pain or tenderness in the face or teeth; and (3) purulent nasal secretions.

Ethmoidal sinusitis usually causes a dull, aching sensation behind the eye. Infection of the frontal and maxillary sinuses generally causes pain over the affected sinus. Ethmoidal sinusitis can spread to the orbit, retro-orbital area, and central nervous system. The headache of sinusitis may be aggravated by bending forward, coughing, or sneezing.

On physical examination, there may be tenderness to palpation and percussion over the involved sinus, and direct visualization of the nasal cavity may show swollen, erythematous mucosa with purulent exudate draining from the ostia. Diminished transillumination of the affected sinus can also be seen. The physical examination should be directed to specifically exclude indications of infectious spread beyond the sinus cavity, as well as complications and confounders in the differential diagnosis.

Diagnosis

Radiography is not recommended for diagnosis in routine cases.[12] Physical examination has moderate ability to identify patients with positive radiographs [summary receiver operating characteristic (SROC) area, 0.74].[14] The radiographic signs of sinusitis are sinus opacity or fluid, with a sensitivity of 0.73 and specificity of 0.80 for radiography when compared to sinus puncture/aspiration as the gold standard.[14] Computed tomography (CT) has a greater ability to define physical characteristics, but its primary role is to diagnose sinusitis when the differential diagnosis is unclear and to define anatomy before surgery.[15] Not all patients with sinus-related symptoms will have CT evidence of abnormality,[16] and conversely, a small number of patients without sinus-related symptoms have abnormalities on CT.[16] Therefore, CT is not routinely indicated for diagnosis, but could be considered in the immunosuppressed or where the diagnosis is not clear.

Cultures of nasopharyngeal secretions are not routinely recommended.[13] However, they can be considered in the immunosuppressed, those who demonstrate any signs of infectious spread external to the sinus cavity, or in those who are systemically toxic.

Differential Diagnosis

The most important points to consider are those diagnoses arising as complications from sinusitis. These include any evidence of infectious extension from the sinus cavity, such as periorbital cellulitis, brain abscess, subdural empyema, meningitis, or cavernous sinus thrombosis. Such patients are usually febrile, extremely ill, may have unstable vital signs, and can demonstrate altered mental status, meningismus, and focal neurologic findings.

The differential diagnosis of patients with signs and symptoms of facial pain include tension headache, migraines, and cluster headache (see Chap. 227). While history and physical examination can usually differentiate these disorders from sinusitis, occasionally they can coexist with sinusitis, making diagnosis more difficult. Dental pain is usually localized to a single tooth, and is exquisitely sensitive to percussion, with few other symptoms to support the diagnosis of sinusitis. History taking should differentiate rhinitis symptoms from mucosal engorgement due to rebound following excessive topical decongestant use.

Treatment

For acute sinusitis with mild symptoms of less than 7 days' duration, symptomatic treatment is recommended.[12] Antibiotics should not be given unless symptoms persist for more than 7 days, or unless symptoms are severe (unilateral facial pain or purulent nasal secretions), regardless of duration of illness.[12] The most narrow-spectrum agent active against the likely pathogens should be selected.

Antimicrobial therapy shortens the symptomatic period by several days[13] and decreases the incidence of respiratory complications.[13] The most cost-effective initial antibiotic choices are amoxicillin or trimethoprim-sulfamethoxazole.[17,18] Cefuroxime or azithromycin are also commonly prescribed. In patients with suspected streptococcal antibiotic resistance, then amoxicillin-clavulanate, or a "respiratory" fluoroquinolone (levofloxacin, gatifloxacin, moxifloxacin, or gemifloxacin) can be considered.[19,20] In chronic sinusitis, recommended antibiotics include amoxicillin-clavulanate, cefuroxime, gatifloxacin, moxifloxacin, gemifloxacin, or clindamycin.

Over-the-counter nasal spray decongestants or antihistamines such as pseudoephedrine, phenylephrine, or oxymetazoline, are commonly used to alleviate symptoms of sinusitis. If topical decongestants are prescribed, they are for limited duration due to rebound mucosal congestion and edema if their use exceeds 5 to 7 days.[21–23] Oral antihistamines may be of use in allergic rhinosinusitis.[21,22] However, in sup-

purative sinusitis, they may result in thickening of secretions with crust formation at the osteomeatal complex.[22]

Steroid nasal sprays, used twice daily, can improve symptoms of acute sinusitis compared to antibiotic treatment alone.[24,25]

Complications

Persistent sinusitis can result in extension of the infectious process into the surrounding tissues. Bony destruction, originating from the frontal sinus, can extend anteriorly. This leads to the development of a doughy, edematous forehead called Potts puffy tumor. If a frontal bone osteomyelitis extends posteriorly, a frontal brain abscess, meningitis, subdural empyema, and epidural abscess can develop. Extension from the ethmoid sinus can result in orbital or periorbital cellulitis. Finally, direct extension from the paranasal sinus to the venous or lymphatic system can cause cavernous sinus thrombosis. All patients suspected of having any extension of infection beyond the paranasal sinuses needs immediate CT or MRI scanning, intravenous antibiotic therapy, and emergent consultation with the appropriate specialist.

Disposition

Most patients with acute sinusitis can be treated as outpatients. Hospitalization is required if there is evidence of infectious spread beyond the sinus cavity, or if there is systemic toxicity. Discharged patients should receive follow-up in 5 to 7 days, with instructions to return to the ED for persistent fever, severe or worsening headache, visual changes, or vomiting.

REFERENCES

1. Shaw CB, Wax MK, Wetmore SJ: Epistaxis: A comparison of treatment. *Otolaryngol Head Neck Surg* 109:60, 1993.
2. Juselius H: Epistaxis: A clinical study of 1724 patients. *J Laryngol Otol* 88:317, 1974.
3. Rubin J, Rood S, Myers E, et al: The management of epistaxis. Self-instructional package. Alexandria VA: American Academy of Otolaryngology-Head and Neck Surgery, 1990.
4. Muller TU: NASA Epistaxis Protocol. February 2002.
5. Herzon FS: Bacteremic and local infections with nasal packing. *Arch Otolarygol* 9:317, 1994.
6. Viducich RA, Blanda MP, Gerson LW: Posterior epistaxis: Clinical features and acute complications. *Ann Emerg Med* 25:592, 1995.
7. Nondapalan V, McIlwain JC: Removal of nasal foreign bodies with a Fogarty biliary balloon catheter. *J Laryngol Otolaryngol* 108:758, 1994.
8. Tong MCF, Ying SY, van Hasselt CA: Nasal foreign bodies in children. *J Pediatr Otorhinolaryngol* 35:207, 1996.
9. Douglas AR: Use of nebulized adrenaline to aid expulsion of intranasal foreign bodies in children. *J Laryngol Otol* 110:559, 1996.
10. Backlin SA: Positive pressure technique for nasal foreign body removal. *Ann Emerg Med* 25:554, 1995.
11. Finkelstein JA: Oral Ambu-bag insufflation to remove unilateral nasal foreign bodies. *Am J Emerg Med* 14:157, 1996.
12. Hickner JM, Bartlett JG, Besser RE, et al: American Academy of Family Physicians, American College of Physicians-American Society of Internal Medicine, Centers for Disease Control, Infectious Diseases Society of America. Principles of appropriate antibiotic use for acute rhinosinusitis in adults. Background. *Ann Intern Med* 134:498, 2001.
13. Kaiser L, Morabia A, Stalder H, et al: Role of nasopharyngeal culture in antibiotic prescription for patients with common cold or acute sinusitis. *Eur J Clin Microbiol Infect Dis* 20:445, 2001.
14. Engels EA, Terrin N, Barza M, et al: Meta-analysis of diagnostic tests for acute sinusitis. *J Clin Epidemiol* 53:852, 2000.
15. Diaz I, Bamberger DM: Acute sinusitis seminars. *Respir Infect* 10:14, 1995.
16. Calhoun KH, Waggenspack GA, Simpson CB, et al: CT evaluation of the paranasal sinuses in symptomatic and asymptomatic populations. *Otolaryngol Head Neck Surg* 104:480, 1991.
17. Benninger MS, Sedory Holzer SE, Lau J: Diagnosis and treatment of uncomplicated acute bacterial rhinosinusitis: Summary of the Agency for

Health Care Policy and Research evidence-based report. *Otolaryngol Head Neck Surg* 122:1, 2000.

18. Gwaltney JM Jr: State-of-the-art: Acute community-acquired sinusitis. *Clin Infect Dis* 23:1209, 1996.

19. Dolor RJ, Witsell DL, Hellkamp AS, et al: Comparison of cefuroxime with or without intranasal fluticasone for the treatment of rhinosinusitis. The CAFFS Trial: A randomized controlled trial. *JAMA* 286:3097, 2001.

20. Siegert R, Gehanno P, Nikolaidis P: A comparison of the safety and efficacy of moxifloxacin and cefuroxime axetil in the treatment of acute bacterial sinusitis in adults. The Sinusitis Study group. *Respir Med* 94:337, 2000.

21. Malm L: Pharmacological background to decongesting and anti-inflammatory treatment of rhinitis and sinusitis. [Review]. *Acta Oto-Laryngologica* 515(Suppl):55, 1994.

22. Mabry RL: Therapeutic agents in the medical management of sinusitis. [Review.] *Otolaryngol Clin North Am* 26:561, 1993.

23. Min YG, Kim HS, Suh SH, et al: Paranasal sinusitis after long-term use of topical nasal decongestants. *Acta Oto-Laryngologica* 116:465, 1996.

24. Meltzer EO, Charous BL, Busse WW, et al: Added relief in the treatment of acute recurrent sinusitis with adjunctive mometasone furoate nasal spray. The Nasonex Sinusitis Group. *J Allergy Clin Immunol* 106:630, 2000.

25. Naval AS, Settipane GA, Pedinoff A, et al, and the Nasonex Sinusitis Group: Effective dose range of mometasone furoate nasal spray in the treatment of acute rhinosinusitis. *Ann Allergy Asthma Immunol* 89:271, 2002.

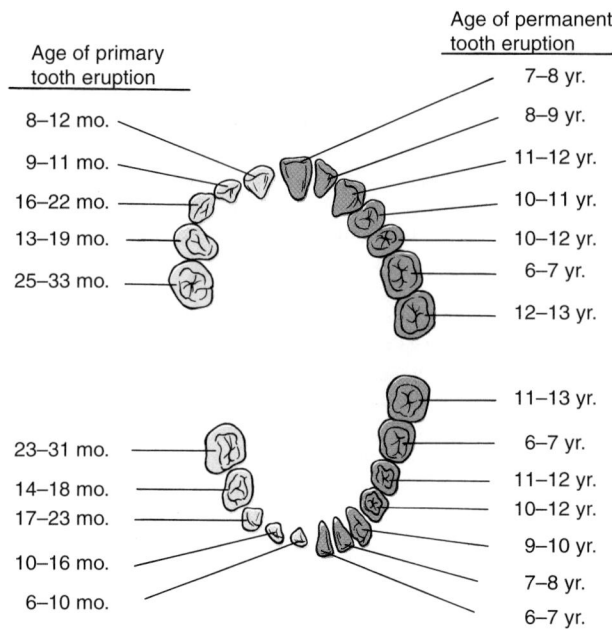

Age of primary tooth eruption

8–12 mo.
9–11 mo.
16–22 mo.
13–19 mo.
25–33 mo.

23–31 mo.
14–18 mo.
17–23 mo.
10–16 mo.
6–10 mo.

Age of permanent tooth eruption

7–8 yr.
8–9 yr.
11–12 yr.
10–11 yr.
10–12 yr.
6–7 yr.
12–13 yr.

11–13 yr.
6–7 yr.
11–12 yr.
10–12 yr.
9–10 yr.
7–8 yr.
6–7 yr.

FIG. 242-1. Normal eruptive patterns of the primary and permanent dentition.

ORAL AND DENTAL EMERGENCIES
Ronald W. Beaudreau

Oral emergencies generally can be divided into three categories: 1) orofacial pain, 2) orofacial trauma, specifically dentoalveolar trauma, and 3) hemorrhage. Early manifestations of many systemic illnesses are evident in the oral environment and may provide clues to the diagnosis of systemic illnesses. Oral lesions may cause pain or anxiety, and it is important that the emergency physician be familiar with common oral pathology and its management.

ORAL AND DENTAL ANATOMY

The normal adult dentition consists of 32 permanent teeth. The adult dentition has four types of teeth: 8 incisors, 4 canines, 8 premolars, and 12 molars. The primary or deciduous dentition consists of 20 teeth of three types: 8 incisors, 4 canines, and 8 molars. Figure 242-1 shows the eruptive pattern of both the primary and permanent dentition. Each tooth type is designed for a specific function in the process of mastication. Incisors are used for biting and cutting, canines and premolars for ripping, and molars for grinding. Figure 242-2 illustrates one commonly used tooth numbering system; however, description by the emergency physician of the tooth type and location is appropriate. Mastication is an important initial step in the digestive process and thus nutrition. The dentition is also important in the development of the mandible and maxilla and aesthetic development of the midface.

Anatomy of the Teeth

Table 242-1 lists commonly used dental nomenclature. A tooth consists largely of *dentin,* which surrounds the *pulp,* or neurovascular supply of the tooth (Figure 242-3). Dentin is a homogeneous material produced by pulpal odontoblasts throughout life. It is deposited as a system of microtubules filled with odontoblastic processes and extracellular fluid. The *crown,* or the visible portion of tooth, consists of a thick *enamel* layer overlying the dentin. Enamel, the hardest substance in the human body, consists largely of hydroxyapatite and is produced by ameloblasts prior to eruption of the tooth into the mouth. The *root* portion of the tooth extends into the alveolar bone and is covered with a thin layer of *cementum.*

The Normal Periodontium

The periodontium, or attachment apparatus, is essential for maintaining the integrity of the dentoalveolar unit. The attachment apparatus consists of a gingival component and a periodontal component. The gingival component includes the junctional epithelium, gingival tissue, and gingival fibers. The periodontal component includes the periodontal ligament, alveolar bone, and cementum of the root of the tooth. The periodontal ligament consists of collagen fibers that extend from the alveolar bone to the root of the tooth, adhering to the cementum via a hemidesmosomal attachment. The latter component forms the majority of the attachment apparatus, and the former aids primarily in maintaining the integrity of the periodontal ligament. Disease states such as gingivitis and periodontal disease weaken and destroy the attachment apparatus, resulting in tooth mobility and tooth loss.[1]

Gingival tissue is keratinized stratified squamous epithelium. It can be divided into the free gingival margin and the attached gingiva. The free gingiva is the portion that forms the 2- to 3-mm-deep *gingival sulcus* in the disease-free state. The attached gingiva adheres firmly to the underlying alveolar bone. The nonkeratinized alveolar mucosa extends from the attached gingiva to the vestibule and floor of the mouth. The mucosal tissue of the cheeks, lips, and floor of the mouth is also comprised of nonkeratinized squamous epithelium.[1]

OROFACIAL PAIN

Pain of Odontogenic Origin

TOOTH ERUPTION   Discomfort is commonly associated with the eruption of primary or deciduous teeth in infants. Irritability, drooling, and decreased intake are commonly associated findings. An associated low-grade fever (37.9°C/100.2°F) and diarrhea are more controversial findings. No scientific data support an association of teething, fever, and diarrhea. One must be careful in attributing either to tooth eruption. Other sources for fever must be carefully sought.[2] Table 242-2 lists common causes of orofacial pain.

As with the primary dentition, eruption of permanent teeth, especially third molars, or *wisdom teeth,* may result in significant pain. Gingival irritation and inflammation associated with tooth eruption

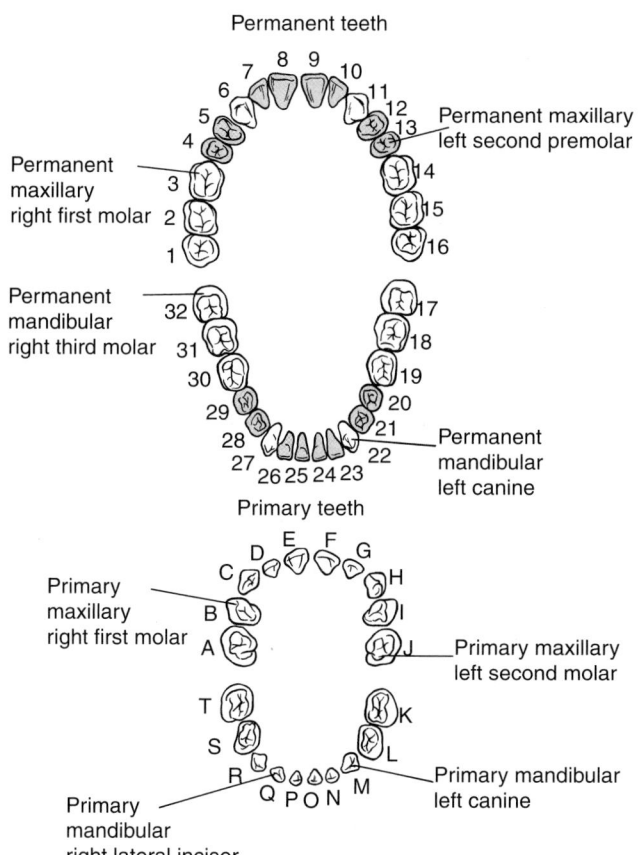

FIG. 242-2. Identification of teeth.

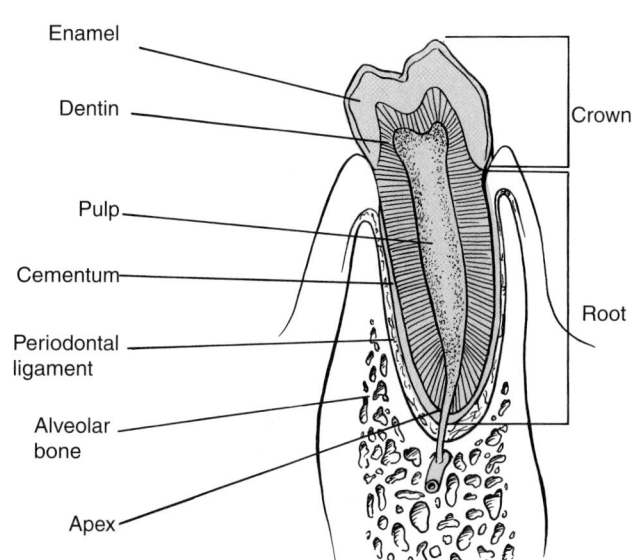

FIG. 242-3. The dental anatomic unit and attachment apparatus.

rinses, and analgesic therapy with nonsteroidal anti-inflammatory drugs (NSAIDs) and opiate preparations as appropriate. Referral to a general dentist or an oral and maxillofacial surgeon within 24 to 48 h is essential. If pericoronitis is related to trauma from an opposing tooth during mastication, as is frequently the case with third molars, concomitant extraction of the opposing tooth and antibiotic therapy will bring marked relief within 24 h. Definitive treatment is extraction of the associated tooth by a general dentist or oral and maxillofacial surgeon.

are common and must be distinguished from *pericoronitis.* Pericoronitis is inflammation of the *operculum,* or the gingival tissue overlying the occlusal surface of an erupting tooth. Impaction of food and debris beneath the operculum results in a severe inflammatory response. Without intervention this progressive inflammatory process will result in frank infection. Because of the close proximity of the masticator space (comprised of the masseteric space, pterygomandibular space, and the superficial and deep temporalis space) to third molars, associated trismus is common and portends the potential for extension into the communicating parapharyngeal spaces. Treatment consists of appropriate antibiotic therapy with penicillin VK 500 mg PO qid, erythromycin 250 mg PO qid, or clindamycin 300 mg PO qid, local irrigation of food and debris from underneath the operculum, saline mouth

TABLE 242-1   Commonly Used Dental Terminology

Anatomically descriptive terms for tooth surfaces

Interproximal	The surface between two adjacent teeth
Mesial	The interproximal surface facing anteriorly or toward the midline
Distal	The interproximal surface facing posteriorly or away from the midline
Occlusal	The chewing surface
Facial	Toward the face, a general term applicable to all teeth
Labial	Toward the lips, specific to the anterior teeth
Buccal	Toward the cheek, specific to the posterior teeth
Palatal	Toward the palate, specific to the maxillary teeth
Lingual	Toward the tongue, specific to the mandibular teeth
Apical	Toward the tip of the root of the tooth
Radicular	Associated with the root, especially the apical region
Coronal	Associated with the crown of the tooth
Incisal	Toward the biting edge of incisors
Cervical	Related to the junction of the crown and root of the tooth

TABLE 242-2   Differential Diagnosis of Orofacial Pain

Odontogenic origin	
Dental caries	Pericoronitis
Reversible pulpitis	Postrestorative pain
Irreversible pulpitis	Postextraction discomfort
Pulpal necrosis and abscess	Postextraction alveolar osteitis
Dentinal sensitivity	Bruxism
Tooth eruption	Cervical erosion
Periodontal pathology	
Gingivitis	Periodontal abscess
Periodontal disease	Acute necrotizing gingivostomatitis
Orofacial trauma	
Dental fractures	Facial fractures
Subtle enamel cracks	Alveolar ridge fractures
Ellis fractures	Soft tissue lacerations
Dental luxation and avulsion	Traumatic ulcers
Infection	
Oral candidiasis	Hand, foot, and mouth disease
Herpes simplex types 1 and 2	Sexually transmitted diseases
Varicella-zoster, primary	Mycobacterial infections
and secondary	Mumps
Herpangina	
Malignancies	
Squamous cell carcinoma	Leukemia
Kaposi sarcoma	Graft-versus-host disease
Lymphoma	Melanoma
Other etiologies	
Cranial neuralgias	Vesiculoulcerative disease
Stomatitis and mucositis	Lichen planus
Uremia	Cicatricial pemphigoid
Vitamin deficiency	Pemphigus vulgaris
Other	Erythema multiforme
Erythema migrans	Crohn disease
Pyogenic granuloma	Behçet syndrome

DENTAL CARIES AND PULPAL PATHOLOGY   *Dental caries* represents the loss of integrity of the tooth enamel secondary to dissolution of hydroxyapatite from prolonged exposure to the acidic metabolic by-products of plaque bacteria. Caries most commonly occurs in areas where plaque accumulates such as pits and fissures of the occlusal surface, interproximally, and along the gingival margins. When a sufficient breach of enamel integrity has occurred, sensitivity to cold or sweet stimulus may result. With dentinal involvement, carious progression occurs more rapidly, spreading along dentinal microtubules. At this stage, direct communication between the oral environment and the vital dental pulp has been established, and inflammatory changes in the pulpal tissue are evident histologically.

The pulpal inflammatory process is initially reversible, but with continued stimuli, the pulp's ability to respond and repair is jeopardized. *Irreversible pulpitis* can be distinguished from *reversible pulpitis* by the duration of symptoms. Both require a stimulus to initiate a painful response; however, in reversible pulpitis, the duration of pain is short, lasting seconds, as compared with irreversible pulpitis, in which the pain may last for minutes to hours. The most common stimulus is thermal, although sweet or sour stimuli also can elicit a painful response. Spontaneous odontogenic pain most frequently represents pulpal death or necrosis. Pain elicited with heat stimulus is most commonly associated with pulpal necrosis. Determining a particular tooth's position in this continuum of disease is impractical for the emergency physician. Treatment focuses on providing adequate analgesia and referral to a general dentist. The definitive treatment for irreversible pulpitis and pulpal necrosis is root canal therapy or dental extraction.

PERIRADICULAR PATHOLOGY   The most common cause of severe odontogenic pain is periapical pathology. *Periapical granuloma,* more appropriately termed *periradicular periodontitis,* is the most common periapical lesion. This lesion is not a true granuloma but rather slowly expanding granulation tissue associated with the root apex. Most commonly, periradicular periodontitis is a result of pulpal inflammation or necrosis, but it can be associated with trauma. *Periapical* or *radicular cyst* and *periradicular abscess* are clinically and radiographically indistinguishable from periradicular periodontitis, yet histologically separate entities. A periapical cyst has an epithelial lining originating embryologically from the rest of Malassez, and a periradicular abscess merely represents the accumulation of associated inflammatory cell. All three lesions are only associated with teeth with severely inflamed or necrotic pulps and may cause significant pain. Radiographically, these periapical lesions appear as a slight widening of the periodontal ligament space, a thinning of the lamina dura, or a frank radiolucent area associated with the root apex on a periapical dental radiograph (Figure 242-4). Radiographic evaluation with a Panorex panoramic x-ray machine is rarely useful for identification of all but the most extensive periradicular lesions, but can be important in identifying other more significant painful osseous pathology.

Pain of dental origin may be diffuse in nature, presenting as a headache, sinus pain, eye pain, or jaw or neck pain, or may be localized to a single tooth. One must remember to consider myocardial infarction as an etiology of jaw pain. Identification of the offending tooth is best accomplished by eliciting pain with percussion of the suspected teeth with a dental mirror handle or similar metallic object. A small swelling of the gingiva with a draining fistula adjacent to the affected tooth is known as a *parulis,* and can help identify the involved tooth. Erosion of a periradicular abscess through the cortical bone and subperiosteal extension results in intraoral or facial swelling and fluctuance that, if possible should be incised and drained intraorally. The emergency physician should treat dental abscesses or other periapical lesions with oral antibiotics such as penicillin VK 500 mg PO qid, clindamycin 300 mg PO qid, or erythromycin 500 mg PO qid, and should provide adequate analgesia with an NSAID. Opioid analgesia

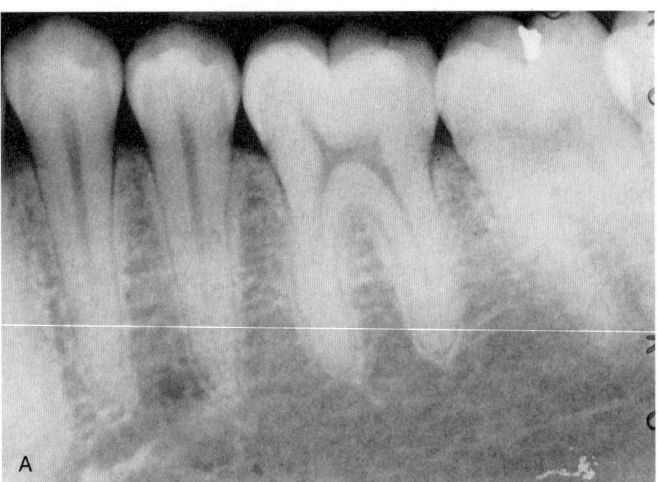

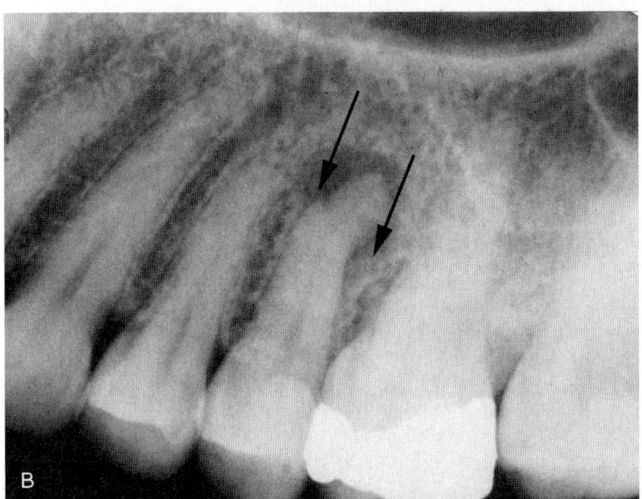

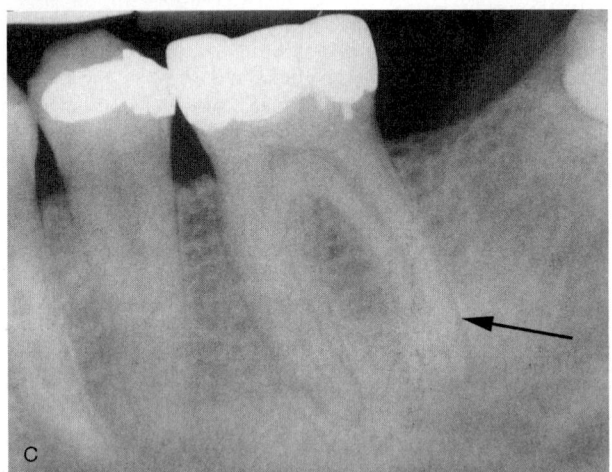

FIG. 242-4. A. The radiographic appearance of a healthy tooth with a normal periodontal ligament space and distinct lamina dura compared with the radiographic appearance of a periapical abscess, periradicular periodontitis, and periradicular cyst. **B.** A periapical radiolucency. **C.** Subtle radiographic loss of the periapical lamina dura and widening of the periodontal ligament space. (Courtesy of Gary M. Beaudreau, DMD.)

may be indicated in the first 24 to 48 h. Prompt referral to a dentist for definitive treatment such as root canal therapy or extraction is indicated.

FACIAL CELLULITIS   Spread of odontogenic infections into the various facial spaces is relatively common. Buccal extension of a periapical infection of the mandibular teeth will involve the buccinator space. Maxillary labial extension of infection primarily will involve the infraorbital space. Perforation through the lingual cortical bone of mandibular molars, particularly the second and third molars, usually occurs below the mylohyoid ridge and involves the submandibular space. Lingual spread of periapical infections associated with mandibular anterior teeth will affect the lingual space. The submandibular space and lingual space communicate with each other at the posterior border of the mylohyoid muscle.

Cellulitis of bilateral submandibular spaces and the lingual space is called *Ludwig angina* (see Chap. 243) and is potentially life-threatening. Clinically, Ludwig angina is a rapidly spreading cellulitis that results in brawny induration of the suprahyoid region and elevation of the tongue. Involvement of the floor of the mouth pushes the tongue posteriorly. As these spaces and the masticator spaces ultimately communicate with the parapharyngeal space, involvement of the epiglottis is not uncommon. As a result, airway compromise is the immediate primary concern. The primary focus of initial management is maintenance of a patent airway. Timely intravenous administration of high-dose penicillin and metronidazole or cefoxitin is essential. An aminoglycoside may be added to extend coverage, and in the penicillin-sensitive person, clindamycin may be substituted. Immediate oral and maxillofacial surgical consultation and hospitalization for incision and drainage and intubation as indicated are necessary.

Infection of the infraorbital space may have a potentially devastating outcome if retrograde spread via the ophthalmic veins occurs, and the cavernous sinus becomes involved. *Cavernous sinus thrombosis* presents as an infraorbital or periorbital cellulitis with rapidly developing meningeal signs, sepsis, and coma. Early recognition and treatment with a high-dose IV antibiotic as above are essential in decreasing morbidity and mortality.

POSTEXTRACTION ALVEOLAR OSTEITIS   Pain in the initial 24 to 48 h after dental extraction, termed *periosteitis*, is common and responds well to analgesics. Depending on the tooth removed, density of the bone, and amount of associated trauma that occurred during extraction, significant discomfort can occur. *Postextraction alveolar osteitis*, or *dry socket*, usually occurs on the second or third postoperative day and is associated with exquisite oral pain. Displacement of the clot from the socket or fibrinolytic dissolution of the clot results in exposure of the alveolar bone to the oral environment. This initiates an inflammatory response resulting in a localized osteomyelitis of the exposed bone. Risk factors for developing postextraction alveolar osteitis include smoking, preexisting pericoronitis or periodontal disease, a traumatic extraction, a prior history of alveolar osteitis, and hormone replacement therapy.[3]

The incidence of postextraction alveolar osteitis is 2 to 5 percent of all extractions but is considerably higher (20 to 35 percent) among impacted third molar extractions. Dental radiographs should be taken to ensure the absence of a retained root tip or other foreign body. Thorough irrigation of the dental socket with sterile normal saline and packing it with oil of cloves- or eugenol-impregnated gauze results in an almost immediate improvement in level of comfort. Dental anesthesia may be necessary to adequately irrigate and pack a dry socket. Antibiotic therapy is indicated in the most severe cases, and daily packing changes are important. Thus, referral to a dentist within 24 h is indicated.[3,4]

Managing postoperative dentoalveolar sequelae is in the realm of emergency medicine. Postoperative pain requiring analgesics, is a common presentation. Pain immediately postoperative is most commonly related to the trauma of surgery. Postoperative edema such as with extraction of third molars peaks within the first 24 to 48 h and is best managed with ice packs and elevation of the head of the bed to 30 degrees. Trismus, also common postoperatively, can result from infection, direct injury to the temporomandibular joint, injury to the muscles of mastication during administration of the inferior alveolar nerve block or during the surgery, and most commonly, normal perioperative inflammation. Trismus peaks in the first 24 h and usually decreases thereafter unless an infective process is the etiology. Postoperative trismus persisting for greater than 1 week will usually require stretching exercises prescribed by the oral and maxillofacial surgeon.[3,4]

POSTRESTORATIVE PAIN   Pain may occur after a dental restorative procedure. Normal trauma from mechanical instrumentation of the tooth or direct exposure of the pulpal tissue during instrumentation may result in pain. Pain associated primarily with mastication may be a result of improper occlusion of the new restoration. After endodontic therapy, patients may experience exquisite pain secondary to instrumentation or a buildup of gaseous pressure in the pulp chamber. Providing analgesia and referral to the patient's general dentist are the treatment of choice.

Periodontal Pathology

PERIODONTAL DISEASE   Gingival inflammation and bleeding, or *gingivitis,* results from the accumulation of plaque along the gingival margins. Hormonal variations of puberty, adolescence, and pregnancy, as well as many medications such as phenytoin, may exacerbate gingival inflammation. As the inflammatory process progresses, destruction of the periodontal attachment apparatus occurs, and the gingival sulcus deepens, resulting in periodontal pockets and *periodontitis.* Periodontal pockets create a favorable environment for plaque accumulation, maturation, and mineralization into *calculus.* Further destruction of the periodontal attachment results. Eventually, sufficient bone loss causes tooth mobility and tooth loss.[1,5]

The pathogenesis of periodontal disease is uncertain, but there is a very strong association between adult periodontitis and *Bacteroides gingivalis.* Many other specific bacteria have been shown to have a role in periodontitis. Destruction of tissue collagens, proteoglycans, and the connective tissue matrix is a major feature of gingivitis and periodontitis. Three theories for the etiology of this destruction have been proposed. Tissue destruction may occur as a result of the direct effects of bacterial plaque and their metabolic products, an accelerated host immune response, or immune deficiencies involving neutrophil function or the autologous mixed lymphocyte response.[1,5]

Four distinctive types of periodontal disease have been identified. These include adult, rapidly progressing, juvenile, and prepubertal periodontitis.[5] Etiology, age and gender predilection, and clinical course of disease vary by type. A definite association between juvenile periodontitis and *Actinobacillus actinomycetemcomitans* exists. More severe and rapidly progressing periodontitis, especially those types affecting a younger population such as the prepubertal and juvenile periodontitis, appears to be associated with decreased neutrophil chemotaxis or phagocytosis. Systemic illnesses such as human immunodeficiency virus (HIV) infection, diabetes, lazy leukocyte syndrome, Down syndrome, and cyclic neutropenia are associated with severe periodontal disease.[1]

Periodontal disease usually progresses painlessly but may present as gingival bleeding or tender, swollen gingival tissue. Treatment is directed at slowing or arresting the progression of disease primarily by the removal of plaque and its by-products.[1] Antibiotics may play a role in treatment. Referral to a dentist for definitive treatment is indicated because the treatment involves extensive dental cleaning, instruction and improvement in oral hygiene, and in some cases, periodontal surgery.

PERIODONTAL ABSCESS When plaque and debris are entrapped in the periodontal pocket, a periodontal abscess may form, resulting in severe pain. Small periodontal abscesses respond to local therapy with warm saline rinses and antibiotics such as penicillin VK 500 mg PO qid or erythromycin 250 mg PO qid. Larger periodontal abscesses require incision and drainage. Saline mouth rinses four times a day are useful. Analgesics are essential.

ACUTE NECROTIZING ULCERATIVE GINGIVITIS Acute necrotizing ulcerative gingivitis (ANUG) is an aggressively destructive process (Figure 242-5). Also known as *Vincent disease* or *trench mouth,* it is part of a spectrum of disease ranging from localized ulceration of the gingiva to often fatal noma, in which localized ulceration and necrosis spread to the adjacent tissues of the cheeks, lips, and underlying facial bones.[6,7] The diagnostic triad includes pain, ulcerated or "punched out" interdental papillae, and gingival bleeding. Secondary signs include fetid breath, pseudomembrane formation, "wooden teeth" feeling, foul metallic taste, tooth mobility, lymphadenopathy, fever, and malaise.[7,8]

The differential diagnosis for ANUG is quite extensive, but herpes gingivostomatitis is most difficult to differentiate. Herpes gingivostomatitis usually has smaller vesicular eruptions, less bleeding, more systemic signs, and lack of interdental papilla involvement.[7,8]

The etiology of ANUG is still poorly understood. It appears to be an opportunistic infection in a host with lowered resistance. It is believed that suppression of the humoral and cell-mediated immune response in HIV infection, severe malnourishment, and perhaps stress may be responsible for a lowered host resistance. Anaerobic bacteria such as *Treponema, Selenomonas, Fusobacterium,* and *Prevotella* are uniformly identified. These bacteria appear to invade otherwise healthy tissue, resulting in an aggressively destructive disease process.[7,8]

The most important predisposing factor is HIV infection. Previous necrotizing gingivitis infection is the second most important predisposing factor. Other contributing factors include poor oral hygiene, unusual emotional stress, poor diet, inadequate sleep, white heritage, age less than 21 years, poor socioeconomic status, recent illness, alcohol use, tobacco use, acatalasia, and various infections such as malaria, measles, and intestinal parasites.[7,8]

Treatment consists primarily of bacterial control. Chlorhexidine oral rinses bid, professional debridement and scaling, and adjunctive antibiotic therapy with metronidazole 250 mg PO tid are the mainstay of treatment. Reduction in pain can be expected within 24 h of institution of this regimen. Identification and resolution of the predisposing factors, and supportive therapy with a soft diet rich in protein, vitamins, and fluids are important in establishing and maintaining a disease-free state.[7]

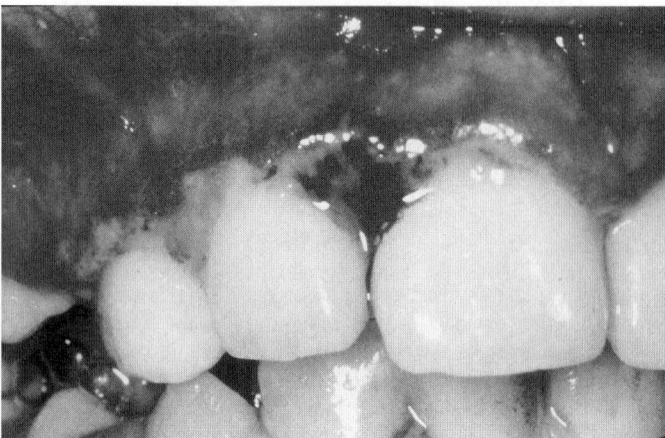

FIG. 242-5. Acute necrotizing ulcerative gingivitis. (Courtesy of Philip J. Hanes, DDS.)

Cranial Neuralgias

Trigeminal neuralgia is the most common of the cranial neuralgias. Others include postherpetic neuralgia, glossopharyngeal and vagal neuralgia, and superior laryngeal neuralgia. Trigeminal neuralgia is undoubtedly one of the most painful entities involving the face. Most commonly affecting adults 30 to 60 years of age, females constitute 60 percent of the patients. Trigeminal neuralgia is almost always unilateral, following the anatomic distribution of the involved cranial nerve. The maxillary branch of the fifth cranial nerve is most commonly affected. Recurrent episodes of excruciating, electric shock like paroxysmal pain of short duration, separated by pain-free periods are characteristic. Associated contraction of the facial and masticatory muscles is typical, resulting in the term *tic douloureux.* Physical stimulation of a trigger point is the usual inciting event.[9]

The pathogenesis of trigeminal neuralgia is still uncertain. Diagnosis is clinical, requiring the exclusion of organic pathology such as acoustic neuroma or a nasopharyngeal carcinoma. Thus referral to a neurologist is important.[9]

Trigeminal neuralgia may respond well to the administration of carbamazepine (100 mg PO bid initially and gradually increasing as needed to a maximum dose of 1200 mg daily). Surgery is reserved for patients who do not respond to medications.[9]

Nonparoxysmal pain of neuropathic origin may develop 1) in patients who have had long-standing neuralgias, 2) secondary to surgical trauma along the distribution of the affected nerve branch, and 3) in association with viral infections, drugs, or heavy metal intoxication. Other neuropathies such as alcoholic and diabetic sensory neuropathies also may affect the oral cavity.

SOFT TISSUE LESIONS OF THE ORAL CAVITY

Lesions of the oral mucosa are common and, when symptomatic or noticed by patients, may require identification and treatment by the emergency physician. Treatment depends on the appropriate diagnosis. Thus familiarization with common oral pathology is important.

Oral Candidiasis

Candidiasis commonly affects the oral cavity. Many healthy adults harbor candidal microorganisms. Many predisposing factors influence the development of oral candidiasis. These include the extremes of age, intraoral prosthetic devices such as dentures, malnourished states, associated mucosal disorders, concurrent infections, antibiotics, and immunocompromised conditions such as acquired immunodeficiency syndrome (AIDS), transplant recipients, radiation therapy, and chronic immunosuppressive therapy. Three oral clinical types have been described. The most common type is the pseudomembranous type, or thrush with white, curdlike plaques. These plaques can be easily scraped off to reveal an underlying erythematous mucosal base. The second type is atrophic or erythematous and usually involves the dorsum of the tongue. Atrophy of the filiform papillae is seen. Finally, the lesions of hyperplastic candidiasis are raised white plaques that can only be partially removed with scraping due to deeper infiltration into the underlying tissue. Perioral candidiasis, presenting as angular cheilitis or scaling patches of the perioral facial tissues is common. Treatment is with topical oral antifungal agents such as nystatin oral suspension 500,000 units qid or systemic agents such as fluconazole 100 to 200 mg PO per d.[6,10]

Aphthous Stomatitis

Aphthous stomatitis or ulceration is one of the most common oral lesions, affecting 20 percent of the normal population (Figure 242-6). Evidence suggests that the etiology appears to be a cell-mediated immune response to a yet unidentified triggering agent. Three etiologic

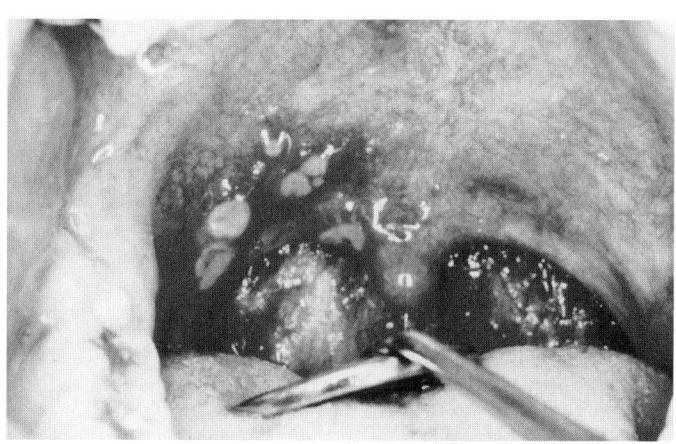

FIG. 242-6. Aphthous stomatitis. (Courtesy of Baldev Singh, BDS, PhD.)

factors are known to predispose aphthous ulcer formation: an immune imbalance, a breach in the mucosal barrier, and an allergic response. Aphthous ulceration involves the nonkeratinized epithelium, especially the labial and buccal mucosa, and begins as an erythematous macule that ulcerates and forms a central fibropurulent eschar. Lesions measure from 2 to 3 mm to several centimeters in diameter, are painful, and frequently are multiple. They usually resolve spontaneously in 10 to 14 days. Aphthous stomatitis occurs in a major and minor form. The major form has larger, deeper ulcers that take up to 6 weeks to heal. A third form, called *herpetiforme aphthae,* has up to 100 ulcers, each 1 to 2 mm in diameter, and takes 7 to 10 days to heal. Treatment consists of topical corticosteroids such as betamethasone syrup or 0.01 percent dexamethasone elixir as a mouth rinse. Fluocinonide 0.05% gel applied topically to isolated lesions is acceptable. Resolution typically occurs 2 days after therapy. Aphthous major is more resistant to therapy and may require intralesional steroid injection or systemic steroid therapy.[11]

Herpes Simplex

Herpes simplex type 1 most commonly affects the oral cavity. Herpes simplex type 2 can occur orally and is clinically indistinguishable. The primary infection, herpes gingivostomatitis, causes acute painful ulcerations on the gingiva and mucosal surfaces. Fever and lymphadenopathy are commonly associated findings and may occur up to 3 days prior to the appearance of oral lesions. Vesicular lesions appear and rupture after 1 to 2 days, leaving painful ulcers that heal gradually over 1 to 2 weeks. Secondary infection affects mostly the lips but may affect the hard palate and attached gingiva. The virus is harbored in sensory ganglion such as the gasserian ganglion of the trigeminal nerve. Periodic stresses activate the virus from its normally dormant state and results in recurrent lesions along the sensory distribution of the nerve. A prodrome of burning or tingling frequently occurs 1 to 2 days preceding outbreak of the characteristic vesicular lesion. Vesicles rupture within 2 to 3 days, forming small, shallow ulcers that heal in 6 to 10 days. Treatment is usually palliative; however, antiviral therapy with acyclovir 400 mg PO tid or valacyclovir 500 mg PO bid for 5 days initiated during the prodromal phase lessens the severity and duration of the ulceration.[6]

Varicella-Zoster

The varicella-zoster virus causes chickenpox (see Chap. 135) in its primary infection, resulting in the typical vesicular eruption. Vesicular involvement of the oropharynx is common and may precede skin involvement. Special care in maintaining adequate hydration is important when oral lesions are present.

Herpes zoster (see Chap. 143) occurs along the distribution of the trigeminal nerve 15 to 20 percent of the time. Typically beginning as a 1- to 4-day prodrome of exquisite pain in the area innervated by the affected nerve and may be mistaken for a simple headache or toothache. Vesicular eruptions characteristically occur unilaterally, not crossing the midline, and last 7 to 10 days. Isolated intraoral lesions can occur but are not common.

Involvement of the ophthalmic branch of the trigeminal nerve requires urgent ophthalmologic consultation.[6]

Herpangina

Herpangina is most commonly caused by coxsackievirus group A, types 1 to 6, 8, 10, and 22. Usually occurring in the summer and autumn, herpangina presents with a sudden onset of high fever, sore throat, headache, and malaise followed by eruption of oral vesicles 1 to 2 mm in size within 24 to 48 h. The vesicles quickly rupture, leaving numerous shallow, painful ulcers. The soft palate, uvula, posterior pharynx, and tonsillar pillars are usually affected, sparing the buccal mucosa, tongue, and gingiva. The disease lasts 7 to 10 days and can be distinguished from herpetic gingivostomatitis by the lack of gingival involvement.[6]

Hand, Foot, and Mouth Disease

Coxsackievirus type A16 and, occasionally, types A4, A5, A9, and A10 are associated with hand, foot, and mouth disease (see Chap. 135). This entity is characterized by the development of a few small vesicles on the tongue, gingiva, soft palate, and buccal mucosa. These vesicles rupture, resulting in painful, shallow ulcers with a surrounding red halo. The buttocks, palms, and plantar surfaces of the feet may be affected. Fever is usually of short duration, and the disease lasts 5 to 8 days. Treatment is supportive.[6]

Traumatic Lesions

Traumatic ulcers are a result of direct trauma to epithelial tissue. Common sources of trauma include rough or jagged edges on teeth or restorations, ill-fitting dentures, oral hygiene mishaps, and burns to the hard or soft palate secondary to hot foods. Removal of persistent sources of trauma is essential; otherwise, treatment is palliative.

A pyogenic granuloma is a common, benign proliferation of connective tissue in response to local trauma or irritation. It occurs primarily on the gingiva. Despite its name, this lesion is not a true granuloma but rather an accumulation of granulation tissue. A specific pyogenic granuloma occurring in pregnancy is referred to as a *pregnancy tumor* (Figure 242-7). This tumor is benign and usually recurs if removed during pregnancy. If the tumor does not regress 2 to 3 months postpartum, definitive removal is indicated.

Medication-Related Soft Tissue Abnormalities

Gingival hyperplasia is associated with many commonly used medications (Figure 242-8). Approximately 50 percent of patients on phenytoin will develop significant gingival hyperplasia. Many other medications, such as cyclosporine and calcium channel blockers, especially nifedipine, are known to cause gingival hyperplasia. Concomitant use of two such medications results in accelerated gingival proliferation. Enlargement begins in the interdental papillae. The clinical and histologic characteristics of gingival hyperplasia related to phenytoin, cyclosporine, and calcium channel blockers appear to be identical. The clinical appearance of the gingival tissue depends on oral hygiene and secondary inflammation. In the absence of inflammation, gingival proliferation results in dense tissue, normal in coloration, with a smooth, stippled, or granular texture. Inflammation causes edematous changes and an erythematous coloration. Inflamed

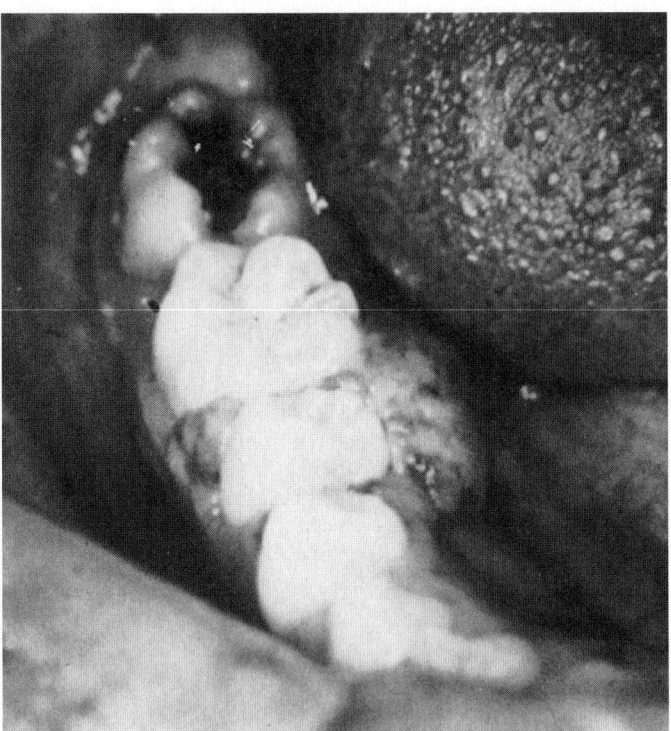

FIG. 242-7. Pyogenic granuloma.

tissue bleeds readily. Histologically, an increase in collagen fibers, in fibroblasts, and in glycosaminoglycans is seen. Epithelial acanthosis also occurs. Although the etiology of drug-related gingival hyperplasia remains unclear, poor oral hygiene clearly increases its likelihood and severity. Treatment includes fastidious oral hygiene to slow the hyperplasia and gingivectomy in advance cases.[12]

Many other medications are known to cause abnormalities of the oral mucosa or dental structures. Allergic mucositis, erythema multiforme, and fixed drug-type reactions are examples. Xerostomia and associated mucosal alterations are a side effect of many medications such as anticholinergics, antidepressants, and antihistamines.[1] Stomatitis or mucosal ulcerations secondary to the use of common chemotherapeutic agents is also common.

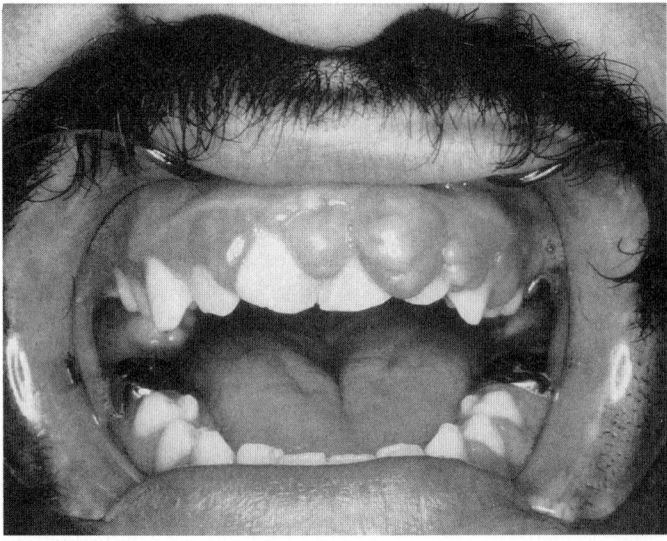

FIG. 242-8. Gingival hyperplasia secondary to cyclosporine. (Courtesy of Philip J. Hanes, DDS, MS.)

Sexually Transmitted Diseases

Many sexually transmitted diseases can affect the oral cavity. With oral–genital contact, the oral mucosa is as susceptible to the transmission of sexually transmitted diseases as the urogenital mucosa. Gonorrhea most commonly causes a pharyngitis involving the uvula and tonsils and may present with or without pustules or exudates. Oral herpes type 1 and type 2 infections are clinically indistinguishable. Human papillomavirus, associated with HPV-6, -11, and -45, is most commonly associated with *condyloma acuminatum,* or *venereal warts,* and can result in similar oral lesions.[6,13]

The primary chancre of syphilis can occur orally. Chancre of the lip is the most common oral site involved. Tongue involvement is next in frequency, followed closely by the tonsils. An oral chancre is similar in appearance to its genital counterpart. In secondary syphilis, oral lesions are common and frequently accompany cutaneous lesions. They are usually multiple, oval-shaped, slightly raised ulcers or erosions covered with a gray membrane. Condyloma lata rarely occur intraorally.[6,13]

Treatment of sexually transmitted diseases of the oral cavity is the same as for genital involvement. The diagnosis of oral sexually transmitted diseases requires maintaining an appropriate level of suspicion. Treatment of the sexual partner is essential to assure reinfection does not occur.

Lesions of the Tongue

Many systemic conditions and local stimuli affect the appearance of the tongue. Many systemic conditions, various vitamins deficiencies, and iron-deficiency anemia cause atrophy of the filiform papillae, resulting in a smooth erythematous appearance. Occurrence of ectopic thyroid tissue on the midline posterior portion of the tongue is called a *lingual thyroid* and is a common finding. Some common conditions affecting the tongue are discussed below.

ERYTHEMA MIGRANS   Erythema migrans, geographic tongue, or benign migratory glossitis is a common benign finding on oral examination, occurring in 1 to 3 percent of the population. Females are affected twice as often as males. The typically multiple, well-demarcated zones of erythema on the tongue are caused by atrophy of the filiform papillae. The lesions concentrate on the tip and lateral borders of the tongue and heal in several days, only to quickly reappear in other areas. These lesions usually are asymptomatic; however, a burning sensation or sensitivity to hot or spicy foods has been described. Etiology is yet unknown; however, fluctuations with stress and menstrual cycle occur. Generally, treatment is not indicated because this entity is benign. Reassurance of patients is usually sufficient. In patients in whom discomfort is a major factor, oral topical steroids such as fluocinonide gel applied several times daily may provide relief.[14]

MEDIAN RHOMBOID GLOSSITIS   Median rhomboid glossitis is believed to be a developmental defect of the dorsal surface of the tongue. It appears as a small 1- by 2-cm ovoid erythematous area just anterior to the circumvallate papillae. The area is devoid of papillae and usually asymptomatic. No treatment is necessary.

STRAWBERRY TONGUE   Strawberry tongue is associated with erythrogenic, toxin-producing *Streptococcus pyogenes.* Clinically, the tongue has prominent red spots on a white-coated background. Microscopically, the fungiform papillae are hyperemic with a smooth glossy surface. Treatment is with antibiotics directed at group A streptococci.

Leukoplakia and Erythroplakia

Leukoplakia is a white patch or plaque that cannot be scraped off and cannot be classified as any other disease. Leukoplakia is the most common oral precancer; however, only 2 to 4 percent of leukoplakic lesions show dysplastic changes. Etiology is unknown, but tobacco, alcohol, ultraviolet radiation, candidiasis, human papillomavirus, tertiary syphilis, and trauma have all been implicated. The most common intraoral site involved is the buccal mucosa. Other sites of involvement include the hard and soft palates, maxillary gingiva, and lip mucosa. Biopsy is mandatory for all persistent leukoplakic lesions. Leukoplakic lesions of the floor of the mouth, tongue, and vermilion border are most likely associated with malignancy. Lesions demonstrating dysplastic changes warrant removal.

Erythroplakia is defined as a red patch that similarly cannot be clinically or pathologically characterized as any other disease. Although erythroplakia is far less common than leukoplakia, it has a greater potential for dysplastic changes.

Oral Cancer

Oral cancer accounts for 2 to 4 percent of the cancers in the United States.[15] More than 90 percent of all oral malignancies are squamous cell carcinoma. Lymphomas, Kaposi sarcoma, and melanoma comprise most of the remainder. Several intrinsic and extrinsic etiologic factors for oral squamous cell carcinoma have been identified. Extrinsic factors include tobacco use, especially chewing tobacco or snuff; excessive alcohol consumption; and sunlight exposure (Figure 242-9). Intrinsic factors include general malnutrition and chronic iron-deficiency anemia. Specific etiologic factors play varying roles in oncogenesis. Oral candidiasis, especially the hyperplastic form, immunosuppressive states such as HIV infection, and oncogenic viruses such as human papillomavirus, herpes simplex virus, and various adenoviruses and retroviruses may play some role in the etiology of oral cancer.

Oral squamous cell carcinoma has four common morphologic presentations. It can be exophytic with an irregular surface, or ulcerative, with irregular depressions and rolled borders. Malignant leukoplakic and erythroplakic lesions are believed to represent squamous cell carcinomas that have yet to form a mass or ulcerate.

The most common site involved in oral cancer is the tongue, particularly the posterolateral border, accounting for approximately 50 percent of oral cancers in the United States. Cancer of the floor of the mouth accounts for nearly 35 percent. Cancer of the lips is common and usually secondary to sunlight exposure. Table 242-3 lists the common signs and symptoms of oral cancer; unfortunately, oral cancer is generally painless, and patients are often unaware of the presence of a mass until it is advanced.[16] Early diagnosis is the key to successful treatment of oral squamous cell carcinoma. All ulcers, erythroplakic lesions, and leukoplakic lesions of the oral cavity that do not respond to palliative treatment in 10 to 14 days warrant biopsy.

Treatment depends on site of involvement and staging of disease. It consists primarily of wide radical excision, radiation therapy, or a combination of the two. Adjunctive chemotherapy has been used to aid in tumor debulking. The prognosis depends on site and tumor stage, but an overall 5-year survival rate for patients with lesions that have not metastasized is 76 percent; overall 5-year survival is 41 percent when cervical nodes are involved, and 9 percent when metastasis below the clavicle has occurred.

Other

Fordyce granules, commonly occurring on the vermillion border of the lips and buccal mucosa, are slightly elevated, cream-colored spots that represent ectopic sebaceous glands. *Linea alba* is a white line on the buccal mucosa at the level of the occlusal surface. It is caused by normal friction from the facial surfaces of the teeth during mastication. Firm exophytic enlargements along the lingual surface of the mandible *(torus mandibularis)* or the maxillary hard palate *(torus palatinus)* are benign exostoses. The etiology is unknown, but no therapeutic intervention is re-

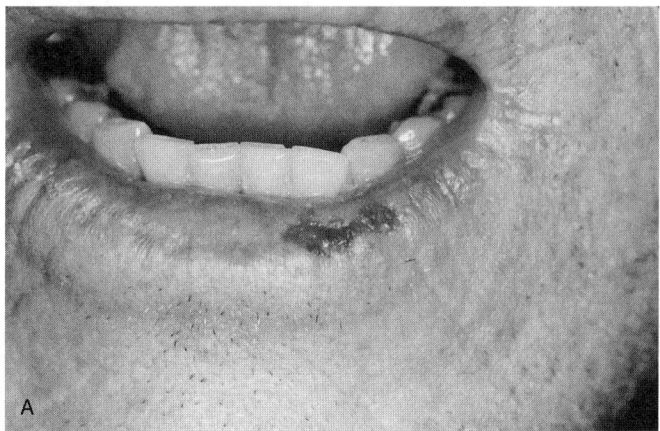

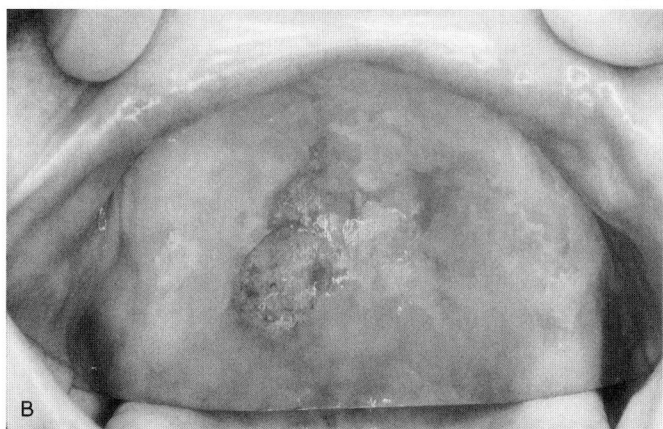

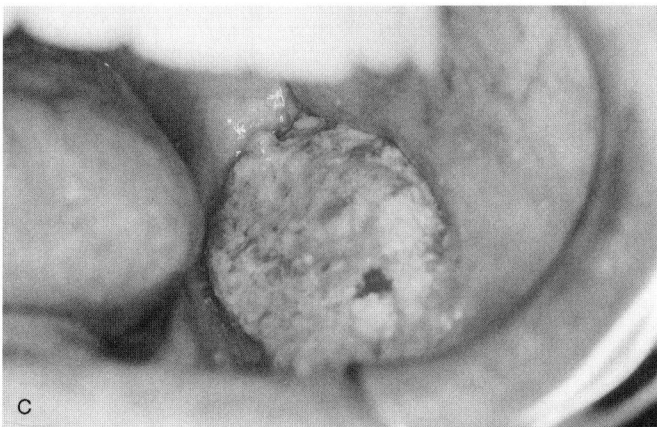

FIG. 242-9. Oral squamous cell carcinoma. **A.** Squamous cell carcinoma of the lip secondary to sun exposure. **B.** Squamous cell carcinoma of the hard palate. **C.** Verrucous carcinoma secondary to dipping snuff. (Courtesy of H. Anthony Neil, DDS.)

quired. Many other disease entities such as pemphigoid, pemphigus, lichen planus, and erythema multiforme affect the oral soft tissues.

OROFACIAL TRAUMA

Dentoalveolar Trauma

The most common dentoalveolar mechanism of injury is falls. Sporting injuries, fights, and motor vehicle collisions account for most of the remainder. Injury to the maxillary central incisors accounts for 70 percent of dental injuries. Management of dentoalveolar trauma

TABLE 242-3   Signs and Symptoms of Oral Cancer

Signs
   Nonhealing ulcer: can be in form of crater with elevated,
      indurated margins
   Bleeding: resulting from ulcerations
   Lymphadenopathy
   Rigidity: lesions fixed to surrounding tissue
   Induration: hardness of the lesion
   Functional interference: such as speech and mastication
Symptoms
   Pain
      Secondary to ulceration
      Secondary to trauma related to functional interferences
   Parathesias
   Drooling: secondary to functional interferences

Source: Reproduced with permission from Marder MZ: The standard of care for oral diagnosis as it relates to oral cancer. *Compend Contin Educ Dent* 19:569, 1998.

depends on the extent of tooth and alveolar involvement, the degree of development of the apex of the tooth, and the age of the patient. In injuries in younger patients, especially those who are younger than 12 years of age, the pulp of anterior teeth is quite large and dental fractures involving the pulp are common. Fortunately, in this age group the apex of the root also is usually incompletely formed, allowing for a greater pulpal regenerative capability. As one ages, more dentin is formed. Thus, in older patients, the pulp chamber may be very small and pulpal exposure highly unlikely. Involvement of the root of the tooth compromises the attachment apparatus and thus the ability of a dentist to adequately restore the tooth to function.

DENTAL FRACTURES   A simple classification of dental fractures is the Ellis classification, which is shown in Figure 242-10. The goal of the emergency treatment of a fractured tooth is maintaining pulpal vitality. The proximity of the fracture to the pulp and the length of time before treatment are most important in determining outcome. Treatment is aimed at sealing the dentinal tubules and creating a barrier between the dental pulp and the oral environment. In properly treated uncomplicated dental fractures, 1 to 2 percent of the affected pulps undergo necrosis. Because pulpal necrosis is a process, it can occur at any time after trauma, and serial follow-up with a dentist is recommended.[17,18]

Ellis class I fractures involve the enamel portion of the tooth only. Generally, no emergent treatment of these fractures is indicated, except

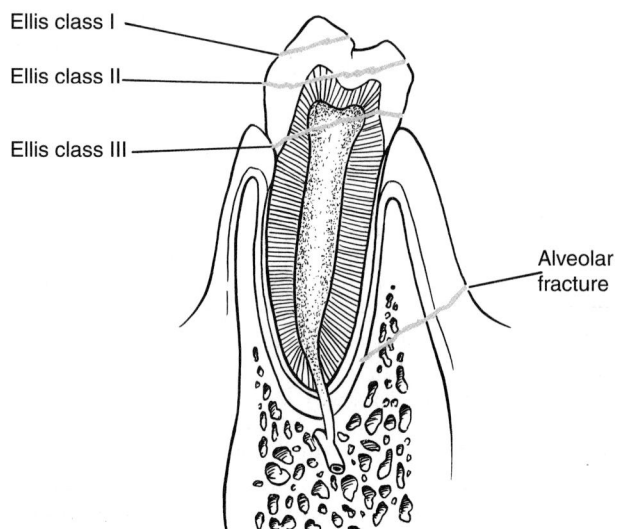

Ellis class I
Ellis class II
Ellis class III
Alveolar fracture

FIG. 242-10. Ellis classification for fractures of anterior teeth.

to smooth sharp corners that may irritate the tongue or mucosa. Referral to a general dentist for aesthetic repair depends on the degree of cosmetic concern of the patient.[17,18]

Ellis class II fractures involve the dentin of the tooth and require intervention. These fractures account for 70 percent of tooth fractures. Generally, patients express sensitivity to hot or cold stimuli as well as air passing over the expose surface during breathing. The Ellis class II fracture can be identified both by the patient's symptoms and visualization of exposed dentin, which is a creamy yellow color compared with the whiter enamel. Because dentin is microtubular in structure, communication between the oral environment and the dental pulp is established with exposure of the dentin. The thickness of remaining dentin determines the rate of pulpal contamination. Greater than 2 mm of remaining dentin is felt to offer some protection to the pulpal tissue. Microorganism contamination of the pulp, oral irritants, or desiccation from mouth breathing initiates an inflammatory process in the pulpal tissue. A delay in treatment increases the likelihood of pulpal necrosis. Thus it is the responsibility of the emergency physician not only to identify such a fracture but also to cover the exposed dentin to decrease pulpal contamination. This is best achieved using a glass ionomer dental cement that is easily mixed according to the manufacturer's instructions and carefully applied to the dried exposed dentin. Referral to a dentist within 24 h is mandatory to best ensure tooth vitality.[17,18]

In Ellis class III fractures, exposure of the pulp has occurred. On wiping the fractured surface dry with sterile gauze, blood originating from the pulp of the tooth is easily identified. One should attempt to cover the exposed dentin with a glass ionomer cement or calcium hydroxide base as in class II fractures until urgent dental evaluation can occur. If the pulpal exposure is extremely small, placing a glass ionomer or calcium hydroxide base is adequate until dental evaluation within 24 h. Prompt appropriate treatment lessens the likelihood of pulpal necrosis by minimizing pulpal contamination. For all but the smallest pulpal exposures, definitive treatment is endodontic or root canal therapy. Oral analgesics should be prescribed and topical analgesics avoided.[17,18]

Root fractures account for 5 percent of all injuries of the permanent dentition. Extraction of the coronal segment is required. If less than one-third of the root is involved, a dentist can perform root canal therapy, and restoration of the tooth may be possible. Careful attention must be paid to identifying fractures of the root because they can be clinically obscure.[18]

CONCUSSIONS, LUXATIONS, AND AVULSIONS   The same forces that cause dental fractures may result in loosening of a tooth from the attachment apparatus. Careful evaluation of the teeth for tenderness, malpositioning, or mobility must be performed. Luxations account for nearly 50 percent of injuries to teeth. Five distinct types of luxations have been described. 1) *Concussion* injuries are defined as injury to the supporting structures of a tooth with clinical tenderness to percussion but no mobility. 2) *Subluxation* is defined as an injury to the attachment apparatus resulting in mobility without clinical or radiographic evidence of dislodgment of the tooth. 3) *Extrusive luxation* is defined as partial avulsion or dislodgment of a tooth from the alveolar bone. 4) *Lateral luxation* is defined as displacement of a tooth laterally with concomitant fracture of the alveolar bone. 5) *Intrusive luxation* is defined as displacement of a tooth into its socket with associated alveolar fracture. Treatment of luxations depends on the tooth involved, the severity of injury, and the presence of associated root fracture and/or significant associated alveolar fracture.[17]

A concussive injury to a tooth represents a minor injury. The degree of tenderness to percussion determines the treatment. Stabilizing the tooth by splinting it to adjacent teeth is not indicated. Management of pain with NSAIDs, soft diet, and referral to a dentist to confirm the diagnosis and exclude more severe injury, are the most appropriate courses of action for the emergency physician. Removal of the occlusal forces from the tooth by a dentist may aid in comfort and healing. Similarly, a subluxed tooth generally does not require splinting. Again, removal from occlusion by a general dentist may be beneficial. Subluxation represents a more significant injury and is associated with a higher incidence of subsequent pulpal necrosis.

An extrusive luxation requires repositioning the tooth in its original position and splinting to stabilize the tooth during healing. Repositioning the tooth may require local anesthesia. Firm, gentle pressure usually will reposition the tooth. If a clot has formed apical to the tooth, then more aggressive manipulation may be required. A flexible wire splint placed by a dentist provides ideal stabilization. In the ED, a temporary splint with Coe-Pak periodontal dressing (Figure 242-11), as described by Medford,[19] is acceptable until the patient can see a dentist or oral and maxillofacial surgeon within 24 h. Care must be taken to avoid excess material placement, especially on the occlusal surface, because interference in occlusion will place stresses on the tooth during mastication. Splinting should be maintained for 1 to 2 weeks. Close follow-up by a dentist is necessary.

A lateral luxation represents a more extensive injury and is associated with crazing or fracture of the surrounding alveolar bone. Repositioning of the tooth is generally more difficult. It usually can be accomplished by manipulating the displaced tooth with the thumb and forefinger. Once the apex has been dislodged from its locked-in position labially, apically directed axial pressure will reposition the tooth. Intraarch stabilization is necessary for a minimum of 2 weeks. Temporary splinting with Coe-Pak periodontal dressing is acceptable if a minimal associated alveolar fractured occurred. Otherwise, splinting by an oral and maxillofacial surgeon or general dentist in the ED is mandatory.

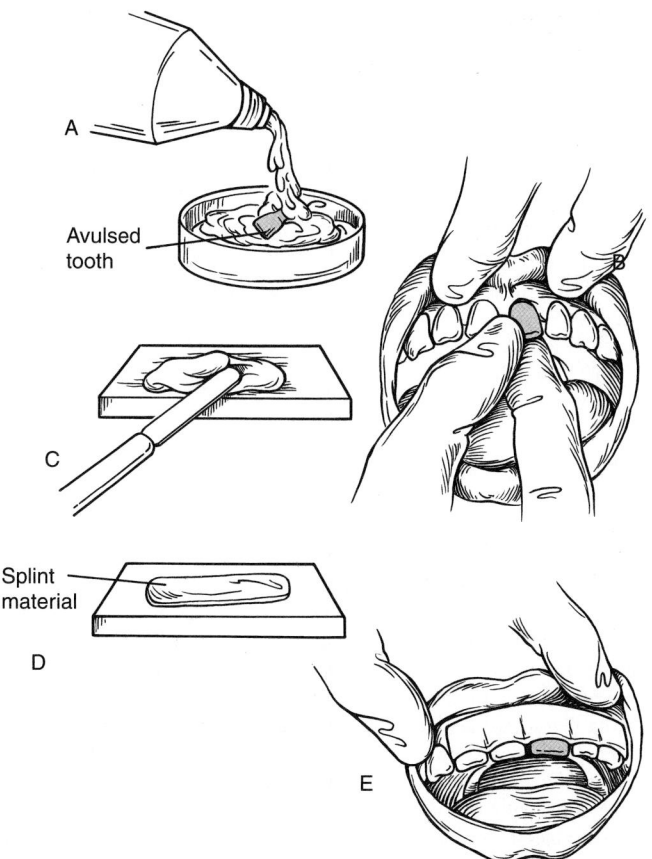

FIG. 242-11. Reimplantation and stabilization of an avulsed tooth. **A.** Tooth is rinsed. **B.** Tooth is placed back into socket. **C.** Splint material is ready for application. **D.** Packing is molded over reimplanted tooth and two adjacent teeth to each side.

Intrusive luxations are the most serious because significant damage to the alveolar socket and periodontal ligament occurs. Root resorption is common as a result of damage to the periodontal ligament. Recommended treatment is allowing the tooth to erupt on its own or to orthodontically extrude the tooth over 3 to 4 weeks.

Total displacement of a tooth from its socket, or *avulsion,* accounts for up to 16 percent of all injuries to teeth. It is necessary to reimplant avulsed permanent teeth as soon as possible. Reimplantation is possible if performed within 2 to 3 h. To minimize this time, ideally, the patient or health care provider at the scene should reimplant the tooth. The tooth should be rinsed with sterile normal saline or tap water to remove debris. Care should be taken to handle only the crown portion of the tooth, and it should be reimplanted immediately into the socket. If this is not possible, or if the risk of aspiration is high, such as in a child or a patient with a decreased level of consciousness, then the tooth should be transported with the patient to the ED. Acceptable transport media include isotonic solutions such as Hank solution, sterile saline, and milk. Commercial preparations of Hank solution such as Save-A-Tooth (TPS, Biologic Rescue Products, Inc.) are available and come with a useful transport container as part of the system. If the avulsed tooth was not recovered, radiographs to ensure that the tooth was not aspirated are indicated.[20–22]

Survival of the periodontal ligament fibers that remain attached to the root of an avulsed tooth is key to successful reimplantation. Milk is an acceptable storage medium because of its osmolarity and essential concentration of calcium and magnesium ions. Hank solution, a pH-balanced cell culture medium, is the best transport medium and has been found to maintain periodontal ligament cell viability for up to 4 to 6 h. It also has been found that Hank solution can help to restore cell viability in a tooth that has been avulsed longer than 20 and 60 min.[21,22]

In the ED, prior to reimplantation, the tooth should be thoroughly rinsed clean of dirt and debris with sterile saline or preferably Hank solution. The root of the tooth should not be scrubbed, and care should be taken not to disrupt existing periodontal fibers. If an avulsed tooth with an open apex has been dry for less than 20 min, then the prognosis for reestablishing a vital pulp is good. If the apex is completely closed, then revitalization is not possible. If the tooth has been dry from 20 to 60 min regardless of apices, it is recommended that the tooth be soaked in Hank balanced salt solution for 30 min. This has been found to decrease the chance of ankylosis. For an avulsed tooth that has been dry for greater than 60 min, the periodontal cells are dead, and the goal is to reduce root resorption. It is recommended that the tooth be soaked in citric acid for 5 min, then 2 percent stannous fluoride, and finally doxycycline for 5 min prior to reimplantation.[20]

Preparation of the dental socket plays little role in the success or failure of the reimplanted tooth. The socket is prepared by carefully removing the clot and irrigating gently with sterile normal saline. As little manipulation as possible of the socket should occur. Local anesthesia is usually required. Reimplantation is accomplished with firm pressure and having the patient bite on gauze until more permanent stabilization can be arranged. Anterior teeth are most commonly affected, and Figure 242-12 illustrates the morphology of the maxillary central incisor to assist reimplantation in the proper orientation. Early improper reimplantation holds a higher success rate for tooth salvage than delayed reimplantation resulting from waiting for an oral and maxillofacial surgeon. Stabilization by an oral and maxillofacial surgeon or using a temporary method such as Coe-Pak periodontal dressing is necessary.[20–22]

Avulsion or luxation of primary teeth is treated differently from that of permanent teeth. Thus identification of primary teeth in patients aged 6 to 12 years when the dentition is mixed is essential. Avulsed primary teeth are never reimplanted. More severe luxations in primary teeth generally require extraction of the tooth. Repositioning or reimplanting primary teeth risks injuring the underlying permanent teeth and thus is avoided. Intruded primary teeth are an exception and

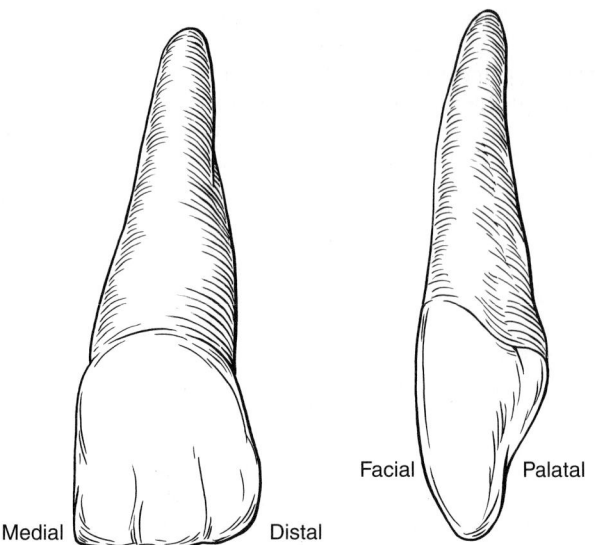

FIG. 242-12. Illustration of a maxillary left central incisor. Note that the part of the tooth facing medially comes to more of a right angle at the incisal edge than occurs distally. The facial portion of the tooth is more convex.

generally are left alone to reerupt into normal position. Referral to a general dentist for follow-up is essential to ensure optimal long-term outcome.[17,20]

Posttraumatic sequelae are variable. Pulp canal obliteration, pulpal necrosis, internal external resorption of the root, and ankylosis may occur. The severity of luxation or avulsion is the most important determining factor in sequela occurrence. Transient apical breakdown occurs with all type of luxations but is especially common with extrusive and lateral luxations. More than 50 percent of extrusively luxated teeth undergo pulpal necrosis within 1.5 years of the traumatic event. Close dental follow-up is essential for early identification of these sequelae.

Significant force must occur to dislodge or fracture teeth; consequently, associated alveolar ridge fracture is common. Care to ensure the integrity of the maxilla and mandible is also important. Stabilization of repositioned or reimplanted teeth is essential for optimal results. This is best accomplished with semi rigid fixation placed by a general dentist or oral surgeon. Stabilization is maintained for 1 to 2 weeks depending on the involvement of alveolar bone. With significant alveolar ridge fracture, segments may require intermaxillary stabilization for up to 6 weeks in order to ensure adequate healing.[17,20]

Soft Tissue Trauma

Traumatic injuries to the soft tissue of the oral cavity are common. Oral lacerations can involve any of the soft tissues of the mouth. Large intraoral lacerations (>1 cm) are susceptible to ulceration and secondary infection and tend to heal in a fibrotic mass. Intraoral lacerations should be inspected carefully for foreign material, including tooth fragments, and irrigated well with sterile NS. Retained foreign bodies serve as a nidus for infection and can result in need for later surgical removal and poor aesthetic outcome. Crushed and nonviable tissue should be debrided. Close approximation of the wound edges rather than a tissue seal is desired to allow drainage. Resorbable suture material such as 4-0 chromic is generally used. Black silk (4-0) is easier to use but requires removal in 7 to 10 days. When resorbable sutures are used, care should be taken to place the sutures so that the knots are buried. Prophylactic antibiotics generally are not indicated except with the most extensive lacerations. Forty-eight-hour follow-up is necessary to monitor healing.

Lacerations of the lips and tongue require special consideration. Care should be taken in wound-edge approximation of lacerations on the dorsum of the tongue because reepithelialization across the wound edge is important. If the edges are not well approximated, the epithelia will migrate downward and will result in an epithelial cleft and a bifid appearance. This is both a cosmetic and a functional problem requiring revision. Small tongue lacerations in children, where the edges remain approximated, do not need to be sutured. Bleeding can be controlled with pressure using gauzes. Extensive tongue lacerations in children require procedural sedation and may be best referred for repair.

Lip lacerations are a potential cosmetic problem, so careful closure is essential. In lacerations involving the vermilion border, alignment of the border is important and should be completed first. The portion of the laceration extraoral to the wet–dry line of the lip and involving the skin of the face should be closed with 6-0 nylon monofilament. The intraoral portion of the laceration is repaired in the same manner as any oral laceration. Because of the musculature of the lips, any deep laceration requires closure of the deep layers using a 4-0 resorbable suture material to decrease the likelihood of the wound edges opening on removal of the suture. As with any laceration involving the face or other aesthetic areas, sutures should be removed as early as possible, generally in 5 days, so as to decrease iatrogenic scarring from the suture material. Careful daily cleansing of the wound and application of a triple-antibiotic ointment makes suture removal easier and improves the aesthetic results.

Controversy concerning closure of through-and-through lip laceration exists. Some advocate leaving the intraoral portion of the laceration open; however, it is my recommendation that mucosal lacerations larger than 1 cm be repaired. Generally, the intraoral component should be repaired first, and then, from an extraoral approach, the laceration should be cleansed and irrigated aggressively. A deep layer of sutures may be necessary in large lacerations. The skin then should be closed aesthetically. Prophylactic antibiotics such as penicillin VK or erythromycin 250 mg PO qid for about 5 days are indicated.

Laceration of the maxillary labial frenulum, unless unusually large, does not require repair. These lacerations can be very painful, so adequate analgesia must be prescribed. Because of the vascularity of adjacent tissue, lacerations to the lingual frenulum usually do need to be repaired. Resorbable suture such as 4-0 chromic is appropriate.

Other soft tissue injuries commonly occur. Intraoral contusions and ecchymoses are prevalent with facial trauma. Ecchymoses and petechial hemorrhages to the soft palate, uvula, and pharynx from direct or indirect trauma are common. Treatment is mainly palliative, with reassurance to the patient and NSAIDs for discomfort.

HEMORRHAGE

Spontaneous Hemorrhage

Spontaneous gingival hemorrhage is not uncommon. A history of recent dental therapy such as periodontal scaling or curettage is important because resulting hemorrhage after scaling is easily controlled with peroxide mouth rinses or direct gingival pressure A careful medical history must be obtained in order to eliminate systemic diseases such as clotting factor deficiencies, leukemia, and end-stage liver disease as the etiology. Excessive anticoagulation may present as spontaneous gingival bleeding. The need for laboratory evaluation depends on a careful history and physical examination. Treatment depends on the specific cause of bleeding in the event that local measures are unsuccessful.

Postoperative Bleeding

Postextraction bleeding is not uncommon. Displacement of the clot may result in recurrent or continued bleeding. Generally, firm pressure applied to the extraction site is adequate to control bleeding. This is best accomplished by neatly folding a 2- × 2-in. gauze pad and placing it over the extraction site, applying firm pressure by clenching firmly with the opposing teeth. This pressure must be held firmly, not a chewing action, for 20 min or until hemostasis is complete. If direct pressure is not successful, then application of Gelfoam, Avitene, or Surgicel into the socket may provide a matrix for clot formation. Sutures should be used for holding such agents in place or to close the gingiva over the socket. The gingiva should not be closed under pressure, especially along the suture line, since this may result in necrosis of the gingival flap. If these methods are unsuccessful, then oral and maxillofacial surgical consultation becomes necessary.

ORAL MANIFESTATIONS OF SYSTEMIC DISEASES

Many diseases have common oral manifestations. In some cases, oral findings may be among the first signs and symptoms of disease. Diseases with oral manifestations are so wide-ranging that only a few of the more important entities will be discussed.

Leukemia

Common oral findings in leukemia include spontaneous gingival hemorrhaging and small petechial hemorrhages or bruising of the oral soft tissue secondary to thrombocytopenia. Leukemic patients are more prone to oral candidiasis, herpetic infections, and neutropenic ulceration. These ulcers are typically deep, punched-out lesions with a gray-white necrotic base. They occur most commonly after chemotherapeutics, related to mucosal trauma or opportunistic infections. Acute leukemias, particularly acute monocytic and myelogenous subtypes, cause infiltration of leukemic cells into oral soft tissue, especially gingival tissue, resulting in swollen, boggy hyperplastic gingivitis. Gingival lesions can be a result of direct infiltration, as shown in Figure 242-13, or a result of drug toxicity, from graft-versus-host disease, or secondary to marrow or lymphoid tissue depression.[23]

Acquired Immunodeficiency Syndrome

There are numerous oral manifestations of HIV infection. Primary HIV infection, occurring from 1 to 6 weeks after contact, is an acute viral syndrome but may have associated intraoral findings such as a sore throat, mucosal erythema, and focal ulceration. Persistent generalized lymphadenopathy, particularly of the cervical lymph nodes, is present in 70 percent of otherwise asymptomatic HIV-infected patients. The presentation of AIDS is highly variable, and numerous oral manifestations can occur. Oropharyngeal candidiasis is the most common oral finding and may lead to the initial diagnosis of AIDS. HIV-related gingivitis, more recently termed linear gingival erythema, is distinctive, presenting as a 2- to 3-mm linear band of erythema along the gingival free margin. Periodontitis among the HIV-infected population is common and usually more aggressive and painful in its presentation. Such necrotizing ulcerative periodontitis is distinguished from acute necrotizing ulcerative gingivitis, which is also a common finding, by its distribution and microbiology. Viruses such as herpes simplex virus, varicella-zoster virus, cytomegalovirus, and Epstein–Barr are fairly common and produce more significant disease when present in the immunocompromised patient. Hairy leukoplakia, a somewhat distinctive hyperkeratotic and epithelial hyperplastic lesions on the lateral borders of the tongue, is the second most common oral manifestation of HIV and strongly suggests HIV infection. Oral hairy leukoplakia is thought to be an Epstein–Barr virus-induced epithelial hyperplasia. Kaposi sarcoma, associated with human herpes virus type 8, is the most common malignancy associated with AIDS. It appears orally as a nonblanching brown to purplish macule or papule affecting most commonly the gingiva or hard palate. Lymphoma, primarily non-Hodgkin lymphoma, is the second most commonly associated cancer. All of these common oral findings in HIV are related to advancing immune suppression. With the concurrent use of newer therapeutic agents such as the nonnucleoside inhibitors, protease inhibitors, and the nucleoside inhibitors, fewer oral manifestations of HIV are occurring.[24]

REFERENCES

1. Williams RC: Periodontal disease. *New Engl J Med* 322:373, 1990.
2. Jaber L, Cohen I, Mor A: Fever associated with teething. *Arch Dis Child* 67:234, 1992.
3. Colby RC: The general practitioner's perspective of the etiology, prevention, and treatment of dry socket. *Gen Dent* 45:461, 1997.
4. Garibaldi JA: Dentoalveolar surgical sequelae. *Compend Contin Educ Dent* 19:407, 1998.
5. Suzuki JB: Diagnosis and classification of periodontal disease. *Dent Clin North Am* 32:195, 1988.
6. Laskaris G: Oral manifestations of infectious diseases. *Dent Clin North Am* 40:395, 1996.
7. Horning GM: Necrotizing gingivostomatitis: NUG to noma. *Compend Contin Educ Dent* 17:951, 1996.
8. Horning GM, Cohen ME: Necrotizing ulcerative gingivitis, periodontitis, and stomatitis: Clinical staging and predisposing factors. *J Periodontol* 66:990, 1995.
9. Donlon WC, Jacobson AL, Truta MP: Neuralgia. *Otolaryngol Clin North Am* 22:1145, 1989.
10. Fotos PG, Vincent SD, Hellstein MAJ: Oral candidiasis. *Oral Surg Oral Med Oral Pathol* 74:41, 1992.
11. Vincent SD, Lilly GE: Clinical, historic, therapeutic features of aphthous stomatitis: Literature review and open clinical trial employing steroids. *Oral Surg Oral Med Oral Pathol* 74:79, 1992.
12. Dongari A, McDonnell HT, Langlais RP: Drug-induced gingival overgrowth. *Oral Surg Oral Med Oral Pathol* 76:543, 1993.
13. Fiumara NJ: Venereal disease of the oral cavity. *J Oral Med* 31:36, 1976.
14. Espelid M, Bang G, Johannessen AC, et al: Geographic stomatitis: Report of 6 cases. *J Oral Pathol Med* 20:425, 1991.
15. Landis SH, Murray T, Bolden S, et al: Cancer statistics, 1998. *CA Cancer J Clin* 48:6,1998.
16. Marder MZ: The standard of care for oral diagnosis as it relates to oral cancer. *Compend Contin Educ Dent* 19:569, 1998.
17. Dumsha TC: Luxation injuries. *Dent Clin North Am* 39:79, 1995.
18. Rauschenberger CR, Hovland EJ: Clinical management of crown fractures. *Dent Clin North Am* 39:25, 1995.
19. Medford HM: Temporary stabilization of avulsed teeth. *Ann Emerg Med* 11:490, 1982.
20. Trope M: Clinical management of the avulsed tooth. *Dent Clin North Am* 39:93, 1995.
21. Blomlof L: Milk and saliva as possible storage media for traumatically exarticulated teeth prior to replantation. *Swed Dent J* 8:1, 1981.

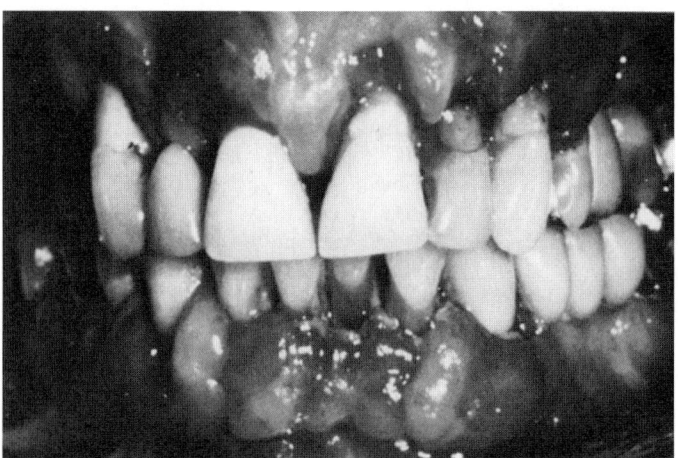

FIG. 242-13. Oral manifestations of leukemia.

22. Lindskog S, Blomlof L: Influence of osmolality and composition of some storage media on human periodontal ligament cells. *Acta Odontol Scand* 40:435, 1982.

23. Barrett AP: Gingival lesions in leukemia: A classification. *J Periodontol* 55:585, 1984.

24. Patton L, Van der Horst C: Oral infections and other manifestations of HIV disease. *Infect Dis Clin North Am* 13:789, 1999.

INFECTIONS AND DISORDERS OF THE NECK AND UPPER AIRWAY
Carol G. Shores

This chapter discusses conditions that can obstruct the upper airway. These disorders must be recognized quickly because early intubation may be lifesaving. Infections of the neck and upper airway include pharyngitis/tonsillitis, peritonsillar abscess, epiglottitis, retropharyngeal abscess, and dental abscess. Cancers, congenital neck masses, ranulas, and mucoceles present as masses in the neck and upper airway. Noninfectious causes of airway obstruction include posttonsillectomy hemorrhage, airway and esophageal foreign bodies, laryngeal papillomatosis, neck and facial trauma, and angioedema. If there is a possibility of surgical intervention in the neck, the patient should receive nothing by mouth (NPO) after arrival at the emergency department.

NECK AND UPPER AIRWAY INFECTIONS

Pharyngitis/Tonsillitis

Pharyngitis in children is discussed in Chap. 121. Pharyngitis in adults is usually infectious, and viral pharyngitis is the most common (Table 243-1). Group A β-hemolytic streptococcus (GABHS) is the most common bacterial organism causing pharyngitis, but rare cases of chlamydial and mycoplasmal pharyngitis have been reported. Noninflammatory conditions such as systemic lupus erythematosus, pemphigoid, or Behçet disease also can cause pharyngitis.

In the vast majority of patients, acute pharyngitis is a self-limiting illness that does not require specific antimicrobial therapy. Patients with pharyngitis should receive symptomatic treatment including gargling with warm saltwater, drinking warm liquids, antipyretics, analgesics, and rest. Dexamethasone 4 mg PO qd can be used for symptomatic relief,[1] and patients unable to tolerate oral fluids or who become dehydrated should be given intravenous fluids.

VIRAL PHARYNGITIS   Viral pharyngitis generally displays a vesicular and petechial pattern on the soft palate and tonsils, is associated with rhinorrhea, but is without tonsillar exudate or cervical adenopathy. Most cases of viral pharyngitis require no specific diagnostic testing. There are three notable exceptions: influenza (see Chap. 143), infectious mononucleosis (see Chap. 143), and acute retroviral syndrome (see Chap. 144). More than 70 percent of primary infections with HIV-1 are associated with acute pharyngitis. Symptoms of pharyngitis develop 2 to 4 weeks after exposure[2,3] and resolve within 2 weeks. Early treatment may decrease the viral load and lead to enhanced immune response, making recognition of acute retroviral syndrome important.[3]

GABHS PHARYNGITIS   *Streptococcus pyogenes* (GABHS) is responsible for 5 to 15 percent of pharyngitis in adults.[4] Virulent strains of GABHS are associated with acute rheumatic fever (ARF) or acute glomerulonephritis.[5] Because of these sequelae, as well as local complications of untreated infection such as peritonsillar abscess, early diagnosis and treatment are important.

After an incubation period of 2 to 5 days, patients develop the sudden onset of sore throat, painful swallowing, chills, and fever. Headache, nausea, and vomiting are common associated symptoms. Signs and symptoms of GABHS pharyngitis include marked erythema of the tonsils and tonsillar pillars; tonsillar exudate; enlarged, tender anterior cervical lymph nodes; and uvular edema. Patients tend to have fever, myalgias, and malaise but not rhinorrhea.

The Centers for Disease Control and Prevention (CDC) lists four criteria for GABHS pharyngitis: 1) tonsillar exudate, 2) tender anterior cervical adenopathy, 3) absence of cough, and 4) history of fever.[6] The CDC recommends no antibiotic treatment for patients with none or only one of these criteria. For patients with two or more criteria, three strategies can be used: 1) Test patients with two, three, or four criteria using a rapid antigen test, and limit antibiotic therapy to patients with positive test results; 2) test patients with two or three criteria using a rapid antigen test, and limit antibiotic therapy to patients with a positive test result or with all four criteria; or 3) do not use any diagnostic tests, and limit antibiotic therapy to patients with three or four criteria. Although throat cultures may be indicated to investigate GABHS outbreaks or antibiotic resistance, they are not recommended for routine evaluation of adult pharyngitis.[7]

Drug resistance is a growing problem and is related directly to the overuse of antibiotics. GABHS is rarely resistant to penicillin, which remains the recommended first-line drug for this disease.[4,7,8] Adults should receive a single intramuscular dose of 1.2 million units of benzathine penicillin G or 500 mg of penicillin VK PO twice or three times daily for 10 days. Erythromycin is the recommended alternative for penicillin-allergic patients. Close contacts and family members should be screened and treated promptly if they become symptomatic or have a positive rapid antigen test.

Several other bacteria can cause pharyngitis, although these infections are not common (see Table 243-1). If non-GABHS bacterial pharyngitis is suspected clinically, the microbiology laboratory should be notified because many of these bacteria require special growth media and will not be identified on routine throat culture. *Neisseria gonorrhoeae* pharyngitis occurs rarely independently of genital infection and is treated by the same antibiotics as genital infections. Diphtheria is caused by *Corynebacterium diphtheriae* and is rare in well-immunized populations. It is characterized by a slow onset of mild to moderate pharyngeal discomfort and low-grade fever. On physical examination, a gray membrane is seen firmly adherent to the tonsillar or pharyngeal surface and may extend to the uvula, soft palate, pharynx and larynx.

FUNGAL PHARYNGITIS   *Candida albicans* can produce painful oropharyngeal moniliasis, or thrush. This is particularly common after a course of antibiotics upsets microbial interactions or if the patient is immunocompromised. Oropharyngeal moniliasis presents with a white, cheesy exudate that can be scraped off an erythematous base. Nystatin oral suspension or clotrimazole troches are usually effective. Immunocompromised patients can develop candidal esophagitis and may require systemic therapy with fluconazole. Other forms of fungal pharyngitis are rare.

All types of pharyngitis can lead to suppurative complications, including cervical lymphadenitis, peritonsillar abscess, retropharyngeal abscess, sinusitis, and otitis media.

Peritonsillar Abscess

Peritonsillar abscess is the most frequently occurring deep-space infection of the head and neck.[9] It is a collection of purulent material between the tonsillar capsule and the superior constrictor and palatopharyngeus muscles (Figure 243-1). The progression from local cellulitis to abscess can occur despite antibiotic administration. Risk factors include chronic tonsillitis, multiple trials of oral antibiotics, and previous peritonsillar abscess. Peritonsillar abscess is most common during the second and third decades and can be bilateral.[10,11] Cultures of ab-

TABLE 243-1   Viral and Bacterial Causes of Pharyngitis

Pathogen	Syndrome/Disease	Signs and Symptoms	Percent
Viral			
Rhinovirus and coronavirus	Common cold	Nonexudative; mild to moderate pharyngeal pain; rhinorrhea; odynophagia, fever, myalgia and malaise uncommon	≥25
Adenovirus	Pharyngoconjunctival fever	More common in summer; fever; malaise; HA; dizziness; conjunctivitis	5
Herpes simplex virus (Chap. 150)	Gingivitis, stomatitis	Vesicles and shallow ulcers of the palate; tender cervical adenopathy	4
Parainfluenza virus	Common cold, croup	Otitis media; cough	2
Influenza virus (Chap. 150)	Influenza	Abrupt onset; fever; chills; myalgia; HA; anorexia; severe pharyngeal pain	2
Coxsackievirus A	Herpangina	Soft palate and tonsillar pillar vesicles; fever; severe pharyngeal pain	<1
Epstein-Barr virus (Chap. 150)	Infectious mononucleosis	Fever; tender cervical adenopathy; HA; malaise; splenomegaly	<1
Cytomegalovirus	Infectious mononucleosis	Pharyngitis less severe than with EBV	<1
HIV-1	Acute retroviral syndrome	Similar to mononucleosis; nonexudative pharyngitis; truncal exanthem; aseptic meningitis	<1
Bacterial			
Streptococcus pyogenes (GABHS)	Pharyngitis/tonsillitis, scarlet fever	Fever; fiery red pharynx with patchy grey/yellow exudate; uvula edema; tender cervical adenopathy; rhinorrhea and cough uncommon	5–15
Group C beta-hemolytic streptococcus	Pharyngitis/tonsillitis	Similar to GABHS, but usually less severe	5–10
Mixed anaerobic infection	Pharyngitis (Vincent angina)	Halitosis; purulent exudate	<1
Neisseria gonorrhoeae	Pharyngitis	Mild pharyngitis; usually concurrent genital infection	<1
Corynebacterium diphtheriae	Diphtheria	Slow onset; mild pharyngeal pain; firmly adherent gray tonsillar or pharyngeal membrane	<1
Arcanobacterium haemolyticum	Pharyngitis, scarlatiniform rash	Exudative pharyngitis; extremity and trunk erythematous maculopapular rash	<1
Yersinia enterocolitica	Pharyngitis, enterocolitis	Exudative pharyngitis; fever; cervical adenapathy; abdominal pain ± diarrhea; high mortality	<1
Treponema pallidum	Secondary syphilis	Silvery gray, superficial OP/OC erosions with erythematous base; other typical signs and symptoms; highly contagious	<1
Unknown			>30

Abbreviations: EBV = Epstein-Barr virus; GABHS = group A beta-hemolytic streptococcus; HA = headache; HIV = human immunodeficiency virus; OP/OC = oropharynx and oral cavity.
Source: Adapted from Mandell et al,[2] with permission.

scess aspirates characteristically produce a mixture of aerobic and anaerobic flora, but specific identification of the infecting bacterium is not usually needed for treatment.[9]

Symptoms of a peritonsillar abscess include fever, malaise, "hot-potato voice," sore throat, odynophagia, dysphagia, and otalgia. Signs include trismus, inferior and medial displacement of the infected tonsil(s), contralateral deflection of the swollen uvula, palatal edema, tender cervical lymphadenopathy, drooling, and dehydration (see Figure 243-1). Although easily diagnosed with a neck computed tomographic (CT) scan (with contrast material, Figure 243-2) or ultrasound, aspiration of purulent material with an 18-gauge needle is usually sufficient for diagnosis. The differential diagnosis of a peritonsillar abscess includes cellulitis, infectious mononucleosis, herpes simplex tonsillitis, retropharyngeal abscess, neoplasm, foreign body, and internal artery carotid aneurysm.

The cornerstone of treatment is drainage of the abscess by needle aspiration,[11] incision and drainage (I&D), or rarely, immediate tonsillectomy. Choice of treatment depends on clinical symptoms, degree of patient cooperation, history of previous of tonsil disease, and patient reliability. Needle aspiration is the least invasive, and 85 percent of patients will be treated effectively after a single needle aspiration.[9] Only needle aspiration will be discussed here.

Needle aspiration should be performed by an individual trained in the technique. Prior to aspiration, lidocaine spray or gel or benzocaine-

tetracaine spray (Cetacaine) is used to topically anesthetize the overlying mucosa. Then 1 to 2 mL of lidocaine with epinephrine is injected into the mucosa of the anterior tonsillar pillar using a 25-gauge needle (Figure 243-3). Once adequate anesthesia is achieved, an 18-gauge needle should be introduced just lateral to the tonsil, approximately halfway between the base of the uvula and the maxillary alveolar ridge, until the abscess cavity is encountered. The abscess then should be aspirated. **The needle should penetrate no more than 1 cm because the internal carotid artery usually lies laterally and posterior to the posterior edge of the tonsil.** Often, multiple aspirations may be required to find the abscess. A contrast CT scan of the neck is recommended when the results of needle aspiration are negative and a parapharyngeal or retropharyngeal space process is suspected.

Following needle aspiration, 10 days of high-dose penicillin or clindamycin for penicillin-allergic patients is the treatment of choice. Follow-up is needed within 24 h of aspiration. If the patient is not improving, consider repeating the aspiration, otolaryngologic consultation for I&D or tonsillectomy, obtaining a CT scan to confirm the diagnosis, or change antibiotics to ampicillin-clavulanic acid, clindamycin, or cefuroxime plus metronidazole.

Complications of a peritonsillar abscess include airway obstruction, rupture of the abscess with aspiration of the contents, cavernous sinus thrombosis, epiglottitis, septicemia, endocarditis, retropharyngeal abscess, and mediastinitis.

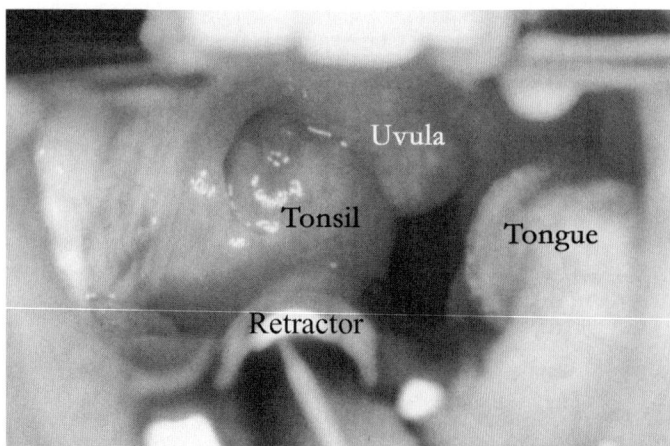

FIG. 243-1. Open-mouth view with retractor on tongue in a patient demonstrating medial right tonsillar displacement, palatal edema, and uvula deviation consistent with a peritonsillar abscess.

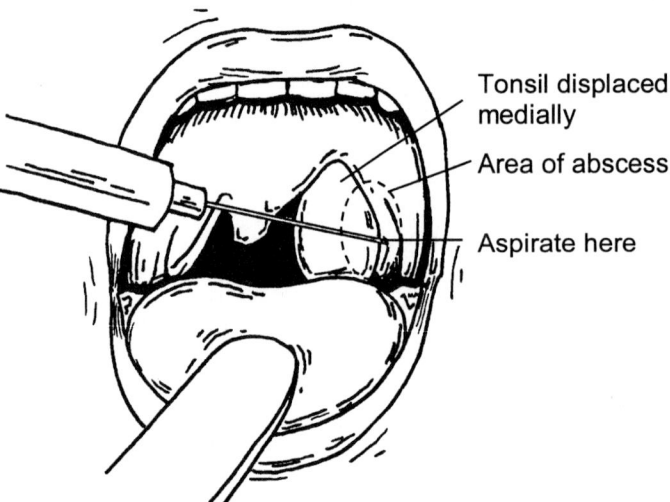

FIG. 243-3. Peritonsillar abscess, demonstrating location for aspiration.

Epiglottitis

Epiglottitis can lead to rapid, unpredictable airway obstruction. It is an inflammatory condition, usually infectious, primarily of the epiglottis but often including the entire supraglottic region. Because of this, many clinicians prefer the term *supraglottitis.*

Since most children are inoculated against *Haemophilus influenzae,* most cases of epiglottitis are now seen in adults with a mean age of 46 years.[12–14] Epiglottitis can be caused by bacteria (most commonly *Haemophilus influenzae* type b, *Streptococcus* species, *Staphylococcus* species), viruses, and fungi, although most frequently no organism can be isolated.[15]

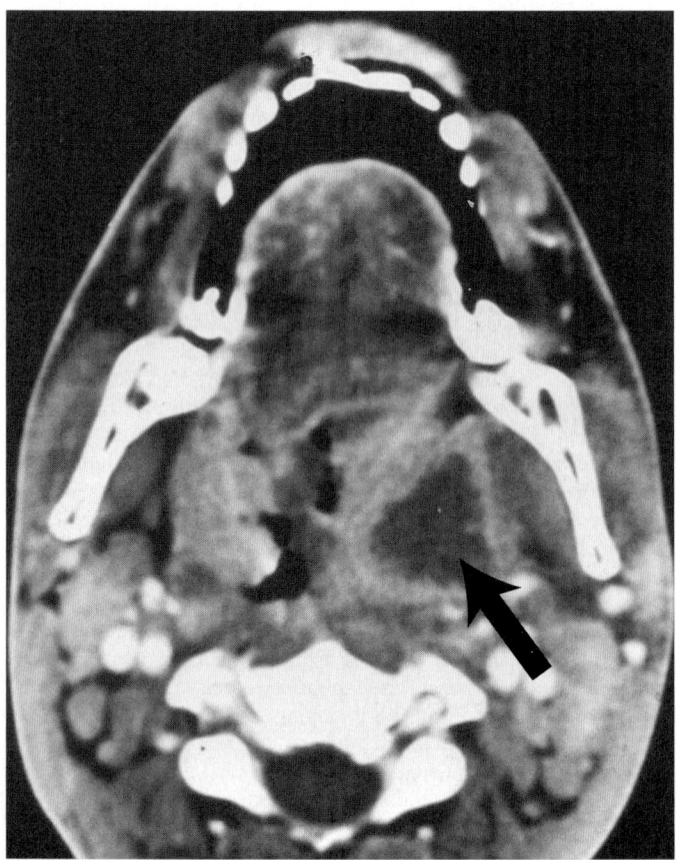

FIG. 243-2. Axial CT of a left peritonsillar abscess.

Patients with epiglottitis typically present with a 1- to 2-day history of worsening dysphagia and odynophagia and dyspnea, particularly in the supine position. Symptoms include fever, tachycardia, cervical adenopathy, drooling, and pain with gentle palpation of the larynx and upper trachea. Stridor is primarily inspiratory and is softer and lower-pitched than in croup. Patients often position themselves sitting up, leaning forward, mouth open, head extended, and panting. Thick oropharyngeal secretions are commonly present, with little or no cough.

Diagnosis is made by history, clinical examination, radiographs, and laryngoscopy. Lateral cervical soft tissue radiographs demonstrate obliteration of the vallecula, swelling of the aryepiglottic folds, edema of the prevertebral and retropharyngeal soft tissues, and ballooning of the hypopharynx (Figure 243-4). The epiglottis appears enlarged and thumb-shaped. Direct fiberoptic examination can confirm the diagnosis in adults if necessary but should be done with extreme caution to avoid sudden, unpredictable airway obstruction.

Patients with suspected epiglottitis require immediate otolaryngologic consultation, and the emergency physician must be prepared to establish a definitive airway. Patients should never be left unattended and should be kept sitting up. Initial treatment consists of supplemental *humidified* oxygen, intravenous hydration, cardiac monitoring, pulse oximetry, and intravenous antibiotics. Humidification and hydration minimize crusting in the airway and can help decrease the risk for sudden airway blockage. Heliox can be given to temporarily decrease airway resistance.

In adults, the need for intubation usually can be determined by fiberoptic examination of the supraglottis. This is generally accomplished by awake fiberoptic intubation in the operating room, with preparations for immediate awake tracheostomy or cricothyrotomy. In cases of airway obstruction in the emergency department, endotracheal intubation must be attempted, but the physician should be prepared for a very difficult intubation secondary to the swollen, distorted anatomy. In the case of intubation failure, the last resorts for preserving the airway in adult and pediatric patients are cricothyrotomy and needle cricothyrotomy, respectively.

Current antibiotic recommendations are cefuroxime as the first-line drug. Alternative antibiotics include ampicillin-sulbactam, cefotaxime, ceftriaxone, or trovafloxacin if the patient has a history of penicillin anaphylaxis.[16] Steroids are used empirically by many otolaryngologists to decrease airway inflammation and edema.

Retropharyngeal Abscess

The retropharyngeal space extends from the base of the skull to the tracheal bifurcation. The two paramedial chains of lymph nodes

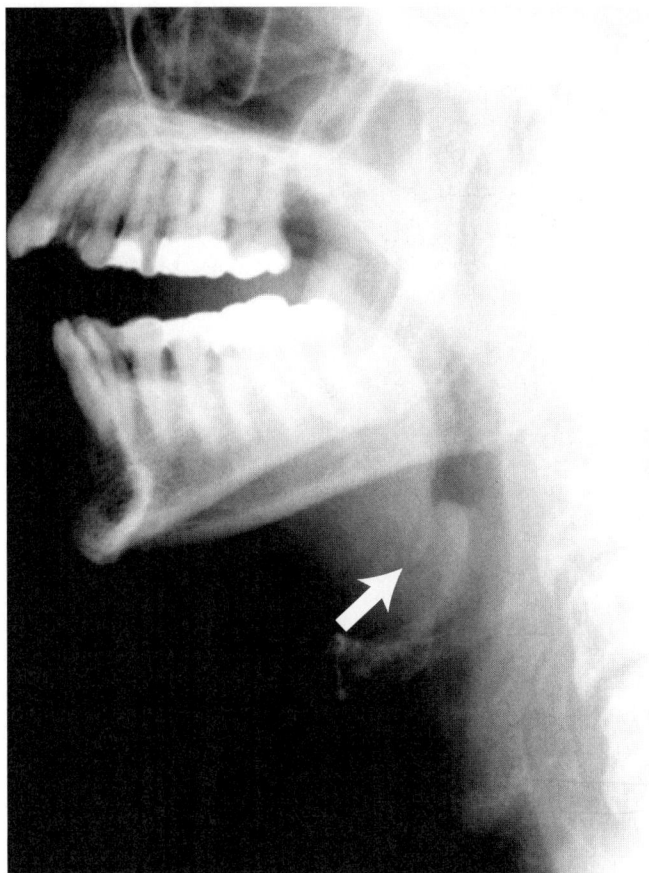

FIG. 243-4. Lateral radiograph demonstrating thumbprinting of the epiglottis consistent with epiglottitis.

(nodes of Rouviere), which drain the nasopharynx, adenoids, and posterior nasal sinuses, can be found within this space. In children, retropharyngeal abscesses usually are suppurative changes within a lymph node, with the primary infection elsewhere in the head and neck. In adults, however, a retropharyngeal abscess is generally the direct extension of purulent debris from an adjacent site, such as Ludwig angina. Therefore, retropharyngeal abscess in an adult is more likely to extend into the mediastinum.[17]

Signs and symptoms include fever, dysphagia, neck pain, limitation of cervical motion, cervical lymphadenopathy, sore throat, poor oral intake, muffled voice, and respiratory distress. Stridor and neck edema are likely in children but not adults. The intense inflammation and swelling associated with a retropharyngeal abscess can lead to inflammatory torticollis, which is unilateral spasm of the sternocleidomastoid muscle, causing posturing of the head with the occiput rotated toward the affected side.

Cultures from retropharyngeal abscesses are usually polymicrobial. The most common aerobic species isolated are *Streptococcus viridans* and *S. pyogenes.* Most of the staphylococcal species isolated are β-lactamase-producing. *Bacteroides* and *Peptostreptococcus* are the most commonly isolated anaerobes.[18]

A contrast-enhanced CT scan of the neck is the "gold standard" for diagnosis of a retropharyngeal abscess. A lateral soft-tissue radiograph of the neck taken during inspiration with moderate cervical extension can demonstrate thickening and protrusion of the retropharyngeal wall. However, even a small degree of flexion in children normally causes a marked forward bulge of the posterior pharyngeal wall that can be misleading. If the diagnosis is strongly suspected, patients should not be sent unobserved for CT scanning, though the potential for airway compromise may be minimal.[17]

All patients with retropharyngeal abscess should have immediate otolaryngologic consultation. Intravenous hydration and antibiotic treatment should be started in the emergency department until the patient can be brought to the operating room for transoral or transcervical incision and drainage. Although a few patients with small abscess cavities may be managed with intravenous antibiotics alone, most patients will require surgical intervention. Clindamycin or ampicillin-sulbactam is recommended.[17,18]

Catastrophic complications from retropharyngeal abscess include extension of the infection into the mediastinum and upper airway asphyxia from direct pressure or sudden rupture of the abscess.

Dental Abscesses, Ludwig Angina, and Deep Neck Abscesses

If an odontogenic abscess is untreated, the abscess can break through cortical bone of the mandible and spread into soft tissue spaces. This discussion will be limited to spread into the sublingual and submandibular spaces, whereas masticator space abscesses are discussed in Chap. 240.

The mylohyoid muscle forms a sling in the floor of the mouth and attaches along a line on the medial surface of the mandible. The sublingual space is superficial to the mylohyoid, whereas the submandibular space is deep to it. Since the roots of the premolars and first molars usually do not extend below the mylohyoid line, medial spread of apical abscesses from these teeth generally causes sublingual abscesses. Third molar infections generally lead to submandibular abscess, whereas second molar infections can lead to either. Clinically, infections of the sublingual space cause marked floor of mouth edema with little extraoral swelling. Submandibular space abscesses lead to edema spreading from the inferior edge of the mandible to the digastric region and inferiorly to the hyoid bone.

Ludwig angina is an infection of submental, sublingual, and submandibular spaces causing elevation and posterior displacement of the tongue and tense induration between the hyoid bone and the genu of the mandible. Patients usually present with poor dental hygiene, dysphagia, odynophagia, trismus, and edema of the upper midline neck and marked floor of mouth edema. The tongue can rapidly become posteriorly displaced, leading to airway compromise. Early signs and symptoms of imminent airway collapse may be subtle, and many patients with Ludwig angina will require awake fiberoptic intubation or awake tracheostomy.[19] Stridor, difficulty managing secretions, anxiety, and cyanosis are late signs and require emergency airway management.

Dental abscesses may spread into the deep neck spaces, including the parapharyngeal, retropharyngeal, and prevertebral spaces. Presenting symptoms include a neck mass, trismus, fever, leukocytosis, dysphagia, and dyspnea. A contrast-enhanced neck CT scan is diagnostic and also aids in surgical management.

Odontogenic abscesses are caused by *Streptococcus* spp. and oral anaerobes. In an uncomplicated infection in an immunocompetant host, culture is not necessary. Treatment includes incision and drainage with intravenous antibiotics (penicillin, clindamycin, and ampicillin-sulbactam are the preferred choices).

NECK AND UPPER AIRWAY MASSES

Intraoral or Intrapharyngeal Masses

Benign lesions usually are covered with normal-appearing mucosa and are nontender and long-standing. Mucoceles (no epithelial lining) and mucus retention cysts (epithelial lined) arise from minor salivary glands found throughout the oral cavity and are treated with excision or marsupialization. A ranula is a mucus retention cyst of the sublingual gland, and when it extends through the mylohyoid muscle into the neck, it is called a *plunging ranula*. Papillomas are sessile, warty-appearing lesions that frequently occur on the soft palate and anterior tonsillar pillars and are treated with surgical excision. Laryngeal papillomas can cause life-threatening airway obstruction and are discussed below. Palatine torus and mandibular torus are exostoses of the palate and mandible. Both are bony, smooth, painless masses covered with normal mucosa that slowly enlarge over many years. Usually, no treatment is needed.

Squamous cell carcinoma is the most common malignancy of the upper airway and generally presents with dysphagia, odynophagia, otalgia, weight loss, and/or neck mass in a patient with a significant smoking and/or alcohol history. The tumors are usually ulcerative lesions found anywhere in the upper airway. Patients with stridor and a suspected mass lesion should be evaluated by a bedside nasopharyngeal fiberoptic examination *prior* to CT scanning to avoid airway compromise when placed supine for the CT scan. The airway should be managed with humidified oxygen and awake fiberoptic intubation versus awake tracheostomy in the operating room.

Lymphomas of Waldeyer ring present with dysphagia and a muffled voice and can be complicated by infection. Posttransplant lymphoproliferative disorder can present with a similar picture.[20]

Neck Masses

Neck masses can result from congenital, infectious, or neoplastic disorders. Enlargement may lead to airway compromise, dehydration secondary to dysphagia and odynophagia, or systemic progression of a local infection. The patient's age aids in the diagnosis (Table 243-2). Neck masses in infants and children represent benign conditions in the majority of cases and include branchial cleft abnormalities, thyroglossal duct cysts, lymphangiomas, hemangiomas, or benign lymphadenopathy.[21] Each of these may become acutely infected and presents initially as a painful mass associated with skin erythema, leukocytosis, and fever.

Branchial cleft cysts are round, smooth, and mobile and not tender unless they become infected. They are located along the anterior border of the sternocleidomastoid muscle (Figure 243-5). In contrast, thyroglossal duct cysts are found in a subhyoid position, within 2 cm of midline (Figure 243-6). These cysts commonly enlarge after an upper respiratory illness and, on examination, are soft, mobile, and frequently have a bluish hue.

TABLE 243-2   Neck Masses by Age

INFANT
Hemangioma
Lymphangioma
Branchial cleft cyst
Rhabdomyosarcoma

CHILD
Reactive lymphadenopathy
Branchial cleft cyst
Thyroglossal duct cyst

YOUNG ADULT
Reactive lymphadenopathy
Mononucleosis
Hodgkin disease
Branchial cleft cyst
Thyroglossal duct cyst

ADULT
Salivary gland or parotid infection or neoplasm
Oral cavity neoplasm
Metastatic carcinoma
Lymphoma
Thyroid disorder

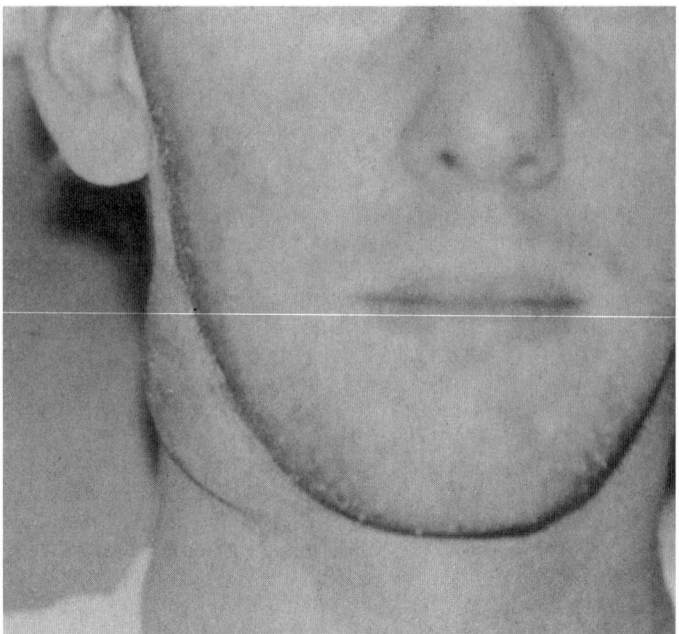

FIG. 243-5. Lateral neck mass in an adolescent demonstrates an infected branchial cleft cyst. It can be found anatomically along the sternocleidomastoid muscle.

Neck masses in adolescents and young adults are caused most commonly by infection or neoplasm. Cervical lymphadenopathy, malaise, and pharyngitis are the symptom complex for mononucleosis. A single, large, inflamed anterolateral neck mass in this age group that develops after an upper respiratory infection suggests a branchial cleft cyst. Young adults with multiple, rubbery low-neck masses, night sweats, fever, and malaise may have Hodgkin disease or lymphoma, whereas generalized adenopathy suggests HIV disease.

In patients older than age 40, 75 percent of neck masses are neoplastic.[22] The most common cause of a unilateral neck mass is squamous cell carcinoma of the upper aerodigestive tract, metastatic to cervical lymph nodes. Other common neoplasms are tumors of the parotid or submandibular gland, thyroid gland, and lymphoma. Neoplastic lymph nodes usually feel firm and, although initially mobile, become fixed to surrounding structures as the cancer invades. Neoplastic nodes can become acutely infected and present as a neck abscess. Diffuse nodular thyroid enlargement that is present for many years suggests a simple goiter, whereas a solitary thyroid nodule, although usually benign, may represent thyroid cancer. Infectious lymphadenopathy can be seen in adults, and infectious nodes can sometimes be differentiated from their malignant counterparts by their soft and occasionally fluctuant texture.

Prominent normal structures can be mistaken for abnormalities. Normal lymph nodes can be up to 1 cm in diameter, except the jugulodigastric node, which can be up to 1.5 cm. Normal submandibular glands may be ptotic and asymmetrical. A pulsatile carotid bulb or the transverse process of the first cervical vertebra can be quite prominent in a thin neck.

The history often helps to limit the differential diagnosis. Infectious processes usually develop over hours to days and have associated pain, redness, warmth, and fever. Patients often have a preceding upper respiratory tract or dental infection. Infected congenital cysts may have enlarged on earlier occasions and resolved with antibiotics. Salivary gland infections often wax and wane, are exacerbated by eating, and may cause a foul taste in the mouth as the gland decompresses. Hodgkin disease and lymphomas are associated with night sweats, malaise, itching, and/or fever. Neoplastic disease usually occurs in adults with a history of smoking and alcohol abuse.

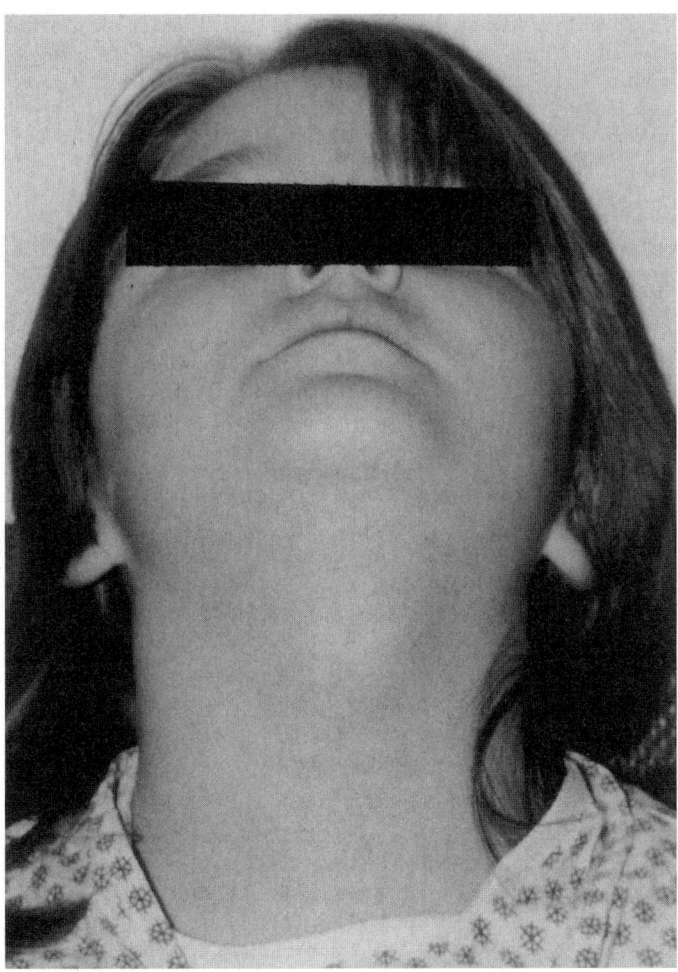

FIG. 243-6. Midline mass in an adolescent demonstrating a thyroglossal duct cyst.

Further evaluation of a neck mass depends on the history and physical examination. Patients with airway compromise or significant dysphagia and odynophagia should be evaluated by nasopharyngoscopy *prior* to CT scan. Laboratory studies are guided by physical findings and the likely differential diagnosis. CT scan with contrast will delineate the extent of the mass and likely will be required for consultation or surgical intervention. Treatment depends on the differential diagnosis. If no airway compromise or dehydration is present, the patient should be scheduled to return as an outpatient for further evaluation. Empirical antibiotic therapy is used for inflammatory nodes, usually with cephalexin, amoxicillin, or clindamycin, and most will resolve within 2 weeks. Sialoadenitis requires staphylococcal coverage.

POTENTIAL AIRWAY OBSTRUCTION

Posttonsillectomy Bleeding

Postoperative bleeding is a well-known complication of tonsillectomy that can lead to death from airway obstruction or hemorrhagic shock. The incidence ranges from 1 to 6 percent, with approximately half requiring surgical intervention for control of bleeding.[23,24]

Although bleeding can be seen within 24 h of surgery, most hemorrhage occurs between postoperative days 5 and 10. There is a significantly higher incidence of bleeding in patients between 21 and 30 years of age,[24] and hemorrhage is less common in children under the age of 6.[25]

Posttonsillectomy bleeding can be fatal and requires prompt intervention with control of the airway. An otolaryngologist should be con-

sulted early. The patient should be maintained NPO, monitored with pulse oximetry, and kept upright. Intravenous access should be obtained, and blood should be drawn for a CBC, coagulation studies, and type and crossmatch. Direct pressure can be applied to the bleeding tonsillar bed using a tonsillar pack or a 4 × 4 gauze with a suture through it to prevent loss of the pack into the airway. Pressure exerted on the lateral pharyngeal wall, avoiding midline manipulation, will decrease stimulation of the gag reflex. The packs can be moistened with thrombin or an equivolume solution of 1:1000 epinephrine and 1 percent lidocaine. Massive bleeding is rare, but when it occurs, intubation may be the only means of protecting the airway. This is always difficult, with oropharyngeal edema from recent surgery and blood obscuring visualization of the cords. Plans should be made for an emergent cricothyrotomy prior to attempting intubation.

Pressure alone can be adequate for control of posttonsillectomy hemorrhage until the otolaryngologist arrives. Alternatively, if a bleeding site can be visualized, bleeding may be cauterized with silver nitrate after local infiltration with 1 percent lidocaine with 1:100,000 epinephrine. Otolaryngologic consultation in the emergency department is always needed because patients may have a second or even third posttonsillectomy hemorrhage,[24] and surgery or endovascular embolization may be necessary for definitive control.[26]

Foreign Bodies of the Aerodigestive Tract

Foreign bodies in the upper aerodigestive tract can be life-threatening, and morbidity and mortality increase with delay in diagnosis. In the year 2000, 160 children younger than 15 years of age died from obstruction of the respiratory tract associated with inhaled or ingested foreign bodies, and 17,537 were treated in emergency departments.[27] Adults usually present soon after ingestion or aspiration of a foreign body and are able to provide a history of the event. Pediatric foreign-body aspiration or ingestion usually presents with a history of a choking episode, frequently with cyanosis, followed by dysphagia, wheezing, and/or coughing. However, 60 percent of children exhibit mild or absent signs and symptoms at presentation to the emergency department.[28]

Esophageal foreign bodies lead to dysphagia, odynophagia, drooling, wheezing, and cough. In adults, food boluses are the most common esophageal foreign body, and the signs, symptoms, and history generally make the diagnosis obvious.[29] In children, coins are most common.[28] See Chap. 76 for detailed discussion of esophageal foreign bodies, including disk battery ingestion.

Retained esophageal foreign bodies can present weeks to years after ingestion and lead to bronchoesophageal fistula, mediastinitis, and fatal aortoesophageal fistula.[30] Symptoms are subtle and include excess salivation, new-onset asthma, and recurrent upper respiratory infections.

There are three stages of signs and symptoms of pulmonary foreign-body aspiration: 1) a choking episode with or without cyanosis and followed by paroxysms of coughing, stridor, wheezing, and unilateral reduced breath sounds, 2) an asymptomatic interval, and 3) recurrent unilateral pneumonia and/or wheezing, worsening or new-onset asthma, and croup.[31]

Food is the most common aspirated foreign body in children, with the most common offenders being nuts, carrot, and popcorn.[31] Sudden death is associated with the aspiration of balloons, hot dogs, and grapes.[32] Chest x-rays frequently are normal, but findings suggesting a foreign body include unilateral hyperexpansion and lobar atelectasis or pneumonia.[33] All suspected foreign-body aspirations require bronchoscopic evaluation. See Chap. 133 for further discussion of foreign-body aspiration in children.

Recurrent Respiratory Papillomatosis

Recurrent respiratory papillomatosis is found in two age groups: children as young as 2 months with a peak onset at age 3 to 4 years and adults with an onset in the third decade of life or later. Recurrent respiratory papillomatosis is caused by infection with papillomavirus types 6 and 11, with maternal transmission in children and sexual transmission in adults. In both age groups, it can present with chronic cough, hoarseness, stridor, and/or dyspnea. The disease is usually recurrent despite multiple surgical excisions, and many patients presenting with an acute exacerbation will have a known history.[34] However, patients with new-onset respiratory papillomatosis can present to the emergency department with acute stridor and require timely diagnosis.

Papillomas are usually found at the glottis and are exophytic, wart-like lesions without ulceration. Their outline may be seen on soft tissue x-rays of the neck, and they are visualized by nasopharyngoscopy. An urgent otolaryngologic consult should be obtained in patients with a known diagnosis or symptoms suspicious for recurrent respiratory papillomatosis. Humidified oxygen or heliox may temporize an urgent airway, and intubation should only be attempted in the emergency department if absolutely needed.

Laryngeal Trauma

External laryngeal trauma is a rare but potentially lethal injury occurring in approximately 1 in every 137,000 inpatient admissions.[35] Blunt and penetrating neck trauma are discussed in Chap. 258. Blunt trauma to the larynx occurs primarily as the result of motor vehicle accidents (dashboard injuries), personal assaults, or sports injuries. The basic mechanism for blunt external injury is compression of the larynx on the anterior cervical bodies. Injuries include endolaryngeal mucosal tears, cartilaginous fractures, and dislocations of the cricoarytenoid joints. The clothesline injury is a form of blunt laryngeal trauma that typically occurs when the victim is riding a motorcycle or snowmobile and the neck strikes a linear stationary object, such as a wire fence or tree limb. The transfer of such a large amount of force to the neck crushes the thyroid cartilage and may cause laryngotracheal separation. Asphyxiation often occurs at the scene, and survivors of such injuries may have an airway held together precariously by mucous membranes bridging the cartilage. If this injury is suspected, the patient should undergo emergent tracheostomy without attempted intubation.

The signs and symptoms of laryngeal trauma include hoarseness, anterior neck pain to palpation, dyspnea, stridor, dysphagia, cough, and/or hemoptysis. Injuries may be asymptomatic initially, except for a subtle change in voice. With more significant or worsening injury, pain, dyspnea, or cough develop, and subcutaneous emphysema may become evident. When the laryngeal lumen is severely compromised, aphonia and apnea may occur, signaling the need for immediate establishment of an alternative airway.

If the airway is stable, a thorough physical examination of the neck and larynx is required. Bleeding, expanding hematomas, bruits, and loss of pulses are signs associated with vascular injury. Flexible fiberoptic nasopharyngolaryngoscopy with the patient sitting upright allows immediate assessment of airway integrity and should be done before CT scan of the neck. In patients with adequate airways, CT examination can delineate the extent of injury.[36] Cervical spine radiographs should be performed to evaluate for vertebral injury, a common concurrent injury.

The two primary goals in the management of acute laryngeal trauma are preservation of life by maintaining the airway and restoration of function. There is some controversy regarding the best way to establish an alternative airway in blunt laryngeal trauma. If the lumen of the laryngeal airway is compromised by ecchymosis and edema but there is no gross disruption of the laryngeal mucosa or displacement of the arytenoids and the tracheal lumen can be identified, then the airway may be secured by intubation or with an endotracheal tube advanced over a flexible bronchoscope.[37] When the laryngeal lumen cannot be visualized because of gross anatomic disruption or edema and hemorrhage, urgent tracheostomy is the preferred method of controlling the airway and avoiding further injury to the larynx. An emergent

tracheotomy is performed through a midline vertical skin incision, and the trachea should be entered at a level lower than usual (fourth or fifth tracheal ring). Cricothyrotomy may be difficult because of cervical emphysema and swelling and should be avoided if possible in suspected laryngeal trauma because it may further injure the subglottis.[38]

Angioedema of the Upper Airway

Angioedema is a nondemarcated swelling of the dermal or submucosal layers of the skin or mucosa. It is usually nonpruritic but can be painful. Angioedema of the upper airway can have sudden onset and rapid progression. There are four main etiologies: 1) congenital or acquired loss of C1 esterase inhibitor, 2) IgE-mediated type I allergic reaction to food, drug, or environmental exposure, 3) adverse reaction to angiotensin-converting enzyme (ACE) inhibitor therapy, and 4) idiopathic. A known diagnosis can direct therapy, but many patients with angioedema have no obvious cause at presentation.

C1 esterase inhibitor is the main regulator of the activation steps of the classical complement pathway, and its genetic deficiency is the cause of hereditary angioedema (HAE).[39] The diagnosis should be suspected in patients with a history of recurrent peripheral angioedema and abdominal pain. Forty percent of patients experience the onset of symptoms before age 5 and 75 percent before age 15. The disease is autosomal dominant, so many patients have a family history of recurrent angioedema. Diagnosis is confirmed by measuring blood levels of C1 and C4 esterase inhibitor, although these tests usually cannot be obtained during an acute emergency department visit.[40] Patients with HAE respond poorly to the usual treatments of angioedema outlined below. Epinephrine can produce some improvement in early acute attacks. Fresh frozen plasma (FFP) replaces the missing inhibitor protein and can improve symptoms. However, a few patients may become more edematous after FFP, and it is not recommended in life-threatening laryngeal edema. Patients with life-threatening edema should undergo fiberoptic intubation with preparation for an emergent surgical airway. Attacks can be prevented with long-term use of acetylated artificial androgens, so patients with suspected HAE should be referred for follow-up to their primary care physicians. Several medications, including estrogens and ACE inhibitors, increase the severity and frequency of HAE attacks, and patients should be advised to stop these.

The use of ACE inhibitors is associated with upper airway angioedema.[41] Sixty percent of cases occur in the first week after starting the drug, but ACE inhibitor-related angioedema can occur after years of treatment. The estimated incidence is 0.1 to 0.2 percent and is more common in African-Americans.[41] Patients must be withdrawn from ACE inhibitors immediately and warned not to use them again.

Treatment of upper airway angioedema usually is empirical. Intravenous access should be established and the airway examined with fiberoptic nasopharyngoscopy as soon as possible. For severe symptoms, epinephrine 1:1000 solution can be given SC in a dose of 0.01 mg/kg, not to exceed 0.3 mg, or the same dose can be administered by inhalation as racemic epinephrine. The dose can be repeated every 15 to 20 min as needed. Classically, diphenhydramine is given IV at 1 to 2 mg/kg, up to a maximum of 50 mg. If the airway is stable, 10 mg of cetirizine can be given PO instead, resulting in less sedation. Methylprednisolone 40 to 125 mg IV should be given, although steroids will not be effective for several hours. If nasopharyngoscopy demonstrates laryngotracheal edema, the patient should be admitted. If there is no airway edema, the patient can be discharged after several hours observation demonstrates clinical improvement.

Uvula Edema

Isolated uvula edema, sometimes referred to as Quincke edema, is a rare presentation of upper airway edema. It is usually caused by the same etiologic factors as upper airway angioedema, but can be associated with upper airway infections such as peritonsillar abscess, or rare epiglottitis. It can also be idiopathic or associated with drugs such as NSAIDs or ACE inhibitors. If it is an isolated finding, and symptoms are uncomfortable to the patient, dexamethasone, 4 mg IV or PO, can be given as a single dose in the ED.

REFERENCES

1. Wei J, Kasperbauer J, Weaver A, Boggust A: Efficacy of single-dose dexamethasone as adjuvant therapy for acute pharyngitis. *Laryngoscope* 112:87, 2002.
2. Mandell GL, Bennett JE, Dolin R (eds): *Principles and Practice of Infectious Diseases,* 5th ed. Philadelphia, Churchill Livingstone, 2000, pp. 1404-1406.
3. Panel on Clinical Practices for Treatment of HIV Infection, convened by the Department of Health and Human Services and the Henry J. Kaiser Family Foundation and American Academy of Pediatrics: Guidelines for the use of antiretroviral agents in HIV-infected adults and adolescents. Available at http://www.hivatis.org; accessed February 4, 2002.
4. Cooper RJ, Hoffman JR, Bartlett JG, et al: Principles of appropriate antibiotic use for acute pharyngitis in adults: Background. *Ann Intern Med* 134:509, 2001.
5. Stollerman GH: Rheumatic fever in the 21st century. *Clin Infect Dis* 33:806, 2001.
6. Centor RM, Witherspoon JM, Dalton HP, et al: The diagnosis of strep throat in adults in the emergency room. *Med Decis Making* 1:239, 1981.
7. Snow V, Mottur-Pilson C, Cooper RJ, Hoffman JR: Principles of appropriate antibiotic use for acute pharyngitis in adults. *Ann Intern Med* 134:506, 2001.
8. Schwartz B, Marcy SM, Phillips WR, et al: Pharyngitis: Principles of judicious use of antimicrobial agents. *Pediatrics* 101(suppl):171, 1998.
9. Herzon F: Peritonsillar abscess, in Gates G (ed): *Current Therapy in Otolaryngology-Head and Neck Surgery.* St Louis, Mosby, 1998, pp. 418-421.
10. Matsuda A, Tanaka H, Kanaya T, et al: Peritonsillar abscess: A study of 724 cases in Japan. *Ear Nose Throat J* 81:384, 2002.
11. Schraff S, McGinn JD, Derkay CS: Peritonsillar abscess in children: A 10-year review of diagnosis and managment. *Int J Pediatr Otolaryngol* 57:213, 2001.
12. Garpenholt O, Hugosson S, Fredlund H, et al: Epiglottitis in Sweden before and after introduction of vaccination against *Haemophilus influenzae* type b. *Pediatr Infect Dis J* 18:490, 1999.
13. Senior BA, Radkowski D, MacArthur C, et al: Changing patterns in pediatric supraglottitis: A multi-institutional review, 1980 to 1992. *Laryngoscope* 104:1314, 1994.
14. Nakamura H, Tanaka H, Matsuda A, et al: Acute epiglottitis: A review of 80 patients. *J Laryngol Otol* 115:31, 2001.
15. Trollfors B, Nylen O, Carenfelt C, et al: Aetiology of acute epiglottitis in adults. *Scand J Infect Dis* 30:49, 1998.
16. Fairbanks D (ed): *Pocket Guide to Antimicrobial Therapy in Otolaryngology-Head and Neck Surgery.* Alexandria, VA, American Academy of Otolaryngology-Head and Neck Surgery, 2001.
17. Kirse DJ, Roberson DW: Surgical management of retropharyngeal space infections in children. *Laryngoscope* 111:1413, 2001.
18. Asmar BI: Bacteriology of retropharyngeal abscess in children. *Pediatr Infect Dis J* 9:595, 1990.
19. Ludwig's angina: A review of current airway management. *Arch Otolaryngol Head Neck Surgery* 125:596, 1999.
20. Nalesnik MA: Clinicopathologic characteristics of post-transplant lymphoproliferative disorders. *Recent Results Cancer Res* 159:9, 2002.
21. Connolly AA, MacKenzie K: Paediatric neck masses: A diagnostic dilemma. *J Laryngol Otol* 111:541, 1997.
22. Gleeson M, Herbert A, Richards A: Managment of lateral neck masses in adults. *Br Medical J* 320:1521, 2000.
23. Bhattacharyya N: Evaluation of post-tonsillectomy bleeding in the adult population. *Ear Nose Throat J* 80:544, 2001.
24. Wei JL, Beatty CW, Gustafson RO: Evaluation of posttonsillectomy hemorrhage and risk factors. *Otolaryngol Head Neck Surg* 123:229, 2000.
25. Windfuhr JP, Chen YS: Hemorrhage following pediatric tonsillectomy before puberty. *Int J Pediatr Otolaryngol* 58:197, 2001.
26. Opatowksy MJ, Browne JD, McGuirt WF, Morris PP: Endovascular treatment of hemorrhage after tonsillectomy in children. *AJNR* 22:713, 2001.
27. Centers for Disease Control and Prevention: Nonfatal choking-related episodes amoung children-United States, 2001. *MMWR* 51:945, 2002.
28. Reilly J, Thompson J, MacArthur C, et al: Pediatric aerodigestive foreign body injuries are complications related to timeliness of diagnosis. *Laryngoscope* 107:17, 1997.
29. Mosca S, Manes G, Martino R, et al: Endoscopic management of foreign bodies in the upper gastrointestinal tract: Report on a series of 414 patients. *Endoscopy* 33:692, 2001.
30. Gilchrist BF, Valerie EP, Nguyen M, et al: Pearls and perils in the management of prolonged, peculiar penetrating esophageal foreign bodies in children. *J Pediatr Surg* 32:1429, 1997.
31. Tan HK, Brown K, McGill T, et al: Airway foreign bodies (FB): A 10-year review. *Int J Pediatr Otolaryngol* 56: 91, 2000.
32. Lifschultz BD, Donoghue ER: Deaths due to foreign body aspiration in children: The continuing hazard of toy ballons. *J Forens Sci* 41:247, 1996.
33. Zerella JT, Dimler M, McGill LC, Pippus KJ: Foreign body aspiration in children: Value of radiography and complications of bronchoscopy. *J Pediatr Surg* 33:1651, 1998.
34. Green GE, Bauman NM, Smith RJ: Pathogenesis and treatment of juvenile onset recurrent respiratory papillomatosis. *Otolaryngol Clin North Am* 33:187, 2000.
35. Jewett BS, Shockley WW, Rutledge R: External laryngeal trauma analysis of 392 patients. *Arch Otolaryngol Head Neck Surgery* 125:877, 1999.
36. Lupetin AR, Hollander M, Rao VM: CT evaluation of laryngotracheal trauma. *Semin Musculoskelet Radiol* 2:105, 1998.
37. Vassiliu P, Baker J, Henderson S, et al: Aerodigestive injuries of the neck. *Am Surg* 6:75, 2001.
38. Chagnon F, Mulder D: Layrngotracheal trauma. *Chest Surg Clinic North Am* 6:733, 1996.
39. Fay A, Abinun M: Current management of hereditary antioedema (C'1 esterase inhibitor deficiency). *J Clin Pathol* 55:266, 2002.
40. Gompels MM, Lock RJ, Morgan JE, et al: A multicentre evaluation of the diagnostic efficiency of serological investigations for C1 inhibitor deficiency. *J Clin Pathol* 55:145, 2002.
41. Vleeming W, van Amsterdam JGC, Stricker BHC, de Wildt DJ: ACE inhibitor-induced angioedema: Incidence, prevention and management. *Drug Saf* 18:171, 1998.

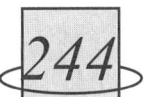

COMPLICATIONS OF AIRWAY DEVICES

Carol G. Shores

Theresa A. Hackeling

Rudolph J. Triana, Jr.

This chapter discusses complications of airway devices, focusing on endotracheal tubes, tracheostomy tubes, laryngeal stents, and alternative speech devices.

ENDOTRACHEAL TUBES

Acute complications of endotracheal intubation range from minor to catastrophic. Minor complications include lip lacerations, corneal abrasions,[1] dental fractures, and tongue injuries, and are all avoidable with proper technique. More serious complications of endotracheal intubation include damage to the soft tissues of the larynx or pharynx and dislocation of the arytenoid cartilage. Repetitive or blind intubation attempts are more likely to result in this type of injury. Mucosal tears may present early with immediate bleeding and subcutaneous emphysema, or late with septic shock.[2] If the endotracheal tube tip is placed in the soft tissue of the neck through a mucosal tear, bag ventilation will be very difficult and will likely result in subcutaneous emphysema with pneumothorax. All efforts to ventilate though the tube should be stopped and consideration given to an emergent surgical airway. Tracheal injuries are much more common in women, perhaps because of the use of improperly large tubes.[3] Mucosal injuries usually require immediate surgical repair by an otolaryngologist. See Chap. 19 for review of other complications of endotracheal intubation.

The endotracheal tube itself may be the source of complications.[4] Airway obstruction can result from kinking or biting the tube or inspissated secretions within the tube. In addition, an overinflated cuff may herniate over the end of the tube and obstruct it. If the obstruction cannot be cleared by suctioning or modification of tube position, the tube must be replaced.

TRACHEOSTOMY TUBES

A standard adult tracheostomy is a surgical procedure in which an opening is created between cartilaginous rings in the trachea and the skin of the neck is usually sutured to the anterior tracheal wall (Figure 244-1). In pediatric and some adult tracheotomies, a vertical incision is made through two or three tracheal rings and the lateral edges are tagged with temporary stay sutures. These sutures are usually removed before the patient leaves the hospital.

Skills needed for tracheostomy management in the ED include replacement of an uncuffed with a cuffed tracheostomy tube for mechanical ventilation, replacement after accidental decannulation, correction of tube obstruction, and control of bleeding or infection at the tracheostomy site (Figure 244-2). Key information in managing a tracheostomy includes why and when the procedure was performed and what type of tracheostomy tube is currently being used. Determine if the patient *can be orally intubated* if needed. **Patients who have undergone a laryngectomy or who have tumors or scarring that occlude the upper airway cannot be orally intubated.**

There are many types of tracheostomy tubes available, including tubes made of plastic, silicone, nylon, and metal. Most hospitals stock only a few types of tracheostomy tubes and emergency physicians should be familiar with the types available at their institution. Tra-

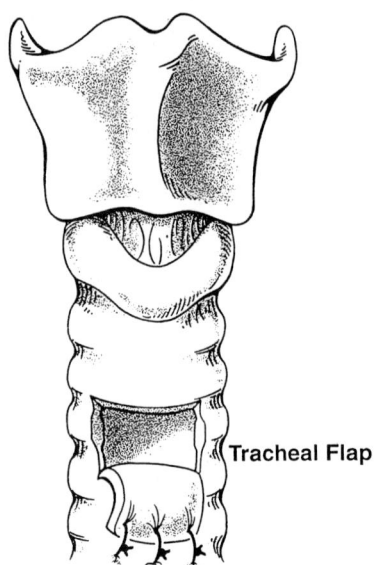

FIG. 244-1. Creation of a tracheal flap.

cheostomy tubes can vary in diameter, total length, and the length before and after the curve and the presence or absence of a cuff (Figure 244-3). The tracheostomy tube cuff is similar that of an endotracheal tube. Most adult tracheostomy tubes have a removable inner cannula, which allows secretions to be cleared from the lumen without removing the entire tube from the trachea. Both disposable and reusable inner cannulas are available. In any adult tracheostomy patient, it is ad-

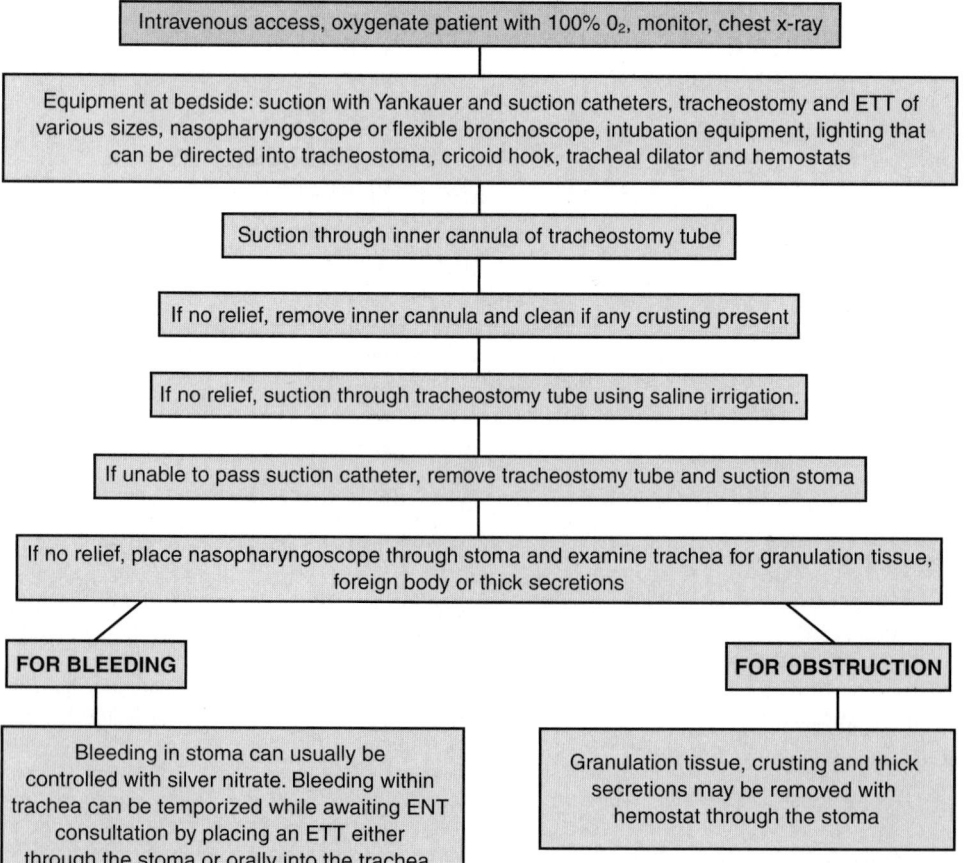

FIG. 244-2. Steps in assessing a tracheostomy patient with respiratory distress. ENT = ear, nose, and throat specialist; ETT = endotracheal tube.

Intravenous access, oxygenate patient with 100% O₂, monitor, chest x-ray

Equipment at bedside: suction with Yankauer and suction catheters, tracheostomy and ETT of various sizes, nasopharyngoscope or flexible bronchoscope, intubation equipment, lighting that can be directed into tracheostoma, cricoid hook, tracheal dilator and hemostats

Suction through inner cannula of tracheostomy tube

If no relief, remove inner cannula and clean if any crusting present

If no relief, suction through tracheostomy tube using saline irrigation.

If unable to pass suction catheter, remove tracheostomy tube and suction stoma

If no relief, place nasopharyngoscope through stoma and examine trachea for granulation tissue, foreign body or thick secretions

FOR BLEEDING

Bleeding in stoma can usually be controlled with silver nitrate. Bleeding within trachea can be temporized while awaiting ENT consultation by placing an ETT either through the stoma or orally into the trachea, then inflate the cuff at the site of bleeding.

FOR OBSTRUCTION

Granulation tissue, crusting and thick secretions may be removed with hemostat through the stoma

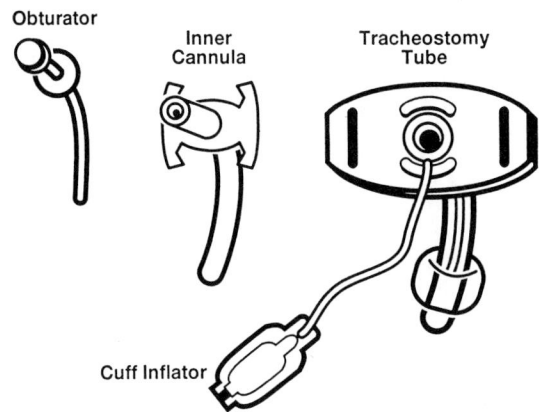

FIG. 244-3. Common components of most tracheostomy tube sets.

visable to remove and examine the inner cannula for crusting or obstruction. Both disposable and reusable inner cannulas can be cleaned with hydrogen peroxide by using a small brush and warm tap water. Because the correct size of disposable inner cannula is rarely available in the ED, the existing inner cannula should be temporarily reused or the entire tracheostomy tube changed. **Pediatric tracheostomy tubes never have an inner cannula because of the small inner diameter;** consequently, the entire tube must be removed for cleaning. The size of the tracheostomy tube is usually defined by the inner diameter, ranging in adults from 5 to 10 mm, and in pediatric tubes from 2.5 to 6.5 mm. Most pediatric and adult tracheostomy tubes have a 15-mm standard respiratory connection that may be used with ventilator tubing and a bag-valve device.

Fenestrated tracheostomy tubes have an opening along the dorsal surface of the body of the tube. The fenestration allows the passage of air through the tracheostomy tube to the vocal cords so the patient can speak. Tubes must be carefully fitted to provide alignment of the fenestration within the trachea with no contact of the fenestration to either the anterior neck tract or the posterior tracheal wall. When the fenestration contacts these structures, slight respiratory movement of the tube will lead to granulation tissue formation. The granulation tissue can extend into the fenestration, leading to bleeding, obstruction, and difficulty removing the tracheostomy tube. If any difficulty is encountered removing a fenestrated tracheostomy tube, otolaryngologic consultation is needed.

Changing a Tracheostomy Tube

The amount of difficulty encountered when changing a tracheostomy tube depends on when the procedure was performed and on patient anatomy. **If the tracheostomy is less than 7 days old, the tract will not be mature and manipulation may easily create a false passage within the soft tissue of the neck. In addition, a tract may easily collapse at any time in patients with obese necks or neck masses.** If the situation is not emergent, and the tracheostomy is less than 7 days old, tracheostomy tubes should be changed by an otolaryngologist or a surgeon familiar with the procedure.

An uneventful tracheostomy change depends on adequate preparation and is best accomplished with an assistant. The spontaneously breathing, stable patient can easily breathe through a patent tracheostoma without the tube in place, so there is no reason to rush through this procedure. The needed equipment is listed in Table 244-1. If a cuffed tube is used, test the balloon before use and make sure the balloon is completely deflated before insertion. If needed, the cricoid hook can be inserted just under the cricoid and used to lift and stabilize the trachea. The dilator is particularly useful if a larger tube is to be inserted, although dilation may require injection of local anesthesia and consideration of otolaryngologic consultation. The physi-

TABLE 244-1   Equipment Needed to Change a Tracheostomy Tube

Suction device with both a Yankauer tip and suction catheters that fit inside the tracheostomy tube
Good lighting directed into the tracheostoma
An appropriate size tracheostomy tube with obturator in place
Another tracheostomy tube one size smaller than planned
Tracheostomy tube tie
Cricoid hook and tracheal dilator (if physician is familiar with their use)

cian should be familiar with both the cricoid hook and tracheal dilator before using them. When the obturator is placed in the tracheostomy tube, the tube presents a solid, rounded end that is less likely to damage the neck soft tissue during tube insertion (see Figure 244-3). To minimize soft tissue damage, obturators should be used whenever a tracheostomy tube is replaced.

After all of the equipment is in place, the patient is placed supine with a shoulder roll to extend the neck, the old tube is removed, the stoma suctioned gently and examined. In most cases, the opening in the trachea and the posterior tracheal wall can be visualized. Gently direct the fresh tube into the opening, curving it downward into the trachea (Figure 244-4). This movement should be smooth and gentle. If resistance is met, the tube is likely caught on the cartilaginous tracheal wall. Remove the tube and reexamine the stoma, then place the tube directly into the tracheal opening. If the tube still cannot be placed, consider placing the smaller tracheostomy tube. However, a smaller tube will also be shorter, and may not be long enough for the patient's neck. Correct tube position can verified by inserting a suction catheter into the tube. It should easily pass beyond the length of the tracheostomy tube without resistance. If there is a question about placement, a nasopharyngoscope or flexible bronchoscope can be passed through the tube for direct visualization of placement, or an x-ray obtained.

Patients who present with accidental decannulation and are in no distress can have the tracheostomy tube replaced as described above. **If the tube has been out for several hours, the stoma may begin to close and dilation may be needed prior to tube insertion.** If this is the case, and if the stoma is small and/or the tracheostomy is the patient's only airway, otolaryngologic consultation should be considered for tube replacement.

Tracheostomy Tube Obstruction

Although problems with the tracheostomy may be the cause of respiratory distress, all other causes should be considered and if the tracheostomy is found to be patent and in the airway, it should be left in place. Tracheostomy tube obstruction with mucous plugging is a

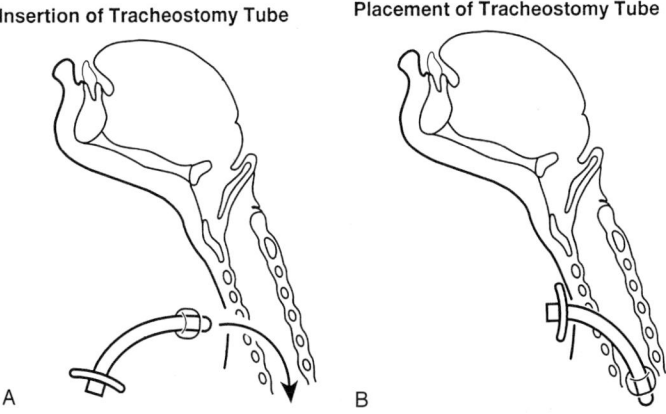

Insertion of Tracheostomy Tube   **Placement of Tracheostomy Tube**

A   B

FIG. 244-4. Insertion and placement of the tracheostomy tube. Cuffed tubes should be inserted with the cuff deflated.

common complication of this airway device. Secretions may act by a ball-valve mechanism, allowing air in but restricting exhalation. As outlined in Figure 244-2, suctioning may relieve the obstruction. However, the inner cannula of the tracheostomy tube and sometimes the entire tracheostomy tube may need to be removed and cleaned. Preoxygenation and placement of sterile saline solution into the trachea will to aid in suctioning. Prolonged use of large suction catheters without preoxygenation will cause hypoxemia.

Mechanical Ventilation with a Tracheostomy Tube

If the patient requires mechanical ventilation, an uncuffed tracheostomy tube will have a large air leak. If the patient cannot be effectively ventilated with an uncuffed tube, it should be replaced with a cuffed tube. If a tracheostomy tube is not readily available, an endotracheal tube may be inserted into the stoma in order to maintain airway security. If the stoma cannot be cannulated, the patient may be orotracheally intubated in order to secure the airway.

Laryngectomy Patients

Laryngectomy patients cannot be orally intubated. The only access to the tracheal bronchial tree in laryngectomy patients is through the neck. Occasionally, laryngectomy patients will wear a laryngectomy tube in their stoma, similar in appearance to a tracheostomy tube. **Laryngectomy patients can be distinguished from tracheostomy patients by history and physical examination, and by the fact that laryngectomy patients are unable to vocalize (or breathe) when the laryngectomy tube is occluded.**

Tracheostomy Dislodgement

The tracheostomy tube may be dislodged from the trachea, but not from the neck. In this case, a suction catheter cannot be passed through the tube and tracheostomy tube may extrinsically compress the trachea (Figure 244-5). In this circumstance, the entire tracheostomy tube should be immediately removed. When attempting to properly reinsert the tracheostomy tube, it may be difficult to accurately identify the actual tracheal stoma. A nasopharyngoscope should be inserted into the visible stoma in an attempt to identify the tracheal opening. If the latter still cannot be identified, otolaryngologic consultation is needed. If the patient cannot maintain the airway, oral intubation will be needed while awaiting the otolaryngologist.

Tracheostomy Site Infection

Indwelling tracheostomy tubes are contaminated with normal, and sometimes pathogenic, flora. Stomal skin infection, tracheitis, and bronchitis can be a recurring problem. *Staphylococcus aureus, Pseudomonas,* and *Candida* are often identified and broad-spectrum antibiotics are indicated in the setting of clinical disease. Dressing changes with gauze soaked in 0.25 percent acetic acid are effective for local wound infections.

Bleeding

Bleeding can occur immediately after a tracheostomy and in the late postoperative period.[5] Sources of hemorrhage include granulation tissue in the stoma or trachea, and erosion of thyroid vessels or the gland itself, the tracheal wall (frequently from suction trauma), or the innominate artery. Slow bleeding originating from the stoma may be controlled by packing the site with saline soaked gauze. If this is ineffective, the tube should be removed and the stoma and tracheal wall examined. Local bleeding can be controlled with silver nitrate or electrocautery. With more brisk bleeding, the tracheostomy tube should be replaced with a cuffed endotracheal tube with the cuff below the bleeding site. An endotracheal tube is preferred, as it is difficult to examine the site around the flange of a tracheostomy tube.

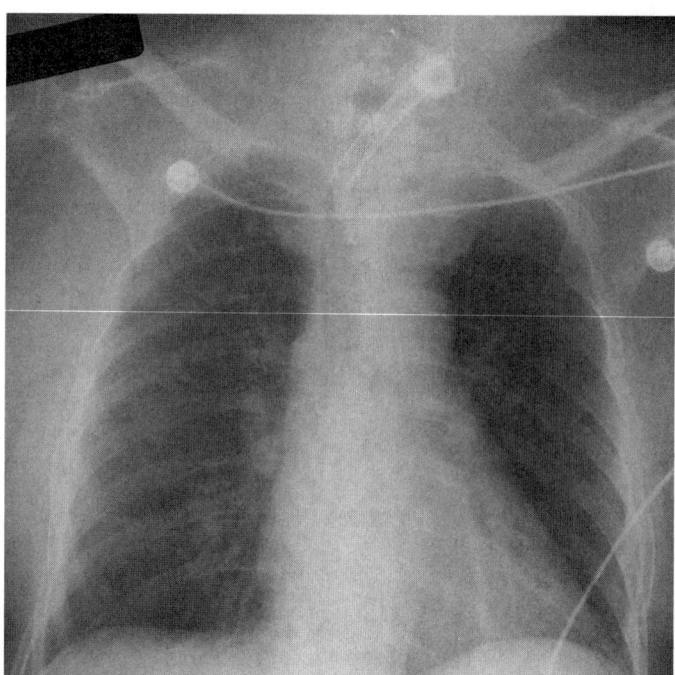

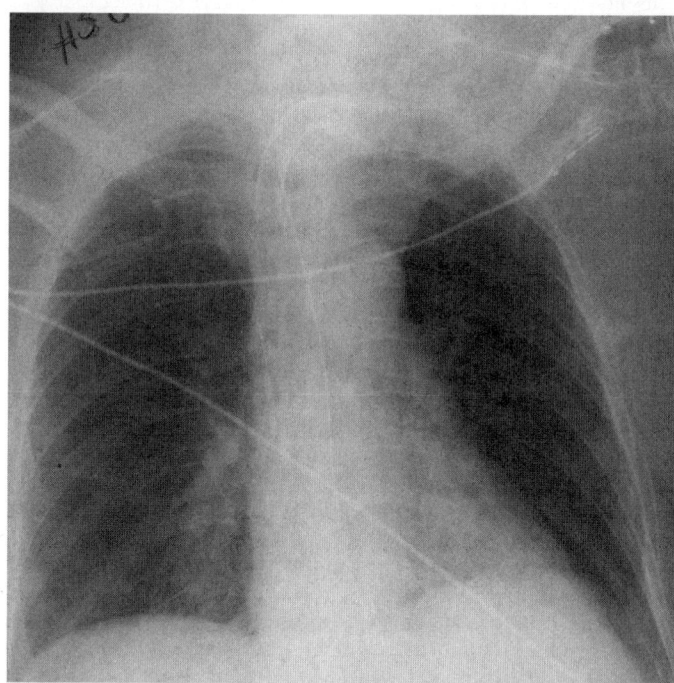

FIG. 244-5. **A.** Patient with a large goiter and a no. 4 Shiley tracheostomy tube with the tip of the tube outside the trachea and compressing the tracheal wall. **B.** Same patient with a longer no. 6 Shiley tracheostomy tube with the tip of the tube inside the trachea.

Tracheo-innominate artery fistula is a rare but life-threatening complication of tracheostomy.[6] Bleeding results from direct pressure of the tip of the tracheal cannula against the innominate artery (Figure 244-6). Maneuvers to control brisk bleeding while planning operative intervention include local digital pressure, hyperinflation of the cuff, and mild traction of the tube with manual pressure. Some patients may present with a sentinel bleed or hemoptysis. Such bleeding may be mild to severe and should not be taken lightly, because the potential exists for sudden massive hemorrhage. Immediate otolaryngologic consultation is required, and operative repair is lifesaving.

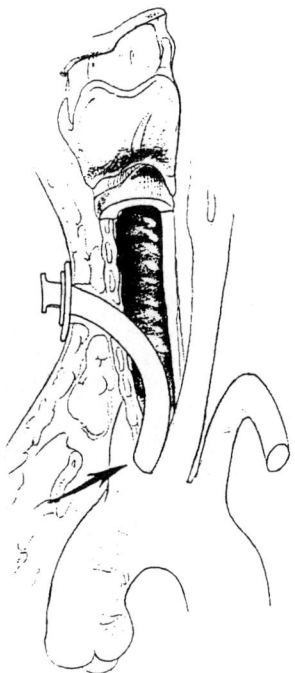

FIG. 244-6. The *arrow* points to the position of the tracheostomy tube in relation to the innominate artery. This close approximation facilitates creation of a tracheo-innominate fistula.

Tracheal Stenosis

Tracheal stenosis can present weeks to months after decannulation and results from mucosal necrosis and subsequent scarring. Signs and symptoms include dyspnea, wheezing, stridor, and the inability to clear secretions. A chest radiograph may demonstrate the narrowed airway. Medical treatment includes humidified oxygen, nebulized racemic epinephrine, and early administration of steroids. Operative treatment involves rigid bronchoscopy with laser excision of the scar bands, and stenting or tracheal reconstruction in more severe cases. Immediate otolaryngologic consultation is warranted.

LARYNGEAL STENTS

The surgical management of severe laryngotracheal stenosis often employs the insertion of tracheal stents for various periods of time. Placement of an endolaryngeal stent renders a patient tracheostomy dependent until the stent is removed, a result of blockage of the airway at the laryngeal level by the solid stent (Figure 244-7). Stents and their associated tracheostomy tubes should only be removed by surgeons familiar with their placement. There are many different endolaryngeal

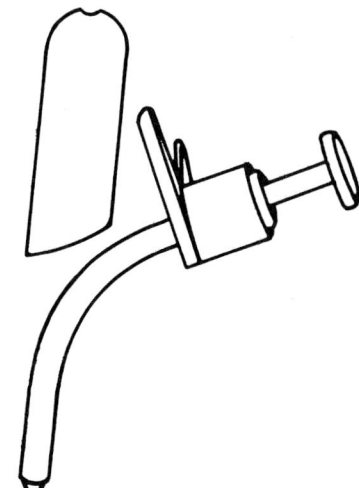

FIG. 244-7. Relation of the tracheostomy tube to the laryngeal stent. The stent lies within the lumen of the trachea, superior to the tracheostomy tube.

stent designs and materials, including silastic molds secured by cutaneous buttons, a stent secured by a strap that exits the tracheal stoma and is attached to the skin, the Aboulker stent complex (a metal tracheostomy tube wired to a silastic stent used in pediatric airway reconstruction), and the Montgomery T-tube stent (Figure 244-8). Although endolaryngeal stents are secured by buttons or straps, a known complication of these devices is dislodgment. If a stent becomes dislodged but the tracheostomy tube remains in position, airway security is usually not an issue. The operating surgeon should be notified when extrusion or dislodgment of any stent occurs.

The Montgomery T-tube configuration is commonly used in adult laryngotracheal reconstruction.[7] It is a modification of a tracheostomy tube that does not have an inner cannula. Humidification and suctioning of the T tube is essential to prevent mucous plugging. Airway obstruction should be addressed by first suctioning both the upper and lower limbs of the T tube (see Figure 244-8). If suctioning both limbs of the T tube does not relieve the obstruction, the T tube can be removed and the trachea cannulated with an appropriately sized tracheostomy tube or an endotracheal tube.

SPEECH DEVICES

The Passy-Muir valve is a one-way valve that fits directly over the opening of an uncuffed tracheostomy tube and allows the patient hands-free speech. When the patient inhales, the valve opens and allows air to pass into the trachea and lungs. Speech is created when the

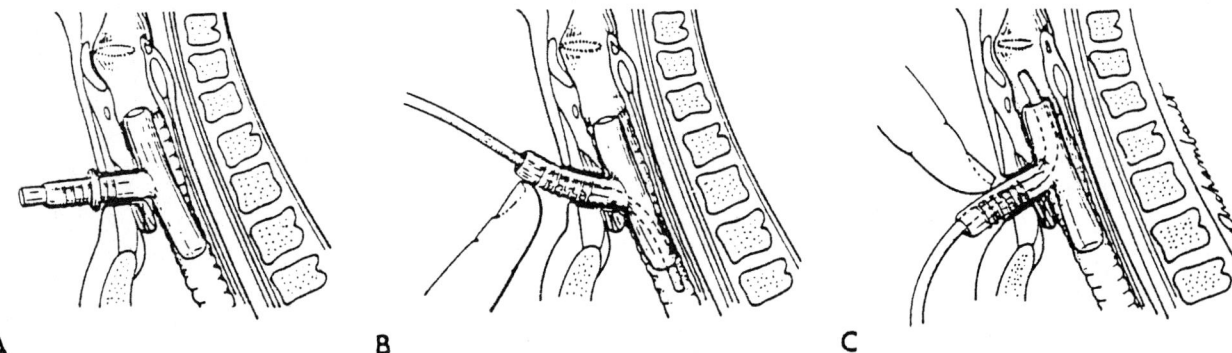

A **B** **C**

FIG. 244-8. Suctioning is required of both the upper and lower limbs of the Montgomery T tube. If necessary the entire T tube can be removed.

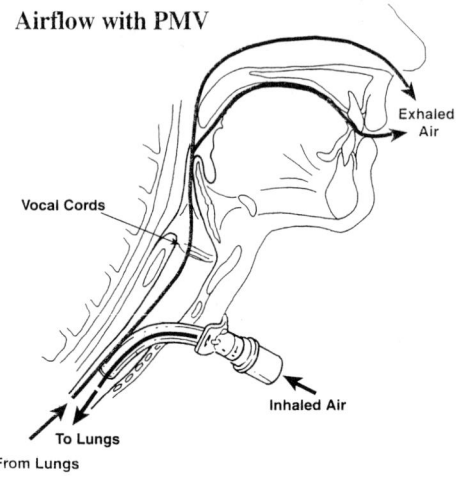

Airflow with PMV

Airflow with PMV on Tracheostomy Tube.

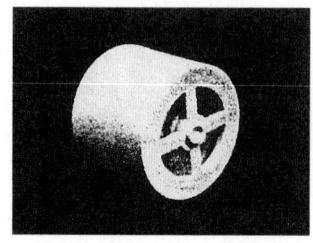 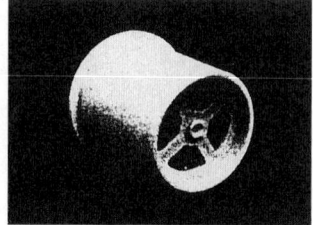

Passey-Muir Valve

FIG. 244-9. The Passy-Muir valve is a one-way valve that fits directly on the opening of the tracheostomy tube. Speech is created when the patient exhales as air is passed up through the vocal cords and out the mouth.

patient exhales hard enough to close the Passy-Muir valve and the air is thus directed around the tracheostomy tube and through the vocal cords (Figure 244-9). Because the patient exhales around the tracheostomy tube, a Passy-Muir valve should never be used with a cuffed tube. If a patient with a Passy-Muir valve develops signs of airway obstruction or an inability to speak, the speaking device should be removed from the tracheostomy tube so that air can pass freely during both inhalation and exhalation. If this does not relieve symptoms, check the tracheostomy tube itself for obstruction.

Speech in post laryngectomy patients has dramatically improved with the use of the tracheo-esophageal prosthesis. This one-way valve is surgically placed between the posterior wall of the tracheal stoma and the anterior wall of the cervical esophagus. To speak, patients exhale while occluding the stoma with their thumb, thus forcing the exhaled air into the esophagus. The air vibrates the esophagus (as a belch does) and the resultant tone is used to provide speech.

Two common complications with tracheo-esophageal prostheses are valve aspiration or extrusion. Aspiration results in persistent cough and respiratory distress. Chest x-ray should be done to visualize the radiopaque valve. Otolaryngologic consultation is indicated if there is suspicion of aspiration, as well as if the prosthesis is dislodged. The tracheo-esophageal puncture site will close quickly after the tube is

dislodged, and can be maintained by insertion of a Foley or red rubber catheter. This should not be attempted if the puncture is less than 2 weeks old, as a false passage may be formed in the neck.

REFERENCES

1. Roth S, Thisted R, Erikson J, Black S, Schreider B: Eye injuries after nonocular surgery. A study of 60,965 anesthetics from 1988 to 1992. *Anesthesiology* 85:1020, 1996.
2. Jougon J, Cantini O, Delcambre F, Minniti et al: Esophageal perforation: Life-threatening complication of endotracheal intubation. *Eur J Cardiothorac Surg* 20:7, 2001.
3. Chen E, Logman Z, Glass P, Bilfinger T: A case of tracheal injury after emergent endotracheal intubation: A review of the literature and causalities. *Anesth Analg* 93:1270, 2001.
4. Dunn P, Goulet R: Endotracheal tubes and airway appliances. *Int Anesthesiol Clin* 38:65, 2000.
5. Goldenberg D, Ari E, Golz A, et al: Tracheotomy complications: A retrospective study of 1130 cases. *Otolaryngol Head Neck Surg* 123:495, 2000.
6. Gelman JJ, Aro M, Weiss SM: Tracheo-innominate artery fistula. *J Am Coll Surg* 179:626, 1994.
7. Montgomery WW, Montgomery SK: Manual for use of Montgomery laryngeal, tracheal and esophageal prostheses: Update 1990. *Ann Otol Rhinol Laryngol Suppl* 150:2, 1990.

APPROACH TO
THE DERMATOLOGIC PATIENT
IN THE EMERGENCY DEPARTMENT

William J. Brady

Andrew D. Perron

Marcus L. Martin

The dermatologic syndromes seen in the emergency department span the spectrum of cutaneous disease. Most skin lesions involve infections, irritants, and allergies.[1] Fortunately, few presentations represent life- or limb-threatening skin disorders. Visual diagnosis with the use of pattern recognition is the key to cutaneous diagnosis. The recommended approach to the patient with skin disease in the emergency department (assuming resuscitation or stabilization is not required) is to:

1. Determine the chief complaint
2. Obtain a brief history (duration, rate of progression, and location of lesions)
3. Perform the dermatologic examination (morphology and distribution)
4. Formulate the differential diagnosis based on lesion morphology and distribution
5. Elicit additional concerns from the history (associated complaints, comorbidity, medications, or exposures) and include or exclude syndromes in the differential based on this information
6. Perform ancillary investigations, if necessary
7. Obtain dermatologic consultation, if necessary, and arrange for appropriate referral (primary care or dermatologic)

DIAGNOSTIC APPROACH

The History

Determine the chief complaint and obtain a brief history (discomfort, duration, rate of progression, and location of lesions). The secondary history should include issues relating to the lesion: morphology, evolutionary nature, rate of progression, and distribution. Associated systemic complaints and mucosal systems must be identified. Ask about exposures to medications (over-the-counter, prescription, and illicit), immunizations, toxins, chemicals, foods, animals, insects, plants, and ill contacts. Sexual history, if appropriate, and medical and family histories should be reviewed. Asking about medication use, sun exposure, or particular food ingestion also may yield helpful information.

The Examination

The dermatologic physical examination must be performed on the disrobed patient in a room with adequate lighting. All skin and mucosal surfaces must be inspected, including hair, nails, scalp, and mucous membranes. Then the specific skin lesions must be inspected. A magnifying lens and a portable lamp are helpful for conducting the examination.

The skin should be examined in a systematic, methodical, orderly process. The distribution, pattern, arrangement, morphology, extent, and evolutionary changes of the lesions must be determined. *Distribution* is the location of the skin findings, and the *pattern* is the anatomic, functional, and physiologic arrangements of the lesions. For example, a unilateral band-like arrangement of lesions on the thorax

suggests varicella-zoster infection. Skin diseases often present with a predilection for certain body areas; as such, location will assist in narrowing the diagnostic possibilities. From the anatomic perspective, the skin surfaces that are usually considered as separate areas of distribution include scalp, hair, face, eyelids, mouth, trunk, axilla, perineum, extremities, and nails; the extremities may be further subdivided into upper versus lower, proximal versus distal, wrists versus ankles, and hands versus feet (Figure 245-1). Rashes on exposed portions of the skin should prompt inquiries about sun exposure, jewelry, or topical agents. Refer to Table 245-1 for a differential diagnosis of skin lesions as a function of location. The clinician can use the "burn rule of 9's" (see Chap. 199, "Thermal Burns") to estimate the degree of skin involvement in disorders with widespread distribution. This calculation also may be used to determine the amount of topical medication required for a specific treatment course.

Lesion arrangement refers to the symmetry and configuration. Bilateral symmetry suggests a systemic internal event or symmetric external exposure, as seen in erythema multiforme, with plaque-like lesions on the flexor surfaces of the extremities or contact dermatitis related to a lotion application. An asymmetric arrangement supports a localized process. *Configuration* may apply to a single lesion with reference to its individual features or, alternatively, to multiple lesions and their relation to one another. For instance, internal configuration is illustrated by the relation between the central papule relative to the erythematous ring in the target lesion of erythema multiforme; on the total-body scale, configuration is demonstrated by clustering of lesions in a herpes virus infection or by a linear arrangement as with a reaction from poison ivy or oak. Other terms used to describe the lesion configuration are listed in Table 245-2.

Recognition of the primary lesion is vital in establishing the diagnosis. The primary lesion is the one that has not been altered by secondary issues, including healing, complicating infection, medication application, or scratching. Examples of primary skin lesions are macules, papules, nodules, tumors, cysts, plaques, wheals, vesicles, bullae, and pustules. Secondary lesions have had their appearance altered due to disease evolution or various external factors, as noted above, and include crusts, scales, fissures, erosions, ulcerations, excoriations, atrophy, scarring, and lichenification. See Table 245-3 for a listing with descriptions of the various morphologic descriptors of dermatologic lesions; refer to Tables 245-4 and 245-5 for a differential diagnosis of the various skin disorders relative to primary and secondary lesion morphologies.

Diagnostic Techniques

The KOH preparation is used in patients with suspected molluscum contagiosum and dermatophytic infections. The test is performed on loose skin scales, nail pairings, subungual debris, short residual hairs, or small pearly globules (from a molluscum body). Test steps are as follows:

1. Place material on the slide, gently crush it, and mix it with two drops of 20 percent KOH
2. Warm but do not boil the specimen and then let it sit for 10 min (thick scrapings may need 20 min)
3. Remove excess solution by placing a paper towel at the corner of the slide
4. Place a coverslip for thick specimens with gentle pressure to compress the material adequately for viewing

The material is then viewed under a microscope at low power, with the condenser and light at low levels. As the slide is scanned, rapidly focus

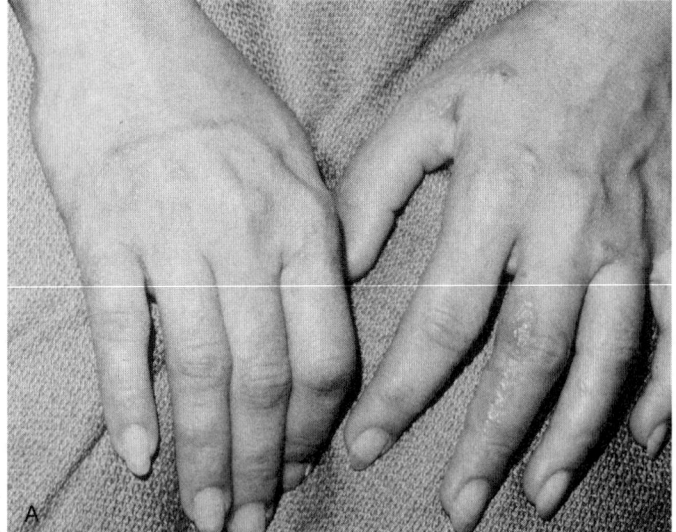

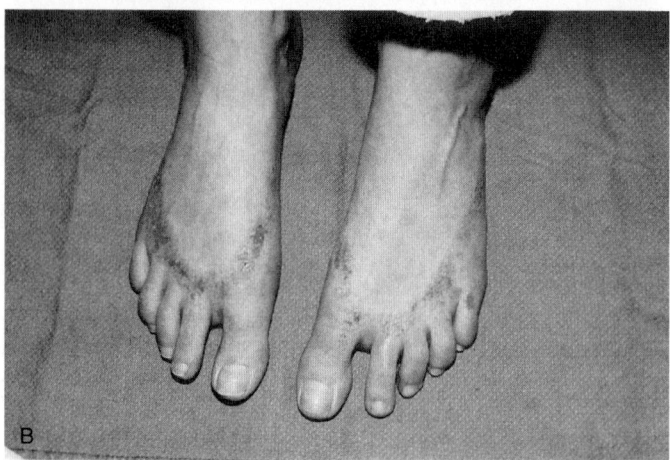

FIG. 245-1. Allergic contact dermatitis. **A.** Allergic contact dermatitis from exposure to poison ivy. Erythema, vesiculation and bullae are present on the fingers and the dorsal surfaces of the hands. Note the linear streak across the right hand. This finding is a diagnostic clue for rhus contact dermatitis (poison ivy). **B.** Allergic contact dermatitis to the straps of sandals. Erythema, scale and excoriations are noted in a symmetric patterned distribution matching to this patient's footwear.

up and down. True hyphae are long, branching, green rods of constant width that cross the borders of epithelial cells. Molluscum bodies are oval discs with homogeneous cytoplasm. In hair fragments, the organisms appear as small, round spores packed closely within the hair shaft.

Scabies and lice preparations are useful in patients with possible infestation. In scabies infestations, the rash itself may resemble other dermatologic syndromes; microscopic analysis will confirm the diagnosis. The donor site for skin specimen selection is very important. The best sites include burrows (10-mm, elongated papule with a pustule or vesicle) and papules on the fingers, wrists, and elbows. Within the vesicle or pustule, a small black dot is noted, which is the mite. The point of the scalpel is scraped across the lesion while holding the skin taut; the mite is then removed. A single drop of mineral oil may be applied to the blade to ensure that the scrapings adhere to the instrument. The material is then placed on the microscope slide with an additional drop of mineral oil; gentle pressure on the coverslip will flatten thick specimens. Using low power, the slide is scanned for presence of the mite, eggs, or feces. Mites are eight-legged creatures that are easily identified on thin smears; thick specimens may require additional

TABLE 245-1   Differential Diagnosis Relative to Lesion Distribution and Pattern

Pattern	Differential Diagnosis
Flexural (flexor areas of skin)	Atopic dermatitis, candidiasis, eczema, ichthyosis
Sun exposure (face, upper thorax, distal extremities)	Sunburn, photosensitive drug eruption, photosensitive dermatitis, systemic lupus erythematosus, viral exanthem, porphyria
Acrodermatitis (distal extremities)	Viral exanthem, atopic or contact dermatitides, eczema, Rocky Mountain spotted fever, gonococcemia
Pityriasis rosea (anterior and posterior thorax)	Pityriasis rosea, secondary syphilis, drug eruption, atopic or contact dermatitis, psoriasis
Clothing covered (thorax and distal lower extremities)	Contact dermatitis, psoriasis, folliculitis
Acneiform (face and upper thorax)	Acne, drug-induced acne, irritant dermatitides

viewing to look for the mite. Additional findings supportive of the diagnosis include eggs (smooth ovals) and feces (clusters of red-brown pellets). Lice are usually found on the scalp, eyelashes, and pubic areas and may be visible to the unaided eye. Moving objects in the area should be grasped with forceps and placed on a slide and viewed under low power. Head lice are long and thin, whereas pubic lice are shorter and broad.

The Tzanck smear, useful in blistering disorders, assists in establishing the diagnosis of a herpes infection: herpes simplex, herpes zoster, and varicella. The choice material for examination is obtained from the base of a recently unroofed lesion; purulent fluid at the base of the lesion is removed with a scalpel and placed on a microscope slide. The material is allowed to air dry and then is stained with Giemsa or Wright stain. Using low power, the slide is scanned for epithelial cells. Multinucleated giant cells, indicative of a herpes infec-

TABLE 245-2   Lesion Configuration Descriptors

Descriptor	Configuration
Annular	Ring-like or pertaining to the outer edge
Arcuate	Curved or pertaining to the curve
Circinate	Circular
Confluent	Blending together
Discoid	Solid, round, slightly raised or pertaining to a disk
Discrete	Separate or individual
Grouped	Clustered
Guttate	Scattered
Gyrate	Coiled or winding
Herpetiform	Creeping
Iris	Concentric circles
Linear	In a line
Polycyclic	Overlapping circles or borders of irregular curves
Retiform	Net-like
Serpiginous	Snake-like
Dermatomal	Belt-like or limited to one side of the body in anatomic dermatome

TABLE 245-3 Lesion Morphology

Descriptor	Morphology	Lesion Nature	Height Relative to Adjacent Skin
Erosion	Ruptured vesicle or bulla with denuded epidermis	Secondary	Depressed
Excoriation	Linear erosion	Secondary	Flat
Fissure	Linear cracks on skin surface	Secondary	Flat
Ulcer	Epidermal or dermal tissue loss	Secondary	Depressed
Macule	Flat, circumscribed discoloration ≤1 cm in diameter; color varies	Primary	Flat
Petechiae	Nonblanching purple spots <2 mm in diameter	Primary	Flat
Sclerosis	Firm, indurated skin	Secondary	Flat or elevated
Telangiectasia	Small, blanchable superficial capillaries	Primary	Flat
Purpura	Nonblanching purple discoloration of the skin	Primary	Flat
Abscess	Tender, erythematous, fluctuant nodule	Primary	Elevated
Cyst	Sack containing liquid or semisolid material	Primary	Elevated
Nodule	Palpable solid lesion <1 cm in diameter	Primary	Elevated
Tumor	Palpable solid lesion >1 cm in diameter	Primary	Elevated
Scar	Sclerotic area of skin	Secondary	Flat or elevated
Wheal	Transient, edematous papule or plaque with peripheral erythema	Primary	Flat or elevated
Vesicle	Circumscribed, thin-walled, elevated blister <5 mm in diameter	Primary	Elevated
Bulla	Circumscribed, thin-walled, elevated blister >5 mm in diameter	Primary	Elevated
Pustule	Vesicle containing purulent fluid	Primary	Elevated
Papule	Elevated, solid, palpable lesion <1 cm in diameter; color varies	Primary	Elevated
Plaque	Flat-topped elevation formed by confluence of papules >0.5 cm in diameter	Primary	Elevated
Comedo	Papule with an impacted pilosebaceous unit	Primary	Elevated

tion, are a syncytium of epidermal cells with multiple overlapping nuclei. The presence of the multinucleated giant cell does not distinguish between herpes simplex, herpes zoster, and varicella syndromes. Wood light examination is helpful in several different situations, including erythrasma (a superficial *Corynebacterium* infection of moist skin in the groin, axilla, and web spaces), tinea versicolor (a superficial fungal infection), certain pseudomonal skin infections, and porphyria cutanea tarda. Wood light is an ultraviolet source that emits light at a wavelength of 365 nm. The following fluorescent findings are noted in these conditions: erythrasma, red or pink; tinea versicolor, green or yellow; pseudomonas, yellow or green; and porphyria cutanea, orange or yellow (urine only). Other laboratory investigations are of limited value; selected tests are listed in Table 245-6 with the respective dermatologic disease.

TREATMENT

In general, the maxim "if it's dry, wet it, and if it's wet, dry it" applies to the initial therapy of many rashes. Water, protein, and lipid losses characterize dry skin diseases. Emollient creams and lotions restore water and lipids to the epidermis, hasten the healing process, and reduce pruritus and pain. Emollients are moisturizers that reduce skin dryness and decrease skin friction and the sensation of tightness. In patients with chronic drying dermatitides, ointments are best, particularly in the winter months. In warm climates, less viscous, less oily preparations, such as a cream, are better tolerated. Open wet dressings using tap water or normal saline not only reduce discomfort due to the dry-

ing but also clean the skin by painlessly loosening crusts and exudates. The various wet cutaneous syndromes involve similar protein and lipid losses due to excessive flow of transudative or exudative fluid from the diseased skin with leaching of the complex macromolecules of the epithelial cells. Drying agents retard this flow of fluid and associated biologic materials from the body, thus assisting in the curative process.

Corticosteroids

Urticaria, angioedema, and toxicodendron dermatitis (rhus, poison ivy, or poison oak) and other contact or allergic dermatitides are potential indications for systemic corticosteroids. Other dermatologic syndromes, such as erythema multiforme, toxic epidermal necrolysis, and vasculitis, are best treated with systemic steroids only after consultation with a dermatologist. In one study, small bursts of prednisone (40 mg daily for 4 days) markedly reduced the pruritus and hastened the clinical improvement of urticaria.[2] Patients with poison ivy or oak who require systemic steroids should be treated with oral prednisone (1 mg/kg body weight) with a slow 2- to 3-week taper. Other contact or allergic dermatitides may benefit from an abbreviated course (4 days) of oral prednisone. **However, oral corticosteroids are relatively contraindicated, or must be used with great care, in those with diabetes, hypertension, active peptic ulcer disease, psychiatric disease, and immunodeficiency.** Close follow-up is needed if oral corticosteroids are prescribed to these patients.

Topical corticosteroids are powerful and useful tools in the management of dermatologic disease. Numerous agents are available for

TABLE 245-4 Differential Diagnosis of Selected Skin Disorders Relative to Primary Lesion Morphology*

Lesion Morphology	Differential Considerations
Macule	Drug eruption (fixed or photosensitive), nevus, tattoo (ink), lice infestation, rheumatic fever, syphilis (secondary), viral exanthem erythema multiforme, toxic or infectious erythemas, meningococcemia (early), external trauma (ecchymosis), vitiligo, tinea versicolor, cellulitis (early)
Papule	Acne, basal cell carcinoma, melanoma, nevus, warts, molluscum contagiosum, skin tags, atopic dermatitis, urticaria, eczema, folliculitis, insect bites, vasculitis, psoriasis, scabies, toxicodendron dermatitis (poison ivy, oak, sumac), erythema multiforme, varicella (early), gonococcemia
Plaque	Eczema, pityriasis rosea, tinea corporis and versicolor, psoriasis, seborrheic dermatitis, urticaria, syphilis (secondary), erythema multiforme
Nodule	Basal cell, squamous cell, or metastatic carcinoma, melanoma, erythema nodosum, furuncle, lipoma, warts
Wheal	Urticaria, angioedema, insect bites, erythema multiforme
Pustule	Acne, folliculitis, gonococcemia, hidradenitis suppurativa, herpetic infection (herpes simplex, herpes zoster, varicella), impetigo, psoriasis, rosacea, pyoderma gangrenosum
Vesicle	Herpetic infection (herpes simplex, herpes zoster, varicella), impetigo, toxicodendron dermatitis (poison ivy, oak, sumac), thermal burn, friction blister, toxic epidermal necrolysis, bullous pemphigoid, pemphigus vulgaris
Bulla	Bullous impetigo, toxicodendron dermatitis (poison ivy, oak, sumac), thermal burn, friction blister, toxic epidermal necrolysis, bullous pemphigoid, pemphigus vulgaris

*This list is not exhaustive, but it represents the more common syndromes likely to be encountered by the emergency physician.

TABLE 245-5 Differential Diagnosis of Selected Skin Disorders Relative to Secondary Lesion Morphology*

Lesion Morphology	Differential Considerations
Scales	Psoriasis, pityriasis rosea, toxic and infectious erythemas, syphilis (secondary), dermatophytic infection (tinea), tinea versicolor, xerosis (dry skin), thermal burn (first degree)
Crusts	Eczema, dermatophytic infection (tinea), impetigo, contact dermatitis, insect bite
Erosions	Candidiasis, dermatophytic infection (tinea), eczema, toxic epidermal necrolysis, toxic-infectious erythemas, erythema multiforme, primary blistering disorders (bullous pemphigoid and pemphigus vulgaris), brown recluse spider envenomation
Ulcers	Aphthous lesions, chancroid, decubitus ulcer, thermal or friction injury, subacute or chronic ischemia, malignancy, chancre (primary syphilis), primary blistering disorders (bullous pemphigoid and pemphigus vulgaris), brown recluse spider envenomation, pyoderma gangrenosum, stasis ulcer, factitial

*This list is not exhaustive, but it represents the more common syndromes likely to be encountered by the emergency physician.

to a maximum of 2.5 percent. Hydrocortisone is safe and may be used on most body surfaces, including the face, genitalia, flexure creases, and intertriginous zones; it also is safe for use in infants and children. For the treatment of diseases involving the palms and soles, hydrocortisone is a poor choice, because the thickened skin does not allow adequate penetration of this relatively low-potency steroid. Corticosteroids of moderate potency, including triamcinolone acetonide and fluocinoline acetonide, are useful in severely inflamed skin and on the thicker skin of the scalp, trunk, extensor surfaces, palms, and soles. These agents should not be applied to the face or genitals or used in the infant. **Fluorinated steroids should not be prescribed to pregnant women.** See Table 245-8 for recommendations of corticosteroid potency relative to dermatologic disease.

Different skin surfaces respond differently to topical corticosteroid therapy; this different response rate varies relative to the absorption of the steroid into the deeper tissues. The relatively thin skin surfaces of the face respond very rapidly to the use of group 7 agents, whereas the thicker skin of the palms and soles requires a highly potent steroid. Irritations that resolve with an effective, higher potency application when using a low-potency agent include raw, inflamed skin (such skin more rapidly and readily absorbs medication), treatment regions involving skin surfaces in frequent contact, such as intertriginous areas (the apposition of two skin surfaces produces enhanced absorption of drug, similar to the effect to an occlusive dressing), and areas of skin surfaces enclosed under tight clothing, such as the diaper area (enhanced absorption of the agent due to the occlusive effect of the

TABLE 245-6 Selected Laboratory Investigations Useful in the Diagnosis of Dermatologic Disease

Laboratory Test	Dermatologic Disease
Sedimentation rate	Leukocytoclastic vasculitis
Urinalysis (active sediment)	Leukocytoclastic vasculitis
Microbiologic studies	Infectious syndromes (toxic and infectious erythemas, tick-borne illnesses, sexually transmitted diseases, etc.)
Platelet count and coagulation studies	Purpuric and petechial states

use. They differ in concentration, base components, and cost. Familiarity with a single agent in each potency class is sufficient to safely and effectively treat any steroid-responsive skin ailment. Corticosteroid potency or strength (i.e., the anti-inflammatory property) is measured by the agent's ability to induce vasoconstriction. Agents' strengths are rated by vasoconstricting ability on a scale of one to seven, with lower scale numbers correlating with more potent corticosteroids: group 1 agents are the most powerful corticosteroids, and group 7 medications are the least potent. Refer to Table 245-7 for a listing of topical corticosteroid agents relative to group potencies. Marked variation in potency is seen among various corticosteroids, whereas much less difference in strength is encountered for individual agents at different concentrations. Many corticosteroids are fluorinated. Fluorination greatly increases the potency but also increases the risk of adverse reactions and should not be used in pregnancy.

Use of the appropriate-strength topical steroid is strongly encouraged at the start of therapy. The use of a less powerful agent is not likely to spare the patient from potential adverse effect or produce adequate control of the disease. Hydrocortisone, perhaps the most frequently used topical corticosteroid in the outpatient setting, is available over the counter in strengths up to 1 percent and by prescription

TABLE 245-7   Listing of Topical Corticosteroid Agents Relative to Group Potencies*

Group	Generic Name	Trade Name (Preparation)	Potency (%)	Tube Size
1	Clobetasol propionate	Temovate (cream/ointment/gel)	0.05	15, 30, 45, 60 g
	Betamethasone dipropionate	Diprolene (lotion/ointment/gel)	0.05	15, 45 g
2	Halcinonide	Halog (cream/ointment/solution)	0.1	15, 30, 60, 240 g
	Fluocinonide	Lidex (cream/ointment/gel/solution)	0.05	15, 30, 60, 120 g
	Desoximetasone	Topicort (cream/ointment/gel)	0.25	15, 60, 120 g
3	Betamethasone dipropionate	Alphatrex (cream/lotion) Maxivate (lotion)	0.05	15, 45 g
	Triamcinolone acetonide	Aristocort (cream/ointment) Kenalog (cream/ointment) Trymex (cream)	0.5	15, 240 g
4	Triamcinolone acetonide	Aristocort (ointment) Kenalog (ointment) Trymex (ointment)	0.1	15, 60, 240 g
	Halcinonide	Halog (cream/ointment)	0.025	15, 60, 240 g
	Mometasone furoate	Elocon (cream/lotion)	0.1	15, 45
5	Triamcinolone acetonide	Aristocort (cream) Kenalog (cream/lotion) Trymex (cream)	0.1	15, 60, 240, 2520 g
	Flurandrenolide	Cordran (ointment)	0.025	30, 60 g
6	Triamcinolone acetonide	Aristocort (cream) Kenalog (cream/lotion) Trymex (cream)	0.025	15, 60, 240, 2520 g
7	Hydrocortisone	Hytone (cream/lotion/ointment)	1, 2.5	1, 2, 4 oz

*Preparations are listed by potency: Group 1 is most potent, and group 7 is least potent.

garment). In general, lower potency agents are acceptable in these situations.

The application of creams, ointments, gels, and lotions is relatively straightforward. The medication, applied in thin layers, should be massaged daily into the skin, as directed. Washing the skin before corticosteroid application is unnecessary. Patients should be advised to follow directions closely, early and late in the treatment course. Early application with extra medication per dose or more frequent medication administrations is not desired; likewise, a reduced frequency of application or a decreased amount of medication as the disease process responds to therapy can cause relapse. Optimum application regimens have not been determined for topical corticosteroids in most dermatologic syndromes. The more potent agents are best applied two to three times daily for 1 to 2 weeks followed by a drug-free week; additional therapy may be required as determined by the disease and by the particular patient's response to the initial therapy. Agents from the less potent steroid groups may be applied three times daily for 2 to 4 weeks followed by a 7-day steroid-free period.

The prescription of the correct amount of topical steroid is at times difficult. The burn rule of 9's may be used to estimate the amount of topical corticosteroid to prescribe. Calculate the percentage of body surface area requiring therapy and then multiply the percentage by a correction factor of 30. This calculation will provide the amount of topical corticosteroid in grams for a single application. Next, determine the number of administration required in the treatment course. For example, a thrice-daily regimen for a duration of 10 days ultimately requires 30 applications. The number of applications is multiplied by the amount required for a single use. In general, 9 g of topical steroid will cover 9 percent of the body surface area in a thrice-daily application for 1 day. Refer to Table 245-9 for a description of topical corticosteroid amount to be dispensed relative to the coverage area and duration of therapy.

Tachyphylaxis refers to the decrease in responsiveness to a drug as a result of enzyme-mediated events. The term is used in relation to topical corticosteroids in reference to acute tolerance to the vasoconstricting ability. In general, vasoconstriction has been demonstrated to decrease progressively over time after a topical steroid has been applied. Such reductions in strength due to tolerance are encountered as soon as 4 days into the treatment course in all potency groups but are felt to be more important in groups 1 and 2. A reasonable strategy to counter the development of tachyphylaxis is the use of interrupted application schedules; such an interrupted treatment course might include an initial thrice-daily application for 2 weeks, followed by 1 week without using the drug and a repeat of the cycle.

TABLE 245-8   Recommendations of Corticosteroid Potency Relative to Dermatologic Disease

Groups 1 and 2	Groups 3-5	Groups 6 and 7
Psoriasis Eczema, of hand (severe) Poison ivy (severe) Atopic dermatitis (severe)	Atopic dermatitis Stasis dermatitis Seborrheic dermatitis Tinea Scabies Nonspecific dermatitis, of face (severe)	Nonspecific dermatitis, of face, eyelids, and perineum

TABLE 245-9   Amount of Corticosteroid Cream to Dispense*

Body Area	Suggested Potency	Amount to Dispense (g)
Face	Low	45
Arm	Intermediate or low	90
Leg	Intermediate or low	180
Hand or foot	Intermediate or low	45
Forearm	Intermediate or low	45
Chest or back	Intermediate or low	180

*Based on thrice-daily applications for 10 days of therapy.

Antihistamine Agents

Antihistamines (H_1 antagonists) are used frequently in the management of dermatologic disease, particularly in the control of pruritus. These agents include the first-generation antihistamines, such as diphenhydramine and hydroxyzine. These H_1 antagonists may be used PO, IM, or IV. The second-generation antihistamine agents, including astemizole, cetirizine, fexofenadine, and loratadine, are newer agents that may be used in certain circumstances. In general, the newer antihistamines offer the advantages of reduced dosing frequency and less sedative effect, but they are more costly. Comparisons of these new medications with hydroxyzine are generally favorable but not in dramatic terms; comparisons among these second-generation agents do not demonstrate significant differences.[3,4] The use of topical antihistamine preparations is discouraged, because these agents are readily absorbed; dosing is therefore difficult to predict. Accidental overdosage may result in the patient who aggressively applies the preparation or is also using similar oral agents. Refer to Table 245-10 for suggested dosing, administration schedules, and routes of therapy for these antihistamines. H_2 antagonists (ranitidine or famotidine) also have demonstrated some benefit in the patient with an allergic-mediated event, in particular urticaria.

Numerous other antipruritic therapies are recommended, including Domeboro solution (aluminum sulfate diluted 1:10 with water) soaks, potassium permanganate baths, and oatmeal baths.

Antimicrobial Agents

Topical antibacterial agents are used primarily as adjuncts to wound dressings; these agents rarely are useful as primary therapy for superficial bacterial infections of the skin. The exception to this statement is topical mupirocin, which is reportedly as effective as oral antimicrobial agents in the management of impetigo. Concerning wound dressings, the agents commonly used include polymyxin B, bacitracin, neomycin, and silver sulfadiazine. Suggested benefits of these medications include reduced adherence of bandaging material to the wound, reduced coagulum, and decreased bacterial colonization. The impact on the rate of wound healing and the prevention of wound infection are less well characterized. Another use of topical antibacterial agents is the treatment of aphthous stomatitis with oral tetracycline

rinses. Systemic antibiotic therapy is useful in certain dermatologic syndromes and is discussed in other chapters.

Various topical antifungal agents are available for the treatment of candida and the dermatophytic infections. The imidazole and polyene classes of agents are the most commonly used in outpatient medicine. Members of the imidazole class include clotrimazole, miconazole, and ketoconazole, and the polyenes are represented by nystatin and amphotericin B. In general, the imidazoles are effective against yeasts and dermatophytes, whereas the polyenes are useful only in the treatment of candidal infections. Because of diagnostic confusion that may arise in the fungal etiology of the superficial infection, polyene agents are best avoided; imidazole agents will treat all such superficial fungal infections. Dermatophytic and yeast infections should be treated for prolonged periods to reduce the possibility of recurrence; in general, a 2- to 4-week period of therapy is advised. In cases involving significant discomfort, combination agents composed of imidazole and corticosteroid agents reduce discomfort and eradicate the organism. Selenium sulfide shampoo is effective against tinea versicolor when applied daily for 30 min for 14 days.

Acyclovir has been used extensively in patients with various herpes virus infections, including acute varicella, varicella zoster virus infections ("shingles"), and herpes simplex infections. Valacyclovir[5] and famciclovir[6] are acceptable therapies.[7] In general, these agents do not offer significant advantages over acyclovir, with the exception of reduced dosing frequency, perhaps by increasing compliance and, therefore, the possibility of an improved outcome.

Infestations with lice are treated with topical lindane, 1 percent permethrin, or pyrethrins. These agents are reasonably effective against adult lice but are less useful against the unhatched eggs (nits). Consequently, a second application 5 to 10 days after the initial treatment should clear the new generation of lice, which was not affected by the first use. **Central nervous system toxicity has been reported in small infants treated with lindane, so permethrin or pyrethrins should be used in children.** Scabies also may be treated with one overnight application of lindane or 5 percent permethrin covering the entire non-hair-bearing skin surface.

Topical Agent Vehicle Considerations

The *vehicle,* or medication base, is the substance in which the active ingredient is dispersed. The base determines the rate at which the active ingredient is absorbed through the skin. Components of some bases may cause irritation or allergy. Creams, a mixture of oils, water, and preservative, are white in color and greasy in texture. Creams are the most versatile vehicle and can be applied to any body surface area; they are particularly useful in the intertriginous areas. Creams are best used for acute therapy only; chronic application may cause excessive drying. Ointments are composed of greases such as petroleum jelly and are free of preservative; little water is added to this vehicle. This vehicle is translucent and, when applied to the skin, remains greasy. This greasy consistency may aid in the lubrication in particularly dry lesions. In general, ointment vehicles allow deeper tissue penetration when compared with the cream base. Ointments also are occlusive, providing very thorough coverage with deep tissue penetration and allowing little movement in moisture and other material into and out of the skin. Acute exudative syndromes and intertriginous areas of the body should not be treated with topical steroids using the ointment vehicle. Gels are greaseless mixtures of propylene glycol and water and at times includes alcohol. Gels have a translucent appearance and are described as "sticky." Alcohol-containing gels are best for acute exudative lesions, such as poison ivy dermatitis, whereas alcohol-free combinations should be applied to dry, scaling conditions. In denuded areas, the alcohol component may cause discomfort. Gels are of particular use in the scalp area; their presence does not alter the arrangement of the hair and is therefore more tolerable for the patient from the cosmetic perspective. Solutions or lotions may contain water or alco-

TABLE 245-10   Antihistamines Useful in the Management of Dermatologic Disease

Medication (Trade Name)	Adult Dose	Pediatric Dose
Diphenhydramine (Benadryl)	25–50 mg PO/IV/IM q6h	4–6 mg/kg per 24 h PO/IV/IM q6–8h, maximum 200 mg/24 h
Hydroxyzine (multiple names)	25–100 mg PO/IV q8h	2–4 mg/kg per 24 h PO/IV q8–12h, maximum 200 mg/24 h
Astemizole* (Hismanal)	10 mg PO q24h	10 mg PO q24h†
Cetirizine* (Zyrtec)	5–10 mg PO q24h	5–10 mg PO q24h†
Fexofenadine* (Allegra)	60 mg PO q12h	Not recommended‡
Loratadine* (Claritin)	10 mg PO q24h	10 mg PO q24h†

*Indication limited to chronic idiopathic urticaria (see package inserts for details).
†Pediatric use is recommended only in children 6 years or older (see package inserts for details).
‡Pediatric use not recommended according to package insert.

hols in addition to other agents. They are clear or milky in appearance; with their liquid consistency, they are best applied to the scalp and other dense hair-bearing areas without leaving significant residue on the hair. In denuded areas, the alcohol component may cause discomfort. Guidelines for specialty consultation or hospital admission are similar. First, extensive skin involvement by erythroderma, bullae, or a palpable purpura suggests the need for rapid emergency department consultation followed by hospital admission. However, certain dermatologic syndromes typically present with generalized involvement and do not require specialty care; classic examples are urticaria and angioedema, acute varicella, and toxicodendron dermatitis. If the diagnosis is in question in the patient with a generalized rash, consider the need for dermatologic consultation.

General medical concerns that might prompt consultation and admission include cardiorespiratory instability, the systemic signs and symptoms, multisystem involvement, significant comorbidity, patient's age, poor home environment, or the need for the initiation of aggressive medical therapy.

REFERENCES

1. Feldman SR, Fleischer AB, McConnell RC: Most common dermatologic problems identified by internists, 1990–1994. *Arch Intern Med* 158:726, 1998.
2. Pollack CV, Romano TJ: Outpatient management of acute urticaria: The role of prednisone. *Ann Emerg Med* 26:547, 1995.
3. Tharp MD: Cetirizine: A new therapeutic alternative for chronic urticaria. *Cutis* 58:94, 1996.
4. Goldsmith P, Dowd PM: The new H$_1$ antihistamines. *Dermatol Clin* 11:87, 1993.
5. Acosta EP, Fletcher CV: Valacyclovir. *Ann Pharmacother* 31:185, 1997.
6. Crumpacker C: The pharmacological profile of famciclovir. *Semin Dermatol* 15(suppl):14, 1996.
7. Stein GE: Pharmacology of new antiherpes agents: Famciclovir and valacyclovir. *J Am Pharm Assoc (Wash)* NS37:157, 1997.

246 SERIOUS GENERALIZED SKIN DISORDERS

William J. Brady

Andrew D. Perron

Daniel J. DeBehnke

This chapter describes selected serious generalized skin disorders in adults and discusses their dermatologic diagnosis and treatment. Discussed are erythema multiforme, toxic epidermal necrolysis (TEN), the toxic infectious erythemas, disseminated viral infections, Rocky Mountain spotted fever (RMSF), meningococcemia, purpura fulminans, and the systemic bullous diseases.

ERYTHEMA MULTIFORME

Erythema multiforme (EM) is an acute inflammatory skin disease presenting across a spectrum. It ranges from a localized papular eruption of the skin (EM minor) to a severe, multisystem illness (EM major) with widespread vesiculobullous lesions and erosions of the mucous membranes, known as Stevens-Johnson syndrome (SJS). The disorder strikes all age groups, with the highest incidence in young adults (age range 20 to 40 years), affects males twice as often as females, and occurs commonly in the spring and fall. Infection, especially mycoplasma and herpes simplex virus (HSV), drugs, especially antibiotics and anticonvulsants, and malignancies are common precipitating factors. However, there is no identifiable etiology in approximately 50 percent of cases.[1]

The pathogenesis of EM remains largely unknown. Most likely, it is the result of a hypersensitivity reaction with the demonstration of immunoglobulin and complement components in the cutaneous microvasculature on immunofluorescence studies of skin biopsy specimens, circulating immune complexes in the serum, and mononuclear cell infiltrate on histologic examination.[1,2]

Patients frequently experience malaise, fever, myalgias, and arthralgias. Diffuse pruritus or a generalized burning sensation can occur before the skin develops lesions. The morphologic configuration of the lesions is quite variable, hence the descriptor *multiforme*. Maculopapular (Figure 246-1A, **Plate 10**) and target (iris, Figure 246-1B, **Plate 11**) lesions are the most characteristic. Erythematous papules appear symmetrically on the dorsum of the hands and feet and on the extensor surfaces of the extremities. The maculopapule evolves into the classic target lesion during the next 24 to 48 h. As the maculopapule enlarges, the central area becomes cyanotic, occasionally accompanied by central purpura or a vesicle. Urticarial plaques also may occur with or without the iris lesion in a similar distribution. Vesiculobullous lesions, which may be pruritic and painful, develop within preexisting maculopapules or plaques, usually on the extensor surface of the arms and legs, less frequently involving the trunk. Vesiculobullous lesions are found most often on mucosal surfaces, including the mouth, eyes, vagina, urethra, and anus; they may also be seen on the trunk. Ocular involvement occurs in approximately 10 percent of patients with EM minor, whereas ophthalmologic lesions in almost 75 percent of patients with SJS.

The various lesions (Table 246-1) develop in successive crops during a 2- to 4-week period, and crops heal over 5 to 7 days. Scarring is rarely a problem except in cases of secondary infection or in heavily pigmented patients in whom hypopigmentation or hyperpigmentation may occur. Recurrence may be noted on repeat exposure to the etiologic agent, a special concern in cases associated with HSV infection or medication use.[3] The rate of EM recurrence is very high in children with HSV infection. For example, 75 percent of children with a history of HSV-related EM experienced EM recurrence after HSV reactivation.[3] Fluid and electrolyte disorders and secondary infection from cutaneous sites represent the most frequent complications and the most common causes of death in the EM patient. The differential diagnosis of EM includes herpetic (herpes simplex virus and varicella zoster virus) infection, vasculitis, TEN, various primary blistering disorders (pemphigus and pemphigoid), urticaria, Kawasaki disease, and the toxic and infectious erythemas.

Outpatient treatment of EM minor with topical corticosteroids is possible, but steroids should not be applied to eroded areas of the skin. Dermatologic consultation may be required; close follow-up with the primary care doctor is advised. Those patients with extensive disease, systemic toxicity, and/or mucous membrane involvement require hospitalization, optimally in the intensive care or burn unit setting.

Systemic steroids are commonly used and provide symptomatic relief, but are of unproven benefit in influencing the duration and outcome of EM.[4] Many authorities recommend a short, intensive steroid course of prednisone, 60 to 80 mg per d PO in divided doses, particularly in drug-related cases, with abrupt cessation in 3 to 5 days if no favorable response is noted. Systemic analgesic agents and antihistamines provide symptomatic relief. Stomatitis is treated with diphenhydramine and viscous lidocaine mouth rinses. Caution is advised with oral lidocaine due to its remarkable efficacy and related neurotoxicity if excessively applied. Blisters are treated with cool, wet Burow's solution (5% aluminum acetate) compresses. Ocular involvement should be monitored by an ophthalmologist; unfortunately, burst steroid therapy does not appear to reduce the chance of development or significance of existing ocular lesions. Acyclovir may reduce recurrence of HSV infection and, therefore, lessen the potential for another bout of EM; prolonged, prophylactic acyclovir therapy may reduce the chance of recurrent EM related to HSV.[3] Erythema multiforme, in particular SJS, has significant morbidity and a mortality of approximately 10 percent despite aggressive therapy.

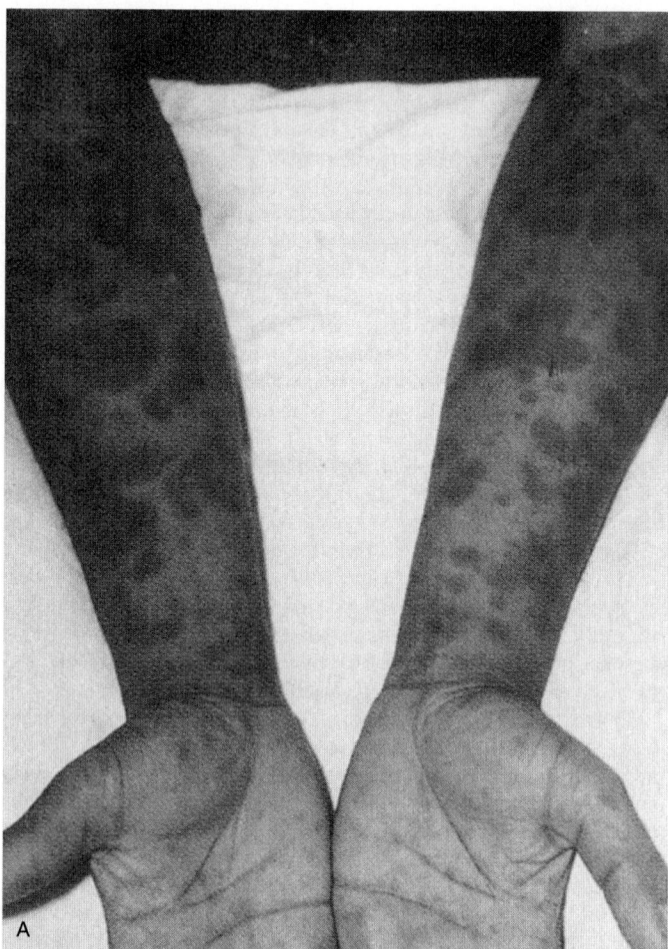

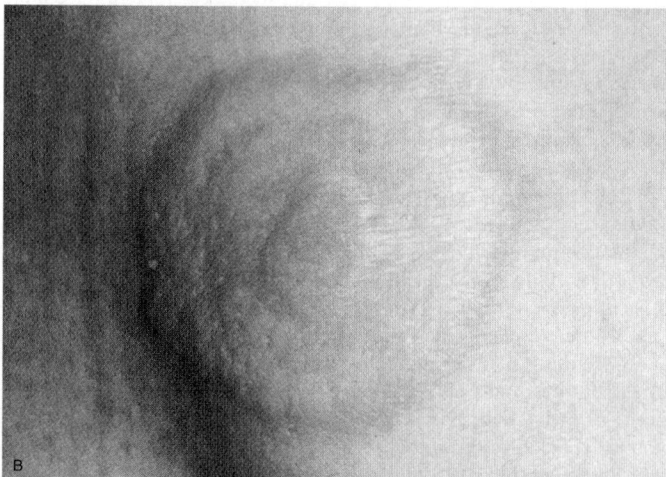

FIG. 246-1. A. (PLATE 10). Erythema multiforme. Symmetrical, plaque-like lesions involve the flexor surface of the upper extremities; these lesions may be misdiagnosed as the immunoglobulin G-mediated urticarial allergic reaction. Also note the erythematous macules on the palms. **B. (PLATE 11).** Iris or target lesion, a finding strongly suggestive of erythema multiforme. This iris lesion is composed of a central bullous lesion with a dusky, edematous center and an erythematous halo. (Reprinted with permission from Brady W, DeBehnke D, Crosby D: Dermatologic emergencies. *Am J Emerg Med* 12:217, 1994.)

TOXIC EPIDERMAL NECROLYSIS

Toxic epidermal necrolysis is an explosive dermatosis characterized by tender erythema, bullae formation, and subsequent exfoliation. Pa-

TABLE 246-1   Lesions of Erythema Multiforme

Erythematous papule or macule
Maculopapule
Iris (or target) lesion
Urticarial lesion
Vesiculobullous
Mucous membrane involvement

tients may be systemically ill on presentation. Many authorities consider the SJS variant of EM and TEN as the same process.[2] Toxic epidermal necrolysis is found in all age groups without predilection to sex. The syndrome has multiple possible etiologies, with medications representing the most common cause.[1,2,5] Sulfa and penicillin antibiotics, anticonvulsants, and oxicam nonsteroidal anti-inflammatory drugs are the most frequent drug triggers for TEN.[6,7] Other causes include malignancy and human immunodeficiency virus.[5] In many cases, an etiology is not found.

The pathogenesis is poorly understood and may be partly an immunologic and partly a genetic predisposition. The tendency to develop TEN may be linked to a highly specific genetic defect in the detoxification of the culprit drug or its reactive metabolites.[8] Human lymphocyte antigen typing also has suggested a possible genetic predisposition.

Patients with TEN often present with a 1- to 2-week prodrome of malaise, anorexia, arthralgias, fever, or upper respiratory infection symptoms. Skin tenderness, pruritus, tingling, or burning may be found at this time. Skin signs (Table 246-2) begin with a warm erythema, initially involving only the eyes, nose, mouth, and genitalia, but later becoming generalized. The erythematous areas become tender and confluent within hours. Flaccid, ill-defined bullae then appear within the areas of erythema. Lateral pressure with a finger on normal skin adjacent to a bullous lesion dislodges the epidermis, producing denuded dermis and demonstrating Nikolsky sign. The bullae form along the cleavage plane between the epidermis and the dermis. The epidermis is then shed in large sheets, leaving raw, denuded areas of exposed dermis. The average time of onset after exposure to the inciting agent is 2 weeks. Cutaneous extension follows an unpredictable time course, ranging from 24 h to 15 days, with a minority of severe cases demonstrating rapid, extensive involvement within 24 h.

Perilabial blistering and erosive lesions are disfiguring and often impair adequate oral intake, contributing to hypovolemia. Ocular complications include purulent conjunctivitis, painful erosions, and potential blindness. Anogenital lesions are common. Additional mucous membrane involvement includes the gastrointestinal, urinary, and respiratory tracts. The two major complications and leading causes of death in TEN are infection and hypovolemia with electrolyte disorders. A broad range of pathogens is usually found, with staphylococcal and pseudomonal species predominating. The mortality rate has been reported as being between 25 and 30 percent. These clinical variables are associated with poor prognosis: advanced age, extensive disease, idiopathic nature, multiple medication use, steroid therapy, azotemia, hyperglycemia, leukopenia, and thrombocytopenia.[6] The differential diagnosis of TEN includes staphylococcal scalded skin syndrome (SSSS), EM, toxic shock syndrome (TSS; staphylococcal and streptococcal), exfoliative drug reactions, primary blistering disorders (pemphigus and pemphigoid), and Kawasaki syndrome.

TABLE 246-2   Lesions of Toxic Epidermal Necrolysis

Warm, tender erythroderma
Vesicle
Bulla
Vesiculobullous
Exfoliation
Mucous membrane involvement

Management of TEN requires hospitalization in a critical care setting or, optimally, a burn unit.[6] In most cases, therapy is similar to the approach for the burn patient. Immediate concerns center on the airway, because sloughing of airway and respiratory epithelium can occur. Hypovolemia and electrolyte abnormalities should be corrected. Prompt, aggressive antibiotic administration is necessary in suspected or documented infection; initial prophylactic antibiotics are not recommended by most. The advice of the burn center should be followed for any topical dressings that are applied before transfer.

EXFOLIATIVE DERMATITIS

Exfoliative dermatitis, a cutaneous reaction produced in response to a drug or a chemical agent or to an underlying systemic or cutaneous disease, is a condition in which most or all of the skin surface is involved with a scaly erythematous dermatitis. Males are affected twice as often as females, and most patients are older than 40 years. The mechanisms responsible are not known, although drug-induced exfoliative dermatitis may be mediated by an increased activity of sensitized suppressor or cytotoxic T lymphocytes.

Exfoliative dermatitis can have an abrupt onset, particularly when related to a drug, contact allergen, or malignancy, whereas exacerbations related to an underlying cutaneous disorder usually evolve more slowly. In many cases, exfoliative dermatitis tends to be a chronic condition, with a mean duration of 5 years, when related to a chronic illness; a shorter course often follows suppression of the underlying dermatosis, discontinuation of causative drugs, or avoidance of allergen. Idiopathic and chronic disease-related exfoliative dermatitis can continue for 20 or more years; death is rare.

Generalized erythema and warmth are noted, similar to TEN, but skin tenderness is usually lacking. Erythema is accompanied by scaling or flaking, and the patient often complains of pruritus and skin tightness (Figure 246-2, **Plate 12**). The process usually begins on the face and upper trunk with progression to other skin surfaces. The patient usually has a low-grade fever. Excessive heat loss and hypothermia can complicate erythroderma. Widespread cutaneous vasodilation may result in high-output congestive heart failure. The disruption of the epidermis results in increased transepidermal water loss, and continued exfoliation can result in significant protein loss and negative nitrogen balance. Chronic inflammatory exfoliation produces many changes, such as dystrophic nails, thinning scalp and body hair, and patchy or diffuse pigmentation changes.

The differential diagnosis of exfoliative dermatitis includes SSSS, EM, TEN, TSS (staphylococcal and streptococcal), and Kawasaki disease. Considerable effort must be made to determine the underlying etiology, including evaluation for underlying malignancy, and biopsy of involved skin. Patients generally require emergent dermatologic consultation and admission. Hypothermia and hypovolemia should be corrected, and systemic corticosteroids are often given after consultation.

TOXIC INFECTIOUS ERYTHEMAS

A number of infectious syndromes caused by toxigenic bacteria with toxin-mediated dermatologic manifestations have been described, including TSS, streptococcal toxic shock syndrome (STSS), SSSS, bullous impetigo, and scarlet fever. In certain cases, the bacteria are colonizers with the disease resulting only from the toxin (e.g., TSS); in other instances, the toxigenic organism produces infection with clinical manifestations developing from the infectious process and the presence of the toxin (e.g., STSS, SSSS, bullous impetigo, and scarlet fever).

Toxic Shock Syndrome

The general features and management of TSS are discussed in Chap. 142, and the dermatologic features are discussed below. The dermatologic hallmark of TSS is nonpruritic, blanching macular erythroderma, a characteristic feature and a major criterion for the diagnosis (Figure 246-3, **Plate 13**). The erythroderma is usually diffuse, although it may be confined to the extremities or trunk and may resemble sunburn. The rash may be subtle and is often missed in heavily pigmented patients or when the patient is examined in a poorly illuminated room. Erythroderma may resolve in 3 to 5 days, and a fine desquamation of the hands and feet follows in 5 to 14 days. Other dermatologic manifestations include conjunctival and mucosal hyperemia, petechiae, alopecia, and fingernail loss. Refer to Table 142-1 for the case definition of TSS. The differential diagnosis is broad and includes scarlet fever, RMSF, leptospirosis, rubeola, meningococcemia, STSS, SSSS, Kawasaki syndrome, TEN, SJS, gram-negative sepsis, and exfoliative drug eruptions.

Streptococcal Toxic Shock Syndrome

Streptococcal TSS is an uncommon clinical syndrome that involves multiple organ systems with fever, hypotension, and skin findings.[10] The causative agent of this clinical disorder is *Streptococcus pyogenes* (group A *Streptococcus*). Streptococcal species produce extracellular

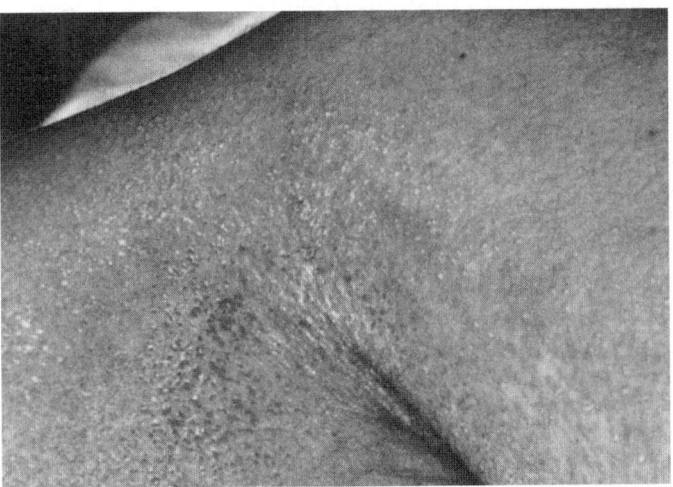

FIG. 246-3. (PLATE 13). Blanching, nonpruritic erythroderma with a "rough" texture in a patient with toxic shock syndrome. (Reprinted with permission from Brady W, DeBehnke D, Crosby D: Dermatologic emergencies. *Am J Emerg Med* 12:217, 1994.)

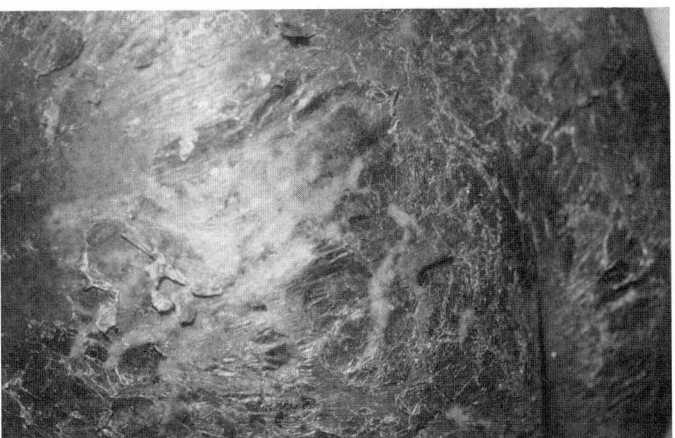

FIG. 246-2. (PLATE 12). Exfoliative dermatitis demonstrated by generalized, warm erythema accompanied by scaling or flaking.

proteins called *streptococcal pyrogenic exotoxins*. Invasive soft tissue streptococcal infection, such as cellulitis, myositis, or fasciitis, is a common factor in the etiology of STSS.

The clinical presentation of STSS includes fever, hypotension, skin edema, and erythema, or bullae (Figure 246-4, **Plate 14**). Subsequent desquamation occurs less commonly than during staphylococcal TSS. The same major and minor criteria used for the diagnosis of staphylococcal TSS can be helpful in identifying patients with STSS. According to a consensus document,[11] clinical features must include isolation of group A streptococci *(S. pyogenes)* and hypoperfusion and evidence of multisystem dysfunction. Because up to 75 percent of cases of STSS have associated soft tissue infection, a thorough skin examination for the site of infection is warranted. Palpate muscle groups for tenderness, indicating possible myositis or fasciitis, and evaluate for secondary compartment syndrome. Treatment is oxygenation and fluid resuscitation. Because soft tissue infection plays a large role in STSS, aggressive management of infection is essential. The site of infection should be identified, incised, and drained, and nonviable tissue should be debrided. Parenteral nafcillin, oxacillin, or vancomycin or a first-generation cephalosporin are often given as initial therapy.

Staphylococcal Scalded Skin Syndrome

Staphylococcal scalded skin syndrome develops in patients with clinically inapparent staphylococcal infections caused by an exotoxin produced by *Staphylococcus aureus*. It occurs primarily in infants and young children and in immunosuppressed adults or those with renal insufficiency. The exotoxins involved, collectively known as *exfoliatin,* are elaborated by the bacteria, released into the circulation, and cause acantholysis and intraepidermal cleavage of the skin.[12]

An episode of SSSS frequently begins as a clinically inapparent staphylococcal infection of the conjunctiva, nasopharynx, or umbilicus. The disease course can be divided into three phases: initial (erythroderma), exfoliative, and desquamation (recovery). Initially, the patient (or parent) notes the sudden appearance of a tender erythroderma, usually diffuse, although localized disease has been described. The involved skin may have a sandpaper texture. Tender erythema is prominent in the perioral, periorbital, and groin regions and in the skin creases of the neck, axilla, popliteal, and antecubital areas. The mucous membranes are spared. The exfoliative stage begins on the second day of the illness. The erythematous skin wrinkles and peels off at sites of minor trauma or with minimal lateral pressure with the examiner's fingertip, illustrating the positive Nikolsky sign (also found in TEN). Large, flaccid, fluid-filled bullae and vesicles then appear. These lesions easily rupture and are shed in large sheets; the underlying tissue resembles scalded skin and rapidly desiccates. After 3 to

5 days of illness, the involved skin desquamates, leaving normal skin in 7 to 10 days. The differential diagnosis for SSSS includes TEN, TSS, exfoliative drug eruptions, and localized bullous impetigo.

Management includes fluid resuscitation, correction of electrolyte abnormalities, and identification and treatment of the source of the toxigenic staphylococcus with oxacillin or vancomycin. Corticosteroids are not recommended.

DISSEMINATED VIRAL INFECTIONS

Infectious Exanthems

Many viral infections are associated with generalized morbilliform cutaneous eruptions. The list is exhaustive but most commonly include adenoviruses, cytomegalovirus, coxsackie and echoviruses, Epstein-Barr virus, hepatitis B virus, human herpesvirus 6, paramyxovirus, respiratory syncytial virus, rotaviruses, rubella virus, and human immunodeficiency virus. Other agents associated with generalized eruptions include mycoplasma, *Borrelia* spp., *Legionella, Leptospira, Listeria,* meningococci, rickettsiae, and *Treponema pallidum.* Erythematous macules and papules or, less often, vesicles and petechiae usually develop centrally, sparing the palms and soles. Diagnosis and differential diagnosis are based on history and physical examination. Drug eruption should always be considered in the differential. Skin lesions usually resolve in 7 to 10 days and are treated symptomatically.

Herpes Zoster

Varicella zoster infections, also referred to as *shingles* or *zoster,* represent reactivation of the previously dormant virus, *Herpesvirus varicellae,* in a patient with an altered immune response. At reactivation, the virus travels down specific sensory nerves to the skin, resulting in skin manifestations of shingles. Patients with lymphoma, leukemia, or diabetes mellitus and who are immunocompromised are at risk for reactivated or disseminated infection.

The rash of herpes zoster consists of clusters of vesicles and papules grouped on an erythematous base (Table 246-3). Vesicles initially appear clear but become cloudy or purulent over several days. They eventually rupture and crust over. The lesions usually appear along an individual dermatome (Figure 246-5, **Plate 15**); less often, adjacent dermatomes are involved. The lesion clusters are usually discrete and separated by normal skin; in the severe case, the cluster may become confluent along the dermatome. Approximately 60 percent of all zoster infections involve the trunk, followed by the head, extremity, and perineal regions in decreasing incidence.[13] Unilateral involvement that abruptly halts at the midline is helpful in correctly identifying the rash; occasionally, a few lesions appear immediately beyond the midline. Involvement of the nose should prompt evaluation for corneal involvement (Figure 246-6, **Plate 16**).

Approximately one-half of cases with varicella zoster infection, in particular those patients with acquired immunodeficiency syndrome (AIDS) or reticuloendothelial malignancy, experience viremia and may exhibit solitary lesions, usually fewer than 30 scattered across the body. Patients with AIDS, using immunosuppressive medications, or with active reticuloendothelial malignancy more often demonstrate true dissemination in which widespread vesicular lesions are distrib-

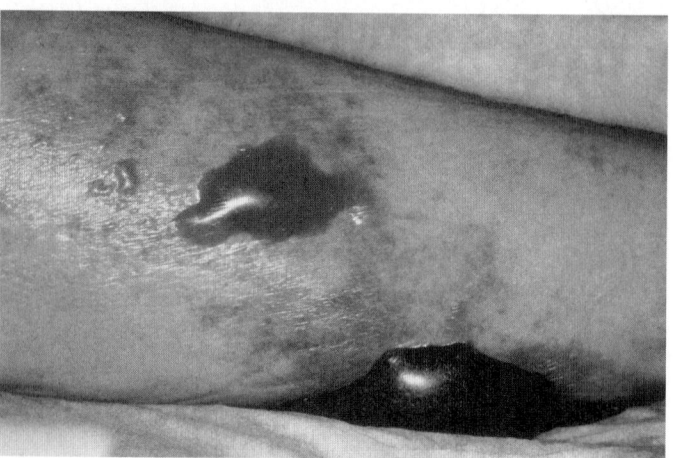

FIG. 246-4. (PLATE 14). Large bullous lesions on the lower extremity in a patient with streptococcal toxic shock.

TABLE 246-3 Lesions of Varicella Zoster (Shingles)

Close grouping or clustering of lesions
Arrayed on an erythematous base
Papulovesicles with clear or purulent fluid
Ultimate ulcer formation with crusting
Lesions vary in size

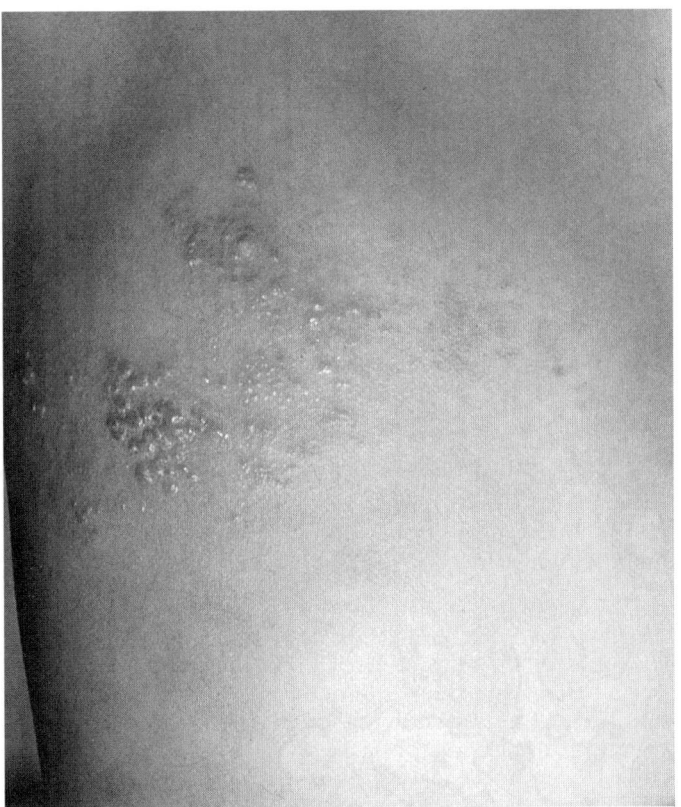

FIG. 246-5. (PLATE 15). Single dermatomal involvement in a patient with herpes zoster infection in a thoracic distribution.

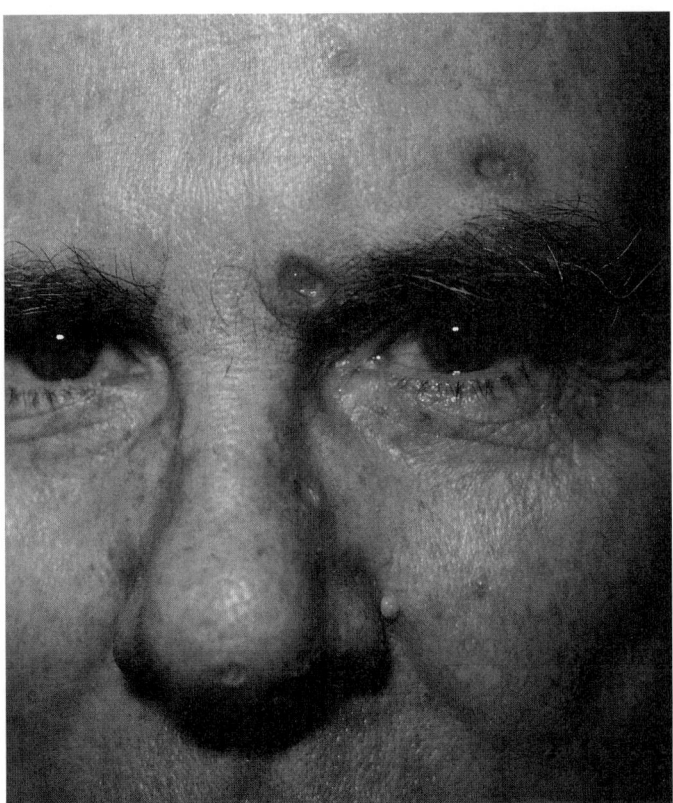

FIG. 246-6. (PLATE 16). Herpes zoster ophthalmic infection. Facial zoster involving the ophthalmic branch of the fifth cranial nerve with nasal lesions strongly suggestive of corneal infection.

uted evenly across the trunk, extremities, and head. In fact, patients with Hodgkin disease are particularly prone to dissemination, with 15 to 50 percent of cases demonstrating involvement of the skin, lungs, and central nervous system. Patients with disseminated herpes zoster infection require admission and treatment with parenteral antiviral therapy.

Herpes Simplex and Eczema Herpeticum

The vast majority of HSV type 1 or type 2 infections involve only localized areas of skin or mucous membranes. In neonates and in adults with atopic dermatitis, malignancy, immunosuppression, and AIDS, the HSV infection may disseminate, resulting in widespread vesicles, pustules, and ulcerations and causing multisystem involvement. The neonate may acquire the infection in utero due to maternal infection during pregnancy or during delivery. Adults undergoing chemotherapy or transplant recipients who are HSV seropositive may reactivate HSV and develop disseminated disease. Patients with atopic dermatitis are also at risk of disseminated disease, which is called *eczema herpeticum.*

The vesicular rash, initially present in some form in up to 70 percent of patients, ranges from the scattered vesicle to full-body distribution. Lesions are vesicular, of similar size, 2 to 3 mm in diameter, clustered together in groups, and arrayed on an erythematous base (Figure 246-7, **Plate 17**). The lesions frequently umbilicate. Occasionally, the disseminated forms of HSV present cutaneously with different lesion morphology and appearance. Rather than grouped, the lesions may occur singly with a widespread distribution; the lesions also may appear as pustules with purulent blister fluid. Bacterial superinfection is common. Regardless of their initial appearance, the lesions will ulcerate with crusting. A Tzanck preparation, in which fluid from an intact vesicle is applied to a microscope slide and stained with Wright or Giemsa stain, often demonstrates multinucleated giant cells.

If necessary, cultures of vesicle fluid can be obtained for confirmatory diagnosis. The patient's course may be complicated soon after by multiorgan failure. Treatment is admission to a critical care unit with parenteral antiviral therapy and antibiotics for bacterial superinfection.

Eczema herpeticum is an association of two common conditions, atopic dermatitis and HSV infection. The most severe forms of eczema herpeticum tend to occur in the young infant and the immunocompromised adult patient. Lesions appear initially in the area of the preexisting dermatitis but eventually may disseminate. The underlying atopic dermatitis and bacterial superinfection may alter lesion appearance. Dermatologic consultation is usually necessary to aid in disposition decisions. Selected cases of local eczema herpeticum can be managed in the outpatient setting with oral acyclovir and antibiotics. More severe or disseminated cases require admission.

DISSEMINATED GONOCOCCAL INFECTION

About 2 percent of patients with mucosal genitourinary infection will develop disseminated gonococcal infection (DGI). Risk factors for dissemination are not well known, but asymptomatic local disease and active menses seem to be associated in some way. Up to 75 percent of patients with DGI were diagnosed in late pregnancy, the immediate postpartum period, or within 1 week of the onset of menses. Disseminated disease, once common in women, is noted currently to occur with increased frequency in men. Disease manifestations result from organism and immune complex dissemination. Fever, arthralgias, and multiple papular, vesicular, or pustular skin lesions characterize gonococcemia. The rash develops on the extensor surfaces of the wrists, palms, and hands and the dorsal aspects of the ankles and feet. The lesions, usually numbering fewer than 10 to 20, initially appear as small red papules or maculopapules (Figure 246-8, **Plate 18**) with a petechial component and an erythematous periphery. Lesions resolve rapidly or evolve into vesicles with purulent fluid, which develop gray

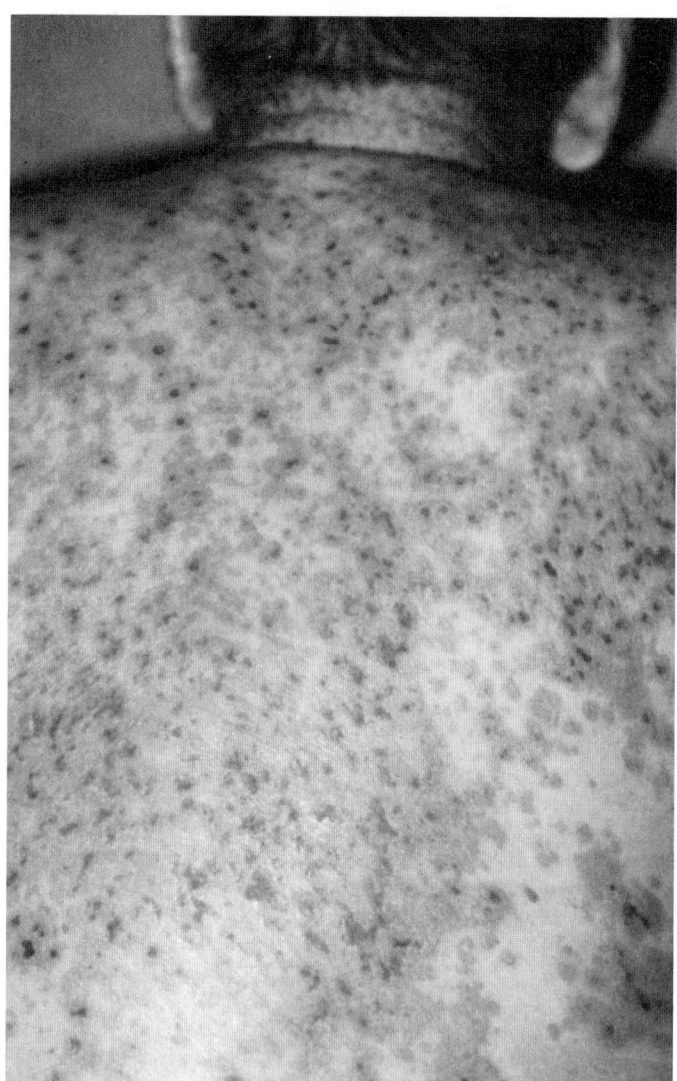

FIG. 246-7. (PLATE 17). Disseminated herpes simplex virus infection in an immunocompromised adult patient; note the widespread distribution of vesicular lesions on an erythematous base.

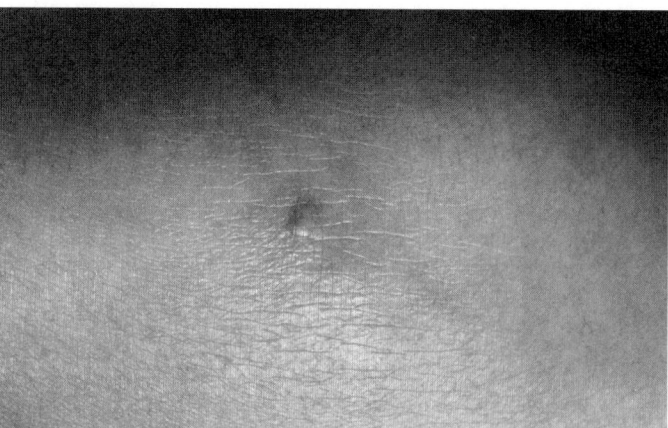

FIG. 246-8. (PLATE 18). Disseminated gonococcal infection in a sexually active adult female. The maculopapule has a petechial component and an erythematous periphery on the extensor surface of the wrist.

necrotic centers. The necrotic center is theorized to be the embolic focus of the gonococcal organism. Ultimately, the lesions become hemorrhagic.

The differential diagnosis includes other petechial syndromes, including RMSF, meningococcemia, staphylococcal acute endocarditis, vasculitides (in particular Henoch-Schönlein purpura and leukocytoclastic vasculitis), enteroviral infections, bacterial sepsis (gram-positive and gram-negative) with disseminated intravascular coagulation, and typhus. The distribution of the rash is similar to that encountered in the RMSF patient, initially seen on the wrists and ankles. The number of lesions in the DGI arthritis-dermatitis patient, however, is markedly smaller compared with the total lesion count in cases of RMSF and meningococcemia. Further, the rash of DGI is pustular rather than obviously petechial and hemorrhagic, as are the lesions of RMSF and meningococcemia. Moreover, the DGI patient usually does not demonstrate systemic toxicity, as commonly seen in patients with RMSF or meningococcemia. Reiter syndrome may be confused with the gonococcal arthritis-dermatitis syndrome. Patients with Reiter syndrome present with urethritis, conjunctivitis, arthritis, and a psoriasis-like cutaneous eruption; patients with Reiter syndrome do not demonstrate petechiae, macules, papules, or maculopapules.

The diagnosis of DGI is made in the sexually active patient with complaints of tenosynovitis, arthralgias, and the appropriate dermato-

logic findings. Gram stain of fluid from unroofed lesions may demonstrate *Neisseria gonorrhoeae*. Blood cultures may be positive with an increased yield in the early phase of illness with active bacteremia, and urethral or cervical specimens can be obtained for culture or gonococcal antigen. Cultures of the various mucosal surfaces (i.e., cervical and vaginal) are frequently sterile in the patient with disseminated disease states. Antimicrobial agents of choice include ceftriaxone and ciprofloxacin; spectinomycin may be used in patients with intolerance to the initial treatment choices. Treatment regimens include ceftriaxone 1 g IV daily for seven doses or parenteral ciprofloxacin over a similar duration.

ROCKY MOUNTAIN SPOTTED FEVER

Rocky Mountain spotted fever, a potentially fatal multisystem illness caused by *Rickettsia rickettsii*, is introduced to humans via the tick vector. Without adequate, timely management, the mortality rate increases to 50 percent. After introduction of the organism to body tissues, it disseminates through the blood stream and invades vascular endothelium, causing a necrotizing vasculitis. Constitutional symptoms of fever, headache, and myalgias develop about 1 week after exposure. The rash in classic RMSF is evident 4 days (range, 1 to 15 days) after the onset of fever and other symptoms. In a minority of patients, usually the adult, the rash is not noted during the entire disease course. This entity, Rocky Mountain "spotless" fever, occurs in approximately 15 percent of cases.

The rash first appears on the wrists and ankles and rapidly spreads to the palms and soles (Figure 246-9, **Plate 19**). As the rash moves centrally, the proximal extremities, trunk, and face are involved. The skin lesions at onset are described as discrete macules or maculopapules that blanch with pressure. The initial lesions evolve into petechiae over 2 to 4 days, fade slowly over 2 to 3 weeks, and heal occasionally with resultant hyperpigmentation. Rarely, the petechiae may coalesce into ecchymotic areas with eventual gangrene of the distal extremities, nose, ear lobes, scrotum, and vulva-purpura fulminans. For further discussion of the treatment of this and other tick-borne diseases, see Chap. 151.

MENINGOCOCCEMIA

Meningococcemia is a potentially fatal infectious illness caused by the gram-negative diplococcus *Neisseria meningitidis*. Meningococcal disease presents across a wide clinical spectrum in the acute and chronic forms. The acute entities include pharyngitis, meningitis, and bacteremia. Meningococci are present in the nasopharynx of 2 to

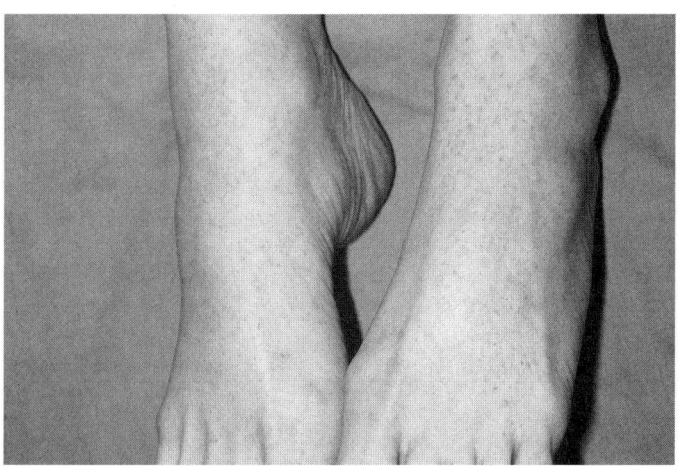

FIG. 246-9. (PLATE 19). A patient with Rocky Mountain spotted fever with petechiae on the ankles.

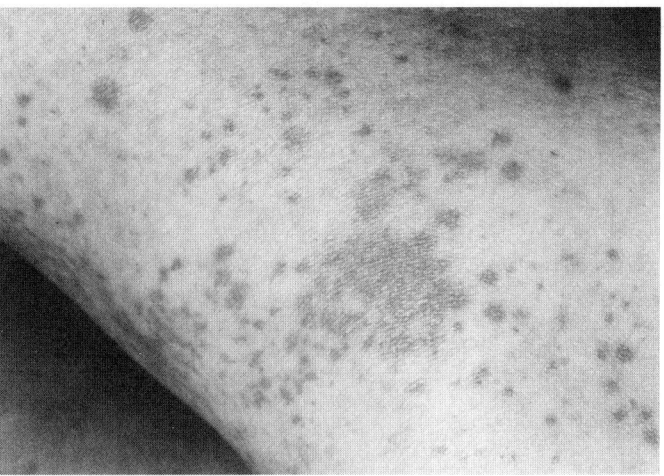

FIG. 246-10. (PLATE 20). Early findings of meningococcemia with petechiae evolving into purpuric lesions. (Reprinted with permission from Brady W, DeBehnke D, Crosby D: Dermatologic emergencies. *Am J Emerg Med* 12:217, 1994.)

20 percent of the general population (the carrier state); during epidemics, the organism is found in up to 30 percent of people without evidence of active disease.

The illness usually strikes patients younger than 20 years, with the vast majority of cases occurring in children and infants younger than 5 years. Epidemic outbreaks occur when a particularly virulent strain of the organism is introduced into a closed, confined population. The highest rates of infection are reported in the winter and spring months, although sporadic cases appear throughout the year. The organism is transmitted through aerosolized droplets of respiratory secretions from asymptomatic carriers and less frequently from actively infected patients. The mortality rate ranges from 5 to 28 percent, although most patients treated appropriately early in the disease course recover. Patients with acute meningococcal infection who exhibit signs of circulatory insufficiency, a peripheral white blood cell count of fewer than 10,000 cells/μL, or a coagulopathy have a high probability of developing organ system failure followed by death.[14]

After exposure to the organism, clinical infection develops usually within 3 to 4 days (range, 2 to 10 days) and progresses rapidly to severe illness. The patient may complain of severe headache, sudden fever, altered mental status, nausea, vomiting, myalgias, arthralgia, and a stiff neck. A rash is frequently noted on presentation and is an invaluable clue to the correct diagnosis early in the disease course. The dermatologic manifestations include petechia, urticaria, hemorrhagic vesicles, macules, and/or maculopapules (Figure 246-10, **Plate 20**). The classic petechial lesions are found on the extremities and trunk but also are noted on the palms, soles, head, and mucous membranes. The petechiae evolve into palpable purpura with gray necrotic centers, a pathognomic finding for meningococcal infection. The skin findings result from the organism's invasion and destruction of the endothelium. Histopathologic analysis shows an infectious vasculitis.

Fulminant meningococcal disease is found in fewer than 5 percent of patients and presents with sudden prostration, petechiae with areas of ecchymosis, and distributive shock. This rapidly progressive version of meningococcemia is complicated by purpura fulminans, a severe form of disseminated intravascular coagulation. Large ecchymotic areas (usually the extremities, acral portions of the face, and genitalia) become necrotic or gangrenous.[14]

The diagnosis of acute meningococcal disease relies on recognition of an ill-appearing patient with an associated petechial rash and the nonspecific symptoms of fever, headache, altered sensorium, and body aches. Additional historical points, physical findings, and laboratory results supportive of the diagnosis include known exposure to active disease, rapid progression of nonspecific symptoms with the associated petechial rash, Gram stain of skin lesions or cerebral spinal fluid demonstrating gram-negative intracellular diplococci, and latex

agglutination of the cerebrospinal fluid. The differential diagnosis includes RMSF, TSS, acute gonococcemia, bacterial endocarditis, vasculitis (Henoch-Schönlein purpura or leukocytoclastic vasculitis), enteroviral infections, and bacterial sepsis (gram-positive and gram-negative) with disseminated intravascular coagulation.

Antibiotics must be given as soon as possible in a patient suspected of acute disease. In adults, an appropriate agent is ceftriaxone; due to the increased prevalence of cephalosporin-resistant pneumococcus, parenteral vancomycin also is given, often empirically.

PURPURA FULMINANS

Purpura fulminans is a rare vascular disorder characterized by fever, shock, multiorgan failure, and the rapid development of hemorrhagic skin necrosis. It is associated with dermal vascular thrombosis resulting from vascular collapse and disseminated intravascular coagulation. Purpura fulminans can result from hereditary or acquired protein C deficiency, activated protein C resistance, or protein S deficiency. It may also result from any condition that causes disseminated intravascular coagulation.

Purpura fulminans presents with the dermatologic triad of widespread ecchymoses, hemorrhagic bullae (Figure 246-11, **Plate 21**), and epidermal necrosis. Commonly, cyanosis with initial ecchymoses and ultimate necrosis of the tip of the nose, ears, and genitalia frequently occur; in general, distal tissue areas with end circulation are affected. Large confluent ecchymoses can develop, often on the extremities, from distal to proximal, and on the perineum, buttocks, and abdomen. The extremities are often involved symmetrically. Treatment is directed at the underlying cause.

BULLOUS DISEASES (PEMPHIGUS VULGARIS AND BULLOUS PEMPHIGOID)

Pemphigus vulgaris (PV) is a generalized, mucocutaneous, autoimmune, blistering eruption with a grave prognosis characterized by intraepidermal acantholytic blistering. Bullous pemphigoid (BP) is a generalized mucocutaneous blistering disease of the elderly, with an average age of 70 years at the time of initial diagnosis. Although the blisters are deeper in the skin than in PV (below the epidermal basement membrane), the prognosis of BP is better with less associated comorbidity and a significantly more rapid response to therapy. Refer to Table 246-4 for a listing of the skin lesions seen in these bullous diseases.

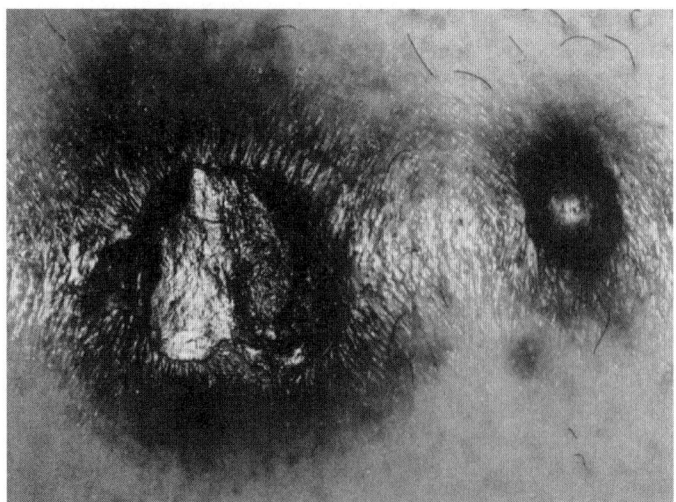

FIG. 246-11. (PLATE 21). Purpura fulminans with hemorrhagic bullae. (Reprinted with permission from Tangoren IA et al: Ecchymoses and epidermal necrosis in a 75-year-old man with bacteremia. *J Crit Illness* 13:108, 1998.)

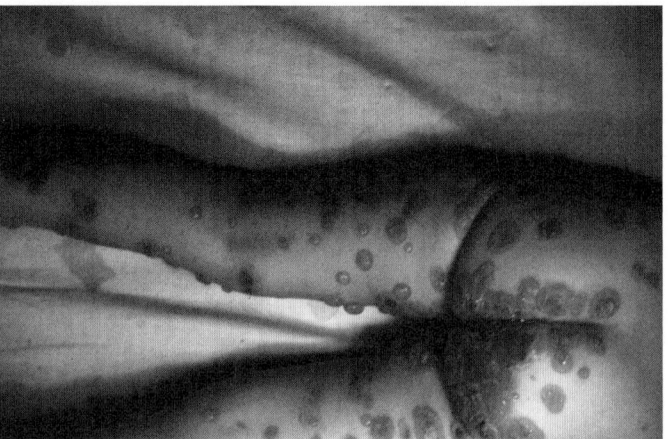

FIG. 246-12. (PLATE 22). Scattered bullous lesions intermixed with erosions and painful inflammatory plaques.

The primary lesions of PV are vesicles or bullae (Figure 246-12, **Plate 22**) that vary in diameter from less than 1 cm to several centimeters; they commonly first affect the head, trunk, and mucous membranes. The blisters are usually clear and tense, originating from normal skin or atop an erythematous or urticarial plaque. Within two to three days, the bullae become turbid and flaccid. Rupture soon follows, producing painful, denuded areas. These erosions are slow to heal and prone to secondary infection. Nikolsky sign is invariably positive in PV and absent in other autoimmune blistering diseases. Mucous membranes are affected in 95 percent of PV patients; in as many as 25 percent, the mucous membranes are the primary sites of involvement. Blisters on mucous membranes are more transitory than blisters on the skin in that they are more vulnerable to rupture; this is particularly true in the mouth, where ragged ulcerative lesions readily develop after inadvertent biting of the tissues.

Bullous pemphigoid is characterized by the presence of tense blisters (up to 10 cm in diameter) that arise from normal skin or from erythematous or urticarial plaques; ulceration with tissue loss follows. Sites of predilection include the intertriginous and flexural areas. Pruritus, occasionally accompanied by a burning sensation, is noted with the appearance of the blistering. Lesions of the oral cavity occur in BP, but with less consistency and severity than in PV. Because the blisters in the oral cavity rupture very easily and heal without scarring, involvement in the mouth is often overlooked. Oral involvement may occur in as many as 40 percent of patients. It is unusual for oral mucosal lesions to precede the cutaneous eruption, as in PV.

The differential diagnosis of PV and BP includes the vesiculobullous diseases; dermatologic consultation is required for diagnosis.

Limited oral intake and accelerated protein, fluid, and electrolyte losses through the involved skin can rapidly lead to hypoalbuminemia, with significant hypovolemia and electrolyte disturbances in PV and BP; therefore, dermatologic consultation is advised for treatment and disposition.

TABLE 246-4   Lesions of the Bullous Diseases

Large, flaccid bullae
Nikolsky sign
Ulcers
Exfoliation
Mucous membrane involvement

REFERENCES

1. Rzany B, Hering O, Mockenhaupt M, et al: Histopathological and epidemiological characteristics of patients with erythema exudativum multiforme major, Stevens-Johnson syndrome and toxic epidermal necrolysis. *Br J Dermatol* 135:6, 1996.
2. Paquet P, Pierard GE: Erythema multiforme and toxic epidermal necrolysis: A comparative study. *Am J Dermatopathol* 19:127, 1997.
3. Weston WL, Morelli JG: Herpes simplex virus-associated erythema multiforme in prepubertal children. *Arch Pediatr Adolesc Med* 151:1014, 1997.
4. Kakourou T, Klontza D, Soteropoulou F, Kattamis C: Corticosteroid treatment of erythema multiforme major (Stevens-Johnson syndrome) in children. *Eur J Pediatr* 156:90, 1997.
5. Porteous DM, Berger TG: Severe cutaneous drug reactions (Stevens-Johnson syndrome and toxic epidermal necrolysis) in human immunodeficiency virus infection. *Arch Dermatol* 127:740, 1991.
6. Kelemen JJ, Cioffi WG, McManus WF, et al: Burn center care for patients with toxic epidermal necrolysis. *J Am Coll Surg* 180:273, 1995.
7. Roujeau JC, Kelly JP, Naldi L, et al: Medication use and the risk of Stevens-Johnson syndrome or toxic epidermal necrolysis. *New Engl J Med* 333:1600, 1995.
8. Wolkenstein P, Charue D, Laurent P, et al: Metabolic predisposition to cutaneous adverse drug reactions: Role in toxic epidermal necrolysis caused by sulfonamides and anticonvulsants. *Arch Dermatol* 131:544, 1995.
9. Hoge CW, Schwartz B, Talkington DF, et al: National Centers for Disease Control and Prevention: The changing epidemiology of invasive group A streptococcal infections and the emergence of streptococcal toxic shock-like syndrome: A retrospective population-based study. *JAMA* 269:384, 1993.
10. The Working Group in Severe Streptococcal Infections: Defining the group A streptococcal toxic shock syndrome: Rationale and consensus definition. *JAMA* 269:390, 1993.
11. Resnick SD: Staphylococcal toxin-mediated syndromes in childhood. *Semin Dermatol* 11:11, 1992.
12. Goh CL, Khoo L: A retrospective study of the clinical presentation and outcome of herpes zoster in a tertiary dermatology outpatient referral clinic. *Int J Dermatol* 36:667, 1997.
13. Algren JT, Lal S, Cutliff SA, et al: Predictors of outcome in acute meningococcal infection in children. *Crit Care Med* 21:447, 1993.

DISORDERS OF THE FACE AND SCALP
Dean Morrell

Lisa May

The list of cutaneous disorders affecting the face and scalp is quite long. This chapter focuses on those disorders that are more specific to this distribution and likely to be encountered in an acute care setting.

ACNEIFORM ERUPTIONS

Although acne vulgaris is a common chronic problem that likely would not be encountered as a chief complaint in the ED setting, several acneiform eruptions may develop with alarming clinical presentations, prompting a patient to seek immediate attention. As these disorders are uncommon and require a dermatologic consultation, they are discussed only briefly. These disorders include acne fulminans, pyoderma faciale, dissecting cellulitis of the scalp, and acne keloidalis.

Acne fulminans is a severe form of cystic acne with ulcerating cysts. It most commonly affects the chest and back of young males. Severe scarring may result. It may have systemic associations including fever, myalgias, arthralgias, malaise, and anorexia. Treatment includes systemic corticosteroids and isotretinoin (Accutane). As isotretinoin has potentially severe side effects, including devastating teratogenicity in women who become pregnant while on this medication, it should be administered only by those familiar with the use of isotretinoin and able to follow the patient during the entire course of therapy.

Pyoderma faciale is an inflammatory cystic acneiform eruption on the central face of young women. Comedones are absent. Scarring is likely to result and thus treatment should be instituted rapidly. Treatment consists of systemic corticosteroids and isotretinoin. Again, a dermatology consultation is recommended.

Dissecting cellulitis of the scalp is an inflammatory and scarring disease of the scalp and neck. It is most commonly seen in young African American males. Clinically, the disease begins with boggy tender nodules on the scalp and neck. The nodules suppurate and develop sinus tracts. Hair loss develops over these nodules, and with time, a permanent scarring alopecia results. The etiology is unknown. It may be seen in association with acne conglobata and hidradenitis suppurativa, where together these three diseases are referred to as the follicular occlusion triad. Treatment is difficult and often unsuccessful. Therapy includes topical and systemic antibiotics; topical, intralesional, or oral corticosteroids; isotretinoin; and excision. Therapy is best managed by a dermatologist.

Acne keloidalis is a perifollicular inflammatory process of the scalp resulting in hypertrophic and keloid scarring. The exact etiology is unknown. It is most common in African Americans, and it is more common in males than females. The primary lesions are follicular-based papules and pustules on the occipital scalp. The individual keloidal papules enlarge and coalesce to form keloidal plaques with an associated scarring alopecia. Treatment includes topical antibiotics such as clindamycin solution (Cleocin-T solution), topical corticosteroids such as fluocinonide (Lidex) solution, and oral antibiotics such as tetracycline. Repeated intralesional corticosteroids may help relieve pruritus and pain, and soften keloidal plaques. Surgical excision and laser excision are often unsatisfactory.

SEBORRHEIC DERMATITIS

Because seborrheic dermatitis is such a common disorder, its recognition and management are important in any clinical setting, including the ED. Although the exact etiology is unclear, the yeast, *Pityrosporum ovale,* may play a role in the pathogenesis of this disease.

Clinical Features

Clinically, one sees erythema and waxy scale in the skin folds and hair-bearing areas of the face, scalp, chest, and groin. Common sites of involvement include the scalp, the pinna of the ear, the posterior auricular sulcus, the eyebrows, and the alar grooves of the nose. Itching is quite variable but usually mild. Any age may be affected, but the elderly and debilitated are more likely to have extensive involvement. In newborns, seborrheic dermatitis is often referred to as cradle cap. Extensive seborrheic dermatitis that is poorly responsive to treatment may be seen in association with HIV.

Diagnosis

Diagnosis is based on clinical examination. A skin biopsy is rarely necessary. The differential diagnosis includes tinea capitis, psoriasis of the scalp, rosacea, and cutaneous lupus erythematosus. Seborrheic dermatitis is diffuse and rarely associated with hair loss; thus, if hair loss is present or the eruption is focal, fungal cultures should be obtained to exclude tinea capitis. As seborrheic dermatitis is uncommon between infancy and puberty, tinea capitis should always be excluded in this age group. Rosacea and seborrheic dermatitis may overlap, but if the predominant features are inflammatory papules and pustules, the patient should be treated for rosacea.

Treatment

Therapy is aimed at controlling the disease; treatment is not curative. Initial treatment should consist of an antidandruff shampoo containing zinc pyrithione (Head and Shoulders), selenium sulfide (Selsun Blue), salicylic acid (Neutrogena T-Sal), or tar (Polytar or Neutrogena T-Gel). Nizoral shampoo can also be used and is now available over the counter. The shampoo should be lathered into the scalp and left on for 5 to 10 min before rinsing. Shampooing should be performed three times a week. A topical corticosteroid such as fluocinonide solution may be applied to the scalp in severe cases. For the face, hydrocortisone 1 or 2.5 percent applied bid should be the initial management. The use of higher-potency topical corticosteroids on the face can lead to the development of perioral dermatitis and should be avoided. Patients should treat the seborrheic dermatitis until clear, and then as needed.

ERYSIPELAS AND FACIAL CELLULITIS

Erysipelas and cellulitis are infections of the dermis and subcutis with erysipelas being more superficial than cellulitis. The distinction between the two is subtle and therapeutically irrelevant. Erysipelas is more likely to occur in the young and in the elderly.

Cellulitis may be a primary process or it may complicate another dermatosis. On the face, it may begin at a site of minor trauma that is often inapparent. Group A streptococcus is the most likely cause of erysipelas. *Haemophilus influenzae* may be a causative organism in children; although this is not as common because of the widespread use of the *H. influenzae* type b vaccine. *Staphylococcal* spp. and *Streptococcal* spp. are the most likely pathogens of cellulitis.

Clinical Features

Erysipelas and cellulitis of the face presents as a hot, bright red, tender, indurated plaque (Figure 247-1). The area of involvement is sharply demarcated and expands peripherally. They do not clear centrally. Vesicles or bullae may be present. They may be unilateral or bilateral. When unilateral, erysipelas and cellulitis need to be distinguished from early herpes zoster infection. When bilateral, they may be mistaken for the malar eruption of systemic lupus erythematosus.

Fever and lymphadenopathy are often present. Periorbital cellulitis can be associated with orbital cellulitis and has the risk of developing an orbital abscess, cerebral abscess, or meningitis.

Diagnosis

Diagnosis is based on clinical presentation. A biopsy is rarely necessary and often not helpful. Needle aspiration of the leading edge for culture has a low yield. A complete blood count and blood cultures should be performed to exclude bacteremia. An imaging study and an ophthalmologic consultation should evaluate periorbital cellulitis.

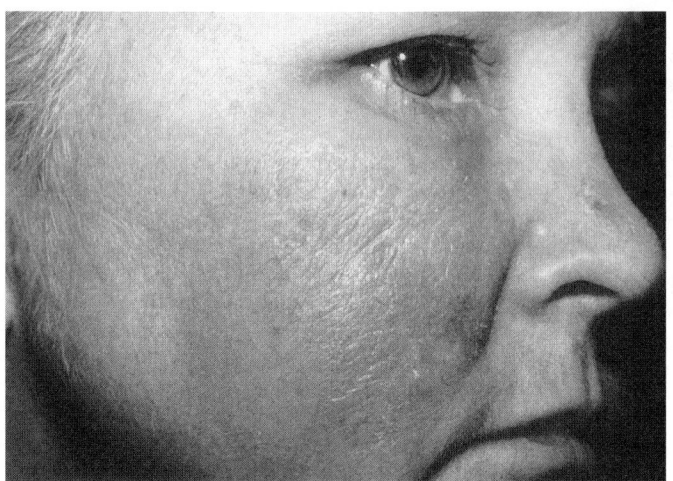

FIG. 247-1. Facial cellulitis. Erythema and edema involve the cheek, nasal bridge, and the upper and lower eyelids.

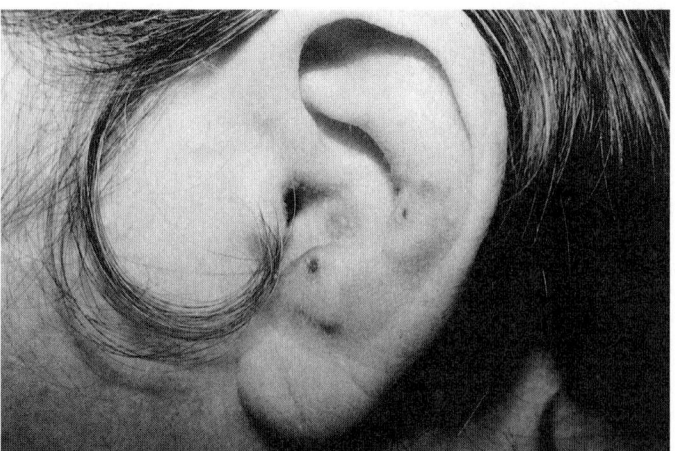

FIG. 247-2. Herpes zoster infection. This example demonstrates clustered intact vesicles and crusts of the pinna and external auditory canal. Patients with this distribution are at risk of developing Ramsay Hunt syndrome with facial nerve involvement resulting in Bell palsy.

Treatment

Cellulitis or erysipelas of the face warrants parenteral therapy in an inpatient setting. Unless history is suggestive of an unusual organism, therapy should be directed toward *Staphylococcal* spp. and *Streptococcal* spp. in adults. Coverage should include these organisms and *H. influenzae* in children. Again, an immediate ophthalmology consultation should be obtained if there is any question of orbital involvement.

HERPES ZOSTER INFECTION

Herpes zoster infections ("shingles") can occur anywhere on the body but most commonly involve the thoracic dermatomes. Involvement of the trigeminal nerve occurs in about 10 percent of herpes zoster infections. Involvement of the face and scalp has the most potentially serious sequelae and thus is discussed here.

Clinical Features

Herpes zoster results from reactivation of latent varicella-zoster virus (VZV). The initial eruption of varicella-zoster virus is chickenpox. Pain or dysesthesia precedes the eruption by 3 to 5 days. Erythematous papules progress to clusters of vesicles with an erythematous base. The vesicles crust in about 1 week. Generalized eruptions may occur in immunocompromised patients.

Any of three branches of the trigeminal nerve may be involved on the face. Involvement of the ophthalmic branch (V1), especially with vesicles on the tip of the nose indicative of involvement of the nasociliary branch, is of serious concern. Involvement of this area raises the possibility of developing keratitis. Therefore, an ophthalmology consult should be obtained.

The virus may spread to motor root ganglia, resulting in motor weakness or paralysis. Ramsay Hunt syndrome results from facial and auditory nerve involvement. The cutaneous eruption consists of zoster lesions in the external auditory canal (Figure 247-2) and on tympanic membrane. Bell palsy and possible deafness or vertigo may result.

Diagnosis

The differential diagnosis includes herpes simplex infections, impetigo, and contact dermatitis. A Tzanck preparation and a viral culture can confirm the diagnosis. The yield is higher when the tests are performed on early intact vesicles. A Tzanck preparation allows for visualization of multinucleated giant cells. It is useful to determine if an eruption is viral in origin; however it is unable to distinguish between herpes simplex and varicella-zoster viruses. Viral culture should be obtained by opening a vesicle and scraping the base of a vesicle onto a synthetic (not cotton) swab to be placed in viral culture media. Growth may take as long as 1 week.

Again, ophthalmic nerve involvement requires an ophthalmology consultation to exclude ocular complications.

Treatment

Antiviral medications are helpful if given within the first 72 h after the eruption begins. Antiviral therapy can shorten the time to healing, decrease new lesion formation, and possibly decrease the pain and duration of postherpetic neuralgia. Acyclovir (800 mg PO five times per day for 7 days), famciclovir (500 mg PO tid for 7 days), or valacyclovir (1 g PO tid for 7 days) are recommended outpatient regimens.

Symptomatic treatment includes Domeboro solution compresses, 1:40 dilution for 15 min qid, followed by Polysporin ointment or Silvadene cream. Analgesics are often necessary as well.

HERPES SIMPLEX VIRUS INFECTIONS

Clinical Features

Herpes simplex virus (HSV) type 1 most commonly occurs on the face. Initial infection occurs during childhood or adolescence and varies in its presentation. Many individuals experience mild symptoms while a few experience a debilitating eruption. Recurrences tend to be mild and occur primarily on the lips, in the nose, and in the oral cavity.

The typical lesions of HSV are painful, grouped vesicles with an erythematous base. The primary eruption may be preceded by constitutional symptoms. The characteristic primary eruption is a gingivostomatitis with herpetic lesions on the lips and in the oral cavity. It may persist for weeks. The differential diagnosis includes erythema multiforme, Coxsackie virus, varicella zoster virus, idiopathic aphthae, and, rarely, Behçet disease and pemphigus vulgaris.

Recurrent HSV is typically seen as herpes labialis ("fever blisters" or "cold sores"). The individual often experiences a prodrome of localized tingling or burning several hours before the onset of the eruption. The herpetic lesion usually occurs along the lip margin and completely heals within 10 days. Ultraviolet light, fever, or local trauma can induce these eruptions.

Diagnosis

The diagnosis is established in the same manner as that for herpes zoster with a positive Tzanck preparation and viral culture.

Treatment

Treatment for primary HSV gingivostomatitis includes symptomatic treatment, as mentioned previously for herpes zoster infections, including compresses and topical antibiotics. If mild, oral antiviral medications are not necessary; in more severe cases, use acyclovir (200 mg PO five times per day for 5 days). Immunocompromised patients with severe involvement require hospitalization for intravenous acyclovir. Treatment can continue for up to 10 days if lesions have not crusted. Recurrent HSV does not require oral antiviral therapy. Patients with recurrent disease should be instructed to avoid triggers, especially the sun, by using sunscreen and a lip balm with ultraviolet light protection.

ECZEMA HERPETICUM

In individuals with cutaneous diseases, most commonly atopic dermatitis, HSV or VZV can infect the dermatitic skin. This disorder is referred to as eczema herpeticum or Kaposi varicelliform eruption. Initially, the infection may be mistaken as an exacerbation or impetiginization of the dermatitis. Pustules and punched-out erosions develop. Constitutional symptoms and adenopathy are usually present. Dissemination of the virus is possible; mortality reports in this disorder are as high as 10 percent. Furthermore, scarring may be extensive if the viral infection is not treated early and aggressively.

An immediate dermatology consultation is warranted if this diagnosis is entertained. Depending on the extent of involvement, oral or intravenous acyclovir should be used. The underlying cutaneous disease requires aggressive treatment as well.

OTHER INFECTIOUS DISEASES OF THE FACE

In children, impetigo on the face is common, as is dermatophyte infections (tinea faciei and tinea barbae). Staphylococcal folliculitis is also seen on the face. The face and scalp are also a common site of involvement in secondary syphilis in which individuals develop "moth-eaten" alopecia, scaly or moist papules around the nose and at the angles of the mouth. Flat warts are frequently seen in males as a result of spreading the virus by shaving. Numerous molluscum contagiosum on the face of an adolescent or adult are suggestive of HIV.

CUTANEOUS LUPUS ERYTHEMATOSUS

Lupus erythematosus is a connective tissue disease of uncertain etiology. It may be a systemic disease with many organ systems involved or confined exclusively to the skin. Cutaneous lupus erythematosus can be divided into three major types: acute cutaneous lupus, subacute cutaneous lupus, and chronic cutaneous lupus. All three types may occur on the face. This section focuses on the malar rash of acute cutaneous lupus and the discoid lesions of chronic cutaneous lupus erythematosus.

Acute Cutaneous Lupus Erythematosus

The classic eruption of acute cutaneous lupus is the malar or butterfly rash. In most cases, this eruption is associated with systemic disease. It usually occurs simultaneously with the onset or flare of systemic lupus erythematosus (SLE). This eruption is induced by ultraviolet radiation. The malar rash is more common in whites than in African Americans.

Clinically, the malar rash consists of erythema on the medial cheeks and across the bridge of the nose. Induration, scale, or telangiectasias may be present. Occasionally, the eyelids may be involved, which makes the eruption difficult to distinguish from heliotrope rash of dermatomyositis.

Diagnosis is based on clinical examination and the presence of other systemic symptoms suggestive of SLE. This eruption is by no means specific for lupus erythematosus. The differential diagnosis includes rosacea, erysipelas, dermatomyositis, seborrheic dermatitis, medication-induced photosensitivity, polymorphous light eruption, and allergic contact dermatitis. Skin biopsy may be helpful especially if the diagnosis is in question. Initial laboratory evaluation includes a complete blood count, chemistry profile to include blood urea nitrogen (BUN) and creatinine, urinalysis with evaluation of urine sediment, antinuclear antibodies, double-stranded DNA, and complement.

If the diagnosis of SLE is likely, a rheumatology consultation should be obtained for further evaluation and management. The urgency of this consultation is dependent on the patient's systemic complaints. If other signs or symptoms of SLE are not present, the other entities in the differential diagnosis should be explored. A nonemergent consultation with a dermatologist is recommended.

Chronic Cutaneous Lupus Erythematosus

Chronic cutaneous lupus erythematosus is referred to as discoid lupus erythematosus (DLE). It is an eruption that results in scarring and pigmentary changes in the skin. DLE is most commonly seen in African Americans. Only 10 percent of patients with this type of lupus develop systemic disease.

Clinically, the lesions of DLE occur in a photodistributed area, especially on the face, ears, scalp, and neck. The lesions begin as erythematous or hyperpigmented papules or plaques that enlarge leaving central depigmentation (Figure 247-3). Follicular plugging may be visible, especially in ear lesions. On the scalp, a scarring alopecia with typical discoid lesions may occur. More extensive involvement of the trunk and extremities is more likely to be associated with systemic disease.

The lesions of DLE are quite characteristic and the diagnosis can often be made clinically. A skin biopsy is performed to confirm the diagnosis or to make a diagnosis in atypical clinical presentations. As DLE is a chronic disease and individuals suspected of having this disorder should be referred to a dermatologist for long-term management.

PHOTOSENSITIVITY

The types of reactions to ultraviolet light are varied. In many disorders, ultraviolet light aggravates, but does not cause, the disease. Examples

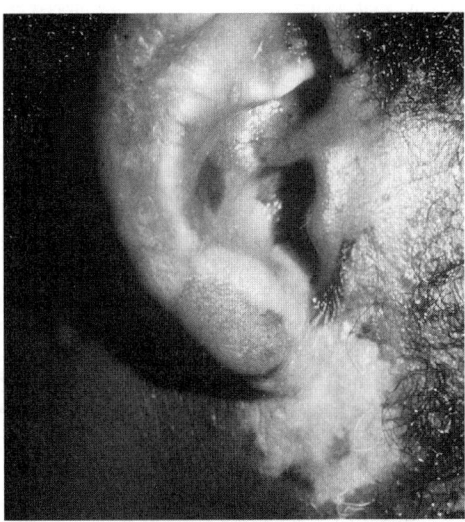

FIG. 247-3. Discoid lupus erythematosus. The external ear and preauricular cheek is a common site of involvement. Central depigmentation with surrounding erythema and hyperpigmentation is typical of discoid lupus erythematosus.

of this type of reaction include lupus erythematosus, porphyria cutanea tarda, dermatitis associated with niacin deficiency (pellagra), and recurrence of HSV. Other disorders are caused primarily by the sun. The most common is a sunburn reaction. Sunburn reaction, exogenously induced photosensitivity, and polymorphous light eruption are discussed here.

Sunburn

A sunburn reaction is the inflammatory response to skin injury as a result of ultraviolet radiation. It may be minimal with little discomfort to the patient, or it may be severe with extensive blistering. Individuals with fair skin, light eyes, and naturally light hair color are more susceptible to sunburns; however, even darker pigmented skin can develop skin injury with large enough ultraviolet light exposure.

The sunburn reaction begins 2 to 6 h after exposure and peaks in 1 to 3 days. Erythema and warmth in sun-exposed areas occurs. Vesiculation may result that is equivalent to a second-degree burn.

The most important part of treatment is prevention. Avoid the midday sun, apply sunscreen liberally and frequently [ultraviolet A (UVA) and B (UVB) protection with sun protection factor (SPF) 15 to 30], wear protective clothing, and seek shade. Sunburns can be treated symptomatically with nonsteroidal anti-inflammatory drugs (NSAIDs), with tepid baths, and by applying topical antibiotics to areas of vesiculation. Emollients may be soothing but will not prevent eventual exfoliation. Individuals should also be advised to avoid the sun until the eruption resolves.

Exogenous Photosensitivity Disorders

These disorders result from topical application or ingestion of an agent that causes the skin to be more sensitive to ultraviolet light. Photosensitivity disorders may be phototoxic or photoallergic. The clinical differences are subtle and do not impact on acute management.

Topical photosensitizers usually result in a cutaneous eruption at their sites of application. Ultraviolet exposure is necessary for the eruption to occur. Furocoumarins are the most common group of agents causing topical photoeruptions. Lime juice applied to the skin, fragrances, figs, celery, and parsnips are examples of furocoumarins. Other topically applied agents causing photosensitivity include *para*-aminobenzoic acid (PABA) esters, topical psoralen, musk ambrette, and salicylanilide antibacterials. The typical clinical eruption is a severe sunburn-like reaction, often with vesiculation. Often a linear appearance suggests that an externally applied substance is the culprit.

Numerous ingested substances can result in a photosensitivity eruption as well (Table 247-1). Because these agents are ingested and distributed throughout the body, the eruption involves all sun-exposed areas. The characteristic distribution of a photosensitivity eruption is the face, posterior neck, dorsal hands, and extensor arms. Certain areas including the creases of the eyelids, the upper lip, the submental anterior neck, and the posterior auricular neck are spared.

TABLE 247-1 Medications Commonly Causing Photosensitivity Eruptions

Amiodarone*
Chlorpromazine
Chloroquine/hydroxychloroquine
Furosemide
Nonsteroidal anti-inflammatory drugs (NSAIDs)
Psoralen
Sulfonamides
Sulfonylreas
Tetracyclines
Thiazides

*Amiodarone also causes a slate-gray pigmentation of the face. Pigmentation is reversible after drug discontinuation.

The diagnosis is based on identifying the offending agent. If the diagnosis is unclear, other photosensitivity disorders, such as lupus erythematosus and polymorphous light eruption, should be excluded. Photopatch testing performed by a dermatologist or allergist may be helpful in identifying the photosensitizing agent.

The causative agent should be discontinued, if possible. Initial management includes topical corticosteroids and management similar to a sunburn reaction. The patient should avoid the sun until the eruption has cleared completely.

CONTACT DERMATITIS OF THE FACE

Two types of contact allergies are likely to result on the face. The first is the result of an aerosolized allergen. The second is direct physical contact that is most prominent on the sensitive skin of the face.

Clinically, allergic contact dermatitis resulting from an aerosolized allergen presents as erythema or scale with or without vesiculation. The involvement is diffuse with upper and lower eyelids affected. This distribution is in contrast with photosensitive eruptions in which non-sun-exposed areas, such as the upper eyelids and the upper lip, are spared. Direct allergic contact dermatitis tends to be most prominent on the most sensitive skin, such as the eyelids. Examples of aerosolized contactants include rhus (poison ivy, poison oak) when the plant has been burned. Examples of common contactants affecting the face include nickel, nail polishes, toothpaste, preservatives in make-up, contact lens solutions, eyeglasses, and hair care products. Chemical-splash injuries are a common cause of facial-irritant contact dermatitis. A thorough history is necessary to uncover the offending agent. Referral to a dermatologist or allergist may be necessary if the history is unrevealing.

Avoiding the offending agent is the most crucial part of treatment. Medical treatment will be of little value if the offending agent is not removed from the patient's environment. Depending on the severity, topical or oral corticosteroids and oral antihistamines are used in medical management. Domeboro solution (aluminum sulfate and calcium acetate) compresses can be beneficial as well. Only short duration (3 to 5 days) of low to medium potency (hydrocortisone valerate 0.2%) topical corticosteroids should be used on the face. Careful application around the eyes is important because topical corticosteroid use has been implicated in causing cataracts and glaucoma. Oftentimes, extensive and severe periocular involvement requires oral prednisone.

HAIR LOSS

Hair loss can be a very alarming event leading to visits to an ED. The causes of hair loss are numerous and are typically divided into scarring and nonscarring alopecia. Nonscarring alopecia may be reversible where as scarring alopecia is rarely reversible. Table 247-2 lists the differential diagnoses for alopecia. Several of the more common types are discussed here.

Tinea Capitis

Tinea capitis is a dermatophyte infection of the scalp. It is most commonly seen in children, particularly African American children.

Clinically one sees areas of alopecia with broken-off hairs and scale at the periphery. The alopecia is patchy and usually nonscarring (Figure 247-4). Occasionally, tinea capitis is associated with an intense inflammatory response. This is manifested as a boggy, tender, indurated plaque with superficial pustules and overlying alopecia. This is referred to as a kerion, and it may result in permanent scarring and alopecia.

Diagnosis is based on a positive potassium hydroxide preparation or positive fungal culture. A potassium hydroxide preparation of the hair is necessary; scraping only the scalp rarely gives a positive potassium hydroxide examination. Culture is often necessary to establish or

TABLE 247-2   Differential Diagnosis of Alopecia

Nonscarring	Scarring
Alopecia areata	Kerion tinea capitis
Secondary syphilis	Herpes zoster infection
Traumatic alopecia	Dissecting cellulitis of the scalp
Trichotillomania	Folliculitis decalvans
Traction alopecia	Acne keloidalis
Contact dermatitis	Discoid lupus erythematosus
Androgenic alopecia	Lichen planopilaris
Thyroid disorders	Morphea
Telogen effluvium	Sarcoidosis
Medications	Scleroderma
Hair shaft abnormalities	Tumors (squamous cell carcinoma, basal cell carcinoma, melanoma, metastatic disease, cylindroma, lymphoma)

confirm the diagnosis. Wood light examination is becoming less helpful as the current types of dermatophytes fail to fluoresce.

The current first-line therapy is griseofulvin. Topical treatment alone is not affective. Ultramicrosized griseofulvin at doses of 15 to 20 mg/kg per d with meals is recommended. Individuals should be treated for 8 weeks, at which time the patient should be reevaluated to determine whether therapy should be continued longer. Nizoral shampoo at least three times per week is recommended, in addition to griseofulvin, in order to decrease contagiousness.

Other family members, especially children, and other close contacts, such as classmates at school or day care, also should be evaluated. Other affected members should be treated simultaneously to prevent reinfection. Follow-up is crucial and should be stressed as persistent infection may only manifest as scale and go unrecognized by caregivers. Follow-up should be with a primary care provider or a dermatologist.

Alopecia Areata

Alopecia areata (Figure 247-5) is disease of unknown etiology that results in nonscarring alopecia. Clinically, one will lose round patches of hair, leaving behind smooth, bald skin. Inflammation or scale is not present. Any hair-bearing area may be affected, but the scalp is the most common site of involvement. Rarely, patients lose all of their scalp or body hair; these are referred to as alopecia totalis and alopecia universalis, respectively. Diagnosis is based on clinical examination. "Exclamation point" hairs may be noted at the periphery. Alopecia areata may be associated with hyperthyroidism; thus, checking a thyroid-stimulating hormone is warranted. Secondary syphilis may result in patchy alopecia described as "moth-eaten" alopecia. Often, scale is present. If secondary syphilis is suspected by history, a screening test, such as an rapid plasma reagent (RPR) or Venereal Disease Research Laboratory (VDRL), should be performed.

Localized alopecia areata usually resolves spontaneously within 12 months. Extensive disease is less likely to resolve. If the disease is extensive, rapidly progressive, or of significant cosmetic concern, the patient should be referred to a dermatologist for treatment. Multiple therapies have been reported including topical, intralesional, and, rarely, systemic corticosteroids; anthralin; contact sensitizers such as dichloronitrobenzene; and photochemotherapy. None is universally successful, and all have potential complications; thus, only those health care providers who can follow the patient long-term to monitor for potential benefit and complications should administer therapy.

Telogen Effluvium

Telogen effluvium is hair loss resulting from a major stressful event. This may include pregnancy and delivery, major surgery, major illness usually requiring hospitalization, or crash diets. The event causes hair to arrest in the telogen growth phase of the hair. Two to 3 months after the event, when new hairs are growing, the telogen hairs are shed. The patient often notices hair clogging the shower drain or numerous hairs on the pillow upon rising in the morning. The patient and the patient's family notice appreciable thinning that is sudden and often quite alarming. Diagnosis is based on diffuse hair loss in the appropriate clinical setting. A related disorder is anagen effluvium, which is secondary to systemic chemotherapeutic agents. Patients should be reassured that complete hair loss is unlikely and actually heralds new hair growth.

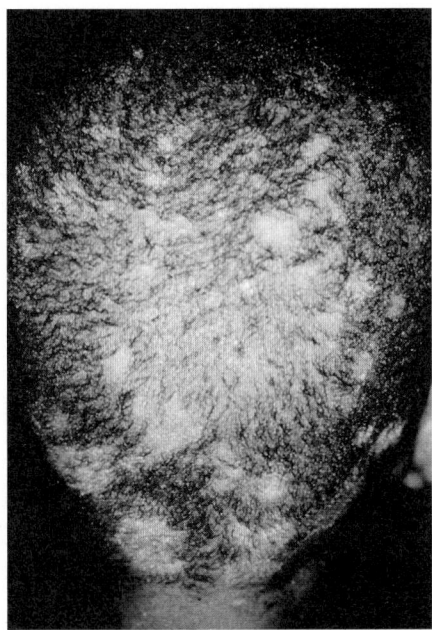

FIG. 247-4. Tinea capitis. Patchy areas of hair loss with broken-off hairs and scale is characteristic of tinea capitis.

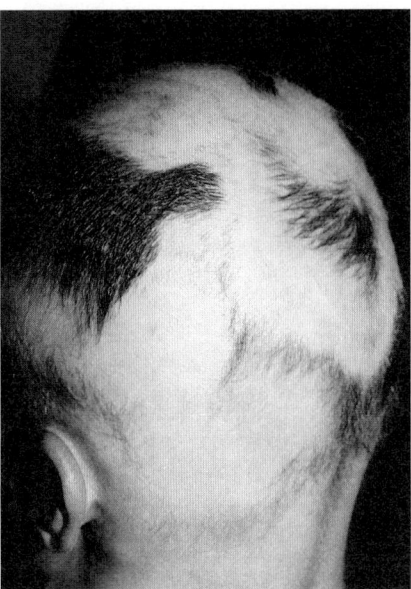

FIG. 247-5. Alopecia areata. This patient's hair loss results in areas of complete balding. The etiology is unknown.

248 DISORDERS OF THE HANDS, FEET, AND EXTREMITIES

Dean Morrell

Lisa May

Dermatologic conditions affecting the hands, feet, and extremities encompass a great majority of skin diseases. This chapter focuses on the disorders that are most likely encountered in an acute care setting. For a comprehensive review of the subject, the reader is referred to standard dermatology texts.

TINEA PEDIS AND TINEA MANUUM

Tinea pedis is a fungal infection of the feet, often referred to as athlete's foot. Tinea manuum is a dermatophyte infection of the hand. It is often unilateral and associated with tinea pedis. Tinea pedis is very common and usually begins in early adulthood. It is rare in children. Men are more often affected than women. Predisposing factors include hot, humid weather, excessive sweating, and occlusive footwear.

Pathophysiology

Dermatophyte infections result from invasion of the stratum corneum by dermatophytes. *Trichophyton rubrum, Trichophyton mentagrophytes,* and *Epidermophyton floccosum* are the most common organisms causing tinea pedis/manuum. *T. mentagrophytes* is most likely to cause inflammatory bullous tinea pedis. Dermatophyte infections are transmitted from person-to-person or from animal-to-person via fomites or direct contact.

Clinical Features

There are three main types of tinea pedis. The most common type of tinea pedis is the interdigital type. This type manifests as maceration and scale in the web spaces between the toes. Ulceration may even be present in severe cases with secondary bacterial and candidal infection (Figure 248-1).

The second type, which is also seen in tinea manuum, presents as chronic, dry scales with little, if any, inflammation on the palmar or plantar surfaces. It often extends to the medial and lateral aspects of the feet but not the dorsal surface. When present on the feet in this distribution, it is often described as a moccasin distribution. Polycyclic or annular patterns may be seen. Maceration between the toes is com-

mon. Onychomycosis may be present with numerous, but usually not all, nails having onycholysis (separation of the nail from the nail bed), and thick subungual debris. Oftentimes, if one hand is involved, both feet are involved as well. It is unclear why the other hand is spared in this "two foot, one hand" type of fungal infection (Figure 248-2).

The third type of fungal infection presents as an acute, painful, pruritic vesicular eruption on the palms or soles. Erythema is a prominent feature. Toenails and web spaces are usually not involved.

Diagnosis

Diagnosis is based on clinical examination and identification of fungal elements on a potassium hydroxide preparation or with fungal culture. Involvement between the toes and dystrophic toenails support the diagnosis of a fungal infection. However, psoriasis, and even chronic hand and foot dermatitis, can involve the web spaces and can cause dystrophic nails.

Although a potassium hydroxide (KOH) examination appears to be a simple test, it is often difficult to perform and interpret by inexperienced clinicians. Even in experienced hands, the KOH examination may have a low yield in the noninflammatory type of tinea pedis/manuum. To perform a KOH examination, the area to be scraped (the peripheral scaling margin or vesicle roof) is cleaned with an alcohol swab. With a no. 15 scalpel blade, the scale is scraped onto a glass slide. A coverslip is then placed over the specimen and a drop of 10 percent potassium hydroxide solution is placed at the edge of the coverslip and allowed to diffuse under the coverslip. The specimen is then heated gently under an alcohol flame to aid in dissolving the keratin of the squamous cells. The specimen is then viewed under 10× magnification. Hyphae appear as light-green, thin strands that cross over cells and have branches (Figure 248-3).

If a positive KOH examination cannot be obtained, scraping of scale can be sent to the laboratory for KOH examination and fungal culture.

Treatment

If a positive KOH examination is obtained, nonbullous tinea pedis and manuum can be treated with topical antifungal agents. Imidazole antifungal agents such as clotrimazole (Lotrimin and Mycelex), miconazole (Micatin and Monistat), ketoconazole (Nizoral), or econazole (Spectazole) cream should be used twice a day. Treatment should be continued for 1 week after clearing has occurred. Although econazole cream is more expensive, it is preferred for interdigital tinea pedis as

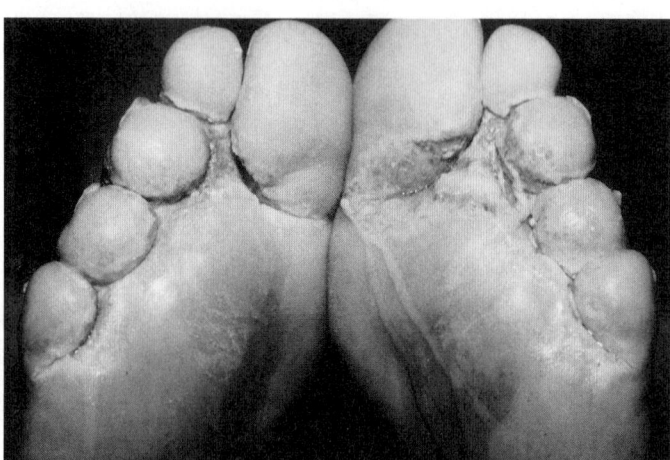

FIG. 248-1. Ulcerative interdigital tinea pedis. Secondary bacterial and/or *Candida* infection complicate this case of interdigital tinea pedis. This eruption is quite painful and debilitating.

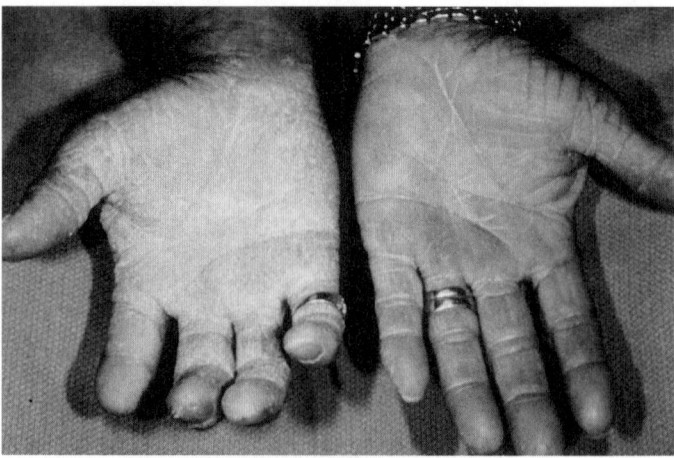

FIG. 248-2. Tinea manuum. The right hand has a markedly scaly palm while the left hand is uninvolved. This presentation is typical of tinea manuum. The feet would likely be involved as well.

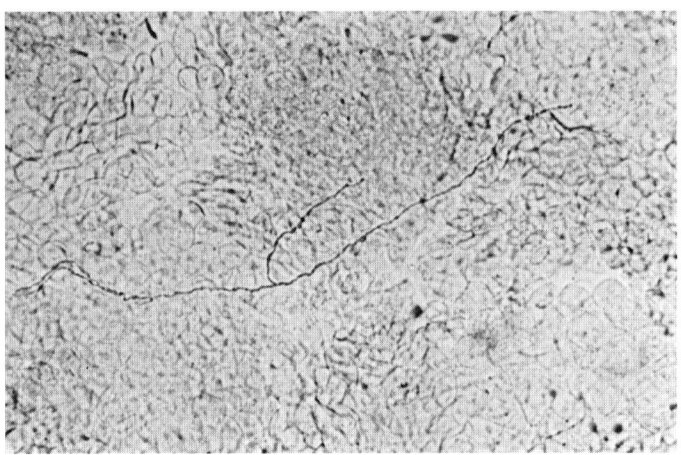

FIG. 248-3. Positive potassium hydroxide (KOH) examination. Viewed under 10× magnification, long, thin branching hyphae are seen.

it has antibacterial properties to treat secondary bacterial (often corynebacterium) infection. Topical terbinafine (Lamisil) cream is a fungicidal agent. It is nonprescription and is used once a day.

Patients should be warned that tinea pedis is often a chronic disease and that recurrences are common. Recurrences or failure to clear with topical medications may warrant treatment with oral agents, and referral to a primary care provider or dermatologist. Patients and physicians should be aware that topical agents do not treat nail infections. Thus, if a patient desires treatment of onychomycosis as well, an oral agent such as itraconazole, fluconazole, or terbinafine is needed, but is best managed by the primary care physician.

If a positive KOH cannot be obtained, but the clinical examination is highly suspicious for a fungal infection, empiric therapy is reasonable. As positive KOH examinations are difficult to obtain after treatment has started, scrapings for fungal cultures should be obtained before beginning therapy, as culture results (whether positive or negative) can help the follow-up physician choose the most appropriate therapy.

Bullous tinea pedis often does not respond to topical treatment. For mild cases, a topical agent can be tried initially. In more severe cases, oral antifungal treatment is necessary. Itraconazole 200 mg PO qd for 14 days or terbinafine 250 mg PO qd for 14 days are effective. The prescribing physician should be familiar with the potential drug interactions and the uncommon but serious side effects (hepatotoxicity and erythema multiforme/toxic epidermal necrolysis) prior to prescribing these medications.

Hands and feet should be kept as dry as possible. After bathing, web spaces should be thoroughly dried. A hair dryer may be helpful for drying. Socks should be changed anytime they become wet with sweat. Shoes and socks should be removed when possible. If the eruption is not clear in 4 to 6 weeks, dermatology referral is needed.

HAND AND FOOT DERMATITIS

Hand and foot dermatitis simply means inflammation of the skin of the hands and/or feet. The term is used to encompass several more specific disorders. These include allergic contact dermatitis, irritant contact dermatitis, dyshidrosis, and atopic dermatitis of the hands.

Pathophysiology

As this term relates to several different diagnoses, the pathophysiology is based on the specific disorder. Allergic contact dermatitis is a delayed hypersensitivity reaction to one of many possible allergens. On the hands, allergens may include rhus (poison ivy/poison oak), nickel, chromate, and rubber components of gloves. Some of the more common agents that cause allergic contact dermatitis on the foot are rhus, rubber accelerators found in shoes, dyes in leather and socks, and dichromates used in tanning leather.

Irritant contact dermatitis is an immediate nonimmunologic response from chemical damage to the skin. Strong irritants such as acids or phenol may cause severe immediate irritation ("chemical burn"). Weaker irritants including soaps, detergents, friction, and cold, dry air cause a more chronic dermatitis.

The cause of dyshidrosis is unknown. It tends to occur equally in men and women during early to mid adulthood (ages 20 to 40 years).

Atopic dermatitis is more often a disease of infancy and childhood; however, persistence into adulthood is possible. Hand or foot involvement is usually not the only cutaneous finding.

Clinical Features

In acute allergic contact dermatitis, erythema with papules, vesicles, and/or bullae is present. Pruritus is intense and excoriations are present. Chronic allergic contact dermatitis has less prominent vesiculation and more scale, lichenification, and fissuring.

Distribution is the most helpful clue to aid in diagnosis. When the hands or feet are involved in allergic contact dermatitis, the eruption tends to be present on the dorsal surfaces sparing the palms, soles, and web spaces. The thick stratum corneum of the palms and soles prevents penetration of potential allergens. Distribution with linear streaks suggests a plant allergy such as rhus (poison ivy or oak) hypersensitivity (Figure 248-4A). Sharp demarcation of footwear indicates a reaction to a component of the patient's shoes (Figure 248-4B). An eruption also present behind the earlobes, around the neck or at the site of a pant snap suggests a possible nickel allergy.

Irritant dermatitis resulting from a strong irritant like an acid or alkali initially begins as immediate burning in the exposed area. Vesiculation and bullae formation with surrounding erythema follow. In severe reactions, necrosis and ulceration may even be present. Eruptions often occur from accidental exposure. Irritant dermatitis from weaker agents presents as erythema, scale, and fissuring. Vesiculation is less prominent, and often is not present. Irritant contact dermatitis is a common problem in occupations that require frequent handwashing or water exposure, such as health care workers, bartenders, and housewives.

Dyshidrosis initially begins as very small, deep-seated, pruritic vesicles on the lateral aspects and the volar surfaces of the palms and soles. The dorsal surface of the distal phalanges may also become involved. A key feature separating this disorder from other dermatitides is the lack of erythema at the onset. Over time, the vesicles may form pustules or desquamate to leave small collarettes of scales. In chronic cases, erythema and scales become more prominent and may be difficult to distinguish from other forms of hand and foot dermatitis.

Atopic dermatitis of the hands and feet often presents as erythematous, pruritic scaly patches with prominent involvement of the dorsal surfaces as well as the palms and soles. Chronic atopic dermatitis will also have hyperpigmentation and lichenification and fissuring. Oftentimes, other areas of the body are involved. Common areas of involvement include the antecubital and popliteal fossae, the posterior neck, and the wrists and ankles.

Diagnosis

The diagnosis is clinical. Differentiation between the above-mentioned disorders, however, may be extremely difficult or impossible. More than one disorder may be present at a time, such as atopic dermatitis complicated by irritant dermatitis. One should try to elicit an occupational or hobby history that may indicate a specific causative agent. A history of an atopic diathesis (atopic dermatitis, allergic asthma, allergic rhinitis) in the patient or other family members should be sought as well. If an allergen is suspected, referral to a dermatologist for skin patch testing can help determine the exact agent responsible. A fungal

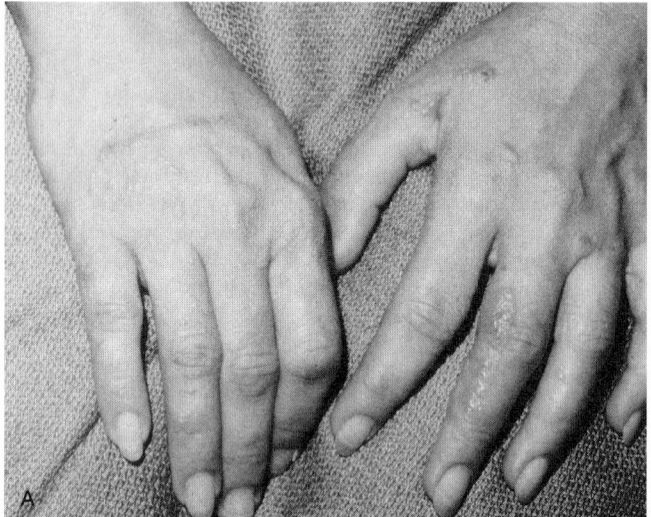

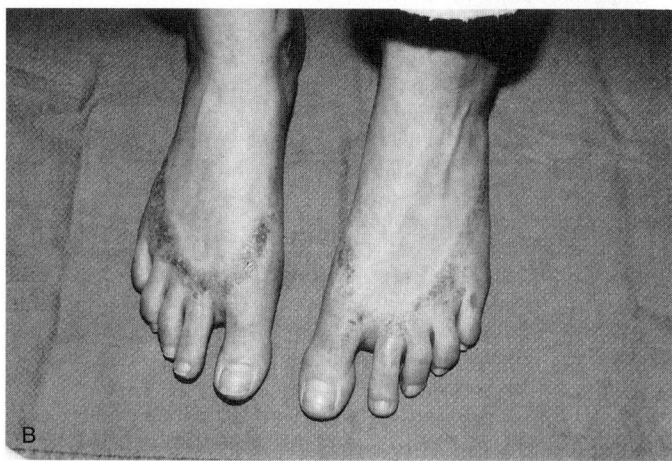

FIG. 248-4. Allergic contact dermatitis. **A.** Allergic contact dermatitis from exposure to poison ivy. Erythema, vesiculation and bullae are present on the fingers and the dorsal surfaces of the hands. Note the linear streak across the right hand. This finding is a diagnostic clue for rhus contact dermatitis (poison ivy). **B.** Allergic contact dermatitis to the straps of sandals. Erythema, scale, and excoriations are noted in a symmetric patterned distribution matching to this patient's footwear.

infection should always be considered in the differential diagnosis. A potassium hydroxide preparation can exclude this possibility. A dermatophytid eruption is another possibility. In this disorder, the hands break out in a dermatitic eruption as a result of a dermatophyte infection of the feet. Checking the patient's feet should be part of the clinical examination. Finally, psoriasis, lichen planus, pityriasis rubra pilaris, keratodermas, and autoimmune bullous diseases should be considered in the differential diagnosis. Rarely is a biopsy indicated, as it cannot differentiate between the different types of dermatitis.

Treatment

Offending agents should be removed. All antihistamine, anesthetic, antibiotic, and anti-itch creams should be stopped as they may cause a second allergy. In addition, water, soaps, detergents, and lotions should be avoided, as they may be irritating. The hands or feet should be well protected when performing any potentially irritating activities such as housecleaning, gardening, or hobbies using glues or chemicals. Friction should be avoided as well. Lubrication with products such as petroleum jelly, Eucerin cream, or Aquaphor ointment should be used frequently and liberally.

Acute eruptions with vesiculation can be treated with an astringent soak. The most commonly used astringent is aluminum acetate (Burow solution) (5% aluminum acetate). One Domeboro (aluminum sulfate and calcium acetate) powder packet or tablet is mixed with 1 pint of water and then applied with a towel or gauze to the affected area for 15 to 20 min qid. A high-potency topical corticosteroid such as fluocinonide (Lidex) ointment is then applied two to three times a day. Weaker nonfluorinated topical corticosteroids, such as hydrocortisone 2.5 percent or desonide, should be used on the face and skin folds. Antihistamines are also valuable, especially to relieve nighttime pruritus. Hydroxyzine (Atarax) 25 to 50 mg every 6 h should be tried initially. In severe cases with debilitating eruptions, systemic glucocorticoids are indicated. In allergic contact dermatitis secondary to rhus, oral prednisone beginning at 40 to 60 mg with a 2- to 3-week taper is recommended. Shorter courses of prednisone can result in relapse. Relative contraindications to prednisone use include diabetes, hypertension, active peptic ulcer disease, psychiatric disease, and immunodeficiency. If prednisone is prescribed to such patients, close follow-up is necessary.

Chronic eruptions should be treated with high-potency topical corticosteroids two to three times a day. Ointments are preferred as they help with lubrication. Hydroxyzine can provide symptomatic relief from itching. Systemic glucocorticoids should be avoided in chronic cases. Although they may provide temporary relief, rebound disease after cessation of the glucocorticoid is common. Furthermore, patients become overly dependent on this medication and the chronic effects of corticosteroid therapy then become an issue.

Severe irritant contact dermatitis with skin necrosis should be treated in a similar manner as a thermal burn. Debridement, and even skin grafting, may be necessary. Immediate referral to burn specialists or a burn center is warranted.

Hospitalization is rarely indicated except in instances of severe chemical burns. Follow up with a primary care physician or dermatologist is needed if the diagnosis is uncertain, if the eruption does not clear in three to four weeks, if systemic glucocorticoids are begun in the emergency department, or if patch testing is necessary. Chronic dermatitis should be seen by a primary care physician or dermatologist in 2 to 3 weeks to assess the need for prolonged treatment and to follow for possible complications of topical corticosteroids.

PSORIASIS

Psoriasis vulgaris or plaque-type psoriasis may involve only the palms and soles, but often extends to other areas especially the elbows, knees, scalp, and gluteal cleft. If pustules are present, the disorder is called pustular psoriasis.

Pathophysiology

Psoriasis is an inherited disease in which the principal abnormality is a shortening of the keratinocyte cell cycle resulting in an overproduction of cells up to 28 times normal. The causes underlying this rapid cell cycle are not clear; however, immunologic factors play a complex role in this process.

Clinical Features

In psoriasis vulgaris, erythema, scales, and fissures are seen in discrete plaques on the palms or soles (Figure 248-5A). Extensive disease may extend over the entire palms, soles, and dorsal surfaces of the hands or feet. Onycholysis (separation of the nail plate from the nail bed), nail pits, and yellow discoloration of the nails help support the diagnosis of psoriasis. Hand and foot dermatitis, lichen simplex chronicus, and Reiter syndrome should be included in the differential diagnosis.

In pustular psoriasis of the palms and soles, erythema, minimal scale, and numerous sterile pustules are seen. The pustules are in var-

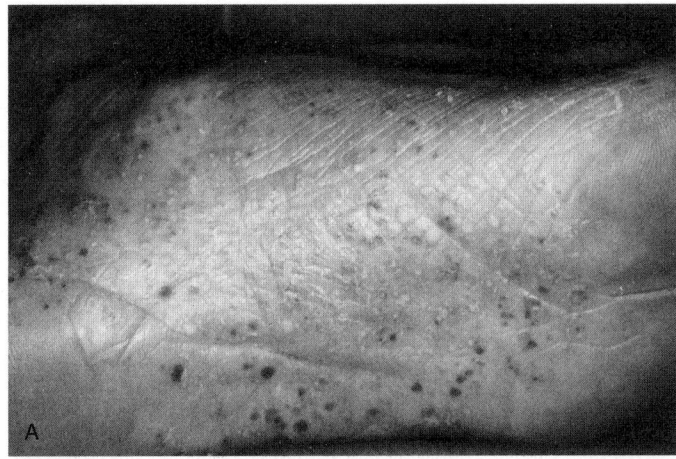

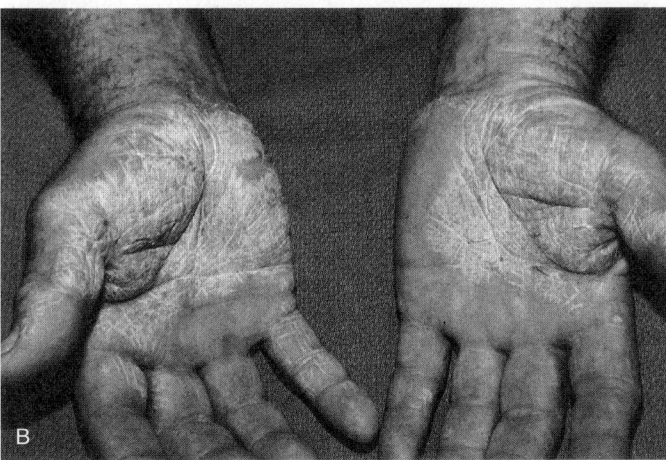

FIG. 248-5. Psoriasis. **A.** In plaque-type psoriasis, erythematous plaques with thick scale are present on the palms. Hand dermatitis and lichen simplex chronicus may be difficult to differentiate clinically from this type of psoriasis. **B.** Pustules in various stages of evolution are seen in this typical example of palmoplantar pustulosis.

ious stages of evolution from small pustules to larger confluent "lakes of pus" to crusts to rings of scale (Figure 248-5B). It is most commonly seen bilaterally in the instep of the foot and the thenar and hypothenar eminences of the hands. The differential diagnosis includes tinea pedis or manuum, *Staphylococcus aureus* infection, herpes simplex infection, and dyshidrosis.

Diagnosis

Complete examination of the skin focusing on the sites commonly affected by psoriasis including the elbows, knees, scalp, lower back, gluteal cleft, and nails may reveal other areas of involvement to aid in diagnosing psoriasis. If no other psoriatic plaques are noted, differentiation from hand and foot dermatitis can be difficult. A biopsy may be helpful in this instance. A KOH examination should be performed to exclude a dermatophyte infection. Bacterial and viral cultures should be obtained when disease is localized to one area.

Treatment

Initial treatment includes the use of topical corticosteroids, tar preparations, and lubrication. A tar solution containing 1 teaspoon of a tar emulsion such as Balnetar or Zetar in a quart of water, should be used to soak the palms and soles for 15 to 20 min bid. Application of a high- or ultrahigh-potency topical corticosteroid such as fluocinonide

(Lidex), clobetasol propionate 0.05 percent (Temovate), or betamethasone dipropionate (Diprolene) 0.05 percent ointment follows this soak. Liberal use of emollients such as petroleum jelly, Aquaphor healing ointment, or Eucerin cream should be encouraged.

The disease is chronic and slow to respond to treatment. Psoriasis of the palms and soles is exceedingly difficult to treat. Because of the chronicity of this disorder, follow-up with a dermatologist within 4 weeks is recommended. Other treatments, such as acitretin (Soriatane), psoralen-ultraviolet light A, or methotrexate, can be instituted by the dermatologist.

LICHEN SIMPLEX CHRONICUS

Lichen simplex chronicus (LSC) is an extremely pruritic eruption that can involve any part of the body. Most commonly, the ankles, lower extremities, neck, scrotum, and vulva are involved. In LSC, the inciting event is often unknown. The pruritus is intense, thus leading to scratching. Scratching intensifies the itching, which then perpetuates the scratching.

Clinical Features

LSC presents as a one or several intensely pruritic well-demarcated plaques. As a result of chronic scratching and rubbing, lichenification is the prominent feature (see Figure 249-3). Erythema, hyperpigmentation, and excoriations are also present. Scale is minimal. The ankles, shins, dorsal feet, and hands may be affected.

Diagnosis

The diagnosis is based on history and clinical examination. The differential diagnosis includes a dermatophyte infection, nummular eczema, psoriasis, and squamous cell carcinoma. A KOH examination is helpful to rule out a dermatophyte infection. Psoriasis oftentimes involves numerous areas of the body, most commonly the elbows, knees, the lower back, the gluteal cleft, and the scalp. Psoriasis tends to have less pruritus, less lichenification, and more silvery scale. Nummular eczema is characterized by more lesions and less lichenification. If the diagnosis is in question, a skin biopsy is suggested.

Treatment

Interrupting the scratch-itch cycle is the most important aspect of treatment. High-potency topical corticosteroids such as fluocinonide (Lidex) ointment should be applied to the plaque two to three times a day. Antihistamines should be used for pruritus and nighttime sedation. Diphenhydramine or hydroxyzine 25 to 100 mg every 6 h is recommended.

The chronicity of the disease and its slow response to treatment should be discussed with the patient. Furthermore, the sedating nature of antihistamines and their avoidance when driving or operating heavy machinery should also be discussed. Follow-up with a primary care provider or a dermatologist should be arranged in 4 to 6 weeks, especially if response to treatment has been minimal.

VENOUS STASIS DERMATITIS AND VENOUS LEG ULCERS

The vast majority of leg ulcers are venous stasis ulcers resulting from chronic venous insufficiency.

Pathophysiology

Chronic venous insufficiency is the cause of stasis dermatitis and venous leg ulcers. Chronic venous insufficiency is usually caused by episodes of phlebitis or varicose veins. This results in poor venous return from the lower extremities leading to increased hydrostatic pressure and lower extremity edema. It is most common on the medial ankle where the inferior perforate connects the superior and deep venous systems and the hydrostatic pressures are the greatest.

Clinical Features

Dependent edema, erythema, and orange-brown hyperpigmentation characterize early stasis dermatitis. The medial distal legs and the pretibial leg are the areas most frequently affected. More chronic and severe cases may have bright weepy erythema and even ulceration (Figure 248-6, **Plate 23**). Like other dermatitic processes, pruritus is common. Bacterial infection may complicate stasis dermatitis. The presence of honey-colored crust and pustules suggest secondary bacterial infection. Cellulitis and lymphangitis may even be present.

Stasis ulcers often begin within areas of stasis dermatitis. The medial and lateral malleolus and the medial aspect of the calf are the most common sites of involvement. The ulcer often has an aching quality with dependency. The ulcer has a punched out appearance with orange-brown hyperpigmentation at the borders and a moist pink base. Peripheral pulses are usually present.

Diagnosis

Diagnosis of stasis dermatitis is based on the history and physical examination. Other disorders to consider include allergic contact dermatitis (especially to topical preparations used to treat underlying stasis changes), lichen simplex chronicus, and xerotic dermatitis. Especially in association with acute exacerbation, secondary infection with *Staphylococcus aureus* should be excluded with a bacterial culture.

Stasis ulcers are also diagnosed on the basis of a history and physical examination. Bacterial cultures should be obtained if secondary bacterial infection is suspected. The differential diagnosis of leg ulcers is quite long and broad. If the ulcer does not have the clinical findings mentioned above, other diagnoses should be considered, and appropri-

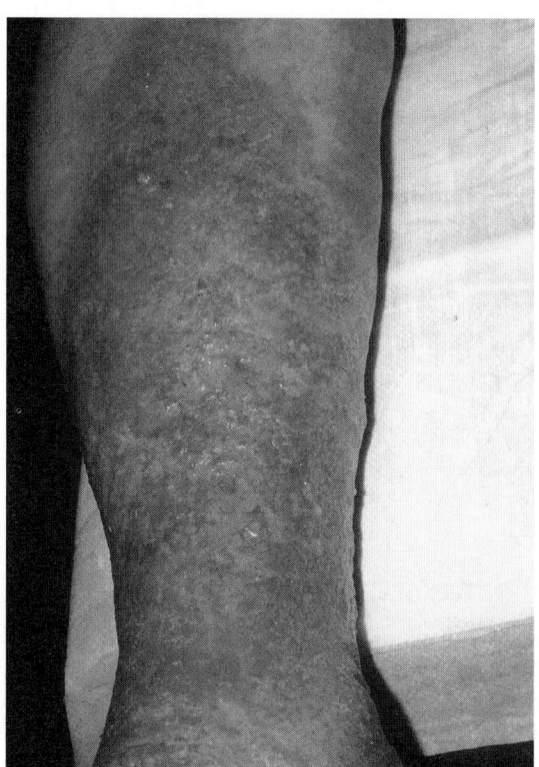

FIG. 248-6. (PLATE 23). Stasis dermatitis. Note the surrounding red-brown pigmentation and the central weepy erythema on the pretibial leg.

ate history sought and tests performed. This is particularly important for certain disorders, such as arterial ulcerations, pyoderma gangrenosum, and polyarteritis nodosa, that require immediate attention. For instance, if peripheral pulses are absent and the patient has a history of claudication, vascular blood flow studies should be performed to exclude arterial ulcers. If the patient reports a rapidly developing ulcer that began as a pustule or erythematous nodule and has violaceous overhanging borders, pyoderma gangrenosum should be suspected. If the diagnosis is in question, consultation with a dermatologist is indicated.

Treatment

Venous hypertension should be reduced by leg elevation and the use of support stockings. Weeping eruptions should be treated with an astringent compress like Domeboro solution. A low- to midpotency topical steroid such as fluocinolone acetonide (Synalar) 0.025 percent cream or hydrocortisone 2.5 percent cream should be used bid. The patient should be told the medication is used to treat the erythema, scale, and pruritus. Hyperpigmentation will not respond to treatment; therefore, the medication should be discontinued when erythema, scale, and pruritus resolve. Oral antihistamines, such as diphenhydramine or hydrozine, should be used for pruritus and for nighttime sedation. Secondary bacterial infection should be treated with cephalexin, dicloxacillin, or ciprofloxacin for 7 to 10 days. Evidence of cellulitis or lymphangitis may require hospitalization for intravenous antibiotics. Topical neomycin, antihistamine creams, and anesthetic creams should be avoided as they may cause allergic contact dermatitis.

Because venous leg ulcers are chronic and slow to heal, ED treatment should focus on treating underlying causes of edema, stasis dermatitis, secondarily infected ulcers, cellulitis, or lymphangitis. Follow-up should be arranged with a dermatologist, with a vascular surgeon, or at a leg ulcer clinic for further treatment.

ERYTHEMA NODOSUM

Erythema nodosum is an inflammatory eruption of the subcutaneous fat. It has numerous possible etiologies. As a result, all age groups can be affected (Figure 248-7, **Plate 24**).

Pathophysiology

Erythema nodosum is classified as a panniculitis, that is, inflammation of the subcutaneous fat. Table 248-1 lists many of the potential causes of erythema nodosum. In approximately 40 percent of cases, the etiology remains unknown.

Clinical Features

Tender, warm, ill-defined erythematous nodules characterize erythema nodosum. It is most commonly seen on the pretibial area of the lower extremities. The upper extremities and trunk can occasionally be involved. Numerous lesions are usually present. Ulceration is not a feature of erythema nodosum and suggests the possibility of another type of panniculitis.

Diagnosis

Clinical examination is characteristic of a panniculitis. Individual lesions may be mistaken for bacterial cellulitis; however, the nodular component supports the diagnosis of erythema nodosum. If a presumed bacterial cellulitis has no obvious portal of bacterial entry, erythema nodosum should be considered in the differential diagnosis. If the diagnosis is unclear, a deep punch biopsy or an incisional biopsy including subcutaneous fat is indicated. After the diagnosis of erythema nodosum is established, one must search for possible etiologies.

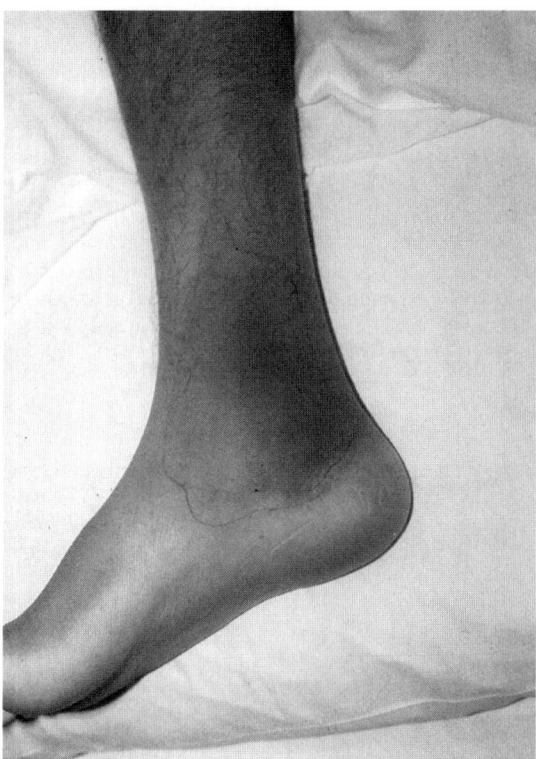

FIG. 248-7. (PLATE 24). Erythema nodosum. An erythematous indurated nodule is seen. This patient's disease was initially diagnosed as cellulitis. However, after no response to antibiotics, a biopsy confirmed the diagnosis of erythema nodosum. Most patients with erythema nodosum will have multiple lesions.

The history may suggest possible causes (see Table 248-1). Further evaluation, as directed by history and physical findings, may include a throat culture, a stool culture, a complete blood count, a chest radiograph to rule out sarcoidosis, and placement of a purified protein derivative (PPD).

Treatment

Therapy focuses on treatment of the underlying cause. If such a cause is not clearly established, symptomatic relief can be obtained with bedrest, leg elevation, and nonsteroidal anti-inflammatory agents. These measures can be instituted in the emergency department until the patient can be seen by dermatologist. Other treatments, including oral potassium iodide and systemic corticosteroids, may be required; however, they should not be started until the etiology is established.

PYOGENIC GRANULOMA

A pyogenic granuloma is a benign proliferation of immature capillaries occurring at the site of minor skin trauma. The name is a misnomer as it is neither an infection nor a granuloma. It most commonly occurs in children, young adults, and pregnant women. In pregnant women, it is called granuloma gravidarum.

Clinical Features

A pyogenic granuloma initially presents as a bright red, shiny papule with a thin collarette of hyperkeratosis. It may be ulcerated and tends to bleed profusely with minor injury. Later, the lesion reepithelializes and becomes a dull red to purple color. Although these lesions can occur anywhere on the body, the extremities, especially the hands, are the most common sites of involvement. The differential diagnosis includes

TABLE 248-1   Causes of Erythema Nodosum

Infectious
Fungal
Blastomycosis
Coccidioidomycosis
Histoplasmosis
Dermatophyte
Bacterial
Streptococcal infections
Campylobacter
Yersinia sp.
Tuberculosis
Leprosy
Parasitic
Leishmaniasis
Toxoplasmosis
Viral
Herpes simplex
Infectious mononucleosis
Pharmacologic
Sulfonamides
Oral contraceptive pills
Penicillin
Bromides
Vaccines
Sarcoidosis
Inflammatory bowel disease
Pregnancy
Behçet syndrome
Leukemia and lymphoma
Idiopathic

amelanotic melanoma, squamous cell carcinoma, bacillary angiomatosis, and cutaneous metastasis.

Diagnosis

The diagnosis is often suspected on clinical grounds; however, a biopsy of the lesion should be performed to confirm the diagnosis and to exclude the above-mentioned disorders, especially an amelanotic melanoma. These two disorders can be indistinguishable by clinical examination alone.

Treatment

Referral to a dermatologist for biopsy is indicated. If the lesion is bleeding profusely in the acute setting, hemostasis can be obtained with pressure and chemical or electrocautery. Destruction of the lesion, excision, or a shave biopsy followed by laser therapy or electrodesiccation and curettage are the treatments of choice. Lesions will rarely resolve completely without treatment.

OTHER DISORDERS AFFECTING THE HANDS AND FEET

Several other generalized skin disorders have classic clinical findings on the palms and soles. Some of these disorders are discussed in more detail in Chap. 246.

Erythema multiforme has characteristic findings on the palms and soles. The lesions are erythematous macules with a violaceous, dusky or bullous center. They are commonly referred to as target or iris lesions. Discovering such lesions should incite a search for similar lesions on the rest of the body, hemorrhagic erosions on the mucosal surfaces, and conjunctival hemorrhage in the eyes.

Secondary syphilis also has characteristic palm and sole lesions. These lesions are asymptomatic red-brown to brown macules on the palms and soles. Although patients with darker pigmented skin may

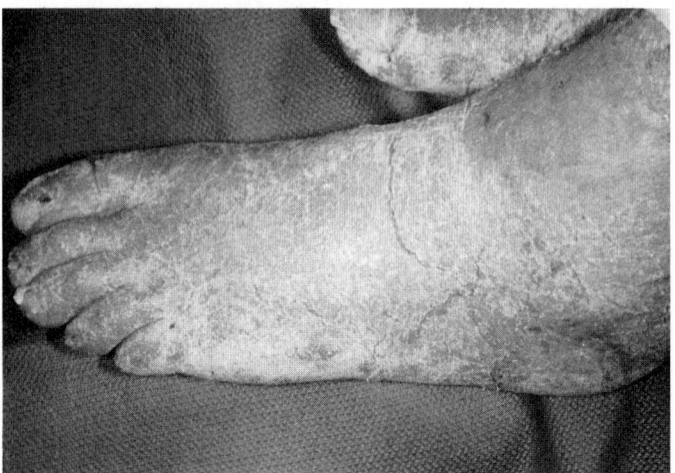

FIG. 248-8. Crusted scabies. The thick scale, erythema, and exudate resemble a foot dermatitis. This disorder should not be forgotten when presented with a patient with extremely pruritic scaly eruption. Crusted scabies is more common in immunocompromised and debilitated patients.

have several hyperpigmented macules as a normal finding, recent onset or failure of the patient to recall such lesions should increase suspicion for secondary syphilis. Appropriate laboratory serology should then be obtained.

Rocky Mountain spotted fever may also present initially with palm or sole lesions, which begin as blanching erythematous macules that later become nonblanching petechial lesions. Lesions start distally and spread proximally.

Kawasaki disease, scarlet fever, and toxic shock syndrome may all have palmar erythema as a prominent feature. The palms and soles will desquamate as these diseases progress.

Furthermore, when considering pruritic eruptions of the extremities, one must always think about scabies. The hands, feet, and elbows along with the groin are the most common areas of involvement. Diagnostic burrows will most likely be found in the hyperkeratotic skin of the palms and soles particularly along the web spaces and the wrist. When the scabetic mite burden becomes quite high, crusted scabies results. Thick hyperkeratosis resembling dermatitis results (Figure 248-8). See Chap. 250 for further discussion.

Finally, all the major types of skin cancer including malignant melanoma, squamous cell carcinoma, and basal cell carcinoma can occur on the extremities.

249 DISORDERS OF THE GROIN AND SKIN FOLDS
Dean Morrell
Lisa May

The skin folds of the body include the groin, intergluteal cleft, axilla, inframammary folds, and pannus folds. The skin folds have unique characteristics that set them apart from other regions of the body. For one, these areas are almost continuously occluded. As a result, scale does not develop; maceration and fissuring develop instead. This alters the appearance of papulosquamous diseases and inflammatory processes in this region. The occlusion also allows for the development of a warm, moist environment favorable to the growth of fungi, yeast, and bacteria. Finally, the skin folds—in particular, the groin, intergluteal cleft, and the axilla—are the major sites in the body of apocrine glands. Thus, certain disease processes of these structures such

as hidradenitis suppurativa occur predominantly in this area. Although many skin diseases can affect the skin folds to some degree, this chapter focuses on common disorders where skin fold eruptions are the main cutaneous finding.

TINEA CRURIS

Tinea cruris is a fungal infection of the groin commonly called jock itch. It is very common in males, uncommon in females, and exceedingly rare in children. Tinea cruris results from invasion of the stratum corneum by the dermatophyte types of fungi. It is transmitted from person to person via fomites and from animal (usually kittens or puppies) to person via direct contact or fomites.

Clinical Features

One sees erythema with a peripheral annular slightly scaly edge in the groin and extending onto the inner thighs (Figure 249-1) and even the buttocks. The penis and scrotum are not affected. This feature is important in distinguishing tinea cruris from other eruptions in the groin as most other eruptions will affect the scrotum.

Other common disorders to be included in the differential diagnosis include candidiasis, erythrasma, lichen simplex chronicus, allergic and irritant contact dermatitis, and extramammary Paget disease. Table 249-1 provides a more extensive list of inflammatory processes of the intertriginous areas. See the description under "Candida Intertrigo" below for a comparison of the features of these disorders.

Diagnosis

The diagnosis is established by a positive potassium hydroxide (KOH) examination. A KOH preparation will demonstrate branching hyphae (see Figure 248-3). If a KOH examination is negative, one of the other above-mentioned disorders should be considered.

Treatment

Antifungal creams such as clotrimazole (Lotrimin or Mycelex), ketoconazole (Nizoral), or econazole (Spectazole) twice a day is the initial treatment. Clotrimazole is suggested initially as it is of low cost and is nonprescription. Spectazole also has antibacterial properties and is preferred if maceration is present. Treatment also includes keeping the affected area as cool and dry as possible. Wearing loose-fitting clothing is recommended. Antifungal powders such as Zeasorb AF should be used on a daily basis to prevent recurrences. The patient should fol-

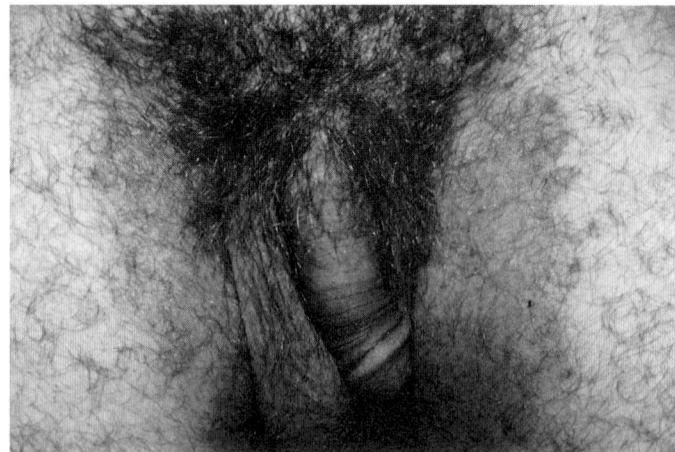

FIG. 249-1. Tinea cruris. Erythema with a more prominent, arciform leading edge on the inner thighs is typical of tinea cruris.

TABLE 249-1   Inflammatory Disorders of the Skin Folds

Infectious
   Tinea cruris
   Candida intertrigo
   Erythrasma
Dermatitis
   Seborrheic dermatitis
   Intertrigo/irritant contact dermatitis
   Allergic contact dermatitis
   Atopic dermatitis
   Lichen simplex chronicus
Psoriasis
Infestations
   Scabies
   Pediculosis pubis
Neoplasia
   Bowen disease (squamous cell carcinoma in situ)
   Extramammary Paget disease
   Histiocytosis X (in diaper dermatitis)
Hidradenitis suppurativa
Cutaneous Crohn disease
Hailey-Hailey disease (benign familial pemphigus)
Darier disease
Lymphogranuloma venereum
Granuloma inguinale
Acrodermatitis enteropathica (zinc, biotin, or essential fatty acid deficiency)

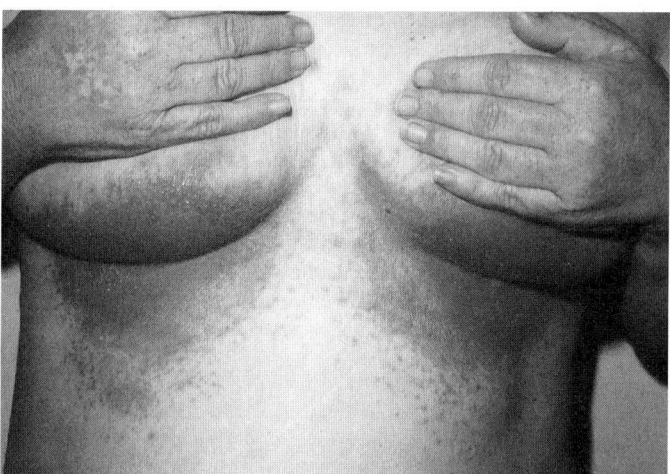

FIG. 249-2. Candida intertrigo. Note the bright-red erythema, erosions, and satellite papules and pustules in this striking example of inframammary candida intertrigo. A KOH examination will confirm the diagnosis.

low up with a primary care provider or dermatologist if the eruption has not resolved in 4 to 6 weeks.

CANDIDA INTERTRIGO

Candidal infections of the skin favor moist, occluded areas of the body. Although any skin fold may be involved, superficial candida infections are commonly seen in the diaper area of infants, the vulva and groin of women, the glans penis (balanitis) in uncircumcised males, and the inframammary and pannus folds of obese patients. Antibiotic therapy, systemic corticosteroid therapy, urinary or fecal incontinence, immunocompromised states, and obesity are predisposing factors. Women with vulvar or inner thigh involvement will often have vaginal candidiasis as well. Frequently, intertrigo is multifactorial with candida complicating other inflammatory intertriginous disorders.

Clinical Features

The typical presentation is erythema and maceration with surrounding small erythematous papules or pustules (Figure 249-2). These satellite pustules are a characteristic finding differentiating candida intertrigo from other inflammatory disorders affecting the skin folds. Patients will complain of burning or itching. The other inflammatory disorders listed in Table 249-1 should be considered in the differential diagnosis.

Diagnosis

The rim of satellite pustules helps to distinguish candida intertrigo from other eruptions of the skin folds. A KOH preparation of the pustules or a leading edge scale may demonstrate short hyphae and spores, but these may be difficult to find in cases with just erythema and maceration. If candida is suspected but not visualized on KOH preparation, and the diagnosis is in question, a fungal culture should be obtained. A thorough evaluation should be done if a primary disorder is resulting in secondary *Candida* infection.

Treatment

Keeping the affected area dry and cool is a cornerstone of treatment. After bathing, air drying or drying with a hair dryer should be en-

couraged. Clothing should be loose and lightweight. Astringent solutions such as (Burow solution, 5% aluminum acetate) aid in drying weepy inflamed eruptions. One Domeboro powder packet or tablet is mixed with 1 pint of water, then applied with a towel or gauze to the affected area for 10 to 15 min bid. A topical antifungal cream such as clotrimazole, ketoconazole (Nizoral), or econazole (Spectazole) should be applied bid. Spectazole is also antibacterial but is more expensive. The addition of hydrocortisone 1 percent cream bid can speed symptomatic relief and healing. Furthermore, drying powders, such as Zeasorb AF, should be used on a daily basis.

Patients with vulvar candidiasis should be evaluated for candida vaginitis and treated appropriately if found. Patients with candida balanitis often have a female sexual partner with candida vaginitis, so this person should be evaluated and treated as well. In infants or in adults with urinary or fecal incontinence, diapers or sanitary pads should be changed frequently. Zinc oxide paste applied over the antifungal agent provides a barrier to the irritation of urine and feces.

NONINFECTIOUS INTERTRIGO

Intertrigo is an irritant dermatitis of the skin folds resulting from moisture, heat, friction, and irritating substances like urine and feces. Intertrigo is common in the skin folds of obese patients where sweating and maceration occur. It is also a frequent occurrence in the diaper area of infants where it is referred to as diaper dermatitis.

Clinical Features

Intertrigo presents as erythema, maceration, and fissures in the occluded area of skin folds, especially the groin and inframammary fold. Satellite papules and pustules are absent. Burning and pruritus are present.

Diagnosis

Intertrigo is a diagnosis of exclusion. Other causes of skin fold erythema and fissuring such as candida intertrigo, erythrasma, tinea cruris, allergic contact dermatitis, seborrheic dermatitis, inverse psoriasis, and extramammary Paget disease must be considered. Differentiating candida intertrigo from inflammatory intertrigo can be difficult. Candida intertrigo will have satellite pustules as a prominent feature. If positive, a KOH examination supports the diagnosis of candida intertrigo. A negative KOH examination, however, does not exclude this possibility, as yeast is difficult to obtain and visualize with this procedure. A scraping of peripheral scale or a pustule to send for fungal culture is suggested.

Clinically, irritant dermatitis cannot always be distinguished from allergic contact dermatitis. A history should be taken to uncover any possible contact allergens or irritants such as neomycin-containing ointments, anesthetic creams, diphenhydramine cream, deodorants, feminine hygiene sprays, or other lotions, solutions, or home remedies.

Complete skin examination will help to uncover other signs of seborrheic dermatitis or psoriasis. Furthermore, extramammary Paget disease and Bowen disease (squamous cell carcinoma in situ) may be clinically indistinguishable from intertrigo—they may even be secondarily infected with *Candida*.

Treatment

As this eruption results from irritation by moisture, heat, and friction, these factors should be eliminated. Keeping the areas dry and cool is helpful. The patient should avoid tight-fitting clothing, especially undergarments. Weight loss can help as well. All potential irritants should be avoided. In diaper dermatitis, disposable diapers are preferred because of their highly absorbent properties. Diapers should be changed frequently, and periods free of diaper wear to dry and cool the affected skin is recommended. Zinc oxide paste provides an excellent barrier to urine and fecal material.

It is a common occurrence for the practitioner to be uncertain of the diagnosis. As a result, treatment is often aimed at both anticandidal and anti-inflammatory therapy. Several pitfalls of this approach exist. First, if used alone, topical corticosteroids can cause persistence or worsening of candida intertrigo. Second, the commonly prescribed combination medications, Lotrisone and Mycolog, contain a high-potency fluorinated corticosteroid. The occlusive nature of skin folds allows for better and deeper penetration of these high-potency corticosteroids, resulting in an increased risk of steroid-induced atrophy and striae. If combination therapy is warranted, Vytone-HC 1 percent (Vioform and 1 percent hydrocortisone) has anticandidal effects with a mild topical corticosteroid more appropriate for use in the intertriginous areas.

For moist, weepy intertrigo, astringent compresses can be used. Domeboro compresses, as described above for candida intertrigo, are recommended.

Secondary bacterial impetiginization can occur and should be treated with oral antibiotics with staphylococcal and streptococcal coverage.

Little or no response to therapy are indications to biopsy the affected area to exclude the serious diagnoses listed above.

SEBORRHEIC DERMATITIS

Seborrheic dermatitis is one of the most common skin disorders. It most notably affects the scalp ("dandruff") and creases of the face and ears; however, other skin folds such as the intergluteal cleft, groin, the axilla, inframammary folds, and the umbilicus can be affected. Severe and extensive seborrheic dermatitis is more common in debilitated patients, patients with HIV, and patients with Parkinson disease.

The exact cause of seborrheic dermatitis is unknown. Overgrowth of *Pityrosporon ovale,* a yeast that normally inhabits hair follicles and sebaceous ducts, with resultant inflammatory response is implicated.

Clinical Features

Seborrheic dermatitis of the scalp and skin folds of the face presents as erythema with a waxy yellow scale. When seborrheic dermatitis affects other skin folds, erythema and maceration are noted. Extension of the eruption onto the pubic area and central chest may be seen.

Diagnosis

The diagnosis is made on clinical examination of the skin folds with special attention to the scalp and creases of the face. Without examination of the face and scalp, the groin or other skin fold involvement is hard to differentiate from the other inflammatory disorders such as candida intertrigo, inverse psoriasis, allergic contact dermatitis, or erythrasma.

Treatment

Treatment can relieving signs and symptoms but there is no cure. The eruption will return after treatment ceases. Shampoos can be used on the scalp and other hair-bearing areas. These include shampoos containing zinc pyrithione (Head and Shoulders), selenium sulfide (Selsun or extra-strength Head and Shoulders), salicylic acid (Neutrogena T-Sal), or tar preparations (Neutrogena T-Gel). Nizoral shampoo can be effective as well and is now available over-the-counter. Seborrheic dermatitis is very responsive to low-potency corticosteroids. Hydrocortisone 1 percent cream can be used in mild cases, while hydrocortisone 2.5 percent cream or desonide (DesOwen) cream or lotion may be required initially in more severe cases. If these initial treatment options fail, dermatology referral is recommended.

LICHEN SIMPLEX CHRONICUS

The scrotum, vulva, and perianal area are common sites of involvement with lichen simplex chronicus. Clinically, lichenification, hyperpigmentation, and excoriation are prominent features (Figure 249-3). Treatment is the same as for lichen simplex chronicus in other areas except that low-potency corticosteroid (hydrocortisone 2.5 percent or desonide) ointments should be used. In cases of perianal lichen simplex chronicus, patients should be instructed to cleanse the perianal area thoroughly to remove fecal debris and tissue paper that may be irritating. Witch hazel pads are recommended for cleansing.

SEXUALLY TRANSMITTED DISEASES

Sexually transmitted diseases can occur in the intergluteal cleft, the perianal area, and the groin with or without genital involvement. The chancre of primary syphilis, condyloma lata, condyloma acuminata, or primary or recurrent herpes simplex virus should be considered. Pediculosis pubis ("crabs") and scabies can cause pruritic excoriated eruptions of the groin and axilla. The clinical findings in granuloma inguinale and lymphogranuloma venereum predominate in the inguinal folds.

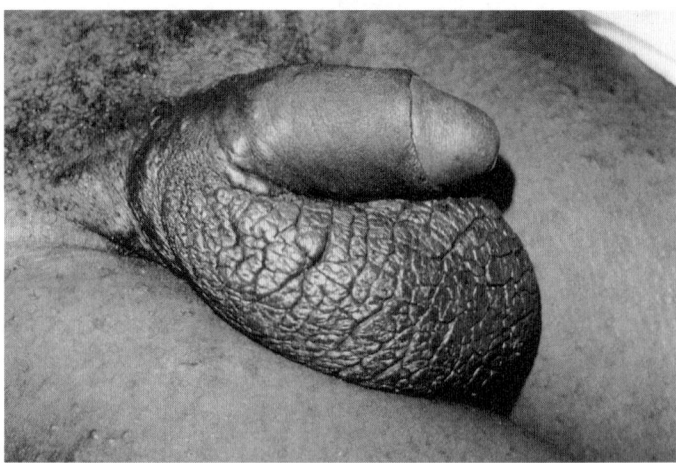

FIG. 249-3. Lichen simplex chronicus. Pronounced lichenification and hyperpigmentation is typical of lichen simplex chronicus. The scrotum is a common site of involvement.

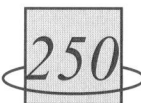

250

INFESTATIONS
Dean Morrell
Lisa May

HUMAN SCABIES

Human scabies is an infestation of the skin by *Sarcoptes scabiei*. Human scabies occurs worldwide and affects all races and social classes. The mite is transmitted from person to person by close physical contact. Although children and young adults are most commonly affected, infestation can occur at any age.

The scabetic mite resides in a burrow within the stratum corneum. Most individuals have an average of 12 mites at any given time. When the mite burden becomes high, numbering in the millions, a form of involvement called crusted scabies develops. It is most commonly seen in association with an immunocompromised state, particularly HIV, mental retardation, dementia, or physical disability. The time from infestation to clinical symptoms is about 3 to 4 weeks.

Clinical Features

Scabies tends to be an extremely pruritic eruption, often disturbing sleep (except crusted scabies, which tends to have minimal associated pruritus). The most common sites of involvement include the hands, feet, flexural surfaces of the elbows and knees, umbilicus, groin, and genitals. Facial involvement is usually seen only in infants. The pathognomonic lesion, or burrow, is a fine erythematous linear or curved lesion with central scale (Figure 250-1). Burrows are most often visible in the web spaces of the fingers, the lateral aspects of the fingers, the volar surface of the wrists, the instep of the foot, and the shaft of the penis. Often, however, burrows are not present, especially in patients with excellent hygiene. Excoriations and pruritic papules may be the only visible cutaneous feature. Vesicles are often seen in infants and young children.

In crusted scabies (see Figure 248-8), one develops thick, dirty-appearing hyperkeratosis on the hands and feet. The nails are often affected as well. Because of the large mite burden, this form of scabies is highly contagious.

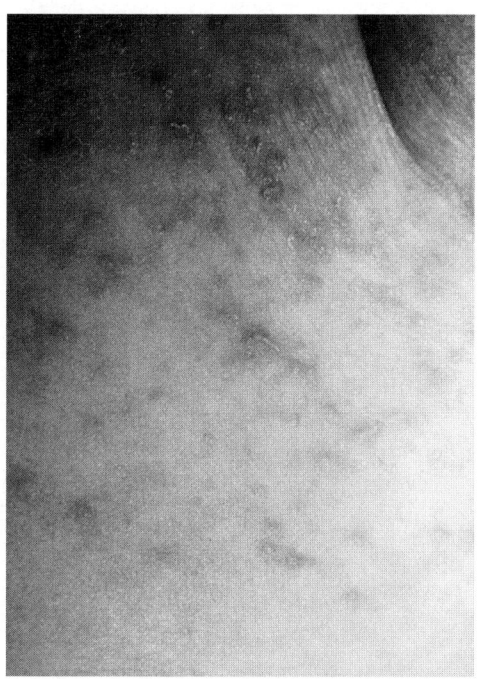

FIG. 250-1. Human scabies. Numerous scabetic burrows are visible near the axilla of this infant infested with scabies.

Diagnosis

The diagnosis is based on a high clinical suspicion and a positive scabies preparation. The diagnosis should be entertained when more than one family member itches. Other disorders to consider in the differential diagnosis include other bite reactions, body lice, atopic dermatitis, neurotic excoriations, and delusions of parasitosis. Suspected cases of scabies should be confirmed by performing a scabies preparation. To perform a scabies preparation, one scrapes or superficially shaves a lesion (preferably a burrow) with a no. 15 blade. The sample is placed on a glass slide, covered with immersion oil and a cover slip, and examined under the microscope. Mites, eggs, or scybala (feces) will be visible (Figure 250-2). When possible, the diagnosis should be confirmed with a scraping prior to treatment.

Treatment

Topical scabicides are the treatments of choice. The topical preparation should be applied from the neck down to the feet, with special attention paid to applying the lotion around and under fingernails, in the web spaces of the fingers and toes, and in the umbilicus.

Permethrin 5 percent cream (Elimite) and lindane 1 percent lotion (Kwell) are equally effective. Either preparation should be left on overnight and rinsed off the following morning. Lindane is easier to apply and less expensive than permethrin, but lindane resistance has been reported. Lindane is neurotoxic to infants, children, and pregnant women, and is contraindicated in those groups. Patients with extensive involvement should be treated again in 1 week.

All household members and sexual contacts at high risk of acquiring scabies should be treated concurrently, even if they are asymptomatic, because a delay from the time of infestation to the development of symptoms exists. Nursing homes, institutions, hospital staff, and schools should be notified, and any symptomatic individuals should be treated. Bed linens, towels, and clothing should be washed and dried in a dryer on high heat.

Antihistamines, such as diphenhydramine or hydroxyzine, should be prescribed for pruritus. A mid-potency topical corticosteroid may also provide relief from itching. Clinically evident secondary bacterial infection should be treated with an antistaphylococcal agent.

Itching may take weeks to subside. Persistence of lesions or itching after 2 weeks requires referral and retreatment.

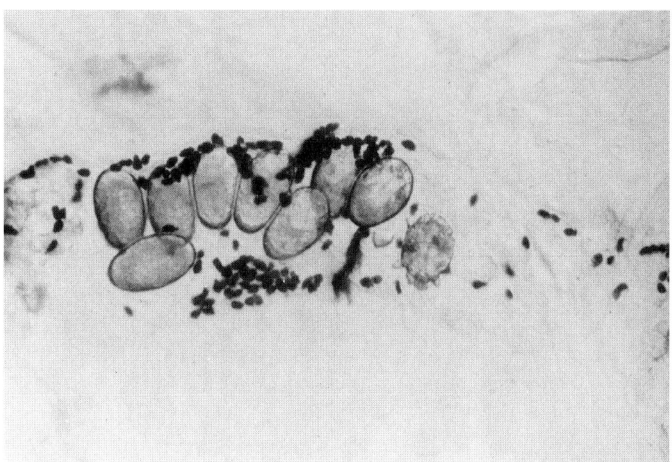

FIG. 250-2. Scabies preparation. The immature mite, ova, and scybala (fecal pellets) are present in this scraping of a burrow. The presence of any one of these elements is considered a positive scabies preparation result.

PEDICULOSIS

Pediculosis capitis (head lice) is an infestation of the hair and scalp by the mite *Pediculus capitis. Pediculus corporis* is the body louse, and pubic lice is an infestation of the pubic hair by *Phthirus pubis.*

Head Lice

This disorder is most commonly seen in school-aged children or in children attending day-care centers. However, any age group can be affected. It is very uncommon in African Americans. The louse is passed from person to person via close contact. The organism may live away from a host on furniture, clothing, linens, hats, or hairbrushes for several weeks, and thus may be passed to another who comes in contact with these articles. Head lice feed off human blood and therefore remain close to the scalp. When the louse lays its eggs, the ova, or nits, are cemented to the hair shaft. The ova hatch within 7 days. The ova encasement remains attached to the hair shaft and grows out with the hair. By the time the nits are a distance of 1 cm or more away from scalp, they have hatched.

CLINICAL FEATURES   Itching may be mild or quite intense. The occiput and posterior neck are common sites of pruritus, and excoriations on the neck may be noted.

DIAGNOSIS   The diagnosis is made on clinical inspection of the scalp for lice and nits (Figure 250-3). Unlike flakes of scale, which can easily be moved up and down the hair shaft, nits are firmly attached to the shaft. If the diagnosis is in question, suspected organisms or ova can be viewed underneath a microscope.

TREATMENT   Two important aspects of treatment should be addressed: treating the current infection and preventing reinfestation. Several agents may be used to treat the infestation. Permethrin 1 percent (Nix) rinse should be used as first-line therapy. Unlike lindane and pyrethrins, permethrin is ovicidal as well as pediculicidal. After shampooing, the treatment should be applied to the scalp for 10 min. For cosmetic reasons, nits can be removed by rinsing the hair in a 50 percent vinegar solution and then combing the hair with a fine-toothed comb.

To prevent reinfestation, all close contacts should be examined and affected individuals treated, including family members, classmates at school or day care, roommates, or health care workers in an institutional setting. Schools and day-care centers should be notified so that appropriate measures can be undertaken to evaluate other individuals.

Clothing, hats, and bed linens should be washed with hot water and dried in a dryer on high heat for 20 to 30 min. Carpets and sofas should be thoroughly vacuumed. Hairbrushes should be washed in hot water with the pediculicide product.

Patients should be reexamined in 7 to 10 days.

Pediculosis Pubis

In general, pubic lice is a sexually transmitted disease. Affected individuals should be evaluated for other sexually transmitted diseases. In children, the possibility of sexual abuse should be considered. Rarely, it may be passed from person to person via infested clothing, bed linens, and so on.

As with head lice, the main complaint is itching, which may vary in intensity. Pubic hair of the groin is most commonly infested, but body hair and eyelashes may be affected as well. Close inspection reveals the lice and nits (Figure 250-4).

Treatment is the same as for head lice. Permethrin (Nix) is the preferred initial therapy and should be applied to the affected area for 10 min and then rinsed. Eyelash infestations should be treated by manually removing as many lice and nits as possible, and then applying petrolatum to the lashes two to three times a day for 10 days.

Pediculosis Corporis

Body lice are currently uncommon in the United States. Infestation is more likely to occur in persons with poor hygiene or overcrowded living conditions. The lice reside on hair-bearing areas of the body but attach their nits to clothing. The lice and nits can survive as long as 30 days without contact with a human host. Clinically, the bite is often not perceived by an individual, but leaves a pruritic red urticarial papule. This lesion is not distinguishable from other bite reactions. A clue to diagnosis is that areas not covered by clothing, such as the face and hands, are usually spared. A high index of suspicion is needed, especially in patients with poor hygiene. Close inspection of clothing reveals nits, especially along clothing seams.

The body louse is the vector for epidemic typhus fever *(Rickettsia prowazekii),* trench fever *(Rickettsia quintana),* and relapsing fever *(Borrelia recurrentis).*

Treatment is as for head or pubic lice. Because the nits can survive long periods without human contact, infested clothing and linens should be destroyed. If they are not destroyed, recommendations include washing and drying on hot cycles and ironing the seams of the textiles. Oral antihistamines and topical corticosteroids may be necessary when itching is severe. Secondary infection, if present, should be treated.

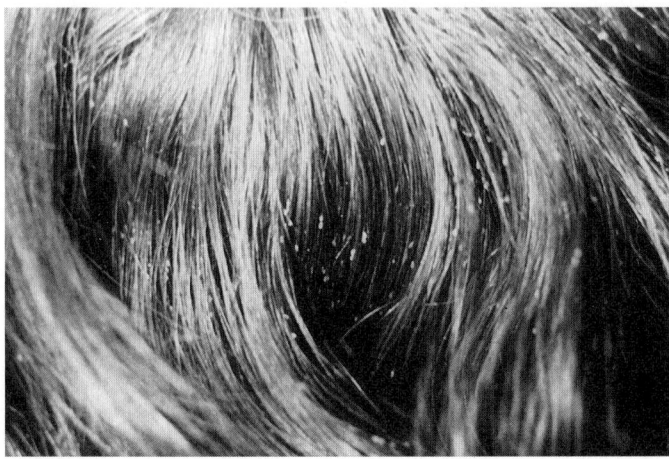

FIG. 250-3. Head lice. Nits are clearly visible, firmly attached to the hair shafts.

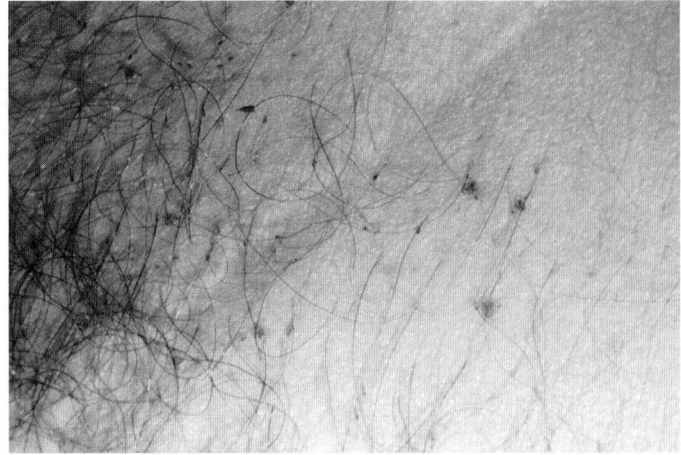

FIG. 250-4. Pubic lice. Pubic lice are seen on the skin surface, and nits are attached to the pubic hairs.

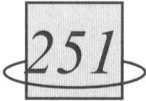

251

INITIAL APPROACH TO TRAUMA
Edward E. Cornwell III

Recent cataclysmic events have made Americans more cognizant of the need for trauma systems and trauma centers. Yet, it is the everyday "unspectacular" injuries that account for nearly 150,000 deaths each year. Injury is the fourth leading killer of Americans and the single greatest cause of death before the age of 45 years.[1] The predominant causes of death following trauma (i.e., head, chest, and major vascular injuries) imply that the organization of trauma centers and trauma systems should be predicated on the concepts of rapid triage, diagnosis, and therapeutic intervention.[2]

TRAUMA SYSTEMS AND TIMELY TRIAGE

The importance of a systems approach to trauma care becomes clear when the timing of death occurring secondary to traumatic injuries is considered.[3] The pattern of mortality takes on roughly a trimodal distribution where three peak occurrences are seen. The *first peak* occurs in the prehospital setting, largely a result of devastating head and major vascular injuries. Efforts to reduce deaths in this setting are largely societal, complex, and multidisciplinary, and include such multifaceted activities as drunk driving laws; safe road construction; seat belt, helmet, and airbag laws; and violence-prevention activities such as counseling, education and outreach efforts, handgun control, and dissemination of conflict resolution skills.[4,5] A *second peak* incidence of deaths as a result of traumatic injuries occurs in the early minutes and hours after a patient's arrival at the hospital. Deaths in this peak are largely a result of major head, chest, and abdominal injuries. The most important function of a trauma system is to decrease deaths in this phase by rapid transport of patients to the most appropriate facility and prompt resuscitation and identification of injuries requiring surgical intervention. The *third peak* in the trimodal distribution of deaths occurs in the intensive care unit, where the sequelae of organ hypoperfusion experienced in the early postinjury period are seen. Specifically, patients who have survived the initial injury, transport, and operative resuscitation die in this setting as a result of the systemic inflammatory response syndrome and multisystem organ failure.

In recognition of the need to establish a system in which injured patients are rapidly triaged to the most appropriate setting, Congress passed the Trauma Care Systems Planning and Development Act of 1991.[6] This Act required the development of a Model Trauma Care System Plan to be used as a reference document for each state to develop its system. Recent appropriations for this originally unfunded mandate have allowed a growing number of states to initiate the development of a comprehensive trauma system. Ultimately, each state must determine the appropriate facility for various types of injuries, and some states have come to rely on a verification process offered by the American College of Surgeons in order to designate certain hospitals as trauma centers.[2] Table 251-1 lists examples of requirements of various levels of trauma centers. In addition to the listed essentials, a trauma center must have all the required features of lower-level trauma centers. An effective trauma program requires the teamwork of emergency medicine, trauma surgery, and trauma care subspecialists.

In short, trauma centers are verified on the basis of commitment of personnel and resources needed to maintain a state of readiness to receive critically injured patients. A well-functioning trauma system ensures that not only are there appropriately designated trauma centers

but that there are also specific triage criteria to designate which patients should be transported to these centers (Table 251-2).

PRIMARY SURVEY

In accordance with the principles of advanced trauma life support, injured patients are assessed and treated in a fashion that establishes priorities based on their presenting vital signs, mental status, and injury mechanism.[7] The initial approach to trauma care is a process that consists of an initial primary assessment, rapid resuscitation, and a more thorough secondary survey followed by diagnostic tests and ultimate disposition constitutes (Table 251-3).

When available, a history obtained from a patient, witnesses, or prehospital provider may provide important information regarding circumstances of the injury (single-car accident, a fall, exposure, smoke inhalation), preexisting medical conditions (depression, cardiac disease, pregnancy), or medications (steroids, β-blockers) that may suggest certain patterns of injury or the physiologic response to injury.

A *primary survey* is undertaken quickly with the goal of identifying and treating life-threatening conditions. Specific lethal problems (discussed in further detail below) that should be identified immediately and addressed during the primary survey are airway obstruction, tension pneumothorax, massive hemorrhage, open pneumothorax, flail chest, and cardiac tamponade. The assessment of the ABCs (airway, breathing, and circulation) is such that evidence for or against the presence of these conditions is sought. During the primary survey, the following are quickly assessed:

*A*irway maintenance with C-spine control
*B*reathing/ventilation
*C*irculation with hemorrhage control
Neurologic *d*isability
*E*xposure, where the patient is completely undressed

Some specific points are emphasized regarding the various components of the trauma evaluation.

Airway with Cervical Spine Control

Rapid assessment for airway patency includes inspecting for foreign bodies or maxillofacial fractures that may result in airway obstruction. The chin-lift or jaw-thrust maneuver or the insertion of an oral or nasal airway is a first response for the patient making inadequate respiratory effort. A two-person technique whenever possible is suggested, where one devotes undivided attention to maintaining in-line immobilization and preventing excessive movement of the cervical spine. Comatose patients (Glasgow Coma Scale score 3 to 8; see "Disability" below) should be intubated tracheally to protect the airway and to prevent the secondary brain injury that occurs with hypoxemia. Logrolling and pharyngeal suction may be necessary to prevent aspiration if the patient vomits. Patients whose anatomy or severe maxillofacial injury precludes endotracheal intubation may require a surgical airway by means of cricothyroidotomy. Agitated trauma patients suffering from head injury, hypoxia, or drug- or alcohol-induced delirium may present a danger to themselves. In these circumstances, paralyzing agents such as succinylcholine or vecuronium, along with a small dose of diazepam or midazolam, may be necessary to enable safe airway management. See Chap. 19 for details, dosages, and techniques.

The issue of cervical spine (C-spine) clearance is one that has received much attention in the recent past. Ultimately, "clearance" of a C-spine is both a radiologic and a clinical undertaking. This implies that

TABLE 251-1 Essential Characteristics of Levels I, II, III and IV Trauma Centers

Level I (not required of levels II, III, and IV trauma centers)
  24-h availability of all surgical subspecialties (including cardiac surgery/ bypass capability)
  Neuroradiology, hemodialysis available 24 h
  Program that establishes and monitors effect of injury prevention/education efforts
  Organized trauma research program
Level II (not required of levels III and IV trauma centers)
  Cardiology, ophthalmology, plastic surgery, gynecologic surgery available
  Operating room ready 24 h a day
  Neurosurgery department in hospital
  Trauma multidisciplinary quality assurance committee
Level III (not required of level IV trauma centers)
  Trauma and emergency medicine services
  24-h radiology capability
  Pulse oximetry, central venous and arterial catheter monitoring capability
  Thermal control equipment for blood and fluids
  Published on-call schedule for surgeons, subspecialists
  Trauma registry
Level IV
  Initial care capabilities only
  Mechanism for prompt transfer
  Transfer agreements and protocols

patients who do not demonstrate evidence of bony fractures or subluxation on x-ray may still have significant injuries that are not appreciated if they cannot cooperate with a thorough physical examination. On the other hand, precious time should not be expended on multiple views in patients who have critical head, thoracic, and abdominal injuries that may require rapid intervention. In these patients, after a cross-table lateral view of the C-spine, the cervical collar should be left in place until the patient ultimately can cooperate with the clinical examination or undergo more sophisticated studies [e.g., computed tomography (CT) scans or magnetic resonance imaging (MRI) of the spine].

Finally, the practice of obtaining multiple C-spine x-rays in awake, alert patients with normal examinations (no pain or tenderness with the

TABLE 251-2 Maryland Criteria for Mandatory Transport to a Trauma Center

Abnormal vital signs (GCS <14 or systolic BP <90) (respiratory rate <10 or >29)
Multiple-system trauma
Penetrating wound to
  Head, neck, or torso
  Gunshot wound(s) to extremities proximal to elbow and knee
  An extremity with neurovascular compromise
CNS injury (head, spine)
Suspected pelvic fracture
Mechanism of injury
  Vehicular deformity
  Intrusion into passenger compartment greater than 12 in
  Major vehicular deformity greater than 20 in
Ejection
Entrapment
Falls greater than three times the patient's height
Fatality in same passenger compartment
Rapid deceleration
Auto–pedestrian/auto–bicycle injury with significant impact (>5 mi/h)
Vehicular rollover
Exposure to blast/explosion

Abbreviations: BP = blood pressure; CNS = central nervous system; GCS = Glasgow Coma Scale.
Source: Adapted from The Maryland Medical Protocols for Emergency Medical Services Providers. Maryland Institute for Emergency Medical Services Systems, 2003, p 121.

TABLE 251-3 A Step-by-Step Procedure for Trauma Resuscitation

1. *Notification by Prehospital Personnel:* The receiving emergency department should be informed about:
  Airway patency
  Pulse and respirations
  Level of consciousness
  Immobilization
  Mechanism of injury and blood loss at the scene
  Anatomic sites of apparent injury
2. *Preparation for Receiving the Trauma Victim*
  Assign tasks to team members
  Check and prepare vital equipment
  Summon surgical consultant and other team members not present
3. *Primary Survey:* The most immediately lethal injuries are taken care of as they are identified.
  Airway
    Clear airway: chin lift, suction, finger sweep
    Protect airway
      Depressed level of consciousness of bleeding, tracheal intubation without neck movement
    Surgical airway
  Breathing
    Ventilate with 100% oxygen
    Check thorax and neck
      Deviated trachea
      Tension pneumothorax (intervention—needle decompression)
      Chest wounds and chest wall motion
      Sucking chest wound (intervention—occlusive dressing)
      Neck and chest crepitation
      Multiple broken ribs
      Fractured sternum
      Pneumothorax
    Listen for breath sounds
      Correct tracheal tube placement?
      Hemopneumothorax?
        Chest tube(s)—38-Fr
        Collect blood for autotransfusion
  Circulation
    Apply pressure to sites of external exsanguination
    Assure that two large-bore IVs established
      Begin with rapid infusion of warm crystalloid solution
      If arm sites unavailable, insert a large central line or perform a saphenous cutdown at the ankle
    Assess for blood volume status
      Radial and carotid pulse, BP determination
      Jugular venous filling
      Quality of heart tones
    Beck triad present?
      Pericardiocentesis or echocardiogram
      Decompress tamponade
        Pericardiocentesis
        Thoracotomy with pericardiotomy
    Hypovolemia
      After 2 L of crystalloid begin blood infusion if still hypovolemic; in children use two 20-mL/kg boluses then 10-mL/kg blood boluses if still unstable
    Near-term pregnant patient—place roll under right hip
  Disability
    Brief neurologic examination
      Pupil size and reactivity
      Limb movement
      Glasgow Coma Scale
  Exposure
    Completely disrobe the patient
    Logroll to inspect back
  Continuing resuscitation
    Monitor fluid administration
      Consider central line for CVP monitoring
      Use fetal heart rate as indicator in pregnant women
      Record all events

(Continued)

TABLE 251-3   A Step-by-Step Procedure for Trauma Resuscitation *(Continued)*

4. *Secondary Survey:* A thorough search for injuries is carried out in order to set further priorities.

    Trauma series x-rays: lateral cervical spine, supine chest, AP pelvis

    Head-to-toe examination looking and feeling; quickly bring problems under control as they are discovered

        Scalp wound bleeding controlled with Raney clips

        Hemotympanum?

        Facial stability?

        Epistaxis tamponaded with balloons if severe

        Avulsed teeth, broken jaw?

        Penetrating injuries?

        Abdominal distention and tenderness?

        Pelvic stability?

        Perineal laceration/hematoma?

        Urethral meatus blood?

        Rectal examination for tone, blood, and prostate position

        Bimanual vaginal examination

        Peripheral pulses

        Deformities, open fractures

        Reflexes, sensation

    Large gastric tube $\geq$18-Fr inserted

    Foley catheter inserted

        Blood?

        Pregnancy test

    Logroll the patient to feel and see the back, flanks, and buttocks if not already done

    Splint unstable fractures/dislocations

    Assure that tetanus prophylaxis is given

    Consult with surgeon regarding further tests or immediate need for surgery or preferred IV medications; consider:

        Emergency thoracotomy to provide aortic compression of cross-clamping

        Aortogram or upright chest x-ray to rule out ruptured aorta

        Cystogram if pelvic fracture present or blood in urine

        IVP or enhanced CT scan of the abdomen

        FAST or diagnostic peritoneal lavage

        Head CT scan

        IV mannitol for neurologic decompensation

        IV steroids for possible spinal cord injury

        IV antibiotics for possible ruptured abdominal viscus

        IV antibiotics for perineal, vaginal, or rectal lacerations

        Pelvic arteriogram and embolization for pelvic hemorrhage

Abbreviations: CVP = central venous pressure; FAST = focused assessment with sonography for trauma; IVP = intravenous pyelography.

neck in neutral position and rotated in all four directions) is excessive. A large multicenter study, the National Emergency X-Radiography Utilization Study (NEXUS) has helped to develop clinical screening criteria that will spare the time and expense of cervical films.[8] The screening criteria that obviate need for C-spine imaging are:

1. No posterior midline C-spine tenderness
2. No evidence of intoxication
3. Alert mental status
4. No focal neurologic deficits
5. No painful distracting injuries

In a cohort of 34,069 patients with 578 clinically significant C-spine injuries, these criteria had a 99.6 percent sensitivity and 99.9 percent negative predictive value.

Breathing

With the patient breathing or now intubated and ventilated with 100 percent oxygen, the thorax and neck should be inspected, auscultated, and palpated to detect abnormalities such as a deviated trachea (tension pneumothorax); crepitus (pneumothorax); paradoxical movement of a chest wall segment (flail chest); sucking chest wound; fractured sternum; and absence of breath sounds on either side of the chest (pneumothorax, tension pneumothorax, massive pneumothorax). Possible interventions here include application of an occlusive dressing to a sucking chest wound, needle thoracostomy for tension pneumothorax, withdrawal of the endotracheal tube from the right mainstem bronchus; reintubation of the trachea if no breath sounds are heard, and insertion of large chest tubes (38-Fr) to relieve hemopneumothorax. Evacuated blood should be collected in an autotransfusion device. The volume of blood that returns should be noted immediately, because 1500 mL of hemorrhage may require a thoracotomy.

Circulation with Hemorrhage Control

Hemorrhagic shock, a common cause of postinjury death, should be assumed to be present in any hypotensive trauma patient until proven otherwise. Direct pressure should be used to control obvious external bleeding, and a rapid assessment of hemodynamic status is essential during the primary survey. This includes evaluation of level of consciousness, skin color, and presence and magnitude of peripheral pulses. Attention should be paid to the specifics of heart rate and blood pulse pressure (systolic minus diastolic blood pressure), particularly in young, previously healthy trauma patients (Table 251-4).

Not all hemorrhage produces hemorrhagic shock, and the unsuspecting clinician may fail to appreciate ongoing hemorrhage with blood loss of up to 30 percent of the circulating blood volume.[7] While class I hemorrhage (loss of up to 15 percent of circulating blood volume) is associated with minimal symptoms in most patients and is clearly not shock, class III hemorrhage associated with gross hypotension is readily appreciated as a state of hypoperfusion. Yet consider a young, healthy male trauma victim who has lost 25 percent of circulating blood volume (class II hemorrhage) and had a preinjury blood pressure of 130/70 mm Hg and a pulse rate of 60 beats/min. If this patient experiences a 50 percent increase in his pulse rate (to a rate of 90 beats/min) and a greater than 50 percent decrement of his pulse pressure (from 130/70 mm Hg pulse pressure of 60 beats/min to 116/90 mm Hg pulse pressure of 26 beats/min), the unsuspecting clinician may assume that the patient is "hemodynamically stable." A false sense of security may lead to delays in aggressively pursuing the source of bleeding (ultrasound, peritoneal lavage, operative exploration). From this example it should be clear that the practice of omitting diastolic blood pressures (and reporting "116/palpable," thus omitting the pulse pressure) is potentially hazardous. The alert, suspicious clinician identifies hemorrhage before it reaches the class III category of obvious shock.

Two large intravenous lines should be established and blood obtained for laboratory studies. While there are varying preferences, a percutaneous large line in the groin for unstable patients in whom upper extremity veins are not available is appropriate. This is so because subclavian lines are potentially dangerous in the hypovolemic patient with upper body trauma, saphenous vein cutdown at the ankle may not be appropriate for the patient with an injured lower extremity, and complications encountered from the femoral venous line may be minimized if the line is removed quickly on completion of resuscitation in the early postoperative period. Unstable patients without an obvious indication for surgery should be assessed for their response to 2 L of rapid infusion of crystalloids. If there is not marked improvement, type O blood should be transfused (O-negative for females of childbearing age). Auscultation for breath sounds and heart sounds and inspection of neck veins are included in the assessment of circulation because two major causes of hypotension may be present in trauma patients with minimal blood loss: *cardiac tamponade* (hypotension, agitation, distended neck veins, muffled heart sounds) and *tension pneumothorax* (hypotension, distended neck veins, absent breath sounds, deviated trachea, tympanic percussion of chest wall).

Echocardiography and abdominal ultrasonography, now becoming available in many emergency departments, are rapid, noninvasive ways to assess for fluid in the pericardium and peritoneal cavity.[9] This

TABLE 251-4 Estimated Fluid and Blood Losses Based on Patient's Initial Presentation

	Class I	Class II	Class III	Class IV
Blood loss (mL)*	Up to 750	750–1500	1500–2000	>2000
Blood loss (percent blood volume)	Up to 15	15–30	30–40	40
Pulse rate	<100	100–120	120–140	>140
Blood pressure	Normal	Normal	Decreased	Decreased
Pulse pressure (mm Hg)	Normal or increased	Decreased	Decreased	Decreased

*Assumes a 70-kg patient with a preinjury circulating blood volume of 5 L.

allows rapid determination of the bleeding source in the unstable multiply injured patient.

A discussion of the long-standing controversies involving *fluid resuscitation* is beyond the scope of this chapter. However, reference must be made to a landmark paper published by Bickell and associates.[10] In their prospective, randomized study of victims of penetrating torso injuries in Houston, patients were randomized to receiving immediate intravenous fluid resuscitation versus withholding fluid until operative intervention could be undertaken. A lower mortality was identified among the group with delayed fluid resuscitation, prompting the authors to speculate that giving fluids before operative control could be achieved is harmful. However one interprets this study, the fact that there were inordinate delays (sometimes >50 min) between hospital arrival and surgical intervention should help achieve consensus around at least one concept: the importance of rapid triage of critically injured patients, particularly those with penetrating trauma, to an appropriate trauma center. One is hard-pressed to identify any beneficial interventions that would justify a delay in rapid transport.

The inability, after nearly three decades, to demonstrate an unequivocal advantage of colloid therapy (which is more expensive than crystalloids) has led to near-universal acceptance of a balanced salt crystalloid (NS or LR) as the fluid of choice for initial resuscitation.

Disability

An abbreviated neurologic evaluation should now be performed, including level of consciousness, pupil size and reactivity, and motor function. The Glasgow Coma Scale (GCS) (see Table 255-2) should be used to quantify the patient's level of consciousness: possible scores range from 3 (no response) to 15 (high response on all measures). Despite the common comorbid presence of drug and alcohol abuse in trauma patients, it is only safe to assume that patients presenting with a GCS score of less than 15 and an appropriate mechanism have a head injury until proven otherwise. The GCS can be used to determine the severity of injury (minor injury GCS 13 and 14, moderate injury GCS 9 to 12, severe injury–coma GCS 3 to 8) and therefore the urgency with which the CT scan is obtained. New head injury guidelines have been formulated by an evidence-based methodology performed by the Brain Trauma Foundation in conjunction with the American Association of Neurological Surgeons.[11,12] Among the updated recommendations are 1) a suggested guideline for the placement of devices for intracranial pressure (ICP) monitoring for head-injured patients with GCS scores of 3 to 8 and a traumatic intracranial lesion and 2) concerns about prolonged prophylactic hyperventilation in the absence of an identified increase in ICP. The result of these two recommendations produces a heightened emphasis on the importance of the head CT scan. Only a head CT scan would identify the intracranial lesion that would lead to placement of an ICP catheter, and it is only with identification of such an increase in ICP that prolonged hyperventilation (until recently a practice routinely taught) can be justified. Accordingly, patients who are comatose after head injury should be intubated with in-line neck immobilization and transported to the CT scanner with the same sense of urgency that a hypotensive patient with a gunshot wound to the abdomen would be rushed to the operating room.

Exposure

No primary survey is complete without thoroughly disrobing the patient and examining the total body surface area carefully for otherwise hidden bruises, lacerations, impaled foreign bodies, and open fractures. If hemodynamically stable and if the airway is ensured, the patient should be logrolled, with one attendant assigned to maintain cervical stabilization. Check the back and thoracic and lumbar spine for tenderness. Check the gluteal cleft and perineum for injury. When the examination is completed, the patient should be covered with warm blankets to prevent hypothermia.

When derangements in any of the components of the primary survey are identified, treatment is undertaken immediately. Once the primary survey is complete, securing of the airway, intravenous catheters as well as urinary and gastric catheters, and monitors should be achieved. At this point a *secondary survey,* a more thorough head-to-toe evaluation, is undertaken. It should be stressed that the secondary survey is not initiated until the primary survey (ABCs) is assessed to be adequate and resuscitation has been initiated.

SPECIFIC INJURIES OF IMPORTANCE

Having discussed the initial assessment of the injured patient, emphasis is placed on specific injuries of importance. These injuries are critical in that they are identified during the primary survey, represent impending demise, and require an immediate response.

Traumatic Arrests

In most emergency medical systems, paramedics transport patients without vital signs to a hospital while CPR is initiated (unless obvious signs of death are present). On arrival to the ED, a critical decision must be made regarding the level of intervention. A series analyzing 862 patients undergoing ED thoracotomy at a regional trauma center yields interesting information.[13] The overall number of neurologically intact survivors was 3.9 percent. Among patients with blunt trauma and no vital signs in the field there were no survivors. This is a consistent finding among other series, and clearly ED thoracotomy for this group of patients should be abandoned. The greatest proportion of neurologically intact survivors was among patients with stab wounds to the chest. Further analysis revealed that survival rate was 23 percent among thoracic stab wound victims with vital signs in the field, and 38 percent among those who were moribund but had some vital signs on arrival to the ED. Therefore, the strongest recommendation for ED thoracotomy can be made for victims with penetrating chest trauma with witnessed signs of life in transport or in the ED and at least cardiac electrical activity on arrival.[13–15] More liberal indications (although not with total consensus) would include victims with abdominal trauma with cardiac electrical activity, in whom thoracotomy is performed for resuscitation and aortic cross-clamping before operating room laparotomy (rather than for hemorrhage control), and patients with blunt torso trauma who have some vital signs on arrival. Patients with blunt trauma and absent vital signs or sign of life on arrival should not undergo thoracotomy.

Severe Head Trauma

Head trauma with coma (GCS 3 to 8) suggests that rapid assessment of the intracranial injury must be undertaken and the patient should be intubated for airway protection and to avoid secondary brain injury associated with hypoxemia. These patients present a dilemma, because ultimately they may be found to have anything ranging from a normal head CT scan to a devastating, nonsurvivable brain injury. The challenge is to quickly identify patients with intracranial injuries that may benefit from neurosurgical evacuation. In such cases, minutes may make a difference in the ultimate patient outcome. Accordingly, all nonessential procedures (i.e., those that do not address a problem discovered during the primary survey) should be prioritized to a time after the head CT is performed. The patient is intubated with in-line neck immobilization, and the C-spine collar is reapplied. A rapid chest x-ray may be justifiable to exclude pneumothorax and to assess endotracheal tube placement, particularly if the film can be developed as the patient is being transported to the CT scan suite. This implies that in the well-run trauma center the critically multisystem-injured patient has ongoing diagnostic workup and therapeutic resuscitation occurring in a smooth transition between ED, x-ray suite, operating room, and postoperative intensive care setting.

Tension Pneumothorax, Open Pneumothorax, and Massive Hemothorax

These are all diagnoses that should be made during the primary survey and subsequently require rapid placement of a chest tube. Absent breath sounds on the side of a gunshot wound, stab wound, or chest wall ecchymosis (associated with tympany in the case of pneumothorax and percussion dullness in the case of hemothorax) in a patient with respiratory distress and tachycardia suggest the diagnosis. These are discussed in detail in Chap. 259.

Abdominal Gunshot Wounds with Hypotension

This deserves special mention. Palpation tenderness elicited on ED admission identifies the need for surgery and should prompt *immediate transport to the operating room* without further workup. Placement of nasogastric, urinary, and intravenous catheters should proceed in the operating room as the patient is being prepared for general anesthesia. The importance of time is emphasized because of the large amount of hemorrhage necessary (>2 L in the 70-kg patient) to produce severe hypotension in a young, previously healthy patient.[7] A false sense of security with these patients brought on by the absence of hypotension is hazardous.

Deeply Impaled Objects

Deeply impaled objects of the chest and abdomen should be left in situ and the patient rapidly transported to the operating room for surgical removal under direct vision to ensure hemostasis.[16] The object can be shortened to facilitate transport.

SECONDARY SURVEY

While resuscitation continues, a secondary survey should be undertaken. The secondary survey is a rapid but thorough physical examination for the purpose of identifying as many injuries as possible. With this information, the resuscitating physician and his or her surgical colleagues can set logical priorities for evaluation and management. Frequent assessments of the patient's blood pressure, pulse rate, and central venous pressure should continue.

The examination is conducted in a head-to-toe fashion, beginning with the scalp. Scalp lacerations can bleed profusely. This bleeding can be controlled with plastic Raney clips that grasp the full thickness of the scalp and galea. The tympanic membranes should be visualized to detect hemotympanum, and the pupil examination should be repeated. If epistaxis is a problem, a balloon-tipped urinary catheter or a nasal balloon should be inserted to provide posterior tamponade. The examination continues over the neck and thorax. A lateral cervical spine x-ray (if not already obtained), a chest x-ray, and an anteroposterior pelvic x-ray should be obtained while the secondary survey continues. A gastric tube should be inserted into the stomach and connected to suction. When there is facial trauma or basilar skull fracture, the gastric tube should be inserted through the mouth rather than the nose. The urinary meatus, scrotum, and perineum are inspected for the presence of blood, hematoma, or laceration.

A rectal examination is done, noting sphincter function and whether the prostate is boggy or displaced. Rectal blood should be noted. If the prostate is normal and there is no blood at the urethral meatus, a urinary drainage catheter can be placed in the bladder. If a urethral injury is suspected (meatal blood present), a urethrogram should be obtained prior to passing the catheter. If the prostate is displaced, it should be assumed that the urethra is disrupted. Catheterization should not be attempted if the urethra is injured. The urine should be examined for blood. If the patient is a woman of childbearing age, a pregnancy test should be obtained. If there is vaginal bleeding, a manual and speculum examination is necessary to identify a possible vaginal laceration in the presence of a pelvic fracture. Palpate all peripheral pulses. The patient should be logrolled to either side while keeping the neck immobilized so that every inch of the patient's body is seen and felt. The extremities should be evaluated for fracture and soft tissue injury. Peripheral pulses should be felt. A more thorough neurologic examination can now be done, carefully checking motor and sensory function.

There are many conditions that may be delayed or not evident during the secondary survey unless specifically sought. The secondary survey should be directed toward evidence of the presence or absence of the following conditions: tracheal disruption, aortic disruption, esophageal disruption, pulmonary contusion, cardiac contusion, and diaphragmatic hernia. The latter five are discussed in Chap. 259.

Some of these are not evident even with diligent search during the secondary survey. Vigilance should be maintained during the ED visit, observation period, and any subsequent hospital stay for delayed presentations. Although usually not life-threatening, missed conditions are most likely to be orthopedic in nature. Careful consideration of extremity orthopedic injuries can be easily overlooked in patients whose presentations require a multitrauma evaluation.

Radiographic Imaging

In patients who are not rapidly transported to the operating suite or the CT scanner after the initial assessment, standard radiographic imaging includes *lateral C-spine, chest,* and *pelvic radiographs.* The chest x-ray and pelvic films image the three regions (left hemithorax, right hemithorax, and extraperitoneal pelvis) outside the true peritoneal cavity that can accommodate volumes of hemorrhage sufficient to produce gross hypotension. X-rays in penetrating trauma are dictated by bullet entry site and include a chest x-ray for patients with torso penetrating trauma and appropriate extremity films to exclude fractures in patients with penetrating extremity injuries.

Echocardiography has become a useful diagnostic tool for emergency physicians and trauma surgeons.[17] A focused abdominal sonographic examination for trauma (FAST) is a rapid diagnostic tool performed with a 3.5-MHz transducer that assesses for fluid in 1) the pericardium, 2) the hepatorenal recess of Morrison (a common location for blood in patients with hemoperitoneum), 3) the pelvis around the bladder, and 4) the perisplenic region. Abdominal sonography in the trauma patient is rapidly supplanting *diagnostic peritoneal lavage* as the procedure of choice to detect hemoperitoneum in the unstable trauma patient for whom transport to the CT suite is unsafe.[9]

DISPOSITION

Options include moving the patient to the operating room, admission to the hospital, or transfer to another facility. The primary and secondary survey must have been completed, and a gastric tube and a urinary drainage catheter should be in place unless a urethral injury was detected. In most urban level I hospitals, the trauma surgeon should have been present for the secondary survey and should assume direction of the diagnostic workup and disposition of the case at that time. In rural hospitals that transfer severe trauma cases, the resuscitating physician should relate all the physical findings discovered during the primary and secondary surveys to the physician receiving the patient. Laboratory results, x-rays, and the flow sheet showing blood pressure, pulse, fluids infused, urine output, gastric output, and neurologic findings should accompany the patient. If a diagnostic peritoneal lavage was performed, a sample of the lavage fluid should accompany the patient. A patient who is being transported to another facility should be accompanied by personnel capable of administering fluids and monitoring vital signs and pupillary changes. Mannitol should be available if there is neurologic deterioration en route.

The hallmark of trauma care in patients without obvious indications for surgery identified on the initial assessment is *serial examination*. An *observation area* is extremely useful for these patients. Such an area (typically with nursing care provisions analogous to those of an intermediate care unit in most hospitals) allows for serial observations of 1) patients with closed head trauma who have regained consciousness but who require repeat neurologic examinations; 2) patients with penetrating abdominal wounds (stab wounds or tangential gunshot wounds) who require repeat abdominal examinations; 3) patients receiving repeat chest x-rays for penetrating chest trauma without pneumothoraces; 4) patients with blunt abdominal trauma with normal physical examination on initial evaluation; and 5) patients with documented blunt injuries to the liver, spleen, or kidney who are clinically stable and are being managed nonoperatively. An observation area for these patients should allow for more rapid triage from the ED and for serial evaluations of multiple patients in a convenient setting and should provide for rapid transport to the operating room in patients whose clinical examination deteriorates.

REFERENCES

1. Committee on Injury Prevention and Control Division of Health Promotion and Disease Prevention, in Bonnie RJ, Fulco CE, Liverman CT (eds): *Reducing the Burden of Injury. Advancing Prevention and Treatment.* Washington, DC: National Academy Press, 1999.
2. American College of Surgeons Committee on Trauma: *Resources for Optimal Care of the Injured Patient: 1999.* Chicago: American College of Surgeons, 1998.
3. Mann NC, Mullins RJ, MacKenzie EJ, et al: Systematic review of published evidence regarding trauma system effectiveness. *J Trauma* 47:S25, 1999.
4. Cornwell EE III, Jacobs D, Walker M, et al: National Medical Association Surgical Section: Position paper on violence prevention: A resolution of trauma surgeons caring for victims of violence. *JAMA* 273:1788, 1995.
5. Cornwell EE III, Berne TV, Belzberg H, et al: Health care crisis from a trauma center perspective: The L.A. story. *JAMA* 276(12):940, 1996.
6. General Accounting Office: *Trauma Care: Life-Saving System Threatened by Unreimbursed Costs and Other Factors. Report to the Chairman, Subcommittee on Health for Families and the Uninsured, Committee on Finance, U.S. Senate.* Washington, DC: GAO (HRD-91-57), 1991.
7. American College of Surgeons Committee on Trauma: *Advanced Trauma Life Support for Doctors, Instructor Course Manual,* 6th ed. Chicago: American College of Surgeons, 1997.
8. Hoffman JR, Mower WR, Wolfson AB, et al: Validity of a set of clinical criteria to rule out injury to the cervical spine in patients with blunt trauma. *New Engl J Med* 343:343, 2000.
9. McKenney GS, Ochsner MG, Schmidt JA, et al: Can ultrasound replace diagnostic peritoneal lavage in the assessment of blunt trauma? *J Trauma* 37:439, 1994.
10. Bickell WH, Wall MJ Jr, Pepe PE, et al: Immediate versus delayed fluid resuscitation for hypotensive patients with penetrating torso injuries. *New Engl J Med* 331:1105, 1994.
11. Brain Trauma Foundation: Indications for intracranial pressure monitoring. *J Neurotrauma* 13:667, 1997.
12. Brain Trauma Foundation: The use of hyperventilation in the acute management of severe traumatic brain injury. *J Neurotrauma* 13:699, 1997.
13. Branney SW, Moore EE, Feldhaus KM, Wolfe RE: Critical analysis of two decades of experience with postinjury emergency department thoracotomy in a regional trauma center. *J Trauma* 45(1):87, 1998.
14. Esposito TJ, Jurkovich GJ, Rice CL, et al: Reappraisal of emergency room thoracotomy in a changing environment. *J Trauma* 31:881, 1991.
15. Velmahos GC, Degiannis E, Souter I, et al: Outcome of a strict policy on emergency department thoracotomies. *Arch Surg* 130:774, 1995.
16. Cartwright AJ, Taams KO, Unsworth-White MJ, et al: Suicidal nonfatal impalement injury of the thorax. *Ann Thorac Surg* 72:1364, 2001.
17. Rozycki GS, Ochsner MG, Frankel HL, et al: A prospective study of surgeon-performed ultrasound as the initial diagnostic modality for injured patient assessment. *J Trauma* 39:492, 1995.

PEDIATRIC TRAUMA
William E. Hauda II

Trauma is the leading cause of death and disability in children over 1 year of age. The most common reason for injury is a motor vehicle crash. Because children have different anatomy and physiology, the management of injuries in children differs in some respects from that of adults. Knowledge of these differences is crucial for emergency physicians to provide expedient and effective care to injured children. Many injuries can be initially managed in a general hospital ED, but care of the most seriously injured children requires prompt triage and transportation to a designated pediatric trauma center.

EPIDEMIOLOGY

Head injury is the most frequent cause of traumatic death in children.[1] Motor vehicle injuries are the leading cause of death among children over the age of 1 year, accounting for 18 percent of all deaths and 37 percent of all deaths due to trauma.[2] Motor vehicle crashes are also the most frequent cause of injury.[1] Alcohol use by a driver is a factor in almost 25 percent of these crashes.[3] Under the age of 1 year, suffocation is the most common cause of death due to injury.[2] The other leading causes of death are drowning, fire/burn, and firearms. Death rates for boys over the age of 5 is twice the rate for girls.[2] Children who are economically disadvantaged are 2.6 times more likely to die from trauma.

Homicide accounts for about 25 percent of pediatric deaths. Infants are 10 times more likely to die from homicide than are children 5 to 9 years of age.[2] Rates of death from injury among children have declined over the past 10 years in the United States in all categories except for firearms, suffocation, and poisoning.

TRAUMA RESUSCITATION PRIORITIES

The priorities in managing children with traumatic injuries do not differ from those of injured adults (see Chap. 251). Injuries and conditions that require immediate lifesaving intervention are treated during the primary survey (Table 252-1). All other conditions are identified and managed during the secondary survey.

A team approach will help to minimize confusion during the initial resuscitation. Tasks for individual members of the team include airway management, cervical spine stabilization, intravascular line placement, assessment of the child by system, and preparation and admin-

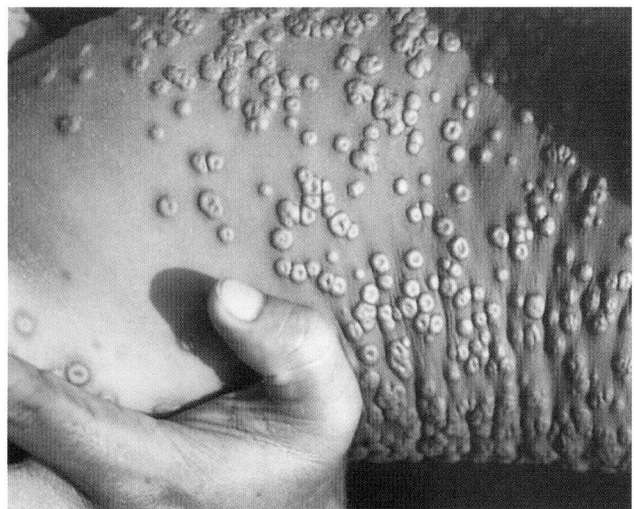

PLATE 1 Smallpox lesions on skin of trunk. [Reprinted with permission from Public Health Images Library (PHIL) ID #284, Centers for Disease Control and Prevention.]

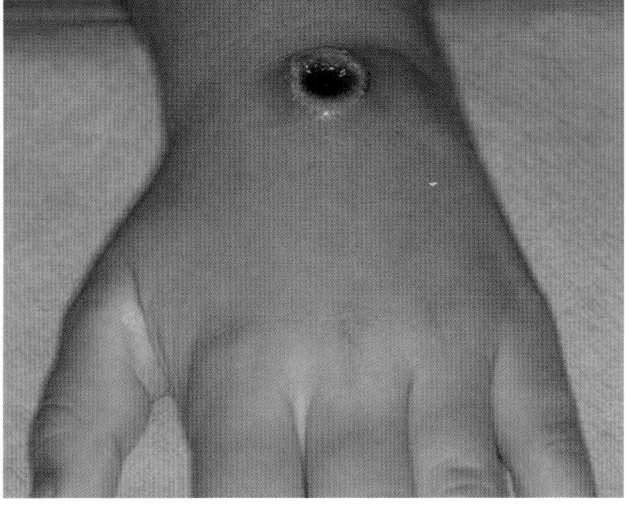

PLATE 2 (Fig. 135-7). Cutaneous anthrax in a 9-year-old girl. [Reproduced with permission from DOIA (Dermatology Online Atlas) University Erlangen, Department of Dermatology, Nürnberg, Germany, www.dermis.net/index_e.htm.]

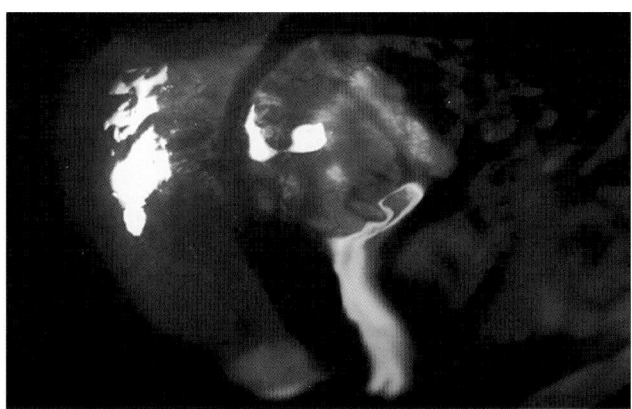

PLATE 3 (Fig. 238-8). Positive Seidel test showing aqueous leaking through a full-thickness corneal wound. Aqueous will turn fluorescein lime-green under a cobalt-blue light as it oozes through the wound while being observed at the slit lamp.

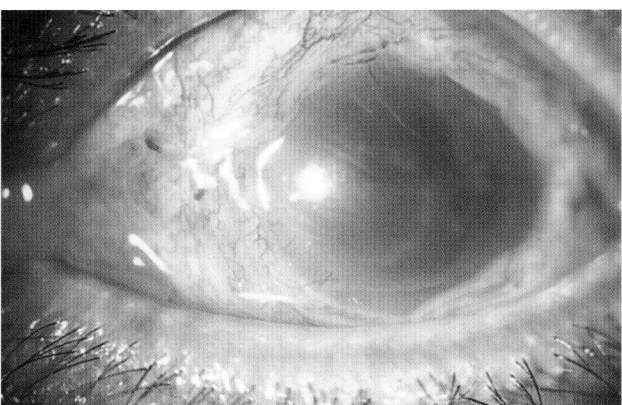

PLATE 4 (Fig. 238-9). Hyphema secondary to blunt trauma. Note the blood filling the lower half of the anterior chamber and hazy appearance of cornea suggesting increased IOP.

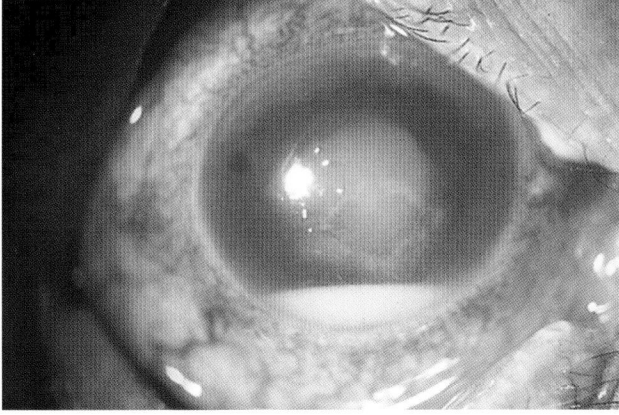

PLATE 5 (Fig. 238-10). Corneal ulcer with hypopyon. The ulcer is seen as a shaggy white corneal infiltrate surrounding the borders of the epithelial defect. The hypopyon represents the accumulation of white cells layering out in the lower one-sixth of the anterior chamber.

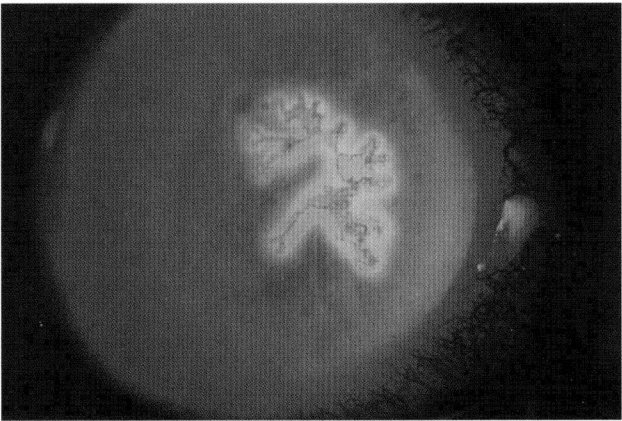

PLATE 6 (Fig. 238-11). Herpes simplex corneal dendrite seen with fluorescein staining and cobalt-blue light.

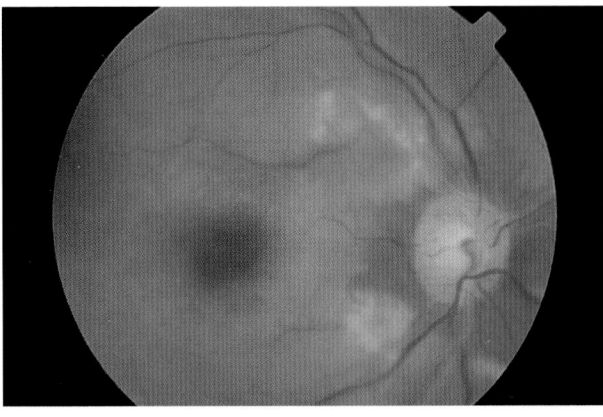

PLATE 7 (Fig. 238-17). Central retinal artery occlusion. Note macular "cherry red spot" and retinal pallor between macula and disc. The retinal veins appear normal size, but the arteries are barely visible and attenuated.

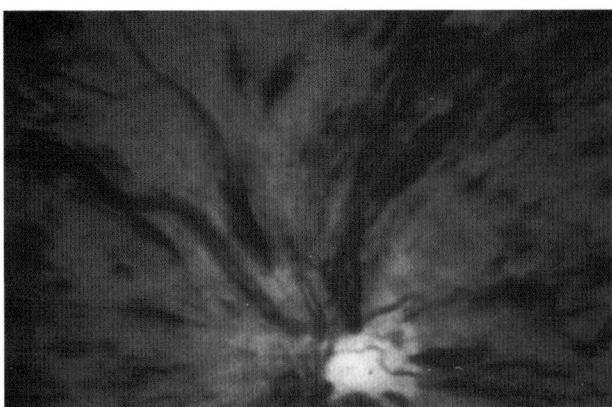

PLATE 8 (Fig. 238-18). Central retinal vein occlusion "blood and thunder fundus." Note diffuse retinal hemorrhages in all retina quadrants and blurred disc margins.

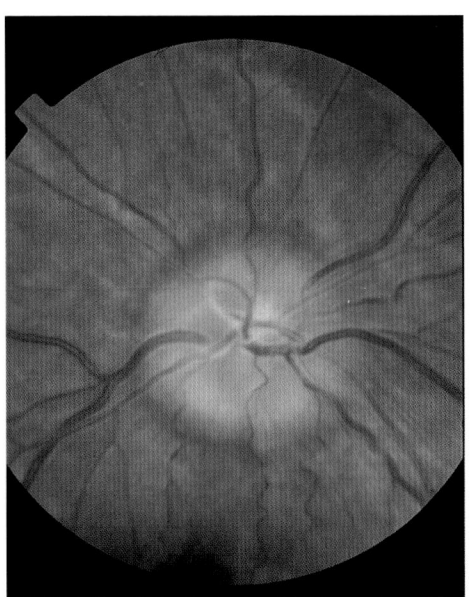

◀ **PLATE 9 (Fig. 238-22).** Optic nerve head edema. Vascular congestion, elevation of the nerve head, and blurred disk margins are characteristically seen in papilledema, papillitis, and compressive lesions of the optic nerve.

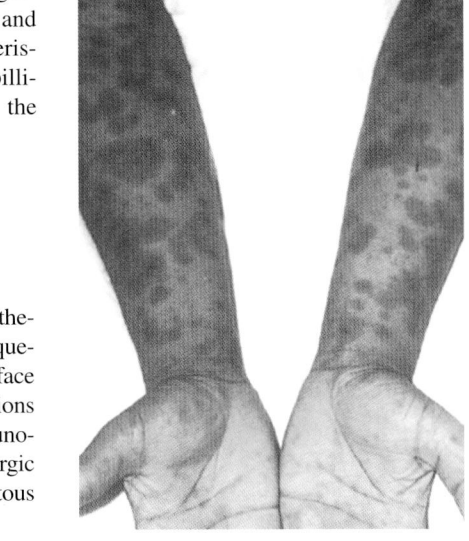

▶ **PLATE 10 (Fig. 246-1A).** Erythema multiforme. Symmetrical, plaque-like lesions involve the flexor surface of the upper extremities; these lesions may be misdiagnosed as the immunoglobulin G-mediated urticarial allergic reaction. Also note the erythematous macules on the palms.

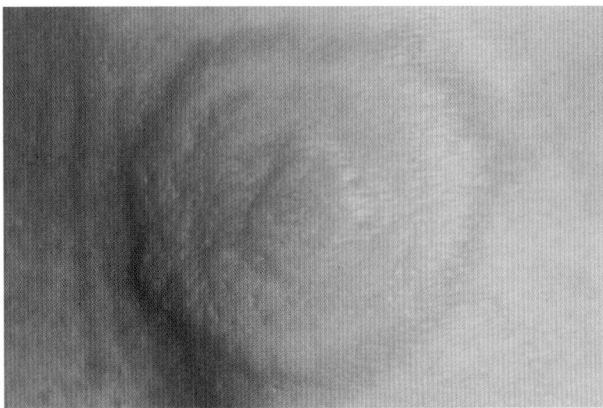

PLATE 11 (Fig. 246-1B). Iris or target lesion, a finding strongly suggestive of erythema multiforme. This iris lesion is composed of a central bullous lesion with a dusky, edematous center and an erythematous halo. (Reprinted with permission from Brady W, DeBehnke D, Crosby D: Dermatologic emergencies. *Am J Emerg Med* 12:217, 1994.)

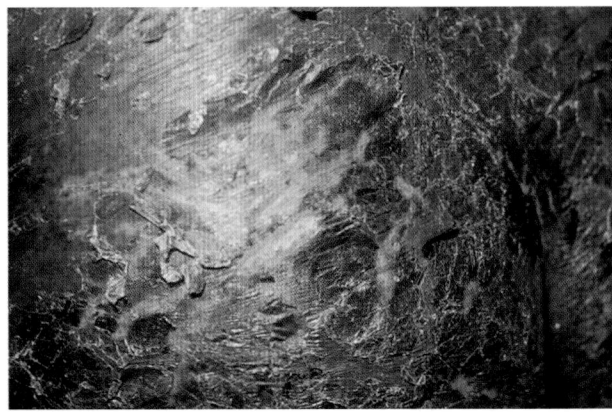

PLATE 12 (Fig. 246-2). Exfoliative dermatitis demonstrated by generalized, warm erythema accompanied by scaling or flaking.

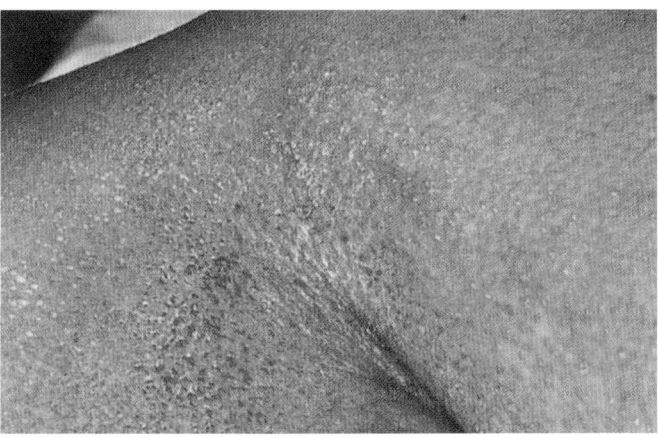

PLATE 13 (Fig. 246-3). Blanching, nonpruritic erythroderma with a "rough" texture in a patient with toxic shock syndrome. (Reprinted with permission from Brady W, DeBehnke D, Crosby D: Dermatologic emergencies. *Am J Emerg Med* 12:217, 1994.)

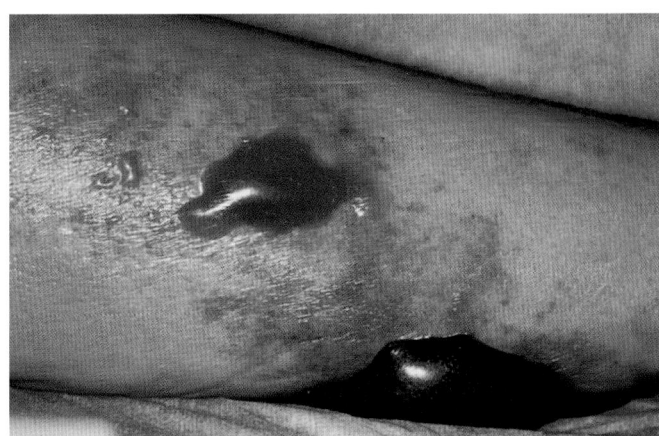

PLATE 14 (Fig. 246-4). Large bullous lesions on the lower extremity in a patient with streptococcal toxic shock.

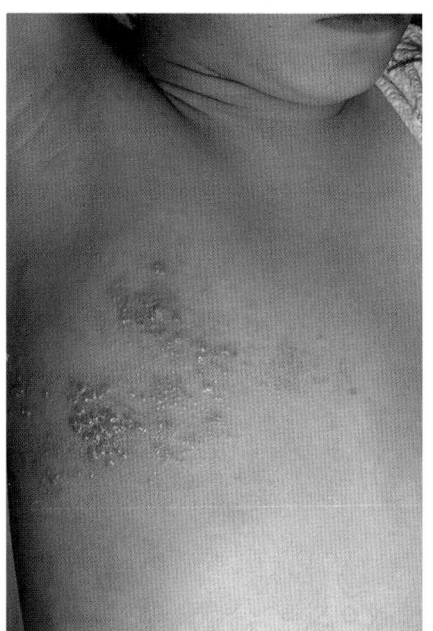

PLATE 15 (Fig. 246-5). Single dermatomal involvement in a patient with herpes zoster infection in a thoracic distribution.

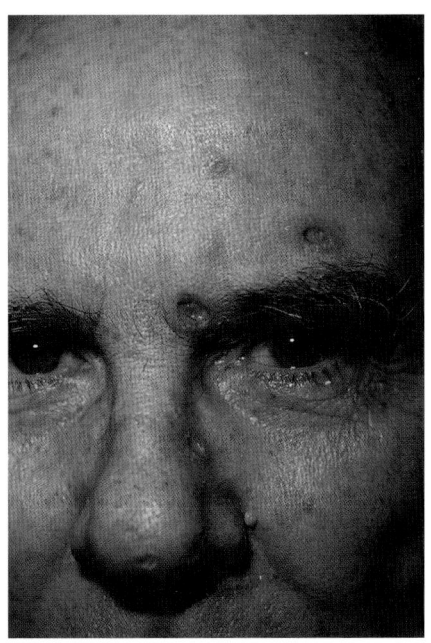

PLATE 16 (Fig. 246-6). Herpes zoster ophthalmic infection. Facial zoster involving the ophthalmic branch of the fifth cranial nerve with nasal lesions strongly suggestive of corneal infection.

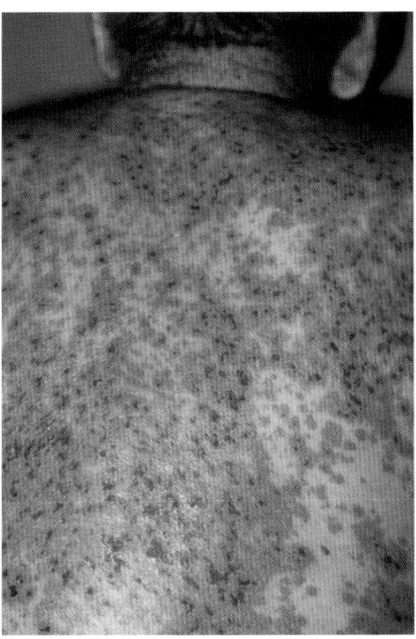

PLATE 17 (Fig. 246-7). Disseminated herpes simplex virus infection in an immunocompromised adult patient; note the widespread distribution of vesicular lesions on an erythematous base.

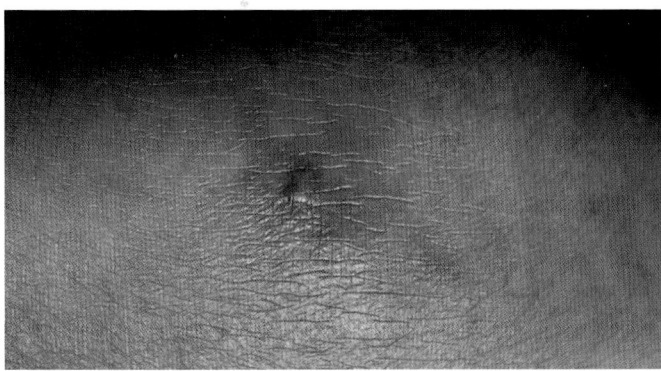

PLATE 18 (Fig. 246-8). Disseminated gonococcal infection in a sexually active adult female. The maculopapule has a petechial component and an erythematous periphery on the extensor surface of the wrist.

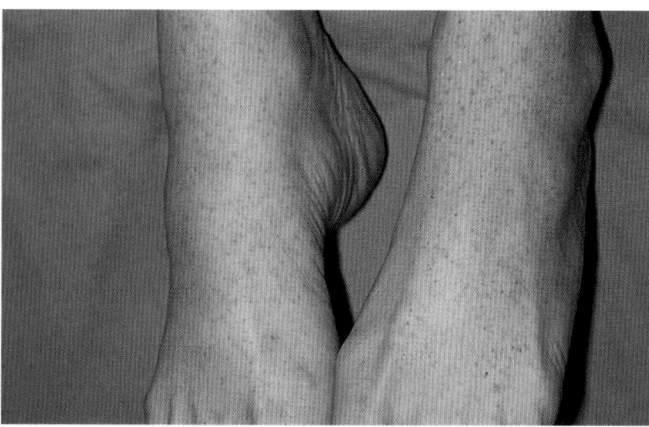

PLATE 19 (Fig. 246-9). A patient with Rocky Mountain spotted fever with petechiae on the ankles.

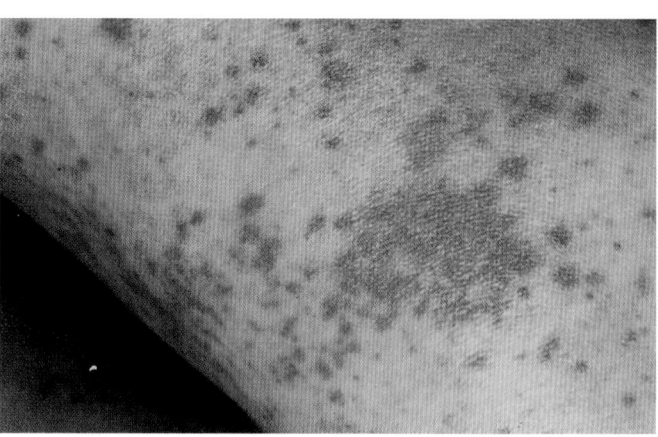

PLATE 20 (Fig. 246-10). Early findings of meningococcemia with petechiae evolving into purpuric lesions. (Reprinted with permission from Brady W, DeBehnke D, Crosby D: Dermatologic emergencies. *Am J Emerg Med* 12:217, 1994.)

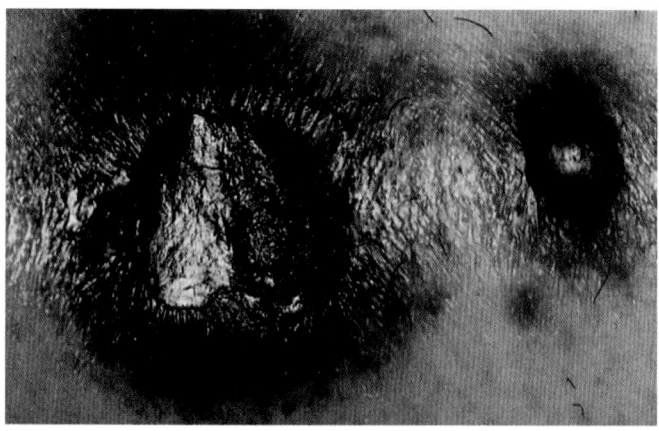

PLATE 21 (Fig. 246-11). Purpura fulminans with hemorrhagic bullae. (Reprinted with permission from Tangoren IA et al: Ecchymoses and epidermal necrosis in a 75-year-old man with bacteremia. *J Crit Illness* 13:108, 1998.)

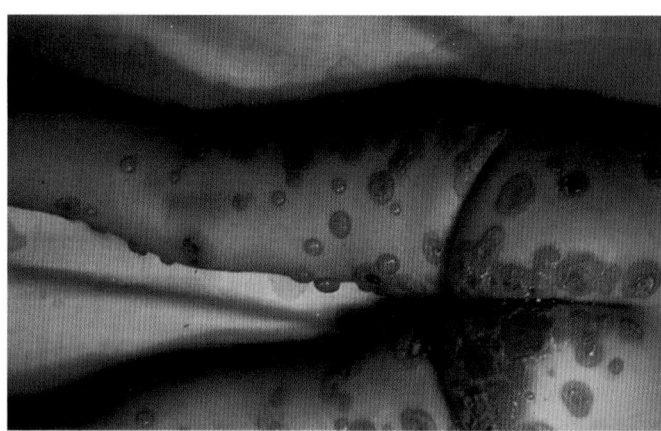

PLATE 22 (Fig. 246-12). Scattered bullous lesions intermixed with erosions and painful inflammatory plaques.

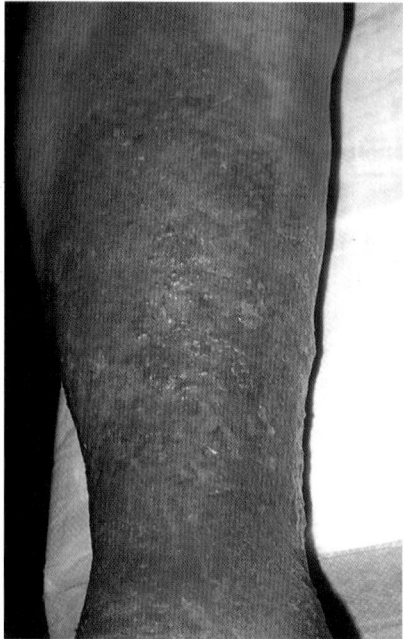

◄ **PLATE 23 (Fig. 248-6).** Stasis dermatitis. Note the surrounding red-brown pigmentation and the central weepy erythema on the pretibial leg.

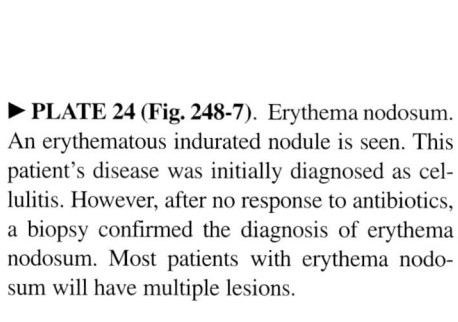

▶ **PLATE 24 (Fig. 248-7).** Erythema nodosum. An erythematous indurated nodule is seen. This patient's disease was initially diagnosed as cellulitis. However, after no response to antibiotics, a biopsy confirmed the diagnosis of erythema nodosum. Most patients with erythema nodosum will have multiple lesions.

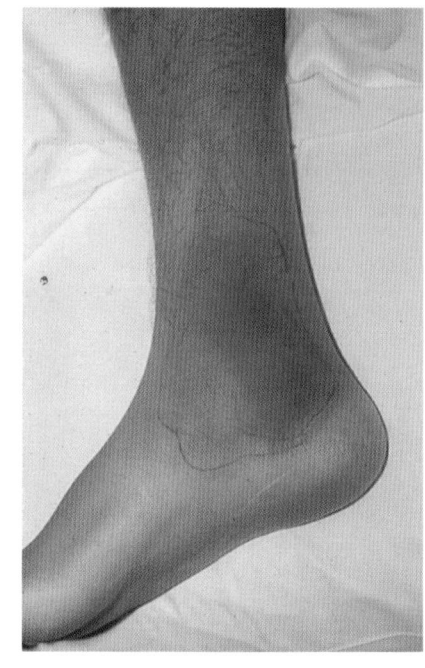

TABLE 252-1 Primary Survey Goals

Identify	Intervene
Airway	
Airway obstruction	Open airway, remove obstruction
Breathing	
Apnea	Positive pressure ventilation
Hypoxia	Supplemental oxygen administration
Tension pneumothorax	Needle thoracostomy, tube thoracostomy
Massive hemothorax	Tube thoracostomy
Open pneumothorax	Occlusive dressing, tube thoracostomy
Circulation	
Shock	Fluid bolus, blood products
Pericardial tamponade	Fluid bolus, pericardiocentesis, thoracotomy
Cardiac arrest	Thoracotomy if penetrating trauma
Disability	
Spinal cord injury	Immobilization, steroids
Cerebral herniation	Hyperventilation, mannitol
Exposure	
Hypothermia	Warmed fluids, external warming
Exsanguinating hemorrhage	Direct pressure, air splints

istration of medications and fluids. A team leader not directly involved in patient care can facilitate the overall management of the patient because that person is not dedicated to a particular task.

Airway

The most important step in trauma care for children is airway intervention. Proficient management of a child's airway requires an understanding of the anatomy of children, basic airway techniques, principles of pediatric intubation, and methods for establishing a surgical airway. All these are covered in detail in Chap. 15. Ketamine should not be used in children with head injury because it causes increased cerebral blood flow and can increase intracranial pressure.

Cervical Spine

The cervical spine must be immobilized for head injury and suspected spinal injury until cervical spine injury can be excluded. No studies have been completed in children to reliably predict which patients require immobilization. Some criteria include spinal pain or tenderness, significant multiple system trauma, severe head or facial trauma, numbness or weakness in any extremity, loss of consciousness, significant distracting injury, and altered mental status with the possibility of trauma. In one study of 102 cases of pediatric spine injuries, 40 percent were associated with head injury.[4] A properly fitting rigid collar should be used. Because a collar does not provide complete immobilization, the head should be secured to the spine board by using towel rolls or commercially available head blocks and tape applied across the forehead and under the chin of the collar.[5,6] If a collar is not used, tape should not be applied under the chin, because this may prevent the mouth from opening. The child's body is secured to the board by straps or wide cloth tape. Blanket rolls should be placed on either side of the child to prevent lateral movement of the child if logrolling becomes necessary to clear the airway. Clearance of the child's cervical spine by clinical or radiographic methods should be delayed until the primary survey is completed.

Breathing

All trauma patients should receive supplemental oxygen. Assessment of breathing should identify inadequate oxygenation or ventilation or the potential for deterioration. Children with respiratory failure should

have positive-pressure ventilation (PPV) (e.g., bag-valve-mask) started immediately. PPV may change an innocuous pneumothorax into a compromising injury, so patients must be actively monitored for such changes. If the presence of a small pneumothorax is already known, a tube thoracostomy may be appropriate early in the resuscitation efforts. Cyanosis, agitation, poor capillary refill, bradycardia, and desaturation on pulse oximetry are signs of hypoxemia. Signs of inadequate ventilation in the young child include tachypnea, nasal flaring, grunting, retractions, and stridor or wheezing. Auscultation of the chest can identify a large pneumothorax or hemothorax. Because breath sounds are easily transmitted across a small chest, they should be assessed in both axillae. If signs of inadequate oxygenation do not improve rapidly with high-flow oxygen administration, then PPV must be started.

TENSION PNEUMOTHORAX   The classic presentation of a tension pneumothorax is absent ipsilateral breath sounds, ipsilateral tympany, relatively fixed expanded ipsilateral chest wall, hypotension, and jugular venous distention due to high intrathoracic pressures. If tension pneumothorax is suspected during the primary survey, a catheter decompression should be performed without radiographic confirmation. Tube thoracostomy can be placed later.

MASSIVE HEMOTHORAX   The classic presentation of a massive hemothorax is absent ipsilateral breath sounds, ipsilateral dullness to percussion, poor to absent ipsilateral chest wall motion with ventilation, and hypotension. Jugular venous distention is unlikely because the circulatory volume is low. Tube thoracostomy is needed for effective management. Operative thoracotomy should be considered if the initial drainage is greater than 15 mL/kg or the chest tube output exceeds 4 mL/kg per h.

OPEN PNEUMOTHORAX   The skin wound of an open pneumothorax should be occluded on three sides with a dressing of petrolatum gauze, a plastic sheet, or a commercially available device such as an Ashermann Chest Seal. If the dressing is completely occlusive, an open pneumothorax may be converted to tension pneumothorax. Leaving one side of the dressing open to act as a flutter valve will minimize the development of a tension pneumothorax. A tube thoracostomy need only be performed after completing the primary survey.

Circulation

Signs of shock include tachycardia, cool extremities, altered level of consciousness, weak distal pulses, low urine output, and capillary refill time longer than 3 s. Capillary refill in children can be prolonged by hypothermia.

For shock, crystalloid fluid boluses of 20 mL/kg are given rapidly. If three boluses of crystalloid fail to correct signs of shock, then blood (packed red blood cells) should be given using 10-mL/kg boluses.

CARDIAC ARREST   Absent pulses in a child with traumatic injuries portends a poor outcome. In children with penetrating chest or abdominal trauma, a resuscitative thoracotomy can be lifesaving if vital signs were recently lost. In children with arrest from blunt trauma, the outcome is always death.[7] Standard advanced cardiac life-support algorithms are followed, but most injured children will have asystole or pulseless electrical activity if in traumatic cardiac arrest. Treatment includes early administration of blood products and rapid correction of life-threatening injuries.

CARDIAC TAMPONADE AND AORTIC RUPTURE   These conditions are rare in children. Most commonly they result from penetrating trauma or severe blunt trauma.[8] Cardiac tamponade is suggested by the Beck triad of hypotension, muffled heart sounds, and jugular venous distention. Diagnosis of tamponade can be confirmed by echocardiography prior to treatment. Initial fluid boluses may be temporizing, but pericardiocentesis and resuscitative thoracotomy can be lifesaving. Management of aortic rupture is the same as in adults.

VASCULAR ACCESS Achieving vascular access is one of the most difficult tasks in an injured child. In a child, placing a single functioning intravenous line is often considered a success. Ideally two lines are placed so that blood and medications or fluids can be given simultaneously. Consideration should be given to early intraosseous line placement, because any fluids, medications, or blood products can be given through this line. The femoral vein is the next easiest site because of the identifiable landmarks and the relative ease of the procedure compared with other locations for central venous lines in children (see Chap. 21).

Disability

Level of consciousness is assessed using either the Glasgow Coma Scale (GCS) or the AVPU system, wherein the child's consciousness is rated as (present or absent): *A*lert, responds to *V*erbal stimuli, responds to *P*ainful stimuli, or is *U*nresponsive. The GCS is commonly used in trauma databases, and lower scores have been associated with increased mortality. An arbitrary cutoff of 8 is often quoted as the score that should prompt endotracheal intubation in trauma patients. This point has been chosen because the mortality rate is greatly increased with scores below this level, and children with low scores appear to benefit from intubation.[9] The AVPU system is recommended by the American Heart Association due to its ease of use.[10]

Examination of cranial nerves and pupillary responsiveness is next, and examination of the motor strength of each limb concludes the disability examination. Gross strength is all that is noted during the primary survey, so that paralysis from a spinal cord or central neurologic event is recognized. If a spinal cord injury is strongly suspected, then intravenous steroids are recommended[11] (see "Spinal Trauma," below).

Exposure

The final part of the primary survey serves to identify any important wounds and to detect and correct hypothermia. Actively bleeding wounds or penetrating wounds will direct the priority of actions taken during the resuscitation and secondary survey. Bleeding is controlled by direct pressure, using air splints on the extremities if needed. A rectal temperature should be obtained. Children become hypothermic much more easily than adults due to their high body surface area. Hypothermia can develop in the emergency department despite a seemingly comfortable ambient temperature. Whenever possible, keep the child covered and use external warming devices. Warm fluids to 40°C (104.0°F) if large amounts of intravenous fluids or blood products are used.

Prehospital Considerations

Standards for prehospital pediatric care have been developing slowly. Many pediatric patients are being treated in systems that lack the experience and standards of care that are needed to manage children appropriately. Intravenous access is the prehospital advanced life-support intervention that is most often performed, although the beneficial effects may be rare. Intravenous success rates are as high as 93 percent. Airway management, however, is often more difficult, with many studies showing success rates from 57 to 79 percent, far lower than the success rates with adult patients. Minimizing scene times is an important issue in pediatric trauma management. Placing intravenous lines en route to the hospital unless a prolonged extrication is required can shorten field times.

POSTRESUSCITATION PRIORITIES

Secondary Survey

The goal of the secondary survey is to identify all other injuries to a trauma patient. It does not begin until the completion of the primary survey. All body areas are completely examined. Resuscitation priorities are established, and any life-threatening injuries should already have been managed. Any needed x-rays, laboratory studies, or diagnostic procedures in the ED are also performed during this phase.

The presence of family will often be helpful to calm and console frightened and injured children. Additionally, during this phase a complete history should be obtained using the AMPLE format (*A*llergies, *M*edications, *P*ast medical history, time of *L*ast meal, and *E*vents leading up to the injury).

Stabilization

In this phase, all of the child's injuries are managed definitively, or the child is stabilized sufficiently to allow safe transfer to a facility that can provide a higher level of care. Continual reassessment is crucial, because some injuries may only be manifest over time, and complications from therapeutic interventions can occur. Emphasis is placed on monitoring the airway and circulation. Endotracheal tube dislodgment, development of a pneumothorax, regurgitation of stomach contents, occult hemorrhage causing shock, and worsening neurologic function are important to continue to anticipate. Careful monitoring of fluid administration will prevent inadvertent overhydration. Analgesia and sedation should be appropriately given, as pain treatment is often neglected in children.

Referral to a Pediatric Center

Pediatric trauma center designation is done by a governmental authority, and the requirements vary from state to state.

Several capabilities define the ideal for the pediatric trauma center.[13] The hospital should have a dedicated pediatric trauma service directed by a pediatric trauma surgeon. Comprehensive pediatric services should be available from scene care to rehabilitation and reintegration into the family and society. The trauma team should be immediately available at all times and be capable of treating at least two patients simultaneously. Other pediatric specialists should be on site or immediately available, including emergency medicine, anesthesiology, neurosurgery, radiology, orthopedics, pediatric intensive care, and nursing. A pediatric intensive care unit is essential.

Use of trauma triage scores can help identify a child who needs a more experienced team for care. However, not all scoring systems are easy to use. Two common scores used are the pediatric trauma score (PTS) and revised trauma score (RTS) (Tables 252-2 and 252-3). Advantages of these scores over other systems are that they include physiologic variables instead of relying only on anatomic variables. Higher

TABLE 252-2 Pediatric Trauma Score

	−1	+1	+2
Size (kg)	<10	10–20	>20
Airway	Unmaintained	Maintained	Normal
Systolic blood pressure (mm Hg)	<50	50–90	>90
Level of consciousness	Comatose	Altered	Awake
Wounds	Major open	Minor open	None
Skeletal trauma	Open/multiple	Closed	None

TABLE 252-3   Revised Trauma Score

Number	Glasgow Coma Score	Systolic Blood Pressure	Respiratory Rate
4	13–15	>89	10–29
3	9–12	76–89	>29
2	6–8	50–75	6–9
1	4–5	1–49	1–5
0	3	0	0

numbers are associated with a higher likelihood of survival, and thus a reduced need for trauma center care. A child with an RTS of less than 12 or a PTS of less than 8 should be taken to a trauma center.[14]

Some common indications for transfer to a pediatric trauma center are listed in Table 252-4.[15] Even low-level falls (0.68 m, or 27 in.) can cause serious injury, especially with a hard impact surface,[16] and intracranial injuries are frequently associated with low-level falls.[17] Therefore low fall height does not necessarily exclude the need for specialized pediatric trauma care.

Transfer to a pediatric trauma center is best done by a pediatric transport team or a critical care transport team with some pediatric experience (pediatric nurse or pediatrician) traveling with the child (see Chap. 4).

SPECIFIC PEDIATRIC INJURIES

Head Trauma

Cerebral trauma is the leading cause of death due to injury in children. Most of these deaths occur outside of the hospital. The most common mechanisms of injury differ by age. Falls, even low-height falls,[16] are the most frequent cause in children less than 2 years of age. Preschoolers also are most frequently injured in falls, but motor vehicle crashes account for 25 percent. In school-age children, falls and motor vehicle crashes occur with equal frequency. Lastly, in adolescents, sports injuries and motor vehicle crashes are about equal.

Children frequently have head injuries because of several factors. A child's head encompasses a relatively larger proportion of body mass and area. The bones of the neck are not fully developed, so the head is attached on a largely ligamentous connection. The incompletely myelinated brain is more susceptible to shear forces during trauma. Because of cartilage in the skull and the presence of open sutures, young children are better able to tolerate increased intracranial pressure than are adolescents and adults.

CLINICAL FINDINGS   Most children will have suffered a mild head injury and present with no or few symptoms in the ED. Common symptoms associated with head injury include vomiting, headache,

TABLE 252-4   Indications for Transfer to a Pediatric Trauma Center

Mechanism of injury	Ejected from motor vehicle Fall from low- or higher-level height[15,16] Prolonged extrication Death of another occupant in motor vehicle
Anatomic injury	Multiple severe trauma More than three long-bone fractures Spinal fractures or spinal cord injury Amputations Severe head or facial trauma Penetrating head, chest, or abdominal trauma

Source: Adapted from Harris et al,[13] with permission.

and lethargy. For children with more significant cerebral injuries, the signs and symptoms are not markedly different from those for adults. The most difficult aspect of evaluation is often the neurologic examination. It is difficult to ascertain inappropriate behavior or mental status, particularly in the very young. Level of consciousness can be rated by the AVPU system or the GCS. A pupillary exam can identify impending herniation even in a child without distress. Asymmetry of spontaneous movements is, of course, a telling sign, while older children can then be asked to move their fingers and toes. Sensory function should be assessed by withdrawal from pain or the ability to feel touch in older children. In young children, look for signs of fontanel fullness (increased intracranial pressure; ICP) or retinal hemorrhages (shaken baby syndrome).

INCREASED INTRACRANIAL PRESSURE   Signs of increased ICP in children are most commonly vomiting, dizziness, headache, irritability, and decreased level of consciousness. Management is not remarkably different from adult management of acutely increased ICP. As in adults, aggressive hyperventilation in children has been associated with worsened cerebral ischemia as compared with more moderate hyperventilation in head-injured children.[18] Children with suspected increased ICP should be mildly hyperventilated ($Paco_2$ 30 to 34 mm Hg) and should have their hemodynamic status maximized with fluids and blood to correct shock. Fluid restriction should not be an acute consideration. To optimize venous drainage, the head of the bed should be elevated to 20° to 30°, and the neck should be straight. Intravenous mannitol in a dose of 0.5 to 1.0 g/kg can be used to lower ICP. Mannitol may acutely lower ICP by removal of free water and decreased blood viscosity. Local preferences will dictate practice. Furosemide (1.0 mg/kg) may decrease edema as well. To date, no studies have shown steroids to be helpful.[19] ICP monitoring is generally done to monitor and treat increased ICP, but its effect on ultimate outcome is as yet uncertain.[19]

POSTTRAUMATIC SEIZURES   Seizures following traumatic head injury are relatively uncommon, occurring in about 5 percent of hospitalized patients.[20] About half will never have a seizure again. Of the remaining half, 50 percent have rare seizures and 50 percent have frequent seizures. Children with loss of consciousness, lower GCS, longer duration of coma, and computed tomography (CT) scan abnormalities are at increased risk for seizures. Intracranial injuries most commonly seen are subdural hemorrhages, depressed skull fractures, and intracranial lacerations.[20] Only 50 percent of children with posttraumatic seizures will have abnormalities on CT scanning.[20] Use of anticonvulsant medication as prophylaxis in the absence of a seizure or following a single seizure is controversial. Children with two or more seizures, or seizures lasting more than a few minutes, should receive anticonvulsant therapy. Prophylactic anticonvulsant therapy should be strongly considered in a child with a GCS under 8, even if no seizures have yet occurred, because the risk of developing acute posttraumatic seizures is high and many of these children already have high ICPs that will increase further with a seizure.[20]

Phenytoin or fosphenytoin is used to treat acute seizures. Dosage is the same (10 to 20 mg/kg intravenous load) except that fosphenytoin is measured in phenytoin equivalents. Acute seizures should be managed with a benzodiazepine such as lorazepam, midazolam, or diazepam.

As with adults, proximity of seizure to the event predicts long-term likelihood of epilepsy. Immediate seizures are least likely to result in long-term sequelae.[20]

RADIOGRAPHY   The primary goal of patient evaluation is to identify traumatic brain injury and to identify intracranial injuries that require surgical intervention. Radiographic studies such as CT and MRI can assist in making this diagnosis.

There are no good predictors for intracranial injury in children <2 years of age. The best predictors seem to be 1) any neurologic abnormality, 2) any altered mental status, 3) any scalp abnormalities (contusion, abrasion, laceration, cephalohematoma), and 4) vomiting.[21] Young children can tolerate increased ICP because sutures are not fused, but once sutures reach their maximal excursion, ICP rises very quickly. CT is the imaging modality of choice. Skull films are better to identify fractures, but the identification of a skull fracture requires CT scanning. The absence of skull fracture does not exclude intracranial injury. Skull films may be indicated in addition to CT scanning for penetrating injury (such as dog bite) or suspected foreign body.

Recommendations for radiographic evaluation of children over 2 years of age who were previously healthy with an isolated minor closed head injury and who are medically evaluated within 24 h of injury were published by the American Academy of Pediatrics and the American Academy of Family Physicians.[22] Children excluded from this practice parameter include children with multiple trauma, unobserved loss of consciousness, suspected cervical spine injury, history of bleeding diathesis, neurologic disorders aggravated by trauma (such as arteriovenous malformations), suspected nonaccidental trauma, and a significant language barrier. A child having a minor closed head injury is defined as a child with a normal mental status, a normal neurologic examination, and no signs suggestive of skull fracture. If the child suffered no loss of consciousness at the time of injury, then no imaging is felt necessary by these authors. If the child suffered a brief loss of consciousness, then observation and CT scan are felt appropriate. A CT scan is also indicated in children who fall into a moderate- or high-risk category (Table 252-5).[22]

For children less than 2 years of age, risks for intracranial injury have not been validated. A higher threshold for CT evaluation should be used in this age group,[23] especially in falls from low heights.[16]

MANAGEMENT   Children in the negligible- to low-risk categories with a normal evaluation can be safely discharged home (assuming no homebound risks) for 24-h observation and follow-up with the primary care provider.[24] Discharge instructions should clearly state the need to return to the ED if any symptoms in the moderate-risk category occur. Children in the moderate- and high-risk categories should be admitted with NS referral as appropriate for skull fracture, persistent neurologic findings, or abnormal CT. See Chap. 255 for detailed discussion of head injury.

Children with any LOC or any symptoms after head injuries from sports should be kept out of play for 1 week and reevaluated before return to play.[25]

Spinal Trauma

Spinal trauma is relatively uncommon in young children, and is more commonly seen in adolescents.[26] Cervical spine injuries predominate, although thoracic and lumbar injuries also occur (as in the lap-belt syndrome). Motor vehicle crashes are the most common reason for spinal injury, followed by falls and sports events. In young children, falls predominate, and in older children motor vehicle crashes predominate. Due to increased flexibility of the spine and spinal column in younger children, fractures and dislocations rarely occur with minor trauma, and spinal cord injury without radiographic abnormality (SCIWORA) can occur. Adolescents more commonly have fracture patterns similar to those of adults. Also, 50 percent of spinal injuries and 67 percent of cervical spinal injuries in children under the age of 12 occur between the occiput and C2. By comparison, adolescents and adults more commonly experience lower cervical spine injuries.[26] Younger children also less frequently have thoracic or lumbar injuries. Part of the reason for this pattern of injury is that an immature child's spine and an adult's spine have several differences (Table 252-6).

Children with incomplete spinal cord deficits have a better prognosis for improvement of neurologic condition than those children with complete spinal cord injuries. Children with spinal cord trauma have a higher mortality rate than adults.

CLINICAL FINDINGS   Presentation is related to the presence or absence of a spinal cord injury. Children with fractures only will have pain, tenderness, or overlying soft tissue injury. Children with spinal cord injuries with or without fracture will have paresthesias, paralysis, and other findings based upon the level or type of spinal cord injury (see Chap. 256).

Over 50 percent of children with SCIWORA have a delayed onset of paralysis, sometimes up to 4 days.[27] Many of these children have transient paresthesias, numbness, or weakness at the time of or shortly after the injury. Because most spinal injuries fail to improve substantially, even in children, the most important factor in prognosis is the initial neurologic status.[27] Children with fractures and neurologic symptoms do worse than children with SCIWORA alone.[27] Despite advances in imaging, SCIWORA remains a problem.[28]

RADIOGRAPHY   Decision algorithms for cervical spine imaging have been based upon adult patient populations. In the National Emergency X-Radiography Utilization Study (NEXUS), the authors showed that in the presence of all of the following one may safely forgo cervical spine radiography: absence of tenderness at the posterior midline of the cervical spine, absence of focal neurologic deficit, normal level of alertness, no evidence of intoxication, and absence of clinically apparent pain that might distract the patient from pain of a cervical spine injury.[29] Only 2.5 percent of the studied patients were 8 years of age or younger in this study, however. In young children, fear and agitation from cervical spine immobilization and the absence of comforting caregivers may make the NEXUS criteria difficult to apply. Until more conclusive pediatric studies can be accomplished, cervical spine imaging in children should be accomplished for the following: 1) moderate- or high-risk head injury; 2) multiple trauma; 3) signs or symptoms of spine injury; 4) mechanism of injury for spine injury; 5) altered mental status or focal neurologic findings; and 6) distracting painful injury with possible mechanism for spine injury. Images should include at a minimum three views: lateral, anteroposterior, and odontoid. The single lateral cervical spine radiograph has been shown to miss fractures and result in a delay in diagnosis.[30]

TABLE 252-5   Risk Groups for Pediatric Head Injury*

NEGLIGIBLE	LOW RISK†	MODERATE–HIGH RISK
Normal exam	Normal exam	Children <2 years old
No symptoms	LOC <1 min	Altered mental status
No LOC	Amnesia	Persistent vomiting
	Headache	LOC >1 min
	Vomiting	Seizures
	Lethargy	Facial injury
		Multiple trauma
		Abnormal examination
Observation	CT scan	CT scan
	Observation	Referral as indicated

*Defined as ages 2–20 years; previously healthy; isolated head injury.
†Risk of positive CT up to 7 percent.
Source: Adapted from http://www.aap.org/policy/ac9858.html.

TABLE 252-6   Characteristics of the Spinal Column in Children

Ligamentous laxity
Underdevelopment of supporting muscles
Partially ossified vertebrae
Wedge-shaped vertebrae
Horizontal facet joints
Higher fulcrum of flexion
Instability of atlantooccipital joint

CT scanning of the cervical spine is also an acceptable alternative, especially if a head CT scan is also being obtained.

Up to 66 percent of spinal cord injuries in children have no radiographic abnormality and thus fall under the rubric of SCIWORA.[27] Widening of the prevertebral soft tissues to 8 mm or more in front of C2 or more than 75 percent of the adjacent vertebral body width is considered abnormal. In infants, however, this becomes less reliable.

Occult fractures and misinterpretation of plain films do occur, so if there is any doubt, a CT scan should be obtained. If the child had paresthesias, numbness, or weakness, or currently has neurologic symptoms, a CT scan is also recommended.[27] If all radiographs are negative but the diagnosis of SCIWORA is being entertained, then an MRI should be obtained. The role of flexion and extension lateral cervical spine x-rays is controversial. They should not be obtained if there are neurologic signs or symptoms. Anytime the diagnosis of SCIWORA is considered, the child requires a neurosurgical consultation from the ED and admission for observation.[27] Cervical spine immobilization should be maintained throughout this entire procedure.

MANAGEMENT   Treatment of spinal cord injuries in the prehospital and ED settings consists of immobilization, diagnosis of the specific injury, and, possibly, steroid administration. Prehospital personnel must be instructed that an infant's relatively large head may cause the neck to flex in the standard supine position, so they require padding behind the shoulders. Steroids can be given if there is evidence of a neurologic deficit. The loading dose is 30 mg/kg of methylprednisolone.[11] Steroids should be started within 8 h of the injury. Those who receive steroids within 3 h should be maintained on steroids for 24 h. Those who receive steroids 3 to 8 h after the injury require maintenance for 48 h. The maintenance dose is 5.4 mg/kg per h. The maintenance dose is initiated 45 min after the initial bolus. Children with a spinal cord injury require immediate neurosurgical consultation. If a spinal fracture is also present, a pediatric orthopedist should also be consulted.

Chest Trauma

Children, with their relatively compliant chest walls, may not show external evidence of serious intrathoracic trauma. Blunt trauma occurs more frequently than penetrating trauma and may be equally as serious. Isolated chest trauma in children carries a 4 to 12 percent mortality rate. Most children with chest trauma will have other significant injuries. In a multiply-injured child, death is 10 times more likely if chest trauma is present.[31] Penetrating chest injuries are becoming more frequent as the number of firearm injuries steadily increases in the United States. Children under the age of 12 are more likely to be injured in unintentional crossfire and require a longer hospitalization than adolescents and adults.

Evaluation of a patient who has evidence of, or who has a good mechanism for, chest injury should include a thorough physical examination to look for bony defects, crepitus, paradoxical chest movement, and unequal breath sounds. A chest x-ray should be taken. To minimize interruption of the resuscitation, a supine chest x-ray can be initially obtained. A rib fracture is a sensitive indicator of serious underlying injury. The most common injury is pulmonary contusion, but this may not be visible on the early ED chest x-ray.[31]

Most injuries requiring emergent treatment can be identified on the standard supine anteroposterior chest x-ray. Mediastinal widening is common on supine chest x-rays, but aortic injury is rare in children who survive to the ED.[8] An upright chest x-ray, preferably using posteroanterior technique, will often obviate the need for additional studies. Aortography is still considered essential to exclude aortic injury when suspected, although contrast-enhanced spiral CT scanning may also identify aortic injury. If an abdominal CT scan is obtained, additional occult chest injuries are often detected.

Tube thoracostomy alone is usually sufficient management for pneumothorax or hemothorax (same size tube for either), both of which are uncommonly associated with blunt trauma in children. Other specific injuries should be managed as outlined in the primary survey section. Emergent thoracotomy should be performed selectively as with adults. Survival from pulseless arrest at the scene or en route to the ED is rare in both blunt and penetrating trauma.[11] Only children who have sustained penetrating trauma and experience a loss of vital signs in the ED should have a resuscitative thoracotomy performed. In all other cases, the attempt is futile and the financial costs are high.[7]

Abdominal Trauma

DIAGNOSIS   The physical examination of a child's abdomen is frequently misleading in the detection of intraabdominal injury. Children with severe injuries can have minimal physical findings, while other children may have serious occult injuries. Physical examination is not a sensitive indicator of abdominal injury. In most children with abdominal symptoms or a mechanism of injury to the abdomen, a CT scan should be obtained.

Diagnostic peritoneal lavage (DPL) is accurate in the identification of serious intraabdominal injury in children,[32] but it has largely been replaced by abdominal CT scanning. Advantages of CT scanning include its noninvasiveness and the ability to visualize the retroperitoneum. Disadvantages of CT scanning include time spent in radiology away from the trauma room, lower accuracy for hollow organ and pancreatic injury, and radiation exposure. Indications for obtaining a CT scan in children include abdominal tenderness, abdominal distention, abdominal bruising, hematuria, vomiting, neurologic obtundation, dropping or low hematocrit, and absent bowel sounds.[33] CT scan and operative findings correlate well with splenic injury grade level.[34] Normal CT findings in blunt trauma are strongly predictive of both no future deterioration and no need for future operative intervention.[33] Subtle CT findings such as unexplained peritoneal fluid, bowel wall enhancement, duodenal hematoma, and bowel wall thickening are associated with bowel trauma.[33,35]

Ultrasound examination of the abdomen may be useful,[36] but currently there is insufficient reported experience to recommend its routine use in the evaluation of pediatric trauma patients[37] or for ultrasound to serve as a substitute for CT.

Splenic Trauma

The spleen is the most commonly injured abdominal organ in children. Children are more likely to be hemodynamically stable than adults, even with the same degree of splenic injury.[34] Children with splenic injuries are more likely to be managed nonoperatively than adults.[34] Several reasons are thought to explain this difference. The spleen in children has a thicker capsule. There are larger amounts of elastin and smooth muscle in both the capsule and the splenic vessels. Children tend to have lower-velocity injuries and overall lower Injury Severity Scores.[34]

Children who are more likely to require operative intervention include those with a higher Injury Severity Score, an injury sustained in a motor vehicle crash, or a greater amount of hemoperitoneum. Any child who requires a splenectomy should receive pneumococcal vaccine to prevent postsplenectomy sepsis.

Hepatic Trauma

The liver is the second most commonly injured abdominal organ in children. Similar to splenic trauma, these injuries can often be managed conservatively. The rate of fatal hemorrhage is higher with hepatic injury than with splenic injury. Diagnosis is often made by abdominal CT scanning in stable trauma patients. Unstable patients often require operative intervention to control hemorrhage.

Pancreatic Trauma

Although pancreatic trauma is uncommon in children, trauma is the most common cause of acute pancreatitis. Handlebar injuries are the most common mechanism of injury and often cause isolated pancreatic trauma.[38] A high index of suspicion is required because symptoms are often delayed and morbidity is related to delay in diagnosis. Serum amylase levels are often elevated, but the degree of elevation does not correlate with the degree of pancreatic injury.[38] CT scanning has at best an 85 percent sensitivity to identify pancreatic injury in the acute setting.[38] Sensitivity is highest when both oral and IV contrast are used. Children with abdominal pain and an elevated serum amylase require an abdominal CT scan and should be hospitalized for observation even if the CT scan findings are normal.[38] Complications of pancreatic injury include pseudocyst formation, acute pancreatitis, and relapsing pancreatitis.

Bowel Trauma

Intestinal injuries occur in less than 5 percent of children with blunt abdominal trauma. The jejunum is most frequently injured, followed by the ileum and cecum. The duodenum is particularly prone to the development of hematomas in the wall, leading to obstruction. The physical examination is often quoted as being unreliable in diagnosing bowel injury following blunt trauma. Children with abdominal wall injuries (bruising or abrasions), tenderness on palpation, or a mechanism of a direct blow to the abdomen require further investigation to exclude bowel injury. In hemodynamically stable patients, a contrast-enhanced CT scan can often increase the suspicion of a bowel injury. CT scans are diagnostic for bowel injury in a minority of cases. Pneumoperitoneum or extravasation of enteral contrast is considered diagnostic of bowel injury and requires immediate laparotomy. Nondiagnostic findings include free peritoneal fluid without solid organ injury and bowel wall enhancement or thickening. A child with a tender abdomen and these nondiagnostic but suggestive radiographic findings requires an exploratory laparotomy or DPL to exclude an intestinal perforation.[39] Complications of bowel injury include peritonitis, obstruction, and intestinal structures.

Bowel injury is associated with seat-belt use in less than 5 percent of children admitted to trauma centers. A particular entity, the lap-belt complex, consists of intestinal or mesenteric injury with a concomitant lumbar spine injury due to a lap belt. It has also been shown to occur with three-point restraints (lap belt/shoulder-harness restraints) when the lap belt is incorrectly positioned over the abdomen. The intraabdominal injury often occurs at the midlumbar level. Most commonly, the jejunum is injured. Any child with a lumbar fracture or an anterior abdominal bruise from a seat belt must have a thorough search for intraabdominal injury. If a spinal injury is present, but the CT scan is negative, the child should be admitted for observation and serial examinations.

Pelvic and Genitourinary Trauma

Trauma to the genitourinary (GU) tract should be considered in all children with multiple trauma, a pelvic fracture, or injury to the flank, back, or groin. GU injuries are uncommon in children. Symptoms and physical findings are often nonspecific, including back pain, abdominal pain, hypotension, and abdominal wall trauma. Pelvic fractures, particularly anterior ring fractures, are associated with urethral and bladder injury. Children are less likely to die of hemorrhage from a pelvic fracture than are adults. Often, other coexisting injuries mask the signs and symptoms of GU trauma in a multiply injured child.

Hematuria is considered the hallmark finding in GU trauma, although it is a nonspecific finding. The degree of hematuria does correlate with the severity of injury, although renal pedicle disruption can be associated with no hematuria.[40] The radiographic evaluation of an injured child with hematuria is based on clinical presentation. Children with gross hematuria or more than 20 RBCs/hpf and unstable vital signs or the emergent need for operative intervention for other injuries require an intravenous pyelogram (IVP) in the ED. Children who have hematuria of more than 10 RBCs/hpf and stable vital signs should have CT of the abdomen performed. Asymptomatic microscopic hematuria in children with blunt trauma and no apparent injuries is a low-yield indication for emergent abdominal CT scanning. These cases can be followed as outpatients.

Cystourethrography is required on all patients with suspected lower urinary tract injuries (for example, blood at the urethral meatus, high prostate, or anterior pelvic fracture). Straddle injuries account for 20 percent of the cases of urethral injury (motor vehicle crashes account for most of the other 80 percent). Straddle injuries are also associated with pubic fractures, testicular injuries, and labial or scrotal hematomas and lacerations. Sexual abuse should be considered in a girl with a straddle injury and a history that does not seem compatible with the injury.

ACKNOWLEDGMENT

Thanks to Dr. Doug Trocenski for his assistance in this manuscript.

REFERENCES

1. Rhodes M, Smith S, Boorse D: Pediatric trauma patients in an "adult" trauma center. *J Trauma* 35:384, 1993.
2. Fingerhut LA, Warner M: *Injury Chartbook, Heath, United States,* 1996–97. Hyattsville, MD: National Center for Health Statistics, 1997.
3. Centers for Disease Control and Prevention (CDC): Alcohol related traffic fatalities involving children: United States, 1985–1996. *MMWR* 46:1130, 1997.
4. Eleraky MA, Theodore N, Adams M, et al: Pediatric cervical spine injuries: Report of 102 cases and review of the literature. *J Neurosurg* 92(1 Suppl):7, 2000.
5. Treloar DJ, Nypaver M: Angulation of the pediatric cervical spine with and without cervical collar. *Pediatr Emerg Care* 13:5, 1997.
6. Huerta C, Griffith R, Joyce SM: Cervical spine stabilization in pediatric patients. Evaluation of current techniques. *Ann Emerg Med* 18:427, 1989.
7. Sheikh AA, Culbertson CB: Emergency department thoracotomy in children: Rationale for selective application. *J Trauma* 34:322, 1993.
8. Karny-Jones R, Hoffer E, Meissner M, et al: Management of traumatic rupture of the thoracic aorta in pediatric patients. *Ann Thorac Surg* 75:1513, 2003.
9. White JR, Farukhi Z, Bull C, et al: Predictors of outcome in severely head-injured children. *Crit Care Med* 29:534, 2001.
10. *Textbook of Pediatric Advanced Life Support.* Dallas: American Heart Association, 2002.
11. Bracken MD, Shepard MJ, Holford TR, et al: Administration of methylprednisolone for 24 or 48 hours in the treatment of acute spinal cord injury. *JAMA* 20:1597, 1997.
12. Alexander J, Manno M: Underuse of analgesia in very young pediatric patients with isolated painful injuries. *Ann Emerg Med* 41:617, 2003.
13. Harris BH, Barlow BA, Ballantine TV, et al: American Pediatric Surgical Association principles of pediatric trauma care. *J Pediatr Surg* 27:423, 1992.
14. Marcin JP, Pollack MM: Triage scoring systems, severity of illness measures, and mortality prediction models in pediatric trauma. *Crit Care Med* 30(11):S457, 2002.
15. Hall JR, Reyes HM, Meller JL, et al: The outcome for children with blunt trauma is best at a pediatric trauma center. *J Pediatr Surg* 31:72, 1996.
16. Bertocci GE, Pierce MC, Deemer E, et al: Using test-dummy experiments to investigate pediatric injury risk in simulated short-distance falls. *Arch Pediatr Adolesc Med* 157:480, 2003.
17. Murray JA, Chen D, Velmahos GC, et al: Pediatric falls: Is height a predictor of injury and outcome? *Am Surgeon* 66:863, 2000.
18. Skippen P, Seear M, Poskitt K, et al: Effect of hyperventilation on regional cerebral blood flow in head-injured children. *Crit Care Med* 25:1402, 1997.
19. Wasserberg J: Treating head injuries. *BMJ* 325:454, 2002.
20. Lewis RJ, Lee L, Inkelis SH, et al: Clinical predictors of post-traumatic seizures in children with head trauma. *Ann Emerg Med* 22:1114, 1993.

21. Greenes DS, Schutzman SA, et al: Clinical significance of scalp abnormalities in asymptomatic head-injured infants. *Pediatr Emerg Care* 17:88, 2001.

22. Committee on Quality Improvement, American Academy of Pediatrics: The management of minor closed head injury in children. *Pediatrics* 104:1407, 1999.

23. Schutzman SA, Barnes P, Duhaime AC, et al: Evaluation and management of children younger than two years old with apparently minor head trauma: Proposed guidelines. *Pediatrics* 107:983, 2001.

24. Spencer MT, Baron BJ, Sinert R, et al: Necessity of hospital admission for pediatric minor head injury. *Am J Emerg Med* 21:111, 2003.

25. AAP: Sports Shorts. Guidelines for Pediatricians. *Head Injuries* (issue 1), Feb. 2000.

26. Hadley MN, Zabramski JM, Browner CM, et al: Pediatric spinal trauma: Review of 122 cases of spinal cord and vertebral column injuries. *J Neurosurg* 68:18, 1998.

27. Pang D, Wilberger JE: Spinal cord injury without radiographic abnormalities in children. *J Neurosurg* 57:114, 1982.

28. Brown RL, Brunn MA, Garcia VF: Cervical spine injuries in children: A review of 103 patients treated consecutively at a level 1 pediatric trauma center. *J Pediatr Surg* 36:1107, 2001.

29. Hoffman JR, Mower WR, Wolfson AB, et al: Validity of a set of clinical criteria to rule out injury to the cervical spine in patients with blunt trauma. *New Engl J Med* 343:94, 2000.

30. Dietrich AM, Ginn-Pease ME, Bartkowski HM, et al: Pediatric cervical spine fractures: Predominately subtle presentation. *J Pediatr Surg* 26:995, 1991.

31. Peclet MH, Newman KD, Eichelberger MR, et al: Thoracic trauma in children: An indicator of increased mortality. *J Pediatr Surg* 25:961, 1990.

32. Rothenberg S, Moore EE, Marx JA, et al: Selective management of blunt abdominal trauma in children: The role of peritoneal lavage. *J Trauma* 27:1101, 1987.

33. Ruess L, Sivit CJ, Eichelberger MR, et al: Blunt abdominal trauma in children: Impact of CT on operative and nonoperative management. *AJR* 169:1011, 1997.

34. Powell M, Courcoulas A, Gardner M, et al: Management of blunt splenic trauma: Significant differences between adults and children. *Surgery* 122:654, 1997.

35. Desai KM, Derword IG, Minkes RK, et al: Blunt duodenal injuries in children. *J Trauma* 54(4): 640, 2003.

36. Katz S, Lazar L, Rathaus V, et al: Can ultrasonography replace computed tomography in the initial assessment of children with blunt abdominal trauma? *J Pediatr Surg* 31:649, 1996.

37. Miller MT, Pasquale MD, Bromberg WJ, et al: Not so FAST. *J Trauma* 54(1)52, 2003.

38. Arkovitz MS, Johnson N, Garcia VF: Pancreatic trauma in children: Mechanisms of injury. *J Trauma* 42:49, 1997.

39. Jerby BL, Attorri RJ, Morton D Jr: Blunt intestinal injury in children: The role of the physical examination. *J Pediatr Surg* 32:580, 1997.

40. Abou-Jaoude WA, Sugarman JM, Fallat ME, et al: Indicators of genitourinary tract injury or anomaly in cases of pediatric blunt trauma. *J Pediatr Surg* 31:86, 1996.

253 GERIATRIC TRAUMA
O. John Ma
Stephen W. Meldon

Although the elderly experience the same type of trauma that younger individuals do, there are differences in the incidence and patterns of injury, and age-related changes may produce a diminished physiologic reserve.

EPIDEMIOLOGY

Persons 65 years of age and older represent a large and growing segment of the population. In 1997, more than 34 million people, 12.7 percent of the total population, were 65 years of age or older.[1] This represents a 21.3 percent increase in this segment of the population

from the 1980 census figures. The Census Bureau projects that those older than 65 years will increase to 52 million by 2020 and to 80 million by 2050 (representing 20 percent of the total population).[1] The number of people older than 85 years of age also are growing at an accelerated pace, with estimates that they will number 14 million by the year 2040.[1]

While persons older than 65 years of age represent 12 percent of the population, they account for 36 percent of all ambulance transports, 25 percent of hospitalizations, and 25 percent of total trauma costs.[2] Geriatric trauma patients represent between 8 and 12 percent of the general trauma population. While male trauma victims are predominant in the younger age groups, males and females are equally represented in the geriatric trauma population.[3] Trauma ranks as the seventh leading cause of death in this age group, although the rate per 100,000 is 92, as compared with 35.7 for all age groups.[3] Although the elderly are less likely to be involved in trauma as compared to other age groups, they are more likely to have fatal outcomes when they are injured. Approximately 28 percent of deaths due to accidental causes involve persons 65 years and older. Also, the elderly have the highest population-based mortality rate of any age group.[2]

Definitions

Defining the term "elderly" is a difficult task because it involves both chronologic and physiologic components. The literature has divided the elderly population into two groups: the "young old" (65 to 80 years of age) and the "old old" (80 years of age and older).[2] Although this is a somewhat arbitrary division, it is helpful in interpreting the literature of geriatric trauma.

One of the difficulties in describing the elderly population is the potential discrepancy between chronologic age and physiologic age. Chronologic age is the actual number of years the individual has lived. Physiologic age describes the actual functional capacity of the patients' organ systems in a physiologic sense. Physiologic reserve describes the various levels of functioning of the patients' organ systems that allows them to compensate for traumatic derangement. Comorbid disease states such as diabetes mellitus, coronary artery disease, arthritis, renal disease, and pulmonary disease can decrease the physiologic reserve of certain patients, which makes it more difficult for them to recover from injury.[4]

PATHOPHYSIOLOGY

Common Mechanisms of Injury

The elderly will experience similar types of injuries that younger individuals do. There are differences, however, in the incidence and patterns of injury for elderly patients compared to younger persons.

Falls

Falls are the most common cause of injury in patients over 65 years of age.[5,6] Fifty percent of elderly persons who fall do so repeatedly. Most individuals who fall will do so on a level surface and most will suffer an isolated orthopedic injury.[3,7] Falls are reported as the underlying cause of 9500 deaths each year in patients older than age of 65 years. Many falls in the elderly population occur in residential institutions such as nursing homes. In the >85-year-old age group, 20 percent of fatal falls occur in nursing homes.[7]

There are age-related changes in postural stability, balance, motor strength, coordination, and reaction time that make the elderly more prone to tripping and falling, and may explain the increased incidence of falls. Also, decreased visual acuity and increased memory loss can cause the patient difficulty in recognizing and avoiding environmental hazards. Acute, preexisting, and chronic diseases also may lead to falls.

Syncope has been implicated in many cases of elderly patients who fall and this may be secondary to dysrhythmias, venous pooling, autonomic derangement, hypoxia, anemia, or hypoglycemia. Other contributing factors include alcohol and medications, most notably sedative, antihypertensive, antidepressant, diuretic, and hypoglycemic agents.[7]

Motor Vehicle Crashes

Motor vehicle crashes rank as the second leading mechanism of injury that brings elderly patients to a trauma center in the United States, and are the most common mechanism for fatal incidents in elderly persons through 80 years of age.[2] Data show that the crash fatality rate among the elderly is considerably higher than for younger age groups.[8] As noted above, similar effects of acute and chronic medical conditions can influence the incidence of motor vehicle crashes. Older persons may have decreased cerebral and motor skills and memory and judgment losses that can compound the difficulty in operating a motor vehicle. Older drivers also are more likely to have decreased auditory or visual acuity, which may make it more difficult to recognize dangerous traffic situations. Furthermore, decreased strength and slower reaction times may hinder an individual's ability to respond to a hazardous traffic situation.[2] Older drivers are more likely to be involved in crashes during daylight hours, in good weather, at intersections, and those involving two vehicles.

Pedestrian-Motor Vehicle Collisions

The elderly are second only to children as victims of pedestrian–motor vehicle collisions. The 65-year-and-older age group accounts for 22 percent of pedestrian–automobile fatalities in the United States.[3] Elderly pedestrians struck by a motor vehicle are much more likely to die than are struck younger pedestrians. Pedestrian–motor vehicle collisions are one of the most lethal mechanisms of injury in this age group, with a 53 percent case-fatality rate.[3] A number of factors contribute to the increased risk of older persons becoming victims of pedestrian-vehicle collisions. Reduced peripheral vision and decreased hearing may limit access to information needed to make rational decisions about crossing the street. Cognitive, memory, and judgment skills are often diminished, and may increase the risk of older pedestrians being struck by automobiles. Postural changes due to musculoskeletal decline may lead to kyphosis, which results in difficulty in lifting the head to see and obey traffic signals. Traffic signals operate at a crossing rate of 4 feet per second, an insufficient amount for some elderly to safely cross some intersections.[2]

Burns

The elderly constitute between 13 and 20 percent of admissions to burn units, but have the highest case fatality of any age group. The majority of burn injuries in this age group are a result of careless activity in the home setting and are a result of either flame injuries from smoking or cooking or tub scald injuries. The elderly have a higher fatality rate than do younger adults with the same extent of burn, and even nonmajor burns (less than 20 percent body surface area) may be significant. Increasing age, male gender, burn size, presence of full-thickness burn, and presence of inhalation injury contribute to mortality.[9] The relationship between higher age and increased burn mortality has been long recognized, and geriatric patients with burns of 70 percent or greater usually do not survive, even with aggressive management. The Baux Index, a simple addition of age and percentage body surface area burned, has continuing prognostic value. A Baux Index of 75 represents a severe burn and an index of 100 is usually fatal.[9]

Violence

While the overall increase in violent crimes in the United States has not spared the elderly, related injury is generally lower in this demo-graphic group. Violent assaults account for 6 percent of trauma admissions in the elderly, as compared with 25 percent in a younger cohort.[5] Elderly persons are seen as ideal targets for robberies because they may possess various age-related physical deficiencies. Just as in the younger population, ethanol consumption by the assailant or victim has been found to be involved in the majority of fatal assaults. Emergency physicians also should have a heightened suspicion for elder or parental abuse in the geriatric trauma patient (see Chap. 300).

CLINICAL FEATURES

Out-of-Hospital Considerations

Following injury, older patients have higher admission rates, longer hospital stays, increased long-term morbidity, and higher mortality rates despite lower injury severity.[10] Emergency medical services (EMS) providers should recognize that seemingly minor trauma mechanisms, such as low-level falls and low-speed motor vehicle crashes, may result in significant injury to older persons. For these reasons, it has been recommended that the threshold for scene triage or transfer to a trauma center be lower for elderly patients than for younger patients.

Despite these recommendations, there is evidence that elderly patients are disproportionately underrepresented at trauma centers.[11,11a] Whether this is secondary to minor injury mechanisms, an initial assessment that underestimates the severity of their trauma, existing prehospital triage protocols or a bias against aggressively treating elderly patients is not clear. Most trauma protocols typically rely on anatomic and physiologic criteria to mandate transfer to a trauma center, and patient age greater than 55 years is often listed as one of several comorbid conditions that should be considered. Consideration of patient age should be a component of out-of-hospital trauma protocols that direct the triage and transport of injured patients.

History

Because elderly patients may have a significant past medical history that impacts their trauma care, obtaining a precise history is vital. Often, the time frame for obtaining information about the traumatic event, past medical history, medications, and allergies is quite short. Medical records and consultation with the patient's family physician may be helpful. Family members also may be able to provide information regarding the traumatic event and the patient's previous level of function. Medications must be carefully listed, as many elderly patients are on cardiac agents, diuretics, psychotropic agents, and anticoagulants.

Vital Signs

The clinician should not be led into a false sense of security by "normal" vital signs. In a study by Scalea and coinvestigators, 8 of 15 geriatric blunt trauma patients initially considered to be hemodynamically "stable" had cardiac outputs less than 3.5 L/min and none had an adequate response to volume loading. Of 7 patients with a normal cardiac output, 5 had inadequate oxygen delivery.[12]

There is progressive stiffening of the myocardium with age that results in a decreased effectiveness of the pumping mechanism. An 80-year-old will have approximately 50 percent of the cardiac output of a 20-year-old, even without significant atherosclerotic coronary artery disease. The myocardium also becomes less sensitive to endogenous and exogenous catecholamines. Conduction defects may be exacerbated by the stress of illness or trauma. A normal tachycardic response to pain, hypovolemia, or anxiety may be absent or blunted in the elderly trauma patient. Medications such as β-blockers may mask tachycardia and hinder the evaluation of the elderly patient. Blood pressures also may be misleading because the prevalence of preexisting hypertension in this age group approaches 70 percent. Emergency physicians should be wary of a "normal" heart rate and blood pressure in the geriatric trauma victim.

DIAGNOSIS AND DIFFERENTIAL

As in all trauma patients, the primary survey should be initiated expeditiously. Special attention should be paid to anatomic variation that may make airway management more difficult. These include the presence of dentures (which may occlude the airway), cervical arthritis (which adds danger to extending the neck), or temporomandibular joint arthritis (which may hinder mouth opening).

A thorough secondary survey is essential to uncover less-serious injuries. These injuries, which include various orthopedic and "minor" head trauma, may not be severe enough to cause problems during the initial resuscitation, but cumulatively may cause significant morbidity and mortality. An important point to note is that patients with no apparent life-threatening injuries can actually have potentially fatal injuries if there is some degree of limited physiologic reserve. Seemingly stable geriatric trauma patients can deteriorate rapidly and without warning.

RECOGNITION AND DIAGNOSIS OF COMMON INJURY PATTERNS

Head Injury

With aging, the brain undergoes progressive atrophy and decreases in size by about 10 percent between the ages of 30 and 70 years.[13] Subtle changes in cognition, memory, and data acquisition may confound the emergency physician's evaluation of the elderly patient's mental status. When evaluating the patient's mental status during the neurologic examination, it would be a grave error to assume that alterations in mental status are due solely to any underlying dementia or senility.

In a 1978 study, elderly persons experienced a much lower incidence of epidural hematomas than the general population.[13] This was attributed to the relatively more dense fibrous bond between the dura mater and the inner table of the skull in older individuals. There is, however, a higher incidence of subdural hematomas in elderly patients. As the brain mass decreases with advancing age, there is greater stretching and tension of the bridging veins that pass from the brain to the dural sinuses. The increased "dead space" within the skull may delay symptoms of intracranial bleeding. More liberal indications for computed tomography (CT) scanning of the head are justified.

Cervical Spine Injuries

Spine injuries may be difficult to evaluate in geriatric patients. Cognitive problems or brain injury may make the clinical evaluation of the spine more difficult. A careful history from the patient or family will provide valuable information regarding the presence of previous neurologic deficits. The Canadian C-Spine Rule for radiography in alert and stable patients following blunt head/neck trauma identified age (≥65 years) as a high risk factor for C-spine injury, even among those with stable vital signs and Glasgow Coma Scale score of 15.[14] Thus, C-spine imaging in all such elderly patients is warranted.

One study found the incidence of cervical spine injury to be twice as great in geriatric patients as it was in a younger cohort of blunt trauma patients. Odontoid fractures were particularly common in geriatric patients, accounting for 20 percent of geriatric cervical spine fractures, as compared with 5 percent of nongeriatric fractures.[15] When the elderly trauma patient presents with neck pain, emergency physicians need to place special emphasis on maintaining cervical immobilization until the cervical spine is properly assessed. Because underlying cervical arthritis may obscure fracture lines, the elderly patient with persistent neck pain and negative plain radiographs should undergo CT scanning of the cervical spine.

Preexisting cervical spine pathology, such as osteoarthritis, may predispose elderly patients to spinal cord injuries. With hyperextension injuries, elderly patients may develop a central cord syndrome. This injury should be suspected in patients with upper greater than lower extremity weakness and sensory loss.

Chest Trauma

Chest trauma, both minor and severe, can compromise elderly individuals. In blunt trauma, rib fractures are the most common injury found. The pain associated with rib fractures, along with any decreased physiologic reserve, may predispose patients to respiratory complications.[2] More severe thoracic injuries, such as hemopneumothorax, pulmonary contusion, flail chest, and cardiac contusion, can quickly lead to decompensation in elderly individuals whose baseline oxygenation status may already be diminished.

Geriatric patients are more susceptible to the development of hypoxia and respiratory infections following trauma. In the elderly, diminished elasticity of the lungs along with progressive changes in the chest wall can lead to a reduction in pulmonary compliance and in the ability to cough effectively. Total lung surface area decreases as alveolar and small airway support diminishes with advancing age. There also is reduced mucociliary clearance of foreign material and bacteria and increased colonization of the oropharynx with gram-negative organisms. All of these factors result in an increased risk for nosocomial gram-negative pneumonia.[2]

The main therapeutic goal is aggressively maintaining adequate oxygen delivery. Frequent arterial blood gas analysis may provide early insight into elderly patients' respiratory function and reserve. Prompt tracheal intubation and use of mechanical ventilation should be considered in patients with more severe injuries, respiratory rates greater than 40 breaths per minute, or when the partial pressure of arterial oxygen (Pao_2) is <60 mm Hg or the partial pressure of carbon dioxide in arterial gas (Pao_2) is >50 mm Hg. While nonventilatory therapy helps to prevent respiratory infections and is always desirable, early mechanical ventilation may avert the disastrous results associated with hypoxia.[2]

Chest trauma alone does not necessarily forecast a bleak outcome. In one series, most patients with blunt chest injuries were discharged home to their preinjury level of independence.[2]

Abdominal Trauma

Significant abdominal injuries are diagnosed in approximately one-third of geriatric trauma patients.[2] The abdominal examination in elderly patients is notoriously unreliable as compared to younger patients. Even with an initially benign physical examination, emergency physicians must have a high index of suspicion for intraabdominal injuries in patients who have associated pelvic and lower rib cage fractures. For older patients, the adhesions associated with previous abdominal surgical procedures may increase the risk of performing diagnostic peritoneal lavage in the emergency department.[2] Therefore, CT scanning with contrast is a valuable diagnostic test. It is important to ensure adequate hydration and baseline assessment of renal function prior to the contrast load for the CT scan. Some patients may be volume depleted as a consequence of medications such as diuretics. Hypovolemia coupled with contrast administration may exacerbate underlying renal pathology.[2] For unstable patients, and especially those with multiple scars on the abdominal wall from previous procedures, the focused assessment with sonography for trauma (FAST) examination is the ideal diagnostic study to detect free intraperitoneal fluid. In prospective studies by emergency physicians and trauma surgeons, ultrasonography has been demonstrated to be highly sensitive and specific for the identification of free intraperitoneal fluid. It also is rapid, portable, noninvasive, and easily repeatable.

Orthopedic Injuries

HIP FRACTURES   Many elderly patients are predisposed to orthopedic injuries as a consequence of skeletal osteopenic and osteoporotic changes. Hip fracture is the single most common diagnosis that leads to hospitalization in all age groups in the United States. Hip fractures occur primarily in four areas: intertrochanteric, transcervical, subcapital, and subtrochanteric. Intertrochanteric fractures are the most common, followed by transcervical fractures.[2] Bleeding from closed pelvic and long-bone fractures can cause hypovolemia in elderly patients. Timely orthopedic consultation, evaluation, and treatment with open reduction and internal fixation should be coordinated with the diagnosis and management of other injuries.

LONG-BONE FRACTURES   Long-bone fractures of the femur, tibia, and humerus may produce a loss of mobility with a resulting decrease in the independent lifestyle of elderly patients.[16] Geriatric patients who present with femoral fractures have been found to have a significantly higher rate of preexisting medical conditions than patients with proximal humeral fractures.[16] Early orthopedic consultation for placing intramedullary rods may result in earlier mobilization.

UPPER EXTREMITY INJURIES   Falls on the outstretched hand increase the risk for Colles fractures. After the diagnosis is confirmed by radiographs, these fractures can usually be treated with closed reduction and immobilization. The incidence of humeral head and surgical neck fractures in elderly patients also are increased by falls on the outstretched hand or elbow.[16] Localized tenderness, swelling, and ecchymosis of the proximal humerus are characteristic signs of these injuries. Early orthopedic consultation and treatment with a shoulder immobilizer or surgical fixation should be arranged. Social services may need to be contacted to arrange for assistance with routine daily activities for some elderly patients being discharged home after an orthopedic injury.

EMERGENCY DEPARTMENT MANAGEMENT AND DISPOSITION

Special Management Principles

The work by Scalea and coinvestigators demonstrated that trauma physicians frequently fail to recognize the severity of hemodynamic instability in geriatric patients. Therefore, early invasive monitoring has been advocated to help physicians assess the elderly patient's hemodynamic status. Scalea and colleagues showed that by reducing the time to invasive monitoring in elderly trauma patients from 5.5 h to 2.2 h (thus recognizing and appropriately treating occult shock), the survival rate increased from 7 to 53 percent. Survival was likely improved secondary to enhanced oxygen delivery through the use of adequate volume loading and inotropic support.[12]

The insertion of invasive monitoring lines may not be a frequent occurrence in many emergency departments because of institutional practice and availability of equipment. Thus, every effort should be made by emergency physicians to expedite emergency department care of elderly trauma patients and prevent unnecessary delays. In the emergency department evaluation of blunt trauma patients, the chest radiograph, cervical spine series, and pelvic radiographs are necessary diagnostic tests during the secondary survey. Only a few radiologic studies, such as emergent head and abdominal computed tomography scans, should take precedence over obtaining vital information from invasive monitoring. Elderly trauma patients may benefit the most from an expeditious transfer to the intensive care unit for further mon-itoring so that hemodynamic status can be more adequately assessed. After assurance that hemodynamic status has been stabilized, patients can be transported back to the radiology suite for further plain radiographic studies.

In the emergency department, one must make critical management decisions regarding volume resuscitation without the benefit of sophisticated invasive monitoring devices. Geriatric trauma patients can decompensate from overly aggressive volume repletion just as quickly as they can with inadequate resuscitation. Elderly patients with underlying coronary artery disease and cerebrovascular disease are at a much greater risk of suffering the consequences of ischemia to vital organs when they become hypotensive after trauma. During the initial resuscitative phase, crystalloid, while the primary option, should be administered judiciously because elderly patients with diminished cardiac compliance are more susceptible to volume overload.

Serial crystalloid fluid boluses of 250 to 500 mL should be administered, with frequent monitoring of blood pressure, pulmonary examination, and urinary output. Strong consideration should be made for early and more liberal use of red blood cell transfusion. Depending on the type of injury and severity of blood loss, switching to blood transfusion after 1 to 2 L of crystalloid resuscitation should be considered. This practice early in the resuscitation may enhance oxygen delivery and help to minimize tissue ischemia.

Prevention, Prognosis, and Outcome

For elderly patients who are discharged home after sustaining an injury from a fall, a home safety assessment should be encouraged, through social services or the primary care physician, to help prevent future falls. Chronic medications that may adversely affect the vestibular system, cause profound sedation, or produce postural hypotension, should be identified; patients can then discuss alternative therapies or dosages with their primary care physicians.[7] When providing a prescription for new medication, select drugs that are the least centrally acting, least associated with postural hypotension, and have the shortest duration of action.

Among geriatric trauma patients who are hospitalized, the mortality rate has been reported to be between 15 and 30 percent. These figures far exceed the mortality rate of 4 to 8 percent found in younger patients.[2] In general, late trauma deaths from multiple organ failure and sepsis occur more often in the elderly. Geriatric patients also are more likely to die following minor traumatic events.[6]

Several markers for poor outcome in elderly trauma victims have been determined. Age greater than 75 years, Glasgow Coma Scale score less than 7, presence of shock upon admission, severe head injury, and the development of sepsis are associated with worse outcome and higher mortality figures.[17] Although the Injury Severity Score (ISS) correlates with mortality rates, it does not fully capture the potential for mortality in this age group. For example, mortality rates for minor trauma (ISS <10) and nonmajor trauma (ISS <15) may be significant in the elderly. Survival probabilities that use ISS also perform less well with low-level falls than with other injury patterns. In the older trauma patient, the number of injuries, and not just the body system with most severe injuries, is a strong and independent contributor to mortality.[18] Comorbidities are common in this age group; however, studies addressing preexisting diseases and trauma mortality in this age group are equivocal and the magnitude of the effect is uncertain. Several studies indicate that preexisting diseases clearly affect trauma outcomes. Other studies, however, have not shown a clear correlation between preexisting diseases and trauma mortality. Explanation for these divergent results may be found in the results of Richmond and coinvestigators.[18] They noted that the presence of preexisting comorbid medical conditions increased the odds of experiencing a complication greater than threefold. Complications themselves were a significant predictor of mortality. For example, cardiovascular complications tripled and pulmonary complications doubled the mortality risk.

The ultimate goal in the care of elderly trauma patients is to return them to their preinjury state of function. Recent data suggest that immediately after discharge, one-third of trauma survivors return to independent living, one-third return to dependent status but living at home, and one-third require nursing home facilities. In the long term, almost 90 percent of trauma survivors ultimately return home and a majority return to independent living.[17,19] Increasing age, total number of injuries, injury to extremities, injuries as a result of falls, and lower functional levels predict discharge to a skilled nursing facility.[18]

In light of investigations showing that elderly patients often return to preexisting health status after trauma and the value of early invasive monitoring, it appears that **aggressive resuscitation efforts for geriatric trauma patients are warranted.**

REFERENCES

1. U.S. Bureau of Census: *Current Population Reports, Special Studies, 65+ in the United States,* pp. 23–190. Available at http://www.census.gov/prod/1/pop/p23-190/p23-190.html. Last accessed April 28, 2003.
2. Schwab CW, Kauder DR: Trauma in the geriatric patient. *Arch Surg* 127:701, 1992.
3. Schiller WR, Knox R, Chleborad W: A five-year experience with severe injuries in elderly patients. *Accid Anal Prev* 27:167, 1995.
4. Morris JA, MacKenzie EJ, Edelstein SL: The effect of pre-existing conditions on mortality in trauma patients. *JAMA* 263:1942, 1990.
5. Osler T, Hales K, Baack B, et al: Trauma in the elderly. *Am J Surg* 156:537, 1988.
6. Smith DP, Enderson BL, Maull KI: Trauma in the elderly: Determinants of outcome. *South Med J* 83:171, 1990.
7. Tinetti ME, Speechley M: Prevention of falls among the elderly. *New Engl J Med* 320:1055, 1989.
8. Li G, Baker SP, Longlois JA, et al: Are female drivers safer? An application of the decomposition method. *Epidemiology* 9:379, 1998.
9. Hammond J, Ward CG: Burns in octogenarians. *South Med J* 84:1316, 1991.
10. Finelli FC, Johnsson J, Champion HR, et al: A case control study for major trauma in geriatric patients. *J Trauma* 29:541, 1989.
11. Meldon SW, Reilly M, Drew BL, et al: Trauma in the very elderly: A community-based study of outcomes at trauma and non-trauma centers. *J Trauma* 52:79, 2002.
11a. Ma MH, MacKenzie EJ, Alcorta R, Kelen GD: Compliance with prehospital triage protocols for major trauma patients. *J Trauma* 46:168, 1999.
12. Scalea TM, Simon HM, Duncan AO, et al: Geriatric blunt trauma: Improved survival with early invasive monitoring. *J Trauma* 30:129, 1990.
13. Kirkpatrick JB, Pearson J: Fatal cerebral injury in the elderly. *J Am Geriatr Soc* 26:489, 1978.
14. Stiell IG, Wells GA, Vandemheen KL, et al: The Canadian C-Spine Rule for radiography in alert and stable trauma patients. *JAMA* 286:1841, 2001.
15. Touger M, Gennis P, Nathanson N, et al: Validity of a decision rule to reduce cervical spine radiography in elderly patients with blunt trauma. *Ann Emerg Med* 40:287, 2002.
16. Sartoretti C, Sartoretti-Schefer S, Ruckert R, et al: Comorbid conditions in old patients with femur fractures. *J Trauma* 43:570, 1997.
17. van Aalst JA, Morris JA, Yates HK, et al: Severely injured geriatric patients return to independent living: A study of factors influencing function and independence. *J Trauma* 31:1096, 1991.
18. Richmond TS, Kauder D, Strumpf N, et al: Characteristics and outcomes of serious traumatic injury in older adults. *J Am Geriatr Soc* 50:215, 2002.
19. DeMaria EJ, Kenney PR, Merriam MA, et al: Aggressive trauma care benefits the elderly. *J Trauma* 27:1200, 1987.

254

TRAUMA IN PREGNANCY
Nelson Tang
Drew White

Trauma remains the leading cause of nonobstetric morbidity and mortality in pregnant women. The conventional paradigm that fetal survival depends wholly on maternal stabilization and well-being is fundamentally accurate. It has become increasingly apparent, however, that in traumatic events (particularly apparently minor ones), the severity of maternal injuries may be a poor predictor of fetal distress and outcome.[1–3] Successful outcomes for both mother and fetus require a collaborative effort among the prehospital provider, emergency physician, trauma surgeon, obstetrician, and neonatologist.

EPIDEMIOLOGY

It has been consistently estimated that significant trauma complicates 6 to 8 percent of all pregnancies.[1] Trauma during pregnancy is associated with an increased risk of preterm labor, placental abruption, fetal-maternal hemorrhage, and pregnancy loss. The maternal trauma-related mortality rate does not appear to be different from that of nonpregnant women.[4] Substance abuse has previously been shown to be a contributing factor, with one study finding a positive toxicology screen in up to 16 percent of patients tested.[5]

The most common cause of blunt abdominal trauma is motor vehicle crashes, accounting for up to 70 percent of acute injuries. This is followed by falls and direct assault in decreasing order of frequency.[1,6] The incidence of falls appears to increase with advancement of pregnancies, presumably due to alterations in maternal balance and coordination. Even minor abdominal trauma can result in fetal demise. Up to 5 percent with minor trauma may experience abruption. The role of domestic violence during pregnancy is of significant concern, with one large series describing more than 31 percent of trauma in pregnant women as intentional injuries, and most studies cite rates of violence during pregnancy at 4 to 8 percent.[7] As many as 88 percent of those cases may involve the husband or boyfriend as the perpetrator.[8]

Penetrating injuries are less common than blunt trauma during pregnancy. Gunshot wounds are the most common form of penetrating trauma. Some of these injuries may be self-inflicted and represent attempts to terminate pregnancies. Fetal mortality rates in penetrating injuries are as high as 70 percent. While the rate of maternal visceral injuries is 19 to 38 percent, there remains a 60 to 90 percent chance of fetal injury. This is presumably due to the protective effect of the gravid uterus on maternal viscera.

INJURY PREVENTION

Substantial evidence has demonstrated that motor vehicle seat belt use during pregnancy helps protect both the mother and the fetus, and current recommendations suggest that safety belts be worn throughout pregnancy. One study found that the best predictors of fetal loss or adverse outcome were crash severity and lack of, or improper, seat belt use.[9] The American College of Obstetricians and Gynecologists (ACOG) and the National Highway Traffic Safety Administration (NHTSA) recommend that the lap belt be placed as low as possible under the gravid uterus (across both the anterior superior iliac spines and the pubic symphysis) and that the shoulder harness be positioned snugly between the breasts but off to the side of the uterus. According to the NHTSA, seatbelt use in the general public increased to its highest level ever of 75 percent in 2002,[10] but the most recent studies in pregnant patients showed that 46 percent of pregnant patients involved in motor vehicle crashes were not wearing seat belts.[11]

One leading panel of expert physicians on the subject has recommended that air bags not be disconnected for pregnant women.[12] While there is a risk of injury to the more proximally located gravid uterus, it is also known that the leading cause of fetal death in motor vehicle crashes is maternal death. With the pregnant woman properly seated as far away as possible from an airbag, the benefits of these restraint devices currently appear to outweigh the apparent risks.

PHYSIOLOGIC CHANGES OF PREGNANCY

Physiologic changes in pregnancy are discussed in detail in Chap. 104. In addition to the normal physiologic changes associated with pregnancy, non-trauma related complications of pregnancy must also be considered. Conditions such as pregnancy-induced hypertension, placenta previa, preeclampsia, and eclampsia may significantly alter the presentation and complicate evaluation and treatment in the setting of trauma (see Chap. 106).

Maternal blood volume begins to expand at approximately week 10 of gestation and peaks at about a 45 percent increase from baseline at week 28, resulting in a state of hypervolemia. Red cell mass increases to a lesser extent, leading to the relative physiologic anemia of pregnancy. Cardiac output is increased by 1.0 to 1.5 L/min at week 10 of pregnancy, and remains elevated until the end of pregnancy. Heart rate in the mother is generally increased by 10 to 20 beats/min in the second trimester, accompanied by decreases in systolic and diastolic blood pressures of 10 to 15 mm Hg.

The relative hypervolemic state can mislead the clinician during maternal resuscitation in trauma and make clinical findings difficult to interpret. A pregnant woman may lose 30 to 35 percent of circulating blood volume before manifesting hypotension or clinical signs of shock.[1] Uterine arteries constrict, resulting in diminished fetal blood flow and tissue oxygenation, before significant evidence of maternal hypovolemia appears.

After week 12 of gestation, the uterus becomes an intra-abdominal organ, removing it from the relative protection of the maternal pelvis and making it more susceptible to direct injuries. The bladder also moves anteriorly into the abdomen in the third trimester of pregnancy, increasing its susceptibility to injury. Uterine blood flow may increase to upward of 600 mL/min, making severe maternal hemorrhage from uterine injury possible. The gravid uterus also causes passive stretching of the abdominal wall and peritoneum as it enlarges and may lead to diminished sensitivity to injury and irritation from intraperitoneal blood. At or about weeks 18 to 20 of gestation, the expanding mass of the gravid uterus may lead to the "supine hypotension syndrome," in which venous return and cardiac output are diminished by compression of the maternal inferior vena cava in the supine position. The enlarging uterus may additionally cause engorgement of lower extremity and lower abdominal vessels, predisposing the patient to severe retroperitoneal hemorrhages with acute injuries to these areas. Placement of intravenous lines in the groin and lower extremity should be avoided if possible because of inferior vena cava compression by the uterus and to avoid pooling in engorged or injured pelvic veins.

As pregnancy progresses, the diaphragm is elevated by as much as 4 cm and tidal volume increases by 40 percent as residual volume diminishes by 25 percent. Functional residual capacity is similarly decreased, and the compensatory increase in ventilation typically results in respiratory alkalosis. Serum pH is usually maintained at normal values by renal compensation. These changes may significantly impair the ability of a pregnant trauma patient to compensate for respiratory compromise. Diaphragmatic elevation should also be considered when thoracostomy tube placement is indicated during maternal resuscitation.

The gastrointestinal tract demonstrates diminished motility, and there is delayed gastric emptying during pregnancy. This increases the likelihood of gastroesophageal reflux and the potential for aspiration from acute injuries as well as from resuscitative interventions, including endotracheal intubation. The small bowel is moved upward in the abdomen by the enlarging uterus, protecting the small bowel to some degree from lower abdominal injuries. It does, however, increase the chance of complex bowel injuries in penetrating trauma of the upper abdomen.[6] The liver is typically unaffected by pregnancy, and the most common etiology of abdominal hemorrhage remains splenic injury, as in nonpregnant patients.

MATERNAL AND FETAL INJURIES

Direct fetal injury is relatively rare in blunt abdominal trauma during the first trimester of pregnancy. When fetal injuries do occur, they are typically seen later in gestation and tend to involve the fetal skull and brain. These injuries are frequently sustained in association with fractures to the maternal pelvis when the fetal head is engaged. When the uterus is penetrated by a sharp object or projectile, the fetus has a high probability of sustaining injury.

Uterine rupture is a relatively uncommon complication of blunt trauma sustained during pregnancy. Its incidence has been reported to be 0.6 to 1.0 percent of injuries in pregnancy, and is more likely to occur during the late second and third trimesters and when there is direct and forceful impact upon the uterus.[6,13] The fetal mortality rate in such cases is nearly 100 percent, whereas maternal mortality is less than 10 percent. The presentation of uterine rupture may be quite nonspecific, but loss of the palpable uterine contour, ease of palpation of fetal parts, or radiologic evidence of abnormal fetal location is suggestive of the diagnosis.

Uterine irritability and the onset of preterm labor may be precipitated by acute abdominal trauma during pregnancy. Numerous reports have noted the management of premature labor in pregnant trauma patients with tocolytic agents, but their use has not been generally recommended and requires individualization. Tocolytic agents have numerous adverse side effects, such as fetal and maternal tachycardia, which may complicate the evaluation of trauma patients. Additionally, their use may further impair the ability to diagnose other significant traumatic injuries, specifically placental abruption. If tocolytics are considered, an obstetrician should be consulted prior to administration.

Second only to maternal death, abruptio placentae is the most common cause of fetal death. Abruptio placentae complicates 1 to 5 percent of minor injuries during pregnancy and up to 40 to 50 percent of major trauma.[6] Placental abruption has been described as being caused by the deformation of the elastic uterus around the relatively inelastic placenta, and is independent of placental location. Further exacerbated by increased intrauterine pressures, shear forces are applied to the placental base, leading to separation from the uterine wall. Findings consistent with abruptio placentae include abdominal pain, vaginal bleeding, and tetanic uterine contractions, classically described as painful vaginal bleeding in the third trimester. Placental abruption may also lead to the introduction of placental products into the maternal circulation, stimulating disseminated intravascular coagulation (DIC) or amniotic fluid embolism. The correlation and predictive value of DIC with respect to fetal mortality remains unsettled.[8,14]

The incidence of fetal-maternal hemorrhage (fetal red blood cells entering the maternal bloodstream) in trauma during pregnancy is four to five times that which occurs in pregnancies not complicated by injury.[6] Fetal-maternal hemorrhage occurs in over 30 percent of significant trauma in pregnant patients and is implicated in the sensitization and subsequent isoimmunization of Rh-negative patients. Fetal hemorrhage itself poses the direct risks of fetal hypovolemia, anemia, distress, and death. Anterior placental location appears to be associated with an increased risk of fetal-maternal hemorrhage.

EMERGENCY TREATMENT

Prehospital Care

An effort to ascertain the possibility of pregnancy should be made during the initial evaluation of all acutely injured women of childbearing age. As in the care of all trauma victims, initial priorities remain the ABCs of resuscitation directed at the mother. All pregnant trauma patients should receive supplemental oxygen, as the gravida becomes less able to compensate for hypoxia. Similarly, early intubation must be considered when indicated by the nature or severity of injuries. Peripheral intravenous lines with crystalloid infusions should be initiated in the prehospital setting.

For pregnant patients beyond 20 weeks of gestation who must be transported in the supine position or in whom spinal immobilization is indicated, a wedge should be placed under the right hip area, tilting the patient approximately 30 degrees toward her left side, to avoid hypotension from inferior vena cava compression by the gravid uterus. Alternatively, the uterus may be manually maneuvered to the left side of the abdomen by transport personnel. Pneumatic antishock trousers are rarely used now, but if considered in a pregnant patient, the abdominal compartment must not be inflated, because that may cause uteroplacental compression and impair venous return to the heart. An integral part of the prehospital role in trauma management is triage to an appropriate hospital. If pregnancy in a trauma patient is identified or suspected, transport should be initiated to a designated trauma center with sufficient capabilities to manage both mother and fetus. Advance notification of the receiving facility should be made to enable the assembly of the appropriate hospital personnel to continue the resuscitation and management efforts.

Emergency Department Management

Upon arrival in the emergency department, the prehospital resuscitative measures already undertaken should be reviewed and continued as appropriate. Since maternal stability and survival offer the best chance for fetal well-being, **initial efforts must be directed toward the adequate resuscitation of the mother prior to evaluation of the fetus.** No critical interventions or diagnostic procedures should be withheld from the treatment of pregnant trauma patients out of concerns for potential adverse fetal consequences. A trauma surgeon and obstetrician should be involved early in the evaluation and management of a significantly traumatized pregnant patient.

Volume Resuscitation

The initial sequence of trauma resuscitation is unchanged in the emergency treatment of an injured pregnant patient. The patient is kept in the left lateral decubitus position to the extent possible to minimize vena caval compression. Since aortocaval compression has also been demonstrated to decrease the effectiveness of chest compressions, maneuvers such as a lateral tilt or manual displacement of the uterus should also be performed during CPR.[16] Securing the airway and ensuring the adequacy of ventilation in addition to the administration of supplemental oxygenation are of primary concern. Gastric tube decompression must be performed early, since delayed stomach emptying makes the possibility of aspiration a particular concern during pregnancy. Sources of hemorrhage should be identified and controlled, because maternal blood loss and hypovolemia occur at the expense of fetal hypoperfusion. Adequate large-bore vascular access is essential, and crystalloid infusions may need to be adjusted upward by as much as 50 percent to account for the additional plasma volume in pregnancy.

The use of vasopressor agents poses a risk of impaired uterine perfusion and should not be initiated until adequate volume replacement has been administered. Their use should not be restricted, however, if required for maternal resuscitation. Initial laboratory studies include complete blood counts, blood typing, and Rh status, as well as coagulation profiles with fibrin degradation products and fibrinogen to determine the possibility of DIC. Low serum bicarbonate levels have been shown to be associated with adverse fetal outcomes, and routine determination of the levels may be of predictive value.[1] After the primary trauma survey, an organized and methodical secondary system survey must be performed to ensure the identification of all potential injuries.

Gestational Age Assessment

Attention should next be turned to the evaluation of the gravid abdomen and fetus. Gestational age can be assessed rapidly by palpating uterine fundal height. At week 12 of gestation the uterine fundus may be palpated at or about the level of the pubic symphysis, and at approximately week 20 it may be felt at about the level of the umbilicus. The abdomen and uterus should be examined for evidence of injury as well as palpated for uterine tenderness or contractions.

Pelvic Examination

If abdominal or pelvic trauma is suspected, a sterile pelvic examination is indicated to inspect for injuries of the lower genital tract, vaginal bleeding, or rupture of amniotic membranes. Fluid with a pH of 7 in the vaginal canal is suggestive of amniotic fluid, whereas a pH of 5 is consistent with vaginal secretions. A branchlike pattern upon drying of vaginal fluid on a microscope slide or "ferning" is also diagnostic of amniotic fluid.

Fetomaternal Hemorrhage

Fetomaternal hemorrhage (FMH) should be suspected if there is uterine tenderness, uterine contractions, vaginal bleeding, or in the presence of direct or indirect maternal abdominal trauma. The occurrence and degree of FMH can be assessed by the Apt test or the Kleihauer-Betke (KB) test. The Apt test is a qualitative determination of the presence of fetal hemoglobin in maternal blood. The KB test applies acid elution to an aliquot of maternal blood, and then maternal and fetal red blood cells are counted under the microscope. An extrapolation is then made to the volume of FMH. Neither test is available on an emergency basis, however, and the KB test has poor sensitivity to detect <5 μL of FMH. The recognition of FMH is important because if the mother is Rh-negative and the fetus is Rh-positive, as little as 0.1 μL of fetal blood can sensitize the mother[15] and endanger this and subsequent pregnancies.

Rh°D Immune Globulin

The American College of Obstetricians and Gynecologists recommends that consideration be given to administering Rh°D immune globulin (Rhogam, BayRhoD, MICRhoGAM, WinRho) to all unsensitized D-negative (Rh-negative) pregnant women with abdominal trauma.[6] Exceptions are 1) prior maternal sensitization; 2) a known Rh-negative fetus; 3) or a known Rh-negative father. History of the latter is often unreliable or unavailable. Rh°D immune globulin protects against Rh isoimmunization if given within 72 h of FMH.

DOSAGE There is no uniform agreement on the dose, but two options are available: **50 μg for gestation 12 weeks or less and 300 μg for gestation 13 weeks or more OR 300 μg for all gestational ages.** The rationale for the lower dose for 12 weeks or less gestation is that the total fetal blood volume at 12 weeks gestation is about 4.2 μL, and a 50-μg dose will be effective for up to 5 μL of FMH. A 300-μg dose will protect up to 30 μL of FMH.

The obstetrician can best determine if doses larger than 300 μg should be administered. The 72-h window for Rh°D immune globulin administration allows for more thorough FMH testing in the hospital.

Tetanus Prophylaxis

Tetanus prophylaxis has no deleterious fetal effects and should be routinely administered as indicated following trauma. Given that the tetanus antibody crosses the placenta, it can also reduce the incidence of neonatal tetanus.

Diagnostic Imaging

The use of diagnostic radiologic imaging in the emergency treatment of pregnant trauma patients adheres to the fundamental principles of trauma management. While the judicious acquisition of studies is indicated to minimize fetal exposure to the potential effects of ionizing radiation (see Radiation Exposure to Uterus/Fetus, Table 105-3), no tests should be withheld if they are necessary for appropriate maternal evaluation and treatment. The principal concerns regarding radiation exposure in utero are the possibilities of childhood neoplasia, fetal loss, congenital malformations, and microcephaly.[17] Thus studies should be limited to those that are essential, as radiation exposure sequelae are cumulative.

The greatest risk to fetal viability is within the first 2 weeks following conception, and the highest potential for malformation is during embryonic organogenesis from 2 to 8 weeks after conception.[17] Adverse fetal effects due to radiation exposure are negligible from doses of less than 10 rad. The standard trauma plain radiographs, such as cervical spine, chest, and pelvis films, deliver significantly less than 1 rad each.[17] Fetal exposure can be further decreased by appropriate shielding of the maternal abdomen and pelvis during many studies.

Abdominopelvic CT scanning, pelvic angiography, and pelvic fluoroscopy result in the highest delivered doses of radiation. The amount is typically 2 to 5 rad, with some variation due to equipment quality, techniques used, and duration of study.[17] A recent study demonstrated that the sensitivity and specificity of abdominal ultrasound for the evaluation of abdominal trauma in pregnancy is similar to that in nonpregnant patients.[18] Radiation exposure in CT may be reduced by performing modified studies and the use of dose-reducing techniques, such as decreasing the number of imaging slices obtained.[17] Diagnostic evaluations with magnetic resonance imaging and ventilation-perfusion scanning have not been reported to cause adverse pregnancy outcomes. Potential effects of contrast agents have not been definitively studied, and their use requires individualization.

DPL and Laparotomy

The indications for emergent laparotomy remain unchanged in the evaluation of pregnant trauma patients. Similarly, diagnostic peritoneal lavage (DPL) is an effective modality for the evaluation of intra-abdominal injuries from acute trauma. DPL should be performed with an open, supraumbilical technique in patients with evidence of a gravid uterus. The fetus appears to tolerate surgery and anesthesia well if adequate oxygenation and uterine perfusion are maintained.[6] The performance of emergent DPL and surgery have not been shown to have an association with fetal loss, and these procedures should not be withheld out of concern for fetal compromise when indicated in trauma.[1] Additionally, a large multi-institutional retrospective review has shown that emergent cesarean delivery results in a fetal survival rate as high as 75 percent when gestation is at or greater than 26 weeks, fetal heart tones are present on admission, and the procedure is performed at the earliest indication of fetal distress.[3]

Fetal Assessment

A rapid assessment of fetal condition should be initiated with auscultation of fetal heart tones to determine fetal viability and identify fetal distress. Assessment of fetal heart tones may be augmented by use of a Doppler stethoscope or ultrasound. It has been suggested that fetal viability in the setting of trauma is directly related to the presence or absence of fetal heart tones on presentation, and that if these are confirmed absent, then the remainder of treatment efforts be directed solely at maternal resuscitation.[3] Normal fetal heart rates are in the range of 120 to 160 beats/min. The most likely cause of fetal bradycardia is acute hypoxia. In acute injuries, maternal hypotension, hypothermia, respiratory compromise, or placental abruption are likely etiologies. Similarly, in the setting of acute trauma, the finding of fetal tachycardia may also represent a hypoxic or hypovolemic state.

The use of bedside ultrasound has become an increasingly valuable adjunct to initial trauma assessment and management. Portable ultrasound in this setting has been shown to be rapid, noninvasive, and facilitates serial examinations.[19] In cases of trauma during pregnancy, ultrasonography may also be of particular value in the evaluation of general fetal condition. Fetal size and estimated gestational age, the presence of fetal heart motion, fetal activity or demise, placental location, and amniotic fluid volume can be assessed.[20] The efficacy of ul-

trasound, however, for the diagnosis of specific trauma-related injuries remains unproven. Several reports have suggested the relative inability of ultrasound to diagnose uterine rupture or fetal-placental injuries, and its sensitivity is insufficient to exclude the diagnosis of placental abruption.[17,20] The intra-abdominal anatomic distortions of late third-trimester pregnancy may further limit the diagnostic capability of ultrasound in acute trauma.

In the management of blunt trauma during pregnancy, external fetal monitoring is indicated for gestational age estimated beyond 20 weeks and is more predictive than ultrasound for abruptio placentae. The initiation of fetal tocodynamometry is recommended at the earliest possible stage of evaluation following maternal stabilization, preferably in the emergency department with obstetric consultation, because abruptio placentae usually becomes apparent shortly after the injury. Fetal monitoring is utilized to assess both uterine contractile activity as well as fetal heart rate. Beyond the viable gestational age of 23 weeks, the presence of fetal tachycardia, lack of beat-to-beat or long-term variability, or late decelerations on tocodynamometry are diagnostic of fetal distress and may be indications for emergent cesarean delivery.

The identification of frequent uterine activity on external fetal monitoring has been shown to be a sensitive predictor of abruptio placentae beyond 20 weeks of gestation. In a major prospective study, no cases of abruptio placentae were identified if there were fewer than 8 contractions per h during the first 4 h of tocodynamometry. A minimum of 4 h of external tocodynamometric monitoring of the potentially viable fetus appears to be predictive of immediate adverse pregnancy outcomes and is indicated for all pregnant patients evaluated for trauma, even those without obvious abdominal injury. Patients demonstrating 3 to 7 contractions per h or persistent uterine irritability should have tocodynamometry extended to a minimum of 24 h. They may subsequently be safely discharged if uterine contractions abate and other reasons for further evaluation do not exist. Patients with fewer than 3 contractions per h during an initial 4-h observation period can be safely discharged in conjunction with the consulting obstetrician. This approach has been shown to have the same pregnancy outcomes among discharged patients when compared with uninjured controls.

PERIMORTEM CESAREAN DELIVERY

The need to perform perimortem cesarean delivery in cases of maternal cardiac arrest arises extremely rarely. Nevertheless, it involves complex ethical, medical, and emotional considerations. The largest review of reported attempts to date in the literature revealed fewer than 200 successful fetal outcomes from the procedure.[22] The time to delivery from the onset of maternal arrest was found to be critical to fetal survival with good neurologic outcome. Excellent outcomes were reported when delivery took place within 5 min of maternal death. Survival was unlikely if delivery occurred after 20 min of maternal arrest. It has since been recommended that the procedure be performed after 4 min of maternal resuscitation, such that the fetus will be delivered within a total of 5 min from initiation of CPR.[22] Successful out-of-hospital perimortem cesarean delivery has been reported, although with a prolonged interval between maternal collapse and delivery and severe neurologic deficits in the infant.

Consideration of perimortem cesarean delivery must be made only after immediate and optimal advanced maternal cardiopulmonary resuscitative measures have been instituted. The procedure may be attempted in gestations estimated at beyond 23 weeks. Full maternal resuscitation must continue unabated while preparing for and during the actual delivery. It is universally recommended that the procedure be performed rapidly with the most readily available materials, and that a single vertical incision be made to enter the peritoneum, followed by a vertical uterine incision to deliver the fetus. Successful maternal revival following fetal delivery has been reported. Improved venous return to the central circulation, increased maternal oxygen delivery following removal of the high uterine demand, and decreased pooling of blood in the uteroplacental circulation have all been suggested as explanations.

DISPOSITION

The decision to admit or discharge after the emergency assessment and management of a pregnant trauma patient is ultimately based on the nature and severity of presenting injuries. Patients suffering severe multisystem trauma will have their further care and management assumed by trauma surgeons and consultant obstetricians. Even in cases of seemingly minor but potentially significant injuries, admission to a trauma service capable of further observation and management is appropriate. Patients who demonstrate evidence of fetal distress or uterine irritability during the initial assessment require admission under the extended evaluation and care of an obstetrician capable of emergency delivery as necessary. Patients who must be transferred to other facilities for definitive trauma or obstetric care must be appropriately stabilized prior to transfer, with provisions for an appropriate level of care during transport. There must be strict adherence to transfer policies that comply with federal regulations. Clearly, the ongoing need for an interdisciplinary approach to patient management in such cases remains even after admission.

Although external fetal monitoring may be initiated in the emergency department with consultation, the monitoring is typically continued in the labor and delivery suite under the direction of an obstetrician. If the extended period of monitoring demonstrates no evidence to suggest fetal or maternal injury or distress, the patient may be discharged. Upon discharge, the patient must be carefully advised to seek medical attention immediately if she should develop abdominal pain or cramping, vaginal bleeding, leakage of fluid, or perception of diminished fetal activity. The decision to discharge an injured pregnant patient from the emergency department must be made carefully. A high index of suspicion should be maintained for occult injuries as well as a low threshold for obstetric consultation when indicated. To screen for the possibility of interpersonal violence, a thorough social services evaluation or referral should be made in all but the most obvious cases of accidental injury. Adequate obstetric follow-up care must be ensured for all pregnant trauma patients when discharged from the emergency department.

REFERENCES

1. Scorpio RJ, Esposito TJ, Smith LG, et al: Blunt trauma during pregnancy: Factors affecting fetal outcome. *J Trauma* 32:213, 1992.
2. Biester EM, Tomich PG, Esposito TJ, et al: Trauma in pregnancy: Normal Revised Trauma Score in relation to other markers of maternofetal status— A preliminary study. *Am J Obstet Gynecol* 176:1206, 1997.
3. Morris JA, Rosenbower TJ, Jurkovich GJ, et al: Infant survival after cesarean section for trauma. *Ann Surg* 223:481, 1996.
4. Esposito TJ, Gens DR, Smith LG, et al: Trauma during pregnancy: A review of 79 cases. *Arch Surg* 126:1073, 1991.
5. Esposito TJ, Gens DR, Smith LG, et al: Evaluation of blunt trauma occurring during pregnancy. *J Trauma* 29:1628, 1989.
6. Obstetric aspects of trauma management. *Am Coll Obstet Gynecol Educ Bull* 251:1, 1998.
7. Gazmararian JA, Lazorick S, Spitz AM, et al: Prevalence of violence against pregnant women. *JAMA* 275:1915, 1996.
8. Poole GV, Martin JN, Perry KG Jr, et al: Trauma in pregnancy: The role of interpersonal violence. *Am J Obstet Gynecol* 174:1873, 1996.
9. Pearlman MD, Klinich KD, Schneider LW, et al: A comprehensive program to improve safety for pregnant women and fetuses in motor vehicle crashes: A preliminary report. *Am J Obstet Gynecol* 182:1554, 2000.
10. U.S. Department of Transportation, National Highway Traffic Safety Administration press release 58-02, September 9, 2002 [NHTSA Website]. Available at: http://www.nhtsa.gov/nhtsa/announce/press/pressdisplay.cfm?year=2002&filename=pr58-02.html. Accessed October 25, 2002.
11. Shah KH, Simons RK, Holbrook T, et al: Trauma in pregnancy: Maternal and fetal outcomes. *J Trauma* 45:83, 1998.
12. National Conference on Medical Indications for Air Bag Disconnection. George Washington University Medical Center. Final report, 1997 [NHTSA web site]. Available at: www.nhtsa.gov/airbags/air%20bag%2orpt.html. Accessed April 30, 2003.
13. Astarita DC, Feldman B: Seat belt placement resulting in uterine rupture. *J Trauma* 42:738, 1997.
14. Ali J, Yeo A, Gana TJ, et al: Predictors of fetal mortality in pregnant trauma patients. *J Trauma* 42:782, 1997.
15. Mollison PL: Clinical aspects of Rh immunization. *Am J Clin Pathol* 60:287, 1973.
16. Towery R, English P, Wisner D: Evaluation of pregnant women after blunt injury. *J Trauma* 35:731, 1993.
17. Goldman SM, Wagner LK: Radiologic management of abdominal trauma in pregnancy. *Am J Radiol* 166:763, 1996.
18. Goodwin H, Holmes JF, Wisner DH: Abdominal ultrasound examination in pregnant blunt trauma patients. *J Trauma* 50:689, 2001.
19. Nordenholz KE, Rubin MA, Gularte GG, et al: Ultrasound in the evaluation and management of blunt abdominal trauma. *Ann Emerg Med* 29:357, 1997.
20. Ma OJ, Mateer JR, DeBehnke DJ: Use of ultrasonography for the evaluation of pregnant trauma patients. *J Trauma* 40:665, 1996.
21. Katz VL, Dotters DJ, Droegemueller W: Perimortem cesarean delivery. *Obstet Gynecol* 68:571, 1986.

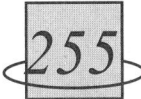

HEAD INJURY

Thomas D. Kirsch
Christopher A. Lipinski

EPIDEMIOLOGY

Injuries are the leading cause of death in persons younger than 45 years old with approximately one-third of these deaths a result of head trauma. Traumatic brain injury (TBI) results from either direct or indirect forces to the brain matter. Direct injury is immediate and caused by the force of an object striking or penetrating the head. Indirect injuries from acceleration/deceleration forces are generated by the variable movements of different areas of the brain against one another and by the impact of the brain against the skull.

Annually, in the United States, there are approximately 1.5 million nonfatal TBIs, 370,000 persons hospitalized as a result of a TBI, and 52,000 persons who die from TBI.[1] TBI also leads to 80,000 annual cases of residual neurologic disability. The costs for treatment of both acute and chronic TBI are estimated to be $4 billion dollars annually.[2]

The peak incidence of TBI occurs in males between the ages of 15 and 24 years, but ethanol-intoxicated individuals, the elderly, and young children are at increased risk of TBI because of underlying anatomic and physiologic factors. The cause of TBI varies greatly by age and demographic factors. For example, for 15- to 24-year-olds the leading cause is gunshot wounds, while for those older than age 65 years it is falls.

ANATOMY

The outermost layer, the scalp, is composed of five layers: skin, subcutaneous tissue, galea, areolar tissue, and the pericranium. Because of the rich blood supply, the scalp has a major role in temperature regulation, being capable of liberating 50 percent of our total body heat. This same generous blood supply, combined with the loose areolar connection to the pericranium, can lead to severe blood loss after injury.

The calvaria or skull is a rigid container made up of eight major bones. These bones are composed of two solid layers separated by cancellous bone, which adds rigidity and strength. The cranial sutures between bones initially serve as expansion joints, but eventually fuse, halting expandability in adults.

Because the basilar skull is the exit and entry point for the cranial nerves and blood vessels basilar fractures places these structures at risk. The *inion* is the anatomic meeting point of the frontal, sphenoid, temporal, and parietal bones. Fractures of the skull at this point can disrupt the underlying middle meningeal artery, leading to epidural hematoma.

The adult brain weighs between 1300 and 1500 g and occupies 80 percent of the total volume of the skull. The brain's three basic structures—the cerebral hemispheres, the cerebellum, and the brainstem—are divided by two major fixed dura attachments. The *falx cerebri* vertically separates the cerebral hemispheres down to the brainstem. The *tentorium cerebelli* separates the cerebellum and brainstem from the cerebrum at the base of the skull. The inner edge of the tentorium cerebelli is the site of the most common brain herniation syndrome, uncal herniation. The cerebrum is further anatomically divided into major lobes named after the bones overlying them: frontal, temporal, parietal, occipital. The cortices encase the deeper brain structures such as the basal ganglia, the major systems integration site. The cerebellum occupies the posterior cranial fossa, and is responsible to pattern motor memory and balance. The brainstem contains the cranial nerve nuclei and the inflow and outflow functional somatic tracts.

The brain is covered with multiple anatomic layers and potential spaces. The outermost layer, the *dura mater,* is firmly adhered to the inner skull and has fixed attachments at the cranial sutures. At some edges of dural reflections, the dura separates into two layers and forms channels called the dural venous sinuses, which serve to drain blood and cerebrospinal fluid from the brain. Underneath the dura mater is a thinner connective tissue layer called the *arachnoid mater.* The arachnoid mater perforates the dura mater at the venous sinuses where it forms arachnoid granulations. The arachnoid granulations serve as filtration and drainage points for the cerebrospinal fluid. The arachnoid mater is loosely adhered to the pia mater making possible the potential subarachnoid space. The *pia mater* is closely associated with the gray matter of the brain and is the innermost layer. Between the arachnoid and the pia is the *subarachnoid space,* where cerebrospinal fluid (CSF) circulates. In the average adult, there is 150 mL of CSF surrounding the brain and spinal cord. Approximately 500 mL of CFS is produced in the choroid plexus of the lateral ventricles each day.

Several subarachnoid spaces known as *cisternae* surround the brain and correspond to large cortical surface irregularities. These include the ambient, prepontine, supracerebellar, cerebellomedullary, interpeduncular, superior, and magna. There are four spaces contained within the brain known as *ventricles:* two lateral ventricles (separated by the septum pellucidum), a third ventricle, and a fourth ventricle. These CSF-containing spaces communicate by foramina: Monroe (between the lateral and third ventricle), aqueduct of Sylvius (between the third and fourth ventricle), and foramen of Luschka and Magendie (outlets from the fourth ventricle into the cerebellomedullary cistern and cisterna magna).

PATHOPHYSIOLOGY

Acute brain injury is usually divided into primary and secondary phases. In the case of traumatic brain injury, the acute or primary phase describes the cellular injury and death that are a direct result of force of the injury. Primary cell death is irreversible and only preventing the injury event and mitigation of the injury forces on the brain reduce morbidity and mortality.

Secondary injury cascades can extend the damage to cells that are not initially irreversibly damaged. In the hours to weeks after the injury, local tissue ischemia from compressive forces or vascular injury lead to secondary cellular death. Prevention of the ischemia and hypoxia are the main therapeutic goals for treating patients with TBI.

Normal Physiology

The cerebrovascular system delivers energy substrates and oxygen while simultaneously removing the byproducts of metabolism. The brain accounts for only 2 percent of total body weight, but consumes 20 percent of the body's total oxygen requirement and 15 percent of total cardiac output. Maintaining adequate brain tissue perfusion is critical to avoid secondary brain injury. The cerebral perfusion pressure (CPP) is the difference between inflow and outflow (ΔP) and is essentially the driving pressure for cerebral blood flow (CBF). Estimates of CPP assume that the relevant inflow pressure is equivalent to the mean arterial pressure (MAP) and the outflow is related to intracranial pressure (ICP). The ICP is used to estimate outflow pressure because the venous system is collapsible at the entry point into the sinuses and changes in this outflow pressure occurs in parallel with increases in the ICP. The CPP is calculated in lieu of CBF:

$$CPP = MAP - ICP$$

The local adjustment of CBF within the brain microcirculation that result from changes in arterial pressure is termed "autoregulation." Autoregulation of CBF is functional with CPP between 50 and 150 mm Hg, but is often lost in patients with TBI where normal relationship between flow and perfusion may be affected. A pressure-volume relationship occurs in the brain microvasculature that illustrates cerebral autoregulation (Figure 255-1). Under normal circumstances the major regulatory mechanisms of CBF are the partial pressure of carbon dioxide (Pco_2), blood pressure, and blood pH. Hypotension or hypoventilation leads to increased Pco_2 and decreased pH. Under these circumstances, the cerebral vasculature dilates to increase CBF and deliver more oxygen. Hypertension, hypocarbia, and alkalosis cause vasoconstriction. Decreased partial pressure of oxygen (Po_2) also leads to increased CBF by causing cerebral vasodilation.

Pressure-Volume Relationship in Brain Injury

Circulation to the brain is vulnerable to conditions that increase the intracranial volume. Normal ICP is less than 15 mm Hg and is determined by the volume of the three intracranial compartments: the brain parenchyma (~1300 mL in the adult), cerebrospinal fluid (100 to 150 mL), and intravascular blood (100 to 150 mL). When one compartment expands there must be a compensatory reduction in the volume of another or the ICP will increase.

When the ICP is outside its normal range autoregulation is lost, and the CBF follows a more linear passive-pressure relationship to CPP. As a result, normal cerebral blood flow may not be restored until the CPP is increased to greater than 90 mm Hg.[3] Cerebral blood flow is generally maintained when the CPP is above 60 to 70 mm Hg in the setting of hypotension and elevated ICP. This CPP level is considered the lower limit of autoregulation, below which local control of CBF cannot be adjusted to maintain flow adequate for function.

Rapid rises in the ICP that cause compression of the brain can lead to a phenomenon known as the *Cushing reflex* (hypertension, bradycardia, and respiratory irregularity). This triad is classic for an acute rise in ICP, but is seen in only one-third of cases, and is more common in children than adults.

Mechanisms of Secondary Cellular Death

Neurons that survive the primary insult face several secondary injury mechanisms that are characterized as *excitotoxicity, oxidative stress, inflammation,* and *apoptosis* (programmed cell death).

Immediately following the acute injury event there is a decrease in the production of ATP, affecting ATP-dependent processes. This results in influx of sodium and water leading to cellular edema, cellular acidosis from anaerobic metabolism, and calcium influx with the release of the excitatory amino acid glutamate. Glutamate is the central initiator of excitotoxicity, leading to multiple lethal reactions that alter the structural and functional integrity of the cell. If the tissue is reperfused, the damage is compounded as free radicals are produced (oxidative stress). Iron-dependent lipid peroxidation products lead to further membrane damage.

FIG. 255-1. Normal cerebral blood flow (CBF) autoregulation curve and the abnormal curve with TBI. Normal autoregulatory control *(black line)* maintains a relatively constant CBF over a broad range of mean arterial pressure (MAP). Loss of autoregulation results in a more linear relationship between CBF and MAP, potentially resulting in increased edema and intracranial pressure (ICP) *(red line)*. Increases in ICP may result in a net loss in CBF.

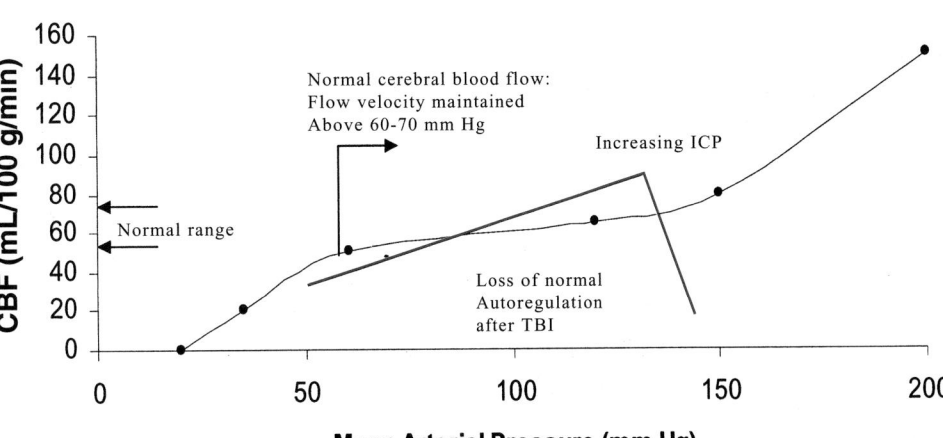

The local production of cytokines causes the inflammatory component of secondary injury. Migration of neutrophils, monocytes, and macrophages into the site of injury amplifies the injury to surviving cells. These cells contribute to the oxidative stress and inflammatory cascades by releasing proteases, free radicals, and vasoconstrictive mediators.

Finally, cells that escape early death may die from an endogenous mechanisms of cell death, broadly called *apoptosis*. The cellular triggers and mediators of apoptosis are beginning to be defined. Treatments that disrupt these secondary cellular injury pathways are still being developed, so the primary clinical treatment remains the prevention of increased ICP, ischemia, and hypoxia.

INITIAL EVALUATION AND MANAGEMENT

Because preventing secondary brain injury is the major goal of TBI management, correcting or preventing hypoxemia, hypotension, anemia, hyperglycemia, and hyperthermia, and evacuation of intracranial masses is critically important. Hypotension [systolic blood pressure (SBP) <90 mm Hg] and hypoxemia (Pao$_2$ <60) are associated with a doubling of TBI mortality.[3] Anemia (hematocrit <30 percent) also leads to increased mortality because of decreased oxygen-carrying capacity.

Airway control with cervical spine stabilization, breathing, and circulation are the first priorities for all trauma patients. Only then can a neurologic and mental status examination be conducted to evaluate disability. Early recognition and treatment of hypoxemia, hypotension, and anemia are essential.

Prehospital Care

The care of the head-injured patient begins with emergency medical services (EMS) personnel in the prehospital setting. In addition to the ABCs (airway, breathing, circulation), assessing the history of the event and the patient's condition and mental status immediately after the injury is important. Hypoxia and hypotension need to be identified and corrected rapidly on the scene. There is no indication for prehospital hyperventilation or use of mannitol for patients with TBI.

ED Resuscitation

Important historical points include the mechanism of injury, the patient's condition before and after the trauma, the past medical history, and the recent use of drugs or alcohol. Important information regarding the condition after the injury includes the length of the loss of consciousness, vomiting, and if seizure activity occurred. A history of anticoagulant use or a coagulopathy should be determined. As with all patients with altered mental status, the potential for other injuries such as hypothermia, inhalation injuries, and toxic exposures should be investigated.

AIRWAY AND BREATHING   Hypoxia increases mortality from TBI, therefore aggressive airway and breathing management is needed. All patients with severe TBI require intubation and ventilation initially with 100 percent O$_2$. In-line cervical spine stabilization is essential until cervical spine injury or fracture is definitively excluded. Orotracheal rapid-sequence intubation (RSI) using appropriate agents optimizes the patient's physiology, prevents increased ICP, and has the lowest complication rate (see Chap. 19). The ideal induction agent should both blunt the increase in ICP and yet not decrease the MAP. Because some of the drugs commonly used for RSI (Table 255-1) cause hypotension, strict attention needs to be paid to assure hemodynamic stability during the procedure.

Lidocaine has been used as a pretreatment agent because of its potential to prevent hemodynamic changes and elevation of intracranial pressure, but recent reports question its utility.[4] A defasciculating dose of succinylcholine (0.1 mg/kg IV), vecuronium (0.01 mg/kg IV), or pancuronium (0.01 mg/kg IV) given 2 to 3 min prior to succinylcholine has been used to prevent RSI-induced increases in ICP, but again, to date there are no clinical trials that demonstrate improved outcome with preinduction agents.

Barbiturates decrease ICP and decrease cerebral metabolic oxygen demand. Therefore, a short-acting barbiturate can be used as an induction agent. Thiopental (3 to 5 mg/kg IV) has a rapid onset and is

TABLE 255-1   Recommended Agents for Rapid Sequence Intubation of Patients with Severe TBI

Preinduction agents* (prevent ICP elevation)
  Succinylcholine 0.1 mg/kg IV *or*
  Vecuronium 0.01 mg/kg IV or pancuronium 0.01 mg/kg IV
Induction agents (sedative/hypnotics and analgesia)
  Thiopental 3–5 mg/kg IV (normotensive) or 0.5–1.0 mg/kg IV
    (hypotensive)
  Fentanyl 3–5 μg/kg IV
  Propofol 1–4 mg/kg IV
Neuromuscular blocking agents (long-acting agents are not recommended
  for TBI patients)
  • Succinylcholine 1.0–1.5 mg/kg IV

*Not clinically validated to improve outcome in TBI patients.

short-acting. Because thiopental is a cardiovascular depressant, patients who are hypotensive should receive only 0.5 to 1 mg/kg or another inducting agent, such as etomidate (0.3 mg/kg). Ketamine has traditionally been avoided as it was thought to cause ICP elevation; however, some studies have shown a decrease in ICP when ventilation is controlled. There is renewed interest in ketamine because it blocks potentially deleterious amino acid [*N*-methyl-D-aspartate (NMDA)] receptors in the brain.[5] Further study in the ED, however, is warranted before a recommendation can be made.

The use of etomidate (0.3 mg/kg) for induction in the ED has not been studied extensively. Those studies that have looked at the effects of etomidate administration on ICP and CPP (in either the intensive care unit or operating room) in head-injured patients have been inconclusive, with mixed reports.[6]

Propofol as an induction agent has several theoretical benefits (rapid onset/recovery and minimal hemodynamic effects). Propofol is commonly used for RSI in the operating setting; however, few reports exist for use in the ED for severely head-injured patients.

Neuromuscular blocking drugs (NMBDs) are used to facilitate airway control and to prevent complications without increasing ICP. The use of NMBDs prevents any meaningful neurologic exam and limits the ability to detect changes in the condition of the patient (e.g., seizure). Therefore the shortest-acting agent, succinylcholine is usually chosen.

RSI techniques should also be used for comatose patients, who are susceptible to increases in ICP with laryngoscope and intubation. Nasotracheal intubation is not specifically contraindicated in TBI, but it should rarely be used because of its higher complication rate, lower success rate, and potential for marked increase in ICP. In the presence of a basilar skull fracture, nasotracheal intubation also leads to an increased risk of meningitis.

CIRCULATION Improved blood pressure resuscitation decreases mortality for patients with severe TBI.[7] Therefore, aggressive fluid resuscitation may be required to prevent hypotension and secondary brain injury. Adequate fluid resuscitation has not been shown to increase ICP and guidelines recommend that the MAP be maintained at 90 mm Hg (systolic blood pressure of 120 to 140 mm Hg) to achieve adequate cerebral perfusion.[8] Isolated head injury rarely produces hypotension, except as a preterminal event. Hypovolemic shock may be seen in infants because of epidural bleeding or subgaleal hematoma or with massive blood loss from scalp lacerations in any age group. If fluid resuscitation is not effective, vasopressors should be used to maintain MAP at 90 mm Hg to preserve CPP. External and internal bleeding need to be controlled quickly and the hematocrit should be maintained above 30 percent.

Hypertension is a critical finding and must be assumed to be an indicator of increased ICP in a patient with a head injury. This *Cushing reflex* requires immediate measures to decrease the intracranial pressure. If hypertension exists independent of increased ICP, then the systemic pressure should be lowered by no more than 30 percent of the MAP by using labetalol.

DISABILITY AND THE NEUROLOGIC EXAMINATION The neurologic examination that is part of the primary survey describes the patient's level of consciousness with the AVPU system: *alert*, responds to *verbal* stimuli, responds to *painful* stimuli, or *unresponsive*. This same assessment provides most of the information needed to calculate the Glasgow Coma Scale (Table 255-2). The GCS is only one component of a complete neurologic examination. The best possible neurologic examination should be conducted as soon as the initial resuscitation is complete, to serve as a baseline for subsequent serial examinations and to dictate treatment.

The GCS was developed as a standardized scoring system to allow reliable interobserver neurologic assessment of patients with TBI. An accurate GCS score is used to direct treatment and predict outcome. Accurate GCS scores can only be obtained after resuscitation, and prior to sedation or intubation. The postresuscitation GCS is based upon three factors: eye opening, verbal function, and motor function. When assessing the GCS in the severely obtunded, noxious stimuli need to be delivered in the form of nailbed pressure on both sides of the body or severe sternal pressure. This is important for grading the depth of disability at the level of more rudimentary reflexes. The best response from each category is added for a score of 3 to 15. The GCS for intubated patients cannot be assessed for verbal response, and paralyzed patients cannot be assessed at all. For nonintubated, nonsedated postresuscitation patients **a GCS of less than 9 is considered a severe TBI, moderate is 9 to 13, and mild is 14 to 15.**

The other important aspect of the neurologic examination is pupil assessment (size, reactivity, and anisocoria). In an unresponsive patient a single fixed and dilated pupil may indicate an ipsilateral intracranial hematoma with uncal herniation that requires rapid operative decompression. Direct ocular trauma should also be considered. Bilateral fixed and dilated pupils suggest increased ICP with poor

TABLE 255-2 The Glasgow Coma Scale for All Age Groups

	4 years to Adult	Child <4 years	Infant
Eye Opening			
4	Spontaneous	Spontaneous	Spontaneous
3	To speech	To speech	To speech
2	To pain	To pain	To pain
1	No response	No response	No response
Verbal Response			
5	Alert and oriented	Oriented, social, speaks, interacts	Coos, babbles
4	Disoriented conversation	Confused speech, disoriented, consolable, aware	Irritable cry
3	Speaking but nonsensical	Inappropriate words, inconsolable, unaware	Cries to pain
2	Moans or unintelligible sounds	Incomprehensible, agitated, restless, unaware	Moans to pain
1	No response	No response	No response
Motor Response			
6	Follows commands	Normal, spontaneous movements	Normal, spontaneous moves
5	Localizes pain	Localizes pain	Withdraws to touch
4	Movement or withdrawal to pain	Withdraws to pain	Withdraws to pain
3	Decorticate flexion	Decorticate flexion	Decorticate flexion
2	Decerebrate extension	Decerebrate extension	Decerebrate extension
1	No response	No response	No response
3–15			

Note: GCS reporting should be modified for intubated and paralyzed patients.

brain perfusion, bilateral uncal herniation, drug effect or severe hypoxia, whereas bilateral pinpoint pupils suggest either opiate use or a pontine lesion.

Altered motor function can indicate brain, spinal cord, or peripheral nerve injuries. Movement in unresponsive patients is assessed by noxious stimuli to a nail bed in all extremities. Decorticate posturing (upper extremity flexion and lower extremity extension) indicates an injury above the midbrain. Decerebrate posturing (arm extension and internal rotation with wrist and finger flexion and internal rotation and extension of the lower extremities) is from a more caudal injury and predicts a worse outcome. For completely unresponsive patients, the respiratory pattern and eye movements will provide information regarding brainstem function. Oculovestibular (cold calorics) and oculocephalic (doll's eyes) responses are not checked until the cervical spine has been fully cleared.

After the primary survey a secondary survey is needed to identify other significant injuries.

THE CLINICAL SPECTRUM OF TBI

Mild Traumatic Brain Injury

Severity grading of TBI uses the GCS score to categorize patients based on their potential outcomes. Mild TBI has traditionally included head-injured patients with a history of loss of consciousness, amnesia or loss of memory to the event, any change in mental status at the time of event, and/or persistent or transient focal neurological deficit. The convention has been to include patients with GCS scores of 13 to 15 in to the mild group, which accounts for most TBI patients. However, because of the wide variation in outcomes those previously described as "mild head injury," are further subdivided into "low risk," "medium risk" or "high risk" mild head injury.[8] Low-risk mild-injury patients include those with a GCS of 15 without a history of loss of consciousness, amnesia, vomiting, or diffuse headache. The risk for intracranial hematoma requiring surgical evacuation is less than 0.1 percent. Medium-risk patients have a GCS of 15 along with one or more of the following: loss of consciousness, amnesia, vomiting, or diffuse headache. These patients have a 1 to 3 percent risk of intracranial hematoma requiring surgical evacuation and CT scans should be obtained for such patients. If computed tomography (CT) is not available, skull x-rays are recommended, and those patients with fractures should be placed in the *high-risk* category and be emergently trans-

ferred to a facility with neurosurgical availability (Figure 255-2). The medium-risk mild TBI group includes those patients meeting diagnostic criteria for postconcussion syndrome (PCS).

High-risk mild head-injury patients are those with an admission GCS of 14 or 15, with a skull fracture and/or neurologic deficits. As many as 10 percent of the patients in this *high-risk* mild TBI group will require surgical evacuation of intracranial hematomas. Patients with coagulopathy, drug or alcohol consumption, previous neurosurgical procedures, epilepsy, or age greater than 60 years should be included in the high-risk group independent of their clinical presentation.

The rate of injury findings on brain CT scans increases within this mild injury group as a function of the GCS.[9] Regardless of the need for neurosurgical intervention, nearly 10 percent of high-risk, mild TBI patients with a GCS of 15 will have a positive brain CT, as compared to 40 percent in those with a GCS of 13.[9]

Mild TBI patients with a GCS of 15, no indication for head CT or a negative CT, and adequate supervision may be safely discharged home from the emergency department. Those patients with a GCS of 14 and a negative head CT should be observed for 6 to 12 h for deterioration (accumulation of edema, seizure, etc.). Those patients with a positive CT scan or persistent neurologic findings require neurosurgical consultation and hospital admission (Figure 255-3).

Moderate Traumatic Brain Injury

Moderate TBI (GCS 9 to 13) accounts for approximately 10 percent of patients with head injuries. Mortality rates for patients with isolated moderate TBI is less than 20 percent, but long-term disability is as high as 50 percent. Overall, 40 percent of moderate TBI patients have a finding on CT scan and 8 percent require neurosurgical intervention.[10] Patients with moderate TBI should be admitted to try to prevent deterioration from secondary brain injury and progression to severe TBI (Figure 255-4). Most patients in this category should be intubated, receive neurosurgical consultation, and admission to a monitored unit.

Severe Traumatic Brain Injury

In severe TBI (GCS <9), mortality approaches 40 percent, with most deaths occurring within 48 h. Less than 10 percent of these patients make even a moderate recovery. The management of patients with severe TBI has three primary goals: to identify other life-threatening

FIG. 255-2. Algorithm for imaging patients with mild TBI.

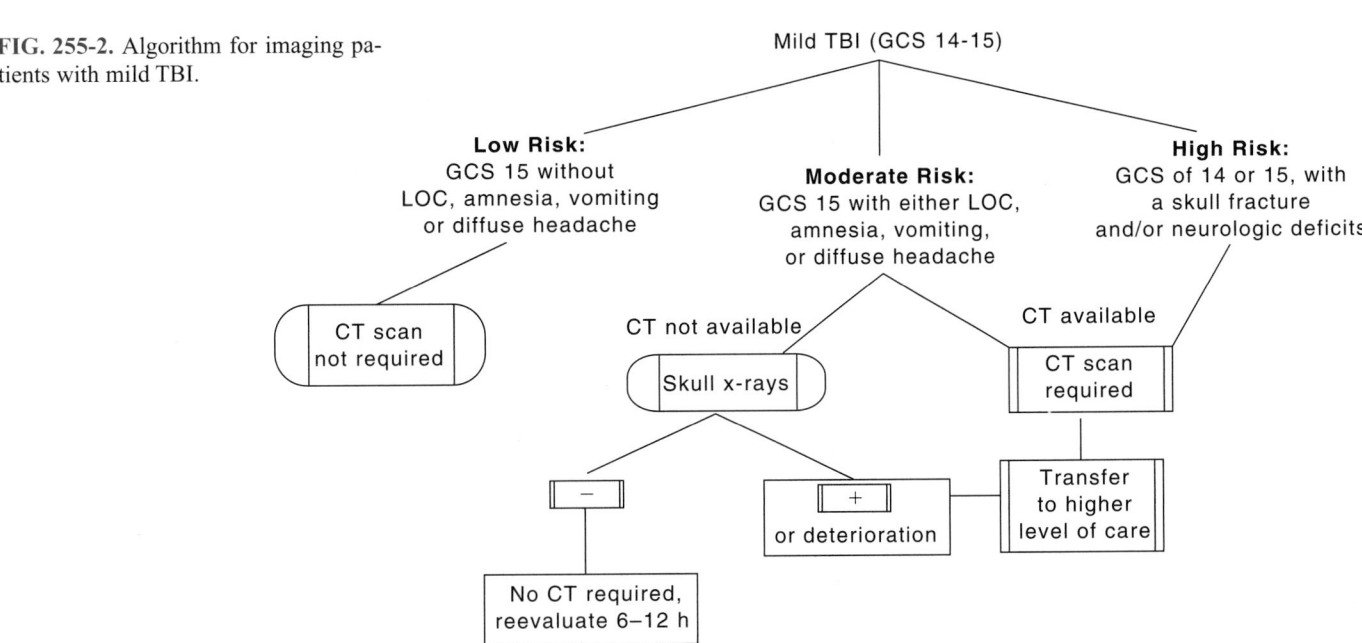

Mild TBI (GCS 14-15)

Low Risk:
GCS 15 without
LOC, amnesia, vomiting
or diffuse headache

Moderate Risk:
GCS 15 with either LOC,
amnesia, vomiting,
or diffuse headache

High Risk:
GCS of 14 or 15, with
a skull fracture
and/or neurologic deficits

CT scan
not required

CT not available

CT available

Skull x-rays

CT scan
required

−

+

or deterioration

Transfer
to higher
level of care

No CT required,
reevaluate 6–12 h

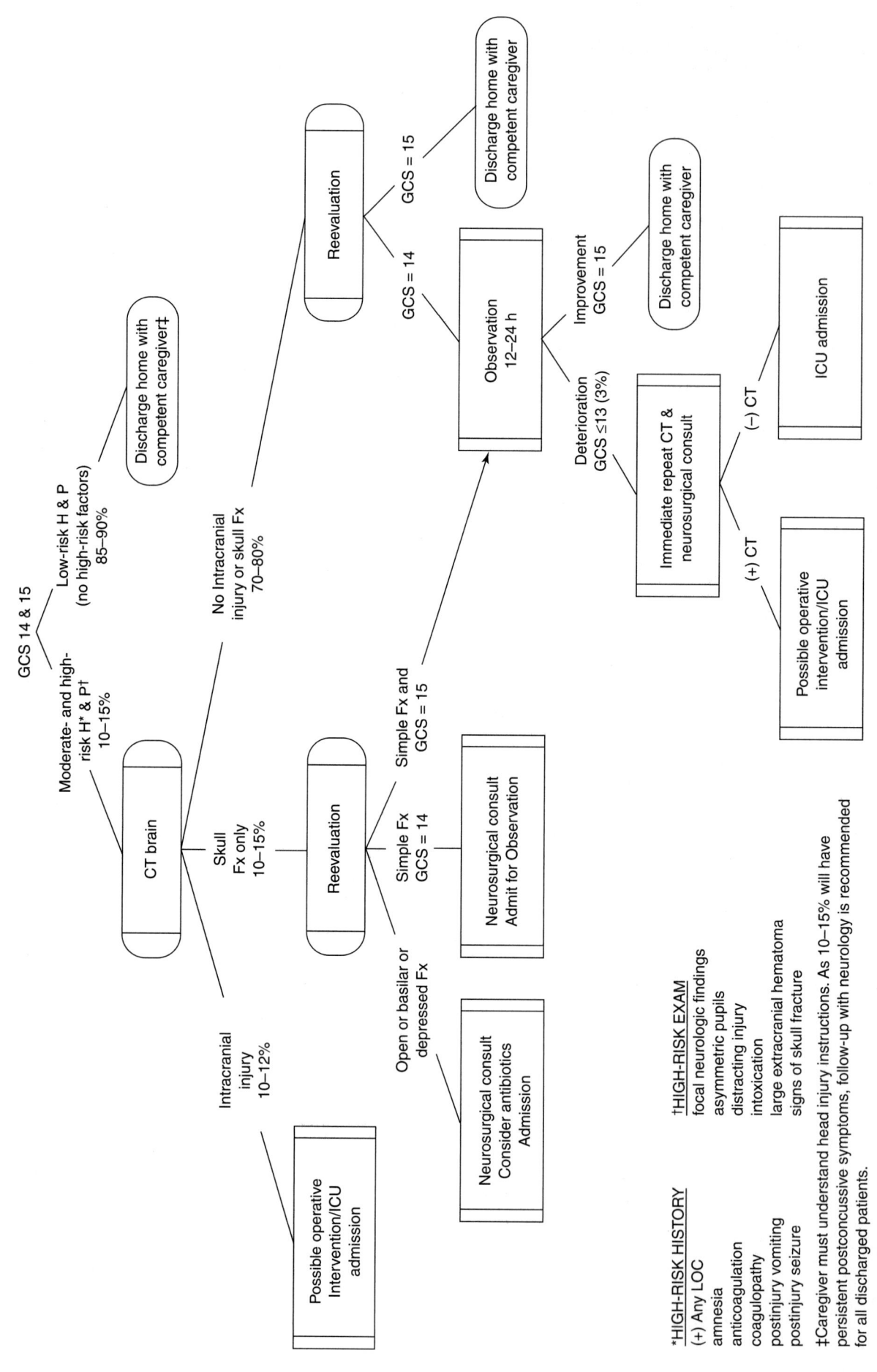

GCS 14 & 15

Moderate- and high-risk H* & Pt
10–15%

Low-risk H & P
(no high-risk factors)
85–90%

Discharge home with
competent caregiver‡

CT brain

Intracranial
injury
10–12%

Skull
Fx only
10–15%

No Intracranial
injury or skull Fx
70–80%

Possible operative
Intervention/ICU
admission

Reevaluation

Open or basilar or
depressed Fx

Simple Fx
GCS = 14

Simple Fx and
GCS = 15

Reevaluation

GCS = 14

GCS = 15

Discharge home with
competent caregiver

Neurosurgical consult
Consider antibiotics
Admission

Neurosurgical consult
Admit for Observation

Observation
12–24 h

Improvement
GCS = 15

Deterioration
GCS ≤13 (3%)

Discharge home with
competent caregiver

Immediate repeat CT &
neurosurgical consult

(+) CT

(–) CT

Possible operative
intervention/ICU
admission

ICU admission

*HIGH-RISK HISTORY
(+) Any LOC
amnesia
anticoagulation
coagulopathy
postinjury vomiting
postinjury seizure

†HIGH-RISK EXAM
focal neurologic findings
asymmetric pupils
distracting injury
intoxication
large extracranial hematoma
signs of skull fracture

‡Caregiver must understand head injury instructions. As 10–15% will have
persistent postconcussive symptoms, follow-up with neurology is recommended
for all discharged patients.

FIG. 255-3. Algorithm for the evaluation and treatment of mild brain injury.

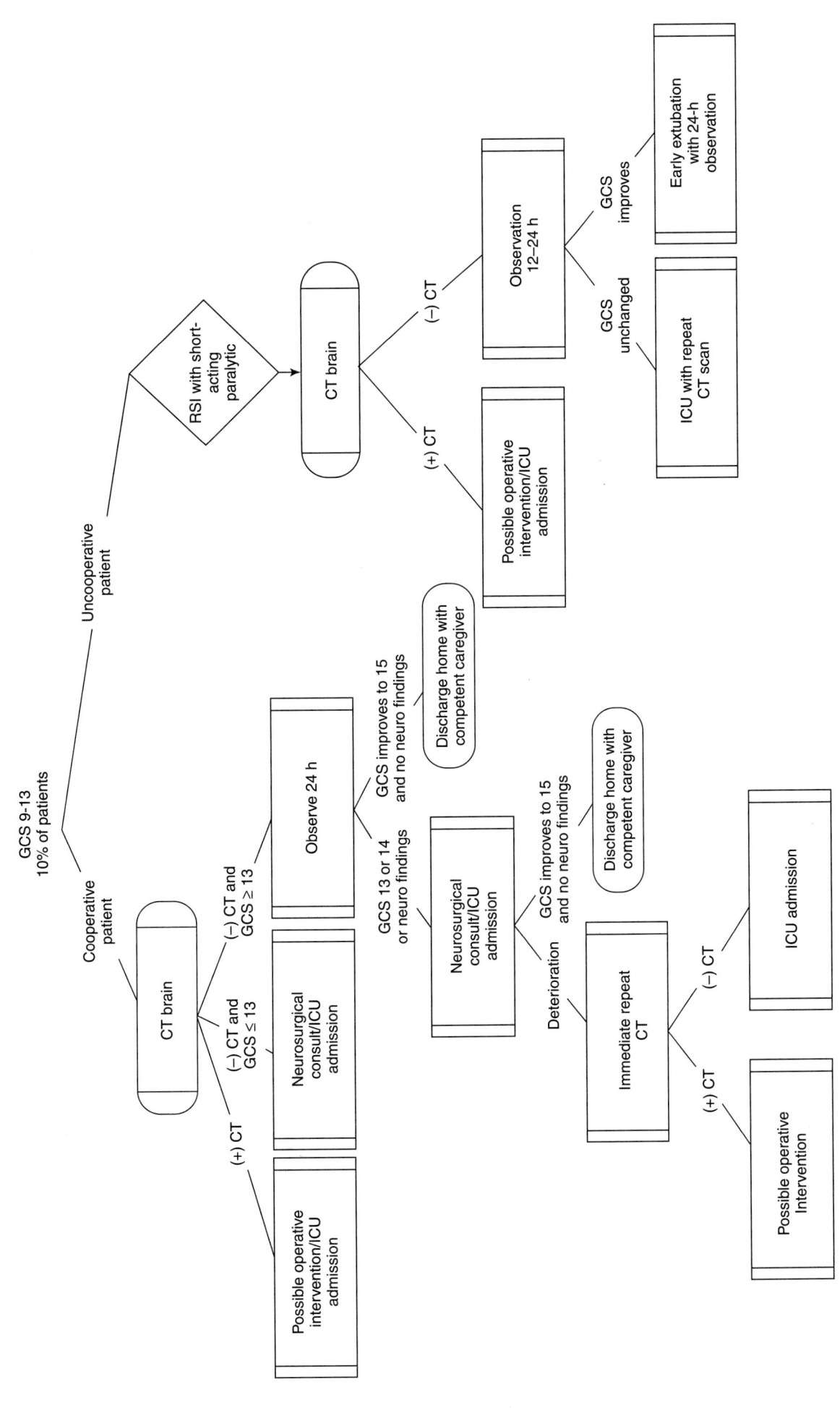

FIG. 255-4. Algorithm for the evaluation and treatment of moderate brain injury.

injuries, to prevent further secondary brain injury, and to identify treatable mass lesions. All patients with severe TBI require a CT scan and should be admitted to an intensive care unit in a hospital with neurosurgical capabilities (Figure 255-5).

DIAGNOSTIC RADIOGRAPHY FOR TBI

All patients with moderate to severe TBI require urgent head CT scans after stabilization. Delays in obtaining a CT scan can lead to a cata-

strophic delay in emergent neurosurgical interventions. Therefore, **if a patient with TBI is uncooperative or combative, RSI is often the best option.** If this is undertaken, a GCS score and the best neurologic exam possible should be performed prior to intubation. Sedation alone should be used infrequently as it is often ineffective and may put patients at risk for further injury or aspiration. Other means to control agitated patients with TBI include haloperidol (5 to 10 mg IM or IV, may repeat), midazolam (1 to 2 mg IV), and propofol (20 mg every 10 s to desired effect). A CT scan is generally diagnostic but there have been

FIG. 255-5. Algorithm for the evaluation and treatment of severe brain injury.

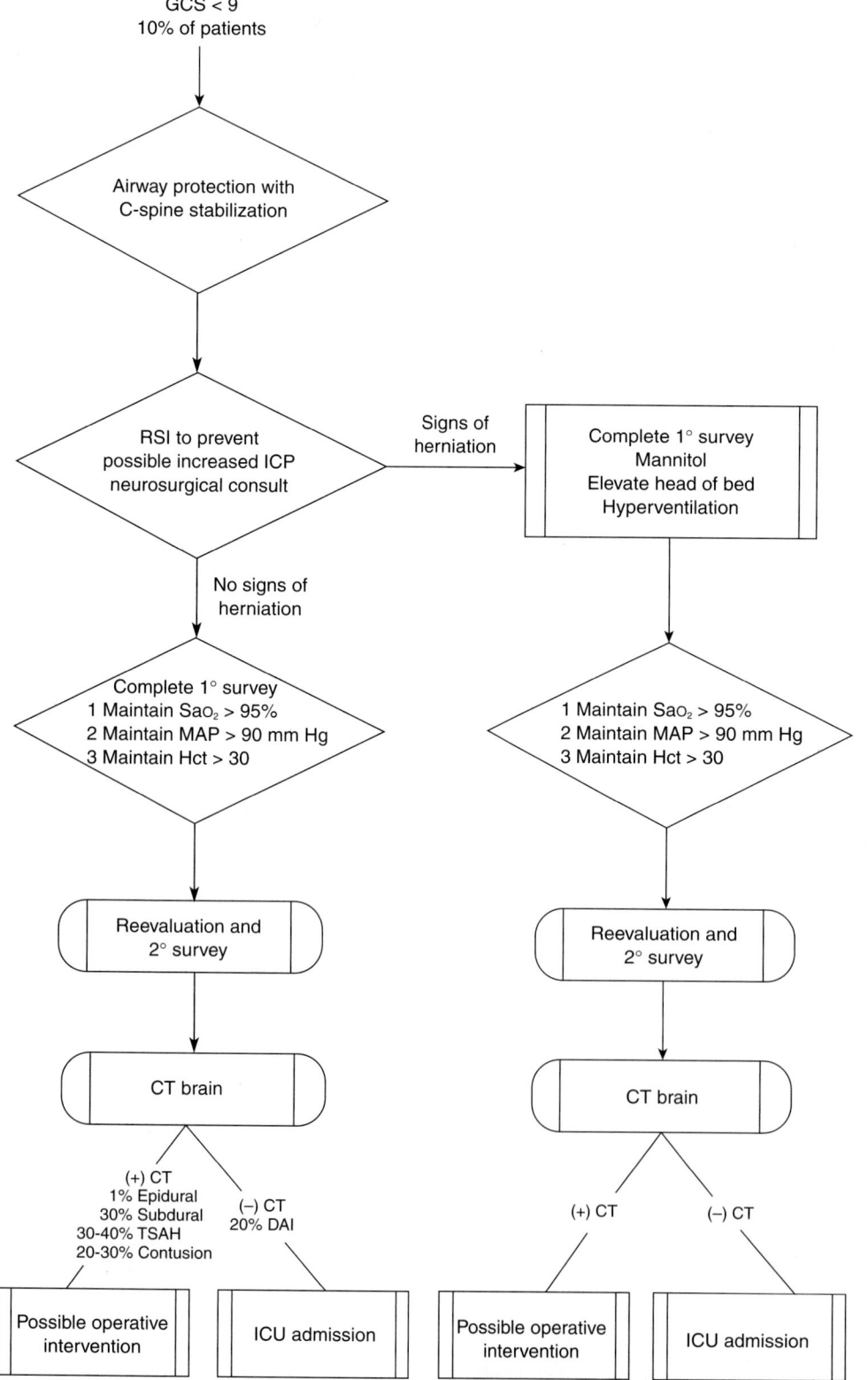

reports of delayed intracranial hematomas, especially subdural hematomas, for patients with nonfocal neurologic examinations with negative initial CT scans.[11]

CT of the head is indicated for all patients with a GCS of 14 or less. There are numerous factors that dictate the need for a CT in patients with a GCS of 15 (Table 255-3). In addition, liberal use of head CT in patients of older than 60 years of age is recommended.[12]

INCREASED ICP AFTER TBI

An intracranial pressure of greater than 20 to 25 mm Hg in the TBI patient increases subsequent morbidity and mortality. In the ED, ICP monitoring is rarely available, therefore physical findings must be used to identify increased ICP and to direct therapy. Indicators of increased ICP include signs of transtentorial herniation (unilateral or bilateral dilated pupils, hemiparesis, motor posturing) and progressive neurologic deterioration (as determined by repetitive AVPU and GCS examinations). Several strategies may be used to lower ICP. All patients with severe TBI and evidence of increased ICP should have the head of the bed elevated to 30 degrees, volume resuscitation to a MAP of 90 mm Hg or a 30 percent reduction in MAP if hypertensive, and maintenance of arterial oxygenation. After these steps mannitol should be used.

Mannitol

Mannitol is the best osmotic agent to reduce ICP. It has beneficial effects on the ICP, CBF, CPP, and brain metabolism. Additionally, mannitol is known to scavenge free radicals. It reduces ICP within 30 min and lasts variably up to 6 to 8 h. Mannitol has the additional benefit of expanding volume, initially reducing hypotension, and improving the blood's oxygen-carrying capacity. Mannitol is administered by repetitive bolus (0.25 g/kg to 1 g/kg), not by constant infusion. Because there is no dose-dependent effect seen with mannitol, some authors advocate the lower range of the suggested dose. Mannitol will lead to a net intravascular volume loss because of its diuretic effect, therefore adequate glomerular filtration rate (GFR) hemodynamic and input-output monitoring is required to maintain euvolemia.

Hyperventilation

Hyperventilation is no longer recommended as a prophylactic intervention during the first 24 h after a severe TBI.[14] Nor is hyperventilation below a PaO$_2$ of 25 mm Hg ever indicated. Hyperventilation does reduce the ICP, but the vasoconstriction caused by reducing carbon dioxide (CO$_2$) levels also leads to cerebral ischemia. Hyperventilation is still used as a last resort for hospitalized patients with signs of increasing ICP despite other therapeutic measures. In this case it is a temporary measure and the PaO$_2$ is monitored closely to maintain the range of 30 to 35 mm Hg.

TABLE 255-3   Indications for CT Scanning for Patients with Mild TBI

Signs
    A Glasgow Coma Scale 13–14
    A skull fracture or large subgaleal swelling
    Focal neurologic findings
    Unexplained asymmetric pupils
    Distracting injuries or intoxication
Symptoms
    A reported loss of consciousness or posttraumatic seizure
    A history of coagulopathy
    Continued diffuse headache
    Amnesia
    Vomiting

Other Modalities

Initiation of barbiturate coma is not indicated in the ED, but there is evidence that it may be considered for hemodynamically stable patients with severe TBI who have continued increased ICP despite other therapies. The recommended dose of pentobarbital is 10 mg/kg over 30 min.

There is some indication that prophylactic anticonvulsants reduce the occurrence of early post-traumatic seizures, but no evidence that these drugs improve long-term outcome. They should be used in consultation with a neurosurgeon. There is no indication to use steroids for the treatment of TBI or increased ICP.[13]

Intracranial Pressure Monitoring

Internal monitoring of ICP should be initiated on all patients with evidence of increased ICP, herniation, and a GCS score of less than 9. This treatment has the most favorable risk:benefit ratio. A ventricular catheter offers the best method to directly monitor ICP and thus calculate CPP. Increases in the ICP above 20 to 25 mm Hg may be reduced by CSF drainage. If CSF drainage is not effective in reducing ICP, then mannitol should be administered, (assuming adequate MAP).

TREATMENT OF SPECIFIC HEAD INJURIES

Scalp Lacerations

Scalp lacerations can lead to massive blood loss. Scalp hemorrhages should be controlled as rapidly as possible. If direct pressure is not effective, lidocaine with epinephrine can be infiltrated locally, and vessels can be clamped or ligated. Wounds should be carefully examined prior to closure for underlying fractures and galeal lacerations. Large galeal disruptions should be repaired, but small ones can be left alone.

Skull Fractures

All patients suspected or found to have a skull fracture require a head CT scan (see Table 255-3). Skull fractures are usually categorized by location (basilar vs. the skull convexity), pattern (linear, depressed, or comminuted) and whether they are open or closed. A careful examination and wound exploration of scalp lacerations is needed to identify a skull fracture in the patient without a loss of consciousness or neurologic findings. Complicated skull fractures include those that are open or depressed, those that involve a sinus, and those that cause intracranial air (pneumocephalus).

LINEAR AND COMMINUTED FRACTURES   The management of linear and simple comminuted skull fractures is the same. Isolated fractures with an overlying laceration require careful evaluation, cleaning, and repair. Wounds should be explored gently so as not to drive bone fragments into the brain. The use of prophylactic antibiotics following an open skull fracture is controversial and should be discussed with the neurosurgeon.

Particular care should be taken in evaluating fractures that cross the middle meningeal artery or a major venous sinus. Linear occipital fractures also have higher intracerebral complication rates. Fractures that are depressed beyond the outer table of the skull require operative repair.

BASILAR SKULL FRACTURE   The most common basilar skull fracture involves the petrous portion of the temporal bone, the external auditory canal, and the tympanic membrane. It is commonly associated with a torn dura leading to CSF leakage from the ear. Signs and symptoms associated with basilar skull fractures include CSF otorrhea or rhinorrhea, mastoid ecchymosis (Battle sign), periorbital ecchymoses (raccoon eyes), hemotympanum, vertigo, decreased hearing or deafness, and seventh nerve palsy. Periorbital and mastoid ecchymoses develop gradually over hours after an injury and are often absent in the ED. CSF leaks are difficult to diagnose. A simple but nonsensitive test for a basilar skull fracture with a CSF leak is to see if the fluid leaves a single or double ring when dripped onto a paper towel. Leaking fluid can also be tested for a specific CSF protein, transferrin. Patients with a basilar skull fracture should be hospitalized.

Patients with CSF fistulas can develop meningitis. Prophylactic antibiotics reduce the incidence of meningitis for patients with basilar skull fractures, thus prophylactic antibiotics in those patients with a basilar skull fracture is recommended.[14] Administration of antibiotics should be done in consultation with a neurosurgeon who will be following the patient. If prophylactic antibiotics are instituted, they should have broad coverage with good penetration into the meninges. A third-generation cephalosporin such as ceftriaxone at 1 to 2 g per day is a reasonable choice.

Brain Herniation

There are four major brain herniation syndromes: uncal and central transtentorial, cerebellotonsillar, and upward posterior fossa. The most common is uncal and it occurs when the uncus of the temporal lobe is displaced inferiorly through the medial edge of the tentorium (Figure 255-6). This is usually caused by an expanding lesion in the temporal lobe or lateral middle fossa. Uncal transtentorial herniation leads to compression of the third cranial (occulomotor) nerve, causing an ipsilateral fixed and dilated pupil. Further herniation compresses the pyramidal tract leading to contralateral motor paralysis. In some cases, the pupillary changes are contralateral, or motor changes are ipsilateral.

Central transtentorial herniation is less common and occurs with midline lesions in the frontal or occipital lobes, or in the vertex. The most prominent symptoms are initial bilateral pinpoint pupils, bilateral Babinski signs, and increased muscle tone. Fixed midpoint pupils follow along with prolonged hyperventilation and decorticate posturing.

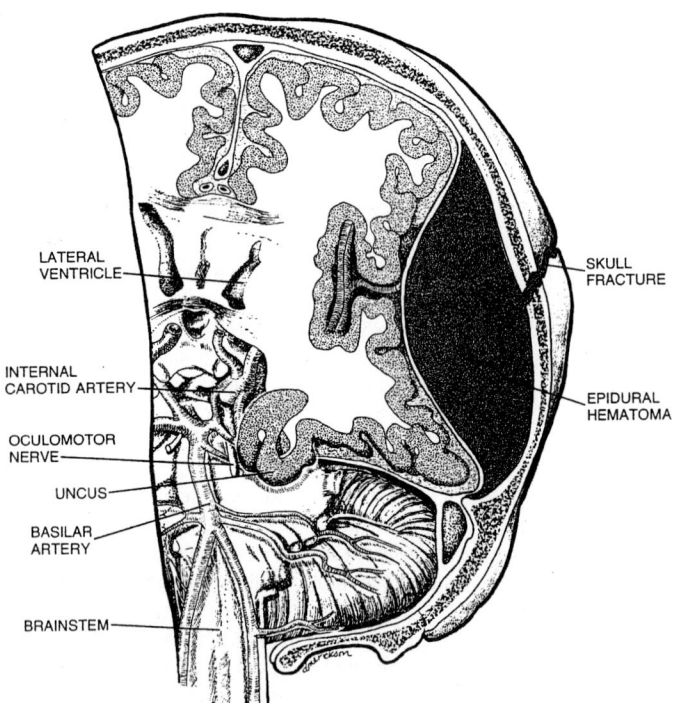

FIG. 255-6. Anterior view of a transtentorial uncal herniation caused by a large hematoma under a skull fracture.

Cerebellotonsillar herniation occurs when the cerebellar tonsils herniate through the foramen magnum. This causes pinpoint pupils, flaccid paralysis, and sudden death. Upward transtentorial herniation results from a posterior fossa lesion and leads to a conjugate downward gaze with absence of vertical eye movements, pinpoint pupils, and rapid death.

When all other methods to control the ICP have failed, patients with signs of herniation may need emergency decompression by trephination ("burr holes"). CT scanning before attempting trephination is recommended to localize the lesion and direct the decompression site. If CT scan is unavailable, or the patient is unstable for CT because of signs of rapidly progressive neurologic deterioration and herniation, then emergency department trephination should be considered.

Cerebral Contusion/Intracerebral Hemorrhage

Contusions are one of the most frequent types of TBI. Contusions most commonly occur in the subfrontal cortex, in the frontal and temporal lobes, and, occasionally, in the occipital lobes. They are often associated with a subarachnoid hemorrhage. Contusions may occur at the site of the blunt trauma or the opposite site of the brain, known as a "contre-coup" injury.

Intracerebral hemorrhage can occur days after significant blunt trauma, often at the site of resolving contusions. This complication is more common with patients with a coagulopathy. CT scans in the immediate postinjury phase can be normal.

Subarachnoid Hemorrhage

Traumatic subarachnoid hemorrhage (tSAH) results from the disruption of subarachnoid vessels and presents with blood in the CSF (Figure 255-7). Patients can present with mild to severe TBI. Those with isolated tSAH often present with a headache and photophobia and mild meningeal signs. tSAH is probably the most common CT abnormality in patients with moderate to severe TBI. Patients with a tSAH are twice as likely to suffer from death, persistent vegetative state, or severe disability. Early development of tSAH (42 percent) represents a trifold mortality risk (42 vs. 14 percent), as compared to those without tSAH.[15] The amount of blood seen on the CT scan is inversely related to the presenting GCS and percent of patients with a positive outcome. Some tSAH can be missed on early CT scans. Generally, scans performed 6 to 8 h after injury are more sensitive for detecting tSAH. Unfortunately, findings may be delayed in a few patients. Careful follow-up instructions, referral for reexamination by a physician, and discharge in the care of a competent adult are necessary, even with a normal CT scan.

The use of nimodipine in patients with tSAH reduces the likelihood of death or severe disability by 55 percent as compared to placebo.[16] Nimodipine should be started as soon as possible after stabilization at 2 mg per h for 7 to 10 days followed by 360 mg daily until day 21. Patient with tSAH requires immediate neurosurgical consultation and admission to an intensive care unit.

Epidural Hematoma

Epidural hematomas are the result of blood collecting in the potential space between the skull and the dura mater (Figure 255-8). Most epidural hematomas result from blunt trauma to the temporal or temporoparietal area with an associated skull fracture and middle meningeal arterial disruption. Occasionally, trauma to the parieto-occipital region or the posterior fossa causes tears of the venous sinuses with epidural hematomas. Almost all epidural hematomas are associated with skull fractures, and some will have additional cerebral lesions.

The classic history of an epidural hematoma is a lucent period following immediate loss of consciousness after significant blunt head

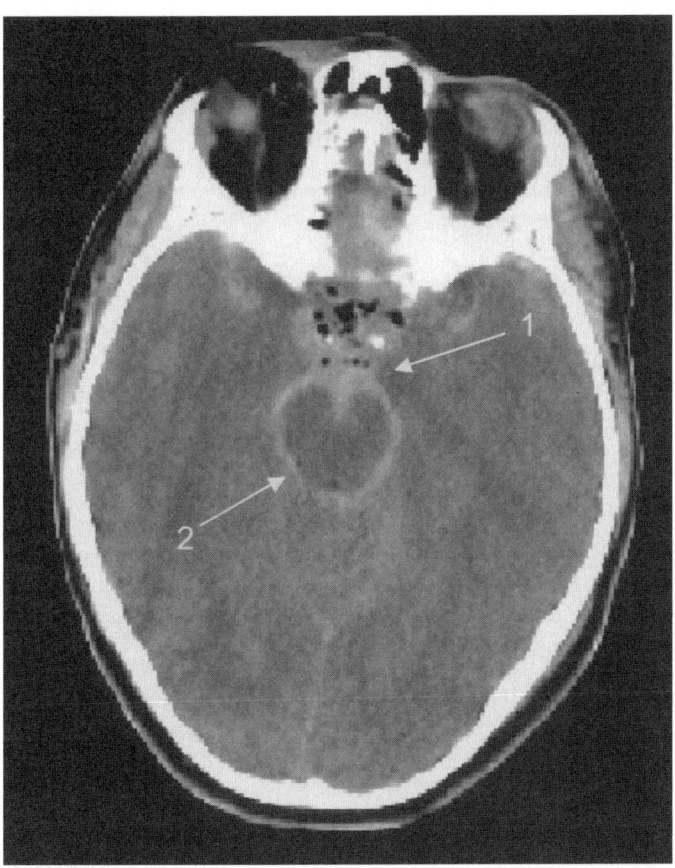

FIG. 255-7. Computed tomography scan illustrating a subarachnoid hemorrhage. *Arrow 1* illustrates prepontine cisternal blood and *arrow 2* represents blood in the ambient cistern.

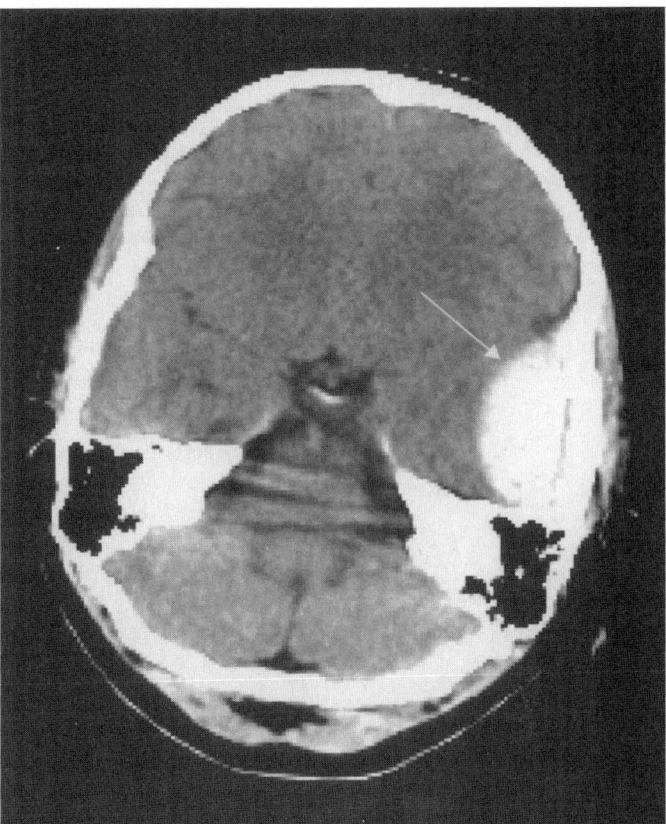

FIG. 255-8. Computed tomography scan illustrating a lenticular epidural hematoma. Note that the hematoma does not cross the suture lines.

trauma. The patient then awakens prior to again falling unconscious. This clinical pattern occurs in a minority of cases. Most patients either never lose consciousness or never regain consciousness after the injury. The diagnosis of an epidural hematoma is based on CT scan and physical findings. On CT scans, epidural hematomas appear biconvex (football shaped), typically in the temporal region.

The high-pressure arterial bleeding of an epidural hematoma can lead to herniation within hours after an injury. Therefore, early recognition and evacuation is key to reduce morbidity and mortality. Bilateral emergency department trephination (burr holes) is only indicated if definitive neurosurgical care is not available. Full recovery can be expected if the hematoma is evacuated prior to herniation or the development of neurologic deficits.

Subdural Hematoma

Subdural hematomas (SDHs) are caused by sudden acceleration-deceleration of brain parenchyma with subsequent tearing of the bridging veins. This results in blood clots forming between the dura mater and the arachnoid (Figure 255-9). Brains with extensive atrophy, as in the elderly and in alcoholics, are more susceptible to subdural hematomas. Children younger than age 2 years are also at increased risk of subdural hematomas. This is related to transfer of the force that limits the risk of sustaining epidural hematomas.

Blood tends to collect more slowly than in epidural hematomas because of its venous origin. However, SDHs are often associated with other brain injuries.

Traditionally, subdural hematomas have been classified as acute, subacute, or chronic, depending on time they present. Acute SDH symptoms usually develop within 14 days of the injury. After 2 weeks,

patients are defined as having a chronic SDH. There is no specific clinical syndrome associated with a subdural hematoma. Acute cases usually present immediately after severe trauma and often the victim is unconscious. Chronic subdural hematomas may present in the elderly or in alcoholics with vague complaints or mental status changes. These patients often do not recall an injury. On CT scan, acute SDHs are hyperdense (white), crescent-shaped lesions that cross suture lines. Subacute SDHs are isodense and more difficult to identify. A CT scan with intravenous contrast can assist in identifying a subacute SDH. A chronic SDH appears hypodense (dark) as the iron in the blood is phagocytized.

The definitive treatment of subdural hematomas depends on the type and on associated brain injuries. Mortality and the need for surgical repair are greater for acute and subacute SDH. Chronic subdurals hematomas can sometimes be managed without surgery depending of the severity of the symptoms. Table 255-4 compares intracranial hematomas.

Diffuse Axonal Injury

Diffuse axonal injury (DAI) is the disruption of axonal fibers in the white matter and brainstem. Shearing forces on the neurons generated by sudden deceleration cause DAI. Classically, DAI is seen after blunt trauma, such as from a motor vehicle accident. In infants, the "shaken-baby syndrome" is a well-described tragic cause.

Injury occurs immediately and is essentially irreversible. There is a rapid or immediate increase in ICP. Patients present unresponsive. The state may be prolonged or permanent until death. A CT scan of a patient with DAI may be normal, but the classic CT demonstrates hemorrhagic injury to the mostly the deep structures of the brain. The

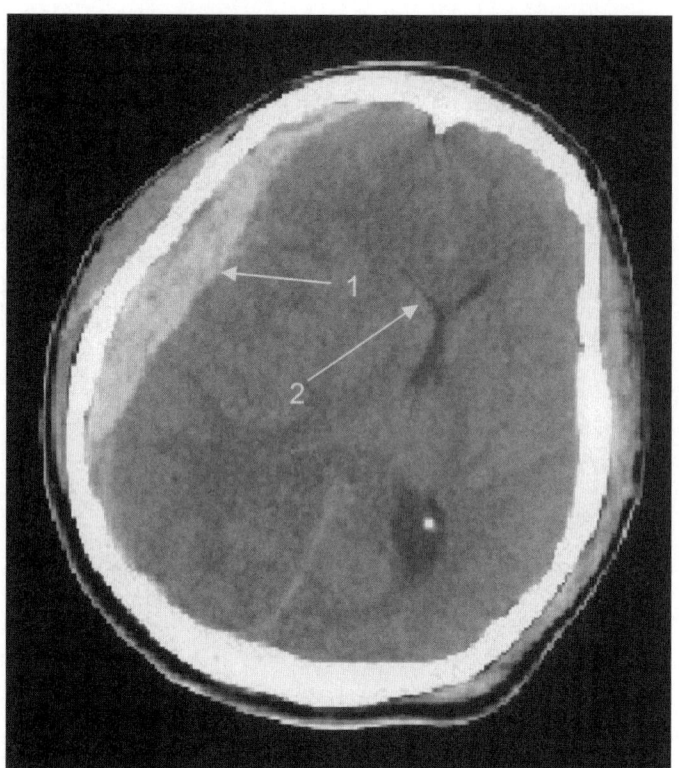

FIG. 255-9. Computed tomography scan of a subdural hematoma (*arrow 1*). Note that the hematoma crosses the suture lines. *Arrow 2* demonstrates midline shift.

treatment options for DAI are very limited, but attempt to prevent secondary damage by reducing cerebral edema.

Penetrating Injury

As a bullet passes through the brain, it creates a cavity three to four times greater than its diameter (see Chap. 264). Direct penetration of the bullet through the brain substance and the transfer of kinetic energy cause the majority of the destruction. The GCS can be used to predict the prognosis of unintoxicated patients with a gunshot wound to the brain. Patients with a GCS >8 and reactive pupils have a 25 percent mortality risk, while those with a GCS <5 approach 100 percent

mortality. All patients with a penetrating gunshot wound to the brain should be intubated and treated with prophylactic antibiotics.

Stab wounds have very low energy and impart only direct damage to the area contacted by the penetrating object. This results in a much lower morbidity and mortality than from gunshot wounds. Essentially all patients sustain penetrating injury require admission, broad-spectrum antibiotics and operative intervention. Impaled objects should be left in place until surgical removal.

COMPLICATIONS/LONG-TERM PROBLEMS

Seizures

The reported incidence of early posttraumatic seizures ranges from 2 to 5 percent, but this incidence rises to near 30 percent in children, alcoholics, and those with intracranial hematomas. A significant association exists between early posttraumatic seizures and unfavorable outcome, but this association is small by comparison to subdural hematoma and cerebral contusion.[17] Prophylactic antiepileptic drugs given after TBI decreases the incidence of early posttraumatic seizures, but there has been no observed reduction in the occurrence of late-seizures, death, or neurologic disability.[18] Thus, at the present time, **use of prophylactic antiepileptic drugs is not supported by the literature.** Acute management of early posttraumatic seizures is the same as for managing any seizure in the ED, but requires close hemodynamic monitoring to prevent antiepileptic drug-induced hypotension or hypoventilation.

Concussion and Postconcussive Syndrome

Concussion is defined as any alteration of cerebral function caused by a force to the head resulting in one or more of the following: a brief loss of consciousness; light-headedness; vertigo; headache; nausea; vomiting; photophobia; cognitive and memory dysfunction; tinnitus; blurred vision; difficulty concentrating; amnesia; fatigue; personality change; or a balance disturbance.[19] In 30 to 80 percent of patients with TBI, symptoms will remain 3 months postinjury; in 15 percent of patients, symptoms will remain at 1 year.[20] Persistence of these signs or symptoms has been termed "postconcussion syndrome" (PCS) (Table 255-5). Prior to discharge from the ED patients should be warned that their symptoms usually clear, but the time needed is generally weeks to months. In addition, they should be referred to a neurologist for long-term care.

Postconcussive syndrome patients continue to have complaints such as headaches, dizziness, inability to concentrate, and memory changes. After 1 year, 85 to 90 percent of these patients recover. The remaining

TABLE 255-4   Intracranial Hematomas

	Type of Patient	Anatomic Location	CT Findings	Common Cause	Classic Symptoms
Epidural	Young, rare in the elderly and age <2 years	Potential space between skull and dura mater	Biconvex, football-shaped hematoma	Skull fracture with tear of the middle meningeal artery	Immediate LOC with a "lucid" period prior to deterioration (only occurs in about 20%)
Subdural	More risk for the elderly and alcoholics	Space between dura mater and arachnoid	Crescent- or sickle-shaped hematoma	Acceleration–deceleration with tearing of the bridging veins	Acute: rapid LOC–lucid period possible Chronic: altered MS and behavior with gradual decrease in consciousness
Subarachnoid	Any age group following blunt trauma	Subarachnoid	Blood in the basilar cisterns and hemispheric sulci and fissures	Acceleration–deceleration with tearing of the subarachnoid vessels	Mild to moderate TBI with meningeal signs and symptoms
Contusion/ intracerebral hematoma	Any age group following blunt trauma	Usually anterior temporal or posterior frontal lobe	May be normal initially with delayed bleed	Severe or penetrating trauma; shaken-baby syndrome	Symptoms range from normal to unconscious

Abbreviations: LOC = loss of consciousness; MS = mental state; TBI = traumatic brain injury.

TABLE 255-5 Postconcussion Syndrome: Complex Involving Somatic, Cognitive, and Affective Symptoms

Somatic
    Headache
    Sleep disturbance
    Nausea
    Sensitivity to photostimuli
    Dizziness/vertigo
    Fatigue
Cognitive
    Memory dysfunction
    Concentration difficulty
    Attention deficit
Affective
    Depression
    Anxiety
    Irritability
    Emotional lability

Note: At 3 months 30–80% are symptomatic; at 1 year 15% are symptomatic.

patients have "persistent postconcussion syndrome" (PPCS). Risk factors for patients PPCS are female sex, ongoing litigation, and low socioeconomic status. While all PCS and PPCS patients should be referred to their primary physicians or neurologist, amitriptyline at 25 to 50 mg PO per d helps with headaches, depression, and insomnia.

Sports-related concussions are common injuries, but their true incidence is greatly underreported. Sports most commonly associated with concussion are boxing, football, soccer, baseball, and basketball. The management of any patient with TBI or concussion is the same as described above. However, for the athlete with a concussion, special consideration must be made for their safe return to a sporting activity. Neurophysiologic assessment instruments are typically used in the hours following TBI and then repeated 5 days after the injury. Some of the tools used for this assessment include the Trail-making test, Stroop test, and the Digit span from the Wechsler Memory Scale, Revised.[19] **When athletes present with symptoms of concussion, they should be referred for testing prior to being cleared to return to sports.**

Infections

Several factors increase the risk for infections following a head injury. Skull fractures and CSF leaks are risk factors for meningitis. In addition to central nervous system (CNS) infections, intubated patients on neuromuscular blockade have longer intensive care unit stays, an increased risk for aspiration pneumonias, and tend toward sepsis. Because of controversies regarding use of prophylactic antibiotics, consultation with the neurosurgeon or intensivist should be obtained prior to their administration.

Patients who present with a history of a skull fracture and fever or other symptoms of meningitis should be treated with antibiotics immediately. The source of infection depends on the time since the injury. In the first 72 h after a head injury, pneumococcus is generally the cause. After that, gram-negative organisms and *Staphylococcus aureus* become more common. Patients should be given vancomycin (1 g IV q12h) and a third-generation cephalosporin, such as ceftazidime 1 g IV q8h, until cultures confirm the cause.

REFERENCES

1. Thurman DJ, Alverson C, Dunn KA, et al: Traumatic brain injury in the United States: A public health perspective. *J Head Trauma Rehabil* 14(6):602, 1999.
2. Wax W, McKenzie EJ, Rice DP: Head injuries: Costs and consequences. *J Head Trauma Rehabil* 6:76, 1991.
3. Chestnut RM, Marshall LF, Klauber MR, et al: The role of secondary brain injury in determining outcome from severe head injury. *J Trauma* 34:216, 1993.
4. Robinson N, Clancy M: In patients with head injury undergoing rapid sequence intubation, does pretreatment with intravenous lignocaine/lidocaine lead to an improved neurological outcome? A review of the literature. *Emerg Med J* 18(6):453, 2001.
5. Albanese J: Ketamine decreases intracranial pressure and electroencephalographic activity in traumatic brain injury patients during propofol sedation. *Anesthesiology* 87(6):1328, 1997.
6. Modica PA: Intracranial pressure during induction of anaesthesia and tracheal intubation with etomidate-induced EEG burst suppression. *Can J Anaesth* 39(3):236, 1992.
7. Vassar MJ, Fischer, RP, O'Brien PE, et al: A multicenter trial for resuscitation of injured patients with 7.5 percent sodium chloride: The effect of added dextrose 70. *Arch Surg* 128:1003, 1993.
8. Servadei F, Teasdale G, Merry G, Neurotraumatology Committee of the World Federation of Neurosurgical Societies: Defining acute mild head injury in adults: A proposal based on prognostic factors, diagnosis, and management. *J Neurotrauma* 18(7):657, 2001.
9. Iverson GL, Lovell MR, Smith S, Franzen MD: Prevalence of abnormal CT scans following mild head injury. *Brain Inj* 14(12):1057, 2000.
10. Stein SC, Ross SE: Moderate head injury: A guide to initial management. *J Neurosurg* 77:562, 1992.
11. Snoey ER, Levitt MA: Delayed diagnosis of subdural hematoma following normal computed tomography scan. *Ann Emerg Med* 23:1127, 1994.
12. Arienta C, Caroli M, Balbi S: Management of head-injured patients in the emergency department: A practical protocol. *Surg Neurol* 48:213, 1997.
13. Bullock RM, et al: Management and prognosis of severe traumatic brain injury, part I, Guidelines for the management of severe traumatic brain injury. *J Neurotrauma* 17:451, 2000.
14. Friedman JA, Ebersold MJ, Quast LM: Post-traumatic cerebrospinal fluid leakage. *World J Surg* 25(8):1062, 2001.
15. Servadei F, Murray GD, Teasdale GM, et al: Traumatic subarachnoid hemorrhage: Demographic and clinical study of 750 patients from the European brain injury consortium survey of head injuries. *Neurosurgery* 50(2):261, 2002.
16. Harders A, Kakarieka A, Braakman R: Traumatic subarachnoid hemorrhage and its treatment with nimodipine. *J Neurosurg* 85:82, 1996.
17. Wiedemayer H, Triesch K, Schafer H, Stolke D: Early seizures following non-penetrating traumatic brain injury in adults: Risk factors and clinical significance. *Brain Inj* 16(4):323, 2002.
18. Schierhout G, Roberts I: Anti-epileptic drugs for preventing seizures following acute traumatic brain injury [review]. *Cochrane Database Syst Rev* (2):CD, 2003. http://www.update-software.com/abstracts/a6000173shtm. (Accessed May 30, 2003)
19. Wojtys EM, Hovda D, Landry G, et al: Concussion in sports. *Am J Sports Med* 27(5):676, 1999.
20. Alves W, Macciocchi S, Barth J: Postconcussive symptoms after uncomplicated mild head injury. *J Head Trauma Rehabil* 8:48, 1993.

SPINAL CORD INJURIES
Bonny J. Baron
Thomas M. Scalea

EPIDEMIOLOGY

Spinal injuries are probably the most devastating of all trauma-related injuries. The incidence of traumatic spinal cord injury (SCI) in the United States is estimated to be 30 cases per million population at risk. Thus, 8000 to 10,000 new cases can be expected annually. The actual incidence is probably higher. Minor injuries are often not reported, and those associated with trauma fatalities may go unnoticed. SCI is predominantly a disease of young men. The most comprehensive data available indicates the mean age has been reported as 33.5 years,[1] with a male-to-female predominance of 4 to 1. Spinal injury occurs more frequently on weekends and holidays and during summer months. The majority (90 percent) of cases are caused by blunt trauma with most of these from motor vehicle crashes.

FUNCTIONAL ANATOMY

The vertebral column serves as the central supporting structure for the head and trunk and provides bony protection for the spinal cord. It consists of 33 vertebrae: 7 cervical, 12 thoracic, 5 lumbar, 5 sacral (fused to form the sacrum), and 4 coccygeal, which are usually fused.

Vertebrae

In accordance with their weight-bearing function, the vertebrae become larger toward the lower end of the column, but all are built on the same fundamental plan. A typical vertebra is composed of a body anteriorly and a vertebral arch posteriorly (Figure 256-1). Between the body and arch is the vertebral foramen through which the spinal cord runs. The vertebral arch is made up of two pedicles, two laminae, and seven processes (one spinous, two transverse, and four articular). The spine has the potential to move in flexion, extension, lateral flexion, rotation, or circumduction (combination of all movements). The articular processes form synovial joints that act as pivots of the spinal column. The orientation of these articular facet joints changes at different levels of the spine. Differences in orientation of the facet joints account for variations in motion of specific regions of the vertebral column. A series of ligaments serve to maintain the alignment of the spinal column. The anterior and posterior longitudinal ligaments run along the vertebral bodies. Surrounding the vertebral arch are the ligamentum flavum and the supraspinous, interspinous, intertransverse, and capsular ligaments. The intervertebral disks lie between adjacent vertebral bodies. Each disk consists of a peripheral annulus fibrosus and a central nucleus pulposus. The annulus fibrosus is composed of fibrocartilage. The nucleus pulposus is a semifluid, gelatinous structure made up of water and cartilage fibers. With advancing age, the proportion of water decreases and fibrocartilage increases. The disks act as shock absorbers to distribute axial load. When compressive forces exceed the absorptive capacity of the disk, the annulus fibrosus ruptures, allowing the nucleus pulposus to protrude into the vertebral canal. This may result in spinal nerve or spinal cord compression.

Spinal Stability

The determination of spinal stability is an important factor in the evaluation of the injured spine. White and Panjabi define stability as the ability of the spine to limit patterns of displacement under physiologic loads so as not to damage or irritate the spinal cord or nerve roots and

to prevent incapacitating deformity or pain because of structural changes.[2] Computed tomography (CT) evaluation applied to the Denis three-column system for classification of thoracolumbar injuries can be used to assess spinal stability.[3] The anterior column is formed by the anterior part of the vertebral body, the anterior annulus fibrosus, and the anterior longitudinal ligament. The middle column is formed by the posterior wall of the vertebral body, the posterior annulus fibrosus, and the posterior longitudinal ligament. The posterior column includes the bony complex of the posterior vertebral arch and the posterior ligamentous complex. For an injury to be unstable, there must be disruption of at least two columns. In evaluating stability, it is also important to include the degree of compression of the vertebral body. Vertebral body compressions of more than 50 percent are generally considered unstable.

Thoracic and Lumbar Spine

The thoracic spine is a rigid segment. The additional support provided by its articulation with the rib cage imparts a stiffness 2.5 times that of the ligamentous spine alone. Relative to other regions of the vertebral column, a large force is necessary to overcome the intrinsic stability of the thoracic spine. While injury to the thoracic spine is less common than in other regions, when it does occur it is usually significant. The spinal canal is narrower than that found in either the cervical or lumbar spine. The large spinal cord diameter relative to canal diameter increases the risk of cord injury. When cord injuries occur, most are neurologically complete (see discussion later). Of additional importance is the association between fractures of the thoracic spine and severe pulmonary injuries, including mediastinal hemorrhage. Patients with blunt chest trauma and mediastinal widening should be evaluated for both aortic and thoracic spine injuries.[4]

The spine is divided into alternating mobile and fixed segments. The thoracolumbar junction (T11-L2) is considered a transitional zone between the fixed thoracic and mobile lumbar regions. This distinction is important because the transitional zones sustain the greatest amount of stress during motion, and these are the areas most vulnerable to traumatic injuries. In addition to this change in bony anatomy, the thoracolumbar junction serves as the level of transition from the end of the spinal cord (about L1) to the nerve roots of the cauda equina. Relative to the thoracic spine, the width of the spinal canal is greater. Despite a large number of vertebral injuries at the thoracolumbar junction, most are associated with normal neurologic examinations or incomplete neurologic findings.

Relative to the thoracic and thoracolumbar regions, the lower lumbar spine is the most mobile. Isolated fractures of the lower lumbar spine rarely result in complete neurologic injuries. When neurologic injuries occur, they are usually complete cauda equina lesions or isolated nerve root injuries.

Sacrum and Coccyx

The sacrum supports the lumbar vertebral column and transmits loads from the trunk to the pelvic girdle and into the lower limbs. The upper border articulates with the fifth lumbar vertebra. The inferior border articulates with the coccyx. Laterally, the sacrum articulates with the iliac bones to form the sacroiliac joints. The vertebral foramina together form the sacral canal. The sacral canal contains the nerve roots of the lumbar, sacral, and coccygeal spinal nerves and the filum terminale.

The coccyx, which articulates with the sacrum, consists of four vertebrae fused together. Except for the first vertebra, the remaining coccygeal vertebrae consist of bodies only.

Injuries of the sacral spine and nerve roots are very unusual. When they occur, they are frequently associated with fractures of the pelvis. There are multiple different classification schemes of sacral fractures that help to predict neurologic deficits and establish treatment proto-

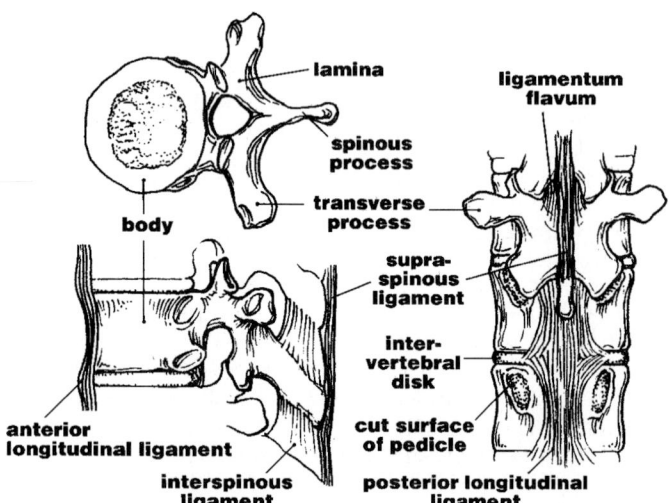

FIG. 256-1. Vertebra. Each vertebra consists of a vertebral body and posterior element. Vertebrae are stabilized by an anterior longitudinal ligament, posterior ligament, and interspinous ligament.

cols. In general, transverse fractures through the body are most significant in that they cause injury to part or all of the cauda equina. Longitudinal fractures may cause radiculopathy. If there is involvement of the central sacral canal, however, bowel or bladder dysfunction may also occur.[5] Careful neurologic evaluation is essential. Motor and sensory evaluation of the sacral nerve roots should be performed. Rectal examination will assess anal sphincter tone and the bulbocavernosus reflex.

Coccygeal injuries are usually associated with direct falls onto the buttocks. Patients typically describe intense pain with sitting and straining. Diagnosis of fracture is made on rectal examination. Pain will be elicited with motion of the coccyx. X-rays are not needed to diagnose coccygeal fractures. Treatment is symptomatic, and includes analgesics and use of a rubber doughnut pillow.

Spinal Cord

The spinal cord is a cylindrical structure that begins at the foramen magnum, where it is continuous with the medulla oblongata of the brain. Inferiorly, it terminates in the tapered conus medullaris at the lower border of the first lumbar vertebra. The conus is continued at its apex by a prolongation of the pia mater, the filum terminale, which extends to the base of the coccyx. The spinal cord gives rise to 31 pairs of spinal nerves: 8 cervical, 12 thoracic, 5 lumbar, 5 sacral, and 1 coccygeal. Each spinal nerve emerges through the intervertebral foramen corresponding to the appropriate spinal cord level. There is disproportionate growth in the length of the spinal cord and the vertebral column. As a result of this inequality, the length of the nerve roots increases progressively from above downward. The lower nerve roots, inferior to the conus medullaris, form an array of nerves around the filum terminale; this is called the *cauda equina*.

MECHANISM OF INJURY

Motor vehicle crashes are the principal cause of traumatic injury to the spinal cord. Other etiologies, in descending order of frequency, include falls, gunshot wounds, and injuries secondary to sports or recreational activities.

Fractures of the spine can be divided into minor and major injuries. Minor injuries are those that are localized to part of a column and do not cause instability. These fractures often result from direct blunt trauma to the posterior elements of the spine. Minor injuries include isolated fractures of the transverse, spinous, and articular processes. Major spinal injuries can be classified into four categories: 1) compression (wedge) fractures; 2) burst fractures; 3) flexion-distraction (seat belt-type injuries); and 4) fracture/dislocations.

Compression fractures result from axial loading and flexion, with subsequent failure of the anterior column (Figure 256-2). The middle column remains intact. These injuries are usually stable unless they are greater than 50 percent. They are unlikely to be directly responsible for neurologic damage.

Burst fractures occur following failure of the vertebral body under axial load (Figure 256-3). In contrast to compression fractures, both the anterior and middle columns fail. There is retropulsion of bone and disk fragments into the canal. This may cause spinal cord compression.

Flexion-distraction injuries are commonly seen following seat belt-type injuries, particularly where lap belts alone are used (Figure 256-4). The seat belt serves as the axis of rotation during distraction, and there is failure of both the posterior and middle columns. The intact anterior column prevents subluxation. Typical radiographic findings reveal increased height of the posterior vertebral body, fracture of the posterior wall of the vertebral body, and posterior opening of the disk space.

Fracture-dislocations are the most damaging of injuries (Figure 256-5). Compression, flexion, distraction, rotation, or shearing forces lead to failure of all three columns. The end result is subluxation or dislocation.

Blunt Injury

MOTOR VEHICLE-RELATED INJURIES   Motor vehicle crashes usually result in acceleration-deceleration injuries. The cervical spine is the most susceptible to injury by this mechanism, but the thoracic and lumbar regions are also at risk. The majority of victims are involved in low-impact crashes. Most commonly, the soft tissues are injured. Patients complain of pain in the posterior neck and back. High-speed, high-energy crashes are more likely to result in structural damage to the spine. Lap-only seat belts are associated with thoracolumbar injuries.

Pedestrians struck by vehicles and motorcyclists are at considerable risk for multiple skeletal injuries, including spinal injuries.

Obvious neurologic deficits mandate emergent treatment for an unstable injury. In the absence of deficits, the mechanism of injury with an understanding of the forces involved should guide management. When in doubt, it is best initially to overtreat and overstudy in order to avoid missing a significant injury.

Falls

Falls from a height are associated with fractures of the lower extremities, pelvis, and spine. Scalea et al. studied 161 patients who fell from a height of one or more stories, nearly one-fourth of whom suffered spine fractures.[6] Of the latter, 74 percent sustained a major compression or burst fracture. The most common site of injury was the thoracolumbar junction. A thorough neurologic evaluation must be part of the early assessment of patients with vertical deceleration injury. All patients must be presumed to have unstable spine fractures until proven otherwise.

Sports Injuries

Spinal injuries occur in both contact and noncontact sports. The specific injury is related to the mechanism, the force involved, and the point of application of the force, rather than to the specific sport. The majority of injuries are self-limiting soft tissue injuries. Injuries at the level of the disk result in disk herniation or degeneration. Those that occur at the level of the bone can range from minimal avulsion-type fractures to compressions or fracture dislocations. Most bony injuries are not associated with neurologic sequelae. Rarely, however, sports injuries do result in significant neurologic compromise. When neurologic impairment occurs, it is usually secondary to direct axial forces. Catastrophic injuries have been associated with football, water sports (especially diving), gymnastics, rugby, and ice hockey.[7]

Penetrating Injury

The majority of penetrating spinal cord lesions are caused by gunshot wounds. These wounds may be localized to the spine or may involve transperitoneal trajectories. The spinal cord may be injured by direct contact with the bullet, by bony fragments, or from concussive forces.[8] Most gunshot wounds result in stable vertebral injuries, although cord lesions are often complete. Stabbing injuries are much less common. These may be inflicted by a variety of implements including knives, axes, ice picks, screwdrivers, and glass fragments. The majority of stab wounds involve incomplete Brown–Séquard lesions of the thoracic cord. Among incomplete spinal injuries, these have the best prognosis. The prognosis for patients with stab injuries to the spine and incomplete paralysis is significantly better than that for patients with gunshot wounds to the spine and a similar extent of paralysis.

CLINICAL FEATURES

Damage to the spinal cord is the result of two types of injury. First is the direct mechanical injury from traumatic impact. This insult sets

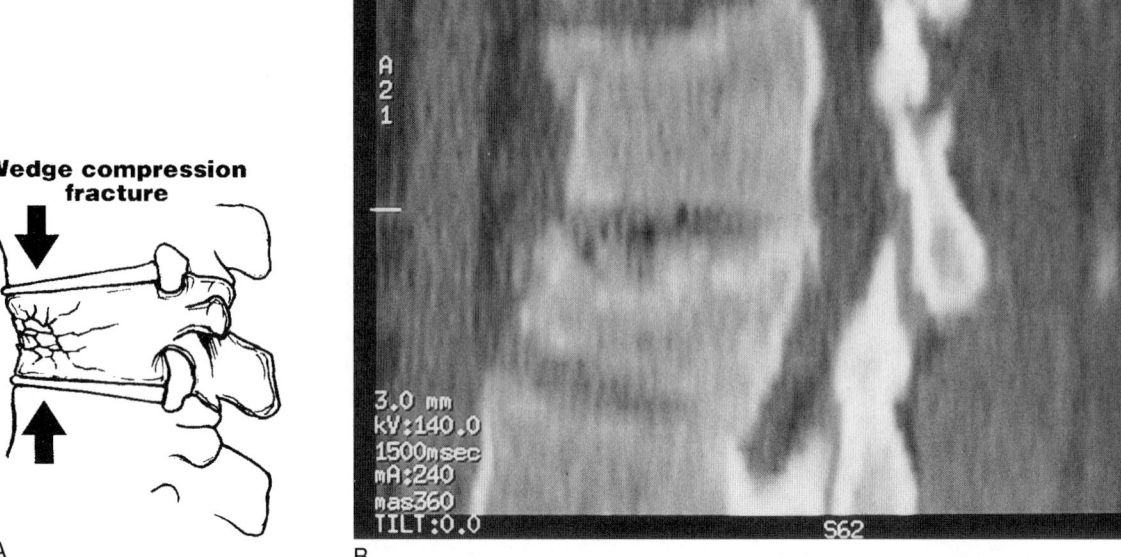

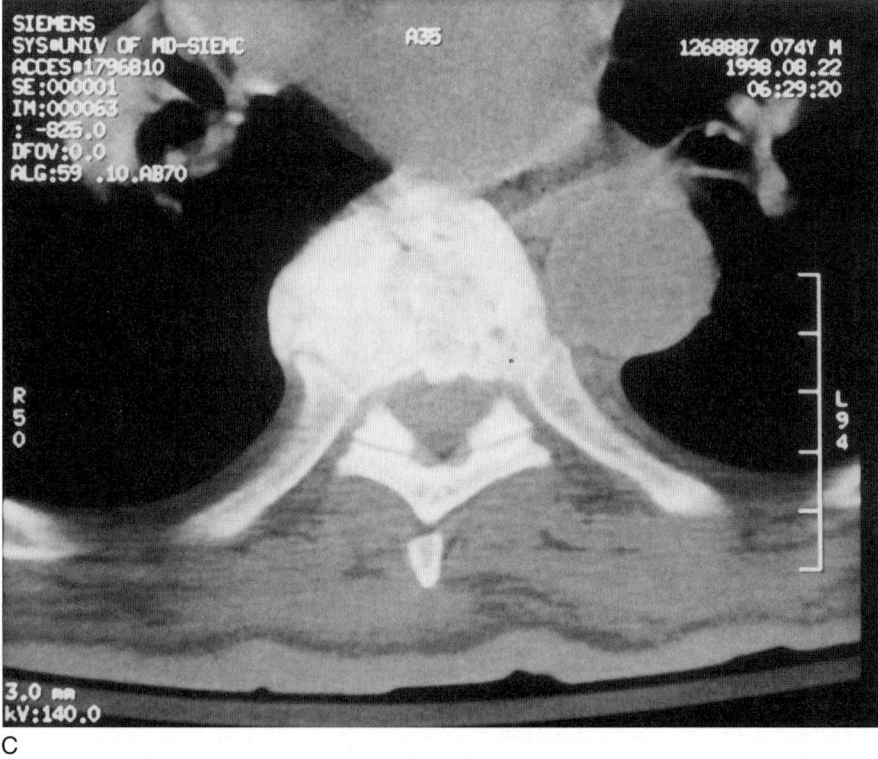

FIG. 256-2. Wedge compression fractures are often caused by axial unloading with failure of the anterior column. **A.** Schematic of a compression fracture. **B.** Lateral reconstruction CT scan demonstrates the anterior wedging. **C.** Axial CT scan demonstrates the anterior wedging and vertebral body fracture. Note the lack of retropulsion of elements into the spinal canal.

into motion a series of vascular and chemical processes that lead to secondary injury. The initial phase is characterized by hemorrhage into the cord and formation of edema at the injured site and surrounding region. Local spinal cord blood flow is diminished owing to vasospasm and thrombosis of the small arterioles within the gray and white matter. Extension of edema may further compromise blood flow and increase ischemia. A secondary tissue degeneration phase begins within hours of injury. This is associated with the release of membrane-destabilizing enzymes, mediators of inflammation, and disturbance of

electrophysiologic coupling by disruption of calcium channel pathways. Lipid peroxidation and hydrolysis appear to play a major role in this secondary phase of spinal cord injury.

Spinal Cord Lesions

It is important to distinguish between complete and incomplete spinal cord injuries. The severity of injury determines the prognosis for recovery of function. The American Spinal Injury Association defines a

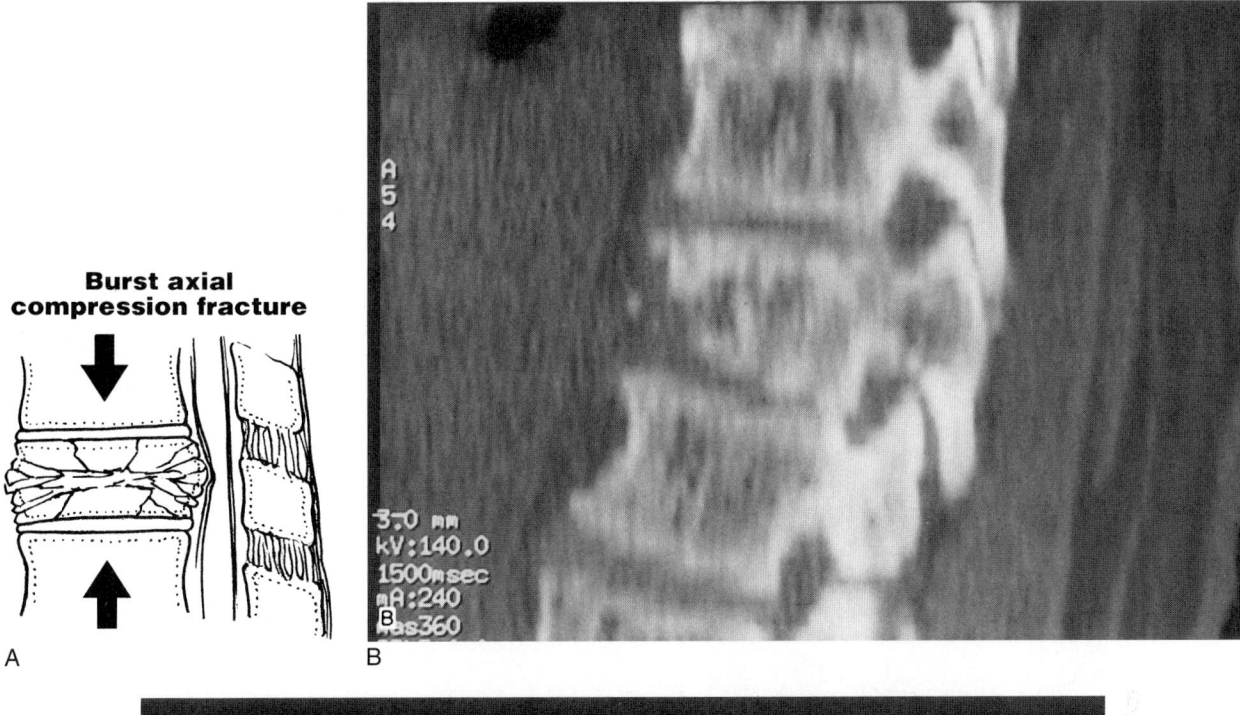

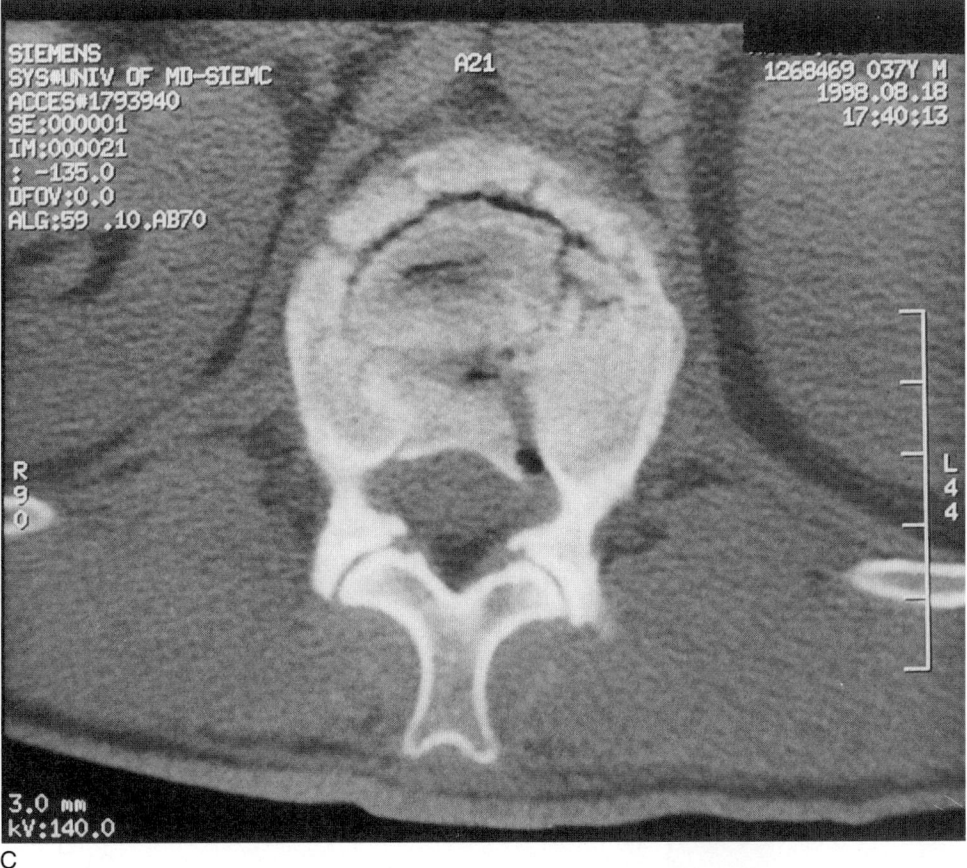

FIG. 256-3. Burst fractures are also caused by axial loading. Both anterior and middle columns have failed. **A.** Schematic of the forces transmitted. **B.** Lateral reconstruction CT scan demonstrates failure of both the anterior and middle columns. **C.** Axial CT scan demonstrates the burst vertebral body. Note the retropulsion of elements into the spinal canal.

complete neurologic lesion as the absence of sensory and motor function below the level of injury. This includes loss of function to the level of the lowest sacral segment. In contrast, a lesion is incomplete if sensory, motor, or both functions are partially present below the neurologic level of injury. This may consist only of sacral sensation at the anal mucocutaneous junction or voluntary contraction of the external anal sphincter upon digital examination.[3] In assessing neurologic function, spinal shock must be considered. Patients in spinal shock lose all reflex activities. This generally resolves over 24 to 48 h, with the return of the bulbocavernosus reflex occurring first. Lesions

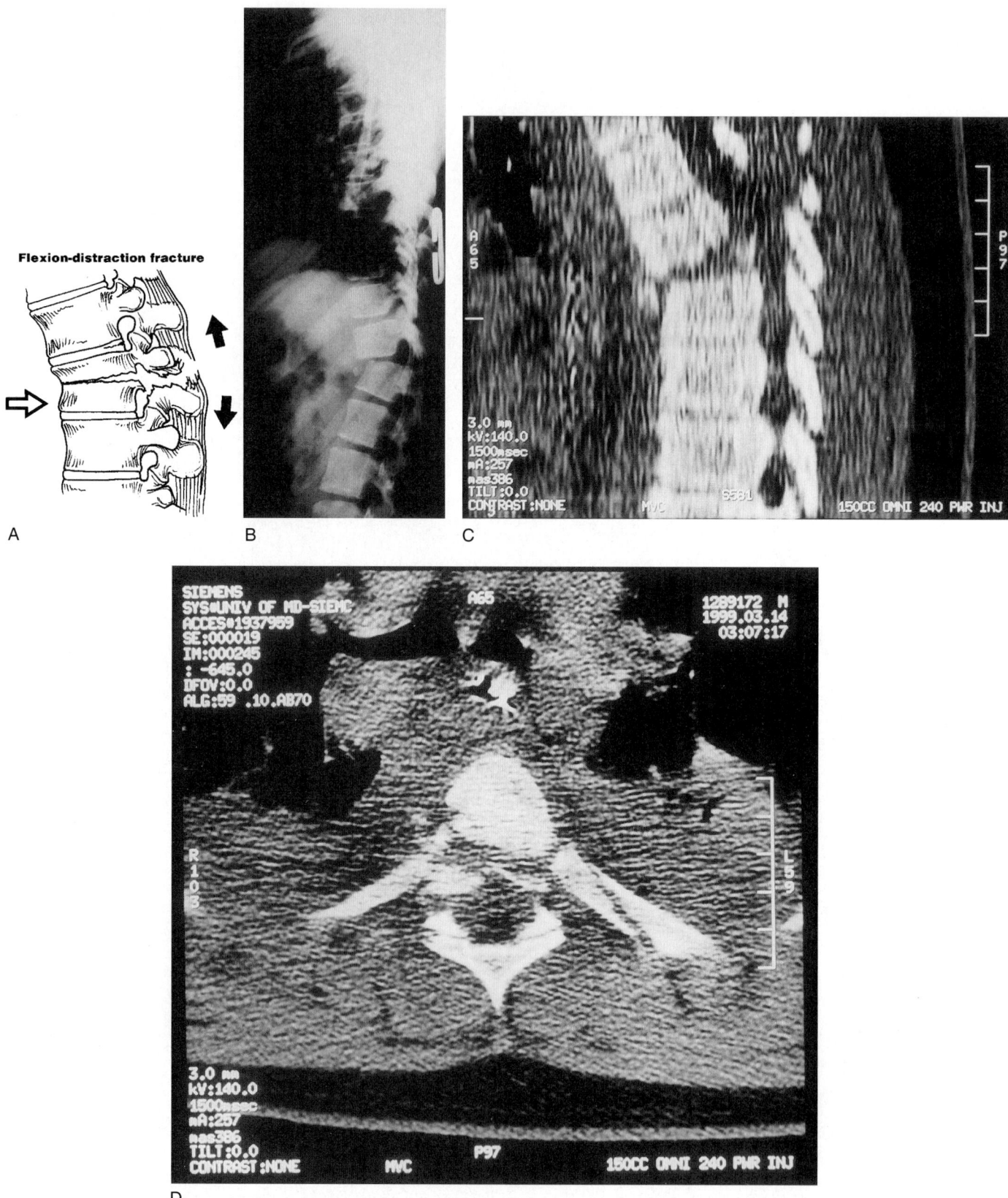

FIG. 256-4. Flexion-distraction injuries involve rotation of forces. This results in failure of both the posterior and middle columns. **A.** Schematic of the forces transmitted. **B.** Lateral view of plain film demonstrating a flexion distraction injury. **C.** Lateral CT reconstruction confirming the pattern, also demonstrating posterior opening of the disk space. **D.** Axial CT scan shows loss of the middle column with fracture through the lateral elements.

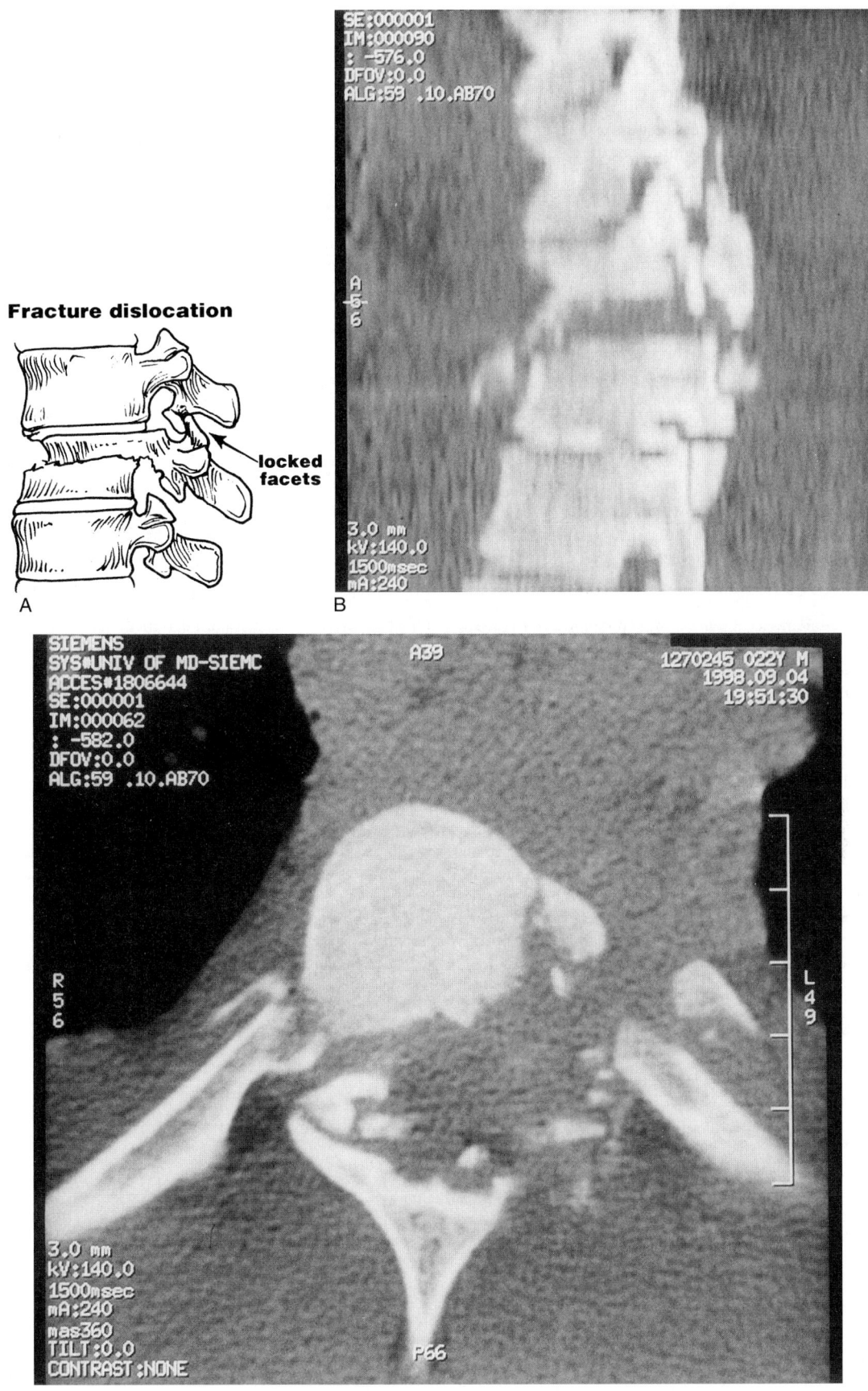

FIG. 256-5. Fracture dislocations are the most damaging of injuries leading to failure of all three columns. **A.** Demonstrates these injuries schematically. **B.** Lateral CT reconstruction demonstrates loss of all three columns. **C.** Axial CT scan demonstrates the dislocation and displacement of the vertebral body.

cannot be deemed complete until spinal shock has resolved. Complete lesions have a minimal chance of functional motor recovery. Patients with incomplete lesions are expected to have at least some degree of recovery.

Clinical syndromes classify incomplete spinal cord lesions. Damage to specific sections of the spinal cord results in predictable physical findings (Table 256-1). A discussion of the anatomy may be helpful.

A large number of descending and ascending tracts have been identified in the spinal cord. The three most important of these in terms of neuroanatomic localization of cord lesions are the corticospinal tracts, spinothalamic tracts, and dorsal (posterior) columns.

The corticospinal tract is a descending motor pathway. Its fibers descend from the cerebral cortex through the internal capsule and the middle of the crus cerebri. The tract then breaks up into bundles in the pons and finally collects into a discrete bundle, forming the pyramid of the medulla. In the lower medulla, approximately 90 percent of the fibers cross (decussate) to the side opposite that of their origin and descend through the spinal cord as the lateral corticospinal tract. These fibers synapse on lower motor neurons in the spinal cord. The 10 percent of corticospinal fibers that do not decussate in the medulla descend in the anterior funiculus of the cervical and upper thoracic cord levels as the ventral corticospinal tract. Damage to the corticospinal tract neurons (upper motor neurons) in the spinal cord results in ipsilateral clinical findings such as muscle weakness, spasticity, increased deep tendon reflexes, and a Babinski sign.

The two major ascending pathways that transmit sensory information are the spinothalamic tracts and the dorsal columns. The first neurons of both of these afferent systems begin as sensory receptors situated in the skin and stretch receptors of muscles. Their cell bodies are located in the dorsal root ganglia of the spinal nerves. The spinothalamic tract transmits pain and temperature sensation. As the axons of the first neurons enter the spinal cord, most rise one or two levels before entering the dorsal gray of the spinal cord, where they synapse with the second neuron of the spinothalamic tract. The second neuron immediately crosses the midline in the anterior commissure of the spinal cord and ascends in the anterolateral funiculus as the lateral spinothalamic tract. When the spinothalamic tract is damaged in the spinal cord, the patient experiences loss of pain and temperature sensation in the contralateral half of the body. The (pain and temperature) sensory loss begins one or two segments below the level of the lesion. The dorsal columns transmit vibration and proprioceptive information. Neurons enter the spinal cord proximal to pain and temperature neurons. They differ from pain and temperature neurons in that they do not immediately synapse. Instead, these axons enter the ipsilateral dorsal column and do not synapse until they reach the gracile or cuneate nuclei of the medulla. From these nuclei, fibers cross the midline and ascend in the medial lemniscus to the thalamus. Injury to one side of the dorsal columns will result in ipsilateral loss of vibration and position sense. The sensory loss begins at the level of the lesion. Light touch is transmitted through both the spinothalamic tracts and the dorsal columns. Therefore, light touch is not completely lost unless there is damage to both the spinothalamic tracts and the dorsal columns.

Concerning the spinal nerves and their relationship to the vertebrae, each spinal nerve is named for its adjacent vertebral body. Because there is an additional pair of spinal nerve roots compared to the number of vertebral bodies, the first seven spinal nerves are named for the first seven cervical vertebrae, each exiting through the intervertebral foramen above its corresponding vertebral body. The spinal nerve exiting below C7, however, is referred to as the C8 spinal nerve, although no eighth cervical vertebra exists. All subsequent nerve roots, beginning with T1, exit below the vertebral body for which they are named.

During fetal development, the downward growth of the vertebral column is greater than that of the spinal cord. Because the adult spinal cord ends as the conus medullaris at the level of the lower border of the first lumbar vertebra, the lumbar and sacral nerve roots must continue inferiorly below the termination of the spinal cord to exit from their respective intervertebral foramina. These nerve roots form the cauda equina. A potential consequence of this arrangement is that injury to a single lower vertebra can involve multiple nerve roots in the cauda equina. For example, an injury at the L3 vertebra can involve the L3 nerve root as well as the lower nerve roots that are progressing to a level caudal to the L3 vertebra.

Anterior Cord Syndrome

The anterior cord syndrome results from damage to the corticospinal and spinothalamic pathways, with preservation of posterior column function. This is manifest by loss of motor function and pain and temperature sensation distal to the lesion. Only vibration, position, and crude touch are preserved. This syndrome may occur following direct injury to the anterior spinal cord. Flexion of the cervical spine may result in cord contusion or bone injury with secondary cord injury. Alternatively, thrombosis of the anterior spinal artery can cause ischemic injury to the anterior cord. Immediate evaluation with CT or magnetic

TABLE 256-1 Spinal Cord Syndromes

Syndrome	Etiology	Symptoms	Prognosis
Anterior cord	Direct anterior cord compression Flexion of cervical spine Thrombosis of anterior spinal artery	Complete paralysis below the lesion with loss of pain and temperature sensation Preservation of proprioception and vibratory function	Poor
Central cord	Hyperextension injuries Disruption of blood flow to the spinal cord Cervical spinal stenosis	Quadriparesis—greater in the upper extremities than the lower extremities. Some loss of pain and temperature sensation, also greater in the upper extremities	Good
Brown-Séquard	Transverse hemisection of the spinal cord Unilateral cord compression	Ipsilateral spastic paresis, loss of proprioception and vibratory sensation and contralateral loss of pain and temperature sensation	Good
Cauda equina	Peripheral nerve injury	Variable motor and sensory loss in the lower extremities, sciatica, bowel/bladder dysfunction and "saddle anesthesia"	Good
Spinal shock	Partial or complete injury usually at the T6 level and above	Areflexia, loss of sensation, and flaccid paralysis below the level of the lesion; a flaccid bladder and loss of rectal tone; bradycarda and hypotension	Complete lesions have a poor prognosis Incomplete lesions have some degree of recovery

resonance imaging (MRI) may reveal an extrinsic mass that is amenable to surgical decompression. The overall prognosis for recovery of function historically has been poor and remains so today.[9]

Central Cord Syndrome

The central cord syndrome is usually seen in older patients with preexisting cervical spondylosis who sustain a hyperextension injury. The injury preferentially involves the central portion of the cord more than the peripheral. The centrally located fibers of the corticospinal and spinothalamic tracts are affected. The neural tracts providing function to the upper extremities are most medial in position. The thoracic, lower extremity, and sacral fibers have a more lateral distribution. Clinically, patients present with decreased strength, and to a lesser degree, decreased pain and temperature sensation, more in the upper than the lower extremities. Spastic paraparesis or spastic quadriparesis can also be seen. The majority will have bowel and bladder control, although this may be impaired in the more severe cases. Prognosis for recovery of function is good; however, most patients do not regain fine motor use of their upper extremities.[9]

Brown–Séquard Syndrome

The Brown–Séquard syndrome results from hemisection of the cord. It is manifest by ipsilateral loss of motor function, proprioception, and vibratory sensation, and contralateral loss of pain and temperature sensation. The most common cause of this syndrome is penetrating injury. It can also be caused by lateral cord compression secondary to disk protrusion, hematomas, bone injury, or tumors. Of all of the incomplete cord lesions, this has the best prognosis for recovery.[9]

Cauda Equina Syndrome

The cauda equina is composed entirely of lumbar, sacral, and coccygeal nerve roots. An injury in this region produces a peripheral nerve injury rather than a direct injury to the spinal cord. Symptoms may include variable motor and sensory loss in the lower extremities, sciatica, bowel and bladder dysfunction, and "saddle anesthesia" (loss of pain sensation over the perineum). Because peripheral nerves possess the ability to regenerate, the prognosis for recovery is better than that for spinal cord lesions.

GENERAL APPROACH

Prehospital Care

The prehospital treatment of patients with spinal cord injury involves recognition of patients at risk, triage to an appropriate facility, and early care. All patients who have complaints of neck or back pain or who have tenderness on prehospital assessment must be presumed to have a spine injury until proven otherwise. Traditionally, all patients with significant injury above the clavicle are also presumed to have cervical spine injury regardless of related complaints. All patients with neurologic complaints must be presumed to have a spinal cord injury. Sometimes this is obvious, as in a patient with flaccid paraplegia. More often, symptoms are much more subtle (numbness or tingling in an extremity). Appropriate triage is imperative, as the results of the treatment for spinal cord injury are somewhat time related. Therefore, initial triage to a center that is capable of rapid diagnostics and therapeutics is essential to optimize outcome following spinal cord injury.

Triage can be difficult. Patients may be asymptomatic or may have suffered a concomitant head injury that makes them unable to describe their injuries and hence does not allow for neurologic assessment in the field. Other injuries may preclude accurate neurologic assessment. The mechanism of injury is an important criterion on which prehospital providers can rely. High-speed or rollover vehicular accidents, falls from a substantial height (injuries to the thoracolumbar junction), and diving and surfing accidents typically produce cervical spine injuries. Any patient at risk by mechanism of injury must be presumed to have a spinal cord injury. While this may result in a substantial rate of overtriage, the consequences of undertriage can be devastating.

Prehospital care for spinal injuries involves immobilization of the entire spine and initial fluid therapy as proposed by the American College of Surgeons.[10] Patients should be transported completely immobilized. The entire cervical spine can be immobilized with a rigid cervical collar supplemented with sandbags and tape. The thoracic and lumbar spine can be immobilized using a long backboard. Patients are "papoosed" onto the boards to maintain spinal alignment. While there is little scientific evidence to support any single target for systolic or mean arterial blood pressure in patients with spinal cord injuries, a mean arterial pressure of 65 to 70 mm Hg seems a reasonable target. Optimal perfusion of the spinal cord is one of the therapies that can be implemented in the field to lessen the chances of secondary spinal injury.

All efforts should be made to rapidly deliver patients with symptomatic spinal injuries to the areawide spine center. Delays engendered by transport to a different site can result in morbidity. Clearly, patients who are not hemodynamically stable must be taken to the closest available hospital.

Emergency Department Stabilization

ED evaluation should not differ substantially from any patient with multiple injuries (see Chap. 251). Consideration should be given to immediate airway control in patients with cervical spine injuries no matter how apparently stable at the time of presentation. The higher the level of spinal injury, the more compelling the indication for early airway intervention. The roots of the phrenic nerve, which supply the diaphragm, emerge at the third, fourth, and fifth cervical vertebral levels. Thus, **any patient with an injury at C5 or above should be intubated.** It may be prudent to intubate parents with cervical cord lesions even below this level. Significant spinal cord edema may progress rostrally to involve the roots of the phrenic nerve. Many patients can initially support ventilatory function utilizing intercostal muscles or abdominal breathing, but they eventually tire and then develop respiratory failure. As the evaluation process for these patients often involves transport outside of the ED, the authors feel strongly that early airway control is the safest route. Patients who develop respiratory failure in the CT scanner or the MRI suite may suffer respiratory arrest before it can be recognized and the airway secured.

AIRWAY   It is important to perform a complete neurologic assessment, if possible, before patients are intubated and sedated. The spine must be kept immobilized while the airway is managed. In general, this is accomplished using orotracheal intubation with in-line cervical stabilization (without distraction force) and cricoid pressure. Nasal intubation can be performed in patients while maintaining spine immobilization, although it is not a preferred method because nasal intubation is generally a blind technique. Virtually all patients with potential cervical spine trauma require sedation before nasal intubation can be accomplished; but if respirations become substantially depressed, nasotracheal intubation may not be possible. If patients are inadequately prepared, they may resist intubation. Motion of an unstable fracture can worsen spinal injury. If patients are oversedated, they may become hypoxic and lose the ability to protect the airway. Also, nasal intubation is performed with a smaller endotracheal tube, which can compromise respiratory therapy later during the hospitalization. Fiberoptic bronchoscopy may later be required for diagnostic purposes, particularly in those with pulmonary injuries or significant atelectasis, to facilitate removal of inspissated mucous plugs or blood. A relatively large endotracheal tube (8 mm or greater in size) is needed during fiberoptic bronchoscopy to ensure that ventilation is not compromised during the procedure. An 8-mm endotracheal tube is often too large for nasotracheal intubation. In addition, the limiting factor in minimizing tube size is the increasing respiratory resistance to gas flow imposing increased work for the patient with each spontaneous breath. Thus, the work of breathing is greater with tubes of 6 to 7 mm internal diameter, sometimes used for nasal intubation, than with tubes of 8 mm or greater internal diameter. The most limiting aspect of nasal intubation is the inability to move the cervical spine to attain the "sniff" position, optimal for the procedure. Finally, nasal intubation increases the risk of sinusitis.

If nasal intubation is selected, fiberoptic guidance is a useful technique. While the concerns of nasal intubation remain, with fiberoptic guidance, it is not a blind technique.

HYPOTENSION   Following airway stabilization, hemodynamic stability is the most pressing concern. Fluid therapy is generally the treatment of choice to support cardiovascular functioning. Patients with spinal cord injuries often present with hypotension, which must be differentiated as to its cause: spinal cord injury, blood loss, cardiac injury, or a combination. Injury to the spinal cord at the level of the cervical or thoracic vertebrae causes sympathetic denervation. There is a loss of α-adrenergic tone and dilatation of the arterial and venous vessels. Elimination of sympathetic arterial tone results in decreased systemic vascular resistance. Loss of sympathetic innervation to the heart (T1 through T4 cord levels) leaves the parasympathetic cardiac innervation via the vagus nerve unopposed, resulting in bradycardia. While it is true that neurogenic shock is associated with bradycardia, it should never be assumed that a patient with hypotension and bradycardia is suffering from isolated neurogenic shock. Vital signs are often nonspecific. Patients with neurogenic shock may have concomitant hemorrhagic shock and may not be able to mount a tachycardic response. **Blood loss must be presumed to be the cause of hypotension until proven otherwise.** In general, patients with neurogenic shock are warm, peripherally vasodilated, and bradycardic. They seem to tolerate hypotension relatively well. This makes some sense, as peripheral oxygen delivery is presumably normal. They have incurred mechanical sympathectomy, thus cardiovascular function is not impaired.

The mechanism of injury is important in determining whether hypotension is from spinal cord injury or blood loss. Factors other than spinal cord injury (mostly blood loss) are responsible at least in part for the hypotension seen in patients with blunt trauma.[11] More than 90 percent of hypotensive patients with penetrating spinal cord injury have blood loss to at least partly explain their hypotension.[12]

In all patients, a rapid search for potential blood loss should be undertaken. A chest x-ray will usually identify blood loss within the thorax. Retroperitoneal blood loss can come from concomitant pelvic fractures or may be secondary to lumbar arterial bleeding from spine fractures, especially in patients with substantial falls from a height. Every patient with a spinal fracture should have an abdominal diagnostic investigation. In hemodynamically unstable patients, CT scanning is often impractical; therefore ultrasonography or diagnostic peritoneal lavage should be used. Retroperitoneal bleeding should be suspected in patients without evidence of intraabdominal blood loss who develop abdominal distention or tenderness.[6] Plain x-rays that demonstrate spinal fractures should help with the diagnosis. Angiography may be necessary for both diagnosis and treatment of active bleeding.

NEUROLOGIC EXAMINATION   Once patients are stabilized and other life-threatening injuries have been excluded or treated, a detailed neurologic examination should be performed. Details of history include whether the patient has had a loss of consciousness. A patient who was asymptomatic in the field and has neurologic deterioration in the ED requires emergent therapy. The presence of neck or back pain, or urinary or fecal incontinence clearly defines the patient at risk for spinal cord injury.

Physical examination should delineate the level of spinal cord injury (Figure 256-6). A complete initial neurologic examination must

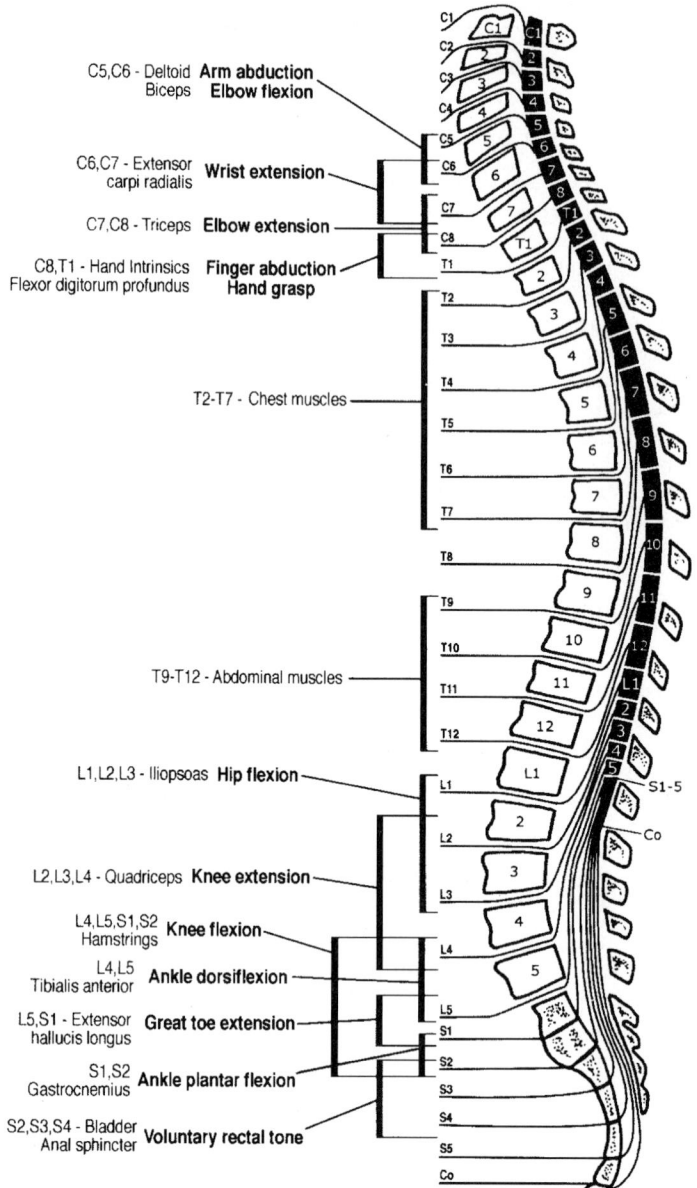

FIG. 256-6. Spinal cord level. This level can be delineated by physical examination, including a detailed neurologic examination.

be documented for appropriate comparison should a patient deteriorate later. The presence or absence of neck or back tenderness should be noted. Motor function for muscle groups should be tested and recorded on a scale of 0 to 5 (Table 256-2). The level of sensory loss should be determined. Gross proprioception or vibratory function must be investigated to examine posterior column function. Deep tendon reflexes should be tested. Anogenital reflexes should also be tested, because "sacral sparing" with preservation of the reflexes denotes an incomplete spinal cord level even if the patient has complete sensory and motor loss. To test the bulbocavernosus reflex, the penis is squeezed to determine whether the anal sphincter simultaneously contracts. Rectal tone can be assessed at the same time. Priapism implies a complete spinal cord injury. The cremasteric reflex is tested by running a pin or a blunt instrument up the medial aspect of the thigh. If the scrotum rises, there is some spinal cord integrity. The area around the anus should be tested with a pin. An "anal wink" (contraction of the anal musculature) indicates at least some sacral sparing.

TABLE 256-2 Motor Grading System

0	No active contraction
1	Trace visible or palpable contraction
2	Movement with gravity eliminated
3	Movement against gravity
4	Movement against gravity plus resistance
5	Normal power

Diagnostic Imaging

Certainly one of the real dilemmas facing the clinician in the ED is identifying which patient requires evaluation for a potential spinal cord injury (Figure 256-7). Blind application of expensive diagnostic testing risks inappropriately increasing the cost of medical care and potentially rendering resources unavailable to other patients. Diagnostic testing must evaluate the possibility of injury to both bone and spinal cord. It is difficult to limit diagnostic testing to those who obviously require it. For example, removing a collar or allowing a patient to walk with an unstable spine risks converting a patient with no spinal cord injury to one with a complete level. Thus, it is prudent to completely image and evaluate all patients with the possibility of spinal cord pathology.

C-SPINE In general, an x-ray of the cervical spine is part of the standard triage for blunt trauma. Patients with possible head or neck trauma who are not fully alert [Glasgow Coma Scale (GCS) <15] should have imaging of their cervical spines. The frequency of cervical spine injury in association with blunt head trauma is approximately 2 to 5 percent. However, it increases to almost 9 percent in patients with significant head injury, defined as a GCS score <10.[13]

The utility of plain films of the cervical spine in patients who are alert, oriented, and have no neck or back pain or tenderness is questionable. The National Emergency X-Radiography Utilization Study (NEXUS) group identified five clinical criteria (absence of midline cervical tenderness; normal level of alertness; no evidence of intoxication; absence of focal neurologic deficit; absence of painful distracting injury) as factors that should be present to eliminate the performance of cervical radiographs.[14] The NEXUS criteria were 99 percent sensitive for detecting clinically significant cervical spine (C-spine) injuries. The specificity of the criteria, however, was only 12.9 percent, raising concerns that use of the NEXUS criteria would actually increase the use of radiography. The "Canadian C-Spine Rule for Radiography" was subsequently developed for alert, stable trauma patients to further reduce practice variation and inefficiency in ED use of C-spine radiography.[15] The Canadian Rule consists of three questions: 1) Are there any high-risk factors that mandate radiography? 2) Are there any low-risk factors that would allow a safe assessment of range of motion? and 3) Is the patient able to actively rotate the neck 45 degrees to the left and to the right? High-risk factors include age 65 years or older, a dangerous mechanism of injury (fall from a height of ≥1 m; an axial loading injury; high-speed motor vehicle crash, rollover, or ejection; motorized recreational vehicle or bicycle collision), or the presence of paresthesias in the extremities. Low-risk factors include simple rear-end motor vehicle crashes, patient able to sit up in the ED, patient ambulatory at any time, delayed onset of neck pain, or the absence of midline cervical tenderness. The Canadian C-Spine Rule had 100 percent sensitivity and 42.5 percent specificity for identifying patients with "clinically important" cervical spine injuries. Stiell et al. suggest that their rule could significantly reduce the use of C-spine radiographs ordered for alert, stable trauma patients.

The "gold standard" for the identification of bony cervical injury includes three views of the cervical spine: anteroposterior (AP), lateral, and odontoid. They allow for imaging of the entire cervical spine. It is important that all seven cervical vertebrae be imaged, including the junction between the seventh cervical and the first thoracic vertebrae. A single lateral cervical spine film will identify 90 percent of injuries to bone and ligaments.[16] The film must be examined for the presence or absence of prevertebral swelling. The prevertebral space anterior to C3 should be less than 5 mm. The predental space should be less than 3 mm. The open-mouth odontoid view will identify many of the remaining abnormalities. Cervical immobilization must be maintained until the patient also has an AP and open-mouth odontoid

FIG. 256-7. Algorithm for blunt spinal trauma.

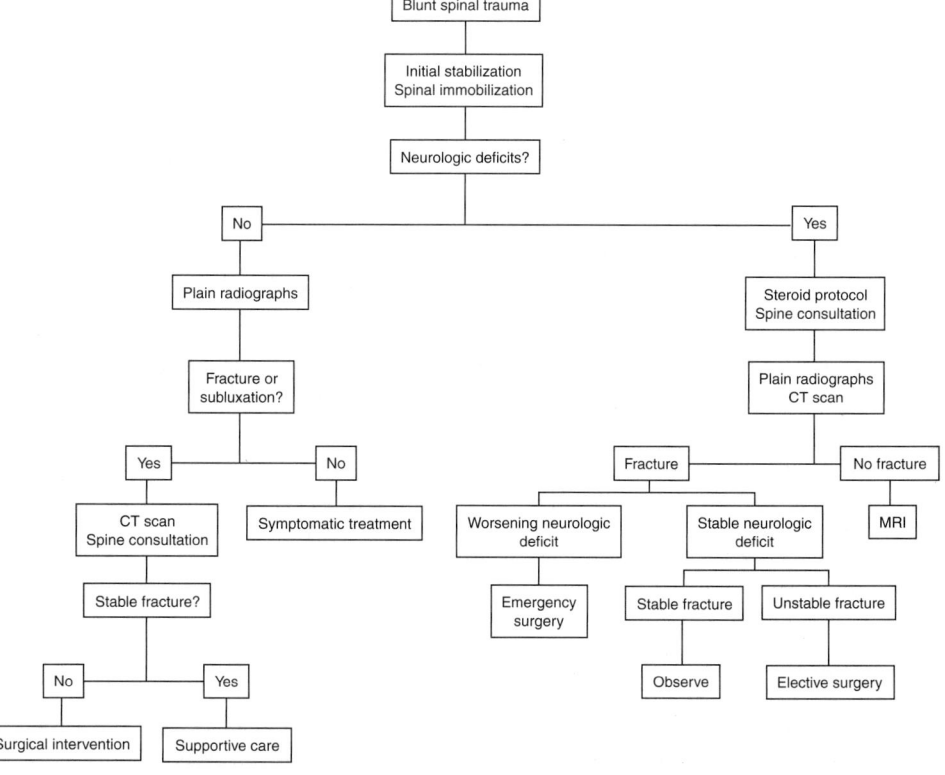

view. If the initial lateral view is normal and the patient is neurologically intact, the AP and open-mouth views can be delayed until other injuries are adequately stabilized. The combination of lateral, AP, and odontoid views is generally adequate to identify or at least raise the suspicion of cervical spine injury.

Alternatively, CT scanning can be used to visualize the entire cervical spine. Patients can have a cervical spine injury even with normal plain films. The current trend in many trauma centers is to CT the entire C-spine. Plain films are poor for imaging C_1 and C_2. The only possible advantage to plain films is for visualization of prevertebral swelling and spinous process. Further, visualization of the entire cervical spine via plain films often can be problematic. Patients' body habitus or the presence of upper-extremity injuries may limit the clinician's ability to pull on the arms, a maneuver necessary to visualize all seven vertebral bodies. An alternative is a swimmer's view, which is aimed through the axilla in an attempt to image the lower cervical spine. Oblique views (45 degrees) can also be obtained. These views have the added advantage of showing the neural foramina well. They demonstrate the pedicles as well as the laminae, which should stack like shingles on a roof. Plain and even CT films of the neck may not identify patients with pure ligamentous injuries. In these patients, ligaments are disrupted but the spine spontaneously reduces to a normal position. Motion, however, risks neurologic injury.

Flexion and extension views demonstrate the degree of spinal column stability. In general, these views are obtained when patients have pain or tenderness but normal plain films. They can only be obtained in a fully awake, unsedated, cooperative patient. The patient carefully and slowly flexes and extends the neck. Motion should be limited by increasing pain or the appearance of any neurologic symptomatology. A stepoff of 3.7 mm or an angulation of greater than 11 degrees denotes cervical spine instability.[17] It is possible to have ligamentous injury even with normal flexion/extension films, because muscle tone can splint the bones in a stable configuration. Most patients in this latter category note pain improvement with analgesics after a few days.

Reliable patients without a substantial mechanism of injury with persistent pain but normal radiographs, including flexion/extension views, can be discharged in a hard collar with outpatient follow-up in 3 to 5 days. Most patients' symptoms will resolve over a few days. A patient with persistent symptoms will require additional outpatient workup. Unreliable patients or those with a significant mechanism of injury or risk factors, such as advanced age, should undergo MRI although this is rarely indicated as part of the initial investigation.

THORACOLUMBAR SPINE Plain films of the thoracic and lumbar spine are the initial examinations generally used to image these spinal levels. Many of the same principles used for cervical spine imaging are important for thoracic and lumbar imaging. All patients with a mechanism of injury, those with complaints of back pain, and those who have tenderness on physical examination must be assumed to have a fracture of the thoracic or lumbar spine. They must be kept immobilized. AP and lateral films are generally obtained and examined for abnormality. In general, the lateral x-rays are much more easily obtained with patients still on a backboard. Skin breakdown and pressure sores can develop very quickly, particularly in obese patients. Our goal is to remove patients from the backboard in less than 2 h. Patients can then be nursed supine in a bed as long as they are logrolled. **A standard hospital mattress provides adequate spinal support.** However, patients must be carefully moved and care must be taken to keep spinal immobilization complete in transfers from bed to stretcher. It may be helpful to place patients back on a backboard for the transportation phases of their care. Alternatively, a scoop stretcher may be used for transport.

It can be difficult to image the upper thoracic spine adequately, even if maximal power of the x-ray beam is used. One alternative is to clear the reliable patient by physical examination. Unreliable or unexaminable patients with a concerning mechanism should be logrolled

until the thoracic spine can be appropriately evaluated. Patients with point tenderness and normal films are a special subset. CT scanning can be useful in this subset, although the yield is low. The thoracic spine has inherent stability from the rib cage. Few fractures in these patients will be unstable. Alternatively, patients can be treated with analgesics and investigated selectively if symptoms persist.

More recently, CT has assumed a much more important role in the imaging of spine injuries. Plain films can be imperfect and may miss a number of such patients. Newer-generation helical scanning is rapid, and CT allows for a complete three-dimensional imaging of bony structures. CT scanning is indicated in almost all patients with proven bony spinal injury, subluxations, for patients with neurologic deficits but no apparent abnormalities on plain films, those with severe neck or back pain and normal plain films, and those in whom the thoracic and lumbar spine should be examined to define the anatomy of a fracture and the extent of impingement on the spinal canal. CT can reveal the exact anatomy of an osseous injury, the extent of spinal canal impingement by bone fragments, and the stability of an injury. CT scans are indicated for all patients with fractures that can be seen on plain films. CT is especially useful when the lower cervical spine cannot be adequately visualized on plain films because of overlying soft tissues.

MRI MRI is not as sensitive as CT for detecting or delineating bone injuries. MRI is superb at defining neurologic, muscular, and soft tissue injury. It is the diagnostic test of choice for describing the anatomy of nerve injury. Entities such as herniated disks or spinal cord contusions are easily seen on MRI. Many of these require only supportive therapy. However, some require acute surgical intervention. Early identification helps plan therapy. MRI may also be used to identify ligamentous injury. MRI is indicated in patients with neurologic findings with no clear explanation following plain films and CT scanning. CT myelography is an alternative when MRI is unavailable and immediate diagnosis of a neurologic lesion is required. If the patient is neurologically stable and MRI is unavailable, delayed MRI and/or transfer to a tertiary care facility may be appropriate.

The determination of a spinal column injury at one level should prompt imaging of the remainder of the spine. Approximately 10 percent of patients with spine fracture in one segment will have a second fracture in another. Often plain films will suffice, but multilevel CT scanning and/or MRI may be necessary to investigate such patients completely.

TREATMENT

The goals of treatment are to prevent secondary injury, alleviate cord compression, and establish spinal stability. Spinal immobilization must be maintained, and movement kept to a minimum.

Once the patient is stabilized, it should be determined whether the patient has a neurologic deficit and/or the spinal column is unstable. If either of those conditions exists, subspecialty consultation should be requested emergently. The consultant, be it a neurosurgeon or orthopedic surgeon, must have the opportunity to perform a detailed neurologic examination early in the patient's course, so as to optimize outcome. In a few cases, this will be impossible if the patient requires intubation. Patients with progressive neurologic deterioration require urgent surgical intervention. The method of stabilization (collar or traction) must be determined, as must the need for further CT or MRI imaging.

Corticosteroids

Although controversial, the use of high-dose methylprednisolone presently remains the standard of care for the treatment of blunt spinal cord injury in the US. The National Acute Spinal Cord Injury Study (NASCIS) group conducted a series of multi-institutional studies to evaluate the efficacy of methylprednisolone in spinal trauma.[18]

Methylprednisolone infusion resulted in improvement of both motor and sensory function in patients with complete and incomplete neurologic lesions. This positive outcome was dependent upon dosage of steroids and time of administration. The current recommended steroid protocol for victims of spinal injury with neurologic deficits is as follows:

1. Treatment must be started within 8 h of injury.
2. Methylprednisolone (30 mg/kg) bolus administered IV over 15 min.
3. This is followed by a 45-min pause.
4. A maintenance infusion of methylprednisolone (5.4 mg/kg per h) is continued for 23 h.

NASCIS evaluated only blunt spinal cord injury. Patients with penetrating injuries were excluded from the study. **Massive steroid therapy has not been shown to be effective in penetrating spinal cord injury,** and in fact may impair recovery of neurologic function.[19]

The major neuroprotective mechanism by which high-dose methylprednisolone is believed to work is its inhibition of free radical-induced lipid peroxidation. Other proposed beneficial actions include its ability to increase levels of spinal cord blood flow, increase extracellular calcium, and prevent loss of potassium from injured cord tissue. Methylprednisolone is advocated in preference to other steroids because it crosses cell membranes more rapidly and completely.

Recent studies question the validity of the NASCIS trials and the effectiveness of high-dose steroid therapy in patients with spinal cord injury.[20,21] Potential complications associated with prolonged, high-dose steroids such as pneumonia, sepsis, wound infection, thromboembolism, gastrointestinal bleeding, and delayed healing are a frequently cited concern; however whether any of these concerns relate to a 23-h protocol has not been investigated to date.

Penetrating Injury

Treatment goals are the same for penetrating and blunt spinal injury. There are, however, additional considerations in penetrating trauma. Figure 256-8 shows an approach for gunshot wounds. Optimal treatment of these injuries has been the subject of debate. One concern is that of infectious complications related to the presence of foreign bodies. Additional contamination is associated with transperitoneal and transintestinal trajectories of gunshot wounds to the spine. Intravenous antibiotics should be given in the ED. Surgical débridement with laminectomy has not proven effective in reducing the incidence of infectious complications, as most are managed nonoperatively. If the patient requires laparotomy for abdominal trauma, irrigation and débridement of the spinal injury through the missile tract may be appropriate.[8]

As with blunt trauma, there is general agreement that progressive neurologic deficits warrant surgical decompression. The indication for removal of bullet and bone fragments in those patients with nonprogressive neurologic deficits is less clear. Wound location may determine the need for surgical intervention. Bullet removal does not significantly improve the neurologic status of patients with stable cervical and thoracic spinal cord lesions. In contrast, bullet removal from the thoracolumbar spine may significantly improve motor recovery in both complete and incomplete injuries.[22] Most gunshot wounds to the spine following penetrating trauma are stable and require only symptomatic treatment with a supportive orthosis and analgesics.

Patients who present with stab wounds to the spinal region with no neurologic deficits should receive antibiotics and local wound care. Plain films and/or CT scan may be performed to evaluate for a retained foreign body, but the literature is controversial as to whether or

FIG. 256-8. Algorithm for gunshot to spine.

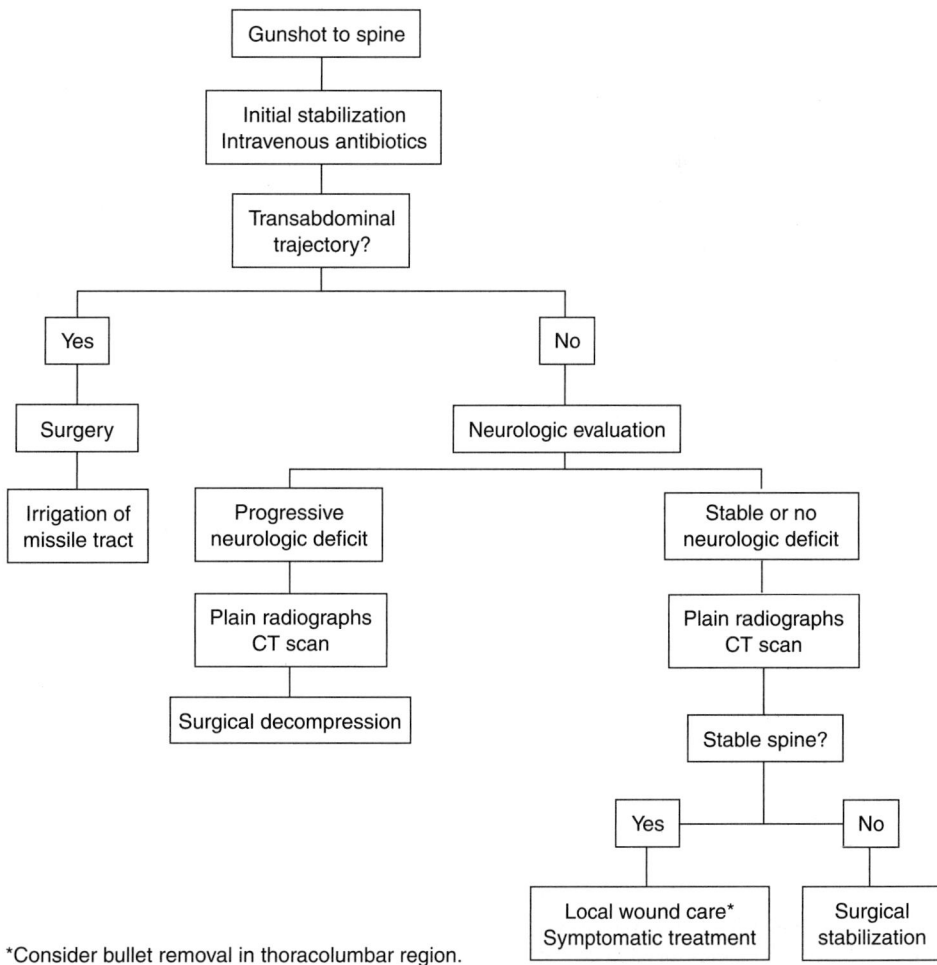

*Consider bullet removal in thoracolumbar region.

not to surgically remove the blade if there are no or stable neurologic deficits. If no metallic foreign bodies are present, neurologic deficits are best evaluated with MRI. Progressive neurologic deficits are generally treated surgically.

Chap. 258 details approaches to stab wounds to the neck. Significant spinal injuries are related to direct penetration of spinal cord neural elements, spinal infarction, or, rarely, from a spinal epidural hematoma. Vertebral instability is not an issue per se. Delayed deficits are rare. When they do occur, they are related to retained fragment of blade within the spinal canal.

Nonoperative Spinal Stabilization

The goal of stabilization is to reduce deformities and then restrict motion and maintain alignment. In the cervical spine, it is important to determine the adequacy of cervical bony reduction. Subluxations are generally reduced using Gardner–Wells tongs, which are placed into the soft tissue of the temples under local anesthesia. The location and type of injury determine the amount of weight applied. The upper cervical spine generally requires less weight for traction than the lower cervical spine. Depending upon location, initial weight should be started at 5 to 10 lb. Weight should be increased in 2.5- to 5-lb increments. Ideally, this should be done under fluoroscopic guidance. If fluoroscopy is unavailable, radiographs and neurologic examinations should be performed after each increment of weight. The radiographs should be evaluated for alignment of the spinal column and to ensure that overdistraction has not occurred. Neurologic performance can improve if reduction is achieved. Inability to achieve adequate reduction is an indication for early spinal decompression and fusion.

Spinal orthoses are used to immobilize well-reduced cervical fractures. The cervical spine is the region most effectively stabilized by external splinting devices. There is less soft tissue separating the brace from the spine at this level. In addition, some braces can be solidly secured by fixation points at the cranium and the thoracic cage. Cervical orthoses consist of cervical and cervicothoracic types. Cervical collars fit around the neck and contour to the mandible and occiput. They restrict flexion and extension in the middle and lower cervical spine. Lateral bending and rotational movements, however, are poorly controlled. Examples of cervical orthoses include the hard collar, the Philadelphia collar, and the Miami J collar. Cervicothoracic braces provide additional support. The "gold standard" is the halo cervical immobilizer, which provides the most rigid stabilization. Consisting of a halo ring pinned to the skull, a vest, and upright posts, it can be used for traction and reduction of unstable fractures as well as immobilization.

Immobilization of the upper thoracic spine by orthoses is difficult. Fortunately, an intact rib cage and sternum provide relative stability. Although brace immobilization is not always necessary in the treatment of these fractures, braces can provide additional comfort. Thoracic corsets provide minimal control of motion and are appropriate only for minor injuries. Jewett and Taylor braces provide intermediate control of spinal motion. Maximum limitation of motion is provided by the Risser jacket and the body cast.

The thoracolumbar junction and lower lumbar regions are also difficult to immobilize externally. Splints are limited by lack of an adequate caudal fixation point. The functions of most thoracolumbosacral orthoses are the following: to create an awareness and remind the patient to restrict movements, to support the abdomen and relieve some of the load on the lumbosacral spine, to provide some restriction of motion of the upper lumbar and thoracolumbar spine by three-point fixation, and to reduce lumbar lordosis in order to provide a straighter, more comfortable lower back.

Complications of external immobilization devices include pain, pressure, muscle weakness and disuse atrophy, venous compromise, psychological dependence, ineffective stabilization, and pin-site complications (halo vest) (see Chap. 236 for ED evaluation).

Operative Management of Spine Injuries

The indication for operative stabilization is somewhat controversial and varies from institution to institution. Those favoring an aggressive approach stress the importance of early mobilization of the multiply injured patient as it helps decrease pulmonary problems, skin breakdown, deep venous thrombosis, and pulmonary embolus. Rigid fixation may also decrease time in hospital as well as long-term pain and deformities.

Those advocating a nonoperative approach point out the possibility of worsening neurologic performance by operative manipulation. In addition, the long-term results with operative intervention may not be substantially better than with nonoperative therapy.

All would agree that progressive neurologic deterioration is an indication for urgent surgery. In addition, spinal instability should most often be managed operatively even in the case of a complete spinal cord level. This helps prevent long-term deformity.

REFERENCES

1. Burney RE, Maio RF, Maynard F, et al: Incidence, characteristics, and outcome of spinal cord injury at trauma centers in North America. *Arch Surg* 128:596, 1993.
2. White AA, Panjabi MM: *Clinical Biomechanics of the Spine,* 3rd ed. Philadelphia, Lippincott, 1990.
3. Denis F: The three column spine and its significance in the classification of acute thoracolumbar spinal injuries. *Spine* 8:817, 1983.
4. Woodring JH, Lee C, Jenkins K: Spinal fractures in blunt chest trauma. *J Trauma* 28:789, 1988.
5. Denis F, Davis S, Comfort T: Sacral fractures: An important problem. Retrospective analysis of 236 cases. *Clin Orthop* 227:67, 1988.
6. Scalea T, Goldstein A, Phillips T, et al: An analysis of 161 falls from a height: The "jumper syndrome." *J Trauma* 26:706, 1986.
7. Tall RL, De Valut W: Spinal injury in sport: Epidemiologic considerations. *Clin Sports Med* 12:441, 1993.
8. Kihtir T, Ivatury RR, Simon R, et al: Management of transperitoneal gunshot wounds of the spine. *J Trauma* 31:1579, 1991.
9. Bosch A, Stauffer ES, Nickel VL: Incomplete traumatic quadriplegia: A ten-year review. *JAMA* 216:473, 1971.
10. American College of Surgeons: *The Advanced Trauma Life Support Course.* Chicago, American College of Surgeons, 2003.
11. Soderstrom C, McArdle DQ, Ducker TB, Militello PR: The diagnosis of intra-abdominal injury in patients with cervical cord trauma. *J Trauma* 23:1061, 1983.
12. Zipnick R, Scalea TM, Trooskin SZ, et al: Hemodynamic responses to penetrating spinal cord injuries. *J Trauma* 35:578, 1993.
13. Bayless P, Ray VG: Incidence of cervical spine injuries in association with blunt head trauma. *Am J Emerg Med* 7:139, 1989.
14. Hoffman JR, Mower WR, Wolfson AB, et al: Validity of a set of clinical criteria to rule out injury to the cervical spine in patients with blunt trauma. *New Engl J Med* 343:94, 2000.
15. Stiell IG, Wells GA, Vandemheen KL, et al: The Canadian C-spine rule for radiography in alert and stable trauma patients. *JAMA* 286:1841, 2001.
16. MacDonald RL, Schwartz ML, Mirich D, et al: Diagnosis of cervical spine injury in motor vehicle crash victims: How many x-rays are enough? *J Trauma* 30(4):392, 1990.
17. Panjabi MM, Tech D, White AA: Basic biomechanics of the spine. *Neurosurgery* 7:76, 1980.
18. Bracken MB, Shepard MJ, Collins WF, et al: A randomized, controlled trial of methylprednisolone or naloxone in the treatment of acute spinal cord injury: Results of the second national acute spinal cord injury study. *New Engl J Med* 322:1405, 1990.
19. Prendergast MR, Saxe JM, Ledgerwood AM, et al: Massive steroids do not reduce the zone of injury after penetrating spinal cord injury. *J Trauma* 37:576, 1994.
20. Nesathurai S: Steroids and spinal cord injury: Revisiting the NASCIS 2 and NASCIS 3 trials. *J Trauma* 45:1088, 1998.
21. Short DJ, El Masry WS, Jones PW: High-dose methylprednisolone in the management of acute spinal cord injury—A systematic review from a clinical perspective. *Spinal Cord* 38:273, 2000.
22. Waters RL, Adkins RH: The effects of removal of bullet fragments retained in the spinal canal. A collaborative study by the National Spinal Cord Injury Model Systems. *Spine* 16:934, 1991.

MAXILLOFACIAL TRAUMA
Nael Hasan
Stephen A. Colucciello

ETIOLOGY/INCIDENCE

Up to 60 percent of patients with severe facial injuries have multisystem trauma and have potential for airway compromise. The etiology of facial fractures varies between urban and rural environments. Penetrating trauma and assault-related injuries are more common in cities, whereas motor vehicle crash (MVC), sporting, and other recreational injuries are seen frequently in rural hospitals. In community emergency departments, fractures of the nose and mandible are most common; in trauma centers, however, midface and zygomatic injuries are more frequent. Domestic violence and elder and child abuse are important causes of facial trauma. Facial injury accounts for the majority of emergency department visits related to domestic violence. As many as one-fourth of women with facial trauma are victims of domestic violence.[1] **If a woman has an orbital fracture, the likelihood of sexual assault or domestic violence rises** to more than 30 percent.[2] Falls are also an important cause of facial injury in the very young and the elderly.

Potential injuries associated with facial trauma are those of the head, cervical spine, and eye. As many as 20 to 50 percent of victims of facial trauma sustain concurrent brain injury, especially those with upper face and midface fractures.

Although most series show no increased incidence in cervical spine injury with facial trauma (1–4 percent), this is of statistical interest only. One must consider possible spinal injury in all patients with significant or suspected maxillofacial fractures because it takes considerable force to shatter the midface or upper face. Factors that may increase the likelihood of cervical spine injury in this population are older age, MVCs, and concomitant brain injury.[3] Maxillofacial trauma by itself can be a "distracting injury" that masks cervical spine injury. Always exclude cervical spine injury clinically and/or radiographically in such patients. One study has linked carotid artery injury to severe facial trauma.[4]

Periorbital fractures may be associated with globe disruption or blindness. The dangerous triad of limited extraocular movement, limited visual acuity, and limited visual fields should be evaluated in all patients with facial injuries.

Blindness occurs in 0.5 to 3 percent of patients with facial fractures and is most frequent in patients with Le Fort III (2.2 percent), Le Fort II (0.64 percent), and zygomatic fractures (0.45 percent).[5] MVCs and gunshot injuries are responsible for most cases of visual loss.

In addition to the physical consequences of facial trauma, there are psychological costs as well. More than one-quarter of patients with significant facial trauma may develop posttraumatic stress disorder.[6]

ANATOMY

The facial buttresses, bony arches joined by suture lines, provide vertical and horizontal support. The main purpose of these buttresses is to withstand vertical stresses associated with mastication, accomplished by the strong zygomaticomaxillary buttress laterally and the frontal process of the maxilla medially. In contrast, the horizontal support is weak and consists of the superior orbital rims, orbital floor, and hard palate. Hence frontal, lateral, and oblique forces tend to produce facial fractures. Sutures linking these facial bones rupture in predictable fashion during trauma. Knowledge of their location enables one to palpate these sutures to detect diastasis or tenderness.

Sutures found at borders of the sphenoid wings, pterygoid plate, and the zygomatic arch anchor the face to the skull. These are the structures disrupted in Le Fort injuries (Figure 257-1). The most complex aspect of facial anatomy is the orbit, an elaborate structure comprised of seven different bones: maxilla, zygoma, frontal, sphenoid, palatine, ethmoid, and lacrimal. Between these bones lie the orbital foramina, through which course cranial nerves II, III, and VI and branches of cranial nerve V. The weakest portions of the orbit are the floor and medial wall, which are the thickness of an eggshell. Rupture of orbital bones may compress the fissures and cause blindness through traction, rupture, or compression of the optic nerves.

PREHOSPITAL CARE

The major concern in prehospital care is control of the airway. In severe midfacial injuries, loss of bony support may result in both collapse of the pharynx and loss of periorbital stability, making use of the bag-valve mask problematic. A nasal airway or laryngeal mask airway (LMA) can help splint the upper airway, as well as sitting the patient up or leaning the patient forward if needed, always being conscious of potential cervical spine injury. The mouth should be cleared of any foreign body or debris and suctioned of blood. The tongue may block the airway, and a jaw thrust or modified chin lift without neck extension often relieves the obstruction. With severe mandible fractures, these maneuvers may not elevate the tongue, necessitating other techniques (see "Airway," below). Prehospital providers should immobilize the cervical spine using standard indications. If there is copious bleeding and massive facial injury, early notification allows the emergency department to prepare for a difficult airway.

EMERGENCY MANAGEMENT: RESUSCITATION

The compelling and sometimes grotesque nature of facial injuries must not distract physicians from following the routine, sequential trauma protocol. The most urgent complication of facial trauma is not shock but airway compromise, particularly with midfacial and lower facial trauma. Prior to detailed evaluation, some presentations require immediate attention, as detailed below.

Airway

Simple intervention, such as the chin lift without neck extension, jaw thrust, and oropharyngeal suctioning, often clears the airway. In mandibular fractures, however, loss of bony support may result in a *flail mandible,* leaving the tongue to obstruct the airway. In this case, the mouth should be opened and the tongue pulled forward with a gauze pad, towel clip, or a large suture placed through the anterior tongue. When the cervical spine has been cleared, clinically or radiographically, it is best to allow the patient to sit up and lean forward and to give the patient a tonsil-tip suction. This position may be lifesaving in patients with significant mandible fractures. Patients who do not respond to simple maneuvers may require intubation.

Intubation Considerations

Because the cribriform plate may be disrupted, avoid nasotracheal intubation in patients with midface trauma. Nasotracheal intubation can result in nasocranial intubation or dramatic nasal hemorrhage. Admittedly, these complications are rare, and some patients have been intubated successfully using the nasotracheal route. Nonetheless, orotracheal intubation is preferred and is often successful even with severely distorted facial anatomy.

Rapid-sequence intubation carries particular risk in facial trauma. These dangers include the failure to intubate and subsequent failure to ventilate with a bag-valve mask. Before paralyzing any patient, evaluate the degree of difficulty anticipated for mask ventilation. Patients with distortion of the maxilla or mandible may be impossible to bag because the mask will not fit tightly on an unstable face.

In such cases, consider an awake intubation. Options include sedation with a benzodiazepine, ketamine, or other induction agent in a

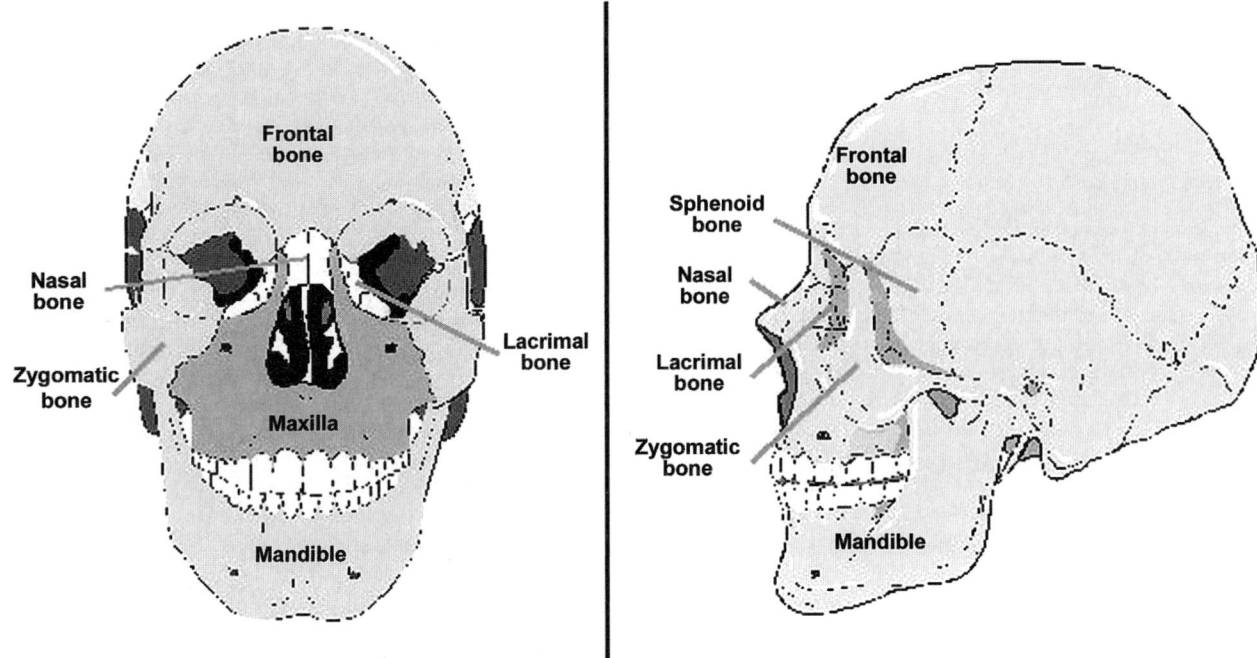

FIG. 257-1. Coronal and lateral facial bone anatomy. [Reprinted with permission from Isenhour J, Colucciello S: Maxillofacial trauma, in Ferrera P et al (eds): *Trauma Management*. St. Louis: Mosby, 2000.]

dose that minimizes respiratory depression. If a patient with severe maxillofacial trauma is given paralytics, prepare for immediate backup cricothyroidotomy. *Preparation* in this case implies more than locating a surgical tray: It extends to povidone-iodine on the neck, a ready blade, an opened cricothyroidotomy tray, and a tracheostomy tube at the bedside. The LMA has emerged as an excellent bridge to intubation or surgical airway in the operative theater, provided the hypopharynx remains intact. Some authors describe creative approaches to intubation in facial trauma. Fiberoptic intubation with patients in the semiprone position may be useful in penetrating injuries of the face. The traditional supine intubating position may be impossible with a ruined maxilla that falls into the airway. Such airways may clear when a patient lies on his or her side (although this may be both awkward and disconcerting to the physician).

Other alternatives include percutaneous transtracheal ventilation and retrograde intubation as a temporizing measure. Both require considerable preparation, and the most dependable alternative airway is surgical. Emergency cricothyroidotomy, being faster and associated with fewer complications, is preferable to emergency tracheostomy.

Hemorrhage Control

Patients rarely develop shock from facial bleeding.[7] In hypotensive patients, other sources of blood loss, such as intrathoracic, intra-abdominal, and retroperitoneal hemorrhage, should be sought. Maxillofacial bleeding is controlled with direct pressure. Clamping in wounds is avoided because important structures such as the facial nerve or parotid duct may be injured. Severe pharyngeal bleeding may require packing of the pharynx and hypopharynx around a cuffed endotracheal tube. In patients with Le Fort fractures, manual reduction of the face should stem bleeding. Grasp the anterior hard palate at the maxillary arch, and realign the fragments.

Severe nasal bleeding requires direct pressure to the nares or combined posterior and anterior packing, taking care not to inadvertently pack the cranium. In the case of massive nasopharyngeal bleeding, a balloon-tipped urinary catheter placed along the floor of the nose and inflated with saline may be lifesaving. Nasopharyngeal dual-lumen balloons and packs impregnated with procoagulant factors are also available commercially for this purpose.

Once the airway is secure and gross hemorrhage controlled, the potential existence of other life threats in the chest, abdomen, and pelvis are sought.

HISTORY

It is important to determine the mechanism and time of injury and to assess for loss of consciousness. The addition of airbags to automobiles is associated with less severe maxillofacial injuries compared with either seatbelt use alone or no restraint.[8] Allergies and tetanus status are standard inquires.

The following essential three face-oriented questions target eye involvement, injury to facial nerves, and alignment of central and lower face:

"How is your vision?"
"Is any part of your face numb?"
"Are your teeth meeting normally?"

Monocular double vision occurs with lens dislocation or with corneal or retinal injury, whereas binocular double vision implies dysfunction of the extraocular muscles or nerves. Pain on eye movement suggests injury to the orbit or globe.

If the mechanism of injury is not an MVC, ask women about domestic violence. Although a victim of domestic violence may tell the triage nurse that she fell or "ran into a door," many patients reveal the true etiology if questioned directly by a physician. Child abuse and elder abuse are important considerations when patients at the extremes of age present with facial trauma. **More than half of all abused children are injured in the head, face, mouth, or neck.**[9]

PHYSICAL EXAMINATION

Inspection

The patient is viewed initially from the front. Facial elongation occurs with high-grade Le Fort fractures (the so-called donkey face). Next, the face is viewed from above looking down (bird's-eye view) and from below up (worm's-eye view). These perspectives reveal subtle asymmetries. Because posttraumatic Bell palsy occurs with fractures of the temporal bone, particular attention should be paid to the cranial nerve. Ecchymoses around the eyes (raccoon's eyes) and over the mastoid area (Battle sign) are associated with basilar skull fracture. These findings usually develop over several hours and often are absent on admission despite serious facial trauma. Raccoon's eyes can be seen with nasoethmoidal-orbital injuries, Le Fort fractures, and frontal bone fractures, as well as with direct periorbital and nasal trauma.

Palpation

Palpation will disclose the majority of facial fractures. The entire face should be palpated carefully for tenderness, bony crepitus, and subcutaneous air. The presence of subcutaneous air is pathognomonic for fracture of a sinus wall or nose.

Particular attention should be paid to vulnerable sutures such as those on the infraorbital rim and the zygomaticofrontal suture located on the upper lateral aspect of the orbit. Simultaneous palpation of the zygomatic arches will reveal any asymmetry. The best way to distinguish tenderness of the soft tissues of the cheek from bony tenderness is by intraoral palpation. A gloved finger is placed inside the patient's mouth and on the buccal surface of the upper molars (outside the teeth). The examining finger is placed under the zygomatic arch. This method will identify displacement or collapse of the arch.

To assess facial stability, with the patient's mouth open, the maxillary arch is grasped (*not* the central incisors—which might pull out). Le Fort fractures are best diagnosed by rocking the maxillary arch and simultaneously feeling the central face for movement with the opposite hand.

Although anesthesia of the face may be secondary to nerve contusion, it often signifies a fracture. Damage to the infraorbital nerve (often due to blowout or rim fractures) results in anesthesia of the ipsilateral upper lip, nasal mucosa at the vestibule, lower eyelid, and maxillary teeth. Lower lip and lower dental anesthesia can occur with mandibular fractures.

Periorbital and Orbital Examination

The eye examination deserves particular attention, especially when there is periorbital injury. The examination should be performed early during the emergency department encounter, before progressive lid edema prevents appropriate examination. If lids are already swollen, lid retractors help visualize the globe. The bird's-eye and worm's-eye views help detect exophthalmos or enophthalmos.

The pupil is examined for reactivity and whether the pupils line up in the horizontal plane. A teardrop-shaped pupil indicates a ruptured or otherwise penetrated globe in patients without preexisting iridectomy. Hyphema may be apparent only when the patient is sitting. The presence of a hyphema correlates with significant visual loss. The Snellen chart, either standard or hand-held, if feasible to administer, should be used to document visual acuity. If the patient cannot see the chart, record finger counting or, barring that, the presence or absence of light perception. Early recognition of traumatic optic neuropathy should trigger an emergency consultation because timely decompressive surgery may prevent blindness.

The best way to detect damage to the optic nerve or retina (afferent defect) is the swinging-flashlight test. An abnormal pupil (Marcus Gunn) initially dilates (rather than constricts) when first exposed to a light that swings between both eyes.

Subconjunctival hemorrhage is often present with periorbital fractures, and lateral hemorrhage frequently accompanies zygomatic fractures. Soft tissue bruising provides other important clues.

With severe periorbital trauma, it is important to measure the distance between the medial canthi. In average adults, the intercanthal distance should be 35 to 40 mm—or approximately the width of a patient's eye.

Widening of this distance is called *telecanthus* and portends serious orbital injury. In patients with telecanthus, the bridge of the nose appears wide, but the distance between the pupils is unchanged. This is usually seen with nasoethmoidal-orbital trauma. A more serious condition known as *hypertelorism* occurs when the interpupillary distance increases. In this case, the orbits are dislocated and literally "blown apart." This devastating injury usually results in blindness.

Extraocular motions must be evaluated for restriction. Fractures of the zygomatic and infraorbital floor frequently cause diplopia, especially on upward gaze. Significant pain with extraocular motions provides a clue to occult injury.

Palpate the entire orbit for tenderness, subcutaneous air, and deformity. Inexperienced physicians frequently neglect the superior and lateral rims. Despite no palpable external deformity, fractures of the orbit occur quite often as a result of transmission of traumatic forces from the thicker external bone to the thinner and weaker bone of the orbital wall and floor.

Bimanual Palpation Test

One of the most important concerns is the status of the medial orbital area (the nasoethmoidal-orbital complex). Consider this injury if the medial canthus is tender or if the patient has telecanthus. When suspected, the bimanual nasal palpation test is a helpful adjunct (Figure 257-2).

To perform this test, the nose is anesthetized with either cocaine or lidocaine. A clamp or long cotton swab is then inserted into nose. The clamp or swab is pressed intranasally against the medial orbital rim (just inside the medial canthus). Simultaneously, the other hand is pressed against the medial canthus. If the bone moves, the complex is fractured. With telecanthus or severe medial canthal tenderness, this test may be omitted in favor of primary computed tomographic (CT) scanning.

Penetrating Injuries

With periorbital penetrating injuries, consider occult globe penetration. When the orbital septum is violated, fat protrudes from the wound, signaling possible globe perforation. Injuries to the medial third of the eyelids should be considered high risk for damage to the lacrimal apparatus. Lid lacerations should be evaluated for disruption of levator palpebral muscle and tarsal plate.

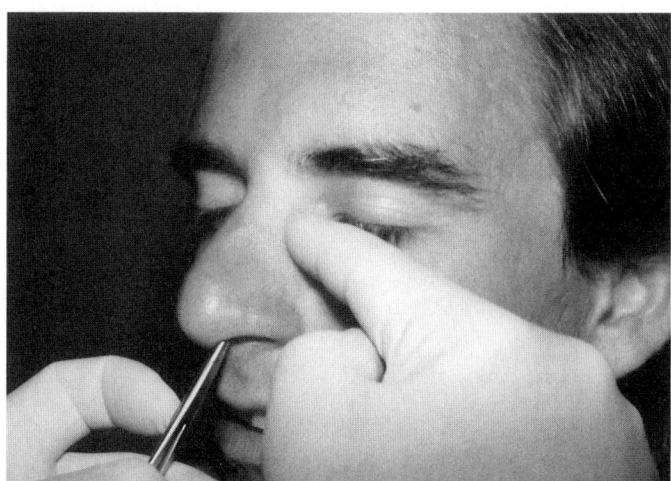

FIG. 257-2. Intranasal palpation test. [Reprinted with permission from Isenhour J, Colucciello S: Maxillofacial trauma, in Ferrera P et al (eds): *Trauma Management.* St. Louis: Mosby, 2000.]

Nose

The nose is inspected from various angles to detect any deformity. Posttraumatic edema often obscures nasal deviation. The patient can assist in the examination by identifying preexisting nasal deformity. Palpation will detect crepitus, subtle deformity, and subcutaneous air. The two most important potential findings are septal hematoma and cerebrospinal fluid (CSF) rhinorrhea. Septal hematoma appears as a bluish, bulging mass on a widened septum. If there is a doubt, the septum can be palpated with a cotton swab to appreciate the doughy swelling.

CSF mixed with blood forms a double ring or *halo sign* when dropped on a paper towel or a bed sheet. This occurs because blood and CSF have different diffusion properties. This finding is *not* specific for CSF and will occur with trauma-related rhinorrhea. Both CSF and simple rhinorrhea can contain glucose.[10]

Ears

The pinna is inspected for subperichondral hematoma. The ear canals should be inspected for lacerations and CSF leak. Hemotympanum appears as a purple (not red), often bulging eardrum. Tympanic membrane ruptures are also seen in conjunction with fractures of the mandibular condyle. In the presence of a basilar skull fracture, the mastoid area may be ecchymotic (Battle sign.)

Oral and Mandibular Examination

During inspection, the jaw is observed for any deviation, which results from either a condylar fracture or dislocation. Malocclusion may indicate Le Fort fractures, and patients may be unable to close the mouth due to premature occlusion of the molars. Zygomatic fractures also prevent jaw closure if the bone fragment either presses against the masseter or impinges on the coronoid process of the mandible. Fracture-associated nerve injury may result in anesthesia of the lips and gingiva.

An intraoral examination may reveal significant pathology. The examination should include manipulation of each tooth, a search for intraoral lacerations, and stress of the mandible. Essentially all fractures can be detected or excluded by both palpating and stressing the jaw. By placing a finger in the external ear canal while a patient opens and closes the mouth, one can palpate the mandibular condyle during jaw motion.

Tongue-Blade Test

The tongue blade, or spatula, test is a useful technique to detect mandibular fractures (Figure 257-3). Although unnecessary in patients with an obvious fracture, it enables physicians to determine the need for x-rays in patients with jaw pain and no obvious instability. The patient should be asked to bite down forcefully on a tongue blade. The physician then twists the tongue blade in an attempt to break the blade. Patients with a broken jaw will reflexively open their mouth, whereas those with an intact mandible will break the blade. In one study, this test was more than 95 percent sensitive and nearly 65 percent specific for mandibular fracture.[11]

IMAGING

The choice and timing of radiographic studies depend on the clinical stability of the patient. Management of head, chest, and abdominal trauma takes precedence over facial imaging. In the critically injured, diagnostic imaging of the face, including a CT scan, may be deferred for days, until the patient's condition has stabilized.

It is not always clear which patients require facial imaging. In one study, physical examination alone detected 90 percent of clinically significant fractures.[12] However, management was altered in 17 percent of patients based on either CT scan or plain films.[12]

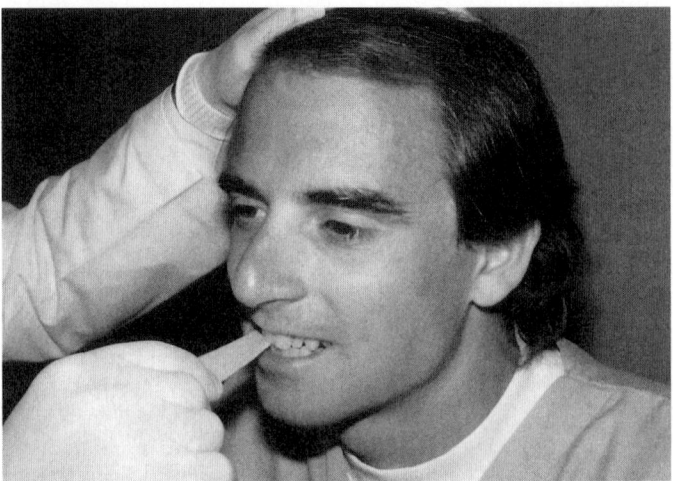

FIG. 257-3. Tongue blade test. [Reprinted with permission from Isenhour J, Colucciello S: Maxillofacial trauma, in Ferrera P, et al (eds): *Trauma Management.* St. Louis: Mosby, 2000.]

Plain Films

Plain films are useful screens for maxillofacial injury and are available in all hospitals. For the uninitiated, the numerous overlapping lines and complex shadows make interpretation challenging. However, becoming adept at reading plain films of the face (in particular the Waters view) can be a time-saving and cost-effective screening tool.[13]

One of the most useful approaches is to assess symmetry. Consider the right and left sides as mirror images. Assymetry is sought for lucencies or shadows, sutures and sinuses. The film is further examined for bony integrity and subcutaneous air. While air-fluid levels in the sinuses may occur with acute sinusitis, in the presence of trauma they are nearly pathognomonic for sinus fracture. Clouding of a sinus may be secondary to soft tissue swelling or due to complete filling of the sinus with blood. When seen in the superior aspect of the maxillary sinus, a soft tissue density may represent herniation of orbital contents through the orbital floor (Figure 257-4).

Radiographic Views of the Face

The Waters or occipital-mental view is the single most valuable study of the midface. Several recent studies have found a single Waters view to be as sensitive as the entire plain-film facial series.[13,14] In one prospective study, the Waters view identified all significant facial fractures, and CT scan of the face was used only to further delineate complex injuries.[15] It evaluates continuity of orbital rims, provides an initial diagnosis of blowout fractures, and will demonstrate air/fluid levels in the maxillary sinus.

The posteroanterior (PA or Caldwell) view, which best details the bones of the upper face, confirms ethmoidal and frontal sinus fractures, as well as lateral orbital injuries.

Cross-table or upright lateral views are difficult to read and are not very helpful. On occasion, they suggest elongation of the face in Le Fort injuries or disruption of the posterior sinus wall. Look for air-fluid levels in sphenoid or ethmoidal sinuses.

The submental-vertex view, known colloquially as the "jug handle" or zygomatic arch view, shows the base of the skull and the zygomatic arches. It may be the only film necessary for suspected arch fractures.

The Towne view is useful for evaluating the mandibular ramus and condyles, as well as the base of the skull. Regarding the mandible, if a Panorex view is unavailable, a four-view mandibular plain-film series can serve as an adequate substitute.[16]

Computed Tomography

CT scans provide a conclusive diagnosis of complex maxillofacial fractures. Its greatest utility lies in evaluating patients with known or

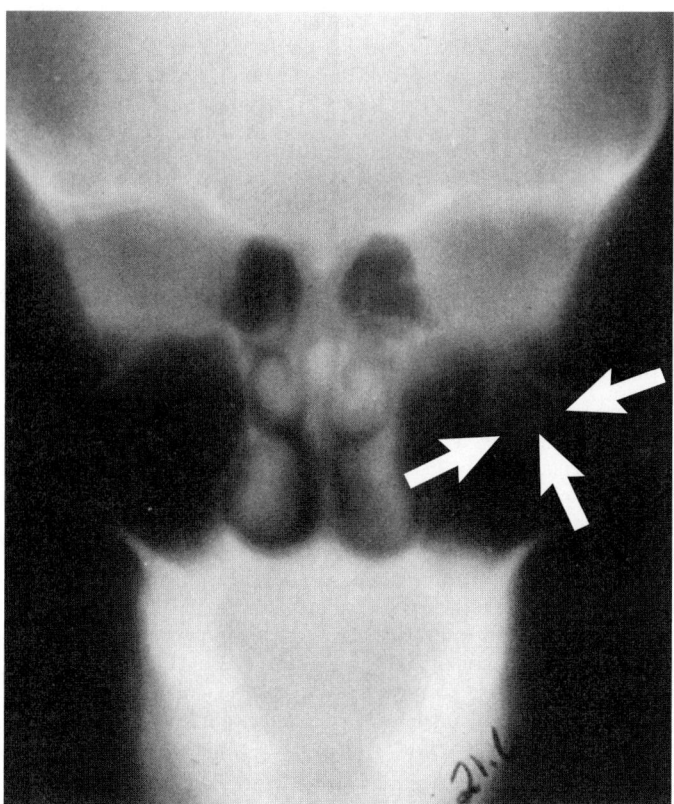

FIG. 257-4. Orbital tomogram showing classical "teardrop" herniation of orbital tissue into the maxillary sinus *(arrows)*.

suspected periorbital and midface fractures. Scans are especially useful to evaluate the globe and orbital fissures. Specialized views—such coronal, sagittal, or parasagittal cuts, thin-slice scans, and three-dimensional reconstruction—are useful in particular circumstances. In general, the slices should be in a plane 90 degrees to that of the suspected fracture—not parallel to the fracture line. A three-dimensional CT scan is superior to a two-dimensional CT scan for serious midface fractures, such as tripod and complex maxillary fractures.

Multiply injured patients, who are intubated, unconscious, or sedated, frequently have significant and unsuspected facial fractures. If they require a CT scan of the head, consider adding a scan of the face for clinically stable patients. Slightly more than 10 percent of such patients may have unsuspected facial fractures needing surgical repair. However, an unstable patient with severe concomitant injuries should not receive a facial scan if it delays emergency surgery.

Computed tomography with various manipulations, such as coronal and axial views, is essential for management of particular complex fractures. However, plain films still have an important role in screening for maxillofacial injury. In stable patients, physical examination along with a single Waters view may be enough for identifying maxillofacial fractures, augmented by CT scanning as needed.[15] In the case of clinically obvious, complex facial injuries (in particular, periorbital and midface fractures), plain films may be eliminated and computed tomography performed directly. Coronal films should be ordered for periorbital fractures, and thin-slice scans may be appropriate in this area.

Magnetic Resonance Imaging

Magnetic resonance imaging (MRI) is useful to consultants who wish to visualize the soft tissues of the face, particularly the optic nerve or retrobulbar hemorrhage. MRI does *not* adequately delineate fractures, however. It does not have a defined role in emergency department evaluation.

SPECIFIC FACIAL FRACTURES

Frontal Sinus/Frontal Bone Fractures

This injury commonly results from a direct blow to the frontal bone with a blunt object—classically a lead pipe or brick. This fracture is frequently associated with intracranial injury secondary to disruption of the posterior table of the sinus. Dural tears are frequent, and patients may have associated injuries to the orbital roof (leading to blindness), as well as to the brain.[17] Late complications include cranial empyema or mucopyoceles. Mucopyoceles are collections of pus and mucus that occur when fractures block the nasal frontal duct, preventing sinus drainage.

Physical examination may reveal disruption or crepitance of the supraorbital rims or subcutaneous emphysema. Fractures often are overlooked because of traditional prohibitions against skull films for head trauma. Patients with a suggestive mechanism or examination benefit from skull films or a Caldwell view of the face. If a depressed or posterior wall fracture is seen on plain film, a CT scan is required. Patients with hard signs of a frontal bone fracture (subcutaneous air, bony step-off, etc.) require only a CT scan.

Consultation with an otolaryngologist or a neurosurgeon is advised regarding antibiotic use in patients with frontal sinus fractures. Many specialists recommend antibiotics that cover common sinus pathogens, although the literature lacks definitive evidence on this issue. Frequently prescribed antibiotics include first-generation cephalosporins, amoxicillin-clavulanate, erythromycin, and trimethoprim-sulfamethoxazole. Patients with depressed fractures or those who have posterior wall involvement require intravenous antibiotics, admission, and consultation. Those with isolated fracture of the anterior wall may be treated as outpatients.

Nasoethmoidal-Orbital Injuries

Suspect nasoethmoidal-orbital injuries in those with trauma to the bridge of the nose or medial orbital wall (see Figure 257-1). The mechanism of injury is usually dramatic, and these fractures are frequently associated with lacrimal disruption and dural tears. Patients may complain of pain on eye movement, and physical examination may reveal traumatic telecanthus or epiphora (tears spilling over the lid).

If the medial canthus is tender, the intranasal palpation test is performed (see Figure 257-2) and examined for CSF rhinorrhea. If the examination is suggestive, order a CT scan of the face to include coronal sections and thin axial slices through the medial orbital wall.

If a nasoethmoidal-orbital fracture is present, consultation with a maxillofacial surgeon is in order.

Orbital Fractures

Blowout fractures are the most common orbital fractures. These injuries occur when a blunt object strikes the globe, resulting in expansion of orbital contents and subsequent rupture through the bony floor. A direct blow to the orbital rim also will result in a blowout. Four clinical findings suggest the diagnosis:

Rare patients may have enophthalmos, or sunken globe, when a large section is ruptured.

Infraorbital anesthesia is a more common finding and develops when the infraorbital nerve is contused by the initial trauma or when compressed by bony fragments. Anesthesia of the maxillary teeth and upper lip is more reliable than numbness over the cheek.

Diplopia, particularly on upward gaze that usually indicates inferior rectus muscle entrapment, is another important clinical finding. However, the etiology of diplopia may be multifactorial and does not necessarily imply entrapment of extraocular muscles. Other causes include direct muscle injury, damage to the third nerve, or entrapment of periorbital fat. CT scanning and consultation are necessary for patients with posttraumatic diplopia.

Occasionally, a step-off deformity can be palpated over the intraorbital rim. Subcutaneous emphysema is pathognomonic for fracture into a sinus or nasal antrum.

Plain films are useful in the diagnosis of blowout fractures. The "hanging teardrop" sign is seen with herniation of orbital fat into the maxillary sinus, whereas the "open bomb-bay door" sign results from bone fragments that protrude into the sinus. Air-fluid levels in the maxillary sinus are seen frequently in association with these signs.

Once a blowout fracture is suspected or confirmed either radiographically or clinically (i.e., diplopia or subcutaneous air), obtain a CT scan with coronal sections to determine the surface area of the broken floor.

There is significant controversy as to the timing and necessity of orbital floor repair. All fractures, including those with diplopia and entrapment, may have repair delayed for 1 to 2 weeks.[18] Some specialists use a CT scan to determine the need for surgery, whereas others repair the orbit only if there is enophthalmos or persistent diplopia.

Many consultants recommend antibiotics active against sinus pathogens for patients with subcutaneous emphysema. Patients with fractures into the sinus should avoid blowing their nose to prevent accumulation of subcutaneous and intraorbital air.

In rare circumstances, malignant periorbital emphysema may jeopardize vision by injuring the retina or optic nerve. In such cases, emergency cantholysis may salvage the patient's vision. In patients with massive emphysema and no evidence of an open globe, measure the intraocular pressure. If the pressure is significantly elevated, immediately consult an ophthalmologist and discuss the need for an emergency cantholysis.

Orbital Fissure Syndromes

The oculomotor and ophthalmic divisions of the trigeminal nerve course through the superior orbital fissure. A fracture of the orbit involving this canal compresses these nerves, leading to the superior orbital fissure syndrome. This condition is characterized by paralysis of extraocular motions, ptosis, and periorbital anesthesia.

A more serious variant is the orbital apex syndrome, which involves the optic nerve. Patients with the orbital apex syndrome have all the aspects of the superior orbital fissure syndrome plus blindness or decrease in visual acuity. The swinging-flashlight test and visual acuity testing are crucial to the diagnosis. Patients with these syndromes need emergent ophthalmic intervention to save their vision. Although few emergency practioners have experience, cantholysis can be considered an emergency department procedure if there is significant retrobulbar hemorrhage and marked increase in intraocular pressure. It involves anesthetizing and then crushing the lateral canthal fold to achieve hemostasis. The lateral canthal ligament is cut, and the lids spring apart, relieving intraocular pressure.

Nasal Fractures

Isolated nasal fractures are discussed in Chap. 240.

Zygomatic Fractures

Zygoma fractures occur in two major patterns. The most serious injury is the tripod fracture, whereas the most common is the arch fracture. The zygoma forms a tripod that abuts the frontal, maxillary, and temporal bones. The classic tripod fracture involves the infraorbital rim, a diastasis of the zygomaticofrontal suture, and disruption of the zygomaticotemporal junction at the arch. The fragment may drop and pull the lateral canthus, causing the eye to "tilt." Later, the cheek will flatten, but edema usually obscures this finding in the emergency department.

A significant percentage of patients with large lateral subconjunctival hematomas have associated zygomatic injury. Either trismus or an open bite will appear if the zygoma impinges on the masseter or coronoid process. Plain films, consisting of the "jug handle" or arch view, are adequate for suspected arch fractures, and the Waters view can screen for tripod injury. Order CT scans for tripod fractures that are diagnosed or suggested by plain films. In patients in whom tripod fractures are unmistakable on physical examination, plain films are superfluous, and the patients should go directly to CT scan. The scans delineate injury to the orbital floor and guide surgical planning.

Patients with tripod fractures require admission for open reduction and internal fixation of displaced fragments. Those with fractures of the arch may be scheduled for outpatient elevation and repair.

Maxillary Fractures

Fractures of the maxilla are high-energy injuries. An impact 100 times the force of gravity is required to break the midface. Accordingly, these patients often have significant multisystem trauma. Many require resuscitation and admission.

On physical examination, a patient may have malocclusion, an open bite, facial lengthening, CSF rhinorrhea, or periorbital ecchymosis. Le Fort fractures are best diagnosed by grasping and rocking the hard palate. In most cases, parts of the midface will shift with this maneuver, but greenstick and impacted fractures may be immobile. Although the classic fracture patterns are diagrammed in this text (Figure 257-5), in clinical practice, fracture patterns are often mixed, with a low-grade Le Fort on one side and a higher grade on the other.

In Le Fort I, a transverse fracture separates the body of the maxilla from the lower portion of the pterygoid plate and nasal septum. With stress of the maxilla, only the hard palate and upper teeth move. A pyramidal fracture of the central maxilla and the palate defines a Le Fort II injury. Facial tugging moves the nose but not the eyes. Le Fort III, also called *craniofacial disjunction,* occurs when the complete facial

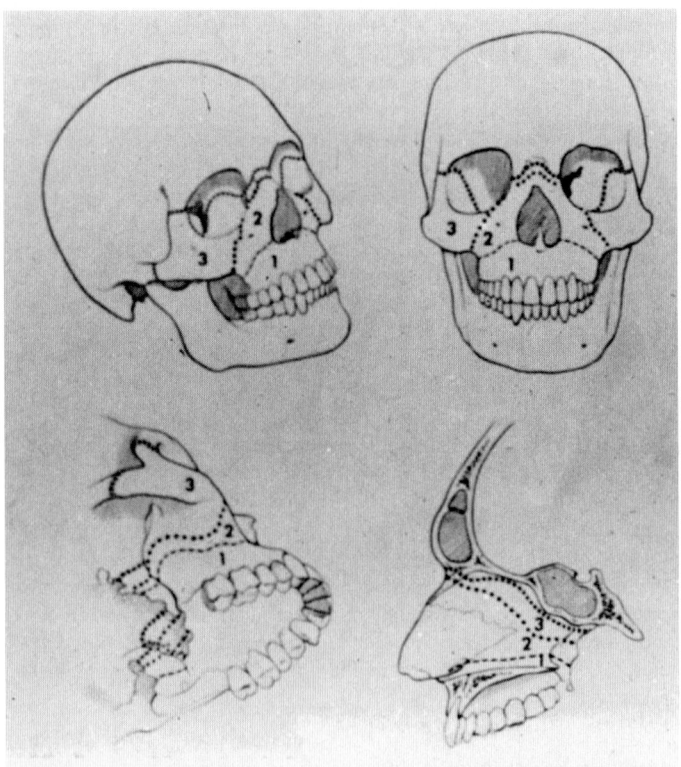

FIG. 257-5. Schematic of midfacial fracture lines: Le Fort I, II, and III are represented by Figures 257-1, 2, and 3 respectively. [Reprinted with permission from Dingman RO, Natvig P: *Surgery of Facial Fractures.* Philadelphia: Saunders, 1964, p 248.]

skeleton separates from the skull. The fracture extends through the frontozygomatic suture lines, across the orbit, and through the base of the nose and ethmoid region. The entire face, including most of both orbits, shifts with mobilization. The Le Fort IV fracture (not initially described by Le Fort) involves the frontal bone as well as the midface.

These catastrophic injuries often require aggressive airway control and frequently intubation. Look for associated injuries, especially intracranial, spinal, thoracic, and abdominal. A test of visual acuity is especially important for patients with Le Fort fractures. CT scans of the face may be ordered in conjunction with a brain CT scan in clinically stable patients. Patients with complex maxillary fractures require admission for open reduction and internal fixation. Even if surgery is delayed, admission is prudent to monitor these often multiply injured victims.

Mandibular Fractures

After nasal bone injury, mandibular fractures are the second most common facial fracture. Assaults and falls on the chin are responsible for most injuries. Because of its ring shape, fractures are often multiple. Most injuries are to the body, angle, and condylar process. An impact to the point of the jaw may transmit forces through the condyles that can fracture the temporal bone and rupture the eardrum.

History and physical examination will detect nearly all injuries. Malocclusion and pain on jaw movement are clues. Intraoral lacerations suggest that a fracture is open. Gingival lacerations may be hidden between the teeth. Ecchymosis under the tongue is a sensitive finding for mandibular fracture, and fracture-induced injury to the mandibular nerve produces anesthesia of the lower lip.

Patients with normal occlusion and a negative tongue-blade test rarely require imaging studies. Radiography may include Panorex, Towne, and lateral oblique views. If the symphysis is involved, occlusal films may be helpful. Sometimes plain films are normal despite a condylar fracture. If films are normal, but clinical suspicion remains high, a CT scan of the condyles may show a fracture.

Patients with open fractures require admission and IV antibiotics. Penicillin G (2-4 million units IV) or clindamycin (600 to 900 mg IV) are considered the drugs of choice, but first-generation cephalosporins are a good alternative. Patients may be made more comfortable with a Barton bandage, which is an Ace bandage wrapped around the jaw and head. This prevents excessive jaw movement. Many patients with closed fractures may be managed as outpatients after consultation with an oral surgeon.

Temporomandibular Joint Dislocation

Temporomandibular joint dislocation and reduction are discussed in Chap. 240, "Face and Jaw Emergencies."

PEDIATRIC INJURIES

Etiology

Suspicion of nonaccidental trauma in cases of pediatric maxillofacial injury should be high. Associated skull fractures, a torn frenulum, and facial bruising may signify child abuse. Children with facial injuries should be undressed completely and examined for other stigmata of nonaccidental trauma. Some may require a radiographic skeletal survey to detect occult or prior trauma.

Fracture Patterns

Fracture patterns relate to developmental anatomy. Young children have a higher incidence of frontal bone injury due to its prominence. Infants and toddlers almost never suffer midface fractures. The dearth of maxillary fractures under age 6 is due to the lack of sinuses in the midface. It is these sinuses that weaken the facial buttresses and predispose adults and adolescents to Le Fort injury. As the child grows, the sinuses pneumatize, and fractures shift to the midface and lower face. By ages 12 to 15, the fracture pattern resembles that in adults.

Associated Injuries

Children with facial trauma also have dissimilar associated injuries than adults. Because the pediatric skull is more prominent, children have a higher incidence of intracranial injuries. In addition, the dynamics of cervical injury vary between children and adults. Children are more likely to suffer an upper, rather than lower, cervical spine injury and are also prone to spinal cord injury without radiographic abnormality (SCIWORA).

Airway Management

A young child's airway is subject to subglottic stenosis and tracheomalacia. For this reason, avoid cricothyroidotomy in children younger than age 12. Intubation is the definitive airway of choice in children who need emergency airway management. If intubation is impossible, appropriately sized LMA or percutaneous transtracheal jet ventilation provides temporary airway control until a formal tracheotomy is feasible. See Chap. 15 for a discussion of pediatric airway management.

Complications and Timing of Follow-Up

Because subsequent facial growth may be asymmetrical, pediatric facial fractures can lead to serious cosmetic deformities. Subcondylar fractures of the jaw and displaced nasal fractures are of particular concern in children under age 5. Condylar fractures in this age group predispose children to facial deformity, micrognathia, and ankylosis of the TMJ. Consultation is essential.

Early follow-up is important in all pediatric facial fractures because a child's facial skeleton heals faster than that of an adult. Within a week, early callous formation makes delayed reduction troublesome.

REFERENCES

1. Ochs HA, Neuenschwander MC, Dodson TB: Are head, neck and facial injuries markers of domestic violence? *J Am Dent Assoc* 127:757, 1996.
2. Hartzell KN, Botek AA, Goldberg SH: Orbital fractures in women due to sexual assault and domestic violence. *Ophthalmology* 103:953, 1996.
3. Hackl W, Hausberger K, Sailer R, et al: Prevalence of cervical spine injuries in patients with facial trauma. *Oral Surg Oral Med Oral Path Oral Radiol Endod* 92:370, 2001.
4. Marciani RD, Israel S: Diagnosis of blunt carotid injury in patients with facial trauma. *Oral Surg Oral Med Oral Pathol Oral Radiol Endod* 83:5, 1997.
5. Zachariades N, Papavassiliou D, Christopoulos P: Blindness after facial trauma. *Oral Surg Oral Med Oral Pathol Oral Radiol Endod* 81:34, 1996.
6. Bisson JI, Shepherd JP, Dhutia M: Psychological sequelae of facial trauma. *J Trauma* 43:496, 1997.
7. Tung TC, Tseng WS, Chen CT, et al: Acute life-threatening injuries in facial fracture patients: A review of 1025 patients. *J Trauma* 49:420, 2000.
8. Major MS, Macgregor A, Bumpous JM: Patterns of maxillofacial injuries as a function of automobile restraint use. *Laryngoscope* 110:608, 2000.
9. Haug RH, Foss J: Maxillofacial injuries in the pediatric patient. *Oral Surg Oral Med Oral Pathol Oral Radiol Endod* 90:126, 2000.
10. Steedman DJ, Gordon M: CSF Rhinorrhoeae: Significance of the glucose oxidase strip. *Injury* 18(5):327, 1987.
11. Alonso LL, Purcell TB: Accuracy of the tongue blade test in patients with suspected mandibular fracture. *J Emerg Med* 13:297, 1995.
12. Thai KN, Hummel RP III, Kitzmiller WJ, Luchette FA: The role of computed tomographic scanning in the management of facial trauma. *J Trauma* 43:214, 1997.
13. Sidebottom AJ, Lord TC: Single view radiographic screening of midfacial trauma. *Int J Oral Maxillofac Surg* 27:356, 1998.

14. Pogrel MA, Podlesh SW, Goldman KE: Efficacy of a single occipitomental radiograph to screen for midfacial fractures. *J Oral Maxillofac Surg* 58:24, 2000.
15. Goh SH, Low BY: Radiologic screening for midfacial fractures: A single 30-degree occipitomental view is enough. *J Trauma* 52:688, 2002.
16. Guss DA, Clark RF, Peitz T, et al: Pantomography vs mandibular series for the detection of mandibular fractures. *Acad Emerg Med* 7:141, 2000.
17. Martello JY, Vasconez HC: Supraorbital roof fractures: A formidable entity with which to contend. *Ann Plast Surg* 38:223, 1997.
18. Courtney DJ, Thomas S, Whitfield PH: Isolated orbital blowout fractures: Survey and review. *Br J Oral Maxillofac Surg* 38:496, 2000.

258 PENETRATING AND BLUNT NECK TRAUMA
Bonny J. Baron

The optimal management of patients with blunt or penetrating neck injuries is challenging. Seemingly minor injuries can quickly become life-threatening. Missed injuries and delayed diagnosis can result in serious complications and death. While ultimate management goals are the same, each mechanism has its own special considerations.

EPIDEMIOLOGY

There are a paucity of data regarding the epidemiology of blunt and penetrating neck trauma. The demographics are expected to mirror those of other trauma victims, particularly in urban settings. There is a predominance of young males, especially those in the 21- to 30-year-old age group. The incidence of gunshot versus stab wounds varies from study to study. Penetrating neck trauma is associated with a high incidence of simultaneous injuries to other systems. Multiple injuries occur approximately half the time.[1] Serious injuries following blunt trauma are not as common and probably are underreported because many are not recognized initially. About half of blunt neck trauma is related to motor vehicle crashes.

ANATOMY

The neck contains a high concentration of vascular, aerodigestive, and spinal structures in a relatively confined space. Other susceptible structures include the thyroid and parathyroid glands, the lower cranial nerves, the brachial plexus, and the thoracic duct. Many of these structures are in close proximity to the skin and therefore are vulnerable to injury. Only the spinal cord has bony protection.

There are several anatomic classifications of the neck. Traditionally, anatomists have defined the neck in terms of anterior and posterior triangles, as divided by the sternocleidomastoid muscle (Figure 258-1). The anterior triangle is bounded by the midline of the neck, the lower border of the mandible, and the anterior border of the sternocleidomastoid muscle. Within this anterior triangle are most major vascular and aerodigestive structures: carotid artery, internal jugular vein, vagus nerve, thyroid gland, larynx, trachea, and esophagus. The boundaries of the posterior triangle are the middle third of the clavicle, the anterior border of the trapezius muscle, and the posterior border of the sternocleidomastoid muscle. The posterior triangle has few vital structures, except at its base, where the subclavian artery and brachial plexus are located.

An alternative anatomic classification divides the neck into three zones (Figure 258-2). This classification was established to guide the clinician in the diagnostic and therapeutic management of penetrating injuries. Various authors have defined the zones differently. The most widely used classification is that of Roon and Christensen.[2] By their definition, zone I extends from the clavicles to the cricoid cartilage. Zone I includes the vertebral and proximal carotid arteries, major thoracic ves-

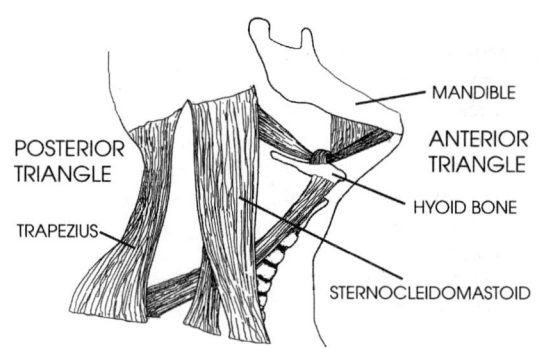

FIG. 258-1. Triangles of the neck.

sels, superior mediastinum, lungs, esophagus, trachea, thoracic duct, and spinal cord. Zone II extends from the inferior margin of the cricoid cartilage cephalad to the angle of the mandible. Injuries in zone II may involve the carotid and vertebral arteries, jugular veins, esophagus, trachea, larynx, and spinal cord. Zone III is located between the angle of the mandible and the base of the skull. The distal carotid and vertebral arteries, pharynx, and spinal cord are all at risk of injury in zone III.

The structures of the neck are supported by a series of fascial layers (Figure 258-3). The superficial fascia surrounds the platysma muscle. This thin muscle covers the entire anterior triangle and the anteroinferior aspect of the posterior triangle. The platysma is the most superficial structure beneath the skin and subcutaneous tissue, and it serves as an important planar landmark when evaluating penetrating neck injuries. Beneath the platysma is the deep cervical fascia, a series of fascial compartments that support the muscles, vessels, and viscera of the neck. The deep cervical fascia divides into the investing, pretracheal, and prevertebral layers. The investing layer splits to enclose the sternocleidomastoid and trapezius muscles. The pretracheal layer attaches to the thyroid and cricoid cartilage and blends with the pericardium in the thoracic cavity. The prevertebral layer covers the prevertebral muscles and blends with the axillary sheath, which encloses the subclavian vessels. All three layers of the deep cervical fascia combine to form the carotid sheath. The tight facial compartments provide a tamponade effect, which limits potential for external bleeding from vascular injuries. Bleeding within these narrow compartments, however, can result in extrinsic airway compression and compromise.

INITIAL MANAGEMENT

The initial approach to patients with neck injury is performed according to Advanced Trauma Life Support (ATLS) protocols.[3] A directed

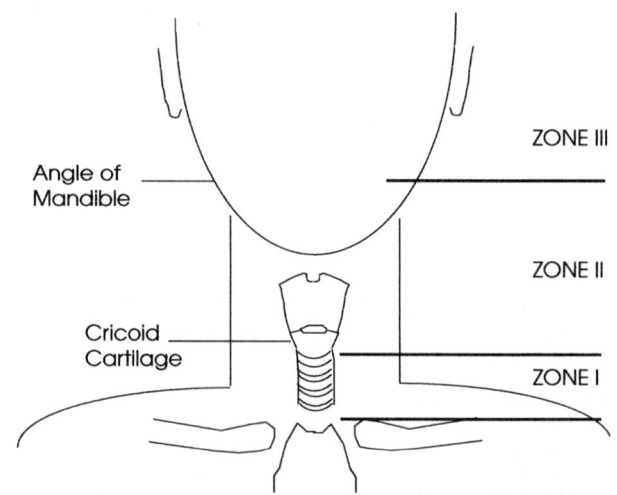

FIG. 258-2. Zones of the neck.

FIG. 258-3. Fascial layers of the neck.

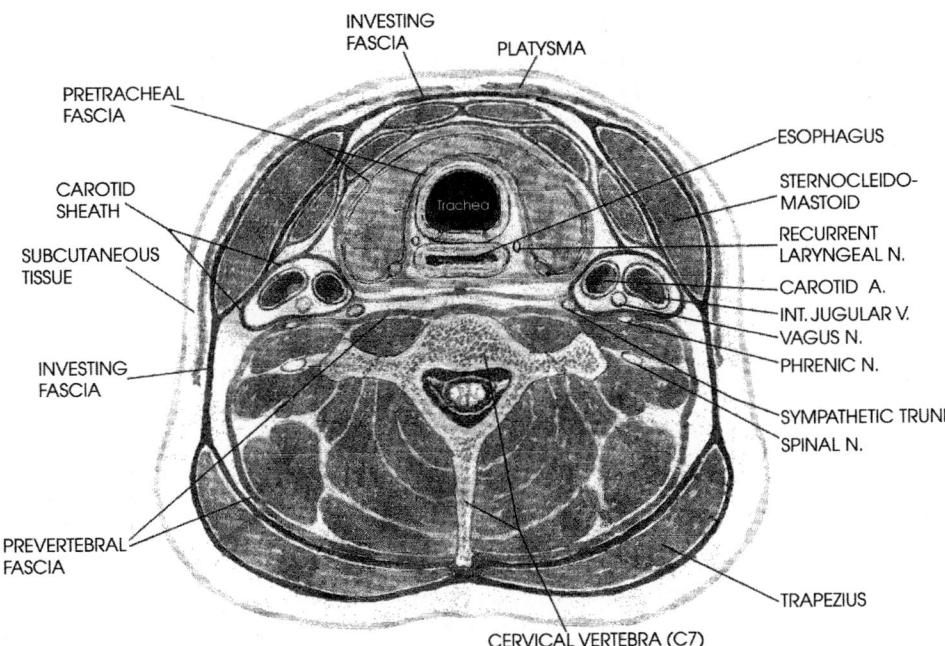

INVESTING FASCIA
PLATYSMA
PRETRACHEAL FASCIA
ESOPHAGUS
CAROTID SHEATH
STERNOCLEIDO-MASTOID
SUBCUTANEOUS TISSUE
RECURRENT LARYNGEAL N.
CAROTID A.
INT. JUGULAR V.
VAGUS N.
INVESTING FASCIA
PHRENIC N.
SYMPATHETIC TRUNK
SPINAL N.
Trachea
PREVERTEBRAL FASCIA
TRAPEZIUS
CERVICAL VERTEBRA (C7)

primary survey, resuscitation, and secondary survey should be performed expeditiously. Once the initial evaluation is completed, decisions concerning optimal diagnostic studies and definitive care are made.

Airway

Neck injuries can create some of the greatest challenges to airway management. All clinicians agree that any patient with acute respiratory distress, airway compromise from blood or secretions, massive subcutaneous emphysema, tracheal shift, or severe alteration in mental status should have early airway intervention. Controversy arises when presented with patients who have significant injury mechanisms without any immediate evidence of vascular injury or airway compromise. There are no published data that definitively outline the optimal approach in such patients. It is important to realize how quickly blood or air dissecting into fascial compartments can distort normal anatomy. Once this occurs, airway management becomes difficult, if not impossible. *In experienced hands, the risk of performing an unnecessary intubation is minimal compared with the potential morbidity of a difficult intubation with respiratory distress and a distorted airway.* It is particularly important to establish a definitive airway before a patient leaves the monitored setting of the emergency department for diagnostic studies. In most cases, orotracheal intubation with rapid-sequence induction can be used.

If unsuccessful, the cricothyroidotomy is generally the next procedure of choice in adults. When performing a cricothyroidotomy, care must be taken to avoid dislodging a contained hematoma. The integrity of the larynx should be evaluated prior to any intubation attempts, particularly in cases of blunt trauma. Intubation of a patient with a fractured larynx may result in complete transection or create a false passage, necessitating a tracheostomy. If there is any doubt regarding the integrity of the larynx, proceeding directly to a tracheostomy may be the best option. Occasionally, a tracheostomy site will be created by the injury itself. An existing tracheostomy may be intubated as a lifesaving means of securing the airway.[4] In all cases of blunt or penetrating neck trauma in which a cervical spine fracture is suspected, the cervical spine should be immobilized in the neutral position.

Breathing

All patients should receive high-flow oxygen and be monitored continuously by pulse oximetry. Proximity of the base of the neck and the

thorax predisposes simultaneous injury to both regions. Difficulty ventilating a patient is indicative of either upper airway or thoracic injuries. Unequal breath sounds and asymmetric chest movement are signs of inadequate ventilation. These signs are associated with a pneumo- or hemothorax. Tracheal deviation may accompany a tension pneumothorax.

Circulation

Active bleeding is controlled by direct pressure at the site of injury. Do not clamp bleeding vessels because additional damage to vascular or nervous structures may result. One should avoid placing intravenous access at a location where the intravenous fluid would flow toward the site of injury (e.g., internal jugular or subclavian vein injury) and extravasate. Nasogastric tubes should be avoided during the initial resuscitation. Gagging and retching induced during nasogastric tube insertion could dislodge a clot and cause hemorrhage from a vascular injury.

Disability

Neurologic deficits may indicate direct nerve or spinal cord injury, or they may result from cerebral ischemia caused by vascular injury. Early evaluation determining the presence or absence of deficits is important, particularly because patients are rapidly sedated and paralyzed for airway control.

Initial Radiographic Evaluation

The first radiographic study should be a lateral C-spine view. This should be followed by an anteroposterior (AP) view, if possible, which may help to quickly determine whether the trajectory of a penetrating injury is transcervical. In cases of penetrating trauma, radiographs are evaluated for fractures and retained foreign bodies. Although the path of a missile is never known with certainty, localizing a bullet may suggest a transcervical trajectory. In both blunt and penetrating trauma, the soft tissues should be examined for hematomas, air-column obstruction or deviation, subcutaneous emphysema, or retropharyngeal thickening. A chest radiograph must be obtained to evaluate for the presence of a pneumothorax, hemothorax, or air in the mediastinum.

Complete Evaluation

A complete history and thorough physical examination should be completed as time allows. Information obtained from prehospital personnel should include mechanism of injury, symptoms, hemodynamic stability, and amount of blood loss at the scene. Once in the emergency department, if possible, the patient should be questioned about neck pain, difficulty breathing, dysphagia, odynophagia, hoarseness, hematemesis, hemoptysis, and any neurologic deficits. Examination of the neck requires a search for clinical signs of vascular, aerodigestive, and neurologic injuries. These include arterial bleeding, large or expanding hematomas, diminished pulses or bruits, lateralizing signs, tracheal deviation, air bubbling through the wound, saliva in the wound, subcutaneous emphysema, and evidence of cranial nerve injuries. These clinical signs can be divided into hard and soft signs of injury[5] (Table 258-1). All signs require diagnostic investigation, but hard signs are more often associated with significant injury.

PENETRATING INJURY

Mechanisms of penetrating injury can be categorized as stab, gunshot, shotgun, or miscellaneous sharp implements. All mechanisms have potential for causing serious injury. Seemingly innocuous wounds may involve multiple structures. Gunshot wounds cause damage both from the bullet itself and from the blast effect. In addition, the path of a bullet is unpredictable. Localizing a bullet will not delineate which structures it has traversed or disrupted. If the bullet has crossed the midline of the neck, however, there is a higher probability of injury. Transcervical gunshot wounds are twice as likely to cause injuries to vital structures in the neck as are gunshot wounds that do not cross the midline.[6] Damage caused by shotguns depends largely on weapon-victim range and type of weapon and shot used. Multiple pellets scattered across all three zones of the neck characterize these wounds. Although the course of stab wounds is more limited than that of gunshot wounds, there is still clear potential for major injury.

Despite differences in mechanism, treatment principles are the same. Initial stabilization is always the primary concern. Once this is accomplished, attention is turned to examination of the wound itself. *If the platysma muscle is clearly intact, local wound repair is all that is required.* If the platysma has been violated, it must be assumed that significant injury has occurred. *Neck wounds must never be probed beneath the platysma so as to avoid disrupting hemostasis.* The next priority is establishing wound location and determining which zones are involved. Vital structures at risk for injury can then be identified. Careful physical examination may reveal hard and soft signs of injury.

TABLE 258-1   Signs and Symptoms of Neck Injury

Hard Signs	Soft Signs
Hypotension in Emergency Department	Hypotension in field
Active arterial bleeding	History of arterial bleeding
Diminished carotid pulse	Tracheal deviation
Expanding hematoma	Nonexpanding large hematoma
Thrill/bruit	Apical capping on chest radiograph
Lateralizing signs	Stridor
Hemothorax >1000 mL	Hoarseness
Air or bubbling in wound	Vocal cord paralysis
Hemoptysis	Subcutaneous emphysema
Hematemesis	Seventh cranial nerve injury
	Unexplained bradycardia (without CNS injury)

A diagnostic plan that will evaluate vulnerable structures is then implemented.

Consultation

If the platysma is violated, immediate surgical consultation is indicated. Similarly, early involvement of radiologists will facilitate a nonoperative diagnostic workup. A team approach will expedite stabilization, diagnosis, and definitive treatment. If the treating facility is unable to provide adequate diagnostic and surgical support, transfer should occur expeditiously after initial stabilization.

Diagnosis and Management

There is general agreement that patients who are hemodynamically unstable or have obvious aerodigestive injury require immediate surgical intervention. In those who are stable, the diagnostic approach is determined by the location of the wound. Nonoperative studies are used to identify injuries in zones I and III. Vascular control is often difficult to obtain in these zones. Zone I injuries requiring operative repair need a thoracic surgical approach to gain proximal vascular control, especially for arterial injuries. Both proximal and distal vascular control is obtained easily in zone II. For zone III, proximal control of arterial injury actually is gained in zone II. More distal injury presents a difficult problem in zone III. Disarticulation of the mandible may be required for adequate exposure. Given these technical difficulties, routine exploration of zones I and III is not indicated. Both these zones should be studied with angiography because physical examination is not always reliable in identifying vascular injuries.[7] Zone I also requires diagnostic evaluation of the esophagus because early injuries are often asymptomatic. The operative difficulties encountered in zones I and III usually are not a problem in zone II.

Controversy surrounds the management of stable patients with zone II injuries. Literature supports both mandatory exploration of all injuries that penetrate the platysma and selective operation based on diagnostic studies. Mandatory exploration was popularized during World War II because this intervention led to markedly reduced morbidity and mortality. Advocates of mandatory exploration describe low complication rates following negative operations, as well as significant morbidity associated with missed injuries. There is also concern that diagnostic modalities that are used to detect aerodigestive injuries are inaccurate. Opponents of mandatory exploration cite its high negative exploration rate. In addition, an injury may be missed during surgical exploration. Alternatively, an injury may be discovered that is difficult to control surgically, such as a vertebral artery injury. Surgical exploration alone is often technically difficult with these injuries, particularly if the vascular anatomy and possible vertebral artery anomalies are not identified first by angiogram. Angiography helps clarify management. Complete occlusion of a vertebral artery in an asymptomatic patient with a normal contralateral vertebral artery and no evidence of a distal arteriovenous (AV) fistula usually is managed conservatively. The patient with active arterial bleeding, AV fistula, or pseudoaneurysm of the vertebral artery is preferably treated by percutaneous transcatheter embolization of the proximal and distal vertebral artery. On occasion, angiographic procedures are used during surgery to aid in obtaining vascular control. Obviously, if angiography is unavailable or unsuccessful, surgical exploration and repair are performed. Selective management results in minimal nontherapeutic operations and spares the patient a surgical scar. No definitive evidence exists to establish one treatment paradigm as being more cost-effective than the other.

Further controversy in the management of zone II injuries focuses on the diagnostic role of physical examination. Some advocate observation alone in asymptomatic patients with zone II injuries.[8,9] Studies supporting this management have mostly been retrospective or had small sample sizes. Missed arterial and esophageal injuries have been demonstrated in asymptomatic patients.[5,7] Clinical signs and symptoms have low sensitivity, specificity, and predictive value.[5,7,10] In addition, multiply injured patients may have associated injuries that make physical examination of the neck less reliable. Selective exploration should be based on the results of diagnostic studies. This will decrease the rate of negative explorations yet avoid missing injuries. Evaluation of zone II injuries routinely should include vascular and esophageal evaluation.

Angiography is currently the "gold standard" for evaluating vascular injury and also can be therapeutic. Duplex sonography is being used with increasing frequency. It is noninvasive, but it is operator-dependent, and its sensitivity at detecting small lesions or intimal flaps is not yet established.

Esophageal evaluation must be performed in all patients because esophageal injuries with trauma in zones I and II are notoriously asymptomatic initially. Delayed treatment of esophageal perforations will result in neck space infections and mediastinitis. Ideally, evaluation should include both an esophagram and esophagoscopy. Using this combination of studies, the sensitivity of detecting injury is increased to nearly 100 percent.[11] Flexible, rather than rigid, esophagoscopy is the current procedure of choice.

Laryngotracheal injuries are of concern in zones I and II. Significant laryngotracheal injuries are rarely occult. Diagnosis is usually easy due to the anterior and superficial position of the trachea. Air bubbling through the wound, dyspnea, stridor, hemoptysis, and subcutaneous emphysema are the most common signs and symptoms. Although optimal management is controversial, diagnostic evaluation with laryngoscopy and bronchoscopy generally is reserved for those who are symptomatic.

In summary, stable patients with zone I injuries should undergo angiography and esophagram and/or esophagoscopy. Those with zone III injuries should undergo angiography. Patients with zone II injuries can undergo mandatory exploration or be evaluated with angiography and esophagram and/or esophagoscopy. Patients with symptoms suggestive of laryngotracheal injury require laryngoscopy and bronchoscopy (Figure 258-4). Despite the presence of a single wound, multiple zones may be involved. This happens most often when the injury is caused by a gunshot. Diagnostic evaluation should be liberal and account for all structures that may have been in the pathway of a trajectory.

Preliminary studies suggest that helical computed tomographic (CT) scan will have an important future role in the diagnostic algorithm for penetrating neck injuries. Helical CT scan can be used in selected, stable patients as a screening test to visualize the trajectory of the penetrating injury and its proximity to vital structures. If objective evidence suggests proximity to vital structures, only then would more invasive tests be performed to fully define the injury.[12] In addition, Munera and colleagues[13] prospectively compared helical CT angiogram (HCTA) with conventional angiography for the evaluation of penetrating vascular injuries of the neck. This group found HCTA to have 90 percent sensitivity and 100 percent specificity for detection of major carotid and vertebral arterial injuries. There are some technical limitations to HCTA. HCTA is limited in detecting low zone I and high zone III injuries. A suboptimal bolus of contrast dye can limit vascular evaluation and obscure small lesions. Studies may be limited by streak artifact caused by metallic foreign bodies. Future prospective studies will help to define the optimal use for helical CT in the diagnosis of penetrating neck injuries.

It is important to recognize that diagnostic evaluation depends to a large extent on the institution and its personnel. Available resources often determine the optimal diagnostic regimen.

Pediatric Considerations

Initial management of children is identical to that of adults. In children, however, certain predisposing factors may alter the diagnostic evaluation. The diagnostic process itself may be associated with significant morbidity. Young children often must be anesthetized to undergo diagnostic procedures. Angiography is technically more difficult due to the smaller vessel size. Hall and colleagues[14] have suggested observation alone in asymptomatic children with zone II penetrating injuries. Hall cautions that this practice should only be followed if close, active observation by skilled consultants can be performed and operative facilities are immediately available.

BLUNT INJURY

Blunt neck trauma is rare. The head, shoulders, and chest offer protection to the neck when it is in the neutral position. Hyperextension, hyperflexion, rotation, and direct blows contribute to blunt injuries. Most commonly, injury results from motor vehicle collisions in which the extended neck strikes the steering wheel or dashboard.[15] Shearing forces from shoulder safety belts are also responsible for injury. Motorcycles, snowmobiles, and all-terrain vehicles have been implicated in "clothesline injuries." These occur when the exposed neck strikes a stationary cord. They are associated with severe laryngotracheal and esophageal injuries. Other mechanisms include direct blows sustained during sports (e.g., football, karate, or hockey), handlebar injuries from bicycles, assaults, and strangulation.[16]

Although uncommon, blunt cervical trauma can be lethal or can result in significant morbidity. Symptoms are often minimal or delayed, and the diagnosis can easily be overlooked. Head, facial, and cervical spine injuries frequently accompany blunt neck trauma. Symptoms of vascular or aerodigestive injuries may be misinterpreted in the context of these associated injuries. Signs and symptoms or a significant injury mechanism mandate aggressive diagnostic evaluation and admission for observation. As with penetrating trauma, surgical consultants should be involved in the initial assessment and management of all patients.

Laryngotracheal Injury

Laryngotracheal injury can range from soft tissue edema and ecchymosis to mucosal lacerations, vocal cord avulsion, fractures of the thyroid and cricoid cartilage, recurrent laryngeal nerve laceration, or complete laryngotracheal disruption. Classic symptoms include dysphonia, hoarseness, dysphagia, odynophagia, dyspnea, pain, hemoptysis, and stridor. Signs of injury include tenderness, subcutaneous emphysema, deformities, contusions, and tracheal deviation. Unfortunately, in contrast to penetrating tracheal trauma, which is frequently associated with signs and symptoms, blunt injury may present with few or no signs.

Establishing an airway is the initial focus in management. Opinions vary as to the optimal method of achieving airway control. Some advocate endotracheal intubation by the most experienced personnel. Others recommend immediate tracheostomy. Those advocating tracheostomy believe that attempts at intubation may result in a false passage, adding further injury to an already compromised airway.

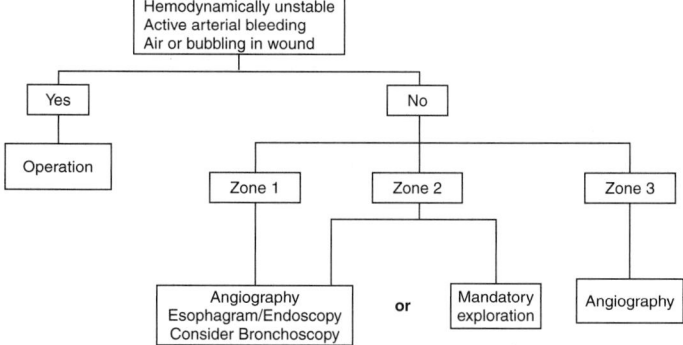

FIG. 258-4. Management of penetrating neck injury.

Cricothyroidotomy should be avoided because this may worsen laryngeal injury. Any patient with suspected laryngotracheal injury should undergo chest, cervical spine, and soft tissue lateral neck radiographs. Subcutaneous emphysema, narrowing of the subglottic airway, and hyoid bone fractures may be seen on radiographs. Diagnostic workup will then focus on identification of specific injuries. Laryngoscopy and bronchoscopy will evaluate vocal cord function, luminal integrity, and level of injury. A CT scan is indicated in hemodynamically stable patients with secure airways. CT scan delineates the type and degree of injury and is helpful in deciding which injuries can be managed conservatively and which require immediate operative intervention.

Pharyngoesophageal Injury

Blunt pharyngoesophageal injuries generally present with few or no symptoms. As with penetrating trauma, untreated, these perforations lead to life-threatening infections. Pharyngoesophageal injuries usually are associated with laryngotracheal injuries. Laryngotracheal injuries should prompt diagnostic evaluation of the esophagus with esophagram and esophagoscopy.

Vascular Injury

High suspicion of injury, coupled with early diagnosis and treatment of carotid injuries, improves outcome. Injuries are often missed because there is a delay in the onset of signs and symptoms, and when these signs do develop, they are often attributed to an associated head injury rather than a vascular injury. Any movement that distracts or compresses the artery can create injury. Five mechanisms of injury have been described:

Hyperextension with compression of the artery against the transverse process of the cervical spine
Hyperflexion, with compression of the artery between the mandible and the spine
Direct blows
Intraoral trauma
Basilar skull fracture causing tearing of the intracranial portion of the carotid artery[17]

Two different lesions may occur following blunt trauma. A pseudoaneurysm may form,[18] or the vessel wall may dissect and cause secondary thrombosis, resulting in distal emboli or occlusion.[19] Clinical findings associated with closed carotid injury include neck hematomas, bruits, pulse deficits, ipsilateral Horner syndrome, transient ischemic attacks, and contralateral motor or sensory deficits. Neurologic symptoms may develop immediately, or they may be delayed for several weeks. Outcome may be compromised once a deficit develops. The first step in diagnosis is a head CT scan to eliminate closed-head injury as the cause of symptoms. This should be followed by angiographic evaluation of the carotid arteries. Once the diagnosis of carotid injury is confirmed, the first line of treatment is anticoagulation. The rationale for systemic anticoagulation is to minimize clot formation at the site of intimal injury, decrease further propagation of the clot that has formed, and prevent embolization of clot from any pseudoaneurysm sac.[20] Medical management has been shown to provide good results in patients with minimal neurologic deficits. Patients with severe neurologic deficits on initial examination may benefit from surgical intervention.

There are several cases in the literature of vertebral injury following chiropractic neck manipulation. Cases of severe neurologic deficit following vertebral artery injury also have been reported with Yoga exercises, calisthenics, archery, and painting a ceiling.[21,22] All mechanisms of injury involve either cervical hyperextension, excessive contralateral rotation, or most commonly, both. The vertebral arteries are susceptible to mechanical injury because of their relationship to neighboring bony structures and ligaments. Traumatic intimal disrup-

tion may lead to complete thrombotic occlusion, subintimal hematoma, dissection, or pseudoaneurysm formation. Distal branch occlusions may result from dissecting aneurysms, thrombus propagation from the neck, or thromboembolism. Patients may be asymptomatic, or they may have transitory or delayed neurologic symptoms. Symptoms vary from neck pain and occipital headache to Wallenberg syndrome and lethal stroke. Wallenberg syndrome (lateral medullary infarction syndrome) may include ipsilateral facial loss of pain and temperature; isolated loss of cranial nerves V, IX, X, and XI; cerebellar ataxia; Horner syndrome; and (body) contralateral loss of pain and temperature sensation. Sudden death, quadriplegia, and "locked-in syndrome" (quadriplegia with loss of all lower cranial nerves) also have been described. Cerebral arteriography should be performed for any suspicion of vertebral artery injury. Anticoagulation and platelet aggregation inhibition are recommended, but the efficacy of this therapy has not been clearly established.

STRANGULATION

Significant external pressure applied to the neck results in strangulation. This is caused by hanging, ligature strangulation, manual strangulation, and postural strangulation. Circumstances surrounding strangulation injuries include homicides or assaults, suicides, accidents, and judicial executions. Depending on the method used, death from strangulation may occur by one of three mechanisms: injury to the spinal cord and brainstem, mechanical constriction of the neck structures, and cardiac arrest.[23] These are explained below.

Pathophysiology

Hanging occurs when pressure is exerted on the neck and then tightened by the weight of the victim's body. Hangings in which the body is suspended and the feet do not touch the ground are termed *complete.* These generally occur with judicial hangings. All other positions of the body, when the feet are in contact with the ground, are referred to as *incomplete.* The mechanism of death may differ depending on the method of hanging. If a victim drops a distance equal to his or her height, death usually results from fracture of the upper cervical spine (hangman's fracture) and transection of the spinal cord. If a hanging is incomplete or the victim drops a distance less than his or her height, the cervical spine is spared. Constriction causes jugular venous obstruction, stagnant cerebral blood flow, and brain ischemia. Loss of consciousness results. Muscle tone decreases, and compression of vital structures increases. Complete arterial occlusion and/or airway compromise result in death. Alternatively, cardiac arrest may occur due to carotid sinus stimulation and increased vagal tone.

In ligature and manual strangulation, the constricting force is external, but the weight of the body and head play no part. Postural strangulation is seen in infants. This results when the victim's neck is placed over an object, and the weight of the body adds pressure to the neck. In all these methods of strangulation, death probably results from airway obstruction (suffocation) or vascular occlusion, as described previously in incomplete hangings.

Fracture of the thyroid cartilage, hyoid bone, and larynx is associated with strangulation. Traumatic edema of the larynx and supraglottic tissue leads to airway compromise. Delayed mortality is often due to neurogenic pulmonary edema and aspiration pneumonia. Cerebral anoxia may cause neurologic damage. Neurologic deficits are not always immediately apparent and may develop over time. Long-term psychiatric manifestations include psychosis, Korsakoff syndrome, amnesia, and progressive dementia.

Clinical Presentation

Abrasions, ecchymosis, and a brownish compression groove may be apparent. A rise in venous pressure above the ligature can lead to the formation of Tardieu spots. These petechial hemorrhages can best be seen in the skin and subconjunctival areas. Patients may complain of painful swallowing. Severe hoarseness and stridor are suggestive of an impending airway obstruction.

Treatment

Treatment is directed at airway, respiratory, cardiac, neurologic, and psychiatric complications. Endotracheal intubation should be performed if airway problems or respiratory abnormalities are evident. As noted earlier, *cervical spine fracture or instability is all but impossible except in judicial-style hangings,* where a significant free-fall drop is designed to cause a death resulting in vertebral fracture. Thus, *for most suicidal and accidental hangings, cervical spine immobilization is unnecessary.* Neurogenic pulmonary complications are best treated with controlled ventilation and positive end-expiratory pressure (PEEP). Cardiac monitoring is essential for the identification and management of dysrhythmias. Cerebral edema and increased intracranial pressure can be difficult to treat and often require intracranial pressure monitoring to direct the use of hyperventilation, diuretics, and fluid restriction. Psychiatric support is often necessary in long-term survivors.

A high level of suspicion must be maintained in all patients who sustain compression injuries to the neck. Admission for 24 h is warranted to observe for delayed airway obstruction.

REFERENCES

1. Irish JC, Hekkenberg R, Gullane PJ, et al: Penetrating and blunt neck trauma: 10-year review of a Canadian experience. *Can J Surg* 40:33, 1997.
2. Roon AJ, Christensen N: Evaluation and treatment of penetrating cervical injuries. *J Trauma* 19:391, 1979.
3. American College of Surgeons, Committee on Trauma: *Advanced Trauma Life Support Course* (Student Manual), 6th ed. Chicago, ACS, 1997.
4. Shearer VE, Giesecke AH: Airway management for patients with penetrating neck trauma: A retrospective study. *Anesth Analg* 77:1135, 1993.
5. Baron BJ, Sinert RH, Kohl L, et al: The value of physical examination in penetrating neck trauma. *Acad Emerg Med* 4:347, 1997.
6. Demetriades D, Theodorou D, Cornwell E, et al: Transcervical gunshot injuries: Mandatory operation is not necessary. *J Trauma* 40:758, 1996.
7. Sclafani SJA, Cavaliere G, Atweh N, et al: The role of angiography in penetrating neck trauma. *J Trauma* 31:557, 1991.
8. Jurkovich GJ, Zingarelli W, Wallace J, et al: Penetrating neck trauma: Diagnostic studies in the asymptomatic patient. *J Trauma* 25:819, 1985.
9. Atteberry LR, Dennis JW, Menawat SS, et al: Physical examination alone is safe and accurate for evaluation of vascular injuries in penetrating zone II neck trauma. *J Am Coll Surg* 179:657, 1994.
10. Apffelstaedt JP, Muller R: Results of mandatory exploration for penetrating neck trauma. *World J Surg* 18:917, 1994.
11. Weigelt JA, Thal ER, Snyder WH, et al: Diagnosis of penetrating cervical esophageal injuries. *Am J Surg* 154:619, 1987.
12. Gracias VH, Reilly PM, Philpott J, et al: Computed tomography in the evaluation of penetrating neck trauma: A preliminary study. *Arch Surg* 136:1231, 2001.
13. Munera F, Soto JA, Palacio D, et al: Diagnosis of arterial injuries caused by penetrating trauma to the neck: Comparison of helical CT angiography and conventional angiography. *Radiology* 216:356, 2000.
14. Hall JR, Reyes HM, Meller JL: Penetrating zone II neck injuries in children. *J Trauma* 31:1614, 1991.
15. Reece GP, Shatney CH: Blunt injuries of the cervical trachea: Review of 51 patients. *South Med J* 81:1542, 1988.
16. Fuhrman GM, Stieg FH, Buerk CA: Blunt laryngeal trauma: Classification and management protocol. *J Trauma* 30:87, 1990.
17. Li MS, Smith BM, Espinosa J, et al: Nonpenetrating trauma to the carotid artery: Seven cases and a literature review. *J Trauma* 36:265, 1994.
18. Sharma P, Rajani M, Mishra N, et al: Extracranial carotid artery aneurysms following accidental injury: Ten years' experience. *Clin Radiol* 43:162, 1991.
19. Watridge CB, Muhlbauer MS, Lowery RD: Traumatic carotid artery dissection: Diagnosis and treatment. *J Neurosurg* 71:854, 1989.
20. Fabian TC, Patton JH, Croce MA, et al: Blunt carotid injury: Importance of early diagnosis and anticoagulant therapy. *Ann Surg* 223:513, 1996.
21. Schellhas KP, Latchaw RE, Wendling LR, et al: Vertebrobasilar injuries following cervical manipulation. *JAMA* 244:1450, 1980.
22. Raskind R, North CM: Vertebral artery injuries following chiropractic cervical spine manipulation: Case reports. *Angiology* 41:445, 1990.
23. Iserson KV: Strangulation: A review of ligature, manual, and postural neck compression injuries. *Ann Emerg Med* 13:179, 1984.

259

THORACIC TRAUMA

Timothy G. Buchman
Bruce L. Hall
William M. Bowling
Gabor D. Kelen

INTRODUCTION

Thoracic trauma accounts for up to a quarter of civilian trauma deaths. Recent advances may reduce the deaths attributable to misdiagnosis, late diagnosis, and the secondary stress of highly invasive therapies. Hospital mortality is quite low (<5 percent) for isolated chest injuries and rises to about 33 percent in severe multisystem injuries.

Mechanism of injury predicts clinical course and outcome. In most cases, penetrating injuries that do not violate the pleura can be managed as simple lacerations or punctures. Penetrating injuries that violate the pleura typically result in a pneumothorax. Hemothorax accompanies pneumothorax in 75 percent of such cases. With the exception of very small pneumothoraces, tube thoracostomy is indicated and is nearly always sufficient therapy. Fewer than one in twenty will require thoracotomy. If the trajectory appears to traverse the diaphragm, suspicion of intra-abdominal injury prompts laparotomy or at least laparoscopy.

Blunt trauma causes injury by several mechanisms: compression (organ rupture), direct trauma (e.g., fracture), and acceleration/deceleration forces (vessel shear and tear). The severity of the injury predicts clinical course and outcome.[1] Patients with blunt injury may or may not require thoracostomy to drain a hemopneumothorax, but many will require intubation and mechanical ventilation and will sustain complications of injury and therapy such as pneumonia. In general, victims of penetrating injuries who survive to reach hospital often have smoother, shorter courses than those who have sustained blunt injuries.

CHEST WALL, BRONCHI, LUNGS, AND DIAPHRAGM

Patients with chest trauma who develop acute, severe respiratory distress have a high mortality rate. In our level I trauma center, about 10 percent of patients admitted with chest trauma require endotracheal intubation soon after entrance to the ED. If shock is also present in addition to the respiratory distress, 75 percent will die. In patients with blunt chest trauma, the most frequent factors associated with acute respiratory distress include shock, coma, multiple rib fractures, and hemopneumothorax (Table 259-1). In patients with penetrating trauma, respiratory distress is usually associated with severe shock or hemopneumothorax (Table 259-2), but the latter is quickly relieved by tube thoracostomy.

Initial Resuscitation, Airway Control, and Ventilation

Initial resuscitation and airway management are discussed in detail in Chaps. 19 and 251. If the patient is making little or no effort to breathe, central nervous system dysfunction due to head trauma, drugs, or spinal cord injury is the most likely problem. If the patient is attempting to breathe but is moving little or no air, upper airway obstruction should be suspected. Auscultation of the neck to detect abnormal or absent air movement can be diagnostic.

TABLE 259-1   Injuries in Patients with Respiratory Failure after Blunt Chest Trauma

Injury	Incidence, %	Mortality Rate, %
Flail chest/multiple rib fracture	75	52
Hemopneumothorax	55	39
Lung contusion	39	45
Extremity fracture	30	53
Intra-abdominal	23	46
Intracranial	23	46
Myocardial contusion	13	57
Diaphragm	9	20
Paraplegia	4	100
Other	7	100

Source: Wilson RF, Gibson DEB, Antonenko D: Shock and acute respiratory failure after chest trauma. *J Trauma* 17:167, 1977.

If the patient is attempting to breathe and the upper airway appears to be intact but the breath sounds are poor, thoracic problems such as flail chest, hemopneumothorax, diaphragmatic injury, or parenchymal lung damage are more likely. Each of these has specific therapies. However, respiratory distress that is not immediately relieved (within a minute or two) by specific intervention should prompt the physician to secure the airway (intubation or surgical airway) and mechanically ventilate the patient with pure oxygen.

CARDIAC ARREST DURING OR JUST AFTER ENDOTRACHEAL IN-TUBATION   Although Rotondo and associates[2] have pointed out that urgent paralysis and intubation of trauma patients who are combative or have complex injuries is relatively safe, cardiac decompensation can occur. Table 259-3 lists common causes for cardiac arrest during intubation. If the patient has poor venous return because of hypovolemia, ventilation with excessive pressures can further reduce venous return and cause cardiac arrest. Hypovolemic patients should probably be ventilated with tidal volumes of only 5 to 8 mL/kg at 10 to 14 times per min until venous return is improved.

If there is a lung injury or if there are fragile subpleural blebs, overzealous insufflation can cause a tension pneumothorax, further reducing venous return. Ventilatory pressure exceeding 50 to 60 cm H_2O damages normal lungs. Excessive hyperventilation can also cause severe alkalosis, shifting the oxyhemoglobin saturation curve to the left, a state that impairs unloading of oxygen at the tissue level. Any patient with a lung injury, especially with hemoptysis, is at risk for developing a systemic air embolus, particularly if high ventilatory pressures are used.

TABLE 259-2   Injuries in Patients with Respiratory Failure after Penetrating Chest Trauma

Injury	Incidence, %	Mortality Rate, %
Lung	55	69
Intra-abdominal	36	83
Heart	29	63
Hemopneumothorax	18	42
Diaphragm	17	64
Chest wall	8	60
Extremity vessels	8	20
Other	41	63

Source: Wilson RF, Gibson DEB, Antonenko D: Shock and acute respiratory failure after chest trauma. *J Trauma* 17:167, 1977.

TABLE 259-3   Causes of Cardiac Arrest with Endotracheal Intubation Complicating Trauma Evaluation

Inadequate preintubation oxygenation and ventilation
Esophageal intubation
Intubation of the right (or left) main bronchus
Excess ventilation, further reducing venous return
Development of a tension pneumothorax
Systemic air embolism (especially with lung injury)
Vasovagal response (rare)
Sudden development of severe respiratory alkalosis (from aggressive manual ventilation)

Vasovagal responses are rare in injured patients. Bag-valve-mask ventilation can distend the stomach. Unexplained bradycardia temporally associated either with bag-assisted ventilation or temporary malposition of a tube intended for the trachea into the esophagus should prompt immediate gastric decompression with a nasogastric tube, verification that oxygen is being delivered to the lungs, and exclusion of a tension pneumothorax.

Initial Survey

Specific life-threatening thoracic injuries should be suspected, diagnosed, and treated during the initial survey. These are airway obstruction (noted above), tension pneumothorax, cardiac tamponade, massive hemothorax, open pneumothorax, and flail chest. In the past, cardiac tamponade and massive hemothorax were difficult to recognize. Today, immediate ultrasound examination facilitates making these two important diagnoses.[3,4]

Although skilled operators may diagnose simple pneumothorax with ultrasound, most depend on a chest radiograph.

TENSION PNEUMOTHORAX   The diagnosis of tension pneumothorax should be suspected based on physical examination alone. The presentation includes dyspnea, hypoperfusion, distended neck veins, diminished or absent breath sounds on the affected side, a hyperresonant percussion note on the affected side, and tracheal deviation to the opposite side. Hyperexpansion of the chest wall with poor respiratory excursion may be present on the affected side. Not all elements of the presentation need be present to suspect the diagnosis. Noise in the resuscitation area makes the percussion note difficult to hear. Distention of the neck veins may be absent in the face of hypovolemia.

If a tension pneumothorax is suspected, the next intervention must be the insertion of a small cannula (typically a 14-gauge IV catheter) through the chest wall into the pleural space to convert the tension pneumothorax into an open pneumothorax. Any point in the superior, anterior, or lateral chest wall may be selected. Once the tension pneumothorax is decompressed (a hiss of gas exiting the pleural space may be audible), the patient's perfusion often improves within seconds. The initial survey should be completed and a chest tube (tube thoracostomy) inserted on the side of the tension pneumothorax as soon as practicable, prior to the first chest radiograph. Lack of improvement following decompression means that another cause of hypoperfusion should be sought immediately. If the neck veins of a patient in shock remain distended once tension pneumothorax has been excluded, cardiac tamponade from pericardial blood (pericardial tamponade) must be suspected, diagnosed, and treated immediately.

PERICARDIAL TAMPONADE (CARDIAC TAMPONADE)   Both blunt and penetrating thoracic injuries have the potential to cause blood to accumulate in the pericardium. Although stab wounds to the mid-chest are the most common cause, blunt compressive forces to the anterior heart can rupture the right atrium or its appendage while maintaining enough filling of the right ventricle to sustain life for a short interval. In either case, blood fills the poorly compliant pericardial sac, with pressure increasing sharply as each small increment of fluid accumulates.

The presentation of tamponade is similar to that of tension pneumothorax: both lesions cause obstruction of venous return to the heart. In addition to hypoperfusion and distended neck veins, the patient with tamponade may have muffled heart tones. Breath sounds should be audible bilaterally and the trachea should lie in the midline. ECG amplitude may be diminished.

While the initial treatment of tamponade is emergency pericardiocentesis (described later), immediate surgical intervention will be required to control the bleeding. An intravenous bolus of fluid to transiently increase the pressure filling the right atrium is helpful to increase cardiac output for a minute or two. If there is any ambiguity about the diagnosis, immediate bedside ultrasound will readily identify fluid in the pericardial sac and often can identify paradoxical septal motion. Ultrasound visualization can be conducted while preparations are being made for the pericardiocentesis and/or immediate surgical intervention. The poorly compliant pericardium, although full and under pressure from the blood within, casts a rather ordinary shadow on the chest x-ray. As little as 150 to 200 mL of blood may result in cardiac tamponade. Therefore, chest radiographs cannot be used to exclude this life-threatening diagnosis.

If surgery cannot be performed immediately, a cannula can be placed within the pericardial sac for serial aspirations as surgical preparations are being made. Aspiration of only 5 to 10 mL of fluid can substantially improve cardiac performance—again a consequence of the rigidity of the pericardium.

MASSIVE HEMOTHORAX   Each hemithorax can potentially hold about 40 to 50 percent of the circulating blood volume. While the hemithorax is ordinarily filled with air, a small amount of blood, and the tissues of the lung, blood can accumulate rapidly in the pleural space. A massive hemothorax in an adult is defined as 1500 mL or more—i.e., about two-thirds of the available space in the hemithorax is occupied by blood.

Massive hemothorax is life threatening by three mechanisms. First, the acute hypovolemia renders preload inadequate to sustain effective left ventricular function. Second, the collapsed lung promotes hypoxia by disturbing ventilation-perfusion matching. Third, the pressure of the hemothorax compresses the vena cava (further impairing preload) and the pulmonary parenchyma, raising pulmonary vascular resistance.

If a radiograph of the chest has been obtained, the diagnosis of a massive hemothorax can be made if the aerated lung is completely surrounded by fluid (blood). However, these patients are often in deep shock and a radiograph may unnecessarily delay therapy. Here again, quick bedside ultrasound can reveal a layer of fluid between the chest wall and the lung. If a radiograph has been obtained, care should be taken to verify that the opaque hemithorax is not the consequence of intubation of the contralateral main stem bronchus. In the latter case, repositioning of the endotracheal tube above the carina will often reveal that the diagnosis of massive hemothorax was in error.

Immediate tube thoracostomy is required to initially manage the massive hemothorax. Surgical repair must be performed emergently; delay can be fatal. Common causes of massive hemothorax include injury to the lung parenchyma, to an intercostal artery, and to the internal mammary artery.

Patients with "ordinary" hemothorax will occasionally drain a moderate amount of blood, but then rebleed or continue to bleed. If there is evidence of ongoing hemorrhage after initial drainage exceeding 600 mL/6 h (i.e., 100 mL/h for 6 h, 300 mL/h for 2 h, or 600 mL/h for 1 h), a "massive hemothorax equivalent" is diagnosed. In such cases of rebleeding/ongoing bleeding, "conservative" management suggests thoracotomy, although occasional patients may be managed nonoperatively.

Since massive hemothorax is by definition associated with accumulation and subsequent drainage of large volumes of potentially "clean" blood, it is desirable to at least collect the effluent into an autotransfusion-prepared device. The decision to proceed with autotransfusion must be based on the patient's condition and the probability that the blood is free from contamination by enteral pathogens from an occult injury to the gastrointestinal tract.

OPEN PNEUMOTHORAX   Open pneumothorax (discussed in detail later) is an open communication between the outer chest wall and the pleural space. Respiratory distress is due to inability to ventilate the affected side. The injury is sometimes referred to as a "sucking chest wound" because of the sound produced as air moves through the wound. Air entry is diminished on the affected side, and chest wall motion is less dynamic. The injury is very often associated with a hemothorax. The initial maneuver in the field or the ED is to cover the wound with a three-sided dressing so that air can escape but not enter through the wound. Complete occlusion may convert the injury into a tension pneumothorax.

FLAIL CHEST   The term *flail chest* refers to a free-floating segment of ribs that are no longer connected to the rest of the thorax. This entity is also described in detail later in this chapter. During the initial survey, the examiner must search for segmental paradoxical chest wall motion, which is easy to miss if not specifically sought. Air entry will be diminished on the affected side. Jugular venous pressure may be intermittently increased in rhythm with respirations due to *pendelluft* (see below).

Ventilatory Support

In patients with chest trauma, impaired ventilation that persists in spite of measures to ensure an open airway, relief of chest wall pain, and drainage of hemopneumothorax is an indication for ventilatory support. Respiratory failure associated with a flail chest is best treated by early endotracheal intubation and ventilatory assistance, particularly if there are associated injuries, and even if the patient's breathing initially seems adequate. Ventilatory assistance should also be strongly considered if the patient is in shock, has had multiple injuries, is comatose, requires multiple transfusions, is elderly, or has preexisting pulmonary disease. A respiratory rate greater than 30 to 35 breaths per min, a vital capacity less than 10 to 15 mL/kg, and/or a negative inspiratory force (NIF) less than 25 to 30 cm H_2O can also be considered early indications for ventilatory support.

All trauma patients should be monitored by pulse oximetry. In patients with severe chest trauma, an arterial blood gas should be drawn soon after admission and at regular intervals thereafter. Metabolic acidosis with insufficient respiratory compensation is another indication for ventilatory support. Although there are several formulas relating the expected change in Pco_2 to the magnitude of the decrease in HCO_3^-, the simplest approach is to expect a 1:1 relationship. For each milliequivalent per liter decrease in HCO_3^-, ventilatory response should result in a decrease of Pco_2 of 1 mm Hg. Thus in the face of metabolic acidosis, "Pco_2 less than 40 mm Hg" may still be inappropriately high (see Chap. 25 for a detailed discussion).

When used properly, pulse oximetry can also reduce the need for arterial blood gas (ABG) determinations; however, since the Sao_2 indicated by the pulse oximeter is often 2 to 3 percent higher than that seen with ABG, one should try to keep the saturation above 92 to 93 percent.

Shock

At the same time that one is ensuring adequate ventilation, efforts should be directed toward rapidly restoring a more than adequate tissue perfusion. Resuscitation to physiologic endpoints such as splanchnic perfusion is necessary for optimal outcomes and may require extraordinary resuscitative measures.[5]

Other preliminary studies indicate that capnometry to determine the end-tidal P_{CO_2} (P_{ETCO_2}), particularly if combined with Pa_{CO_2} determinations so one can determine the arterial-end tidal CO_2 difference [P (a – ET) CO_2] can also help monitor the adequacy of tissue perfusion ventilation. In general, a persistent P_{ETCO_2} <28 mm Hg or P (a – ET) CO_2 >10 mm Hg is an indication of a poor prognosis.

If hypovolemic hypotension is present in patients with blunt chest trauma, it is most likely due to pelvic or extremity fractures, intraabdominal injuries, and/or intrathoracic bleeding. In patients with penetrating chest trauma, the cause of shock will most often be the intrathoracic injury. The most frequent sources of intrathoracic bleeding are lung, heart, great vessels, and intercostal or internal mammary arteries. Up to one-half may have extrathoracic injuries contributing to the shock. When this occurs, it is most likely due to intra-abdominal bleeding, which often has a delayed diagnosis. The delay is due to the fact that blood flows down the pressure gradient from the abdomen to the pleural space. Thus abdominal bleeding can present as a hemothorax.

TREATMENT

Fluids Failure to correct hypotension within 15 to 30 min greatly increases the mortality rate. In previously healthy patients requiring massive transfusions but having hypotension for less than 30 min, the mortality rate has averaged about 10 percent. However, if the hypotension is present for more than 30 min, the mortality rises to almost 50 percent. If the patient has preexisting disease or is over 65 years of age, the mortality with massive transfusions plus prolonged hypotension exceeds 90 percent.

To provide fluids rapidly in hypotensive patients, one usually needs at least two large-gauge intravenous catheters. If peripheral veins are not readily available, one may be forced to cannulate the subclavian or internal jugular veins. **If subclavian venous cannulation is required, it should be performed on the side of the injury.** If one side of a chest is injured and the other lung is collapsed during insertion of a central intravenous line, impaired function of both lungs could be rapidly fatal. Many prefer to cannulate the right internal jugular vein regardless of the side of injury, due to the much more favorable geometry and the relatively lower risk of pneumothorax. A corollary to this observation is that failure to cannulate a central vein of one hemithorax requires an intervening chest radiograph to exclude hemopneumothorax prior to attempting venous cannulation on the other side.

Peripheral veins may be collapsed, unavailable, or inadequate. Especially in patients with thoracic trauma (and because of the activity required at the chest to deal with the direct consequence of that trauma), femoral venous cannulation is a preferred route of access for infusion of fluids. Seldinger technique (i.e., catheter over a guidewire) is usually used to insert a short, fat cannula, such as an introducer of the kind otherwise used in conjunction with pulmonary artery catheters.

The goal is to stabilize the intravascular volume long enough to definitively manage the bleeding, and only then to volume replete the patient. Rapid resuscitation prior to control of the source can increase the rate and volume of blood loss, worsening hypothermia, immune suppression, and even mortality. Stopping the bleeding is the ultimate priority.

Chest Tube and Thoracotomy A large hemothorax or hemopneumothorax can seriously interfere with ventilation and venous return; consequently, it should be evacuated as rapidly as possible. If the vital signs deteriorate as the blood is being evacuated, in spite of the rapid infusion of IV fluids, the patient may be exsanguinating via the chest tube because the tamponading effect of the hemothorax has been lost. In this unique circumstance, the chest tube should be clamped and the patient taken directly to the operating room for an emergency thoracotomy.

Cardiac Arrest

EXTERNAL MASSAGE   In patients with cardiac arrest due to chest trauma, **external cardiac massage is generally of no value and may in fact be harmful.** Since the trauma patient suffering cardiac arrest is generally hypovolemic, external massage is usually ineffective and may actually cause significant additional injury to the heart, liver, lungs, or great vessels. In addition, forced ventilation and external cardiac compression may result in air emboli in the coronary arteries.

THORACOTOMY AND INTERNAL (OPEN) MASSAGE   Resuscitative thoracotomy can be helpful in carefully selected patients (see below). Patients with blunt thoracic injuries who arrive in the ED without signs of life should be declared dead.

The decision to perform a thoracotomy or alternately determine that resuscitation is futile, must of course be made in short order under highly stressful circumstances. Fortunately, data based on the presence of vital signs[6] or signs of life (SOL)[6,7] are available to guide the decision. Unfortunately, different studies use different definitions of these terms. Branney and colleagues[6] use the presence of a palpable pulse (at least carotid) and measurable/palpable blood pressure as evidence of vital signs. Rhee and associates use pupillary response and spontaneous ventilatory effort as evidence of SOL,[7] while the American College of Surgeons Committee on Trauma contain all elements of the former two as indications of SOL.[8] Others have included electrical cardiac activity, respiratory effort, corneal reflex, gag reflex, and extremity motion within the definition of SOL, making comparison of studies difficult. The Committee on Trauma's practice guidelines are based on a 24-year review (1966–1999) of 167,000 references.[8] The final recommendations are based on a review of more than 8300 emergency department resuscitations. There were no class I (prospective, randomized) trials.

Essentially **for all blunt injuries (thoracic, abdominal, or multiple), thoracotomy is indicated only if there were SOL at least on patient arrival** (even if they were subsequently lost in the ED). There is no chance of survival in the absence of SOL at the scene.[6–8] Survival among those who lose SOL at the scene or in transit is approximately 2.5 percent (presumably due to effective CPR and prehospital resuscitation measures). Slightly more (4.0 percent) of those who are hemodynamically unstable or lose SOL in the ED survive. Results in children and adults are similar. There is no difference whether the injuries are thoracic, abdominal, or multiple. These data may even be optimistic as publications likely reflect best experiences.

Patients with penetrating wounds have a significantly better chance of surviving with benefit of thoracotomy.[6–8] Overall, patients with stab wounds (15 percent survival)[6] are more likely to benefit than those with gunshot wounds (GSWs) (4 percent survival).[6,7] The American College of Surgeons Committee on Trauma also has practice guidelines regarding indications for thoracotomy for penetrating wounds. **If there were no vital signs at the scene, thoracotomy is not indicated** unless basic resuscitative measures are effective. Survival rates in such patients with GSWs are exceedingly poor (about 1 percent), but fair for those with stab wounds (9 percent).[6] Patients who lose their vital signs at the scene or in transit should have a thoracotomy performed, particularly for cardiac chest wounds, and as an adjunct in treating abdominal vascular injuries, as a reasonable rate of survival for both GSWs (16 percent) and stab wounds (23 percent) can be expected.[6] Among these patients cardiac injuries, especially stab wounds associated with tamponade, have the best prognosis, with survival as high as 29 percent.[6] In this group, thoracotomy can be employed to differentiate cardiac from other injuries. As in blunt trauma, those who arrive with SOL, even if later lost in the ED, should have a thoracotomy. Survival rates in this group are as high as 38 percent for stab wounds, but remain low (14 percent) for GSWs.[6] Pediatric experience is similar.[8]

A high rate of good neurologic outcomes (76 to 92 percent) can be expected among those who survive thoracotomy, with uniformly better prognosis for those with penetrating injuries.[6–8] A detailed description of thoracotomy is beyond the scope of this chapter.

Open cardiac massage is usually performed through an anterolateral incision in the fifth intercostal space on the side of the injury (Figures 259-1 and 259-2). The pericardium is opened vertically 1 to 2 cm anterior to the phrenic nerve. The thoracic incision allows direct inspection of the heart, control of bleeding sites in the chest, and complete evacuation of any pericardial tamponade or hemopneumothorax. In addition, a left thoracotomy allows the physician to compress or clamp the descending thoracic aorta.

Since about 60 percent of the cardiac output normally goes to the tissues below the diaphragm, clamping of the descending thoracic aorta can increase coronary and carotid blood flow almost threefold. If the arterial systolic blood pressure does not rise to 90 mm Hg within 5 to 10 min of aortic cross-clamping, further resuscitation will probably be of no avail. On the other hand, if the proximal aortic pressure rises above 160 to 180 mm Hg in a previously normotensive individual, both the brain and left ventricle are at risk.

Diagnosis of Thoracic Injuries

SYMPTOMS   The most frequent symptoms of thoracic trauma are chest pain and shortness of breath. The pain is usually well localized to the involved area of the chest wall, but sometimes it is referred to the abdomen, neck, shoulder, or arms. Dyspnea and tachypnea are nonspecific and may also be caused by anxiety or pain from other injuries.

PHYSICAL EXAMINATION   A thorough physical examination, directed toward detecting the potential presence of the six major conditions to be sought during the primary survey, can be performed rapidly. There should not be an excessive reliance on chest x-rays. In particular, tension pneumothorax should be diagnosed and treated before obtaining a chest x-ray.

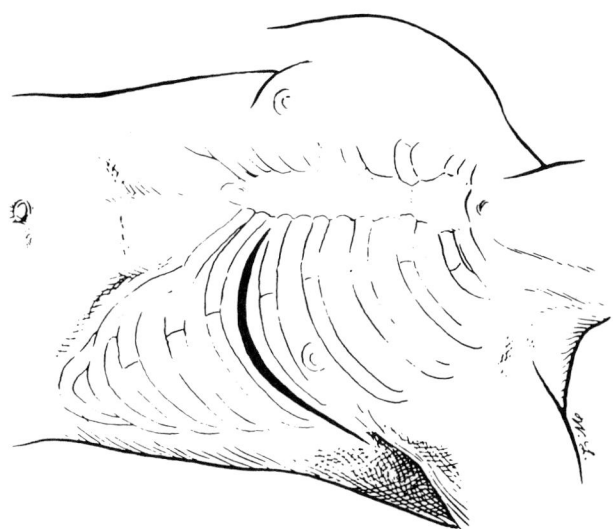

FIG. 259-1. Emergency thoracotomy to treat a stab wound of the heart or to perform open cardiac massage is usually done through an anterolateral thoracotomy approach. The incision extends along the fifth intercostal space with the skin incision placed in the inframammary crease. It extends from just lateral to the sternum to the midaxillary line. (Reproduced with permission from Geller ER: *Shock and Resuscitation*. New York: McGraw-Hill, 1993.)

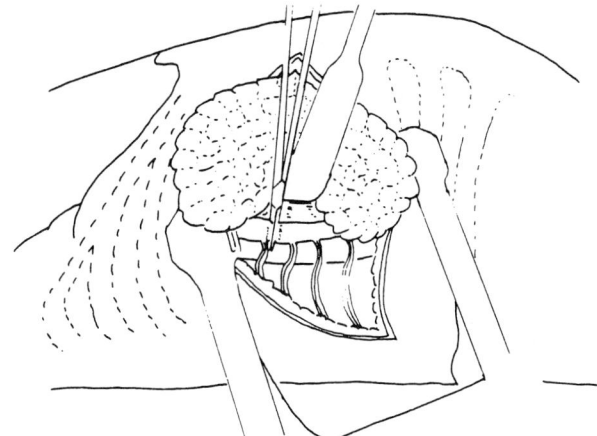

FIG. 259-2. If the descending thoracic aorta is to be cross-clamped, it is best done under direct vision. To accomplish this, the anterior thoracotomy must be large and the incision opened as widely as possible. The left lung is pulled up anteriorly as far as possible by an assistant standing at the right side of the table. The pleura and fascia anterior to the aorta are thin, but the tissue between the aorta and the vertebral column is often rather tough and must be incised to get around the aorta properly. A straight clamp is often easier to put around the aorta than a curved clamp, and is less likely to rupture the intercostal vessels. (Reproduced with permission from Geller ER: *Shock and Resuscitation*. New York: McGraw-Hill, 1993.)

Inspection

CHEST WALL   The chest wall is inspected for contusions, abrasions, and other signs of trauma such as a seat belt imprint sign. In addition, signs of paradoxical segments (flail chest), intrathoracic bleeding, and open (sucking) chest wounds are sought. The paradoxical motion of a flail chest may be minimal when the patient is first seen, especially if it involves the lateral or posterior thorax.

However, some penetrating wounds are open only intermittently and may not be discovered until or unless the patient makes increased ventilatory efforts.

NECK   Distended neck veins, especially when the patient is sitting upright, may indicate the presence of pericardial tamponade, tension pneumothorax, cardiac failure, or air embolism. However, distended neck veins may not appear until hypovolemia has been at least partially corrected. If the face and neck are cyanotic and swollen, severe damage to the superior mediastinum with occlusion or compression of the superior vena cava should be suspected. Subcutaneous emphysema from a torn bronchus or laceration of the lung can cause severe swelling of the neck and face.

ABDOMEN   A scaphoid abdomen may indicate a diaphragmatic injury with herniation of abdominal contents into the chest. Excessive abdominal movement during breathing may indicate chest wall damage that might not otherwise be apparent. A rocking-horse type of ventilation may indicate a high spinal cord injury with paralysis of intercostal muscles.

PALPATION   Palpation of the chest should begin with determining whether the trachea is midline or displaced. Palpation of the chest wall may reveal areas of localized tenderness or crepitus from fractured ribs or subcutaneous emphysema. Well-localized and consistent tenderness over ribs should be considered to be due to rib fractures, even if the initial x-rays appear to be normal.

Motion of a portion of the sternum or severe localized tenderness may be the only objective evidence of a fractured sternum. When a patient is coughing or straining, palpation can sometimes detect abnormal motion of an unstable portion of the chest wall better than visual inspection.

Percussion   Percussion of the chest wall can be of some help in differentiating between a hemothorax and pneumothorax. Dullness to percussion over one side of the chest following trauma may be the first evidence that a hemothorax is present, which may be missed if the chest x-ray is taken while the patient is lying supine. Hyperresonance may indicate the presence of a pneumothorax.

If the pericardial cavity is greatly distended by an effusion or tamponade, the area of cardiac dullness may extend beyond the midclavicular line on the left or the sternal border on the right. This sign is especially helpful if the point of maximal impulse is located more than an inch inside the left border of cardiac dullness. However, lack of extended cardiac dullness does not exclude tamponade.

Auscultation   Initial auscultation should always focus on the axillae, where the distance from the skin to pulmonary parenchyma is least and therefore breath sounds are most readily heard. Later the chest may be auscultated systematically and thoroughly. If the breath sounds are equal bilaterally, the major bronchi are probably intact.

The presence of bowel sounds high in the chest may be the first indication of a diaphragmatic injury. Decreased breath sounds on one side usually indicate the presence of hemothorax or pneumothorax, but this may also occur if the endotracheal tube is in too far and only one lung is being ventilated. Before inserting a chest tube in such patients, the position of the endotracheal tube should be evaluated, and if appropriate, repositioned so that it is no deeper than 21 cm for adult women and 23 cm for adult men. Occasionally, persistently decreased breath sounds on one side are due to a bronchial foreign body or ruptured bronchus.

Imaging   Bedside ultrasound can give early clues to life-threatening diagnoses such as hemothorax and pericardial tamponade. Chest radiographs, especially upright inspiration and expiration views, can verify the presence of pneumothoraces and hemothoraces as well as identifying rib fractures, pulmonary contusions, and diaphragmatic rupture. Computed tomography (CT) of the chest is becoming standard in all major blunt torso trauma.[9]

Injuries to the Chest Wall

SOFT TISSUE INJURIES

Bleeding   Probing of a penetrating chest wound to determine its depth or direction can be deceptive and dangerous. If bleeding from chest wall musculature persists after 5 min of local pressure, it is preferred to inspect the depths of the wound in the operating room and use ligatures to control the bleeding and carefully close the wound.

Open (Sucking) Chest Wounds   Small open chest wounds can act as one-way valves, allowing air to enter during inspiration, but none to leave during expiration, thereby causing an expanding pneumothorax. This not only reduces tidal volume, but can also interfere with venous return. If the open chest wound exceeds two-thirds the area of the trachea, air will preferentially enter the pleural cavity through the chest wall opening rather than through the tracheobronchial tree into the lungs.

Sucking wounds of the chest should be covered immediately by a sterile petrolatum gauze, and a chest tube should be inserted simultaneously at a separate site to relieve the consequent pneumothorax. Although often advised, **a chest tube should not be inserted through the trauma wound,** because it is then likely to follow the missile or knife tract into the lung or diaphragm. In the prehospital setting, the occlusive dressing is fastened to the skin on only three sides, in order to allow air to escape during exhalation, but none to enter during inhalation.

Tissue Loss   Injuries caused by close-range shotgun blasts or high-powered rifles may destroy such large volumes of chest wall that it may be impossible to close the chest in the usual manner. Intubation and mechanical ventilation are required until the defect is definitively closed.

Subcutaneous Emphysema   Subcutaneous emphysema usually develops because air from lung parenchyma or the tracheobronchial tree gains access to the chest wall through an opening in the parietal pleura. The air may also reach the chest wall from an interstitial lung injury by dissecting back along the bronchi into the hilum and mediastinum and then into the extrapleural spaces. Extensive subcutaneous emphysema suggests an injury to the pharynx, larynx, or esophagus.

Patients with subcutaneous emphysema should be presumed to have an underlying pneumothorax, even if it is not visible on the chest x-ray. If the patient requires a general anesthetic or is to be placed on a ventilator, a chest tube should be inserted on the involved side(s). If subcutaneous emphysema is severe, a major bronchial injury should be suspected and sought by bronchoscopy.

Very rarely, linear incisions into the subcutaneous space of the chest wall are used to relieve massive subcutaneous emphysema. Once the initiating cause is controlled, subcutaneous emphysema usually disappears over a period of several days.

BONY INJURIES

Clavicular Fractures   Isolated clavicular fractures due to blunt trauma are usually uncomplicated. Occasionally, however, direct trauma produces sharp fragments that may injure the subclavian vein and produce a moderately large hematoma or venous thrombosis. Rarely, excess callus that forms later at the site of a clavicular fracture may press against the subclavian artery or brachial plexus, producing a thoracic outlet syndrome.

Rib Fractures

SIMPLE FRACTURES   Rib fractures should be assumed to be present in any patient who has localized pain and tenderness over one or more ribs after chest trauma. Up to 50 percent of rib fractures (especially those involving the anterior and lateral portions of the first five ribs) may not be apparent on x-ray, particularly for the first few days after injury. Furthermore, injuries to the cartilaginous portions of the ribs may never be appreciated on x-ray.

The principal diagnostic goal with clinically suspected rib fractures is the detection of significant complications: hemopneumothorax, pulmonary contusion, or major vascular injury. If there is a suspicion of a pneumothorax that is not seen on the initial chest x-ray, the pneumothorax may be better appreciated on expiratory films, on which a pneumothorax is better visualized. If the patient has severe trauma, if the rib fractures have sharp fragments, or if the patient has other injuries, serial chest roentgenograms (every 6 to 12 h for 24 to 48 h) should be obtained.

The pain of rib fractures can greatly interfere with ventilation. Strapping the chest with adhesive tape or a rib belt is more likely to predispose to atelectasis and pneumonia and is not recommended. Probably the best analgesic for mild to moderate chest wall pain is the combination of an opioid and an NSAID.

If the patient is admitted, an intercostal nerve block with a long-acting agent such as bupivacaine will relieve pain of muscle spasm and ventilation for 6 to 12 h. Intrapleural catheters for administration of local anesthetics can also relieve chest wall pain quite well. Epidural analgesia usually works even better,[10] but in many hospitals this requires admission to a step-down or intensive care unit (ICU) for monitoring.

FIRST- AND SECOND-RIB FRACTURES With the exception of direct trauma, as from a hammer blow, it takes great force to fracture the first and second ribs. It is frequently associated with significant injuries such as blunt myocardial injury (formerly referred to as myocardial contusion), bronchial tears, or a major vascular injury. There is conflicting evidence in the literature as to whether first- or second-rib fractures are more likely to be associated with mortality. Nevertheless, 15 to 30 percent of cases of either fracture type is associated with poor outcome, usually from head injury or rupture of a major vessel.

MULTIPLE RIB FRACTURES If a patient with fractured ribs, especially ribs 9, 10, and 11, becomes hypotensive and does not have a large hemothorax or tension pneumothorax, intra-abdominal bleeding from the liver or spleen should be suspected. In major trauma, it is wise to image the abdomen with CT if multiple lower ribs are fractured.

In general, it is wise to hospitalize patients with fractured ribs for at least 24 to 48 h if they cannot cough and clear their secretions adequately, especially if they are elderly or have preexisting pulmonary disease. Admitting the patient also provides time to observe the patient for associated injuries that might not be apparent initially. Aspiration pneumonitis and fat embolism often do not become apparent clinically or on chest x-ray for at least 24 to 48 h.

Flail Chest

PATHOPHYSIOLOGY Segmental fractures (i.e., fractures in two or more locations on the same rib) of three or more adjacent ribs anteriorly or laterally often result in an unstable chest wall and the phenomenon known as flail chest. This injury is characterized by a paradoxical inward movement of the involved portion of the chest wall during spontaneous inspiration and outward movement during expiration.

Although the paradoxical motion of the involved chest wall can greatly increase the work of breathing, the main cause of the hypoxemia is the underlying lung contusion. In the past, pendelluft (a ventilatory phenomenon referring to movement of air back and forth between the injured and uninjured lungs with each breath) was considered to be an important cause of the hypoxemia. However, pendelluft is probably significant only when the upper airway is partially obstructed.

Immediately after the injury, little flail may be apparent. Later, as fluid moves into the area of the pulmonary contusion, lung compliance falls, and more pressure is needed to inflate the lungs. The increasing pressure differential between intrathoracic and atmospheric pressure may then overcome the resistance of the muscles attached to the fractured ribs, thereby allowing the involved chest wall to develop increasing paradox. In addition, the patient may fatigue rapidly because of the decreased efficiency of ventilation and increased muscular effort. Thus a vicious cycle of decreasing efficiency of ventilation, increasing fatigue, and hypoxemia may develop. In some instances, the increasing ventilatory fatigue can result in a sudden respiratory arrest.

TREATMENT OF FLAIL CHEST Historically, belts and adhesive tape were applied to strap and stabilize the chest. These interventions actually inhibit expansion of the chest and thereby aggravate the atelectasis of the underlying lung. The preferred intervention is analgesia adequate to allow the patient to fully expand the underlying lung, with a goal of improving ventilation and pulmonary toilet.

Patients with mild to moderate flail chest and little or no underlying pulmonary contusion or associated injuries can often be managed without a ventilator, by 1) relief of pain by analgesics or intercostal nerve block, 2) frequent coughing and chest physiotherapy, and 3) restriction of IV fluids to prevent volume overload. However, ventilatory support should be provided if, in spite of this regimen, the arterial P_{O_2} remains less than 80 mm Hg on supplemental oxygen.

Indications for early ventilatory support of patients with flail chest include shock, three or more associated injuries, severe head injury, comorbid pulmonary disease, fracture of eight or more ribs, or age greater than 65 years. Early (prophylactic) ventilatory assistance in patients with flail chest and one or two additional injuries may reduce mortality to about 7 percent. This is in sharp contrast to a mortality rate of 69 percent in similar patients in whom ventilatory assistance is delayed until there is clinical evidence of respiratory failure. Demand-based ventilatory support such as pressure-support ventilation can be used in most simple cases. Where there is underlying pulmonary contusion, bronchopleural fistula, or a combination, high-frequency oscillation (using, for example, the SensorMedics 3100 series ventilators) may splint the alveoli open while minimizing air leakage.

A controversial area in the management of flail chest is the role of surgical fixation of the fractured ribs or the sternum. The aim is to reduce the need for ventilatory assistance. However, this same objective can often be achieved with improved pain relief and ventilatory support. Although some European and Asian surgeons have claimed significant reductions in mortality and morbidity with surgical fixation of the flail chest, it is performed only infrequently in the United States.[11,12]

STERNAL FRACTURES Historically, fracture of the sternum had long been considered associated with motor vehicle collisions (MVCs) and a marker of serious and life-threatening injury, particularly cardiovascular injury. Mortality rates as high as 45 percent were reported. However, a large study of patients with sternal fractures collected over 6½ years found that the incidence of sternal fracture as a result of MVCs was only 3 percent.[13] This series had a very low incidence of cardiac dysrhythmias requiring treatment (1.5 percent), and a low mortality rate (0.7 percent).

The variability in the data likely reflect diverse definitions of blunt myocardial injury (BMI). Accumulating evidence suggests that sternal fracture is not an indicator of significant blunt myocardial injury.[14,15] Authors of a small retrospective study have offered an algorithm to use in the consideration of BMI.[15] Patients with blunt chest trauma without sternal fractures whose vital signs and ECG are normal require no further consideration of BMI. Patients with normal vital signs and ECG with sternal fractures should have repeat ECG in 6 h. If unchanged, then no further work-up for BMI is required.[15]

TRAUMATIC ASPHYXIA Sudden, severe crushing of the chest may cause subconjunctival hemorrhage or petechiae together with vascular engorgement; edema; and cyanosis of the head, neck, and upper extremities. This clinical picture appears to be due to an abrupt sustained rise in superior vena caval pressure and concurrent closure of the airway after deep inspiration. Although these patients often look moribund initially, neurologic impairment is usually only temporary, and long-term morbidity is due primarily to associated injuries.[16]

Injury to the Lungs

PULMONARY CONTUSION Pulmonary contusions, defined as direct damage to the lung resulting in both hemorrhage and edema in the absence of a pulmonary laceration, are a significant source of severe morbidity and mortality following penetrating and blunt trauma. While such trauma has long been recognized to be a source of deranged physiology, new diagnostic techniques, including CT, have made recognition of this common problem much more frequent. Prompt recognition and therapy can be life-saving. The most typical cause of pulmonary contusion is a compression-decompression injury to the chest. In high-speed automobile crashes, airbags can attenuate but do not entirely prevent this injury.

Pathophysiology There appear to be two significant stages in the pathophysiology of pulmonary contusion. The first is related to the direct injury, while the second is related to the resuscitative measures directed at associated injuries that ultimately prove harmful to the lung, in particular the administration of IV fluid. Administration of fluid in the setting of unilateral pulmonary contusion can cause extravasation of fluid into the contralateral (uninjured) lung, probably in association with reflex attempts to increase blood flow through this uninjured lung. The mechanism appears to be a fall in pulmonary vascular resistance in the uninjured lung, causing pressures exerted by the right heart to increase hydrostatic pressure in the capillaries, high enough to force both blood and fluid out of those capillaries into the interstitium and alveoli. Unfortunately, the process is self-perpetuating because as each proximate segment of lung sees the full force of the right heart activity, it becomes functionally congested and contused, and the process continues to the next uninjured segment of lung.

Intrapulmonary shunting is increased, resistance to airflow is increased, the elasticity of the lungs is reduced, and respiratory work is markedly increased. Thus the patient becomes hypoxic, hypercarbic, and acidotic. Adaptive increases in cardiac output are usually insufficient to overcome the hypoxic process and cardiopulmonary decompensation can occur very quickly.

Diagnosis   Areas of opacification of the lung seen on the chest x-ray within 6 h of blunt trauma are usually considered to be pulmonary contusions. The lung changes with aspiration pneumonia and fat embolism are not usually seen on chest x-rays for at least 12 to 24 h. The extent of the lung injury seen at thoracotomy or autopsy or on CT scan is usually much greater than suspected from chest x-rays.

Treatment   Treatment primarily involves maintenance of adequate ventilation. Chest physiotherapy, intercostal nerve blocks, epidural analgesia, and nasotracheal suction are used as needed to ensure that the patient takes deep breaths and coughs adequately. If ventilatory assistance is required, care should be taken not to overstretch the normal alveoli, which are preferentially inflated. Patients with extensive pulmonary contusion who may need mechanical stenting of most alveoli throughout the ventilatory cycle may be well-served with high-frequency oscillation. An important determinant of the need for mechanical ventilation is the volume of contused lung. Patients with involvement of less than 18 percent of total lung volume (about one lobe) do not require such support, whereas patients with more than 28 percent of total lung volume involved in the contusion predictably require such support. Premorbid health status and associated injuries can, of course, affect the threshold for mechanical ventilation in either direction.

Patients who have a severe unilateral lung injury and are responding poorly to conventional mechanical ventilation may benefit from synchronous independent lung ventilation (SILV) provided through a double-lumen endobronchial catheter. This rarely used technique helps prevent overinflation of the normal lung and underinflation of the damaged, poorly compliant lung.

In severe pulmonary contusion, ordinary mechanical ventilation may be insufficient to reverse the hypoxemia. The first maneuver should be to place the good lung "down" by turning the patient to the decubitus position to improve ventilation/perfusion matching. Failing this, consideration should be given to chemical paralysis and institution either of pressure-controlled inverse-ratio ventilation, or (if available) high-frequency oscillation. Both modes cause hemodynamic changes that require experience and invasive monitoring for effective management. However, the airway pressures sustained in effective high-frequency oscillation are typically lower than those required to perform pressure-controlled inverse-ratio ventilation. For this reason, high-frequency oscillation may be favored.

HEMOTHORAX

Etiology   Hemothorax requiring a thoracotomy is most frequently caused by bleeding from lung injuries, but is required in fewer than 5 percent of patients admitted with chest trauma. The compressing effect of the shed blood, the high concentration of thromboplastin in the lungs, and the low pulmonary arterial pressure combine to help reduce bleeding from torn lung parenchyma. The other causes of severe and/or continuing intrathoracic bleeding include damage to the great vessels of the chest or intercostal or internal mammary arteries.

Pathophysiology   If there is more than 300 to 500 mL of blood in the pleural cavity, it should be removed as completely and rapidly as possible. Large clots can act as a local anticoagulant by releasing fibrinolysins and fibrinogenolysins from their surface. A large hemothorax also restricts ventilation and venous return. Bleeding from multiple small intrathoracic vessels often stops fairly rapidly after the hemothorax is completely evacuated.

Diagnosis   A hemothorax should be suspected following trauma if the breath sounds are reduced and the chest is dull to percussion on the involved side. Fluid collections greater than 200 to 300 mL can usually be seen on good upright or decubitus radiographs of the chest. However, if the patient is supine, more than 1000 mL of blood may easily be missed because it may only produce a mild to moderate diffuse haziness on that side. Use of ultrasound trauma to detect hemothorax is increasingly accepted. Even so, plain chest x-rays give much more additional information.

Treatment   If the hemothorax is judged large enough to drain, a chest tube should be used. Needle aspiration of a hemothorax is usually incomplete and may cause a pneumothorax or infection of the hemothorax. Tube thoracostomy remains the mainstay of care.

CHEST TUBE (TUBE THORACOSTOMY) TECHNIQUE   Detailed description of thoracostomy tube placement is beyond the scope of this chapter. A few important aspects are provided here. Chest tubes for treatment of traumatic pneumothorax or hemothorax are usually inserted in the anterior axillary line just behind the lateral edge of the pectoralis major muscle. For a pneumothorax the tube should be directed as high and anteriorly as possible without the tip pressing on the mediastinum. For a hemothorax, the tube is usually inserted at the level of the nipple and directed posteriorly and laterally.

We prefer the skin incision to be at least 1 to 2 cm below the interspace through which the tube will be placed. A large clamp is then inserted through the intercostal muscles in the next higher intercostal space, with care taken to prevent the tip of the clamp from penetrating the lung (Figure 259-3A). The resulting oblique tunnel through the subcutaneous tissue and intercostal muscles usually closes promptly after the chest tube is removed, thereby reducing the chances of recurrent pneumothorax.

Once the clamp is pushed through the internal intercostal fascia, it is opened to enlarge the hole to approximately 1.5 to 2 cm. A finger is inserted along the top of the clamp through the hole to verify the position within the thorax and to make sure the lung is not adherent to the chest wall (Figure 259-3B). This is particularly important if a chest x-ray has not been taken or if the x-ray does not clearly show that the lung is away from the chest wall.

For a simple pneumothorax, a 24F or 28F chest tube can be inserted. For a hemothorax, a 32F to 40F chest tube is preferred. When in doubt, the larger tube should be chosen for trauma situations. Smaller tubes may not drain blood adequately. The tube is advanced at least until the last side hole is 2.5 to 5 cm (1 to 2 in.) inside the chest wall.

The open end of the tube is attached to a combination fluid-collection water-seal suction device, such as the Pleur-evac, with 20- to 30-cm H_2O suction. If a significant hemothorax is known to be present or if a large amount of blood starts to drain immediately, consideration should be given to collection of blood in a heparinized autotransfusion device so that it can be returned to the patient either directly or after washing the red blood cells in saline.

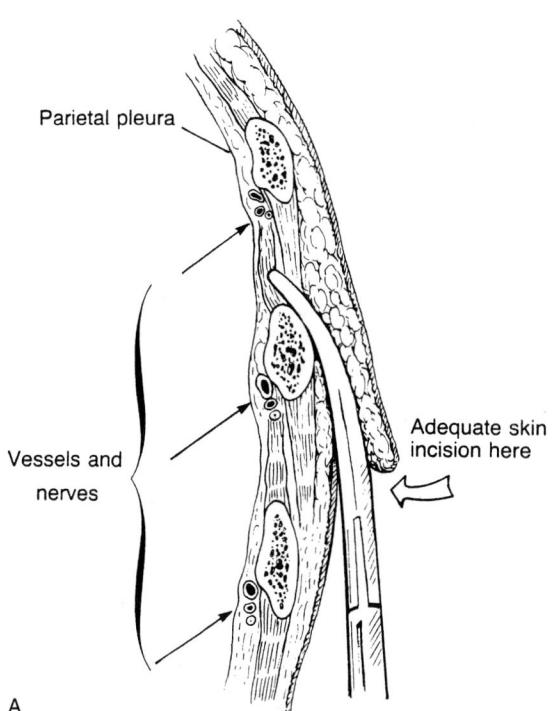

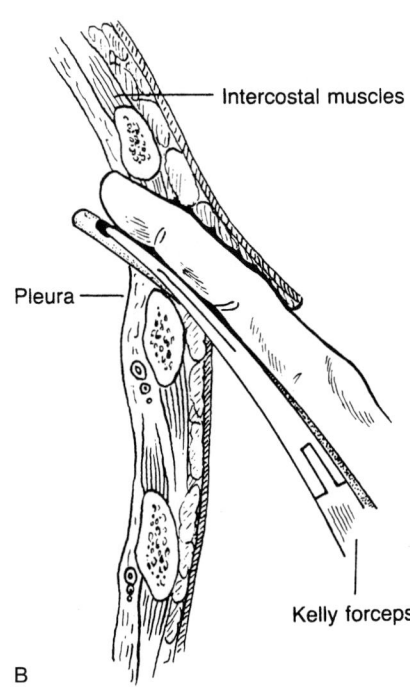

FIG. 259-3A. The clamp is inserted through the incision and is tunneled up to the next intercostal space. (Reproduced with permission from Roberts JR, Hedges JR: *Clinical Procedures in Emergency Medicine,* 2d ed. Philadelphia, PA: WB Saunders, 1991.)

FIG. 259-3B. Using the finger as a guide, one places the tip into the pleural cavity. The pleura is punctured just above the rib to avoid intercostal vessels and nerves. (Reproduced with permission from Roberts JR, Hedges JR: *Clinical Procedures in Emergency Medicine,* 2d ed. Philadelphia, PA: WB Saunders, 1991.)

The intrathoracic position of the chest tube and its last hole and the amount of air or fluid remaining in the pleural cavity should be checked with a chest x-ray as soon as possible after the tube is inserted. If there is a significant air leak, the chest films are best done as portables at the patient's bedside so as not to risk the development of a tension pneumothorax while the patient is off suction en route to the x-ray department.

If the patient is sent to the radiology department, the chest tube should not be clamped because any continuing air leakage can rapidly collapse the lung and/or cause a tension pneumothorax. While the tube is unclamped, the water-seal bottle should be kept 1 to 2 ft lower than the patient's chest.

Serial chest auscultation, chest x-rays, and careful recording of the volume of blood loss and the amount of air leakage are important guides to the functioning of chest tubes. If a chest tube becomes blocked and a significant pneumothorax or hemothorax is still present, the tube should be replaced. This can often be done easily through the same incision. Irrigating an occluded chest tube or passing a Fogarty catheter through it in an effort to reestablish its patency is seldom effective and almost certainly increases the risk of infection. If the chest tube is functional and well placed but a decubitus film shows a shift of some of the pleural fluid, the hemothorax is partially clotted; another chest tube placed with ultrasound guidance may be helpful. If a significant hemothorax persists, early evacuation of the clotted blood via thoracoscopy can prevent atelectasis.

If a chest tube is inserted for pneumothorax, is left in place on suction for at least 24 h after all air leaks have stopped. If it is inserted for bleeding, it is left in place until the drainage is serous and less than 200 mL/24 h.[17] However, if the patient is mechanically ventilated, many physicians prefer to keep the chest tubes in place in case a new pneumothorax suddenly develops.

When the tube is to be removed, the patient is asked to take a deep breath and bear down, as in a Valsalva maneuver, to produce maximum intrathoracic pressure and lung volume. The patient should be in full inspiration when the tube is pulled. An involuntary reflex due to pleu-

ral pain while the tube is being pulled may rapidly suck in several hundred milliliters of air just as the tube is being removed, necessitating reinsertion of another tube. Following removal of the chest tube, a chest x-ray should be obtained to rule out a recurrent pneumothorax. Another chest x-ray should be obtained 12 to 24 h later to confirm continued complete expansion of the lungs.

Although there continues to be controversy about the need for prophylactic antibiotics in patients requiring a chest tube for a traumatic hemothorax and/or pneumothorax, a recent study showed a reduction in the incidence of pneumonia and/or empyema when antibiotics were given until the chest tubes were removed.[18] Studies suggest that giving antibiotics for just 24 h is adequate,[19] and one study suggests that only one dose of antibiotic need be given when thoracostomy tubes are required following penetrating trauma.[20] More important than antibiotics, however, is adherence to a protocol for placement, maintenance, and early removal of chest tubes placed for simple thoracic trauma when there is no other indication for antibiotics. Where such protocols exist and are followed, a single dose of an antibiotic at the time of tube placement may well suffice to limit subsequent infections to an irreducible minimum.

THORACOTOMY Most patients with intrathoracic bleeding can be treated adequately by intravenous administration of fluids and evacuation of the hemothorax with a chest tube. Fewer than 5 percent will require operative management. Massive hemothorax mandates operation (see earlier discussion). Selection of management approach must be made by the most qualified surgeon in the context of available resources.

Occasionally, when the chest tube is initially inserted, blood emerges at an alarmingly rapid rate. If the patient's condition improves as the blood is being removed, continuing drainage of the blood and observation of the patient are in order. However, if the patient's vital signs deteriorate as the blood is being removed, loss of the tamponading effect of the hemothorax has probably allowed serious bleeding from the lung to recur. Consequently, the patient should be taken directly to surgery.

PNEUMOTHORAX

Pathophysiology Collections of air or blood within the pleural cavity reduce vital capacity and increase intrathoracic pressure, thereby decreasing minute ventilation and venous return to the heart. During inspiration, the negative intrapleural pressure increases the tendency for air or blood to leak into the pleural cavity through any wound in the lung or chest wall. If there is any obstruction of the upper airway or if the patient has chronic obstructive lung disease, additional air may be forced into the pleural cavity during expiration, increasing the likelihood of tension pneumothorax with intrapleural pressures exceeding atmospheric pressure.

Diagnosis Failure to obtain a chest x-ray soon after admission and again in 4 to 8 h may result in missing significant intrathoracic injuries. The presence of a chest injury is usually readily apparent from the history and physical examination; however, accurate assessment of the damage, especially to intrathoracic organs, often requires serial chest x-rays and/or a CT scan.

A pneumothorax is not likely to cause severe symptoms unless it 1) is a tension pneumothorax, 2) occupies more than 40 percent of one hemithorax—about 2.5 cm from the chest wall in an adult, or 3) occurs in a patient with shock or preexisting cardiopulmonary disease. If there is a suspicion of a pneumothorax but it is not clearly seen on the first chest roentgenogram, repeat films during exhalation may be helpful. Apical-lordotic films may allow better visualization of an apical pneumothorax. Occasionally, a pneumothorax after a stab wound is delayed for more than 12 h. Consequently, serial chest x-rays every 6 h for 12 to 24 h are indicated in selected patients. In a recent study of 4106 patients with initially asymptomatic stab wounds of the chest, Ordog and associates found that 12 percent of the patients required a tube thoracostomy for a delayed hemothorax or pneumothorax.[21] Current accepted practice is to observe the patient and repeat the film in 6 h. If no pneumothorax is noted on the repeat film, and there are no other concerns, the patient can be discharged.

One should assume that a tension pneumothorax is present and begin treatment without waiting for a chest x-ray if the patient has 1) severe respiratory distress, 2) decreased breath sounds and hyperresonance on one side of the chest, 3) distended neck veins, and 4) deviation of the trachea away from the involved side. Insertion of a large needle into the involved side through the second intercostal space in the midclavicular line is indicated and may help confirm the diagnosis and provide temporary relief while a chest tube is inserted.

A small pneumothorax (less than 1.0 cm wide and confined to the upper third of the chest) that is unchanged on two chest roentgenograms taken 4 to 6 h apart in an otherwise healthy individual can usually be treated by observation alone. However, in most instances after trauma, a chest tube or small catheter should be inserted as a precautionary measure, especially if the patient cannot continue to be observed closely or requires intubation and mechanical ventilation.

Occasionally a small pneumothorax is not apparent on chest x-rays but is seen on a CT scan of the chest or abdomen. This is referred to as an *occult pneumothorax*. Chest tube drainage of an occult pneumothorax is not required unless the patient requires mechanical ventilation.[22,23]

If only a pneumothorax is present, a small (24F or smaller) chest tube may be inserted anteriorly in the second intercostal space in the midclavicular line. However, a high midaxillary tube is generally preferable. We believe it is safest to avoid trocar techniques and insert chest tubes using a large hemostat. Catheter aspiration of a simple pneumothorax (CASP) is most suitable for the treatment of iatrogenic pneumothoraces caused by needles or catheters. It has no role in trauma care.

Complications In general, a small- or moderate-sized pneumothorax does not cause problems unless there is a continuing air leak or the patient has other trauma or preexisting cardiopulmonary disease. Also, a continuing air leak does not usually result in complications provided the lung is completely expanded. However, if a combination of a pneumothorax and continued air leak is allowed to exist for more than 24 to 48 h, the incidence of empyema and bronchopleural fistula is greatly increased.

The most frequent reasons for failure to evacuate a pneumothorax rapidly and to completely expand the lungs are 1) improper connections or leaks in the external tubing or water-seal collection apparatus, 2) improper position of the chest tube(s), 3) occlusion of bronchial by secretions or a foreign body, 4) a tear of one of the large bronchi, or 5) a large tear of the lung parenchyma. If a pneumothorax persists in spite of one or two well-placed chest tubes and there is a large leak, emergency bronchoscopy should be performed to clear the bronchi and identify any damage to the tracheobronchial tree that may need repair. High-frequency oscillation is indicated for bronchopleural fistula and may substantially slow the leak. Continued large air leakage and failure of the lung to expand adequately in spite of these measures is an indication for early thoracotomy to control the air leak.

PNEUMOMEDIASTINUM
Subcutaneous emphysema in the neck or the presence of a crunching sound (Hamman sign) over the heart during systole suggests the presence of a pneumomediastinum. The diagnosis is usually readily apparent on CT scans. It can easily be missed on chest x-rays. Traumatic pneumomediastinum is of itself usually asymptomatic, but one must look closely for an injury to the larynx, trachea, major bronchi, pharynx, or esophagus. Although foreign body aspiration has occasionally been linked to pneumomediastinum in children, and although severe trauma can potentially cause both aspiration and pneumomediastinum, pneumomediastinum in the setting of thoracic injury is much more likely to be due to the other causes listed.

PULMONARY HEMATOMAS
Pulmonary hematomas are parenchymal tears filled with blood. These generally resolve spontaneously over a few weeks; however, if they become infected, they can form lung abscesses that may be very difficult to manage. These hematomas are more likely to become infected if a thoracotomy is performed, if there is prolonged chest tube drainage of the pleural cavity, and/or if prolonged ventilatory assistance is required.

PULMONARY LACERATIONS WITH HEMOPNEUMOTHORAX
Major hemorrhage from lacerations of the lung following blunt trauma are usually caused by the sharp ends of fractured ribs. Occasionally they may be caused by tearing of the lung at pleural adhesions during rapid deceleration injuries. Very rarely the adhesions themselves are quite vascular, and a torn adhesion will bleed enough to cause shock.

SYSTEMIC AIR EMBOLISM
In patients with penetrating chest wounds, and particularly those with hemoptysis, positive-pressure ventilation must be used with great care. High ventilatory pressures, especially over 50 cm H_2O, may force air from an injured bronchus into an adjacent injured vessel, producing systemic air emboli. This may account for many of the severe dysrhythmias or central nervous system (CNS) changes that occur when patients with penetrating chest wounds are intubated and ventilated. One should be particularly concerned about causing systemic air emboli if the patient has hemoptysis.

If systemic air embolism occurs, the head should be lowered, and an immediate thoracotomy should be performed to clamp the injured area of lung and then aspirate air from the heart and ascending aorta. Open cardiac massage with clamping of the ascending aorta may help push air through the coronary arteries. Cardiopulmonary bypass should be instituted promptly if available.

INTRABRONCHIAL BLEEDING
Intrabronchial bleeding is poorly tolerated and can rapidly cause death from severe hypoxemia by flooding dependent alveoli. Patients with intrabronchial blood tend to die from "drowning" rather than from hypovolemia.

In patients with hemoptysis due to trauma, the uninvolved lung should be kept as free of blood as possible and nasotracheal suction and bronchoscopy used as often as necessary. If the bleeding is severe, a double-lumen endotracheal (Carlen) tube can sometimes be used to confine the bleeding to one lung. If a Carlen or similar split-function tube is not available or cannot be inserted, one may insert an endotracheal tube over a flexible bronchoscope into the unaffected main-stem bronchus.

ASPIRATION   Aspiration of gastric contents is quite common after severe trauma, especially if the patient is unconscious. If it is recognized promptly, immediate bronchoscopy should be performed to remove any residual food particles. Immediate irrigation of the tracheobronchial tree with buffered saline or a bicarbonate solution may also help reduce the severity of the chemical pneumonitis, but the value of such irrigation is controversial.

Radiologic changes are usually delayed for more than 12 to 24 h. If an opaque foreign body is aspirated into the tracheobronchial tree, it is usually readily diagnosed on x-ray. However, radiolucent foreign bodies are easily missed. Inspiratory and expiratory chest films may help diagnosis of a one-way valve effect due to a foreign body by demonstrating failure of one lung to empty properly during expiration. Occasionally, a foreign body can remain lodged in various bronchi, causing repeated pulmonary infections or hemoptysis for years before being discovered. Persistent or recurrent cough, atelectasis, or pneumonia after trauma should be indications for bronchoscopy and/or bronchography.

Tracheobronchial Injury

LOWER TRACHEA AND MAJOR BRONCHI   Most injuries to major bronchi are due to rapid deceleration and shearing of more mobile bronchi from relatively fixed proximal structures. However, forced expiration against a closed glottis and/or compression against the vertebral column may cause bursting of these structures.

The most common presenting signs and symptoms are dyspnea, hemoptysis, subcutaneous emphysema, Hamman sign, and sternal tenderness. A large pneumothorax, pneumomediastinum, deep cervical emphysema, and an endotracheal tube balloon with a round appearance on chest roentgenograms may suggest tracheobronchial injury. Approximately 10 percent are almost completely asymptomatic.

Most tracheobronchial injuries occur within 2 cm of the carina or at the origin of lobar bronchi. The air leak (bronchopleural fistula) following tube thoracostomy is continuous and massive. Either rigid or fiberoptic bronchoscopy can be used to make the diagnosis. High-frequency oscillation is the ventilator modality of choice to maintain gas exchange and expand the alveoli in the face of the massive gas leak.

Lacerations of the bronchi involving more than a third of the circumference should be surgically repaired because they tend to eventually cause severe bronchial stenosis with repeated pulmonary infections or complete atelectasis. Untreated tracheal tears may result in severe mediastinitis.

Those patients who survive a tracheal transection generally have their injury in the cervical trachea and have no associated injuries. Intrathoracic tracheal transection is usually associated with two or more major injuries and is almost invariably fatal. Concurrent esophageal injuries occur in almost 25 percent of penetrating tracheobronchial injuries and are easily missed unless esophagoscopy or contrast studies are also performed.

CERVICAL TRACHEAL INJURIES   Injuries to the cervical trachea from blunt trauma usually occur at the junction of the trachea and cricoid cartilage. This is most frequently caused when the anterior neck strikes the dashboard in an automobile accident. Evidence of trauma to the neck with subcutaneous emphysema should arouse sus-

picion of this injury. Inspiratory stridor usually indicates a 70 to 80 percent upper airway obstruction. However, cricotracheal separation is often only suspected when an endotracheal tube or bronchoscope cannot be inserted past the cricoid cartilage.

If the patient has a laceration of the trachea that is small and high, it may be managed simply by performing a tracheostomy below the injury. All lacerations of the trachea should be repaired.

Diaphragmatic Injury

ETIOLOGY   In urban centers, diaphragmatic injuries are caused most frequently by penetrating trauma, particularly gunshot wounds of the lower chest or upper abdomen. Rupture due to blunt trauma is much less frequent and occurs in less than 5 percent of patients hospitalized with chest trauma. If there is a fracture of the pelvis, the incidence increases.

Because of the protective effect of the liver on the right and the possible increased weakness of the left posterolateral diaphragm, it was previously believed that 80 to 90 percent of the diaphragmatic injuries following blunt trauma occur in that area. However, in the series of Brown and Richardson,[24] the incidence of right- and left-sided diaphragmatic rupture was almost equal. The discrepancy can be explained by the fact that some right-sided injuries are overlooked owing to the liver blocking herniation of abdominal contents.

NATURAL HISTORY   The initial signs and symptoms are often masked by other injuries and occur late unless the diaphragmatic lesion is large. Over time, sometimes even years, a large amount of viscera can gradually work up into the chest through small diaphragmatic tears. The intrathoracic bowel may then become obstructed or strangulated or cause severe compression of the adjacent lung, a phenomenon we have referred to as *tension enterothorax*.

DIAGNOSIS   With penetrating trauma, the diagnosis of diaphragmatic injury is often made only intraoperatively. However, if the entrance wound is in the abdomen and there is evidence of an intrathoracic injury or foreign body, one can assume that the missile or knife has traversed the diaphragm. In the series just mentioned, 59 percent of the patients with diaphragmatic injuries had diagnostic chest x-rays. However, eight of nine peritoneal lavages done in these patients were negative.[24] In the only positive lavage, the lavage fluid drained out through a previously placed chest tube.

With blunt trauma, any abnormality of the diaphragm or lower lung fields on chest x-ray should arouse suspicion of a diaphragmatic tear. Often, a nasogastric tube is seen to go into the abdomen and then back up into the chest because the stomach has passed through a diaphragmatic tear.

Techniques for diagnosing the less obvious diaphragmatic injuries include upper gastrointestinal (GI) series, looking for displacement of viscera into the chest, and CT scan with contrast. Still, many diaphragmatic injuries are diagnosed only during a thoracotomy or laparotomy. Subtle diaphragmatic injuries can be difficult to diagnose, particularly on the right.

THERAPY   Laparotomy is necessary to repair the diaphragm. Thoracotomy may be necessary for associated chest injury, resuscitation, delayed repair of the diaphragm, or management of thoracic complications. Recently there have been several reports of repair using thoracoscopy techniques.

HEART

Penetrating Injury to the Heart

The many factors affecting survival from penetrating injury to the heart include the weapon used, the size of the myocardial injury, the injured cardiac chamber, coronary artery damage, the presence of tamponade, associated injuries, and the time taken to reach the hospital. Every patient with penetrating chest injury anywhere near the heart and shock on admission should be considered as having a cardiac injury until proven otherwise. The converse is not true, since about one-third of patients who arrive in an ED alive and are subsequently proven to have a penetrating cardiac wound have near-normal vital signs. With early aggressive resuscitation and surgery, up to one-third of patients arriving in a trauma center in extremis with a cardiac injury can be saved. In patients brought to the operating room with signs of life and a recordable blood pressure, the survival rate is about 75 percent.[25]

Prognosis in penetrating cardiac injury correlates with cardiovascular status on presentation. Those patients who reach the ED with near-normal vital signs typically have good outcomes, while few who lose signs of life during transport or on arrival to the ED survive with intact neurologic function. Patients who have no signs of life in the field are not candidates for resuscitative efforts.

PATHOPHYSIOLOGY   Penetrating wounds of the heart are usually rapidly fatal, generally because of massive hemorrhage; fewer than one-fourth of the patients with this injury reach the hospital alive. Patients surviving more than 15 to 30 min usually have either a small wound or some component of pericardial tamponade. In a sense, pericardial tamponade is a two-edged sword; although it may prolong life by reducing the initial blood loss, the tamponade itself can be fatal by interfering with diastolic filling of the heart.

DIAGNOSIS

Clinical Features   All patients in shock with a penetrating wound of the chest between the midclavicular line on the right and the anterior axillary line on the left should be considered to have a cardiac injury until proven otherwise. If the only problem is tamponade and the patient is not hypovolemic, Beck triad may be present: distended neck veins, hypotension, and muffled heart tones. The last is the least reliable sign, even with a large acute pericardial tamponade, which seldom is more than 200 mL.

Since patients with penetrating heart wounds are usually hypotensive, the neck veins will generally not distend until the blood volume is at least partially restored. On the other hand, chest injuries can cause the patient to breathe abnormally or strain, thereby causing neck vein distention in the normovolemic patient even in the absence of tamponade. Other causes of Beck triad include tension pneumothorax, myocardial dysfunction, and systemic air embolism.

Tamponade may also cause two Kussmaul signs. One is increased distention of neck veins during inspiration and the other is pulsus paradoxus. Paradoxical pulse is characterized by a drop in systolic blood pressure of more than 10 to 15 mm Hg during normal spontaneous inspiration. The amount of paradox may be further increased by hypovolemia.

Invasive Monitoring   While the obstruction to cardiac venous return is usually evident on physical examination and by the finding of distended neck veins, occasionally a central venous catheter may be required to confirm the elevated central venous pressure in the setting of hypoperfusion. Patients in extremis should undergo diagnostic pericardiocentesis in lieu of central venous pressure following insertion of a central venous catheter.

X-Rays   The pericardium is noncompliant. Whereas an obviously globular cardiac silhouette may suggest tamponade as the cause of hypoperfusion, the converse is not true; **most patients with acute tamponade have very ordinary-appearing cardiac silhouettes.**

Electrocardiography   Electrocardiography (ECG) changes following cardiac injury are usually nonspecific. ST-T wave changes may indicate pericardial irritation or may reflect associated ischemia or hypoxia.

Echocardiography   Transthoracic echocardiography (TTE) is now the diagnostic procedure of choice. TTE performed by both emergency physicians and trauma surgeons has been shown to be successful in the detection of pericardial fluid. Performed in the ED, TTE results in more rapid diagnosis and faster time to surgical intervention, as well as improved survival and neurologic outcome.[26] The presence of a hemothorax may limit the ability of TTE to detect occult cardiac injuries;[27] however, there are simple methods to distinguish hemothorax from pericardial fluid by using different views.

In experienced hands, transesophageal echocardiography (TEE) is an efficient diagnostic tool, provided that the patient is already intubated and ventilated, the probe can be inserted quickly, and an experienced operator is immediately available.

Diagnostic Pericardiocentesis

ACCURACY   Pericardiocentesis is useful as a diagnostic tool only in cases in which the patient is in extremis and the possibility of tamponade must be excluded within seconds. In Demetriades' series, the incidence of false-negative pericardiocentesis was 80 percent and the incidence of false-positives was 33 percent.[20] In addition to its inaccuracy, attempts at pericardiocentesis may injure the heart or cause dangerous delays in needed surgery.

TECHNIQUE   Again, the scope of this chapter allows discussion of only a few details. The paraxiphoid approach is commonly used. An 18-gauge, 10-cm spinal needle attached to a stopcock and then to a 20-mL syringe is usually used. Continuous ECG monitoring should be used if possible. Use of ultrasound guidance of the needle increases accuracy,[28] and is a class I ACC/AHA recommendation for critically injured patients.[29] If this technique is not available or the operator is experienced, the V lead of the ECG can be attached to the metal pericardiocentesis needle using an insulated wire with alligator clips on both ends.

Most authors direct the needle toward the left scapula tip; however, directing the needle toward the right scapula is more likely to parallel the right border of the heart and is less likely to penetrate the right ventricle (Figure 259-4).

One should aspirate every 1 to 2 mm as the needle is advanced. One can insert a stylet or inject 0.5 to 1.0 mL of saline solution at intervals to be certain that the needle is not plugged. The needle is then carefully advanced until 1) ultrasound indicates correct placement, 2) blood is obtained, 3) cardiac pulsations are felt, or 4) the ECG shows an abrupt change.

Generally, a large portion of the blood in the pericardial cavity is clotted. Consequently, one can usually remove only a few milliliters of blood without manipulating the needle. If 20 mL of blood can be drawn out easily and rapidly, it usually indicates that the blood is being aspirated from the right ventricle.

If an immediate thoracotomy is not possible in a patient with a positive pericardiocentesis, a plastic catheter (inserted over a needle or Seldinger wire) can be left in place for continuous drainage of intrapericardial blood until the cardiac wound can be surgically repaired.

COMPLICATIONS   The pericardiocentesis needle can perforate the right ventricle or a coronary artery and cause tamponade as a consequence of the procedure itself. Dysrhythmias may also occur. A falsely negative pericardiocentesis may delay needed surgery.

Pericardial Windows   If the patient has been hemodynamically stable and echocardiography is either not available or equivocal, an alternative method for diagnosing pericardial tamponade is a subxiphoid pericardial window. This should be performed in the operating room under general anesthesia.

TREATMENT

Fluid Replacement   It is essential that patients with penetrating wounds of the chest have two or more large intravenous lines in place,

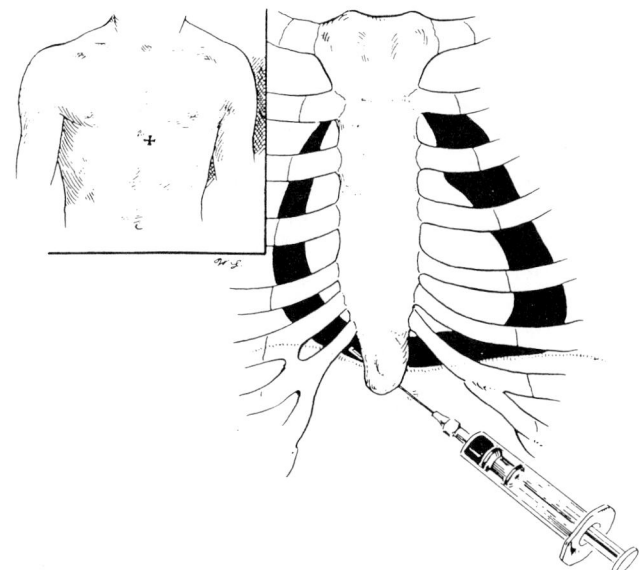

FIG. 259-4. The paraxiphoid technique for pericardiocentesis is usually performed with the needle directed toward the left shoulder or left scapula tip. *However,* if one aims toward the tip of the right scapula, the needle tends to go parallel to the lateral border of the right heart and is less apt to penetrate the coronary artery or myocardium. [Reproduced with permission from Wilson RF: Injury to the heart and great vessels, in Henning RS (ed): *Critical Care Cardiology.* New York, NY: Churchill Livingstone, 1989.]

with at least one line in a groin or leg vein in the event that the superior vena cava or one of its major branches is injured. It is particularly important to have an adequate or increased blood volume if hypovolemia or tamponade is present. If tamponade is present with an elevated central venous pressure, one should administer further fluid and blood to improve venous return to the heart while moving the patient to an operating room.

Pericardiocentesis   Pericardiocentesis in diagnosed tamponade is therapeutic. Patients who are in shock and may have a cardiac injury should have an emergency thoracotomy as soon as possible. If it is not possible to perform an emergency thoracotomy promptly, continuing pericardiocentesis to relieve the suspected tamponade should be attempted.

Removal of as little as 5 to 10 mL of blood from the pericardial sac may increase stroke volume by 25 to 50 percent, with a dramatic improvement in cardiac output and blood pressure.

Thoracotomy   Conservative management of penetrating heart injury requires prompt surgical exploration and repair. Only in the rarest circumstance, a highly selected, stable patient with a tiny penetrating cardiac injury, as by a needle or ice pick, may be successfully treated without surgery. However, all patients with hemodynamic instability and a suspected injury to the heart should have an immediate resuscitative thoracotomy.

Blunt Injury to the Heart

ETIOLOGY AND MECHANISMS OF INJURY   The most common cause of blunt cardiac trauma is a high-speed motor vehicle accident. However, myocardial injury has been documented in accidents involving vehicles going less than 20 mph. Other causes include direct blows to the chest, industrial crush injuries, falls from heights, blast injuries, and athletic trauma.

The heart is suspended relatively freely from the great vessels within the chest cavity, and this mobility plus its location between the

sternum and the thoracic vertebrae make it susceptible to injury as a result of several mechanisms: 1) sudden horizontal acceleration and/or deceleration, causing the heart to impact against the sternum and vertebrae; 2) a compression between the sternum and vertebrae following a direct forceful blow to the chest; 3) a sudden increase in intrathoracic and intracardiac pressures, causing disruption of the myocardium or cardiac valves; 4) a "hydraulic ram effect," with compression of the abdomen forcibly displacing abdominal viscera against the heart with sudden great force; and 5) strenuous or prolonged cardiac massage, particularly if done through the intact chest wall.

TYPES OF INJURIES   Blunt trauma to the heart can cause a wide spectrum of injuries, including 1) rupture of an outer chamber wall, with resulting death from tamponade or bleeding; 2) septal rupture; 3) valvular injuries (aortic valve is the most common); 4) direct myocardial injury (contusion); 5) laceration or thrombosis of coronary arteries; and 6) pericardial injury.

DIAGNOSTIC PROBLEMS   Blunt cardiac trauma can be very difficult to detect. The victim may have experienced severe multiple-system trauma, overshadowing the presence of a cardiac injury. In addition, the forces that produce blunt cardiac trauma may cause little or no external evidence of injury. Therefore, a history of moderate to severe chest or upper abdominal injury, even without abnormalities on physical examination, should make one suspect cardiac injury (Table 259-4).

BLUNT MYOCARDIAL INJURY (BMI)

Terminology   There has been great confusion regarding the appropriate appellation for cardiac injuries related to blunt trauma. The terms *cardiac* (or *myocardial*) *contusion, cardiac* (or *myocardial*) *concussion, blunt myocardial injury,* and *blunt cardiac injury* have all been proposed. Certainly there is a spectrum of injuries to the heart for which the term *blunt cardiac injury* would be appropriate, if not very specific. *Myocardial concussion,* sometimes referred to as *commotio cordis,* suggests no obvious gross or microscopic pathology to explain the phenomenon. However, sudden death from dysrhythmia can occur. The initiating mechanism is usually from a sudden direct force to the chest, while an individual is participating in contact sports (e.g., karate, hockey, etc.).[30] The term *myocardial contusion,* although somewhat out of favor currently, may in fact have a pathologic definition indicating

TABLE 259-4   Clues to Diagnosis of Blunt Cardiac Injury

History
    High-speed motor vehicle accident
    Crush steering wheel
    Angina-like chest pain
Physical examination
    Tachycardia out of proportion to other findings
    Any dysrhythmia
    Any part of Beck triad
    Evidence of severe anterior chest injury
    Any evidence of heart failure
Radiography
    Fractured sternum or first two ribs
    Widened pericardial silhouette
Laboratory
    Elevated CPK-MB levels
ECG
    Dysrhythmias or conduction disturbance
    Elevated ST segments
Other studies
    Impaired motion of anterior heart on two-dimensional echocardiogram or
        radionuclide angiography
    Pulmonary artery catheter monitoring showing elevated pulmonary artery
        wedge pressure, low cardiac output, and/or poor response to fluid

anatomic injury. The term BMI, a more encompassing term although not universally accepted, has come into vogue, since *myocardial contusion* rarely exists in the strictest sense, but is often associated with other injuries (e.g., coronary artery thrombosis, infarction related to hypotension). Also, the underlying pathologic definition is less important than determining the cardiac risk profile of patients with blunt chest trauma.

Pathologic Changes   The pathologic changes seen in the myocardium typically include subendocardial hemorrhage and a much larger area of focal myocardial edema, interstitial hemorrhage, and myocytolysis with infiltrates of polymorphonuclear leukocytes. The areas most frequently involved are 1) the anterior right ventricular wall, 2) the anterior interventricular septum, and 3) the anterior-apical left ventricle.

Additional myocardial injury may occur if there are concomitant intimal tears or compression from adjacent hemorrhage and edema. Indeed, some feel that much of the myocardial injury seen is due to redistribution of coronary blood flow. Very occasionally, transient hypotension may cause complete occlusion of a previously diseased coronary artery.

Usually there is complete clinical recovery with minimal residual scarring within 3 to 6 weeks of a myocardial contusion. However, in rare cases with severe transmural injury, a ventricular aneurysm may develop.

Physiologic Changes   In addition to rhythm and conduction disturbances, some reduction in cardiac output can be found in most victims studied. The degree of cardiac depression is directly related to the mass of contused myocardium. Screening tests, such as the ECG and CK-MB isoenzymes, usually do not accurately indicate the severity of the injury, nor are they predictive of major morbidity or mortality.

Most patients with myocardial contusions have relatively little problem. However, occasionally there is a problem with a dysrhythmia, especially premature ventricular contractions (PVCs), atrial fibrillation, or a conduction defect, or there is clinical evidence of heart failure. Such problems are most apt to occur in patients with preexisting cardiac disease, prolonged general anesthetics, or hypotension because of other injuries.

Diagnosis   Overall, significant BMI is an unlikely injury. A recent meta-analysis of studies of blunt cardiac trauma revealed that fewer than 3 percent of over 2200 patients in 25 prospective studies developed a cardiac complication (defined as requiring treatment or intervention).[31] Most of these were ECG abnormalities (ventricular ectopy, supraventricular dysrhythmias, symptomatic bradycardia). The most frequent cardiac rhythm finding, sinus tachycardia, was not considered, as it did not require specific treatment. ECG abnormalities requiring treatment were independently associated with cardiac complications.[31]

Methods to diagnose myocardial injury have long been controversial. The variation in sensitivity reported for the various diagnostic tests has two origins. First, the tests require subjective interpretation. Second, there is no gold standard for comparison. Since diagnostic criteria (and even terminology) have not been agreed upon, the focus has appropriately become predicting the likelihood of adverse events.

CLINICAL FEATURES   Any patient involved in a motor vehicle crash involving speeds exceeding 35 mph and having any chest symptoms or signs should be suspected of having a BMI. Rarely, a patient with BMI will have angina-like pain that is not relieved by nitroglycerin.

Tachycardia disproportionate to the degree of trauma or blood loss may be the first sign of a BMI. Occasionally, an irregular rhythm due to atrial fibrillation or multiple premature atrial or ventricular contractions may be noted. Differentiation from an acute myocardial infarction in older individuals may be difficult in the ED.

RADIOLOGIC EXAMINATION   The chest x-ray has its greatest value in the recognition of associated injuries. The closest x-ray correlates of

BMI include pulmonary contusion and fractures (of the first two ribs, the clavicles, or the sternum). Sternal fractures are no longer considered to have specific importance.[14,15]

Cardiac tamponade usually does not cause an enlarged cardiac silhouette, but a widened azygos vein is suggestive of this diagnosis.

ELECTROCARDIOGRAPHY   As with other tests applied in suspected BMI, the value of the ECG is controversial. Suggestions have ranged from a single ED-based ECG to 72 h of continuous ECG monitoring. A recent study of 71 patients with blunt chest trauma (not requiring admission to an intensive care unit) revealed that the initial ECG was predictive of subsequent clinically significant ECG events.[32] Still, an initially normal ECG does not exclude the development of a clinically significant cardiac event, since most abnormalities will develop over 24 h.[32] The most frequent ECG abnormality is sinus tachycardia, although this finding does not suggest increased risk in and of itself. Significant ECG findings include injury pattern, tachydysrhythmias, ST-T wave abnormalities, and ectopy—particularly premature ventricular contractions.

One reasonable approach is to obtain an initial 12-lead ECG. If normal, then the patient must be monitored for 4 to 6 h. If there are no untoward events, patients can be safely discharged.[33] If the ECG is abnormal but there is no hemodynamic instability, the patient should be admitted to a monitored setting, with the 12-lead ECG repeated in 24 h. Some authorities suggest an intervening ECG at 6 and 12 h. Hemodynamic instability suggests the need for an aggressive diagnostic approach (see below). If at any time the ECG is abnormal (or changed) or if there is ectopy or dysrhythmia, cardiac monitoring should be continued and a cardiology consult obtained.

CARDIAC ENZYMES   Initially there was considerable controversy regarding the value of CK-MB determination. Its certainly appeared that CK-MB determinations were of questionable value and likely only to confuse, as they appeared to be of insufficient specificity and sensitivity.[34] Further, elevated MB fractions in this setting do not correlate with the clinical course.

Determination of cardiac troponins has been advocated as a laboratory criterion,[35] and has even been proposed as the gold standard for the diagnosis of BMI. In particular, troponin I may have greater specificity for myocardial injury than troponin T, CK-MB or myoglobin. Experimental animal data appear to show that troponin I and T release kinetics are associated with the degree of blunt trauma force. Significant myocardial injury can occur without significant troponin release.[36] Also, due to the complex kinetics of troponin release, serial assessment may be required.[37] Finally, troponin release could be related to ischemic consequences of hemorrhage and shock in severely injured patients.[38]

ECHOCARDIOGRAPHY   A recent detailed review concludes that echocardiography does not appear to be useful as a primary screening modality in the identification of patients likely to develop complications from myocardial injury. It may well be the most sensitive test, but observed wall motion abnormalities often resolve and are usually clinically insignificant. However, patients who do develop cardiac complications may benefit from echocardiographic evaluation. Thus the current recommendation is to use echocardiography in selected patients who demonstrate cardiac dysrhythmias or dysfunction.[38] While myocardial wall motion abnormalities may be present in stable patients with blunt chest trauma, this finding alone does not seem to predict the likelihood of a complication.

Treatment   Although occasional patients will require treatment of heart failure or rhythm or conduction disturbances, specific treatment interventions are seldom required.

Supplemental oxygen should be administered as needed to maintain Pao_2 above 80 mm Hg, and analgesics should be given as needed to reduce excessive pain. Coronary vasodilators should not be used unless the patient has suspected preexisting coronary artery disease. Cardiac dysrhythmias should be diagnosed and treated appropriately. Prophylaxis against dysrhythmias is not indicated. Low cardiac output or hypotension should be treated with fluids or inotropic agents as indicated, with prompt ultrasound evaluation to exclude tamponade.

In the absence of dysrhythmias or hemodynamic instability, patients with BMI can safely undergo surgical procedures so long as continuous hemodynamic monitoring (invasive or sonographic) is used. If the patient remains in a low-output state despite adequate fluid resuscitation, inotropic support, and correction of any mechanical problems such as tamponade, use of an intra-aortic balloon counterpulsation device should be considered.

There is some question as to whether patients with a myocardial contusion and an intramural thrombus seen on two-dimensional echocardiography should have prophylactic anticoagulation if not otherwise contraindicated. In limited studies, patients with echocardiographically proven right ventricular thrombi did not develop subsequent systemic or pulmonary embolization. Furthermore, anticoagulation is contraindicated in most cases of multiple trauma because of the potential for severe hemorrhage.

OTHER BLUNT CARDIAC INJURIES   The underlying etiology for other significant blunt cardiac injuries will rarely be apparent in the ED. Ninety percent of those with cardiac rupture die at the scene. The few that arrive stable will deteriorate suddenly and resuscitation will be unsuccessful. If recognized, immediate thoracotomy is the only hope. Similarly, patients with septal defects (may be evidenced on typical ECG pattern) are unlikely to survive. Other injuries include valvular rupture and mitral papillary muscle rupture. The latter usually results in death within a few days. Direct injury to the coronary arteries is rare, but may cause tamponade or intrathoracic bleeding. Immediate repair is required. Delayed development of hemopericardium or effusion can occur even without evidence of BMI. Small infusions are usually asymptomatic and resolve.

FOLLOW-UP   It is important that patients with proven or suspected cardiac injury be closely observed, not only throughout their hospital stay but also later, for undiagnosed injuries or complications. One should consider posttraumatic pericarditis, ventricular septal defect, valvular defects, and ventricular aneurysms.

PERICARDIAL INFLAMMATION SYNDROME

Etiology and Pathogenesis   The cause of pericardial inflammation following unplanned or planned (surgical) injury remains obscure. It may be a delayed hypersensitivity reaction to the presence of damaged myocardium in the pericardial cavity.

Diagnosis   This syndrome should be considered in individuals who develop chest pain, fever, and pleural or pericardial effusions 2 to 4 weeks after cardiac trauma (or surgery). Patients may also have friction rubs, arthralgia, and pulmonary infiltrates. The blood count often shows a leukocytosis, and the ECG will often show ST-T wave changes consistent with pericarditis.

Treatment   Treatment is primarily symptomatic. Nonsteroidal anti-inflammatory medications and rest can often reduce symptoms dramatically within 12 to 24 h, but glucocorticoids are occasionally required. Rarely, drainage of pleural or pericardial fluid may be required to relieve symptoms or rule out other problems.

GREAT VESSELS OF THE CHEST

Penetrating Trauma

Of the patients who reach the hospital with penetrating chest wounds and require admission, only 5 to 15 percent require a thoracotomy, but up to 25 percent of the patients having such surgery have an injury to a great vessel. The survival rate with stab wounds is generally much higher than with gunshot wounds. Small knife wounds are often rapidly sealed off by surrounding tissue, especially vascular adventitia. This limits the amount of blood loss, particularly after hypotension develops. If the knife stays in place, it may temporarily seal the involved vessel.

The factors that determine the amount of tissue destruction caused by a bullet are discussed in Chap. 264.

TYPES OF VASCULAR INJURIES   Simple lacerations are the most common injuries of the great arteries of the chest. They cause exsanguination, tamponade, hemothorax, and/or air embolism. Other vascular injuries include AV fistulas and false aneurysms, which may not be apparent for days or even months. Pulmonary AV fistulas after penetrating chest trauma are said to be extremely rare.

DIAGNOSIS

History   Unless the patient had signs of life in the field or in the ED, resuscitative efforts are not indicated. As previously discussed, the decision is based on history alone.

The size of a knife, its length, and the angle of penetration may suggest the vessels or organs most likely to be injured. If there are two skin wounds, it is helpful to know whether they represent two entrance wounds or an exit and an entrance wound. In some instances, a bullet that entered the chest without exiting is not evident on chest or abdominal x-rays because it is in lateral subcutaneous tissues or has entered a major vessel and has embolized. It is also helpful to know, if possible, the caliber of the bullet and whether it was a high-velocity missile (>1000 ft/s). In the case of shotgun wounds, the size and spread of the projectiles can be helpful in predicting injury—small shot (e.g., birdshot) that is dispersed with wounds several centimeters apart tend to be low-energy projectiles that do not penetrate deeply. Conversely, a single large wound containing a few larger projectiles (e.g., 00 buckshot) signals massive tissue destruction within.

Physical Examination   Close inspection including lifting the skin edge with a forceps may be useful to determine the general trajectory. **Under no circumstances should the wound be deeply probed to determine depth.**

A large upper mediastinal hematoma may cause an acute superior vena caval syndrome, tracheal compression, and/or respiratory distress. Occasionally, a decreased upper extremity pulse may be noted. Unfortunately patients with injuries to major vessels at the thoracic inlet may have none of the usual diagnostic signs of significant vascular injury.

One should auscultate the entire chest for bruits after a penetrating injury. A systolic bruit, particularly over the back or upper chest, should make one suspect a false aneurysm involving one of the great vessels. A continuous bruit suggests an AV fistula. A millwheel murmur, thought to be due to the churning of air in the heart, may be diagnostic of air embolism. Loss of a peripheral pulse caused by an embolization of a bullet from a thoracic vascular injury is rarely but occasionally seen.

Radiography

PLAIN RADIOGRAPHS   The surface wounds should be marked. Evidence of cervical or supraclavicular swelling or widening of the upper mediastinal silhouette or chest x-ray is often present in patients with injury to brachiocephalic vessels. A "fuzzy" foreign body (bullet) can be an important radiologic sign, and is not due to poor radiologic technique. Because foreign bodies tend to pulsate when they lie next to major vessels, their margins may appear indistinct on chest films. Therefore a fuzzy foreign body contiguous with clear mediastinal structures on chest films can be an important x-ray clue to a vascular injury.

TRAJECTORY VS. EMBOLIZATION Bullets entering large systemic veins or the right heart can embolize to the lungs, whereas bullets entering the pulmonary veins or left heart can embolize to major systemic arteries. Some of these emboli cause no symptoms or signs and cannot be found except with multiple x-rays. If the missile appears distant from the anticipated trajectory, embolization should be suspected. The other explanation for missiles off trajectory is gravity: low-velocity bullets that violate the pleural space but are not trapped in lung parenchyma often fall to the "lowest" place in the hemithorax, namely the posterior costophrenic recess. In AP radiographic projection, the missile appears to be intra-abdominal, but triangulation with the lateral projection discloses the true location and can avoid needless laparotomy.

COMPUTED TOMOGRAPHY SCAN   Newer multidetector CT scans acquire data so rapidly that breath-holding is possible, greatly increasing the quality of the image. In combination with computer-controlled contrast injection, low pitch spiral data acquisition, and multiplanar subtractive reconstruction, CT angiography is used increasingly as a rapid screening tool. Caution and high-level supervision should be exercised in transporting marginal patients to the CT scanner, where management of decompensation is difficult and rarely successful.

ARTERIOGRAM   Indeed, before exploring penetrating injuries of the thoracic inlet in hemodynamically stable patients, one should obtain a preoperative image to visualize the arch of the aorta and its major branches. Aortography is still considered by some to be the definitive study for evaluating injury to the aorta.

VENOGRAMS   Venograms to identify major vascular injuries in the chest are seldom performed. A patient who is actively bleeding from a major venous injury is usually explored emergently because of unstable vital signs or continued blood loss through chest tubes.

CONTRAST SWALLOWS   A contrast swallow may be performed on a stable patient if there is concern about an associated esophageal injury. Water-soluble contrast is used first, but may miss up to half of esophageal leaks. Barium swallows have fewer false-negatives but can cause a worse mediastinitis if a perforation is present.

Endoscopy   With penetrating wounds of the chest or lower neck in hemodynamically stable patients, it may be prudent to perform bronchoscopy and esophagoscopy to rule out an injury to the aerodigestive tract. Such studies should be deferred until the patient is hemodynamically stable.

Ultrasound   Controversy persists regarding the evaluation of hemodynamically stable patients with transmediastinal gunshot wounds. The goal is the determination of trajectory to identify or exclude wounds to the heart, esophagus, and trachea. The combination of CT scan, contrast swallow, and transesophageal echocardiography to evaluate trajectory probably represents the current choice of many trauma surgeons.

TREATMENT

Initial Resuscitation   The standard ABCs (airway, breathing, circulation) of initial resuscitation should be followed aggressively if the patient is in shock. One of the problems occasionally seen with injuries to vessels in the thoracic outlet is massive mediastinal hematoma formation with resulting tracheal compression. Consequently, **early endotracheal intubation should be performed**. Tracheostomy should be avoided in patients with injuries at the thoracic inlet, at least initially, because of the possibility of precipitating massive bleeding from an otherwise controlled hematoma.

If the patient is in severe shock (systolic blood pressure <60 mm Hg), surgery should be performed promptly and aggressive fluid replacement should not be employed to a target blood pressure around 90 mm Hg. If the shock is persistent, the patient is rushed to the operating room. If cardiac arrest appears imminent, an immediate resuscitative thoracotomy should be performed there to control bleeding, provide internal cardiac massage, and cross-clamp the descending thoracic aorta as needed.

If rapid control of the bleeding sites and cross-clamping of the descending thoracic aortic arch do not raise the systolic blood pressure to at least 90 mm Hg within 5 min, terminal cardiovascular failure is present; almost all of these patients will die in the operating room regardless of effort.

Blunt Trauma to the Great Vessels of the Chest

The mechanical factors responsible for traumatic rupture of the thoracic aorta and its major branches are probably somewhat different for each anatomic area, but include shearing stress, bending stress, and torsion stress.

The aortic injury tends to progress from the intima out toward the adventitia. The adventitia, which has the lowest elastic limit, seems to withstand these stresses better than the intima or media.

Of the patients who reach a hospital and survive for 1 h, about half die within 24 h, and three-quarters die within 7 days. Of the remainder, most die within the next 1 to 3 months. Diagnosis and treatment can therefore be lifesaving.

At least 90 percent of blunt aortic injuries in patients who reach the hospital alive occur in the isthmus of the aorta, between the left subclavian artery and the ligamentum arteriosum.

DIAGNOSIS

History   The single most important factor in establishing the diagnosis of acute traumatic rupture of the aorta (TRA) is a high index of suspicion (Table 259-5), particularly in anyone who has sustained sudden severe deceleration or a high-speed impact from the side.

Patients with TRA usually complain primarily of their associated injuries and generally have no symptoms related to the aortic injury itself. The most common complaint that may be due to the aortic injury itself is retrosternal or interscapular pain. Recurrence or exacerbation of the pain, particularly if associated with a rise in blood pressure (which may be due to excess fluid administration or inadequate pain control), may herald an impending rupture of the pseudoaneurysm. Less frequent symptoms, due primarily to pressure from the associated hematoma, include dysphagia, stridor, dyspnea, or hoarseness.

Physical Examination   In many reports, at least one-third of the patients with blunt trauma to the aorta have no external evidence of thoracic injury at the time of the initial physical examination.

Physical findings that suggest aortic injury include 1) an acute onset of upper extremity hypertension, 2) difference in pulse amplitude between the upper and lower extremities, and 3) the presence of a harsh systolic murmur over the precordium or posterior interscapular

TABLE 259-5   Clinical Factors Suggesting Possible Traumatic Rupture of the Aorta

High-speed deceleration injury or side impact
Multiple rib fractures or flail chest
Pulse deficits
Hypertension
Systolic murmur over back
Hoarseness without laryngeal injury
Superior vena caval syndrome

area. Upper extremity hypertension has occurred in 31 to 43 percent of the patients reported in the literature, and has been attributed to compression of the aortic lumen by a periaortic hematoma. However, the hypertension may also be secondary to stretching or stimulation of special receptors located in the vicinity of the aortic isthmus. If the torn intima and media form a flap that acts as a ball valve, partial or complete aortic obstruction can occur. With partial obstruction, an "acute coarctation syndrome" can develop, with hypertension in the upper extremities and weak pulses or hypotension in the lower extremities. A systolic murmur, thought to be caused by turbulent blood flow across the area of transection, is found in fewer than 30 percent of the patients. If complete aortic obstruction occurs, anuria and paraplegia can develop almost immediately. Other, less frequently encountered physical findings include hoarseness, voice change, superior vena cava syndrome, swelling at the base of the neck, and paraplegia.

Plain Chest X-Ray   The original report by Gundry and colleagues, of radiographic findings in traumatic rupture of the aorta (TRA)[39](Table 259-6), is still helpful. Widened mediastinum visualized on an upright chest radiograph remains the most sensitive and specific finding in patients subsequently shown to have TRA. Secondary signs, which are less predictive, include: esophageal deviation, obscuration of the aortic knob, and loss of the paraspinal stripe.

One of the main reasons that many unnecessary aortograms are performed is a technically poor chest x-ray. The upper mediastinum tends to appear wider than normal if the chest x-ray is taken: 1) anteroposteriorly (AP) rather than posteroanteriorly (PA), 2) with the patient less than 3.25 ft (100 cm) from the origin of the x-ray beam, 3) with the patient lying flat, and 4) with poor inspiration.

The most accurate radiographic sign of TRA is usually deviation of the esophagus more than 1 to 2 cm to the right of the spinous process of T4. Patients in whom the esophagus is deviated less than 1.0 cm from the midline are unlikely to have a TRA. A nasogastric tube in a normal position virtually excludes TRA. Blurring or obscuration of the aortic knob or descending aorta is almost as accurate an indication of TRA. Studies have shown that patients with a normal aortic contour and no evidence of deviation of the trachea or nasogastric tube to the right on the chest x-ray do not have TRA.

Other chest x-ray signs include displacement of the left main stem bronchus more than 40° below the horizontal, obliteration of the usual clear space between the aortic knob and the left pulmonary artery (apical cap), widening of the right paratracheal stripe, and displacement of the right paraspinous interface.

The paratracheal stripe is a linear structure just to the right of the tracheal air column. It extends from the thoracic inlet to the proximal right bronchus and normally measures less than 5 mm in thickness at a level 2 cm above the azygos vein. If the paratracheal stripe is more than 5 mm wide and/or is deviated to the right, this may be another sign of mediastinal hemorrhage.

The paraspinal lines lie between the pleura and the lung, projected away from the lateral margin of the thoracic spine. The right paraspinal line is usually not visible on routine chest x-rays, but if it is seen and if it is displaced to the right in the absence of spinal or sternal fractures, it may be of some diagnostic value.

The left paraspinal line may be distinguished from the image of the descending aorta by the fact that it is not continuous with the aortic knob. When displaced more than one-half the distance from the spine to the left margin of the descending aorta without spinal or sternal fractures, the displacement is almost certainly due to a periaortic hematoma.

It is now very controversial whether fractures of the first or second ribs are associated with a significantly increased incidence of TRA.

One should not assume that a TRA has been ruled out if the initial chest x-ray is normal, because in up to one-third of cases, characteristic x-ray changes may not be apparent until several hours after the injury. Two-thirds of patients above 65 years of age with TRA may not show mediastinal widening. Consequently, serial chest films should be taken in any patient with severe chest trauma at 6- to 12-h intervals during the first day and then daily for at least the next 3 days. Indeed, the circumstances of the trauma in such individuals should be the main indication for ordering an aortogram.

Transesophageal Ultrasound   Unlike aortography, CT, or magnetic resonance imaging (MRI), transesophageal echocardiography (TEE) can be safely performed in hemodynamically unstable patients.

The thoracic aorta is not readily imaged by transthoracic ultrasound. However, the entire thoracic aorta can be imaged by TEE. TEE can be performed in less than 30 min compared to aortography, which requires over 75 min on average. Data on sensitivity and specificity of TEE is study-dependent on local factors such as patient population, limited study enrollment, operator type (cardiologists, surgeons, and radiologists), and experience. However, in at least one study, TEE and CT were equivalent in detecting blunt aortic injury requiring surgical repair, but had the advantage of diagnosing associated injuries such as to the innominate artery, and could identify lesions to the intima and media not identifiable on CT.[40]

The complication rate from TEE is very low, with esophageal perforation (perhaps the most feared complication) being on the order of 2 to 3 per 10,000.

CT Scans   Technical advances in instrumentation and technique are so rapid that an ongoing dialogue between emergency physicians and radiologists at the facility is necessary to understand local capabilities. Reports in the literature more than 2 to 3 years old tend to underestimate the sensitivity and specificity of current CT diagnosis. The sole contraindication to CT evaluation is hemodynamic instability. CT has become the predominant screening tool in many trauma centers.

TABLE 259-6   Reliability of Selected Clinical and Radiographic Criteria in the Detection of Traumatic Rupture of the Aorta*†

Radiographic or Clinical Finding	Correlation with TRA	Sensitivity	Specificity	Accuracy
Widened mediastinum (under 65 years old)	$p = .001$	0.95	0.82	0.84
Widened mediastinum (all ages)	$p = .001$	0.80	0.82	0.82
Murmur	$p = .002$	0.32	0.93	0.84
Pneumothorax/pulmonary contusion	$p = .07$	0.22	0.67	0.51
Hemothorax	$p = .21$	0.25	0.88	0.81
First/second rib fracture	$p = .39$	0.36	0.73	0.68

*All other clinical and radiographic criteria were less useful in detecting TRA.
†Sensitivity = TP/(TP + FN); Specificity = TN/(TN + FP); Accuracy = (TP + TN)/All tests.
Source: From Gundry,[39] with permission.

Magnetic Resonance Imaging MRI is a technically seductive method for investigating injuries to the aorta and great vessels. MRI has certainly emerged as the preferred tool for the evaluation of dissecting aneurysms of the thoracic aorta. Given the conditions required for current-generation imaging, the role of MRI in the evaluation of blunt thoracic injuries remains indeterminate at best.

Aortography Although aortography is still considered by some to be the gold standard for the diagnosis of TRA, it is positive in only about 10 percent of patients in whom injuries are suspected based on plain films. Further, it is an invasive procedure that requires 1 to 2 h.

A patient who is in shock from a suspected TRA or who has a rapidly expanding mediastinal hematoma should be taken directly to the operating room without undergoing aortography.

Although it is often thought that there is relatively little risk to angiography, the overall complication rate has remained steady at about 25 percent,[41,42] although the rates of amputation (0.1 percent) or death (0.3 percent) resulting from transfemoral studies is relatively low. If angiography is done in a hospital where relatively few cases are done each year, the incidence of complications can be increased up to 32-fold. It should be remembered that occasional false-negatives occur with aortography.

TREATMENT Although it is essential to resuscitate severely injured patients aggressively and to correct hypotension and hypoxemia rapidly, **the patient with a TRA should not be allowed to develop a systolic blood pressure over 120 mm Hg or to perform a Valsalva maneuver.** Endotracheal intubation can likewise cause gagging and coughing. In addition to the standard paralytic and sedative drugs administered during rapid-sequence intubation, preemptive intravenous administration of lidocaine (1 mg/kg) to attenuate the vascular and bronchial responses prior to laryngoscopy may be advisable in patients with suspected or proven TRA. Fluid administration should be watched carefully, and administration of sedatives, analgesics, vasodilators, and beta-adrenergic blockers may be required to keep the patient's systolic blood pressure at safe levels. Nasogastric intubation should be undertaken with caution owing to the transient spikes in blood pressure should the patient cough and gag during insertion.

Since 1958, emergency repair has become the accepted standard for care. More recently, three alternatives have emerged: endovascular stenting; initial aggressive medical control of blood pressure, with delayed repair; and prolonged observation with careful BP control in some patients with small unsuspected injuries seen only on high-resolution CT scan.

Special Considerations in Less Frequent Great Vessel Injuries

ASCENDING AORTA Very few patients with ascending aortic injury survive long enough for the diagnosis to be established and repair to be carried out. These injuries are frequently associated with cardiac rupture or severe myocardial contusion, and the aortic tears are multiple in up to 15 to 20 percent. Most victims have been hit by or thrown from moving vehicles or have fallen from great heights.

Thoracic aortic injuries distal to the isthmus should be suspected with severe chest trauma in which a lower thoracic vertebra is severely crushed.

DESCENDING AORTA Injuries to the descending aorta are uncommon. The presentations include paraplegia (owing to injuries to vessels supplying the spinal cord), mesenteric ischemia, anuria, or lower extremity ischemia. Contrast-enhanced CT scans may show a false channel, pseudoaneurysm, or extravasation into perivascular tissues. Cardiopulmonary bypass may be required for surgical management. The more distal the injury, the better the anticipated outcome-provided that the patient does not exsanguinate prior to repair. If the injury lies between the renal arteries and the aortic bifurcation, endovascular stenting may be considered. Otherwise, traditional open repair should be performed immediately.

INNOMINATE ARTERY In patients reaching the hospital alive, blunt injuries of the innominate artery are second in frequency only to rupture of the aorta at the isthmus.

Making a diagnosis of blunt injury to the innominate artery can be very difficult because there are no characteristic physical findings except for some diminution of the right radial or brachial pulse, which occurs in about 50 percent of the patients. Signs and symptoms of distal ischemia are uncommon. Occasionally, a systolic murmur may draw attention to a possible lesion in this area.

The chest x-ray findings are somewhat similar to those seen with TRA, but the mediastinal hematoma tends to be higher and the trachea and esophagus may be pushed to the left. Although aortography remains the standard diagnostic technique, CT angiography is now widely used, at least as a screening tool.

Subclavian Artery Although a subclavian artery is occasionally avulsed at its origin because of sudden deceleration, direct trauma to the distal artery with intimal damage and occlusion associated with fractures of the first rib or clavicle are more likely. Shoulder restraints that are loose may be a major factor in causing this injury.

The most important sign of a subclavian occlusion is absence of a radial pulse. In the patient with only a partial laceration and no occlusion, the radial pulse may be preserved. Other physical findings that are highly suggestive of subclavian artery rupture are a pulsatile mass or a bruit in the root of the neck. Occasionally a patient may develop an acute subclavian steal syndrome if the subclavian artery occludes proximal to the origin of the vertebral artery.

Up to 60 percent of patients with blunt injury to the subclavian artery, especially from motor vehicle accidents, will also have some damage to the brachial plexus. Horner syndrome often indicates avulsion of nerve roots from the spinal cord.

The chest x-ray with subclavian artery injuries may show the presence of a widened superior mediastinum without obscuration of the aortic knob. CT angiography can be diagnostic. An angiogram usually shows occlusion, but a pseudoaneurysm is occasionally found.

The treatment of acute subclavian artery injury is usually immediate repair. However, in certain high-risk patients who are doing poorly, occlusion by an interventional radiologist may be the treatment of choice. If the artery is already occluded, observation may be all that is required. The collateral circulation to the distal portions of the vessel is usually very good. However, if there has been severe blunt trauma to the shoulder girdle, many of the collateral vessels may be damaged, resulting in critical ischemia of the hand or upper extremity gangrene in about 30 percent.

ESOPHAGEAL AND THORACIC DUCT INJURIES

Esophageal Injuries

Lacerations of the esophagus occur most frequently during endoscopic biopsy or dilatation of a narrowed or obstructed esophagus. The esophagus can also be injured by swallowed foreign bodies. Injury to the thoracic esophagus is seen only rarely in patients who reach the hospital alive.

If esophageal injury is suspected, an esophagogram should be obtained. **The initial study should be performed using water-soluble contrast,** since extravasation of barium into the mediastinum can complicate mediastinitis. However, a negative water-soluble contrast study should always be confirmed with a barium study owing to the former's relatively high false-negative rate. Small leaks of water-soluble contrast may be better visualized on CT scan, which should be performed prior to a barium study.

Flexible esophagoscopy is being performed increasingly for diagnosis but may miss occasional injuries, even if combined with an esophagogram. **Neither barium nor water-soluble contrast will interfere with a subsequent esophagoscopy.** Some prefer rigid esophagoscopy in combination with bronchoscopy to rule out associated tracheobronchial injuries.

In spite of all our technical and nutritional advances in recent years, the mortality rate for esophageal injuries ranges from 5 to 25 percent for those treated definitively within 12 h, and 25 to 66 percent for those treated after 24 h.

Thoracic Duct Injuries

Thoracic duct injuries should be suspected in patients with penetrating trauma to near the left proximal subclavian vein. The diagnosis is unlikely to be made in the ED and usually discovered at time of surgical exploration and repair.

REFERENCES

1. Richter M, Kettek C, Otte D et al: Correlation between crash severity, injury severity and clinical course in car occupants with thoracic trauma: A technical and medical study. *J Trauma Injury Infect Crit Care* 50:10, 2001.
2. Rotondo MF, McGonigal MD, Schwab CW, et al: Urgent paralysis and intubation of trauma patients: Is it safe? *J Trauma* 34:242, 1993.
3. Dulchavsky SA, Schwarz KL, Kirkpatrick AW, et al: Prospective evaluation of thoracic ultrasound in the detection of pneumothorax. *J Trauma Injury Infect Crit Care* 50:201, 2001.
4. Carrillo EH, Guinn BJ, Ali AT, et al: Transthoracic ultrasonography is an alternative to subxyphoid ultrasonography for the diagnosis of hemopericardium in penetrating precordial trauma. *Am J Surg* 179:34, 2000.
5. Kirton OC, Windsor J, Wedderburn R, et al: Failure of splanchnic resuscitation in the acutely injured trauma patient correlates with multiple organ system failure and length of stay in the ICU. *Chest* 113:1064, 1998.
6. Branney SW, Moore EE, Feldhaus KM, et al: Critical analysis of two decades of experience with postinjury emergency department thoracotomy in a regional trauma center. *J Trauma* 45:87, 1998.
7. Rhee PM, Acosta J, Bridgeman A, et al: Survival after emergency department thoracotomy: Review of published data from the past 25 years. *J Am Coll Surg* 190:288, 2000.
8. Working Group, Ad Hoc Subcommittee on Outcomes, American College of Surgeons Committee on Trauma: Practice management guidelines for emergency department thoracotomy. *J Am Coll Surg* 193:303, 2001.
9. Exadaktylos AK, Sclabas G, Schmid SW, et al: Do we really need routine computed tomographic scanning in the primary evaluation of blunt chest trauma in patients with "normal" chest radiograph? *J Trauma Injury Infect Crit Care* 51:1173, 2001.
10. Luchette FA, Radfshar MR, Kaiser R, et al: Prospective evaluation of epidural versus intrapleural catheters for analgesia in chest wall trauma. *J Trauma* 35:165, 1993.
11. Galan G, Penalver JC, Paris E, et al: Blunt chest injuries in 1696 patients. *Eur J Cardiothorac Surg* 6:284, 1992.
12. Tanaka H, Yukioka T, Yamaguti Y, et al: Surgical stabilization or internal pneumatic stabilization? A prospective randomized study of management of severe flail chest patients. *J Trauma Injury Infect Crit Care* 52:727, 2002.
13. Brookes JG, Dunn RJ, Rogers IR: Sternal fractures: A retrospective analysis of 272 cases. *J Trauma* 35:46, 1993.
14. Wright SW: Myth of the dangerous sternal fracture. *Ann Emerg Med* 22:1589, 1993.
15. Chiu WC, D'amelio LF, Hammond JS: Sternal fractures in blunt chest trauma: A practical algorithm for management. *Am J Emerg Med* 15:252, 1997.
16. Jongewaard WR, Cogbill TH, Landercasper J: Neurologic consequences of traumatic asphyxia. *J Trauma* 32:28, 1992.
17. Younes RN, Gross JL, Aguiar S, et al: When to remove a chest tube? A randomized study with subsequent prospective consecutive validation. *J Am Coll Surg* 195:658, 2002.
18. Gonzalez RP, Holevar MR: Role of prophylactic antibiotics for tube thoracostomy in chest trauma. *Am Surg* 64:617, 1998.
19. Cant PJ, Smyth S, Smart DO: Antibiotic prophylaxis is indicated for chest stab wounds requiring closed tube thoracostomy. *Br J Surg* 80:464, 1993.
20. Demetriades D, Breckon V, Breckon C, et al: Antibiotic prophylaxis in penetrating injuries of the chest. *Ann R Coll Surg Engl* 73:348, 1991.
21. Ordog GJ, Wasserberger J, Balasubramanium S, et al: Asymptomatic stab wounds of the chest. *J Trauma* 36:680, 1994.
22. Collins JC, Levine G, Waxman K: Occult traumatic pneumothorax: Immediate tube thoracostomy versus expectant management. *Am Surg* 58:743, 1992.
23. Enderson BL, Abdalla R, Frame SB, et al: Tube thoracostomy for occult pneumothorax: A prospective randomized study of its use. *J Trauma* 35:726, 1993.
24. Brown GL, Richardson JD: Traumatic diaphragmatic hernia. *Ann Thorac Surg* 39:172, 1985.
25. Tyburski JG, Astra L, Wilson RF, et al: Factors affecting prognosis with penetrating wounds of the heart. *J Trauma Injury Infect Crit Care* 48:587, 2000.
26. Plummer D, Brunette D, Asinger R, et al: Emergency department echocardiography improves outcome in penetrating cardiac injury. *Ann Emerg Med* 21:709, 1992.
27. Meyer DM, Jessen ME, Grayburn PA: Use of echocardiography to detect occult cardiac injury after penetrating thoracic trauma: A prospective study. *J Trauma* 39:902, 1995.
28. Armstrong G, Cardon L, Vilkomerson D, et al: Localization of needle tip with color Doppler during pericardiocentesis: In vitro validation and initial clinical application. *J Am Soc Echocardiogr* 14:29, 2001.
29. ACC/AHA Cardiology Guideline Summaries, in Braunwald E (ed): *Heart Disease: A Textbook of Cardiovascular Medicine,* 6 ed. Philadelphia, WB Saunders, 101(101), 2001.
30. Maron BJ, Gohman TE, Kyle SB, et al: Clinical profile and spectrum of commotio cordis. *JAMA* 287:1142, 2002.
31. Maenza RL, Seaberg D, D'Amico F: A meta-analysis of blunt cardiac trauma: Ending myocardial confusion. *Am J Emerg Med* 14:237, 1996.
32. Fulda GJ: An evaluation of serum troponin T and signal-averaged electrocardiography in predicting electrocardiographic abnormalities after blunt chest trauma. *J Trauma* 43:304, 1997.
33. Foil MB, Mackersie RC, Furst SR, et al: The asymptomatic patient with suspected myocardial contusion. *Am J Surg* 160:638, 1990.
34. Biffl WA, Moore FA, Moore EE, et al: Cardiac enzymes are irrelevant in the patient with suspected myocardial contusion. *Am J Surg* 169:523, 1994.
35. Adams JE, Davila-Roman VGH, Bessey PQ, et al: Improved detection of cardiac contusion with cardiac troponin-I. *Am Heart J* 131:308, 1996.
36. Ferjani M, Droc G, Dreux S, et al: Circulating cardiac troponin T in myocardial contusion. *Chest* 111:427, 1997.
37. Bertinchant JP, Polge A, Mohty D, et al: Evaluation of incidence, clinical significance, and prognostic value of circulating cardiac troponin I and T elevation in hemodynamically stable patients with suspected myocardial contusion after blunt chest trauma. *J Trauma Injury Infect Crit Care* 48: 924, 2000.
38. Edouard AR, Benoist JF, Cosson C, et al: Circulating cardiac troponin I in trauma patients without cardiac contusion. *Intens Care Med* 24:569, 1998.
39. Gundry SR, Williams S, Burney RE: Indications for aortography in blunt thoracic trauma. A reassessment. *J Trauma* 22:664, 1982.
40. Vignon P, Boncoeur MP, François B, et al: Comparison of multiplane transesophageal echocardiography and contrast-enhanced helical CT in the diagnosis of blunt traumatic cardiovascular injuries. *Anesthesiology* 94:615, 2001.
41. Waugh JR, Sacharias N: Arteriographic complications in the DSA eras. *Radiology* 182:243, 1992.
42. Young N, Chi KK, Ajaka J, et al: Complications with outpatient angiography and interventional procedures. *Cardiovasc Intervent Radiol* 25:123, 2002.

ABDOMINAL INJURIES
Thomas M. Scalea
Sharon A. Boswell

PATHOPHYSIOLOGY OF INJURY

Abdominal trauma generally is divided into two types: blunt and penetrating. This is somewhat simplistic. For instance, patients can suffer both blunt and penetrating trauma simultaneously. Patients involved in motor vehicle crashes may be impaled on objects at the same time. In addition, people who are shot or stabbed may also be assaulted at the same time.

Blunt Trauma

Blunt trauma is the most common mechanism of injury seen in the United States. This diffuse injury pattern puts all abdominal organs at risk for injury. The biomechanics of blunt injury involve a compression or crushing by direct energy transmission. If the compressive, shearing, or stretching forces exceed tissue tolerance limits, they are disrupted. This may result in injury to solid viscera (i.e., liver or spleen) or rupture of hollow viscera (i.e., the gastrointestinal tract).

Injury also can result from the movement of organs within the body. Some organs are rigidly fixed, whereas others are more mobile. Injury is particularly common in areas of transition before fixed and mobile organs. Examples include mesenteric or small-bowel injuries, particularly at the ligament of Treitz or at the junction of the distal small bowel and right colon.

Falls from a height produce a unique pattern of injury. Injury severity is a function of distance, the surface on which the victim lands, and whether the fall is broken. Intraabdominal injuries are uncommon and hollow visceral rupture is most common.[1] Retroperitoneal injuries with significant blood loss, however, are common because force is transmitted up the axial skeleton.

Pedestrians struck by cars are completely unprotected and all force is applied directly to the patient's body. Motorcyclists or bicyclists generally are protected only by a helmet.

Penetrating Trauma

Stab wounds directly injure tissue as the blade passes through the body. External examination of the wound may underestimate internal damage and cannot define the trajectory of the blade. Any stab wound in the lower chest, pelvis, flank, or back has caused abdominal injury until proven otherwise.

Gunshot wounds injure in several ways. Bullets may injure organs directly, via secondary missiles such as bone or bullet fragments or from energy transmitted from the bullet. Bullets designed to break apart once they enter a victim cause much more tissue destruction than a bullet that remains intact.

Entrance and exit wounds can approximate the missile trajectory. Plain radiographs help to localize the foreign body, allowing prediction of organs at risk. Unfortunately, bullets may not travel in a straight line. Thus all structures in any proximity to the presumed trajectory must be considered injured (see Chap. 264).

DIAGNOSING ABDOMINAL INJURY

Solid Visceral Injuries

Solid visceral injuries usually produce symptoms by blood loss. Patients often develop hypotension.[2] Some patients develop tachycardia, skin changes, and mental confusion with blood loss.[2] These signs are highly nonspecific. Young patients may lose 50 to 60 percent of their blood volume and be asymptomatic.[3] Thus, assuming that a stable patient does not have an intraabdominal injury is hazardous.

Abdominal tenderness, distention, and/or tympany may not be present until patients have nearly exsanguinated into their abdomen. Some patients develop tenderness early with hemoperitoneum. Others, however, remain asymptomatic for many hours or days. Use of physical examination alone will lead to an unacceptable rate of missed injuries.

Gastrointestinal Injuries

Hollow visceral injuries produce symptoms by the combination of blood loss and peritoneal contamination. Perforation of the stomach, small bowel, or colon is often accompanied by some blood loss such as from a concomitant mesenteric injury. Gastrointestinal contamination will produce physical findings over a period of time. Patients with trau-

matic brain injuries or intoxication may not demonstrate physical findings initially. In addition, patients with substantial injuries elsewhere may be distracted from their abdominal pain for a number of hours.

Gastric injuries produce symptoms by chemical irritation when acidic contents are spilled into the abdominal cavity. This often occurs early in the treatment course but may take more time if patients are on H_2 blockers. Small-bowel and colonic injuries elicit symptoms because bacterial content produces suppurative peritonitis. Inflammation may take 6 to 8 h to develop.

Retroperitoneal Injuries

As with intraabdominal injuries, symptoms and physical findings of retroperitoneal injuries may be subtle or completely absent initially. Occasionally, retroperitoneal injuries do produce abdominal pain, even if they are relatively insignificant, such as a small retroperitoneal hematoma.

Duodenal injuries also can be asymptomatic at the time of presentation. Duodenal wall hematomas can produce relative gastric outlet obstruction with abdominal pain, nausea, and vomiting (Figure 260-1). Duodenal rupture is usually contained within the retroperitoneum. This may present with abdominal pain, fever, and tenderness, though they may take hours or even days to become clinically obvious. Duodenal rupture often occurs from rapid increases in intraluminal pressure when both the pylorus and the proximal small bowel develop spasm, most often occur after high-speed vertical or horizontal decelerating trauma.

Pancreatic injuries often accompany rapid decelerating injury. Pancreatic transection usually occurs in the midbody as the pancreas is displaced against the vertebral column. Thus, unrestrained drivers who hit the steering column or bicyclists who hit the handlebars are at special risk for pancreatic injury.

The diagnosis of pancreatic injury can be elusive. Patients can have few symptoms initially. There are no biochemical or radiographic markers pathognomonic for the diagnosis. Elevations in serum amylase are nonspecific. Computed tomography (CT) scanning may be normal initially. Relatively small pancreatic injuries can become symptomatic days later. Leakage of activated pancreatic enzymes from the pancreas can produce retroperitoneal autodigestion. These also can become superinfected with bacteria, producing a retroperitoneal abscess.

Urologic injuries may occur with abdominal trauma, but are discussed in detail in Chap. 262.

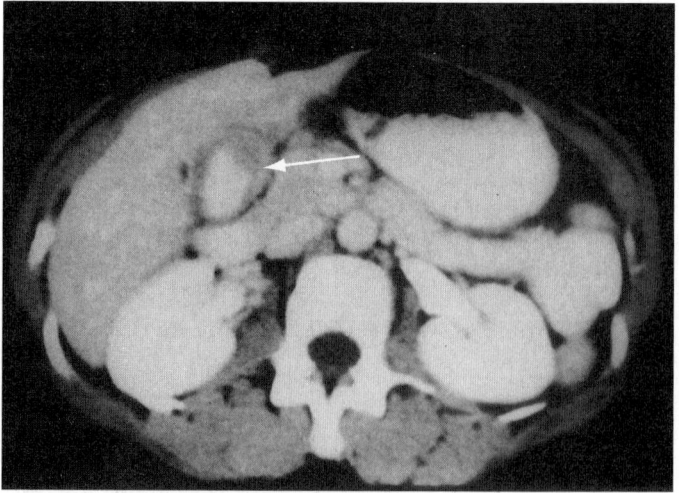

FIG. 260-1. Duodenal injury. Computed tomography (CT) scan demonstrating duodenal hematoma. Note the partial obstruction of the duodenum with an intramural hematoma. The injury resolved with nasogastric decompression and a short period of intravenous nutrition.

Diaphragmatic Injuries

A plain film of the chest demonstrating viscera in the chest or a nasogastric tube coiled in the thorax definitively diagnoses a diaphragm injury. More often, chest x-ray findings are subtle or absent. Diagnostic peritoneal lavage (DPL) can be helpful, particularly if the DPL fluid exits via a concomitantly placed chest tube or if follow-up chest x-ray demonstrates a new pleural effusion. Both helical CT and magnetic resonance imaging (MRI) can be helpful in diagnosing a diaphragmatic injury.[4] Occasionally, cavitary endoscopy or laparotomy are necessary to make the diagnosis.

ABDOMINAL EVALUATION AFTER BLUNT TRAUMA

A multiplicity of diagnostic modalities exist to evaluate the abdomen. No test is foolproof, and each must be used in conjunction with an assessment of stability, associated injuries, and physical findings.

Who Needs Evaluation?

All patients undergo initial physical examination. Unfortunately, this is often inadequate to make the diagnosis of abdominal injury. As a minimum, the following category of patients should undergo evaluation:

1. Presence of abdominal pain, tenderness, or distention
2. Mechanism of injury and prehospital details suggest potential for injury
3. Lower chest or pelvic injury
4. High-speed collisions or collisions where there has been substantial deformity to the vehicle (particularly if the patient was unrestrained)
5. Motor vehicle crashes with fatalities or those in which there were others with substantial injuries
6. Unprotected injury (i.e., motorcycle crashes)
7. Inability to tolerate a delayed diagnosis (e.g., the elderly, those with significant comorbid diseases)
8. Presence of distracting injuries (e.g., long-bone fractures)
9. Decreased level of consciousness/altered sensorium
10. Pain-masking drugs (e.g., ethanol, opiates)

Techniques of Evaluation

In the past, diagnostics were designed merely to document that an abdominal injury existed. Organ-specific diagnosis was made at the time of surgery, and all patients with abdominal injury underwent laparotomy. A large number of patients are now managed nonoperatively. Table 260-1 details the available diagnostic testing used for blunt abdominal trauma. Some specific comments, however, are necessary.

Physical Examination

The abdomen should be examined for signs of injury such as abrasions or contusions. This should include the flank, back, and lower chest, as well as the anterior abdomen.

A single physical examination is insensitive. Serial physical examinations increase the utility in identifying intraabdominal injury. These must be performed by the same senior-level clinician and should span a period of time of at least 16 to 24 h. The patient must be awake, alert, and reliable. While there is little science describing this technique, we suggest that physical examination must be performed at least every 30 min for the first 4 h, hourly for an additional 4 to 6 h, and every 2 to 4 h for the remainder of the 24-h observation period. This should be accompanied by frequent hematocrit determinations and measurement of vital signs.

Plain Radiographs

Plain radiographs have an extremely limited use in patients with blunt abdominal trauma. They are incapable of making the diagnosis of hemoperitoneum. Even patients with hollow visceral injury often have normal radiographs. Occasionally, a chest x-ray will show free air under the diaphragm. However, routine use of plain films of the abdomen is not cost-effective.

Pelvic films, on the other hand, are standard in the evaluation process. Patients with pelvic fractures have a high-energy mechanism. This mandates rapid abdominal evaluation to avoid confusing retroperitoneal bleeding, common with pelvic fracture, with intraabdominal blood loss. In addition, patients with thoracolumbar spine fractures must have abdominal evaluation. Intravenous pyelography (IVP) has been replaced by CT. Retrograde urethrography is useful in males with pelvic fractures to exclude urethral injury.

Screening Examinations for Abdominal Injury

Both DPL and ultrasonic abdominal evaluation can screen for hemoperitoneum after blunt trauma. Both examinations identify the presence or absence of blood in the abdomen but can make no determination as to the etiology of the hemoperitoneum. DPL is rapid, safe, and inexpensive. There is approximately a 1 percent incidence of major complication. DPL can be performed using either an open or a closed technique (Figures 260-2 and 260-3). We prefer closed percutaneous DPL because the complication rate is no different from the more cumbersome open technique. An immediately positive tap is defined as the aspiration of 10 mL of free-flowing blood. If the tap is negative, 1 L of saline is instilled and the abdomen drained by gravity. Some authors recommend that 250 mL of return is necessary.[5] One hundred thousand red blood cells per μL is considered a positive lavage in blunt trauma. Thus, only 25 mL of blood must accumulate in the abdomen (assuming complete mixing) for DPL to be positive.

Laparotomy based solely on a positive DPL for red cells results in a nontherapeutic procedure approximately 30 percent of the time.[6] Minimal injury can easily produce a hemoperitoneum sufficient to render DPL positive. Determining white cell count in the DPL effluent is nonspecific.[7] In addition, biochemical assays such as liver function tests or amylase determination are nonspecific. Decision on laparotomy should be made based on the patient's hemodynamics and associated injuries in concert with the DPL. A patient with a positive DPL who is stable and does not have peritonitis is still a candidate for nonoperative management.

Focused assessment with sonography for trauma (FAST) is a rapid screen for intraabdominal injury and can be performed in less than 3 min. Like DPL, it can determine the presence of hemoperitoneum.

TABLE 260-1 Diagnostic Testing

Techniques	Easy	Rapid	Sensitive	Specific	Retroperitoneum	Expensive	Repeatable	Invasive	Transport from ED
Physical examination	Yes	Yes	No	No	No	No	Yes	No	No
DPL	Yes	Yes	Yes	Not at all	No	No	No	Yes	No
FAST	Yes	Yes	Yes	Not at all	No	No	Yes	No	No
CT	No	No	Yes	Yes	Yes	Yes	Yes	IV contrast	Yes

Abbreviations: CT = computed tomography; DPL = diagnostic peritoneal lavage; FAST = focused assessment with sonography for trauma.

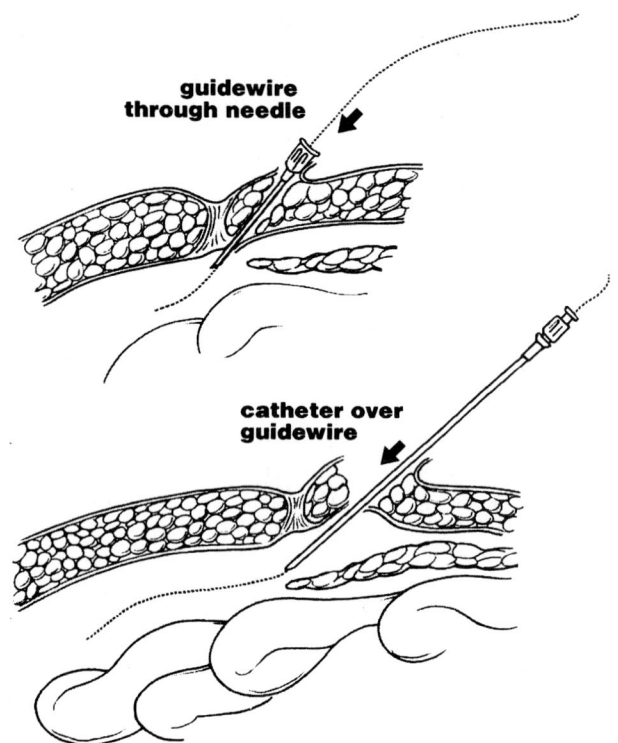

FIG. 260-2. Closed diagnostic peritoneal lavage (DPL). Closed percutaneous DPL is an effective manner of evaluating the abdomen for hemoperitoneum. A needle is inserted two finger breadths below the umbilicus after infiltration with local lidocaine with epinephrine. A guidewire can be then inserted into the abdomen and the peritoneal lavage catheter inserted over the guidewire. One liter of fluid is instilled and the abdomen is then drained.

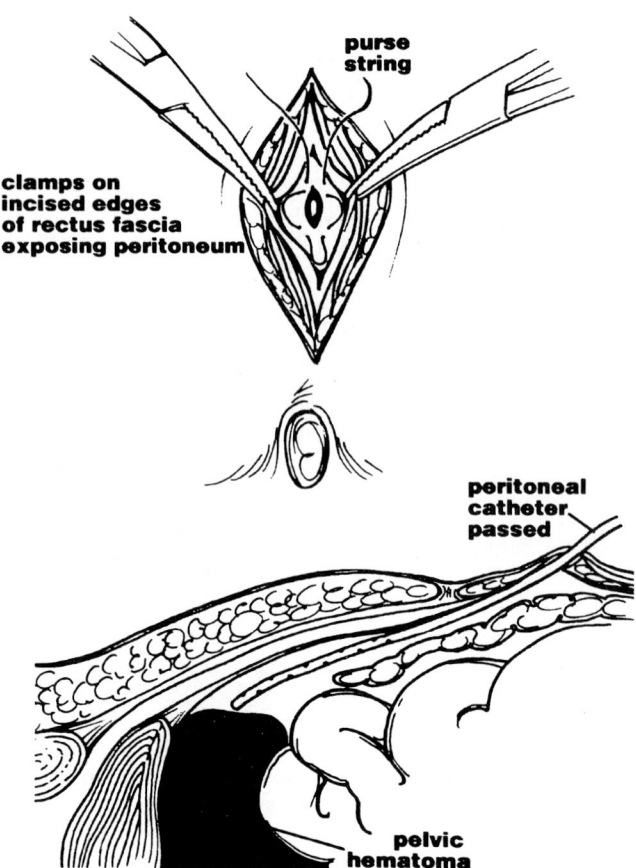

FIG. 260-3. Open diagnostic peritoneal lavage. Open diagnostic peritoneal lavage (DPL) is a surgical procedure requiring some expertise. An incision is made under local anesthetic and can be performed in an infraumbilical or supraumbilical location. **Patients with pelvic fractures must have their DPL performed open and above the umbilicus.** An incision is made through the skin and subcutaneous tissue under local anesthesia. The fascia is opened and a purse-string suture placed in the peritoneum. The peritoneum is then opened within the purse-string suture and the catheter passed into the peritoneal cavity. Fluid is infused and returned as with a closed DPL.

FAST is clearly operator-dependent and requires true expertise for reliable use. Like DPL, FAST is ineffective for imaging the retroperitoneum.

The amount of fluid necessary for a positive FAST remains unclear. In general, several hundred cubic centimeters of fluid/blood are necessary to be clearly visible using FAST.[8] Like DPL, FAST cannot determine the etiology of the fluid.

FAST is generally performed in four areas: perisplenic, perihepatic, pelvic, and pericardial. No matter which organ is injured, the perihepatic view is most commonly positive. Blood pools in Morison pouch, the most dependent portion of the abdomen. The pericardial views can be extremely helpful, although pericardial tamponade is rare after blunt abdominal injury.

The ability of FAST to determine the need for laparotomy is questionable. McKinney et al. have encouraging data that suggest that their scoring system can predict the need for laparotomy.[9] Unlike DPL, FAST can be repeated.

Clearly, FAST has limitations. Its ability to detect small amounts of fluid is questionable, even in skilled hands. In addition, a single FAST cannot absolutely exclude intraabdominal injury. A recent international consensus conference concluded that **prudent evaluation would involve two FAST exams performed at least 6 h apart** supplemented with serial physical exams to avoid missing an injury.[10]

ORGAN-SPECIFIC DIAGNOSIS

Only CT scanning can make the diagnosis of organ-specific abdominal injury. CT scanning images both the abdomen and the retroperitoneum. It is the diagnostic test of choice to investigate the duodenum and pancreas. It can diagnose urinary extravasation and images the ureters. CT can quantitate the amount of blood in the abdomen.

The disadvantages of CT are the expense and time required to perform the scan. In some centers, the CT scanner is some distance away

from the ED. This limits its use, particularly in critically ill patients. The oral contrast material often produces nausea and vomiting and must be administered while the spine remains immobilized. The intravenous contrast material has a small incidence of allergic reactions. Some advocate that oral contrast is unnecessary for abdominal CT during the initial assessment.[11] This requires further study before it is likely to gain widespread acceptance.

There are some patients who require CT scanning despite a normal FAST. Chiu et al. have shown that 28 percent of selected patients may have intraabdominal solid visceral injury without hemoperitoneum.[12] These include those with abrasions or tenderness in the lower chest, abdomen, or pelvis. Other findings mandating CT are pelvic fractures or thoracolumbar spine fractures.

EVALUATION OF THE ABDOMEN AFTER PENETRATING TRAUMA

Stab Wounds

Mandatory exploration, a policy used in the 1960s and early 1970s, has largely been abandoned, as it yields unacceptably high rates of nontherapeutic laparotomy. Feliciano and Renz described significant complication rates for nontherapeutic trauma laparotomy.[13]

Diagnostic modalities available for the evaluation of patients with stab wounds to the anterior abdomen include physical examination, DPL, and local wound exploration.

Physical examination may fail to suggest injury for the reasons stated for blunt trauma. Serial physical exams, on the other hand, are accurate in the evaluation of patients with abdominal stab wounds.[14] This must be considered with all the provisos mentioned above.

Closed percutaneous DPL is an excellent technique for evaluating patients with anterior abdominal stab wounds. It is performed exactly as used for blunt trauma. There is some controversy as to the amount of red cells required for a positive DPL for stab wounds. The lower the threshold for a positive cell count, the higher is the rate of nontherapeutic laparotomy, but the lower is the rate of missed injury. The converse is also true. Most centers set between 10,000 and 20,000 red blood cells/μL as a threshold for laparotomy. The accuracy increases from approximately 78 to 90 percent as the threshold for positivity decreases. Any patient who undergoes DPL must be observed in the hospital for at least 12 to 24 h.

Local wound exploration accurately evaluates the abdomen after a stab wound (Figure 260-4). This is a surgical procedure that requires proper lighting, instruments, and local anesthesia. **Digital probing of the wound or radiographic trajectograms with contrast material are unwise.** Both are inaccurate and lead to both nontherapeutic laparotomy and missed injuries.

If local wound exploration demonstrates no violation of the anterior fascia, the patient can be discharged home. If local wound exploration demonstrates fascial violation, several options exist. Diagnostic exploration is reasonable as the rate of nontherapeutic laparotomy will be relatively low. Positive local wound explorations can also be followed by DPL. If DPL fluid does not exit the wound or is negative by cell count, the patient can be observed.

It is often difficult to follow the trajectory of a stab wound. If the clinician is not completely comfortable that this has been a technically satisfactory procedure, one must abandon the use of local wound exploration and use another form of evaluation. Our preference would be to use DPL in this setting.

Gunshot Wounds

The most important consideration with anterior abdominal gunshot wounds is to determine whether the missile traversed the peritoneal cavity. Patients with transabdominal gunshot wounds virtually all have

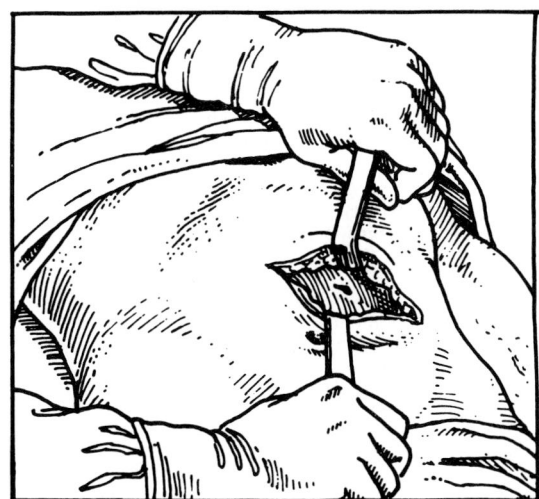

FIG. 260-4. Local wound exploration. Local wound exploration is the appropriate way to evaluate the abdomen after a stab wound. This is a surgical procedure requiring expertise, proper instrumentation, and lights. It is an appropriate diagnostic technique only for patients with anterior abdominal stab wounds. The stab wound is widened and explored down to the level of the fascia. A determination can be made whether the anterior fascia and/or posterior fascia has been violated.

intraabdominal injury requiring surgery. Most often, this can be determined by estimating trajectory. Thus, a hole both in the anterior and posterior abdomen clearly defines a transabdominal trajectory. In the event of a single entrance, a plain film of the chest, pelvis, and/or abdomen often can determine trajectory. A lateral film may be helpful.

Occasionally, in the case of tangential injuries or multiple gunshot wounds, it may be impossible to clearly determine trajectory. It often may be safest to simply explore these patients. While not perfect, surgical exploration at least ensures that a potentially life-threatening injury will not be missed. The second option is to carefully observe the patient with frequent physical examinations and laboratory values. The last option is to perform a peritoneal lavage. There are virtually no data that determine the correct threshold for red blood cell positivity in patients with gunshot wounds. The only purpose is to determine whether the missile traversed the abdominal cavity. Thus, we generally set the threshold very low and explore patients if there is even a pink tinge to the effluent or the red blood cell count is 5000/μL or greater.

Penetrating trauma to the flank and back can be investigated with contrast-enhanced CT enema using oral, intravenous, and rectal contrast agents and managed nonoperatively (see Chap. 261 for details).

CT scanning is now being used to evaluate injuries to the anterior abdomen as well. It can easily make the diagnosis of transabdominal trajectory by demonstrating free air or fluid,[15] but cannot accurately define the organs injured. Patients with a positive CT scan should have diagnostic laparotomy.

Likewise, FAST is now being used for penetrating trauma. A positive FAST has a positive predictive value of >90 percent.[16] A negative FAST, however, cannot exclude injury. Further investigation is necessary.

MANAGEMENT OF ABDOMINAL INJURY

Laparotomy

Laparotomy is the "gold standard" therapy for intraabdominal injuries. It is definitive, rarely misses an injury, and allows for complete evaluation of the abdomen and retroperitoneum. Table 260-2 describes generally accepted indications for exploratory laparotomy. Certainly all patients with hypotension, abdominal wall disruption, or peritonitis mandate surgical exploration. In addition, the presence of extraluminal, intraabdominal, or retroperitoneal air either on plain film or CT should prompt surgical exploration. Finally, organ-specific diagnosis on CT often will mandate exploration. Examples include pancreatic injury, duodenal injury, renal injury with urine leak outside Gerota fascia, or a bowel injury.

Some patients have the diagnosis of injury made but are hemodynamically stable with a normal physical examination. Examples include patients with a positive DPL or FAST or patients with a CT-diagnosed splenic or hepatic injury. Clearly, some of these patients can be managed nonoperatively. In smaller centers or community hospitals, these patients may be best served by surgical exploration. In tertiary care centers, some of these patients can be managed nonoperatively.

Many patients with fluid seen on CT scan without a solid visceral injury have a trivial liver or splenic injury that is missed on CT. Unfortunately, others will have mesenteric injuries and/or small-bowel injuries. Often the safest course is exploration to avoid late diagnosis of GI perforation or ischemia. Careful observation and/or repeat CT can also be used.

NONOPERATIVE MANAGEMENT OF BLUNT TRAUMA

The evolution of nonoperative therapy has been greatly advanced by the evolution of CT. CT makes the diagnosis of solid visceral injury and often can rule out other injuries requiring surgery. Solid visceral injuries can be graded as to severity.

TABLE 260-2   Indications for Laparotomy

	Blunt	Penetrating
Absolute	Anterior abdominal injury and hypotension Abdominal wall disruption Peritonitis Free air on chest x-ray CT-diagnosed injury requiring surgery, i.e., pancreatic transection; duodenal rupture	Injury to abdomen, back, and flank with hypotension Abdominal tenderness GI evisceration Positive DPL (GSW) High suspicion for transabdominal trajectory CT-diagnosed injury requiring surgery, i.e., ureter or pancreas
Relative	Positive DPL or FAST in stable patient Solid visceral injury in stable patient Hemoperitoneum on CT without clear source	Positive local wound exploration (SW)

Unfortunately, CT grading may not agree with intraoperative observation and does not always predict the success of nonoperative therapy.[17,18] CT precisely reveals the status of the internal parenchyma but not three-dimensional injury anatomy. Operative grading provides an excellent three-dimensional view of the organ, but may underestimate internal damage. CT is a single snapshot in time, not a dynamic assessment.

As patients age, the capsule of the spleen and liver weakens. Parenchymal changes may occur as well. Accordingly, nonoperative management of even very severe injuries is the norm in children. Failure rates are much higher in adults. As patients age, the consequences of rebleeding increase.

Over the last several years, several technologic advances have increased the sophistication of nonoperative management. The increased resolution of helical CT can identify vascular injuries (i.e., pseudo-aneurysms or atrioventricular fistulas) or active extravasation of contrast. Angiography can also diagnose intraparenchymal vascular injury and evaluate the possibility of ongoing blood loss. Patients without vascular injury usually can be managed nonoperatively. In patients in whom vascular injury is diagnosed, percutaneous transcatheter embolization with either stainless steel coils or Gelfoam pledgets can arrest hemorrhage with a high degree of reliability.

Nonoperative Management of Hepatic Injury

Several recent large series have documented successful nonoperative treatment in 90 percent of patients who are hemodynamically stable at presentation.[19] Liver injuries are most commonly classified according to the system described by the American Association for the Surgery of Trauma (AAST) (Table 260-3). Complications of nonoperative management of hepatic injuries include delayed bleeding, bile leak, intraabdominal sepsis, and missed intraabdominal injuries. These are relatively rare and occurred in only 5 percent of the largest series of nonoperative management of liver injuries.[19] However, the vast majority of complications occurred in higher-grade injuries.

Today, many of these complications can be managed nonoperatively as well. Angiography with selective embolization can treat delayed blood loss from hepatic injuries. Percutaneous drainage can treat "bilomas" or hepatic abscesses. Endoscopic retrograde cholangiopancreatography (ERCP) can decompress clots from the biliary tree and stent intraparenchymal hepatic ductal injury. Recently, Carrillo et al. reviewed 135 patients managed nonoperatively.[20] Thirty-two patients developed complications requiring intervention, with most of these patients having high-grade injuries. A combination of these techniques successfully managed these complications nonoperatively 85 percent of the time.

Nonoperative Management of Splenic Injury

Nonoperative management of splenic injuries in adults has a failure rate as high as 20 percent. This relatively high failure rate has prompted some authors to advocate limiting nonoperative management to patients under 55 years of age and those with a CT injury grade no higher than 3 (Table 260-4).

The addition of angiography to the treatment algorithm has radically changed the nature of nonoperative management for splenic injury. First reported by Sclafani et al., sequential DPL, CT, and angiog-

TABLE 260-3   American Association for the Surgery of Trauma (AAST) Liver Injury Scale

Grade*	Injury Description
I. Hematoma Laceration	Subcapsular, nonexpanding, <10 cm surface area Capsular tear, nonbleeding, <1 cm parenchymal depth
II. Hematoma Laceration	Subcapsular, nonexpanding, 10–50 percent surface area; intraparenchymal, nonexpanding, <10 cm in diameter Capsular tear, active bleeding; 1–3 cm parenchymal depth, <10 cm in length
III. Hematoma Laceration	Subcapsular, >50 percent surface area or expanding; ruptured subcapsular hematoma with active bleeding; intraparenchymal hematoma, >10 cm or expanding >3 cm parenchymal depth
IV. Hematoma Laceration	Ruptured intraparenchymal hematoma with active bleeding Parenchymal disruption involving 25–75 percent of hepatic lobe or 1–3 Couinaud's segments within a single lobe
V. Laceration Vascular	Parenchymal disruption involving >75 percent of hepatic lobe or >3 Couinaud's segments within a single lobe Juxtahepatic venous injuries, i.e., retrohepatic vena cava/central major hepatic veins
VI. Vascular	Hepatic avulsion

*Advance one grade for multiple injuries, up to grade III.

TABLE 260-4   American Association for the Surgery of Trauma (AAST) Spleen Injury Scale (1994 Revision)

Grade*	Injury Description
I. Hematoma Laceration	Subcapsular, nonexpanding, <10 percent surface area Capsular tear, nonbleeding, <1 cm parenchymal depth
II. Hematoma Laceration	Subcapsular, nonexpanding, 10–50 percent surface area; intraparenchymal, nonexpanding, <5 cm in diameter Capsular tear, active bleeding; 1–3 cm parenchymal depth, which does not involve a trabecular vessel
III. Hematoma Laceration	Subcapsular, >50 percent surface area or expanding; ruptured subcapsular hematoma with active bleeding; intraparenchymal hematoma, >5 cm or expanding >3 cm parenchymal depth or involving trabecular vessels
IV. Hematoma Laceration	Ruptured intraparenchymal hematoma with active bleeding Laceration involving segmental or hilar vessels producing major devascularization (>25 percent of spleen)
V. Laceration Vascular	Completely shattered spleen Hilar vascular injury that devascularizes spleen

*Advance one grade for multiple injuries up to grade III.

raphy was used as a management algorithm in the care of patients with blunt trauma.[17] Stable patients with a positive DPL underwent CT. All patients with CT-diagnosed splenic injury were then treated angiographically. All vascular injuries identified at the time of angiography were treated with proximal coil embolization. Proximal embolization, similarly to splenic artery ligation, decreases the pressure head to the spleen, allowing for spontaneous hemostasis. Splenic viability and immune function are preserved by collateral vessels via the pancreatic branches of the splenic artery, the short gastric vessels, and collaterals from the superior mesenteric artery. In 150 patients, splenic salvage rate was 98 percent.[17] Most important, a negative splenic arteriogram predicted successful nonoperative management.

Initial CT scan may miss a splenic pseudoaneurysm in 75 percent of the patients with this pathology. Thus, follow-up CT even in asymptomatic patients is important.

While higher-grade injuries have an increased likelihood of vascular injury identified,[17,21] more than 10 percent of patients with grade 1 injuries have vascular injuries identified and embolized at the time of angiography.[17] Thus, reliance on CT grading to predict the success of nonoperative therapy may be insufficient. Alternatively, early, liberal use of angiography should help to identify patients with vascular injuries. Either of these techniques (i.e., follow-up CT, early angiography) appears to decrease the incidence of delayed splenic rupture. This often presents at 7 to 10 days in patients who were stable initially following the diagnosis of splenic injury.

The early series cited above[17,21] did not have a large proportion of high-grade splenic injuries contained within them. Recently, the authors prospectively evaluated a series of 120 patients with a large proportion of CT grade 3 and 4 injuries.[22] All patients diagnosed with splenic injuries underwent early angiography. The presence of a vascular abnormality correlated with grading. The higher the grade, the more likely the patient was to have vascular injury at the time of angiography. These were treated with a combination of proximal coil and subselective embolotechniques (Figure 260-5). Nonoperative management was successful more than 90 percent of the time, although some patients required repeat angiography and/or embolization.

Nonoperative management for splenic injuries is certainly a safe and effective technique. However, this must involve a committed team of emergency physicians, surgeons, and invasive radiologists to safely manage patients with high-grade injuries nonoperatively. Coil embolization is a safe technique and an effective method of hemostasis. These innovative techniques should be performed in a tertiary care center under strict protocol in order to be managed safely.

REFERENCES

1. Scalea TM, Goldstein AS, Phillips TF, et al: An analysis of 161 falls from a height: The "jumper syndrome." *J Trauma* 26:706, 1986.
2. American College of Surgeons, Committee on Trauma: *Advanced Life Support Course, Student Manual.* ACS, 1993.
3. Scalea TM, Holman M, Fourtes M, et al: Central venous blood oxygen saturation: An early, accurate measurement of volume during hemorrhage. *J Trauma* 28:725, 1988.
4. Shanmuganathan K, Mirvis SE, White CS, Pomertanz SM: MR imaging evaluation of hemidiaphragms in acute blunt trauma: Experience with 16 patients. *AJR* 167:397, 1996.
5. Saunders CJ, Battistella FD, Whetzel TP, Stokes RB: Percutaneous diagnostic peritoneal lavage using a Veress needle versus an open technique: A prospective randomized trial. *J Trauma* 44:883, 1998.
6. Goldstein AS, Scalfani SJA, Kupterstein NH, et al: The diagnostic superiority of computed tomography. *J Trauma* 25:939, 1985.
7. Otomo Y, Henmi H, Mashiko K, et al: New diagnostic peritoneal lavage criteria for diagnosis of intestinal injury. *J Trauma* 44:991, 1998.
8. Branney SW, Wolfe RE, Moore EE, et al: Quantitative sensitivity of ultrasound in detecting free intraperitoneal fluid. *J Trauma* 39:375, 1995.
9. McKinney MG, Lentz K, Nunez D, et al: Can ultrasound replace diagnostic peritoneal lavage in the assessment of blunt trauma? *J Trauma* 37:439, 1994.
10. Glaser K, Ischmelitsch J, Kluiger P, et al: Ultrasonography in the management of blunt abdominal and thoracic trauma. *Arch Surg* 129:742, 1994.
11. Tsang BD, Panacek EA, Brant WE, Wisner DH: Effect of oral contrast administration for abdominal computed tomography in the evaluation of acute blunt trauma. *Ann Emerg Med* 30:7, 1997.
12. Chiu WC, Cushing BM, Rodriquez A, et al: Abdominal injuries without hemoperitoneum: A potential limitation of focused abdominal sonography for trauma (FAST). *J Trauma* 42:617, 1997.
13. Renz BM, Feliciano DV: Unnecessary laparotomies for trauma: A prospective study of morbidity. *J Trauma* 38:350, 1995.
14. Zubowski R, Nallathambi M, Ivatury R, Stahl W: Selective conservatism in abdominal stab wounds: The efficacy of serial physical examination. *J Trauma* 28:1665, 1988.
15. Chiu WC, Shanmuganathan K, Mirvis SE, Scalea TM: Determining the need for laparotomy in penetrating torso trauma: A prospective study with triple-contrast abdominopelvic computed tomography. *J Trauma* 51:860, 2001.
16. Udobi K, Rodriguez A, Chiu WC, Scalea TM: The role of ultrasonography in penetrating abdominal trauma: A prospective clinical study. *J Trauma* 50:475, 2001.
17. Sclafani SJA, Shaftan GW, Scalea TM, et al: Nonoperative salvage of computer tomograph–diagnosed splenic injuries: Utilization of angiography for triage and embolization for hemostasis. *J Trauma* 39:818, 1995.
18. Mirvis SE, Whitley NO, Gens DR: Blunt splenic trauma in adults: CT-based classification and correlation with prognosis and treatment. *Radiology* 171:133, 1989.
19. Pachter HL, Knudson MM, Esrig B, et al: Status of nonoperative management of blunt hepatic injuries in 1995: A multicenter experience with 404 patients. *J Trauma* 40:31, 1996.

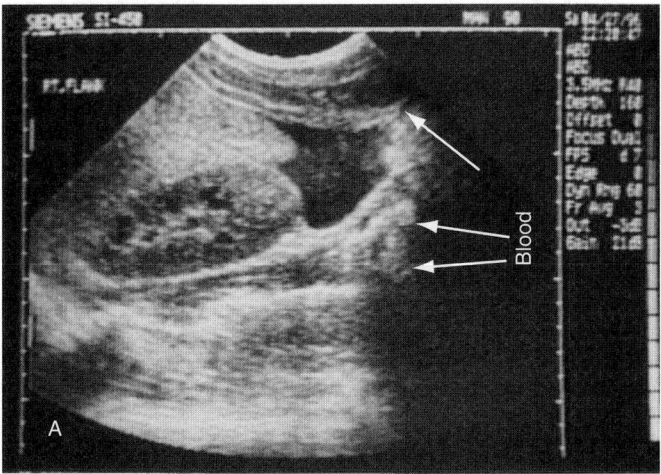

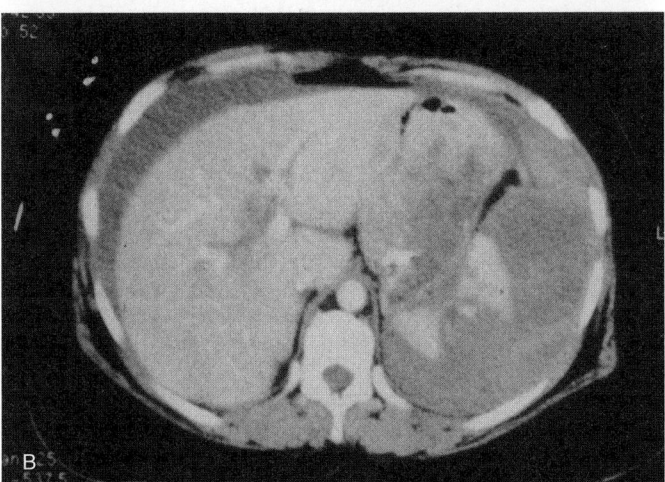

FIG. 260-5. Nonoperative management of splenic injuries. **A.** FAST (focused assessment with sonography for trauma) in this 21-year-old female with blunt abdominal trauma clearly demonstrates hemoperitoneum. **B.** The patient remains hemodynamically stable and CT scan demonstrates a grade 4 splenic injury.

20. Carrillo EH, Spain DA, Wohltmann CD, et al: Interventional techniques are useful adjuncts in nonoperative management of hepatic injuries. *J Trauma* 46:619, 1999.
21. Davis KA, Fabian TC, Croce MA: Improved success in nonoperative management of blunt splenic injuries: Embolization of splenic artery pseudoaneurysms. *J Trauma* 44:1008, 1998.
22. Haan J, Scott J, Boyd-Kranis R, et al: Admission angiography for blunt splenic injury: Advantages and pitfalls. *J Trauma* 51:1161, 2001.

PENETRATING TRAUMA TO THE FLANK AND BUTTOCK
261
Alasdair K. T. Conn

Penetrating injuries to the flank and buttock challenge the physician because of the possibility of missed injuries to retroperitoneal structures. Gunshot and stab wounds in these areas must be evaluated carefully to determine whether there is retroperitoneal injury with intraperitoneal or vascular injury that might mandate immediate surgical intervention. Evaluation is difficult; the retroperitoneal structures are well protected by dense layers of musculature and the spine. There is significant risk of missed injury and delay in diagnosis. Fortunately, an increased armamentarium of diagnostic testing assists in timely diagnosis and allows for selective conservative management. The choice of management, conservative or operative, is determined based on the emergency evaluation, making the emergency physician's input essential to a correct decision and a clinically successful outcome. Penetrating injuries to the buttock are relatively uncommon, and some trauma centers report as few as three to five patients with this type of injury per year. Trauma centers in urban settings have reported 50 to 80 patients per year. With appropriate management, the mortality is low, but case reports indicate that there is a potential for a missed injury to the bowel or major vessels, especially with shotgun or high-velocity gunshot wounds, unless the clinician is vigilant in the emergency evaluation. This chapter outlines the evaluation of patients who present to the emergency department with penetrating trauma to the flank or to the buttock.

PENETRATING TRAUMA TO THE FLANK

Pathophysiology

The flank is the area between the anterior and posterior axillary lines, superiorly bordered by the sixth rib and inferiorly bordered by the iliac crest. Although a penetrating wound to the flank can produce intraperitoneal injury with the associated physical findings of peritonitis or hemoperitoneum with shock, it is possible that a penetrating flank wound only injures the retroperitoneal organs. A delay in diagnosis of duodenal, colonic, rectal, renal, pancreatic, or major vascular injuries may result in the late appearance of septic or hemorrhagic shock.

The path of a gunshot or stab wound to the flank may track superiorly. Bullets may ricochet off the bony structures of the spine and produce a unique bullet path and injury pattern. Other intra-abdominal organs may be injured, such as the stomach or pancreas, the diaphragm, and intrathoracic organs. Inferior tracking will jeopardize the lower gastrointestinal (GI) tract and colon. Treatment of these specific organ injuries is covered elsewhere in this text.

Clinical Features

Patients with penetrating trauma to the flank should be resuscitated and evaluated according to standard resuscitative protocols. Initial resuscitative efforts should be directed toward the primary survey (see Chap. 251). Information regarding the mechanism of injury, how

much time has passed since the traumatic event, and the nature of the weapon should be obtained and recorded. In the case of a gunshot wound, the nature of the gun (e.g., shotgun, handgun, BB gun) and the range between the gun and the patient at time of the gun's discharge should be ascertained and noted in the emergency record. Following stabilization, an attempt should be made to find an exit wound, and a bullet path should be reconstructed. Baseline laboratory and radiologic data, including a hemogram, chest radiograph, urinalysis, and rectal examination with testing for occult blood, should be performed on all patients. In the presence of peritonitis, IV fluid and broad-spectrum antibiotics (e.g., ampicillin 0.5–2 g IV every 6 h, gentamycin 1.0–1.7 mg/kg IV every 8 h, metronidazole 15 mg/kg IV × 1 and then 7.5 mg/kg IV every 6 h) should be administered and urgent surgical consultation obtained. Multiple regimens are available, but coverage for gram-negative aerobic and anaerobic organisms is required. A suitable regime of antibiotics is ampicillin, gentamycin, and metronidazole initiated in the emergency department. Most patients are stable and will require additional diagnostic modalities.

Diagnosis

BEDSIDE ULTRASOUND   In a patient with a penetrating wound to the flank, portable bedside ultrasonography can be used to determine if there is fluid in the abdominal cavity. In the absence of a preexisting medical condition (such as cirrhosis with ascites), such information may be invaluable. Although the sensitivity and specificity vary with the type of equipment used and the experience of the operator, fluid collections of 600 mL should be detected easily by the emergency physician.[1] For a patient with a gunshot wound, this may be sufficient to recommend an operative approach. For a patient with a stab wound, this indicates a significant intra-abdominal injury, even if the patient is hemodynamically stable. Operative intervention is sometimes delayed pending further adjunctive diagnostic measures. A recent study indicates that this should be a screening study only—the positive predictive value being 90 percent, but the negative predictive value being only 60 percent.[2]

WOUND EXPLORATION   Although local wound exploration under adequate local anesthesia using sterile technique is of value in anterior abdominal wounds, it is only of limited value in wounds of the flank. If local exploration demonstrates that the injury does not penetrate beyond fascia or muscle, the wound may be closed safely and the patient discharged from the emergency department with appropriate follow-up instructions. With deeper penetrating injuries, it is difficult to determine the extent of injury with local wound exploration. More information usually can be obtained by computed tomographic (CT) scanning. Deep wound exploration often leads to further hemorrhage and tissue damage and is of limited value. It is difficult, if not impossible, to ascertain the exact depth of a stab wound from deep wound exploration.

DIAGNOSTIC PERITONEAL LAVAGE   Appropriately performed, diagnostic peritoneal lavage (DPL) is highly accurate in determining the presence of intraperitoneal injury, but it does not detect injuries restricted to the retroperitoneum. (For details of the technique and criteria, see Chap. 260.) In most institutions, the use of DPL for a stable patient has been replaced by CT scanning. In an unstable patient, DPL can be performed (especially if portable ultrasound is not immediately available) to rapidly detect the presence (or absence) of hemoperitoneum.

COMPUTED TOMOGRAPHY   In many centers, CT has become the diagnostic modality of choice in patients who present hemodynamically stable following a penetrating flank trauma.[3–5] Double (oral Gastrografin and intravenous) contrast or triple (oral, intravenous, and rectal) contrast is used; rectal contrast should be used if there is even a remote likelihood of a rectal or sigmoid injury. Cooperation with the radiologist is essential because fine "cuts" through the site of injury may be required to delineate the injury tract. Particular attention should be paid to the presence of intraperitoneal fluid and any edema of the bowel wall. The latter may represent bowel perforation, even without evident leakage of the contrast material.[6]

CT scanning is of particular use in stab wounds to the flank in which the patient is hemodynamically stable. The diagnostic accuracy has been reported at 97.9 percent for CT scanning.[7] Other studies[8,9] validate this figure with a 97 percent accuracy in predicting the need for laparotomy.

The majority of patients with identified injury will be found to have retroperitoneal hematoma without bowel or solid-organ damage. Rarely, a hematoma around one of the major blood vessels or the pancreas is evident, requiring further diagnostic testing such as angiography, venography, or endoscopic retrograde cholangiopancreatogram (ERCP). Occasionally, a gunshot wound may be observed to pass extraperitoneally, but concerns about blast effect may lead to the decision to perform laparoscopy.

Treatment

The treatment of penetrating trauma to the flank remains somewhat controversial, although there is a tendency toward more conservative management. Celiotomy is generally reserved for patients with hemorrhagic shock, peritonitis, evisceration, transabdominal missile path, and intraperitoneal free air. At the time of surgery, all intraperitoneal and retroperitoneal organ structures should be evaluated according to standard operative procedures.

Although some surgeons still advocate mandatory exploratory laparotomy in an effort to detect all injuries early, most surgeons now advocate selective management with early CT scanning, which allows many injuries to be managed by close observation. Using this conservative approach, celiotomy rates have been decreasing from 100 percent to approximately 30 percent, with the incidence of positive laparotomy rising from 15 percent to approximately 80 percent, without increases in untoward outcome.[10] Using this approach, the risks associated with the negative laparotomy (early: hemorrhage and infection; late: complications and small bowel obstruction) as well as added expense are avoided. Many recent reviews support this selective management approach.

Exploratory laparotomy is performed most commonly for flank gunshot wounds. Many flank stab wounds can be safely managed conservatively. In the case of high-velocity gunshot wounds, blast effect must be considered. Depending on the exact location and type of injury, consideration of the blast effect may lead to exploratory laparotomy if there is concern about bowel, bladder, or vascular integrity. Laparoscopy also may be used to determine the extent of intraperitoneal injury. A surgeon experienced in laparoscopy should perform this procedure because bowel injuries may be difficult to detect.

With CT scanning, the exact depth of a stab wound often can be determined. Decision algorithms based on low-risk flank stab wounds (penetration superficial to the deep fascia) or high-risk flank stab wounds (penetration beyond the deep fascia) have been developed and appear to be justified clinically.[11] Hemodynamically stable patients with stab wounds to the flank can be risk-stratified based on these contrast-enhanced CT findings. Low-risk patients may be discharged immediately from the emergency department. High-risk patients require surgical consultation and should be admitted to the hospital, but in many cases a discharge decision can be made within 24 h.

PENETRATING BUTTOCK INJURIES

Pathophysiology

Penetrating trauma to the buttock may be either from gunshot wounds or stab wounds. Gunshot wounds have the greatest potential for injury because the thick musculature and fat over the buttocks normally pro-

tects the gastrointestinal, genitourinary, and neurologic systems from injury in all except the deepest penetrating trauma from stab wounds. With gunshot wounds, the risk of intraperitoneal injury is much higher and may necessitate immediate exploratory celiotomy. Injured systems requiring operative intervention are the lower GI tract, the lower genitourinary (GU) tract, and rarely, a vascular injury. Vascular injury to gluteal or internal iliac arteries has been reported from gluteal-penetrating wounds and may lead to exsanguinating external hemorrhage.[12] An intrapelvic injury also may cause injury to the internal iliac vessels with hypovolemic shock; this will require early operative intervention. A delay in diagnosis of colonic or rectal injury will contribute to increased mortality and morbidity. From the civilian trauma literature, approximately 30 percent of patients who present with gunshot wounds to the buttock require surgery. Factors associated with surgical intervention include findings of peritonitis, a positive finding at sigmoidoscopy, gross blood in the urine, entrance wound above the level of the greater trochanters, and a transpelvic (as opposed to extrapelvic) bullet course.[13–15] In contradistinction, stab wounds to the buttock infrequently require laparotomy.

Diagnosis and Management

Initial approaches to trauma resuscitation should be followed, as noted earlier. Local wound exploration is of limited value, primarily to detect gross foreign bodies. Attention should be paid to the abdominal examination. If there is indication of peritonitis or of a gunshot wound with a transabdominal missile path, emergent surgical consultation should be obtained, broad spectrum antibiotics given intravenously, and preparations made for an exploratory laparotomy. Baseline hemogram, urinalysis, and rectal examination should be performed on all patients. If there is any concern about injury to the rectum because of blood being noted on rectal examination or because of the trajectory of the bullet, proctosigmoidoscopy should be performed.[15] A cystourethrogram should be obtained on patients when there is blood on urinalysis or the proximity of the wound to the GI tract is a concern. This can be performed either as a separate study or in conjunction with CT scanning with rectal and intravenous contrast material and clamping of the urethral catheter to obtain a CT cystogram. If the CT scan demonstrates a pelvic hematoma, angiography or venography may be indicated to document a significant vascular injury. In all patients, the peripheral pulses in the lower extremities should be examined looking for decreased pulses or pallor as evidence of a proximal injury. Neurologic examination of the lower extremities searching for any injury to the sciatic or femoral nerve also should be performed on all patients. Buttock wounds rarely cause damage to the sciatic plexus or femoral plexus. Injury could include transsection, partial transsection, or stretch injury secondary to the trauma. The presence of any symptomatic signs requires appropriate consultation. The signs of peritonitis, intrapelvic or transabdominal missile path, and intraperitoneal free air warrant immediate celiotomy.

REFERENCES

1. Branney SW, Wolfe RE, Moore EE, et al: Quantitative sensitivity of ultrasound in detecting free intraperitoneal fluid. *J Trauma* 39(2): 375, 1995.
2. Udobi KF, Rodriguez A, Chiu WC: Role of ultrasonography in penetrating abdominal trauma: A prospective clinical study. *J Trauma* 50(3):475, 2001.
3. Easter DW, Shackford SR, Mattrey RF: A prospective, randomized comparison of computed tomography with conventional diagnostic methods in the evaluation of penetrating injuries to the back and flank. *Arch Surg* 126(9):1115, 1991.
4. Kirton OC, Wint D, Thrasher B, et al: Stab wounds to the back and flank in the hemodynamically stable patient: A decision algorithm based on contrast-enhanced computed tomography with colonic opacification. *Am J Surg* 173(3):189, 1997.
5. Ginzburg E, Carrillo EH, Kopelman T, et al: The role of computed tomography in selective management of gunshot wounds to the abdomen. *J Trauma* 45(6):1005, 1998.

6. Himmelman RG, Martin M, Gilkey S, et al: Triple-contrast CT scans in penetrating back and flank trauma. *J Trauma* 31(6):852, 1991.

7. Albrecht RM, Vigil A, Schermer CR, et al: Stab wounds to the back/flank in hemodynamically stable patients: Evaluation using triple-contrast computed tomography. *Am Surg* 65(7):683–687; Discussion 687, 1999.

8. Shanmuganathan K, Mirvis SE, Chiu WC, et al: Triple-contrast helical CT in penetrating torso trauma: A prospective study to determine peritoneal violation and the need for laparotomy. *AJR* 177(6):1247, 2001.

9. Chiu WC, Shanmuganathan K, Mirvis SE, Scalea TM: Determining the need for laparotomy in penetrating torso trauma: A prospective study using triple-contrast enhanced abdominopelvic computed tomography. *J Trauma* 51(5):860, 2001.

10. Boyle EM Jr, Maier RV, Salazar JD, et al: Diagnosis of injuries after stab wounds to the back and flank. *J Trauma* 42(2):260, 1997.

11. Velmahos GC, Demetriades D, Cornwell EE, et al: Gunshot wounds to the buttocks: Predicting the need for operation. *Dis Colon Rectum* 40(3):307, 1997.

12. McCarthy MC, Lowdermilk GA, Canal DF, et al: Prediction of injury caused by penetrating wounds to the abdomen, flank and back. *Arch Surg* 126(8):962, 1991.

13. DiGiacomo JC, Schwab CW, Rotondo MF, et al: Gluteal gunshot wounds: Who warrants exploration? *J Trauma* 37(4):622, 1994.

14. Ferraro FJ, Livingston DH, Odom J, et al: The role of sigmoidoscopy in the management of gunshot wounds to the buttocks. *Am Surg* 59(6):350, 1997.

15. Mercer DW, Buckman RF Jr, Sood R, et al: Anatomic considerations in penetrating gluteal wounds. *Arch Surg* 127(4):407, 1992.

262 GENITOURINARY TRAUMA
Frederick Levy
Gabor D. Kelen

EPIDEMIOLOGY

Injuries to the genitourinary system occur in approximately 2 to 5 percent of adult trauma victims. The vast majority of these injuries are a result of blunt trauma. More than 80 percent of those with injuries to the kidney have other concurrent injuries; approximately a third of those injuries are life-threatening. Consequently, detection of injury to the genitourinary system may be overlooked.

Approximately 80 percent of the urogenital injuries involve the kidney, and approximately 10 percent involve the bladder. Patients with anatomic anomalies, including tumor and hydronephrosis, appear more susceptible to renal injury. Significant ureteral injuries are relatively rare and are usually associated with penetrating trauma. Significant urethral injuries most often occur in males and are usually associated with pelvic fracture. Accurate overall estimates for children are not available, but it appears that approximately 10 percent of pediatric patients with blunt abdominal trauma have genitourinary system injury. This increased percentage in children may reflect the absence of periadipose tissue and the large size of the kidneys relative to overall body size.[1]

CLINICAL APPROACH

Chap. 251 discusses the overall approach to trauma. Only issues specific to genitourinary trauma are discussed here.

Genitourinary system injuries rarely require immediate intervention. Investigation of renal injuries should not supersede evaluation of more life-threatening injuries. For example, with a pelvic fracture, determining the need for pelvic angiography is more important than determining whether a urethral injury exists. The patient may well die from a sheared major artery, whereas an injured urethra will never require immediate attention. The retrograde introduction of dye will render subsequent pelvic angiography very difficult, if not impossible.

During the detailed secondary survey, a concerted effort should be made to closely inspect the perineum. Blood on the underwear is an important finding. In both male and female patients, the folds of the buttocks should be spread in search of perineal lacerations, which often denote an open pelvic fracture. Such lacerations should not be probed lest a clot be disrupted and exsanguinating hemorrhage result. During the rectal examination, sphincter tone, the position of the prostate gland, and presence of any blood should be noted. If the prostate is riding high or feels boggy, there has been a disruption of the membranous urethra.

In males, the scrotum is palpated and inspected for ecchymoses, laceration, and testicular disruption. Simultaneously, the length of the penis is palpated to inspect for blood at the meatus. In females, the vaginal introitus is inspected for lacerations and hematomas. These findings are often associated with pelvic fractures in which a displaced fracture fragment may cause a vaginal laceration or urethral disruption. If there is any evidence or likelihood of trauma in this area, a bimanual vaginal examination is required. If there is blood in the vagina, a speculum examination is necessary to exclude vaginal laceration.

During the secondary survey, the trauma series x-rays are obtained and often include an anteroposterior view of the pelvis. The presence of a pelvic fracture has important implications in the workup of genitourinary injuries. Patients with pelvic fractures have a higher incidence of mortality and often have concomitant extraperitoneal bladder injuries.

Generally, no urinary catheter should be introduced until the urine can be evaluated for hematuria. However, the placement of a urinary catheter for monitoring of urine output may be required in severely injured patients who cannot void. Often times, catheter placement will reveal the first signs of genitourinary injury. If there is doubt and placement of a catheter is emergent, a suprapubic approach may be the most prudent. In menstruating women, a specimen obtained with a catheter is likely to offer more accurate urinalysis than a spontaneously voided specimen.

The standard hematology and serum chemistry results are generally not helpful in determining the presence or degree of renal injury in the acute setting.

Detection of Specific Injuries

The need to determine the existence of specific injuries is based on the clinical elements obtained in the history, physical examination, and plain films, and to some extent, on the age of the patient. Table 262-1 lists some key elements that should prompt the consideration of further evaluation of renal tract injury. The approach to evaluation is dependent on the following: blunt versus penetrating trauma, the presence of gross or microscopic hematuria, associated injuries, mechanism of injury, hemodynamic stability, and age of the patient.[2] Renal injuries require staging for appropriate management (Table 262-2).[3] Staging is usually accomplished through use of an imaging modality, but sometimes exploration is required (see below).

TABLE 262-1 Key Clinical Findings Associated with Renal System Injury

Acceleration or deceleration injury (renal pedical)
Lower rib fractures (kidney)
Fracture lower thoracic or upper lumbar spine
Pelvic fracture (urethra)
Abdominal trauma
Flank ecchymosis, tenderness, mass (kidney)
Straddle injuries (urethra)
Penetrating trauma (in vicinity of any part of the renal system)
Penile scrotal or perineal hematoma (urethra)
Gross hematuria
Microscopic hematuria in certain circumstances (see text)
Abnormally positioned prostate (posterior urethra)
Blood at penile meatus (urethra)

TABLE 262-2   Grading of Renal Injuries[4]

Grade	Injury	Treatment
I	Contusion (microscopic or gross hematuria, with normal urologic study results) Subscapular, nonexpanding hematoma without laceration	Observation, spontoneous resolution
II	Parenchymal laceration <1.0 cm depth limited to cortex, no extravasation Nonexpanding hematoma, confined to retroperitoneum	Observation, spontoneous resolution
III	Parenchymal laceration >1 cm depth with extravasation or collecting system rupture	Observation or surgery
IV	Laceration extending through to collecting system Vascular pedical injury, hemorrhage contained	Surgery
V	Shattered kidney Avulsed hilum (devascularized kidney)	Surgery

TABLE 262-3   Selection of Diagnostic Imaging for Suspected Renal System Injury

Imaging Study	Suspected Injury
Retrograde urethrogram or cystogram	Urethral injury
CT (with IV contrast)	Renal injury (staging) Ureteral injury
Cystogram, plain film (retrograde)	Bladder injury
CT cystogram (retrograde)	Bladder injury
"One-shot" IVP	Unstable patients taken to operating room
IVP	Alternative to CT in unstable patients Ureteral injury
Angiogram or venogram	Pedicle injuries, venous disruption
Retrograde pyelogram	Renal pelvis disruption

Abbreviations: CT = computed tomography; IVP = intravenous pyelogram.

BLUNT TRAUMA

Physical Exam Findings as a Clue to Injury Localization

MEATAL BLOOD   Blood at the meatus is associated with urethral injuries. Urethral injuries are almost exclusively seen in males. Posterior urethral injuries are commonly associated with pelvic fractures. A superiorly displaced prostate indicates disruption of the posterior urethra. Anterior urethral injuries are associated with straddle injuries and instrumentation.

When meatal blood is noted, a urinary catheter should not be placed in order to prevent the conversion of a partial urethral laceration into a complete transection. A retrograde urethrogram is virtually mandatory in this setting in order to make the diagnosis and to minimize the chances of long-term complications of a urethral transection (i.e., urethral strictures and urinary incontinence).

HEMATURIA   For the purposes of trauma, microscopic hematuria is defined as more than five red blood cells (RBCs) per high-power field (hpf). A 10-mL specimen must be centrifuged for 5 min at 2000 revolutions for an accurate assessment. Gross hematuria is, of course, readily visible blood. Reddish urine, per se, does not necessarily indicate hematuria; several medications and toxic substances may cause discoloration. Results of a dipstick evaluation may be erroneous because myoglobin, a frequent finding in patients with rhabdomyolysis as a consequence of major trauma, reacts with the reagent.

The initially voided urine may provide clues as to the location of injury. When possible, at least two specimens (initial stream and terminal stream) should be obtained. Initial hematuria suggests injury to the distal system (i.e., urethra or prostate). Terminal hematuria suggests bladder neck injury. Continuous hematuria suggests upper renal system (bladder, ureter, or kidney) injury.

Gross hematuria may occur from injury virtually anywhere in the genitourinary renal tract. The finding of gross hematuria mandates a diagnostic imaging study that is chosen based on other findings (Table 262-3). For example, in the presence of pelvic fractures, gross hematuria should raise the possibility of bladder or urethral injury. Almost 95 percent of bladder injuries are associated with gross hematuria.

All patients in whom microscopic hematuria is found with concurrent nonrenal injuries and those with hemodynamic instability should

have a diagnostic imaging study, as discussed below. In such patients, computed tomography (CT) is often impractical. A "one-shot" intravenous pyelogram (IVP) can be obtained in the operating room.

Many studies demonstrate that, **in adult patients with blunt trauma, the degree of hematuria does not correspond to the degree of injury.** Gross hematuria may be seen with relatively minor renal contusions, whereas microscopic hematuria (or even no hematuria) may be seen in renovascular injuries. However, in the absence of significant hemodynamic compromise, isolated microscopic hematuria is unlikely to represent significant blunt injury. While there is no clinically validated or generally accepted upper limit of microscopic hematuria beyond which imaging is done, many physicians do not image patients where the degree of microscopic hematuria is ≤50 RBCs/hpf. A review of several major studies addressing this question concluded that isolated microscopic hematuria indicates significant injury in approximately 1 in 500 patients with such a finding.[2] Thus, the current consensus is that adult patients with isolated microscopic hematuria do not require further imaging studies. There are three exceptions. When the mechanism of trauma involves rapid deceleration, renal pedicle injuries may ensue but can present with minimal (or even no) hematuria. Also, hematuria in a patient with even transient hypotension should not be considered an isolated finding.

Special Considerations

RAPID DECELERATION FORCES   Rapid deceleration injuries may result in renal pedicle and vascular injuries. Such injuries result in high mortality rates, but, fortunately, they are quite rare, occurring in less than 1 percent of blunt renal trauma. However, hematuria, the clue to renal injury, may not be present. Accordingly, patients whose mechanism of injury is from forces of rapid deceleration should have a renovascular imaging study. Because pedicle injuries virtually always occur in association with other significant injuries,[4] other indications for radiographic evaluation are likely. Many such patients have other indications for surgical exploration.

PEDIATRIC BLUNT TRAUMA   Hematuria following blunt trauma may have different significance in the pediatric population.[5,6] Unlike the situation in adults, the degree of hematuria does seem to correlate with the degree of injury.[4] Many advocate that pediatric patients with any degree of hematuria, even if hemodynamically stable, should undergo imaging studies.[7,8] However, **pediatric patients with less than 50 RBCs/hpf do not appear to have significant injuries.**[1,4] Thus, it appears appropriate to perform imaging studies on only those patients with significant hematuria, as defined above.[2] The most recent experience suggests that all grades of renal injury in stable children can be managed conservatively.[6] Other standards for imaging studies for pediatric patients remain similar to those for adults.

Imaging Techniques for Diagnosing Genitourinary Blunt Trauma Injury

The following should be considered when ordering studies in the trauma patient: 1) intravenous contrast agents can cause false-positive scan results for blood; 2) the total quantity of contrast required may limit the number of contrast studies, especially with shock; 3) hypotensive patients are at risk for developing contrast-induced acute renal failure; 4) abdominal CT reveals more information but requires a hemodynamically stable condition; and 5) an intraoperative IVP during an emergency laparotomy may be needed to determine the status of the contralateral kidney. Table 262-3 provides a guideline for the selection of diagnostic imaging modalities.

ULTRASONOGRAPHY   Ultrasonographic examination of the right upper quadrant (Morrison pouch) and the left upper quadrant (splenorenal recess) is part of the focused assessment with sonography for trauma (FAST) examination (see Chaps. 251 and 303) but has little accepted role to date in the initial detection (or exclusion) of significant renal injury in the United States. Certain conditions, such as patient position, obesity, fractured ribs, and overlying bowel gas make such examinations difficult to perform. Furthermore, sonography reveals nothing about renal function.

PLAIN FILM   Plain films are helpful in determining likelihood of renal trauma when abnormalities such as lower rib fractures, lower thoracic and upper lumbar spinal fractures, and pelvic fractures are seen. Loss of the psoas shadow or scoliosis may suggest injury. However, plain films are inappropriate for evaluating the renal tract.

COMPUTED TOMOGRAPHY   Indications for imaging the kidneys following blunt trauma include gross hematuria, hematuria with multiple injuries or hemodynamic instability, and mechanisms that include rapid deceleration (Table 262-4). When renal injury is suspected, CT is considered superior to other imaging modalities, including sonography, angiography, and IVP. CT is most likely to allow appropriate staging of renal injury (see Table 262-2) and has several advantages. CT is a noninvasive modality with superior imaging detail that allows detection of even minor injuries and minimal extravasation, estimation of extent of hematoma, and simultaneous evaluation of other organs. In the last decade, the use of helical (spiral) CT scanning has enhanced the sensitivity of detecting renal injury, primarily by eliminating the phenomenon of respiratory misregistration. In children with hematuria, CT is the radiographic study of choice in evaluating renal injuries because a significant nonrenal intraabdominal injury is more likely than a renal injury.

The major disadvantage of CT scanning is that it can be performed only in a stable patient. Other disadvantages are cost and the difficulty in detecting vascular, particularly venous, injury.

TABLE 262-4   Clinical Indications for Contrast CT of the Upper Urinary Tract

1. Patients with hematuria with/without shock.
2. Hemodynamically stable with microscopic hematuria who have other indications for a CT of the abdomen/pelvis.
3. Hemodynamically stable patients with microscopic hematuria with clinical evidence of major blunt flank trauma.
4. Patients with any degree of hematuria following penetrating flank injuries.

Source: Tze MW, Spencer JA: The role of CT in the management of adult urinary tract trauma. *Clin Radiol* 56:276, 2001.

Certain considerations should be kept in mind. Routine abdominal CT evaluation often stops at the iliac crests. In situations where lower ureter or bladder trauma is under consideration, the examination should be extended to the pelvis. Also, contrast enhancement is usually indicated for appropriate evaluation. Both oral and intravenous contrast material is often given when other intraabdominal trauma is under consideration. However, if enhanced CT is required to image the kidneys and collecting system appropriately, gastrointestinal contrast studies may need to be delayed to allow accurate interpretation.

MAGNETIC RESONANCE IMAGING   Magnetic resonance imaging (MRI) is generally not a first-line imaging modality. However, its accuracy appears to be similar to that of CT. It may prove useful in stable patients who have dye allergy or patients with equivocal findings on CT.

ANGIOGRAPHY   Angiography has largely been replaced by CT. It still has a role when vascular injury is suspected and remains the gold standard for detecting renal venous injury. Arteriography may be indicated in selected patients when no renal function is evident on IVP or CT. Other indications include penetrating trauma where the likelihood of vascular injury is high, and when embolization is considered for persistent or delayed hemorrhage. It should be kept in mind that the kidney can tolerate only 4 to 6 h of warm ischemia. Arteriographic confirmation may cause an undue delay.

RADIONUCLIDE IMAGING   Radionuclide imaging has a very limited role now, given the superiority of CT. It may still be useful in patients with iodinated dye allergy in whom technetium-99m (^{99m}Tc) glucoheptonate can be safely used.

INTRAVENOUS PYELOGRAM   Formal IVP with or without tomograms can be used in stable patients if CT is unavailable. However, it is not the ideal study in the trauma setting, given the need for quality imaging. If used, the dose of contrast material needs to be greater than the standard 1 mL/kg to account for hemodilution for intravenous fluid administration and possible impaired renal perfusion. The recommendation is 2 mL/kg up to 150 mL of 60 percent iodinated contrast. In patients with a history of allergy, a nonionic agent, such as iohexol, can be used. Alternatively, noncontrast CT, radionuclide imaging, or MRI may offer satisfactory results.

IVP remains the mainstay of diagnosing ureteral injuries, although it is not infallible.[9] Extravasation of dye is the classic finding, although on occasion there is absence or delay of contrast in the distal collecting system. However, many are now using spiral CT to diagnose ureteral injuries because it offers the advantage of viewing the entire retroperitoneal space and has the ability to detect urinomas.

A "one-shot" IVP can be obtained in unstable patients in the emergency department or operating room, although there continues to be some controversy surrounding the need for a single-shot study. Certain authors suggest that the single-shot IVP can often give the surgeon valuable information, not only about the presence of a contralateral kidney, but about which renal injuries may be safely observed.[10] Others suggest that the utility of this test is limited to those patients who present with either flank wound or hematuria.[11]

The technique entails injecting 2 mL/kg intravenous contrast material about 5 min before the film is taken. However, if the patient's blood pressure is 70 mm Hg or less, the kidneys may not concentrate the contrast material and are more susceptible to dye-related injury.

CYSTOGRAPHY   For suspected bladder injuries, plain-film cystogram is classically used. Approximately 300 to 500 mL (5 mL/kg in children) of contrast media is instilled retrograde into the bladder under gravity from 2 ft (60 cm) above the patient. At a height of 2 ft, the intravesical pressure generated approximates the physiologic voiding pressure. Unless adequate bladder pressure is generated, the cystogram may be falsely negative. Ideally, the procedure is performed under fluoroscopy to avoid filling the peritoneal cavity with contrast material in the event of a tear. A film of the distended bladder is taken, and a postdrainage view is obtained to note any extravasation not evident on the initial film. Some authorities suggest that the bladder be "washed out" with saline solution prior to obtaining the post-"wash-out" view.

Although some authors continue to advocate clamping a urinary catheter to allow antegrade filling of the bladder,[12] retrograde cystography is felt to be more accurate in detecting bladder injuries, presumably because retrograde filling is not dependent on progressive dilution of contrast material.[13] CT cystogram may be preferred in patients who require intravenous contrast-enhanced CT imaging for other indications.[14] However, contrast material must still be injected retrograde. Postvoiding scans are generally not required because CT allows full imaging of the retrovesicular space.

A prospective investigation studying indications for cystography in blunt trauma with hematuria or pelvic fracture concluded that it was appropriate and cost effective to restrict this procedure to patients with gross hematuria only.[15] The authors contend that patients with pelvic fracture and microscopic hematuria do not routinely require cystography.

Urethral injuries are also investigated by retrograde cystography. **An unlubricated urinary catheter is placed** approximately 2 to 3 cm into the navicular fossa of the distal urethra, and the balloon is inflated with 1 to 3 mL water. Approximately 20 to 30 mL of contrast material is injected. An oblique view is obtained. The entire length of the urethra is seen on the plain film when the x-ray is taken as the last 10 mL of the contrast solution is injected. Occasionally, a patient may be transferred from another facility with an indwelling urethral catheter in place. A retrograde urethrogram can still be performed without removing the catheter, by injecting contrast solution into the urethra through a small feeding tube placed adjacent to the urethral catheter.

Urethral injuries should not be investigated in cases of pelvic trauma until it is certain that pelvic angiography or embolization is not required. Also, if the prostate gland was grossly displaced on rectal examination, the urethra is transected, and a retrograde study is not needed, at least not during the initial evaluation.

CONTRAST STUDIES When both upper and lower tract injuries are suspected, imaging needs to be approached with particular attention to order. While the most serious potential injury should guide the order of obtaining images, **oral contrast material should generally not be given before an IVP or cystogram** because gastrointestinal contrast may obscure important findings. Patients with potential bladder injuries may require a retrograde urethrogram to evaluate possible urethral disruption first. If injury is noted, cystography can be accomplished by suprapubic puncture.

Situations in which contrast is best avoided and risk of contrast nephropathy are discussed in Chap. 302.

IMAGING CONSIDERATIONS FOR OTHER CONDITIONS A perinephric hematoma may initially be difficult to distinguish from a urinoma. A delayed CT image may demonstrate contrast, indicating a urinoma. Patients with such perinephric collections can be followed with ultrasonographic studies. A nuclear ^{99m}Tc renal scan can also detect a persistent urine leak.

Significant adrenal injuries are relatively rare. Adrenal hematomas may be found in up to 3 percent of patients with blunt abdominal trauma. They are usually associated with other significant thoracic and abdominal injuries. Adrenal hematomas can be followed by CT or sonography and usually resolve over a few months. Long-term sequelae are unlikely.

PENETRATING TRAUMA

Approximately 10 percent of patients with renal injury related to stab wounds may not manifest hematuria. Thus, appropriate evaluation depends on clinical suspicion, the weapon involved, and patient characteristics. Generally, all stable patients with penetrating trauma with the potential of genitourinary system injury should undergo imaging studies. Hematuria, microscopic or gross, does not correlate with injury from penetrating trauma.[16]

The choice of imaging depends on the vicinity of the trauma. The presence of penetrating trauma alone mandates further evaluation.

Penetrating ureteral injuries are usually a result of bullet wounds. Again, hematuria is not a reliable finding in this setting. Imaging is required for penetrating injuries near ureters. Contusions from secondary energy forces related to bullets cannot be detected by imaging. They may come to light during surgical exploration.

Penetrating bladder injuries are usually accompanied by gross hematuria. As with other penetrating trauma, in the absence of hematuria, the need to perform imaging studies is driven by clinical concern.

Choice of Diagnostic Imaging for Penetrating Renal Trauma

CT with intravenous contrast material remains the primary imaging modality for penetrating trauma to the kidneys. It usually shows appropriate detail of injury to inform management decisions. Several studies have shown utility for staging even penetrating injuries, allowing nonoperative management in selected patients (i.e., those with minor injury).[17,18]

As with blunt trauma, sonography has no accepted role for detection or staging of renal injury in the United States at this time.

Ureteral injuries can be assessed by IVP or CT with contrast. Extravasation indicates injury. CT has the added advantage of being able to evaluate the extent of extravasation and other intraabdominal injuries. As with blunt trauma, cystography (plain film or CT) is required to evaluate penetrating injuries of the bladder. Unstable patients who require emergency laparotomy can undergo a "one-shot" IVP while in the operating room.

SPECIFIC INJURIES

Renal Injuries

The kidneys are well protected in the retroperitoneal location, being surrounded by bulky musculature, fascia, and lower ribs. Considerable force is generally necessary to cause significant renal injury. Fractured ribs, vertebral transverse process fractures, flank bruises or hematomas, and hematuria may indicate injury. Contusions account for most (92 percent) renal injuries, with renal lacerations (5 percent), renal pedicle injuries (2 percent), and renal ruptures or shattered kidneys (1 percent) accounting for the rest.

RENAL CONTUSION This relatively minor injury includes renal parenchymal ecchymosis, minor lacerations, and subcapsular hematomas with an intact renal capsule. Results of the IVP are usually normal. The CT may reveal edema with microextravasation of contrast material within the renal parenchyma. Subcapsular hematoma appears as a flattened portion of the renal cortex compressed by the hematoma under the renal capsule.

RENAL LACERATION Renal lacerations are classified as either minor cortical lacerations that do not involve the medulla or collecting system, or major renal lacerations that extend deep into the corticomedullary junction or collecting system (see Table 262-2). The resulting perirenal hematoma may fill the perirenal space before it is tamponaded by the Gerota fascia. Radiographic studies demonstrate disruption of the renal outline, a perirenal hematoma, and possibly extravasation of contrast material adjacent to the kidney.

RENAL PEDICLE INJURY   Renal pedicle injuries include lacerations and thrombosis of the renal artery, renal vein, and their branches. These injuries result from high-velocity deceleration injuries and penetrating trauma. In blunt trauma, the most common renal pedicle injury is thrombosis of the renal artery, which follows tearing of the intima with intact adventitial and medial layers. There is bruising surrounding the renal artery, but no perirenal hematoma is found in renal pedicle lacerations. When the renal artery is occluded or divided, the IVP shows nonfunction, and the arteriogram reveals renal artery occlusion or bleeding. In such injuries, CT demonstrates a thin rim of contrast material just below the renal capsule. This represents blood flow through the capsular arteries to the subcapsular cortex ("rim sign").

Renal vein thrombosis results in delayed renal function and parenchymal swelling in the absence of ureteral obstruction.

RENAL RUPTURE   A large expanding perirenal hematoma accompanies renal rupture, and the patient becomes clinically unstable from continued bleeding. Radiographic studies reveal multiple deep lacerations, devitalized kidney fragments, and extravasation of contrast.

RENAL PELVIS RUPTURE   Ruptures of the renal pelvis result in extravasation of urine into the perirenal space and along the psoas muscle. Renal pelvis ruptures are rare and are often associated with congenital renal anomalies. Radiographic studies reveal a normally functioning kidney, filling of the calyceal system, and extravasation of contrast without visualization of the ureter. Renal pelvis ruptures are often misdiagnosed as small renal lacerations. If the diagnosis is delayed, the patient may develop high fever, increased abdominal pain, and tenderness as the extravasation of urine continues into the retroperitoneal space. Sepsis may ensue. The diagnosis of renal pelvis rupture is confirmed by retrograde pyelogram.

Ureteral Injuries

Ureteral injuries are the rarest of all genitourinary injuries and are usually the result of penetrating trauma (Figure 262-1). Blunt trauma, however, can induce a rupture at or just below the ureteropelvic junction as a result of hyperextension of the spine with the distal ureter fixed at the trigone of the bladder. Blast effects from gunshot wounds may cause microvascular thrombosis in the ureteral wall, delayed

ureteral necrosis, and urinary fistula formation. Diagnosis is sometimes delayed. If the ureter is completely transected, hematuria may be absent.[10] IVP is likely to miss such injuries.[10] Enhanced CT or a retrograde pyelogram may be required for detection.

Bladder Injuries

The bladder is an intra-abdominal organ in children, but is situated deep in the bony pelvis in adults. It is protected from all but the most severe injuries to the abdomen and pelvis. Bladder injuries are the second most common injury to the genitourinary tract after renal injuries and are usually associated with blunt trauma and pelvic fracture. Penetrating bladder injuries are often associated with injuries to other abdominal and pelvic organs.

BLADDER CONTUSION   Bladder contusion is bruising of the bladder wall and resultant hematuria. A cystogram demonstrates an intact bladder outline. With a fractured pelvis, a large hematoma often results inside the bony pelvis, causing displacement of the bladder superiorly and laterally (Figure 262-2). This finding can serve as an indicator of pelvic hemorrhage. Large bladder hematomas also alter the architecture of the bladder, which takes on the shape of an inverted pear, hence the term "pear-shaped" bladder. Hematomas are best detected by CT.

BLADDER RUPTURE   There are two types of bladder ruptures. *Intraperitoneal* bladder rupture is usually a burst injury of a full bladder resulting in a 1-in laceration in the dome posteriorly, the only portion of the dome covered by the peritoneum. In this type of injury, urine is spilled into the peritoneal cavity. *Extraperitoneal* bladder rupture is more common. The rupture is usually located at the bladder neck. Associated pelvic ring fractures predominate. The classic triad includes abdominal pain and tenderness, hematuria (usually gross), and inability to void. If the rupture is intraperitoneal, there may be peritonitis. Kehr sign (pain referred to the shoulder), suggesting blood or urine irritating the diaphragm, may be a clue. Patients in whom bladder injury is suspected but who are unable to void spontaneously should have a retrograde or suprapubic catheter placed. Retrograde catheter placement should be avoided until urethral disruption has been ruled out.

Bladder injuries are best diagnosed by cystogram or CT cystogram (see above). Gross extravasation indicates rupture. Intraperitoneal rupture

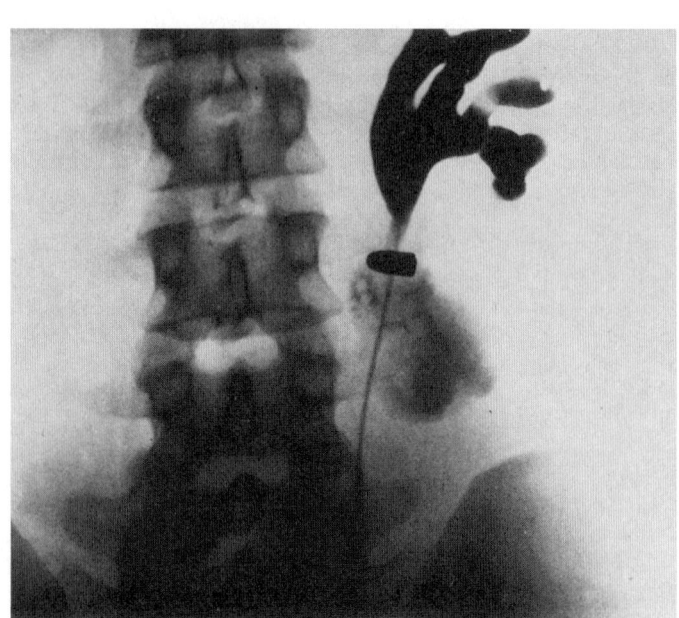

FIG. 262-1. Rare ureteral injury from a gunshot wound, with extravasation of contrast material on retrograde pyelogram.

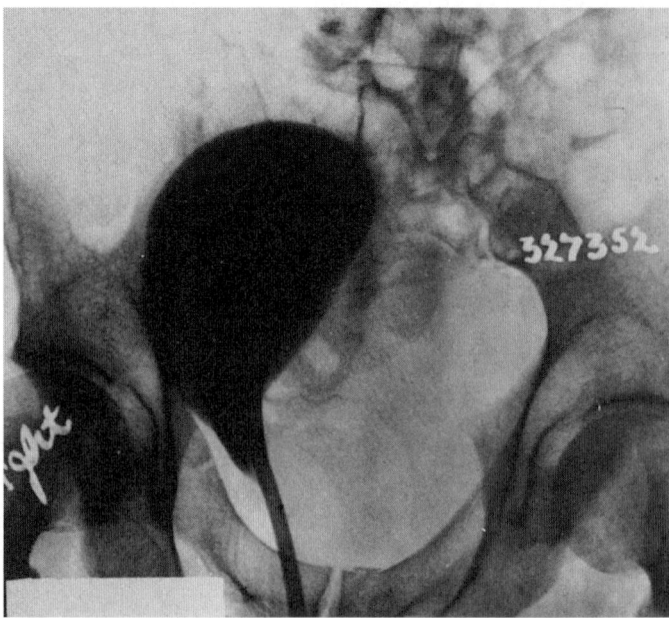

FIG. 262-2. Bladder contusion and displacement from pelvic hematoma.

is demonstrated by extravasation of contrast material in the cul-de-sac posterior to the bladder, along the paracolic gutters, and between the loops of intestine above the bladder. In extraperitoneal bladder rupture, the cystogram shows flamelike extravasation of contrast material streaking into the perivesical tissues. The wash-out film (not necessary with CT cystogram) is helpful when the extravasation is predominantly behind the bladder and obscured by contrast material in the full-bladder film of the cystogram. An irregular outline of an intact bladder may indicate contusion, hematoma, or an incomplete tear. Cystoscopy is not considered useful in this setting due to the gross hematuria and clot formation.[2]

Urethral Injuries

Urethral injuries in males occur in the posterior (prostatomembranous) urethra and in the anterior (bulbous and penile) urethra. Posterior urethral injuries are associated with pelvic fractures. Digital rectal and perineal examinations reveal the presence of a perineal hematoma or high-riding detached prostate, which is associated with complete posterior urethral disruption. Anterior urethral injuries result from direct blows to the urethra (e.g., fall-astride injuries, straddle injuries, or kicks) or from instrumentation, and in conjunction with a penile fracture. Examination reveals the classic "butterfly" perineal hematoma, limited by the attachments of the fascia lata.

In anterior urethral contusions, there is blood at the external urinary meatus, but the retrograde urethrogram findings are normal. In partial anterior urethral lacerations, the retrograde urethrogram reveals contrast extravasation at the site of injury and contrast material outlining the urethra proximal to the site of injury (Figure 262-3). In complete anterior urethral lacerations, the retrograde urethrogram reveals contrast extravasation at the site of injury without contrast proximal to the site of injury.

Female urethral injuries should be suspected in extensive pelvic fractures. Most female urethral injuries present with vaginal bleeding. Careful vaginal and endoscopic examination should be undertaken, even when the patient has menstrual bleeding or an indwelling tampon. Delayed diagnosis has resulted in labial edema, necrotizing fasciitis, and sepsis.

MANAGEMENT OF UPPER GENITOURINARY SYSTEM INJURIES

Patients with isolated microscopic hematuria (5 to 50 RBCs/hpf) in whom imaging was not indicated may be discharged from the emergency department. Strenuous activity should be proscribed. Follow-up urinalysis should be obtained in 1 to 2 weeks.

Renal

Grades I and II renal injuries (see Table 262-2) are usually managed nonoperatively. If there are no other medical considerations, such patients can be treated similarly to those with isolated hematuria. Renal contusions almost always resolve without sequelae unless there is a preexisting renal lesion, such as hydronephrosis, cyst, or tumor. Almost all minor lacerations heal without sequelae with conservative management.

Patients with grades III and IV injuries should be admitted to the hospital. Most of these patients will have other compelling reasons to be admitted or be taken to the operating room. Many hemodynamically stable adult patients with clearly delineated grade III and even grade IV injuries can still be managed nonoperatively.[19,20] Interestingly, most of these patients have retroperitoneal penetrating renal injuries.

Many centers attempt nonoperative management for all stable children unless the renal injury is particularly severe or the child fails conservative therapy.[6,21]

Exploration itself is not without consequence, because it may accentuate considerable hemorrhage. Neither the volume of blood replacement nor the degree of extravasation is an indication for exploration in itself.[2] However, if exploration is undertaken for the evaluation of other injuries, repair of renal injuries is usually undertaken. If conservative management is attempted, frequent reassessment is required, and there should be a low threshold for ordering reimaging studies. Conservative management includes bed rest, hydration, serial hematocrit determinations, monitoring of vital signs, and serial urine specimens to assess the degree of hematuria. Patients with gross hematuria remain at bed rest until the gross hematuria resolves, and remain at limited activity until microscopic hematuria resolves.

Table 262-5 lists indications for operative management.[2] Renal rupture is usually explored and nephrectomy usually required. Most, but not all, penetrating injuries are explored. The only widely accepted absolute indication for surgical exploration of a renal injury is persistent retroperitoneal bleeding with hemodynamic instability. As noted, CT may allow adequate staging even for penetrating injuries.[17,18] If the patient has other injuries warranting abdominal exploration, an intraoperative IVP may assist in determining the necessity for retroperitoneal exploration while also giving information regarding function of the contralateral kidney.

Renal pedicle injuries are usually associated with multiple life-threatening injuries, and the safest surgical option is nephrectomy. In a stable patient with an isolated renal pedicle injury, repair should be undertaken within 12 h of the injury if a viable kidney is to result. Thrombosis of segmental arteries is treated conservatively.

Ureter

Ureteral injuries are managed intraoperatively. Unfortunately, not all ureteral injuries are found at the time of injury. Delayed presentations

TABLE 262-5 Indications for Operative Exploration or Intervention in Renal Injury

Uncontrolled renal hemorrhage
Penetrating injuries
Inadequate staging
Multiple kidney lacerations
Shattered (ruptured) kidney
Avulsed major renal vessel
Pulsatile or expanding hematoma found on abdominal exploration
Vascular injuries*
Extensive extravasation

*Only those found early (see the text).
Source: Moore EE, Shackford SR, Pachter HL, et al: Organ injury scaling: Spleen, liver, kidney. *J Trauma* 29:1664, 1989.

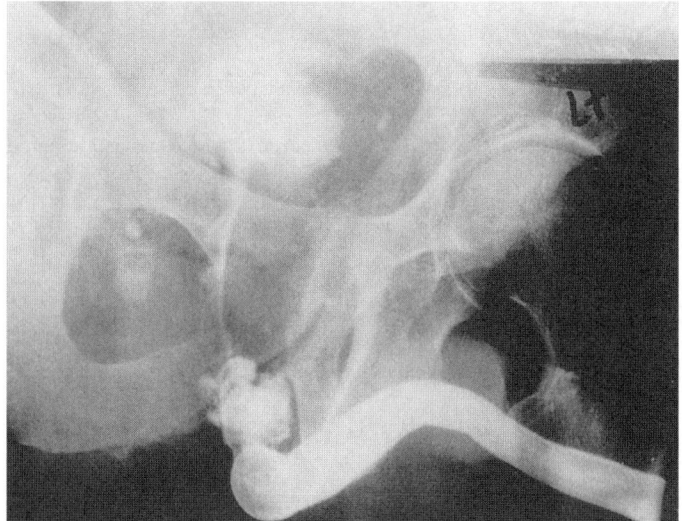

FIG. 262-3. Partial urethral laceration, with contrast extravasation at the site of injury and outlining the prostatic urethra and bladder.

include infection, including sepsis, and urinoma formation. Contusions are missed by imaging studies, but, if noted at the time of exploration, can be managed expectantly or with placement of an internal stent.

MANAGEMENT OF LOWER GENITOURINARY SYSTEM INJURIES

Bladder

Incomplete bladder lacerations can be managed by catheter placement and observation. Contusions require no specific intervention. Intraperitoneal rupture and penetrating injuries require operative intervention. Extraperitoneal bladder ruptures are treated with urethral catheter drainage alone. In such cases, the catheter remains indwelling for 10 to 14 days, and the cystogram is repeated to verify healing before the urethral catheter is removed. Rarely, persistent urinary extravasation is seen, with a bony fragment remaining in the bladder wall or a pelvic fixation impinging upon the bladder.

Urethra

Anterior contusion heals with conservative management, with or without a urethral catheter, depending on whether the patient can void. Partial anterior urethral lacerations are managed with an indwelling urethral catheter (placed coaxially over a guide wire under fluoroscopic control) or with a suprapubic cystostomy. Complete lacerations of the anterior urethra are repaired surgically with debridement and end-to-end anastomosis over a urethral catheter.

Surgical repair is usually deferred for posterior urethral injuries. Suprapubic cystostomy is favored by most for bladder drainage. Partial posterior urethral lacerations are managed with a urethral catheter placed coaxially over a guide wire under fluoroscopic control or with a suprapubic catheter. In complete posterior urethral lacerations, the management remains controversial. The injury is managed with primary realignment of the lacerated urethra or with suprapubic cystostomy alone. Stricture formation occurs with both techniques. However, the subsequent urethral stricture in patients with primary realignment tends to be less extensive. The advantage of suprapubic cystostomy alone, especially in an unstable patient, is its simplicity. The impotence and incontinence rates are thought to be related to the extent of injury and are the same for both techniques.

In women, a layer repair of the urethral and associated vaginal injuries is performed over a urethral catheter. The voiding phase of the repeat cystogram is essential in confirming complete urethral healing.

The Full-Bladder Dilemma

Emergency physicians in nontrauma centers may encounter patients with a urethral injury precluding bladder catheterization but with a full urinary bladder. Such a patient may have to be transferred many miles to reach a center with a urologic service. Spontaneous or conscious bladder contraction may ensue, with spillage of urine into the perivesical space, increasing the risk of infection. Guidewire-aided placement of a temporary suprapubic catheter into the bladder can alleviate this problem. Using the Seldinger-technique, a large-bore central venous catheter or cavity drainage catheter may provide temporary relief. The exploring needle is inserted perpendicularly about two finger breadths above the symphysis pubis. The guidewire is inserted when urine returns. The catheter selected should be long enough to coil within the bladder so that it remains in the lumen of the bladder when it is empty. Because the bladder may be displaced by a large hematoma or extravasated urine, it is advisable to inject a few milliliters of contrast material into the bladder while obtaining an x-ray to confirm that the catheter is actually in the bladder.

Testicular and Scrotal Injuries

The mobility of the testicle, cremaster muscle contraction, and the tough capsule of the testis (tunica albuginea) are responsible for the infrequent rate of injury to the testis. A direct blow to the testis impinging it against the symphysis pubis is the primary cause of blunt testicular injury. Blunt testicular injuries are either contusions or ruptures. Rarely, traumatic dislocation of the testicle to the inguinal canal has been reported. In testicular contusions or ruptures, the tunica vaginalis sac fills with blood (hematocele) and appears as a large, blue, tender scrotal mass. Penetrating injuries to the scrotum through the tunica vaginalis require exploration. Bilateral testicular injuries are often seen in penetrating trauma. Testicular ultrasonography studies with colored Doppler studies can help to delineate the extent of testicular trauma and are quite reliable in diagnosing ruptured testes.

Most testicular injuries can be managed conservatively with nonsteroidal anti-inflammatory drugs, ice, elevation, scrotal support, and appropriate urologic follow up.

For more severe injuries, early exploration, evacuation of blood clots, and repair of testicular rupture tend to result in an earlier return to normal activity, decreased hematoma infection, and less testicular atrophy than does conservative management. Testicular salvage following penetrating trauma is on the order of 35 percent.[22]

Scrotal skin avulsion is managed by housing the testicle in the remaining scrotal skin even though the reconstruction places the skin under tension. Usually the scrotum returns to nearly normal size within a few months. In complete scrotal skin loss, the testicles are placed in pouches in the inner thighs.

Injuries to the Penis

Injuries to the penis range from small contusions to degloving injuries or amputations. Self-inflicted injuries include vacuum cleaner injuries and blade injuries. Vacuum cleaners cause extensive injury to the glans penis and some loss of the urethra, requiring débridement of devitalized tissue and reconstruction. Amputation of the penis is managed by reimplantation or local repair. Reimplantation is preferable if the distal penis is in satisfactory condition, and the ischemia time is less than 12 to 18 h. Loss of penile skin by avulsion injury or burns is managed by split-thickness skin grafts after the denuded penis is clean and sterile. The avulsed skin should not be reapplied, for it invariably becomes necrotic and infected, and must be subsequently removed.

Traumatic rupture of the corpus cavernosum of the penis or fracture of the penis occurs when the erect penis impacts forcibly on a hard object (sexual partner's pubis or the floor), receives a direct blow, or is subjected to abnormal bending. A cracking sound is heard, followed by penile pain, immediate detumescence, rapid swelling, discoloration, and distention. Urethral injuries may accompany penile ruptures. Penile ruptures are managed by immediate surgical evacuation of blood clot and repair of the torn tunica albuginea of the corpus cavernosum and urethra.

Zipper injury to the penis is caused when the penile skin is trapped in the trouser zipper. Mineral oil and lidocaine infiltration are useful in freeing the penile skin from the zipper. Otherwise, wire-cutting or bone-cutting pliers are used to divide the median bar (or diamond) of the zipper, which causes the zipper to fall apart, freeing the penile skin.

Contusions of the perineum or penis, which can result from straddle or toilet seat injuries, are treated conservatively with cold packs, rest, and elevation. If the patient is unable to void, catheter drainage is elected.

REFERENCES

1. Perez-Brayfield MR, Gatti JM, Smith EA, et al: Blunt traumatic hematuria in children. Is a simplified algorithm justified? *J Urol* 167:2545, 2002.
2. Ahn JH, Morey AF, McAninch JW: Workup and management of traumatic hematuria. *Emerg Med Clin North Am* 16:145, 1998.

3. Moore EE, Shackford SR, Pachter HL, et al: Organ injury scaling: Spleen, liver, kidney. *J Trauma* 29:1664, 1989.

4. Morey AF, Bruce JE, McAninch JW: Efficacy of radiographic imaging in pediatric blunt renal trauma. *J Urol* 156:2014, 1996.

5. Abou-Jaoude WA, Sugarman JM, Fallat ME, et al: Indicators of genitourinary tract injury or anomaly in cases of pediatric blunt trauma. *J Pediatr Surg* 31:86, 1996.

6. Margenthaler JA, Weber TR, Keller MS, et al: Blunt renal trauma in children: Experience with conservative management at a pediatric trauma center. *J Trauma* 52:929, 2002.

7. Brown SL, Haas C, Dinchman KH, et al: Radiologic evaluation of pediatric blunt renal trauma in patients with microscopic hematuria. *World J Surg* 25:1557, 2001.

8. Wessel LM, Scholz S, Jester I, et al: Management of kidney injuries in children with blunt abdominal trauma. *J Pediatr Surg* 35:1327, 2000.

9. Brandes SB, Chelsky MJ, Buckman RF, et al: Ureteral injuries from penetrating trauma. *J Trauma* 36:745, 1994.

10. Morey AF, McAninch JW, Tiller BK, et al: Single-shot intraoperative excretory urography for the immediate evaluation of renal trauma. *J Urol* 161:1091, 1999.

11. Nagy KK, Brenneman FD, Krosner SM, et al: Routine preoperative "one-shot" intravenous pyelogram is not indicated in all patients with abdominal trauma. *J Am Coll Surg* 185:530, 1997.

12. Sivit CJ, Cutting JP, Eichelberger MR, et al: CT diagnosis and localization of rupture of the bladder in children with blunt abdominal trauma: Significance of contrast material extravasation in the pelvis. *AJR* 164:1243, 1995.

13. Peng MY, Parisky YR, Cornwell EE III, et al: CT cystography versus conventional cystography in evaluation of bladder injury. *AJR* 173:1271, 1999.

14. Deck AJ, Shaves S, Talner L, et al: Computerized tomography cystography for the diagnosis of traumatic bladder rupture. *J Urol* 164:44, 2000.

15. Fuhrman GM, Simmons GT, Davidson BS, Buerk CA: The single indication for cystography in blunt trauma. *Am Surg* 59:335, 1993.

16. Medina D, Lavery R, Ross SE, et al: Ureteral trauma: Preoperative studies neither predict injury nor prevent missed injury. *J Am Coll Surg* 186:641, 1998.

17. Thall EH, Stone NN, Cheng DL, et al: Conservative management of penetrating and blunt type III renal injuries. *Br J Urol* 77:513, 1996.

18. Velmahos GC, Demetriades D, Cornwell EE III, et al: Selective management of renal gunshot wounds. *Br J Surg* 85:1121, 1998.

19. Goldman SM: Upper urinary tract trauma. *World J Urol* 16:62, 1998.

20. Mansi MK, Alkhudar WK: Conservative management with percutaneous intervention of major blunt renal injuries. *Am J Emerg Med* 7:633, 1997.

21. Wessel LM, Scholz S, Jester I, et al: Management of kidney injuries in children with blunt abdominal trauma. *J Pediatr Surg* 35:1326, 2000.

22. Cline KJ: Penetrating trauma to the male external genitalia. *J Trauma* 44:492, 1998.

PENETRATING TRAUMA TO THE EXTREMITIES

Alan M. Kumar
Richard D. Zane

Emergent management of penetrating extremity injuries is an evolving and controversial subject. Recent advances in surgical technique enable arterial repair with an extremely low rate of postoperative thrombosis, making the recognition and rapid treatment of arterial injury of paramount importance. Associated injury to soft tissue, nerve, and bony structures is now the primary determinants of limb salvage. Emergency physicians play a crucial role in the management of penetrating extremity injuries by identifying injuries early and promptly initiating care crucial to limb rescue. Unnecessary delays in treatment can lead to irreversible limb ischemia and subsequent limb loss.

EPIDEMIOLOGY

In the past 10 years, there has been a surge in the number of violent crimes associated with firearm usage. Gun-related assaults, robberies, and murders have risen by 59 percent since 1987. Penetrating trauma accounts for up to 82 percent of all vascular injuries to the extremities. Gunshot and shotgun wounds account for nearly 65 percent of penetrating vascular extremity injuries, and stab wounds account for approximately 15 percent. Of patients presenting with gunshot wounds, 20 to 40 percent have extremity involvement, either isolated or in combination with other injuries. In 1950, a patient with a penetrating extremity injury with vascular involvement had a 50 percent chance of leaving the hospital with an amputated limb. With recent advances in emergency care, vascular surgery, invasive radiology, and the science of thrombosis, penetrating extremity injury results in amputation in fewer than 5 percent.[1] Despite this improved diagnosis, there is still a 15 to 40 percent long-term morbidity due to other complications, such as nerve damage, fractures, wound infections, open joint injuries, and compartment syndromes.[2]

PATHOPHYSIOLOGY

Gunshot and stab wounds account for the largest percentage of penetrating extremity injuries. Gunshot and blast injuries often present a diagnostic and management dilemma. A basic understanding of wound ballistics will enable astute clinicians to better plan the clinical management of patients who sustain a gunshot wound to an extremity. Diagnostic and treatment modalities as well as outcome differ with the type and severity of the injury. Although the damage from a stab wound can be relatively predictable with a good knowledge of clinical anatomy, the tissue damage inflicted by a missile or blast depends on a variety of factors (see Chap. 264).

DIAGNOSIS AND MANAGEMENT

After the initial trauma resuscitation and primary and secondary surveys are complete, specific points of the victim's past medical history should be examined: preexisting vascular and neuromuscular deficits, and the events surrounding the injury, such as the type of gun and number of shots. An extremely careful and thorough physical examination is needed to identify significant injuries rapidly and to determine whether immediate surgical intervention is necessary or which, if any, diagnostic studies are indicated. This may be challenging in the presence of other serious trauma or distracting injuries.

The presentation of penetrating vascular injury varies widely. Prompt recognition of arterial injury is one of the fundamental goals of management. The presence and volume of the distal pulses in the affected extremity should be noted and compared with the unaffected limb. Ankle-brachial indices (ABIs) should be calculated on the affected and unaffected limbs (method described below). The color, temperature, and capillary refill time are important clinical indicators of more subtle injury to underlying vessels. Examination should also look for signs of compartment syndrome. Capillary refill alone is an unpredictable marker of vascular injury but may be useful in conjunction with other modalities. Only a small minority of patients (fewer than 6 percent) will present with classic "hard" signs of arterial injury (Table 263-1). These patients require expeditious operative management or, under certain circumstances, angiography (Figure 263-1). A surgeon should be involved in the management of these patients as soon as possible. Patients with "soft" signs (Table 263-1) of arterial vascular trauma can usually be managed without surgical intervention on an inpatient surgical service.[3] Controversy surrounds the management of the patient with a wound in proximity to a major vascular structure but without clinical evidence of arterial injury. Historically, patients with these types of injuries were all surgically explored, which yielded a large number of negative exploratory surgeries, and thus angiography became popular. Angiography based on proximity alone yields abnormalities in 10 to 20 percent of the cases, with less than 2 percent requiring surgical intervention. Current practice regarding penetrating injuries in proximity to major vessels without any signs of

TABLE 263-1   Clinical Manifestations of Extremity Vascular Trauma

Hard signs
    Absent or diminished distal pulses
    Obvious arterial bleeding
    Large expanding or pulsatile hematoma
    Audible bruit
    Palpable thrill
    Distal ischemia (pain, pallor, paralysis, paresthesias, coolness)
Soft signs
    Small, stable hematoma
    Injury to anatomically related nerve
    Unexplained hypotension
    History of hemorrhage
    Proximity of injury to major vascular structures
    Complex fracture

vascular injury is to observe patients with clinically silent arterial injury. The natural course in these cases is likely benign, and these patients can be safely observed with serial examinations.

Duplex ultrasound has become a popular modality in the management of proximity injuries without evidence of arterial injury. Recent advances in duplex ultrasonography have shown highly accurate rates of detecting occult arterial injury (see below). Some clinicians use duplex ultrasound to distinguish between patients who require observation and those who can safely be discharged home.

Although patients with venous trauma can bleed profusely, management by either ligation or reanastomosis often yields similar results.[4] Asymptomatic venous injury rarely results in long-term morbidity. During the initial trauma resuscitation, attempts should not be made to clamp or ligate bleeding vessels in an attempt to control bleeding. Nerves are bundled with vascular structures and can be easily damaged by blind clamping or ligation. Profuse bleeding should be initially controlled with direct pressure.

Although arterial injury is the most dramatic result of penetrating extremity injury and represents the most immediate life threat, injuries to major nerves are the most likely to lead to long-term disability. Fortunately, 70 percent of peripheral nerve injuries noted during the initial examination recover completely within 6 months of the initial injury. A neuromuscular examination of the extremities should indicate both muscular and sensory function (Table 263-2) and check for evidence of compartment syndrome. Patients with suspected nerve, orthopedic, vascular injury or compartment syndrome should be immediately evaluated by surgical subspecialists.

The size and shape of the wounds, and soft tissue and obvious bony deformities, should be noted and thoroughly examined. Pain on palpation or movement of an extremity is suspicious for an underlying fracture. Penetrating trauma near a joint should be evaluated thoroughly for damage to the joint capsule, as associated long-term morbidity is significant. Radiologic evidence of air in a joint is evidence of joint penetration. Patients with obvious bony or joint capsule injury should be evaluated by an orthopedic surgeon. The majority of orthopedic surgeons will undertake arthroscopic exploration and "wash out" an involved major joint. Joint sepsis and destruction, rapid chondrolysis, and loss of anatomic contours can lead to long-term morbidity in the form of posttraumatic degenerative arthritis and decreased or total loss of flexibility. Metal fragments left in the joint space may dissolve in the synovial fluid, resulting in lead toxicity. Patients with penetrating injury proximal to or overlying a major joint without obvious joint penetration and without fracture can be splinted and discharged with 24 h orthopedic follow-up. Most orthopedic authors recommend discharging these patients on oral antibiotics, although the rationale has not been clearly established. Bony fractures as a result of penetrating injury are treated as open fractures. The injury is surgically debrided and the patient admitted for intravenous antibiotics.

Wound management is of great importance in the proper healing of penetrating injuries. Careful treatment is, however, just one important factor in decreasing the rate of wound infection. Bacterial inoculum, tissue devitalization, blood supply, time to presentation and treatment, presence of foreign bodies, and host immune status all play a role in the final outcome. Irrigation of wounds with either normal saline or

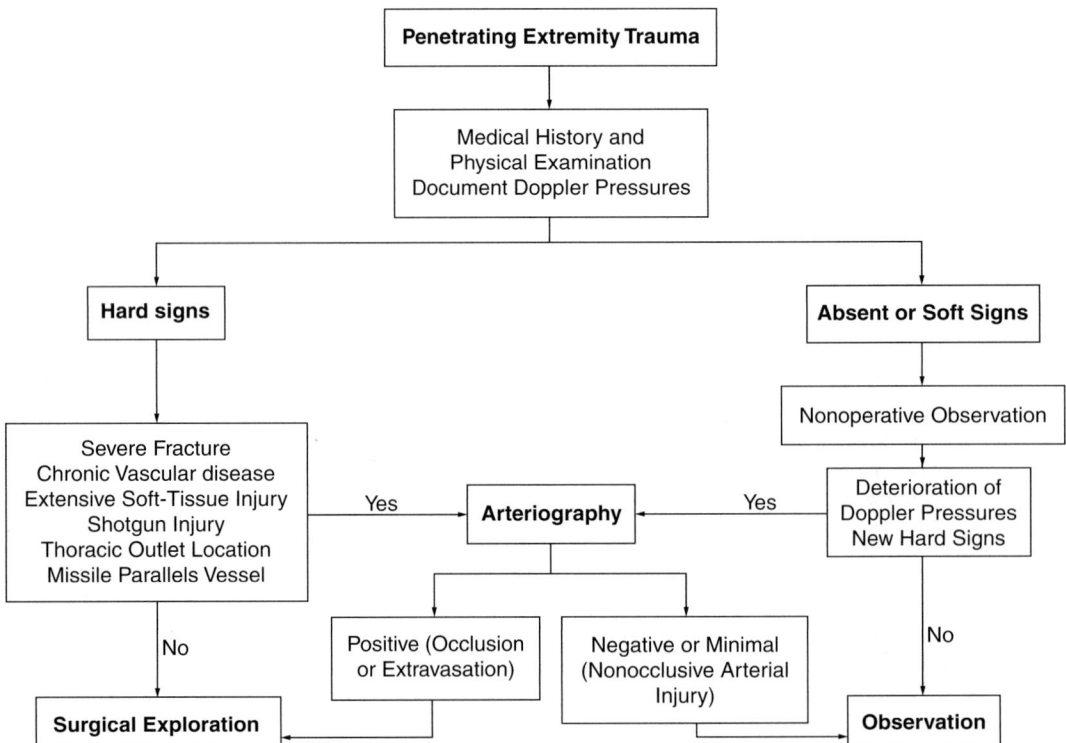

FIG. 263-1. Algorithm for the evaluation of an injured extremity for vascular trauma. (Adapted from Frykberg ER: Advances in diagnosis and treatment of extremity trauma. *Surg Clin North Am* 75:207, 1995.)

TABLE 263-2   Clinical Examination of the Nerves of the Extremities

Nerve	Test of Motor Function	Test for Sensation
Axillary (C5–6)	Arm abduction Arm internal, external rotation	Lateral aspect of shoulder
Musculocutaneous (C5–6)	Forearm flexion	Lateral forearm
Radial (C5–8)	Forearm, wrist, and finger extension	Dorsoradial hand, thumb
Median (C6–T1)	Wrist flexion, finger adduction	Volar aspect of thumb and index finger
Ulnar (C7–T1)	Finger abduction	Volar aspect of little finger
Femoral (L1–L4)	Knee extension	
Obturator (L2–L4)	Hip adduction	
Superior gluteal (L4–S1)	Hip abduction	
Sciatic (L4–S3)	Knee flexion	
Deep peroneal (L4–S1)	Ankle and great toe dorsiflexion	
Superficial peroneal (L5–S1)	Foot eversion	
Tibial (L5–S2)	Ankle plantar flexion	
Posterior tibial (L5–S2)	Great toe plantar flexion	
Spinal L4		Medial calf
Spinal L5		Dorsal foot
Spinal S1		Lateral plantar foot

1% povidone-iodine solution at high pressure until removal of all visible contaminants or at least 250 mL is recommended to reduce bacterial counts. More vigorous and lengthy irrigation might be needed for heavily contaminated wounds. In wounds older than 3 to 4 h, host defenses can actually prevent further reduction in bacterial counts and gentle scrubbing of the wound is recommended.

Soft tissue foreign bodies present a special dilemma. If the wound is not completely visualized, radiographic studies are often necessary. Materials such as glass, metal, gravel, or bone are usually visible on plain films and can be localized using this technique. Organic materials such as wood are more difficult to isolate using this method and ultrasound has become an increasingly useful modality in their localization. However, object size, density compared to surrounding tissue, orientation, depth, and the presence of devitalized tissue and air can limit the effectiveness of either of these radiographic techniques. CT scanning is more accurate in finding both radiolucent and opaque foreign bodies. Once localized, the decision to remove a foreign body is dependent on many factors. The exploration of tissue necessary to find the foreign body can further damage tissue and increase risk of infection. The size of the object, along with its composition, should also be considered. Organic materials tend to be more reactive and have a higher risk of causing infection. Inert substances such as bullet fragments and glass are less likely to cause these reactions. The chance that a bullet may migrate into vital structures or the possibility of embolism if it is near a vessel makes removal of the foreign body more important.

The decision to close a wound depends on the presentation and degree of contamination. If it is associated with bony injury, the wound should be considered an open fracture and the patient admitted for surgical debridement. Wounds that have little contamination and

are amenable to irrigation can be closed if close follow-up can be arranged. Patients with delayed presentations, contaminated wounds, soft tissue foreign bodies, or extensive tissue destruction would likely benefit from delayed primary closure after 72 to 96 h if there are no signs of infection at that time. The role of antibiotics remains controversial in penetrating extremity trauma. They are not beneficial in low risk injuries but may have a role in special situations such as hand injuries, patients with compromised immune systems, significant tissue damage or contamination, and joint or bony involvement.[5]

DIAGNOSTIC MODALITIES

Radiographic Studies

Plain films, including anteroposterior and lateral views, of the involved extremities should be obtained in all cases. Oblique views may also offer additional information. **It is important that the joints above and below the suspected injury site be imaged.** Five general types of fracture patterns are created from bullets (Figure 263-2). A drill hole pattern from penetration of cancellous bone is often seen in sites such as the proximal humerus, pelvis, and distal femur. These fractures have less communition than those in cortical bone because cancellous bone is more porous and less dense. Unicortical fractures of the metaphysis on long bones are often seen with bullet impact on a tangential plane. The majority of gunshot fractures of the diaphysis are comminuted, and the degree of communition depends on the amount of energy transfer from the penetrating missile. Spiral fractures distant from the site of impact on the bone can occur if the bone is under a degree of torsional stress. There have also been reports of

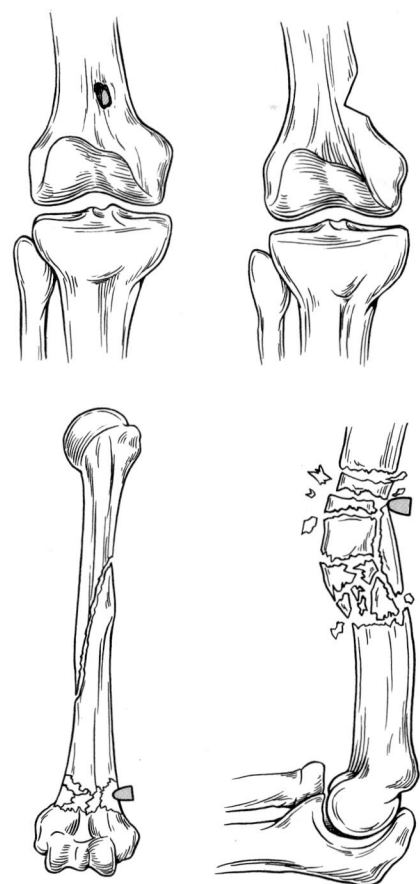

FIG. 263-2. Types of fracture patterns created by bullets: drill hole, unicortical, distant spiral, comminuted. The fifth type seen is a simple fracture.

simple fractures of long bones caused by indirect damage from the temporary cavity. It is also important to note whether a joint has been penetrated, because this complication changes patient management. **In the case of shotgun or blast injury, it is important to image the extremity distal to the injury** in order to detect any pellets that may have embolized (Figures 263-3A and B).

Computed tomography is considered helpful in selected cases before definitive orthopedic care. It can help diagnose bony pathology and determine if intraarticular fractures, fragments, or foreign bodies are present.

Magnetic resonance imaging is not commonly used for penetrating extremity trauma. Angiography can be used to delineate the extent, nature, and location of vascular injuries with special situations such as shotgun wounds, multiple or severe fractures, chronic vascular disease, thoracic outlet wounds, or extensive soft tissue injury. The widespread availability and accuracy of angiography led it to become the

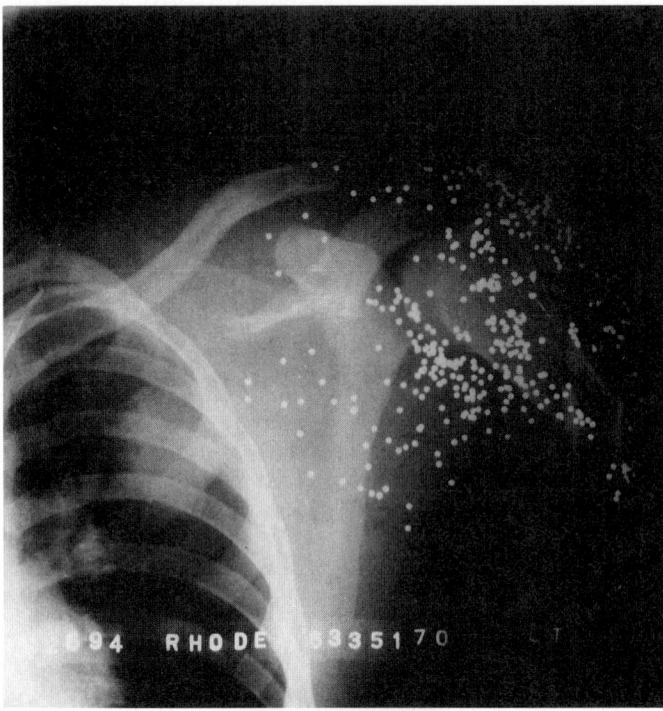

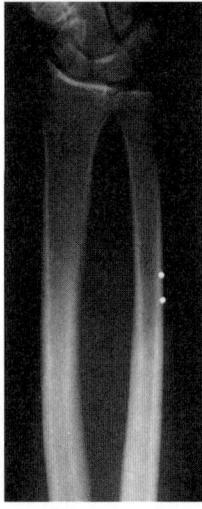

FIG. 263-3. A. Gunshot wound to the shoulder and axilla. **B.** Actual embolization of shotgun pellet, illustrating importance of obtaining images of the extremity distal to such injuries.

"gold standard" in the evaluation of patients with wounds in proximity to major neurovascular bundles. Arteriography for the evaluation of proximity injuries in patients without hard signs of injury reveals normal results in 80 to 90 percent, with a complication rate of 1 to 2 percent from the procedure. Recent studies have shown that occult vascular injuries can exist without hard clinical findings in up to 23 percent of patients. Among these, however, fewer than 2 percent have surgically important lesions. Still, with observation and a careful examination, positive findings will eventually be more evident and the wounds subsequently repaired without increased morbidity.[6–9]

The algorithm presented in Figure 263-1 outlines the approach to vascular injuries. In the presence of hard signs of vascular injury on clinical examination, immediate surgery is indicated in some conditions, without a preoperative angiogram. However, certain injuries are still best evaluated by angiography prior to surgical intervention. The need for angiography in patients with soft signs of vascular injury is still a matter of some debate among surgeons and radiologists. However, current practice in most centers is to observe patients with soft signs and conduct serial examinations. Angiography and surgery are delayed until there is clinical evidence of arterial injury.

Digital subtraction angiography has also been used in evaluation of vascular trauma with accuracy similar to standard techniques but is less reliable in detecting intimal disruption. The test requires a cooperative patient, because it is extremely sensitive to motion artifact.[3]

Ankle Brachial Indices

Doppler devices are used to determine wrist or ankle brachial indices (ABIs). Diagnostic accuracy has been reported to be as high as 95 percent, but sensitivity and specificity vary depending on whether the classification of abnormal is set at a ratio of 1.0 or 0.9.[9,10] This test does not reliably detect nonocclusive arterial disease, such as intimal flaps and pseudoaneurysms. It can augment the clinical examination by objectively confirming the subjective impression of a diminished pulse in a patient under observation. To perform accurate ABIs, it is important to place the patient in supine position and measure the systolic blood pressure in all four extremities. To measure an ankle systolic pressure, a standard adult blood pressure cuff should be snugly wrapped around the ankle just above the malleoli. While using the Doppler flowmeter to monitor the signal from the posterior of the anterior tibial artery, distal to the cuff, inflate the cuff to a pressure approximately 30 mm Hg above the systolic pressure to occlude flow temporarily. As the cuff is slowly deflated (2 to 5 mm Hg/s), the pressure at which the Doppler flow signal is heard should be noted and recorded as the ankle systolic pressure. To assure accuracy, the upper extremity systolic blood pressure should be measured by using a Doppler flowmeter, as well. An ABI is then calculated by dividing the ankle systolic blood pressure by the greater of the two systolic upper extremity blood pressures. An ABI of greater than 1.0 is normal. An ABI of 0.5 to 0.9 is indicative of injury to a single arterial segment. An ABI of less than 0.5 is indicative of severe arterial injury or injury to multiple arterial segments. A difference of greater than 20 mm Hg between the upper extremity blood pressures is indicative of upper extremity arterial injury. Underlying conditions, such as preexisting peripheral vascular disease or severe hypothermia, can also affect the accuracy of the ABI.

Duplex Ultrasonography

Duplex ultrasonography has a diagnostic accuracy of 96 to 98 percent and can image extremity vessels with as much resolution as contrast angiography. Advantages over angiography include an increased safety profile and rapid results. However, it is highly operator dependent and has not been tested in patients with severely injured extremities with open wounds or fractures, large hematomas, bulky dressings, or traction devices.[1,3,10]

DISPOSITION

Patients with hard signs of arterial injury are not a diagnostic dilemma. These patients require surgical intervention or, at the very least, expedient surgical evaluation and angiography. Patients with soft signs of arterial injury require inpatient observation. Patients with penetrating extremity injury, no signs of arterial injury, no bony or nervous injury, minimal soft tissue defect, and no signs of developing compartment syndrome can be safely discharged home with close follow-up after a period of observation and serial examinations. There is no consensus on the ideal observation time, but the current literature describes times from 3 to 12 h. Wound exploration in the emergency department should be reserved for those patients with suspected foreign bodies in the wound, for ligamentous involvement, or for control of minor venous bleeding. Wound exploration to control arterial or major venous bleeding should be done in the operating room. The general principles of wound management, including tetanus prophylaxis, apply here. Although controversial, there is no proven rule for prophylactic antibiotics unless a wound is contaminated or patients have an underlying preexisting condition that would predispose to infection.

REFERENCES

1. Conrad MF, Patton JH Jr, Parikshak M, Kralovich KA: Evaluation of vascular injury in penetrating extremity trauma: Angiographers stay home. *Am Surg* 68:269, 2002.
2. Hull JB: Management of gunshot fractures of the extremities. *J Trauma* 40(suppl):193, 1996.
3. Mandracchia VJ, Buddecke DE Jr, Statler TK, Nelson ScC: Related articles gunshot wounds to the lower extremity. A comprehensive review. *Clin Podiatr Med Surg* 16:597, 1999.
4. Schmidt-Matthiesen A, Roding H, Windolf J, et al: A prospective, randomised comparison of single vs. multiple dose antibiotic prophylaxis in penetrating trauma. *Chemotherapy* 45:380, 1999.
5. Gonzalez RP, Falimirski ME: The utility of physical examination in proximity penetrating extremity trauma. *Am Surg* 65:784, 1999.
6. American College of Emergency Physicians: Clinical policy for the initial approach to patients presenting with penetrating extremity trauma. *Ann Emeg Med* 33:612, 1999.
7. Feliciano DV, Herskowitz K, O'Gorman RB, et al: Management of vascular injuries in the lower extremities. *J Trauma* 28:319, 1988.
8. Gates JD: Penetrating wounds of the extremities: Methods of identifying arterial injury. *Orthop Rev* 10(suppl):2, 1994.
9. Nassoura ZE, Ivatury RR, Simon RJ, et al: A reassessment of Doppler pressure indices in the detection of arterial lesions in proximity penetrating injuries of extremities: A prospective study. *Am J Emerg Med* 14:151, 1996.
10. Bergstein JM, Blair JF, Edwards J, et al: Pitfalls in the use of color-flow duplex ultrasound for screening of suspected arterial injuries in penetrating extremities. *J Trauma* 33:395, 1992.

WOUND BALLISTICS

Jeremy J. Hollerman
Martin L. Fackler

GENERAL CONCEPTS

The medical literature is full of erroneous articles classifying gunshot wounds based on bullet velocity. Other bullet and tissue characteristics are at least as important as velocity.[1–3] Bullet *mass,* which is related to diameter and length, is a major determinant of how deeply the bullet will penetrate tissue. Bullet *construction* (such as whether the bullet is solid lead with no bullet jacket, is partially jacketed, or has a full metal jacket) is a primary determinant of whether the bullet will deform or fragment. Bullet shape and center of mass (which determine how soon it will yaw in its path through tissue), the *thickness of the body part*

wounded (determining whether the bullet has a long enough path through tissue to deform or yaw) (Figure 264-1), *tissue type* struck (e.g., femur versus lung), tissue elasticity, density, specific gravity, and internal cohesiveness [which determine how well the tissue will withstand tissue stretch (temporary cavitation) forces] are all important, in addition to bullet *velocity,* in determining the nature of the wound produced. The amount of kinetic energy "deposited" or "retained" in a victim wounded by a projectile is not a reliable predictor of wound severity,[4] and muzzle energy is not a reliable indicator of bullet performance.

An understanding of wound ballistics enables physicians to evaluate and treat missile wounds without repeating the errors of conventional wisdom. Based on common misconceptions about wound ballistics, many papers have suggested harmful and unnecessary treatment for gunshot wounds. An example of such an unnecessary and harmful recommendation is that for mandatory surgical excision of the tissue surrounding the bullet track (the path of the projectile through tissue) whenever an extremity wound is caused by a high-velocity bullet. This is based on the belief that these tissues will become necrotic. Clinical experience and research show this to be false.[5]

WOUNDING POTENTIAL

Every moving bullet has a maximum wounding potential determined by its mass and velocity. Bullets of equal wounding potential may produce wounds of very different severity depending on bullet shape, internal and external construction, and which tissues they traverse.

Bullets with equal wounding potential often do not produce similar wounds. A heavier, slower bullet crushes more tissue but induces less temporary cavitation; most of the wounding potential of a lighter, faster bullet is likely to be used up forming a larger temporary cavity, but this bullet leaves a smaller permanent cavity (crushes less tissue).[4,6] The heavier, slower bullet causes a more severe wound in elastic tissue than the lighter, faster bullet, which uses up much of its wounding potential producing tissue stretch (temporary cavitation). This tissue stretch may be absorbed with little or no ill effect by elastic tissue such as lung or muscle. In less elastic tissue such as liver or brain, the temporary cavity produced by the lighter, faster bullet can produce a more severe wound. Penetration depth will be less with the lighter, faster bullet, and critical structures such as the heart may not be reached.

MECHANISMS OF WOUNDING

Both missile and tissue characteristics determine the nature of the wound. Missile characteristics are partly inherent (mass, shape, and construction) and are partly conferred by the weapon (longitudinal and rotational velocity). Tissue characteristics (elasticity, density, and anatomic relationships) also strongly affect the nature of the wound. The severity of a bullet wound is influenced by the bullet's orientation during its flight through tissue and by whether the bullet fragments[4] and/or deforms (into the typical mushroom shape of expanding hollow-point or soft-point bullets).

Two major mechanisms of wounding occur: the *crushing* of the tissue struck by the projectile (forming the permanent cavity) and the radial *stretching* of the projectile path walls (forming a temporary cavity) (see Figure 264-1). In addition, a sonic pressure wave precedes the projectile through tissue. The sonic pressure wave plays no part in wounding.[7]

Crushing of Tissue

A missile crushes the tissue it strikes, thereby creating a permanent wound channel (permanent cavity). If the bullet is traveling with its pointed end forward and its long axis parallel to the longitudinal axis

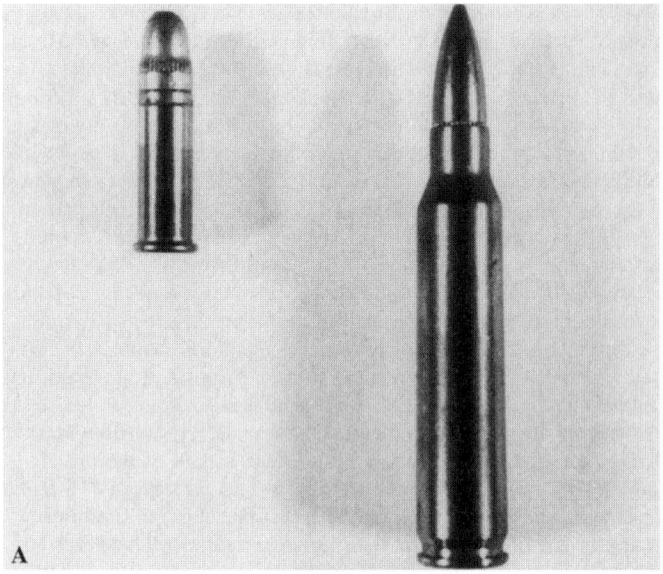

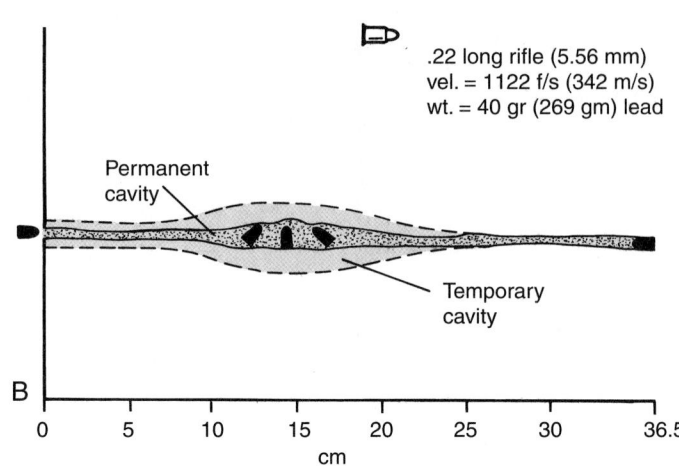

.22 long rifle (5.56 mm)
vel. = 1122 f/s (342 m/s)
wt. = 40 gr (269 gm) lead

Permanent
cavity

Temporary
cavity

B

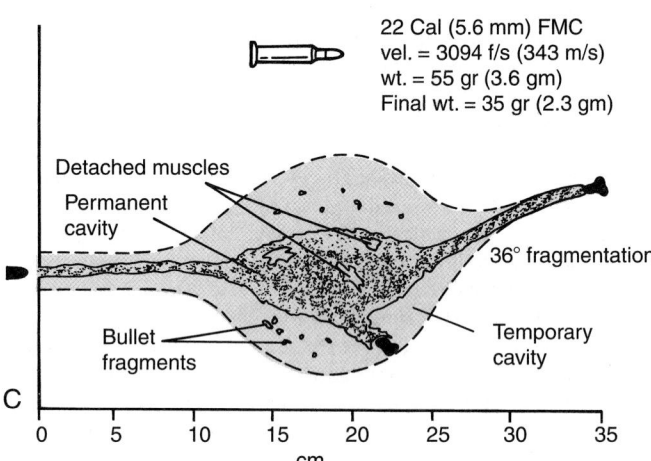

22 Cal (5.6 mm) FMC
vel. = 3094 f/s (343 m/s)
wt. = 55 gr (3.6 gm)
Final wt. = 35 gr (2.3 gm)

Detached muscles
Permanent
cavity

36° fragmentation

Bullet
fragments

Temporary
cavity

C

FIG. 264-1. A. A .22 long-rifle round *(left)* and an M16 round *(right).* **B, C.** Wound profiles of the same .22 long-rifle (**B**) and .224 caliber M-193 round of the M16A1 rifle (**C**). [Full metal case (FMC) is a synonym for full metal jacket (FMJ), the type of bullet used in the military.] This figure shows that caliber (bullet diameter in decimals of an inch or in millimeters) is only one indicator of wounding potential and not a very good one. Because of much higher velocity [3094 ft/s (943 m/s), as opposed to 1122 ft/s (342 m/s) for the .22 long-rifle bullet], because it fragments in tissue, and because of greater bullet mass, the M16 bullet has the potential to cause a much more severe wound if the anatomic part struck is sufficiently thick. Note that in the gelatin block, both the permanent cavity and the temporary cavity caused by the M16 bullet are much larger than those of the .22 long-rifle bullet. As is usual for a nondeforming bullet, the temporary and permanent cavities caused by the .22 long-rifle bullet are largest when the bullet is at 90 degrees of yaw. (Reproduced with permission from Hollerman et al.)[1]

of flight (0 degrees of yaw, the angle between the long axis of the bullet and its path of flight), it crushes a tube of tissue approximately equal to its diameter. When the bullet yaws to 90 degrees, the entire long axis of the bullet strikes tissue. The amount of tissue crushed may be three times greater than at 0 degrees of yaw.

When striking soft tissue with sufficient velocity, soft-point and hollow-point bullets deform into a mushroom shape. This increases surface area and the amount of tissue crushed. For most big-game hunting, such bullets are mandated by law. This is to increase the probability of prompt lethality rather than the creation of a disabling but nonlethal wound causing an animal prolonged suffering. If the mushroomed diameter is 2.5 times greater than the initial diameter of the bullet, the area of tissue crushed by the bullet is 6.25 times greater than the amount that would have been crushed by the undeformed bullet.

Bullet fragmentation also increases the volume of tissue crushed.[1,4] After bullet fragmentation, bullet surface area is increased, and much more tissue is crushed. For large handgun (e.g., .44 magnum) and rifle bullets, the striking of bone is one of the causes of early bullet fragmentation.

Comminuted fracture may be created by rifle and large handgun bullets striking bone. Bone fragments can become secondary missiles, crushing tissue. Many handgun bullets are unable to fragment bone

significantly. When a large bone is struck, it is likely that the bullet will expend its wounding potential in the victim and will not exit.

Bullet fragments and secondary missiles, such as bone fragments, teeth, or coins propelled by contact with the bullet are likely to increase the severity of the wound. Multiple perforations weaken tissue and create focal points for stress (stress risers). Tissue tears are particularly likely to occur at stress risers during temporary cavitation stretch.[4]

Unjacketed lead bullets cannot be driven faster than about 2000 ft/s (610 m/s) without some of the lead stripping off in the barrel. This is avoided if a jacket made of a harder metal (such as copper or a copper alloy) is used to surround the lead. The jacket of a military bullet completely covers the bullet tip (a full metal jacket). Civilians often use hollow-point or soft-point bullets. Hollow-point bullets have a hole in the jacket at the bullet tip, and soft-point bullets have some of the lead core of the bullet exposed at the bullet tip. These constructions weaken the bullet tip, causing it to flatten on impact. This flattening often greatly exceeds bullet diameter, resulting in a mushroom-shaped projectile.

The hollow-point and soft-point bullets used by civilians are often more damaging to tissue than are military bullets fired from rounds otherwise configured identically.[1,4,8] Because of this, wounds produced by civilian hunting rifles, shotguns, and large-caliber handguns are usually more severe than wounds produced by military-rifle bullets of the same mass and velocity.[8]

Hollow-point and soft-point bullets either deform into a mushroom shape or stay undeformed. Up to one-third of hollow-point and soft-point handgun bullets fail to deform into a mushroom shape, usually due to insufficient bullet velocity or an excessively stiff or thick bullet jacket that prevents deformation.

When the tip of a hollow-point bullet is plugged with material such as clothing or drywall, bullet expansion into a mushroom shape in tissue is usually delayed and sometimes prevented. This causes deeper penetration of tissue, sometimes resulting in a perforating wound (having both and entrance and an exit). This may result in the injury of bystanders. Some recent handgun bullets have designs attempting to overcome this problem.

Projectiles penetrate more deeply as projectile velocity is increased, but only up to the point where velocity becomes sufficiently high to deform the projectile. Penetration decreases markedly from that point on. The greater the bullet diameter expansion from mushrooming, the less is the depth of penetration.[9]

There is a critical range of velocity for each handgun hollow-point and soft-point bullet within which the bullet may perform as expected. Below this velocity range, the bullet will have insufficient velocity to mushroom on impact, and at velocities above this range, the bullet may fragment after impact, resulting in many light bullet pieces crushing tissue at a superficial depth.

Military full metal jacket bullets do not flatten at the bullet tip; i.e., they do not mushroom. Sometimes they can break and fragment as a result of yawing to 90 degrees. The stress on the bullet as its long axis strikes tissue causes the sides of the bullet to flatten as if the bullet had been squeezed in a vise. If the bullet breaks, it usually will do so at the cannelure, a circular groove around the bullet where it is crimped into the cartridge case. Although the M-193 military bullet of the M16 rifle fragments in soft tissue wounds with a characteristic pattern depending on range,[10] most other full metal jacket military bullets, such as those fired from the AK-47, AK-74, and the NATO 7.62-mm rifle (U.S. version), do not fragment unless they strike a large bone.

If a bullet is jacketed, the bullet jacket usually cannot be distinguished from the lead core on standard radiographs because the entire bullet is metallic density. Sometimes, as the bullet deforms or fragments, the bullet jacket separates from the bullet and is visible on a radiograph. It is often less dense than the bullet fragments and may have a distinctive shape.

In extremity wounds, when a radiograph reveals an undeformed bullet lying in the soft tissues and no fracture is present, tissue disruption is usually minor. If a major vessel or nerve is divided, however, even a simple wound can have a severe effect on the patient.

Wounding is like real estate: Location is the most important factor. A bullet of low wounding potential can cause a severe wound if it passes through a vital structure such as the spinal cord.

Temporary Cavitation (Tissue Stretch)

Fired from an appropriate, well-designed weapon, a bullet flies in air with its nose pointed forward; it yaws only 1 to 3 degrees. Yaw occurs around the bullet's center of mass. In pointed rifle bullets, the center of mass is behind the midpoint of the bullet's long axis. Although the bullet's most naturally stable in-flight orientation would be with its heaviest part (its base) forward, for aerodynamically efficient flight, it must fly point forward.

During flight, a bullet is stabilized against yaw by the spin imparted to it by the spiral grooves (rifling) in the gun barrel. The longer (and heavier) the bullet in relation to its diameter, the more rapidly it must be rotated to avoid significant yaw in flight. A gun barrel in-

tended to fire a heavier bullet has rifling that makes a full turn in fewer inches of barrel length than the rifling in a barrel intended for a shorter, lighter bullet of the same caliber. This will cause a faster rate of bullet spin.

A gun with a shorter barrel generally will produce a bullet of lower velocity than would a weapon with a longer barrel when firing the same round. With shorter barrel length, the expanding gasses of the burning gunpowder have less time to accelerate the bullet before they are discharged into the atmosphere. A .22 long-rifle round fired in a rifle will produce a bullet with up to 300 ft/s more velocity than would the same round fired in a handgun.

Although the bullet's spin is adequate to stabilize it against yaw in its flight through air, it is not adequate to stabilize it in its path through tissue because of the higher density of the medium. If it does not deform, a pointed bullet eventually yaws to a base-forward position (180 degrees of yaw). Expanding bullets lose the physical stimulus to yaw because, after mushrooming, their heaviest part is forward.

As a bullet passes through 90 degrees of yaw or after it deforms into a mushroom shape, it is crushing its maximal amount of tissue (unless it fragments, which will crush more). It is slowed down rapidly as its wounding potential is used up. The bullet creates a splash-type force in tissue, which spreads out radially. This force creates the temporary cavity. This aspect of the wounding process is analogous to the splash of a diver entering the water.

If a diver enters the water very straight and pointed forward (similar to a bullet at 0 degrees of yaw), the splash may be minimal. If the diver does a belly-flop (similar to a bullet at 90 degrees of yaw), a large splash is induced. In tissue, this splash, the temporary cavity, produces localized blunt trauma.[6]

The maximal size of the temporary cavity occurs several milliseconds after the bullet has passed through the tissue. Because forces follow paths of least resistance, temporary cavitation is likely to be asymmetric and spread out through tissue planes.

The temporary cavity caused by common handgun bullets is generally too small to be a significant wounding factor in all but the most sensitive tissues (brain and liver). Center-fire rifle bullets and large handgun bullets (e.g., .44 magnum) often induce a large temporary cavity [10- to 25-cm (4- to 10-in.) diameter] in tissue. This can be a significant wounding factor depending on the characteristics of the tissue in which it forms.

Near-water-density, less elastic tissue (such as brain, liver, or spleen), fluid-filled organs (including the heart, bladder, and gastrointestinal tract), and dense tissue (such as bone) may be damaged severely when a large temporary cavity displaces them or forms within them. More elastic tissue (such as skeletal muscle) and lower-density elastic tissue (such as lung) are less affected by the formation of a temporary cavity. Because of these tissue differences, transmitted blunt trauma from temporary cavitation caused by a bullet traveling 800 to 950 m/s can cause a more severe pulmonary contusion when the bullet traverses the chest wall musculature than the pulmonary contusion it would have caused if it passed through the lung.

Although the formation of a large temporary cavity often has devastating effects in the brain or liver, its effect in wounds of the extremities frequently has been exaggerated.[11] Fracture of large bones not hit by the bullet and tearing of major vessels or nerves by the temporary cavity are mentioned often in the literature but are rare in clinical experience. This includes a systematic review of 1400 rifle wounds sustained in the Vietnam conflict and analyzed in the Wound Data and Munitions Effectiveness Team (WDMET) study (R. F. Bellamy, personal communication). Most of the permanent damage done in wounds of the extremities is the result of structures being hit by the intact bullet, bullet fragments, or secondary missiles. As in all blunt trauma, shear forces develop and tear structures at points where one side is fixed and the other side is free to move. The temporary cavity is no exception.[6] In the unlikely event that the blunt trauma caused by the temporary cavity tears a vessel wall, this is particularly likely to occur at the vessel origin.

BALLISTIC PROPERTIES AND THE WOUND PRODUCED

Animal experiments using military-rifle bullets[5] have clearly disproved the assertion that all tissue exposed to temporary cavitation is destroyed. Not only does the 14-cm-diameter temporary cavity produced by an AK-74 bullet not destroy a great amount of muscle, but the sizable stellate exit wound it causes in the uncomplicated thigh wound ensures excellent wound drainage, which assists healing.[5] A history that the wound was caused by a high-velocity bullet does not mandate radical excision of the wound path.[11]

The characteristics of the wounded tissue; the thickness of the body part; the point in the path of the bullet at which deformation into a mushroom shape or yaw or fragmentation occurs; and other factors strongly influence the wound produced.

Experiments with ballistic gelatin (which reproduces the projectile deformation and penetration depth of living animal muscle) have shown that most full metal jacket rifle bullets yaw significantly only at tissue depths greater than the diameter of human extremities.

In the first 12 cm (the average thickness of an adult human thigh) of a soft tissue wound path, there is often little or no difference between the wounding effect of low- and high-velocity bullets when the high-velocity bullet is of the military full metal jacket type. This is particularly true of the relatively heavier military-rifle bullets such as those fired by the AK-47 and NATO 7.62-mm (U.S. version) rifle. A wound of an extremity caused by an AK-47 bullet that does not hit bone is often similar to a handgun bullet wound. No matter how high its velocity, if a nondeforming, heavy bullet does not break, fragment, or hit a large bone, it may exit an extremity with much of its wounding potential unspent. These same bullets are often lethal in chest or abdominal wounds because the trunk is thicker than an extremity and allows the bullet a sufficiently long path through tissue to yaw. Maximal temporary cavitation induced by the AK-47 bullet usually occurs at a tissue depth of 28 cm, much greater than the diameter of a human extremity.

A soft-point or hollow-point bullet fired from a civilian center-fire rifle deforms soon after entering tissue and produces a much more severe extremity wound than will a military full metal jacket bullet that does not break and fragment.

The more recently developed, smaller-caliber AK-74 fires a bullet that is lighter than the AK-47 bullet and yaws earlier.[12] Its maximal temporary cavity occurs at a tissue depth of 11 cm. Extremity wounds from the AK-74 can be expected to be more severe than those from the AK-47.[12] The lighter, smaller AK-74 round allows a soldier to carry many more rounds of ammunition. This was the primary motivation for development of the M16 and the AK-74.

Caliber

Caliber (bullet diameter in decimals of an inch or in millimeters) is only one indicator of wounding potential but not a very good one (see Figure 264-1). Caliber indicates bullet diameter but not bullet length and therefore does not disclose bullet mass. Caliber also is independent of bullet velocity and bullet construction.

Unfortunately, commonly used weapon and bullet designations are often misleading. As an example, the .38 special and the .357 magnum use bullets that have the same diameter [.357 in. (9.07 mm)] (Table 264-1). The longer cartridge case of the magnum can hold more powder, giving the bullet higher velocity and greater wounding potential.

Gunshot Fractures

Handgun wounds of the extremities yield characteristic fracture patterns. Frequently seen are divot fractures of cortical bone, drill-hole fractures, butterfly fractures, and double butterfly fractures.[3] Nondisplaced fracture lines sometimes radiate from these defects. These usually heal well. The bullet hole itself can act as a stress riser. Spiral fractures extending proximally or distally from the bullet hole may result from the dissipation of stress forces at the bullet hole. Occasionally, remote spiral fractures at some distance proximal or distal to the bony gunshot wound also occur, probably because of the presence of stress risers, such as vascular channels in the bone, and the fact hat the bone was under load and often torsional stress at the time of impact.[13]

In gunshot fractures from rifles and large handguns, a greater extent of comminution may be seen. These fractures often have complications because of the soft tissue damage these bullets cause.[3] The vascular compromise associated with these comminuted gunshot fractures increases the likelihood of delayed union or nonunion of the fracture. Wound infections are more common in this group. Early fasciotomy to prevent compartment syndrome is important, when needed.

At some hospitals, outpatient treatment is being used successfully for extremity fractures caused by handguns if no significant neurologic or vascular compromise has occurred.

Trunk Wounds

Bullets are not sterilized by the heat of firing. They can carry bacteria from the body surface or body organs, such as a perforated colon, deep into the wound.

In trunk wounds, an analysis of the bullet path is mandatory to determine whether a laparotomy is needed. Two radiographs in planes separated by 90 degrees, computed tomography (CT), clinical examination, and peritoneal lavage are all useful. Abdominal CT is more accurate if performed before peritoneal lavage. If peritoneal penetration by a bullet is suspected, laparotomy is indicated. The morbidity and mortality rates of an exploratory laparotomy that shows no significant intra-abdominal injury are low compared with those of missed intestinal injury. CT is useful, especially when an exclusively body wall or retroperitoneal path is suspected. CT has largely replaced excretory urography as the preferred means of evaluating the urinary tract after penetrating trauma.

Any bullet wound below the nipple line should raise the question of whether the diaphragm or abdomen has been penetrated. CT sometimes can be used to make this determination. Laparotomy is required if peritoneal penetration cannot be excluded.

Whenever a gunshot wound traverses the midline of the neck or the mediastinum, perforation of the esophagus should be suspected. Esophageal evaluation should not be overlooked after angiographic evaluation of the neck or chest.

Head Wounds

In skull wounds, as elsewhere in bone gunshot fractures, inward beveling of the calvarial defect at the bullet entrance and outward beveling of the skull at the exit wound are typical.[2,14] This is due partly to the geometry of the skull and partly to the bullet-bone interaction. Characteristic fracture patterns of the skull can be used to identify entrance and exit wounds.[14] When there is a cranial exit wound, skull fractures propagate across the calvarium faster than the bullet travels through the brain, producing characteristic patterns of fracture. These fracture patterns sometimes allow differentiation of entrance and exit wounds.[14] Radial fractures often spread out in a star pattern from the entrance and to a lesser extent from the exit holes in the skull. Concentric heaving fractures may occur, connecting the arcs of the radial fractures around both the entrance and exit holes, if sufficient temporary cavitation forces are generated inside the brain to cause significant outwardly directed tissue splash forces inside the skull, pushing

TABLE 264-1   Cartridge Case Name and Actual Bullet Diameter Used

Cartridge Cases	Actual Bullet Diameter (Inches)
Of common interest:	
32 Auto (ACP)	.312
380 Auto (ACP)	.355
9-mm Luger (9-mm Parabellum)	.355
38 Super	.355 or .357
38 Special	.357
357 Magnum	.357
44 Special	.4295
44 Magnum	.4295
444 Marlin	.4295
Others of interest:	
22 Hornet	.223 and .224
218 Bee	.224
219 Donaldson Wasp	.224
219 Zipper	.224
221 Remington Fireball	.224
222 Remington	.224
221 Remington Magnum	.224
223 Remington	.224
224 Weatherby Magnum	.224
225 Winchester	.224
22-250 Remington	.224
220 Swift	.224
243 Winchester	.243
244 Remington/6-mm Remington	.243
240 Weatherby Magnum	.243
256 Winchester Magnum	.257
250/300 Savage	.257
257 Roberts	.257
25/06 Remington	.257
257 Weatherby Magnum	.257
30-06	.308
30-30 Winchester	.308
30 M1 Carbine	.308
7.62-mm × 39-mm (AK-47)	.308
30/40 Krag	.308
7.5-mm × 55-mm Swiss (Schmidt-Rubin)	.308
300 Savage	.308
7.62-mm Russian	.308
308 Winchester	.308
7.62-mm NATO	.308
30-06 Springfield	.308
300 H & M Magnum	.308
30-338	.308
300 Winchester Magnum	.308
308 Norma Magnum	.308
300 Weatherby Magnum	.308
303 British	.311
7.65-mm Mauser	.311
7.7-mm Japanese	.311

Note: Often, both the numerical designation associated with the bullet and the cartridge case do not reflect exact measurements. As an example, the 44 Remington Magnum Pistol cartridge is 0.456 inch in diameter at its distal end and uses a bullet with a 0.43-inch diameter.[25] Both the .38 special and the .357 magnum use bullets that have the same diameter [0.357 in (9.07 mm)]. These bullets are often exactly the same weight. When trying to determine bullet type from a radiograph, in addition to correcting for magnification or deformation, one must look up actual bullet diameter rather than relying on the bullet name for its size.
Abbreviation: ACP = Automatic Colt Pistol.
Sources: Adapted from refs. 24 and 25.

out the calvarium.[14] Because a fracture will not cross a preexisting fracture line, the temporal sequence of the occurrence of the fractures sometimes can be determined from the pattern of the fractures.

Brain, whose tissue properties include near-water density, very little elasticity, and poor tissue cohesiveness, is extremely sensitive to temporary cavitation forces. When disrupted by such forces, severe brain injury often results. In addition to the relative lack of elasticity of brain tissue, its enclosure in the rigid cranial vault magnifies brain disruption by temporary cavitation forces.

Pellet Wounds

Compared with a pointed rifle bullet, spherical pellets slow rapidly in their flight through air or tissue. The entire wounding potential of a shot pellet at its entrance velocity is likely to be delivered to the target tissue, often with no exit wound. At close range (less than 3 m), shotgun pellets remain tightly clustered. Therefore, shot pellet size makes little difference because the entire load of the pellets functions as a unit, with a velocity virtually equal to muzzle velocity. Shotgun wounds at ranges of less than 5 m consist of multiple parallel wound channels. This grossly disrupts the blood supply to tissue between the wound channels.

The most severe civilian firearm wounds typically seen are those inflicted by a shotgun from close range. After a close-range or contact shotgun wound to the trunk, external examination of the patient, particularly after adequate volume resuscitation, often does not disclose the severity of the internal injuries present.

Major neural injury after shotgun wounding of the extremities may be more important than fracture or major vascular injury in determining the final outcome.[15]

During surgical exploration of a close-range shotgun wound, it is important to search for wadding, casing debris, the plastic shot cup, and surface materials carried into the wound (e.g., clothing, glass, or wood). Many of these are radiolucent.[3]

Diagnosing long-range injury based on the pattern of pellet spread is sometimes problematic. When shotgun pellets are tightly clustered or widely spread out, close-range injury or long-range injury (respectively) is usually suspected. However, in close-range injuries, the *billiard-ball effect* may cause considerable pellet spread.[16] When the tightly clustered group of shot at close range contacts the skin, the pellets at the front of the group are slowed. The pellets behind them in the group strike the pellets in front, with an effect like a billiard-ball break. This causes much more pellet spread in tissue than would be expected at close range. On radiographs, particularly in trunk wounds, this effect can simulate the pellet spread of a longer-range injury.[16] This pitfall can be avoided if the skin physical examination is correlated with the radiologic findings. If there is only one entrance wound hole, it is a close-range injury. If the distribution of the multiple skin entrance wounds is the same as the pellet spread on the radiograph, the injury occurred at longer range.

Recently manufactured BB guns and air guns that fire small pellets have considerably higher muzzle velocity [600 ft/s (183 m/s) or more] than older guns of this type. Penetrating injuries from these weapons are sometimes fatal. These air guns should not be considered toys. It is possible for a patient who has been shot with a BB pellet that has penetrated the scalp, skull, and brain to think that only a scalp wound is present.[17]

ASSESSMENT OF MISSILE TYPE AND LOCATION IN THE BODY

As in all of radiology, localization requires two views at 90 degrees or a tomographic image. CT of the head and body is often useful for analysis of bullet path.[3]

The CT digital scout radiograph, which can be used for missile localization, usually can be taken in anteroposterior and lateral projections without moving the patient. The ability to manipulate the display window and center enables visualization of bullets seen through dense structures such as the shoulders and pelvis.

Assessment of Missile Type

On a radiograph, assessment of missile caliber is difficult because of magnification and missile deformation. If an undeformed bullet is seen in two views at 90 degrees and its degree of magnification is known, the approximate caliber of the bullet can be determined. Some bullets are difficult to distinguish because their diameter is similar to others (see Table 264-1). Sometimes deformed bullets can be characterized accurately radiologically for intact bullet caliber and weight.[18]

Many radiographs show only fragments of the bullet and do not enable determination of the type of weapon and projectile that caused the wound. However, certain bullets deform or fragment in a characteristic pattern (such as the M16 military bullet, the Winchester Black Talon or SXT handgun bullets, and the .357 magnum 125-grain Remington semijacketed soft-point bullet) that can be used to identify them. Deformation of large lead shotgun pellets (e.g., 00 buckshot) after contact with bone can cause these to be confused with deformed bullet fragments.

MISSILE EMBOLIZATION

It always must be ascertained that the path from the entrance wound is consistent with the bullet's current location because a bullet may have reached its present location by embolization. Arterial and venous embolization of bullets and shotgun pellets, as well as bullet movement within the subarachnoid space in the head and spine, have been reported. It is generally accepted that a missile freely floating within a cardiac chamber should be removed to prevent embolization. Missiles clearly embedded in chamber walls are relatively safe.[19] Missile size does not seem to be especially important because all sizes can produce morbidity after embolization. Two-dimensional echocardiography may be useful in determining whether a missile is embedded in a chamber wall. CT (particularly high-speed CT) and magnetic resonance imaging for nonmagnetic missiles also have a role. On chest radiographs, blurring of the margins of a pericardiac missile or fragment is a reason to suspect that the missile is in or next to the heart.[16] Bullets and pellets have embolized from the heart to the head during CPR, causing stroke.

Whenever a bullet is not found on radiographs of the body part predicted based on the entrance wound, the bullet's location is not currently known, and there is no exit wound, additional radiographs or fluoroscopy to find the bullet are mandatory. Immediately before surgery for missile removal, repeat radiographic confirmation of the exact location of the missile is usually indicated.

Interventional radiologic techniques are useful in bullet removal, including the removal of intravascular and intrarenal bullets. Significant deformation of an intravascular bullet is a relative contraindication to retrieval using a transarterial catheter because of potential damage to the vessel intima. Arthroscopy sometimes can be used for removing bullets from joints, especially the knee.

Most bullets follow straight paths through the body, but sometimes, even in the absence of embolization, a bullet, particularly a handgun bullet, will not. It may ricochet off body structures, especially bone, or may follow fascial or tissue planes. Bullets traveling less than 1100 ft/s (335 m/s) are the ones most likely to be deflected by anatomic structures or to follow tissue planes. Bullet shape also influences the tendency to be deflected.

Far more common than bullet displacement by embolization from where it came to rest in the body at the end of its path is bullet movement due to the effect of gravity on a bullet that ends up free in the pleural space or peritoneal cavity.

LEAD FRAGMENTS AND LEAD POISONING

Lead fragments in soft tissue usually become encapsulated with fibrous tissue and do not cause problems. Bullet-induced lead poisoning is most common with intra-articular, disk space, and bursal locations

of bullet fragments because of the solubility of lead in synovial fluid.[20,21] Lead fragments in the brain are usually relatively benign unless they are copper-plated (as are many civilian .22 caliber bullets).[22] Copper-plated lead pellets produced a sterile abscess or granuloma in the brain of cats surgically implanted with missiles of this type.[22] This can be associated with downward migration of the missile, resorption of copper from the surface of the missile, progressive neurologic deficit, and sometimes death of the cat. These findings were absent in cats whose brains were implanted with uncoated lead pellets.

Intra-articular fragments should be removed to avoid both the mechanical trauma and the destructive synovitis lead can cause.[20] Significant damage to the articular cartilage visible at surgery may be present as a result of lead synovitis, even when radiographs remain normal except for bullet fragments.[20] If large fragments are present in the joint, they can cause severe mechanical trauma during motion. This motion can lead to further lead fragmentation.

Whether lead poisoning occurs depends largely on the surface area of the retained lead particles and their location in the body.[21] Sometimes the onset of clinical lead poisoning can be quite rapid, but usually it takes years.

Patients with retained lead pellets or lead bullet fragments should be advised that, on rare occasions, a fragment may erode into a bursa or joint space and cause lead poisoning. They should be assured that lead poisoning poses a threat *only if unrecognized and untreated*. They should be cautioned to inform their physician of the retained lead any time they seek treatment for problems such as headache, abdominal pain, personality change, or bizarre neurologic symptoms. Once the possibility of lead poisoning is considered, it can be easily confirmed or excluded simply by determining the blood lead level.

EVIDENTIARY CONCERNS

Physicians must be aware of the importance of preserving evidence in patients being resuscitated after penetrating trauma. Do not cut through bullet holes or knife holes in clothing when removing it. Do not incise through skin wounds unless absolutely necessary. To preserve powder marks, do not scrub wounds unless necessary. Take photographs, when possible, prior to initiating wound treatment.

Emergency departments must have a protocol for collecting clothing and other evidence so that it can be documented that it was always under surveillance or otherwise kept in such a way that tampering could not occur. Do not describe wounds as entry or exit wounds; instead, describe the appearance of wounds in detail, without interpretation. Describe the location, size, and shape of all gunshot wounds. Include the presence or absence of a soot ring, skin or subcutaneous tissue tattooing with gunpowder, or the presence of subcutaneous gas (such as from a contact wound with injection into the subcutaneous tissues of gases from burning gunpowder). When a bullet or fragment is encountered, do not pick it up with a metallic clamp so that ballistic markings can be interpreted without the possibility that marks were made later with a surgical instrument. Prehospital personnel should receive similar instruction relative to preserving evidence at the scene. The history of the episode can be useful if the number of shots fired or the position of the victim relative to the assailant was observed.

The sharp bullet jacket edges that some soft-point and hollow-point handgun bullets have when they are deformed into a mushroom shape should be avoided. Infectious diseases such as hepatitis and HIV can pass from the victim to the health care provider as a result of skin punctures from these sharp edges.

Some emergency medicine residency programs now include a course in forensic medicine.[23]

REFERENCES

1. Hollerman JJ, Fackler ML, Coldwell DM, Ben-Menachem Y: Gunshot wounds: 1. Bullets, ballistics and mechanisms of injury. *AJR* 155:685, 1990.

2. Hollerman JJ, Fackler ML: Gunshot wounds: Radiology and wound ballistics. *Emerg Radiol* 2:171, 1995.

3. Hollerman JJ, Fackler ML, Coldwell DM, Ben-Menachem Y: Gunshot wounds: 2. Radiology. *AJR* 155:691, 1990.

4. Fackler ML, Surinchak JS, Malinowski JA, Bowen RE: Bullet fragmentation: A major cause of tissue disruption. *J Trauma* 24:35, 1984.

5. Fackler ML, Breteau JPL, Courbil LJ, et al: Open wound drainage versus wound excision in treating the modern assault rifle wound. *Surgery* 105:576, 1989.

6. Hollerman JJ: Wound ballistics is a model of the pathophysiology of all blunt and penetrating trauma. *Emerg Radiol* 5:279, 1998.

7. Harvey EN, Korr IM, Oster G, McMillen JH: Secondary damage in wounding due to pressure changes accompanying the passage of high-velocity missiles. *Surgery* 21:218, 1947.

8. DeMuth WE Jr: Bullet velocity and design as determinants of wounding capability: An experimental study. *J Trauma* 6:222, 1966.

9. Wolberg EJ: Performance of the Winchester 9-mm 147-grain subsonic jacketed hollow point bullet in human tissue and tissue simulant. *J Int Wound Ballistics Assoc* 1:10, 1991.

10. Fackler ML: Wounding patterns of military rifle bullets. *Int Defense Rev* 22:59, 1989.

11. Fackler ML: Wound ballistics: A review of common misconceptions. *JAMA* 259:2730, 1988.

12. Fackler ML, Surinchak JS, Malinowski JA, Bowen RE: Wounding potential of the Russian AK-74 assault rifle. *J Trauma* 24:263, 1984.

13. Smith HW, Wheatley KK Jr: Biomechanics of femur fractures secondary to gunshot wounds. *J Trauma* 24:970, 1984.

14. Smith OC, Berryman HE, Lahren CH: Cranial fracture patterns and estimate of direction from low velocity gunshot wounds. *J Forensic Sci* 32:1416, 1987.

15. Deitch EA, Grimes WR: Experience with 112 shotgun wounds of the extremities. *J Trauma* 24:600, 1984.

16. Messmer JM, Fierro MF: Radiologic forensic investigation of fatal gunshot wounds. *Radiographics* 6:457, 1986.

17. Lucas RM, Mitterer D: Pneumatic firearm injuries: Trivial trauma or perilous pitfalls? *J Emerg Med* 8:433, 1990.

18. Bixler RP, Ahrens CR, Rossi RP, Thickman D: Bullet identification with radiography. *Radiology* 178:563, 1991.

19. Robison RJ, Brown JW, Caldwell R, et al: Management of asymptomatic intracardiac missiles using echocardiography. *J Trauma* 28:1402, 1988.

20. Sclafani SJA, Vuletin JC, Twersky J: Lead arthropathy: Arthritis caused by retained intra-articular bullets. *Radiology* 156:299, 1985.

21. Linden MA, Manton WI, Stewart RM, et al: Lead poisoning from retained bullets: Pathogenesis, diagnosis, and management. *Ann Surg* 195:305, 1982.

22. Sights WP, Bye RJ: The fate of retained intracerebral shotgun pellets: An experimental study. *J Neurosurg* 33:646, 1970.

23. Smock WS: Development of a clinical forensic medicine curriculum for emergency physicians in the USA. *J Clin Forensic Med* 1:27, 1994.

24. *Sierra Rifle Reloading Manual,* 3d ed. Santa Fe Springs, CA, Sierra Bullets, 1989.

25. *Sierra Handgun Reloading Manual,* 3d ed. Santa Fe Springs, CA, Sierra Bullets, 1989.

FORENSICS
David R. Fowler
John E. Smialek

Good medical practice obligates physician/health care providers in EDs to serve as an interface between patients and the state within the context of the public health, legal, and justice systems. To comply with these additional responsibilities, physicians must be aware of local public health and legal obligations, for example infectious reporting requirements in Maryland,[1] and must be able to recognize patterns of injury. Observations must be appropriately documented and evidence must be processed in a manner consistent with legal standards.[2]

Each ED should provide its physicians with a standard protocol for responding to state-imposed legal and public health[1] requirements. As an example, all states impose an obligation to report certain infectious diseases[1] (also see Chap. 153) and many states also require reporting of certain injuries to state social services or law enforcement agencies. Generally, these reporting requirements are centered on the vulnerable patients such as children,[3] the elderly, and victims of domestic violence. Reporting laws for other types of injuries vary from state to state. There may be obligations to report gunshot wounds, knife wounds, assaults, and burns.

It is important that the physician also take a proper history from the patient and other reporting witnesses, which must include a statement regarding the origin of the injury. These statements must be documented verbatim for several reasons. First, they may be self-serving and the explanation may change upon subsequent reflection. Second, such statements are of legal significance and are admissible in subsequent legal proceedings where they will be analyzed in minute detail.

In addition to obtaining this initial history, the physician must also provide a physical examination of the injury and documentation of that examination before the injury is altered by healing or medical treatment. It is critical that this be documented in detail, because in those surviving their injuries, this becomes the only medicolegal information collected. Other diagnostic and documentary tools, such as x-ray, should supplement the physical examination. The legal significance of injury assessment also warrants documentation of the injury by photograph. Therefore, an autofocus, Polaroid, or digital camera should be standard equipment in every ED.

SURVEILLANCE

ED physicians must also recognize their pivotal role in emerging diseases surveillance for bioterrorist events. Persons who present first to emergency departments might fall under medical examiner jurisdiction if they die suddenly and unexpectedly without a clear diagnosis. Examples include West Nile encephalitis in New York[4] and the recent anthrax deaths.[5] Any death that results from the deliberate dissemination of an otherwise natural disease is also a homicide and must be reported to the medical examiner/coroner. Other examples of unexplained deaths include the series of cyanide-laced acetaminophen deaths. Syndromic surveillance is likely to become a primary tool in early identification of emerging diseases and bioterrorism.

PATTERNS OF INJURY

Classification

Injuries may be classified in a variety of ways. Mode of production is one classification that includes blunt force, sharp force, missile, heat, electricity, and chemicals. Injuries may also be categorized according to the circumstances in which they were inflicted. Such circumstances are accidental, suicidal, or homicidal. Wounds may also be characterized as surgical or ritual, depending on the setting in which these wounds are sustained. However, the most useful classification is based on the components of the injury pattern. Injuries consist of one or a combination of several types of tissue damage (Table 265-1).

TABLE 265-1 Types of Tissue Damage from Injury

Abrasion
Bruise
Contusion
Laceration/tear
Stab/cut
Bite
Burn
Missile penetration
Strangulation

Abrasion

An *abrasion* is the damage inflicted on the superficial layers of the skin (epidermis) by friction or pressure. An abrasion may be sustained by sliding on a rough carpet, producing what is commonly called a *rug burn.* A much more extreme version of an abrasion is the injury produced when a pedestrian is knocked to the pavement by an automobile, sustaining extensive friction injuries to the skin on various parts of the body. These injuries are commonly called *road burn* or *road rash.* While abrasions may be lacking in specific detail to allow an instrument of causation to be identified, some abrasion patterns may be very specific (imprint abrasions). These may include the abrasions resulting from a rope used as a ligature around the neck or extremities and rubbed against the skin, called *ligature marks.* Abrasions can also be caused by the irregular surface of the shoe sole or by an electrical cord used as a whip (Figure 265-1).

Bruise (Ecchymosis)

An *external bruise* represents bleeding beneath the skin. If sufficient bleeding occurs to create a lump, this is called a *hematoma.* Such injuries result from direct force applied to the skin surface, resulting in the tearing of subcutaneous blood vessels. The pattern of bleeding may be circular, surrounding a central bleeding point where the blow has stretched and torn a blood vessel wall. When multiple blood vessels are torn because of the use of a specific instrument, the bleeding pattern may conform to the outline of that instrument. For example, a blow inflicted with a human fist can produce multiple circular bruises in a pattern that conforms to the tips of the knuckles (Figure 265-2). Similarly, pressure from fingertips, such as occurs when someone grabs another by the arm, may produce several circular to oval bruises.

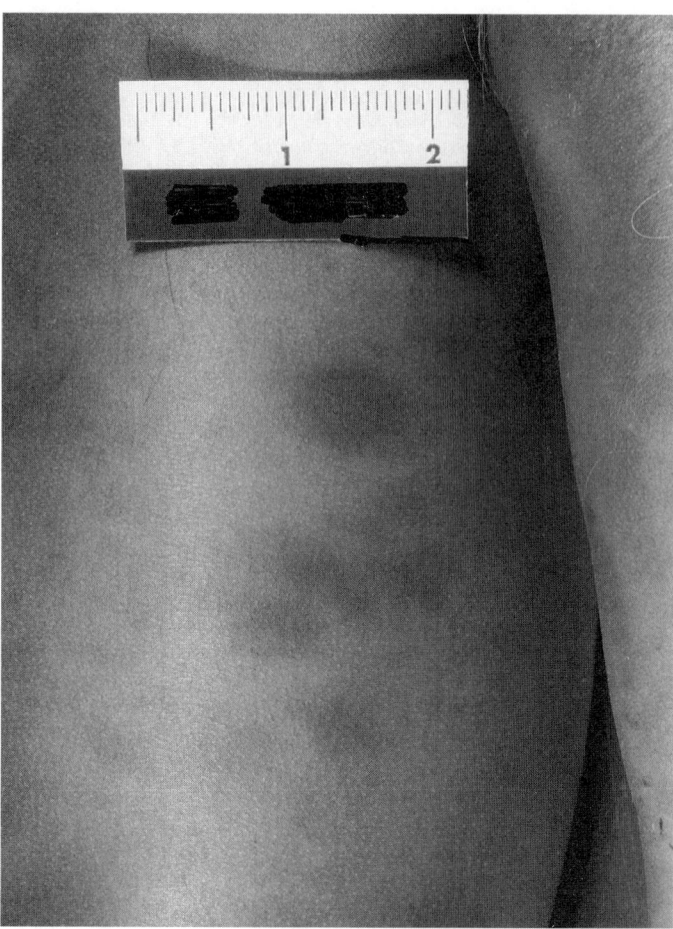

FIG. 265-2. Bruise pattern from knuckles.

In contrast, a strike with a police baton can produce parallel linear bruises conforming to the diameter of the baton (Figure 265-3).

Contusion

When sufficient force is applied to the surface of the body, the combination of friction or pressure and tearing of underlying blood vessels produces a bruise with an overlying abrasion. The term commonly used for this injury pattern is *contusion,* although some individuals use it interchangeably with bruise. Contusions and bruises have different appearances, depending on the pigmentation of the person's skin and the age of the injury. A bruise or contusion that is dark red or purple with well-defined margins is consistent with having been inflicted less than 48 h prior to examination. In contrast, a bruise or contusion that is yellow or brown or whose margins have begun to fade is certainly older than 48 h.

Laceration/Tear

A *laceration* is a tear of the skin caused by blunt force and not a sharp instrument. Depending on the amount of force used, the tear may be confined to the dermis or may extend through the full thickness of the skin. An example of an injury confined to the dermis is overstretching (Figure 265-4). A full-thickness laceration extends into the subcutaneous tissue. When the injury is examined, *bridging* by intact blood vessels may be evident (Figure 265-5). The resilience of elastic walled structures, such as arteries, allows them to maintain their integrity despite a blunt-force impact that tears the adjacent skin.

Because a laceration is usually the result of a crushing force, the margins of the laceration will show the effects of the pressure crush-

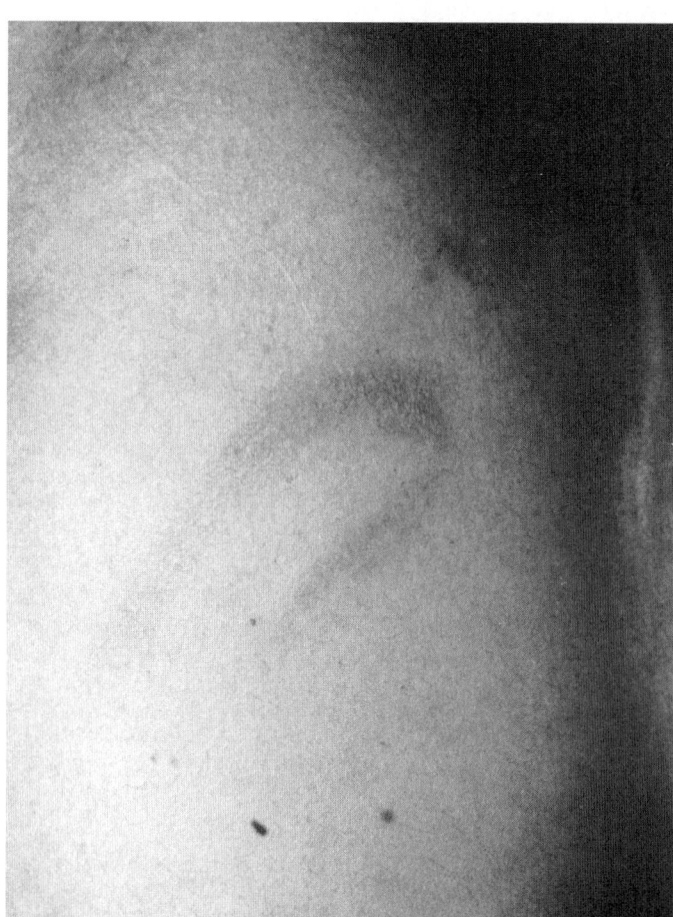

FIG. 265-1. Abrasion caused by electric cord.

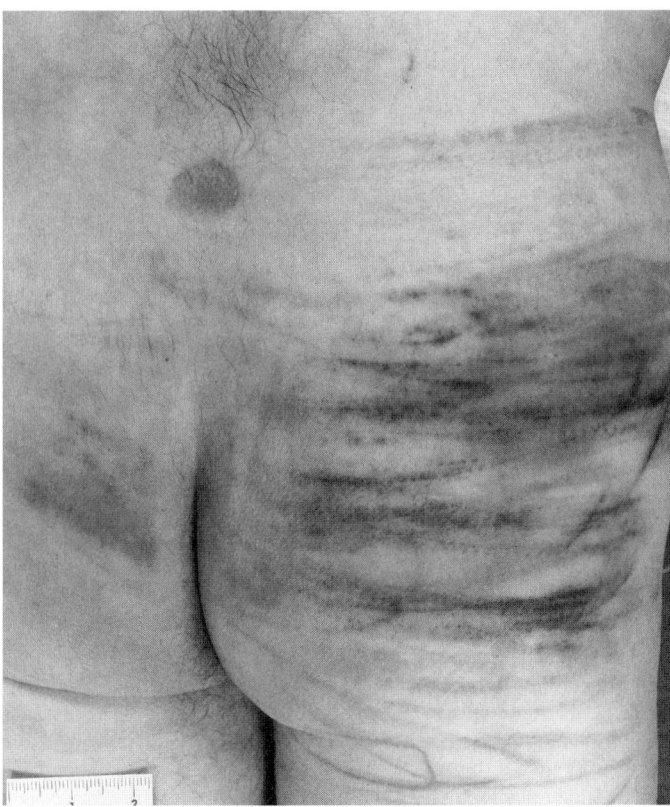

FIG. 265-3. Parallel linear bruises from police baton.

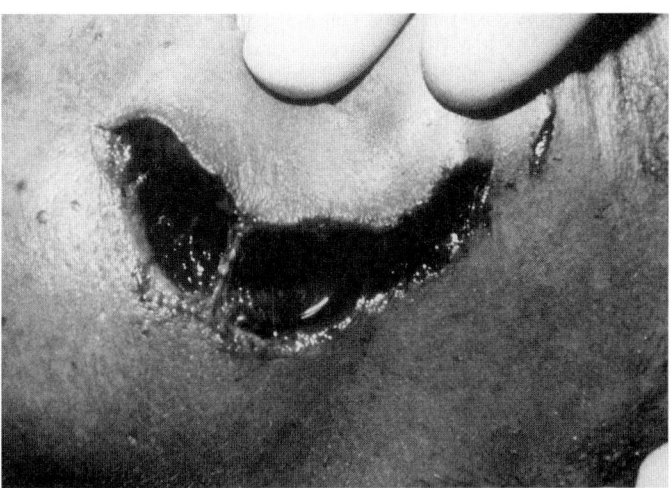

FIG. 265-5. Full-thickness laceration with "bridging" by intact blood vessels.

ing the epidermal layer or skin surface. Depending on the instrument causing the injury, a specific imprint may be evident when the margins of the laceration are reapposed. A laceration can also be called a tear but should never be called a cut, which implies the application of something other than blunt force. A common type of laceration occurs in protuberant areas of the body such as the elbow, knee, or eyebrow, where a fall against a hard surface such as a floor or pavement may result in the crushing of the skin against the underlying bone. Because the crushed skin margins may be nonviable, simple suturing of such a laceration without débridement may not result in healing by first intention.

Because lacerations often result from contact with a foreign object, residue from this object may be left within the wound. Recognition

and recovery of particles of concrete, brick, or sand may be very helpful in the determination of whether an injury resulted from impact with an object such as a rock or the butt of a handgun (Figure 265-6). This information should be included in the description of the injury.

Stab/Cut

A *stab* or *cut* is an injury inflicted on the skin by contact with a sharp object. Laceration (see above) is not the correct term to use when describing cuts, as it specifically means tearing of the skin. Knife blades, shards of glass, and fragments of metal can penetrate the skin and leave a cutting pattern that will vary depending on the movement of the injured party and the object causing the injury. The sharp edge

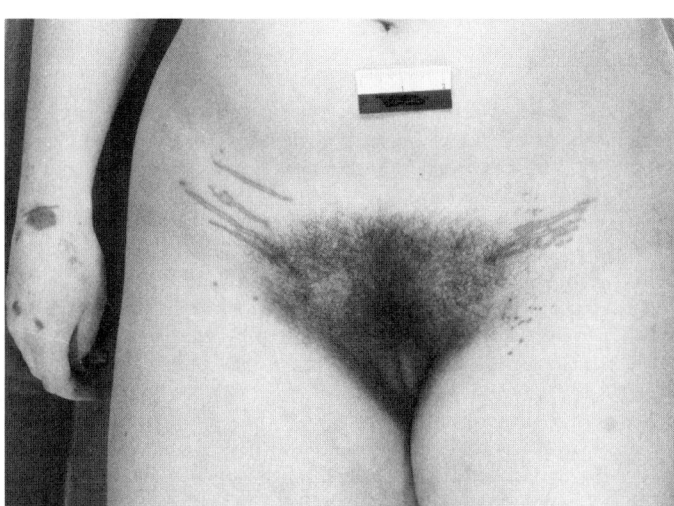

FIG. 265-4. "Overstretching" type laceration confined to the dermis.

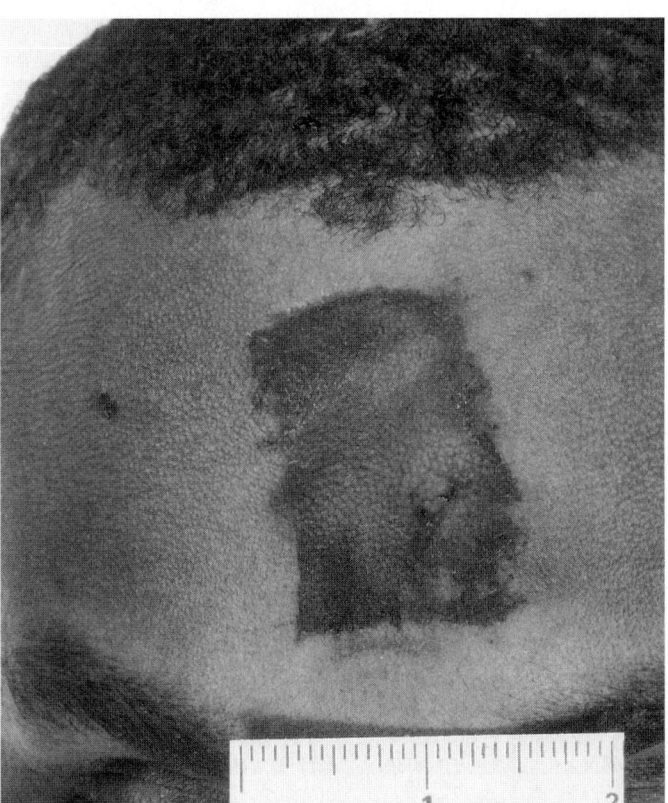

FIG. 265-6. Revealing pattern, suggesting that injury was caused by butt of a handgun.

of these objects severs structures in the skin, leaving no evidence of bridging such as that seen in lacerations. Depending on the shape of the sharp object, the cut edges will be abraded accordingly while the ends of the wound may be squared or pointed (Figure 265-7). Unique abrasions found around a stab wound may represent the effect of the hilt of a knife blade striking the skin (see Figure 265-7). Examination of the stab-wound track may reveal particles of the offending weapon, and such particles should be retained as evidence to assist in the identification of a weapon. The location of specific stabs or cutting wounds may suggest the manner in which they were inflicted. For example, cuts or stabs on the inner (volar) side of the wrist or forearm are consistent with efforts of individuals trying to protect themselves from an assailant by raising their arm in front of their body in a defensive posture. Forensic pathologists call these defense wounds.

To properly evaluate the wound characteristics of cutting or stabbing wounds, the wound edges must be reapposed. The reapposition counteracts the effect of elastofibro-retraction and allows the physician to observe the wound as it occurred. It also enables the physician to identify abraded margins, as well as patterns of squared ends or pointed ends. A *squared end* results from the noncutting or blunt edge of a knife blade, whereas a *pointed end* results from contact with the sharp edge of a blade. The physician should use transparent tape to hold the edges of the wound together while the wound is photographed. This practice can be extremely valuable in the comparison of the wound with a suspected weapon (Figure 265-8).

Another example of a patterned abrasion injury is the one caused by fragments of automobile glass. These characteristic wound patterns in human skin can enable the physician to identify whether the glass causing the injury is from a windshield or side auto window. The side window consists of tempered glass that breaks into 5-mm cubes, causing right-angle cuts to the left side of the face of the driver of the vehicle sustaining a driver-side impact. They may also be found on the right side of the face of passenger of a vehicle sustaining a passenger-side impact (Figure 265-9A). Recognizing these patterns and their location can be useful in establishing who was driving the vehicle at the time of the collision. Cuts from windshield glass are distinguishable from side-impact injuries. Windshield glass, which consists of thin layers of laminated glass, breaks into tiny splinters that produce superficial, parallel, linear cuts (Figure 265-9B).

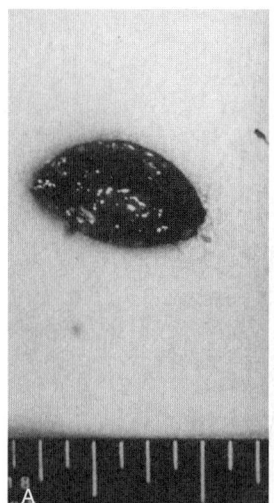
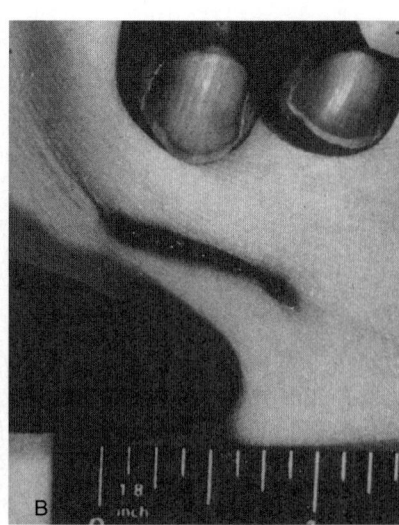

FIG. 265-8. Transparent tape applied over wound may aid in reconstruction and identification or verification of weapon.

Bite

Contact between human mouth and/or teeth and skin will leave evidence of the amount of force used in the contact as well as material (saliva) and/or teeth marks that can lead to the identification of the biter. Love bites or hickeys (suction injuries) result when there is extended oral contact with the skin of a partner involving sucking or biting. Hickeys are typically seen on the neck but may occur on any part of the body and usually exhibit no evidence of damage to the subepidermal layers, although discoloration from tissue fluid leakage may occur. On the other hand, *love bites,* and bites inflicted during a struggle, usually damage the dermis, leaving a partial or complete pattern of the dentition of the biter (Figure 265-10). Not only can this bite pattern be used for comparison with the dental pattern of the suspect, but also the recognition of the bite mark sustained during an attack should alert a physician to protect the skin surrounded by the bite pattern so that it can be swabbed to obtain saliva containing DNA material. A DNA profile can be compared with that of a suspect, providing almost 100 percent accuracy of identification. The most severe form of human bite is one that extends through the dermis into the subcutaneous tissue and results in the loss of blood. Thus, one can grade bite marks as first degree (mild), second degree (moderate), or third degree (severe). Using this grading system, a love bite would be considered in the mild category, whereas one similar to that occurring during a recent notorious boxing match as third degree (severe).

Burn

Injuries of the skin resulting from contact with electrical energy, extreme heat, heated objects, or certain chemicals often exhibit characteristic patterns. For example, immersion of a child's buttock in 60°C (140°F) water will result in second-degree burns to the immersed skin. The resulting burn pattern will show a characteristic line of demarcation that represents the amount of skin immersed in the hot water (Figure 265-11). Similarly, contact of the skin with electrical current can result in a central area of necrosis characteristically seen as black, charred tissue surrounded by a pale zone with a bright-red peripheral margin.

Tremendous electrical force contained in a lightning strike may produce relatively little in the way of external evidence and may include only singeing of hair or slight charring of skin where contact occurs. An arborization or fernlike pattern of redness may be seen on the skin of fatally injured victims. A possible result of contact with a lightning strike is magnetization of certain metal articles on the victim's body.

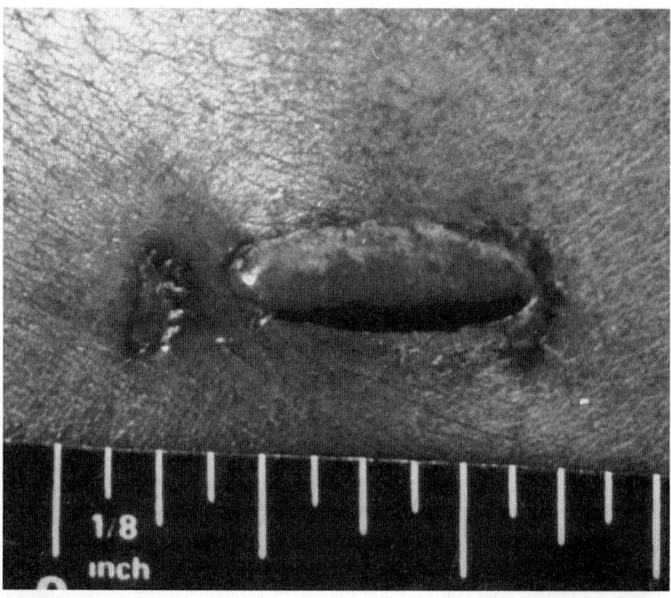

FIG. 265-7. Abrasion and bruise around periphery of stab wound suggesting cause is blunt trauma from hilt of a knife blade.

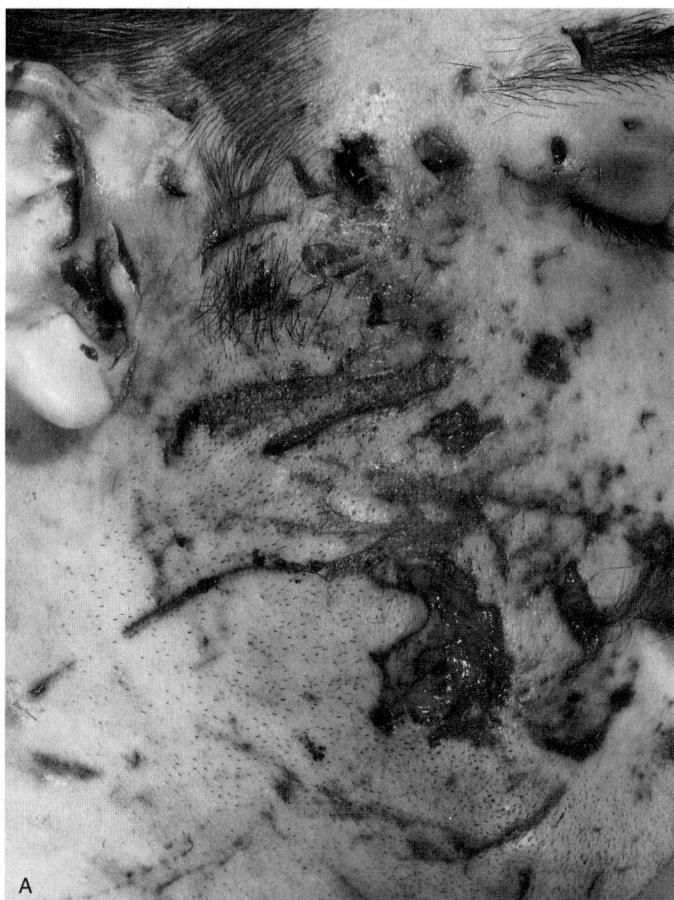

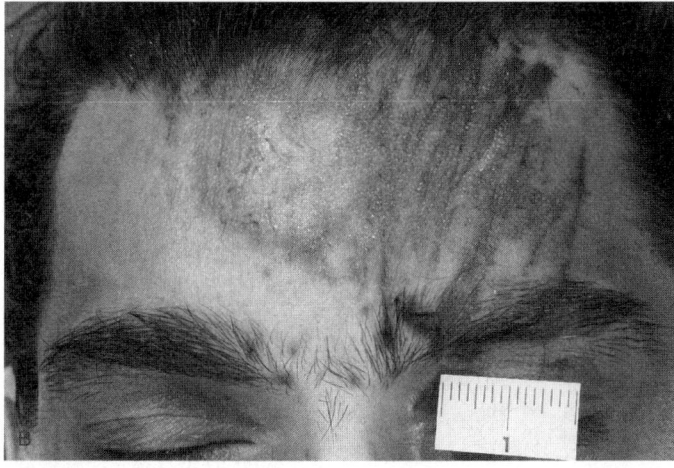

FIG. 265-9. A. Right-angle lacerations from side window glass of car made of tempered glass that brakes into 5-mm cubes. **B.** Linear lacerations and abrasions from windshield glass that brakes into tiny splinters.

Missile Penetration

The entrance wound of a skin penetration caused by a high-speed missile (such as a bullet) or a low-speed missile (such as an arrow) is circular, oval, or triangular, with a circumferential rim of abrasion. This abrasion pattern, produced by the friction sustained by the skin margins in contact with the missile, enables a physician to identify which hole is the exit and which is the entrance in a through-and-through gunshot wound. The outer skin edges of an exit wound do not come in contact with the missile and therefore do not sustain friction damage

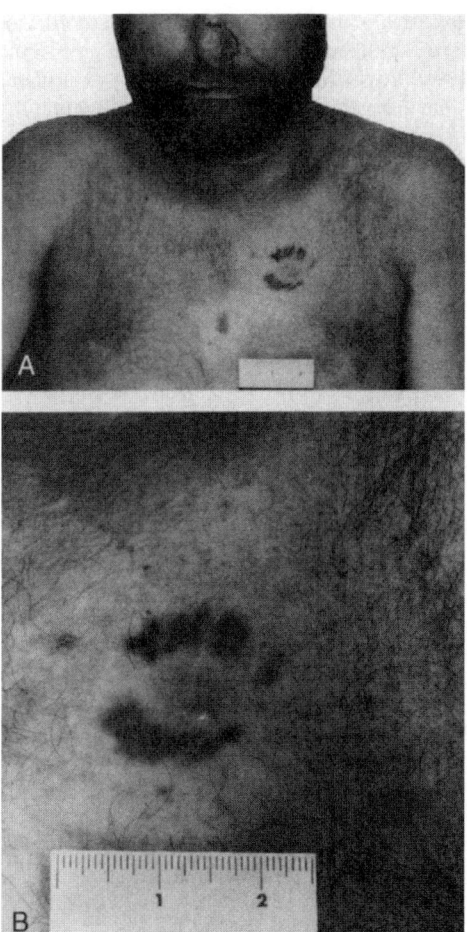

FIG. 265-10. Human bite revealing pattern of dentition.

and do not exhibit this rim of abrasion. However, if a person is wearing tight clothing or the skin is resting against a hard, firm surface when the missile exits, the skin around the exit wound may be abraded from contact with this material. This produces a pattern called a *shored exit wound* (Figure 265-12).

The presence of gunpowder residue surrounding a gunshot wound of the skin is a critical finding that needs to be described and documented with photographs before cleansing. The description of the distribution of the gunpowder residue, whether it consists of black smudging (soot) or stippling by particles of gunpowder, should include measurements with photographs. Wound photographs should always have a measurement scale in the field (see Figure 265-2). Clothing soiled with gunpowder residue must be protected and retained for collection by law enforcement agencies for analysis in the crime lab. This type of evidence is used for determining the distance between the muzzle of the weapon firing the bullet and the injured party. Establishing this distance provides one parameter for evaluating the validity of accounts given by each of the parties as to the circumstances of the shooting. For example, one person may allege that there was a struggle and the gun was fired in self-defense, while the other person may say he or she was shot without threatening the shooter in any way.

Identification of the site of the entrance and exit of a gunshot wound path is an important step in the reconstruction of the shooting incident. When these incidents are not fatal, legal action often results, leading to a dispute over the accuracy of accounts given by each of the two parties: the injured party and the shooter.

Physicians without forensic training should avoid giving any opinion regarding a wound being an entrance or exit, or whether firing at close

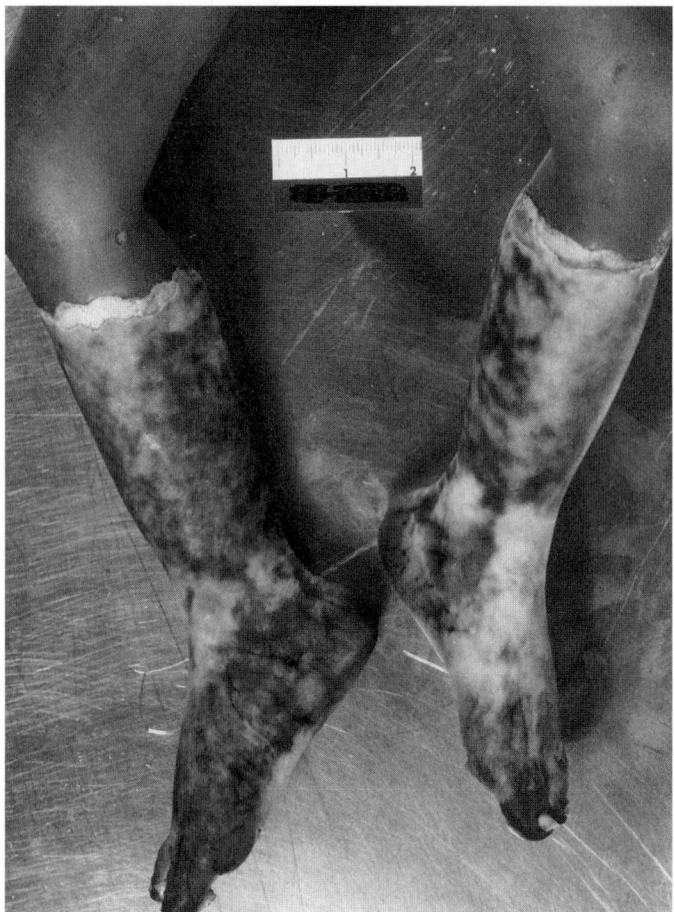

FIG. 265-11. Characteristic line of demarcation secondary immersion burns injury seen in abuse.

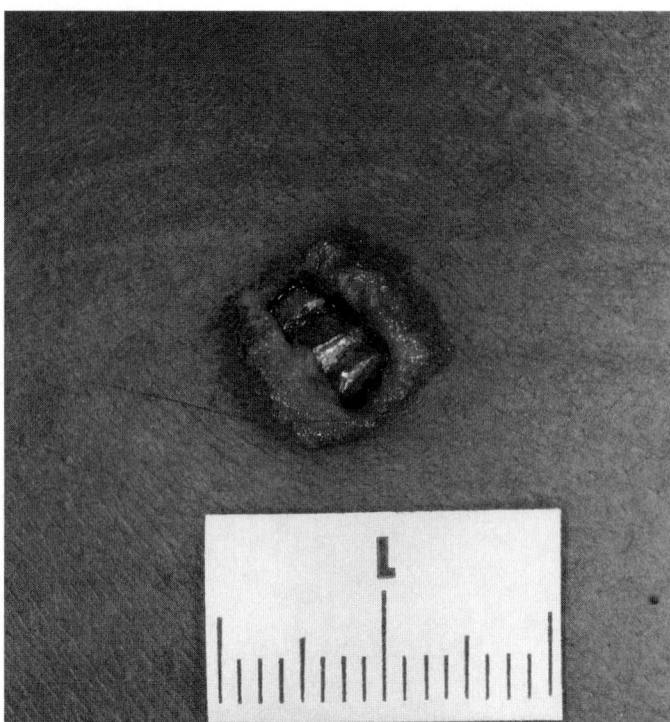

FIG. 265-12. Characteristic "shored exit wound," an abrasion pattern resulting from missile exit when skin is resting against a hard surface.

range or a distance caused it, or whether any type of activity or movement occurred during the shooting or what type of ammunition was used. Rather, physicians should document in as much detail as possible the information set out above for evaluation by those expert in this area.

Strangulation

Attempts to injure or kill a person by strangulation using one's hands, a ligature, or forearm, in a chokehold, may result in skin damage to the neck. For example, in manual strangulation, multiple bruises and scratches typical of contact with hands and fingernails will be seen on a victim's neck. On the other hand, if a ligature is forcefully wrapped around a victim's neck, a band of abrasion approximating the diameter of the ligature will be seen on the skin. Pinpoint hemorrhages, or petechiae, which are dramatically evident in the translucent conjunctival lining of the eyes, are important evidence of strangulation. These hemorrhages, which are the result of ruptured capillaries, occur when the buildup in pressure occurring when venous return from the head and face is obstructed. Because a period of 4 min is required for compression of the blood supply of the brain to result in irreversible neuronal damage and death, it is not surprising that so many attackers let go of their victim before death has occurred. If other forces, such as shooting, stabbing, or beating, are not used, a victim may survive strangulation and appear in the ED, with evidence of neck injury and petechial hemorrhages in the eyes. Such victims should be examined for evidence of sexual assault, and vaginal swabs should be taken for identification with semen and DNA analysis.

The foregoing categories of injuries represent those most commonly seen in a trauma unit or a medical examiner office. However,

readers who wish to become more familiar with the variety and details of injury are referred to several informative forensic medicine texts available in the medical library.

MEDICAL RECORDS

When an injury becomes the subject of a legal proceeding, the medical record documenting that injury and its subsequent treatment becomes a central part of the court deliberations, which may include obtaining testimony from the physician that created that record. The defendant or the accused is entitled to cross-examine that physician to establish or refute the validity of the medical information presented to the court. Physicians must recognize the legal responsibility that society places on them and be prepared to provide competent, professional testimony when required. The proper documentation of injuries includes the description of the details previously specified under *wound pattern*. The use of anatomic diagrams, together with photographs, makes the record more representative of the injuries as a physician saw them and more understandable by the lay members of a court. These items (charts, diagrams, and cameras) should be essential equipment in an ED, and photographs should become part of the permanent medical record.

PRESERVATION AND COLLECTION OF EVIDENCE

Preservation of blood samples, missiles, and debris found in wounds may be extremely valuable in identifying a particular weapon and in tying this weapon to an assailant. However, this evidence is useful only if a proper chain of custody is established. In handling such evidence, EDs should follow a protocol developed in consultation with the local law enforcement agency. The use of a simple envelope that enables a physician to identify the patient, the date the evidence was recovered, where it was recovered from, and to whom it was given, and signed by the physician is adequate for establishing the chain of custody. Use of an appropriate receipt form documenting the transfer of this evidence should be an essential part of the medical record.

REPORT OF DEATH

This chapter is confined to those issues relevant to the assessment of living patients. However, another important responsibility of the emergency physicians is that of notifying the local law enforcement agency, medical examiner, or coroner of a death that constitutes a medical examiner or coroner case.

Statutory language identifies those deaths that require an investigation by a medical examiner/coroner of the circumstances of the death. This enables one to determine whether an autopsy is necessary, which can then be carried out under the same statutory authority. Such deaths are generally those of individuals who die suddenly while not under the immediate care of a physician and any death associated with some type of injury, and usually include a category of any suspicious or unusual death. It should be emphasized that the length of time a patient has been in hospital, or the age of an injury associated with the underlying cause of death, is not a factor in determining whether the death should be reported to the medical examiner/coroner.

For example, the death of a person who sustained paraplegia from a gunshot wound of the back remains a medical examiner case despite the many medical procedures and complications that result from such an injury—even when many years have passed and the victim has died of a complication of paraplegia, such as a chronic urinary tract infection. The evidence of gunshot injury together with the medical treatment and any other intervening events leading up to the eventual death need to be assessed by the medical examiner/coroner. If a chain of events exists, leading from the gunshot wound to the immediate cause of death, then the manner of death would be determined to be homicide.

Death Certification

A death certificate is an important legal document. The information on the document forms the basis of public heath data and provides essential documentation of the cause and manner of death to insurance companies, the legal profession, and family to name but a few. Inaccurate information has many serious consequences, including affecting insurance payments. The information on the document should reflect the sequence of abnormalities that resulted in the death of the individual. This should be done by following the national guidelines.[6] The terminal cause of death is placed on the top line, and then each subsequent line contains the preceding process until the bottom line contains the primary underlying cause of death. This is the disease or injury that started the cascade of events that directly lead to the death. Death certificates also have fields for information on how injuries occurred and these must be completed if the death was due to an injury.

The death certificate must be filled out by the physician who last attended the deceased and must be completed within 24 h of the death. For deaths occurring in the ED, the obligation rests with the attending physician. The certificate usually accompanies the remains to the funeral home. If the case is a medical examiner/coroner case, it is usually appropriate to contact that office immediately after death to obtain a decision on whether or not medical examiner/coroner intends to accept the case. If the case is going to the medical examiner/coroner, that office can inform the physician of local statues, regulations, and protocols. In most medical examiner/coroner cases, the medical examiner/coroner will complete the death certificate.

As with most legal documents, death certificates must be filed out in black ink only, abbreviations, erasures, alterations, white-out, and the like are unacceptable and a certificate with such marks will be returned to the physician.

Certain terms, such as asystole, cardiac arrest, brain death, and arrhythmia, are mechanisms of death that are final physiologic common pathways. These are usually not accepted by the various departments of vital records and will result in a rejected certificate. Other terms such as "_____ failure" (i.e., heart failure, respiratory failure, etc.) will also cause inquiries and must be qualified with the cause of the failure.

REFERENCES

1. Maryland Code: Health-general: Title 18. Disease prevention: Subtitle 1. General responsibilities of secretary: §18-102. Infectious and contagious diseases.
2. McCracken LM: Living forensics: A natural evolution in emergency care. *Accid Emerg Nurs* 7(4):211, 1999.
3. Maryland Code: Family law: Title 5. Children: Subtitle 7. Child abuse and neglect: §5-704. Reporting of abuse or neglect-By health practitioner, police officer, educator, or human service worker.
4. Sampson BA, Ambrosi C, Charlot A, et al: The pathology of human West Nile virus infection. *Hum Pathol* 31:527, 2000.
5. Borio L, Frank D, Mani V, et al: Death due to bioterrorism-related inhalational anthrax: Report of 2 patients *JAMA* 286:2554, 2001.
6. *Physicians' Handbook on Medical Certification of Death.* Hyattsville, MD, U.S. Department of Health and Human Services, Public Health Service, National Center for Health Statistics, September 1987. DHHS Publication No. (PHS) 87.

ADDITION GENERAL REFERENCE TEXTS

DiMaio DJ, DiMaio VJM: *Forensic Pathology.* New York, Elsevier, 1989.
DiMaio VJM: *Gunshot Wounds: Practical Aspects of Firearms, Ballistics and Forensic Techniques.* New York, Elsevier, 1985.
Spitz WU, Fisher RS: *Medicolegal Investigations of Death Investigation,* 3d ed. Springfield, IL, Charles C. Thomas, 1993.

INJURY CONTROL
Arthur L. Kellermann
Debra E. Houry

Injuries account for about one-fourth of emergency department visits nationwide, and they are the most common cause of death for Americans ages 1 to 44.[1] Because injuries disproportionately affect the young, they account for more years of potential life lost before age 65 than all causes of cancer and heart disease *combined*.

Epidemiologic research shows that injuries, like diseases, tend to affect identifiable high-risk groups, follow a predictable chain of events, and therefore are preventable. After an injury occurs, morbidity can be minimized by providing optimal acute care and, subsequently, rehabilitation. This combination of strategies—prevention, acute care, and rehabilitation—is termed *injury control*.

A PUBLIC HEALTH APPROACH

William Haddon developed the classic approach to injury control by identifying the three principal factors of injury (host, vehicle, and environment) and considering each factor in the three temporal phases of an injury-causing event: prior to the event, the event itself, and the postevent phase. This can be portrayed graphically in a *phase-factor matrix* of nine discrete cells.[2] Examining each cell can suggest a variety of strategies to prevent or control injuries. Since its introduction in 1972, the *Haddon matrix,* as it is now known, has proven to be an invaluable tool for injury control.

Haddon also outlined 10 generic injury-control strategies that can be used to break the chain of injury causation[3] (Table 266-1). Examining this list to identify promising approaches to injury control is known as *options analysis.* Certain options lend themselves more easily to one class of injuries than others. The best injury-control strategy is not always the most obvious one. Often a combination of approaches is superior to any single strategy.

The Injury-Control Model

More than a century after yellow fever was controlled by targeting the vector of transmission to prevent the disease, Haddon's work demonstrated

TABLE 266-1   Options Analysis: Strategies with Examples for Injury Control

1. Prevent creation of hazard
   Ban production and sale of assault weapons to civilians
2. Reduce the amount of hazard
   Limit water heater temperature to 47.25°C (125°F)
3. Prevent the release of a hazard that already exists
   Put dangerous medications in "childproof" containers
4. Modify the rate of distribution of release of the hazard from its source
   Require fire-safe cigarettes that cannot easily ignite furniture or bedding
5. Separate, by time or space, the hazard from that which is to be protected
   Construct overpasses or underpasses to eliminate crossing streams of traffic
6. Physically separate, by barriers, the hazard from that which is to be protected.
   Equip cabs with bullet- and knifeproof partitions
7. Modify surfaces and basic structures to minimize injury
   Equip all new cars with driver- and passenger-side air bags
8. Make that which is to be protected more resistant to damage
   Issue bulletproof vests to law enforcement officers and security guards
9. Begin to counter damage already done
   Promote citizen training in first aid and CPR
10. Stabilize, repair, and rehabilitate the injured person
    Implement trauma care systems throughout the United States

Source: From Haddon,[2] with permission.

that many injuries can be controlled by broadening our traditional emphasis on acute care and rehabilitation to include *prevention.* Injury control draws on the expertise of many disciplines, including epidemiology, prevention, biomechanics, acute care, rehabilitation, law, and public administration. Whenever it is practical, prevention should be tried first. If and when prevention is not enough, acute care can minimize further damage from trauma. After a victim is stabilized and his or her injuries have been treated, long-term outcomes can be enhanced by optimal rehabilitation.

Haddon's approach was first applied with great effect to reduce deaths and injuries from car crashes. Prior to his involvement, the federal government poured millions of dollars into costly and largely ineffective media campaigns directed at drivers. Little progress occurred until the National Highway Traffic Safety Administration mandated changes in the design of motor vehicles, as well as the development of safer roadways and driving environments (see "Engineering" below).[4]

These efforts produced one of the greatest public health achievements of the twentieth century. While the number of vehicle miles traveled in the United States has risen annually, today's crash fatality rate is less than one-third that of 1950. If the United States had not launched and maintained its highway traffic safety initiative, the annual toll of motor vehicle crash-related deaths, injuries, and costs would be thousands of lives and billions of dollars higher than it is today.

PREVENTION STRATEGIES

Active and Passive Countermeasures

Preventive countermeasures can be divided into two basic strategies—active and passive. *Active* countermeasures require the conscious cooperation of the individual to be effective. Examples include use of manual safety belts, motorcycle helmets, and child safety seats. *Passive* countermeasures, on the other hand, require little or no cooperation by the person being protected. Examples include automatic air bags, sprinkler systems, floatation hulls on watercraft, and spring-loaded kill switches on lawn mowers. In general, the less a countermeasure relies on the user, the more likely it will provide protection when needed. For example, manual safety belts reduce the risk of death in a car crash by 45 to 55 percent. However, they are effective

only when buckled by the user. In contrast, air bags deploy in serious crashes virtually 100 percent of the time.

The Three E's of Injury Control

Whether active or passive in nature, most injury-prevention efforts fall under one of the three E's of injury control—*e*ducation, *e*nforcement of safety regulations, and *e*ngineering to make products or environments safer.

EDUCATION   Education is often the first approach taken to encourage the public to accept an active countermeasure of proven efficacy. Implicit in its approach is the belief that once people are taught what to do, they will change their behavior to reduce their risk of injury. Driver's education programs, child pedestrian training, and bicycle helmet campaigns are examples of this strategy.

Although public education campaigns are popular and often attract large numbers of volunteers, they rarely result in sustained behavior change. One study evaluated the impact of a campaign to promote bicycle helmet use by children. Although the campaign was launched in several communities, subsequent surveys revealed that the helmet use went up only 1 percent compared with communities without the educational campaigns.[5]

Not all public education efforts have yielded such dismal results. A multistate community action campaign promoting responsible alcohol consumption found that self-reported rates of "having had too much to drink" declined 49 percent and driving when "over the legal limit" decreased 51 percent. More important, assault injuries declined by 43 percent and motor vehicle collisions declined by 10 percent.[6] A hospital-led bicycle helmet-promotion campaign for children reported a 20 percent increase in helmet use and a 10 percent decline in bicycle-related head injuries.[7]

The impact of public education campaigns is blunted by *attenuation of effect.* No matter how powerful, pervasive, and repetitive a safety message may be, there will always be people who never encounter it. Among those who see or hear the message, some will actively reject it. Others will receive the message but be insufficiently motivated to change their behavior. Among those changing their behavior, some will relapse into old habits over time. Others will fail to follow the message on a consistent basis. Finally, not everyone who conscientiously adopts a protective strategy escapes injury.

Educational interventions may be enhanced by incorporating theoretical models that include important determinants of individual behavior.[8] These include a number of personal, community, and political factors. The PRECEDE health-promotion model has been used with some success in planning injury-prevention programs.[9,10] PRECEDE is an acronym for *predisposing, reinforcing,* and *enabling causes in educational diagnosis* and *evaluation.* Predisposing factors are characteristics of a patient, consumer, or community that motivate behavior. Reinforcing factors are rewards or punishments that are anticipated or follow as a consequence of these specific behaviors. Enabling factors are environmental characteristics that facilitate or hinder injury-prevention behaviors. This framework has been used successfully to assess educational needs and select appropriate strategies to encourage bicycle helmet use and prevent child pedestrian injuries.[9,10]

ENFORCEMENT   Unfortunately, **the group most prone to risk-taking behaviors (e.g., adolescent males) is precisely the group least likely to respond to a public education campaigns.** When voluntary acceptance of an effective countermeasure is poor, compliance can be increased by adding the force of law. The impact of "mandatory use" laws can be impressive. Although an educational campaign to promote bicycle helmet use only boosted use by 1 percent in a Maryland county, helmet use went up 26 percent after the state enacted a mandatory helmet law.[5] Motorists in Texas increased restraint use by

15 percent after law enforcement began issuing traffic citations and fines.[11] In comparison, 6 months after Florida repealed its motorcycle helmet law, the number of brain-injured motorcyclists presenting to one trauma center increased from 18 to 35, the number of fatalities increased from 2 to 8, and self-reported helmet use by patients decreased from 83 to 56 percent.[12]

Community education and high-visibility enforcement are needed to obtain maximal benefit from a mandatory use law. In Elmira, New York, an enforcement and publicity campaign promoting the state's seat belt law boosted rates of belt use from 49 to 77 percent. Four months later, use sagged to 66 percent, but it rebounded to 80 percent during a reminder campaign.[13] Mandatory use laws are effective, but they are difficult to enact. People are often quite willing to support measures limiting the ability of others to injure them, but they resist measures that limit their own actions. Speed limits, drunk driving laws, and measures to ban the carrying of weapons on commercial aircraft enjoy broad-based support, but mandatory use of seat belts, motorcycle helmets, and restrictions on the purchase of firearms are less popular. Mandatory use laws often engender spirited resistance from those who perceive these laws as an infringement on "personal freedom."

Political backlash can block promising legislation or ultimately lead to the repeal of a successful law. A survey of Colorado legislators revealed that 96 percent knew that safety belts reduce the risk of death and 87 percent believed that a safety belt law would save lives, but the strongest predictor of a "yes" vote on a mandatory use bill was the impression that their constituents favored the law.[14] Despite overwhelming evidence that motorcycle helmet laws save lives, 26 states repealed their statutes when federal incentives were relaxed in 1976. In these states, motorcycle crash fatality rates subsequently increased 40 percent.[15] As of 2000, only 22 states had universal helmet laws, 28 mandate helmets for young riders, and 3 lack any requirement.[16]

Opponents of mandatory use laws argue that individuals should be permitted to ignore mandatory use laws if they consider the level of risk acceptable to them. Unfortunately, the circle of harm extends far beyond the victim. For example, a motorcyclist or a bicyclist who rides without a helmet faces an increased risk of serious head injury or death. When such individuals are killed or disabled in a crash, their family and loved ones lose companionship, their dependents lose an important source of financial support, their employers lose productivity, and society is required to cover the cost of their care. All of us, either directly or indirectly, pay the costs of preventable injury.

ENGINEERING Many injuries can be prevented by building safer vehicles or modifying the physical environment in which injuries occur. The up-front cost to design and implement an engineering countermeasure often exceeds the up-front cost of educational or an enforcement campaign, but the downstream effect is often greater as well. Engineering is usually more effective than behavioral strategies because it does not require users to permanently and consistently change what they do.

Consider, for example, the lessons learned in highway safety. In contrast to the consistently disappointing results of driver's education, federal standards for motor vehicle construction saved an estimated 37,000 lives between 1975 and 1978 alone. These standards addressed such issues as passenger restraint systems, windshields, fuel tank integrity, and the flammability of interior fabric. Introduction of air bags cut the nation's toll of deaths and injuries due to car crashes even further. Construction of the interstate highway system saved lives as well. Modifications to the driving environment, such as banked curves, divided lanes of traffic, controlled ramps for ingress and egress, elimination of crossing streams of traffic, and the positioning of energy-absorbing pilings in front of fixed obstructions cut the interstate highway death rate to less than half that for other similarly sized roads.

These lessons could be applied to other hazardous products as well. Cigarettes cause more than half of U.S. house fire fatalities. Most fires occur when the smoker falls asleep in bed or leaves a burning cigarette on the arm of a sofa or chair. Television, radio, and print advertisements warning of the dangers of smoking in bed have had little or no impact on this problem. Smoke detectors save lives by warning of an impending catastrophe in time to permit the occupants to evacuate the house but require a concerted effort to encourage people to install and maintain them. Passive engineering of the home environment by installing a residential sprinkler system could be a very effective strategy. Unfortunately, such systems are expensive, rarely available, and often cannot be retrofitted into older homes. A more promising option is to modify the cigarette itself to diminish its potential to ignite furniture or bedding.

Laws that require products to be designed so that their potential to cause harm is diminished can be highly effective. Unfortunately, they are difficult to enact. Manufacturers often oppose such regulations because they fear that they will raise the price of their product and discourage sales. In addition to the issue of personal freedom, concerns are often raised about cost, government interference, and reduced competitiveness with nonregulated manufacturers. If efforts to regulate a hazardous product fail, product liability lawsuits may be the only way to force needed changes in product design.

PRACTICE OF INJURY CONTROL

Step 1: Define the Problem

Population-based data of the incidence and impact of injury are essential to define the scope of the problem and mobilize the resources necessary to achieve change. Public health surveillance is needed to monitor patterns and trends and to evaluate the impact of countermeasures.

Several sources of information can be used for this purpose. Vital records or death certificates are useful to document the impact of injuries on overall rates of mortality, but they do not provide information about nonfatal injuries. Hospital discharge data and trauma registries can provide essential information about cases of major trauma, but population-based data are needed to calculate rates of injury. Furthermore, hospital admission statistics and trauma registry data do not capture patients who are treated and released from the emergency department.

Although injuries that are managed on an outpatient basis generally are assumed to be minor, they can result in significant long-term disability. This is particularly true of head, back, and hand injuries. Patients visiting an emergency department for injury have an increased risk for recurrent injury, especially if their index visit is related to alcohol abuse or violence.

Assignment of external cause-of-injury codes *(E-codes)* to every injury-related emergency department visit can substantially enhance community-based surveillance efforts. Several states mandate E-coding of all hospital admissions, but very few require hospitals to E-code emergency department visits.

Step 2: Identify Causes and Risk Factors

Descriptive studies usually are conducted to determine *who* is injured, *what* kinds of injuries are involved, and *where, when,* and *why* those injuries occur. These data provide essential clues to injury causation and often generate hypotheses that can be investigated with analytical methods.

In some cases, the link between a risk factor and an injury is so strong that no additional research is needed. For example, early studies of automobile injury showed that 50 percent of all fatal crashes and 60 percent of all fatal single-vehicle crashes involved alcohol.[17] In most cases, however, it is necessary to compare the rate of injury among those *with* a risk factor with the rate of injury in an otherwise similar group *without* a risk factor. Cohort, quasi-experimental, or classic experimental studies may be employed to reach a definitive conclusion. When the outcome of interest is rare and exposure to the risk factor(s) of interest can be shown to precede the injury, case-control studies may be employed. Meticulous attention to methodology is essential to generate valid results and control for the effects of confounding variables.

Step 3: Develop and Test Interventions

Once the magnitude of the problem and its associated risk factors are identified, a variety of countermeasures may be considered for implementation. Careful attention must be given to the characteristics of the target population, the feasibility of the countermeasure(s), their acceptability to the target population, and cost. Pilot intervention programs often are helpful to test various strategies. The most promising program can then be selected for widespread implementation.

Community education programs are often tried first because they are relatively easy to initiate, attract motivated volunteers, and are invaluable for raising public awareness. They also can help build public support for legislative changes at a later date. It is essential to take the views and values of the community into consideration at every step of the process. Citizen involvement is crucial to any program's success.

Most programs set milestones and predefined measures of success. For example, a campaign to prevent deaths and injuries in residential fires may identify selected measures of *structure* (number of staff hired, office space, cooperative agreements reached), *process* (number of pamphlets distributed, number of home visits made, total smoke detectors installed), or *outcome* (reductions in the rate of deaths, decline in hospital admissions).

It is not always feasible to demonstrate major impacts on rates of morbidity or mortality with small-scale demonstration projects. When this is the case, surrogate measures may be used to demonstrate program impact. For example, preintervention rates of smoke detector use in a target neighborhood can be compared with rates noted after an educational campaign. Telephone surveys can seek evidence of changes in knowledge, attitudes, and self-reported behavior. Self-reports do not guarantee long-term behavior change, but they confirm that a program is reaching the target group.

Step 4: Implement Effective Interventions and Evaluate Their Impact

Once a program is initiated on a large-scale basis, evaluation data should be collected to demonstrate its impact. Measures of cost-effectiveness (e.g., dollars spent per life saved or injury prevented) are particularly important. It is easy to tabulate the cost of a prevention program, but it is harder to document the savings from "tragedies that did not happen." Program support tends to wane over time, especially when no specific group champions its continuation. During difficult economic times, prevention programs are often the first to go. Without documented evidence of clinical or economic impact, worthy programs can fade into extinction.

THE ROLE OF THE EMERGENCY PHYSICIAN IN INJURY CONTROL

Patient Education

Injury-control measures need not be implemented on a grand scale to make a difference. Emergency physicians can incorporate injury-prevention principles into their clinical practice, although long-term benefit has never been shown.[18]

Special efforts should be made to correct factors that precipitated the injury or contributed to its severity. Otherwise, a patient is likely to return with a more serious injury in the future. A child sustaining a mi-

nor head injury while bike riding should be told to wear his or her bicycle helmet. The unbelted adult who sustained minor injuries in a low-velocity motor vehicle crash deserves a short lecture on the importance of safety belts. An elder who has fallen should be counseled about checking his or her home for loose rugs and other tripping hazards.

However, emergency physicians should consider every emergency department encounter a *teachable moment*.[19] Due to the nature of their work, emergency physicians are more likely to provide acute care to injured patients than any other group of physicians. Therefore, they have a special stake in preventing and controlling injuries. The mother who brings her child to the emergency department for evaluation of an ear infection should leave the department with information about the importance of child safety seats, bicycle helmets, and four-sided fencing around her swimming pool. Emergency physicians have the opportunity to motivate patients to change high-risk behaviors and modify their home environment to decrease injury risk.

Data Collection and Program Evaluation

If current trends toward capitated care continue, the emergency department will become an increasingly important arena for prevention efforts. Until now, the financial incentives of health care have encouraged hospitalization and provision of services. The move toward capitated payment substantially increases the incentive to prevent rather than treat illness and injuries. As the portal of entry for 40 percent of U.S. inpatient admissions, the emergency department can play a key role in monitoring system performance, identifying high-risk groups, reducing the need for expensive inpatient care, and evaluating the impact of community-based prevention programs.

Research

Emergency physicians are ideally positioned to conduct injury surveillance and evaluate countermeasures. They should take the lead in community-based epidemiologic research. Priority areas for research include prevention of pediatric injuries and alcohol-related trauma; evaluation of drunk driving enforcement efforts; reduction of firearm-related injuries, intimate partner violence, and residential fires; and studies of the biomechanics of trauma.

Advocacy

Sometimes evaluation data indicate that a countermeasure is effective but rarely used. When education is not enough to motivate behavioral change, legislation may have a major impact, particularly when coupled with ongoing education efforts and visible enforcement. For example, states with mandatory motorcycle helmet laws report compliance rates as high as 98 percent.

Coalition building is essential in assembling a broad base of support. Physician leadership ensures the success of these efforts. The testimonies of health care providers, surviving family members, and disabled individuals are needed to give the statistics an emotional context and deliver the message in a personal manner. Information on the economic impact of injuries and the cost-effectiveness of countermeasures is also helpful.

Academic emergency physicians have an important role to play in training the next generation of injury-control experts. Research suggests that many medical students lack a fundamental understanding of the principles and practice of injury control.[20] In addition, although 90 percent of emergency medicine residents believe that injury prevention is pertinent to our specialty, the majority do not feel that they received adequate training in injury prevention during residency.[21] Academic emergency physicians can play an important role by emphasizing the importance of injury control to their trainees.

REFERENCES

1. Ventura SJ, Peters KD, Martin JA, Maurer JD: Births and deaths: United States, 1996. *Monthly Vital Statistics Report* 46(1 suppl 2):32, 1997.
2. Haddon W: A logical framework for categorizing highway safety phenomenon and activity. *J Trauma* 12:193, 1972.
3. Haddon W: Energy damage and the ten countermeasure strategies. *J Trauma* 13:321, 1973.
4. Waller JA: Reflections on a half century of injury control. *Am J Public Health* 84:664, 1994.
5. Dannenberg AL, Gielen AC, Beilenson PL, et al: Bicycle hemlmet laws and educational campaigns: An evaluation of strategies to increase children's helmet use. *Am J Public Health* 83:667, 1993.
6. Holder HD, Guenewald PJ, Ponicki WR, et al: Effect of community-based interventions on high-risk drinking and alcohol-related injuries. *JAMA* 284:2341, 2000.
7. Lee AJ, Mann NP, Takriti R: A hospital-led promotion campaign aimed to increase bicycle helmet wearing among children aged 11–15 living in West Berkshire. *Injury Prevention* 6:151, 2000.
8. Gielen AC: Health education and injury control: Integrating approaches. *Health Educ Q* 19:203, 1992.
9. Howat P, Jones S, Hall M, et al: The PRECEDE-PROCEED model: Application to planning a child pedestrian injury prevention program. *Injury Prevention* 3:282, 1997.
10. Hendrickson SG, Becker H: Impact of a theory-based intervention to increase bicycle helmet use in low-income children. *Injury Prevention* 4:126, 1998.
11. Hanfling MJ, Mangus LG, Gill AC et al: A multifaceted approach to improving motor vehicle restraint compliance. *Injury Prevention* 6:125, 2000.
12. Hotz GA, Cohn SM, Popkin C, et al: The impact of a repealed motorcycle helmet law in Miami-Dade County. *J Trauma* 52:469, 2002.
13. Williams AF, Preusser DF, Blomberg RD, Lund AD: Seat belt use law enforcement and publicity in Elmira, New York: A reminder campaign. *Am J Public Health* 77:1450, 1987.
14. Lowenstein SR, Koziol-McLain J, Satterfield G, et al: Facts versus values: Why legislators vote against injury-control laws. *J Trauma* 35:786, 1993.
15. Watson GS, Zador PL, Wilks A: The repeal of helmet use laws and increased motorcyclist mortality in the United States, 1975–1978. *Am J Public Health* 70:579, 1980.
16. Vaca F: Motorcycle helmet law repeal: A tax assessment for the rest of the United States? *Ann Emerg Med* 37:230, 2001.
17. Polen MR, Friendam GD: Automobile injury: Selected risk factors and prevention in the health care setting. *JAMA* 259:76, 1988.
18. Dunn KA, Cline DM, Grant T, et al: Injury-prevention instruction in the emergency department. *Ann Emerg Med* 22:1280, 1993.
19. Todd KH: Air bags and the teachable moment. *Ann Emerg Med* 28:242, 1996.
20. Butler RN, Todd KH, Kellermann AL, et al: Injury-control education in six U.S. medical schools. *Acad Med* 73:524, 1998.
21. Anglin D, Hutson HR, Kyriacou DN: Emergency medicine residents' perspectives on injury prevention. *Ann Emerg Med* 28:41, 1996.

INJURIES TO THE BONES, JOINTS, AND SOFT TISSUE

INITIAL EVALUATION AND MANAGEMENT OF ORTHOPEDIC INJURIES
Jeffrey S. Menkes

CLINICAL PHYSIOLOGY OF FRACTURES

The ability to properly assess and treat skeletal injuries in the emergency department depends to a large extent on understanding the physiologic processes by which fractures are created and by which they heal. Practical knowledge of fracture physiology may provide the index of suspicion needed to diagnose an injury that might otherwise be missed. It also might help prevent or minimize complications and may form the basis for advising the patient regarding the outlook for recovery of function.

How Fractures Occur

Although fractures are sometimes described in terms of the external mechanism creating them, they also may be considered in terms of the physiology involved.

"TYPICAL" FRACTURES   Most fractures are the result of significant trauma to healthy bone. The bony cortex may be disrupted by a variety of forces, including a direct blow, axial loading, angular (bending) forces, torque (twisting) stress, or a combination of these.

PATHOLOGIC FRACTURES   Fractures that occur from relatively minor trauma to diseased or otherwise abnormal bone are termed *pathologic fractures*. This term implies that a preexisting pathologic process has weakened the bone and rendered it susceptible to fracture by forces that, under normal circumstances, would not disrupt the cortex. Common examples of such injuries are fractures through metastatic lytic lesions, fractures through benign bone cysts (as in the humerus of Little League pitchers), and vertebral compression fractures in patients with advanced osteoporosis. Numerous other disease processes may render patients susceptible to pathologic fracture.

Because these injuries often are not associated with a history of significant trauma, subtle pathologic fractures may go undetected unless there is a preexisting index of suspicion based on the knowledge that such injuries can occur.

STRESS FRACTURES   In some cases, bone may undergo a "fatigue" fracture as a result of being subject to uncustomary repetitive forces before the bone and its supporting tissues have had adequate time to accommodate to such forces. An example is the insidious occurrence of a metatarsal shaft fracture in unconditioned foot soldiers (the so-called march fracture). The physiologic principle of stress fracture can be easily envisioned by anyone who has "cut" an aluminum finger splint to the desired length by bending it back and forth. The pliable metal, too hard to cut with ordinary scissors, ultimately gives way in the face of repeated stresses requiring relatively little force.

The processes that render bone susceptible to stress fracture are not generally agreed upon. The important point is that diagnosis depends on a familiarity with the entity, because **x-rays are typically negative early in the patient's course.** Initial diagnosis may be presumptive, based solely on the history and physical findings. Days or weeks may pass before the fracture line or new bone formation becomes visible on x-ray, ultimately confirming the suspicions of the clinician who, hav-

ing made the correct clinical diagnosis, will have treated the patient appropriately from the outset.

SALTER (EPIPHYSEAL) FRACTURES   Fractures involving the physis, the cartilaginous epiphyseal plate near the ends of the long bones of growing children, are called *Salter fractures* after Salter and Harris, the physicians who devised the most popular method of classifying these injuries.[1] The supply of new bone material needed for the elongation of bones during growth is provided by specialized cells within the physis. When growth is completed, the physis transforms into bone, ultimately fusing with the surrounding bone and disappearing as a distinct entity. By definition, Salter fractures cannot occur in fully grown adults.

Any damage to the epiphyseal plate during a child's growth may destroy part or all of its ability to produce new bone substance, resulting in aborted or deformed growth of the bone thereafter. The potential for growth disturbance from an epiphyseal injury is related to the number of years the child has yet to grow (the older the child, the less time remains for deformity to develop) and to the pattern of the fracture line through the epiphyseal area. Classification of Salter fractures and their clinical implications are discussed later in this chapter.

Fracture Healing

The physiology of fracture healing constitutes the basis for many decisions in the emergency department. The judgment as to whether an angulated fracture requires reduction, the choice of treatment modality in relation to the patient's age, and the prognosis for regaining function or being left with residual deformity require familiarity with the short- and long-term aspects of the healing process.

Fracture healing can be described in terms of three phases—inflammatory, reparative, and remodeling—each of which gradually blends into the next.[2]

When a fracture occurs, the microvessels crossing the fracture line are severed, depriving the damaged bone ends of their blood supply. As a result, the bone ends necrose during the ensuing days, triggering a classic inflammatory response. This early phase is brief but creates the tissue environment for the most predominant aspect of fracture healing: the reparative phase.

Granulation tissue soon begins to infiltrate the area. Within this tissue are specialized cells capable of forming collagen, cartilage, and bone, the ingredients of callus, which gradually surrounds the fractured ends and stabilizes them. With time, the callus becomes more densely mineralized.

Meanwhile, the necrotic edges of the fragments are removed by osteoclasts, cells whose specific function is to resorb bone. That is the reason some "hairline" fractures do not appear on x-ray until days after injury. Initially invisible, the diagnostic fracture line appears only after necrotic bone has been resorbed from the area.

The final phase of bone healing, the remodeling phase, is the longest, often lasting years. Remodeling is the tendency of bone to gradually regain its original shape and contour. During this phase, the superfluous portions of callus are resorbed, and new bone is laid down along natural lines of stress. These internal layers, easily visible in x-rays of normal bone, are the bony trabeculae. Formation of trabecular bone is a physiologically efficient process providing maximum strength relative to the amount of bone material used.

The anticipated degree of successful remodeling is related to a number of factors. Young children have a greater capacity for remodeling than adults do. Accordingly, their potential for residual deformity is less, other circumstances being equal. Remodeling is also related to the magnitude and direction of unreduced angulation and to the fracture's location along the bone. Specific predictors of satisfactory remodeling include youth, proximity of the fracture to the end of the bone (but not involving the epiphyseal plate), and direction of angulation coinciding with the plane of natural joint motion.

Clinical decisions regarding the aggressiveness of fracture reduction are directly linked to a knowledge of this physiology. Angulation near the end of a long bone, for example, is more acceptable than angulation near the midshaft. Dorsal or volar angulation at the wrist has a better prognosis than does ulnar or radial angulation, because the natural plane of wrist motion is dorsal to volar. Mild angulation in a 2-year-old child may be left to remodel on its own, whereas the same angulation in an adult may require correction.

ORTHOPEDIC EMERGENCIES

Some types of musculoskeletal trauma deserve special mention, because a delay in their diagnosis or treatment can increase the chance of significant complications or a negative outcome.

Open Fracture

An open fracture (or compound fracture, in older terminology) is a fracture associated with overlying soft tissue injury, creating communication between the fracture site and the external surface of the body. Although *open fracture* may convey the image of grossly exposed bone, the term is equally applicable to a simple puncture wound extending to the depth of an underlying fracture. Such puncture wounds may be created by external forces or by a sharp bone fragment transiently protruding through the skin before receding back beneath the surface.

The most dreaded complication of open fracture is osteomyelitis. Once established, osteomyelitis may result in months or years of pain, disability, medical therapy, surgical procedures, and ultimately, amputation. Although osteomyelitis may be unavoidable in some cases, it becomes less likely when treatment is prompt and meticulous.

Open fractures are sometimes classified by severity, based on the length of the overlying laceration, extent of tissue damage, kinetic energy of the injuring force, and evidence or likelihood of significant contamination. Irrespective of these factors, any open fracture should be promptly and carefully treated. Elements in the care of open fractures are described later in this chapter.

Dislocation and Subluxation

A joint is dislocated when the articular surfaces of the bones that normally meet at the joint have been displaced completely out of contact with one another. This is the most extreme form of subluxation, a condition in which the articular surfaces are nonconcentric to any degree.

The urgency of treating dislocated joints is based on several factors. One is the potential for neurologic or circulatory compromise. The neurovascular bundle passing close to the affected joint is typically "kinked" around the deformity associated with the dislocation. Persistence of this condition can result in a neurologic or vascular deficit that may be temporary if the deformity is reduced promptly but irreversible if treatment is delayed.

Another consideration is that, the longer a joint has been dislocated, the more difficult it may be to reduce and the more likely it is to be unstable after reduction. This is probably due, at least in part, to edema, muscle spasm, and other tissue changes that increase over time.

Dislocation of the hip carries its own particular urgency in addition to those mentioned above: the danger of avascular necrosis of the femoral head. Avascular necrosis occurs because much of the blood supply to the femoral head is delivered through vessels that emerge from the acetabulum. When the joint is dislocated, circulation to the femoral head is disrupted. At some point, the vascular insult becomes irreversible, and bony necrosis is the ultimate result. Although aseptic necrosis may occur despite the clinician's best efforts, its likelihood increases with the time delay until reduction.

Neurovascular Deficit

Naturally, any injury associated with neurologic or vascular compromise, such as may result from a severely deformed fracture, should be addressed as soon as possible. The longer a deficit goes untreated, the longer it is likely to persist and the greater the possibility that it will be irreversible. In some cases, simply reducing a deformity by means of longitudinal traction may restore circulation or nerve function, allowing the remainder of the patient's evaluation and treatment to proceed at a calmer pace.

PREHOSPITAL CARE

With the growing sophistication of emergency medical service (EMS) programs in many areas of the United States, important aspects of early care are more likely to be implemented in a timely manner.

Preliminary Splinting

Effective splinting of the injured extremity is crucial for several reasons: (1) it reduces the patient's pain; (2) it reduces damage to nerves and vessels by preventing them from being repeatedly ground between the fragments or being stretched by increased angulation at the fracture site; (3) it reduces the chance of inadvertently converting a closed fracture to an open one as a sharp bone fragment pokes its way through the skin (considered a mishap of severe consequence, because of the potential for osteomyelitis); and (4) it facilitates patient transport and the taking of x-rays by reducing the pain and manipulation associated with moving the patient from ground to ambulance to emergency department stretcher to x-ray table.

Prehospital Splinting Devices

Many splinting devices are available to EMS systems. For injuries of the wrist or forearm, a foam-padded intravenous board can be wrapped in place, supplemented by a sling. The sling is important, because optimal immobilization includes the joint above and the joint below the fracture. The sling keeps the elbow (the joint above) at rest.

For suspected injuries to the elbow or humerus, a sling-and-swathe arrangement works well. This method involves applying a sling and then binding the affected arm to the thorax with a gauze wrap. An exception to this principle is immobilization of patients with suspected anterior dislocation of the shoulder. Such patients have difficulty adducting the forearm against the thorax, and forcibly binding it there is painful and not recommended. A simple sling is adequate. Injuries to the ankle can be immobilized in a pillow or well-padded cardboard splint. If fracture of the tibial shaft or knee is suspected, the device should extend well above the knee (to immobilize the joint above and the joint below).

Some injuries warrant specialized splints, such as winch-mechanism traction devices for femoral shaft fractures. Although such devices do not immobilize the hip (the joint above), the added element of traction makes this component unnecessary. If a traction device is unavailable, the hip needs to be immobilized, which can be accomplished with military antishock trousers, with all compartments inflated or, less elegantly, by binding the legs together and then binding the patient to a backboard from ankles to thorax.

Other types of splints exist, but their use is controversial. Inflatable plastic splints, for example, are acceptable for injuries to the ankle or wrist but sometimes are used inappropriately for fractures of the humerus or femur. Because these devices normally do not extend above the elbow or knee, they provide inadequate immobilization for such injuries. Also, overinflation of plastic splints may seriously impair circulation. (If the splint cannot be dented by moderate thumb pressure, it is probably overinflated.) Inflatable splints should not be applied over clothing, because underlying wrinkles in the clothing may cause pressure sores in swollen and vulnerable tissue.

Also controversial are nonmalleable aluminum splints, because they are based on the "one size fits all" principle, which some clinicians interpret as "this size fits none." If used, aluminum splints should be very well padded, because their hard surfaces may cause pressure sores. Like any splint, they should immobilize the joint above and the joint below the fracture if they are used for long-bone injuries. For example, an above-knee splint is needed for fracture of the tibial shaft. Aluminum splints should be removed as soon as possible, once a fracture is diagnosed or ruled out. If a fracture is confirmed, the splint should be replaced with another type of immobilization dressing before the patient leaves the emergency department.

Reducing Deformity in the Field

Many EMS programs do not recommend prehospital reduction of deformity of an injured extremity. If the deformity is near a joint (suggesting the possibility of dislocation), this is certainly good advice. Injudicious manipulation may convert a pure dislocation to a fracture-dislocation. Even if a fracture already exists, there will be no way to prove it was not caused by the manipulation.

A circumstance in which prehospital reduction of obvious fractures along the shaft of a long bone can be justified is the absence of a distal pulse. Minutes may count in such cases.

Without a common standard, the indications for reduction of deformity by prehospital personnel ultimately remain at the discretion of the supervising EMS program. If reduction is attempted, it should be performed by means of longitudinal traction.

EMERGENCY DEPARTMENT EVALUATION AND DIFFERENTIAL DIAGNOSIS

The importance of a careful history and physical examination cannot be overstated. Orthopedic diagnosis is sometimes thought of as being as simple as taking an x-ray of the spot where the patient says the pain is. This philosophy is probably more responsible than any other factor for clinicians missing significant injuries.

Although x-ray is an important adjunct, it is not the ultimate diagnostic resource, for the following reasons. The pain of a fracture or even a dislocation may be referred to another area. For example, patients with disruption of the sternoclavicular joint or fracture of the humeral shaft may present complaining of shoulder pain. If the x-ray is based solely on where the patient reports subjective discomfort, then the injury might not be included on the film. The area x-rayed should be determined not only by the patient's chief complaint, but also by systematic palpation looking for subtle deformity or significant point tenderness.

Some fractures or dislocations are apparent only on special x-ray views, which are not part of the standard series for that body part. Such special views will never be ordered unless the clinician has already formulated a presumptive differential diagnosis before x-ray, based on the history and physical findings.

Some injuries may not be radiologically apparent on the first day, regardless of what views are taken. Common examples of such injuries are fracture of the scaphoid (carpal navicular), nondisplaced fracture of the radial head, and stress fracture of a metatarsal. The classic radiologic signs accompanying such injuries, such as the fat-pad sign of the elbow, are not always conveniently present, but suggestive history and findings commonly are. In such cases, the diagnosis of fracture may have to be purely clinical until 7 to 10 days after injury, when enough bony resorption has occurred at the fracture site to reveal a lucency on x-ray. A bone scan may suggest the fracture even sooner, but on the day of injury, there may be no readily available test capable of demonstrating the pathology. Only the clinician's index of suspicion, arrived at through a systematic history and physical examination, will result in proper and timely treatment of a radiologically undemonstrable fracture.

History

The value of history taking in the case of orthopedic injuries is often underestimated. In fact, knowing the precise mechanism of injury or listening carefully to the patient's symptoms may be the key to diagnosing fractures or dislocations. For example, a history of shoulder injury combined with the complaint of dysphagia may be the only clue to the existence of posterior sternoclavicular dislocation. This entity, which causes pressure on the mediastinal structures, often can be demonstrated only by computed tomography and is associated with severe complications if treatment is delayed. Another example is a history of landing flat on the feet from a significant height, which should prompt the clinician to consider fracture of one or both calcanei, in addition to associated tibial plateau, acetabular, and lumbar vertebral compression fractures.

History is often the only means of correctly assessing and treating young children who "just won't use the arm." Such children, who present with a seemingly paralyzed arm ("pseudoparalysis") after being pulled or yanked, may be incorrectly diagnosed as having a brachial plexus injury, when in fact the history and presentation are classic for subluxed radial head, an entity not discernible on x-ray and easily and quickly remedied by a proper reduction maneuver.

A careful history may enable the clinician to diagnose posterior dislocation of the shoulder, another entity commonly missed on routine films. If the patient has (1) experienced a direct blow to the front of the shoulder, (2) landed forward on an outstretched arm, or (3) had a seizure or undergone violent muscle contraction for any other reason (e.g., contact with high-voltage current) and now complains of excruciating shoulder pain and severely limited motion, the diagnosis of posterior dislocation should be entertained. If the implications of the history are not appreciated, then the specific x-ray views needed to demonstrate the injury may never be ordered.

Table 267-1 provides other examples of mechanisms that might lead the clinician to suspect, or presumptively treat for, specific injuries. This is by no means a definitive or exhaustive list. Some of the mechanisms described may produce injuries other than those mentioned. Conversely, the injuries may be produced by mechanisms other than those listed.

Some musculoskeletal injuries or conditions may not necessarily be associated with a history of trauma. Occult fracture of the hip in an osteoporotic individual, occult stress fracture of a metatarsal in someone who has recently done an unusual amount of walking, and slipped capital femoral epiphysis in a preteenager or young adolescent are examples of injuries whose symptoms may be gradual and insidious in onset, unrelated to an isolated traumatic event. Tenderness to palpation or pain on weight bearing or range of motion suggests the possibility of an occult or easily missed fracture. Depending on the index of suspicion, further studies, such as bone scan or magnetic resonance imaging, may be indicated to rule out significant pathologic conditions before the patient is allowed to resume weight bearing.

History taking should not necessarily be limited to orthopedic issues. Depending on the situation, a general medical history should be obtained, because it may have implications for further workup, the potential for complications, or ultimate prognosis for recovery of function. For example, relevant items may include a history of heart disease, anticoagulant medication, falling due to syncope or transient hemiparesis rather than simply stumbling, or an unsteady baseline gait that cannot withstand further impairment.

TABLE 267-1   Mechanisms Associated with Particular Orthopedic Injuries

Mechanism	Possible Injury
Bilateral compression of shoulders	Anterior or posterior sternoclavicular dislocation
Direct blow to medial clavicle	Posterior sternoclavicular dislocation
Fall, landing on point of shoulder	Acromioclavicular separation
Direct blow to anterior shoulder, fall on outstretched arm, seizure or electroconvulsive muscular activity	Posterior dislocation of shoulder
Yanking of infant's or toddler's arm	Subluxed radial head (sometimes misdiagnosed as brachial plexus injury because of pseudoparalysis of arm)
Fall, landing on outstretched arm or with elbow beneath the body	Fracture of radial head (may be occult on initial x-rays)
Wrist hyperextension (forced dorsiflexion)	Fracture of scaphoid (carpal navicular), lunate or perilunar dislocation, Colles fracture
Striking knee against dashboard in high-speed collision	Posterior dislocation of hip
Landing flat on feet from height	Calcaneus fracture (one or both); tibial plateau fracture (one or more); acetabular fracture (one or both); vertebral compression fracture, usually lumbar (one or more)
Ankle inversion force	Fracture of any of the malleoli, fracture of base of fifth metatarsal
Rotatory ankle force	Fracture of any of the malleoli, disruption of the anterior tibiofibular ligament with proximal fibular fracture (Maisonneuve injury)
Inversion, medial or lateral stress to forefoot; axial load on metatarsal heads with ankle plantarflexed	Midfoot dislocation (Lisfranc injury)

Physical Examination

Essential components of the examination for musculoskeletal trauma are (1) inspection for swelling, discoloration, or deformity; (2) assessment of active and passive range of motion of the joints proximal and distal to the injury; (3) palpation for tenderness or subtle deformity; and (4) verification of neurovascular status.

INSPECTION AND RANGE OF MOTION   Gross deformity along the shaft of a long bone is pathognomonic for fracture. The presence of most dislocations or fractures near a joint can be inferred by deformity at the joint, loss of range of motion, and severe pain at rest. An exception is posterior dislocation of the shoulder, which, although intensely painful, may not be accompanied by obvious deformity. Chap. 271 presents a more complete discussion of this entity.

PALPATION   When gross deformity is not present, presumptive orthopedic diagnosis strongly depends on the findings noted on palpation. Palpation will disclose areas of bony step-off and the precise location of point tenderness. If films are ordered before performing this phase of the examination, the wrong area may be x-rayed, because pain is commonly referred to a location distant from the injury site.

The palpation examination should be done systematically and consistently from one patient to the next. The area palpated should extend well beyond the location of the patient's subjective pain. For example, when an injured patient complains of shoulder pain, palpation should begin at the sternoclavicular joint and then proceed along the clavicle, onto the acromioclavicular joint, onto the humeral head, and along the entire humeral shaft. In addition, the scapula should be palpated for tenderness, and the posterior aspect of the shoulder should be palpated for any unnatural prominence that might suggest a posterior dislocation. Injury to any of these areas may be reported by the patient as pain in the shoulder. Only a meticulous palpation examination may protect the clinician from being misled by referred pain and missing a crucial diagnosis.

NEUROVASCULAR ASSESSMENT   When injury involves an extremity, as opposed to the vertebral column, sensorimotor testing should be performed on the basis of *peripheral nerve* function, rather than nerve root and dermatomal distribution (Figure 267-1A, B). In the upper extremity, the radial, median, and ulnar nerves should be tested. When the shoulder is anteriorly dislocated, two additional nerves, the axillary (supplying sensation to the lateral aspect of the shoulder) and the musculocutaneous (supplying sensation to the extensor aspect of the forearm), also should be checked. In the lower extremity, examination of the saphenous (sensory only), peroneal, and tibial nerves should be performed. Neurologic deficit is important to document early, particularly before the patient has undergone any significant manipulation or reduction maneuvers.

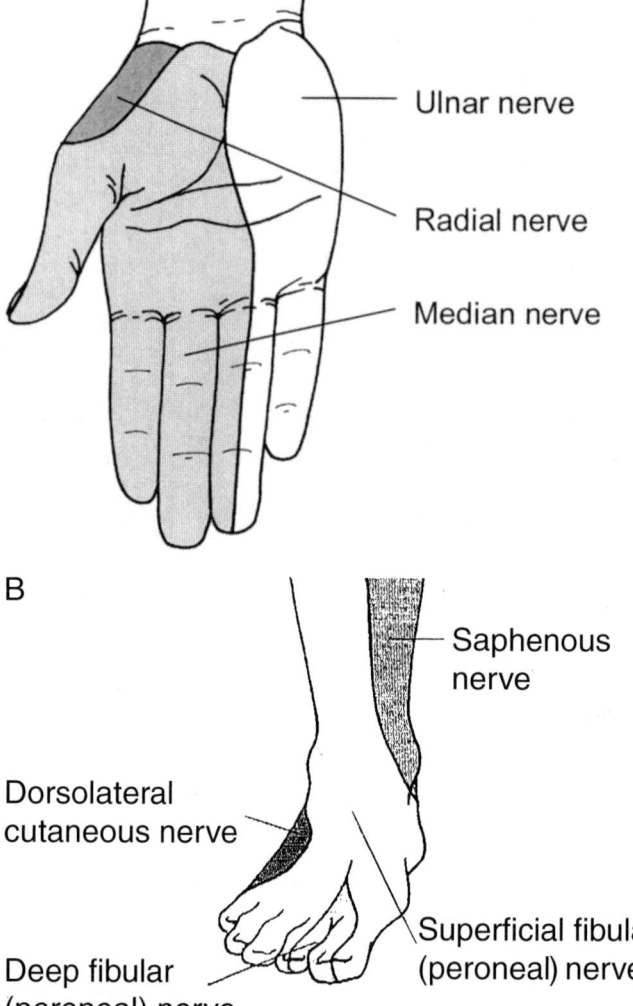

FIG. 267-1. **A.** Peripheral sensory nerve distribution of the hand. **B.** Peripheral sensory nerve distribution of the foot.

Assessment of vascular status also should be performed early. The sooner circulatory compromise is identified and addressed, the better the chance of avoiding tissue ischemia or necrosis. Injuries such as dislocation of the knee (tibiofemoral joint), fracture-dislocation of the ankle, and displaced supracondylar fracture of the elbow in children are commonly associated with vascular occlusion or disruption, with resulting circulatory impairment.

RADIOLOGIC EVALUATION

The area x-rayed and the particular views ordered should be based on the history and physical examination, rather than on where the patient reports subjective pain. **The joint above and the joint below a fracture should be included on the films,** because injury at the proximal or distal joint may coexist with long-bone fractures.

Injuries that may require special views to be visualized include acromioclavicular separation, fracture of the scaphoid, posterior shoulder dislocation, and sternoclavicular dislocation. **Thus formulation of a presumptive diagnosis** *before* **x-ray is crucial. The clinician may never order the specialized views needed to demonstrate a particular injury unless he or she has already anticipated the injury by virtue of the history and physical examination.**

Children who have sustained trauma at or near a joint may need comparison studies of the opposite extremity to differentiate fracture lines from normal epiphyseal plates or ossifying growth centers. This is particularly true for the pediatric elbow, which typically exhibits six separate ossification centers sequentially as the child grows.

Although the clinician may be tempted to base diagnostic and treatment decisions on the radiologist's written report, this is not advisable for at least two reasons. First, a report of negative findings does not rule out significant injury. Fractures of the radial head, scaphoid, or metatarsal shaft, for example, initially may be undetectable on x-ray, even when special views are taken. Second, the terminology used by radiologists to describe malposition of fracture fragments or disrupted joints often differs from the terminology used by orthopedists. Because the emergency physician often will be conferring with an orthopedist regarding the initial management of a patient, and because this interaction commonly involves describing the radiologic appearance of a patient's injury, it is important that the two physicians "speak the same language." This communication might not be achieved by simply relaying the radiologist's written description.

Describing Radiographs

When orthopedic consultation is indicated, proper management of the patient may rest on the emergency physician's accurate description of the x-ray. Often the narrative will influence the orthopedist's decision regarding the need for hospital admission and whether surgical versus nonsurgical management is warranted. In essence, the emergency physician should be able to transmit a virtual copy of the x-ray by means of verbal description.

There are various ways of classifying or categorizing fractures. The method presented in this chapter is intended to be the most practical from the standpoint of effective communication with a consultant who is not physically present.[3]

OPEN VERSUS CLOSED   Although not a radiologic finding per se, this aspect of an injury is among the most important and should be conveyed to the orthopedist before any other. The implications of open fracture are of such significance that this factor alone may determine the patient's immediate care or ultimate disposition.

LOCATION OF THE FRACTURE   Typical reference points used by orthopedists to describe the location of a fracture along the shaft of a long bone are the midshaft, the junction of the proximal and middle thirds, and the junction of the middle and distal thirds. Any fracture

more proximal or distal than these locations may be localized in terms of its distance, in centimeters, from the bone end.

When a fracture extends into the adjacent joint, it is termed *intraarticular.* Intraarticular fractures have special significance because disruption of the joint surface may warrant surgery to restore the joint's contour and prevent subsequent traumatic arthritis. This feature of a fracture line, if present, constitutes important information.

Anatomic bony reference points should be cited when applicable. A fracture just above the condyles of the distal humerus or femur, for example, is most precisely called a *supracondylar* fracture. A fracture running from the greater to the lesser trochanter of the proximal femur is an *intertrochanteric* hip fracture, whereas a fracture just below the trochanters is *subtrochanteric,* and a fracture just above is said to involve the femoral *neck.* The area at or proximal to the coronoid process of the ulna is the *olecranon* and should be referred to as such, rather than simply the proximal ulna. Other bony landmarks include the radial head (proximal), radial styloid (distal), and greater tuberosity of the humerus. Numerous additional examples exist.

ORIENTATION OF THE FRACTURE LINE   The most common orientations of fracture lines are illustrated in Figure 267-2. Torus and greenstick fractures are seen almost exclusively in young children, whose bones are more pliable than those of adults. Note the segmental fracture, which is commonly described incorrectly as a comminuted fracture. To an orthopedist, the term *comminuted* implies splintering or shattering. A single, large, free-floating segment of bone between two well-defined fracture lines is a *segmental fracture.*

DISPLACEMENT AND SEPARATION   *Displacement* refers to the fracture fragments being nonconcentric or offset from each other. It is expressed in terms of direct measurement (4-mm displacement) or in terms of the percentage of the width of the bone (e.g., 50 percent displacement or complete displacement). The direction of displacement is based on the position of the distal fragment in relation to the proximal fragment.

Displacement should not be confused with *separation,* which is the distance two fragments have been pulled apart. Figure 267-3 illustrates principles of displacement and separation.

SHORTENING   Shortening is the amount by which the bone's length has been reduced and is expressed in millimeters or centimeters. Shortening may occur by impaction (telescoping of the fragments into one another) or by the overlap of two completely displaced fragments (Figure 267-4). The latter is referred to by some orthopedists as *overriding.* Because an x-ray affords no depth perception, a fracture that appears impacted on one view must be visualized at an angle 90 degrees from the first to differentiate it from a fracture whose ends are completely displaced and overriding.

Depending on the location of the fracture and the age of the patient, shortening may have long-range functional implications and may have to be corrected by closed manipulation or by surgery.

ANGULATION   Angulation is expressed in terms of two parameters: direction and amount (Figure 267-5). Quantifying the angulation is relatively simple. One need only estimate the amount of "unbending" (expressed in degrees) that would be required to make the fragments parallel.

Describing the direction of angulation is more difficult, because the terminology is less consistent among clinicians. In general, when a fracture is near the midshaft of a long bone, the direction of angulation is the direction of the *apex* of the angle formed by the two fragments. Figures 267-5A and 267-5B show 30 degrees of dorsal angulation. When a fracture is near the end of a bone, however, angulation is described in terms of the direction the *terminal fragment* is deviated. Figure 267-5C also shows 30 degrees of dorsal angulation, even though the apex of the angle formed by the fragments is pointing in the

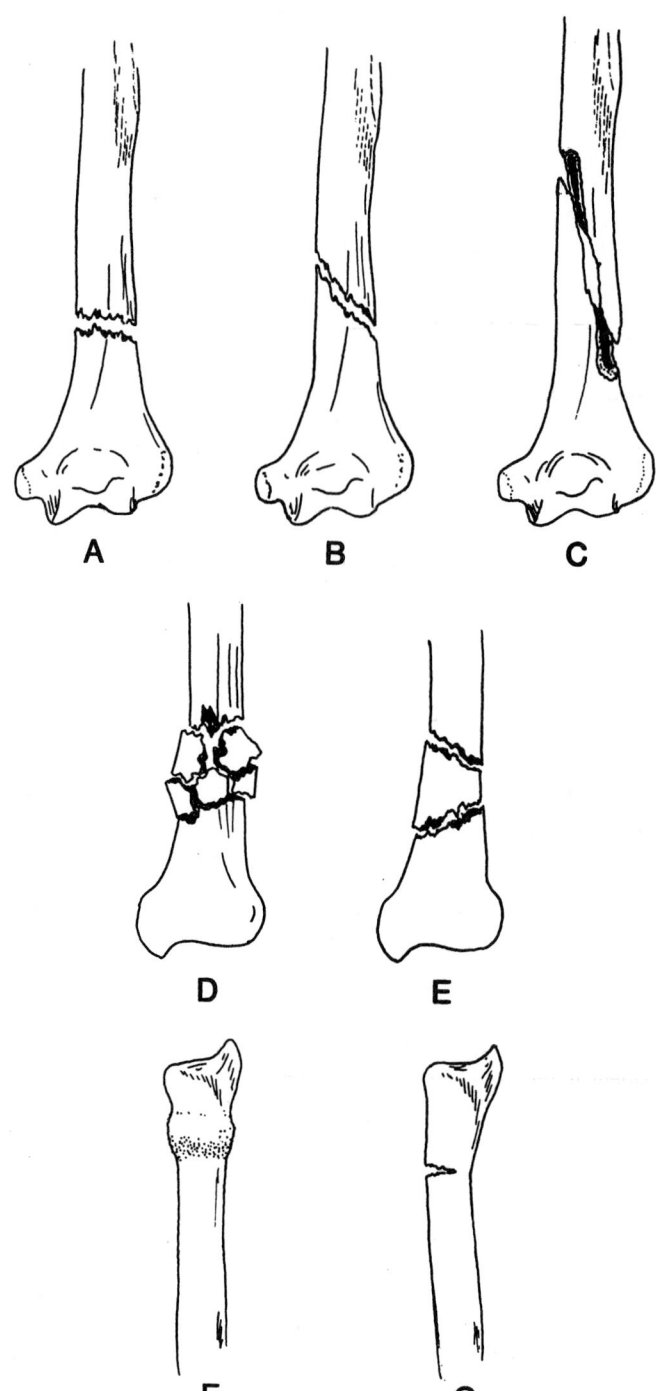

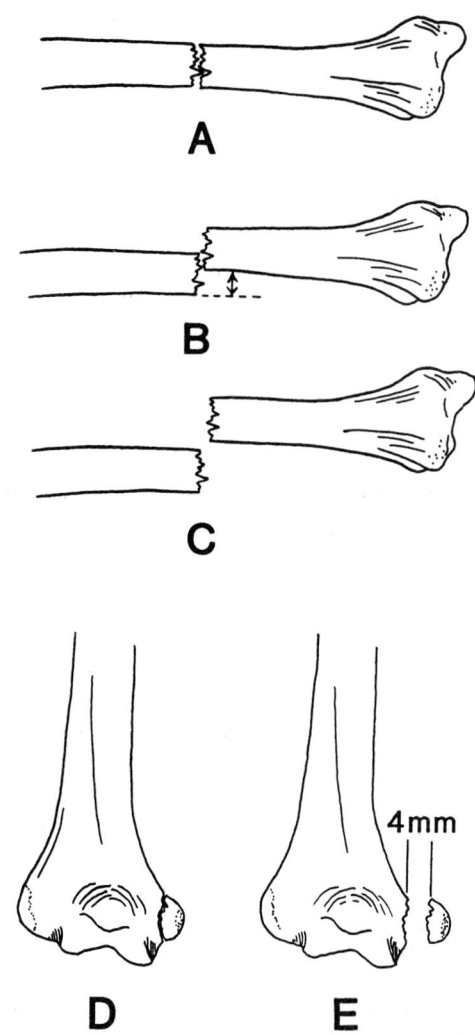

FIG. 267-2. Line orientation. **A.** Transverse. **B.** Oblique. **C.** Spiral. **D.** Comminuted. **E.** Segmental. **F.** Torus. **G.** Greenstick.

FIG. 267-3. Fracture displacement and separation. **A.** No displacement, slight separation. **B.** Fifty percent dorsal displacement. **C.** Complete dorsal displacement. **D.** Nondisplaced, no separation. **E.** A 4-mm separation.

opposite direction from that in the preceding figures. If there is a possibility of ambiguity in the description, specifying the *direction of deviation of the distal fragment* usually can resolve it.

Depending on the anatomic area involved, direction of angulation may be expressed as radial or ulnar, dorsal or volar, anterior or posterior, or lateral or medial.

ROTATIONAL DEFORMITY   Rotational deformity, that is, the extent to which the distal fracture fragment is twisted on its own axis relative to the proximal fragment, is generally not measurable on x-ray and sometimes not even radiologically apparent. This element of fracture description depends on physical examination. Its detection is particu-

larly important in the phalanges of the fingers, where, if rotational deformity goes unrecognized and uncorrected, the affected finger will be malaligned when the hand is closed.

FRACTURE COMBINED WITH DISLOCATION OR SUBLUXATION
Injuries near a joint may involve dislocation or subluxation in combination with a proximate fracture. An example is fracture of one or more ankle malleoli, together with partial or complete displacement of the talus from beneath the tibia. Fracture-dislocations are significant injuries, often requiring surgical intervention. If, in describing the injury, the clinician emphasizes the fracture component but expresses the dislocation or subluxation component as mere displacement, then the full severity may not be appreciated by the orthopedist. Such injuries should be described as *fracture-dislocations* or *fracture-subluxations*.

SALTER FRACTURES   The physiology of Salter fractures, fractures involving the epiphyseal plate at the end of the long bone of a growing child, has already been discussed. Salter fractures are classified into five types, based on the pattern of the fracture line. Because the type generally correlates with the potential for future growth disturbance (and, consequently, with the aggressiveness of treatment required), the ability to classify such injuries based on their x-ray appearance is important.

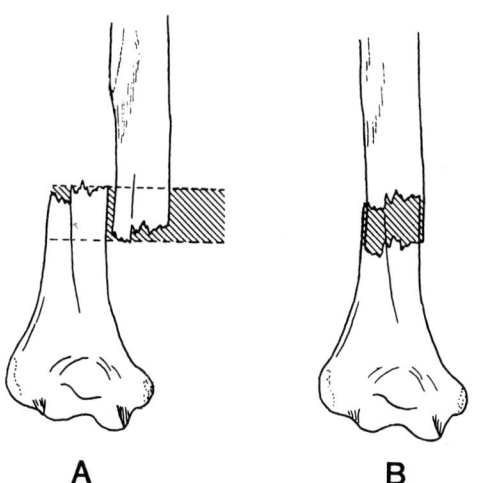

FIG. 267-4. Shortening at fracture site. **A.** Complete displacement with overriding. **B.** Impaction. In both cases, the width of the shaded area represents the amount of shortening.

Perhaps the easiest way to remember the Salter classification system is to think of these injuries not in terms of where the fracture line runs, but in terms of what has been broken off. Figure 267-6 illustrates the anatomy involved. Table 267-2 lists the five types of Salter fractures, which are illustrated in Figure 267-7. The potential for growth disturbance is least for type I and increases with the classification number, the worst prognosis being associated with type V injuries.

Type I and type V Salter fractures may be radiologically undetectable. Type I injuries usually involve little or no separation of the epiphysis from the rest of the bone, and the lucent fracture line is not visible along the equally lucent epiphyseal plate. If the epiphysis and plate slip transversely along the end of the shaft, or if the epiphysis

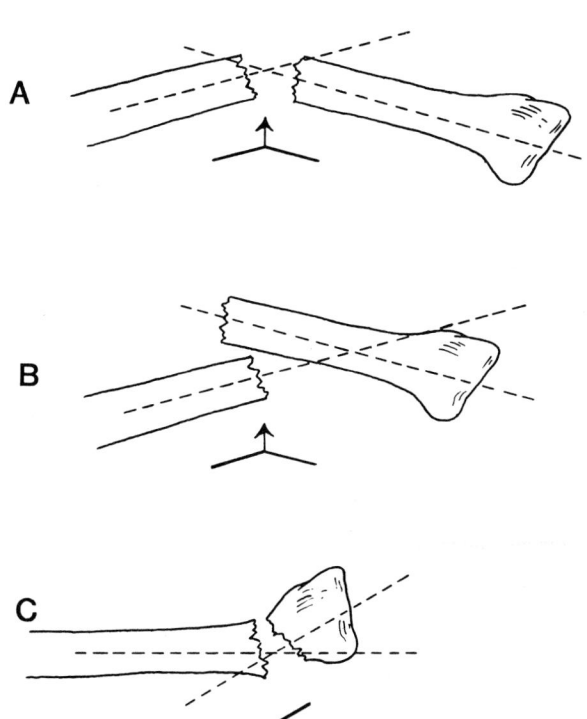

FIG. 267-5. Fracture angulation. All figures depict 30-degree dorsal angulation. **A, B.** Direction is based on the apex of the angle drawn below the figures. **C.** Direction is based on the direction of the terminal fragment.

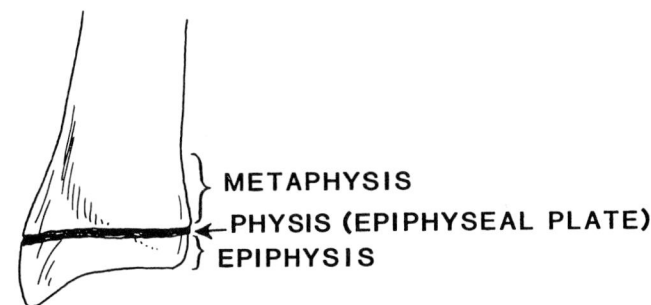

FIG. 267-6. Epiphyseal anatomy.

separates appreciably from the shaft, the abnormality will be visible on x-ray, but these rarely occur with type I injuries. Diagnosis of acute Salter type I fractures is usually clinical, based on the presence of swelling and tenderness in the region of the physis.

Type V injuries may be evident only retrospectively, when growth disturbance first begins to appear. At the time of initial presentation, however, a history of a significant axial loading force, coupled with significant tenderness in the area of the epiphyseal plate, should suggest the possibility of a type V injury. Such injuries should be immobilized and referred for orthopedic follow-up.

TREATMENT IN THE EMERGENCY DEPARTMENT

Control of Pain and Swelling

Measures to reduce swelling should be initiated early. Severe swelling not only intensifies the patient's discomfort but also may delay the application of a definitive immobilization dressing and may make the skin more susceptible to pressure sores. Although sometimes regarded as trivial modalities, the application of cold and elevation are effective in keeping swelling to a minimum or at least preventing its progression. When cold is applied, the skin should be protected from direct contact with ice-cold temperatures.

Parenteral analgesics should be administered as necessary. If the patient is relatively comfortable at rest, medication may not be required. **Analgesics have virtually no effect on the pain of movement or manipulation unless combined with hypnotics or other central nervous system active agents.** Jewelry, watches, or rings that may cause compression as an extremity swells should be removed.

Withholding Oral Intake

Any patient who may be a candidate for prompt surgical fixation, manipulation, or any other procedure under general anesthesia or procedural sedation should not be allowed to eat or drink from the moment of arrival until the need for, and timing of, such a procedure has been ascertained. This seemingly obvious point is commonly overlooked, particularly in a busy emergency department, where the process of clinical evaluation may be prolonged and patient hunger or thirst may develop in the interim.

TABLE 267-2   Description of Salter Fractures

Salter Type	What Is Broken Off
I	The entire epiphysis
II	The entire epiphysis *with* a portion of the metaphysis
III	A portion of the epiphysis
IV	A portion of the epiphysis *with* a portion of the metaphysis
V	Nothing "broken off"; compression injury of the epiphyseal plate

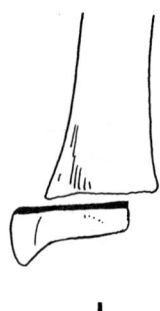 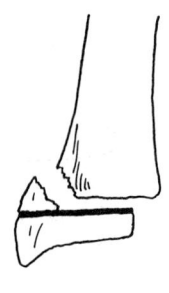 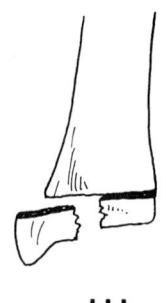 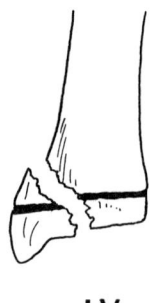 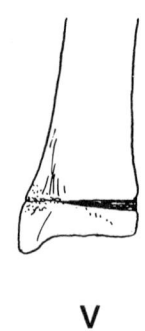

| I | II | III | IV | V |

FIG. 267-7. Epiphyseal fractures based on the classification of Salter and Harris.

Reducing Fracture Deformity

The long-term purpose of reducing significant deformity associated with fractures is restoration of normal appearance and function of the extremity. However, there are short-term reasons for reducing deformity early in the patient's course: (1) alleviating pain, (2) relieving the tension on nerves or vessels that may be stretched as they pass over the deformity, (3) eliminating or significantly minimizing the possibility of inadvertently converting a closed fracture to an open one when the skin is tented by a sharp bony fragment, and (4) restoring circulation to a pulseless distal extremity.

After the patient has been sedated, deformity at or near the midshaft of a long bone is usually easy to reduce with gradual, steady, longitudinal traction. Any rotational deformity should be corrected only after the angular component has been addressed and should be performed while traction is maintained. If reduction is performed as a definitive procedure before immobilization, attention to rotational deformity is particularly important, because of its profound effect on ultimate function. Rotational deformity is much easier to appreciate by examining the patient than by examining the x-ray.

The nearer the deformity is to a joint, the more difficult it may be to correct and the more specialized the reduction maneuver may have to be. Who performs the procedure, the emergency physician or the orthopedist, is determined by a variety of circumstances, some of which may be specific to the particular practice environment. When deformity is associated with circulatory deficit, a true emergency exists, and the anticipated delay until reduction should be considered.

Reducing Dislocations

The techniques used to reduce specific dislocations are discussed in subsequent chapters. In general, prereduction x-rays are advisable, unless circulation is threatened and prompt radiologic evaluation is not available. X-rays are needed because dislocations and fracture-dislocations may have a similar appearance on physical examination, but the techniques used to treat them may be markedly different. An example is simple anterior dislocation of the shoulder, as opposed to the same injury associated with complete fracture through the humeral neck. If the fracture is identified at the outset, the patient will be spared the pain of prolonged unsuccessful reduction attempts, and no question will arise as to exactly when the fracture might have occurred. Even "pure" dislocations may be associated with minute fracture fragments. A prereduction film usually will furnish proof of the preexistence of such fragments.

Of course, there are circumstances in which the potential benefits of a prereduction film may be outweighed by the associated expenditure of time and money. For example, a prereduction film may be omitted in a patient with a history of multiple recurrent dislocations of the shoulder who presents with history, signs, and symptoms typical of another recurrence.

The importance of postreduction films is another consideration. Occasionally a joint may feel to the clinician as though it has been reduced, when in fact it has not. Even when a maneuver is successful, the joint may re-dislocate after the patient leaves the emergency department. There is no way to prove that the joint was in anatomic po-

sition at the time of discharge, without a postreduction film. The obtaining of postreduction films is a matter of judgment and ultimately at the clinician's discretion.

Initial Management of Open Fractures

Open fractures, which may be complicated by subsequent osteomyelitis, warrant prompt and meticulous attention. The most important elements in the treatment of open fractures, aside from tetanus prophylaxis that applies generally to any wound, are irrigation, debridement, and antibiotics provided as soon as is practical. Although irrigation and debridement might be performed in the operating room, antibiotics can be administered in the emergency department.

Early administration of antibiotics can help prevent or reduce the clinical manifestations of bacterial contamination in open fractures.[4–5] The longer the interval between the time of injury and the initiation of antibiotic therapy, the less effective such therapy is likely to be. Exactly what constitutes the ideal antibiotic is controversial. An accepted combination is a first-generation cephalosporin plus an aminoglycoside, but this is by no means the only regimen in use. Aerobic and anaerobic wound cultures can be obtained before antibiotics are administered.

Antibiotics by themselves are not a substitute for irrigation and debridement, both of which have been well demonstrated to be crucial to reducing the incidence of osteomyelitis in open fractures by reducing bacterial contamination and the potential for bacterial colonization.[6–7] Irrigation should be extensive to (1) make the area more visible to inspection for foreign material, (2) float out nonviable tissue or at least float it into the field of vision so it can be removed, and (3) float out contaminated blood clots and bits of tissue. Pulsatile pumps may increase the effectiveness of irrigation provided the stream is not too forceful. Excessive force may pack debris farther into the recesses of the wound.

Debridement of minor wounds that overlie a fracture sometimes may be performed in the emergency department. When tissue damage is moderate or severe, formal debridement and irrigation are commonly performed in the operating room.

ORTHOPEDIC CONSULTATION IN THE EMERGENCY DEPARTMENT

In many cases, such as fracture of the hip, the need for hospital admission and/or orthopedic consultation in the emergency department is obvious. In some situations, however, differences of opinion may exist among emergency physicians and among orthopedists as to whether the patient needs to be seen by an orthopedist in the emergency department, or whether the patient may be treated in preliminary fashion and referred for subsequent definitive orthopedic management. Even patients with injuries that ultimately may require surgical repair, such as an unstable ankle fracture, sometimes may be immobilized and discharged for prompt orthopedic follow-up.

Some entities or situations that may warrant orthopedic consultation while the patient is still in the emergency department are discussed below.

Compartment Syndrome

The physiology and potentially catastrophic consequences of compartment syndrome are described in Chap. 278. In cases of known or suspected compartment syndrome, orthopedic consultation should be obtained promptly. Emergency surgical intervention may be required to try to avert permanent tissue damage and muscle contracture.

Irreducible Dislocation

The emergency physician sometimes may be unable to reduce a dislocation, even with the aid of nerve block or procedural sedation. Although technique is certainly a factor, there may be other reasons closed reduction cannot be accomplished, such as the interposition of soft tissues or the presence of associated fractures. Orthopedic consultation should be sought in such cases. Timely reduction, which sometimes may be achieved only surgically, may help minimize the complications (and shorten the pain) resulting from a dislocated joint.

Circulatory Compromise

Circulatory deficit resulting from musculoskeletal injury warrants prompt orthopedic consultation. Even if circulation has been restored by the emergency physician through the correction of deformity, the orthopedist may wish to investigate the integrity of the involved vessels and should at least be contacted to discuss the case.

Open Fracture

Some open fractures need to be treated aggressively in the operating room. Other types, such as those involving the phalanges, often may be irrigated in the emergency department and referred for follow-up. If there is any question, a discussion with the follow-up orthopedist may result in a mutually agreeable plan of care.

Injuries Requiring Surgical Repair

Whereas some musculoskeletal injuries require operative intervention as soon as possible, others may be treated on a delayed basis. In many cases, orthopedists differ in their preferred approach to the timing of surgery. Orthopedic consultation, at least by telephone, is indicated in cases of musculoskeletal injury that the emergency physician believes may need operative fixation or repair. The orthopedist may then exercise his or her choice to admit the patient right away, or to see the patient in timely follow-up and schedule surgery at that time.

IMMOBILIZATION TECHNIQUES

Immobilization is indicated not only for fractures but also for dislocated joints that have been reduced. When a joint becomes dislocated, the ligaments that had provided its stability are disrupted, and the joint is susceptible to redislocation until healing has occurred.

Whether plaster or fiberglass is used in the dressing depends on a number of factors, including the emergency physician's preference, the philosophy of the orthopedic community, the needs of the patient, and the hospital's resources. Fiberglass has the advantages of being lightweight, fast setting, and resistant to damage by moisture. Ultimately, the clinician should use the material he or she is most comfortable with and can use most skillfully with the best results.

Principles of Splinting

With the exception of the specific chemical substance involved, references to plaster in the following description are equally applicable to fiberglass.

The chemical reaction that causes plaster of paris (calcium sulfate) to crystallize, or set, is initiated by contact with water. The higher the water temperature, the faster the hardening process. However, the setting of plaster is an exothermic chemical reaction, which liberates heat. The faster plaster sets, the more heat it generates. This means that the maximum temperature to which the patient's skin is exposed will be the *additive* result of the water temperature plus the heat released by the plaster. For this reason, severe burns can result when plaster has been immersed in hot water, even though the temperature of the water was not sufficient to cause such burns. Although there is no universally prescribed ideal water temperature, a safe practice is to make the water slightly warmer than room temperature. If steam is visible, the water is almost certainly too hot.

To avoid irritation and minimize the potential for pressure sores, plaster dressings need to include several layers of padding between the plaster and the skin. When longitudinal splints are used, the padding need not be circumferential. Longitudinal padding will effectively protect the skin as long as it slightly exceeds the width and length of the splint. The best way to ensure this is to fashion the dry splint first and then measure the padding over it.

The length of a splint should be sufficient to provide ample leverage to immobilize the injured joint. To immobilize the elbow, for example, a splint should begin distal to the wrist and extend high up the lateral arm, to the level of the humeral neck. To effectively immobilize the ankle, a splint should extend from beneath the metatarsal heads to the high calf. If the fracture is along the midshaft of the distal extremity rather than at a joint, the splint should be long enough to immobilize the joint above and the joint below the fracture.

Splints may be fashioned from the plaster rolls normally used for casting or from prepadded material supplied on a continuous roll, which can be cut to length. When using common plaster rolls, determine the necessary length of the splint by measuring out a single layer along the extremity. Then, on a flat surface, unroll the plaster back and forth over itself to make a multilayered splint. For an adult, the splint should be at least 12 layers thick. Even more layers should be used for children, who typically remain as active as possible and have little regard for protecting the dressing.

When the dry splint has been prepared, measure out several layers of padding over it, making the padding longer and wider than the plaster. After setting the padding aside, grip each end of the splint and immerse it in water, keeping it submerged until bubbling stops (indicating that water has been fully absorbed into the interstices of the material). Then withdraw the splint and remove the excess water by sliding the thumb and index finger along the length of the plaster on each side. (Be sure to use a stripping motion, rather than crumpling or wringing out the dressing, or much of the plaster may be lost.)

The next step, frequently overlooked, is to lay the splint on a flat surface and massage the layers into one another so that they fuse. This creates a strong dressing that is solid on cross section. A splint whose separate layers are still visible on cross section is much weaker.

The padding should now be laid on the plaster and the dressing applied to the extremity, with the padded surface against the skin. An assistant can hold the splint against the extremity while it is wrapped in place with gauze bandage. Make sure the assistant uses the palms, rather than fingertips, when holding the plaster. Hardened finger dents can cause irritation or even pressure sores. If a compressive effect is desired, an elastic bandage may be wrapped over the gauze. (If an elastic bandage is wrapped directly onto plaster without an intervening layer of gauze, it will set into the plaster and lose much of its compressive function.)

While the plaster is setting, the affected joint may need to be held in a particular position. The palms, rather than the fingers, should be used. Once the setting process is well under way, the position of a joint should not be changed, or the dressing may crack and become functionally useless. If the joint has gradually migrated from the desired position, the clinician must decide to accept the current position or remove the dressing and start over. There is no need to feel hesitant about the latter course. Patients generally appreciate a desire for perfection by their clinician.

Types of Immobilization Dressings

The more common immobilization dressings used in the emergency department are discussed below and summarized in Table 267-3.

SHOULDER IMMOBILIZER   This is a removable, Velcro-fastened device that keeps the arm in "sling position" but allows less mobility than a sling (Figure 267-8). A wide band wraps around the thorax. Two cuffs are attached to the thoracic piece, one on the lateral side, which grasps the upper arm, keeping it adducted against the thorax, and one anterior, which grasps the wrist, keeping the forearm against the abdomen. This dressing is suitable for fractures about the shoulder girdle, including clavicle and well-positioned humeral neck fractures, and for reduced shoulder dislocations.

The shoulder immobilizer is also commonly used for acromioclavicular separations, although the ideal dressing for this injury is one that exerts upward pressure on the elbow and downward pressure on the clavicle. Commercial versions of such dressings exist, but they are cumbersome to apply and uncomfortable to wear, leading to noncompliance. A shoulder immobilizer (or sling and swathe) is an acceptable alternative dressing.

ARM SLING   Although it does not provide rigid immobilization, a sling (Figure 267-9) may be used as an adjunct to other splinting techniques for a variety of upper extremity injuries to enhance comfort, reduce motion, and provide some degree of support and elevation to the upper extremity. In some cases, as for nondisplaced fractures of the radial head, it may be used alone, without the need for supplementary immobilization.

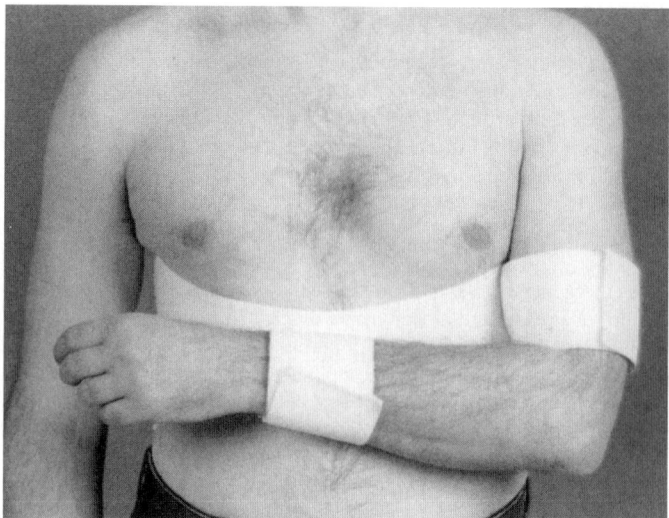

FIG. 267-8. Shoulder immobilizer.

CLAVICLE STRAP (FIGURE-OF-EIGHT BANDAGE)   The figure-of-eight clavicle strap is mentioned only as a historical note. This dressing had long been considered the appropriate immobilization method for fracture of the clavicle, but in fact it is fairly ineffective at maintaining alignment of the fracture fragments.[8] In addition, a clavicle strap may be awkward to apply, may require frequent readjustment, may cause problems related to pressure on the brachial plexus, and is often uncomfortable for the patient. A shoulder immobilizer or a simple sling is a better choice.

LONG-ARM GUTTER SPLINT   A long-arm gutter splint maintains the elbow in flexion, usually at 90 degrees (Figure 267-10). The upper extremity is placed in sling position (elbow flexed and palm facing the abdomen). The splint begins on the ulnar surface of the hand at the metacarpal heads and extends along the ulnar surface of the forearm, past the apex of the elbow, to a spot high on the lateral surface of the upper arm just opposite and below the axillary crease. It should be supplemented with a sling.

TABLE 267-3   Immobilization Devices and Uses

Immobilization Technique	Clinical Application
Shoulder immobilizer	Clavicle fracture Acromioclavicular separation Shoulder dislocation (postreduction) Humeral neck fracture
Sling	A variety of upper extremity injuries, in conjunction with other immobilization techniques; may be used alone for nondisplaced or clinically suspected fracture of the radial head
Long-arm gutter	Elbow fracture or reduced dislocation
Sugar-tong	Wrist or forearm fracture
Short-arm gutter	Metacarpal or proximal phalanx fracture [ulnar gutter for 4th or 5th ray; radial gutter for 2nd (index) or 3rd ray]
Thumb spica	Carpal scaphoid (navicular) fracture (proven or suspected) Thumb metacarpal or proximal thumb phalanx fracture
Knee immobilizer	Patella fracture Knee dislocation, postreduction Tibial plateau fracture Knee ligament injury Suspected meniscal tear (provided the knee can be fully extended)
Posterior ankle mold (consider above-the-knee extension and/or adjunctive use of ankle sugar-tong for unstable ankle injuries)	Ankle dislocation or fracture–dislocation Unstable ankle fracture (high fibula or medial and/or posterior malleolus) Widened medial mortise
Ankle stirrup	Simple ankle sprain Stable lateral malleolus fracture without other ankle involvement

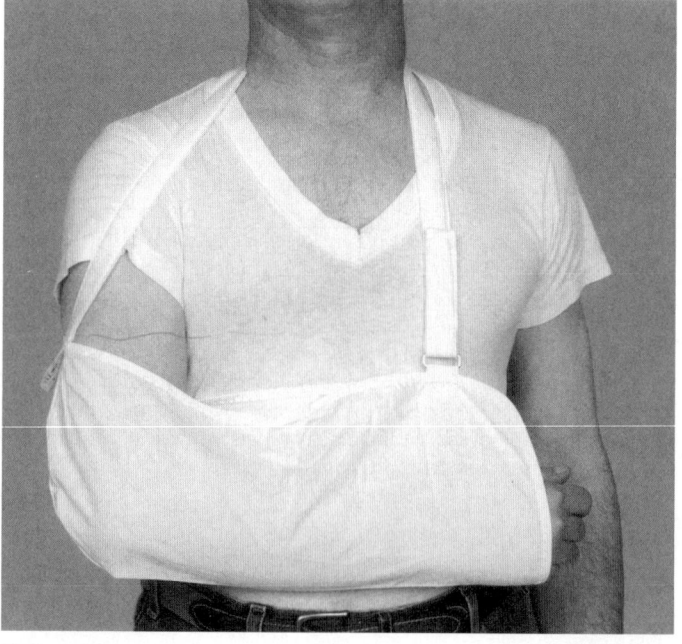

FIG. 267-9. Arm sling.

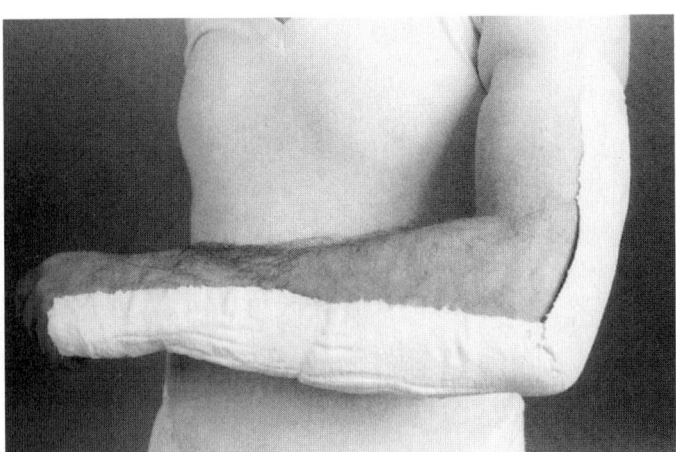

FIG. 267-10. Long-arm ulnar gutter splint.

The most common error associated with fashioning this dressing is insufficient length. If the splint is not carried far enough above the elbow, it will not exert enough leverage to prevent motion of the joint.

The long-arm ulnar gutter is useful for injuries about the elbow, including radial head fractures, nondisplaced supracondylar humeral fractures, and reduced dislocation of the elbow.

SUGAR-TONG SPLINT

The sugar-tong is a plaster splint that prevents motion of the wrist and elbow, including pronation-supination (Figure 267-11). The upper extremity is placed in sling position, as described above. The splint begins on the extensor aspect of the hand at the level of the metacarpal heads and runs along the extensor aspect of the forearm, around the elbow and humeral condyles onto the flexor aspect of the forearm, and ultimately to the palmar aspect of the hand, ending at the level of the metacarpal heads. It is wrapped in place with gauze and often topped off with a compression bandage. It should be supplemented with a sling.

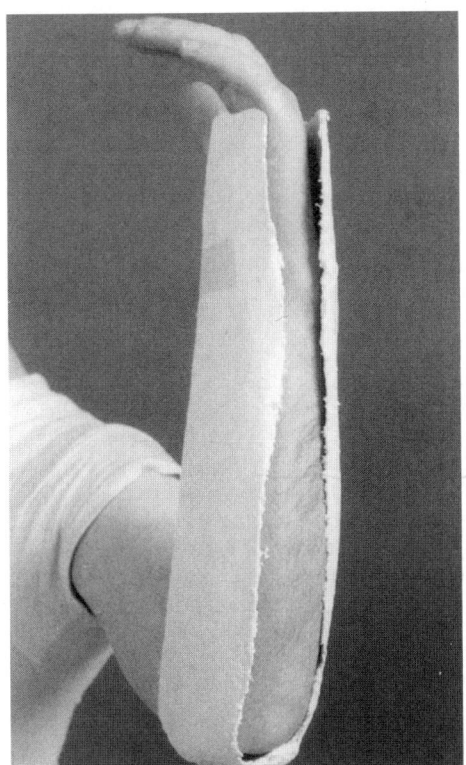

FIG. 267-11. Sugar-tong splint.

Proper length of the sugar-tong dressing is important. Too short a splint will fail to immobilize the wrist. If the dressing is too long, it will impair motion of the metacarpophalangeal joints, leaving them stiff and making the fingers more susceptible to swelling due to immobility.

The sugar-tong splint is appropriate for fractures about the wrist or distal forearm. Some orthopedists use it as a definitive dressing after reduction of wrist fractures.

"COCK-UP" WRIST SPLINT (TO BE AVOIDED)

A "cock-up" splint is a removable device that extends from the distal forearm to the proximal portion of the hand, and it maintains the wrist in a dorsiflexed position. The splint is fastened with Velcro straps. **Cock-up splints should not be used for fractures of the wrist or carpals,** because such injuries with plaster dressings are usually caused by forceful dorsiflexion, and the splint only reproduces the position of injury, imposing considerable pain in the process. Fractures about the wrist are generally immobilized in neutral position. Colles fractures may even be immobilized in palmar flexion after reduction.

"Cock-up" splints may be useful in some situations unrelated to fractures, such as to immobilize the wrist for tendinitis or to support it in the case of wrist drop due to radial nerve palsy. In such instances, dorsiflexion of the wrist will preserve the patient's grip strength.

SHORT-ARM GUTTER SPLINT

A short-arm gutter immobilizes the wrist and the ulnar or radial half of the hand (Figure 267-12). The ulnar gutter, for example, extends along the ulnar surface of the hand and forearm, beginning just proximal to the tip of the fifth finger and ending high onto the forearm. The splint should be wide enough to encompass the fourth and fifth rays (fingers and metacarpals) on the extensor and palmar aspects of the hand. The splint is wrapped in place, with the fourth and fifth fingers bound together but separated by a thin layer of padding to prevent maceration of the skin. The metacarpophalangeal joints and interphalangeal joints should be positioned in gentle flexion. The dressing should be supplemented with a sling.

The short-arm ulnar gutter is useful for fractures of the proximal phalanx of the ring or little finger or for fractures of the fourth or fifth metacarpal (including the common "boxer's fracture"). The counterpart of this splint, the short-arm radial gutter, is designed in similar fashion but extends along the radial surface of the hand and forearm and is used for comparable injuries of the index or middle rays. It is fashioned with a hole that allows the thumb to pass through.

THUMB SPICA

A thumb spica immobilizes the wrist and the thumb (Figure 267-13). The term *spica* applies to any dressing that encompasses a main trunk plus one or more of its branches, in this case, the forearm plus the thumb. It is used for fractures of the scaphoid or for fractures of the thumb metacarpal or proximal phalanx.

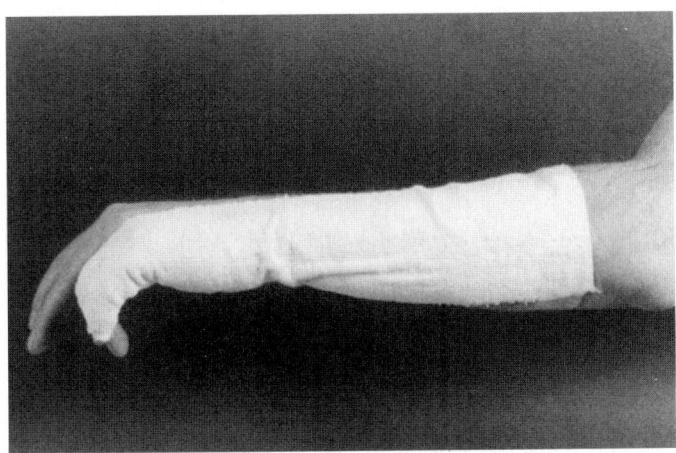

FIG. 267-12. Short-arm ulnar gutter splint.

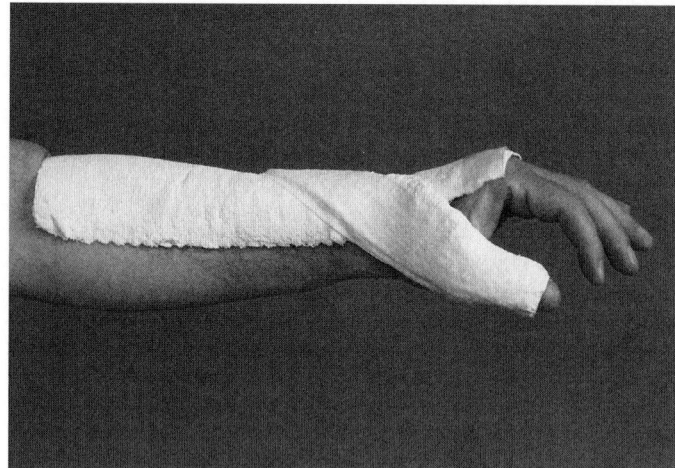

FIG. 267-13. Thumb spica splint.

A thumb spica can be fashioned from one wide plaster splint, but a more effective and better-looking dressing can be made from two separate splints. The wrist piece runs along the extensor aspect of the hand and forearm, beginning at the metacarpal heads and ending just short of the elbow. The more narrow thumb piece, approximately 2 in. wide, extends from the tip of the thumb (which has been padded separately), along the outer aspect of the thumb metacarpal, and onto the extensor aspect of the forearm, well overlapping the first splint. Along their area of contact, the two splints are molded into each other, with no padding between them, to form a sturdy dressing. The plaster is wrapped in place with gauze, and a compression wrap may be added at the clinician's discretion. The dressing is supplemented with a sling.

While the plaster is setting, optimal position can be achieved by keeping the wrist in *neutral* position and having the patient oppose the tips of the thumb and index fingers in the form of an "OK" sign. This preserves thumb-to-index pinch function, thereby minimizing the patient's incapacitation. It also avoids reproducing the position of injury in the case of scaphoid fractures, which are typically caused by forced dorsiflexion of the wrist.

KNEE IMMOBILIZER The knee immobilizer is a removable circumferential device that extends from the thigh to just above the ankle (Figure 267-14). The splint contains longitudinal metal struts and is fastened with Velcro straps.

A knee immobilizer maintains the knee joint in extension, its position of maximum stability. The device is useful for a variety of injuries, including fracture of the lateral or medial tibial plateau, fracture of the patella, meniscal injuries (provided the patient's knee is not locked in partial flexion), and ligamentous strains or tears.

Use of an immobilizer for days to a week or two may result in painful stiffness of the knee joint. For this reason, orthopedic follow-up should occur within about 7 days. If immobilization is indicated beyond that point, the orthopedist may replace the original device with a cast brace or other orthosis that allows controlled and gradually progressive range of motion.

Motion and Strength Exercises for the Knee Joint stiffness and instability due to quadriceps weakness may occur rapidly when an injured knee is immobilized. Patients wearing an immobilizer should be encouraged to remove the device periodically and perform the following exercises.

1. Passive flexion: While sitting on a flat surface, pull upward on the ends of a towel draped beneath the sole of the foot, creating as much knee flexion as possible without undue pain.
2. "Gravity-assisted" flexion: While sitting on the edge of a bed or chair, support the knee in extension, with the well foot beneath the

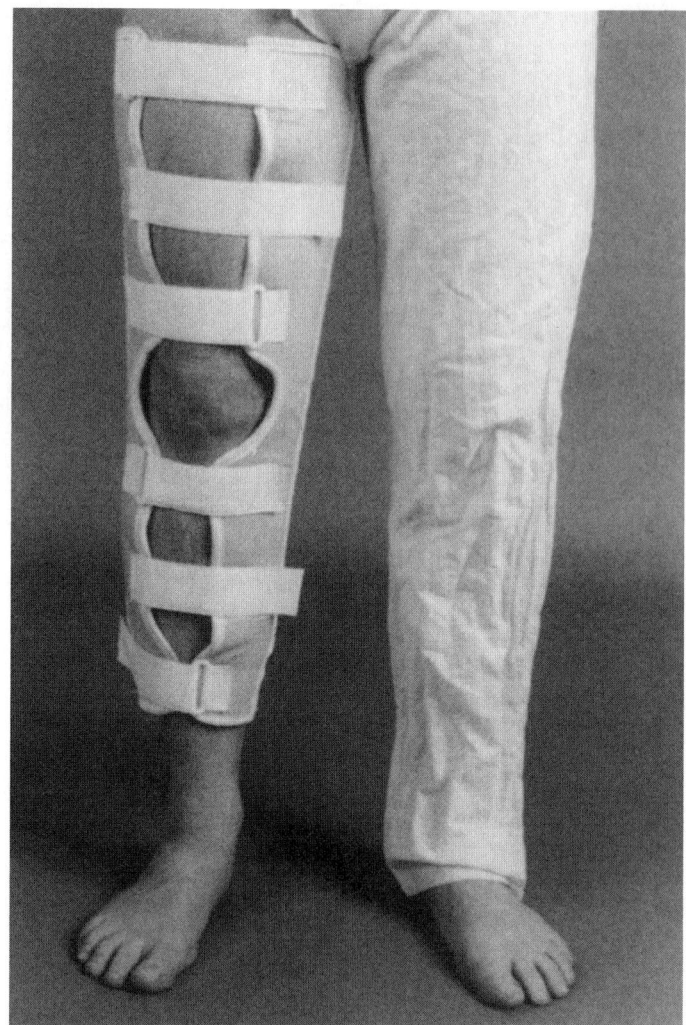

FIG. 267-14. Knee immobilizer.

ankle of the injured extremity, then gradually lower the supporting foot so the injured knee "drops" into flexion. When tolerance is reached, bring the knee back into extension.
3. Quadriceps strengthening: While lying supine with a pillow beneath the knee, actively bring the knee to full extension in a straight leg raise and then relax.

Each of these exercises should be performed as multiple repetitions several times a day.

POSTERIOR ANKLE MOLD A posterior mold is a plaster splint that immobilizes the ankle (Figure 267-15). It begins beneath the metatarsal heads, runs along the plantar aspect of the foot, and continues up the back of the lower leg, ending at high calf. The splint is used for severe sprains or fractures of the ankle. Support may be supplemented by a sugar-tong component running down one side of the leg, beneath the heel, and up the other side. Where the two components overlap, they are molded together. The additional component helps minimize inversion and eversion of the ankle. Even more stability is provided by continuing the posterior splint past the back of the knee to the high posterior thigh and using wider plaster for this area. With the knee slightly flexed, rotational motion at the ankle also will be prevented.

While the plaster is setting, the ankle should be maintained in a position as close as possible to neutral, that is, at 90 degrees to the leg. This facilitates regaining range of motion after the dressing is removed. Because most patients with ankle injuries tend to keep the ankle plantar flexed, the clinician usually will have to maintain passive

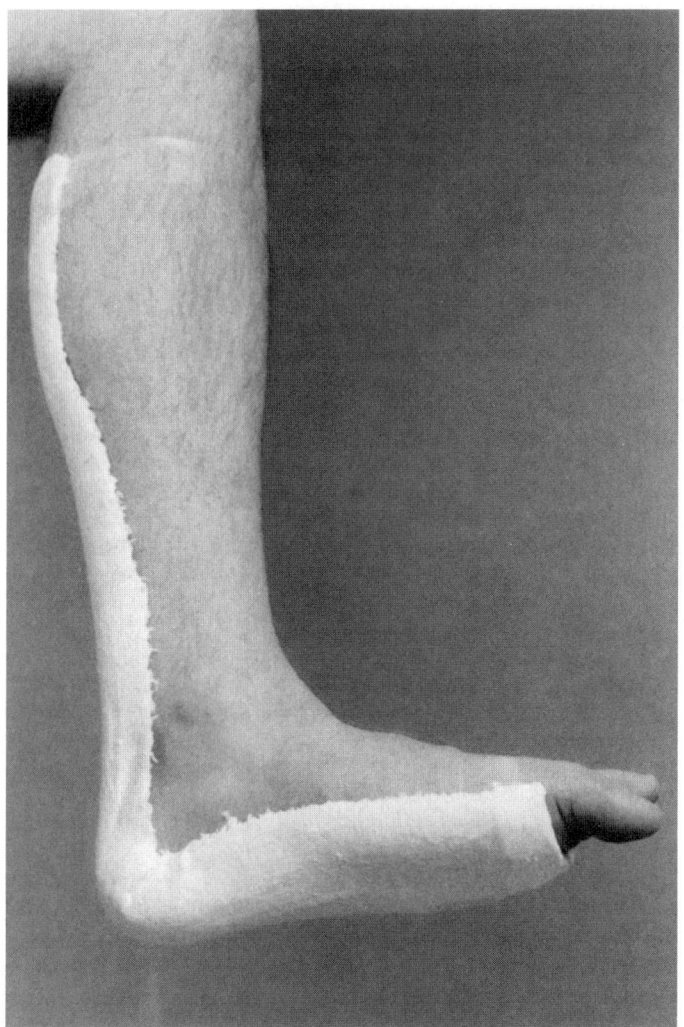

FIG. 267-15. Posterior ankle mold.

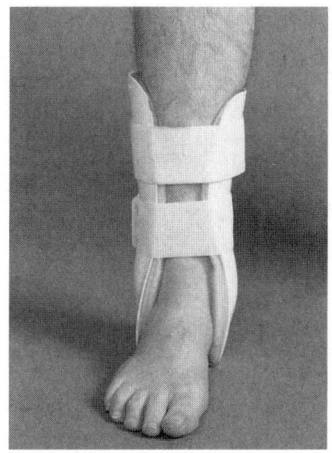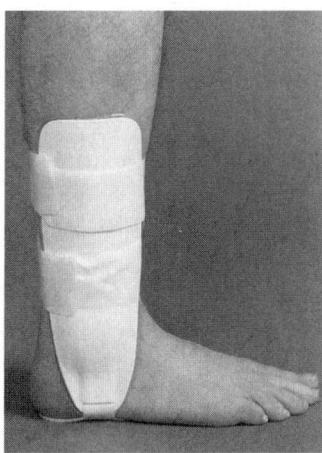

FIG. 267-16. Ankle stirrup.

grasp the medial and lateral aspects of the ankle and lower leg. The final step is to wrap the straps about the posterior and anterior aspects of the dressing.

Motion and Strength Exercises for the Ankle   Exercises to restore range of motion, stability, and balance should be started as soon as possible after an ankle injury.

1. Active dorsiflexion and plantarflexion: When done supine with the foot well elevated, this exercise may also enhance lymphatic drainage, thereby reducing swelling.
2. Passive dorsiflexion: One method for performing this exercise is to stand with the palms braced against the wall and then to bend the knee toward the wall while keeping the entire plantar surface of the foot flat on the floor.
3. Eversion, dorsiflexion, and plantarflexion against resistance: This exercise may be achieved by manually applying a counterforce with a stretchable elastic cord (commercially available). Standing on the toes is another means of resistive plantarflexion.

Each of these exercises should be performed as multiple repetitions several times a day.

ADJUNCTS TO AMBULATION

Crutches

Crutches should be used by patients who can bear little or no weight on an injured lower extremity. Ideal crutch height is one hand width

dorsiflexion by exerting gentle pressure with a palm beneath the sole of the foot. An exception to the 90-degree principle is immobilization for rupture of the Achilles tendon. Patients with this injury should be immobilized in plantar flexion to reduce tension on the tendon.

ANKLE STIRRUP   Easier to apply and less cumbersome for the patient than a posterior mold, the ankle stirrup (Figure 267-16) is useful for ankle sprains and for stable lateral malleolus fractures. The ankle stirrup is essentially an air-padded "sugar-tong" splint held in place by Velcro straps. Unlike the posterior mold, this device is intended for use in conjunction with weight bearing. It limits inversion more effectively than taping, but allows normal plantarflexion and dorsiflexion. This feature and the graduated compressive effect of the air-filled layers may result in less swelling and edema, less joint stiffness, and a faster return to comfortable ambulation than is typically observed after plaster immobilization.[9]

The stirrup may be removed for purposes of bathing or when not bearing weight. If the patient does remove the splint temporarily, a common error when reapplying it is to fail to unwrap the Velcro straps completely—specifically, to leave the straps attached posteriorly, so that the splint is "hinged" along its posterior aspect, like a "book." This may result in the foot persistently slipping forward and out of the splint. The clinician may wish to instruct the patient that the proper way to reapply the splint is to unwrap the straps *all the way around,* so that the sides fall apart bilaterally, with the foot pad acting as the "hinge" on the plantar aspect (Figure 267-17). The foot can then be positioned on the lower pad, and the sides brought together to adequately

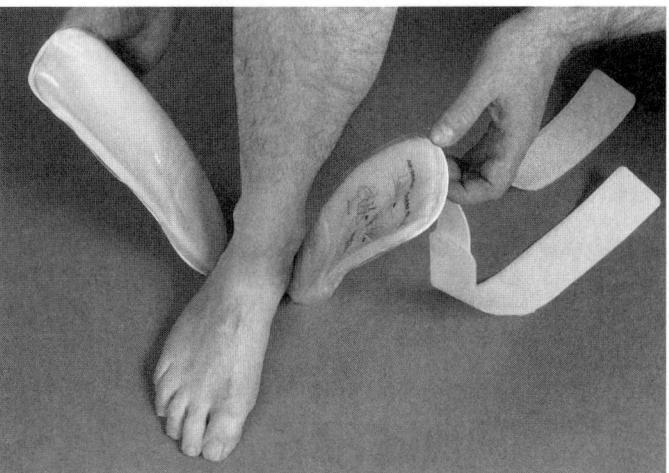

FIG. 267-17. Technique for applying ankle stirrup.

below the axillae. The grip bar should be adjusted to a height at which the elbows are mildly flexed while supporting the body weight. The patient should be instructed to bear the pressure of the pads against the sides of the thorax rather than in the axillae, or brachial plexus injury might result (crutch palsy).

Any of several crutch gaits may be prescribed. With a two-point gait, the patient advances the crutches first and then brings the well leg up to the crutches ("swing-to" gait) or just past the crutches ("swing-through" gait). With a three-point gait, the crutches and the injured extremity are advanced together, and the well extremity is advanced to meet them. The three-point gait results in slower forward progression than does the two-point gait, but it requires less energy. Partial or no weight bearing may be prescribed for the injured extremity, regardless of the gait used.

The method for negotiating stairs is similar for the two- and three-point gaits. To ascend stairs, the patient advances the well extremity up to the next step, followed by the crutches and the injured extremity. To descend stairs, the crutches are lowered first.

Walkers and Canes

Most elderly or infirm patients do not have the strength to use crutches safely. For them, a walker or cane is more suitable. Unfortunately, these devices are more appropriate for partial weight-bearing than for full non-weight-bearing conditions. Elderly patients who can bear no weight on an injured extremity may require initial bedrest and subsequent rehabilitation.

The technique for using a walker is essentially intuitive, with the patient simply lifting it and placing it a short distance ahead and then advancing up to it. In contrast, the technique for using a cane tends to be counterintuitive. Most patients instinctively hold a cane on the same side as the injured extremity. In fact, when the cane is held in the hand on the *well* side, much less strength is required to maintain balance, resulting in an easier and less awkward gait. The patient should be instructed to advance the cane (held on the well side) and the injured extremity simultaneously and then advance the noninjured extremity to meet them.

DISCHARGE INSTRUCTIONS

Continuous elevation of the injured part usually helps minimize swelling and pain. However, most individuals do not realize that, to be effective, elevation must be above the level of the heart. Patients with an injured lower extremity often sit at home or at work with the leg resting on a chair, thinking they are complying with instructions. The patient should understand that the benefits of elevating a lower extremity can be achieved only in a recumbent or near-recumbent position, with the leg supported higher than the rest of the body.

Patients discharged in a lower-extremity plaster dressing should be cautioned not to rest the heel on the floor or any other hard surface. Plaster takes about 24 h to fully set. During this time, prolonged pressure on the heel can gradually create an indentation that may cause significant discomfort or even a pressure sore. This is not a consideration with fiberglass, which sets almost immediately.

If an upper-extremity sugar-tong dressing has been applied, the patient should be instructed to work the fingers (wiggle or wave) as much as possible to minimize stiffness and swelling. The sugar-tong splint should allow full flexion of the metacarpophalangeal joints.

Patients should be advised to monitor the fingers or toes for excessive swelling, decreased sensation, or cyanosis and to be alert for a significant increase in pain. Any of these signs or symptoms warrants a return to the emergency department or prompt evaluation by the follow-up physician.

When crutches, a cane, or a walker is supplied, instruction for use should be provided, and the patient's ability to navigate with such aids should be verified.

FOLLOW-UP

There is no universally prescribed follow-up interval for specific injuries. Orthopedists differ in their opinions as to how soon patients should be seen. In general, patients with unreduced fractures or injuries that may require surgical intervention should be seen within 1 or 2 days.

Sometimes the situation may be discussed with the follow-up physician and an appointment arranged while the patient is still in the emergency department. Alternatively, the emergency physician may instruct the patient to contact the follow-up physician or clinic as soon as possible. If the name of the injury is written on the discharge instruction sheet, the patient can convey it at the time of the call. Based on this information, the follow-up physician can decide when the patient should be seen.

COMPLICATIONS

Complications associated with musculoskeletal injury may be early or delayed and may occur minutes, days, weeks, or even months later.

Neurologic Deficit

Neurologic injury resulting from long-bone fractures or joint dislocations is usually due to traction or pressure on a peripheral nerve or a nerve plexus. Such complications usually manifest themselves early. Recovery may take hours, days, or weeks. Sometimes the injury is irreversible. Prompt reduction of deformity often can prevent, eliminate, or mitigate the effects of neurologic involvement, but it is not a guarantee against permanent deficit.

Vascular Injury

Peripheral vessels that run close to a joint sometimes may be compressed or disrupted when the joint becomes dislocated, as, for example, with dislocation of the ankle or knee (tibiofemoral joint). Loss of peripheral pulse or poor to absent capillary refill calls for expeditious reduction of deformity. Even after reduction, evidence of significant vascular injury may be delayed. Patients who experience tibiofemoral dislocation, for example, often undergo routine postreduction angiography to verify the integrity and patency of the popliteal vessels, regardless of whether a circulatory deficit was noted on initial examination.

Compartment Syndrome

After a fracture or a direct blow to an extremity, there may be extravasation of blood, swelling of muscle tissues, and impairment of venous flow within one or more fascial compartment. The resulting increase in pressure within the limb may lead to circulatory compromise, neurologic damage, and muscle necrosis, known collectively as *compartment syndrome*. This is a true surgical emergency, and early recognition is crucial. Compartment syndrome is discussed in detail in Chap. 278.

Delayed and Late Complications

Patients who have sustained a fracture may be at risk for pulmonary fat embolus, usually originating from the marrow of a large bone, such as the femur. If fat embolism occurs, it is usually within the first few days after injury, rather than in the first hours. This event may have a variable effect on pulmonary function, ranging from mild distress to severe or even fatal respiratory failure.

The most delayed complications of fractures include nonunion, malunion (healing with deformity), joint stiffness, traumatic arthritis of an involved joint, avascular necrosis of one of the bone fragments, and, in the case of open fractures, osteomyelitis.

ACKNOWLEDGMENTS

Original artwork is by Eleanore Denton Rhodes, AMI. Photography is by Joy Miller, BPA., Joe Driscoll, and Kevin Hagan.

REFERENCES

1. Salter RB, Harris WR: Injuries involving the epiphyseal plate. *J Bone Joint Surg* 45A:587, 1963.
2. Buckwalter JA, Einhorn TA, Marsh JL: Bone and joint healing, in Bucholz RW, Heckman JD (eds): *Rockwood and Green's Fractures in Adults,* vol 1, 5th ed. Philadelphia, Lippincott Williams & Wilkins, 2001, p. 245.
3. Schultz RJ: *The Language of Fractures.* Baltimore, Williams & Wilkins, 1972.
4. Braun R, Enzler MA, Rittmann WW: A double-blind clinical trial of prophylactic cloxacillin in open fractures. *J Orthop Trauma* 1:12, 1987.
5. Worlock P, Slack R, Harvey L, Mawhinney R: The prevention of infection in open fractures: An experimental study of the effects of antibiotic therapy. *J Bone Joint Surg* 70A:1341, 1988.
6. Olson SA, Finkeheier, CG, Moehring, HD: Open fractures, in Bucholz RW, Heckman JD (eds): *Rockwood and Green's Fractures in Adults,* vol 1, 5th ed. Philadelphia, Lippincott Williams & Wilkins, 2001, p. 285.
7. Worlock P, Slack R, Harvey L, et al: The prevention of infection in open fractures: An experimental study of the effect of fracture stability. *Injury* 25:31, 1994.
8. Anderson K, Jensen PO, Lauritzen J: Treatment of clavicular fractures: Figure of eight bandage vs. a simple sling. *Acta Orthop Scand* 57:71, 1987.
9. Kannus P, Renstron P. Treatment for acute tears of the lateral ligaments of the ankle: operation, cast, or early controlled mobilization. *J Bone Joint Surg Am* 73:305, 1991.

INJURIES TO THE HAND AND DIGITS
Robert L. Muelleman
Michael C. Wadman

Hand injuries are commonly encountered in the emergency department (ED). The best outcome often depends on an accurate initial evaluation and treatment. This chapter discusses soft tissue injuries distal to the volar wrist crease and fractures distal to the carpal bones.

ANATOMY

The hand consists of 27 bones: 14 phalangeal bones, 5 metacarpal bones, and 8 carpal bones arranged in 5 rays of metacarpals and phalanges having its base at the carpometacarpal (CMC) articulation (Figure 268-1).

The carpal bones are made up of two rows of four bones. They are concave on the volar surface and bridged by flexor retinaculum. This forms the carpal tunnel through which pass the median nerve and the nine long flexor tendons of the fingers. The bases of the second and third CMC articulation are fixed. The thumb, ring, and little finger have mobility at the CMC joint and provide movement that allows for grasp and adaptive movement of the hand.

The soft tissue supporting these bones and joints are the capsular ligamentous structures that give stability, the intrinsic muscles of the hand, and the tendinous structures that generate mobility. The collateral ligaments of the metacarpophalangeal (MP) joints are tightest in flexion (Figure 268-2). The interphalangeal (IP) collaterals are tight throughout the entire range of motion.

The intrinsic muscles of the hand are those that have their origins and insertions within the hand. They consist of the muscle of the thenar and hypothenar eminences, adductor pollicis, the interossei, and the lumbricals (Figure 268-3).

The thenar muscles cover the thumb metacarpal, originate in the flexor retinaculum and carpal bones, and insert at the base of the first metacarpal and first proximal phalanx. The thenar muscles consist of abductor pollicis brevis, opponens pollicis, and flexor pollicis brevis. The median nerve innervates all three. Adductor pollicis is innervated by the ulnar nerve and originates from the second and third metacarpals and inserts in the first proximal phalanx.

The hypothenar group includes opponens digiti minimi, the flexor digiti minimi, and the abductor digiti minimi. These muscles originate in the flexor retinaculum and carpal bones and insert at the proximal phalanx and metacarpal of the little finger. They are innervated by the ulnar nerve.

There are seven interossei. The three palmar and four dorsal interossei lie between the metacarpal bones and originate from them. The palmar interosseus and the palmar portion of the dorsal interosseus have an insertion into the extensor hood. The palmar interosseus adducts the index, ring, and small finger. The dorsal portion of the dorsal interosseus inserts by tendons into the base of the proximal phalanx. The dorsal interosseous muscles abduct the fingers away from the midline. The interossei are innervated by the ulnar nerve (Figure 268-4).

The lumbricals arise from the flexor digitorum profundus tendons in the palm and course radially to the MP joints and reinforce the interosseous lateral band on the radial side of the digit. The lumbricals contribute little to the flexion of the MP joint; however, they contribute to the extension of the IP joints. The lumbricals play a critical role coordinating the flexor and extensor system of the digits. The median nerve innervates the radial two lumbricals, and the ulnar nerve innervates the ulnar two.

The extensor tendons course over the dorsal side of the forearm, wrist, and hand. Nine extensor tendons pass under the extensor retinaculum and separate into six compartments. In the dorsum of the hand, the extensors digitorum communis are connected by junctura. **Because of this, a complete tendon laceration proximal to the junctura may still result in normal extensor function.** In the finger, the extensor expansion divides into a central slip that attaches to the middle phalanx and into two lateral bands that join with the tendons of the lumbricals and interosseous muscles and that attach to the base of the distal phalanx.

The flexor tendons course over the volar side of the forearm, wrist, and hand. Flexor carpi radialis, flexor carpi ulnaris, and palmaris longus primarily flex the wrist. The remaining nine tendons pass through the carpal tunnel. One tendon goes to the base of the distal phalanx of the thumb. The other four digits have two tendons each. The flexor digitorum superficialis (FDS) inserts into the middle phalanx and flexes all the joints it crosses. The flexor digitorum profundus (FDP) runs deep to FDS until the level of the MP joint where FDS bifurcates. FDP inserts at the base of the distal phalanx and acts primarily to flex the distal interphalangeal (DIP) joint as well as all other joints flexed by FDS (Figure 268-5). Unlike the extensor tendons, the flexor tendons are enclosed in synovial sheaths, making them prone to deep space infections.

The hand and digits have dual blood supplies with contributions from the radial and ulnar arteries. The blood supply of the proximal portion of the hand is composed of a series of deep and superficial arches on the palmar and dorsal side. The blood supply of the fingers is distributed by the digital arteries that arise from the superficial palmar arch (see Figures 268-3 and 268-6).

The radial, ulnar, and median nerves innervate the hand (Figure 268-7). In the hand, the median and ulnar nerves have mixed motor and sensory function. The radial nerve (C5-T1) just has sensory function to the dorsal radial aspect of the hand. The ulnar nerve (C7-T1) supplies sensory function to the ulnar one and one-half fingers and motor function to the hypothenar muscles, ulnar two lumbricals, interossei, adductor pollicis, and the deep head of the flexor pollicis longus. The median nerve (C5-T1) supplies sensory function to the thumb and radial two and one-half fingers and motor function to abductor pollicis brevis, superficial head of flexor pollicis brevis, and

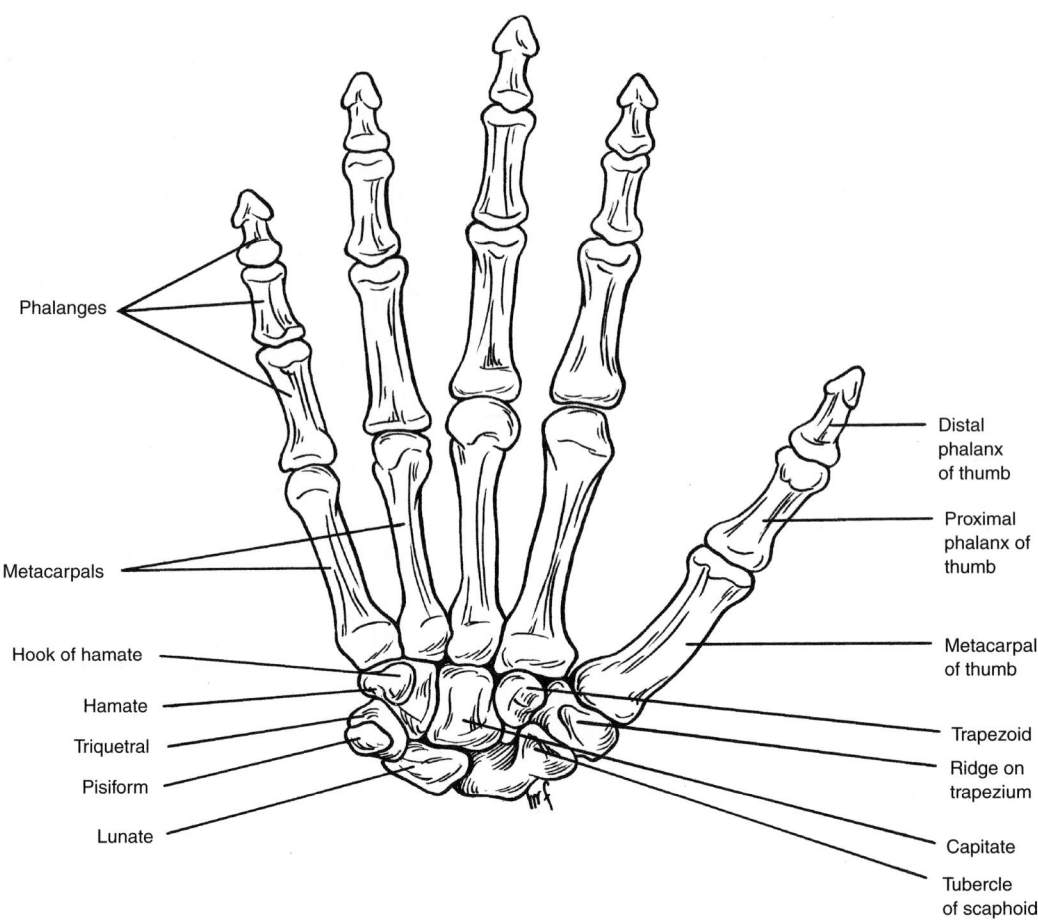

FIG. 268-1. Bones of the hand.

opponens pollicis. As the digital nerves course through the palm, they are superficial structures and are the structures most often injured, so that digital nerve sensation and two-point discrimination should be routinely assessed when evaluating lacerations of the palm (Figure 268-8). The palm is often called "no-man's-land" because penetrating injuries in this area are so difficult to evaluate and treat. Careful neu-

rovascular testing of the hand and digits is necessary for all palmar injuries that involve more than the skin, and hand consultation is advised if the extent of injury is uncertain. In the digits, digital nerves divide into volar and dorsal branches to supply sensation to the fingers. Knowing their location is important to properly perform a digital block (see Figure 268-3).

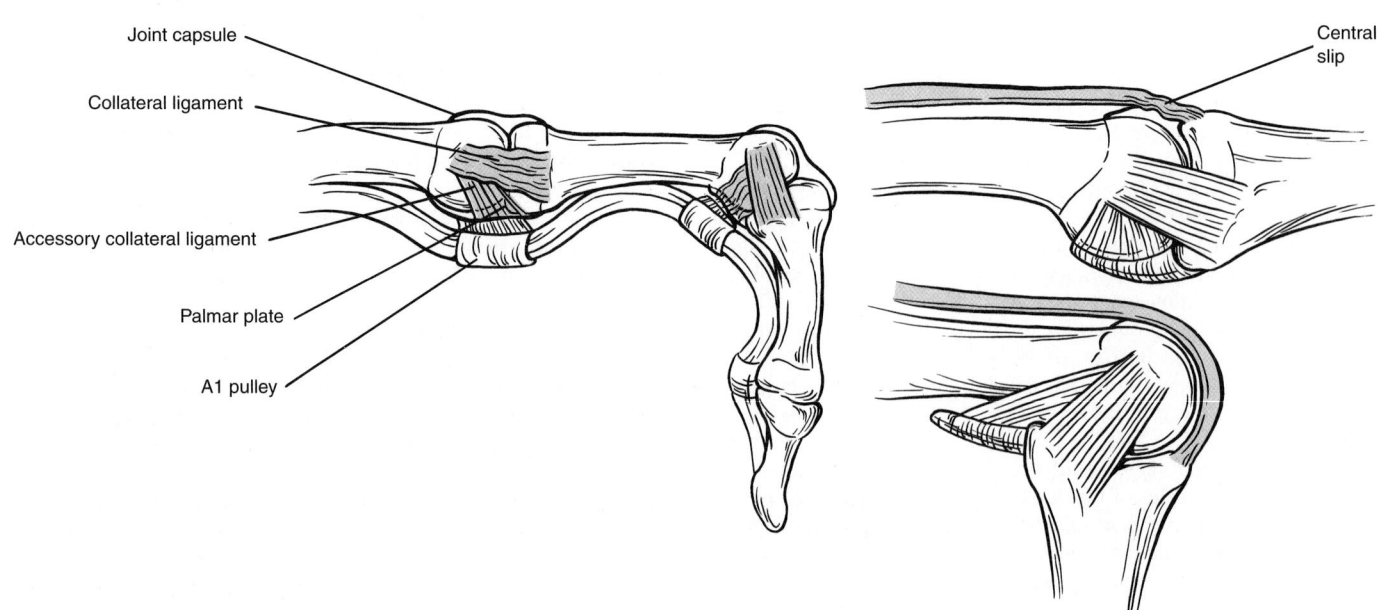

FIG. 268-2. Ligament attachments of the metacarpophalangeal and interphalangeal joints.

FIG. 268-3. Anterior view of the hand showing relationship of muscles and tendon sheaths.

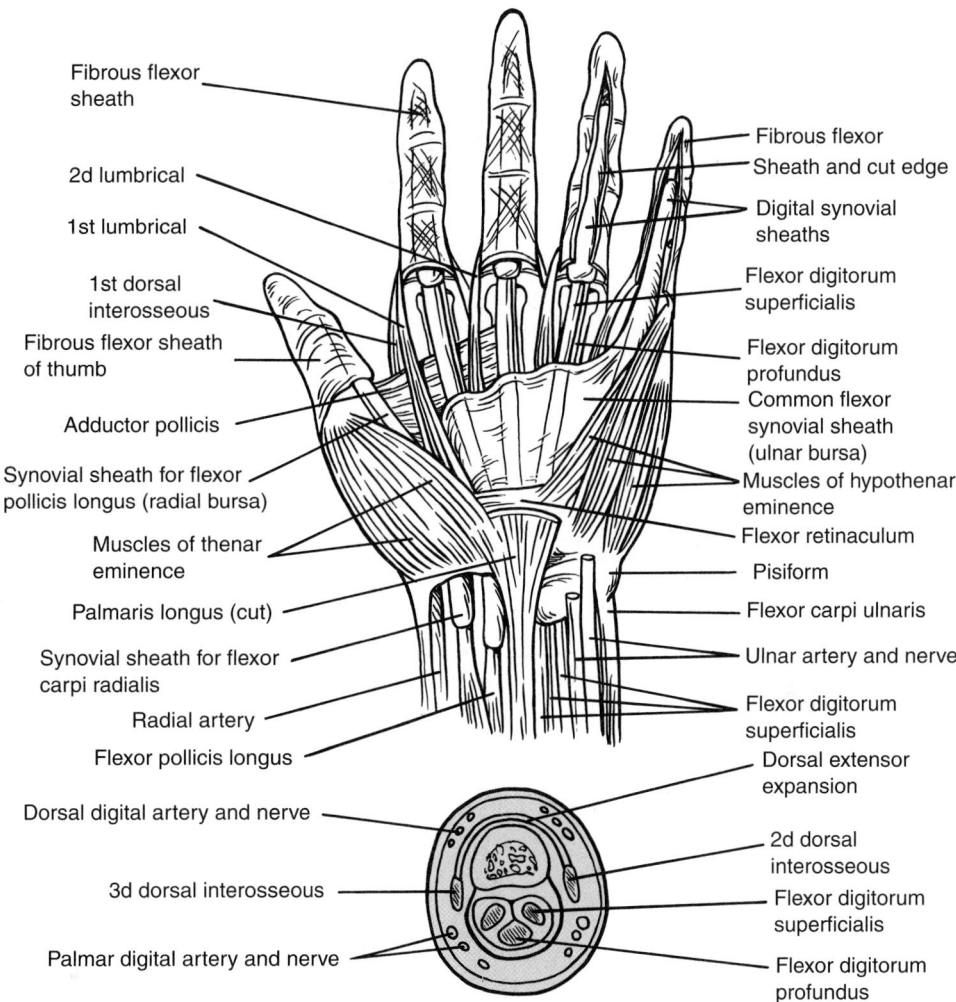

Fibrous flexor sheath

2d lumbrical

1st lumbrical

1st dorsal interosseous

Fibrous flexor sheath of thumb

Adductor pollicis

Synovial sheath for flexor pollicis longus (radial bursa)

Muscles of thenar eminence

Palmaris longus (cut)

Synovial sheath for flexor carpi radialis

Radial artery

Flexor pollicis longus

Dorsal digital artery and nerve

3d dorsal interosseous

Palmar digital artery and nerve

Fibrous flexor Sheath and cut edge

Digital synovial sheaths

Flexor digitorum superficialis

Flexor digitorum profundus

Common flexor synovial sheath (ulnar bursa)

Muscles of hypothenar eminence

Flexor retinaculum

Pisiform

Flexor carpi ulnaris

Ulnar artery and nerve

Flexor digitorum superficialis

Dorsal extensor expansion

2d dorsal interosseous

Flexor digitorum superficialis

Flexor digitorum profundus

PRINCIPLES OF EVALUATION

It is important not to let a visually striking hand injury delay the identification and treatment of other potentially life-threatening injuries. After hemorrhage control, assessment involves a detailed history, general hand examination, testing of nerves and tendons, anesthesia, and direct wound inspection. Comparison with the uninjured hand is helpful, especially to identify partial motor or sensory deficits.

History

The history should include the time and cause of injury as well as the possibility of associated crush, burn, or chemical exposure. The position of the hand at the time of injury should be determined. **Injuries with the digits in flexion may result in retraction of the cut end of the tendon when the digit is examined in neutral position.** The patient's occupation, avocations, prior hand injuries, and handedness should be documented because they are important indicators of the functional impact of the injury.

General Hand Examination

The general examination should detail the extent of injury by documenting the amount of devascularization, status of the skin, posture of the fingers, and presence of deformity or active bleeding. Bilateral grip strength should be checked.

Both hands should be compared when assessing motor, sensory, and tendon function to better assess baseline function. Range of motion and strength should be tested against resistance. Have the patient make a clenched fist to observe the orientation of the middle and distal phalanxes. They should be oriented parallel to each other with the nails positioned in the same plane when the fist is clenched. Then, starting with the fingers extended, the patient should draw the fingertips together, so that the tip of the thumb contacts the tips of the other four digits. This is a gross estimation of intact median, ulnar, and radial nerve motor function. Pincer function should also be routinely tested. Have the patient tightly grasp a piece of paper between the thumb and index finger. Weakness suggests median nerve or ulnar collateral ligament disruption, depending on the mechanism of injury being evaluated. Circulation is assessed by regional pulses and capillary refill.[1]

NERVE TESTING   To test the median nerve, have the patient flex the distal phalanx of the thumb against resistance. Test opposition by touching the tip of the thumb to the tip of the little finger. The patient may be able to accomplish this range of motion with loss of median nerve function due to compensation with muscle groups innervated by the ulnar nerve, but **the patient will be unable to oppose against resistance if median nerve function is lost.** Finally, test thumb abduction by placing the hand palm up and raising the thumb to the perpendicular while palpating the belly of the abductor pollicis muscle to insure it is contracting.

To test the ulnar nerve, spread the fingers apart against resistance and then push them together against resistance. To test the hypothenar muscles (ulnar innervation), extend the fingers and then move the fifth finger away from the others. To test thumb adduction (the ulnar nerve innervates the adductor pollicis muscles), bring the thumb tightly against the side of the index finger. Adductor strength can be further

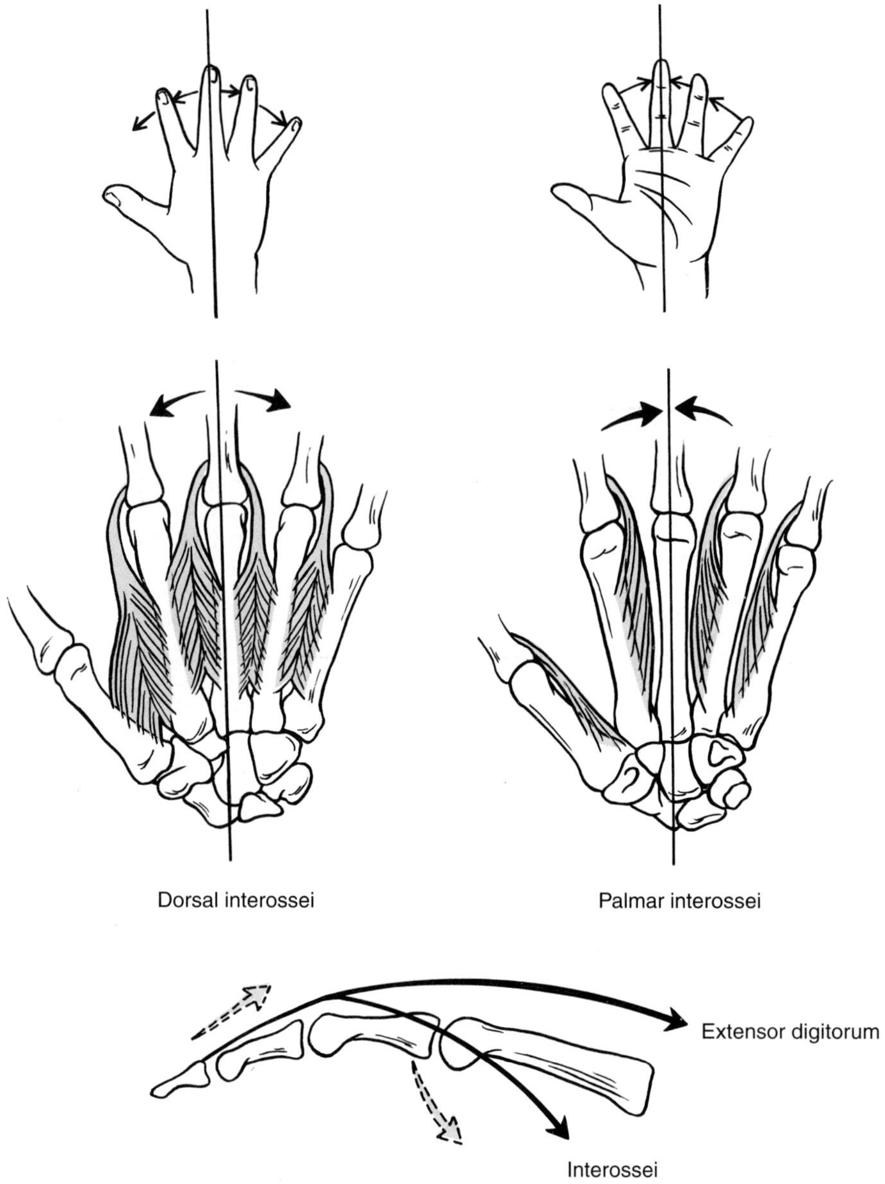

FIG. 268-4. Origins, insertions, and actions of the palmar and dorsal interossei.

Dorsal interossei

Palmar interossei

Extensor digitorum

Interossei

tested by interposing a piece of paper between the thumb and the side of the index finger and then trying to pull the paper away. To test the radial nerve, extend the fingers and wrist. With the thumb in the hitchhiking position, test its resistance to further extension.

Sensation is determined by two-point discrimination. **Normal two-point discrimination is <6 mm at the fingertips and is often <2 mm. Both injured and noninjured fingers must be compared.** Because patients are likely to guess correctly by chance, hand specialists recommend repeating two-point discrimination testing two to four times on each side of the digit. At least 80 percent accuracy is considered acceptable. Less than 80 percent or indeterminate accuracy suggests the possibility of digital nerve injury. A sensory deficit implies a potential digital artery laceration because of the close proximity of the two.

TESTING OF TENDONS   In assessing tendon function, full range of motion of each tendon against resistance should be assessed and compared with the uninjured side. It is important to test resistance because **up to 90 percent of a tendon can be lacerated with preservation of range of motion without resistance.** In addition, digit extension is also accomplished by the juncturae tendinum on the dorsum of the hand, so with lacerations of the extensor digitorum communis the

digits can be extended, but not against resistance. Pain along the course of the tendon during resistance testing suggests a partial laceration even if strength appears adequate. Patients can distinguish deep pain of tendon laceration from the superficial pain of lacerated skin. FDP is tested by flexing the DIP against resistance, while the MP and proximal interphalangeal (PIP) are held in extension. Flexing the PIP against resistance while the remaining fingers are held in full extension tests FDS. Each finger must be tested separately. The variable anatomy associated with the FDS to the small finger may lead to a falsely positive result. A modified version of this test, allowing simultaneous ring and small finger flexion, increases the sensitivity of FDS testing.

Anesthesia and Direct Wound Examination

Anesthesia and direct wound inspection is necessary because partial tendon lacerations or intraarticular injuries are not always readily apparent. Sensation and range of motion should be tested before anesthesia. A bloodless field can be facilitated by milking the digit proximally and then applying a local tourniquet or Penrose drain around the base of the digit. The tourniquet should not be stretched to more than 150 percent of its length, and it can be held in place with a hemostat.

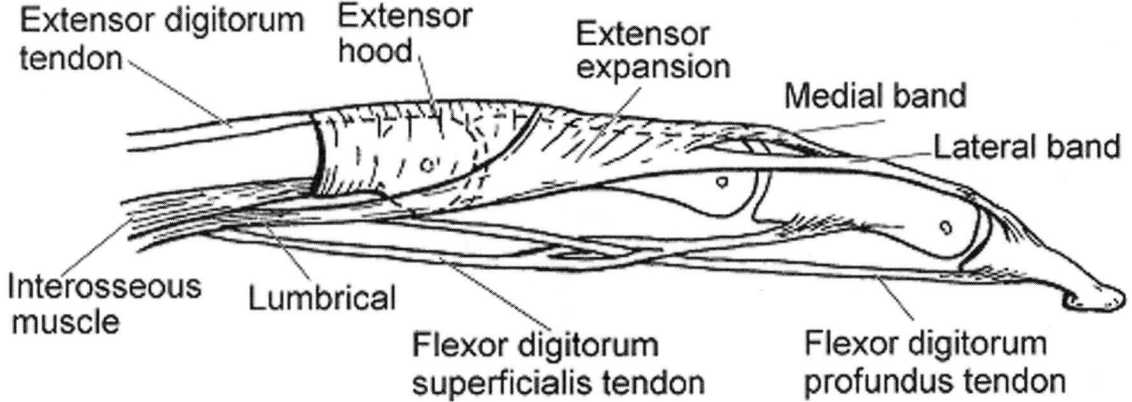

FIG. 268-5. Extensor and flexor tendons of the digits.

The digit can be milked by wrapping another Penrose drain circumferentially around the entire digit, going from distal to proximal or by reconfiguring a 4 × 4 in gauze dressing into a narrow band and wrapping that circumferentially around the entire digit. Only moderate compression should be used to avoid compression injury to the digit. The tourniquet should not be left in place for more than 20 min. Contaminated wounds should be copiously irrigated with normal saline, and antibiotics should be administered. Tetanus toxoid should be administered as needed.

Radiographs, Consultation, and Disposition

Radiologic evaluation should include at a minimum a posteroanterior (PA), lateral, and oblique projection. Similar projections are used for the digits, except that the x-ray beam is centered over the digits. Ac-

tual or suspected injuries of tendons and nerves should be referred to a hand specialist. Whether consultation is provided in the emergency department or in follow-up (1 to 3 days) depends on local resources. Injuries requiring immediate and delayed follow-up by a hand surgeon are listed in Tables 268-1 and 268-2, respectively. Table 268-3 provides guidelines for adequate immobilization and follow-up for specific hand injuries referred for delayed hand surgery evaluation. Often the skin can be closed, the hand splinted in the position of function, and at follow-up the wound can be extended, explored, and definitive repair performed by the hand specialist. Most hand specialists prefer to do definitive repair within a 3- to 5-day window after acute injury. While most injuries involving less than 20 percent of the tendon are not surgically repaired, hand specialist follow-up and rehabilitation are still necessary to accurately determine the extent of injury, minimize scarring and tendon contraction, and minimize neuroma formation.

FIG. 268-6. The dual blood supply to the hands and digits.

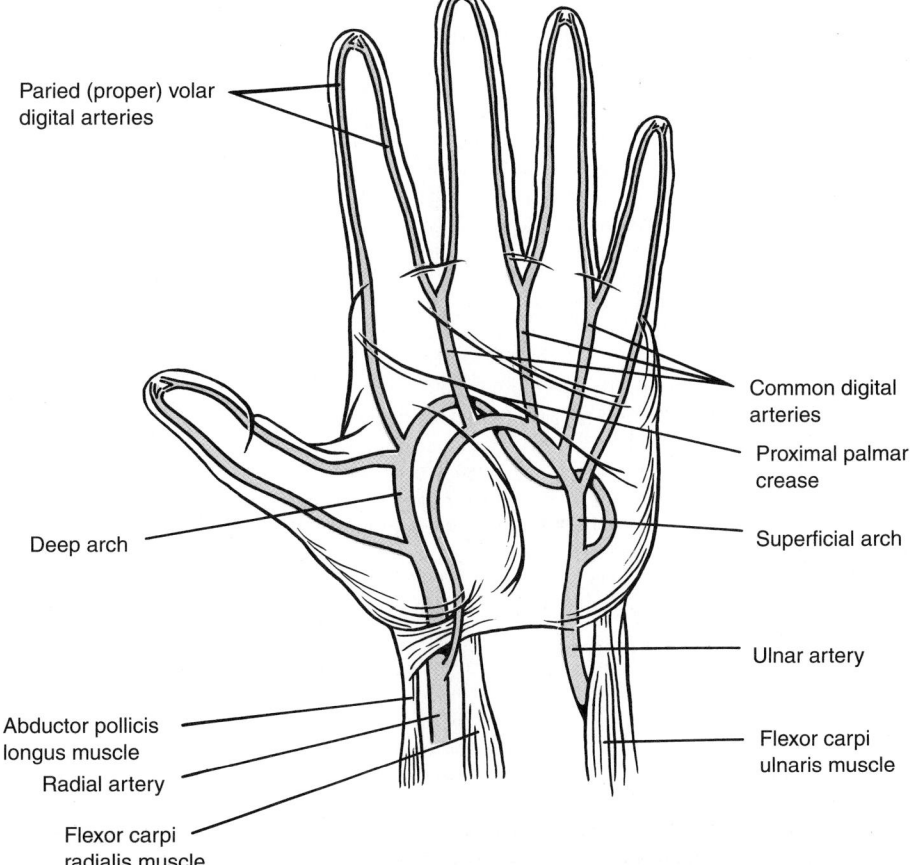

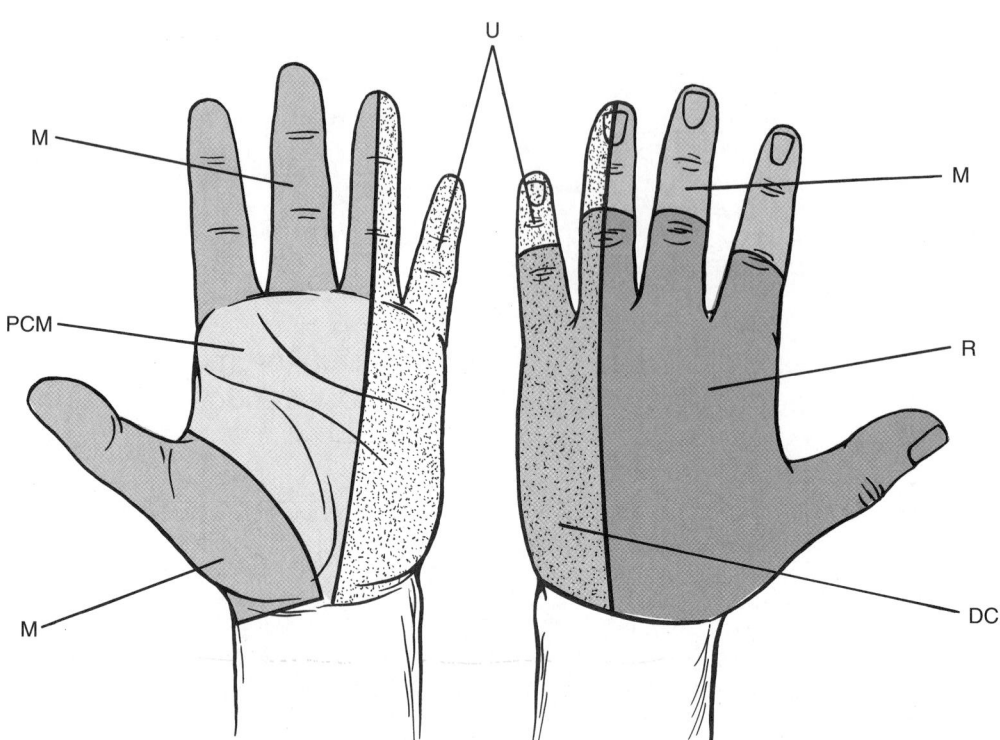

FIG. 268-7. The cutaneous nerve supply in the hand. DCU = dorsal branch of ulnar nerve; M = median; PCM = palmar branch of median nerve; R = radial; U = ulnar.

For patients with hand or digit lacerations that are sutured in the emergency department, and where there is no suspicion of neurovascular or tendon injury, follow-up evaluation and suture removal in the emergency department should always include repeat hand examination to make sure that significant injuries have not been missed.

TENDON INJURIES

Flexor Tendons

The most common cause of flexor tendon injury is a laceration. Flexor tendon lacerations can be subtle; however, the careful examiner will identify these injuries. A distal-to-proximal five-zone (I–V) classification system for flexor tendon injuries has been developed based on location, treatment considerations, and prognosis.[2]

ZONE I   Extends from the insertion of FDS to the profundus tendon. Patients with these injuries lose flexion at the DIP. Retrieval of the proximal tendon is often difficult.

ZONE II   Involves the portion of the digital canal occupied by both FDS and FDP (see Figure 268-5). The close proximity of these tendons makes it essential for exact repair with minimal operative trauma. This region is often referred to as "no-man's-land" because of the frequent poor outcomes prior to the 1960s when improved repair techniques were developed. Lacerations in this zone are common, and partial lacerations are more common then complete.

ZONE III   Extends from the distal edge of the carpal tunnel to the proximal edge of the flexor sheath. The lumbrical muscles originate from FDP in this region. Outcomes are generally favorable.

ZONE IV   Involves the carpal tunnel and related structures. The area must be explored carefully because so many vital structures go through the carpal tunnel. Isolated injuries are the exception.

ZONE V   Involves injuries to tendons proximal to the carpal tunnel. Injuries here tend to be severe and often involve multiple tendons as well as the median or ulnar nerve. It is essential to search for all major structures.

A hand surgeon should repair flexor tendon lacerations. Primary repair should occur within 12 h. Secondary repair can occur up to 4 weeks after the injury.

Another type of flexor tendon injury is the avulsion of FDP from its insertion in the distal phalanx. This can occur from a grasping motion against high-speed resistance. The patient will be unable to flex the distal phalanx. Prognosis depends on the size of the bony fragment, the length of time from injury to repair, and the blood supply to the tendon.

Extensor Tendons

The extensor tendons are the most common site of tendon injuries because of the superficial nature of the tendons on the dorsum of the hand. A separate zone classification system (I–VIII) has been developed for assessing injury patterns, repair techniques, and rehabilitation.[13]

ZONE I   Involves the area over the distal phalanx and DIP. Injury can occur from blunt or sharp trauma. Complete laceration or rupture of the tendon at this level will result in the DIP joint flexed 40 degrees. **This injury after blunt trauma is often referred to as "mallet finger," and it is the most common tendon injury in athletes.** This injury has been classified as type I if there is tendon only rupture, type II if there is a small avulsion fracture, and type III if greater than 25 percent of the articular surface is involved. Types I and II can be treated with the DIP joint immobilized in slight hyperextension continuously for 6 to 10 weeks. Some hand surgeons may prefer operative treatment. Controversy exists whether treatment of type III injuries should be conservative or operative. Chronic untreated mallet finger may develop a **swan-neck deformity** (Figure 268-9). This is caused when the lateral bands are displaced proximally and dorsally, resulting in increased extension forces on the PIP joint.

ZONE II   Involves the area over the middle phalanx. Injuries are usually a result of laceration. Treatment is similar to zone I injuries.

FIG. 268-8. Relationship of nerves, arteries, tendons, and muscles in the hand.

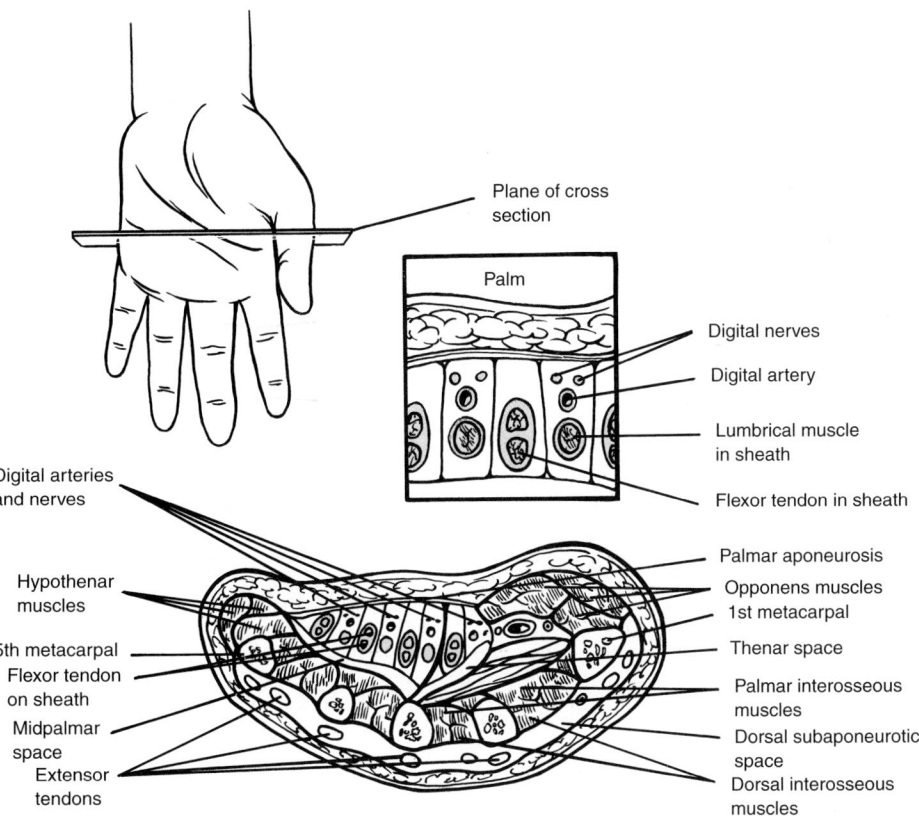

ZONE III   Involves the area over the PIP. The central tendon is the most commonly injured structure. Complete disruption of the central tendon may result in the volar displacement of the lateral bands, causing them to be flexors, along with the unopposed FDP. Additionally, the extensor hood retracts, causing extension of the MP and the DIP joints, resulting in the **boutonnière deformity** (Figure 268-10). Closed injuries are treated with the PIP joint immobilized in extension for 5 to 6 weeks.

ZONE IV   Involves the area over the proximal phalanx. These injuries have clinical findings similar to zone III injuries. Often these injuries are less problematic because the joint is not involved and the tendon at this level is broad and flat.

ZONE V   Involves the area over the MP. Open injuries to this area should be considered human bites until proven otherwise. Wounds from human bites should have delayed repair when free from infection. Clean wounds can be repaired primarily.

ZONE VI   Involves the area over the dorsum of the hand. Because the tendons in this area are so superficial, even minor-appearing lacerations may be associated with one or more tendon injuries. If the laceration is proximal to the junctura tendineae, the patient may be able to extend the involved MP joint, because weak extensor forces are transmitted to the junctura from adjacent extensor tendons.

ZONE VII   Involves the area over the wrist. Repair here can be difficult because of the presence of the extensor retinaculum. This thick, fibrous structure on the dorsum of the wrist contains 12 extensor tendons and 6 retinacular compartments that are lined with synovium.

ZONE VIII   Involves the area of the distal forearm. Injuries to this area require a thorough exploration to identify all injured structures. The tendons frequently retract into the forearm and must be retrieved and repaired. As a general principle, lacerations of less than 25 percent don't require repair; 25 to 50 percent need simple suture repair, and greater than 50 percent need repair with a modified Kessler or similar technique. After repairs in zones V through VII, splinting should occur with the wrist in 15-degree extension, the MP joint in 15-degree flexion, and the IP in 15-degree flexion in the involved and adjacent digit.

LIGAMENT AND DISLOCATION INJURIES

Soft tissue injuries to the hand are extremely common. Accurate diagnosis and treatment are important to avoid complications such as joint luxatio, loss of motion, chronic pain, and deformity.

DIP

Dislocations of the DIP joint are uncommon because of the firm attachments of the skin and subcutaneous tissue to the underlying bone

TABLE 268-1   Immediate Hand Surgery Consultation Guidelines

Vascular injury with signs of tissue ischemia or poorly controlled hemorrhage
Irreducible dislocations
Grossly contaminated wounds
Severe crush injury
Compartment syndrome
High pressure injection injury
Hand/finger amputation

TABLE 268-2   Delayed Hand Surgery Consultation Guidelines

Extensor/flexor tendon laceration (if not repaired in ED)
Flexor digitorum profundus rupture (closed)
Nerve injury (proximal to mid middle phalanx)
Fractures
Dislocations
Ligamentous injuries with instability

TABLE 268-3 Immobilization and Follow-Up Guidelines

Injury	Splint	Duration	Referral
Ligamentous injuries			
Thumb MP UCL rupture			
Partial tears	Thumb spica, IP free to flex	2 weeks	1 week
Complete or equivocal	Thumb spica (presurgical repair)	—	2–3 days
Tendon injuries			
Mallet finger	Dorsal splint, full extension at DIP	8 weeks	1 week
Flexor tendon laceration	Dorsal splint, 30-degree wrist flex, 70-degree MCP flexion, 30–45-degree PIP flexion (presurgical repair)	—	1 day
Dislocations			
DIP	Dorsal splint, full extension	2 weeks	1 week
PIP			
Stable/postreduction	Dorsal splint, 30-degree PIP flexion	2 weeks	1 week
Unstable/postreduction	Dorsal splint, 30-degree PIP flexion	2 weeks	2–3 days
MP	Buddy-taping	2 weeks	1 week
CMC	Dorsal–volar splint	2 weeks	2–3 days
Thumb IP	Dorsal splint, full extension	2 weeks	1 week
Thumb MP	Thumb spica	2 weeks	1 week
Fractures			
Distal phalanx	Volar or hairpin splint not immobilizing PIP	2 weeks	2 weeks
Middle/proximal phalanx			
Stable/nondisplaced	Buddy-taping/dynamic splinting	2 weeks	1 week
Nonstable/displaced	Radial/ulnar gutter, 90-degree MP flexion, <15–20-degree PIP flexion, <5–10-degree DIP flexion	2 weeks	1 week
Thumb proximal phalanx	Thumb spica	2 weeks	1 week
Metacarpal			
Index, middle	Radial gutter, 20-degree wrist flexion, 90-degree MP flexion, PIP left mobile	2 weeks	1 week
Ring, small	Ulnar gutter, 20-degree wrist flexion, 90-degree MP flexion, PIP left mobile	2 weeks	1 week
Thumb metacarpal	Thumb spica	2 weeks	1 week
Extraarticular	Thumb spica for initial immobilization (presurgical repair)		
Intraarticular		—	2–3 days

Abbreviations: CMC = carpometacarpal; DIP = distal interphalangeal; IP = interphalangeal; MP = metacarpophalangeal; PIP = proximal interphalangeal; UCL = ulnar collateral ligament.

by osteocutaneous fibers. There is additional stability of the flexor and extensor tendons. When they do occur, they are usually dorsal. Longitudinal traction and hyperextension, followed by direct dorsal pressure to the base of the distal phalanx, accomplish reduction after digital nerve block. Irreducible cases may be due to the entrapment of an avulsion fracture, profundus tendon, or volar plate.

PIP

Dislocations of the PIP joint are one of the most common ligamentous injuries of the hand. The mechanism is usually due to axial load and hyperextension. Dorsal dislocation occurs when the volar plate ruptures. Lateral dislocations occur when one of the collateral ligaments ruptures with at least a partial avulsion of the volar plate from the middle phalanx. The digit is usually ulnarly deviated because the radial collateral ligament is six times more likely than the ulnar collateral ligament to rupture. Volar dislocations are rare. Dorsal dislocations are reduced similarly to DIP dorsal dislocations. After reduction, active motion and strength is tested. If testing is normal, the joint

should be splinted at 30-degree flexion for 3 weeks. If the joint is irreducible or there is evidence of complete ligamentous disruption, operative repair is required.

MP

Dislocations of the MP joint are less common than at the PIP joint. The mechanism is usually due to hyperextension forces that rupture the volar plate causing dorsal dislocation. In simple dislocations (subluxation), the joint appears to be hyperextended 60 to 90 degrees and the articular surfaces are still in contact. Reduction here does not involve hyperextension because it might convert a simple dislocation into a complex one. Reduction is performed with the wrist flexed to relax the flexor tendon and applying pressure over the dorsum of the proximal phalanx in a distal and volar direction. After reduction, the MP joint should be splinted in flexion. Complex dislocations appear

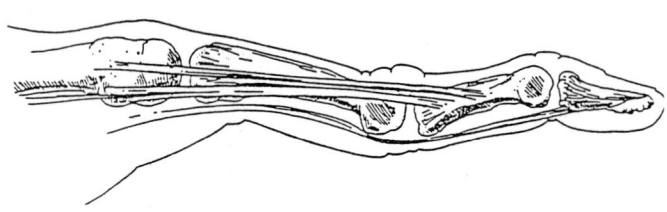

FIG. 268-9. Swan-neck deformity.

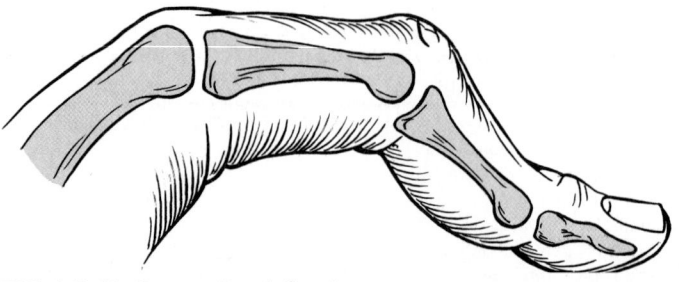

FIG. 268-10. Boutonnière deformity.

less deformed. Because the volar plate is interposed in the MP joint space, closed reduction is usually not possible. Volar dislocations are rare and usually require operative reduction.

CMC

Dislocations of the carpometacarpal joint are uncommon because the joint is supported by strong dorsal, volar, and interosseous ligaments and are reinforced by the broad insertions of the wrist flexions and extensors. The cause is usually a result of high-speed mechanisms such as motor vehicle crashes, falls, crushes, or clenched fist trauma. If a dislocation occurs, it is usually dorsal with associated fracture. Reduction of dorsal CMC dislocations can be attempted after regional anesthesia with traction and flexion with simultaneous longitudinal pressure on the metacarpal base. Early referral after reduction is needed to determine if further fixation is needed.

Thumb IP

Dislocations of the thumb IP are rare but, if present, usually open. The mechanism is usually hyperextension with rupture of the volar plate. Reduction is similar to the IP joints of the other digits. After reduction, the joint should be immobilized 3 weeks in mild flexion.

Thumb MP

Dislocations of the MP joint of the thumb are usually dorsal from a hyperextension force causing rupture of the volar plate. The dislocation may be simple or complex. Reduction, after radial nerve block, is accomplished with pressure directed distally on the base of the proximal phalanx with the metacarpal flexed and abducted.

Thumb MP Collateral Ligament Rupture

Rupture of the ulnar collateral ligament (gamekeeper's thumb, skier's thumb) occurs when the mechanism causes radial deviation (abduction) of the MP joint. The tear usually occurs at the insertion into the proximal phalanx. Often significant injury to the dorsal capsule and volar plate occurs. **Hand surgery referral is recommended for all patients with weakness of pincer function and point tenderness at the volar-ulnar aspect of the thumb MCP joint** resulting from a forced abduction mechanism of injury. For patients with normal radiographs, abduction stress testing of the ulnar collateral ligament may be performed to provide additional clinical information. The examiner tests the thumb MCP, both in full extension and 30-degree flexion, by stabilizing the metacarpal with one hand while applying lateral (radial) stress on the proximal phalanx with the other. More than 40 degrees radial angulation indicates complete rupture and requires surgical consultation. Repair is best accomplished within 1 week. Radial collateral ligament rupture is not as common, and the mechanism is forced adduction.

Thumb CMC

Isolated thumb CMC dislocation is rare compared to the more common Bennett fracture dislocation. These are easy to reduce but unstable after reduction. After reduction, a thumb spica splint should be applied. These injuries should have a surgical referral for a decision on operative repair.

FRACTURES

Distal Phalanx

Fractures of the distal phalanx account for 15 to 30 percent of all hand fractures. Mechanisms are usually from crush or shearing forces. The fractures can be classified as tuft, shaft, or intraarticular. Tuft fractures can be associated with nail bed lacerations. Fractures at the base may be associated with flexor or extensor tendon involvement. Generally, these fractures are treated as soft tissue injuries with protective splinting.

Proximal and Middle Phalanx

The proximal phalanx has no tendinous attachments, therefore fractures frequently have volar angulation from the forces of the extensor and interosseous muscles. The middle phalanx has the FDS insert on the entire volar surface and the extensor tendon insert at the proximal base; therefore, fractures at the base have dorsal angulation and fractures at the neck result in volar angulation. A direct blow mechanism usually causes a transverse or comminuted fracture, while a twisting mechanism will more often result in a spiral fracture. Most often these fractures are stable and nondisplaced and can be treated with early protected motion by buddy taping. Unstable fractures amenable to closed reduction can be splinted from the elbow to the DIP with the wrist at 20-degree extension and the MP joint in 90-degree flexion. Midshaft transverse fractures, spiral fractures, and intraarticular fractures often require internal fixation.

Metacarpal (II to V) Fractures

The second and third metacarpals are relatively immobile, and fractures require anatomic reduction. The fourth and fifth metacarpals have 15- to 20-degree AP motion, which allows for some compensation. Metacarpal fractures are categorized as head, neck, shaft, or base fractures.

HEAD Fractures of the metacarpal head are usually caused by a direct blow, crush, or missile. These fractures are distal to the insertion of the collateral ligaments and are often comminuted. If a laceration is present, a human bite must be considered. Treatment consists of ice, elevation, and immobilization with referral to a hand surgeon.

NECK Fractures of the metacarpal neck are usually caused by a direct impaction force. A fracture of the fifth metacarpal neck is often referred to as a boxer's fracture. These fractures are usually unstable with volar angulation. **Angulation of less than 20 degrees in the fourth and 40 degrees in the fifth metacarpal will not result in functional impairment. If greater angulation in these metacarpals occur, reduction should be attempted. In the second and third metacarpal, angulation of <15 degrees is acceptable.** These fractures should be splinted with the wrist in 20-degree extension and the MP flexed at 90 degrees. Fractures of the second or third metacarpal that are significantly displaced or angulated require anatomic reduction and surgical fixation.

SHAFT A direct blow usually injures fractures in this region. Rotational deformity and shortening are more likely in shaft fractures than in neck fractures. If manipulative reduction is necessary, operative fixation is usually indicated.

BASE Fractures at the base of the metacarpal are usually caused by a direct blow or axial force. They are often associated with carpal bone fractures. Fractures at the base of the fourth and fifth metacarpal can result in paralysis of the motor branch of the ulnar nerve.

Thumb Metacarpal

Because of the mobility of the thumb metacarpal, shaft fractures are uncommon. Fractures usually involve the base.

EXTRAARTICULAR Extraarticular fractures are caused by a direct blow or impaction mechanism. The mobility of the CMC joint can allow for 20-degree angular deformity. Angulation greater than this requires reduction and thumb spica splint for 4 weeks. Spiral fractures often require fixation.

INTRAARTICULAR   Intraarticular fractures are caused by impaction from striking a fixed object. Two fracture types have been described.

Bennett Fracture   A Bennett fracture is an intraarticular fracture with associated subluxation or dislocation at the CMC joint. The ulnar portion of the metacarpal usually remains in place. The distal portion usually subluxes radially and dorsally from the pull of abduction pollicis longus and the adductor pollicis. Treatment includes thumb spica splint and surgical referral.

Rolando Fracture   A Rolando fracture is an intraarticular comminuted fracture at the base of the metacarpal. The mechanism of injury is similar to the Bennett fracture, but less common. Treatment includes thumb spica splint and surgical consultation.

COMPARTMENT SYNDROME

Crush injury of the hand, with or without associated fracture, may result in compartment syndrome. The involved compartments of the hand include the thenar, hypothenar, adductor pollicis, and four interossei. Edema of tissues or hemorrhage within any of these compartments may lead to elevated pressures that result in tissue necrosis and subsequent loss of hand function due to contracture if not diagnosed and treated in a timely and appropriate manner.[3]

Signs and symptoms of compartment syndrome typically include pain and paresthesias early, with paralysis and pulselessness occurring later in the course of the ischemic injury. Hand compartment syndromes, however, may lack paresthesias and the extremely subtle motor deficits and difficulty in assessing response to passive stretch on physical examination make the diagnosis more elusive than at other anatomic sites. Pain, the most consistent clinical sign, is often described as deep, constant, poorly localized, and disproportionate to clinical findings. Physical examination findings suggestive of hand compartment syndrome include "intrinsic minus" position at rest (MCP extended with PIP slightly flexed), pain with passive stretch of the involved compartmental muscles (interosseous: performed with MCP extended and PIP fully flexed with slight radial and ulnar deviation; thenar, hypothenar: performed by extension of MCP), and tense swelling of the affected compartment.

Diagnosis is usually confirmed by compartment pressure measurement, but this procedure is more difficult in the relatively small compartments of the hand and may yield misleading results. In the setting of severe crush injury with signs and symptoms suggestive of compartment syndrome, emergent hand surgeon consultation for fasciotomy is mandatory.

HIGH-PRESSURE INJECTION INJURY

A high-risk injury to the hand that initially appears benign is the injection of certain substances under high pressures into the soft tissues of the hand (often 2000 to 10,000 psi). Often occurring in the industrial setting, the operator of the high-pressure device typically attempts to test or clean the nozzle with his nondominant hand and inadvertently injects the substance. The initial dissipation of kinetic energy through the soft tissues of the hand and the subsequent chemical inflammation both produce tissue edema and resultant ischemia of tissue. The most commonly injected substances include grease, paint, hydraulic fluid, diesel fuel, paint thinner, and water. Of the most commonly injected substances, paint, especially oil-based paint, triggers a more intense inflammatory response that contributes to the overall risk for significant ischemic injury and consequent amputation.

The benign appearance of the small injection site puncture wound in the immediate postinjection period may mislead the clinician, and his-

torical information must dictate treatment/disposition decisions. With time, the digit becomes edematous, pale, and severely tender to palpation suggesting the ischemic injury of compartment syndrome. Pressure to areas surrounding the wound may express the injected substance.

Plain radiographs of the injected hand and adjacent forearm provide valuable information as radio-opaque substances, such as lead-based paints or grease, or subcutaneous emphysema may delineate the extent of the injection.

Definitive treatment of high-pressure injection injuries is early surgical decompression and debridement of injected areas. The emergency physician must recognize the injury as a surgical emergency and obtain immediate hand surgery consultation, immobilize and elevate the affected hand, administer tetanus prophylaxis and broad-spectrum antibiotics, and provide adequate analgesia.[4-6]

REFERENCES

1. Smith P (ed): *Lister's the Hand: Diagnosis and Indications,* 4th ed. London, Churchill Livingstone, 2002.
2. Hart RG, Kutz JE: Flexor tendon injuries of the hand. *Emerg Med Clin North Am* 11(3):621, 1993.
3. Kleinert HE, Verdan C: Report of the Committee on tendon injuries. *J Hand Surg* 8:795, 1983.
4. Del Pinal F, Herrero F, Jado E, et al: Acute hand compartment syndromes after closed crush: A reappraisal. *Plast Reconstr Surg* 110(5):1232, 2002.
5. Schnall SB, Mirzayan R: High pressure injection injuries to the hand. *Hand Clin* 15(2);245, 1999.
6. Vasilevski D, Noorbergen M, Depierreux M, et al: High pressure injection injuries to the hand. *Am J Emerg Med* 8(7);820, 2000.

WRIST INJURIES
Dennis T. Uehara
Dean Wolanyk
Robert H. Escarza

The wrist comprises the area from the distal radius and ulna to the carpometacarpal joints. It is a complex unit with articulations among the eight carpal bones and the distal radius and ulna. Wrist injuries are common and clinical diagnosis is often difficult. Even subtle injuries may lead to significant impairment if not properly diagnosed and treated. Therefore an understanding of the functional anatomy, mechanisms of injury, and clinical evaluations are needed for proper diagnosis and treatment.

ANATOMY

The distal radius is the only forearm bone that articulates directly with the carpal bones (scaphoid and lunate). The distal radius has three articular surfaces: radiocarpal, distal radioulnar, and the triangular fibrocartilage complex (TFCC). The radiocarpal surface is concave and tilted in two planes. It has an ulnar inclination or tilt of 15 to 25 degrees in the frontal plane and a volar tilt of 10 to 15 degrees in the sagittal plane. The ulna is separated from the carpal bones by the triangular fibrocartilage complex, the main stabilizer of the distal radioulnar joint (DRUJ), on its distal end. The TFCC forms a smooth, continuous, ulnarly directed extension of the distal radial surface and supports the lunate and triquetrum on the distal ulna. The distal radius has a concave sigmoid notch as its ulnar aspect that articulates with the curvature of the ulnar head, permitting rotation of the wrist during pronation/supination of the forearm. The distal radioulnar joint is also supported by dorsal and volar radioulnar ligaments that merge with the TFCC.[1]

The eight carpal bones are arranged in two rows (Figure 269-1). The distal row (trapezium, trapezoid, capitate, and hamate) is joined tightly together and to the adjoining metacarpals. This row is quite sta-

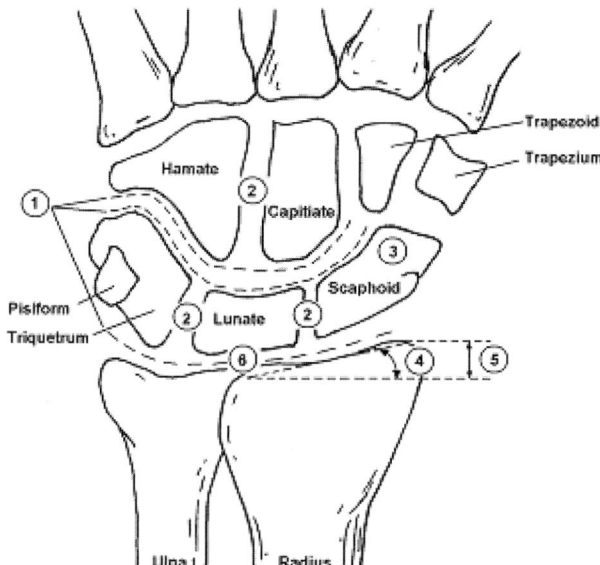

FIG. 269-1. Key elements on a normal posteroanterior view. (1) The carpal bones are arranged in two rows forming three smooth arcs. (2) The carpal bones are separated by a uniform 1- to 2-mm space. (3) The scaphoid is elongated. (4) The radius has an ulnar inclination of 13 to 30 degrees. (5) The radial styloid projects 8 to 18 mm, with an average of 13 mm. (6) Half the lunate articulates with the radius, with equal length over the ulna (neutral ulnar variance).

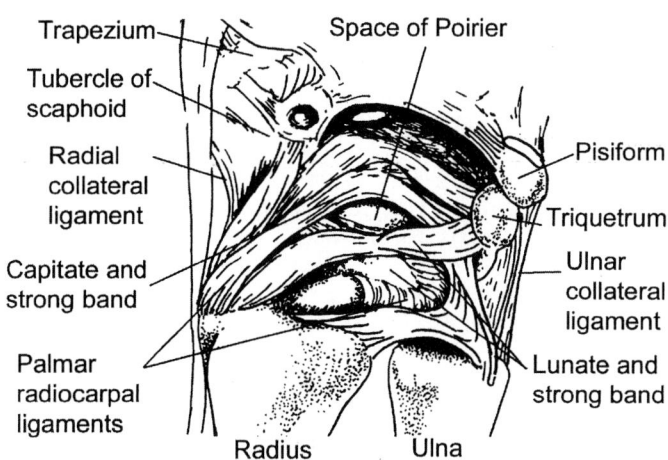

FIG. 269-2. The space of Poirier is inherently weak and is the site of disruption in perilunate and lunate dislocations.

ble, moving together with the metacarpals as a unit in a relatively stable arch. The proximal carpal row (scaphoid, lunate, triquetrum, and pisiform) is also arranged in an arch between the distal radius and distal carpal row. This proximal row functions as a mobile link or "intercalated segment" in this arrangement, and by virtue of this position is potentially unstable. The scaphoid holds a unique position, acting as a stabilizing strut and linking the proximal and distal carpal rows at the radial aspect of the wrist. This position explains the scaphoid's greater propensity for injury.

Wrist motion is produced by forearm muscles that insert onto the bases of the metacarpals. There are no direct tendon insertions on the carpal bones (except for the pisiform, a sesamoid bone of the flexor carpi ulnaris). The carpal bones move passively in response to hand position. Although the radiocarpal joint is often referred to as the "wrist joint," it is important to realize that wrist motion is nearly equally divided between the radiocarpal and midcarpal joints. This is best appreciated when viewing carpal movement from the sagittal view. During flexion and extension of the wrist, each row moves in the same direction with similar degrees of angulation.

The carpal bones are stabilized to one another by intrinsic ligaments and to the bones of the forearm by extrinsic ligaments. The key extrinsic ligaments are arranged in three arcades, two of which are volar and one dorsal. The two volar ligaments are arranged in two inverted-V shaped arches. The apex of one arch inserts on the lunate supporting the proximal carpal row, while the other arch reaches to the distal carpal row, inserting on the capitate. The area between these two palmar arches is inherently weak and is known as the space of Poirier (Figure 269-2). This space lies at the junction of the capitate and lunate and widens upon dorsiflexion of the wrist. Forceful dorsiflexion may tear the capsule here and produce a lunate or perilunate dislocation. The single dorsal arcade has its origins on the rim and styloid of the radius on one side and distal ulna/TFCC on the other. This ligament is less important for wrist stability, acting as a sling across the dorsum of the wrist.[2]

The intrinsic ligaments are largely responsible for holding the carpal bones together as a kinematic unit in their respective carpal rows. The intrinsic ligaments of the mobile proximal carpal row are particularly important because of their greater propensity for injury. The intrinsic ligaments of the proximal carpal row are named after the respective carpal bones they connect: the scapholunate and triquetrolunate. The palmar flexed posture of the scaphoid produces a flexion torque on the lunate that is counterbalanced by an extension torque from the triquetrum. Unfortunately, this delicate balance is lost if either ligament is disrupted, producing a dorsal or volar tilt of the proximal carpal row and carpal instability.

CLINICAL ASSESSMENT

Mechanism of injury is an often ignored but helpful aspect of the evaluation of wrist injuries.[3] Age affects the maturity of the bones and predisposes patients to certain types of injury. Children are more likely to sustain injuries to the immature, weaker epiphyseal plate or metaphysis of the radius, sparing the still-cartilaginous carpal bones. Young adults, particularly those with active lifestyles, are more likely to be injured with greater force and disrupt either the scaphoid, proximal row intrinsic ligaments, or distal radial metaphysis. In the elderly, the weak point is the brittle distal radial metaphysis, resulting in a Colles' fracture, often with intra-articular involvement.

Most injuries are caused by a fall on an outstretched hand. Impact on the thenar eminence is more likely to injure the scaphoid and its supporting ligaments. An impact on the hypothenar eminence is likely to cause injury to the triquetrum, pisiform, and their supporting ligaments.

Pinpointing areas of tenderness and correlating them to anatomic landmarks of the wrist will help determine what structure may be injured, and the best way to evaluate it is with radiography. The most noteworthy landmark on the dorsum of the wrist is the "anatomic snuffbox." The scaphoid is palpable within this triangle formed by the bony radial styloid at its proximal base, the extensor pollicis brevis tendon at its radial aspect, and the extensor pollicis longus tendon at its ulnar aspect. The extensor pollicis longus tendon wraps around a bony prominence of the distal radius, known as Lister's tubercle. The area immediately distal to this point marks the location of the scapholunate joint. Immediately ulnar to the scapholunate joint is a palpable indentation in the center of the wrist. This is the location of the lunate and capitate, which are palpable as they rise out of this space during wrist flexion. The ulnar styloid is the bony prominence on the ulnar aspect of the wrist. The triquetrum and triangular fibrocartilage complex are located just distal to this prominence.

The crease noted on the volar aspect of the wrist marks the location of the proximal carpal row. The scaphotrapezium joint is palpable at the base of the thenar eminence. The pisiform is the palpable bony prominence at the base of the hypothenar eminence. The hook of the hamate is palpable in the soft tissue distal and radial to the pisiform.

RADIOGRAPHY

Clinical examination should dictate which radiographic views to order to support a diagnosis. Standard views of the wrist include posteroanterior (PA), lateral, and oblique views. These views are adequate in the majority of cases; however, other projections may be necessary to profile specific carpal injuries.[4,5]

The key to interpreting the radiograph is to first ensure proper positioning, then identify specific features on each projection. On a properly positioned PA view, the distal radius and ulna should not overlap at their distal articulation, and the axis of the third metacarpal should parallel that of the radius. In addition to looking for disruption of the bony cortex, key elements on the PA view are illustrated in Figure 269-1.

On the PA view, three smooth arcs outline the articular surfaces at the radiocarpal and midcarpal joints. Two of these arcs are formed by the proximal and distal surfaces of the scaphoid, lunate, and triquetrum. The third arc is formed by the proximal articular surface of the capitate and hamate in the midcarpal joint. Any distortion of these lines implies a possible fracture, dislocation, or subluxation at the site.

The carpal bones fit together much like a jigsaw puzzle, with the pieces separated by a uniform 1 to 2 mm space. This space is increased or obliterated with ligament disruption, carpal instability patterns, or fracture/dislocations. This occurs most often around the lunate at the scapholunate and capitolunate joints.

The scaphoid has an elongated shape in its normal, palmarly flexed position. Fractures or ligament disruption may cause further palmar rotation, causing the scaphoid to appear shortened on the PA view. Injuries to the scaphoid also may obscure the "scaphoid fat stripe," a linear or triangular, radiolucent collection of fat distal to the radial styloid and parallel to the radial border of the scaphoid.[6]

Unfortunately, incorrect positioning can produce overlap patterns that can be misinterpreted as pathologic. For example, radial deviation of the wrist causes normal physiologic rotation of the proximal carpal row, obliterating the capitolunate space. At the same time, the scaphoid that should appear elongated on the PA view appears shorter as it rotates palmarly, and can be confused with a rotary subluxation of the scaphoid.

The radial styloid should project 8 to 18 mm beyond the distal radioulnar joint and create an ulnar inclination of 13 to 30 degrees on the PA view. Distal radius fractures can alter these measurements. At the distal radioulnar joint, the ulna and adjacent portion of the radius should be of equal length, and the distal radius should articulate with at least half the lunate. The extrinsic ligaments along with the TFCC prevent ulnar translocation (migration of the carpal bones down the ulnar tilt of the radiocarpal surface). The lunate would have less contact and support from the radius if ulnar translocation were present. A shorter ulna (negative ulnar variance) also provides less support to the lunate and increases potential shear stress to the lunate, predisposing the lunate to injury.

The lateral radiograph is important for determining carpal alignment and degree of fracture angulation. Again, the first step is assuring that the wrist is properly positioned on the radiograph. The radius and ulna should completely overlap one another, and the radial styloid should be centered over the distal radial articular surface. The key elements are illustrated in Figure 269-3A.

The axis of the radius, lunate, and capitate is collinear on the lateral view. If the articular surfaces of these bones were highlighted, they would appear as three consecutive C's. This provides a simple radiographic assessment of wrist dislocation. Measurement of the capitolunate and scapholunate angles is a more precise assessment of carpal alignment. The axis of the capitate, lunate, and scaphoid runs through the center of their proximal and distal articular surfaces. The axis of the lunate and capitate should nearly overlap and form an angle that is less than 10 to 20 degrees. The scaphoid is normally palmar-flexed on the lateral view; its axis should form an angle between 30 and

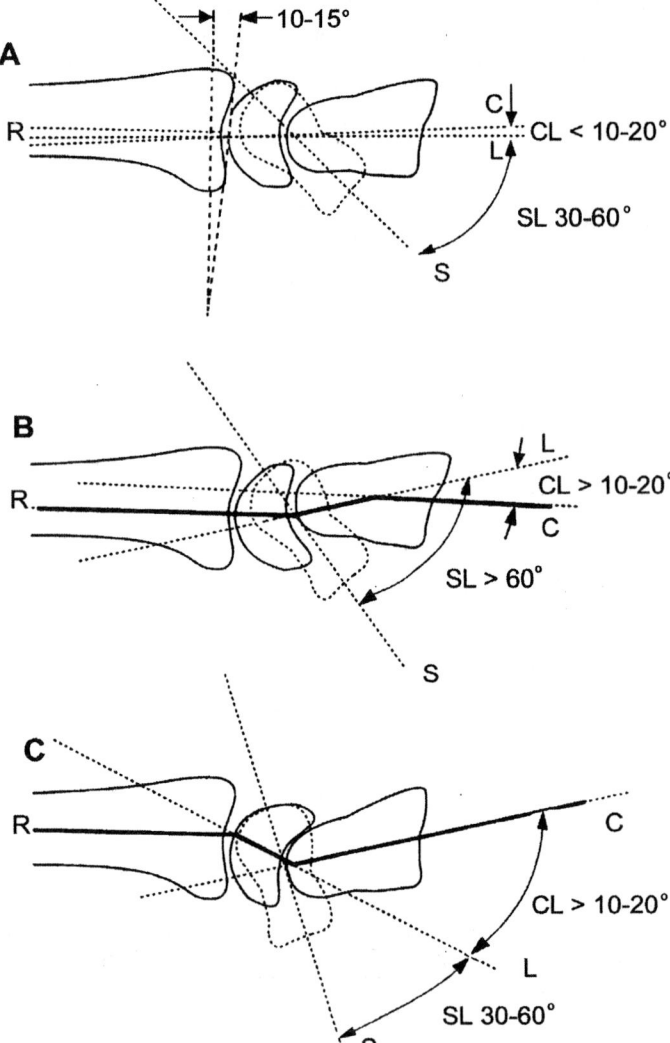

FIG. 269-3. **A.** Normal wrist. (1) Axis of the radius, lunate, and capitate are collinear (three C's sign). (2) The capitolunate (CL) angle is less than 10 to 20 degrees. (3) The scapholunate (SL) angle is between 30 and 60 degrees. (4) The radial volar tilt is 10 to 15 degrees. **B.** Dorsal intercalated segment instability (DISI). The lunate tilts dorsal and slides palmar, increasing the capitolunate angle. The scaphoid tilts more palmar and increases the scapholunate angle. The axes of the radius, lunate, and capitate take on a zigzag pattern (dark line). **C.** Volar intercalated segment instability (VISI). The lunate tilts palmar and the capitolunate angle increases, but the scapholunate angle is maintained. The zigzag pattern is in the opposite direction.

60 degrees with the lunate. Deviation from either of these angles suggests ligament disruption and carpal instability patterns (Figures 269-3B and 269-3C).

Fracture of the distal radius is the most common fracture in the wrist.[7] While a displaced fracture is the obvious deformity, the alteration of the normal volar tilt of 10 to 15 degrees of the distal radial articular surface has greater long-term consequences for wrist function. The shape of the distal radius, distal ulna, and TFCC has a significant influence on carpal alignment and movement.

Other radiographic views profile specific areas of the wrist. Oblique views are performed in either partial pronation or supination, and project the scaphotrapezium joint or pisiform away from overlapping adjacent carpal bones. The scaphoid view is a cone-down PA view of the scaphoid in ulnar deviation. This position extends the normal flexed posture of the scaphoid so that the bone is projected lengthwise. This view may assist in detecting subtle fractures and should be used whenever scaphoid injury is suspected. The carpal tunnel view is a tangential view through the carpal tunnel and is helpful in visualizing the pisiform and hook of the hamate. Motion studies are dynamic views in flexion, extension, and radial and ulnar deviation. These views examine carpal movement relative to one another, and stress the intercarpal ligaments for laxity, characterized by widening of the intercarpal space. Likewise, the grip compression or fist view is a stress view in the PA projection of the tightly clenched fist. The capitate is pushed into the proximal carpal row and forces the carpal bones apart if intrinsic ligaments are disrupted.

LIGAMENTOUS INJURIES

The lunate is located in the middle of the wrist, so it is not surprising that the majority of ligamentous injuries are centered on the lunate. These injuries usually result from forceful dorsiflexion of the wrist, most often from a fall on an outstretched hand. The various injuries occur sequentially depending on the degree of force, and range from isolated tears to perilunate and lunate dislocations.[8]

Scapholunate Ligament Instability

The scapholunate ligament is the intrinsic ligament that binds the scaphoid and lunate. Since the scaphoid bridges the proximal and distal carpal rows, it is not surprising that the scapholunate ligament has a marked propensity for injury and is the most commonly injured ligament of the wrist. Injury most often is from a fall on an outstretched hand with impact on the thenar eminence. Patients will complain of pain and swelling on the radial side of the wrist, and often a "clicking" sensation with wrist movement. Examination reveals localized tenderness on the dorsum of the wrist in the area immediately distal to Lister's tubercle. Ballottement of the scaphoid may also produce pain in this area.

This injury is often referred to by the various radiographic appearances it may take. There are three different radiographic signs that may occur separately or in combination with one another. Scapholunate dissociation is a widening of the scapholunate joint space of more than 3 mm on the PA view (Figure 269-4). This has been called the "Terry Thomas sign,"[9] named after a British comedian with a notable dental diastema between his upper front incisors. If it is not apparent on routine views, a grip-compression view or motion study may be necessary to demonstrate the abnormal gap. These maneuvers are particularly helpful in identifying an incomplete tear of the ligament. Rotary subluxation of the scaphoid is another abnormality that often accompanies scapholunate dissociation. A torn scapholunate ligament can cause the scaphoid to tilt more palmar and increase the scapholunate angle to greater than 60 degrees on the lateral view. On the PA view, the scaphoid tilts toward the observer so that it appears shorter as it is viewed more on its end. This causes the circular cortex of the bone to become more prominent and appear as a ring, known as the "cortical ring sign." A third radiographic abnormality is a carpal instability pattern known as dorsal intercalated segment instability (DISI; see Figure 269-3B). The normal flexed posture of the scaphoid produces a flexion torque on the lunate that is counterbalanced by an extension torque from the triquetrum. When the scapholunate ligament is torn, this balance is disrupted. The lunate tilts dorsal from the unopposed extension torque from the triquetrum, while the scaphoid tilts more palmar (rotary subluxation of the scaphoid) because it has lost support from the lunate. The dorsal tilt of the lunate also causes a slight flexion tilt of the capitate. In the lateral view, the normal collinear arrangement of the axes of the capitate, lunate, and radius are replaced by a characteristic zigzag pattern. Both the scapholunate and capitolunate angles are increased. The concept of the proximal carpal row being the middle link or "intercalated segment" in this system, combined with the lunate's pathological dorsal tilt and zigzag pattern, is how this abnormality came to be named "dorsal intercalated segment instability."[10]

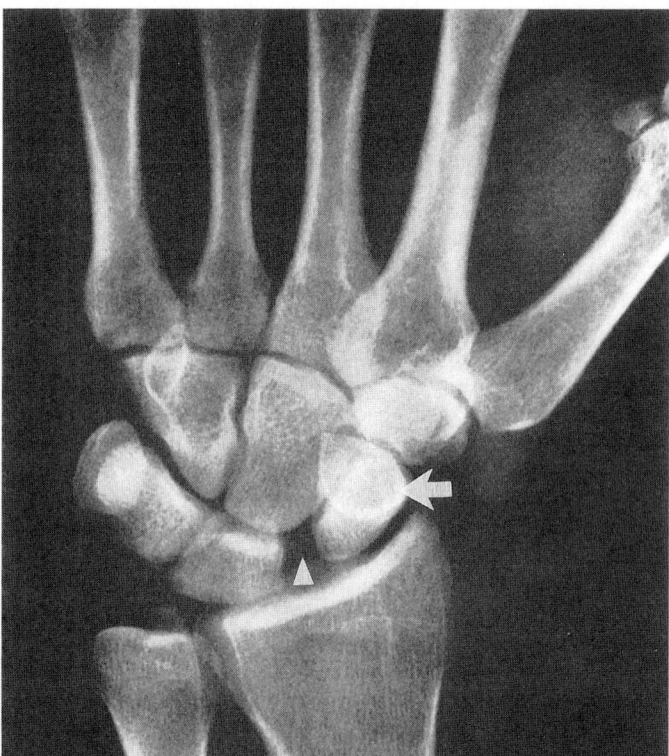

FIG. 269-4. Scapholunate dissociation with accompanying rotary subluxation of the scaphoid. The scaphoid and lunate are separated by a gap of more than 3 mm *(arrowhead)* and the scaphoid appears shorter from rotation with a dense ring *(cortical ring sign, arrow).*

These injuries are treated acutely with a radial gutter splint or short arm volar posterior mold. Appropriate orthopedic referral is necessary because these injuries require either closed reduction with percutaneous pinning, or open reduction and internal repair of the ligament.[8] Early, severe degenerative arthritis is a possible sequela if left untreated.

Triquetrolunate Ligament Instability

The triquetrolunate ligament binds the triquetrum and lunate on the ulnar aspect of the wrist. Injury to this ligament is the ulnar equivalent of the scapholunate ligament injury. Triquetrolunate ligament injury occurs much less often and is more stable. This injury most often results from falls on the outstretched, dorsiflexed hand with impact on the hypothenar eminence. There will be localized tenderness on the ulnar aspect of the wrist just distal to the ulna. Ballottement of the triquetrum may produce a painful clicking sensation.

Complete disruption of this ligament removes the ability of the triquetrum to counterbalance the flexion torque from the palmar-flexed scaphoid. The lunate hence tilts palmar, and the capitate extends slightly in response. A zigzag pattern in the opposite direction of the scapholunate injury is produced. The capitolunate angle is increased more than 10 to 20 degrees; however, the scapholunate angle is unaffected because the scapholunate ligament is still intact. The lateral radiograph reveals the "volar intercalated segment instability (VISI)" pattern (Figures 269-3C and 269-5). The PA view may reveal a widening of the triquetrolunate joint space and obliteration of the capitolunate joint space because of the volar tilt of the lunate.

These injuries are treated acutely with an ulnar gutter splint or short arm posterior mold and referred to an orthopedist. Immobilization in a cast for 6 to 8 weeks, followed by a protective splint is sufficient in most cases. Open reduction and internal fixation is generally reserved for chronic injuries. Unrecognized injuries can result in early degenerative arthritis and a chronically painful wrist.

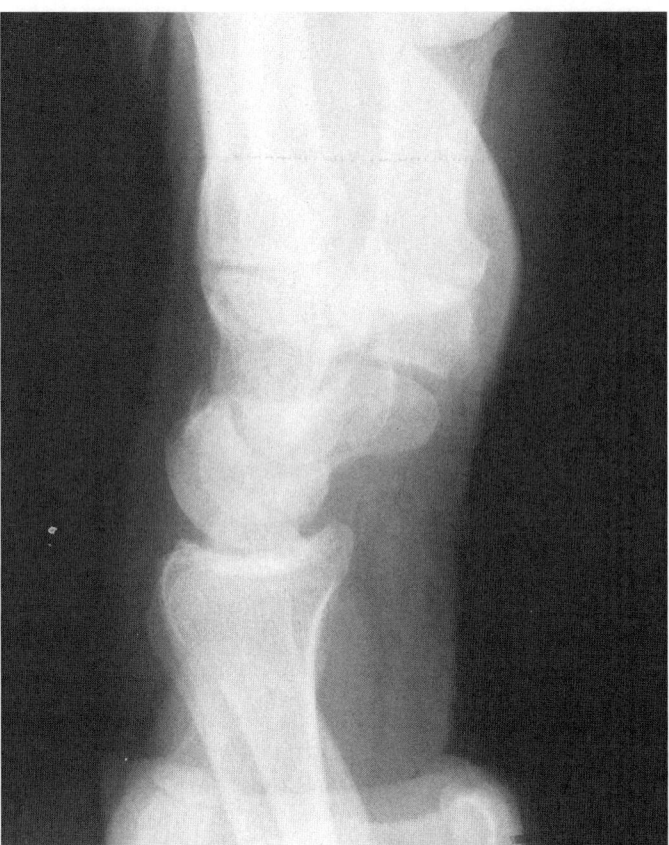

FIG. 269-5. Volar intercalated segment instability (VISI).

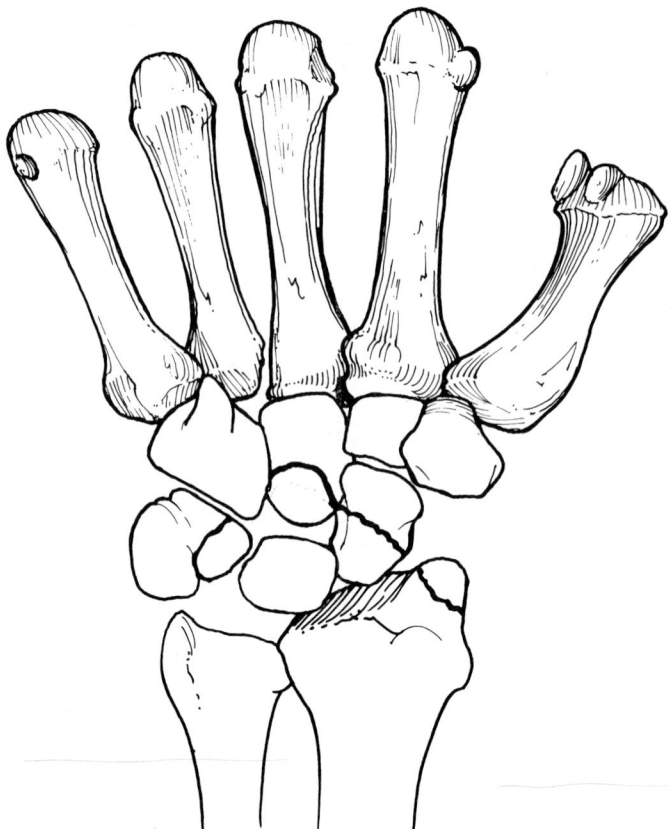

FIG. 269-6. Perilunate and lunate dislocations can fracture any of the carpal bones that surround the lunate in an arc pattern.

Perilunate and Lunate Dislocations

Perilunate and lunate dislocations represent the final stages of midcarpal ligament disruption. Much like the scapholunate and lunatotriquetral injuries, these injuries are also the result of forceful dorsiflexion and impact on the outstretched hand, but usually with much greater force, such as a fall from height or impact from a motor vehicle collision. The injury can begin on either side of the lunate, but typically begins on the radial aspect, tearing the scapholunate ligament. It progresses around the lunate in a semicircular fashion, tearing the volar ligament arcade at the radiocapitate ligament.[11] Remember that the extrinsic ligaments form two strong volar arcades with an inherently weak area between them that widens with dorsiflexion of the wrist (see Figure 269-2). This space of Poirier lies at the junction of the lunate and capitate. This space is opened further as additional loading disrupts the lunatotriquetral ligament. In addition to ligament disruption, any number of carpal bones may fracture along an arc around the lunate (Figure 269-6). If sufficient force is applied, the ligaments and carpal bones around the lunate are stripped away. The capitate is displaced posterior to the lunate, producing a perilunate dislocation. If the capitate rebounds with sufficient force, it can push the lunate off the radius and into the palm, creating a lunate dislocation. These injuries are all part of a continuous spectrum of ligament disruption.

On clinical examination, there is often generalized swelling, pain, and tenderness. However, a gross deformity, typical of many other joint dislocations, is often absent and may be misleading. Radiographic interpretation is the key to diagnosis. The perilunate dislocation is best appreciated on the lateral view. The linear arrangement of the three C's sign is disrupted with the capitate, represented by the third C, displaced posterior to the lunate. The lunate retains its contact with the radius. The scapholunate and capitolunate angles are increased. On the PA view, the three smooth arcs are disrupted and the capitolunate joint space is oblit-

erated as the bones overlap one another. The scapholunate and triquetrolunate joint space may either be increased because of torn ligaments, or obliterated by rotation of the fractured carpal fragments. The scaphoid will appear shortened from rotary subluxation or fracture. A perilunate dislocation may also overshadow any associated carpal bone fracture. The scaphoid and capitate are most often involved, so it is prudent to carefully inspect these bones for fractures. These fractures are designated by adding the prefix "trans-" to the carpal bone name (e.g., transscaphoid perilunate dislocation) (Figures 269-7A and 269-7B).

A lunate dislocation has many similar and several distinct radiographic features when compared to a perilunate dislocation. On the PA view, the lunate has a triangular shape ("piece-of-pie" sign) that is pathognomonic for lunate dislocation (Figure 269-8A). On the lateral view, it also disrupts the three C's sign. The lunate (represented by the middle C) is pushed off the radius into the palm. This has been called the "spilled teacup" sign because it resembles a cup spilling in the direction of the palm (Figure 269-8B). The capitate may rebound back and even rest on the radius. The signs of ligament disruption and the associated carpal bone fractures described with perilunate injuries may also be present.

All patients with perilunate or lunate dislocations require emergency orthopedic consultation. Treatment is determined by the extent of the injury. Closed reduction and long-arm splint immobilization is appropriate for reducible dislocations. Open, unstable, and irreducible dislocations require open reduction and internal fixation, with repair of the ligaments and fractures. Some orthopedists operate on all peri-lunate and lunate dislocations. The complications include development of carpal instability patterns that lead to early degenerative arthritis, delayed union, malunion, nonunion, avascular necrosis, and occasionally, median nerve compression from the volar dislocation of the lunate into the carpal tunnel.

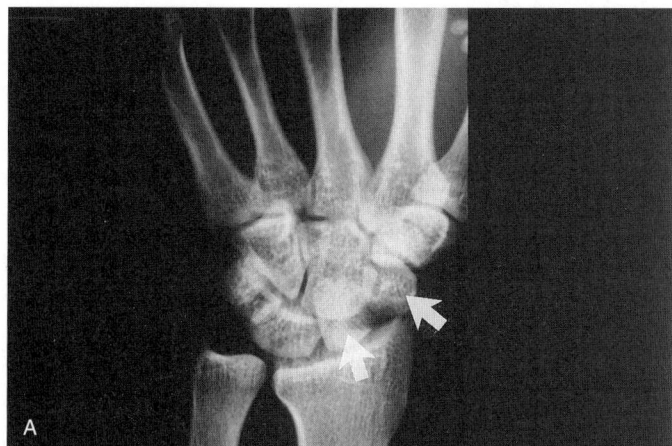

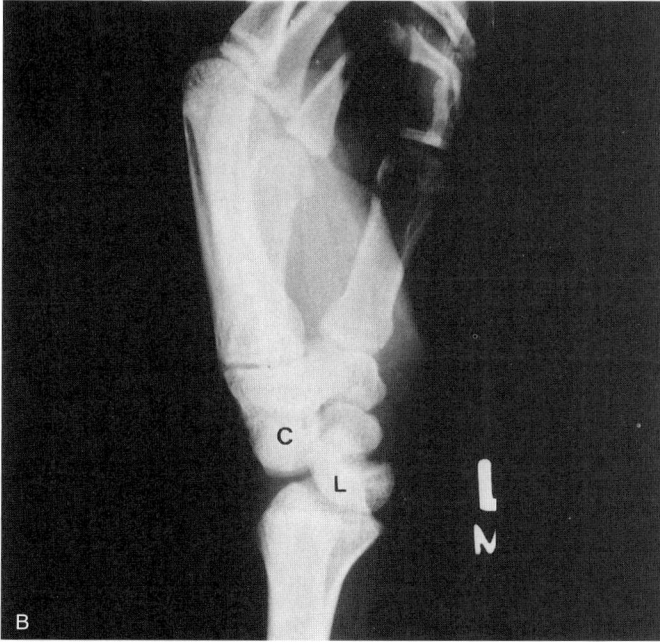

FIG. 269-7. Transscaphoid perilunate dislocation. **A.** PA view shows subtle overlap of the lunate and capitate. A displaced scaphoid fracture is present *(arrows)*. **B.** Lateral view shows lunate (L) maintaining contact with the radius while the capitate (C) is positioned posterior to the lunate. (Reproduced with permission from Chin HW, Visotsky J: Ligamentous wrist injuries. *Emerg Med Clin North Am* 11:3, 1993.)

CARPAL BONE FRACTURES

Carpal bone fractures account for 7 to 10 percent of all hand injuries. Unfortunately, they are among the most commonly missed wrist injuries. It is important that a high index of suspicion be maintained and a focused examination used to recognize these injuries. The following carpal fractures are listed in descending order of occurrence.

Scaphoid Fracture

The scaphoid is an oblong bone that has the unique role of linking and stabilizing the two rows of carpal bones. Because of this anatomy, it also transmits compression forces from the hand to the forearm, which unfortunately increases its propensity for injury, making it the most common carpal bone fracture. The injuries usually result from a fall on an outstretched dorsiflexed hand or by an axial load directed along the thumb's metacarpal. There is pain along the radial side of the wrist and localized tenderness in the anatomic snuffbox. Examining the wrist in

ulnar deviation exposes more of the scaphoid to direct palpation in the anatomic snuffbox. Eliciting pain in this area when the patient resists supination or pronation of the hand, or pain with axial pressure directed along the thumb's metacarpal, is also suggestive of injury.

Standard and scaphoid views should be carefully examined for any cortical disruption (Figure 269-9). The scaphoid view profiles the bone lengthwise and may assist in detecting subtle fractures. Distortion of a soft tissue fat stripe that lies adjacent to the radial side of the scaphoid is also suggestive of injury. Two-thirds of the fractures occur at the waist or middle third of the bone, 16 to 28 percent in the proximal third, and 10 percent in the distal third. A scaphoid fracture may also have an associated injury in 12 percent of cases, involving either the radius, neighboring carpals, a carpal instability pattern, or dislocation.

A scaphoid fracture can develop avascular necrosis of the proximal fracture segment that can lead to disabling arthritis.[12] Since the vascular supply to the scaphoid enters the distal portion of the bone through small branches off the radial artery and the palmar and superficial arteries, a fracture can easily disrupt the blood supply to the proximal segment. In general, the more proximal, oblique, or displaced the fracture, the greater the risk of developing avascular necrosis. A scaphoid fracture is considered unstable if it is oblique; if there is as little as 1 mm of displacement; if there is rotation or comminution; or if a carpal instability pattern is present. Two-thirds of the scaphoid's surface is also articular. This only adds to the scaphoid's problems, because articular fractures are more difficult to heal. Thus the main complications of improperly healed scaphoid fractures are avascular necrosis, delayed union, nonunion, malunion, and subsequent early degenerative arthritis.

Because 10 percent of initial radiographs fail to detect a fracture, initial treatment should be directed by clinical suspicion until follow-up studies can exclude the diagnosis. Nondisplaced fractures and those that are only clinically suspected can be treated in a short-arm thumb spica splint. Splinting in dorsiflexion and radial deviation helps to compress the fracture fragments. Patients with unstable fractures should be placed in a long-arm thumb spica splint and should be seen promptly by an orthopedic surgeon for definitive treatment.

Arthroscopic surgery is a promising alternative in acute management of scaphoid fractures. The repair reunites the two fracture fragments with a cannulated screw. The procedure is minimally invasive and allows early use of the hand, markedly decreasing the adverse effects of immobilization, such as muscle atrophy, articular cartilage breakdown, and osteopenia.

Triquetrum Fractures

Triquetrum fractures are either dorsal avulsion fractures or fractures through the body. Avulsion fractures are produced when a twisting motion of the hand is suddenly resisted, or a hyperextension shear stress pushes the hamate or ulnar styloid against the triquetrum. Fractures of the body occur from direct trauma and are seen in association with perilunate and lunate dislocations (part of the arc fractures). There will be localized tenderness over the dorsum of the wrist in the area immediately distal to the ulnar styloid. The dorsal avulsion fracture is best seen on the lateral view or an oblique view in partial pronation. It appears as a tiny flake of bone on the dorsum of the triquetrum. Triquetrum body fractures are usually nondisplaced because numerous ligaments encase the bone. These are best seen on the PA view. Nonunion is possible, but avascular necrosis has not been reported.

Patients with a dorsal avulsion fracture have an excellent prognosis for full recovery. Symptomatic patients are treated with a wrist splint for 1 to 2 weeks. Asymptomatic or minimally symptomatic patients may be treated with early range of motion. Stable body fractures are treated in a cast for 6 weeks. Unstable body fractures (>1 mm displacement) and those associated with perilunate/lunate dislocations may require internal fixation, either percutaneous or open. Patients with triquetrum body fractures should be referred to an orthopedist.

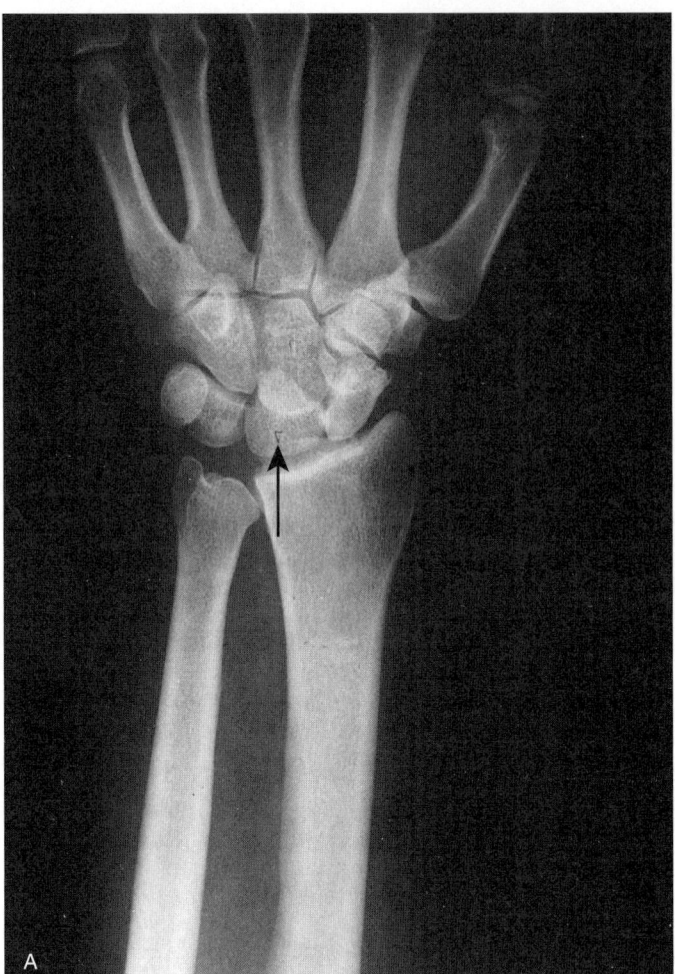
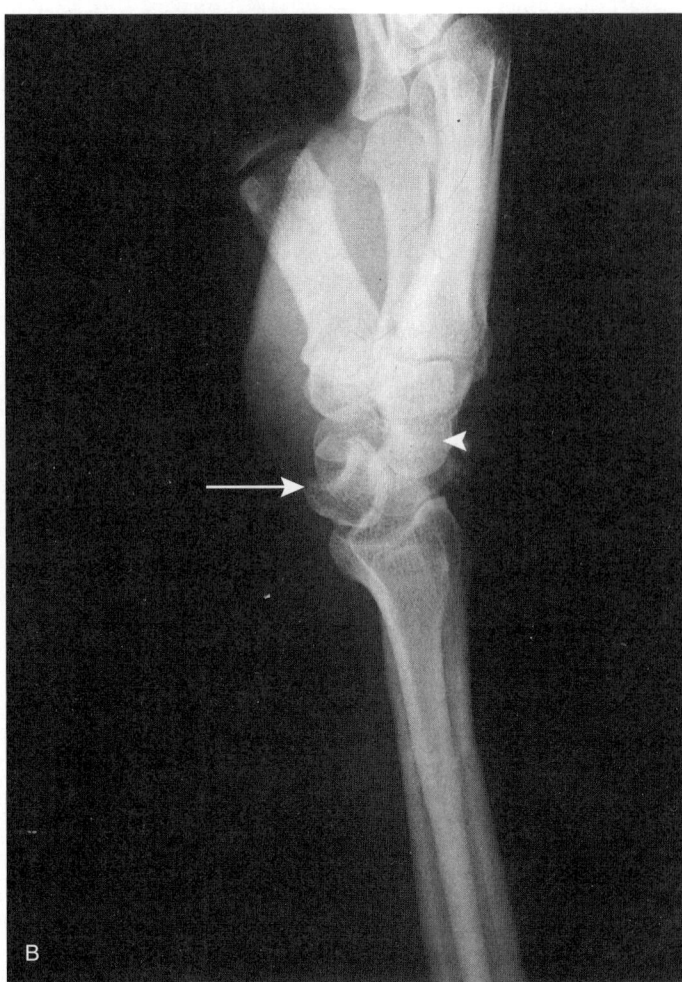

FIG. 269-8. Lunate dislocation. **A.** PA view demonstrates pathognomonic triangular shape of the lunate *(piece-of-pie sign, arrow)*. **B.** Lateral view shows the lunate tilting into the palm *(spilled teacup sign, arrow)* and the capitate positioned posterior to the lunate *(arrowhead)*. Note associated scaphoid and triquetrum fractures. (Reproduced with permission from Chin HW, Visotsky J: Ligamentous wrist injuries. *Emerg Med Clin North Am* 11:3, 1993.)

Lunate Fracture

Lunate fractures generally occur in association with other carpal injuries. It is rare to have an isolated lunate injury. Like many other carpal injuries, it usually is the result of a fall on the outstretched hand. There will be localized tenderness in the middle of the wrist. The lu-

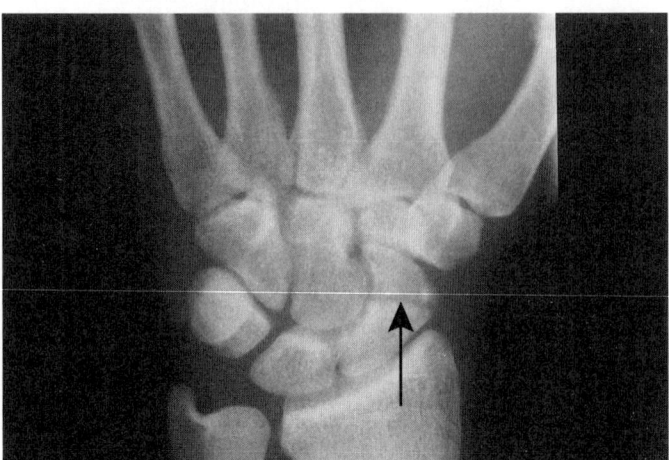

FIG. 269-9. Scaphoid fracture in the middle third or waist *(arrow)*.

nate is present in the shallow indentation on the mid-dorsum of the wrist. If the wrist is flexed, the lunate is easily palpable as it rises out of the floor of this indentation. Axial pressure applied along the third metacarpal ray may also elicit pain in this same area and is suggestive of injury. Like the scaphoid, the lunate's blood supply enters through the distal end. A fracture risks producing avascular necrosis in the proximal portion. Because the lunate is nestled in the middle of the wrist, overlap with other carpal bones may make it difficult to identify an injury on a plain radiograph. Clinical suspicion should dictate the acute treatment. A thumb spica splint should be applied until further evaluation is made by the orthopedist. MRI and CT to identify occult fractures have replaced tomography and bone scans. The major complication is avascular necrosis (Kienböck disease), that can lead to lunate collapse, osteoarthritis, chronic pain, and decreased grip strength. Repetitive trauma to the lunate can also produce microfractures of the bone and subsequent osteonecrosis. Individuals with ulnar negative variance are at increased risk of developing Kienböck disease, because a shorter ulna provides less support to the lunate.

Trapezium Fracture

The trapezium is a saddle-shaped bone that is adjacent to the thumb metacarpal. Injuries are produced by a direct blow to the thumb or from a dorsiflexion and radial deviation force. Fractures occur either at the trapezial ridge or body and are often intraarticular. Vertical fractures occur and are analogous to a Bennett's fracture (an intra-articular proximal thumb metacarpal fracture). Examination reveals painful thumb movement and a weak pinch. There is tenderness at the apex of the anatomic snuffbox and at the base of the thenar eminence. This injury is best profiled on a 20-degree pronated oblique view. The major complication is nonunion.

Emergency treatment of nondisplaced fractures is in a thumb spica splint. Displaced fractures >1 mm or diastasis >2 mm require surgery, either percutaneous or open reduction and internal fixation.

Pisiform Fracture

The pisiform is a sesamoid bone within the flexor carpi ulnaris tendon. It is positioned immediately volar to the triquetrum and is the palpable bony prominence at the base of the hypothenar eminence. Injuries usually result from a fall directed on the hypothenar eminence. There will be localized tenderness on the pisiform itself. If the wrist is flexed, the pisiform can be grasped and palpated between the examiner's fingers. This should elicit pain. Because the pisiform and hook of the hamate form the bony walls of Guyon's canal that contains the ulnar nerve and artery, it is important to exclude injury to them. Radiographs in partial supination, or the carpal tunnel view, are optimal because they remove the overlap with the triquetrum that is present on standard views (Figure 269-10).[13] The pisiform is the last carpal bone to ossify; it is usually complete by age 12. Before this age, multiple ossification centers in the pisiform may be confused with a fracture; however, these will have smoother margins and lack the perfect jigsaw-puzzle fit seen with fracture fragments. After age 12, any radiographic lines suggest fractures.

Emergency treatment of pisiform fractures is either in a compression dressing or in a splint in 30 degrees of flexion and ulnar deviation that relaxes the tension from the flexor carpi ulnaris. These fractures have an excellent prognosis.

Hamate Fracture

Hamate fractures may involve the body of the hamate, the hook of the hamate, or any of its articular surfaces. Body fractures are rare and are generally associated with fracture-dislocations of the fourth or fifth metacarpals. Most hamate fractures involve the hamate hook, which is

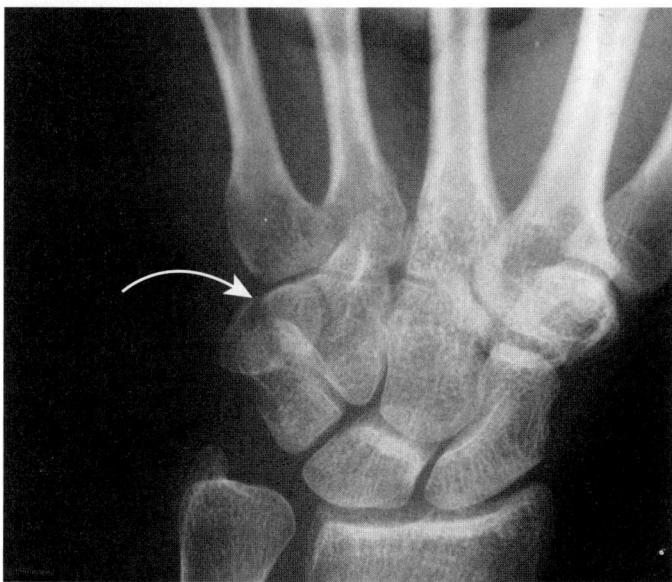

FIG. 269-10. Pisiform fracture. PA view with a thin lucency in the center of the bone *(arrow)*. (Reproduced with permission from Chin HW, Visotsky J: Wrist fractures. *Emerg Med Clin North Am* 11:3, 1993.)

a small bony prominence on its volar aspect. The classic mechanism is an interrupted swing with a golf club, bat, or racquet. The handle impacts against the hypothenar eminence and compresses the bone. The hook of the hamate is palpable in the soft tissue of the hypothenar eminence, distal and radial to the pisiform. There will be localized tenderness here. Standard and carpal tunnel views are necessary to visualize the fracture. Occult fractures may be identified by bone scan or computed tomography.

Hamate hook fractures are treated with a compression dressing or splint. Nonunion is common and excision of the bone may be necessary. Injury to Guyon canal and the ulnar nerve or artery are potential complications. Nondisplaced body fractures are treated by splint immobilization. Displaced body fractures are unstable and are surgically treated. Emergency treatment is splint immobilization and orthopedic referral.

Capitate Fracture

The capitate is the largest carpal bone. It is an elongated bone with a large proximal head that articulates with the lunate; the midportion is the neck; and the distal end, or body, articulates with the third metacarpal. Capitate fractures most often occur in the neck, and usually occur in conjunction with a scaphoid fracture. This association of scaphoid and capitate fractures is called the "scaphocapitate syndrome." Isolated capitate fractures are rare. These injuries result from forceful dorsiflexion of the hand with impact on the radial side. The scaphoid is fractured first, followed by the capitate through its neck. This can continue around the lunate, creating other so-called arc fractures (see Figure 269-6), and eventually a perilunate or lunate dislocation. Like the scaphoid and lunate, the capitate's blood supply enters through the distal end. Thus capitate fractures also share the same legacy of potential avascular necrosis of the proximal fracture segment.

Physical examination reveals diffuse swelling and tenderness over the capitate, just proximal to the third metacarpal. The capitate neck fractures are best seen on the lateral radiograph. The head of the capitate should be carefully noted because it can rotate as much as 180 degrees. Unfortunately, capitate fractures are most often overlooked because the accompanying scaphoid fracture or perilunate/lunate dislocation overshadows it. Complications include avascular necrosis, delayed union, nonunion, and malunion.

Emergency treatment of undisplaced, isolated capitate fractures is splint immobilization and early orthopedic referral. Most capitate fractures, however, are displaced or associated with the scaphocapitate syndrome, and require closed or open reduction and internal fixation.

Trapezoid Fracture

This is an extremely rare fracture, accounting for only 1 percent of all carpal fractures. The injury results from an axial load onto the index metacarpal. There will be tenderness on the radial side that is augmented by applying pressure along the index metacarpal ray. These injuries are difficult to see on standard radiographs, and CT or MRI may be necessary to visualize it. Emergency treatment is in a thumb spica splint.

DISTAL RADIUS AND ULNA FRACTURES

Fractures of the distal metaphysis of the radius and ulna are among the most common injuries affecting the wrist. Among the factors that influence the type and amount of displacement of the fracture are the point and direction of impact, the degree of force, and the patient's age (Table 269-1).

In general, the thinner cortices of the elderly make them more likely to sustain extraarticular fractures, whereas younger adults often sustain more complicated intraarticular fractures.

TABLE 269-1   Radiographic Appearance of Distal Radius Fractures

Colles fracture
    Dorsal angulation of the plane of the distal radius
    Distal radius fragment is displaced proximally and dorsally
    Radial displacement of the carpus
    Ulnar styloid may be fractured
Smith fracture
    Volar angulation of the plane of the distal radius
    Distal radius fragment is displaced proximally and volarly
    Radial displacement of the carpus
    The fracture line extends obliquely from the dorsal surface to the volar surface 1–2 cm proximal to the articular surface
Barton fracture
    Volar and proximal displacement of a large fragment of radial articular surface
    Volar displacement of the carpus
    Radial styloid may be fractured

Colles Fracture

Colles fracture results most often from a fall on the outstretched hand. This mechanism produces a distal radial metaphysis fracture that is dorsally angulated and displaced proximally and dorsally. Compression forces on the dorsal side often produce dorsal comminution of bone. The fracture line may also comminute and extend into the radioulnar or radiocarpal joint ("die-punch" fracture). A fracture of the ulnar styloid is often present and may be suggestive of injury to the TFCC.

The wrist has the characteristic dorsiflexion, or "dinner-fork," deformity. Patients may complain of palmar paresthesias from tension or pressure on the median nerve. Posteroanterior radiographs reveal a distal metaphyseal fracture of the radius that often appears shortened from the angulation or comminution of the bone. The lateral view provides the best view of the dorsal angulation and comminution. In general, potentially unstable fractures have more than 20 degrees of angulation, intra-articular involvement, marked comminution, or more than a centimeter of shortening. These injuries are more likely to develop loss of reduction, distal radioulnar joint instability, radiocarpal instability patterns, and subsequent arthritis.

Stable fractures may be treated with a compression dressing and splint until they can be evaluated by an orthopedic surgeon. Otherwise, closed reduction is performed, with traction provided by finger traps while the fracture fragment is pushed distal and palmar and the patient's forearm is held firmly. The goal is to restore the volar tilt, radial inclination, and proper length to the radius. This is particularly important in younger patients. The volar tilt ideally should be restored to its normal position, but a minimum of neutral or zero degrees of angulation is acceptable.

Although most Colles fractures can be treated with closed reduction and cast immobilization, those that are unstable, severely comminuted, or intra-articular may require casting with pinning, external fixation with possible bone grafting, or open reduction and internal fixation. Good to excellent results are achieved in 56 to 81 percent of patients with these more aggressive treatment alternatives. All open and neurovascularly compromised fractures require prompt evaluation by the orthopedic surgeon.

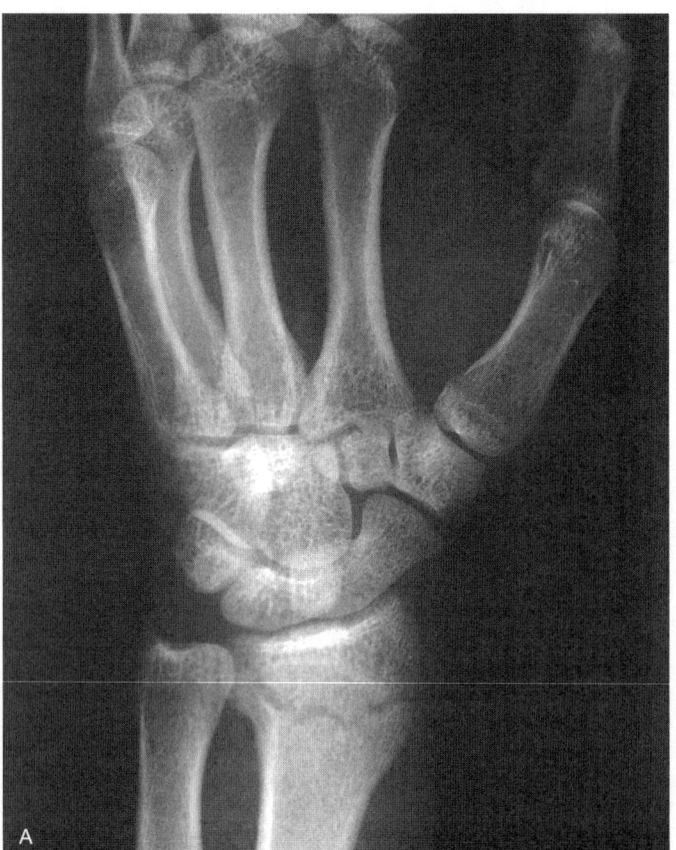
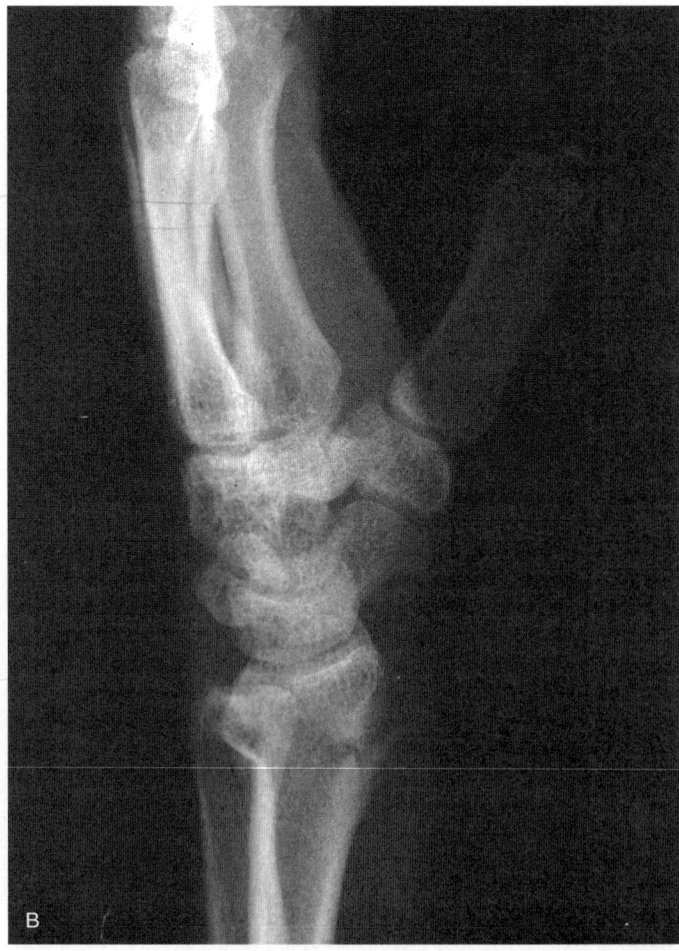

FIG. 269-11. Colles fracture. PA **(A)** and lateral **(B)** views of the wrist, demonstrating typical radiographic findings.

Complications include malunion, median nerve injuries, TFCC injuries, secondary radioulnar and radiocarpal instability patterns, and arthritis. These complications can produce a weak, stiff, and painful wrist.

Smith Fracture

distal end breaks inward

Smith fracture, or "reverse Colles fracture," is a volar angulated fracture of the distal radius. This results from a fall or direct blow on the dorsum of the hand and wrist, or from a fall on the outstretched hand in supination that then shifts into a pronated position. The hand is displaced palmar and produces a "garden-spade deformity" on physical examination. The posteroanterior radiograph looks much like the Colles fracture, with a distal metaphyseal radius fracture that may be shortened and comminuted. The lateral radiograph shows the volar angulated and displaced fracture (Figure 269-12).

The treatment objectives and complications are much like those seen with the Colles fracture. In this case, however, the angulation is volar rather than dorsal.

Barton Fracture

Barton fractures are dorsal or volar rim fractures of the distal radius. The dorsal rim fractures result from a dorsiflexion and pronation force, whereas the less common volar rim fracture is produced by a fall on the outstretched hand in supination. These injuries are often fracture dislocations or subluxations, because the carpus or hand is frequently displaced in the direction of the fracture. Accompanying ligamentous injuries create radiocarpal instability. This is often not fully appreciated in the acute setting, but can lead to various secondary carpal instability patterns and premature degenerative arthritis. The posteroanterior radiograph often shows a comminuted fracture of the distal radial metaphysis. The lateral view reveals an intra-articular fracture of the volar or dorsal rim of the radius, which may be accompanied by carpal subluxation in the same direction (Figure 269-13).

Minimally displaced fractures can be treated acutely in a splint until evaluation by an orthopedist. Unstable fractures involving more than 50 percent of the radial articular surface or those with accompanying carpal subluxation, require open reduction and internal fixation.

Radial Styloid Fracture

A force directed along the radial side of the hand can produce a transverse or oblique fracture that runs from the scaphoid fossa to the metaphysis of the radius. It is best seen on the posteroanterior radiograph as a thin, lucent line beneath the radial styloid. Because the major carpal ligaments along the radial side of the wrist insert on the radial styloid, displacement of this fracture can produce carpal instability. Displaced fractures often require open reduction and internal fixation. Displacement of as little as 3 mm is often associated with accompanying scapholunate dissociation. Failure to recognize these intercarpal ligament tears adds to the potential for subsequent posttraumatic arthritis.

Ulnar Styloid Fracture

Forced radial deviation, dorsiflexion, and rotatory stress fracture the ulnar styloid. The ulnar styloid fracture may be isolated or may accompany other injuries, such as Colles fracture. Avulsion fractures are rarely clinically significant, the major consideration being the associated radial soft tissue and bony injuries. Displaced ulnar base fractures can be intra-articular and be associated with tears of the TFCC, which is the main stabilizer of the distal radioulnar joint. These patients complain of a painful clicking or locking sensation in the wrist. If the distal radioulnar joint (DRUJ) is stable, ulnar styloid fractures are treated acutely in an ulnar gutter splint in slight ulnar deviation and neutral positioning of the wrist. If there is any question about stability, these patients should be referred acutely for surgical evaluation. Arthrograms or MRI imaging may be necessary to delineate the full extent of these injuries.

Distal Radioulnar Joint Disruption

Distal radioulnar joint (DRUJ) disruption is generally seen with intra-articular or distal radial shaft fractures (Galeazzi fracture-dislocation; see Chap. 270),[14] or with fractures of both bones of the forearm. These more apparent injuries often overshadow distal radioulnar joint disruption, and unfortunately cause these injuries to remain unrecognized until subsequent pain and diminished wrist movement are appreciated.

Isolated radioulnar joint dislocations are uncommon and are unrecognized acutely in as many as 50 percent of cases. Dorsal dislocation of the ulna results most often from falls on the wrist in hyperpronation. The rare volar dislocation results from forced hypersupination of the wrist. Patients with disruption of the distal radioulnar joint present with pain at the DRUJ, weak grip, and restricted range of motion, especially pronation and supination. The ulnar head is prominent, but this can be quite subtle and easily overlooked.

The posteroanterior radiograph reveals narrowing and overlap of the distal radioulnar joint. The lateral radiograph demonstrates either volar or dorsal displacement of the ulna, which is normally centered and overlapping the radius. Because slight oblique positioning of the wrist can produce a misleading appearance of ulnar displacement, it is crucial that a properly positioned lateral view be obtained. A true lateral view should have superimposition of the four ulnar metacarpals, superimposition of the proximal pole of the scaphoid with the lunate and triquetrum, and the radial styloid centered over its distal articular

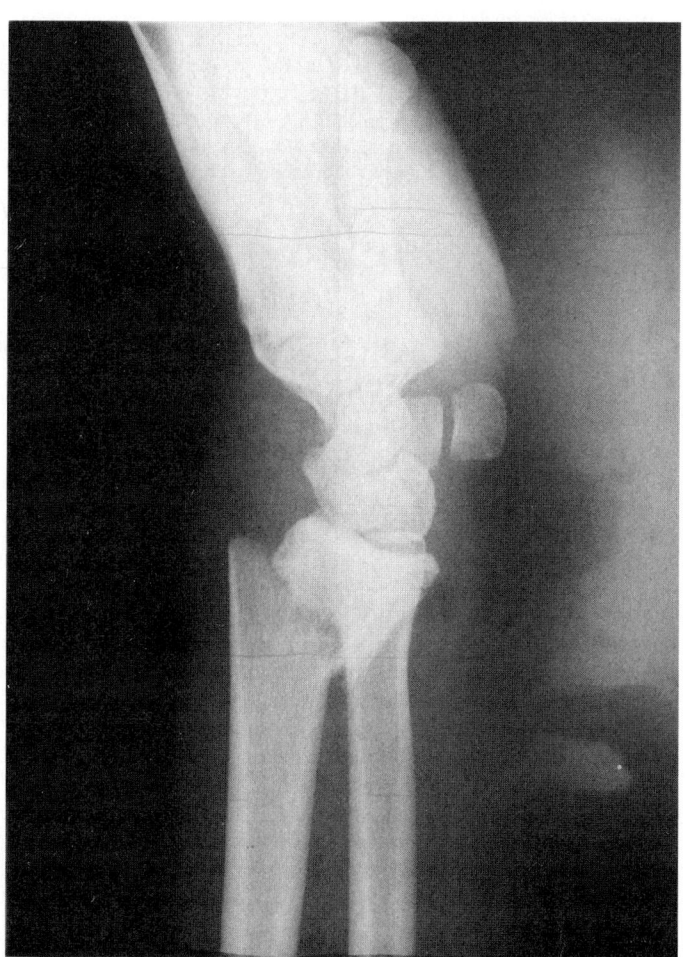

FIG. 269-12. Smith fracture.

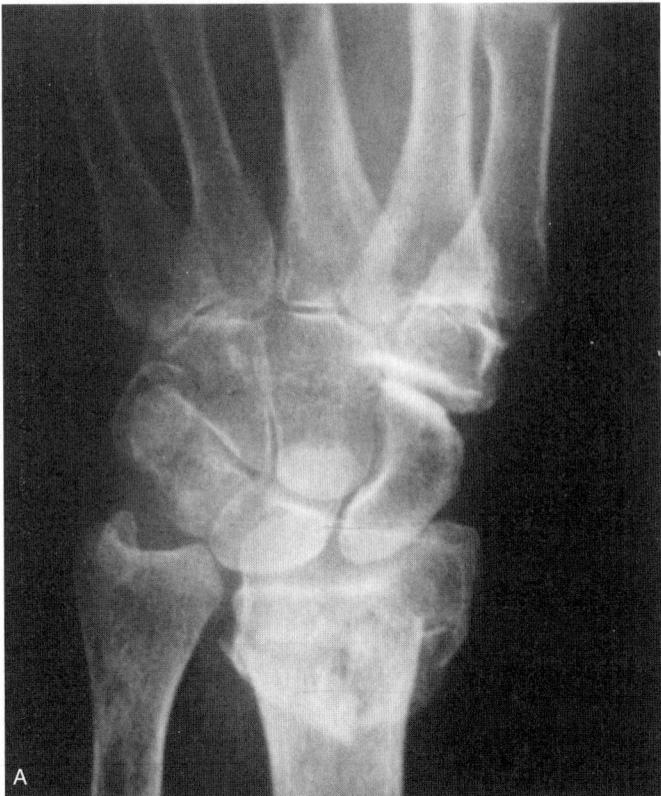

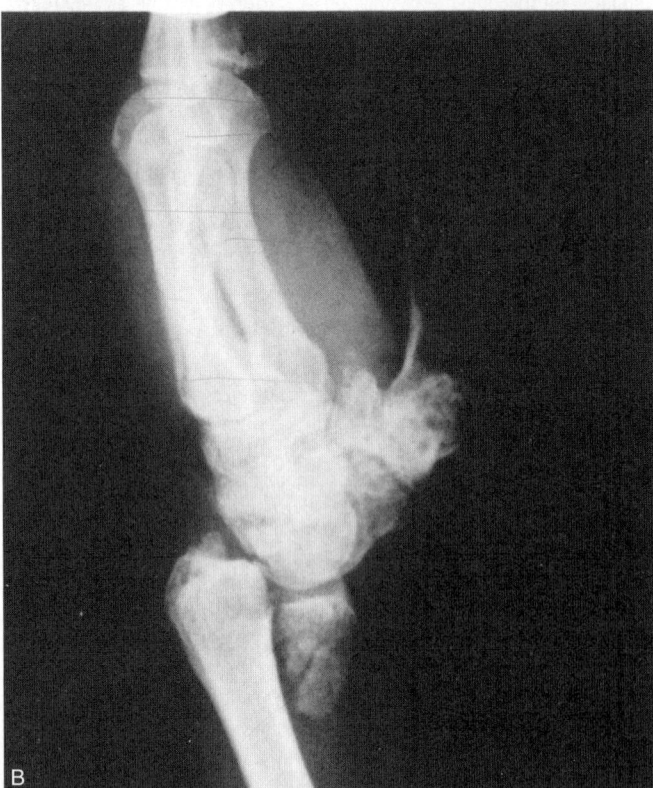

FIG. 269-13. Volar Barton fracture. **A.** Posteroanterior view. **B.** Lateral view. (Reproduced with permission from Chin HW, Visotsky J: Wrist fractures. *Emerg Med Clin North Am* 11:3, 1993.)

surface. CT scanning may be necessary to establish the diagnosis if plain films are inconclusive.

Immobilizing the wrist in supination reduces dorsal dislocations, whereas volar dislocations are placed in pronation. Patients with acute DRUJ disruption are referred acutely for orthopedic follow up. These injuries unfortunately have a high recurrence rate, particularly if there are delays in diagnosis, and may require reconstructive surgery.

ACKNOWLEDGMENT

The authors wish to acknowledge the contributions of Harold Chin, MD, to previous editions of this chapter.

REFERENCES

1. Berger RA: The anatomy and ligaments of the wrist and distal radioulnar joints. *Clin Orthop Related Res* 383:32, 2001.
2. Adams BD, Samani JE, Holley KA: Triangular fibrocartilage injury: A laboratory model. *J Hand Surg [Am]* 21:189, 1996.
3. Ritchie JV, Munter DW: Emergency department evaluation and treatment of wrist injuries. *Emerg Med Clin North Am* 17:823, 1999.
4. Gilbert TJ, Cohen M: Imaging of acute injuries to the wrist and hand. *Radiol Clin North Am* 35:701, 1997.
5. Goldfarb CA, Yuming Y, Gilula LA, et al: Wrist fractures: What the clinician wants to know. *Radiology* 219:11, 2001.
6. Terry DW, Ramin JE: The navicular fat stripes: A useful roentgen feature for evaluating wrist trauma. *AJR* 124:24, 1975.
7. Sherman GM, Seitz WH: Fractures and dislocations of the wrist. *Curr Opinion Orthop* 10:237, 1999.
8. Meldon SW, Hargarten SW: Ligamentous injuries of the wrist. *J Emerg Med* 13:217, 1995.
9. Frankel VH: The Terry Thomas Sign. *Clin Orthop* 135:311, 1978.
10. Gelberman RH, Cooney WP, Szabo RM: Carpal instability. *J Bone Joint Surg* 82A:578, 2000.
11. Perron AD, Brady WJ, Keats TE, et al: Orthopedic pitfalls in the ED: Lunate and perilunate injuries. *Am J Emerg Med* 19:157, 2001.
12. Krasin E, Goldwirth M, Gold A, et al: Review of the current methods in the diagnosis and treatment of scaphoid fractures. *Postgrad Med J* 77:235, 2001.
13. Lacey JD, Hodge JC: Pisiform and hamulus fractures: Easily missed wrist fractures diagnosed on a reverse oblique radiograph. *J Emerg Med* 16:445, 1998.
14. Perron AD, Hersh RE, Brady WJ, et al: Orthopedic pitfalls in the ED: Galeazzi and Monteggia fracture-dislocation. *Am J Emerg Med* 19:225, 2001.

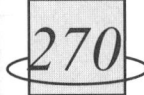

INJURIES TO THE ELBOW AND FOREARM

Arthur F. Proust

Jason H. Bredenkamp

Dennis T. Uehara

ELBOW

Elbow Dislocation

The elbow with its ulnohumeral articulation is one of the most stable joints in the body. The inherent stability in the flexion-extension plane is augmented by the muscular attachments and collateral ligaments. Because of this stability, surgical repair for acute instability is usually not required, and chronic dislocations are unusual. Despite this, however, dislocations of the elbow are commonly seen, and rank third in large-joint dislocations, after glenohumeral and patellofemoral dislocations. Additionally, fractures of the coronoid process, radial head, medial epicondyle, or olecranon may be associated with an elbow dislocation, complicating its treatment.

There are five general types of elbow dislocations: (1) posterior, (2) anterior, (3) medial, (4) lateral, and (5) divergent. The vast majority of elbow dislocations are posterior; the others are rare. The mechanism of injury is usually due to a fall on the outstretched hand.

Clinically, the patient presents with the elbow in 45 degrees of flexion. The olecranon is prominent posteriorly, and the deformity resembles a displaced supracondylar fracture. If the patient is seen immediately after the injury, the bony landmarks can be identified. Later, however, the swelling may be quite severe, with no possibility of evaluating the injury topographically. The first priority of care is to assess neurovascular status, with specific attention to the brachial artery and the ulnar, radial, and median nerves, as these structures are the most vulnerable to entrapment. The examination must be performed before and after manipulation, since neurovascular complications occur in 8 to 21 percent of patients, the most frequent being injury to the ulnar nerve. Vascular complications occur in 5 to 13 percent of elbow dislocations, with brachial artery injury the most common.[1] Absence of a radial pulse before reduction, an open dislocation, and other systemic injuries (such as those of the head, chest, and abdomen) are significantly associated with arterial injury.[2,3]

Radiographically, on the lateral view, both the ulna and radius are displaced posteriorly (Figure 270-1). In the anteroposterior view, there may be lateral or medial displacement, with the ulna and radius in their normal relationship to each other. A search for associated fractures should be performed. In a child, a fracture of the medial epicondyle is most commonly seen. In adults, fractures of the coronoid process, radial head, capitellum, or olecranon may occur. Initially, these fractures should only be noted, with primary attention focused on the dislocation.

After adequate sedation, closed reduction is accomplished by gentle longitudinal traction on the wrist and forearm (Figure 270-2). An assistant applies countertraction on the arm. Any medial or lateral displacement is corrected with the other hand. Downward pressure on the proximal forearm helps to disengage the coronoid process from the olecranon fossa. Distal traction is continued, and the elbow is flexed. With reduction, a palpable "clunk" is felt as the olecranon is seated in the humeral articular surface. The elbow is then moved through its full range of motion (ROM) to assess stability. If full smooth passive ROM is not possible, the postreduction radiograph should be examined for entrapment of the medial epicondyle, especially common in children (Figure 270-3). Instability in extension suggests associated fractures or disruption of the capsule. Entrapped soft tissue and/or loose intra-articular fragments indicate the need for open reduction.

After reduction, the elbow is placed in a plaster splint from the axilla to the base of the fingers with the elbow in at least 90 degrees of flexion. Because of the soft-tissue trauma and subsequent edema, cylinder casts should not be placed. A neurovascular follow-up examination should be obtained the following day. Treatment with an early ROM program after 1 to 2 weeks of splinting generally leads to favorable results.

Appropriate treatment of elbow dislocations requires adequate reduction and recognition of neurovascular complications, associated fractures, and postreduction instability. If there is any question of neurovascular compromise, the patient should be admitted for observation. Immediate orthopedic consultation should be sought with irreducible dislocations, neurovascular compromise, joint capsule disruption, associated fractures, and open dislocations. Potential late complications include posttraumatic stiffness, posterolateral joint instability, ectopic ossification, and occult distal radioulnar joint disruption.

Fractures about the Elbow

Fractures about the elbow include fractures of the intercondylar areas, supracondyles, epicondyles, condyles, trochlea, capitulum, and radial head.[4]

INTERCONDYLAR T OR Y FRACTURES Intercondylar fractures, in which the condylar fragments are separated, are much more common in adults than in children. Any distal humerus fracture in an adult

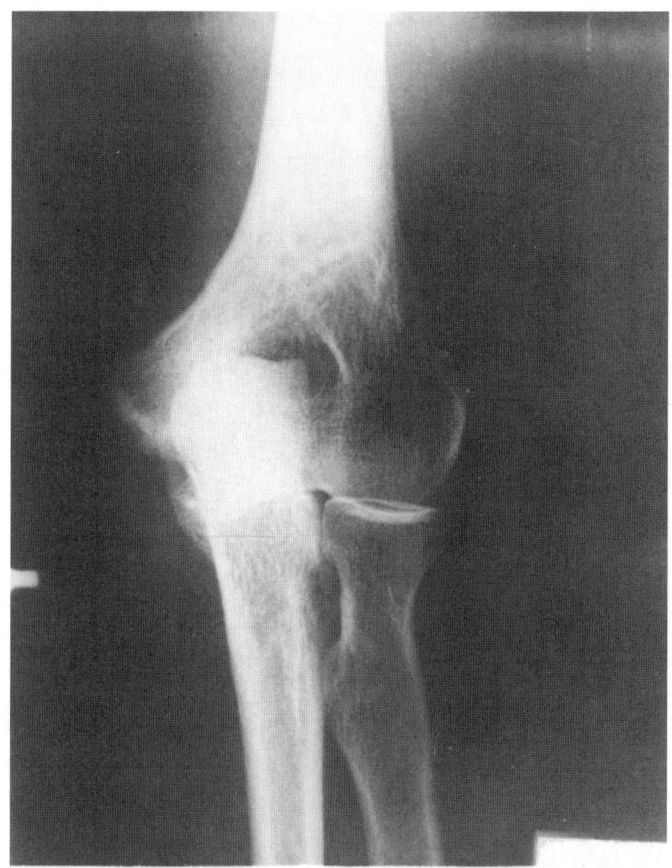
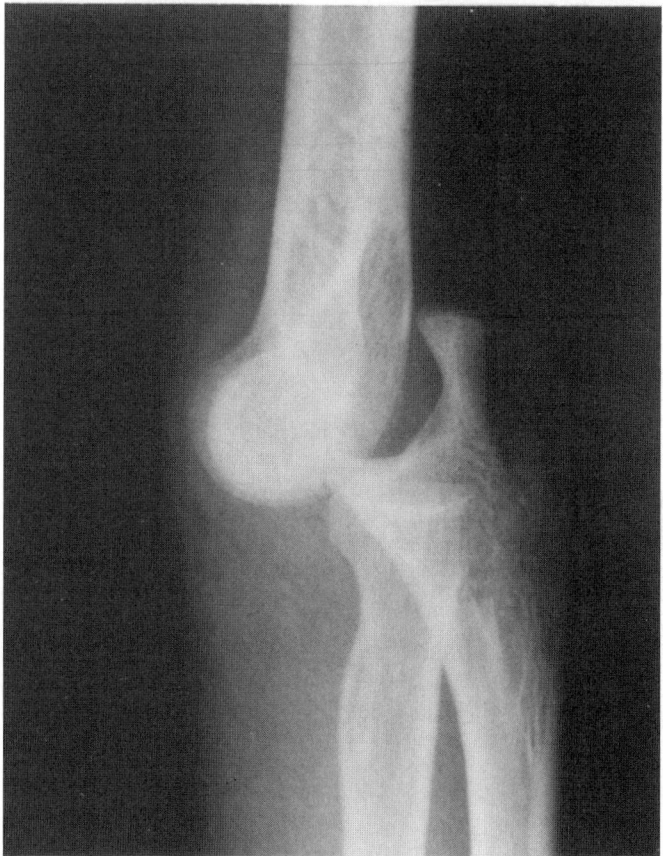

FIG. 270-1. Posterior dislocation of the elbow, on posteroanterior and lateral views.

A

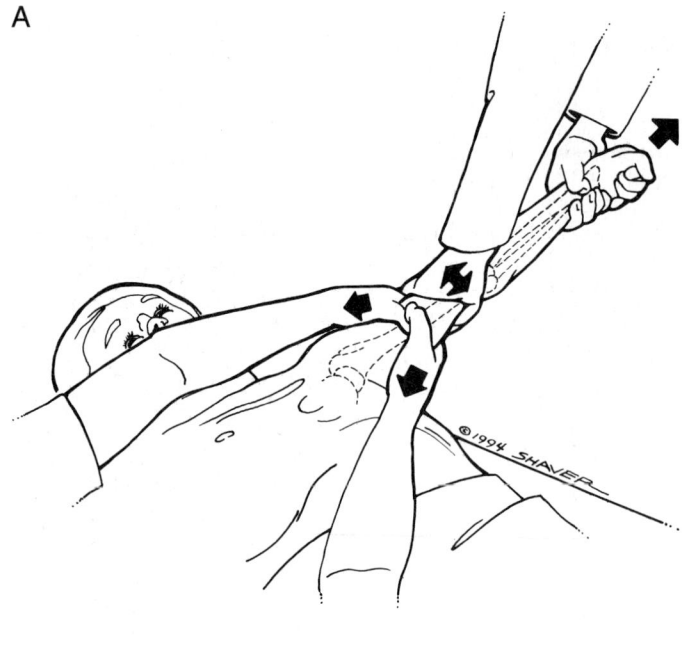

B

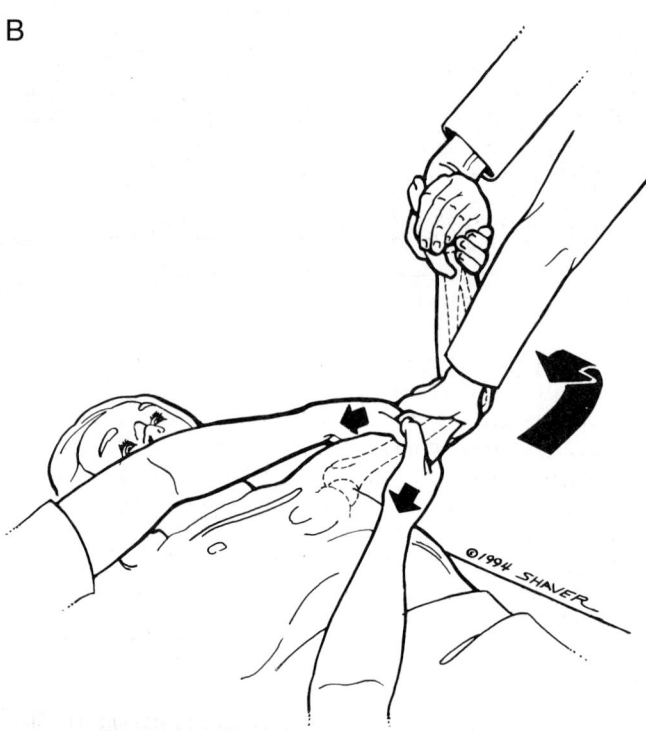

FIG. 270-2. Reduction of posterior elbow dislocation. **A.** Operator applies gentle traction as assistant applies countertraction. Displacement is corrected with the other hand. Downward pressure on the proximal forearm disengages the coronoid process from the olecranon fossa. **B.** Distal traction is continued as the elbow is flexed.

should initially be assumed to be intercondylar rather than supracondylar (Figure 270-4). A careful search should be made for a fracture line separating the condyles from each other and from the humerus. This distinguishes intercondylar T or Y fractures from other fractures of the distal humerus.

The mechanism of injury is a force directed against the posterior elbow, driving the olecranon against the humeral articular surface, separating the condyles and producing the typical fracture. These fractures are associated with severe soft-tissue injuries. Treatment in the

young is directed at anatomic reduction. In older patients with severe injuries, treatment is often directed at reestablishing articular surface congruity. If this cannot be achieved by closed methods, then the integrity of the articular surface is restored by an open reduction. As in supracondylar fractures, patients with severe edema or displaced fractures should be admitted.

SUPRACONDYLAR FRACTURES Supracondylar fractures of the humerus are common and account for 60 percent of all fractures of the elbow in children. Ninety-five percent of these extra-articular fractures are displaced posteriorly as a result of an extension force. When the mechanism of injury is due to a flexion force, the much less common anterior displacement occurs. There can also be various degrees of abduction, adduction, and rotation of the distal fragment.[5]

Extension-Type Supracondylar Fractures In an extension-type fracture, the patient will have significant edema and tenderness at the elbow. The olecranon is prominent, and there is a depression proximally over the area of the triceps muscle. This appearance may be easily mistaken for a posterior elbow dislocation.

Extension-type supracondylar fractures are classified into three types. Type I fractures are undisplaced. Type II fractures are displaced and have cortical contact. Type III fractures are subdivided into posterolateral and posteromedial fractures based on displacement and have no cortical contact.

Radiographs may reveal a fat-pad sign in undisplaced fractures (Figure 270-5).[6] Fat from the olecranon fossa is displaced posteriorly (posterior fat pad) by hemarthrosis, and the anterior fat pad may be quite prominent. Normally, a posterior fat pad is not visible, and an anterior fat pad may be visible as a thin lucent stripe. Abnormal fat pads may also be seen with nontraumatic joint effusions. In addition, they may be absent in severe trauma that disrupts the joint capsule and allows intra-articular fluid to extravasate. In some undisplaced fractures, the fracture line may not be seen, with **the fat-pad sign being the only evidence of injury. Treatment should be initiated as though a fracture were identified,** with splint immobilization and orthopedic consultation. In displaced fractures, the anteroposterior radiograph usually reveals a transverse fracture line. More severely displaced fractures may show medial or lateral displacement or rotation along the axis of the humerus (Figure 270-6). The lateral radiograph will reveal the fracture line extending obliquely from posterior proximal to anterior distal. The distal fragment will be displaced proximally and posteriorly.

Treatment of undisplaced or type I fractures consists of plaster immobilization. Type II and type III displaced fractures are treated by closed methods followed by pin fixation. The current major indications for open reduction are vascular insufficiency with a probable entrapped brachial artery in the fracture site or an irreducible fracture. Patients with displaced fractures or severe edema should be admitted for observation of neurovascular status.

Flexion-Type Supracondylar Fractures Flexion-type fractures occur in fewer than 5 percent of supracondylar fractures. The mechanism is direct anterior force against a flexed elbow. This results in anterior displacement of the distal fragment. Since the mechanism is direct force, these fractures are often open.

Radiographs reveal an oblique fracture from anterior proximal to posterior distal. The distal fragment is anterior to the humerus.

Management consists of closed reduction and plaster immobilization or surgery if reduction cannot be maintained by closed methods.

Complications of Supracondylar Fractures There are numerous complications of supracondylar fractures, including nerve and vascular injuries and those occurring late, such as nonunion, malunion, myositis ossificans, and loss of motion.

Neurologic complications have an incidence of 7 percent and are the result of traction, direct trauma, or nerve ischemia. Posteromedial

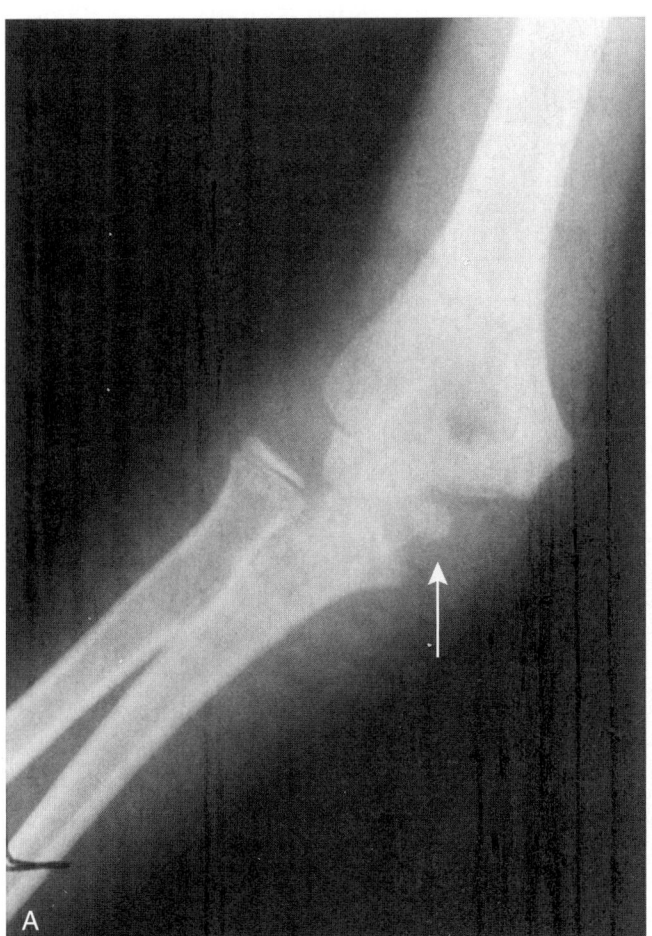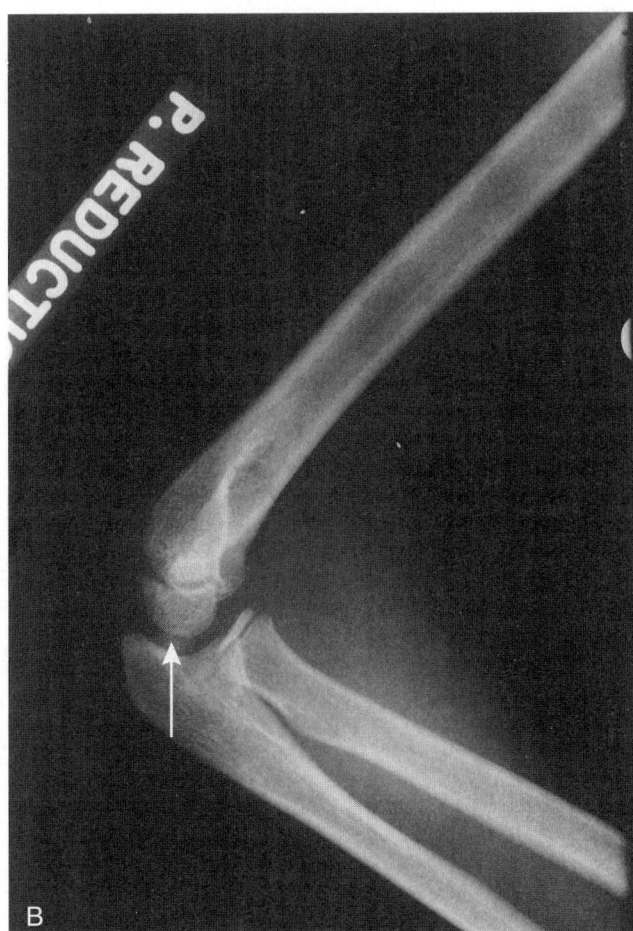

FIG. 270-3. Postreduction radiograph of a posterior elbow dislocation. The medial epicondyle is fragmented in the joint space and is seen in the anteroposterior **(A)** and lateral **(B)** radiographs *(arrow).*

displacement involves the radial nerve and posterolateral displacement usually affects the median nerve. Ulnar nerve injuries are uncommon; the highest incidence has been reported from pin placement. A high incidence of anterior interosseous nerve injuries has also been noted with supracondylar fractures. This nerve arises from the median nerve and innervates the flexor pollicis longus, the radial part of the flexor digitorum profundus, and the pronator quadratus. Since there is no sensory component to the anterior interosseous nerve, identification of the injury can be made only by specific muscle testing. Testing consists of flexion at the index finger distal interphalangeal and thumb interphalangeal joints. The mechanism of injury is usually traction and/or contusion. Complete transection is rare, and entrapment within the fracture occurs only occasionally. Joist and colleagues[5] noted all patients regained full flexion and strength after 4 to 17 weeks.

Acute vascular injuries must always be suspected in patients with supracondylar fractures. Absence of a radial pulse is common in children. This is most frequently due to transient arterial spasm. Rarely, there is a partial or complete transection of the brachial artery, an intimal tear and thrombosis, or entrapment within the fracture fragment.

The most serious complication is **Volkmann's ischemic contracture.** This classically occurs following a supracondylar fracture. Postischemic swelling, producing increased pressure within the enclosed osteofascial forearm compartment, reduces capillary blood perfusion below the level necessary for tissue viability. If unrelieved, the end result is muscle and nerve necrosis, and eventual replacement by fibrotic tissue, producing a contracture. Refusal to open the hand in children, pain with passive extension of the fingers, and forearm tenderness are signs of impending Volkmann's ischemia. It is now well understood

that the mere lack of a radial pulse does not indicate ischemia unless accompanied by these signs.

Treatment of supracondylar fractures with absent radial pulse begins with closed reduction and percutaneous pinning. Extremities still without a pulse and with signs of ischemia are taken to the operating room for fasciotomy and/or brachial artery exploration. Extremities without a pulse and no signs of ischemia may be treated in one of three ways: (1) close observation, (2) observation for 24 to 36 h followed by arteriography and surgery if indicated, or (3) immediate surgical exploration.

DISTAL HUMERUS FRACTURES The distal humerus can be imagined as two columns of bone that end in the medial and lateral condyles (Figure 270-7). The flared proximal portions of the condyles are the epicondyles. The epicondyles are nonarticulating surfaces that serve as sites of origin for forearm, wrist, and digit flexors and pronators (medial), and extensors and supinators (lateral). The distal aspects of the condyles are the articular surfaces. Medially, the trochlea articulates with the olecranon to form a uniaxial hinge joint, and laterally, the capitellum abuts the radial head to form a pivot joint. Between the condyles is the coronoid fossa anteriorly and the olecranon fossa posteriorly. These allow for full flexion and extension of the ulna. Additionally, the radial fossa lies just proximal to the capitellum anteriorly and permits full flexion of the radius.

Several important neurovascular structures lie in close proximity to the distal humerus, and evaluation of their function is essential. These include the brachial artery, which is palpable just medial to the distal biceps tendon in the antecubital fossa, and the radial, median, and ulnar nerves. The latter is palpable as a cord just posterior to

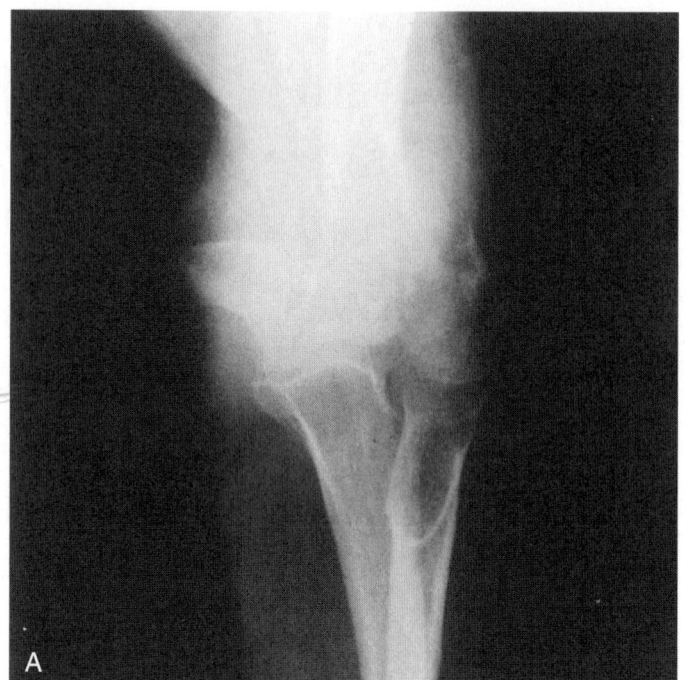

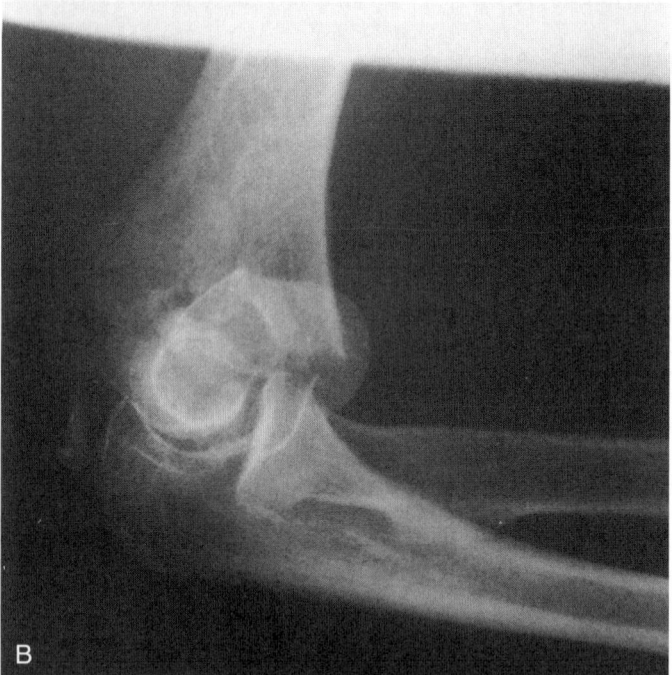

FIG. 270-4. Comminuted displaced and rotated intercondylar fracture (type IV). **A.** Posteroanterior view. **B.** Lateral view.

the medial epicondyle and is vulnerable to injury with lacerations over this area. Sensory and motor function of each individual nerve should be assessed.

Standard radiographs of the elbow may have subtle findings, especially in the pediatric population. Knowledge of the age at which ossification centers appear is critical (see Chap. 136).

Routine emergency department care of distal humerus fractures includes immobilization, ice, elevation, analgesics, and orthopedic referral within 24 h if no neurovascular compromise, or in the emergency department if the latter is present.

Epicondyle Fractures *Lateral epicondyle fractures* almost never occur, since the anatomic position of the condyle reduces the exposure to direct

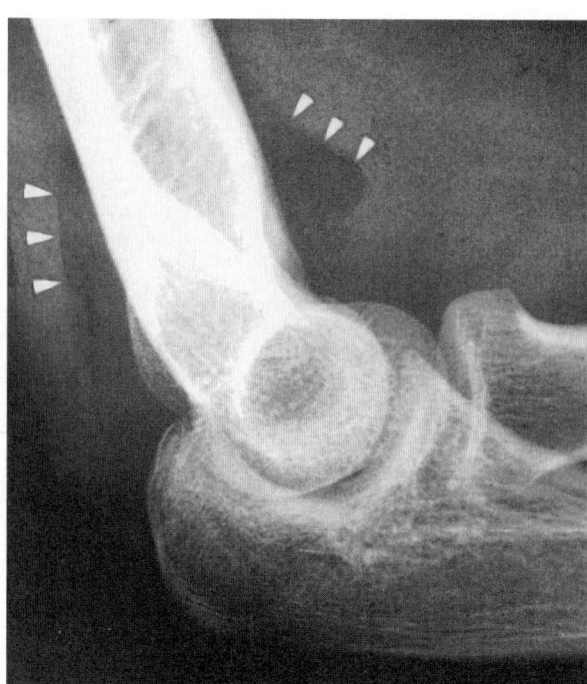

FIG. 270-5. Anterior and posterior fat pad signs.

blows, resulting instead in fractures of the lateral condyle. When they do occur, these fractures are usually avulsion fractures and may be treated by immobilization with the elbow flexed to 90 degrees and the forearm in supination. The patient is referred to an orthopedist within 1 week.

Isolated medial epicondyle fractures are considered extraarticular injuries and usually occur in children and adolescents. Mechanisms include a posterior elbow dislocation, repeated valgus stress, such as throwing a baseball (Little League elbow), or a direct blow. If there is an associated tear of the medial collateral ligament, the epicondyle itself may become entrapped in the joint space. Patients present with pain over the medial elbow that is exacerbated by supination of the forearm and flexion of the forearm, wrist, and digits. Edema and tenderness are noted in the same area. Standard radiographs should be obtained with special attention to any intraarticular fragment. Careful examination of ulnar nerve function is needed. Nondisplaced or minimally displaced medial epicondyle fractures are treated nonoperatively, with early motion. Fragment displacement greater than 1 cm or valgus instability are generally treated by internal fixation.

Emergency department management consists of immobilization of the forearm in flexion and pronation, and the wrists in flexion.

Condyle Fractures *Lateral condyle fractures* occur in children and are more common than their medial counterpart.[7] They result from a direct blow to the lateral elbow or from varus stress with the forearm extended, as in a fall on an outstretched hand. Patients complain of pain in the lateral elbow, and swelling is noted in the same area.

Medial condyle fractures are uncommon and are mostly limited to children. Mechanism of injury is from either a transmitted force from the ulna, such as a fall on an outstretched hand, or excessive valgus stress. Pain and swelling medially are prominent findings. The injury is often confused with the more common medial epicondyle fracture for two reasons. First, the mechanism and examination findings are similar. Second, because the trochlea ossification center does not appear until age 9 to 10 years, it is often missed on radiographs.

Complications of lateral and medial epicondyle fractures are frequent and include nonunion, cubitus valgus or varus deformity, ulnar nerve palsy, and avascular necrosis.[8] Careful neurovascular assessment is needed for these injuries. Because surgical correction is generally preferred, emergent orthopedic consultation is generally recommended for both lateral and medial epicondylar fractures.

FIG. 270-6. Type III displaced supra-condylar fracture. The distal fragment is displaced posteriorly, proximally, and medially. The proximal fragment is displaced anteriorly and distally.

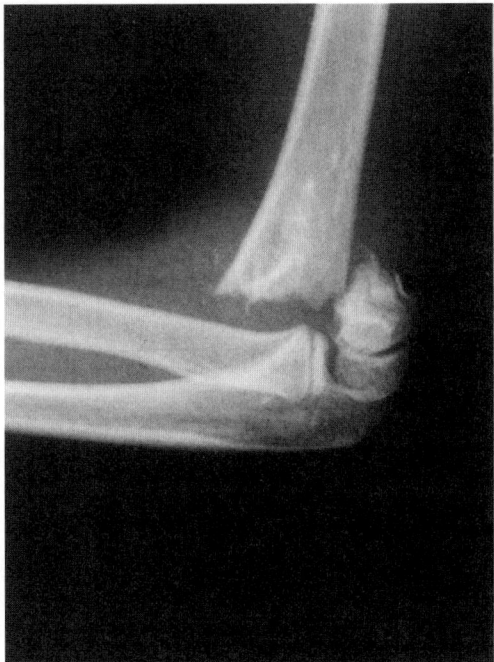

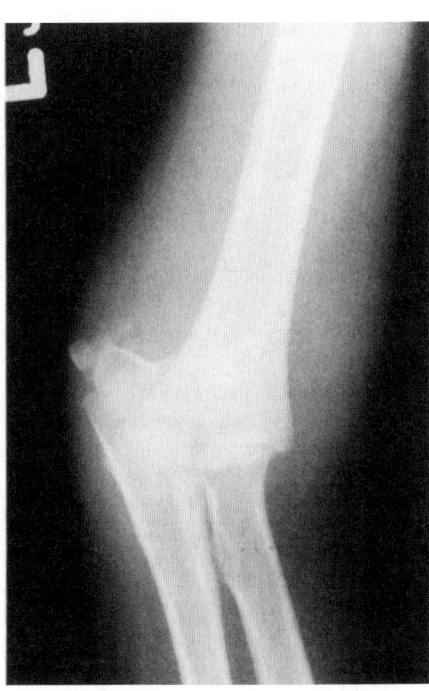

ARTICULAR SURFACE FRACTURES

Trochlea Fractures Isolated trochlea fractures are rare, and they are more often associated with other elbow injuries, such as posterior elbow dislocations. Physical findings usually include swelling, tenderness, and limited movement of the elbow joint. Radiographic findings can be subtle, and ultrasound or magnetic resonance imaging may be required for diagnosis. Complications are common and include limited flexion and extension, elbow joint instability, avascular necrosis, nonunion, and arthritis. Surgical repair is usually indicated.

Capitellum Fractures Isolated capitellum fractures are rare. They are usually associated with radial head fractures. Pain and tenderness are present over the lateral elbow, and examination reveals swelling, lateral tenderness, and limitation of flexion and extension. If pain and tenderness are present medially, injury to the medial collateral ligament

FIG. 270-7. Elbow anatomy.

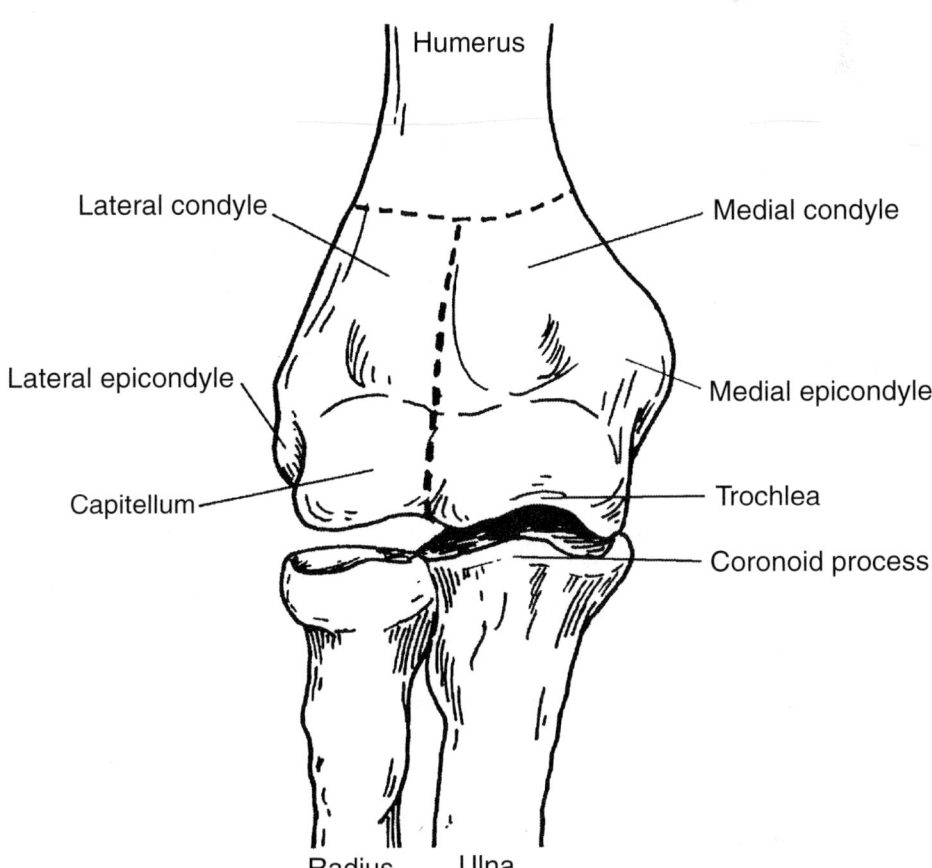

should be suspected. Radiographic findings may be subtle and are best seen on a lateral view. The capitellum has no tendinous or ligamentous attachments, so many fractures are nondisplaced. A radial head-capitellum view can be helpful in addition to standard views. Definitive care is surgical and complications are similar to those of trochlea fractures.

Radial Head Fractures   The radial head is located just distal to the lateral epicondyle. It can be palpated by rotating the forearm while flexed. It articulates with the capitellum and the lesser sigmoid notch of the ulna to form a pivot joint. The radial head serves as a stabilizer of the elbow against valgus stress, along with the medial collateral ligament, and against longitudinal forces.

Radial head fractures are the most common fractures of the elbow. They result from a fall on an outstretched hand causing the radial head to be driven into the capitellum. Associated injuries are common and may include capitellum, olecranon, and coronoid fractures, medial collateral ligament injury, medial epicondyle avulsion fracture secondary to valgus stress, and elbow dislocation. A specific associated injury, the *Essex-Lopresti lesion,* occurs when there is disruption of the triangular fibrocartilage of the wrist and the interosseous membrane between the radius and ulna, causing pain in the wrist and forearm. The result is a distal radioulnar joint dissociation, which can cause migration of the radius proximally if radial head excision is performed.

Radial head fractures cause pain in the lateral elbow, especially with pronation and supination of the forearm. On examination, there may be swelling laterally and tenderness with palpation of the radial head. On standard elbow radiographs, radial head fractures may be subtle. Additional images, including obliques and a radial head-capitellum view, may be helpful. Furthermore, two radiographic clues can aid in the diagnosis. **The first is the radiocapitellar line. On lateral films, a line drawn from the center of the radial shaft should transect the radial head and capitellum (Figure 270-8).** This is especially helpful in children whose epiphysis has not fused. **The other clue is the appearance of an abnormal fat pad (see Figure 270-5).**

Nondisplaced fractures with no mobility restrictions can be treated conservatively with immobilization. For these, emergency department treatment consists of sling immobilization with the elbow in flexion, ice, elevation, analgesics, and referral to an orthopedic surgeon within 1 week. For displaced fractures or those with restricted range of motion, surgical repair is generally indicated, and orthopedic referral in 24 h is needed. Complications of radial head fracture include chronic pain and restricted range of motion at the elbow.

PROXIMAL ULNA FRACTURES   The distal humerus articulates with the proximal ulna to form a uniaxial hinge joint, which allows flexion and extension of the forearm and provides some intrinsic stability. The

trochlea of the humerus rests in the greater sigmoid (semilunar) notch of the ulna. The anterior projection of the notch is the coronoid, and the posterior prominence, which is easily palpable, is the olecranon. The brachialis muscle inserts at the coronoid, and the triceps muscle inserts at the olecranon. A subtendinous bursa separates the triceps tendon from the olecranon, and a subcutaneous bursa lies just distal to the tendinous insertion. The latter frequently becomes inflamed. All proximal ulna fractures are considered intra-articular.

Coronoid Fractures   Coronoid fractures are uncommon and usually associated with posterior elbow dislocations as the trochlea is driven into the coronoid, or as an isolated injury secondary to elbow hyperextension. There is pain, swelling, and tenderness over the antecubital fossa. Radiographic visualization is best with lateral and oblique films.

If elbow dislocation is present, careful neurovascular examination should be done prior to and after reduction, with special emphasis on the ulnar nerve (see elbow dislocation above). Emergency department treatment should include immobilization with the elbow in flexion and the forearm in supination, ice, elevation, analgesics, and referral to an orthopedic surgeon within 24 h. Severe fractures or those associated with joint instability require open reduction and internal fixation, and frequently have poor outcomes.

Olecranon Fractures   The olecranon is usually fractured by direct trauma, or by a fall on an outstretched hand with the elbow in flexion. Associated injuries are common, including open wounds, dislocations, other fractures (especially of the radial head), and ulnar nerve injury. Pain is present over the posterior elbow and examination reveals swelling, tenderness, and occasionally crepitus. Because the triceps muscle inserts at the olecranon, triceps function is usually compromised when tested by forearm extension. **Ulnar nerve injury is common, and therefore a careful neurologic examination is needed.** Lateral films offer the best view of the olecranon. In adolescents, the epiphysis ossifies by age 11 and fuses by age 16, so comparison films and the appearance of an abnormal fat pad can aid in the diagnosis.

Emergency department treatment should include immobilization with the elbow in flexion forearm neutral, ice, elevation, analgesics, and referral to an orthopedist in 24 h. Nondisplaced fractures (less than 2 mm in both flexion and extension) can be treated conservatively with immobilization, but all others require surgical repair.

FOREARM FRACTURES

The radius and ulna are joined together along their entire length by a fibrous interosseous membrane, and touch only at their ends to form the complex proximal and distal radioulnar joints. The ulna is a comparatively straight bone, whereas the radius has an important outward bowing. During the motions of supination and pronation, the radius rotates around the relatively fixed ulna. Because these bones have such a close relationship to one another, injury to either will have a direct impact on the other. A displaced or angulated fracture of one bone typically disrupts the other or causes a dislocation at the proximal or distal radioulnar joint, such as in the Monteggia and Galeazzi fracture-dislocations.

The radius and ulna are also under the influence of numerous muscle groups, such as those that supinate and pronate. The biceps brachii and the supinator insert on the proximal radius and are the powerful supinators of the forearm. The pronator teres inserts on the radial shaft and exerts a pronating force. Radius fractures that are located between these muscle groups will result in marked displacement of the bone, with supination of the proximal segment and pronation of the distal portion. However, if the fracture is distal to the insertion of the pronator teres, these forces tend to neutralize one another and result in less rotational deformity. When considering treatment of these fractures, careful attention must be paid to the maintenance of length and align-

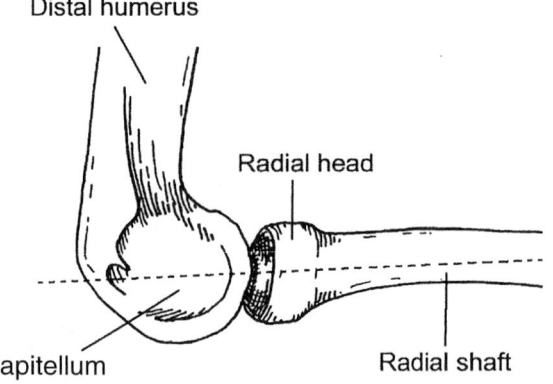

Distal humerus

Radial head

Capitellum

Radial shaft

FIG. 270-8. The radiocapitellar line. On lateral views a line drawn through the center of the radius transects the radial head and middle third of the capitellum. This relationship is lost even in subtle fractures.

ment. Also, the lateral bow of the radius must be preserved to allow full pronation and supination after healing.

The neuroanatomy is most easily understood by appreciating the neural control of the most basic components of wrist and finger movement (Figure 270-9). The radial nerve travels over the lateral epicondyle and supplies the muscles of wrist extension before it gives off a branch, the posterior interosseous nerve. This branch travels around the proximal radius and controls the muscles of finger and thumb extension. The remainder of the radial nerve is purely sensory and innervates the posterior aspect of the hand from the thumb to radial half of the ring finger. Thus the proximal portion of the radial nerve controls the more proximal function of wrist extension, the distal branch (posterior interosseus nerve) controls the more distal function of finger extension, and another branch is purely sensory. Therefore, an isolated injury (e.g., to the posterior interosseous branch) would affect finger extension but spare wrist extension and sensation to the dorsum of the hand. **The single best test of radial nerve motor function is to have the patient extend both the wrist and fingers against resistance. Sensation is tested over the dorsum of the thumb index web space.**

The median nerve controls the basic movements of wrist and finger flexion and sensation on the volar surface of the hand from the thumb to the radial half of the ring finger. The proximal portion of the median nerve innervates the muscles that control wrist flexion and the flexor digitorum superficialis before it gives off the anterior interosseous nerve. This branch controls portions of the remaining deep finger flexors: flexor digitorum profundus, flexor pollicis longus, and pronator quadratus. The remaining portion of the median nerve provides sensation to most of the volar surface of the hand plus a motor branch to the thenar muscles of the thumb (recurrent branch of the median nerve). The median nerve is evaluated by assessing each of these distal branches. **A simple test of anterior interosseous nerve function is the ability to make a circle, or "OK" sign, with the thumb and index finger. Abduction of the thumb (recurrent branch of the median nerve) and intact sensation on the radial side of the palm complete the evaluation of the median nerve.**

The ulnar nerve provides innervation to forearm muscles, but more important, it controls the intrinsic muscles of the hand and provides sensation to the little finger and the ulnar half of the ring finger. The ability to abduct the index finger against resistance (palpate the first interosseous muscle) and two-point discrimination over the tip of the little finger are easy tests of ulnar nerve function.

In adults, solitary fractures of the forearm are uncommon due to the close relationship of the radius and ulna. The fibrous interconnection

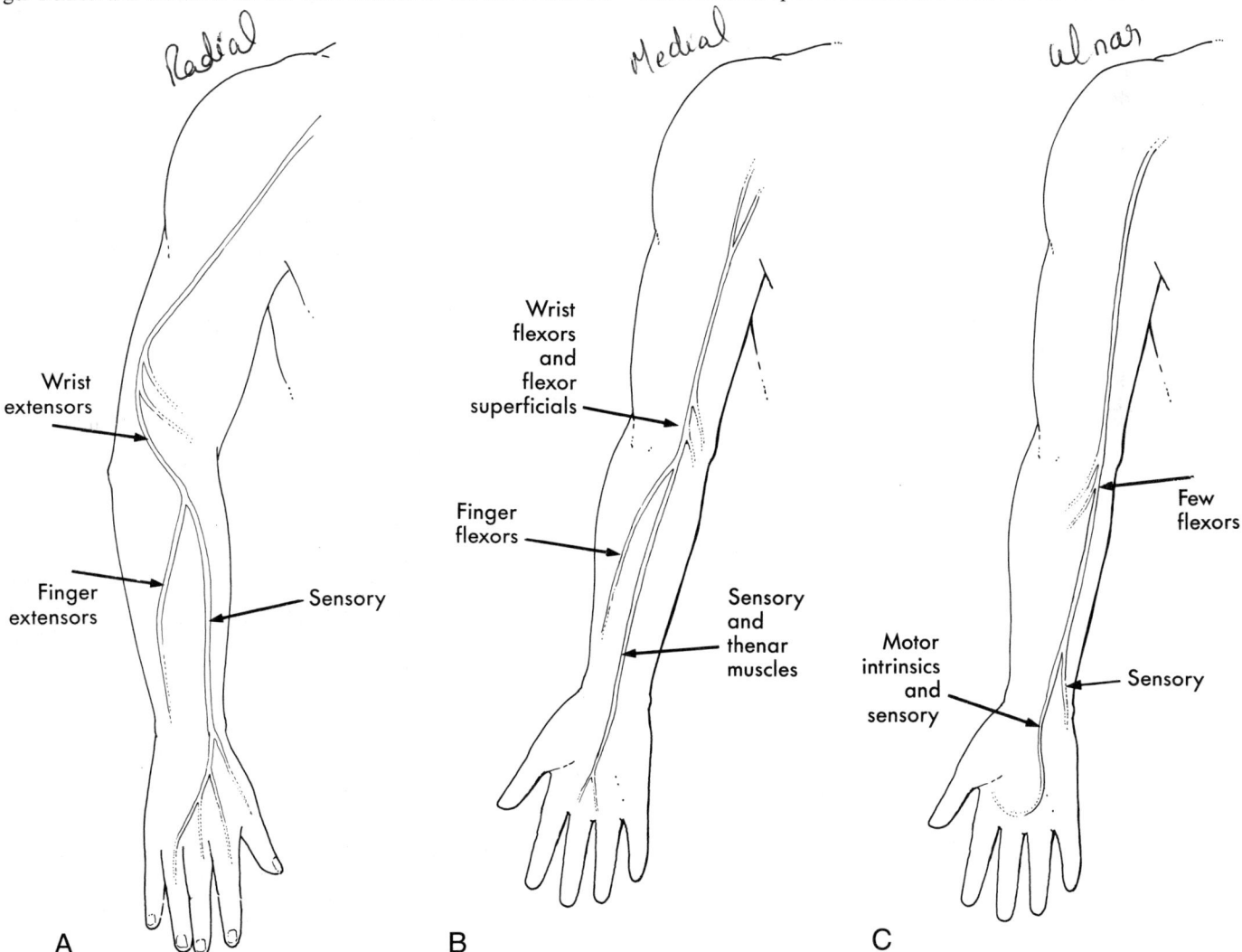

FIG. 270-9. **A.** The radial nerve controls wrist extension before branching into the posterior interosseous nerve. **B.** The median nerve controls wrist flexion and the flexor digitorum superficialis before branching into the anterior interosseous nerve (which controls the deep finger flexors in the forearm) and a branch that innervates the thenar muscles and provides sensation to most of the palm. **C.** The ulnar nerve controls the intrinsic muscles and provides sensation to the ulnar side of the hand. [Reproduced with permission from Chin HW, Propp DA, Orban DJ: Forearm and wrist, in Rosen P, Barkin RM, et al (eds): *Emergency Medicine Concepts and Clinical Practice,* 3d ed. Vol 1. St. Louis: Mosby–Year Book, 1992.]

between the radius and ulna transmits traumatic energy above and below the injury. Thus fractures usually occur at two or more sites or involve a fracture of one bone with a ligamentous injury, with or without an associated joint dislocation. Because distant structures are commonly injured, the clinician must examine joints above and below the involved bones both clinically and radiologically. This occurrence is usually present with significantly angulated injuries.

Fractures of Both Radius and Ulna

A great amount of force is necessary to fracture both the radius and ulna. This injury occurs most often from vehicular trauma, falls from a height, or a direct blow to the forearm. The magnitude of the force determines the type of injury. A moderate force produces transverse or mildly oblique fractures. Comminuted and segmental fractures are produced by a high-impact force. As one might expect, these fractures are often displaced. Open fractures of the radius and ulna are second only to tibia fractures because of the subcutaneous location of the entire ulna and the distal portion of the radius.

Nondisplaced fractures of both bones are exceedingly rare because the force necessary to produce the injury is also sufficient to displace it. Examination reveals swelling, deformity, and tenderness of the forearm. Careful assessment of the neurovascular status is needed. Nerve injuries can be seen with severe open fractures, but fortunately are uncommon with most closed injuries. Because of the excellent collateral circulation of the forearm, vascular compromise is generally not a major problem if either the radial or ulnar circulation is intact.

The fractures are clearly visible on the radiographs. The amount and degree of angulation, displacement, and shortening should be noted. Changes in rotational alignment may be subtle. A rough estimate of rotational alignment can be made by noting the normal orientation of various bony prominences of these bones. On the anteroposterior radiograph, the radial styloid and radial (bicipital) tuberosity normally point in opposite directions, whereas the ulnar styloid and coronoid process do so on the lateral view. A change in this arrangement suggests rotation malalignment. Since these bones are also oblong rather than circular in their cross-sectional appearance, a sudden change in the bone's width at the fracture site is another clue to a rotational deformity. The wrist and elbow may also be x-rayed because of the likelihood of an associated dislocation or articular fracture.

Treatment depends upon the type of fracture. Torus or greenstick fractures in children can be treated with plaster immobilization. All other fractures in children or adults require operative reduction and internal or external fixation.

Complications include reduced ability to supinate and pronate, osteomyelitis, nonunion, malunion, neurovascular injury, and compartment syndrome. Recognizing the development of a compartment syndrome is particularly important to prevent debilitating ischemic or Volkmann's contractures of the forearm. The diagnostic findings are palpable induration of the area, pain with passive movement of the fingers, and pain that appears to be disproportionate to the physical findings. The presence of a palpable pulse does not exclude the diagnosis of compartment syndrome. Alterations in sensation and the pulse are late findings. Direct measurements of elevated compartment pressures confirm the diagnosis. Urgent fasciotomy is required, ideally within 8 h of the onset of symptoms.

Ulna Fractures

ISOLATED ULNA FRACTURE (NIGHTSTICK FRACTURE) Isolated fractures of the ulna most often result from direct blows to the forearm. A fracture resulting from the natural response to raise the forearm in defense of a blow from a club is referred to as a *nightstick fracture*. Undisplaced fractures are immobilized in a long-arm splint and closely followed for subsequent displacement of the fracture.

Displaced fractures are those with greater than 10 degrees of angulation or displacement of more than 50 percent of the width of the bone at the site of the fracture. Open reduction and internal fixation with a compression plate and screws are necessary to prevent angulation, loss of length, and rotational deformity. These injuries should be closely scrutinized for any possible radius fracture or dislocation.

MONTEGGIA FRACTURE-DISLOCATION Fracture of the ulnar shaft with a radial head dislocation is often referred to as *Monteggia fracture-dislocation* (Figure 270-10). It is very easy to miss the associated radial head dislocation.[9] Fractures are classified into four types, depending on the location of the ulna fracture and the direction of the radial head dislocation (Table 270-1). Most typical is a diaphyseal fracture in the proximal third of the ulna with an anterior dislocation of the radial head (60 percent of cases). Clinically, there is considerable pain and swelling at the elbow. The radial head may be palpable in an anterolateral or posterolateral location. The forearm may appear shortened and angulated. The ulnar fracture is clearly visible and may overshadow the less obvious radial head dislocation. As a rule, the radial head normally points to the capitellum in all radiographic views of the elbow. In a Monteggia fracture, the apex of the ulna fracture points in the direction of the radial head dislocation.

Monteggia fracture-dislocations are generally treated with open reduction and internal fixation of the ulna and closed reduction of the radial head dislocation, although children may be treated by closed reduction of both bones and long-arm cast immobilization. Complications include nonunion, redislocation, infection, and paralysis of the posterior interosseus nerve, a deep branch of the radial nerve (remember that the nerve wraps around the proximal radius).

Radius Fractures

FRACTURES OF THE PROXIMAL TWO-THIRDS OF THE RADIUS Radius fractures can be divided into those that are proximal and those that are distal to the junction of the middle and distal thirds of the bone. Excluding radial head fractures, isolated fractures of the proximal two-thirds of the radius are rare because the radius is relatively well protected from direct blows by the ulna and surrounding forearm musculature. Undisplaced fractures are rare; these are treated with cast immobilization. Fractures of the proximal two-thirds of the radius are often displaced by both the force of the injury and the action of the supinators and pronators on the radius. They require internal fixation to prevent rotational deformity. Compartment syndrome is rare with these fractures. Most complications involve malunion or nonunion because of inadequate or lost reduction.

FRACTURES OF THE DISTAL ONE-THIRD OF THE RADIUS (GALEAZZI FRACTURE) Fractures of the distal third of the radial shaft are produced by falls on the outstretched hand in forced pronation or by a direct blow. Much like the Monteggia fracture-dislocation, the distal radial shaft fracture is often associated with a distal radioulnar joint dislocation, hence the name *reverse Monteggia fracture* or, more commonly, *Galeazzi fracture*. There is localized tenderness and swelling over the distal radius and wrist. The radius fracture is usually short oblique or transverse with dorsal lateral angulation. The distal radioulnar joint injury can be subtle. Radiographs may show only a slightly increased distal radioulnar joint space on the anteroposterior view. On the lateral view, the ulna is displaced dorsally. This injury is treated by open reduction and internal fixation of the radius fracture. Complications include infection, nonunion, and malunion. Injuries to the ulnar nerve and anterior interosseous branch of the median nerve have been reported, but usually heal spontaneously. If the radius heals with a rotational deformity, there may be pain at the distal radioulnar joint with extreme pronation and supination.

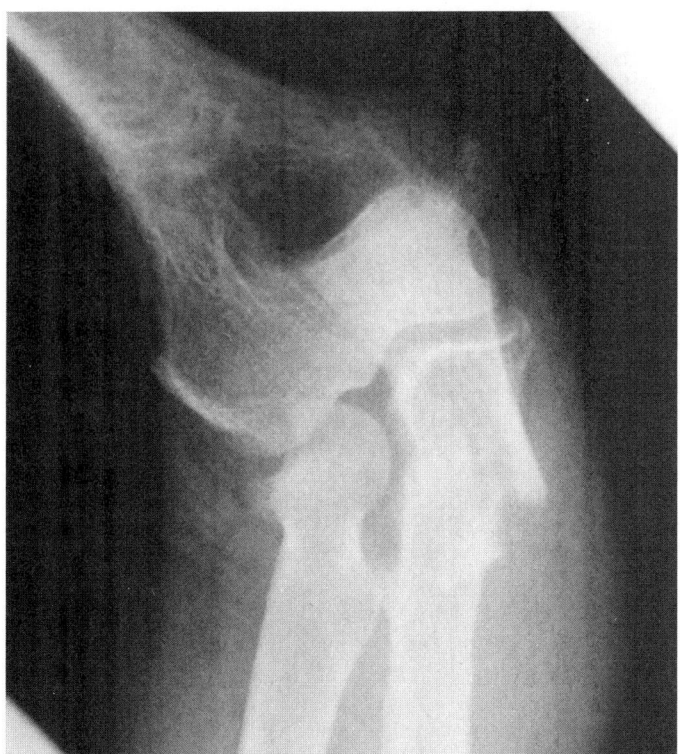

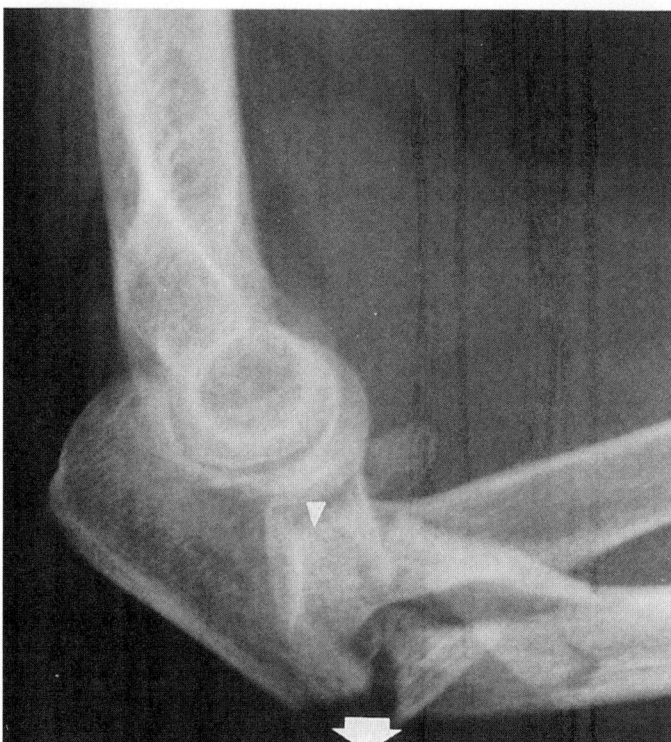

FIG. 270-10. Type II Monteggia fracture-dislocation. The angulation of the comminuted fracture of the proximal ulna *(arrow)* points in the direction of the radial head dislocation *(arrowhead)*.

BICEPS AND TRICEPS RUPTURE

Biceps Rupture

The biceps muscle has two proximal heads. The long head originates at the supraglenoid tubercle of the scapula and superior labrum of the

TABLE 270-1 Bado Classification of Monteggia Fracture-Dislocation

Type I:	60% Fracture of the proximal or middle third of the ulna with anterior dislocation of the radial head (fracture apex anterior)
Type II:	Fracture of the proximal or middle third of the ulna with posterior dislocation of the radial head (fracture apex posterior)
Type III:	Fracture of the ulna distal to the coronoid process with lateral dislocation of the radial head
Type IV:	Fracture of the proximal or middle third of the ulna and fracture of the proximal third of the radius with the anterior dislocation of the radial head

glenohumeral joint, and then travels through the capsule of the shoulder and along the intertubercle (bicipital) groove of the humerus (Figure 270-11). The short head originates at the coracoid process of the scapula. The distal attachments are to the radial tuberosity and forearm via the bicipital aponeurosis. A bicipitoradial bursa lies adjacent to the radial tuberosity. The biceps muscle is innervated by the musculocutaneous nerve (C5, C6), and functions to flex the supinated forearm and supinate the flexed forearm.

The vast majority of all injuries to the biceps are proximal, and nearly all involve the proximal long head. Injuries are usually the result of repetitive microtrauma and overuse. Steroids, whether injected locally or used systemically, can accelerate the breakdown of tendons. Rupture of the biceps tendon usually occurs in middle-aged to older individuals with a history of chronic bicipital tenosynovitis when there is sudden or prolonged contraction against resistance. A snap or pop is usually described and pain is present in the anterior shoulder. Examination of the anterior shoulder will reveal swelling, tenderness, and often crepitus over the bicipital groove. Flexion of the forearm, best accomplished with the arm abducted and externally rotated, will elicit pain and may produce a mid arm "ball," which represents the distally retracted biceps muscle. Comparing arms for

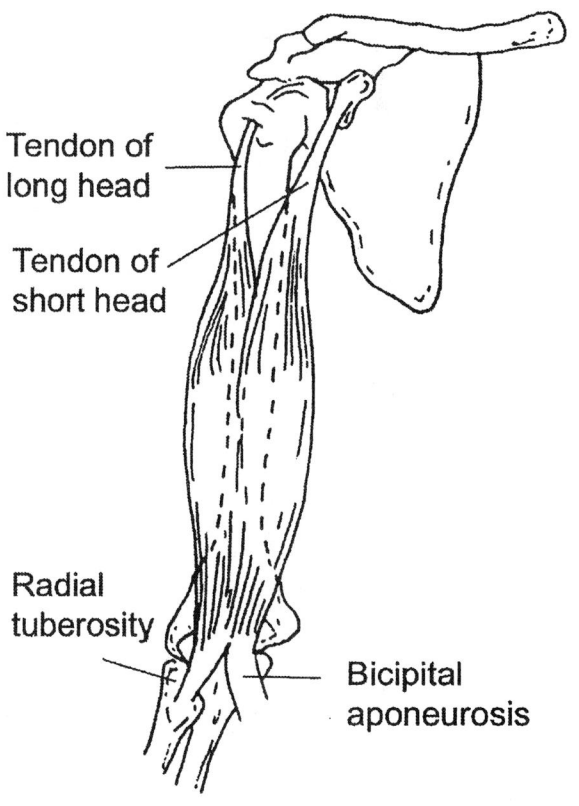

FIG. 270-11. Biceps muscle anatomy.

symmetry helps. Loss of strength is minimal due to the function of the brachialis and supinators. Radiographs of the shoulder should be obtained as avulsion fractures occasionally occur.

General emergency department treatment includes sling, ice, analgesics, and referral to an orthopedic surgeon for definitive care. Surgical repair is usually recommended for young, active patients. A conservative approach with immobilization may be adequate for elderly patients whose activities of daily living are not significantly compromised by the injury.

Distal biceps injuries are quite rare.[10,11] Complete ruptures of the tendon are most common in middle-aged men and usually involve the dominant extremity. Partial tears are seen in men and women. Mechanism of injury is similar to that of proximal injuries. With rupture of the distal biceps, pain is felt in the antecubital fossa, with swelling, ecchymosis, and tenderness to palpation noted on examination. Inability to palpate the distal biceps tendon in the antecubital fossa and a mid arm "ball" indicate a distal rupture. Strength loss, especially supination, is usually greater than with proximal ruptures. Radiographs should be obtained to search for an associated avulsion fracture. While most complete distal ruptures are diagnosed clinically, magnetic resonance imaging and ultrasound can aid in confirming the diagnosis of partial tears.[12]

Emergency department treatment includes sling, ice, analgesics, and referral to an orthopedic surgeon for definitive care. Without surgical repair of complete ruptures, supination strength is decreased by approximately 50 percent and flexion strength by almost 30 percent. Therefore, in young active individuals, most authorities recommend surgical repair.

Triceps Rupture

The triceps muscle has three proximal heads. The long head originates at the infraglenoid tubercle of the scapula, the lateral head on the posterior surface of the humerus superior to the radial (spiral) groove, and the medial head inferior to the radial groove (Figure 270-12). The triceps inserts at the olecranon. A subtendinous bursa separates the triceps from the olecranon, and a subcutaneous bursa lies just distal to the tendinous insertion. The latter frequently becomes inflamed. The triceps muscle is innervated by the radial nerve (C6, C7, C8) and is the sole extensor of the forearm. Additionally, it also aids in extension and adduction of the arm, and the long head stabilizes the head of the humerus in abduction.

Injury to the triceps is rare and almost always occurs distally. Rupture is more common in young men and results from either a fall on an outstretched hand causing a forceful flexion of an extended forearm, or a direct blow to the olecranon. Spontaneous ruptures from systemic illnesses, particularly hyperparathyroidism, have also been reported. With rupture of the triceps, pain is present in the posterior elbow. Examination of the elbow reveals swelling and tenderness posteriorly just proximal to the olecranon. A sulcus with a more proximal mass, representing the retracted triceps muscle, may be palpated. With partial tears some degree of function remains, whereas with complete ruptures, the ability to extend the forearm is lost. A modified Thompson test can be used to evaluate triceps function. The upper extremity is positioned such that the arm is supported and the forearm is hanging in a relaxed position with 90 degrees of flexion. Squeezing the triceps muscle should produce extension of the forearm unless a complete rupture is present. Radiographs are needed, as avulsion fractures of the olecranon are common.[13] Ultrasound and magnetic resonance imaging may aid in diagnosis, especially of partial tears.

Emergency department treatment includes sling, ice, analgesics, and referral to an orthopedic surgeon for definitive care. Complete ruptures require surgical repair, while most partial tears can be treated conservatively with immobilization.

ACKNOWLEDGMENT

The authors wish to recognize the contributions of Harold Chin, MD, in previous editions of this chapter.

REFERENCES

1. Platz A, Heinzelmann M, Ertel W, Trentz O: Posterior elbow dislocation with associated vascular injury after blunt trauma. *J Trauma* 46: 948, 1999.
2. Cohen MS, Hastings H: Acute elbow dislocation: Evaluation and management. *J Am Acad Orthop Surg* 6:15, 1998.
3. Hildebrand KA, Patterson SD, King GJ: Acute elbow dislocations: Simple and complex. *Orthop Clin North Am* 30:63, 1999.
4. Kuntz DG Jr, Baratz ME: Fractures of the elbow. *Orthop Clin North Am* 30:37, 1999.
5. Joist A, Joosten U, Wetterkamp D, et al: Anterior interosseous nerve compression after supracondylar fracture of the humerus: A metaanalysis. *J Neurosurg* 90:1053, 1999.
6. Villarin LA, Belk KE, Freid R: Emergency department evaluation and treatment of elbow and forearm injuries. *Emerg Med Clin North Am* 17:843, 1999.
7. Mirsky EC, Karas EH, Weiner LS: Lateral condyle fractures in children: Evaluation of classification and treatment. *J Orthop Trauma* 11:117, 1997.
8. Lins RE, Simovitch RW, Waters PM: Pediatric elbow trauma. *Orthop Clin North Am* 30:119, 1999.
9. Perron AD, Hersh RE, Brady WJ, Keats TE: Orthopedic pitfalls in the ED: Galeazzi and Monteggia fracture-dislocation. *Am J Emerg Med* 19:225, 2001.
10. Baker BE, Bierwagen D: Rupture of the distal tendon of the biceps brachii. *J Bone Joint Surg* 67-A:414, 1985.
11. Bernstein AD, Breslow MJ, Jazrawi LM: Distal biceps tendon ruptures: A historical perspective and current concepts. *Am J Orthop* 30:193, 2001.
12. Miller TT, Adler RS: Sonography of tears of the distal biceps tendon. *AJR* 175:1081, 2000.
13. Viegas SF: Avulsion of the triceps tendon. *Orthop Rev* 19:533, 1990.

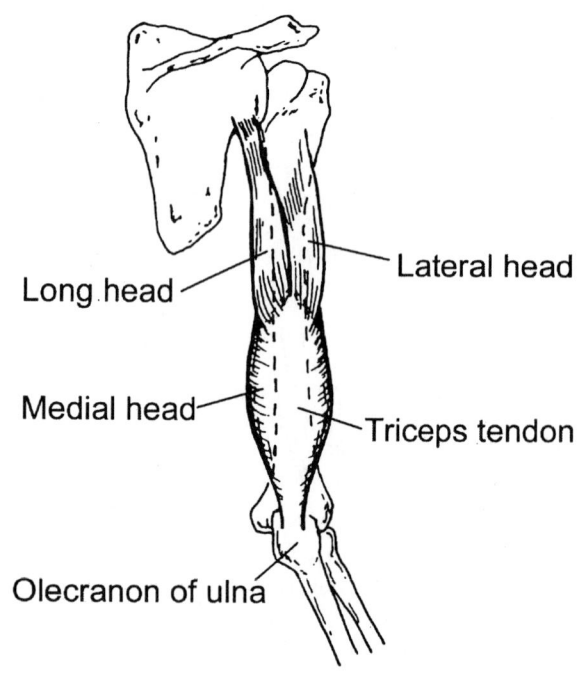

Triceps brachii

FIG. 270-12. Triceps muscle anatomy.

271 INJURIES TO THE SHOULDER COMPLEX AND HUMERUS

Dennis T. Uehara
John P. Rudzinski

Function of the upper extremity is intimately dependent on the shoulder complex. Movement is accomplished through an intricate mechanism with integration of muscles, ligaments, osseous components, and a system of joints all working in harmony. Through its joint system, which consists of four joints, the sternoclavicular, glenohumeral, acromioclavicular, and scapulothoracic, the upper extremity is able to move through a complex and wide range of motion. The following discussion focuses on the major soft tissue and osseous components of the shoulder complex and humerus and those injuries that create loss of motion, instability, and pain.

STERNOCLAVICULAR DISLOCATIONS

The sternoclavicular joint is the most frequently moved nonaxial joint of the body because almost any movement of the upper extremity is transferred proximally to this joint. It also has the least amount of bony stability of any major joint because less than half of the medial end of the clavicle actually articulates with the upper sternum. Joint stability therefore depends on the integrity of the surrounding ligaments, which give the sternoclavicular joint surprising strength. As a result, the majority of injuries to this area are simple sprains, dislocations being uncommon.

A sprain of the sternoclavicular joint can result from the shoulder being forced forward suddenly or from a medially directed force applied to the shoulder. Pain and swelling are localized to the joint, and treatment is symptomatic with ice, sling, and analgesics. Differential diagnosis should include consideration of septic arthritis, especially in intravenous drug abusers.

Sternoclavicular dislocations are uncommon, accounting for only 3 percent of a series of 1603 shoulder girdle injuries. Dislocations usually result from motor vehicle accidents or sports injuries, but spontaneous dislocations have been reported. Posterior sternoclavicular joint dislocations are much less common than anterior dislocations. A posterior dislocation may result from a direct blow or from an indirect force to the shoulder if the shoulder is rolled forward at the time of impact. An anterior sternoclavicular joint dislocation may result from the same indirect force if the shoulder is rolled backward at the time of impact. Of note is that the medial clavicular epiphysis is the last epiphysis of the body to appear radiographically (age 18) and the last to close (age 22 to 25). As a result, physeal injuries in this age group can easily be misdiagnosed as a dislocation.

Patients with a sternoclavicular joint dislocation have severe pain that is exacerbated by arm motion and when in the supine position. The shoulder appears shortened and rolled forward. On examination, anterior dislocations have a prominent medial clavicle end that is visible and palpable anterior to the sternum. In posterior dislocations, the medial clavicle end is less visible and not palpable, and the patient may have signs and symptoms of impingement of the superior mediastinal contents. Routine radiographs may not be diagnostic, although specialized views or tomograms may be helpful. Computed tomography (CT) is the imaging procedure of choice.

Closed reduction of anterior sternoclavicular joint dislocations is usually attempted with the patient supine and with a sandbag or pad between the shoulders. Direct pressure over the clavicle may reduce the dislocation. The patient is usually discharged in a figure-of-eight clavicle harness. Unfortunately, many anterior dislocations prove unstable and recur as soon as direct pressure is released. Patients may subsequently undergo open reduction, or the position of the deformity may be accepted and no further treatment rendered.

In posterior dislocations, life-threatening injuries to adjacent structures may result in a pneumothorax or in compression or laceration of the great vessels, trachea, or esophagus. Local swelling may obscure any deformity, and routine radiographs are often not conclusive, making diagnosis difficult. Additional injuries should be aggressively sought and addressed. Orthopedists may attempt closed reduction, with thoracic surgical back-up. A towel clip is often used to grasp and pull the medial clavicle forward and back into place. Open reduction may be necessary.

CLAVICLE

Clavicle fractures account for nearly half of significant injuries to the shoulder girdle and are the most common fracture of childhood, with almost half of these injuries occurring by the age of 7. The clavicle functions as a strut, connecting the shoulder girdle to the trunk, and provides support and mobility for upper extremity function. The clavicle also protects the adjacent lung, brachial plexus, and subclavian and brachial blood vessels.

The most common mechanism of injury is a blow to the shoulder. Transmission of the compressive force results in a buckling of the clavicle, which fractures once a critical force is achieved. Children will often have a greenstick or buckle-type fracture or a bowing deformity without a definite fracture. Open fractures, from extreme tenting and piercing of the overlying skin, may occasionally be seen.

Eighty percent of clavicle fractures involve the middle third, 15 percent the distal third, and 5 percent the medial third. Patients typically present with swelling, deformity, and tenderness localized to the clavicle. The arm is slumped inward and downward and is supported by the other extremity. Routine clavicle radiographs may miss fractures due to overlap of surrounding structures, particularly with fractures at either end of the bone. Diagnosis may require CT.

Numerous forms of treatment have been described for this common injury. Simple immobilization with a sling is often successful, with displaced fractures often treated with a figure-of-eight brace. A shoulder spica or open reduction may be required for severely displaced fractures, poor patient compliance, or for complications. Healing may occur as rapidly as 2 weeks for infants, with most adults healing in a 4- to 6-week period. The nonunion rate varies from 0.1 to 15 percent.[1] Factors associated with nonunion are marked initial displacement and shortening.[2] Delayed internal fixation is sometimes done for severely displaced clavicle fractures with functional disability.[1,2]

Although the vast majority of these fractures have a benign course, serious associated injuries and complications may occasionally occur. Penetrating or blunt trauma may result in associated lung, neurovascular, or first-rib injuries. Injury to the adjacent vascular structures, usually the subclavian artery, subclavian vein, internal jugular vein, or axillary artery, may be life-threatening. **Distal clavicle fractures with displacement typically are associated with rupture of the coracoclavicular ligament and may require operative intervention to avoid nonunion. Medial clavicle fractures may be associated with intrathoracic injuries or develop late complications, such as arthritis.** Significant callus formation may result in subsequent compression of adjacent neurovascular structures and is cosmetically deforming.

SCAPULA

The scapula links the axial skeleton to the upper extremity and serves as a stabilizing platform for motion of the arm. Fracture of the scapula is infrequent, accounting for less than 1 percent of all fractures. Due to the high energy typically required to fracture this protected bone, there is a greater than 80 percent association of injuries to the ipsilateral lung, thoracic cage, and shoulder girdle.

Significant scapular injury occurs most frequently in men between 25 and 40 years of age, usually as a result of motor vehicle accidents, falls, or other severe trauma. The mechanism of injury is from a direct blow, trauma to the shoulder sometimes with injury of the acromion or coracoid, or a fall on the outstretched arm. An indirect axial load transmitted by the outstretched arm may result in a scapular neck fracture, while the indirect force of a shoulder dislocation may result in fracture of the glenoid. Scapular fractures may be classified by their anatomic location: body, glenoid neck, intraarticular glenoid, spine, coracoid, and acromion (Figure 271-1). Fractures of the body and glenoid neck are the most common.

A patient with an isolated scapular fracture typically will present with localized tenderness over the scapula and the ipsilateral arm held in adduction. The shoulder may have a flattened appearance. Radiographs consisting of an anteroposterior shoulder, lateral scapula, and axillary views will identify most fractures. However, scapula fractures are often associated with other significant injuries, and hence diagnosis may be delayed or initially missed entirely. In Ada and Miller's series,[3] 96 percent of scapular fractures had associated injuries, of which rib fractures were the most common, followed by pulmonary, humeral head, and shoulder girdle injuries. Other injuries may include neurovascular, abdominal, and spine trauma.

Rarely, significant trauma may result in scapulothoracic dissociation. This syndrome consists of lateral scapular displacement, clavicular disruption, and severe soft-tissue injury. This injury is sometimes associated with brachial plexus avulsion, subclavian artery disruption, or both. Its presence may be suspected by neurovascular findings or by lateral displacement of the scapula visualized on a nonrotated chest radiograph.

The vast majority of scapular fractures are treated nonsurgically, with a sling for immobilization, ice, analgesics, and early range-of-motion exercises. Surgical intervention may be necessary for significant or displaced articular fractures of the glenoid, angulated glenoid neck fractures, acromial fractures associated with a rotator cuff tear, and some coracoid fractures. Fractures of the glenoid, acromion, or coracoid are more likely to be associated with long-term disability.

Complications of scapular fractures themselves are uncommon. Although many of these fractures heal with some degree of malunion, typically this does not result in significant disability. Most long-term disability is a result of other, associated injuries.

ACROMIOCLAVICULAR JOINT INJURIES

Injuries to the acromioclavicular joint are commonly seen in emergency practice. Although they may occur in any age group, the majority occur in young, active males. Emergency management consists of identifying the severity of injury, recognizing associated injuries, and managing selected patients as outpatients.

Anatomy

The acromioclavicular joint is a diarthrodial joint that, together with the sternoclavicular joint, connects the upper extremity to the axial skeleton. The support of the acromioclavicular joint is through the acromioclavicular and coracoclavicular ligaments and the strong attachment of the trapezius and deltoid muscles (Figure 271-2). The acromioclavicular joint is surrounded by a thin capsule, which is reinforced by the acromioclavicular ligaments. The superior fibers of this ligament blend with the fascia of the trapezius and deltoid muscles, which attach to the clavicle and acromion. The acromioclavicular ligaments provide horizontal stability to the joint. The tough coracoclavicular ligaments consist of two parts, the more lateral trapezoid and the medial conoid. They attach the distal inferior clavicle to the coracoid process of the scapula. The coracoclavicular ligament is the major suspensory ligament of the upper extremity and provides vertical stability to the acromioclavicular joint.

Mechanism of Injury

The mechanism of injury is usually direct trauma to the acromioclavicular joint from a fall with the arm adducted, as typically may occur in a sporting activity. An indirect mechanism is a fall on the outstretched hand with transmission of force to the acromioclavicular joint. The result is that the scapula and shoulder girdle are driven inferiorly while the clavicle remains in its normal position. This is confirmed by observing the opposite clavicle, which is at the same level as the injured one.

Clinical Features

The diagnosis of acromioclavicular joint injuries is made clinically. The typical mechanism of injury, as well as tenderness and deformity at the acromioclavicular joint, is confirmatory. Radiographs are useful for identifying other fractures and determining the severity of injury. Acromioclavicular radiographs should specifically be ordered because

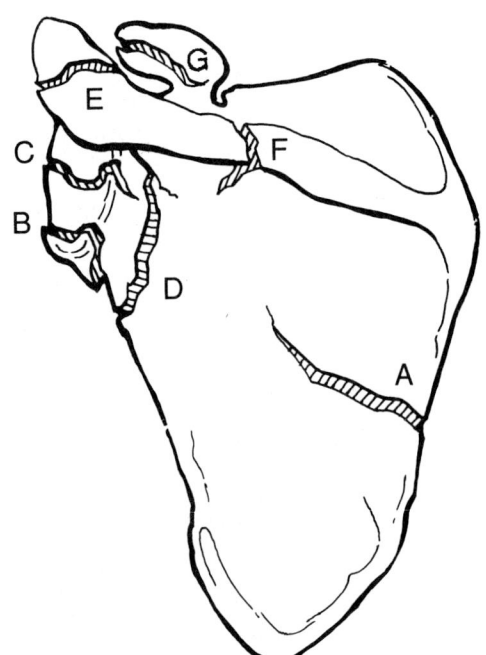

FIG. 271-1. Sites of scapula fractures. **A.** Body. **B.** Glenoid rim. **C.** Intraarticular glenoid. **D.** Neck. **E.** Acromion. **F.** Spine. **G.** Coracoid.

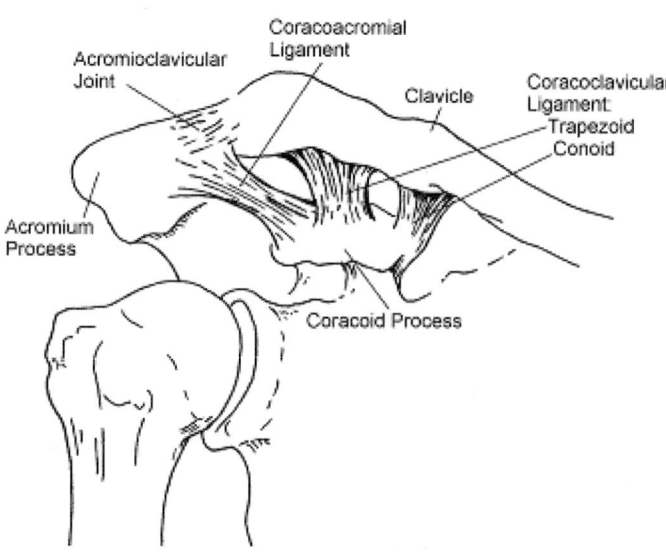

FIG. 271-2. Anatomy of the acromioclavicular joint.

they require only one-third to one-half the penetration of standard shoulder films. Shoulder technique will overpenetrate the acromioclavicular joint, and small fractures may be missed. Although standard acromioclavicular radiographs are generally sufficient, an axillary view is required to identify posterior clavicular dislocation (type IV, see below). Routine use of stress radiographs has been standard practice; Bossart and colleagues[4] have called this practice into question. Their study suggests that stress radiographs are of low yield and that their routine use should be abandoned. Although some agree, others disagree, citing occult type III (see below) injuries that can be unmasked only with stress radiographs.

Classification of Injury

The classification of acromioclavicular joint injuries classically describes three types of injuries. Rockwood describes three others (Figure 271-3). Types I, II, and III are common; types IV, V, and VI are rare. The anatomic injury, radiographic findings, and physical findings are summarized in Table 271-1.

Treatment

Treatment of type I injuries consists of rest, ice, analgesics, and immobilization, followed by early range-of-motion exercises.[5] Most agree that type II injuries should be similarly treated. Various straps and braces have been used to reduce the dislocation, but none have proven successful. A simple sling remains the most convenient and ef-

fective. Prognosis for type I and II injuries is excellent, with only a small percentage who develop late symptoms requiring excision of the distal clavicle. Treatment of type III injuries is controversial, with proponents for both conservative and operative philosophies.[6] A trend, however, reveals a shift to conservative treatment with sling immobilization. Both strategies have yielded good results in selected patients, with the specific management operator-dependent. Treatment decisions are based on such factors as age, occupation, and activity level. Types IV, V, and VI are severe injuries, and most authors recommend surgical repair. Because other injuries are associated with these more severe forms of acromioclavicular joint injuries (especially type VI), a careful clinical and radiographic examination must be performed.

DISLOCATION OF THE GLENOHUMERAL JOINT

Anterior dislocations of the glenohumeral joint are the most common major joint dislocations. Posterior dislocations are described, but occur in less than 2 percent of cases. Other dislocations include inferior (luxatio erecta) and superior (very rare). Neurovascular examination should always be done before and after reduction.

Anterior Glenohumeral Dislocations

There are four types of anterior dislocations. In subcoracoid dislocation, the most common type, the humeral head is displaced anterior to the glenoid and inferior to the coracoid. In a subglenoid dislocation, the humeral head lies inferior and anterior to the glenoid fossa. In a

FIG. 271-3. Classification of acromioclavicular joint injuries. (Reproduced with permission from Rockwood CA, Green DP, Bucholz RW: *Rockwood & Green's Fractures in Adults,* 3d ed. Philadelphia, PA: Lippincott, 1991.)

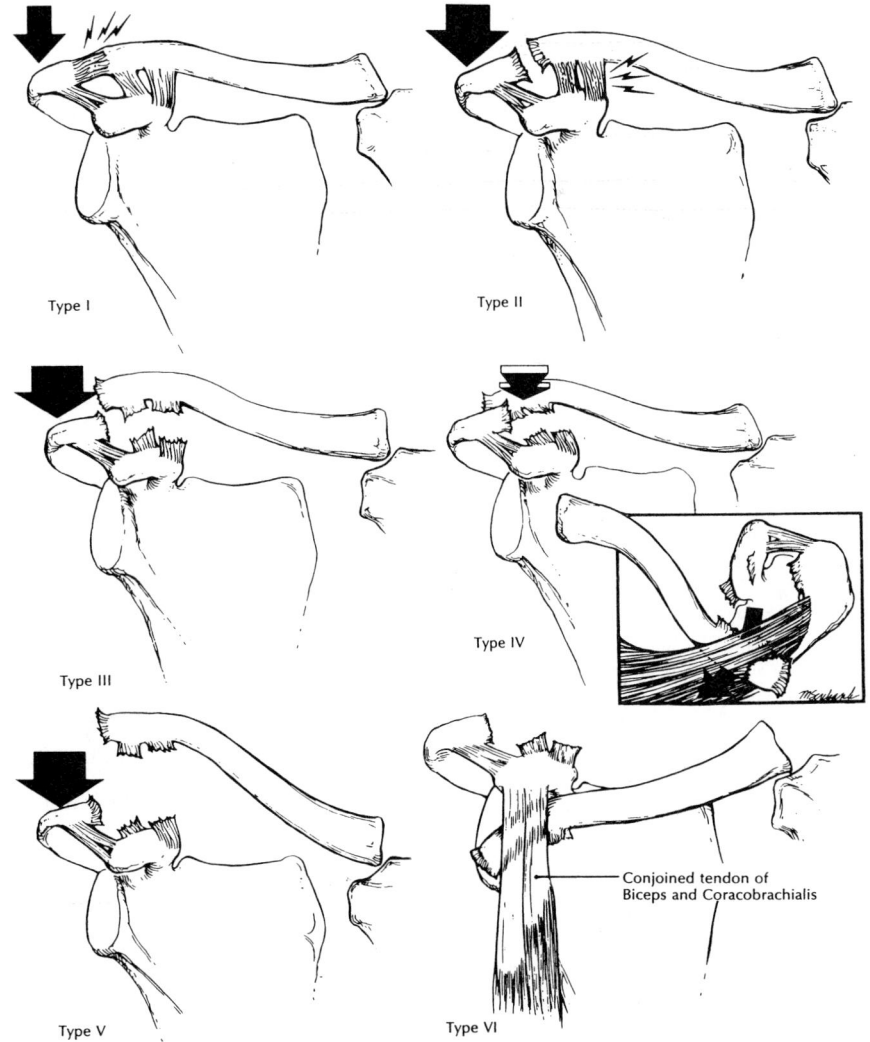

Type I

Type II

Type III

Type IV

Type V

Type VI

Conjoined tendon of Biceps and Coracobrachialis

TABLE 271-1   Classification and Physical Findings in Acromioclavicular Joint Injuries

Type	Injury	Radiograph	Examination
I	Sprained acromioclavicular ligaments	Normal	Tenderness over acromioclavicular joint
II	Acromioclavicular ligaments ruptured; coracoclavicular ligaments sprained	Slight widening of acromioclavicular joint; clavicle elevated 25–50% above acromion; may be slight widening of the coracoclavicular interspace	Tenderness and mild step-off deformity of acromioclavicular joint
III	Acromioclavicular ligaments ruptured; coracoclavicular ligaments ruptured; deltoid and trapezius muscles detached	Acromioclavicular joint dislocated 100%; coracoclavicular interspace widened 25–100%	Distal end of clavicle prominent; shoulder droops
IV	Rupture of all supporting structures; clavicle displaced posteriorly in or through the trapezius	May appear similar to type II and III; axillary radiograph required to visualize posterior dislocation	Possible posterior displacement of clavicle
V	Rupture of all supporting structures (more severe form of type III injury)	Acromioclavicular joint dislocated; generally 200–300% disparity of coracoclavicular interspace compared to normal shoulder	More pain; gross deformity of clavicle
VI	Acromioclavicular ligaments disrupted; coracoclavicular ligaments may be disrupted; deltoid, and trapezius muscles disrupted	Acromioclavicular joint dislocated; clavicle displaced inferiorly	Severe swelling; multiple associated injuries

subclavicular dislocation, the head of the humerus is displaced medial to the coracoid below the clavicle. In the very rare intrathoracic dislocation, the head of the humerus lies between the ribs and thoracic cavity.

The mechanism of injury may be direct force, but an indirect force is more common. The combination of abduction, extension, and external rotation with sufficient force will cause an anterior dislocation.

The patient is usually in severe pain. The arm is in slight abduction and external rotation. The shoulder is "squared off," lacking the normal rounded contour. The patient resists abduction and internal rotation. The humeral head can often be palpated anteriorly. Because neurovascular injuries occur, a careful examination must be performed. The axillary nerve is most commonly injured. This nerve may be tested by pinprick sensation over the skin of the deltoid muscle.

Anteroposterior and scapular lateral or "Y" radiographs should be obtained before reduction is attempted. Although the anteroposterior radiograph will reveal the dislocation, the scapular Y radiograph will indicate the direction of dislocation: anterior or posterior. Bony injuries reported in the literature include fractures of the anterior glenoid lip, greater tuberosity, coracoid, and acromion, and compression fractures of the humeral head (Hill-Sachs lesion).

Many reduction techniques have been described.[7] The three main categories are traction, leverage, and scapular manipulation.[8] Success rates are between 70 and 96 percent regardless of technique. The use of conscious sedation is recommended, but any reduction technique may be attempted without medication when performed slowly and atraumatically. It is important for the physician to be comfortable with two or three techniques in case of a failed first attempt. Considerations in selection of a technique include ease of performance, effectiveness, as little trauma and pain as possible, requirement for medication, number of assistants, and time for procedure.

HIPPOCRATIC (MODIFIED) A modification of the Hippocratic method uses traction-countertraction (Figure 271-4). The patient is supine with the arm abducted and elbow flexed at 90 degrees. A sheet is tied and placed across the thorax of the patient and then around the waist of the assistant. Another sheet is tied and placed around the forearm of the patient at the elbow and the waist of the physician. The physician gradually applies traction as the assistant provides countertraction. Gentle internal and external rotation or outward pressure on the proximal humerus may aid reduction.

STIMSON The patient is placed prone on a gurney with the dislocated extremity hanging over the side and a 10 lb. weight attached to

the wrist. Complete muscle relaxation is required. Reduction occurs in 20 to 30 min.

Although safe, effective, and easy to learn, the time involved and constant monitoring by a nurse are drawbacks to this technique.

MILCH The patient is supine. The physician slowly abducts and externally rotates the arm to the overhead position (Figure 271-5). With the elbow fully extended, traction is applied. With the other hand, pressure may be placed on the humeral head to manipulate it over the lip of the glenoid.

This technique is well tolerated by the patient, effective, and atraumatic. It is the technique of choice for many physicians.

SCAPULAR MANIPULATION The patient is positioned with weights in the same manner as the Stimson technique (Figure 271-6). After adequate sedation, the physician pushes the tip of the scapula medially using the thumbs, while stabilizing the superior aspect with the cephalad hand.

Physicians have found this technique relatively painless, fast, and in one study 96 percent successful.[9]

EXTERNAL ROTATION The patient is supine with the arm adducted to the patient's side. With the elbow at 90° of flexion, the arm is slowly externally rotated. No longitudinal traction is applied. It is important to perform the movement slowly to allow time for spasm and pain to

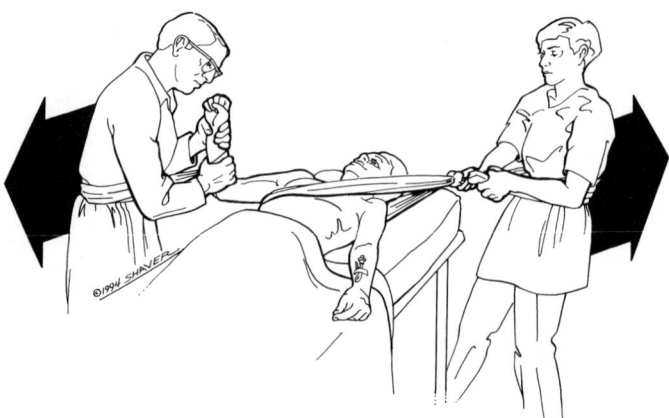

FIG. 271-4. Modified Hippocratic technique.

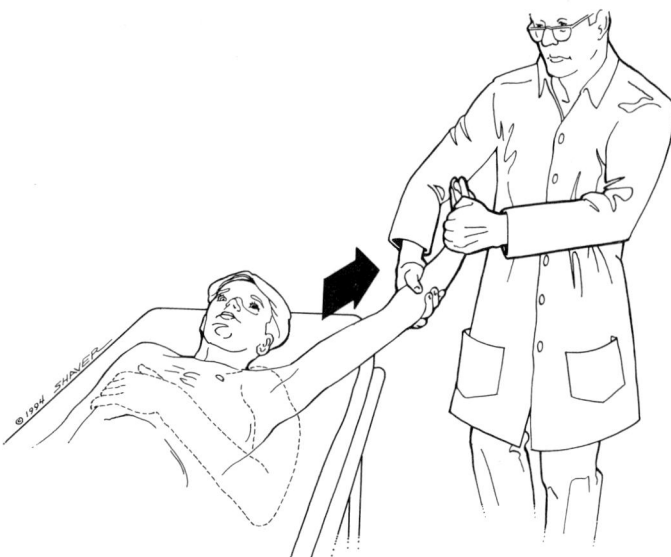

FIG. 271-5. Milch technique.

resolve. Reduction is usually complete prior to reaching the coronal plane and is often not noted either by the patient or physician. This method has been reported to be 78 percent successful, relatively atraumatic, safe, and easily learned.

COMPLICATIONS   Complications are frequently encountered in patients with anterior glenohumeral dislocations.[10] The most common complication is recurrent dislocation, which is age dependent. Those patients less than 20 years of age may have a greater than 90 percent recurrence; those older than 40 years have a 10 to 15 percent recurrence.[10,11] The high recurrence rate in younger patients is thought to be related to the higher incidence in this group of avulsions of the anterior inferior glenohumeral ligament, the major anterior stabilizer of the glenohumeral joint (Bankart lesion). Early surgical repair, open or arthroscopic, may significantly decrease the recurrence rate. Younger patients with first-time shoulder dislocations should be referred for orthopedic evaluation.[12–14] Other complications include fractures and injuries to nerves and to the rotator cuff. Vascular injuries are rare, but when they occur tend to involve the axillary artery in elderly patients. Clinical findings of vascular injury include absent radial pulse, axillary hematoma, bruising of the lateral chest wall, and an axillary bruit.

Bony injuries are common and include fractures of the humeral head (Hill-Sachs lesion), anterior glenoid lip, and greater tuberosity. Neural injuries occur in 10 to 25 percent of acute dislocations. Of these injuries, which are the result of traction neuropraxia, most occur in the axillary nerve. This injury is temporary and resolves spontaneously. The common test of sensation over the skin of the deltoid muscle may not be reliable, with only an electromyogram providing an accurate evaluation. Other nerves injured are the radial, ulnar, median, musculocutaneous, and brachial plexus.[10]

A frequent but often missed injury is a tear of the rotator cuff. The rotator cuff weakens with advancing age, and as many as 86 percent of patients older than 40 years with an anterior dislocation have an associated rotator cuff tear. Pain or weakness 2 to 4 weeks after a glenohumeral dislocation is an indication for imaging such as MR or arthrogram. Early diagnosis is important since prompt surgery yields the best results.

Posterior Glenohumeral Dislocations

Posterior dislocation may occur with the humeral head in the subacromial (most commonly with the humeral head posterior to the glenoid and inferior to the acromion), subglenoid, or subspinous. The latter two are rare.

The usual mechanism is an indirect force that produces forceful internal rotation and adduction. This may occur during a fall or from violent muscle contraction due to a seizure or electric shock. Direct force to the anterior shoulder can also produce a posterior dislocation.

Posterior dislocations are reported to be commonly missed. Thus a careful examination and radiographic evaluation are essential. Clinical findings include the following:

1. The arm is adducted and internally rotated.
2. The anterior shoulder is flat and the posterior aspect full.
3. The coracoid process is prominent.
4. The patient will not allow external rotation or abduction because of severe pain.

Although the anteroposterior radiograph is helpful, the scapular Y radiograph is diagnostic. In this radiograph, the humeral head is seen in a posterior position.

Since severe pain and muscle spasms are the norm, muscle relaxation and analgesia are paramount. The reduction is performed with the patient supine. Traction is applied to the adducted arm in the long axis of the humerus. An assistant gently pushes the humeral head anteriorly into the glenoid fossa.

Most complications are fractures, including fractures of the posterior glenoid rim, humeral head (reversed Hill-Sachs deformity), humeral shaft, and lesser tuberosity. Neurovascular and rotator cuff tears are less common than in anterior dislocations.

Inferior Dislocations (Luxatio Erecta)

Although inferior dislocation is a rare injury, it is one that will be seen in a busy emergency practice. It is always a severe injury and is associated with significant soft-tissue trauma or fracture. The mechanism of injury is a hyperabduction force, which levers the neck of the humerus against the acromion. As the force continues the inferior capsule tears, and the humeral head is forced out inferiorly.

The patient is in severe pain. The humerus is fully abducted, the elbow is flexed, and the patient's hand is on or behind the head. The humeral head can be palpated on the lateral chest wall. This clinical presentation is difficult to mistake for another condition.

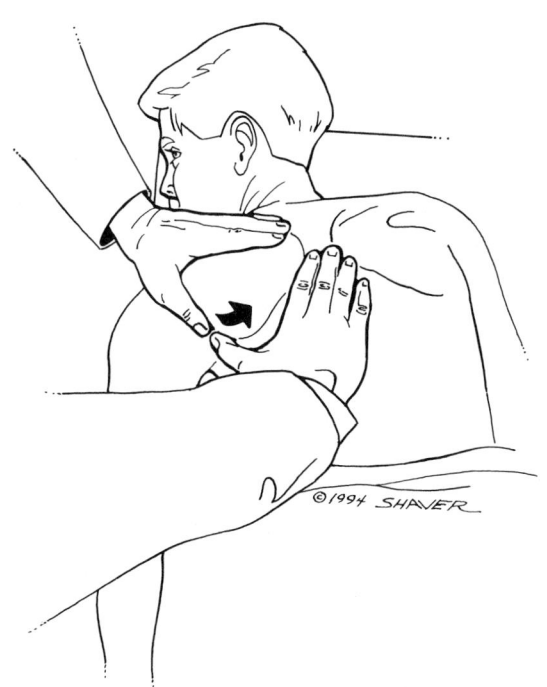

FIG. 271-6. Scapular manipulation technique.

Reduction consists of traction in an upward and outward direction in line with the humerus (Figure 271-7). The assistant applies counter-traction. Reduction is signaled by a "clunk." The arm is then brought to the patient's side and immobilized in a shoulder immobilizer.

Complications include severe soft-tissue injuries and fractures of the proximal humerus. The rotator cuff, which is always detached, re-quires orthopedic follow-up. Neurovascular compression injuries are usually found, but almost always resolve following reduction. When the humeral head is buttonholed through the inferior capsule, the dis-location is irreducible, and operative reduction is required.

HUMERUS FRACTURES

Proximal Humerus

Fractures of the proximal humerus typically occur in elderly osteoporotic patients through an indirect mechanism, such as a fall on an outstretched hand with the elbow extended. Simple, one-part fractures without signif-icant displacement can be initially managed by the emergency physician, but the remainder have significant displacement and are a challenge to correctly diagnose and treat. Fortunately, the shoulder joint has an intrin-sic reserve of range of motion, which can often provide a surprisingly functional outcome despite seemingly crippling injuries.

The proximal humerus is composed of the articular segment, the greater and lesser tuberosities, and the proximal humeral shaft. Mus-cles of the rotator cuff insert on the humeral tuberosities, and the bi-ceps tendon travels between them. The humeral circumflex arteries en-ter in the area of the bicipital groove and the tuberosities to supply blood flow to the articular segment.

Patients with fractures typically present with pain, swelling, and tenderness about the shoulder. Crepitus and ecchymosis may be pres-ent, and the arm is held closely against the chest wall. A neu-rovascular examination should be performed, since the brachial plexus and axillary arteries are near the coracoid process and not uncom-monly injured. The axillary nerve is the most commonly injured nerve, and sensation over the skin of the deltoid muscle should be tested rou-tinely. Injury to the axillary artery is the most common vascular injury and may be suggested by paresthesias, pallor, pulselessness, or an expanding hematoma. Vascular injuries may occur with even trivial trauma in atherosclerotic elderly patients.

Radiographs consisting of anteroposterior, lateral shoulder, and ax-illary views will correctly diagnose most proximal humerus fractures. Fractures of the articular surface may be suggested by a fat fluid level or by a superior joint hematoma that appears to push the humerus downward in the joint as a "pseudosubluxation." A transthoracic lat-eral radiograph, tomograms, CT scan, and magnetic resonance imag-ing scan may also be of value.

The Neer classification system uses the relationship of the proxi-mal humerus segments (greater and lesser tuberosities, anatomic neck, and surgical neck) to guide the management of these fractures. **Sig-nificant fragment displacement is defined as greater than 1 cm separation or greater than 45 degrees of angulation between frag-ments.** The number of fracture fragments significantly displaced de-termines the classification in the Neer system (Figure 271-8).

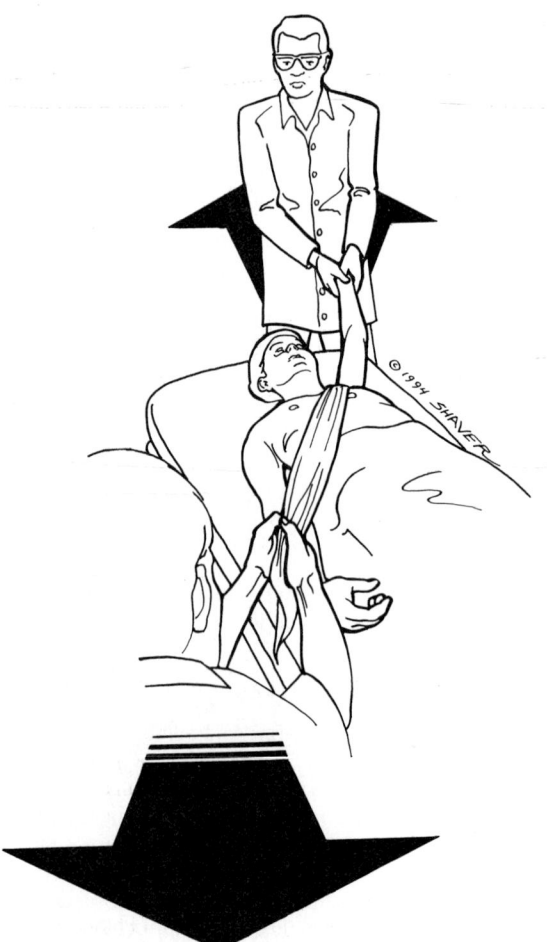

FIG. 271-7. Reduction of luxatio erecta.

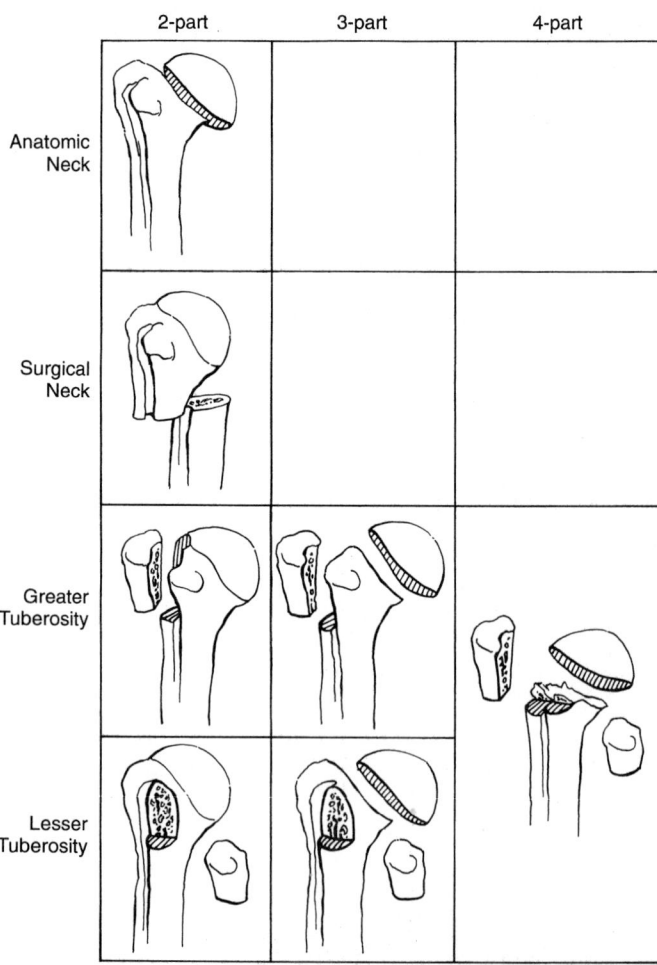

FIG. 271-8. The Neer classification system for displaced proximal humerus fractures.

A one-part fracture under the Neer system may have any number of fracture lines, but no major segment is significantly displaced. The surrounding soft tissue and periosteum hold fracture fragments together. Treatment generally consists of immobilization with a sling and swathe or collar and cuff, ice, analgesics, and referral. Early exercise is important to avoid adhesive capsulitis. The overall prognosis is generally good.

Proximal humerus fractures with significant displacement and/or angulation between fracture fragments are classified as multipart fractures under the Neer system. Treatment considerations include integrity of the blood supply, integrity of the rotator cuff, likelihood of union, associated dislocations and neurovascular injuries, and the functionality of the patient. These fractures are more frequently associated with complications and are often difficult to manage. Closed reduction, intraoperative treatment, or a combination of the two may be necessary.[15] Emergent orthopedic consultation for multipart fractures facilitates subsequent reduction and referral.

Any fracture involving the anatomic neck or the articular surface may result in compromise of the blood supply to the articular segment. Ischemic necrosis of the articular segment may ultimately require insertion of a humeral head prosthesis for these relatively uncommon fractures. Greater tuberosity fractures accompany up to 15 percent of anterior shoulder dislocations. Significant displacement of a greater tuberosity fragment implies a concomitant rotator cuff tear, with surgical repair often necessary for the active patient. Fracture of the lesser tuberosity should alert the examiner to a potential posterior shoulder dislocation. Significantly angulated surgical neck fractures are at risk for neurovascular damage (axillary neurovascular structures and brachial plexus) and should be immediately immobilized and radiographed in the position of presentation. Children may have significant displacement or separation of the proximal humeral epiphysis and may require exact reduction if near skeletal maturity. A shoulder spica is often used after reduction.

Humeral Shaft

Fractures of the humeral shaft occur in a bimodal age distribution, with peaks in the third and seventh decades of life, representing active young men and osteoporotic elderly women, respectively. The most common site of fracture is the middle third. **Neurovascular injuries are a common complication of these fractures and are due to the anatomy of the upper extremity.** Displacement of fracture fragments is common as a result of the insertions and actions of the various muscles (deltoid, biceps, triceps, supraspinatus, and pectoralis major) that act on the upper arm (Figure 271-9).

Humeral shaft fractures may be caused by a direct blow that produces a bending force, which results in a transverse fracture. They may also be caused by an indirect mechanism, such as a fall on the outstretched hand that produces a torsion force, resulting in a spiral fracture. A combination of bending and torsion forces results in an oblique fracture, sometimes with comminution, producing the "butterfly" fragment. The humerus is also a common site of pathologic fractures, especially from metastatic breast cancer.

Clinical examination reveals localized tenderness, swelling, pain, and abnormal mobility or crepitus on palpation. Displaced fractures are associated with shortening of the upper extremity. Attention must be given to the initial neurovascular status, and reevaluation must be performed, especially after manipulation. Radiographs should include two views of the humerus, and consideration should be given to radiographic examination of the shoulder and elbow as well. The vast majority of closed fractures of the shaft of the humerus are managed nonoperatively. The treatment of uncomplicated fractures includes immobilization, ice, analgesia, and referral. Closed treatment options include the coaptation splint (sugar tong), a hanging cast, functional bracing, and external fixation. A simple sling and swathe are adequate for most emergency management. Some surgeons favor internal fixation for patients with transverse fracture lines, very proximal or very distal humerus fractures, pathologic fractures, multiple trauma, and fractures associated with neurovascular injuries.

Complications include injury to the brachial artery or vein, or the radial, ulnar, or median nerves. A radial nerve injury, which is the most common, may be manifested by a wrist drop and altered sensation at the dorsal first web space. The incidence of radial nerve palsy ranges from 10 to 20 percent. **Fractures of the distal third are particularly prone to entrapment of the radial nerve, either as a result of the**

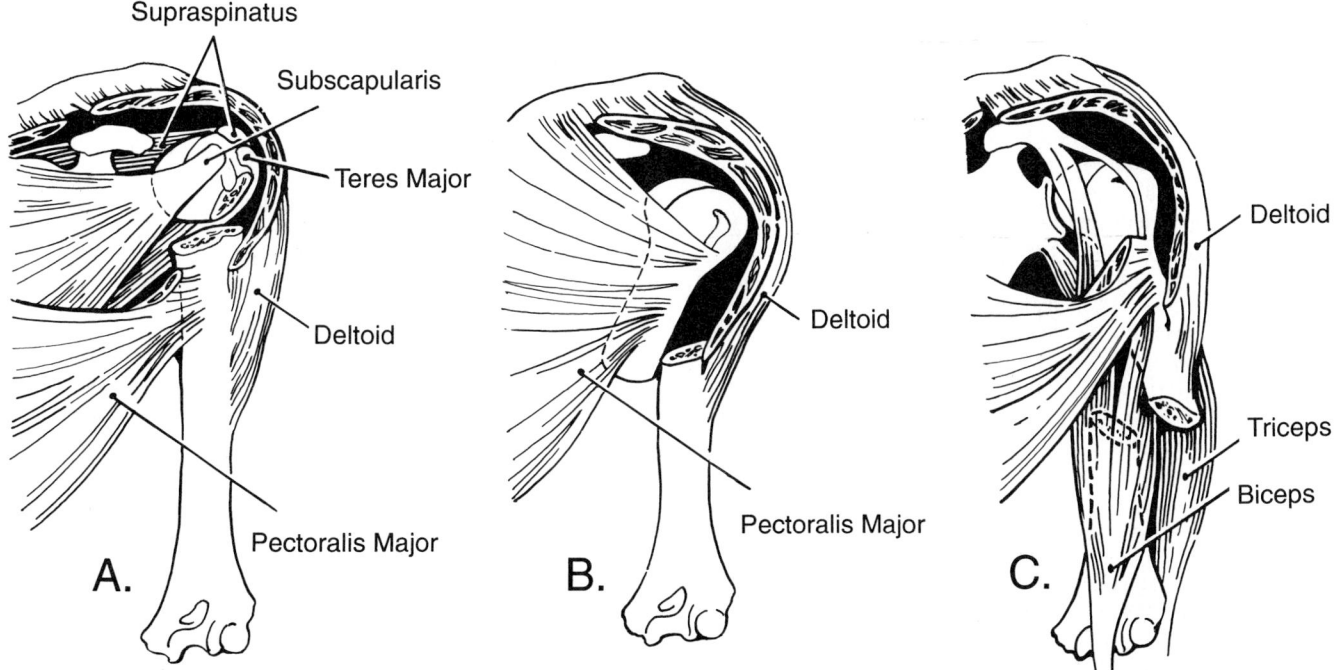

FIG. 271-9. The actions of the muscles inserting on the humeral shaft determine fracture angulation and displacement. Humeral fractures anterior view: **A.** Angulation of fragments with fracture line distal to rotator cuff insertion. **B.** Angulation of fragments with fracture line distal to pectoralis major insertion. **C.** Angulation of fragments with fracture line distal to deltoid insertion.

initial injury or after closed reduction. The majority of patients have eventual return of nerve function without operative intervention.

BRACHIAL PLEXUS INJURIES

The brachial plexus originates from the fourth through eighth cervical and first thoracic nerve roots, and a knowledge of its anatomy is crucial. At the lateral border of the interscalene triangle, formed by the anterior and middle scalene muscles, the fifth and sixth cervical (C5 and C6) nerve roots form the upper trunk of the plexus, the root of C7 the middle trunk, and the roots of C8 and T1 the lower trunk. Upon reaching the clavicle, each trunk then divides into anterior and posterior divisions. Lateral to the first rib, the anterior divisions of the upper and middle trunks combine to form the lateral cord, the anterior division of the lower trunk forms the medial cord, and all posterior divisions combine to form the posterior cord. Then, lateral to the pectoralis minor, these cords further divide into the peripheral nerves of the upper extremity: median, ulnar, musculocutaneous, axillary, and radial. Injuries to the brachial plexus can occur from penetrating, compression, or traction injuries. Traction injuries from high-speed motor vehicle crashes are the most common emergency presentation, with an overall incidence of brachial plexus injuries ranging from 0.67 to 1.3 percent. The nerves are stretched longitudinally, typically by a mechanism in which there is simultaneous traction of the arm and opposite distraction of the head.[16] Motorcycle crashes have a much higher incidence of brachial plexus injuries, due to the forces applied to an unprotected body.

The initial presentation of brachial plexus injuries in such patients is often overshadowed by their associated injuries. The most common of these is closed head injury, with chest trauma, fractures of nearby structures (clavicle, scapula, and long bones), shoulder dislocation, and trauma to the subclavian or neck vessels also frequently encountered. Significant swelling and soft tissue injury to the neck and shoulder girdle suggest traumatic forces sufficient to injure the brachial plexus. The accumulation of cerebrospinal fluid from avulsed spinal roots may cause swelling in the posterior triangle. Horner's sign may be present due to adjacent ganglion damage. However, brachial plexus injury may not be clinically apparent until a responsive patient can indicate the extent of motor and sensory deficits, days to weeks after initial stabilization and treatment. Arm pain that is constant and burning in character is common. Upper limb and shoulder girdle motor and sensory deficits define the extent of damage to the brachial plexus. Adduction and internal rotation of the shoulder indicates weakness of the deltoid and infraspinatus muscles (C5), while elbow extension is due to weakness of the biceps (C6), and flexion of the digits and wrists is due to weakness of the extensors (C7).

Magnetic resonance imaging and CT myelography are common radiographic imaging procedures. Electromyographic and nerve conduction velocity studies may aid in diagnosis, and surgical exploration of the area may be necessary. The delineation of pre- and postganglionic injury may not be possible until wallerian degeneration is completed 2 weeks after injury.

Treatment and prognosis[17] will depend on the location and extent of nerve damage. Complete supraclavicular traction injuries with rupture of the nerve roots from the spinal cord may be the most devastating of all lesions of the peripheral nerves. A multidisciplinary approach with nerve transfers and long-term physical therapy may provide surprisingly good functional outcomes. In general, early neurosurgical consultation and timely referral to a facility capable of handling the complex multiple trauma patient will result in the best outcome.

REFERENCES

1. Chu CM, Wang SJ, Lin LC: Fixation of mid-third clavicular fractures with Knowles pins: 78 patients followed for 2-7 years. *Acta Orthop Scand* 73:134, 2002.
2. Wick M, Muller EJ, Kollig E, et al: Midshaft fractures of the clavicle with a shortening of more than 2 cm predisposes to nonunion. *Arch Orthop Trauma Surg* 121:2072, 2001.
3. Ada JR, Miller ME: Scapular fractures. *Clin Orthop* 269:174, 1991.
4. Bossart PJ, Joyce SM, Manaster BJ, et al: Lack of efficacy of "weighted" radiographs in diagnosing acute acromioclavicular separation. *Ann Emerg Med* 17:20, 1988.
5. Cox JS: Current method of treatment of acromioclavicular joint dislocations. *Orthopedics* 15:1041, 1992.
6. Schlegel TF, Burks RT, Robin LD, et al: A prospective evaluation of untreated acute grade III acromioclavicular separations. *Am J Sports Med* 29:699, 2001.
7. Riebel GD, McCabe JB: Anterior shoulder dislocation: A review of reduction techniques. *Am J Emerg Med* 9:180, 1991.
8. Wen DY: Therapeutics: Current concepts in the treatment of anterior shoulder dislocations. *Am J Emerg Med* 17:401, 1999.
9. Kothari RU, Dronen SC: Prospective evaluation of the scapular manipulation technique in reducing anterior shoulder dislocation. *Ann Emerg Med* 21:1349, 1992.
10. Beeson MS: Complications of shoulder dislocation. *Am J Emerg Med* 17: 288, 1999.
11. Warme WJ, Arciero RA, Taylor DC: Anterior shoulder instability in sports: Current management recommendations. *Sports Med* 28:209, 1999.
12. Cleeman E, Flatow EL: Conservative management of shoulder injuries: Shoulder dislocations in the young patient. *Orthop Clin North Am* 31:217, 2000.
13. Styaner LR, Cummings J, Andersen J, et al: Conservative management of shoulder injuries: Shoulder dislocations in patients older than 40 years of age. *Orthop Clin North Am* 31:231, 2000.
14. Walton J, Paxinos A, Tzannes A, et al: The unstable shoulder in the adolescent athlete. *Am J Sports Med* 30:758, 2002.
15. Williams G, Wong K: Two-part and three-part fractures. *Orthop Clin North Am* 31:1, 2000.
16. Birch R: Injuries to the brachial plexus. *Neurosurg Clin North Am* 12:285, 2001.
17. Terzis J, Papakonstantinou K: The surgical treatment of brachial plexus injuries in adults. *Plast Reconstr Surg* 106:1097, 2000.

INJURIES TO THE SPINE
James L. Larson, Jr.

Injuries to the spine are due to blunt trauma in about 90 percent of cases. The most common injury mechanism is a motor vehicle accident, followed by assaults, mostly gunshot wounds, falls, and sporting accidents. The cervical spine is the most common site for injury (61 percent), followed by the thoracolumbar junction (19 percent), the thoracic spine (16 percent), and the lumbosacral spine (4 percent).[1] This chapter discusses the radiologic identification and evaluation of spinal injuries. A thorough discussion of resuscitation, assessment, neurologic evaluation, and treatment are covered in Chaps. 35 and 256.

EVALUATION

Resuscitation and Spinal Immobilization

Injuries to the spine and spinal cord are frequently associated with other injuries. Initial resuscitation of the patient with multiple injuries from trauma focuses on airway, breathing, and circulation (the ABCs). The patient with a potential spine injury should undergo immobilization to prevent deterioration during resuscitation. Patients who are at high risk for spinal injury include those who have had automobile and motorcycle accidents, falls, and diving accidents. Any patients complaining of neck pain, weakness, paresthesias, or paralysis should be considered to have a spinal cord injury. A patient with a history of trauma and an altered level of consciousness should always be treated as if a spinal cord injury were present.

Spinal immobilization is important to prevent secondary injury. The components of spinal immobilization include a long spine board, a semirigid cervical spine collar, and "sandbags" or other devices to limit head and neck motion. Athletes wearing helmets and shoulder pads should be immobilized in their equipment. Removal should occur in the emergency department after radiographic evaluation.[2]

Cervical collars vary in their ability to restrict movement. In general, cervical spine collars alone reduce flexion and extension movement somewhat and are ineffective in limiting lateral movement. The process for moving a patient onto a spine board or for examination of the back involves a "log-roll." One person is required to maintain the head and neck in neutral position while a minimum of two other people gently roll the patient. The person holding the head directs the team to avoid nonsynchronous motion. Manual in-line stabilization using a dedicated person to hold the head and neck in a neutral position is superior to the use of a cervical collar alone. During proper in-line stabilization, no traction is applied to the head and spine. Axial traction is discouraged, because it can cause distraction of cervical spine fractures.

RADIOGRAPHIC EVALUATION

Clinical Clearance

The use of clinical criteria to "clear" the cervical spine and avoid unnecessary radiographs in selected trauma patients has been examined by two large, multicenter studies. The NEXUS group prospectively validated five criteria (Table 272-1) in blunt trauma patients. The criteria have a sensitivity of 99.6 percent for detecting clinically significant cervical spine injury.[3] A second large study is currently under way to validate the Canadian C-spine decision rule for cervical spine trauma.[4]

Plain Cervical Spine Radiographs

Cervical spine radiographs are often the initial screening test for cervical spine injury. A cervical spine series consists of a lateral view, an anteroposterior (AP) view, and an odontoid view. The lateral view radiograph detects 70 to 80 percent of traumatic cervical spine injuries.[5] The lateral view should include the cervothoracic junction, because 20 percent of cervical spine fractures will occur at C7.[6] Gentle traction on the upper extremities may move the shoulders out of the way and improve C7-T1 visualization. Another radiographic technique for defining the bony anatomy of the cervicothoracic junction is the "swimmer's" view. The lateral view should be inspected methodically to detect abnormalities (Table 272-2). Alignment should be evaluated by following anatomic lines (Figure 272-1). There should be no step-offs or breaks in the lines. The anterior longitudinal ligament line follows the anterior surface of the vertebral bodies. This line should follow the normal lordotic curve of the spine. The line of the posterior longitudinal ligament runs along the posterior bodies of the vertebrae and is immediately anterior to the spinal cord. A change of 11 degrees or more in the angle of this line at an interspace should be considered evidence of ligamentous injury (Figure 272-2). The spinolaminar line is formed by the junction of the lamina with the spinous process at each vertebra. Fractures of the odontoid or C2 pedicles can be detected by examining the spinolaminar line. The spinolaminar line connecting

TABLE 272-1   NEXUS Criteria for Cervical Spine Radiography

According to NEXUS low-risk criteria, cervical spine radiography can be omitted for trauma patients only if they exhibit *all* of the following criteria:
No posterior midline cervical spine tenderness
No evidence of intoxication
Normal level of alertness
No focal neurologic deficit
No painful distracting injuries

TABLE 272-2   Criteria for Clearing the Cervical Spine Cross-Table Lateral View

All seven vertebral bodies must be clearly seen, including the C7–T1 junction
Evaluate proper alignment of the posterior cervical line and the four lordotic curves; anterior longitudinal ligament line, posterior longitudinal ligament line, spinolaminal line, and tips of spinous processes
Evaluate the predental space (3 mm in adults, 4–5 mm in children)
Evaluate each vertebra for fracture and increased or decreased density (e.g., suggestive of a compression fracture, metastatic lesion, osteoporosis)
Evaluate the intervertebral and interspinous processes (abrupt angulation of more than 11 degrees at a single interspace is abnormal)
Evaluate for fanning of the spinous processes, suggestive of posterior ligament disruption
Evaluate the prevertebral soft tissue distance
   <7 mm at C2 or <5 mm at C3–C4 is considered normal
   In children <2 y, the prevertebral space may appear widened if the film is obtained during expiration
Evaluate the atlantooccipital region for possible dislocation

Source: Van Hare RS: The ring of C2 and evaluation of the cross-table lateral view of the cervical spine. *Ann Emerg Med* 21:733, 1992.

C1 with C3 should pass within 1 mm of the spinolaminar junction of C2. Displacement of more than 1 mm suggests anterior or posterior displacement of the odontoid, or a hangman's fracture (Figure 272-3). The last line is the line connecting the tips of the spinous processes.

Examination of the soft tissues of the neck may be helpful in defining injury. Injury to the cervical spine can cause hematomas and edema that increase the size of the prevertebral space as seen on the lateral view radiograph. Prevertebral soft tissue distances greater than 7 mm at C2 or 21 mm at C6 result in a sensitivity of 53 percent and specificity of 95 percent for detecting spinal injury.[7]

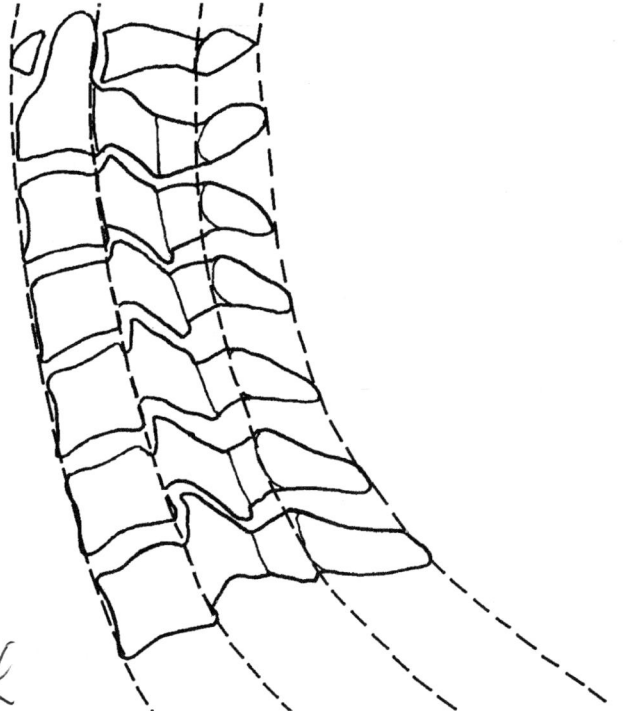

| Anterior Longitudinal Ligament Line | Posterior Longitudinal Ligament Line | Spino-Laminal Line | Spinous Processes Line |

FIG. 272-1. Alignment of the lateral cervical spine.

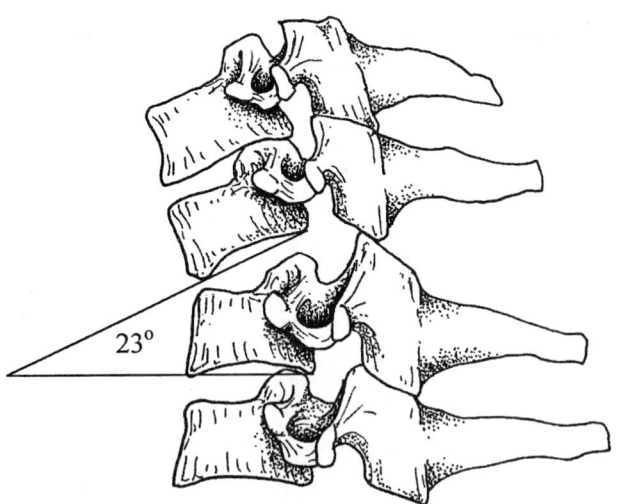

FIG. 272-2. Angulation relative to the posterior longitudinal ligament. (Reproduced with permission from Galli RL, Spaite DW, Simon RR: *Emergency Orthopedics: The Spine.* Norwalk, CT, Appleton & Lange, 1989, p. 9.)

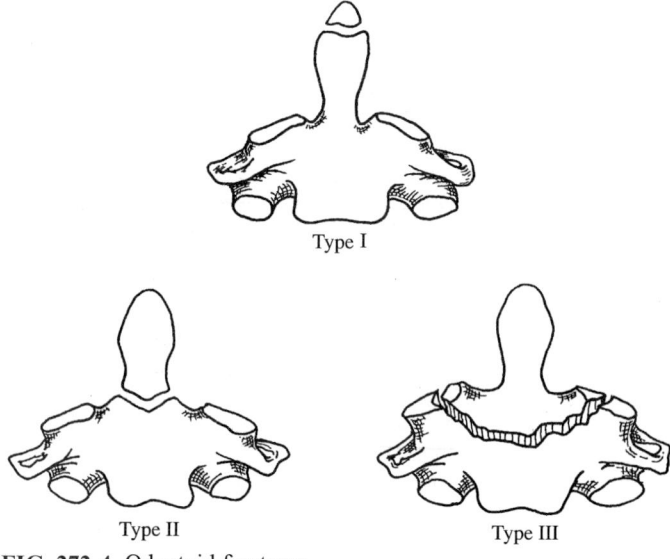

FIG. 272-4. Odontoid fractures.

The AP view is used to examine for angulation of the lateral cortex of the articular masses as compared with superior or inferior neighbors. In addition, the spinous processes can be seen on end, and abnormal widening or malalignment may indicate a hyperflexion sprain or interfacetal dislocation.

The odontoid or open-mouth view shows the odontoid and its relation to the lateral masses of C1. The dens should be centered between the lateral masses, and the lateral masses of C1 should be directly over the lateral portions of C2. Rotation of the head may cause some displacement of the lateral masses and asymmetry of the relation of the dens and C1. Rotation can be detected by using the space between the central incisors as a reference point, which should be in the midline in an unrotated view. Possible fracture lines through the dens should be sought (Figure 272-4).

Plain radiography is a screening tool and cannot detect all injuries. In the largest cervical spine study to date, an adequate three-view cervical spine series had a sensitivity of 89.4 percent for detecting at least one lesion in an injured patient.[8] Additional radiographic studies may be needed to detect injury when clinical suspicion is present.

Computed Tomography

Computed tomography (CT) is indicated in any major fracture or dislocation of the spine. Computed tomography can improve the detection of fractures in areas poorly visualized by plain radiography—these areas comprise the C1, C2, C6, and C7 vertebrae. Figures 272-5 and 272-6 show the benefit of CT in evaluating the upper cervical spine. Computed tomography is indicated if clinical suspicion for occult fracture exists after normal plain radiographs of the spine. Screening helical CT combined with a single lateral view in lieu of plain radiography is cost effective and accurate in groups at high risk for cervical spinal injury.[9] (Table 272-3) It is also helpful for evaluating the cervical spine in the elderly or those with prior spinal surgery or underlying spinal disease. Computed tomography is less useful for purely soft tissue injuries seen with ligamentous disruption.

Magnetic Resonance Imaging

Magnetic resonance imaging (MRI) is better than CT for defining the soft tissue injury seen with spinal fractures and is indicated in all patients who have neurologic deficits from a spinal cord injury. Magnetic resonance imaging can evaluate the epidural space for herniated intervertebral disks, hematoma, and bone fragments and can image the

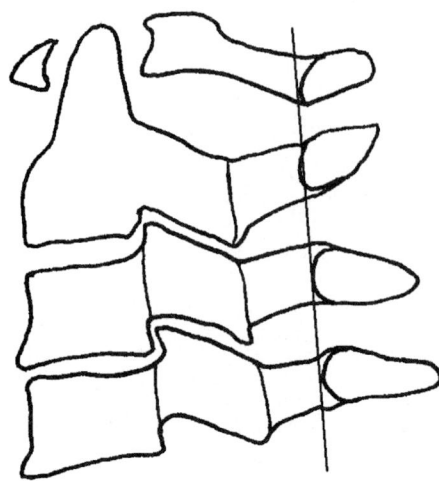

FIG. 272-3. Spinolaminar alignment. (Reproduced with permission from Galli RL, Spaite DW, Simon RR: *Emergency Orthopedics: The Spine.* Norwalk, CT, Appleton & Lange, 1989, p. 9.)

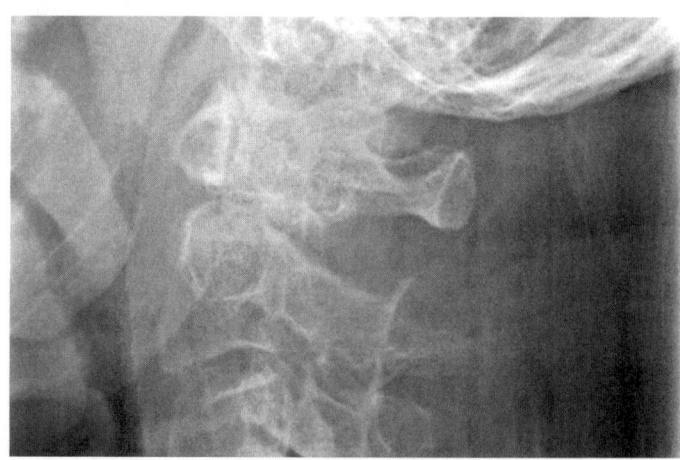

FIG. 272-5. Subtle fracture of dens on lateral C-spine film.

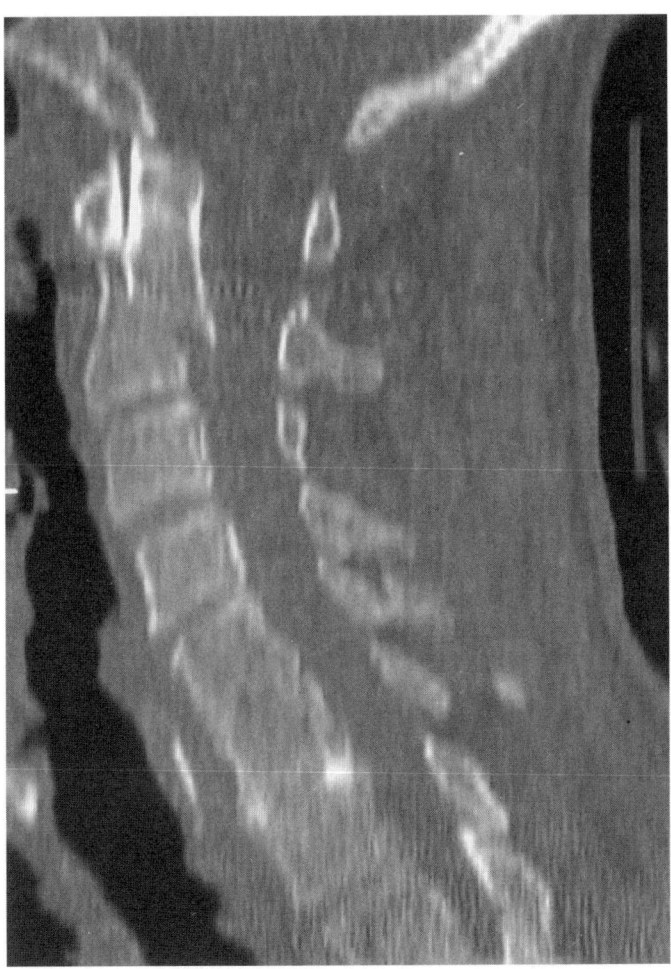

FIG. 272-6. Sagittal computed tomography of dens fracture.

spinal cord for edema, hemorrhage, or laceration. Magnetic resonance imaging is more time consuming than CT and should be used only for patients who are hemodynamically stable.

Flexion-Extension Views

An injury to the ligamentous structures of the spine may occur without a bony fracture. If the initial radiographs show no evidence of fracture but are suggestive of subluxation, or if suspicion of a ligamentous injury exists, flexion and extension views may be performed. However, their indications and even some measurement parameters are controversial. Anterior subluxation injuries are exacerbated in flexion and reduced in extension. Flexion-extension films should be per-

TABLE 272-3 High-Risk Criteria for Selection of Use of Screening Cervical Computed Tomography

Mechanism
   High-speed motor vehicle collision (≥35 mph combined impact)
   Fall from height (≥10 ft)
   Pedestrian struck by car
Evaluation
   Significant closed-head injury or intracranial hemorrhage
   Unconscious at time of examination
   Neurologic symptoms or signs referred to the cervical spine

Source: Blackmore CC, Mann FA, Wilson AJ: Helical CT in the primary trauma evaluation of the cervical spine: An evidence-based approach. *Skeletal Radiol* 29:632, 2000.

formed only in awake, cooperative patients and should be halted at the point when they cause the patient pain. The pain associated with cervical spinal injuries may prevent adequate flexion and extension. Some authorities do not recommend flexion-extension views at the time of initial evaluation and opt for acute MRI or delayed flexion-extension testing.[10] The patient should wear a well-fitting cervical collar until the delayed flexion-extension testing is performed.

CERVICAL SPINE INJURIES

Upper Cervical Spine (Occiput, C1, C2)

ANATOMY The upper cervical spine (occiput, C1, and C2) is anatomically and functionally distinct from the lower cervical spine (C3 to C7). The upper cervical spine is designed for rotary motion. C1 (atlas) is a ring structure with large lateral masses which articulate with the skull and vertebral column. C2 (axis) is composed of a body with an anterior projection (dens) that articulates with the anterior inner surface of C1. The dens is stabilized to C1 by the transverse ligament.

OCCIPITOATLANTAL DISSOCIATION In occipitoatlantal dissociation, the skull may be displaced anteriorly or posteriorly or distracted from the cervical spine. Occipitoatlantal dissociation frequently results in death. Severe occipitoatlantal dissociation is easily detected on the lateral radiograph. Occipitoatlantal subluxation is more difficult to detect on radiographs. Harris described a method for detecting occipitoatlantal injury.[11] The basion-axial interval can be measured in most lateral radiographs. This is the distance between the basion (the tip of the clivus) and a line extending from the posterior cortex of C2. The basion-axial interval should not exceed 12 mm (Figure 272-7A). The basion-dental interval is the distance between the basion and the superior cortex of the dens. This distance also should be less than 12 mm (see Figure 272-7B).[11] Atlantooccipital injuries are extremely unstable.

C1 (Atlas) Fractures

JEFFERSON FRACTURE The Jefferson fracture is usually produced when the cervical spine is subjected to an axial load due to a direct blow to the top of the head. The occipital condyles are displaced downward and produce a burst fracture by driving the lateral masses of C1

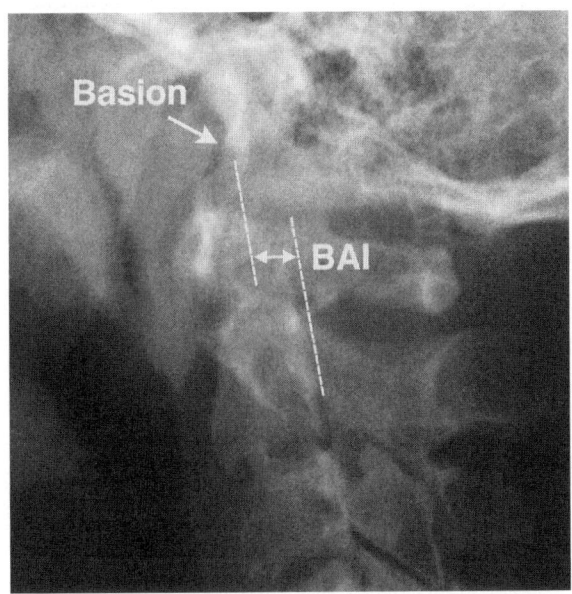

FIG. 272-7A. Basion-axial interval (BAI).

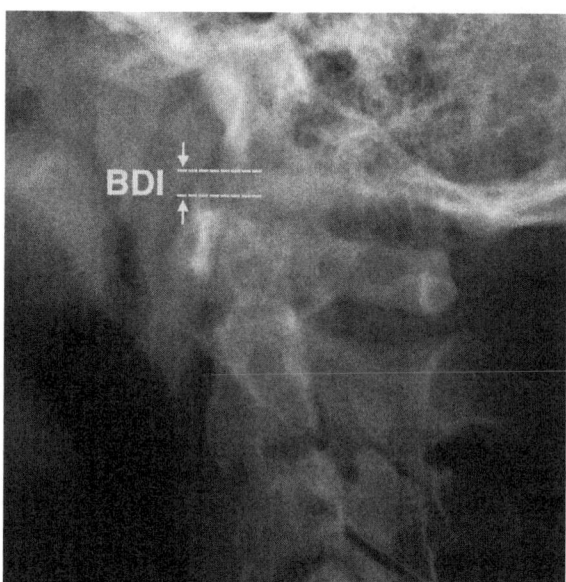

FIG. 272-7B. Basion-dental interval (BDI).

apart (Figure 272-8). The lateral masses will be displaced laterally on the open-mouth odontoid radiograph. A fracture through one lateral mass will cause unilateral displacement on the open-mouth view. Instability is likely if the lateral masses are displaced significantly. If the displacement of the lateral masses on each side added together is greater than 7 mm, rupture of the transverse ligament is likely.

TRANSVERSE LIGAMENT DISRUPTION   The transverse ligament is located anteriorly on the inside of the ring of C1 and runs along the posterior surface of the dens. The transverse ligament is crucial to maintaining the stability of the first and second vertebrae. Pure ligamentous rupture without an associated fracture can occur in older patients with a direct blow to the occiput, as would occur in a fall. Without a fracture present, radiographic diagnosis relies on identifying the atlantodens interval, also known as the *predental space*, which is viewed on the lateral x-ray. The space is between the posterior aspect of the anterior arch of C1 and the anterior border of the odontoid. The space should be 3 mm or less in adults. **More than 3 mm of space implies damage to the transverse ligament; more than 5 mm implies rupture of the transverse ligament.** Immediate specialist consultation is necessary for these injuries.

AVULSION FRACTURE OF THE ANTERIOR ARCH OF THE ATLAS
A hyperextension injury may avulse the inferior pole of the anterior

tubercle of C1. This is most readily detected on the lateral view (Figure 272-9). The presence of perivertebral soft tissue swelling and absence of cortication distinguish it from the ununited secondary ossification center of the inferior pole of the tubercle. A fracture involving the entire anterior arch is unstable.

C2 (Axis) Fractures

ODONTOID FRACTURES   Fractures of the odontoid are usually due to major forces and frequently involve other injuries to the cervical spine and multisystem trauma. Awake patients usually will complain of immediate and severe high cervical pain with muscle spasm aggravated by movement. The pain may not be severe and can radiate to the occiput of the head. Neurologic injury presents in 18 to 25 percent of cases. This can range from minimal sensory or motor loss to quadriplegia. Classification of odontoid fractures relies on identifying the level of injury. Type I fractures are avulsions of the tip. The transverse ligament remains attached to the dens, the fracture is stable, and the injury carries a good prognosis. Type II fractures occur at the junction of the odontoid and the body of C2. This is the most common odontoid fracture. Type III odontoid fractures occur through the superior portion of C2 at the base of the dens (see Figure 272-4).

HANGMAN'S FRACTURE (TRAUMATIC SPONDYLOLITHESIS OF THE AXIS)   The hangman's fracture is located in the pedicles of C2, with C2 displacing anteriorly on C3 (Figure 272-10). The fracture is caused by an extension mechanism and is seen in judicial hangings. Suicidal hangings do not usually cause the extreme hyperextension seen in judicial hangings and do not cause a hangman's fracture. The same fracture is seen in motor vehicle and diving accidents, where sudden hyperextension forces are applied in deceleration. Owing to the large diameter of the spinal canal at the level of C2, even displacement of C2 on C3 may not cause neurologic injury, and patients may be neurologically intact. This injury is unstable.

Lower Cervical Spine (C3 to C7)

ANATOMY   An understanding of the anatomy of the cervical spine is essential to the classification of injuries. For the purpose of understanding how mechanisms of injury affect the spine, consider the spine as consisting of three columns.[12] The anterior column resists compression (flexion) with the vertebral centrum and intervertebral disk and resists distraction (extension) with the anterior longitudinal ligament and the anterior annulus fibrosis. The middle column resists compression through the posterior vertebral body wall and resists distraction by the posterior longitudinal ligament and the posterior annu-

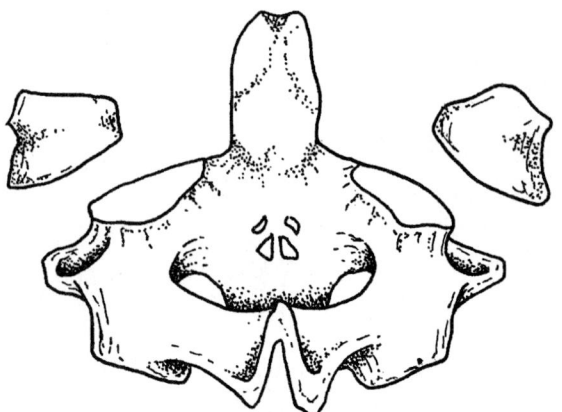

FIG. 272-8. Jefferson fracture.

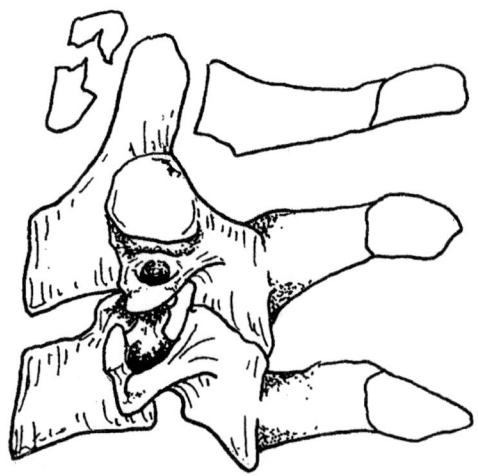

FIG. 272-9. Avulsion fracture of the anterior arch of the atlas.

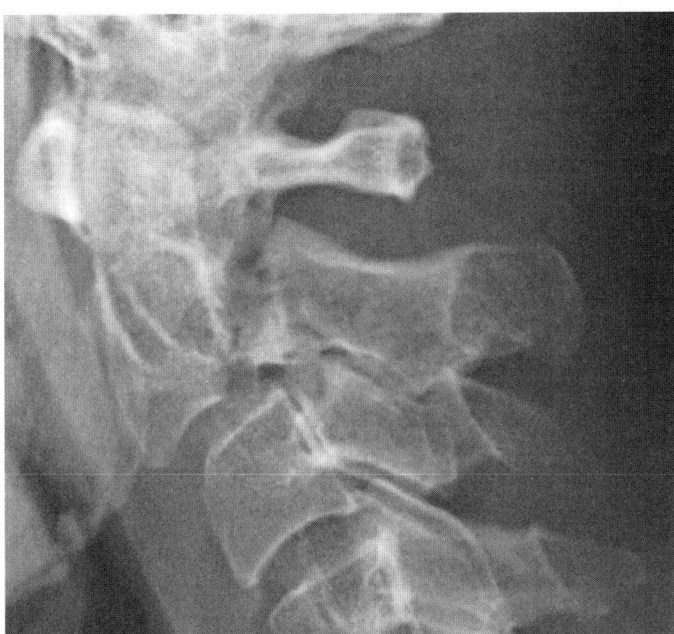

FIG. 272-10. "Hangman's" fracture.

TABLE 272-4   Cervical Spine Injuries: Mechanism of Injury

Flexion
Anterior subluxation (hyperflexion sprain)
Bilateral interfacetal dislocation
Simple wedge (compression) fracture
Clay-shoveler's (coal-shoveler's) fracture
Flexion teardrop fracture
Flexion–rotation
Unilateral interfacetal dislocation
Pillar fracture
Fracture or separation (pedicolaminar fracture)
Vertical compression
Jefferson burst fracture of atlas
Burst (bursting, dispersion, axial-loading) fracture
Hyperextension
Hyperextension dislocation
Avulsion fracture of anterior arch of atlas
Extension teardrop fracture
Fracture of posterior arch of atlas
Laminar fracture
Traumatic spondylolisthesis ("hangman's" fracture)
Lateral flexion
Uncinate process fracture
Injuries caused by diverse or poorly understood mechanisms
Occipitoatlantal dissociation
Occipital condylar fractures
Dens fractures

Source: Harris J: Spine, including soft tissue of the pharynx and neck, in Harris J, Harris W (eds): *The Radiology of Emergency Medicine,* 4th ed. Baltimore, Lippincott Williams & Wilkins, 2000, p. 137.

lus fibrosis. The posterior column resists compression through the facet joints and lateral masses and resists distraction through the facet joint capsules and intraspinous ligaments.[13]

UNSTABLE FRACTURES   The three-column model of the spine is useful when assessing for the stability of fractures. Instability of the anterior column can occur when the anterior 20 percent of the vertebral body is damaged by compression causing a teardrop fracture.[14] Loss of 25 percent or more of the vertebral body height also is a marker of failure.[15] Loss of integrity of the posterior wall of a vertebral body is a marker for instability in the middle column. Radiographic findings include widening of pedicles, loss of more than 25 percent of posterior vertebral body height, and the presence of sagittal plane fracture lines through the posterior vertebral body cortex.[16] Instability of the posterior column is the result of damage to the facet complex.[13]

The ligaments providing stability to the spine can be damaged without causing radiographic abnormalities. Determining stability can involve dynamic testing (flexion-extension), MRI, and other investigations. Determination of stability should be left to the spine consultant.

MECHANISM OF INJURY   The forces that lead to cervical spine injury have been studied in laboratory settings. These experiments have associated specific patterns of injury with the initial dominant force present at the time of injury. A classification system for describing cervical spine injuries based on the biomechanical force responsible for the injury has been proposed by Harris[11] (Table 272-4). A description of selected cervical spinal fractures based on this classification follows.

Mechanism: Hyperflexion

ANTERIOR SUBLUXATION   Anterior subluxation is also known as *hyperflexion sprain.* The posterior ligamentous structures fail, because of the hyperflexion of the cervical spine. A pure subluxation injury has no associated fractures. Radiographic findings can include a "fanning," or widening, of the spinous processes at the level of injury. The disc space may be widened posteriorly and narrowed anteriorly. Abrupt angulation change of more than 11 degrees at a single interspace may also signal an injury[16] (see Figure 272-2).

Cervical spine radiographs may be normal or only demonstrate soft tissue swelling if the hyperflexion sprain has not caused a fracture and the subluxation has been reduced. Pain on movement, or neurologic findings, should prompt CT scanning or MRI for diagnosis.

CLAY-SHOVELER'S FRACTURE   An avulsion of the spinous process of the lower cervical vertebrae, classically C7, is known as a clay-shoveler's fracture (Figure 272-11). Intense flexion against contracted posterior erector spinal muscles causes avulsion of the spinous process. An isolated clay-shoveler's fracture is mechanically stable.[11]

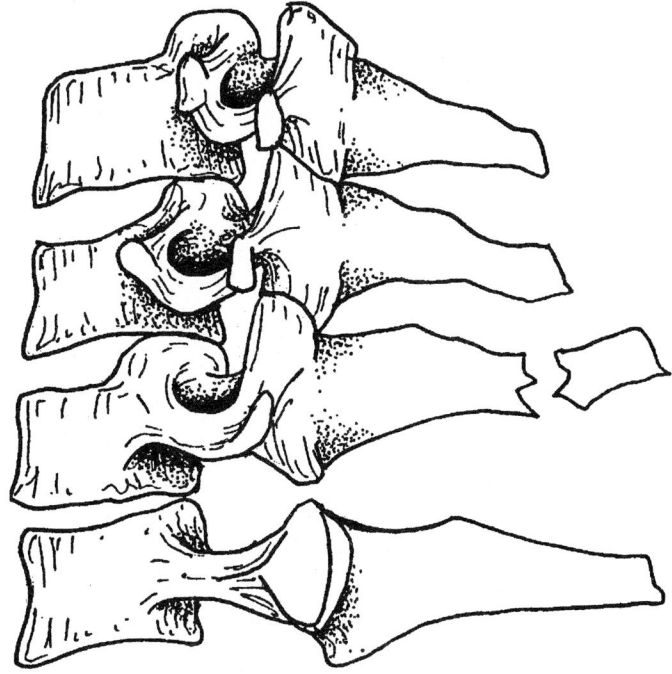

FIG. 272-11. Clay-shoveler's fracture.

SIMPLE WEDGE FRACTURE A wedge fracture of a vertebra is caused by compression between two other vertebrae. The superior end plate fractures while the inferior surface of the vertebra remains intact (Figure 272-12). The posterior ligaments may be disrupted, leading to an increase in the distance between spinous processes. Posterior element disruption makes the injury unstable. The simple wedge fracture is differentiated from a burst fracture by the absence of a vertical fracture of the vertebral body.

FLEXION TEARDROP FRACTURE Extreme flexion can cause the flexion teardrop fracture (Figure 272-13). The associated anterior cord syndrome is due to impingement of the spinal cord by the fracture hyperkyphosis. There is complete disruption of all ligamentous structures at the level of the injury. The "teardrop" is the anteroinferior portion of the vertebral body, which is separated and displaced from the remaining portion of the vertebra. This injury is mechanically unstable.[11]

BILATERAL INTERFACETAL DISLOCATION Bilateral interfacetal dislocation (BID) occurs when disruption to all ligamentous structures due to hyperflexion allows the articular masses of the involved vertebra to dislocate superiorly and anteriorly over into the intervertebral foramen inferior to the involved vertebra (Figures 272-14 and 272-15). Radiographically, the vertebra can be seen dislocated anteriorly to at least 50 percent its width. The injury is mechanically unstable and usually presents with neurologic findings.[11] A "perched" vertebra is seen in partial BID, when the articular masses of the involved vertebra are perched on the superior articular processes of the subjacent vertebra. This configuration is also mechanically unstable but may not present with neurologic compromise.[10] Using the term *locked facets* to describe a BID is misleading, because the injury is unstable.

Mechanism: Flexion and Rotation

UNILATERAL INTERFACETAL DISLOCATION Simultaneous forces of flexion and rotation can produce a unilateral facet dislocation. The articular mass and inferior facet on one side of the vertebra are anteriorly dislocated (Figure 272-16). Radiographically, the AP view will reveal the rotation, because the spinous processes will not be projected directly over one another. The affected spinous process will point toward the side of the vertebra that is dislocated. The involved vertebra will be displaced anteriorly less than 50 percent of the width of a vertebra on the lateral view. The dislocation is mechanically stable unless there is a fracture at the base of the inferior articular mass of the dislocated vertebra or a fracture of the superior articular mass of the inferior vertebra.

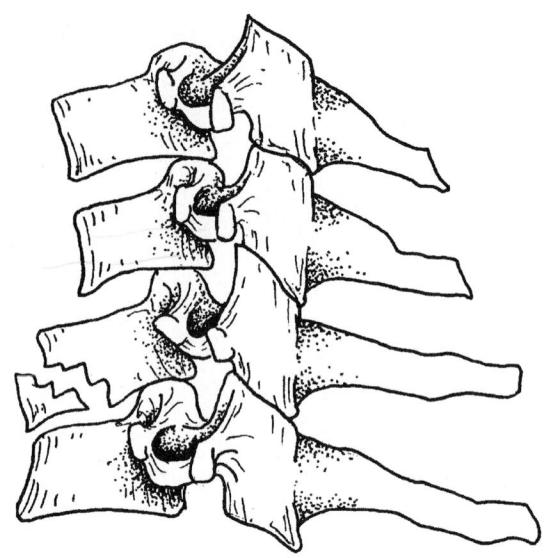

FIG. 272-13. Flexion teardrop fracture.

Mechanism: Extension and Rotation

PILLAR FRACTURE Extension and rotation can cause impaction of a superior vertebra on the articular mass of its inferior neighbor. The resultant vertical or oblique fracture of the articular mass is called a *pillar fracture* (Figure 272-17). The adjacent lamina and pedicle remain intact. The lateral view may show a "double-outline" sign at the level

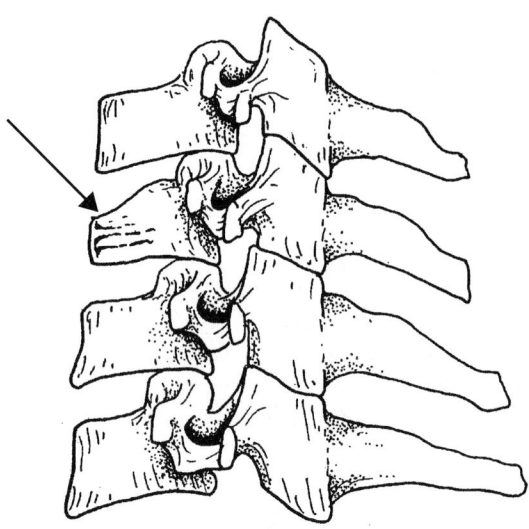

FIG. 272-12. Wedge fracture.

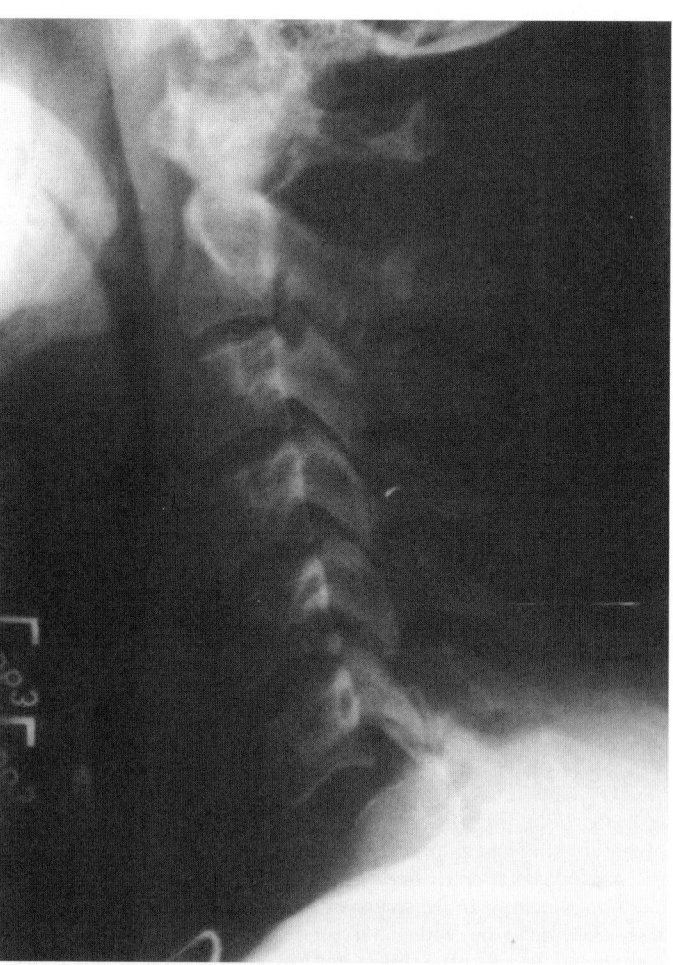

FIG. 272-14. Bilateral interfacetal dislocation between C6 and C7.

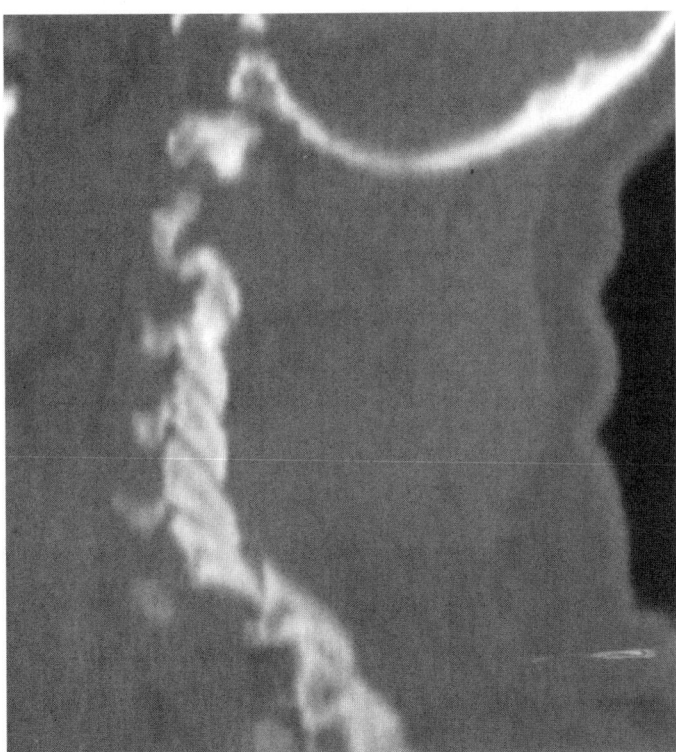

FIG. 272-15. Sagittal computed tomography of bilateral interfacetal dislocation between C6 and C7 showing jumped facet.

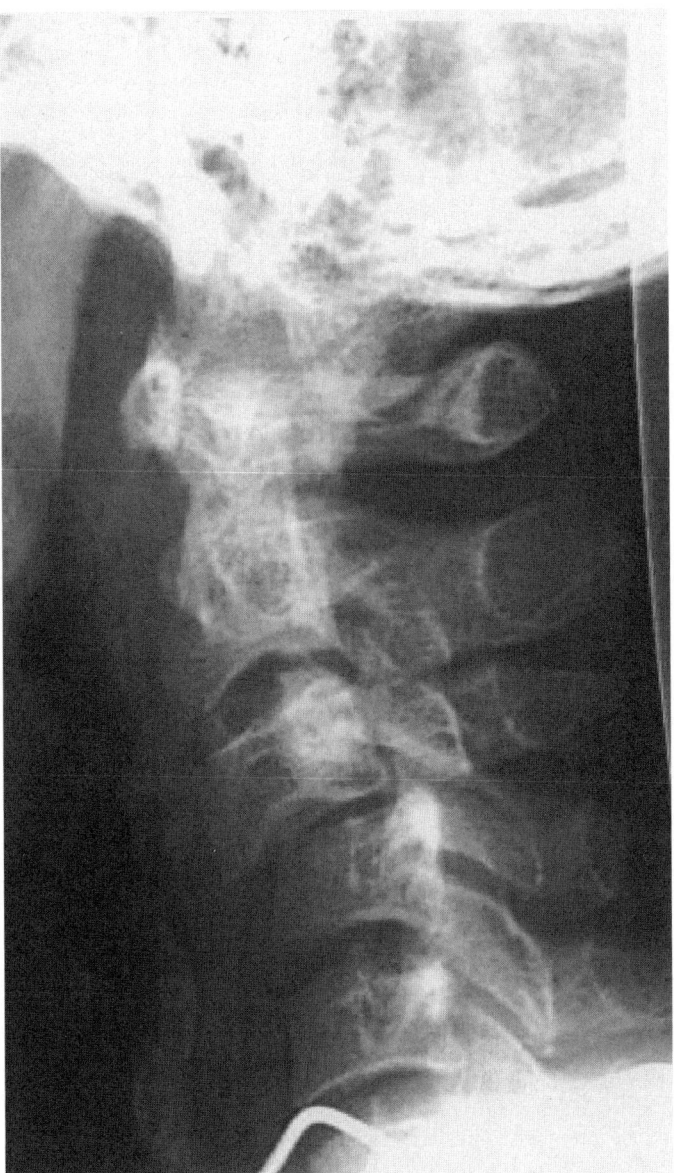

FIG. 272-16. Unilateral facet dislocation.

of the injury. This can be differentiated from the normal lateral radiograph, in which the articular masses are imposed on one another and one radiographic density is seen. The double outline occurs when the fractured articular mass is displaced posteriorly and causes two radiographic shadows. The AP projection will show an abnormality of the lateral column and a fracture at the level of the injury. The fracture is considered stable.

FRACTURE SEPARATION   Harris described the fracture and separation as a pedicolaminar fracture, because it involves fractures of the pedicle and lamina.[11] There are different degrees of fracture, ranging from fractures without displacement to disruption of the anterior longitudinal ligament and disk rupture. The lateral radiograph may show rotation of the involved articular mass as compared with the uninvolved lateral mass at the level of the injury. Anterior listhesis may be seen in more severe mechanisms. The AP view may show disruption of the lateral column.

Mechanism: Vertical Compression Injuries

BURST FRACTURE   A direct axial load causes a burst fracture of the lower cervical spine. The axial force causes the vertebra to burst, with fragments displacing in all directions (Figure 272-18). The spinal cord may be injured if a fragment enters the spinal canal. The lateral radiograph may show a fracture of the superior and inferior vertebral end plates and retropulsion of the posterior segment of the vertebra into the spinal canal. The AP view will show a vertical fracture and widening of the interpedicular distance. This injury is unstable.

Mechanism: Hyperextension Injuries

HYPEREXTENSION DISLOCATION   A hyperextension injury involves a complete tear of the anterior longitudinal ligament and intervertebral disk, with disruption of the posterior ligamentous complex.

Facial trauma with a central cord syndrome is the most common clinical presentation. In the lateral cervical spine film, the vertebrae may be normally aligned, because the dislocation will be reduced. Diffuse prevertebral soft tissue swelling is usually present. Other signs include a disk-space widening anteriorly or a fracture of the anteroinferior end plate of the vertebrae.[11] If the patient has no neurologic deficit and no evidence of fracture, CT or MRI is generally used to confirm ligamentous disruption.

EXTENSION TEARDROP FRACTURE   A hyperextension mechanism may cause the anterior longitudinal ligament to avulse the inferior portion of the anterior vertebral body at its insertion (Figure 272-19). The height of the fragment usually exceeds its width. This fracture is more common in older patients with osteoporosis. The extension teardrop fracture is unstable in extension.

LAMINAR FRACTURE   Isolated laminar fractures are caused by hyperextension and may be subtle on plain radiographs. Associated spinous process fractures may be present. Computed tomography is required to define the extent of spinal cord involvement.

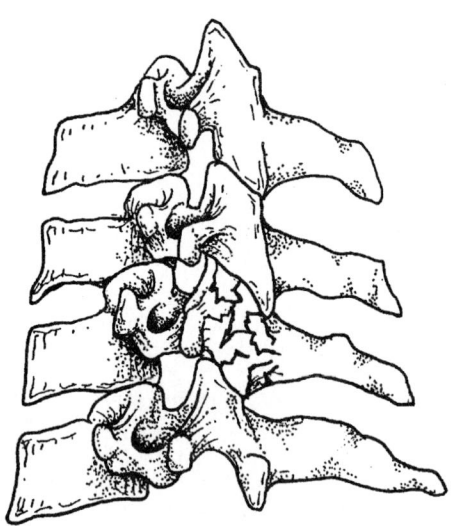

FIG. 272-17. Pillar fracture.

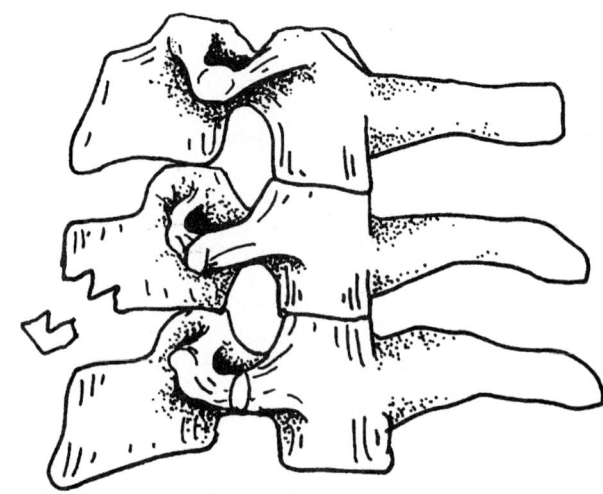

FIG. 272-19. Extension teardrop fracture.

Mechanism: Lateral Flexion

UNCINATE PROCESS FRACTURE   Pure lateral flexion is rare in most mechanisms of injury. Lateral flexion can cause a transverse fracture at the base of the uncinate process as the lateral aspect of the superior vertebral body fractures the inferior uncinate process. During the initial injury, the degree of lateral neck flexion is limited, because the head strikes the shoulder. This fracture may be seen in the AP or lateral view.

Spinal Cord Injury without Radiographic Abnormality

Spinal cord injury without radiographic abnormality (SCIWORA) is used to describe the condition of neurologic abnormality after injury but without fractures or bony malalignment on plain radiographs.[17] Initially described in children, it also occurs in adults but is rare in both age groups.[18] In one large study, only about 3 percent of those with spinal cord injury had SCIWORA.[18]

Neurologic findings are variable and can include central cord syndrome. Diagnosis is by MRI, with the most common findings of central disc herniation, spinal stenosis, intramedullary hematoma or contusion, and cord edema.

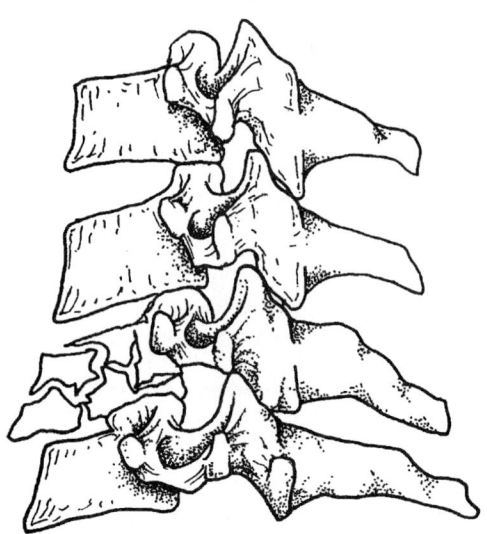

FIG. 272-18. Burst fracture.

THORACOLUMBAR SPINE INJURIES

Anatomy

The thoracolumbar spine is relatively more protected and stable than the cervical spine. Vertebrae T1 through T10 are fixed, owing to their articulation with the thoracic cage. Large forces are required to fracture thoracic vertebrae, and neurologic abnormalities are common. The mobility of the thoracolumbar junction predisposes it to injury. The thoracolumbar junction is second only to the cervical spine in frequency of injury. The spinal cord ends at approximately L1 at the conus medullaris. The individual nerve roots extending from the conus medullaris constitute the cauda equina. These nerve roots are less susceptible to damage and neurologic injury, because trauma to the lower lumbar and sacral segments occurs less often and is less severe. McAfee and associates classified thoracolumbar spine injuries into major and minor fractures[19] (Table 272-5). A discussion of the classification follows.

Major Fractures and Dislocations

WEDGE COMPRESSION FRACTURES   These fractures are the result of flexion causing compression of the anterior body of the vertebra. Plain radiographs demonstrate loss of anterior height in the traumatized vertebra. The posterior height and cortex are intact. Computed tomography should be performed to define the stability of the posterior elements and determine whether there is involvement of the neural canal. These fractures are not usually associated with neurologic

TABLE 272-5   Classification of Thoracolumbar Spine Injury

Major Injuries*	Minor Injuries†
Wedge compression fractures	Transverse process fracture
Chance fractures	Spinous process fracture
Burst fractures	Pars interarticularis fracture
Flexion distraction injuries	
Translational injuries	

*Assume to be unstable; should be cared for at a center with orthopedic or neurosurgical spine specialists.
†Implies isolated fracture with no neurologic deficits; generally are stable.
Source: Savitsky E, Votey S: Emergency department approach to acute thoracolumbar spine injury. *J Emerg Med* 15:49, 1997.

compromise but should be treated as unstable until evaluation is complete.

BURST FRACTURE   A flexion mechanism causing anterior vertebral compression with involvement of the posterior cortex defines the burst fracture. Lateral plain radiography will show the loss of anterior and posterior height; AP views will show an increase in the interpedicular distance; and CT will define the extent of the injury (Figure 272-20). The burst fracture should be considered unstable.

CHANCE FRACTURE   A Chance fracture is caused by a flexion around an axis anterior to the anterior spinal longitudinal ligament. A high-speed motor vehicle accident with the occupant in a lap belt will produce this mechanism. The Chance fracture involves the spinous process, lamina, transverse processes, pedicles, and vertebral body.[20] The lateral radiograph will show the fracture through the posterior elements and vertebral body. Computed tomography may help to define the injury but can miss it if the fracture is in the same plane as the scan. The Chance fracture should be considered unstable.

FLEXION AND DISTRACTION INJURIES   A flexion-distraction mechanism places the anterior portions of the spine under compression while distracting the posterior elements. The lateral radiograph shows loss of height in the anterior portion of the vertebra, with increased interspinous spaces posteriorly ("fanning"). Computed tomography and specialist consultation are recommended. This injury is unstable.

TRANSLATION INJURIES   Translational injuries are the result of large shear forces that cause complete disruption of spine stability.

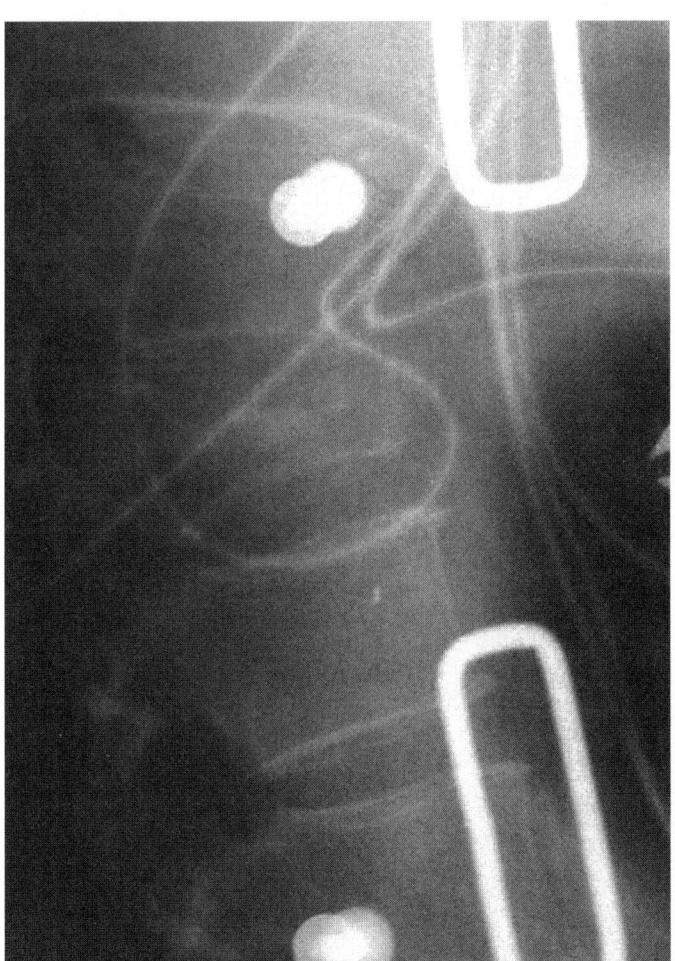

FIG. 272-20. T12 burst fracture.

The lateral radiograph will show translation of one or more vertebral segments on subsequent segments. Associated neurologic injury is common.

MINOR FRACTURES   Minor fractures include spinous process fractures, transverse process fractures, and pars interarticularis fractures. Minor fractures that have no additional spinal or visceral injuries and associated neurologic compromise are considered stable. Computed tomography is needed to evaluate the extent of injury and to exclude concomitant major fractures.

Consultation and Disposition

The differentiation of spinal injuries as "stable" or "unstable" is not a useful categorization for the emergency physician. Acute bony or ligamentous injuries and injuries with actual or suspected neurologic deficits are best referred to the spinal surgeon to institute proper acute treatment, ensure absence of additional associated spinal injuries, determine appropriate disposition, and ensure follow-up care, which can minimize the development of delayed instability and pain syndromes.

Patients should remain in spinal immobilization until definitive diagnosis and evaluation of CT and MRI are made by the spinal surgeon.

REFERENCES

1. Fife D, Kraus J: Anatomic location of spinal cord injury relationship to the cause of injury. *Spine* 11:2, 1986.
2. Kleiner DM, Almquist JL, Bailes J, et al: *Prehospital Care of the Spine-Injured Athlete.* Dallas, TX, National Athletic Trainers' Association, 2001.
3. Hoffman JR, Mower WR, Wolfson AB, et al: Validity of a set of clinical criteria to rule out injury to the cervical spine in patients with blunt trauma. *New Engl J Med* 343:94, 2000.
4. Stiell IG, Wells GA, Vandemheen KL, et al: The Canadian c-spine rule for radiography in alert and stable trauma patients. *JAMA* 286:1841, 2001.
5. Blahd WH, Iserson KV, Bjelland JC, et al: Efficacy of the post-traumatic cross table lateral view of the cervical spine. *J Emerg Med* 2:243, 1985.
6. Goldberg W, Mueller C, Panacek E, et al: Distribution and patterns of blunt traumatic cervical spine injury. *Ann Emerg Med* 38:17, 2001.
7. Matar LD, Doyle AJ: Prevertebral soft-tissue measurements in cervical spine injury. *Australas Radiol* 41:229, 1997.
8. Mower WR, Hoffman JR, Pollack CV, et al: Use of plain radiography to screen for cervical spine injuries. *Ann Emerg Med* 38:1, 2001.
9. Blackmore CC, Mann FA, Wilson AJ: Helical CT in the primary trauma evaluation of the cervical spine: An evidence-based approach. *Skeletal Radiol* 29:632, 2000.
10. Crim JR, Moore K, Brodke D: Clearance of the cervical spine in multi-trauma patients: The role of advanced imaging. *Semin Ultrasound CT MRI* 22:283, 2001.
11. Harris J: Spine, including soft tissues of the pharynx and neck, in Harris J, Harris W (eds): *The Radiology of Emergency Medicine,* 4th ed. Philadelphia, Lippincott Williams & Wilkins, 2000, p. 137.
12. Denis F: Spinal instability as defined by the three column spine concept in acute spinal trauma. *Clin Orthop Rel Res* 189:65, 1983.
13. Stauffer ES, MacMillan M: Fractures and dislocations of the cervical spine, in Rockwood CA, Green DP (eds): *Rockwood and Green's Fractures in Adults,* 5th ed. Philadelphia, Lippincott Williams & Wilkins, 2000.
14. Allen BL, Ferguson RL, Lehmann TR: A mechanistic classification of closed, indirect fractures and dislocations of the lower cervical spine. *Spine* 7:1, 1982.
15. Mazur JM, Stauffer ED: Unrecognized spinal instability associated with seemingly "simple" cervical compression fractures. *Spine* 8:687, 1983.
16. White AA III, Punjabi MM: *Clinical Biomechanics of the Spine,* 2d ed. Philadelphia, Lippincott, 1990.
17. Gupta SK, Khosla RK, Sharma BS, et al: Spinal cord injury without radiographic abnormality in adults. *Spinal Cord* 38:129, 2000.
18. Hendey GW, Wolfon AB, Mower WR, et al, and the National Emergency X-Radiography Utilization Study Group: Spinal cord injury without

radiographic abnormality: Results of the National Emergency X-Radiography Utilization Study in Blunt Cervical Trauma. *J Trauma* 53:1198, 2002.

19. McAfee PC, Hansen YA, Fredrickson BE, et al: The value of computed tomography in thoracolumbar fractures. *J Bone Joint Surg* 65A:461, 1983.

20. Smith WS, Kaufer H: Patterns and mechanisms of lumbar injuries associated with lap seat belts. *J Bone Joint Surg* 51A:239, 1969.

TRAUMA TO THE PELVIS, HIP, AND FEMUR

Mark T. Steele
Stefanie R. Ellison

TRAUMA TO THE PELVIS

Pelvic fractures and associated injuries are a frequent cause of morbidity from blunt trauma sustained in automobile accidents. Most pelvic fractures are secondary to automobile passenger or pedestrian accidents, but are also the result of minor falls in older persons and from major falls or industrial accidents. This chapter discusses the most common fractures of the pelvis, femur, and hip, the mechanisms of injury, radiologic evaluation, and treatment.

ANATOMY AND BIOMECHANICS

The major functions of the pelvis are protection, support, and hematopoiesis. The pelvis consists of the two innominate bones, which are made up of the ilium, ischium, and pubis; the sacrum; and the coccyx. The two innominate bones and sacrum form a ring structure, which is the basis of pelvic stability. This stability is dependent on the strong posterior sacroiliac, sacrotuberous, and sacrospinous ligaments (Figure 273-1). Any single break in the ring will yield a stable injury without significant risk of displacement. An injury with two breaks in the ring is unstable with the risk of displacement. The iliopectineal, or arcuate line, divides the pelvis into the upper, or false, pelvis, which is part of the abdomen, and the lower, true pelvis. In addition, this line constitutes the major portion of the femorosacral arch, which, along with the subsidiary tie arch (bodies of pubic bones and superior rami), supports the body in the erect position. In the sitting position, the weight-bearing forces are transmitted by the ischiosacral arch augmented by its tie arch, the pubic bones, inferior pubic rami, and ischial rami. The tie arches fracture first, especially at the symphysis pubis, pubic rami, and just lateral to the sacroiliac (SI) joints. Incorporated in the pelvic structure are five joints that allow some movement in the

bony ring. The lumbosacral, SI, and sacrococcygeal joints, and the symphysis pubis allow little movement. The acetabulum is a ball-and-socket joint that is divided into three portions: the iliac portion, or superior dome, is the chief weight-bearing surface; the inner wall consists of the pubis, and is thin and easily fractured; and the posterior acetabulum is derived from the thick ischium.

The pelvis is extremely vascular, a fact that is significant in pelvic fractures. The nerve supply through the pelvis is derived from the lumbar and sacral plexuses. Injury to the pelvis may produce deficits at any level from the nerve root to small peripheral branches.

The lower urinary tract is contained in the pelvis (Figure 273-2). In the adult, the bladder lies behind the symphysis and pubic bones, and the peritoneum covers the dome and base posteriorly. The location of the bladder and the degree of peritoneal reflection are determined by urine content. The lower gastrointestinal tract housed in the pelvis includes a small portion of the descending colon, the sigmoid colon, the rectum, and the anus. In women, the uterus and vagina are also housed in the bony pelvis.

Clinical Evaluation

HISTORY   All victims of serious or multiple trauma should be considered to have fractures of the pelvis. A patient with a suspected pelvic fracture should be questioned about details of the accident to determine the mechanism of injury and the prehospital evaluation and treatment. The patient should be specifically questioned to determine areas of pain, last urination or defecation, present bladder sensation, and the last solid and fluid intake. In addition, the time of the last menses or the presence of pregnancy, current medications, and allergies should be ascertained.

PHYSICAL EXAMINATION   Symptoms and signs of pelvic injuries vary from local pain and tenderness, especially with walking, to pelvic instability and severe shock. On inspection, look for perineal and pelvic edema, ecchymoses, lacerations, and deformities. Look for hematomas above the inguinal ligament or over the scrotum (Destot sign). Roll the patient over, if appropriate, and examine the areas overlying the sacrum and coccyx. On palpation feel for irregularities, crepitance, or movement at the iliac crests, pubic rami, and ischial rami. The clinical examination in awake and alert trauma patients is very sensitive in diagnosing a pelvic fracture. Palpation of a bony prominence or large hematoma or tenderness along the fracture line is possible by rectal examination (Earle sign). Compress the pelvis lateral to medial through the iliac crests, anterior to posterior through the symphysis pubis, and anterior to posterior through the iliac crests. Compress the greater trochanters and determine the range of motion

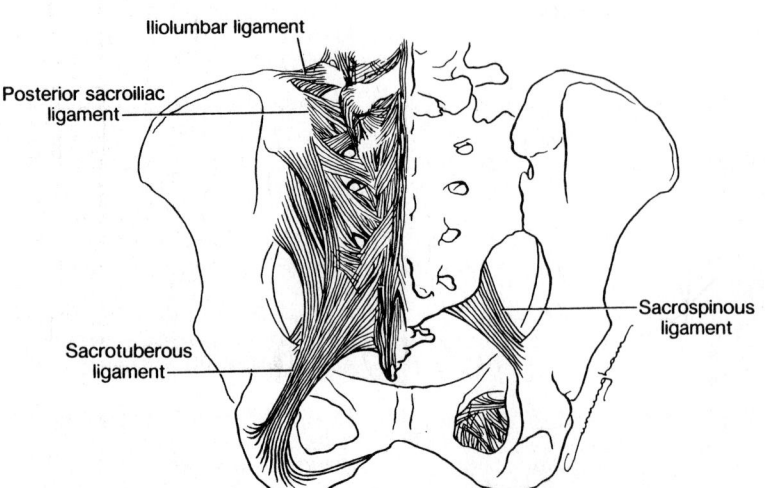

Iliolumbar ligament

Posterior sacroiliac ligament

Sacrotuberous ligament

Sacrospinous ligament

FIG. 273-1. The major posterior stabilizing structures of the pelvic ring, that is, the posterior tension band of the pelvis, include the iliolumbar ligament, the posterior sacroiliac ligaments, the sacrospinous ligaments, and the sacrotuberous ligaments. [Reproduced with permission from Tile M, Kellam J, Helfet DL (eds): Anatomy, in *Fractures of the Pelvis and Acetabulum.* Baltimore: Williams & Wilkins, 1984, p 11.]

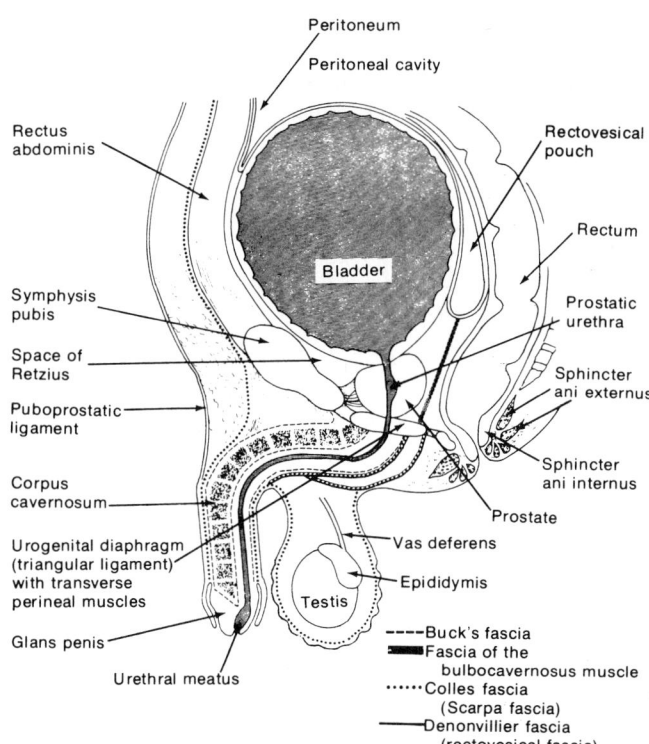

Peritoneum

Peritoneal cavity

Rectus abdominis

Rectovesical pouch

Rectum

Bladder

Symphysis pubis

Prostatic urethra

Space of Retzius

Sphincter ani externus

Puboprostatic ligament

Sphincter ani internus

Corpus cavernosum

Prostate

Vas deferens

Urogenital diaphragm (triangular ligament) with transverse perineal muscles

Epididymis

Testis

Glans penis

Urethral meatus

----Buck's fascia
Fascia of the bulbocavernosus muscle
······Colles fascia (Scarpa fascia)
Denonvillier fascia (rectovesical fascia)

FIG. 273-2. Sagittal section of the male pelvis showing the relation of the full bladder. [Reproduced with permission from Kane WJ: Fractures of the pelvis, in Rockwood CA Jr, Green DP (eds): *Fractures.* Vol. 2. Philadelphia: Lippincott, 1975, pp 916, 917.]

of the hips.[1] On rectal examination, superior or posterior displacement of the prostate, or rectal injuries are indicative of intraperitoneal and urologic injury. Proctoscopic examination may be required to fully assess for the presence of rectal tears. Decrease in anal sphincter tone may suggest neurologic injury, and blood at the urethral meatus may suggest urologic injury. Pelvic examination should be carefully performed in women to detect the presence of blood or lacerations that suggest the possibility of open fracture. Carefully evaluate neurovascular function. If a pelvic fracture is found, assume intraabdominal, retroperitoneal, gynecologic, and urologic injuries until proven otherwise.

RADIOLOGIC EVALUATION Stabilization of the patient takes priority over obtaining x-ray films. Unnecessary movement may produce further injury or cause more blood loss. After stabilization, roentgenographic evaluation of the pelvis is a must in all unconscious patients who have sustained multiple injuries. Lower extremity long bone fractures, as well as pelvic symptoms or signs, are also indications for

roentgenograms. A standard anteroposterior (AP) view of the pelvis is indicated in the presence of multisystem blunt trauma or if pelvic fracture is suspected. If additional studies are needed, lateral views, AP views of either hemipelvis, internal and external oblique views of the hemipelvis, or inlet and outlet views of the pelvis may be done. An inlet view shows anterior-posterior displacement of ring fractures (Figures 273-3 and 273-4). An outlet view shows superior-inferior displacement. Oblique views of the hemipelvis are true AP and lateral views of the acetabulum. Tomography, computed tomography (CT) scans, and special studies may be needed to fully evaluate and manage patients, particularly for acetabular and sacral fractures. CT is superior to plain radiography in assessing the posterior pelvic arch and acetabulum and has the added advantage of being able to identify the presence or absence of ongoing pelvic hemorrhage.[2] Angiography or venography may be necessary to determine a source of bleeding. The patient's condition must dictate what is done and when.

Classification and Treatment of Pelvic Fractures

BREAK IN THE PELVIC RING Pelvic fractures include those that involve a break in the pelvic ring, fractures of a single bone without a break in the pelvic ring, and acetabular fractures. Pelvic fractures involving a break in the pelvic ring can be complex and therefore difficult to classify. These injuries range from low-energy stable fractures to high-energy unstable patterns. The most clinically useful classification, by Young, is presented in Table 273-1.[3] It differentiates fracture patterns based on mechanism of injury and direction of causative force. Incidence of complications (i.e., urogenital and vascular) is correlated with the fracture pattern, making identification of the type more clinically significant and useful.

Three main types of patterns have been identified. The first and most-common mechanism, lateral compression (LC) (Figures 273-5 through 273-9), accounts for close to half the injuries. Motor vehicle accidents in which a car is broadsided or a pedestrian struck from the side are examples. Anteroposterior compression (APC), or open book fractures (Figures 273-10, 273-11, and 273-12), is the second type, accounting for approximately 25 percent of injuries. Head-on motor vehicle accidents are the classic example. The least-common mechanism is vertical shear (VS) (Figure 273-13), which is typified by a fall or jump from a height, accounting for approximately 5 percent of fractures. A combination of other injury patterns make up the other 20 to 25 percent of injuries.

The different injury types may be suggested by history, but can also be differentiated radiographically. The alignment of pubic rami fractures is one such clue to the mechanism and direction of force. Horizontal fractures suggest lateral compression injury, whereas vertical ones point to an anteroposterior direction of force. If there is sacroiliac joint diastasis and an associated crush fracture of the sacrum, then the injury is a result of lateral compression. Central hip dislocations

FIG. 273-3. A. Anatomic appearance in the inlet projection. **B.** Radiologic appearance in the inlet projection. [Reproduced with permission from Tile M, Kellam J, Helfet DL (eds): Assessment, in *Fractures of the Pelvis and Acetabulum.* Baltimore: Williams & Wilkins, 1984, p 63.]

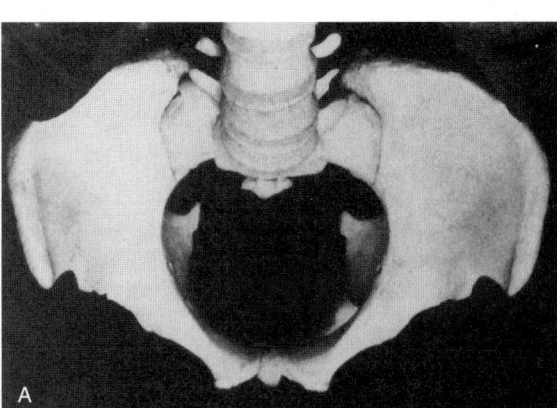

A

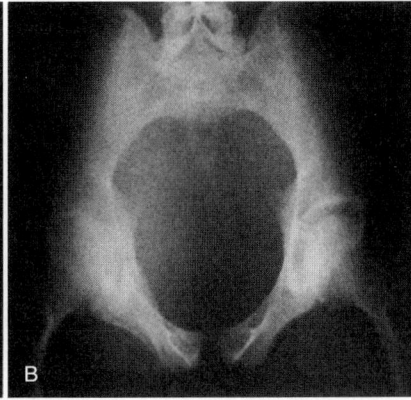

B

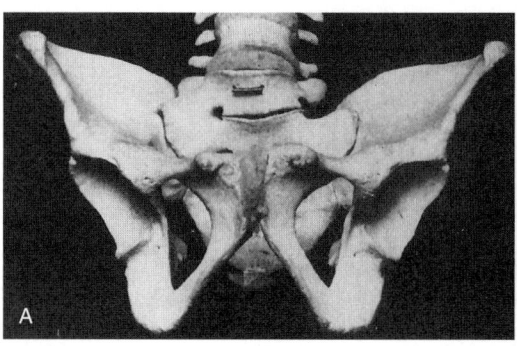
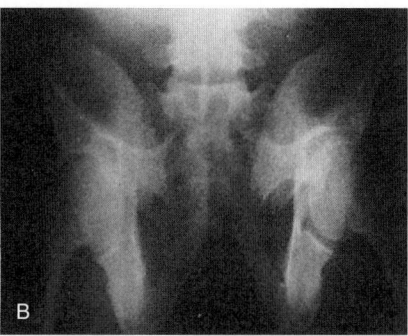

FIG. 273-4. A. Anatomic appearance in the outlet projection. **B.** Radiologic appearance in the outlet projection. [Reproduced with permission from Tile M, Kellam J, Helfet DL (eds): Assessment, in *Fractures of the Pelvis and Acetabulum.* Baltimore: Williams & Wilkins, 1984, p 64.]

suggest a lateral compression mechanism, whereas posterior dislocation suggests an anteroposterior force. With vertical shear patterns, fractures are vertical in alignment with vertical displacement of fragments. Based on the recognition of the fracture pattern, one can then predict the likelihood of severe hemorrhage or urogenital injury (Table 273-2).

Mortality usually is a result of associated injuries, although pelvic hemorrhage is also a contributor. Mortality rates approach 25 percent for severe APC and VS injuries, whereas it is approximately 13 percent with LC injuries. Mortality is reduced with early fracture fixation and patient mobilization.[4] In addition to mortality, the fracture type and severity can also predict the organ injury pattern and resuscitation needs. The treatment of LC-I and APC-I injuries consists of a few days of bedrest followed by protected weight-bearing. LC-II and III, APC II and III, and VS injuries typically require open reduction and internal fixation within 5 to 14 days of injury.[3] The long-term outcome/disability following open reduction and internal fixation of unstable pelvic fractures is generally fair, with 75 percent of patients having some mild disability and approximately 75 percent of those employed preinjury returning to their preinjury occupations.[5]

True open-book-type fractures with an intact posterior ring have the greatest potential benefit from anterior external fixator placement. Stabilization decreases the volume of the pelvis with resultant tam-

ponade of hemorrhage.[6] The tamponade effect is less if the posterior arch of the pelvis has been disrupted. Anterior stabilization should be considered in hemodynamically unstable patients with unstable pelvic fractures.[7,8]

AVULSION AND SINGLE BONE FRACTURES For fractures of the anterior superior iliac spine, anterior inferior iliac spine, ischial tuberosity, pubic ramus, body of the ischium, iliac wing, sacrum, or coccyx, refer to Figures 273-14 and 273-15 and Table 273-3.

ACETABULAR FRACTURES Acetabular fractures are usually secondary to automobile accidents. The fracture force is either transmitted laterally through the hip or through the femur as with a knee-versus-dashboard mechanism. Acetabular fractures are seen commonly with other injuries including femur, hip fractures and dislocations, and knee injuries. The roentgenographic anatomy of acetabular fractures is shown in Figure 273-16. There are five simple types of fractures as classified by Judet-Letournel, and nearly all are associated with hip dislocations; posterior wall, posterior column, anterior wall, anterior column, and transverse[9] (see Figure 273-17 and Table 273-4). In addition, combinations of any of these fractures can occur and are classified as complex acetabular fractures. If an acetabular fracture is suspected, it can best be evaluated with an anteroposterior film, a 45-degree iliac oblique, and a 45-degree obturator oblique view; together known as *Judet views.*

Posterior Wall Fracture The mechanism of injury in a posterior fracture is direct trauma to a flexed knee and hip. Anteroposterior and lateral radiologic views easily demonstrate the posterior acetabular fracture with the posterior hip dislocation. The fracture only involves the posterior border of the acetabulum.

Posterior Column Fracture In this fracture, the posterior column of the acetabulum is completely detached. The fracture originates at the

TABLE 273-1 Injury Classification Keys According to the Young System

Category	Distinguishing Characteristics
LC	Transverse fracture of pubic rami, ipsilateral or contralateral to posterior injury I—Sacral compression on side of impact II—Crescent (iliac wing) fracture on side of impact III—LC-1 or LC-II injury on side of impact; contralateral open-book (APC) injury
APC	Symphyseal diastasis and/or longitudinal rami fractures I—*Slight* widening of pubic symphysis and/or anterior SI joint; stretched but intact anterior SI, sacrotuberous, and sacrospinous ligaments; intact posterior SI ligaments II—Widened anterior SI joint; disrupted anterior SI, sacrotuberous, and sacrospinous ligaments; intact posterior SI ligaments III—Complete SI joint disruption with lateral displacement; disrupted anterior SI, sacrotuberous, and sacrospinous ligaments; disrupted posterior SI ligaments
VS	Symphyseal diastasis or vertical displacement anteriorly and posteriorly, usually through SI joint, occasionally through the iliac wing and/or sacrum
CM	Combination of other injury patterns, LC/VS being the most common

Abbreviations: APC = anteroposterior compression; CM = combination; LC = lateral compression; SI = sacroiliac; VS = vertical shear.

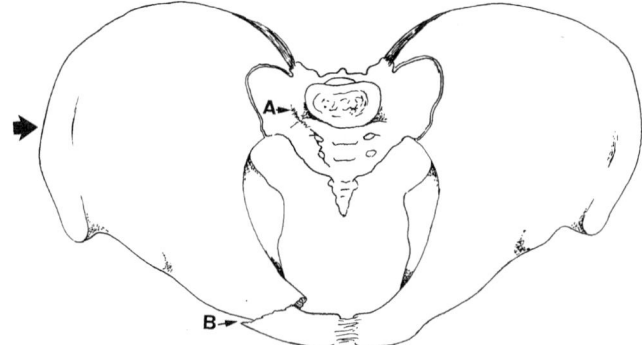

FIG. 273-5. Type I lateral compression fracture: The lateral force is applied posteriorly *(arrow).* This causes a crush effect on the sacroiliac joint, which may be visible radiographically as a sacral fracture *(A).* The characteristic fracture pattern of the pubic rami will be seen *(B).* No ligamentous injury is seen.

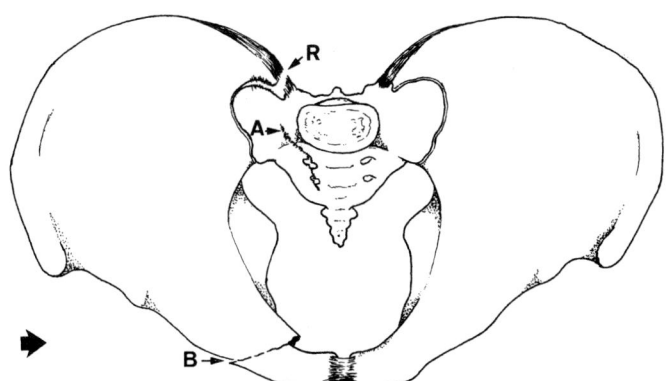

FIG. 273-6. Type II lateral compression fracture: The force is applied anteriorly *(arrow)*, causing the typical anterior public rami fractures *(B)*. In this case, however, rotation of the pelvis around the anterior sacral margin may occur, causing rupture of the posterior sacroiliac ligaments *(R)*. A crush fracture of the sacrum may also be seen *(A)*.

greater sciatic notch, traverses through the weight-bearing portion of the acetabulum, and exits through the obturator foramen. On x-ray the AP view shows medial displacement of the femoral head and sciatic buttress. The ilioischial line is also clearly disrupted. The oblique view is best to identify this fracture. Complications are sciatic nerve injury, which may occur in up to 40 percent of this fracture type, and femoral fractures. CT scan is an invaluable tool for evaluating this fracture and determining if operative or nonoperative treatment is required.

Anterior Wall Fracture   This fracture originates at the anterior inferior iliac spine, passes inferiorly through the junction of the articular dome and the superior ramus. It results from a lateral force applied to the greater trochanter with the hip externally rotated. On x-ray the iliopectineal line is disrupted and involvement of the weight-bearing dome can be seen. The most common complication is sciatic nerve injury.

Anterior Column Fracture   This fracture extends from the middle of the pubic ramus through to any point exiting the anterior segment of the iliac crest. The iliac oblique view reveals disruption of the iliopectineal line and the weight-bearing dome of the acetabulum. CT scan can be useful in evaluating this fracture.

Transverse Fracture   This fracture extends transversely from the anterior to the posterior column. It may or may not include the weight-bearing portion of the dome. The ischial ring remains intact in this fracture. The mechanism is force lateral to medial over the greater trochanter, or force posterior to anterior on the posterior pelvis with

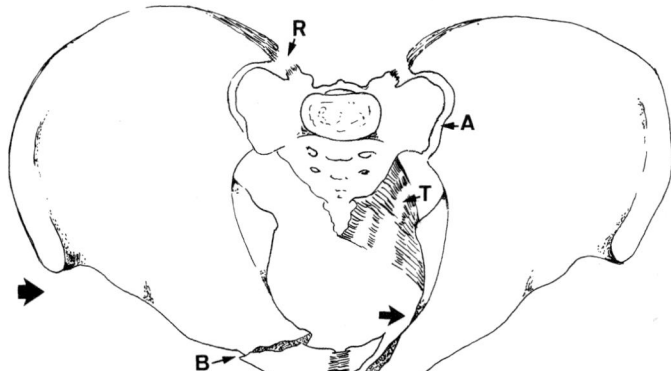

FIG. 273-8. Type III lateral compression fracture: The force is applied laterally *(arrow)*, causing internal rotation of the anterior hemipelvis. Continuing through to the contralateral hemipelvis *(arrow)*, the force causes it to rotate externally. The result is a pattern of lateral compression on the ipsilateral side, with apparent anteroposterior compression on the contralateral side. *(A)* This results in rupture of the posterior sacroiliac ligaments on the ipsilateral side *(R)* and sacrospinous/sacrotuberous complex *(T)* and anterior ligaments on the contralateral side. *(B)* Typical public rami fractures are to be expected.

the hip flexed. An AP x-ray film clearly demonstrates the fracture with a central hip dislocation.

Early orthopedic consultation and hospital admission is indicated for patients with acetabular fractures. Nondisplaced fractures may be treated with bedrest and analgesics. Early reduction and internal fixation is indicated for displaced fractures. Significant long-term disability is associated with acetabular fractures.

Complications of Pelvic Fractures

Acute complications of associated injuries include hemorrhage, urogynecologic injury, rectal injury, ruptured diaphragm, and nerve root injury.

HEMORRHAGE   Hemorrhage is a common cause of death in patients with pelvic injuries. Retroperitoneal bleeding is an inevitable complication, and up to 4 L of blood can be accommodated in this space until vascular pressure is overcome and tamponade occurs. It is thought that most pelvic bleeding is from the fractures and low-pressure sacral venous plexus. Both small and large vessels, especially the superior gluteal and internal pudendal branches of the internal iliac artery, can also be disrupted, with hemorrhage dissecting from the back to the buttocks.

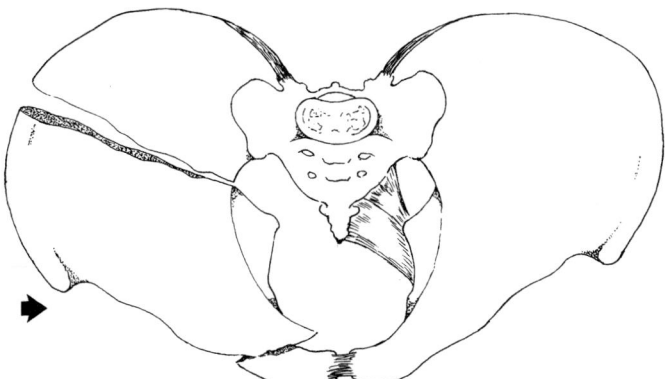

FIG. 273-7. Alternatively (compared to Figure 273-6), a fracture of the iliac wing may occur, which dissipates the rotational forces and thus leaves the posterior ligaments intact.

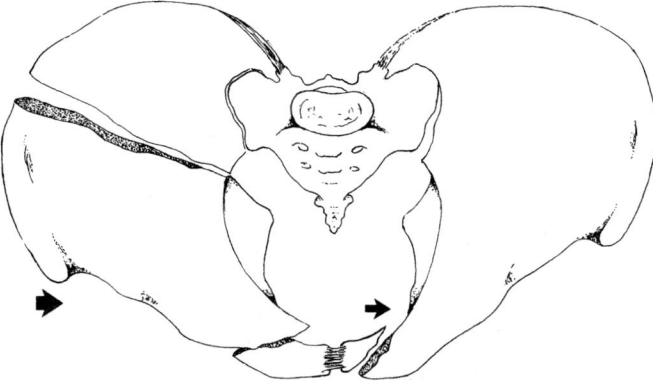

FIG. 273-9. Alternatively (compared to Figure 273-8), as in type II B fractures (Figure 273-7), there may be an iliac wing fracture sparing the posterior sacroiliac joint on the ipsilateral side.

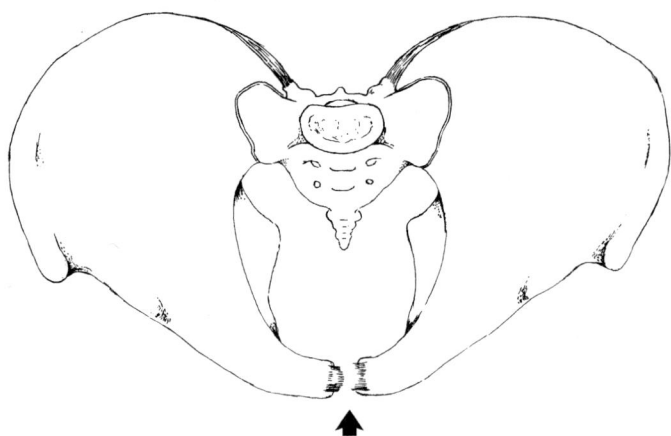

FIG. 273-10. Type I anteroposterior compression fracture: The force is delivered in an anteroposterior direction *(large arrow)*, tending to "open" the pelvis. This gives rise to mild splaying of the symphysis, due to rupture of the anterior sacroiliac ligaments.

General resuscitative measures include massive crystalloid, colloid, and blood replacement. In one series of high-energy pelvic fractures, patients on average required approximately 6 units of blood transfused.[10] The average transfusion requirement for APC injuries was approximately 15 units, VS injuries averaged 9 units, and LC injuries average approximately 3.5 units. Aggressive resuscitation along with treatment of extrapelvic injuries and early or delayed open reduction and internal fixation of the fractures may reduce mortality.[11]

The use of the antishock garment is controversial. It may be helpful in controlling bleeding sites by immobilizing fractures and compressing the pelvis. Disadvantages include decreased visibility and access to the abdomen and lower extremities, and the risk of compartment syndrome with prolonged application. This garment is generally only recommended for pelvic stabilization in the prehospital and ED setting. Reduction and stabilization of the unstable pelvis is reported to be an effective means of controlling hemorrhage.[3] Advanced trauma life support (ATLS) now includes a protocol for pelvic ring fractures that advises use of a bedsheet for pelvic support and stabilization. Reduction may be accomplished in the prehospital setting and the emergency department with external circumferential pressure to stabilize lateral compression, and anterior-posterior compression

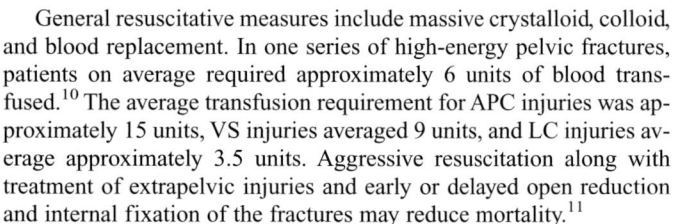

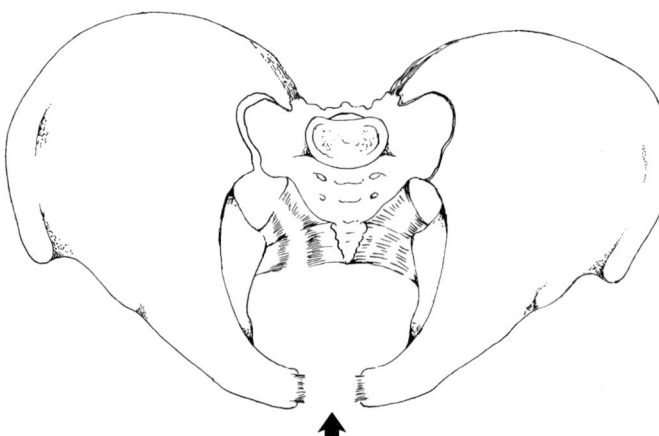

FIG. 273-11. Type II anteroposterior compression fracture: The anteroposterior force vector *(large arrow)* has caused further "opening" of the anterior pelvis, with additional rupture of the anterior sacroiliac, sacrotuberous, and sacrospinous ligaments.

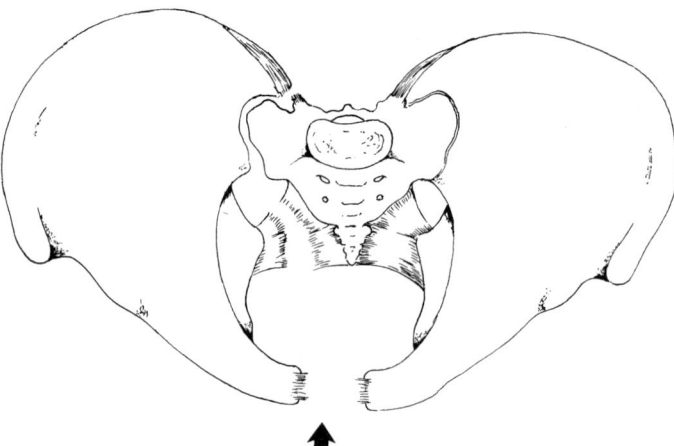

FIG. 273-12. Type III anteroposterior compression fracture: There is total disruption of the sacroiliac joint because of wide "opening" of the pelvis. All supporting ligament groups, including the posterior sacroiliac ligaments, may be disrupted.

for open-book type pelvic fractures. One proposed mechanism suggests that reduction of pelvic volume by the circumferential pressure method decreases the pelvic space for potential bleeding. Another hypothesis is that apposition of the fracture surfaces may decrease bleeding from the fracture itself.[12] Early orthopedic consultation should be considered for placement of external fixator device to help control hemorrhage in patients with persistent hemodynamic instability.

If the patient is exsanguinating, angiography can be done and small arterial bleeding sites controlled by transarterial embolization. Most authorities agree that aggressive fluid and blood replacement is the best initial therapy along with correction of hypothermia and coagulopathy. Placement of an external fixator and laparotomy should also be considered prior to angiography. Overall only about 2 percent of patients with pelvic fracture require embolization and efficacy approaches 100 percent when used.[13] Younger age, shorter time from injury to embolization, and hemodynamic stability are associated with improved survival.

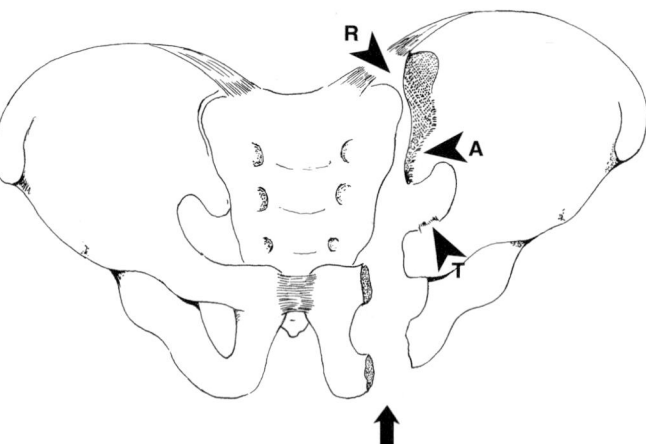

FIG. 273-13. Vertical shear vector: The injury force vector is delivered in a vertical plane *(large arrow)*, causing disruption along this line. Fractures of the pubic rami are usually seen anteriorly, while fractures of the sacrum, sacroiliac joint, or iliac wing are usually seen posteriorly. The fractures are vertical and are associated with vertical displacement of fragments. Ligamentous injury to the posterior *(R)* and anterior *(A)* sacroiliac ligaments may be seen, as well to sacrospinous/sacrotuberous *(T)*, and (possibly) symphysis ligaments.

TABLE 273-2   Local Associated Injuries

	% Occurrence		
	Severe Hemorrhage	Bladder Rupture	Urethral Injury
Lateral compression fractures			
Type I	0.5	4.0	2.0
Type II	36.0	7.0	0.0
Type III	60.0	20.0	20.0
Anteroposterior compression fractures			
Type I	1.0	8.0	12.0
Type II	28.0	11.0	23.0
Type III	53.0	14.0	36.0
Vertical shear fractures	75.0	15.0	25.0
Mixed patterns	58.0	16.0	21.0

Source: Reproduced with permission from Young JWR, Burgess AR: *Radiologic Management of Pelvic Ring Fractures: Systematic Radiologic Diagnosis.* Baltimore: Urban & Schwarzenberg, 1987.

UROGYNECOLOGIC INJURY   Urinary tract injuries are discussed in Chap. 262. Gynecologic injuries are uncommonly associated with pelvic trauma. Vaginal laceration is the most common injury seen with anterior pelvic fractures. A bimanual pelvic examination should be performed on all women with pelvic fractures. If blood is found in a woman of childbearing age, a speculum examination is needed to distinguish menses from laceration. Treatment is irrigation, debridement, and wound repair in the operating room and antibiotic therapy.

A high fetal death rate is associated with pelvic trauma in pregnancy if the mother is in shock; if there is placental, uterine, or direct fetal injury; or if the mother dies. Immediate caesarean section must be considered (see Chap. 254).

RECTAL INJURIES   Rectal injuries are uncommon and are usually associated with urinary injuries and ischial fractures. Diagnosis is by rectal examination or by proctoscopy, during which gross blood is found in the rectum. Treatment includes a diverting colostomy with washout of the distal colon and presacral space drainage. Antibiotics should be given as soon as the injury is discovered.

RUPTURED DIAPHRAGM   Ruptured diaphragm associated with fracture of the pelvis may be more common than previously thought. It may be associated with rib injuries. Suspect the diagnosis with physical findings such as displacement of the heart toward the right, absent breath sounds, or presence of bowel sounds in the chest. Confirmation is by x-ray and CT scan. Diagnosis is difficult if the defect is small.

NERVE ROOT INJURY   Nerve root or peripheral nerve injuries can occur because of traction, pressure from hemorrhage, callus or fibrous tissue, and impingement-laceration by bone fragments. The onset of symptoms and signs may be delayed, but deficits usually follow a nerve root pattern. Lumbar nerve root injuries are associated with SI joint dislocation or fracture. Sacral root injuries are associated with sacral fractures, especially fractures of S1 and S2.

TRAUMA TO THE HIP AND FEMUR

Anatomy

The hip is a ball-and-socket joint made up of the acetabulum and the femur. The hip includes the acetabulum and the proximal femur 2 to 3 inches below the lesser trochanter. The functions of the hip are

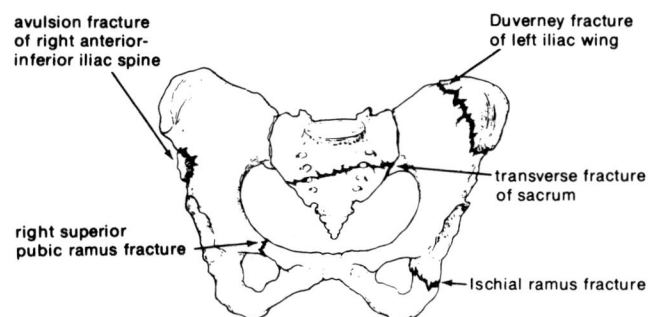

Type I: Fracture of individual bones without break in pelvic ring. Examples shown above.

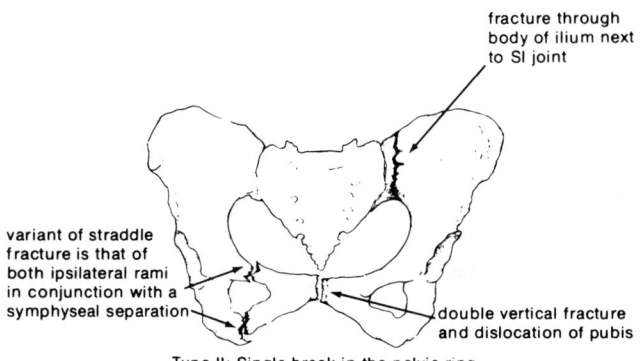

Type II: Single break in the pelvic ring. See examples above.

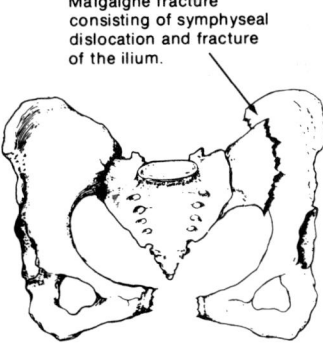

Type III: Double break in pelvic ring.

FIG. 273-14. Pelvic fractures (type I, II, and III) according to classification by Key JA, Conwell HE: *The Management of Fractures, Dislocations, and Sprains,* 4th ed. St. Louis, Mosby, 1946, p 857, as adapted by Kane WJ: Fractures of the pelvis, in Rockwood CA Jr, Green DP (eds): *Fractures in Adults,* 4th ed. Vol. 2. Philadelphia, Lippincott, 1996, p 1119.

weight-bearing and movement. The fibrous capsule that surrounds the joint on all sides is exceedingly strong. It attaches around the acetabulum proximally and runs to the intertrochanteric line distally on the anterior surface. Posteriorly, it falls short of the intertrochanteric crest and inserts on the neck of the femur. It is weakest posteriorly.

The blood supply of the femoral head is derived from nutrient branches of the obturator, medial femoral circumflex, lateral femoral circumflex, and superior and inferior gluteal arteries. These course

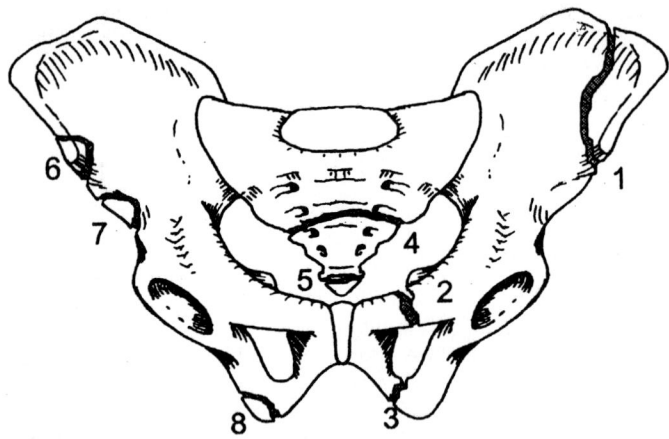

FIG. 273-15. Avulsion fractures of the pelvis. 1. Iliac wing fracture (Duverney fracture). 2. Superior pubic ramus fracture. 3. Inferior pubic ramus fracture. 4. Transverse sacral fracture. 5. Coccyx fracture. 6. Anterior superior iliac spine avulsion. 7. Anterior inferior iliac spine avulsion. 8. Ischial tuberosity avulsion.

beneath the reflection of the capsule on the neck of the femur and also along the ligamentum teres. The capsular vessels are much more important than those of the ligamentum teres.

Clinical Evaluation

PHYSICAL EXAMINATION   The examination of the hip begins with a detailed history and complete examination of the patient. The pelvis and hip are then carefully evaluated. The unclothed, erect patient is inspected for a list, injuries, scars, or asymmetry of the muscles. Gait should be tested, if possible.

If the patient is a trauma victim, after primary survey and initial stabilization observe the position of the extremities, looking for deformities, shortening, rotation, lacerations, or bruises, and test for stability and range of motion. On palpation, feel for irregularities in movement at the iliac crest, pubic rami, and ischial rami. Compress the pelvis lateral to medial through the iliac crest; anterior to posterior through the symphysis pubis; and anterior to posterior through the iliac crest, seeking pain and tenderness. Also, compress the greater trochanters of the hips.

If no significant abnormalities are found, range of motion of the hips should then be studied. If rotation of the hip with the leg in extension is painful all other maneuvers should be done cautiously. If a hip or pelvic fracture or dislocation is identified in a trauma victim, assume that intra-abdominal, retroperitoneal, and urologic injuries have occurred as well, until proven otherwise. Always perform a detailed neurovascular examination and a rectal examination, looking for displacement of the prostate in male patients. Associated femoral shaft fractures should be ruled out.

RADIOLOGIC EVALUATION   Roentgenographic evaluation of the pelvis and hips is a must in all unconscious patients who have sustained multiple injuries. The threshold for obtaining radiographs in demented elderly patients who have sustained minor falls should also be relatively low because those patients may be particularly difficult to evaluate. Lower-extremity long bone fractures, as well as pelvic symptoms or signs, are also indications for these x-ray examinations. The x-ray evaluation should include a standard AP and a lateral view of the pelvis. If further studies are needed, AP views of either hemipelvis, in-

TABLE 273-3   Avulsion and Single Bone Fractures

Fracture	Description/ Mechanism of Injury	Clinical Findings/ Associated Injuries	Treatment	Disposition
Iliac wing (Duverney) fracture	Direct trauma, usually lateral to medial	Swelling, tenderness over iliac wing; abdominal pain; ileus; acetabular fractures; serious injury infrequent	Analgesics, strapping	Discharge with PCP or orthopedic follow-up in 1–2 weeks; admit for open fracture or concerning abdominal examination
Single ramus of pubis or ischium	Fall or direct trauma in elderly; exercise-induced stress fracture in young or in pregnant women	Local pain and tenderness; inability to ambulate; rectal injury	Analgesics, crutches	Discharge with PCP or orthopedic follow-up in 1–2 weeks
Ischium body	Violent, external trauma or from fall in sitting position; least-common fracture	Local pain and tenderness; pain with hamstring movement; rectal injury	Bedrest, analgesics, donut-ring cushion, crutches	Discharge with PCP or orthopedic follow-up in 1–2 weeks
Sacral fracture	Transverse fractures from direct AP trauma; upper transverse fractures from fall in flexed position	Pain on rectal examination; sacral root injury with upper transverse fractures	Bedrest, analgesics	Discharge with orthopedic follow-up 1–2 weeks; early consultation and surgery for neurologic disability
Coccyx fracture	Fall in sitting position; more common in women	Pain, tenderness over sacral region; pain on compression during rectal examination	Bedrest, sitz baths, donut-ring cushion	PCP or orthopedic follow-up in 2–3 weeks; surgical excision of fracture fragment if chronic pain
Anterior superior iliac spine	Forceful sartorius muscle contraction (e.g., adolescent sprinters)	Pain with hip flexion and abduction	NSAIDs, rest abducted and flexed 3–4 weeks, crutches	Discharge with PCP follow-up in 1–2 weeks
Anterior inferior iliac spine	Forceful rectus femoris muscle contraction (e.g., adolescent soccer players)	Pain in groin; pain with hip flexion	NSAIDs, rest in flexion 3–4 weeks	Discharge with PCP follow-up in 1–2 weeks
Ischial tuberosity	Forceful contraction of hamstrings	Pain with sitting or flexing the thigh	NSAIDs, rest, crutches	Discharge with PCP follow-up in 1–2 weeks

Abbreviations: AP = anteroposterior; NSAID = nonsteroidal anti-inflammatory drug; PCP = primary care physician.

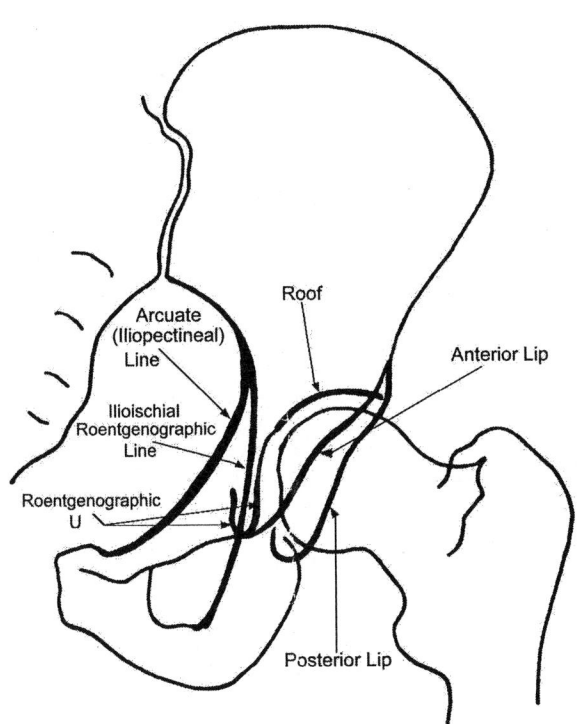

FIG. 273-16. Roentgenographic anatomy of type IV acetabular fractures. (Reproduced with permission from Judet R, Judet J, Letournel E: Fractures of the acetabulum: Classification and surgical approaches for open reduction. *J Bone Joint Surg* 46A:1616, 1964.)

ternal and external oblique views of the hemipelvis as described by Judet and colleagues, or "inlet" and "tilt" views may be done. In certain instances, such views allow better identification and detail of the acetabulum and femoral head and neck. Always inspect not only the hip joint but also the femur and knee when evaluating hip disorders on x-ray films. Disorders to the knee and the femoral shaft often occur with hip injuries. Significant hip pain with weight-bearing following trauma and normal radiographs suggest the possibility of occult fracture, especially at the femoral neck or acetabulum.[14] The patient should be prescribed protected weight-bearing and the emergency

physician should communicate with the patient's primary care provider or orthopedist regarding close follow-up for possible CT or MR hip imaging to rule out occult fracture.[15,16] MR is reliable in detecting occult fractures within 24 h of injury.

Femoral nerve blocks can provide analgesia for hip dislocations, femoral neck fractures, and femoral shaft fractures. See Figure 37-14A and B for the technique.

Classification/Epidemiology of Hip Fractures

The estimated incidence of hip fractures in the United States is approximately 80 per 100,000 population.[17] The incidence increases with age and doubles for each decade past the age of 50 years. The incidence is approximately two to three times higher in women than in men, and fractures are more common in white than in nonwhite women.

The possibility of elder abuse should be considered in all elderly patients with falls and fractures.[18] See Chap. 300 for detailed discussion of elder abuse.

Hip fractures are classified as femoral head and neck (intracapsular) and trochanteric, intertrochanteric, and subtrochanteric (extracapsular) (Figures 273-18, 273-19 and Table 273-5). The prognosis for successful union and restoration of normal function varies considerably with the fracture.

In intracapsular fractures with displacement, the femoral neck vessels are compromised because of a tear or compression secondary to an intracapsular hemarthrosis. The blood supply to the femoral head originates from the medial and lateral femoral circumflex arteries. These arteries form an extracapsular ring that courses inside the capsule at its insertion to the proximal femur. Intracapsular fractures may disrupt blood flow but not the vascular structures. Vessels may kink because of fracture fragments or as a result of tension from the fracture. Urgent anatomic reduction of the fracture may restore flood flow. The blood supply through the ligamentum teres may not be sufficient to nourish the entire femoral head; consequently, avascular necrosis inevitably results (15 to 35 percent overall) unless some of the capsular vessels remain intact.[19] Basilar neck and intertrochanteric fractures below the capsule rarely sever important arteries. Morbidity and mortality associated with hip fractures is primarily a result of patient immobilization and the development of deep venous thrombosis and pulmonary embolus. Even with modern treatment modalities, mortality following hip fracture ranges from 15 to 35 percent within 1 year of

FIG. 273-17. The Judet-Letournel classification of simple acetabular fractures. 1. Posterior wall fracture. 2. Posterior column fracture. 3. Anterior wall fracture. 4. Anterior column fracture. 5. Transverse fracture.

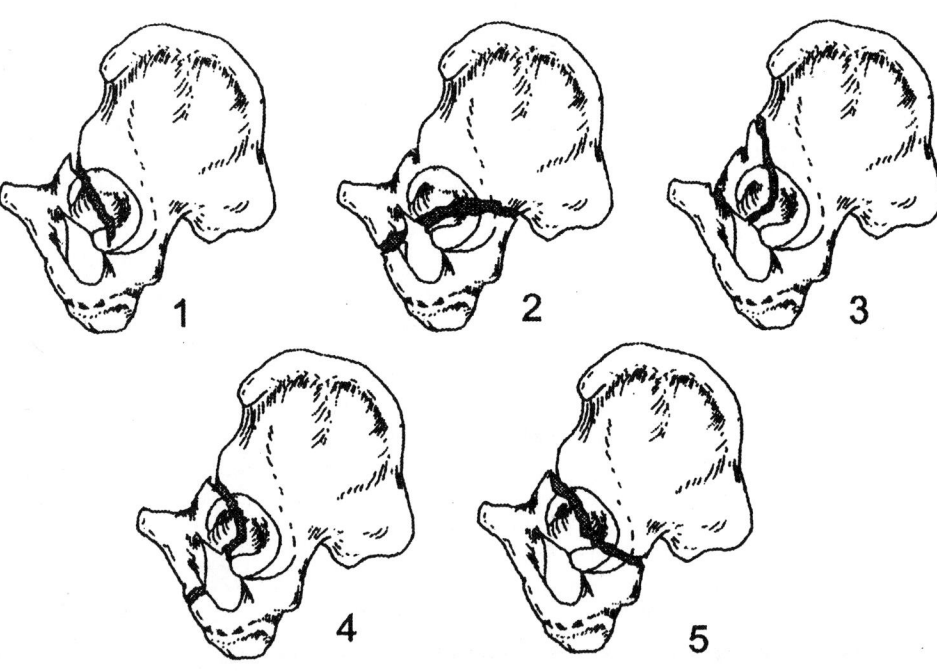

TABLE 273-4   Acetabular Fractures

Hip Fracture	Mechanism	Description	Associated Injuries	Treatment/Disposition
Posterior wall fracture	Direct trauma to flexed hip and knee	Acetabulum fracture	Sciatic nerve injury; femoral fractures	Bedrest, analgesics; early orthopedic consultation, hospital admission
Posterior column fracture	Posteriorly directed force to abducted, flexed leg	Fracture acetabulum through obturator foramen; ischial ring disrupted	Sciatic nerve injury (40%), weight-bearing disrupted	Same as above
Anterior wall fracture	Lateral force to the greater trochanter with hip externally rotated	Fracture extends anterior inferior iliac spine to superior ramus; ischial ring and iliopectineal line disrupted	Weight-bearing disrupted	Same as above
Anterior column fracture	Posterior force to knee with hip abducted and flexed	Fracture from pubic ramus through iliac crest; ischial ring and iliopectineal line disrupted	Weight-bearing disrupted	Same as above
Transverse fracture acetabulum	Force lateral to medial over greater trochanter	Fracture extends anterior to posterior through acetabulum; ischial ring intact	Sciatic nerve injury	Same as above

surgery and 25 to 50 percent of the survivors will not regain their ability to ambulate.[20] Factors predictive of increased mortality include male sex, increased age, dementia, institutionalization, poorly controlled systemic disease, and the development of postoperative complications. There is some evidence that early (<72 h) hip fracture fixation of low impact hip fractures in the elderly reduces morbidity and mortality.[21,22,23]

FEMORAL HEAD FRACTURES   Isolated femoral head fractures occur infrequently. They are usually associated with dislocations of the hip (see Table 273-5). Femoral head fractures occur in 10 to 16 percent of posterior hip dislocations and in 22 to 77 percent of anterior hip dislocations. Fracture types include depressions, flattening, and subchondral fractures of the femoral head. They are usually best seen on radiographs obtained after reduction of a hip dislocation. Shear fractures

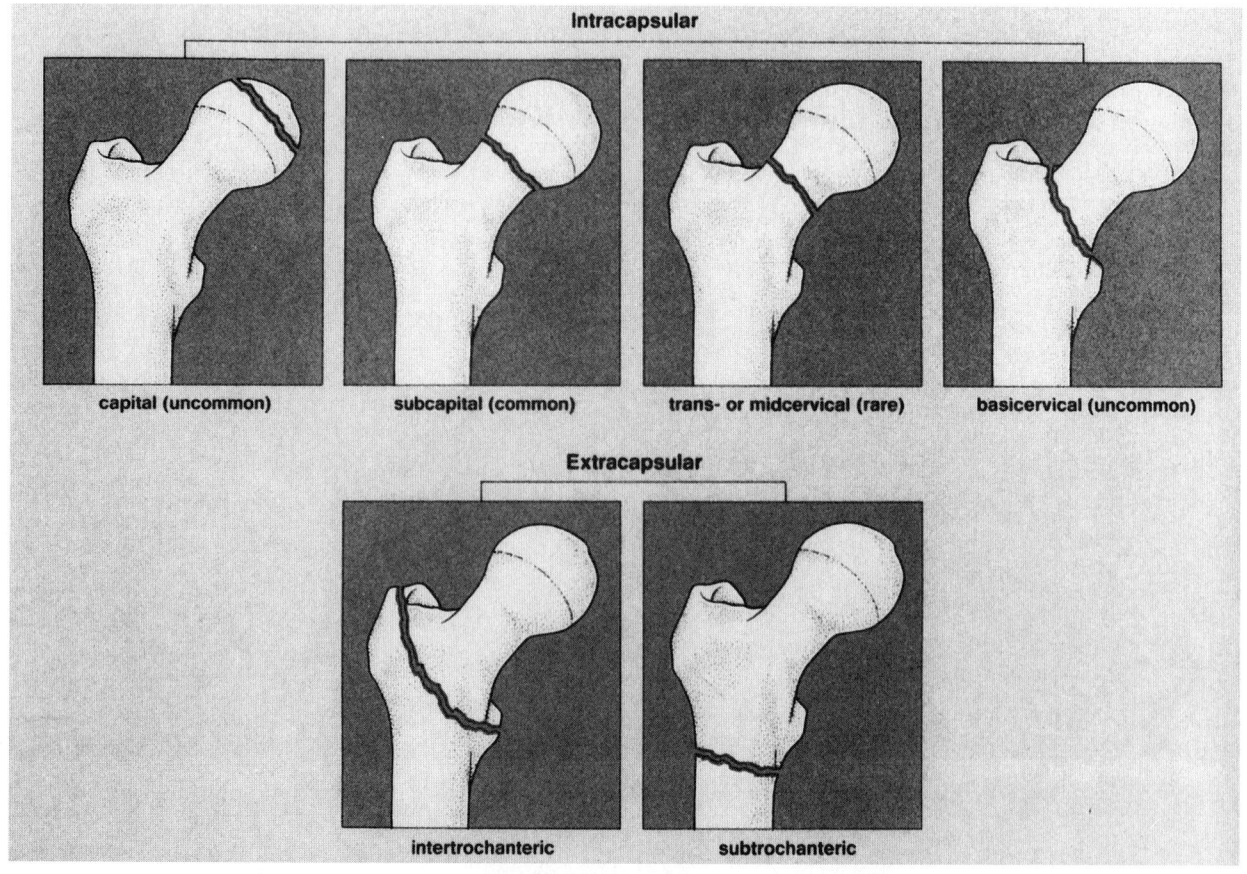

FIG. 273-18. Fractures of the proximal femur are traditionally classified as intracapsular and extracapsular. (Used with permission from Greenspan A: *Orthopedic Radiology.* Philadelphia: JB Lippincott, 1988, p 5.17.)

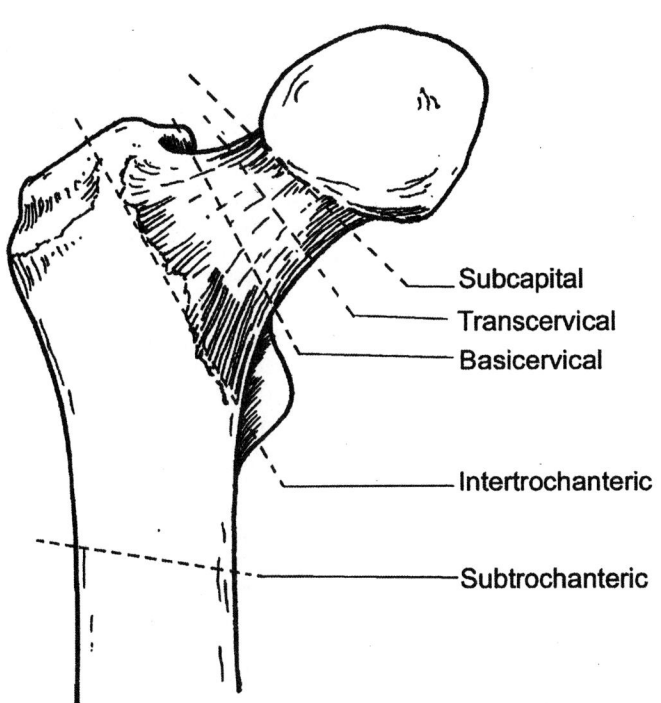

FIG. 273-19. Classification of proximal femur fractures.

of the superior aspect of the femoral head are associated with anterior dislocations, and shear fractures of the inferior femoral head are associated with posterior dislocations.

In most instances, the symptoms and signs are those of the associated dislocation rather than of the fracture itself. The standard AP and lateral x-ray views usually demonstrate the fragment adequately.

Orthopedic consultation should be obtained in the ED for these fractures. Treatment is to reduce the associated dislocation and then at-

tain anatomic reduction of the fracture fragment. Treatment should be limited to a single attempt at closed reduction. If this fails, then open reduction and internal fixation is the next treatment of choice.

Complications are associated with the high-energy trauma that produces the fracture-dislocation, that is, the more comminuted the fracture, the more severe the dislocation and the greater the severity of trauma to the patient. Life-threatening injuries must then be ruled out.

The prognosis is related to the severity of the initial trauma resulting in the dislocation. Poor prognostic indicators include delay between hip dislocation and reduction, repetitive unsuccessful relocation attempts, and associated injuries. Posttraumatic arthritis occurs in up to 50 percent of patients, avascular necrosis in two to 40 percent, and myositis ossificans can also occur.[24]

FEMORAL NECK FRACTURES Femoral neck fractures are commonly seen among older adults, most often because of osteoporosis, and occur more frequently in women than in men. These fractures are rare among the younger population. The cause of such fractures is usually minor trauma secondary to falls (90 percent) or torsion in the patient with osteoporosis or osteomalacia. In younger patients, the high kinetic energy sustained in the major trauma causes a fracture through normal bone with marked soft tissue disruption and comminution. These patients may have associated head, chest, abdominal or other serious concomitant injury. Femoral neck fractures are classified as subcapital, transcervical, and basicervical fractures (see Figure 273-19). Anatomically these fractures are intracapsular and the blood supply may be disrupted as discussed above.

The classification of femoral neck fractures is by fracture displacement. The higher the grade of fracture displacement implies a worse prognosis for healing and repair. The symptoms seen with femoral neck fractures range from complaints of mild pain in the groin or inner thigh in patients with an incomplete fracture, to moderate to severe pain in patients with displaced fractures. Patients who have sustained a fracture without displacement may walk with some limping rather than being completely unable to bear weight. Their only physi-

TABLE 273-5 Proximal Femur Fractures

Fracture	Description/ Mechanism of Injury	Clinical Findings/ Associated Injuries	ED Treatment	Disposition
Femoral head fractures	Superior aspect in anterior dislocations; inferior aspect in posterior dislocations	AVN from dislocation; multisystem injury from high-energy trauma	Analgesics; urgent reduction with anatomic reduction of fracture	ED orthopedic consultation; admission; possible ORIF for difficult reductions
Femoral neck fractures	Primarily from falls; older women with osteroporosis	AVN; nonunion; emboli; infection	Analgesics	ED orthopedic consultation, possibly for ORIF; displaced fractures require surgery; hospitalize all
Trochanteric fractures	Direct trauma; greater trochanter avulsion from forceful contraction of gluteus medius muscle	Pain with abduction; limp	Protective weight-bearing	Orthopedic follow-up 1–2 weeks; possible ORIF if displacement >1 cm
	Lesser trochanter avulsion caused by forceful contraction of iliopsoas muscles (in young gymnasts and dancers)	Pain with flexion, rotation	Bed rest; gradual weight-bearing; NSAIDs	Follow-up 1–2 weeks with PCP or orthopedics; possible ORIF if displacement >2 cm
Intertrochanteric fractures	Falls; primarily in elderly women	Pain, swelling of hip; externally rotated, shortened; AVN; nonunion; infection; thromboembolic disease	Buck traction; analgesics	ED orthopedic consultation for hospital admission; eventual ORIF
Subtrochanteric fractures	Falls, primarily in elderly; high-energy impact to femur in young patients	Severe hemorrhage into thigh; hypovolemic shock; compartment syndrome; fracture or dislocation of joint above or below	Hare or Sager splint; analgesics	ED orthopedic consultation for hospital admission; eventual ORIF

Abbreviations: AVN = avascular necrosis; NSAID = nonsteroidal anti-inflammatory drug; ORIF = open reduction and internal fixation; PCP = primary care physician.

cal findings are minor pain with movement and minimal muscle spasm limiting range of motion. In contrast, displaced fractures cause severe pain, inability to ambulate, limited range of motion, and no palpable movement of the extracapsular head. The patient lies with the extremity in slight external rotation, abduction, and shortening.

Radiographic evaluation is essential in any patient suspected of having a femoral neck fracture. Stress fractures, however, may not become evident on x-ray for days or weeks, so repeat films or bone scans in symptomatic patients are necessary. The standard AP view should have the patient maximally internally rotated to best demonstrate the femoral neck. The AP view should be inspected for a fracture line starting on the superior surface of the neck. These fracture lines routinely become complete within 10 to 14 days. Also, disruption of Shenton line (a smooth curvilinear line along the superior border of the obturator foramen and the medial aspect of the femoral metaphysis) may be appreciated on the AP view in some instances. If there is any concern that the patient has sustained a fracture that is not visible on the initial x-ray examination, the patient should be conservatively treated and x-ray films should be made again in 10 to 14 days; or the physician may order a CT or MRI, which demonstrates the fracture in most instances. In contrast, displaced fractures are obvious on the AP film, but a lateral view should also be done to ascertain the exact position. There is a 10 percent incidence of an ipsilateral femoral shaft fracture, of which 30 percent are missed on initial presentation.[25]

Orthopedic consultation should be obtained in the ED for these fractures. The orthopedic surgeon's goal of treatment for femoral neck fractures is anatomic reduction and stability. Treatment for nondisplaced or impacted fractures is somewhat controversial but usually involves a form of internal fixation. Conservative treatment is generally only considered if the patient is medically unfit for surgery or the fracture is several weeks old and the patient is walking without pain. Displaced fractures definitely require emergency surgery for fixation, especially in the young and active patient. Older patients who are active with good bone stock and reasonable physiologic age may also benefit from open reduction and internal fixation. The older individual with marked osteopenia and a high degree of fracture displacement or existing arthritis should be considered for a total hip arthroplasty.[26]

Skeletal traction is contraindicated with femoral neck fractures because it may further compromise femoral head blood flow.

The complications of femoral neck fractures are significant. They include infections, emboli, nonunion, and avascular necrosis, which is the most feared early complication. Avascular necrosis has an incidence of up to 15 percent in nondisplaced fractures, and rises to near 90 percent with untreated, completely displaced fractures.

TROCHANTERIC FRACTURES   Greater trochanteric fractures are usually caused by avulsions at the insertion of the gluteus medius. In the younger population (7 to 17 years of age), this is a true epiphyseal separation, in contrast to the adult population, in which this is caused by direct trauma. The patient presents with pain, especially with abduction and extension, and a limp. Also, there is tenderness to palpation over the greater trochanter.

Standard AP and lateral x-ray views reveal displacement in the superior-posterior area, or comminution. The treatment is generally conservative with protected weight-bearing recommended until the patient is asymptomatic. Outpatient orthopedic referral is indicated. Orthopedic consultation for possible surgical fixation may be considered for fracture displacement of greater than 1 cm.[27]

Lesser trochanteric fractures caused by an avulsion secondary to a forceful contraction of the iliopsoas are commonly seen in children and young athletic adults, particularly gymnasts and dancers. These patients present with pain during flexion and internal rotation maneuvers. In most instances, the treatment is bedrest and then gradual weight-bearing to regain full activity. Outpatient follow-up by primary care or orthopedics is advised. Full recovery generally occurs within 3 weeks.

If greater than 2-cm displacement is seen on the standard AP and lateral views, then screw fixation by the consulting orthopedic surgeon may be indicated.

INTERTROCHANTERIC FRACTURES   These fractures are defined as extracapsular fractures occurring in a line between the greater and lesser trochanters. Intertrochanteric fractures generally occur in the elderly and are more common in women, again due to the high incidence of osteoporosis. The mechanism of injury is usually a fall or occasionally an automobile accident. It is postulated that a rotational component along with the direct trauma is involved in some instances as well.

Symptoms and signs include pain, swelling of the hip, local ecchymosis, and pain with any hip movement or weight-bearing. Moreover, the extremity is markedly externally rotated and shortened, in contrast to the minimal deformities associated with femoral neck fractures. These fractures are classified as stable or unstable. Stable fractures are defined as ones in which the medial cortices of the neck and femoral fragments abut. X-ray evaluation should include AP and lateral views, with the AP view having as much internal rotation as possible to adequately visualize the neck.

Severe life-threatening injuries must be excluded. The consulting orthopedic physician can then admit the patient to the hospital and perform surgical fixation to attain a stable reduction as soon as possible, although this is not an emergency. Buck traction may temporarily help reduce pain.

The complications and prognosis are related to other associated injuries and prior disease. The overall mortality is approximately 10 to 30 percent. Infection can be a major problem, with an incidence of up to 17 percent.[28] Thromboembolic disease is especially a problem if postoperative mobilization does not occur quickly. Avascular necrosis is rare in these patients, and nonunion is also uncommon. Morbidity is a result of the patient's inability to return to prefracture activity.

SUBTROCHANTERIC FRACTURES   Subtrochanteric fractures may be seen in two different populations. They usually occur secondary to falling in the 40- to 60-year-old patient with osteoporotic or weakened bone. The second population is young persons who have suffered major trauma with significant kinetic energies directed into the femur. These fractures may be an extension of an intertrochanteric or other isolated fracture and are usually classified as stable or unstable, with stable defined as bony contact of the medial and posterior femoral cortices.

The symptoms and signs are similar to those of trochanteric or femoral fractures, with local pain, deformity, swelling, crepitance, and so forth. These patients can lose a large amount of blood into the thigh area and may present in hypovolemic shock. Because this injury is a result of significant trauma, other, more life-threatening injuries must be excluded prior to treatment of this specific fracture.

Standard AP and lateral x-ray views of the hip are necessary to properly assess the fracture. Moreover, x-ray studies of the pelvis, femur, and knee are indicated to rule out associated fractures.

Treatment consists of immobilization with a traction apparatus. Hare (Dyna-Med, Carlsbad, CA) or Sager (Minto Research & Development, Redding, CA) splints (Figures 273-20 and 273-21) may be

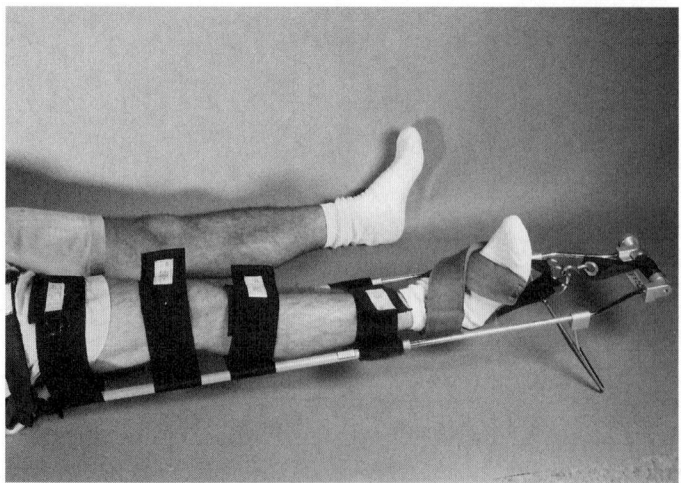

FIG. 273-20. Hare traction splint.

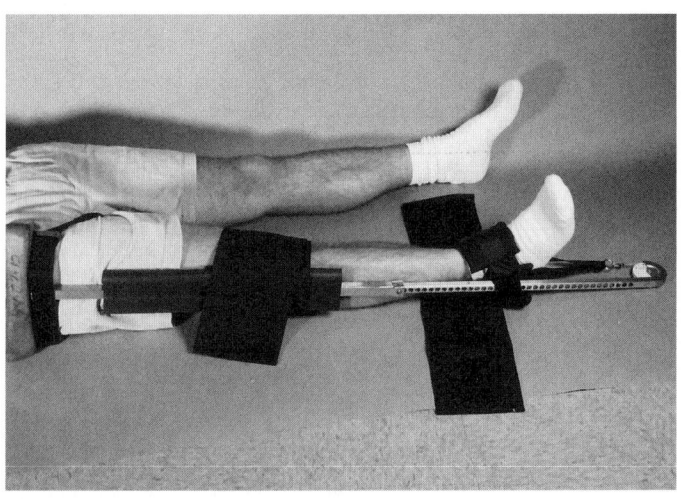

FIG. 273-21. Sager traction splint.

employed in the prehospital setting. Proper evaluation of the entire patient to rule out associated severe injuries should be conducted. After the patient has stabilized and secondary evaluation has occurred, orthopedics should be consulted. Open reduction and internal fixation is generally indicated for fracture management.[29]

The complications are similar to those of intertrochanteric fractures, except that there is a higher incidence of nonunion. Malunion and delayed union occur as well in this population. Prognosis is better for proximal fractures that are not comminuted.

Hip Dislocations

Hip dislocations can be classified as anterior, posterior, and central. Acetabular fracture with central hip dislocation is discussed under acetabular fractures.

ANTERIOR DISLOCATIONS   Approximately 10 percent of hip dislocations are anterior (Figure 273-22A and B), and the majority are secondary to automobile accidents, but they may also result from a fall, or a blow to the back while squatting. In anterior dislocations, the femoral

FIG. 273-22. A. Anterior superior dislocation of the hip. **B.** Inferior dislocations (obturator, thyroid, or perineal). **C.** Clinical appearance of a superior-type anterior dislocation of the hip. **D.** Clinical appearance of an inferior-type dislocation of the hip. [Reproduced with permission from Rockwood CA Jr, Green DP, Bucholz RW (eds): *Fractures in Adults,* 4th ed. Vol. 2. Philadelphia: JB Lippincott, 1996, pp 1757, 1759, 1767, 1768.]

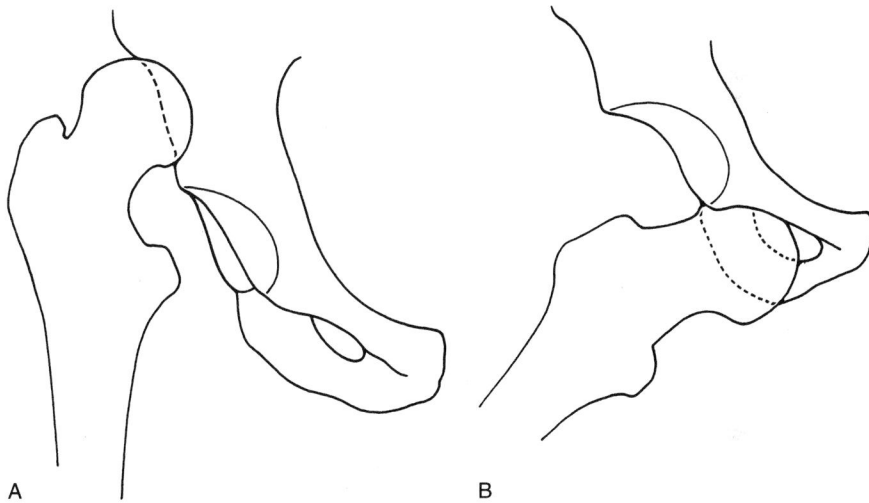

A

B

C

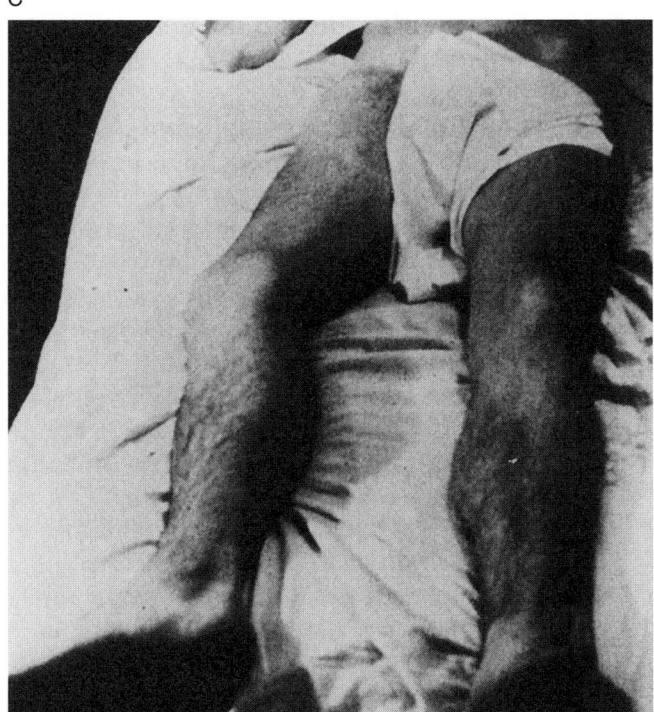

D

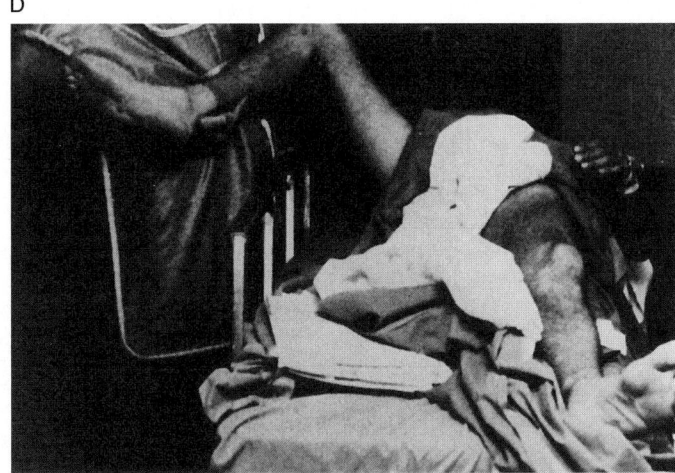

head rests anterior to the coronal plane of the acetabulum. Anterior dislocations can be superior or inferior (obturator, thyroid, perineal) depending on the degree of hip flexion present at the time of injury. If the hip is abducted, externally rotated, and flexed at the time of injury, inferior dislocation occurs. If the hip is abducted, externally rotated, and extended, superior dislocation occurs. The mechanism of injury is forced abduction that causes the femoral head to be levered out through an anterior capsular tear. The affected extremity is in abduction and external rotation. However, the clinical appearance of superior versus inferior dislocations is dramatically different (Figures 273-22C and D). Neurovascular compromise is an unusual, but possible complication.

An AP film of the pelvis easily demonstrates the femoral head to be anterior to the acetabulum. A lateral view illustrates the anterior dislocation more clearly, although it may be difficult to obtain because of the patient's pain.

Hip dislocations are true orthopedic emergencies. Treatment for the dislocation is early closed reduction, usually under conscious sedation in the emergency department. Strong, in-line traction is done with simultaneous flexion and internal rotation (see Figure 273-23). Finally, the hip is abducted once the head clears the rim of the acetabulum. The dislocation should be reduced quickly, within a few hours, because the longer the delay in reduction, the higher the incidence of avascular necrosis. Attempts at reduction in the emergency department should be limited. Difficulties with reduction may be due to occult fracture, or incarcerated tendon or capsule. Early decision for closed reduction under general anesthesia or open reduction should be made with in conjunction with your orthopedic consultant. Postreduction radiographs should be specifically examined for acetabular or femoral head fractures and the possibility of small fragments in the joint not appreciated on the initial films.

POSTERIOR DISLOCATIONS Posterior dislocations (Figure 273-24A) constitute 80 to 90 percent of hip dislocations.[24] They are caused by force applied to a flexed knee, directed posteriorly. Acetabular fractures may result as well. On examination, the extremity is found to be shortened, internally rotated, and adducted (Figure 273-24B). Concomitant life-threatening injuries must be ruled out.

Anteroposterior and lateral x-ray films of the pelvis and hip will reveal the dislocation, but further assessment of the acetabulum and femur must be done to rule out fractures. The oblique views of Judet and colleagues will reveal an acetabular fracture. Also, inferior femoral head fracture will be seen on the AP or oblique view. Hip dislocations are difficult to recognize if there is an associated femoral shaft fracture, so roentgenograms of the pelvis and hips should be routinely obtained in such cases.

The treatment of posterior dislocation without fracture is closed reduction under conscious sedation or general anesthesia, as quickly as possible and always within 6 h. In-line traction, gentle flexion to 90 degrees, and then gentle internal-to-external rotation is done (Allis maneuver, see Figure 273-23). The Stimson maneuver (Figure 273-25) may prove useful in certain situations.

Complications include sciatic nerve injury in approximately 10 percent of the patients and avascular necrosis that increases in direct proportion to the delay in adequate reduction.

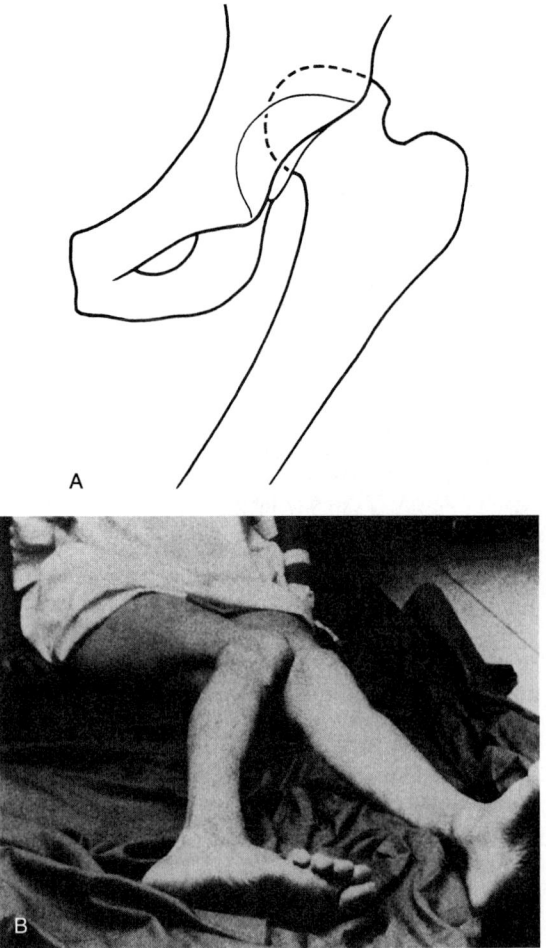

FIG. 273-24. A. Posterior dislocation of the hip. **B.** The clinical appearance of a posterior dislocation of the right hip. [Reproduced with permission from Rockwood CA Jr, Green DP, Bucholz RW (eds): *Fractures in Adults,* 4th ed. Vol. 2. Philadelphia: JB Lippincott, 1996, pp 1761, 1771.].

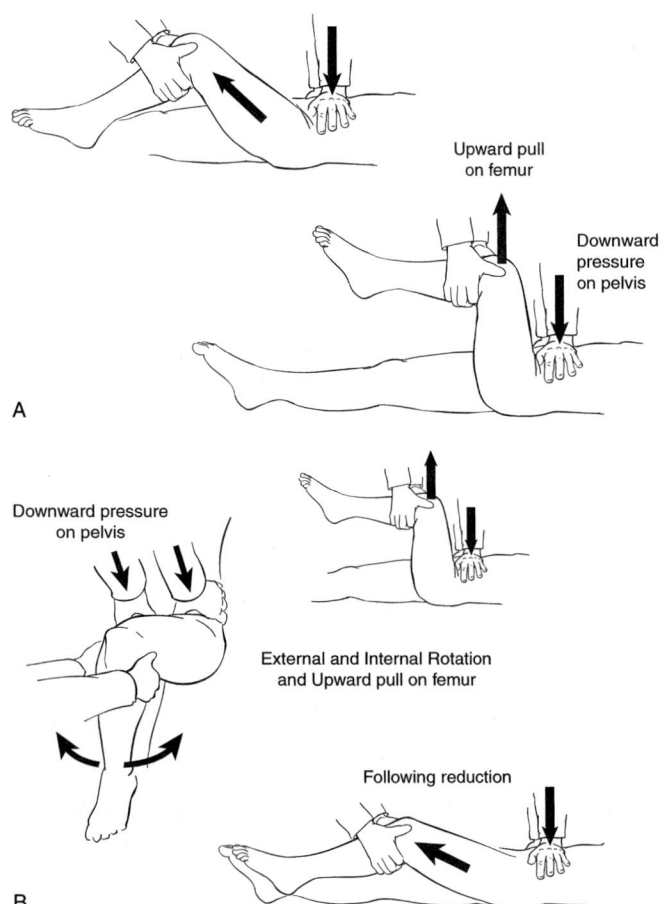

FIG. 273-23. A and **B**. Allis maneuver for reduction of anterior hip dislocation.

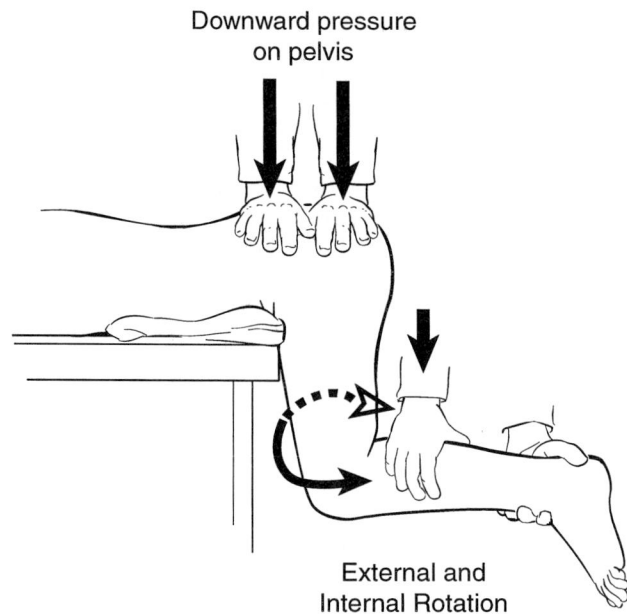

Downward pressure
on pelvis

External and
Internal Rotation

FIG. 273-25. Stimson maneuver for reduction of posterior hip dislocation.

Femoral Shaft Fractures

Fractures of the shaft of the femur most often occur in men during their most active period in life. Falls, industrial and automobile accidents, and gunshot wounds account for the majority of these fractures. Severe, direct trauma may result in transverse fractures (most common) with displacement, oblique or spiral oblique fractures, or badly comminuted segments. Pathologic fractures are uncommon but can occur secondary to metastases (breast, lung, or prostate most common) or rarely secondary to primary bone tumors such as osteogenic sarcoma.

Femoral shaft fractures are generally evident in the field to prehospital personnel because of the shortening, deformity and associated swelling. Initially, basic stabilization of the patient should take place in the field, along with spinal assessment and immobilization. External hemorrhage should be controlled by direct pressure, open wounds covered with a sterile dressing and then neurovascular examination of the extremities performed. It is best to splint the affected extremity with a traction splint at the time of injury. Hare (Dyna-Med, Carlsbad, CA) or Sager (Minto Research & Development, Redding, CA) traction splints can be placed over the trousers, applying traction to a sling around the ankle and forefoot (see Figures 273-20 and 273-21). Traction splints are relatively contraindicated in cases of open fracture with grossly contaminated exposed bone ends or when sciatic nerve injury is probable because traction can exacerbate nerve injury. For the latter, splint placement without application of traction is indicated.

Emergency department management includes basic stabilization of the patient followed by careful neurovascular examination of the affected extremity. Open fractures require broad spectrum antibiotics, debridement, and copious irrigation, generally in the operating room. Radiographs of the femur are generally lower priority in the acute resuscitation phase and parenteral analgesics are generally required if there is no contraindication to their use. Orthopedic consultation should be obtained early and most patients require hospitalization and surgical intervention.

Definitive management options include traction, external fixation, pins and plaster, and internal fixation. The intramedullary interlocking nailing is the method of choice for the treatment of uncomplicated fractures of the midshaft and junction of the upper and middle third of the femur in adults, except where comminution is so extensive that sta-

bility with the rod cannot be maintained.[30] In cases where comminution is severe, either dual-plating or the use of a compression plate device can result in excellent fixation. Open femur fractures require early orthopedic consultation for copious irrigation and debridement in the operating room. These injuries can generally be nailed immediately. In severely contaminated open fractures, external fixation may be the preferred method of treatment.

The overall prognosis of midshaft femur fractures is very good, with most patients being able to return to work within 6 months. Union rates approach 100 percent, with nonunion being very uncommon. Mild degrees of limb shortening or misalignment can result in limp and posttraumatic arthritis.

REFERENCES

1. Gonzalez RP, Fried PQ, Bukhalo M: The utility of clinical examination in screening for pelvic fractures in blunt trauma. *J Am Coll Surg* 194(2):121, 2002.
2. Cerva DS Jr, Mirvic SE, Shanmuganathan K, et al: Detection of bleeding in patients with major pelvic fractures: Value of contrast-enhanced CT. *AJR* 166:131, 1996.
3. Jones AL, Burgess AR: Fractures of the pelvic ring, in Bucholz RW, Heckman JD (eds): *Rockwood and Green's Fractures in Adults*, 5th ed. Philadelphia, JB Lippincott, 2001, pp 1471.
4. Riemer BL, Butterfield SL, Diamond DL, et al: Acute mortality associated with injuries to the pelvic ring: The role of early patient mobilization and external fixation. *J Trauma* 35:671, 1993.
5. Gruen GS, Leit ME, Gruen RJ, et al: Functional outcome of patients with unstable pelvic ring fractures stabilized with open reduction and internal fixation. *J Trauma* 39:838, 1995.
6. Yang AP, Iannacone WM: External fixation for pelvic ring disruptions. *Orthop Clin North Am* 28:331, 1997.
7. Routt ML Jr, Simonian PT, Swiontkowski MF: Stabilization of pelvic ring fractures. *Orthop Clin North Am* 28:369, 1997.
8. Wolinsky PR: Assessment and management of pelvic fracture in the hemody-namically unstable patient. *Orthop Clin North Am* 28:321, 1997.
9. Perry DC, DeLong W: Acetabular fractures. *Orthop Clin North Am* 28(3):405, 1997.
10. Burgess AR, Eastridge BJ, Young JW, Ellison TS: Pelvic ring disruptions: Effective classification system and treatment protocols. *J Trauma* 30:848, 1990.
11. Gruen GS, Leit ME, Gruen RJ, et al: The acute management of hemodynamically unstable multiple trauma patients with pelvic ring fractures. *J Trauma* 36:706, 1994.
12. Simpson T, Krieg JC, Heuer F, Bottlang M: Stabilization of pelvic ring disruptions with a circumferential sheet. *J Trauma* 52:158, 2002.
13. Agolini SF, Shah K, Jaffe J, et al: Arterial embolization is a rapid and effective technique for controlling pelvic fracture hemorrhage. *J Trauma* 43:395, 1997.
14. Lindberg EF, Macias D, Gipe BT: Clinically occult presentation of comminuted intertrochanteric hip fractures. *Ann Emerg Med* 21:1511, 1992.
15. Alba E, Youngberg R: Occult fractures of the femoral neck. *Am J Emerg Med* 10:64, 1992.
16. Pandey R, McNally E, Ali A, Bulstrode C: The role of MRI in the diagnosis of occult hip fractures. *Injury* 29:61, 1998.
17. Zuckerman JD: Hip fracture. *New Engl J Med* 334:1519, 1996.
18. Kleinschmidt KC: Elder abuse: A review. *Ann Emerg Med* 30:463, 1997.
19. Schmidt AH, Swiontkowski MF: Femoral neck fractures. *Orthop Clin North Am* 33:97, 2002.
20. Ahmad LA, Eckhoff DG, Kramer AM: Outcome studies of hip fractures: A functional viewpoint. *Orthop Rev* 23:19, 1994.
21. Rogers FB, Shackford SR, Keller MS: Early fixation reduces morbidity and mortality in elderly patients with hip fractures from low-impact falls. *J Trauma* 39:261, 1995.
22. Bredahl C, Nyholm B, Hindsholm KB: Mortality after hip fracture: Results of operation within 12 h of admission. *Injury* 23:83, 1992.
23. Fox HJ, Pooler J, Prothero D, et al: Factors affecting the outcome after proximal femoral fractures. *Injury* 25:2977, 1994.
24. Tornetta P: Hip dislocations and fractures of the femoral head, in Bucholz RW, Heckman JD (eds): *Rockwood and Green's Fractures in Adults*, 5th ed. Philadelphia, JB Lippincott, 2001, p 1547.

25. Bernstein SM, Zinar DM, et al: Ipsilateral hip and femoral shaft fractures. *Clin Orthop* 296:168, 1993.
26. Shah AK, Eissler J, Radomisli T: Algorithms for the treatment of femoral neck fractures. *Clin Orthop* 399:28, 2002.
27. Kovol KJ, Zuckerman JD: Intertrochanteric fractures, in Bucholz RW, Heckman JD (eds): *Rockwood and Green's Fractures in Adults,* 5th ed. Philadelphia, JB Lippincott, 2001, p 1661.
28. Lyons AR: Clinical outcomes and treatment of hip fractures. *Am J Med* 103:51S, 1997.
29. DeLong WG Jr: Subtrochanteric fractures, in Bucholz RW, Heckman JD (eds): *Rockwood and Green's Fractures in Adults,* 5th ed. Philadelphia, JB Lippincott, 2001, p 1673.
30. Starr AJ, Bucholz RW: Fractures of the shaft of the femur, in Bucholz RW, Heckman JD (eds): *Rockwood and Green's Fractures in Adults,* 5th ed. Philadelphia, JB Lippincott, 2001, p 1696.

KNEE INJURIES

Mark T. Steele
Jeffrey N. Glaspy

Injuries to the knee are common in our exercise and sports-oriented society. Because the knee is essential for ambulation, one must be familiar with the examination of the normal and abnormal knee to be able to recognize, treat, and appropriately refer specific injuries. This chapter deals with examination of the knee and with recognition of fractures and dislocations of the patella; fractures of femoral condyles; fractures of the tibial spines, tuberosity, and plateaus; ligamentous and meniscal injuries of the knee joint; knee dislocation; quadriceps and patellar tendon ruptures; patellar tendinitis and chondromalacia patellae; penetrating injuries and foreign bodies; total knee replacement and postarthroscopy problems; and osteochondritis dissecans.

An accurate diagnosis of the injured knee is required before proper treatment can be instituted. The first examination is usually the easiest to perform and may be the most valid because the patient does not anticipate pain and therefore does not guard, and involuntary muscular spasm, and because inflammation and effusion causing further limitation of the examination may not yet have occurred.

EXAMINATION

The examination of the knee is divided into five phases: history, observation, inspection, palpation, and stress testing.

The current mechanism of injury as well as any prior serious injuries or surgical procedures frequently clarifies subtleties in the examination, allowing a more accurate diagnosis and appropriate treatment.

The patient should be examined while walking, if possible, and in both the sitting and lying positions. Take note of the gait, muscular development, functional range of motion, and the ability of the patient to extend the flexed knee against minimal resistance.

The knee should be inspected for swelling, ecchymoses, effusion, masses, patella location and size, muscle mass, erythema, and evidence of local trauma. With the patient supine, note whether leg lengths are equal or unequal. Lastly, ask the patient to perform the best possible active range of motion.

Initially the neurovascular status of the leg should be noted. As with all orthopedic examinations, the noninjured or normal knee should be compared with the injured knee during all aspects of the examination, but especially during palpation and stress testing. When palpating the knee, begin in the nontender areas and work toward the tender area so that the patient does not guard or become apprehensive. The patella and patellar facets, as well as the femoral and tibial condyles, should be palpated for pain and crepitance. Effusion, tenderness, increased temperature, strength, sensation, and location of pulses should be noted.

Examine the patella for size, shape, and location with the knee in flexion; check mobility with the knee in extension. The patella should be compressed to check for pain as well as moved laterally and medially to ascertain possible subluxation. The popliteal space should be palpated for masses, swelling, and pulses. Both the medial and lateral joint lines should be palpated because tenderness at those locations suggests the possibility of meniscal injury. Palpation of the medial and lateral collateral ligaments should also be performed with tenderness, again suggesting the possibility of injury.

The final phase of the examination of the knee is stress testing (also see "Ligamentous and Meniscal Injuries" below). This is the most difficult aspect of the examination, although potentially the most informative. The patient must be reassured and relaxed and made as comfortable as possible. This may require allowing the leg to hang over the side of the bed with the bed supporting the posterior thigh rather than the physician holding the leg, as is usually done during stress testing. The uninjured, hopefully normal, opposite knee should be examined first to determine the patient's normal laxity. A brief summary of the instabilities and tests to demonstrate them are presented in the section on ligamentous and meniscal injuries.

RADIOGRAPHIC EVALUATION

The Ottawa Knee Rules (Table 274-1) for determining the need for x-rays have proven sensitive for fracture[1] and have resulted in reduced emergency department waiting times and costs. The Pittsburgh Knee Rules (Table 274-2) are similar and recently were prospectively shown to be as sensitive, but more specific than the Ottawa Rules.[2] They also have the added advantage of being applicable to both children and adults. A recent evaluation[3] suggested that point tenderness is not a good predictor of knee fracture in children. This study suggested that applying a rule of an inability to bear weight and inability to flex the knee to 90 degrees would decrease x-rays ordered by 75 percent without any missed fractures.

Anteroposterior, lateral, and oblique radiographs are typically obtained if x-rays are determined to be necessary.[4] Fat fluid levels (lipohemarthrosis) may be identified on a lateral view of the knee which is suggestive of intra-articular fracture.[5] Oblique views are particularly helpful at detecting subtle tibial plateau fractures (internal oblique view is best to visualize lateral plateau, external oblique film best to visualize medial plateau). A tunnel or intercondylar view provides a clear view of the intercondylar region and is particularly useful in identifying tibial spine fractures. The sunrise (skyline, axial, or tangential) view is most useful in detecting nondisplaced vertical or marginal fractures of the patella which may be missed with the conventional three views. The sunrise view is indicated if patellar subluxation or fracture is suspected. Computerized tomography (CT) scanning may be necessary to fully delineate the extent of tibial plateau fractures.[6] Magnetic resonance imaging (MRI) is also helpful in this regard, having the added benefit of being able to assess soft tissue injury (i.e., ligamentous and meniscal).

FRACTURES

Fractures of the Patella

Fractures of the patella occur from a direct blow such as with the knee striking a car dashboard in a motor vehicle accident, a fall on the

TABLE 274-1 Ottawa Knee Rules: X-ray if One Criterion Is Present[1]

Patient older than 55 years
Tenderness at the head of the fibula
Isolated tenderness of the patella
Inability to flex knee to 90 degrees
Inability to transfer weight for four steps both immediately after the injury and in the ED

TABLE 274-2 Pittsburgh Knee Rules[2]

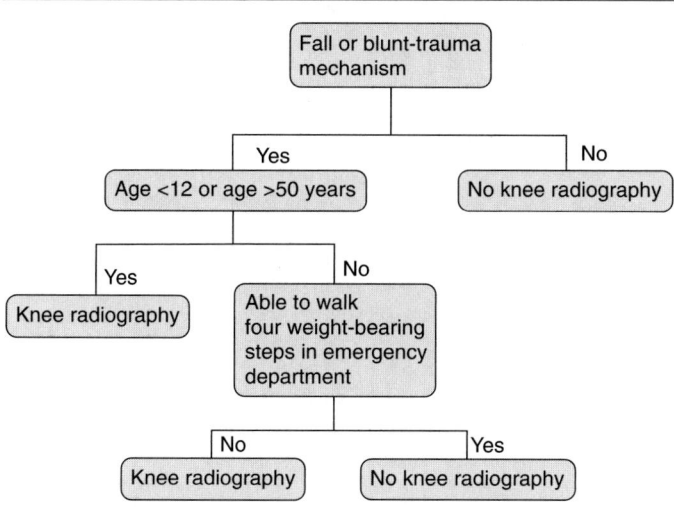

flexed knee, or forceful contraction of the quadriceps muscles, which can occur with falling or stumbling. Fractures may be transverse, comminuted, or of the avulsion type, when the quadriceps or patellar tendon pulls off a small portion of the patella (Figure 274-1).

Transverse fractures of the patella are most common, followed by stellate and comminuted fractures.[7] Patients with nondisplaced fractures may be ambulatory. Physical examination reveals focal patellar tenderness, swelling, and effusion. The integrity of the extensor mechanism of the knee should be checked by having the patient perform a straight-leg raise against gravity. Transverse fractures are more likely to be displaced and have a disrupted extensor mechanism. Differential diagnosis of patellar fractures radiographically includes bipartite patella. This condition involves the superior lateral corner of the patella, is typically bilateral, and is differentiated from fracture by its smooth cortical margins.

A nondisplaced fracture of the patella with an intact extensor mechanism is initially treated in the emergency department with a knee immobilizer, ice, elevation, and nonsteroidal anti-inflammatory drugs and/or opioid analgesics. Such fractures are generally treated in a long leg cast for a total of 6 weeks of immobilization.[7] During this period the patient should be encouraged to walk on crutches initially, with partial weight bearing progressing to full weight bearing as tolerated. Fractures that are displaced greater than 3 mm, or that are asso-

ciated with the disruption of the extensor mechanism, require early referral to orthopedics for open reduction and internal fixation.[7] This generally consists of tension-band wiring of the patella and suturing of the retinaculum. Severely comminuted fractures may be treated surgically by removal of smaller fragments (or all fragments if they are small) and suturing of the quadriceps and patellar tendons. All open fractures must be debrided and irrigated by orthopedics in the operating room, and antistaphylococcal antibiotics should be administered. The overall prognosis for patellar fractures is good.[7]

Fractures of Femoral Condyles

Fractures of the femoral condyles account for 4 percent of femur fractures and include supracondylar, intercondylar, condylar, and distal femoral epiphyseal fractures (Figure 274-2). Most often, these injuries are secondary to direct trauma from a fall with axial loading or a blow to the distal femur. Examination reveals pain, swelling, deformity, rotation, shortening, and an inability to ambulate. Although neurovascular injuries are uncommon, the potential for popliteal artery injury exists so the status of distal sensation and pulses must be checked. The space between the first and second toe, innervated by the deep peroneal nerve, should be tested for sensation. In addition, a search for ipsilateral hip dislocation or fractures, and damage to the quadriceps apparatus must be made. Incomplete or nondisplaced fractures in any age group and stable impacted fractures in the elderly can be treated with cast immobilization.[7] Open reduction and internal fixation is generally required for displaced fractures or if there is any degree of joint incongruity present.[8] Therefore, leg splinting and orthopedic consultation is essential. The overall progress of these injuries is fair. Complications include deep venous thrombosis, fat embolus syndrome, delayed or malunion, and the subsequent development of osteoarthritis.

Fractures of the Tibial Spines and Tuberosity

Although isolated injuries of the tibial spine are uncommon, they usually result in cruciate ligament insufficiency. The injury is most often

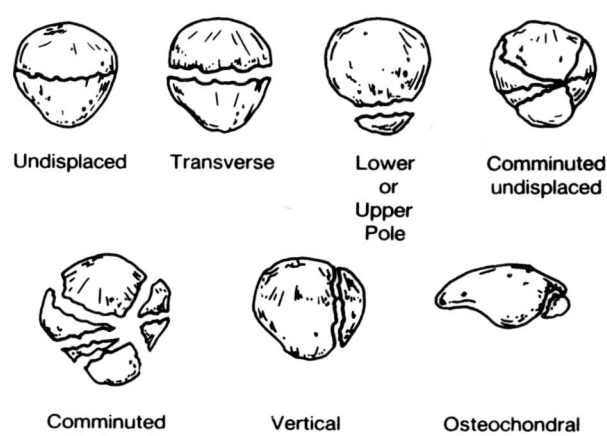

FIG. 274-1. Classification of patellar fractures. [Reproduced with permission from Hohl M, Johnson EE, Wiss DA: Fractures of the knee, in Rockwood CA Jr, Green DP, Bucholz RW (eds): *Fractures in Adults,* 3d ed. Vol. 2. Philadelphia, JB Lippincott, 1991, p 1765.]

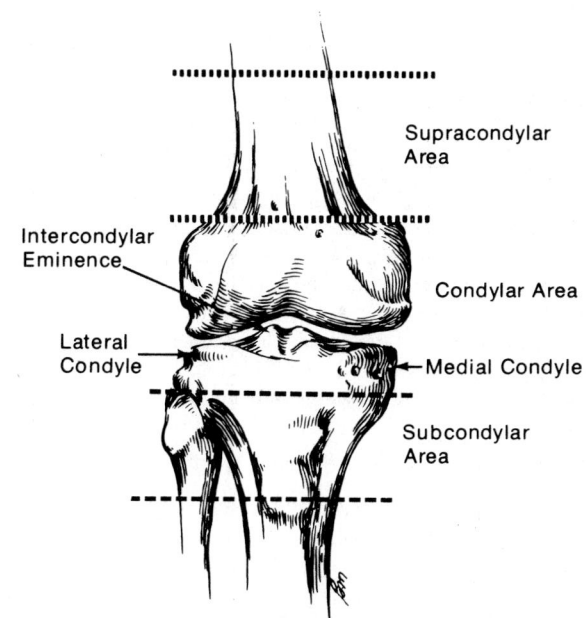

FIG. 274-2. The supracondylar and condylar areas of the femur, and the medial and subcondylar areas of the tibia. [Modified with permission from Hohl M, Larson RL: Fractures and dislocations of the knee, in Rockwood CA Jr, Green DP (eds): *Fractures.* Vol. 2. Philadelphia, JB Lippincott, 1975, pp 1132, 1147.]

caused by a force directed against the flexed proximal tibia in an anterior or posterior direction, resulting in incomplete avulsion of the tibial spine, with or without displacement, or complete fracture of the spine. Vehicular and sporting accidents are the most common causes of these injuries.[7] Fracture of the anterior tibial spine is about tenfold more common than fracture of the posterior spine. Examination shows a painful, swollen knee, secondary to hemarthrosis, inability to extend fully, and a positive Lachman sign (see "Ligamentous and Meniscal Injuries" below). If the fracture is incomplete or nondisplaced, it should be immobilized in full extension in a knee immobilizer. Protected weight bearing and outpatient orthopedic follow-up within a few days to a week is advised. Complete, displaced fractures require early orthopedic consultation and often need open reduction, and internal fixation.

The quadriceps mechanism inserts on the tibial tubercle. A sudden force to the flexed knee with the quadriceps muscle contracted may result in a complete or incomplete avulsion of the tibial tubercle. The fracture line may extend into the joint. Examination reveals pain and tenderness over the proximal anterior tibia with pain on passive or active extension. If the avulsion is small or nondisplaced, the fragment may be maintained in position by immobilization; otherwise, open reduction and internal fixation are necessary.[7]

Fractures of the Tibial Plateaus

Fractures of the tibial plateaus are seen more commonly in the older population and can be very difficult to detect. They are produced by valgus or varus forces combined with axial loading, which drives the femoral condyles into the articulating surface of the tibia. A fall from a height or the leg being struck by the bumper of a car are common causes of these fractures.[9] Both medial and lateral plateaus may be fractured simultaneously, although the lateral plateau is more often fractured.[7] Direct trauma to the lateral aspect of the knee may account for the preponderance of lateral tibial plateau fractures. The patient presents with painful swelling of the knee and limitation of motion. Radiographs may demonstrate a fracture but often only show a lipohemarthrosis on the lateral view. Careful review of the x-rays is essential. Ligamentous instability may be present in up to one-third of those injuries. Anterior cruciate and medial collateral ligament injuries are associated with lateral plateau fractures whereas posterior cruciate and lateral collateral ligament injuries occur with medial plateau fractures.[7] If one plateau is fractured but not displaced, treatment in a knee immobilizer, without weight bearing, is indicated with outpatient orthopedic follow-up scheduled within a few days to a week. Long-term treatment of these nondisplaced fractures consists of a long leg cast and prolonged non-weight bearing. Depression of the articular surface necessitates early orthopedic consultation and open reduction and elevation of the bony fragment. The treatment goal is precise reconstruction of the articular surfaces to allow for early range of motion so as to minimize the development of osteoarthritis.[7] Potential complications of those fractures include popliteal artery injury with high-energy displaced fractures, the development of deep venous thrombosis, and osteoarthritis. The prognosis for these injuries is fair.

LIGAMENTOUS AND MENISCAL INJURIES

The knee joint depends on ligaments and muscles for support (Figure 274-3). It is frequently subjected to injuries from traumatic forces while extended or in various stages of flexion. These traumatic forces include abduction, flexion, and internal rotation of the femur on the tibia; adduction, flexion, and external rotation of the femur on the tibia; hyperextension; and anteroposterior displacement. By far the most common are abduction, flexion, and internal rotation of the femur on the tibia, which produce injuries to the medial side of the knee. Injuries to the lateral side of the knee are produced by adduction, flexion, and external rotation. Such forces may result in a strain or rup-

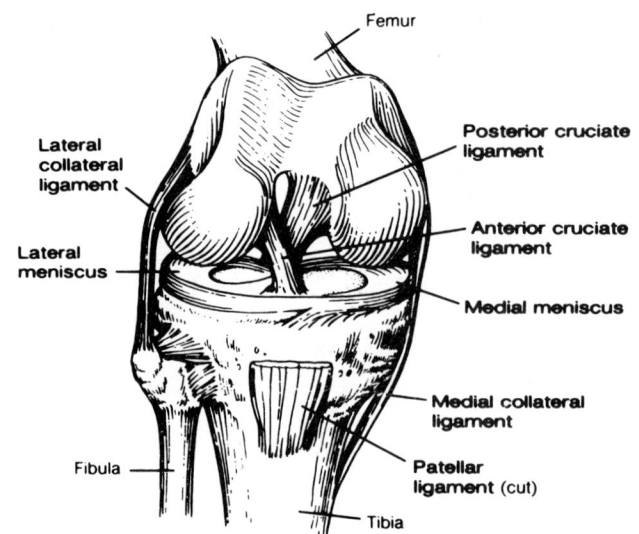

FIG. 274-3. Ligaments of the right knee joint. The articular capsule and the patella have been removed. (Reproduced with permission from Spencer AP, Mason EB: *Human Anatomy and Physiology.* Menlo Park, CA: Benjamin/Cummings, 1979, p 174.)

ture of the medial or lateral collateral ligaments, the anterior or posterior cruciate ligaments, the capsular structures, or a tear in the medial or lateral meniscus, singularly or in combination. Functional instability of the knee is determined by stress testing, which may demonstrate abnormal laxity when properly done. Solomon et al. reviewed the literature and analyzed the reported sensitivity, specificity, and positive and negative likelihood ratios for diagnosis of ligamentous and meniscal injury.[10] Table 274-3 summarizes the reported results from this study.

Initial stress testing is an abduction or valgus deformity (Figure 274-4) applied to the knee, which is in approximately 30 degrees of flexion, to determine the integrity of the medial capsular and ligamentous structures. The medial collateral ligament supplies the majority of restraint to valgus deformities of the knee in all stages of flexion. A varus or adduction force is then applied to the lateral aspect of the knee, again with approximately 30 degrees of flexion, to ascertain the integrity of the lateral structures. The lateral collateral ligament, similar to the medial collateral ligament, is the major restraint to varus laxity on the knee at all positions of flexion. If there is a demonstrated laxity of greater than 1 cm without a firm end point as compared to the other knee, there is a complete rupture of the medial or lateral collateral ligament.[11] If there is laxity with a firm end point or a laxity of less than 1 cm, an incomplete or partial tear is present. If there is no demonstrated instability but there is pain, the patient has suffered a strain in the ligamentous structures tested. The patient who is unstable with the varus or valgus test performed with 30 degrees of flexion should be brought into full extension, if possible, and similar maneuvers carried out. Medial instability in full extension indicates a severe lesion involving the cruciate ligaments and posterior capsule along with the medial ligaments. Lateral instability in extension likewise indicates a severe injury that may involve the posterolateral corner of the knee as well as the cruciate ligaments. Peroneal nerve injuries may also occur in lateral injuries. Although these tests may aid in the diagnosis of medial collateral ligament and lateral collateral ligament injuries, there are no adequate published reports to comment on their sensitivity and specificity.[10]

Injury to the *anterior cruciate ligament* may be the most common ligamentous injury today.[11] The mechanism of injury is usually noncontact; a deceleration, hyperextension, or marked internal rotation of the tibia on the femur results in an injury to the cruciate. This injury is often associated with a "pop" and swelling that develops within hours.

TABLE 274-3   Reliability of Physical Exam for Diagnosis of Knee Ligament and Meniscus Injuries

Structure	Maneuver	Mean Sensitivity (Range)	Mean Specificity (Range)	Positive Likelihood Ratio (95% CI)	Negative Likelihood Ratio (95% CI)	Comments
ACL	Composite exam*	82% (62–100)	94% (56–100)	25 (2.1–306)	0.04 (0.01–0.48)	When limited to acute injury (one study), 62% sensitivity and 56% specificity.
	Anterior drawer	62% (9–93)	67% (23–100)	3.8 (0.7–22.0)	0.3 (0.05–1.5)	Variability of studies may be due to small sample sizes.
	Lachman's test	84% (60–100)	100% (100)	42 (2.7–651)	0.1 (0.0–0.4)	Only one study commented on specificity. Therefore specificity and likelihood ratios may be inaccurate.
	Lateral pivot shift	38% (27–95)	N/A	N/A	N/A	No study commented on specificity.
PCL	Composite exam*	95.5% (91–100)	89.5% (80–99)	21 (2.1–205)	0.05 (0.01–0.50)	Results limited to two studies.
	Posterior drawer	55% (51–86)	N/A	N/A	N/A	No study commented on specificity.
MCL/LCL	N/A	N/A	N/A	N/A	N/A	No study was identified that adequately examined diagnostic accuracy for these injuries.
Meniscal injury	Composite exam*	77% (64–82)	81% (78–84)	N/A	N/A	Only three of five studies commented on specificity.
	Joint-line tenderness	79% (76–85)	15% (11–43)	0.9 (0.8–1.0)	1.1 (1.0–1.3)	Only two of four studies included acute injury and all four included chronic injuries; consequently, applicability to ED is limited.
	McMurray test	53% (29–63)	59% (29–100)	1.3 (0.9–1.7)	0.8 (0.6–1.1)	

*These studies reported the "composite exam" without giving data on the specific examination maneuvers.
Abbreviations: ACL = anterior cruciate ligament; CI = confidence interval; LCL = lateral collateral ligament; MCL = medial collateral ligament; N/A = not applicable; PCL = posterior cruciate ligament.
Source: Adapted from Solomon DH, Simel DL, Bates DW, et al: Does this patient have a torn meniscus or ligament of the knee? Value of physical exam. *JAMA* 286:1610, 2001.

This pop is considered pathognomonic for anterior cruciate injury.[12] There may be an associated medial meniscal tear as well. Such a mechanism of injury combined with the presence of a traumatic effusion is very suggestive of a disruption of the anterior cruciate ligament.

The diagnosis of the anterior cruciate ligament injury is ascertained by using the Lachman test (Figure 274-5), the anterior drawer sign (Figure 274-6), and the pivot shift (Figure 274-7).[13] Although the anterior drawer sign has been used for a long time, the sensitivity is only approximately 62 percent (see Table 274-3). The maneuver is done with 45-degree flexion at the hip and 90 degrees of flexion at the knee. The physician then attempts to forwardly displace the tibia from the femur. A displacement of greater than 6 mm as compared to the normal, opposite knee indicates that there has been an injury to the anterior cruciate ligament. There are false-negatives associated with this maneuver. The Lachman test is a much more sensitive test, with a re-

ported sensitivity of 84 percent.[10,11] The examiner places the knee in 20 degrees of flexion by resting it on a pillow and stabilizes the femur above the knee with his or her nondominant hand. The dominant hand is placed behind the leg at the level of the tibial tubercle, and the examiner introduces an anterior force, attempting to displace the tibia forward. If a displacement of greater than 5 mm as compared to the opposite knee occurs, or if there is a soft, mushy end point, then a tear in the anterior cruciate ligament has occurred. Although this examination is more sensitive than the anterior drawer and able to identify partial tears in the anterior cruciate ligament when the examiner is skilled, it is difficult to perform on patients with large legs. The pivot shift is the third maneuver by which the examiner can determine the integrity of the anterior cruciate ligament. The pivot shift is easily performed once the examiner is familiar with it, but it may be somewhat painful to the patient. While the patient is supine and relaxed, the examiner

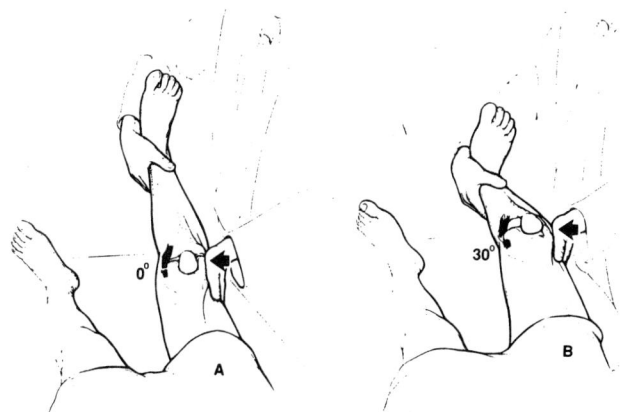

FIG. 274-4. Valgus stress in full extension (**A**) and in 30 degrees of flexion (**B**). (Reproduced with permission from Scott WN: *Ligament and Extensor Mechanism Injuries of the Knee: Diagnosis and Treatment.* St. Louis: Mosby-Year Book, 1991, p 91.)

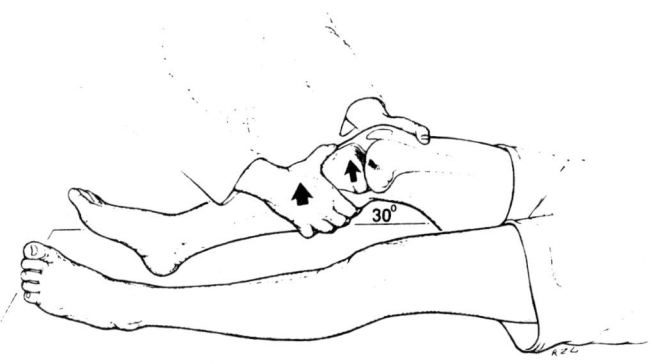

FIG. 274-5. The Lachman test is performed with the knee flexed between 15 degrees and 30 degrees. (Reproduced with permission from Scott WN: *Ligament and Extensor Mechanism Injuries of the Knee: Diagnosis and Treatment.* St. Louis: Mosby-Year Book, 1991, p 94.)

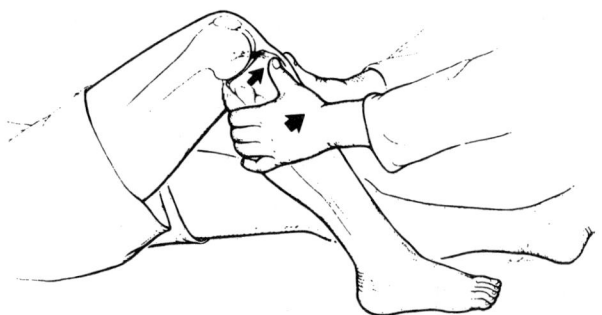

FIG. 274-6. Anterior drawer test. (Reproduced with permission from Scott WN: *Ligament and Extensor Mechanism Injuries of the Knee: Diagnosis and Treatment.* St. Louis: Mosby-Year Book, 1991, p 95.)

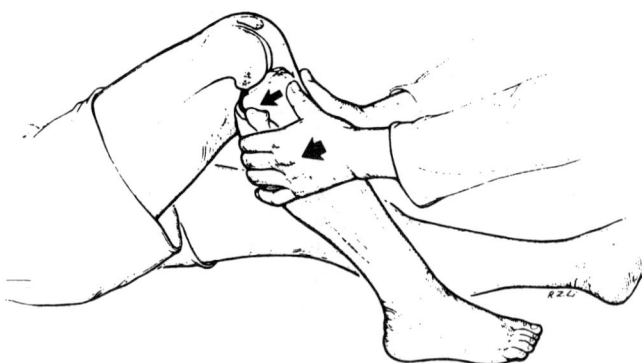

FIG. 274-8. Posterior drawer test. (Reproduced with permission from Scott WN: *Ligament and Extensor Mechanism Injuries of the Knee: Diagnosis and Treatment.* St. Louis: Mosby-Year Book, 1991, p 97.)

lifts the heel of the foot to approximately 45 degrees of hip flexion with the knee fully extended. The opposite hand grasps the knee with the thumb behind the fibular head. The examiner then internally rotates the ankle and knee, applies a valgus force to the knee, and flexes the knee. If an anterior subluxation of the tibia is present, a sudden visible, audible, and palpable reduction of the subluxation occurs at about 20 to 40 degrees of flexion. This indicates a deficit in the anterior cruciate ligament, which is required to stabilize the knee in this position. There are other tests described in the literature to determine the integrity of the anterior cruciate ligament, including the jerk test and dynamic extension testing.

The *posterior cruciate ligament* can also suffer an isolated injury or be injured in combination with other ligamentous structures of the knee. In contrast to anterior cruciate injuries, isolated posterior cruciate injuries are seen much less frequently. The posterior cruciate ligament provides initial resistance to posterior translation at all angles of flexion of the knee. The mechanism of injury then is usually an anterior to posterior force applied to the tibia or lower leg. Posterior cruciate injuries are seen in association with other ligamentous injuries when a serious injury has occurred to the knee. A deficit in this ligament is determined by the posterior drawer test (Figure 274-8). The knee is examined with flexion at the hip and at the knee as described for the anterior drawer sign. The physician applies a posterior force to

the tibial tubercle. If there is displacement posteriorly, then the examiner can diagnose an injury to this ligament. The physician might also notice a posterior sag or drop back of the tibial tubercle because of loss of integrity of the posterior cruciate when observing the knee with 45-degree flexion at the hip and 90-degree flexion at the knee. This test can be misleading, however, if there is a straight anterior instability resulting in a subluxation of the knee forward. This abnormal position would give the physician the false impression of too much posterior play when performing the posterior drawer test because the knee would be reduced to its normal anatomic alignment from the forwardly subluxed position. Although the posterior drawer test has only a 55 percent sensitivity, the composite history and physical exam is much more accurate in the diagnosis of posterior cruciate ligament injuries (see Table 274-3).[10]

Combined instabilities of the knee are often seen, especially in athletes. Anteromedial and anterolateral instability are the two that occur most frequently. They result from external rotation and abduction or adduction forces placed on the knee. Virtually any combination of medial and lateral instabilities of the knee can occur, however.

One knee injury that is especially difficult to detect is injury to the posterolateral structures. Posterolateral instability usually involves a *tear of the popliteus-arcuate complex,* which may occur in combination with lateral ligament injury and possible anterior or posterior cruciate ligament injury. Isolated injuries to the popliteus-arcuate complex can occur themselves but are rare. Isolated posterolateral instability is demonstrated by testing at 0 to 30 degrees of flexion for maximal posterior translation, and at 90 degrees of flexion for maximal external rotation as compared to the normal opposite knee. Further testing to determine the integrity of the lateral collateral ligament and anterior or posterior cruciate ligaments must be done as well.

Most ligamentous injuries of the knee present with hemarthroses. **In fact, approximately 75 percent of all hemarthroses are caused by disruption of the anterior cruciate ligament.**[11] Serious ligament injuries, however, may present with minimal pain and no hemarthrosis because of complete disruption of the ligamentous and capsular fibers, allowing leakage of the blood into the soft tissue spaces. Hemarthrosis can also be caused by osteochondral fractures or fractures that extend into the joint line or peripheral meniscal tears. Traumatic hemarthroses usually occur within minutes to hours of injury, in contrast to chronic effusions of the knee because of synovial inflammation, which occur 1 to 2 days after strenuous use of the joint.

Plain radiographs in ligamentous injuries are typically normal or only reveal an effusion. An avulsion fracture at the site of attachment of the lateral capsular ligament on the lateral tibial condyle (Segond fracture) is a marker for anterior cruciate ligament rupture.[14] Cortical avulsion of the medial tibial plateau (very uncommon) is associated with tears of the posterior cruciate ligament and medial meniscus.[15] Continued refinements in MRI have resulted in high-quality images of

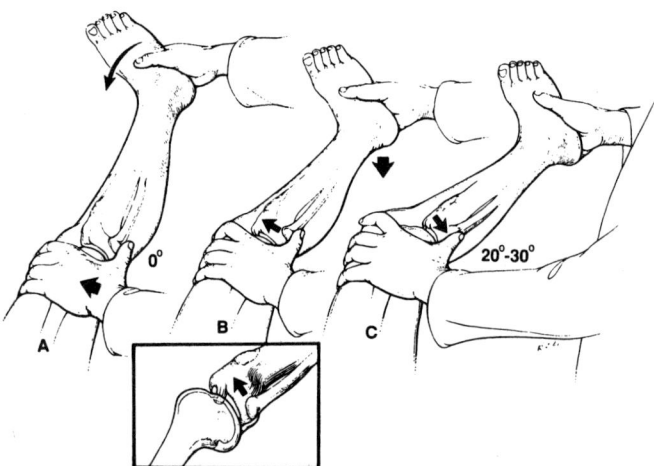

FIG. 274-7. In the pivot shift of Galway and MacIntosh, the test is done with the knee in full extension with application of a valgus and internal rotation stress. The "clunk" of reduction is felt in the first 20 degrees to 30 degrees of flexion. (Reproduced with permission from Scott WN: *Ligament and Extensor Mechanism Injuries of the Knee: Diagnosis and Treatment.* St. Louis: Mosby-Year Book, 1991, p 95.)

the ligamentous and meniscal structures of the knee, resulting in an accuracy rate of close to 90 percent for meniscal and cruciate ligament disruption.[7] The ordering of this examination, however, is typically done by the patient's primary care provider or orthopedist in follow-up.

Stable injuries involving a single ligament with minor strain can be managed with a knee immobilizer, ice packs, elevation, nonsteroidal anti-inflammatory agents, and ambulation as soon as is comfortable for the patient.[16] **When knee immobilizers are placed, the patient must be instructed to perform daily range of motion exercises to avoid contracture and maintain mobility.** These complications are more common in the elderly and can occur after only a few days of immobilization. While there is no universally accepted regimen for range of motion exercise, one regimen is to first apply ice to relieve pain, and then to perform 10 to 20 knee flexion-extensions (no weights should be added) three or four times a day. These injuries should be referred to an orthopedic surgeon or to the patient's primary care provider within the next few days to a week for follow-up examination. Complete rupture of an isolated ligament can generally be treated conservatively in the same fashion with quadriceps strengthening, range of motion exercises, and functional bracing being part of the follow-up care.[12] Professional athletes with single ligament ruptures or patients with more than one ligament torn and an unstable knee necessitate immediate orthopedic consultation so that definitive surgical management can be planned.

Arthrocentesis may be of therapeutic benefit in patients with large, tense effusions of the knee; however, good evidence has not been reported. Wallman and Carley performed a literature review to ascertain whether aspiration improves symptoms in patient's with acute traumatic hemarthrosis and found no relevant articles.[17] Furthermore, recurrence of the effusion following aspiration is common. Arthrocentesis may be of assistance diagnostically if the etiology of the effusion is not clearly due to trauma. **The presence of blood and glistening fat globules is pathognomonic of lipohemarthrosis, which indicates intraarticular knee fracture.** The major complication of arthrocentesis is septic arthritis.

Meniscal Injuries

Meniscal injuries of the knee occur by themselves or in combination with ligamentous injuries. For example, anterior cruciate injuries are commonly associated with meniscal injuries. Cutting, squatting, or twisting maneuvers may cause injury to the meniscus. The medial meniscus is approximately twice as likely as the lateral meniscus to be injured. Four-fifths of the tears involve the peripheral posterior aspect of the meniscus.[18] Many maneuvers have been described in the literature to determine whether a meniscus has been injured. Most of these tests, however, have an unacceptable specificity and sensitivity (see Table 274-3). Although the diagnosis of a meniscal tear is difficult to make in certain patients, a combination of a suggestive history and physical findings on examination should lead the emergency physician to consider the diagnosis. On questioning the patient, the physician should ask if the patient experiences locking of the knee joint on either flexion or extension that is painful and limits further activity. This sign clearly points to the diagnosis of a torn meniscus. Effusions that occur after activity; a sensation of popping, clicking, or snapping; a feeling of an unstable joint, especially with activity; or tenderness in the anterior joint space after excessive activity suggests the diagnosis of a meniscal tear.

When performing a physical examination, a physician should attempt to identify atrophy of the quadriceps muscle because of disuse and joint-line tenderness, which is very suggestive. Various maneuvers, such as McMurray test or the grind test, are useful but, as mentioned earlier, are positive only about 50 percent of the time.[19] If a tentative diagnosis of a meniscal tear is considered, referral to an orthopedic surgeon or the patient's primary care provider is warranted. Nonsteroidal anti-inflammatory agents and partial weight bearing are

advised pending follow-up. Definitive diagnosis can be made by MRI or arthroscopy with the latter having the advantage of allowing for definitive surgical treatment (usually partial meniscectomy or meniscal repair).

The patient who presents to the emergency department with a locked knee can experience a great deal of pain along with loss of mobility. Following conscious sedation, one can attempt to unlock the knee by positioning the patient with the leg hanging over the edge of the table with the knee in 90 degrees or greater of flexion. After a period of relaxation, the physician can apply longitudinal traction to the knee with internal and external rotation in an attempt to unlock the joint. If this maneuver is unsuccessful, consultation with the orthopedic surgeon is recommended.

Knee Dislocation

Knee dislocation (Figure 274-9) is a result of tremendous ligamentous disruption due to hyperextension, direct posterior force applied to the anterior tibia, force to the fibula or medial femur, force to the tibia or lateral femur, or rotatory force resulting in anterior, posterior lateral, medial, or rotatory dislocation. This injury typically occurs following sporting accidents and falls and posterior dislocation is most common. With posterior dislocation, there is complete disruption of the anterior and posterior cruciate ligaments and the posterior joint capsule. The extensor mechanism of the knee may also be disrupted and should be checked postreduction. Because of knee instability, reduction very often occurs spontaneously. A severely unstable knee in multiple directions is suspicious for a spontaneously reduced knee dislocation. Suspicion of the injury is important because of the high incidence of associated complications, including popliteal artery injury and peroneal nerve injury (mostly with posterolateral dislocations), in addition to ligamentous and meniscal injury.

Early reduction of the dislocation employing longitudinal traction is essential. Neurovascular status of the extremity should be documented pre- and postreduction. Hospitalization is required and orthopedic consultation should be obtained immediately.

Controversy exists regarding when to obtain arteriography in patients with knee dislocation. Because of the high incidence of popliteal artery injury (up to one-third of patients) and poor outcomes related to delays in vascular reconstruction, some authors recommend arteriography for all confirmed knee dislocations.[20] Others suggest that clinical examination alone is reliable in identifying patients requiring

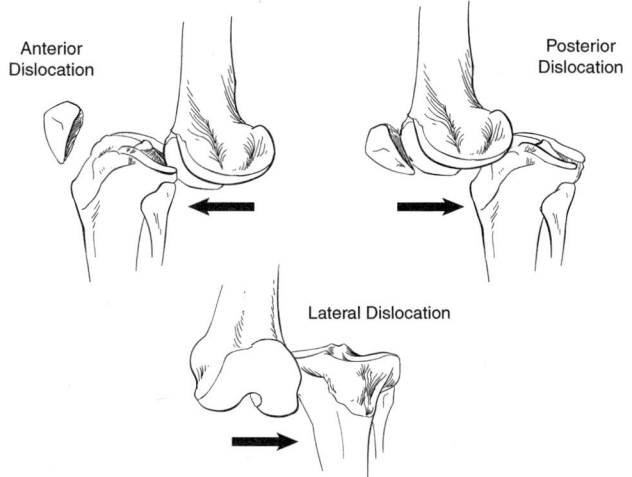

FIG. 274-9. Types of dislocations: Anterior; Posterior; and Lateral. (Reproduced with permission from DePalma AF: *Management of Fractures and Dislocations: An Atlas.* Philadelphia: WB Saunders, 1970, p 1621.)

arteriography and/or surgical intervention.[21] Patients with an absent pulse or other signs of vascular injury (i.e., bruit, distal ischemia) require immediate vascular surgical consultation for surgical exploration. Patients with an absent pulse prereduction with return of a pulse postreduction probably necessitate arteriography.[22] Patients with normal pulses pre- and postreduction along with normal Doppler pressure indices (ankle-brachial index) can probably be safely observed in the hospital with serial vascular examinations. Presence of normal distal pulses, however, does not preclude occult popliteal artery injury.[23] As a result, if any doubt exists, arteriography should be performed.

Patella Dislocation

Dislocation of the patella usually occurs from a twisting injury on the extended knee and is more common in women. The patella is displaced laterally over the lateral condyle, resulting in pain and deformity of the knee (Figure 274-10). Tearing of the medial knee joint capsule often occurs. Reduction is accomplished following conscious sedation by flexing the hip, hyperextending the knee, and sliding the patella back into place. This results in immediate relief of pain, but further soreness from capsular injury persists for a period of time. The patella and knee should be x-rayed to rule out a fracture, and the knee should be immobilized after reduction. Follow-up with a primary care provider or orthopedist within 1 to 2 weeks is suggested. Partial weight bearing progressing to full weight bearing, nonsteroidal anti-inflammatory agents, and isometric quadriceps strengthening exercises are also indicated. Recurrent lateral dislocation of the patella occurs in approximately 15 percent of patients, and superior, horizontal, and intercondylar dislocations require referral to an orthopedic surgeon for possible surgical intervention.

Quadriceps/Patellar Tendon Rupture

Rupture of the quadriceps or patellar tendons can occur from forceful contraction of the quadriceps muscle or falling on a flexed knee. Patel-

lar tendon rupture occurs most commonly in individuals younger than age 40 years with a history of tendinitis or past steroid injections. Quadriceps tendon rupture is most frequent in the older than 40 years age group.[7] There is significant pain, diffuse swelling, and the patient is unable to extend a flexed knee against mild resistance in both instances. Depending on the tendon ruptured, a defect may be palpable above or below the patella (Figure 274-12). A "high-riding patella" may be seen on the lateral x-ray of the knee with patellar tendon rupture (Figure 274-11). The treatment is surgical repair of the involved tendon[24] within the first 7 to 10 days following rupture to achieve the best results. Orthopedic consultation in the emergency department is indicated.

Osteochondritis Dissecans

Osteochondritis dissecans is a disorder in which a segment of articular cartilage and subchondral bone become partially or totally separated from the underlying bone. It is a rare condition of unknown etiology that has been thought to result from acute or chronic trauma. It typically is found in adolescents, is generally unilateral, and most often involves the non-weight-bearing lateral aspect of the medial femoral condyle. Patients generally complain of pain and swelling but typically do not recall any specific incident of trauma. The condition can be diagnosed on routine radiographs with tunnel views being particularly helpful. Treatment is conservative with protective weight bearing if the epiphyses are still open. If the epiphyses are closed and the fragments are detached, the prognosis for healing is poor. Arthroscopy for the retrieval of loose bodies or arthrotomy for pinning or bone grafting of the detached lesions is suggested in this instance.[25]

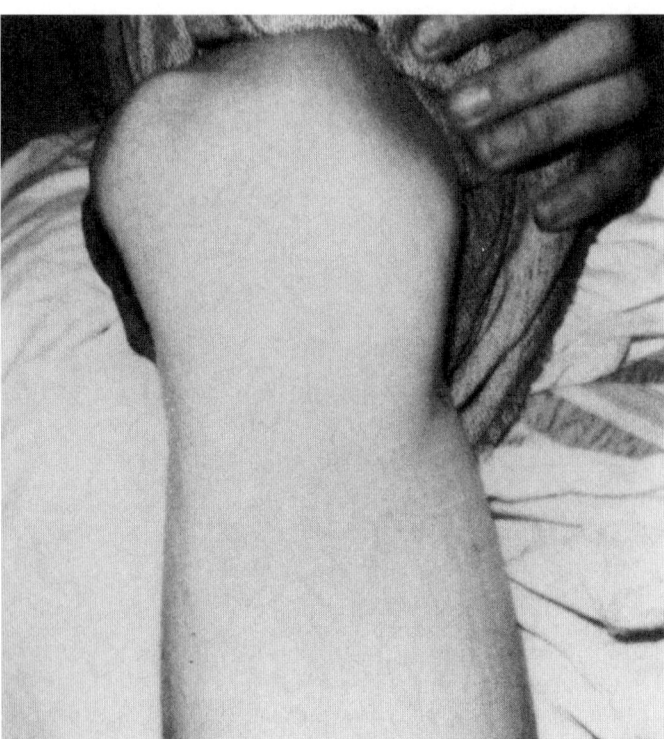

FIG. 274-10. Lateral dislocation of the right patella. [Reproduced with permission from Lyman JI, Ervin ME: Management of common dislocations, in Roberts JR, Hedges JR (eds): *Clinical Procedures in Emergency Medicine.* Philadelphia: WB Saunders, 1985, p 634.]

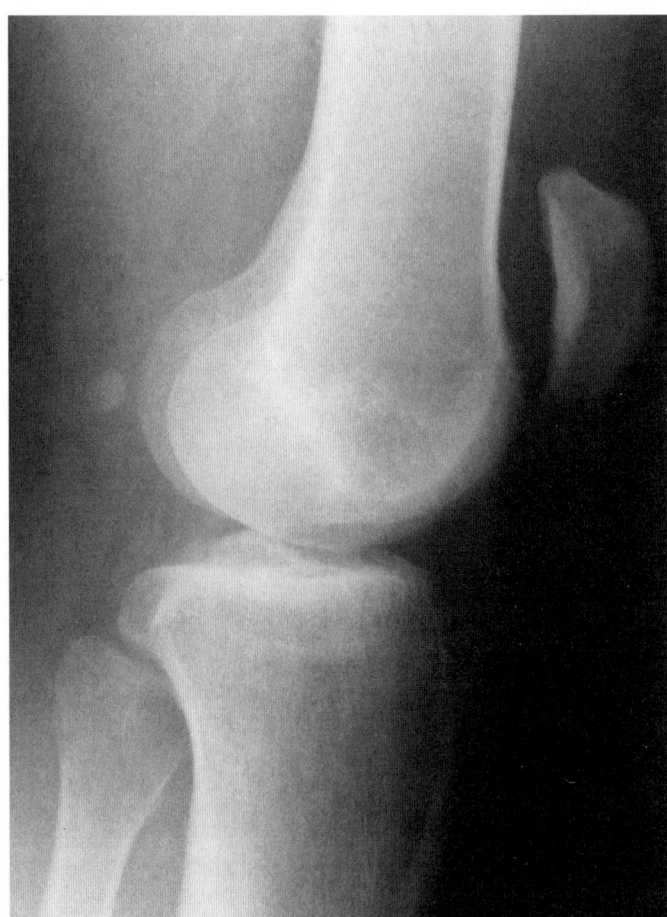

FIG. 274-11. Patella alta.

FIG. 274-12. Right patella tendon rupture. Note the depression distal to the patella.

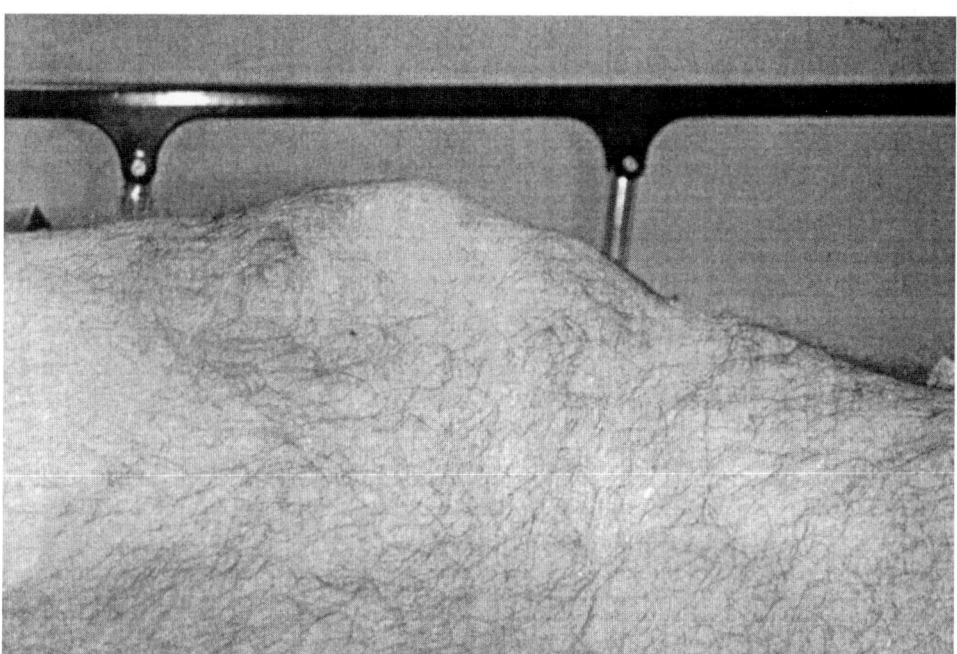

Osteonecrosis

Osteonecrosis is a bony infarction caused by disruption of blood supply to the bone. Osteonecrosis is divided into two main categories, primary (spontaneous, idiopathic) and secondary. The etiology of primary osteonecrosis remains unknown. Secondary causes include steroid therapy, systemic lupus erythematosus, alcoholism, sickle cell disease, and renal transplantation. Patients with osteonecrosis are typically elderly women who present with acute knee pain. The weight-bearing surface of the medial femoral condyle of the knee is the most common site of involvement. Physical examination generally reveals tenderness over the involved femoral condyle or tibial compartment. Secondary osteonecrosis occurs in a younger age group. Plain radiographs are typically normal early in the course of the disease but magnetic resonance scanning is diagnostic. Initial treatment is nonoperative and consists of protected weight bearing and the use of nonsteroidal anti-inflammatory drugs. The outcome of the disease depends on the percentage of the weight-bearing surface of the joint involved. Treatment options for advanced stages of the disease include arthroscopic debridement, curettage or drilling of the lesion, bone grafting, high tibial osteotomy, use of osteochondral allografts, and total knee arthroplasty.[26]

Patellar Tendinitis

Also known as "jumpers knee," patellar tendinitis is primarily seen in runners, basketball and volleyball players, and high jumpers. Pain is referred to the area of the patellar tendon and is worsened when going from sitting to standing or when running up hills. Point tenderness can be found at the distal aspect of the patella or proximal part of the patellar tendon. Treatment consists of heat, nonsteroidal anti-inflammatory agents, and quadriceps strengthening exercises. Steroid injections predispose to tendon rupture so should be avoided.

Chondromalacia Patellae

Chondromalacia patellae is an overuse syndrome of the articular cartilage of the patella. The condition is caused by patellofemoral malalignment, which leads to a tracking abnormality of the patella, placing excessive lateral pressure on the articular cartilage. It is most common in young, active women and the pain is generally localized to

the region of the anterior knee. Stair climbing and rising from a chair exacerbate the pain.

Two tests may aid in the diagnosis. The patellar compression test is performed by pushing the patella distal in the trochlear groove with the knee extended and quadriceps muscles tightened. This maneuver elicits pain. The apprehension test is performed on a relaxed leg. When the patella is pushed laterally, the quadriceps muscles contract in anticipation of pain. Treatment of this condition consists of rest, nonsteroidal anti-inflammatory medication, and quadriceps strengthening exercises.[27]

Postarthroscopy Presentations

Patients may rarely present to the emergency department following arthroscopy secondary to pain and swelling. Effusions are common following arthroscopy, but joint infection is very uncommon. Diagnostic arthrocentesis should be performed if joint infection is suspected. Arthrocentesis may be helpful therapeutically for large tense effusions. Intraarticular injection of bupivacaine and morphine after traumatic knee injuries and arthroscopy reduces the need for systemic analgesia, but morphine is more effective and can provide relief longer.[28]

Penetrating Knee Injury/Joint Foreign Bodies

If the knee joint has clearly been violated as a consequence of penetrating injury, orthopedic consultation should be obtained for joint irrigation in the operating room. If penetration is suspected, but is in doubt, injection of the joint with sterile methylene blue can help to confirm the diagnosis. Extravasation of dye indicates penetration and the need for irrigation. **Remember that the history obtained must recreate the position of the knee when the penetrating injury occurred.** Many occupational injuries occur with the knee flexed, but the joint is examined with the knee resting in extension. Failure to anticipate the trajectory of injury with the knee flexed could lead to misdiagnosis and failure to anticipate joint penetration.

Radiopaque foreign bodies (i.e., metal, glass) will visualize on conventional radiographs. In general, foreign bodies in the knee joint need to be removed. A bullet in the joint can destroy the cartilage and lead poisoning can occur.[29] A bullet lodged in the bone only, however, does not necessitate removal. Antibiotics to cover streptococci and staphylococci are generally indicated for both penetrating knee wounds and foreign bodies. Tetanus prophylaxis should be administered if indicated.

REFERENCES

1. Stiell IG, Wells GA, Hoag RH, et al: Implementation of the Ottawa Knee Rules for the use of radiography in acute knee injuries. *JAMA* 278:2075, 1997.
2. Seaberg DC, Yealy DM, Lukens T, et al: Multicenter comparison of two clinical decision rules for the use of radiography in acute, high-risk knee injuries. *Ann Emerg Med* 32:8, 1998.
3. Cohen DM, Jasser JW, Kean JR, Smith GA: Clinical criteria for using radiography for children with acute knee injuries. *Pediatr Emerg Care* 14:185, 1998.
4. Gray SD, Kaplan PA, Dussault RG, et al: Acute knee trauma: How many plain films are necessary for the initial examination? *Skeletal Radiol* 26:298, 1997.
5. Lugo-Olivieri CH, Scott WW Jr, Zehovni EA: Fluid-fluid levels in injured knees: Do they always represent lipohemarthrosis? *Radiology* 198:499, 1996.
6. Walker CW, Moore TE: Imaging of skeletal and soft tissue injuries in and around the knee. *Radiol Clin North Am* 35:631, 1997.
7. Wiss DA, Watson JT, Johnson EE: Fractures of the knee, in Rockwood CA Jr, Green DP, Bucholz RW, Heckman JD (eds): *Fractures in Adults*, 4th ed. Philadelphia, JB Lippincott, 1996, p 1919.
8. Schatzker J: Fractures of the distal femur revisited. *Clin Orthop* 347:43, 1998.
9. Watson JT: High-energy fractures of the tibial plateau. *Orthop Clin North Am* 25:723, 1994.
10. Solomon DH, Simel DL, Bates DW, et al: Does this patient have a torn meniscus or ligament of the knee? Value of the physical examination. *JAMA* 286:1610, 2001.
11. Swenson TM, Harrer CD: Knee ligament injuries: Current concepts. *Orthop Clin North Am* 26:529, 1995.
12. Scuderi GR, Scott WN, Install JN: Injuries of the knee, in Rockwood CA Jr, Green DP, Bucholz RW, Heckman JD (eds): *Fractures in Adults*, 4th ed. Philadelphia, JB Lippincott, 1996, p 2001.
13. Scott WN: *Ligament and Extensor Mechanism Injuries of the Knee: Diagnosis and Treatment.* St. Louis, Mosby-Year Book, 1991, p 87.
14. Kerr HD: Segond fracture, hemarthrosis, and anterior ligament disruption. *J Emerg Med* 8:29, 1990.
15. Hall FM, Hochman MG: Medial Segond-type fracture: Cortical avulsion off the medial tibial plateau associated with tears of the posterior cruciate ligament and medial meniscus. *Skeletal Radiol* 26:553, 1997.
16. Hughston JC: *Knee Ligaments: Injury and Repair.* St. Louis, Mosby-Year Book, 1993.
17. Wallman P, Carley S: Aspiration of acute traumatic knee hemarthrosis. *Emerg Med J* 19:50, 2002.
18. Hardin GT, Farr J, Bach BR Jr: Meniscal tears: Diagnosis, evaluation, and treatment. *Orthop Rev* 21:1311, 1992.
19. Evans PJ, Bell GD, Frank C: Prospective evaluation of the McMurray test. *Am J Sports Med* 21:604, 1993.
20. Dennis JW, Jagger C, Butcher JL, et al: Reassessing the role of arteriograms in the management of posterior knee dislocations. *J Trauma* 35:692, 1993.
21. Kendall RW, Taylor DC, Salvian AJ, O'Brien PJ: The role of arteriography in assessing vascular injuries associated with dislocations of the knee. *J Trauma* 35:875, 1993.
22. Merrill KD: Knee dislocation with vascular injuries. *Orthop Clin North Am* 25:707, 1994.
23. Gable DR, Allen JW, Richardson JD: Blunt popliteal artery injury: Is physical examination enough for evaluation? *J Trauma* 43:541, 1997.
24. Haas SB, Callaway H: Disruptions of the extensor mechanism. *Orthop Clin North Am* 23:687, 1992.
25. Garrett JC: Osteochondritis dissecans. *Clin Sports Med* 10:569, 1991.
26. Patel DV, Breazeale NM, Behr CT, et al: Osteonecrosis of the knee: Current clinical concepts. *Knee Surg Sports Traumatol Arthrosc* 6:2, 1998.
27. Zappala FG, Taffel CB, Senderi GR: Rehabilitation of patellofemoral joint disorders. *Orthop Clin North Am* 23:555, 1992.
28. VanNess SA, Gittiris ME: Comparison of intra-articular morphine and bupivacaine following knee arthroscopy. *Orthop Rev* 23:743, 1994.
29. Bolanos AA, Demizio JP Jr, Vigorita VJ, Bryk E: Lead poisoning from an intra-articular shotgun pellet in the knee treated with arthroscopic extraction and chelation therapy. A case report. *J Bone Joint Surg* 78:422, 1996.

LEG INJURIES
Paul R. Haller

Lower leg injuries are common. The tibia is the most common long bone fractured. Significant soft tissue injuries to the leg can also occur. Documentation of the history and the physical examination are crucial to the proper evaluation of lower leg injuries.[1] A knowledge of the anatomy aids in the interpretation of findings.

ANATOMY

Bone

Support for weight bearing is provided primarily by the tibia, a bone triangular in cross section that lies subcutaneously in the anterior aspect of the leg. Although it is in harm's way, it has a thick cortex and significant force is required to fracture it. Proximally, the tibia is splayed out to form the medial and lateral plateaus that articulate with the femoral condyles. The lateral plateau is higher and smaller than the medial and is more susceptible to fracture. The distal tibia articulates with the fibula laterally and the talus inferiorly. This articulation is supported by the ankle syndesmosis, a series of ligaments that lie inferior to the interosseous membrane. The fibula lies lateral and posterior to the tibia. Its smaller diameter allows it to be broken with less force than the tibia. Patients can remain ambulatory after a fibula fracture, because it bears little weight. The tibia and fibula are connected by a dense interosseous membrane.

Compartments

The cylinder of the lower leg is divided into four chambers or compartments by bone and dense layers of fascia. It is useful to describe the neurovascular and muscular anatomy in terms of the position of the nerves and muscles in these four compartments, the anterior, lateral, superficial posterior, and deep posterior compartments. The *anterior compartment* is bordered by the tibia medially, the interosseous ligament posteriorly, and the anterior crural septum on its lateral aspect. It contains the muscles that dorsiflex the ankles and toes. The anterior tibial artery runs through this compartment before becoming the dorsal pedal artery of the foot. The deep peroneal nerve that also traverses this compartment supplies motor function to the dorsal flexors of the foot and toes. It provides sensory innervation to the web space of the first and second toes. The *lateral compartment* is circumscribed by the anterior peroneal septum, the fibula, and the posterior peroneal septum. It houses the superficial peroneal nerve, which is sensory to the lateral dorsum of the foot, and motor control for the muscles within the compartment that evert the foot. The peroneal nerve runs just lateral to the fibular head, where it is exposed to direct trauma. The *superficial posterior compartment* contains muscles that plantar flex the ankle (gastrocnemius, soleus, and plantaris). The sural nerve runs through it before providing sensory innervation to the lateral heel. No major arteries traverse this compartment. The *deep posterior compartment* contains muscle groups that plantar flex the toes. The tibial nerve provides motor control to these muscles and sensation for the sole of the foot. This compartment also contains the posterior tibial artery, whose pulse can be felt posterior to the medial malleolus of the ankle. The physical findings produced by increased pressure within each compartment are tabulated in Chap. 278.

EVALUATION

Leg injuries are initially evaluated with a directed history, including the amount and type of violence that occurred. The history may also give clues about nontraumatic soft tissue injuries. On examination, nerves should be evaluated by checking sensation in the web space, lateral heel, and sole of the foot. Motor tests should include the ability to plantar and dorsal flex the foot, as well as to evert the foot. The extent of soft tissue injury is evaluated visually and by palpating the muscle groups. The tibia and fibula should be palpated along their entire lengths. The popliteal, dorsal pedal, and posterior tibial pulses should be palpated. An absent or decreased pulse may indicate the need for urgent fracture reduction and vascular evaluation. Patients with tibial shaft fractures are unable to bear weight or lift their foot off of the cart. Patients with fibular fractures alone are often able to bear weight.

Simple anteroposterior and lateral x-rays of the leg that include the knee and ankle are sufficient to evaluate leg injuries. If ankle or knee injuries are suspected, then further x-ray evaluation is needed. If a tibial shaft fracture is suspected, the leg should be splinted with a radiolucent device to control pain and prevent further soft tissue damage prior to obtaining films. Check pulses, movement, and sensation before and after moving the leg.

TREATMENT

Detailed attention to soft tissue injuries is critical to treating lower leg injuries properly. Often it is the extent of such injury, rather than the fracture itself, that determines the outcome. Wounds should be cleansed and debrided of loose tissue and foreign material. Tetanus immunization should be given, if indicated. Splinting of fractures will prevent further damage to soft tissue caused by movement of the sharp bone fragments. Carefully palpate the compartments to detect any possible compartment syndrome. If suspected, inform the consulting surgeon so that appropriate priorities can be set in the management of the injury. Parenteral antibiotics should be administered in open-fracture cases.

COMPLICATIONS

Wounds that are not adequately cleansed and debrided are very prone to infection, an event not preventable by the use of antibiotics alone. Patients with compartment syndromes may develop permanent disability if the syndromes are not suspected or diagnosed. Fractures that are not adequately aligned or immobilized heal poorly or not at all. If a vascular injury is not urgently repaired, amputation can result.

SPECIFIC INJURIES

Fibula Fractures

Most fibular shaft fractures occur in the setting of a tibia fracture, in which case, treatment and expected outcome are determined by the injury to the tibia. Isolated fibula fractures usually result from a direct blow. They are relatively uncommon. Because this bone only bears 15 percent of the body weight, patients are often able to walk despite the fracture. Proximal fibula fractures are often the result of external rotation, whereas distal fibula fractures usually result from internal rotation. A low velocity injury leading to a fibula fracture can be treated with immobilization using elastic wrap (distal fibula) or a knee immobilizer (proximal fibula). More impressive pain and disability can be treated with crutches and casting, or splinting. Nonunion is uncommon.

Repetitive trauma, particularly in runners beginning their training, may result in a stress fracture of the distal fibula. Radiographs in stress fractures are often normal initially, with a fracture being detected either by bone scan acutely, or by repeat x-ray 1 to 2 weeks after the event. Pain medication, cessation of the causative activity, and ice and elevation are recommended.

Tibia Fractures

A significant amount of force must be applied to the tibia in one of three ways for a fracture to occur. A torsional injury occurs when the body rotates on a planted foot. This low-energy force often results in a spiral fracture. A bending force on the tibia often produces a transverse or short oblique fracture line. Direct force, such as a crush injury, may result from a blow from a baseball bat. The scant amount of tissue between the tibia and the skin results in little protection of the shaft from direct blow.

The goal of treatment of tibial fractures is to avoid infection, obtain bony union, and restore function. Most closed fractures that are minimally displaced can be treated with reduction and immobilization by an orthopedist. If pain control is adequate, and the patient reliable, discharge from the emergency department to home is possible. Injuries with more than minimal displacement require orthopedic evaluation for reduction and immobilization of the fragments. Patients often require admission for pain control, further fracture care, and observation for the possibility of compartment syndrome.

An open fracture of the tibial shaft requires prompt consultation by an orthopedist while the other associated injuries are addressed. The management and expected outcome of an open tibia fracture is determined by a number of factors. Wounds with small lacerations (<1 cm), minimal muscle contusion, and simple transversal fracture lines have <5 percent incidence of infection, and generally heal within 20 weeks. Injuries that involve more extensive soft tissue damage to the muscle, skin, and vascular system from crush injuries or high-velocity violence have up to 25 percent infection rate, and take up to twice as long to heal. Severe injury may result in amputation. Thus, factors that assist in the evaluation of the patient with an open tibial shaft fracture include (1) general health of the patient and presence of other injuries; (2) pattern of fracture line; (3) number of fracture fragments; (4) whether the fibula is intact or fractured; (5) extent of soft tissue damage; (6) amount of contamination of the wound; and (7) presence of vascular compromise.

ED evaluation of open injuries includes prompt immobilization of the fractured extremity, along with sterile coverage of the wound. Often this must be done in conjunction with the care of the other injuries the patient has sustained. Intravenous antibiotics should be administered in the emergency department. This may be first-generation cephalosporin for low-energy injuries without significant soft tissue damage. More severely injured extremities may benefit from broader coverage, such as that offered by ticarcillin-clavulanate. Treatment includes prompt irrigation and debridement of the wound in the operating room.

Achilles Tendon Rupture

When the soleus and gastrocnemius muscles contract, the Achilles tendon pulls up the calcaneus, plantar flexing the foot. Rupture often occurs in sports settings, especially in poorly conditioned players. Forceful plantar flexion results in rupture of the tendon. A popping sound is heard by the patient, who then has difficulty ambulating. This injury is also likely to occur in individuals who have rheumatoid arthritis, lupus erythematosus, have received quinolone antibiotics, or prior steroid injection of the tendon.[2,3] It frequently ruptures 2 to 6 cm above its attachment to the calcaneus, where it has its poorest vascular supply. A gap may be palpated at this point, and a dent may be visible. Achilles tendon function should be checked when patients complain of injuries to the ankle or heel. The Thompson-Doherty test is performed by squeezing the midportion of the calf of the patient lying in the prone position. An intact Achilles tendon is demonstrated by a plantar flexion of the foot. Another test is to have the patient walk on his or her toes. The diagnosis does not usually require imaging, but ultrasonography, computed tomography, or magnetic resonance imaging can be helpful in ambiguous cases. In the emergency department, the patient should be splinted in neutral position with a Robert Jones splint, with prompt referral to an orthopedist. Crutches will be needed for ambulation.

Gastrocnemius Rupture

The medial head of the gastrocnemius is frequently injured during athletic events. A forceful plantar flexion of the foot, often with an extended knee, results in partial tear or rupture of the medial head of the gastrocnemius near its origin on the distal femur. This may be the result of a fall on a plantar-flexed foot or the sudden plantar flexion that occurs in the back leg of an athlete serving a tennis ball. Predisposing factors include inadequate stretching, prior muscle injury, and advanced age.

The athlete feels a sudden sharp pain on the medial aspect of the proximal gastrocnemius. It is painful to ambulate and plantar flexion is uncomfortable. On examination, the proximal medial calf is tender, and may be swollen and bruised. Walking on tiptoes is possible, but uncomfortable. The history is similar to that of Achilles tendon rupture, but the pain and tenderness are more proximal, and the Thompson test is negative in patients with gastrocnemius muscle rupture. Rupture of a Baker cyst should also be considered in the diagnosis, along with deep vein thrombosis.

Treatment typically consists of immobilization with a posterior splint, crutches for ambulation, ice, and pain medications. A mild rupture may be treated simply with rest and non-weight bearing.

Shin Splints

The term *shin splints* describes pain over the medial or anterior tibia that occurs with exertion and is relieved by rest. The cause is microtears of the muscular fibers at their point of bony attachment. Pain is often described as burning during running, or aching after exercise is completed. The only physical finding may be tenderness to the anterior or medial tibial surfaces. Radiographs may be useful to detect a stress fracture of the tibia, but a bone scan is more sensitive to diagnose stress fracture. Treatment of shin splints consists of cessation of the offending activity, orthotics to decrease excessive pronation, and strengthening and flexibility programs.

Osgood-Schlatter Disease

This lesion is typically seen in athletic teenagers of both genders. Football, soccer, basketball, gymnastics, and ballet can cause this injury. The anatomic lesion is the partial separation of the tibial tuberosity at the insertion of the patellar tendon. In about one-fourth of cases, it is a bilateral process. Palpation of the tibial tuberosity reveals tenderness and induration. A lateral x-ray of the proximal tibia with the knee flexed 30 degrees reveals an elevation of the distal portion of the tubercle off of the tibia. Alternatively, ultrasonography can be used for diagnosis. Cold compresses, anti-inflammatory drugs, and stopping the offending activity is standard treatment. Follow-up with an orthopedist is advisable for this sometimes chronic condition.

REFERENCES

1. Russell TA: Fractures of the tibia and fibula, in Rockwood CA Jr, Green DP (eds): *Fractures in Adults,* 5th ed. Philadelphia, Lippincott-Raven, 2000.
2. Cetti R, Junge J, Vyberg M: Spontaneous rupture of the Achilles tendon is preceded by widespread and bilateral tendon damage and ipsilateral inflammation. *Acta Orthop Scand* 74:78, 2003.
3. Greene BL: Physical therapy management of fluoroquinolone-induced Achilles tendinopathy. *Phys Ther* 82:1224, 2002.

ANKLE INJURIES
John A. Michael
Ian G. Stiell

EPIDEMIOLOGY

Injuries to the ankle are a common presenting complaint in EDs. Most patients are younger than 40 years and are equally distributed between males and females. Fractures, most commonly of the lateral malleolus, are seen in 15 percent of these patients.[1,2] For patients younger than 50 years, fractures are more common in men; for those older than 50 years, fractures are more common in women. Fracture-dislocations are more common in women.

ANATOMY

The ankle joint bears the weight of the body. An understanding of ankle injuries depends not only on a thorough knowledge of the anatomy of the joint but also on the mechanism of force that caused the injury.

The proximal part of the joint, or mortise, is comprised of the distal fibula and the tibia. This part fits on top of the talus, or plafond, the distal part of the joint. These three bones are bound together by three groups of ligaments. Bony stability is provided by the medial and lateral malleoli extending over the plafond. Ligamentous stability is provided by the lateral ligament complex, the medial deltoid ligament, and the syndesmosis. The lateral malleolus is attached to the anterior and posterior aspects of the talus and to the calcaneus, respectively, by the anterior talofibular, posterior talofibular, and calcaneofibular ligaments. The medial collateral or deltoid ligament is a thick triangular band of tissue that originates on the medial malleolus. The superficial fibers insert on the navicular, the sustentaculum of the calcaneus, and the talus, and a deep set of fibers inserts on the medial aspect of the talus. The syndesmosis is a group of four distinct ligaments that attach the distal fibula to the tibia just above the plafond (Figure 276-1).

The ankle joint is sometimes described as having a range of motion in only the plantar and dorsiflexion plane; however, a small degree of medial and lateral movement does occur. The four groups of muscles that serve the ankle joint are supplied by branches of the sciatic nerve. Dorsiflexion is accomplished by tibialis anterior, extensor digitorum longus, and extensor hallucis longus muscles that run over the anterior aspect of the joint. On the medial side of the joint, the tibialis posterior, flexor digitorum longus, and flexor hallucis longus run behind the medial malleolus and contribute to inversion of the joint. Laterally, running behind the distal fibula, the peroneus and brevis muscles contribute to eversion and plantar flexion. These two peroneal tendons share a common synovial sheath that is held in place by a groove on the posterior aspect of the lateral malleolus and the superior retinaculum. Plantar flexion is provided by the soleus and gastrocnemius muscles. The blood supply of the foot is served by branches of the popliteal artery.

Almost all injuries of the ankle joint are due to an abnormal motion of the talus within the mortise. Motion of the talus causes a stress on the malleoli and the ligaments, thus causing injury. If the injury allows shifting of the position of the talar dome within the mortise, then the injury has the potential to be unstable. Fractures above the plafond may be unstable, and injuries that cause disruption on both sides of the joint are unstable. Instability can result from a fracture of a malleolus and rupture of a ligament, fracture of both malleoli, or rupture of both ligaments. The definition of instability is usually made radiographically, because it is difficult to make a satisfactory functional examination in an acutely injured ankle. Essentially, if there is an asymmetry in the gap between the talar dome and the two malleoli on the talus view of the ankle, then the injury is presumed to be unstable (Figure 276-2).

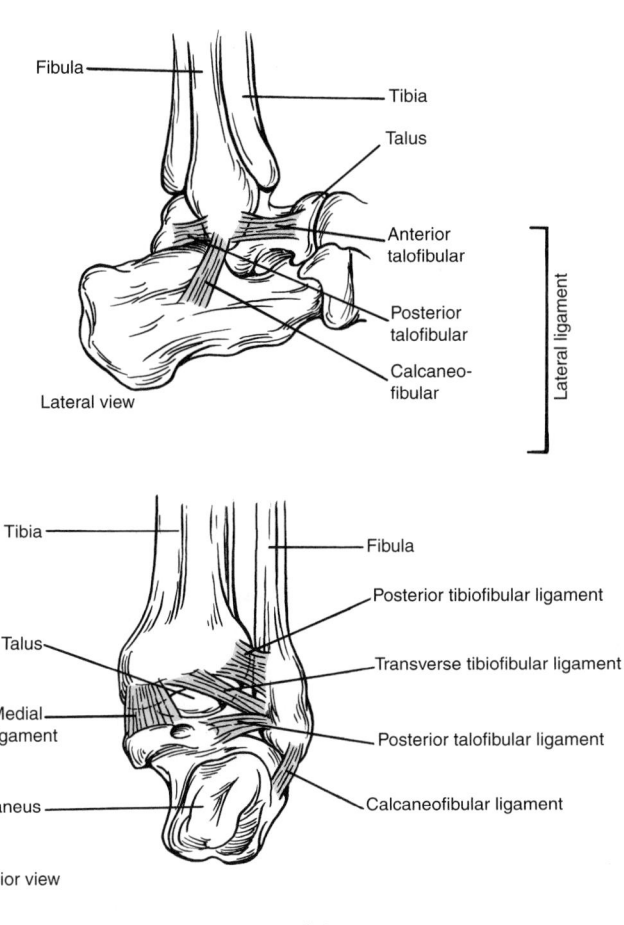

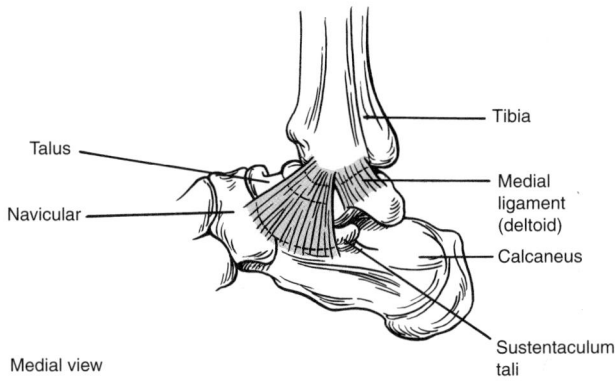

FIG. 276-1. Anatomy of the ankle joint.

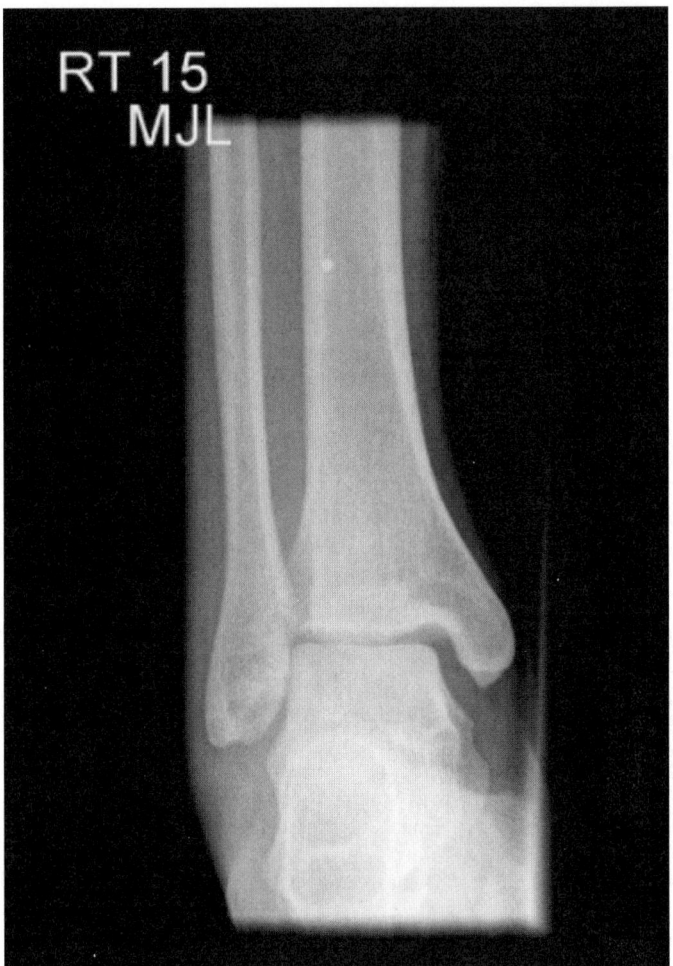

FIG. 276-2. X-ray of widened mortise.

EVALUATION

History

Although knowledge of the mechanism of the injury is important, many patients cannot recollect the exact movement that caused the injury. The classification systems used to describe ankle injuries use the direction of the deforming force to describe the potential injury. This information is useful, but, to emergency physicians, the circumstances surrounding the injury are of greater importance in consideration of other injuries. The potential for associated injuries is greater in an individual who has jumped from a 12-ft fence than in a basketball player who came down on one foot from a hoop jump. Likewise, an elderly woman is more likely to have a second injury when she trips on a curbstone and falls to the pavement on an outstretched hand. The treatment of patients who have chronic medical conditions, such as diabetes or peripheral vascular disease, which can cause sensory deficits, or who

are on chronic immunosuppressive therapy has to be approached with caution. A normal-appearing ankle or minimal tenderness on examination does not exclude the necessity of further evaluation. The ability to bear weight immediately after an injury, with subsequent increase in pain and swelling as the patient continues to ambulate, suggests a sprain rather than a fracture. The time of the injury and previous bony or soft tissue injuries to the ankle need to be documented.

Physical Examination

Once significant swelling has taken place, the examination of the ankle becomes more difficult. This difficulty may be temporized in the busy ED by the application of ice at triage and getting the patient to elevate the foot. Although tempting, the patient should not be examined in a wheelchair, but on a stretcher.

It is critical to examine the joint above and below the injury. Note the position, swelling, and skin integrity of the injured ankle. Ask the patient to plantar and dorsiflex the ankle actively and then put the ankle through a passive range of motion. Soft tissue injuries are more likely when there is a significant difference between the passive and active ranges of motion.

Palpate the area of obvious injury last: Hurt the patient initially and any cooperation will rapidly diminish. Tenderness of the knee, the fibular head, or the proximal fibular shaft suggests a fibulotibialis ligament tear or a Maisonneuve fracture. Compress the fibula toward the tibia just above the midpoint of the calf to exclude clinically an isolated syndesmotic sprain. Starting at least 6 cm proximally, palpate the posterior aspects of lateral and medial malleoli to the distal tips of the shaft.

Examine the Achilles tendon. If there is tenderness or a defect, perform the Thompson test. With the patient prone on a stretcher, squeeze the calf: loss of plantar flexion indicates a complete rupture of the tendon.

Palpate the midfoot and hindfoot over the calcaneus, the tarsals, and the base of the fifth metacarpal. Patients can complain of an ankle injury when they have actually injured the foot or the Achilles tendon. Injuries to these structures are not excluded with the three-view ankle series.

Perform a neurovascular examination, which includes palpation of the dorsalis pedis and posterior tibial pulse and capillary refill. Check the foot for motor and sensory impairment. If the patient cannot plantar flex the great toe, suspect a peroneal nerve injury; if the patient cannot dorsiflex the toes, then suspect a tibial nerve injury. These nerves are rarely injured in ankle injuries. Ask the patient to walk four steps: if the patient can transfer weight from one foot to the other and the findings on physical examination as outlined above are normal, the likelihood of a significant fracture is nil.

IMAGING

The Ottawa Ankle Rules have provided a significant advance in the evaluation of ankle injuries in the ED. Previous studies suggested that not all patients who present to the ED need radiographs.[3] The Ottawa Ankle Rules were derived from an initial series of studies[4–6] and then were prospectively validated.[1,7,8] These studies involved more than 9000 patient encounters and 200 emergency physicians. Two other studies by the same group found the implementation of the rules to be cost-effective and that, once taught, emergency physicians continue to use them.[9,10] Although these studies were carried out in eight academic and community EDs in Canada, other studies at independent sites in the United States,[11,12] the United Kingdom,[13] and France[2] have validated their use. In addition, it has been demonstrated that nurses at triage can apply the rules successfully.[11,13] Only two studies failed to replicate these results,[14,15] but these studies were found to have a flawed methodology or did not accurately assess the rules as developed.

The rules are simple to apply and are illustrated in Figure 276-3. The rules can be used on patients with an injury to the ankle, which is clinically broadly defined as the area of the distal leg and the midfoot

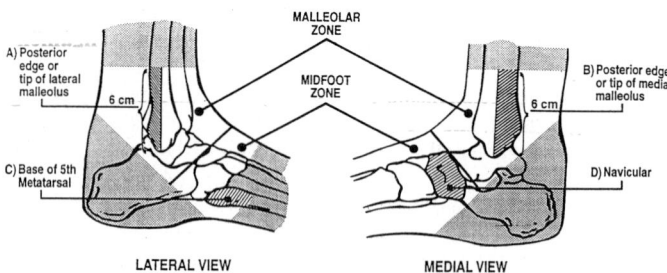

FIG. 276-3. Ottawa Ankle Rules for ankle and midfoot injuries.

subject to twisting injuries. Mechanisms of injury include twisting, direct blunt trauma, and falls. **The Ottawa Ankle Rules were not developed for patients younger than 18 years.** Clinical judgment should prevail if the examination is unreliable due to lack of cooperation, intoxication, distracting injuries, or a diminished sensation in the leg. To assess the ability to bear weight, ask the patient to take four steps. If the patient can complete two transfers to the injured ankle, then the patient passes the test.

Various objections that have been raised in the United States to applying these rules include, but are not limited to, the malpractice potential of missing any fracture, however insignificant; the patient's expectation of a radiograph and perception of a full assessment; and the physician's perception that the proportion of patients with fractures who present with ankle injuries is higher in the United States. Communication with the patient, such as an explanation of the thoroughness of the clinical examination, and the fact that a chip fracture, if missed, is treated like a sprain, is often effective. The saving of time and money for the patients should help them to accept the completeness of the evaluation. In addition, studies done in the United States showed a similar 15 percent fracture rate as demonstrated in Canada, the United Kingdom, France, and Scandinavia.

An excellent review of radiologic subtleties in the diagnosis of extremity injuries is found in Weissman.[16] The use of computed tomography and magnetic resonance imaging in the assessment of ankle injuries, although useful, is not a common practice in the ED.

INJURIES, TREATMENT, AND PROGNOSIS

Soft Tissue

LIGAMENTOUS SPRAINS

Lateral Ligament Complex Sprains of the lateral ankle are the most common ankle injury, and most are minor. The classification systems for ligamentous injuries to the lateral ankle are quite confusing. Older texts described a purely anatomic classification scheme, whereas more recent articles described a more functional system. These two classification systems are probably of little value to emergency physicians. A much more useful approach divides the injuries into two groups: stable and potentially unstable or unstable.[17] If stress testing can be accomplished in the ED and the findings are normal, then the patient has a stable lateral ankle sprain and can be so treated. If results on stress testing are clearly abnormal or indeterminate because of excessive swelling or pain, then the sprain should be treated as unstable.

Treatment of lateral ankle sprains has been controversial. However, a review of more recent literature included some fairly well-performed prospective studies.[18–21] Most of these studies treated patients with grade 2 or 3 ankle sprains with compression, rest, and cryotherapy for 24 to 72 h. They then usually compared two treatment groups: (1) weight bearing with an ankle brace that allows plantar-dorsiflexion while resisting inversion and (2) eversion and plaster immobilization for up to 6 weeks. Patients in the early-mobilization groups returned to work or sport earlier than did the immobilization groups, but at late follow-up there were no differences in outcomes. In addition, direct comparisons of operative repair with cast, cast alone, and early controlled mobilization of acute grade 3 ankle sprains suggested no difference in long-term outcome.[22]

The data indicate that individuals with stable and unstable ankle sprains, who are unable to bear weight easily, should be treated with rest, ice, compression, and elevation (RICE) for 24 to 72 h, depending on the amount of swelling and degree of pain. Individuals who can easily bear weight and have a stable joint probably need no more than simple analgesics and an elastic bandage, near-normal activity with no sports involvement or prolonged walking, and follow-up in 1 week if they still have discomfort. Patients who are unable to bear weight in the ED but appear to have a stable joint can be given an ankle brace and be told to apply it in 24 to 72 h and to follow up with their primary care physician or orthopedist within 1 week for a repeat evaluation. Patients who clearly have an unstable joint should be referred to an orthopedic surgeon, with consideration of a posterior mold. Timing of consultation depends on local preferences, but it would be prudent to establish communication early, because the ultimate decision on the method of treatment lies with the orthopedic surgeon.

Medial Ligament Complex An isolated sprain of the deltoid ligament is rare and usually associated with a fibular fracture or significant tear of the tibial-fibular syndesmosis resulting from an eversion stress. When there is significant medial malleolus tenderness and swelling, Maisonneuve fracture is suspected, and careful attention should be paid to the proximal fibula and fibular shaft. If the radiographs of the ankle and the fibula are negative, then a significant syndesmosis tear should be suspected. Patients with this type of injury should be treated with RICE and early referral to an orthopedist.

Tibiofibular Syndesmotic Complex These injuries are usually associated with a hyperdorsiflexion injury. The talus moves in a superior direction and separates the fibula and tibia, resulting in a partial or complete rupture of the syndesmosis. Patients usually complain of pain just above the plafond. These are significant injuries with prolonged recovery time and should be treated with RICE and early consultation.

An excellent review of deltoid ligament, syndesmosis, and other "atypical ankle sprains" can be found in the work by Clanton and Porter.[17]

PROGNOSIS OF LIGAMENTOUS INJURIES The long-term complications of ankle sprains include functional instability (a subjective sensation of giving way without mechanical instability), mechanical instability (a demonstrable laxity), chronic pain, stiffness, and recurrent swelling. The documented incidence of complications is highly variable, from 6 to 40 percent.[19] The long-term sequelae can be reduced with early rehabilitation. Physical therapy should be directed initially at active and passive range-of-motion exercises followed by early mobilization, strengthening exercises, proprioceptive training, and restoration of normal activity.

STRAINS AND CONTUSIONS Strains are injuries to muscles or tendons and usually are not associated with a specific injury but rather are due to repetitive stress. The stress can be due to overuse secondary to athletic activity or to poorly fitting footwear. Treatment includes simple analgesics (anti-inflammatory medications may be beneficial), rest, identification and correction of provocative factors, and specific rehabilitative exercises. Contusions are usually caused by direct trauma, typically from a baseball or a hockey puck. Fractures are rare and usually are of the bone cortex only. Treatment is symptomatic with simple analgesics and ice.

PERONEAL TENDON SUBLUXATIONS AND DISLOCATIONS These injuries can be easily misdiagnosed as lateral ankle sprains. The mechanism is described by a sudden hyperdorsiflexion of the foot while the peroneal tendons are taut in eversion. This injury most often is associated with skiing. The superior retinaculum holding the peroneal tendons in place is stripped off the posterolateral malleolus. In more severe injuries, a small avulsion fracture is noted on a radiograph, and the peroneal tendons dislocate or, more often, sublux anteriorly over the distal tip of the fibula. Consider this injury when tenderness and ecchymosis over the posterior edge of the lateral malleolus are noted in the absence of tenderness over the anterior talofibular ligament. It is important to consider this diagnosis in the acute setting: the treatment is frequently operative repair of the retinaculum.[17]

ACHILLES TENDON RUPTURES These injuries are most common in sedentary males engaging in a weekend of sporting activity and are a result of sudden plantar flexion of the foot. Treatment is individual, although the tendency is toward operative repair of the tendon in individuals who want full return to all activities.

Fractures and Dislocations

CLASSIFICATION SCHEMES There are multiple classifications of ankle fractures. The more complex use the position of the foot at the time of injury and the deforming force. These classifications are useful in predicting associated injuries. In the Lauge-Hansen classification system, the first word refers to the position and the second word refers to the force. The Danis-Weber classification is based on the level of the fracture of the fibula. Proximal fractures of the fibula are associated with damage to the syndesmosis and the increased likelihood of an unstable fracture. There are three types of injury in this classification scheme: type A (fracture of the fibula below the syndesmosis) is a supination injury and corresponds to the Lauge-Hansen type of supination and adduction injury; type B (fibular fracture at the level of the syndesmosis) is associated with an external rotation force and corresponds with the supination and eversion injury of Lauge-Hansen; and type C (fibular fracture above the syndesmosis) is associated with an external rotation and abduction force and corresponds with the pronation and eversion or abduction Lauge-Hansen injuries. The AO classification system amplifies the Danis-Weber system by subdividing each classification type into three subtypes to better describe associated medial injuries. The simplest classification system is based on radiographic appearance. This scheme is commonly employed and uses the terms *unimalleolar, bimalleolar,* and *trimalleolar* to describe fractures of the ankle.

Although it is important to have a basic understanding of these classification systems, the most essential aspects of ankle injuries to appreciate is the stability of the injury and the exclusion of associated injuries (Table 276-1).

TREATMENT All fractures of the ankle, with the exception of fibular avulsion fractures, require immobilization by cast alone or surgical reduction with subsequent casting. **Avulsion fractures are treated as stable ankle sprains if they are minimally displaced, smaller than 3 mm in diameter, and there is no indication of a medial ligamentous injury.** The treatment goal with all other ankle fractures is to restore the anatomic relationship of the ankle, maintain reduction during the healing process, and institute early mobilization of the ankle. To obtain these goals, the talus has to be anatomically positioned in the mortise, the joint line has to be parallel to the ground, and the articular surface has to be smooth. The means to attain this goal depends not only on the type of fracture but also on the age and athletic expectations of the patient. Local preferences also may play a role in this decision. Most fractures, with the exception of unimalleolar injuries, require open reduction and fixation. The Maisonneuve fracture (AO types C2 and C3), although considered an unstable injury, can generally be treated with cast immobilization for 6 to 8 weeks, depending on the stability of the syndesmosis.[15] The Bosworth fracture, a rare variation of the Maisonneuve fracture in which the proximal fibula gets trapped behind the tibia, usually requires operative reduction. The debate over the necessity of operative treatment for unimalleolar fractures with associated syndesmosis and deltoid ligamentous injuries is complex and beyond the scope of this chapter. Stable fibular fractures are treated with a short leg-walking cast for 6 weeks.

The timing of consultation is discussed below. In the interim, fractures should be splinted with a posterior mold and kept non-weight bearing in all cases and elevated with application of ice in many cases. The analgesic need of the patient should be addressed. There is absolutely no basis for the practice of withholding analgesics until operative consent is obtained.

TABLE 276-1   Associated and Occult Injuries of the Ankle

Injury	Clinical Suspicion	Confirmatory Test
Important to identify in the ED		
Fracture of base of fifth metatarsal	Examine lateral foot, tenderness to palpation	Anteroposterior foot radiograph
Maisonneuve fracture	Examine proximal fibula and shaft, tenderness to palpation	Fibula radiograph
Peroneal tendon dislocation	Palpable anterior tendon dislocation or subluxation	Clinical examination
Usually identified in follow-up of ankle sprains		
Osteochondral injuries	Diffuse ankle swelling, passive plantar flexion	Ankle mortise view/CT
Syndesmosis tear	Significant ankle pain, positive squeeze test	Widened mortise with weight bearing
Anterior calcaneal process fracture	Tenderness more inferioanterior than a typical ankle sprain	Lateral ankle radiograph/CT
Lateral talar process fracture	Tenderness just distal to the tip of fibula	Ankle mortise view/CT
Os trigonum	Tenderness anterior to Achilles tendon	Lateral ankle radiograph

Abbreviation: CT = computed tomography.

OSTEOCHONDRAL FRACTURES   Osteochondral fractures are due to acute trauma or repetitive stress. These injuries vary from a deformation of the cartilage overlying the talar dome to a free-floating avulsion fracture. The staging and treatment of these lesions are complex, and orthopedic consultation is required. Treatment can involve excision or cast immobilization for up to 6 weeks.[17]

PROGNOSIS OF ANKLE FRACTURES   Early complications and sequelae of ankle fractures are several and include skin necrosis and osteomyelitis in the short term and chronic pain, osteoarthritis, malunion, nonunion, and reflex sympathetic dystrophy in the long term. Although most of these problems are rare, postreduction arthritis can complicate up to 30 percent of fractures.

FRACTURE-DISLOCATIONS AND OPEN FRACTURES   Dislocations of the ankle joint can occur in one of four planes and are frequently associated with a fracture. The posterior dislocation is most common and happens usually when the foot is plantar flexed and a backward force is applied. The injury is usually associated with rupture of the tibiofibular ligaments or fracture of the lateral malleolus. The anterior dislocation occurs with a dorsiflexed foot and fracture of the anterior aspect of the tibia. Lateral displacement is accompanied by ligamentous disruption and fracture of either or both malleoli. The talus can be displaced upward with a significant impaction. There will be an associated fracture of the talar dome or tibial plafond and disruption of the syndesmosis.

Patients with fracture-dislocations of the ankle are at considerable risk of neurovascular compromise and conversion of a closed fracture to an open one. Under most circumstances, the reduction of fracture-dislocations is left to an orthopedic surgeon. However, if there is vascular compromise, indicated by absent pulses and a cool dusky foot or tenting of the skin caused by fractured bone, the emergency physician should perform the reduction. Do not delay reduction to obtain radiographs. If possible, place the patient on the stretcher, with the affected foot hanging over the side with a flexed knee. This position forces the leg into external rotation and the foot into internal rotation. It also gives the physician the advantage of gravity. Administer adequate intravenous analgesia with the appropriate cardiorespiratory monitoring. The heel and foot should be grasped with both hands (with an assistant stabilizing the proximal leg), and downward traction and rotation should be applied in the opposite direction of the mechanism of the injury. Little force is required. A splint is applied once distal perfusion is restored and the foot is again elevated. Irreducible fractures are quite rare and, of course, require open reduction.

Protect open fractures from further contamination by applying a wet, sterile dressing over the wound with a gauze roll. No studies have substantiated the application of Betadine-soaked gauze to the lacera-tion site. Splint the injury until radiographs and definitive treatment are available. Tetanus-diphtheria toxoid is given as necessary, and tetanus immunoglobulin is considered if the wound is grossly contaminated. The antibiotic of choice is cephalexin, and an aminoglycoside is added if the wound is grossly contaminated. Consider clindamycin for patients with penicillin allergy.

TIMING OF CONSULTATION

No set of rigid rules for the timing of orthopedic consultation exists to guide emergency physicians for specific ankle injuries. Although it may be reasonable to request an in-person orthopedic consultation in an academic center at 3 o'clock in the morning for a stable ankle fracture, this will not endear a community-based emergency physician to his or her orthopedic colleagues. Although it may be perfectly acceptable for an emergency physician in some countries to apply a circular short leg cast to an AO type A1 fracture and arrange follow-up, this approach would not be common practice in other locales (Table 276-2).

EMERGENCY DEPARTMENT TREATMENT ISSUES

Pharmacotherapy

The need for analgesia should always be addressed. Because individual perception of pain varies, a simple ankle sprain may require only an elastic bandage or acetaminophen in most patients, whereas some will require oral narcotics. **Studies have suggested that there is no benefit of using nonsteroidal anti-inflammatory drugs in the treatment of ankle fractures.**[23] Patients who are in significant distress or who should be kept nonoral because of anticipated surgery require parenteral analgesia.

Immobilization

Noncircular cast immobilization can be accomplished with a Jones bandage or a posterior mold.

A Jones bandage has more padding and probably is more comfortable for patients with severe bruising and swelling, but may not accomplish the same degree of immobilization as a posterior mold. The patient should be supine on a stretcher. Apply two to three layers of abdominal pads, extending from the distal foot to just below the knee, and hold the pads in place with 4-in. elastic bandages. A 4-in. cotton cast padding can be applied, in place of the abdominal pads, in a circular fashion overlapping by at least 50 percent with a minimum of three complete layers. The Jones bandage should not be used for more than a couple of days.

A posterior mold is most easily applied if the patient is prone on a stretcher with the knee flexed to 90 degrees. Most EDs have prepack-

TABLE 276-2 Timing of Consultation

Immediate Consultation in ED	Deferred Consultation*	Within 1 Week
All open fractures	Stable unimalleolar fractures	Potentially unstable sprains
All fracture dislocations	Unstable ligamentous injuries	
All dislocations	Acute peroneal dislocations	
All trimalleolar fractures†	Pediatric Salter I, II	
All bimalleolar fractures†		
Unstable unimalleolar fractures†		
Pediatric Salter III, IV, V†		
Maisonneuve fractures†		

*Implies that communication is established at time of diagnosis and specific time of consultation has been set.
†Consultation can be delayed in the ED in fractures without neurovascular compromise and appropriate splinting.

aged padded splint material available. For extra padding, apply a single layer of 4-in. cotton cast padding from the toes to the knee, followed by the fiberglass splint (Figure 276-4). If more support is required, especially in the setting of an unstable joint, another slab can be added to provide additional medial and lateral support.

Size the patient, if necessary, for crutches and instruct in their appropriate use. For a weight-bearing patient, a cast shoe can be applied.

Ankle Braces and Cast Boots

Several different ankle braces (which allow dorsoplantar flexion but do not allow inversion or eversion of the ankle) are available. These devices vary from complex applications of athletic tape to lace-up splints and inflatable plastic stirrup-type braces (see Chap. 267). Although few studies have compared these braces, it is clear that any device that speeds mobilization and weight bearing will promote early return to full function.[2,19] A recent useful addition is the cast boot. This appliance, which resembles a ski boot, is easily applied and molds to the joint by inflatable air bladders. It can be used with significant ankle sprains, nondisplaced metatarsal fractures, and stable ankle fractures.

Cryotherapy and Other Modalities

Ice packs have been shown to limit swelling and decrease pain. The pack is applied directly to the ankle or the splint and is left on for 20 min at a time. It can be repeated every few hours. Ultrasound has not been shown to promote healing.[24]

REFERENCES

1. Stiell IG, McKnight RD, Greenberg GH, et al: Interobserver agreement in the examination of acute injury patients. *Am J Emerg Med* 10:14, 1992.
2. Auleley G-R, Ravaud P, Giraudeau B, et al: Implementation of the Ottawa Ankle Rules in France. *JAMA* 277:1935, 1997.
3. Auletta AG, Conway WF, Hayes CW, et al: Indications for radiography in patients with acute ankle injuries: Role of the physical examination. *AJR* 157:789, 1991.
4. Stiell I, Wells G, Laupacis A, et al: Multicentre trial to introduce the Ottawa Ankle Rules for use of radiography in acute ankle injuries. *BMJ* 311:594, 1995.
5. Stiell IG, McDowell I, Nair RC, et al: Use of radiography in acute ankle injuries: Physicians' attitudes and practice. *CMAJ* 147:1671, 1992.
6. Stiell IG, Greenberg GH, McKnight RD, et al: Decision rules for the use of radiography in acute ankle injuries. *JAMA* 269:1127, 1993.
7. Stiell IG, McKnight RD, Greenberg GH, et al: Implementation of the Ottawa Ankle Rules. *JAMA* 271:827, 1994.
8. Stiell IG, Greenberg GH, McKnight RD, et al: A study to develop clinical decision rules for the use of radiography in acute ankle injuries. *Ann Emerg Med* 21:384, 1992.
9. Anis AH, Stiell IG, Stewart DG, et al: Cost-effectiveness analysis of the Ottawa Ankle Rules. *Ann Emerg Med* 26:422, 1995.
10. Verbeek PR, Stiell IG, Hebert G, et al: Ankle radiograph utilization after learning a decision rule: A 12-month follow-up. *Acad Emerg Med* 4:776, 1997.
11. Pigman EC, Klug RK, Sanford S, et al: Evaluation of the Ottawa clinical decision rules for the use of radiography in acute ankle and midfoot injuries in the emergency department: An independent site assessment. *Ann Emerg Med* 24:41, 1994.
12. Verma S, Hamilton K, Hawkins HH, et al: Clinical application of the Ottawa Ankle Rules for the use of radiography in acute ankle injuries: An independent site assessment. *AJR* 169:825, 1997.
13. Salt P, Clancy M: Implementation of the Ottawa Ankle Rules by nurses working in an accident and emergency department. *J Accid Emerg Med* 14:363, 1997.
14. Lucchesi GM, Cerasani C, Jackson RE, et al: Sensitivity of Ottawa Ankle Rules. *Ann Emerg Med* 26:1, 1995.
15. Kerr L, Kelly AM, Grant J, et al: Failed validation of a clinical decision rule for the use of radiography in acute ankle injury. *N Z Med J* 107:294, 1994.
16. Weissman BN: The radiologic diagnosis of subtle extremity injuries. *Emerg Med Clin North Am* 3:600, 1985.
17. Clanton TO, Porter DA: Primary care of foot and ankle injuries in the athlete. *Clin Sports Med* 16:435, 1997.
18. Kerkhoffs GM, Rowe BH, Assendelft WJ, et al: Immobilisation for ankle sprains. A systematic review. *Arch Orthop Trauma Surg* 121:462, 2001.

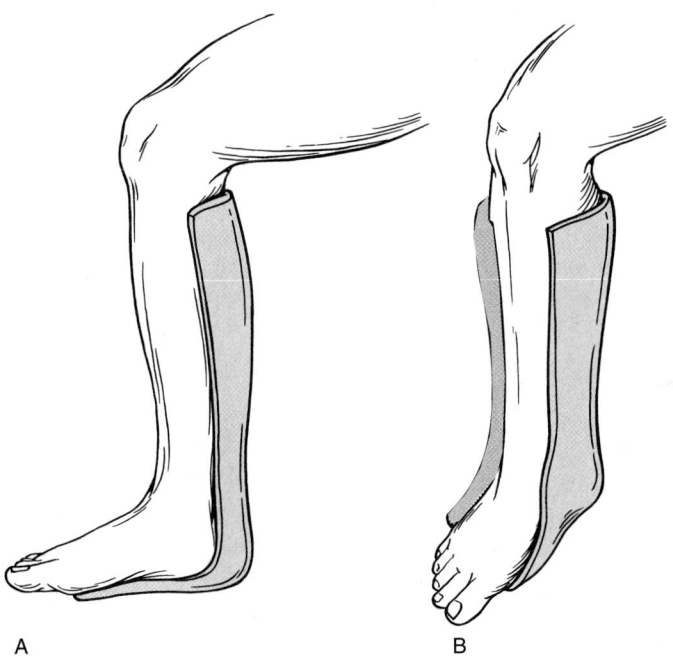

A B

FIG. 276-4. Short-leg posterior splint without (**A**) and with (**B**) a stirrup splint.

19. Konradsen L, Holmer P, Sondergaard L: Early mobilizing treatment for grade III ankle ligament injuries. *Foot Ankle* 12:69, 1991.
20. Karlsson J, Eriksson BI, Sward L: Early functional treatment for acute ligament injuries of the ankle. *Scand J Med Sci Sports* 6:341, 1996.
21. Kerkhoffs GM, Struijs PA, Marti RK, et al: Different functional treatment strategies for acute lateral ligament injuries in adults. *Cochrane Database Syst Rev* 3:CD002938, 2002.
22. Munk B, Holm-Christensen K, Lind T: Long-term outcome after ruptured lateral ankle ligaments. *Acta Orthop Scand* 66:452, 1995.
23. Dupont M, Beliveau P, Theiriault G: The efficacy of antiinflammatory medication in the treatment of the acutely sprained ankle. *Am J Sports Med* 15:41, 1987.
24. Van Der Windt DA, Van Der Heijden GJ, Van Den Berg SG, et al: Ultrasound therapy of acute ankle sprains. *Cochrane Database Syst Rev* 1:CD001250, 2002.

277 FOOT INJURIES
John A. Michael
Ian G. Stiell

The foot is a complex, highly evolved structure that bears the weight of the body and acts as a lever to propel the body forward while walking or running. It is designed to carry the body over varied terrain with little apparent difficulty. Although most injuries are minor and heal with time, undertreated and unrecognized injuries can result in significant long-term pain and disability. Radiographs are sometimes difficult to interpret, and seemingly minor abnormalities can be associated with a significant injury.

ANATOMY

Chopart and Lisfranc joints divide the foot into three regions. The talus and the calcaneum comprise the hindfoot. The midfoot contains the cuneiforms, the cuboid, and the navicular. The metatarsals and the phalanges make up the forefoot (Figure 277-1). The foot consists of 28 bones and 57 articular surfaces. Numerous intrinsic muscles and ligaments contribute to the integrity of the foot's structure. The biomechanical specifics of the foot involved in ambulation are extremely complex. In general, eversion and inversion occur about the subtalar and calcaneus tarsal joints, whereas adduction and abduction and flexion and extension occur about the metatarsophalangeal and interphalangeal joints, respectively.

The body weight when standing is distributed about the heel to the rear and the five metatarsal heads to the front. The curved shape of the foot is held in position by three arches. The shape of the bones, the arrangement of the ligaments, and the tone of the muscles maintain the position of the arches. The plantar aponeurosis covers the sole of the foot and is a strong band of fascia that originates on the medial side of the calcaneum and fuses with the fibrous sheaths of the phalanges.

The blood supply of the foot comes from branches of the popliteal artery. The anterior tibial artery serves the dorsum of the foot, and its branch, the dorsalis pedis, can be palpated over the dorsum of the midfoot. Branches of the posterior tibial and the peroneal arteries serve the sole. The motor and sensory nerves of the foot include branches of the femoral and sciatic nerves and include branches of the saphenous, sural (sensory), and deep and superficial peroneal nerves (sensory and motor) (see Figure 267-1B).

The essential parts of the anatomy of concern include, but are not limited to, the following. The first metatarsal bears twice the weight as any other metatarsal, and injuries to this bone require a more conservative approach. The blood supply to the foot is tenuous, and major fractures of the talus and subtalar dislocations are complicated by avascular necrosis. The base of the second metatarsal is the "keystone"

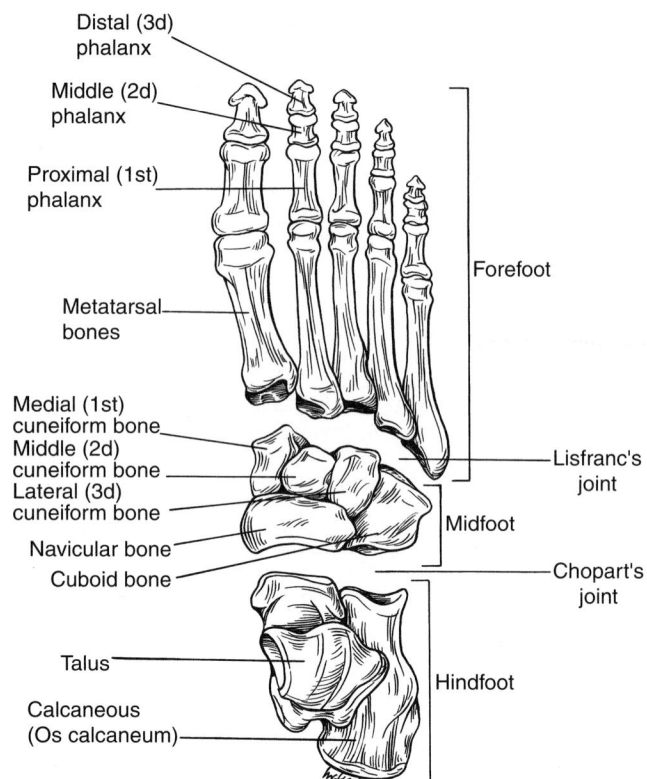

FIG. 277-1. Bony anatomy of the foot.

of the Lisfranc complex, and any injury to this area has to be carefully evaluated.

EVALUATION

History

As with all injuries, it is important to obtain an adequate history. Many injuries to the foot are associated with significant forces or falls from a height, and other injuries have to be sought. In general, most foot injuries are caused by direct or twisting forces. Twisting forces are associated with avulsion-type injuries and are generally more minor than the injuries caused by direct trauma. Previous injuries, general medical condition, and repetitive mechanisms are important to elicit from the patient. Increasing inability to ambulate after an injury and increasing pain may be suggestive of a minor sprain or of an impending vascular catastrophe. Special care should be paid to puncture wounds. Consider the type of shoes worn, the possibility of a foreign body, and the potential of tetanus.

Physical Examination

Elevation of the foot and the application of ice at triage will facilitate the physical examination. The patient should be examined on a stretcher. Examination of the foot includes an ankle examination (see Chap. 276, "Ankle Injuries"). The foot should be inspected for any loss of skin integrity, deformity, and swelling and ecchymosis. Passive range of motion should be assessed and compared with the uninjured foot. Palpate the Achilles tendon, the calcaneum, the dorsum of the midfoot, and then the metatarsals and phalanges. Pay special attention to the base of the fifth metatarsal and the area over the base of the second metatarsal. Actively move the various joints of the foot through their ranges of motion. Next, grasp two adjacent metatarsal heads and move them in opposite dorsoplantar directions. If the foregoing examination does not suggest a specific injury, observe the patient ambulating. Normal findings on examination and the ability to complete several weight transfers to the injured foot essentially exclude a significant injury.

IMAGING

Patients with normal findings on examination of the hindfoot and forefoot and on examination of the ankle and midfoot (see Figure 276-3 for the Ottawa Ankle Rules) probably do not need radiographs. Clinical judgment should always prevail in the decision-making process. Abnormal findings on examination mandate a complete, three-view, standard foot series. If there is pain about the heel, an axial view of the calcaneum should be added. The lateral view of the foot and the axial view of the calcaneum are important in excluding hindfoot injuries, whereas the anteroposterior and oblique projections are more useful in delineating midfoot and forefoot injuries.

Other plain radiographic views, bone scans, and computed tomographic (CT) scans are seldom used by emergency physicians in the evaluation of foot injuries. Emergency physicians, however, occasionally should order CT scans of the foot to exclude a subtle diastasis (>1 mm) at the Lisfranc joint.

INJURIES AND TREATMENT

Acute Soft Tissue Injuries

Puncture wounds are discussed in Chap. 46. Complicated foot infections, gunshot wounds to the foot, and many lawn mower injuries require consultation and/or operative debridement.[1,2] The latter two open injuries require a careful search for associated vascular and tendon injuries, radiographs to document foreign-body presence and bony involvement, consideration of tetanus vaccine and immunoglobulin administration, aggressive wound irrigation, analgesics, and antibiotics in most cases. Do not rely on the presence of fever, abnormal radiographs, or elevated white cell counts and erythrocyte sedimentation rates to exclude the diagnosis of osteomyelitis.[3,4]

TURF TOE   Forced hyperextension of the first proxima phalanx causes a sprain or tear of the metatarsophalangeal joint capsule with dorsal subluxation. The injury is usually associated with repetitive push-off mechanism from a hard surface. The initial treatment is conservative, with analgesics and a supportive shoe to prevent further dorsiflexion. Orthopedic referral is needed for continued pain.

PLANTAR FASCIA RUPTURE   This is a tear in the plantar fascia at the point of insertion on the calcaneum. Patients describe a sudden pop and pain that is usually associated with sudden plantar flexion of the foot. Treatment is nonoperative.

TENDON RUPTURES   Acute ruptures of the tendons of the foot are rare and usually associated with penetrating or lacerating injuries. Extensor and flexor hallucis tendon injuries are repaired primarily. The treatment of other tendon transections is controversial.

CRUSH INJURIES AND COMPARTMENT SYNDROME   Injuries caused by crush-type mechanisms without associated skin or bone injuries may appear innocuous. These injuries, however, place the foot at risk for the development of compartment syndrome. Compartment syndrome should be suspected when there is pain out of proportion to the injury. Typically, the foot is tensely swollen, and the pain is not relieved by elevation and is increased by passive dorsiflexion of the big toe. Paresthesias may be present, but pedal pulses and capillary refill are often preserved. If compartment syndrome is suspected, intracom-

partmental pressures must be measured. There are multiple compartments in the foot. The measure of pressure in these small compartments is technically difficult, and orthopedic consultation may be necessary to exclude this diagnosis. Immediate fasciotomy is required once the diagnosis is confirmed.

Fractures and Dislocations

HINDFOOT   Talar fractures are uncommon. Minor avulsion fractures of the neck, body, and lateral process are usually treated with a posterior slab, crutches, and orthopedic follow-up. Os trigonum and transchondral talar dome fractures are difficult to identify in the emergency department and sometimes are diagnosed in the follow-up of "ankle sprains." Major fractures of the talar neck and body are associated with severe dorsiflexion and axial forces. These injuries often require open reduction and merit immediate orthopedic consultation. These fractures are frequently complicated by avascular necrosis.

Peritalar or subtalar dislocations are rare. In this injury, the calcaneus talar and talonavicular joints are disrupted, and the tibiotalar joint remains intact. Although the dislocation can occur in any direction, medial dislocation is by far the most common and is the result of a severe rotational-inversion force. These injuries require immediate orthopedic consultation and emergent reduction. Closed reduction sometimes can be accomplished by using conscious sedation in the emergency department, although frequently a general or regional anesthetic in the operating room is required.

An axial load to the heel, caused by a fall from a height, is the mechanism associated with most fractures of the calcaneum. These injuries are frequently associated with other injuries, most commonly vertebral column, forearm, and other lower extremity fractures. Fractures should be categorized as intra-articular or extra-articular.

Although the more common subtalar, intra-articular fractures are usually obvious on the lateral foot radiograph, some compression fractures may be subtle. When this injury is suspected by mechanism or examination, carefully examine the radiograph by using the measurement of Boehler angle. **If the angle is smaller than 20 degrees, suspect a fracture** (Figure 277-2). The criterion for open reduction of these fractures is controversial, with CT scanning playing an important diagnostic and preoperative planning role. Seek immediate orthopedic consultation. In the interim, apply a well-padded posterior splint, elevate the foot, and address analgesic needs. Comminuted fractures of the calcaneum can be extremely painful. **The incidence of compartment syndrome with these fractures is high.**

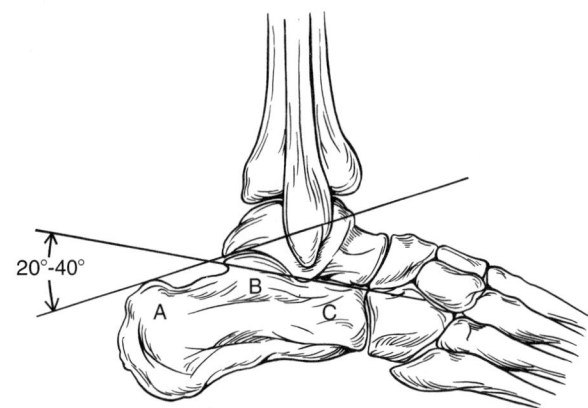

FIG. 277-2. Boehler angle is formed by two lines, one between the posterior tuberosity *(A)* and the apex of the posterior facet *(B)*, and the other between the apex of the posterior facet *(B)* and the apex of the anterior process *(C)*. An angle smaller than 20 degrees suggests a calcaneal compression fracture.

Extra-articular fractures are less common and usually associated with a rotational mechanism and an axial load. Included are fractures of the tuberosity, the sustentaculum tali, anterior process avulsion, and extra-articular oblique body fractures. Most nondisplaced fractures can be treated conservatively with a posterior slab, crutches, and early orthopedic consultation.

MIDFOOT   Isolated fractures of the navicular, cuboid, and cuneiforms are uncommon and difficult to identify on radiograph. Fractures of the navicular are most common and can involve the tuberosity, the dorsal surface, and the body. Isolated fractures of the cuboid and cuneiforms are extremely rare, and an associated injury to the Lisfranc joint should be sought. Most isolated injuries of the tarsal bones are treated conservatively.

The six-bone tarsometatarsal complex is known as the *Lisfranc joint*. Injuries to this joint are not uncommon, and unfortunately up to 20 percent of these injuries are missed in the emergency department.[5] The plantar ecchymosis sign, a bruise on the plantar surface of the midfoot, is suggested as an occult sign of an injury.[6] The force required and the mechanism of injury are varied and can range from a seemingly minor rotational force to a severe axial load, as seen in an automobile accident. The great majority of injuries to the Lisfranc joint are associated with fractures, usually of the metatarsals, the cuboid, or the cuneiforms. **A fracture of the base of the second metatarsal is pathognomonic of a disruption of the Lisfranc ligamentous complex** (Figure 277-3). The Lisfranc injury is classified by the direction of the dislocation. A divergent dislocation describes metatarsals splayed in medial and lateral directions, usually between the first and second metatarsals. In isolated dislocations, one or more metatarsals are displaced from the rest. In homolateral dislocations, all five metatarsals are displaced in the same direction, either laterally or medially. Suspect this injury if there is point tenderness over the midfoot or when there is laxity between the first and second metatarsals in a dorsal-to-plantar direction. Diagnosis is made radiographically on the anteroposterior view when there is a gap larger than 1 mm between the bases of the first and second metatarsals. Other radiographic signs

are loss of alignment of the medial edge of the base of the second metatarsal with the medial edge of the middle cuneiform on the anteroposterior or oblique view; loss of alignment of the lateral border of the third metacarpal shaft with the lateral border of the lateral cuneiform on the oblique view; or loss of alignment of the medial border of the fourth metatarsal with the medial border of the cuboid on the oblique view (Figure 277-4).[5] Weight-bearing radiographs have been suggested to make the diagnosis, but recent studies have suggested that CT scanning is the imaging modality of choice.[7] Injuries to the Lisfranc joint frequently require open reduction and fixation or percutaneous placement of Kirschner wires and non-weightbearing for several weeks. These injuries are complicated by dorsalis pedis artery damage in the short term and degenerative arthritis and chronic pain in the long term.

FOREFOOT   Metatarsal fractures are associated most often with a crush or more occasionally with a twisting injury. Metatarsal fractures are divided into shaft and neck fractures. Nondisplaced shaft injuries are usually treated conservatively with a walking cast or an orthopedic shoe. An exception is a fracture of the first metatarsal shaft. Keep this injury non-weight bearing. Likewise, displaced shaft fractures of the middle metatarsals can be treated with closed reduction, followed by immobilization in a cast and non-weight bearing for 6 weeks. A displaced first metatarsal fracture often will require an open reduction and fixation. Metatarsal neck fractures generally follow the treatment of shaft fractures, but postreduction instability of displaced neck fractures is not uncommon, and open fixation is sometimes required.

Fifth metatarsal fractures are the most common of the metatarsal fractures. Shaft fractures usually can be treated conservatively, as above. **The Jones fracture is described as a transverse fracture through the base of the fifth metatarsal 10 to 20 mm distal to the proximal part of the metatarsal (Figure 277-5). This fracture is fre-**

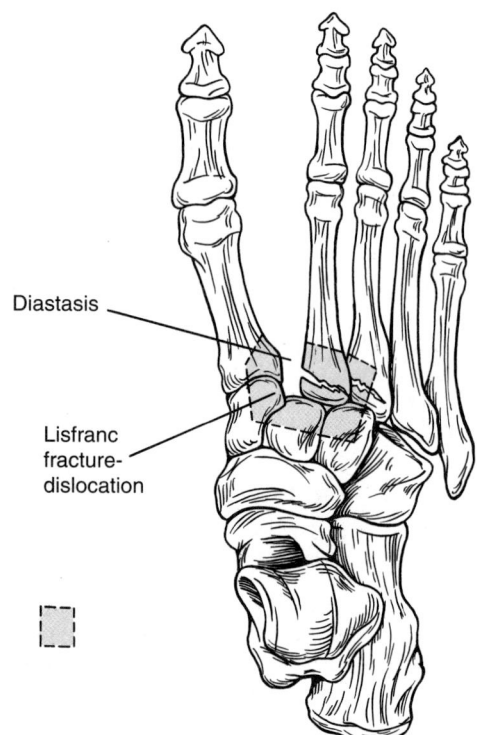

Diastasis

Lisfranc fracture-dislocation

FIG. 277-3. Fracture of the base of the second metatarsal.

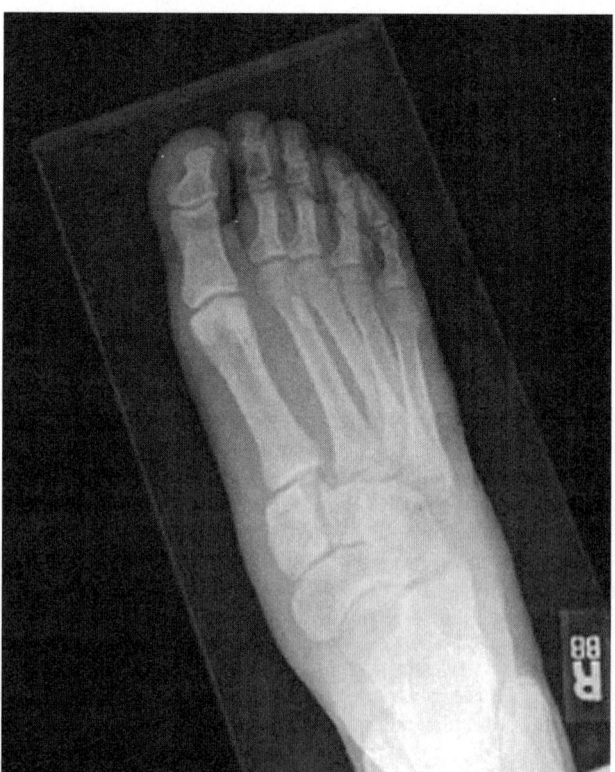

FIG. 277-4. Radiograph of Lisfranc fracture with large gap between the bases of the first and second metatarsals and malalignment of the second, third, and fourth metatarsals with the middle cuneiform, lateral cuneiform, and cuboid, respectively.

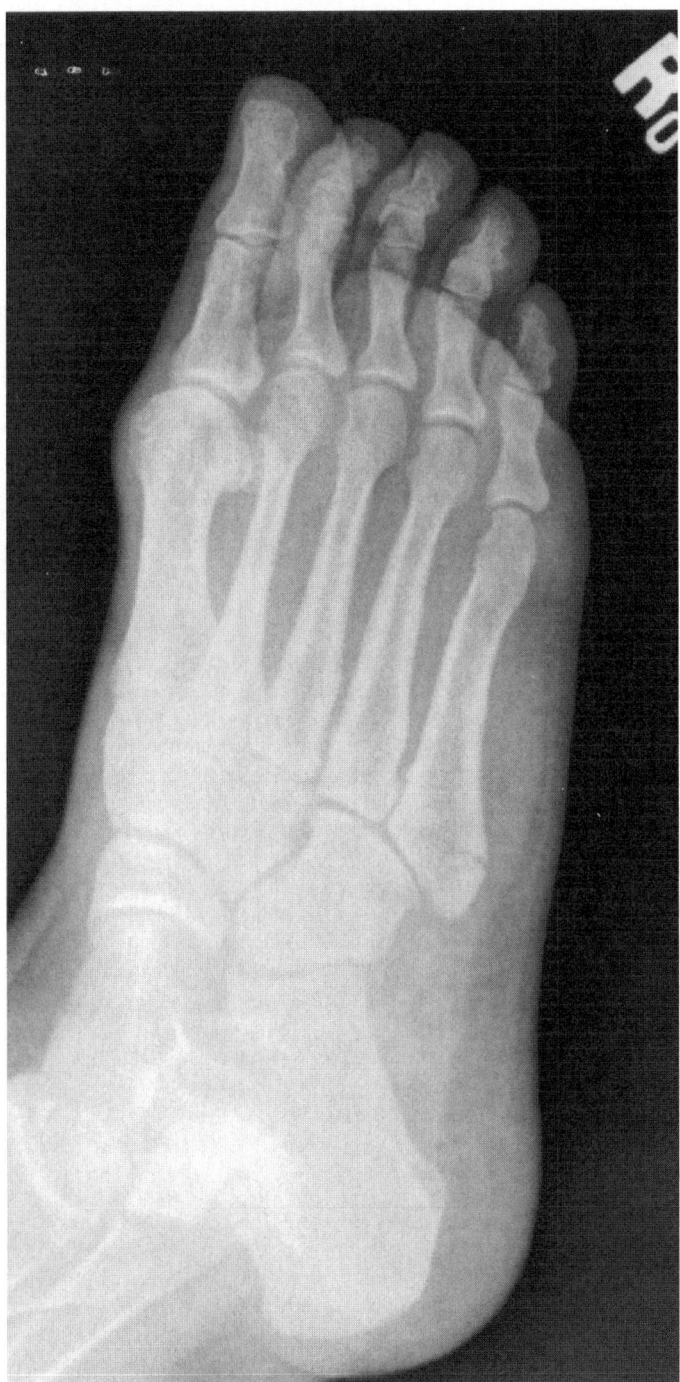

FIG. 277-5. Radiograph of a Jones fracture.

quently complicated by nonunion or malunion and should be treated with a non-weight-bearing cast for 6 weeks. The "pseudo-Jones" is an avulsion fracture of the tuberosity of the base proximal to the articulation between the bases of the fourth and fifth metatarsals. It can be treated with a cast shoe (Figure 277-6).

Most nondisplaced phalangeal fractures can be treated conservatively with "buddy taping" and, occasionally, a cast shoe. Address the patient's analgesic need and arrange orthopedic consultation on a pro re nata basis. Advise against prolonged ambulation or standing in the first week. Displaced fractures can be manipulated into position by using a digital block and manual traction. Some investigators advocate open reduction of some displaced fractures, especially of the big toe.

Most dislocations of the forefoot involve the distal interphalangeal and posterior interphalangeal joints of the second through fifth toes.

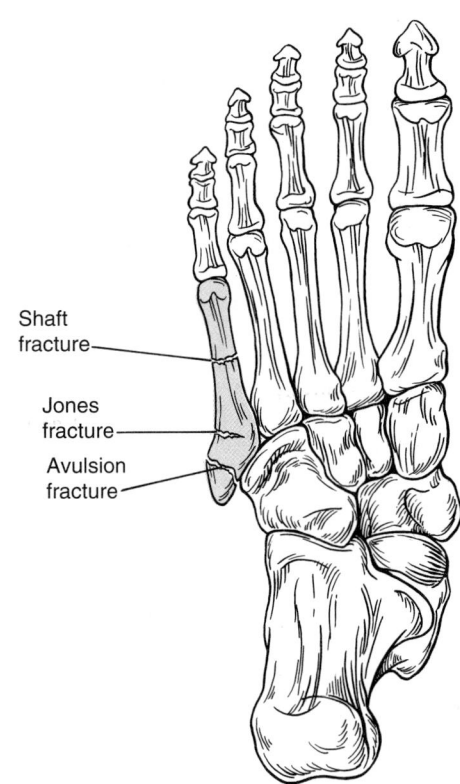

FIG. 277-6. Fractures of the fifth metatarsal.

These injuries can be easily reduced by manual traction and treated with buddy taping, as needed. Dislocations of the big toe are rare, occasionally difficult to reduce, and require walking-cast immobilization for 3 weeks.

OPEN FRACTURES

Open fractures of the foot require immediate orthopedic consultation. In the interim, protect open fractures from further contamination by applying a wet, sterile dressing over the wound with a gauze roll. Splint the injury until definitive treatment is available. Consider tetanus immunoglobulin if the wound is grossly contaminated. The antibiotic of choice is cephalexin and add an aminoglycoside if the wound is grossly contaminated. Consider clindamycin for patients with a penicillin allergy. If there is going to be a significant delay to operative management, the wound should be irrigated.

TIMING OF CONSULTATION

Like ankle injuries, no set of rigid rules for the timing of orthopedic consultation exists to guide emergency physicians for each specific foot injury. In Table 277-1 a general guideline is set forth. Timing of consultation will vary with local preferences.

EMERGENCY DEPARTMENT TREATMENT ISSUES

Analgesia

The need for analgesia should always be addressed by the emergency physician. Because individual perception of pain varies, a fifth metatarsal tuberosity fracture may require acetaminophen and a cast shoe in most patients, whereas others will require hydrocodone or oxycodone with acetaminophen. Patients who are in significant distress, or who should be kept nonoral because of anticipated surgery, require parenteral analgesia.

TABLE 277-1   Timing of Consultation for Foot Injuries

Immediate Consultation in Emergency Department	Deferred Consultation*	Within 1 Week	PRN
All open fractures	Extra-articular calcaneus fractures	Avulsion fractures, calcaneus	Pseudo-Jones fracture
All fracture dislocations	First metatarsal fractures	Avulsion fractures, tarsal	Phalangeal fractures
Major talar neck and body fractures†	Displaced metatarsal shaft	Metatarsal fractures	Phalangeal dislocations
Intra-articular calcaneus fractures†	True Jones fractures	Pediatric metatarsal fractures	Soft tissue injuries
All Lisfranc injuries†	Tendon ruptures and lacerations	Ruptured plantar fascia	
Most gunshot wounds	Retained foreign bodies		
Suspected compartment syndrome			

*Implies that communication is established at time of diagnosis and that the specific time of consultation has been set.
†Consultation can be delayed in the emergency department in fractures without neurovascular compromise and with appropriate splinting.

Immobilization

Most fractures of the foot can be splinted by a posterior slab or a Jones bandage (the appropriate method of application is discussed in Chap. 276, "Ankle Injuries"). Cast shoes, variably called orthopedic, Reece, or post-op shoes, are useful in splinting minor foot fractures when the patient is allowed to bear weight on the injured extremity. Cast shoes also can be applied over a posterior splint to allow weight bearing. Apply an appropriately sized piece of felt or cotton padding between the two phalanges when they are being buddy taped.

Cryotherapy

Ice packs have been shown to limit swelling and decrease pain.[8]

REFERENCES

1. Boucree JB, Gabriel RA, Lezine-Hanna JT: Gunshot wounds to the foot. *Orthop Clin North Am* 26:191, 1995.
2. Anger DM, Ledbetter BR, Stasikelis PJ, et al: Injuries of the foot related to the use of lawn mowers. *J Bone Joint Surg [Am]* 77:719, 1995.
3. Laughlin TJ, Armstrong DG, Caporusso J, et al: Soft tissue and bone infections from puncture wounds in children. *West J Med* 166:126, 1997.
4. Lavery LA, Harkless LB, Ashry HR, et al: Puncture wounds: Normal laboratory values in the face of severe infection in diabetics and non-diabetics. *Am J Med* 101:521, 1996.
5. Englanoff G, Anglin D, Hutson HR: Lisfranc fracture-dislocation: A frequently missed diagnosis in the emergency department. *Ann Emerg Med* 26:229, 1995.
6. Preidler KW, Peicha L, Lajtai G, et al: Conventional radiography, CT, MR imaging in patients with hyperflexion injuries of the foot: Diagnostic accuracy in detection of bony and ligamentous changes. *AJR* 173:1673, 1999.
7. Ross G, Cronin R, Hauzenblaus J, et al: Plantar ecchymosis sign: A clinical aid to diagnosis of occult Lisfranc tarsometatarsal injuries. *J Orthop Trauma* 10:119, 1996.
8. Ogilvie-Harris DJ, Gilbart M: Treatment modalities for soft tissue injuries of the ankle: A critical review. *Clin J Sport Med* 5:175, 1995.

COMPARTMENT SYNDROMES
278 Paul R. Haller

Compartment syndrome occurs when tissue pressures in a confined space rise to the point of compromising perfusion. The resulting tissue hypoxia causes damage to the structures coursing through that compartment. Particularly susceptible to this ischemia are the nerves and muscles. Prolonged muscle hypoxia leads to necrosis and permanent posttraumatic muscle contracture: Volkmann's ischemia. The goal of the clinician is to diagnose elevated tissue pressures promptly so measures can be taken to reduce the pressures, thereby preventing nerve dysfunction or muscle death.

PATHOPHYSIOLOGY

Normal tissue perfusion is dependent on an adequate difference between arterial and venous pressures at the capillary level. When pressure within a compartment increases, tissue perfusion is compromised either by loss of vasomotor tone of the arterioles, or collapse of the thin-walled veins. When muscles become ischemic, histamine-like substances act locally to dilate the capillary bed and increase endothelial permeability. The resulting transudation of plasma causes erythrocyte sludging and a further decreasing of microvascular flow.

Elevated compartment pressure results from either extrinsic forces constricting the compartment (i.e., a circular cast that is too tight), or from an increase in the volume of the contents of the compartment. Compartment volume may increase secondary to a hematoma that has formed within a compartment, or may be due to edema accumulating after reperfusion of ischemic muscle after its vascular supply has been restored (Table 278-1).

Normal tissue pressure is about zero and usually less than 10 mm Hg. Capillary blood flow within the compartment is compromised at pressures greater than about 20 mm Hg, and muscle and nerves are at risk for ischemic necrosis at pressures greater than about 30 to 40 mm Hg. Of the tissues within the compartments, nerve is most sensitive, followed by muscle tissue.

Blood flow through arteries, arterioles, and collaterals is not compromised significantly at these pressures. Nevertheless, tissues within the compartment that are dependent on the nutrient capillaries become ischemic and then necrotic if the compartment pressure is not reduced promptly. By the time that distal pulses are reduced, muscle necrosis has occurred. Ischemic muscles hurt, and this pain is exacerbated by active muscle contraction and by passive stretching of the muscle.

COMPARTMENTS

A compartment is a structure made up of an outer perimeter dense enough to limit swelling within it. This perimeter is made up of a com-

TABLE 278-1   Common Causes of Compartment Syndrome

Orthopedic	Tibial fractures
	Forearm fractures
Vascular	Ischemic-reperfusion injury
	Hemorrhage
Iatrogenic	Vascular puncture in anticoagulated patients
	Intravenous/intra-arterial drug injection
	Constructive casts
Soft tissue injury	Prolonged limb compression
	Crush injury
	Burns

bination of bone and dense connective tissue such as interosseous membranes. Compartments in the body that have elastic enough borders to permit some stretching (such as the upper arm or upper leg) are less likely to undergo elevation of tissue pressures.

Upper Extremity

The upper arm has an anterior and a posterior compartment. The anterior compartment contains the biceps and brachialis muscles, and the ulnar, median, and radial nerves (Figure 278-1). The posterior compartment contains the triceps muscle. Fortunately, the compartments of the upper arm are relatively roomy, and compartment syndromes are uncommon in this location.

The forearm is the portion of the upper extremity most prone to compartment syndrome. An interosseous membrane, along with the radius and ulna, separate the volar compartment from the dorsal (Figure 278-2). The dorsal compartment contains the radial nerve and the wrist and finger extensors. The volar compartment of the forearm envelops the wrist and finger flexors, the radial and ulnar arteries, along with the median and ulnar nerves (Table 278-2).

There are four compartments in the hand: thenar, hypothenar, central, and interossei (Figure 278-3). The thenar and hypothenar compartments contain the intrinsic muscles of the thumb and little finger, respectively. The interosseous muscles of the hand are contained in their own compartments.

Lower Extremity

There are three gluteal compartments of the buttocks. One contains the tensor muscle of the fascia lata, another the gluteus medius and minimus, and the third the gluteus maximus. The sciatic nerve lies adjacent to the gluteus maximus and can be compressed by it.

The thigh has three compartments: the anterior, medial, and posterior. The anterior compartment contains the vastus lateralis, the vastus intermedius, and the vastus medialis muscles, as well as the sartorius and rectus femoris muscles. The femoral artery and nerve also traverse the anterior thigh compartment. The medial compartment contains the adductor longus, the adductor brevis, and the adductor magnus muscles, plus the gracilis muscle. The posterior compartment contains the semimembranosus, the semitendinosus, and the biceps femoris muscles. The sciatic nerve also traverses the posterior compartment.

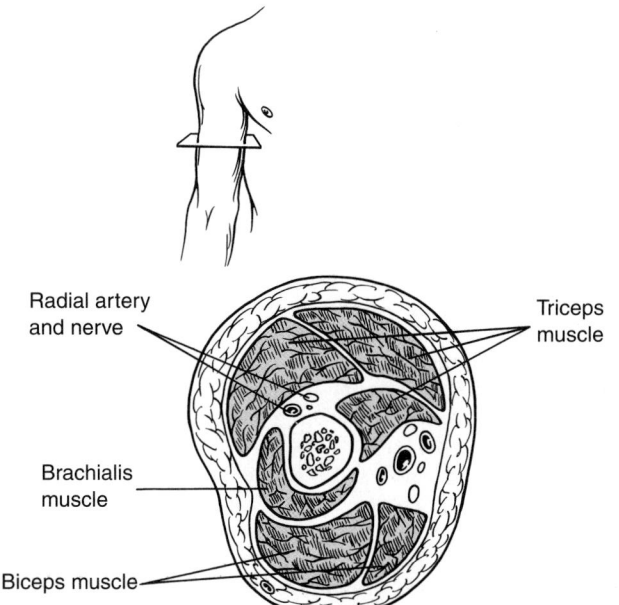

FIG. 278-1. The biceps-brachialis *(anterior)* and triceps *(posterior)* compartments of the right arm.

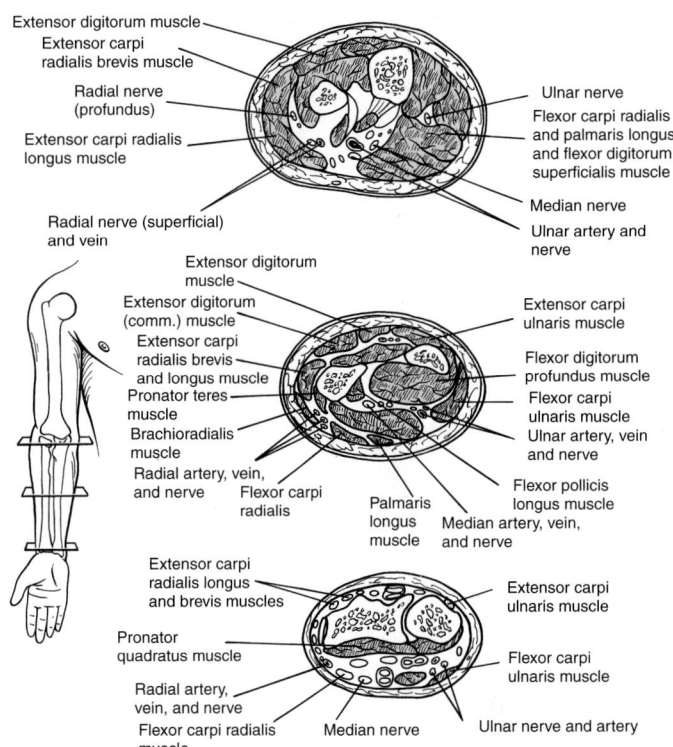

FIG. 278-2. Forearm compartments: transverse sections through the right forearm at various levels.

The leg has four compartments (Figure 278-4 and Table 278-3). The interosseous membrane, forming a plane that spans from the tibia to the fibula, forms one wall of the anterior compartment; the tibia and fibula form the lateral and medial walls of this compartment. The anterior compartment contains the extensor muscles of the toes, the anterior tibial artery, and the deep peroneal nerve. This compartment is most susceptible to compartment syndrome. The lateral compartment of the leg is described by the fibula, along with the intermuscular septum that projects anteriorly and posteriorly from the fibula's edges. The lateral compartment contains the peroneal muscles which evert the foot and the superficial peroneal nerve, which innervates these muscles and is sensory to the lateral dorsum of the foot.

The posterior aspect of the lower leg is divided into a superficial compartment (containing gastrocnemius and soleus muscles), and a deep compartment. The transverse intermuscular septum is the sheet that separates them. The deep posterior compartment contains the flexor muscles of the foot, the tibial artery, and the tibial and peroneal nerves.

The four compartments of the foot are the medial, lateral, central, and interosseous, similar to the compartments of the hand.

CLINICAL FEATURES

Two classic sets of findings are based upon the letter *P: P*ain (out of proportion to findings), *P*aresthesia (decreased sensation to pinprick, light touch, or two-point discrimination), *P*ain with *P*assive *S*tretch (PPS), and *P*aresis[1]; or *P*ain, *P*allor, and Pulseless *P*aralysis.

TABLE 278-2   Anatomy of the Forearm

Compartment	Muscles	Vessels	Nerves
Volar forearm	Wrist & finger flexors	Radial artery Ulnar artery	Median & ulnar
Dorsal forearm	Wrist & finger extenders		Radial

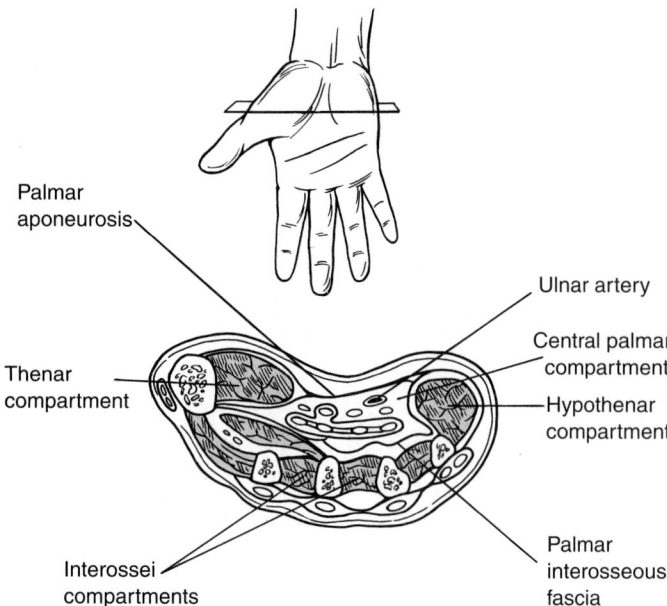

FIG. 278-3. Hand compartments: transverse section through the right hand.

The history in a patient with compartment syndrome usually involves trauma. This may be due to a direct blow to the muscle in the compartment. Hematoma formation in the compartment or induced edema may elevate the pressure. Force sufficient to cause a fracture is often present, but compartment syndrome may occur without fracture. If the vascular supply to a muscle group has been disrupted, as is seen with a knee dislocation, the muscles may become edematous and increase in volume after vascular supply has been restored.[1]

Pain is an early and almost universal finding in an alert patient with compartment syndrome. The pain of tissue ischemia is described as deep, unremitting, and poorly localized. This pain is difficult to control with the normal dosages of narcotics used to treat fractures. The pain of compartment syndrome is exacerbated when the muscle group within the compartment is stretched, either passively or actively.

Another early sign is paresthesia in the cutaneous distribution of the nerves coursing through the affected compartment. Sensory disturbance generally precedes motor dysfunction. Pulselessness is either a late finding or is not present at all, since large arteries that course

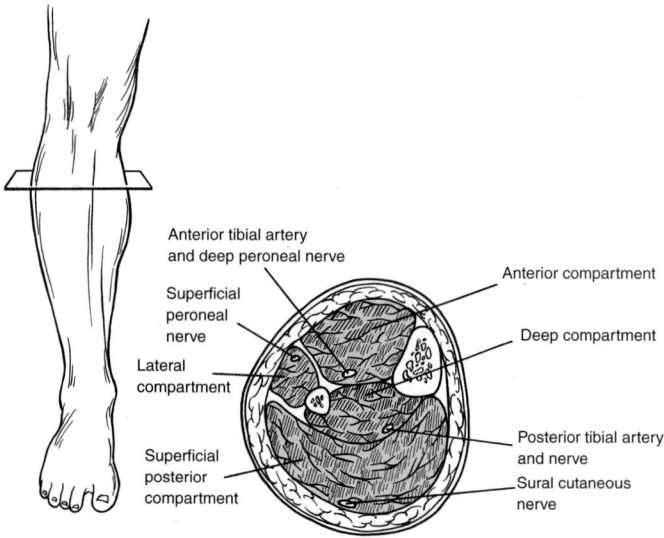

FIG. 278-4. The four compartments of the leg.

through a compartment remain patent even with prolonged and dramatic tissue pressure elevation. For paralysis to occur, the affected limb must be ischemic for some time, and permanent damage may well have already occurred.

Palpation of a compartment will increase pain in an alert patient. The compartment may feel tense. Stretching of the muscles in the compartment also exacerbates pain.

A recent meta-analysis was able to identify only four useful articles reporting clinical findings of compartment syndrome.[2] The sensitivity, specificity, positive predictive value, and negative predictive value of each individual finding were as follows: pain: 0.19, 0.97, 0.14, 0.998; paresthesia: 0.13, 0.98, 0.15, 0.98; pain with passive stretch: 0.19, 0.97, 0.14, 0.98; and paresis: 0.13, 0.97, 0.11, 0.98. Therefore the absence of any of the findings is helpful to exclude the diagnosis. In the presence of any one clinical finding, the likelihood of the diagnosis of compartment syndrome is about 25 percent (19 to 26 percent); with any two findings 68 percent; with any three findings 93 percent; and with all four, 98 percent. The sensitivity of clinical findings is under 20 percent, positive predictive value about 15 percent, specificity 97 percent, and negative predictive value 98 percent.[1] The clinical features of compartment syndrome are more useful by their absence, which can exclude the diagnosis.

If compartment syndrome is suspected, constricting cases or circular dressings must be removed immediately. The pressure within the compartment should be measured.

Pressure Measurement

When compartment syndrome is suspected, the tissue pressures should be measured.[3] Commercial kits are available, such as the Stic Catheter (Stryker Instruments, Kalamazoo, MI). The apparatus consists of a fluid-filled syringe attached to a needle. The side-ported needle is inserted into the compartment and a small amount of saline is injected to ascertain that the needle does not rest against fibrous tissue. A pressure monitor that is attached between the needle and the syringe detects the pressure in the compartment. Normal compartment pressure is 0 mm Hg. When the system is initially flushed after insertion, the pressure reading will overshoot as resistance to flow and inertia are overcome.

An accurate measurement of the compartment pressure will then be displayed. Care must be taken to be sure that the apparatus is level. The accuracy of the needle and transducer can be verified by holding it level and open to the atmosphere; it should read zero.

The needle should be placed in the suspect compartment near the site of the fracture or where the compartment seems most tense. The highest pressures within a compartment are within 5 cm of the fracture site.

Compartments in the hand and foot are small, and elevated pressures there are difficult to detect. Often, the decision to perform a fasciotomy is made solely on clinical grounds.[4]

TREATMENT

The definitive treatment of compartment syndrome is fasciotomy.

A surgical incision is made along the length of the compartment to relieve the pressure. The wound is left open. Several days later, after resolution of the edema, the patient returns to the operating room for closure of the wound.

Compartment pressures of <15 mm Hg are safe. Pressures between 20 and 30 mm Hg may cause damage if they persist for several hours. Levels in this range may be closely followed clinically with repeat pressure measurements. Pressures of 30 to 40 mm Hg are generally considered grounds for emergent fasciotomy. Injuries resulting in an inability to closely follow borderline elevations in compartment pressures may be an indication for fasciotomy.

TABLE 278-3   Anatomy of the Leg

Compartment	Muscles	Vessels	Nerves	Sensory Distribution
Anterior	Extensor muscles of toes	Anterior tibial artery	Deep peroneal nerve	Web space of first & second toes
Deep posterior	Deep flexor muscles	Posterior tibial artery	Tibial nerve Peroneal nerve	Heel
Superficial posterior	Superficial flexor muscles (gastrocnemius and soleus)			
Lateral	Peroneal muscles		Superficial peroneal nerve	Lateral dorsum of foot

REFERENCES

1. Velhamos GC, Toutouzas KG: Vascular trauma and compartment syndromes. *Surg Clin North Am* 82:1, 2002.
2. Ulmer T: The clinical diagnosis of compartment syndrome of the lower leg: Are clinical findings predictive of the disorder? *J Orthop Trauma* 16:572, 2002.
3. Tiwara A, Haq AI, Myint F, et al: Acute compartment syndromes. *Br J Surg* 89:397, 2002.
4. Perry MD, Manoli II A: Foot compartment syndrome. *Orthop Clin North Am* 32:1, 2001.

RHABDOMYOLYSIS
Francis L. Counselman

PATHOPHYSIOLOGY

Rhabdomyolysis is a syndrome characterized by injury to skeletal muscle with subsequent release of intracellular contents. These contents include myoglobin, creatine phosphokinase (CK), aldolase, lactate dehydrogenase, serum glutamic oxaloacetic transaminase, and potassium. Although numerous causes of rhabdomyolysis have been described, the common terminal event appears to involve the disruption of the Na^+K^+ ATPase pump and calcium transport, resulting in increased intracellular calcium and subsequent muscle cell necrosis. In addition, calcium activates phospholipase A_2 and various vasoactive molecules and proteases and the production of free oxygen radicals.[1]

Several classification systems have been developed to characterize the numerous causes of rhabdomyolysis. None of these systems is universally recognized, and each has its limitations. In addition, many patients have multiple causes of rhabdomyolysis (e.g., alcohol abuse and hypokalemia). Table 279-1 lists commonly recognized causes. **In general, the most common causes of rhabdomyolysis in adults appear to be alcohol and drug abuse, toxin ingestion, trauma, infection, strenuous physical activity, and heat-related illness.** In the pediatric population, rhabdomyolysis is an uncommon disorder.[2] In one study of pediatric patients, the most common causes of nonrecurrent rhabdomyolysis were trauma, nonketotic hyperosmolar coma, viral myositis, dystonia, and malignant hyperthermia.[3] For adult and pediatric patients, inherited metabolic disorders should be suspected in recurrent episodes of rhabdomyolysis, especially if associated with exercise intolerance.

Patients in coma are at risk for development of rhabdomyolysis due to immobility from unrelieved pressure on gravity-dependent body parts. In one study, the most common positions leading to rhabdomyolysis were the lateral decubitus, lithotomy, sitting, knee-to-chest, and prone positions.[4] Alcohol consumption can result in rhabdomyolysis secondary to coma-induced muscle compression and a direct toxic effect. Nutritional compromise, hypokalemia, hypomagnesemia, and hypophosphatemia, all common in alcoholics, increase the risk of rhabdomyolysis. Alcohol and drugs are thought to play a role in up to 80 percent of cases of rhabdomyolysis in adults.[5–7] Drugs of abuse that have commonly been implicated in acute rhabdomyolysis include cocaine, amphetamines (including "Ecstasy"), lysergic acid diethylamide, heroin, and phencyclidine. Common medications associated with the development of rhabdomyolysis include diuretics, lipid-lowering agents (e.g., statins and clofibrate), narcotics, theophylline, corticosteroids, benzodiazepines, phenothiazines, and tricyclic antidepressants.

Viral and bacterial infections have been known to cause rhabdomyolysis. Influenza virus is the most frequently cited infectious cause, and *Legionella* is the most frequently reported bacterial cause of rhabdomyolysis.[8] Strenuous physical activity, as seen in athletes, military recruits, and outdoor laborers, is a common cause of rhabdomyolysis. Factors that increase the risk in this group of patients include poor physical conditioning, inadequate fluid intake, high ambient temperatures, and high humidity levels.[9]

CLINICAL FEATURES

The presenting symptoms of rhabdomyolysis are usually acute in onset and include myalgias, stiffness, weakness, malaise, low-grade fever, and dark (usually brown) urine. Symptoms relating to the musculoskeletal system, however, may be present in only 50 percent of cases.[5] Nausea, vomiting, abdominal pain, and tachycardia can occur in severe rhabdomyolysis. On occasion, mental status changes are present secondary to urea-induced encephalopathy. Swelling and tenderness of the involved muscle groups and hemorrhagic discoloration of overlying skin may be observed, but only in a minority of cases. Muscle swelling may not become apparent until after rehydration with intravenous fluids. The muscle groups involved may be localized or diffuse, depending on the etiology. Commonly, the postural muscles of the thighs, calves, and the lower back are involved. An important point to remember is that acute rhabdomyolysis may be present without any of these signs or symptoms, and the patient may have essentially normal findings on physical examination. For this reason, the diagnosis often is made only after soliciting a historical clue (e.g., recent cocaine use) or finding an elevated serum CK or the presence of myoglobinuria on routine laboratory testing.

DIAGNOSIS

An elevated serum CK level is the most sensitive and reliable indicator of muscle injury. The degree of CK elevation correlates with the amount of muscle injury and the severity of illness, but not the development of renal failure or other morbidity. Most investigators consider a fivefold or greater increase in serum CK, without cardiac or brain injury, as the requirement for making the diagnosis of rhabdomyolysis. In general, serum CK begins to rise approximately 2 to 12 h after the onset of muscle injury, peaks within 24 to 72 h, and then declines at the relatively constant rate of 39 percent of the previous day's value.[5] Ongoing muscle necrosis should be suspected in patients with elevated CK values that fail to decrease in this manner. The isoenzyme CK-MM (found in skeletal and cardiac muscle) is responsible in large part for the elevation in serum CK. The CK-MB fraction (found primarily in cardiac but also in skeletal muscle) also may be elevated but should not exceed 5 percent of the total CK level.

TABLE 279-1   Common Causes of Rhabdomyolysis

Direct muscle injury	*Shigella*
Crush	*Staphylococcus aureus*
Electrical or lightning injury	*Streptococcus pneumoniae*
Drugs of abuse	Viral
Amphetamines (including Ecstasy)	Coxsackie virus
Caffeine	Cytomegalovirus
Cocaine	Epstein-Barr virus
Ethanol	Enterovirus
Heroin	Hepatitis
Lysergic acid diethylamide	Herpes simplex virus
Methamphetamines	Human immunodeficiency virus
Opiates	Influenza (A and B)
Phencyclidine	Rotavirus
Excessive muscular activity	Ischemic injury
Contact sports	Compartment syndrome
Delirium tremens	Compression
Dystonia	Medications
Psychosis	Barbiturates
Seizures	Benzodiazepines
Sports and basic training	Clofibrate
Genetic disorders	Colchicine
Glycolysis and glycogenolysis disorders	Corticosteroids
Fatty acid oxidation disorders	Isoniazid
Mitochondrial and respiratory chain metabolism disorders	Lithium
Immunologic diseases	Monoamine oxidase inhibitors
Dermatomyositis	Narcotics
Polymyositis	Neuroleptic agents
Infection	Phenothiazines
Bacterial	Salicylates
Clostridium	Serotonergic agents
Group A B-hemolytic *Streptococcus*	Statins
Legionnaires' disease	Theophylline
Salmonella	Tricyclic antidepressants

Myoglobin is an oxygen-binding protein found in skeletal and cardiac muscles and is involved in oxidative metabolism. Myoglobin elevation occurs before CK elevation after muscle injury and then is rapidly cleared from the plasma through renal excretion and metabolism to bilirubin. Myoglobin enters the urine when the plasma concentration exceeds 1.5 mg/dL and causes the typical reddish brown discoloration when urine myoglobin exceeds 100 mg/dL.[5] Because myoglobin contains heme, qualitative tests such as the dipstick (which uses the orthotoluidine reaction) does not differentiate between hemoglobin, myoglobin, and red blood cells. Therefore, suspect myoglobinuria when the urine dipstick is positive for blood, but no red blood cells are present on microscopic examination. Radioimmunoassay is slightly more sensitive than the dipstick technique in identifying myoglobinuria, but usually is not necessary. Because myoglobin levels may return to normal within 1 to 6 h after the onset of muscle necrosis, the absence of an elevated serum myoglobin or of myoglobinuria does not exclude the diagnosis. In one study, 26 percent of patients with rhabdomyolysis did not have myoglobinuria.[5]

Other laboratory studies may be useful to identify the common complications of rhabdomyolysis and the underlying etiology. Electrolytes, calcium, phosphorus, and uric acid levels should be determined to identify hyperkalemia, abnormal calcium and phosphorus levels, and hyperuricemia. A urinalysis should be performed on all patients. Serum creatinine and blood urea nitrogen are useful as a baseline and to identify acute renal failure. Because disseminated intravascular coagulation (DIC) is a complication, all patients suspected of rhabdomyolysis should have a baseline complete blood cell count and DIC screen (e.g., prothrombin time, partial thromboplastin time, fibrin split products, and fibrinogen). Other common laboratory findings in rhabdomyolysis include elevated levels of aldolase, lactate dehydrogenase, urea, creatine, and aminotransferases. Magnetic reso-

nance imaging, especially when using gadolinium enhancement, has recently been shown to be very effective in localizing rhabdomyolysis and is more sensitive than computed tomography or ultrasound in detecting abnormal muscle (e.g., edema and inflammation).[10] Further laboratory testing to identify the underlying cause(s) of rhabdomyolysis should be based on the medical history and clinical presentation.

COMPLICATIONS

The complications of rhabdomyolysis include acute renal failure (ARF), metabolic derangements, DIC, and mechanical complications (e.g., compartment syndrome or peripheral neuropathy; Table 279-2). Acute renal failure is the most serious complication of rhabdomyolysis. Although rhabdomyolysis is thought to account for up to 10 percent of all cases of ARF,[11] the incidence of this complication in rhabdomyolysis is less clear. It is estimated that between 0[12] and 50[13] percent of patients with rhabdomyolysis develop ARF, with 33 percent being the most often quoted figure.[5] This wide range probably reflects the multifactorial etiology necessary for the development of ARF. Factors known to contribute to rhabdomyolysis-induced ARF include hypovolemia, acidosis or aciduria, tubular obstruction, and the nephrotoxic effects of myoglobin. Renal tubular obstruction occurs secondary to precipitation of uric acid and myoglobin. Ferrihemate, the breakdown product of myoglobin, is responsible for the direct toxic effect on the kidneys. This effect, however, appears to occur only in the presence of hypovolemia and aciduria (pH < 5.6). The ARF may be oliguric (most common) or nonoliguric. The need for dialysis, serum potassium and calcium levels, and mortality rates appear to be similar for rhabdomyolysis-induced and non-rhabdomyolysis-induced ARF. Patients with rhabdomyolysis-induced ARF, however, have higher serum uric acid and anion gap levels.[5] Neither the presence of myo-

TABLE 279-2   Complications of Rhabdomyolysis

Acute renal failure

Metabolic derangements
   Hypercalcemia (late)
   Hyperkalemia
   Hyperphosphatemia
   Hyperuricemia
   Hypocalcemia
   Hypophosphatemia (late)
Disseminated intravascular coagulation
Mechanical complications
   Compartment syndrome
   Peripheral neuropathy

globinuria nor the degree of CK elevation is predictive of which patients are at risk for developing ARF.

The serum potassium level is elevated in 10 to 40 percent of cases, due to release of potassium from injured skeletal muscle.[5,14] Renal function, however, appears to be the most important determinant of the degree of elevation. Hyperkalemia can be a significant complication of rhabdomyolysis if acute renal failure occurs.

Elevated uric acid levels can occur, especially in crush injures, due to release of muscle adenosine nucleotides and subsequent conversion to uric acid by the liver. Uric acid levels usually correlate with serum CK levels.

In rhabdomyolysis, serum phosphorus levels initially may be elevated, due to its leakage from injured muscle. Later in the disease course, mild hypophosphatemia may be seen but rarely requires treatment. Hypocalcemia, the most common metabolic complication, occurs early in rhabdomyolysis and is usually asymptomatic. It has been attributed to the deposition of calcium salts in necrotic muscle, due to the hyperphosphatemia and decreased levels of 1,25-dihydroxycholecalciferol. These soft tissue calcifications sometimes can be observed on x-ray of the involved limb muscles. The hypocalcemia can occur, however, without elevated levels of phosphorus. Later, as calcium is mobilized from damaged muscle, serum calcium levels rise and symptomatic hypercalcemia may be observed.

Disseminated intravascular coagulation occurs in severe rhabdomyolysis and can result in hemorrhagic complications. The DIC usually resolves spontaneously within several days.

The mechanical complications of rhabdomyolysis consist of compartment syndrome and peripheral nerve injury. Compartment syndrome occurs secondary to marked swelling and edema of the involved muscle groups. Characteristic signs and symptoms include pain, paresthesias, paralysis, pallor, and pulselessness. Of these, a sensory deficit is the most reliable physical finding.[15] Presence of a pulse is not helpful in excluding the diagnosis. If the intracompartmental pressures exceed 30 to 35 mm Hg, fasciotomy should be considered. The associated muscle swelling also may cause pressure on peripheral nerves, resulting in neuronal ischemia and causing paraesthesias or paralysis. Nerve injury is often proximal, and multiple nerves may be involved in the same extremity.[16] These peripheral neuropathies usually resolve within a few days or weeks, although, in a minority of patients, they can be permanent.

TREATMENT

Prehospital Care

For victims of crush injury or patients strongly suspected of having rhabdomyolysis and prolonged extrication and transport times, intravenous rehydration with NS should be initiated as soon as possible. Recently, a volume replenishment protocol for victims of crush injuries has been proposed.[17] Once a limb is extricated, intravenous NS should be initiated at 1 L/h. After extrication, continue intravenous NS at 500 mL, alternating with D5NS, at 1 L/h. Potassium- or lactate-containing solutions should be avoided. The addition of sodium bicarbonate to each liter of crystalloid may be considered, but there are no controlled studies in the prehospital setting to confirm its benefit.

Emergency Department

Once in the emergency department, aggressive intravenous rehydration remains the mainstay of therapy. This treatment should be continued for the first 24 to 72 h. Curry and colleagues recommended rapid correction of the fluid deficit with intravenous crystalloids followed by infusion of 2.5 mL/kg per h, with the goal of maintaining a minimum urine output of 2 mL/kg per h.[18] Others recommend a goal of 200 to 300 mL of urine output each hour. Sodium bicarbonate, one ampule (44 mEq) added to 1 L of $\frac{1}{2}$NS or two to three ampules (88 to 132 mEq) in D5W to run at a rate of 100 mL/h, has been recommended to maintain a urine pH of 6.5 or above to prevent the development of ARF.[6] Alkalinization is not without risks, however, because it can exacerbate the hypocalcemia observed in rhabdomyolysis.

To assist in diuresis, 20 percent mannitol is commonly recommended, although there are no prospective studies on its benefit. This solution may be given as 1 g/kg IV over 30 min,[18] or as 25 g IV initially, followed by 5 g/h IV, for a total of 120 g/day. Proposed benefits of mannitol include increased renal blood flow and glomerular filtration rate; hyperosmotic pull of fluid from the interstitial compartment, counterbalancing hypovolemia, and reducing muscle swelling and nerve compression; increased urinary flow and flushing of myoglobin; and the scavenging of free radicals.[1,17] Mannitol should be given only after volume replacement and avoided in patients with oliguria. The use of loop diuretics (e.g., furosemide) in rhabdomyolysis is controversial, with some researchers recommending their use[6,14] and others opposing it because loop diuretics acidify the urine.[8] Despite appropriate treatment, dialysis may be necessary to treat rhabdomyolysis-induced ARF.

All patients should have a Foley catheter placed to monitor urine output. Patients should be placed on a cardiac monitor, because of the risk of dysrhythmias secondary to metabolic complications. For patients with heart disease, comorbid conditions, or preexisting renal disease or for elderly patients, hemodynamic monitoring may be necessary to avoid fluid overload. Serial measurements of urine pH, arterial pH, electrolytes, CK, calcium, phosphorus, blood urea nitrogen, and creatinine should be performed.

Hypocalcemia observed early in rhabdomyolysis usually requires no treatment. Calcium should be given only to treat hyperkalemia-induced cardiotoxicity or profound signs and symptoms of hypocalcemia. In contrast, hypercalcemia is frequently symptomatic and normally responds to saline diuresis and intravenous furosemide. Hyperphosphatemia should be treated with oral phosphate binders when serum levels exceed 7 mg/dL. Similarly, the hypophosphatemia, which may occur late in rhabdomyolysis, requires treatment only when the serum level is below 1 mg/dL. Hyperkalemia, which is usually most severe in the first 12 to 36 h after muscle injury, can be significant when associated with ARF. Treatment should be initiated to prevent cardiac complications. Traditional insulin and glucose therapy, although recommended, may not be as effective in rhabdomyolysis-induced hyperkalemia. The use of ion-exchange resins (e.g., sodium polystyrene sulfonate) is effective, as is dialysis.

Avoid the use of prostaglandin inhibitors such as nonsteroidal anti-inflammatory agents, because of their vasoconstrictive effects on the kidney. Most importantly, treat the underlying etiology of the rhabdomyolysis.

DISPOSITION

All patients with suspected rhabdomyolysis require admission for intravenous hydration, diuresis, management of complications, and treatment of the underlying etiology. For at least the initial 24 to 48 h, these patients probably should be admitted to a monitored bed to identify dysrhythmias secondary to the metabolic complications. The nephrology service should be consulted to evaluate the need for dialysis for all patients presenting with ARF or symptomatic hyperkalemia unresponsive to therapy.

REFERENCES

1. Vanholder R, Sever MS, Ekrem E, et al: Rhabdomyolysis. *J Am Soc Nephrol* 11:1553, 2000.
2. Ng Y-T, Johnson HM: Clinical rhabdomyolysis. *J Paediatr Child Health* 36:397, 2000.
3. Watemberg N, Leshner RL, Arrmstrong BA, et al: Acute pediatric rhabdomyolysis. *J Child Neurol* 15:222, 2000.
4. Szewczyk D, Ovadia P, Abdullah F, et al: Pressure-induced rhabdomyolysis and acute renal failure. *J Trauma* 44:384, 1998.
5. Gabow PA, Kaehny WD, Kelleher SP: The spectrum of rhabdomyolysis. *Medicine (Baltimore)* 61:141, 1982.
6. Richards JR: Rhabdomyolysis and drugs of abuse. *J Emerg Med* 19:51, 2000.
7. Warren JD, Blumbergs PC, Thompson PD: Rhabdomyolysis: A review. *Muscle Nerve* 25:332, 2002.
8. David WS: Myoglobinuria. *Neurol Clin* 18:215, 2000.
9. Line RL, Rust GS: Acute exertional rhabdomyolysis. *Am Fam Phys* 52:2712, 1995.
10. Kakuda W, Naritomi H, Miyashita K, et al: Rhabdomyolysis lesions showing magnetic resonance contrast enhancement. *J Neuroimaging* 9:182, 1999.
11. Veenstra J, Smit WM, Krediet RT, et al: Relationship between elevated creatine phosphokinase and the clinical spectrum of rhabdomyolysis. *Nephrol Dial Transplant* 9:637, 1994.
12. Sinert R, Kohl L, Rainone T, et al: Exercise-induced rhabdomyolysis. *Ann Emerg Med* 23:1301, 1994.
13. Feinfeld DA, Cheng JT, Beysolow TD, et al: A prospective study of urine and serum myoglobin levels in patients with acute rhabdomyolysis. *Clin Nephrol* 38:193, 1992.
14. Knochel JP: Rhabdomyolysis and myoglobinuria. *Annu Rev Med* 33:435, 1982.
15. Moore RE, Friedman RJ: Current concepts and pathophysiology in diagnosis of compartment syndromes. *J Emerg Med* 7:657, 1989.
16. Shields RW, Root RE, Wilbourn AJ: Compartment syndromes and compression neuropathies in coma. *Neurology* 36:1370, 1986.
17. Abassi ZA, Hoffman A, Better OS: Acute renal failure complicating muscle crush injury. *Semin Nephrol* 18:558, 1998.
18. Curry SC, Chang D, Connor D: Drug- and toxin-induced rhabdomyolysis. *Ann Emerg Med* 18:1068, 1989.

280 ORTHOPEDIC DEVICES AND RECONSTRUCTIONS
Scott S. Kelley
Carroll P. Jones

Orthopedic surgery requires a wide variety of implants to reconstruct the musculoskeletal system (Table 280-1). Processes ranging from traumatic soft tissue disruption to degenerative arthritis may affect multiple anatomic areas. Each area has unique mechanical requirements, and the universal goal of surgical intervention is to provide painless musculoskeletal function. Implants are used for joint and ligament reconstructions, soft tissue repairs, and fusion and fracture fixation. The purpose of an orthopedic device dictates whether its role is temporary or permanent.

This chapter reviews potential problems with orthopedic implants. Postoperative complications related to orthopedic devices that are commonly seen in an emergency department, including implant failure, loss of fixation, nonunion, and infection, are also discussed.

COMMON ORTHOPEDIC IMPLANTS STABILIZING BONE TO BONE

Internal Fixation

PLATES AND SCREWS Plates with screws are used to provide stability while fractures and osteotomies heal or arthrodeses fuse. The variety of shapes and sizes fit different areas of the skeleton. They share the common function of stabilizing bone in an anatomically acceptable position while it heals. To perform this function, the plate must be securely attached to bone with multiple screws. When managing fractures with plates, the bones are often placed in direct contact, and healing usually occurs without the large amount of callus formation seen with casting or intramedullary nailing (Figure 280-1A, B). Therefore, it is often difficult to determine when fracture union is complete, and it is not uncommon for the fracture line to be visible more than 1 year after surgery (Figure 280-2).

Complications Wound infection is the most common early complication. Superficial infections usually are amenable to antibiotics. In contrast, deep wound sepsis often requires surgical debridement. Nonunion of the fracture is a late complication, which may be related to a deep chronic infection.

Plate-and-screw constructs are simply temporizing measures. If the bone does not heal, the plate eventually will break or the screws will pull out of the bone (Figure 280-3). Plates and screws sometimes are removed after the fracture has healed, and the bone is then at risk for refracture for approximately 3 months (often through a screw hole).

RIGID INTRAMEDULLARY RODS A rigid, single intramedullary rod is the most common implant used to treat femoral and tibial shaft fractures (Figure 280-4) and, occasionally, selective humeral fractures. They are also used to stabilize osteotomies and arthrodeses. The rigidity of the fracture immobilization is less than that with plates and screws; therefore, the healing process involves visible callus formation at the fracture site (Figure 280-5).

Although the designs of modern intramedullary rods have been standardized, there are several different techniques for their application. An entry site for the rod is first established at the end (usually proximal) of the bone, through a small skin incision. Closed fractures typically are reduced with manipulation under fluoroscopic guidance; the fracture hematoma and periosteum are left undisturbed, resulting in high union rates. Open fractures may be reduced directly through the wound but heal less reliably than closed injuries, because of the soft tissue disruption and compromised vascularity of the bone. Before passing the rod across the reduced fracture, the intramedullary canal is usually mechanically reamed to a size slightly larger than the nail, thus facilitating passage of a larger rod and potentially stimulating healing by generating bone debris. Occasionally, for the sake of preserving the endosteal blood supply of the bone and to avoid creating fat emboli, an unreamed nail is used. After the insertion of the rod, interlocking screws usually are added to provide rotational stability at the fracture or osteotomy and to maintain the appropriate length of the bone (see Figure 280-4). Rarely, the rod is placed without interlocking screws. Partly locking the rod (screws at one end only) is a technique sometimes used to allow compression at the fracture while controlling migration of the nail.

FLEXIBLE INTRAMEDULLARY RODS Multiple flexible intramedullary rods are gaining popularity for the treatment of pediatric

TABLE 280-1   Common Orthopedic Implants, Expected Time to Heal, and Radiographic Guidelines to Assess for Potential Complications

Implants	Time to Heal	Ideal Radiograph	Radiographic Evidence of Failure
Bone to bone			
Internal fixation	6–8 wk		
Plates/screws (Figure 280-1)			
Intramedullary rods		Bone-to-bone opposition	Broken hardware (Figures 280-3 and 280-7)
Rigid (Figure 280-4)		Bridging bone or callus (Figure 280-5)*	Screw/wire pullout
Flexible (Figure 280-6)		Intact hardware	Gross change in alignment
Tension band/cerclage wires (Figures 280-9 and 280-10)		Adequate alignment	Interval displacement of fracture (Figure 280-7)
Percutaneous pins (Figure 280-11)	3–8 wk		
External fixation (Figure 280-12)	8–12 wk		
Spine implants	6–9 mo		
Tension band wires (Figure 280-13)		Maintained alignment	Migrated hardware
Plates/screws (Figures 280-14 and 280-16)		Intact hardware	Dislodged hooks (Figure 280-20)
Cages (Figure 280-15)		Fusion mass	Broken hardware (Figure 280-21)
Rods (Figures 280-17 and 280-18)			
Pedicle screws (Figure 280-19)			
Soft tissue to bone			
Interference screws (Figure 280-22)	6–8 wk	Well fixed in bone	Usually no radiographic abnormality†
Suture anchors (Figure 280-23)			Screw/anchor pullout (rare)
Arthroplasty			
Hemiarthroplasty (Figure 280-24)	6 wk (uncemented)	Reduced joint (biplanar views)	Periprosthetic fracture (Figure 280-10)
Total joint arthroplasty (Figure 280-25)		Appropriate alignment	Dislocation (Figure 280-26)
			Change in implant position (Figure 280-27)
			Complete radiolucent line around implant

*Rigidly fixed fractures with plate/screws often heal with minimal callus.
†Failure of soft tissue fixation is best detected clinically.

long bone fractures. These devices can be inserted through a small hole created in the side of the metaphysis to avoid injury to open growth plates (Figure 280-6). Because flexible rod fixation is less stable than rigid intramedullary nailing, it is seldom used for the slower healing adult population. Another advantage of this technique for pediatric patients is the avoidance of cumbersome external immobilization (i.e., spica casts), which allows early joint range of motion.

Complications   Infection is a relatively uncommon early complication and occurs in 1 to 2 percent of closed fractures treated with intramedullary rods and perioperative antibiotics. Open fractures treated with intramedullary nails, however, have an infection rate up to 25 percent.

Largely related to their central location, rods have a greater mechanical strength than do plates and screws. Rare implant failures usually occur at interlocking screws or holes. However, they also may fail (usually after 1 year) by breaking at an unhealed fracture site (Figure 280-7). Because open fractures treated with intramedullary rods have higher nonunion rates than closed fractures, hardware failure is also more common.

A noninterlocked nail may work its way back out of the bone and irritate surrounding soft tissue. The multiple, small, flexible rods are notorious for this problem and often become palpable under the skin (Figure 280-8).

TENSION BAND AND CERCLAGE WIRES   Tension band wires often are used to reapproximate and stabilize structures that have fractured under tension. Examples are greater tuberosity avulsions of the proximal humerus and olecranon fractures (Figure 280-9A, B). They often are applied in a "figure-of-eight" fashion through a drill hole placed in the bone distal to the fracture, and then around and deep to the tendinous attachment on the avulsed fragment.

Internal cerclage wires are used to approximate bone fragments to each other, with or without a plate. This technique is advantageous in situations when screw fixation is not feasible. For example, cerclage wires are commonly used to stabilize fractures around a prosthetic stem, in combination with a plate (Figure 280-10A, B).

Complications   Patients may present with a painful bursitis over prominent wires, especially when the hardware is in a superficial location (i.e., olecranon tension band). Occasionally, wire perforation occurs through thin overlying skin. As with all types of internal fixation, hardware failure (wire breakage) may occur before bony union.

PERCUTANEOUS PINS   Small smooth or threaded percutaneous pins (Figure 280-11A, B) often are used in the small bones of the hand or foot to add stability while fracture union occurs. The hand and foot possess an excellent blood supply, which usually results in early union. The pins are usually cut off outside the skin, so that they may be removed between 3 and 8 weeks postoperatively.

Complications   As with external fixation pins, one of the most common complications of using percutaneous fixation is pin tract infection. These infections usually resolve after removing the pin, but removal should be done only after consultation with an orthopedist. A course of oral antibiotics also may be necessary.

Pin migration and breakage, easily detected radiographically, are also common.

External Fixation

The external fixator is divided into two components: the fixation pins (or wires) and the external frame. The threaded pins (or wires) are in-

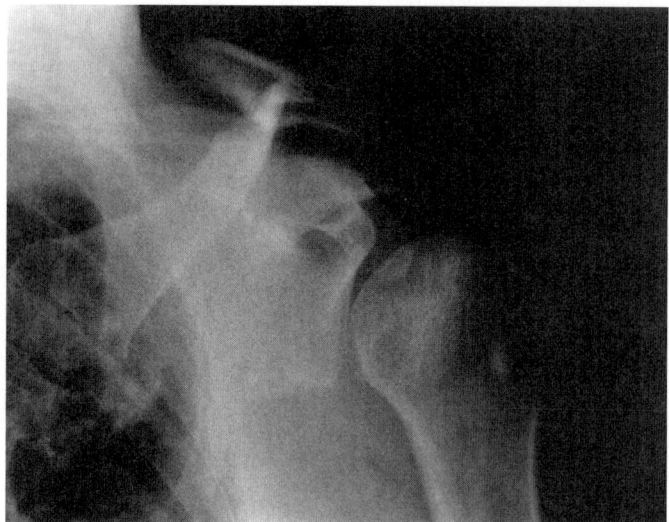

A

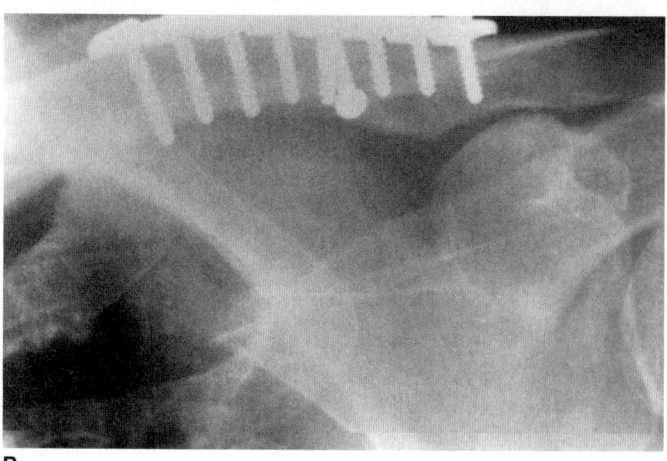

B

FIG. 280-1. A. This clavicle fracture was rigidly fixed with a plate and screws. **B.** The fracture is healing without significant callus formation.

serted into each fragment proximal and distal to the fracture (Figure 280-12) or osteotomy. When connected to the frame, they are able to hold the bone so that union occurs.

External fixators are preferentially used to stabilize open fractures (over cast immobilization), allowing the physician easier access to the soft tissue injury. External fixators are also used to temporarily stabilize an extremity or pelvis while life- or limb-threatening surgery is performed. Certain types of closed injuries, such as distal radius fractures, may be treated with external fixation, often in combination with percutaneous pins.

In addition to fracture fixation, uses of external fixators include stabilization of arthrodeses and osteotomies. Complex wire and ring (Ilizarov) fixators are commonly used to lengthen bones and correct angular deformities.

COMPLICATIONS Because external fixation is often chosen for severe open fractures (which have a higher rate of complications), emergency department visits are more frequent. Patients may present with increased redness, swelling, or drainage at the previous open wound site or at the pin sites. If a deep wound infection is suspected, the skin should be prepared and cultures obtained by aspiration or swab (before antibiotics are administered). The treating orthopaedist should be contacted.

Releasing the skin around the pin with a scalpel, after adequate local anesthesia, may easily treat superficial pin tract infections. Oral antibiotics should be given empirically. Even in the absence of infection,

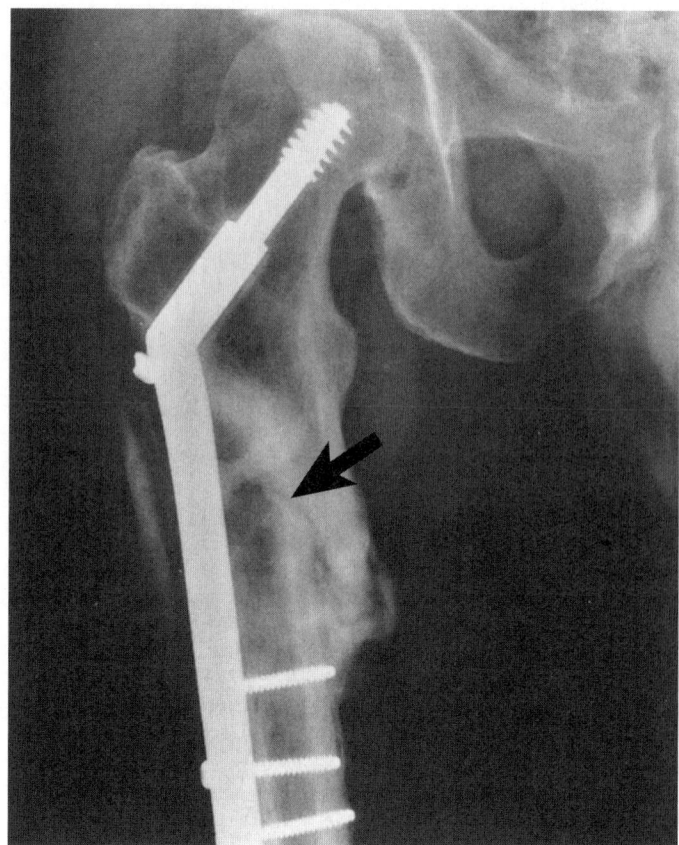

FIG. 280-2. This femur fracture has rigidly healed at 1 year, but the fracture line *(arrow)* is still present.

loosening of the fixator pins in the bone commonly occurs after their application.

The clamps connecting the pins to the frame also may loosen. This loosening may result in instability or loss of reduction at the fracture site, which is usually detectable clinically (unstable fractures are painful when stressed) or radiographically.

Spine Implants

Cervical Spine The cervical spine is unique from the rest of the vertebral column due to its vulnerable location relative to the skull. This relation allows for a unique stabilization method, halo fixation. A halo is a ring external fixator that is rigidly attached to the outer skull table with pins. Usually, four rods are used to connect this ring to a well-molded plastic or plaster body jacket. The halo limits the motion of the cervical spine, allowing fractures to heal or arthrodeses to unite.

Similar to internal fixation used in the extremities, common cervical implants include posterior tension band wires (Figure 280-13) and, more recently, plates and screws (Figure 280-14). In addition, bone grafts may be used as structural biologic implants to facilitate single- or multilevel cervical fusions.

A relatively new device used to achieve single-level fusions in the spine is the cage. Cages are hollow cylindrical devices, typically titanium, that are inserted between two vertebral bodies in the disc space, usually from an anterior approach (Figure 280-15). In addition to providing stability and restoration of the disc height, the structure of cages serves as a delivery system for bone graft, which can be packed into its hollow center.

COMPLICATIONS Similar to other types of external fixation, the most common complication of halo fixation is pin tract infection. In-

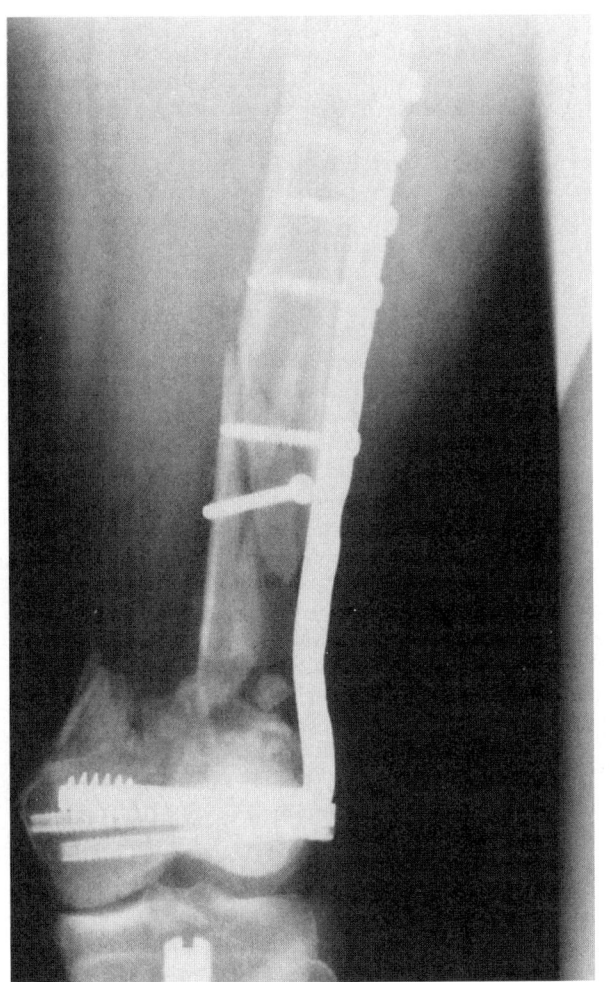

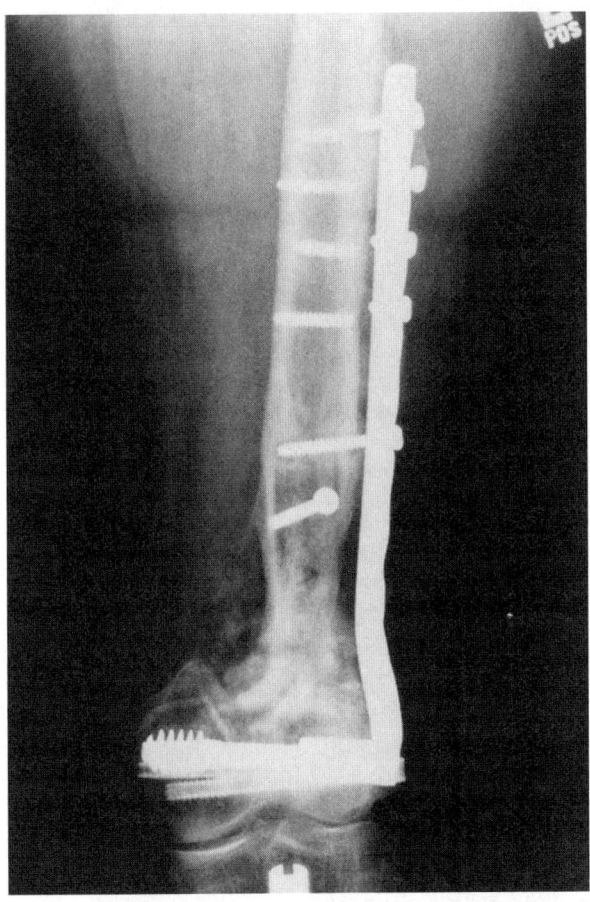

A

B

FIG. 280-3. A. This severely comminuted, open distal femur fracture was fixed with a plate and screws. **B.** Despite bone grafting, the screws broke before the fracture healed.

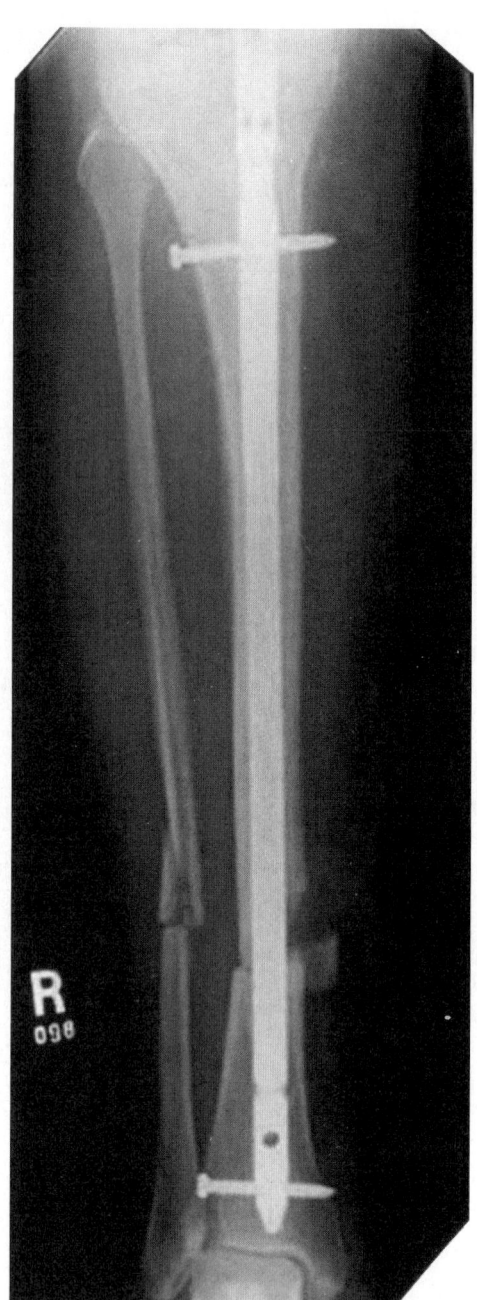

FIG. 280-4. This tibia fracture was stabilized with a rigid intramedullary rod. Proximal and distal interlock screws were placed to control length and rotation.

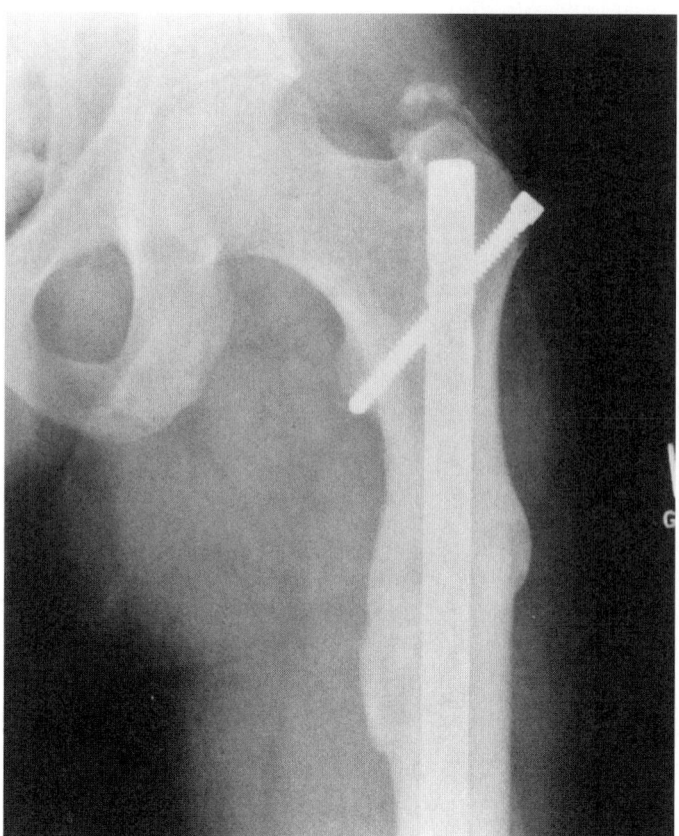

FIG. 280-5. A large callus formation at the fracture site.

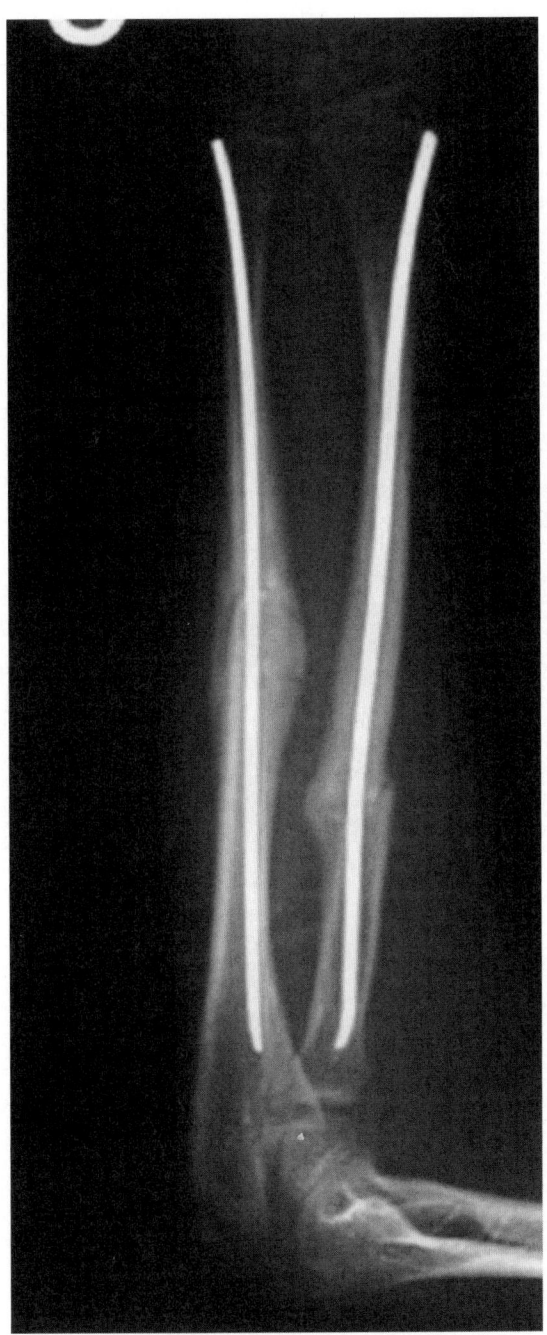

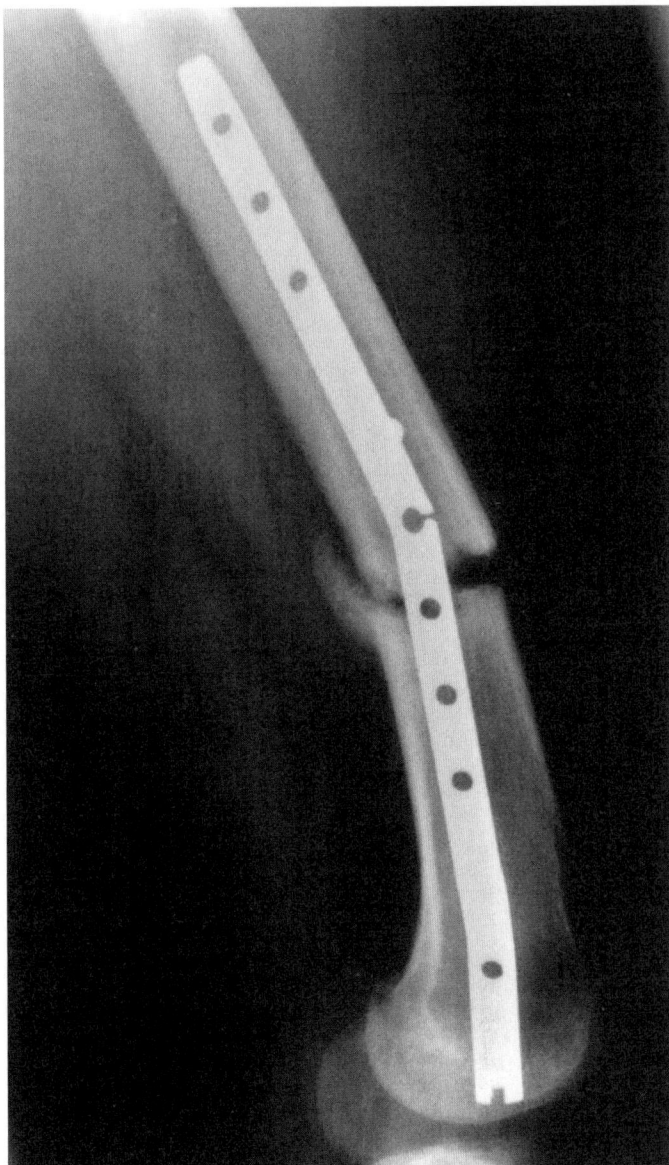

FIG. 280-7. This distal femoral intramedullary nail broke before fracture union occurred. There is also gross change in the alignment of the fracture.

FIG. 280-6. Flexible intramedullary rods were inserted through the metaphyses to treat this pediatric forearm fracture.

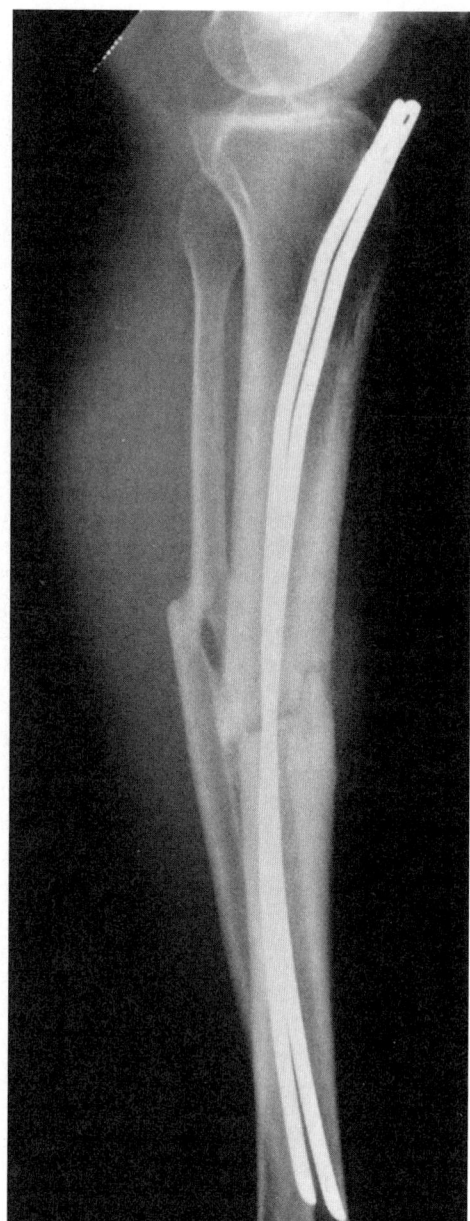

FIG. 280-8. These flexible rods "backed out" of the bone and were prominent just under the skin.

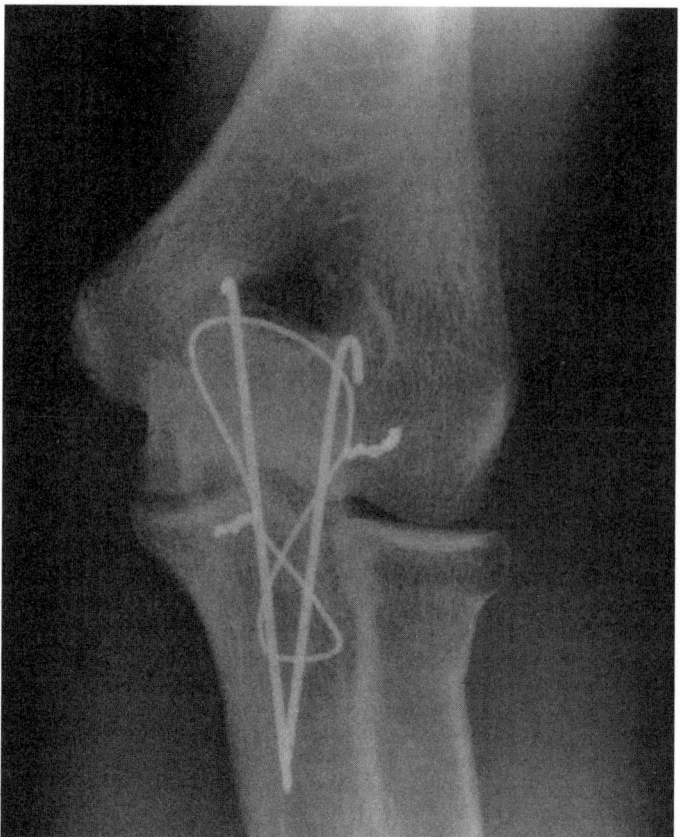

A

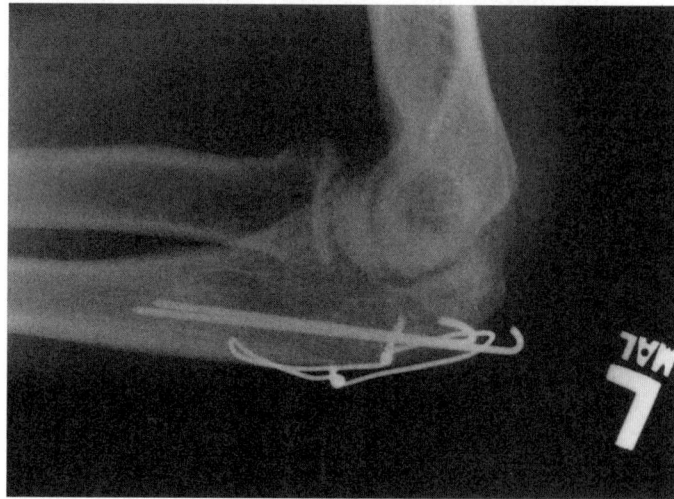

B

FIG. 280-9. A and **B.** A tension band wire and two smooth pins were used to stabilize this olecranon fracture.

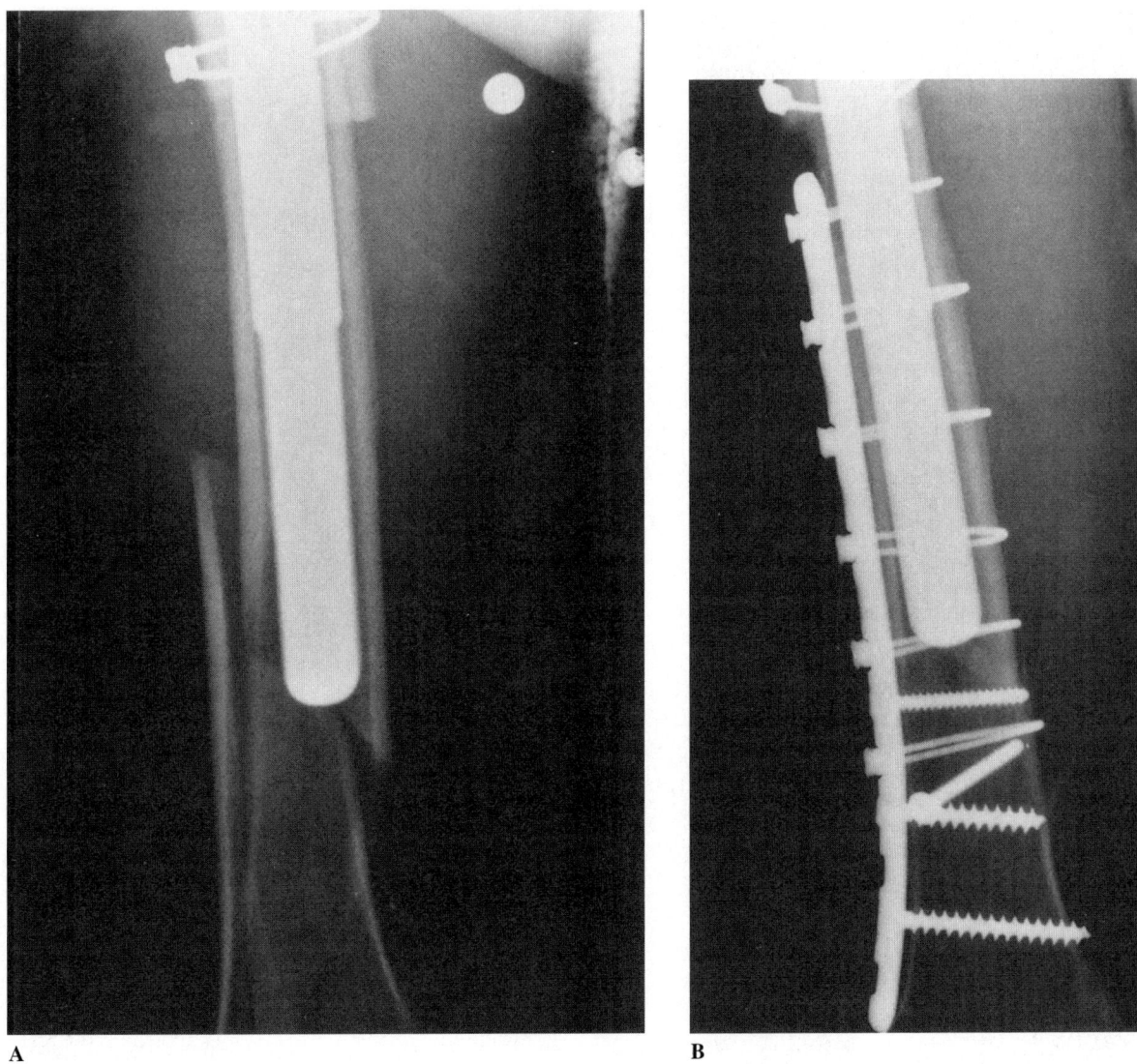

A   B

FIG. 280-10. A and **B.** This periprosthetic femur fracture was stabilized with a plate, cerclage wires, and screws.

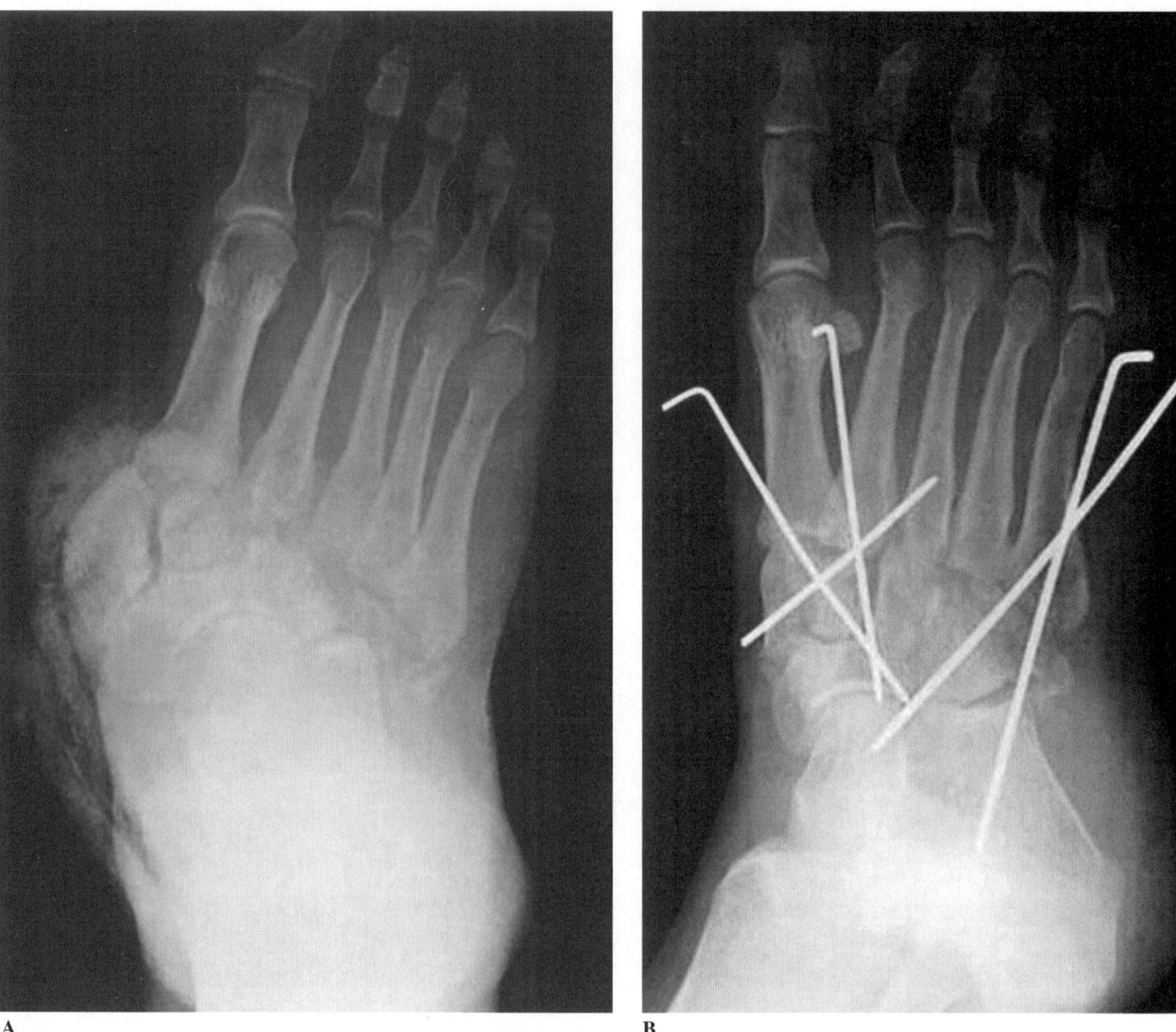

A   **B**

FIG. 280-11. A and **B.** Smooth percutaneous pins were used to stabilize this foot with multiple metatarsal fracture-dislocations.

fected pins are usually removed and a new pin is placed in an alternative site. Loose pins should rarely (if ever) be tightened, because of the risk of inner skull table penetration and resultant meningitis.

The internal implants will fail if the vertebrae fail to unite. A potentially devastating complication of spinal implants is migration of the hardware into the spinal canal, which can be detected radiographically.

Thoracolumbar Spine   Although there are many different spinal instrumentation systems, the basic concepts are simple. Rigid internal fixation is used to limit motion between vertebral segments and allow healing or fusion to occur. Similar to the cervical spine, this may be achieved with plates and screws (Figure 280-16), tension band wires, and cages (see Figure 280-15). Implants unique to the thoracolumbar spine include rods combined with hooks, wires, or screws (pedicle screws from T12 to the sacrum).

Rods are used in the spine to provide stability for fusions. Applications include the treatment of traumatic instability, arthrodesis for degenerative arthritis, and fusions for scoliosis.

Most advances in spinal instrumentation arose from the treatment of childhood scoliosis. One of the earliest constructs was the Harrington rod-and-hook system, which was introduced in 1960. Two major lessons were learned in the development of this system: (1) extremely durable materials are needed to avoid hardware failure, and (2) even

the most rigid instrumentation will fail if fusion does not occur. Modifications to this system may include a combination of hooks, screws, and wire (Figure 280-17) and have resulted in improved fixation and correction of deformity, higher fusion rates, and, subsequently, less failure of the hardware. A different system consisting of smooth metal rods placed along the posterior aspect of the spine and wired to each segment, rather than using hooks (Figure 280-18), is commonly used to correct neuromuscular scoliotic deformities. These extremely rigid constructs do not require postoperative bracing.

One drawback of rod-and-hook and rod-and-wire systems is the need for the implant to immobilize a large number of vertebral levels to achieve adequate fixation for fusion. This problem has been addressed by pedicle screws placed directly into the vertebral body, which are then connected to a rigid rod or plate (Figure 280-19). Because the screw passes through the posterior and anterior spinal elements, excellent fixation is obtained and fewer segments need to be immobilized.

COMPLICATIONS   Early emergency department visits usually involve wound problems. Diagnosis of an infection is supported by the presence of wound drainage, severe pain, an increased erythrocyte sedimentation rate, and, less frequently, an elevated temperature and white blood cell count. Although early implant failure is uncommon,

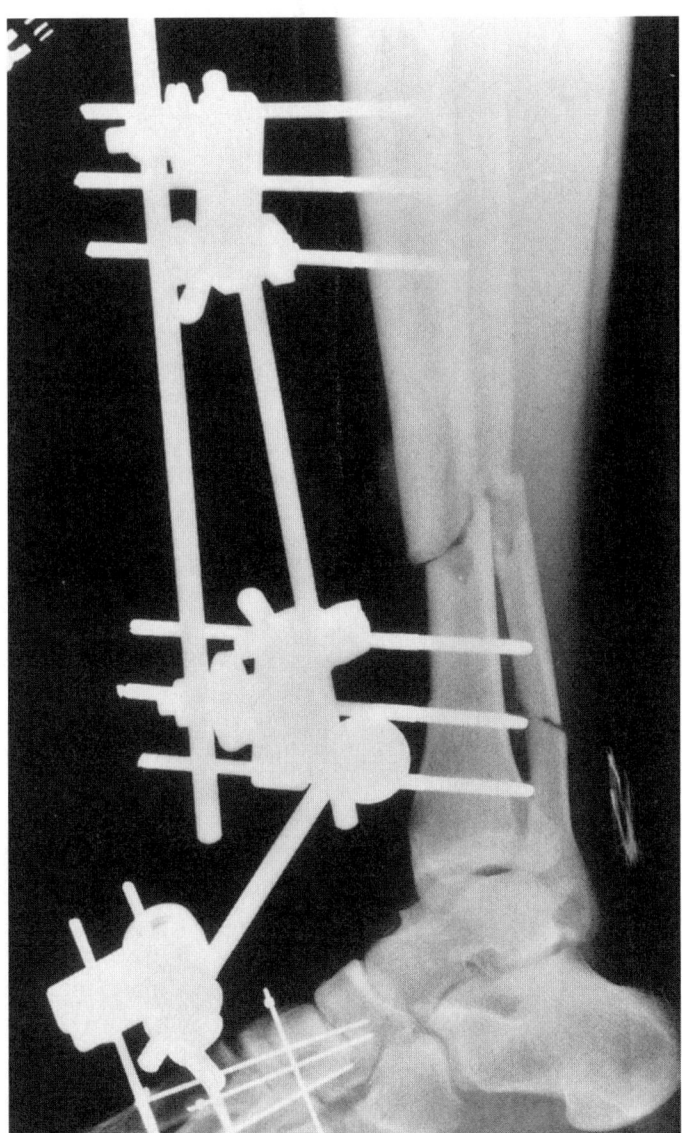

FIG. 280-12. An external fixator was used to stabilize this open tibia fracture and allow access to the soft tissue wound. Note the percutaneous pins in the foot.

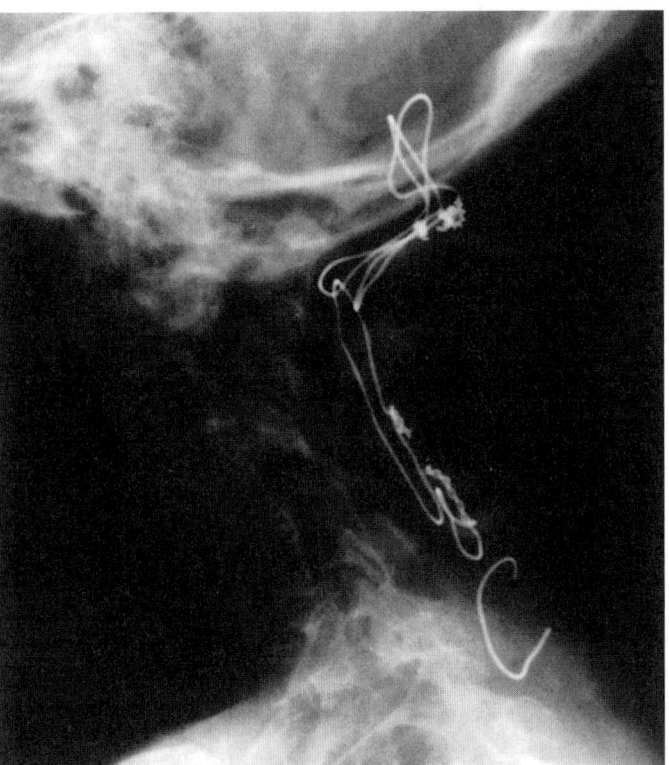

FIG. 280-13. This patient underwent posterior fusion of the entire cervical spine with multiple tension band wires.

failure of fixation may occur in the acute postoperative period. Harrington-type hook implants may disengage from the spine, and the patient may experience an acute "pop" and increase in pain. A lateral radiograph will demonstrate a hook disengaged from, and no longer under, the vertebral lamina (Figure 280-20A, B).

Rod breakage is usually a late occurrence (more than 3 to 6 months postoperatively) due to failure of the fusion to prevent motion. A broken rod should be clearly visible on standard anteroposterior and lateral radiograph views (Figure 280-21). Complaints of back pain from spine surgery patients are commonly encountered in the emergency department. If there is no clear evidence of a postoperative complication, narcotics should be given sparingly. Communication with the orthopedic surgeon is often helpful in the management of patients with chronic pain.

COMMON ORTHOPEDIC IMPLANTS STABILIZING SOFT TISSUE TO BONE

The fitness craze of the past 20 years has led to a larger number of sports-related injuries and has resulted in more surgery performed for repairing avulsed ligaments and tendons to bone. Reconstructions using autogenous and allogenic graft implants are also more common

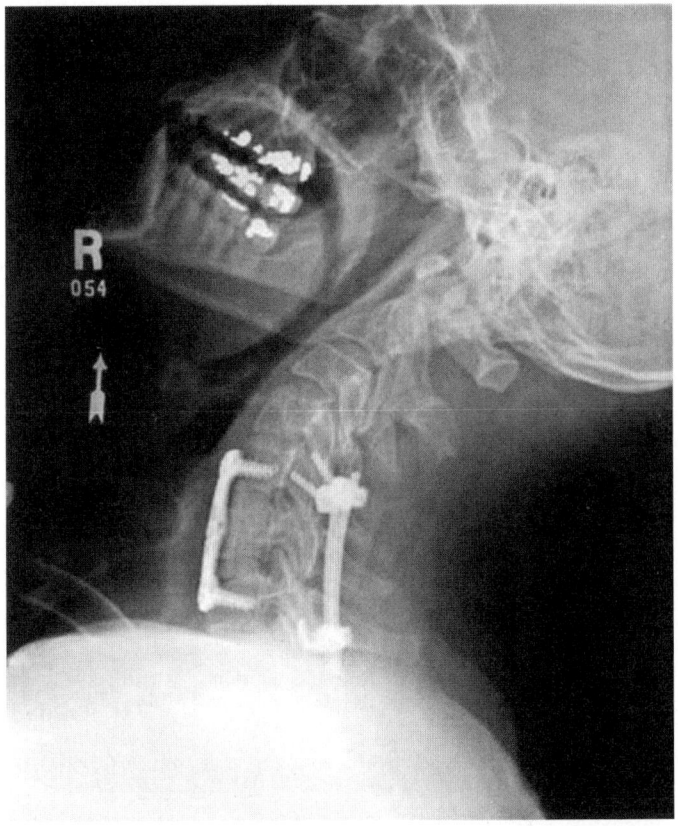

FIG. 280-14. An anterior cervical plate and screws and posterior rod instrumentation were used to stabilize this cervical burst fracture.

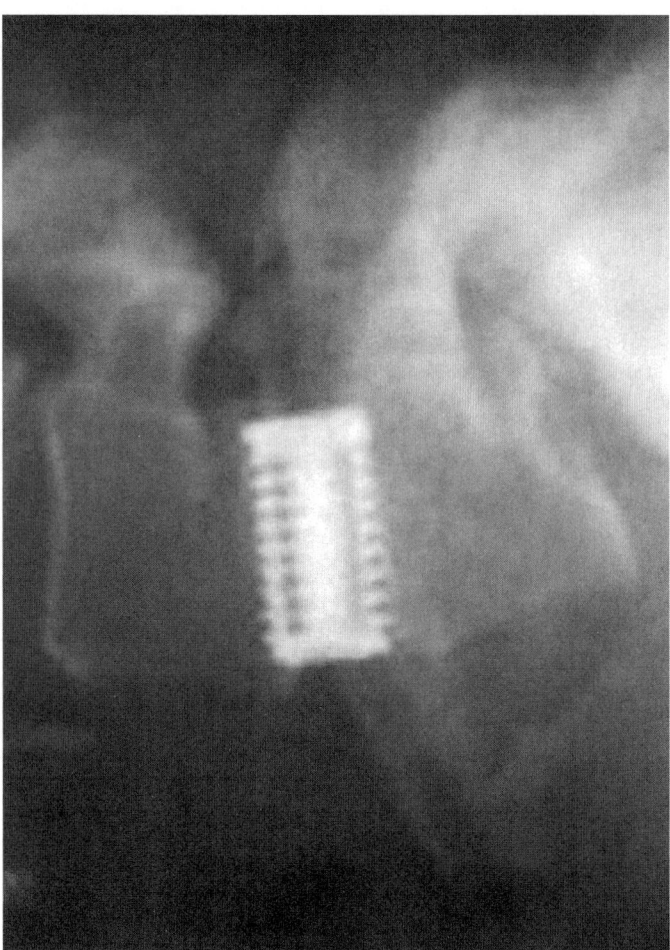

FIG. 280-15. This titanium cage was placed in the disc space between L4 and L5 to achieve single-level lumbar spine fusion.

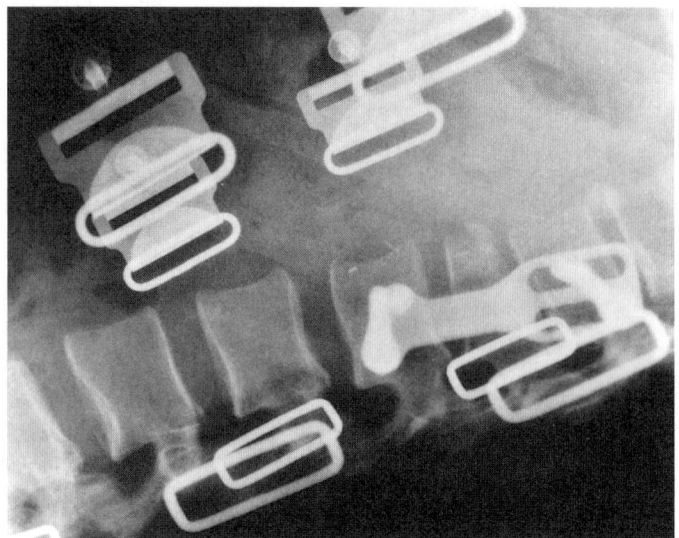

FIG. 280-16. An anterior spinal plate and screws were used to stabilize this lumbar burst fracture. The numerous buckles are part of a molded plastic orthosis, which adds additional support.

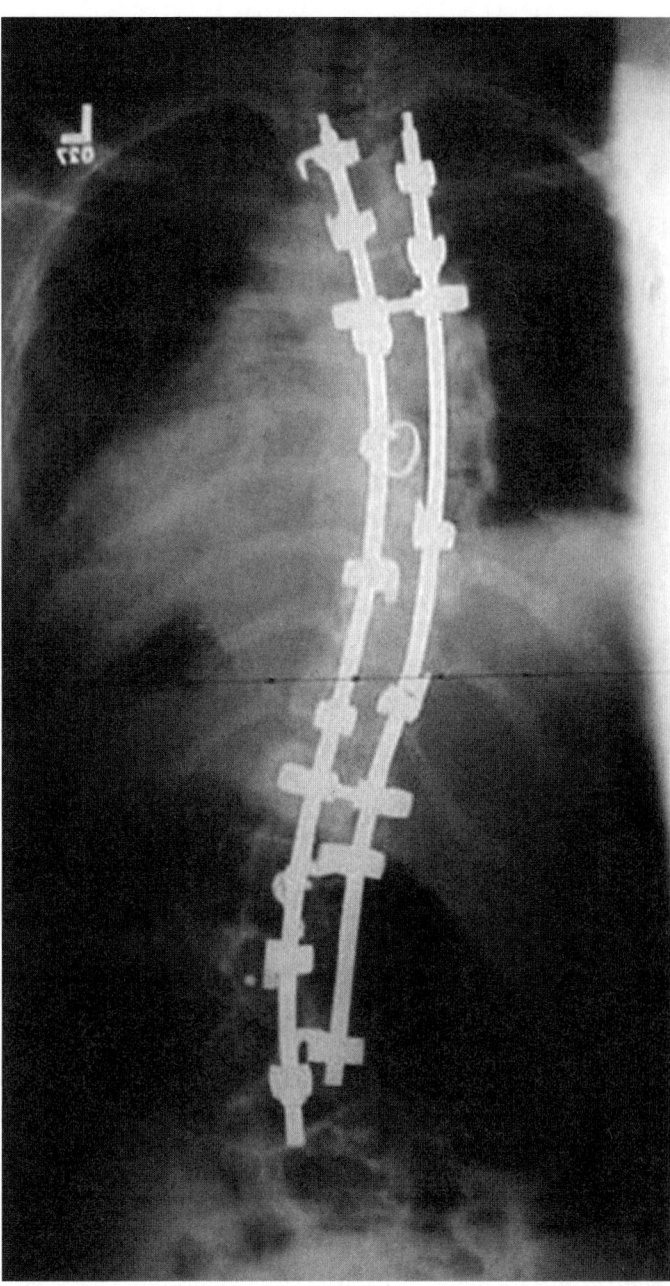

FIG. 280-17. A rod-and-hook construct was used to provide stability for a posterior spinal fusion in this patient with idiopathic scoliosis.

and must be stabilized while they heal to the host bone. Thousands of anterior cruciate ligament reconstructions are performed each year in the United States. The ruptured ligament may be replaced with harvested hamstring tendons or part of the patella tendon still connected at each end to a bone block from the patella and the tibia. Cadaveric graft tissues are also used. These reconstructions improve knee stability and protect the menisci from future injuries.

The graft may be stabilized to bone with heavy sutures or with a metallic implant. Grafts that do not have attached bone (i.e., hamstring tendon) are stabilized with heavy nonabsorbable suture tied to a screw, staple, or "button." The free bone-patella-bone grafts are typically stabilized with interference screws that are placed parallel to the graft bone in the tunnel. The threads engage and secure the graft bone to the host bone (Figure 280-22A, B).

Tendon avulsions are often repaired back to their insertion on the bone. This may be accomplished by drilling small holes in the bone, through which the suture can be threaded and tied. More recently, special

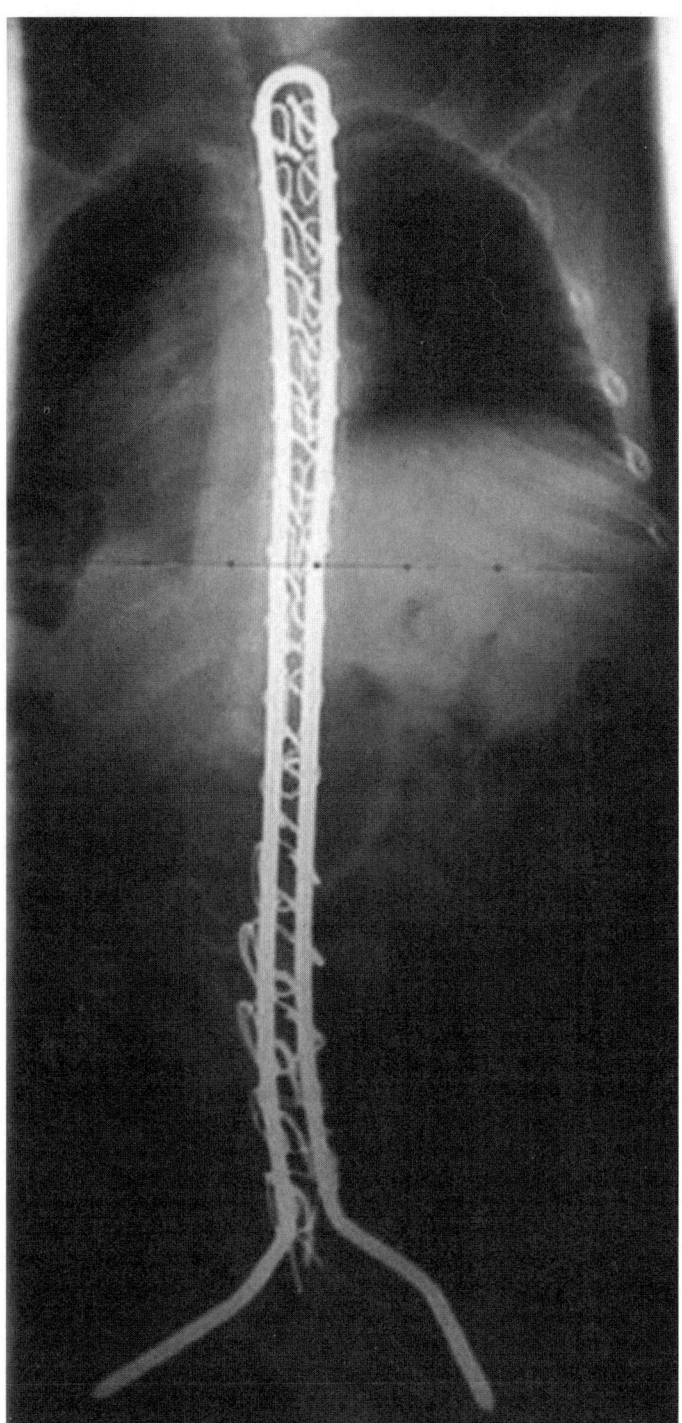

FIG. 280-18. A rod with segmental sublaminar wires was used to provide stability for a posterior spinal fusion for neuromuscular scoliosis. The ends of the rods insert into the pelvis for additional stability.

suture anchors and screws have been developed that are drilled into the bone. The attached suture is then used to reapproximate the tendon to its insertion on the bone. These devices are commonly used around the shoulder and have greatly simplified surgical techniques (Figure 280-23).

Complications

Although rare, postoperative infection (presenting as increased pain and low-grade fever) is a catastrophic early complication of ligament reconstructions. Immediate surgical debridement is usually indicated.

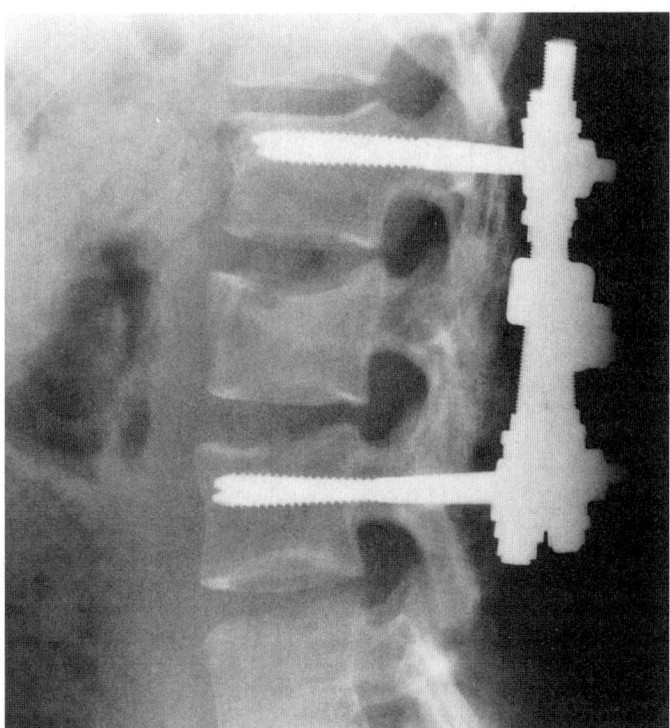

FIG. 280-19. The fracture has been reduced and stabilized with pedicle screws attached to posterior bars.

A more common complication of soft tissue-stabilizing implants is loss of fixation. This may occur through failure of the suture or the bone-to-implant interface. Suture anchors and interference screws usually do not pull out of the bone or migrate. Because radiographs are often normal, the diagnosis of a failed soft tissue-to-bone procedure is made clinically (history and physical examination).

Often an athlete will present to an emergency department with an injury to a previously reconstructed knee. The reconstructed anterior cruciate ligament may be reinjured in the same manner as the original ligament, or the patient may sustain an injury to a different structure, such as the meniscus. Great psychological stress may accompany reinjury, and this diagnosis should therefore be communicated by an orthopedist. If surgery was performed less than 6 weeks previously, the knee examination also should be deferred to the treating orthopedist, because the graft itself may not have fully healed to bone. Placement of a knee immobilizer is usually a simple temporizing measure if orthopedic evaluation can be arranged to occur within days. The orthopedist often is unable to perform an optimal clinical examination until 7 to 10 days after the injury, but earlier referral may be necessary to quell the patient's anxiety. If orthopaedic evaluation is delayed 7 to 10 days, then cold therapy, gentle active range-of-motion exercises, and nonsteroidal anti-inflammatory drugs may be beneficial.

TOTAL JOINT ARTHROPLASTY

Prosthetic replacement of damaged joints is common in the United States. They have been designed for almost every joint of the upper and lower extremities. The weight-bearing joints of the lower extremity must tolerate much higher forces than the joints of the upper extremity. Fortunately, the bones of the lower extremity are much larger, which allows for better fixation of the prosthetic devices.

Prosthetic Types

Joint arthroplasties are divided into total (complete) joint arthroplasty and hemiarthroplasty (partial), based on whether both sides or one side

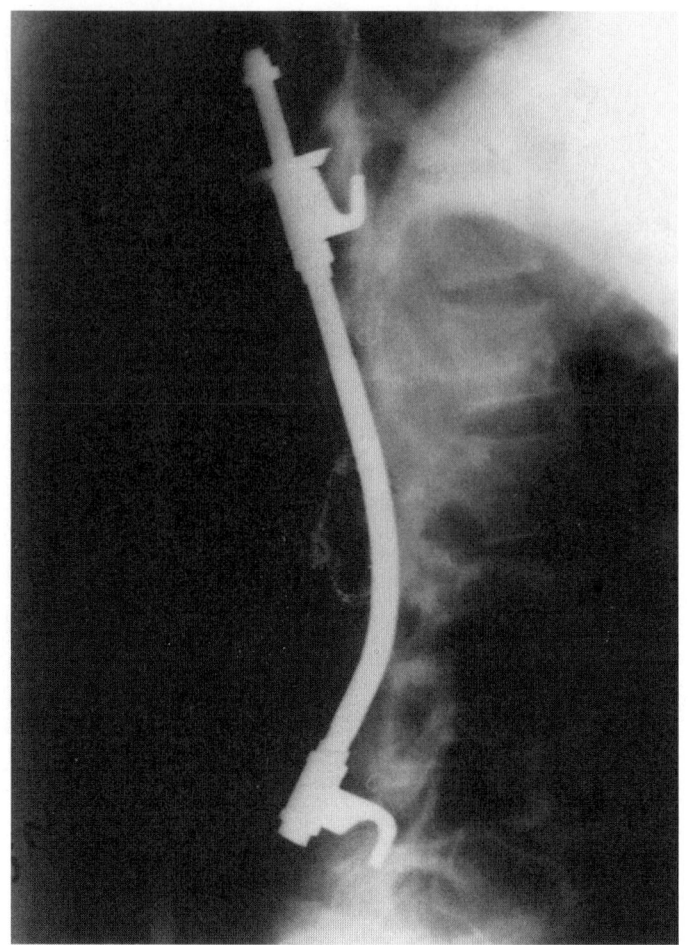

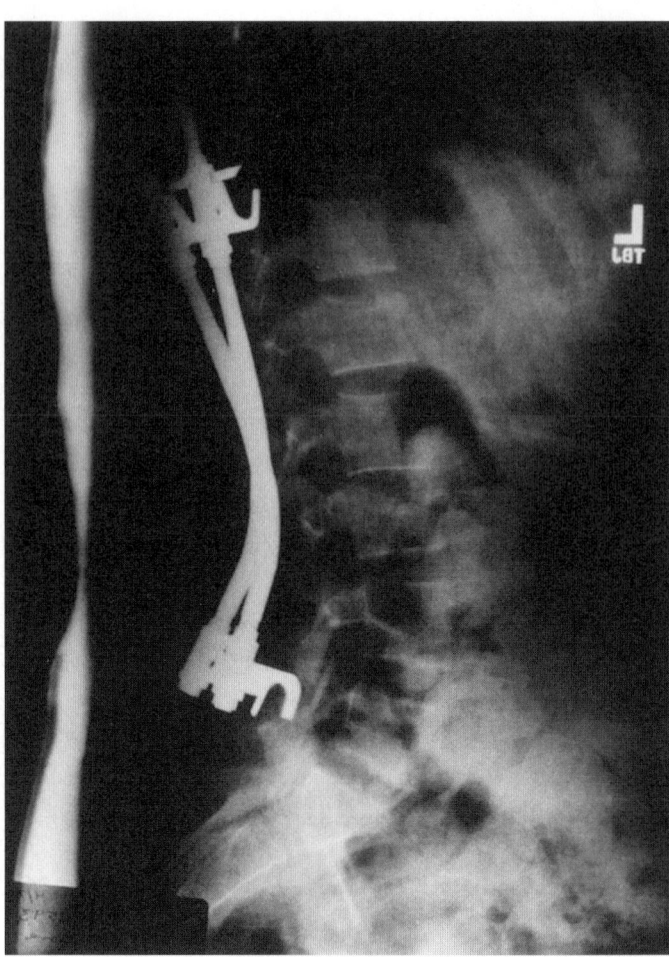

A

B

FIG. 280-20. A. This hook-and-rod system was used to stabilize a lumbar burst fracture. **B.** The patient noted a "pop" with forward bending, and the lateral radiograph confirms that the top hook was disengaged.

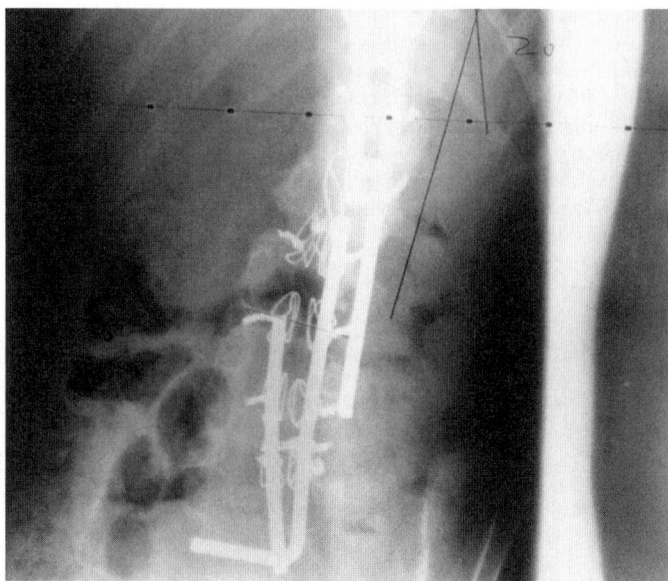

FIG. 280-21. This double rod construct broke before fusion.

of the joint is replaced, respectively. Hemiarthroplasties are used most often to replace the humeral or femoral head because of a displaced fracture (Figure 280-24). The prosthetic head is attached to a stem that is inserted into the intramedullary canal.

Sir John Charnley popularized total joint arthroplasty for the treatment of hip arthritis. The most common hip replacement has a metal femoral prosthesis that articulates with a plastic acetabular cup, which usually has a metal backing that is secured to the pelvis (Figure 280-25). Metal-on-plastic prostheses are now used to replace almost every other extremity joint, including the knee, shoulder, elbow, wrist, ankle, and, infrequently, the small bones of the hand and feet.

Total joints may be constrained but are more frequently stabilized by the patient's native joint ligaments and tendons. The rate of loosening from the bone is higher with constrained implants, which are designed with the two components locked together. These designs are used primarily for revision surgery when soft tissue loss and attenuation increase the risk of dislocation. The exception is the elbow, where primary (first time) constrained prostheses are often used, because the surgical exposure violates significant stabilizing structures.

Two methods of fixing the prosthesis to the bone may be used. The implant may be press-fit by wedging the implant into the gross bone structure. Additional stability can be achieved with a special surface

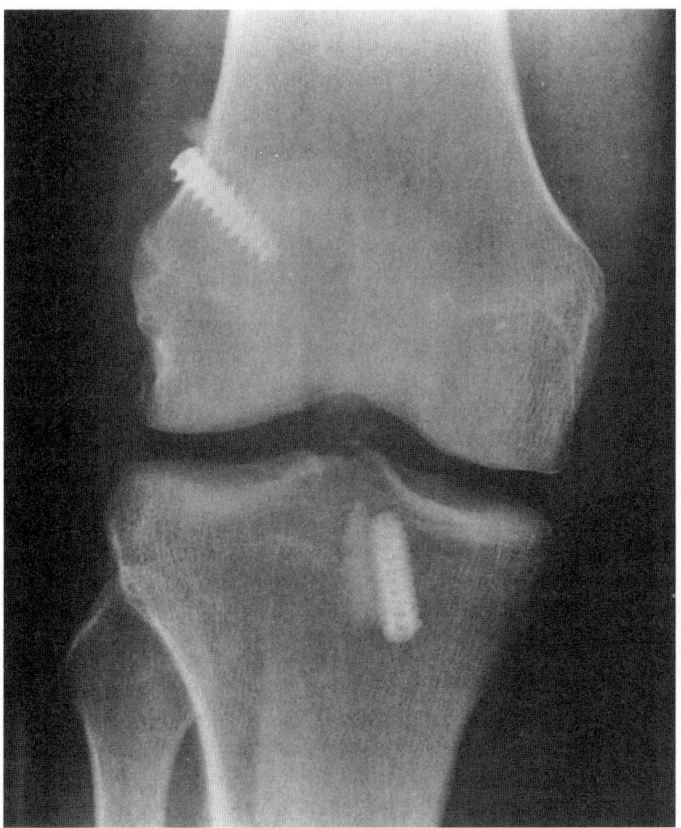

A

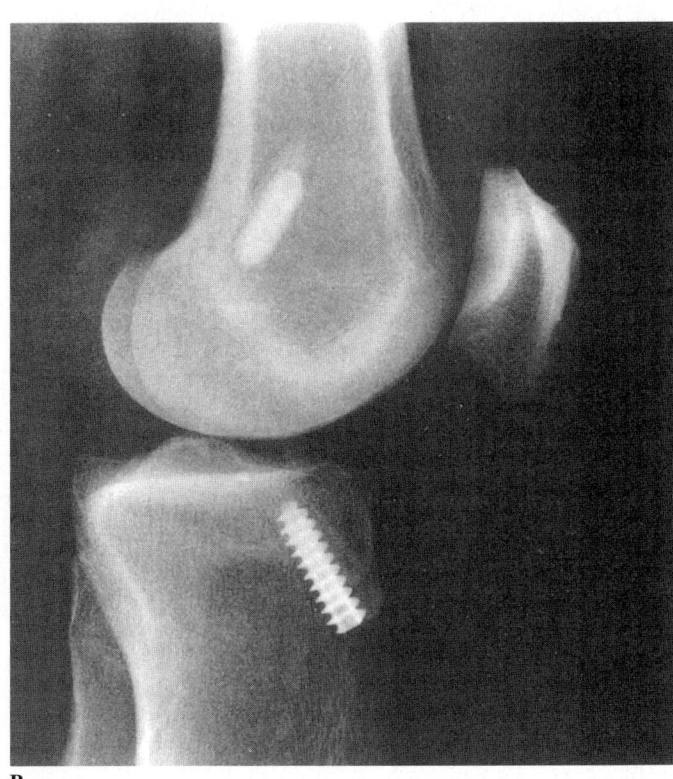

B

FIG. 280-22. A and **B.** These interference screws rigidly fix a bone-patellar-bone autograft used for an ACL reconstruction.

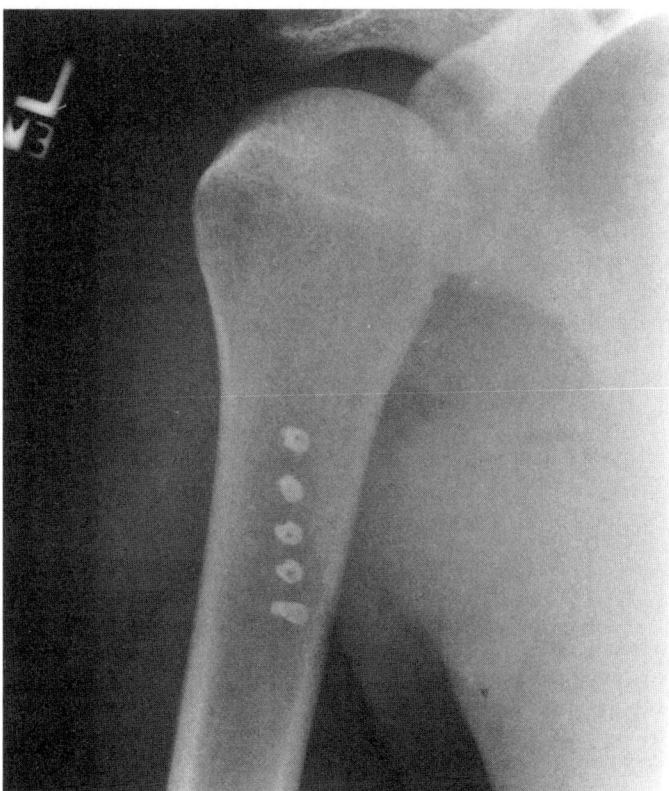

FIG. 280-23. These metal-anchored sutures were used to repair a ruptured pectoralis major insertion to the proximal humerus.

coating, which allows the bone to grow directly onto the prosthesis. The second method of fixation is polymethylmethacrylate cement, which stabilizes the bone and the implant in a similar manner that mortar secures a post in a hole.

The results of modern joint arthroplasty are excellent. Currently, total hip and total knee arthroplasty have a greater than 90 percent success rate at 15- to 20-year follow-up.

Complications

When a patient presents with new onset of periprosthetic pain, dislocation, periprosthetic fracture, implant loosening, or infection should be suspected.

It is possible for nonconstrained and constrained implants to dislocate. The diagnosis is usually obvious but should be confirmed with biplane radiographs. One view may not clearly show the dislocation and appear deceptively normal (Figure 280-26A, B). Because many of today's implants are modular (i.e., snap together in the operating room), relocation should not be attempted without discussion with an orthopedic surgeon. Disassembly of modular prosthesis during attempted closed reduction has been reported. Dislocated constrained implants are rarely amenable to reduction in the emergency department, and these designs often require open reduction in the operating room.

Modern alloys have greatly reduced the incidence of prosthetic breakage. More commonly, the bone around the prosthesis fractures (see Figure 280-10). Once the emergency medicine physician makes the diagnosis of a periprosthetic or prosthetic fracture, an orthopedist should be consulted.

Implant loosening is the most common long-term complication of joint arthroplasty, but it is usually characterized by insidious onset of pain and rarely presents to the emergency department. Although pros-

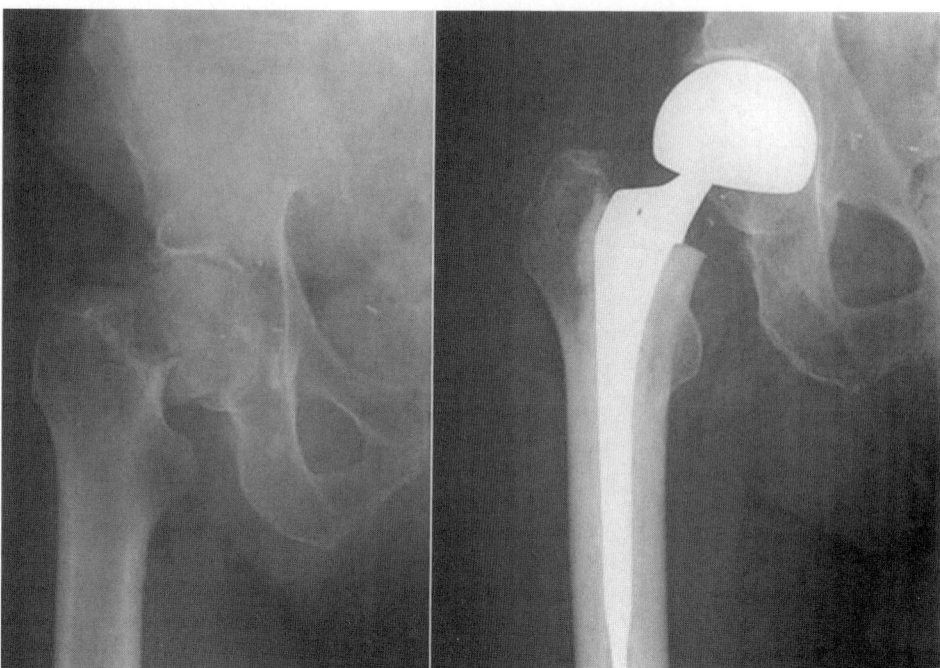

FIG. 280-24. A cemented hemiarthroplasty was used to treat this displaced femoral neck fracture.

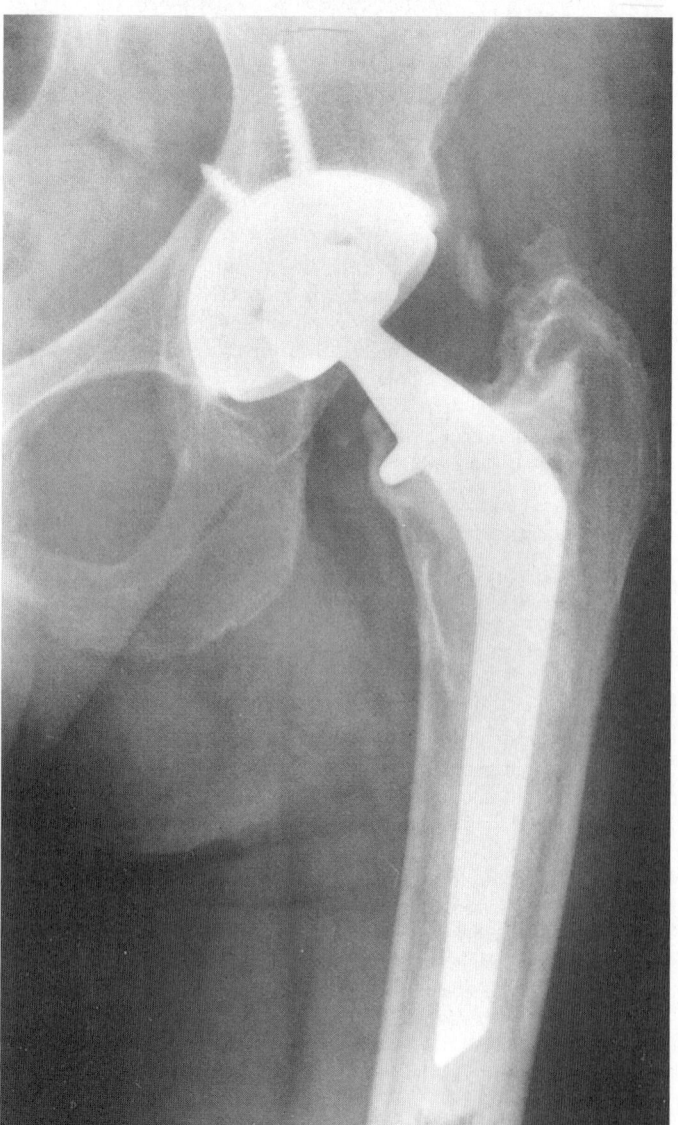

FIG. 280-25. This "hybrid" total hip arthroplasty has a cemented femoral component and an uncemented acetabular component that is also fixed with screws.

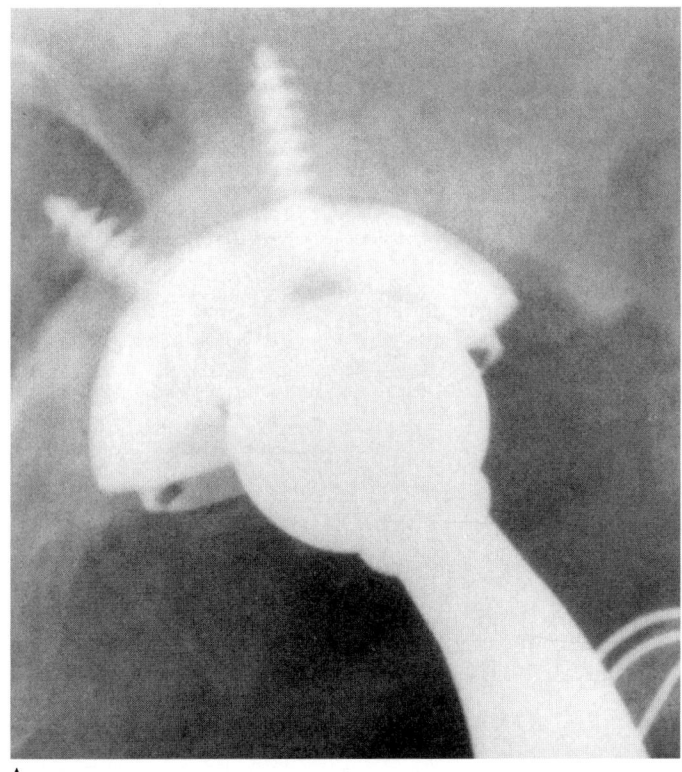
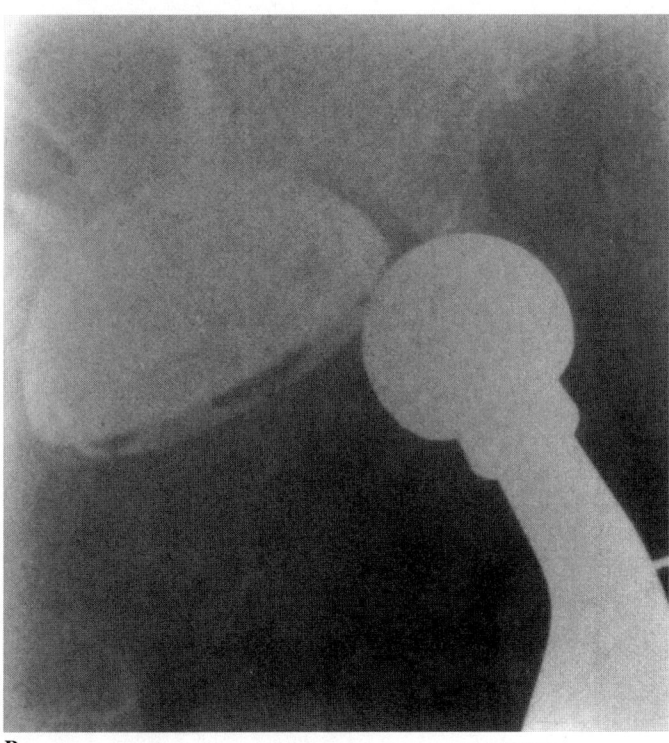

A　　　　　　　　　　　　　　　　　　　　　　**B**

FIG. 280-26. **A** and **B.** This patient's total hip arthroplasty is dislocated. The slight asymmetry on the first view was not detected, and additional radiographs were needed to diagnose the dislocation.

thetic loosening most often is not related to infection, deep wound sepsis may be the cause and should be considered. Radiographic criteria for loosening reported in the orthopedic literature include migration of the implant (Figure 280-27), lytic destruction of bone around the prosthesis, or a complete radiolucent line around the bone-to-prosthetic construct interface.

Infection of a total joint arthroplasty is a catastrophic event. Deep infection typically presents with wound drainage, intractable pain, and increases in the erythrocyte sedimentation rate or C-reactive protein. It is rarely associated with systemic symptoms, and blood cultures are usually negative. Aspiration of the joint should be performed before administration of antibiotics and never without a surgeon's approval. It is possible for an aseptic implant to be infected by a needle aspiration. Infections after primary arthroplasties now have an incidence of less than 1 percent when using modern sterile techniques.

The emergency department physician is more likely to see a patient with a history of a joint infection previously treated with a one- or two-stage debridement. Because one-stage revisions (or simple debridements) for infected arthroplasties are associated with higher recurrence rates, this information has prognostic value and should be sought from the patient.

Other serious complications of total joint arthroplasties involve the soft tissue structures around the joint. Ligaments holding the joint together can disrupt, causing instability of the joint. Tendons that pass around the joint can rupture, leading to loss of function of the joint. If diagnosed early, they can often be repaired with an excellent result.

Complications of Upper Extremity Arthroplasties

The prosthetic elbow joint has more frequent complications than other commonly replaced joints. Even in the best centers, infection rates of 10 percent or greater are not uncommon. This infection rate may be due to the thin soft tissue over the posterior elbow. High loosening rates of elbow prostheses may be related to the frequent use of constrained designs and the limited bone available for fixation.

The shoulder's humeral component is extremely durable. The glenoid component is prone to failure because of its small bone surface area for fixation. Dislocation of the shoulder can be diagnosed only with a true anteroposterior and an axillary or transscapular lateral radiograph. Acute loss of motor power may be the result of a rotator cuff tear.

Complications of Lower Extremity Arthroplasty

Ankle arthroplasty has had limited success in the past because the small bones of the hindfoot do not allow adequate fixation to withstand the high forces placed across the ankle joint. More recently, improved designs have demonstrated better short-term results.

The knee has excellent inherent ligamentous stability, and minimally constrained implants are usually used. Although not as common as in the shoulder or hip, it is possible for these implants to dislocate. Instability can develop in knee arthroplasties if a ligament (such as the medial collateral) is disrupted. Diagnosis is by the same examination methods used on unreplaced knees. Disruption of the quadriceps mechanism is a devastating complication and must be considered if the patient is unable to perform a straight leg raise. When the patella tendon ruptures, repair rates are extremely poor, especially if not diagnosed and treated early.

The hip, like the shoulder, may be replaced with a hemi- or total arthroplasty. The acetabulum usually is not replaced in fracture management but is almost always resurfaced for arthritis. The hip is the most common joint arthroplasty to dislocate. Dislocation is confirmed by biplane radiographs. Because these prostheses are often modular, great care should be used during relocation. Reattachment of the trochanter after the occasional transtrochanteric surgical approach is usually performed with wire. These wires commonly break during the healing process but are not usually a problem.

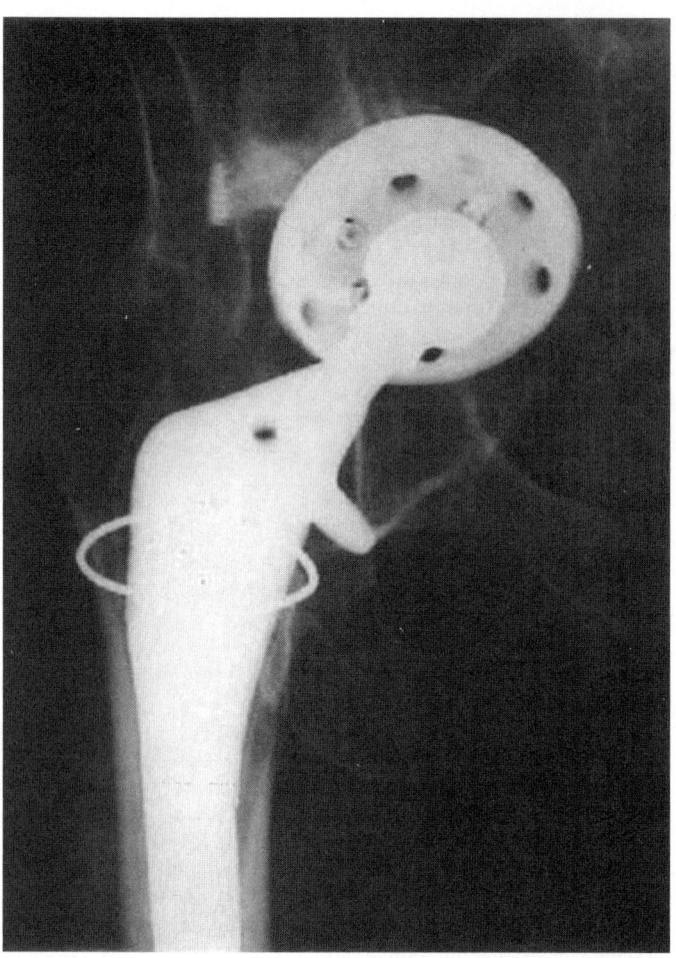

FIG. 280-27. The acetabular component loosened and has migrated into the pelvis.

BIBLIOGRAPHY

Browner BD, Jupiter JB, et al: *Skeletal Trauma,* 2nd ed. Philadelphia, Saunders, 1998.

Chapman MW: *Operative Orthopaedics,* 2nd ed. Philadelphia, Lippincott, 1993.

Delee J, Drez D: *Orthopaedic Sports Medicine,* 2nd ed Philadelphia, Saunders, 2003.

Green DP: *Operative Hand Surgery,* 4th ed. New York, Churchill Livingstone, 1999.

Morrey BF: *Joint Replacement Arthroplasty.* New York, Churchill Livingstone, 1991.

Muller ME, Allgower M, et al: *Manual of Internal Fixation,* 3rd ed. Berlin, Springer-Verlag, 1991.

Rockwood CA Jr, Green DP, et al: *Fractures in Adults,* 5th ed. Philadelphia, Lippincott Williams & Wilkins, 2001.

Rothman RH, Simeone FA, Herkowitz, H: *The Spine,* 4th ed. Philadelphia, Saunders, 1999.

NONTRAUMATIC MUSCULOSKELETAL DISORDERS

NECK PAIN
William J. Frohna

The causes of neck pain include trauma and biomechanical injuries, degeneration, inflammation (arthritides), infection (e.g., discitis, meningitis, epidural abscess), and infiltration (e.g., metastatic carcinoma, spinal cord tumors, osteoid osteoma).[1,2] In most cases of neck pain, no specific etiology can be identified.[1] A knowledge of cervical spine anatomy and a complete history and physical examination, focusing on the presence or absence of neurologic signs, are needed to identify pathologic causes and prevent complications.

ANATOMY

The cervical spine consists of seven vertebrae. The upper cervical spine (occipitoatlantoaxial complex) is unique and is made up of the base of the skull, atlas (C1), axis (C2), and several strong ligaments. The atlas (C1) supports the occipital condyles in its lateral masses. This articulation allows for flexion and extension but no rotation. The articular surfaces of the atlas (C1) and axis (C2) are convex to each other and allow flexion, extension, and especially rotation to occur. The transverse, accessory, and alar ligaments are the primary stabilizing ligaments of the occipitoatlantoaxial complex. The mid and lower cervical spine (C3 to C7) consists of vertebrae which are similar in size and shape. These vertebral bodies articulate with each other via their superior and inferior articular processes, enabling limited rotation and lateral flexion. The transverse processes of each of the cervical vertebrae are perforated by a foramen through which the vertebral vessels pass. Topographically, the first cervical vertebra is located immediately behind the angle of the mandible, the transverse process of the atlas is positioned between the angle of the mandible and the mastoid process, the hyoid bone is anterior to the level of C3, the thyroid cartilage is anterior to C4, and the cricoid cartilage is at the level of the sixth cervical vertebra.

The muscles of the neck are compartmentalized into seven fascial planes. These planes normally enable pain-free movement of one muscle group on the other. Following acute neck trauma, petechial hemorrhages and edema within these same fascial planes may produce limited motion associated with complaints of stiffness, pain, and swelling.

The stable but flexible cervical spine is linked by both ligaments and disks. Because of major structural differences, the cervical disks are less likely than lumbar disks to prolapse. The cervical spine is more mobile, the superincumbent weight is less, the nucleus pulposus is located more anteriorly, and unlike the lumbar spine, the annulus is reinforced posteriorly in its entire width by the posterior longitudinal ligament.

The eight paired cervical spinal roots exit the intervertebral foramina between the superior and inferior pedicles, except for the first cervical roots. The nerve roots exit the spinal canal above the level of the same numbered vertebra, with the exception of the C8 nerve root, which exits at the C7-T1 interspace.[3] Unique to the cervical spinal roots, the ventral and dorsal roots are separate at the neural foramina in over half of cases. Therefore isolated irritation of the dorsal (sensory) root posteriorly by an osteophyte may produce only sensory complaints. Similarly, ventral root (motor) compromise by a degenerative or herniated disk may produce only painless, progressive weakness.

The sinuvertebral nerves from the dorsal root reenter the intervertebral foramina, supplying sensory innervation to the ligaments of the spinal canal. Anteriorly, they supply the posterior longitudinal ligament and posteriorly the ligamentum flavum, meninges, and associated vessels. Ascending and descending branches supply the zygoapophyseal joints and provide position sense.

CLINICAL FEATURES

In general, it is helpful to classify patients with neck pain into two groups: (1) those with pain arising mainly from the joints and associated ligaments and muscles of the neck, and (2) those with neck pain and *radiculopathy* (signs and symptoms attributable to a single nerve root) and/or *myelopathy* (signs or symptoms due to a spinal cord lesion, stenosis, or compression).[1,4] Most patients do not exhibit either radiculopathy or myelopathy, but the course and treatment for those who do may be quite different from those patients with isolated neck pain.[4]

History

Ask about onset, duration, and location of the neck pain; recent or remote trauma, associated symptoms; stiffness; deformity; neurologic complaints (e.g., weakness, changes in sensation, gait, or vision); constitutional symptoms such as fever, anorexia, and weight loss; and comorbid conditions such as arthritis, cancer, and infections.[1] Several rheumatologic conditions predispose to neck pain and instability of the atlantoaxial (C1-C2) joint. Rheumatoid arthritis, ankylosing spondylitis, and psoriatic spondyloarthropathy may involve the C1-C2 joint and damage the transverse ligament and erode the odontoid process. Subluxation may occur spontaneously or following a trivial injury. Morning stiffness may signify arthritic joints, unremitting night pain may indicate a malignant process, and fever and night sweats suggest an infection.[3] Identify precipitating and palliative factors, maneuvers, or activities. Inquire about prior episodes of neck pain, past diagnostic studies, and treatment. Determine the character of pain and its distribution. Patients with radiculopathy often complain of sharp, burning, intense pain that radiates to the trapezius, periscapular area, or down the arm.[1] Weakness or paresthesias may develop weeks after pain onset.[4] Patients with myelopathy may have neck pain that progresses insidiously and may complain of clumsy hands, gait disturbances, and sexual or bladder dysfunction.[4] Table 281-1 summarizes important differences in symptoms between mechanical neck pain and neck pain associated with radiculopathy or myelopathy.[1]

Physical Examination

The physical examination should begin with a general assessment of the patient, noting evidence of weight loss, pallor, adenopathy, and abnormalities of posture, movement, and facial expression.[1] Pain may cause splinting of the head on the shoulders during position change. Active and passive movement should be assessed, including rotation (chin to shoulder), lateral flexion (ear to shoulder), and flexion-extension. Most mechanical causes of neck pain result in asymmetric lesions and asymmetrically limited or painful movements.[1] Inflammatory or neoplastic disorders are typically more widespread, with pain and movement restriction being more symmetric.[1] When localized ipsilateral neck pain is felt toward the side of head movement, zygoapophyseal joint irritability is suspected. *Spurling sign* (gentle pressure applied to the patient's head during extension and lateral rotation) may reproduce radicular pain with radiation into the ipsilateral upper extremity. The *abduction relief sign,* performed by having the

TABLE 281-1   Symptoms and History Associated with Neck Pain

Group 1: Cervical Problems Arising Mainly from Neck Joints and Associated Ligaments and Muscles	Group 2: Cervical Problems Involving the Cervical Nerve Roots or the Spinal Cord
Patients complain of pain and stiffness	Patients complain of significant root pain
Pain is a deep, dull aching sensation and often episodic	Pain is sharp and intense and is often described as a burning sensation
Patients have a history of excessive or unaccustomed activity or of sustaining an awkward posture	Pain may radiate to the trapezial and periscapular areas or down the arm
There is no history of specific injury	Patients complain of numbness and motor weakness in a myotomial distribution
Ligament and muscle pain are localized and asymmetic	
Pain from upper cervical segments is referred toward the head; pain from lower segments, to the upper limb girdle	Headache may occur if the upper cervical roots are involved
Symptoms are aggravated by neck movement and relieved by rest	Symptoms often become more severe with neck hyperextension

Source: Reproduced with permission from Tsang.[1]

patient place the hand of the affected upper extremity on the top of his or her head to obtain relief, may indicate soft disc protrusion causing radicular pain.[3] When neck pain occurs on the side away from head movement, a ligamentous or muscular source for the pain is suspected as these structures are stretched.

Further assessment should include palpation of the structures of the head and neck and a thorough musculoskeletal and neurologic examination. Palpate the posterior cervical triangle, the supraclavicular fossa, carotid sheaths, and the anterior neck. C5-C6 root lesions often elicit tenderness over the brachial plexus at Erb's point in the supraclavicular fossa, whereas a C8-T1 root lesion may cause tenderness over the ulnar nerve at the elbow.

Pathology in the lymph nodes, salivary glands, or thyroid gland may result in neck pain. Auscultation of the carotid and the subclavian arteries may demonstrate bruits, in the former associated with potential cerebral insufficiency and in the latter with thoracic outlet or vascular steal syndrome. The temporal artery should be examined for signs of inflammation, as temporal arteritis may be the cause of neck and shoulder pain.

Sensory symptoms of pain or dysesthesias are difficult to evaluate, particularly when motor signs are absent. This is often the case in cervical spinal radiculopathies. The discrete separation of the motor and sensory roots at the cervical neural foramina is the explanation for motor sparing despite severe sensory symptoms. For example, C7 root irritability without motor weakness can present as aching at the medial to middle scapular border, aching in the myotome distribution to the chest, axilla, or triceps, or as numbness or tingling in the middle finger.

Early cervical spinal myelopathies can only be recognized if the examiner looks for them by performing a complete neurologic examina-

tion. Findings in patients with myelopathy include hyperreflexia, a positive Babinski sign, clonus, gait disturbance, sexual or bladder dysfunction, lower extremity weakness, impaired fine hand movement, and upper and lower extremity spasticity. In the patient with cord compression, the clinician may elicit *Lhermitte sign,* an electric-like shock radiating down the spine and often into the extremities, with neck flexion. *Hoffman sign* indicates an upper motor neuron lesion and is performed by flicking the tip of the middle finger as the hand is relaxed in a neutral position. A positive response is flexion of the thumb and index finger in a pinching motion.[3]

Table 281-2 summarizes the sensory, motor, and reflex findings in cervical radiculopathy. This information should be used to determine the level of motor and sensory involvement, and to compare findings in the affected and unaffected sides. Bilateral or multilevel involvement usually implies serious pathology.[1]

Imaging Studies

The need for radiographs depends on the clinical condition suspected and the duration of neck pain. Acute (days to weeks), uncomplicated, nonradicular, nonmyelopathic, atraumatic neck pain typically requires no imaging studies, as the cause is likely benign and the treatment is conservative.[1,4] Obtain three-view cervical spine films in patients with chronic (weeks to months) neck pain with or without a history of trauma, those with neck pain and a prior history of malignancy or remote neck surgery,[5] and in those with neck pain and preexisting spinal disorders such as rheumatoid arthritis, ankylosing spondylitis, and psoriatic spondyloarthropathy. Films are obtained to identify bone destruction or cervical spine instability.

TABLE 281-2   Signs and Symptoms of Cervical Radiculopathy

Disk Space	Cervical Root	Pain Complaint	Sensory Abnormality	Motor Weakness	Altered Reflex
C1-C2	C2	Neck, scalp	Scalp		
C4-C5	C5	Neck, shoulder, upper arm	Shoulder	Infraspinatus, deltoid, biceps	Reduced biceps reflex
C5-C6	C6	Neck, shoulder, upper medial, scapular area, proximal forearm, thumb, index finger	Thumb and index finger, lateral forearm	Deltoid, biceps, pronator teres, wrist extensors	Reduced biceps and brachioradialis reflex
C6-C7	C7	Neck, posterior arm, dorsum proximal forearm, chest, medial third of scapula, middle finger	Middle finger, forearm	Triceps, pronator teres	Reduced triceps reflex
C7-T1	C8	Neck, posterior arm, ulnar side of forearm, medial inferior scapular border, medial hand, ring, and little fingers	Ring and little fingers	Triceps, flexor carpi ulnaris, hand intrinsics	Reduced triceps reflex

If degenerative disease is suspected, oblique views of the cervical spine can identify foraminal narrowing. Flexion-extension films may be useful if instability is suspected. Patients with normal radiographs, patients with radiographic evidence of cervical spondylosis and no neck instability (degenerative changes manifested by osteophyte formation, disc space narrowing, and facet disease), or patients with radiographic evidence of previous trauma *and* no neurologic signs or symptoms need no further imaging.[5] **Magnetic resonance imaging (MRI) is indicated for those patients with neurologic signs or symptoms regardless of the plain film findings.**[5] MRI is also indicated when plain radiographs reveal bone or disc margin destruction, if there is cervical instability, and (with intravenous contrast) if epidural abscess is suspected.[5] CT myelography is recommended when contraindications to MRI exist.

ETIOLOGY

Cervical Soft Tissue Injury

Soft tissue neck injury is also known as hyperextension strain, acceleration-deceleration injury, hyperextension-hyperflexion injury, neck strain, neck sprain, and whiplash. The most common precipitating events are motor vehicle collisions, falls, sports injuries, and work-related injuries. Acute and chronic pain may develop secondary to trauma to the richly innervated structures of the neck and cervical muscle groups. The forces applied during motor vehicle crashes are multiple and depend on the position of the head and neck as well as the type of accident. Typically, whiplash injury results from sudden acceleration-deceleration trauma that occurs when an unaware victim in a stationary vehicle is struck from behind. Patients often complain of pain and stiffness and examination may reveal tender paracervical muscles with decreased range of motion. Typically, pain is delayed for a number of hours following an accident.

Other uncommon and highly variable postinjury complaints include headache, vertigo or dizziness, spatial instability, dysphagia, or hoarseness. Headache can occur from stretching and tearing of occipital muscles and the occipital nerve. The cause of vertigo is unknown, but it could be due to brainstem contusion, vertebral artery dissection, trauma to sympathetic fibers that accompany vertebral arteries, vertebral artery insufficiency secondary to atherosclerosis, or osteophytic compression of the vertebral arteries. Patients may describe true vertigo, or a feeling of "sliding" or "veering" with changes of direction. Any neurologic findings after whiplash injury should be evaluated for brain or spinal cord injury or vertebral artery dissection.[6,7] Dysphagia or hoarseness are symptoms of severe blunt neck or laryngeal injury and require thorough evaluation.

The most devastating complication of hyperflexion-hyperextension injury is the central cord syndrome, which may occur in the presence of cervical spondylosis, spinal stenosis, ankylosing spondylitis, or disk herniation. There may be no radiographic evidence of spinal trauma. Physical examination findings of central cord syndrome include weakness that is disproportionately greater in the upper extremities than the lower extremities, and it can be accompanied by variable sensory loss (see Chap. 272, for further discussion).

The NEXUS criteria can be followed to determine indications for cervical spine imaging after such injuries (see Chaps. 256 and 272 for detailed discussion of spine injuries.)

Cervical Disk Herniations

Cervical disk herniations occur as the nucleus pulposus protrudes through the posterior annulus fibrosis, producing either an acute radiculopathy or occasionally a myelopathy. Protrusions are usually confined by the posterior longitudinal ligament, but can occasionally extrude through this ligament as free fragments. Direct posterior ruptures, although infrequent, can produce progressive myelopathy, whereas the more common posterolateral herniations can cause acute cervical radiculopathy. Disk prolapse is more common in males, occurring most often in the fourth decade. The levels of most frequent involvement are C5-C6 (C6 root) usually right sided, and C6-C7 (C7 root), usually left sided. C6 root compression accounts for 20 percent of cases, while C7 root compression accounts for 70 percent of cervical disk herniation cases.[4]

The symptoms of an acute cervical disk prolapse include neck pain, headache, pain referred to the shoulder and along the medial scapular border, and dermatome pain and dysesthesia in the spinal root distribution to the shoulder and arm. Motor signs include fasciculations, atrophy and weakness in the dermatome distribution of the spinal root, loss of deep tendon reflexes, and with cervical myelopathy, lower extremity hyperreflexia, Babinski sign, and rarely loss of sphincter control. Cervical hyperextension and lateral flexion to the symptomatic side (Spurling sign) may replicate the symptoms, as can a Valsalva maneuver, whereas manual cervical distraction in flexion alleviates them. A thorough physical examination, including strength, sensory, and reflex testing, easily delineates the level of root involvement (see Table 281-2).

Cervical spine radiographs are often more useful in these syndromes for what they fail to reveal rather than what they demonstrate. Magnetic resonance imaging is necessary for diagnosis.

Cervical Spondylosis and Stenosis

Cervical spondylosis is a progressive, degenerative condition that often presents either as a loss of cervical flexibility, neck pain, occipital neuralgia, radicular pain, or occasionally as progressive myelopathy. There is progressive degeneration of the discs, ligaments, facet joints (zygoapophyseal joints), and uncovertebral joints (joints of Luschka).[3] Other common clinical terms used for this condition are osteoarthritis of the neck and degenerative disk disease. From a radiographic standpoint, cervical spondylosis may be diagnosed if any of three findings are present: osteophytes, disc space narrowing, and facet disease.[5] However, there is a high prevalence of cervical spondylosis in asymptomatic individuals, and care must be taken in ascribing painful syndromes to distinct anatomic abnormalities.[3] Degenerative disk disease predisposes to progressive osteoarthrosis of the cervical spine, joint instability, and incongruous joint motion during neck movement. Spondylosis most commonly occurs at the C5-C6 and C6-C7 levels.

Osteophytic spurs can encroach posteriorly on the spinal canal, producing cervical myelopathy; laterally on the intervertebral foramen, producing cervical radiculopathy; and anteriorly on the esophagus, producing dysphagia. Spurious osteophytes may also produce Horner's syndrome, vertebrobasilar symptoms, severe radicular symptoms without associated neck pain, painless upper extremity myotome weakness, and chest pain mimicking angina. Neurologic findings (radiculopathy or myelopathy) may be gradual in onset unless there is a history of recent trauma.

The combination of a congenitally narrowed spinal canal further compromised by a vertebral osteophytic bar anteriorly and a buckling ligamentum flavum posteriorly, increases the risk of myelopathy secondary to cervical spinal stenosis as the diameter of the spinal canal is reduced to less than 13 mm. Cervical spinal stenosis can also occur in about 20 percent of patients with lumbar spinal stenosis.

Cancer

Metastatic cancer should be in the differential diagnosis of the patient who presents with chronic neck pain, even though a past history of cancer is lacking. The complaint of unremitting night pain may be indicative of a malignant process.[3] Lung, breast, and prostate cancers as well as lymphoma and multiple myeloma may involve the cervical spine causing neck pain.[4] Although most cases of epidural cord compression occur in the thoracic spine (70 percent), approximately 10 percent involve the cervical spine.[8] Myelopathy, typically caused by disk or degenerative disease, is rarely caused by metastatic tumors.[4] Plain films of the cervical spine may reveal destruction of the vertebral bodies and pedicles, lytic lesions of the pedicles, and pathologic compression fractures.[4] Cancer patients with radiographic evidence of bone or disc margin destruction should undergo magnetic resonance imaging.[5] Imaging of the cervical spine with CT scan or tomograms should be considered in the patient with questionable findings on plain film.

Myofascial Pain Syndrome

Myofascial pain syndrome (MPS) is a cause of chronic neck pain and is often confused with radiculopathy. Although it has been defined as pain persisting more than several months, MPS may present acutely, especially after trauma, with typical clinical characteristics.[9] Psychological distress and specific personality traits contribute to the conversion of emotional distress into bodily complaints and focus on the body so that nonpainful sensations are perceived as painful.[9] The location of pain may help in discriminating MPS from true radicular pain. MPS patients often complain of pain in the neck, scapula, and shoulder and in a nondermatomal radiation into the upper extremity. On physical examination, the MPS patient will not have neurologic abnormalities, while the patient with radiculopathy may exhibit weakness or an altered deep tendon reflex. Patients with MPS have tender spots, "trigger points," that may be found on palpation of the head, neck, shoulder, and scapular region. Because cervical spine abnormalities develop with age in the asymptomatic population, radiographic findings cannot be relied upon to verify the source of neck pain or upper extremity complaints. Imaging of the MPS patient reveals either nonspecific degenerative or disc changes that do not correlate with the clinically suspected site.[9]

Other Conditions

Epidural abscess, osteomyelitis, and temporal arteritis are infectious and inflammatory causes of neck pain. Cervical spinal epidural hematoma often presents with neck pain followed by symptoms and signs of cord compression. Pain from ischemic heart disease may radiate into the neck and shoulder. Peripheral nerve involvement, such as carpal tunnel syndrome, may present as a C6-C7 sensory radiculopathy, while multiple sclerosis, amyotrophic lateral sclerosis (ALS), subacute combined degeneration, and syrinx are in the differential of myelopathy.[4]

TREATMENT

Treatment issues can be divided into three categories: neck pain, neck and arm pain (radiculopathy), and myelopathy.[3] There is little evidence-based material to support many of the recommended physical medicine modalities [traction, thermotherapy, electrical stimulation, massage, electromyographic biofeedback, transcutaneous electrical nerve stimulation (TENS), and therapeutic ultrasound].[10,11] However, individual patients may indeed benefit from one or more of these therapies.

Neck Pain

Most cases of neck pain without clear underlying pathology will improve with minimal intervention. The patient should be advised to avoid activities that produce pain. Initial medications may include nonsteroidal anti-inflammatory drugs, muscle relaxants, and for significant pain, a short course of oral opiates. Follow-up with the primary physician should be encouraged to assess the need for physical or manual therapies. In patients with chronic neck pain (>12 weeks

duration), The Philadelphia Panel[10] recommends the use of proprioceptive and therapeutic exercises.

Patients with acute neck pain following an acceleration-deceleration (whiplash) injury may benefit from a similar pharmacologic regimen as that described above. There is insufficient data to recommend corticosteroid treatment for whiplash injuries.[12,13] Rest and immobilization using collars are not recommended ("rest makes rusty") and usual activities should be maintained.[14]

Treatment of neck pain in patients with a predisposing rheumatologic or neoplastic condition will depend on whether or not there is cervical spine instability (C1/C2) and/or evidence of cord compression. Pain medications and consideration of a course of oral glucocorticoids may be considered as first-line treatment if neither instability nor cord compression is present. Admission and neurosurgical consultation should be undertaken if either complication is present.

Therapy for neck pain from myofascial pain syndrome should address both muscular tension and psychobehavioral issues.[9] Initial treatment includes nonsteroidal anti-inflammatory drugs, muscle relaxants, and short-course opioid analgesics for severe symptoms. Follow-up with the primary care physician is needed to arrange optimal therapies.

Radiculopathy

Most authors recommend a trial of conservative treatment as long as there is no evidence of myelopathy.[3] Initial treatment consists of activity modification, oral medications, and immobilization with a soft cervical collar. The patient should be encouraged to follow-up closely with their primary physician for consideration of specialist consultation, electrodiagnostic evaluation, and additional rehabilitation interventions. Oral medications may include anti-inflammatory agents, opioid analgesics, and muscle relaxants. A course of steroids, oral (e.g., methylprednisolone self-weaning dose pack) or epidural, may be useful in the acute phase of radicular pain.[3] If the symptoms and signs of acute cervical root compression fail to respond to conservative treatment or recur, surgery may be recommended if imaging demonstrates concordant findings. Indications for hospital admission include:

1. Intractable radicular pain unresponsive to treatment
2. Progressive upper extremity weakness, especially in the C7 distribution
3. Acute or progressive symptoms or signs of myelopathy

Myelopathy

Treatment decisions for patients with symptoms and signs of cord compression should be made in conjunction with specialists. Cervical spondylotic myelopathy is the condition causing the greatest amount of impairment and disability in the continuum of spondylosis.[3] Myelopathy is the most common cause of spastic paraparesis in patients older than 55 years of age, thus paralleling the time course of spondylosis.[3] The patient with myelopathy should be referred to a neurosurgeon for consideration of decompressive surgery. Additional therapeutic considerations will depend on the time course of symptoms and signs and etiology, but should be made in conjunction with a neurosurgeon.

Acknowledgement to Myron M. LaBar, author of this chapter in the 2nd through 5th editions.

REFERENCES

1. Tsang I: Rheumatology: 12. Pain in the neck. *CMAJ* 164:1182, 2001.
2. Croft PR, Lewis M, Papageorgiou AC, et al: Risk factors for neck pain: A longitudinal study in the general population. *Pain* 93:317, 2001.
3. Levy HI: Cervical pain syndromes: Primary care diagnosis and management. *Comp Ther* 26:82, 2000.

4. Kriss TC, Kriss VM: Neck Pain—Primary care work-up of acute and chronic symptoms. *Geriatrics* 55:47, 2000.

5. Daffner RH, Dalinka MK, Alazraki N, et al: American College of Radiology ACR Appropriateness Criteria 2000: Chronic neck pain. *Radiology* 215(Suppl):345, 2000.

6. Chong CL, Ooi, SB: Neck pain after minor neck trauma—is it always neck sprain? *Eur J Emerg Med* 7:147, 2000.

7. Sim E, Vaccaro AR, Barzalanovich A, et al: The effects of staged static cervical flexion-distraction deformities on the patency of the vertebral arterial vasculature. *Spine* 25:2180, 2000.

8. Byrne TN: Spinal cord compression from epidural metastases. *New Engl J Med* 327:614, 1992.

9. Pawl RP: Chronic neck syndromes: An update. *Comp Ther* 25:278, 1999.

10. The Philadelphia Panel: Philadelphia Panel evidence-based clinical practice guidelines on selected rehabilitation interventions for neck pain. *Phys Ther* 81:1701, 2001.

11. Gross AR, Aker PD, Goldsmith CH, et al: Physical medicine modalities for mechanical neck disorders (Cochrane Review), in: *The Cochrane Library* 3, 2002. Oxford: Update Software.

12. Bracken MB: Steroids for acute spinal cord injury (Cochrane Review), in: *The Cochrane Library* 3, 2002. Oxford: Update Software.

13. Petterson K, Toolanen G: High dose methylprednisone prevents extensive sick-leave after whiplash injury. A prospective randomized double blind study. *Spine* 23:984, 1998.

14. Verhagens AP, Peeters CGM, de Bie RA, et al: Conservative treatment for whiplash (Cochrane Review), in: *The Cochrane Library* 3, 2002. Oxford: Update Software.

282 THORACIC AND LUMBAR PAIN SYNDROMES
David Della-Giustina
Marco Coppola

INTRODUCTION

Back pain is second only to upper respiratory tract infection as a symptom-related reason for visits to primary care physicians.[1,2] It is the most common cause of work-related disability in persons younger than 45 years of age and the second most common cause of temporary disability for all ages.[1,2] The majority of patients that present to the ED with back pain have a nonspecific etiology that has no life-threatening or neurologically impairing concerns. However, due to the high volume of ED patients with back pain, one can develop an indifference to this complaint and potentially overlook serious causes for the symptoms. The best approach to this complaint is to perform a systematic evaluation based on *risk factors* in the history and physical examination and let this guide one's approach in terms of diagnostic testing and management (Table 282-1).

CLINICAL EVALUATION

[handwritten: acute < 6 wks / sub acute 6–12 wks / chro > 12 wks]

History

The history should focus on the risk factors for serious disease, which includes duration of symptoms, age, pain location, trauma history, systemic symptoms, specific pain features, neurologic deficits, and past medical history.

DURATION OF SYMPTOMS   Back pain is categorized into three groups based on the duration of symptoms: acute is less than 6 weeks, subacute is pain continuing between 6 and 12 weeks, and chronic is pain more than 12 weeks.[3] Pain lasting greater than 6 weeks is a risk factor for specific problems as most episodes of nonspecific back pain (80 to 90 percent) resolve within 6 weeks.[2,4]

PATIENT AGE   Patients under age 18 and over age 50 have a higher likelihood of a serious cause for back pain. In both of these age groups, back pain is more likely to be caused by tumor or infection than in the 18 to 50 age group. Patients younger than 18 have a higher incidence of congenital and bony abnormalities such as spondylolysis, spondylolisthesis, and Scheuermann kyphosis. In those aged 50 and older, nonmechanical causes such as a rupturing abdominal aortic aneurysm and other intra-abdominal processes are more common.

LOCATION OF THE PAIN   Pain that originates from muscular, ligamentous, vertebral, or disk disease without nerve involvement is located primarily in the back, possibly with radiation into the buttocks or thighs. Sciatica is radicular pain in the distribution of a lumbar or sacral nerve root and is often accompanied by sensory or motor deficits.[3] It occurs in only 1 percent of patients with back pain.[3,5] Sciatica is associated with disk herniation or nerve root impingement below the L3 nerve root. This is based on the dermatomal distribution of the nerve roots and the fact that the pain associated with nerve root impingement radiates along the entire pathway of the nerve. Ninety-five percent of herniated disks occur at the L4-L5 or the L5-S1 lumbar disk spaces, impinging on the L5 or S1 nerve roots, respectively.[3]

HISTORY OF TRAUMA   History of major trauma is a risk factor for fracture and should prompt one to order plain radiographs of the involved spine. One special situation involves elderly patients who may sustain a vertebral fracture with even minor trauma such as falling from standing or from sitting in a chair. This is due to the bony changes with aging, predominantly osteoporosis. Thus a history of minor trauma in an elderly patient with back pain suggests fracture and warrants ordering plain radiographs.

SYSTEMIC COMPLAINTS   Systemic symptoms such as fever, chills, night sweats, malaise, and an undesired weight loss suggest infection or malignancy. These symptoms are more worrisome for infection if the patient has any of the following risk factors: recent bacterial infection, especially urinary tract infection or pneumonia; recent genitourinary or gastrointestinal procedure; immunocompromised status; or injection drug use. Injection drug use is a substantial risk factor for spinal infection, and one should follow the axiom that back pain

TABLE 282-1   Summary of Risk Factors in Back Pain

	Concern
Historical Risk Factors	
Pain >6 weeks	Tumor, infection
Age <18, >50	Congenital anomaly, tumor
Major trauma	Fracture
Minor trauma in elderly	Fracture
History of cancer	Tumor
Fever and rigors	Infection
Weight loss	Tumor, infection
Injection drug use	Infection
Immunocompromise	Infection
Night pain	Tumor, infection
Unremitting pain, even when supine	Tumor, infection
Incontinence	Epidural compression
Saddle anesthesia	Epidural compression
Severe/progressive neurologic deficit	Epidural compression
Physical Risk Factors	
Fever	Infection
Patient writhing in pain	Infection
Unexpected anal sphincter laxity	Epidural compression
Perianal/perineal sensory loss	Epidural compression
Major motor weakness	Nerve root or epidural compression
Positive straight leg raise test	Herniated disk

in a patient who is an injection drug user is vertebral osteomyelitis or epidural abscess until proven otherwise.

However, it is important to review the abdomen, chest, and urinary system to avoid overlooking extraspinal disease processes referring or radiating to the back. The most serious of these is a rupturing abdominal aortic aneurysm. Other potential causes of pain referred to the back include pancreatitis, a posterior lower lobe pneumonia, nephrolithiasis, and renal infarct.

ATYPICAL PAIN FEATURES   Most patients with a benign etiology for their back symptoms complain of a dull, aching pain that generally worsens with movement but improves with rest and lying still. Risk factors for tumor and infection include pain that occurs at night, often awakening the patient from sleep, or is unrelenting despite appropriate use of analgesics and rest. Pain suspicious for disk herniation is that which is worsened by coughing, Valsalva maneuver, or sitting, and is relieved by lying in the supine position.[1,3,5] Spinal stenosis is associated with bilateral sciatic pain that is worsened by activities such as walking, prolonged standing, and back extension, and is relieved by rest and forward flexion. In the authors' experience, night pain and unrelenting pain are worrisome symptoms that are commonly overlooked in the evaluation of patients with back pain.

ASSOCIATED NEUROLOGIC DEFICITS   Most patients with non-specific back pain have no associated neurologic deficits or complaints. Any neurologic deficit is a risk factor for structural back disorders. Neurologic complaints such as paresthesias, numbness, weakness, and gait disturbances must be further addressed in the history and delineated in the physical examination to determine whether the symptoms involve single or multiple nerve roots. Bowel or bladder incontinence is a symptom worrisome for an epidural compression syndrome such as spinal cord compression, cauda equina syndrome, or conus medullaris syndrome. If a patient presents with back pain and a history of urinary incontinence (acute or chronic), but an otherwise completely normal history and evaluation, measure the postvoid residual volume. A large postvoid residual volume (e.g., >100 mL) indicates overflow incontinence, which in the setting of low back pain suggests neurologic compromise and an epidural compression syndrome.[6]

PAST MEDICAL HISTORY   History of cancer is a risk factor as back pain is the initial symptom in the majority of those with spinal metastases. Malignant neoplasm is the most common systemic disease affecting the spine. Approximately 80 percent of the patients with this diagnosis are over age 50.[6] Patients with a history of cancer of the breast, lung, thyroid, kidney, or prostate, and those with a history of myeloma, lymphoma, or sarcoma are at highest risk for metastatic disease to the spine.[7] However, only one-third of patients diagnosed with spinal malignancy have a known history of cancer.[6] Thus one must rely on other symptoms such as unremitting pain, night pain, and weight loss to direct one to further diagnostic testing to make this diagnosis.

Physical Examination

The physical examination does not need to be comprehensive, but is must be focused on ruling out risk factors and identifying neurologic deficits.

VITAL SIGNS   Fever is a risk factor for infection. Unfortunately, the sensitivity of fever is low, varying from 27 percent for tuberculous osteomyelitis to 50 percent for pyogenic osteomyelitis and 83 percent for spinal epidural abscess.[6] Approximately 2 percent of patients with non-specific back pain will present with fever that is not due to a spinal infection. In these cases it is usually attributed to a concomitant viral illness.[6] However, the first concern is for a spinal infection until it is ruled out by further history, physical examination, and possibly diagnostic testing.

GENERAL APPEARANCE   Patients with a benign source of back pain are generally most comfortable when lying still. In patients with severe or excessive pain, consider acute spinal infection, abdominal aortic aneurysm, or nephrolithiasis.

ABDOMEN   Examine the abdomen of all patients with back pain. The examination should include auscultation for bruits and palpation for masses, tenderness, and an enlarged aorta.

BACK   Examine the back for signs of underlying disease. Erythema, warmth, and purulent drainage are consistent with infection. Contusion and swelling are concerning for trauma. Palpate the back and percuss the vertebral bodies. Point tenderness to percussion is found with fractures and bacterial infection, with a sensitivity of 86 percent and specificity of 60 percent for infection.[6]

The final portion of the back examination consists of straight leg raise testing. With the patient lying supine, passively lift each leg separately to approximately 70 degrees in an attempt to reproduce the pain (Figure 282-1). A positive straight leg raise test results in a re-

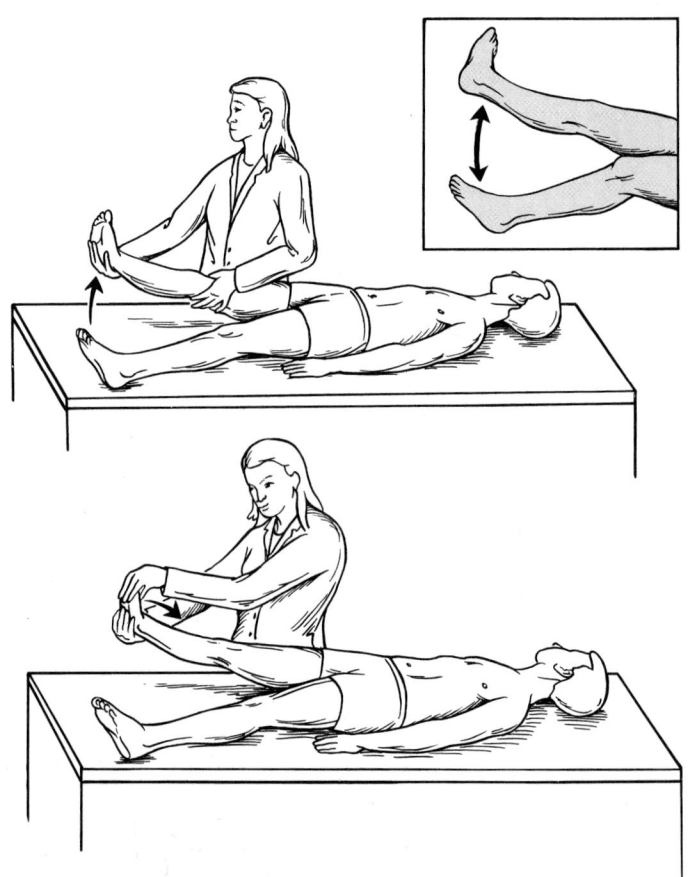

FIG. 282-1. Instructions for the straight leg raising (SLR) test. 1. Ask the patient to lie as straight as possible on a table in the supine position. 2. With one hand placed above the knee of the leg being examined, exert enough firm pressure to keep the knee fully extended. Ask the patient to relax. 3. With the other hand cupped under the heel, slowly raise the straight limb. Tell the patient "If this bothers you, let me know, and I will stop." 4. Monitor for any movement of the pelvis before complaints are elicited. True sciatic tension should elicit complaints before the hamstrings are stretched enough to move the pelvis. 5. Estimate the degree of leg elevation that elicits complaint from the patient. Then determine the most distal area of discomfort: back, hip, thigh, knee, or below the knee. 6. While holding the leg at the limit of straight leg raising, dorsiflex the ankle. Note whether this aggravates the pain. Internal rotation of the limb can also increase the tension on the sciatic nerve roots.

production of the patient's sciatic pain or a radicular pain into the affected leg below the knee. The radicular pain is worsened by ankle dorsiflexion and improved with ankle plantar flexion or decreasing the elevation. Reproduction of the patient's back pain or pain in the gluteal or hamstring area does not constitute a positive result. An important point regarding the straight leg raise test is that it can be easily and surreptitiously confirmed from the seated position with similar leg extension and foot dorsiflexion (Figure 282-2). Straight leg raise testing is a screening examination for herniated nucleus pulposus (disk). A positive straight leg raise test is approximately 80 percent sensitive for a L4-L5 or L5-S1 herniated disk. Radicular pain down the affected leg when lifting the asymptomatic leg is called a positive crossed straight leg raise test. A positive result is highly specific, but insensitive for nerve root compression by a herniated disk.[2,3,5]

NEUROLOGIC EXAMINATION The neurologic examination is the most important aspect of the physical examination. It is directed to detecting deficits in each of the specific spinal nerve roots. Sensation may be tested by using light touch initially, followed more formally by pinprick, temperature, proprioception, and vibration testing if there are any questions regarding diminished sensation. Next one assesses strength, with a focus on those muscle groups innervated by individual nerve roots (Figure 282-3). Specifically, individually test the ankle dorsiflexors (L4), extensor hallucis longus (great toe dorsiflexion) (L5), and ankle plantar flexors (S1/S2). Finally, evaluate the patellar (L3-L4), Achilles (S1), and Babinski reflexes. There is no easily obtainable reflex for the L5 nerve root. Babinski sign is an abnormal reflex that appears when upper motor neuron innervation through the corticospinal tract is lost. A positive Babinski sign is extension of the great toe and abduction of the other toes with plantar stimulation, rather than the normal flexion response.

Digital rectal examination should be performed in those patients with any risk factors, especially those with neurologic complaints, and in those with severe pain. The test is performed to evaluate for rectal sphincter tone and sensation, the presence of prostatic and rectal masses, and to rule out perirectal abscess. Poor rectal tone in association with back pain and saddle anesthesia indicates an epidural compression syndrome.

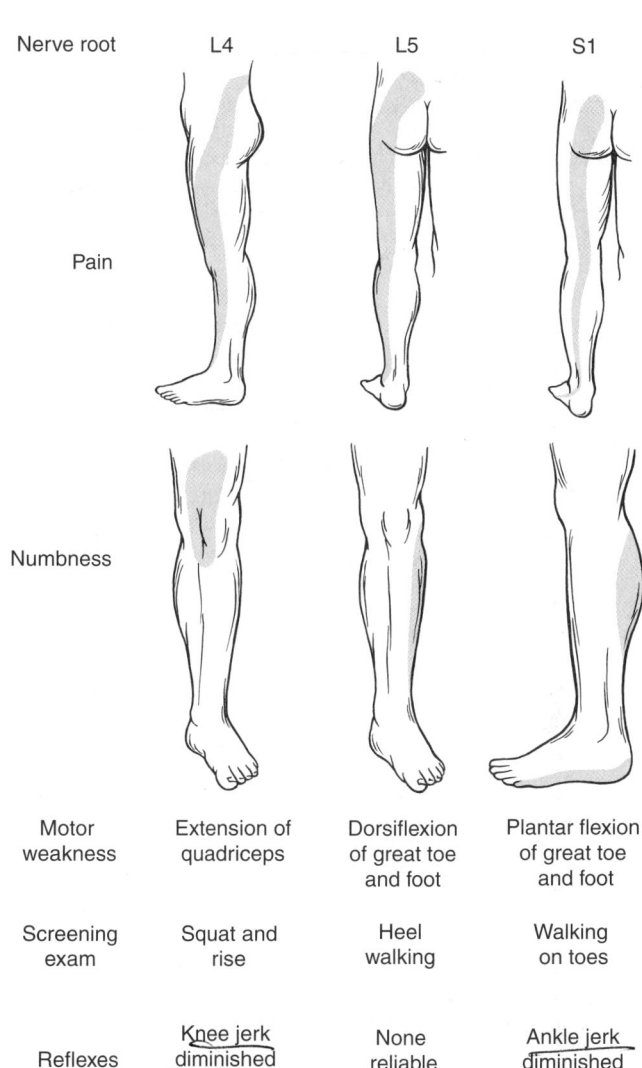

FIG. 282-3. Testing for lumbar nerve root compromise.

DIAGNOSTIC TESTING

Laboratory Testing

Laboratory testing is indicated if one has concern for infection, tumor, or rheumatologic causes of the back pain. Order a CBC, erythrocyte sedimentation rate (ESR), and urinalysis (UA). With infection, the white blood cell count may be normal or elevated. However, the ESR is invariably elevated, even in those with immunocompromise.[8,9,10] The C-reactive protein is also elevated. The ESR will also be elevated in patients with a rheumatologic etiology of their symptoms, as well as in the majority of patients with neoplastic disease of the spine.[11] Urinalysis is obtained to rule out urinary tract infection as an infectious source for seeding of the spine and to rule out renal disease being referred to the back.

Radiographic Imaging

PLAIN SPINAL RADIOGRAPHS Plain spinal radiographs can be considered when one suspects fracture, tumor, or infection. In ordering these images, only anteroposterior and lateral views are necessary. The cone-down L5-S1 and oblique views rarely add clinically useful information while more than doubling gonadal radiation exposure and cost.[3]

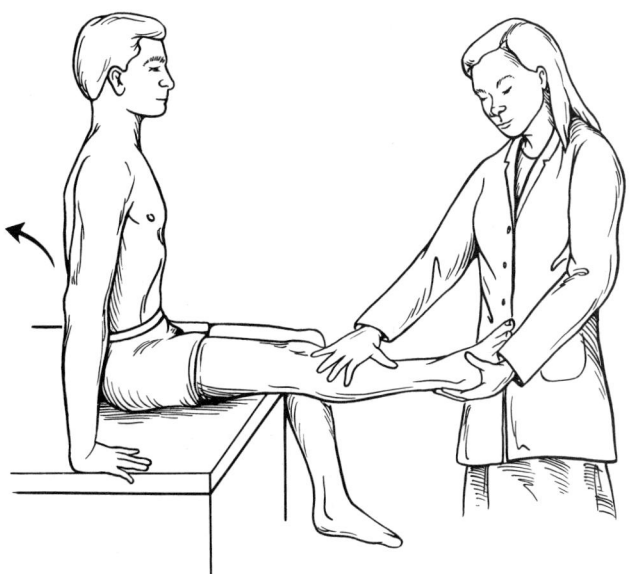

FIG. 282-2. Instructions for sitting knee extension test. With the patient sitting on a table, both hip and knees flexed at 90 degrees, slowly extend the knee as if evaluating the patella or bottom of the foot. This maneuver stretches nerve roots as much as a moderate degree of supine SLR.

MRI   MRI is the definitive imaging modality in most emergent situations involving back pain. It offers the best resolution for lesions in the vertebral bodies, spinal canal, spinal cord, and disk disease. It is the gold-standard study in cases of suspected spinal infection, neoplasm, and epidural compression syndromes. Furthermore, its routine or urgent use is indicated in evaluating for neoplastic processes of the entire spine and disk disease, or when the patient's symptoms fail to resolve after 6 to 8 weeks.[2,12]

CT SCAN   CT scanning is most useful in evaluating vertebral fractures, the facet joints, and the posterior elements of the spine. It shows good detail of the vertebral bodies, but has poor resolution of the spinal canal and spinal cord in comparison to MRI. Because of its widespread availability, it is useful in those settings in which MRI is either unavailable or unsuitable. In the setting of suspected spinal canal or cord involvement, such as epidural abscess or compression, CT myelography is the best substitute when MRI is unavailable.[13]

DIFFERENTIAL DIAGNOSIS AND MANAGEMENT

Nonspecific Back Pain

The majority of patients seen in the ED with acute back pain will receive this diagnosis. This is a symptom complex that has countless names, including back strain/sprain, mechanical back pain, and lumbago. However, because strain and/or sprain have never been histopathologically documented in these patients, a more accurate diagnosis is idiopathic or nonspecific back pain. Nonspecific back pain is the authors' choice, especially since up to 85 percent of these patients will never be given a more precise diagnosis.[2]

SYMPTOMS AND DIAGNOSIS   The patient with nonspecific back pain typically complains of mild to moderate pain that is aggravated with movement and relieved with rest. While the typical mechanism is usually minor exertion or lifting, the patient may not recall any remarkable etiology. The history and physical examination generally reveal an absence of risk factors, or if any risk factors are present, the diagnostic evaluation is normal.

MANAGEMENT   The management strategy for nonspecific back pain is multifaceted, including activity, analgesia, manipulation, and other physical modalities. First, patients should be monitored for 4 to 6 weeks for improvement of their symptoms before embarking on a diagnostic evaluation, because 80 to 90 percent will resolve on their own within this time period.[14] Thus, watchful waiting avoids wasting time, money, and unnecessary radiation exposure to the patient. This point should be discussed with the patient, as they commonly expect to have plain spinal radiographs, at a minimum, obtained for their symptoms in the ED.

The therapeutic value of activity has gained significant recognition as a cornerstone of management. While bed rest had been previously advocated, it has been demonstrated that patients who resume their normal activities to the extent tolerable recover more rapidly than those on 2 or 7 days of bed rest or those who performed back-mobilizing exercises.[3,15] Thus, patients should continue with their daily activities as much as possible, using pain as the limiting factor. Withhold exercise programs until the acute painful episode has resolved or improved significantly.

The foundation of pharmacologic therapy is acetaminophen and NSAIDs. Acetaminophen is an excellent first-line agent and there is no evidence that NSAIDs are more effective for symptomatic relief. However, most physicians use NSAIDs. Most NSAIDs are equally efficacious for back pain, yet there are significant differences in the side effect profiles and toxicity.[16,17] In one review, ibuprofen was the least toxic of the twelve studied, particularly with regard to upper GI bleeding.[17] Since there is a linear relationship between dose and toxicity, the lowest dose possible should be used in patients at risk. In those patients at risk for GI bleeding, the addition of misoprostol or omeprazole can reduce the risk.[17] The NSAID ketorolac is no more effective than oral ibuprofen in patients with musculoskeletal pain, but it has a higher rate of side effects.

We recommend using acetaminophen in combination with NSAIDs or as the sole initial agent when treating patients at higher risk for adverse effects of NSAIDs, such as the elderly and patients with renal disease or peptic ulcers. One regimen is acetaminophen 650 to 975 mg q 4 to 6 h, either alone or in conjunction with either ibuprofen 800 mg tid, or naproxen 250 to 500 mg bid.

Opioid analgesics should be offered to patients with moderate to severe pain, but for a limited (1 to 2 weeks) duration. When prescribing opioid analgesic combinations that include acetaminophen, warn patients not to combine them with other acetaminophen products.

Muscle relaxants are useful for treating back pain, especially when accompanied by muscular spasms. Muscle relaxants such as diazepam 5 to 10 mg q 6 to 8 h, and methocarbamol 1000 to 1500 mg qid, are effective. Although their efficacy appears equal to NSAIDs, there does not appear to be any additional pain relief or synergistic benefit when used in combination with them.[16] Corticosteroids taken systemically, injected locally or into the epidural space, have no role in the treatment of nonspecific back pain.[16]

Manipulative therapy, while not generally an ED treatment, is one of the more controversial treatment options for back pain. Recent research showed that acute manipulation is no better than physical therapy and only slightly better in terms of patient satisfaction than giving the patient a one-dollar educational booklet.[18] Furthermore, manipulation fared no better than standard medical therapy in terms of clinical outcome.[19] Consequently, we question the utility and cost-effectiveness of manipulative therapy and do not recommend it in patients with acute back pain.

Other physical modalities include traction, diathermy, cutaneous laser treatment, exercise, ultrasound treatment, and transcutaneous electrical nerve stimulation. None of these have any proven efficacy in the treatment of acute low back symptoms. The application of heat or ice may provide temporary symptomatic relief in some patients.

Chronic Nonspecific Back Pain

There is a higher concern for serious disease in patients with ongoing or intermittent symptoms for months to years. The best approach is to review the past evaluation to ensure that it has been complete and that abnormalities have not been overlooked. Specifically, review laboratory testing and plain spinal radiographs. If the evaluation has been incomplete, then complete it in the ED at that visit. If the evaluation has been thorough and negative, then treat as described for nonspecific back pain. If opioid analgesics are needed, prescribe them for only a week or so, until a primary care physician can assume care.

Sciatica

While sciatica only affects 1 percent of all patients with back pain, it is present in 95 percent of patients with a symptomatic herniated disk.[3] Although disk herniation is the most common cause of sciatica, other etiologies to consider include intraspinal tumor or infection, foraminal stenosis, extraspinal plexus compression, piriformis syndrome, and lumbar canal stenosis (spinal stenosis).

Disk Herniation

SYMPTOMS AND DIAGNOSIS   Patients who present with sciatica due to a herniated disk generally complain more about the radicular symptoms than the back pain. Because more than 95 percent of disk herniations occur at the L4-L5 (L5 nerve root) or L5-S1 (S1 nerve root) level, the radicular pain extends below the knee in the dermatomal distribution of the nerve root.[2,3] The remaining 5 percent of patients are usually older patients who have a relatively increased risk of disk herniation at the L2-L3 (L3 nerve root) and L3-L4 (L4 nerve root) levels. The physical examination generally demonstrates localization of pain and a neurologic deficit in a unilateral single nerve root, usually L5 or S1, and frequently a positive result on straight leg raise testing.

If the patient has no risk factors in the history and physical examination for serious disease other than sciatica, treat conservatively and do not perform any diagnostic tests in the ED.[1–3,5,13,14] If the patient has a demonstrable neurologic deficit, then one may consider obtaining plain radiographs to rule out other possible causes for symptoms such as tumor, fracture, spondylolisthesis, and infection. It is the authors' practice not to obtain any plain radiographs in this setting. If the patient returns to the ED for a worsening condition or the sciatica fails to improve, then an MRI is indicated. However, if the symptoms have not progressed rapidly or the symptoms are not severe, the MRI can be ordered routinely or urgently but not emergently.

MANAGEMENT   The treatment of patients with herniated disk is similar to that of patients with lumbosacral strain. Routine daily activity is as good as 2 weeks of bed rest in terms of intensity of pain, bothersomeness of symptoms, and functional status.[20] The use of analgesics (acetaminophen, NSAIDs, and narcotics) and muscle relaxants is the same as that described for lumbosacral strain. Interestingly, NSAIDs are less effective in treating the symptoms than they are in treating lumbosacral strain.[16]

Corticosteroid therapy for herniated disk has a limited benefit. Specifically, epidural corticosteroid injection has been shown to have a minor reduction in leg pain and sensory deficits in comparison to placebo. However, the improvement in symptoms is not associated with any significant functional benefit nor does it reduce the need for surgery.[16,21] Although epidural steroid injection is not an ED procedure, it offers an alternative for the moderately to severely symptomatic patient in follow-up. Local and systemic administration of corticosteroids has not been proven beneficial in herniated disk.

Manipulation is not recommended for the routine management of symptoms from herniated disk.[3,14] Other physical modalities have not been shown to be useful in managing sciatica, although as in the case of lumbosacral strain, application of heat or ice may provide temporary relief.

Most patients with a herniated disk may be treated and monitored by their primary care physician without specialist referral. Approximately 80 percent of patients will ultimately improve with nonsurgical therapy, with more than 50 percent recovering in 6 weeks.[1–3] Most spine surgeons agree that surgery is appropriate only when all three of the following criteria are met:

1. Definitive evidence of herniation as demonstrated by an imaging study
2. This evidence exists in conjunction with a corresponding clinical picture and neurologic deficit
3. Conservative treatment for 4 to 6 weeks fails to produce improvement

The major benefit of surgery is to cure the sciatica and the neurologic deficits. Approximately 70 percent of patients who undergo surgery obtain relief of their back pain.[5] Emergency decompressive surgery is required only in patients with acute epidural compression syndromes. Conservative nonsurgical treatment has been compared with surgery for herniated disks in two studies. The results showed that patients who underwent surgery had improved function and fewer symptoms at 1 and 2 years postoperatively, compared with those treated conservatively; however, by 4 and 10 years postoperatively, both groups had comparable results.[2,3]

Spinal Stenosis

Spinal stenosis is a narrowing of any part of the lumbar spine, including the spinal canal, nerve root canal, and intervertebral foramina, that that may occur at single or multiple spinal levels. Degenerative disease causes narrowing and compression of vascular and neural structures. It is a cause of chronic back pain, generally over a period of years, which may have associated sciatica. The symptoms, which usually begin in the sixth decade, include low back pain that is aggravated by prolonged standing and spinal extension, and is relieved by rest and forward flexion. Typically, symptomatic patients present with low back and lower extremity pain with walking that is symptomatically similar to vascular claudication. This symptom is termed pseudoclaudication. Pseudoclaudication, which occurs in 60 percent of patients with spinal stenosis, is pain of the lateral legs that occurs with walking and is relieved with rest. It is called pseudoclaudication because it is caused by neurologic compression, not arterial occlusion. Physical examination findings are often absent. The diagnosis is made by history with confirmation by CT scan or MRI. Referral to a spine surgeon is indicated to determine if surgery can be beneficial. Symptomatic treatment is as for chronic back pain.

Ankylosing Spondylitis

Ankylosing spondylitis is an autoimmune arthritis that primarily affects the spine and pelvis. It has been also associated with HLA B-27, trauma, and infection. It most commonly occurs in patients under age 40 with a 3:1 male predilection. Patients complain of awakening with low back pain and stiffness that improves throughout the day with mild activity, as well as other constitutional symptoms such as malaise and fatigue. The diagnosis is made by history in individuals with symptoms longer than 3 months' duration. Radiographic studies demonstrate sacroiliitis and squaring of the vertebral bodies, the so-called "bamboo spine." Patients are treated symptomatically with NSAIDs and should be referred to a rheumatologist for further management.

Epidural Compression Syndromes

Epidural compression syndrome is a collective term encompassing spinal cord compression, cauda equina syndrome, and conus medullaris syndrome. This term is used to group these syndromes together for two reasons. First, the presentation for these syndromes is similar, except for the level of the neurologic deficit. Secondly, the initial evaluation and management for these syndromes is similar, until the actual diagnosis is known.

While the diagnosis of a complete epidural compression is obvious, the challenge to emergency physicians is in detecting those patients with early signs and symptoms. The initial differential diagnosis is broad and includes most conditions that cause weakness, sensory changes, or autonomic dysfunction. The history and physical examination will enable one to narrow the differential to a compressive lesion of the spinal cord or cauda equina.

Possible causes of epidural compression include spinal canal hemorrhage, tumors of the spine or epidural space, spinal canal infections, and massive midline disk herniation. Transverse myelitis is a noncompressive condition that may present exactly like a compressive lesion of the spinal cord.[7]

The history for patients with epidural compression usually includes back pain with associated neurologic deficits, incontinence, and sciatica in one or both legs. The duration of symptoms does not help differentiate these syndromes from benign causes of back pain. Important features are a history of malignancy and a rapid progression of neurologic symptoms, especially bilateral symptoms.

The physical examination findings vary depending on the level of compression and the amount and area of the spinal cord or cauda equina that is compressed. The most common finding in cauda equina syndrome is urinary retention with overflow incontinence, with a sensitivity of 90 percent and a specificity of about 95 percent.[6] Other common findings for epidural compression include weakness or stiffness in the lower extremities, paresthesias or sensory deficits, gait difficulty, and abnormal results on straight leg raising.[2] The most common sensory deficit occurs over the buttocks, posterosuperior thighs, and perineal regions, and is commonly called "saddle anesthesia." Anal sphincter tone is decreased in 60 to 80 percent of cases.[6]

When one clinically suspects epidural compression, especially due to tumor, treat the patient with dexamethasone 10 mg IV before obtaining any confirmatory tests.[21] This is done in an attempt to minimize progression of the compression, edema, and the resultant neurologic damage. The reason to treat before determining a definitive diagnosis is because the diagnostic evaluation may take several hours or longer, and there may be a progression of the neurologic deficit while the patient is waiting.

After the patient has received dexamethasone, obtain an emergent MRI of the spine. If investigating the possibility of epidural compression due to neoplasm, obtain an MRI of the entire spine, as 10 percent of patients with vertebral metastases have additional silent epidural metastases, which would be missed by a localized imaging study.[22] The presence of tumors remote from the symptomatic site may change patient management. Additionally, the neurologic examination may falsely localize the spinal lesion(s), and limited regional MRI may not detect the lesion. If one suspects a pure cauda equina syndrome, then it is reasonable to obtain a localized MRI.

The functional clinical outcome for epidural compression from tumor depends on patient symptoms at presentation. Patients who cannot walk before treatment rarely walk again. Those who are too weak to walk without assistance but who are not paraplegic have a 50 percent chance of walking again. Those who are able to walk when treatment begins are likely to remain ambulatory.[22] Of those patients who require a catheter for urinary retention before treatment, 82 percent will continue to require the urinary catheter after treatment.[23]

Spinal Infections

Spinal infections are very serious but uncommon causes of back pain. Infections are often associated with immunocompromised states such as cancer, diabetes, organ transplant, and injection drug use. Patients with spinal infections usually have had prolonged symptoms, and in greater than 50 percent, the symptoms have been present for greater than 3 months.[12] The principal symptom is pain, which is present in almost all patients.

Physical examination demonstrates fever in approximately 50 percent of patients and vertebral body tenderness to percussion. Laboratory evaluation usually shows an elevated WBC count, although this may be normal, and the erythrocyte sedimentation rate is universally elevated. Blood cultures are positive in approximately 40 percent of cases of osteomyelitis, and even higher in patients with epidural abscess. In osteomyelitis, plain radiographs will be normal until the process has had sufficient time to demineralize the bone, which can range from 2 to 8 weeks. The most common radiographic abnormalities with vertebral osteomyelitis are bony destruction, irregularity of vertebral end plates, and disk space narrowing. In epidural abscess, the plain films will be normal unless there is a concomitant vertebral osteomyelitis. MRI is the gold standard imaging study to make the diagnosis of these spinal infections.

The treatment of epidural abscess is primarily surgical and requires emergent evaluation and treatment by a spine surgeon. The treatment for vertebral osteomyelitis is primarily medical, consisting of 6 weeks of intravenous antibiotics, followed by a 4- to 8-week course of oral antibiotics. However, in treating vertebral osteomyelitis, consultation with a spine surgeon is important and should be performed prior to the administration of antibiotics, as they may wish to obtain core bone biopsies, and prior antibiotic therapy may result in negative culture results. However, one should not withhold antibiotic therapy unless specifically directed by the spine surgeon. The remainder of treatment is symptomatic, with bed rest and immobilization commonly employed, along with appropriate analgesia.

SPECIAL SITUATIONS

Back Pain in the Patient with a History of Cancer

The patient with a history of cancer who presents with back pain is a unique situation due to the possibility of spinal metastases. The best way to approach these patients is by dividing them into three groups based on their symptoms.

GROUP I: PATIENTS WITH NEW OR PROGRESSIVE SYMPTOMS Group I includes patients with new or progressing signs or symptoms of epidural compression that have been present for several hours to several days. These symptoms may include new urinary urgency or incontinence, paresthesias, numbness, weakness, gait disturbances, absent reflexes, or the involvement of two or more nerve roots. Treat this group with immediate corticosteroid therapy, and obtain an emergent MRI as you would for other patients with epidural compression.[22]

GROUP II: PATIENTS WITH STABLE SYMPTOMS Group II includes those patients with stable symptoms or signs that have been present for several days to several weeks. These signs include an isolated Babinski sign or radiculopathy without other neurologic deficits or evidence of cord compression. Radiculopathy is characterized by radicular pain, weakness, sensory changes, or reflex changes involving only one nerve root. Involvement of more than one nerve root places the patients into group I. Evaluation and treatment are similar to those for group I. The major difference is that patients with stable symptoms do not require immediate MRI, although evaluation within 24 h is advisable. If one does not obtain an MRI from the ED, then one should obtain plain films of the involved area to look for evidence of metastatic disease. If there is evidence of metastatic disease on the plain films, obtain an MRI in the ED. We recommend initiating dexamethasone 10 mg orally while awaiting definitive diagnostic evaluation.[22] We feel the side effects of 1 to 2 days of dexamethasone are negligible in comparison to the potential benefit.

GROUP III: PATIENTS WITHOUT NEUROLOGIC SIGNS OR SYMPTOMS Group III includes those patients with back pain only, without any neurologic signs or symptoms. In the ED, obtain plain radiographs of the involved spine that include anteroposterior (AP) and lateral views. If any focal bony lesions are discovered, obtain an MRI of the entire spine. Note that normal findings on plain radiographs do not rule out epidural metastases. In fact, more than 60 percent of patients with lymphoma and epidural metastases have normal plain radiographs.[22] If patients have negative plain films, they should be followed-up by their primary physician within 5 to 7 days to ensure improvement and no worsening in their symptoms.

REFERENCES

1. Mazanec D: Back Pain: Medical evaluation and therapy. *Cleve Clin J Med* 62:163, 1995.
2. Deyo R, Weinstein J: Primary care: Low back pain. *New Engl J Med* 344:363, 2001.
3. Frymoyer J: Back pain and sciatica. *New Engl J Med* 318:291, 1988.
4. Hanley E: Distinguish the specific from the non-specific low back pain. *Bull Hosp Jt Dis Orthop Inst* 55:195, 1996.
5. Deyo RA, Loeser JD, Bigos SJ: Herniated intervertebral disk. *Ann Intern Med* 112:598, 1990.
6. Deyo RA, Rainville J, Kent DL: What can the history and physical examination tell us about low back pain? *JAMA* 286:760, 1992.

7. Schmidt R, Markovchick V: Nontraumatic spinal cord compression. *J Emerg Med* 10:189, 1992.

8. Wisneski R: Infectious disease of the spine. Diagnostic and treatment considerations. *Orthop Clin North Am* 22:491, 1991.

9. Baker AS, Ojemann RG, Swartz MN, et al: Spinal epidural abscess. *New Engl J Med* 293:463, 1975.

10. Chelsom J, Solberg CO: Vertebral osteomyelitis at a Norwegian University hospital 1987–97. Clinical features, laboratory findings, and outcome. *Scand J Infect Dis* 30:147, 1998.

11. Deyo RA, Diehl AK: Cancer as a cause of back pain. *Gen Intern Med* 3:230, 1988.

12. Rothman S: The diagnosis of infections of the spine by modern imaging techniques. *Orthop Clin North Am* 27:15, 1996.

13. Deen HG: Diagnosis and management of lumbar disk disease. *Mayo Clin Proc* 71:283, 1996.

14. Bigos S, Bowyer O, Braen G, et al: Acute Low Back Problems in Adults. Clinical Practice Guideline. Quick Reference Guide Number 14. Rockville, MD, Agency for Health Care Policy and Research, December 1994. U.S. Dept of Health and Human Services, Public Health Service publication AHCPR 95–0643.

15. Malmivaara A, Hakkinen U, Aro T, et al: The treatment of acute low back pain-bed rest, exercise, or ordinary activity. *New Engl J Med* 332:321, 1995.

16. Deyo RA: Drug therapy for back pain. Which drugs help which patients? *Spine* 21:2840, 1996.

17. Gotzsche P: Non-steroidal anti-inflammatory drugs. *BMJ* 2320:1058, 2000.

18. Cherkin D, Deyo R, Battie, M et al: A comparison of physical therapy, chiropractic manipulation, and provision of an educational booklet for the treatment of patients with low back pain. *New Engl J Med* 339:1021, 1998.

19. Andersson GB, Lucente T, Davis AM, et al: A comparison of osteopathic spinal manipulation with standard care for patients with low back pain. *N Engl J Med* 341:1426, 1999.

20. Vroomen P, de Krom M, Wilmink J, et al: Lack of effectiveness of bed rest for sciatica. *New Engl J Med* 340:418, 1999.

21. Carette S, Leclaire R, Marcoux S, et al: Epidural corticosteroid injections for sciatica due to herniated nucleus pulposus. *New Engl J Med* 336: 1634, 1997.

22. Portenoy R, Lipton R, Foley K: Back pain in the cancer patient: An algorithm for evaluation and management. *Neurology* 37:134, 1987.

23. Helweg–Larsen S: Clinical outcome in metastatic spinal cord compression: A prospective study of 153 patients. *Acta Neurol Scand* 94:269, 1996.

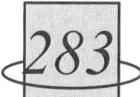

283 SHOULDER PAIN

David Della-Giustina
Benjamin Harrison
D. Monte Hunter

Injuries involving the rotator cuff are the most common cause of shoulder pain.[1] While these injuries can be acute, they more commonly occur from chronic overuse. Overuse can produce pathologic changes in the rotator cuff structures that progress along the continuum starting with subacromial bursitis from mechanical irritation, progressing to rotator cuff tendinitis, and eventually leading to partial- and full-thickness rotator cuff tears. Laborers who work with their arms above the horizontal and athletes of all ages, especially throwers, swimmers, and racquet sports enthusiasts, are the most susceptible to chronic overuse injuries. Acute injuries to the rotator cuff usually require significant trauma such as extreme forced hyperabduction or hyperextension of the upper extremity.

Conditions affecting other intrinsic structures of the shoulder complex can also cause pain. Additionally, extrinsic disorders can refer pain to the shoulder and must be considered in the differential diagnosis. A focused history and physical examination carried out with an understanding of the complex anatomy and function of the shoulder is essential in determining the source of shoulder pain. Establishing the proper diagnosis, initiating the appropriate treatment, and making timely referrals for follow-up are critical in preserving the function and mobility of the shoulder.

FUNCTIONAL ANATOMY

The shoulder is designed for mobility rather than stability.[2] Its functions are to help position the hand and upper extremity for accurate and efficient use, and to provide strength and power to upper extremity movements. To meet the many demands placed on it, the shoulder uses three bones, four joints, and a specialized set of soft tissues consisting of muscles, tendons, ligaments, and bursae.

Bones and Joints

The humerus, clavicle, and scapula make up the bony structures of the shoulder complex. The scapula has two bony extensions, the coracoid and the acromion, which help protect the rotator cuff and play important roles in shoulder function.

The four joints of the shoulder are the glenohumeral, acromioclavicular, sternoclavicular, and scapulothoracic. The glenohumeral joint is a ball-and-socket joint and is the central axis of shoulder motion. While the glenohumeral joint is the most mobile joint in the body, it is the least stable. To help improve its stability, this joint relies on three components. The first is the glenoid labrum, which is a fibrous ring of tissue encircling the glenoid cavity. The glenoid labrum increases the surface contact area of the humeral head within the relatively shallow glenoid fossa. The second component consists of three glenohumeral ligaments, which aid stability by reinforcing the joint capsule. Finally, four specialized muscles, known as the rotator cuff, encompass the glenohumeral joint and provide significant stability during motion.

The sternoclavicular and acromioclavicular joints work together to contribute to glenohumeral motion. Rotation at the acromioclavicular joint and elevation at the sternoclavicular joint allow complete arm elevation. The scapulothoracic joint represents the articulation of the scapula on the posterior wall of the thorax. Scapular motion is essential for overall shoulder motion: every degree of scapulothoracic motion allows two degrees of glenohumeral motion.

Muscles

The deltoid, which drapes the shoulder complex and forms its contour, acts as a powerful and independent elevator of the arm. Along with the pectoralis, the deltoid is the major mover of the upper extremity.

The rotator cuff consists of four muscles: supraspinatus, infraspinatus, teres minor, and subscapularis. All originate on the scapula, traverse the glenohumeral joint, and insert on the proximal humerus. The rotator cuff functions primarily as a dynamic stabilizer of the glenohumeral joint. The rotator cuff muscles also contribute significantly to the power of the upper extremity, providing 30 to 50 percent of the power in abduction and 90 percent in external rotation (Figures 283-1 and 283-2).

The supraspinatus originates on the posterior and superior aspect of the scapula, passes beneath the acromion, and inserts on the great tuberosity of the humerus. It initiates arm elevation and abducts the shoulder. It also balances the power of the deltoid, keeping the humerus centered in the glenoid during deltoid contraction. The infraspinatus originates on the posterior scapula just inferior to the scapular spine. It inserts on the posterior aspect of the greater tuberosity and acts primarily as an external rotator of the arm (see Figure 283-1). The teres minor originates on the lateral border of the scapula just inferior to the infraspinatus and inserts on the posterior aspect of the humerus. It works with the infraspinatus to provide external rotation (see Figure 283-1). The subscapularis is the only rotator cuff muscle that arises from the anterior aspect of the scapula. It attaches to the lesser tuberosity of the humerus and provides internal rotation of the arm (see Figure 283-2).

The long head of the biceps tendon, although not formally considered part of the rotator cuff, assists in rotator cuff function. This tendon courses superiorly in the bicipital groove of the humerus between

Posterior

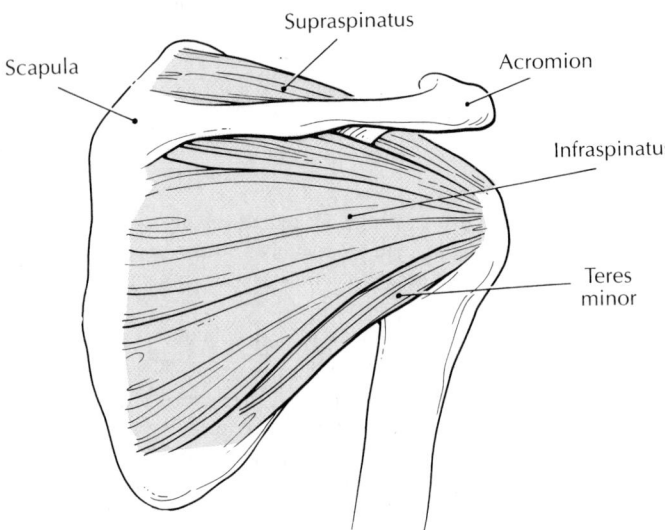

FIG. 283-1. Posterior view of shoulder illustrating rotator cuff muscles.

the greater and lesser tuberosities, passes between the subscapularis and supraspinatus tendons, and penetrates the glenohumeral joint to insert on the labrum (see Figure 283-2). During arm elevation, the tendon of the long head of the biceps depresses the humeral head, helping it remain centered in the glenoid.

Bursae

The bursae facilitate motion between the components of the shoulder. There are eight identifiable bursae in the shoulder complex. However, only the large subacromial bursa is clinically significant. The subacromial bursa is extra-articular; its roof adheres to the undersurface of the deltoid, and its floor to the underlying rotator cuff. This bursa, lubricated by synovial fluid and surrounded by a layer of peribursal fat, aids in a smooth, frictionless motion between the rotator cuff and adjacent structures.

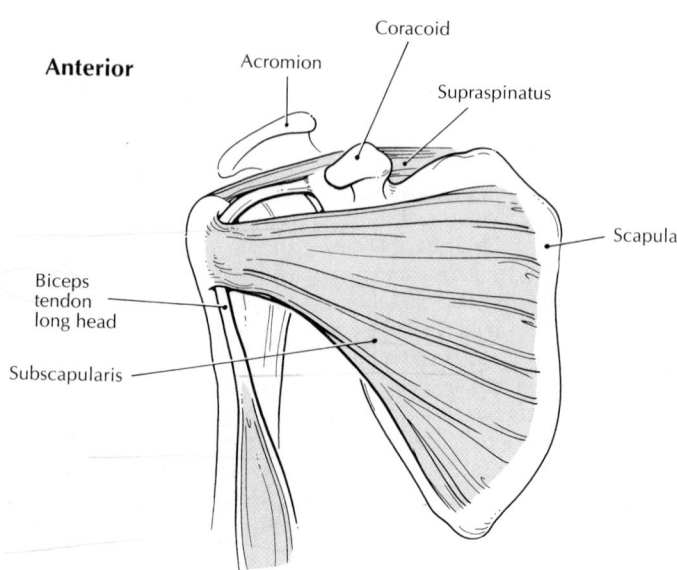

FIG. 283-2. Anterior view of shoulder illustrating supraspinatus and long head of biceps.

Coracoacromial Arch

The coracoacromial arch is an important anatomic concept in understanding shoulder pathology. The arch is formed by the coracoid posteriorly, by the acromion anteriorly, and by the coracoacromial ligament, which forms the anterior roof of the arch (Figure 283-3). The humeral head provides the floor of the arch. This arch defines the space within which the tendons of the rotator cuff, the tendon of the long head of the biceps, and the subacromial bursa must function.

IMPINGEMENT SYNDROME

(Subacromial Bursitis, Rotator Cuff Tendinitis, Supraspinatus Tendinitis, Painful Arc Syndrome)

Repetitive overhead use of the arm or movement of the shoulder above the horizontal causes encroachment of the subacromial space by the humeral head (Figure 283-4). This results in a loss of the normal gliding mechanism between the rotator cuff and related soft tissues within the coracoacromial arch.

Impingement syndrome refers to the pathologic changes that occur to the rotator cuff, subacromial bursa, and other soft tissues within the coracoacromial arch due to this repetitive compression.[3] In the past, these symptoms were referred to separately as subacromial bursitis, rotator cuff tendinitis, supraspinatus tendinitis, and painful arc syndrome. However, impingement syndrome is the current terminology that encompasses all of these previous terms and pathologic processes. Impingement syndrome is the leading cause of shoulder pain and dysfunction.

Pathophysiology

Repetitive impingement of the bursa, rotator cuff, and biceps tendon produces pathologic changes in these structures that evolve in a progressive pattern classified in three stages. In stage 1, reversible edema

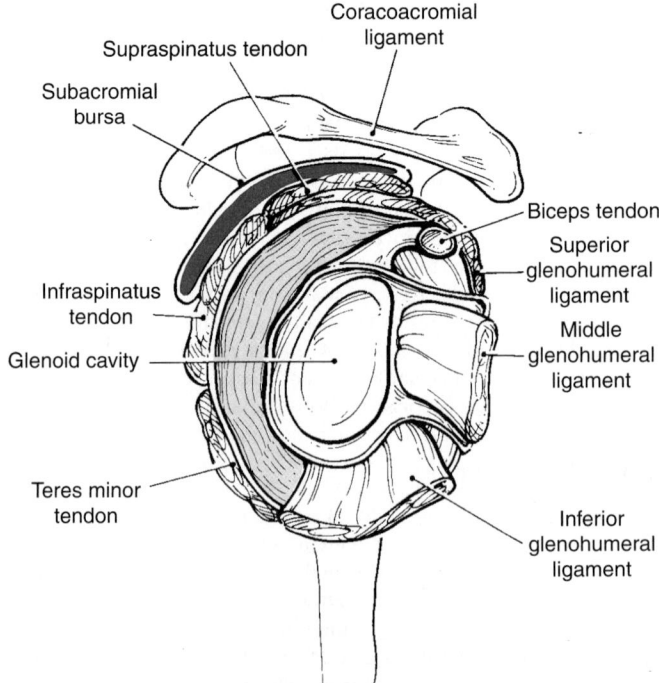

FIG. 283-3. Lateral view of shoulder illustrating coracoacromial arch with rotator cuff and subacromial bursa.

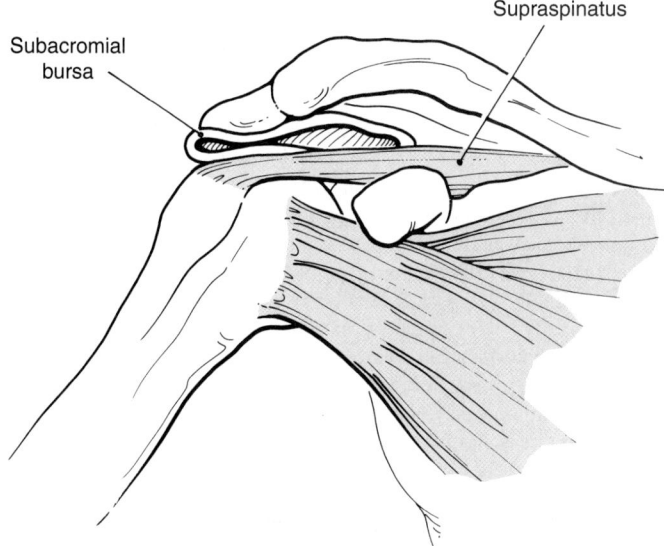

FIG. 283-4. Impingement of subacromial bursa and rotator cuff.

and hemorrhage about the rotator cuff occurs. While this stage can occur at any age, it is classically seen in young athletes under age 25 who engage in sports that require excessive overhead use of the shoulder. During this stage, patients complain of a dull ache over the anterolateral shoulder that is aggravated by activity and improved by rest. The clinical course at this point is typically reversible with rest, activity modification with avoidance of the aggravating activity, antiinflammatory agents, and ice.

If patients continue the aggravating activities and do not follow the prescribed treatment, then the repeated mechanical trauma from the impingement can progress to stage 2. In stage 2, the edema and hemorrhage progress to tendinitis of the rotator cuff with subsequent fibrosis and thickening of the tendons of the rotator cuff and bursa. This stage is typically seen in patients between the ages of 25 and 40. However, it is the prolonged duration (weeks to months) or recurrence of symptoms that is most useful in making this diagnosis. During this stage, patients will complain of a recurrent or chronic aching pain with daily activities, vigorous activity, and night pain. The nocturnal pain is a deep aching pain that interferes with sleep and especially occurs when the patient lies on that shoulder or sleeps with his or her arms overhead. Treatment is conservative as for stage 1. Continued overuse can lead to stage 3. Stage 3 consists of rotator cuff tears, rupture of the long head of the biceps, and subacromial spurs. Patients at this stage have a history of progressive symptoms and disability and often require surgical decompression of the subacromial space.

Some of the earliest and more significant pathologic changes in the rotator cuff due to impingement occur near the humeral insertion of the supraspinatus tendon. This area, called the critical zone, is affected early because it is a relatively avascular site. Repetitive compression in this area causes a relative ischemia, which leads to tissue degeneration over time and ultimately tissue failure.[3]

Physical Examination

On examination, disuse atrophy of the shoulder musculature may be present if symptoms have been chronic (stages 2 and 3). Palpation of the rotator cuff insertion at the lateral aspect of the proximal humerus will usually produce pain and tenderness. During range-of-motion maneuvers, fibrosis and scarring within the tendon can cause crepitus. A sensation of catching also may be present if scar tissue is trapped beneath the acromion. Rotator cuff strength testing will reveal mild to moderate weakness. Pain will usually be present when resistance is applied. The individual muscles of the rotator cuff can be isolated and

tested individually. *To test the supraspinatus,* abduct the arm to 90° and place it forward 30° with the thumb pointed down in the so-called "empty beer can" position (Figure 283-5). Pain or weakness against resistance in this position suggests injury to the supraspinatus. *To test the infraspinatus and the teres minor,* externally rotate the shoulder with the patient's arm against the body, and the elbow bent to 90° and the forearm in neutral position. Stabilize the elbow against the patient's waist and instruct the patient to rotate the arm outward. *To test the subscapularis,* maintain the elbow flexed to 90° and fixed against the patient's body, and have the patient rotate the arm inward around the front of the body against resistance.

Specific maneuvers on physical examination test for signs of impingement by compressing the rotator cuff and bursa between the humeral head and coracoacromial arch. In the classic impingement maneuver of Neer, the examiner prevents scapular rotation with one hand, while raising the patient's straightened arm smoothly in full forward flexion to overhead. This maneuver impinges the critical zone of the rotator cuff and bursa between the undersurface of the acromion and the greater tuberosity of the humerus. A second test, Hawkins impingement test (Figure 283-6), requires the examiner to position the patient's arm in 90° of abduction and 90° of elbow flexion. Rotation of the arm inwardly across the front of the patient with internal rotation of the shoulder compresses the cuff and bursa between the humeral head and coracoacromial ligament. These tests are considered positive if they reproduce pain, but cannot be used to stage the impingement as they elicit symptoms in all three stages.

Radiography

Radiography plays a minor role in the diagnosis of impingement syndrome, as it is primarily a clinical diagnosis. However, early radiographic signs include nonspecific sclerosis and cyst formation of the greater tuberosity of the humerus or osteoarthritis of the acromioclavicular joint. These findings are seen with impingement syndrome, but are nonspecific.[3] A specific but late finding is that of an anterior acromial enthesophyte (spur).[3] This spur may be seen on the anteroposterior shoulder radiograph.

Emergency Department Treatment

The goals of treatment of impingement syndrome are twofold: to reduce pain and inflammation and, more importantly, to prevent progression of

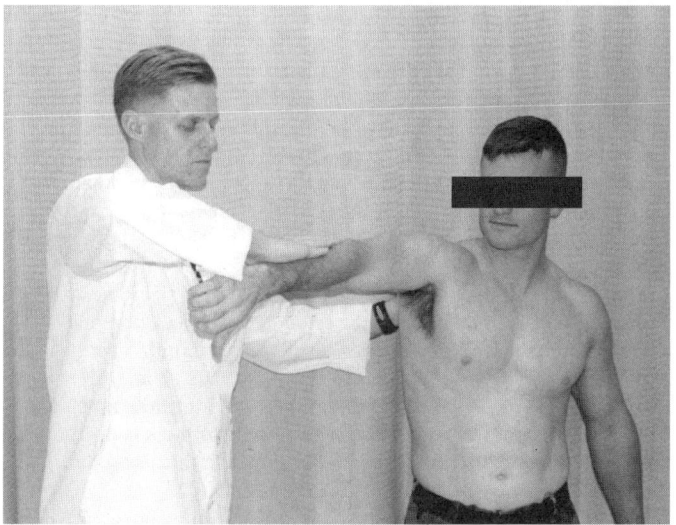

FIG. 283-5. The "empty beer can" position, which isolates the supraspinatus tendon on physical examination.

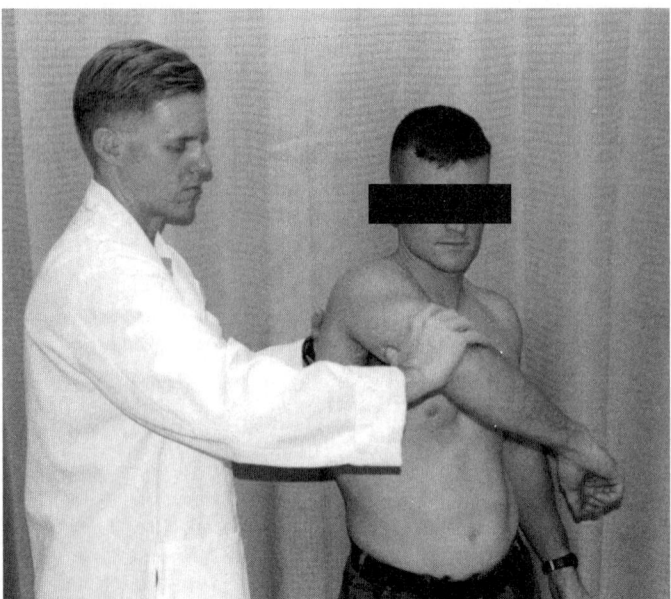

FIG. 283-6. Hawkins impingement test. The examiner positions the patient's shoulder at 90° of abduction and 90° of elbow flexion. The examiner then rotates the shoulder internally and brings the arm across the front of the patient.

the process. Regardless of the stage of impingement identified, a conservative treatment program should include the following:

1. *Relative rest and activity modification.* The patient should avoid the aggravating activity and minimize all overhead activities. While brief periods of support with a sling may be prescribed, complete immobilization should be avoided whenever possible. At a minimum, the patient should perform range-of-motion exercises (see below) three to four times daily to minimize the chance of developing adhesive capsulitis.

2. *Medication to reduce pain and inflammation.* Analgesics are often required to control pain during stage 2 and 3 impingement. Nonsteroidal anti-inflammatory drugs (NSAIDs) should be prescribed for a 7 to 21 day course. Short-term opioid analgesics will be needed for moderate to severe pain.

3. *Cryotherapy.* The application of ice to the affected shoulder for 10 to 15 min two to three times daily can have analgesic effects and is thought to reduce local inflammation and edema.

4. *Gentle range of motion.* Two simple exercises can help the patient maintain glenohumeral motion. Pendulum swings are done with the patient slightly bent at the waist with the arm hanging freely in front of the body. Gentle arcs of motion in both a clockwise and counterclockwise direction to the level of pain tolerance can be carried out for 5 to 10 min three to four times daily. The size of the arcs should increase daily as symptoms allow. Have the patient stand sideways an arm's length from a wall, and walk the fingers up the wall to the level of pain tolerance, and repeat three to four times daily.

5. *Stretching and strengthening.* Stretching and strengthening exercises are best prescribed by the primary care physician or orthopedist, carried out under the supervision of a physical therapist.

6. *Corticosteroid injections.* While local corticosteroid injections into the subacromial space can be effective for pain relief, adverse effects include muscular atrophy, weakness, and further tissue degeneration. Injection directly into the substance of the tendon can lead to necrosis and rupture. Injection is best left to the primary care physician or orthopedist.

7. *Follow-up.* Clinical follow-up is usually recommended after 7 to 14 days.

ROTATOR CUFF TEARS

Rotator cuff tears present with acute shoulder pain and are either due to acute traumatic injury, chronic injury, or an acute extension of a chronic injury to the rotator cuff tendons. Chronic rotator cuff tears account for 90 percent of all rotator cuff tears, and are almost always due to progressive degeneration of stage 3 impingement. Healthy rotator cuff tendons are resistant to acute injury unless weakened by some other factor such as age, repetitive stress such as that seen in swimmers or baseball pitchers, steroid injections, or impingement. Acute rotator cuff tears account for only 10 percent of all rotator cuff tears and usually occur as a result of significant trauma. Traumatic causes typically involve forced or extreme hyperabduction or hyperextension, such as from a fall on an outstretched arm, lifting a heavy object, or catching a heavy object as it falls. Glenohumeral dislocations are also a common cause of acute rotator cuff tears, and the incidence of such tears rises significantly in patients over age 40 with shoulder dislocations.

Rotator cuff tears are further classified as full thickness or partial thickness. Partial-thickness tears are twice as common as full-thickness tears and most commonly occur on the inferior aspect of the tendon. Partial-thickness rotator cuff tears are more likely to occur from an acute injury, especially in younger patients. The type and extent of the tear have significant implications for the ultimate treatment and prognosis. Full-thickness tears usually require surgical treatment, whereas partial thickness tears often respond to a trial of conservative management.

As previously described, the critical zone of the rotator cuff is near the humeral insertion of the tendon. Repetitive compression and impingement cause ischemia in this area, and over time this area degenerates and ultimately tears. The supraspinatus, due to its location within the coracoacromial arch, is the most commonly affected tendon of the rotator cuff. The critical zone is the most common site of all rotator cuff tears (Figure 283-7).

Acute traumatic rotator cuff tears in a healthy tendon require a significant force. The tensile strength of a normal tendon is greater than that of bone; therefore, a bony avulsion injury of the humerus is much more common than an isolated rotator cuff tear following acute trauma.

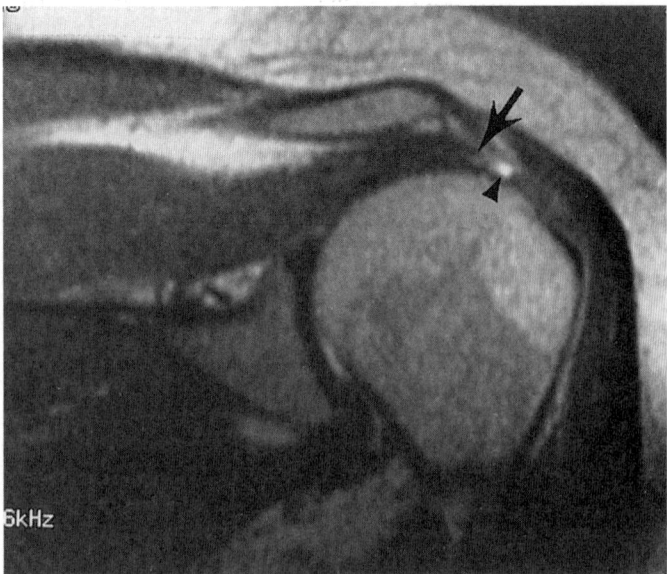

FIG. 283-7. Rotator cuff tear. MRI coronal image of shoulder reveals tear in supraspinatus tendon at the critical zone *(arrow)* with edema *(arrowhead).*

Clinical Features

Patients with rotator cuff tears are almost always older than 40 years of age; rotator cuff tears in the young are rare. The clinical features of a chronic rotator cuff tear differ from those of an acute tear. Only about half of patients with chronic rotator cuff tears recall specific trauma or an event associated with the onset of pain and the trauma is usually not significant. Patients more commonly report a history of gradual and progressive pain, which initially is described as worse at night. The pain eventually becomes persistent. The pain may be described as diffuse, but is commonly localized to the lateral aspect of the upper arm. The patient may report flares of bursitis and tendinitis that initially responded to rest, anti-inflammatory agents, and glucocorticoid injections. As the rotator cuff weakens, the frequency, intensity, and duration of the symptoms increase and are less responsive to the usual treatments. Shoulder dysfunction progressively worsens and interferes with work, recreation, and normal daily activities. Arm elevation, external rotation, and lifting even light objects worsen the symptoms.

With acute injuries, such as a fall or catching a heavy object, the patient may report a "tearing" sensation in the shoulder followed by severe pain and inability to raise the arm. An acute rotator cuff tear will produce immediate significant pain and disability. Asymmetry may be noted due to significant local swelling. Active motion will be limited, with inability to abduct or externally rotate the arm against even minimal resistance. The drop arm test (see below) is positive and impingement signs are typically positive, but testing for them may not be practical after an acute injury.

On examination, disuse atrophy may be present in patients with chronic rotator cuff tears. Palpation may produce discomfort at the lateral aspect of the upper arm or in the subacromial region. The rent test, which is used to assess for complete rotator cuff tears, is sensitive and specific in experienced hands. The examiner places one hand on the patient's relaxed flexed elbow while using the other hand to palpate the rotator cuff (anterior to the acromion through the deltoid). A soft tissue defect (cuff tear) and eminence (greater tuberosity of the humerus) are palpable as the arm is brought into full extension with gentle internal and external rotation. This test is more applicable to patients with chronic pain since patients with acute injuries may not tolerate the test due to a limited, painful range of motion.[4]

Active and passive range of motion of the glenohumeral joint and motor strength of the rotator cuff muscles should be evaluated. Most patients with rotator cuff tears will have weakness and pain of abduction, elevation, and most commonly, external rotation. *The drop arm test* is positive if the patient is unable to hold or lower a fully extended arm at 90 degrees shoulder abduction without dropping it. Crepitus and pain are usually present on range-of-motion testing.

Radiographic Findings

Routine shoulder radiographs are generally indicated in all patients with shoulder pain presenting for the first time to the ED, although they only occasionally give additional diagnostic information. Most often they reveal findings associated with chronic rotator cuff pathology: sclerosis of the humeral head, degenerative joint disease of the acromioclavicular joint, osteophytes on the undersurface of the acromion and/or clavicle, and a hooked acromion. The most specific radiographic sign for large rotator cuff tears is a narrowing of the acromiohumeral space (<7 mm).[3]

No radiographic findings are diagnostic of an acute rotator cuff tear and the diagnosis should rely on clinical findings. The peribursal fat plane (curvilinear radiolucency about the lateral humeral margin on internal rotation views) may be obliterated. With a large tear, the humeral head can "buttonhole" through the defect in the rotator cuff and assume a position superior to the glenoid, but this is rarely appreciated. Small avulsion fractures of the humerus, at the rotator cuff insertion, may also rarely be seen. For patients presenting with acute traumatic conditions and impaired range of motion of the shoulder, a scapular Y-view or an axillary lateral view should be included to rule out glenohumeral dislocation.[5]

While often not readily available to the practicing emergency physician, MRI, ultrasonography, and arthrography are the most sensitive modalities for detecting rotator cuff tears. All tend to underestimate the extent of the tear, but are commonly used by specialists to further evaluate these lesions.[6]

Emergency Department Care

Practically speaking, it may be very difficult to distinguish a full-thickness tear from a partial-thickness tear, or to even distinguish a rotator cuff injury from other inflammatory rotator cuff conditions. The basic goals of emergency care for suspected rotator cuff injuries are to provide support, protection, pain relief, and most importantly to help prevent further dysfunction and disability. An arm sling can provide support and comfort until the acute symptoms subside. Prolonged immobilization should be avoided. NSAIDs, opiate analgesics, ice, and gentle range-of-motion exercises (such as pendulum swings and walking the fingers up the wall) should be prescribed until follow-up.

Following acute injuries, any evidence or suspicion of neurovascular compromise requires immediate orthopedic consultation. Patients with an acute rotator cuff tear (with or without a history of chronic symptoms) and those with significant disability should receive referral to an orthopedist within a week. Complete rotator cuff tears usually require surgical repair, and functional results are better if repair is carried out within 3 weeks of injury, before retraction, fibrosis, tendon degeneration, and muscular atrophy have occurred.

Partial-thickness or chronic tears may respond to conservative measures more so than acute injuries; however, early referral is still warranted for further diagnostic evaluation, rehabilitation, and consideration for surgical repair.

CALCIFIC TENDINITIS

Pathophysiology

Calcific tendinitis is a self-limiting disorder characterized by the deposition of calcium hydroxyapatite crystals within one or more tendons of the rotator cuff. In time, the calcium deposition undergoes painful spontaneous resorption with subsequent healing of the tendon. Primary tendon degeneration as a result of chronic repetitive microtrauma, age, or tissue hypoxia has been postulated to be the primary cause of this disorder. The underlying cause of the deposits, however, remains uncertain, and calcific tendinitis has not been definitively linked to any generalized disorders or to rotator cuff tears. The supraspinatus is by far the most commonly affected tendon, with calcium deposition usually occurring in the critical zone of the tendon (1 to 2 cm proximal to its insertion on the humerus). Any of the rotator cuff tendons as well as the tendon of the long head of the biceps may be affected.

As calcification occurs over a period of time, the patients are generally asymptomatic but may experience mild pain at rest or at night. Abduction pain and a "catching" sensation may be present on movement. During the *resorptive phase,* incapacitating pain can occur from vascular proliferation, formation of granulation tissue, and calcium crystal extravasation into the subacromial bursa.

Symptoms are usually self-limited, lasting 1 to 2 weeks in most cases. Symptoms may produce variable levels of pain and shoulder dysfunction and last several months *(postcalcific period).* Adhesive capsulitis is the most common complication of calcific tendinitis and may be responsible for more chronic symptoms as well.[7]

Clinical Features

Middle-aged patients are most commonly affected, and this process is rarely seen in patients over 70. Females are slightly more likely to be affected than males, and calcification is often present bilaterally.

The onset of pain typically coincides with the resorption of the calcium deposit rather than the formation of it. Symptomatic patients experience sudden onset of shoulder pain, usually at rest, and any shoulder motion reproduces significant pain. The pain is often worse at night and interferes with sleep.

During an acute attack with intense pain, patients hold their arm across their body and often are reluctant to move it. Laboratory testing is unnecessary as it is usually normal in most patients. A point of maximum tenderness may be palpated over the proximal humerus near the tendinous insertion of the rotator cuff. Active and passive range of motion of the glenohumeral joint is usually limited to varying degrees. Flexion, extension, abduction, and internal/external rotation of this joint should be documented. Muscle atrophy and crepitus may also be present.

Radiographic Findings

Routine shoulder radiographs may reveal calcific deposits, and anteroposterior views with the humerus in the neutral position as well as in internal and external rotation may increase sensitivity. During the initial formative phase, calcium deposits are usually dense and well-defined if visualized. The presence of visible calcifications, however, is not necessarily specific for this disorder. Calcification in the rotator cuff tendons is found on radiographs in approximately 7 percent of patients older than age 30 with shoulder pain. In asymptomatic patients between 31 and 40, 10 to 20 percent demonstrate rotator cuff calcification on routine radiographs. Of these patients, only 35 to 45 percent will eventually become symptomatic. Conversely, most patients presenting to the ED will most likely be experiencing acute pain during the resorptive phase, when calcium deposits are ill-defined and less visible.

Emergency Department Treatment

Treatment is similar to that for impingement syndrome. During an acute attack, NSAIDs, opioid analgesics, and ice help calm the intense pain. Resting the shoulder with a sling for brief periods of immobilization may be utilized, but prolonged immobilization should be avoided to prevent loss of motion. The patient should be instructed to rest the shoulder in abduction on the back of a chair as often as is tolerable. Sleeping with a pillow beneath the axilla can also help prevent restricted motion. Local heat application may be used once acute symptoms have diminished. Gentle and progressive range-of-motion exercises should be emphasized and encouraged. Physical therapy is indicated in patients with more chronic cases who have significantly limited range of motion of the shoulder.

There is controversy regarding the effectiveness of subacromial corticosteroid injection,[7] so this is best left to the primary care physician or orthopedist. Therapeutic ultrasonography, transcutaneous electrical nerve stimulation (TENS), and oral steroid administration are other modalities that can be prescribed by the primary care physician.[8]

The patient should follow-up with an orthopedist within a week. Calcific tendinitis is a self-limited process in the vast majority of cases. Surgical removal of the calcium deposit is usually considered only after all conservative measures have been exhausted.

ADHESIVE CAPSULITIS

Adhesive capsulitis, commonly referred to as the *frozen shoulder syndrome,* begins as painful inflammation of the glenohumeral joint, followed by eventual fibrosis of the joint capsule and restriction of shoulder motion. Primary or idiopathic adhesive capsulitis is associated with a wide variety of unrelated conditions, including postmenopause, diabetes, thyroid disease, pulmonary neoplasms, and autoimmune disorders. Secondary adhesive capsulitis has similar clinical and pathologic findings, but results from a known cause, such as prolonged immobilization after trauma, surgery, or stroke, or a primary inflammatory condition of the shoulder such as impingement syndrome or bicipital tendinitis. The condition resolves with conservative therapy in most patients, although some are left with residual pain or stiffness.

Pathophysiology

Four stages of this disorder have been described based on arthroscopic and clinical findings correlated with pathologic changes of the capsule. However, controversy exists with regard to the classification of adhesive capsulitis, and patients do not necessarily follow these stages in a uniform fashion.[9]

Stage 1, which occurs during the first 2 to 3 months, is marked by acute synovial inflammation with limitation of shoulder movement due to pain. Stage 2 *(freezing stage),* which occurs from months 3 to 9, is characterized by decreased shoulder motion from capsular thickening and scarring, and chronic pain. In stage 3 *(frozen stage),* which occurs from months 9 to 15, the pain has diminished to a low level, but there is a more fibrotic and thick capsule and continued significantly decreased flexion, abduction, and internal/external rotation. Stage 4 *(thawing stage),* which generally occurs after 15 months, is associated with minimal pain and progressive improvement in the range of motion of the shoulder.[9]

Clinical Features

Pain is described typically as diffuse and aching, is poorly localized, and often extends down the upper arm. The pain is often described as worse at night and is also present at rest, especially in earlier stages. A painful stiffened shoulder is the hallmark finding on examination. Active and passive range of motion are limited, especially in abduction and in internal/external rotation. Disuse atrophy may be present. Pain is not usually reproducible by palpation, but is present at the limits of motion. Impingement testing is difficult due to restricted motion. Posterior glenohumeral dislocation must always be considered in the patient with restricted motion of the shoulder in an appropriate clinical scenario.

Radiographic Findings

There are no specific radiographic findings other than disuse osteopenia in long-standing cases. Radiographs should be ordered to exclude other disorders, such as posterior glenohumeral dislocation after trauma or seizure.

Emergency Department Treatment

The overall goals of treatment, regardless of stage, are to reduce pain and initiate restoration of motion and function. NSAIDs, analgesics, ice, and progressive range-of-motion exercises should be prescribed in the ED. Shoulder immobilization with a sling should be avoided unless absolutely necessary. If administered in those early stage 1 patients with severe pain, its use should be discontinued as soon as possible to prevent increased loss of motion due to further capsular restriction.

Follow-up should be provided with the primary care physician or orthopedist in 1 week for initiation of physical therapy and consideration of steroid injection.

DISORDERS OF THE BICEPS TENDON

Pathophysiology

Disorders of the biceps tendon can be a source of shoulder pain for patients and may result from progressive impingement or from isolated tendon inflammation or injury. The tendon of the long head of the biceps lies anterior and superior to the humeral head as it courses through the bicipital groove before inserting into the superior aspect of the glenoid labrum (see Figures 283-2 and 283-3). The tendon may become inflamed, subluxed out of the bicipital groove, or rupture altogether. Acute traumatic ruptures of the bicipital tendon are discussed in Chap. 271.

Clinical Features

Bicipital tendinitis presents as acute, intense, localized pain at the anterior aspect of the shoulder. Palpation of the tendon within the bicipital groove reproduces the intense pain. Forearm supination, one of the main actions of the biceps, will also reproduce pain, especially when resistance is applied. *Speed test* identifies biceps tendon weakness or inflammation. A downward force is applied to the patient's forearm with the thumb in an upright position. The patient's shoulder is flexed 60 degrees and the elbow is fully extended. A positive result is indicated by palpable pain in the affected shoulder's biceps groove as the examiner resists forearm supination by the patient, although muscle weakness may also be elicited in cases of muscle injury or rupture. *Yergason test* (Figure 283-8) also may be used to diagnose biceps tendinitis. The examiner similarly resists patient forearm supination with the shoulder adducted and elbow flexed at 90 degrees. A positive test elicits pain at the proximal bicipital groove.

The tendon may sublux or momentarily dislocate from the bicipital groove if the transhumeral ligament, which forms the roof of the groove, tears from degeneration or acute trauma. Resisted forearm supination may cause subluxation that is palpable and accompanied by a painful popping sensation as the tendon subluxes.

Rupture of the biceps tendon is almost always proximal, and as with rotator cuff injury, is due to microtears and other age-related degenerative changes in this area of the tendon. In younger patients, mild trauma may cause complete rupture of the biceps tendon and is heralded by an audible snap or pop followed by severe pain. On examination, the classic finding is described as a "Popeye" deformity caused by distal contraction of the muscle belly. Supination is weak on muscle testing but elbow flexion remains strong because of the presence of other intact elbow flexors (short head of biceps and brachialis muscles).

Emergency Department Treatment

Tendinitis and subluxation are managed conservatively with brief use of a sling as needed for support and comfort. Analgesics and anti-

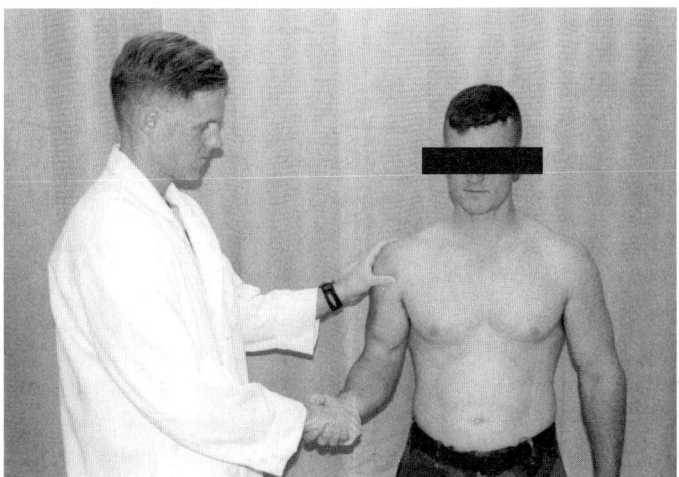

FIG. 283-8. Yergason test is used to identify bicipital tendinitis. With the patient's elbow flexed at 90°, the examiner palpates the bicipital groove as the patient attempts forearm supination against resistance. Pain or instability at the proximal bicipital groove indicates biceps tendinitis or tendon subluxation.

inflammatory agents may be used in conjunction with relative rest, use of ice for 10 to 15 min several times daily, and elevation to reduce swelling. Early mobilization with stretching exercises should be initiated with close follow-up scheduled with the patient's primary provider.

Bicipital tendinitis usually resolves with conservative therapy. Follow-up with the primary provider within 1 week will suffice. Orthopedic consultation should be reserved for severe cases or those that fail to respond to a conservative treatment regimen. Decompressive surgery and biceps tenodesis are options for this subset of patients.[10] Bicipital tendon rupture often requires surgical repair so orthopedic referral in 24 to 48 h is best.

OSTEOARTHRITIS

Since the glenohumeral joint is non-weight-bearing, primary osteoarthritis is rare. When it does occur, presentation is similar to that of degenerative disease in other joints; the patient experiences gradual and progressive onset of pain, which is worse with motion and better with rest. This usually occurs concurrently with degenerative disease of the acromioclavicular joint.

Secondary osteoarthritis is more common and usually associated with a previous fracture, recurrent dislocations, or with an underlying rheumatologic, metabolic, or endocrinologic disorder. ED care of both primary and secondary arthritis includes analgesics, anti-inflammatory agents, and gentle exercises to preserve range of motion. Referral should be made for further evaluation of possible underlying rheumatologic or inflammatory conditions.

DIFFERENTIAL DIAGNOSIS OF SHOULDER PAIN

Although disorders of the rotator cuff and other intrinsic structures of the shoulder are the most common cause of shoulder pain, extrinsic conditions outside the shoulder complex can refer pain to the shoulder. The differential diagnosis includes disorders of the cervical spine, brachial plexus injuries, axillary artery thrombosis, suprascapular nerve injury, thoracic outlet syndrome, Pancoast tumor, and miscellaneous thoracoabdominal disorders.

The neck is the most common source of pain referred to the shoulder. Degenerative disease of the cervical spine, degenerative disk disease, and herniated nucleus pulposus can all refer pain to the shoulder. The patient with a C5-C6 herniated disk may present with pain very similar to that due to rotator cuff disease. Careful and thorough examination of the cervical spine and a complete neurovascular examination should be included in the evaluation of any patient with shoulder pain. See Chap. 281 for discussion of neck pain.

Brachial plexus injury can cause pain referred to the shoulder and can produce weakness and atrophy in the muscles of the shoulder within weeks of injury. Radiographic evaluation of the cervical spine should be included in the ED evaluation of patients with suspected brachial plexus injury or involvement. *Brachial plexus neuritis* is uncommon but can be very painful. It is presumed to be of viral origin. The inflammation of the brachial plexus can lead to weakness and atrophy of the muscles of the shoulder complex within weeks following the onset of pain. Brachial plexus neuritis is usually self-limiting. Referral to a neurologist should be arranged if this disorder is suspected.

The most serious vascular injury that can cause shoulder pain is *acute thrombosis of the axillary artery*. Repetitive mechanical trauma or explosive stress from lifting heavy objects can compress and contuse the intimal lining of the axillary artery, predisposing the artery to thrombosis.

Compression of the suprascapular nerve can cause shoulder pain. This nerve originates from the brachial plexus distal C5-C6 nerve roots and courses posteriorly to the suprascapular notch. It can become entrapped beneath the transverse ligament at the level of the suprascapular notch. Traction injuries from explosive movements can also injure the nerve. On examination, infraspinatus atrophy and associated weakness and external rotation will typically be found. The initial treatment is conservative. Electromyographic and nerve conduction velocity studies will reveal the extent and location of nerve injury. Surgery for decompression is considered if conservative measures fail.

Compression of the brachial plexus and blood vessels proximal to the shoulder, *the thoracic outlet syndrome,* can cause shoulder pain. Women in the childbearing years are affected three times more commonly than men. The medial trunk of the brachial plexus is most commonly affected, and the symptoms usually involve pain that radiates through the shoulder to the medial forearm and occasionally to the small and ring ringers. Patients can usually identify motions that reproduce the symptoms. Radiographic evaluation may reveal evidence of a prior clavicle fracture with malunion, or the presence of a cervical rib band, which compress the brachial plexus. Surgical decompression may be considered if the symptoms are debilitating or refractory to conservative measures.

Pancoast tumor may compress the brachial plexus against the chest wall and cause shoulder pain. The patient may experience local or radicular shoulder pain or sense a fullness in the supraclavicular fossa.

Finally, a large number of *thoracoabdominal disorders* can cause shoulder pain. These include myocardial ischemia and infarction, pneumonia, and pulmonary embolism and infarction. Any thoracic or abdominal disorder that irritates the diaphragm can also cause referred shoulder pain. Abdominal disorders that can cause shoulder pain include biliary tract disease, splenic injury or inflammation, perforated viscus, or ruptured ectopic pregnancy.

REFERENCES

1. Stevenson JH, Trojian T: Evaluation of shoulder pain. *J Fam Pract* 51:605, 2002.
2. Blake R, Hoffman J: Emergency department evaluation and treatment of the shoulder and humerus. *Emerg Med Clin North Am* 17:859, 1999.
3. Resnick D (ed): *Diagnosis of Bone and Joint Disorders.* Philadelphia, WB Saunders, 2002.
4. Wolf E, Agrawal V: Transdeltoid palpation (the rent test) in the diagnosis of rotator cuff tears. *J Shoulder Elbow Surg* 10:470, 2001.
5. Soohoo N, Rosen P: Diagnosis and treatment of rotator cuff tears in the emergency department. *J Emerg Med* 14:309, 1996.
6. Bryant L, Shnier R, Bryant C: A comparison of clinical estimation, ultrasonography, magnetic resonance imaging, and arthroscopy in determining the size of rotator cuff tears. *J Shoulder Elbow Surg* 11:219, 2002.
7. Speed CA, Hazleman BL: Calcific tendinitis of the shoulder. *New Engl J Med* 340:1582, 1999.
8. Wainner RS, Hasz M: Management of acute calcific tendinitis of the shoulder. *J Orthop Sports Phys Ther* 27:231, 1998.
9. Hannafin JA, Chiaia TA: Adhesive capsulitis: A treatment approach. *Clin Orthop* 372:95, 2000.
10. Curtis AS, Snyder SJ: Evaluation and treatment of biceps tendon pathology. *Orthop Clin North Am* 24:33, 1993.

EMERGENCIES IN SYSTEMIC RHEUMATIC DISEASES

284

Richard C. Chandler
Mary Chester Morgan Wasko

Systemic rheumatologic diseases rarely cause life-threatening illness, and when they do, it usually results from internal organ damage, such as alveolar hemorrhage in SLE or aortic arch dissection in temporal arteritis.[1] Alternatively, life-threatening illness may be a complication of treatment itself, such as infection in the setting of immunosuppression, or gastrointestinal hemorrhage complicating nonsteroidal anti-inflammatory drug (NSAID) use. Either can lead to serious morbidity and increased mortality if not recognized and managed promptly.

This chapter discusses rheumatologic emergencies from an organ-system, rather than disease-oriented, perspective. Table 284-1 highlights emergent musculoskeletal complaints that warrant prompt evaluation, along with a differential diagnosis for each.

RHEUMATIC EMERGENCIES ASSOCIATED WITH RISK OF MORTALITY

The Airway and Respiratory System

Systemic rheumatologic diseases may cause life-threatening respiratory compromise by airway obstruction or respiratory failure (Table 284-2).[2] Relapsing polychondritis is an inflammatory disease affecting cartilage that usually begins with the abrupt onset of pain, redness, and swelling of the ears or the nose. The airway is affected in roughly half of patients, causing inflammation, destruction, and ultimate collapse of tracheobronchial cartilage with airway obstruction. Patients report throat tenderness over cartilaginous structures and hoarseness. Less commonly, they experience shortness of breath, cough, or stridor. Repeated exacerbations ultimately may cause asphyxiation. Patients should be hospitalized for careful observation and high-dose cortico-steroids during acute exacerbations. In severe cases, emergency tracheostomy may be necessary.

Up to 25 percent of patients with rheumatoid arthritis (RA) may have cricoarytenoid joint involvement with associated pain which is aggravated by swallowing/speaking and which may be referred to the ear. Severe involvement of the cricoarytenoid joint may lead to hoarseness, stridor, and airway obstruction, mandating emergent laryngoscopy and/or tracheostomy.

In addition to airway obstruction, respiratory muscles may be impaired by inflammatory muscle disease, leading to respiratory failure. Patients with dermatomyositis and polymyositis may be too weak to generate intercostal retractions, so nasal flaring may be the only indi-

TABLE 284-1 Emergent Musculoskeletal Clinical Signs and Symptoms

Feature	Differential Diagnosis
History of significant trauma	Soft tissue injury, internal derangement, or fracture
Hot, swollen joint	Infection, systemic rheumatic disease, gout, pseudogout
Constitutional signs and symptoms (e.g., fever, weight loss, malaise)	Infection, sepsis, systemic rheumatic disease, malignancy
Weakness:	
Focal	Focal nerve lesion (compartment syndrome, entrapment neuropathy, mononeuritis multiplex, motor neuron disease, radiculopathy*)
Diffuse	Myositis, metabolic myopathy, toxin, paraneoplastic syndrome, degenerative neuromuscular disorder, myelopathy,* transverse myelitis
Neurogenic pain (burning, numbness, paresthesia):	
Asymmetric	Radiculopathy,* reflex sympathetic dystrophy, entrapment neuropathy
Symmetric	Myelopathy,* peripheral neuropathy
Claudication pain pattern	Peripheral vascular disease, giant cell arteritis (jaw pain), lumbar spinal stenosis

*Radiculopathy and myelopathy may be due to infectious, neoplastic, or mechanical processes.

Source: From American College of Rheumatology Ad Hoc Committee on Clinical Guidelines: Guidelines for the Initial Evaluation of the Adult Patient with Acute Musculoskeletal Symptoms. *Arthritis Rheum* 39(1):2, 1996, with permission.

TABLE 284-2   Respiratory Manifestations of Rheumatic Diseases

Disease	Common	Infrequent	Rare
SLE	Serositis, effusion	Infiltrate	Hemorrhage, "shrinking lungs," fibrosis
RA	Nodules, effusion	Pulmonary fibrosis	Cricoarytenoid obstruction
Spondyloarthropathies		Pulmonary fibrosis	Pulmonary infiltrates, ARDS
Relapsing polychondritis	Airway obstruction	Tracheobronchial collapse	
Polymyositis and dermatomyositis		Hypoventilation with hypoxemia, respiratory failure Interstitial pneumonitis	
Scleroderma	Pulmonary fibrosis	Pulmonary hypertension	
Vasculitides Wegener granulomatosis	Sinusitis, nasal ulcers, pulmonary nodules, infiltrate, bronchospasm, hemoptysis	Hemorrhage	
Polyarteritis nodosa		Peripheral infiltrate	Interstitial pneumonitis

Abbreviations: ARDS = acute respiratory distress syndrome; RA = rheumatoid arthritis; SLE = systemic lupus erythematosus.

cator of respiratory insufficiency. Unless aspiration pneumonitis is present, chest x-rays are usually normal or show a "high-riding" diaphragm. Admission for patients with inflammatory muscle disease and signs of respiratory distress is advised in anticipation of the possible need for intubation. The clinical course can be followed at bedside with measurements of peak inspiratory force and expiratory flow rate or volume. Respiratory failure is predictable with peak inspiratory effort of less than 30 percent of predicted or vital capacity of less than 50 percent of predicted.

Pleuritic chest pain is uncommon in RA, but in SLE up to 50 percent of patients have symptomatic pleurisy during the course of their disease.[3] Pleural effusions are common across the spectrum of rheumatic disease. Rheumatic, infectious, and malignant effusions are often exudative and either polymorphonuclear or mononuclear cells may predominate. In the patient without renal insufficiency, NSAIDs (e.g., indomethacin 25 to 50 mg tid) usually prove beneficial. Prednisone 10 mg PO tid is useful for patients failing this regimen.

Other serious pulmonary complications may be associated with other rheumatologic diseases. Pulmonary hemorrhage can complicate Goodpasture disease, SLE, hypersensitivity vasculitis, and Wegener granulomatosis. Ankylosing spondylitis, scleroderma, and rarely RA and other rheumatic diseases can lead to pulmonary fibrosis. Patients may present with abrupt decompensation after a history of a well-tolerated slow decline. In polymyositis, however, interstitial pneumonitis may develop with quiescent muscle disease, progress rapidly, and result in fulminant respiratory failure. Patients with acute respiratory insufficiency should be hospitalized to exclude infection and be treated with aggressive immunosuppression.

Cardiac Diseases

Pericarditis is one of the most common cardiac disorders associated with rheumatic diseases, especially in RA and juvenile rheumatoid arthritis (JRA).[4,5] SLE often causes symptomatic pericarditis, particularly in the elderly, and may be associated with symptoms of a flare such as a rash, oral ulcers, or joint pain. Symptoms tend to be consistent from one flare to the next, and therefore a thorough review of systems is important. The diagnoses of malignancy and infection should be considered in symptomatic pericarditis. Treatment with NSAIDS or indomethacin is similar to that for pleurisy. Complications of pericarditis, such as pericardial tamponade and constrictive pericarditis, are uncommon in RA and SLE.

While therapy has greatly improved long-term survival in SLE, late mortality from premature atherosclerotic disease is increasing. Pre-

cordial chest pain in SLE is not always due to serositis or costochondritis, particularly with long-standing disease, and myocardial ischemia should always be considered in the differential diagnosis.

Myocardial infarction (MI) in rheumatic diseases is not usually related to underlying disease. The noteworthy exceptions are Kawasaki disease and polyarteritis nodosa (PAN). PAN is a form of vasculitis affecting small to medium caliber arteries of the skin (nodular, urticarial, or multiform rashes), gut (abdominal angina), and kidneys (hypertension, hematuria). Coronary arteries are commonly involved.

Acute rheumatic fever (ARF) remains an important cause of pancarditis. ARF follows group A streptococcal pharyngitis within a few weeks. It is heralded by fever and acute polyarthritis in adults or migratory arthritis in children. A few patients have a more insidious onset. Signs of ARF include the presence of subcutaneous nodules, chorea, or erythema marginatum, but only a third of patients will have one of these manifestations. Diagnosis is based on documenting the clinical involvement and antecedent streptococcal infection. The throat should be cultured and antistreptolysin O (ASO) or streptozyme titers determined at intervals to document a fourfold change in titer over a month. Other baseline tests include chest radiography, echocardiography, and ECGs to monitor the carditis; and acute phase reactants such as the erythrocyte sedimentation rate (ESR) and C-reactive protein (CRP). The fever and arthritis usually respond to salicylate therapy, but salicylates should be held until the diagnosis is clear. Patients should be placed at bed rest until clinical and laboratory parameters begin to normalize.

Other diseases are associated with migratory arthritis (Table 284-3). Bacterial endocarditis or septicemia due to common bacterial pathogens and the prodromal phase of pulmonary mycoplasma or fungal infections may cause migratory joint pain. Children with Henoch-Schönlein purpura and cefaclor serum sickness often have migratory articular and periarticular involvement. Stage II Lyme disease can be manifested by migratory articular involvement, with individual joints resolving over hours to days. Often young adults with polyarthritis are empirically treated with intravenous penicillin for disseminated gonococcus (GC). The arthritis of ARF does not respond to antibiotic therapy; therefore prompt improvement suggests the diagnosis of GC.

Valvular heart disease is a recognized extra-articular manifestation of the seronegative spondyloarthropathies, particularly in patients with HLA-B27-positive ankylosing spondylitis.[6] Fibrotic changes of the aortic valve are usually asymptomatic, with dysfunction occurring more often in patients with longstanding, severe disease. Scar tissue also may impair cardiac conduction, leading to atrioventricular block. Relapsing polychondritis can result in aortic insufficiency and aortic

TABLE 284-3   Conditions Associated with Migratory Arthritis

Rheumatic fever
Subacute bacterial endocarditis
Henoch-Schönlein purpura
Cefaclor hypersensitivity (children)
Septicemia: staphylococcal, streptococcal, meningococcal, gonococcal
Pulmonary infection: *Mycoplasma,* histoplasmosis, coccidioidomycosis
Lyme disease

aneurysm. Table 284-4 summarizes cardiac involvement in rheumatic diseases.

Adrenal Insufficiency

Patients with steroid-dependent rheumatic diseases are at risk for adrenal insufficiency either from unexpected medical or traumatic stressors, or from abrupt cessation of prescribed steroid medication. Common symptoms of acute adrenal insufficiency include hypotension, lethargy, mental status changes, and hypoglycemia (see Chap. 217). Patients known to be steroid dependent and exhibiting signs of acute adrenal insufficiency should be treated with IV NS solution, glucose, and hydrocortisone 100 mg IV unless diagnostic evaluation for another cause of adrenal insufficiency is necessary. In that case, dexamethasone 4 mg IV should be substituted for hydrocortisone as dexamethasone does not interfere with an ACTH suppression test or cortisol level. Rarely, patients treated with steroids in the past 18 months develop adrenal insufficiency. They may have early symptoms of weakness, depression, fatigue, and postural dizziness, or late life-threatening vomiting. The serum chemistries usually do not reveal hyponatremia or hyperkalemia in patients with adrenal insufficiency after prednisone withdrawal because that steroid has no mineralo-corticoid activity. If the diagnosis is uncertain, prior to steroid administration a cortisol level should be drawn in the ED. Under stress, normally-functioning adrenal glands generate a cortisol level in excess of 20 μg/dL.

RHEUMATIC PRESENTATIONS WITH HIGH RISK OF MORBIDITY

The Cervical Spine and Spinal Cord

Cervical spine disease and its neurologic risk is well-recognized in rheumatoid arthritis and ankylosing spondylitis. In RA, pannus for-

mation and destruction of ligamentous supporting structures may lead to atlantoaxial subluxation.[7] An atlantodental distance in excess of the normal 3.5 mm seen in a lateral flexion view suggests instability (in children under 12, 4 mm of widening is normal). Cord compression may occur acutely following a trivial injury or be more insidious. Subtle clues include a change in bowel or bladder function, new weakness, numbness, or paresthesias. Instability may lead to posterior subluxation of the odontoid, causing vertigo or other complaints relating to vertebral insufficiency. Lhermitte sign, an electric shock sensation radiating down the back on neck flexion, is a classic indication of cervical spine instability. Strength may be difficult to assess in an RA patient, so subtle differences in reflexes are particularly informative. Plain films, cervical spine CT scan, or MRI are indicated depending on the clinical findings.

The ankylosed, inflexible cervical spine in a patient with a seronegative spondyloarthropathy (e.g., ankylosing spondylitis) is susceptible to fracture with minor trauma.[8] A forcible blow from behind may result in new neck pain in an ankylosed area. The complaint of new neck pain requires a careful history and examination, with attention to possible trauma to the neck and evidence of peripheral nerve damage. Fractures are most commonly transverse through a disc space, leading to greater risk of dislocation and cord compression.

Intubation of patients with possible rheumatic cervical spine disease should be accomplished by the most experienced clinician available. Atlantoaxial instability should be assumed, and the neck stabilized during intubation.

Spinal cord injury can also be caused by transverse myelitis in SLE, or by an anterior spinal artery syndrome in patients with other rheumatic diseases.[9] The anterior spinal artery is a direct branch of the aorta; dissection of the aorta, vasculitis, or embolism can impair blood supply to the anterior cord and produce a clinical picture distinct from transverse myelitis or metastatic tumor by sparing of posterior column function (position sense and vibration).

The Eye

Temporal arteritis (TA), also called giant cell arteritis (GCA), must be correctly diagnosed and promptly treated to prevent the complication of sudden and irreversible blindness.[10] TA occurs in up to 30 percent of patients with polymyalgia rheumatica (PMR), a related systemic illness that affects middle-elderly aged individuals who usually present with unexplained anemia, fatigue, and proximal limb/girdle pain. TA is a granulomatous arteritis of the thoracic aorta and its branches; the vasculitis and ischemia in this distribution induce characteristic signs and symptoms: new headache, tender scalp, fluctuating vision, diminution or loss of a brachial pulse, jaw claudication while chewing or talking, and constitutional symptoms. The ESR is usually (but not always) elevated >50 mm/h, as is the CRP >2.45 mg/dL, and using both studies increases diagnostic specificity. Prodromal changes in vision almost always precede blindness. A high index of suspicion is critical when evaluating anyone older than 50 with a new headache, fluctuating vision, or jaw, tongue, or upper extremity claudication. The diagnosis of TA is established by temporal artery biopsy, but treatment with prednisone 60 mg/d should be instituted prior to biopsy if the diagnosis is likely. Immediate treatment of suspected TA may prevent blindness, yet does not seem to affect biopsy outcome if the biopsy is done within a week. Treatment of PMR requires lower doses of prednisone, in the 10- to -20-mg/d range.

Sjögren syndrome, a lymphocytic infiltration of the lacrimal and salivary glands causing dry eyes and dry mouth, may complicate many rheumatic diseases or occur independently.[11] It predisposes the patient to corneal irritation, ulceration, and superimposed infection.

In RA, a red eye requires careful evaluation.[12] Under bright natural light, examination can reveal the difference between episcleritis, which is usually self-limiting, and scleritis, which can be an emergency. Episcleritis is a painless injection of the episcleral vessels,

TABLE 284-4   Cardiac Manifestations of Rheumatic Diseases

Disease	Common	Infrequent	Rare
Systemic lupus erythematosus	Pericarditis	Angina, myocarditis	Tamponade, constrictive pericarditis
Ankylosing spondylitis		Aortic stenosis/ insufficiency, dissection	Drop attacks
Relapsing polychondritis		Aortic insufficiency, dissection	
Polymyositis and dermatomyositis		Arrhythmias, myocarditis	
Scleroderma		Myocardial fibrosis, arrhythmias	Cor pulmonale
Vasculitides		Angina, myocardial infarction, pericarditis	

giving the eye a pink-red appearance; it rarely impairs vision. As it is self-limiting, no therapy is indicated. Scleritis causes exquisite ocular tenderness and the eye has a deep purplish discoloration. Visual impairment and scleral thinning with rupture are feared outcomes. High-dose steroids and intensive ophthalmologic management are required.

Hypertension

Hypertension is associated with PAN, Wegener granulomatosus, or SLE with renal involvement, as well as RA with drug-induced renal toxicity (e.g., nephritis, or renal papillary necrosis). Hypertension is a concerning complication of systemic sclerosis (scleroderma), and hypertensive renal crisis was the leading cause of death in scleroderma until the advent of angiotensin-converting enzyme (ACE) inhibitors.[13] The most susceptible patients have rapidly progressive skin changes and present within the first few years of diagnosis with complaints related to hypertension. Laboratory studies reveal rapidly progressive renal insufficiency and frequently a microangiopathic hemolytic anemia and thrombocytopenia. Hypertension results from sclerosis and impaired renal glomerular perfusion, causing hyperreninemia. Dehydration from gastroenteritis or diuretics may precipitate the crisis. Patients should be hospitalized and promptly treated with captopril. Any intervention such as diuretics that might exacerbate volume contraction and the underlying pathophysiology should be avoided.

The Kidney

Most systemic rheumatic diseases can affect kidney function.[14] Glomerulonephritis is a major determinant of morbidity in patients with lupus and Wegener granulomatosis. Urinalysis abnormalities (hematuria, proteinuria) and hypertension are apparent before serum creatinine rises. Patients with lupus and nephrotic syndrome can develop renal vein thrombosis due to urinary loss of antithrombin III; presenting with flank pain and proteinuria. In diffuse scleroderma, renal dysfunction secondary to hypertension and microangiopathy typically develops rapidly over days to a few weeks.

Occasionally, a patient with active polymyositis or metabolic muscle disease develops acute renal insufficiency due to rhabdomyolysis. In metabolic muscle disease, myalgias and muscle breakdown can be triggered by exercise. Myoglobinuria should be suspected when the urine is brown and the urinary dipstick detects hemoglobin but no red blood cells are seen on microscopic examination. In contrast to a hemolytic state, the serum is clear, creatine phosphokinase is elevated, and haptoglobin is normal. Patients should be hydrated with normal saline to restore intravascular loss that accompanies muscle necrosis. Furosemide and mannitol also are indicated to preserve urinary output (see Chap. 279).

A final consideration is medication nephrotoxicity. Patients, particularly the elderly, treated with nonsteroidal anti-inflammatory drugs can develop renal insufficiency and fluid retention on the basis of alteration in renal blood flow; this is mediated by prostaglandin inhibition (see Chap. 172). A decline in renal function in any rheumatic disease patient should prompt a search for remediable causes of renal dysfunction, either related to drug therapy or to the rheumatic disease itself.

REFERENCES

1. Halla J: Rheumatologic emergencies. *Bull Rheum Dis* 46:4, 1997.
2. Bandi V, Munnur U, Braman SS: Airway problems in patients with rheumatologic disorders. *Crit Care Clin* 18:749, 2002.
3. Wang DY: Diagnosis and management of lupus pleuritis. *Curr Opin Pulm Med* 8:312, 202.
4. Kitas G, Banks MJ, Bacon PA: Cardiac involvement in rheumatoid disease. *Clin Med* 1:18, 2001.
5. Guedes C, Bianchi-Fior P, Cormier B, et al: Cardiac manifestations of rheumatoid arthritis: A case-control transesophageal echocardiography study in 30 patients. *Arthritis Rheum* 45:129, 2001.
6. Lautermann D, Braun J: Ankylosing spondylitis—cardiac manifestations. *Clin Exp Rheumatol* 20(6 Suppl 28):S11, 2002.
7. Laiho K, Kaarela K, Kauppi M: Cervical spine disorders in patients with rheumatoid arthritis and secondary amyloidosis. *Clin Rheumatol* 21:227, 2002.
8. Exner G, Botel U, Kluger P, et al: Treatment of fracture and complication of cervical spine with ankylosing spondylitis. *Spinal Cord* 36:377, 1998.
9. Williams F, Chinn S, Hughes G, et al: Critical illness in systemic lupus erythematosus and the antiphospholipid syndrome. *Ann Rheum Dis* 61:414, 2002.
10. Salvarani C, Cantini F, Boiardi L, Hunder GG: Polymyalgia rheumatica and giant-cell arteritis. *New Engl J Med* 347:261, 2002.
11. Afshari NA, Afshari MA, Foster CS: Inflammatory conditions of the eye associated with rheumatic diseases. *Curr Rheumatol Rep* 3:453, 2001.
12. Hamideh F, Prete PE: Ophthalmologic manifestations of rheumatic diseases. *Semin Arthritis Rheum* 30:217, 2001.
13. Cossio M, Menon Y, Wilson W, deBoisblanc BP: Life-threatening complications of systemic sclerosis. *Crit Care Clin* 18:819, 2002.
14. Yorgin PD: Renal manifestations of rheumatic diseases affecting adolescents. *Adolesc Med* 9:127, 1998.

NONTRAUMATIC DISORDERS OF THE HAND
285
Mark W. Fourre

HAND INFECTIONS

Infection is most commonly introduced by an injury to the dermis. The infection initially may remain superficial, as a cellulitis, or localized, as a paronychia or felon. Left untreated, infections ultimately will spread along anatomic planes or to adjacent compartments in the hand. Deeper injuries may directly seed underlying structures, giving rise to rapidly spreading infections such as those seen with closed-fist injuries or cat bites. Rarely, hematogenous seeding may be the source of hand infections.[1,3]

A directed history should be obtained to delineate a likely cause of the infection. Patients who present with systemic symptoms secondary to a hand infection are seriously ill, and parenteral antibiotics with inpatient management is indicated. A history of chronic illness or immunodeficiency should alert the physician to the possibility of atypical pathogens.[2,3]

Since hand infections tend to disseminate along anatomic compartments and planes, the physical examination should be directed at defining the anatomic limits of the infection. The examiner should document if the process involves the skin, subcutaneous tissues, fascial spaces, tendon, joint, or bone. If deep structures of the hand are involved, emergent consultation with a hand specialist is indicated because treatment likely will involve inpatient care and drainage in the operating room.

With the exception of superficial cellulitis, hand infections are surgical problems that must be managed using accepted surgical principles. First, if there is pus, drain it. Superficial and discrete infections, such as paronychia and felons, can be drained in the ED. All other infections involving deep structures in the hand should be treated in the operating room by a hand surgeon. Second, immobilize and elevate the extremity. This will rest the hand, reduce inflammation, avoid secondary injury, and limit anatomic extension of the infection. Immobilization is accomplished by applying a bulky hand dressing and splinting the hand in a position of function: the wrist at 15 to 30 degrees of extension, the metacarpophalangeal (MCP) joints at 50 to 90 degrees of flexion, and the interphalangeal (IP) joints at 5 to 15 degrees of flexion (Figure 285-1). The hand may be elevated on pillows or suspended using stockinet. Third, broad-spectrum antibiotics should be initiated (Table 285-1). Finally, serial examinations should be performed to ensure that an effective management plan has been instituted. If the

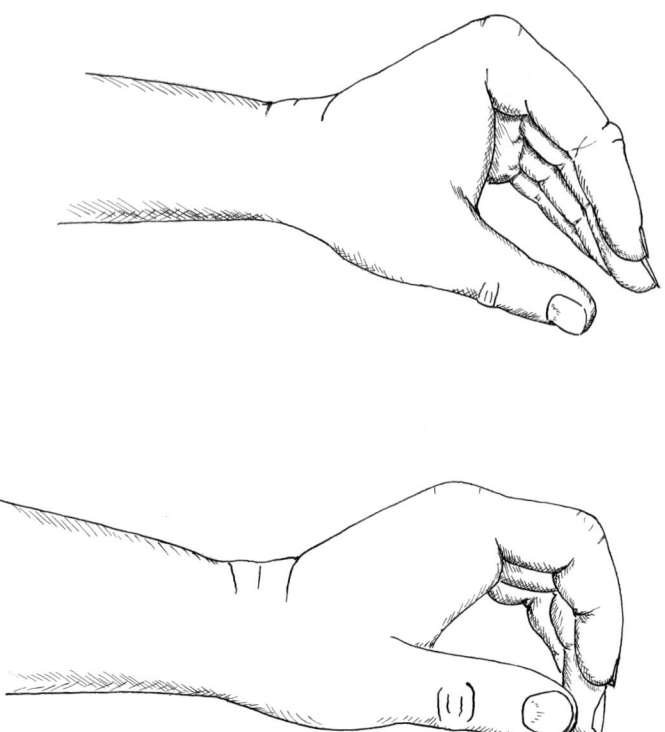

FIG. 285-1. Positioning the hand during immobilization. Top position is used when splints are applied in fractures or severe sprains. Bottom position is position of function used when applying a soft bulky dressing.

patient is not admitted to the hospital, timely and appropriate follow-up must be arranged by the emergency physician.

Pathophysiology

The bacterial etiology of hand infections depends on the source of the offending inoculum. Since *Staphylococcus* and *Streptococcus* species routinely colonize the skin, they are the bacteria most frequently isolated from hand infections. Polymicrobial infections, including anaerobes, are common.

Injection drug users typically present with abscesses or deep space infections secondary to *Staphylococcus aureus*. Infections are most commonly caused by direct introduction of a contaminated needle through inadequately cleaned skin, but hematogenous spread from bacterial endocarditis should also be considered. Paronychia and felons are commonly caused by minor trauma associated with chewing fingernails or exposing minor injuries to saliva. Most of these infections are polymicrobial in origin, with most harboring anaerobic bacteria.

Bacteria found in infections caused by animal bites reflect the oral flora of the involved species. This encompasses a broad range of bacteria, including gram-positive, anaerobic, and gram-negative organisms. In human bites, *Eikenella corrodens* is a common pathogen. *Eikenella* is sensitive to penicillin and ampicillin, but is relatively resistant to numerous antibiotics, including first-generation cephalosporins, nafcillin, and clindamycin. Therefore, an aminopenicillin with a beta-lactamase inhibitor or a first-generation cephalosporin in combination with penicillin is required for prophylactic antibiotic coverage for human bites and for treatment of hand infections caused by human bites (see Table 285–1). Cat and dog bites may harbor *Pasteurella multocida,* which typically produces an aggressive, rapidly spreading cellulitis that quickly becomes suppurative. *Pasteurella* is also sensitive to penicillin and ampicillin, and antibiotic coverage is the same as that indicated for human bites. Initial antibiotic coverage is reviewed in Table 285-1. For a complete discussion on animal bites, see Chap. 47.

Patients with diabetes or acquired immunodeficiency syndrome (AIDS) may harbor atypical infections caused by *Mycobacterium* or *Candida albicans*. Patients who are immunocompromised or asplenic may be at risk for rapidly progressive and fatal infections. Aggressive intervention is indicated in these settings.

Cellulitis

Cellulitis is the most superficial of hand infections and may be treated definitively with oral antibiotics if diagnosed early. Diagnosis is made by documenting erythema, warmth, and edema in the affected portion of the hand. The examiner must document lack of involvement of any deeper structures in the hand. Specifically, range of motion of the digits, hand, or wrist should not be uncomfortable for the patient, and palpation of the deeper structures of the hand should not produce any tenderness.

TABLE 285-1 Initial Antibiotic Coverage for Common Hand Infections

Infection	Initial Antibiotic	Likely Organisms	Comments
Cellulitis	First-generation cephalosporin (cephalexin) *or* antistaphylococcal penicillin (amoxicillin-clavulanate, dicloxacillin)	*S. pyogenes, S. aureus*	Consider vancomycin for intravenous drug abusers
Felon/paronychia	First-generation cephalosporin (cephalexin) *or* antistaphylococcal penicillin (amoxicillin-clavulanate, dicloxacillin)	Polymicrobial, *S. aureus,* anaerobes	Antibiotics indicated for infections with associated localized cellulitis
Flexor tenosynovitis	Aminopenicillin with a β-lactamase inhibitor (ampicillin/sulbactam) *or* first-generation cephalosporin (cefazolin) and penicillin	*S. aureus,* streptococci, anaerobes, gram-negatives	Parenteral antibiotics are indicated; consider ceftriaxone for *N. gonorrhoeae*
Deep space infection	Aminopenicillin with a β-lactamase inhibitor (ampicillin/sulbactam) *or* first-generation cephalosporin (cefazolin) and penicillin	*S. aureus,* streptococci, anaerobes, gram-negatives	Inpatient management
Animal bites (including human)	Aminopenicillin with a β-lactamase inhibitor (ampicillin/sulbactam) *or* first-generation cephalosporin (cefazolin) and penicillin	*S. aureus,* streptococci, *E. corrodens* (human), *Pasteurella multocida* (cat), anaerobes and gram-negatives	All animal bite wounds should receive prophylactic oral antibiotics
Herpetic whitlow	None, unless secondary bacterial contamination is present	Herpes simplex	Consider acyclovir, no surgical drainage is indicated

The most common offending organism is *Streptococcus pyogenes,* although *S. aureus* and other pathogens are identified occasionally. An antistaphylococcal penicillin or first-generation cephalosporin is recommended for initial treatment (see Table 285-1). For more extensive involvement, parenteral antibiotics should be instituted. Inpatient management should be reserved for patients who are immunocompromised or systemically ill and for rapidly spreading infections.

The hand should be immobilized in a position of function, and the patient should keep the hand elevated as much as possible. Finally, close follow-up should be arranged, with reexamination in approximately 24 h.

Flexor Tenosynovitis

Flexor tenosynovitis is a surgical emergency. Failure to accurately diagnose and manage flexor tenosynovitis will lead to loss of function of the digit and eventually loss of function of the entire hand. Diagnosis is made by recognizing the four classic clinical findings described by Kanavel: tenderness over the flexor tendon sheath, symmetric swelling of the finger, pain with passive extension, and a flexed posture of the involved digit at rest.[3]

The infection usually is associated with penetrating trauma of the affected area, although the patient may be unaware of this injury. *Staphylococcus* is the most common bacterium isolated; however, infections often harbor anaerobes and are routinely polymicrobial in origin. Suspect disseminated *Neisseria gonorrhoeae* in a patient with a recent history consistent with a sexually transmitted disease.

Initiate treatment with parenteral antibiotics (see Table 285-1). Vancomycin should be considered for injection drug abusers because they may harbor methicillin-resistant *S. aureus* (MRSA). Any spontaneous exudate from the infection should be sent for Gram stain and culture with sensitivities.

The hand should be immobilized and elevated, and a hand surgeon should be consulted from the ED. If the infection is identified early in its course, conservative (e.g., nonoperative) therapy may be indicated initially. The patient would then be treated with parenteral antibiotics, immobilization, elevation, and reevaluation within 24 h. The decision to manage the patient without operative intervention must be made in conjunction with the hand surgeon.

Deep Space Infections

The hand offers numerous compartments in which infections may propagate and migrate. The volar surface of the hand encompasses many potential spaces that may become infected by direct inoculation or spread from surrounding structures. These include the thenar space, the midpalmar space, the radial bursa, and the ulna bursa (Figures 285-2 and 285-3).

The volar aspect of the hand is covered by the tough and relatively fixed tissues of the palm; the veins and lymphatics course through the softer tissues on the dorsum of the hand; thus, regardless of the precise anatomic site of infection or inflammation, the dorsum of the hand will always swell whenever there is an inflammatory process. For this reason, a deep space infection initially may be misdiagnosed as a cellulitis over the dorsum of the hand if the practitioner does not obtain a thorough history and conduct a complete examination, including palpation of the volar surface of the hand to elicit tenderness, induration, or fluctuance, as well as doing a sensory evaluation. Since these compartments are contiguous with the flexor tendons of the hand, range of motion of the digits often produces significant pain for the patient.

Occasionally, infections will arise in the web space. These "collar button" abscesses present with pain and swelling of the web space, causing separation of the affected digits. Examination reveals induration or fluctuance in the dorsal and/or volar web space, along with erythema, warmth, and tenderness. *S. aureus* and *Streptococcus* species are the most common organisms isolated.[3]

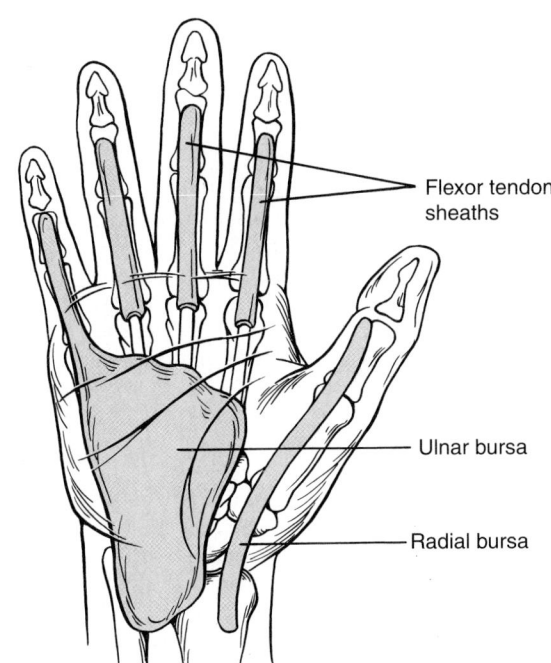

FIG. 285-2. Anatomy. Flexor tendon infections may travel quickly along established anatomic planes and spread quickly to the ulnar and radial bursae.

Give parenteral antibiotics (see Table 285-1), and immobilize and elevate the hand. The patient likely will require analgesia while in the ED. Emergent evaluation by a hand surgeon is required because drainage of the infection should be undertaken in the operating room.

Infections from Closed-Fist Injuries

The most common human bite infection of the hand is the result of striking another individual's teeth with a clenched fist. Because of the

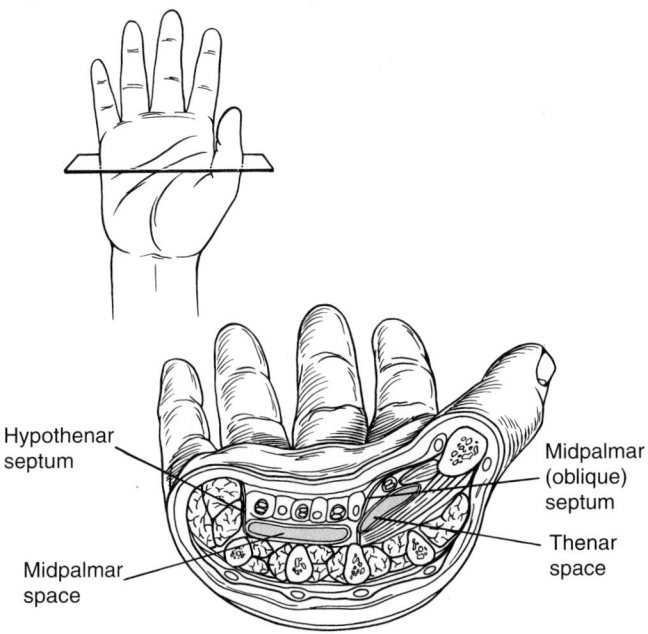

FIG. 285-3. Deep palmar spaces. The midpalmar and thenar spaces are deep structures of the hand. The proximity to vital structures necessitates an aggressive management course including parenteral antibiotics and referral to a hand surgeon for drainage.

force associated with the contact and the penetrating nature of the human incisor, these infections tend to occur on multiple planes, and infection spreads rapidly to adjacent compartments. Skin, extensor tendons, joint space, bone, and surrounding deep spaces often are involved because the inoculum of saliva may traverse all these structures.

The physical examination should document the extent of the infection. Hand x-rays are indicated because closed-fist injuries are often associated with fractures, or may contain tooth fragments. The most common organisms reflect the natural flora of the mouth and include *Streptococcus* species, *S. aureus*, anaerobes, *E. corrodens*, and *Neisseria* species. Antibiotics should be initiated in the ED and a hand surgeon consulted (see Table 285-1). The wound should be irrigated in the operating room and left open. The hand should be immobilized in the position of function and elevated.

Paronychia

Paronychia is an infection of the lateral nail fold or perionychium, occasionally extending to the cuticle or eponychium. It is usually caused by minor trauma such as nail biting, manicures, or hangnails. The infection starts as a small area of induration that may be erythematous and tender. Most paronychia contain both aerobic and anaerobic bacteria. *S. aureus* and *Streptococcus* species are the most common aerobic bacteria cultured. Chronic paronychia may occur, particularly in patients who are immunocompromised. Consider atypical bacterial or fungal infections such as with *C. albicans* in these cases.[4]

If no fluctuance is identified, the paronychia may be treated with warm soaks, elevation, and antibiotics (see Table 285-1). Early intervention may prevent the need for surgical drainage. After suppuration has occurred, the infection will exhibit either fluctuance or identifiable pus that will necessitate drainage. Minor infections can be treated with elevation of the perionychium or eponychium with a flat probe or no. 11 blade (Figure 285-4). This procedure sometimes can be performed without placing a digital block or providing analgesia.

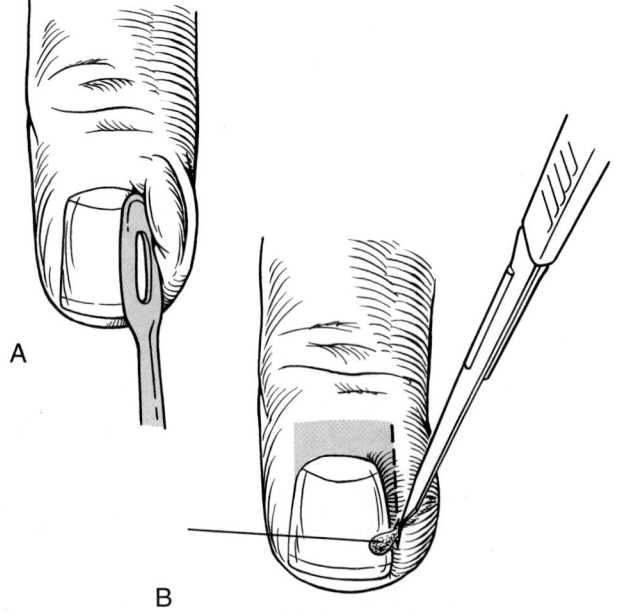

FIG. 285-4. Paronychia. **A.** The eponychial fold is elevated using a flat probe or no. 11 blade in order to allow the wound to drain. **B.** Alternatively, for more extensive infections, a no. 11 blade may be used to incise the area of greatest fluctuance directly into the eponychium. The wound may then be gently probed with a small clamp to ensure drainage.

More extensive infections that do not communicate directly with the nail fold may require digital block and incision directly into the area of greatest fluctuance. Severe infections with pus beneath the nail require removal of a portion of the lateral or proximal nail to ensure adequate drainage. Rarely, a free-floating nail will be encountered on a bed of pus, necessitating removal of the entire nail.

Following incision and drainage, keep the hand elevated and immobilized. Warm soaks may be initiated to keep the wound open and clean. The patient should be scheduled for reevaluation in 24 to 48 h. If cellulitis is present, a short course of antibiotics should be prescribed.

Felon

A felon is a subcutaneous pyogenic infection of the pulp space of the distal finger or thumb. The septa of the finger pad produce multiple individual compartments and confine the infection under pressure. The patient presents with marked throbbing pain and a red, tense distal pulp space. Infection typically begins with minor trauma to the dermis overlying the finger pad. With time, the bacterial infection gradually spreads between septae, forming multiple compartmentalized abscesses. Left untreated, the infection may spread to the flexor tendon sheath and the interphalangeal joints, or eventually osteomyelitis may develop. Do not mistake a felon for pulp erythema secondary to a paronychia or herpetic whitlow.[5,6]

S. aureus is the most common organism, but *Streptococcus* species, anaerobes, and gram-negative organisms are frequently encountered. A Gram stain and culture should be obtained because these infections may be difficult to eradicate, and chronic infections may be caused by atypical organisms. If osteomyelitis has developed, positive identification of the offending organism is necessary because long-term antibiotic therapy will be indicated.

If the finger pad is swollen and tense, or if there is any palpable fluctuance, drainage is necessary. A digital block using a long-acting anesthetic such as bupivacaine should be used because postoperative discomfort is considerable (see Chap. 37). Most felons can be drained adequately with a limited incision and drainage procedure.

A unilateral longitudinal approach is the most frequently used technique because it spares the sensate volar pad and achieves adequate drainage (Figure 285-5A). A no. 11 blade is introduced lateral to the felon and is directed across the finger until pus is encountered. The incision should be extended to ensure adequate drainage, although it should not extend to the distal interphalangeal (DIP) flexor crease. Also, the incision should not carry through the distal end of the finger pad because this would likely cause instability and loss of sensation to the distal fingertip. A small clamp may be used to bluntly dissect septa to ensure complete drainage. If the wound is large enough, a small wick may be placed to encourage continued drainage.

If the felon is pointing toward the volar fat pad, a longitudinal volar approach may be used, as depicted in Figure 285-5B. Care should be exercised to avoid extending the incision to the flexor crease of the DIP joint. More extensive incisions such as the fishmouth, hockey stick, and through-and-through incisions are rarely if ever indicated. These incisions are routinely associated with loss of sensation to the fingertip and instability of the finger pad.

Following drainage, the wound should be irrigated and then dressed with a dry, sterile dressing. The patient should be instructed to keep the extremity elevated, and the wound should be reevaluated in 24 to 48 h. Warm soaks may be initiated to keep the wound clean and promote continued drainage.

Most felons have significant associated cellulitis that should be treated with oral antibiotics. A first-generation cephalosporin or antistaphylococcal penicillin should be prescribed for 7 to 10 days or until the infection has abated. Felons not responding to treatments outlined above should be referred to a hand specialist for more definitive management and long-term follow-up.

Herpetic Whitlow

Herpetic whitlow is a viral infection of the distal finger caused by the herpes simplex virus, usually from contact with oral herpetic infections. Herpetic whitlow in children tends to be associated with gingivostomatitis and herpes simplex virus type 1 (HSV-1), whereas adults most commonly harbor herpes simplex virus type 2 (HSV-2). Health care professionals are at especially high risk for this infection.[7]

The patient will present with a burning, pruritic sensation similar to all herpes simplex infections. On examination, the lesion is erythematous and tender, with vesicular bullae (Figure 285-6). The finger may be indurated, but is not tense, as is seen in a felon. Do not mistake herpetic whitlow for a felon because incision and drainage may result in increased morbidity and prolonged failure to heal. If there is any question concerning the diagnosis of herpetic whitlow, a vesicle may be unroofed, and the drainage fluid may be used for a Tzanck smear to confirm the diagnosis.

Treatment consists of immobilization, elevation, and pain medication. Antiviral agents such as acyclovir or valacyclovir may shorten the duration and have been shown to prevent recurrent infections. The patient must be instructed in the management of the infection, and the finger should be kept in a clean dressing to prevent autoinoculation or spread of the herpes infection to other individuals.

NONINFECTIOUS INFLAMMATORY STATES OF THE HAND

Noninfectious inflammatory states of the hand often present as an acute exacerbation of symptoms related to recent overuse, either in the workplace or at home. Inflammatory states of joints and tendons can be markedly painful, and may be difficult to distinguish from acute septic arthritis or suppurative tenosynovitis. If the diagnosis is in doubt, treat for infection, and consult a hand specialist.

If an inflammatory state is confidently diagnosed, the patient initially should be treated with conservative measures. These include rest, immobilization, elevation, and initiation of anti-inflammatory agents.

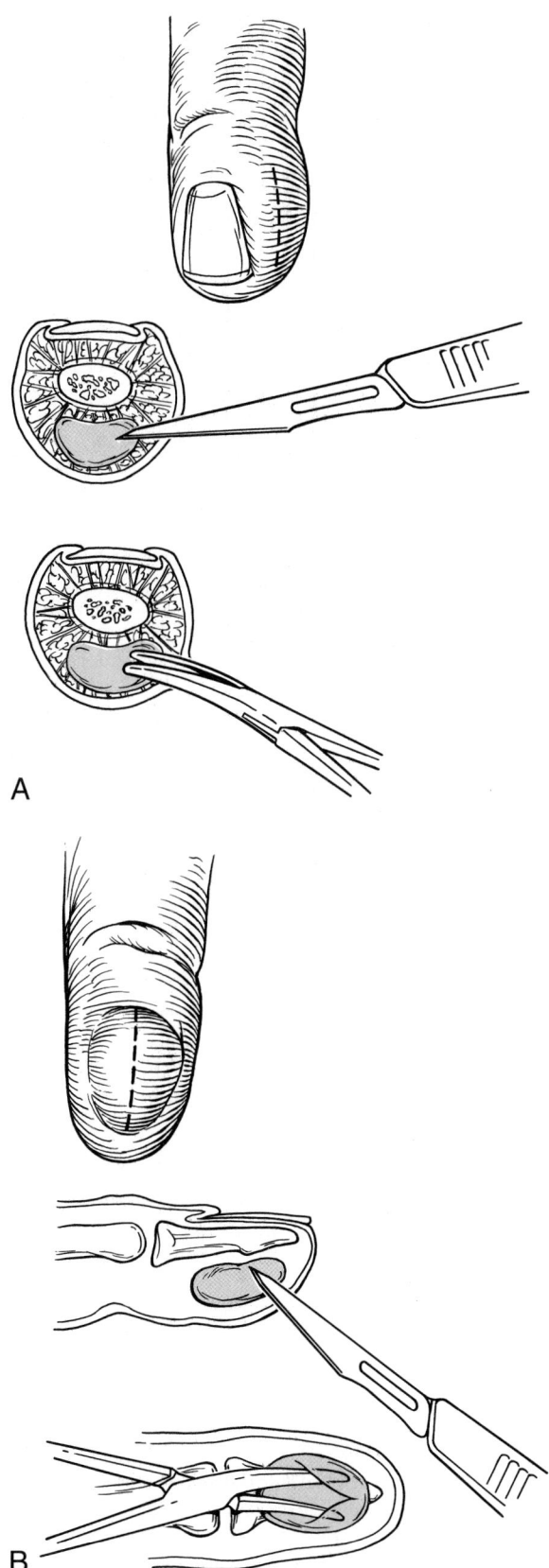

FIG. 285-5. Felon. **A.** The unilateral longitudinal approach is the most frequently used method for draining felons. This approach minimizes interference with sensate areas of the finger pad. **B.** If the felon is pointing toward the volar surface of the finger pad, the longitudinal volar approach may be used.

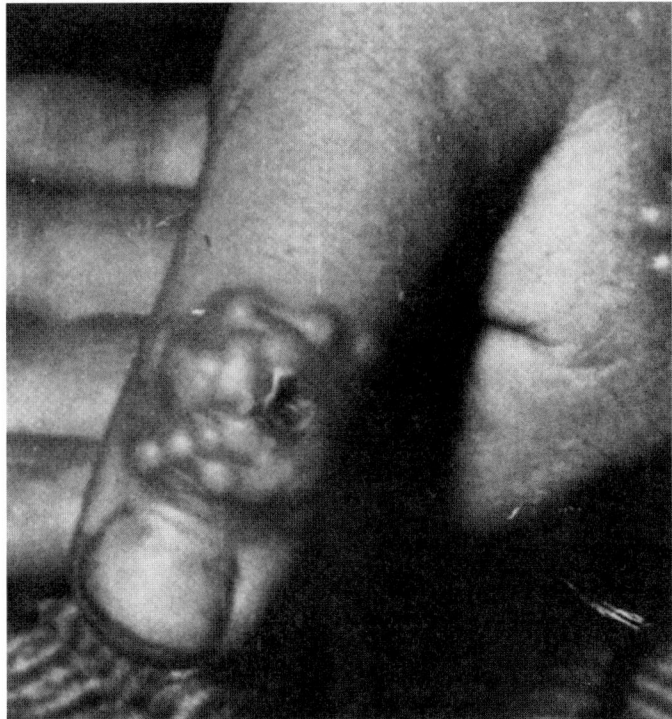

FIG. 285-6. Herpetic whitlow. (Reproduced with permission from Domonkos AN: *Andrews' Diseases of the Skin.* Philadelphia: Saunders, 1971).

Tendinitis and Tenosynovitis

Inflammatory tendinitis may involve the flexor or extensor tendons of the hand. Most often, the patient is able to recount a history of repetitive motion directly affecting the inflamed tendon. Palpation of the tendon produces tenderness. Active or passive movement of the tendon produces significant pain.

Treatment is splinting in the position of function with elevation of the affected area, and nonsteroidal anti-inflammatory agents. Patients should be referred to their primary care physician or a hand surgeon for follow-up. The patient also should be directed to return to the ED for worsening pain, increased swelling, or any signs of infection, including fever and erythema.

Trigger Finger

Tenosynovitis can develop in the flexor sheaths of the fingers and thumb. Scarring or inflammation may cause the tendon to become nodular, which results in friction and catching between the tendon and its sheath, usually in the vicinity of the A1 pulley at the volar crease at the base of each digit. This is referred to as *stenosing tenosynovitis,* or *trigger finger.* The patient experiences binding of the tendon, usually as the finger extends, relieved by a painful "snap" as the tendon clears the obstruction. Occasionally, this condition may progress to the point that the finger locks, usually in flexion. Early stages of trigger finger have been treated successfully with depot steroid injection into the tendon sheath, although there may be recurrence. Surgical division of the A1 pulley is usually curative.

De Quervain's Stenosing Tenosynovitis

De Quervain's tenosynovitis is a common condition that occurs in patients who have experienced excessive use of the thumb. Often no plausible cause can be found. This is a tenosynovitis of the extensor pollicis brevis and abductor pollicis tendons, where they lie in the groove of the radial styloid.

The patient presents with pain along the radial aspect of the wrist that extends into the forearm. The definitive examination that confirms the diagnosis is the Finkelstein test (Figure 285-7), in which the patient grasps the thumb in the palm of the hand and the examiner ulnar deviates the thumb and hand. This produces sharp pain along the involved tendons.

The thumb and wrist should be immobilized with a splint. Instruct the patient to remove the splint briefly each day and perform range-of-motion exercises to prevent joint stiffness. Anti-inflammatory medication should be prescribed for 10 to 14 days. Recurrence of this condition is not uncommon, particularly when related to occupational stress. Persistent cases should be referred to a hand surgeon.

Carpal Tunnel Syndrome

Carpal tunnel syndrome is a peripheral mononeuropathy that involves entrapment of the median nerve in the carpal canal or tunnel, which is covered by the tense transverse carpal ligament. Whenever a condition causes swelling in the carpal tunnel, the median nerve is compressed, causing paresthesias that extend into the index and long fingers, the radial aspect of the ring finger, and along the palmar aspect of the thumb. The patient often complains of awakening at night with burning pain and tingling in the hand, or numbness when driving a car or maintaining the wrist in prolonged flexion.

Direct trauma to the wrist may exacerbate symptoms; however, a more common scenario involves overuse syndromes in which the patient recounts a history of repeated flexion and extension of the wrist that results in edema in the carpal tunnel. Edematous conditions such as pregnancy and congestive heart failure may acutely exacerbate symptoms in patients with a predisposition for carpal tunnel syndrome. It is also common in diabetes and rheumatoid arthritis.

Tinel sign may support the diagnosis and involves tapping the volar aspect of the wrist over the median nerve. A positive sign produces paresthesias that extend into the index and long finger. Phalen sign is more sensitive (50 percent) and specific (75 percent), and involves flexing the wrist maximally and holding it in this position for at least 1 min. The patient complains of tingling and numbness along the median nerve distribution. Both signs are subject to false-positive and false-negative results and electrodiagnostic techniques may be required to confirm the diagnosis.[8,9]

The presence of median nerve motor deficit requires emergency hand consultation. Otherwise, initial treatment is a volar splint to maintain the wrist in neutral position, and nonsteroidal anti-inflammatory agents. Surgery may be needed if symptoms do not improve, so referral to a hand surgeon is needed.

Dupuytren Contracture

Dupuytren contracture is a poorly understood disorder resulting in fibroplastic changes of the subcutaneous tissues of the palm and volar aspect of the fingers. There appears to be a genetic component, and the condition is found most commonly in men of northern European descent. This process eventually may lead to tethering and joint contracture. Firm longitudinal thickening and nodularity of the superficial tissues usually are readily appreciated. The diagnosis is made by identifying a nodule in the palm, usually at the distal palmar crease of the ring or small finger, which is held in the classic flexion contracture. This condition should be referred to a skilled hand specialist because surgical excision of the fibrotic bands is usually palliative.

Ganglion Cysts

A ganglion or synovial cyst is a cystic collection of synovial fluid within a joint or tendon sheath. It is one of the most common conditions of the wrist and hand. Clinically, the patient presents with a tender cystic swelling over or near a tendon sheath. Common locations are the dorsal and volar wrist, flexor surface of the metacarpophalangeal joint, or the base of the nail. Involvement of the thumb may appear as generalized thumb pain, pain with movement, and edema. Treatment is pain control and nonsteroidal anti-inflammatory agents. About one-third of cysts resolve spontaneously. Referral to a hand surgeon is indicated for persistent or recurrent pain, or cosmetic deformity. Treatment options include cyst aspiration, corticosteroid injection, or occasionally, surgical excision.

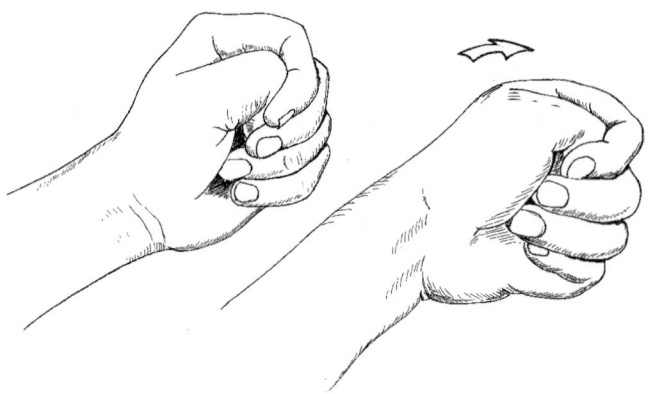

FIG. 285-7. The Finkelstein test. The thumb is cupped in the closed fist and ulnar deviation reproduces pain along the extensor pollicis and abductor pollicis.

REFERENCES

1. Hausman MR, Lisser SP: Hand infections. *Orthop Clin North Am* 5:171, 1992.
2. Kour AK, Looi KP, Phone MH, et al: Hand infections in patients with diabetes. *Clin Orthop* 331:238, 1996.
3. Moran GJ, Talan DA: Hand infections. *Emerg Med Clin North Am* 11:601, 1993.
4. Brook I: Aerobic and anaerobic microbiology of paronychia. *Ann Emerg Med* 19:994, 1990.
5. Dahir K (ed): *The Hand: Primary Care of Common Problems,* 2d ed. New York, Churchill-Livingstone, 1990.
6. Concannon MJ (ed): *Common Hand Problems in Primary Care.* Philadelphia: Hanley & Belfus, 1999.
7. Laskin OL: Acyclovir and suppression of frequently recurring herpetic whitlow. *Ann Emerg Med* 102:494, 1985.
8. Atroshi I, Gummesson MS, Johnsson R, et al: Prevalence of carpal tunnel syndrome in a general population. *JAMA* 282:153, 1999.
9. Novak M: Carpal tunnel syndrome. *Lippincott's Primary Care Pract* 4:642, 2000.

286 ACUTE DISORDERS OF THE JOINTS AND BURSAE
John H. Burton

Acute disorders of the joints affect a collection of patients with diseases that span a vast spectrum of age, acuity, and etiologies. Emergency physicians must differentiate conditions that require immediate attention from those that require less urgent therapy. A careful, methodical process utilizing certain unifying approaches within the clinical history, physical examination, laboratory evaluation, and radiographic assessment will lead to appropriate diagnosis, treatment, and disposition.

CLINICAL FEATURES

Many pathways provoke acute joint complaints: degradation and degeneration of articular cartilage (osteoarthritis), deposition of immune complexes or immune-system-related phenomena (rheumatoid arthritis, rheumatic fever, and gonococcal arthritis), crystal-induced inflammation (gout and pseudogout), seronegative spondyloarthropathies (ankylosing spondylitis and Reiter syndrome), and bacterial invasion (septic or Lyme arthritis) or viral invasion (viral arthritis). These processes impact joint capsules and surfaces, resulting in a cascade of reactive and inflammatory events.

The most useful tool for evaluation of joint disorders is evaluation of synovial fluid. Table 286-1 lists the diagnostic characteristics of synovial fluid. However, joint aspiration may be difficult or impossible in smaller joints or those with minimal effusions. Identifying the distribution and number of affected joints is also useful for diagnosis (Table 286-2). A migratory pattern of joint involvement may be helpful as well (Table 286-3).[1]

Patient age and gender are aids to diagnosis. Although no clinical pattern is diagnostic, certain general observations are helpful. Septic arthritis is important in infants and children,[2] with typical affecting organisms characteristic of age and development (Table 286-4). Additionally, a number of infectious and inflammatory processes are unique to childhood (see Chap. 136 for detailed discussion).[2] In teen and adult years, sexual activity results in an increase in prevalence of gonococcal arthritis and Reiter syndrome associated with chlamydial urethritis.[3]

Crystal-induced arthritides commonly affect middle-aged adults. Gout is the most common inflammatory joint disease in men over age 40.[4] The classic gout patient is a middle-aged man with an acute monoarthritis. Women, however, are generally spared the onset of gout until later middle age but can develop polyarticular involvement.[4]

As age progresses, the incidence of rheumatoid and osteoarthritis increases. Whereas osteoarthritis is a disease of older adults (over age 60), rheumatoid arthritis tends to strike earlier with a predilection for women three to four times that of men.[1] Additionally, rheumatoid arthritis classically demonstrates a progressive course with additive, polyarticular involvement of symmetric joints.[5]

DIAGNOSIS

Examination of Synovial Fluid

Joint fluid should routinely be analyzed for culture, Gram stain, leukocyte count with differential, and a wet preparation for crystals.[6] Glucose and lactate levels may be assessed as well. Cultures should include those for gonococci and anaerobes, when appropriate. Certain disease mechanisms are associated with classic joint aspirate findings (see Table 286-1).

Laboratory Tests

In the acute setting, few tests other than the joint aspirate contribute meaningfully to the diagnostic evaluation. Although the erythrocyte sedimentation rate (ESR) is frequently elevated in a number of acute inflammatory and reactive arthritides (septic, gonococcal, crystal-induced, spondyloarthropathies, and rheumatoid and Lyme arthritis),[7] the ESR is neither specific nor sufficiently sensitive for disease or as a marker for disease progression. The most applicable use for ESR in children and young infants in whom ESR sensitivity has been reported as 90 percent in the face of septic arthritis.[8]

TABLE 286-1 Examination of Synovial Fluid

	Normal	Noninflammatory	Inflammatory	Septic
Clarity	Transparent	Transparent	Cloudy	Cloudy
Color	Clear	Yellow	Yellow	Yellow
WBC/μL	<200	<200–2000	200–50,000	>50,000
PMNs (%)*	<25	<25	>50	>50
Culture	Negative	Negative	Negative	>50% positive
Crystals	None	None	Multiple or none	None
Associated conditions		Osteoarthritis, trauma, rheumatic fever	Gout, pseudogout, spondyloarthropathies, RA, Lyme disease, SLE	Nongonococcal or gonococcal septic arthritis

*The white blood cell count (WBC) and percent polymorphonuclear leukocytes (PMNs) are affected by a number of factors, including disease progression, affecting organism, and host immune status. The joint aspirate WBC and PMNs should be considered part of a continuum for each disease, particularly septic arthritis, and should be correlated with other clinical information. RA = rheumatoid arthritis; SLE = systemic lupus erythematosus.

TABLE 286-2 Classification of Arthritis by Number of Affected Joints

Number of Joints	Differential Considerations
1 = Monoarthritis	Trauma-induced arthritis Infection/septic arthritis Crystal-induced (gout, pseudogout) Osteoarthritis (acute) Lyme disease Avascular necrosis Tumor
2–3 = Oligoarthritis	Lyme disease Reiter syndrome Ankylosing spondylitis Gonococcal arthritis Rheumatic fever
>3 = Polyarthritis	Rheumatoid arthritis Systemic lupus erythematosus Viral arthritis Osteoarthritis (chronic)

TABLE 286-4 Commonly Encountered Organisms in the Septic Arthritis Patient

Patient/ Condition	Expected Organisms	Antibiotic Considerations
Neonates and infants	*Staphylococcus*, gram-negative bacteria, group B *Streptococcus*, *Candida*	Nafcillin* plus aminoglycoside or third-generation cephalosporin, ampicillin-sulbactam
Children <5 years	*Staphylococcus*, *Streptococcus*, *Haemophilus influenzae*	Nafcillin* plus cefuroxime, ampicillin-sulbactam
Older children and healthy adults	*Staphylococcus*, *Neisseria gonorrhoeae*, *Streptococcus*	Nafcillin* plus third-generation cephalosporin, ampicillin-sulbactam
Involvement of the foot	*Staphylococcus*, *Pseudomonas*	Nafcillin* plus ceftazidime or aminoglycoside
Intravenous drug users	*Staphylococcus*, gram-negative bacilli	Nafcillin* plus aminoglycoside, ampicillin-sulbactam
Sickle-cell patients	*Salmonella*	Ciprofloxacin, ofloxacin, or ceftriaxone

*First-generation cephalosporin may be substituted for penicillinase-resistant penicillin. Vancomycin should be employed for treatment of suspected methicillin-resistant staphylococci.

Conversely, the white blood cell count (WBC) also has poor sensitivity and specificity for septic arthritis. Notably, in pediatric septic arthritis, the total WBC is reported as 30 to 60 percent sensitive, with a left shift of the differential approaching 66 percent sensitivity.[8] Similar findings have been described in the adult population.[9]

Blood cultures have limited utility although they are routine for possible septic arthritis. Cultures should be drawn prior to antibiotic therapy. Blood cultures have demonstrated sensitivities of 23 and 40 percent, in adults and children, respectively.[9,10]

Additional laboratory assessment may be required for follow-up, including Lyme titer, rheumatoid factor, antinuclear antibodies, antineutrophil cytoplasmic antibodies, HLA-B27 tissue typing, lupus anticoagulant, and repeat synovial fluid analysis.

Radiology

Radiographs of an inflamed joint should be obtained when trauma, tumor, ankylosing spondylitis, avascular necrosis, or osteomyelitis are in the differential diagnosis. Radiographic evidence of osteomyelitis has been noted to follow symptom onset by 7 to 14 days.[1] Radioisotope scanning is not usually required for emergency department diagnosis, but can be useful to detect osteomyelitis, occult fracture, avascular necrosis, or tumor.

ARTHROCENTESIS

Accurate diagnosis of articular problems often depends on aspiration and examination of synovial fluid from the affected joint(s) (see Table 286-1).

Technique for Preparation of Selected Arthrocentesis Site

The skin overlying the affected joint should be free of cellulitis or impetigo in order to avoid contamination of the joint space during arthrocentesis. Other relative contraindications to joint aspiration are co-

TABLE 286-3 Common Joint Disorders Displaying a Migratory Distribution Pattern

Gonococcal arthritis
Acute rheumatic fever
Lyme disease
Viral arthritis
Systemic lupus erythematosus

agulopathy, hemarthrosis in hemophiliac patients before factor replacement, and the presence of a prosthetic joint. However, if the concern for septic arthritis is high, arthrocentesis may be performed in these settings after consultation.

The technique for preparation of any selected joint begins with overlying skin preparation and proper anesthesia. A large area overlying and adjacent to the affected joint is cleansed with povidone-iodine solution. After air drying, the skin is cleaned with an alcohol wipe to remove the povidone-iodine solution from the skin surface. This prevents the introduction of the povidone-iodine antiseptic into the joint, which can result in chemical irritation, or sterilization of the aspiration sample. Sterile drapes are then placed over the site.

Anesthesia is accomplished with infiltration of a local anesthetic by using a 25- to 30-gauge needle. Intra-articular injection of anesthetic should be avoided, because it can inhibit bacterial growth and may result in a spuriously negative culture in an early septic joint.[9]

A large-bore needle (18 or 19 gauge) should be used for aspiration of the joint. Smaller joints may require a smaller-bore needle to enter the joint space. The anticipated volume of fluid within the joint space should direct the selection of syringe size. As much synovial fluid should be removed as possible to optimize diagnosis and relieve pain from joint capsule distention. Aspirated fluid should promptly be sent for appropriate studies, including culture, Gram stain, leukocyte count with differential, and crystal analysis.

Recent reports have documented ultrasound-assisted arthrocentesis by emergency physicians.[11,12] Ultrasound should not be utilized to determine if arthrocentesis is indicated, but rather as an adjunct to assist localization and aspiration of joint fluid.

Shoulder

ANTERIOR APPROACH   Insert the needle just lateral to the coracoid process. This technique is performed with the patient sitting in an upright position, facing the examiner. The needle is directed posteriorly between the coracoid process and the humeral head. Because of the difficulty in locating the coracoid process, a posterior approach to the glenohumeral joint may be preferable in some patients.

POSTERIOR APPROACH   Sit the patient upright with his or her back toward you. The spine of the scapula is palpated to its lateral limit: the acromion. The posterolateral corner of the acromion is located. The point for needle insertion lies 1 cm inferior and 1 cm medial to the posterolateral corner of the acromion (Figure 286-1). A $1\frac{1}{2}$-in. needle is directed anterior and medial toward the presumed position of the coracoid process. The glenohumeral joint is located at a depth of approximately 1 to $1\frac{1}{2}$ in.

Elbow

A lateral approach to the elbow is used. Place the elbow in 90 degree flexion, resting on a table, with the hand prone. Locate the radial head, lateral epicondyle of the distal humerus, and the lateral aspect of the olecranon tip. These three landmarks form the anconeus triangle. The center of this triangle is the site for needle entry into the skin. The needle should be directed medial and perpendicular to the radius (Figure 286-2).

Wrist

Landmarks for wrist arthrocentesis are palpable with the wrist in a neutral position. Noted landmarks are the radial tubercle of the distal radius, the anatomic snuff-box, the extensor pollicis longus tendon, and the common extensor tendon of the index finger (Figure 286-3). The needle should be inserted perpendicular to the skin slightly ulnar to the radial tubercle and the anatomic snuff-box between the extensor pollicis longus and the common extensor tendons.

Hip

Hip arthrocentesis may be performed via an anterior or medial approach. Due to the belief that patients, particularly children, with a

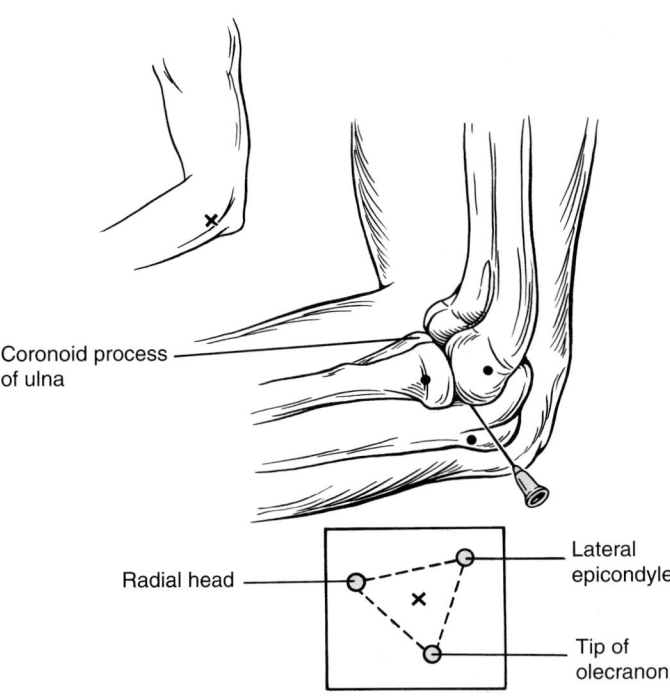

FIG. 286-2. Arthrocentesis of the elbow.

septic hip should undergo open surgical assessment and drainage, an orthopedic consultant will generally perform this procedure.[2] Controversy exists regarding the utility of ultrasound, bone scan, or magnetic resonance imaging as a screening test prior to open surgical evaluation.[13,14] Immediate consultation with orthopedics is therefore desirable when a diagnosis of septic hip arthritis is considered.

Knee

The knee joint can be entered either medial or lateral to the patella. With the patient supine, the knee should be fully extended and the quadriceps muscle relaxed. The midpoint of the patella is identified. The insertion point of the needle is located approximately 1 cm inferior to the patellar edge, either lateral (Figure 286-4) or medial (Figure 286-5) to the middle of the patella. The needle should be directed posterior to the patella and horizontally toward the joint space. Compression applied over the joint

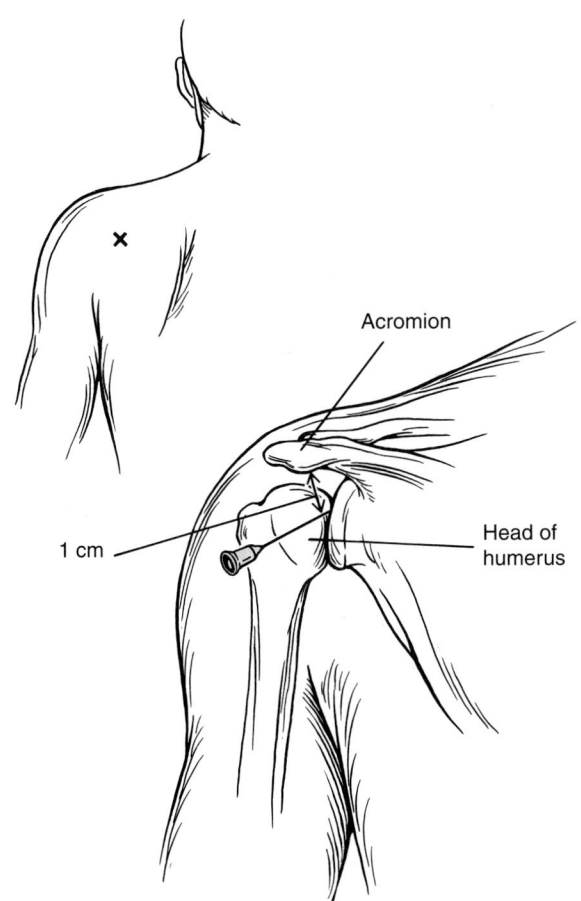

FIG. 286-1. Arthrocentesis of the shoulder, posterior approach.

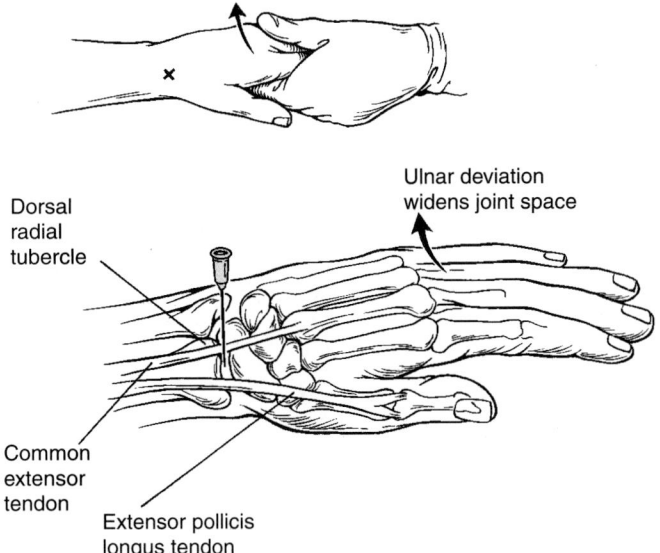

FIG. 286-3. Arthrocentesis of the wrist.

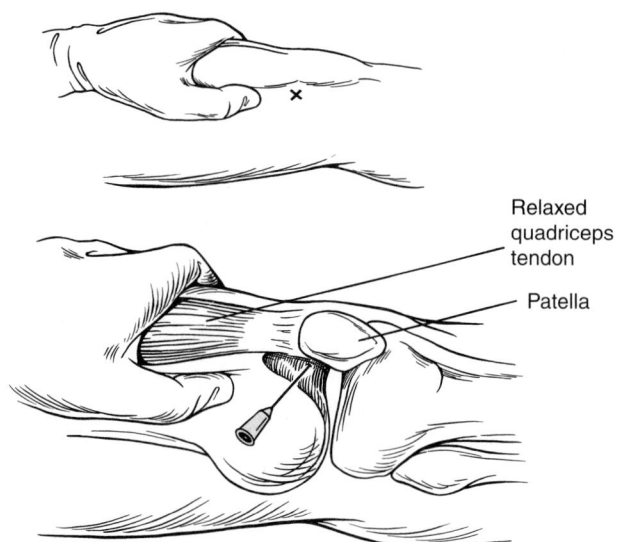

FIG. 286-4. Arthrocentesis of the knee, lateral approach.

space or "milking" of the bursae, on the patellar side opposite the needle insertion site, may facilitate aspiration.

Ankle

Ankle arthrocentesis may be performed at either the subtalar joint (lateral approach) (Figure 286-6) or the tibiotalar joint (medial approach) (Figure 286-7). The subtalar joint is entered just below the tip of the lateral malleolus with the foot perpendicular to the leg. The needle should be directed medially toward the joint space.

The tibiotalar joint is approached with the patient supine and the foot initially perpendicular to the leg. This position facilitates the location of a sulcus lateral to the medial malleolus and medial to the tibialis anterior and extensor hallucis longus tendons (see Figure 286-7). The foot is then plantar flexed with the needle entering the skin over-

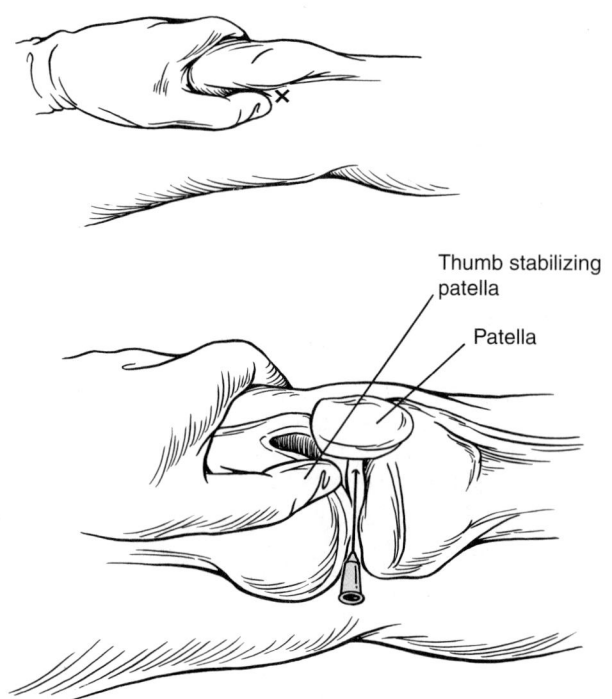

FIG. 286-5. Arthrocentesis of the knee, medial approach.

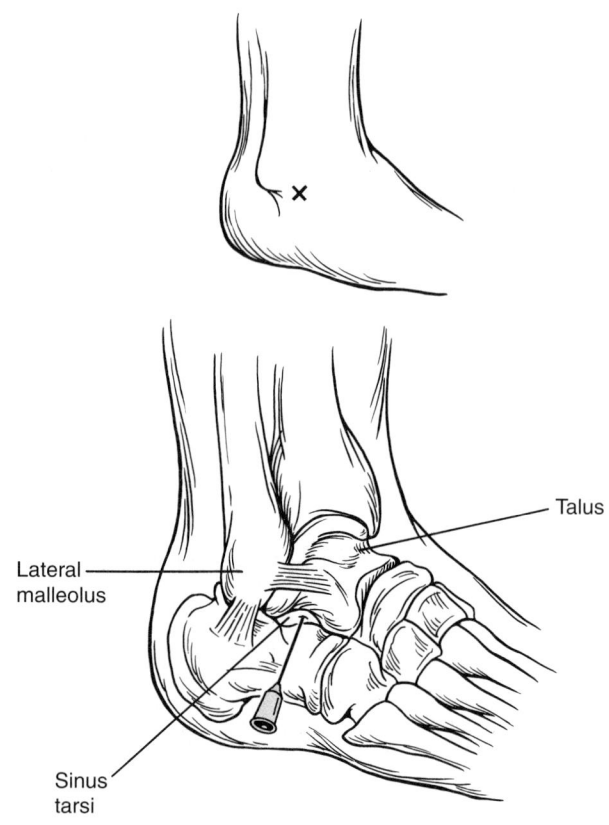

FIG. 286-6. Arthrocentesis of the ankle, lateral approach.

lying the sulcus. The needle should be angled slightly cephalad as it passes between the medial malleolus and the tibialis anterior tendon.

SPECIFIC CONDITIONS

Traumatic Arthritis

Traumatic hemarthrosis has a high association with ligamentous injury or an intra-articular fracture. Effusions following trauma may range from small to large, painful fluid collections that impede range of motion. Aspiration of very large traumatic effusions will provide pain relief and increase range of motion. Treatment of traumatic hemarthrosis consists of immobilization, ice, and elevation of the affected joint. In the absence of a fracture or significantly unstable joint requiring immediate orthopedic evaluation, follow-up is needed for possible ligamentous and articular injuries.

Spontaneous hemarthrosis usually indicates underlying systemic illness and should trigger a search for primary or secondary coagulopathies. Hemophiliacs should receive specific clotting factor replacement (see Chap. 220), and joint aspiration for acute hemarthrosis in hemophilia is controversial, but recommended by some for large bleeds if done during the first 12 h.[15] Follow-up and/or consultation should be provided with hematology and orthopedics.

Nongonococcal Septic Arthritis

Three mechanisms can lead to septic arthritis: (1) hematogenous spread of bacteria, (2) migration of bacteria from a focus contiguous to a joint, and (3) direct inoculation of bacteria into the joint.

Septic arthritis is a medical emergency. A rampant bacterial infection with a normal inflammatory response can destroy a joint within days. The involved joint can become exquisitely painful over a few hours. On examination, effusions may be scant, with significant splinting and resistance to movement.

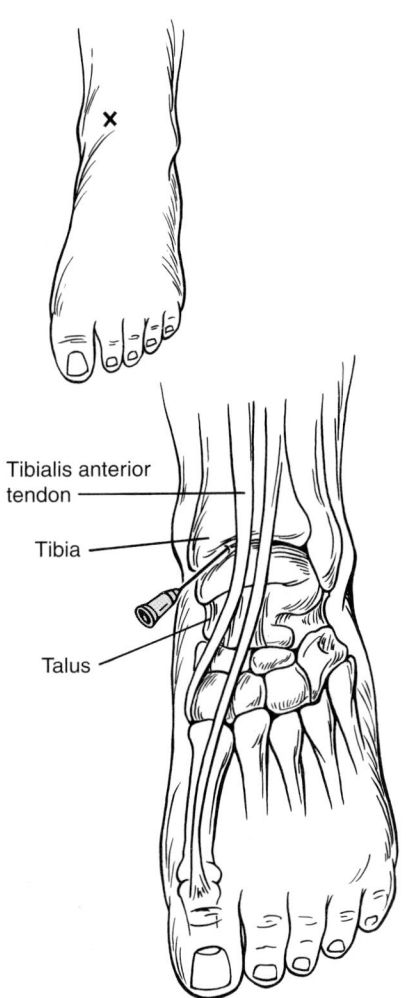

FIG. 286-7. Arthrocentesis of the ankle, medial approach.

Although the classic bacterial arthritis patient is described as febrile with chills and rigors, a 10-year retrospective review of 43 adult patients noted presence of fever or rigors in only 40 and 21 percent of patients, respectively.[9] Thus the absence of constitutional symptoms should not preclude a septic arthritis diagnosis. A suspicion for a bacterial infection should always guide clinical decision making when approaching patients with monarthritis.

After joint aspiration, if septic arthritis cannot be excluded, the patient should be admitted for pain control and parenteral antibiotics until synovial culture results are available. Consultation with orthopedics or infectious disease is desirable. Repeat closed-needle aspiration, arthroscopy, or open surgical drainage may be required, depending on a number of factors, including consultant preference, patient age, affected joint, and likelihood of septic source.

Gonococcal Arthritis

Gonococcal arthritis is the most common cause of septic arthritis in adolescents and young adults.[2] Joint infection will typically have a prodromal phase in which migratory arthritis and tenosynovitis predominate before pain and swelling settle on one or more septic joints. Vesiculopustular lesions, especially on the fingers, may be found.

Synovial fluid cultures are often negative in gonococcal arthritis, with only 25 to 50 percent of cases yielding positive identification of the organism. Cultures of the posterior pharynx, urethra, cervix, and rectum prior to antibiotic treatment may increase the culture yield.[2]

Treatment for gonococcal arthritis follows the same principles as treatment for nongonococcal septic arthritis. *Neisseria gonorrhoeae,*

in the setting of arthritis, remains sensitive to penicillin, and extended antibiotic coverage is typically not required following identification of the organism.

Crystal-Induced Synovitis (Gout and Pseudogout)

Crystal-induced synovitis is primarily an illness of middle-aged and elderly adults. Uric acid (gout) and calcium pyrophosphate (pseudogout) are the two most common crystalline agents, with gout representing the most common form of inflammatory joint disease in men older than age 40.[4] Patients typically present with joint pain that acutely evolves over hours, as in acute gout attack, or over a single day, as in pseudogout. An acute gout or pseudogout attack often follows trauma, surgery, a significant illness, or change in medications that results in an abrupt change in uric acid levels. Crystalline involvement of joints has a predilection for the lower extremities. Although the first metatarsophalangeal joint is a classic focus for acute gout, no joint is the exclusive site of involvement for either crystal.

The diagnosis of a crystal-induced synovitis is by joint aspiration and identification of crystals through a polarizing microscope. Uric acid crystals appear needle-shaped and blue when the source of light is perpendicular to the crystal. Calcium pyrophosphate is yellow in this alignment, with a rhomboid shape. Crystals should be located within phagocytes from aspirates of synovial fluid or inflamed tissues adjacent to the affected joint.

Serum uric acid levels have limited utility in diagnosis, as up to 30 percent of patients will have normal uric acid levels during an acute gout attack.[4] The joint aspirate WBC is often high with gout, approaching $100,000/\mu L$ in some cases.[4] However, the presence of crystals, absence of findings on Gram stain or culture and frequently, the dramatic response to nonsteroidal anti-inflammatory drugs (NSAIDs) will clarify the diagnosis. When the diagnosis of a septic joint cannot be excluded, hospital admission until cultures and/or clinical response clarify the diagnosis is the safest course of action.

When the diagnosis of gout or pseudogout is established, an NSAID, such as indomethacin, is standard first-line therapy. All NSAID dosing should be adjusted for renal function and continue for approximately 1 week. For patients with normal renal function, the initial dose of indomethacin is 50 mg. Therapy is continued three times a day for 3 to 5 days. Substantial pain relief typically occurs within 2 h of NSAID administration.[16] Additional treatment for pseudogout is typically not required.

Colchicine, although not often necessary, may also be employed as an alternative in the treatment of acute gout. Oral colchicine is typically administered at a dose of 0.6 mg/h until intolerable side effects (vomiting or diarrhea) or efficacy ensues. Intravenous administration of colchicine can be associated with serious side effects, with risks such as bone marrow suppression, neuropathy, myopathy, and death. Consequently, intravenous colchicine is limited to a single dose of 1 to 2 mg administered slowly over 1 h in an established intravenous line.[17]

Patient disposition is determined by consideration of effective analgesia and the inclusion or elimination of septic arthritis as a diagnosis in the patient evaluation. Once the symptoms of an acute crystal-induced synovitis episode have resolved, long-term control may be achieved with reduction or elimination of gout-inducing agents (diuretics, aspirin, or cyclosporine) and treatment with prophylactic drugs, such as allopurinol or probenecid.

Lyme Disease

The arthritic manifestations associated with Lyme disease occur in the weeks, months, or years following the primary, stage I infection. Typically, a monarticular or oligoarticular, asymmetric involvement of joints is noted, with brief exacerbations followed by complete remission. Large joints are most often affected.[18] A migratory pattern of oligoarthritis may be noted, in addition to brief attacks of bursitis and tendonitis.

Arthrocentesis yields an inflammatory synovial fluid, usually with negative cultures.[18] The diagnosis of Lyme arthritis is initially suspected in patients residing in, or with a recent visit to, an endemic area. A history of tick bite or erythema chronicum migrans (ECM) rash is helpful but often absent. In patients with no history of rash, tick bite, or endemic location, a constellation of characteristic stage II and stage III findings—such as fatigue, neurologic abnormalities, and/or cardiac conduction disturbances—may be helpful in establishing the diagnosis. Ultimately, definitive diagnosis requires the history or presence of the ECM rash, multi-organ system involvement, or laboratory confirmation through enzyme-linked immunosorbent assay, immunofluorescent antibody titer, or isolation of the *Borrelia burgdorferi* spirochete from a clinical specimen.

Given the difficulty of making a definitive diagnosis in many patients, treatment of suspected Lyme arthritis is often initiated on the grounds of high clinical suspicion. Treatment is administered for 3 to 4 weeks, with a number of antibiotics recognized as effective, including doxycycline, penicillin G, amoxicillin, or ceftriaxone. Intravenous antibiotic therapy is reserved for those patients with more severe presentations.

Rheumatoid Arthritis

Rheumatoid arthritis is distinguished by its symmetric, polyarticular involvement, with noted sparing of the distal interphalangeal (DIP) joints. Patients will describe stiffness of the joints occurring after prolonged periods of inactivity (morning stiffness). Multisystem involvement is characteristic, and depression, fatigue, and generalized myalgias are also common. Extra-articular symptoms and signs include pericarditis, myocarditis, pleural effusion, pneumonitis, and mononeuritis multiplex syndrome.

Articular involvement is noted for symmetric, painful, tender joints. A "boggy," slightly edematous synovium may be palpated. Sparing of the DIP joints is the rule, with an additive involvement of affected joints during the course of the illness. Arthrocentesis of synovial fluid is typically noted for an inflammatory profile.

Treatment during an acute exacerbation is directed at reducing pain and inflammation. Salicylates or other NSAIDs are the cornerstone of treatment, with immobilization providing added relief from joint movement pain. Corticosteroids may be utilized for brief periods, with long-term therapy using agents such as antimalarials, gold, and methotrexate.

Osteoarthritis

Osteoarthritis is distinguished from rheumatoid arthritis by a lack of constitutional symptoms and/or multisystem involvement. Destruction of joints in osteoarthritis may involve the DIP joints, with less dramatic symmetric, polyarticular exacerbations. Although osteoarthritis is a chronic, polyarticular disease, patients may present with an acute monoarthritis exacerbation, typically of the knee. Effusions are small and difficult to aspirate. If fluid is aspirated, it is noninflammatory.

Radiographs contribute to the diagnosis of osteoarthritis, demonstrating characteristic joint space narrowing due to destruction of articular cartilage. Treatment, as in rheumatoid arthritis, involves rest of affected joints and the use of salicylates or NSAIDs. Because of the noninflammatory and destructive nature of osteoarthritis, corticosteroids are not used in the disease. Disease progression often necessitates total joint replacement.

Reiter Syndrome

Reiter syndrome, or reactive arthritis, is a seronegative spondyloarthropathy characterized by an acute, asymmetric oligoarthritis preceded 2 to 6 weeks earlier by an infectious illness. **The classic triad of Reiter syndrome is arthritis, urethritis, and conjunctivitis. A history of all three components is not necessary for diagnosis.** *Chlamydia* or *Ureaplasma* are common inciting agents, particularly with regard

to a precipitating urethritis. Diarrhea has also become recognized as an entity that may precipitate a reactive arthritis. A history of recent diarrhea or enteric infection while traveling abroad may suggest a recent *Salmonella* or *Shigella* infection as an inciting factor for the disease.[3]

Joint involvement is typically found in the lower extremities, particularly the heels of the feet. A diffuse swelling of an entire digit (sausage digit) may be found as well, but is not specific to Reiter syndrome alone.[1] Synovial fluid aspirates demonstrate an inflammatory profile. Treatment is supportive with emphasis on pain control and NSAID therapy. Antibiotics have not been found to be useful.

Ankylosing Spondylitis

Another of the seronegative spondyloarthropathies—ankylosing spondylitis—demonstrates an arthritic predilection for the spine and pelvis. Ankylosing spondylitis is similar to rheumatoid arthritis in its association with morning stiffness and multisystem involvement with constitutional symptoms such as malaise, weakness, and fatigue. However, ankylosing spondylitis is clearly differentiated in its association with hereditary factors, particularly the HLA-B27 antigen and negative rheumatoid factor.

Ankylosing spondylitis is suspected in individuals younger than age 40 who note insidious onset of symptoms that improve with exercise, are associated with morning stiffness, and last longer than 3 months. Radiographic findings, in addition to genetic predisposition, are helpful in the diagnosis of ankylosing spondylitis. Squaring of the vertebral bodies (bamboo spine) and sacroiliitis are some of the more classic findings. Treatment consists of pain control with short-term and long-term management with NSAIDs.

BURSITIS

The term *bursitis* refers to any acute or chronic inflammatory process involving one of the more than 150 bursae identified throughout the human body.[19] Bursitis is classified by etiology, body location, and presence of infection. Etiologic entities include trauma, crystal-induced, rheumatoid, and idiopathic forms. Presence of infection is noted by classification as septic or nonseptic. *Staphylococcus aureus* accounts for the majority of identified infectious agents, but *Staphylococcus epidermidis* and *Streptococcus* species are also encountered.

Bursitis is a relatively common condition, due to the number of bursae and the minimal trauma required to initiate a clinically evident process. The affected site is determined by the activity precipitating the event and/or the relatively superficial location of many bursae. Certain entities are frequently associated with occupations or activities that precipitate their occurrence: "carpet layer's knee" (prepatellar bursitis) or "student's elbow" (olecranon bursitis).

General principles of management include restraint from further trauma/injury, elevation, and a compressive dressing. Drug therapy with NSAIDs is the primary pharmacotherapeutic intervention. Injection of the affected bursa with steroids is controversial and should be avoided when septic bursitis cannot be excluded.

Septic bursitis generally responds well to oral antibiotics, with emphasis on coverage of *Staphylococcus* and *Streptococcus* species. Selected patients will require more aggressive interventions, including admission to hospital, administration of parenteral antibiotics, incision and debridement, and open irrigation. These patients typically have more advanced, purulent infection within the bursa, extensive spread of infection/cellulitis to surrounding soft tissues, suspected joint involvement, or failure to respond to oral antibiotics and outpatient interventions.

Specific Conditions

OLECRANON BURSITIS   The olecranon bursa overlies the olecranon process on the extensor surface of the elbow. Patients with olecranon bursitis present with a tense, edematous bursa that is often tender to palpation. Pain elicited with range of motion at the elbow is minor until the motion tightens and compresses the distended overlying bursa. The bursa is frequently erythematous and warm.

Distinguishing nonseptic bursitis from the septic and crystal-induced forms is a clinical challenge. Patients with crystal-induced bursitis will often demonstrate gouty tophi overlying the elbow extensor surface. Presence of crystals in bursal fluid analysis is diagnostic.

Septic bursitis and nonseptic bursitis are difficult to distinguish. No definitive conclusion can be reached solely on the basis of physical examination findings or history, although one report has noted the utility of surface temperature comparison of the affected bursa with the unaffected side.[19] These authors reported a temperature difference exceeding 2.1°C to be highly predictive of a septic bursal fluid aspirate.

Most authors advocate the importance of aspirating bursal fluid,[19–22] which is performed both for diagnostic and therapeutic purposes. Bursal fluid, like joint aspirates, demonstrates characteristic findings (Table 286-5). The utility of any one finding is limited, however, and the culture represents the definitive test for presence or absence of infection.

Aspiration of olecranon bursitis fluid is undertaken by means of a lateral approach to the affected bursa. As in joint aspirates, a sterile technique should be utilized, with evacuation of as much fluid as possible.

Management of patients with olecranon bursitis follows the aforementioned general bursitis management principles. When a septic bursitis is definitively excluded, a steroid injected into the bursa may expedite resolution of inflammation.[22] However, a septic process usually cannot be excluded during the initial evaluation of an acute olecranon bursitis. As a consequence, utilization of steroid injection should be approached with caution.

Antibiotic treatment is usually effective with a 14-day course of oral antibiotic therapy.[19,21] Selected patients who may require parenteral therapy or operative management are generally distinguished by their toxic appearance, systemic signs of infection, extensive cellulitis to surrounding tissues, failure of outpatient interventions, or immunocompromised host status.

PREPATELLAR BURSITIS   Prepatellar bursitis may affect any of the four bursae surrounding the extensor aspect of the knee. As in other bursitis conditions, a history of overuse or trauma to the prepatellar area is often elicited.[19] Clinical findings are consistent with those of olecranon bursitis.

TABLE 286-5   Characteristics of Bursal Fluid in Patients with Septic and Nonseptic Olecranon and Prepatellar Bursitis

	Septic	Traumatic and Idiopathic	Crystal Induced
Appearance	Purulent; may be straw colored or serosanguineous	Straw colored, serosanguineous, or bloody	Straw colored to bloody
Leukocytes/μL	1500–300,000; mean 75,000	50–11,000; mean 1100	1000–6000; mean 2900
Differential count	Predominantly PMNs	Predominantly mononuclear	Highly variable
Ratio bursal fluid to serum glucose	<50%	>50%	Unknown
Gram stain	Positive in 70%	Negative	Negative
Crystals present	No	No	Yes
Culture results	Positive	Negative	Negative

Source: From McAfee and Smith,[19] with permission.

Aspiration of prepatellar bursal fluid should be accomplished using either a medial or lateral approach to the affected bursa. Treatment emphasizes conservative management and occasionally requires antibiotic therapy or admission following the same approach as outlined for patients with septic olecranon bursitis.

REFERENCES

1. Barth WF: Office evaluation of the patient with musculoskeletal complaints. *Am J Med* 102(Suppl 1A):3S, 1997.
2. Shaw BA, Kasser JR: Acute septic arthritis in infancy and childhood. *Clin Orthop* 257:212, 1990.
3. Pinals RS: Polyarthritis and fever. *New Engl J Med* 330:769, 1994.
4. Joseph J, McGrath H: Gout or "pseudogout": How to differentiate crystal-induced arthropathies. *Geriatrics* 50:33, 1995.
5. Harris ED Jr: Rheumatoid arthritis. Pathophysiology and implications for therapy. *New Engl J Med* 322:1277, 1990.
6. Schmerling RH, Delbanco TL, Tosteson ANA, et al: Synovial fluid tests: What should be ordered? *JAMA* 264:1009, 1990.
7. Malleson PN: Management of childhood arthritis: Part 1. Acute arthritis. *Arch Dis Child* 76:460, 1997.
8. Del Beccaro MA, Champoux AN, Bockers T, et al: Septic arthritis versus transient synovitis of the hip: The value of screening laboratory tests. *Ann Emerg Med* 21:1418, 1992.
9. Schlapbach P: Bacterial arthritis: Are fever, rigors, leucocytosis and blood cultures of diagnostic value? *Clin Rheumatol* 9:69, 1990.
10. Wilson NIL, DiPaola M: Acute septic arthritis in infancy and childhood. *J Bone Joint Surg [Br]* 68:584, 1986.
11. Roy S, Dewitz A, Paul I: Ultrasound-assisted ankle arthrocentesis. *Am J Emerg Med* 17:300, 1999.
12. Smith SW: Emergency physician-performed ultrasonography-guided hip arthrocentesis. *Acad Emerg Med* 6:84, 1999.
13. Fink AM, Berman L, Edwards D, et al: Immediate ultrasound guided aspiration and prevention of hospital admission. *Arch Dis Child* 72:110, 1995.
14. Alexander JE, Seibert JJ, Aronson J, et al: A protocol of plain radiographs, hip ultrasound, and triple phase bone scans in the evaluation of the painful pediatric hip. *Clin Pediatr (Phila)* 27:175, 1988.
15. Rodriguez-Merchan EC: Articular bleeding (hemarthrosis) in hemophilia, an orthopaedist's point of view, www.wfh.org, World Federation of Hemophilia) accessed July, 2003.
16. Shrestha M, Morgan DL, Moreden JM, et al: Randomized double-blind comparison of the analgesic efficacy of intramuscular ketorolac and oral indomethacin in the treatment of acute gouty arthritis. *Ann Emerg Med* 26:682, 1995.
17. Emmerson, BT: The management of gout. *New Engl J Med* 334:445, 1996.
18. Gerber MA, Zemel LS, Shapiro ED: Lyme arthritis in children: Clinical epidemiology and long-term outcomes. *Pediatrics* 102:905, 1998.
19. McAfee JH, Smith DL: Olecranon and prepatellar bursitis: Diagnosis and treatment. *West J Med* 149:607, 1988.
20. Smith DL, McAfee JH, Lucas LM, et al: Septic and nonseptic olecranon bursitis: Utility of the surface temperature probe in the early differentiation of septic and nonseptic cases. *Arch Intern Med* 149:1581, 1989.
21. Ho G, Tice AD, Kaplan SR: Septic bursitis in the prepatellar and olecranon bursae: An analysis of 25 cases. *Ann Intern Med* 89:21, 1978.
22. Smith DL, McAfee JH, Lucas LM, et al: Treatment of nonseptic olecranon bursitis: A controlled, blinded prospective trial. *Arch Intern Med* 149:2527, 1989.

SOFT TISSUE PROBLEMS OF THE FOOT
Frantz R. Melio

Foot problems are common human afflictions. This chapter discusses the common foot disorders that are likely to present to the ED. Patients with chronic or complicated foot problems generally should be referred to a dermatologist, orthopedist, general surgeon, or podiatrist, depending on disease and local resources.

CORNS AND CALLUSES

Pressure or irritation causes focal hyperkeratotic lesions of the skin of the foot. The cause of these lesions can be external (poorly fitted shoe) or internal (bunion). These areas of epidermal accumulation are called *calluses*. Calluses serve a protective function and should not be treated if they are not painful. Calluses grow outward but are soon pushed inward by continued pressure and become corns. Corns also develop in areas of scarring and between toes. Corns are classified as hard or soft. Hard corns are seen over bony protuberances where the skin is dry. Soft corns are seen between toes where the skin is moist. Corns may be painful or painless, but pressure on the corn usually produces pain. Corns interrupt the normal dermal lines and can thus be differentiated from calluses. Hard corns may resemble warts; however, when pared, warts bleed and corns do not. Soft corns resemble tinea, which often leads to misdiagnosis and mistreatment.[1,2]

Treatment of symptomatic lesions consists of paring with a no. 15 blade scalpel and application of a pad on or around the lesion to relieve pressure. Avoiding constrictive footwear is also important. The use of keratolytic agents is controversial. Patients should be referred to a podiatrist, since therapy includes repeated paring and possibly surgery to correct any underlying source of pressure.[1,2]

Keratotic lesions may be an indication of more severe underlying disease, deformity, local foot disorder, or mechanical problem. Other causes of keratotic lesions include syphilis, psoriasis, arsenic poisoning, rosacea, lichen planus, basal cell nevus syndrome, and rarely, malignancies.[2]

PLANTAR WARTS

Plantar warts are caused by the human papillomavirus. These warts are fairly common and contagious. They may be painful and are usually found over bony prominences. Single lesions are endophytic and hyperkeratotic. A mother-daughter wart is similar to a single lesion except for a small vesicular satellite lesion. Mosaic warts are often painless, closely grouped, and may coalesce. Diagnosis is usually made clinically. There are many therapeutic options. Treatment is complicated by the fact that many of these lesions will resorb spontaneously within 2 years. Plantar warts may require prolonged treatment so referral to a dermatologist or podiatrist is best.[1–3]

TINEA PEDIS AND ONYCHOMYCOSIS

Tinea pedis and onychomycosis are discussed in Chap. 248, "Disorders of the Hands, Feet, and Extremities."

ONYCHOCRYPTOSIS (INGROWN TOENAIL)

Ingrown toenails occur when a segment of the nail plate penetrates the nail sulcus and subcutaneous tissue. Curvature of the nail plate is the most common predisposing factor. The lesion usually occurs as a result of external trauma or self-treatment. Onychocryptosis is characterized by inflammation, swelling, and infection of the medial or lateral aspect of the toenail. The great toe is the most commonly affected. Protracted infection may result in periungual ulcerative granulation. In patients with underlying diabetes or arterial insufficiency, cellulitis, ulceration, and necrosis may lead to amputation if treatment is delayed. If infection is not present at the time of presentation, simple elevation of the nail with placement of a wisp of cotton between the nail plate and the skin, daily foot soaks, and avoidance of pressure on the nail is usually sufficient treatment. Another option, if no infection is present, is to remove a small spicule of the offending nail. A digital block is placed (see Chap. 37). The area is cleaned, and the skin is prepared for surgical procedure. An oblique portion of the affected nail is trimmed about one- to two-thirds of the way back to the posterior nail fold. The nail groove should then be debrided, and a nonadherent dressing placed[2,4] (Figure 287-1).

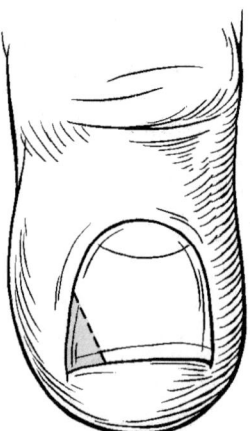

FIG. 287-1. Partial toenail removal.

If granulation or infection is present, then partial removal of the nail plate is indicated. This is performed by first placing a digital block, and preparing the area for a surgical procedure. The entire affected area, one-quarter or less of the nail plate, is cut longitudinally (base to tip), including the portion of the nail beneath the cuticle. English anvil scissors or a nail splitter are the optimal instruments for cutting the nail. The affected cut portion of the nail is then grasped with a hemostat and, using a rocking motion, removed from the nail groove. The nail groove is then debrided[4] (Figure 287-2). Once the procedure is completed, a nonadherent gauze or antibiotic ointment should be placed on the wound. A bulky dressing should then be placed on the toe. The wound should be checked in 24 to 48 h.[4]

OTHER NAIL LESIONS

Other common toenail afflictions include paronychia and subungual hematoma, which are treated similarly to when they occur in the fingers. Hyperkeratotic toenails can be a problem in the elderly. These may become so severe as to affect gait and cause ulcerations and infections. Patients with these lesions require referral for repeated trimming or nail plate removal.[2]

BURSITIS

There are many bursae in the foot, all of which may become a source of pain. Pathologic bursae can be divided into noninflammatory, inflam-

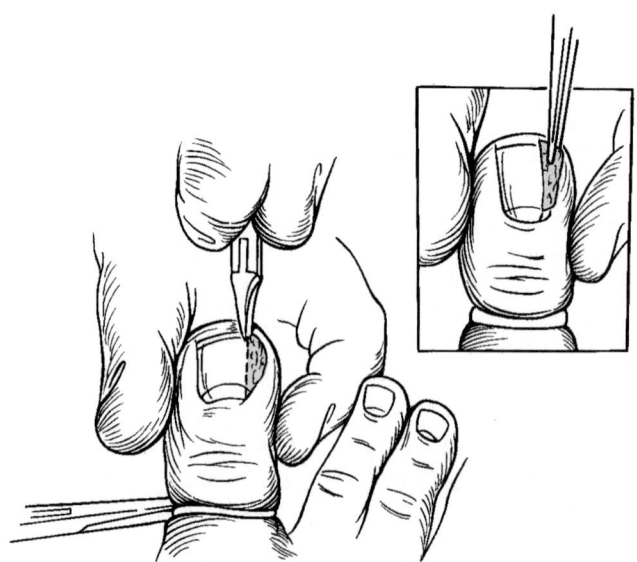

FIG. 287-2. Partial toenail removal (infection present).

matory, suppurative, and calcified. Noninflammatory bursae are usually pressure-induced and are found over bony prominences. Inflammatory bursae are commonly due to gout, or rheumatoid arthritis. Suppurative bursitis is due to the invasion of the bursae, usually from adjacent wounds, by pyogenic organisms (primarily staphylococcal species). Acute bursitis can lead to the formation of a hygroma or calcified bursae. In severe cases, pressure on bursae can lead to fistula and ulcer formation. Diagnosis of these lesions is dependent on analysis of bursal fluid, which can be obtained by large-bore needle aspiration. Fluid should be sent for cell count; protein, glucose, and lactate (elevated in septic bursitis) levels; crystal analysis; and Gram stain as well as culture (since initial Gram stains are often negative). Treatment of the bursitis depends on its cause. In all cases one should avoid further pressure to the area by instructing the patients to avoid putting weight on the affected foot. Septic bursitis should be initially treated with a penicillinase-resistant semisynthetic penicillin while awaiting culture results. Repeated aspiration or incision and drainage may become necessary.[5]

PLANTAR FASCIITIS

Plantar fasciitis is an inflammation of the plantar aponeurosis. The plantar fascia's main function is to anchor the plantar skin to the bone, thus protecting the longitudinal arch of the foot. The cause of plantar fasciitis is usually overuse in the physically active patient or in the patient unaccustomed to activity. Other causes include abnormal joint mechanics, tightness of the Achilles tendon, shoes with poor cushioning, abnormal foot position and anatomy, and obesity. In the younger patient, autoimmune and rheumatic diseases can lead to this entity. Patients present with pain on the plantar surface of the foot that is worse on arising and after physical activity. Examination usually reveals a point of deep tenderness at the anterior medial aspect of the calcaneus, the point of attachment of the plantar fascia. Ultrasound and magnetic resonance imaging (MRI) may aid in diagnosis. Plantar fasciitis is generally a self-limited disease. Short-term treatment consists of rest, ice, nonsteroidal anti-inflammatory drugs (NSAIDs), heel and arch support shoe inserts, and dorsiflexion night splints (molded ankle-foot orthosis that holds the plantar fascia and Achilles tendon stretched). Patients should be taught Achilles tendon stretching exercises and be told to avoid walking barefoot on hard surfaces. In severe cases, a short-leg walking cast may be applied to unload and rest the plantar fascia. Glucocorticoid injections are associated with plantar fascia rupture, and are usually best left to the orthopedist.[1,6] Patients should be referred to a podiatrist, orthopedist, or primary care physician for follow-up care.[1,6]

TARSAL TUNNEL SYNDROME

Tarsal tunnel syndrome is a compression neuropathy of the posterior tibial nerve that causes foot and heel pain. After coursing inferiorly to the medial malleolus, the posterior tibial nerve enters the tarsal tunnel. The plantar aspect of the tarsal tunnel is bound by the talus and calcaneus bones, and by the tibialis posterior, flexor hallucis longus, and flexor digitorum longus. The dorsal aspect is bound by the inelastic flexor retinaculum, which extends from the medial malleolus to the calcaneus to the abductor hallucis muscle.

Nerve compression may be intrinsic or extrinsic. In the setting of overuse, running and activities requiring restrictive footwear (e.g., ski boots, skates) have been implicated. The edema of pregnancy, post-traumatic fibrosis, ganglion cysts, osteophytes, and tumors may also be a precipitant. Hyperpronation (inward rotation) while running makes the nerve more vulnerable both to direct trauma from stretch and to indirect trauma from inflammation of the surrounding structures resulting in compression.[7]

Pain or dysesthesia is noted at the medial malleolus, the heel (calcaneal branch), and sole (medial or lateral plantar branch), depending on the site and severity of compression. Distal calf pain may result due to retrograde radiation (Valleix phenomenon). Similar to carpal tunnel syndrome, the pain is often worse at night. More advanced disease may result in weak toe flexion. Tinel sign is positive inferior to the medial malleolus. Simultaneous dorsiflexion and eversion of the ankle exacerbates symptoms. Diagnosis is aided by nerve conduction studies or MRI.

The differential diagnosis includes plantar fasciitis and, if limited to the heel, Achilles tendinitis. Plantar fasciitis will cause point tenderness over the plantar heel and worse pain upon morning standing. Tarsal tunnel syndrome causes greater medial heel and arch pain, due to involvement of the abductor hallucis muscle. Tarsal tunnel pain worsens with ambulation throughout the day. In addition, tarsal tunnel syndrome may produce distal calf pain, whereas fasciitis does not.

Initial treatment includes avoidance of the exacerbating activities and use of NSAIDs. If there is no improvement or symptoms recur after a few weeks, then orthopedic evaluation and treatment, which includes electromyographic studies, steroid injection, orthotic devices, or surgery, are recommended.[7]

GANGLIONS

A ganglion is a common benign synovial cyst. Ganglions are often clinically asymptomatic. Ganglions are 1.5 to 2.5 cm in diameter and are often attached to a joint capsule or tendon sheath. Although ganglions typically occur in the wrist or hand, they may also occur in the foot. These lesions typically arise in the anterolateral aspect of the ankle, but can occur in many areas of the foot. The pathogenesis of these lesions is unknown. The two most popular theories are (1) that they are produced by herniation of the tendon sheath, and (2) that they arise from focal myxomatous degeneration of collagenous tissues caused by trauma. Ganglions may appear suddenly or gradually, may enlarge and diminish in size, and may be painful or asymptomatic. On examination one notes a firm, usually nontender, cystic lesion. Diagnosis is usually made clinically, although ultrasound and MRI are useful if there is any question of the diagnosis. Aspiration and instillation of glucocorticoids by an orthopedist leads to the complete resolution of ganglions in some cases, with surgical excision required for persistence.[8]

TENDON LESIONS

Tendon lesions usually require referral and/or consultation with a podiatrist or orthopedist to aid in treatment decisions (Figures 287-3 and 287-4). Tenosynovitis and tendinitis may occur in the foot, usually due to overuse. Patients present with pain over the involved tendon. The flexor hallucis longus, posterior tibialis, and Achilles tendon are most commonly involved. Treatment consists of rest, ice, and oral NSAIDs.[9]

Tendon lacerations are usually traumatic. The usual mechanism of injury is a cut to the dorsal or plantar aspect of the foot. Tendon lacerations should be explored and repaired if the ends of the tendon are visible in the wound. The foot should be casted in dorsiflexion after the repair of extensor tendons, and in equinus after repair of flexor tendons. Unfortunately, tendon repairs in the foot have a relatively high complication and disability rate. Specialty consultation is appropriate.[9]

Spontaneous rupture of the Achilles, tibialis anterior, and posterior tibialis tendons is fairly common. Diagnosis and proper treatment of tendon ruptures is aided by ultrasound or MRI studies. Orthopedic consultation should be obtained to aid in proper therapeutic decisions. Achilles tendon ruptures are usually due to forceful dorsiflexion and occur more commonly in males. Patients present with pain, a palpable defect in the area of the tendon, and inability to stand on tiptoes. Squeezing the calf of the prone patient whose knee is flexed at 90° will normally cause the foot to plantar flex (Thompson test). This response will be absent in patients with Achilles tendon ruptures. Treatment is generally surgical in younger patients and conservative (casting in equinus) in older patients.[9]

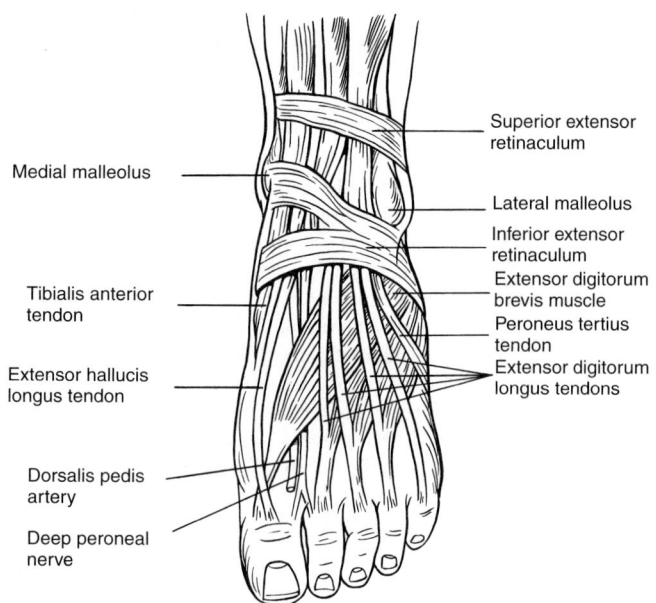

FIG. 287-3. Tendons of the foot, anterior view.

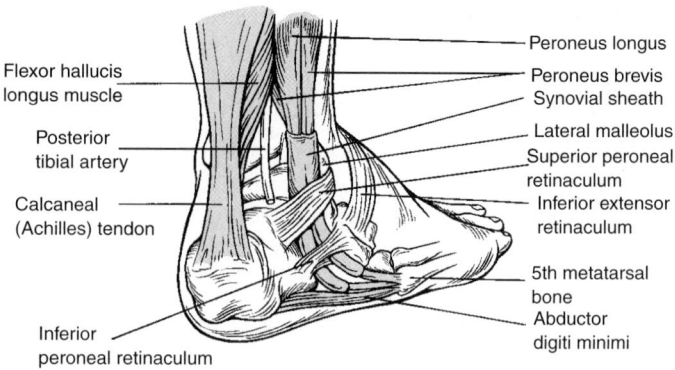

A Lateral

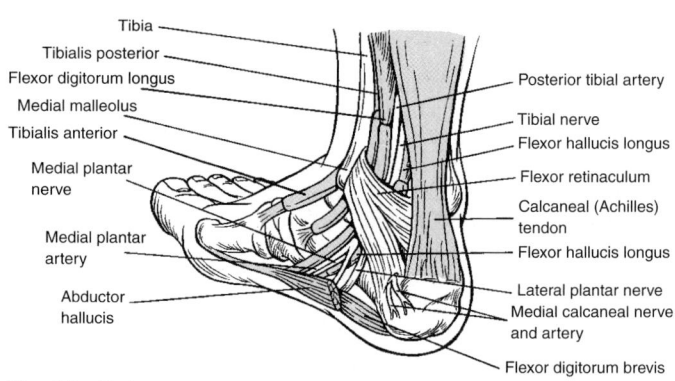

B Medial

FIG. 287-4. Tendons of the foot, posterior view.

Ruptures of the anterior tibialis tendon are rare. These usually occur after the fourth decade and are not excessively painful. Patients present with varying degrees of foot drop and a palpable defect distal to the ankle joint in the area of the tendon. In most cases, disability is minimal and surgery is not necessary.[9]

Spontaneous ruptures of the posterior tibialis tendon also occur after the fourth decade. Two-thirds of these cases occur in women. The presentation is usually chronic and insidious. Patients notice a gradual flattening of their arch, with modest discomfort and swelling over the medial ankle. Examination reveals absence of the tendon's normal prominence and weakness on inversion of the foot. Patients find it impossible to stand on tiptoes. Treatment may be conservative or surgical, depending on the duration of the tear and activity of the patient.[9]

Flexor hallucis longus tenosynovitis classically affects ballet dancers, but can also be seen in runners and nonathletes. Presentation is similar to plantar fasciitis and tarsal tunnel syndrome. Posteromedial ankle pain, medial arch pain, and a positive Tinel sign are seen. Management is often surgical. Flexor hallucis longus rupture presents as a loss of plantar flexion of the great toe. This lesion must be repaired in ballet dancers but not in the nonathlete.[9]

Disruption of the peroneal retinaculum can occur as a result of direct trauma during dorsiflexion of the foot. Besides pain localized to the peroneal tendon behind the lateral malleolus, the patient complains of a clicking when walking as the tendon subluxes. Peroneal tendon injuries may lead to lateral ankle instability. Treatment is generally surgical repair.[9]

PLANTAR INTERDIGITAL NEUROMA (MORTON NEUROMA)

Neuromas may form in a plantar digital nerve, usually proximal to its bifurcation. These neuromas may occur in any of the digital nerves but are most common in the third interspace. The cause of these lesions is thought to be local irritation of the nerve due to entrapment, usually from tight-fitting shoes. Women between the ages of 25 and 50 years are the most commonly affected group. Patients present with pain located in the area of the metatarsal head. The pain is described as burning, cramping, or aching. Pain is worsened by ambulation and resolved by rest and removal of shoes. The pain may radiate to the affected toes, and patients may note numbness in the toes. Pain is usually easily reproduced upon palpation of the area, and at times a mass is felt. Diagnosis is usually made clinically, but nerve conduction studies, electromyograms, ultrasounds, and MRI may be helpful at times. Conservative treatment consists of wearing wide shoes with good metatarsal head supports and metatarsal head off-loading inserts. Local glucocorticoid injections can sometimes be curative. Conservative therapy is often unsuccessful, and patients may ultimately require neurolysis or surgical intervention.[10]

COMPARTMENT SYNDROME

Compartment syndromes have been more commonly described to affect the arms and legs (see Chap. 278 for further discussion). Nine compartments have been identified in the foot. Compartment syndrome occurs when an elevation of tissue pressure within one of these nonyielding fascial compartments impedes vascular flow. In the foot, the cause of compartment syndrome is usually a high-energy injury associated with multiple fractures. Crush injuries are more likely to cause compartment syndrome than are penetrating injuries. Compartment syndromes have been reported in association with foot and ankle fractures, burns, contusions, bleeding disorders, postischemic swelling after arterial injury or thrombosis, venous obstruction, exercise, and prolonged pressure to the affected area. There have also been reports of chronic compartment syndromes due to overuse. Patients typically present with severe acute pain that is worsened on active or passive movement, swelling, paresthesias, and neurovascular deficits. The only reliable method to diagnose compartment syndrome is by obtaining intracompartmental pressures. Once the diagnosis is made, fasciotomy should be performed emergently. The sequelae of compartment syndrome range from transient neurologic compromise to complete myoneural necrosis, fibrosis, and ischemic contractures. The prognosis of compartment syndrome is directly related to the time delay in diagnosis and treatment.[11]

PLANTAR FIBROMATOSIS

Plantar fibromatosis, or Dupuytren contracture of the plantar fascia, does not occur as commonly as in the hand. Plantar fibromatosis is a disorder of fibrous tissue proliferation, which slowly invades the skin and soft tissues. Presentation is generally in adolescence or young adulthood. Patients present with small (0.5 to 1.0 cm), asymptomatic, palpable, slowly enlarging, fixed, firm masses on the plantar aspect of one or both feet. These lesions tend to be in the non-weight-bearing areas of the foot. Toe contractures do not occur. Lesions have a tendency to reabsorb spontaneously. Diagnosis is aided by the use of MRI. Treatment is conservative, and only rarely is surgery indicated. Patients should be referred to the appropriate consultant for continued care.[12]

FOOT ULCERS

Foot ulcers can generally be classified as neuropathic or ischemic by the predominant etiologic factor and clinical features. Infection can be a complicating factor in either type of ulcer. Diabetics are prone to both types of ulcers and in addition are more apt to develop infections. It has been estimated that proper foot care in diabetics (including prophylaxis and treatment of foot ulcers) could reduce the number of lower limb amputations by 44 to 80 percent.[13]

Venous stasis ulcers of the lower extremity are discussed in Chap. 247. The following sections discuss ischemic and neuropathic ulcers of the feet.

Ischemic ulcers are secondary to vascular compromise, usually due to atherosclerosis of larger vessels. Ulcers rarely develop due to problems with the microcirculation. These ulcers are seen in the setting of a cool foot, dependent rubor, pallor on elevation, atrophic shiny skin, and diminished pulses. Patients may complain of symptoms of intermittent claudication and leg or foot pain in the supine position, relieved by dependency. If the underlying vascular disease is corrected, these ulcers usually heal quickly. Without reconstructive surgery, the prognosis is poor and amputation is often inevitable.[13,14]

Neuropathic ulcers are essentially pressure ulcers. Patients at risk are those with absent or distorted foot sensation. These include patients with diabetes, leprosy, tabes dorsalis, and other congenital or acquired neuropathies. Their feet are prone to ischemia from pressure by ill-fitting shoes, foreign bodies, abnormal bony prominences, and most commonly from the daily stresses of walking. The ulcers are usually well circumscribed with surrounding white callus-like material. The foot (if there is no underlying vascular disease) has normal temperature, color, and pulses. Defects in touch, pressure, or proprioception are noted on examination. Motor weakness and muscular atrophy may also be present. These changes can lead to abnormal gait and foot anatomy. Autonomic neuropathy leads to dry, cracked and callus skin from decreased perspiration. Disruption of the protective skin barrier may lead to infection.[13,14]

Once an ulcer becomes infected, two aspects of therapy are essential for healing: thorough debridement and complete pressure relief. Debridement must be aggressive; wet-to-dry dressing changes are not sufficient. Once debridement is completed, the role of wet-to-dry dressing is controversial. These dressings may promote drying of the ulcer and eschar formation. Foot soaks have not been shown to be of benefit. Relief of pressure is accomplished by either complete bed rest or by total contact casting.[13–15]

Antibiotics and often admission are warranted for the treatment of infected ulcers. Infections can be categorized as non-limb-threatening, limb-threatening, and life-threatening. Non-life-threatening infections can usually be treated in an outpatient setting. These infections are superficial infections with purulent drainage and minimal (less than 2 cm extension from the portal of entry) or absent cellulitis. There are no signs of systemic toxicity. Limb- or life-threatening infections require hospitalization. Limb-threatening infections involve ulceration into the deep tissues, extensive purulent drainage, advanced cellulitis, lymphangitis, and systemic toxicity. Significant ischemia and gangrene may be present. Life-threatening infections have the same findings as limb-threatening infections, but in addition are accompanied by septic shock, bacteremia, osteomyelitis, or marked gangrene and necrosis.

Infections are usually polymicrobial. The most common organisms of non-limb-threatening infections are *Staphylococcus aureus* and group A and B streptococci. Limb-threatening and life-threatening infections are often due to *S. aureus*, *Streptococci*, *Enterococcus*, Gram-negative bacilli (including *Proteus* spp., *Klebsiella* spp., *E. coli*, and *Pseudomonas* spp.), and anaerobic organisms (particularly *Bacteroides* and *Peptostreptococci*). Superficial cultures of infected ulcers are unreliable. Cultures should be obtained of any purulent drainage and of aspirates from fluctuant areas. Antibiotics should initially be broad-spectrum to cover the wide variety of possible infective organisms. Choices depend on the severity of infection (Table 287-1). Abscesses should be incised and drained. X-rays should be considered if there is any suspicion of subcutaneous gas, foreign body, osteomyelitis, and Charcot foot. MRI and bone scan may be indicated to determine the presence of osteomyelitis. Palpation of bone in the depths of infected pedal ulcers has been shown to strongly correlate with osteomyelitis.

With diabetics, a serum glucose level should be obtained, as it is often elevated. Patients with nonhealing foot ulcers should be referred for evaluation and treatment. The underlying etiology of the ulcers include vascular, diabetic, or other systemic disease, including malignancies. Recent advances in the treatment of foot ulcers include recombinant human growth factor (becaplermin gel), granulocyte colony-stimulating factor, platelet releasate, and human skin equivalents. Hyperbaric oxygen has been advocated by some as beneficial in the treatment of both infected and noninfected foot ulcers.[13–16]

MALIGNANT MELANOMA

The incidence of malignant melanoma is increasing, thus making consideration of this disease process important. Malignant melanoma of the foot accounts for up to 15 percent of all cutaneous melanomas. Melanomas can present as an atypical, pigmented, or nonhealing lesion of the foot, including the nail. These malignancies often imitate more common foot disorders such as fungal infections and plantar warts. Since prognosis is directly related to early diagnosis, a high index of suspicion must be maintained. Acral lentiginous melanoma is

TABLE 287-1 Selected Empirical Antimicrobial Regimens for Foot Infections in Patients with Diabetes Mellitus*

Non-limb-threatening infection: Oral regimen
  Cephalexin or other first-generation cephalosporin
  Clindamycin
  Dicloxacillin
  Amoxicillin-clavulanate
  Extended-spectrum fluoroquinolone (e.g., levofloxacin)
Limb-threatening infection: Parenteral regimen
  Ampicillin-sulbactam
  Ticarcillin-clavulanate
  Piperacillin-tazobactam
  Cefoxitin or cefotetan
  Extended-spectrum fluoroquinolone + clindamycin
  Aztreonam + clindamycin
Life-threatening infection: Parenteral regimen
  Imipenem-cilastin or meropenem or trovafloxacin + vancomycin
  Metronidazole + aztreonam + vancomycin

*These regimens may require adjustment if the patient has a history of allergies or if there are clinical or epidemiologic factors suggesting unusual pathogens. Doses should be commensurate with the severity of infection, with adjustment for renal or hepatic dysfunction when indicated.
Source: From Temple[14] and Gilbert,[16] with permission.

an aggressive malignant tumor that more commonly affects noncaucasians. This tumor has a predilection for the plantar surface of the foot. It may present with atypical features leading to a delay in diagnosis and poor outcome. All skin lesions that are either atypical or not healing despite treatment should be referred for biopsy.[17]

REFERENCES

1. Bedinghaus JM, Niedfeldt MW: Over-the-counter foot remedies. *Am Fam Physician* 64:791, 2001.
2. Birrer RB, Dellacorte MP: Skin and nail disorders of the foot. *Emerg Med* 25:27, 1993.
3. Glover MG: Plantar warts. *Foot Ankle* 11:172, 1990.
4. Malusky LP: Podiatric procedures, in Roberts JR, Hedges JR (eds): *Clinical Procedures in Emergency Medicine,* 3d ed. Philadelphia, Saunders, 1998.
5. Hernandez PA, Hernandez WA, Hernandez A: Clinical aspects of bursae and tendon sheaths of the foot. *J Am Podiatr Med Assoc* 81:366, 1991.
6. Young CC, Rutherford DS, Niedfeldt MW: Treatment of plantar fasciitis. *Am Fam Physician* 64:570, 2001.
7. Reade BM, Longo DC, Keller MC: Tarsal tunnel syndrome. *Clin Podiatr Med Surg* 18:395, 2001.
8. Wu KK: Ganglions of the foot. *J Foot Ankle Surg* 32:343, 1993.
9. Coughlin MJ: Disorders of tendons, in Coughlin MJ, Mann RA (eds): *Surgery of the Foot and Ankle,* 7th ed. St. Louis, Mosby, 1999, p. 786.
10. Wu KK: Morton neuroma and metatarsalgia. *Curr Opin Rheumatol* 12:131, 2000.
11. Perry MD, Manoli A II: Foot compartment syndrome. *Orthop Clin North Am* 32:103, 2001.
12. Lee TH, Wapner KL, Hecht PJ: Plantar fibromatosis. *J Bone Joint Surg* 75A:1080, 1993.
13. Sumpio BE: Foot ulcers. *New Engl J Med* 343:787, 2000.
14. Temple ME, Nahata MC: Pharmacotherapy of lower limb diabetic ulcers. *J Am Geriatr Soc* 48:822, 2000.
15. Kantor J, Margolis DJ: Treatment options for diabetic neuropathic foot ulcers: A cost-effectiveness analysis. *Dermatol Surg* 27:347, 2001.
16. Gilbert DN, Moellering RC, Sande MA: *The Sanford Guide to Antimicrobial Therapy,* 33d ed. Hyde Park, VT: Jeb C. Sanford, 2003, p. 10.
17. Franke W, Neumann NJ, Ruzicka T, et al: Plantar malignant melanoma—A challenge for early recognition. *Melanoma Res* 10:571, 2000.

BEHAVIORAL DISORDERS: CLINICAL FEATURES
Douglas A. Rund

Estimates of the proportion of emergency department patients who present with a psychiatric disorder range from a few percent to over a third. This variability is due in part due to differences in patient population and the community's use of alternatives for psychiatric crisis intervention.

When patients are screened for mental disorders including substance abuse, many have unrecognized psychopathology that is relevant to their assessment and treatment in the emergency setting. Subgroups of the emergency patient population at higher risk for psychiatric disorders include those who are self-referred for nonurgent, nonspecific, vague medical or social problems, and the "after midnight" group of emergency department patients who have been shown to have a higher prevalence of psychiatric illness than those presenting during the daytime. Sometimes, psychiatric disorders clearly make up the primary reason for an individual's presentation to an emergency department. In other cases, psychiatric disorders lead to injury and illness.[1] In contrast, psychiatric disorders may form part of the current or past medical history of a patient, yet possess little importance for the immediate clinical condition.

In studies that report categories of psychiatric illness seen in the emergency department, the most prominent diagnoses are substance abuse, affective disorders, anxiety disorders, antisocial personality disorder, and severe cognitive impairment. Among repeat users of the emergency department, persons with schizophrenia are overrepresented.

DIAGNOSIS

In the assessment of patients presenting with psychiatric symptoms, as with other medical conditions encountered in the emergency department, promptly stabilize the patient's acute psychiatric condition and evaluate the major complaint.[2] Formulating a specific diagnosis is not as important as determining if the patient is harmful to him- or herself or others and needs hospitalization. The determination that an individual is suicidal and in need of protection and hospitalization, for instance, is more important than deciding whether that person suffers from schizophrenia or psychotic depression.

Nevertheless, provisional psychiatric diagnoses can be made in the emergency department. Recognition of specific behavioral syndromes can assist in evaluating the presenting complaint, pursuing associated symptoms, and determining treatment and disposition. Emergency physicians should be sufficiently familiar with commonly seen psychiatric illnesses to describe their predominant clinical features.

Structured Diagnostic Criteria

The current official diagnostic nomenclature, most recently published in 2000 by the American Psychiatric Association, is the *Diagnostic and Statistical Manual of Mental Disorders,* fourth edition (text revision), commonly known as *DSM-IV-TR.*[3] A copy of *DSM-IV-TR* should be available for reference in the emergency department, because it contains the list of criteria for each disorder and additional material on demographics, associated symptoms and syndromes, and differential diagnosis.

Multiaxial Diagnostic System

The *DSM-IV* diagnoses are made on a multiaxial system in which each axis refers to a different domain of information. This system aids in making a comprehensive assessment, organizing complex clinical information, and communicating between professionals. Axis I disorders comprise the clinical syndromes of mental disorders. Conditions listed under axis II are the personality disorders and developmental disorders, including mental retardation, which may underlie the more florid axis I syndrome. Axis III concerns general medical conditions. Axis IV consists of psychosocial and environmental stressors or problems. Axis V relates global, overall functioning (Table 288-1). Knowledge of this multi-axial system may facilitate an understanding of medical records, psychiatric consultants' notes, and interaction with consulting psychiatrists or psychosocial personnel. For instance, a patient with previous medical records containing *DSM-IV* diagnoses of axis I (alcohol intoxication), axis II (antisocial personality disorder), and axis III (scalp laceration) should be recognized as likely to display features of the axis II personality disorder, although the patient's chief complaint may be a new problem.

PSYCHIATRIC SYNDROMES (AXIS I DISORDERS)

The major categories of axis I disorders covered in this chapter are listed in Table 288-2. A useful strategy for making a *DSM-IV* diagnosis is to classify the primary feature into a major category, consider possible nonpsychiatric etiologies for the complaint, and then use the decision trees in Appendix B of *DSM-IV* to identify the appropriate diagnosis. The decision trees guide the clinician who is unfamiliar with the intricacies of the criteria within a category to identify the features that distinguish closely related conditions. An example of the decision tree for evaluating acute psychosis is shown in Figure 288-1.

Delirium, Dementia, Amnestic, and Other Cognitive Disorders

This group of syndromes is characterized by a clinically significant deficit in cognitive or memory function due to a general medical condition. There are several distinct and common causes of organic brain syndromes in which the causative factor is known, for example, vascular dementia and alcohol withdrawal delirium. In these cases, the specific diagnosis is listed in *DSM-IV.* In other cases, the etiologic factor should be specified with the descriptor "due to [general medical disorder or substance]," for example, "delirium due to hepatic encephalopathy."

DEMENTIA   The essential clinical feature of *dementia* is a pervasive disturbance of cognitive functioning in several areas, including memory, abstract thinking, judgment, personality, and other higher cortical functions such as language. If clouding of consciousness is present, then the patient does not have solely a dementing illness but has *delirium* or intoxication. The presence of global cognitive impairment may be detected by a bedside cognitive examination, such as the Mini-Mental Status Examination[4] (see Chap. 289), and additional confirmatory history should be gathered from an informant, such as a family member. Memory disturbance is usually the earliest sign to be apparent to others, and, unless it is very mild, it can be easily identified by examination. Such an examination asks the patient to retain, recall, and register information such as a list of words. The examiner may ask the patient to remember three words (*tree, pen,* and *book*) and repeat them back immediately and in 5 min.

Patients with dementia may be brought to the emergency department after having been found wandering away from home or an institution. Because the onset of most forms of dementia is slow and gradual, presentation to the emergency department often occurs only when some acute

TABLE 288-1   Multiaxial Psychiatric Assessment

Axis I	Mental disorders Clinical and other psychiatric conditions that may be a focus of clinical attention
Axis II	Personality disorders and mental retardation
Axis III	General medical conditions Medical conditions that are relevant to the understanding or management of the case
Axis IV	Psychosocial and environmental problems
Axis V	Global assessment of functioning

Source: Adapted from the American Psychiatric Association: *Diagnostic and Statistical Manual of Mental Disorders,* 4th ed. Washington, D.C., American Psychiatric Association, 2000.

worsening of mental status occurs, which may be the result of a superimposed medical illness, adverse drug effect, or environmental change. The demented patient's diminished intellectual and physiologic resources allow abrupt worsening of function with the addition of such stressors.

Early in the course of dementia, anxiety, depression,[5] or psychosis may dominate the clinical picture and obscure cognitive dysfunction. **For this reason, a high degree of clinical suspicion of dementia should be maintained when evaluating an elderly patient with no prior psychiatric history who presents with new psychiatric problems.** Demented persons are also prone to unrecognized physical illness, because of inability to perceive or describe symptoms. Careful examination and appropriate laboratory testing are always indicated in the initial and ongoing evaluation of such patients.

Dementia is not synonymous with the previous designation of "chronic organic brain syndrome," which implies irreversibility. Common causes of potentially reversible dementia include metabolic and endocrine disorders, polypharmacy, and depression. Often, especially in elderly patients, depression may present with prominent cognitive impairment, a condition erroneously labeled "pseudodementia," but more accurately called *dementia of depression.* A relatively acute onset, prominent mood changes, and vegetative disturbances such as loss of appetite and weight, sleep disturbance, or expressions of guilt or suicidal ideation point to depression as the cause. In these situations, treatment of the mood disorder may lead to resolution of the cognitive impairment, although recent studies indicate that many such patients have evidence of brain dysfunction and only partial treatment response.

DELIRIUM   Like dementia, *delirium* is characterized by global impairment in cognitive function but is distinguished from it in two major ways.[6] **In delirium, the patient has clouding of consciousness, a reduction in the awareness of the external environment (manifest as difficulty sustaining attention), varying degrees of alertness ranging from drowsiness to stupor, and sensory misperception.**

The primary distinguishing feature of delirium is the course that is typically acute, with rapid deterioration in hours or days, rather than in months as with dementia. Also, the severity of delirium fluctuates over the course of hours; the patient may appear normal at one time and

TABLE 288-2   Axis I Disorders

Delirium dementia, and amnestic and other cognitive disorders
Substance induced disorders
Mental disorders due to a general medical condition
Schizophrenia and other psychotic disorders
Mood disorders
Anxiety disorders
Somatoform disorders
Factitious disorders
Dissociative disorders
Eating disorders
Adjustment disorders

wildly agitated a few hours later. Extreme changes in psychomotor activity, ranging from restlessness and hyperactivity to stupor, are frequent in delirium but uncommon in dementia except in the later stages when a delirious state may be superimposed. Hallucinations, often visual, are common in delirium. They typically have a vivid quality to which the patient reacts strongly. The hallucinations contrast with the visual hallucinations seen by psychotic patients, which often are described and experienced indifferently.

Substance-Induced Disorders

INTOXICATION   When recent ingestion of a specific exogenous substance produces maladaptive behavior and impairment of judgment, perception, attention, emotional control, or psychomotor activity, and the patient does not display features of delirium, hallucinosis, or other organic brain syndromes, a diagnosis of *intoxication* is made. When the offending substance is known, it should be specified (e.g., alcohol intoxication or amphetamine intoxication). The specific features of intoxication syndromes commonly seen in the emergency department are described in greater detail in the section on toxicology.

As a general rule, the diagnosis of intoxication can be rather easy when laboratory analysis reveals the type and amount of intoxicant circulating in the system. The clinical features of alcohol intoxication are familiar to experienced emergency physicians and range from impaired judgment and coordination through ataxia, lethargy, and coma. When repeated episodes of intoxication occur within a brief period, the individual by definition has a substance abuse disorder, and the additional diagnosis is made. A urine toxicology screening test and a blood alcohol level are most useful in evaluating patients with new onset psychiatric symptoms and often are required as part of the evaluation assessment of patients admitted to psychiatric facilities.

WITHDRAWAL   *Withdrawal* can follow cessation or reduction in use of a substance of abuse. The category signifies a syndrome characteristic of withdrawal from that particular drug, when the clinical syndrome does not satisfy the criteria for delirium or another organic brain syndrome. For example, mild forms of alcohol withdrawal would be classified here, but if the patient is confused, hallucinating, and agitated, a diagnosis of alcohol withdrawal delirium is indicated. The diagnosis is made by identification of the withdrawal syndrome and evidence of recent use of the substance in a pattern sufficient to produce withdrawal when the amount ingested is decreased. Specific withdrawal patterns depend on the agent customarily used.

Alcohol withdrawal, for instance, includes up to four stages: autonomic hyperactivity (sweating, tachycardia; 6 to 8 h after cessation of drinking), hallucinations (24 h after withdrawal), major motor seizures (1 to 2 days), and global confusion (3 to 5 days after last use of alcohol). Some withdrawal syndromes, particularly from alcohol or barbiturates, can be life-threatening.

Mental Disorders Due to a General Medical Condition

The *DSM-IV* has implemented a major change in the classification of psychiatric symptoms caused by medical conditions. The previous terminology of "organic brain syndrome" and the subtypes organic mood disorder and organic delusional disorder, for example, have been eliminated, because of the implication that the "functional" mental disorders are unrelated to biologic changes in brain function.

Using *DSM-IV,* when there is evidence that a psychiatric disturbance is a direct physiologic consequence of a general medical condition or substance, the mental disorder is specified as "due to" the medical problem, for example, "major depression due to hypothyroidism."

Schizophrenia and Other Psychotic Disorders

Schizophrenia and related disorders are marked by the presence of psychotic symptoms, primarily delusions and hallucinations. *Delu-*

FIG. 288-1. Decision tree for evaluating psychosis.

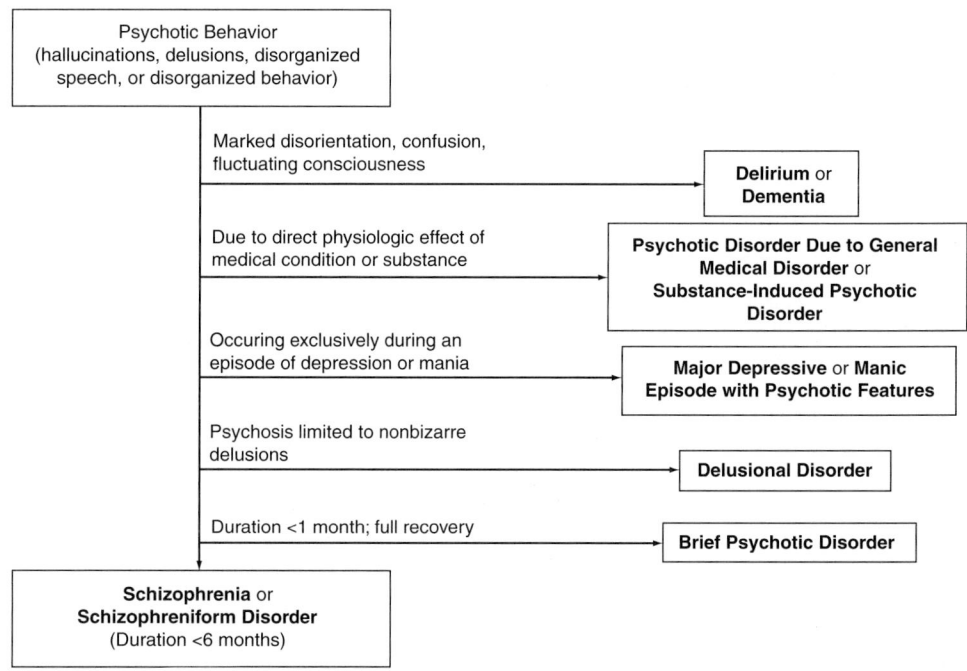

sions are defined as fixed false beliefs that are not amenable to arguments or facts to the contrary and that are not shared by others of similar cultural background. Common delusions are of several types. *Persecutory delusions* are those in which one believes that one is being attacked, followed, harassed, or conspired against. *Grandiose delusions* are those that involve themes of special powers or abilities. *Bizarre delusions* are those with patently absurd content, such as believing that one's thoughts are controlled by extraterrestrial beings. *Hallucinations* are false perceptions experienced in a sensory modality and occurring in clear consciousness. Auditory hallucinations are the most common, followed in order of prevalence by visual, tactile, olfactory, and gustatory; the presence of the latter, nonauditory hallucinations suggests a medical, not psychiatric, cause of psychosis (such as alcohol withdrawal). The most prevalent psychosis is *schizophrenia,* described in detail in the next section. The other psychotic disorders, discussed briefly, are less common. A decision tree helpful in evaluating psychotic symptoms is presented in Figure 288-1.

SCHIZOPHRENIA   Schizophrenia is one of the most serious public health problems in the world, affecting just under 1 percent of the world's population. The essential features are a deterioration in functioning, characteristic active-phase symptoms (hallucinations, delusions, disorganized speech, disorganized behavior, and catatonic behavior), negative symptoms (blunted affect, emotional withdrawal, lack of spontaneity, anhedonia, or attentional impairment), cognitive impairment manifested by loose associations or incoherence for at least 1 month, and the relative absence of a mood disorder. Research has established the importance of genetic factors in its cause, and schizophrenia is most likely a group of disorders of different etiologies that shares a final common pathway, much as is the case with mental retardation. It is a brain disease, and there is no evidence that psychosocial stressors or poor parenting is responsible for the cause of the illness, although these may have a profound effect on the patient's adaptation to this usually chronic disorder.

Symptoms of schizophrenia usually begin in late adolescence or early adulthood, although the onset can occur at any age. The childhood history of schizophrenics often is marked by shyness, oddness or eccentric behavior, school difficulties, or paranoid behaviors, but such features are not always present. A prodromal phase, in which a gradual deterioration of function is noted, usually precedes the development of active delusions or hallucinations. Such deterioration usually includes the worsening of social withdrawal or the new onset of social

withdrawal, odd behavior or speech, and difficulty in functioning in school or work. Patients or their families rarely seek care until the onset of the active phase of psychosis. Schizophrenics seldom seek care at all, because they lack insight; they do not realize that their perceptions, thoughts, and behavior are abnormal.

Typical, or older, antipsychotic drugs (such as haloperidol) usually reduce the severity of positive symptoms (delusions and hallucinations). Other manifestations of schizophrenia less responsive to typical antipsychotics include negative symptoms (lack of volition, blunting of emotion, anhedonia, and inattention). Such symptoms result in lasting impairment in self-care, work, and social relations. Newer, "atypical," antipsychotic agents (such as risperidone, olanzapine, clozapine and ziprasidone) seem to have a greater effect in improving the negative and positive symptoms.

Disorganization of thinking and behavior characterizes schizophrenia. Disheveled appearance and grooming, bizarre behavior, poor judgment, and loosening of associations indicate such disorganization. *Loosening of associations* refers to a loss of the normal logical connections between one thought and the next; the schizophrenic patient's speech is often vague, rambling, disjointed, or nonsensical. Fantastic experiences and bizarre ideas are described in an indifferent manner and unchanging facial expression.

Common reasons for persons with schizophrenia to come to the emergency department include worsening of psychosis resulting from stress or noncompliance with medication, suicidal behavior, violence (often as a result of paranoid thinking), and extrapyramidal side effects of neuroleptic drugs. Schizophrenics constitute a large share of the chronic homeless population and may be brought in by authorities, in a confused state, obviously unable to attend to their basic needs. Their poor judgment and disorganization may lead to disregard for medical problems, so attention must be given to their physical status and the psychiatric problem.

SCHIZOPHRENIFORM DISORDER   *Schizophreniform disorder* is diagnosed when the patient meets the criteria for schizophrenia but the symptoms have been continuously present for less than 6 months. A rapid onset over a few days and good premorbid functioning are more common than in schizophrenia.

BRIEF PSYCHOTIC DISORDER   Some individuals may become acutely psychotic after exposure to an extremely traumatic life experience. If such a psychosis lasts for less than 4 weeks, it is termed a *brief psychotic disorder*. Precipitants of the psychosis include the death of a loved one or a life-threatening situation such as combat or a natural disaster. Emotional turmoil, confusion, and extremely bizarre behavior and speech are common.

Mood Disorders

The mood disorders are the most prevalent of the major psychiatric disorders, affecting about 10 to 15 percent of the general population at some time in their lives. Depressive disorders are the major cause of completed suicide. An unsuccessful attempt may bring the patient to the emergency department. Mood disorders, substance abuse, and anxiety disorders are the most common psychiatric diagnoses in emergency patients.

Mood, or *affective,* disorders differ from the normal extremes of sadness and happiness in that characteristic clusters of psychological and vegetative symptoms (depressive or manic syndrome) are present, and functioning is impaired. Any of the features of schizophrenia such as delusions, hallucinations, or disorganization may be present, but if a full depressive or manic syndrome exists, a diagnosis of a psychotic mood disorder is required. Another important characteristic of affective disorders is that they tend to be episodic, with periods of remission and normal function.

MAJOR DEPRESSION The essential features of *major depression* are a persistent sad or depressed (dysphoric) mood or pervasive loss of interest in usual activities lasting for at least 2 weeks. Associated psychological symptoms include guilt over past deeds, self-reproach, feelings of worthlessness or hopelessness, inability to experience pleasure, and recurrent thought of death or suicide. "Vegetative symptoms" involve physiologic functioning and include loss of appetite and weight, sleep disturbance, fatigue, inability to concentrate, and psychomotor agitation or retardation. The depression may begin gradually or rapidly but usually will have been present for several weeks before the patient comes for treatment.

When the patient complains of the full spectrum of depression symptoms, the diagnosis of major depression is easy to make, but when the chief complaint is a single symptom such as insomnia or fatigue, it will be necessary to elicit the other symptoms of major depression to make the diagnosis. Somatic complaints such as vague pain or weakness may be part of major depression, as may generalized anxiety. A useful screening mnemonic is presented in Figure 288-2.

Major depression is more common in women, persons with a family history of depression or suicide, and individuals with medical or other psychiatric illnesses. When a medical disorder or drug produces a depressive syndrome through a presumed biologic effect on the brain, the diagnosis should be "depression due to [the offending condition]." Major depression is often superimposed on other mental disorders such as substance abuse, personality disorders, and anxiety disorders; and such conditions are frequently comorbid conditions. Depression in the elderly may go unrecognized by the emergency physician. Screening tools for depression recognition in the geriatric population can be helpful in diagnosis.

In	Interest
S	Sleep
A	Appetite
D	Depressed mood
C	Concentration
A	Activity
G	Guilt
E	Energy
S	Suicide

FIG. 288-2. In SAD CAGES. A screening mnemonic for major depression. (Reprinted with permission from Rund DA, Hutzler JC: *Emergency Psychiatry.* St. Louis, Mosby, 1983.)

Primary mood disorders tend to display more biologic features, are more familial, and respond better to somatic antidepressant treatment than do mood disorders due to medical disorders. The lifetime risk of suicide in patients with major depression is 15 percent, so prompt and aggressive treatment is strongly indicated. Major depression is often recurrent, so certain patients must be maintained on long-term treatment to prevent relapse.

BIPOLAR DISORDER Bipolar disorder, previously termed *manic-depressive illness,* is characterized by the occurrence of mania cycling with periods of depression. A full manic syndrome is one of the most striking and distinctive conditions in clinical practice. The essential disturbance in mood is one of elation or irritability. Manic patients feel "on top of the world," expansive, and energetic. The state is precarious, however, and the patient may quickly become argumentative, hostile, irritable, and sarcastic, especially when their plans are thwarted.

The vegetative signs of mania are a decreased need for sleep, increased activity, rapid pressured speech, and racing thoughts. Manics may have grandiose ideas, such as unrealistic plans to start a business or run for public office, and if the grandiosity reaches delusional proportions, such patients may believe themselves to be famous, fabulously wealthy, or blessed with special powers and abilities. Poor judgment in spending money and sexual behavior may lead to problems that prompt manics' families to seek treatment for them, because manics usually lack insight into their abnormal condition and deny that anything is wrong. For this reason, reports from informants such as relatives often reveal important information to substantiate the diagnosis. Because patients who have had a manic episode almost invariably have depressions at some time (the other "pole" of bipolar disorder), a history of depression also may help in diagnosis.

The disorder is equally common in men and women, and the onset is usually in the third and fourth decades. Complications include suicide, substance abuse (excessive alcohol use is common during the manic phase), and marital and occupational disruptions. The course of bipolar disorder is episodic, with the duration, frequency, and regularity of the episodes varying greatly. Depressive episodes are more frequent than manic episodes.

DYSTHYMIC DISORDER *Dysthymic disorder* is a more chronic and less severe form of depressive illness and was previously termed *depressive neurosis.* Depressed mood must have been present most of the day, more days than not, for at least 2 years. Psychotic features are not seen, and these patients often have a life-long gloomy, pessimistic outlook. Women are affected more often than men, and the onset is typically in childhood, adolescence, or early adulthood.

Associated personality disorders and substance abuse are common. When vegetative symptoms are present, they are usually less severe than with major depression. Major depression may be superimposed on dysthymia, often in association with stressful life events. When major depression complicates dysthymia, the patient may be brought in for evaluation, because of the severity of symptoms or treatment after a suicide attempt.

Anxiety Disorders

The *anxiety disorders* are mental disorders in which apprehension, fears, and excessive worry dominate the psychological life of the individual. Pathologic degrees of anxiety are accompanied by different degrees of autonomic activity (sweating, tachycardia, or dizziness) out of proportion to any real danger or threat. Because anxiety is a ubiquitous condition and frequently associated with medical illness, depression, neurologic syndromes, and psychoses, a diagnosis of a primary anxiety disorder should be made by exclusion of other causes.

Anxiety disorders are diagnosed in 4 to 8 percent of the general population and are diagnosed more often in women than in men. Because of the physical nature of certain symptoms associated with anxiety disorders, patients often seek treatment and evaluation in medical rather than psychiatric settings.

PANIC DISORDER Patients who experience recurrent attacks of severe anxiety are said to suffer from *panic disorder.* For detailed discussion, see Chap. 292. A panic attack consists of a sudden extreme surge of anxiety and dread accompanied by autonomic signs, including palpitations, tachycardia, shortness of breath, chest tightness, dizziness, sweating, and tremulousness. The symptoms develop over a few minutes at most and may be unprovoked or occur with a phobic stimulus, such as a crowded store. After the attacks begin, some patients start to avoid situations that seem to precipitate the panic (phobic avoidance). When activities are severely limited, the complication of *agoraphobia* is diagnosed. In agoraphobia, the patient tends to avoid situations where ready escape or assistance during an attack is not possible. The frequency and severity of panic attacks wax and wane, but the illness is generally chronic.

GENERALIZED ANXIETY DISORDER When anxiety attacks are absent but the patient complains of persistent worry, tension, or free-floating anxiety, a diagnosis of generalized anxiety disorder should be considered. This condition lasts at least 6 months and is characterized by apprehensive worrying, muscle tension, insomnia, irritability, restlessness, jumpiness, or distractibility. Muscle tension may be so severe that the patient actually experiences diffuse muscular pain. Associated autonomic symptoms include the cardiopulmonary, gastrointestinal, and neurologic symptoms seen in panic attacks. In generalized anxiety disorder, such symptoms occur more continuously and chronically than in panic disorder.

PHOBIC DISORDERS Phobic disorders, other than agoraphobia, are an unusual cause of self-referral to the emergency department. In phobias, the anxiety symptoms are recognized as excessive and occur when the patient is exposed to, or anticipates exposure to, a specific situation, which then leads to avoidance of the stimulus to a degree that it interferes with the patient's life. In social phobia, the situation involves having the attention of others drawn to the patient. Such activities as public speaking or meeting strangers create a fear that the patient will be embarrassed in some way. Specific phobias are quite common; they involve fear of a very specific stimulus, such as animals, heights, dark, or flying.

OTHER ANXIETY DISORDERS *Posttraumatic stress disorder* is an anxiety reaction to a severe psychosocial stressor, usually life threatening, such as military combat, fire, rape, or natural disaster. Symptoms involve repetitive and intrusive memories of the event, nightmares, emotional numbing, survivor guilt, and different degrees of depression and anxiety. Substance abuse appears to be a frequent complication.

Obsessive-compulsive disorder is a mental disorder in which the patient experiences intrusive thoughts or images that cannot be eliminated from the mind. Typical thoughts involve images of graphic violence to self or others, contamination, or perverse sexual behavior that the patient would not carry out but nevertheless obsessively fantasizes about. To control the obsessive thoughts, the individual may engage in compulsive behavior or rituals, such as excessive washing, repetitive checking, or counting. When the obsessions and compulsions occupy a great deal of time, the patient may become significantly disabled and seek psychiatric attention. The sense of helplessness and the impairment can lead to the development of depression, which also leads the patient to seek help.

Somatoform Disorders

Many patients have particular complaints or symptoms for which no medical explanation can be identified. When a physical cause has been clearly eliminated, and the complaint is not delusional or occurring in the context of a depression or anxiety disorder, somatoform disorders may be considered. When the complaint involves a loss of function, usually in the neurologic system (e.g., paralysis, blindness, or numbness) and psychological factors are deemed etiologic, a *conversion disorder* may be present. Conversion disorders are much more common in culturally and psychologically unsophisticated persons. This diagnosis should be made with extreme caution, if at all, in the emergency department, because studies indicate that many patients diagnosed with conversion disorder eventually develop signs of a physical disorder explaining the symptom. For further discussion, see Chap. 293.

Some patients have a wide variety of complaints and long complicated histories of medical problems that have no apparent medical cause. Such individuals may have *somatization disorder,* a disorder beginning in the teens and twenties, usually in women, and leading to considerable unnecessary diagnostic and surgical intervention. The prototypical patient is a middle-aged woman who describes a "positive review of systems" in a dramatic and confusing way. As with conversion disorder, a firm diagnosis of somatization disorder should not be made on the basis of one visit to the emergency department, but the identification of somatizing behavior is useful for future reference, because patients frequently make repeated contacts with medical providers.

Hypochondriasis may be diagnosed when the patient is preoccupied with fears of serious illness, fears that persist despite appropriate medical evaluation and reassurance.

When pain is the sole complaint and the intensity and secondary disability are unexplained by a known physical ailment, a diagnosis of *pain disorder* may be considered.

Dissociative Disorders

The dissociative disorders comprise a group of uncommon and poorly understood conditions in which the central feature is a sudden alteration in the normal integration of identity and consciousness. The dissociation often occurs under severe stress and may or may not be recurrent, although it is rarely permanent. The forms of dissociative state relevant to emergency practice are *psychogenic amnesia,* a temporary loss of memory for important personal details that is not due to an organic cause, and *psychogenic fugue,* in which a similar loss of memory and assumption of new identity are accompanied by travel away from home. Dissociative disorders are difficult to distinguish from *malingering,* in which the individual in pursuit of a clear goal, such as avoiding incarceration or military duty, may consciously feign amnesia. As always, organic causes, such as drug intoxication, or loss of memory, such as that resulting from transient global amnesia, must be ruled out.

Other conditions in this category include *multiple personality disorder* and *depersonalization disorder.*

PERSONALITY (AXIS II) DISORDERS

Personality refers to an enduring pattern of perceiving, relating to, and reacting to one's environment and interpersonal relationships. When a pattern of behavior is lifelong, not limited to periods of illness, and causes significant impairment in social and occupational functioning or considerable distress, a *personality disorder* is present. Some individuals are painfully aware of the consequences of their behavior but are unable to alter these fundamental ways of dealing with their world. Most patients who are seen clinically in medical and psychiatric settings who are diagnosed with a personality disorder lack a clear awareness of how their behavior alienates others or aggravates their own stress. Even when such insight is possible, actual personality change is unlikely.

The patient presenting with a personality disorder often may be recognized by the characteristic effect the interaction has on the physician

TABLE 288-3 Behavioral Characteristics that Suggest Various Clusters of Personality Disorders

Behavior	Personality Disorder Group
Eccentric, odd, isolated, withdrawn, suspicious, inhibited, no friends, overly sensitive	Paranoid, schizoid, schizotypal
Emotional, dramatic, angry, seductive, impulsive, erratic	Antisocial, histrionic, borderline, narcissistic
Anxious, fearful, nervous, cautious	Dependent, avoidant, obsessive-compulsive

Sources: Rund DA, Hutzler JC: *Emergency Psychiatry.* St. Louis, CV Mosby, 1983; American Psychiatric Association: *Diagnostic and Statistical Manual of Mental Disorders,* 4th ed. Washington, D.C., American Psychiatric Association, 2000.

and medical staff. Antisocial patients, for instance, are disliked immediately; they seem to be in control of their behavior, unlike psychotic or depressed patients, but nonetheless have repeatedly engaged in maladaptive behavior. The patient may be seen as using the emergency department for some vague, or obvious, goal. These disorders are the most common secondary diagnosis in the malingerer.

The emergency physician seldom needs to decide which of the personality disorders relates appropriately to the patient. General categories of personality disorders are grouped in Table 288-3. When such features are present and seem to be interfering with some important aspect of the patient's life, personality disorder can be suspected. The presenting complaint should be evaluated appropriately, because patients with well-established character disorders still develop bona fide medical illnesses.

The personality disorder that constitutes a disproportionate share of emergency visits is *antisocial personality disorder.* The patient shows a continuous pattern of maladaptive behavior displaying disregard for the rights of others in a variety of ways: criminal behavior, fighting, lying, abuse and neglect of dependents and spouses, financial irresponsibility, recklessness, and inability to sustain enduring attachments to others.

The sociopathic behavior begins before the age of 15 years, but the diagnosis may not be made until after the age of 18 years. Sociopathy is much more frequent in males, in lower socioeconomic classes, and in relatives of alcoholics and sociopaths. Alcohol and drug abuse, imprisonment, multiple divorces, traumatic injury, accidental and violent deaths, and poor medical compliance are common complications.

Management of the antisocial patient in the emergency department is often frustrating, but anger toward the patient can be minimized and the interaction hastened along by setting firm limits on behavior, focusing on the chief complaint, and providing the patient with necessary information about the medical problem at hand. No effective psychiatric intervention can be forced on the patient, although certain patients may benefit from substance abuse treatment, psychotherapy, or organized religion when motivated to make changes in their lives. Fortunately, the most violent and disruptive behavior of many antisocials seems to "burn out" in the late twenties or after, although their adjustment to society often continues to be marginal.

REFERENCES

1. Broderick KB, Lerner EB, et al: Emergency physician practices and requirements regarding the medical screening examination of psychiatric patients. *Acad Emerg Med* 9:88, 2002.
2. Jagoda A, Riggio S: Psychiatric emergencies. *Emerg Med Clin North Am* 18:173, 2002.
3. American Psychiatric Association: *Diagnostic and Statistical Manual of Mental Disorders,* 4th ed. Washington, D.C., American Psychiatric Association, 2000.
4. Lamarre CJ, Patten SB: Evaluation of the modified mini-mental state examination in a general psychiatric population. *Can J Psychiatry* 36:507, 1991.
5. Meldon SW, Emerman CL, Schubert D: Recognition of depression in geriatric ED patients by emergency physicians. *Ann Emerg Med* 30:4, 1997.
6. Samuels SC, Evers MM: Delirium: Pragmatic guidance for managing a common, confounding and sometime lethal condition. *Geriatrics* 57:33, 2002.

289 BEHAVIORAL DISORDERS: EMERGENCY ASSESSMENT

Douglas A. Rund
Jeffery C. Hutzler

This chapter presents the principles of medical and psychiatric evaluation of patients with behavior disorders and reviews the management of suicidal and violent patients. The majority of psychiatric patient visits to emergency departments occur during the evening and at night when psychiatric services are limited; therefore, the hospital must be staffed at off-hours with adequate personnel adept at handling patients who are suicidal, violent, psychotic, or otherwise distraught.

Situations that require emergency stabilization include potential or actual homicidal or suicidal behavior,[1] or rapidly progressive medical conditions resulting in disturbed behavior (e.g., hypoglycemia, meningitis, or other causes of delirium).

A decision strategy for emergency psychiatric assessment should follow this sequence of questions: (1) Is the patient stable or unstable? (2) Does the patient have a serious medical condition that is causing abnormal behavior or thought processes? (3) If the cause of changes in behavior is not the result of an underlying medical condition, it will be primarily *psychiatric* or *functional.* What is the diagnosis and severity? (4) Is a psychiatric consultation necessary? (5) When should the patient be forcibly detained for emergency evaluation?

SAFETY ISSUES

Violent behavior demands immediate restraint. Hospital security forces and police are best equipped and best trained to subdue violent patients with the least chance of staff or patient injury. Further discussion of contemporary restraint practices is provided in Chap. 301. Pharmacological treatment of violent or agitated patients is discussed in Chap. 290.

Patients who are threatening or who demonstrate actual or potential violent behavior should be disrobed, gowned, and searched for weapons. Seemingly innocuous objects such as belts or belt buckles, which can be used to inflict self-injury or injury to others, should be removed.

Patients whose behavior suggests the potential for violence should be approached cautiously and with a nonthreatening attitude, with adequate security force nearby. The physician should also stay distant from the patient, avoid excessive eye contact, and maintain a somewhat submissive posture and tone of voice. Ideally, the physician should stand in a location that neither threatens the patient nor blocks the exit of the patient or the physician from the room. Allow the patient to ventilate feelings verbally. Setting limits on acceptable behavior and making neutral comments may diffuse a potentially violent situation. Adequate force nearby should be visible to the patient, and the patient should clearly be told that uncontrollable behavior will result in restraint. Patients who are actually or potentially dangerous to themselves or to others will generally need psychiatric admission.

A patient expressing suicidal ideation requires specific measures for protection. All dangerous objects are removed from the patient and the treatment room. Staff members, or a reliable family member, should accompany the patient if it necessary to leave the examining room. Some institutions have members of the security staff available to provide supervision. Patients expressing suicidal ideation should not be allowed to leave the emergency department before medical or psychiatric evaluation.

History

The important elements of history taking include documentation of behavioral change, identification of important medical symptoms, determination of medical comorbidities, and medication/drug history.

The changed behavior is a good starting point for inquiry. Sudden onset of major changes in behavior, mood, or thought in a previously normal patient, or definite deterioration in a patient with a chronic behavioral disorder, should stimulate evaluation for an underlying medical or neurologic disorder. A sudden change in behavior, especially in a patient older than age 40 years, is an important indicator of a new and correctable disease process. The most important information about behavioral changes will come from the patient's family. If the family is unavailable, friends or coworkers should be contacted and questioned. The source may be able to report substance abuse or compliance with medication, and can describe the level of previous functioning. Family and social history may identify stressors in the patient's environment that are either a direct cause of changes in behavior or accentuate any responses to underlying disease. To help identify patterns of relapse, determine the history of previous psychiatric illness and treatment. All personal history should be corroborated by family members when possible. The physician should compare his or her own direct observations of the patient's behavior with reports from the patient's family and friends.

Neurologic symptoms associated with the behavioral changes should be explored. Such symptoms include fainting, dizziness, disorientation, impairment of speech, confusion, loss of consciousness, headaches, and difficulty performing routine tasks.

Medical comorbidities must be identified, as psychiatric patients often develop medical illnesses producing changes in behavior.

Specifically ask about fever, head trauma, human immunodeficiency virus (HIV) risk factors, and toxic ingestions or overdose.

Ask about the use of prescription and over-the-counter drugs, especially sedative-hypnotics, stimulants, psychotropic agents, anticonvulsants, anticholinergic agents, angiotensin-converting enzyme inhibitors, beta-blockers, corticosteroids, fluoroquinolone antibiotics, H_2-receptor blockers, opioids, salicylates, selective serotonin reuptake inhibitors, thiazide diuretics, and antiparkinsonian agents.[2] Over-the-counter analgesics or herbals containing salicylates, anticholinergics, antihistamines, or bromides may produce delirium or toxic psychosis. Alcohol[3] and street drugs such as phencyclidine, lysergic acid diethylamide (LSD), mescaline, amphetamines, and cocaine can produce a toxic psychosis. Hypnosedatives such as barbiturates and benzodiazepines may produce a confusional state or delirium both with intoxication and withdrawal.

Patients with chronic mental illness have a higher incidence of alcohol abuse than the general population. The syndromes associated with alcohol abuse which can result in altered behavior include intoxication, withdrawal, delirium, hallucinosis, alcohol amnestic disorder, paranoid behavior, and dementia. Alcohol screening tests are useful in disturbed patients even when the odor of ethanol is not present.

Mental Status Examination

The objective of the mental status examination is to distinguish psychiatric (functional) from medical (organic) disorders. A great deal of the information obtained in mental status examinations becomes evident through patient observation and the initial patient interview (Table 289-1). Important components of the mental status examination include level of consciousness, spontaneous speech, spontaneous behavior, physical appearance, the relaying of history information, attention, and language comprehension. Another tool to detect dementia

TABLE 289-1   Mental Status in the Emergency Department: An Outline

Behavior
What is the patient doing?
Affect
What feelings is the patient displaying?
Orientation
Does the patient know what is happening, where, and when?
Language
Is the patient understanding and being understood?
Memory
Can the patient recall historical details, recent and remote?
Thought content
Is the patient reporting beliefs that make little sense?
Perceptual abnormalities
Is the patient experiencing unusual sensory phenomena?
Judgment
Is the patient able to make rational decisions?

or delirium is the Mini-Mental Status Examination (MMSE), described in Chap. 307, Figure 307-2. An abnormal mental status examination suggests a medical (organic) basis for abnormal thought or behavior. Lability of affect, the necessity to repeat simple questions, irritability, disorientation, and lack of cooperation are some signs of organic dysfunction.

Documentation of the patient's orientation should include an assessment of attention, ability to concentrate on a specific task, and the traditional evaluation of person, place, and time. The patient should be asked the day, month, year, and place where he or she is presently being examined. Impaired language performance, including difficulty with speech, reading, writing, and word finding, may indicate a neurologic disorder. Memory is often divided into three categories: immediate, recent, and remote. Immediate memory is tested by asking a patient to repeat a series of digits (usually five) forward and backward. Recent memory can be tested by asking the patient to repeat three unrelated words (e.g., tree, apple, bicycle) immediately and then again after 3 to 5 min. The patient should be able to restate these after 3 to 5 min. The patient may also be asked about events that have occurred in the last few hours. Remote memory can be tested by asking about previous addresses, occupations, or historical events from an early period in the patient's life. Tests of memory should include details of significant personal, national, and international historical events. Investigation of higher cognitive functions includes assessment of a patient's general command of information; mental calculation, especially subtraction, such as serial sevens; and spelling of words forward and backward (such as world). Patients with organic disease often have difficulty spelling backward or performing serial calculation. The patient's affect or outward display of emotion should be evaluated for sadness, euphoria, and anxiety. This may help distinguish between cognitive disturbance induced by depressive disorders and dementia due to significant cerebral pathology. An examiner can draw some conclusions regarding a patient's thought processes during the patient's own telling of his or her history.

Disordered thought processes include paranoid or grandiose delusions, fixed false beliefs, and delusional denial of illness. Such beliefs should be compared with reports from family and friends.

Visual hallucinations do occur in functional psychotic illnesses (schizophrenia or affective disorder), but most often result from organic disease. A patient with visual hallucinations should always be assumed to have organic pathology until proven otherwise.

Judgment may be impaired in organic disease, and historical evidence of faulty judgment should be elicited. Insight about judgment can be gained by asking a patient how he or she would deal with day-to-day problems, such as finding the way home from the hospital.

Finally, the examiner should test for specific focal neurologic deficits, including apraxias, agnosias, right-left disorientation, aphasias, and inability to follow complex spoken and written commands. Such signs may or may not occur in association with other localizing neurological signs, such as asymmetric reflexes, paresthesia, or hemiparesis. Ask the patient to "draw a clock face." The physician can draw a circle on a piece of paper and ask the patient to fill in the numbers on the paper to look like a clock face. If the patient can put in the numbers correctly in a clock face, he or she should then be asked to put the hands at the position to read a specific time (e.g., 10:30). If the patient cannot do these tasks, organic disease is present.

Accurately diagnosing and understanding behavioral emergencies in the elderly is difficult but important. Syndromes include confusion, agitation, psychosis, and behavioral regression. Detailed discussion is provided in Chap. 307.

Physical Examination

The objectives of physical examination are to identify medical disorders that may cause or have an impact on behavior and to identify the presence of medical problems that may need special care in, or are inappropriate for, management in a psychiatric setting. A limited physical examination should be conducted on every patient.[4-7] Vital signs, including temperature, should be obtained on all psychiatric patients. Abnormal vital signs should not automatically be dismissed as secondary to anxiety or stress, but should be investigated.

The extent of the physical examination depends to some extent on the patient's age,[8,9] the nature of the chief psychiatric complaint, psychosocial history, and the existence of medical comorbidities. Patients with abnormal vital signs, abnormal mental status examination, psychosis, mental retardation, and the elderly usually require a more complete physical examination, including assessment of chest, heart, and abdomen. Examine all patients for signs of trauma to the head, face, and neck, and carefully reconstruct the mechanism of injury. In the homeless, or in those with exposure, check extremities for frostbite. Examine for needle tracks. Neurologic examination typically includes an assessment of cranial nerves, gait, mental status, and general motor function and strength.

Laboratory Evaluation

Laboratory testing depends upon findings from the history, mental status examination, and physical examination.

A urine toxicology screen and blood alcohol level are two of the most commonly required tests for patients transferred to, or admitted to, psychiatric facilities from the emergency department. However, these tests may be most helpful when the cause of abnormal thought or behavior is unknown.

Consultation and Referral

In the ideal setting, all emergency departments would have psychiatric consultation available at all times. However, in many instances, the emergency physician will have to rely on more-limited resources. In many instances, following initial screening, disposition can be made to a variety of secondary sources of evaluation and treatment. Judgments regarding referral depend on assessment of a patient's likelihood of becoming violent toward self or others. Clues that suggest potential violence include hostile behavior, verbal aggressiveness, or statements about violent intent. Such patients need immediate hospitalization. Marked disorientation and confusion require evaluation for organic components. In the absence of such indications, referral can be made to a psychiatrist or a psychiatric facility. Results of the emergency department medical and psychiatric evaluation should be summarized in writing and provided to the consultant. The patient should receive clear discharge instructions and should have a follow-up interval for any medical or surgical disorders that were identified. Documentation of a thorough evaluation of these risk factors is important.

SUICIDE

Suicide continues to be a major cause of death throughout the world and a leading cause of death among the young. There seem to be epidemiologic differences between suicide attempters and suicide completers. Suicide completers, for instance, are more likely than attempters to be older, male, living alone, or physically ill. Such patients are at high risk and need to be carefully assessed. The ratio of attempted suicides to completed suicide is estimated to be approximately 40:1.

A suicide attempt is not a common accompaniment of the "downward" portion of the normal mood swings occasionally experienced by everyone. Only approximately 2 percent of the general population have seriously considered taking their lives and only approximately 1 percent have actually attempted suicide. Therefore, suicide attempters must be taken seriously. The attitude of the staff should be empathic; steps to insure patient safety in the emergency department should be instituted, including supervision and removal of potentially dangerous objects; and following medical management, the assessment of suicide risk should be carefully evaluated and documented.

Suicidal thinking is more frequent among women than among men and is associated with a clinical depression, social isolation, undesirable life events, and early parental loss. Suicidal thinking may precede an actual attempt by many months and may persist long after improvement in mental status and personal relationships.

Negative attitudes toward the suicide attempter have been documented among all types of emergency personnel: paramedics, nurses, and emergency physicians. A negative attitude intensifies a patient's already low self-esteem, thus increasing the risk of subsequent suicide and making it difficult to establish a therapeutic relationship.

Schizophrenia, substance abuse, and depression are psychiatric diagnoses that place a suicidal patient at relatively high risk. Personality disorder and adjustment disorder implying a transient situational disturbance are frequent diagnoses in suicide attempters and are generally associated with relatively lower completion risk than the major psychiatric illnesses noted previously. However, patients with these latter disorders still show a higher risk of completed suicide than the general population.

Drug overdose accounts for the overwhelming majority of all contemporary suicide attempts. Drugs used for suicide attempts tend to parallel prevailing prescribing patterns. Toxicity of the agent and the lethal intent of the patient help assess the relative risk. A patient taking a large dose of amitriptyline would be considered at greater risk than someone taking a few antihistamine tablets. Some patients may be relatively unaware of a drug's potential toxicity, however, and such knowledge and their continuing intent to die must be assessed by questions such as, "Were you surprised to find yourself alive after taking the overdose?"

Violent attempts (shooting, jumping, hanging) are generally considered serious and a high-risk factor for a future attempt. A number of reports have described a "wrist-cutting syndrome" in young, unmarried women whose self-mutilation, although repetitive, has traditionally been thought to be less serious in lethal intent than other situations. Such acts usually have been carried out in a state of mounting tension with depersonalization followed by relief after self-mutilation. A significant number of "wrist slashers," or self-mutilators, however, whose cases have been followed for 5 to 6 years, have committed suicide.

In determining suicide risk, a general rule is that the risk of a successful suicide rises with advancing age. Men are two to three times more likely than women to complete suicide, whereas women are two or three times more likely than men to attempt suicide. Patients who are single, divorced, separated, widowed, or unemployed are at higher risk than those who are married and employed.

A psychotic patient who attempts suicide requires careful observation, whatever restraint necessary, and evaluation by a psychiatrist. A psychotic patient may respond unpredictably to distorted perceptions in a fearful or driven manner.

Secondary gain is a term that indicates that while the primary motive for a suicide attempt appears to be death, the attempt may meet another need such as attention or a plea for emotional help. When such needs are met by the attempt, a secondary gain is achieved and the risk of subsequent suicide attempt is lessened momentarily. It is dangerous, however, to assume that secondary gain is the cause of a suicide attempt with an initial evaluation in an emergency department. All suicide behaviors should be taken seriously.

Perhaps the most important part of the assessment of the suicide attempter is a determination of the patient's feelings and thoughts at the time of the interview.[10] The patient who experiences helplessness, exhaustion, overwhelming depression, and a clear expression of intent to die certainly remains at high risk. If a patient expresses continuation of such feelings at the time of the interview, the physician has sufficient evidence that the patient needs psychiatric consultation immediately. Some patients, however, seem to equate self-injury with other forms of emotional discharge, such as crying, talking to a friend, or becoming inebriated. They do not perceive the event as an attempt to end their life. When asked about their feelings at the time of the attempt, such patients may indicate that they were angry or vengeful. Attitudes and affect that generally indicate a good prognosis at the time of the interview are anger, remorse, or embarrassment. A patient who sits quietly, refusing to provide additional information to an examiner, should be considered at high risk. Feelings of hopelessness, helplessness, or exhaustion seem to be among the clearest indicators of long-term suicidal risk in patients hospitalized at one time for depression.[11]

Patient disposition can be aided by estimating the lethality of the attempt and the likelihood of rescue. When there is a high likelihood of rescue and low lethality, a patient is considered at lower risk than in the reverse situation. A patient who makes a hanging attempt in a desolate wooded area is at greater risk than a person who takes a handful of relatively nontoxic pills in front of witnesses.

Patients who have made previous suicide attempts have traditionally been considered to be at greater risk for future suicide. Prior attempts seem a particularly ominous sign, particularly if the intensity and apparent lethality of the suicide attempts escalate with each subsequent attempt.

A "no harm contract"[12] is very useful in the emergency department in evaluating suicidal risk. The "no harm contract" is a verbal or written agreement, initiated by the emergency physician or psychiatrist, in which the suicidal patient is asked to agree not to harm or kill himself or herself for a particular period of time. This can be therapeutic, helping to reveal the intent of the patient and reduce it. It can also be diagnostic in assessing the nature and severity of a patient's suicidality. It can uncover specific issues precipitating suicidal thoughts and the ability of the patient to contract for safety. Such a contract has no legal implications, however. The most important aspect of the patient's record is the clear documentation by the physician that the patient is or is not an imminent risk to self or others, and why or why not. A very difficult decision in the emergency department is when to discharge a child or adolescent patient who has expressed suicidal thoughts or behavior. Consideration of the following criteria is suggested before discharging a child or adolescent patient[13] with suicidal ideation or behavior from the emergency department:

1. The patient must not be imminently suicidal.
2. The patient must be medically stable.
3. The patient and the parents agree to return to the emergency department if suicidal intent recurs.
4. The patient must not be intoxicated, delirious, or demented.
5. Potentially lethal means of self-harm have been removed.
6. Treatment of underlying psychiatric diagnoses has been arranged.
7. Acute precipitants to the crisis have been addressed and attempts been undertaken to resolve them.

8. The physician believes that the patient and family will follow through on treatment recommendations.
9. The patient's caregivers and social supports are in agreement with the discharge plans. All of these conditions should be documented.

Adolescents who complete suicide are more likely to have had histories of substance or drug abuse, disruptive disorders, anxiety, mood disorder, or schizophrenia. Precipitating events are usually stressors such as disciplinary crises, being in trouble with the law or at school, or the loss of a relationship. Gender identity concerns are also a precipitant. Table 289-2 summarizes high-risk and low-risk suicide profiles.

Disposition

High-risk patients whose suicide intent is strong and immediate require immediate psychiatric hospitalization. Moderate-risk patients are those who present in a serious suicidal crisis, but who, because of a positive response to initial intervention and favorable social support, are not judged to be in immediate danger. Hospitalization can often be avoided with such patients, provided practical outpatient treatment can be established immediately. Such determinations are most often made in concert with a psychiatric consultant. Available means of suicide,

TABLE 289-2 Evaluation of Suicide Risk in Adults and Adolescents

Demographic and Social Profile	High Risk	Lower Risk
Gender	Male	Female
Marital status	Separated, divorced, or widowed	Married
Family history	Chaotic, conflictual Family history of suicide	Stable
Job	Unemployed	Employed
Relationships	Recent conflict or loss of a relationship	Stable relationships
School	In disciplinary trouble	No disciplinary problems
Religion	Weak or no suicide taboo	Strong taboo against suicide
Health		
Physical	Acute or chronic illness	Good health
	Excessive drug or alcohol use	Little or no drug or alcohol use
Mental	Depression (Sig ECAPS)*	No depression
	Schizophrenia or bipolar history	No psychosis
	Panic disorder	Minimal anxiety
	Disruptive behavior	Directable, oriented
	Feelings of helplessness or hopelessness	Has hope
Suicide ideation	Frequent, intense, prolonged	Infrequent, low intensity, transient
Suicide attempts	Repeated attempts	No prior attempts
	Realistic plan	No plan
	High risk	High likelihood of rescue
	Guilt	Embarrassment about suicide ideation
	Continuing wish to die	No continuing wish to die
Other	Lack of concern	Good insight
	Unsupportive family	Concerned family
	Socially isolated	Socially integrated

*Sig ECAPS is an aid to remembering 8 symptoms of depression: S-sleep disturbance; I-loss of interest; G-guilt; E-loss of energy; C-inability to concentrate; A-loss of appetite; P-psychomotor slowing; S-suicidal thoughts.

such as firearms or drug supplies, should be removed from the patient's access, and any psychotropic medication should be prescribed conservatively (usually no more than a 2-week supply). It is important to have a family member take charge of a patient's medications.

Before discharging a patient, the physician must be certain that the patient has a good social support system in place. The support system usually includes a place to live and family or friends who will support the patient emotionally, and that one or more of these people will be with the patient for the next 24 h.

Low-risk patients frequently present with suicidal threats or minor attempts that occur in the context of a clearly definable external crisis. Social support is usually available and responsive. However, because many attempts that appear trivial on first glance are found to have more serious implications on closer examination, all patients presenting following a suicide attempt should be carefully assessed. If there is any question about the safety of discharging a suicidal patient, and psychiatric consultation is not immediately available, the patient should be hospitalized.

REFERENCES

1. Centers for Disease Control: Nonfatal self-inflicted injuries treated in hospital emergency departments—United States, 2000. *MMWR* 51(20):429, 2002.
2. Drugs that may cause psychiatric symptoms. *Med Lett* 44:59, 2002.
3. D'Onofrio GD, Degutis LC: Preventive care in the emergency department: Screening and brief intervention for alcohol problems in the emergency department, a systematic review. *Acad Emerg Med* 9(6):627, 2002.
4. Tintinalli JE, Peacock FW, Wright MA: Emergency medical evaluation of psychiatric patients. *Ann Emerg Med* 22(4):859, 1994.
5. Reeves RR, Pendarvis EJ, Kimble R: Unrecognized medical emergencies admitted to psychiatric units. *Am J Emerg Med* 18 (4):391, 2000.
6. Marsh C: Psychiatric presentations of medical illness. *Psychiatr Clin North Am* 20(1):181, 1997.
7. Korn CS, Currier GW, Henderson SO: Medical clearance of psychiatric patients without medical complaints in the emergency department. *J Emerg Med* 18(2):173, 2000.
8. Hustey F, Meldon SW: The prevalence and documentation of impaired mental status in elderly emergency department patients. *Ann Emerg Med* 39(3):248, 2002.
9. Fabacher DA, Roccio-Robak N, McErlean MA, Verdile VP: Validation of a brief screening tool to detect depression in elderly ED patients. *Am J Emerg Med* 20(2):99, 2002.
10. Maser JD, Akisal HS, Schettler P, et al: Can temperament identify affectively ill patients who engage in lethal or near-lethal behavior? A 14-year prospective Study. *Suicide Life Threat Behav* 32(1):10, 2002.
11. Jamison UR, Baldessarini RJ: Effects of medical interventions on suicidal behavior. *J Clin Psychiatry* 60(Suppl 2):3, 1999.
12. Stanford EJ, Goetz RR, Bloom JD: The no harm contract in the emergency assessment of suicidal risk. *J Clin Psychiatry* 55:344, 1994.
13. Schaffer D, Craft L: Methods of adolescent suicide prevention. *J Clin Psychiatry* 60(Suppl 2):70, 1999.

PSYCHOTROPIC MEDICATIONS
Richard A. Nockowitz
Douglas A. Rund

The emergency physician should be familiar with the emergency indications, common side effects, toxic reactions, and common interactions of the psychotropic medications. Caution in prescribing is the rule. Patients with medical disorders, a history of serious side effects with psychotropic medication, or apparent need for more than one psychoactive medication usually require psychiatric consultation.

There are four major classes of psychotropic medications dealt with here: antipsychotics, anxiolytics/sedative-hypnotics, antidepressants, and mood stabilizers such as lithium and anticonvulsants. There

are multiple indications for several of these medications, particularly the antidepressants and anticonvulsants. However, only the antipsychotic and anxiolytic classes have undisputed emergency utility.

Antidepressants and lithium are rarely prescribed by the emergency physician, primarily because they have long latencies of action and multiple side effects and require careful long-term monitoring. Only in exceptional circumstances, in consultation with a psychiatrist who agrees to provide follow-up care, might the emergency physician elect to initiate antidepressant or lithium therapy. Extensive pretreatment evaluation and detailed patient education weigh heavily against prescribing lithium, monoamine oxidase inhibitors (MAOIs), or heterocyclic antidepressants in the emergency department.

ANTIPSYCHOTICS (NEUROLEPTICS)

Indications

Because antipsychotic medications are symptom-specific (not disease-specific), they are useful in nearly all psychoses, whether primary (a result of psychiatric illness) or secondary (substance-induced or because of a general medical condition). In the emergency setting, they are most often indicated to control agitated or psychotic behavior that constitutes an imminent danger to the patient or others.

A known allergy to a specific antipsychotic medication is a contraindication to its use and to use of other antipsychotic medications of the same class. Most patients who claim to be allergic to antipsychotic medications, however, actually describe a history of acute dystonic reactions when questioned more carefully.

Guidelines and Rapid Tranquilization

Low-potency antipsychotics (Table 290-1) such as chlorpromazine and thioridazine may cause significant hypotension and thus are rarely used in emergency medicine. High-potency antipsychotics such

TABLE 290-1   Commonly Used Antipsychotic Agents

Generic Name	Brand Name	Approximate Equivalent Dose, mg	Relative Potency
Phenothiazines			
Aliphatic			
Chlorpromazine	Thorazine	100	Low
Triflupromazine	Vesprine	30	Low
Piperidines			
Mesoridazine	Serentil	50	Intermediate
Thioridazine	Mellaril	100	Intermediate
Piperazines			
Acetophenazine	Tindal	15	Intermediate
Perphenazine	Trilafon	10	Intermediate
Trifluoperazine	Stelazine	5	High
Fluphenazine	Prolixin, Permitil	2	High
Thioxanthines			
Aliphatic			
Chlorprothixene	Taractan	100	Low
Piperazine			
Thiothixene	Navane	4	High
Dibenzapine			
Loxapine	Loxitane, Daxolin	15	Intermediate
Dihydroindolones			
Molindone	Moban	10	Intermediate
Butyrophenones			
Haloperidol	Haldol	2	High
Droperidol	Inapsine (for injection)	2	High

as haloperidol and fluphenazine have relatively few anticholinergic and alpha-blocking effects and are remarkably safe, even at high doses. They have traditionally been the emergency antipsychotic agents of choice.

Haloperidol is given IV but only the IM use is U.S. Food and Drug Administration (USDA) approved. One advantage of using haloperidol IV is the relatively low incidence of extrapyramidal side effects compared with the incidence seen with IM or oral routes of administration. The onset of action of IM haloperidol is typically 10 to 20 min. Haloperidol can cause extrapyramidal symptoms and signs and should not be given to those with Parkinson disease or other movement disorders, anticholinergic toxicity, or phencyclidine (PCP) overdose. It is not recommended in pregnant or nursing women. The initial dosage of oral or IM haloperidol ranges from 1 to 5 mg in adults. Lower initial doses are used if the patient is elderly, debilitated, brain injured or has AIDS.

Rapid Tranquilization

Rapid tranquilization is a method of pharmacologic management of acute agitation or psychosis using a high-potency neuroleptic such as haloperidol IV or IM (Table 290-2). The combination of a neuroleptic, haloperidol, and a benzodiazepine anxiolytic, lorazepam is often used and may be more effective in combination than either single agent used alone.[1] Oral dosing is acceptable and enables the patient to participate in the initial care plan. Parenteral administration may be the only available route, however, if the patient will not accept oral medication. For rapid tranquilization, certain target behavioral features such as agitation, violent behavior, or hostility are identified. An initial dose of 2 to 5 mg is given IM. Symptoms are reevaluated in 30 to 45 min and the dose may be repeated if target symptoms continue. The dosage may be repeated in another 30 to 45 min and symptoms reevaluated. Psychiatric evaluation and consultation should be obtained during the process. A general rule is that no more than six doses are given in the first 24 h of treatment.

Another technique for rapid tranquilization is to begin with haloperidol 2 mg in adults and double the dose every 45 min until the symptoms are controlled, the patient is calmed, or the behavior is stabilized. In this approach one does not think of the dosages as cumulative but rather determines the one single dose that effectively treats the symptoms. Once this is accomplished, use the particular effective dose on an "as needed" basis each time the patient's symptoms reappear.

Lorazepam is a benzodiazepine with a wide therapeutic index, rapid onset of action, and ease of administration by the parenteral or oral route. Lorazepam is the only benzodiazepine that can be reliably administered IM, and its oral and parenteral potencies do not greatly differ, allowing for ease in dosage calculation. Benzodiazepines are the preferred agents for the treatment of agitation associated with co-caine intoxication and alcohol withdrawal. An initial dose of lorazepam 2 mg IM or IV is typically administered to adults and 1 to 2 mg is typically administered to the elderly. The dose can be repeated in a half hour. Lorazepam and haloperidol may be mixed in the same syringe (typically combined as lorazepam 2 mg and haloperidol 5 mg). There is a synergistic effect between the two medications. Additionally, the benzodiazepine may prevent the potential extrapyramidal problems that occasionally occur with neuroleptic use.

Droperidol is a butyrophenone derivative similar to haloperidol that has been used extensively in emergency department for the treatment of acute agitation and violent behavior. Traditional doses of droperidol range from 2.5 to 5 mg given IM or IV. Side effects include dystonia, akathisia, and hypotension, which are usually managed with IV fluids. Reports of QT prolongation and torsades de pointes resulted in official warning regarding its use, even though recent reports suggest safety and efficacy when used in appropriate dosages in the ED.[2–5]

Side Effects

Antipsychotics block dopamine receptors throughout the central nervous system (CNS). Dopamine receptor blockade in the mesolimbic areas accounts for their antipsychotic properties. Dopamine blockade in the nigrostriatal tract is responsible for the majority of motor side effects, including acute dystonias, akathisia, and Parkinson syndrome.

ACUTE DYSTONIA Acute dystonias, which usually occur in young males during the trial phase of antipsychotic treatment, are probably the most common side effect of antipsychotic medications seen in the ED. Muscle spasms of the neck, face, and back are the most common dystonias, but oculogyric crisis and even laryngospasm may also occur. When a drug history is not carefully obtained, dystonias are often misdiagnosed as primary neurologic illnesses (seizures, meningitis, tetanus, etc.). Treatment with either benztropine 1 to 2 mg IV or diphenhydramine 50 to 100 mg IV rapidly corrects the dystonia. Dystonias often recur, however, even if the antipsychotic is decreased or discontinued, unless an antiparkinsonian drug such as benztropine, 1 mg PO two to four times daily, is administered over the next several days.

AKATHISIA Akathisia, a sensation of motor restlessness with a subjective desire to move, can begin several days to several weeks after initiation of antipsychotic treatment. Often misdiagnosed as anxiety or exacerbation of psychiatric illness, akathisia is aggravated by subsequent increases in antipsychotic dosage. Other coexisting extrapyramidal effects, such as cogwheel rigidity and shuffling gait, suggest antipsychotic effect, but these signs are not invariably present. Management can be difficult, but some useful strategies are known. If possible, the dosage of the antipsychotic should be decreased. The best treatment is probably administration of β-blockers. Propanolol 30 to 60 mg per d is a good starting dose. Some patients need 90 to 180 mg/d per d as blood pressure and heart rate allow. Antiparkinsonian or anticholinergic drugs such as benztropine 1 mg PO 2 to 4 times daily may also afford some relief. In refractory cases, the antipsychotic may need to be changed to an atypical agent, as discussed below.

PARKINSONISM Antipsychotic-induced Parkinson syndrome is particularly common in the elderly and usually begins in the first month of treatment. A complete Parkinson syndrome—including bradykinesia, resting tremor, cogwheel rigidity, shuffling gait, masked facies, and drooling—can occur, but often only one or two features of the syndrome are obvious. Antipsychotic dosage reduction and/or anticholinergic medication is usually effective.

Whereas antidopaminergic extrapyramidal side effects (EPS) such as acute dystonia, akathisia, and parkinsonism occur more often with high-potency neuroleptics, anticholinergic and antiadrenergic effects are more commonly seen with low-potency neuroleptics. Both anticholinergic and

---

TABLE 290-2   Management of Acute Agitation or Violent Behavior Using Rapid Tranquilization

1. Identify target symptoms to be brought under control: violent or agitated behavior, hostility, tension.
2. Identify contraindications to haloperidol (previous allergy, pregnancy, overdose with anticholinergics, Parkinson disease or other movement disorders, PCP toxicity).
3. If no contraindications, administer haloperidol IM (or IV)
   Haloperidol: 1–2 mg in the elderly
           5 mg in normal sized adult
   Lorazepam: 1–2 mg in the elderly
           2–4 mg in normal sized adult
4. Observe patient for 30–45 min for resolution of target symptoms and behavioral control.
5. Repeat dosing at 30–45 min if symptoms not under control.
6. Usually reassess after 3 doses of medication. Obtain psychiatric consultation. No more than 6 doses usually given in 24 h.

alpha-blocking effects are dose-related and much more common in the elderly.

ANTICHOLINERGIC EFFECTS   Anticholinergic effects range from mild sedation to delirium. Peripheral manifestations may include dry mouth and skin, blurred vision, urinary retention, constipation, paralytic ileus, cardiac dysrhythmias, and exacerbation of narrow-angle glaucoma. The central anticholinergic syndrome is characterized by dilated pupils, dysarthria, and an agitated delirium. Discontinuation of the antipsychotic and institution of supportive measures is the most prudent therapy.

CARDIOVASCULAR EFFECTS   Cardiovascular side effects are seen almost exclusively with low-potency antipsychotics. The exception to this is the rare occurrence of torsades de pointes caused by high dosages of high-potency neuroleptics such as haloperidol and droperidol. The majority of reported cases occurred in the context of a prolonged QT_c interval (≥ 500 ms) prior to starting the medicine or prolongation of the QT_c by greater than 25 percent consequent to initiating haldol or droperidol. Thus underlying presence of such QT_c prolongation should caution the physician about further use of the medicine. α-Adrenergic blockade and a negative inotropic effect on the myocardium may cause pronounced orthostatic hypotension and, rarely, cardiovascular collapse. Usually the hypotension can be easily managed with intravenous fluid. In severe cases, vasopressor support may be required.

NEUROLEPTIC MALIGNANT SYNDROME   Neuroleptic malignant syndrome (NMS) is an uncommon idiosyncratic reaction to neuroleptic drugs manifested by rigidity, fever, autonomic instability (tachycardia, diaphoresis, and blood pressure abnormalities), and a confusional state. Elevation of creatinine phosphokinase, aldolase, the white blood cell count, and liver function tests are often seen. While high-potency antipsychotics may be more likely to cause the disorder, all antipsychotics are potential offenders. NMS is a medical emergency and has a mortality rate as high as 20 percent. Management includes immediate discontinuation of the antipsychotic medication, hydration, and meticulous supportive treatment in an intensive care setting. Anticholinergic medications are not helpful and may worsen the condition by further impairing centrally mediated temperature regulation. Medications such as dantrolene sodium or bromocriptine are sometimes used to relieve the rigidity. See Chap. 159 for a detailed discussion.

Overdose

While antipsychotics are rarely fatal when taken alone, overdose can present some unique management problems. With the exception of thioridazine (Mellaril), antipsychotics are potent antiemetics. Agents with β-agonist activity such as isoproterenol are contraindicated for cardiovascular support because β-stimulated vasodilatation may worsen hypotension. Extrapyramidal effects may also be prominent in antipsychotic overdosage and are best treated with diphenhydramine (Benadryl) 50 to 100 mg IV.

ATYPICAL AGENTS

Clozapine

Clozapine is an "atypical" antipsychotic medication in that it is preferentially more active at limbic than at striatal dopamine receptors and causes few or no EPS. Unfortunately, it may produce agranulocytosis, so its use is reserved for patients with schizophrenia unresponsive to standard agents and for those suffering from severe EPS or tardive dyskinesia with the standard agents. Use of clozapine requires weekly CBCs the first 6 months of use and then every 2 weeks after that. Any

white blood cell count less than 3500 requires closer monitoring, whereas a white blood cell count less than 2000 or absolute granulocyte count less than 1000 mandates immediate discontinuation of the drug and consultation with a hematologist. Fever may be a side effect during the first few weeks of therapy and should prompt an immediate CBC. If the CBC is normal, the fever will typically reverse. Clozapine is strongly sedating, strongly anticholinergic, and has considerable hypotensive effects. It also poses a substantial risk for inducing seizures, particularly when higher doses are used. Respiratory depression and arrest have been rarely reported, and there is a suggestion that coprescription of a benzodiazepine may increase the risk for this side effect.

Commonly reported features of overdose include altered sensorium (drowsiness, delirium, and coma), tachycardia, hypotension, respiratory depression and failure, hypersalivation, and seizures. Management, in addition to administration of activated charcoal, is symptomatic and supportive. Epinephrine and its derivatives should be avoided, as should antidysrhythmics such as procainamide and quinidine. Close surveillance, including cardiac and vital sign monitoring, should continue for several days because of risk of delayed toxic effects. Fatal overdosages have been reported, usually at dosages greater than 2500 mg.

Risperidone

Risperidone is another "atypical" antipsychotic medication whose pharmacologic profile of potent serotonin ($5\text{-}HT_2$) antagonism and moderate dopamine (D_2) antagonism probably accounts for its relatively lower risk of EPS. Unlike clozapine, it does not have increased risk of agranulocytosis. Common side effects include sedation, insomnia, constipation, and weight gain. Cardiovascular effects may include small, short-term increases in heart rate, accompanied by reduced systolic/diastolic blood pressure, orthostatic hypotension, and QT-interval prolongation. Seizures have been reported in 0.3 percent of patients.

Features of overdose generally reflect exaggerated pharmacologic effects: drowsiness, sedation, tachycardia, hypotension, EPS, prolonged QT, widened QRS and, in several instances, seizure. Management is basically supportive. Cardiovascular monitoring is imperative. Should antidysrhythmic therapy be required, agents such as disopyramide, procainamide, and quinidine, which have the potential for QT-prolonging effects, should be avoided. As with more traditional antipsychotics, agents that may worsen effects of β-adrenergic blockade, such as bretylium, epinephrine, and dopamine, should also be avoided. An IM preparation of risperidone is currently available for emergency use. Although proven effective for controlling acute agitation, it is this author's opinion that it is a second-line agent due to its cost. The inexpensive traditional neuroleptics described earlier are very effective and relatively safe, with potential side effects that are easily recognized and managed.

Olanzapine

Olanzapine has a chemical profile very similar to that of clozapine and thus causes little or no EPS. It also has the advantage of not being known to cause agranulocytosis and thus does not require monitoring of the white blood count. Its main adverse effects can include considerable weight gain, sedation, and mild anticholinergic activity. There is limited experience at this time about effects of overdose, but exacerbation of brain side effects such as somnolence and anticholinergic signs would be expected. At the time of this writing, an intramuscular form of olanzapine is about to come to market. There is an intramuscular preparation of olanzapine being tested at the time of this writing. Although likely to be effective for controlling agitation, the above comments for risperidone about its place in emergency medicine hold true for this medication as well.

Quetiapine

Quetiapine (Seroquel) is yet another atypical antipsychotic agent and, like the others, is characterized by a high 5-HT$_2$/D$_2$ binding ratio, responsible for its low incidence of EPS, while maintaining its antipsychotic effect. It has a high affinity for histaminic and α-adrenergic receptors, however, causing prominent adverse effects of sedation, orthostatic hypotension, and some dizziness. Again, experience is limited about effects of quetiapine in overdose.

Ziprasidone

Ziprasidone (Geodon), the most recent atypical antipsychotic available in the U.S. market, has similar receptor binding to risperidone. There is also an intramuscular preparation being used, which some say could eventually replace haloperidol as the agent of choice in the acute management of the agitated psychotic patient.[6,7] Ziprasidone has a similar side effect profile to risperidone. Some advise that ziprasidone should be reserved for cases where a typical antipsychotic cannot be used. The initial dose of ziprasidone is 20 mg IM. A second dose of 20 mg can be given in 4 h raising questions about the emergency physician's ability to "titrate" the dose as one does with haloperidol.

The atypical agents also have the potential to cause QT$_c$ prolongation and therefore carry the theoretical risk of related complications, as reported for the older agents.

ANXIOLYTICS

Indications

Severe emotional distress may indicate a need for psychotropic medication, even if the patient is not psychotic or an imminent threat to him- or herself or others. While not a substitute for psychotherapy, short-term anxiolytic therapy may be particularly beneficial in the anxious, agitated patient during a psychosocial crisis. Anxiolytics are also indicated for acute panic reactions unresponsive to reassurance.

Anxiolytics have utility in medical and surgical emergencies as well. Nonpsychiatric uses include facilitation of cooperation and muscle relaxation during painful procedures; controlling seizures; treating alcohol, sedative, or hypnotic withdrawal; and allaying anxiety when a painful procedure such as surgery has been delayed.

Benzodiazepines are contraindicated in patients with known hypersensitivity to benzodiazepines and in acute, narrow-angle glaucoma. Pregnancy, particularly in the first trimester, is a relative contraindication.

Guidelines

Before prescribing anxiolytics, the emergency physician should try to rule out any serious underlying psychiatric illness. Because agitation and anxiety may indicate incipient psychosis or major affective disorder, anxiolytics should be used with extreme caution in patients with a history of major psychiatric illness. The possibility that a patient may be feigning illness to procure controlled substances should also be considered.

Benzodiazepines are very effective anxiolytics with a high therapeutic index. Nonbenzodiazepine anxiolytics (e.g., barbiturates and propanediols) have low therapeutic indices and high addiction potential. Except in the rare case of an allergy to benzodiazepines, nonbenzodiazepine anxiolytics have little use in modern psychopharmacology. Buspirone hydrochloride (BuSpar), an atypical anxiolytic medication that does not interact with the benzodiazepine–γ-aminobutyric acid (GABA) receptor complex, has a delayed onset of action of days to weeks, which makes it impractical for use in emergent situations. Because it does not have cross-tolerance with other sedative/hypnotics or alcohol, it is not useful in treatment of sedative/hypnotic or alcohol withdrawal.

Certain benzodiazepines have relatively long half-lives (Table 290-3), including diazepam, chlordiazepoxide, flurazepam, and prazepam. Agents with long half-lives gradually accumulate in the body and thus have a greater potential for causing sedation and confusion, particularly in the elderly. For short-term use, these agents may benefit the young, healthy person in crisis who complains of insomnia but who is also anxious during the day. A single bedtime dose both induces sleep and has a mild anxiolytic effect the following day. For the most part, however, with the exception of the use of diazepam in seizures, short-acting benzodiazepines such as lorazepam, oxazepam, and alprazolam are the preferred agents in emergency medicine. Alprazolam, 0.25 to 0.50 mg PO, is a particularly effective treatment in acute panic attack. Lorazepam, an agent with very low cardiopulmonary toxicity, is particularly well suited for emergency use. Dosages of 1 to 2 mg PO or IM are usually effective. Only midazolam, a very short-acting agent, and lorazepam have reliable intramuscular absorption. As with all benzodiazepines, dosage adjustments may be necessary: higher dosages may be required in patients with histories of alcohol or sedative/hypnotic abuse; lower dosages in patients with hepatic disease or severe debilitation. Because they potentiate other CNS depressants, benzodiazepines should be used with extreme caution in intoxicated patients. Benzodiazepines particularly suppress hypoxic respiratory drive and should be used with caution in patients with hypercarbia, especially if the patient is also receiving supplemental oxygen.

Side Effects

Benzodiazepine side effects are usually mild and easily treated. Drowsiness, decreased mental alertness, sedation, and ataxia are the most common side effects. Such effects can usually be managed conservatively by decreasing the dose and advising the patient to avoid potentially hazardous activities, such as driving or operating dangerous machinery. Excessive sedation and overdose can be reversed with flumazenil by giving 0.2 mg IV over 15 to 30 s and then 0.2 to 0.4 mg every 30 to 60 s up to 3 mg total dose, depending on the circumstances. Its use should be limited due to potential for significant adverse events. This is contraindicated, however, in mixed overdoses and chronic benzodiazepine use. Infrequent paradoxical responses to benzodiazepines of insomnia and agitation are more common in the elderly and require discontinuation of the medication. Because benzodiazepines have abuse potential and high street value, the emergency physician should never prescribe more than a week's supply.

TABLE 290-3   Commonly Used Benzodiazepines

Generic Name	Brand Name	Approximate Half-Life, h	Usual Total Oral Dose, mg
ANXIOLYTICS*			
Alprazolam	Xanax	12	1–6
Chlorazepate	Tranxene	48	15–60
Chlordiazepoxide	Librium	20	15–60
Diazepam	Valium	35	15–60
Lorazepam	Ativan	16	2–6
Midazolam	Versed	2	‡
Oxazepam	Serax	15	20–60
Prazepam	Centrax	15†, 100†	20–60
HYPNOTICS			
Flurazepam	Dalmane	2†, 72†	15–30 qhs
Temazepam	Restoril	15	15–30 qhs
Trizolam	Halcion	2	0.125–0.5 qhs

*Anxiolytics are administered in divided doses, usually three or four times daily.

†Flurazepam and prazepam have active metabolites with long half-lives.

‡Midazolam is available for parenteral use only.

HETEROCYCLIC ANTIDEPRESSANTS

Although tricyclic antidepressants (named for their three-ring structure) were first synthesized in the nineteenth century, their antidepressant properties were not recognized until the late 1950s. Since that time, other "cyclic" antidepressant agents have been formulated thus creating need for the more general term *heterocyclic* (Table 290-4). The therapeutic effect of heterocyclic antidepressants (HCAs) is believed to be related to secondary downregulation of norepinephrine and serotonin postsynaptic receptors after initial blockade of presynaptic reuptake of norepinephrine and serotonin. HCAs are primarily indicated for major depression, but may also be effective for dysthymic disorder, panic disorder, agoraphobia, obsessive compulsive disorder, enuresis, and school phobia. As previously advised, initiation of HCA therapy in the emergency department is not routinely recommended.

Side Effects

HCAs have low therapeutic indices. Side effects are common and often occur with customary dosages, even though serum levels may be within the designated therapeutic range. The majority of side effects are either anticholinergic or cardiotoxic.

ANTICHOLINERGIC EFFECTS   Anticholinergic side effects are the most common. They are particularly likely to occur with concomitant use of other drugs with anticholinergic properties, such as low-potency antipsychotics, antiparkinsonian agents, antihistamines, and over-the-counter sleeping remedies. Both peripheral and central effects may occur. Peripheral effects include dry mouth, metallic taste, blurred vision, constipation, paralytic ileus, urinary retention, tachycardia, and exacerbation of narrow-angle glaucoma. Central effects include sedation, mydriasis, agitation, and delirium. Mild to moderately severe anticholinergic effects may be managed by dosage reduction, change to a medication with fewer anticholinergic properties, or addition of urecholine, 10 to 25 mg PO three times daily. For acute urinary retention, urecholine, 2.5 to 5 mg may be given SC.

CARDIOVASCULAR EFFECTS   Cardiac side effects of HCAs may include nonspecific T-wave changes, prolonged QT interval, varying degrees of atrioventricular block, and atrial and ventricular dysrhythmias. Orthostatic hypotension from α-adrenergic blockade may be significant, particularly in the elderly (see Chaps. 158 and 159).

HCA therapy may also be complicated by allergic obstructive jaundice, decreased seizure threshold (especially with maprotiline, clomipramine, and amoxapine), and, very rarely, agranulocytosis.

TABLE 290-4   Commonly Used Heterocyclic Antidepressants

Generic Name	Brand Name	Usual Dose mg/d
TRICYCLICS		
Amitriptyline	Amitril, Elavil, Endep	75–200
Amoxapine	Asendin	100–300
Desipramine	Norpramin, Pertofrane	75–200
Doxepin	Adapin, Curetin, Sinequan	75–200
Imipramine	Janimine, Presamine, SK-Pramine, Tofranil	75–200
Nortriptyline	Aventyl, Pamelor	40–150
Pritriptyline	Vivactil	15–40
Trimipramine	Surmontil	75–200
OTHERS		
Maprotiline	Ludiomil	100–150
Trazodone	Desyrel	100–200

Trazodone has little in common with other HCAs. It lacks significant anticholinergic or cardiac conduction effects but may be associated with marked sedation, ventricular dysrhythmias, and significant orthostatic hypotension. It may also cause priapism.

MONOAMINE OXIDASE INHIBITORS

Monoamine oxidase catalyzes the oxidation of biogenic amines (tyramine, serotonin, dopamine, and norepinephrine) throughout the body. The therapeutic effect of MAOIs is probably related to their ability to increase norepinephrine and serotonin in the CNS. They are recommended for atypical major depressive episodes, characterized by hyperphagia, hypersomnolence, reversed diurnal variation (worse in the evening), emotional lability, so-called leaden paralysis (heavy leaden feelings in arms or legs), and rejection hypersensitivity. They are also occasionally useful in selected cases of HCA-refractory major depression and panic disorder. Only two agents in this class, phenelzine and tranylcypromine, are commonly used in the United States. As with HCAs, initiation of therapy in the emergency department is not recommended. The physician who initiates MAOI therapy must have firmly established an appropriate indication for use and provided the patient with extensive counseling about toxic interactions with numerous medications and foods.

Side Effects

In general, MAOIs have fewer side effects than do HCAs. Orthostatic hypotension, although occasionally severe, usually responds to supportive therapy. CNS irritability, including agitation, motor restlessness, and insomnia, is managed by dosage reduction or addition of a benzodiazepine. Occasionally, MAOIs, like other antidepressant medications, actually precipitate a manic episode. Autonomic side effects, such as dry mouth, constipation, urinary retention, and delayed ejaculation, sometimes occur but are usually mild.

MAOIs block oxidative deamination of tyramine and may precipitate a hypertensive crisis when certain drugs, such as sympathomimetic amines, levodopa (L-dopa), narcotics, or HCAs, or tyramine-containing foods are ingested. Common tyramine-containing foods include aged cheese, beer, wine, pickled herring, yeast extracts, chopped liver, yogurt, sour cream, and fava beans. The onset of the crisis is usually heralded by a severe headache. While hypertension is potentially the most serious effect, cardiac dysrhythmias, restlessness, diaphoresis, mydriasis, and vomiting may also occur. Beta-blocking agents are contraindicated, because they may intensify vasoconstriction and worsen hypertension. Although death may occur from hypertensive intracranial hemorrhage, the vast majority of patients recover completely from the hypertensive episode within a few hours. The MAOI can be restarted the following day after dietary counseling is reinforced.

Drug-drug interactions often complicate MAOI therapy. MAOIs potentiate the actions of sympathomimetics, anticholinergics, and oral hypoglycemics. They also inhibit metabolic degradation of alcohol, barbiturates, and narcotics. When combined with meperidine, MAOIs may cause a variety of adverse effects, including hypotension, hypertension, fever, and neuromuscular irritability. While the interactions listed are among the most common, the list is far from exhaustive. More comprehensive accounts may be found in standard references.

SELECTIVE SEROTONIN REUPTAKE INHIBITORS

Since the introduction of fluoxetine in 1988, the selective serotonin reuptake inhibitors (SSRIs) have become the most commonly prescribed antidepressants in the United States. Other SSRIs currently available include sertraline, paroxetine, fluvoxamine, citalopram, and escitalopram. SSRIs are primarily indicated for treatment of major depressive episodes but are also useful in dysthymia and in anxiety disorders, including generalized anxiety disorder, panic disorder, and obsessive-compulsive disorder. Because of their favorable side effect profile and relative safety in overdose, some have argued that institution of an SSRI by an emergency department physician may occasionally be appropriate if (1) the patient can be assessed to rule out general medical causes for the depression, (2) ongoing substance abuse can be ruled out, and (3) the patient can be followed in the emergency setting until picked up by another health care provider. However, this rationale has rightly been questioned because of the concern over SSRIs and other antidepressants precipitating mania. The detection of bipolar disorder, because of its many variations and subtle forms, requires evaluation by an experienced psychiatrist. All antidepressants carry some degree of risk for precipitating a manic or mixed episode in a patient predisposed to bipolar illness.

Side Effects

SSRIs lack the anticholinergic and cardiac effects typical of the HCAs, although there are several reports of symptomatic bradycardia with fluoxetine. The side-effect profile of SSRIs reflect their potent serotonin antagonism. Among the most common side effects are headaches, dizziness, sexual dysfunction, nausea, diarrhea, insomnia, and agitation. Less-common side effects are akithisia and apathy syndrome. A significant advantage of SSRIs is their high therapeutic index and associated low lethality, even when large quantities are ingested acutely.

An SSRI discontinuation syndrome has become apparent, more commonly with agents having a shorter half-life (e.g., sertraline, paroxetine). It typically presents several days after cessation of one drug and is characterized by a flulike syndrome, including nausea, vomiting, fatigue, myalgias, vertigo, headache, insomnia, and sometimes paresthesias. Treatment is to reinstate SSRI therapy and taper more gradually.

A serotonin syndrome with SSRIs can occur when SSRIs are combined with other serotonergic medications such as the MAOIs. The syndrome is manifest by both CNS (restlessness, tremor, myoclonus, hyperreflexia, and seizures) and gastrointestinal (nausea, vomiting, diarrhea) irritability. Consequently, SSRIs or any medication that enhances serotonin levels should not be combined with MAOIs. Treatment of the serotonin syndrome consists of discontinuing the serotonergic agents and providing supportive care.

NEWER "COMBINATION" ANTIDEPRESSANTS

Whereas most tricyclic antidepressants enhance norepinephrine levels, SSRIs enhance serotonin levels, and psychostimulants (a category not discussed here) enhance dopamine levels. The newer antidepressants evidence "combinations" of these effects through various mechanisms. Examples of this include venlafaxine, bupropion, nefazodone, and mirtazapine.

Venlafaxine (Effexor)

Venlafaxine, which is structurally distinct from other antidepressants, is conceptually a combination of a tricyclic and an SSRI in that it enhances both serotonin and norepinephrine (as well as dopamine slightly) through reuptake blockade. Its advantages are relative freedom from medication interactions and no significant affinity for muscarinic, histaminic, and α-adrenergic receptors. Although lack of blockade for various receptors improves its side-effect profile somewhat, common complaints include agitation and insomnia, nausea, occasional dizziness, constipation, and sweating. Potential problems associated with venlafaxine include dose-related, sustained hypertension and the growing awareness of a significant discontinuation syndrome

requiring very slow tapering of the drug. The hypertension needs to be monitored and may require lowering of the medication. The discontinuation syndrome can be significant. It usually occurs within days to 2 weeks after lowering or stopping the drug and is similar to SSRI discontinuation symptoms. It can be treated with an SSRI or by increasing the venlafaxine and tapering it more slowly. Venlafaxine should not be used in combination with an MAOI.

Bupropion (Wellbutrin)

Bupropion is also structurally unique and works by initiating reuptake inhibition of both norepinephrine and dopamine, the former more than the latter. It also interacts with few other medications and has a favorable side-effect profile because of its minimal anticholinergic and antihistaminic effects. It is also being used as an aid in smoking cessation.[8]

Common side effects include some initial restlessness and insomnia that typically resolves within 2 weeks. It is noted for having the lowest incidence of sexual side effects, which are common with other antidepressants, including SSRIs. In fact, when bupropion is added for SSRI-induced sexual dysfunction, sexual functioning improves in many patients. One concern with this drug had been a dose-related increase in the incidence of seizures. However, further study has shown no higher incidence at usual therapeutic dosages compared with other antidepressants. Caution should be taken when using this drug in patients with bulimia or metabolic disturbances predisposing to seizures. Likewise, individual doses greater than 200 mg and daily dosages greater than 400 mg should be avoided. Combination with an MAOI is to be avoided as well. Bupropion may be the least likely of all antidepressants to precipitate a switch into mania.

Nefazodone (Serzone)

Nefazodone inhibits serotonin reuptake inhibitors and blocks postsynaptic 5-HT$_2$ receptors at the same time. It is similar chemically to trazodone but possesses less α-adrenergic blockade. Common side effects are dizziness, headache, dry mouth, and nausea. Some patients also have problems with orthostatic hypotension and drowsiness. Anxiety is less of a problem with this drug than with SSRIs, and sexual side effects are less common. It may be particularly useful for depression-associated insomnia.

Mirtazapine (Remeron)

Mirtazapine antagonizes inhibitory norepinephrine autoreceptors and heteroreceptors, causing increased release of norepinephrine and serotonin. The main side effects are somnolence, increased appetite, weight gain, and dizziness. Although serotonin enhancement is one of this drug's end results, it is via a very different mechanism, and the typical SSRI side effects are usually minimal. Given the limited clinical experience with this relatively new medication, effects of overdose are not well known.

MOOD STABILIZERS

Although lithium has been the mainstay of bipolar disorder (manic depression) treatment for years, anticonvulsants such as carbamazepine, oxcarbamazepine, valproic acid, gabapentin, lamotrigine, tiagabine, and topiramate have come to play an increasingly important role in the management of this and other neuropsychiatric disturbances.

Lithium

Lithium carbonate is indicated for both acute mania and maintenance therapy in bipolar disorder. It is also useful in some cases of major depression (both unipolar and bipolar), and in some disorders characterized by episodic explosive outbursts or self-mutilation. Its mechanism of action is not exactly known, although it may relate to reducing dopaminergic function, enhancing serotonergic function, or reducing "excessive signaling" by the phosphatidylinositol system. The extensive pretreatment evaluation and long latency of action preclude the use of lithium as an emergency psychotropic medication. The emergency physician should be aware, however, of its side effects and signs of toxicity (see Chap. 162).

SIDE EFFECTS Patients vary widely in susceptibility to lithium side effects. While most of the serious adverse effects are associated with toxic serum levels, mild side effects such as gastrointestinal distress, dry mouth, excessive thirst, fine tremors, mild polyuria, and peripheral edema are often seen even when serum levels lie within the designated therapeutic range. This is particularly common during the first few weeks of therapy. Many of the more chronic side effects, including polyuria, nephrogenic diabetes insipidus, benign diffuse goiter, hypothyroidism, skin rashes and ulcerations, psoriasis, and leukocytosis without a left shift, appear unrelated to serum lithium levels. Underlying neurologic illness, dehydration, salt-restricted diets, and childbirth predispose to both minor and major side effects.

TOXICITY AND OVERDOSE The severity of lithium toxicity is related to both the serum lithium level and the duration of the elevated level. Even in acute overdose, symptoms may not be fully apparent for up to 48 h. As a general rule, lithium toxicity is rare at serum levels of less than 2 mEq/L. Early signs of toxicity include nausea and vomiting, dysarthria, lethargy, and a coarse hand tremor. As toxicity worsens, neurologic symptoms increase. Ataxia, myasthenia, incoordination, hyperreflexia, muscle fasciculation, blurred vision, and scotomas may develop. Eventually, confusion, choreoathetosis, myoclonus, and seizures occur, and the patient may finally become comatose. Cardiovascular toxicity is unusual at serum levels of less than 4 mEq/L. In addition to nonspecific T-wave changes, high lithium levels may be associated with hypotension, atrioventricular conduction defects, ventricular tachydysrhythmias, and eventually complete cardiovascular collapse.

Because lithium toxicity may result in permanent neurologic sequelae, it should be considered a medical emergency. Chap. 162 discusses management of lithium overdose.[9]

Anticonvulsants

These drugs all act through different mechanisms, such as enhanced GABA inhibitory function or decreased glutamate and aspartate excitatory release, all of which ultimately result in neuronal relaxation or stabilization. They have come to be used for mood stabilization in rapid-cycling, cyclothymic, and mixed states of bipolar illness. Recent studies demonstrate the superiority of anticonvulsants over lithium for such indications. Other uses are for impulsive aggression, behavioral disturbances in head-injured patients and in patients exhibiting self-injurious behavior, and even for the irritability commonly seen in severe personality disorders. The side effects of carbamazepine and valproic acid are well known from their use as anticonvulsants.

Gabapentin is well tolerated, has few drug interactions, and does not need blood-level monitoring. It may be titrated quickly and may be useful for patients already on multiple medications or with hepatic impairment. The main disadvantages are drowsiness, ataxia, and nausea at high dosages.

Lamotrigine is also well tolerated, with few adverse behavioral or cognitive effects. It does have some drug interactions (carbamazepine, valproate) and risk of potentially severe and fatal rash such as Stevens-Johnson syndrome and toxic epidermal necrolysis. The rash is more common in children and seems to be related to starting at too high a dosage, titrating too rapidly, and concomitant valproate therapy. Such a rash dictates immediate cessation of the medication in almost all circumstances. There may be additive toxicity with carbamazepine as well, causing more ataxia and dizziness than when used alone.[10]

At the time of this writing, experience is growing with the various anticonvulsants for anxiety, mood, behavioral, and other psychiatric issues.

REFERENCES

1. Battaglia J, Moss S, Rush J, et al: Haloperidol, lorazepam or both for psychotic agitation. *Am J Emerg Med* 15(4):335, 1997.
2. Chase PB, Biros MH: A retrospective review of the use and safety of droperidol in a large, high-risk, inner-city emergency department patient population. *Acad Emerg Med* 9(1):1402, 2002.
3. Horowitz BZ, Bizovi K, Moreno R: Droperidol—Behind the black box warning. *Acad Emerg Med* 9(6):615, 2002.
4. Richman PB, Allegra J, Eskin B, et al: A randomized clinical trial to assess the efficacy of intramuscular droperidol for the treatment of acute migraine headache. *Am J Emerg Med* 20(1):39, 2002.
5. Droperidol and arrhythmias. *Med Lett* 44:53,2002.
6. Brook S, Lucey JV, Gunn KP: Intramuscular ziprasidone compared with intramuscular haloperidol in the treatment of acute psychosis. Ziprasidone IM Study Group. *J Clin Psychiatry* 61(12):933, 2000.
7. Daniel DG: Ziprasidone: Comprehensive overview and clinical use of a novel antipsychotic. *Expert Opin Invest Drugs* 9(4):819, 2001.
8. Hughs JR, Goldstein MG, Hurt RD: Recent advances in the pharmacotherapy of smoking. *JAMA* 281(1):72, 1999.
9. Marangell LB, Martinez JM, Silver JM, et al. (eds): *Concise Guide to Psychopharmacology.* Arlington, VA: American Psychiatric Association, 2002, www.appi.org.
10. Abramowicz M (ed): Drugs that may cause psychiatric symptoms. *Med Lett* 44:59, 2002.

291

ANOREXIA NERVOSA AND BULIMIA NERVOSA
Alexander H. Sackeyfio
Susan J. Gottlieb

Anorexia nervosa and bulimia nervosa have reached epidemic proportions in the last 10 years. These diseases were once viewed as purely psychological in nature. However, increasing evidence has confirmed that both disorders involve physical complications, and knowledge of and ability to treat the medical complications that accompany eating disorders are crucial for the patient's well-being.

In the United States, eating disorders affect approximately 5 to 10 percent of adolescent girls and young women, and up to 1 percent of males. Eating disorders are now recognized across all socioeconomic and racial groups, in patients between the ages of 8 and 80 years.[1] The onset of anorexia is usually between 12 years of age and the mid-thirties, with a bimodal distribution of ages 13 to 14 and 17 to 18. Bulimia usually begins between the ages of 17 and 25. The onset of both disorders has been reported in older persons.

Anorexia, with its resulting starvation syndrome, is more likely to be recognized than the commoner bulimia, which is frequently concealed from both family and physician. Table 291-1 lists the signs and symptoms that suggest a diagnosis of anorexia, and Table 291-2 lists the signs and symptoms of bulimia.

TABLE 291-1 Clues to Undiagnosed Anorexia Nervosa

Unexplained growth retardation
Unexplained primary amenorrhea
Weight loss of unknown origin
Unexplained hypercholesterolemia or carotenemia in a thin person
Exercise abuse
Membership in a vulnerable vocation group (see Table 291-2)

TABLE 291-2 Signs and Symptoms of Bulimia in Adolescents and Young Adults

Hypokalemia of unknown cause or complications of hypokalemia
Metabolic acidosis, related to laxative abuse/excessive exercise
Parotid gland or submandibular gland enlargement; esophagitis; esophageal bleeding or rupture
Large unexplained weight fluctuations or weight loss
Unexplained elevations of serum amylase
Unexplained secondary amenorrhea
Extensive loss of dental enamel or severe caries onset[7]
Scars on the knuckles of the hand from induced vomiting[15]
Juvenile diabetes mellitus
Other disorders of impulse control (alcoholism, drug abuse, borderline personality)
Member of predisposed vocational group: models, ballet students or professionals, wrestlers, jockeys, athletes[16]

Source: Wells LA, Sadowski CA: Bulimia nervosa: An update and treatment recommendations. *Curr Opin Pediatr* 13:591, 2001.

Anorexic patients[2] may present with one or all of the following:

1. Refusal to maintain body weight over a minimum normal weight for age and height; for example, weight loss or failure to make expected weight gain during a period of growth, leading to body weight 15 percent below normal.
2. Intense fear of becoming obese even when underweight.
3. Disturbance in the way in which body weight, shape, or size is perceived. For example, the obviously underweight or even emaciated patient may complain of being fat, or may believe that one area of the body is "too fat."
4. Absence of at least three consecutive expected menstrual cycles (primary or secondary amenorrhea).

A diagnosis of bulimia[2] is suggested by the following:

1. A minimum average of two episodes of binge eating (rapid consumption of a large amount of food in a short period of time) per week for at least 3 months.
2. During the eating binges, there is a feeling of lack of control over the eating behavior.
3. The individual regularly engages in self-induced vomiting, use of laxatives, strict dieting, fasting, or vigorous exercising in order to prevent weight gain.
4. Persistent overconcern with body shape and weight.

Another diagnosis[2] to be considered is *eating disorder, not otherwise specified.* It is characterized by:

1. For females, all criteria for anorexia except that the patient is still menstruating.
2. All criteria for anorexia except normal weight.
3. All criteria for bulimia but lower frequency or duration.
4. Regular use of compensatory weight control measures after eating a small amount of food.
5. Chewing/spitting out, but not swallowing, large amounts of food.
6. Binge-eating disorder.

The diagnosis of an eating disorder should be considered in a premenarchal patient who engages in potentially unhealthy weight-control practices and/or demonstrates obsessive thinking about food, weight, and height, especially if there is a delay in the maturation for gender and age.

ETIOLOGY

Anorexia nervosa and bulimia nervosa are found in societies that consider fat people as beautiful, attractive, and desirable, not just in societies that emphasize a drive for thinness and firm bodies. Etiologic factors include biological vulnerability, family issues and societal pressures.[3] There is an increased rate in monozygotic twins and in first-degree relatives.

Personality factors that increase susceptibility to anorexia nervosa and bulimia nervosa include perfectionism, obsessive-compulsive disorder, symmetry and exactness and harm avoidance.[4,5] Dysfunctional family dynamics are more common in patients with eating disorders than in controls.

Other factors linked to increased incidence of eating disorders include early menarche, which is also associated with not living with biological father for more than 1 year during childhood. Trauma or stress in early life can increase sensitivity of the anterior pituitary and increased risk for depression and eating disorders.

Neurotransmitters and neuropeptides are also implicated in the predisposition and perpetuation of eating disorders. Serotonin, which is known to be involved in feeding, moods and obsessions, impulse control, and harm avoidance, has been extensively studied. Anorexia is seen as a hyperserotonergic state and bulimia as a hyperserotonergic state.

Anorexia most often begins during adolescence. Normal physiologic changes that are preparation for the reproductive function, namely an increase in total body fat (up to 200 percent in adolescent females) as well as the accumulation of fat around the chest and hips, are perceived as "fatness," and the adolescent begins to diet to lose the unwanted weight. Various reasons have been proposed for the progression of "normal" dieting into an eating disorder. Some feel that for the anorexic, restriction of eating serves as a part of a general need to control impulses and disturbing feelings. Others have suggested that the central problems might be an avoidance of adulthood, an emergent panic related to the challenge of late adolescence and the loss of the security enjoyed by the child and early adolescent.[3,4]

Bulimics have an intense need for approval, a high self-expectation, and a poor body image. Bingeing provides escape from boredom, anger, and loneliness, and is sometimes a preferred social experience, especially when interpersonal intimacy has been elusive. Purging only adds to an already negative self-image. Binge eating in bulimics almost always begins as a response to hunger from dieting and weight loss. Late in the syndrome, binge eating becomes generalized to deal with emotional distress.[3,4]

DIFFERENTIAL DIAGNOSIS

The differential diagnosis includes both psychiatric and medical disorders. Schizophrenics can present with an aversion to eating and sometimes with eating and purging. In depressive illness, anorexia and hyperphagia can be part of the presenting symptoms. Hysterics, inadequate personality disorders, and patients with borderline personality disorders may also exhibit eating disorders.

A number of medical disorders should be considered, including superior mesenteric artery syndrome, inflammatory bowel disease, chronic hepatitis, Addison's disease, diabetes, hyperthyroidism, hyperemesis gravidarum, tuberculosis, and malignancy. Eating disorders may coexist with other conditions, such as adolescent diabetes.

PATHOPHYSIOLOGY

Eating disorders are associated with a number of physiologic changes (Tables 291-3 and 291-4).

Cachetic patients are relatively well adapted to their chronically deprived, mildly catabolic state. The hypothalamus is affected by low fat intake and that disturbs the reproductive, metabolic, growth and neurohypophyseal hormones. There is an associated fall in metabolic rate, protein levels are preserved and cell-mediated immunity tends to be normal.[6]

Self-induced vomiting results in various disorders. Dental problems[7] are caused by gastric acid regurgitation into the oral cavity. In

TABLE 291-3 Physiologic Changes Associated with Eating Disorders

Hematologic
   Normochromic normocytic anemia
   Leukopenia with relative lymphocytosis
   Low sedimentation rate
   Reduced C3 complement
Biochemical
   Hypokalemia
   Hyponatremia
   Hypomagnesemia
   Hypocalcemia
   Hypophosphatemia
   Osteoporosis
Carbohydrate metabolism
   Lower serum insulin levels
   High serum glucagon levels
   Starvation ketosis and hypoglycemia
   Abnormal glucose tolerance as a consequence of fasting
   Hypercholesterolemia
Endocrine
   Normal T4, low T3
   Elevated serum corticol without diurnal variation
   Lower serum LH, FSH, and estradiol
   Low total urinary estrogens
   Increased growth hormone
   Pseudo Bartter syndrome (laxative and diuretic abusers)
   Decreased ADH secretion (diabetes insipidus)
   Decreased peripheral adrenergic activity with normal adrenomedullary
      function
Cutaneous[15]
   Xerosis
   Cheilitis
   Hypertrichosis
   Alopecia
   Dry scalp hair
   Acral coldness or cyanosis
   Periungual erythema
   Gingivitis
   Brittle nails
   Hand calluses
   Bruising

Abbreviations: ADH = antidiuretic hormone; FSH = follicle-stimulating hormone; LH = luteinizing hormone.

TABLE 291-4 Clinical Effects of Eating Disorders

Cardiac: arrhythmias, cardiac arrest, orthostatic hypotension, Q-T prolongation,[17] nonspecific electrocardiogram changes
Gastrointestinal: constipation, ileus, exacerbation of hepatic encephalopathy
Metabolic: glucose intolerance, hypokalemic metabolic alkalosis
Neuromuscular/orthopedic: hypo- or areflexia, paralysis, peripheral neuropathy, respiratory depression, rhabdomyolysis, weakness, pathologic fractures[18]
Renal: decreased urinary concentrating ability; polyuria and polydipsia, nephropathy; myoglobinuria (caused by rhabdomyolysis)

addition, the oral hygiene of most anorexics is poor, and the vigorous brushing often done by bulimics aggravates dental problems. Poor oral hygiene, together with dietary deficiencies and dehydration of the soft tissue of the mouth, can cause gingivitis and dental erosion.

Parotid and submandibular gland enlargement is often seen. Oral lacerations and contusions, and callous formations on knuckles from stimulating the gag reflex, are common. Dysphagia, hematemesis, and, rarely, rupture of the esophagus, subcutaneous emphysema, or pneumomediastinum can occur following excessive purging. Easy bruising because of loss of bile salts and poor absorption of vitamin K is another complication. Severe hypokalemia and hypovolemia often accompany recurrent vomiting. Ipecac abuse can cause dermatomyositis-like syndrome and cardiomyopathy. Hyperamylasemia, probably of salivary gland origin, is associated with purging episodes.

Laxative abuse produces weight loss mainly by dehydration and hypokalemia. Common nonspecific complaints of laxative abuse include constipation, diarrhea, abdominal cramping, and bloating. Severe potassium depletion as a result of chronic laxative abuse and intense physical exercise may contribute to rhabdomyolysis. Specific effects include melanosis coli and cathartic colon. In cathartic colon, the colon is converted into an inert tube incapable of propelling the fecal stream without large doses of laxatives. This condition is not entirely reversible and may require colectomy. Brownish gray hyperpig-

mented areas on the skin are reported as complications of phenolphthalein-containing laxatives (Correctol, Ex-Lax).

Diuretic abuse results in dehydration and multiple serum abnormalities including hypokalemia, hypercalcemia, hyperuricemia, hypomagnesemia, and hyponatremia.

Binge eating after a period of starvation can result in acute gastric distention and/or pancreatitis. Postbinge pancreatitis has a reported 10 percent mortality rate.

Periods of starvation result in hypoglycemia, which is a poor prognostic indicator. Hypoglycemia is often associated with hypothermia, coma, and infections, and may be fatal. Starvation leads to low insulin levels that are insensitive to both glucose and amino acid infusion. Gastric distention and reduced gastric emptying produce enhanced satiation and prolonged intermeal intervals. Food has been demonstrated to remain in the stomachs of anorexics for up to 24 h.

Starvation causes a decreased hypoxic ventilatory drive, decreased vital capacity, tidal volume, and minute ventilation. In addition, the surfactant pool is reduced, resulting in "stiffer" lungs with a greater tendency to collapse. The muscles of ventilation are affected by starvation, causing reduced diaphragm mass and respiratory muscle weakness.

Cardiovascular changes include brady- and tachyarrhythmias caused by cardiomyopathy or electrolyte abnormalities. ST-T wave changes, and Q-T interval prolongation, may be evident. Decreased peripheral adrenergic activity with normal adrenomedullary function results in bradycardia and orthostatic hypotension.

Dermatologic changes include pedal or pretibial edema, with or without hypoalbuminemia; excessive loss of subcutaneous fat; brittle hair and nails; pellagra or scurvy; and petechiae or purpura.

Peripheral neuropathy, most likely a product of chronic malnutrition, is a notable complication. Localized compression neuropathies secondary to subcutaneous tissue loss can also develop. Some patients experience paresthesias of the fingers and toes. Deep tendon reflexes may be diminished, and gross motor coordination may be impaired.

Anorexics are especially likely to be compulsive exercisers. Stress fractures[8] in the feet, march hemoglobinuria, and various musculoskeletal overuse syndromes have been identified in our institution as complications of compulsive exercise.

Osteoporosis is common in anorexics. It usually affects the femur, radius, and spine in decreasing frequency. Estrogen deficiency is not a major causative factor. Any patient with an eating disorder who has been amenorrheic and low in weight for more than a year should undergo bone density studies. We have seen a femur fracture in a young anorexic who tripped on a rug.[8]

Adolescent diabetics induce ketosis by skipping insulin for a day or two to lose weight; sometimes they overeat and increase insulin in compensation. The abuse of insulin and food can lead to severe metabolic consequences. Young diabetics with frequent hospitalizations should be evaluated for a coexisting eating disorder.

PSYCHOLOGICAL PRESENTATIONS

In addition to the presenting physical symptoms, psychological manifestations may also be detected on emergency evaluation. Depression, including suicidal ideation, is the primary psychological complication of eating disorders. Other psychological manifestations include obsessive-compulsive personality traits, with rumination about food, calories, and weight. Ritualistic eating and exercising behavior are also evident. Perfectionistic striving often results in deterioration of friendships and leisure activities.

Impulse control disorder is a psychological complication of eating disorders more commonly seen in bulimics than anorexics. Other behavioral manifestations include shoplifting and stealing, sexual promiscuity, drug and alcohol abuse, and self-mutilation.

PROGNOSIS

As with most mental illnesses, the earlier the onset, detection, and treatment the better the prognosis. There is a large variation in outcome. Some studies report longer term improvement in 30 to 50 percent of patients,[9,10] but in most, it is a chronic disorder. Eating disorders can have potentially irreversible effects on the physical and emotional growth in adolescents. There is evidence suggesting improved outcome with early treatment and therefore the threshold for intervention should be lower than in adults. Behaviors may remain constant or the patient may improve briefly and return to the eating disorder during stressful times. Psychological immaturity persists in approximately 50 percent of the patients, with difficulties in social adjustment, and one-third of patients continue to have problems with eating. Chronicity increases the risk of morbidity.

In spite of the advances in the understanding of anorexia and bulimia nervosa, eating disorders are still associated with significant long-term morbidity and mortality. Mortality figures range from 2 to 5 percent to a high of 18 percent. Abnormally low albumin levels and low body weight (≤60 percent ideal body weight) best predicts a lethal course. High creatinine and uric acid levels predict chronicity in anorectics.[11] Death may result from suicide, starvation, metabolic catastrophe, infection, and cardiac insufficiency. Agents used to induce weight loss may lead to fatal complications.

TREATMENT

Emergency management of the patient with an eating disorder consists of volume repletion and correction of electrolyte imbalance. Fluid and nutritional replacement should be gradual. Cachectic patients do not secrete inducible enzymes, such as lipase or lactase. They have reduced gastric emptying and atrophy of small intestinal villi. Aggressive refeeding can lead to hypertonic dehydration, hypernatremia, prerenal azotemia, and refeeding pancreatitis. Caloric requirements should be advanced slowly. The refeeding syndrome, with severe cardiopulmonary and neurologic complications, has been described in anorexics and is associated with rapid electrolyte shifts, hypophosphatemia, hypokalemia, and hypomagnesemia. Anorexics usually present with bradycardia and the pulse rate may be the simplest noninvasive way to monitor fluid replacement. Closely monitor the electrocardiogram, serum and urine electrolytes, phosphorus, and magnesium.

Hospitalization is suggested for the following conditions:

1. Weight loss greater than 30 percent over 3 months
2. Severe metabolic disturbance
3. Depression severe enough to be at risk for suicide
4. Severe bingeing and purging
5. Failure to maintain outpatient weight contract
6. Psychosis
7. Family crisis
8. Need to confront patient and family denial
9. Need for initiation of therapy (individual, family, and/or pharmacotherapy)
10. Complex differential diagnosis

A period of about 48 h in an inpatient setting is essential to determine the extent and severity of the illness an its complications. An eating disorders unit or medical floor with involvement of a multidisciplinary psychiatric and internal medicine team is advised.

A variety of medications have been used in eating disorders, including H_1 antagonists (cyproheptadine), selective serotonin reuptake inhibitor and cyclic antidepressants, and atypical antipsychotics (olanzapine).[12–14] The sense of bloating or uncomfortable fullness as anorexics begin refeeding is usually related to delayed gastric emptying and can be helped by taking metoclopramide before meals.

The selective serotonin reuptake inhibitors are the mainstay of pharmacologic treatment in bulimia. Naltrexone and odansetron have been reported as useful in some cases.

A trial of outpatient psychological treatment can be attempted if food restriction and weight loss are of less than 3 months' duration, and if there is a very positive family support system. Referral to a local health professional who specializes in the treatment of eating disorders or to a self-help group can be obtained by contacting the following national organizations:

National Association of Anorexia Nervosa and Associated
  Disorders (ANAD)
PO Box 7
Highland Park, IL 60035
1.847.831.3438
www.healthtouch.com/leve11/leaflets/anad/anad001.htm

Anorexia Nervosa and Related Eating Disorders, Inc. (ANRED)
PO Box 5102
Eugene, OR 97405
1.541.344.1144
www.anred.com

American Anorexia/Bulimia Association, Inc. (AABA)
165 W. 46th Street, #1108
New York, NY 07666
1.212.575.6200
http://members.aol.com/AmanBu

National Eating Disorders Organization (NEDO)
6655 S. Yale Avenue
Tulsa, OK 74136
1.918.481.4044
www.laureate.com

Academy for Eating Disorders; Montefiore Medical Center
  (AED)
111 East 210th Street
Bronx, NY 10467
1.718.920.6782
www.acadeatdis.org

REFERENCES

1. Kotler LA, Cohen P, Davies M, et al: Longitudinal relationships between child, adolescent, and adult eating disorders. *J Am Acad Child Adolesc Psychiatry* 40:1434, 2001.
2. American Psychiatric Association: *Diagnostic and Statistical Manual of Mental Disorders,* 4th ed. Washington, DC, American Psychiatric Association, 1994.
3. Polivy J, Herman CP: Causes of eating disorders. *Annu Rev Psychol* 53:187, 2002.
4. Kaye, WH, Klump KL, Frank GK, et al: Anorexia and bulimia nervosa. *Annu Rev Med* 51:299, 2000.
5. Milos G, Spindler A, Ruggiero G, et al: Comorbidity of obsessive-compulsive disorders and duration of eating disorders. *Int J Eat Disord* 31:284, 2002.
6. Garner DM, Sackeyfio AH: *Eating Disorders: Handbook of Behavioral Therapy in Psychiatric Setting.* 1993, p 477.
7. Little JW: Eating disorders; dental implications. *Oral Surg Oral Med Oral Pathol Oral Radiol Endod* 93:138, 2002.
8. LaBan MM, Wilkins JC, Sackeyfio AH, Taylor RS: Osteoporotic stress fractures in anorexia nervosa. *Arch Phys Med Rehabil* 76;884, 1996.

9. Steinhausen HC: The outcome of anorexia nervosa in the 20th century. *Am J Psychiatry* 159:1284, 2002.

10. Lowe B, Zipfel S, Buchholz C, et al: Long-term outcome of anorexia nervosa in a prospective 21-year followup study. *Psychol Med* 31:881, 2001.

11. Herzog W, Deter HC, Fiehn W, Petzold E: Medical findings and predictors of long-term physical outcome in anorexia nervosa: A prospective, 12-year follow-up study. *Psychol Med* 27:269, 1997.

12. Santonastaso P, Friederici S, Favaro A: Sertraline in the treatment of restricting anorexia nervosa; an open controlled trial. *J Child Adolesc Psychopharmacol* 11:143, 2001.

13. Kaye WH, Nagata T, Weltzin TE, et al: Double-blind placebo-controlled administration of fluoxetine in restricting-and restricting-purging-type anorexia nervosa. *Biol Psychiatry* 49:644, 2001.

14. Mitchell JE, Peterson CB, Myers T, et al: Combining pharmacotherapy and psychotherapy in the treatment of patients with eating disorders. *Psychiatr Clin North Am* 24:315, 2001.

15. Hediger, C, Rost B, Itin P: Cutaneous manifestations in anorexia nervosa. *J Suisse Med* 130:565, 2002.

16. Byrne S, McLean N: Eating disorders in athletes: A review of the literature. *J Sci Med Sport* 4:145, 2001.

17. Galetta F, Franzoni F, Cupisti A, et al: QT interval dispersion in young women with anorexia nervosa. *J Pediatr* 140:456, 2002.

18. Heer M, Mika C, Grzella I, et al: Changes in bone turnover in patients with anorexia nervosa during eleven weeks of inpatient dietary treatment. *Clin Chem* 48:754, 2002.

292 PANIC DISORDER
Linda M. Nicholas
Ann E. Maloney
Susan L. Siegfreid

Panic disorder is a common, often chronic, condition characterized by recurrent, spontaneous panic attacks. Panic attacks are short-lived episodes of anxiety or intense fear, accompanied by a range of somatic symptoms, which may include tachycardia, tachypnea, dyspnea, chest tightness, weakness, nausea, dizziness, and paresthesias. Panic disorder may occur with or without agoraphobia, a condition typified by avoidance of places or situations associated with anxiety. Panic disorder with agoraphobia may be severely disabling, because patients may be incapable of functioning socially or occupationally.

Because many of the symptoms of panic overlap with those of acute medical illness, the first point of contact for patients with panic disorder is often the emergency room.

When compared with patients who had other psychiatric or medical problems, patients with panic disorder had the highest rates of use of emergency department services.[1] Increased use can precede the diagnosis of panic disorder by up to 10 years.[2] Although progress is made in diagnosis and treatment, as many as 50 percent who have the disorder are undiagnosed.

EPIDEMIOLOGY

Panic disorder is relatively common, with national lifetime and 12-month prevalences of 3.5 and 2.5 percent,[3] respectively, and a cross-national lifetime prevalence of 1.6 to 2.2 percent.[4] The age of onset is usually from late adolescence to the mid-30s. The incidence may have a bimodal distribution, with the first peak in late adolescence, followed by a second, smaller peak in the mid-30s.[5]

Women are two to three times more likely than men to develop panic disorder. There is some evidence that panic attacks may remit during pregnancy, only to be exacerbated in the postpartum period.[6,7] Cultural factors may play a role in the presentation of panic disorder. Sleep paralysis and hypertension are common symptoms of panic disorder in the African American population.[8] *Ataque de nervios* is an anxiety syndrome in Hispanic cultures that, at times, has a similar presentation to panic disorder.[9]

PATHOPHYSIOLOGY

The etiology basis of panic disorder is unknown. It is most likely multifactorial in origin, with genetic, behavioral, and biological underpinnings.[10]

Genetic or Familial

First-degree relatives of patients with panic disorder have a four- to sevenfold increased risk of developing the disorder,[6] and monozygotic twins have a higher concordance than dizygotic twins for panic disorder.[7,11]

Behavioral

Cognitive-behavioral theorists have proposed that panic disorder is a learned response to interoceptive cues. Heightened awareness of body functions and/or cognitive misinterpretation of these cues are postulated to trigger a conditioned fear response.[12] Anticipatory anxiety and agoraphobia develop as a person begins to associate panic attacks with a particular place or situation.

Biological

Neurobiological research into the etiology of panic disorder uses two main approaches: studies that use provocative ("panicogenic") substances and studies that use known pharmacologic treatments. These approaches have implicated multiple neurotransmitters or neuropeptides, including norepinephrine, serotonin (5-hydroxytryptamine), γ-aminobutyric acid (GABA), and cholecystokinin (CCK), among others.

NOREPINEPHRINE   Panic disorder patients are generally hypersensitive to carbon dioxide inhalation.[13] One model has been proposed that carbon dioxide stimulates the locus ceruleus, which contains noradrenergic neurons, and induces panic by stimulating norepinephrine release.[14] In addition, there is some evidence for impaired receptor sensitivity in panic disorder.[13]

SEROTONIN   Two agents have been reported to provoke panic attacks via effects on serotonergic receptors. Fenfluramine and *m*-chlorophenylpiperazine cause panic in challenge tests.[13] Theories that have attempted to explain the results of these tests and incorporate the known efficacy of serotonergic agents in treating panic disorder include the following hypotheses: increased sensitivity of postsynaptic receptors, decreased or increased central nervous system serotonin activity, and interactions between serotonin and norepinephrine, GABA, or CCK.[13]

CHOLECYSTOKININ   Recently, much attention has been given to the neuropeptide, CCK, as an important mediator in panic disorder. It is present in many of the neuroanatomic areas thought to be involved in panic disorder, including the cerebral cortex, hippocampus, and brainstem. A tetrapeptide form of CCK causes panic when administered to panic disorder patients and its effects are attenuated by imipramine, a tricyclic antidepressant with efficacy in treating panic.[15] There are also close interactions between CCK and GABA, between serotonin and dopamine, and between endogenous opioids and the excitatory amino acid, glutamate.[15]

The mechanisms by which the provocative agents sodium lactate, yohimbine, and caffeine, which reproducibly induce panic in patients with panic disorder, cause panic attacks are not known.

CLINICAL FEATURES

The cardinal features of panic disorder are recurrent, unexpected panic attacks and persistent worry about having another attack and/or its potential implications, such as heralding a serious medical illness. Panic attacks are of sudden onset and include feelings of apprehension, fear, and discomfort; these attacks are relatively brief in duration, with a peak within about 10 min and resolution within 1 h. The attacks are accompanied by characteristic somatic and/or cognitive symptoms.[5] Somatic symptoms are referable to the major organ systems in the body. Cardiovascular complaints include palpitations and tachycardia or chest pain and discomfort. Respiratory symptoms of shortness of breath or the sensation of being smothered are common. A choking sensation, nausea, and gastric distress comprise most gastrointestinal complaints. Neurologic symptoms include dizziness, unsteadiness, lightheadedness, faintness, trembling, shaking, or paresthesias. Sweating, hot flushes, or chills are also common. Cognitive symptoms include feelings of unreality about or being detached from one's environment (derealization) or one's self (depersonalization) and the fear of going crazy, losing control, or dying.[5] Some patients alter their behavior to minimize their risk of having more panic attacks, even to the point of becoming fearful of leaving their home and being in places or situations where escape or finding help would be difficult if a panic attack occurred (agoraphobia).[5]

DIAGNOSIS

For a diagnosis of panic disorder, the patient must have recurrent, unexpected panic attacks followed by at least 1 month of persistent fear of having additional attacks, worry about the implications or consequence (e.g., going crazy, having a heart attack), or a significant change in behavior.[5] The panic attacks must not be better accounted for by another psychiatric or medical disorder (Table 292-1). The patient's age, presenting symptoms, time course of symptom development and resolution, and lack of other identifiable medical causes are often helpful in considering the differential diagnosis of a panic attack.[16] Care must be taken to identify victims of domestic violence, who often present with psychiatric complaints. When screening suggests domestic violence, safety planning and referrals for counseling should be provided.

Psychiatric Differential Diagnosis

A panic attack is an episode of intense fear that develops abruptly and reaches a peak within 10 min. During a panic attack, at least 4 of 13 characteristic symptoms must be present, as listed in Table 292-2. Panic attacks are characterized in the *Diagnostic and Statistical Manual of Mental Disorders,* 4th edition, as unexpected (uncued), situationally bound (cued; i.e., always occurring with exposure to a specific trigger), or situationally predisposed (i.e., likely to occur with exposure to a given situation). Situationally bound or predisposed panic attacks may occur in association with a wide range of psychiatric disorders, including social phobia, specific phobia, acute or posttraumatic stress disorder, separation anxiety disorder, obsessive-compulsive disorder, and depressive disorders. The occurrence of spontaneous or unexpected panic attacks is necessary for a diagnosis of panic disorder. The patient always should be questioned about situations triggering the attacks. It is often useful to ask patients if their panic attacks occur "out of the blue" or to inquire if they are ever awakened by panic attacks.

Medical Differential Diagnosis

A patient presenting to the emergency department with multiple somatic complaints consistent with a panic attack, even if they are known to have panic disorder, should have a thorough history, physical examination, and, when indicated, other specific tests performed to rule out medical causes. The differential diagnosis is quite extensive, and panic disorder is often a diagnosis of exclusion.

The clinician should carefully review the patient's concurrent medical problems and prescribed and over-the-counter medications, because some medical conditions and/or treatments can provoke anxiety and overt panic attacks. Substance intoxication and withdrawal states

TABLE 292-1   Medical Differential Diagnosis of Panic

Cardiovascular
  Angina
  Myocardial infarction
  Mitral valve prolapse
  Congestive heart failure
  Premature atrial contractions
Pulmonary
  Hyperventilation
  Asthma
  Pulmonary embolus
Endocrine
  Hyperthyroidism
  Hypoglycemia
  Hyponatremia
  Pheochromocytoma
  Carcinoid syndrome
  Cushing syndrome
Neurologic
  Migraines
  Ménière disease
  Complex partial seizures
  Transient ischemic attacks
Drug induced
  Caffeine
  Cocaine
  Sympathomimetics
  Theophylline
  Thyroid preparations
  Selective serotonin reuptake inhibitors
  Cannabis
  Corticosteroids
  β-Agonists
  Triptans
  Nicotine
  Yohimbine
  Hallucinogens
  Anticholinergics
  Drug withdrawal
Alcohol
  Barbiturates
  Benzodiazepines
  Opiates
  β-Antagonists
Psychiatric
  Posttraumatic stress disorder
  Depressive disorders
  Other anxiety disorders
Psychosocial
  Partner violence
  Sexual abuse or assault
  Other situational stressors

also may induce panic. A history of caffeine use is important, because panic patients often are exquisitely sensitive to methylxanthines. A brief psychosocial history should include questions regarding substance use and recent or ongoing psychosocial stressors that may be exacerbating or precipitating panic attacks. Table 292-1 contains a partial list of medical diagnoses and substance-induced states that may present with symptoms similar to those of panic disorder.

Physical examination findings in panic patients most commonly are transient tachycardia and mildly elevated systolic blood pressure. Laboratory findings, when present, are most consistent with hyperventilation with low levels of sodium bicarbonate. In general, most patients with panic disorder will have a negative medical workup.

ASSOCIATIONS

Panic disorder is closely associated with other psychiatric and medical conditions. Comorbid psychiatric disorders include depression in up to

TABLE 292-2   Symptoms of a Panic Attack

Somatic Symptoms	Cognitive Symptoms
Palpitations, pounding heart or tachycardia	Fear of losing control
Sweating	Fear of dying
Sensations of shortness of breath or smothering	Derealization (feeling of unreality) or depersonalization (feeling detached from oneself)
Trembling or shaking	
Feeling of choking	
Chest pain or discomfort	
Nausea or abdominal distress	
Feeling dizzy, unsteady, lightheaded, or faint	
Paresthesias	
Chills or hot flashes	

50 to 65 percent, other mood disorders, substance abuse and dependence, other anxiety disorders, and personality disorders.[5] Certain medical conditions have been associated with panic disorder but are unrelated to its etiology. Panic disorder has well-documented associations with mitral valve prolapse and asthma.[5] Other medical conditions, such as idiopathic cardiomyopathy, hypertension, atypical chest pain without evidence of coronary artery disease, irritable bowel syndrome, chronic obstructive pulmonary disease, Parkinson disease, and migraine headaches, have been associated with panic attacks.[17]

COURSE

The course of panic disorder is variable in frequency and severity. Some patients suffer only intermittent attacks, whereas others have attacks almost continuously. In general, the course of the illness is chronic, with a pattern of waxing and waning. Panic disorder patients also can have situationally predisposed attacks when exposed to certain cues or triggers, limited symptom panic attacks in which fewer than 4 of the 13 recognized diagnostic somatic or cognitive symptoms occur, and nocturnal panic attacks. A 4- to 6-year follow-up study of patients from a tertiary care setting after treatment showed that 30 percent were asymptomatic, 40 to 50 percent were improved, and 20 to 30 percent remained the same or were worse.[18] Lifetime rates of suicide attempts are similar for patients with uncomplicated panic disorder and uncomplicated major depression (7 and 7.9 percent, respectively), whereas rates for patients with comorbid panic disorder and depression were 19.5 percent.[19]

Patients with panic symptoms should always be asked about suicidal feelings. It is imperative that panic disorder be diagnosed and appropriately treated to prevent significant morbidity and mortality.

TREATMENT

Treatment of panic disorder starts with recognition of the illness. Ballenger proposed that the following screening question be used in patients for rapid identification: "Have you experienced brief periods for seconds or minutes of an overwhelming panic or terror which was accompanied by racing heart, shortness of breath or dizziness?"[20] Once a diagnosis of panic disorder is made, the next step is to educate patients while providing reassurance that they are not dying or going crazy and emphasizing that it is an illness that can be treated effectively. Instruction on avoidance of triggers for panic attacks can reduce the long-term sequelae.[21]

Cognitive behavioral therapy (CBT) and pharmacotherapy are effective treatment modalities for panic disorder.[22] Choice of treatment is based on an individual assessment of risks, benefits, efficacy, availability, acuity, and patient preference. Cognitive behavioral therapy and pharmacotherapy, with the exception of benzodiazepines, take at least 4 weeks for most patients to notice significant benefit. If there is no improvement within 6 to 8 weeks of a particular treatment, often a different treatment is required or combined CBT and medication is used.

Cognitive Behavioral Treatment

Cognitive behavioral therapy involves education about the disorder, symptom and thought records, learning anxiety management skills (e.g., breathing retraining), changing cognitions associated with panic attacks (cognitive restructuring), and exposure (with response prevention) to feared situations, usually by using a hierarchy created by the patient and therapist.[22]

Medications

Four classes of drugs have been found to be effective in treating panic disorder: selective serotonin reuptake inhibitors (SSRIs), tricyclic antidepressants (TCAs), monoamine oxidase inhibitors (MAOIs), and benzodiazepines. Tables 292-3 through 292-6 list some of the advantages and disadvantages of each class. Drugs found to be ineffective include bupropion, Ludiomil, deprenyl, buspirone, β antagonists, and barbiturates.

ANTIDEPRESSANTS   Antidepressants are considered by many to be the mainstay of treatment for panic disorder, because the potential complications of abuse, dependence, and withdrawal are not associated with their use. In addition, antidepressants may be beneficial in treating comorbid mood and anxiety disorders, including posttraumatic stress disorder and premenstrual dysphoric disorder. Due to safety considerations and side-effect profiles, SSRIs are considered the drugs of choice. Although sexual side effects may be problematic with these antidepressant classes, SSRIs lack the anticholinergic side effects, cardiovascular effects, and toxicity in overdose associated with TCAs or MAOIs.

When initiating treatment with SSRIs and TCAs, the starting dose should be lower than that used to treat depression, because panic disorder patients often are extremely sensitive to side effects. It is helpful to advise patients that they may temporarily notice some increased anxiety or activation when initiating treatment or increasing the dose. Patients also should be told that it might take several weeks before there are noticeable benefits.

Monoamine oxidase inhibitors are used much less frequently now and are reserved as second-line treatment due to the dietary restrictions and risk of hypertensive crisis.[22] Reversible monoamine oxidase inhibitors, which do not require adherence to a tyramine-free diet, are effective for treating panic and phobic symptoms.[23,24] However, reversible monoamine oxidase inhibitors are not currently approved for use in the United States.

TABLE 292-3   Selective Serotonin Reuptake Inhibitors

Advantages	Disadvantages
Single daily dose	Delayed onset
Antidepressant effects	Early anxiogenic effect
Safety	Sexual side effects
Benign side-effect profile	Requires dose titration
No abuse potential	
Effective	

TABLE 292-4   Tricyclic Antidepressants

Advantages	Disadvantages
Single daily dose	Delayed onset
Antidepressant effects	Anticholinergic effects
Well studied	Postural hypotension
Generics available	Sexual side effects
No abuse potential	Weight gain
Effective	Initial stimulation
	Dangerous in overdose

TABLE 292-6   Benzodiazepines

Advantages	Disadvantages
Rapid onset	Discontinuation reactions
Effective	Sedation
Well tolerated	Multiple daily dosing
General antianxiety effects	Abuse potential
Relatively safe in overdose	Fall risk
Generics available	Cognitive slowing risk
Tolerance rare for panic effects	Dose escalation by patient
	Disinhibition (paradoxic reaction) in some patients

BENZODIAZEPINES   For patients in whom more rapid control of panic symptoms is necessary, such as those who are unable to fulfill expected major psychosocial obligations (work, school, etc.), benzodiazepines may be the drug of choice. Alprazolam has been the most extensively studied benzodiazepine and is currently the only one approved by the U.S. Food and Drug Administration for treatment of panic disorder. It may be initiated at a dose of 0.5 mg qid. In double-blind studies, alprazolam, in the 5- to 6-mg per d dosage range, reduced panic attack frequency, anticipatory anxiety, phobic avoidance, and disability.[22] Studies suggested that diazepam, lorazepam, and clonazepam in equivalent doses also may be effective in treating panic disorder (i.e., clonazepam 0.25 to 0.5 mg by mouth twice daily, with most patients responding well to 1 to 3 mg per d).

Benzodiazepines also may be administered acutely for a patient who is having a panic attack, regardless of the etiology of the panic. These drugs should be used with caution in patients with a respiratory disorder or who have a history of substance abuse or dependence. Caution also should be used in the elderly in whom there is concern for falls, cognitive slowing, or drug interactions due to polypharmacy.

It may be beneficial to initiate treatment with an antidepressant and a benzodiazepine, with the goal to later taper or minimize the benzodiazepine dose as the antidepressant begins to control symptoms. Tapering is required, because abrupt withdrawal can lead to seizures or delirium. A controlled trial of alprazolam as an adjunct to imipramine during the first 4 to 6 weeks of treatment demonstrated that patients receiving both drugs have a more rapid therapeutic response.[25] However, 10 of 17 patients were unable to discontinue the alprazolam in 2 weeks after the treatment period. Thus, the benefits of a rapid response must be weighed against the risk of difficulty in discontinuing the benzodiazepine.

Selective serotonin reuptake inhibitors and CBT are currently the treatments of choice for panic disorder, whereas benzodiazepines are extremely effective for short-term relief.

Cognitive-behavioral therapy and pharmacologic treatment, with the exception of benzodiazepines, take at least 4 weeks for most patients to notice significant benefit. If there is no improvement within 6 to 8 weeks of a particular treatment, often a different treatment is required, or combined CBT and medication is used. Acute treatment usually lasts at least 12 weeks. If medication is being used, often a taper and discontinuation is attempted after 1 year of maintenance treatment. It is unclear whether further CBT sessions ("booster sessions") are beneficial in prevention of relapse. Relapse is treated with CBT and/or medication.

DISPOSITION

Usually, treatment for panic disorder can be initiated in an outpatient setting. If a patient is already being treated for panic disorder, it is optimal to consult with the treating physician before initiating or changing medication. The clinician may wish to seek a psychiatric consultation while the patient is in the emergency department or refer the patient to the primary care physician or a psychiatrist for follow-up care.

Patients who are suicidal or who are so incapacitated that they cannot care for themselves require psychiatric hospitalization. In such cases, a psychiatric evaluation is necessary to determine the extent of dangerousness and need for inpatient treatment.

REFERENCES

1. Klerman GL, Weissman MM, Ouellette R, et al: Panic attacks in the community: Social morbidity and health care utilization. *JAMA* 265:742, 1991.
2. Simpson RJ, Kazmierczak T, Power KG, et al: Controlled comparison of the characteristics of patients with panic disorder. *Br J Gen Pract* 44:352, 1994.
3. Kessler RC, McGonagle KA, Zhao S, et al: Lifetime and 12-month prevalence of DSM-III-R psychiatric disorders in the United States. Results from the National Comorbidity Survey. *Arch Gen Psychiatry* 51:8, 1994.
4. Weissman MM, Bland RC, Canino GJ, et al: The cross-national epidemiology of panic disorder. *Arch Gen Psychiatry* 54:305, 1997.
5. American Psychiatric Association: *Diagnostic and Statistical Manual of Mental Disorders,* 4th ed. Washington, DC, American Psychiatric Association, 1994.
6. George DT, Landenheim JA, Nutt D: Effect of pregnancy on panic attacks. *Am J Psychiatry* 44:1078, 1987.
7. Cohen LS, Sichel DA, Dimmock JA, et al: Postpartum course in women with preexisting panic disorder. *J Clin Psychiatry* 55:289, 1994.
8. Bell CC, Hildreth CJ, Jenkins EJ, et al: The relationship of isolated sleep paralysis and panic disorder to hypertension. *J Natl Med Assoc* 80:289, 1988.
9. Liebowitz MR, Salman E, Justino CM, et al: Ataque de nervios and panic disorder. *Am J Psychiatry* 151:871, 1994.
10. Knowles JA, Weissman MM: Panic disorder and agoraphobia, in Oldham JM, Riba MB (eds): *American Psychiatric Press Review of Psychiatry.* Vol 14. Washington, DC: American Psychiatric Press, 1995, p. 383.
11. Perna G, Caldirola D, Arancio C, et al: Panic attacks: A twin study. *Psychiatr Res* 15:69, 1997.

TABLE 292-5   Monoamine Oxidase Inhibitors

Advantages	Disadvantages
Single daily dose	Delayed onset
Antidepressant effects	Drug interactions
Well studied	Dietary restrictions
Effective	Hypertensive crisis risk
No abuse potential	Sexual side effects
	Weight gain
	Initial stimulation
	Dangerous in overdose

12. Barlow DH, Cohen AS, Waddell MT, et al: Panic and generalized anxiety disorder: nature and treatment. *Behav Ther* 15:431, 1984.
13. Bourin M, Baker GB, Bradwejn J: Neurobiology of panic disorder. *J Psychosom Res* 44:163, 1998.
14. Klein DF, Gorman JM: A model of panic and agoraphobic development. *Acta Psychiatr Scand* 335:87, 1987.
15. Bradwejn J, Koszycki D: Imipramine antagonizes the panicogenic effects of CCK-4 in panic disorder patients. *Am J Psychiatry* 15:261, 1994.
16. Zunn LS: Panic disorder: Diagnosis and treatment in emergency medicine. *Ann Emerg Med* 30:92, 1997.
17. Zaubler TS, Katon W: Panic disorder in the medical setting. *J Psychosom Res* 44:25, 1998.
18. Katschnig H, Amering M, Stolk JM, et al: Predictors of quality of life in a long-term follow-up study of panic disorder patients after a clinical drug trial. *Psychopharmacol Bull* 32:149, 1996.
19. Johnson J, Weissman MM, Klerman GL: Panic disorder, comorbidity, and suicide attempts. *Arch Gen Psychiatry* 47:805, 1990.
20. Ballenger JC: Treatment of panic disorder in the general medical setting. *J Psychosom Res* 44:5, 1998.
21. Swinson RP, Soulios C, Cox BJ, et al: Brief treatment of emergency room patients with panic attacks. *Am J Psychiatry* 149:944, 1992.
22. American Psychiatric Association: Practice guideline for the treatment of patients with panic disorder. *Am J Psychiatry* 155(suppl), 1998, pp. 1–34.
23. Bakish D, Saxena BM, Bowen R, et al: Reversible monoamine oxidase inhibitors in panic disorder. *Clin Neuropsychopharmacol* 16(suppl 2):S77, 1993.
24. Garcia-Borreguero D, Lauer CJ, et al: Brofaramine in panic disorder: a pilot study with a new reversible inhibitor of monoamine oxidase-A. *Pharmacopsychiatry* 25:261, 1992.
25. Woods S, Nagy LM, Koleszar AS, et al: Controlled trial of alprazolam supplementation during imipramine treatment of panic disorder. *J Clin Psychopharmacol* 12:32, 1991.

CONVERSION DISORDER
Gregory P. Moore
Kenneth C. Jackimczyk

For a diagnosis of conversion disorder to be made, the following five criteria must be met:[1]

1. A symptom is expressed in which there is a change or loss of physical function suggesting a physical disorder.
2. The patient has experienced a recent psychological stressor or conflict.
3. The patient unconsciously produces the symptom.
4. The symptom cannot be explained by a known organic etiology or culturally sanctioned response pattern.
5. The symptom is not limited to pain or sexual dysfunction.

PATHOPHYSIOLOGY

An illustrative example involves the case of a young wife who is scheduled to visit her debilitated father in the hospital. His recent diagnosis of cancer has left her distraught, and the sight of him depresses her greatly. On the morning of her visit, she suddenly becomes blind.

This example typifies a conversion disorder in which conflict is caused by the patient's intense, but psychically unacceptable, urge to avoid a required action (in this case, visiting her father). The physical symptom (blindness) allows expression of the urge (how can she drive there if she is blind?) without consciously confronting the feelings that led to the wish. At the same time, the symptom imposes morbidity as a punishment for the wish. Often, the presenting symptom will have a symbolic relationship to the conflict, but this is not always the case. In this case, the sight of her father is distressing, and therefore loss of sight is the chief complaint.

Conversion disorders are often thought of as nonverbal exertions of control on the environment. Two mechanisms are responsible for the symptoms. The first is *primary gain,* in which the symptom allows patients to avoid confronting their uncomfortable feelings. The second is *secondary gain,* in which uncomfortable situations are avoided and support is given that might not normally be available. In our example, secondary gain would occur if the patient's husband then stayed home from work to tend to his "blind" wife.

Conversion disorders are described as rare, with an annual incidence in outpatient psychiatric settings of 0.01 to 0.02 percent. An incidence of 5 to 16 percent among inpatients with psychiatric consultations has been noted. Most agree that the incidence is declining. Cases predominantly involve neurologic and orthopedic manifestations and are seen in the military during times of war, in victims of industrial accidents, and in victims of violence. Conversion disorders are much more frequent in women, accounting for up to 80 percent of cases in some series, than in men. The most common ages of presentation are adolescence or early childhood, although other age groups are affected. Conversion disorders are more prevalent in rural, lower socioeconomic, and less educated populations. Other predisposing factors include medical illness, depression, anxiety, schizophrenia, somatization disorder, dependent personality disorder (5 to 21 percent of patients), borderline personality disorder, and passive aggressive personality disorder.[2,3]

CLINICAL FEATURES

Conversion disorders usually present as a single symptom with a sudden onset related to a severe stress. Precise history taking should focus on how the problem affects the patient and the surrounding events at time of onset. It may be necessary to interview the patient and family separately to confirm diagnostic suspicions. The most reliable diagnostic criterion for conversion disorder is a history of the disorder or a somatization disorder (each found in one-third of cases). Symptoms may vary in cases of recurrence.[2–4] Motor complaints, usually involving voluntary muscles, are more common than sensory complaints.[2–4]

Classic symptoms of conversion disorders include paralysis, aphonia, seizures, coordination disturbances, akinesia, dyskinesia, blindness, tunnel vision, anosmia, anesthesia, and paresthesia. Pseudoseizures represent 10 to 40 percent of conversion disorders referred to psychiatrists. Patients may describe their condition with surprising lack of concern, considering the severity of the symptom *(la belle indifférence).* This was previously thought to be a hallmark of the disorder, but it is absent in about half of cases and is found just as often in patients with organic disease. It is no longer considered diagnostic.[2,5]

Diagnosis is made first and foremost by ruling out organic pathology. Absence of a medical condition does not necessarily support the diagnosis of conversion disorder, because the appropriate psychological criteria also must be met. Suspicion for the disorder should arise when no physical findings related to the symptom are found or the examination is not consistent with known anatomic or pathophysiologic states. Several techniques that can be used in the physical examination are helpful in testing for true neurologic deficits (Table 293-1). Appropriate laboratory and ancillary studies should be ordered to confirm suspected organic disease. However, it is important to remember that organic disease may be present concurrently with conversion disorder.[6]

DIFFERENTIAL DIAGNOSIS

Careful history taking and physical examination should be used to rule out neurologic disease. A high index of suspicion should be maintained for physical disorders that have a vague onset, such as systemic lupus erythematosus, multiple sclerosis, polymyositis, Lyme disease, and drug toxicity or poisoning. Schizophrenia and depression may have associated conversion disorders. In somatization disorders, the symptoms are more chronic and involve multiple organ systems. With

TABLE 293-1   Physical Examination Techniques Used to Distinguish True Neurologic Deficits and Conversion Disorder

Function	Techique
Sensation	
Yes–no test	Patient closes eyes and responds *yes* or *no* to touch stimulus. *No* response in numb area favors conversion disorder.
Bowlus and Currier test	Patient extends crossed arms with thumbs pointed down and palms facing together. Fingers (but no thumbs) are interlocked, and then hands are rotated inward toward chest. The distortion of body position makes false responses to sensory stimuli difficult.
Strength test	Patient closes eyes. Test "strength" by touching finger to be moved. True lack of sensation would not allow patient to ascertain finger to be moved.
Pain	
Gray test	With abdominal pain due to psychological factors, the patient will close eyes during palpation. In pain of organic basis, the patient is more likely to watch the examiner's hand to anticipate pain.
Motor	
Drop test	When a patient with paralysis of nonorganic etiology lifts a thumb, the affected limb will drop more slowly or fall with exaggerated speed as compared with the unaffected limb. In addition, an extremity dropped from above the face will miss it.
Stretch reflex test	Patient contracts a muscle at maximum strength while counteraction is provided. The examiner suddenly jerks the muscle into extension. This will produce a stretch reflex that reveals the patient's true muscle strength.
Thigh adductor test	Examiner places hands against the inner thighs of the patient who is told to adduct the normal leg against resistance. With pseudoparalysis, the other leg will adduct.
Hoover test	Examiner's hands cup both heels of the patient who is asked to elevate the normal leg. With pseudoparalysis the other leg will push downward. Absence of downward pressure of the normal leg when the patient is instructed to lift the weak leg indicates noncompliance.
Sternomastoid test	Patient with conversion hemiplegia cannot turn head to the weak side.
Coma	
Corneal reflex	Corneal reflexes remain intact in an awake patient.
Bell phenomenon	Eyes divert upward when lids are opened, whereas eyes remain in neutral position in true coma.
Lid closing	In true coma, lids when opened close rapidly initially and then more slowly as lids descend. Awake patients will have lids stay open, snap shut, or flutter.
Seizures	
Corneal reflex	Usually intact in pseudoseizure.
Abdominal musculature	Palpation of abdominal musculature reveals lack of contractions with pseudoseizure.
Blindness	
Opticokinetic drum	Rotating drum with alternating black and white stripes or piece of tape with alternating black and white sections pulled laterally in front of a patient's open eyes will produce nystagmus in a patient with intact vision.

Source: Purcell TB: The somatic patient. *Emerg Clin North Am* 9:137, 1991.

hypochondriasis, patients are usually without loss of function and display the conviction that some terrible undiscovered illness is present. Hypochondriacal patients will be overly concerned with symptoms. In cases of factitious symptoms, usually associated with malingering, patients will consciously complain about symptoms to get out of an undesirable duty or to receive sympathy or undeserved compensation. Such patients rarely have neurologic complaints. Amobarbital interviews have been used to diagnose conversion disorder and coexisting diagnoses. The interviews also may be therapeutic.[7]

TREATMENT AND PROGNOSIS

The patient is devoid of insight that the symptoms have no organic cause. Confronting the patient and insisting that nothing "real" is wrong is not helpful in alleviating symptoms and may worsen the patient's condition. The symptoms should be neither trivialized nor reinforced. If the precipitating factor is identified, correction of the situation should be attempted. Meanwhile, the patient should receive reassurance that no serious medical problem has been identified. If the results of initial testing and the examination are negative, it should be suggested to the patient that the symptoms will resolve. Nonspecific supportive therapy should be prescribed. For instance, in the example cited at the beginning of this chapter, it could be suggested that the patient visit her father less often, call daily instead, and have her husband accompany her to the hospital. She should expect the blindness to resolve if she follows this course.[2,8]

Referral is mandatory. Patients with conversion disorders may need repetitive reassurance and suggestions that symptoms will resolve before returning to full function. Periodic follow-up is also important to monitor for subtle organic disease. Between 25 and 50 percent of patients diagnosed with conversion disorders later develop serious organic conditions.[2,9] A recent study of 85 patients with a diagnosis of conversion disorder found that 12 percent had a neurologic problem.[10] Factors that increased the likelihood of an organic etiology were older age, longer symptoms, suspicion of a neurologic problem, and use of medication.[10] Other investigators, in reporting six cases of severe neurologic pathology in patients diagnosed as having conversion disorder, highlighted six errors in evaluation of conversion disorder patients (Table 293-2).[11] Use of magnetic resonance imaging led to the correct diagnosis in five of those cases.[11] Most conversion disorders are brief and quickly resolve. Favorable prognostic factors are lack of other psychiatric disorders, sudden severe stress as a precipitating cause, and absence of medical problems. Some cases are resistant and require hypnosis or amobarbital interview for resolution. The interview should be coordinated by the primary care provider. Lorazepam has been found to be helpful in the management of this condition. Approximately 25 percent of patients will have another episode over the ensuing 1 to 6 years, which may involve the same or a new symptom complex.[2,9]

Some patients develop a chronic form of the disorder with complications, including contractures and atrophy of muscle groups. In addition, unnecessary diagnostic tests may lead to iatrogenic complications.

TABLE 293-2   Errors and Cautions in the Diagnosis of Conversion Disorders

Errors
- A finding in the evaluation is "unbelievable"
- A finding has "never been seen before" by the examiner
- A finding is nonanatomic
- The examination is inconsistent, effort is poor, classic feigning signs are present (see Table 293-1)
- The patient exhibits *la belle indifférence*
- There is an "obvious" psychologic explanation

Cautions
- Neurologic symptoms can be bizarre
- A physician's "neurologic clinical experience" may be limited
- A physician may be unfamiliar with true anatomic pathology
- There are many reasons for inconsistent effort, including neurologic pathology and examiner input
- *La belle indifférence* may be the expression of neurologic problems or due simply to individual variation
- Physicians often fall into the trap of jumping to a psychological explanation for a confusing entity

Source: Glick TH, Workman MD, Gaufberg SV: Suspected conversion disorder: Foreseeable risks and avoidable errors. *Adac Emerg Med* 7:1272, 2000.

REFERENCES

1. American Psychiatric Association: *Diagnostic and Statistical Manual of Mental Disorders,* 4th ed, rev. Washington, DC, American Psychiatric Association, 1994.
2. Sadock BS, Sadock VA: Conversion disorder, in Sadock, BJ, Sadock VA (eds): *Kaplan and Sadock's Comprehensive Textbook of Psychiatry,* 7th ed. Baltimore, Lippincott, Williams & Wilkins, 2000, p 642.
3. Binzer M, Andersen PM, Kullgren G: Clinical characteristics of patients with motor disability due to conversion disorder: A prospective control group study. *J Neurol Neurosurg Psychiatry* 63:83, 1997.
4. Dula DJ, DeNaples L: Emergency department presentation of patients with conversion disorder. *Acad Emerg Med* 2:120, 1995.
5. Lazare A: Conversion symptoms. *New Engl J Med* 305:745, 1981.
6. Purcell TB: The somatic patient. *Emerg Clin North Am* 9:137, 1991.
7. Fackler SM, Anfinson TJ, Rand JA: Serial sodium Amytal interviews in the clinical setting. *Psychosomatics* 38:558, 1997.
8. Silver FW: Management of conversion disorder. *Am J Phys Med Rehabil* 75:134, 1996.
9. Hafeiz HV: Hysterical conversion: A prognostic study. *Br J Psychiatry* 136:548, 1980.
10. Moene FC, Landberg EH, Hoogduin KA, et al: Organic syndromes diagnosed as conversion disorder: Identification and frequency in a study of 85 patients. *J Pyschosom Res* 49:7, 2000.
11. Glick TH, Workman MD, Gaufberg SV: Suspected conversion disorder: Foreseeable risks and avoidable errors. *Acad Emerg Med* 7:1272, 2000.

294   NOTIFYING THE LIVING OF DEATH
James Brown
Glenn Hamilton

Of the 90+ million ED visits in 1995, a total of 339,000 (0.4 percent) deaths occurred in the department.[1] The timing and nature of death are often unexpected and traumatic to the survivors. In one study, 65 percent of ED deaths were considered unexpected versus 7 percent of inpatient deaths. Compounding this difficult, acute situation is the fact that the ED staff generally have no prior relationship with the patient or the family.

Death notification training is deficient throughout medical education. Medical students question how well they are prepared to tell a family about death. One-half of emergency physicians report training in death notification during medical school and only one-third during

residency. Seventy percent of ED physicians find death notification to be emotionally draining. Without proper training, this role is even more difficult.[2] Educational programs involving videotaping of death notifications and role playing can assist physicians in developing the necessary skills.[3,4] The ED staff can become desensitized or preoccupied with moving on to the living patients who are waiting. One-fourth of families describe the ED staff as cold, unsympathetic, and not reassuring.[5]

PREPARING FOR NOTIFICATION

An organized approach is essential (Table 294-1). A secluded area close to the ED should be available for the family and friends. This area should include a telephone with long-distance access to allow the contact of relatives and friends. If the family arrives while resuscitation efforts are continuing, a physician or trained member of the hospital staff should inform them of the resuscitation and its progress. Families who wish to be present at the resuscitation should be allowed to be (see below, and Chap. 17). Updates should be given frequently (every 5 to 10 min) until the effort concludes.[6] Sharing information and empathy during this time allows family members to become knowledgeably prepared for the potential outcome.

After leaving the resuscitation room, the physician must mentally "change gears" within 15 to 30 s. It is important to collect one's thoughts and organize the presentation. If clothing is soiled, it should be changed before the notification. An appropriate amount of time for family discussion is allotted. Other tasks in the department are delegated to others, or families are informed of the reason for delay. Advance information about which family members are present and their preparation is obtained whenever possible. It is best not to go alone. If clergy or social services support is not present or will not be available in a timely fashion, the nursing staff can be enlisted.

TELLING THE SURVIVORS

It is the physician's responsibility to inform family members of the death.[7] Upon entering the room, the physician should introduce the team to the patient's family. The leading family member is identified, and all parties, including the physician, are seated, if possible. Sitting minimizes the chance of trauma occurring from fainting or falling and signals the family that the physician will remain as long as necessary. The deceased should be addressed by name. The family is then given a very brief summary of the patient's response to treatment, if any. This should be done in plain language, without medical jargon. Providing unnecessary or lengthy detail before announcing the death can rouse false hopes and cause extreme anxiety.

After these few brief phrases, the family is told that the patient has died and sympathy is expressed. To avoid confusion, terms such as *passed on* or *no longer with us* should not be used. Once the initial statement is made, allow a brief period for the initial grief response (30 to 60 s). The physician may give physical comfort to the family if the physician is comfortable doing so.

After the initial pause, asking the most stable survivor for a perception of the event allows the initial presentation of information to conclude. Families may receive some comfort from statements that the patient suffered no pain (if appropriate) and that everything possible was done. They are told that the coroner or medical examiner and their private physician will be contacted. They are also told that the physician will return to answer any questions they may have.[8]

GRIEF REACTION

Individual responses to the death of a loved one vary greatly. The initial response has been described as a "psychic pain spike." It lasts only a brief period, usually 5 to 15 min. During this period, the family can make no decisions. Once this period of acute grief has ended, the fam-

TABLE 294-1   Sequence of Events

Preparation	Private area or room is prepared. The family is gathered. The family advised of ongoing efforts, if any. Social services or the chaplain is contacted. The physician prepares mentally and physically.
Notification	Introduce yourself and identify family members. Sit down with the family. Give a brief synopsis of events to date. Tell the family that the patient has died.
Grief response	Give physical comfort, if able. Do not move away. After the initial response, ask a question about the patient. Reassure the family that no suffering was involved, if appropriate. Support other physicians and emergency medical service personnel when possible. Stand up. Advise the family that you will contact the family physician and coroner. Leave the room.
Viewing the body	Allow the family to view the deceased. Do not force a viewing. The body is prepared before viewing. A staff member accompanies family.
Concluding process	Express condolences. Ask family members whether thay have questions. Inquire about an autopsy and organ donation. Sign papers. Identify those at risk for pathologic grief. Avoid prescribing sedatives. Arrange follow-up as appropriate. Tell the family when to leave.

Sources: Hamilton GC: Sudden death in the ED: Telling the living. *Ann Emerg Med* 17:382, 1988; Walters DT: Family grief in the emergency department. *Emerg Med Clin North Am* 9:189, 1991.

ily members will progress through other reactions: denial, anger, and/or guilt.[9]

Denial may be expressed as disbelief. The family may insist on viewing the deceased, and this should be done when possible.[9] Denial may be a protective mechanism, giving the mind time to absorb the situation. It is accepted and tolerated patiently, allowing the bereaved some time to adjust.

Anger may be directed at the physician or staff. Accusations of negligence or statements about what should have been done may be made. Although difficult to accept, the physician must see these as expressions of grief. This anger is often misplaced guilt at causing or failing to prevent the death. Unconscious frustration with the deceased for abandoning the bereaved can find its outlet in anger directed at others. A defensive posture on the part of the physician is counterproductive. Reflecting the family members' feelings back to them and not taking the outbursts personally is the best response. Eventually the anger will dissipate, allowing the family to move on with their grief. The physician's handling of this immediate response is an important step in facilitating grief.

Guilt is nearly universal. There may be issues between the deceased and the bereaved that can no longer be resolved. It is important to intercept the survivor's self-accusations and to address the components of the survivor's guilt when possible. Exoneration by the physician can be very comforting.

The emotional response depends on the cultural background of the bereaved. Responses vary from hysterical crying to cold distraction. Regardless of the initial response, the bereaved must be allowed to express their feelings. The physician's response to these expressions is one of calm and silence. If possible, gently touching the bereaved can be more important than any words. Clichés such as "It's God's will" or "Life must go on" should be avoided.[9]

Normal grieving lasts 6 to 8 months. Physical symptoms include headache, irritability, fatigue, insomnia, restlessness, dyspnea, or anorexia. Emotional symptoms include guilt, denial, anger, depression, difficulty concentrating, lack of organization, and preoccupation with the deceased. These symptoms become pathologic grief if they persist over a prolonged period or with heightened intensity. Other manifestations of pathologic grief may include an exacerbating or remitting pattern of grief or signs of physical disability. Pathologic grief can be seen with multiple symptoms, including apathy, panic attacks, overactivity, hostility with paranoia, suppression of hostility with resultant flat affect, depression, or symptoms resembling those of the deceased.

Recognition of survivors at risk for or manifesting pathologic grief allows for early intervention. Risk factors for pathologic grief include sudden or unexpected death; death of an infant, child, or spouse; death involving suicide or homicide; or death where the survivor contributed to it. A surviving spouse with children may not have time to mourn appropriately. Those spouses with a high-conflict relationship, long duration of marriage, or a dependent relationship on the deceased are

particularly at risk. In the 2 years after losing a spouse older than 50 years, the risk of the survivor dying is increased over fourfold.

Physicians may be asked to provide sedatives, tranquilizers, or sleeping medications for the bereaved. The grieving process requires active work on the part of the bereaved. The survivors must learn to adjust to the absence of the deceased, form new relationships, and live in their environment without their loved one. This process is delayed by tranquilizing medications. Their use is to be avoided except in cases of pathologic grief and then only as part of comprehensive psychotherapy. Requests for medication should be countered with empathy and reassurance.

VIEWING THE BODY

After the initial grief reaction, the family should be offered an opportunity to view the body of the deceased, without pressuring them to do so. Failure to view the body may prolong the process by not permitting the survivors to believe the person is really dead. Whereas most find viewing the body to be a helpful experience, those who do not express no regret about their decision.[5]

The body is prepared before viewing. Blood and body secretions are cleaned off. The eyes are closed, and the body is covered except for the hands and face. If permitted by the circumstances and local protocol, tubes and catheters are removed. If disfigurement has occurred, these areas are bandaged. The family is warned about the temperature and color changes of the deceased. The body is placed in a smaller room, away from the treatment area, to give the mourners more privacy. The physician, clergy, or nursing staff accompanies the family to provide support or answer questions. The family is encouraged to speak to and touch the deceased, if they wish. A family member may wish to be alone with the deceased. This is permitted in appropriate circumstances; a staff member should remain close by for support. The deceased should be referred to by name or "him" or "her" and never by "it" or "the body."[7,9]

CONCLUDING PROCESS

Even after the family has an opportunity to view the body, several important processes remain. Now is the time to make requests for autopsy and organ donation. Any signing of papers is done at this time, and copies are given to the family. Any further questions are addressed at this time. Arrangements for funeral home and release of the body are made. The family is told that the patient's private physician will be contacted.[7] The physician and staff should be sympathetic but not apologetic. Families may misinterpret such expressions as an admission of guilt. Expressions such as, "You have my sympathy," or "I know this is very hard for you," are superior to, "I'm sorry."[7]

As in any other emergency encounter, follow-up arrangements conclude the visit. The survivors are educated about common grief symptoms. They are told to expect these as a normal part of grieving. At the minimum, the family should have the name and number of a staff member who can provide further information or answer questions that may arise.[7] Most researchers recommend a follow-up phone call or letter within 1 week and again in 2 months. One facility has established a program in which the staff sends a sympathy card, phone calls are made periodically during the year after the death, and the attending physician sends a letter explaining the autopsy findings.[2]

Finally, the family is told that it is time to leave. Survivors are frequently so overwhelmed with events that they do not know when to leave. They are escorted to the door and again given reassurance. Suggestions are made about contacting other friends or family for notification and funeral preparations.

SPECIAL CONSIDERATIONS

Long-Distance Notification

Telephone death notification is never ideal. If the survivors have not been notified of their family member's arrival in the ED, then initiate telephone contact. The caller should identify him- or herself and establish the identity of the survivor. The survivor is told that the relative or friend is severely injured or ill and that he or she must come to the hospital immediately. Instruct the survivor to drive carefully.[9]

There are times when distance, environmental, or other factors make physical notification inadvisable. One study showed that many survivors prefer to be notified by telephone if the driving time exceeded 1 h. Notification should not be rushed but should proceed in the same fashion as if done in person. The notification should not be forced; if the family member seems unprepared, offer to speak with another family member in the home or another relative. After the notification is made, if the survivor is alone, offer to contact some supporting person. If the survivor appears suicidal, local police may need to be contacted. If no adult is present, ask the oldest child how to contact an adult relative. Assure the child that an adult will be in contact shortly. Depending on the circumstances (distance, time of day, weather), the survivor should be instructed to come to the hospital driven by some supporter.

Coroner's Cases

In most states, the coroner and/or medical examiner has the responsibility to investigate the cause of death within a particular jurisdiction. Cases the medical examiner may choose for further investigation include those of a sudden, mysterious, unusual, or unnatural nature. Deaths with a possible public health danger, deaths in police custody or in prison, or violent death (including those resulting from motor vehicle crashes) are also cases for the medical examiner. Autopsy is usually performed in these cases, and the family is informed. Organ donation may still be possible, in consultation with the medical examiner.[7] Before viewing of the body by the family, resuscitative lines and tubes must be left in place. Except in very unusual circumstances, such as homicide, the viewing of the deceased can take place.

Autopsy

Autopsy rates have continued to decline in the United States, for a number of reasons. The Joint Commission on Accreditation of Hospitals eliminated its minimum autopsy rate of 20 percent in 1971.

Findings from autopsies can clarify premortem diagnoses or aid in the diagnosis of new diseases. Autopsies can assist in the grieving process by demonstrating to the family that they did not contribute to the death. Despite physicians' fears that the autopsy will lead to increased liability exposure, postmortem examinations are used more often as a defense.

Public misperceptions concerning autopsy abound. Some of the misperceptions are that diagnostic tests are infallible; autopsy disturbs the patient's "peace"; bodily mutilation occurs; funeral arrangements will be delayed; it is too late to accomplish anything positive; there are religious prohibitions; the family never gets the results; and if an autopsy is necessary, one will be requested.

The most senior physician involved with the case should approach the family with the request for autopsy. Specific points to be discussed include that the autopsy is done by specialists in pathology (an analogy to surgery may be helpful); specific determination of cause of death may help to dispel any doubt the family has; funeral arrangements will not be disturbed; and no mutilation occurs. If the family is concerned about religious prohibitions, they can be reassured that autopsy is not prohibited by most major religions and can be encouraged to consult with the chaplain. The physician requesting the autopsy must be aware of local and institutional policies regarding billing and payment for autopsies. Many teaching institutions consider the autopsy as part of comprehensive care and do not submit a charge. However, there is great variation in policies in community, state, and municipal hospitals, and insurance policies may not pay for an autopsy, so the patient's family should be informed about possible costs when they make their decision.[7]

Organ Donation

Although actually harvesting organs in the ED is a rare event, many organs can be harvested up to 24 h after death, if the body is refrigerated within 4 h of death. These harvestable organs include tissues such as cornea, bone, skin, tendon, fascia, cartilage, saphenous vein, and heart valves. Contraindications to donation include age older than 80 years, death from infectious disease, cancer (although corneas may still be donated), or toxic exposure.[10] Organs have been harvested successfully despite fatal exposures to cocaine, ethanol, carbon monoxide, lead, and barbiturates. Consultation with a toxicologist is recommended in these circumstances.[7,11]

There are several barriers to tissue procurement in the ED. One study showed that only 43 percent of families were approached, with a successful donation rate of 12 percent. Reasons given for not approaching families included a coroner's investigation (35 percent), family not available (20 percent), family too upset (18 percent), deceased medically unsuitable (14 percent), and no patient identification (12 percent). Time constraints are another barrier to successfully obtaining donation. Limited time to develop rapport with families and to allow them to come to terms with the death, along with a busy staff, have been cited as reasons for unsuccessful donation efforts.[10]

The appropriate time to make a request for organ donation is after the family has viewed the body. At this point, an interval has occurred from the actual notification, and the bereaved have had time to come to accept the death as real. A premature request for organ donation may leave the family with doubts about the resuscitative efforts. The family is informed that they are not charged for any procedures related to the donation and that no alteration in the appearance of the deceased occurs.

Viewing Resuscitation

The presence of family during resuscitation is somewhat controversial. Traditionally, family members were excluded from the resuscitation area. More recent data have challenged this practice. Families believe they have a right to be present and that they should be asked. Most of those present at a resuscitation feel that the process helped them adapt to the death and that their presence benefited the deceased.[12] Postresuscitation psychological testing of family members present at a resuscitation found no harm and a trend toward benefit for the survivors.[13] Out-of-hospital resuscitations have occurred for years in the presence of family members. The American Heart Association in its 2000 guidelines has recommended offering the option of viewing resuscitation to families.[14]

Conversely, health care providers remain opposed to this practice. Concerns listed include interference in the resuscitation, offering false hope to the family while cardiopulmonary resuscitation continues, fainting or other medical deterioration of witnesses, discomfort or anxiety of team members, and medicolegal conflicts.[15,16] Despite such anecdotal reports, the overwhelming body of evidence suggests a reasoned policy of allowing the family to view resuscitation.

Deaths of Children

Regardless of the etiology of the child's death, survivors are at increased risk of pathologic grief. Divorce is common after the death of a child. Parents of deceased children display a wide range of emotional responses, but anger and guilt with associated despair predominate. These emotions may be related to a sense of failure of the parent's protective role. Both parents are equally devastated and unable to support each other adequately. The need to care for surviving children may not allow time for proper grieving to occur. In particular, a perinatal death with a surviving twin or subsequent pregnancy within months places families at higher risk for pathologic grief responses.

Surviving children are also deeply affected by the death of a sibling. Feelings of abandonment, fear of death, and guilt predominate. If the child wished the sibling dead at a time near the death, the child may believe that the "magical" thinking was causative. Parents, unable to deal with their own grief, may explain the death in misleading or vague terms.

Managing a pediatric death in the ED is the most stressful professional situation most physicians will encounter. Most emergency physicians feel a sense of guilt or inadequacy after a pediatric death, and many will feel impaired for the duration of their shift.[17] The American Academy of Pediatrics and the American College of Emergency Physicians have developed a joint policy on the death of a child in the ED. They recommend a "family-centered and team-oriented approach" to the death of a child.[18]

The autopsy is particularly helpful in cases of pediatric death. It provides an organic, identifiable cause of death, helping to alleviate guilt. It can offer a source of comfort to the family that the knowledge gained may be useful in helping other children. Organ donation is also useful in this fashion.[19] A memory box, containing a lock of the child's hair and impressions of hands and feet, can be of comfort to the grieving parents.[16]

REFERENCES

1. McCaig LF, Stussman BJ. *Advance Data: National Hospital Ambulatory Medical Care Survey: 1996 Emergency Department Summary.* Hyattsville, MD: National Center for Health Statistics, 1997, p. 293.
2. Schmidt TA, Tolle SW: Emergency physician's responses to families following patient death. *Ann Emerg Med* 19:125, 1990.
3. Schmidt TA, Norton RL, Tolle SW: Sudden death in the ED: Educating residents to compassionately inform families. *J Emerg Med* 10:643, 1992.
4. Tolle SW, Cooney TG, Hickam DH: A program to teach residents humanistic skills for notifying survivors of a patient's death. *Acad Med* 64:505, 1989.
5. Parrish GA, Holdren KS, Skiendzielewski JJ, et al: Emergency department experience with sudden death: A survey of survivors. *Ann Emerg Med* 16:792, 1987.
6. Jones WH, Butery M: Sudden death: Survivors' perceptions of their emergency department experience. *J Emerg Nursing* 7:14, 1981.
7. Olsen JC, Buenefe ML, Falco WD: Death in the emergency department. *Ann Emerg Med* 31:758, 1998.
8. Hamilton GC: Sudden death in the ED: Telling the living. *Ann Emerg Med* 17:382, 1988.
9. Edlich RF, Kübler-Ross E: On death and dying in the emergency department. *J Emerg Med* 10:225, 1992.
10. Lewis LM, Martin L, Hoffman T, et al: Tissue and organ procurement in the emergency department setting. *Am J Emerg Med* 11:347, 1993.
11. Leikin JB, Heyn-Lamb R, Aks S, et al: The toxic patient as a potential organ donor. *Am J Emerg Med* 12:151, 1994.
12. Boudreaux ED, Francis JL, Loyacano T: Family presence during invasive procedures and resuscitations in the emergency department: A critical review and suggestions for future research. *Ann Emerg Med* 40:193, 2002.
13. Robinson SM, Mackenzie-Ross S, Campbell Hewson GL, et al: Psychological effect of witnessed resuscitation on bereaved relatives. *Lancet* 352:614, 1998.
14. Guidelines 2000 for cardiopulmonary resuscitation and emergency cardiovascular care. Part 2: Ethical aspects of CPR and ECC. *Circulation* 102:I12, 2000.
15. Tsai E: Should family members be present during cardiopulmonary resuscitation? *N Engl J Med* 346:1019, 2002.
16. Iserson KV: *Grave Words: Notifying Survivors About Sudden, Unexpected Deaths.* Tucson, AZ, Galen Press, 1999.
17. Ahrens WR, Hart RG: Emergency physicians' experience with pediatric death. *Am J Emerg Med* 15:642, 1997.
18. Death of a child in the emergency department, a joint statement by the American Academy of Pediatrics and the American College of Emergency Physicians. *Ann Emerg Med* 40:409, 2002.
19. Beckwith J: The value of the pediatric post mortem examination. *Pediatr Clin North Am* 36:29, 1989.

SUBSTANCE AND ALCOHOL ABUSE

William A. Berk
 Alcoholism and Alcohol Abuse:
 Medical Aspects
Edward Bernstein
Judith Bernstein
Irene Coletsos
Gail D'Onofrio
 Alcohol and Drug Abuse:
 Emergency Department Identification,
 Intervention, and Referral

ALCOHOLISM AND ALCOHOL ABUSE: MEDICAL ASPECTS

Alcoholism is a ubiquitous medical and social problem that crosses social and economic boundaries. Ethanol dependence, defined as regular use resulting in tolerance to the drug and the likelihood of withdrawal symptoms if intake is suspended, is experienced by 4.4 percent of Americans. Ethanol abuse, affecting another 3 percent of the population, is a separate problem marked by social or medical problems that result from inappropriate use of ethanol but without the presence of dependence.[1–2] The lifetime risk for alcohol dependence was recently calculated at 13.3 percent.[3] Examples of ethanol abuse include intermittent bouts of drinking resulting in aggressive or antisocial behavior or driving while intoxicated. Although alcoholism is less common in women than in men, affected women are no less susceptible to medical and traumatic complications.[4]

Although alcoholism by itself does not constitute a medical emergency, alcohol abuse and dependence were found to be important in the presentation of 2.6 million patients to ED visits, or 2.7 percent of all visits.[5] These presentations included trauma, infections, and various entities involving the gastrointestinal tract and central nervous system. Acute alcohol intoxication and other complications of alcohol use, such as hepatitis, pancreatitis, and alcohol withdrawal, frequently result in ED visits. Alcohol is often used with other drugs. Emergency physicians should be able to recognize alcoholism as a contributor to a patient's presenting problems and as an underlying problem requiring care.

Etiology

The pathogenesis of alcoholism is multifactorial, with genetic and environmental inputs. Studies of isolated twins and adopted children and of families in general have confirmed a heritable component to alcoholism that seems greater in men than in women and is greater in identical twins than in fraternal twins. Close relatives of alcoholics have a fourfold risk of alcoholism over controls, even when they are adopted children raised away from their genetic family from birth.

Alcoholism has been defined as a "primary, chronic disease with genetic, psychosocial, and environmental factors influencing its development and manifestations . . . [and] is characterized by impaired control over drinking, preoccupation with the drug ethanol, use of ethanol despite adverse consequences, and distortions in thinking, most notably denial. Each of these symptoms may be continuous or periodic."[2] Male sex, age between 25 and 34 years, poor education, pre-existent psychiatric disorder, and homelessness are common associations; nevertheless, alcoholism is a disorder that crosses all socioeconomic boundaries and involves all age groups. Among the homeless, estimated at 250,000 on any given night and 3 million people per year, 20 to 45 percent are alcoholics. Secondary psychiatric diagnoses, including antisocial personality, mania, and schizophrenia, are more common in alcoholics than in the general population. Suicide attempts and problems with drugs other than ethanol are also common among alcoholics.

The fact that 10 percent of the population have ethanol-related problems means that alcoholism touches most Americans' lives at some time, whether at home, on the road, or in the workplace.

Effects of Alcohol on Health

Ethanol abuse and its association with trauma represent a major public health issue. Forty percent of Americans will be involved in an ethanol-related motor vehicle collision in their lifetimes, and more than 40 percent of fatal motor vehicle accidents are associated with use of ethanol. Those who drink are also at increased risk for accidents within the home and for injuries from assault.

Alcoholics have been estimated on average to have a life span 10 to 15 years shorter than that for moderate drinkers or abstainers.[6] Increased mortality results chiefly from heart and liver disease, cancer, and trauma. Although the occurrence of coronary artery disease is decreased among alcoholics, heavy ethanol use increases the likelihood of hypertension and, hence, hypertensive disease, and itself is a common cause of cardiomyopathy. Ethanol is the most common cause of liver failure in the United States and worldwide. Fatty liver is present in virtually all alcoholics, and 10 to 35 percent develop alcoholic hepatitis. Heavy ethanol use also is associated with increased risk of cancer of the esophagus, stomach, pancreas, liver, and breast.

Chronic toxicity from ethanol abuse may affect nearly every major organ system with serious health consequences (Table 295-1). A detailed discussion of these complications is beyond the scope of this chapter.

There is good evidence that moderate ethanol use may actually promote health (in contrast to tobacco, which is legal but for which there is no safe level of consumption). A large population-based study found that subjects who consumed between one drink a month and one drink a day had a lower mortality rate than did those who drank more or less. This observation is the basis for so-called U-shaped or J-shaped curves of mortality in relation to alcohol consumption, with mortality lowest with moderate rates of consumption, greater with abstinence, and greatest at the highest levels of consumption. Decreased mortality may result from diminished coronary risk among users of ethanol, apparently mediated through increased blood levels of high-density lipoprotein and an antithrombotic effect. Although these effects persist at higher levels of ethanol use, the other deleterious effects of chronic use of the drug outweigh those.

Trauma and the Ethanol-Intoxicated Patient

Alcohol is an important predisposing factor for trauma of all types. The drinker and those in the vicinity of the drinker are at risk: of the

TABLE 295-1   Some Adverse Health Effects Associated with Ethanol Abuse and Dependence

Central nervous system
  Acute intoxication
  Ethanol withdrawal
    Seizures
    Hallucinations
  Wernicke encephalopathy
  Korsakoff psychosis
  Dementia
  Depression, antisocial personality, suicidal ideation
Gastrointestinal
  Esophageal varices
  Erosive gastritis
  Alcoholic hepatitis/liver failure
  Peptic ulcer disease
  Pancreatitis
  Oropharyngeal, esophageal, gastric, hepatic and pancreatic malignancies
Cardiovascular
  Hypertension
  Cardiomyopathy
  Stroke
  Arrhythmias associated with intoxication or withdrawal
Musculoskeletal
  Fractures secondary to ethanol-associated trauma
  Osteopenia
  Myopathy
Endocrine/metabolic
  Testicular atrophy
  Alcoholic ketoacidosis
  Folic acid and thiamine deficiencies
Hematopoietic
  Thrombocytopenia secondary to marrow suppression, folate deficiency, splenic sequestration
  Anemia secondary to marrow suppression, folate deficiency, gastrointestinal bleeding, splenic sequestration
  Leukopenia secondary to marrow suppression, splenic sequestration
Immune
  Bacterial pneumonia
  Tuberculosis
  Hepatitis C
Other
  Fetal alcohol syndrome
  Breast cancer in women

more than 11 million victims of interpersonal trauma seen annually, 25 percent report alcohol use by their assailant,[7] and alcohol abuse as reported by the injured woman is the strongest predictor for acute injury related to domestic violence.[8] The proportion of fatal collisions involving a driver with a blood alcohol level higher than 10 mg/dL dropped from 51 to 41 percent between 1987 and 1996, but then increased by 4.1 percent from 1999 to 2000, when alcohol-related fatalities totaled 16,199. Alcohol-related trauma clearly represents a significant public health problem, with a large impact on emergency medicine practice. In addition, it has been argued that injured alcoholic patients require more observation, testing, and/or treatment than do other trauma patients, because they may be more severely traumatized, they are at higher risk of complications, and intoxication may mask serious injuries. A study of more than 1 million motor vehicle crashes, which attempted to control for safety belt use, vehicle deformation, vehicle speed, and other factors, found that drivers who drank were more likely to suffer a serious injury or death. However, when severity of injury was controlled, chronic alcoholism, but not acute intoxication, was found to be an independent predictor of poor outcome. These findings most likely reflect the comorbidity of underlying organ system dysfunction. Although there is good evidence that stable intoxicated trauma victims, for example, with a Glasgow Coma Score of 15 and nontender abdomens, may be managed conservatively,[9] severely injured and/or severely intoxicated patients can be expected to require more diagnostic and treatment resources than other patients.

Evaluation of intoxicated patients with head injuries is particularly problematic. Serious head injuries are easily overlooked in intoxicated patients, some of whom, especially in inner-city locales, may arrive at the ED with no definite history of trauma and no external signs of head trauma. In our experience, the most common serious error made in management of intoxicated patients is to assume for too long that a depressed or abnormal mental status is secondary to intoxication. Intoxicated patients should undergo computed tomographic (CT) evaluation, if there is a history of head injury and the Glasgow Coma Score is less than 15; for any worsening of mental status while under observation; or if there is no improvement in mental status by 3 h after admission. Once the decision to perform CT has been made, no delay should be allowed due to lack of cooperation by the patient, which may be due to ethanol or concomitant drug use or the effects of head injury. Sedation may be required, with careful attention to airway protection and paralysis and intubation, if necessary.

Hypothermia and Ethanol Intoxication

Many cases of hypothermia during the winter months in urban settings are associated with ethanol use. Many homeless persons are heavy users of ethanol and, on cold nights, may use ethanol to inure themselves to the effects of low temperature. Although the sedative effects of ethanol may result in exposure predisposing to hypothermia, ethanol also directly contributes to body cooling. It depresses central thermoregulatory mechanisms, decreases shivering, and enhances heat loss through vasodilatation. Management of the hypothermic intoxicated patient is similar to that of hypothermia in other patients. Prognosis is related to severity of hypothermia and the presence of underlying diseases, but does not appeared to be adversely affected by ethanol intoxication.

Ethanol Withdrawal

Some alcoholics exhibit one or more symptoms of withdrawal upon discontinuation of ethanol intake. Symptoms and signs include tremor, anxiety, agitation, and signs of autonomic hyperactivity, including cardiac dysrhythmias, and, most frequently, sinus tachycardia or atrial fibrillation. Seizures may occur, and hallucinations, usually visual, reflect moderate to severe withdrawal. Signs and symptoms of withdrawal are most likely to reach peak intensity at 48 h after the patient's last drink. There is wide variation in the timing of onset and peak severity of alcohol withdrawal, which reflects differences in patterns of ethanol intake, individual susceptibility to withdrawal, and concomitant illness. For example, significant withdrawal may occur while alcoholics still have detectable blood ethanol or within a short time after the last drink. These situations likely reflect a recent pattern of decreased but continued intake of ethanol, or alcoholics' common practice of self-treatment with ethanol when symptoms first appear, followed by presentation for seeking medical care if those symptoms fail to resolve.

Because ethanol withdrawal is a syndrome complex, more than one sign is present in most cases. When alcoholic patients present with one sign typical of ethanol withdrawal, other causes should be considered. Seizures in particular are frequently secondary to other causes, most notably recent or remote head trauma, and whether the patient recounts a history. Hallucinations may be secondary to a psychiatric disorder (although these are more likely to be auditory, not visual) or concomitant drug use.

MANAGEMENT   After the diagnosis of alcohol withdrawal is established, an examination for complicating medical conditions or injury should be performed. Patients with alcohol withdrawal are frequently volume depleted and may require crystalloid infusion. If possible, patients should be placed in a quiet area with a minimum of stimulation. For patients who have experienced seizures, **CT examination is indicated when focal seizures have occurred, when a focal neurologic finding is elicited if there has been head trauma, or when the patient has a persistent postictal defect in consciousness.**

The use of benzodiazepines to treat alcohol withdrawal has been validated by many studies.[10] A recent randomized controlled trial found that treatment of patients who have experienced one withdrawal seizure with a small dose of lorazepam is effective in preventing seizure recurrence,[11] adding further evidence for benzodiazepines as the primary treatment of choice for alcohol withdrawal. γ-Aminobutyric acid, carbamazepine, valproic acid, β-blockers, and other agents have been advocated for treatment of alcohol withdrawal,[10] but none has the support of clinical evidence. Phenobarbital is effective, but has no advantage over benzodiazepines, and due to its risk profile, particularly respiratory depression and hypotension, has fallen out of favor. It is still used for control of status epilepticus (see Chap. 225).

The initial dose of lorazepam is 2 to 4 mg intravenously, followed by doses of 2 to 4 mg every 15 to 30 min until a condition of light sedation is attained (Table 295-2). Clinicians should approach treatment of alcohol withdrawal prepared to administer lorazepam repeatedly and in cumulatively large doses. At the same time as primary therapy is initiated for alcohol withdrawal, 1 L of D5NS with 100 mg of thiamine and 4 g of magnesium sulfate is given over 1 to 2 h. Although magnesium has not been shown to be effective against ethanol withdrawal in general, hypomagnesemia has been closely associated with tremor in alcoholics and may play a role in the genesis of seizures.

DISPOSITION   Patients with alcohol withdrawal and complicating medical problems, such as infections or congestive heart failure, should be admitted to the hospital. Patients who fail to respond to one or two doses of sedative medications also should be admitted. **Administration of lorazepam, more than 8 mg, is in most cases an indication for admission** to a nursing unit, where the patient can receive close observation by nursing and physician staffs, and in many hospitals, an intensive care unit. Patients with mild alcohol withdrawal that responds to treatment may be discharged. If they have received phenobarbital, no outpatient prescription is necessary. In any case, the benefit of prescribing outpatient benzodiazepines is doubtful if a patient is likely to resume drinking after discharge from the ED.

The Elderly Patient and Alcohol

Fewer older people drink regularly, and intake among older drinkers is less than that among younger people. Nevertheless, alcohol is a significant problem among the elderly, and alcohol is by far the most common drug-related problem in this age group, as other (illegal) drugs are rarely abused. Moreover, because many physicians are even less likely to consider the possibility of alcohol abuse or alcoholism in older than in younger patients, the diagnosis is often missed. The

TABLE 295-2   Treatment of Alcohol Withdrawal

1. Fluid resuscitation, D5NS or D5LR with 100 mg thiamine/L
2. Lorazepam 2–4 mg IV, followed by 2–4 mg IV q15–30 min until light sedation
3. Magnesium sulfate, 4 gm IV over 1–2 h

significance of the impact that alcohol has on the health of the elderly is made clear by the following: the prevalence of alcohol-related hospitalizations during a recent year for people older than 65 years was 54.7 per 10,000 population for men and 14.8 per 10,000 for women. Alcohol plays a significant role in motor vehicle collisions and other trauma involving the elderly[12] and has a greater impact on health than in younger persons, because mortality and morbidity from all types of trauma is greater among older patients.

Women and Alcohol

Women are less likely than men to abuse alcohol[1–4] and yet are more prone to alcohol-associated health problems, especially cirrhosis. A population-based study found that, among those averaging six or more drinks per day, the relative risk for mortality for women was five times that of men. The reason for this observation is unclear but may be related to the fact that women have virtually no first-pass metabolism of alcohol by gastric alcohol dehydrogenase and a smaller volume of distribution than men, resulting in considerably higher blood alcohol levels after ingestion of a given dose of alcohol.

Women who drink during pregnancy predispose their children to growth retardation in utero, fetal alcohol syndrome, characterized by facial dysmorphology, and mental and growth retardation after birth. Even women who report intake of less than one drink a day are at increased risk to have a child in the bottom decile for weight at birth. Because emergency physicians frequently diagnose pregnancy and patients with alcohol problems are often seen in EDs, emergency physicians are more likely than many physicians to have the opportunity to advise pregnant patients about the risks inherent in using alcohol during pregnancy.

ALCOHOL AND DRUG ABUSE: EMERGENCY DEPARTMENT IDENTIFICATION, INTERVENTION, AND REFERRAL

Emergency Department Recognition of Alcohol and Substance Abuse

Clinical medicine until recently has lacked the social mandate, resources, will, and training necessary to treat alcohol and drug addiction adequately, despite the proven effectiveness of treatment in breaking the cycle of addiction and reducing recidivism, and instead often has deferred to the criminal justice system.[13] Emergency physicians are experts in the stabilization, diagnosis, and treatment of *acute* alcohol and drug emergencies and their secondary complications, but often fail to detect and refer patients for treatment of addiction. Referral rates as low as 13 and 23 percent[14] have been reported among ED patients with documented substance abuse problems. As a result, many ED patients who could be assisted in breaking the cycle of addiction continue to visit the ED with trauma and medical problems. Studies in trauma centers have shown that, although up to 44 percent of patients screen positive for chronic alcohol abuse, fewer than 15 percent of the nation's trauma centers do such screening, and even fewer provide alcohol counseling.[15]

Barriers to detection and referral include insufficient evidence-based knowledge, time constraints, inadequate treatment resources, and a belief that substance abuse is not an appropriate emergency room concern. Emergency physicians have an opportunity to use the ED visit, the "teachable moment," to link patients presenting to the ED with the substance abuse treatment system. Brief educational sessions with emergency medicine residents have resulted in a significant difference in their willingness to discuss substance abuse. After a 4-h didactic training session in screening and brief intervention, use of these skills increased from 17 percent before training to 58 percent compared with a control group in which performance remained the same over time.[16]

Emergency medicine physicians' attitudes also may be based on the incorrect assumption that substance abuse is significantly different from other medical conditions and that it defies treatment. In reality, drug dependence shares many of the same characteristics as those of chronic illnesses. McLellan and colleagues found that the etiology, pathophysiology, and response to treatment (including relapse and adherence rates) in patients with drug and alcohol dependence are similar to those in patients with diseases such as asthma, type II diabetes, and hypertension.[17] Further, treatment works and is associated with reduced health care costs. When substance-abusing patients receive adequate evaluation, medication management, and monitoring, they receive lasting benefits,[17] and a gain of $7 is reported for every dollar invested in treatment; overall, the $200 million spent on treatment resulted in a $1.5 billion savings for California taxpayers.[18]

Effectiveness of Brief Intervention

Chafetz established the effectiveness of screening, detection, and brief intervention four decades ago at Massachusetts General Hospital.[19] A randomized controlled trial among a population consisting primarily of homeless men demonstrated that it was possible to enhance care, even in a hard-to-reach group, by "establishing emotionally meaningful communication with these patients." As a result of this intervention performed by a social worker and psychiatric resident, 65 percent completed a referral to an alcohol clinic as opposed to 1 percent of the control group. Forty percent completed five or more voluntary visits compared with 0 percent of the control subjects who were managed by the ED staff in the routine manner.

Many models for brief intervention have been tested in case controlled or randomized control trials. In 32 of 39 studies reviewed by D'Onofrio and Degutis on the effectiveness of brief counseling for alcohol problems, patients were helped by these interventions.[20] Positive effects included reduced alcohol consumption, lower blood pressure, and fewer sick days.[20] A 48 percent reduction in injuries requiring hospital admission on 3-year follow-up was reported by Gentilello and colleagues in a randomized controlled trial of brief motivational interviewing among alcohol-impaired patients in a trauma center.[15] The elements common to successful trials included feedback, responsibility, advice, menu or choice, empathy, and self-efficacy (FRAMES). A World Health Organization study evaluating heavy problem drinkers across 12 nations with very different cultural orientations and social circumstances reinforced the strength of this counseling method.[21]

In some EDs, social workers, psychologists, addiction specialists, volunteers from Alcoholics Anonymous or Narcotics Anonymous, or health promotion advocates (peer educators) have joined the traditional ED team to assist in screening, using brief intervention techniques, and referring patients to the treatment system, primary health care, and other needed services (e.g., housing, food, clothing, and jobs).

One of the first of these models to report ED data was Project ASSERT at Boston Medical Center,[22] which used trained community outreach workers from cultural backgrounds similar to those of the patients. They interview patients in the ED examining rooms by using a health-needs history to screen for substance abuse and other preventable conditions, and they offer health education and referrals for smoking cessation, domestic violence counseling, and other services. If substance abuse is identified, outreach workers assess readiness to change, negotiate the pros and cons of change, explore treatment options with patients, discuss potential treatment sites, secure placement, and provide taxicab vouchers (if needed) for transportation to a treatment facility.

Use of such a model among 7118 adult ED patients screened for alcohol and drug problems during the first study year resulted in 2931 problem situations detected. Among 245 enrollees who participated in a 90-day follow-up, there was a significant reduction in self-report of problems related to substance abuse, a 45 percent decrease in drug-abuse severity scores, a 67 percent reduction in the number of enrollees using cocaine or crack, a 62 percent reduction in the number using marijuana, a 56 percent reduction in alcohol use, and a 64 percent reduction in binge drinking. More than 50 percent reported that they followed up on a treatment referral. Project ASSERT also has been implemented successfully at Yale New Haven Hospital. During the first year 5812 patients were screened and more than 1500 Brief Negotiated Interviews (BNIs) were performed. Of the 712 patients who were referred to a specialized alcohol and drug treatment center, 41 percent were contacted and 78 percent enrolled in the program.[23]

Diagnostic Criteria

Alcohol use disorders include a spectrum of problems ranging from at-risk drinking to dependence. It is important to identify where patients fall along this continuum, because the intervention may differ. *At-risk drinking* is defined as drinking above certain limits that increases risk for injury and/or illness. Currently the drinker is not experiencing any problems, medical, legal or social. Another term is *hazardous drinking*. If the patient drinks over the recommended limits and is currently experiencing medical, social, or legal issues, that patient is drinking at harmful levels. The National Institute of Alcohol Abuse and Alcoholism (NIAAA) defines at-risk drinking for men no older than 65 years of age to be more than 14 drinks per week or more 4 drinks per occasion. For women or anyone older than 65 years, at-risk drinking is defined as more than 7 drinks per week or more than 3 drinks per occasion. A standard drink is defined as 12 g of pure alcohol, which is equal to one 12-oz bottle of beer or wine cooler, one 5-oz glass of wine, or 1.5 oz of distilled spirits.[24]

According to the American Psychiatric Association criteria (*Diagnostic and Statistical Manual of Mental Disorders,* 4th ed.), the diagnosis of alcohol or substance *dependence* requires that at least three of the following criteria be present during a 12-month period:

1. Tolerance: manifested by the need for markedly increased amounts of substance for intoxication or by a diminished effect with continued use of the same amount.
2. Withdrawal: manifested by withdrawal symptoms or taking a substance (or closely related substitute) to avoid withdrawal.
3. Consuming larger amounts of substance than intended.
4. Persistent or unsuccessful attempts to cut down use.
5. Spending a great deal of time obtaining or consuming the substance or recovering from its effects.
6. Giving up or reducing important social, occupational, or recreational activities.
7. Continuing substance use, despite knowing it caused or will exacerbate a psychological or physical problem.

Screening Methods

Universal screening in the ED for substance abuse requires practitioners to first ask questions that reflect their concern for the patients' overall health and safety. Substance abuse questions should be imbedded among other preventive health issues to reduce stigma. Questions should be asked in a nonjudgmental, matter-of-fact fashion. Questions can be prefaced with a statement such as:

I am going to ask you some very personal questions that I ask all my patients that I hope improve the care I give. You do not have to answer them if you are uncomfortable.

1. Do you wear seat belts every time you are in a car?
2. Do you smoke?
3. Do you drink beer, wine, liquor, or distilled spirits?
4. Do you feel safe in your current relationship?
5. Do you use drugs not prescribed by a physician now and then?

Ask current drinkers:

1. On average, how many days per week do you drink alcohol?
2. On a typical day when you drink, how many drinks do you have?

3. What is the maximum number of drinks you had on any given occasion during the last month?

The NIAAA guidelines also recommend that practitioners proceed with the CAGE questions to assess for severity.[24] The CAGE (Table 295-3), a mnemonic for the questions in the table, has been studied extensively and is easy to remember and use.

A score of 1 or higher requires further assessment. A score of 2 or higher is highly specific for alcohol dependence. Although the CAGE test is designed for assessing lifetime dependency, the questions should be prefaced with the phrase "in the last 12 months" to detect current problems. If the patient presents with alcohol intoxication and clinical evidence of an alcohol-related health problem, it may be better to start with CAGE to prevent resistance or argument on the part of the patient to attempts to quantify alcohol consumption. If patients state that they use illegal drugs or misuse prescription drugs, "use of drugs" can be substituted for "drinking" in the CAGE questions.

Standardized tests, such as the CAGE, have been found to have a higher sensitivity for screening for substance-abusing patients than other diagnostic tools, including saliva tests, breath alcohol testing, breath smell, patient self-report, or presenting complaint. Brief screening instruments are easy to administer, assist in identifying dependent drinkers, and may facilitate the process of matching an individual to the most appropriate treatment resource. In one study, 31 percent of patients presenting to an urban ED had positive results on the CAGE screening test, whereas only 13 percent were biochemically positive for alcohol with a saliva alcohol test.[14]

The CAGE test has been specifically studied for its applicability to the ED.[25] The sensitivity was reported as 75 percent for at-risk drinkers and 76 percent for dependent drinkers. The specificity was 88 percent for at-risk drinkers and 90 percent for dependent drinkers.

If concerns about drugs and alcohol arise based on the screening questions or the presenting problems, a brief intervention should be performed and a referral made once the acute medical issues are addressed.

Intervention Methods

The first principle of intervention is that it comes *to* people, instead of people having to seek it out. The second is that it is timely. The best time for early intervention is the crisis (the teachable moment) that brings the person with an alcohol or drug problem into the system for a medical, social, or criminal justice problem. The entire interaction often can be accomplished in less than 10 to 15 min, and the dialogue can take place at discharge or, ideally, while suturing or casting.

The BNI is a dialogue format that was developed in a busy urban ED for negotiating change in substance-related behaviors.[22] In this method, the practitioner, a nonaddiction specialist, is the facilitator rather than the agent of change. The BNI may result in behavior change for the individual who is at risk and facilitate contact with the treatment system for the individual who is dependent. Through negotiation, patients' needs are tailored to solutions, and patients are matched with treatment modalities they are able to accept.

The BNI is based on the principles of brief motivational interviewing developed by Miller and Rollnick,[26] which are encapsulated in the FRAMES acronym (feedback, responsibility, advice, menu or choice, empathy, and self-efficacy). This intervention is based on a stages-of-change model in which five stages of change with highly predictable

TABLE 295-3 CAGE Questionnaire

C: Have you ever felt that you should *cut* down on your drinking?
A: Have people ever *annoyed* you by criticizing your drinking?
G: Have you ever felt bad or *guilty* about your drinking?
E: Have you ever had a drink first thing in the morning to steady your nerves or get rid of a hangover (*eye opener*)?

patterns are identified: precontemplation, contemplation, preparation, action, and maintenance, with the possibility of setbacks or relapse. Substance abusers are thought to cycle through these five stages in the course of changing their addiction behavior. Intervention techniques have been developed to suit each of these stages and explore with individuals the pros and cons of their behavior. In this process, the interventionist assists the person abusing or dependent on alcohol or drugs to (1) define the problem, (2) identify the abuser's present stage of readiness to change, and (3) move through the stages of change toward recovery.[27]

The BNI consists of the following steps:[28]

1. *Establish rapport and ask the patient's permission to discuss their use of alcohol and drugs.* Establish an atmosphere of positive regard in which the patient is not a problem but a person who has a problem.

2. *Explore the pros and cons of their current use.* Use open-ended questions such as: "Help me to understand what you like about your use of alcohol?" Listen carefully and reflect back what you hear so the patient knows you have understood what is being said. Then inquire what the patient likes less about their use. Explore the importance to the patient of the issues that emerge. Establish which of the pros and cons has the greatest salience to concentrate on those with the highest priority. Explore the patient's level of confidence in making a change.

3. *Use reflective listening* to summarize what you think the patient said to verify your interpretation. "On the one hand, you like the taste, how it helps you to loosen up and forget your problems, and it is something to do when your bored. On the other hand, you said you don't like how you feel the next day, and wrecking your cars in the crash and ending up in the ED is no fun. You also told me you are spending a lot of money on drinking and are concerned about not meeting some responsibilities. So then in the balance, where does that leave you?"

4. *Assess readiness to change on a readiness ruler.* The patient is asked to mark on a drawing of a ruler, with a scale of 1 to 10, how ready they are to change the way they drink.

5. *Negotiate a workable plan* with the patient based on the readiness score (not ready, unsure, or ready) and inner strength and support system. If the patient is ready for change (a score of 8 to 10), then solicit previous experience in trying to quit and brainstorm a menu of options and available resources. If the patient scores in the unsure range (5 to 7), inquire, "Why didn't you mark 4?" This allows the patient to state in their own words why they are less ready and the provider an opportunity to offer positive encouragement. Some patients are unsure about making a change, because they do not feel confident or able. They may lack resources, such as childcare, or fear losing their apartment or job. A list of social services and other resources and referral for further assessment may be more appropriate. If the score is in the not-ready range (1 to 4), ask why they didn't mark 1 and explore what it will take to get more ready. If they are not interested in further discussion, then express concern, offer information about the effects of drugs and alcohol, provide reassurance, and hope and indicate that, if they change their mind, they can call a number on the resource list.

6. *Provide verbal or written feedback and advice* to patients to follow NIAAA guidelines, to avoid alcohol with certain medications, to cut back or stop drinking to address certain health conditions, not to drink or drive, and, if not successful, to seek further assessment.

7. *Document* the negotiated plan in the chart and in the discharge instructions.

The Referral Process

If a patient is ready to accept referral, a staff member familiar with treatment resources can assist the patient with placement. Each ED should post a resource list and provide a handout for patients with the names, addresses, and phone numbers of treatment programs. The U.S. Department of Health and Human Services' Center for Substance Abuse Treatment has an online resource locator (http://findtreatment.samhsa.gov/facilitylocatordoc.htm). The resource list may include specialized facilities for patients with mental illness, inpatient and outpatient detoxification, acupuncture, and methadone maintenance programs, outpatient individual and group counseling, residential communities, Alcoholics and Narcotics Anonymous (ALANON), and programs focused on the needs of women, culture-specific programs, and programs designed for gay, lesbian, and transgendered clients. The American College of Emergency Physicians online tool kit also offers suggestions for setting up such a resource list (www.Acep.org/1,4688,0.html).

If a patient who is injecting drugs is not ready to accept a treatment referral, it may be possible to negotiate contact with a needle exchange program. Such programs have documented effectiveness in reducing the spread of the human immunodeficiency virus[29] and hepatitis B and C and facilitating entry into the drug treatment system.

REFERENCES

1. Secretary of Health and Human Services: *Tenth Special Report to the U.S Congress on Alcohol and Health.* Washington, D.C., U.S. Department of Health and Human Services, U.S. Government Printing Office, 2000.
2. Morse RM, Flavin DK for the Joint Committee of the National Council on Alcoholism and Drug Dependence and the American Society of Addiction Medicine to Study the Definition and Criteria for the Diagnosis of Alcoholism: The definition of alcoholism. *JAMA* 268:1012, 1992.
3. Grant BF: Prevalence and correlates of alcohol use and DSM-IV alcohol dependence in the United States: Results of the National Longitudinal Alcohol Epidemiologic Survey. *J Stud Alcohol* 464:464, 1997.
4. Gentilello LM, Rivara FP, Donovan DM, et al: Alcohol problems in women admitted to a level I trauma center: A gender-based comparison. *J Trauma* 48:108, 2000.
5. Li G, Keyl PM, Rothman R, et al: Epidemiology of alcohol-related emergency department visits. *Acad Emerg Med* 5:788, 1998.
6. Ojesjo L, Hagnell O, Otterbeck L: Mortality in alcoholism among men in the Lundby Community Cohort, Sweden: A forty-year follow-up. *J Stud Alcohol* 59:140, 1998.
7. Whiteman PJ, Hoffman RS, Goldfrank LR: Alcoholism in the emergency department: An epidemiologic study. *Acad Emerg Med* 7:14, 2000.
8. Kyriacou DN, McCabe F, Anglin D et al. Emergency department-based study of risk factors for acute injury from domestic violence against women. *Ann Emerg Med* 31:502, 1998.
9. McCadams JS, Daley BJ, Enderson BL: Does alcohol intoxication alter the assessment and outcome of "observation-status" trauma patients? *Am Surg* 67:1110, 2001.
10. Mayo-Smith MF: Pharmacological management of alcohol withdrawal. A meta-analysis and evidence-based practice guideline. American Society of Addiction Medicine Working Group on Pharmacological Management of Alcohol Withdrawal. *JAMA* 278:144, 1997.
11. D'Onofrio G, Rathlev NK, Ulrich AS, et al: Lorazepam for the prevention of recurrent seizures related to alcohol. *New Engl J Med* 340:915, 1999.
12. Higgins JP, Wright SW, Wrenn KD: Alcohol, the elderly, and motor vehicle crashes. *Am J Emerg Med* 14:265, 1996.
13. Institute of Medicine: *Pathways of Addiction: Opportunities in Drug Abuse Research.* Washington, D.C., National Academy Press, 1996.
14. Bernstein E, Tracey A, Bernstein J, Williams C: Emergency department detection and referral rate for patients with problem drinking. *Subst Abuse* 17:69, 1996.
15. Gentilello LM, Rivara FP, Donovan DM, et al: Alcohol interventions in a trauma center as a means of reducing the risk of injury recurrence. *Ann Surg* 230:473, 1999.
16. D'Onofrio G, Nadel ED, Degutis LC, et al: Improving emergency medicine residents' approach to patients with alcohol problems: A controlled educational trial. *Acad Emerg Med* 40:50, 2002.
17. McLellan AT, Lewis DC, O'Brien CP, Kleber HD: Drug dependence, a chronic medical illness. *JAMA* 284:1689, 2000.
18. Gerstein DR, Harwood HJ, Sutter N, et al: *Evaluating Recovery Services: The California Drug and Alcohol Treatment Assessment.* Sacramento, State of California Department of Alcohol and Drug Programs, 1994.

19. Chafetz ME, Blane HT, Abram HS, et al: Establishing treatment relations with alcoholics. *Nerv Ment Dis* 134:395, 1962.
20. D'Onofrio GD, Degutis LC: Preventive care in the emergency department: Screening and brief intervention for alcohol problems in the emergency department: a systemic review. *Acad Emerg Med* 9:627, 2002.
21. WHO Brief Intervention Study Group: A cross-national trial of brief interventions with heavy drinkers. *Am J Public Health* 86:948, 1996.
22. Bernstein E, Bernstein J, Levenson S: Project ASSERT: An ED-based intervention to increase access to primary care, preventive services, and the substance abuse treatment system. *Ann Emerg Med* 30:181, 1997.
23. D'Onofrio G, Mascia R, Razzak J, Degutis LC. Utilizing health promotion advocates for selected health risk screening and intervention in the ED. *Acad Emerg Med* 8:543, 2001.
24. National Institute of Alcohol Abuse and Alcoholism: *The Physician's Guide to Helping Patients with Alcohol Problems.* National Institutes of Health Publication 95-3769. Washington, D.C., U.S. Department of Health and Human Services, Public Health Service, 1995.
25. Cherpital CJ: Screening for alcohol problems in the emergency department. *Ann Emerg Med* 26:158, 1995.
26. Miller WR, Rollnick S: *Motivational Interviewing: Preparing People to Change Addictive Behaviors.* New York, Guilford, 2002.
27. Rollnick S, Mason P, Butler C: *Health Behavior Change: A Guide for Practitioners.* Edinburgh, Churchill Livingstone. 1999.
28. D'Onofrio G, Bernstein E, Bernstein J, Woolard RH, et al: Patients with alcohol problems in the emergency department, Part 2: Intervention and Referral. *Acad Emerg Med* 5:1210, 1998.
29. Hurley SF, Jolley DJ, Kaldor JM: Effectiveness of needle-exchange programmes for prevention of HIV infection. *Lancet* 349:1797, 1997.

PHYSICIAN WELL-BEING
Sanford H. Koltonow

Physician well-being is an important personal and professional issue.[1] When distracted by unmet needs, one may lose the edge necessary to manage multiple patients, bring forth one's skills and knowledge, and be decisive. The practice of medicine is a sacred privilege that also contains risks to the equanimity of the provider that often are not apparent.

The practice of emergency medicine requires a large knowledge base and advanced cognitive and interpersonal skills. Not quite as obvious is the need for excellent *intrapersonal* skills. Situations arise that conflict with one's personal values and produce intense feelings of uneasiness. To remain effective, coping methods need to be used that are adaptive and resolve conflict. The thought that one can meet *all* of a patient's needs ignores one's own needs for supports and limits. Physicians who understand their attitudes toward work and their profession can make reasonable choices about structuring their work. Those who understand their needs and abilities in relation to others can function more effectively as members of health care teams and as members of families.

Stress is necessary as a force that motivates. When excess stress becomes detrimental, it is more appropriately called *distress.* Much like Starling's law, each individual has his or her own curve with a point beyond which further stress causes less, rather than more, output.

Burnout is a state of physical, emotional, and mental exhaustion that occurs as a result of intense involvement with people over long periods in emotionally demanding situations. Physicians suffering from burnout often refer to a sense of lack of accomplishment in their work. As the stress syndrome progresses, providers attempt to decrease their contact with patients and staff, become less respectful listeners, and order more tests and referrals. They may behave rudely and be quick to anger, argue, and blame. Burnout within a department or organization usually is experienced as increased turnover, absenteeism, poor morale, and patient dissatisfaction. Burnout symptoms in their extreme form are characterized by physical depletion and chronic fatigue, feelings of helplessness and hopelessness, and the development of negative attitudes toward self, work, life, and others. Among physicians, symptoms of burnout are thought to be potential precursors of more severe manifestations of impairment, including alcoholism, drug abuse, and suicidal ideation.

Emergency physicians practice in an environment that can foster burnout. Critical decisions must be made with incomplete information. Noises, smells, crowding, children, families, terminal illnesses, substance abusers, psychiatric patients, police, and criminals are part of the everyday clinical work. The ED, the historical safety net for unmet needs, faces unrelenting demands for an ever-widening range of services. It is easy to become overwhelmed.

The American Medical Association defines an impaired physician as "one who is unable to practice medicine with reasonable skill and safety because of physical or mental illness, including deterioration though the aging process, loss of motor skill, or excessive use . . . of drugs, including alcohol." Various estimates of impairment range from 7 to 13 percent. Well before attrition occurs, there are warning signs that, with awareness, can be identified and remedied before a patient's care and a physician's status are threatened.

Suicide, the ultimate manifestation of impairment, accounts for one-third of the premature deaths among physicians. The percentage is higher for women, in particular young women. Annually, more than 100 physicians complete suicide.

BURNOUT

Burnout is a condition born of good intentions. Doctors who fall prey to it are, for the most part, individuals who have striven for perfection.[2] It grows from unrealistic goal setting. Burnout is fostered by common personality characteristics of those who choose and succeed in emergency medicine. Near-compulsive overachievement,[3–4] denial of one's limits, a low level of trust, distant interpersonal relationships, and independent self-sufficiency are common. An effect is that the processing of deep feelings is repressed. Instead of addressing their own symptoms of personal stress, *physicians tend to project feelings* of irritability, anger, and frustration on others: patients, nurses, and their families.

The ability to dissociate one's feelings from one's work is an adaptive coping mechanism for working with contagious disease and dangerous situations, but it can help physicians ignore their own vulnerabilities. They may not recognize the toll that a lifestyle of little sleep, poor diet, and little time for recreation or reflection may be having on them and their families. Dissociation becomes deadly when the "it can't happen to me" philosophy is used to justify increasing alcohol and drug consumption or other self-destructive behaviors.[5]

Fear of incompetence is nearly universal among physicians and is the source of many of the stressors related to medical decision making. When dealing with other people's lives, mistakes can have life-threatening ramifications. If one cannot accept his or her limits and the possibility of making a mistake, one must (at least hope to) be perfect and all-knowing, a situation that promotes arrogance and a strong need to defend against perceived criticism. Even symbolic challenges, perhaps by someone asking a question about care or interjecting a different opinion, can strike deep at defense mechanisms, frequently resulting in inappropriate physician behavior.

PROFESSIONAL ENVIRONMENTAL STRESSORS

Stressors arising from nonmedical issues within the professional environment and from a physician's personal environment can compound the difficulties in providing quality emergency care. Career satisfaction has been found to correlate with the following issues: (1) control over working conditions, (2) hospital administrative support, (3) having time for family and personal life, and (4) departmental security.

Death and Dying

Death and dying involve physicians in sharing one of a family's most personal and powerful events. Emergency physicians need to become comfortable exploring patient's wishes and informing families of unexpected death and morbidity, because they will be called on to do so often. Empathy requires emotional energy. Speaking with a grieving family forces a physician to face system and personal conflicts.

The need of the patient and family for compassion is a difficult process to rush. There are questions from loved ones about the events leading up to a death that must be dealt with empathically to facilitate the grieving process. Offering understanding, comfort, compassion, and solace can be an important source of satisfaction for physicians. Often, deaths resurrect powerful feelings in physicians, based on prior personal experiences.

Some difficulties of physicians may stem from the belief that a physician's career represents the battle against death and disease. Facing a surviving family or counseling a dying patient may symbolize "failure" in that battle. In addition, a physician can become a target for misplaced anger and denial.

Malpractice Litigation

Universally, physicians feel the need to expend significant resources to prevent malpractice litigation (as opposed to the resources used to prevent malpractice). For those unfamiliar with the process, a medical malpractice lawsuit can be frightening.[6] It seems to strike at one's very being and self-worth. Many physicians will respond with disbelief, then anger, and finally depression. The process of meetings, testimony, and eventually the trial can be dehumanizing. The single factor most predictive of a dysfunctional response is the experience of isolation. Embarrassment and self-doubt can cause avoidance of one's very sources of support. Colleagues' responses may reinforce a physician's feeling of shame. Knowing the physician is busy preparing a defense, colleagues may change their referral and social patterns, which can be interpreted as judgment about the facts of the case.

Self-doubt frequently carries over to one's personal life. For reasons of not wanting to bring home the pain or from feelings of shame for getting named in a lawsuit, many physicians withdraw from their spouses and families, furthering their isolation.

PERSONAL ENVIRONMENTAL STRESSORS

Sleep Deprivation

Shift work and scheduling difficulties are the most common sources of stress, career dissatisfaction, and attrition in emergency medicine. Circadian principles acknowledge the body's natural rhythms and can help in integrating one's work schedule with one's personal life and promote quality sleep and, thus, health.[7]

SLEEP PHYSIOLOGY   Sleep occurs in discrete stages. The bulk of delta sleep or *slow wave sleep* (SWS) occurs early in the sleep period. There is an increase in SWS in subjects who perform challenging intellectual tasks. Slow wave sleep is thought to be vital for *physical* recuperation. Those deprived of SWS often complain of fatigue and muscle aches.

Rapid eye movement (REM) *sleep* is characterized by rapid conjugate eye movements, a change in the electroencephalogram to a pattern similar to wakefulness, and the occurrence of dreams. Those with shorter sleep periods will have REM deprivation, which is difficult to make up. Rapid eye movement sleep is thought to be vital for *psychological* well-being. Those deprived of it complain of irritability and moodiness. They also score higher on testing of aggressive behavior. Rapid eye movement sleep also may be important in the consolidation of complex learning. Experimental subjects deprived only of REM

sleep but allowed the other phases begin displaying a thought disorder reminiscent of psychosis within 3 to 4 days.

Humans have a 25-h circadian clock. Many physiologic functions follow circadian patterns that can be transposed by keeping experimental subjects awake at night and sleeping during the day. This process is known as *entrainment* of the circadian rhythm. Many circadian patterns have been demonstrated to be sensitive to entrainment, including alertness. The duration of the sleep period depends more on the phase of the circadian rhythm than on the prior period of wakefulness. This partly explains why those working short stretches of nights sleep fewer hours during the daytime than those working night shifts regularly, leading to REM sleep deprivation.

Many physicians attempt to use pharmaceuticals to assist them in falling asleep. Essentially all decrease the proportion of REM sleep. Stimulants, including nicotine and caffeine, impede onset of sleep and normal sleep stage progression.

Studies on sleep deprivation show that the ability to perform challenging intellectual tasks is slowed but otherwise relatively unchanged; however, motivation to perform routine tasks is diminished. Because the quality of emergency medical practice often depends on properly performing routine tasks that may follow prolonged periods of intellectual exertion, physicians who work different shifts need to schedule themselves in ways that minimize risk to patients.

SUPPORTIVE STRATEGIES   When planning shift rotations, it is healthier to rotate forward (from days to afternoons to early mornings), because the human circadian rhythm is 25 h long. Many physicians favor 12-h shifts to increase the number of days off. **When rotating shifts, however, it takes longer to reset the biologic clock across a 12-h change than across an 8-h change** (Table 296-1).

The circadian "gold standard" is not to change shifts at all, but those working only night shifts must maintain a daytime sleep pattern, even during days off, to avoid re-entrainment to a daytime pattern. Working nights for long periods is difficult due to pressures to participate in daytime family and social activities or to be involved regularly in administrative activities.

There is a compromise known as *anchor sleep,* which minimizes circadian disruption. **By sleeping a block of at least 4 h at the same time every day, one tends to anchor the circadian rhythm.** It can be

TABLE 296-1   Strategies and Recommendations to Assist in the Health of Shift Workers

Given the right set of circumstances, the best strategy is to work the same shift all of the time and keep the same sleep pattern.

For those unable to maintain consistent sleep patterns, use compromise strategies such as anchor sleep and napping to mitigate circadian disruptions.

Rotate all shifts in a clockwise direction, with at least 1-month minimum time per rotation.

One or two night shifts in a row causes minimal circadian disruption.

Sleep in a quiet, darkened room, minimizing disruptions. When working nights, give the work schedule to likely daytime callers.

Start the awake period with a high-protein meal and switch to complex carbohydrates toward bedtime. Avoid caffeine and high-calorie, high-fat snack food before sleep. Eat meals regularly.

Use bright light (more than 10,000 lux) for 2 h after rising, as an adjunct for entraining to new shifts.

Get regular exercise. Vigorous aerobic exercise after rising may diminish the time needed to adjust to new shifts. Avoid heavy exertion before attempting to sleep.

Work with family and friends to plan regular quality time together.

Do not try to live a day-shift lifestyle while working night shifts. Hold administrative meetings early in the morning or late in the afternoon when working night shifts. Respect the circadian rights of those working nights by excusing them from meetings held during the day.

Source: Adapted with permission from Whitehead DC, Thomas HR, Slapper DM: A rational approach to shift work in emergency medicine. *Ann Emerg Med* 21:1250, 1992.

useful for permanent nightshift workers during their days off or during short periods of irregular shift work, making it easier to return to "normal" sleep patterns.

Social life is important for shift workers. Maintaining close ties with family and friends helps to relieve stress and mitigates the sense of temporal isolation that shift workers face. Planning for quality social time is as vital as planning for work.

Family

It has long been known that supportive, intimate relationships can improve stress management, improve mood, and encourage healthy living. Good relationships also are associated with a decrease in somatic symptoms, less depression, increased life span, and greater job satisfaction. The personality characteristics chosen by and supported in medicine often conflict with intimacy, family, and self-care priorities. With the increasing complexity of a physician's clinical and administrative schedule, social and community obligations, and the spouse's and children's interests, it is the family as a unit that is most likely to suffer.

Specific hardships are associated with being in a relationship with a physician.[8] Two-physician families are becoming more common, with their own specific pressures. Living with the persistent demands of medicine, most physician couples live for the future, convinced that eventually there will be time to spend together. The couple unconsciously assumes that the delay will not endanger the quality of the relationship and that the relationship will remain as fresh and intense as the day it was postponed.

Complex defense mechanisms, learned in the milieu of the emotional and physical fatigue of training and practice, frequently lead to a blunting of one's ability to respond to deep personal feelings. The most common complaint from physicians' families entering counseling is that the physician member is emotionally unreachable, if not physically absent.

Physicians become professionally comfortable being decisive and responsible. Rarely are the feelings or opinions of others welcomed; physicians merely give "orders." As experts, they know what is best for patients. This behavior is commonly carried over to the home. The physician is tired, communication falters, and compromise is one sided as the family member decides to "let it go; at least he's [or she's] finally home." Arrogance is enabled. Conflict is postponed until crisis develops.

Spouses can benefit from a support organization. The aim is to assist in understanding medical stress, share coping mechanisms, reduce isolation, and understand their own role in the patterns that shape their intimate relationships.

If a physician provides medical treatment to his or her family, the care given can be unsuitable, either excessive or inadequate. A physician cannot remain objective in assessing loved ones, and it is most often inappropriate to try. The physician and his or her family deserve as complete and thorough an evaluation as would be provided to patients arriving at their ED.

Aging

Aging sometimes makes it physically difficult to do all that is required. Changes in the shift rotations are more difficult. Visual and hearing acuity may suffer. It may be difficult to accommodate medical problems or medication schedules.

Career transitions are available in many specialties, but, as a new specialty, emergency medicine does not have as much experience in tailoring the practice to accommodate older physicians.

STRATEGIES FOR WELL-BEING

Table 296-2 lists the author's principles for promoting personal well-being. The overriding tenets are self-awareness and self-responsibility.

TABLE 296-2 Principles for Promotion of Physician Well-Being

Commit to being aware of your stresses and anxieties. Relate to stress as a challenge to overcome, not as something intolerable with power over your life.

Maintain perspective. Don't take yourself too seriously. Develop a separate identity, one not dependent on your role as a physician.

Allow yourself space to be human. Realize medicine is not the cause of your problems or unhappiness—you are free to choose the lifestyle and work environment. Confront the options.

Be here now. If your family, religion, community, or other activity is actually a priority, spend time with it. Your family deserves planned blocks of time that are sacrosanct.

Focus on the intrinsic rewards of medicine: altruism, interest in the science, the challenge of the patients who need your skills, and stimulation by the broad range of people with whom you work. There are rewards in medicine you find motivating. If these are not apparent, then this is an area in need of exploration.

Develop networks with your peers. Don't allow yourself to become isolated.

Support systems need to be acceptable to all concerned and not threaten professional status. You must have personal and professional confidants and accurate feedback. Learn to recognize maladaptive coping mechanisms in yourself and colleagues.

Expose students and residents to psychotherapists, who can establish scientific and interpersonal credibility. This exposure can facilitate their personal use during times of crisis.

Be certain there is adequate staffing provided to afford relief, time-off, and backup in times of crisis.

Care for yourself by attending to your physical health:
  Make necessary provisions to assure adequate, quality sleep.
  Get regular exercise, control your weight, and pay attention to your diet.
  Provide for your relaxation. This is different from leisure.
  See your doctor(s) and follow *their* instructions.

No individual or institution created your conflicts or can resolve them. However, one can mold the environment until it best suits one's needs. Choices and alternatives always exist.[9]

Self-Assessment

During a particularly difficult period, most people know they feel stressed and may not be functioning as efficiently as usual. Frequently, this is attributed to a difficult patient, a busy shift, or a particular personal stressor outside of one's control. Self-awareness enables individuals to begin to appreciate their patterns of response from a wider perspective. Paradoxically, some physicians, when faced with the disillusionment of a lifestyle not realized, use denial and cling harder to their original motives.

Table 296-3 lists some questions to be used as a starting point to assess one's own emotional fatigue. If several of the answers are affirmative, perhaps this is evidence of divergence between personal values and career activities. This divergence may motivate you to seek feedback from a trusted source.

TABLE 296-3 Questions for Self-Assessment

Do you find the old ways of coping are not as reliable as they once were?

Do you find yourself becoming cynical about your colleagues or the "system"?

Do you waste time at work, dreading to see patients or slowed by indecision?

Are you drinking, eating, or smoking more than is normal for you?

Is your self-esteem unduly affected by criticism?

Have you lost the intrigue with medicine?

Do you feel helpless over the loss of control in the direction that medicine is taking?

Do you have continuous problems with insomnia, fatigue, or depression?

Do you feel lonely or isolated? Do you avoid others so they don't see how unhappy you are?

Principles of Management

Common methods for overcoming professional fatigue use time management, support systems, debriefing and relaxation, administrative training, and physical self-care. Regardless of the validity of the need, one cannot say *yes* to one commitment without saying *no* to something else. A process of *value clarification* helps identify those obligations one is willing to commit to and provides a starting point for determining personal priorities. One then should set life's major goals in all areas—physical, mental, financial, spiritual, and social—according to the individual's most meaningful objectives.

Develop relationships with peers that go beyond the immediate clinical issues. Listen and provide emotional support and challenge. Be the one to take the risk of talking about the things that are felt but ignored. Share the social reality of what living and practicing in current society is like by sharing thoughts, feelings, and strategies. The fear that someone may discover one's vulnerabilities needs to be resisted. Such a fear encourages low levels of trust in peers and tends to isolate one from the social supports needed in times of crisis.

Concern for the well-being of medical trainees must be constantly modeled in training. Many trainees do not have the advantage of *mentors* who share with them their mistakes, let down their guard, and demonstrate that a lack of perfection does not mean incompetence. Such mentors demonstrate that a mistake is compatible with excellence and compassionate care. Errors in problem solving can be used to improve learned behavior. A faculty that can mentor on personal and professional humility is the best prevention against medical arrogance.

Well-being committees within hospital or medical societies can provide education and referral to other resources. Lines of communication are opened as physicians learn coping techniques that others have found effective. Topics to present to the medical staff include value clarification, goal setting, time management, grieving, and reframing. A well-being committee is different from professional assistance programs for impaired, disabled, or "troubled" physicians, although these programs should complement one another.

The *critical incident stress debriefing* team is an approach that attempts to reduce the severity of poststress disorders by intervention at the time of occurrence. Personnel who have experienced a critical or anxiety-provoking situation are debriefed as a group. The process is facilitated by experienced group leaders of similar professional background in conjunction with mental health professionals. The goal is to intercede before unhealthy reactions have time to be fully incorporated. Each individual is asked to describe what he or she saw, heard, and felt. The debriefing becomes a setting to share experiences and counter isolation. Participants are given the message that the discomfort they are encountering is a normal reaction to an abnormal experience. It also allows the opportunity to identify those individuals who may need further assistance.

Rapport

In emergency situations, one often does not have the benefit of an ongoing doctor-patient relationship. There are some easy things that emergency physicians can do to build rapport and trust. Most revolve around communicating the perception of listening and caring. Physicians should greet patients by name and introduce themselves, shaking hands when appropriate. Emergency physicians should sit down whenever possible; regardless of how long physicians actually remain in the room, patients perceive it as much longer. When touching patients, do so gently with an air of caring. Respect a patient's privacy by closing curtains and exposing only that which is necessary. When clinically appropriate, listen to a patient's overall agenda, because it may save time. Do not use complex language. If a patient is lying down, sit or bend down and put your eyes at the patient's level. Set expectations for a patient with the first encounter, for examples, "results will be back in 2 h, and I'll be back to discuss them then," or "I have a critical patient to care for but you'll be next." Finding a small need that you can fulfill (e.g., a glass of water, a pillow, a phone call) will help establish rapport.

Conflict Resolution

Conflict resolution skills are important in emergency medicine for interactions with patients, peers, physicians in other specialties, and other hospital staff. The issues of conflict differ, but the dynamics are similar.

Demanding patients or families are best handled by acknowledging their expectations and attempting compromise. Sometimes, it is effective to acknowledge that the patient has been heard and his or her perspective considered, and the physician has a different perspective and position. Although firmness may be necessary, rarely will anything be gained by hostility or by confrontation.

Administrators, nurses, and consultants may be other sources of conflict; often, ongoing personality conflicts exist, provoked by the intensity of the work environment. One needs to focus on finding the "common ground," which is the patient's needs.

Not every conflict is a battle that must be won. Healthy conflict resolution requires physicians to know when to stand up and when to negotiate or retreat.

Malpractice Litigation Support

More than 95 percent of physicians react to being sued with periods of emotional distress. Malpractice litigation stress support groups can be developed or may exist in state medical societies. The groups consist of risk management professionals who describe what to expect at each step and clarify the meaning of legal terms and physicians with prior experience who share their experiences. Family members also may participate and can provide insight into the process their family is experiencing and their emotional responses.

Physical Health

Most physicians do not get regular preventive health care, likely due to the tremendous time constraints of practice and a denial of one's vulnerability to illness. Either way, a physician can wind up caring less for self than for the patients.

Exercise and proper diet help maintain physical health and relieve emotional tension. In addition, setting aside the time for one's own health, within one's busy schedule and conflicting priorities, confirms with action the belief that caring for oneself is an important use of time.

Relaxation Techniques

Relaxation is quiet time that allows for personal reflection, integration, and planning.

Relaxation is different from leisure, although leisure activity is an important way to achieve balance. The stressors of leisure activity, such as sports, outdoor activities, hobbies, or special skills, are enjoyable in part because they are so different from the common stressors of professional life. Leisure activity will also often involve family and friends.

Relaxation is also different from doing nothing. Relaxation increases awareness and focuses the mind while resting the body. It is a time to be present, to reflect, and to process experiences and feelings. Systematic relaxation requires concentration and deliberate mental activity. It will lead to lower arousal and release of strain. Many techniques are available for relaxation, including meditation, progressive muscle relaxation, selective awareness, self-hypnosis, somatics, yoga, breath control, and biofeedback. Audiotapes are available to help guide one conveniently through the learning process. For some, religious thought and introspection may fulfill the need for relaxation.

IDENTIFICATION OF IMPAIRMENT

Emergency physicians frequently feel temporarily emotionally overwhelmed. These feelings become maladaptive when they become established behaviors (Table 296-4).

Detecting impairment in others is difficult.[5] Psychologically and chemically impaired professionals are often able to delay notice by protecting their job performance at the expense of every other dimension of their lives. The common signs of uncharacteristic behavior are frequently ignored. Family, neighbors, friends, and coworkers may become involved in *enabling* impaired behaviors. Physicians feel that they are experts capable of treating their own problems, because they have received training in pharmacology and psychiatry.

Intervention is almost always required with impaired physicians, because of the massive denial and other defense mechanisms they employ. Shame, embarrassment, fear, and guilt keep many health care workers from consciously accepting that they are not in control until confronted by trusted colleagues or, more commonly, authorities. Intervention requires referral to individuals with *specialized training.*

The seriousness of the emotional impact of confrontation on the sick physician must be appreciated; it is critical to anticipate and prevent the possibility of a suicide[10] or bodily harm by accident or trauma. These possibilities are not uncommon, particularly among impaired health professionals.

RESOURCES

1. The Institute for the Study of Health and Illness is a nonprofit educational and research foundation focused on, among other things, the professional development of physicians who serve people with life-threatening illnesses. Directed by Rachel Remen, M.D., it offers books, tapes, and category I CME credit at small retreats that focus on topics such as loss, grief, personal limitation, impotence, isolation, and the examination of goals, values, and meanings. (Contact: ISHI, P.O. Box 316, Bolinas, CA 94924.)

2. The Society and Center for Professional Well-Being of Durham, North Carolina, is a professional educational and consultative organization offering programs in value clarification, practice assessment, mediation, conflict resolution, and support group development. (Contact: Dr. John-Henry Pfifferling, telephone 1-919-489-9167.)

3. The Talbot-Marsh recovery program for substance abuse and psychiatric disabilities in Atlanta, Georgia, specializes in treating health care professionals and is nationally recognized as a model for extended outpatient treatment of substance-abusing physicians. (Telephone 1-800-445-4232.)

4. The Menninger Clinic of Topeka, Kansas, provides individual, marital, and family therapy and is a major psychoanalytic training program. It also sponsors educational workshops in a retreat setting in Estes Park, Colorado, for one week each July. Designed specifically for physician couples, it focuses on the problem of balancing the demands of medical practice with the needs for self and family. (Contact: P.O. Box 829, Topeka, KS 66601; telephone 1-800-288-7377.)

5. The American College of Emergency Physicians, Society for Academic Emergency Medicine (SAEM), and other medical societies provide state-of-the-art educational resources. Most of the topics in this chapter have been included in their presentations. The American College of Emergency Physicians has a membership section on well-being, which one may join for the informational newsletters of articles by other members and to become active in supporting such issues with the college. (Contact: Well-Being Section, American College of Emergency Physicians, P.O. Box 619911, Dallas, TX 75261-9911.)

6. The American Medical Association's Department of Mental Health has established the Physician's Health Foundation. Its purpose is to provide financial assistance for physicians disabled from any cause, including psychological or chemical impairment and human immunodeficiency virus. The foundation also supports research, focused education and retraining programs, job placement, and the International Conference on Physician Health. (Contact: Elaine Tejeck, telephone 1-312-464-5073.)

TABLE 296-4 Possible Signs and Symptoms of Burnout

Using home time only as time to rest, with withdrawal from family
    activities
"Acting out" behavior on spouse, family members, nurses, and staff
Chronic complaining, cynicism, blaming others
Dreading to see patients
Writing short, ambiguous charts; quality assurance or utilization review
    notice of inappropriate or unintelligible comments
Request frequent consultations
Inappropriate anger toward medicine, patients, staff, authority
Overprescribing to a patient's symptoms
Sharing personal problems with patients, blurring of boundaries
Degrading of peers, backbiting, questioning motives of others
Frequent illness, unexplained absence, and patterns of late arrival or early
    departures
Frequent job changes
Excessive "toys" that become time-consuming obsessions, such as computers,
    boats, and planes
Spending nonwork time at the practice without apparent reason
Unusual number of patient complaints
Passive–aggressive response to change

REFERENCES

1. Andrew LB, Pollack ML: *Wellness for Emergency Physicians.* Dallas, American College of Emergency Physicians, 1995.
2. McCranie EW, Brandsma JM: Personality antecedents of burnout among middle-aged physicians. *Behav Med* 14:30, 1988.
3. Gabbard G: The role of compulsiveness in the normal physician. *JAMA* 254:2926, 1985.
4. Gabbard G, Menninger RW: The psychology of postponement in the medical marriage. *JAMA* 261:2378, 1989.
5. Hughes PH, Brandenburg N: Prevalence of substance use among US physicians. *JAMA* 267:2333, 1992.
6. Charles SC: Coping with a medical malpractice suit. *West J Med* 174:55, 2001.
7. Whitehead DC, Thomas HR, Slapper DR: A rational approach to shift work in emergency medicine. *Ann Emerg Med* 21:1250, 1992.
8. Myers MF: *Doctors' Marriages—A Look at Their Problems and Solutions,* 2nd ed. New York, Plenum, 1994.
9. Novack DH: Calibrating the physician, personal awareness and effective patient care. *JAMA* 278:502, 1997.
10. Sonneck G, Wagner R: Suicide and burnout of physicians. *Omega* 33:255, 1996.

CHILD ABUSE AND NEGLECT
Carol D. Berkowitz

SPECTRUM OF CHILD ABUSE AND NEGLECT

The concept of child maltreatment, defined as harm to a child because of abnormal child-rearing practices, is a broadening of the initial description of the battered child syndrome. *Child maltreatment* is an all-inclusive term covering physical abuse; sexual abuse; emotional abuse; parental substance abuse; physical, nutritional, and emotional neglect; supervisional neglect; and Munchausen syndrome by proxy.[1]

The ease with which physicians are able to recognize these disorders in part depends on their knowledge of normal children and normal development. The physical stigmata of maltreatment are characteristic, although the findings of neglect and sexual abuse are more subtle than those of gross physical trauma.

CHILD NEGLECT

Child neglect includes physical and emotional neglect. Neglect results from failure of the child's caregiver to provide adequate clothing, shelter, food, health care, and/or schooling. Children who are the victims of neglect may appear in the ED dirty, improperly clothed, and unimmunized. Their medical problems may not have been attended to in a timely manner. They may have suffered from burns or fractures because of inadequate supervision. Child neglect from early infancy also can result in the syndrome of failure to thrive (FTT). This syndrome usually affects children younger than 3 years, although older children who remain in a non-nurturing environment show similar manifestations.

The FTT patient is often brought to the emergency department because of other medical problems, such as intercurrent infections; skin rashes, in particular severe monilial diaper dermatitis; or acute gastroenteritis.

The history of the acute illness may not alert the physician to the chronic nature of the underlying problem. The physical examination provides the clue to the diagnosis of longstanding malnutrition. Overall physical care and hygiene are frequently poor. Infants have very little subcutaneous tissue. The ribs protrude prominently through the skin, and the skin of the buttocks hangs in loose folds. There may be alopecia over a flattened occiput, reflecting that the baby has been allowed to lie on its back all day. Muscle tone is usually increased (although sometimes these babies are hypotonic). This increased tone is most notable in the lower extremities, and infants may manifest scissoring, similar to infants with cerebral palsy.[2]

Infants with FTT also show distinct behavioral characteristics. They are wide-eyed and wary. If brought in close proximity to the examiner's face, they may purposely turn away to avoid eye contact. They become irritable if interpersonal interaction is pursued. They are difficult to console and are not cuddly. They prefer inanimate over animate objects and spend much time with their hands in their mouths. When left alone, they assume a "straphanger's position," with their arms flexed at the elbows and extended over their shoulders.

Weights and lengths should be plotted on the appropriate growth curves. In general, weight is more adversely affected than length, although this depends on the duration of the neglect. This may be reflected in a body mass index [weight (kg)/height (m^2)] below the fifth percentile. Likewise, longstanding neglect results in a diminution in the rate of the growth of the head.

In addition to observing for these physical signs, physicians should obtain certain historical information, including the birth weight (to assess the rate of growth); any maternal use of cigarettes, alcohol, and/or drugs during pregnancy; previous hospitalizations; and the parental stature. A full social service assessment also should be obtained, although this is usually done by a medical social worker.

Infants suspected of suffering from significant environmental FTT should be admitted to the hospital. Weight gain in the hospital is felt to be the sine qua non of environmental FTT. Most infants gain weight within 1 to 2 weeks after admission; in addition, the hospitalization enables a more extensive social service assessment while the infant is in a protected environment. A skeletal survey of the long bones should be carried out to detect any evidence of physical abuse.[3]

Children older than 2 to 3 years with environmental neglect are termed *psychosocial dwarfs*. Their short stature is a more prominent finding than their low weight. These children manifest a classic triad of short stature, bizarre voracious appetite (eating from trash cans), and a disturbed home situation. They are frequently hyperactive and have delayed or unintelligible speech. Psychosocial dwarfs have been studied endocrinologically and have been found to have low to normal levels of growth hormone that fail to increase with stimulation of insulin or arginine. These children also should be admitted for evaluation and initiation of appropriate social intervention. The endocrinologic disturbances rapidly reverse after hospitalization or placement in a foster home.

MUNCHAUSEN SYNDROME BY PROXY

Munchausen syndrome by proxy (MSBP) is a relatively uncommon form of child abuse in which a parent induces or fabricates an illness in a child to secure for himself or herself prolonged contact with health care providers. Children with MSBP may arrive at the emergency department with reported symptoms such as bleeding, seizures, altered mental status, apnea, diarrhea, vomiting, fever, rash, or multiple organ system involvement. These symptoms may result from administration of agents such as warfarin or ipecac.[4,5] Often the cases are medically perplexing, and families frequently move from hospital to hospital, seemingly in search of diagnosis. Children with MSBP are often subject to multiple unnecessary tests as physicians seek to uncover the etiology of the disorder. The parent (the biologic mother in 98 percent of cases) encourages the staff to do more diagnostic procedures and often seems uncharacteristically happy if a test is positive.

Social service and psychologic evaluation is mandatory in the evaluation and management of these children, who should be admitted to the hospital to ensure their safety and to institute needed therapy. Covert video surveillance has been used in some centers to document a parent's invasive actions.

SEXUAL ABUSE

Victims of prior child sexual abuse are frequently difficult for inexperienced physicians to assess, because of an unfamiliarity with the normal prepubertal genital examination. Children who have been sexually abused are brought to the ED because of a disclosure about the abuse or because of other symptoms such as those referable to the genitourinary tract, including vaginal discharge, vaginal bleeding, dysuria, urinary tract infections, or urethral discharge; behavior disturbances, including excessive masturbation, genital fondling, or other sexually oriented or provocative behavior; encopresis; regression; nightmares; and unrelated complaints.[6] Approximately 15 percent of children diagnosed in an ED as victims of sexual abuse in one report had unrelated complaints such as abdominal pain, asthma, and sore throat.

Children who are sexually abused rarely disclose their abuse until time has elapsed from the acute episode. Children who are seen immediately after an assault should be evaluated for evidence of acute injuries and for the presence of forensic material, such as semen or other bodily secretions that may provide DNA evidence.[7]

More often, several years have elapsed since the abuse was initiated, although it may be ongoing. Children 8 to 11 years of age frequently disclose that they have been victims of sexual abuse for a significant period. The assailant is known to the child in more than 90 percent of cases.

A medical history should be obtained from all children being evaluated for sexual abuse. Because evidence of the abuse may not be apparent until the child is examined, the physician may have to obtain additional medical history information after the physical assessment. The record of the medical history should include pertinent statements about whether the child has any underlying condition or has undergone any previous procedures that might cause changes in the anogenital area. Genitourinary surgery or trauma would be particularly important to note.

The child should be questioned directly about what happened. The child's name for genitalia and other body parts should be recorded, and all statements that the child makes concerning the abuse should be recorded verbatim. The demands of a busy ED may make it difficult for physicians to conduct a detailed and sensitive interview. In such cases, a hospital social worker should be consulted.

Examining physicians must maintain a high index of suspicion of sexual abuse when evaluating children who have anogenital or behavioral complaints. The physical assessment should include an evaluation of the child's overall well-being and a general physical examination. The skin should be examined for bruises. Nongenital physical injuries are unusual, even after acute abuse. Rarely, there may be grip marks on the forearms or puncture wounds on the inner aspects of the lips caused by a slap to the face. The age of the child and the degree of sexual development should be noted.

The genital examination should be confined to a careful inspection of the genitalia and perianal area. In general, there is no need for a speculum examination unless the victim is an older adolescent or unless perforating vaginal trauma is suspected. Likewise, sedation is rarely needed, and most children can be reassured verbally if they are at all apprehensive. Careful inspection of the external genitalia is sufficient to establish physical evidence of genital injury. The examination is sometimes augmented by the use of a colposcope to enable detection of subtle changes in the hymen. The colposcope also facilitates photographing the external genital area. However, most EDs are not equipped with a colposcope, and this instrument is, in fact, not critical to an adequate assessment of the anogenital area. Magnification can easily be achieved with the use of handheld lenses. Toluidine blue dye applied to the genital area also may detect subtle acute injuries. The use of digital cameras, which may be available in the emergency department, may permit photographs, which can then be reviewed by more experienced examiners.

Many different positions have been used to facilitate the examination. Infants may be seated on their parents' laps. Children are easily examined supine on the examining table with their legs in a frog-leg position. Some physicians also place all children in a prone knee-to-chest position to help fully assess the contour and homogeneity of the hymen. Placing a child in "stirrups" is usually unnecessary unless she is obese or has achieved adult stature.[8]

The normal prepubescent girl has full labia majora and small thin labia minora. The vaginal opening is covered by the hymen, a fine reddish-orange, thin-edged membrane. The thickness and color of the hymen varies as a function of age. It is normally thick during infancy and again with the onset of puberty. In between, it is thinner, most of-

ten annular or crescentic, and smooth edged. The hymenal orifice can be measured, although there is a range of variation depending on the child's age, size, position, and degree of relaxation. The significance of the diameter of the hymenal orifice as an indication of prior vaginal penetration is questioned by most experts. Trauma may result in changes such as hymenal notches, also referred to as *concavities* or *clefts*. Concavities at the 6-o'clock position are associated with prior penetrating trauma. Attenuation or reduction in the amount of hymenal tissue may lead to a gaping opening. Irregularities in the contour, in particular deep notches, are also associated with prior injury. Scarring, as demonstrated by marked alteration in the vascular pattern (white areas or swirling vascularity), is another sign of healed injury. In contrast, erythema may be secondary to irritation, inflammation, and/or chronic manipulation and is not specific for abuse.[9]

Physical findings indicative of a sexually transmitted disease should also be noted, including a vaginal discharge, warts consistent with condylomata acuminata or condylomata lata, and vesicles or ulcers consistent with herpes genitalia.

It is critically important for emergency physicians to be aware that the absence of physical findings does not preclude abuse. There are many sexually abusive activities (such as oral-to-genital contact) that would not be expected to produce scarring trauma. In addition, as is true elsewhere in the body, injuries can heal without residual scarring.

The genital examination in the sexually victimized young boy is less revealing. Rarely, there may be bite marks on the penis or scrotum. There may be a urethral discharge; the penis may become erect without tactile stimulation and remain erect.

The perianal examination is often more revealing, although it too may be completely normal in the case of acute or chronic sodomy. Acute penetration may produce no changes or may be associated with fissures, abrasions, hematomas, and changes in tone, including both dilatation and anal spasm. In the young female patient, anal penetration is easier than vaginal penetration, and changes in this area may be seen. Anal fissures or tags may be noted. The perianal folds, or rugae, may be thickened in some areas, thinned out in others, and distorted. The perianal skin may be lichenified and thickened secondary to frictional rubbing. Anal tone may be reduced when there has been repeated prior anal penetration. However, stool in the rectal ampulla may lead to similar dilatation, and one should be careful to note the presence or absence of stool.[10]

The laboratory evaluation of sexually abused children should include cultures of the throat, vagina (or urethra), and rectum for gonorrhea and a culture from the vagina (or urethra) for *Chlamydia*. Rapid antigen assays are not considered reliable forensic evidence in prepubescent children. A serologic test for syphilis is indicated if there is clinical evidence of syphilis, a history of syphilis in the assailant, or the presence of another sexually transmitted disease. Testing for the human immunodeficiency virus should be done only after appropriate counseling and if there is reason to suspect infection.

A suspicion of child sexual abuse mandates that a report be filed with child protective services or law enforcement agencies. These agencies will pursue an investigation and attempt to ensure that the child is placed in a protected environment.

Although there is the likelihood that the child may be removed from the home, a return appointment for follow-up of cultures for sexually transmitted diseases and a referral for psychologic counseling should be given.

PHYSICAL ABUSE

The spectrum of injuries and presenting complaints in children who have been intentionally traumatized is wide. Familiarity with this spectrum enables physicians in the ED to arrive at the correct diagnosis in a timely manner. Two-thirds of the victims of physical abuse are younger than 3 years, and one-third are younger than 6 months. The physical vulnerability of such small children is easy to understand.

A report published in 1999 noted that nearly one-third of infants and young children presenting to the ED with abusive head trauma had been previously evaluated (mean time, 7 days) and the diagnosis had been missed.[11]

Historical data may raise suspicions of inflicted trauma. A history that is inconsistent with the nature or the extent of the injuries (e.g., a fractured femur in an infant from a fall off a bed), a history that keeps changing as to the circumstances surrounding the injury, a discrepancy between the story the child gives and the story the caretaker gives, a history of previous trauma in the patient or siblings, or a delay in seeking medical attention should raise one's index of suspicion of physical abuse. Knowledge of normal motor development assists physicians in determining the likelihood that an injury happened in the stated manner. Children younger than 6 months are incapable of inducing accidents or accidentally ingesting any drugs or poisons. The evaluating physician should record the developmental milestones the child has achieved, e.g., the age of sitting unsupported, walking. A recent study showed that developmental milestones were recorded in none of the emergency department visits in which physical abuse was suspected.[12] Parental behavior in the ED should be observed, and it should be noted if the parents appear intoxicated or under the influence of drugs. The level of parental concern about the injury also should be noted.

Toddlers and older children should be questioned about the circumstances of the injury, and the comments should be recorded verbatim on the record. These statements are frequently admissible in court under exceptions to the hearsay rule and may help establish the diagnosis of child abuse.

The physical examination should note the child's overall hygiene and well-being. Normal children, especially toddlers who are just learning how to walk, may have multiple ecchymoses over the anterior shins, the forehead, and other bony prominences. Most falls result in bruises on only one body surface. Bruises over multiple areas, especially the low back, buttocks, thighs, cheeks, ear pinnae, neck, ankles, wrists, corners of the mouth, and lips, suggest physical abuse. Hand prints may be observed, or there may be uniform but bizarre bruises caused by belts, buckles, cords, or blunt instruments.[13] Bites produce bruising in a characteristic oval pattern, with teeth indentations along the periphery. Bites with an intercanine diameter larger than 3 cm have been inflicted by an adult. Bites should be photographed and swabbed for forensic evidence (saliva). Lacerations of the frenulum or oral mucosa may be present, especially in infants who have been force-fed. Lacerations and abrasions in the genital area are seen in toddlers who are "punished" because of toilet-training accidents.

Estimating the duration of a bruise by the color of the lesion is imprecise. Often, no discoloration is noted initially, although the bruised area may be swollen and tender. Within a day or two, the lesion may become reddish-blue, and this may last for about 5 days. The color changes to green, then to yellow, and finally to brown before resolving. Variability in the appearance of color changes does exist and depends on the size and depth of the hematoma.[14]

Children with multiple bruises should be evaluated with a complete blood cell count, a differential blood count, and coagulation studies, including a platelet count, a prothrombin time, and a partial thromboplastin time. Occasionally, a child with leukemia, aplastic anemia, hemophilia, or thrombocytopenia is brought for evaluation because of multiple bruises.

Burns constitute another form of inflicted injuries. These may be scald burns caused by immersion in hot water. Such burns do not conform to a splash configuration; rather, an entire hand or foot ("glove-and-stocking" pattern) may be involved. There is sharp demarcation of the burn margin. The buttocks may be burned during toilet-training "punishment" by immersion in a bathtub filled with hot water. Knees, anterior thighs, feet, and portions of the abdomen are spared, and the buttocks and genitalia are scalded. Cigarette burns leave small (approximately 5 mm) circumferential scab-covered injuries. These le-

sions may resemble impetigo, as do scald injuries, which may resemble bullous impetigo. A culture of material from these lesions differentiates the burn from the infection. Other inflicted burns can result from forced contact with metal objects, such as an iron, curling iron, or heater grid.

Skeletal injuries may be detected when a child presents with unexplained swelling of an extremity or refusal to walk or to use an extremity. Fractures may take any form, but spiral fractures, caused by torsion (twisting) of a long bone, and metaphyseal chip fractures suggest inflicted injury, especially when present in infants younger than 6 months. Skeletal surveys, referred to as a *trauma series* (or *trauma x*), should be obtained. These include films of all long bones, the ribs, the clavicles, the fingers, the toes, the pelvis, and the skull. They may reveal periosteal elevation secondary to new bone formation at sites of previous microfractures or periosteal injury; multiple fractures at different stages of healing; fractures at unusual sites such as the ribs, the lateral clavicle, the sternum, or the scapula; or repeated fractures to the same site. Such x-ray findings support the diagnosis of child abuse. Sometimes, bone scans will reveal fractures not readily apparent on x-rays.[15]

Head injuries are a serious and potentially lethal form of child abuse.[16] Infants with significant intracranial hemorrhage may have no apparent external injuries and may present with vomiting, irritability, apnea, or seizures. Intracranial hemorrhages may result from vigorous shaking of the infant or from thrusting the infant down onto a surface, such as a mattress. This is referred to as *shaken baby* or *shaken impact syndrome*. Older children may have been beaten about the head or face. Changes in mental status should therefore be evaluated by head computed tomography if there is any suspicion of abuse. Bruises around the ears, eyes, and cheeks and swelling of the scalp secondary to subgaleal hematomas or underlying skull fractures may be noted. Funduscopic examination may reveal retinal hemorrhages, which are usually associated with subdural hematomas. Retin Cam, a wide-field digital ophthalmic camera, allows for photodocumentation of the fundus. Such equipment is not readily available in most emergency departments but may be found in some hospitals with a neonatal intensive care unit. Ophthalmologic consultation is appropriate in cases of suspected abusive head trauma.[17,18] Intracranial hemorrhages may result from direct trauma to the skull or severe shaking of the child. These children should be evaluated with computed tomography, and coagulation studies should be performed to rule out underlying coagulopathies. Magnetic resonance imaging studies are also being used to help differentiate recent from older intracranial bleeding episodes and are the preferred imaging modality in children without symptoms of acute head injury. Additional eye injuries caused by trauma may include hyphema, lens dislocation, and retinal detachment.

Injuries to the abdomen are equally serious and are a common cause of death from child abuse. Symptoms include recurrent vomiting, abdominal pain and tenderness, diminished bowel sounds, and/or abdominal distention. A history of injury and bruising of the overlying skin may be absent. Abdominal x-ray films may reveal a distended stomach with a "double-bubble sign" secondary to a duodenal hematoma. Diffuse distention also may be noted. Laboratory studies may reveal anemia, an elevated amylase level from traumatic pancreatitis, or hematuria from kidney trauma. Other abdominal injuries caused by trauma may include hepatic or splenic rupture, intestinal perforation, or rupture of intra-abdominal blood vessels.

Any serious injury in a child younger than 5 years, especially in the absence of a witnessed event, should be viewed with suspicion. Other injuries that may suggest child abuse include those the child states were inflicted by another, were self-inflicted, or were inflicted by an unknown assailant.

The behavioral interaction between the child, the parent, and the physician may provide supportive evidence of the diagnosis of abuse. These children are often very compliant and submissive. They do not resist the medical examiner and readily submit to painful procedures such as blood drawing. They are overly affectionate to the medical staff, frequently preferring the nurse or the physician to the parent. Sometimes, they are protective of the abusing parent, try to foster to his or her needs, and lie to cover up the true nature of the injury.

Parental behavior is less uniform, but certain distinct characteristics may be noted. The parents may not interact with the child in a comforting or supportive manner during the examination. They may become angry at the physician early in the course of the evaluation and may refuse diagnostic studies. They may appear to be intoxicated or under the influence of drugs. They may have brought the child in for seemingly minor complaints and ignored the major injuries or lesions. They may insist on hospital admission of the child for these minor problems and may readily confess they can no longer cope with the child. They may express fear of losing control.

The social service assessment may reveal an unstable home situation, with frequent moves, poor parental support systems, low parental self-esteem (often caused by battering during their own childhood), parental substance abuse, and/or domestic violence. This adds further supportive evidence of a high-risk situation.

MANAGEMENT

Once the medical assessment has been completed, the physician must initiate the appropriate treatment. The medical management should be guided by the physical findings. Frequently, hospitalization is needed.

Although the specifics of the laws surrounding child abuse and neglect differ from state to state, every state does require that suspected cases be reported.[19] A verbal report is made initially to the police department and/or the child protection agency of the locality in which the abuse has occurred. Law enforcement officers often appear in the ED, especially if the child does not require hospitalization. The child may be removed from the home and placed in protective custody, taken to a juvenile facility, placed temporarily with other relatives, or placed in a foster shelter home. The final disposition is dependent on a court hearing. The physician is also required to complete an official report detailing the specifics of the evaluation and giving his or her diagnostic opinion as to the reasons the injuries or neglect are nonaccidental. The report should use nontechnical terms, e.g., *bruise* instead of *ecchymosis,* so the law enforcement and social service workers can understand the extent of the injuries.

Physicians are sometimes hesitant to report suspected cases. They are not "100 percent" certain. They are fearful of the parental response to the report. They are concerned about removing a child from the natural home. It is important to remember that physicians are required by law to report all suspected cases of abuse and neglect. Failure to report suspected cases can result in misdemeanor charges and lead to a fine or imprisonment. In addition, physicians are protected by the law from legal retaliation by the parents.

Parental anger is a natural response to the filing of a report of suspected child abuse. The physician should refrain from being accusatory. Instead, the physician should note his or her concern about the child's well-being and advise the family that a physician is required by law to report any suspicions. The physician should verbally acknowledge the anger but persist in the role of child advocate. This job is facilitated in hospitals that have child abuse teams available to assist physicians in the ED.

REFERENCES

1. Reece RM: *Child Abuse: Medical Diagnosis and Management.* Philadelphia, Lea and Febiger, 1994.
2. Berkowitz CD: Failure to thrive, in Berkowitz CD (ed): *Pediatrics: A Primary Care Approach,* 2nd ed. Philadelphia, WB Saunders, 2000, p 481.
3. Merten DF, Carpenter BLM: Radiologic imaging of inflicted injury in the child abuse syndrome. *Pediatr Clin North Am* 37:815, 1990.
4. Rosenberg DA: Web of deceit: A literature review of Munchausen syndrome by proxy. *Child Abuse Negl* 11:547, 1987.
5. Ayoub CC, Schreier HA, Alexander R: Munchausen by proxy: Special focus issue. *Child Maltreat* 7:103, 2002.
6. Seidel JS, Elvik SL, Berkowitz CD, et al: Presentation and evaluation of sexual misuse in the emergency department. *Pediatr Emerg Care* 2:157, 1986.
7. Ledray LE, Netzel L: DNA evidence collection. *J Emerg Nurs* 23:156,1997.
8. McCann L, Voris J, Simon M, et al: Comparison of genital examination techniques in prepubertal children. *Pediatrics* 85:182, 1990.
9. McCann J, Wells R, Simon M, et al: Genital findings in prepubescent girls selected for non-abuse: A descriptive study. *Pediatrics* 86:428, 1990.
10. McCann J: Perianal findings in prepubertal children selected for non abuse: A descriptive study. *Child Abuse Negl* 13:179, 1989.
11. Jenny C, Hymel KP, Ritzen A, et al: Analysis of missed cases of abusive head trauma. *JAMA* 281:621, 1999.
12. Limbos MA, Berkowitz CD: Documentation of child physical abuse: How far have we come? *Pediatrics* 102:53, 1998.
13. Berkowitz CD: Pediatric abuse: New patterns of injury. *Emerg Med Clin North Am* 13:321, 1995.
14. Stephenson T, Bialas Y: Estimation of the age of bruising. *Arch Dis Child* 74:53, 1996.
15. Kleinman PK (ed): *Diagnostic Imaging of Child Abuse,* 2d ed. Baltimore, Williams and Wilkins, 1998.
16. Alexander, R, Sato Y, Smith W, Bennett T: Incidence of impact trauma with cranial injuries ascribed to shaking. *Am J Dis Child* 144:724, 1990.
17. Levin AV: Retinal hemorrhages and child abuse. *Recent Adv Paediatr* 18:151, 2000.
18. Budenz DL, Faber MG, Mirchandani HG, et al: Ocular and optic nerve hemorrhages in abused infants with intracranial injuries. *Ophthalmology* 101:559, 1994.
19. Forman DL: *Every Parent's Guide to the Law.* San Diego, Harcourt, Brace, 1998.

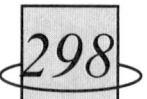

298 FEMALE AND MALE SEXUAL ASSAULT
Kim M. Feldhaus

EPIDEMIOLOGY

Sexual assault accounts for nearly 1 percent of all violent crimes reported in the 2001 U.S. Uniform Crimes Report.[1] Authorities believe that as few as one in three cases are reported to law enforcement.[2] Most sexual assaults are committed by a person known to the victim, whether a current or former partner, relative, friend, or first-time acquaintance.[3–5] The vast majority of information and statistics available relate to female rape victims. Only recently has male sexual assault been recognized and reported; the estimated incidence of male sexual assault is approximately 10 percent of all sexual assaults.[2]

Rape is a violent crime motivated by the need for power and control or by anger. Of victims who seek medical care following the sexual assault, general body trauma is present in 45 to 67 percent.[3,6,7] Rates of documented genital injury in sexual assault patients range from 9 to 45 percent; higher rates are documented if staining techniques or colposcopic magnification is used.[8,9] However, genital injuries are not an inevitable consequence of rape, and lack of genital injuries does not imply consensual intercourse. Evidence of semen or sperm has been documented in up to 45 percent of victims without evidence of injury on examination.[3]

The physician's responsibility is to provide for the patient's physical and psychological well-being first and then, if the patient consents, to provide police with corroborative forensic evidence. Victims should be encouraged to undergo an evidentiary examination as soon as possible because critical evidence may be lost if this examination is delayed. The victim may later choose not to proceed through the criminal justice system, but collection of forensic evidence does not commit him or her to seek prosecution.

CLINICAL FEATURES

The Female Rape Examination

HISTORY   The purpose of the history is to obtain data tactfully about the assault, along with a pertinent past medical history, in order to provide proper medical care. The victims should not have to relive every detail of the assault, and in fact, an extensive detailed history may hinder subsequent prosecution.[10–12] A professional, caring manner should be conveyed, and the history should be obtained in private.

Assault History

1. *Who?* Did the victim know the assailant? Was it a single assailant or multiple? Ask about their identity and race, and document in the medical records.
2. *What happened?* Was the victim physically assaulted? With what (e.g., gun, bat, or fist), and where? Delineate actual or attempted vaginal, anal, or oral penetration. Did ejaculation occur? If so, where? Was a foreign object used? Was a condom used? This information will direct the physical examination to areas of potential injury.
2. *When?* When did the assault occur? Most authorities caution that the chances of finding forensic evidence greater than 72 h after the assault are slim, and therefore, a forensic examination should not be performed. Emergency contraception is most effective when started within 72 h of the assault.
4. *Where?* Where did the assault occur? Corroborating evidence may be found based on the location of the assault.
5. *Suspicion of drug-facilitated rape?*[13] Was there a period of amnesia? A history of being out drinking and then suddenly feeling very intoxicated? A history of waking up naked? Of waking up with genital or pelvic soreness?
6. *Douche, shower, or change of clothing?* Any of these activities performed prior to seeking medical attention may decrease the probability of sperm or acid phosphatase recovery, as well as other bits of trace evidence.

Medical History

1. *Last menstrual period? Birth control method?* This will help to determine pregnancy risk.
2. *Last consensual intercourse?* If the patient has had consensual intercourse within the last 3 to 4 days, it may confuse laboratory analysis of sperm, acid phosphatase, and genetic typing.
3. *Allergies and prior medical history?* This information is necessary before prescribing antibiotics or pregnancy prophylaxis.
4. *Prior sexual assault?* Has this ever happened to the victim before?

PHYSICAL EXAMINATION   The physical examination should be performed thoroughly and compassionately. Document a general medical examination, including vital signs and level of consciousness. Bruises, lacerations, or other signs of trauma should be described in detail using a body map. Carefully inspect the victim's face, oral cavity, neck, breasts, wrist, thighs, and buttocks. Areas of tenderness should be recorded. Inspect the perineum for bruising, abrasions, and lacerations. A speculum examination should be performed, noting any vaginal discharge, vaginal abrasions, cervical abrasions, and cervical lacerations. Examine the rectum for abrasions or lacerations. The routine use of anoscopy following anal assault increases the detection of trauma.[14] If blood is present on rectal examination, anoscopy or sigmoidoscopy should be performed to look for the bleeding source.[14]

Toluidine blue can be used to detect small vulvar lacerations, since lacerations expose the deeper dermis, containing nuclei that absorb this stain.[8,10–12] Prior to inserting the speculum, the dye is applied to the perineum with gauze and wiped away with lubricating jelly. Lac-

erations are demonstrated by a linear blue stain. The magnification provided by a colposcope also has increased the documentation of genital injuries, especially injuries to the posterior fourchette.[9]

EVIDENTIARY EXAMINATION   Forensic evidence collection is performed within 72 h of the assault and serves legal purposes only. If more than 72 h have elapsed, the patient should still receive a full history, physical examination, documentation of injuries, and treatment for pregnancy and sexually transmitted disease (STD) prophylaxis.

Informed consent is required prior to evidence collection, and a system to maintain "chain of evidence" is essential. Most hospitals have a prepackaged rape kit (Table 298-1) with equipment and directions. Not every piece of the forensic evidence kit needs to be used every time; the collection of evidence should be tailored to the specifics of the assault. Follow the directions carefully to avoid evidence being declared inadmissible in court due to irregularities. The least invasive procedures should be performed first, and unnecessary duplication of procedures should be avoided.

Clothing worn during the assault or since the assault should be collected because it often reveals signs of a struggle (torn collar, missing buttons, etc.) Examining the skin with a Wood's lamp will reveal semen stains on a patient's body. These areas should be swabbed with a moistened cotton-tipped applicator. Microscopic examination of wet mounts (from vaginal, oral, or anal samples) for the presence of sperm should be left to forensic scientists.[4,10,15] If there is a concern for drug-facilitated sexual assault, urine should be obtained for drug testing. This testing should be done by law enforcement to preserve chain of evidence, and victims should be informed that any previous volitional, recreational drug use (such as cocaine or marijuana) also may be revealed in the toxicologic screening.[12,13] The urine sample should be refrigerated after receipt by law enforcement in order to preserve the detection of drugs of abuse.

The Male Rape Examination

History taking is similar to that in the female rape examination. The physical examination must be tailored to the particulars of the assault. Victims of oral penetration require a careful examination of the oral cavity; pharyngeal edema or mucosal lacerations may be found. Swabs should be taken of buccal and gingival areas if an oral assault occurred. In cases of anal assault, inspect the anus externally for signs of trauma, and perform anoscopy.[14] Up to two-thirds of victims will have minor genital injuries such as perineal contusions, anal fissures, or rectal mucosal tears.[14] Obtain a rectal swab or a rectal aspirate in cases

TABLE 298-1   Forensic Evidence Kit Contents

Control samples from victim
   Head hair samples
   Saliva sample
   Blood sample
   Pubic hair samples
Samples to identify assailant
   Skin swabbing for assailant's saliva
   Fingernail scrapings or clipping
   Pubic hair combing
   Trace evidence
Evidence for proof of recent sexual contact
   Oral, vaginal, and/or anal swabs for semen
   Wet mounts of oral, vaginal, and/or anal swabs for sperm
   Skin swabbing for semen
Evidence for proof of force or coercion
   Documentation of injuries found on exam
   Fingernail scrapings or clippings
   Urine or blood for toxicologic testing
   All clothing

Source: From Patel and Minshall[11] and Ferris and Sandercock.[15]

of anal assault for evidentiary purposes. Sterile saline can be injected into the rectum, allowed to equilibrate, and then aspirated.[11] Swabs from the victim's penis should be collected and examined for saliva if there is a history of oral copulation.

FORENSIC LABORATORY EVALUATION

The definition of rape is legal, not medical, and contains three elements: (1) any degree of carnal knowledge, (2) nonconsent-unless the victim is a minor, intoxicated, or mentally incompetent, in which case they are deemed unable to give consent, and (3) compulsion or fear of great harm.[10–12]

Proof of recent sexual contact includes the presence of sperm on wet mounts and the identification of acid phosphatase or other seminal products in any oral, anal, or vaginal cavity swabbing. Proof of force can be substantiated by documentation of injuries or a struggle (i.e., clothing evidence) or by the victim's statements regarding threats or coercion. Evidence that can help identify the assailant includes trace evidence (such as foreign hair) and DNA analysis or ABO secretor status typing of blood, saliva, or semen.[15]

Evidence of Semen

Historically, the courts and legal professions have placed a high significance on sperm or seminal fluid detection as confirmatory evidence for rape.[15] The detection of sperm depends on several factors, including time lapse between the assault and the physical examination, whether the assailant is azoospermic or has had a vasectomy, whether the assailant ejaculated, whether the victim douched prior to examination, and whether she has had consensual intercourse in the previous 72 h.[10–12,15] Previous studies suggest that one-quarter to one-third of sexual assault victims will have sperm detected as part of the evidentiary examination.[15] Evidence of seminal fluid (presence of spermatozoa or high levels of acid phosphatase or presence of p30 prostate specific antigen) is found in 38 to 48 percent of cases.[3,7]

Genetic Typing and DNA Analysis

Genetic typing helps to narrow the field of suspects but cannot specify an individual. Forensic analysis of evidence is used to determine genetic markers for the victim, the evidence, and the possible assailants. Determining blood type and secretor status can be used to exclude a potential assailant if his genetic typing does not match that of the evidence. DNA typing can be used to characterize an individual's unique genetic material and distinguish two individuals statistically. This typing can be performed on very small samples of evidence, as well as on old or decomposing samples.

All evidence collected from a victim should be labeled carefully with the victim's name, the type and source of the evidence, the date and time of collection, and the name of the person who collected the evidence. Following instructions for proper collection and storage of evidence is critical to producing optimal laboratory results.[11,12]

CORRELATES WITH PROSECUTION

Several studies have examined the relationship between victim characteristics, assault characteristics, and forensic evidence and the legal outcome of an individual case.[6,7,16] Successful prosecution has been associated with younger victims, victims who had evidence of trauma on examination, and cases where a weapon was used.[6] The presence of a known assailant, a history of multiple assailants, or evidence of trauma can increase the odds that charges will be filed by law enforcement.[7] Charges were filed three times more often in cases where forensic evidence was collected as compared with cases where a forensic evaluation was not performed, regardless of the results of the evidence collection.[7] There is a gradient association between the severity

of overall trauma (both genital and general body trauma) found on examination and the odds of charges being filed by law enforcement, as well as the odds of a conviction being secured.[7] A recent Canadian study reported no statistically significant relationships between legal evidence collected and the filing of charges in cases of sexual assault. However, many nonmedical variables such as the victim's age, use of alcohol, and relationship between victim and assailant were statistically associated with the filing charges.[16]

TREATMENT

Treatment of the rape victim includes, first and foremost, management of any physical injuries and psychological needs according to standards of care. This is followed by pregnancy prophylaxis and STD and human immunodeficiency virus (HIV) prophylaxis. Recent research suggests that many sexual assault victims are not receiving the full complement of treatment for pregnancy prevention and for STDs.[17] Drug or alcohol screens should be obtained only if medically indicated and if the results will influence treatment.

Pregnancy Prophylaxis

A pregnancy test should be obtained on all female rape victims of childbearing age in order to identify any preexisting pregnancy, and a negative pregnancy test should be documented before providing postcoital contraception. Contraceptives are pregnancy category X, and although a postcoital dose in very early pregnancy is not anticipated to have teratogenic effects, all women who receive postcoital contraception should have gynecologic follow-up in case pregnancy occurs. Although the risk of pregnancy after an isolated sexual encounter during nonfertile periods of the menstrual cycle is thought to be less than 1 percent, it is significantly higher at midcycle. Approximately 5 percent of all sexual assault victims become pregnant as a result of the assault.[5,18] As of this writing, there are several oral medication options for postcoital emergency contraception[19] (Table 298-2). The pooled failure rate of postcoital contraception is 3 percent or less. It should be given within 72 h.

The exact mechanism of action of emergency postcoital contraception is unclear, but it is thought that the agents act primarily to inhibit or disrupt ovulation or possibly to inhibit fertilization or implantation. Emergency contraception is not effective once implantation has occurred, and it will not disrupt an existing pregnancy. Common side effects include nausea and vomiting. Rates of nausea and vomiting for progestin-only medications are reported to be less than with combination pills.

Sexually Transmitted Disease Prophylaxis

Most of the literature demonstrates poor compliance of sexual assault patients with follow-up.[20] Therefore, prophylaxis for STDs should be given to all.[12,21] The current guidelines from the Centers for Disease Control and Prevention (CDC) recommend prophylaxis against gonorrhea, *Chlamydia, Trichomonas,* and bacterial vaginosis.[21] The CDC also recommends postexposure vaccination for hepatitis B, with the first dose administered at the time of the initial examination.[21] A negative pregnancy test should be documented prior to administering antibiotics because a positive pregnancy test will alter the choice of antibiotics. See Chap. 141 for further information on treatment of STDs. Table 298-3 presents the current CDC guidelines for antibiotic choices

TABLE 298-2   Postcoital Contraception*

Plan B (levonorgestrel) 1 tab initially then 1 in 12 h
Preven (ethinyl estradiol and levonorgestrel) 2 tabs initially then 2 in 12 h
Ovral (ethinyl estradiol and norgestrel) 2 tabs initially then 2 in 12 h

*Medication for nausea also should be prescribed.

TABLE 298-3   Treatment of Sexually Transmitted Diseases Following Sexual Assault

1. **Recommended regimens for gonorrhea prophylaxis:**
   Ceftriaxone (125 mg IM in a single dose)
   Alternative regimens:
   Cefixime 400 mg PO in a single dose
   or
   Ciprofloxacin 500 mg PO in a single dose
   or
   Ofloxacin 400 mg PO in a single dose
   If pregnant:
   Ceftriaxone 125 mg IM in a single dose (avoid fluoroquinolones and tetracyclines)
   plus
2. **Recommended regimens for *Chlamydia* prophylaxis:**
   Azithromycin 1 g PO in a single dose
   or
   Doxycycline 100 mg PO twice a day for 7 days
   Alternative regimens:
   Ofloxacin 300 mg PO twice a day for 7 days
   or
   Erythromycin base 500 mg PO four times a day for 7 days
   or
   Erythromycin ethylsuccinate 800 mg PO four times a day for 7 days
   If pregnant:
   Erythromycin base 500 mg PO four times a day for 7 days
   or
   Amoxicillin 500 mg PO three times a day for 7 days (avoid fluoroquinolones and tetracyclines)
   plus
3. **Recommended regimens for trichomoniasis and bacterial vaginosis prophylaxis:**
   Metronidazole 2 g PO in a single dose
   If pregnant with symptomatic bacterial vaginosis:
   Metronidazole 250 mg PO three times a day for 7 days
   or
   Clindamycin 300 mg PO two times a day for 7 days (avoid topical metronidazole gel or clindamycin cream)
   If pregnant with symptomatic trichomoniasis:
   Metronidazole 2 g PO in a single dose
   If pregnant and asymptomatic:
   Controversy exists regarding use of oral metronidazole in first trimester. Untreated BV and trichomoniasis have been associated with adverse pregnancy outcomes. Consult with patient's primary obstetrician regarding close follow-up or prophylactic treatment with metronidazole
   plus
4. **Recommended regimens for hepatitis B prophylaxis:**
   Hepatitis B vaccine at time of initial examination
   Follow-up doses of vaccine at 1–2 months and 4–6 months
   Hepatitis B immunoglobin not routinely administered.

Source: Centers for Disease Control: Sexually transmitted diseases treatment guidelines, 2002. *MMWR* 51(RR-6):1–80, May 10, 2002.

and hepatitis B vaccination. Administration of hepatitis B immunglobulin (HBIG) generally is not recommended but may be considered in a high-risk situation (assailant with known hepatitis B positivity or in a high-risk group). For those in a high-risk situation who have been vaccinated, a booster and HBIG should be given only if antibody titers are inadequate.[21]

Counseling and Testing for HIV

The true risk of contracting HIV from a single sexual encounter is unknown but believed to be low.[12,21,22] Estimated rates are felt to be highest with receptive, unprotected anal intercourse (0.008-0.032 infections per episode with an HIV-positive partner); the risk with receptive vaginal intercourse is 0.005 to 0.0015 infections per episode.[22–24] Circumstances of a specific assault may change the probability of HIV transmission: type of assault, presence of trauma,

viral load in the ejaculate, preexisting presence of a genital lesion or sexually transmitted infection in the assailant or victim, ejaculation on mucous membranes, and a history of multiple assaults.[21–23] Besides the uncertainty of HIV transmission after sexual assault, other factors complicate decision making about postexposure prophylaxis (PEP): potential inability to identify or test the assailant for HIV, expense of PEP, side effects of medication (e.g., nausea, vomiting, and anorexia in up to 50 percent of patients), the need for repetitive laboratory testing, the usual time delay between assault and initiation of PEP, and the need to provide follow-up with physicians familiar with PEP for HIV.[23,24] Extrapolating from the CDC guidelines for occupational PEP and from data regarding the benefits of PEP, PEP for HIV can be "recommended" for victims with the highest-risk exposures and should be "considered" for victims with moderate-risk exposures. Routine PEP following sexual assault by an assailant whose HIV status is unknown is not recommended[23,24] (Table 298-4).

If PEP is offered, the victim should be aware of the unknown efficacy and known toxicities of antiretroviral agents as well as the need for close follow-up and strict compliance with the regiment. The guidelines for occupational mucous membrane exposure should be followed, and treatment should be begun within 72 h.[22,24] Consultation with an HIV or infectious disease specialist is encouraged. See Chap. 154 regarding occupational exposure guidelines.

FOLLOW-UP CARE

Ideally, counseling for sexual assault patients should be available 24 h a day in the emergency department. Often, a rape counselor will precede the physician in assessing a victim, preparing him or her for the examination, and provide moral support. Multidisciplinary *sexual assault response teams* are common in some areas of the country and work to provide coordinated, sensitive care of the sexual assault victim, including addressing medical, legal, and psychological needs.[12,25–28] If no social worker or rape counselor is available when a sexual assault victim arrives, the physician should provide information on local rape counseling centers where the patient may seek further care.

Follow-up medical care is needed to ensure that any injuries have healed properly and to ensure the effectiveness of the pregnancy prophylaxis and STD treatment. A male rape victim should be referred to

TABLE 298-4   Probability of HIV Transmission Based on Type of Sexual Assault

High: Recommend PEP
   Unprotected receptive anal intercourse with known HIV+ assailant
   Unprotected receptive anal intercourse with an assailant of unknown HIV status from a high-risk population (estimated to have a 30% or greater risk of HIV infection)
Moderate: Consider PEP
   Unprotected vaginal intercourse with a known HIV+ assailant
   Unprotected receptive anal intercourse with an assailant of unknown HIV status from an intermediate-risk population (estimated to have a 10–30% risk of HIV infection)
Low: Inform patient of PEP
   Unprotected vaginal intercourse with an assailant of unknown HIV status from a low-risk population
   Unprotected receptive anal intercourse with an assailant of unknown HIV status from a low-risk population
   Oral sex without ejaculation (risk of transmission from oral sex with ejaculation is unknown)
Recommended PEP: Inform patient that expected benefits of PEP outweigh risks and that PEP is advisable.
Consider PEP: Inform patient and tailor decision to clinical situation and patient desires.
Inform patient: Explain benefits and risks of PEP but advise patient that risk of infection is low and probably outweighed by toxicity and cost of PEP.

Source: From Moran[23] and Lurie et al.[24]

a urologist or a proctologist. Young children should be referred to a pediatrician for evaluation. These follow-up instructions should be explained clearly in a written aftercare information sheet because victims often recall very little of their emergency department encounter.[12,25]

REFERENCES

1. U.S. Department of Justice, Federal Bureau of Investigation, Uniform Crime Reports: *Crime in the United States,* 2001. Washington, U.S. Government Printing Office, 2001.
2. U.S. Department of Justice, Bureau of Justice Statistics: *Rape and Sexual Assault: Reporting to the Police and Medical Attention,* 1992–2000. NCJ 194530. Washington, U.S. Government Printing Office, 2002.
3. Riggs N, Houry D, Long G, et al: Analysis of 1,076 cases of sexual assault. *Ann Emerg Med* 35(4):358, 2000.
4. Feldhaus KM, Houry D, Kaminsky R: Lifetime sexual assault prevalence rates and reporting practices in an emergency department population. *Ann Emerg Med* 36(1)23, 2000.
5. Resnick HS, Holmes MM, Kilpatrick DG, et al: Predictors of post-rape medical care in a national sample of women. *Am J Prevent Med* 19(4):214, 2000.
6. Gray-Eurom K, Seaberg DC, Wears RL: The prosecution of sexual assault cases: correlation with forensic evidence. *Ann Emerg Med* 39(1):39, 2002.
7. McGregor MJ, Du Mont J, Myhr TL: Sexual assault forensic medical examination: is evidence related to successful prosecution? *Ann Emerg Med* 39(6):639, 2002.
8. Lincoln C: Genital injury: Is it significant? A review of the literature. *Med Sci Law* 41(3):206, 2001.
9. Slaughter L, Brown CR, Crowley S, et al: Patterns of genital injury in female sexual assault victims. *Am J Obstet Gynecol* 176(3):609, 1997.
10. DeLahunta EA, Baram DA: Sexual assault. *Clin Obstet Gynecol* 40(3):648, 1997.
11. Patel M, Minshall L: Management of sexual assault. *Emerg Med Clin North Am* 19(3):817, 2001.
12. American College of Emergency Physicians, Emergency Medicine Practice Committee: *Evaluation and Management of the Sexually Assaulted or Sexually Abused Patient. Dallas, American College of Emergency Physicians,* June 1999.
13. Anglin D, Spears KL, Hutson HR: Flunitrazepam and its involvement in date or acquaintance rape. *Acad Emerg Med* 4(4):323, 1997.
14. Ernst AA, Green E, Ferguson MT, et al: The utility of anoscopy and colposcopy in the evaluation of male sexual assault victims. *Ann Emerg Med* 36(5):432, 2000.
15. Ferris LE, Sandercock J: The sensitivity of forensic tests for rape. *Med Law* 17(3):333, 1998.
16. Du Mont J, Parnis D: Sexual assault and legal resolution: Querying the medical collection of forensic evidence. *Med Law* 19(4):779, 2000.
17. Amey AL, Bishai D: Measuring the quality of medical care for women who experience sexual assault with data from the National Hospital Ambulatory Medical Care Survey. *Ann Emerg Med* 39(6):631, 2002.
18. Holmes MM, Resnick HS, Kilpatrick DG, et al: Rape-related pregnancy: Estimates and descriptive characteristics from a national sample of women. *Am J Obstet Gynecol* 175(2):320,1996; discussion, 324.
19. Mendez MN: Emergency contraception: A review of current oral options. *West J Med* 176(3):188, 2002.
20. Holmes MM, Resnick HS, Frampton D: Follow-up of sexual assault victims. *Am J Obstet Gynecol* 179(2):336, 1998.
21. Centers for Disease Control and Prevention: Sexually transmitted diseases treatment guidelines 2002. *MMWR* 51(RR-6):1, 2002.
22. Bamberger JD, Waldo CR, Gerberding JL, et al: Postexposure prophylaxis for human immunodeficiency virus (HIV) infection following sexual assault. *Am J Med* 106(3):323, 1999.
23. Moran GJ: Pharmacologic management of HIV/STD exposure. *Emerg Med Clin North Am* 18(4):829, 2000.
24. Lurie P, Miller S, Hecht F, et al: Postexposure prophylaxis after nonoccupational HIV exposure: Clinical, ethical, and policy considerations. *JAMA* 280(20):1769, 1998.
25. Ledray LE: SANE development and operation guide. *J Emerg Nurs* 24(2):197, 1998.
26. Ledray L: Sexual assault nurse examiner (SANE) programs. *J Emerg Nurs* 22(5):460, 1996.
27. Ciancone AC, Wilson C, Collette R, et al: Sexual assault nurse examiner programs in the United States. *Ann Emerg Med* 35(4):353, 2000.
28. U.S. Department of Justice, Office of Justice Programs: *Sexual Assault Nurse Examiner Programs: Improving the Community Response to Sexual Assault Victims.* NCJ 185690. Washington, U.S. Government Printing Office, 2001.

299 INTIMATE PARTNER VIOLENCE AND ABUSE
Patricia R. Salber

Intimate partner violence is defined as a pattern of assaultive, coercive behaviors that may include inflicted physical injury, psychological abuse, sexual assault, progressive social isolation, stalking, deprivation, intimidation, and threats. These behaviors are perpetrated by someone who is, was, or wishes to be involved in an intimate or dating relationship with an adult or adolescent victim and are aimed at establishing control by one partner over the other.[1]

The term *intimate partner violence and abuse* (IPVA) should be used instead of older terms such as *spousal abuse, wife battering,* or *domestic violence,* because IPVA more accurately reflects the fact that this type of abuse occurs not only in adult heterosexual married relationships but also in cohabiting, separated, gay and lesbian relationships, and adolescent dating relationships.

Intimate partner violence and abuse occurs in every race, ethnicity, culture, geographic area, and religious group, and it affects individuals from all socioeconomic and educational backgrounds.[2–4] Male victimization also occurs.

Effects extend beyond the victim. Children who grow up in violent homes may be physically or emotionally abused or neglected, and witnessing violence can have short- and long-term adverse health consequences.[5,6] About 30 to 60 percent of reported cases of spousal abuse also report child abuse.[7] Children also can be incidentally injured or injured when they try to intervene in the struggle.[8] Children exposed to violence in the home may develop significant behavioral difficulties, including depression, abusive behaviors, or drug abuse. Perpetrators of violence, in particular severe violence, may be at risk for suicide, committing murder or suicide, or being murdered by a family member.[9]

Unless a history of IPVA is specifically sought and responded to during health care encounters, IPVA may go unrecognized and untreated. The consequences may be further intimate partner violence and abuse-related injury, illness or death.

EPIDEMIOLOGY

In 1999, a reported 671,110 women and girls older than 12 years experienced murder, rape, sexual assault, robbery, aggravated assault, and simple assault at the hands of an intimate. This figure is substantially lower than the 875,340 reported in 1998 and more than 40 percent lower than the 1.1 million reported in 1993. In addition, 120,100 men were reported as victimized by intimates in 1999, down from 157,330 in 1998.[10]

Risk factors for IPVA include female sex, age between 16 and 24 years, low income household, relationship status of separated rather than divorced or married, and children younger than 3 years in the home.[6,10] Women aged 16 to 24 years experienced violence by intimates at a rate of approximately 16 in 1000, compared with an overall rate of about 6 in 1000. Ninety-six percent of female intimate partner violence victimization occurs between the ages of 16 to 49 years, especially in low income households, although IPVA rates are still significant in households earning $50,000 or more.

Black and white females experience intimate partner violence at similar rates for every age group except 20 to 24 years, in which rates in black women are higher than those in white women. Rates for Hispanic women are lower than those for black and white women; however, rates of victimization follow a similar age distribution.[10]

Of the 1642 people murdered by intimates in 1999, 1218, or 74 percent, were women.[11] An intimate was responsible for 32 percent of all murders of women compared with 4 percent of male homicides. The rate of IPVA murders has been declining since 1976, with the rate of decline substantially greater for males. Approximately 60 percent of IPVA homicides are committed with a gun.[12] Between 1993 and 1998, about two-thirds of reported female and male victims of IPVA were physically attacked. Those in the remaining third were victims of threats or attempted violence. Fifty percent of female victims of IPVA were injured by their attackers compared with 32 percent of male victims.[3]

EMERGENCY DEPARTMENT DIAGNOSIS

Overall, an estimated 5 million visits each year to the ED are made because of IPVA.[13] Between 4 and 15 percent of women seen in EDs are there because of symptoms related to IPVA, with 2 to 4 percent presenting with acute IPVA trauma.[14–16] In addition, more than 50 percent of women seen in EDs have experienced IPVA at some point in their lives.[14]

The responsibilities of the ED team include:[17]

1. Identification of IPVA
2. Validation of the victim's experience
3. Assessment of immediate risk and safety planning
4. Referral to IPVA experts
5. Medical record documentation

IDENTIFICATION

There are myriad presentations of IPVA, including injuries; chronic pain syndromes; obstetric and gynecologic manifestations, including rape, sexually transmitted diseases, and complications of pregnancy; mental health presentations, including anxiety, hyperventilation, panic disorders, posttraumatic stress disorder, dissociation, phobias, suicide attempts,[18] and complications of alcohol and other substance abuse. There are no "typical" presentations of IPVA in the ED, but there are important historical and examination features that suggest IPVA.

Certain Characteristic Injuries Characteristic injuries include fingernail scratches, bite marks, cigarette burns, bruises suggesting strangulation, and rope burns.

Injuries Suggesting a Defensive Posture Forearm bruises or fractures may be sustained when women try to fend off blows to the face or chest.

Central Pattern of Injury Examples of central patterns are injuries to the head, neck, face, and thorax and abdominal injuries in pregnant women.

An Extent or Type of Injury Inconsistent with the Patient's Explanation Such injuries include multiple abrasions and contusions to different anatomic sites inconsistent with the mechanism of injury.

Multiple Injuries in Various Stages of Healing These may be reported as "accidents" or "clumsiness."

Substantial Delay Between the Time of Injury and the Presentation for Treatment Victims may wait several days before seeking medical care for injuries. They may seek care for minor or resolving injuries.

Visits for Vague or Minor Complaints Without Evidence of Physiologic Abnormality This pattern may include frequent ED visits for a variety of injuries or illnesses, including chronic pelvic pain and other chronic pain syndromes.

Suicide Attempts Women who attempt or commit suicide often have a history of IPVA.[18]

Obstetric and Gynecologic Presentations Sexual coercion and rape occur in some IPVA relationships. The result may be unwanted pregnancies and sexually transmitted diseases, including human immunodeficiency virus.[19] Complications related to pregnancy, including complications of abdominal trauma, smoking or alcohol and drug use, low maternal weight gain, and neglect of prenatal care, are other features associated with IPVA.[20]

Partner's Behavior Partners accompanying victims of IPVA may provide clues to the diagnosis by exhibiting controlling or abusive behavior. Further, the victim may appear frightened of her partner or refuse to answer questions and instead defer all responses to the partner.

SCREENING FOR IPVA

Because the features of IPVA are so varied, many experts recommend routine screening for IPVA for all adolescent and adult women who present to the ED.[16,21,22] National screening consensus guidelines have been published and are available online at http://www.fvpf.org.[23] At a minimum, the ED staff should screen all non-critically ill adolescent and adult patients and mothers of children seen in the ED for current exposure to IPVA. Because of the known adverse long-term impacts of IPVA on health, when time permits, screening for lifetime exposure should be considered.

Screening should be conducted by providers educated about the dynamics of IPVA and the safety and autonomy of abused patients. Screening should be conducted in a safe and private environment with direct and nonjudgmental language. If translators are required, it is best to use individuals who have no connection to the patient and, if possible, who have had education about the dynamics of abuse. Documentation of screening, its results, safety assessment, and any interventions, including referrals and required reporting, should be clearly charted.

Screening guidelines for adolescent and adult patients are summarized in Table 299-1. Sample verbal screening questions are listed in Table 299-2.

TREATMENT GOALS

If ED staff feel that the immediate goal is to "place the victim in a shelter" or "have the attacker arrested," they are bound to become frustrated. Ensuring the safety of the woman and her children is the foremost goal. It is the woman, however, who must make the ultimate determination of whether it is safe to return home. By providing women with information about IPVA, risks, and options, the physician will help the woman decide what is best for her and her family.

Validation: Providing Confirmation and Support

Patients must be told that violence, abuse, and intimidation are not a part of normal, healthy relationships. The victim's reports and experiences should be acknowledged and believed. Let victims know that you take the situation seriously and that you are concerned about the health and safety of her and her children. Victims also should be told explicitly that they have done nothing that warrants the violence and abuse. It is the perpetrator whose behavior is unacceptable. Finally, make it clear that ED personnel can help victims contact IPVA experts (trained social workers or IPVA advocates) who can help them develop

TABLE 299-1 Summary of National Consensus Guidelines for Screening for Intimate Partner Violence and Abuse in the Emergency Department

Screening	Assessment	Intervention	Documentation	Referral and Follow-Up

Routinely screen at every visit
Screen for current abuse and if time allows, screen for past history of abuse
Privately (one on one) or with nonrelated trained interpreter
Ask: What happened? When did it happen? Where did it happen? Who did this?
Respect patient decision to disclose or not
Discuss any required reporting
Include screening questions on intake forms
	Assess immediate safety
	Assess health impact of abuse
	Assess pattern of abuse
	Danger and lethality assessment
	If the danger assessment is positive, assess for suicide and homicide
		Careful listening and support
		"I'm concerned for your health and safety"
		"You are not alone"
		"Help is available"
		"It is not your fault"
		"You don't deserve it"
		"What happened to you can affect your health"
		Provide DV information and materials
		"What can I do for you?"
		Provide a safety plan
		Offer services to DV advocate, social work, police, shelter, etc.
			Legible, full signature, maintain confidentiality of records
			Abuse history:
			  Subjective information: patient states…
			  Objective information: detailed description of patient's appearance, behavioral indicators, injuries and health complaints
			Use of rape kits where appropriate
			Results of physical examination
			Use of body maps
			Photography (with patient's consent)
			Radiology, laboratory findings, collection of forensic evidence: clothes, debris, etc.
			Any materials and referrals offered
			Results of health and safety assessments
				Check if patient has a PCP to follow up with or refer to PCP, mental health provider, social worker, or DV advocate
				Obtain permission to notify provider
				Know current phone numbers for:
				  DV programs
				  Legal services
				  Children's programs
				  Mental health services
				  Law enforcement
				  Substance abuse
				  Transportation
				  Local clergy or other community organizations

Abbreviations: DV = domestic violence; PCP = primary care physician.
Source: National Consensus Guidelines on Identifying and Responding to Domestic Violence Victimization in Health Care Settings. San Francisco, Family Violence Prevention Fund, 2002.

the logistics of leaving the relationship or assist with other safety strategies, if the victim chooses to stay in the relationship.

The validation process, in and of itself, has been documented to be a turning point for victims by helping them to begin to plan for a life without IPVA. Therefore, validation should be considered a treatment goal for each IPVA encounter.[24,25]

Safety Assessment

High risk indicators of a potentially lethal situation include escalation in the frequency or severity of violence; the threat or actual use of weapons, in particular firearms; obsession with the victim; hostage taking; stalking; and homicide or suicide threats or attempts and evidence of violent behavior outside the home. Other risk factors for serious injury or death include substance abuse, especially with drugs, such as crack cocaine or amphetamines, that are associated with an increase in violent behaviors.[26]

The most dangerous periods for victims of IPVA are during the time of abuse disclosure and during attempts to leave the relationship. Some victims feel safer remaining in the violent relationship rather than leaving without adequate planning for safe departure.[26] If lethality risk is high, it is important that victims have an opportunity to speak with IPVA experts, such as hospital-based social workers or community-based advocates, before discharge from the ED. Hospital admission of the victim or children is another option in high-risk situations in which there is no other way to ensure safety.

Referral to IPVA Experts

Victims of IPVA should be referred to IPVA experts, such as hospital social workers or community-based IPVA advocates, who can help the victim assess the situation, understand options, plan for safety, and arrange safe shelter. Community advocates are typically on-call or

available by telephone. If it is not possible or necessary that a personal contact be made before discharge from the ED, the victims should be given up-to-date information about IPVA services in the community, so that follow-up can be arranged later at the patient's discretion. The IPVA advocates should not be asked to call the patient directly unless the patient agrees, because calls to the home could jeopardize the patient's safety.

Resources for health care providers to prepare their practices for optimal response to IPVA are available from the following organizations:

1. Physicians for a Violence-free Society: www.pvs.org
2. Family Violence Prevention Fund's National Health Resources Center on Domestic Violence: www.endabuse.org/health
3. National Domestic Violence Hotline: 1-800-799-SAFE (7233)

ED Record Documentation

Documentation should include whether IPVA was identified by routine screening or by voluntary patient statements. With voluntary statements, it is better to record a description of the abuse in the victim's own words (e.g., "the patient states her boyfriend, Jim Smith, struck her in the eye with his closed fist"). Avoid using legalistic jargon, such as "the patient alleges her husband hit her," because it can be interpreted during legal proceedings that the recorder doubted the veracity of the statement.

Record episodes of past and current abuse. Include dates, times, locations, details of incidents, and the names of any witnesses, if possible. Describe the patient's appearance and demeanor and any visible injuries. Use a body map and photographs to supplement the written description, particularly for documentation of injuries, such as scalp hematoma hidden by hair and soft tissue injuries that are not yet discolored. Collect relevant forensic evidence, such as saliva from bite wounds and semen (using a rape kit), if sexual assault has occurred.

TABLE 299-2 Sample Oral Questions to Screen for Intimate Partner Violence and Abuse

Framing questions: Sometimes it feels awkward to suddenly introduce the subject of abuse, particularly if there are no obvious indications a woman is being abused. The following questions are examples of ways providers can introduce the issue.

We now know intimate partner violence and abuse is a very common problem. It is harmful to your health and the health of your family members. Are you in a relationship where your partner threatens to harm you, insults you, belittles you, or hits, kicks, or slaps you?

Because partner violence is common in women's lives, I now ask every woman I see in the emergency department if she has been physically, sexually, or emotionally abused.

I don't know if this is a problem for you, but many of the women I see as patients are dealing with abusive relationships. Some are too afraid or uncomfortable to bring it up themselves, so I ask about it routinely.

Some women think they deserve abuse because they have not lived up to their partners' expectations, but no matter what someone has or hasn't done, no one deserves to be beaten or emotionally abused.

Because so many women I see in my practice are involved with someone who hits them, threatens them, continually puts them down, or tries to control them, I routinely ask all of my patients about abuse.

Many of the lesbian and gay men we see here are hurt by their partners. Does your partner every try to hurt you?

Direct questions: However one initially raises the issue of intimate partner violence and abuse, it is important to include direct and specific questions.

Did someone hit you? Who was it? Was it your partner or husband?

Has your partner or ex-partner ever hit you or physically hurt you? Has he ever threatened to hurt you or someone close to you?

I'm concerned that your symptoms may have been caused by someone hurting you. Has someone been hurting you?

Does your partner ever try to control you by threatening to hurt you or your family?

Has your partner ever forced you to have sex when you didn't want to? Has he ever refused to practice safe sex?

Has your freedom been restricted or are you kept from doing things that are important to you (like going to school, working, or seeing your friends or family)?

Does your partner frequently belittle you, insult you, and blame you?

Do you feel controlled or isolated by your partner?

Do you ever feel afraid of your partner? Do you feel you are in danger? Is it safe for you to go home?

Is your partner jealous? Does he frequently accuse you of infidelity?

Indirect questions: In some clinical settings, it may be appropriate to start the inquiry with an indirect question before proceeding to more direct questions. The following questions are examples of this approach.

Have you been under any stress lately? Are you having any problems with your partner? Do you ever argue or fight? Do the fights ever become physical? Are you ever afraid? Have you ever gotten hurt?

You seem to be concerned about your partner. Can you tell me more about that? Does he ever act in ways that frighten you?

You mentioned that your partner loses his temper with the children. Can you tell me more about that? Has he ever hit or threatened to physically harm you or the children?

How are things going in your relationship or marriage? All couples argue sometimes. Are you having fights? Do you fight physically?

You mentioned that your partner drinks alcohol (or uses drugs). How does he act when he is intoxicated? Does his behavior ever frighten you? Does he ever become violent?

Like all other couples, gay couples have various ways of resolving their conflicts. How do you and your partner deal with conflicts? What happens when you disagree? What happens when your partner doesn't get his (her) way?

Source: Salber P, Taliaferro E: *The Physicians' Guide to Domestic Violence.* Volcano, CA, Volcano Press, 1995.

Record the results of any relevant laboratory or diagnostic imaging studies.

LEGAL CONSIDERATIONS

Reporting to Law Enforcement

Most states have laws that require health care providers to report injuries resulting from firearms, knives, or other weapons. Twenty-three states have reporting requirements for injuries resulting from crimes (IPVA is a crime in all 50 states); seven states have statutes that specifically require health providers to report injuries resulting from IPVA. The specifics of the reporting requirements vary from state to state, and the adequacy of response by the police to reporting varies by jurisdiction. Inadequate or inappropriate response to the reports (e.g., informing the perpetrator of the report without provision for safety of the victim) can increase the risk of harm to victims. ED personnel should be aware of reporting requirements and police response in their area. In addition, victims of IPVA must be apprised not only of the requirement to make a police report but also of possible ramifications.

Medicolegal Liability

DUTY TO CARE As routine IPVA screening, intervention, documentation, and referral become widely recognized in the medical literature and in the medical community as the standard of care, the risk

that health care providers who fail to meet this standard may be found liable increases. A recent ED case, although settled out of court, has heightened awareness of the issue in the legal community.[27]

DUTY TO WARN Victims of IPVA should be asked routinely whether they have suicidal or homicidal ideation. Such ideation, particularly if accompanied by a concrete plan of action, should trigger immediate consultation with a mental health provider. All physicians have a duty to warn potential victims if they become aware of a patient's intent to harm a third party. If commitment to a psychiatric facility is planned, the third party is protected and does not have to be warned.[28]

PREPARING THE ED FOR OPTIMAL RESPONSE TO IPVA

EDs should take the following steps to prepare for optimal IPVA response:

1. Place multicultural, multilingual brochures and posters in examination rooms and other areas of the hospital that provide information about IPVA and its impact on victims and other family members and provide information about community-based programs that provide services to victims.
2. Implement a routine screening protocol that addresses training of ED personnel, confidential interviewing, and appropriate interventions, including validation and referral.
3. Establish an IPVA continuous quality improvement program that assesses adherence to recommended screening and intervention strategies.

4. Form close relationships with hospital- and/or community-based IPVA experts to ensure appropriate referral practices.
5. Establish a program in the ED and other hospital facilities that addresses IPVA.

REFERENCES

1. *Preventing Domestic Violence: Clinical Guidelines on Routine Screening.* San Francisco, Family Violence Prevention Fund, 1999.
2. Watts C, Zimmerman C: Violence against women: Global scope and magnitude. *Lancet* 359:1232, 2002.
3. Rennison CM, Welchans S: *Intimate Partner Violence.* Bureau of Justice Statistics Special Report, NCJ 178247, 1-11. May 2000, revised January 31, 2002.
4. Haile-Miriam T, Smith J: Domestic violence against women in the international community. *Emerg Med Clin North Am* 17:617, 1999.
5. Felitti VJ, Anda RF, Nordenberg D, et al: Relationship of childhood abuse and household dysfunction to many of the leading causes of death in adults. *Am J Prev Med* 14:245, 1998.
6. Duffy SJ, McGrath ME, Becker BM, et al: Mothers with histories of domestic violence in a pediatric emergency department. *Pediatrics* 103:1007, 1999.
7. Edelson JL: The overlap between child maltreatment and woman battering. *Violence Against Women* 5:134, 1999.
8. Fantuzzo J, Boruch R, Beriama A, et al: Domestic violence and children: Prevalence and risk in five major US cities. *J Am Acad Child Adolesc Psychiatry* 36:122, 1997.
9. Connor KR, Cerulli C, Caine ED: Threatened and attempted suicide by partner-violent male respondents petitioned to family violence court. *Violence Vict* 17:115, 2002.
10. Rennison CM: *Intimate Partner Violence and Age of Victim, 1993–1999.* Bureau of Justice Statistics Special Report, NCJ 187635. October 2001, revised November 28, 2001.
11. Bureau of Justice Statistics, US Department of Justice: *Homicide Trends in the US: Intimate Homicide.* Available at: http://www.ojp.usdoj.gov/bjs/homicide/intimates.htm. Updated January 4, 2001.
12. Kellerman A, Heron S: Firearms and family violence. *Emerg Clin North Am* 17:699, 1999.
13. Abbott J, Johnson R, Koziol-McLain J, Lowenstein SR: Domestic violence against women: Incidence and prevalence in an emergency department population. *JAMA* 273:1763, 1995.
14. Dearwater SR, Coben JH, Campbell JC, et al: Prevalence of intimate partner abuse in women treated at community hospital emergency departments. *JAMA* 280:433, 1998.
15. Ernst AA, Weiss SJ: Intimate partner violence from the emergency medicine perspective. *Women Health* 35:71, 2002.
16. Gerbert B, Lee D, Durborow N, Salber PR (eds): How health care providers help battered women: The survivor's perspective. *Women Health* 29:115, 1999.
17. Gerbert B, Moe J, Caspers N, et al: Physicians' response to victims of domestic violence: Toward a model of care. *Women Health* 35:1, 2002.
18. Kaplan ML, Asnis GN, Lipschitz DS, Chomey P: Suicidal behavior and abuse in psychiatric outpatients. *Compr Psychiatry* 36:229, 1995.
19. El-Bassel N, Gilbert L, Krishnan S, et al: Partner violence and sexual HIV-risk behaviors among women in an inner-city emergency department. *Violence Vict* 13:377, 1998.
20. Petersen R, Gazmararian JA, Spitz AM, et al: Violence and adverse pregnancy outcomes: A review of the literature and directions for future research. *Am J Prev Med* 13:366, 1997.
21. Abbott J: Injuries and illnesses of domestic violence. *Ann Emerg Med* 29:781, 1997.
22. Fanslow JL, Norton RN, Spinola CG: Indicators of assault-related injuries among women presenting to the emergency department. *Ann Emerg Med* 32:341, 1998.
23. *National Consensus Guidelines on Identifying and Responding to Domestic Violence Victimization in Health Care Settings.* San Francisco, Family Violence Prevention Fund, 2002.
24. Rodriguez MA, Quiroga SS, Bauer HM: Breaking the silence: Battered women's perspectives on medical care. *Arch Fam Med* 15:153, 1996.
25. Gerbert B, Abercrombie P, Caspers N, et al: How health care providers help battered women: The survivor's perspective. *Women Health* 29:115, 1999.
26. Campbell J: *Assessing Dangerousness: Potential for Further Violence of Sexual Offenders, Batterers, and Child Abusers.* Newbury Park, CA, Sage Publications, 1995.
27. Brown-Cranstoun J: Kringen v Boslough and Saint Vincent Hospital: A new trend for healthcare professionals who treat victims of domestic violence? *J Health Law* 35:629, 2000.
28. Warshaw C: Identification, assessment and intervention with victims of domestic violence, in Abercrombie P, Caspers N, *Improving the Health Care Response to Violence: A Resource Manual for Health Care Providers.* San Francisco, Family Violence Prevention Fund, 1998, p. 78.

300 ABUSE IN THE ELDERLY AND IMPAIRED
Ellen H. Taliaferro

Abuse continues to be an underrecognized and underreported cause of morbidity and mortality in the elderly. Historical information often remains undetected during medical evaluation, and social stigmata surround the problem. About 3 percent of the elderly population experiences abuse or neglect.[1] This number is significant, because the number of elderly in the United States is growing. By the year 2020, about 20 percent of the U.S. population will be 65 years or older. Detection of elder abuse and neglect is contingent on physicians' awareness of the problem and the ability to recognize risk factors. Community emergency medical services[2] and emergency departments[3] also should play a role in the identification of elder abuse.

The American College of Emergency Physicians adopted a policy statement on the management of elder abuse and neglect.[4] This statement contains the following recommendations:

1. Emergency departments should have written protocols on the recognition and treatment of elder abuse.
2. Hospitals should have appropriate ancillary staff and other resources readily available to help in the assessment and disposition of those individuals who may be abused or neglected. The hospital staff should be educated in local laws governing the reporting of such incidents and in defusing potentially hostile situations.
3. Hospitals and emergency departments should establish relationships with agencies that oversee the management and investigation of elder abuse.
4. In jurisdictions that have mandatory reporting requirements, persons reporting in good faith should be immune from liability for compliance.
5. Further research should be conducted in epidemiology, detection, prevention, and management of elder abuse and neglect; standardized definitions of elder abuse developed by the National Center on Elder Abuse should facilitate research in this area.

The National Center on Elder Abuse[5] has defined seven types of elder abuse (Table 300-1). In addition, there are three basic categories of elder abuse: (1) domestic elder abuse that occurs in the home, (2) institutional elder abuse, and (3) self-neglect or self-abuse. In most states, statutes provide the definitions of these different categories of elder abuse. Neglect can be intentional or unintentional. Unintentional neglect may occur through ignorance or inability to provide care.

SOCIAL AND ENVIRONMENTAL RISKS FOR ELDER ABUSE

In general, elderly victims are socially isolated from family and friends, but many live with their abuser. When abuse occurs, the abuser is often dependent on the victim for housing and financial, social, and emotional support. Caretakers usually attempt to provide ac-

TABLE 300-1   Elder Abuse Definitions (Category 1A)

Types of Abuse	Definitions	Examples
Physical	Injury or harm intending to cause suffering, pain, or impairment	Slapping, biting, burning, pushing, improper or use of restraint
Sexual	Nonconsensual sexual involvement of any kind	Rape; sexual threats or innuendoes
Emotional or psychological	Inflicting anguish, pain, or distress, verbally or nonverbally	Threats to institutionalize or withhold medicine, food, or water
Financial or material exploitation	Illegal or improper use of funds, property, or assets	Stealing, forgery, financial coercion, or blackmail
Neglect	Refusal or failure of caregiver to fulfill obligations or duties	Not providing food, clothing, medicine, shelter, supervision, or social support
Abandonment	Desertion by custodian or caregiver who has assumed responsibility for care	
Self-neglect	Failure of the older person to provide for own mental and medical care	

Source: National Center on Elder Abuse. Available at: http://www.elderabusecenter.org.

ceptable and appropriate care. However, when the caregiver is overwhelmed, frustrated, or resentful of the responsibilities involved in the task of caring for a less than fully independent elder, abuse or neglect may occur.

Certain conditions tend to set the stage for abuse or neglect. Functional disability and worsening cognitive impairment of the aging individual, especially an acute decline, are risk factors associated with elder mistreatment.[6]

Abuse is associated more with personality problems of the caregiver than with situational stress.[7] In general, abusers are heavily dependent individuals. Caretakers who are disabled, alcohol- or drug-dependent, cognitively impaired, or mentally ill are also at risk for abusive or neglectful behavior.

CLINICAL FEATURES

Mistreatment or neglect of elderly patients may be difficult to recognize. It occurs most commonly in residential settings. The problem is complicated by the fact that, when abuse is suspected, it may be difficult to secure confirmation from the patient. The patient may welcome and be relieved by the physician's concern and identification. However, embarrassment, fear of abandonment, fear of retaliation, and fear of nursing home placement can prompt the patient to deny the physician's concerns. The history and physical examination are excellent tools to identify elder abuse.[8]

History taking should focus on: (1) detecting the presence of caretaker mental illness, mental retardation, dementia, or drug or alcohol abuse; (2) family history of violence; (3) caretaker dependence on the elder patient for housing, finances, or emotional support; (4) patient isolation, as reflected by the fact that the patient does not have the opportunity to relate with people or to pursue activities and interests in a manner that the patient chooses; (5) whether the patient and suspected abuser are living together; and (6) recent occurrence of stressful life events, such as loss of job, moving, or death of a loved one for the caretaker.[9]

Important historical information concerning the patient should include dependency needs. Problems such as mental confusion, immobility, and need for assistance with hygiene can be associated with neglect. Eliciting a history of cognitive impairment is essential, because abused victims have been found to have significantly greater cognitive impairment than nonabused elderly patients. Abused patients also have a traumatic history of problematic behavior such as incontinence, nocturnal shouting, wandering, or paranoia.[1]

An important direct question to put to the patient is, "Are you happy at home, or have you experienced any recent changes in mood or sleeping or eating patterns?" Look also for the sudden onset of be-

havioral signs and symptoms that suggest victimization: depression, fear, withdrawal, confusion, anxiety, low self-esteem, or helplessness.

Other historical indicators of abuse or neglect include a pattern of "physician shopping," unexplained delay in seeking treatment, lack of medical care, a series of missed medical appointments, previous unexplained injuries, explanation of past injuries inconsistent with medical findings, and previous reports of similar injuries.

The **physical examination** begins with an observation of the interaction between the patient and accompanying caretakers. The following findings suggest abuse:

1. The patient appears fearful of his or her companion.
2. There are conflicting accounts of the injury or illness between the patient and caretaker.
3. There is an absence of assistance from the caretaker.
4. The caretaker displays an attitude of indifference or anger toward the patient.
5. The caretaker is overly concerned with the costs of treatment needed by the patient.
6. The caretaker denies the patient the chance to interact privately with the physician.

The mental status examination should try to elicit signs and symptoms of confusion or disorientation. If such signs are present, it is important to seek an underlying cause, especially if they are new, because they may represent underlying medical disorders or may be reflective of intentional or unintentional medication abuse or misuse resulting from abuse or neglect.

The general physical examination should focus on detecting signs and symptoms of poor personal hygiene, inappropriate or soiled clothing, dehydration, malnutrition, and worsening decubiti. Specific injuries suggestive of abuse are unexplained fractures or dislocations, unexplained lacerations or abrasions, burns in unusual locations or of unusual shapes, unexplained injuries to the head or face, the presence of sexually transmitted diseases, and unexplained bruises.

Detection and diagnosis of elder abuse depends on being open to what is reported by the patient or others. Without such openness, reported abuse may be dismissed as paranoia, dementia, or patient noncompliance. A high index of suspicion is necessary. Otherwise, signs of abuse and neglect may be erroneously ascribed to frequent falls, accidental medication errors, failure to thrive, or the normal decline with aging.

There is no substitute for direct questioning when inquiring about abuse. In one report,[10] 33 percent of abused victims stated on initial presentation to the emergency department that they were involved in an abusive relationship. Another 6 percent of abuse cases were detected by eliciting information from other informants. The remaining cases were elicited by physical examination (43 percent) or by social service evaluation during hospitalization (19 percent).

TREATMENT

Elder abuse treatment is twofold. First, ED treatment of the injuries and illnesses resulting from abuse or neglect must be specific for the injuries and illnesses detected. Second, detection of elder abuse or neglect must be aimed at intervention. Therefore, all treatment, whether delivered in the emergency department or the hospital, for the victim and the victim's caregiver, should be on the basis of multidisciplinary assessment and may result in admission of the elderly patient to an extended-care facility.

Intervention includes the resolution of disposition problems brought about through caregiver exhaustion, the inability of patients to care for themselves in the community, and abandonment by individuals and institutions. Intervention requires a complex array of skills. For example, the serious problem of drug and alcohol abuse among the elderly must be recognized and addressed by emergency department staff. Physical problems often disguise the existence of a problem of substance abuse.

In cases of proven or strongly suspected elder abuse or neglect, intervention must include the involvement of adult protective services.[5,11,12] All 50 states have passed legislation aimed at protecting elderly victims of domestic abuse and neglect and establishing adult protective services programs. Forty-two states have mandatory reporting laws directed toward health care and social service professionals. The National Center on Elder Abuse provides a listing of telephone numbers for elder abuse reporting in the 50 states and Puerto Rico.[5] They also provide a nationwide reporting hotline called Eldercare Locator (1-800-677-1116, verified November 2002). Overall, about 20 percent of reports are from health professionals, 15 percent from service providers, 16 percent from family or relatives, and the remaining 50 percent from friends, neighbors, clergy, bankers, and others. In addition, since 1975, the Older American Act has required each state to have a long-term care ombudsman program to investigate nursing home care complaints.

DISPOSITION

Elderly patients with problems requiring hospital admission should be admitted to the appropriate medical service, and the department of social services should be consulted for evaluation. Patients who do not medically require admission may need to be admitted for protective placement if they cannot be safely discharged to their caretakers or returned to their institutional setting. Clinical strategies to stop abuse include hospitalization, close monitoring through office visits, and home nursing. Patients must not be returned to their living situations if there is any doubt about their safety. A formal safety assessment can be requested from professionals, such as a hospital-based social worker or an on-call community-based elder abuse counselor. It is important to remember that abuse or neglect may occur when a caregiver is overwhelmed, frustrated, or resentful of the responsibilities involved in taking care of the patient. Caregivers should be provided with intervention options, such as arranging for home care, respite, or counseling and should be given advice as to the appropriate care for their family members.

The serious problem of drug and alcohol abuse among the elderly must be recognized by ED staff and addressed through appropriate referrals. Communities with geriatric treatment centers provide a valuable resource for patients identified through emergency department visits.

Referrals also should include specific available services, such as "Meals on Wheels," home health aides, visiting nurses, transportation, emergency shelter, legal aid, and medical and mental health services.

REFERENCES

1. Jones JS, Holstege C, Holstege H: Elder abuse and neglect: Understanding the causes and potential risk factors. *Am J Emerg Med* 15:579, 1997.
2. Werfel PA: When seniors suffer. Elder abuse emerges as a new EMS dilemma. *J Emerg Med Serv* 26:48, 2001.
3. Fulmer T, Paveza G, Abraham I, et al: Elder neglect assessment in the emergency department. *J Emerg Med* 26:436, 2000.
4. American College of Emergency Physicians: Policy statement: Management of elder abuse and neglect. *Ann Emerg Med* 31:149, 1998.
5. National Center on Elder Abuse. http://www.elderabusecenter.org.
6. Clarke ME, Pierson W: Management of elder abuse in the emergency department. *Emerg Med Clin North Am* 17:631, 1999.
7. Lachs MS, Williams C, O'Brien S, et al: Risk factors for reported elder abuse and neglect: A nine-year observational cohort study. *Gerontologist* 37:469, 1997.
8. Marshall CE, Benton D, Brazier JM: Elder abuse. Using clinical tools to identify clues of mistreatment. *Geriatrics* 55:42, 2000.
9. Pillemer K, Finkelhor D: Causes of elder abuse: Caregiver stress versus problem relatives. *Am J Orthopsychiatry* 59:179, 1989.
10. Kleinschmidt K: Elder abuse: A review. *Ann Emerg Med* 30:463, 1997.
11. Jones J, Dougherty J, Schelble D, et al: Emergency department protocol for the diagnosis and evaluation of geriatric abuse. *Ann Emerg Med* 17:1006, 1988.
12. Capezuti E, Brush BL, Lawson WT III: Reporting elder mistreatment. *J Gerontol Nurs* 23:24, 1997.

301 | VIOLENCE IN THE EMERGENCY DEPARTMENT
Marshall C. McCoy

Violence once threatened only law enforcement personnel among those dealing with the public. Now it has spread into the health care arena. No health care providers are more at risk for violence than those involved with the first-line care of patients. Prehospital care providers have shown an increasing fear of violent calls and admit that violent encounters contribute to high levels of burnout.[1] Mock and coworkers found that violence occurs in 5 percent of emergency medical services runs, and an additional 14 percent of calls are precipitated by violence.[2] Recent surveys of ED residents have shown that one of their primary concerns is for their safety while working in the ED.[3] Although comprehensive data addressing the problem are still being collected from ED personnel, urban and rural hospitals are reporting a higher incidence of potential and actual violent episodes in their EDs.[4]

By its nature, the ED has an atmosphere of controlled chaos. EDs provide unlimited and unrestricted access and have readily available drugs. They are frequented by those who are fatigued or hungry, and they accommodate family and friends of critically ill patients who have heightened levels of frustration and anxiety. Furthermore, EDs are frequented by substance abusers who are often violent. Other factors that may predispose the ED to violence are increasing waiting times, staff shortages, overcrowding, patient financial problems, and the high expectations of the patients.

About 50 percent of all health services providers will be involved in a violent episode in their career. In a 1988 survey of 127 teaching hospitals, 32 percent of respondents had at least one verbal threat daily, 25 percent reported using restraints at least once daily, and 18 percent had at least one threat from a weapon monthly. Unfortunately, 7 percent reported a death related to ED violence in the past 5 years. Of the institutions responding, 35 percent lacked 24-h ED security, and of the 9 respondents who reported a death, 55 percent lacked 24-h security.[5]

Close to 5 percent of all emergency psychiatric patients have weapons on their person. One study using metal detectors to screen all ED patients over a 6-month period found 33 hand guns, 1324 knives,

97 mace-type canisters, and various other items considered dangerous to the patient and staff.[6] The presence of metal detectors in an ED appears to improve feelings of safety and protection.[7] Preventive measures often are not employed until after a violent event occurs.

RECOGNIZING THE VIOLENT PATIENT

Most perpetrators of violence are males with a history of substance abuse. Education, ethnicity, marital status, and diagnosis are not reliable predictors. However, these factors may lead to frustration and anxiety for both the staff and the patient, increasing the likelihood of a violent encounter.

The most obvious predictor of potential violence is the patient's history. Any patient with a past history of violent behavior must be handled cautiously. Trivializing a patient's threat, no matter how subtle, may be the cause of unrecognized violence escalation in its early stages. Every patient exhibiting violent or threatening behavior should have a thorough physical and mental status examination. This may require some form of control (restraints or sedation) before an examination can be completed.[8] Using family members, friends, therapists, and/or medical records as a source of history may be valuable. The examining physician needs to differentiate between an organic and a functional cause of the disordered behavior. The treatment of an underlying disorder may completely remove any threat, such as the administration of intravenous glucose to a disoriented, aggressive hypoglycemic patient. The organic diseases most likely involved in a violent episode are those related to drugs and withdrawal syndrome(s), especially delirium tremens. According to the American Psychiatric Association, the presence of any one of the following indicators should prompt a search for an organic etiology: a patient older than 40 years of age with no previous psychiatric history; disorientation, lethargy, or stupor; abnormal vital signs; visual hallucinations; or illusions. A thorough evaluation should include laboratory work, toxicology screening, electrocardiograms, and in some cases, computed tomographic (CT) scans and lumbar puncture.

The most common functional disorder related to violent behavior is schizophrenia, especially in patients in paranoid subgroups or with personality disorders.

PRODROMES OF VIOLENCE

In most cases, violent behavior does not erupt suddenly. Therefore, recognition of the prodromes of violence and the phases of escalation is necessary. The first is the anxiety phase, followed by defensiveness, and then physical aggression.[9] Each phase should evoke a professional response that is proportionate to the patient's behavior. There may be overlap of phases.

Phase 1: Anxiety

The first level of behavior seen in a potentially violent patient is anxiety. Patients, but also their family and visitors who have been waiting for long periods, exhibit anxiety. In general, the signs of increasing anxiety are indicated by body language. Movements that seem to have no purpose other than to expend energy may be the first clue. These may include pacing, wringing of hands, clenching of fists, unwillingness to stay in the treatment area, or a disheveled appearance. Speech may be pressured and loud. Questions such as "Why am I here?" or "How long is this going to take?" may be asked. It is not necessarily what is said but the manner of speech that suggests anxiety. One of the most common reasons for escalation of behavior beyond anxiety is that the staff ignores these signals rather than acknowledging and responding to them in a constructive way. The appropriate response to the anxiety phase is the development of some type of rapport. Time (a precious commodity to emergency staff and physicians) is usually all that is needed. Listening to the patient's concerns and addressing them

appropriately may be all that is required to diffuse the situation. Dismissing or ignoring the patient, family, or visitors will only cause more anxiety. Most patients are fearful of a loss of control and usually welcome the opportunity to politely vent their feelings. The patient must be treated honestly and with respect and empathy. Simple courtesy will go a long way toward establishing rapport and preventing future problems. Be supportive with responses that acknowledge the patient's feelings, such as "I understand why you are angry." A peace offering of food or drink also may help. Do not be judgmental. Concentrate on what the patient is saying, and do not feign attention. Restating what the patient has just said may help clarify the patient's complaints and allow the patient to continue venting. Remain on the topic and, above all, remain calm. This will help the patient feel more in control.

Phase 2: Defensiveness

The next level in the continuum of violent behavior is defensiveness. A patient may present to the emergency department in this stage, having passed the anxiety stage outside the hospital At this point, the patient's behavior is volatile and becomes verbally abusive and profane, often with associated body posturing. Verbal attacks may be directed to staff members or others in the department and may include statements about age, gender, weight, or heritage. The patient's behaviors are irrational and often have nothing to do with why the patient presented to the ED. The patient is losing control and may feel helpless. If the patient is restrained, feelings of helplessness may be further magnified.

The goal is to prevent total loss of control by the patient. This goal is achieved by setting reasonable limits and by offering the patient a choice. One must be firm in tone and action but professional and calm. Do not overreact or make false promises. The patient must have reasonable limits set and be made aware of the consequences of continued aggression. Limits must be simple, clear, enforceable, and consistent. No consequence should be stated if it is not enforceable. Giving the patient reasonable choices helps diffuse the situation and makes the patient feel rewarded for good behavior. If the situation continues to deteriorate, the patient should be isolated. A show of force by uniformed security personnel may then be in order. Although this may cause further deterioration of behavior, this is the exception, not the rule.

Phase 3: Physical Aggression

The third level is physical aggression. The patient is totally out of control, and no amount of verbal intervention is effective. The physically aggressive patient must be confronted and controlled physically, for the safety of the violent patient, other patients, visitors, and staff. When all other interventions have failed, no further negotiation is warranted. Physical control of a patient requires personnel skilled in the technique and should never be attempted single-handedly. Using appropriate restraint enables the staff to provide necessary care for a violent patient. Physical control is implemented not for punitive reasons but in the interest of patient care and safety for others.

RESTRAINT AND SECLUSION

The philosophy of any institution should be to limit the use of restraints or seclusion to situations where less restrictive interventions have failed and the clinical appropriateness is clearly justified. A *restraint* is defined as any device, including manual holds, that is attached or adjacent to the patient's body that cannot be removed easily and restricts freedom of movement or normal access to one's body. *Seclusion* is the involuntary confinement of a person in a room or area so that the person is physically prevented from leaving. The purpose of restraints or seclusion is to ensure the safety of patients and others or prevent damage to property, never for punitive reasons, convenience, or when a patient may be medically compromised by their use.

Health care providers and administrative personnel should familiarize themselves with the Acute Medical and Surgical Care Restraint Standards and the Behavioral Health Care Restraint and Seclusion Standards[10] as set forth by the Joint Commission on Accreditation of Health Care Organizations (JCAHO) and the Center for Medicare/Medicaid Services (CMS). These standards and their interpretations are ever-changing, so periodic review is necessary.

In general, the Acute Medical and Surgical Care Restraint Standards are used to promote healing, e.g., patients who will compromise their medical care by self-removal of an endotracheal or intravenous tube. Essentially all other clinical justifications for restraint will fall under the standards used for behavioral health care. It is important to note that these standards are invoked regardless of the patient's location within an institution.

In the case of physical restraint, each institution should have policies and procedures that document when restraints can be used, who can order restraints, how patients are monitored in restraints, and mechanisms for the review of their use. Any documents should begin with the clinical indications for restraint and the alternatives that were attempted and deemed to be ineffective.

According to the JCAHO, only licensed independent practitioners (LIPs) can order restraints. However, often the LIP is not present when the need for restraint is determined. Therefore, trained caregivers may institute the restraint, and an LIP must perform a face-to-face evaluation within 1 h of restraint use. A written order must be obtained that includes the type of restraint, reason for restraint, and time limit of the order.[10] Any written or verbal order is limited to 1 h for children younger than age 9, 2 h for individuals aged 9 to 17 years, and 4 h for individuals aged 18 and older.[11]

Early release from the restraint before the time-limited order has expired may be initiated by trained providers if the patient demonstrates a reduction in the condition that led to the restraint. For patients in restraints or seclusion, continuous monitoring is required. Those in restraints require evaluation every 15 min, and this should include examination for signs of injury associated with the restraints, nutrition, hydration, circulation and range of motion in the extremities, vital signs, hygiene and elimination, physical comfort, psychologic status, and readiness for discontinuation of the restraints. Since approaching or awakening a restrained patient every 15 min may cause further agitation, evaluation may not necessarily include all the former parameters, but as many as practical should be performed. Patients in seclusion must be observed continuously for the first hour, after which audio or video equipment may be used, but it must be monitored continuously.

Seclusion generally has been considered a better alternative to restraints because it allows some freedom of movement and is medically safer. In adolescents and robust adults, however, free use of the extremities, combined with their strength, may be dangerous, and the isolation and sense of rejection may be psychologically harmful.[12] Seclusion rooms require walls that cannot be damaged by combative patients, safety windows for continuous monitoring, appropriate lighting, and calming colors.

Once the decision to restrain a patient is made, appropriate personnel must be assembled. A trained security person or hospital staff member should act as the team leader because untrained personnel may cause undue harm to the patient or staff. Soft restraints should never be used on a truly violent patient. One should explain the reason for restraint to the patient, and once restrained, the patient should never be abandoned. No patient for whom restraints were necessary should be allowed to leave the ED against medical advice. If necessary, contacting hospital legal authorities may be helpful. In general, if a patient is brought to the ED in handcuffs, he or she should remain in handcuffs until the threat of violence and medical condition are assessed. Remember that many an escape has taken place in a hospital setting.

MEDICATIONS

Some patients are too violent, even when restrained, to perform an adequate evaluation. In these patients, the use of medications can be a safe and effective means to manage violent behavior. Rapid tranquilization is the delivery of medications in a titrated fashion to gain control of aggressive patients. Antipsychotic agents and benzodiazepines, alone or in combination, are the most frequently used medications. Each can be given IM, IV, or PO, giving the physician alternatives in delivery methods depending on the patient's condition. Intramuscular injection is usually the route of choice because these medications are absorbed rapidly. Moreover, attempting intravenous access on a violent patient can be dangerous.

Haloperidol (Haldol) is currently the antipsychotic of choice. In an adult, a 5-mg IM injection has rapid onset and can be repeated as needed to obtain the desired effect. In the elderly, the starting dosage should be lowered to 1 or 2 mg. Few patients will have extrapyramidal side effects, but if they occur, they are easily treated with benztropine or diphenhydramine. Haloperidol also has fewer side effects than older antipsychotics such as chlorpromazine (Thorazine) or thioridazine (Mellaril), which are more sedating and can cause hypotension and anticholinergic effects

Benzodiazepines are more sedating then the antipsychotics but have no extrapyramidal side effects. Lorazepam is an excellent choice due to its rapid onset. Doses of lorazepam 2 to 4 mg IM or IV are effective in most patients, but additional doses may be needed in withdrawal syndromes or extremely agitated patients. The use of benzodiazepines in combination with haloperidol is also effective and has a more rapid onset of effect and reduces the number of subsequent injections needed.

Droperidol, a sedative-hypnotic with antiemetic properties, also has been used for violent patients. Doses of 2.5 mg IM or IV are absorbed rapidly but can be heavily sedating. Rare cases of QT-interval prolongation with resulting torsades de pointes have been reported in patients receiving droperidol.[13] However, the causal relationship between QT prolongation and droperidol is questioned.[14] Therefore, droperidol could be used in patients in whom benefits outweigh the potential risks.

VIOLENCE PREVENTION

The single best way to handle a violent patient or curtail the potential for violence in the ED is by prevention. Careful planning of the work area, cooperation with hospital security personnel, and training of all ED personnel to recognize violent patients are critical.

Interviews of the potentially violent patient should be conducted in a safe, calm environment. Seclusion rooms for interviewing patients should be safe for both the patient and the interviewer. Solid walls with sturdy, heavy furniture that cannot be lifted should be used. Lighting should be able to be dimmed or brightened, depending on the circumstance. No free-standing objects, such as ashtrays, pictures, or pencils, should be allowed because they all could become potential weapons. The room exit should be clear of obstruction and readily available to the interviewer. Panic buttons may be installed or signals developed to be used in the event of threatening behavior on the part of the patient. If violent aggression does develop, the room should be large enough for a team of security personnel to safely overcome the patient without undue harm.

Deterrence is also a preventive technique. Signs outside the ED should clearly state that weapons of any type are not permitted, and trained hospital security personnel should be visible to everyone entering the emergency department. The use of metal detectors and x-ray machines for personal articles, such as handbags, may allow for easy screening of those entering the treatment area. Carefully placed monitors and alarm buttons also may be warranted. However, metal detectors, monitors, and alarms are only a part of an overall security system and complement personnel training in the management of potential and actual violent situations.[15,16]

The education of ED personnel is the most important factor in curbing violence in the ED.[17] Several national programs, such as that offered by the National Crisis Prevention Institute (http://www.crisisprevention.com/program/nci:html), are invaluable in teaching a basic understanding of violent behavior, its recognition and management, and basic self-defense against violent patients. Educational seminars conduced by security personnel and law enforcement officials also may be of benefit.

REFERENCES

1. Tintinalli JE, McCoy M: Violent patients and the prehospital provider. *Ann Emerg Med* 22:1276, 1993.
2. Mock EF, Wrenn KD, Wright SW, et al: Prospective field study of violence in emergency medical service calls. *Ann Emerg Med* 32:33, 1998.
3. Anglin D, Kyriacou DN, Hudson HR: Resident's perspective on violence and personal safety in the emergency department. *Ann Emerg Med* 23:1082, 1994.
4. Allison DJ, Matthews RT: Hot spot: Planning, design, and construction is the right remedy for ED dangers. *Health Facilities Monogr* 11(3):38, 1998.
5. Lavoie FW, Carter GL, Danzel DF, Berg RL: Emergency department violence in United States' teaching hospitals. *Ann Emerg Med* 17:1227, 1988.
6. Dubin WR, Tarduff K, Maler G: Overcoming danger with violent patients: Guidelines for safe and effective management. *Emergency Medicine Reports* 13(14), 1992.
7. Mattox EA, Wright SW, Bracilowski AC: Metal detectors in the pediatric emergency department: Patient attitudes and national prevalence. *Pediatr Emerg Care* 16(3):163, 2000.
8. *Seclusion and Restraint: The Psychiatric Uses.* Washington, Task Force Report 22, American Psychiatric Association, 1985.
9. *Nonviolent Crisis Intervention Workbook.* Brookfield, WI, National Crisis Prevention Institute, 1987.
10. Joint Commission on Accreditation of Healthcare Organizations: *Comprehensive Accreditation Manual for Hospitals,* Update 1. Austin, TX, JCAHO, 2002.
11. Health Care Financing Administration: Hospital condition of participation in Medicare and Medicaid. *Fed Reg* 64:127, 1999.
12. Practice parameter for the prevention and management of aggressive behavior in child and adolescent psychiatric institutions, with special reference to seclusion and restraint. *J Am Acad Child Adolesc Psychiatry* 41(2):45, 2002.
13. Lawrence KR, Nasraway SA: Conduction disturbances associated with administration of butytrophenone antipsychotic in the critically ill: A review of the literature. *Pharmacotherapy* 17(3), 1997.
14. Kao LW, Kirk MA, Evers SJ, et al: Droperidol, QT prolongation, and sudden death: What is the evidence? *Ann Emerg Med* 41(4):559, 2003.
15. Thompson B, Nunn J, Kramer I, et al: Disarming the department: Weapon screening and improved security to create a safer emergency department environment. *Ann Emerg Med* 17:419, 1988.
16. Rankins RC, Hendey GW: Effect of a security system on violent incidents and hidden weapons in the emergency department. *Ann Emerg Med* 33:6, 676, 1999.
17. Fernandes CMB, Raboud JM, Christenson JM, et al: The effect of an education program on violence in the emergency department. *Ann Emerg Med* 39:47, 2002.

CONTRAST STUDIES
John Eng

Iodinated intravascular contrast agents significantly improve the visualization of structures in many radiologic examinations, and millions of doses are administered each year in the United States for this purpose. While it is always advisable to discuss the need for iodinated contrast agents with a radiologist on a case-by-case basis, some general indications are offered here. Throughout this chapter, *contrast agent* refers to iodinated intravascular contrast material unless otherwise indicated.

IODINATED INTRAVASCULAR CONTRAST AGENTS

Mechanism of Action

Iodinated intravascular contrast agents are water-soluble molecules that contain several radiodense iodine atoms per molecule. Following injection, contrast agents remain in the vascular space for only a short time (initial-pass $t_{1/2}$ 1–3 min) and are distributed rapidly into the extracellular space. With normal renal function, the $t_{1/2}$ of elimination is approximately 2 h. Contrast agents do not enter the intracellular space or cross an intact blood-brain barrier. They are excreted rapidly by the kidney via glomerular filtration without tubular resorption.

Since the radiodense iodine atoms absorb more x-rays than do biologic tissues, contrast agents appear white (like the bones, which are also radiodense) if they are present in high enough concentration during examinations made with x-rays (radiographs). Contrast agents are visible on arteriography during the short time they are in high concentration in the vascular space. They are visible in the urinary tract during intravenous urography (IVU), after excretion by the kidney. Because of its ability to discriminate subtle differences in radiodensity, computed tomography (CT) shows the presence of contrast agents in all tissue compartments even though they may be present in relatively low concentration (compared with arteriography or radiography).

Types of Agents

Contrast agents are classified according to osmolality (Table 302-1). High-osmolality agents have been in clinical use since the 1950s, and they are often called *ionic* contrast agents because they are all organic salts (Figure 302-1). Low-osmolality agents have been in use since 1986, and they are commonly called *nonionic* agents because all but one are organic molecules without electronic charge (Figure 302-2). A number of studies have demonstrated that low-osmolality contrast agents are associated with at least a 50 percent reduction in the incidence of both minor and severe reactions (see Table 302-1). Fatal reactions are rare.[1] Anecdotally, injection of low-osmolality agents is associated with less subjective effects, such as flushing, heat, chemical taste, and osmotic diuresis. Currently in the United States, low-osmolality contrast agents cost on average five to six times more than an equivalent dose of a high-osmolality agent. The use of low-osmolality contrast agents is surrounded by some controversy due to the significant cost differential for a relatively modest difference in incidence of severe reactions, which are rare. The controversy has subsided somewhat as the price of low-osmolality agents has slowly decreased since their introduction.

Types of Contrast Reactions

Contrast reactions can be divided into three categories: anaphylactoid, chemotoxic, and vasovagal (Table 302-2). Anaphylactoid reactions occur idiosyncratically, and they mimic allergic or anaphylactic reactions and shock. Anaphylactoid contrast reactions have no known consistent pathophysiologic mechanism. They may involve one or more of the following mechanisms: histamine release, complement activation, hapten formation, contact sensitivity, endovascular reactions, and central nervous system factors. However, unlike true immunoallergic or anaphylactic reactions, they do not involve IgE mediation. An increased risk of anaphylactoid contrast reaction is associated with a history of asthma, food or drug allergy, or a previous contrast reaction. Low-osmolality agents are associated with a lower risk of anaphylactoid contrast reaction.

Chemotoxic reactions are related to osmotoxic and other chemical effects of contrast agents. The pathophysiologic mechanisms for chemotoxicity are not well understood, but its occurrence is less idiosyncratic. Since many of the chemotoxic cardiovascular reactions, such as dysrhythmia and pulmonary edema, occur primarily with coronary artery injections, their occurrence in the emergency department setting is probably of less concern than in the cardiac catheterization suite.

Contrast agents also can cause vasovagal reactions, a result of increased vagal tone of the heart and blood vessels of unknown etiology but thought to be related to the central nervous system. In addition to being caused by contrast agents, vasovagal reactions also may be caused by the circumstances surrounding their administration, such as fear, anxiety, or discomfort from needle puncture.

RISK ASSESSMENT AND PATIENT PREPARATION

There are no absolute contraindications for receiving intravascular contrast agents. Certain clinical conditions either increase the risk of developing a contrast reaction or increase the severity of the reaction should one develop. Risk assessment and, in some cases, preventive measures should be performed prior to contrast agent administration. Considerations for patient preparation are summarized in Table 302-3, and additional comments are offered below.

History of Allergy

A history of asthma or severe allergy (e.g., anaphylaxis) to one or more allergens is associated with an increased risk of a contrast reaction. Patients with a history of asthma may have a fivefold greater risk of an adverse reaction than the general population, and a history of allergy may double the risk.[2] A history of reaction during a previous contrast agent administration is associated with a three- to eightfold greater risk of a subsequent adverse reaction than in the general population.[2]

Renal Disease

Classically, the risk factors for developing renal insufficiency from contrast agents are preexisting renal insufficiency (creatinine level > 1.5 mg/mL), diabetes mellitus, volume depletion, use of diuretics in cardiovascular disease, advanced age (>70 years), multiple myeloma, hypertension, and hyperuricemia.[3] More recent studies have shown that the most significant risk is associated with the coexistence of diabetes *and* renal insufficiency.[4]

TABLE 302-1   Comparison of High- and Low-Osmolality Contrast Agents

Characteristic	High-Osmolality Agent (Ionic)	Low-Osmolality Agent (Nonionic)
Approximate osmolality relative to serum	5	2*
Overall incidence of adverse reaction	5–8%	1–2%
Incidence of severe reaction	1–2 per 1000	1–2 per 10,000
Incidence of fatal reaction	1/40,000–1/250,000	1/200,000–1/500,000
Relative cost	1	5–6

*One nonionic agent, iodixanol (Visipaque), is isosmolar.

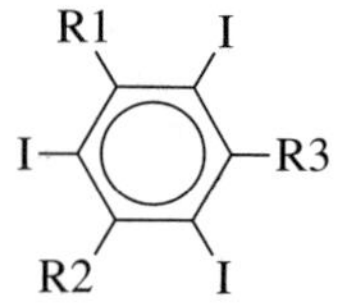

FIG. 302-2. The basic chemical structure of a nonionic, low-osmolality contrast agent. There are five such agents currently on the market, each with a different R group: iohexol (Omnipaque), iopamidol (Isovue), iopromide (Ultravist), ioversol (Optiray), and ioxilan (Oxilan). All the R groups contain multiple hydroxyl groups for solubility. A sixth low-osmolality agent, iodixanol (Visipaque), chemically links two of the basic structures to further reduce osmolality. A seventh agent, ioxaglate (Hexabrix), has a different chemical structure (not shown) that is unique because it is both ionic and low osmolality.

As a preventive measure, patients with preexisting renal insufficiency, diabetes, or volume depletion should receive hydration in the form of ½NS at 100 mL/h beginning 12 h before and continuing 12 h after contrast agent administration. In patients with end-stage renal failure receiving chronic dialysis, the contrast agent and extra fluid must be removed by dialysis, but the dialysis does not need to be performed emergently[5] unless there is significant underlying cardiac dysfunction (and thus increased risk of direct cardiac chemotoxicity). In patients with chronic renal failure, there is some evidence that acetylcysteine given orally beginning the day before contrast agent administration can reduce the risk of developing acute contrast-agent-induced renal failure,[6,7] but this is not currently considered standard practice.

Cardiac Disease

Patients with significant cardiac disease appear to be at increased risk for contrast reactions. Significant cardiac disease includes severe angina pectoris, congestive heart failure, severe valvular disease, primary pulmonary hypertension, and cardiomyopathy.

Metformin Therapy

Metformin (Glucophage) is an oral antihyperglycemic agent used to treat non-insulin-dependent diabetes mellitus. Development of potentially fatal lactic acidosis is a rare adverse effect of metformin and may occur if contrast-induced renal insufficiency (itself a rare event) develops. Therefore, metformin should be discontinued at the time of contrast agent administration and withheld for 48 h afterward. The drug may be restarted after the patient's renal function is rechecked and found to be normal.[8]

Anxiety

There is some evidence that severe contrast reactions may be partially mediated by anxiety. Therefore, an anxious patient should be reassured and calmed prior to contrast injection.

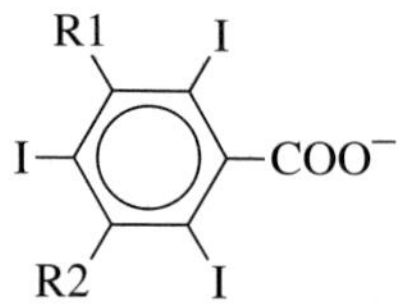

FIG. 302-1. The general chemical structure of the anion of a high-osmolality contrast agent. The R groups are either diatrizoate or iothalamate, depending on the manufacturer. The corresponding cation is either sodium or meglumine.

Other Diseases

In patients with pheochromocytoma, pretreatment with phentolamine, an α-adrenergic antagonist, is recommended prior to contrast agent administration. In a nonstabilized patient with recent seizures, pretreatment with diazepam may be advisable.[2] Convulsions or seizures following contrast agent administration may be due to a lowering of the seizure threshold, or they may be a final result of a severe hypotensive or vasovagal reaction.[4]

As mentioned earlier, hyperuricemia and dysproteinemias, such as multiple myeloma, are associated with an increased risk of contrast-induced renal insufficiency, but there is conflicting evidence regarding the strength of this relationship. Similarly, some studies suggest that sickle cell trait and disease are also associated with an increased risk of contrast reaction, but the significance of the relationship is unclear.

Premedication

Premedication with a steroid regimen has been shown in some studies to reduce the overall incidence of contrast reactions to both high- and low-osmolality agents. However, no controlled studies have been performed to determine whether premedication reduces the incidence of *severe* reactions. Most institutions prescribe premedication if there is a history of a significant (more than nausea, vomiting, or a few hives) reaction to a previous contrast agent injection.[9] Some institutions also premedicate if there is a history of severe allergy to any substance. There are no standard indications or protocols for premedication. Two commonly prescribed premedication regimens are listed in Table 302-4.[10,11]

TABLE 302-2   Classification of Contrast Reactions

Reaction Type	Signs and Symptoms
Anaphylactoid	
Generalized urticaria	Hives (generalized)
Laryngeal or facial edema	Stridor, facial swelling
Bronchospasm	Wheezing, dyspnea
Cardiovascular collapse (shock)	Hypotension, sinus tachycardia
Chemotoxic	
Renal tubular injury	Rising creatinine
Cardiac dysrhythmia	Electrocardiographic changes
Cardiac impairment	Pulmonary edema
Neurotoxicity	Seizure
Mild reactions	Nausea, emesis, warmth, dizziness, headache, pallor, flushing, shaking, chills, diaphoresis, hives (localized), altered taste, pruritus
Vasovagal	Hypotension, sinus bradycardia

TABLE 302-3   Summary of Patient Preparation Prior to Intravascular Administration of Iodinated Contrast Agents

Item for Consideration	Action
Clinical history	Elicit any history of allergy, asthma, previous use of contrast material, renal insufficiency, diabetes, cardiac disease, seizures, metformin therapy
Creatinine level	Obtain in patients with suspected renal dysfunction only (see Table 302-5)
Hydration	Consider in patients with renal insufficiency, diabetes, volume depletion
Premedication	Prescribe for patients with history of contrast allergy and possibly patients with history of severe allergy to a substance other than contrast material (see Table 302-4)
Selection of low-osmolality agent	Refer to American College of Radiology guidelines (see Table 302-6)

Serum Creatinine

A baseline serum creatinine level should be determined prior to contrast agent injection for patients with suspected renal dysfunction or considered at increased risk for contrast-induced nephrotoxicity[4] (Table 302-5). **Determination of the serum creatinine level is not necessary in patients without suspected renal dysfunction.** Furthermore, in cases of suspected renal dysfunction, clinical judgment may determine that an urgently needed contrast-enhanced examination should not be delayed by determination of the serum creatinine level.

Selective Use of Low-Osmolality Agents

Because of their lower incidence of reactions, low-osmolality agents are used by many institutions with selected patients at higher risk for developing a contrast reaction. The American College of Radiology has suggested guidelines for the selective use of low-osmolality agents[4] (Table 302-6). These guidelines are the result of a consensus and are not evidence-based because it is difficult to study severe contrast reactions due to their rarity. Some practices have elected to use low-osmolality agents exclusively, especially since they are generally better tolerated by patients (e.g., less nausea, vomiting, flushing, and heat sensation).

INDICATIONS FOR INTRAVASCULAR CONTRAST AGENTS

An intravascular contrast agent is required to visualize vascular structures in arteriography, venography, and vascular CT (e.g., aorta and pulmonary arteries). An intravascular contrast agent is also required to visualize the urinary tract in an IVU. In such cases, decisions regarding the use of intravascular contrast agents are linked to the decision to perform the examination. Aside from these indications, decisions

TABLE 302-4   Commonly Prescribed Regimens for Premedication Prior to Contrast Administration

Regimen	Dosage
1	Methylprednisolone (Medrol) 32 mg PO 12 h and 2 h before contrast injection
2	Prednisone 50 mg PO 13 h, 7 h, and 1 h before contrast injection, *and* Diphenhydramine (Benadryl) 50 mg PO 1 h before contrast injection

Source: Regimen 1 from Lasser et al[10] and regimen 2 from Greenberger and Patterson,[11] with permission.

TABLE 302-5   Recommendations for Obtaining Serum Creatinine Level Prior to Administration of Intravascular Iodinated Contrast Agents

History of "kidney disease" as an adult, including tumor and transplant
Family history of kidney failure
Insulin-dependent diabetes mellitus of 2 years' duration or greater
Non-insulin-dependent diabetes mellitus of over 5 years' duration (if on diabetic medication for that period)
Paraproteinemia syndromes or diseases (e.g., myeloma)
Collagen vascular disease
Patients taking certain medications: metformin (Glucophage), nonsteroidal anti-inflammatory drugs, or nephrotoxic antibiotics (e.g., aminoglycosides)

Source: American College of Radiology,[4] with permission.

regarding the use of contrast agents usually arise in the context of nonvascular CT. Although highly desirable in many situations, contrast enhancement is not *absolutely* required for nonvascular CT and may not add much to the emergency department evaluation in many situations. While the potential imaging benefits versus the risks of contrast-enhanced CT always should be discussed with a radiologist on a case-by-case basis, some general guidelines are offered below (Table 302-7).

Vascular Computed Tomography

As with conventional angiography, an intravascular contrast agent is required for CT evaluation of vascular structures. In the emergency department, such an examination is done most commonly to evaluate the aorta for trauma, dissection, or aneurysm. If the clinical suspicion is high, initial evaluation with conventional aortography should be considered instead of CT because, in such cases, aortography (requiring additional doses of a contrast agent) probably would be performed whether or not the CT findings are positive.

Helical CT (a high-speed form of CT) has been used in conjunction with rapid contrast injection to perform CT pulmonary arteriography as an alternative to conventional arteriography for the detection of pulmonary embolism. A scintigraphic ventilation-perfusion scan may be performed as a screening study prior to either type of pulmonary arteriography (usually prior to conventional arteriography). If results of the ventilation-perfusion scan are normal or near normal and the a priori probability is also low, pulmonary embolism is excluded, and in most cases, further evaluation with a contrast study is unnecessary (see Chap. 56).

TABLE 302-6   American College of Radiology Suggested Guidelines for the Selective Use of Iodinated Intravascular Low-Osmolality Contrast Agents

Patients with a history of any previous adverse reaction to intravascular iodinated contrast material, with the exception of a sensation of heat, flushing, or a single episode of nausea or vomiting
Patients with asthma
Patients with a previous serious allergic reaction to materials other than contrast agents
Patients with known cardiac dysfunction, including recent or potentially imminent cardiac decompensation, severe dysrhythmias, unstable angina pectoris, recent myocardial infarction, and pulmonary hypertension
Patients with renal insufficiency (particularly those with diabetes)
Patients with generalized severe debilitation, as determined by a physician
Patients at high risk for contrast extravasation
Any other circumstances where, after due consideration, the radiologist believes there is a specific indication for the use of low-osmolality contrast material, examples of which include but are not restricted to
   (1) sickle cell disease,
   (2) patients at increased risk for aspiration,
   (3) patients who are very anxious about the contrast procedure or who request or demand the use of low-osmolality contrast material, and
   (4) patients in whom the risk factors cannot be satisfactorily established

Source: American College of Radiology,[4] with permission.

TABLE 302-7 Indications for Iodinated Intravascular Contrast Agents

Required
  Arteriography
  Venography
  Intravenous urography
  Vascular CT (CT aortography for injury, dissection, aneurysm; CT
    pulmonary arteriography for embolism)
Highly desirable but *not absolutely* required
  CT for trauma to abnormal or pelvic organs
  CT for abdominal or pelvic abscess
  CT for appendicitis or diverticulitis
  CT for bowel obstruction
  CT for orbital infection
Not indicated
  Musculoskeletal CT for trauma (e.g., face, spine, pelvis)
  Cranial CT for trauma or acute neurologic symptoms
  Abdominal CT for urolithiasis

Intravenous Urography and Urolithiasis

The intravenous urography (IVU), or intravenous pyelogram, is the classic study for the evaluation of ureteral obstruction due to urolithiasis. During an IVU, contrast material excreted by the kidney visibly flows in the urinary tract up to the level of obstruction. If the obstruction is partial, its severity may be estimated. However, the obstructing calculus is not always visualized. More recently, non-contrast-enhanced helical CT has been applied to detect ureteral calculi directly in the setting of suspected obstruction.[12,13] The size and location of the calculus, which indicate the likelihood of spontaneous passage, can be determined accurately. However, the degree of functional obstruction cannot be evaluated without contrast agent administration. Therefore, non-contrast-enhanced CT is less helpful in evaluating a patient with known calculi who presents with new symptoms.

Renal ultrasound is often requested in the evaluation of suspected acute ureteral obstruction. In such a setting, ultrasound is usually *not* helpful because (1) hydronephrosis may be absent in early acute ureteral obstruction, (2) a dilated renal collecting system may be due to causes other than acute ureteral obstruction, and (3) the detection of calculi within the kidney does not necessarily imply obstruction by a more distal calculus.

Abdominal Trauma

Intravenous contrast agents are indicated in all CT examinations performed to detect intra-abdominal injuries from blunt trauma, including liver laceration, splenic laceration, renal trauma, bowel hematoma, pancreatic fracture, ureteral injury, and bladder perforation. Intravenous contrast agents differentiate normal organ parenchyma from hematoma within an area of injury. In patients for whom the risk of administering intravenous contrast agents is thought to be too great, non-contrast-enhanced CT is probably still of benefit, but small to moderate intra-abdominal injuries may be missed, especially if there is no associated intraperitoneal fluid from hemorrhage. Because of the importance of intravenous contrast, some institutions proceed with contrast agent injection (using a low-osmolality agent) in all patients undergoing emergent abdominal CT regardless of past medical history. With such a policy, it is felt that the imaging benefits of contrast enhancement combined with an emergency situation outweigh any possible risk of adverse reaction.

In the setting of penetrating trauma to the back or flank, an intravenous contrast agent is administered as part of the triple-contrast CT, the other two types of contrast being orally and rectally administered. Triple-contrast CT should be reserved for patients who have a wound that penetrates the muscular fascia, are clinically stable, and have no obvious signs of intraperitoneal or other internal injury.[14] In such patients, intravascular contrast imaging is required to detect renal and vascular injuries, and rectal administration of contrast material is particularly important for detecting subtle colonic injury.

Acute Abdomen

Intravenous contrast enhancement is indicated for all CT examinations performed for the evaluation of acute abdomen. Acute abdominal conditions for which CT is commonly performed include appendicitis, diverticulitis, intra-abdominal abscess, and bowel obstruction. While intravenous contrast material enhances the visualization of all these conditions, its role is not as great as in CT for abdominal trauma. For example, mesenteric inflammation is detectable in the absence of intravenous contrast enhancement in the case of appendicitis or diverticulitis. Furthermore, intravenous contrast enhancement is not involved directly in detection of the complications of acute gastrointestinal inflammation, such as bowel obstruction, abscess formation, and bowel perforation. One cause of an acute abdomen, bowel ischemia, is an exception, in that intravenous contrast enhancement plays a major role in its detection, especially when strangulation is present.

The role of intravenous contrast enhancement in the detection of intra-abdominal abscess is somewhat controversial. Thorough filling and opacification of bowel loops by an oral contrast agent is arguably more important than the use of intravenous contrast agents in optimal CT evaluation for the presence of intra-abdominal abscess. As in other pathologic processes in the female pelvis, radiologic evaluation of intrapelvic abscess in a female usually should begin with transabdominal and endovaginal ultrasound rather than CT. The uterus and ovaries are almost always better visualized by endovaginal ultrasound.

For the diagnosis of appendicitis in children, ultrasound with graded compression is an accurate alternative to contrast-enhanced CT.[15] The technique is rapid and requires no intravascular contrast material. Its main disadvantage is the requirement of a sonographer skilled in the specific technique of examining the appendix.

Focused helical CT of the appendix without intravenous contrast enhancement has been shown to be a cost-effective method of evaluating patients with clinically suspected appendicitis.[16] This examination is performed with both oral and rectal contrast material but without intravenous contrast agents, and images of only the axial levels surrounding the appendix are obtained.[17] A focused CT examination of the appendix should be considered only if the primary clinical question is the presence or absence of appendicitis. Evaluation for other intra-abdominal pathologic conditions may be limited in this type of focused CT examination.

Cranial Computed Tomography

Contrast-enhanced cranial CT is not often utilized in the emergency setting. Abnormalities detected only by contrast-enhanced cranial CT, such as meningitis, some subacute infarcts, and small metastases, rarely change the immediate diagnostic workup and treatment and are more appropriately evaluated with magnetic resonance imaging (MRI). In the case of infarction, administration of a contrast agent may exacerbate the patient's clinical condition. However, CT cranial angiography sometimes has a role in stroke diagnosis and treatment. Intravenous contrast material may obscure intracranial hemorrhage, especially in the subarachnoid space.

Skeletal Trauma

Since bone appears much denser on CT than does even intravascular contrast material, imaging of the skeletal system does not require contrast agent injection. Emergent skeletal CT is performed most often to evaluate fracture of the axial skeleton. Intravenous contrast enhancement may be necessary to detect concomitant injury of the abdominal or pelvic organs.

CT of the spine, particularly of the lumbar spine, following administration of *intrathecal* contrast material is performed occasionally for the evaluation of back pain. This procedure, CT myelography, essentially has been replaced by MRI, which provides significantly better visualization of the spinal cord, nerve roots, and intervertebral disks. CT myelography should be performed only in special cases, such as preoperative evaluation and planning.

IODINATED GASTROINTESTINAL CONTRAST AGENTS

In most nonemergent fluoroscopic studies of the gastrointestinal tract, oral or rectal barium sulfate contrast material is preferred over iodinated contrast material (e.g., Gastrografin, Gastroview, Hypaque) because barium demonstrates the mucosa in greater detail and is less susceptible to dilution. However, iodinated contrast agents are indicated in many emergent situations in which barium contrast material is contraindicated: (1) suspected or potential bowel perforation (including trauma or abscess), (2) administration before gastrointestinal surgery or endoscopy, and (3) evaluation of the position of percutaneously placed bowel catheters. Iodinated contrast agents are appropriate in these situations because they are reabsorbed rapidly from the peritoneal and interstitial spaces.[4] If a fluoroscopic study with iodinated contrast material does not demonstrate a suspected perforation, many radiologists repeat the study using barium to look for small leaks, which are often more apparent with barium than with iodinated contrast agents.

For gastrointestinal studies involving iodinated contrast material, low-osmolality agents are indicated in the following situations: (1) oral administration in patients who are at risk for aspiration because contrast-induced pulmonary edema is less with low-osmolality agents and (2) patients with fluid or electrolyte imbalances because low-osmolality agents cause less dilution and fluid shifts into the bowel lumen.[4]

Following oral or rectal administration, a small amount of iodinated contrast agent (approximately 1–2 percent) is absorbed by the bowel and excreted into the urine.[4] Therefore, the risk of developing an anaphylactoid contrast reaction is theoretically the same as it is for intravascular administration, and the same preprocedural evaluation and precautions apply. However, moderate or severe contrast reactions are reported only very rarely following oral or rectal administration of iodinated contrast agents. Therefore, the actual risk may be lower than that for intravascular administration. These comments are also applicable to administration of iodinated contrast material into the bladder or male urethra for the evaluation of trauma. In such examinations, it is likely that absorption of the contrast agent is even less than in the gastrointestinal tract.

The administration of oral or rectal contrast material is important in a number of indications for abdominal CT, particularly those involving the detection of fluid collections, such as abscesses, that may be confused with a fluid-filled bowel loop. Unlike fluoroscopic studies, gastrointestinal CT studies entail no significant difference in diagnostic quality between barium and iodinated contrast agents because only very dilute gastrointestinal contrast material is required. Therefore, high-osmolality iodinated contrast agents may be used routinely for emergent CT evaluation of the gastrointestinal tract.

DIAGNOSIS AND TREATMENT OF CONTRAST REACTIONS

The great majority of adverse effects from contrast agents are mild or moderate events that are not life-threatening and require only observation, reassurance, and general supportive measures. However, vigilance must be maintained because most severe contrast reactions begin with mild to moderate symptoms and signs. The vigilance need not be prolonged because essentially all life-threatening contrast reactions occur immediately or within 15 min of injection.

From a clinical perspective, acute reactions to contrast agents can be classified in the following types: (1) nausea and/or vomiting, (2) urticaria (hives) without respiratory symptoms, (3) bronchospasm (wheezing) without cutaneous or cardiovascular manifestations, (4) isolated hypotension, (5) vagal reaction, (6) isolated laryngeal edema, and (7) generalized anaphylactoid reaction.[2,4] Clinically, an anaphylactoid reaction is characterized by a severe or rapidly accelerating combination of one or more of the following: bronchospasm, generalized urticaria, angioedema, laryngeal spasm or edema, and hypotension with tachycardia (shock). Table 302-8 presents one

TABLE 302-8   Guidelines for the Diagnosis and Treatment of Contrast Reactions

Signs and Symptoms	Treatment	Treatment Interval	Treatment Precautions
Nausea and/or vomiting			
Transient	Supportive observation		
Severe, protracted	Prochlorperazine 5–10 mg IV or IM	Every 3–4 h	Give slowly; drowsiness
Urticaria			
Scattered, transient	Supportive observation		
Scattered, protracted	Diphenhydramine 25–50 mg PO/IV/IM	Every 2–3 h	Drowsiness, hypotension
Severe	Cimetidine 300 mg IV *or* Ranitidine 50 mg IV	Every 6–8 h	Give slowly; drowsiness
Profound, diffuse edema	See anaphylactoid reaction		
Bronchospasm (wheezing)	O$_2$ 6 L/min by mask; pulse oximeter		
Isolated wheezing	Albuterol inhaler 2 puffs or nebulized treatment	Every 4–6 h	Proper inhalation technique (use of spacer)
Moderate or severe	See anaphylactoid reaction (below)		
Hypotension, isolated	O$_2$ 6 L/min by mask		
Sinus tachycardia (shock)	NS 1–2 L IV bolus *or* LR 1–2 L IV bolus *and* If poorly responsive, see anaphylactoid reaction (below)	Per blood pressure and urine output	Fluid overload
Sinus bradycardia (vagal)	Atropine 0.6–1.0 mg IV *and* IV fluids as for sinus tachycardia	Every 3–5 min up to 3 mg total	Monitor pulse rate; fluid overload
Laryngeal or facial edema (stridor)	See anaphylactoid reaction (below)		
Anaphylactoid reaction	O$_2$ 6 L/min by mask; pulse oximeter		
Moderate	Epinephrine 1:1000 0.1–0.3 mL SC (0.1–0.3 mg)	Every 10–15 min up to 1 mL	Patients on β-blockers, may experience hypotension due to unopposed α-adrenergic stimulation
Accelerating or severe	Epinephrine 1:10,000 1 mL IV (0.1 mg) over 5–10 min	Every 5–10 min up to 10 mL	

Source: Modified from Bush and Swanson[2] and American College of Radiology,[4] with permission.

approach to the treatment of acute contrast reactions. Contrast reactions also may have nonspecific manifestations, such as pulmonary edema, angina, seizure, or hypertensive urgency. Such reactions should be treated with standard therapies and protocols (see Chap. 34).

REFERENCES

1. Lasser EC, Lyon SG, Berry CC: Reports on contrast media reactions: Analysis of data from reports to the U.S. Food and Drug Administration. *Radiology* 203:605, 1997.
2. Bush WH, Swanson DP: Acute reactions to intravascular contrast media: Types, risk factors, recognition, and specific treatment. *AJR* 157:1153, 1991.
3. Katzberg RW: Urography into the twenty-first century: New contrast media, renal handling, imaging characteristics, and nephrotoxicity. *Radiology* 204:297, 1997.
4. American College of Radiology: *Manual on Contrast Media,* Edition 4.1. Reston, VA, American College of Radiology, 2001.
5. Younathan CM, Kande JV, Cook MD, et al: Dialysis is not indicated immediately after administration of nonionic contrast agents in patients with end-stage renal disease treated by maintenance dialysis. *AJR* 163:969, 1994.
6. Tepel M, van der Giet M, Schwarzfeld C, et al: Prevention of radiographic-contrast-agent-induced reductions in renal function by acetylcysteine. *New Engl J Med* 343:180, 2000.
7. Kay J, Chow WH, Chan TM, et al: Acetylcysteine for prevention of acute deterioration of renal function following elective coronary angiography and intervention: A randomized controlled trial. *JAMA* 289:553, 2003.
8. Morcos SK, Thomsen HS: European Society of Urogenital Radiology guidelines on administering contrast media. *Abdom Imaging* 28:187, 2003.
9. Cohan RH, Ellis JH, Dunnick NR: Use of low-osmolar agents and premedication to reduce the frequency of adverse reactions to radiographic contrast media: A survey of the Society of Uroradiology. *Radiology* 194:357, 1995.
10. Lasser EC, Berry CC, Tainer LB, et al: Pretreatment with corticosteroids to alleviate reactions to intravenous contrast material. *New Engl J Med* 317:845, 1987.
11. Greenberger PA, Patterson R: The prevention of immediate generalized reactions to radiocontrast media in high-risk patients. *J Allergy Clin Immunol* 87:867, 1991.
12. Smith RC, Verga M, McCarthy S, et al: Diagnosis of acute flank pain: Value of unenhanced helical CT. *AJR* 166:97, 1996.
13. Sommer FG, Jeffrey RB, Rubin GD, et al: Detection of ureteral calculi in patients with suspected renal colic: Value of reformatted noncontrast helical CT. *AJR* 165:509, 1995.
14. Boyle EM, Maier RV, Salazar JD, et al: Diagnosis of injuries after stab wounds to the back and flank. *J Trauma* 42:260, 1997.
15. Kaiser S, Frenckner B, Jorulf HK: Suspected appendicitis in children: US and CT—A prospective randomized study. *Radiology* 223:633, 2002.
16. Rao PM, Rhea JT, Novelline RA, et al: Effect of computed tomography of the appendix on treatment of patients and use of hospital resources. *New Engl J Med* 338:141, 1998.
17. Rao PM, Rhea JT, Novelline RA, et al: Helical CT technique for the diagnosis of appendicitis: Prospective evaluation of a focused appendix CT examination. *Radiology* 202:139, 1997.

PRINCIPLES OF EMERGENCY DEPARTMENT SONOGRAPHY
Scott W. Melanson
Michael B. Heller

Emergency ultrasonography examinations should usually be restricted to those areas that are amenable to the type of limited, goal-directed examinations described in this chapter and in textbooks on emergency ultrasonography. Any abnormality noted on a bedside examination that the examiner cannot explain should be further evaluated with formal ultrasonography or another imaging modality.

At this time, only a half-dozen ED applications are firmly established as a major contribution to daily practice (see Table 303-1). The first four of these are life-threatening, time-sensitive conditions for which the bedside ultrasonographic examination provides rapid, easily interpreted information that is often unavailable in a timely manner by any other means. The other two applications, for suspected obstructive renal disease and acute gallbladder pathology, are ordinarily not acutely life-threatening but are so common and so amenable to ultrasonography studies that they have gained widespread acceptance as primary indications. Other potential applications (not reviewed in detail) include determination of urinary bladder postvoid residual volume, soft tissue foreign body detection, deep venous thrombosis (DVT) evaluation, soft tissue abscess evaluation, and vascular access.

FUNDAMENTALS

The ultrasonographic image is created electronically from high-frequency sound waves generated by the transducer (or probe), which also receives the reflected waves. The time required for the reflection of each structure determines its depth on the image, and the intensity of the reflection determines its shade on a black-to-white scale. A perfect reflector of ultrasound waves appears white and is referred to as *hyperechoic.* A perfect transmitter of ultrasound waves has no reflection and appears black, or *anechoic.* A great advantage of ultrasonography is that most structures, particularly those not well visualized by standard radiography, have intermediate echogenicity that is quite characteristic and allows for identification of normal and abnormal organs and tissues.

An important factor in determining the quality of the image is the frequency of the transducer employed: the lower the frequency, the greater the depth of penetration but the lower the resolution. For all the primary ED indications (except endovaginal ultrasound), a general-purpose probe of approximately 3.5 MHz is appropriate and will allow visualization even in obese patients. A 5-MHz probe can be used in thin adults or pediatric patients, providing better resolution. Some of the specialized applications, including many vascular and procedural uses (Table 303-2), require higher-frequency probes for adequate sonographic examination.

Color Doppler technology provides information on blood-flow characteristics of vascular structures by superimposing colors over the normal grayscale image. The displayed colors, which range from red to blue, indicate the direction and velocity of blood flow relative to the transducer. While this technology is helpful in identifying vascular structures, it is not necessary for any of the primary ED applications of ultrasonography.

An important limitation of ultrasonography is that even small amounts of air (e.g., in bowel loops and pneumoperitoneum) preclude effective visualization distal to the gas. Bone, too, is poorly imaged by ultrasound (compared to plain x-ray), and finding appropriate acoustic windows that avoid these problems is one of the skills required of the emergency sonologist.

TABLE 303-1   Primary Indications for Emergency Department Ultrasonography

Indication	Key Sonographic Finding
Abdominal aortic aneurysms	Aortic diameter >3 cm
Trauma evaluation	Hemoperitoneum
First-trimester pregnancy	Intrauterine pregnancy
Cardiac evaluation	Cardiac activity, pericardial fluid
Obstructive uropathy	Hydronephrosis
Gallbladder disease	Gallstones, sonographic Murphy sign*

*See the text for full details of sonographic findings.

TABLE 303-2   Examples of Specialized Applications for Emergency Department Ultrasonography

Appendicitis
Ascites evaluation
Cardiac wall motion abnormalities
Deep venous thrombosis
Pelvic masses
Pleural fluid visualization
Procedural applications
    Abscess drainage
    Foreign-body removal
    Suprapubic aspiration
    Vascular access

Orientation

Certain arbitrary but generally accepted conventions are used for creating and displaying ultrasonographic images. The skin-transducer interface is placed at the top of the image. Each transducer has a mark of some sort, which is used for left-right orientation. The *marker always points to the left side of the screen, as viewed from in front.* When scanning in the transverse plane, the physician points the marker groove to the patient's right side, and the image is displayed as a cross section from the patient's feet (Figure 303-1). For longitudinal or sagittal views, the *marker points to the patient's head.* The image then appears with the most cephalad portion on the left (Figure 303-2).

    The transmission of ultrasound waves is blocked by highly echogenic structures (e.g., gallstones), resulting in a relatively anechoic area distal to the echogenic structure. This effect is known as *acoustic shadowing. Acoustic enhancement* occurs distal to an anechoic, fluid-filled structure, such as the gallbladder. The area distal to the anechoic structure has increased echogenicity because of the greater number of ultrasound waves reaching this area through the anechoic structure. Examples of these phenomena are present in almost every ultrasonographic image. However, the many other technical factors that influence the creation of ultrasonographic images and artifacts are beyond the scope of this discussion. Two of the most common and useful are illustrated in Figure 303-3.

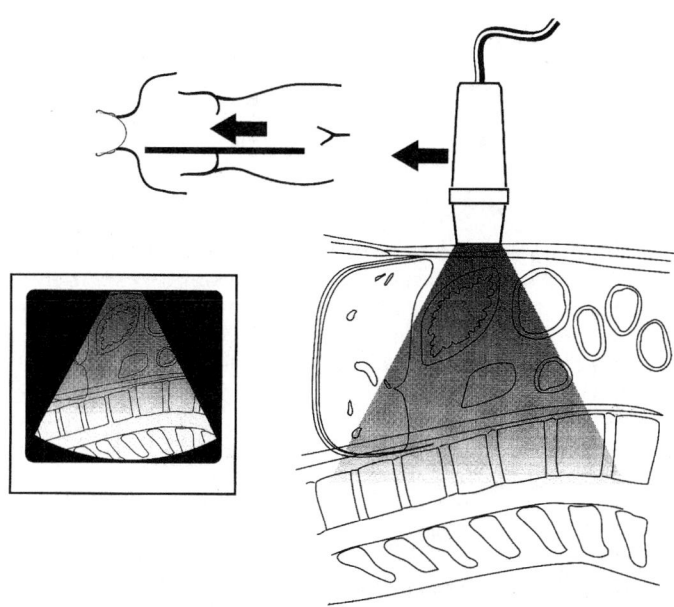

FIG. 303-2. Longitudinal ultrasonographic image. The marker dot on the probe is directed toward the patient's head. [Reproduced with permission from Heller M, Jehle D (eds): *Ultrasound in Emergency Medicine.* Philadelphia, Saunders, 1995.]

Characteristics of the Emergency Department Ultrasonography Examination

The ED ultrasonography examination is significantly different from the formal sonography that is performed in the radiology suite. The most important distinction is that the ED examination is very focused. Five of the six examinations seek only one primary finding: a yes-or-no answer (see Table 303-1). This generally allows the examination to be performed in a single position (supine) and within only a few minutes. Also, the ED examination can be more interactive. The physician can use the patient's response and clinical findings together with the ultrasound image to aid in interpretation.

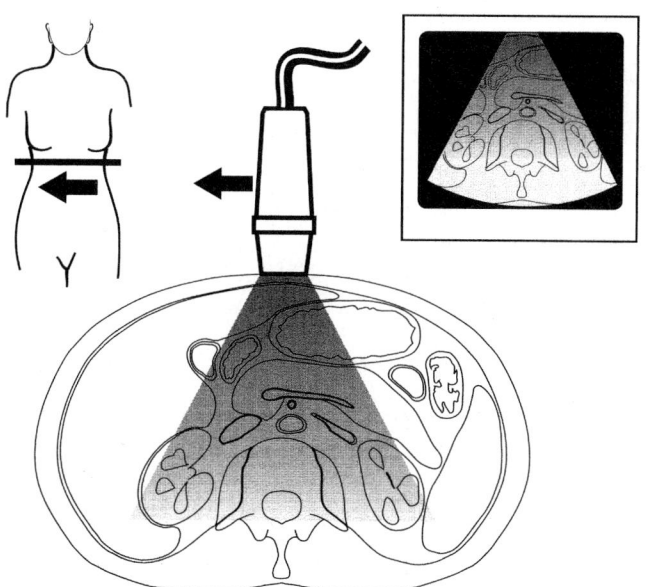

FIG. 303-1. Transverse ultrasonographic image. This is obtained by directing the marker dot on the probe toward the patient's right side. [Reproduced with permission from Heller M, Jehle D (eds): *Ultrasound in Emergency Medicine.* Philadelphia, Saunders, 1995.]

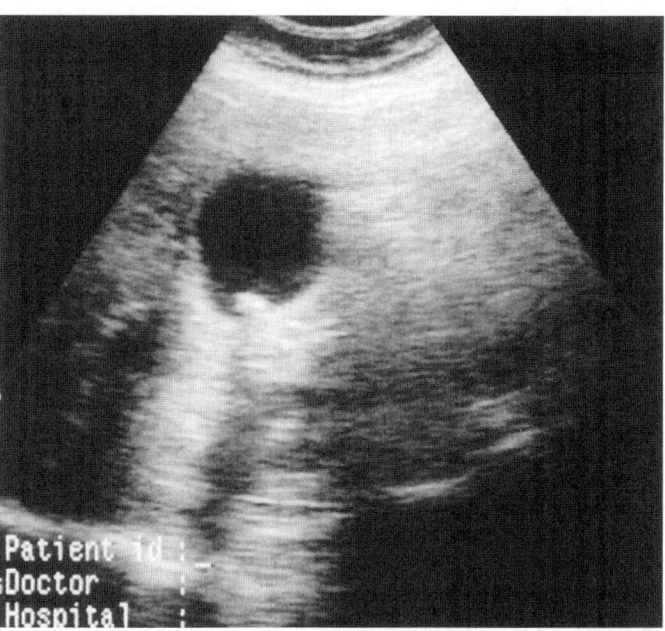

FIG. 303-3. Acoustic shadow created by solitary gallstone. Acoustic enhancement increased ecogenicity distal to the gallbladder is also well documented.

The ED applications described are usually performed with relatively modest, very portable, non-Doppler units. The addition of Doppler technology, which allows for evaluation of function (flow) as well as form (anatomy), can be expected to significantly expand the utility of bedside emergency ultrasound during the next decade.

PRIMARY INDICATIONS

Primary applications are those examinations that are critically time-dependent and/or of such nature that the information gained is likely to be of major benefit to the patient and physician (see Table 303-1). These examinations each involve looking for only a few easily recognized findings. The straightforward, limited nature of these examinations allows emergency physicians to perform them with less-formal training than the imaging specialist, occasionally under severe time constraints.

Abdominal Aortic Aneurysm

Ultrasonography is as accurate as computed tomography (CT) and more accurate than angiography in measuring aneurysmal diameter.[1] Specific indications for ultrasonographic evaluation of the aorta include abdominal pain in hypotensive patients and elderly patients with unexplained back, flank, or abdominal pain.

SONOGRAPHIC CONSIDERATIONS   The aorta is located in the midline of the abdomen, to the left of the inferior vena cava (IVC), just anterior to the spine and posterior to all other abdominal contents (Figure 303-4). The aorta normally tapers as it progresses distally, and any diameter greater than 3 cm is abnormal. An ultrasonographic examination that images the aorta from the diaphragm to its distal bifurcation is extremely accurate at confirming or refuting the diagnosis of abdominal aortic aneurysm (AAA). Although pressure on the transducer usually displaces intervening bowel gas, complete visualization is sometimes impossible. Such examinations are considered indeterminate.

With experience, it is generally not difficult to differentiate the aorta from the IVC (see Figure 303-4). The IVC, usually to the right of the aorta, has thinner walls and changes remarkably in size with probe pressure and the Valsalva maneuver. Both the aorta and the IVC are pulsatile, although the gentle, undulating pulsation of the IVC can, with experience, be differentiated from the forceful, centripetal aortic pulsation.

The primary sonographic finding of AAA is an aortic diameter greater than 3 cm. When AAA is suspected, the aorta should be imaged in the transverse and sagittal planes from the diaphragm to its bifurcation at the level of the umbilicus. Transverse images measured horizontally from outside wall to outside wall are the most reliable in accurately determining true aortic size. Echogenic thrombus within the outer margins of AAAs is very common, and care must be taken to identify the outer limits of the aortic wall (Figure 303-5). While ultrasonography is very accurate in measuring AAA size, it is often impossible to determine sonographically whether the AAA has ruptured, because rupture most often occurs into the retroperitoneal space. A hypoechoic retroperitoneal hematoma may be seen but is often very difficult to identify. AAA rupture into the peritoneal space is usually fatal.

Renal Colic

Intravenous pyelogram (IVP), spiral CT, and ultrasonography are all used in evaluating patients thought to have renal colic (see Chap. 96). Bedside ultrasonography often allows a much more rapid diagnosis and disposition of ED patients than either IVP or spiral CT, and there are situations where the use of contrast material or iodizing radiation is unwise (e.g., pregnancy, renal insufficiency, and volume depletion). False-negative sonographic results occur, but the sonographic appearance of hydronephrosis in the appropriate clinical setting aids in diagnosis, and negative findings on examination should lead to an alternative diagnosis. Renal colic without hydronephrosis remains in the differential diagnosis.

SONOGRAPHIC CONSIDERATIONS   A standard 3.5-MHz probe is generally used for renal scanning, but a 5-MHz transducer can be used with better resolution in thin adults and children. The right kidney is best visualized in the anterior to midaxillary line over the lower ribs, but a subcostal approach can sometimes be successful in imaging the kidneys, avoiding the distraction of rib shadows. The left kidney is more difficult to see because of overlying bowel and stomach and the

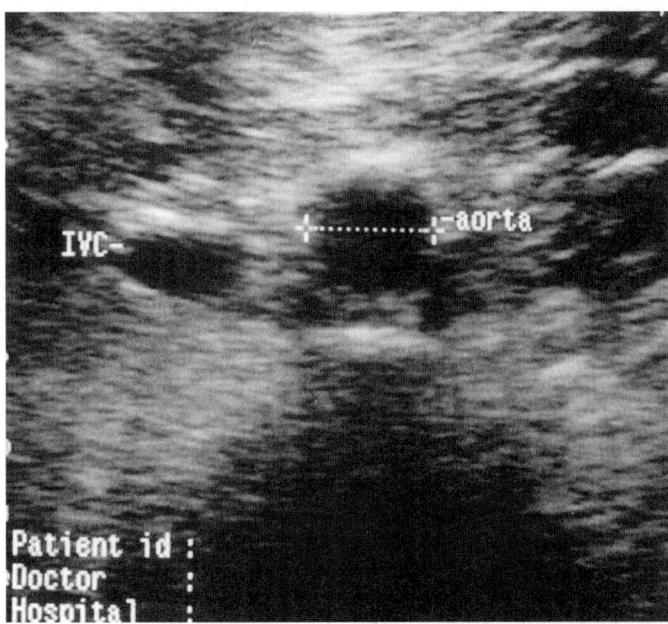

FIG. 303-4. Transverse view of a normal abdominal aorta and inferior vena cava (IVC). The vertebral body is represented by the large hypoechoic area in the far field.

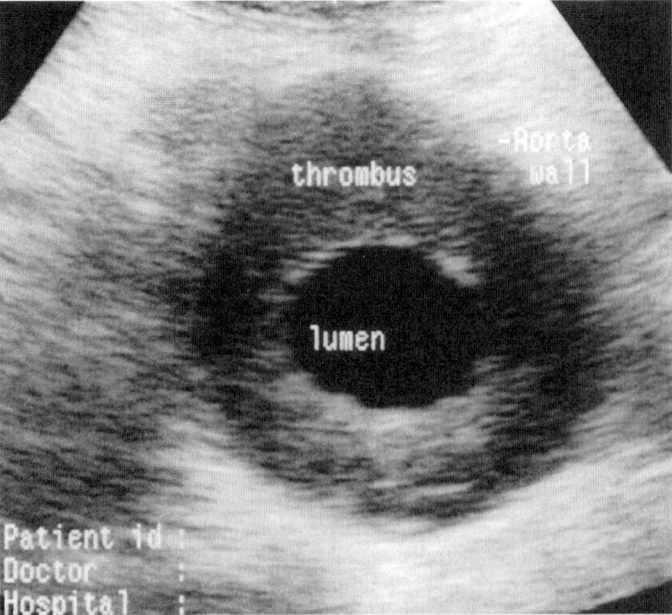

FIG. 303-5. Abdominal aortic aneurysm with intraluminal thrombus.

absence of the liver, which acts as an acoustic window, but is perfectly amenable to ED visualization as well. The best initial approach to the left kidney is somewhat more dorsally, in the posterior axillary line over the lower ribs. Occasionally, a posterior thoracic approach is necessary to adequately visualize the kidneys. Deep inspiration lowers the diaphragm and may move the kidneys caudally into a more easily visualized location. To fully evaluate the kidneys for hydronephrosis, both longitudinal and transverse images should be obtained, and both kidneys should be scanned with each examination.

The kidneys are retroperitoneal organs measuring approximately 12 cm in length and 5 cm in width, and are divided into two sonographically distinct areas: the renal cortex and the renal sinus. The renal cortex occupies the periphery of the kidney and has an echogenicity similar to that of the liver or spleen. The renal sinus appears as a central echogenic stripe within the kidney and includes the collecting system as well as major vessels of the hilum (Figure 303-6). Renal medullary pyramids appear hypoechoic relative to the cortex and are triangular in shape, occurring at the junction of the cortex and the more echogenic renal sinus. When the urine produced in a kidney flows freely into the bladder, there is no appreciable urine within the renal sinus, and therefore no significant anechoic space within the hilum. Obstruction of urine outflow from a calculus results in the development of hydronephrosis, which appears as an anechoic fluid collection within the echogenic renal sinus (Figure 303-7). Hydronephrosis can be graded from mild, with minimal separation of the sinus echoes, to severe, manifested by extensive separation of the central echoes, with renal parenchymal thinning.

Renal cysts occur commonly and can be confused with hydronephrosis. Renal cysts are thin-walled, round, anechoic structures with distal acoustic enhancement that typically occur in the periphery of the kidney and lack the more echogenic border typical of the collecting system, as seen with hydronephrosis.

The urolith (calculus) causing the obstruction most often lodges at the ureterovesicular junction, the ureteropelvic junction, or the pelvic brim. While stones at the ureterovesicular junction can occasionally be seen sonographically through the bladder window, **calculi are usually not identified by sonographic examinations.** One study found that the ureteral calculi were identified by ultrasonography in only 19 percent of patients with documented stones, whereas spiral CT and IVP were able to identify 94 and 52 percent, respectively. Hydronephrosis was identified sonographically in 73 percent of the patients with

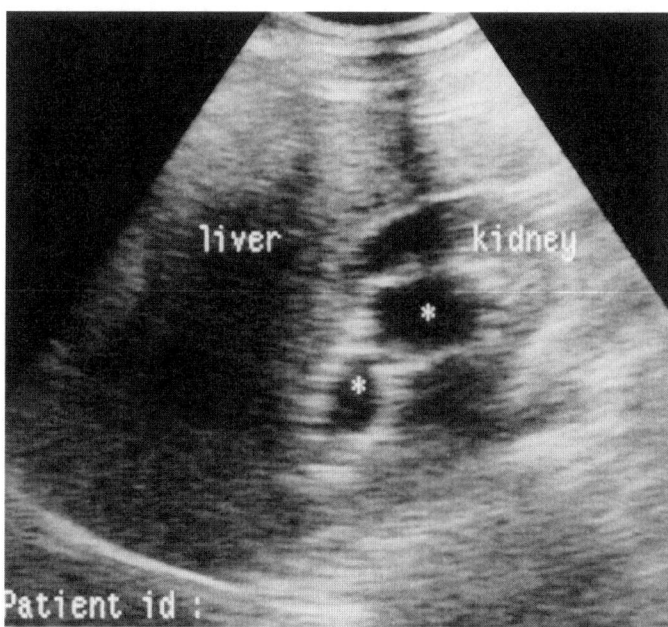

FIG. 303-7. Hydronephrosis of the right kidney with distended renal collecting system (*).

ureteral calculi.[2] In another study, emergency physicians performed bedside renal ultrasonography after a 500-mL bolus of NS in 108 patients suspected of having renal colic. When used in conjunction with the history and a kidney-ureter-bladder film, the emergency physicians were able to diagnose renal colic with a sensitivity of 97 percent. The specificity and accuracy were 59 and 83 percent, respectively.[3] It is possible that the fluid loading the patients received prior to the ultrasonographic studies resulted in a number of the false-positive results that contributed to the low specificity.

Hydronephrosis occurs in more than 65 percent of pregnant women, peaking between 24 and 28 weeks of gestation. This is believed to be caused by mechanical pressure of the enlarged uterus on the ureters and is usually more pronounced in the right kidney. This condition resolves within several weeks of delivery. False-positive scan results are also seen with overly vigorous hydration or a very full bladder. Peripelvic cysts and extrarenal pelvis are two fairly common conditions that may also cause confusion.

Gallbladder Disease

Ultrasonography is generally accepted to be the modality of choice in the evaluation of biliary disease.[4] Greater than 90 percent of biliary disease is calculous in origin, and, regardless of composition, even the smallest of gallstones are visible sonographically. Conversely, only 15 percent of gallstones are visible with standard radiographs.

SONOGRAPHIC CONSIDERATIONS   The gallbladder is an ideal organ for sonographic evaluation. This cystic structure is typically filled with anechoic bile and can be imaged through the liver, an excellent acoustic window. The gallbladder can be imaged in the right upper quadrant over the lower ribs or just below the costal margin. Deep inspiration moves the gallbladder caudally, often facilitating its visualization. The gallbladder varies in size, being smallest after fatty meals and largest after fasting, but it is typically 7 to 10 cm in length and 2 to 3 cm in width. The absence of reflective surfaces within the gallbladder results in distal acoustic enhancement. With experience and high-quality equipment, it is possible to visualize the common bile duct, especially when dilated, and this finding may be of considerable clinical import.

The primary sonographic finding in biliary disease is gallstones. Gallstones appear as bright, echogenic foci within the gallbladder and

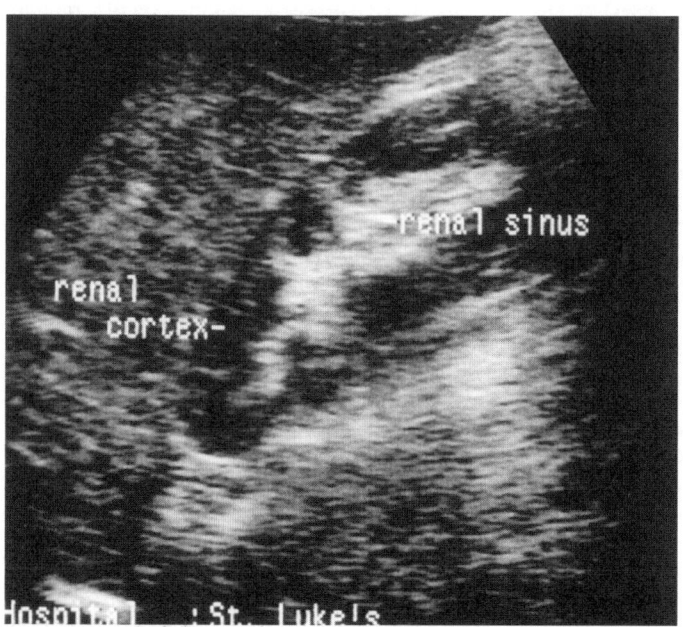

FIG. 303-6. Normal appearance of the right kidney.

move with changes in position unless impacted (Figure 303-8). A minority of gallstones float within the bile. Symptomatic gallstones may be very small in relation to the volume of the gallbladder, and a thorough search of the organ is mandatory. To ensure this, the patient should be instructed to halt inspiration when the gallbladder is well visualized. During this breath holding, the entire gallbladder should be visualized in one axis, sweeping from one side of the gallbladder to the other. This should be repeated with scanning done 90 degrees to the axis of the first scanning plane, thus obtaining both sagittal and transverse images. *Acoustic shadows* appear as anechoic lines distal to the echogenic stones. These shadows are caused by the blockage of ultrasound wave transmission distal to the stone and are helpful in identifying stones, often being more readily identified than the gallstone itself. Gallbladder polyps can mimic the appearance of gallstones, but do not change position upon moving the patient and do not create acoustic shadows.

A second extremely important sonographic finding of biliary disease is a positive sonographic Murphy sign. **The sonographic Murphy sign is considered positive when the point of maximal tenderness to transducer pressure is directly over the sonographically located gallbladder.** A positive sonographic Murphy sign in the presence of cholelithiasis is reported to have a 92 percent positive predictive value for symptomatic gallbladder disease. Gallbladder wall thickening, defined as proximal gallbladder wall thickness greater than 3 mm, occurs in 50 to 75 percent of patients with acute cholecystitis, but this finding is not specific for cholecystitis. Edematous states, as well as such conditions as liver disease, AIDS, ascites, renal disease, and the postprandial state, can also result in gallbladder wall thickening. Gallbladder sludge is nearly always abnormal in the ambulatory patient, suggesting biliary disease. Sludge is composed of calcium bilirubinate and cholesterol granules, and generally form a bile-sludge layer within the gallbladder and does not create acoustic shadows (Figure 303-9). Finally, a fluid collection around the gallbladder, or pericholecystic fluid, is evidence of marked inflammation and often of perforation. This is usually seen in patients with other clinical and sonographic evidence of cholecystitis.

In summary, the sonographic signs of biliary disease are gallstones, sonographic Murphy sign, gallbladder wall thickening, gallbladder sludge, and pericholecystic fluid. The combination of a positive sonographic Murphy sign and any of the other sonographic findings described is highly reliable in diagnosing acute gallbladder disease. In

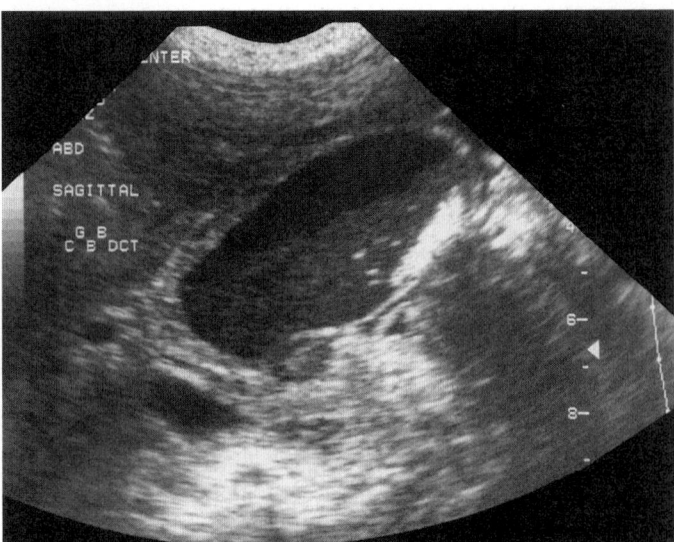

FIG. 303-9. Gallbladder sludge. The sludge is seen to layer out in the gallbladder. Multiple gallstones are also present. [Reproduced with permission from Heller M, Jehle D (eds): *Ultrasound in Emergency Medicine.* Philadelphia, Saunders, 1995.]

fact, the presence of any two of the sonographic signs in the appropriate clinical setting is highly suggestive of the disease. Completely normal examination findings, including a negative sonographic Murphy sign, are reliable in excluding symptomatic gallbladder disease.

Focused Abdominal Sonography for Trauma (FAST)

Abdominal CT scanning remains an important tool in evaluating trauma, with an accuracy of more than 90 percent in detecting presence of intra-abdominal injuries. However, CT is expensive and requires a hemodynamically stable, cooperative patient. It also involves contrast-medium administration and ionizing radiation. Diagnostic peritoneal lavage (DPL) has sensitivities greater than 90 percent for hemoperitoneum. However, up to one-third of laparotomies performed on the basis of positive DPL findings are unnecessary. As little as 20 mL of blood mixed with the standard liter of peritoneal lavage fluid will result in a positive DPL (100,000 red blood cells per cubic millimeter). In addition, this invasive procedure requires significant time and causes complications in up to 5 percent of patients.

Focused abdominal sonography for trauma (FAST) has proven to be a valuable tool in the evaluation of trauma victims. More than two dozen studies in European and North American centers have demonstrated that ED sonography has an accuracy similar to that of DPL for the detection of hemoperitoneum but has several advantages: it is more rapid (generally completed in under 5 min), requires no preparations (e.g., nasogastric tube and urinary drainage catheter), has no contraindications, and is noninvasive. While ultrasonography cannot reliably identify intraabdominal organ injuries (as can CT), it is accurate in predicting the need for laparotomy in trauma patients. Large studies have found the sensitivity of ultrasonography to be 86 percent or higher with specificities of 98 percent or higher,[5] depending on the gold standards employed. Some studies have used the need for a therapeutic laparotomy as the gold standard, whereas others have used the presence of any intra-abdominal injury or blood on CT as the gold standard, regardless of need for laparotomy (see Chap. 259 for further discussion). Subcutaneous emphysema and marked obesity can impair the ability of ultrasonography to image the abdomen, but it is uncommon that they prevent an adequate FAST examination. Training for as little as 2 to 8 h has been sufficient for emergency physicians and surgeons to learn the FAST examination,[6] and it has completely replaced DPL in many centers.

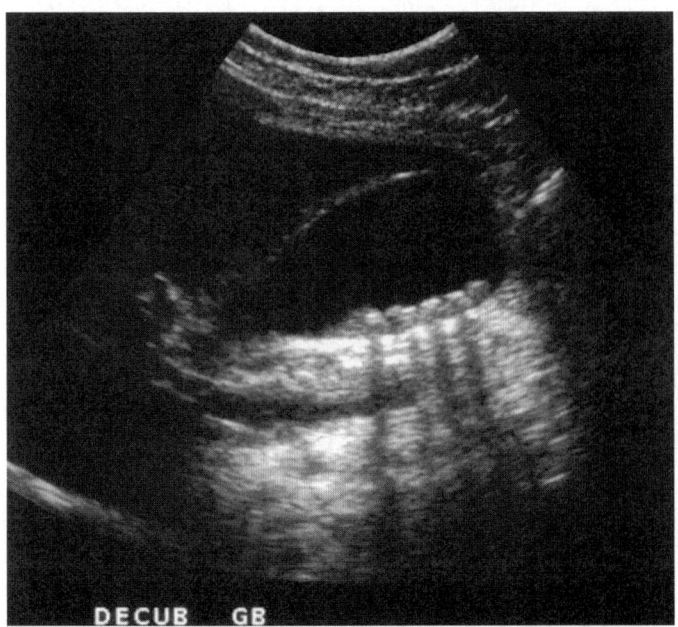

FIG. 303-8. Multiple dependent gallstones with acoustic shadowing.

SONOGRAPHIC CONSIDERATIONS The primary finding in the FAST examination is anechoic fluid collections (blood) within the peritoneal cavity. Figure 303-10 shows the four standard views of the trauma ultrasonographic examination. The right upper quadrant view, the easiest of the FAST examination views to visualize, is obtained by imaging over the lower rib cage in the area of the anterior to midaxillary line with the marker dot pointed cephalad. The liver, kidney, and Morison pouch are examined (Figure 303-11). The Morison pouch is a potential space between the Gerota fascia of the kidney and the Glisson capsule of the liver, and is usually devoid of fluid. Because the Morison pouch is one of the most posterior compartments of the supine abdomen, blood tends to accumulate in this space, creating an easily identified anechoic stripe (Figure 303-12). Organ lesions, while not reliably identified by ultrasonography, may appear as anechoic areas within the organ or as echogenic foci. The left upper quadrant view examines the potential space between the spleen and the kidney, the splenorenal space (Figure 303-13). This view is obtained by placing the transducer in the mid to posterior axillary line over the lower left costal margin. Again, blood will appear as an anechoic stripe between the spleen and kidney. While not routine, placing the patient into a Trendelenburg position may increase the amount of blood in the upper abdomen, facilitating sonographic identification of blood in both the right and left upper quadrant. Both upper abdominal views are also capable of identifying hemothorax, where the anechoic fluid collection appears above the diaphragm. Studies have found ultrasound to be at least as accurate as chest x-ray in identifying hemothorax.[7,8] The pelvis is the most dependent location within the intraperitoneal cavity in a supine patient, explaining why hemoperitoneum commonly collects in this location. The pelvic view seeks to identify intraperitoneal blood in the potential space between the rectum and uterus (pouch of Douglas) or its homologue in the male, the rectovesicular space. As with the other views, blood here appears as a fluid collection between two adjacent soft tissue structures (Figure 303-14). Unclotted intraperitoneal blood is anechoic, with sharp borders against the peritoneal confines. The pelvic view is facilitated by a full bladder, which can be produced by instilling 250 mL of NS via a urinary drainage catheter. The full bladder acts as an acoustic window, optimizing the view of the pelvic structures. As little as 250 mL of intraperitoneal

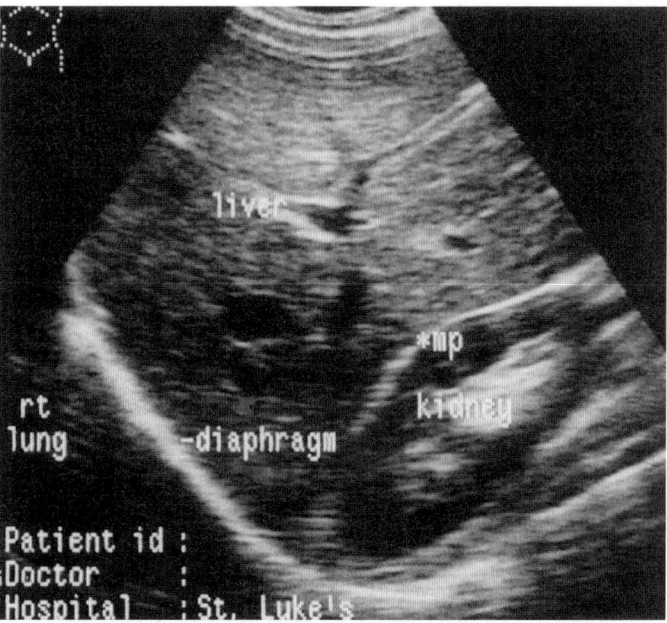

FIG. 303-11. Normal ultrasonographic image of the right upper quadrant demonstrating an absence of fluid in Morison pouch *(mp)*.

blood should be routinely noted with ultrasound; even smaller collections can often be identified.

The last view, that of the subcostal area, examines the heart for evidence of pericardial fluid collections, which would suggest cardiac injury (Figure 303-15). Rapid ultrasonographic evaluation of the heart has resulted in faster times to diagnosis and to surgical intervention, as well as improved survival rates and neurologic outcomes in patients with penetrating cardiac injuries.[9] It is occasionally necessary to differentiate pleural from pericardial fluid. Any fluid collection that follows the contours of the heart and is surrounded by the echogenic pericardium is pericardial fluid. There is no pleural reflection between the liver and heart; the subcostal view will therefore demonstrate pericardial, but not

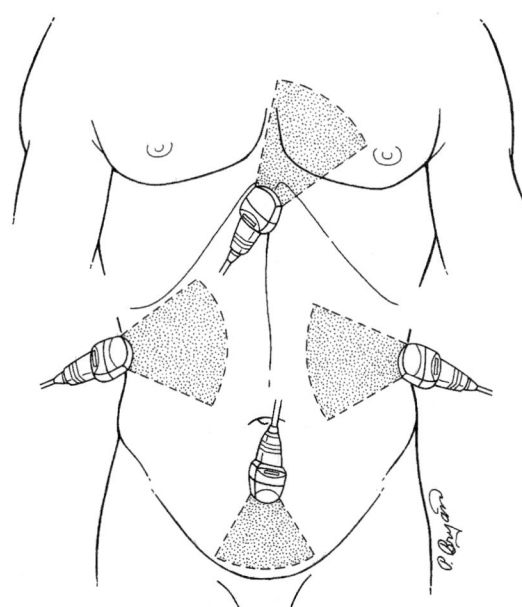

FIG. 303-10. Standard four views of the FAST examination. (Reproduced with permission from Sisley AC, Rozycki GS, Ballard RB, et al: Rapid detection of traumatic effusion using surgeon-performed ultrasonography. *J Trauma* 44:291, 1998.)

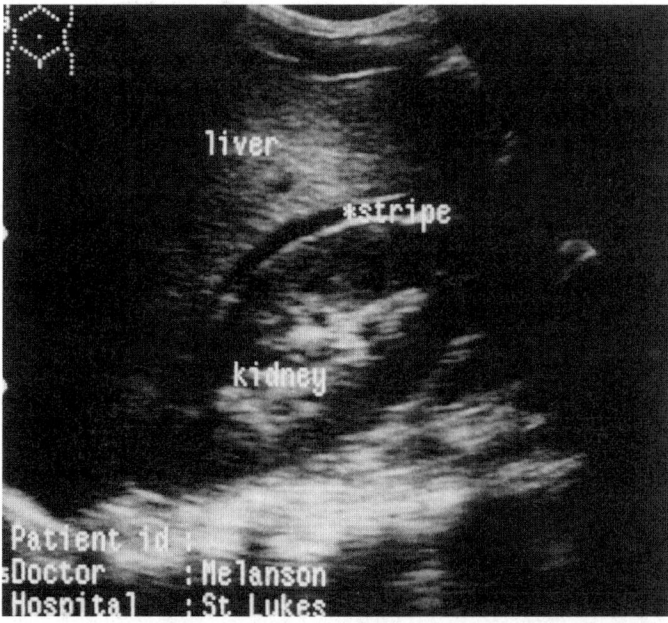

FIG. 303-12. Positive right upper quadrant FAST examination findings. Note "stripe" of fluid in Morison pouch.

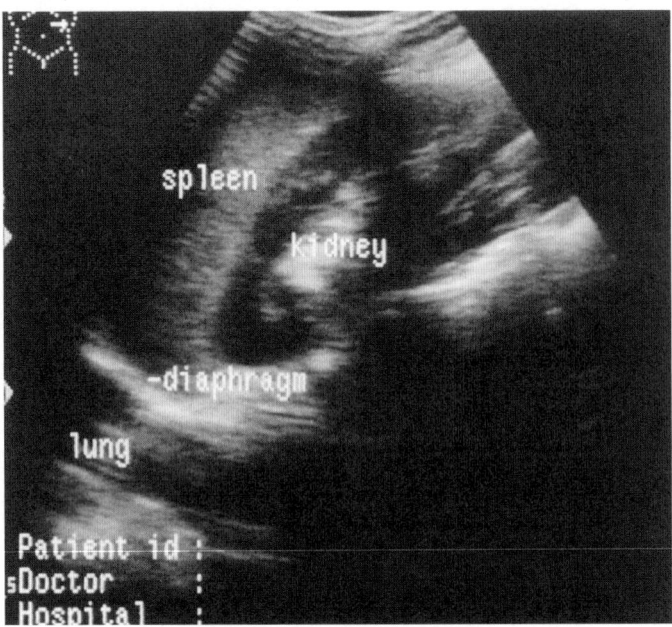

FIG. 303-13. Normal findings on left upper quadrant ultrasonogram. The potential space between the kidney and spleen is devoid of anechoic fluid.

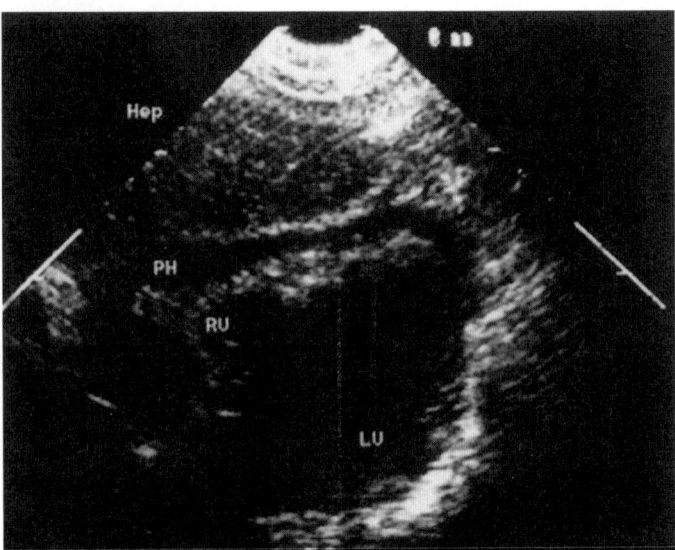

FIG. 303-15. Subcostal echocardiogram demonstrating pericardial hemorrhage (PH). Hep = hepatic parenchyma; LV = left ventricle; RV = right ventricle. [Reproduced with permission from Heller M, Jehle D (eds): *Ultrasound in Emergency Medicine.* Philadelphia, Saunders, 1995.]

pleural, fluid. Blood within the pericardial space can appear anechoic but may be partially echogenic, depending on the degree of clotting and defibrination that occurs.

First-Trimester Pregnancy Evaluation

No set of historical factors, signs, or symptoms can accurately identify patients with ectopic pregnancy, and no laboratory tests are diagnostic of this condition. Sonographically identifying an intrauterine pregnancy can markedly reduce the possibility of ectopic pregnancy because heterotopic pregnancies (concurrent intrauterine and ectopic pregnancies) occur with an incidence of less than 1:30,000 pregnan-

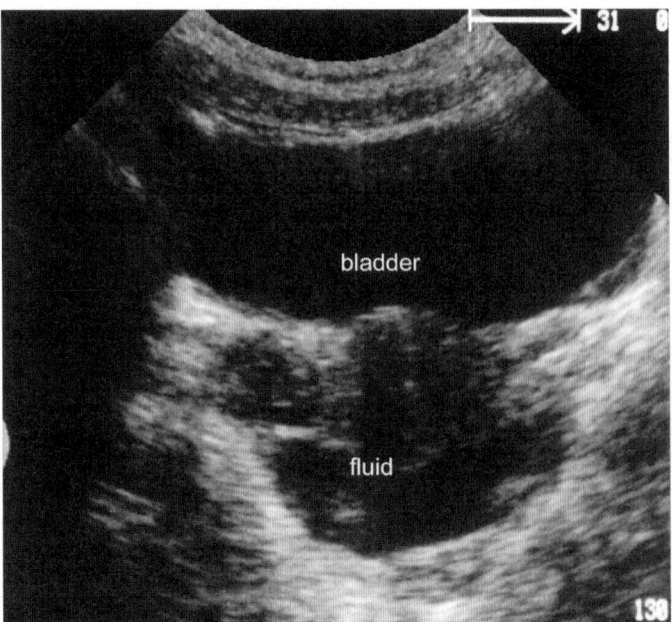

FIG. 303-14. Positive pelvic FAST examination findings. An anechoic fluid collection is seen distal to the large fluid-filled bladder.

cies, except for infertility or in vitro fertilization patients, who must be managed in concert with their obstetrician.

When ultrasonography is used only in selected first-trimester ED patients (rather than all patients), 40 to 50 percent of the ectopic pregnancies are not identified. Approximately one-half of these ectopic pregnancies are ruptured at the time of diagnosis, which increases the risk of morbidity and mortality while decreasing the likelihood of subsequent normal pregnancy.[10] Ultrasonographic evaluation of *all* first-trimester pregnant patients presenting to the ED with any abdominal or pelvic pain, vaginal bleeding, or risk factors for ectopic pregnancy has been recommended. Such an approach markedly decreases the frequency of delayed diagnoses and ectopic rupture at the time of diagnosis.[11] Emergency physicians have been proven capable of performing pelvic sonography in the evaluation of women at risk for ectopic pregnancy with an accuracy similar to that of obstetrics-gynecology consultants. Furthermore, when an emergency physician performed the sonography, the patients were dispositioned much more quickly than when the ultrasonogram was performed by an obstetrics-gynecology consultant (60 vs. 180 min).[12]

SONOGRAPHIC CONSIDERATIONS   This material is covered in detail in Chap. 103.

Cardiac Ultrasonography

Two-dimensional echocardiography has become an invaluable tool in the evaluation of cardiac anatomy and function. Echocardiography is capable of evaluating myocardial wall motion, valve function, the great vessels, and pericardial fluid collections. The examination of these structures can be technically demanding, requiring specialized transducers and specialized training. Applications of bedside ultrasonography by emergency physicians is therefore limited to critically time-dependent diagnoses that can be recognized by emergency physicians with a modicum of training and the standard ultrasonography equipment available in the ED. The evaluation of cardiac trauma, pulseless electrical activity (PEA), and pericardial tamponade are such applications. The sonographic findings of interest in such settings are pericardial fluid collections and myocardial wall activity.

The use of ultrasonography in the evaluation of potential cardiac trauma was discussed earlier in the section on the FAST examination. Both blunt and penetrating trauma can result in hemopericardium, which can be rapidly diagnosed with ultrasound (see Figure 303-15). Electromechanical dissociation is a cause of PEA that has an extremely poor prognosis. An echocardiogram demonstrating a flaccid, inactive heart in a patient with PEA suggests very little chance of survival. In contrast, a hyperdynamic heart with small right-heart dimensions suggests hypovolemia, a readily treatable condition. Cardiac tamponade can be very difficult to diagnose at the bedside without the assistance of ultrasonography. Echocardiography provides a means of rapidly determining whether a pericardial fluid collection is present, without which there can be no tamponade.

A number of windows used to sonographically evaluate the cardiac structures have been described. The *subcostal view* is the most useful to emergency physicians. This view can be obtained while other procedures are being performed with a 3.5-MHz transducer. Other views are best obtained using specialized transducer heads with small footprints (the surface area of the portion of the transducer that comes into contact with the patient) in order to image between the ribs. The subcostal view, obtained by placing the transducer in the area of the xiphoid process aiming toward the left shoulder, provides visualization of all four cardiac chambers. As always, structures that are closest to the transducer appear at the top of the image monitor; the liver, therefore, appears uppermost on the monitor, with the right atrium adjacent to it. The left atrium and ventricle appear closest to the bottom of the screen.

Other views used to evaluate cardiac structure include the left parasternal short-axis (LPSA), the left parasternal long-axis (LPLA), and the apical views. The *parasternal window* is obtained by placing the transducer between the second and fourth intercostal spaces adjacent to the sternum. In the LPLA, the ultrasound beam is directed in a plane parallel to a line drawn from the right shoulder to the left hip. This view images the aortic valve, proximal ascending aorta, and left ventricle well. The LPSA view is obtained by rotating the transducer 90 degrees, so that the beam is parallel to a line drawn from the left shoulder to the right hip. Here the left ventricle appears as a round, thick-walled chamber, and the right ventricle appears more anteriorly in a crescent shape. The LPSA view is best used to image the mitral valve, papillary muscles, and aortic valve. The *apical view* is obtained by placing the transducer over the point of maximal cardiac impulse on the precordium (the apex) with the beam directed to the right shoulder. This view allows for the assessment of chamber size and the identification of aneurysms and intracardiac masses. The emergency physician can generally obtain the information necessary for the bedside indications mentioned above by using only the subcostal view. The other views described may provide added information if the examiner has the appropriate equipment and training.

SONOGRAPHIC CONSIDERATIONS The echocardiographic evaluation of cardiac tamponade requires little training and can be rapidly performed at the bedside. The subcostal view should visualize any pericardial fluid collection large enough to result in tamponade. The pericardium is a dense, fibrous, echogenic sac that surrounds the heart. The pericardial space contains less than 50 mL of pericardial fluid under normal circumstances. Pericardial effusions appear as echo-free areas within the pericardial space. Small pericardial effusions (<100 mL) usually occupy a dependent position in the pericardial sac, while large effusions (>300 mL) are present both anteriorly and posteriorly. Whether a pericardial fluid collection affects cardiac function depends on such variables as the amount of fluid present, the rate of formation, and the underlying condition of the pericardium (diseased or not). Intrapericardial pressure rises abruptly after 80 to 200 mL of fluid has collected rapidly in the previously normal pericardial space. Early sonographic signs of increased intrapericardial pressure include right atrial and right ventricular collapse in diastole,

but these findings are not always appreciable during the ED sonographic examination.

The interpretation of an echocardiographic finding of pericardial fluid collection must incorporate the clinical status of the patient. While the absence of a pericardial fluid collection excludes the diagnosis of cardiac tamponade, the mere presence of a pericardial fluid collection in an unstable patient is not diagnostic of pericardial tamponade. When pericardiocentesis is deemed necessary, sonographic localization of the heart will assist in determining the best approach for the procedure.

The patient with PEA (i.e., electrical cardiac activity without a palpable pulse) can be suffering from a wide variety of conditions, some fatal, some easily treated. Ultrasonography greatly assists in the rapid diagnosis and treatment of such patients. The sonographic examination is straightforward. Cardiopulmonary resuscitation should be stopped briefly during the ultrasound examination. Any of the standard cardiac windows can be used, but the subcostal view has the advantages of easy imaging with standard ultrasonographic transducers and lack of interference with other procedures. Once visualized, the ventricles and valves are examined for evidence of activity. A patient in true electromechanical dissociation has no demonstrable cardiac activity. Several treatable causes of PEA can be diagnosed with a sonogram and appropriate treatment instituted. The ventricles of a hypovolemic patient contract vigorously, while the right-heart dimensions are diminished. Cardiac tamponade, another treatable cause of PEA, can also be easily diagnosed with echocardiography, as discussed above.

OTHER EMERGENCY DEPARTMENT APPLICATIONS

Formal radiology department ultrasonography studies have been helpful in a great number of conditions beyond those already discussed. Emergency physicians, given the appropriate time, training, and equipment could technically perform any of these examinations at the bedside. This section discusses some applications that have been used by emergency physicians but are not now considered primary indications.

Deep Venous Thrombosis

Compression ultrasonography has been performed by emergency physicians to evaluate ED patients suspected of having lower-extremity DVT.[13] Such studies detect venous thrombosis based on the fact that a vein filled with thrombus is not compressible, whereas normal veins can be easily compressed. An examination of the lower extremity for DVTs, therefore, consists of sonographically identifying the common femoral vein and artery and proceeding distally to the trifurcation of the popliteal vein, imaging the veins at 3- to 5-cm intervals. The inability to compress a vein by transducer pressure is diagnostic of DVT in the portion of the vein being imaged. Echogenic thrombus is occasionally visualized within the vein, but slow-flowing blood may have a similar appearance, making this finding nonspecific. Compression ultrasonography has both a sensitivity and a specificity of approximately 95 percent in venographically proven proximal leg DVTs, but the test is not accurate for identifying calf DVTs. Because approximately 20 percent of calf DVTs propagate to the proximal leg, repeat studies of the lower extremity are recommended in patients suspected of having a DVT found to have negative findings on compression ultrasound study. (See Chap. 56 for a detailed discussion.)

Visualization of Bladder and Fluid Collections

Ultrasonography excels at identifying fluid collections, and a number of possible ED applications use this property. Unless devoid of urine, the bladder is very easy to identify by ultrasonography, and most ultrasonography machines have the capability to estimate bladder volume based on easily performed measurements. The invasive and painful procedure of catheterizing the bladder to determine postvoid residual volume can often be obviated by ultrasonography. Furthermore, suprapubic bladder catheterizations and aspirations are easier and more likely to be successful when guided by ultrasonography. Identifying abscesses is another area where ultrasonography can be of assistance. With the use of high-frequency transducers (7.5 to 10 MHz), the presence or absence of fluid collections within subcutaneous masses can be determined. If an abscess is present, the depth of the abscess and surrounding structures (e.g., vessels) can be identified. The fluid within the abscess appears anechoic or has scattered echoes within a hypoechoic collection, representing necrotic debris. Just as ultrasonography can identify hemothoraces, it can identify even small pleural effusions and guide aspiration attempts.

Procedural Uses

In addition to the bladder aspiration, mentioned above, there are several other procedural applications for ultrasonography in the ED. While plain-film radiography or fluoroscopy is very accurate at identifying radiopaque foreign bodies, other objects, such as wood, can be very difficult to identify in a wound. Ultrasonography is capable of identifying wooden objects as small as 2.5 by 1.0 mm in soft tissue and is also capable of identifying metal, plastic, glass, and vegetable matter.[14,15] With high-frequency probes (7.5 to 10 MHz), foreign bodies appear echogenic, often with acoustic shadowing. With a small wound that is not amenable to exploration, it is acceptable to image directly over the potential entry site with the transducer and gel.

Sonography may also be used to assist in the percutaneous placement of central venous catheters.[16] Studies have found that the use of ultrasonography to guide this procedure results in a decreased failure rate and lowers the overall incidence of complications.[17] Here, a 7.5- to 10-MHz probe identifies the location of the vein to be cannulated (e.g., internal jugular vein), and then the percutaneous puncture can be performed with accurate knowledge of the location of the vein. The vein is seen to compress considerably before puncture occurs.

Appendicitis

The sonographic evaluation of patients suspected of harboring acute appendicitis is mentioned here primarily as a cautionary note. The finding of a noncompressible appendix greater than 6 mm in diameter has been found to be helpful in making the diagnosis of appendicitis in the appropriate clinical setting.[18] However, several aspects of this examination make it particularly unsuited for performance by emergency physicians. This examination is generally quite time-consuming, requires specialized training and experience, and can be very difficult technically. The diagnosis of appendicitis is also not as critically time dependent, as are such entities as ruptured AAA or hemoperitoneum in a trauma patient, and generally is best left in the hands of sonologists trained in this technique. Other potential uses for bedside ultrasonography in the ED can be found in standard emergency sonography texts.[19,20]

REFERENCES

1. Kuhn M, Bonnin RL, Davey MJ, et al: Emergency department ultrasound scanning for abdominal aortic aneurysm: Accessible, accurate, and advantageous. *Ann Emerg Med* 36:219, 2000.
2. Yilmaz S, Sindel T, Arslan G, et al: Renal colic: Comparison of spiral CT, US and IVU in the detection of ureteral calculi. *Eur Radiol* 8:212, 1998.
3. Henderson SO, Hoffner RJ, Aragona JL, et al: Bedside emergency department ultrasonography plus radiography of the kidneys, ureters, and bladder vs intravenous pyelography in the evaluation of suspected ureteral colic. *Acad Emerg Med* 5:666, 1998.
4. Simmons MZ: Pitfalls in ultrasound of the gallbladder and biliary tract. *Ultrasound Q* 14:2, 1998.
5. Dolich MO, McKenney MG, Varela JE, et al: 2576 ultrasounds for blunt abdominal trauma. *J Trauma* 50:108, 2001.
6. Thomas B, Falcone RE, Vasquez D, et al: Ultrasound evaluation of blunt abdominal trauma: Program implementation, initial experience, and learning curve. *J Trauma* 42:384, 1997.
7. Sisley AC, Rozycki GS, Ballard RB, et al: Rapid detection of traumatic effusion using surgeon-performed ultrasonography. *J Trauma* 44:291, 1998.
8. Ma OJ, Mateer JR: Trauma ultrasound examination versus chest radiograph in the detection of hemothorax. *Ann Emerg Med* 29:312, 1997.
9. Rozycki GS, Feliciano DV, Schmidt JA: The role of surgeon-performed ultrasound in patients with possible cardiac wounds. *Ann Surg* 223:737, 1996.
10. Stovall TG, Kellerman AL, Ling FW, Buster JE: Emergency department diagnosis of ectopic pregnancy. *Ann Emerg Med* 19:1098, 1990.
11. Mateer JR, Valley VT, Aiman EJ, et al: Outcome analysis of a protocol including bedside endovaginal sonography in patients at risk for ectopic pregnancy. *Ann Emerg Med* 27:283, 1996.
12. Shih C: Effect of emergency physician-performed pelvic sonography on length of stay in the emergency department. *Ann Emerg Med* 29:348, 1997.
13. Blaivas M, Lambert MJ, Harwood RA, et al: Lower-extremity Doppler for deep venous thrombosis—Can emergency physicians be accurate and fast? *Acad Emerg Med* 7:120, 2000.
14. Jacobson JA, Powell A, Craig JG, et al: Wooden foreign bodies in soft tissue: Detection at US. *Radiology* 206:45, 1998.
15. Orlinsky M, Knittel P, Feit T, et al: The comparative accuracy of radiolucent foreign body detection using ultrasonography. *Am J Emerg Med* 18:401, 2000.
16. Keenan SP: Use of ultrasound to place central lines. *J Crit Care* 17:126, 2002.
17. Randolph AG, Cook DJ, Gonzales CA, Pribble CG: Ultrasound guidance for placement of central venous catheters: A meta-analysis of the literature. *Crit Care Med* 24:2053, 1996.
18. Zielke A, Hasse C, Sitter H, Rothmund M: Influence of ultrasound on clinical decision making in acute appendicitis: A prospective study. *Eur J Surg* 164:201, 1998.
19. Heller M, Jehle D: *Ultrasound in Emergency Medicine.* West Seneca, NY, Center Page, 2002.
20. Ma OJ, Mateer JR: *Emergency Ultrasound.* New York, McGraw-Hill, 2002.

304 PRINCIPLES OF EMERGENCY DEPARTMENT USE OF COMPUTED TOMOGRAPHY
Stephanie B. Abbuhl

BASIC PHYSICS AND TERMINOLOGY

Computed tomography (CT) is a technique that creates cross-sectional images with the use of x-rays and computerized image reconstruction. The patient passes through a gantry that contains an x-ray tube on one side and a set of detectors on the other. The gantry rotates around the patient, obtaining information from the detectors that is then analyzed by computer and displayed as an image. The image information can be manipulated by the computer to display a greater spectrum of densities than can be displayed on conventional x-ray film.

Image Formation and CT Numbers

The various shades of gray that make up a CT image are determined by the density of a structure and the amount of x-ray energy that passes through it. This phenomenon is referred to as the *attenuation* of the x-ray. The degree of beam attenuation on a CT image is quantified and expressed in Hounsfield units (HU), which are also referred to as CT numbers. Attenuation values span a range of 4000 CT numbers, from air at -1000 HU to cortical bone at $+3000$ HU, and water is assigned the density of approximately 0 HU.

In conventional CT, each cross-sectional slice through a patient's body has a thickness, referred to as its *z axis*. The data are divided further into tiny cubes of equal volume called *voxels* (volume elements). Each voxel is assigned a CT number that is determined by the degree to which the material in that voxel absorbed the x-ray beam. The two-dimensional CT image is formed by displaying the front face of each voxel, termed a *pixel* (picture element), in a composite matrix. The most common matrix size of CT scanners is 512 rows of pixels by 512 columns, or a total of 262,144 pixels[1] (Figure 304-1).

Volume Averaging

Certain factors affect the accuracy of the Hounsfield units and the accuracy of the image. The degree of linear attenuation and the resultant CT number are determined by the average density of the material within that voxel. Therefore, when a voxel is filled with several structures (or the structure of interest is smaller than the voxel), the voxel is assigned a CT number or Hounsfield unit that is subject to the *volume averaging* artifact. If the resolution of a very small structure is important, decreasing the scan thickness will improve accuracy. However, the benefits of thinner sections must be considered with the risk of a higher radiation dose to the patient with the increased number of slices. Scanning protocols are designed to balance image resolution with acceptable radiation dose.

Image Noise

Although thinner sections increase image resolution, some of the advantages are lost due to increased image *noise,* also known as *quantum mottle.* Image noise is due to an insufficient number of x-ray photons reaching the detectors, resulting in a grainy image. Image noise can be reduced by increasing the radiation dose, but a compromise between radiation exposure and image noise determines the quantitative x-ray dose.

Window and Level

Window width and *window level* are display settings that can be manipulated to optimize the appearance of the image. Selecting a window

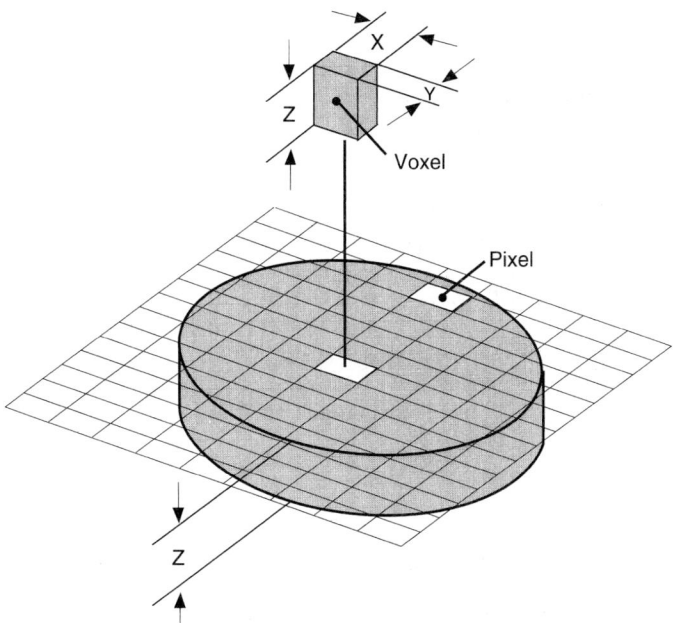

FIG. 304-1. The gray disc represents a cross-sectional slice corresponding to the patient. To create an image, the patient's data are segmented. A pixel is a two-dimensional square. A voxel incorporates the thickness of the slice and is a three-dimensional cube. (Reproduced from Romans: *Introduction to Computed Tomography,* p. 4, 25, 29. Philadelphia, Lippincott, Williams & Wilkins, 1995).

width determines the range of CT numbers that will be represented on a specific image. The computer assigns different shades of gray to CT numbers that fall within the selected range. Computed tomography numbers that are above the chosen range will appear white, and numbers below the chosen range will appear black. By increasing the window width, a greater range of CT numbers is assigned to a shade of gray. This technique is used when it is desirable to view a variety of tissues that vary greatly in density (e.g., lung). The disadvantage to wider windows (400 to 2000 HU) is that subtle differences in density will not be visualized.[1]

When the goal is to visualize a section of anatomy with minor discrepancies in tissue density, narrow window width is chosen (50 to 400 HU). A good example of the use of narrow window width is in the brain, where there is little difference in tissue densities; nevertheless, with the higher contrast achieved with a narrow window, white and gray matter can be differentiated.

Window level determines the CT number that will be the center of the gray scale. The window level is generally set at the same value as the average attenuation number of the tissue of interest.

The image from a single data set can be displayed at different window widths and levels to highlight various tissues of interest. For example, in chest CT, settings that optimize the image of the soft tissue mediastinal structures use a moderate window width (e.g., 350 HU) centered at a level just above water (e.g., +30 HU). However, this setting does not allow visualization of the details of the lungs (Figure 304-2A). In contrast, lung settings use a wide window (e.g., 1400 HU) and a low level (e.g., −600 HU) to center the gray scale so it includes air densities (see Figure 304-2B). To optimize the image of a bony structure, a wide window (e.g., 1500 HU) and a higher level (e.g., +305 HU) would be used to center the gray scale toward higher-density tissues (Figure 304-3).

SCANNER GENERATION

The terms *first-generation through fourth-generation scanners* are used to represent the developments in technology that relate the configuration of the x-ray tube to the detectors. The first-generation scanners, which are no longer in use, had a thin x-ray beam pass linearly over the patient in a 180-degree arc, followed by a single detector on the opposite side.[2] Scanning time was very lengthy. Second-generation scanners used multiple detectors and a fan-shaped x-ray beam that continued to pass linearly across the patient before rotating. Scan times improved but were still very long.

Third-generation scanners represented a significant advance in technology, and scan times were greatly reduced. This design incorporates a fan-shaped beam and a detector array, and both move in a circle within the gantry. With the use of a rotating detector, all the readings that make up a view can be recorded at the same time.[1]

Fourth-generation scanners have a detector array that is fixed and positioned in a complete circle within the gantry. The x-ray tube produces a fan-shaped beam that rotates around the patient. Scan times are theoretically shorter than with third-generation scanners, but as of this writing, few fourth-generation scanners have been installed.[2]

SPIRAL COMPUTED TOMOGRAPHY

The greatest technologic advance came with the advent of spiral or helical scanning. Rather than scanning with the traditional axial method, where the slices lie parallel to one another, spiral scanning obtains data continually in a spiral fashion. There is a continually rotating x-ray gantry and continuous table movement. This continual movement was achieved by a critical advance in hardware technology with the introduction of slip-ring interfaces in gantry construction, allowing for continuous rotation of the source detector assembly.[3] With conventional CT, a patient is required to hold the breath for each additional slice. When a patient breathes to different depths with each

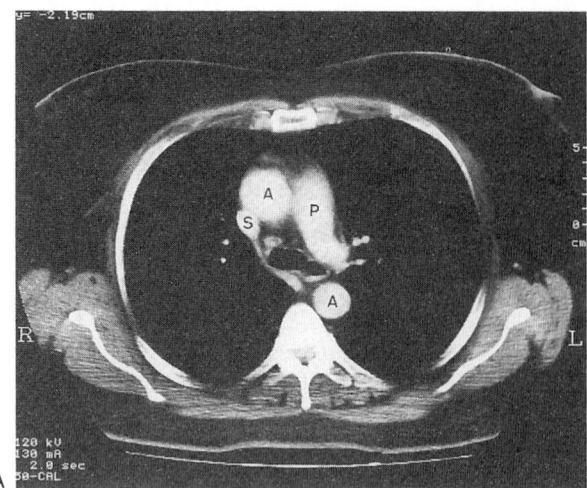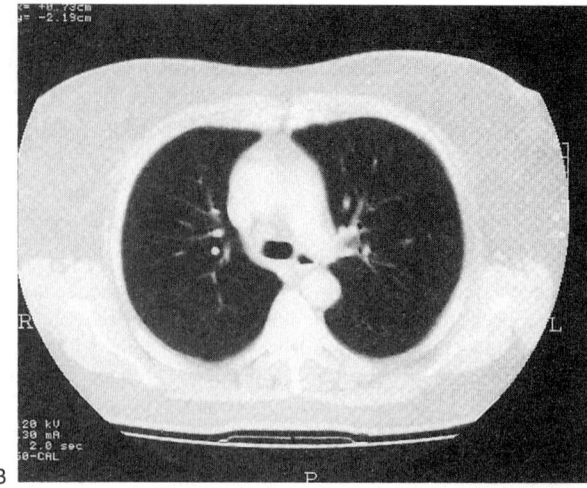

FIG. 304-2. Computed tomography windows. **A.** Mediastinal window. The mediastinal anatomy is well shown; no lung detail can be seen. A = aorta; P = pulmonary artery; S = superior vena cava. **B.** Lung window. The vascular anatomy of the lungs is now well seen. (Reprinted by permission from Lisle D: *Imaging for Students,* p 82. London, Hodder Arnold, 1997).

slice, lesions as large as 1 cm can be missed as a result of slice *misregistration* (Figure 304-4). In a typical spiral scanner, 60 images can be acquired in 1 min or less. There is less breath holding (often just once) and thus less likelihood of slice misregistration.

Because spiral scans are acquired at a slight slant, computer software must adjust for the angle by averaging the data. This statistical method of processing the data is referred to as *interpolation* (linear and nonlinear). The evolution of mathematical software processes enabling missing data to be estimated in helical data sets also has been critical to the advancement and success of spiral CT.[3] There is, however, a small decrease in resolution inherent to interpolation (Figure 304-5).

The term *pitch* refers to the relation of table speed to slice thickness. If pitch is set at 1:1, the table will move at a speed that allows the gantry to rotate once for every slice thickness chosen. For example, with slice thickness at 5 mm, the table moves at a speed that allows the gantry to rotate once every 5 mm of table travel. If the pitch is adjusted to 2:1 and the slice thickness is maintained at 5 mm, the tube rotates only once for every 10 mm of table motion. Pitch sometimes is adjusted toward 2:1, which, in essence, "stretches the spring" and fewer data are acquired.[1] Pitch usually is set at close to 1:1 but may be increased when it is important to cover a long anatomic area in a very short time, as with CT angiography.

Spiral CT scanning has optimized the delivery of IV contrast. The rapid speed of the scanning technique allows for much finer control over which phase of IV contrast enhancement is imaged and allows for the possibility of obtaining more information from a single bolus of contrast. For example, in the abdomen, images can be obtained during the hepatic arterial, portal venous, and equilibrium phases. Delayed images are also easily and rapidly obtained when enhancement characteristics of certain lesions need to be visualized or when the urinary excretory phase must be imaged. This capability is used widely in trauma, where major organ lacerations and active bleeding sites are best visualized during early phases of contrast enhancement, whereas bladder perforation may be better imaged on delayed contrast imaging.

The major advantages of helical scanning over conventional scanning are:

Volumetric data acquisition is obtained rapidly.
Less contrast material is needed because of increased scanning speed.
Images can be retrospectively reconstructed at any desired interval or thickness or may be overlapping without rescanning the patient.

Respiratory, cardiac, and other motion artifacts are reduced.
The continuous nature of the data allows high-quality three-dimensional and multiplanar reconstruction.

Although the advantages of spiral CT predominate, there are some disadvantages:

If pitch (relation of table speed to slice thickness) is increased from 1:1 toward 2:1, image resolution can be lost.
When scanning very large patients, there will be increased image noise if the milliampere setting cannot be maintained. Scanners differ with regard to weight limitations, although the average maximum patient weight is approximately 140 to 160 kg (300 to 350 lb).
Some image resolution may be lost due to the interpolation required to process spiral data.
Contrast material injection must be timed precisely, although this problem has been minimized with the use of established contrast protocols and power injectors.
Children and uncooperative adults need sedation and thus close monitoring.

Spiral CT scanners continue to have the capability of acquiring axial images. For example, at some institutions, CT protocols for cervical spine trauma use a spiral CT scanner to obtain axial images, because of the potential improvement in image resolution in this anatomic area.

An important issue raised by the advent of spiral CT is what constitutes an appropriate examination archive. At this point, because of the enormous space required to store all the information, most CT scanners delete the raw data soon after the scan is acquired. Thus, it is important to select the reconstruction interval quickly and appropriately so that the opportunity is not lost to request additional reformatted images before the raw data are deleted.

Multidetector Spiral CT

Within the past decade, there have been major advances in spiral CT technology, including the incorporation of multidetector arrays to replace the single-slice systems. Multidetector CT (MDCT) scanners provide up to 4 to 16 simultaneous channels of data acquisition, allowing imaging over long distances using thin collimation, faster than with standard spiral CT. When combined with quicker gantry rotation times (0.5 s for one 360-degree rotation), a MDCT can scan an entire

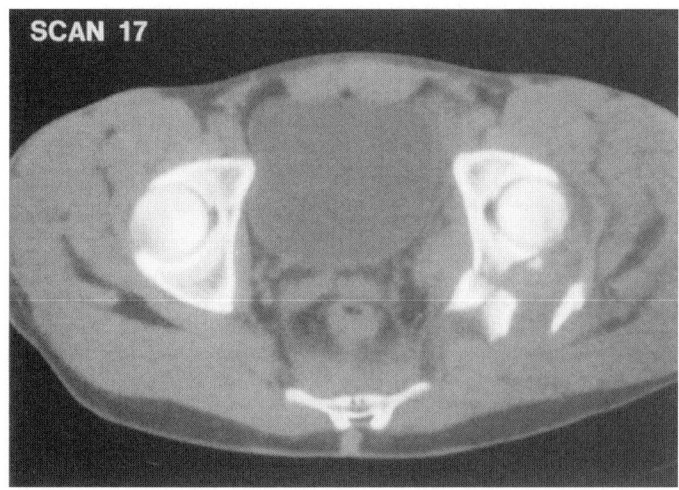

A

B

FIG. 304-3. Computed tomography at window and level settings different from those shown in Figure 304-2. A posterior wall fracture of the left acetabulum is shown at settings for bone **(A)** and for soft tissue **(B).** The wider window and higher level of the bone settings enable better visualization of bone detail but make all soft tissue structures nearly the same shade of gray. Soft tissue settings allow examination for hemarthrosis and adjacent soft tissue hematoma. (Courtesy of Jeremy J. Hollerman, MD).

abdomen and pelvis, using 1-mm collimation, in a single breath hold of 30 to 35 s.[4]

The faster data acquisition capability of MDCT has enabled even more specialized contrast examinations, including early and late arterial phases, parenchymal phase, and delayed phase, after a bolus administration of IV contrast. The use of MDCT for imaging the thoracic aorta, for example, typically will result in superior image quality, because the scans are usually acquired with a narrower section thickness and in a shorter period. In addition, the shorter scan time results in a substantial reduction in the amount of contrast required.[5] Multidetector CT technology and the sophisticated software for data visualization and analysis also have led to multiplanar and three-dimensional reconstruction capability, surface and volume renderings, and perspective internal renderings (virtual endoscopy).[6]

Multidetector CT scans do not fundamentally alter the radiation dose when compared with spiral CT. However, when thinner slices are acquired, the radiation dose must be increased to maintain a favorable signal-to-noise ratio.[6] Radiation burden always should be considered when deliberating the risks and benefits of the various imaging modalities.

Electron Beam Tomography

Electron beam tomography, or ultrafast CT, is available in only a few centers in the country and relies on a beam of electrons hitting a large stationary anode with the patient situated at the center. The images have a high resolution and the data acquisition time is extremely short (e.g., 50 to 100 ms).[6] Ultrafast CT has been used most for cardiovascular applications, including the demonstration of coronary artery calcification and stenosis,[7] pericardial problems, and aortic dissection.[6]

GENERAL USES AND LIMITATIONS

As CT technology has advanced, the role of CT in the ED has increased enormously. A CT scanner is in, or adjacent to, many EDs today, in recognition of its fundamental utility and to minimize patient transport. The only real disadvantages of CT are its relatively high cost and the use of ionizing radiation. However, in some situations, the radiation dose received is less than that for plain films, as may be the case for lumbar sacral spine plain film versus CT. Standard charges for conventional and spiral CT are the same. Head CT continues to be the primary imaging study for screening ED patients acutely, in particular for detection of acute hemorrhage, trauma, and cerebrovascular accident. Magnetic resonance imaging, however, may have a role when posterior fossa pathology or subtle parenchymal abnormalities are suspected. In general, CT is the imaging study of choice for the examination of the retroperitoneum and for many disorders of the abdomen and pelvis. At many

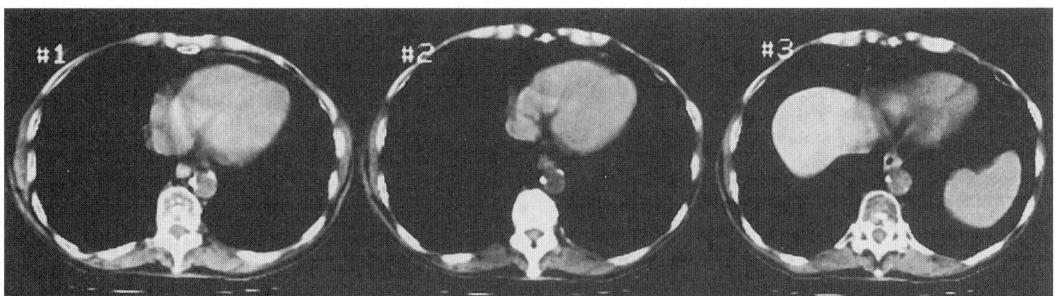

FIG. 304-4. Slice misregistration caused by a patient's breathing. Each consecutive slice was 10 mm or more inferior, but the second image appears as the most superior. Lesions as large as 1 cm can be missed as a result of slice misregistration. (Reproduced from Romans: *Introduction to Computed Tomography,* p. 4, 25, 29. Philadelphia, Lippincott, Williams & Wilkins, 1995).

METHODS OF DAT

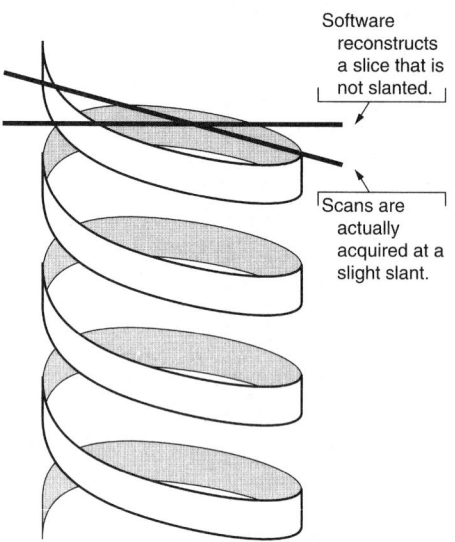

Software reconstructs a slice that is not slanted.

Scans are actually acquired at a slight slant.

FIG. 304-5. Spiral scans are acquired at a slight slant, because of the continuous motion of the x-ray tube and table. By interpolating the data, the computer creates an image that is not slanted. This process increases the effective slice thickness and causes some loss of image resolution. The more pronounced the slant, the more interpolation is required. The slant is affected by selected slice thickness and pitch. (Reproduced from Romans: *Introduction to Computed Tomography,* p. 4, 25, 29. Philadelphia, Lippincott, Williams & Wilkins, 1995).

institutions, spiral CT has become the primary imaging modality for detection of acute appendicitis[8] and ureteral calculi. It is also the modality of choice for many disorders of the mediastinum and lungs. Fractures and other bone pathologies are often best visualized with CT, and it is excellent for detecting cervical spine, pelvic, and facial bone fractures.

Only a few areas of the body are poorly imaged with CT. The pituitary fossa and the posterior intracranial fossa can be difficult to visualize, because the adjacent bony structures cause significant streak artifact, particularly with older scanners. Magnetic resonance imaging is the preferred study in these anatomic areas. Computed tomography is not sensitive in differentiating spinal cord or nerve roots from cerebrospinal fluid unless contrast has been injected into the cerebrospinal fluid space (CT myelogram). Magnetic resonance imaging is the imaging study of choice to evaluate the spinal cord.

Although spiral scanning data can be reformatted into high-quality sagittal and coronal plane images, conventional CT usually is limited to the axial (transverse) plane. There are anatomic areas (such as the head and ankles) that can be positioned in the gantry of conventional CT scanners to obtain direct coronal images.

The role of CT in the evaluation of all potential ED presentations is beyond the scope of this chapter. The reader is referred to specific chapters of chief complaints or diagnoses for a discussion of the potential value of CT for each topic.

THE USE OF CONTRAST

Contrast materials for CT examinations can be administered via oral, rectal, intravenous, intraarterial, intraarticular, or intrathecal routes, and usage changes according to the examination desired. In general, contrast usage in the ED is limited to the oral and/or IV routes.

Oral Contrast

Oral contrast agents are used for most CT examinations of the abdomen and pelvis to ensure adequate contrast opacification and dis-

tention of the bowel, which are necessary to enhance the appearance of the bowel wall to detect hematoma, edema, mass, or laceration. Enhancement usually is achieved with *positive* contrast agents, such as iodine-based and barium-based agents. At times, however, *negative* contrast is optimal in the upper gastrointestinal tract and is achieved by using an oral water preparation. Water is helpful, for example, when the indication for abdominal CT is to evaluate the pancreas in a patient with jaundice. Occasionally, distention of the upper gastrointestinal tract also can be achieved by the additional administration of effervescent granules that cause gas formation within the bowel lumen. It is important that the radiologist and/or technician know the purpose of the study so that the correct oral preparation is ordered. It is much more common to administer water-soluble iodinated oral agents to ED and trauma patients to avoid complications from extravasation of barium agents.

The iodine-based oral contrast used for CT is very dilute compared with the full-strength iodine-based contrast used for conventional radiography (upper gastrointestinal and barium enema series). Full-strength solutions may cause artifacts on CT, because of their high density. Whereas full-strength iodine-based contrast aspiration may cause life-threatening pneumonitis, the dilute contrast used for CT poses much less risk. Nonetheless, use of this agent should be avoided, or it should be used with caution in patients at risk for aspiration. If oral contrast is necessary in a patient with a known iodine allergy and a known gastrointestinal tract disorder, a dilute barium sulfate suspension should be administered instead.

Administering oral contrast takes approximately 2 h in a patient with a normal transit time if the entire bowel needs to be opacified. For example, intralumenal contrast must be present in the right colon to evaluate a patient adequately for possible appendicitis. For evaluating certain upper abdominal conditions, an additional 200 mL of oral contrast should be given just before scanning, to opacify the stomach and proximal small bowel. Not infrequently, an ED patient has nausea and vomiting, and a nasogastric tube and antiemetics are required to facilitate the oral contrast administration. Some contrast protocols use rectally administered contrast. The terms *double contrast* and *triple contrast* usually refer to the possible combined routes (oral, rectal, or vascular), but in some situations may refer to the concentration.

Intravenous Contrast

Intravenous contrast is used frequently for emergency CT studies, because it creates a more detailed image of many structures, in particular the abdominal, pelvic, and retroperitoneal organs. The contrast material causes beam attenuation that is directly related to the iodine concentration achieved by the vascular supply to that tissue. Abnormal tissue, whether due to a malignant, inflammatory, or infectious etiology, has contrast enhancement patterns different from normal tissue and may appear avascular, hypovascular, isodense, or hypervascular. Images can be obtained at various phases after contrast administration. Depending on the diagnosis in question, the study should be tailored to acquire data at the appropriate time (Figure 304-6).

In certain circumstances, it may be necessary to perform noncontrast and contrast CT scans. Scans to evaluate patients with potential urinary tract calculi must be performed initially without IV contrast, because the presence of contrast can easily obscure any renal stones present. In addition, an obstructing ureteral calculus is usually detected on an unenhanced CT study. However, IV contrast can be useful to determine the exact level of ureteral obstruction or to determine whether a pelvic calcification lies within the ureter. It also may provide information on the function of the kidneys and other potential diagnoses. In general, the best way to optimize any study is to discuss the purpose of the CT adequately with the radiologist and/or technician performing the study.

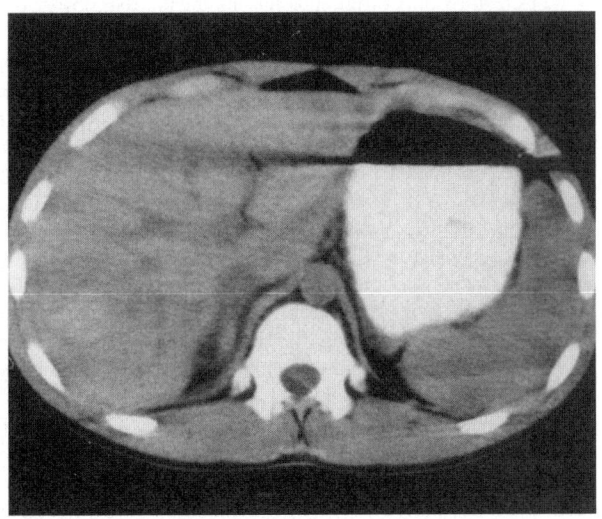

A

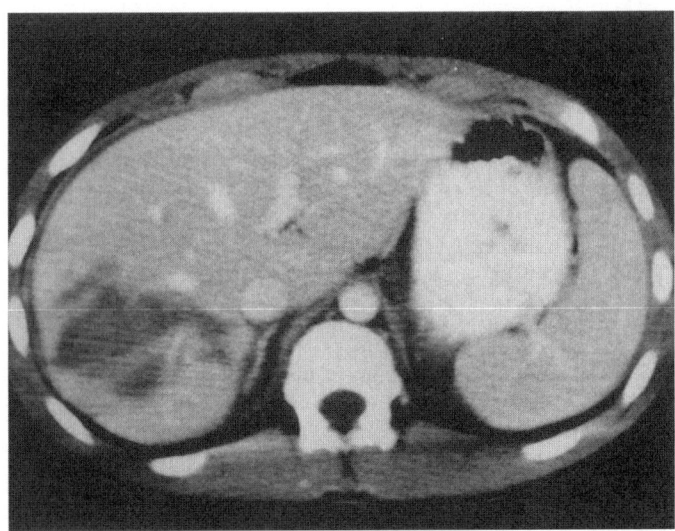

B

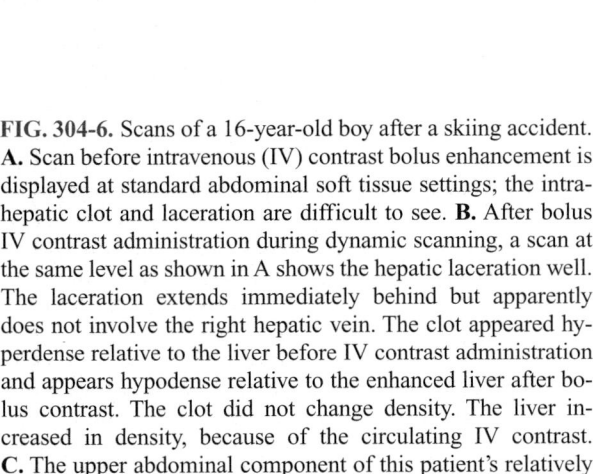

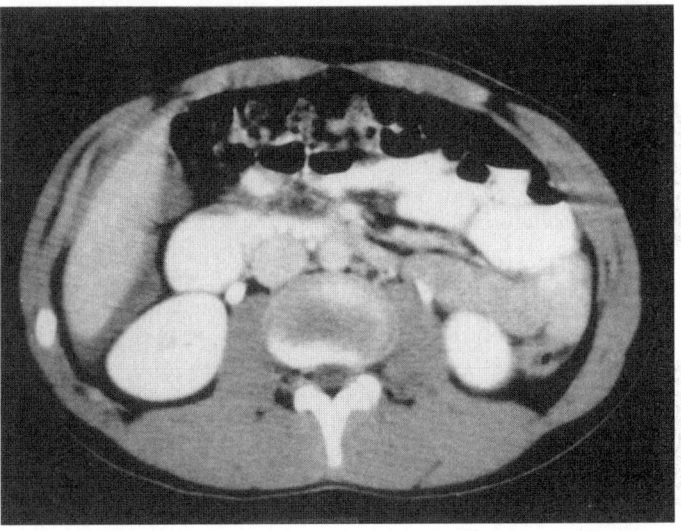

C

FIG. 304-6. Scans of a 16-year-old boy after a skiing accident. **A.** Scan before intravenous (IV) contrast bolus enhancement is displayed at standard abdominal soft tissue settings; the intrahepatic clot and laceration are difficult to see. **B.** After bolus IV contrast administration during dynamic scanning, a scan at the same level as shown in A shows the hepatic laceration well. The laceration extends immediately behind but apparently does not involve the right hepatic vein. The clot appeared hyperdense relative to the liver before IV contrast administration and appears hypodense relative to the enhanced liver after bolus contrast. The clot did not change density. The liver increased in density, because of the circulating IV contrast. **C.** The upper abdominal component of this patient's relatively small hemoperitoneum is seen as blood in Morison's pouch (the right posterior subhepatic space between the liver and kidney). (Courtesy of Jeremy J. Hollerman, MD).

REFERENCES

1. Romans LE: *Introduction to Computed Tomography.* Media, PA, Williams & Wilkins, 1995.
2. Napel SA: Basic principles of spiral CT, in Fishman EK, Jeffrey RB Jr (eds): *Spiral CT: Principles, Techniques and Clinical Applications.* New York, Raven, 1995, p. 1.
3. Brink JA: Technical aspects of helical (spiral) CT. *Radiol Clin North Am* 33:825, 1995.
4. Mortele KJ, McTavish J, Ros PR: Current techniques of computed tomography: Helical CT, multidetector CT, and 3D reconstruction. *Clin Liver Dis* 6:29, 2002.
5. Rubin GD, Shiau MC, Leung AN, et al: Aorta and iliac arteries: Single versus multidetector-row helical CT angiography. *Radiology* 215:670, 2000.
6. Grainger RG, Allison D, Adam A, Dixon A (eds): *Grainger and Allison's Diagnostic Radiology: A Textbook of Medical Imaging,* 4th ed. London, Churchill Livingstone, 2001.
7. Achenbach S, Moshage W, Ropers D, et al: Value of electron-beam computed tomography for the noninvasive detection of high-grade coronary-artery stenoses and occlusions. *New Engl J Med* 339:1964, 1998.
8. Rao PM, Rhea JT, Novelline RA, et al: Effect of computed tomography of the appendix on treatment of patients and the use of hospital resources. *New Engl J Med* 338:141, 1998.

MAGNETIC RESONANCE IMAGING: PRINCIPLES AND SOME APPLICATIONS
Irwin D. Weisman

The significant advances in imaging technology of recent years have dramatically expedited diagnosis and improved outcomes in emergency department patients, and magnetic resonance imaging (MRI) has been at the forefront. In just a short time, it has become a major adjunct for neurologic and musculoskeletal evaluation.

Magnetic resonance imaging has the following major advantages:

1. Like ultrasound, it does not use ionizing radiation and no short-term or long-term side effects have been demonstrated. This is in contrast to the high-energy ionizing radiation of computed tomography (CT) and other x-ray methods, which produce small but finite biologic damage that may have long-term carcinogenic implications. Because of this consideration, where applicable, MRI should be preferred over CT and tomography in the pediatric and childbearing female populations.

2. It produces variable-thickness, two-dimensional slices in any orientation through the body part of interest, thus optimizing visualization of tissues and their interfaces. With few exceptions, CT is restricted to a scan plane[1] that is transverse to the long axis of the body.

3. Because of the different physical principles underlying magnetic resonance (as opposed to x-rays), it provides better contrast resolution and tissue discrimination in many areas compared with x-rays or ultrasound. For example, spinal cord, bone marrow, muscles, and tendons are better visualized with MRI than with CT. As a result, MRI is replacing invasive methods such as myelography, arthrography, and increasingly, catheter angiography.

MRI is a specific application of nuclear magnetic resonance to medical imaging.[1,2] Nuclear magnetic resonance was discovered simultaneously in 1946 by Bloch and colleagues at Stanford University[3] and by Purcell and colleagues at Harvard University.[4] Bloch and Purcell shared the Nobel Prize in 1952 for their outstanding contribution to the physical sciences.

PHYSICAL BASIS

The nuclei of hydrogen in water and fat molecules behave like small spinning bar magnets. When placed in a strong uniform magnetic field (greater than 0.01 tesla or 100 gauss), they execute a circular motion, or precession, weakly aligning to form a net nuclear polarization nearly parallel to the external magnetic field. If a short pulse of radio frequency (rf) energy (radio wave) is applied that is precisely tuned to the precession frequency of the water and fat proton nuclear magnets, the nuclei absorb a small amount of energy, change their alignment, and then gradually return to their previous equilibrium positions. In responding to the radio wave, the net nuclear magnetization generates a small voltage: the nuclear magnetic resonance signal. This can be detected and recorded electronically.

Two parameters, T1 and T2, also known as longitudinal and transverse relaxation times respectively, govern the behavior of the electronic signal detected. The relaxation times are a function of the immediate environment of the resonating protons and vary in the different biologic tissues. For example, free water exhibits long T1 and T2 values and fat exhibits short T1 and relatively short T2 values. Image generation requires a large number of repetitions of the sequence that produces the nuclear resonance signal. The time between repetitions is called TR. For technical reasons, a two-pulse sequence is used to generate a particular type of signal called a spin echo. The spacing between pulses is labeled TE/2, and an echo occurs at a time TE. There are important relationships between the intensity of the nuclear magnetic resonance echo and TR, T1, TE, and T2. Based on the effects of the different relaxation times (T1 and T2), two types of imaging are carried out. Short repetition times (TR) between successive cycles of rf excitation pulses and short echo times (TE) produce stronger signals from tissues with relatively short T1 times, such as fat, especially bone marrow. Hence, weighting favoring short T1 results from pulse sequences using short TR and short TE. On the other hand, longer TRs eliminate much of the T1 signal difference between fat and water, so that further manipulation of the rf pulse spacing (longer TE) will enhance signals from tissues with long T2 times, such as edema fluid. Long TR, TE pulse sequences preferentially weight long T2 tissues. Thus, the two basic methods of MRI scanning are labeled T1-weighted and T2-weighted imaging.

To construct an image from the tissue-specific signals of an object (for example, a patient), it is necessary to apply small, spatially inhomogeneous, three-dimensional magnetic fields called gradients. They modify the signal decay of the nuclear magnetization and spatially tag the hydrogen nuclear magnets in the object for mapping the image. The actual reconstruction of an image is complex, just as in CT scanning, and requires a relatively fast computer with a large memory.

The ultimate result is a two-dimensional, medically diagnostic, cross-sectional body image that is displayed on a video monitor and recorded on film or digitally stored on a hard disk or magnetic tape as a permanent record. In most gray-scale imaging formats, the strongest signal corresponds to maximum brightness on the black-and-white monitor. Therefore, in heavily T2-weighted images, water appears bright, whereas fat appears intermediate gray. On the other hand, on T1-weighted images, fat appears bright and water appears dark (Figure 305-1). Another commonly used basic imaging mode is proton density weighting, crudely described as a balance between T1 and T2 weighting. Table 305-1 lists the expected signal intensities for several biologic tissues in these three cases. Many newer and more sophisticated imaging pulse sequences have evolved from this imaging framework, such as chemical fat suppression, inversion recovery, short T1 inversion recovery (STIR), fluid attenuation inversion recovery (FLAIR), gradient echo recall, magnetization transfer, rapid acquisition with relaxation enhancement (RARE), echo planar, and diffusion gradient. For a more complete discussion of the technical aspects and clinical applications of MRI, readers are referred to more specialized texts.[5,6]

The physical basis of image formation using MRI is quite different from CT, which is based on differential x-ray absorption coefficients. Even though both are tomographic imaging techniques, the meaning of bright and dark signals in MRI is relative to the pulse sequence eliciting them and has very little resemblance to the contrast in CT.

The core of an MRI system is the large magnet needed to generate the strong, constant, and uniform magnetic field, as well as the magnetic gradients. The magnet is composed of coils of a special superconducting wire that loses all resistance to electrical current when submerged in liquid helium. At this temperature, $-269°C$ ($-450°F$), the coils can handle the relatively large currents of electricity required to produce the magnetic field. A specially designed, thermally insulated container encloses the magnet coils and the liquid helium. The liquid slowly boils away and must be replaced at regular intervals. The magnet is housed in a special room containing steel sheets and copper screen, which shield the system against interference by steel and radio waves on the outside and vice versa. The other components of the system, consisting of a radio transmitter, a sophisticated rf receiver, and a high-speed large-memory computer, are located near the operator's console just outside the room.

SAFETY

The only hazard associated with diagnostic x-rays is the effect on biological tissue of ionizing radiation, but this is well known and documented. Although no definite long-term harmful effects have been attributed to MRI, there are known potential safety concerns that need to be addressed (Table 305-2). In a few cases, the large static magnetic field could be a health hazard to the patient,[7-9] necessitating the use of alternative diagnostic methods such as ultrasound or CT. Internal cardiac pacemakers may be converted to an abnormal asynchronous mode by the magnetic field. Certain types of steel cerebral aneurysm clips (ferromagnetic as opposed to nonmagnetic stainless steel) may be subject to strong forces, with the potential of harming the brain. Small steel slivers embedded in the eye (occasionally seen in asymptomatic sheet metal workers or welders) could injure the retina and cause blindness. Life-support equipment containing magnetic steel will be strongly attracted into the magnetic field, threatening both the patient and the system. Injuries from unsecured apparatus have been known to occur.

Cochlear implants may be damaged or cause unacceptable injury due to eddy current heating effects. Patients in any of the aforementioned categories cannot be scanned with MRI. There are other devices, such as implantable cardiac defibrillators, neurostimulators, and bone growth stimulators that may malfunction in the presence of high magnetic fields. Certain prosthetic heart valves contain nearly magnetic stainless steel components that are subject to strong forces when placed in powerful magnetic fields. However, it has been pointed out

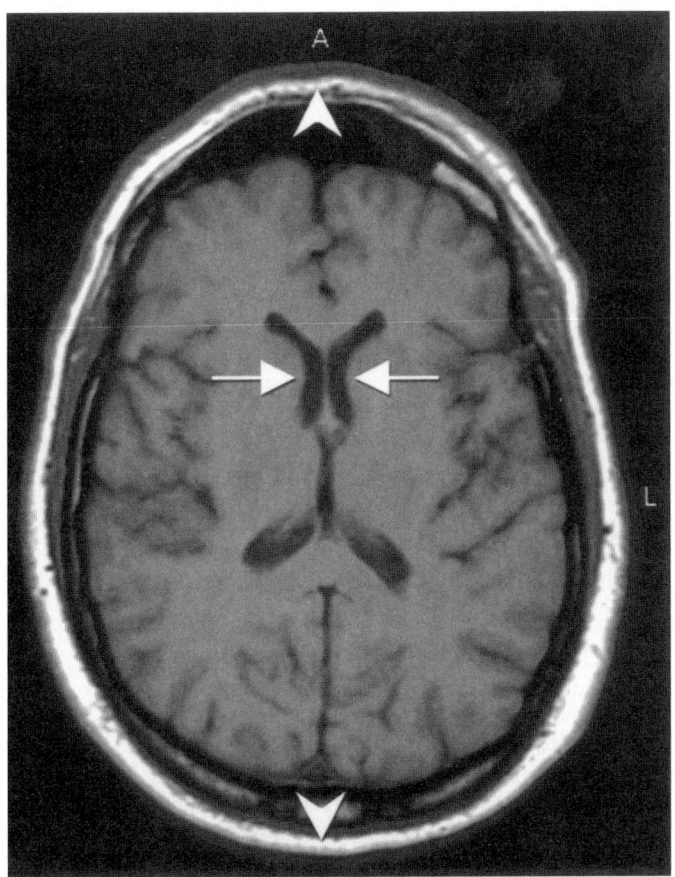
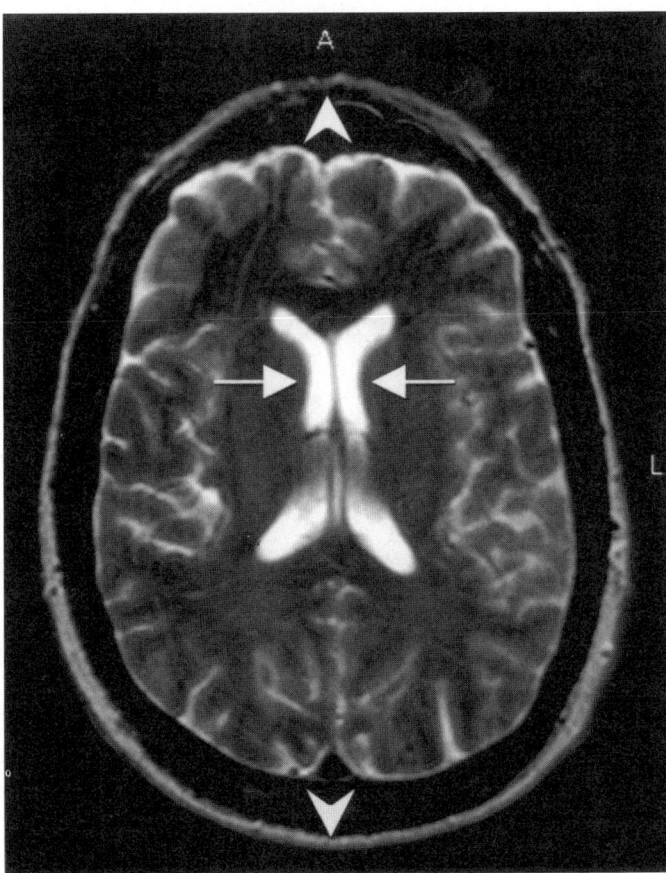

A   B

FIG. 305-1. Examples of T1-weighted and T2-weighted magnetic resonance images. **A.** T1-weighted axial image: note that the cerebrospinal fluid in the lateral ventricles of the brain (*white arrows*), which is essentially water with a long T1, appears dark, whereas the subcutaneous fat around the calvarium with a short T1 appears bright (*white arrowhead*). **B.** T2-weighted axial image of the same brain as in **A.** Note that the CSF, which has a long T2, now appears bright, whereas the surrounding subcutaneous fat with its shorter T2 is intermediate in brightness.

that the stress placed on the valve by the heart itself exceeds that generated by even high-field magnets, and hence this is only a relative contraindication to MRI scanning.

The pulsed radio waves and time-varying magnetic field gradients induce electric currents, which are a source of heat energy that is deposited within the body. Software programs built into the computers restrict the frequency of pulsing so that the maximum allowable power deposition averaged over the whole patient is never exceeded. Occasionally, superficial burns have been reported when a patient's skin has come into direct contact with uninsulated wire leads near the transmitter coils, but taking proper precautions prevent this from happening.

The complete examination takes from 30 to 60 min, is painless, and is well tolerated by most patients. It does require suspension of all motion (except for breathing) for periods ranging from a few seconds to 15 min at a time, depending on the particular pulse sequence. Some patients are claustrophobic and have difficulty with the examination. Most problems of this nature are satisfactorily treated with minor tranquilizers administered orally. Some of these patients may need to be

referred to open architecture, less confining low-field MR scanners with possible reduced diagnostic sensitivity. Patients heavier than 140 kg (300 lb) may be over the weight limit for most high field scanners (>0.5 T). However, they can usually be accommodated in the low-field magnets because of the less restrictive environment. Infants, younger pediatric patients, and agitated adults need to be sedated as in CT, because any motion degrades the MRI scan. Development of MR-compatible pulsed oximeters has made sedation more routine.

Some minor precautions are necessary. Magnetically encoded plastic cards, such as credit, cash, and parking cards, may be damaged when they come within a certain distance of the magnetic field. Some watches with steel parts and hearing aids (and their batteries) are vulnerable to damage. Any ferromagnetic steel objects are potentially lethal missiles if carried into the magnet room. Patients need to leave such objects outside the scanning room. Deaths and at least one case of blindness have been reported in connection with the above-mentioned hazards.[7] Another minor hazard is the loud noise produced by the gradient coils, which has the potential to produce long-term

TABLE 305-1   Tissue Appearance in Magnetic Resonance Imaging

Weight	TR (ms)	TE (ms)	Fat	Water	Muscle	Ligament	Bone Cortex
T1	300–600	20–30	Bright	Dark	Intermediate	Dark	Dark
Proton density	2000–6000	10–40	Intermediate	Intermediate	Intermediate	Dark	Dark
T2	2000–6000	60–120	Intermediate	Bright	Intermediate	Dark	Dark

Note: Above values for TR and TE are relative and not absolute.

TABLE 305-2   Emergency Department Patients in the Magnetic Resonance Environment

Device/Equipment	Action/Substitute
Pulse monitoring	MR-compatible pulse monitor*
Blood oxygenation	MR-compatible blood oxygen monitor*
Blood pressure	MR-compatible blood pressure device*
Oxygen therapy	Wall O$_2$ in the MR suite, or aluminum MR oxygen cylinders
Medication infusion pumps	Multiple high-pressure extension tubings, to place the infusion pump outside of the high-gauss magnetic field
Anesthesia pump	MR-compatible anesthesia pump*
Swan-Ganz catheters	Not MR compatible
External fixation devices, halo devices	Some compatible; consult with MR personnel and provide type/manufacturer
Electrocardiogram monitoring	Diagnostic waveforms are not available in the MR environment; low-level capability for identifying prominent arthymias is available

*Available from MR department personnel.
Abbreviation: MR = magnetic resonance.
Source: Courtesy of D. Bluemke.

hearing loss. This can be addressed by offering the patients earplugs or other noise-attenuating devices.

In summary, patients with implanted cardiac pacemakers, defibrillators, ferromagnetic cerebral aneurysm clips, or cochlear electronic devices, should not have MRI examinations. It is difficult to compose a complete list of preclusion to MRI as the arena of MR safety continues to expand and become more complex with proliferation of more sophisticated implant and monitoring devices. These issues have been addressed recently with further updates.[7,9] The list is constantly being modified (extended or contracted) as technology changes and as clinicians gain more experience with implantable systems.[7–9]

APPLICATIONS

MRI has been widely applied to the brain and spinal cord,[10] where it provides images that are superior in diagnostic quality to those obtained with CT. Furthermore, this information can be obtained with less risk to patients because CT myelography requires intrathecal contrast agents for a specific diagnosis. Although special intravenous contrast agents are frequently required to improve the sensitivity of MRI, they have been associated with much less toxicity (including decreased incidence of renal failure) and reactions as compared with the intravenous CT contrast agents. However, some precautions are advised, especially in cases of established asthma and early pregnancy.[7,9] Recent developments in echo planar and diffusion imaging make it possible to diagnose cytotoxic cerebral edema almost immediately after an acute ischemic event, even earlier than with CT or conventional MRI. This has obvious implications with the advent of more aggressive fibrinolytic therapy aimed at early salvage of brain tissue after strokes. Figure 305-2 demonstrates an acute pontine infarct shown by MRI that takes advantage of diffusion imaging. CT is notoriously insensitive in this area of the brain.

Except in the cases of acute intracerebral hemorrhage, skull fracture, and some calcified brain lesions, MRI may completely replace CT of the head. The exact role of MRI versus CT in trauma and degenerative disease of the spine is still evolving.

CT visualizes fracture fragment relationships and bone detail more optimally, but MRI visualizes the soft tissues with better resolution. Because of its sensitivity to marrow and trabecular bone changes, MRI is more accurate in detecting acute fractures, especially in the hips and knees where CT and plain film findings may sometimes be equivocal.

MRI has been useful in examining the chest and abdomen (especially the chest wall, mediastinum, liver, spleen, adrenals, pulmonary arteries, and aorta), but has played a lesser role compared with CT because of respiratory motion and heart pulsation artifacts that degrade anatomic delineation of critical structures. They can be compensated for to some degree

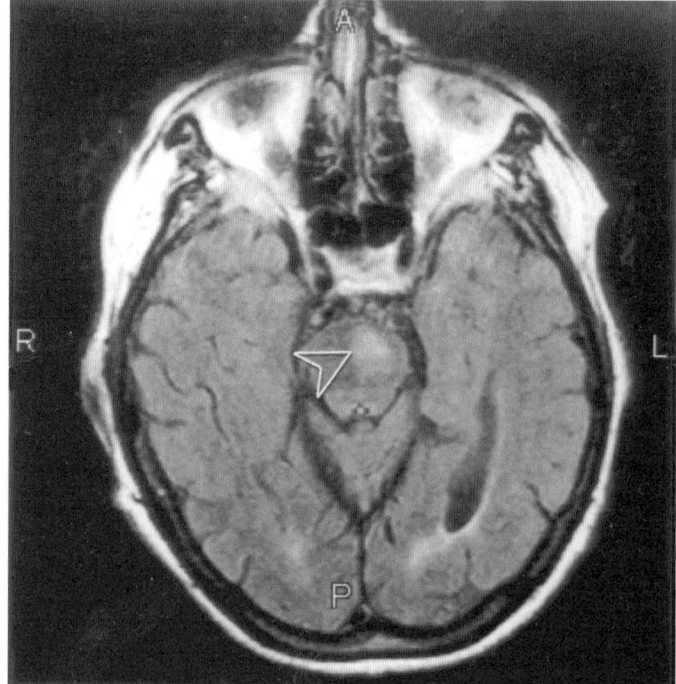

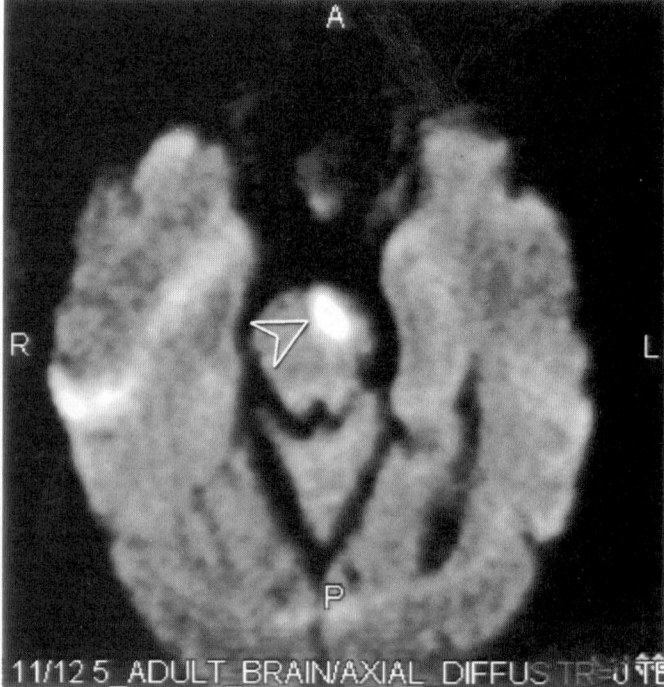

A   B

FIG. 305-2. Acute pontine infarct. **A.** FLAIR (fluid attenuated inversion recovery) axial image of the brainstem demonstrates a questionable area of increased signal in the left pons (*white arrowhead*). **B.** Diffusion axial image through the same region as the image in **A** delineates a hyperintense signal (*white arrowhead*) indicating a focus of restricted diffusion most consistent with an acute pontine infarct.

with electrocardiograph and respiratory gating and associated electronic manipulation, but the methods are cumbersome and difficult to implement with an acutely ill patient. A recent innovation is the introduction of breath-hold MR cholangiography for the noninvasive evaluation of the biliary and pancreatic ducts.[11] It has had limited application to cooperative patients with biliary or pancreatic disease not amenable to ultrasound, CT, or other conventional methods. There has also been progress in cardiac MRI,[5,12] but introduction of these methods into the emergency practice are currently limited due to cost, availability, and reproducibility.

MRI has a major role in other areas of the musculoskeletal system,[6] especially the knee, shoulder, hip, and temporomandibular joints. Although MRI is not indicated for most acute fractures, it may be preferred in the diagnosis of rotator cuff tear of the shoulder, internal derangement of the knee (meniscus, tendon, and ligament tears), tendon or soft tissue injury to any of the small joints, soft tissue injury in the spine, and posttraumatic avascular necrosis of any bone. In addition, carpal tunnel syndrome has been evaluated using MRI. Figure 305-3 demonstrates a meniscus tear in the knee. Before MRI, arthrography,

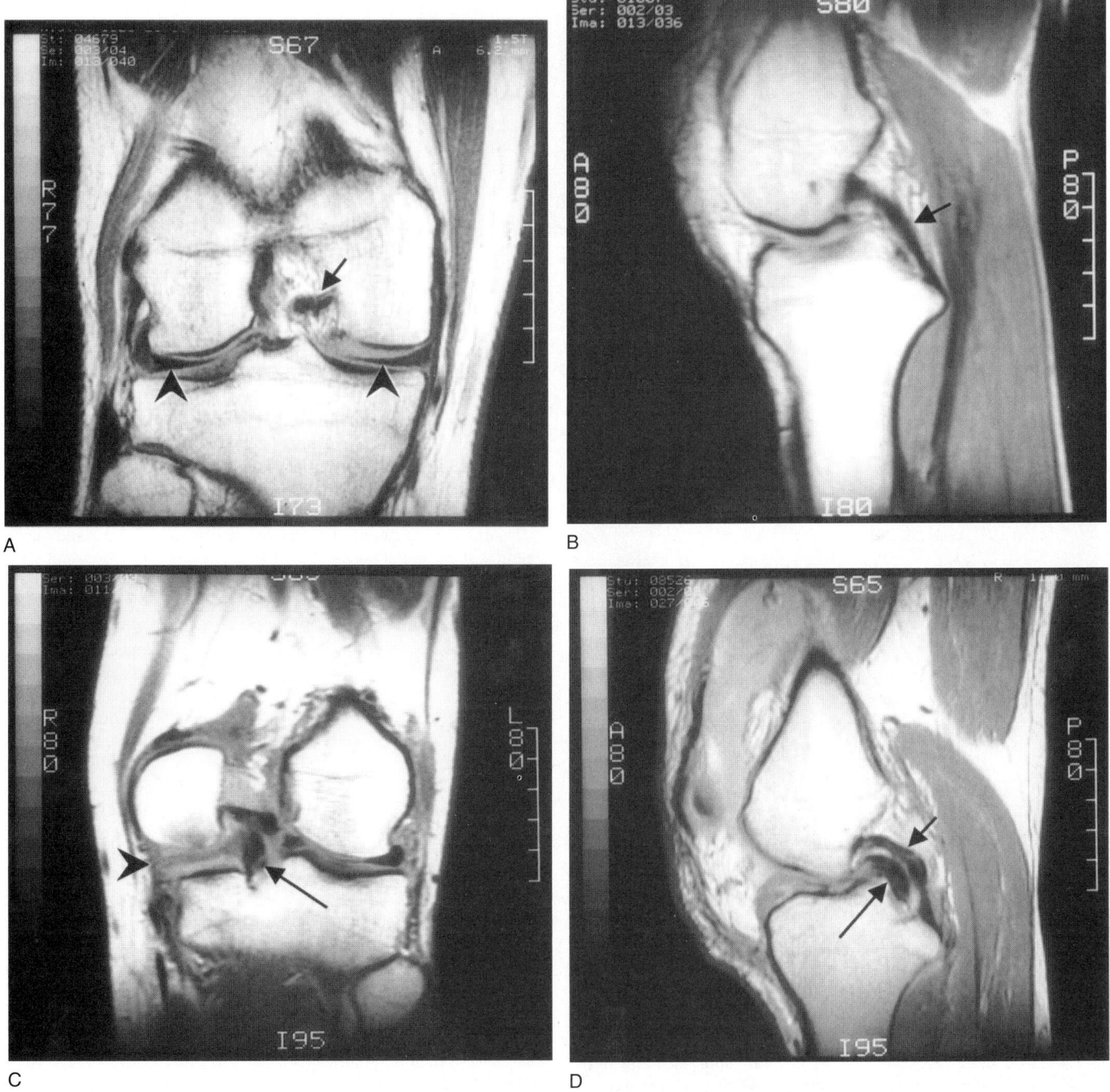

FIG. 305-3. Bucket-handle meniscal tear. **A.** Normal medial and lateral menisci and **B.** normal posterior cruciate ligament in the intercondylar notch as demonstrated on magnetic resonance proton-density (partial T2 weighting) coronal and sagittal images. The menisci are the dark triangular structures in **A** marked with arrowheads. The normal posterior cruciate ligament is shown as a small black arrow in **A** and **B. C.** Proton-density coronal scan showing a large complex tear involving the posterior horn of the medial meniscus (*black arrowhead*) with most of the fragment displaced into the intercondylar notch (the "bucket-handle," *long black arrow*) inferior to the normal posterior cruciate ligament. **D.** Sagittal proton-density image showing the meniscal fragment (*long black arrow*) displaced under the posterior cruciate ligament (*short black arrow*) and having a similar appearance ("double PCL sign"). Not shown is the "bucket" part of the meniscus, which stays attached to the medial tibia.

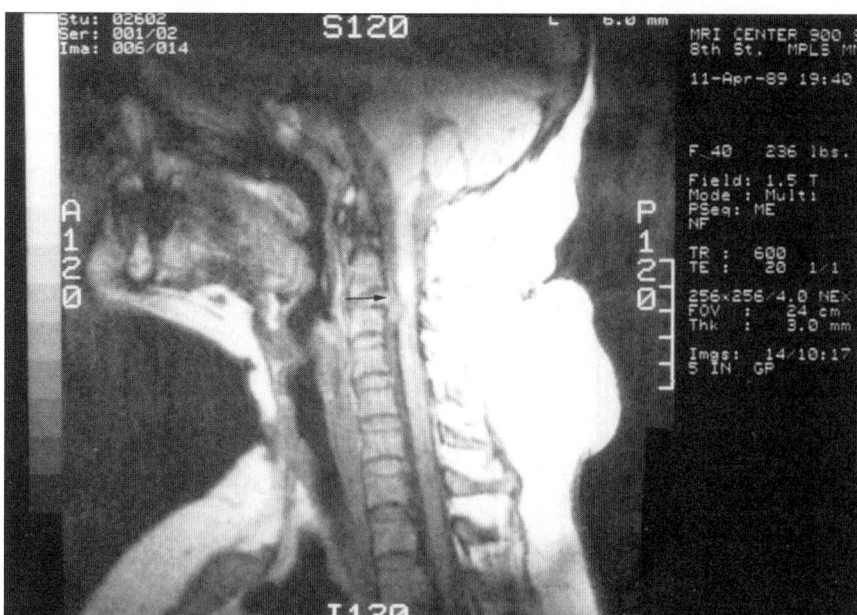

FIG. 305-4. Cervical spinal cord compression. T1-weighted sagittal magnetic resonance imaging demonstrates moderate spinal cord compression by an acute traumatically herniated disk at the C2-3 level (*arrow*). The patient was in a motor vehicle accident and also suffered associated bilateral C2 pedicle fractures.

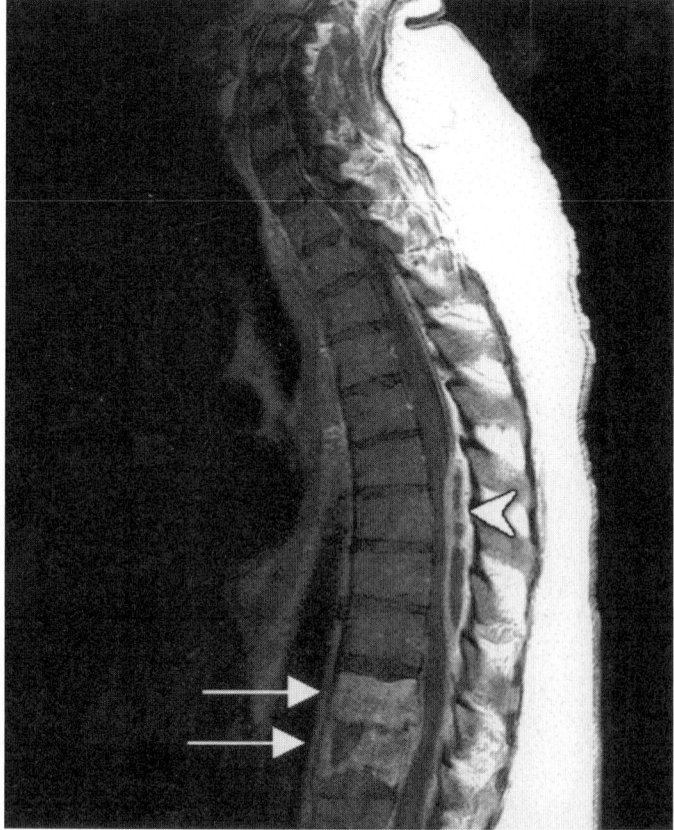

FIG. 305-5. Thoracic spinal cord compression due to osteomyelitis/discitis and epidural abscess. T1-weighted fat suppressed and intravenous gadolinium contrast-enhanced sagittal image of the thoracic spine demonstrates abnormal signal in the vertebral bodies of T10 and T11 with associated disk space and end plate destruction (*white arrows*) consistent with discitis and osteomyelitis. There is an epidural abscess with an enhancing capsule (*white arrowhead*) posterior to the vertebral bodies of T6-T9, which compresses the thoracic spinal cord anterior to the abscess.

which involves injection of contrast agents into the joint, was used to detect cartilage injuries. This type of examination is not only painful but carries a small but measurable risk of infection and contrast reaction. MRI of these joints is painless and only requires that the patient be able to hold still for a moderate length of time. The information obtained in the knee and hips exceeds what can be obtained using other methods. In the hips, MRI has proven to be the most reliable method for detecting avascular necrosis.

In problematic cases, MRI has detected stress fractures and occult fractures in the small bones of the hand. Even though it does not visualize cortex, any break in the medullary cancellous bone can be readily detected.

The sequelae of soft tissue musculoskeletal trauma, such as complete muscular or tendon tears, hemorrhage, and edema, are very easily diagnosed with MRI. Even injuries to the medium-sized nerves and brachial plexus can be demonstrated.[13,14]

MRI has also been used to study infection in bone and soft tissues, where in many cases it has been superior to modalities such as nuclear medicine and CT.[15,16] However, if the patient has a metallic prosthesis in the region of the abnormality, rf currents or magnetic field inhomogeneities due to the metal induce artifacts in the MRI scan reduce the sensitivity. This is even more of a problem in CT, where x-ray scattering from the prosthesis may completely obliterate the scan. In such cases only nuclear medicine studies may be useful, in particular indium[111] tagged to white blood cells.

MRI is extremely sensitive and specific in detecting metastatic disease in bone when questions arise after a positive bone scan. MRI is neither practical nor cost effective to use for whole body surveys, but when applied to specific lesions, the anatomic information expedites diagnosis.

CT continues to be the modality of choice for suspected head, spine, and abdominal injuries, because it is quick, more widely available, and more compatible with life-support equipment. Although MRI-compatible respirators and pulsed oximeters are now available, most standard life-support equipment either contains magnetic steel components or sensitive electronics that will not operate properly in the presence of rf or large static or dynamic magnetic fields. MRI is used in an elective setting after a patient has been stabilized and there is time to address the less acute problems.

MRI IN THE EMERGENT SETTING

At present there are two areas where MRI is the procedure of choice in the acute setting: (1) evaluation of suspected spinal cord compression from any cause, and (2) radiographically occult femoral intertrochanteric and neck fractures. In both cases, the unique ability to form images in axial, coronal, or sagittal planes gives MRI a distinct advantage. Another major factor is the superb contrast resolution of MRI that facilitates detection of spinal cord injury or fracture through cancellous bone of the hip. Figure 305-4 demonstrates an example of cervical cord compression resulting from a traumatically herniated disk. Thoracic cord compression due to infection is shown in Figure 305-5. Figure 305-6 is an example of an occult femoral intertrochanteric fracture best demonstrated on MRI. Small studies[17,18] have confirmed higher sensitivity and specificity for MRI as compared with radionuclide bone scanning, tomography, and CT in the detection of occult fractures, especially in the femoral head and neck.

Another potential area for MRI evaluation in the acute setting is aortic dissection. MRI is superior to contrast-enhanced CT and possibly transesophageal ultrasound in delineating the aortic intimal flap. Unfortunately, many of these patients are unstable hemodynamically and are agitated, requiring life support and sedation. Thus few, if any, are good candidates for MRI. As more MRI-compatible life-support and monitoring equipment becomes available, this situation will change.

Finally, a second potential application is in pediatric fractures[19] when there may be significant injury to unossified cartilage around open growth plates. Fractures through cartilage are not seen on plain films but are easily identified on MRI.

One innovation—the development of low and very low magnetic field imaging systems—may have some impact on emergency departments. Most of the hazards previously delineated apply to high-field systems. In low-field systems, in which the magnetic flux density is less in magnitude and more restricted in spatial extent, it is easier to accommodate life-support equipment. The design of these units allows more access to the patient and reduces the chances of interference with the proper operation of the life-support electronics. Thus installation of a low-field MRI scanner in the emergency department becomes more feasible. However, because of theoretical considerations, signal to noise is much less (i.e., less signal) at low field. Therefore there may be trade-off in diagnostic quality of the scans. Some signal can be recovered with optimal design of the software and hardware, but this remains a controversial area. There may be a place for low-field MRI in the emergent setting in the evaluation of subacute intracerebral hemorrhage and brain edema.

MR angiography, which (except for innocuous intravenous contrast) is noninvasive, has been evolving slowly and improving steadily.[5] It may eventually be the method of choice in the emergent evaluation of suspected subarachnoid hemorrhage or in leaking aortic aneurysms. An example of an intravenous contrast MR angiogram delineating a subclavian "steal" syndrome is shown in Figure 305-7.

MRI continues to evolve with more potential applications to emergency medicine in addition to its role in spinal cord compression, radiographically occult fractures, and acute aortic dissection. The new areas are diffusion imaging (to detect early strokes), noninvasive cerebral and body MRI angiography, and in the future cardiac and pulmonary MRI angiography. Taking advantage of its compatibility with life-support equipment, further development of a low magnetic field system with improved signal to noise might accelerate introduction of the above applications into emergency medicine practice.

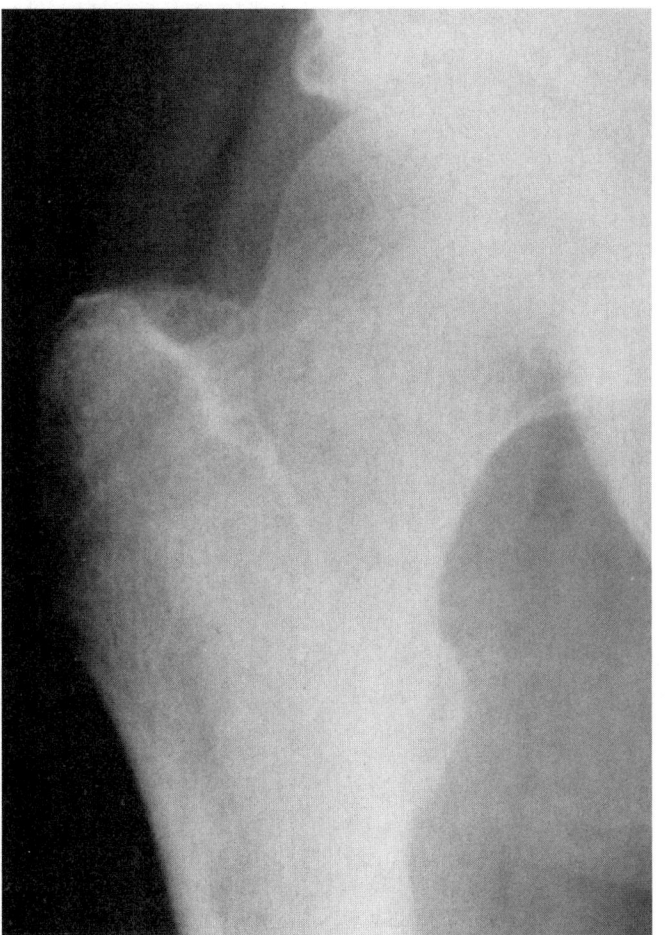

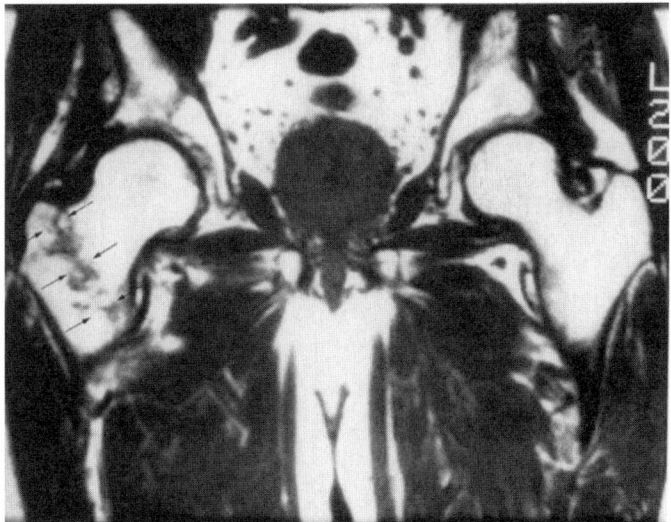

FIG. 305-6. Occult hip fracture. **A.** Anteroposterior radiograph of a 55-year-old patient on steroids who had right hip pain after a fall. No fracture is evident. **B.** T1-weighted coronal magnetic resonance scan of the same hip clearly demonstrates a nondisplaced intertrochanteric femoral shaft fracture (*arrows*).

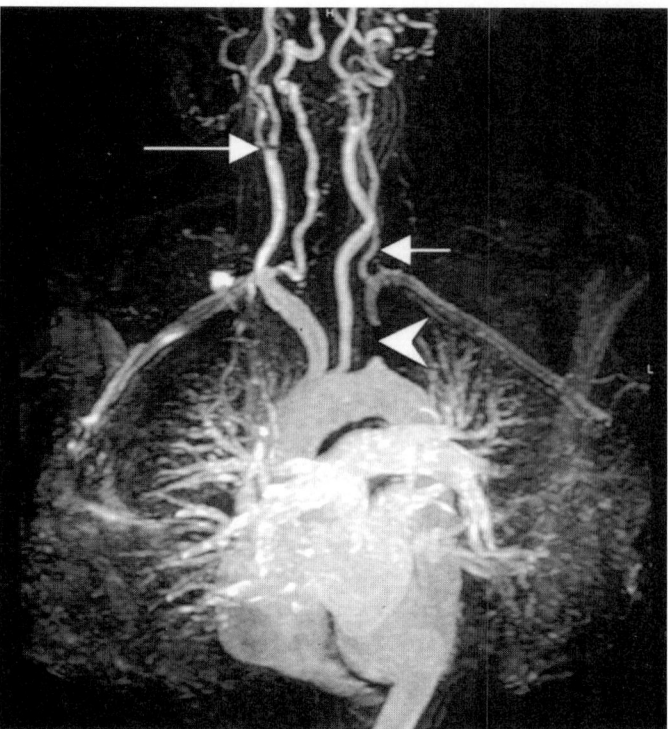

FIG. 305-7. Intravenous contrast-enhanced magnetic resonance angiogram of the aorta and great vessels delineates the major lesion of a subclavian "steal" syndrome. Image of the aortic arch and great vessels reconstructed from computer generated maximum-intensity projection data after a three-dimensional volume acquisition following an injected intravenous bolus of a gadolinium chelate. A long segmental subtotal occlusion of the proximal left subclavian (*solid white arrowhead*) predisposes the patient to a subclavian steal situation. In that case, blood needed to supply the left arm is "stolen" from the brain via reversed flow in the left vertebral artery (*short white arrow*). There is a second major lesion, a significant stenosis in the right internal carotid artery (*long white arrow*).

REFERENCES

1. Lauterbur PC: Image formation by induced local interactions: Example employing nuclear magnetic resonance. *Nature* 242:190, 1973.
2. Kumar A, Welti D, Ernst RR: NMR Fourier zeugmatography. *J Magn Reson* 18:69, 1975.
3. Bloch F, Hansen WW, Packard M: Nuclear induction. *Phys Rev* 69:127, 1946.
4. Purcell EM, Torrey HC, Pound RV: Resonance absorption by nuclear magnetic moments in a solid. *Phys Rev* 69:37, 1946.
5. Stark DD, Bradley WG Jr (eds): *Magnetic Resonance Imaging,* 3d ed. St. Louis, Mosby, 1999.
6. Stoller DW (ed): *Magnetic Resonance Imaging in Orthopaedics and Sports Medicine.* Philadelphia, Lippincott-Raven, 1997.
7. Kanal E (ed): *Practical MR Safety Considerations for Physicians, Physicists, and Technologists.* Oak Brook, IL, Radiological Society of North America, 2001.
8. Shellock FG. *Pocket Guide to MR Procedures and Metallic Objects: Update 1999.* Philadelphia, Lippincott Williams & Wilkins, 1999.
9. Kanal E, Borgstede JP, Barkovich AJ, et al: American College of Radiology White Paper on MR Safety. *AJR* 178:1335, 2002.
10. Atlas SW (ed): *Magnetic Resonance of the Brain and Spine,* 3d ed. Philadelphia, Lippincott Williams & Wilkins, 2002.
11. Fulcher AS, Turner MA, Capps GW, et al: Half-Fourier RARE MR cholangiopancreatography: Experience in 300 subjects. *Radiology* 207:21, 1998.
12. Manning WJ, Pennell DJ (eds): *Cardiovascular Magnetic Resonance.* Philadelphia, Churchill Livingstone, 2002.
13. Wittenberg KH, Adkins MC: MR imaging of nontraumatic brachial plexopathies: Frequency and spectrum of findings. *Radiographics* 20:1023, 2000.
14. Kneeland JB, Kellman GM, Middleton WD, et al: Diagnosis of diseases of the supraclavicular region by use of MR imaging. *AJR* 148:1149, 1987.
15. Erdman WA, Tamburro F, Jayson HT, et al: Osteomyelitis: Characteristics and pitfalls of diagnosis with MR imaging. *Radiology* 180:533, 1991.
16. Ledermann HP, Morrison WB, Schweitzer ME: MR image analysis of pedal osteomyelitis: Distribution, patterns of spread, and frequency of associated ulceration and septic arthritis. *Radiology* 223:747, 2002.
17. Deutsch AL, Mink JH, Waxman AD: Occult fractures of the proximal femur: MR imaging. *Radiology* 170:113, 1989.
18. Quinn SF, McCarthy JL: Prospective evaluation of patients with suspected hip fracture and indeterminate radiographs: Use of T1-weighted MR images. *Radiology* 187:469, 1993.
19. Jaramillo D, Shapiro F: Musculoskeletal trauma in children. *MRI Clin North Am* 6:521, 1998.

INJECTION DRUG USERS
Brigitte M. Baumann
Suzanne M. Shepherd

The practice of injection drug use and the lifestyle of the injection drug user (IDU), place the individual at risk for a wide variety of infectious and noninfectious complications.[1] In addition to an increased risk of the human immunodeficiency virus (HIV), hepatitis, and sexually transmitted diseases, the IDU's lifestyle is also associated with an increased risk of trauma. The high incidence of homelessness, nutritional deficiencies, smoking and alcohol use, and mental illness further compromise this population's health.

Approximately 2.4 million individuals in the United States have used heroin at some point in their lives, with nearly 130,000 having used it within the past 30 days.[2] The ED is a common point of entry to health care for many IDUs, with an estimated 14 percent of all drug-related ED episodes involving heroin. Between 1991 and 1996, heroin-related ED episodes more than doubled (from 35,898 to 73,846) and in youths aged 12 to 17 years, heroin-related episodes nearly quadrupled.[2] To adequately evaluate IDUs, health care providers should be aware of the drugs used in their catchment area as well as their street names. Patients should be asked about drug type(s) and amount, preparation of materials for injection (e.g., licking needles or use of saliva or tap/toilet water for drug reconstitution), reuse of needles, needle sharing, use of antibiotics, and coincident illness. Socioeconomic issues such as the IDU's ability to purchase medications and return for follow-up should also be addressed when making dispositions. The IDU should receive nonjudgmental instruction in measures to reduce the risk of complications and infections. Finally, drug rehabilitation (even as a referral) should always be offered.

PATHOPHYSIOLOGY

In addition to placing patients at greater risk for immunocompromising infections such as HIV and hepatitis, IDU itself has been associated with immune dysfunction. Exaggerated and atypical lymphocytosis, diminished lymphocyte responsiveness to mitogenic stimulation, hypergammaglobulinemia, increased opsonin production, high levels of circulating immune complexes, and reticuloendothelial abnormalities, have been found. Because of this immune stimulation, false-positive syphilis serology, positive Coombs tests, and thrombotic thrombocytopenic purpura have all been described in this population. Given immune dysfunction, febrile IDUs should be suspected of having infections, even when the fever is low grade and with normal/near-normal white blood counts and erythrocyte sedimentation rates.[3]

CLINICAL FEATURES

Complications of the IDU may be obvious, such as a painful mass caused by a skin abscess. However, constitutional symptoms such as weakness, anorexia, body pains, weight loss, and fever are common and may be the only subtle sign(s) of serious underlying disease (Table 306-1).

Fever

Fever is part of the presenting complaint in the majority of ED visits by IDUs and is associated with infection in more than two-thirds of patients.[4] Prospective studies of febrile IDUs have found bacteremia in up to 42 percent, pneumonia in 26 to 38 percent, and endocarditis in up to 13 percent of patients.[4] Neither clinical judgment nor derived predictive rules were reliable in identifying those with serious underlying causes of fever.[4]

Noninfectious causes of fever include acute toxic reactions to substances of abuse, reactions to injected adulterants, and withdrawal syndromes. Cocaine and amphetamines can cause fevers acutely, occasionally in excess of 40°C (104°F). Adulterants used to dilute active substances may also cause dramatic febrile reactions accompanied by alteration in mental status and leukocytosis. One syndrome known as "cotton fever" is associated with the use of cotton balls as filters for drug suspensions. Patients with cotton fever develop a flulike syndrome within hours after injection. Physical findings may include tachypnea, tachycardia, abdominal pain, and inflammatory retinal nodules. Chest radiographs are typically normal, but may demonstrate inflammatory pulmonary granulomata. This syndrome spontaneously resolves within 24 h. While the cause remains unclear, it has been proposed that the acute symptoms are caused by either endotoxin from gram-negative rods introduced by injection or by the pyrogenic effect of injected cotton particulate matter. Patients withdrawing from barbiturates or heroin also may appear acutely ill, with chest and abdominal pain, diaphoresis, tachycardia, and fever.

Because no reliable markers are available to exclude serious illness in the febrile IDU, common practice has been to obtain blood cultures and admit such patients for observation, awaiting culture results. In clinically well patients for whom follow-up can be ensured, outpatient evaluation is reasonable as long as an adequate cultures are obtained.

Dyspnea

A wide range of both infectious and noninfectious causes may produce dyspnea and cough in IDUs. Pneumonia in IDUs is typically community-acquired. However, other infectious causes for dyspnea include opportunistic infections and septic pulmonary emboli from right-sided endocarditis. The febrile IDU presenting with dyspnea, cough, or an abnormal chest radiograph should be placed in respiratory isolation until tuberculosis has been excluded and/or an alternative diagnosis is found.[5]

Noninfectious causes of dyspnea include pneumothorax, hemothorax, toxic reactions to injected substances, and hypersensitivity reaction. Pneumo- and hemothorax are seen most commonly with the practice of "pocket shooting," when drug users inject into veins in the supraclavicular fossa to access the subclavian, jugular, or brachiocephalic vein. Talc lung is a syndrome of progressive respiratory distress and diffuse interstitial infiltrates caused by the injection of the adulterant talc.[6] Hypersensitivity reactions, associated with both heroin and cocaine injection, present with cough and wheezing and typically respond to inhaled β-agonist therapy. Noncardiogenic pulmonary edema is associated with both heroin and cocaine use. Patients may complain of dyspnea or have a low pulse oximetry reading, with the chest radiograph revealing diffuse alveolar infiltrates; treatment is supportive. Finally, septic, air, or needle fragment emboli can produce dyspnea.[7]

Altered Mental Status

Drug intoxication or withdrawal, stroke syndromes, hypoxia, delayed leukoencephalopathy, infectious diseases, mycotic aneurysms, and secondary trauma from either loss of consciousness and fall or drug-related violence may all cause altered mental status in the IDU. Central nervous system (CNS) infections may be a result of embolic complications of distant infections (e.g., endocarditis) or of extensions of local infections (e.g., vertebral osteomyelitis). Infections commonly

TABLE 306-1 Evaluation of Injection Drug Users in the Emergency Department

Presenting Symptom	Other Findings	Possible Diagnoses	Ancillary Tests
Fever alone	Needle and track marks Heart murmur Rales and rhonchi Hypoxia	Pneumonia Endocarditis Occult bacteremia	Chest radiograph Blood cultures Urinalysis Erythrocyte sedimentation rate Echocardiogram
Fever and nausea/vomiting Rigors Abdominal pain	Diaphoresis Recent injection	Drug withdrawal "Cotton fever"	CBC Blood cultures
Fever and dyspnea/cough	Rales/rhonchi Purulent sputum Hypoxia	Bacterial pneumonia Atypical pneumonia Opportunistic pneumonia	Chest radiograph Blood cultures Sputum culture and Gram stain
Fever and weakness Weight loss Anorexia Night sweats Diarrhea	Cachexia Oral thrush	HIV infection Tuberculosis Hepatitis B and C	HIV serology Blood cultures Chest radiograph Sputum for AFB stain and culture Hepatitis serology
Fever and back pain	Heart murmur Focal neurologic signs Flank tenderness	Osteomyelitis Epidural abscess Endocarditis Renal abscess	Blood cultures Erythrocyte sedimentation rate Bone radiographs CT or MRI Urinalysis
Dyspnea/cough	Expiratory wheezes Rales/rhonchi Fever Pleuritic chest pain	Hypersensitivity reaction Noncardiogenic pulmonary edema Pneumonia Septic pulmonary emboli Talc reaction	Chest radiograph Spirometry Echocardiogram Consider blood cultures
Painful limb	Localized erythema Tenderness Localized bruit Muscle pain/swelling Fever	Cellulitis Abscess Pseudoaneurysm Myositis Fasciitis Retained foreign body	Wound cultures Soft tissue radiographs CT Doppler ultrasonography Consider blood cultures
Altered mental status	Obtundation Focal neurologic signs Meningismus Seizure	Drug overdose/intoxication Drug withdrawal CNS lesion Meningitis Tetanus	CT scan Drug screen Lumbar puncture Consider blood cultures
Eye pain/vision loss	Periorbital vesicles Subconjunctival lesions Keratitis Iridocyclitis Retinitis	Herpes zoster Kaposi's sarcoma Keratoconjunctivitis sicca Herpes simplex CMV Varicella zoster Toxoplasmosis Syphilis Fungal infection	

Abbreviations: AFB = acid-fast bacillus; CBC = complete blood cell count; CMV = cytomegalovirus; CNS = central nervous system; CT = computed tomography; MRI = magnetic resonance imaging.

seen in this population include epidural abscess, bacterial and fungal meningitis, and brain abscess. Meningococcus, pneumococcus, and *Staphylococcus aureus* spreading from a primary endocarditis are the common causes for bacterial meningitis. Opportunistic organisms are common in the patient with coincident HIV infection.

Stroke syndromes may be secondary to low-flow states during heroin intoxication, hypertensive hemorrhage from amphetamines, phencyclidine, or cocaine, and embolized vegetations from infectious endocarditis. Delayed leukoencephalopathies, both hypoxic and non-hypoxic, have been reported in IDUs, but are rare.

Back Pain

Back pain may be the result of an epidural abscess, vertebral os-teomyelitis, or complications from trauma. In patients with coincident

HIV, opportunistic infections may present with a more indolent course. Nontraumatic focal back pain usually requires imagining studies such as computed tomography (CT) and magnetic resonance imaging (MRI) to evaluate for possible infection.

SPECIFIC INFECTIONS

HIV

The use of intravenous drugs plays a major role in the acquisition and transmission of HIV.[8] In the United States, the proportion of HIV cases directly attributable to intravenous drug use is estimated at 50 percent, and HIV seroprevalence rates in IDUs range from 10 to 65 percent. The proportion of HIV cases caused by intravenous drug use increased from 17 to 27 percent from the 1980s to the early 1990s, thought to be largely a result of increasing use of intravenous cocaine. In addition to widespread needle sharing, cocaine's highly addictive properties and short duration of effect encourage frequent injections.

The prevalence of HIV in IDUs has expanded the spectrum of diseases associated with intravenous drug use to include those typically associated with HIV infection. While AIDS-defining illnesses in intravenous drug users are similar in spectrum to those in nonintravenous drug users, the distribution of such diseases appears to be different. IDUs have proportionately more cryptococcal disease, *Pneumocystis carinii* pneumonia, tuberculosis, and wasting syndrome, and significantly less cytomegalovirus (CMV) infection, non-Hodgkin lymphoma, and Kaposi sarcoma.[8] Overall, IDUs generally have a less complicated course than do homosexual HIV patients. However, this advantage is lost by unnecessary complications caused by their psychiatric disorders, noncompliance, and concealment of signs of disease, all of which lead to worse outcomes from infections.

Endocarditis

The incidence of endocarditis in the IDU is estimated to be 40 times that of the general population, or approximately 1 case in 500 IDUs. Unlike the general population, endocarditis in IDUs is typically right-sided (50 to 76 percent), with 40 to 69 percent of cases involving the tricuspid valve, 20 to 30 percent involving the mitral and aortic valves, and 5 to 42 percent involving multiple valves.[3,9] The pathogenesis of right-sided endocarditis in IDUs is thought to be dependent on four factors: (1) endothelial damage; (2) specific interactions between microorganisms and valvular location; (3) degree of bacterial load; and (4) host immune status.[4]

Patients with IDU-related endocarditis usually have no evidence of prior valve damage, a common risk factor for endocarditis in non-IDUs. It is thought that the IDU contributes to endocardial damage via mechanical and ischemic mechanisms. Mechanical damage is caused by both direct bombardment with particulate matter (talc or other diluents) and by increased right-sided pressure gradients and turbulence as a consequence of drug-induced pulmonary hypertension. The tricuspid valve is particularly susceptible to mechanical damage because it is the first valve exposed to these substances. Additional endothelial damage may be caused by chronic valvular inflammation due to frequent antigenic exposure. An increased risk of endocarditis in intravenous cocaine users is attributed to a the greater frequency of injections (increased mechanical damage), less chance of needle sterilization because cocaine does not need to be heated in order to go into solution, and the greater likelihood of needle sharing. An alternative explanation is that the vasoconstrictive properties of cocaine may cause interstitial or endothelial damage which predisposes to infection.

Specific interactions between valvular location and infecting organisms may account for the prevalence of right-sided *Staphylococcus aureus* and *Pseudomonas aeruginosa* endocarditis. *S. aureus* is the most common pathogen in isolated tricuspid valve endocarditis, accounting for 50 to 60 percent of cases among IDUs. *S. aureus* possesses unique surface proteins that enable it to adhere to host tissue. In addition, IDUs are postulated to have a greater expression of matrix molecules that bind to the microbial surface components recognizing adhesive matrix molecules found on injected particulate matter. This increased affinity as well as *S. aureus'* protective fibrin coat enhances vegetation formation and prevents host clearance. Pseudomonas endocarditis is more prevalent in IDUs because of the frequent use of tap or toilet water in the preparation of the street drugs pentazocine and tripelennamine.[3]

Bacterial load is related to the risk of endocarditis in a "dose-response" fashion. The fact that cocaine, which has a shorter half-life than heroin and requires more frequent dosing, is associated with more cases of endocarditis may be related to increased mechanical damage and greater frequencies of bacteremia. Immunologic dysregulation with hypergammaglobulinemia, high levels of circulating immune complexes, exaggerated lymphocytosis as well as atypical lymphocytosis is thought to play a role in the increased risk of endocarditis. In IDUs with HIV, low CD4$^+$ T-cell counts increase the risk for endocarditis sixfold.[3]

Presenting signs and symptoms in IDUs with endocarditis include fever, cardiac murmur (>50% of patients), cough, pleuritic chest pain, and hemoptysis. Right-sided murmurs, which vary with respiration, are typically pathologic and more specific for the diagnosis.[9] In those with right-sided endocarditis and septic pulmonary emboli, pulmonary complaints, infiltrates on chest radiographs, and moderate hypoxia have been described in more than one-third of patients, and may mislead the physician to identify the lung as the primary source of infection. Pyuria and hematuria are ascribed to glomerulonephritis, embolic renal infarction, and perinephric abscess.

Blood cultures will be positive in more than 98 percent of IDU-related endocarditis patients if three to five sets are obtained. True culture-negative endocarditis in the setting of high clinical suspicion and careful laboratory procedure is rare. *S. aureus* has been isolated from blood cultures in more than 50 percent, and up to one-third of these isolates, particularly those from large urban areas, are methicillin resistant.[10] *Streptococcus* is the second most frequently reported isolate, particularly *S. viridans.* Unlike *S. aureus,* streptococci are more likely to involve left-sided structures.

Other less-commonly isolated organisms include enterococci and gram-negative bacteria, particularly *P. aeruginosa, Serratia marcescens,* and *Klebsiella pneumoniae.* Atypical organisms usually reflect local environmental pathogens or drug-injecting habits. For example, licking needles prior to injection has been implicated in *Eikenella corrodens, Haemophilus parainfluenzae, Bacteroides* sp., and *Neisseria* sp. infections. Up to 20 percent of IDU-related endocarditis is polymicrobial in nature. Although rare, fungal endocarditis has been reported, with *Candida parapsilosis* accounting for over half of all isolates.

Diagnosis generally requires microbial isolation from a blood culture and/or the ability to demonstrate typical lesions on echocardiography.[9] The classic findings of embolic phenomena, Janeway lesions and Roth spots, are usually not observed unless the infection is advanced. A complete blood count (CBC), chest radiograph, and urinalysis will usually demonstrate abnormalities, although no single result is specific for endocarditis. Typical radiographic findings include infiltrates consistent with septic emboli, pneumonia, or congestive heart failure.

Transthoracic echocardiography (TEE) is the most sensitive imaging modality for demonstrating vegetations, myocardial and ring abscesses, and tricuspid valve involvement in IDU-related endocarditis and will reveal diagnostic cardiac lesions in up to 80 percent of patients. While the accuracy of TEE is clear, the timing of the study is not. Some authors advocate early imaging to confirm the diagnosis, while others advocate reserving imaging on those with positive blood cultures, to determine response to therapy and plan treatment.

Attempts to develop criteria that prospectively identify endocarditis in the IDU with reasonable certainty have failed.[4] At least two sets of blood cultures should be obtained in patients with suspected endocarditis, followed by hospital admission. The need for empirical antibiotic therapy should be determined by the patient's clinical stability and ability to wait for initial blood culture results. Initial treatment should be directed against *S. aureus* and *Streptococcus* spp., with consideration of local sensitivities and pathogens. Vancomycin or nafcillin and gentamicin are often initial therapy. The addition of an aminoglycoside has been shown to shorten the duration of bacteremia and duration of treatment in patients with *S. aureus* infections. Although 4 to 6 weeks of antibiotic therapy is standard, excellent cure rates have been achieved with only 2 weeks of an isoxazolyl-penicillin (e.g., cloxacillin) and an aminoglycoside in patients with right-sided endocarditis caused by sensitive *S. aureus.*[11]

Complications of endocarditis include pump failure, dysrhythmias, and pulmonary and systemic emboli. Mortality is related to vegetation location and size, response to antibiotics, and therapeutic compliance.

Left-sided endocarditis is more likely to be complicated by left-sided heart failure, septic cerebral and systemic emboli, and the need for surgery. Overall mortality for IDU-related left-sided endocarditis is 14 to 21 percent. In patients with right-sided endocarditis, the noteworthy complication is septic pulmonary emboli in 30 to 60 percent. Most complications related to right-sided endocarditis may be managed medically, and the prognosis is excellent with overall mortality rates 2 to 7 percent.

Pulmonary Infections

Community-acquired pneumonia caused by *S. pneumoniae* and *H. influenzae* is the most common pulmonary infection in the IDU.[12] However, patients are at high risk for aspiration pneumonia, tuberculosis, and, in HIV-positive patients, opportunistic infections from *P. carinii*, cytomegalovirus, and atypical mycobacteria.[12] Extrapulmonary tuberculosis affecting the cervical lymph nodes, CNS, bone, abdomen, genitourinary system, pericardium, skin, and the eyes, as well as drug resistance, are also more common in the IDU. In those IDUs with septic emboli or endocarditis, *S. aureus* must be considered. Aspiration pneumonia should be considered in those with a history of depressed level of consciousness and/or radiographic infiltrate in the posterior or basal lung segments. Because of the risk of atypical infection, coincident bacteremia, and endocarditis, admission to the hospital is recommended, and respiratory isolation should be maintained until tuberculosis is excluded.

Skin and Soft Tissue Infections

Unique features of skin infections in the IDU include a high rate of skin and pharyngeal colonization with *S. aureus* and streptococcal species, and the high frequency with which cutaneous abscesses are caused by oral flora.[13,14] Conflicting evidence exists as to whether HIV seropositivity confers additional risk for the development of skin abscesses.[14] The IDU will self-inject, often multiple times a day, with nonsterile needles, which may be licked prior to injection. Tap water, toilet water, or saliva often are used to dissolve narcotics, and each has been implicated in harboring causative organisms in both skin and blood-borne infections. Female gender is associated with an increased incidence of skin infections because of a relatively high rate of skin injection (skin popping).

Local infections of the skin and soft tissue include cellulitis, subcutaneous abscesses, septic phlebitis, necrotizing fasciitis, Fournier's gangrene, gas gangrene, and pyomyositis. Cellulitis is typically caused by *S. aureus* and *Streptococcus* spp. Cultures from cutaneous abscesses are often polymicrobial, with aerobic gram-negative rods, anaerobic cocci, and bacilli.[13] Quinine, used to "cut" heroin, may increase the risk of abscess formation. The extensive interconnected abscesses produced by skin-popping provide ideal growth conditions for *Clostridium botulinum* and *C. tetani*. Broken needles lodged in the skin are foreign bodies that potentiate infection. Groin injection has been associated with local gangrene, as well as with the development of rapidly progressive and fatal Fournier gangrene. Cutaneous abscesses in the neck may involve the carotid triangle and produce airway obstruction, vocal cord paralysis, and laryngeal edema.

Presenting signs and symptoms of cutaneous infections, including pyomyositis, are fever, pain, localized erythema, and edema. The painful area should be carefully inspected for fluctuance, crepitance, and lymphangitis. Infections over venipuncture sites suggest infected pseudoaneurysms. Pulsatile masses must be imaged with ultrasonography prior to incision and drainage, as attempts to aspirate or incise and drain an infected pseudoaneurysm can result in significant hemorrhage. Angiography may be required to identify vasospasm, thrombosis, emboli, mycotic aneurysms, or septic hematomas. Plain radiographs can demonstrate air in the soft tissues. Computed tomography delineates the involvement of other structures and the extent of deep abscesses, especially in complex areas such as the neck. Whenever crepitus or subcutaneous air is detected or deep tissue or muscle involvement is suspected clinically, a surgical consultation for possible exploration or debridement is appropriate. Wound botulism and tetanus have been reported in IDUs, and tetanus immunization status should be updated appropriately.[15,16]

IDUs with superficial cellulitis without evidence of systemic involvement can be managed as outpatients with oral antibiotics to cover streptococci and staphylococci. Febrile or toxic-appearing patients, or those not responding to outpatient treatment, require hospital admission. Blood and wound cultures should be obtained, and broad-spectrum intravenous antibiotics initiated pending culture results. Coverage should include penicillinase-resistant synthetic penicillin or vancomycin plus an antipseudomonal aminoglycoside, antipseudomonal penicillin, or cephalosporin. Surgical consultation is indicated for deep tissue and necrotizing soft tissue infections.

Vascular Infections

Vascular injury associated with IDU includes inadvertent arterial injection with resultant vasospasm or thrombosis, septic thrombophlebitis, venous and arterial pseudoaneurysms, and infected hematomas. Arterial injection rarely results in major vessel occlusion; instead, pain, edema, and patchy mottling of the affected limb caused by ischemia occur. Tissue necrosis and gangrene are the consequence of persistent focal ischemia, the etiology of which is thought to be a combination of vasospasm, embolization of particulate matter, and endothelial injury leading to thrombosis and vasculitis.[17]

When limb ischemia is suspected, a vascular surgeon should determine if either surgical intervention or intraarterial thrombolysis is indicated. However, the majority of cases involve distal vessels, and treatment is limited to heparin and supportive care. Limb edema can progress to compartment syndrome, which may require fasciotomy, or rhabdomyolysis.

Infected pseudoaneurysm is a commonly reported vascular complication in IDUs and is most often reported in the femoral, followed by the radial and brachial arteries.[17,18] Venous pseudoaneurysms are relatively rare and are usually secondary to septic phlebitis, with the femoral vein most often involved. Patients typically present with fever and a painful mass. Although similar in gross appearance to an abscess, the presence of pulsations and a bruit suggest this diagnosis. Because of the disastrous hemorrhagic consequences of attempted incision and drainage or medical management with a course of antibiotics, all painful masses, particularly in the groin, should be imaged. Treatment for infected pseudoaneurysm usually involves resection of the infected vessel. Appropriate broad-spectrum antibiotics should be initiated in the ED. Revascularization at the time of resection of the pseudoaneurysm may be necessary.[18]

Bone and Joint Infections

Bone and joint infections usually occur from either contiguous spread from an overlying skin or soft tissue infection, or secondary to hematogenous spread from a distant site. In contrast to the general population in which *S. aureus* predominates, infecting microorganisms in the IDU tend to be unusual, with *Candida* and gram-negative organisms the most common. In IDUs, osteomyelitis is seen more frequently in the axial skeleton than in the extremities.

Pyogenic infections predominate in bones and joints. Earlier studies in IDU-related osteomyelitis or septic arthritis found a high likelihood of polymicrobial or uncommon organisms; however, recent studies demonstrate an increasing frequency of *S. aureus* and *Streptococcus* groups A and G bone infections in IDUs. Because of the high incidence sexually transmitted diseases in this population, gonococcal arthritis and tenosynovitis should also be considered. *E. corrodens* osteomyelitis has been reported in IDUs who lick their needles prior to injection.

Nonpyogenic organisms may cause osteomyelitis and septic arthritis in IDUs. Mycobacterial infections usually involve the ribs and vertebral column (Pott disease). These infections present with night sweats, fevers, weight loss, and localized pain. *Candida* spp. has been reported in as high as 20 percent of IDU-related osteomyelitis patients. Candidal infections are postulated to be hematogenous in origin. Some patients report an initial flulike syndrome lasting 3 to 4 days, followed by the appearance of metastatic lesions involving the skin, eye (chorioretinitis and endophthalmitis), and the bones and joints several days to weeks later. Rarely, *Aspergillus* spp. may cause osteomyelitis of the sternum in IDUs.

IDU-related osteomyelitis involves the vertebral column in approximately 50 percent of cases, particularly the lumbar segments, followed by the sternoclavicular joint in approximately 18 percent of cases, and the extremities, particularly around the hip and knee joints, in 17 percent of cases. Vertebral osteomyelitis usually presents with localized pain and tenderness to palpation over the involved bone and a soft tissue mass may be palpable. Symptoms may be present for days in the case of bacterial infections to weeks in the case of fungal or mycobacterial infections. Many patients both fever and leukocytosis and an elevated erythrocyte sedimentation rate (ESR) and C-reactive protein are helpful, if present, but their absence does not exclude these infections. Drainage from contiguous abscesses should be cultured. Biopsy or needle aspiration of joint space and bony infections may be necessary, especially in the case of unusual or fastidious organisms, such as *Mycobacterium, Candida,* or *Eikenella.* Appropriate imaging for osteomyelitis will vary by institution; however, MRI, CT, and radionuclide bone scans are used. Patients with osteomyelitis warrant admission. Unless the patient appears septic or coincident endocarditis is a concern, antibiotic administration should be based on culture results and is typically required for 4 to 6 weeks.

Septic arthritis in the IDU usually involves the knee or hip. Sternoclavicular infectious arthritis, well described in this population, strongly suggests IDU. Patients often will note a recent history of trauma to the area, but causality has yet to be proven. Patients will describe pain, localized tenderness, and swelling at the sites. The ESR is usually elevated, and fever and leukocytosis may be present. Up to 80 percent of patients will have normal plain radiographs; however, joint space widening, articular surface erosion, and surrounding soft tissue infection may be noted. Bone scans are often positive early in the process, and these infections also may be delineated with CT or MRI. The most sensitive but nonspecific finding on synovial fluid analysis is a white blood cell count greater than 20,000/µL, with a neutrophil predominance. Synovial fluid Gram stain may aid in antibiotic selection. Immobilization, physical therapy, therapeutic arthrocentesis, and occasionally open drainage may be warranted.

Hepatic Disease

The IDU can develop liver disease, including cirrhosis, from both parenterally and sexually transmitted hepatitis A, B, C, G, and non A-G viruses, as well as the delta virus.[19] More than 80 percent of IDUs are estimated to have had hepatitis, with the majority of cases caused by hepatitis B and C. These patients frequently progress to chronic active hepatitis. When an IDU patient presents with a clinical syndrome suggestive of acute hepatitis, appropriate laboratory testing includes serum transaminases, bilirubin levels, alkaline phosphatase, prothrombin time, and serologic testing. If other significant disease can be excluded, most can be managed as outpatients. Admission criteria include inability to tolerate oral intake, toxicity, and prolonged prothrombin time. Patients should be counseled on both sexual contact and needle exposure and should be encouraged to inform all sexual and needle partners and household contacts of exposure. Seronegative patients should receive hepatitis B and A immunization.

Ophthalmologic Infections

Ophthalmologic infections in the IDU are usually the result of hematogenous seeding from a primary source of infection, such as endocarditis, or of opportunistic infections associated with HIV disease.[20] Bacterial endophthalmitis often presents acutely, with pain, redness, lid swelling, and decrease in visual acuity. Inflammation is usually present in both anterior and posterior chambers. White-centered, flame-shaped hemorrhages (Roth spots), cotton wool exudates, and macular holes may be present. *S. aureus* is the most commonly isolated organism, followed by *Streptococcus* sp. Treatment involves subconjunctival and systemic antibiotic therapy; surgical intervention may be needed.

Fungal endophthalmitis, usually caused by *Candida,* is more common than bacterial endophthalmitis. Symptoms include blurred vision, pain, and decreased visual acuity and can progress over days to weeks. White cotton-like lesions are seen on the choroid retina, with vitreous haziness. Uveitis, papillitis, and vitreitis also have been reported. Since 1980, a marked increase in *Candida* sp. infections has been reported in IDUs who use brown heroin. *Candida* chorioretinitis or endophthalmitis is characterized by the appearance of a high fever, followed in 3 to 4 days by ocular symptoms, cutaneous lesions, and costochondral involvement. Aspergillosis is the second most common fungal cause of endophthalmitis in IDUs, producing ocular symptoms and signs without cutaneous or musculoskeletal involvement. The prognosis for fungal endophthalmitis depends on prompt diagnosis and treatment. Fungal endophthalmitis secondary to *Torulopsis, Helminthosporium,* and *Penicillium* spp. also has been reported in IDUs. In IDUs with HIV, cytomegalovirus, toxoplasmosis retinitis, and choroidal *Cryptococcus* and *Mycobacterium avium intracellulare* infections have been reported.

REFERENCES

1. Sanchez-Carbonell X, Vilaregut A: A 10-year follow-up study on the health status of heroin addicts based on official registers. *Addiction* 96: 1777, 2001.
2. National Institute on Drug Abuse: *Epidemiologic Trends in Drug Abuse* Vol. 1. *Highlights and Executive Summary, Community Epidemiology Work Group.* NIH Pub. No. 00-4739. Washington, DC, Superintendent of Documents, 2000.
3. Frontera JA, Gradon JD: Right-side endocarditis in injection drug users: Review of proposed mechanisms of pathogenesis. *Clin Infect Dis* 30: 374, 2000.
4. Weisse AB, Heller DR, Schimentoi RJ, et al: The febrile parenteral drug user: A prospective study in 121 patients. *Am J Med* 94:274, 1993.
5. Tattevin P, Casalino E, Fleury L, et al: The validity of medical history, classic symptoms, and chest radiographs in predicting pulmonary tuberculosis: Derivation of a pulmonary tuberculosis prediction model. *Chest* 115: 1248, 1999.
6. Ward S, Heyneman LE, Reittner P, et al: Talcosis associated with IV abuse of oral medications: CT findings. *AJR* 174:789, 2000.
7. Ngaage DL, Cowen ME: Right ventricular needle embolus in an injecting drug user: The need for early removal. *Emerg Med J* 18:500, 2001.
8. Cohn JA: HIV-1 infection in injection drug users. *Infect Dis Clin North Am* 16:745, 2002.
9. Netzer RO, Zollinger E, Seiler C, Cerny A: Infective endocarditis: Clinical spectrum, presentation and outcome. An analysis of 212 cases 1980–1995. *Heart* 84:25, 2000.
10. Fleisch F, Zbinden R, Vanoli C, et al: Epidemic spread of a single clone of methicillin-resistant *Staphylococcus aureus* among injection drug users in Zurich, Switzerland. *Clin Infect Dis* 32:581, 2001.
11. Fortun J, Navas E, Martinez-Beltran J, et al: Short-course therapy for right-side endocarditis due to *Staphylococcus aureus* in drug abusers: Cloxacillin versus glycopeptides in combination with gentamicin. *Clin Infect Dis* 33: 120, 2001.
12. Hind CR: Pulmonary complications of intravenous drug misuse. 1. Epidemiology and non-infectious complications. 2. Infective and HIV related complications. *Thorax* 45:891, 957, 1990.
13. Summanen PH, Talan DA, Strong C, et al: Bacteriology of skin and soft-tissue infections: Comparison of infections in intravenous drug users and individuals with no history of intravenous drug use. *Clin Infect Dis* 20(Suppl 2):S279, 1995.

14. Murphy EL, DeVita D, Liu H, et al: Risk factors for skin and soft tissue abscesses among injection drug users: A case-control study. *Clin Infect Dis* 33:35, 2001.

15. Passaro DJ, Werner SB, McGee J, et al: Wound botulism associated with black tar heroin among injecting drug users. *JAMA* 279:859, 1998.

16. Centers for Disease Control and Prevention: Tetanus among injecting-drug users—California, 1997. *MMWR* 47:149, 1998.

17. Woodburn KR, Murie JA: Vascular complications of injecting drug misuse. *Br J Surg* 83:1329, 1996.

18. Levi N, Rordam P, Jensen LP, Schroeder TV: Femoral pseudoaneurysms in drug addicts. *Eur J Vasc Endovasc Surg* 13:361, 1997.

19. Lemberg BD, Shaw-Stiffel TA: Hepatitic disease in injection drug users. *Infect Dis Clin North Am* 16:667, 2002.

20. Kim RW, Juzych MS, Eliott D: Ocular manifestations of injection drug use. *Infect Dis Clin North Am* 16:607, 2002.

THE ELDER PATIENT
Arthur B. Sanders

Older patients represent a special population for emergency medicine. The approach that focuses on one chief complaint and develops a differential diagnosis based on life-threatening and common diseases may miss significant conditions in older persons. Older patients are more time-consuming, more difficult to evaluate, and use more resources than do younger adult patients. The complexity of their presentations and dispositions, as well as communication problems with the patients, their families, and primary care providers, all make the ED evaluation of elderly persons more difficult as compared with younger adult patients.[1] The physiology of aging results in altered disease presentations, altered pharmacodynamics, and decreased functional reserve, as well as social problems, which must be dealt with in the setting of a busy ED.

EPIDEMIOLOGY

The elderly population in the United States is growing rapidly, with projected increases from 200 percent for the 65- to 74-year-old segment, 300 percent for the 75- to 84-year-old segment, and more than 500 percent for those older than age 85 years by the year 2050. Approximately 12 percent of the population was 65 years of age or older in 1990, whereas 20 percent of the population (or 55 million persons) will be 65 years of age or older by the year 2030. As noted, the oldest elderly, those age 85 years and older, are the most rapidly increasing segment of the elderly population. This is also the population with the most health problems and in greatest need for health care. There is great variability in the physiologic age of individual patients. A 55-year-old with multiple chronic diseases and poor physiologic reserve may have a physiologic age much older than a healthy 80-year-old.

In 1995, almost 16 percent of ED visits were made by patients age 65 years and older, and 46 percent were admitted to the hospital.[2] Older patients spend more time in the ED, require more ancillary tests, and are more likely to be admitted to critical care units as compared to younger patients. The National Center for Health Statistics (NCHS) 2000 survey documents that persons aged 75 years and older had 64.8 ED visits per 100 persons per year, twice the rate for younger persons.[3] The rate of ambulance use increased with age, with 43 percent of persons age 75 and older taking ambulance transport to the ED.[3]

PATHOPHYSIOLOGY

The basic principles of geriatric emergency medicine have been defined (Table 307-1). Older patients often present with ambiguous complaints, such as not feeling right, feeling weak, or not doing usual

TABLE 307-1   Principles of Geriatric Emergency Medicine

1. The patient's presentation is frequently complex.
2. Common diseases present atypically in this age group.
3. The confounding effects of comorbid diseases must be considered.
4. Polypharmacy is common and may be a factor in presentation, diagnosis, and management.
5. Recognition of the possibility for cognitive impairment is important.
6. Some diagnostic tests may have different normal values.
7. The likelihood of decreased functional reserve must be anticipated.
8. Social support systems may not be adequate, and patients may need to rely on caregivers.
9. A knowledge of baseline functional status is essential for evaluating new complaints.
10. Health problems must be evaluated for associated psychosocial adjustment.
11. The emergency department encounter is an opportunity to assess important conditions in a patient's personal life.

Source: Reproduced with permission from Sanders AB, Witzke DB, Jones JS, et al: Principles of care and application of geriatric emergency care model, in Sanders AB (ed): *Emergency Care of the Elder Person.* St. Louis, Beverly Cracom Publications, 1996, p 59.

activities. Vague complaints, such as general weakness or functional decline, may indicate important diseases, such as sepsis, subdural hematoma, or myocardial infarction. Assessment of functional status can be used for classifying and evaluating these complaints.

Common diseases often present atypically in older persons, resulting in missed diagnoses unless physicians understand and suspect the atypical presentations in this population. For example, consider two common presenting complaints—chest pain and abdominal pain—and common diagnoses for each—myocardial infarction and acute appendicitis. Fewer than half of patients 85 years of age and older will present with chest pain as a symptom of acute myocardial infarction.[4] Instead, patients present atypically with dyspnea, syncope, weakness, or dizziness.[4] Older patients with acute appendicitis are often diagnosed late and have a high perforation rate.[5] A large percent of patients with appendicitis are diagnosed more than 48 h after the onset of symptoms, with up to 20 percent diagnosed after 3 days. The abdominal pain is vague, and the symptoms may be poorly localized. Classic patterns of pain and accompanying symptoms, such as nausea and vomiting, are present in only a minority of older patients with acute appendicitis. Older patients with acute abdominal conditions commonly lack physical findings of guarding or rebound.[6]

Older patients frequently will have confounding comorbid diseases, and emergency physicians should evaluate whether the presenting complaint reflects an exacerbation of one of the comorbid diseases or a new disease process. Comorbid diseases, especially those treated with multiple medications, may also affect the management and disposition of patients.

Older adults take an average of more than four prescription drugs and more than two over-the-counter drugs each day. Approximately 30 percent of older persons will develop adverse medication effects, and they are twice as likely as younger adults to have adverse effects. Adverse medication effects account for approximately 5 percent of hospital admissions. The number of medications that a patient takes is directly related to the chance of adverse drug effects. Normal aging results in a loss of cardiac, pulmonary, hepatic, and renal functional reserve.[7] Thus, the margin of error decreases for many medications, such as nonsteroidal anti-inflammatory drugs. The distribution of drugs changes with age; as lean body mass decreases, the larger proportion of adipose tissue increases the volume of distribution of drugs, such as benzodiazepines, phenytoin, barbiturates, and phenothiazines, and prolongs their duration of action. Drug clearance depends primarily on hepatic and renal function. The decreased renal function with age may affect drugs such as digoxin and the aminoglycoside antibiotics. Drug receptor interactions also play a role in pharmacodynamics. Older persons have an increased sensitivity to warfarin and benzodiazepines. Common complications of medications or drug interactions include delirium, depression, functional decline, worsening dementia, orthostatic hypotension, weakness, dizziness, falls, and incontinence. The impact of new medications prescribed in emergency departments, such as anticholinergics, sedatives, and diuretics, as well as adverse interactions with current medicines, should be anticipated.[8]

Older persons frequently have cognitive impairment that may not be recognized by health care providers.[9] Cognitive impairment includes both acute confusional states (delirium) and dementia. Abnormal cognitive states in older patients affect the reliability of the history and impact disposition planning. Acute cognitive impairment can be an important symptom of sepsis, congestive heart failure, metabolic abnormality, adverse drug effect, or subdural hematoma. When older ED patients are screened for cognitive impairment, 30 to 40 percent of those who have no previous history of impairment will have abnormal cognition based on formal mental status exams.[9] Approximately 10 percent of patients will meet formal criteria for delirium, which should be considered a symptom of a medical emergency. Formal tools for evaluation of cognition are recommended later in this chapter.

Accurate laboratory test interpretation requires a knowledge of which "normal" values are altered with aging. Although many laboratories control for age variations in neonates and children, few list control values for older patients. For example, laboratory parameters such as the sedimentation rate, glucose and creatinine levels, and arterial blood oxygen tension change with physiologic aging.

The likelihood of decreased functional reserve should be anticipated in older persons. Most patients are asymptomatic until they are stressed or reach a critical threshold in which symptoms are manifested. Most organ functions decline with age. Resting cardiac output decreases at approximately 1 percent per year after age 30 years. Pulmonary, renal, neurologic, and immunologic functions also decrease with age. Chronologic and physiologic age, however, may vary considerably, depending on genetics, environment, health behaviors, diet, tobacco use, alcohol use, exercise, and stress. When older persons are stressed, for example, by extreme heat or cold, their regulatory mechanisms are not as effective as when they are not so stressed.

Older persons should be viewed in the context of their home environment and social support network. Simply addressing an injury or illness may not be adequate. More than 20 percent report a change in their ability to care for themselves following their ED visit. An independent-living 80-year-old woman who sprains her ankle may become incapacitated. Enlisting the help of a social service network and of home health providers will ensure that such patients are able to carry on the functions of daily living. In addition, many older persons need to rely on caretakers, so an assessment of the caretaker's ability to help the patient is important. Is the caretaker an elderly spouse who will predictably injure himself or herself in trying to lift a patient who is incapacitated by a new injury? Elder abuse and neglect is a significant issue that should be assessed by questioning the patient and caretaker separately (see Chap. 300).[10]

The emergency health care professional can play a key role in screening for such important conditions such as elder abuse, depression, alcoholism, malnutrition, incontinence, falls, and immunizations. In a multicenter study in which patients were screened, almost 80 percent of older patients demonstrated a problem in one or more of these areas.[11]

SPECIFIC ISSUES

Altered Mental Status

Of ED older patients with no prior history of cognitive problems, 30 to 40 percent will meet the criteria for either delirium or cognitive dysfunction, and this is often unsuspected by the physician.[9] Consequently, older patients should be routinely screened for cognitive dys-

function. The simplest screening tool is evaluation for orientation and three-item recall. If no problem is detected, no further testing need be done. If the screen is failed, further testing can be done. The Confusion Assessment Method (CAM) scale is a useful tool for the emergency physician (Figure 307-1). Using the CAM scale, the patient is evaluated for (1) acute onset, (2) fluctuating course, (3) inattention, (4) disorganized thinking, and (5) altered level of consciousness. These factors are assessed through the ED history and observation, as well as structured questions such as three-item recall, stating the days of the week or months of the year backward. Patients who present with inattention—either acute onset or fluctuating course—and disorganized thinking or altered level of consciousness should be considered to have delirium and evaluated for acute medical problems as the cause. Cognitive function can be further assessed with formal mental status tools such as the Mini-Mental Status Exam (MMSE). These scales are useful because they are widely accepted as indicative of cognitive dysfunction and can be followed by different clinicians over time (Figure 307-2).

Delirium, dementia, or decreased level of consciousness are usually obvious on history and physical examination. The Glasgow Coma Scale is useful for classifying a decreased level of consciousness. Acute mental status changes in older patients represent a medical emergency of presumed organic cause requiring diagnostic tests to determine the etiology.[12] The differential diagnosis includes a large number of disorders such as pneumonia, urosepsis, electrolyte imbalance, medication reaction, or congestive heart failure, which can cause a decrease in mental status.

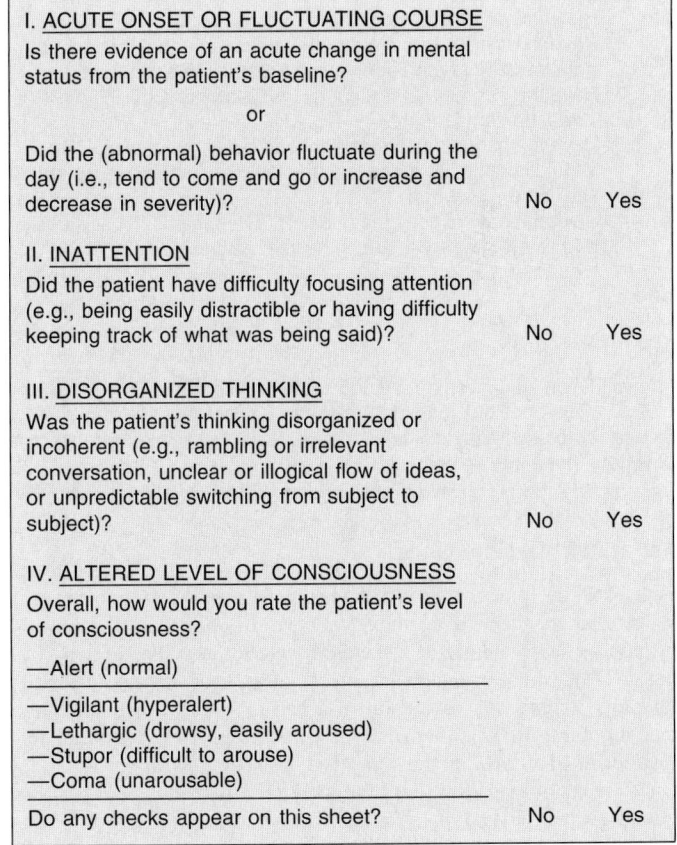

FIG. 307-1. Confusion Assessment Method (CAM) worksheet. The diagnosis of delirium is suggested with the presence of the first two criteria and either the third or fourth criteria. (Reproduced with permission from Inouye SK, van Dyck CH, Alessi CA, et al: Clarifying confusion: The confusion assessment methods—A new method for detection of delirium. *Ann Intern Med* 113:941, 1990.)

Add points for each correct response.   Score   Points

Orientation

1. What is the: Year?   _____   1
                    Season?   _____   1
                    Date?   _____   1
                    Day?   _____   1
                    Month?   _____   1

2. Where are we?   State?   _____   1
                    County?   _____   1
                    Town or city?   _____   1
                    Hospital?   _____   1
                    Floor?   _____   1

Registration

3. Name three objects, taking one second to say each. Then ask the   _____   3
   patient to repeat all three after you have said them.

   Give one point for each correct answer. Repeat the answers until
   patient learns all three.

Attention and calculation

4. Serial sevens. Give one point for each correct answer. Stop after five _____   5
   answers. Alternate: Spell WORLD backwards.

Recall

5. Ask for names of three objects learned in question 3. Give one point   _____   3
   for each correct answer.

Language

6. Point to a pencil and a watch. Have the patient name them as you   _____   2
   point.
7. Have the patient repeat "No ifs, ands, or buts."   _____   1
8. Have the patient follow a three-stage command: "Take a paper in your   _____   3
   right hand. Fold the paper in half. Put the paper on the floor."
9. Have the patient read and obey the following: 'CLOSE YOUR EYES.'   _____   1
   (Write it in large letters.)
10. Have the patient write a sentence of his or her choice. (The sentence   _____   1
    should contain a subject and an object and should make sense. Ignore
    spelling errors when scoring.)
11. Have the patient copy the design. (Give one point if all sides and   _____   1
    angles are preserved and if the intersecting sides form
    a quadrangle.)

                                                            _____ = Total   30

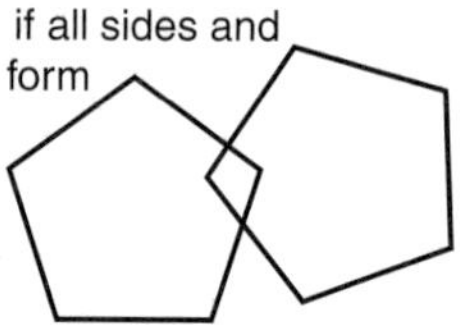

In validation studies using a cutoff score of 23 or below, the MMSE has a sensitivity of 87%, a specificity of 82%, a false-positive ratio of 39.4%, and a false-negative ratio of 4.7%. These ratios refer to the MMSE's capacity to accurately distinguish patients with clinically diagnosed dementia or delirium from patients without these syndromes.

FIG. 307-2. Mini-Mental Status Examination (MMSE). (Courtesy of Marshall Folstein. Reproduced with permission from Folstein MF, Folstein S, McHugh PR: Mini-Mental State Examination: A practical method for grading cognitive state of patients for the clinician. *J Psychiatr Res* 12:189, 1975.)

Functional Decline

Functional decline represents a change in a patient's ability to perform tasks of independent living and is not a part of normal aging. This can be assessed with the use of a standard scale for activities of daily living (ADL), which evaluates a patient's ability for bathing, dressing, toileting, transferring (in or out of a bed or chair), continence, and feeding (Table 307-2). The patient is asked whether he or she can perform each of these functions with no assistance, with partial assistance, or cannot perform these functions. If a patient cannot perform these basic activities of daily living, then a caregiver is necessary. Deterioration in ADL generally follows an orderly progressive pattern of bathing, dressing, toileting (including continence), transferring, and feeding. When this pattern is not seen, such as deterioration in feeding before the others, organic disease should be suspected. Another scale, the instrumental activities of daily living (IADL), assesses more sophisticated skills, such as telephone use, walking, shopping, preparing meals, housework, handiwork, laundry, taking medicines, and handling finances (see Table 307-2). It is best to use these formal scales in evaluating older patients and assessing changes over time. Acute functional decline represents an acute medical syndrome that needs appropriate workup and treatment (Figure 307-3). The differential diagnosis for functional decline includes serious diseases such as myocardial infarction, sepsis, and subdural hematoma, as well as adverse drug reactions. Patients will often present with a vague symptom, such as weakness, that on further questioning and use of the scale is noted to be functional decline. A functional assessment in the ED can be used to guide decision making regarding hospitalization, discharge planning, and future health care needs.[13]

Trauma

Trauma is a major cause of morbidity and mortality among older persons. Although fewer than 20 percent of trauma patients are 65 years of age or older, older patients represent 28 percent of trauma deaths.[14]

**TABLE 307-2 Activities of Daily Living (ADL)
and Instrumental Activities of Daily Living (IADL) Scales**

Activities of Daily Living (ADL) Scale (Katz et al)	Instrumental Activities of Daily Living (IADL) Scale (Lawton and Brody)
Bathing	Telephone use
Dressing	Walking
Toileting	Shopping
Transfer	Preparing meals
Continence	Housework
Feeding	Handiwork
	Laundry
	Take medicines
	Manage finances

Sources: Reproduced with permission from Katz S, Ford AB, Moskowitz RW, et al: Studies in illness in the aged. The index of ADL: A standardized measure of biologic and psychosocial function. *JAMA* 185:914, 1963; and from Lawton MP, Brody EM: Assessment of older people: Self-maintaining and instrumental activities of daily living. *Gerontologist* 9:179, 1969.

They are more likely to have significant complications and prolonged hospitalizations because of their decreased functional reserve. Falls are the most common mechanism of injury for older persons, followed by motor vehicle crashes and pedestrian accidents. Regardless of injury severity or mechanism of injury, mortality starts to increase for patients at 50 years of age and continues to increase with increasing age. The major challenge for emergency physicians who treat older patients with multisystem trauma is that the standard physiologic indices, such as blood pressure and pulse, often remain within normal limits until the patient deteriorates acutely. Occult shock must be strongly suspected in all older patients who experience significant trauma. Early hemodynamic monitoring of older trauma patients can detect occult shock early in the course and improve the chance of survival (see Chap. 253).[14]

Falls

Falls are not a normal part of aging.[15] A fall is a symptom, and emergency physicians need to assess both the cause and the consequences

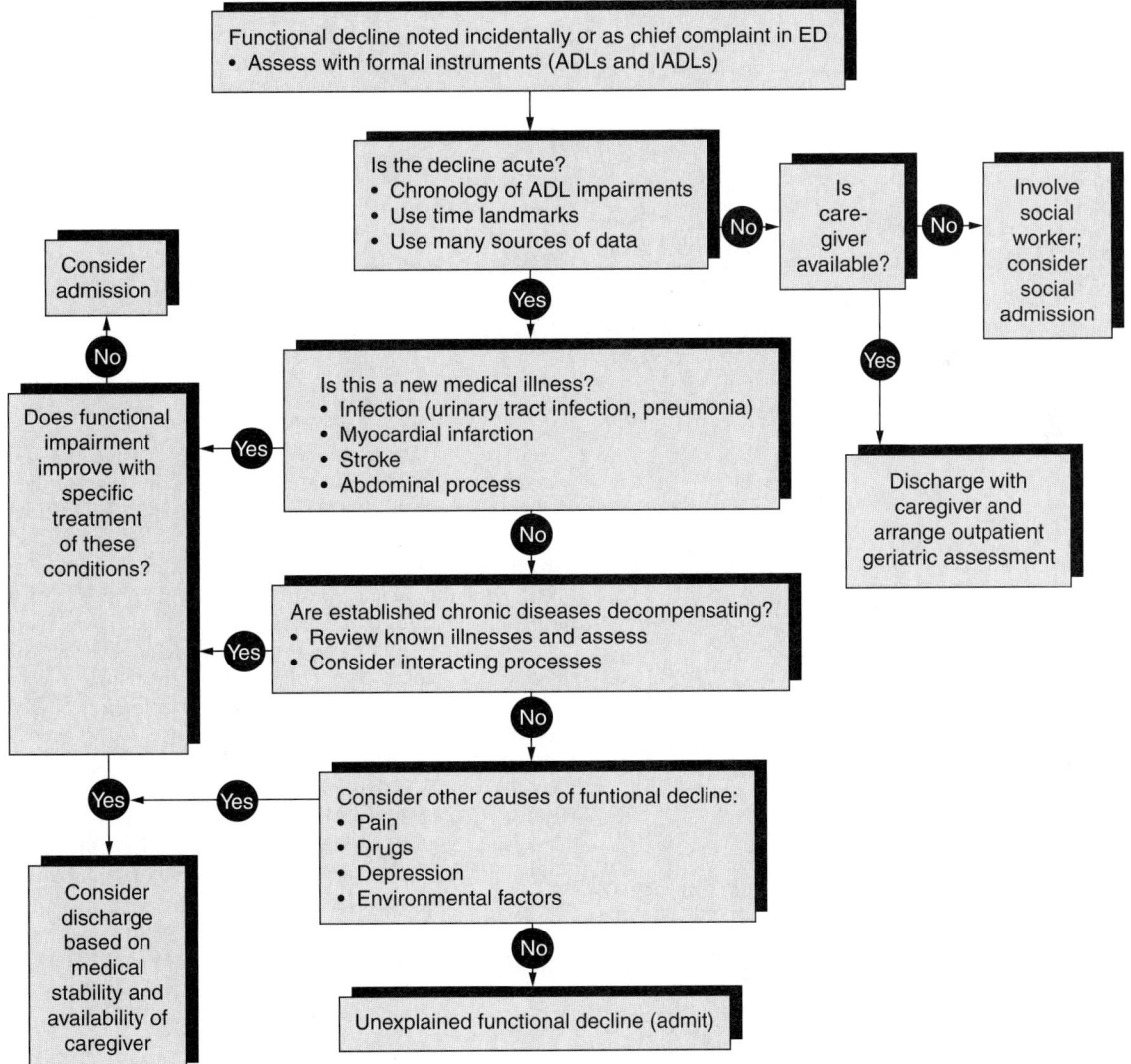

FIG. 307-3. Algorithm for the evaluation and management of functional decline in elderly patients. *Abbreviations:* ADL = activities of daily living scale; IADL = instrumental activities of daily living scale. [Reproduced with permission from Lachs MS: Functional decline, in Sanders AB (ed): *Emergency Care of the Elder Person.* St. Louis, Beverly Cracom Publications, 1996, pp 143.]

of the fall.[16] The causes of a fall may include acute or chronic diseases, medications, and environmental factors. Consequences of a fall include injury and fear of falling, resulting in a decrease in activities. A fall can represent a sentinel event in an older person's life and result in a downward spiral of decreased activities, leading to death. As many as 50 percent of older patients admitted to the hospital after a fall die within 1 year. An emergency physician should obtain the history of what caused the fall and determine whether further ED screening tests (electrocardiography, computed tomography, laboratory tests, social service consultation, etc.) need to be done to evaluate the cause. The patient should then be informed about fall assessment programs that decrease the incidence and morbidity from falls.

Infections

Multiple factors as well as changes in the immune system with age are responsible for the increased susceptibility to infection in the elderly.[17] In addition, older persons will have atypical disease presentations of sepsis. Focal symptoms or signs of infection may be lacking. Instead, patients may present with isolated fever or nonspecific symptoms of anorexia, weakness, fatigue, and functional decline as the only evidence of infection. Hypothermia may be evident instead of fever. The most common sites of infection include the lungs, urinary tract, abdomen, and skin. Urinary tract infections in the elderly encompass of broader spectrum of potential pathogen, and is complicated by comorbidities, the frequent present of baseline asymptomatic bacteruria, and the lack of pyuria as a accurate predictor of urinary infection.[18]

Bacteremia and occult bacterial infection are common in the febrile elderly. Mellors and coworkers identified the following multivariate predictors of bacteremia and occult bacterial infection in febrile adults without localizing symptoms or signs: (1) age older than 50 years; (2) diabetes; (3) white blood cell count (WBC) greater than 15,000/μL; (4) neutrophil band count greater than 1500/μL; and (5) erythrocyte sedimentation rate greater than 30 mm/h.[19] Patients with one or two of these factors had a seven- to eightfold relative risk for bacteremia or focal bacterial infection. Other studies in the febrile elderly have also found that leukocytosis and "left shift" on the WBC differential was also associated with a two- to threefold greater likelihood of bacterial infection.

DISPOSITION

For all the foregoing reasons, elderly patients in the ED are more likely to require hospital admission for their illness or injury than are younger patients. When discharged from an ED, elderly patients may not fully understand the instructions, may not be able to obtain and take prescribed medications, may not be able to access appropriate follow-up, or may not be able to care for their personal needs during the period of illness. An elderly patient's family, friends, and social support system should be informed and involved before the patient leaves the ED.

REFERENCES

1. McNamara RM, Rousseau E, Sanders AB: Geriatric emergency medicine: A survey of practicing emergency physicians. *Ann Emerg Med* 21:796, 1992.
2. Strange GR, Chen EH: Use of emergency departments by elder patients: A five-year follow up study. *Acad Emerg Med* 5:1157, 1998.
3. McCraig LF: *National Hospital Ambulatory Medical Care Survey: 2000 Emergency Department Summary.* Washington, DC, National Center for Health Statistics, Centers for Disease Control and Prevention, US Department of Health and Human Services, 2002.
4. Gregoratos G: Clinical manifestation of acute myocardial infarction in older patients. *Am J Geriatr Cardiol* 10:345, 2001.
5. Kraemer M, Franke C, Ohmann C, et al: Acute appendicitis in late adulthood: Incidence, presentation, and outcome. Results of a prospective multicenter acute abdominal pain study and a review of the literature. *Langenbecks Arch Surg* 385:470, 2000.
6. Sanson TG, O'Keefe KP: Evaluation of abdominal pain in the elderly. *Emerg Med Clin North Am* 14:615, 1996.
7. Herrlinger C, Klotz U: Drug metabolism and drug interactions in the elderly. *Best Pract Res Clin Gastroenterol* 15:897, 2001.
8. Chin MH, Wand LC, Jin L, et al: Appropriateness of medication selection for older persons in an urban academic emergency department. *Acad Emerg Med* 6:1232, 1999.
9. Naughton BJ, Moran MB, Kadah H, et al: Delirium and other cognitive impairment in older adults in an emergency department. *Ann Emerg Med* 25: 751, 1995.
10. Kleinschmidt KC: Elder abuse: A review. *Ann Emerg Med* 30:463, 1997.
11. Gerson LW, Rousseau E, Hogan J, et al: A multicenter study of case findings in elderly emergency department patients. *Acad Emerg Med* 2:729, 1995.
12. O'Keefe KP, Sanson TG: Elderly patients with altered mental status. *Emerg Med Clin North Am* 16:701, 1998.
13. Lee V, Ross B, Tracy B: Functional assessment of older patients in an emergency department. *Can J Occup Ther* 68:121, 2001.
14. Mandavia D, Newton K: Geriatric trauma. *Emerg Med Clin North Am* 16:257, 1998.
15. Tinetti ME: Clinical practice. Preventing falls in elderly persons. *New Engl J Med* 348:42, 2003.
16. Weigand JV, Gerson LW: Preventive care in the emergency department: Should emergency departments institute a falls prevention program for elder patients? A systematic review. *Acad Emerg Med* 8:823, 2001.
17. Gavazzi G, Krause KH: Aging and infection. *Lancet Infect Dis* 2:659, 2002.
18. Shortliffe LM, McCue JD: Urinary tract infections at age extremes: Pediatrics and geriatrics. *Am J Med* 113(suppl 1A):55S, 2002.
19. Mellors JW, Horwitz RI, Harvey MR, Horwitz SM: A simple index to identify occult bacterial infection in adults with unexplained fever. *Arch Intern Med* 147:666, 1987.

ADULTS WITH PHYSICAL DISABILITIES
Paul J.W. Tawney
John N. Oh

Many individuals live with significant impairments and disabilities; an estimated 5 to 10 percent of the total population of the United States has major disabilities. Persons with disabilities seeking medical care in an ED may present with problems that are specific to their impairment or with signs and symptoms different from those that would occur in a nondisabled patient. An important principle in evaluating disabled adults is to remember that the individual who is disabled is not unable, and every effort should be made to obtain the history directly from the patient. Do not automatically direct questions to persons with the disabled individual without first finding out whether the patient is capable of giving accurate responses. Sit down to get at eye level with a patient in a wheelchair. Make an effort to use a dysphasic or dysarthric patient's communication system so that they may tell their story. After emergency care is rendered, referral of patients with physical and cognitive impairment to a physiatrist (a physical medicine and rehabilitation physician) is appropriate for comprehensive management of functional deficits.

SPINAL CORD INJURY

Autonomic Dysreflexia

Patients with spinal cord injuries at or above the T6 level are at risk for developing autonomic dysreflexia (also called autonomic hyperreflexia).[1,2] This reflex is initiated by a noxious stimulus from below the level of the patient's spinal cord lesion. Intact sensory neurons below the level of the lesion transmit a message up the spinothalamic tract and posterior columns, where interconnections stimulate the intermediolateral gray matter neurons, producing sympathetic outflow from spinal cord levels between T6 and L2, releasing norepinephrine, β-hydroxylase, and dopamine. This sympathetic reflex is relatively unopposed because the normal inhibitory impulses that would prevent it originate above T6 and are blocked at the level of injury.[2]

The sympathetic response produces a rise in blood pressure, vasoconstriction, skin pallor, and piloerection below the level of the lesion. Intact carotid and aortic arch baroreceptors detect the hypertension, producing increased parasympathetic activity in the vagus nerve causing bradycardia and, above the level of the lesion, profuse sweating, vasodilation, and skin flushing.[1,2]

Common signs and symptoms of autonomic dysreflexia are a pounding headache, nasal congestion, a feeling of apprehension or anxiety, visual changes, and most significant, a marked increase in systolic and diastolic blood pressure above baseline.[1,2] Patients with spinal cord injury at or above the T6 level often have lower baseline systolic blood pressures, in the 90- to 110-mm Hg range. Therefore, blood pressure elevations of 20 to 40 mm Hg or systolic pressures of 130 to 150 mm Hg are significant. Acute elevation in blood pressure is the most worrisome and potentially life-threatening manifestation of this syndrome.

A variety of stimuli can produce an acute episode of autonomic dysreflexia. The most common causes usually involve the urinary system: bladder distention, urinary tract infection, and kidney stones. The second most common reasons involve the colon: fecal impaction or bowel distention. However, any noxious stimulus below the level of injury can lead to autonomic dysreflexia, including peptic ulcers, appendicitis, and gallstones, fractures, deep venous thrombosis (DVT), pressure ulcers, ingrown toenails, tight-fitting clothing, sunburns, blisters, heterotopic ossification, sexual intercourse, pregnancy, and labor and delivery.

Treatment begins with monitoring and controlling the patient's blood pressure. If possible, the patient should sit up to lower blood pressure.[2,3] All constrictive clothing items should be loosened. If the systolic blood pressure is above 150 mm Hg, an antihypertensive agent with a rapid onset and short duration should be used.[3] Nitroprusside and nitrates are the most commonly used agents. More aggressive treatment should be undertaken if these agents do not adequately correct the elevated blood pressure.

After assessment of the blood pressure, the bladder should be checked for distention and infection.[2,3] If the patient does not already have a urinary catheter, one should be placed. The stimulus of catheterization may add to the autonomic reflex, and lidocaine jelly should be used in the urethra prior to catheter insertion if it is readily available, but its lack should not delay the placement of the catheter. If the patient already has an indwelling urinary or suprapubic catheter, it should be checked for obstruction and proper placement. The bladder can be gently irrigated through the catheter with body-temperature normal saline solution to check for obstruction and improper placement. Urine should be sent for urinalysis and culture.

If symptoms persist, the physician should suspect fecal impaction.[1,2] Prior to the rectal examination, the patient's blood pressure should be managed, and the anal opening should be anesthetized with lidocaine jelly placed into the rectum for 5 min before beginning the examination.[1,2] The patient's blood pressure should be monitored to ensure that the hypertension is not aggravated during this procedure, since rectal examination can exacerbate autonomic dysreflexia. If the blood pressure increases, stop the examination, instill more anesthetic agent, and wait additional time. If the bladder or bowel does not appear to be the cause of the patient's symptoms, a search for other causes should be undertaken.

Following relief of an acute episode, patients should be monitored for at least 2 h after resolution to ensure that there is no recurrence.[3] Patients with bladder distention do not routinely require discharge with an indwelling urinary catheter. It is best to discuss that option with the patient's physician. If the patient responds poorly or the cause has not been identified, the patient may be admitted for more aggres-

sive pharmacologic control of blood pressure and a more thorough investigation of the cause.[1-3] The Clinical Practice Guideline for Acute Management of Autonomic Dysreflexia available through the Paralyzed Veterans of America (www.pva.org) is highly recommended.

Urinary Tract Infection

A urinary tract infection should be suspected when a spinal-cord-injured patient presents with fever, discomfort over the kidney or bladder, worsening spasticity, development of urinary incontinence, autonomic dysreflexia, cloudy or foul-smelling urine, a change in energy level, or a feeling of apprehension.[4] Unless there are confounding factors, the urinalysis shows pyuria and significant bacteriuria. In a patient with the above-mentioned symptoms and signs and pyuria, empiric treatment for urinary tract infection should be initiated. Absence of pyuria makes the diagnosis less likely but does not completely exclude it. Conversely, pyuria in an asymptomatic patient with spinal cord injury does not warrant treatment. Pyuria without infection can occur from irritation of the bladder wall in patients with indwelling catheters and in those who use intermittent catheterization.[5]

Significant bacteriuria for the spinal-cord-injured population is defined according to the method used for bladder emptying. For women who can spontaneously void, significant bacteriuria is defined as greater than 100,000 colony-forming units (CFUs) of bacteria per milliliter. For men who spontaneously void or use condom catheters, greater than 10,000 CFUs/mL is considered significant. For both women and men who use intermittent catheterization, greater than 100 CFUs/mL indicates significant bacteriuria. For patients with indwelling urethral or suprapubic catheters, any detectable level of bacteriuria is significant.[4]

Urinary tract infections in the spinal-cord-injured population are considered complicated urinary tract infections.[6] Antibiotics with broader-spectrum coverage should be used, since such organisms as *Proteus, Klebsiella, Pseudomonas, Serratia, Providencia,* enterococci, and *Staphylococcus* are more common. Because of the higher risk of upper-tract infection, 7 to 14 days of treatment should be considered.[4-6]

Asymptomatic bacteriuria is very common in patients with a neurogenic bladder and requires periodic or indwelling catheterization. Asymptomatic bacteriuria should not be routinely treated.[4,5]

Acute Abdomen

Classic signs of the acute abdomen are often missing in patients with spinal cord injury.[7] The diagnosis of perforated peptic ulcer, intestinal obstruction, appendicitis, peritonitis, cholecystitis, and renal abscess is often delayed because the classic findings of abdominal muscle rigidity, rebound, abdominal tenderness, fever, and leukocytosis may not be present. In patients with spinal cord injury, other signs and symptoms suggestive of an acute abdomen are autonomic dysreflexia, referred scapular tip pain, abdominal distention, change in muscle spasticity, nausea and vomiting, and a sense of apprehension.[7] A high index of suspicion, along with laboratory and imaging tests, is necessary to avoid missing the diagnosis.[8] One confounding factor is that urinary tract infections may present with similar signs and symptoms. Thus the finding of pyuria or bacteriuria alone should not be used to exclude the diagnosis of an acute abdomen. While abdominal radiographs are also useful in the diagnosis of intestinal obstruction, many patients with spinal cord injury have chronic dysmotility problems and have baseline increased bowel gas and air-fluid levels that may mimic a mechanical obstruction. Ultrasound, radiologic studies using radiocontrast media, and computed tomography (CT) imaging studies are often required for correct diagnosis in such patients.[8]

Syringomyelia

Posttraumatic syringomyelia may present months to years after a spinal cord injury.[9,10] This process produces a cystic cavitation of the central cord that may extend over several levels. Ascending sensory level (i.e., a decrease or loss of sensation above the preexisting sensory level) and pain are the most common presenting symptoms. Motor weakness, a change in spasticity, and a change in deep-tendon reflexes may also be seen. Magnetic resonance imaging is the imaging study of choice for making the diagnosis of syringomyelia. Surgery is indicated in progressive neurologic deterioration.

Immobilization Hypercalcemia

Risk factors for immobilization hypercalcemia include age less than 21 years, complete neurologic injuries, cervical injuries, prolonged immobilization, and dehydration.[11] Presenting symptoms include anorexia, nausea, headache, malaise, and depression in mild cases. In more severe cases, patients may have persistent nausea and vomiting, gastric dilatation, fecal impaction, and abdominal pain. Microscopic calcium deposition in the kidney may impair its ability to concentrate urine, leading to polyuria and polydipsia. Patients may also develop cardiac dysrhythmias and seizures.[12]

The pathophysiology of immobilization hypercalcemia is thought to be due to the combination of increased bone resorption and the inability of the kidneys to excrete the excess calcium. Compared to other age groups, adolescents are at higher risk due to a higher-than-normal bone turnover rate and more total bone mineral.[11,12] Immobilization causes a decrease in osteoblastic activity in the weight-bearing bones and an increased rate of bone resorption. Together, these factors lead to a higher-than-normal serum calcium level during prolonged periods of immobilization. In most cases, the kidneys can usually excrete the calcium, but in some patients this ability breaks down.

Treating immobilization hypercalcemia starts with hydration and diuresis with NS solution 2 to 3 L/d with the addition of furosemide. Calcitonin in doses of 1 to 4 IU/kg SC every 12 h can also effectively reduce the serum calcium level.[11,12]

Heterotopic Ossification

Heterotopic ossification (HO) is the formation of bone in the soft tissues.[13] The mechanisms of the formation of heterotopic bone are not precisely known. In spinal-cord-injured patients, it is more common among those with spasticity. Symptoms may present as early as 1 month after injury. Pain is prominent in other patients with HO but is often absent in spinal-cord-injured patients. For spinal-cord-injured patients, the most common symptom of HO is a decreased range of motion. Other findings are a change in spasticity, fever, erythema, joint effusion, and swelling.[13] The differential diagnosis includes DVT, infection, and tumor. Sometimes HO and DVT are seen together.

The incidence of HO in spinal-cord-injured patients has been reported to be 16 to 53 percent. The most common sites are the hip, knee, femur, and shoulder. Plain radiograph findings are often negative in the early stages of HO. The gold standard for diagnosis is the three-phase bone scan. Serum alkaline phosphatase (ALP) levels have been used as a screening test for HO, since developing bone produces ALP. However, this is a nonspecific test indicating increased bone metabolic activity, which may occur in fractures or tumors.

Treatment for HO is usually disodium etidronate 20 mg/kg per d for 2 weeks followed by 10 mg/kg per day for 10 weeks, along with gentle physical therapy. Referral to a physiatrist (a physician specializing in the care of patients with disabilities) or other spinal-cord-injury specialist is recommended to institute and monitor treatment.

Leg Pain

If a patient with spinal cord injury or a brain injury presents with a swollen and painful leg, the differential diagnosis includes trauma (e.g., contusion, sprain, or fracture), spasticity, DVT, heterotopic ossification, and reflex sympathetic dystrophy.[1] For those individuals who have impaired sensation, language, or cognition that might hinder the history and physical examination, a high index of suspicion and liberal use of ancillary studies are critical. Plain radiographs are usually adequate for evaluating trauma. For those who have suffered from a recent spinal cord injury (within 8 weeks), the risk of deep vein thrombosis is substantial, most likely from venous stasis. Signs and symptoms include swelling, pain, and warmth. Noninvasive venous studies (duplex Doppler) are usually adequate for evaluating DVT.

Another likely cause of leg pain is spasticity. This condition is often chronic in nature, but certain noxious stimuli may acutely worsen the symptoms. Such causes include infections (UTI, upper respiratory infections, pneumonia, gastroenteritis, etc.), trauma, and stress. Initial treatment is to identify and eliminate these causes. Baclofen is the first line for medicinal treatment and should be started at a dose of 5 mg PO tid, and titrated upward according to symptoms. If the patient does not respond to baclofen, tizanidine, diazepam, and dantrolene may be tried. Once the patient is stabilized, a referral to a physiatrist or other specialist in the care of patients with spinal cord injury should be arranged.

BRAIN INJURY

Posttraumatic Hydrocephalus

Patients with a history of traumatic brain injury may present to the emergency department with the complaint of changing functional status, including psychomotor slowing, cognitive decline, change in gait, and loss of continence.[14] An evaluation for possible infectious or metabolic causes must be undertaken, but a CT scan of the head is critical to evaluate for posttraumatic hydrocephalus.[14,15] A CT scan revealing periventricular lucency, diminishing sulci, and dilatation of the ventricles suggests posttraumatic hydrocephalus. Consultation with a neurosurgeon for appropriate treatment options, such as shunting, should be undertaken.

REFERENCES

1. McKinley WO, Gittler MS, Kirshblum SC, et al: Spinal cord injury medicine. 2. Medical complications after spinal cord injury: Identification and management. *Arch Phys Med Rehabil* 83(Suppl 1):S58, S90, 2002.
2. Karlsson AK: Autonomic dysreflexia. *Spinal Cord* 37:383, 1999.
3. Consortium for Spinal Cord Medicine: Acute management of autonomic dysreflexia: Individuals with spinal cord injury presenting to health-care facilities. *J Spinal Cord Med* 25(Suppl 1):S67, 2002.
4. Siroky MB: Pathogenesis of bacteriuria and infection in the spinal cord injured patient. *Am J Med* 113(Suppl 1A):67S, 2002.
5. Biering-Sorensen F: Urinary tract infection in individuals with spinal cord lesion. *Curr Opin Urol* 12:45, 2002.
6. Biering-Sorenson F, Bagi P, Hoiby N: Urinary tract infections in patients with spinal cord lesions: Treatment and prevention. *Drugs* 61:1275, 2001.
7. Bar-On Z, Ohry A: The acute abdomen in spinal cord injury individuals. *Paraplegia* 33:704, 1995.
8. Miller BJ, Geraghty TJ, Wong CH, et al: Outcome of the acute abdomen in patients with previous spinal cord injury. *Aust N Z J Surg* 71:407, 2001.
9. Vannemreddy SS, Rowed DW, Bharatwal N: Posttraumatic syringomyelia: Predisposing factors. *Br J Neurosurg* 16:276, 2002.
10. Schurch B, Wichmann W, Rossier AB: Post-traumatic syringomyelia (cystic myelopathy): A prospective study of 449 patients with spinal cord injury. *J Neurol Neurosurg Psychiatry* 60:61, 1996.
11. Mechanick JI, Brett EM: Endocrine and metabolic issues in the management of the chronically critically ill patient. *Crit Care Clin* 18:619, 2002.
12. Maynard FM: Immobilization hypercalcemia following spinal cord injury. *Arch Phys Med Rehabil* 67:41, 1986.
13. van Kuijk AA, Geurts AC, van Kuppevelt HJ: Neurogenic heterotopic ossification in spinal cord injury. *Spinal Cord* 40:313, 2002.
14. Brandstater ME, Bontke CF, Cobble ND, et al: Rehabilitation in brain disorders. 4. Specific disorders. *Arch Phys Med Rehabil* 72(4-S):S332, 1991.
15. Guyot LL, Michael DB: Post-traumatic hydrocephalus. *Neurol Res* 22:25, 2000.

THE MENTALLY RETARDED ADULT
Linmarie Sikich

Evaluating a developmentally disabled adult in the ED poses a number of challenges, including accurately assessing the ability of the individual to communicate his or her complaints, the ability to make an accurate diagnosis in the absence of sufficient historical information, and the recognition of unusual presentations of common disorders. In addition, 25 percent of individuals with developmental disabilities appear to have significantly increased pain thresholds that result in reduced responses to illnesses and to physical examinations.[1] Such pain insensitivity may limit recognition of medical problems (e.g., intestinal obstruction) until late in the disease process, with potentially catastrophic consequences. Treatment of developmentally disabled individuals is also complicated by questions about guardianship, decreased ability of the patient to understand the treatment recommendations, and often, inadequate preventative and routine medical care. However, it is essential that health care providers overcome these obstacles to provide care to this special population that has difficulty advocating for itself.

EPIDEMIOLOGY

The primary developmental disability is mental retardation, defined as significant cognitive (IQ less than 70) and functional delays with onset before adulthood. Over 40 percent of individuals with mental retardation have associated medical conditions. Typically, the lower the patient's IQ, the more likely a specific etiology of the mental retardation can be identified. Etiologic factors implicated in mental retardation may be prenatal, perinatal, postnatal, or traumatic. Genetic factors account for 7 to 15 percent of all mental retardation; there are 500 genetic syndromes known to be associated with mental retardation.[2] Depending on the etiology, some medical problems are associated with specific mental retardation syndromes (Table 309-1).[3–5]

About 6 million individuals in the United States and 150 million in the world (2.5 percent of the population) have mental retardation. Two other developmental disorders, autism spectrum disorders and language disabilities, are also important for health care providers to recognize. Many autistic individuals have tactile defensiveness and become very agitated when they are touched, which complicates physical examination. People with either autism or language disorder often have difficulty communicating their symptoms and understanding, appropriately generalizing, and responding to information about suggested medical treatments, regardless of their level of cognitive functioning.

Over the past 20 to 30 years there has been a movement in the United States to remove developmentally disabled individuals from institutional settings and care for them in the community. About 89 percent of American adults with mental retardation currently are in the community. However, adults with mental retardation who were moved from an institutional setting to the community had a 51 percent greater mortality rate than those who remained in the institution,[6] although this may not be generalizable to all communities.[7] The caretakers of individuals with developmental disabilities who have recently moved may lack adequate knowledge of the patient's baseline and past medical history.[8]

GENERAL APPROACH

The general approach consists of avoiding overstimulation, gathering specific and collateral information, assessing the patient's ability to communicate, performing a physical examination, and obtaining appropriate ancillary studies.

Individuals with intellectual disabilities should be evaluated in an area with as few distractions as possible by a limited number of health care providers.[9]

TABLE 309-1   Medical Problems Associated with Specific Mental Retardation Syndromes

Syndrome	Incidence	% MR	Common Medical Problems
Down	1/1000	4–12	Atlantoaxial instability; obesity; leukemia; dementia; sleep apnea; hypothyroidism; diabetes; cataracts; hearing loss; congenital heart disease
Fragile X	0.67/1000	1–6	Seizures; mitral valve prolapse; dilated great arteries; otitis
Fetal alcohol	2/1000	10	Seizures; congenital heart disease; eye problems; hearing loss
Prader-Willi	0.1/1000	0.4	Obesity; sleep apnea; hypoventilation; diabetes; inability to vomit; hypertension; ischemic heart disease
Williams	0.1/1000	0.4	Hypertension; supravalvular aortic stenosis; ulcers; renal artery stenosis; urethral stenosis; diverticulitis; vesicoureteral reflux; hypercalcemia
Lesch-Nyhan	0.02/1000	0.08	Severe self-injurious behavior; sudden death; gout; renal calculi; renal failure
Tuberous sclerosis	0.1/1000	0.4	Brain and skin tubers; seizures; rhabdomyomas of heart; angiomyolipomas of kidney; renal failure
Cerebral palsy	3/1000	12–30	Pain; contractures; seizures; respiratory and urinary tract infections

Abbreviation: MR = Mental retardation.

Determine the patient's specific baseline behaviors in the following areas: (1) communication, (2) environmental awareness, (3) motor activity, (4) urinary and bowel habits, (5) sleep pattern, (6) appetite, and (7) use of assistive devices such as glasses or hearing aids. Acute disease processes in individuals with developmental disabilities often present as nonspecific changes in routine activities rather than focal complaints. Obtain a complete past medical history, an accurate list of medications, and history of prior adverse medical reactions. Frequently used medications and associated side effects are shown in Table 309-2. Next, determine the patient's living situation. Even relatively minor changes in routine or caretakers can have a dramatic impact on the functioning of some developmentally disabled individuals. Ask both the patient and caretakers about possible physical or sexual abuse. Rates of sexual assault in girls with developmental disabilities appear to be two- to fivefold higher than in typically developing girls.[10] Also identify resources for appropriate follow-up care within the community. Finally, determine whether the patient has a guardian, or if not, if the patient is capable of making decisions about medical care.

The evaluation of developmentally disabled patients usually requires collateral information from parents, group home staff, or social service agency staff. The extent and importance of such information increases as the developmentally disabled patient's ability to communicate decreases. Ask the collateral source explicitly how much they know or have in writing, and whether there are others with more information who can be contacted by phone. When possible, written collateral information should be reviewed prior to seeing the patient. Such information often clarifies the patient's usual level of cognitive functioning and communication, past medical history, current medications, and longitudinal vital signs.

TABLE 309-2 Frequently Used Medications and Side Effects

Medications	Frequency of Use*	Important Side Effects
Psychotropics	44%	
Antipsychotics		Extrapyramidal symptoms; neuroleptic malignant syndrome; dystonia can affect swallowing and breathing; sedation; orthostatic hypotension; weight gain; constipation
SSRIs		Gastrointestinal distress; agitation; insomnia; sedation
Benzodiazepines		Sedation; disinhibition; agitation; delirium
Anticholinergics		Blurry vision; urinary retention; constipation
Lithium		Hypothyroidism; delirium; cardiac arrhythmias
Anticonvulsants	30–50%	Sedation; delirium; ataxia
Carbamazepine		Blood dyscrasias; rashes; constipation; lowers other drug levels
Lamotrigine		Severe rashes
Cardiovascular	25%	Overdosage may lead to cardiotoxicity
Laxatives	20%	Vitamin deficiencies
Bronchodilators	14%	Agitation; decreased bone mineralization
Analgesics	12%	Renal problems; anemia
Histamine blockers	10%	Psychosis
Thyroid supplements	8%	Psychosis; agitation; hot flashes; odd skin sensations

Abbreviation: SSRI = Selective serotonin reuptake inhibitor.
Source: Data from Cooper SA: Clinical study of the effects of age on the physical health of adults with mental retardation. *Am J Ment Retard* 102:582, 1998.

Assess the Individual's Ability to Communicate

Developmentally disabled individuals have a broad range of cognitive and communicative abilities. Approach patients in a manner consistent with their abilities and be sensitive to and respectful of their thoughts and feelings. About 85 percent of mentally retarded individuals are mildly impaired and typically function at about a fifth-grade level. They can generally provide relevant history and describe many of their symptoms. They are also likely to understand simple written directions. About 10 percent of mentally retarded adults are moderately affected; they function at the level of a preschool child, are likely to be able to follow commands, and may be able to answer simple questions. The remaining 5 percent are likely to have no expressive language, although they sometimes can follow simple commands. Individuals with autism or language disabilities often have significantly more communication impairments than cognitive limitations.

Patients should be directly interviewed in addition to gaining information from collateral sources. If individuals are verbal, attempt open-ended rather than yes/no questions. It is also helpful to ask higher-functioning individuals to repeat back information to make sure they have understood. Many mentally retarded individuals have particular difficulties with time and causality concepts. Nonverbal patients may be able to point in response to simple questions.

A thorough physical examination is needed because sufficient history is often not available to focus the examination. However, examination may be difficult in patients with extreme agitation or tactile defensiveness. The physician should thoroughly explain and (when possible) demonstrate all procedures prior to performing them. If not

medically contraindicated, it may be helpful to offer the patient food or distractions. A familiar person should be present during the examination and for any procedures. If the patient is still too anxious to allow an evaluation, an anxiolytic may be indicated or assistance may be required to briefly hold the patient. During the exam, special attention should be given to all body orifices because objects are often inserted into these areas without the caretakers' knowledge. Vital signs should be obtained when the patient is calm.

Ancillary studies should be obtained as appropriate. If there are no localizing symptoms or physical signs, complete blood cell count, electrolytes, liver function tests, urinalysis, and serum drug levels may be necessary.[11]

FREQUENTLY ENCOUNTERED PROBLEMS

The incidence of medical problems is greater in individuals with developmental disabilities than in the general population. These differences are most pronounced for individuals with severe to profound mental retardation. For individuals with mild cognitive limitations, the rate of chronic medical problems increases significantly after age 30. Chronic medical problems in the mentally retarded population include seizures; nonischemic heart disease, gastrointestinal problems, and pulmonary disease (in individuals younger than 50); and osteoporosis, arthritis, sensory impairment, and dementia (in the elderly).[12–16] Emergency department visits are most often precipitated by infections (35 percent), trauma (33 percent), seizures (15 percent), and gastrointestinal concerns (5 percent).[12] In addition, agitation frequently leads to ED evaluations. Most often, mortality is related to respiratory or cardiovascular events, though bowel perforation and seizures are also common.[14,15]

Infections

Infections are common in the developmentally disabled population. Aspiration is common in individuals with oral-motor dyspraxias, esophageal reflux, and tube feedings. Urinary tract infections are common, partially due to neurogenic bladder, limited mobility, and poor hygiene. Because individuals may not initially recognize or describe dysuria, they are at greater risk for pyelonephritis. With a history of repeated urinary tract infections, it is important to exclude congenital malformations of the urinary system. Skin infections, dental caries, and periodontal disease are also common.

Injuries

Injuries may be self-inflicted, accidental, or result from assault. Minor trauma can result in fractures because patients are more likely to be osteopenic.[17] The majority of injuries that mentally retarded individuals experience are the result of self-injurious behaviors. Although self-injurious behaviors may be self-stimulating, medical and environmental precipitants are often identified if the self-injurious behaviors are of sudden onset. Bosch and colleagues found that in 28 percent of their patients, treatment of previously undiagnosed, painful medical conditions resulted in significant reductions in self-injurious behaviors.[18] Constipation, gastroesophageal reflux, and peptic ulcer disease were the most common disorders. In these cases, there had often been a cyclic pattern to the self-injurious behaviors or a recent exacerbation. Similarly, increased self-injurious behaviors are often associated with anxiety. If no medical or environmental precipitants for these behaviors can be identified, it may be useful to treat individuals with selective serotonin reuptake inhibitors (SSRIs). Naltrexone or atypical antipsychotics may also be useful. Protective behavioral measures such as a helmet to prevent head-banging may be needed to avoid further injury.

Neurologic Problems

SEIZURES Thirty to 50 percent of all developmentally delayed individuals have seizure disorders. Often, an individual experiences several different types of seizures. The mortality associated with seizures is 2 to 3 times greater among individuals with mental retardation than among those with normal intelligence.[19] The priorities are to ensure adequate oxygenation, stop the seizure, and identify seizure precipitants. Seizures are commonly precipitated by a change in medication. Unintentional medication changes may occur when a person with mental retardation moves to a new living situation, because a medication has been forgotten or given incorrectly. Other common seizure precipitants are addition of new medications that alter the seizure threshold or infection.

DELIRIUM Developmentally disabled individuals appear to be particularly vulnerable to delirium. Typically, caretakers will describe a relatively acute change in mental status. Visual and tactile hallucinations and agitation are not uncommon. Most often, the delirium results from infection or drug toxicity. The latter may occur at low medication doses. Toxicity may also be precipitated by interactions with other medications. For instance, erythromycin and fluoxetine slow the metabolism of several anticonvulsants. Anticonvulsants and anticholinergics frequently cause delirium. Less often, delirium results from metabolic disturbances including hyperglycemia, hypothyroidism, hypoxia, or vitamin or cofactor deficiencies (e.g., carnitine in individuals treated with valproic acid).

SPINAL CORD COMPRESSION DUE TO ATLANTOAXIAL INSTABILITY **Individuals with mental retardation, especially Down syndrome, often have atlantoaxial instability as a result of connective tissue laxity and anomalies of the atlas and axis.** The spinal cord is vulnerable to compression with neck flexion or extension. Intubation, tracheal suctioning, laryngoscopy, bronchoscopy, and dental work are examples of procedures that can result in neck flexion and cord compression. Chronic atlantoaxial instability can also cause more subtle neurologic manifestations, such as easy fatigability, difficulties in walking, neck pain, limited neck mobility, torticollis, clumsiness, sensory deficits, incontinence, and spasticity. These symptoms may progress to paralysis or even death. Most individuals have had symptoms for more than a month prior to their diagnosis. Rarely, sudden subluxation has occurred when there was a sudden change in momentum, as in motor vehicle accidents.[20] Treatment of atlantoaxial instability usually involves surgical stabilization.

Gastrointestinal Disorders

Erosive esophagitis and ulcers are common causes of gastrointestinal bleeding in patients with developmental disabilities. About 40 percent of mentally retarded individuals have severe constipation, often with overflow diarrhea and infrequently with rectal tears. Treatment must include both acute and long-term measures. Pica is present in many individuals, about 10 percent of whom will develop bezoars or intestinal obstruction.

Psychiatric Disorders

Psychiatric disorders are estimated to afflict up to 50 percent of the developmentally disabled population. Emergency visits are usually precipitated by aggression or extreme agitation. In such cases, benzodiazepines or low-dose, low-potency antipsychotics, may be acutely helpful in controlling the patient's behavior sufficiently to proceed with an evaluation. Undiagnosed, painful medical problems, including severe constipation, are common causes of behavior problems.[12] Sleep apnea or anxiety can also be manifest as increased irritability. Anxiety may result from environmental factors, such as change in caretaker or uncorrected sensory deficits, posttraumatic stress disorder, or panic attacks. Akathisia, a dose-related side-effect syndrome caused by both typical and atypical antipsychotics, is manifest as agitation and hyperactivity. Akathisia should be considered if there is a history of worsening agitation with increased antipsychotic medications. This disorder usually responds to propranolol. Finally, agitation may occur in response to psychotic symptoms. Catatonic behavior may reflect delirium, depression, or status epilepticus with absence or partial-complex seizures. Mood disorders typically present with changes in the patient's sleep, appetite, and activity level.

REFERENCES

1. Biersdorff KK: Incidence of significantly altered pain experience among individuals with developmental disabilities. *Am J Ment Retard* 98:619, 1994.
2. Murphy CC, Boyle C, Schendel D, et al: Epidemiology of mental retardation in children. *Ment Retard Dev Disabil Res Rev* 4:6, 1998.
3. Yeargin-Allsopp M, Murphy CC, Cordero JF, et al: Reported biomedical causes and associated medical conditions for mental retardation among 10-year-old children, metropolitan Atlanta, 1985 to 1987. *Develop Med Child Neurol* 39:142, 1997.
4. Gilberg C: *Clinical Child Neuropsychiatry.* Cambridge, England: Cambridge University Press, 1995.
5. Abel EL, Sokol RJ: Fetal alcohol syndrome is now the leading cause of mental retardation. *Lancet* 2:1222, 1986.
6. Strauss D, Shavelle R, Baumeister A, et al: Mortality in persons with developmental disabilities after transfer into community care. *Am J Ment Retard* 102:569, 1998.
7. Borthwick-Duffy S, Widaman KF, Grossman HJ: Mortality research, placement, and risk of death: Basic research, the media, and public policy. *Ment Retard* 36:416, 1998.
8. Minihan PM, Dean DH, Lyons CM: Managing the care of patients with mental retardation: A survey of physicians. *Ment Retard* 31:239, 1993.
9. Grossman SA, Richards CF, Anglin D, et al: Caring for the patient with mental retardation in the emergency department. *Ann Emerg Med* 35:69, 2000.
10. Chamberlain A, Rauh J, Passer A, et al: Issues in fertility control for mentally retarded female adolescents: I. Sexual activity, sexual abuse, and contraception. *Pediatrics* 73:445, 1984.
11. Ryan R, Sunada K: Medical evaluation of persons with mental retardation referred for psychiatric assessment. *Gen Hosp Psychiatry* 19:274, 1997.
12. Tyler CV, Bourguet C: Primary care of adults with mental retardation. *J Fam Pract* 44:487, 1997.
13. Patja K, Iivanainen M, Vesala H, et al: Life expectancy of people with intellectual disability: A 35-year follow-up study. *J Intellect Disabil Res* 44:591, 2000.
14. Strauss D, Anderson TW, Shavelle R, et al: Causes of death of persons with developmental disabilities: Comparison of institutional and community residents. *Ment Retard* 36:386, 1998.
15. Patja K, Molsa P, Iivanainen M: Cause-specific mortality of people with intellectual disability in a population-based, 35-year follow-up study. *J Intellect Disabil Res* 45:30, 2001.
16. Kapell D, Nightingale B, Rodriquez A, et al: Prevalence of chronic medical conditions in adults with mental retardation: Comparison with the general population. *Ment Retard* 36:269, 1998.
17. Center J, Beane H, McElduff A: People with mental retardation have an increased prevalence of osteoporosis: A population study. *Am J Ment Retard* 103:19, 1998.
18. Bosch J, Van Dyke DC, Smith SM, et al: Role of medical conditions in the exacerbation of self-injurious behavior: An exploratory study. *Ment Retard* 35:124, 1997.
19. Wakamoto H, Nagao H, Hayasi M, et al: Long-term medical, educational, and social prognosis of childhood-onset epilepsy: A population-based study in a rural district of Japan. *Brain Dev* 22:246, 2000.
20. American Academy of Pediatrics Committee on Sports Medicine and Fitness: Atlantoaxial instability in Down syndrome: Subject review. *Pediatrics* 96:151, 1995.

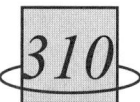

THE HOMELESS PATIENT
Rama B. Rao
Lewis R. Goldfrank

Homelessness is a social problem of epidemic proportions worldwide.[1] In the United States alone, estimates of the homeless population range between 3 and 13.5 million, and as much as 7.4 percent of the general population will experience homelessness in their lifetime. Homelessness affects a diverse population of all ethnic groups and includes both urban and rural families, the elderly, children, veterans, migrant farm workers, mentally ill persons, and persons with substance use disorders. Minority groups are overrepresented in this population, most likely due to disparities in economic opportunities. Causes of homelessness are related to divorce or separation, domestic violence, pregnancy, adolescent runaways, substance use, eviction, acute or chronic unemployment, and the deinstitutionalization of persons with mental illness. A disparity between the need for low-income housing and its availability has also contributed to the epidemic of homelessness.

Homelessness has been defined in a variety of ways, including living on the street, in shelters that provide temporary residence, or in single-room occupancy hotels with shared bathrooms. The consequences of homelessness are profound. Homeless adults have an age-adjusted mortality rate nearly four times higher than that of the general population, with a median age of death of 44.[2] Infant mortality rates among homeless mothers are more than twice those for nonpoor, domiciled mothers, and 50 percent higher than those for poor domiciled mothers. The effects of homelessness on children may be profound, with a higher incidence of acute illnesses and medical treatment.[3] Other risks important to homeless populations include communicable diseases, environmental exposures to extreme heat or cold, and traumatic injury due to violent encounters, foraging for food, and seeking shelter.[4] These factors contribute greatly to acute medical illness among the homeless. Some of the increased risks are associated with poverty, and others are specific to undomiciled patients. Chronic illnesses, such as hypertension and diabetes, are neglected or poorly managed due to desperate living circumstances. Homeless individuals often delay care of minor medical problems until they become severe or unbearable.

The ED is often used as a primary source of medical care for acute and nonacute illnesses of the homeless.[5-7] Homeless persons have emergency department utilization rates that are 1.5 to 3 times that of the general population, with up to 20 percent reporting that the emergency department was their sole source of medical care.[7] Outpatient community- and shelter-based clinics provide medical care in a limited fashion and can lead to ED referral for more extensive evaluation and management. In some cities, homeless patients may arrive by police or emergency medical services because of extreme weather emergencies or other health and safety mandates. All of these factors make knowledge of this population important to emergency physicians. The management of the homeless patient is complex, and similarities to the domiciled patient are limited. Decision analysis for this vulnerable population is distinctly different and admission criteria are uniquely dependent on the environment.

CARE AND EVALUATION

Homeless patients may have both specific and nonspecific medical complaints. Once the primary reason for the visit is addressed, a thorough examination of the entire body, including the skin and particularly the feet, should be considered. This is especially necessary for the homeless patient who is disheveled, intoxicated, or has a significant psychosis. A valuable medical history may include the last evaluation for tuberculosis exposure, tetanus immunization status, vaccination status in children, psychiatric history, history of chemical dependence, and potential for substance withdrawal while receiving care in the ED. A social history may include family support, precipitants of homelessness, and prior contact with a social worker.

SPECIAL MEDICAL CONSIDERATIONS

General Hygiene

Homeless persons have limited access to facilities for maintaining hygiene, and regular bathing and daily dental care may be severely impaired. The emergency physician should closely inspect all of the skin, lower extremities, and perineum as part of the routine evaluation of all homeless patients.

Lower Extremity Diseases

Homeless patients have a variety of lower extremity disorders. Such patients may spend a disproportionate amount of time with their legs in a dependent position while sleeping upright or ambulating for extended periods. The poverty associated with homelessness may prevent some patients from obtaining socks and shoes that are seasonally appropriate and well fitting. Ulcers and wounds from lack of foot protection, blisters from poorly fitting shoes, or bites from rodents or insects may occur.

Some homeless patients may not have an available change of footwear or a place to change and bathe. Socks and shoes may not be removed for days to weeks for reasons such as warmth, fear that footwear may be stolen, embarrassment, or coexisting mental illness. These factors, along with limitations on hygiene, predispose to fungal infections, which can be treated with topical or oral therapy. Also of concern in this population is the condition known as trench foot. Protracted exposure to moisture around the foot (usually from wet or sweaty socks) leads to absorption of water into the stratum corneum. Over 1 to 2 days, such exposure causes inflammatory changes that result in foot pain and skin breakdown. Bacterial superinfection with *Corynebacterium* species and *Pseudomonas* species can ensue. In the absence of superinfection, analgesia, leg elevation, and drying are adequate to treat the earliest stages of trench foot. In colder climates, frostbite from formation of ice crystals in the tissues is a serious threat to limbs, ears, and nose. Careful in-hospital management is warranted, since the environmental risks persist as long as the patient remains homeless, and compliance with treatment may be difficult if not impossible.

Patients predisposed to peripheral vascular disease can have exacerbation of their illness due to inadequate nutrition, poor protein status, alcoholism and substance use, use of tobacco, and inability to elevate the legs while sleeping upright. The resulting edema can lead to chronic venous stasis ulcers. The ulcers can become infected with common skin flora or even maggots (fly larvae). For uninfected ulcers, the use of venous support garments, such as Unna boots, is a valuable management tool. Unna boots are impregnated with antibiotic ointment and require less frequent changes. Patients with infected ulcers require admission. The erythema associated with cellulitis may be difficult to distinguish from deep venous thrombosis or venous stasis changes. When the diagnosis is unclear, an evaluation of venous flow should be undertaken. For lesions infected with maggots, chloroform is a traditional therapy for deinfestation. Chloroform may not be available due to safety issues of combustibility. Ethyl chloride is an alternative. Ironically, maggots survive by ingesting necrotic tissue, keeping ulcers clean and well debrided. Once deinfestation is completed, close follow-up is mandatory, since natural debridement via fly larvae is terminated. Maggot infestation is a grave sign of serious neglect and suggests the inability to manage a clinical plan outside a supervised setting.

All homeless patients need education to minimize the risk of trench foot and fungal infections. Patients should be told to change or remove all footwear when environmental conditions allow, examine the feet, and attempt to find a place to rest where their legs may be elevated. Injection drug users should be warned about the risk of skin infection from drug administration into the extremities. Community resources, which can provide clean, dry socks and well-fitting shoes, should be identified. Such preventive measures are especially important for diabetic patients and those who suffer from peripheral neuropathies.

Infections

Homeless patients develop common community-acquired respiratory infections, but tuberculosis is also a threat.[5] The incidence of tuberculosis increases dramatically when people live under crowded conditions and when patients are immunosuppressed from diseases such as AIDS, malnutrition, or alcoholism. Multiple studies of various homeless populations confirm the high incidence and prevalence of tuberculosis in homeless patients. For homeless patients, compliance with a treatment regimen for an exposure to tuberculosis may be limited. Daily, directly observed therapy programs have been very successful by using incentives to organize therapy and decrease the risk of tuberculosis transmission.

Homeless patients in shelters or other group living arrangements are also at higher risk than are domiciled patients for communicable skin diseases, such as pediculosis (lice), scabies, and impetigo. Deinfestation of lice and scabies is problematic for patients, since bathing facilities and the ability to wash and change clothing are limited. Patients may return to the environment where infestation originally occurred, and they are at high risk for reinfestation. A dermatologic disease known as bacillary angiomatosis-peliosis has been identified in homeless patients exposed to lice.[8] The causative organism is *Bartonella quintana,* and the condition can be treated effectively with macrolide antibiotics. *Bartonella quintana* infections may also cause trench fever, endocarditis, and chronic bacteremia in the homeless.[9]

The living conditions of the impoverished can place them at risk for other infections. Diarrheal illness from the ingestion of improperly preserved or discarded food has been poorly studied, but has been described by homeless patients and is particularly problematic when access to toilet facilities is limited. Fecal-oral transmission of illness is also increased.

Sexually transmitted diseases are prevalent in homeless individuals who engage in sexual activity voluntarily or by coercion to obtain food, shelter, cash, or other goods. Money for prophylactic condoms or other forms of contraception is limited, unavailable, or a low priority for survival. These problems, in addition to injection drug use, have lead to epidemic rates of HIV among the homeless. Discrimination and disability from HIV disease are also implicated as a cause of homelessness.

The management of HIV disease is complicated for both patients and medical practitioners even under ideal circumstances. Newer drug regimens, which include multiple medications, are expensive and depend on a reliable dosing schedule and follow-up. The use of reverse transcriptase and protease inhibitors may depend on the ability of patients to comply with therapy.[10]

Hospital admission of homeless patients with diseases such as varicella or hepatitis may be necessary to avoid infections in shelters or other public areas in which the homeless may congregate.

Compliance

Prioritization of other life-sustaining activities, such as finding food or shelter, may interfere with compliance to medical regimens or follow-up despite the intention to do so.[11] Money may be unavailable for prescriptions. Even hospital-dispensed medications may be traded for cash or other items perceived as more essential, depending on the patient's level of despair and how well the patient understands the consequences of forgoing treatment. Some items necessary for treatment, such as insulin syringes or other medications, are valuable for illicit

use and are at risk of theft. Agents such as insulin may lose their efficacy and safety when stored improperly. It may be impossible to refrigerate medications. A regular dosing medication schedule is complicated and nearly impossible in a lifestyle devoid of daily routines.

Lack of medical insurance may limit patient access to primary care for follow-up. Negotiating eligibility for various types of state and federal medical coverage is usually complicated, but may be of tremendous benefit to patients with chronic illnesses, for which poverty potentially thwarts adequate management. Patients should be referred to social workers familiar with eligibility requirements and processing. Unfortunately, even eligible patients may require several visits to social-services agencies to establish medical coverage, and this process alone may be too complex and demeaning to complete.

Other barriers to care include lack of transportation or mental illness. The precarious existence of such patients must be considered with compassion, and they should be treated with a medical regimen that accommodates the limitations of their social situation. For example, patients dependent on soup kitchens should have appointments arranged that would not limit access to mealtimes. Shelter-based drop-in clinic systems may be more realistic than tightly scheduled appointments.

SPECIAL POPULATIONS

Women and Children

Women and children comprise a rapidly increasing proportion of the homeless population. Women may present for routine medical problems or as a result of domestic violence or rape, for which they are at particularly high risk.[12] Some women may resort to prostitution to support themselves or their children. Preventive gynecologic care is often inadequate and extends from inadequate screening for cervical cancer and venereal diseases to insufficient or absent prenatal care. The consequences are devastating. Children born to homeless mothers often have lower birth weights, higher rates of prematurity, and higher rates of infant mortality. Iron-deficiency anemia, malnutrition, elevated blood lead concentrations, and a higher rate of asthma are found in homeless children, as in other impoverished children, compared to the general population.[3] Unlike impoverished domiciled children, homeless children are more likely to be inadequately immunized and suffer disproportionately from developmental delay or a lack of progression in school. The long-term psychological, social, and educational consequences of homelessness have yet to be rigorously evaluated.

Homeless adolescents, especially runaways, have high rates of alcoholism, illicit substance use, violent encounters, and psychiatric illness. Engaging in sex for survival has resulted in high rates of unplanned pregnancy, sexually transmitted disease, and HIV infection. Patients should be offered a variety of resources, including education regarding safe-sex practices, counseling, and the location and availability of drop-in centers. Social workers, psychiatrists, and adolescent specialists can cooperatively provide support for homeless runaways regardless of their chief medical complaint.

The Elderly

There are few studies of the homeless elderly. Limited, fixed incomes with progressively increasing housing costs account for the displacement of many elderly people from their homes. Another factor may be gradual changes in cognitive and psychosocial performance, which may not be realized on a brief medical examination. For all people at risk, reassessment for organic disease, dementia, and depression is essential to ensure an appropriate care plan.

Substance Use

Patients who are dependent on alcohol or illicit substances should be identified in order to facilitate appropriate disposition. For homeless patients who present intoxicated and sedated, close monitoring of body temperature, blood glucose monitoring, and serial evaluations for arousability should be performed in addition to a thorough physical examination. Whenever possible, a specific history of substance use should be obtained. A specific history of withdrawal from any sedative-hypnotic agent or ethanol should alert the clinician to the need for careful observation while primary evaluation of the chief complaint is undertaken. The patient should be asked whether he or she has a past history of participating in detoxification programs and whether that is a current desire.

Mental Illness

Some homeless patients without documented history of chronic psychiatric illness or substance dependence may present to the ED with psychiatric complaints. The stresses of sustaining life without a home are associated with a variety of diagnoses, including adjustment disorders, substance use, and major depression.[13] Alternatively, some homeless patients have a chronic history of psychiatric illness, including schizophrenia or bipolar disorder, that may be partially responsible for precipitating homelessness.[5] The psychiatric assessment of homeless patients is important to facilitate adequate disposition of medical problems whose management may be compromised by mental illness. In addition, primary pharmacologic therapy can be evaluated or instituted in patients with chronic psychiatric disorders. All patients should have an assessment for fear and risk of suicide as part of the routine screening.

EMERGENCY DEPARTMENT TREATMENT

ED management includes adjuncts to care, such as use of vitamin supplements and food, dispensing medications, updating immunizations, and reviewing documentation of past medical care. Pregnancy status and potential for sexually transmitted diseases should be investigated in homeless women of childbearing age. Appropriate gynecologic care, prenatal care, or family planning services can thus be arranged. Once a diagnosis and treatment plan is defined, patients should be assessed for language barriers, literacy, and capacity to comply with routine care instructions, medical regimens, or follow-up. An old chart may indicate immunization status, forgotten or disregarded health problems, and the ability of homeless patients to establish continuous care. A lower threshold for hospitalization should be maintained for patients with an impaired ability to manage their own care. This decision is easily acceptable if one appreciates how the patient arrived at the condition in question and how difficult, if not impossible, outpatient care may be under certain circumstances. A public health approach to managing communicable diseases should be incorporated into admission criteria. A multidisciplinary approach to care, including social workers and nursing, medical, and psychiatric staff, may offer the most supportive environment for homeless patients. Such compassionate care in the ED, using trained and motivated individuals, will ensure that patients receive essential care, increase patient satisfaction, and reduce the rate of recidivism among frequent users of the ED.[14]

REFERENCES

1. Committee on Health Care for Homeless People, Institute of Medicine: Who are the homeless?, in Committee on Health Care for Homeless People, Institute of Medicine (ed): *Homelessness, Health, and Human Needs.* Washington, National Academy Press, 1988, p 1.
2. Hwang SW: Mortality among men using homeless shelters in Toronto, Ontario. *JAMA* 283:152, 2000.
3. Weinreb L, Goldberg R, Bassuk E, Perloff J: Determinants of health and service use patterns in homeless and low-income housed children. *Pediatrics* 102:554, 1998.
4. Hwang SW, Orav EJ, O'Connell JJ: Causes of death in homeless adults in Boston. *Ann Intern Med* 126:625, 1997.
5. D'Amore J, Hung O, Chiang W, et al: The epidemiology of the homeless population and its impact on an urban emergency department. *Acad Emerg Med* 8:1051, 2001.
6. Kushel MB, Vittinghoff E, Haas JS: Factors associated with the health care utilization of homeless persons. *JAMA* 285:200, 2001.
7. Kushel MB, Perruy S, Bangsberg D, et al: Emergency department use among the homeless and marginally housed: Results from a community base study. *Am J Public Health* 92:778, 2000.
8. Koehler JE, Sanchez MA, Garrido CS, et al: Molecular epidemiology of *Bartonella* infections in patients with bacillary angiomatosis-peliosis. *New Engl J Med* 337:1876, 1997.
9. Foucault C, Barrau K, Brouqui P, et al: *Bartonella quintana* bacteremia among homeless people. *Clin Infect Dis* 35:684, 2002.
10. Bangsberg D, Tulsky JP, Hecht FM, et al: Protease inhibitors in the homeless. *JAMA* 278:63, 1997.
11. Gelberg L, Gallagher TC, Andersen RM, et al: Competing priorities as a barrier to medical care among homeless adults in Los Angeles. *Am J Public Health* 87:217, 1997.
12. Weinreb L, Goldberg R, Perloff J: Health characteristics and medical service patterns of sheltered homeless and low-income housed mothers. *J Gen Intern Med* 13:389, 1998.
13. Lundy JW: The burden of comorbidity among the homeless at a drop-in clinic. *JAAPA* 12:32, 1999.
14. Redelmeier DA, Molin JP, Tibshirani RJ: A randomized trial of compassionate care for the homeless in an emergency department. *Lancet* 345:1131, 1995.

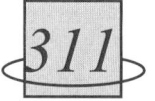

THE MORBIDLY OBESE PATIENT

Robert J. Vissers
Kathleen A. Raftery

Obesity is the condition of an excessive proportion of adipose tissue to total body weight. It is a major health problem, with the prevalence of obesity in the United States doubling in the past 20 years, such that today over half of all adults are estimated to be overweight.[1] Since body fat is difficult to measure in the clinical setting, body mass index (BMI) is frequently utilized. BMI is calculated by dividing the weight in kilograms by the square of the height in meters. A BMI greater than 28 kg/m² defines obesity in both sexes, and morbid obesity is associated with a BMI of 40 kg/m² or greater.

Morbidly obese patients pose a number of challenges for emergency health care providers. Prehospital care may be delayed due to problems in moving and transporting these patients. Appropriate-sized gurneys may not be readily available. Even providing common amenities, such as hospital gowns or bedpans of adequate size, can be difficult. In addition, the ED staff must anticipate and be prepared for challenges in performing technical procedures. Excess tissue makes access to body fluids and body cavities a formidable task, while performing imaging procedures can be difficult or impossible. Morbidly obese patients may also evince changes in cardiopulmonary physiology and patterns of traumatic injury, which add to the complexity of their care.[2]

PATHOPHYSIOLOGY

The etiology of obesity is heterogeneous, including increased caloric intake, a low level of habitual physical activity, a low resting metabolic rate, and possibly high insulin sensitivity.[3] The recent epidemic in developed countries is felt to be more likely due to inactivity than increased caloric intake. The recent discovery of leptin, an antiobesity hormone, has kindled interest in the metabolic pathophysiology of this disease.

Cardiopulmonary Disease

Morbidity and mortality are considerably greater among the obese than in normal-weight patients, and many of the health risks associated with obesity increase progressively and disproportionately with increasing weight.[3] The most significant physiologic disturbances pertain to the cardiopulmonary system.[4]

Coronary artery disease, hypertension, and congestive heart failure are highly correlated with obesity. Both left- and right-sided heart failures are often observed in patients with obesity-hypoventilation syndrome. Obesity has also been linked to depressed left ventricular function even in young, asymptomatic patients.

Obesity is associated with an increased risk of venous thromboembolism, especially after surgery.[5] This is due to several factors found in the obese patient, including decreased levels of circulating antithrombin III, preexisting venous disease, and increased immobility.[3] The obesity-hypoventilation syndrome, also known as the *pickwickian syndrome,* occurs in 5 percent of the morbidly obese. In obese individuals without hypoventilation, disturbances in the ventilation-perfusion relationship are prevalent.[6] Pulmonary hypertension is a common finding, resulting from chronic hypoxemia, hypoxic pulmonary vasoconstriction, and the added contribution of compromised cardiac function.[6]

The vital capacity, total lung capacity, and functional residual volume are reduced by up to 30 percent in morbidly obese patients. The work of breathing is increased due to higher chest wall and airway resistance and functionally flattened diaphragms. When ventilating obese patients, tidal volume may need to be lowered and adjusted based on inflation pressures and blood gases. Positive end-expiratory pressure may prevent end-expiratory airway closure and atelectasis.[3]

Recognition of the increased risk of cardiorespiratory compromise in the morbidly obese patient is crucial, even when the patient presents to the ED with a problem unrelated to the cardiovascular system. The morbidly obese patient who states that he or she can only sleep in the upright position should be maintained in an upright position as much as possible, or in a lateral position with the head up while performing procedures. If the patient must remain supine, elevate the head of a patient who is on a backboard by placing towels under the board and utilize continuous pulse oximetry monitoring.

Pregnancy

Obesity will also complicate pregnancy. Body weight before pregnancy and weight gain during pregnancy both influence labor, and obese women are more likely to require cesarean sections and to experience abnormal labor. In addition, these infants tend to be heavier than those born to nonobese women, increasing the potential for difficult labor and delivery. Other complications such as hypertension, diabetes, preeclampsia, and eclampsia occur with increased frequency in pregnant obese women.

Trauma

Differences in the mechanisms of injury and associated injury patterns have been described, and obesity has been identified as an independent premorbid risk factor in trauma.[2,3,7]

Excessive weight interferes with activities of daily living, therefore increasing the risk of injury. Moreover, the presence of obesity-related diseases such as diabetes, heart disease, and somnolence secondary to sleep apnea may contribute to accidents. A higher incidence of displaced ankle and elbow fractures has been described in obese patients sustaining minimal trauma (stumbling, low-energy falls).[8] Obese patients have also been noted to be less likely to wear seat belts because of poor fit or discomfort.

Obesity appears to protect the blunt trauma victim from head injury, but is associated with a significantly higher incidence of injuries to the chest, primarily rib fractures and pulmonary contusions. It is hypothesized that the larger torso serves as a physiologic airbag, and although this offers some protection from head injury, there is an associated increase in thoracic injury. This may partly explain the dramatically higher mortality rate due to respiratory causes in morbidly obese trauma patients. The impact of morbid obesity on mortality in blunt trauma was seen in a study that found a 42.1 percent mortality rate in severely overweight patients, compared with 5.0 and 8.0 percent in the average and overweight groups.[7]

Despite the logistical difficulties the obese patient presents, the principles of trauma management apply, with necessary spinal precautions and full exposure. The presence of subcutaneous fat obscures physical findings in thoracic and abdominal injuries. The limitations of physical findings are further compounded by poor quality portable chest radiographs in this population. A more aggressive approach to airway management with early intubation and assisted ventilation may be indicated.

The incidence of pelvic fractures is higher in the obese trauma victim. Portable films are often of a poorer quality in the obese patient, therefore clinical suspicion of a pelvic fracture should be pursued by repeat views or computed tomography, despite a negative portable pelvic radiograph.

PROCEDURES

Procedures are more difficult to perform on the obese ED patient (Table 311-1). Landmarks are obscured or nonpalpable, access is often impaired by excessive tissue, and positioning problems are common. Airway management may be difficult, intravenous access delayed, and investigations cumbersome or impossible to obtain in the obese patient. These factors all contribute to inevitable obstructions to rapid assessment and resuscitation. Having alternative approaches readily available is the ideal strategy. The appropriate equipment, such as the right blood pressure cuff, should be easy to access. Extra personnel are often required, and a minimum of six people is usually necessary to transfer the patient, particularly when cervical spine precautions must be maintained.

Airway Management

Obesity may be associated with difficult intubation or bag-valve-mask ventilation, particularly if other predictors of intubation difficulty are present. Obesity alone is not a contraindication to rapid-sequence intubation and this may be the preferred method in most patients. However, in this population it is particularly important to assess and recognize other objective predictors of a difficult intubation (see Chap. 19).

Preoxygenation is critical, since morbidly obese patients will desaturate more quickly than normal-sized adults.[9] Patients should be kept sitting upright or semirecumbent as long as possible prior to intubation. If bag-mask ventilation is required, the obese patient often has reduced pulmonary compliance, which necessitates higher ventilatory pressures. The pop-off valve on the ventilation bag may have to be occluded in order to provide adequate ventilation.

Once the process of intubation is begun, access to the airway is enhanced by elevating both the head and shoulders with towels or by placing a rolled blanket between the scapulae and under the occiput. Elevation of the shoulders allows displacement of the breasts away from the midline. The greater elevation of the head places it in the sniffing position, and creates more space, as the chest wall of the morbidly obese patient may actually obstruct the handle of the laryngoscope. A shorter-than-average handle for the laryngoscope or an adjustable-angle laryngoscope is useful in this situation.

Alternative techniques of airway management such as awake oral intubation or blind nasotracheal intubation may be utilized if difficulty is predicted. Nasotracheal intubation is technically more difficult than orotracheal intubation, but may be relatively advantageous if performed by an experienced physician to intubate a spontaneously breathing patient with a short thick neck. Transtracheal jet ventilation requires higher ventilatory pressures and therefore may be less useful and cause increased barotrauma in the obese patient with decreased pulmonary compliance. The intubating laryngeal mask airway and the

TABLE 311-1   Procedural Problems and Solutions in the Morbidly Obese

Procedure	Problem	Solution
Bag-mask ventilation	Reduced pulmonary compliance	Occlude pop-off valve
Oral intubation	Potentially difficult airway	Objective predictors of difficulty Adjustable angle laryngoscope Double-lumen esophageal-tracheal tube Surgical airway
Sphygmomanometry	Falsely elevated readings	Use larger cuff size
Pulse oximetry	Poor signal	Earlobe probe
Vascular access	Inability to locate vein/artery	Use 3- to 4-in. catheter Patient positioning Ultrasound-facilitated cannulation
Lumbar puncture	Difficulty in palpating landmarks Difficult to obtain cerebrospinal fluid	Upright patient positioning Increase needle length to 5 in.
Diagnostic peritoneal lavage	Accessing peritoneal cavity	Modified Seldinger technique

esophageal-tracheal double-lumen tube are possible rescue devices, and their utility in the morbidly obese patient has been described.[10,11] A fiberoptic bronchoscope can also be used to aid intubation, although visualization may be impaired by circumpharyngeal fat.

Finally, a cricothyrotomy may be indicated if other maneuvers fail. Landmarks may not be appreciated by palpation and the cricothyroid membrane is located approximately four fingerbreadths above the sternal notch. Needle cricothyrotomy is difficult given the anatomy of a morbidly obese patient's neck.

Electrocardiogram Analysis

Host factors such as body mass influence the ease of obtaining and interpreting an electrocardiogram (ECG). Landmarks for lead placement may be difficult to determine, and can result in inaccurate lead placement. Variation in fat deposits surrounding the heart and in the chest wall can lead to inconsistent voltage changes, although in general, obese patients demonstrate loss of voltage.[12] Flattening or inversion of the T wave in the inferior or lateral leads is one consistent change. None of these ECG changes is specific for obesity, and such abnormalities should not be attributed to obesity alone.

Sphygmomanometry

Inadequate cuff width and circumference will artificially elevate pressure readings.[13] However, many morbidly obese patients are hypertensive, and a high pressure reading cannot always be blamed on inappropriate equipment. In order to minimize errors in blood pressure recording, a correct ratio of cuff width to arm circumference, approximately 2:5, should be chosen. The bladder length should be 80 percent of the arm circumference. The ED should stock a variety of sizes of blood pressure cuffs specifically for use in the obese population.

Pulse Oximetry

Tissue thickness can make the transmission of light waves more difficult in the extremely obese, and thus make pulse oximetry readings unreliable. However, pulse oximetry in the moderately obese is generally accurate. In morbidly obese patients, the earlobe could be used instead of the finger for probe placement. Other potential areas of placement include the fifth digit of the hand or foot, the nose, lip, or temporal artery.

Venous Access

Morbidly obese patients are notoriously difficult candidates for intravenous catheterization, venipuncture, or arterial puncture. Anatomy is distorted by subcutaneous fat, and landmark vessels are often not visible or palpable. This leads to multiple attempts, delay in access, and an increased incidence of central line placement, with delays in changing a line after admission. All these factors contribute to a higher rate of complications, such as wound infection, pneumothorax, phlebitis, and thrombosis. In addition, standard 1.5-in. needles or catheters may not be long enough to penetrate the subcutaneous tissue and reach the target vessel; 3- or 4-in. needles and catheters are preferred. Locating the radial or femoral artery in order to obtain a sample for arterial blood gas analysis can also be extremely difficult. It may be necessary to change needle lengths on the prepackaged arterial blood gas syringes.

Various techniques can be employed to improve access to the vessel. Application of heat, light tapping over the vessel, active or passive pumping of the extremity, and application of topical nitroglycerin can be used to encourage vasodilation. Reactive hyperemia can be created by occluding the circulation for 3 to 4 min, then releasing the sphygmomanometer to 10 to 15 mm Hg below the diastolic pressure.

The medial cubital and basilic veins are the first choice in the morbidly obese, since they are large, the antecubital crease is visible, and the skin and subcutaneous tissues are thinner in this area. Branches of the median and basilic veins on the volar surface of the forearm may be too deep to the adipose tissue to be easily accessed. The cephalic vein on the radial aspect of the wrist is a good second choice if it is not also obscured by fat. Another option is the vessels of the dorsum of the hand. The veins of the fingers may be accessible, especially those over the dorsal aspect of the thumb and forefinger. The veins of the feet are usually not good candidates, since they tend to be obscured by fat or changes from peripheral vascular disease. If peripheral veins are not available, a cutdown at the forearm veins or an attempt at cannulation of the external jugular vein may be considered. Venisection at the saphenous vein, a common alternative in patients of normal weight, will be challenging because of excess adipose tissue.

Central line placement can also be challenging.[14] Femoral catheterization is preferred over saphenous venisection in the obese patient with a palpable femoral pulse, and can be facilitated by placing a towel under the ipsilateral buttock and having an assistant retract the panniculus. Subclavian vein cannulation may be preferable to the internal jugular, since the bony landmarks are more easily palpable. The patient is usually placed in the Trendelenburg position; however, this position may be relatively contraindicated in some cases, such as the patient who cannot sleep supine.[3] During subclavian line placement, abduction of the arm (as opposed to the standard recommendation of arm adduction) and retraction of chest tissue away from the clavicle may reduce excessive tissue layers at the site. It is common practice to insert a roll under the shoulders or a pillow lengthwise along the spine to improve access.

Ultrasound can facilitate venous cannulation and arterial puncture, allowing a higher success rate with fewer attempts, because it is performed independent of landmarks.[15]

Lumbar Puncture

A lumbar puncture is most successfully performed in the obese patient in the sitting position. With the patient upright, the midline is easier to estimate and both iliac crests are usually palpable. Bone encountered after only a few centimeters usually represents spinous process, and suggests an adjustment in the vertical plane above or below that point. A deeper bony encounter is likely lamina and requires a medial adjustment. Ultrasonography has been described as an aid to locating the vertebra. Despite the excessive tissue, the standard 3-in. needle is adequate for many obese patients, although this may require pushing the needle hub to the point of dimpling the skin. The 5-in. needle is sometimes needed. Tight intervertebral disk spaces are common in this population. The best choice is a 22- or 24-gauge needle, which allows adequate flow and easier passage and decreases the likelihood of post-puncture headache.

Diagnostic Peritoneal Lavage

Diagnostic peritoneal lavage (DPL) is used for the early recognition of intra-abdominal injury requiring exploratory laparotomy. In many centers, the use of DPL has been supplanted by imaging techniques because of increased accessibility to improved computed tomography (CT) and ultrasonography. However, size and weight restrictions and transport difficulties may preclude the use of CT scanning in the obese trauma victim. Abdominal ultrasonography is also less reliable in the morbidly obese patient. Therefore DPL may be the best available diagnostic approach in these patients.

There are three general DPL techniques: the open, semiopen, and closed. In the open technique, a catheter is passed into the abdominal cavity through a large incision that exposes the peritoneum. Because of the larger incision required, the technical difficulties presented by the panniculus, and a potentially higher rate of wound infection and herniation, morbid obesity has been described as a relative contraindication to this procedure.[16]

Closed DPL using a blind Seldinger technique with an 18-gauge needle has been shown to be as efficient as the open technique, and may represent the method of choice in the obese patient. In patients whose abdominal wall thickness exceeds the reach of the needle, a modified Seldinger technique has been described, in which a 2- to 4-cm incision is carried down to the midline fascia and an 18-gauge needle is then inserted at that point. This procedure was used successfully in six morbidly obese patients whose weight exceeded the weight limit of the CT scanner, typically 350 pounds.[16]

Imaging

Radiographs have limited utility in the morbidly obese. Standard film cassettes are too small to accommodate the entire chest or abdomen, and two or more films may be required. Excessive soft tissue can result in extremely underpenetrated films. Since transport is invariably problematic, morbidly obese patients may need to undergo portable radiography, resulting in lower-quality images.

CT and MRI scans are clearly superior to radiographs, offering better resolution and greater penetration. However, many CT scanners have a weight limit of 300 to 350 lb and a girth limit of 30 in. Most standard MRI scanners have a maximum shoulder-to-shoulder width of 52 in. and a weight limit of 136 to 159 kg (300–350 lb) (Table 311-2). Thus many morbidly obese patients will be excluded from undergoing these studies. There are, however, private companies, veterinary schools, and zoos that have scanners with a larger capacity.

TABLE 311-2 Weight Limits of Standard ED and Imaging Equipment

Wheelchairs (16- to 18-in. width)	118 kg (260 lb)
Wheelchairs (20-in. width)	140 kg (310 lb)
Stretchers	227 kg (500 lb)
Radiology table	136 kg (300 lb)
CT table	136–159 kg (300–350 lb)
MRI table	159 kg (350 lb)

EQUIPMENT PROBLEMS SPECIFIC TO ED CARE

From the time the obese patient enters the waiting area until the time he or she leaves the ED, issues related to the patient's size challenge both personnel and equipment. Waiting-room chairs may be too small. Most wheelchairs also have weight limits and are not designed to safely accommodate patients weighing over 118 kg (260 lb). Gurneys are often too small for the patient if the protective side rails are in place, and without the side rails, the patient is not safe. In addition, collapsible gurneys are not designed to hold the weight of the morbidly obese patient, leading to instability and concomitant patient and staff danger. If they are used, keeping the gurney at a lower height will enhance stability, if the device allows function at this level. Heavy-duty stretchers (one with additional cross-brace supports) and wheelchairs designed to hold patients weighing more than 118 kg (260 lb) are available and should be present in the ED. Metal clamshell transport stretchers are preferable to the standard wooden stretchers for stability, weight-bearing, and unloading of the patient.

The comfort and modesty of morbidly obese patients should be thoughtfully considered during his or her ED stay.[17] The ED should stock oversized hospital gowns. Patients should also be allowed to wear their own night clothing as long as it does not obstruct care.

Any care that requires lifting or turning of the obese patient is difficult, as techniques used for average-sized patients cannot be used. In general, more than two providers should always be utilized to move the patient. Provision of an overhead trapeze will greatly facilitate patient-assisted transfers and should be available in the ED.

REFERENCES

1. National Center for Health Statistics, Centers for Disease Control and Prevention, http://www.cdc.gov, 2002.
2. Boulanger B, Milzman D, Mitchell K, et al: Body habitus as a predictor of injury pattern following blunt trauma. *J Trauma* 33:228, 1992.
3. Varon J, Marik P: Management of the obese critically ill patient. *Crit Care Clin* 17:187, 2001.
4. Ernst ND, Obarzanek E, Clark MB, et al: Cardiovascular health risks related to overweight. *J Am Diet Assoc* 97(7 suppl):S47, 1997.
5. Goldhaber S, Grodstein E, Stampfer M, et al: A prospective study of risk factors for pulmonary embolism in women. *JAMA* 277:642, 1997.
6. Lazarus R, Sparrow D, Weiss S: Effects of obesity and fat distribution on ventilatory function: The normative aging study. *Chest* 111:891, 1997.
7. Choban PS, Weireter L, Maynes C: Obesity and increased mortality in blunt trauma. *J Trauma* 31:1253, 1991.
8. Bostman OM: Body mass index of patients with elbow and ankle fractures requiring surgical treatment. *J Trauma* 37:62, 1994.
9. Berthoud MC, Peacock JE, Reilly CS: Effectiveness of preoxygenation in morbidly obese patients. *Br J Anaesth* 67:464, 1991.
10. Banyai M, Falger S, Roggla M, et al: Emergency intubation with the Combitube in a grossly obese patient with bull neck. *Resuscitation* 26:271, 1993.
11. Levitan RM, Ochroch EA, Stuart S, et al: Use of intubating laryngeal mask airway by medical and nonmedical personnel. *Am J Emerg Med* 18:12, 2000.
12. Alpert MA, Terry BE, Cohen MV, et al: The electrocardiogram in morbid obesity. *Am J Cardiol* 85:908, 2000.
13. Maxwell MH, Waks AU, Schroth PC, et al: Error in blood-pressure measurement due to incorrect cuff size in obese patients. *Lancet* 2:33, 1982.
14. Dronen S, Younger J: Central venous catheterization and central venous pressure monitoring, in Roberts JR, Hedges JR (eds): *Clinical Procedures in Emergency Medicine*, 3d ed. Philadelphia, Saunders, 1998, p 358.

15. Keyes LE, Frazee BW, Snoey ER, et al: Ultrasound-guided brachial and basilic vein cannulation in emergency department patients with difficult intravenous access. *Ann Emerg Med* 34:711, 1999.

16. Ochsner MG, Herr D, Drucker W, et al: A modified Seldinger technique for peritoneal lavage in trauma patients who are obese. *Surg Gynecol Obstet* 173:158, 1991.

17. Wadden TA, Stunkard AJ: Social and psychological consequences of obesity. *Ann Intern Med* 103:1062, 1985.

PATIENT SAFETY IN EMERGENCY MEDICINE

Cherri Hobgood

Pat Croskerry

Robert L. Wears

Armando Hevia

Error in medicine became a national issue with the publication of the Institute of Medicine report *To Err is Human*.[1] This report suggested that errors in medicine were common, costly, and often disregarded by the medical community. When these error rates were considered in terms of human life and health care dollars, both the public and the medical community took notice. Though the accuracy of these numbers has been the subject of debate, they have stimulated an intense evaluation of the current patient safety standards in U.S. health care.[2,3] As a result, the medical community is more aware than ever before of the incidence of medical error in their clinical environments. Medicine's unstated objective to provide the highest quality of care for all our patients and continuously improve the care process has now become a mandate. In this chapter, we will discuss error in the ED, examine why error is prevalent in this clinical environment, and identify principles and practices that can make the ED a safer place for all our patients.

Error is defined by the Institute of Medicine (IOM) as the "failure of a planned action to be completed as intended or the use of a wrong plan to achieve an aim."[1] To date, there are no large prospective studies describing the demographics of error in the ED. Three large retrospective inpatient studies on medical error—the Harvard Medical Practice Study, the Colorado-Utah study, and the Quality in Australian Health Care Study—give some indication of the nature of error in the ED, but are clearly limited by the fact that they only considered error associated with patients admitted from the ED.[4–6] The majority of patients seen in the ED, those that are discharged, are not included. In each of these studies, the ED was responsible for only a small percentage of all adverse events (1.5 to 3 percent), but was consistently identified as the clinical setting with the highest rate of preventable errors with serious consequences. The Harvard Medical Practice Study determined that 3 percent of all injuries due to adverse events in admitted patients occurred in the ED and 25 percent of those resulted in death or disability. Of these serious or fatal injuries, 70 percent were attributed to negligence and 93 percent were deemed preventable.[4] In the Colorado-Utah study, 53 percent of the ED-related events were considered negligent. Of events attributed to emergency physicians, 95 percent were judged as "negligent."[5] In the Quality in Australian Health Care Study, the highest proportion of "highly preventable" adverse event injuries, 82 percent, were found in the ED.[6]

These "highly preventable" and "negligent" error estimates, coupled with the IOM report, caused many emergency physicians to feel singled out and defensive about patient safety in the ED. Patient safety in the ED should be an important focus for emergency physicians regardless of the accuracy of the IOM error rates. The impact of medical errors can be visualized by a graph that shows numbers of encounters per death for different activities (Figure 312-1). The points marked UB and LB show the upper and lower bounds of the IOM estimates

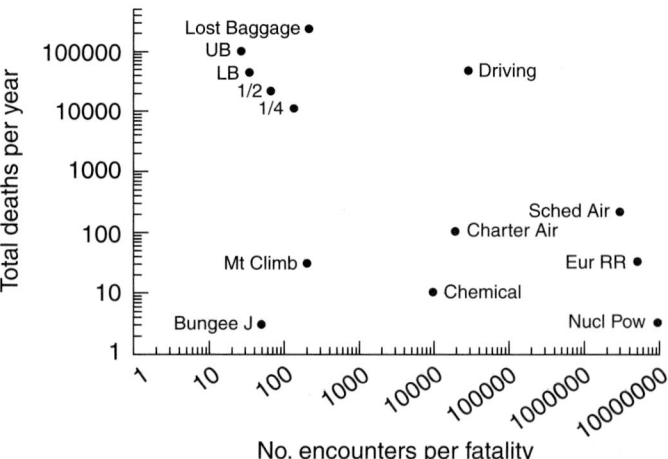

FIG. 312-1. Examples of hazardous activities and their death rates. The Y axis represents the total burden of deaths, and the X axis represents the number of encounters required to produce one death. The points marked UB and LB are the upper and lower bounds of the Institute of Medicine estimates, and the points marked ½ and ¼ are the lower bound divided by 2 and 4, respectively. The lost baggage data point is used as a reference activity of a high-volume process with many opportunities for error to occur. For this reference point the Y axis shows the total number of lost bags per year and the X axis shows the number of bags checked per each bag lost. Bungee J = bungee jumping; Charter Air = charter airline travel; Chemical = chemical industry; Driving = driving an automobile; Eur RR = European rail travel; Lost Baggage = airline industry baggage handling; Mt Climb = mountain climbing; Nucl Pow = nuclear power industry; Sched Air = scheduled commercial airline travel; LB = lower IOM estimate; UB = upper IOM estimate; ½ = half of lower IOM estimate; ¼ = one quarter of lower IOM estimate. (Modified from Amalberti R: The paradoxes of almost totally safe transportation systems. *Safety Sci* 37:109, 2002, and reproduced with permission from Wears R: Human error and adverse events in emergency medicine. *EM Pulse* 7:17, 2002.)

(98,000 and 44,000 deaths, respectively). For those who believe that the estimates are inflated, two other points are graphed: the points marked ½ and ¼ represent the lower estimate divided by 2 or 4, respectively. It should be clear from this exercise that imprecision in the estimates is not terribly material; health care is in very impressive company, even if we postulate that the lower IOM estimate is off by a factor of 4. Health care is closer in both risk and volume to airline baggage handling than any of the other activities shown. Continued debate over the exact number is a waste of time and viewed as self-serving by the public. A recent comment puts the issue in perspective: ". . . criticizing the IOM numbers because they are wrong is like criticizing Columbus because he got lost. It may be true but it misses a larger truth."[3] Because emergency department volumes continue to grow, patient safety efforts that focus on the emergency department will have a substantial impact on improving the quality of health care in the United States.

MODELS OF COGNITIVE PERFORMANCE

The types of errors that occur in the ED environment are not unique to the ED. Medicine arrived late to error analysis and classification; consequently, most error types had already been described in other areas. One of the most widely accepted error classification schemes is based on a model of cognitive performance originated by Rasmussen and Jensen in 1974, and elaborated upon by Reason.[7,8] It described three levels: skill-based, rule-based, and knowledge-based.

Skill-Based

Skill-based cognitive performance refers to actions that are automatic due to a previously acquired skill. They usually happen quickly with little conscious input on the part of the clinician. Their clinical action is based on predefined schemata or preprogrammed instructions. For example, getting dressed or driving a car are actions that require little conscious monitoring, i.e., we do not need to explicitly think about them in order to accomplish them. Similarly, for experienced clinicians, prepping a wound, tying a suture, or starting a central line may require relatively little conscious input. Once the decision to proceed with the process is made, the technical performance of the event is virtually automatic. Some decisions can be relegated to a level of automaticity with practice (which arm goes in which sleeve, or which direction the next knot should be tied). Any departure from this kind of skill-based processing requires either a rules-based or knowledge-based approach to perform the task.

Rules-Based

Rules-based processing involves matching the context and clinical symptoms currently facing the clinician with a known rule. These rules are typically of the form "if X then Y," and can be based on past experience, explicit instructions, or clinical guidelines. For example, decision making can be optimized for some conditions by following empirically-derived clinical decision rules. Thus for a patient with an ankle injury, application of the Ottawa ankle rules results in a decision being made about the need for a radiograph.

Knowledge-Based

When faced with novel or unfamiliar situations, or when rules are not useful, we need to use knowledge-based processing. As with rules-based processing, knowledge-based processing is a conscious process. It refers to what we typically think of as analytic thought. Knowledge-based cognitive behavior involves interpreting and understanding novel situations and problems against a background of specific domain knowledge. This type of decision making is most commonly called into play in situations requiring diagnostic reasoning (e.g., integrating the presenting complaint, past medical history, physical examination, and laboratory findings in a patient with syncope) or in management decisions. This is clinical decision making.

As a provider's clinical performance evolves through training and experience, predictable changes occur in cognitive functioning. With increasing experience, clinical problems become more familiar and less novel, and there will be less demand for knowledge-based function. Consequently, the provider is more likely to use rules- or skill-based functions. The relationship between provider proficiency and probability of error varies for different levels of cognitive performance (Fig. 312-2).

ERROR CLASSIFICATION

Classifying clinical errors based on the three-level model of cognition provides insight into how the error may have occurred and offers a possible means of a reduction (Table 312-1). The major types of errors that flow from this model of cognitive performance are skill-based errors, referred to as slips and lapses, and those of rules- and knowledge-based cognition, known as mistakes.[9] Slips are failures in attention or perception that result in the breakdown of the planned execution of an observable action sequence. These are action errors, often caused by interruptions or a break in the routine of activity performance. Lapses are also skill-based errors however, they are based on a failure of memory that leads to a failure of execution of a plan. Mistakes, on the other hand, usually occur during problem solving.

In rules-based mistakes, the wrong rule is applied. This may occur due either to incorrect rule selection, misapplication of the rule, or in-

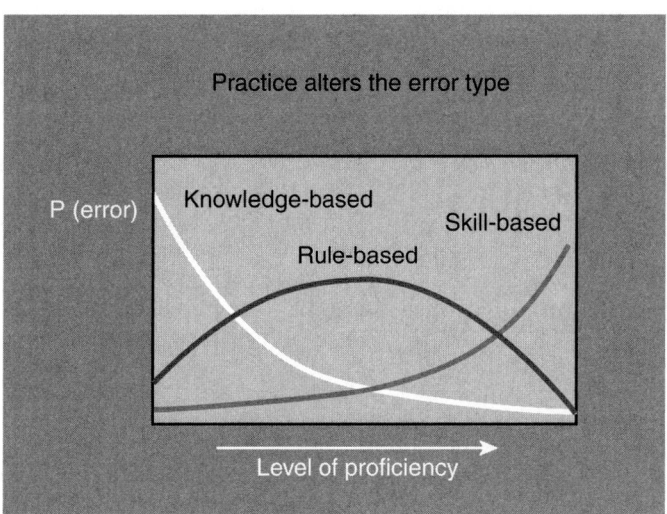

FIG. 312-2. The relationship between errors and provider proficiency according to error type. The Y axis represents the probability of error, while the X axis represents the level of provider proficiency. Knowledge-based errors decline with proficiency. Paradoxically, the more skilled the providers, the more likely they will commit an "absent minded" skill-based error, because performance becomes increasingly automatic. Rules-based errors first increase through an acquisition phase of the rule repertoire, then decrease as their use becomes more finely discriminated. [Reproduced with permission from Reason J: Overview of unsafe acts. Presented at the Second Halifax Symposium on Health Care Error, October 2002, Halifax, Nova Scotia, Canada.]

correct identification of the situation and selection of an incorrect rule. Knowledge-based mistakes are more complicated, but the same processes apply. For example, incomplete or incorrect knowledge, and/or flawed analytical processes may lead to mistakes.

Another useful approach to categorizing error in the ED is to break it down into *procedural, cognitive,* and *affective* types.[10] Procedural error may occur in any of a variety of procedures typically performed in the ED (e.g., suturing, cast application, insertion of chest tube or central line, diagnostic peritoneal lavage, intubation, and others). Procedural competency first depends on a thorough understanding of the

TABLE 312-1   Commonly Used Definitions of Error

Execution error—Failure of a planned action to be completed as intended[1]
Error of planning—Use of a wrong plan to achieve an aim[1]
Adverse event is an injury caused by medical management rather than by the underlying disease or condition of the patient[1]
Preventable adverse events are attributable to error[1]
Negligent adverse events meet the legal criteria for negligence[1]
Slip—a failure in execution of an action sequence, due to a failure of attention or perception; the wrong action is observable[8,9]
Lapse—a failure of execution when the action performed was not the intended action; often related to a failure of memory; the wrong action is not observable[8,9]
Mistake is a planning failure, where actions go as planned, but the plan was bad; these are errors of decision making and judgment; these errors stem from cognitive breakdowns and are often influenced by a number of external system factors[1,8,9,11]
Rules-based errors occur when the wrong rule is chosen due to the misperception of the situation, or the misapplication of rule[9]
Knowledge-based errors occur from a lack of or misapplication of knowledge or a misinterpretation of the situation[9]
Active error/failure—unsafe acts or omissions which result in immediate adverse consequences[9,17]
Latent error/failure—a decision whose consequences may only become evident when it combines with other factors to breach the systems defense or that results in unsafe conditions in which unsafe work occurs[9,17]

process, followed by numerous repetitions to establish a smooth coordination of visual, motor, and haptic skills, and continuing competency depends on maintenance. Cognitive errors, in contrast, are thinking errors. They may arise anywhere within the large domain of decisions emergency clinicians make in the course of management, diagnosis, and disposition of their patients. Affective error occurs when the emotions or affective state of the physician unduly influence the clinical decision-making process. They typically arise from attribution error, countertransference phenomena, or may originate from the endogenous affective state of the clinician. The properties of these three classes of error differ significantly from each other (Table 312-2).

SYSTEMS CAN ENCOURAGE ERRORS

Students of error and human performance believe that *all humans err,* ergo the title of the Institute of Medicine report *To Err is Human.*[1] Error is to be expected, and although a provider is invariably involved when accidents occur in a professional setting, the causes of the error may be out of the individual's control.[11] In fact, the ED's high preventable error rate has been largely attributed to environmental factors such as the complexity inherent in the delivery of emergency care and the variance in work procedures. Therefore, a complete and thorough understanding of the error-prone system will be required to determine the etiology of errors and their correction.

Inevitability and Ubiquity of Error in the ED

It is obvious at even the most casual level of observation that error in the ED is abundant. Unique operating aspects of this microsystem predispose it to a variety of errors (Table 312-3). These are categorized into error-producing conditions (EPCs) and violation-producing behaviors (VPBs).[12] EPCs arise largely from the intrinsic properties of emergency medicine, but also from the design of the system in which it is practiced. Thus intrinsic features include high levels of diagnostic uncertainty associated with an inordinately high decision density, and high cognitive load for ED clinicians. These demands are made more difficult by the clinician's unfamiliarity with most patients, as well as the narrow time windows available for assessing illness. Further diffi-

TABLE 312-2 Comparison of Properties of Procedural, Cognitive, and Affective Errors

Property	ERROR CATEGORY		
	Procedural	Cognitive	Affective
Visibility	High	Low	Moderate
Discreteness*	High	Low	Low
Witnessed	Usually	Not usually	Not usually
Awareness	High	Low	Low
Recorded	Yes	Rarely	No
Temporality	Close	Distant	Distant
Medical nature	High	Low	Very low
Familiarity†	High	Low	Very low
Preventability	High	High but difficult	High but difficult
Root cause analysis	Amenable	Difficult	Very difficult

Discreteness refers to the perceived separateness or isolation of the event from those around it. Procedural errors are often distinct in this fashion, whereas cognitive and affective errors are not.

†*Familiarity* refers to the strength of the clinician's familiarity with the error. Causing a pneumothorax by insertion of a central line is well known to ED physicians, whereas few would be familiar with the etiology of cognitive and affective errors in their decision making.

Source: Reproduced with permission from Croskerry.[10]

TABLE 312-3 Operating Characteristics of the ED Which May Compromise Safety

ERROR-PRODUCING CONDITIONS (EPCs)		
Intrinsic	Systemic	Violation-Producing Behaviors (VPBs)
High levels of diagnostic uncertainty	Poor ED design	Gender
High decision density	Poor equipment design	Risk-taking behavior
High cognitive load	Poor maintenance	Normalization of deviance
Narrow time windows	High communication load	Maladaptive group pressures
Multiple transitions of care	Overcrowding	Maladaptive copying behavior
Multiple interruptions/ distractions	Holding admitted patients in the ED	Underconfidence
Low signal-to-noise ratio	Production pressures	Overconfidence
Surge phenomena	High noise levels	Maladaptive decision styles
Circadian factors dysynchronicity/ fatigue	Inadequate staffing	Authority gradient effects
Novel or infrequently occurring conditions	Incompatible goals	Likelihood of detection
	Poor feedback	Inconvenience
	Inexperience	Safety procedures seen as inconvenient
	Inadequate supervision	

culties arise from frequent interruptions and distractions, surge phenomena (abrupt changes in workload and/or acuity), shift changes and multiple transitions of care, fatigued staff, or staff suffering circadian dysynchronicity due to insufficient recovery time from a shift change. These and other factors may all contribute to uneven, abbreviated, and unsafe care. An especially difficult intrinsic EPC is the low signal-to-noise ratio of some diagnoses that must not be missed [i.e., many serious conditions (signals) that present in the ED such as subarachnoid hemorrhage, aortic dissection, pulmonary embolus, and ectopic pregnancy, are mimicked by a variety of considerably more frequent benign conditions (noise)].

A number of systemic EPCs compromise safety and contribute to error. Insufficient space and beds, suboptimal equipment design and maintenance, and overall inadequacies in ergonomic design of the ED are some common problems. Excessive communication load, noise levels, overcrowding, and production pressures are others. Inexperience and inadequate supervision will compromise performance, as will inadequate staffing levels. The especially poor feedback systems in many EDs compromise good clinical calibration. Occasionally, too, clinicians will be faced with incompatible goals when externally imposed cost-containment conflicts with a patient's therapeutic needs. Ultimately, particular combinations of EPCs may lead to a trade-off (TO) between resource availability (RA) and continuous quality improvement (CQI). The onset of RACQITO signals that a threshold of safety has been crossed.

The other major sources of error are violation-producing behaviors (VPBs), which are mostly due to individual characteristics. Workplace behavior is influenced by gender, personality factors such as the willingness to take risks and deviate from accepted safe operating procedures, underconfidence and overconfidence, responsiveness to authority gradients, and other factors. Impairments in performance may result from personality variables, and maladaptive styles of decision making.[8] For example, "thematic vagabonding" is characterized by moving quickly from one problem to another, avoiding the pursuit of clinical closure. This indecisiveness in the ED is sometimes accomplished by ordering unnecessary tests or other stalling behavior to avoid making a decision. In contrast to vagabonding, "encysting" is the tendency to focus unduly on minor clinical details of a case at the expense of more significant ones. VPBs may be either intentional or erroneous (e.g., deliberately administering a drug by a route that has not been approved, or ordering a drug to be given without being aware that it is contraindicated in certain conditions). Importantly, safety violations may be driven by EPCs and, in some EDs, may be seen as convenient or necessary corner-cutting measures in order to meet the work demand ("normalization of deviance"). A quantitative method for assessing the interaction between EPCs and VPBs in the workplace has been developed by Williams using Human Error Assessment and Reduction Technique (HEART) analysis.[12]

Error arising from EPCs and VPBs occur continuously in most EDs. Under current systems of error monitoring, very little of it will show up in data banks or official reports. Some of the error is inconsequential, while most of that which is significant will be corrected continuously. These corrective actions correspond to the series of slices in Reason's swiss cheese model, which provides the defenses, barriers, and safeguards against potential error achieving realization.[11] The holes in the various slices arise from *active failures* (mostly VPBs) combining with *latent conditions* (mostly EPCs). In an ideal system, there would be no holes in the slices, but any ED will fall far short of the ideal. Under certain conditions (e.g., at RACQITO), the holes in successive barriers all line up, allowing the potential accident with a trajectory through the system, resulting in critical incidents or catastrophes. This will often be the first time that particular parts of the system are brought under close scrutiny, and may be the first time that the impact of active and latent failures is revealed.

CLINICAL DECISION-MAKING ERROR

Understanding clinical decision-making error requires some insight into the processes by which decisions are usually made in the ED. Presently, there is no single model of decision making that adequately applies to the complex variety of clinical situations that prevail in most EDs. The normative Bayesian approach that underpins classical decision theory is useful in the development of certain algorithms and clinical decision rules, but has little practical application in urgent or emergent situations, or in "flesh and blood" decision making. Instead, the dynamic, ambient conditions of the ED are more suited to the features and properties of models derived from both Bounded Rationality and Naturalistic Decision Making (NDM).[13,14]

Bounded rationality simply acknowledges the limitations of human cognitive capability and recognizes that fully rational decisions are rarely attainable. In real situations, rationality is bounded by principles that underlie nonoptimizing adaptive behavior. Thus in the bounded rationality of the ED, with its intrinsic and systemic EPCs, clinicians strive not for completely optimal decisions, but for the best decisions possible under the prevailing circumstances. Similarly, NDM accepts that decision making is driven more by situational variables, which may change over time and may be influenced by resource limitations. It avoids quantitative, analytical strategies, emphasizing instead economy of thought and action, and acknowledging the natural variance of cognitive strategies. Both models are more realistic and accepting of human fallibility and the inevitability of error, and are especially applicable in the specific milieu of the ED.

The density and acuity of decision making is exceptional in emergency medicine. The progress of a patient through the ED is driven by multiple decisions underlying the sequence: assessment–management–diagnosis–treatment–disposition. Invariably, the pivotal feature in the sequence is diagnosis, and the clinical decision making that underpins it is therefore critically important for patient safety. Delayed or missed diagnoses are the ED errors that are most likely to lead to disability and death, and account for about half of all litigation brought against emergency physicians.

There are three major sources of diagnostic error (Table 312-4).[15] The first, *no-fault errors,* arises from a variety of factors: silent, subclinical, or atypical presentations; when little is known about a disease; when patients misrepresent their symptoms for psychiatric or other reasons; when the patient is confusing, inaccurate, or uncooperative; when patients are noncompliant; and from other unknowable

TABLE 312-4   Categories of Diagnostic Failures in the ED

	ERROR TYPE	
No-Fault	Systemic	Cognitive
Confusing, inaccurate, or misleading information from patient	Error-producing conditions*	Knowledge deficiency
Deliberate misrepresentation of illness (malingering)	Laboratory error (preanalytic, analytic, postanalytic)	Incomplete data gathering
Somatization disorder	Inefficient report follow-up	Test misinterpretation
Factitious disorder	Time delays	Cognitive dispositions to respond†
Insufficient medical information available about a new disease	Unavailability of services	
Patient refusal of critical diagnostic tests/procedure/consultation	Poor patient follow-up	
Silent presentation of comorbid illness		

*See Table 312-3.
†See Table 312-5.

factors. The second, *system errors,* occurs largely as a result of EPCs but also includes laboratory errors, equipment failure, or organizational failures such as inadequate follow-up of abnormal test results, unavailability of expertise or particular resources, delays in testing, missed appointments, backlogs, and other inefficiencies. The third, *cognitive errors,* is probably the most devastating of the diagnostic errors. Some cognitive errors arise from faulty data gathering, test interpretation, or incomplete or incorrect knowledge, but the majority appear to arise through a variety of "cognitive dispositions to respond" in certain ways in particular clinical situations.[16] These will be influenced by both EPCs and VPBs.

Many of these cognitive dispositions to respond, or CDRs, have their origins in heuristics. Heuristics are shortcuts, rules of thumb, or any kind of abbreviated thinking that accomplishes fast and efficient decision making. Heuristic thinking characterizes the emergency physician. For the most part heuristics work well, but occasionally they lead to poor outcomes. When they fail, they are typically described in hindsight by terms such as biases, neglect, fallacies, slips, failures, and errors. These CDRs reflect a "cognitive determinism," the tendency to perceive and respond to a clinical situation in a particular way, based on a summation of historical, prevailing, and ambient factors. Thirty CDRs have been described in the context of emergency medicine, and there are probably more (Table 312-5).

The prevalence of CDRs and their adverse influence on decision making is well recognized.[16] Some effort has been directed at undoing

TABLE 312-5   Cognitive Dispositions to Respond (CDR) That May Lead to Adverse Outcomes

Aggregate bias	Gender bias	Psych-out errors
Anchoring	Hindsight bias	Representativeness restraint
Ascertainment bias	Multiple alternatives bias	Search satisfying
Availability	Omission bias	Sutton's slip
Base-rate neglect	Order effects	Triage-cueing
Commission bias	Outcome bias	Unpacking principle
Confirmation bias	Overconfidence bias	Vertical line failure
Diagnosis momentum	Playing the odds	Visceral bias
Fundamental attribution error	Posterior probability error	Ying-yang out
Gambler's fallacy	Premature closure	Zebra retreat

Source: Reproduced with permission from Croskerry.[16]

their effects using specific cognitive debiasing approaches. More recently, metacognitive techniques have been employed, aimed at blocking or modifying the CDR through cognitive forcing strategies.[10] For example, the predictable and catastrophic error of using fibrinolytics in a patient with an acute myocardial infarct mimic (left ventricular aneurysm, benign early repolarization, non-AMI ST-segment elevation, aortic dissection, acute pericarditis) has its origin in a combination of CDRs: *representativeness restraint, anchoring, search satisfying,* and *premature diagnostic closure.* A necessary first step in avoiding this error is to develop an awareness and knowledge of the known CDRs. The second is to recognize the scenario in which the error is likely to occur, and the final step is to apply the cognitive forcing strategy, in this case to metacognitively reflect on competing hypotheses before taking unpropitious action. Considerable further effort will be required to discover and develop additional strategies for minimizing or avoiding the adverse outcomes associated with CDRs.

DEVELOPING A SYSTEMS APPROACH TO PATIENT SAFETY

Critical incident and organizational analysis in health care has been facilitated by integration of knowledge from many different disciplines.[17] *Cognitive science* or *cognitive engineering* provides tools to understand and model cognitive abilities such as perception, learning, language, memory, and problem solving. *Human factors* or *ergonomics* evaluates the specifics of human performance and its interface with the physical environment in which we operate in an effort to maximize user performance. *Systems analysis,* with its background in operations research, models systems and organizations to better understand their functions, including relationships with other systems and subsystems. Each of these approaches has unique attributes and analytic capacity that, when merged, will allow the development of an integrated picture of the ED environment as an environment prone to error.

Vincent and colleagues have proposed a specific safety analysis framework to evaluate adverse incidents in clinical medicine.[17] This framework is designed around a hierarchy of seven types of factors that influence clinical practice (Table 312-6). Ideally, interventions to improve safety should be targeted at each of these factors.[17] It is ironic that interventions at the higher levels, which are more likely to be effective and whose effects are more likely to be long-lasting, are more difficult than short-term, quick fixes at the lower levels.

An important step in selecting or designing corrective interventions is to have some mechanism for finding out when things go wrong and for understanding the ways in which systems of care fail. Thus some form of reporting of incidents (near misses) and accidents

(adverse events), coupled with in-depth investigation of selected episodes, is valuable for guiding interventions. In general, in-depth investigation of a small number of meaningful events tends to be more productive than attempts at comprehensive cataloging of small amounts of information on many events.[18]

Three general strategies for reducing incidents and adverse events exist: prevention, recognition, and mitigation. Prevention of slips, lapses, and mistakes is an attractive strategy; for example, eliminating look-alike drug containers prevents mental slips whereby a nurse picks up one container when intending to pick up another, leading to a wrong drug administration. However, the abundance of such errors is so high that it is virtually certain that some will always occur.[17] The second strategic defense, then, is to make such mishaps easily recognized so they can be corrected before they affect a patient. For example, Australian anesthetists have adopted a convention that paralytic agents are always drawn up in red marked syringes, so that it is obvious to everyone in the room when a paralytic is about to be given.[19] If a worker inadvertently picks up the wrong syringe, it is more likely that someone will recognize in time to intervene. Similarly, the practice of repeating back verbal orders ("check-back"), or calling out medications when they are given, allows greater opportunity for failures to be recognized and dealt with promptly.[20] The third general strategy, mitigation, involves enhancing the ability to recover from problems by preventing or minimizing their damage. For example, bringing a crash cart, airway equipment, and reversing agents to sites where procedural sedation is performed enhances the likelihood that laryngospasm, hypoventilation, or inadvertent oversedation will be successfully managed without patient injury.

At a more specific level, there are several general tactical approaches that can be used in support of any of the three strategies. The first is simplification of processes. The more steps there are in a process, the more likely it is that something in the process will go wrong, even if the individual steps are executed with a high degree of reliability. For example, there is a 12 percent chance that a 25-step process will contain at least one error, even if each step is executed correctly 99.5 percent of the time; reducing the number of steps to 10 cuts the probability of failure to less than 5 percent. In the clinical area, simplification of fibrinolytic dosing regimens has been shown to reduce dosing errors and led to a 30 percent relative reduction in mortality.[21] A second general tactic is the use of constraints or "forcing functions." These are design changes that make it difficult to do the wrong thing. For example, gas connectors on anesthesia machines are designed so that oxygen and nitrous oxide tanks can be attached only to the proper ports, eliminating the chance of a gas mix-up with potentially fatal consequences.

TABLE 312-6 Framework of Factors Influencing Clinical Practice

Factor Type	Influencing Contributory Factors	Example
Institutional context	Economic context, regulatory agenda, legal framework and constraints	Inconsistent or conflicting policies and regulations
Organizational and management factors	Organization structure, priorities, organizational safety culture, financial constraints	Lack of senior leadership commitment to a culture of patient safety
Work environment factors	Staffing levels and skills, workload, shift patterns, support structure	High workload with inadequate staffing
Team factors	Communication, supervision and support, leadership, consistency	Limited communication between staff members
Individual (staff) factors	Skills, competence, training	Lack of basic fund of knowledge
Task factors	Task design, clarity, protocol availability, accuracy of results	No or unclear protocols for routine work
Patient factors	Complexity, acuity, language and communication, social factors	Language barrier

Source: Adapted from Vincent et al.[17]

Advanced technology, particularly automation and computerization, has great potential for improving safety, but carries with it its own set of hazards.[22,23] Introducing new technology into a complex system can increase operational demands. It inevitably changes the nature of work, tending to make easy tasks easier and hard tasks harder. It tends to make systems more brittle; they fail less often, but their failures are more likely to be catastrophic.[24] New technology should be introduced, but introduced carefully, with preparedness to confront and rapidly resolve new and unexpected problems.

External standards organizations can be expected to play a role in suggesting or even mandating specific corrective actions.[25] External regulatory bodies can be important forces for safety, preventing a "race to the bottom" under production pressures, but their actions, although well-intended, can have unforeseen consequences if the recommendations are made without a deep understanding of the nature of work in the emergency department. For example, the Joint Commission on Accreditation of Healthcare Organizations has identified that communication failures leading to delays in therapy are a common cause of sentinel events submitted to it, and the Commission has noted that over half of such cases were "ED-related."[26] In 2002, the Joint Commission issued six safety goals that they expect to be fully implemented as of January 1, 2003, including:[27]

1. Improving accuracy of patient identification, including use of two different patient identifiers and a final verification check before invasive procedures are performed;
2. Improved communication among caregivers, including check-backs for verbal orders and standardization of abbreviations, acronyms, and symbols;
3. Removal of "high alert" medications from treatment areas (mainly concentrated electrolyte solutions);
4. Eliminating wrong-site, wrong-patient, and wrong-procedure failures, using verification processes and marking;
5. Eliminating infusion pumps that permit free flow; and
6. Ensuring that alarms are "sufficiently audible" given the distance and level of competing noise in the treatment area.

While all these goals are laudable, the specific implementations that surveyors will accept are not known. For some, implementation in the emergency department will be a challenge and may produce unintended consequences.

In addition, the Agency for Healthcare Research and Quality has recently reviewed the evidentiary base for a large number of safety-related practices and recommends several for immediate and widespread implementation because they were supported by strong evidence.[28] Several are pertinent to emergency care. The first requires that insertion of central lines should be done under maximum sterile technique (gown, gloves, drape, mask, and cap); that they not be placed blindly, but under ultrasound guidance; and that antibiotic-impregnated catheters be used. The second recommendation was to routinely ask patients to recall and restate what they were told in the process of informed consent, although a close reading suggests this recommendation was based more on ethical grounds than on evidence it improves safety.

Emergency department leaders should expect that external pressure to improve safety in emergency care will continue and they should be constructively engaged in this process. Choosing safety-related interventions for emergency departments is difficult. Little is known in detail about the ways in which emergency care succeeds or fails; superficial learning, resulting in quick fixes, is easy, while the more fundamental lessons are more difficult.[29]

ETHICAL IMPLICATIONS OF ERROR

When an error or a lapse in patient safety occurs, an important component of the process is the disclosure of the event to the patient. Most professional organizations, including the American Medical Association, have ethical standards that require the disclosure of unintended medical outcomes. Specific discussion of medical errors has been vague, leaving the interpretation of disclosure of "significant" error or "appropriate" conditions for disclosure to the discretion of the medical provider. Currently, no official professional organization calls for the complete disclosure of all medical error or defines the conditions under which disclosure must occur. Recent regulatory standards have addressed this ambiguity. In 2001, the Joint Commission required hospitals to document that "patients and, when appropriate, their families are informed about the outcomes of care, including unanticipated outcomes."

The medical literature supports the concept that physicians have an ethical duty to disclose errors to a patient when disclosure furthers the patient's health, respects the patient's autonomy, or enables the patient to be compensated for serious irreparable harm.[30] Similarly, legal duty requires a physician to disclose to the patient the necessary medical information to permit the patient to make an intelligent decision with regard to treatment, and the physician must reveal all that is in the patient's best interest.[31] Much has been written about the conflict between the ethical duty to disclose error and the physician's and patient's personal, financial, psychological, and professional well-being, yet we know little about the actual impact of error disclosure on our patients.[30,31] In a recent ED study of patient preference for medical error disclosure, researchers found that 88 percent of patients would wish to know everything about a mistake, while the remaining 12 percent would want to know about the mistake if it could or did affect their health.[31] These data suggest that despite limited knowledge of the ramifications of disclosure, patients would like to know about medical errors committed during the course of their care. Therefore, disclosure of medical errors should be our goal in an effort to simply tell the truth.

REFERENCES

1. Kohn LT, Corrigan JM, Donaldson MS (eds): *To Err Is Human.* Washington, DC, Institute of Medicine, National Academy Press, 2000.
2. McDonald CJ, Weiner M, Hui SL: Deaths due to medical errors are exaggerated in Institute of Medicine report. *JAMA* 284:93, 2000.
3. Dunn JD, Wears RL: The November special issue on errors (letters). *Acad Emerg Med* 8:686, 2001.
4. Brennan TA, Leape LL, Laird NM, et al: Incidence of adverse events and negligence in hospitalized patients. Results of the Harvard Medical Practice Study I. *New Engl J Med* 324:370, 1991.
5. Thomas EJ, Studdert DM, Burstin HR, et al: Incidence and types of adverse events and negligent care in Utah and Colorado. *Med Care* 38:261, 2000.
6. Wilson RM, Harrison BT, Gibberd RW, et al: An analysis of the causes of adverse events from the Quality in Australian Health Care Study. *Med J Aust* 170:411, 1999.
7. Rasmussen J, Jensen A: Mental procedures in real-life tasks: A case study of electronic troubleshooting. *Ergonomics* 17:293, 1974.
8. Reason J: *Human Error.* Cambridge, UK: Cambridge University Press, 1990.
9. Leape LL: Error in medicine. *JAMA* 272:1151, 1994.
10. Croskerry P: Cognitive forcing strategies in clinical decision making. *Ann Emerg Med* 41:110, 2003.
11. Reason J: Human error: Models and management. *BMJ* 320:768, 2000.
12. Williams JC: Assessing and Reducing the Likelihood of Violation Behavior—A Preliminary Investigation. Proceedings of an International Conference on *The Commercial & Operational Benefits of Probabilistic Safety Assessments.* Institute of Nuclear Engineers. Edinburgh, Scotland, October 1997.
13. Selten R: What is bounded rationality? in Gigerenzer G, Selten R (eds): *Bounded Rationality: The Adaptive Toolbox.* Cambridge, MA: MIT Press, 2001.
14. Klein GA, Orasanu R, Calderwood R, et al: *Decision Making in Action: Models and Methods.* Norwood, NJ, Ablex Publishing, 1993.
15. Graber M, Gordon R, Franklin N: Reducing diagnostic errors in medicine: What's the goal? *Acad Med* 77:981, 2002.
16. Croskerry P: Achieving quality in clinical decision making: Cognitive strategies and detection of bias. *Acad Emerg Med* 9:1184, 2002.

17. Vincent C, Taylor-Adams S, Stanhope N: Framework for analyzing risk and safety in clinical medicine. *BMJ* 316:1154, 1998.

18. Billings CE, Woods DD: Human error in perspective. The patient safety movement. *Postgrad Med* 109:13, 2001.

19. Russell WJ: Getting into the red: A strategic step for safety. *Qual Saf Health Care* 11:107, 2002.

20. Morey JC, Simon R, Jay GD, et al: Error reduction and performance improvement in the emergency department through teamwork training: Evaluation results of the MedTeams project. *Health Serv Res* 37:1553, 2002.

21. Richards CF, Cannon CP: Reducing medication errors: Potential benefits of bolus thrombolytic agents. *Acad Emerg Med* 7:1285, 2000.

22. Bates DW, Leape LL, Cullen DJ, et al: Effect of computerized physician order entry and a team intervention on prevention of serious medication errors. *JAMA* 280:1311, 1998.

23. Rochlin GI: *Trapped in the Net: The Unanticipated Consequences of Computerization.* Princeton, NJ: Princeton University Press, 1997.

24. Dekker S: *The Field Guide to Human Error Investigations.* Aldershot, Hampshire, UK, Ashgate, 2002.

25. Leapfrog Group: Leapfrog initiatives to drive great leaps in patient safety. http://www.leapfroggroup.org/safety1.htm, accessed 17 October 2000.

26. Joint Commission on Accreditation of Healthcare Organizations: Delays in treatment, in *JCAHO Sentinel Event Alert,* 2002.

27. Joint Commission on Accreditation of Healthcare Organizations: 2003 National Patient Safety Goals. Accessed 21 November 2002.

28. Shojania KG, Duncan BW, McDonald KM, et al: *Making Health Care Safer: A Critical Analysis of Patient Safety Practices.* Rockville, MD, Agency for Healthcare Research and Quality, Evidence Report/Technology Assessment No. 43. AHRQ Publication 01-E058, 2001, http://www.ahcpr.gov/clinic/ptsafety/.

29. Choularton R: Complex learning: Organizational learning from disasters. *Safety Sci* 39:61, 2002.

30. Wu AW, Cavanaugh TA, McPhee SJ, et al: To tell the truth: Ethical and practical issues in disclosing medical mistakes to patients. *J Gen Intern Med* 12:770, 1997.

31. Hobgood C, Peck CR, Gilbert B, et al: Medical errors—What and when: What do patients want to know? *Acad Emerg Med* 9:96, 2002.

NOTE: Numbers followed with *f* and *t* refer to figure and table pages.

TABLE 255-2 Glasgow Coma Scale

	4 years to Adult	Child <4 years	Infant
Eye Opening			
4	Spontaneous	Spontaneous	Spontaneous
3	To speech	To speech	To speech
2	To pain	To pain	To pain
1	No response	No response	No response
Verbal Response			
5	Alert and oriented	Oriented, social, speaks, interacts	Coos, babbles
4	Disoriented conversation	Confused speech, disoriented, consolable, aware	Irritable cry
3	Speaking but nonsensical	Inappropriate words, inconsolable, unaware	Cries to pain
2	Moans or unintelligible sounds	Incomprehensible, agitated, restless, unaware	Moans to pain
1	No response	No response	No response
Motor Response			
6	Follows commands	Normal, spontaneous movements	Normal, spontaneous moves
5	Localizes pain	Localizes pain	Withdraws to touch
4	Movement or withdrawal to pain	Withdraws to pain	Withdraws to pain
3	Decorticate flexion	Decorticate flexion	Decorticate flexion
2	Decerebrate extension	Decerebrate extension	Decerebrate extension
1	No response	No response	No response
3–15			

Note: GCS reporting should be modified for intubated and paralyzed patients.

TABLE 274-1 Ottawa Knee Rules

Patient older than 55 years
Tenderness at the head of the fibula
Isolated tenderness of the patella
Inability to flex knee to 90 degrees
Inability to transfer weight for four steps both immediately after the injury and in the ED

TABLE 272-1 NEXUS Criteria

According to NEXUS low-risk criteria, cervical spine radiography can be omitted for trauma patients only if they exhibit *all* of the following criteria:
No posterior midline cervical spine tenderness
No evidence of intoxication
Normal level of alertness
No focal neurologic deficit
No painful distracting injuries

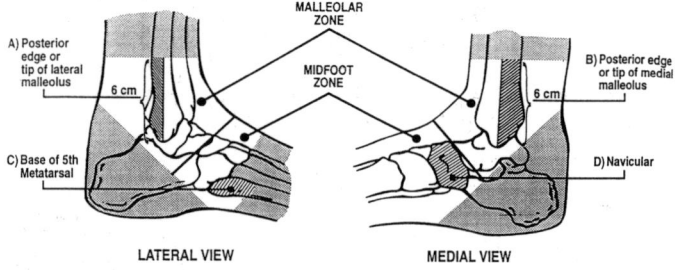

a) An ankle x-ray series is only required if:
There is any pain in malleolar zone and any of these findings:
   i) bone tenderness at A
       OR
   ii) bone tenderness at B
       OR
   iii) inability to bear weight both immediately and in ED

b) A foot x-ray series is only required if:
There is any pain in midfoot zone and any of these findings:
   i) bone tenderness at C
       OR
   ii) bone tenderness at D
       OR
   iii) inability to bear weight both immediately and in ED

FIG. 276-3. Ottawa Ankle Rules.

TABLE 252-2 Pediatric Trauma Score

	−1	+1	+2
Size (kg)	<10	10–20	>20
Airway	Unmaintained	Maintained	Normal
Systolic blood pressure (mm Hg)	<50	50–90	>90
Level of consciousness	Comatose	Altered	Awake
Wounds	Major open	Minor open	None
Skeletal trauma	Open/multiple	Closed	None

TABLE 252-3 Revised Trauma Score

Number	Glasgow Coma Score	Systolic Blood Pressure	Respiratory Rate
4	13–15	>89	10–29
3	9–12	76–89	>29
2	6–8	50–75	6–9
1	4–5	1–49	1–5
0	3	0	0